Infectious Diseases

THIRD EDITION

Infectious Diseases

THIRD EDITION

Edited by

Sherwood L. Gorbach, MD

PROFESSOR OF COMMUNITY HEALTH, MEDICINE, AND MOLECULAR BIOLOGY/MICROBIOLOGY
TUFTS UNIVERSITY SCHOOL OF MEDICINE
ATTENDING PHYSICIAN, TUFTS-NEW ENGLAND MEDICAL CENTER AND
CARITAS ST. ELIZABETH'S MEDICAL CENTER
BOSTON, MASSACHUSETTS

John G. Bartlett, MD

STANHOPE BAYNE JONES PROFESSOR OF MEDICINE
THE JOHNS HOPKINS UNIVERSITY SCHOOL OF MEDICINE
CHIEF, DIVISION OF INFECTIOUS DISEASES
THE JOHNS HOPKINS HOSPITAL
BALTIMORE, MARYLAND

Neil R. Blacklow, MD

CHAIRMAN EMERITUS, DEPARTMENT OF MEDICINE
PROFESSOR OF MEDICINE, MOLECULAR GENETICS AND MICROBIOLOGY
UNIVERSITY OF MASSACHUSETTS MEDICAL SCHOOL
WORCESTER, MASSACHUSETTS;
VISITING PROFESSOR OF MEDICINE
HARVARD MEDICAL SCHOOL
BOSTON, MASSACHUSETTS

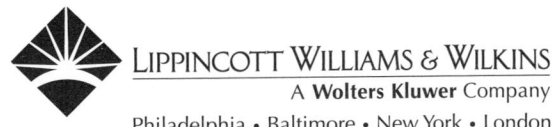

LIPPINCOTT WILLIAMS & WILKINS
A **Wolters Kluwer** Company

Philadelphia • Baltimore • New York • London
Buenos Aires • Hong Kong • Sydney • Tokyo

Acquisitions Editor: James Merritt
Developmental Editor: Joyce Murphy
Manufacturing Manager: Benjamin Rivera
Production Editor: Timothy Prairie
Cover Designer: David Levy
Compositor: TechBooks
Printer: Quebecor World-Taunton

Cover images: *From left to right:* Micrograph of SARS coronavirus (with the permission of Prof. Malik Peiris and Dr. John Nicholls); Gram stain of blood in culture media from patient who died of inhalational anthrax (from Borio L, Frank D, Mani V, et al. Death due to bioterrorism-related inhalational anthrax: report of 2 patients. *JAMA* 2001;286:2554–2559, with permission); last reported naturally occurring case of smallpox in 1977 (courtesy of Dr. Samuel L. Katz); the mosquito is a vector in transmission of many infectious diseases, reportedly responsible for 1 in 7 deaths in the world. *Background: Penicillium notatum* demonstrating antibacterial properties against *Staphylococcus aureus*, as first discovered by Alexander Fleming (from the British Museum).

Printed in the United States of America

9 8 7 6 5 4 3 2 1

Library of Congress Cataloging-in-Publication Data

Infectious diseases / edited by Sherwood L. Gorbach, John G. Bartlett, Neil R. Blacklow.—
3rd ed.
  p. ; cm.
  Includes bibliographical references and index.
  ISBN 0-7817-3371-5 (alk. paper)
  1. Communicable diseases. I. Gorbach, Sherwood L., 1934– II. Bartlett, John G.
III. Blacklow, Neil R.
  [DNLM: 1. Communicable Diseases. 2. Bacterial Infections. 3. Virus Diseases. WC 100
I4033 2004]
RC111.I5128 2004
616.9—dc21   2003047509

Care has been taken to confirm the accuracy of the information presented and to describe generally accepted practices. However, the authors, editors, and publisher are not responsible for errors or omissions or for any consequences from application of the information in this book and make no warranty, expressed or implied, with respect to the contents of the publication.

The authors, editors, and publisher have exerted every effort to ensure that drug selection and dosage set forth in this text are in accordance with current recommendations and practice at the time of publication. However, in view of ongoing research, changes in government regulations, and the constant flow of information relating to drug therapy and drug reactions, the reader is urged to check the package insert for each drug for any change in indications and dosage and for added warnings and precautions. This is particularly important when the recommended agent is a new or infrequently employed drug.

Some drugs and medical devices presented in this publication have Food and Drug Administration (FDA) clearance for limited use in restricted research settings. It is the responsibility of the health care provider to ascertain the FDA status of each drug or device planned for use in their clinical practice.

To Judy, Jean, and Margery,
who supported us in this, and in every other, endeavor;

To our students, house officers,
fellows, and colleagues,
who inspired us to learn and study,
and for whom we have written it down; and

To our patients,
who made it worth the while.

Contents

PART IV
Prevention of Infectious Diseases 371

PART V
Clinical Infections 412

HEAD AND NECK 412

PLEUROPULMONARY 470

CARDIOVASCULAR SYSTEM 552

GASTROINTESTINAL TRACT 597

PART VI
Microbial Agents   1585

Contributing Authors

Fredrick M. Abrahamian, DO, FACEP
Assistant Professor of Medicine
UCLA School of Medicine;
Director of Education
Department of Emergency Medicine
Olive View—UCLA Medical Center
Sylmar, California

David W. K. Acheson, MD, FRCP
Chief Medical Officer
Center for Food Safety and Applied
    Nutrition
Food and Drug Administration
College Park, Maryland

Michelle J. Aifa, PhD
Professor
Department of Medical Microbiology
University of Manitoba;
Assistant Director
Department of Microbiology
St. Boniface General Hospital
Winnipeg, Manitoba
Canada

Ban Mishu Allos, MD
Assistant Professor
Division of Infectious Diseases
Department of Medicine
Vanderbilt University School of
    Medicine
Nashville, Tennessee

Vincent T. Andriole, MD
Professor
Department of Internal Medicine
Yale University School of Medicine;
Attending Physician
Department of Internal Medicine
Yale-New Haven Hospital
New Haven, Connecticut

Adriano Arguedas, MD
Pediatric Infectious Diseases
Instituto Costarricense de Investigaciones
    Clinicas
San Jose, Costa Rica

David M. Asher, MD
Chief
Laboratory of Bacterial, Parasitic, and
    Unconventional Agents
Center for Biologic Evaluation and
    Research
Food and Drug Administration
Rockville, Maryland

Aristides P. Assimacopoulas, MD
Infectious Disease Specialist
Sioux Falls, South Dakota

Robert Austrian, MD, DSc (Hon.)
Professor and Chairman Emeritus
Department of Research Medicine
University of Pennsylvania School of
    Medicine;
Visiting Physician
Department of Medicine
University of Pennsylvania Hospital
Philadelphia, Pennsylvania

John W. Baddley, MD
Assistant Professor
Division of Infectious Diseases
Department of Medicine
University of Alabama at Birmingham;
Attending Physician
Department of Medicine
University of Alabama Hospital
Birmingham, Alabama

Ann Sullivan Baker, MD (Deceased)
Infectious Disease Unit
Harvard Medical School;
Massachusetts General Hospital;
Massachusetts Eye and Ear Infirmary
Boston, Massachusetts

Neil L. Barg, MD
Internal Medicine Associates of Yakima
Yakima, WA

John G. Bartlett, MD
Stanhope Bayne Jones Professor of Medicine
The Johns Hopkins University School of
    Medicine
Chief
Division of Infectious Diseases
The Johns Hopkins Hospital
Baltimore, Maryland

Michael Barza, MD
Professor
Department of Medicine
Tufts University School of Medicine
Boston, Massachusetts;
Chief
Department of Medicine
Caritas Carney Hospital
Dorchester, Massachusetts

Robert E. Baughn, PhD
Professor of Dermatology
Professor of Microbiology and Immunology
Baylor College of Medicine;
Director
Syphilis Research Laboratory
Veterans Affairs Medical Center
Houston, Texas

Jules L. Baum, MD
Emeritus Professor of Ophthalmology
Tufts University School of Medicine
Boston, Massachusetts

Stephen G. Baum, MD
Professor
Department of Medicine, Microbiology, and
    Immunology
Albert Einstein College of Medicine;
Chairman
Department of Medicine
Beth Israel Medical Center
New York, New York

Theodore M. Bayless, MD
Professor of Medicine
Department of Medicine
The Johns Hopkins University School of
    Medicine;
Director
Meyerhoff IBD Center
The Johns Hopkins Hospital
Baltimore, Maryland

Irmgard Behlau, MD
Westfield, New Jersey

Stephanie R. Black, MD
Assistant Professor
Section of Infectious Diseases
Rush Medical College;
Attending Physician
Section of Infectious Diseases
Rush Presbyterian St. Luke's Medical
    Center
Chicago, Illinois

Neil R. Blacklow, MD
Chairman Emeritus, Department of
    Medicine
Professor of Medicine, Molecular Genetics,
    and Microbiology
University of Massachusetts Medical School
Worcester, Massachusetts;
Visiting Professor of Medicine
Harvard Medical School
Boston, Massachusetts

Charles D. Bluestone, MD
Eberly Professor of Pediatric
    Otolaryngology
Department of Otolaryngology
University of Pittsburgh School of Medicine;
Director
Department of Pediatric Otolaryngology
Children's Hospital of Pittsburgh
Pittsburgh, Pennsylvania

Gerald P. Bodey, MD
Professor and Clinical Internist
Department of Infectious Diseases, Infection
    Control, and Employee Health
The University of Texas M. D. Anderson
    Cancer Center
Houston, Texas

Roger C. Bone, MD (Deceased)
Distinguished Professor of Medicine
Rush Medical College
Chicago, Illinois

Fernando Borrego, MD
Assistant Professor
Division of Infectious Diseases
Department of Medicine
Mount Sinai School of Medicine;
Assistant Attending
Division of Infectious Diseases
Department of Medicine
Mount Sinai Hospital
New York, New York

John W. Boslego, MD
Director
Vaccine Infectious Diseases Clinical
    Research
Merck Research Laboratories
West Point, Pennsylvania

Edward J. Bottone, PhD
Professor
Departments of Medicine, Microbiology, and
    Pathology
Mount Sinai School of Medicine;
Director
Consultative Microbiology
Division of Infectious Diseases
The Mount Sinai Hospital
New York, New York

Alain R. Bouckenooghe, MD
Director
Regulatory Affairs Europe
Merck Sharp and Dohme (Europe), Inc.
Brussels, Belgium

Mathijs H. Brentjens, MS, MD
Resident
Department of Dermatology
University of Texas Medical Branch
Galveston, Texas

Claire Broome, MD
Deputy Director
Centers for Disease Control and Prevention
Atlanta, Georgia

Cara Carthel Burns, PhD
Microbiologist
Division of Viral and Rickettsial Diseases
Centers for Disease Control and Prevention
Atlanta, Georgia

Thomas Butler, MD
Professor
Department of Internal Medicine
Chief
Infectious Diseases
Texas Tech University Health Sciences
    Center
Lubbock, Texas

**Michael V. Callahan, MD, MSPH, DTM & H
(U.K.)**
Assistant Professor of International Health
Center for International Health
Boston University School of Public Health;
Division of Infectious Diseases
Massachusetts General Hospital
Boston, Massachusetts

James D. Campbell, MD
Assistant Professor
Department of Pediatrics
University of Maryland Medical School
Baltimore, Maryland

Carlos Carrillo, MD
Principal Professor of Microbiology
Universidad Peruana Cayetano Heredia;
Director
Instituto Nacional de Salud
Lima, Peru

Kenneth G. Castro, MD
Assistant Surgeon General, U.S. Public Health
    Service
Director, Division of Tuberculosis Elimination
National Center for HIV, STD, and TB
    Prevention
Centers for Disease Control and Prevention;
Clinical Assistant Professor of Medicine
Infectious Diseases Program
Grady Health Systems
Atlanta, Georgia

Marsha L. Chaffins, MD
Senior Staff Physician
Department of Dermatology
Henry Ford Hospital
Detroit, Michigan

Richard E. Chaisson, MD
Professor
Departments of Medicine, Epidemiology, and
    International Health
The Johns Hopkins University;
Director
The Johns Hopkins Center for Tuberculosis
    Research
The Johns Hopkins Hospital
Baltimore, Maryland

Sarah H. Cheeseman, MD
Professor
Departments of Medicine, Pediatrics, and
    Molecular Genetics and Microbiology
University of Massachusetts Medical School;
Division of Infectious Diseases and
    Immunology
Department of Medicine
UMASS Memorial Health Care
Worcester, Massachusetts

James E. Childs, ScD
Adjunct Professor
Department of Biology
Emory University
Atlanta, Georgia

Anthony W. Chow, MD
Professor
Division of Infectious Diseases
Department of Medicine
University of British Columbia;
Consultant Physician
Division of Infectious Diseases
Department of Medicine
Vancouver Hospital
Vancouver, British Columbia
Canada

Clay J. Cockerell, MD
Associate Professor
Department of Dermatology
University of Texas Southwestern
Dallas, Texas

Mitchell L. Cohen, MD
Director
Division of Bacterial and Mycotic Diseases
National Center for Infectious Diseases
Centers for Disease Control and Prevention
Atlanta, Georgia

Robert E. Condon, MD, MSc, FNCS
Professor Emeritus
Department of Surgery
The Medical College of Wisconsin
Milwaukee, Wisconsin

Deborah Cotton, MD, MPH
Professor
Department of Medicine
Boston University School of Medicine
Boston, Massachusetts;
Chief
Department of Medical Service
VA Boston Healthcare System
West Roxbury, Massachusetts

William A. Craig, MD
Professor
Department of Medicine
University of Wisconsin;
Consultant
Department of Medicine
William S. Middleton Memorial VA Hospital
Madison, Wisconsin

Burke A. Cunha, MD, MACP
Professor
Department of Medicine
State University of New York School of
    Medicine at Stony Brook
Stony Brook, New York;
Chief
Division of Infectious Diseases
Winthrop-University Hospital
Mineola, New York

Carrie Ann Cusack, MD
Chief Resident
Department of Dermatology
Henry Ford Hospital
Detroit, Michigan

Jennifer S. Daly, MD
Associate Professor
Department of Medicine
University of Massachusetts Medical School;
Clinical Chief
Division of Infectious Diseases and
    Immunology
UMASS Memorial Medical Center
Worcester, Massachusetts

Richard F. D'Amato, PhD
Director
Department of Infectious Diseases
ICON Laboratories, Inc.
Farmingdale, New York

Raymond J. Dattwyler, MD
Professor
Department of Medicine
Center for Infectious Diseases
State University of New York at Stony
    Brook;
Chief of Clinical Immunology
Departments of Medicine and Pediatrics
University Hospital
Stony Brook, New York

Raul Davaro, MD
Assistant Professor and Attending
  Physician
Department of Medicine
University of Massachusetts Medical
  School
Worcester, Massachusetts

George S. Deepe, Jr., MD
Professor
Division of Infectious Diseases
Department of Internal Medicine
University of Cincinnati College of Medicine
Cincinnati, Ohio

Mary Ann DeGroote, MD
Research Faculty
Department of Molecular, Cellular, and
  Developmental Biology
University of Colorado
Boulder, Colorado;
Infectious Disease Consultant
Department of Medicine
Swedish Medical Center
Englewood, Colorado

E. Patchen Dellinger, MD
Professor and Vice-Chairman
Department of Surgery
Chief
Division of General Surgery
University of Washington School of Medicine;
Associate Medical Director
University of Washington Medical Center
Seattle, Washington

David T. Dennis, MD, MPH
Faculty Affiliate
Department of Microbiology
Colorado State University;
Medical Epidemiologist
Division of Vector-Borne Infectious
  Diseases
National Center of Infectious Diseases
Centers for Disease Control and
  Prevention
Fort Collins, Colorado

Stanley C. Deresinski, MD
Clinical Professor
Division of Infectious Diseases
Department of Medicine
Stanford University
Stanford, California;
Associate Chief
Division of Infectious Diseases
Department of Medicine
Santa Clara Valley Medical Center
San Jose, California

Catherine Diamond, MD, MPH
Assistant Professor of Clinical Medicine
Department of Medicine
University of California Irvine Medical
  Center
Orange, California

Arry Dieudonne, MD
Assistant Professor
Department of Pediatrics
UMDNJ/New Jersey Medical School;
Attending Physician
Department of Pediatrics
University Hospital
Newark, New Jersey

William E. Dismukes, MD
Professor and Vice-Chairman
Department of Medicine
Director
Division of Infectious Diseases
University of Alabama at Birmingham;
Attending Physician
Department of Medicine
University of Alabama Hospital
Birmingham, Alabama

Gary V. Doern, MD
Professor
Department of Pathology
University of Iowa College of Medicine;
Director
Clinical Microbiology Laboratories
Department of Pathology
University of Iowa Hospital and Clinics
Iowa City, Iowa

Michael S. Donnenberg, MD
Professor of Medicine
Head
Division of Infectious Diseases
University of Maryland School of Medicine
Baltimore, Maryland

J. Stephen Dumler, MD
Professor
Division of Medical Microbiology
Department of Pathology
The Johns Hopkins University School of
  Medicine;
Director of Parasitology and Molecular
  Microbiology
Division of Medical Microbiology
Department of Pathology
The Johns Hopkins Hospital
Baltimore, Maryland

Herbert L. DuPont, MD
Director
Center for Infectious Diseases
University of Texas-Houston School of Public
  Health;
Mary W. Kelsey Professor
University of Texas-Houston;
H. Irving Schweppe, Jr., Chair and Vice
  Chairman
Department of Medicine
Baylor College of Medicine;
Chief
Internal Medicine
St. Luke's Episcopal Hospital
Houston, Texas

William Jerry Durbin, MD
Professor of Pediatrics and Medicine
Department of Pediatrics
University of Massachusetts Medical School;
Pediatric Residency Director
Department of Pediatrics
UMASS Memorial Health Care
Worcester, Massachusetts

George M. Eliopoulos, MD
Professor
Department of Medicine
Harvard Medical School;
Physician
Division of Infectious Diseases
Department of Medicine
Beth Israel Deaconess Medical Center
Boston, Massachusetts

Richard T. Ellison III, MD
Professor of Medicine, Molecular Genetics,
  and Microbiology
University of Massachusetts Medical
  School
Worcester, Massachusetts

Jerrold J. Ellner, MD
Professor and Chair
Department of Medicine
New Jersey Medical School;
Chief of Medical Service
Department of Medicine
University Hospital
Newark, New Jersey

Lawrence J. Eron, MD
Associate Professor
Department of Medicine
John A. Burns School of Medicine
University of Hawaii;
Infectious Diseases Consultant
Kaiser Moanalua Medical Center
Honolulu, Hawaii

David A. Eschenbach, MD
Professor
Department of Obstetrics and
  Gynecology
University of Washington School of
  Medicine
Seattle, Washington

Joseph J. Esposito, PhD
Coordinator of Collaborative Research and
  Senior Research Scientist
Centers for Disease Control and
  Prevention
Atlanta, Georgia

Max Essex, DVM, PhD
Chairman
Department of Immunology and Infectious
  Diseases
Harvard AIDS Institute
Harvard School of Public Health
Boston, Massachusetts

Michael J. G. Farthing, DSc, MD, FRCP
Professor and Executive Dean
Faculty of Medicine
University of Glasgow
Glasgow, United Kingdom

David S. Feingold, MD
Professor
Department of Dermatology
Tufts University School of Medicine
Boston, Massachusetts

Robert Fekety, MD
Professor Emeritus
Division of Infectious Diseases
Department of Medicine
University of Michigan Medical School
Ann Arbor, Michigan

Kevin P. Fennelly, MD, MPH
Assistant Professor
Department of Medicine
UMDNJ—New Jersey Medical School;
Pulmonary Medicine Consultant
Department of Medicine
University Hospital
Newark, New Jersey

Robert W. Finberg, MD
Chair
Department of Medicine
University of Massachusetts Medical School;
Chief
Department of Medicine
UMASS Memorial Health Care
Worcester, Massachusetts

Douglas A. Finch, MD
Instructor
Department of Medicine
Mount Sinai School of Medicine;
Attending Physician
Section of Infectious Diseases
Bronx Veterans Affairs Medical Center
Bronx, New York

Sydney M. Finegold, MD
Professor
Departments of Medicine, Immunology, and
    Molecular Genetics
UCLA School of Medicine;
Staff Physician
Section of Infectious Diseases
VA Medical Center West Los Angeles
Los Angeles, California

Joyce D. Fingeroth, MD
Associate Professor
Divisions of Infectious Diseases and
    Experimental Medicine
Department of Medicine
Beth Israel Deaconess Medical Center
Harvard Institutes of Medicine
Boston, Massachusetts

Staci Ann Fischer, MD
Assistant Professor
Department of Medicine
Director
Infectious Disease Fellowship
Brown Medical School;
Attending Physician
Department of Medicine
Director
Outpatient Infectious Diseases
Rhode Island Hospital
Providence, Rhode Island

Thomas Foitzik, MD
Associate Professor
Department of Surgery
University of Rostock
Rostock, Germany

Graeme N. Forrest, MBBS
Assistant Professor
Division of Infectious Diseases
Department of Medicine
University of Maryland School of Medicine
Baltimore, Maryland

David O. Freedman, MD
Professor
Division of Geographic Medicine
University of Alabama at Birmingham
Birmingham, Alabama

Thomas R. Gadacz, MD
Moretz-Mansberger Professor and Chair
Department of Surgery
Medical College of Georgia;
Clinical Chief
Department of Surgery
Medical College of Georgia, Inc.
Augusta, Georgia

Pierce Gardner, MD
Professor
Department of Medicine
State University of New York at Stony
    Brook
Stony Brook, New York

Michael A. Gerber, MD
Professor
Department of Pediatrics
University of Cincinnati College of
    Medicine;
Attending Physician
Division of Infectious Diseases
Cincinnati Children's Hospital Medical
    Center
Cincinnati, Ohio

Khalil G. Ghanem, MD
Division of Infectious Diseases
Department of Medicine
The Johns Hopkins University School of
    Medicine
Baltimore, Maryland

David F. Giansiracusa, MD
Professor of Medicine
University of Massachusetts Medical
    School;
Staff Rheumatologist
Department of Medicine
UMASS Memorial Health Care
Worcester, Massachusetts

Laura L. Gibson, MD
Assistant Professor
Departments of Pediatrics and Medicine
University of Massachusetts Medical School;
Division of Infectious Diseases and
    Immunology
Department of Pediatrics and Medicine
UMASS Memorial Health Care
Worcester, Massachusetts

Richard A. Gleckman, MD
St. Joseph's Hospital and Medical Center
Paterson, New Jersey

Richard H. Glew, MD
Vice-Chair for Undergraduate Education and
    Faculty Affairs
Department of Medicine
University of Massachusetts Medical Center;
Active Medical Staff
Division of Infectious Diseases
Department of Medicine
UMASS Memorial Health Care
Worcester, Massachusetts

W. Paul Glezen, MD
Professor
Department of Molecular Virology and
    Microbiology
Baylor College of Medicine;
Attending Pediatrician
Department of Pediatrics
Ben Taub General Hospital
Houston, Texas

Howard S. Gold, MD
Assistant Professor
Harvard Medical School;
Attending Physician
Department of Medicine
Beth Israel Deaconess Medical Center
Boston, Massachusetts

Marcia B. Goldberg, MD
Associate Professor
Department of Medicine
Harvard Medical School;
Associate Physician
Department of Medicine
Massachusetts General Hospital
Boston, Massachusetts

Matthew R. Golden, MD, MPH
Assistant Professor of Medicine
Division of Infectious Diseases
University of Washington;
Attending Physician
Division of Infectious Diseases
Department of Internal Medicine
Harborview Medical Center
Seattle, Washington

Ellie J. C. Goldstein, MD
Clinical Professor of Medicine
UCLA School of Medicine;
Director
R. M. Alden Research Laboratory
Santa Monica, California

Sherwood L. Gorbach, MD
Professor of Community Health, Medicine,
    and Molecular Biology/Microbiology
Tufts University School of Medicine
Attending Physician
Tufts-New England Medical Center and
    Caritas St. Elizabeth's Medical Center
Boston, Massachusetts

Eduardo Gotuzzo, MD, FACP
Principal Professor of Medicine
Universidad Peruana Cayetano Heredia;
Director
Instituto de Medicina Tropical "Alexander
    von Humboldt;"
Chairman
Department of Transmissible Diseases
Hospital Nacional Cayetano Heredia
Lima, Peru

John R. Graybill, MD
Professor
Department of Medicine
University of Texas Health Science Center at
    San Antonio;
Staff Physician
Department of Medicine
University Hospital
San Antonio, Texas

Sharone Green, MD
Associate Professor
Department of Medicine
University of Massachusetts Medical School
Worcester, Massachusetts

Ronald A. Greenfield, MD
Professor and Chief
Section of Infectious Diseases
Department of Medicine
University of Oklahoma Health Sciences
    Center
Oklahoma City, Oklahoma

Michael H. Grieco, MD
Professor Emeritus of Clinical Medicine
Department of Medicine
Columbia University
New York, New York

Diane E. Griffin, MD, PhD
Professor and Chair
Department of Molecular Microbiology and
    Immunology
Bloomberg School of Public Health
The Johns Hopkins University
Baltimore, Maryland

Patricia M. Griffin, MD
Chief
Food Borne Diseases Epidemiology Section
Food Borne and Diarrheal Diseases Branch
Division of Bacterial and Mycotic Diseases
National Center for Infectious Diseases
Centers for Disease Control and
    Prevention
Atlanta, Georgia

Jeffrey K. Griffiths, MD, MPH & TM
Director
Graduate Programs in Public Health
Associate Professor of Family Medicine and
    Community Health and of Medicine
Department of Family Medicine and
    Community Health
Tufts University School of Medicine;
Physician
Division of Geographic Medicine and
    Infectious Diseases
Department of Medicine
Tufts-New England Medical Center
Boston, Massachusetts

Charles Grose, MD
Professor
Department of Pediatrics
University of Iowa College of Medicine;
Director
Division of Infectious Diseases
University of Iowa Hospital
Iowa City, Iowa

Marta A. Guerra, DVM, PhD
Veterinary Epidemiologist
Division of Global Migration and
    Quarantine
Centers for Disease Control and
    Prevention
Atlanta, Georgia

Alejandra C. Gurtman, MD
Associate Professor
Division of Infectious Diseases
Department of Medicine
Mount Sinai School of Medicine;
Attending Physician
Division of Infectious Diseases
Department of Medicine
Mount Sinai Hospital
New York, New York

Susan Hadley, MD
Associate Professor
Department of Medicine
Tufts University School of Medicine;
Staff Physician
Department of Medicine
Tufts-New England Medical Center
Boston, Massachusetts

Scott B. Halstead, MD
Adjunct Professor
Department of Preventive Medicine and
    Biometrics
Uniformed Services University of the Health
    Sciences
Bethesda, Maryland

Neal A. Halsey, MD
Professor
Department of International Health
The Johns Hopkins University;
Staff
Department of Pediatrics, Infectious Disease
The Johns Hopkins Hospital
Baltimore, Maryland

Davidson Hawes Hamer, MD, FACP
Assistant Professor of Medicine and
    Nutrition
Department of Medicine
Friedman School of Nutrition Science and
    Policy
Tufts University;
Director
Traveler's Health Service
Tufts-New England Medical Center
Boston, Massachusetts

Margaret R. Hammerschlag, MD
Professor
Departments of Pediatrics and Medicine
Division of Pediatric Infectious Diseases
SUNY Downstate Medical Center
University Hospital of Brooklyn
Brooklyn, New York

H. Hunter Handsfield, MD
Professor
Division of Infectious Diseases
University of Washington;
Director
Sexually Transmitted Diseases Program
Department of Public Health–Seattle and
    King County
Harborview Medical Center
Seattle, Washington

Alan A. Harris, MD
Professor
Department of Internal Medicine and
    Preventive Medicine
Rush Medical College;
Senior Assistant Chairman and Program
    Director
Hospital Epidemiologist
Department of Internal Medicine
Rush-Presbyterian-St. Luke's Medical
    Center
Chicago, Illinois

Rodrigo Hasbun, MD
Assistant Professor
Adult Infectious Diseases Section
Department of Medicine
Tulane University Health Sciences Center
New Orleans, Louisiana

Charles L. Hatheway, PhD
Chief
Botulism Laboratory
Centers for Disease Control and
    Prevention
National Center for Infectious Diseases
Division of Bacterial and Mycotic
    Diseases
Atlanta, Georgia

Bassam Helou, MD
Chief, Surgical Resident
Department of Surgery
Medical College of Georgia
Augusta, Georgia

Kelly J. Henrickson, MD
Associate Professor
Department of Pediatric Infectious Diseases
Medical College of Wisconsin;
Physician
Department of Pediatric Infectious Diseases
Children's Hospital of Wisconsin
Milwaukee, Wisconsin

John E. Herrmann, PhD
Research Professor
Division of Infectious Diseases
Tufts University School of Veterinary
    Medicine
North Grafton, Massachusetts

David W. Hines, MD
Assistant Professor
Rush Medical College
Chicago, Illinois;
Section Head
Infectious Diseases
Rush/Westlake Hospital
Melrose Park, Illinois

Jan V. Hirschmann, MD
Professor
Department of Medicine
University of Washington School of
    Medicine;
Staff Physician
Department of Medical Service
VA Medical Center
Seattle, Washington

Brian L. Hjelle, MD
Professor
Infectious Disease and Inflammation
    Program
Department of Pathology
University of New Mexico
Albuquerque, New Mexico

John L. Ho, MD
Associate Professor of Medicine and
    Microbiology
Division of International Medicine and
    Infectious Diseases
Department of Medicine
Weill Medical College of Cornell University;
Associate Attending Physician
Department of Medicine
New York–Presbyterian Hospital
New York, New York

Charles H. Hoke, Jr., MD
Colonel
Medical Corps
Director
Military Infectious Diseases Research
    Program
Department of the Army
US Army Medical Research and Materiel
    Command
Fort Detrick, Maryland

Paul D. Holtom, MD
Associate Professor
Department of Clinical Medicine and
    Orthopaedics
Keck School of Medicine
University of Southern California;
Hospital Epidemiologist
LAC and USC Medical Center
Los Angeles, California

Edward W. Hook, III, MD
Professor
Departments of Medicine, Epidemiology, and
    Microbiology
University of Alabama at Birmingham;
Medical Director
Sexually Transmitted Diseases Program
Jefferson County Department of Health
Birmingham, Alabama

C. Robert Horsburgh, Jr., MD
Department of Epidemiology and
    Biostatistics
Boston University Schools of Public Health
    and Medicine
Boston, Massachusetts

Marshall S. Horwitz, MD
Professor and Chairman
Department of Microbiology and
    Immunology
Albert Einstein College of Medicine
Bronx, New York

Walter T. Hughes, MD
Professor
Department of Pediatrics
University of Tennessee College of
    Medicine;
Emeritus Member
Department of Infectious Diseases
St. Jude Children's Research
    Hospital
Memphis, Tennessee

Shirish S. Huprikar, MD
Assistant Professor
Department of Medicine
Mount Sinai School of Medicine;
Attending Physician
Department of Medicine
Mount Sinai Hospital
New York, New York

Newton E. Hyslop, Jr., MD
Professor and Section Chief
Adult Infectious Diseases Section
Department of Medicine
Tulane University Health Sciences
    Center;
Medical Director
HIV/AIDS/Tuberculosis In-Patient
    Service
Charity Hospital of New Orleans
New Orleans, Louisiana

David N. Irani, MD
Assistant Professor
Department of Neurology
The Johns Hopkins University School of
    Medicine
The Johns Hopkins Hospital
Baltimore, Maryland

Michael D. Iseman, MD
Professor
Department of Medicine
University of Colorado School of
    Medicine;
Chief
Mycobacterial Disease Division
Department of Medicine
National Jewish Medical and Research
    Center
Denver, Colorado

Henry D. Isenberg, PhD
Professor
Department of Pathology
Albert Einstein College of Medicine
Bronx, New York;
Director, Infection Control
Chief Emeritus, Microbiology
Departments of Medicine and Pathology
North Shore Long Island Jewish Health
    System
Long Island Jewish Medical Center
New Hyde Park, New York

Hillel Janai, MD
Pediatric Infectious Disease
Private Practice
Arroyo Grande, California

Stephen G. Jenkins, PhD
Clinical Associate Professor
Department of Pathology
Mount Sinai School of Medicine;
Director of Microbiology and Immunology
Department of Pathology
Carolinas Medical Center
Charlotte, North Carolina

Daniel B. Jernigan, MD, MPH
Chief
Epidemiology Section
Division of Healthcare Quality Promotion
National Center for Infectious Diseases
Centers for Disease Control and Prevention
Atlanta, Georgia

Juan Carlos Jimenez, MD
Resident
Department of Surgery
University of California, Irvine
Orange, California

Richard T. Johnson, MD
Distinguished Service Professor
Departments of Neurology, Microbiology,
    and Neuroscience
Bloomberg School of Public Health
The Johns Hopkins University School of
    Medicine;
Neurologist
Department of Neurology
The Johns Hopkins Hospital
Baltimore, Maryland

Warren D. Johnson, Jr., MD
B. H. Kean Professor of Tropical Medicine
Division of International Medicine and
    Infectious Diseases
Department of Medicine
Weill Medical College of Cornell University;
Attending Physician
Department of Medicine
New York–Presbyterian Hospital
New York, New York

Ronald C. Jones, MD
Chief
Department of Surgery
Baylor University Medical Center
Dallas, Texas

Adolf W. Karchmer, MD
Professor
Department of Medicine
Harvard Medical School;
Chief
Division of Infectious Diseases
Department of Medicine
Beth Israel Deaconess Medical Center
Boston, Massachusetts

Dennis L. Kasper, MD
William Ellery Channing Professor
Departments of Medicine, Microbiology, and
    Molecular Genetics
Harvard Medical School;
Director
Channing Laboratory
Department of Medicine
Brigham and Women's Hospital
Boston, Massachusetts

Donald Kaye, MD, MACP
Professor
Department of Medicine
Drexel University College of Medicine
Philadelphia, Pennsylvania

Col. Patrick W. Kelley, MD, DrPH
Director
Board on Global Health
Institute of Medicine
National Academies of Science
Washington, D.C.

Carol A. Kemper, MD, FACP
Clinical Associate Professor
Department of Medicine
Stanford University;
Physician
Santa Clara Valley Medical Center
The Camino Medical Group
San Jose, California

Gerald T. Keusch, MD
Professor of Medicine
Tufts University School of Medicine;
Chief
Division of Geographic Medicine and
    Infectious Diseases
New England Medical Center
Boston, Massachusetts

Olen M. Kew, PhD
Chief
Section of Molecular Virology
Division of Viral and Rickettsial
    Diseases
National Center for Infectious Diseases
Centers for Disease Control and
    Prevention
Atlanta, Georgia

Jay S. Keystone, MD, MSc (CTM), FRCPC
Professor
Department of Medicine
University of Toronto;
Center for Travel and Tropical Medicine
Toronto General Hospital
Toronto, Ontario
Canada

Rachel G. Khadaroo, MD
General Surgery Resident
Department of Surgery
University of Alberta
Edmonton, Alberta
Canada

Ali S. Khan, MD, MPH
Associate Director for Science
Division of Parasitic Diseases
National Center for Infectious Diseases
Centers for Disease Control and
    Prevention
Atlanta, Georgia

Elliott Kieff, MD, PhD
Albee Professor
Departments of Medicine and Microbiology
Harvard University;
Director
Division of Infectious Diseases
Brigham and Women's Hospital
Boston, Massachusetts

Arthur Y. Kim, MD
Clinical and Research Fellow
Department of Medicine
Harvard Medical School;
Graduate Assistant
Department of Infectious Diseases
Massachusetts General Hospital
Boston, Massachusetts

Seung H. Kim, MD
Chief
Department of Pathology
US Army Institute of Surgical Research
    BAMC
San Antonio, Texas

Charles H. King, MD, MS
Associate Professor
Center for Global Heath and Diseases
Case Western Reserve University;
Attending Physician
Department of Medicine
University Hospitals of Cleveland
Cleveland, Ohio

Ernst Klar, MD
Associate Professor
Department of Surgery
University of Heidelberg;
Chief
Department of Surgery
District Hospital
Konstanz, Germany

Bruce S. Klein, MD
Professor
Department of Pediatrics
University of Wisconsin Medical School
Madison, Wisconsin

Jerome O. Klein, MD
Professor
Department of Pediatrics
Boston University School of Medicine;
Vice-Chairman for Academic Affairs
Department of Pediatrics
Boston Medical Center
Boston, Massachusetts

Mark S. Klempner, MD
Assistant Provost for Research
Conrad Wesselhoeft Professor of Medicine
Vice Chair for Research
Department of Medicine
Boston University
Boston, Massachusetts

Stephen A. Klotz, MD
Professor of Medicine
Section of Infectious Diseases
Department of Medicine
University of Arizona;
Physician
Department of Medicine
Southern Arizona VA Health Care System
Tucson, Arizona

Raymond S. Koff, MD
Professor
Department of Medicine
University of Massachusetts Medical School
Worcester, Massachusetts

Tsoline Kojaoghlanian, MD
Fellow
Division of Pediatric Infectious Diseases
Department of Pediatrics
Children's Hospital at Montefiore
Bronx, New York

Brian S. Koll, MD
Associate Professor
Department of Medicine
Albert Einstein College of Medicine;
Associate Attending
Department of Medicine
Beth Israel Medical Center
New York, New York

Dimitrios P. Kontoyiannis, MD, MS, ScD, FACP
Associate Professor
Department of Infectious Diseases
University of Texas MD Anderson Cancer
    Center
Houston, Texas

Venkatarama R. Koppaka, MD, PhD
Clinical Assistant Professor
Division of Pulmonary and Critical Care
    Medicine
Virginia Commonwealth University;
Medical Officer
Division of Tuberculosis Elimination
Centers for Disease Control and Prevention
Atlanta, Georgia

Frederick Koster, MD
Professor
Department of Internal Medicine
University of New Mexico
Albuquerque, New Mexico

Karen L. Kotloff, MD
Professor
Department of Pediatrics
University of Maryland Medical School
Baltimore, Maryland

Calvin M. Kunin, MD
Professor Emeritus
Department of Internal Medicine
Ohio State University
Columbus, Ohio

John R. La Montagne, PhD
Deputy Director
National Institute of Allergy and Infectious
    Diseases
National Institutes of Health
Bethesda, Maryland

Clayton S. Lau, MD
Resident
Department of Urology
Tufts-New England Medical Center
Boston, Massachusetts

William J. Ledger, MD
Professor and Chairman Emeritus
Department of Obstetrics–Gynecology
Weill Medical College of Cornell University;
Senior Attending Physician
Department of Obstetrics–Gynecology
New York Presbyterian Hospital
New York, New York

Patricia C. Lee, MD
Houston, Texas

John M. Leedom, MD
Professor
Department of Medicine
Keck School of Medicine
University of Southern California;
LAC and USC Medical Center
Los Angeles, California

Thomas J. Leipzig, MD
Assistant Professor
Department of Surgery
Indiana University School of Medicine;
Indianapolis Neurosurgical Group, Inc.
Indianapolis, Indiana

Stanley M. Lemon, MD
Professor
Departments of Microbiology and
    Immunology
Dean
Office of the Dean of Medicine
University of Texas Medical Branch
Galveston, Texas

Donald Leung, MD, PhD
Professor
Department of Pediatrics
University of Colorado Health Sciences
    Center;
Head
Division of Pediatric Allergy-Immunology
National Jewish Medical and Research
    Center
Denver, Colorado

Roland A. Levandowski, MD
Supervisory Medical Officer
Division of Viral Products
Center for Biologics Evaluation and
    Research
Bethesda, Maryland

Myron M. Levine, MD, DTPH
Professor
Department of Pediatrics and Medicine
University of Maryland School of
    Medicine
Baltimore, Maryland

Daniel P. Lew, MD
Division of Infectious Diseases
Department of Medicine
Geneva University Hospital
Geneva, Switzerland

Jeffrey M. Lisowski, MD
Assistant Professor
Rush Medical College
Grant Hospital
Chicago, Illinois

Philip D. Lister, PhD
Associate Professor
Department of Medical Microbiology and
    Immunology
Creighton University School of Medicine
Omaha, Nebraska

Nancy Liu, MD
Department of Medicine
UMASS Memorial Medical Center
Worcester, Massachusetts

Diana N. J. Lockwood, MD
Senior Lecturer
London School of Hygiene and Tropical
   Medicine;
Consultant Physician and Leprologist
Hospital for Tropical Diseases
London, United Kingdom

Walter J. Loesche, DMD, PhD
Marcus Ward Professor Emeritus
Department of Microbiology and
   Immunology
University of Michigan School of Medicine
   and School of Dentistry;
Ann Arbor, Michigan

Donald B. Louria, MD
Professor
Department of Preventive Medicine and
   Community Health
University of Medicine and Dentistry of New
   Jersey
Newark, New Jersey

Janine Maenza, MD
Clinical Assistant Professor
Division of Allergy and Infectious
   Diseases
Department of Medicine
University of Washington
Seattle, Washington

James H. Maguire, MD
Division of Infectious Diseases
Brigham and Women's Hospital
Harvard Medical School
Boston, Massachusetts;
Division of Parasitic Diseases
Centers for Disease Control and
   Prevention
Atlanta, Georgia

Adel A. F. Mahmoud, MD, PhD
President
Merck Vaccines
Merck & Co., Inc.
Whitehouse Station, New Jersey

Harry L. Malech, MD
Chief
Laboratory of Host Defenses
National Institute of Allergy and Infectious
   Diseases
National Institutes of Health
Bethesda, Maryland

Joan B. Mannick, MD
Assistant Professor
Department of Medicine
University of Massachusetts Medical
   School;
Physician
Department of Medicine
University of Massachusetts Medical
   Center
Worcester, Massachusetts

Richard B. Markham, MD
Professor
Department of Molecular Microbiology and
   Immunology
Bloomberg School of Public Health
The Johns Hopkins University
Baltimore, Maryland

Melvin I. Marks, MD
Professor and Vice-Chair
Department of Pediatrics
University of California at Irvine Medical
   Center
Irvine, California;
Administrator
Miller Children's Hospital at Long Beach
Long Beach, California

Annette Martin, PhD
Chargée de Recherche
Department of Virology
Institut Pasteur
Paris, France

Henry Masur, MD
Chief
Department of Critical Care Medicine
Clinical Center
National Institutes of Health
Bethesda, Maryland

Glen Eric Mathisen, MD
Clinical Professor of Medicine
Department of Medicine
David Geffen School of Medicine at UCLA
Los Angeles, California;
Chief
Infectious Disease Service
Department of Medicine
Olive View-UCLA Medical Center
Sylmar, California

Els Mathieu, MD, MPH
Medical Epidemiologist
Division of Parasitic Diseases
Centers for Disease Control and
   Prevention
Atlanta, Georgia

Keith P. W. J. McAdam, MD
MRC Laboratories, Fajara
Banjul, The Gambia

William M. McCormack, MD
Professor
Department of Medicine
SUNY Downstate Medical Center
Brooklyn, New York

Joseph E. McDade, PhD
Deputy Director
National Center for Infectious Diseases
Centers for Disease Control and
   Prevention
Atlanta, Georgia

John E. McGowan, Jr., MD
Professor of Epidemiology and Medicine
Department of Infectious Diseases
Emory University
Atlanta, Georgia

Kelly T. McKee, Jr., MD, MPH
Managing Research Physician
U.S. Army Medical Research Institute of
   Infectious Diseases
Fort Detrick, Maryland

Rima McLeod, MD
Jules and Doris Stein RPB Professor and
   Attending Physician
Department of Ophthalmology and Visual
   Sciences
The University of Chicago
Chicago, Illinois

Albert T. McManus, PhD
Senior Scientist
U.S. Army Institute of Surgical Research
Brooke Army Medical Center
San Antonio, Texas

Jennifer H. McQuiston, DVM, MS
Veterinary Epidemiologist
Branch of Viral and Rickettsial Zoonoses
Centers for Disease Control and Prevention
Atlanta, Georgia

H. Cody Meissner, MD
Associate Professor
Department of Pediatrics
Tufts University School of Medicine;
Chief
Division of Infectious Diseases
Tufts-New England Medical Center
Boston, Massachusetts

William G. Merz, PhD
Professor
Department of Pathology
The Johns Hopkins University;
Director
Mycology Lab
Department of Microbiology and Pathology
The Johns Hopkins Hospital
Baltimore, Maryland

Richard D. Meyer, MD
Clinical Professor of Medicine
Department of Medicine
David Geffen School of Medicine at UCLA
Los Angeles, California;
Staff
Department of Medicine
Northridge Hospital Medical Center
Northridge, California

Burt R. Meyers, MD
Professor and Attending Physician
Division of Infectious Diseases
Department of Medicine
Mount Sinai School of Medicine and
   Hospital
New York, New York

Sue M. Mietzner, MS
Research Associate
Special Pathogens Laboratory
VA Medical Center
Pittsburgh, Pennsylvania

Laurence F. Mirels, MD
Department of Medicine
Division of Infectious Diseases and
   Geographic Medicine
Stanford University School of Medicine
Stanford, California;
Department of Medicine
Division of Infectious Diseases
Santa Clara Valley Medical Center;
Infectious Diseases Research Laboratory
California Institute for Medical Research
San Jose, California

Robert C. Moellering, Jr., MD
Herrman Blumgart Professor of Medicine
Harvard Medical School;
Physician-in-Chief
Department of Medicine
Beth Israel Deaconess Medical Center
Boston, Massachusetts

Bernard Moss, MD, PhD
Chief
Laboratory of Viral Diseases
National Institute of Allergy and Infectious
  Diseases
National Institutes of Health
Bethesda, Maryland

Robert R. Muder, MD
Professor
Department of Medicine
University of Pittsburgh;
Hospital Epidemiologist
Section of Infectious Diseases
VA Pittsburgh Healthcare System
Pittsburgh, Pennsylvania

Maurice A. Mufson, MD
Professor and Chair Emeritus
Department of Medicine
Marshall University School of Medicine
Huntington, West Virginia

Timothy F. Murphy, MD
Professor
Departments of Medicine and
  Microbiology
Chief
Division of Infectious Diseases
State University of New York at Buffalo;
Chief
Department of Infectious Diseases
Buffalo VA Medical Center
Buffalo, New York

Barbara E. Murray, MD
Professor and Director
Division of Infectious Diseases
University of Texas Medical School;
Co-Director
Center for the Study of Emerging and
  Re-emerging Pathogens
University of Texas Health Science
  Center-Houston
Houston, Texas

Daniel M. Musher, MD
Professor
Departments of Medicine and Molecular
  Virology and Microbiology
Baylor College of Medicine;
Chief
Division of Infectious Diseases
Medical Care Line
Department of Veterans Affairs
Houston, Texas

G. Balakrish Nair, PhD
Associate Director and Head
Division of Laboratory Sciences
International Center for Diarrheal
  Disease
Center for Health and Population
  Research
Mohakhali, Dhaka
Bangladesh

Avery B. Nathens, MD, PhD, MPH
Associate Professor
Department of Surgery
University of Washington;
Associate Professor
Department of Surgery
Harborview Medical Center
Seattle, Washington

Judith L. Nerad, MD, MS
Assistant Professor
Section of Infectious Diseases
Department of Medicine
Rush Medical College;
Attending Physician
Division of Infectious Diseases
John H. Stroger, Jr., Hospital of Cook County
Chicago, Illinois

Kathleen M. Neuzil, MD, MPH
Associate Professor
Department of Medicine
University of Washington School of Medicine;
Staff Physician
Department of Infectious Diseases
VA Puget Sound Health Care System
Seattle, Washington

Ronald Lee Nichols, MD
William Henderson Professor Emeritus
Departments of Surgery, Microbiology, and
  Immunology
Tulane University School of Medicine;
Senior Visiting Surgeon
Department of Surgery
Medical Center of Louisiana at New Orleans
New Orleans, Louisiana

Richard A. Nitzberg, MD
Assistant Clinical Professor of Surgery
Columbia University Medical School
New York, New York;
Staff Vascular Surgeon
Overlook Hospital
Summit, New Jersey

John Noble, MD
Professor
Department of Medicine
Boston University;
Director
Center for Primary Care
Boston Medical Center
Boston, Massachusetts

Vladimir A. Novitsky, MD, PhD
Research Scientist
Department of Immunology and Infectious
  Diseases
Harvard School of Public Health
Boston, Massachusetts

M. Steven Oberste, PhD
Research Microbiologist
Enterovirus Section
National Center for Infectious Diseases
Centers for Disease Control and Prevention
Atlanta, Georgia

Thomas F. O'Donnell, Jr., MD
Andrews Professor and Chairman
Department of Surgery and Surgeon in Chief
Tufts University School of Medicine
New England Medical Center
Boston, Massachusetts

Pearay L. Ogra, MD
John Sealy Distinguished Chair Professor and
  Chairman (Retired)
Department of Pediatrics
University of Texas Medical Branch
Galveston, Texas;
Professor of Pediatrics
State University of New York at Buffalo
Buffalo, New York

Christopher A. Ohl, MD
Associate Professor of Medicine
Section on Infectious Diseases
Wake Forest University School of
  Medicine;
Medical Director
Center for Antimicrobial Utilization
  Stewardship and Epidemiology
Wake Forest University Baptist Medical
  Center
Winston-Salem, North Carolina

David W. Oldach, MD
Associate Professor
Department of Medicine
University of Maryland School of Medicine;
Investigator
Institute of Human Virology
University of Maryland Biotechnology
  Institutes
Baltimore, Maryland

James M. Oleske, MD, MPH
Professor
Department of Pediatrics
UMDNJ/New Jersey Medical School;
Attending
Department of Pediatrics
University Hospital
Newark, New Jersey

James G. Olson, PhD
Head
Department of Virology
Navy Medical Research Center Detachment
American Embassy
Lima, Peru

Lillian A. Orciari, MS
Microbiologist
WHO Collaborating Center for Reference and
  Research on Rabies
Division of Viral and Rickettsial Diseases
Centers for Disease Control and Prevention
Atlanta, Georgia

Ynes R. Ortega, PhD, MPH
Assistant Professor
Center for Food Safety
University of Georgia
Griffin, Georgia

Michael N. Oxman, MD
Professor
Departments of Medicine and Pathology
University of California, San Diego;
Staff Physician
Department of Infectious Diseases
VA Medical Center
San Diego, California

Christopher D. Paddock, MD
Staff Pathologist
Department of Infectious Disease Pathology
  Activity
Centers for Disease Control and Prevention
Atlanta, Georgia

Mark A. Pallansch, PhD
Chief
Enterovirus Section
National Center for Infectious Diseases
Centers for Disease Control and
  Prevention
Atlanta, Georgia

Darwin L. Palmer, MD
Professor Emeritus
Department of Medicine
University of New Mexico School of Medicine
Albuquerque, New Mexico

Julie Parsonnet, MD
Associate Professor
Departments of Medicine and Health
    Research and Policy
Stanford University School of Medicine
Stanford, California

David C. Perlman, MD
Professor
Department of Medicine
Albert Einstein College of Medicine;
Chief
Department of Infectious Diseases
Beth Israel Singer Division
Beth Israel Medical Center
New York, New York

Robert Pinner, MD
Special Assistant for Surveillance
National Center for Infectious Diseases
Centers for Disease Control and Prevention
Atlanta, Georgia

Yale D. Podnos, MD, MPH
Chief Resident
Department of Surgery
University of California Irvine Medical Center
Orange, California

Matthew Pollack, MD
Professor of Medicine
Head, Infectious Diseases Division
F. Edward Hébert School of Medicine
Uniformed University of the Health
    Sciences;
Attending Staff Physician
Department of Medicine
National Naval Medical Center
Bethesda, Maryland

Richard Jay Pollack, PhD
Instructor
Immunology and Infectious Diseases
Harvard School of Public Health
Boston, Massachusetts

John C. Pottage, Jr., MD
Senior Director
Drug Development
Achillion Pharmaceuticals
New Haven, Connecticut

Susan M. Poutanen, MD, MPH, FRCPC
Senior Infectious Diseases Fellow
Department of Medicine
Division of Infectious Diseases and
    Geographic Medicine
Stanford University Medical Center
Stanford, California

Basil A. Pruitt, Jr., MD
Clinical Professor
Department of Surgery
University of Texas Health Science Center at
    San Antonio;
Staff Surgeon
Division of Trauma Surgery
University Hospital
San Antonio, Texas

Thomas C. Quinn, MD
Professor
Division of Infectious Diseases
Department of Medicine
The Johns Hopkins University
Baltimore, Maryland

C. George Ray, MD
Clinical Professor
Department of Pathology
University of Arizona;
Clinical Pathologist
Department of Pathology
University Medical Center
Tucson, Arizona

Sharon L. Reed, MD
Professor
Department of Pathology and Medicine
University of California, San Diego;
Director
Microbiology Laboratory
University of California San Diego Medical
    Center
San Diego, California

Megan E. Reller, MD
Fellow in Infectious Diseases
Departments of Medicine and Pediatrics
Harvard Medical School;
Fellow in Infectious Diseases
Department of Medicine
Children's Hospital Boston
Boston, Massachusetts

Jack S. Remington, MD
Professor
Department of Medicine
Division of Infectious Diseases and
    Geographic Medicine
Stanford University School of Medicine;
Professor
Department of Medicine
Stanford Hospital
Palo Alto, California

Craig W. Roberts, PhD
Senior Lecturer
Department of Immunology
University of Strathclyde
Glasgow, United Kingdom

Allan R. Ronald, OC, MD, FRSC, FRCPC, MACP
Distinguished Professor Emeritus
Department of Internal Medicine
University of Manitoba;
Consultant
Department of Infectious Diseases
St. Boniface Hospital
Winnipeg, Manitoba
Canada

Noel R. Rose, MD, PhD, FCAP
Professor
Departments of Pathology, Molecular
    Microbiology, and Immunology
The Johns Hopkins University;
Director
Center for Autoimmune Disease
    Research
Departments of Pathology, Molecular
    Microbiology, and Immunology
The Johns Hopkins Hospital
Baltimore, Maryland

Jill R. Rosenthal, MD
Assistant Professor of Dermatology
Tufts University School of Medicine;
Dermatologist and Director of Pediatric
    Dermatology
Department of Medical and Surgical
    Dermatology
New England Medical Center
Boston, Massachusetts

Alan L. Rothman, MD
Professor
Department of Medicine
University of Massachusetts Medical School
Worcester, Massachusetts

Ori D. Rotstein, MD, FRCSC
Professor
Department of Surgery
University of Toronto;
Head
Division of General Surgery
Department of Surgery
University Health Network
Toronto, Ontario
Canada

Donald H. Rubin, MD
Professor
Department of Medicine, Microbiology, and
    Immunology
Vanderbilt University School of Medicine;
Associate Chief of Staff
Department of Research and Development
Nashville VA Medical Center
Nashville, Tennessee

Robert H. Rubin, MD, FACP, FCCP
Osborne Professor of Health Sciences and
    Technology
Department of Medicine
Director
Center for Experimental Pharmacology and
    Therapeutics
Harvard–MIT Division of Health Science and
    Technology;
Associate Director
Division of Infectious Diseases
Brigham and Women's Hospital
Boston, Massachusetts

Charles E. Rupprecht, MD
Chief
Rabies Section
Centers for Disease Control and Prevention
Atlanta, Georgia

David A. Sack, MD
Professor
Department of International Health
The Johns Hopkins Bloomberg School of
    Public Health;
Director
International Center for Diarrheal Disease
    Research
Center for Health and Population Research
Mohakhali, Dhaka
Bangladesh

Majid Sadigh, MD
Associate Clinical Professor
Department of Medicine
Yale University School of Medicine;
Associate Program Director
Department of Medicine
St. Mary's Hospital
Waterbury, Connecticut

Grannum R. Sant, MD
Professor
Department of Urology
Tufts University School of Medicine;
Chairman
Department of Urology
Tufts-New England Medical Center
Boston, Massachusetts

Francisco L. Sapico, MD
Professor Emeritus
Department of Medicine
Keck School of Medicine
University of Southern California;
Former Chief of Infectious Diseases
Department of Medicine
Rancho Los Amigos National Rehabilitation
Center
Downey, California

Dennis R. Schaberg, MD
Professor and Chairman
Department of Medicine
University of Tennessee Health Science
Center
Memphis, Tennessee

Julius Schachter, PhD
Professor
Department of Laboratory Medicine
University of California, San Francisco
San Francisco, California

Peter M. Schantz, VMD, PhD
Epidemiologist
Division of Parasitic Diseases
National Center for Infectious Diseases
Centers for Disease Control and Prevention
Atlanta, Georgia

Gilbert M. Schiff, MD, FACP
Professor Emeritus
Departments of Medicine and of Pediatrics
University of Cincinnati College of Medicine;
Director Emeritus
Gamble Program for Clinical Studies
Division of Infectious Diseases
Department of Pediatrics
Cincinnati Children's Hospital Medical
Center
Cincinnati, Ohio

Patrick M. Schlievert, PhD
Professor
Department of Microbiology
University of Minnesota
Minneapolis, Minnesota

Anne Schuchat, MD
Medical Epidemiologist
Division of Bacterial and Mycotic Diseases
National Center for Infectious Diseases
Centers for Disease Control and Prevention
Atlanta, Georgia

Alan L. Scott, PhD
Professor
Department of Molecular Microbiology and
Immunology
Bloomberg School of Public Health
The Johns Hopkins University
Baltimore, Maryland

Deborah E. Sentochnik, MD
Attending Staff
Infectious Diseases
Lahey Clinic Medical Center
Burlington, Massachusetts

John L. Sever, MD, PhD
Professor of Pediatrics, Obstetrics and
Gynecology, Immunology, Microbiology,
and Tropical Medicine
Department of Pediatrics
The George Washington University Medical
Center
Children's National Medical Center
Washington, DC

Keerti V. Shah, MD, DrPH
Professor
Department of Molecular Microbiology and
Immunology
Bloomberg School of Public Health
The Johns Hopkins University
Baltimore, Maryland

Roger Shapiro, MD
Research Associate
Department of Immunology and Infectious
Diseases
Harvard School of Public Health;
Instructor
Division of Infectious Diseases
Beth Israel Deaconess Medical Center
Boston, Massachusetts

John N. Sheagren, MD
Professor
Department of Medicine
University of Illinois College of Medicine;
Chair
Department of Internal Medicine
Advocate Illinois Masonic Medical Center
Chicago, Illinois

Jonas A. Shulman, MD
Executive Associate Dean
Departments of Medical Education and
Student Affairs
Emory University School of Medicine
Atlanta, Georgia

Anthony Simmons, MD, PhD
Professor
Division of Virology
Department of Pediatrics
University of Texas Medical Branch
Galveston, Texas

David R. Snydman, MD
Professor
Department of Medicine
Tufts University School of Medicine;
Chief
Division of Infectious Diseases
Department of Medicine
Tufts-New England Medical Center
Boston, Massachusetts

Steven F. Solga, MD
Senior Clinical Fellow
Department of Gastroenterology
The Johns Hopkins University School of
Medicine
Baltimore, Maryland

Hans M. L. Spiegel, MD
Assistant Professor
Departments of Pediatrics, Microbiology, and
Tropical Medicine
George Washington University;
Director
Department of Special Immunology Services
Children's National Medical Center
Washington, DC

Andrew Spielman, ScD
Professor
Department of Immunology and Infectious
Diseases
Harvard School of Public Health
Boston, Massachusetts

Walter E. Stamm, MD
Professor and Head
Division of Allergy and Infectious Diseases
Department of Medicine
University of Washington
Seattle, Washington

Lawrence R. Stanberry, MD, PhD
Chair
Department of Pediatrics
University of Texas Medical Branch at
Galveston
Galveston, Texas

Ann E. Stapleton, MD
Associate Professor
Division of Allergy and Infectious Diseases
Department of Medicine
University of Washington Medical Center
Seattle, Washington

Charles R. Sterling, PhD
Professor
Department of Veterinary Science and
Microbiology
University of Arizona
Tucson, Arizona

Gene H. Stollerman, MD
Professor Emeritus
Department of Medicine and Public Health
Boston University
Boston, Massachusetts

David R. Stone, MD
Assistant Professor
Department of Medicine
Tufts University School of Medicine;
Attending Physician
Division of Infectious Diseases
Department of Geographic Medicine
New England Medicine Center
Boston, Massachusetts

Janet E. Stout, PhD
Assistant Professor
Division of Infectious Diseases
Department of Medicine
University of Pittsburgh;
Director
Special Pathogens Laboratory
VA Medical Center
Pittsburgh, Pennsylvania

Stephen E. Straus, MD
Director
National Center for Complementary and
Alternative Medicine
National Institutes of Health
Bethesda, Maryland

Larry J. Strausbaugh, MD
Professor
Department of Medicine
Oregon Health and Science University;
Hospital Epidemiologist
Division of Hospital and Specialty Medicine
VA Medical Center
Portland, Oregon

Alan M. Sugar, MD
Professor
Department of Medicine
Boston University School of Medicine;
Director
HIV/AIDS Program and Infectious Disease
    Consulting Service
Cape Cod Hospital
Hyannis, Massachusetts

Kathryn N. Suh, MD, FRCPC
Assistant Professor
Division of Infectious Diseases
Department of Medicine
Queens University;
Attending Physician
Division of Infectious Diseases
Children's Hospital of Eastern Ontario
Ottawa, Ontario
Canada

John W. Sumner, MD
Microbiologist
Department of Infectious Diseases Pathology
    Activity
Centers for Disease Control and Prevention
Atlanta, Georgia

Morton N. Swartz, MD
Professor
Department of Medicine
Harvard University;
Chief
Jackson Firm
Department of Medicine
Massachusetts General Hospital
Boston, Massachusetts

Richard L. Sweet, MD
Professor
Department of Obstetrics and Gynecology
University of California, Davis
Sacramento, California

Gordon L. Telford, MD
Professor
Department of Surgery
Medical College of Wisconsin;
Chief
Minimally Invasive and Gastrointestinal
    Surgery
Department of Surgery
Froedtert Memorial Lutheran Hospital
Milwaukee, Wisconsin

Fred C. Tenover, PhD, ABMM
Adjunct Professor
Division of Epidemiology
Rollins School of Public Health
Emory University;
Associate Director for Laboratory
    Science
Division of Healthcare Quality
    Promotion
Centers for Disease Control and
    Prevention
Atlanta, Georgia

Kenneth S. Thomson, PhD
Professor
Department of Medical Microbiology and
    Immunology
Creighton University School of
    Medicine
Omaha, Nebraska

Jeremiah Tilles, MD
Professor
Department of Medicine
University of California, Irvine;
Associate Dean
Department of Medicine
University of California Irvine Medical Center
Orange, California

Nina E. Tolkoff-Rubin, MD, FACP
Associate Professor
Department of Nephrology
Harvard Medical School;
Director of ESRD Program
Department of Nephrology
Massachusetts General Hospital
Boston, Massachusetts

Lucy S. Tompkins, MD, PhD
Professor and Chief
Division of Infectious Diseases and
    Geographic Medicine
Department of Medicine
Stanford University School of Medicine;
Medical Director
Department of Hospital Epidemiology and
    Infection Control
Stanford Hospital and Clinics
Stanford, California

Edmund C. Tramont, MD
Professor and Director
Medical Biotechnology Center
University of Maryland Biotechnology
    Center;
Staff
University of Maryland Medical Systems
Baltimore, Maryland

Theodore F. Tsai, MD
Global Medical Affairs
Wyeth
St. Davids, Pennsylvania

Walter W. Tunnessen, Jr., MD
(Deceased)
Senior Vice President
American Board of Pediatrics
Chapel Hill, North Carolina

Stephen K. Tyring, MD, PhD
Professor
Departments of Dermatology and
    Microbiology/Immunology Medicine
University of Texas Medical Branch
Galveston, Texas

Mitchell Wachtel, MD
Pathologist
Department of Pathology
St. Joseph Regional Health Center
Bryan, Texas

Francis A. Waldvogel, MD
Clinical Physician
Department of Internal Medicine
Geneva University Hospital
Geneva, Switzerland

Andrew L. Warshaw, MD
W. Gerald Austen Professor
Department of Surgery
Harvard Medical School;
Surgeon-in-Chief and Chairman
Department of Surgery
Massachusetts General Hospital
Boston, Massachusetts

John A. Weigelt, MD, DVM, MMA
Professor and Vice-Chairman
Department of Surgery
Medical College of Wisconsin
Milwaukee, Wisconsin

Robert A. Weinstein, MD
Professor
Department of Medicine
Rush Medical College;
Chairman
Division of Infectious Diseases
Cook County Hospital
Chicago, Illinois

Harold J. Welch, MD
Assistant Professor
Department of Surgery
Tufts University School of Medicine
Boston, Massachusetts;
Senior Staff Surgeon
Department of Vascular Surgery
Lahey Clinic
Burlington, Massachusetts

Robert C. Welliver, Sr., MD
Professor
Department of Pediatrics
State University of New York;
Co-Director
Department of Infectious Diseases
Women's and Children's Hospital
Buffalo, New York

Michael R. Wessels, MD
Professor
Department of Pediatrics and Medicine
Harvard Medical School;
Chief
Division of Infectious Diseases
Children's Hospital of Boston
Boston, Massachusetts

L. Joseph Wheat, MD
President
Mira Vista Diagnostics
Indianapolis, Indiana

Richard J. Whitley, MD
Professor
Departments of Pediatrics, Microbiology,
    Medicine, and Neurosurgery
University of Alabama at Birmingham
Birmingham, Alabama

David N. Williams, MB, ChB
Professor
Department of Medicine
University of Minnesota Medical
    School;
Assistant Chief
Department of Medicine
Hennepin County Medical Center
Minneapolis, Minnesota

Russell A. Williams, MD
Professor
Department of Surgery
University of California, Irvine;
Vice-Chairman
Department of Surgery
University of California Irvine Medical
    Center
Orange, California

Kaethe Willms, MD
Professor
Department of Microbiology and
    Parasitology
Department of Medicine
Ciudad University
Mexico

Mary E. Wilson, MD, FACP
Associate Professor of Medicine
Harvard Medical School
Associate Professor of Population and
    International Health
Harvard School of Public Health
Boston, Massachusetts;
Consultant
Departments of Infectious Diseases and
    Medicine
Mount Auburn Hospital
Cambridge, Massachusetts

Samuel E. Wilson, MD
Associate Dean and Professor
Department of Surgery
University of California, Irvine;
Surgeon
Department of Surgery
University of California Irvine Medical
    Center
Orange, California

Jerry A. Winkelstein, MD
Eudowood Professor of Pediatrics
Departments of Pediatrics, Medicine, and
    Pathology
The Johns Hopkins University
Director
Division of Immunology
Department of Pediatrics
The Johns Hopkins Hospital
Baltimore, Maryland

Dietmar H. Wittmann, MD, PhD, FACS
Professor Emeritus
Department of Surgery
The Medical College of Wisconsin
Milwaukee, Wisconsin

Martin S. Wolfe, MD, FACP
Clinical Professor
Department of Medicine
Georgetown University Medical School
George Washington University Medical
    School;
Director
Traveler's Medical Service of Washington, DC
Washington, DC

Gary P. Wormser, MD
Professor
Department of Medicine
New York Medical College;
Chief
Division of Infectious Diseases
Department of Medicine
Westchester County Medical Center
Valhalla, New York

Peter F. Wright, MD
Professor
Department of Pediatrics
Vanderbilt University;
Chief
Division of Infectious Diseases
Vanderbilt University Medical Center
Nashville, Tennessee

Kimberly A. Yeung-Yue, MD
Research Fellow
Department of Dermatology
University of Texas Medical Branch
Galveston, Texas

Deborah S. Yokoe, MD, MPH
Assistant Professor
Department of Medicine
Harvard Medical School;
Associate Hospital Epidemiologist
Department of Medicine
Brigham and Women's Hospital
Boston, Massachusetts

Neal S. Young, MD
Chief
Hematology Branch
National Heart, Lung, and Blood Institute
National Institutes of Health
Bethesda, Maryland

John A. Zaia, MD
Professor
Department of Virology
Beckman Research Institute of City of Hope;
Full Member
Department of Pediatrics
City of Hope Comprehensive Cancer Center
Duarte, California

Jonathan M. Zenilman, MD
Professor
Division of Infectious Diseases
Department of Medicine
The Johns Hopkins University School of
    Medicine
Baltimore, Maryland

Stephen H. Zinner, MD
Charles S. Davidson Professor
Department of Medicine
Harvard Medical School;
Chairman
Department of Medicine
Mount Auburn Hospital
Cambridge, Massachusetts

Preface

During the past half century, the frontiers of infection have undergone dramatic expansion. Our predecessors thought of infection as synonymous with contagion. The "fever doctor" treated the classic exanthems, typhoid fever, polio, and meningitis, each of which exacted a costly toll in premature death and disability.

A combination of public health measures, vaccines, and antimicrobial drugs has led to a merciful decline in the traditional contagious diseases. Even the freestanding infectious disease hospitals were eliminated as their censuses fell and the remnants of such units were absorbed into the modern hospital complex.

Yet these developments have not removed infection from the register of human afflictions. Insidious microbes still threaten the well-being of our patients, often in a different venue (acquired in the hospital instead of the community) or in the guise of a modern plague (AIDS). Ironically, advances in surgical techniques, such as the insertion of prosthetic devices and organ transplantation, have virtually created a new field, postoperative infection. Contemporary diagnosis and treatment of infection are no longer the domain of the solitary physician; they now require a cooperative approach that involves multiple specialties and utilizes a vast array of laboratory methods, imaging techniques, pharmacologic agents, and surgical intervention.

The field of infectious diseases has expanded at a rapid rate since the publication of the second edition of this book. As a result, the third edition incorporates many changes that keep pace with the new developments. We have added chapters on bioterrorism, human herpesvirus-8, linezolid and quinupristin-dalfopristin, West Nile virus, food safety, hospital infections, emerging infections, and the diagnostic usefulness of nonspecific laboratory abnormalities. New authors have joined the list of contributors and the chapters of the prior edition have been updated and extensively revised.

We have attempted to select authors with recognized expertise in their subjects. As a result, the list of contributors is a veritable "Who's Who" of contemporary authorities in medical and surgical infections. We are particularly proud of our section on surgical infections (which currently are a significant portion of infection within the hospital), written by surgeons preeminent in their areas of interest. The editors have read and critiqued every chapter. The authors themselves bear the responsibility for their chapters, but they have cooperated fully in meeting the requests of the editors for clarification and expansion.

The reader might note the liberal inclusion of tables and figures. The generous use of illustrative material is intended to highlight the seminal points of the text; in addition, we believe that illustrations render the text more accessible.

Our efforts were supported by an outstanding team at Lippincott Williams & Wilkins, particularly our managing editor, Joyce Murphy, and our production editor, Tim Prairie.

We include herewith a few thoughts on why we who work in this field are so committed to the enterprise of fighting infection. In all candor, most of us admit to the unqualified excitement of the quest, the perceptual challenge, the relentless pursuit of conquest over these microscopic agents of disease. Hans Zinsser captured in words the spirit of this calling in his classic book *Rats, Lice and History* (1935):

> Infectious disease is one of the few genuine adventures left in the world ... however secure and well-regulated life may become, bacteria, protozoa, viruses, infected fleas, ticks, mosquitoes, and bedbugs will always lurk in the shadows ready to pounce when neglect, poverty, famine, or war lets down the defenses. And even in normal times they prey on the weak, the very young and the very old, living along with us, in mysterious obscurity waiting their opportunities. About the only genuine sporting proposition that remains unimpaired by the relentless domestication of a once free-living human species is the war against these ferocious little fellow creatures, which lurk in the dark corners and stalk us in the bodies of rats, mice, and all kinds of domestic animals; which fly and crawl with the insects, and waylay us in our food and drink and even in our love.

The challenge of infection is quite unlike any other in medicine, for it goes beyond the boundaries of knowledge about humankind, requiring a mastery over the biology of the offending microorganism—its habitats; how it lives, feeds, and makes its way in a hostile world; its allies and vectors; its strengths; and most important, its vulnerabilities. Most fields of medicine encourage an anthropocentric image of the world. But an understanding of infectious diseases requires a vision beyond the human biosphere—one that encompasses the ecosystem of microscopic creatures that share our environment.

Yet treating infection is more than an intellectual challenge; it is the added dimension of caring for the victims that is the driving spirit behind these endeavors. Whether in the laboratory, in the epidemiology office, or at the bedside, we physicians all recognize that the focus of our efforts is the hapless patient who suffers from an infectious disease. Fortunately, many infectious agents yield to the appropriate use of an antimicrobial drug or can be prevented by the use of a vaccine or the skillful application of public health measures. We do accept the reality that many microorganisms cannot be treated with current therapies or have established themselves in hosts incapable of mustering sufficient responses in their own defense. And we also recognize, sadly, that many people still succumb to infectious diseases that are either treatable or readily preventable.

Ultimately, the practice of infectious diseases is the art of the possible. The editors and contributors have tried to set down what is known about infections in medicine and surgery in a way that conveys the excitement of the science and the satisfaction that follows the judicious application of appropriate diagnosis, therapy, and preventive measures.

Sherwood L. Gorbach, MD
John G. Bartlett, MD
Neil R. Blacklow, MD

General Principles of Infection

How Microorganisms Cause Disease

CHAPTER 1
Molecular Epidemiology in Infectious Diseases

Susan M. Poutanen and Lucy S. Tompkins

The term *molecular epidemiology* has been used in published literature in the context of infectious diseases as well as other disciplines since the late 1970s and early 1980s (1,2). Since its first published use, it has been defined in a number of different ways and in a number of different contexts, ranging from "[the use of] biochemical techniques for the genetic and phenotypic analysis of viruses" (3) to "the application of sophisticated techniques to the epidemiologic study of biological material" (4). Perhaps the simplest way to define it is to define each component of molecular epidemiology separately (5): *molecular* referring to *molecular biology*, defined as "the branch of biology concerned with the nature and function, at the molecular level, of biological phenomena, such as RNA and DNA, proteins, and other macromolecules" (6); and *epidemiology*, defined as "the study of the distribution and determinants of health-related states or events in specified populations, and the application of this study to control of health problems" (7). In this way, molecular epidemiology can be defined as the application of molecular biology to epidemiology and, specifically with regard to infectious diseases, as the application of molecular biological methods to the study of the distribution and determinants of infectious diseases, with the goal of controlling such diseases.

Although some authors use the term molecular epidemiology to describe a distinct subspecialty of epidemiology, it has been argued that this term should be used instead to describe merely a tool that is used in the discipline of epidemiology (8,9). This latter school of thought pools the term molecular epidemiology with other terms, such as *seroepidemiology* and *biochemical epidemiology*, both of which also describe the application of various tools, that is, serology and biochemistry, respectively, to the discipline of epidemiology. Regardless as to the controversy related to the precise definition of molecular epidemiology, the studies

that have applied molecular techniques to infectious diseases epidemiology have been appreciated as particularly valuable contributions, and molecular epidemiology in general has been recognized as showing great promise in the future (7,10,11).

OVERVIEW OF MOLECULAR METHODS USED IN INFECTIOUS DISEASES EPIDEMIOLOGY

The molecular methods used in infectious diseases epidemiology can be classified into three categories: (a) methods to identify infectious agents; (b) methods to strain type infectious agents (also known as *fingerprinting*); and (c) methods to detect molecular biomarkers reflecting pathogen virulence, host susceptibility, and host response to infectious diseases. These methods have complemented nonmolecular methods and, at times, replaced them altogether. Each of these three categories of molecular methods can be applied to infectious diseases epidemiology as illustrated in the following examples.

Identification of Infectious Agents

Epidemiologic studies in infectious diseases rely on reproducible valid diagnostic assays. In the past, to identify infectious agents, one would rely on culture, enzyme-linked immunosorbent assays, agglutination methods, or monoclonal antibodies. Compared with these conventional methods, molecular methods have reduced the time required to identify the presence of microorganisms in clinical specimens while increasing the sensitivity of doing so and maintaining high specificity. These techniques also facilitate the identification of infectious agents associated with chronic diseases and provide a means to identify nonculturable organisms. Details concerning the molecular techniques used for the detection and identification of infectious agents are discussed in Chapter 14 of this book.

Strain Typing of Infectious Agents

Strain typing is the method used to identify organisms that share the same phenotypic and genotypic traits and that are then, by inference, assumed to be clonally related, that is, genetically identical or closely related to each other. The process of strain typing infectious agents is important in infectious disease epidemiology in a number of ways. It aids infection surveillance and is particularly useful in the identification and investigation of outbreaks. In addition, it facilitates the identification of sources and modes of transmission of infectious agents outside of an outbreak situation. For example, if all isolates obtained from a group of patients have the identical fingerprint, then this suggests either the presence of a common source of the infectious agent, cross-contamination between patients, or the presence of an endemic strain causing frequent infection. Epidemiologic investigation can aid in differentiating between these possibilities.

To be useful, a typing system should have typeability, reproducibility, and high discriminatory power. In other words, it should be able to give an unambiguous result for each organism; it should be able to give the same result each time the same isolate is tested; and it should be able to detect differences among clonally unrelated strains. Conventional phenotypic typing methods, such as biotyping, phage typing, serotyping, and antibiotic susceptibility typing, fall short of meeting these requirements, unlike molecular methods, which have become the typing methods of choice in most epidemiologic studies.

There are many molecular typing methods available, and not all typing methods perform equally well for all species. Unfortunately, because techniques, type nomenclature, reference strains, and species-specific gold standard typing methods have not been standardized for most molecular typing methods, the interpretation and comparison of results obtained by different methods and different laboratories are impeded. Attempts have been made to develop standards and guidelines for the use of molecular typing methods (12–14), but this is an ongoing process needing to be continually updated as more methods are being developed.

Detection of Molecular Biomarkers of Pathogen Virulence, Host Susceptibility, and Host Response to Infectious Diseases

Molecular methods have been used in epidemiologic studies to detect molecular biomarkers of pathogen virulence, host susceptibility, and host response to infectious diseases. Recent innovations in molecular methods, specifically with respect to microarray technology, will likely allow for a considerable expansion in the number and yield of such studies. The information obtained through these studies is likely to be of considerable value in the design of new therapeutic and preventive options regarding infectious diseases.

SPECIFIC MOLECULAR METHODS USED IN INFECTIOUS DISEASES EPIDEMIOLOGY

A summary of molecular methods commonly used in infectious diseases epidemiology is shown in Table 1.1. Descriptions of these molecular methods, along with examples of applications of these methods, are summarized as follows.

Protein-Based Methods

Multilocus enzyme electrophoresis (MLEE) is a protein-based molecular method that has been used primarily as a strain typing method in infectious diseases epidemiology. In this procedure, multiple enzymes from each isolate of interest are subjected to electrophoresis using a starch gel (15). Electrophoresis separates these enzymes (or any group of charged molecules) on the basis of their differing rates of migration in an electric field. Their rates of migration are determined by both the molecular weight of the molecules and their electrical charge. In MLEE, the relative electrophoretic mobility of each enzyme, compared with a standard chosen from a control strain, is detected using staining solutions that include enzyme-specific substrate, coenzymes, cofactors, and a dye. When assessing a specific enzyme,

which should have the same approximate molecular weight for each isolate, the differences in mobility between isolates are assumed to result from charge differences due to amino acid substitution reflecting changes in the underlying DNA encoding the polypeptide. All of the different mobility variants of each enzyme assessed are numbered according to their mobility. In this way, every isolate studied can be described by a series of numbers corresponding to the different mobility variants of each enzyme evaluated. This series of numbers acts as a fingerprint specific to each isolate. An example of an application of MLEE as a typing tool is a study by Norton and colleagues in which a cluster of cases of melioidosis was investigated (16). This study revealed that the molecular type of *Burkholderia pseudomallei* was associated with the clinical presentation of the patient more so than the geographical location of the patient, thereby providing better understanding of the pathogenesis of this infectious disease. However, although MLEE is a useful procedure, the technique is very demanding and has only moderate discriminatory power.

Similar to MLEE, immunoblotting has been used as a strain typing tool in infectious disease epidemiology. In this procedure, bacterial proteins from each isolate of interest are subjected to polyacrylamide gel electrophoresis. These electrophoresed proteins are then transferred onto a nitrocellulose membrane and exposed to specific or broadly reactive antibodies that are detected using commercially available enzyme-labeled antiimmunoglobulins (17). The electrophoretic patterns detected in this way act as fingerprints specific to each isolate. In a study by Mulligan and coworkers, immunoblots were used to type *Staphylococcus aureus* clinical isolates and were found to be useful with good reproducibility and discriminatory power (18). However, one disadvantage of this technique is that the electrophoretic patterns

---

TABLE 1.1.   Molecular Methods Used in Infectious Diseases Epidemiology

Protein-based methods
   Multilocus enzyme electrophoresis (MLEE)
   Immunoblotting
Nonamplifiied nucleic acid–based methods
Plasmid DNA
   Whole plasmid analysis
   Restriction endonuclease analysis (REA) of plasmid DNA
Chromosomal DNA
   Conventional REA
   Restriction fragment length polymorphism (RFLP) analysis using conventional REA gels subjeted to Southern blotting followed by hybridization
   Ribotyping
   Pulsed field gel electrophoresis (PFGE)
   Multilocus sequence typing (MLST)
   Single-locuss sequence typing
Amplified nucleic acid–based methods
Polymerase chain reaction
   Amplification of a single target specific to a pathogen
   RFLP analysis using a single amplified product subjected to endonuclease digestin (PPER-RFLP)
   PCR-ribotyping
   Repetitive element PCR (rep-PCR)
   Arbitrary primed PCR (AP-PCR), also known as randomly amplified polymorphic DNA (RAPD)
Microarray (DNA chip)–based methods
Expression profiling
Genomic profiling
   Matrix-based comparative genomic hybridization
   Sequence variation analysis

can contain a large number of bands, making interpretation of results difficult and subjective.

Nonamplified Nucleic Acid–Based Methods

PLASMID DNA

One of the first nonamplified nucleic acid–based methods used in infectious diseases epidemiology, and specifically strain typing, was plasmid analysis. Plasmids are extrachromosomal DNA that encode a wide variety of genes, including those mediating antimicrobial resistance and virulence. The basis of plasmid analysis is that organisms that are clonally related carry the same number of plasmids, with the same molecular weights and restriction endonuclease patterns (19).

Whole plasmid analysis involves extracting plasmids and subjecting them to agarose gel electrophoresis. Bands can be identified by staining the gel with ethidium bromide and by examining the gel under ultraviolet light. In this way, the number and size of the plasmids carried by an isolate can be determined and compared between isolates. The discriminatory power can be improved by digesting the plasmids with high-frequency restriction endonucleases and electrophoretically analyzing the number and size of the resulting restriction fragments in a technique known as restriction endonuclease analysis (REA) of plasmid DNA. Variations in the REA pattern can results from sequence rearrangement, insertion or deletion of DNA, or base substitution within the endonuclease recognition site. Sexton and associates used whole plasmid analysis and REA of plasmid DNA to type 44 isolates of ampicillin-resistant *Enterococcus* species obtained from hospitalized patients in a tertiary-care teaching hospital over a 2-year period (20). Such typing revealed multiple different unique fingerprints, thereby showing that the source of these strains was multifocal.

In general, plasmid analysis is a relatively easy and inexpensive method with good discriminatory power. However, variations in the plasmid extraction method and the electrophoretic conditions can influence the final plasmid profile. In addition, plasmids can be spontaneously lost from or acquired by an isolate. Furthermore, plasmids can undergo molecular rearrangement or deletion. Moreover, some strains are not typeable by this method given that they do not carry plasmids.

CHROMOSOMAL DNA

Conventional REA of chromosomal DNA is an alternative typing method. Similar to REA of plasmid DNA, REA of chromosomal DNA involves the comparison of the number and the size of electrophoresed fragments produced by digestion of chromosomal DNA with high-frequency restriction endonucleases (21). Through the use of REA as a typing tool, potable water that harbors *Legionella pneumophila* was shown to be an important source of community-acquired legionnaires' disease in a study by Stout and coworkers (22). Although this technique is relatively simple and inexpensive, with all isolates being theoretically typeable, the patterns of fragments can be very difficult to interpret given the large number of bands that may be unresolved or overlapping (21). In addition, one cannot easily differentiate bands that may represent plasmid DNA versus chromosomal DNA.

Restriction fragment length polymorphism (RFLP) refers to the polymorphic nature of the locations of restriction endonuclease sites within defined genetic regions. By transferring electrophoresed DNA fragments from conventional REA gels to a nylon or nitrocellulose membrane (in a method called *Southern blotting*) (23) and hybridizing the membrane-bound nucleic acid to a labeled DNA probe, one can assess polymorphisms within

the specific regions of the chromosome homologous to the hybridization probe. Only those restriction fragments that contain sequences homologous to the hybridization probe are detected. The pattern of the number and sizes of the fragments detected, which is greatly simplified because the probe will combine with only a few genomic fragments, can then be used for strain typing. Thus, RFLP analysis using conventional REA gels subjected to Southern blotting followed by hybridization can help with some of the problems associated with conventional REA alone, specifically those problems related to the difficulty in interpreting fingerprints with large numbers of bands. RFLP analysis using this method, specifically with *Pvu*II as the high-frequency restriction endonuclease and the DNA insertion element IS*6110* as a probe, has been found to be a useful typing method for *Mycobacterium tuberculosis* and has been recommended as the standard typing method in order to facilitate comparison of *M. tuberculosis* strain types across different laboratories (12,24). Figure 1.1 shows an example of RFLP patterns used in a study that investigated all

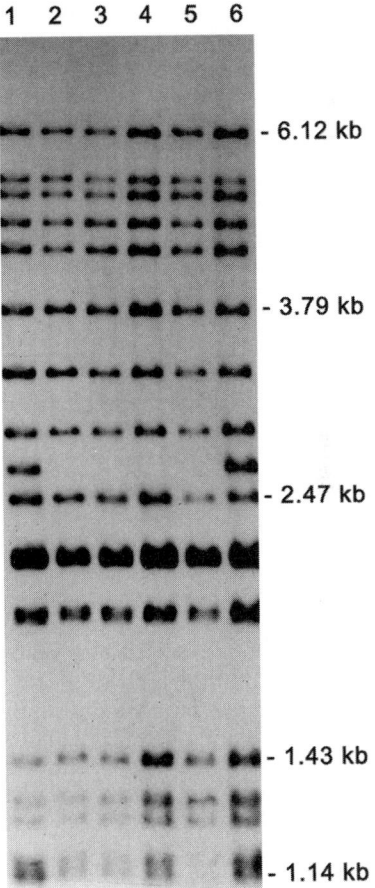

Figure 1.1. Restriction fragment length polymorphism (RFLP) patterns of *Mycobacterium tuberculosis* isolates (using chromosomal DNA digested with *Pvu*II followed by Southern blotting and hybridization with IS*6110*) obtained during a retrospective review of all reported cases of multidrug-resistant tuberculosis occurring in New York City in the early 1990s. The base-pair sizes of selected bands are shown in kilobases. The identical or nearly identical RFLP patterns, as shown here and as seen in 261 other strains, indicated that genetically related strains of *M. tuberculosis* were responsible for a large proportion of the reported cases. Epidemiologic analysis revealed that most of these cases were acquired nosocomially in four New York City hospitals, indicating an extensive multiinstitutional outbreak. (Adapted from Thomas F, Sherman LF, Maw KL, et al. A multiinstitutional outbreak of highly drug-resistant tuberculosis: epidemiology and clinical outcomes. *JAMA* 1996;276[15]:1230, with permission.)

reported cases of multidrug-resistant tuberculosis that occurred in New York City over a 43-month period in the early 1990s (25). Identical or nearly identical RFLP patterns were identified for 267 *M. tuberculosis* strains, indicating that genetically related strains of *M. tuberculosis* were responsible for a large proportion of the reported cases. Epidemiologic analysis revealed that most of these cases were acquired nosocomially in four New York City hospitals during overlapping time periods, indicating the presence of an extensive multiinstitutional outbreak.

Ribotyping is a specific example of RFLP analysis using conventional REA gels subjected to Southern blotting followed by hybridization. It uses ribosomal RNA (rRNA) probes to assess polymorphism in the chromosomal regions containing the rRNA genes (26). One advantage of using rRNA probes is that the genes encoding rRNA contain highly conserved sequences, allowing a probe derived from one species to be used to type all eubacteria. Ribotyping was used in a study by Demarta and colleagues to type strains of *Aeromonas* species isolated from stool of children with gastroenteritis, stool of asymptomatic household contacts, and household environmental fomites in an effort to understand better the determinants of symptomatic *Aeromonas* gastrointestinal disease (27). The *Aeromonas* ribotype found in those with gastroenteritis was identical to that found for *Aeromonas* isolated from asymptomatic household carriers and household environments, suggesting that predisposing factors of the host made individuals prone to symptomatic *Aeromonas* gastrointestinal disease. Despite the fact that ribotyping and RFLP analysis in general, as described previously, have been shown to be a useful typing tool for some organisms, it has been shown that clonally unrelated isolates may demonstrate identical patterns. In addition, the technique is relatively labor intensive and time consuming, and the appropriate restriction endonuclease must be determined for each species.

Pulsed field gel electrophoresis (PFGE) addresses some of these shortcomings (28). Chromosomal DNA is digested with low-frequency restriction endonucleases, creating large DNA fragments (as opposed to digestion with high-frequency restriction endonucleases, creating small fragments as in conventional REA). These large DNA fragments are then resolved with PFGE in which the electric fields are altered, enabling the resolution of large DNA molecules. In this way, patterns involving a limited number of relatively large fragments are created that can be easily identified and compared. PFGE is considered the typing method of choice for most bacterial species because of its typeability, reproducibility, discriminatory power, and ease of comparison among different fingerprints (12). A study by Passaro and associates (29) provides a good example of the use of PFGE as a typing tool complementing standard epidemiologic methodology in an investigation of an outbreak of nosocomial postoperative *Serratia marcescens* infections. This study revealed the source of the outbreak to be a contaminated jar of cream used by a scrub nurse who wore artificial nails. An example of PFGE patterns from this study is shown in Figure 1.2.

Comparative sequencing is an alternative typing method. Two different strategies have been used to provide genotyping data: multilocus sequence typing (MLST) and single-locus sequence typing. MLST compares sequence variation in numerous housekeeping gene targets, whereas single-locus sequence typing compares sequence variation of a single target only (30). MLST, as opposed to single-locus sequence typing, tends to be too labor intensive, time consuming, and costly to use in a clinical setting. In addition, for some subpopulations, genetic variability in the housekeeping targets is limited, and MLST has poor discriminatory power under these circumstances. Nonetheless, for some organisms, such as *S. aureus*, it has been validated as a typing method (31), the results of which have the advan-

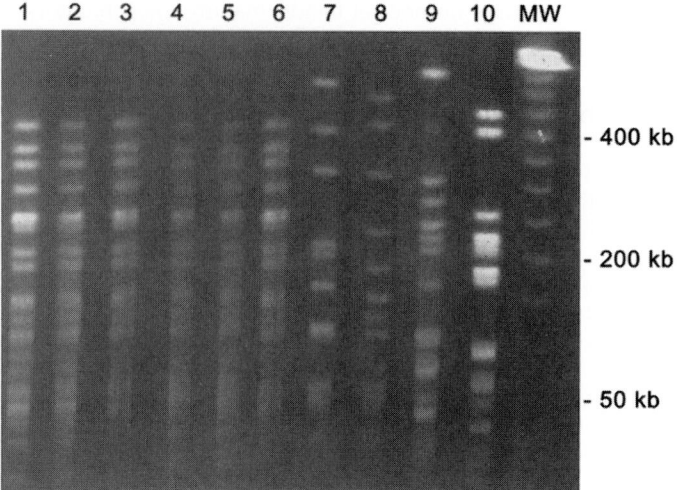

Figure 1.2. Pulsed field gel electrophoresis (PFGE) patterns of *Serratia marcescens* isolates (using chromosomal DNA digested with *Xba*I) obtained in an investigation of an outbreak of nosocomial postoperative *S. marcescens* infections. Lanes 1 through 5 represent isolates obtained from a sample of patients involved in the outbreak. Lane 6 represents the isolate obtained from a contaminated jar of cream that was implicated as being the source of the outbreak through epidemiologic investigation. Lanes 7 through 10 represent epidemiologically unrelated strains of *S. marcescens* included for comparison. The lane labeled MW represents a molecular weight marker (lambda ladder) with base-pair sizes as shown in kilobases. The identical PFGE patterns in lanes 1 through 6 confirm that a single clone of *S. marcescens* was responsible for the outbreak and that the source of the outbreak was likely the contaminated cream that was routinely used by a scrub nurse who wore artificial nails.

tage of being able to be readily compared between different laboratories and across different locations given the unambiguous nature of sequence data. Single-locus sequence typing has also been validated in *S. aureus* to be a useful typing method (30) and has the advantages of being a less costly and time-consuming typing method than MLST while maintaining the advantages of objectivity associated with the use of sequence data.

Amplified Nucleic Acid–Based Methods

POLYMERASE CHAIN REACTION
Polymerase chain reaction (PCR)–based methods have been applied broadly in infectious diseases epidemiology. They have been used to identify and strain type infectious agents. In addition, they have been used to detect biomarkers of pathogen virulence as well as host susceptibility and host response to infectious diseases. The essential feature of PCR is that it can rapidly and exponentially amplify target sequences of DNA that may be present in only very small amounts. It does so by completing multiple consecutive cycles of DNA sequencing (using oligonucleotide primers that flank the target DNA sequence, heat-stable DNA polymerase, and deoxynucleotides) followed by DNA denaturation (using heat) (12). Conventional PCR involves amplification of a single target specific to a pathogen using primers that flank the specific target DNA sequence. The presence or absence of amplified product can be detected by using gel electrophoresis followed by ethidium bromide staining and examination with ultraviolet light. Conventional PCR was used to identify exposure to human papillomavirus (HPV) in a case-control study designed to investigate the determinants of cervical intraepithelial neoplasia (CIN) (32). This study revealed

that the great majority of all grades of CIN can be attributed to HPV infection. Several variations of PCR based methods are also available.

RFLP analysis using a single amplified product subjected to endonuclease digestion (PCR-RFLP) has been applied in a number of situations. In this variant, the amplified product is digested with a frequently cutting restriction endonuclease, and the resultant fragments are separated by electrophoresis and examined with ultraviolet light after ethidium bromide staining (33). The size and number of fragments allows for strain typing. Hibberd and colleagues used PCR-RFLP to amplify the human mannose-binding lectin gene and find variants associated with an increased susceptibility to meningococcal disease (34).

A variant of ribotyping, called *PCR-ribotyping*, is similar to the above method (35). Primers specific for conserved regions of the 16S and 23S rRNA genes are used to amplify the 16S to 23S intergenic spacer regions of rRNA operons that are a potential source of polymorphisms. The products are then separated by electrophoresis and examined with ultraviolet light after ethidium bromide staining. Restriction digestion of the amplified product is not necessary but can be used to increase the number of fragments and improve the discriminatory power of this method. Neal and coworkers used this technique to investigate a cluster of neonatal cases with *S. marcescens* bacteremia (36). They were able to show that the cluster represented cases of pseudobacteremia associated with a contaminated blood glucose/lactate analyzer. A variant of PCR-ribotyping has been used to identify nonculturable pathogens (37,38). For example, the agent of Whipple's disease was identified by amplifying bacterial 16S rRNA genes directly from tissues of patients with Whipple's disease using PCR and primers flanking the 16S rRNA genes (38). The DNA sequence of the products was determined and analyzed for phylogenetic relatedness to other known organisms. In so doing, this bacterium was identified as a gram-positive actinomycete not closely related to any known genus. It was provisionally named *Tropheryma whippelii* (38) and, more recently, formally named *Tropheryma whipplei* (39).

Repetitive element PCR (rep-PCR), another variant of PCR, is based on the fact that many organisms contain specific DNA sequences that are repeated many times throughout their genome (40). In this technique, oligonucleotide primers complementary to these repeated elements are used to amplify intervening DNA. The PCR products are subjected to gel electrophoresis, ethidium bromide staining, and examination under ultraviolet light. Variations in the sizes of the amplified PCR products result from variations in the distance between repeated sequences, thereby allowing one to detect polymorphisms between clonally unrelated strains. Various repetitive sequences have been targeted in rep-PCR, including enterobacterial repetitive intergenic consensus sequences (ERIC), repetitive extragenic palindromic sequences, insertion sequences, and polymorphic guanine/cytosine-rich repetitive sequences (5). An example of an application of this method is a study by Davin-Regli and colleagues in which ERIC-PCR was used to rule out an environmental source related to a cluster of cases of infections due to *Aeromonas hydrophila* (41).

Arbitrarily primed PCR (AP-PCR), also known as randomly amplified polymeric DNA typing (RAPD), is another variation of PCR (42). In this technique, a short primer with an arbitrary sequence that is not directed at a specific DNA sequence is used in a low-stringency PCR that allows the primer to anneal to several nonspecific locations on the target DNA. If two such locations are within a few kilobases of each other and on opposite strands, then amplification can occur. In this way, a set of fragments is generated, and the number and size of the fragments provide the basis for strain typing. This method is relatively simple, rapid, and widely applicable. It also has the additional advantage that

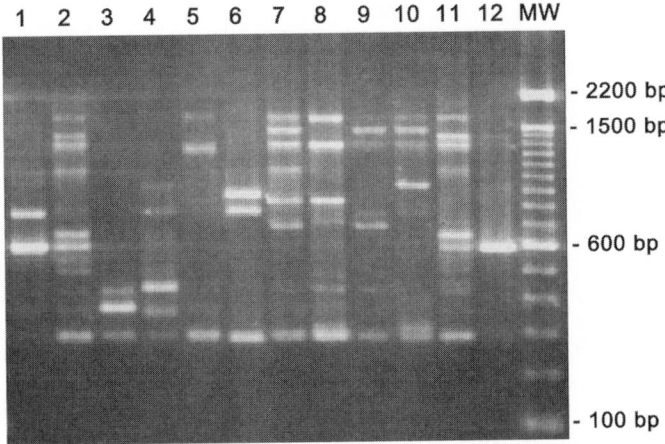

1 2 3 4 5 6 7 8 9 10 11 12 MW

- 2200 bp
- 1500 bp

- 600 bp

- 100 bp

Figure 1.3. Arbitrarily primed polymerase chain reaction (AP-PCR) patterns of a sample of clinical *Clostridium difficile* isolates investigated in a study designed to determine whether nosocomial transmission was responsible for an observed increase in the prevalence of hospitalized patients with *C. difficile*–associated diarrhea. Most of the AP-PCR patterns of the 173 isolates investigated in this study were unique, as illustrated in this figure. The authors concluded that a low frequency of nosocomial transmission was occurring. The lanes labeled MW represent a molecular weight marker (100 base-pair DNA ladder), with base-pair sizes as shown. (Adapted from Wullt M, Laurell MH. Low prevalence of nosocomial *Clostridium difficile* transmission, as determined by comparison of arbitrarily primed PCR and epidemiological data. *J Hosp Infect* 1999;43:269, with permission.)

no prior sequence information about the target is required. AP-PCR has been found to be a useful typing method for *Clostridium difficile* and is considered one of the typing methods of choice for this organism (12). Wullt and associates used this technique in an investigation designed to determine whether nosocomial transmission was responsible for an observed increase in the prevalence of hospitalized patients with *C. difficile*–associated diarrhea (43). Most of the AP-PCR patterns were unique, leading the authors to conclude that a low frequency of nosocomial transmission was occurring. Figure 1.3 shows a sample of these AP-PCR patterns.

Microarray (DNA Chip)–Based Methods

Microarrays, also known as DNA chips, are miniature devices containing libraries of polynucleotides robotically printed on solid supports in such a way that the identity of each polynucleotide is defined by its location. The potential applications of this technology include both expression and genomic profiling (44), helpful in the elucidation of pathogen virulence factors, host susceptibility factors, and host response factors as well as in the identification and typing of infectious agents. Although microarray technology is being used primarily in the setting of research laboratories, it is reasonable to expect that this technology will be standardized for clinical use in the future (45).

EXPRESSION PROFILING

Microarray-based technology can be used to analyze the expression levels of thousands of genes per single experiment, whether human genes or microbial genes, based on which genes have been transcribed to messenger RNA (mRNA) (46). For this application, microarrays are created using gene-specific polynucleotides of interest that are printed on solid supports. Total RNA, including mRNA, from both the test and a reference sample is fluorescently labeled using different fluorochromes for the test sample and the reference sample. The labeled RNA is then

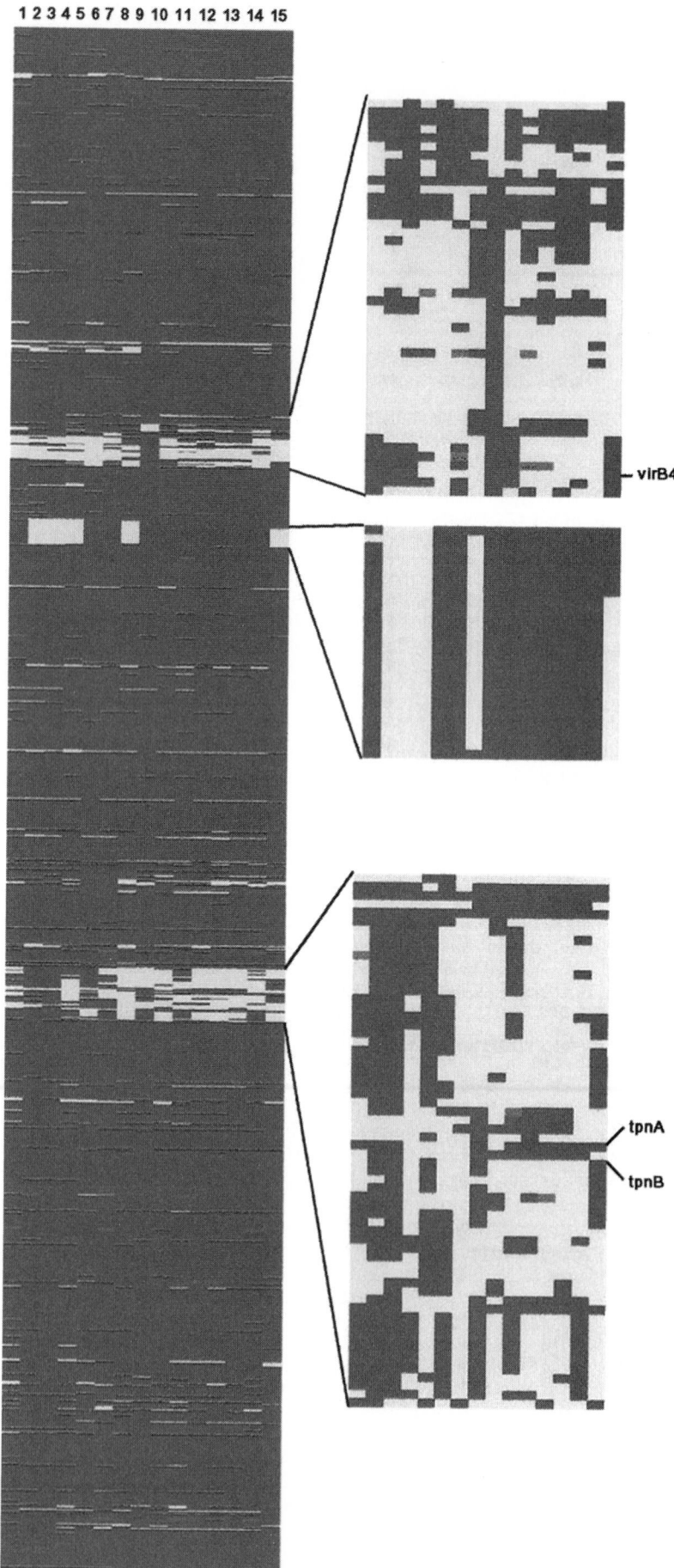

Figure 1.4. Computer-generated image summarizing the results of matrix-based comparative genomic hybridization (CGH) of 15 clinical *Helicobacter pylori* isolates compared with two reference strains. The presence (*dark gray*) or absence (*white*) of genes in the clinical isolates is displayed, with missing data shown in *light gray*. Each column represents one clinical isolate, and each row represents one gene. The identity of the genes is based on their position in the image, with the order of the genes representing that in the *H. pylori* chromosome. Zoomed images of two portions of the image where significant variability in the presence or absence of genes is displayed. The names of selected genes are indicated. Although this technology is currently being used primarily in the setting of research laboratories, it is reasonable to expect that this technology will be standardized for clinical use in the future with applications in infectious diseases epidemiology as described in the text. (Adapted from Salama N, Guillemin, K, McDaniel TK, et al. A whole-genome microarray reveals genetic diversity among *Helicobacter pylori* strains. *Proc Natl Acad Sci USA* 2000;97(26):14670, with permission. Copyright 2000, National Academy of Sciences, USA.)

fragmented, pooled, and allowed to hybridize under stringent conditions to the genes printed on the array. Laser excitation of the incorporated labeled RNA (referred to as *targets*) yields measurable characteristic emissions that can then be imported into software. This software produces a pseudocolored merged image summarizing the levels of expression of each gene for both the test and reference sample based on the measurable emissions. Intensity ratios are used to compare the level of expression of the test sample with that of the reference sample. With regard to the test sample, ratios of more than 1 are indicative of increased levels of gene expression, and ratios of less than 1 are indicative of decreased levels of gene expression relative to the reference sample. In this way, an expression profile can be obtained for a particular infectious agent or host. Coombes and colleagues used this technology to investigate altered gene expression in human endothelial cells in response to *Chlamydia pneumoniae* infections in an attempt to understand better the potential mechanisms of atherogenesis (47). In so doing, the authors defined potential biomarkers of *C. pneumoniae*–specific host response that may be able to be applied in epidemiologic investigations related to the determinants of coronary artery disease (47).

GENOMIC PROFILING

Microarray technology also allows for one to characterize genomic profiles. For example, in matrix-based comparative genomic hybridization (CGH), genomic DNA of interest, whether it is human or microbial, is compared with genomic DNA from a reference genome printed on a microarray. With respect to matrix-based CGH for microbes, the microarray contains gene-specific polynucleotides (with or without intergenic region-specific polynucleotides) representing the genetic sequence from one or more microbial reference strains. Fluorescently labeled whole genomic DNA from clinical isolates is fragmented, hybridized to the chip, and then detected in the same manner as described previously. Computer-generated pictorial summaries reflecting the presence of shared genes/genomic regions between the isolates of interest and the reference strains, as well as the absence of specific genes/genomic regions represented in the isolates of interest compared with the reference strains, are then produced based on the hybridization results. Compared with other nucleic acid–based methods, this technique provides a much more extensive and specific fingerprint of each strain and, in addition, can provide detailed information regarding potential virulence factors in infectious agents. Salama and coworkers used this technique to compare clinical isolates of *Helicobacter pylori* with two sequenced reference strains (48). Seventy-eight percent of the reference strain genes were common to all of the clinical isolates, whereas the remaining 22% were strain-specific genes, missing from at least one clinical strain. As expected, known virulence genes were present in all strains that were known to derive from patients with significant pathology. In addition, cluster analysis identified genes that were clustered with known virulence genes and that may thus represent potential virulence genes themselves. Figure 1.4 shows a computer-generated image summarizing these results. This methodology may ultimately be able to be applied in infectious diseases epidemiology as a means to investigate the determinants of infectious diseases specifically related to microarray-based biomarkers reflecting virulence factors. It may also be used as an extremely sensitive typing tool. Indeed, Kato-Maeda and associates have shown that array-based analysis of small-scale genomic deletions using CGH appears to be a suitable genotyping system for *M. tuberculosis* (49). In addition, epidemiologic studies using matrix-based CGH created with human genomic DNA and analyzed using DNA from persons with and without specific infectious diseases may serve as a useful tool to identify specific host susceptibility factors.

In addition to matrix-based CGH, sequence variation analysis can also be completed using microarray technology (50). Multiple different methods have been developed, and more methods are under intensive development. An example of an application of one of these methods is a study by Kozal and colleagues (51). Through the use of high-density oligonucleotide array sequencing of human immunodeficiency virus type 1 (HIV-1) protease genes, it was found that many of the amino acid changes that are known to contribute to drug resistance occur as natural polymorphisms in isolates from patients who had never received protease inhibitors. This technique may ultimately have other applications as a typing tool in infectious diseases epidemiologic investigations.

SUMMARY

It is clear that the molecular methods developed during the past few decades have proved to be exquisitely useful techniques that permit the examination of many previously unknown facets of the epidemiology of infectious diseases. These methods are extremely sensitive as diagnostic tools enhancing conventional diagnostic techniques and enabling the identification of unculturable pathogens and agents associated with chronic disease. They are exceptionally useful as typing tools aiding surveillance as well as the identification and investigation of outbreaks in addition to helping pinpoint the source and modes of transmission of infectious diseases in nonoutbreak settings. Molecular methods are also extremely useful in the identification and detection of molecular biomarkers reflecting host susceptibility and host response to infectious diseases as well as specific virulence factors associated with infectious agents. With the ongoing development of technology, and in particular with the expansion of applications of microarray technology, many more exciting and important discoveries will surely follow that will be able to be applied to the epidemiology of infectious diseases.

REFERENCES

1. Kilbourne E. The molecular epidemiology of influenza. *J Infectious Dis* 1973;127:478–487.
2. Handsfield H, Totten P, Fennel C, et al. Molecular epidemiology of *Haemophilus ducreyi* infections. *Ann Intern Med* 1981;95:315–318.
3. Oxford J. Biochemical techniques for the genetic and phenotypic analysis of viruses: "molecular epidemiology." *J Hygiene* 1985;94:1–7.
4. Higginson J. The role of the pathologist in environmental medicine and public health. *Am J Pathol* 1977;86:460–484.
5. Foxman B, Riley L. Molecular epidemiology: focus on Infection. *Am J Epidemiol* 2001;153:1135–1141.
6. *Encarta world English dictionary* [North American edition] [On-line]. Microsoft Corporation, 2001. Available: *dictionary.msn.com*
7. *A dictionary of epidemiology.* New York: Oxford University Press, 1995.
8. McMichael AJ. Molecular epidemiology: new pathway or new travelling companion? [Invited commentary]. *Am J Epidemiol* 1994;140:1–11.
9. Hunter DJ. The future of molecular epidemiology. *Int J Epidemiol* 1999;28:S1012–S1014.
10. Jarvis W. Usefulness of molecular epidemiology for outbreak investigations. *Infect Control Hospital Epidemiol* 1994;15:500–503.
11. Vegni F. What relevance do advances in molecular biology and genetics have for epidemiology? High tech needle and thread to sew the web of causation. *Ann Ig* 1997;9:273–279.
12. Tenover F, Arbeit R, Goering R. How to select and interpret molecular strain typing methods for epidemiological studies of bacterial infections: a review for healthcare epidemiologists. *Infect Control Hosp Epidemiol* 1997;18:426–439.
13. Struelens M. Consensus guidelines for appropriate use and evaluation of microbial epidemiologic typing systems. *Clin Microbiol Infect* 1996;2:2–11.
14. Tenover F, Arbeit R, Goering R, et al. Interpreting chromosomal DNA restriction patterns produced by pulsed-field gel electrophoresis: criteria for bacterial strain typing. *J Clin Microbiol* 1995;33:2233–2239.

15. Selander R, Caugant D, Ochman H, et al. Methods of multilocus enzyme electrophoresis for bacterial population genetics and systematics. *Appl Environ Microbiol* 1986;51:873–884.

16. Norton R, Roberts B, Freeman M, et al. Characterization and molecular typing of *Burkholderia pseudomallei*: are disease presentations of melioidosis clonally related? *FEMS Immunol Med Microbiol* 1998;20:37–44.

17. Burnie J, Matthews R. Immunoblot analysis: a new method for fingerprinting hospital pathogens. *J Immunol Methods* 1987;100:41–46.

18. Mulligan M, Kwok R, Citron D, et al. Immunoblots, antimicrobial resistance, and bacteriophage typing of oxacillin-resistant *Staphylococcus aureus*. *J Clin Microbiol* 1988;26:2395–2401.

19. Mayer L. Use of plasmid profiles in epidemiologic surveillance of disease outbreaks and in tracing the transmission of antibiotic resistance. *Clin Microbiol Rev* 1988;1:228–243.

20. Sexton D, Harrel L, Thorpe J, et al. A case-control study of nosocomial ampicillin-resistant enterococcal infection and colonization at a university hospital. *Infect Control Hosp Epidemiol* 1993;14:629–635.

21. Sader HS, Hollis RJ, Pfaller MA. The use of molecular techniques in the epidemiology and control of infectious diseases. *Contemp Issues Clin Microbiol* 1995;15:407–431.

22. Stout JE, Lu VL, Muraca P, et al. Potable water as a cause of sporadic cases of community-acquired legionnaires' disease. *N Engl J Mede* 1992;326.

23. Southern E. Detection of specific sequences among DNA fragments separated by gel electrophoresis. *J Mol Biol* 1975;98:503–517.

24. van Embden J, Cave M, Crawford J, et al. Strain identification of *Mycobacterium tuberculosis* by DNA fingerprinting: recommendations for a standardized methodology. *J Clin Microbiol* 1993;31:406–409.

25. Frieden TR, Sherman LF, Maw KL, et al. A multi-institutional outbreak of highly drug-resistant tuberculosis: epidemiology and clinical outcomes. *JAMA* 1996;276:1229–1235.

26. Stull T, LiPuma J, Edlind T. A broad-spectrum probe for molecular epidemiology of bacteria: ribosomal RNA. *J Infect Dis* 1988;157:280–286.

27. Demarta A, Tonolla M, Caminada A, et al. Epidemiological relationships between *Aeromonas* strains isolated from symptomatic children and household environments as determined by ribotyping. *Eur J Epidemiol* 2000;16:447–453.

28. Lai E, Birren B, Clark S, et al. Pulsed field gel electrophoresis. *Biotechniques* 1989;7:34–42.

29. Passaro DJ, Waring L, Armstrong R, et al. Postoperative *Serratia marcescens* wound infections traced to an out-of-hospital source. *J Infect Dis* 1997;175:992–995.

30. Shopsin B, Kreiswirth BN. Molecular epidemiology of methicillin-resistant *Staphylococcus aureus*. *Emerg Infect Dis* 2001;7:323–326.

31. Enright MC, Day NPJ, Davies CE, et al. Multilocus sequence typing for characterization of methicillin-resistant and methicillin-susceptible clones of *Staphylococcus aureus*. *J Clin Microbiol* 2000;38:1008–1015.

32. Schiffman M, Bauer H, Hoover R, et al. Epidemiologic evidence showing that human papillomavirus infection causes most cervical intraepithelial neoplasia. *J Natl Cancer Inst* 1993;85:958–964.

33. Olive D, Bean P. Principles and applications of methods for DNA-based typing of microbial organisms. *J Clin Microbiol* 1999;37:1661–1669.

34. Hibberd ML, Sumia M, Summerfiled JA, et al. Association of variants of the gene for mannose-binding lectin with susceptibility to meningococcal disease. *Lancet* 1999;353:1049–1053.

35. Kostman J, Alden M, Mair M, et al. A universal approach to bacterial molecular epidemiology by polymerase chain reaction ribotyping. *J Infect Dis* 1995;171:204–208.

36. Neal T, Corkill J, Bennett K, et al. *Serratia marcescens* pseudobacteraemia in neonates associated with a contaminated blood glucose/lactate analyzer confirmed by molecular typing. *J Hosp Infect* 1999;41:219–222.

37. Relman D, Loutit J, Schmidt T, et al. The agent of bacillary angiomatosis: an approach to the identification of uncultured pathogens. *N Engl J Med* 1990;323:1573–1580.

38. Relman D, Schmidt T, MacDermott R, et al. Identification of the uncultured bacillus of Whipple's disease. *N Engl J Med* 1992;327:293–301.

39. La Scola B, Fenollar F, Fournier P-E, et al. Description of *Tropheryma whipplei* gen. nov., sp. nov., the Whipple's disease bacillus. *Int J Syst Evolutionary Microbiol* 2001;51:1471–1479.

40. Versalovic J, Koeuth T, Lupski J. Distribution of repetitive DNA sequences in eubacteria and application to fingerprinting of bacterial genomes. *Nucleic Acids Res* 1991;19:6823–6831.

41. Davin-Regli A, Bollet C, Chamorey E, et al. A cluster of cases of infections due to *Aeromonas hydrophila* revealed by combined RAPD and ERIC-PCR. *J Med Microbiol* 1998;47:499–504.

42. Williams J, Kubelik A, Livak K, et al. DNA polymorphisms amplified by arbitrary primers are useful as genetic markers. *Nucleic Acids Res* 1990;18:6531–6535.

43. Wullt M, Laurell M. Low prevalence of nosocomial *Clostridium difficile* transmission, as determined by comparison of arbitrarily primed PCR and epidemiological data. *J Hosp Infect* 1999;43:265–273.

44. Wilgenbus KK, Lichter P. DNA chip technology *ante portas*. *J Mol Med* 1999;77:761–768.

45. Cummings C, Relman D. Using DNA microarrays to study host-microbe interactions. *Emerg Infect Dis* 2000;6:513–525.

46. Duggan DJ, Bittner M, Chen Y, et al. Expression profiling using cDNA microarrays. *Nat Genet* 1999;21:10–14.

47. Coombes B, Mahony J. cDNA array analysis of altered gene expression in human endothelial cells in response to *Chlamydia pneumoniae* infection. *Infect Immun* 2001;69:1420–1427.

48. Salama N, Guillemin K, McDaniel TK, et al. A whole-genome microarray reveals genetic diversity among *Helicobacter pylori* strains. *Proc Natl Acad Sci USA* 2000;97:14668–16873.

49. Kato-Maeda M, Rhee JT, Gingeras TR, et al. Comparing genomes within the species *Mycobacterium tuberculosis*. *Genome Res* 2001;11:547–554.

50. Tillib SV, Mirzabekov AD. Advances in the analysis of DNA sequence variations using oligonucleotide microchip technology. *Curr Opin Biotechnol* 2001;12:53–58.

51. Kozal M, Shah N, Shen N, et al. Extensive polymorphisms observed in HIV-1 clade B protease gene using high-density oligonucleotide arrays. *Nat Med* 1996;2:753–759.

Host Factors

CHAPTER 2
The Complement System

Jerry A. Winkelstein

Resistance to infection depends on the cooperative efforts of a number of different components of the immune system. One of these, the complement system, plays an important role in the defense against a wide variety of bacterial, viral, and fungal infections in both the nonimmune and immune host. This chapter summarizes current knowledge about the biochemistry and biology of the complement system, its significance in the host's defense against infection, and those clinical situations in which deficiencies of the complement system lead to an increased susceptibility to infection.

BIOCHEMISTRY OF COMPLEMENT

The complement system is composed of a series of plasma proteins and cellular receptors that are important mediators of host defense and inflammation (1). Most of the biologically significant effects of the complement system are mediated by the third component (C3) and the terminal components (C5-9). To subserve their protective and inflammatory functions, however, C3 and C5-9 must first be activated. At least two mechanisms exist by which they can be activated, the classical and alternative pathways (Fig. 2.1).

Activation of the classical pathway is usually initiated by antigen-antibody complexes (2). Antibodies of the appropriate immunoglobulin class (IgG and IgM) and subclass (IgG1, IgG2, and IgG3) bind to antigen and in doing so create an immune complex that in turn binds and activates the first component of complement (C1). The first component of complement is a macromolecular complex composed of three biochemically distinct subcomponents, C1q, C1r, and C1s. The binding of C1q to the Fc portion of immunoglobulin leads to the activation of C1r, which in turn activates C1s. Activated C1s possesses serine esterase activity and is able to cleave the fourth component of complement (C4) into a high-molecular-weight fragment (C4b) and a low-molecular-weight fragment (C4a). The reaction continues with the activation of C2 by C1s. The cleavage of C2 results in the liberation of a small peptide (C2b). The larger fragment,

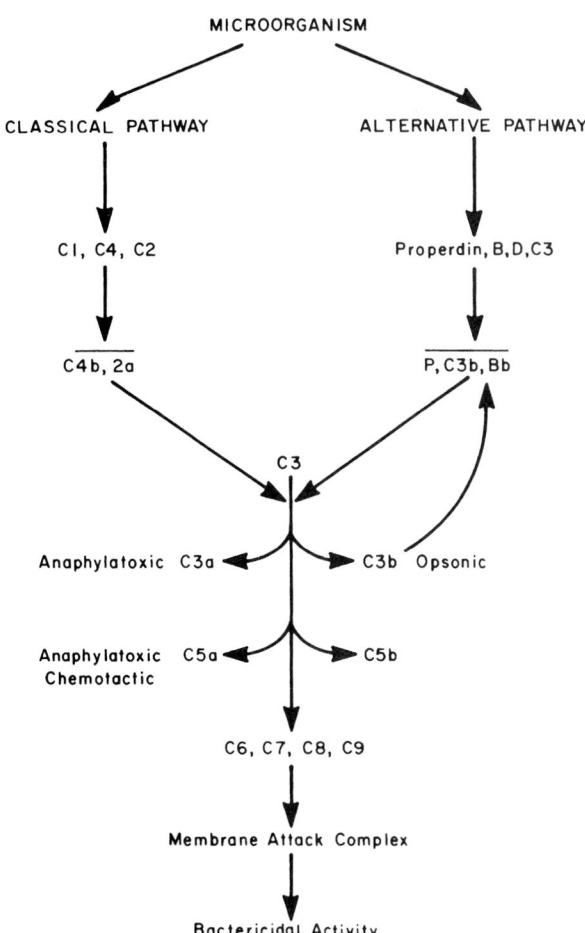

Figure 2.1. The complement system in humans. Microorganisms can activate C3 and the terminal components (C5-9) by either the classical pathway or the alternative pathway. Activation of C3 and the terminal components generates a variety of biologically significant activities important in the host's defense against infection. (From Oski FA, De Angeles C, Feigen R, et al. *Principles and practice of pediatrics*. Philadelphia: JB Lippincott, 1990:837, with permission.)

C2a, then combines with C4b to form a bimolecular enzyme, C4b,2a, which is responsible for activating C3 and assembling C5-9 into the membrane attack complex.

Activation of the alternative pathway begins with the C3 molecule (3). Native C3 contains an internal thiolester. Under normal conditions, there is continuous low-grade hydrolysis of this thiolester to create a molecule [C3(H$_2$O)] that can bind native factor B and allow its cleavage by factor D. Two cleavage products of factor B are generated, a larger product (Bb) and a smaller product (Ba). The association of the hydrolyzed C3 with Bb then creates a C3-cleaving enzyme [C3(H$_2$O),Bb] termed the *priming C3 convertase*, which is responsible for the continuous, low-grade cleavage of C3 and, hence, the generation of nascent C3b. If the nascent C3b binds to a suitable surface, it forms a reversible complex with native factor B, which is then cleaved by factor D to create a highly efficient C3-cleaving enzyme (C3b,Bb), termed the *amplification C3 convertase*. Properdin stabilizes the binding of Bb to C3b, thereby retarding its intrinsic decay.

Whether C3 is activated by the classical or alternative pathway, the C3 is cleaved, generating two fragments of unequal size, C3a and C3b. The smaller fragment, C3a, is released into the fluid phase, where it acts as an anaphylatoxin (see later). The larger fragment, C3b, binds to the surface of cells such as bacte-

ria, where it is able to act as an opsonin (see later) or combine with either of the two C3-cleaving enzymes to create two new enzymes, the alternative pathway (C3b$_2$,Bb) and classical pathway (C4b,2a,3b) C5-cleaving enzymes.

Activation of C5 by either the alternative or the classical pathway C5-cleaving enzymes creates a smaller fragment, C5a, and a larger fragment, C5b. The smaller cleavage product, C5a, is released into the fluid phase, where it possesses anaphylatoxic and chemotactic activity (see later). If C5b combines with native C6 while it is still attached to the C5-cleaving enzymes, it is stabilized and can initiate formation of the membrane attack complex, a multimolecular assembly of C5b, C6, C7, C8, and C9 that is capable of inserting into cell membranes and thereby expressing cytolytic activity (4).

If the activation of the classical or alternative pathway were to proceed in an uncontrolled fashion, this would result in the generation of excessive amounts of the phlogistic fragments of complement, which in turn could cause widespread immunopathological damage to the host. Fortunately, a number of mechanisms act to control the assembly and expression of both the classical and alternative pathway C3-cleaving enzymes. Each of these C3-cleaving enzymes is relatively labile and rapidly undergoes intrinsic decay under physiological conditions. In addition, a number of control proteins inhibit the classical pathway (C1 esterase inhibitor, C4-binding protein, factor I, and decay-accelerating factor) and the alternative pathway (factor H, factor I). Thus, in the usual situation, the activation of C3 and C5-9 proceeds in a controlled fashion and is limited to the immediate vicinity of the initiating substance (e.g., microbial surface or immune complex).

Activation of the classical pathway is usually initiated by antigen-antibody complexes and is therefore considered to be especially important in acquired immunity. However, some enveloped RNA viruses, some *Mycoplasma* species, and certain strains and species of both gram-negative and gram-positive bacteria can bind C1q directly and activate the classical pathway without a requirement for antibody. Activation of the alternative pathway does not usually require the participation of antibody; thus, it is generally viewed as an important mechanism of natural immunity. However, antibody can participate functionally in the activation of the alternative pathway by a variety of particles, such as bacteria and virus-infected cells. Thus, under some circumstances, the classical pathway may function in "natural" immunity, and the alternative pathway may participate in "acquired" immunity (5).

BIOLOGIC CONSEQUENCES OF COMPLEMENT ACTIVATION

Whether C3 and C5-9 are activated by the classical or alternative pathway, they generate a wide variety of biologically significant activities that are important in the host's defense against infection.

The smaller cleavage products of C3 and C5, C3a and C5a, are potent anaphylatoxins (6). They were originally identified through their ability to cause histamine release from basophils and mast cells, promote smooth muscle contraction, and increase vascular permeability. Additional functions of these peptides have been identified and include the ability to aggregate platelets and leukocytes, causing the production and release of arachidonic acid metabolites from them, and the ability to induce neutrophils to produce toxic oxygen metabolites and discharge their granular enzymes (7).

In addition to its anaphylatoxic activities, C5a is a potent chemotactic factor causing the directed movement of polymorphonuclear leukocytes and monocytes toward a focus of microbial invasion (8).

The larger cleavage product of C3, C3b, acts as a potent opsonin when it is fixed to the surface of a microorganism (9). It appears that C3b subserves different opsonic functions, depending on the nature of the phagocytic cell and its state of activation (10). In the case of neutrophils and nonactivated macrophages, C3b promotes attachment of the particle, whereas IgG acts to favor ingestion. In the case of activated macrophages, C3b serves to aid in both attachment and ingestion.

The generation of efficient complement-mediated serum bactericidal activity requires the participation of the entire terminal complement sequence, C5b-9 (11). Only gram-negative bacteria can be killed by complement. The site of action of C5-9 appears to be the outer, lipid membrane of gram-negative organisms.

ROLE OF COMPLEMENT IN HOST DEFENSE

A number of studies have established the biologic significance of the complement system in the host's defense against infection and have also provided valuable insight into the mechanisms by which the complement system exerts its protective effects. Studies in experimental animals have shown that the complement system plays an important role in resistance to a variety of bacteria, viruses, and fungi. For example, animals that have been pharmacologically depleted of C3 or are genetically deficient in C4, C3, or C5 are markedly more susceptible than normal animals to challenge with pneumococcus (12), staphylococcus (13), *Haemophilus influenzae* (14), rabies virus (15), Sindbis virus (16), influenza A virus (17), and *Candida* species (18), to mention just a few.

Other studies have addressed the mechanisms by which the complement system exerts its protective effect. For example, one such study has shown that C3b is responsible for a major portion of serum opsonic activity *in vivo* (12), and another has shown that C5a plays a critical role in the initial migration of polymorphonuclear leukocytes to a focus of invading microorganisms (19).

Finally, the complement system also appears to play an important defensive role in a number of different locations in the body. Not only is complement important in the clearance of microorganisms from the bloodstream (20), but it can also be shown to play an important role in local resistance to pneumonia (21), meningitis (14), and soft tissue infections (13).

PRIMARY COMPLEMENT DEFICIENCY DISEASES

Although most of the genetically determined complement deficiencies are inherited as autosomal recessive disorders, one of them, properdin deficiency, is inherited as an X-linked recessive disorder (Table 2.1), and another, C1 esterase inhibitor deficiency, is inherited as an autosomal dominant disorder. Most patients with genetically determined deficiencies of individual complement components present with an increased susceptibility to infection, rheumatic diseases, or angioedema (22,23). The kinds of infections seen in complement-deficient patients relate to the biologic functions of the missing component. Thus, patients with a deficiency of C3, or with a deficiency of a component in either of the two pathways necessary for the activation of C3, usually have an increased susceptibility to infections caused by bacteria for which C3b-dependent opsonization is an important host defense (e.g., *Streptococcus pneumoniae* and *H. influenzae*). In contrast, patients with deficiencies of C5-9 have normal resistance to the pneumococcus and *H. influenzae* because C3b-mediated opsonization is intact, but they are unusually susceptible to infection with *Neisseria meningitidis* because they lack C5-9–mediated serum bactericidal activity, an important host defense against this organism.

Complement deficiency diseases are more common among patients with certain infectious diseases. For example, a number of studies have shown that about 5% to 15% of patients with systemic meningococcal infections have a genetically determined deficiency of a terminal component (24–26). The prevalence of complement deficiencies appears to be particularly high in patients with infections caused by "uncommon" serogroups (e.g., X, Y, and W135) (27), in patients with meningococcemia caused by unencapsulated organisms (28), in patients with a positive family history of systemic meningococcal infections (29), and in patients with recurrences (26,29). Although patients with complement deficiencies have an increased susceptibility to infection and are more likely to have recurrent infections, if their infections are recognized early, they can usually be treated successfully.

C1q Deficiency

There are two forms of C1q deficiency: one in which C1q cannot be detected by either functional or immunochemical analysis, and another in which immunochemical C1q is present but lacks functional activity (22,23,30). The most common clinical presentation of either form of C1q deficiency has been a lupus-like syndrome. Some patients have also had an increased

	TABLE 2.1. Genetically Determined Complement Deficiencies	
Deficiency	**Inheritance**	**Major clinical manifestations**
C1q	Autosomal recessive	Rheumatic disorders and systemic bacterial infections
C1r/C1s	Autosomal recessive	Rheumatic disorders
C4	Autosomal recessive	Rheumatic disorders and systemic bacterial infections
C2	Autosomal recessive	Rheumatic disorders and systemic bacterial infections
C3	Autosomal recessive	Rheumatic disorders and systemic bacterial infections
C5	Autosomal recessive	Meningococcal sepsis and meningitis
C6	Autosomal recessive	Meningococcal sepsis and meningitis
C7	Autosomal recessive	Meningococcal sepsis and meningitis
C8	Autosomal recessive	Meningococcal sepsis and meningitis
C9	Autosomal recessive	Meningococcal sepsis and meningitis
Factor H	Autosomal recessive	Hemolytic-uremic syndrome
Factor I	Autosomal recessive	Systemic bacterial infections
Properdin	X-linked recessive	Meningococcal sepsis and meningitis

susceptibility to infection as manifested by bacterial sepsis or meningitis.

C1r/C1s Deficiency

Genetically determined deficiencies of C1r are characterized by a marked reduction of C1r (less than 1% of normal) and a moderate reduction of C1s (20% to 50% of normal) (22,23,30). The clinical presentation of C1r/C1s deficiency has included both a lupus-like illness and glomerulonephritis; to this date, an increased susceptibility to infection has not been prominent.

C4 Deficiency

Two loci within the major histocompatibility complex encode for C4, termed C4A and C4B. Patients with total C4 deficiency are homozygous for a double-null C4 haplotype and have severely depressed serum levels of both antigenic and functional C4 (less than 1%) (22,23,31). The predominant clinical manifestation of C4 deficiency has been a systemic lupus erythematosus–like illness, although some patients with C4 deficiency have presented with an increased susceptibility to infection.

Homozygous deficiencies of either C4A or C4B are relatively common, occurring in 1% and 3% of individuals, respectively (31). Although the products of the two loci share some functional, structural, and antigenic characteristics that identify them as C4, they nevertheless differ slightly. For example, C4B possesses about four times the functional activity that C4A does. Studies have shown that homozygous C4B-deficient children have an increased susceptibility to bacteremia or meningitis, presumably because they have to rely on the less functional C4A isotype for the activation of C3 and C5-9 (32).

C2 Deficiency

A deficiency of C2 is the most common of the inherited complement deficiencies (33). The frequency of the gene for C2 deficiency has been estimated between 0.5% and 1% (34), with homozygous deficient individuals occurring as frequently as 1 per 10,000 (33). The clinical manifestations of C2 deficiency have varied. Although some individuals are asymptomatic, most are clinically affected, with an increased susceptibility to infection, rheumatic diseases, or both (22,23). For the most part, the infections have been blood borne and systemic (e.g., sepsis, meningitis, arthritis, and osteomyelitis) and caused by encapsulated bacteria (e.g., pneumococcus, *H. influenzae*). A variety of rheumatic diseases have also been seen in association with C2 deficiency. The most common of these has been a disorder that resembles systemic lupus erythematosus, but glomerulonephritis, dermatomyositis, anaphylactoid purpura, and vasculitis have also been seen.

C3 Deficiency

Patients with C3 deficiency generally have less than 1% of the normal amount of C3 in their serum (22,23,35). Those serum activities directly dependent on C3, or indirectly dependent on C3 because of its role in the activation of C5-9, are markedly reduced. Thus, serum opsonic, chemotactic, and bactericidal activities are either absent or markedly diminished in patients with C3 deficiency. The clinical manifestations of C3 deficiency have included an increased susceptibility to infection and rheumatic disorders (22,23,35). Patients with C3 deficiency have had a variety of infections caused by encapsulated bacteria, including pneumonia,

bacteremia, meningitis, and osteomyelitis. A number of patients have also presented with a clinical picture consistent with systemic lupus erythematosus or membranoproliferative glomerulonephritis.

C5 Deficiency

The sera of patients with C5 deficiency have markedly reduced levels of C5 and are therefore unable to generate normal chemotactic or bactericidal activity (22,23,36). Like patients with deficiencies of the other terminal components, patients with C5 deficiency have usually presented with systemic meningococcal infections.

C6 Deficiency

The only abnormality relating to the complement system in C6-deficient patients is a marked deficiency of serum bactericidal activity (22,23,37). The major clinical manifestation of C6 deficiency has been systemic neisserial infections. Whereas most patients have had meningococcal sepsis and meningitis, a few have had disseminated gonococcal infections.

C7 Deficiency

Only a few patients with C7 deficiency have been identified, and as expected, serum bactericidal activity has been markedly reduced in those patients in whom it has been tested (22,23,38). As with the other deficiencies of terminal components, patients with C7 deficiency have had systemic meningococcal infections or disseminated gonococcal infections.

C8 Deficiency

Native C8 is composed of three chains (α, β, and γ). The α chain and γ chain are covalently linked to form one subunit (C8 α-γ), which is joined by noncovalent bonds to the other subunit composed of the β chain (C8 β). In one form of C8 deficiency, patients lack the C8 α-γ subunit; in the other, the C8-β subunit is deficient (22,23,39). In either case, C8 activity is markedly reduced (less than 1% of normal). The only functional defect in C8-deficient sera is a marked reduction in bactericidal activity. The clinical presentation of C8 deficiency has consisted of systemic meningococcal infections, but systemic lupus erythematosus has also rarely been seen.

C9 Deficiency

Although genetically determined C9 deficiency is rare in the West, it is the most common complement deficiency in Japan (22,23,40). Serum bactericidal activity can be generated by C5b-8 without a requirement for C9, although the rate of killing is significantly reduced. Nevertheless, evidence suggests that patients with C9 deficiency, like patients with deficiencies of the other terminal components, have an increased susceptibility to meningococcal sepsis and meningitis (41).

Factor I Deficiency

Patients with factor I deficiency have uncontrolled activation of C3 by the alternative pathway because, in the absence of factor I, there is no control imposed on the formation and expression of the alternative pathway C3 convertase (42–44). Therefore, they have a secondary consumption of C3 resulting in markedly reduced levels of native C3 in the serum. As expected, those serum activities that depend on C3, either directly or indirectly, such as opsonic, chemotactic, and bactericidal activity, are reduced in patients with factor I deficiency. The most common clinical expression of factor I deficiency is an increased susceptibility to infection (22–23). As with primary C3 deficiency, the organisms most commonly responsible for these infections have been encapsulated bacteria, organisms for which C3 is an important opsonic ligand.

Properdin Deficiency

Properdin deficiency is inherited in an X-linked recessive pattern (22,23) and exists in three different forms. In one form, properdin is undetectable in the serum of affected males (45,46). In a second form, serum properdin is reduced but detectable (47). In a third form, properdin is present in normal amounts but lacks function (48). To this date, the only clinical manifestation of properdin deficiency has been systemic meningococcal infections.

SECONDARY COMPLEMENT DEFICIENCIES

A number of clinical conditions exist in which the complement system is secondarily affected. In some of these, the secondary defect in complement function may be responsible, at least in part, for an increased susceptibility to infection.

The Newborn Infant

Newborn infants are unusually susceptible to a variety of infections. A number of defects in host defense have been identified in these infants, each of which has the potential to contribute to their increased susceptibility to infection (49). Among these, defects in two complement-mediated functions, serum opsonizing and chemotactic activities, have been described (49). The levels of most components of complement are mildly to moderately decreased in full-term infants, averaging between 50% and 80% of adult levels (50). The levels in premature infants are more markedly reduced; in general, the more premature the infant, the more the given component is decreased relative to adult levels. Although the levels of individual components are only moderately reduced in newborns, it is likely that they contribute to the newborn's susceptibility to infection because nearly all components are reduced, and therefore the functional integrity of the complete cascade is impaired (51).

Sickle Cell Disease

Patients with sickle cell disease have an increased susceptibility to bacterial sepsis and meningitis, particularly due to pneumococcus (52). In one study, the risk for acquiring pneumococcal meningitis in children with sickle cell disease was 300 to 500 times that in children without sickle cell disease (53). Children with sickle cell disease have two immunological defects that could contribute to their susceptibility to pneumococcus: functional or anatomic asplenia (54) and decreased serum opsonizing activity (55,56). A number of studies have shown that the decrease in serum opsonizing activity in sickle cell disease is secondary to a functionally significant defect in the alternative pathway (56–58), but the basis for that defect is unclear. It is likely that the decrease in complement-mediated serum opsonizing activity contributes to the increased susceptibility to infection seen in sickle cell disease because these patients have a higher risk for sepsis and meningitis than could be accounted for by splenectomy alone.

C3 Nephritic Factor

Some individuals develop significant and sustained hypocomplementemia that is due to an autoantibody aimed at the alternative pathway C3-cleaving enzyme C3b,Bb (59,60). The autoantibody, termed C3 nephritic factor (C3NeF), binds to the convertase and prolongs its half-life. This, in turn, leads to the persistent activation and consumption of C3 and results in markedly reduced levels of native C3. Nephritic factor was first identified in patients with glomerulonephritis (61) and partial lipodystrophy (62). Subsequently, at least two patients with C3NeF have been identified who have had sepsis and meningitis presumably secondary to their marked decrease in serum C3 levels (63,64).

Burn Patients

Patients with burns typically have many problems with bacterial infections. In one series, more than 50% of deaths in burn-injured patients were related to sepsis (65). A number of studies have shown that components of the complement system are reduced in burn patients in the days immediately after injury (66,67); apparently, the alternative pathway is affected to a greater degree than the classical pathway (67). The decrease in function of the alternative pathway leads to decreased levels of serum opsonic and chemotactic activities (68,69), which in turn could contribute to the marked susceptibility to infection seen in these patients.

LABORATORY ASSESSMENT OF THE COMPLEMENT SYSTEM

Genetically determined deficiencies of the classical activating pathway (C1, C4, and C2), of C3, and of the terminal components (C5, C6, C7, C8, and C9) can be detected by use of antibody-sensitized sheep erythrocytes in a total serum hemolytic complement (CH_{50}) assay. The lysis of sensitized erythrocytes can occur in the absence of C9, although it occurs at a lower rate and to a lesser extent than in the presence of C9. Therefore, a severe deficiency of any of the first eight components leads to a marked reduction in total hemolytic complement activity; a deficiency of C9 results in a CH_{50} that is one third to one half the lower limit of normal.

Deficiencies of factor H, factor I, and properdin can be detected by a hemolytic assay that assesses lysis of rabbit erythrocytes because rabbit erythrocytes are potent activators of the alternative pathway. Obviously, the serum of patients with deficiencies of C3 or C5-9 will also be abnormal when it is tested in the rabbit erythrocyte assay because the lysis of rabbit erythrocytes depends on these components as well as on components of the alternative activating pathway.

The identification of the specific component that is deficient usually rests on both functional and immunochemical tests. In most cases, functional and immunochemical assessment of the specific component shows the deficiency. There are some exceptions, however. For example, one form of C1q deficiency is characterized by dysfunctional proteins that can be detected by immunochemical assays but are markedly reduced in functional activity.

REFERENCES

1. Frank MM. The complement system in host defense and inflammation. *Rev Infect Dis* 1979;1:483.
2. Porter RR, Reid KBM. The biochemistry of complement. *Nature* 1978;275:699.
3. Fearon DT. Activation of the alternative complement pathway. *Crit Rev Immunol* 1979;1:1.

4. Mayer MM, Michaels DW, Ramm LE, et al. Membrane damage by complement. *Crit Rev Immunol* 1981;22:133.

5. Winkelstein JA. Complement and natural immunity. *Clin Immunol Allergy* 1983;3:421.

6. Hugh TE. The structural basis for anaphylatoxin and chemotactic functions of C3a, C4a, and C5a. *Crit Rev Immunol* 1981;22:321.

7. Vogt W. Anaphylatoxins: possible roles in diseases. *Complement* 1986;3:177.

8. Synderman R, Goeta EJ. Molecular and cellular mechanisms of leukocyte chemotaxis. *Science* 1981;213:830.

9. Hostetter MK, Gordon DL. Biochemistry of C3 and related thiolester proteins in infection and inflammation. *Rev Infect Dis* 1987;9:97.

10. Griffin FM. Opsonizations, phagocytosis, and intracellular killing in the complement system. In: Rother K, Till GO, eds. *The complement system.* Springer-Verlag, Berlin, 1988:395–418.

11. Joiner KA. Studies on the mechanism of bacterial resistance to complement-mediated killing and on the mechanisms of action of bactericidal antibody. *Curr Top Microbiol Immunol* 1985;121:99.

12. Winkelstein JA, Smith MR. Shin HS. The role of C3 as an opsonin in the early stages of infection. *Proc Soc Exp Biol Med* 1975;149:397.

13. Easmon CSF, Glynn AA. Comparison of subcutaneous and intraperitoneal staphylococcal infections in normal and complement deficient mice. *Infect Immun* 1976;13:399.

14. Crosson FJ Jr, Winkelstein JA, Moxon ER. Participation of complement in the nonimmune host defense against experimental *Haemophilus influenzae* type b septicemia and meningitis. *Infect Immun* 1976;14:882.

15. Miller A, Morse HC, Winkelstein JA, et al. The role of antibody in recovery from experimental rabies. *J Immunol* 1978;121:321.

16. Hirsch RL, Griffin DE, Winkelstein JA. The effect of complement depletion on the course of Sindbis virus infection in mice. *J Immunol* 1978;121:1276.

17. Hicks JT, Ennis FA, Kim E, et al. The importance of an intact complement pathway in recovery from a primary viral infection: influenza in decomplemented and C5-deficient mice. *J Immunol* 1978;121:1437.

18. Gelfand JA, Hurley DL, Fauci AS, et al. Role of complement in host defense against experimental candidiasis. *J Infect Dis* 1978;138:9.

19. Snyderman R, Phillips JK, Merganhagen SE. Biological activity of complement in vivo: role of C5 in the accumulation of polymorphonuclear leukocytes in inflammatory exudates. *J Exp Med* 1971;134:1131.

20. Hosea SW, Brown EJ, Frank MM. The critical role of complement in experimental pneumococcal sepsis. *J Infect Dis* 1980;142:903.

21. Bakker-Wondenberg IAJM, DeJong-Hoenderop JYT, Michel MF. Efficacy of antimicrobial therapy in experimental pneumococcal pneumonia: effects of impaired phagocytosis. *Infect Immun* 1979;25:366.

22. Ross SC, Densen P. Complement deficiency states and infections: epidemiology, pathogenesis and consequences of neisserial and other infections in an immune deficiency. *Medicine* (Baltimore) 1984;63:243.

23. Figueroa JE, Densen P. Infectious diseases associated with complement deficiencies. *Clin Microbiol Rev* 1991;4:359.

24. Ellison RT, Kohler PH, Curd JG, et al. Prevalence of congenital or acquired complement deficiency in patients with sporadic meningococcal disease. *N Engl J Med* 1983;308:913.

25. Leggiardo RJ, Winkelstein JA. Prevalence of complement deficiencies in children with systemic meningococcal infections. *Pediatr Infect Dis* 1987;6:75.

26. Memo J, Rodriguez-Valverde V, Lamelas JA, et al. Prevalence of deficits of complement components in patients with recurrent meningococcal disease. *J Infect Dis* 1983;148:331.

27. Fijen CAP, Kuijper EJ, Hannema AJ, et al. Complement deficiencies in patients over ten years old with meningococcal disease due to uncommon serogroups. *Lancet* 1989;2:585.

28. Hummel DS, Mocca LF, Frasch CE, et al. Meningitis caused by an unencapsulated strain of *Neisseria meningitidis* in twin infants with C6 deficiency. *J Infect Dis* 1987;155:815.

29. Nielsen HE, Koch C, Magnussen P, et al. Complement deficiencies in selected groups of patients with meningococcal disease. *Scand J Infect Dis* 1989;21:389.

30. Loos M, Heinz HP. Hereditary and acquired complement deficiencies in animals and man: the first component. *Prog Allergy* 1986;39:212.

31. Hauptmann G, Tappeiner G, Schifferli JA. Inherited deficiency of the fourth component of complement. *Immunodeficiency Rev* 1988;1:3.

32. Rowe PC, McLean RH, Wood RA, et al. Association of homozygous C4B deficiency with bacterial meningitis. *J Infect Dis* 1989;160:448.

33. Ruddy S. Hereditary and acquired complement deficiencies in animals and man: the second component. *Prog Allergy* 1986;39:267.

34. Sullivan KE, Petri M, Schmeckpeper B, et al. The prevalence of a mutation that causes C2 deficiency in SLE. *J Rheumatol* 1994;21:6.

35. Singer L, Colten HR, Wetsel RA. Complement C3 deficiency: human, animal, and experimental models. *Pathobiology* 1994;62:14.

36. McCarty GA, Snyderman R. Hereditary and acquired complement deficiencies in animals and man: the fifth component. *Prog Allergy* 1986;39:272.

37. Rother V. Hereditary and acquired complement deficiencies in animals and man: the sixth component. *Prog Allergy* 1986;39:283.

38. Zeitz HJ, Lint TF, Gewurz A, et al. Hereditary and acquired complement deficiencies in animals and man: the seventh component. *Prog Allergy* 1986;39:289.

39. Tedesco F. Hereditary and acquired complement deficiencies in animals and man: the eighth component. *Prog Allergy* 1986;39:295.

40. Lint TF, Gewurz H. Hereditary and acquired complement deficiencies in animals and man: the ninth component. *Prog Allergy* 1986;39:307.

41. Nagata M, Hara T, Aoki T, et al. Inherited deficiency of the ninth component, of complement: an increased risk of meningococcal meningitis. *J Pediatr* 1989;114:260.

42. Abramson N, Alper CA, Lachmann PJ, et al. Deficiency of C3 inactivator in man. *J Immunol* 1971;107:19.

43. Thompson RA, Lachmann PJ. A second case of human C3b inhibitor (KAF) deficiency. *Clin Exp Immunol* 1977;27:23.

44. Barrett DJ, Boyle MDP. Restoration of complement function in vivo by plasma infusion in factor I deficiency. *J Pediatr* 1984;104:76.

45. Sjoholm AG, Braconier JH, Soderstrom C. Properdin deficiency in a family with fulminant meningococcal infections. *Clin Exp Immunol* 1982;50:291.

46. Densen P. Weiler JM, Griffiss IM, et al. Familial properdin deficiency and fatal meninigococcemia: correction of the bactericidal defect by vaccination. *N Engl J Med* 1987;316:922.

47. Sjoholm AG, Soderstrom C, Nilsonn LA. A second variant of properdin deficiency: the detection of properdin at low concentrations in affected males. *Complement Inflamm* 1988;5:130.

48. Sjoholm AG, Kuijper EJ, Tijssen CC, et al. Dysfunctional properdin in a Dutch family with meningococcal disease: *N Engl J Med* 1988;319:33.

49. Miller ME. Host defenses in the human neonate. *Pediatr Clin North Am* 1977;24:413.

50. Johnston RB Jr, Altenburger KM, Atkinson AW Jr, et al. Complement in the newborn infant. *Pediatrics* 1979;64:S781.

51. Winkelstein JA, Kurlandsky LE, Swift AJ. Defective activation of the third component of complement in the sera of newborn infants. *Pediatr Res* 1979;13:1093.

52. Barrett-Connor E. Bacterial infection and sickle cell anemia. *Medicine* (Baltimore) 1971;50:97.

53. Robinson MG, Watson RI. Pneumococcal meningitis in sickle cell anemia. *N Engl J Med* 1966;274:1006.

54. Pearson HA, Spencer RP, Cornelius EA. Functional asplenia in sickle cell anemia. *N Engl J Med* 1969;281:923.

55. Winkelstein JA, Drachman RH. Deficiency of pneumococcal serum opsonizing activity in sickle-cell disease. *N Engl J Med* 1968;279:459.

56. Johnston RB Jr, Newman SL, Struth AG. An abnormality of the alternative pathway of complement activation in sickle cell disease. *N Engl J Med* 1973;288:803.

57. Wilson WA, Thomas EJ, Sissons JEP. Complement activation in asymptomatic patients with sickle cell anemia. *Clin Exp Immunol* 1979;36:130.

58. Koethe SM, Casper JT, Rodney GE. Alternative complement pathway activity in sera from patients with sickle cell disease. *Clin Exp Immunol* 1976;23:56.

59. Daka MR, Fearon DT, Austen KF. C3 nephritic factor: stabilization of fluid phase and, cell bound alternative pathway convertase. *J Immunol* 1976;116:1.

60. Davis AE III, Arnaout MA, Alper CA, et al. Transfer of C3 nephritic factor from mother to fetus: is C3 nephritic factor IgG? *N Engl J Med* 1977;297:144.

61. Spitzer RE, Vallota EH, Forrestal J, et al. Serum C3 lytic system in patients with glomerulonephritis. *Science* 1969;164:436.

62. Sissons JGP, West KJ, Fallows J, et al. Complement abnormalities in lipodystrophy. *N Engl J Med* 1976;294:461.

63. Edwards KM, Alford R, Gemurz H, et al. Recurrent bacterial infections associated with C3 nephritic factor and hypocomplementemia. *N Engl J Med* 1983;308:1138.

64. Thompson RA, Yap PL, Brettle RB, et al. Meningococcal meningitis associated with persistent hypocomplementemia due to circulating nephritic factor. *Clin Exp Immunol* 1983;52:153.

65. Sevitt S. A review of the complications of burns: their origin and importance for illness and death. *J Trauma* 1979;19:358.

66. Bjornson AB, Altemeier WA, Bjornson HS. Complement, opsonins and the immune response to bacterial infection in. burned patients. *Ann Surg* 1980;191:323.

67. Gelfand JA, Donelan M, Burke JF. Preferential activation and depletion of the alternative pathway by burn injury. *Ann Surg* 1983;198:58.

68. Bjornson AB, Alexander JW. Alterations of serum opsonins in patients with severe thermal injury. *J Lab Clin Med* 1974;83:372.

69. Nathenson G, Miller ME, Myers KA, et al. Decreased opsonic and chemotactic activities in sera of postburn patients and partial opsonic restoration with properdin and properdin convertase. *Clin Immunol Immunopathol* 1978;9:269.

CHAPTER 3
Phagocytes: Normal and Abnormal Neutrophil Host Defenses

Mark S. Klempner and Harry L. Malech

ANATOMY

Polymorphonuclear neutrophils (PMNs) are 5 μm in diameter with a distinctive multilobed nucleus and many small granules (1,2) (Fig. 3.1). Neutrophils exit the circulation at sites of inflammation by protruding between endothelial cells (diapedesis), demonstrating ameboid movement and pleomorphic changes in shape during migration in the extravascular tissue. The most distinctive morphologic feature of the mature neutrophil is the multilobed nucleus, typically appearing as two to four distinct lobes connected by thin strands of chromatin. This pattern appears late in myeloid differentiation. With stress or infection, immature neutrophils released from the marrow pool may have nuclei that lack distinct nuclear lobes, instead appearing bandlike, sometimes with a midpoint constriction. These immature neutrophils are often called bands because of the shape of the nucleus. The presence of increased numbers of band forms in the circulating blood (greater than 1% to 2% of the neutrophil count) classically has been thought to be a useful indicator of increased flux of neutrophils from the marrow pool independent of the absolute neutrophil count, and a reliable indicator of infection or other inflammatory process when leukocytosis and fever are absent. Recently the clinical utility of the band count has been called into question relative to other measures of inflammation and infection such as C-reactive protein or measures of inflammatory cytokines (3). Compared with fully mature neutrophils, bands may be less capable of performing functions essential to host defense against microorganisms (4).

Excessive segmentation of the neutrophil nucleus (five or more lobes) may be a manifestation of folate or vitamin B_{12} deficiency. The Pelger-Huët anomaly is an infrequent (1:5,000) autosomal dominant benign inherited trait resulting in neutrophils with distinctive bilobed nuclei that must be distinguished from band forms. This results from mutations in the lamin B receptor (chromosome 1q41-43); and in its very rare homozygous form, neutrophil nuclei are ovoid and the affected homozygotes display varying degrees of developmental delay, epilepsy and skeletal abnormalities (5). Pseudo-Pelger-Huët cells have also been seen as a rare side effect of drugs such as mycophenolate mofetil and ganciclovir, as well as in association with some leukemias and myelodysplastic syndromes. The normal physiologic role for the multilobed nucleus of neutrophils is unknown, but it may allow greater deformation of neutrophils during migration into tissues to sites of inflammation.

Neutrophils contain many small granules at the limit of resolution by light microscopy. Classic descriptions of the granules of neutrophils define two types (6,7). Azurophil (primary) granules are lysosome-like; contain acid hydrolases and many proteases; and are associated with a large number of cationic microbicidal proteins. Some of these such as defensins and bactericidal/permeability increasing (BPI) protein not only exhibit potent antimicrobial properties, but in recombinant form the whole molecule or fragments have the potential to be developed as pharmaceutical agents (8). Azurophil granules are peroxidase-positive, containing a large amount of myeloper-

oxidase (MPO), and are produced mainly at the promyelocyte stage of neutrophil differentiation (Fig. 3.2). Specific (secondary) granules are produced primarily at the myelocyte-metamyelocyte stage of neutrophil differentiation and are three times more numerous than azurophil granules in the mature neutrophil. Neutrophil-specific granules may actually be a group of morphologically similar, but functionally distinct granules which contain distinctive components such as lactoferrin, vitamin B_{12} binding protein, and matrix metalloproteinases (MMP) of which the most prominent is gelatinase B (also known as MMP9) (9). Gelatinase B may play an important role in the tissue damage associated with inflammation, but also may be essential in wound healing. The specific granule membrane appears to contain many integral membrane proteins also found in the plasma membrane, including formylpeptide chemotactic receptors, the CD18 family of integrin adhesion receptors plus adhesion receptors for a number of connective tissue elements. Of note is that even the cytochrome *b*-558 component of the respiratory burst oxidase, which had classically been thought to be a plasma membrane component, is actually sequestered in intracellular vesicles that may be co-incident with a subset of the diverse group in the specific granule compartment (10). Many stimuli cause degranulation of specific granules, a process that results in fusion of specific granule membranes with both the plasma membrane and the forming phagosome. Some of these tissue-degradation enzymes from both specific granules and azurophil granules are also released extracellularly where they may be necessary for neutrophil migration into tissues and the positive features of inflammation and wound healing, but may also result in pathologic tissue damage when release of such enzymes is uncontrolled.

The cytoplasm of unstimulated blood neutrophils contains large amounts of glycogen particles that are visible by electron microscopy. The predominant cellular energy source of neutrophils is anaerobic glycolysis, and stimulated neutrophils at sites of inflammation deplete these glycogen stores. Neutrophils

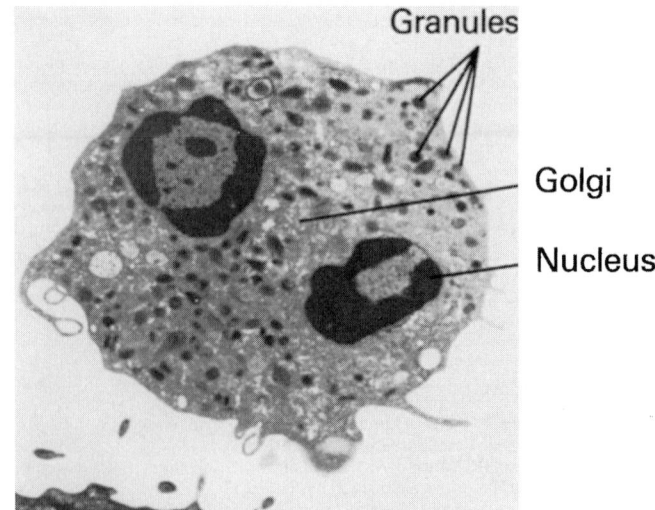

Figure 3.1. Electron micrograph of a human peripheral blood neutrophil. Two lobes of the segmented nucleus and many cytoplasmic granules are the most prominent features of this cell. Without specific staining for peroxidase, it is not possible to accurately distinguish the azurophil granules. However, the specific granules tend to be smaller and less electron dense than the azurophil granules. A portion of the Golgi membranes is evident as vesicular structures near the center of this cell. Just discernible is the grainy appearance of the cytoplasm, representing glycogen particles. (10,000×)

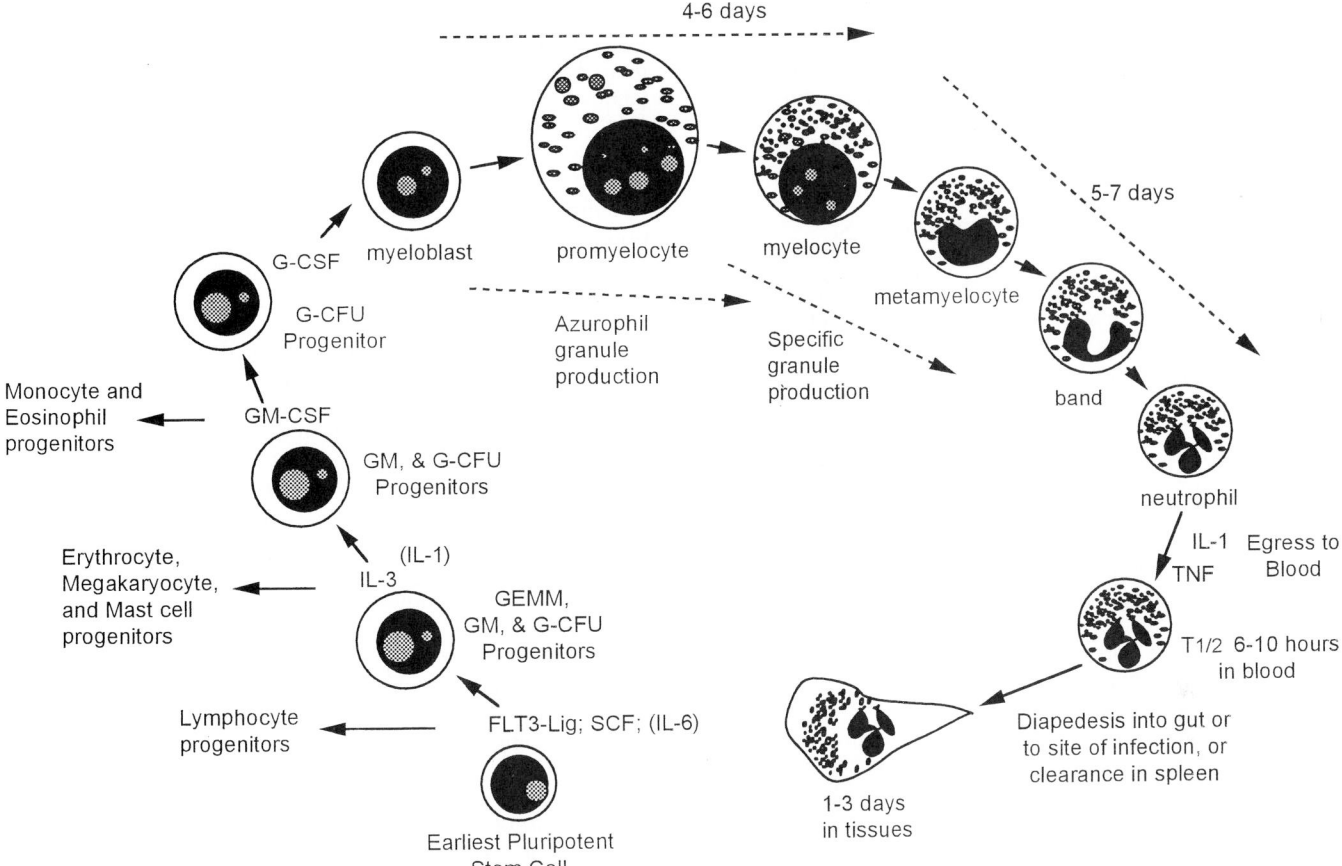

Figure 3.2. The production, differentiation, and distribution of neutrophils. FLT3 ligand, stem cell factor, and possibly interleukin-6 (IL-6), growth factors produced by marrow stroma cells, probably act synergistically to support proliferation of primitive pluripotent stem cells. IL-3, possibly synergistically augmented by IL-1 and other later acting factors, enhances proliferation at a slightly later stage. Granulocyte-macrophage colony-stimulating factor (GM-CSF) appears to act only on monomyeloid precursors; granulocyte colony-stimulating factor (G-CSF) influences neutrophil precursors only. Both GM-CSF and G-CSF are also produced at sites of inflammation and can augment host defense functions of mature neutrophils. In addition, G-CSF and possibly GM-CSF appears to enhance the life span of mature neutrophils, possibly by delaying progression to apoptosis. G-CSF and GM-CSF have a proven role in the treatment of neutropenias or to enhance marrow recovery after transplantation or chemotherapy. Preliminary reports of several studies indicate that G-CSF and GM-CSF may also eventually find a place as useful therapeutic agents to enhance neutrophil host defense function in the setting of severe infections in the elderly or others with impaired host defense, even when neutropenia and compromised marrow function are not factors. By the myeloblast stage of neutrophil differentiation, cells under the influence of G-CSF enter the committed differentiation phase of development. Azurophil and specific granules are synthesized at the stages indicted by the *arrows* above the relevant labels. The overlap of two arrows indicates an overlap in the later stages of azurophil granule production and the earliest stage of specific granule production. When neutrophils are fully mature, they may remain in the marrow for a few days, but these cells are released early under the influence of IL-1 and tumor necrosis factor and possibly other factors in the setting of infections. Neutrophil half-time in the blood is 6 to 10 hours, followed by egress from the blood to the gut or to sites of infection. Neutrophil senescence is an apoptotic process with clearing by the spleen from the blood or by macrophages at other tissue sites. GEMM, Granulocyte-erythrocyte-macrophage-megakaryocyte.

contain few mitochondria. Neutrophils contain relatively few ribosomes but are capable of protein synthesis. Protein synthesis by neutrophils has increasingly been shown to play a more important role in the inflammatory process than was formerly appreciated (11). A variety of interleukins and chemokines are produced by neutrophils in response to infection or other inflammatory stimuli (12–14). In particular, it has been shown that neutrophils not only release stores of pre-synthesized interleukin-8 (IL-8), but that in response to a variety of stimuli are capable of de novo synthesis of very large amounts of IL-8 (15). Because this is a potent chemotactic factor for neutrophils, this is likely an important autologous positive feedback loop to augment neutrophil migration to a site of infection. Further-

more, the final phase of the neutrophil's life cycle involves progression to apoptosis as will be discussed further below. This involves activation of genes encoding proteins important for the apoptotic pathway (16). A prominent Golgi apparatus is present in neutrophils and may be important for recycling of membrane components and processing of newly synthesized proteins. A pair of centrioles with associated microtubule organizing centers is usually found near the Golgi apparatus (17). In resting neutrophils, scant cytoskeletal elements are seen by electron microscopy, but in response to chemoattractants, there is an increase in cortical microfilaments containing F-actin and an increased number and length of microtubules extending radially from the microtubule organizing centers (17). Microfilaments generate the contractile forces responsible for cell motility including migration and phagocytosis (18,19). Microtubules are important for maintaining a stereotypic polarized internal organization of cellular organelles during neutrophil migration and probably play a role in movements of vesicular components (17,20).

GRANULOPOIESIS AND DISTRIBUTION

Myeloid precursors constitute the majority of cells in bone marrow. Neutrophil precursors are distributed in a reticular pattern; most immature forms are found near the bony spicules, and more mature forms are found nearest sinusoids. Neutrophils mature from myeloblasts to mature neutrophils in approximately 10 days, although this can be accelerated by infection or by administration of marrow growth factors such as granulocyte colony-stimulating factor (G-CSF) (21,22). Morphologically mature neutrophils reside in the marrow pool for several additional days before release into the circulation. This marrow pool exceeds the number of neutrophils in the circulation by several-fold. Although G-CSF, IL-1, tumor necrosis factor, and perhaps other inflammatory response cytokines enhance release of both morphologically mature and immature marrow pool neutrophils, the mechanisms controlling release of neutrophils from the marrow in the normal uninfected host have not been firmly established. There is some indirect evidence that chemokine receptor CXCR4, which binds to and mediates chemotaxis toward SDF-1 (CXCL12), produced by marrow stromal cells, could play a role in maintaining immature neutrophils in the marrow, in that G-CSF can inhibit expression of CXCR4 on neutrophils and a specific inhibitor of CXCR4 can stimulate a rapid release of neutrophils from the bone marrow (23,24). However, control of physiology affecting the kinetics and pathway of the last stages of the maturation process of neutrophils in the marrow is likely affected differently by a range of stimuli. For example, marrow pool neutrophils released to the circulation in response to bacterial infection may differ in the expression of some surface markers compared with neutrophils released spontaneously in the normal host. These antigenically immature neutrophils and band forms that are released from the marrow in response to infection or stress appear to be functionally less capable than are mature neutrophils (4).

The normal adult bone marrow produces about 100 billion neutrophils daily. Whereas senescent neutrophils that do not enter the tissues undergo apoptosis and are probably cleared through ingestion by macrophages in the spleen, large numbers of neutrophils migrate into the alimentary tract, providing surveillance protection in the mouth and gut against bacteria breaching the mucosal barrier. Marrow production may be increased to 1 trillion neutrophils per day during serious infection. The normal half-life of circulating neutrophils is 6 to 10 hours and may be shortened to less than 1 hour in severe infection. With ongoing infection, neutrophil precursors mature more rapidly, leading to cells with distinctive characteristics (21,22). Toxic granulation can be seen, corresponding to the presence of an increased number of large primary granules. Döhle bodies consisting of retained ribosome-rich endoplasmic reticulum can also be seen (1).

ACTIVATION OF NEUTROPHILS: SIGNAL TRANSDUCTION PATHWAYS

PMNs circulate in a metabolically quiescent state. Their basal expression of membrane receptors, oxidase components and other markers is considerably less than that seen in activated cells. When neutrophils encounter opsonized microorganisms, products derived from microorganisms, or any of a variety of chemotactic or chemokine molecules released at sites of infection, injury or chronic inflammation, the neutrophil rapidly becomes activated. The cellular changes are so rapid and so profound that the neutrophil has served as one of the prototypic cells used to define the signal transduction pathways common to activation of many cell types. These changes with activation involve the display of additional receptors from internal vesicular stores, whose activation then results in further changes to neutrophils in a stepwise fashion (25).

There has been such an explosion of knowledge about signal transduction pathways in neutrophils that it is not possible in this short section to delineate each of the pathways in detail. At the risk of vast oversimplification of a very complex system, the signal cascades which start at the plasma membrane with receptor binding to a soluble or particulate ligand can be divided either into those signal cascades that start from the group of receptors that signal through the proximate activation of heterotrimeric G-proteins or into those signal cascades that start from a very heterogenous group of receptors that signal through the proximate activation of a tyrosine kinase. The heterotrimeric G-protein activating group includes the receptors for chemotactic factors and chemokines that share the common structural feature of possessing seven transmembrane helix domains, common physiologic regulatory mechanisms and shared features of their intracellular signaling cascade that will be described in this section (26–28). However, the latter group includes a rather diverse group of receptors that defy common structural characterization and include, but are not limited to, the receptors for the Fc domain of immunoglobulins (29–31), the integrin adhesion molecules (32–34), the receptors for growth hormones such as G-CSF and granulocyte-macrophage colony-stimulating factor (GM-CSF) (35–38), receptors for immune hormones such as interferon gamma and tumor necrosis factor alpha (37,39), as well as the receptors for non-chemokine interleukins (38,40). One can now also add to this latter group expression of a number of the toll-like receptors (TLR), which mediate responses to a variety of products of microorganisms (e.g. TLR4 which mediates responses to bacterial lipopolysaccharides or TLR2 which mediates responses to peptidoglycan, and lipoarabinomannan) (35,41). While some receptors from this group (Fc receptors for example) actively trigger such effecter functions as degranulation and activation of the phagocyte oxidase associated with the chemoattractant/chemokine receptor group, the role of others may serve to regulate apoptosis (G-CSF or GM-CSF inhibit apoptosis), to increase display of Fc receptors (interferon gamma), or to increase the subsequent response to chemotactic/chemokine stimuli (TLRs), or to mediate specialized functions such as adherence (integrins). The functions and signal cascades associated with some of these will be discussed in later sections.

Some important non-chemokine chemoattractant receptors found on neutrophils (28,42,43) include receptors for formylmethionyl peptides (products of bacterial protein synthesis), C5a (a byproduct of complement fixation on the surface of microorganisms [opsonization]), as well as leukotriene B4 and platelet-activating factor (which both stimulate neutrophils and are produced by neutrophils at sites of inflammation, providing positive feedback). In general these receptors mediate motility and chemotaxis at lower concentrations of ligand, and extensive degranulation and to a variable degree, activation of oxidase activity at higher concentrations of ligand. Neutrophil responses to the chemoattractant chemokine, IL-8 (CXCL8), mediated by the receptors with high and low affinity for IL-8 (CXCR1 and CXCR2) found on human neutrophils deserve particular note because of the preponderant role played by this chemokine in a process of recruitment of neutrophils to sites of infection and inflammation, a process that includes a strong positive feedback mediated by exuberant production of IL-8 from neutrophils (13–15,44).

Some generalizations can be made about physiology, regulation, and signal transduction cascade associated with the seven transmembrane helix group of chemoattractant and chemokine receptors. As noted above, all interact with any of a variety of heterotrimeric G-proteins (guanosine triphosphate [GTP] binding proteins consisting of a heterogeneous group of alpha, beta and gamma subunits) of the Gi class, where the activated subunit components of the G-protein mediate the next level of the signal cascade. The activation signal from the ligand-receptor complex is limited in time by the triggering of a negative feedback loop involving inactivating kinases that can be specific for each receptor and that phosphorylate the intracellular C-terminal portion of the receptor resulting in binding to proteins called arrestins (45). This specificity is such that the receptor down-regulation following high level ligand exposure is in general limited to a specific receptor, leaving the neutrophil still capable of subsequent response to another ligand. This facilitates stepwise activation of neutrophils as different ligands are encountered during migration to a site of infection or inflammation. The negative-feedback inactivation of a receptor is associated with a decrease in receptor-ligand affinity and with internalization of the receptor-ligand complex into endosomes. Following processing that can involve passage into either a lysosomal compartment or through the Golgi apparatus, receptors may be either degraded or returned to the cell surface where they can be activated again (46).

It is important to note that the metabolic events involved in signal transduction of neutrophils are transient, lasting no more than a few minutes. Equally important is that signals may be asymmetric because of a concentration gradient of ligand. There is some evidence to suggest that the neutrophil magnifies the effects of a ligand concentration gradient by asymmetric amplification of signaling cascades (47). Thus, it is important to appreciate that it is not possible to understand how the signaling cascades to be described below translate into chemotactic responses, for example, without appreciating that there are both temporal transients and asymmetric spatial components to these responses (48). As noted previously, termination of the activation cascade is as important to these temporal and spatial transients as the activation phase. These details are still being defined.

As noted previously, the heterotrimeric G proteins serve as important transducers for ligand-receptor coupling to activation of effector enzymes or ion channels. Important proximal events transduced by the activated G-protein subunits are up-regulation of the activity of phosphoinositide 3-kinase (PI3K) gamma and delta, with activation of phospholipase C (PLC) beta. PI3K mediates synthesis of phosphatidylinositol (3,4,5) triphosphate (PIP3) in the plasma membrane, which itself has signaling properties and also is acted upon by PLC to produce inositol 1,4,5-trisphosphate and diacylglycerol (49,50). These two important secondary products mediate a bifurcating, but interacting metabolic cascade that ultimately activates PMN effecter responses. Diacylglycerol activates protein kinase C delta, which is translocated from the cytosol to the plasma membrane, where it phosphorylates proteins critical to functional responses (51). Phospholipase D1 is also activated as part of this signaling cascade and this enzyme acting on phosphocholine in the plasma membrane becomes the major source of phosphatidic acid which is an important second messenger that intensifies the signals that lead to degranulation and activation of the phagocyte oxidase (52,53). Further metabolism of phospha-

tidic acid to diacylglycerol results in phospholipase D indirectly also being responsible for secondarily for the bulk of production of the diacylglycerol second messenger (54). The inositol 1,4,5-trisphosphate that is formed by the action of phospholipase C leads to an increase in the cytosolic calcium concentration through interaction with specialized intracellular vesicular compartments where calcium is sequestered (55). Positive feedback loops possibly relating to conversion of inositol 1,4,5-trisphosphate to 1,3,4,5-tetrakisphosphate may trigger calcium channels in the plasma membrane to open transiently, facilitating a pulsed flow of additional ionized calcium into the cytosol from the extracellular milieu (56). Calcium binding proteins have been discovered, such as calmodulin or calpain, that serve the roles of detection of the ionized calcium spike and transducing this signal into triggers for actin polymerization associated with locomotion, remodeling of plasma membrane, fusion of granule membranes with the plasma membrane or the forming phagosome, and other events associated with the effecter functions of neutrophils (57,58). While beyond the scope of this short review, a variety of small GTPases including the *rho* sub-family of the *ras* superfamily of regulatory proteins (e.g. *rho, rac*1, *rac*2 and *cdc*42) and *arf* proteins, as well as a variety of tyrosine kinases including the p38 MAP kinase cascade, activation of NF-kappaB, ERK activation of cytoplasmic phospholipase A2 (an important source of arachidonate) all play a part in facilitating neutrophil effecter functions (40,59,60).

ADHERENCE

To get to extravascular sites of infection or inflammation, neutrophils must exit the circulation. Then neutrophils must adhere to extracellular matrix components and at sites of infection must adhere to and phagocytose opsonized microorganisms. The development of monoclonal antibodies directed at a vast array of cell surface epitopes on neutrophils, endothelial cells, platelets and other cells has led to the identification and classification of an equally vast array of groupings of structurally related cell surface molecules mediating adhesion of neutrophils at sites of inflammation and infection (61,62). In many cases the adhesion proteins come in pairs with specific affinity of one member of the pair to the other member mediating adhesion of one type of cell to another or even to specific sites on a cell (for example there are specific receptors on neutrophils that mediate adhesion to the junctional areas between two post-capillary venule endothelial cells) (63,64). In some cases, both members of an adhesion receptor protein pair are found on neutrophils and mediate homotypic adhesion (neutrophils sticking to other neutrophils in the post-capillary venule at a site of infection). In some cases, there is promiscuity with respect to the targets to which a particular adhesion molecule can bind. Furthermore, for some adhesion proteins the binding affinity may be lectin-like in that the other member of the "pair" is a simple or complex carbohydrate moiety that may be found on a large array of proteins (65,66). As with the signaling cascades described above for the chemoattractant/chemokine receptors, a full understanding of the function of neutrophil adhesion molecules must take into account both temporal changes and spatial asymmetries. Not only can adhesion molecules on neutrophils and their adhesion pair targets be distributed asymmetrically, but both the numbers and affinity of adhesion molecules may change. Neutrophils must not only adhere, they must also let go to traverse the endothelium and migrate to sites of infection. Depending on the specific adhesion molecule, these changes may involve increased surface expression from intracellular stores with cellular activation (e.g., as occurs with the CD11b/CD18 integrin), cleavage from the cell surface (e.g., as occurs with L-selectins) or internalization. Adhesion molecules may also be induced to increase or decrease adhesion affinity; events that may involve phosphorylation or dephosphorylation associated with conformational changes in the adhesion molecule (67–69). Table 3.1 lists those adhesion molecules most important for egress of neutrophils from the circulation to sites of infection or inflammation. The importance of these adherence molecules for neutrophil host defense function is emphasized by the frequent, severe infections that occur in patients with inherited defects in adhesion molecules (70–73) (see footnote to Table 3.1). Not included in Table 3.1 are receptors for a variety of other ligands important for adherence to and ingestion of microorganisms (e.g., immunoglobulin Fc receptors or fibronectin receptors).

The current model of the mechanism of neutrophil egress from the circulations still posits the three-step process originally proposed by Springer (61,62) in which neutrophils initially form labile, transient interactions with endothelial cells mediated by selectin binding to sialyl Lewis mucins and encounter higher concentrations of chemoattractants that "activate" integrins, followed by the firm adherence provided by activated integrin binding to the intercellular adhesion molecule members of the immunoglobulin superfamily. This firm adherence allows the neutrophil to stop, spread on the endothelial cell's surface, and then migrate between endothelial cells into the extravascular space. This process of neutrophil egress occurs in the postcapillary venule. This general scheme has been refined as more adhesion molecules have been discovered (69) and as it has been appreciated that specialized adhesion molecules mediate specific parts of this process such as the transit between endothelial cell junctions (63,64).

To understand this process, it is useful to know about the properties of four groups of surface molecules mediating this process. The selectin family of adhesion molecules has an N-terminal domain related to the calcium-dependent lectins that is extended from the cell surface by a variable number of repeating domains with homology to the epidermal growth factor repeat domain. L-selectin is present on neutrophils; P-selectin and E-selectin are found on endothelial cells. The ligand or counterreceptors to which selectins bind are sialyl mucins. Whereas selectins are lectin-like molecules targeting the sialyl Lewis x or sialyl Lewis a carbohydrate moieties, there appears to be some selectivity for specific carbohydrate-rich mucins. For example, P-selectin has selectivity for the P-selectin glycoprotein ligand on the neutrophil surface (65,66,72,73). Selectin-mucin interactions tether the neutrophil to the activated endothelial cell surface, but shear forces of blood flow are capable of breaking these bonds. This results in a slowing of neutrophil passage through the venule as the neutrophil alternately sticks briefly to the endothelium and rolls along it (69).

This rolling with slowed passage through the venule allows more time for chemoattractant factors diffusing from sites of inflammation to interact with specific receptors and activate the neutrophil. This activation results in changes in an $\alpha_1\beta_2$ integrin family of neutrophil adhesion receptors (61,67–69). As indicated in Table 3.1, the three integrin molecules found on neutrophils are heterodimers in which the α-subunit is unique to each integrin (CD11a, CD11b, or CD11c) but the β-subunit is a 95-kDa glycopeptide (CD18) shared by all three integrins. Because these receptors were initially identified by their function, by their size, or by the monoclonal antibody used to identify them, different names in the literature actually refer to the same molecule as indicated in Table 3.1 (62,74). Thus, CD11b/CD18 or complement receptor type 3 (CR3) is the membrane receptor for the opsonic complement fragment iC3b and is a dimer of the 95-kDa common β-chain linked to an α-chain of 185 kDa; CD11a/CD18 or lymphocyte function-associated antigen-1 contains an α-chain of 190 kDa; and the α-chain of CD11c/CD18 or p150,95 is 150

TABLE 3.1. Neutrophil Adhesion Molecules[a]

Neutrophil receptor	Ligand	Function
L-selectin	Sialyl Lewis sulfate-rich mucins	Labile leukocyte-endothelial adhesion mediating rolling
P-selectin glycoprotein ligand (PSGL-1)	P-selectin	Labile leukocyte-endothelial adhesion mediating rolling
Sialyl Lewis x mucins	E-selectin	Early firm leukocyte-endothelial adhesion mediating tethering
CD11a/CD18 (LFA-1)	ICAM-1 (CD54), ICAM-2 (CD102), ICAM-3	Firm but reversible leukocyte-endothelial and leukocyte-leukocyte adhesion
CD11b/CD18 (Mac-1, CR3)	ICAM-1 iC3b, fibrinogen, factor X	Firm but reversible leukocyte-endothelial and leukocyte-leukocyte adhesion; complement binding; phagocytosis
CD11c/CD18 (p150,95)	iC3b, fibrinogen	Complement binding; phagocytosis
ICAM-1	LFA-1, Mac-1	Homotypic reversible neutrophil aggregation
PECAM-1	ICAM-1, PECAM-1	Migration through endothelium and basement membrane

CR3, Complement receptor type 3; ICAM, intercellular adhesion molecule; LFA-1, lymphocyte function-associated antigen-1; Mac-1, heterodimer of the CD11/CD18 complex.
[a]Selectins are lectins mediating early events ("rolling") in neutrophil-endothelial cell interactions. L-selectin is shed from leukocytes during the detachment phase. The ligands are receptors for neutrophil surface adhesion molecules found on endothelial cells (P-selectin and E-selectin, ICAMs, sialyl Lewis), neutrophils (LFA-1, Mac-1), or opsonized microorganisms (iC3b) or at sites of inflammation. LFA-1, Mac-1, and p150,95 are $\alpha_1\beta_2$ integrins mediating firm cell-cell attachments. Enhanced adhesion and then later de-adhesion result from regulatable conformational changes in the integrin molecules. This mediates arrest of rolling with firm attachment to endothelium at a site of inflammation followed by transendothelial migration. ICAMs are members of the immunoglobulin superfamily. ICAM-1 is found on neutrophils and can interact with LFA-1 or MAC-1 on neutrophils to mediate homotypic adhesion (neutrophil aggregation), which serves to pile up a plug of neutrophils attached to endothelium in the postcapillary venule at sites of inflammation. Leukocyte adhesion deficiency type 1 (LAD-1) results from genetic defects in the CD18 gene leading to lack of leukocyte integrin (or in rare instances abnormal integrin function) and impaired transendothelial egress associated with recurrent infections. LAD-2, reported in only a few kindreds, may result from abnormalities of fucose metabolism leading to failure to produce the E-selectin and P-selectin ligands, resulting in clinical features similar to LAD-1.

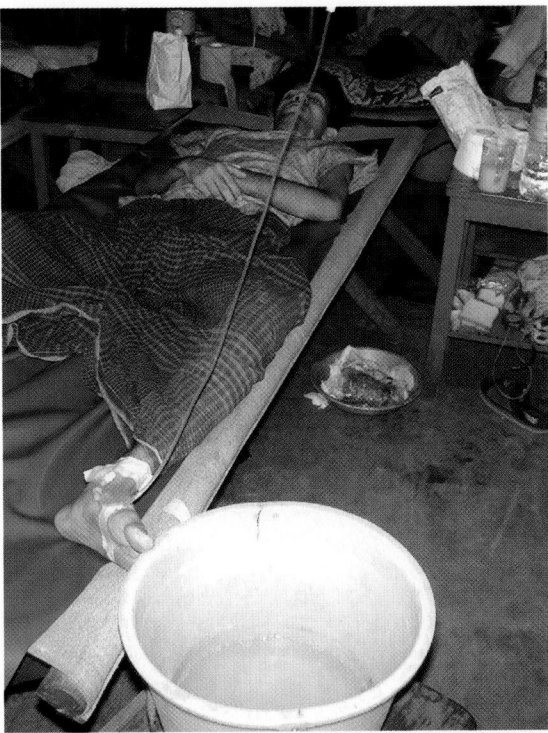

Figure 73.4. Patient excreting large volumes of nonbloody rice-water stool.

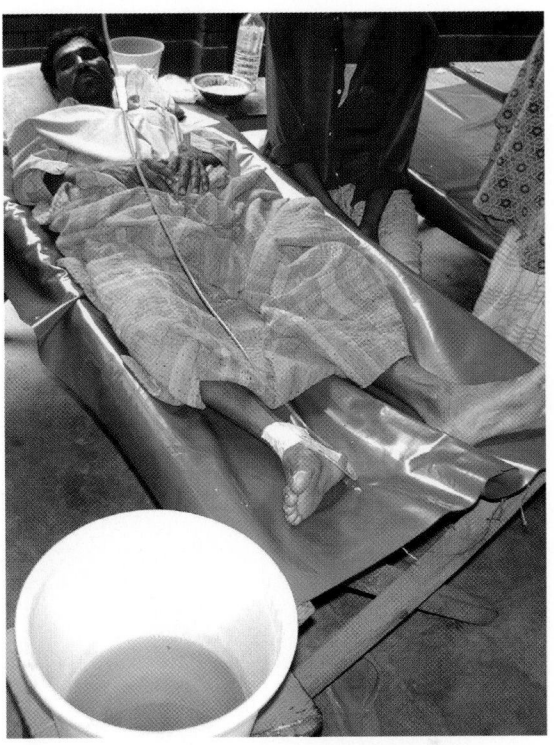

Figure 73.5. Patient excreting "washed meat" stool that is watery but bloody.

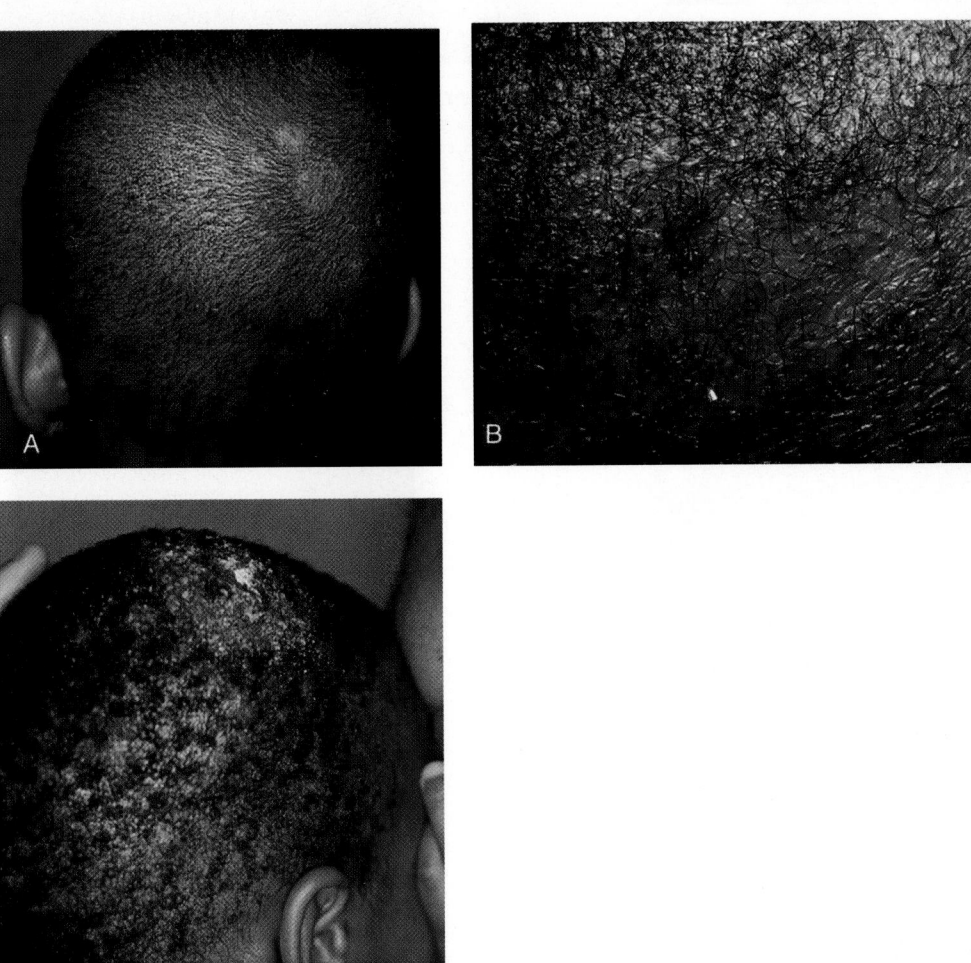

Figure 136.1. Tinea capitis. **A:** Multiple scaly alopecic plaques. **B:** Black-dot tinea capitis. **C:** Kerion with visibly enlarged postauricular lymph node.

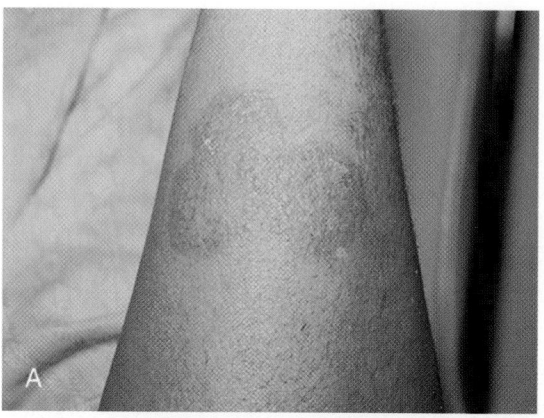

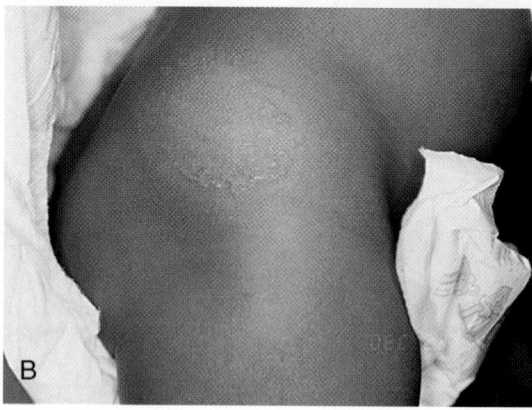

Figure 136.3. Tinea corporis. **A:** Coalescing scaly annular plaques on the forearm. **B:** Annular erythematous plaque on an infant's hip, occluded by the diaper.

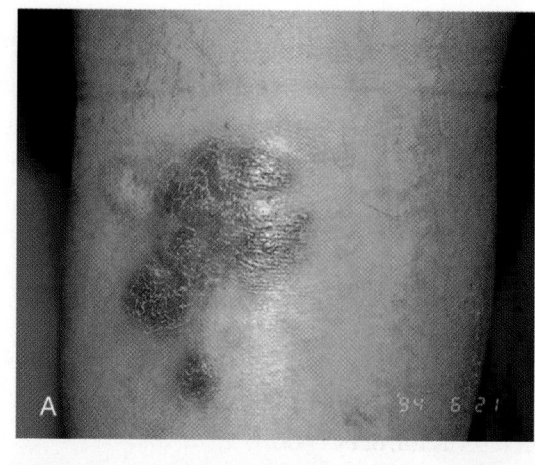

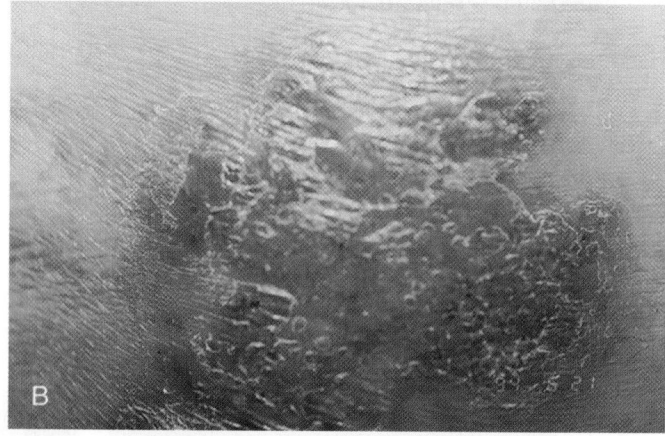

Figure 274.1. Chromoblastomycosis. **A:** Multiple plaques on the lower leg. **B:** Close-up of (A). (Courtesy Nellie Konnikov, M.D., New England Medical Center, Boston, Mass.)

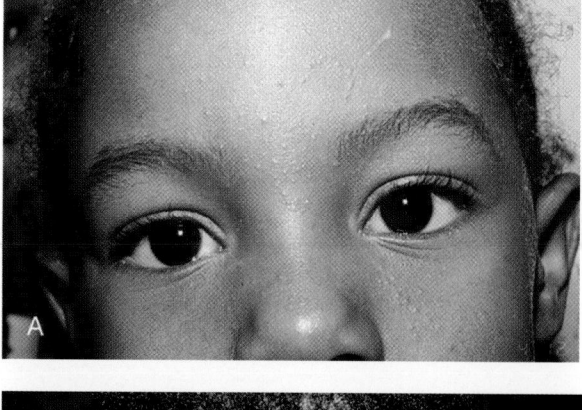

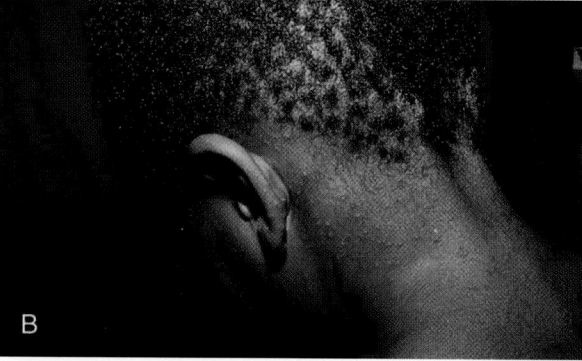

Figure 136.14. Id reaction. **A:** Fine papular eruption on the face in a 3-year-old girl with tinea capitis. **B:** Tinea capitis with fine papular id reaction on the neck.

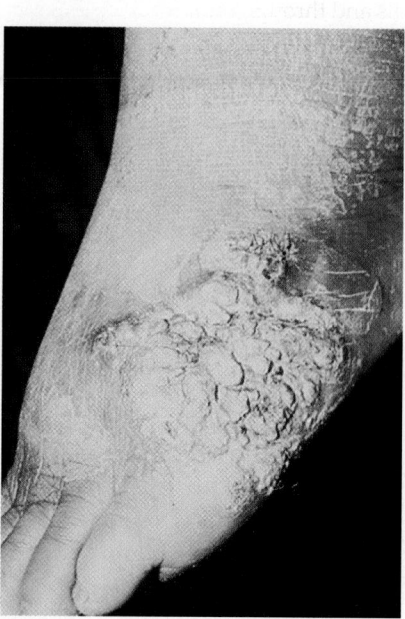

Figure 274.2. Chromoblastomycosis. Verrucous plaques on the lateral aspect of the foot.

kDa. The polypeptide α-chains are all coded on chromosome 16, the β-chain is coded on chromosome 21, and they are assembled into the heterodimer configuration before transport to the plasma membrane (75).

The leukocyte integrins mediate adhesion by binding to specific ligands. In particular, a family of molecules known as intercellular adhesion molecules (ICAMs), which are related to the immunoglobulin superfamily, are important counter-receptors or ligands for the leukocyte integrins (76,77). The specific targets for specific neutrophil integrins are indicated in Table 3.1. Localization of neutrophils at sites of inflammation depends on the dynamics of changes in neutrophil selectin and integrin molecules and endothelial cell adhesion receptors in response to activation by inflammatory cytokines, such as interleukin-1 or tumor necrosis factor, or by endotoxin (lipopolysaccharide) (69). It has been demonstrated that after exposure of neutrophils to chemotactic factors, new epitopes appear on leukocyte integrin molecules associated with increased adherence mediated by the integrins. Monoclonal antibodies directed at these neoepitopes inhibit adherence. This suggests that changes in conformation of integrin receptors probably play an important role in regulating adhesion (78). This regulated integrin adhesion is reversible, allowing the neutrophil to firmly adhere to the endothelium and then to follow a chemotactic gradient through the endothelium into the extravascular space. Adhesion molecules likely interact either directly or through intermediary linker proteins with the actin cytoskeleton and with other membrane components (79). This links adhesion events occurring at the cell surface with effector function processes such as motility, phagosome formation, and asymmetries in the activation of phagocyte oxidase or degranulation.

MIGRATION

Unstimulated neutrophils in the circulation are round and without apparent polarity. Neutrophils stimulated by contact with adherent surfaces or on exposure to chemoattractants demonstrate ameboid movement. There is development of a polarized structure characterized by elongation of the cell and formation of an active pseudopodium. At sites of inflammation, neutrophils adhere to postcapillary venule endothelium, migrating between endothelial cells and through the basement membrane, the latter event likely involving PECAM-1 (CD31) adhesion molecules (80). During migration, there is some secretion of degradative enzymes by neutrophils, possibly serving to facilitate migration through connective tissues (81). In the evolution of the inflammatory response, neutrophils are the first cells to arrive, but these are followed over the next 24 hours by an influx of monocytes as well.

Most of the important seven transmembrane helix chemoattractant receptors and the proximal signal transduction events leading to activation of neutrophil effecter functions were outlined previously in the section on Signal Transduction Pathways. In this section, attention will be focused on the biochemical events connecting the signal transduction cascade with the remodeling of the actin cytoskeleton of neutrophils associated with and required for motility. The motile process in neutrophils involves the formation and retraction of many types of cell surface protrusions, which must coordinate with the formation and severing of adhesive attachments of the neutrophil plasma membrane to other cells and to extracellular matrix elements. Cytoplasmic nonmuscle actin plays a central role in these events, generating motile forces in the neutrophil during migration or phagocytosis (18,19). Neutrophils contain millimolar concentration of actin, much of which is monomeric in resting cells. On activation of neutrophils, there is a fourfold increase in the proportion of this actin incorporated into filaments. Much has been learned about a large number of other proteins interactive with actin to coordinate the proper configuration and timing of actin assembly and disassembly (18,19,82–89).

In the presence of adenosine triphosphate, purified monomeric actin spontaneously forms long filaments (82). This is a polarized process, in which there is preferential addition of monomers to one end of the forming filament. Within the cytoplasm of living cells there is a family of proteins that bind actin monomers, inhibiting their incorporation into filaments. The prototype of this group is profilin (83). There is evidence that membrane phosphatidylinositol phosphates dissociate actin monomer from profilin and increase availability of monomeric actin for spontaneous assembly into filaments (84).

With purified actin, the elongation of actin filaments is energetically favored over the nucleation process required to begin the formation of a new filament. There are a number of proteins in cells that either initiate nucleation or inhibit filament elongation by binding to what should be the rapidly elongating end of the actin filament. This favors the formation of many short filaments over fewer long filaments. Other proteins, such as gelsolin, are capable of severing actin filaments, also favoring an increased number of short filaments (85). Calcium transients occurring during cell activation may enhance the severing activity of gelsolin and nucleating activity of other proteins, creating many short actin filaments (86). As calcium levels decrease, the effect of increased phosphorylation of membrane phosphatidylinositols predominates, resulting in elongation of this increased number of short filaments (90). The mechanical stability of these filaments is further enhanced by actin cross-linking proteins. In leukocytes, the submembranous cortical actin networks tend to be orthogonal. This may be a result of the action of actin-binding protein (nonmuscle filamen), which both links actin filaments to membrane glycoproteins, such as integrins, and promotes right-angle branching of these filaments (91). Many additional proteins participate in linking the upstream signal cascade originating with receptor-ligand stimulation or adhesion events and the regulation of the dynamic processes involved in the reshaping of the actin cytoskeleton required for motility (92). The importance of the *rho* family of GTP-binding proteins in this process has been highlighted by the discovery of a patient with an inherited mutation in *rac*2 that exerts a dominant-negative effect on the activity of *rac*1 and 2. This is associated with a clinically significant defect in neutrophil motility that can be attributed to defects in actin cytoskeleton remodeling (93). More about this inherited defect in neutrophil function will be discussed in later sections of this chapter. A very active current area of investigation involves delineation of how the Wiskott-Aldrich syndrome family of proteins (WASP and N-WASP) are involved in the most distal part of the regulation of cytoskeleton remodeling. The *rho*-related GTPases, *rac* or *cdc*24, interact with the WASP proteins to regulate Arp2/3 complex nucleation of actin polymerization (94–96).

PHAGOCYTOSIS

The process of internalizing particles by cells is termed *phagocytosis* and involves the attachment of the particle to the cell surface, which in turn triggers the extension of a pseudopod to enclose the particle in an endocytic vesicle or phagosome. Specific particle recognition and attachment to the PMN membrane are facilitated by PMN membrane receptors for the Fc portion of immunoglobulin G (IgG) and for cleavage fragments of the third complement component C3. At least three Fc-γ receptors (designated Fc-γ RI to RIII) have been identified; these differ in their molecular structure, affinity for IgG and its subclasses, expression on different cell types, and functional role in promoting particle internalization (97).

Fc-γ RI has the highest affinity for IgG with an association constant (K_a) of approximately 1 to 3×10^{-8} mol/L. This high-affinity Fc-γ receptor is a 72-kDa protein that is present on monocyte/macrophages but not on PMNs (98,99). Strong evidence points to a prominent role for this receptor in phagocytosis and antibody-dependent cellular cytotoxicity by monocyte/macrophages (100). Fc-γ RII, which is expressed on neutrophil membranes, has a lower affinity for binding IgG, and the binding activity differs substantially according to the physical state of the IgG (101). Monomeric IgG1 binds minimally to neutrophils, whereas multimeric IgG binds to the neutrophil Fc-γ RIIA (CD32) with a high affinity (102). This observation explains why circulating neutrophils, which are constantly bathed in serum IgG, do not have their Fc receptors occupied when they encounter an opsonized particle that presents multimers of IgG Fc to the neutrophil surface. In addition to Fc-γ RII, which has a broad electrophoretic mobility with an apparent molecular mass between 50 and 70 kDa, is Fc-γ RIII, with a molecular mass of 40 kDa (103). This Fc receptor is widely distributed on leukocytes, including neutrophils, monocyte/macrophages, platelets, and B cells. Like Fc-γ RII, Fc-γ RIII exhibits a low binding avidity for monomeric IgG but a much higher affinity for IgG aggregates. Fc-γ RIII is the same molecule as CD16 and tethered to the cell membrane by a phosphatidylinositol (PI) linkage. There is some evidence that this low-affinity Fc receptor may mediate early neutrophil recruitment in immune complex-mediated inflammation (104).

Because of the molecular diversity of the Fc receptors and the presence of multiple receptors on the same cells, it has been difficult to assign specific function to the different receptor classes. However, Fc receptor expression is not uniform on all neutrophils and may play a role in the functional heterogeneity of both mature and immature cells (105). Fc-γ RI (not present on neutrophils) Fc-γ RIII (present on neutrophils) signal largely by association with a separate gamma subunit containing a conserved cytoplasmic motif called *ITAM* whose tyrosines are phosphorylated following stimulation. Fc-γ RII signaling does not have a requirement for the gamma subunit. Neutrophils signaling from both Fc-γ RII and Fc-γ RIII require activation of *syk* (a *ras* family tyrosine kinase), which appears to bind both to the gamma subunit and directly to Fc-γ RII (106,107). Activation of phospholipase D1 may be an important downstream target of Fc receptor mediated neutrophil activation (108). Negative feedback of Fc-γ RII mediated responses in monocytes and macrophages, and probably also neutrophils, is accomplished through the Src homology 2 domain-containing inositol 5-phosphatase (SHIP) through mechanisms that are not fully understood (109). SHIP may also modulate phagocytic responses mediated through the complement fragment C3bi receptor (CD11b/CD18) (110).

At least two neutrophil plasma membrane receptors for complement function as opsonin receptors and promote particle attachment to the neutrophil surface. Complement receptor type 1 (CR1 or CD35) binds C3b but not uncleaved C3 and is a glycoprotein with four different allelic forms ranging in molecular mass from 160 to 250 kDa. Homozygotes express CR1 with a single molecular mass, whereas heterozygotes express two CR1 species. No disease has been linked to a specific CR1 phenotype. CR1 is expressed on both neutrophils and monocyte/macrophages, where it mediates attachment of particles coated with C3b (111). It is also expressed on erythrocytes, lym-

phocytes, and glomerular podocytes, where its function is unknown. CR3, which is one of the leukocyte integrins, binds particles coated with iC3b, which is the cleavage fragment of C3b. In addition, several microorganisms and particles such as *Escherichia coli*, *Staphylococcus aureus*, *Histoplasma capsulatum*, and zymosan appear to bind directly to the phagocyte CR3 receptor in the absence of complement (112,113). At least in macrophages, the *E. coli* ligand that binds to CR3 is the lipid A portion of lipopolysaccharide or endotoxin.

A major characteristic of CR1 and CR3 (CD11b/CD18) on phagocytic cells is their regulation by extracellular matrix proteins and soluble mediators. Both the binding affinity and the apparent numbers of CR1 and CR3 receptors are transiently increased when neutrophils are activated by spreading on surfaces coated with fibronectin, serum amyloid P component, or laminin as well as by soluble stimuli, such as the tumor promoter phorbol myristate acetate (61,62,67–69). The increased number of CR3 receptors appears to result from mobilization of an intracellular pool of receptors from specific granules to the plasma membrane, whereas the origin of additional CR1 is not known. Regulation of the binding affinity of CR3 for iC3b-coated particles may involve conversion of low-affinity receptors to higher affinity CR3 by phosphorylation, and this process may be important in the phagocytic capacity of neutrophils in the course of different diseases.

Once the opsonized particle is bound to the phagocyte plasma membrane by CR1, CR3, or Fc receptor, engulfment occurs by the localized extension of a pseudopod. The pseudopod progressively surrounds the particle as membrane receptors engage opsonin molecules on the surface in a process that has been analogized to "zippering up" the particle within the developing phagosome (114). The ionic and biochemical events that propel the peripheral cytoplasm to surround the opsonized particle appear similar to those that propel the whole cell during chemotactic locomotion. Before and after complete closure of the extended pseudopod, cytoplasmic granule movement increases at the base of the phagosome, where the granule membranes of both specific and azurophil granules fuse with the phagosome to form the phagolysosome. This process likely requires a number of specialized proteins that catalyze the fusion of the granule and phagosome membranes (115–118).

MICROBICIDAL MECHANISMS

Oxygen-Independent Killing

For convenience, the microbicidal components bathing the microorganism in the phagolysosome are divided into oxygen-independent and oxygen-dependent categories. The former refers to those factors that contribute to phagocyte killing of microorganisms in an anaerobic environment. Of the nonoxygen-dependent microbicidal factors of phagocytic cells, most attention has focused on granule-associated proteins, because fusion of granules with the phagosome to form the phagolysosome provides a mechanism for exposing the organism to these substances within a closed space (6–12,119). Table 3.2 lists some of the granule-associated proteins of neutrophils and their location within the cell. Borregaard and Cowland provide a more complete list of the granular and vesicular contents of neutrophils, and in addition to the azurophil and specific granule compartments, they also define the contents of rapidly mobilized gelatinase granule and secretory vesicle compartments (119).

Several granule-associated proteins with microbicidal activity have been well characterized. BPI protein is a constituent of

TABLE 3.2. Contents of Human Neutrophil Granules

Type of constituent	Azurophil (primary) granule	Specific (secondary) granule	Other
Antimicrobial enzyme	Lysozyme Myeloperoxidase	Lysozyme	
Antimicrobial peptides and proteins	Bactericidal/permeability increasing protein	Lactoferrin	
		Cathelicidin/hCAP-18	
	Defensins Azurocidin/CAP37/Heparin binding protein		
Enzymes	Acid phosphatase	Cytochrome b-558	Cytochrome b-558
	β-Glucosaminidase		β-Glucosaminidase
	α-Mannosidase		α-Mannosidase
	Arylsulfatase	Gelatinase B/MMP9	Gelatinase B/MMP9
	α-Fucosidase	Histaminase	
	neutrophil serine protease PR3 (proteinase 3)		
	Cathepsin G	Heparinase	
	Cathepsin D		Cathepsin D
	Elastase/MMP12	Sialidase	
	Phospholipase A		
	Histonase		
	Deoxyribonuclease		
	5'-Nucleotidase		
	Collagenase-2/MMP8	Collagenase-2/MMP8	
	β-Glycerophosphatase		
	β-Glucuronidase		β-Glucuronidase
Receptors		iC3b	
		FMLP	
Other	Glycosaminoglycans	Laminin	Laminin
	Chondroitin sulfate	Vitamin B_{12} binding protein	
	Heparin sulfate		

MMPs, matrix metalloproteinases.

PMN azurophil granules that is lethal for many enteric gram-negative organisms but has no activity against gram-positive bacteria, fungi, or eukaryotic cells. BPI protein appears to act by binding to and inserting into the outer membrane of gram-negative bacteria, where it destabilizes the membrane, leading to increased permeability (8). Hydrolysis of bacterial phospholipids and changes in the synthesis of outer membrane proteins also occur early after BPI protein binding. The defensins are a family of polypeptide molecules containing 29 to 34 amino acids that are localized in a subset of the azurophil granules of neutrophils (8). In human PMNs, there are four different defensins designated human neutrophil protein-1, -2, -3, and -4. Similar cysteine-rich antimicrobial peptides have also been isolated from rabbit, rat, and guinea pig leukocytes as well as from Paneth cells in the mouse small intestine. The defensins exhibit broad antimicrobial activity against gram-positive and gram-negative bacteria, fungi, and certain enveloped viruses. They are also cytotoxic for some human and murine cells. As with BPI protein, the mechanism of action of these polypeptides involves destabilization and permeabilization of the target membrane. Other azurophil granule proteins with documented antimicrobial activities have been described (119). Cathelicidin or hCAP-18, is present in specific granules and an antimicrobial C-terminal antimicrobial peptide, LL-37, can be liberated by the action of proteinase 3 (120).

Lysozyme is a well-characterized, small (molecular mass of 14,500), highly cationic protein that cleaves the β-(1,4)-glycosidic linkage between N-acetylglucosamine and N-acetylmuramic acid present in the bacterial cell wall. Although this protein, which is present in both azurophil and specific granules of PMN, rapidly lyses some nonpathogenic gram-positive bacteria (e.g., *Micrococcus lysodeikticus*), most organisms are resistant to the direct microbicidal action of lysozyme because the peptidoglycan is protected either by extensive cross-linking or by the outer membrane of gram-negative organisms. Lactoferrin, a constituent of the specific granules of PMNs, is an iron binding protein that exerts its antimicrobial effect by competing with bacteria for this essential growth factor (121). An acid pH in the phagolysosome contributes to the microbicidal activity of PMNs by directly inhibiting the growth of some bacteria and by promoting the activity of the peroxide-dependent killing mechanism and BPI protein. Within 15 minutes after particle ingestion, the pH in the developing phagosome progressively decreases to pH 4.0 to 6.5. Acidification is due to the action of proton pumps located in the lysosomal and plasma membranes as well as protons released during the respiratory burst. The respirator burst is also connected directly to the non-oxidative killing mechanisms of neutrophils by the observation that the large anionic charge derived from accumulation of superoxide in the phagosome leads to a massive influx of K^+ ions that enter in a pH-dependent fashion. The rise in ionic strength helps to release cationic proteases (see below) from the anionic sulfated proteoglycan matrix in the azurophil granule matrix. This allows the activation of these proteases, which appears necessary for killing and degradation of microorganisms (122). This latter process is essential for resolution of the inflammatory process. In fact this process may be part of the reason that patients with chronic granulomatous disease, who lack the oxidative burst, fail to resolve granulomas.

Neutrophils also contain a very large number of degradation enzymes that probably serve a variety of normal physiologic purposes such as facilitating the migration of neutrophils through tissues, tissue remodeling during wound healing and activation, or degradation of chemotactic factors. As noted previously, these enzymes are also very important in killing and digesting microorganisms. As noted previously, these enzymes particularly the matrix metalloproteinases (gelatinase B/MMP9 and elastase/MMP12 and collagenase 2/MMP-8) (9,123–126) can damage connective tissue and thereby play a role in the pathogenesis of joint damage in osteoarthritis or in the lung damage associated with emphysema.

Oxidative Killing

During phagocytosis or in response to high concentrations of chemoattractants, neutrophils are triggered to produce large amounts of superoxide that dismutates to hydrogen peroxide and other microbicidal oxidants. This response has been called a respiratory burst because of the rapid consumption of oxygen associated with it (Fig. 3.3). When neutrophils, monocytes, or eosinophils are stimulated, a unique nicotinamide adenine dinucleotide phosphate (NADPH) oxidase is activated. Activa-

tion of this oxidase requires assembly of an electron transport chain at the plasma membrane or the membrane of the forming phagosome. Activation of the NADPH oxidase requires the interaction of both membrane and cytoplasmic components (9, 127,128).

Figure 3.3 is a schematic representation of the components of the phagocytic cell NADPH oxidase (10,127–131). Early events in activation result in phosphorylation of several serines in the cationic C-terminal third of the cytoplasmic protein, p47phox (47-kDa phagocyte oxidase protein). This phosphorylation dissociates the internal binding of a proline-rich SH3-binding domain in that region from an SH3 domain in the middle third of the molecule. This allows two uncovered SH3 regions to bind to p67phox and eventually also to interact with another proline-rich SH3-binding domain on the p22phox subunit of the transmembrane cytochrome b-558 (132–135). At the same time *Rac*2, a *Rho*-related member of the *Ras* superfamily of GTPs (59,93,139,140) interacts with an N-terminal region of p67 and the complex of p47phox/p67phox/*rac*2 translocates to the membrane of the forming phagosome to interact with the cytochrome b-558. At the cell membrane, these cytoplasmic factors interact together and with a unique phagocyte flavocytochrome b-558 to form the active oxidase complex (10,127–131,141,142). Flavocytochrome

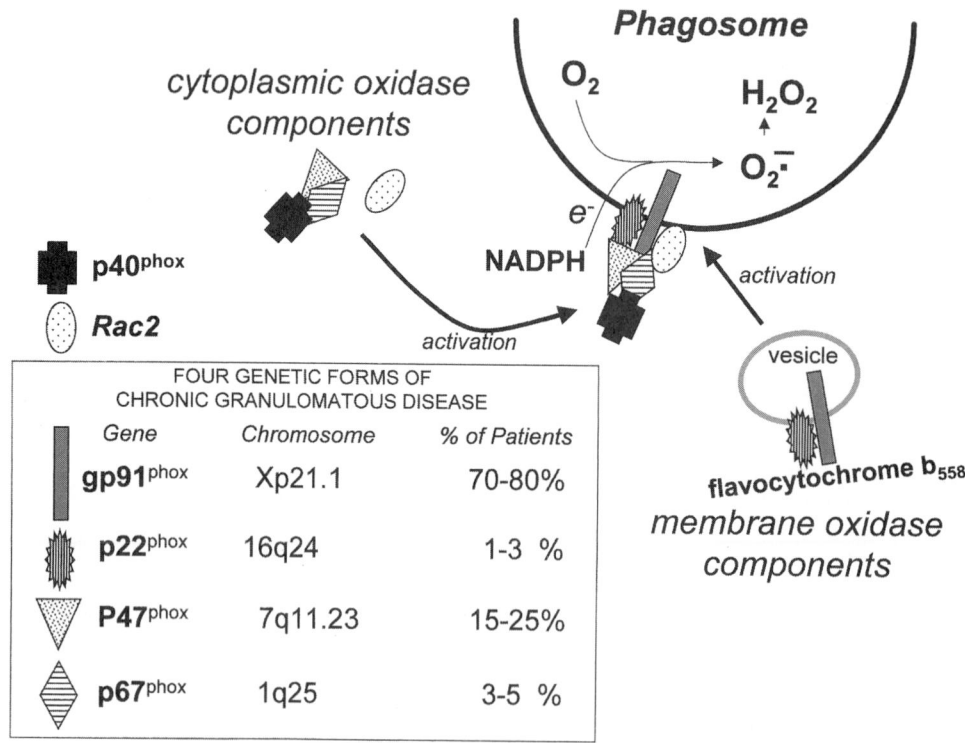

Figure 3.3. Components of the phagocytic cell respiratory burst and the genetic lesions affecting these components in chronic granulomatous disease. The flavocytochrome b-558, consisting of a heterodimer of gp91phox and p22phox, is an integral membrane protein containing flavin, heme, and an NADPH binding site. The p47phox, p40phox, p67phox, and Rac2 (a Rho family guanosine triphosphatase) are cytoplasmic proteins in the resting cell. On activation, the p47phox is multiply phosphorylated and together with the other cytoplasmic factors translocates to the membrane of the forming phagosome; there they interact with the cytoplasmic domain of the flavocytochrome to form the enzymatically active NADPH oxidase. The cytoplasmic surface of the membrane lies beneath the line; above the line indicates the inside of the phagosome or the cell surface. After activation, electrons are transferred from NADPH to molecular oxygen to form superoxide. This breaks down into hydrogen peroxide, which together with chloride anion interacts with myeloperoxidase derived from azurophil granules fusing with the phagosome to form hypochlorous acid. The hydrogen peroxide and hypochlorous acid are the major oxidase-derived microbicidal substances. Chronic granulomatous disease results from mutations in the genes encoding any of the four phox proteins indicated in the box. The chromosome location and frequency of genetic abnormalities are shown in the box.

b-558 is a heterodimer composed of two tightly associated subunits, p22phox and a highly glycosylated transmembrane large subunit gp9lphox (143–146). The gp91phox glycopeptide appears to have flavin and NADPH binding consensus sequences and together with the p22phox peptide coordinates the binding of two heme groups (147,148). This flavin- and heme-containing flavocytochrome has an electron potential of −245 mV and is the terminal electron donor to molecular oxygen, capable of forming superoxide anion. Another cytoplasmic component of the oxidase, p40phox, appears to be associated with a preformed complex with p47phox and p67phox (149). In cell-free reconstructions of the oxidase, the p40phox is not a required component, so its role in oxidase activation *in vivo* is not clearly delineated, but studies suggest that it may serve to stabilize the complex and participate in translocation to the membrane. This concept is supported by the fact that both p47phox and p40phox contain PX domains which bind lipids, particularly phosphoinositides, but may also bind phosphatidic acids. This may serve a role in the translocation to membrane or inducing conformational changes during oxidase activation (150–152).

Although much is now known about the fine structure of the NADPH oxidase components and the molecular basis of the protein-protein interactions leading to oxidase assembly, details of the three-dimensional structure of these proteins and the flow of electrons from NADPH to molecular oxygen remain under study. In addition, the terminal signal events that trigger assembly of these components appear to involve phospholipid mediators and kinases (51,53,153,154), and it is an active area of investigation.

The NADPH substrate for the oxidative burst is supplied by a sudden increase in anaerobic glucose metabolism through the hexose monophosphate shunt. In mildly acidic conditions, superoxide rapidly reacts with water to form hydrogen peroxide. Superoxide dismutase, present in all cellular cytoplasm, further accelerates this reaction. Hydrogen peroxide is a more potent antimicrobial and cytocidal oxidant than is superoxide. Furthermore, in the presence of neutrophil MPO and a halide (Cl^-, Br^-, I^-), the hydrogen peroxide reacts to form hypohalous acids, of which hypochlorous acid is the most abundant (155). Additional reactions may occur to produce free halogens and other reactive compounds. These halous oxidants are extremely potent antimicrobial substances. These oxidants not only damage microorganisms but also enhance the susceptibility of pathogens to some of the nonoxidative antimicrobial substances present in neutrophil granules, including proteases and other degradative enzymes. It is possible to speculate that the anaerobic environment within some abscesses deprives neutrophils of the oxygen necessary to produce this array of antimicrobial substances. As noted previously, it is now known that even activation of the antimicrobial protease systems from granules depends on the ionized potassium flux into phagosomes that is dependent on production of superoxide anion (122). Drainage of abscesses not only removes the bulk of organisms within the abscess but also achieves another important physiologic effect by enhancing neutrophil access to the oxygen that is required for function of the activated oxidase.

Some of the oxidants produced by neutrophils may also damage host tissues. In the presence of iron salts, hydrogen peroxide and superoxide can interact to form hydroxyl radical. Whereas hydroxyl radical does have antimicrobial activity, it is particularly damaging to host tissues (156–158). There is evidence that apolactoferrin present in large amounts in neutrophil specific granules may limit hydroxyl radical formation by sequestering iron. MPO may similarly limit formation of hydroxyl radical by shunting hydrogen peroxide into other reactions more appropriate to host defense (159). Nonetheless, studies using hydroxyl radical scavengers in animals (160) indicate that sufficient hydroxyl radical is formed at sites of inflammation and neutrophil activation to have an impact on the pathophysiologic process of a number of conditions including adult respiratory distress syndrome, myocardial infarction, and autoimmune disorders.

NEUTROPHIL APOPTOSIS

Physiologic control of the potent tissue degrading enzymes from neutrophils is essential, and the histology and physiology of the last phase of neutrophil function, apoptosis, is critical to that process. It had been appreciated by histology that neutrophils in tissues appeared to have two final fates, cellular breakdown with uncontrolled release of neutrophil contents or an involution type of process that is now appreciated as the hallmark of controlled cellular apoptosis in which the neutrophil remains intact, but the nucleus fragments, the cell blebs and shrinks in size and the apoptotic cell is eventually engulfed by tissue macrophages. The former process occurs with some types of inflammation and some types of infections that are associated with tissue damage, while the latter process, if allowed to proceed, controls nonphysiologic tissue damage and exerts positive and even essential effects in processes such as wound healing (161).

Apoptosis is therefore the natural and physiologically preferred last stage of "differentiation" of the neutrophil (16,162) with a distinct histologic appearance associated with activation of known apoptotic pathways such as Fas/Fas ligand and the display on the cell surface of specific receptors that mediate uptake and ingestion by scavenger macrophages (16,163–166). The normal production of oxidants by neutrophils may accelerate the apoptotic process and the granuloma formation associated with the chronic granulomatous disease may in part be related to delayed apoptosis in the absence of oxidant production (167). Both G-CSF and GM-CSF can inhibit apoptotic processes in neutrophils (36), and it is possible to speculate that this could play a role in keeping the marrow pool of neutrophils from progressing to apoptosis as well as prolonging the lifespan of neutrophils at sites of inflammation when these growth factors are produced locally produced from endothelial cells in response to infection (168).

While familial Mediterranean fever is not classically thought of as a neutrophil disorder, in fact the recent discovery that this disorder results from defects in a protein called pyrin, led to the appreciation that domains in that molecule play an important role in neutrophil apoptosis during inflammation (169). Part of the abnormal neutrophil accumulation seen in this and some other newly defined inherited auto-inflammatory disorders may involve a failure of neutrophils to undergo normal apoptosis (170). Although these inherited disorder are not usually thought of as primary disorders of neutrophils it would not be unreasonable to consider them part of the spectrum of disorders of neutrophils included in the sections below.

NEUTROPENIA

Acquired Neutropenia

The peripheral blood neutrophil count is normally 1,500 to 8,000 cells/mm³, but can be as low as 1,000 cells/mm³. There are ethnic differences in what comprises a normal neutrophil count. For example, individuals of African ancestry have a lower mean absolute neutrophil count than individuals of European ancestry (2,500 vs. 3,200 cells/mm³) (171), and studies suggest that this difference may be regulated at the early progenitor cell level in the marrow (172,173). Neutrophil counts in a normal individual are generally constant if that person is observed for several years. There are a number of syndromes other than acute infection that can result in a high neutrophil count, such as that associated with leukocyte adhesion deficiency (LAD, to be discussed), Pelger Huet syndrome (discussed previously), leukemoid reactions (can be from tuberculosis, vasculitis or other autoimmune disorders), leukemia, or rare inherited syndromes (174). Neutrophilia will not be discussed further in this chapter.

A rule of thumb established several decades ago in the setting of chemotherapy-induced neutropenia is that neutrophil counts lower than 1,000 cells/mm³ are associated with some increased risk for infection and that patients with counts below 500 cells/mm³ are at high risk for development of bacterial or fungal infection (175). The risk is further increased in patients with absolute neutrophil counts below 100/mm³. From these initial observations, criteria for treatment of patients with cancer chemotherapy induced neutropenia were developed and con-

tinue to be modified (176–180). These statistical correlations and suggestions for medical intervention were developed in a specific clinical setting, cancer chemotherapy–related neutropenia. The significance of a specific absolute neutrophil count in a patient with an unexplained neutropenia should be tempered by taking into account whether the neutrophil count is decreasing or remaining steady. A decreasing neutrophil count or a significant decrease over steady-state levels, together with a failure to increase counts in the setting of infection or other challenge to bone marrow reserve, carries a higher risk of infection than a low neutrophil count that has remained constant for many months or years and increases significantly in response to infection.

Some causes of inherited and acquired neutropenias are listed in Table 3.3. The most common neutropenias are iatrogenic, resulting from the widespread use of cytotoxic or immunosuppressive therapies for malignant neoplasm or control of autoimmune disorders. These drugs cause neutropenia because they are toxic to rapidly growing cells of the marrow. Cytotoxic chemotherapeutic agents fall into this category, but certain antibiotics such as chloramphenicol, linezolid, trimethoprim-sulfamethoxazole (TMP-SMX), flucytosine, vidarabine, and the antiretroviral drug

TABLE 3.3.   Causes of Inherited and Acquired Neutropenias

Neutropenias	Description
Immune	
Alloimmune neonatal neutropenia	Maternal-fetal neutrophil antigen incompatibility
Primary autoimmune neutropenia	Antineutrophil antibodies
Acquired neutropenia associated with LGL leukemia can be a cyclic neutropenia	Associated with clonal expansion of large granular lymphocytes; may progress to LGL leukemia
Aplastic anemia-agranulocytosis	Cause unknown, possibly drug related
Drug-related autoimmune neutropenia	Drugs as haptens interacting with neutrophils
Secondary to other autoimmune disorders	Lupus erythematosus, Felty syndrome, rheumatoid arthritis
Hypersplenism	
Metabolic "storage" diseases	Gaucher's disease, Fabrey's disease, etc
Some infections or autoimmune diseases	
Infection	
Epstein-Barr virus infection, hepatitis	Direct marrow suppression or immune phenomena
Human immunodeficiency virus infection	
Marrow failure in neonates	Results from overwhelming infection
Acute endotoxinemia neutropenia (transient, not a true neutropenia)	Acute margination of neutrophils in postcapillary venules from bacteremia
Cytotoxic drug effects	
Therapy for cancer, immune disorders, or side effect of other drugs	Direct suppression of progenitors, iatrogenic and most common cause of neutropenia
Inherited neutropenic syndromes	
Familial benign neutropenia	Benign dominant inherited trait with marrow response to infection
Congenital agranulocytosis (Kostmann syndrome)	Apoptosis of precursor cells resulting from mutations in the elastase gene (ELA-2); responsive to granulocyte colony-stimulating factor; progression to leukemia or myelodysplasia 2% per year
Inherited cyclic neutropenia	Periodic apoptosis of progenitors resulting from mutations in the elastase gene (ELA-2); responsive to granulocyte colony-stimulating factor
Abnormal marrow release syndromes (a feature of several rare disorders, e.g., lazy leukocyte syndrome, myelokathexis, WHIM syndrome)	Several different disorders with normal marrow production of neutrophils and failure of release; functional and morphologic abnormalities of neutrophils
Reticular dysgenesis and some other severe combined immunodeficiencies	Defective myeloid and lymphoid series inherited disorder related to the severe combined immunodeficiencies
Shwachman syndrome	Myeloid dysgenesis and pancreatic insufficiency due to mutations in SBDS gene (function unknown) located at 7q11; Fas-mediated precursor apoptosis seen

zidovudine may also cause neutropenia by inhibiting myeloid precursor proliferation. The marrow suppression is generally dose-related and dependent on continued administration of the drug.

Drugs may also cause neutropenia by serving as immune haptens, resulting in sensitization of neutrophils or neutrophil precursors to immune-mediated destruction. Drug-dependent immune neutropenia may appear as early as 7 days after exposure to a drug, but when there has been previous exposure, it may occur after only a few hours of exposure. Although almost any drug can cause this type of immune neutropenia, it is important to consider any of the commonly used antibiotics, particularly sulfa-containing compounds, penicillins, and cephalosporins (181–184). There may be associated fever or eosinophilia, but these signs are often not present. However, all medications, including common over-the-counter drugs, are possible causes of acute idiopathic neutropenia. Drug-induced immune neutropenia can be severe but usually requires only that the sensitizing drug be discontinued. Neutrophil counts usually begin to increase within 5 to 7 days and not longer than 10 days after the drug is stopped. Readministration of the sensitizing drug is usually associated with abrupt decreases in neutrophil counts. Diagnostic challenge with a suspect drug should not be done, because even short periods of neutropenia entail some risk for infection. Drugs can also be associated with aplastic anemia, affecting all formed blood elements, or with agranulocytosis; continued use may result in a prolonged neutropenia that may remit spontaneously but may be permanent. Some substances such as aromatic hydrocarbons (benzene), phenothiazines, phenylbutazone, and oxyphenbutazone, and chloramphenicol have been specifically connected with idiosyncratic reactions resulting in prolonged or permanent neutropenia (185–187).

Acquired neutropenia can be caused by antineutrophil specific antibodies directed at any of a large group of antigens specific to neutrophils (188,189). Many of these antigens represent antigenic variants of the neutrophil IgG Fc receptor Fcgamma RIIIb (190). Antineutrophil antibody immune neutropenias can arise as an autoimmune disorder or may occur in the neonatal period from maternal antibodies that arise by sensitization to neutrophil-specific antigen fetal/maternal incompatibility (191–193). Acquired neutropenia is also associated with viral infections, including human immunodeficiency virus (HIV) infection, though with the advent of potent anti-HIV therapies, the neutropenia seen in this disorder is more commonly related to these antiviral agents. Rarely, acquired neutropenia may be associated with a T-cell large granular lymphocyte clonal disorder that can progress to leukemia (T-LGL). Sometimes this disorder is manifest as an acquired cyclic neutropenia (194,195). In the past this was treated with steroids, but with the appreciation that this is a manifestation of the biologic effects from a lymphocytic neoplasm treatment with chemotherapy may be more appropriate in some cases (196,197).

Neutropenia may be associated with autoimmune disease or metabolic disorders in which there is splenomegaly with trapping and destruction of neutrophils (Felty syndrome, portal hypertension, or lysosomal storage diseases) (198). A transient neutropenia may be seen acutely in gram-negative bacteremia as circulating neutrophils abruptly marginate in response to circulating bacterial endotoxin. Severe infection in a premature infant or an elderly individual may occasionally be related to a more gradual decline in neutrophil counts to neutropenic levels when large numbers of circulating early neutrophil precursors are also seen. This may be evidence of bone marrow failure and, in the setting of severe infection in infants or the elderly, is a grave prognostic sign (199,200).

Hereditary Neutropenia

Reticular dysgenesis is a very rare congenital immunodeficiency, whose gene has not been identified. The disease is classified within the severe combined immunodeficiencies (SCID) group and characterized by impairment of both lymphoid and myeloid cell development that is best treated with bone marrow transplantation (201,202). In addition to reticular dysgenesis, some other disorders in the SCID group can be associated with neutropenia (203). Shwachman-Diamond (or just Shwachman's) syndrome is an autosomal recessive disorder associated with congenital neutropenia and other cytopenias plus pancreatic exocrine insufficiency and skeletal abnormalities (204,205). Approximately one third of cases progress to leukemia. The gene for this disorder has been cloned and is called *SBDS*, located at 7q11 (206). The function of this gene is not yet known.

A severe congenital neutropenia of childhood known as Kostmann's syndrome was originally thought to be related to abnormalities of the receptor for G-CSF, and responds to treatment with G-CSF (207,208). Recently severe congenital neutropenia has been shown to result from mutations in the gene (*ELA2*) at 19p13.3 encoding neutrophil elastase, which is also known as leukocyte elastase, elastase 2, or medullasin (209,210). However, the disease is associated with an underlying genetic instability, because patients develop additional genetic defects during the course of disease, such as G-CSF receptor gene mutations and chromosomal rearrangements, with progression of approximately 2% of cases per year to myeloid leukemia or myelodysplastic syndrome (211,212). Hereditary cyclic neutropenia is a rare autosomal dominant disorder characterized by a remarkably regular 3-week cycle (194,213). This disorder also turns out to be a result of mutations in the *ELA2* gene (elastase) (209,210,214). The mechanism by which mutations in elastase cause these neutropenias is not clear, but may result from the action of abnormal processed mutant protein (215).

General Principles of Evaluation and Management of Neutropenia

In neutropenia, the inflammatory response is modified. The absence of neutrophil accumulation means that pus is not seen and the degree of swelling and redness is decreased. Fever and malaise are more reliable systemic signs of infection, and local signs may be limited to pain, warmth, and limitation of movement. Significant pulmonary infections may be evident despite only minor changes on chest radiographs. On physical examination, it is essential to look for gingivitis and aphthous ulcers, lymphadenitis, rectal abscess or fistula, splenomegaly, and liver tenderness. The skin should be carefully examined for early signs of cutaneous infection. In acute, severe neutropenia, the gastrointestinal and respiratory tracts are common sources of infection, although the site may be difficult to demonstrate. Blood cultures, urine cultures, and complete blood cell count as well as a chest radiograph should be obtained. Other studies should be dictated by history and physical findings. In cases of chronic neutropenia, laboratory studies should include a chest radiograph and possibly liver-spleen scan; complete blood cell count with differential; blood folate, vitamin B_{12}, and copper determinations; serum protein electrophoresis; immunoglobulin levels; and renal and liver function studies. When appropriate, a white blood cell count and differential should be performed at least 3 days a week for an 8-week period to identify any cyclic pattern. A bone marrow aspirate and biopsy specimen for histologic examination and culture are an essential part of the workup in chronic neutropenias, but they may be delayed in some cases of acute neutropenia when the cause is clear and recovery is likely. The clinical setting may determine if this is more likely to be acquired, and if so whether it is a drug toxicity, an immune drug reaction, or an autoimmune-related neutropenia. Although new medications may be more suspect, reactions can develop to chronically administered medication. If appropriate to the setting, as many medications as possible should be discontinued. A lymphocyte phenotype analysis may detect an associated lymphocyte abnormality, such as a large granular lymphocyte monoclonal expansion. Studies to detect antineutrophil antibodies should be obtained. If one of the congenital neutropenias is suspected, specific genetic mutation analysis may be performed. Some of the congenital and acquired neutropenias respond to G-CSF administration, and this should be used if the absolute neutrophil count is consistently or periodically well below 500 cells/mm^3.

For patients with chronic neutropenia, management of infection risk should be dictated by the medical history, although any infection, no matter how minor, should receive prompt attention. Patients whose neutrophil counts generally remain above 500 cells/mm^3 or who show a significant marrow reserve in the setting of infection (or by steroid challenge) and whose history does not reveal major problems with recurrent infections should not receive prophylactic antibiotics and should not limit their activities. Patients with constant or cyclic neutrophil counts below 500 cells/mm^3 who show little marrow reserve response to infection are more susceptible to infection, although a history of infections may differ significantly among individuals with similar degrees of chronic neutropenia. These patients may benefit from prophylactic antibiotics. Oral TMP (160 g)-SMX (800 mg) twice daily is a commonly used regimen. This may be combined with oral itraconazole 200 mg daily for fungal prophylaxis and is well tolerated. Oral quinolones, such as ciprofloxacin 500 mg twice daily, are a reasonable alternative to TMP-SMX. In the setting of cytotoxic chemotherapy with severe persistent neutropenia, the proven effectiveness of TMP-SMX in preventing *Pneumocystis carinii* pneumonia may offer another incentive to use this form of antibacterial prophylaxis. These patients should try to avoid heavy exposure to airborne soil, dust, or decaying organic matter to decrease exposure to *Aspergillus* spores. Restriction of activities or social contacts probably makes little difference in infection risk. Good oral hygiene is essential. In addition to routine dental care, neutropenic patients can decrease gingivitis by using chlorhexidine mouthwash and brushing with hydrogen peroxide–sodium bicarbonate paste.

There is some evidence that in cytotoxic therapy–induced severe acute neutropenia, a simple reverse isolation regimen can be helpful in reducing infection during the neutropenic period. This regimen consists of wearing a facemask and of careful handwashing by staff and visitors. More stringent isolation is probably unnecessary and serves only to impede contact of the patient with family and medical personnel. As noted previously, prophylactic oral TMP-SMX or a quinolone plus itraconazole is useful as is the use of mouthwash.

As noted previously, signs of inflammation are muted with severe neutropenia, so that fever or hypotension and occasionally pain at the site of infection may be the only signs of life-threatening infection. A number of algorithms of using studies of inflammation such as C-reactive protein, and other measures have been developed to determine the likelihood of infection and need to begin broad-spectrum antibiotic therapy (174,179,180). Slight infiltrates on chest radiography may be the only sign of severe pneumonia. Bacteremia without an obvious source of infection is common. When a site of infection can be determined, it is usually the mouth, sinuses, gastrointestinal tract, rectum, lungs, or skin. Bowel wall cellulitis and necrosis can present insidiously

with fever and abdominal pain and is a surgical emergency. Urinary tract infection occurs, but in the absence of instrumentation or anatomic abnormality, it is less common. With neutropenic individuals, it is essential in the presence of fever or other potential sign of infection, including hypotension in the absence of fever, that the patient be evaluated rapidly; that blood, sputum, urine, and other cultures be obtained; and that intravenous administration of broad-spectrum antibiotics be started promptly. The specific regimens chosen often depend on standards for a particular institution, and change as new antimicrobial agents become available. The most important thing is that antibiotic treatment not be delayed by time taken for too many diagnostic measures because rapid treatment with antibiotic most closely correlates with reduction in mortality from infection. Cultures and diagnostic studies must be performed expeditiously, and antibiotic therapy must take precedence over a more extensive evaluation.

INHERITED DEFECTS OF NEUTROPHIL FUNCTION

Leukocyte Adhesion Deficiency

Defects in the gene for the common subunit of the leukocyte adhesion molecules CD11a/CD18 (lymphocyte function-associated antigen-1), CD11b/CD18 (macrophage-1 antigen, CR3), and CD11c/CD18 (p150,95) result in a spectrum of clinical manifestations collectively known as leukocyte adhesion deficiency (LAD), which are inherited in an autosomal recessive pattern (70,71,75,216). This is a rare disorder with frequency of only a few per million or less. A few individuals have been identified with a similar spectrum of clinical features who have defects in fucose metabolism, leading to a failure to produce the carbohydrate ligands required for selectin binding (71–73,217). To distinguish the two types of LAD genetic diseases, the more common (although still rare) inherited adhesion deficiency resulting from mutations in the CD18 gene is designated LAD-1; the selectin ligand defect currently reported in only a few individuals is designated LAD-2.

Most of the following discussion of diagnosis and treatment relates to experience with LAD-1, but many of the clinical features of LAD-2 and approaches to treatment would be similar. However, some features of LAD-2 are unique in that the patients are reported to have craniofacial dysmorphism, neurologic defects, and lack of the red blood cell H antigen, thus manifesting the Bombay (hh) erythrocyte phenotype. The patients have normal levels of CD11/CD18 integrins but appear to have a defect in glycosylation resulting in defective expression of sialyl Lewis x (71–73).

CD18 is encoded on chromosome 21q22.3 and is the site of mutations causing LAD-1. Primary defects in the genes encoding any of the CD11 α-subunit integrins have not been seen. However, proper translation and processing of the CD18 subunit are required for both stability and proper trafficking to cell membrane of any normally synthesized CD11 subunits. Inherited defects in production or structure of CD18 subunit result in instability of the associated CD11 subunits, leading to absent or deficient lymphocyte function-associated antigen, Mac-1 (heterodimer of the CD11b/CD18 complex), and p150,95 at the cell surface. A number of specific mutations have been identified that either impair messenger ribonucleic acid (mRNA) production or alter or prevent posttranslational processing of CD18 to such a degree that detectable leukocyte integrins at the surface of neutrophils are scarce or absent. However, certain mutations lead to production of some functional CD18, leading to low levels (1% to 10%) of integrin molecules on the cell surface. A patient has been described who makes large amounts of a functionally impaired CD18.

The magnitude of the deficiency is reflected in the clinical spectrum of disease. Completely absent expression of the leukocyte adhesion proteins by resting neutrophils results in the severe phenotype in which inflammatory cytokines do not increase their expression and activated T and B cells are also deficient. By immunofluorescence flow cytometry (fluorescence-activated cell sorting [FACS] analysis), neutrophils from patients with a moderate phenotype express between 1% and 10% of the normal amount of CD11a/CD18, CD1lb/CD18, and CD11c/CD18. Currently, an LAD-1 diagnosis is confirmed by demonstrating low or absent levels of these integrins on the surface of neutrophils or lymphocytes by FACS analysis. However, there is unpublished evidence of a CD18 point mutation leading to abnormal integrin function with normal levels of surface antigen associated with a mild LAD-1 phenotype.

The functional abnormalities of neutrophils from patients with LAD-1 are predictably based on the role these molecules play in normal neutrophil function. Cells adhere poorly to endothelial cells or protein-coated surfaces. Adherence-dependent functions, including chemotaxis and aggregation, are deficient in direct relationship to the severity of the integrin deficiency. Particles coated with iC3b, which normally adhere to the CR3 (CD11b/CD18) receptor, fail to bind to or induce phagocytosis or the respiratory burst of LAD-1 neutrophils. Whereas a variety of T- and B-lymphocyte abnormalities have been described in LAD-1, other lymphocyte-adhesive molecules that are expressed normally must be sufficient to account for the fact that patients with LAD-1 do not appear to have a higher frequency of viral or protozoal infections.

Patients with severe LAD-1 experience recurrent, indolent bacterial infections primarily involving the skin, oral and genital mucosa, and respiratory and intestinal tracts. Infections usually begin shortly after birth, often with an episode of omphalitis. One of the hallmarks of severe LAD-1 is delayed separation of the umbilical cord. Infections, especially of the skin, tend to become necrotic with progressively enlarging borders, slow healing, and development of dysplastic scars. The most frequently encountered bacteria are *Staphylococcus aureus* and enteric gram-negative organisms. Like patients with severe neutropenia, patients with severe LAD-1 fail to form pus at sites of infection and are unusually susceptible to fungi such as *Candida* and *Aspergillus*. As with neutropenic patients, redness, heat, and swelling may be absent from an infected site, with only pain and fever indicating the presence and site of infection. Other than specific FACS analysis for integrin levels or specialized studies of neutrophil phagocytosis, aggregation, or spreading on glass or plastic surfaces, the only laboratory sign of severe LAD-1 is a persistent leukocytosis that may reach levels above 100,000 cells/mm^3 during acute infection, although 30,000 to 60,000 cells/mm^3 is more typical. When infection is not present, a persistent baseline neutrophil count above 12,000 cells/mm^3 in a child or young adult with a history of recurrent or unusual infections should include LAD-1 in the differential diagnosis.

Expression of even a small amount of functional leukocyte integrin molecules results in a more moderate phenotype. Although these patients also experience recurrent infections, these infections are usually less frequent and less severe and may begin or be identified later in childhood. However, the spectrum of pathogens causing these problems is similar to that seen in the severe form of LAD-1. Recurrent episodes of sinusitis, otitis, and pneumonia as well as severe gingivitis, periodontitis, and poor dentition have been particularly frequent in these patients. Infections of the lower extremities may result in indolent enlarging and ulcerating lesions that require aggressive and prolonged an-

tibiotics and débridement and may require skin grafting. These infections may become polymicrobial in type and include anaerobic organisms. These ulcers can be very difficult to manage and heal. We have found that local administration of allogeneic granulocytes topically can result in healing of these ulcers, suggesting that products of normal neutrophils may be required for wound healing. The patient's own neutrophils cannot efficiently egress from the circulation to these sites of infection.

Treatment of LAD-1 depends on the severity of the deficiency of leukocyte integrin expression and its associated clinical phenotype. All patients are likely to benefit from prophylaxis with TMP-SMX as noted for treatment of neutropenia. This antibiotic has been successfully used as antibiotic prophylaxis in other pediatric populations with abnormal neutrophil function and is active against the most common organisms causing infections in these patients. Actuarial survival data for patients with moderate LAD-1 ($N = 24$) indicate that approximately 35% survive into the fourth decade. However, earlier recognition of these patients, institution of prophylactic antibiotics, and aggressive treatment of established infection should improve the overall outlook for those with the moderate phenotype. Patients with severe LAD-1 have a poor prognosis, with more than 75% mortality in the first decade. As a result, bone marrow transplantation has become the treatment of choice for these patients with severe LAD-1, and it should be considered early because of the otherwise high mortality of affected individuals in their first year (218). Human leukocyte antigen partially mismatched bone marrow successfully engrafts in these patients, probably due to their abnormal T-cell function, making bone marrow transplantation a particularly attractive treatment. Although gene replacement therapy has not yet resulted in clinical benefit, preliminary feasibility clinical studies have been done (219), and this disease is an ideal candidate because even low levels of expression of CD18 would probably provide clinical benefit.

Disorders of Neutrophil Motility

Recurrent bacterial infections, particularly those associated with gingivitis and aphthous ulcers of the mouth, may be caused by a defect in neutrophil motility. Neutrophil motility can be assessed with use of a number of types of micropore filter chemotactic chambers (220,221). There are now a number of commercial microwell chambers available for this type of assay. In general, neutrophils are placed on one side of a porous filter or well of the agarose and buffer, or any of a number of chemotactic substances are placed on the other side. A normal donor should always be tested at the same time. Because chemotactic assays generally have a wide range of normal distribution, repeated studies may be required to confirm a mild-to-moderate defect; only profound defects of 50% of normal or less are likely to be of clinical significance. It is useful to test the cellular response of the patient to a variety of stimuli such as commercially available formyl methionyl peptide or IL-8.

Although skin windows are sometimes used to assess *in vivo* neutrophil responses, there is such a broad range of normal that this study is best interpreted at a center where large numbers of patients and normal subjects have been tested previously. This study is done by abrading the skin and then taping a sterile glass coverslip to the surface, changing the glass several times in a 24-hour period, and assessing both the number of cells per area and the normal change from predominantly neutrophils at 6 to 8 hours to predominantly monocytes at 24 hours (222).

Given the large number of proteins involved in cellular motility, it was likely that nonlethal inherited defects would be possible in either actin or one of these actin binding proteins that would cause faulty phagocytic cell motility. A number of defects have been defined which affect actin or actin regulating proteins that cause clinically deleterious defects in neutrophil mobility (223). Nunoi and colleagues have described a patient who was heterozygous for a mutant beta actin involving a G-1174 to A substitution, predicting a glutamic acid-364 to lysine substitution in and this was associated with a variety of problems including a defect in neutrophil motility (223,224). Expression of the mutant beta actin in normal cells resulted in defects in actin polymerization and in cell motility, suggesting that the abnormal mutant beta actin affected actin functions in a dominant-negative manner. Howard and colleagues originally described a patient with recurrent infections and a neutrophil motility and actin dysfunction with increased amounts of a 47-kDa protein and decreased amounts of an 89-kDa protein, a defect that they have called NAD 47/89 (225). Further analysis has shown that the overexpressed 47-kDa protein is the same as lymphocyte-specific protein 1 (LSP1). Overexpression of LSP1 could reproduce the excessive F-actin bundles formation and abnormal villus-like morphologic features seen in the patient's neutrophils (226). Furthermore this protein contains known F-actin binding domains, making it likely that overexpression of the p47 LSP1 was responsible for the morphologic and motile abnormalities characteristic of the NAD 47/89 phenotype (227).

The mammalian Rho GTPase family molecule *Rac2* plays an important role in actin remodeling in the lamellipodia of cells, including neutrophils (50,228). A patient has been described who had recurrent infections, a profound defect in neutrophil motility and a moderate defect in neutrophil oxidase activity. This patient was heterozygous for a single base pair change (G to A at nucleotide 169) in the coding sequence of *Rac2*, resulting in an asparagine for aspartic acid mutation at amino acid 57 (D57N). This is in a highly conserved region involved in GTP nucleotide binding. Functional studies showed that the D57N is a dominant-negative *Rac2* functional mutation inhibiting the action of both *Rac2* and *Rac1* in the cell, explaining the degree of defect seen in the heterozygous state (93,229–232).

Patients with inherited neutrophil specific granule deficiency to be described also have a defect in neutrophil chemotaxis *in vitro* and abnormal migration *in vivo* to skin windows. This possibly results from both the failure to release proinflammatory factors and the inability to achieve increase in certain surface receptors that normally accompanies degranulation. Patients with LAD (discussed previously) or with Chédiak-Higashi syndrome (CHS) (to be discussed) also have significant abnormalities of neutrophil migration into tissues.

ABNORMALITIES OF NEUTROPHIL GRANULE FORMATION AND CONTENT

Chédiak-Higashi Syndrome

One of the most profound defects in the formation of intracellular granules occurs in Chédiak-Higashi syndrome (CHS), a rare autosomal recessive hereditary disorder (233–239). The major morphologic abnormality in CHS is the fusion of intracellular granules with each other to form giant granules that are not uniformly distributed in the cytoplasm of the cell. The formation of giant intracellular granules is not limited to leukocytes but is also seen in other granule-containing cells, including platelets, melanocytes (from which abnormally large granules in hair can be seen), renal tubular cells, Schwann cells, thyroid follicle cells, and mast cells and pancreatic acinar cells in animal homologs of CHS. Thus, the function of cells containing the giant granules is impaired. Clinical manifestations of CHS are hypopigmenta-

tion of the skin, eyes, and hair; prolonged bleeding times; easy bruisability; recurrent infections; and abnormal natural killer cell function. The frequency of infections can be variable and in some patients is not a prominent feature. Patients may enter an "accelerated phase" in which a potentially fatal lymphoproliferative lymphoma-like disorder develops. Many patients with CHS undergo transplantation either before or at onset of the accelerated phase. A progressive severe mixed sensorimotor peripheral neuropathy develops in most patients, and nystagmus develops by the end of the second or third decade of life. Bone marrow transplantation does not prevent the neuropathy. It is possible to speculate that the vesicle sorting and formation defect in CHS might affect axonal transport leading to the neuropathy. CHS neutrophils have abnormal large granules and also exhibit a defect in motility.

Complementation studies showed that the genetic lesion in the beige mouse model of CHS is the same as in the human form of CHS and using the mouse information the CHS gene was partially localized (233). The CHS was mapped to chromosome segment lq42.1-q42.2. and cloned (234). The gene responsible for CHS was given the name *LYST* (for lysosomal trafficking regulator gene). Of interest is that this over 430,000 Da gene product has molecular features similar to the yeast vacuolar sorting protein, VPS15 (234). Most patients with CSH have mutations that lead to production of a truncated gene product and this might be the basis for different clinical phenotypes (235,236).

Studies using a yeast two-hybrid system to see what the *LYST* gene product binds to in the cells suggest interactions with known vesicular transport proteins (237). Further study has suggested that *LYST* is only the first of a newly discovered group of proteins called BEACH domain proteins (named after the Beige mouse and CHS) for the shared region (237,239,240).

There is a group of disorders including CHS, Griscelli syndrome, and Hermansky-Pudlak syndrome, which share the features of immunologic defects and pigmentation defect. In addition, the genes involved in their defects all relate to vesicle and granule formation (239).

Clinical management of CHS includes daily oral TMP-SMX prophylaxis. Bone marrow transplantation has been successful in a limited number of individuals to treat or prevent the lymphoproliferative disorder, but this does not treat the peripheral neuropathy. In some of the very early descriptions of this disorder, there were abnormalities of microtubule assembly and that administration of ascorbate (vitamin C) could partially reverse this cellular defect in both beige mice and patients with CHS (242). On that basis it has been suggested that it has become customary to treat patients with CHS vitamin C, but there are no long-term studies studies to demonstrate that this alters the clinical course of this disorder.

Myeloperoxidase Deficiency

Deficiency of the enzyme MPO in the azurophil granules of neutrophils occurs with a prevalence of approximately one in 2,000 individuals, making it the most common neutrophil abnormality by a large margin. Automated white blood cell differential counts that detect peroxidase in neutrophils by flow cytometry enabled the widespread screening of individuals for peroxidase-negative granulocytes, providing accurate prevalence estimates (155,243–246). Inherited and acquired types of MPO deficiency are recognized. Kindred studies have suggested an autosomal recessive pattern of inheritance with variable expression. The structure, organization, and expression of the gene for MPO, which is located on the long arm of chromosome 17, have been characterized (247). There is strong evidence that hereditary MPO deficiency results from both pretranslational and posttranslational abnormalities (248–250). In some patients, the gene for MPO is apparently normal however, there are only trace amounts of MPO mRNA and no proMPO or mature enzyme. Other patients with the same MPO-deficient phenotype express normal amounts of proMPO but no mature enzyme, consistent with the fact that the mutations affect the posttranslational processing of MPO.

Specific mutations have been identified for some individuals with MPO deficiency and these have provided important insights into biosynthesis of MPO (250–254). Analysis of one of these mutations, a change at amino acid 569 from arginine to tryptophan, has been shown to specifically interfere with heme binding, leading to an unstable apoprotein that does not undergo the normal posttranslational processing (253). This is consistent with the early original findings regarding lack of mature protein and trace amounts of larger sized preprocessed peptide in the mature neutrophils from a number of MPO-deficient individuals (246).

Acquired MPO deficiency is most often associated with hematologic disorders, including acute and chronic myelogenous leukemias; myelodysplastic syndrome, refractory megaloblastic anemia, and aplastic anemia. The disappearance of the MPO-deficient phenotype occurs in patients with acute myelogenous leukemia in complete remission, and relapse may be presaged by the reappearance of MPO-deficient malignant cells before leukemic cells are seen in peripheral blood smears. As in most forms of hereditary MPO deficiency, mRNA for MPO may be detectable in leukemic cells that are cytochemically negative for MPO. This may be helpful in the classification of acute leukemias (255–257). Acquired MPO deficiency has also been reported in lead intoxication (258) and ceroid lipofuscinosis and transiently during the neonatal period and pregnancy.

The function of MPO-deficient neutrophils offers some clues to the potential clinical manifestations of MPO deficiency (259). Phagocytosis, chemotaxis, and degranulation are normal, whereas the respiratory burst is often more sustained than in normal neutrophils. Microbicidal activity for bacteria is delayed but not absent. When the kinetics of bacterial killing are examined, MPO-deficient neutrophils are defective for the first 45 minutes but usually reach normal levels by 1 hour. In contrast, killing of *Candida albicans*, *Candida tropicalis*, *Candida stellatoidea*, and *Candida krusei* is absent. *Torulopsis glabrata*, *Candida parapsilosis* and *Candida pseudotropicalis* are killed normally by MPO-deficient neutrophils. These studies indicate the sensitivity of bacteria and some fungi to the MPO-independent microbicidal mechanisms of neutrophils and the complete dependence on the MPO-hydrogen peroxide-halide system for killing some clinically significant *Candida* species (155).

MPO is the most abundant granule protein in the neutrophil and plays an important role in production of hypohalous acids which have antimicrobial properties. As noted previously, following stimulation MPO neutrophils show a higher and more sustained increased production of superoxide and hydrogen peroxide suggesting that the diversion of hydrogen peroxide to other products through the action of MPO may paradoxically reduce impact of the generation of those reactive radicals that cause tissue damage (155). The availability of MPO knockout mice has also allowed more definitive assessment of the physiologic consequences of MPO deficiency, suggesting that lack of MPO can be associated with increased pathology from immune-mediated inflammation (260,261). This is associated with a delay in apoptosis by MPO-deficient neutrophils (262). Although it had been thought that MPO deficiency did not carry significant clinical significance unless other disease such as diabetes was present (244,263), recent epidemiologic assessments of MPO patients (245,259,264) suggests that MPO patients have significantly higher occurrence of severe infections and chronic inflammatory processes, but there may be a protective effect against cardiovascular damage. However, the most recent assessment did not support the suggestion by others that MPO patients might have an increased incidence of cancers. Regarding susceptibility to infection, the current consensus is that majority of patients with isolated MPO deficiency have a sufficiently low incidence of infection that, prophylactic antibiotics should be limited only to those who appear to experience recurrent infections or who have another disorder predisposing to infection (e.g., diabetes).

Specific Granule Deficiency

Because the secondary or specific granules of neutrophils contain a mobilizable store of chemotactic factor receptors (fMLP), adhesion molecules and opsonin receptors (iC3b), and cytochrome *b*, and other components (e.g., gelatinase B, lactoferrin) which all modulate the function of neutrophils, it is not surprising that patients whose neutrophils either lack or are deficient in these granules experience recurrent bacterial infections. Both congenital and acquired forms of specific granule deficiency are recognized. Congenital specific granule deficiency appears to be inherited in an autosomal recessive pattern (265). Neutrophils from neonates (266) and thermally injured patients (267,268) are also deficient in specific granules, and the magnitude of the depletion of these granules correlates with the functional impairment.

Neutrophils that are deficient in specific granules display abnormal chemotaxis *in vivo* and *in vitro*, fail to up-regulate the number of chemotactic receptors after stimulation, have an impaired respiratory burst, and do not kill bacteria normally. Microscopic, protein, mRNA, and DNA studies of leukocytes from patients with the rare inherited form of specific granule deficiency suggest a more complex abnormality than simply a failure to produce specific granules. Not only are neutrophils missing specific granules, but eosinophils are also missing their normal complement of large, eosin-staining cytoplasmic granules, making them difficult to distinguish from neutrophils at the light microscopic level (269). Neutrophils lack seven of the usual proteins found in specific granules including lactoferrin, vitamin B_{12} binding protein, neutrophil procollagenase, and others (270,271). Neutrophil marrow precursors are markedly deficient in the mRNA transcripts for these proteins. Neutrophils are also missing defensins and some other but not all proteins that are usually found in the azurophil granules. For example, they have normal amounts of MPO. The morphologically abnormal eosinophils lack three of the eosinophil-specific granule proteins, eosinophil-cationic protein, eosinophil-derived neurotoxin, and major basic protein (269). Even though there is only a single gene for lactoferrin, these patients make normal amounts of lactoferrin in tears and nasal secretions but, as noted, fail to transcribe mRNA for lactoferrin in myeloid precursors (270). When taken together, all of this information pointed to a genetic defect in some regulatory element involved in gene activation during myeloid differentiation. In the course of studying the effects of knocking out DNA binding regulatory protein genes known to be involved in the late stages of myeloid cell development, it was noticed that a knock-out mouse deficient in the late-acting myeloid differentiation regulator C/EBP(epsilon) had hematologic features similar to human patients with specific granule deficiency (272). This led to the discovery of clinically significant mutations in the C/EBP (epsilon) gene in specific granule deficient patients, and was sufficient to explain their hematologic abnormalities and clinical disease phenotype (273,274).

Patients with congenital specific granule deficiency experience recurrent bacterial infections that usually begin in early childhood. No particular predilection for certain bacterial pathogens has been noted. As with LAD, the inflammatory response at the infected site is often minimal, which underestimates the severity of the infection. Cutaneous, sinopulmonary, and otic infections are the most common. Treatment is directed toward the specific pathogens, and therapy must usually be prolonged. No trials of antibiotic prophylaxis or experimental therapies have been reported, but it has become practice to place these patients on prophylactic TMP-SMX and itraconazole. As seen with patients with LAD, large non-healing ulcers often develop, reflecting not only susceptibility to infections, but probably as with LAD there is a problem with wound healing because of the lack of critical neutrophil enzymes (possibly the absence of gelatinase B in the case of specific granule deficiency).

Chronic Granulomatous Diseases of Childhood

Chronic granulomatous diseases (CGDs) are a group of four inherited disorders resulting from mutations in the genes encoding four of the six subunits of the phagocyte NADPH oxidase shown in Fig. 3.3 (129–131,134,143–146,277,278). All forms of CGD (deficiencies in gp91phox, p47phox, p22phox or p67phox) have a common phenotype characterized by the failure of phagocytic cells to generate superoxide and the derivative microbicidal products hydrogen peroxide and hypochlorous acid, associated with recurrent infections complicated by excessive inflammation and granuloma formation. No patient deficient in p40phox has been reported, and it is not known what phenotype, if any, would result from a defect in that component. In the section on defects in neutrophil motility, a patient heterozygous for a dominant-negative mutation of Rac2 was described (93,229–232). While this patient did suffer from recurrent infections, there was only a modest defect in stimulated phagocyte oxidant production, but had a more profound defect in cell motility that is not seen with CGD. It is perhaps a semantic distinction; however, that patient was not considered to have the CGD phenotype because of the lack of granuloma formation and some other hallmarks of the "classic" CGD.

The establishment of a registry in the United States (279) and ongoing demographic studies from Sweden (280) and Japan (281,282) suggest a frequency of CGD of more than five living patients per million. There is also online access to current catalogued mutations of CGD patients (*www.uta.fi/imt/bioinfo/*) (283). Current mortality for X-linked CGD (gp91phox deficiency) patients is 3% to 5% per year, while that for the p47phox autosomal recessive CGD is approximately 1% to 2% per year. This is a significant improvement from the high rate of early childhood mortality 25 years ago. There are currently more adult patients with CGDs than in the past. This is probably due to improvements in both diagnosis and treatment.

The defect in oxidase activity in CGDs involves neutrophils, monocytes, eosinophils, and certain fixed tissue macrophages. The normal array of microbicidal oxidants is not produced, and these patients are susceptible to recurrent, often life-threatening infections. These patients also tend to form granulomata in all tissues, particularly in lungs, liver, and spleen. Formation of a large granuloma can occasionally obstruct the urinary or gastrointestinal tracts, and granulomatous colitis is also a complication seen in a significant subset of patients (134,278,279).

GENETICS

As noted previously, there are four genetic forms of CGD, one X-linked and the other three autosomal recessive, each resulting from a defect in a distinct component required for activation of the NADPH oxidase. For each genetic form of CGD, the defective or missing gene product, chromosome location, and frequency are indicated in Fig. 3.3 (129,130,134,143–146,278–284). The most common form of CGD is X-linked, resulting from defects in the gene encoding the gp91phox large subunit of flavocytochrome b-558. Many types of distinct defects in this gene in a large number of affected kindreds have been documented, including deletions, inversions, and point mutations (277,283). Depending on the X-linked kindred, gp91phox mRNA transcripts may be present or absent. No flavocytochrome is detectable in most individuals, but a nonfunctional flavocytochrome protein is made in some cases (285,286). A rare autosomal form of CGD resulting from defective gene encoding p22phox is phenotypically similar to the X-linked CGD in that no flavocytochrome b-558 is detectable in most cases, but a nonfunctional protein can be made with certain point mutations (283,287,288). We have found by overdeveloping immunoprotein electrophoresis Western blots that patients with X-linked CGD who have no detectable gp91phox, have a trace amount of p22phox detectable, but that patients who have p22phox autosomal-recessive CGD making no detectable p22phox also have no detectable gp91phox. Thus, it is possible to use the protein electrophoresis Western immunoblot to distinguish these two types of CGD. Thus, normal transcripts for both subunits are required for either translation or stability of the subunits, although the restrictions for p22phox synthesis or stability are not as strict as those for gp91phox in differentiating myeloid cells. The second most common form of CGD affects the cytoplasmic p47phox. With these patients, p47phox transcripts are present, but no p47phox protein is detectable in their phagocytes. Although a number of mutations in this gene have been defined, more than 90% of the mutant alleles have a GT dinucleotide deletion at the start of the second exon (288–291). This mutation results in a frameshift leading to a shortened and unstable protein. The relatively high frequency of a specific mutation in a number of racial groups is unusual without some specific cause. Two pseudogenes highly homologous to the gene encoding p47phox and containing this mutation has been identified. It is likely that recombination of these pseudogenes (gene conversion) with the p47phox gene may account for the high frequency of this mutation (292,293). Another rare genetic form of CGD is a result of mutations identified in the gene encoding the cytoplasmic p67phox protein (284,294–296).

DIAGNOSIS

When CGD is suspected (see diagnostic indicators in following paragraphs), a screening assay should be performed. For more than 25 years, some variation of the nitroblue tetrazolium (NBT) dye reduction slide test has been the standard screening assay (297), but fluorescence-activated cell sorting (FACS) flow cytometric assays have been developed that are rapid and more accurate (286,298,299). Because many hospital laboratories at major medical centers have FACS equipment for lymphocyte phenotype analysis, and the assay is simple to perform, this has become the screening assay of choice. If a diagnosis of CGD is made by use of such screening assays, the results should be confirmed with a quantitative measurement of superoxide output by purified neutrophils using the ferricytochrome *c* reduction assay or a chemoluminescence assay (286,300). Such a quantitative assay is also useful for determining whether the defect in superoxide output is complete or partial because production of 2% or more superoxide relative to normal neutrophils can be associated with a less severe phenotype.

The principle behind the NBT assay is that when neutrophils produce superoxide, the yellow, soluble NBT is reduced to insoluble blue-black formazan, which precipitates on and within activated cells. Normal neutrophils produce a "positive" NBT test result, whereas CGD neutrophils are "negative." A normal control assay should always be done, and more than 95% of neutrophils in that control specimen should be positive. If not, then the test is invalid. It is also important that the assay be run for only 20 minutes before the reaction is terminated. Neutrophils from a few patients with X-linked CGD and many of the patients with the autosomal recessive, p47phox-deficient form of CGD may make trace amounts of superoxide. If the NBT assay is allowed to develop too long, formazan product accumulates in neutrophils from such patients, leading to a falsely "normal" phenotype. These principles (inclusion of a normal control specimen and proper timing of the reaction) also apply to the FACS assay, which measures the oxidation of dihydrorhodamine 123 byproducts of the phagocyte NADPH oxidase. Whereas the NBT test generally involves subjective scoring of formazan precipitate, the FACS assay involves machine-generated quantitative assessment of oxidase production on an individual cell basis.

The screening assay should be performed on both the affected individual and the mother because this may provide an early indication of the genotype. Female carriers of the X-linked form of CGD demonstrate phenotypic mosaicism of oxidase activity between individual neutrophils because of the normal embryonic process of lyonization, or inactivation of one of the two X chromosomes in different myeloid precursor cells. This mosaicism (a mixture of NBT-positive and NBT-negative neutrophils; or two distinct peaks of fluorescent-bright and fluorescent-negative neutrophils in the FACS assay) (286,297–299) is pathognomonic of the X-linked CGD female carrier state. A female carrier can occasionally show extremes of lyonization in which 5% or less of neutrophils are normal or vice versa. The extreme CGD phenotype at the cellular level in these carriers is generally not associated with increased susceptibility to infection. However, X-linked CGD female carriers with less than 5% oxidase normal neutrophils can have infections characteristic of CGD and may be misdiagnosed as having an autosomal recessive form of CGD. The FACS assay is particularly sensitive at detecting neutrophils of the normal phenotype at a level even below 1%, thus revealing the X-linked carrier state in this setting. None of the assays is capable of reliably detecting the X-linked carrier state when lyonization has resulted in 95% or more of the neutrophils having the normal phenotype. Because of this, it is not possible to distinguish this situation from the significant number of cases of X-linked CGD that are a result of new mutations. This distinction has important implications for genetic counseling of the mother regarding the risk for CGD in children of any future pregnancies. Testing of the proband's maternal grandmother and the mother's sisters as well as the proband's siblings can sometimes clarify these issues. Although the etiology is unclear, there is an association of the female carrier state of X-linked CGD with discoid lupus erythematosus, which may hint at the genotype of the proband when it is present (279,301,302).

In specialized centers, protein electrophoretic immunoblot analysis of neutrophils for the presence of oxidase proteins together with cell-free assays of oxidase activation using cytosol and membrane fractions from neutrophils can be used to identify the genetic subtype of most patients with CGD (286). Knowledge of the genetic subtype can be helpful for family genetic counseling and for guiding more detailed mutational analysis at the mRNA and genomic DNA level. However, detailed knowledge of the genotype or specific mutation responsible for the CGD currently does not alter the approach to the clinical care of the patient as outlined later. There is some evidence that as a group, patients with the p47phox autosomal recessive type of CGD, or

patients with any type of CGD genotype in which more than 0.5% of the normal rate of superoxide production occurs, have a better prognosis (279). However, "mild" or "severe" infection history can characterize a particular CGD kindred regardless of other laboratory findings, and the clinical history of even siblings may vary considerably.

Advances in methods for mutational analysis and ease of sequencing together with a strong scientific interest in mapping critical functional domains of the oxidase proteins and identifying mutational "hot spots" have led to mutational analysis of hundreds of CGD patients worldwide (277,283). As noted previously, a portion of this information is contained in a database available through a website (*www.helsinki.fi/science/signal/databases/x-cgdbase*). In addition to the scientific value, mutation analysis is important to patients and families for confirmation of CGD genotype and for prenatal diagnosis. Although gene therapy (to be discussed) is not yet developed as a working therapy for CGD, it is an area of active investigation. If gene therapy is developed for treatment of CGD, it may be important to know the specific mutation responsible for the CGD. Mutation analysis for CGD is currently available only in a small number of research centers, requires considerable time and effort, and may not be successful in identifying all mutations. However, current advances in techniques for identifying mutations and in automation of sequence analysis may eventually make mutation analysis for CGD cheap, rapid, and accurate (285).

CLINICAL MANIFESTATIONS

The clinical presentation of CGD can be varied (134). Testing may be prompted by the knowledge that a sibling or other family member has CGD. A family history of unexplained deaths of infant or young boys may hint at X-linked CGD. However, the severity of the defect can be variable, and infections can be episodic. Particularly with the autosomal recessive forms of CGD, the average age at diagnosis is almost 10 years, considerably later than that seen with X-linked CGD. Increasingly, the medical community has become aware that the first severe infection in a CGD patient may not appear until the middle teen years or even far into adulthood (134,278,279,303). This highlights the importance of screening for CGD in teenagers or adults with even one episode of a type of infection or with a pathogen suggestive of CGD. CGD should be part of the differential diagnosis in patients with unexplained pneumonia with *S. aureus*, *Aspergillus*, *Nocardia*, *Burkholderia* (formerly *Pseudomonas*) *cepacia*, or *Serratia*. These and other organisms that are catalase-positive are particularly pathogenic in patients with CGD. Any child with a pneumonia that does not rapidly resolve with conventional therapy should have a CGD screening assay. Particularly pathognomonic of CGD is an osteomyelitis with *Serratia marcescens* or any type of infection with one of the organisms newly reclassified within the *Burkholderia* group (*B. cepacia*, *B. pseudomallei*, or *B. gladioli*) and relapses with these organisms is common (304,305). It is particularly important to note that *Aspergillus* infection in CGD either may present as an indolent infection associated with a dense infiltrate or may present acutely with severe respiratory distress associated with a panlobular miliary or reticulonodular infiltrate. The latter presentation as a first severe infection in an older child or adult patient not previously known to have CGD may be misdiagnosed as hypersensitivity pneumonitis with potentially fatal consequences when *Aspergillus* is seen in sputum or bronchial lavage. CGD testing and recognition of the invasive nature of this *Aspergillus* infection are critical to institution of appropriate lifesaving therapy (see later) (307,308). In addition to *Aspergillus*, a large number of fungi have been demonstrated to cause infection in patients with CGD (308). *Paecilomyces* is a CGD pathogen (309). However, many microbiology diagnostic laboratories misclassify this organism as a *Penicillium* and thus report it as a contaminant or nonpathogenic species. Therefore, a pneumonia or soft tissue infection from which "*Penicillium*" is the only isolate also should prompt testing for CGD. Unexplained liver abscess is an indication for CGD testing. Needle biopsy of the liver often isolates no organism and surgical removal of large nodular granulomatous lesions in the liver may be required. CGD patients also have an increased susceptibility to *Mycobacterium tuberculosis*, and this infection in a child in populations in which this infection is uncommon is an indication for CGD testing. In *Mycobacterium tuberculosis* endemic parts of the world, this infection can sometimes be one of the most common severe CGD infections. Chronic infections with cytomegalovirus can also be seen in a small subset of CGD patients, particularly those on corticosteroids for management of granulomatous colitis or other granuloma problem, although such infection is not particularly diagnostic of CGD.

In some patients, problems with granuloma formation and other inflammatory manifestations of CGD may predominate over problems with infections (134,310–313). These patients may first present from early childhood through young adulthood with symptoms of partial gastric outlet obstruction or dysphagia resulting from obstructive granuloma of the pylorus or esophagus. Granuloma of the bladder may present as deep pain associated with urination or as acute bladder outlet obstruction (134,314). CGD may occasionally go unrecognized, carrying a diagnosis of inflammatory bowel disease with symptoms of abdominal pain and chronic diarrhea, with or without rectal fissures or abscesses, and with or without radiographic and histologic evidence of a granulomatous process in the small or large intestine (315,316). If such patients should also have an infection of a type or with a pathogen suggestive of CGD, then CGD screening should be done. Inflammatory ocular problems, including a chorioretinitis (317), can be seen in a small subset of patients. An arthritis resembling juvenile rheumatoid arthritis may develop in a few patients (318).

MANAGEMENT: PROPHYLAXIS

Infection prophylaxis is an important element of the care of patients with CGD. Particular attention to oral hygiene can control the gingivitis and aphthous ulcers that affect a subset of (but not all) patients. Use of chlorhexidine mouthwash and/or bicarbonate-hydrogen peroxide–based toothpaste for brushing can help. Prompt local care of cuts and minor skin infections with washing, hydrogen peroxide, and application of topical antibiotic are recommended. The activities and social interactions of children with CGD should not be limited. The only exception is that patients must avoid extremely dusty environments and should specifically not use power mowers, should not dig holes in the ground, and should carefully avoid sites of dispersion of decaying organic material such as spreading animal manure or garden mulch piles. They should also avoid construction sites and should not be near or participate in major renovations of old buildings. All of these activities are associated with high risk for fungal pneumonia, particularly the acute reticulonodular form. Daily prophylactic administration of oral TMP-SMX has been shown to significantly decrease the frequency of bacterial infections (319,320). Oral ciprofloxacin is a good choice to use in sulfa-allergic individuals. The prophylactic daily administration of itraconazole to patients with CGD has been shown to be efficacious as fungus prophylaxis and is well tolerated (321). It has been shown that prophylactic administration of subcutaneously

injected recombinant interferon gamma results in a more than 70% reduction in infection risk in CGD patients, leading to regulatory approval of this treatment (322). This protective effect is additive to the effect of prophylactic antibiotics and appears to be sustained for long periods (323,324). It is currently recommended that all CGD patients receive both prophylactic antibiotics and prophylactic interferon gamma. At the doses of interferon gamma recommended (50 μg/m^2 of body surface, 3 days a week), there are few side effects. Occasional fever, malaise, or headache can be handled with acetaminophen. These symptoms or neutropenia may rarely require dose reduction. The mechanism of protective effect is not understood but relates to partial amelioration of the defect in phagocyte oxidative burst in only a small subset of individuals, and most CGD patients do not have any change in their oxidase activity (325,326). This prophylactic effect has been reproduced in a CGD knock-out mouse model (327). A first manifestation of infection in a patient with CGD receiving prophylactic interferon gamma may be the new appearance of fever associated with dosing of the interferon. This suggests that this fever results from a synergy between the exogenously administered interferon gamma and endogenous cytokines generated as a result of infection. Because interferon gamma administration requires chronic injections and is expensive, common questions are whether certain patients may benefit more than others and whether it could or should be used to treat infection rather than prophylactically. Unfortunately, no studies have been done to answer these two questions.

MANAGEMENT: TREATMENT OF INFECTIONS AND COMPLICATIONS

Despite these maneuvers, patients with CGD may get infections including those that are life threatening. The approach to diagnosis and management of infections in patients with CGD follows many of the general principles applicable to patients with defects in host defense (134). Early recognition of infection, diligent attempts to identify a pathogen, adequate doses of antibiotics, and relatively long courses of treatment ensure the best outcome. In addition, patients with CGD have such extensive granuloma formation associated with infection that in a number of circumstances, partial or complete surgical extirpation of infected tissue is required to effect a cure (134,307,328–330). Infections tend to occur with the catalase-positive pathogens indicated in the previous discussion. Although the frequency of deep fungal infections has not increased, fungal infections now account for more than 50% of total infections seen in patients with CGD (134,307,308,320).

The most common infections are cellulitis and lymphadenitis. These often respond to local care and oral antibiotics, but lymphadenitis may require surgical treatment and intravenous antibiotics. Liver abscess and pneumonia are the most common deep organ infections, followed by infection of bone. Computed tomography (CT) of the chest is far more sensitive for early diagnosis of pneumonia in CGD patients than is chest radiography. Because early diagnosis may allow a shorter course of therapy or oral therapy for resolution, may require shorter hospitalization, and may catch an infection of the lung before spread to ribs or vertebrae, the early use of CT for diagnosis and follow-up is highly recommended. Because the only sign of liver abscess in a CGD patient may be intermittent fever or malaise, or liver abscess may silently complicate major infection elsewhere, CT of the liver is also highly recommended as part of an "infection workup" in a CGD patient. For liver abscess, magnetic resonance imaging actually appears to be more sensitive than CT at picking up additional early lesions and should be performed before proceeding to surgical drainage, but it is often more convenient to obtain liver CT at the time of chest CT in the context of the initial search for the site of a suspected infection.

Infections in lung or liver may occasionally be accompanied by metastatic infection at other sites including bone, spleen, or brain. With *Nocardia* infections, it is particularly important to perform CT of the head and bone scans. It is therefore important to have a low threshold for embarking on a more extensive workup even when a single site of infection is obvious. Bacteremia and meningitis are uncommon; bacteremia is most commonly seen with infection with *Burkholderia* species or other gram-negative organisms. Signs and symptoms of infection may occasionally be limited to malaise or pain. Fever may be absent or intermittent. With pneumonia, the presence of cough and shortness of breath are variable. Neutrophilia is not always present. An increase of the erythrocyte sedimentation rate from some previous baseline value can be a valuable indicator of infection and, when elevated, is a useful parameter to monitor during treatment. The erythrocyte sedimentation rate is a more reliable indicator of infection than is elevation of the white blood cell count.

Identification of a pathogen may often require biopsy for histologic examination and culture. Advances in interventional radiology have made it safe and convenient to perform needle biopsy under CT guidance of lung, liver, or other tissue (308). When histologic identification of a pathogen by cytopathologic examination with special stains is combined with results from microbiology, needle biopsy can identify a pathogen in more than 80% of cases, particularly if repeated biopsy is performed when no organism is found by a first biopsy. Whereas surgical extirpation or débridement of liver abscess (which is generally a solid granulomatous mass with microabscesses) or major bone infection (328–330) continue to be critical for eradication of infection and shortening the time to cure, surgical intervention in pulmonary infections appears to be needed only when there is a large segment of devitalized lung or there is clear spread of infection to bone. Surgical drainage, débridement, or extirpation of nonviable tissue is essential in treatment of extensive infections of lung, liver, or bone. In cases of pneumonia, bronchoscopy is often done, but particularly with fungal infections, it often will not yield a credible pathogen. For this reason, needle biopsy is the preferred diagnostic procedure unless the lesion is not reachable by the transthoracic approach. Infection with more than one pathogen in patients with CGD is not uncommon, particularly in cases of pneumonia. For example, mixed infection with *Aspergillus* species and *Nocardia* or *Burkholderia* species may be seen. Sometimes the second infection may become apparent because it is not covered in the specific treatment for the first identified pathogen.

As noted, pneumonia due to either *Burkholderia* species (particularly *B. cepacia*) or *Aspergillus* species is generally life-threatening in patients with CGD. With *B. cepacia*, patients often have high temperature with shortness of breath. In addition, the infection may progress rapidly in these patients. Furthermore, in many centers, this organism may be highly resistant to many first-line antibiotics. *Aspergillus* pneumonia usually presents with insidious onset, appearing as dense segmental or lobar infiltrates on the chest radiograph (307). Extension to ribs or vertebrae is a grave prognostic sign (134,307). While in the past only amphotericin B or lipid formulations of amphotericin B were available, the availability of voriconazole, which is very active against *Aspergillus* species, has changed the way fungus infection is treated in CGD. We have found this agent to be very effective for deep tissue infections of lung or bone even when treatment is by oral administration. We recommend using the maximum dosing of voriconazole recommended by the manufacturer, and that treatment is at least for 6 weeks. Segmental and

occasionally lobar resection of devitalized tissue is needed when the lesion is very large and there is clear evidence of progression. Extension to bony structures may also require débridement. In some centers, daily granulocyte transfusions may be used, but this should be reserved for situations where progression of the lesion is evident despite appropriate antibiotic therapy because this can lead to HLA sensitization, which both limits the use of future granulocyte transfusion and could interfere with future plans for stem cell transplantation (331). Transfused granulocytes should be ABO matched, should be obtained by centrifugation leukapheresis, and should not be irradiated because this adversely affects oxidase activity (332). There are no studies demonstrating efficacy of granulocyte transfusions in the treatment of CGD patients, but the transfused granulocytes do reach sites of infection, and there is in vitro evidence of synergy of fungal killing by the combination of small numbers of normal neutrophils mixed with a larger number of CGD neutrophils (333). As noted previously, *Aspergillus* pneumonia in CGD patients may present as an acute febrile illness with shortness of breath associated with a miliary infiltrate on the chest radiograph affecting the entire field of both lungs. In this setting, early compromise of oxygenation can be life-threatening. Because this diffusion defect appears to be exacerbated by the exuberant granuloma formation characteristic of CGD, short-term use of steroids at an equivalent of 1 to 1.5 mg/kg of prednisone for 4 or 5 days may be lifesaving. Of course this must be done only under coverage with a potent anti-*Aspergillus* agent such as voriconazole. Although theoretically this might also compromise host defense against the fungal infection, keeping the steroid dosing to less than a week and instituting aggressive antifungal therapy have led to cure of this type of infection in most cases. Antifungal therapy continued for 6 weeks is typically effective for treatment of most fungal pneumonias in CGD, although in practice with oral voriconazole, treatment is often continued until complete radiologic resolution, which can take 8 to 12 weeks.

In approximately 20% of infections in patients with CGD, no organism is isolated despite multiple biopsies and bronchoscopy and even surgical débridement. Empirical therapy for infection should begin with antibacterial therapy aimed at the most likely organisms in that setting. With pneumonias in patients receiving TMP-SMX prophylaxis, *Staphylococcus* is rarely a pathogen and is easy to isolate when it is present. When no organism is isolated, empirical therapy with high-dose intravenous TMP-SMX plus ceftriaxone (or levofloxacin in cephalosporin or sulfa allergic patients) appears to be most successful. If infection progresses with this regimen, then levofloxacin or imipenem-cilastatin can be added. If 10 to 14 days of this approach suggest that the infection is progressing, then empirical antifungal therapy with voriconazole must be initiated after repeated biopsy. In certain settings, such as acute presentation with the reticulonodular, panlobular pattern, it is important to begin voriconazole immediately.

Obstructive granulomata of the gastrointestinal or urinary tract may result from infection or may occur in the absence of any apparent infectious process (134,310–317). Symptoms of gastrointestinal granuloma may include difficulty swallowing, early satiety, unexplained periodic vomiting, or just chronic indolent abdominal pain. The gastrointestinal granulomatous process may occasionally be indistinguishable from Crohn disease or ulcerative colitis, involving chronic diarrhea and abdominal pain, except that it is occurring in a patient with CGD. Instrumentation and biopsy should be done with caution but may be helpful in diagnosis. Because patients with CGD are particularly susceptible to *Clostridium difficile*, this pathogen must be excluded as a cause of the problem. Genitourinary tract granulomata may present as bladder discomfort or pain or as acute bladder outlet obstruction. In this setting, surgical correction of the process should be avoided, because trauma may exacerbate the process. For both the gastrointestinal and the genitourinary obstructive granulomatous processes, if no pathogen is identified, an empirical course of antibiotics is recommended, together with starting a course of steroids. There is probably only a slightly increased infection risk associated with steroid use, but patients should be monitored closely. A dose in the range of 0.5 to at most 1 mg/kg of prednisone daily for 2 weeks is recommended, followed by a taper because CGD obstructive granulomata are often responsive to steroids. The taper should aim at rapidly progressing to an alternate-day regimen, when no steroid is administered on one of the days. The taper can then be extended for several weeks. A patient may rarely need a repeated course or even require long-term alternate-day low doses to prevent repeated obstruction. Sometimes only extraordinarily low alternate-day dosing is required to prevent the problem. In the case of CGD-related colitis with chronic diarrhea, if *C. difficile* is ruled out, a prolonged empirical course of a combination of metronidazole and ciprofloxacin is recommended. This may be combined after a while with a course of steroids in the manner indicated before. In approximately two thirds of cases, this will control the colitis. For the others, this may remain a prolonged intractable problem, often of greater concern to the patient than infection. There is one report of the successful use of cyclosporine in this setting (334). There is also a report of a dramatic response of CGD-related colitis to treatment with G-CSF (335). We have had limited experience with use of infliximab (anti–tumor necrosis factor therapy) to treat Crohn's-like colitis in CGD with good outcome. The concern is that the combination of the transient host defense defect in lymphocyte/macrophage function induced by the infliximab together with the CGD defect in oxidase activity would put the patient at increase risk of infection, so that at this time we recommend limiting this to patients with severe colitis for whom no other treatment options have worked.

FUTURE PROSPECTS FOR BONE MARROW TRANSPLANTATION AND GENE THERAPY

Bone marrow transplantation has been performed for CGD (336–343) and successful engraftment can result in permanent cure of the disorder. Complications of the procedure have included failure of the graft, graft-versus-host disease, and fatal progression of infection present at the time of transplantation. The availability of a human leukocyte antigen-identical matched donor is correlated with much better outcome, and transplantation should be a consideration for a patient with CGD when such a donor is available. On balance, the risks of bone marrow transplantation when there is no fully human leukocyte antigen-identical donor appear to be greater than with conventional therapy. Work is in progress to try to increase the safety of such transplants by using non-myeloablative approaches to conditioning, but such approaches may be associated with a lower rate of engraftment, particularly in children than seen with conventional ablative conditioning transplants (342,343). Advances in transplantation procedures may change this equation and make allogeneic transplantation a more general consideration for patients with CGD.

As noted previously, bone marrow transplantation can cure CGD, and the genes for all four genetic forms of CGD have been cloned. This has raised the theoretical possibility of developing gene therapy for CGD by targeting hematopoietic progenitor cells from CGD with the normal oxidase gene. Preliminary results of phase I human clinical trials of gene therapy for the p47phox-deficient and X-linked (gp91phox deficient) forms of CGD have been reported (344–346). These trials involved one or more cycles of retrovirus-mediated gene transfer into autolo-

gous hematopoietic CD34$^+$ progenitor cells cultured short term ex vivo with a retrovirus vector to transfer corrective CGD genes and then reinfused without any previous conditioning of the recipient to suppress bone marrow. After this infusion of gene-corrected autologous hematopoietic progenitors, small numbers of oxidase-normal granulocytes were detected in the peripheral blood at a level of 1 in 500 to 1 in 30,000 granulocytes for up to 14 months. Although this is an encouraging demonstration of feasibility, it points out that considerable further development of gene therapy techniques is required before any clinical benefit from this technique can be expected. Some promising approaches may involve the use of vectors based on the human immunodeficiency virus (a lentivector), which may better target the primitive non-dividing stem cells (347).

REFERENCES

1. Yawata Y. *Atlas of blood diseases: cytology and histology.* St. Louis: Mosby, 1996.
2. Rich RR, Fleisher TA, Shearer WT, et al, eds. *Clinical immunology: principles and practice.* St. Louis: New York, 2001.
3. Cornbleet PJ. Clinical utility of the band count. *Clin Lab Med* 2002;22:101.
4. Koller M, Wick M, Muhr G. Decreased leukotriene release from neutrophils after severe trauma: role of immature cells. *Inflammation* 2001;25:53.
5. Hoffmann K, Dreger CK, Olins AL, et al. Mutations in the gene encoding the lamin B receptor produce an altered nuclear morphology in granulocytes (Pelger-Huet anomaly). *Nat Genet* 2002;31:410.
6. Dell'Angelica EC, Mullins C, Caplan S, et al. Lysosome-related organelles. *FASEB J* 2000;14:1265.
7. Borregaard N. Development of neutrophil granule diversity. *Ann NY Acad Sci* 1997;832:62.
8. Ganz T, Weiss J. Antimicrobial peptides of phagocytes and epithelia. *Semin Hematol* 1997;34:343.
9. Van den Steen PE, Dubois B, Nelissen I, et al. Biochemistry and molecular biology of gelatinase B or matrix metalloproteinase-9 (MMP-9). *Crit Rev Biochem Mol Biol* 2002;37:375.
10. Karlsson A, Dahlgren C. Assembly and activation of the neutrophil NADPH oxidase in granule membranes. *Antioxid Redox Signal* 2002;4:49.
11. Tomasinsig L, Scocchi M, Di Loreto C, et al. Inducible expression of an antimicrobial peptide of the innate immunity in polymorphonuclear leukocytes. *J Leukoc Biol* 2002;72:1003.
12. Burn TC, Petrovick MS, Hohaus S, et al. Monocyte chemoattractant protein-1 gene is expressed in activated neutrophils and retinoic acid-induced human myeloid cell lines. *Blood* 1994;84:2776.
13. Garcia-Ramallo E, Marques T, Prats N, et al. Resident cell chemokine expression serves as the major mechanism for leukocyte recruitment during local inflammation. *J Immunol* 2002;169:6467.
14. Scapini P, Lapinet-Vera JA, Gasperini S, et al. The neutrophil as a cellular source of chemokines. *Immunol Rev* 2000;177:195.
15. Kuhns DB, Nelson EL, Alvord WG, et al. Fibrinogen induces IL-8 synthesis in human neutrophils stimulated with formyl-methionyl-leucyl-phenylalanine or leukotriene B(4). *J Immunol* 2001;167:2869.
16. Kobayashi SD, Voyich JM, Somerville GA, et al. An apoptosis-differentiation program in human polymorphonuclear leukocytes facilitates resolution of inflammation. *J Leukoc Biol* 2003;73:315.
17. Malech HL, Root RK, Gallin JI. Structural analysis of human neutrophil migration: Centriole, microtubule and microfilament orientation and function during chemotaxis. *J Cell Biol* 1997;75:666.
18. Stossel TP. From signal to pseudopod: how cells control cytoplasmic actin assembly. *J Biol Chem* 1989;264:18261.
19. Glogauer M, Hartwig J, Stossel T. Endocytic protein intersectin-l regulates actin assembly via Cdc42 and N-WASP. *J Cell Biol* 2000;150:785.
20. Eddy RJ, Pierini LM, Maxfield FR. microtubule asymmetry during neutrophil polarization and migration. *Mol Biol Cell* 2002;13:4470.
21. Price TH, Chatta GS, Dale DC. Effect of recombinant granulocyte colony-stimulating factor on neutrophil kinetics in normal young and elderly humans. *Blood* 1996;88:335.
22. Athens JW, Haab OP, Raab SO, et al. Leukokinetic studies. IV The total blood, circulatory and marginal pools and the granulocyte turnover rate in normal subjects. *J Clin Invest* 1961;40:989.
23. Hendrix CW, Flexner C, MacFarland RT, et al. Pharmacokinetics and safety of AMD-3100, a novel antagonist of the CXCR-4 chemokine receptor, in human volunteers. *Antimicrob Agents Chemother* 2000;44:1667.
24. Nagase H, Miyamasu M, Yamaguchi M, et al. Cytokine-mediated regulation of CXCR4 expression in human neutrophils. *J Leukoc Biol* 2002;71:711.
25. Yamashiro S, Kamohara H, Wang JM, et al. Phenotypic and functional change of cytokine-activated neutrophils: inflammatory neutrophils are heterogeneous and enhance adaptive immune responses. *J Leukoc Biol* 2001;69:698.
26. McDermott DH, Murphy PM. Chemokines and their receptors in infectious disease. *Semin Immunopathol* 2000;22:393.

27. Zhelev DV, Alteraifi A. Signaling in the motility responses of the human neutrophil. *Ann Biomed Eng* 2002;30:356.

28. Haribabu B, Richardson RM, Verghese MW, et al. Function and regulation of chemoattractant receptors. *Immunol Res* 2000;22:271.

29. McKenzie SE, Schreiber AD. Fc gamma receptors in phagocytes. *Curr Opin Hematol* 1998;5:16.

30. Strzelecka-Kiliszek A, Kwiatkowska K, Sobota A. Lyn and Syk kinases are sequentially engaged in phagocytosis mediated by Fc gamma R. *J Immunol* 2002;169:6787.

31. Kim MK, Pan XQ, Huang ZY, et al. Fc gamma receptors differ in their structural requirements for interaction with the tyrosine kinase Syk in the initial steps of signaling for phagocytosis. *Clin Immunol* 2001;98:125.

32. Berton G, Lowell CA. Integrin signalling in neutrophils and macrophages. *Cell Signal* 1999;11:621.

33. Turutin DV, Kubareva EA, Pushkareva MA, et al. Activation of NF-kappaB transcription factor in human neutrophils by sulphatides and L-selectin cross-linking. *FEBS Lett* 2003;536:241.

34. Melander F, Andersson T, Dib K. Fgr but not Syk tyrosine kinase is a target for beta2 integrin-induced c-Cbl-mediated ubiquitination in adherent human neutrophils. *Biochem J* 2003;370:687.

35. Kurt-Jones EA, Mandell L, Whitney C, et al. Role of toll-like receptor 2 (TLR2) in neutrophil activation: GM-CSF enhances TLR2 expression and TLR2-mediated interleukin 8 responses in neutrophils. *Blood* 2002;100:1860.

36. Sakamoto C, Suzuki K, Hato F, et al. Antiapoptotic effect of granulocyte colony-stimulating factor, granulocyte-macrophage colony-stimulating factor, and cyclic AMP on human neutrophils: protein synthesis-dependent and protein synthesis-independent mechanisms and the role of the Janus kinase-STAT pathway. *Int J Hematol* 2003;77:60.

37. Scapini P, Nardelli B, Nadali G, et al. G-CSF-stimulated neutrophils are a prominent source of functional BLyS. *J Exp Med* 2003;197:297.

38. Epling-Burnette PK, Garcia R, Bai F, et al. Carboxy-terminal truncated STAT5 is induced by interleukin-2 and GM-CSF in human neutrophils. *Cell Immunol* 2002;217:1.

39. Hoffmeyer F, Witte K, Schmidt RE. The high-affinity Fc gamma RI on PMN: regulation of expression and signal transduction. *Immunology* 1997;92:544.

40. Al-Mohanna F, Saleh S, Parhar RS, et al. IL-12-dependent nuclear factor-kappaB activation leads to de novo synthesis and release of IL-8 and TNF-alpha in human neutrophils. *J Leukoc Biol* 2002;72:995.

41. Sabroe I, Jones EC, Usher LR, Whyte MK, et al. Toll-like receptor (TLR)2 and TLR4 in human peripheral blood granulocytes: a critical role for monocytes in leukocyte lipopolysaccharide responses. *J Immunol* 2002;168:4701.

42. Haribabu B, Zhelev DV, Pridgen BC, et al. Chemoattractant receptors activate distinct pathways for chemotaxis and secretion. Role of G-protein usage. *J Biol Chem* 1999;274:37087.

43. Sumichika H, Sakata K, Sato N, et al. Identification of a potent and orally active non-peptide C5a receptor antagonist. *J Biol Chem* 2002;277:49403.

44. Baggiolini M. Chemokines in pathology and medicine. *J Intern Med* 2001;250:91.

45. Barlic J, Khandaker MH, Mahon E, et al. Beta-arrestins regulate interleukin-8-induced CXCR1 internalization. *J Biol Chem* 1999;274:16287.

46. Koenig JA, Edwardson JM. Endocytosis and recycling of G protein-coupled receptors. *Trends Pharmacol Sci* 1997;18:276.

47. Servant G, Weiner OD, Herzmark P, et al. Polarization of chemoattractant receptor signaling during neutrophil chemotaxis. *Science* 2000;287:1037.

48. Kindzelskii AL, Petty HR. Intracellular calcium waves accompany neutrophil polarization, formylmethionylleucylphenylalanine stimulation, and phagocytosis: a high speed microscopy study. *J Immunol* 2003;170:64.

49. Sadhu C, Masinovsky B, Dick K, et al. Essential role of phosphoinositide 3-kinase delta in neutrophil directional movement. *J Immunol* 2003;170:2647.

50. Srinivasan S, Wang F, Glavas S, et al. Rac and Cdc42 play distinct roles in regulating PI(3,4,5)P3 and polarity during neutrophil chemotaxis. *J Cell Biol* 2003;160:375.

51. Kent JD, Sergeant S, Burns DJ, et al. Identification and regulation of protein kinase C-delta in human neutrophils. *J Immunol* 1996;157:4641.

52. Ktistakis NT, Delon C, Manifava M, et al. Phospholipase D1 and potential targets of its hydrolysis product, phosphatidic acid. *Biochem Soc Trans* 2003;31:94.

53. Palicz A, Foubert TR, Jesaitis AJ, et al. Phosphatidic acid and diacylglycerol directly activate NADPH oxidase by interacting with enzyme components. *J Biol Chem* 2001;276:3090.

54. Melendez AJ, Allen JM. Phospholipase D and immune receptor signalling. *Semin Immunol* 2002;14:49.

55. Krause KH, Campbell KP, Welsh MJ, et al. The calcium signal and neutrophil activation. *Clin Biochem* 1990;23:159.

56. Pittet D, Lew DP, Mayr GW, et al. Chemoattractant receptor promotion of Ca2+ influx across the plasma membrane of HL-60 cells. A role for cytosolic free calcium elevations and inositol 1, 3, 4, 5-tetrakisphosphate production. *J Biol Chem* 1989;264:7251.

57. Verploegen S, van Leeuwen CM, van Deutekom HW, et al. Role of Ca2+/calmodulin regulated signaling pathways in chemoattractant induced neutrophil effector functions. Comparison with the role of phosphotidylinositol-3 kinase. *Eur J Biochem* 2002;269:4625.

58. Dewitt S, Hallett MB. Cytosolic free Ca(2+) changes and calpain activation are required for beta integrin-accelerated phagocytosis by human neutrophils. *J Cell Biol* 2002;159:181.

59. Yamamori T, Inanami O, Sumimoto H, et al. Relationship between p38 mitogen-activated protein kinase and small GTPase Rac for the activation of NADPH oxidase in bovine neutrophils. *Biochem Biophys Res Commun* 2002;293:1571.

60. Kaldi K, Szeberenyi J, Rada BK, et al. Contribution of phopholipase D and a brefeldin A-sensitive ARF to chemoattractant-induced superoxide production and secretion of human neutrophils. *J Leukoc Biol* 2002;71:695.

61. Springer TA. Traffic signals for lymphocyte recirculation and leukocyte emigration: The multistep paradigm. *Cell* 1994;76:301.

62. Diamond MS, Springer TA. A subpopulation of Mac-1 (CD11b/CD18) molecules mediates neutrophil adhesion to ICAM-1 and fibrinogen. *J Cell Biol* 1993;120:545.

63. Ostermann G, Weber KS, Zernecke A, et al. JAM-1 is a ligand of the beta(2) integrin LFA-1 involved in transendothelial migration of leukocytes. *Nat Immunol* 2002;3:151.

64. Luscinskas FW, Ma S, Nusrat A, et al. The role of endothelial cell lateral junctions during leukocyte trafficking. *Immunol Rev* 2002;186:57.

65. Lowe JB. Glycosylation in the control of selectin counter-receptor structure and function. *Immunol Rev* 2002;186:19.

66. Berg EL, Magnani J, Warnock RA, et al. Comparison of L-selectin and E-selectin ligand specificities: the L-selectin can bind the E-selectin ligands sialyl Le(x) and sialyl Le(a). *Biochem Biophys Res Commun* 1992;184:1048.

67. Laudanna C, Kim JY, Constantin G, et al. Rapid leukocyte integrin activation by chemokines. *Immunol Rev* 2002;186:37.

68. Hogg N, Henderson R, Leitinger B, et al. Mechanisms contributing to the activity of integrins on leukocytes. *Immunol Rev* 2002;186:164.

69. Ley K. Integration of inflammatory signals by rolling neutrophils. *Immunol Rev* 2002;186:8.

70. Shaw JM, Al-Shamkhani A, Boxer LA, et al. Characterization of four CD18 mutants in leucocyte adhesion deficient (LAD) patients with differential capacities to support expression and function of the CD11/CD18 integrins LFA-1, Mac-1 and p150,95. *Clin Exp Immunol* 2001;126:311.

71. Bunting M, Harris ES, McIntyre TM, et al. Leukocyte adhesion deficiency syndromes: adhesion and tethering defects involving beta 2 integrins and selectin ligands. *Curr Opin Hematol* 2002;9:30.

72. Etzioni A, Sturla L, Antonellis A, et al. Leukocyte adhesion deficiency (LAD) type II/carbohydrate deficient glycoprotein (CDG) IIc founder effect and genotype/phenotype correlation. *Am J Med Genet* 2002;110:131.

73. Wild MK, Luhn K, Marquardt T, et al. Leukocyte adhesion deficiency II: therapy and genetic defect. *Cells Tissues Organs* 2002;172:161.

74. Sanchez-Madrid F, Nagy JA, Robbins E, et al. A human leukocyte differentiation antigen family with distinct alpha-subunits and a common beta-subunit: the lymphocyte function-associated antigen (LFA-1), the C3bi complement receptor (OKM1/Mac-1), and the p150,95 molecule. *J Exp Med* 1983;158:1785.

75. Marlin SD, Morton CC, Anderson DC, et al. LFA-1 immunodeficiency disease: Definition of the genetic defect and chromosomal mapping of alpha and beta subunits by complementation in hybrid cells. *J Exp Med* 1986;164:855.

76. Rothlein R, Dustin ML, Marlin SD, et al. A human intercellular adhesion molecule (ICAM-1) distinct from LFA-1. *J Immunol* 1986;137:1270.

77. Wang Q, Doerschuk CM. The signaling pathways induced by neutrophil-endothelial cell adhesion. *Antioxid Redox Signal* 2002;4:39.

78. Xia Y, Borland G, Huang J, et al. Function of the lectin domain of Mac-1/complement receptor type 3 (CD11b/CD18) in regulating neutrophil adhesion. *J Immunol* 2002;169:6417.

79. Anderson SI, Hotchin NA, Nash GB. Role of the cytoskeleton in rapid activation of CD11b/CD18 function and its subsequent downregulation in neutrophils. *J Cell Sci* 2000;113:2737.

80. Dangerfield J, Larbi KY, Huang MT, et al. PECAM-1 (CD31) homophilic interaction up-regulates alpha6beta1 on transmigrated neutrophils in vivo and plays a functional role in the ability of alpha6 integrins to mediate leukocyte migration through the perivascular basement membrane. *J Exp Med* 2002;196:1201.

81. Wright DG, Gallin JI. Secretory responses of human neutrophils: exocytosis of specific (secondary) granules by human neutrophils during adherence in vitro and during exudation in vivo. *J Immunol* 1979;123:285.

82. Janmey PA, Hvidt S, Peetermans J, et al. Viscoelasticity of F-actin and F-actin/gelsolin complexes. *Biochemistry* 1988;27:8218.

83. Lind SE, Janmey PA, Chaponnier C, et al. Reversible binding of actin to gelsolin and profilin in human platelet extracts. *J Cell Biol* 1987;105:833.

84. Lassing I, Lindberg U. Specific interaction between phosphatidylinositol 4,5-bisphosphate and profilactin. *Nature* 1985;314:472.

85. Hartwig JH, Chambers KA, Stossel TP. Association of gelsolin with actin filaments and cell membranes of macrophages and platelets. *J Cell Biol* 1989;108:469.

86. Yin HL, Stossel TP. Purification and structural properties of gelsolin, a Ca2+-activated regulatory protein of macrophages. *J Cell Biol* 1980;255:9490.

87. Janmey PA, Ida K, Yin HL, et al. Polyphosphoinositide micelles and polyphosphoinositide-containing vesicles dissociate endogenous gelsolin-actin complex and promote actin assembly from the fast-growing end of actin filaments blocked by gelsolin. *J Biol Chem* 1987;262:12228.

88. Hartwig JH, Shevlin PA. The architecture of actin filaments and the ultrastructural location of actin-binding protein in the periphery of lung macrophages. *J Cell Biol* 1986;103:1007.

89. Gorlin JB, Yamin R, Egan S, et al. Human endothelial actin-binding protein (ABP-280, nonmuscle filamin): a molecular leaf spring. *J Cell Biol* 1990;111:1089.

90. Cunningham CC, Vegners R, Bucki R, et al. Cell permeant polyphosphoinositide-binding peptides that block cell motility and actin assembly. *J Biol Chem* 2001;276:43390.

91. Valmu L, Fagerholm S, Suila H, et al. The cytoskeletal association of CD11/CD18 leukocyte integrins in phorbol ester-activated cells correlates with CD18 phosphorylation. *Eur J Immunol* 1999;29:2107.

92. Watts RG, Howard TH. Role of tropomyosin, alpha-actinin, and actin binding protein 280 in stabilizing Triton insoluble F-actin in basal and chemotactic factor activated neutrophils. *Cell Motil Cytoskeleton* 1994;28:155.

93. Dinauer MC. Regulation of neutrophil function by Rac GTPases. *Curr Opin Hematol* 2003;10:8.

94. Higgs HN, Pollard TD. Activation by Cdc42 and PIP(2) of Wiskott-Aldrich syndrome protein (WASp) stimulates actin nucleation by Arp2/3 complex. *J Cell Biol* 2000;150:1311.

95. Glogauer M, Hartwig J, Stossel T. Two pathways through Cdc42 couple the N-formyl receptor to actin nucleation in permeabilized human neutrophils. *J Cell Biol* 2000;150:785.

96. Snapper SB, Rosen FS. A family of WASPs. *N Engl J Med* 2003;348:350.

97. Indik ZK, Park JG, Hunter S, et al. The molecular dissection of Fc gamma receptor mediated phagocytosis. *Blood* 1995;86:4389.

98. Anderson CL. Isolation of the receptor for IgG from a human monocyte cell line (U937) and from human peripheral blood monocytes. *J Exp Med* 1982;156:1794.

99. Anderson CL, Spence JM, Edwards TS, et al. Characterization of a polyvalent antibody directed against the IgG Fc receptor of human mononuclear phagocytes. *J Immunol* 1985;134:465.

100. Shen L, Guyre PM, Anderson CL, et al. Heteroantibody-mediated cytotoxicity: Antibody to the high affinity Fc receptor for IgG mediates cytotoxicity by human monocytes that is enhanced by interferon-gamma and is not blocked by human IgG. *J Immunol* 1986;137:3378.

101. Fleit HB, Wright SD, Unkeless JC. Human neutrophil Fc gamma receptor distribution and structure. *Proc Natl Acad Sci USA* 1982;79:3275.

102. Kurlander RJ, Batker J. The binding of human immunoglobulin G1 monomer and small, covalently cross-linked polymers of immunoglobulin G1 to human peripheral blood monocytes and polymorphonuclear leukocytes. *J Clin Invest* 1982;69:1.

103. Kulczycki A Jr. Human neutrophils and eosinophils have structurally distinct Fc receptors. *J Immunol* 1984;133:849.

104. Coxon A, Cullere X, Knight S, et al. Fc gamma RIII mediates neutrophil recruitment to immune complexes. A mechanism for neutrophil accumulation in immune-mediated inflammation. *Immunity* 2001;14:693.

105. Klempner MS, Gallin JI. Separation and functional characterization of human neutrophil subpopulations. *Blood* 1978;4:659.

106. Kim MK, Pan XQ, Huang ZY, et al. Fc gamma receptors differ in their structural requirements for interaction with the tyrosine kinase Syk in the initial steps of signaling for phagocytosis. *Clin Immunol* 2001;98:125.

107. Strzelecka-Kiliszek A, Kwiatkowska K, Sobota A. Lyn and Syk kinases are sequentially engaged in phagocytosis mediated by Fc gamma R. *J Immunol* 2002;169:6787.

108. Kusner DJ, Hall CF, Jackson S. Fc gamma receptor-mediated activation of phospholipase D regulates macrophage phagocytosis of IgG-opsonized particles. *J Immunol* 1999;162:2266.

109. Nakamura K, Malykhin A, Coggeshall KM. The Src homology 2 domain-containing inositol 5-phosphatase negatively regulates Fcgamma receptor-mediated phagocytosis through immunoreceptor tyrosine-based activation motif-bearing phagocytic receptors. *Blood* 2002;100:3374.

110. Cox D, Dale BM, Kashiwada M, et al. A regulatory role for Src homology 2 domain-containing inositol 5'-phosphatase (SHIP) in phagocytosis mediated by Fc gamma receptors and complement receptor 3 (alpha(M)beta(2); CD11b/CD18). *J Exp Med* 2001;193:61.

111. Bullock WE, Wright SD. The role of adherence-promoting receptors, CR3, LFA-1, and p150,95 in binding of *Histoplasma capsulatum* by human macrophages. *J Exp Med* 1987;165:195.

112. Wright SD, Jong MTC. Adhesion-promoting receptors on human macrophages recognize *E. coli* by binding to lipopolysaccharide. *J Exp Med* 1986;164:1876.

113. Wright SD, Griffin FM Jr. Activation of phagocytic cells' C3 receptors for phagocytosis. *J Leukoc Biol* 1985;38:327.

114. Griffin FM, Griffin JA, Leider JE, et al. Studies on the mechanism of phagocytosis. I. Requirements for circumferential attachment of particle bound ligands to specific receptors on the macrophage plasma membrane. *J Exp Med* 1975;142:1263.

115. Collins RF, Schreiber AD, Grinstein S, et al. Syntaxins 13 and 7 function at distinct steps during phagocytosis. *J Immunol* 2002;169:3250.

116. Lindmark IM, Karlsson A, Serrander L, et al. Synaptotagmin II could confer Ca(2+) sensitivity to phagocytosis in human neutrophils. *Biochim Biophys Acta* 2002;1590:159.

117. Perskvist N, Roberg K, Kulyte A, et al. Rab5a GTPase regulates fusion between pathogen-containing phagosomes and cytoplasmic organelles in human neutrophils. *J Cell Sci* 2002;115:1321.

118. Smolen JE, Hessler RJ, Nauseef WM, et al. Identification and cloning of the SNARE proteins VAMP-2 and syntaxin-4 from HL-60 cells and human neutrophils. *Inflammation* 2001;25:255.

119. Borregaard N, Cowland JB. Granules of the human neutrophilic polymorphonuclear leukocyte. *Blood* 1997;89:3503.

120. Lehrer RI, Ganz T. Cathelicidins: a family of endogenous antimicrobial peptides. *Curr Opin Hematol* 2002;9:18.

121. Ward PP, Uribe-Luna S, Conneely OM. Lactoferrin and host defense. *Biochem Cell Biol* 2002;80:95.

122. Reeves EP, Lu H, Jacobs HL, et al. Killing activity of neutrophils is mediated through activation of proteases by K+ flux. *Nature* 2002;416:291.

123. Prikk K, Maisi P, Pirila E, et al. Airway obstruction correlates with collagenase-2 (MMP-8) expression and activation in bronchial asthma. *Lab Invest* 2002;82:1535.

124. Ratjen F, Hartog CM, Paul K, et al. Matrix metalloproteases in BAL fluid of patients with cystic fibrosis and their modulation by treatment with dornase alpha. *Thorax* 2002;57:930.

125. Claesson R, Johansson A, Belibasakis G, et al. Release and activation of matrix metalloproteinase 8 from human neutrophils triggered by the leukotoxin of *Actinobacillus actinomycetemcomitans*. *J Periodontal Res* 2002;37:353.

126. Shapiro SD. Proteinases in chronic obstructive pulmonary disease. *Biochem Soc Trans* 2002;30:98.

127. Segal AW, Shatwell KP. The NADPH oxidase of phagocytic leukocytes. *Ann NY Acad Sci* 1997;832:215.

128. Clark RA. Activation of the neutrophil respiratory burst oxidase. *J Infect Dis* 1999;179[Suppl 2]:S309.

129. Lomax KJ, Leto TL, Nunoi H, et al. Recombinant 47-kD cytosol factor restores NADPH oxidase in chronic granulomatous disease [published erratum in *Science* 1989;246:987]. *Science* 1989;245:409.

130. Leto TL, Lomax KJ, Volpp BD, et al. Cloning of a 67K neutrophil oxidase factor with similarity to a noncatalytic region of p60-11. *Science* 1990;248:727.

131. Nunoi H, Rotrosen D, Gallin JI, et al. Two forms of autosomal chronic granulomatous disease lack distinct neutrophil cytosol factors. *Science* 1988;242:1298.

132. Babior BM. The activity of leukocyte NADPH oxidase: regulation by p47PHOX cysteine and serine residues. *Antioxid Redox Signal* 2002;4:35.

133. de Mendez I, Homayounpour N, Leto TL. Specificity of p47phox SH3 domain interactions in NADPH oxidase assembly and activation. *Mol Cell Biol* 1997;17:2177.

134. Segal BH, Leto TL, Gallin JI, et al. Genetic, biochemical, and clinical features of chronic granulomatous disease. *Medicine (Baltimore)* 2000;79:170.

135. de Mendez I, Adams AG, Sokolic RA, et al. Multiple SH3 domain interactions regulate NADPH oxidase assembly in whole cells. *EMBO J* 1996;15:1211.

136. Kwong CH, Malech HL, Rotrosen D, et al. Regulation of the human neutrophil NADPH oxidase by rho-related G-proteins. *Biochemistry* 1993;32:5711.

137. Clark RA, Volpp BD, Leidal KG, et al. Two cytosolic components of the human neutrophil respiratory burst oxidase translocate to the plasma membrane during cell activation. *J Clin Invest* 1990;85:714.

138. Malech HL. Phagocyte oxidative mechanisms. *Curr Opin Hematol* 1993;1:123.

139. Diekmann D, Abo A, Johnston C, et al. Interaction of Rac with p67phox and regulation of phagocytic NADPH oxidase activity. *Science* 1994;265:531.

140. Abo A, Boyhan A, West I, et al. Reconstitution of neutrophil NADPH oxidase activity in the cell-free system by four components: p67-phox, p47-phox, p21rac1, and cytochrome b-245. *J Biol Chem* 1992;267:16767.

141. Cross AR, Jones OT, Harper AM, et al. Oxidation-reduction *properties of the* cytochrome b found in the plasma-membrane fraction of human neutrophils: a possible oxidase in the respiratory burst. *Biochem J* 1981;194:599.

142. Rotrosen D, Yeung CL, Leto, TL, et al. Cytochrome *b*558: The flavin-binding component of the phagocyte NADPH oxidase. *Science* 1992;256:1459.

143. Royer-Pokora B, Kunkel LM, Monaco AP, et al. Cloning the gene for an inherited human disorder-chronic granulomatous disease-on the basis of its chromosome location. *Nature* 1986;322:32.

144. Dinauer MC, Orkin SH, Brown R, et al. The glycoprotein encoded by the X-linked chronic granulomatous disease locus is a component of the neutrophil cytochrome b complex. *Nature* 1987;327:717.

145. Dinauer MC, Orkin SH, Brown R, et al. The glycoprotein encoded by the X-linked chronic granulomatous disease locus is a component of the neutrophil cytochrome b complex. *Nature* 1987;327:717.

146. Teahan C, Rowe P, Parker P, et al. The X-linked chronic granulomatous disease gene codes for the beta-chain of cytochrome b245. *Nature* 1987;327:720.

147. Cross AR, Rae J, Curnutte JT. Cytochrome b-245 of the neutrophil superoxide-generating system contains two nonidentical hemes. Potentiometric studies of a mutant form of gp91phox. *J Biol Chem* 1995;270:17075.

148. Rotrosen D, Kleinberg ME, Nunoi H, et al. Evidence for a functional cytoplasmic domain of phagocyte oxidase cytochrome *b*558. *J Biol Chem* 1990;265:8745.

149. Lapouge K, Smith SJ, Groemping Y, et al. Architecture of the p40-p47-p67phox complex in the resting state of the NADPH oxidase. A central role for p67phox. *J Biol Chem* 2002;277:10121.

150. Zhan Y, Virbasius JV, Song X, et al. The p40phox and p47phox PX domains of NADPH oxidase target cell membranes via direct and indirect recruitment by phosphoinositides. *J Biol Chem* 2002;277:4512.

151. Wientjes FB, Reeves EP, Soskic V, et al. The NADPH oxidase components p47(phox) and p40(phox) bind to moesin through their PX domain. *Biochem Biophys Res Commun* 2001;289:382.

152. Bravo J, Karathanassis D, Pacold CM, et al. The crystal structure of the PX domain from p40(phox) bound to phosphatidylinositol 3-phosphate. *Mol Cell* 2001;8:829.

153. McPhail LC, Qualliotine-Mann D, Agwu DE, et al. Phospholipases and activation of the NADPH oxidase. *Eur J Haematol* 1993;51:294.

154. McPhail LC, Qualliotine-Mann D, Waite KA. Cell-free activation of neutrophil NADPH oxidase by a phosphatidic acid-regulated protein kinase. *Proc Natl Acad Sci USA* 1995;92:7931.

155. Klebanoff SJ. Myeloperoxidase. *Proc Assoc Am Physicians* 1999;111:383.

156. Hirose J, Yamaga M, Kato T, et al. Effects of a hydroxyl radical scavenger, EPC-K1, and neutrophil depletion on reperfusion injury in rat skeletal muscle. *Acta Orthop Scand* 2001;72:404.

157. Shen Z, Wu W, Hazen SL. Activated leukocytes oxidatively damage DNA, RNA, and the nucleotide pool through halide-dependent formation of hydroxyl radical. *Biochemistry* 2000;39:5474.

158. Hampton MB, Kettle AJ, Winterbourn CC. Inside the neutrophil phagosome: oxidants, myeloperoxidase, and bacterial killing. *Blood* 1998;92:3007.

159. Britigan BE, Hassett DJ, Rosen GM, et al. Neutrophil degranulation inhibits potential hydroxyl-radical formation. Relative impact of myeloperoxidase and lactoferrin release on hydroxyl radical production by iron-supplemented neutrophils assessed by spin-trapping techniques. *Biochem J* 1989;264:447.

160. Hatherill JR, Till GO, Bruner LH, et al. Thermal injury, intravascular hemolysis, and toxic oxygen products. *J Clin Invest* 1986;78:629.

161. Sylvia CJ. The role of neutrophil apoptosis in influencing tissue repair. *J Wound Care* 2003;12:13.

162. Kobayashi SD, Voyich JM, Buhl CL, et al. Global changes in gene expression by human polymorphonuclear leukocytes during receptor-mediated phagocytosis: cell fate is regulated at the level of gene expression. *Proc Natl Acad Sci USA* 2002;99:6901.

163. Liles WC, Klebanoff SJ. Regulation of apoptosis in neutrophils—Fas track to death? *J Immunol* 1995;155:3289.

164. Liles WC, Kiener PA, Ledbetter JA, et al. Differential expression of Fas (CD95) and Fas ligand on normal human phagocytes: implications for the regulation of apoptosis in neutrophils. *J Exp Med* 1996;184:429.

165. Teder P, Vandivier RW, Jiang D, et al. Resolution of lung inflammation by CD44. *Science* 2002;296:155.

166. Vivers S, Dransfield I, Hart SP. Role of macrophage CD44 in the disposal of inflammatory cell corpses. *Clin Sci (Lond)* 2002;103:441.

167. Arroyo A, Modriansky M, Serinkan FB, et al. NADPH oxidase-dependent oxidation and externalization of phosphatidylserine during apoptosis in Me2SO-differentiated HL-60 cells. Role in phagocytic clearance. *J Biol Chem* 2002;277:49965.

168. Saba S, Soong G, Greenberg S, et al. Bacterial stimulation of epithelial G-CSF and GM-CSF expression promotes PMN survival in CF airways. *Am J Respir Cell Mol Biol* 2002;27:561.

169. Centola M, Wood G, Frucht DM, et al. The gene for familial Mediterranean fever, MEFV, is expressed in early leukocyte development and is regulated in response to inflammatory mediators. *Blood* 2000;95:3223.

170. Hull KM, Shoham N, Chae JJ, et al. The expanding spectrum of systemic autoinflammatory disorders and their rheumatic manifestations. *Curr Opin Rheumatol* 2003;15:61.

171. Bain BJ, Phillips D, Thomson K, et al. Investigation of the effect of marathon running on leucocyte counts of subjects of different ethnic origins: relevance to the aetiology of ethnic neutropenia. *Br J Haematol* 2000;108:483.

172. Rezvani K, Flanagan AM, Sarma U, et al. Investigation of ethnic neutropenia by assessment of bone marrow colony-forming cells. *Acta Haematol* 2001;105:32.

173. Phillips D, Rezvani K, Bain BJ. Exercise induced mobilization of the marginated granulocyte pool in the investigation of ethnic neutropenia. *J Clin Pathol* 2000;53:481.

174. Kyono W, Coates TD. A practical approach to neutrophil disorders. *Pediatr Clin North Am* 2002;49:929.

175. Bodey GP, Buckley M, Sathe YS, et al. Quantitative relationships between circulating leukocytes and infections in patients with acute leukemia. *Ann Intern Med* 1966;64:328.

176. Hughes WT, Armstrong D, Bodey GP, et al. Guidelines for the use of antimicrobial agents in neutropenic patients with unexplained fever. *J Infect Dis* 1990;161:381.

177. Elting LS, Bodey GP, Keefe BH. Septicemia and shock syndrome due to viridans streptococci: a case-control study of predisposing factors. *Clin Infect Dis* 1992;14:1201.

178. Bochud PY, Calandra T, Francioli P. Bacteremia due to viridans streptococci in neutropenic patients: a review. *Am J Med* 1994;97:256.

179. Hugues WT, Armstrong D, Bodey GP, et al. Guidelines for the use of antimicrobial agents in neutropenic patients with unexplained fever. *Clin Infect Dis* 1997;25:551.

180. Engelhart S, Glasmacher A, Exner M, et al. Surveillance for nosocomial infections and fever of unknown origin among adult hematology-oncology patients. *Infect Control Hosp Epidemiol* 2002;23:244.

181. Murphy MF, Metcalfe P, Grint PCA, et al. Cephalosporin-induced immune neutropenia. *Br J Haematol* 1985;59:9.

182. Palmblad J, Papadaki HA, Eliopoulos G. Acute and chronic neutropenias. What is new? *J Intern Med* 2001;250:476.

183. Bux J. Molecular nature of antigens implicated in immune neutropenias. *Int J Hematol* 2002;76[Suppl 1]:399.

184. Stroncek DF. Drug-induced immune neutropenia. *Transfus Med Rev* 1993;7:268.

185. Parrish DD, Schlosser MJ, Kapeghian JC, et al. Activation of CGS 12094 (prinomide metabolite) to 1,4-benzoquinone by myeloperoxidase: implications for human idiosyncratic agranulocytosis. *Fundam Appl Toxicol* 1997;35:197.

186. Ruiz MA, Augusto LG, Vassallo J, et al. Bone marrow morphology in patients with neutropenia due to chronic exposure to organic solvents (benzene): early lesions. *Pathol Res Pract* 1994;190:151.

187. Lubran MM. Hematologic side effects of drugs. *Ann Clin Lab Sci* 1989;19:114.

188. Bux J. Molecular nature of antigens implicated in immune neutropenias. *Int J Hematol* 2002;76[Suppl 1]:399.

189. Lucas G, Rogers S, de Haas M, et al. Report on the Fourth International Granulocyte Immunology Workshop: progress toward quality assessment. *Transfusion* 2002;42:462.

190. Flesch BK, Doose S, Siebert R, et al. FCGR3 variants and expression of human neutrophil antigen-1a, -1b, and -1c in the populations of northern Germany and Uganda. *Transfusion* 2002;42:469.

191. Lalezari P, Khorshidi M, Petrosova M. Autoimmune neutropenia of infancy. *J Pediatr* 1986;109:764.

192. Taniuchi S, Masuda M, Hasui M, et al. Differential diagnosis and clinical course of autoimmune neutropenia in infancy: comparison with congenital neutropenia. *Acta Paediatr* 2002;91:1179.

193. Bruin MC, von dem Borne AE, Tamminga RY, et al. Neutrophil antibody specificity in different types of childhood autoimmune neutropenia. *Blood* 1999;94:1797.

194. Dale DC, Hammond WP IV. Cyclic neutropenia: a clinical review. *Blood Rev* 1988;2:178.

195. Loughran TP Jr, Hammond WP IV. Adult-onset cyclic neutropenia is a benign neoplasm associated with clonal proliferation of large granular lymphocytes. *J Exp Med* 1986;164:2089.

196. Sternberg A, Eagleton H, Pillai N, et al. Neutropenia and anaemia associated with T-cell large granular lymphocyte leukaemia responds to fludarabine with minimal toxicity. *Br J Haematol* 2003;120:699.

197. Shvidel L, Duksin C, Tzimanis A, et al. Cytokine release by activated T-cells in large granular lymphocytic leukemia associated with autoimmune disorders. *Hematol J* 2002;3:32.

198. Starkebaum G. Chronic neutropenia associated with autoimmune disease. *Semin Hematol* 2002;39:121.

199. Cairo MS. Neutrophil storage pool depletion in neonates with sepsis. *J Pediatr* 1989;114:1064.

200. Schibler KR, Osborne KA, Leung LY, et al. A randomized, placebo-controlled trial of granulocyte colony-stimulating factor administration to newborn infants with neutropenia and clinical signs of early-onset sepsis. *Pediatrics* 1998;102:6.

201. Roper M, Parmley RT, Crist WM, et al. Severe congenital leukopenia (reticular dysgenesis). *Am J Dis Child* 1985;139:832.

202. Bertrand Y, Muller SM, Casanova JL, et al. Reticular dysgenesis: HLA non-identical bone marrow transplants in a series of 10 patients. *Bone Marrow Transplant* 2002;29:759.

203. Cham B, Bonilla MA, Winkelstein J. Neutropenia associated with primary immunodeficiency syndromes. *Semin Hematol* 2002;39:107.

204. Woods WG, Roloff JS, Lukens JN, et al. The occurrence of leukemia in patients with the Shwachman syndrome. *J Pediatr* 1981;99:425.

205. Cipolli M, D'Orazio C, Delmarco A, et al. Shwachman's syndrome: pathomorphosis and long-term outcome. *J Pediatr Gastroenterol Nutr* 1999;29:265.

206. Boocock GR, Morrison JA, Popovic M, et al. Mutations in SBDS are associated with Shwachman-Diamond syndrome. *Nat Genet* 2003;33:97.

207. Kostmann R. Infantile genetic agranulocytosis. A review with presentation of ten new cases. *Acta Paediatr Scand* 1975;64:362.

208. Zeidler C, Boxer L, Dale DC, et al. Management of Kostmann syndrome in the G-CSF era. *Br J Haematol* 2000;109:490.

209. Dale DC, Person RE, Bolyard AA, et al. Mutations in the gene encoding neutrophil elastase in congenital and cyclic neutropenia. *Blood* 2000;96:2317.

210. Aprikyan AA, Dale DC. Mutations in the neutrophil elastase gene in cyclic and congenital neutropenia. *Curr Opin Immunol* 2001;13:535.

211. Zeidler C, Welte K. Kostmann syndrome and severe congenital neutropenia. *Semin Hematol* 2002;39:82.

212. Freedman MH, Bonilla MA, Fier C, et al. Myelodysplasia syndrome and acute myeloid leukemia in patients with congenital neutropenia receiving G-CSF therapy. *Blood* 2000;96:429.

213. Palmer SE, Stephens K, Dale DC. Genetics, phenotype, and natural history of autosomal dominant cyclic hematopoiesis. *Am J Med Genet* 1996;66:413.

214. Horwitz M, Benson KF, Person RE, et al. Mutations in ELA2, encoding neutrophil elastase, define a 21-day biological clock in cyclic haematopoiesis. *Nat Genet* 1999;23:433.

215. Aprikyan AA, Liles WC, Boxer LA, et al. Mutant elastase in pathogenesis of cyclic and severe congenital neutropenia. *J Pediatr Hematol Oncol* 2002;24:784.

216. Roos D, Law SK. Hematologically important mutations: leukocyte adhesion deficiency. *Blood Cells Mol Dis* 2001;27:1000.

217. Etzioni A, Tonetti M. Leukocyte adhesion deficiency II-from A to almost Z. *Immunol Rev* 2000;178:138.

218. Lanfranchi A, Verardi R, Tettoni K, et al. Haploidentical peripheral blood and marrow stem cell transplantation in nine cases of primary immunodeficiency. *Haematologica* 2000;85[Suppl 11]:41.

219. Bauer TR Jr, Hickstein DD: Gene therapy for leukocyte adhesion deficiency. *Curr Opin Mol Ther* 2000 Aug;2(4):383, 2000.

220. Gallin JI, Clark RA, Kimball HR. Granulocyte chemotaxis: an improved assay employing 51-Cr-labelled granulocytes. *J Immunol* 1973;110:233.

221. Capsoni F, Minonzio F, Ongari AM, et al. A new simplified single-filter assay

for 'in vitro' evaluation of chemotaxis of 51 Cr-labeled polymorphonuclear leukocytes. *J Immunol Methods* 1989;120:125.

222. Carletto A, Biasi D, Bambara LM, et al. Studies of skin-window exudate human neutrophils: increased resistance to pentoxifylline of the respiratory burst in primed cells. *Inflammation* 1997;21:191.

223. Nunoi H, Yamazaki T, Kanegasaki S. Neutrophil cytoskeletal disease. *Int J Hematol* 2001;74:119.

224. Nunoi H, Yamazaki T, Tsuchiya H, et al. A heterozygous mutation of beta-actin associated with neutrophil dysfunction and recurrent infection. *Proc Natl Acad Sci USA* 1999;96:8693.

225. Howard T, Li Y, Torres M, et al. The 47-kD protein increased in neutrophil actin dysfunction with 47- and 89-kD protein abnormalities is lymphocyte-specific protein. *Blood* 1994;83:231.

226. Howard TH, Hartwig J, Cunningham C. Lymphocyte-specific protein 1 expression in eukaryotic cells reproduces the morphologic and motile abnormality of NAD 47/89 neutrophils. *Blood* 1998;91:4786.

227. Zhang Q, Li Y, Howard TH. Human lymphocyte-specific protein 1, the protein overexpressed in neutrophil actin dysfunction with 47-kDa and 89-kDa protein abnormalities (NAD 47/89), has multiple F-actin binding domains. *J Immunol* 2000;165:2052.

228. Etienne-Manneville S, Hall A. Rho GTPases in cell biology. *Nature* 2002;420:629.

229. Ambruso DR, Knall C, Abell AN, et al. Human neutrophil immunodeficiency syndrome is associated with an inhibitory Rac2 mutation. *Proc Natl Acad Sci USA* 2000;97:4654.

230. Williams DA, Tao W, Yang F, et al. Dominant negative mutation of the hematopoietic-specific Rho GTPase, Rac2, is associated with a human phagocyte immunodeficiency. *Blood* 2000;96:1646.

231. Kurkchubasche AG, Panepinto JA, Tracy TF Jr, et al. Clinical features of a human Rac2 mutation: a complex neutrophil dysfunction disease. *J Pediatr* 2001;139:141.

232. Gu Y, Williams DA. RAC2 GTPase deficiency and myeloid cell dysfunction in human and mouse. *J Pediatr Hematol Oncol* 2002;24:791.

233. Kingsmore SF, Barbosa MD, Tchernev VT, et al. Positional cloning of the Chediak-Higashi syndrome gene: genetic mapping of the beige locus on mouse chromosome 13. *J Investig Med* 1996;44:454.

234. Nagle DL, Karim MA, Woolf EA, et al. Identification and mutation analysis of the complete gene for Chediak-Higashi syndrome. *Nat Genet* 1996;14:307.

235. Certain S, Barrat F, Pastural E, et al. Protein truncation test of LYST reveals heterogenous mutations in patients with Chediak-Higashi syndrome. *Blood* 2000;95:979.

236. Karim MA, Suzuki K, Fukai K, et al. Apparent genotype-phenotype correlation in childhood, adolescent, and adult Chediak-Higashi syndrome. *Am J Med Genet* 2002;108:16.

237. Tchernev VT, Mansfield TA, Giot L, et al. The Chediak-Higashi protein interacts with SNARE complex and signal transduction proteins. *Mol Med* 2002;8:56.

238. Ward DM, Shiflett SL, Kaplan J. Chediak-Higashi syndrome: a clinical and molecular view of a rare lysosomal storage disorder. *Curr Mol Med* 2002;2:469.

239. Griffiths GM. Albinism and immunity: what's the link? *Curr Mol Med* 2002;2:479.

240. De Lozanne A. The role of BEACH proteins in dictyostelium. *Traffic* 2003;4:6.

241. Boxer LA, Wantanabe AM, Rister M, et al. Correction of leukocyte function in CHS by ascorbate. *N Engl J Med* 1976;295:1041.

242. Gallin JI, Elin RJ, Hubert RT, et al. Efficacy of ascorbic acid in Chédiak-Higashi syndrome: studies in humans and mice. *Blood* 1979;53:226.

243. Nauseef WM. Myeloperoxidase deficiency. *Hematol Oncol Clin North Am* 1988;2:135.

244. Parry MF, Root RK, Metcalf JA, et al. Myeloperoxidase deficiency: prevalence and clinical significance. *Ann Intern Med* 1981;95:483.

245. Kutter D. Prevalence of myeloperoxidase deficiency: population studies using Bayer-Technicon automated hematology. *J Mol Med* 1998;76:669.

246. Nauseef WM, Root RK, Malech HL. Biochemical and immunologic analysis of hereditary myeloperoxidase deficiency. *J Clin Invest* 1983;71:1297.

247. Johnson KR, Nauseef WM. Molecular biology of myeloperoxidase. In: Everse J, Grisham M, eds. *Peroxidases in chemistry and biology.* Boca Raton, FL: CRC Press, 1990:63–83.

248. Nauseef WM. Aberrant restriction endonuclease digests of DNA from subjects with hereditary myeloperoxidase deficiency. *Blood* 1989;3:290.

249. Tobler A, Selsted ME, Miller CW, et al. Evidence of a pretranslational defect in hereditary and acquired myeloperoxidase deficiency. *Blood* 1989;73:1980.

250. Nauseef WM. Insights into myeloperoxidase biosynthesis from its inherited deficiency. *J Mol Med* 1998;76:661.

251. Nauseef WM, Brigham S, Cogley M. Hereditary myeloperoxidase deficiency due to a missense mutation of arginine 569 to tryptophan. *J Biol Chem* 1994;269:1212.

252. Kizaki M, Miller CW, Selsted ME, et al. Myeloperoxidase (MPO) gene mutation in hereditary MPO deficiency. *Blood* 1994;83:1935.

253. Nauseef WM, Cogley M, McCormick S. Effect of the R569W missense mutation on the biosynthesis of myeloperoxidase. *J Biol Chem* 1996;27:9546.

254. Petrides PE. Molecular genetics of peroxidase deficiency. *J Mol Med* 1998;76:688–698.

255. Davey FR, Erber WN, Gatter KC, et al. Abnormal neutrophils in acute myeloid leukemia and myelodysplastic syndrome. *Hum Pathol* 1988;19:454.

256. Hoy A, Leininger-Muller B, Kutter D, et al. Growing significance of myeloperoxidase in non-infectious diseases. *Clin Chem Lab Med* 2002;40:2.

257. Crisan D, David D. Use of myeloperoxidase mRNA in monitoring patients with acute myelogenous leukemia for early detection of circulating blasts. *Mol Diagn* 1996;1:313.

258. Caldwell KC, Taddeini L, Woodburn RL, et al. Induction of myeloperoxidase deficiency in granulocytes in lead-intoxicated dogs. *Blood* 1979;53:588.

259. Kutter D, Devaquet P, Vanderstocken G, et al. Consequences of total and subtotal myeloperoxidase deficiency: risk or benefit? *Acta Haematol* 2000;104:10.

260. Brennan ML, Anderson MM, Shih DM, et al. Increased atherosclerosis in myeloperoxidase-deficient mice. *J Clin Invest* 2001;107:419.

261. Takizawa S, Aratani Y, Fukuyama N, et al. Deficiency of myeloperoxidase increases infarct volume and nitrotyrosine formation in mouse brain. *J Cereb Blood Flow Metab* 2002;22:50.

262. Tsurubuchi T, Aratani Y, Maeda N, et al. Retardation of early-onset PMA-induced apoptosis in mouse neutrophils deficient in myeloperoxidase. *J Leukoc Biol* 2001;70:52.

263. Cech P, Papathanassiou A, Boreaux G, et al. Hereditary myeloperoxidase deficiency. *Blood* 1979;53:403.

264. Lanza F. Clinical manifestation of myeloperoxidase deficiency. *J Mol Med* 1998;76:676.

265. Gallin JI. Neutrophil specific granule deficiency. *Annu Rev Med* 1985;36:263.

266. Falloon J, Gallin JI. Neutrophil granules in health and disease. *J Allergy Clin Immunol* 1986;77:653.

267. Davis J, Dineen P, Gallin JI. Neutrophil degranulation and abnormal chemotaxis after thermal injury. *J Immunol* 1980;124:1467.

268. Wolach B, Coates TD, Hugh TE, et al. Plasma lactoferrin reflects granulocyte activation via complement in burn patients. *J Lab Clin Med* 1984;103:284.

269. Rosenberg HF, Gallin JI. Neutrophil-specific granule deficiency includes eosinophils. *Blood* 1993;82:268.

270. Lomax KJ, Gallin JI, Rotrosen D, et al. Selective defect in myeloid cell lactoferrin gene expression in neutrophil specific granule deficiency. *J Clin Invest* 1989;83:514.

271. Johnston JJ, Boxer LA, Berliner N. Correlation of messenger RNA levels with protein defects in specific granule deficiency. *Blood* 1992;80:2088.

272. Lekstrom-Himes JA. The role of C/EBP(epsilon) in the terminal stages of granulocyte differentiation. *Stem Cells* 2001;19:125.

273. Lekstrom-Himes JA, Dorman SE, Kopar P, et al. Neutrophil-specific granule deficiency results from a novel mutation with loss of function of the transcription factor CCAAT/enhancer binding protein epsilon. *J Exp Med* 1999;189:1847.

274. Gombart AF, Koeffler HP. Neutrophil specific granule deficiency and mutations in the gene encoding transcription factor C/EBP(epsilon). *Curr Opin Hematol* 2002;9:36.

275. Gallin JI, Fletcher MP, Seligmann BE, et al. Human neutrophil-specific granule deficiency: a model to assess the role of neutrophil-specific granules in the evolution of the inflammatory response. *Blood* 1982;59:1317.

276. Malech HL, Bauer TR Jr, Hickstein DD. Prospects for gene therapy of neutrophil defects. *Semin Hematol* 1997;34:355.

277. Roos D, Curnutte JT, Hossle JP, et al. X-CGDbase: A database of X-CGD-causing mutations. *Immunol Today* 1996;17:517.

278. Johnston RB Jr. Clinical aspects of chronic granulomatous disease. *Curr Opin Hematol* 2001;8:17.

279. Winkelstein JA, Marino MC, Johnston RB Jr, et al. Chronic granulomatous disease. Report on a national registry of 368 patients. *Medicine (Baltimore)* 2000;79:155.

280. Ahlin A, de Boer M, Roos D, et al. Prevalence, genetics and clinical presentation of chronic granulomatous disease in Sweden. *Acta Paediatr* 1995;84:1386.

281. Ishibashi F, Nunoi H, Endo F, et al. Statistical and mutational analysis of chronic granulomatous disease in Japan with special reference to gp91-phox and p22-phox deficiency. *Hum Genet* 2000;106:473.

282. Nunoi H, Ishibashi F. Statistical evaluation of chronic granulomatous disease in Japan and basic studies for gene therapy for CGD patients (in Japanese; abstract in English). *Rinsho Byori* 1999;47:658.

283. Valiaho J, Riikonen P, Vihinen M. Novel immunodeficiency data servers. *Immunol Rev* 2000;178:177.

284. Francke U, Hsieh CL, Foellmer BE, et al. Genes for two autosomal recessive forms of chronic granulomatous disease assigned to 1q25 (*NCF2*) and 7q11.23 (*NCF1*). *Am J Hum Genet* 1990;47:483.

285. Jirapongsananuruk O, Niemela JE, Malech HL, et al. CYBB mutation analysis in X-linked chronic granulomatous disease. *Clin Immunol* 2002;104:73.

286. Jirapongsananuruk O, Malech HL, Kuhns DB, et al. Diagnostic paradigm for evaluation of male patients with chronic granulomatous disease, based on the dihydrorhodamine 123 assay. *J Allergy Clin Immunol* 2003;111:374.

287. Dinauer MC, Pierce EA, Bruns GA, et al. Human neutrophil cytochrome *b* light chain (p22-phox). Gene structure, chromosomal location, and mutations in cytochrome-negative autosomal recessive chronic granulomatous disease. *J Clin Invest* 1990;86:1729.

288. Roos D, de Boer M, Kuribayashi F, et al. Mutations in the X-linked and autosomal recessive forms of chronic granulomatous disease. *Blood* 1996;87:1663.

289. Casimir CM, Bu-Ghanuim HN, Rodaway ARF, et al. Autosomal recessive chronic granulomatous disease caused by deletion at a dinucleotide repeat. *Proc Natl Acad Sci USA* 1991;88:2753.

290. Iwata M, Nunoi H, Yamazaki H, et al. Homologous dinucleotide (GT or TG)

deletion in Japanese patients with chronic granulomatous disease with p47-phox deficiency. *Biochem Biophys Res Commun* 1994;199:1372.

291. Vazquez N, Lehrnbecher T, Chen R, et al. Mutational analysis of patients with p47-phox-deficient chronic granulomatous disease: the significance of recombination events between the p47-phox gene (NCF1) and its highly homologous pseudogenes. *Exp Hematol* 2001;29:234.

292. Roesler J, Gorlach A, Rae J, et al. Recombination events between the normal p47-phox gene and a highly homologous pseudogene are the main cause of autosomal recessive chronic granulomatous disease (abstract). *Blood* 1995;86[Suppl 1]:260a.

293. Chanock SJ, Roesler J, Zhan S, et al. Genomic structure of the human p47-phox (NCF1) gene. *Blood Cells Mol Dis* 2000;26:37.

294. Nunoi H, Iwata M, Tatsuzawa S, et al. AG dinucleotide insertion in a patient with chronic granulomatous disease lacking cytosolic 67-k1) protein. *Blood* 1995;86:329.

295. Tanugi-Cholley LC, Issartel JP, Lunardi J, et al. A mutation located at the 5′ splice junction sequence of intron 3 in the p67phox gene causes the lack of p67phox mRNA in a patient with chronic granulomatous disease. *Blood* 1995;85:242.

296. de Boer M, Hilarius-Stokman PM, Hossle JP, et al. Autosomal recessive chronic granulomatous disease with absence of the 67-k1) cytosolic NADPH oxidase component: Identification of mutation and detection of carriers. *Blood* 1994;83:531.

297. Buescher ES, Alling DW, Gallin JI. Use of an X-linked human neutrophil marker to estimate timing of lyonization and size of the dividing stem pool. *J Clin Invest* 1985;76:1581.

298. Vowells SJ, Sekhsaria S, Malech HL, et al. Flow cytometric analysis of the granulocyte respiratory burst: a comparison study of fluorescent probes. *J Immunol Methods* 1995;178:89.

299. Vowells SJ, Fleisher TA, Sekhsaria S, et al. Genotype dependent variability in flow cytometric evaluation of NADPH oxidase function in patients with chronic granulomatous disease. *J Pediatr* 1996;128:104.

300. Weil WM, Linton GF, Whiting-Theobald N, et al. Genetic correction of p67phox deficient chronic granulomatous disease using peripheral blood progenitor cells as a target for retrovirus mediated gene transfer. *Blood* 1997;89:1754.

301. Brandrup F, Koch C, Petri M, et al. Discoid lupus erythematosus-like lesions and stomatitis in female carriers of X-linked chronic granulomatous disease. *Br J Dermatol* 1981;104:495.

302. Rupec RA, Petropoulou T, Belohradsky BH, et al. Lupus erythematosus tumidus and chronic discoid lupus erythematosus in carriers of X-linked chronic granulomatous disease. *Eur J Dermatol* 2000;10:184.

303. Schapiro BL, Newburger PE, Klempner MS, et al. Chronic granulomatous disease presenting in a 69-year-old man. *N Engl J Med* 1991;325:1786.

304. Ross JP, Holland SM, Gill VJ, et al. Severe *Burkholderia (Pseudomonas) gladioli* infection in chronic granulomatous disease: report of two successfully treated cases. *Clin Infect Dis* 1995;21:1291.

305. Lacy DE, Spencer DA, Goldstein A, et al. Chronic granulomatous disease presenting in childhood with *Pseudomonas cepacia* septicaemia. *J Infect* 1993;27:301.

306. Guide SV, Stock F, Gill VJ, et al. Reinfection, rather than persistent infection, in patients with chronic granulomatous disease. *J Infect Dis* 2003;187:845.

307. Segal BH, DeCarlo ES, Kwon-Chung KJ, et al. *Aspergillus nidulans* infection in chronic granulomatous disease. *Medicine (Baltimore)* 1998;77:345.

308. Abati A, Cajigas A, Holland SM, et al. Chronic granulomatous disease of childhood: respiratory cytology. *Diagn Cytopathol* 1996;15:98.

309. Williamson PR, Kwon-Chung KJ, Gallin JI. Successful treatment of *Paecilomyces varioti* infection in a patient with chronic granulomatous disease and a review of *Paecilomyces* species infections. *Clin Infect Dis* 1992;14:1023.

310. Chin TW, Stiehm ER, Falloon J, et al. Corticosteroids in treatment of obstructive lesions of chronic granulomatous disease. *J Pediatr* 1987;111:349.

311. Barton LL, Moussa SL, Villar RG, et al. Gastrointestinal complications of chronic granulomatous disease: case report and literature review. *Clin Pediatr (Phila)* 1998;37:231.

312. Hiller H, Fisher D, Abrahamov A, et al. Esophageal involvement in chronic granulomatous disease. Case report and review. *Pediatr Radiol* 1995;25:308.

313. Hoeffel JC, Tran Minh VA, Pracros JP. Esophageal involvement in chronic granulomatous disease. *Pediatr Radiol* 1996;26:169.

314. Kis E, Verebely T, Meszner Z. Inflammatory pseudotumor of the bladder in chronic granulomatous disease. *Pediatr Nephrol* 2002;17:220.

315. Stopyrowa J, Fyderek K, Sikorska B, et al. Chronic granulomatous disease of childhood: Gastric manifestation and response to salazosulfapyridine therapy. *Eur J Pediatr* 1989;149:28.

316. Fisher JE, Khan AR, Heitlinger L, et al. Chronic granulomatous disease of childhood with acute ulcerative colitis: a unique association. *Pediatr Pathol* 1987;7:91.

317. Goldblatt D, Butcher J, Thrasher AJ, et al. Chorioretinal lesions in patients and carriers of chronic granulomatous disease. *J Pediatr* 1999;134:780.

318. Lee BW, Yap HK. Polyarthritis resembling juvenile rheumatoid arthritis in a girl with chronic granulomatous disease. *Arthritis Rheum* 1994;37:773.

319. Gallin JI. Recent advances in chronic granulomatous disease. *Ann Intern Med* 1983;99:657.

320. Margolis DM, Melnick DA, Alling DW, et al. Trimethoprim-sulfamethoxazole prophylaxis in the management of chronic granulomatous disease. *J Infect Dis* 1990;162:723.

321. Gallin JI, Alling DW, Malech HL, et al. Itraconazole prophylaxis for fungal infections in chronic granulomatous disease of childhood. *N Engl J Med,* 2003 *(in press).*

322. The International Chronic Granulomatous Disease Cooperative Study Group. A phase III study establishing efficacy of recombinant human interferon gamma for infection prophylaxis in chronic granulomatous disease. *N Engl J Med* 1991;324:509.

323. Gallin JI, Farber JM, Holland SM, et al. Interferon-gamma in the management of infectious diseases. *Ann Intern Med* 1995;123:216.

324. Bemiller LS, Roberts DH, Starko KM, et al. Safety and effectiveness of long-term interferon gamma therapy in patients with chronic granulomatous disease. *Blood Cells Mol Dis* 1995;21:239.

325. Sechler JMG, Malech HL, White CJ, et al. Recombinant human interferon-gamma reconstitutes defective phagocyte function in patients with chronic granulomatous disease of childhood. *Proc Natl Acad Sci USA* 1988;85:4874.

326. Ezekowitz RAB, Dinauer MC, Jaffe HS, et al. Partial correction of the phagocyte defect in patients with X-linked chronic granulomatous disease by subcutaneous interferon gamma. *N Engl J Med* 1988;319:146.

327. Jackson SH, Miller GF, Segal BH, et al. IFN-gamma is effective in reducing infections in the mouse model of chronic granulomatous disease (CGD). *J Interferon Cytokine Res* 2001;21:567.

328. Sponseller PD, Malech HL, McCarthy EF Jr, et al. Skeletal involvement in children who have chronic granulomatous disease. *J Bone Joint Surg Am* 1991;73:37.

329. Pogrebniak HW, Gallin JI, Malech HL, et al. Surgical management of pulmonary infections in chronic granulomatous disease of childhood. *Ann Thorac Surg* 1993;55:844.

330. Lublin M, Bartlett DL, Danforth DN, et al. Hepatic abscess in patients with chronic granulomatous disease. *Ann Surg* 2002;235:383.

331. Stroncek DF, Leonard K, Eiber G, et al. Alloimmunization after granulocyte transfusions. *Transfusion* 1996;36:1009.

332. Stroncek DF, Matthews CL, Follmann D, et al. Kinetics of G-CSF-induced granulocyte mobilization in healthy subjects: effects of route of administration and addition of dexamethasone. *Transfusion* 2002;42:597.

333. Rex JH, Bennett JE, Gallin JI, et al. Normal and deficient neutrophils can cooperate to damage *Aspergillus fumigatus* hyphae. *J Infect Dis* 1990;162:523.

334. Rosh JR, Tang HB, Mayer L, et al. Treatment of intractable gastrointestinal manifestations of chronic granulomatous disease with cyclosporin. *J Pediatr* 1995;126:143.

335. Myrup B, Valerius NH, Mortensen PB. Treatment of enteritis in chronic granulomatous disease with granulocyte colony stimulating factor. *Gut* 1998;42:127.

336. Weening RS, Leitz GJ, Seger RA. Recombinant human interferon-gamma in patients with chronic granulomatous disease European follow up study. *Eur J Pediatr* 1995;154:295.

337. Kamani N, August CS, Campbell DE, et al. Marrow transplantation in chronic granulomatous disease: an update with 6-year follow-up. *J Pediatr* 1988;113:697.

338. Rappaport JM, Newburger PE, Golblum RM, et al. Allogeneic bone marrow transplantation for chronic granulomatous disease. *J Pediatr* 1982;101:952.

339. Di Bartolomeo P, Di Girolamo G, Angrilli F, et al. Reconstitution of normal neutrophil function in chronic granulomatous disease by bone marrow transplantation. *Bone Marrow Transplant* 1989;4:695.

340. Hobbs JR, Monteil M, McCluskey DR, et al. Chronic granulomatous disease 100% corrected by displacement bone marrow transplantation from a volunteer unrelated donor. *Eur J Pediatr* 1992;151:806.

341. Watanabe C, Yajima Y, Taguchi T, et al. Successful unrelated bone marrow transplantation for a patient with chronic granulomatous disease and associated resistant pneumonitis and *Aspergillus* osteomyelitis. *Bone Marrow Transplant* 2001;28:83.

342. Seger RA, Gungor T, Belohradsky BH, et al. Treatment of chronic granulomatous disease with myeloablative conditioning and an unmodified hemopoietic allograft: a survey of the European experience, 1985–2000. *Blood* 2002;100:4344.

343. Horwitz ME, Barrett AJ, Brown MR, et al. Treatment of chronic granulomatous disease with nonmyeloablative conditioning and a T-cell-depleted hematopoietic allograft. *N Engl J Med* 2001;344:881.

344. Malech HL, Maples PB, Whiting-Theobald N, et al. Prolonged production of NADPH oxidase-corrected granulocytes after gene therapy of chronic granulomatous disease. *Proc Natl Acad Sci USA* 1997;94:12133.

345. Malech HL. Progress in gene therapy for chronic granulomatous disease. *J Infect Dis* 1999;179[Suppl 2]:S318.

346. Malech HL. Use of serum-free medium with fibronectin fragment enhanced transduction in a system of gas permeable plastic containers to achieve high levels of retrovirus transduction at clinical scale. *Stem Cells* 2000;18:155.

347. Roesler J, Brenner S, Bukovsky AA, et al. Third-generation, self-inactivating gp91(phox) lentivector corrects the oxidase defect in NOD/SCID mouse-repopulating peripheral blood-mobilized CD34+ cells from patients with X-linked chronic granulomatous disease. *Blood* 2002;100:4381.

CHAPTER 4
Cell-Mediated Immunity

Richard B. Markham and Alan L. Scott

Mammals are susceptible to a wide spectrum of pathogenic microorganisms, which, in order to cause disease, must first contact the host and then establish a focus of infection. Pathogens that successfully establish infection and cause disease must overcome three major defensive strategies. The first consists of the physical, anatomical, and molecular barriers that have evolved in mammals to prevent colonization at epithelial and mucosal surfaces. Viruses, bacteria, and parasites that breach this first line of defense are immediately faced with the second line of defense—the cells and molecules of the innate immune system. Innate immunity provides an immediate response mediated by constitutively produced effector mechanisms that engage the pathogen directly with the goal of eliminating the infectious threat. The innate immune response often succeeds in preventing infection, precluding the necessity of further responses. If the pathogen is not eliminated by the cellular and humoral components of the innate immune response, the third phase of host defense is initiated, resulting in the induction of an adaptive immune response mediated by antigen-specific T cells.

Traditionally, cell-mediated immunity has been defined as the segment of an adaptive immune response that can be adoptively transferred only with viable T cells. It has become clear that the cells and molecules of innate immunity play key roles in the initiation and regulation of the adaptive, T-cell–mediated immune responses. Thus, the ontogeny of the cell-mediated immune response that develops as a consequence of a primary exposure to a pathogen can be divided into an immediate, nonspecific, innate phase and a delayed, antigen-specific, adaptive phase. In this chapter, we outline the major cellular and molecular components of the innate and adaptive phases of cell-mediated immunity.

CELLS OF THE INNATE PHASE OF CELL-MEDIATED IMMUNITY

The innate immune response serves two important functions. First, it is the initial, immediate response to viruses, bacteria, and parasites that serves to limit the pathogen's capacity to reproduce. This delay in the expansion of pathogen numbers provides the adaptive immune response the time it needs to tap into its combinatorial repertoire of T-cell and B-cell receptors, to carry out clonal expansion and properly activate antigen-specific effector T cells and B cells. Second, innate immune responses stimulate and influence the qualitative and quantitative nature of the subsequent adaptive responses against the pathogen. In addition to providing a signal that a pathogen is present, the composition of the cells and cytokines generated during the initial stages of innate immunity is a critical determinant of the helper T-cell subtype (T_H1 versus T_H2) and intensity of the antigen-specific cell-mediated immune response that ensues. It is important to note that many of the effector mechanisms used during innate responses to keep microorganisms in check also play important roles during the adaptive phase, during which these same effectors are under the control of cytokines produced by T cells. Macrophages, dendritic cells, and natural killer (NK) cells are the major cellular components of the innate response. Endothelial cells, platelets, mast cells, and fibroblasts are also important sources of regulatory molecules.

Macrophages and Dendritic Cells

Macrophages develop within the bone marrow and are released into the peripheral circulation as monocytes. Once they establish residency in a tissue, the monocytes transform into the mature macrophage (reviewed in reference 1). Monocytes and macrophages constitute a major cellular component of the innate immune response, where they function as phagocytic effector cells that eliminate pathogens (2) and as major sources of cytokines that regulate both innate and adaptive immunity.

Dendritic cells are bone marrow derived and initially circulate as precursors that home to tissues where they reside as immature phagocytic cells (reviewed in reference 3). Following infection or injury, the immature dendritic cells capture antigen and initiate a maturation process that initially results in the induction of cell surface molecules and cytokines important in regulation of effectors of innate immunity such as NK cells. Also as a consequence of antigen exposure, dendritic cells migrate to lymphoid organs, where they mediate the selection, activation, and clonal expansion of the rare antigen-specific T cells that will give rise to the adaptive immune response. Dendritic cells are unique because they are the only antigen-presenting cell capable of inducing a primary immune response. Depending on the specific circumstances of antigen exposure, subsets of dendritic cells are formed that provide T cells with the cytokines and cell–cell interactions required to drive CD4+ T cells down the T_H1 or T_H2 pathways (4). Thus, dendritic cells represent an important link between innate responses and the establishment of antigen-specific adaptive effector and memory responses.

Macrophages and dendritic cells recognize the presence of generic structures that are characteristic of molecules on or released by microbial pathogens. The receptors used to recognize these characteristic structures have been termed *pattern recognition receptors* (5). Examples of pattern recognition receptors include the mannose receptor on macrophages that binds to certain carbohydrates found selectively on bacteria and certain viruses (6) and the toll-like receptor (TLR) family of proteins, including the TLR-4–CD14 complex, which is the receptor for bacterial lipopolysaccharide/endotoxin (LPS) and TLR-9 that recognizes nonmethylated CpG motifs in bacterial deoxyribonucleic acid (DNA) (7,8).

Natural Killer Cells

NK cells are bone marrow–derived cells that participate in innate immune responses against intracellular pathogens and certain tumors. They comprise 15% of the lymphocyte compartment in the peripheral blood and are found in peripheral tissues, including the peritoneal cavity, liver, and placenta (9). Although they have the same basic morphology as T and B cells, NK cells are larger, with characteristic cytoplasmic granules. From the functional standpoint, NK cells exhibit the ability to lyse certain tumor lines *in vitro*, particularly those deficient in class I major histocompatibility complex (MHC), without the need for activation or immunization. Although they are capable of killing appropriate targets without activation, exposure of NK cells to interferons (IFNs), interleukin-12 (IL-12), IL-18, and IL-15 increases their ability to lyse cells up to 100-fold (10,11). In addition, when NK cells are treated with high concentrations of IL-2, they differentiate into lymphokine-activated killer (LAK) cells that demonstrate enhanced cytolytic capacity and a broad target specificity (12). NK cells play a key role in the initial control of infection by a spectrum of intracellular pathogens. Activated NK cells produce large amounts of IFN-γ, which is key in containing viral, bacterial, and protozoan replication during the lag period needed to mobilize and expand antigen-specific T cells. In addition, NK cells have antitumor activity (13). NK cells kill target cells utilizing a perforin-dependent mechanism similar, except for the activation signal, to that described for cytotoxic T cells (14).

Although all of the details of the mechanism used by NK cells to recognize infected, stressed, and abnormal cells have not been defined, it appears that alterations in the molecular composition of the infected cell is involved. NK cells have two classes of receptor that regulate their killing activity: activating or killing receptors and inhibitory receptors. The activating or killing receptors on human NK cells are a complex of molecules with representatives from the immunoglobulin superfamily (CD16, FcγRIII, NKp46, NKp30, and NKp44) and the C-type lectin family (NKG2D). These coexpressed receptors work in consort to produce an activation signal that induces cytotoxic activity. The ligands for the human activating receptor system include the stress-induced, nonpolymorphic class I MHC–like MICA/A (15), the family of UL16-binding proteins (16), and certain viral proteins (13,17). The ligand for CD16, cell-bound immunoglobulin G (IgG), is the dominant interaction through which NK cells participate in antibody-dependent cell-mediated cytotoxicity (ADCC) reactions.

The inhibitory receptors, or killer inhibitory receptors (KIRs; CD158), prevent NK cells from activating and killing self through recognition of unaltered levels of human leukocyte antigen A (HLA-A), HLA-B, and HLA-C. The functional analogues of the KIRs in mice are of molecules in the Ly49 family (18). The products of the 10 distinct genes that encode the KIR family of proteins are all members of the immunoglobulin superfamily, with each member exhibiting the capacity to discriminate between allelic forms of class I MHC (19). Typically, multiple receptors are expressed on each NK cell in a stochastic manner that generates a complex combinatorial repertoire of NK specificities. Through KIRs, NK cells monitor the altered levels of expression of class I MHC molecules on cells undergoing pathological changes. Reduced class I MHC expression is caused by a perturbation of cellular physiology or is a consequence of the immune evasion strategies developed by certain intracellular pathogens to disrupt the processing and presentation of peptide antigens to cytotoxic T cells (20,21).

Although NK cells have been reported to be important for the control of a wide variety of viral pathogens, they appear to be particularly relevant in combating herpesvirus infections (22). NK-cell dysfunction is common in human immunodeficiency virus (HIV)-infected individuals (23,24). In addition to their antiviral activity, murine NK cells have been shown to lyse directly *Trypanosoma cruzi* (25) and *Toxoplasma gondii* (26).

Cells of the Adaptive Phase of Cell-Mediated Immunity

The T lymphocyte, so named because of its obligatory residency in the thymus during development and differentiation, is the central cell in the regulation and expression of cell-mediated immunity. T lymphocytes directly kill infected cells, generate delayed-type hypersensitivity responses, and promote antibody formation. They are also capable of suppressing any or all of these immunological activities. Although all of these actions are carried out by T cells, each individual function is attributable to a distinct subset of T cells with more restricted capabilities that carry characteristic sets of proteins on their surface (27,28).

T cells have been subdivided into distinct functional subsets. Helper/inducer T cells (T_H) facilitate the generation of immune responses by other T cells or B cells (29) and secrete products that promote the antimicrobial activity of phagocytic cells (30) or the direct killing of infected cells (31,32). These cells bear the CD4 protein on their surface. Cytotoxic T cells (T_{CTL}) lyse tumor cells or cells infected with viruses or bacteria (33–35) and carry the CD8 protein on their surface (36).

Antigen Recognition by T Cells

A key element in understanding antigen recognition and subsequent T-cell activation was the observation that most T cells could only recognize foreign antigens when those antigens were presented to the T cell by other cells of the immune system and that this antigen presentation was a cognate interaction that required that the T cell and the cell presenting the antigen be "matched" in their MHC proteins (37–40). The MHC complex is a large genetic locus that encodes highly polymorphic proteins that bind and display the peptides recognized by T cells. The protein products of the MHC locus have been divided into three major classes of molecules and two of these, class I and class II, are important in T-cell activation. Three class I loci have been identified: HLA-A, HLA-B, and HLA-C (H-2K, H-2D, and H-2L in the mouse) (41). Class II genes are encoded in HLA-D, HLA-DR, HLA-DQ, and HLA-DP (I-A and I-E in the mouse) (42). All of these loci are strikingly polymorphic in both humans and the mouse. Class I antigens are the primary antigens recognized as foreign during tissue graft rejection and are also the antigens that must be shared between the classic CD8$^+$ cytotoxic T cell and its target for killing of the target cell to occur (43). Similarly, helper T cells can only be activated by antigen-presenting cells that possess the same class II antigens as the helper cell (38).

Class I antigens are found in varying amounts on virtually every mammalian cell (44). The cellular distribution of class II antigens is more restricted; with expression primarily on the professional antigen-presenting cell monocyte-macrophages (45), dendritic cells (45), and B cells (46). Much smaller quantities of class II antigens are found on activated CD4$^+$ T cells (47), endothelial cells (48), and epithelial cells (49).

The importance of the class I and class II MHC molecules in T-cell immunity derives from the inability of most T cells to be activated by a foreign antigen unless that antigen is physically associated with one of these molecules (Fig. 4.1A). Only peptides, not intact proteins, are capable of associating with the polymorphic regions of MHC products (50–52), which explains the inability of T cells to react to native proteins. The need for an accessory cell to activate T cells derives in part from a requirement for a cell that can take up complex proteins, process them into small peptides, and then noncovalently attach those peptides to MHC proteins, which are subsequently expressed on the cell surface. Contact between the TCR of a specific T cell and the peptide–MHC complex is required for that T cell to be activated (Fig. 4.1A). From the structure of the TCR, it is apparent that only a single receptor is involved in the binding of the MHC gene product–foreign peptide complex, so that interaction between the T-cell receptor (TCR) and the MHC gene product is an integral part of the attachment of the TCR to a foreign peptide.

Not all peptides can bind to the class I or class II molecule of a given individual (53). Selectivity of which peptide binds depends on the allelic forms of the class I and class II proteins produced by that individual. In some cases, none of the peptides that result from processing of a protein will be capable of binding to MHC products of a specific individual, and that individual will then be incapable of generating a T-cell response to those peptides or to the protein from which they were derived. On the other hand, T lymphocytes from two different individuals could appear to be activated by exposure of the immune system to the same complex protein, whereas in fact the T cells from the two individuals are reacting to "processed" peptides derived from different portions of that protein. This issue is particularly important for the development of vaccines that will

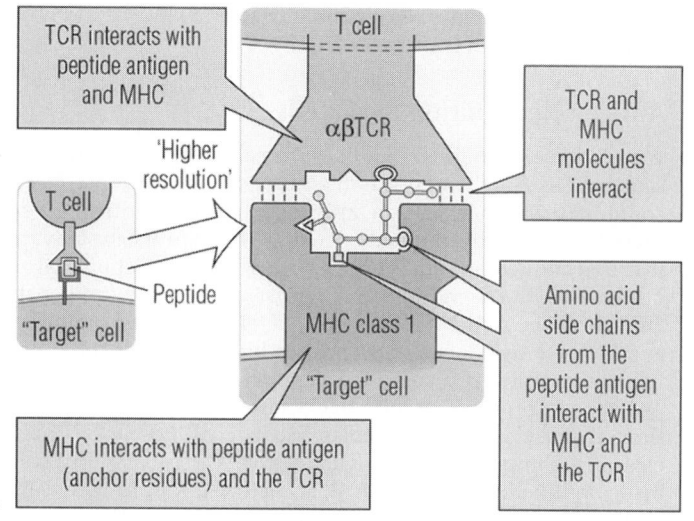

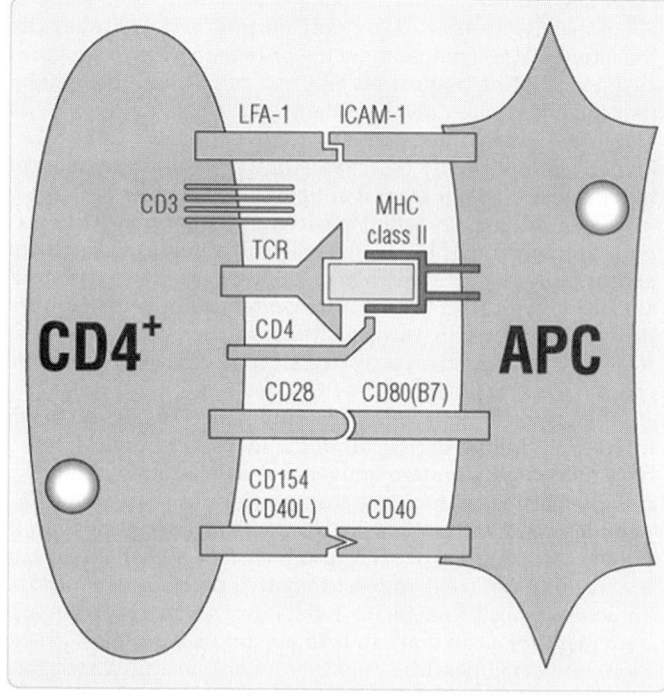

Figure 4.1. A: Presentation of a major histocompatibility complex (MHC)-bound peptide to a T cell. Peptides bound by specific "anchor" residues to MHC molecules on antigen-presenting cells engage the T-cell receptor (TCR) through other residues on the peptide. CD8 or CD4 molecules on the T cell will also react directly with class I or II MHC molecules, respectively, on the antigen-presenting cell (not shown). **B:** Co-stimulatory molecules involved in T-cell activation. Engagement of the TCR is not sufficient to initiate the activation process. Engagement of co-stimulatory molecules by their respective ligands is also required. Engagement of CD28 is critical for T-cell activation, whereas engagement of CD40L enhances the degree of activation. Interactions between intercellular adhesion molecule 1 (ICAM-1) and leukocyte function–associated antigen 1 (LFA-1) stabilize the other receptor-ligand interactions. APC, antigen-presenting cell. (**A** and **B** from Nairn H. *Immunology for medical students.* St. Louis: Mosby, 2002, with permission.)

activate T lymphocytes: any successful vaccine will have to contain proteins that can be processed into peptides that will bind to the wide variety of MHC proteins expressed by diverse human populations.

The discovery that peptides from ultraviolet (UV) radiation–inactivated influenza virus were presented in association with class II antigens, whereas peptides from live virus were pre-

sented in association with class I antigens (54), provided a framework for understanding the differences in antigen processing. This observation suggested that endogenous synthesis of proteins within the cytoplasm of the antigen-presenting cell, as would occur with live virus infection, directed the proteins away from entry into lysosomes and favored their association with class I antigens. The movement of cytosolic peptides to the endoplasmic reticulum from the cytoplasm depends on the activity of two polymorphic transport proteins, termed TAP-1 and TAP-2 (55–57). The polymorphic nature of TAP-1 and TAP-2 and their variable expression in different cells (58) are possible sources of variation in immune responses among different individuals. This association occurs as the class I MHC protein is being synthesized in the endoplasmic reticulum (59). The release of class I proteins from the endoplasmic reticulum requires their association with peptides (60). Under certain conditions, exogenous soluble antigens are capable of moving from the endosome into the cytoplasm and associating with class I MHC, resulting in cross-presentation of a peptide on both class I and class II MHC molecules on the same cell (61).

The importance of self-MHC as a critical component of the antigen recognition system for most classes of T cells is attributed to positive selection of self-MHC–restricted T cells within the thymus during T-cell differentiation. Studies with transgenic mice suggest that T cells with receptors capable of binding to self-MHC continue to mature within the thymus and ultimately populate the peripheral T-cell pools (62). More than 90% of the T cells entering the thymus fail to mature and die there (63), indicating that most T-cell precursors lack the receptors necessary for interacting with self-MHC in a manner that promotes their survival. Somewhat paradoxically, interactions between MHC-expressing thymic epithelial and maturing T lymphocytes are also believed to play a role in eliminating T cells reactive to self-antigens (64). Elimination of such cells is essential to the prevention of autoimmune disease. Whether a cell is destined for preservation or destruction within the thymus may depend on the affinity of the interaction between the T cell and the thymic epithelial cell, with either too low or too high an affinity resulting in death of the T cell.

The T-Cell Receptor

Binding of the TCR to the foreign peptide–MHC complex, in combination with accessory signals provided by antigen-presenting cells, results in clonal expansion of the resting T cell bearing the receptor specific for that peptide–MHC complex (65,66). The prototypical TCR is composed of a disulfide-linked heterodimer of highly variable α and β chains expressed at the surface as a complex with the invariant CD3 chains (67) (Fig. 4.1A). Elegant studies from several laboratories (68–70) demonstrated that the $\alpha\beta$ heterodimer is sufficient to recognize peptide antigen in the context of self-MHC, but the CD3 complex is required for intracellular signaling subsequent to receptor binding (71,72).

At the genomic level, the $\alpha\beta$ TCR is encoded by three α-chain or four β-chain gene segments, with each gene segment composed of a cluster of genes. Diversity is generated by random combinatorial associations of multiple germline gene segments plus junctional diversity generated by the imprecise joining of gene segments during recombination (65). The β chain, for example, is composed of four regions: the variable region (V), the diversity segment (D), the joining region (J), and the constant region (C). There are more than 50 distinct V region genes for the human β chain, and only one of those genes is selected during rearrangement of the V, D, and J genes that will ultimately encode a β chain. Similarly there are about 70 V region genes capable of encoding the V region of a single human α-chain TCR.

About 5% of mature circulating T cells carry an alternate antigen recognition molecule—the $\gamma\delta$ receptor (73,74). The basic structure of the $\gamma\delta$ receptor parallels that of the $\alpha\beta$ receptor, with V, J, and C region gene clusters for the gamma chain and V, J, D and C region gene clusters for the δ chain. The TCR repertoire of $\gamma\delta$ T cells is much more restricted than that of $\alpha\beta$ T cells, and the diversity that does exist tends to be segregated in different tissues (75). Most $\gamma\delta$ T cells lack CD4/CD8 and funcion as non–MHC-restricted cytotoxic T cells (76–78) that can respond directly to cell-bound antigens defined by the presence of structures such as phosphate or alkyl amines mimicking those found in microbial pathogens, such as *Mycobacterium tuberculosis* (79–81).

The binding of the TCR to the MHC–peptide complex is not sufficient to promote T-cell activation and proliferation. Two additional signals are required. First, proper activation of T cells requires the signals provided by cytokines such as IL-2 (see later). Second, concurrent with TCR–peptide–MHC interactions, T cells require additional receptor–ligand interactions at the interface with the antigen-presenting cells, referred to as *co-stimulatory* signals (Fig. 4.1B). Examples of co-stimulatory interactions that lead to T-cell activation include CD28 with B7-1/B7-2, CD40L with CD40 and leukocyte function–associated antigen 1 (LFA-1) with intercellular adhesion molecule 1 (ICAM-1) (reviewed in reference 82). Importantly, other cognate T-cell–antigen-presenting cell interactions, such as CTLA-4 with B7, serve to regulate the degree of T-cell proliferation and activation (83).

Intracellular Events Associated with T-Cell Activation

Binding of antigen to the TCR results in cell differentiation and the secretion of cytokines. Differentiation and secretion are the end products of a complex series of biochemical events that link the TCR on the cell's membrane and the transcription factors that promote gene expression (Fig. 4.2). This movement of signals from cell surface to cell genome requires the conversion of inactive proteins in the cytoplasm to forms that will interact with other cytoplasmic proteins, resulting in a cascade of reactions leading to lymphokine gene expression (84,85). The pathways involved in this process have been reviewed in great detail (86) and will only be summarized here.

The $\alpha\beta$ chains possess a short cytoplasmic tail and therefore depend on the invariant proteins of the CD3 complex to which they are noncovalently linked for their intracellular signaling (87). The proteins that make up the CD3 complex possess cytoplasmic tails that contain sequences referred to as *immunoglobulin receptor family tyrosine-based activation motif* (ITAM). Phosphorylation of signature tyrosine residues within ITAMs occurs rapidly after TCR–antigen–MHC engagement and is mediated by p56 *lck* and p59 *fyn*, which are members of the *src* family of protein tyrosine kinases (PTKs) (88–91). Phosphorylation of the ITAM facilitates binding and activation of another cytoplasmic PTK, termed ZAP-70 (92,93), which, along with the *src* kinases, can then phosphorylate tyrosine residues on an array of additional intracellular proteins involved in T-cell activation.

One target protein for the activity of these kinases is phospholipase lipase C-γ (PLC-γ) (91), which in turn hydrolyses phosphatidylinositol 4,5-biphosphate to biologically active diacylglycerol (DAG) and inositol 1,4,5-triphosphate (IP$_3$). DAG and IP$_3$ act as second messengers activating two distinct pathways. DAG activates protein kinase C (PKC), leading to the phosphorylation-mediated regulation of numerous pathways. IP$_3$ releases calcium from intracellular stores such as the endoplasmic reticulum, which results in the activation of calcium-dependent protein kinases.

In addition to acting on PLC-γ, phosphorylation leads to the activation of a serine-threonine kinase, Raf-1. Raf-1 initiates a cascade of mitogen-activated protein kinases (MAP kinases), which include p38 MAP kinase, ERK1, and ERK2 (94). These kinases activate a series of transcriptional activators, including nuclear factor of activated T cells (NFAT), nuclear factor-κB (NF-κB), and activated protein-1 (AP-1), involved in the expression of cytokine genes. These activated transcription factors bind to promoter regions to regulate gene expression.

The receptor–ligand interactions necessary for T-cell activation require that the relevant molecules that are initially distributed over the cell surface be brought together in close enough proximity to interact. Their coming together into specialized areas of the nonuniform cell membrane, termed *lipid rafts*, facilitates this approximation of interacting molecules. Lipid rafts are cholesterol- and sphingolipid-rich components of the cell membrane that are resistant to detergent solubilization (95,96). The linker for activation of T cells (LAT) is a 36- to 38-kd protein that appears to be particularly important in enabling interactions between certain membrane-bound and cytosolic proteins that are critical to intracellular signaling following TCR engagement (97). When LAT is phosphorylated by ZAP-70, it moves into lipid rafts, where, by facilitating the movement of PLC-γ into the raft, it can bring this molecule into association with its lipid substrates.

Cytokines and Cytokine Receptors

The ability of T lymphocytes to participate in antimicrobial resistance ultimately depends on the secretion of proteins that indirectly promote phagocytosis of microorganisms, directly kill or inhibit the growth of microbes, destroy infected cells, or augment the activity of other cells of the immune response that contribute to antimicrobial activity. The general term used to describe these secreted proteins that affect the behavior of other cells is *cytokine*. Cytokines made by lymphocytes are often referred to as lymphokines or interleukins, and those produced by macrophages as monokines. In this chapter, the generic term cytokine is used.

Cytokines are antigen-independent regulators of cellular proliferation, activation, differentiation, and in some cases, death. They are the soluble mediators of innate and adaptive immunity and the mechanism through which leukocytes communicate with each other and with other cell types. Although each cytokine has a distinctive molecular structure and set of biologic activities, they share a number of properties that are important to keep in mind (98).

- Cytokine synthesis is typically short lived and self-regulating. Most cytokines are produced as a consequence of exposure to antigen; thus, they require ribonucleic acid (RNA) and protein synthesis. Transcription is usually transient, and the messenger RNAs (mRNAs) are unstable; therefore, protein synthesis is also transient. Certain cytokines are additionally regulated at the level of RNA processing and by posttranslational modifications. Once the cytokine is produced, it is rapidly secreted.
- Each cytokine is secreted by a variety of cell types, and it is common for a single cell to produce a number of different cytokines.
- Cytokines act on a variety of different cell types. Cytokines have multiple and varied effects on the same target cell, depending on the activation state of the cell, its cell cycle status, and the presence of other cytokines.
- The ability of cytokines to regulate cellular activity is dependent on the deployment of specific receptors. A single cell can express receptors for multiple cytokines. Typically, these receptors are of high affinity, with binding constants of 10^{10} to 10^{12}. The levels of cytokine receptors are regulated by

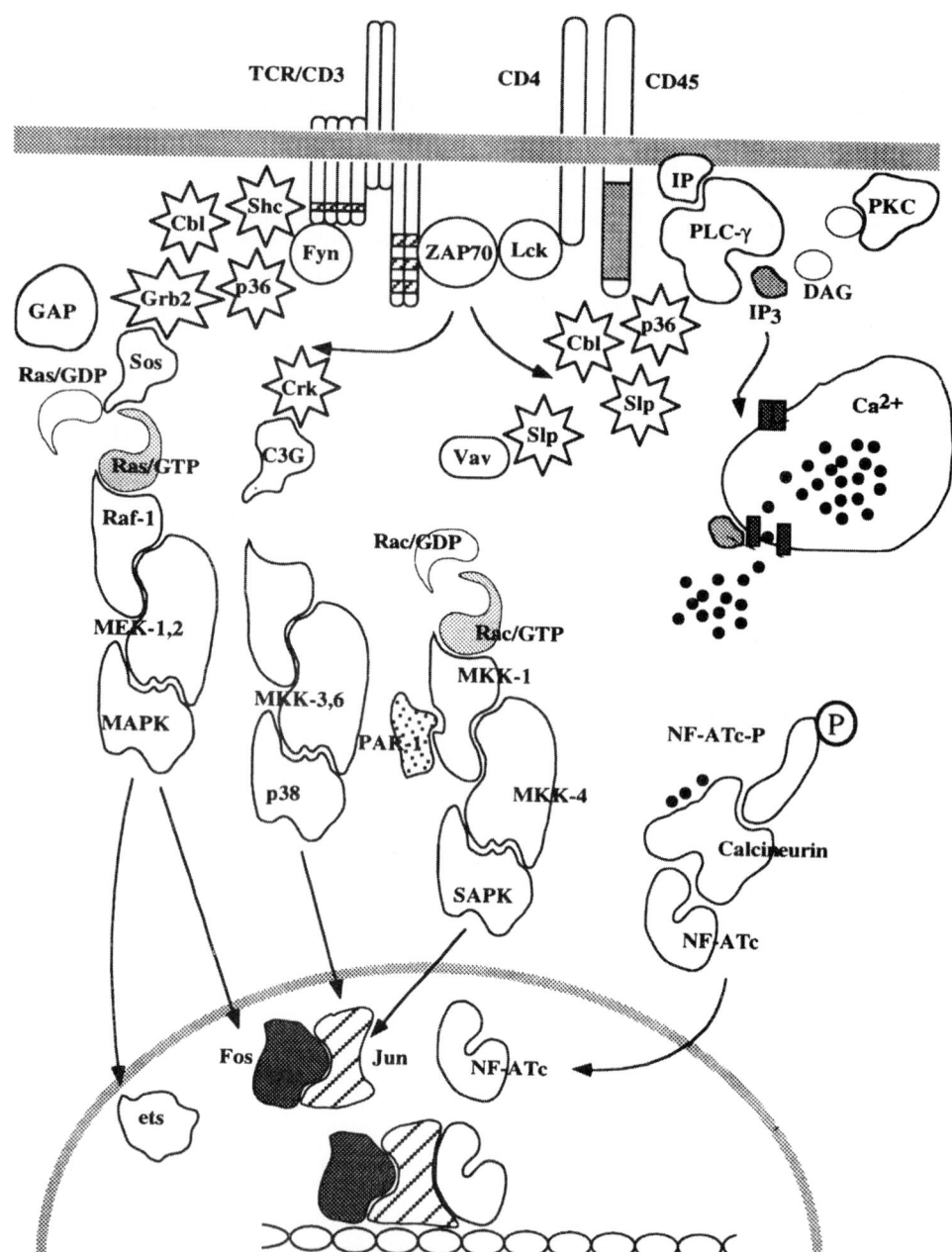

Figure 4.2. Signal induction through the T-cell receptor (TCR). Signals emanate from the TCR. Interaction of the TCR with its ligand induces activation of tyrosine kinases of the *src* and *syk* families, which phosphorylate adaptor proteins and immunoglobulin receptor family tyrosine-based activation motifs (ITAM) in the cytoplasmic tails of the CD3 molecules, recruiting different effector pathways that include small guanosine triphosphate (GTP)-binding proteins and phospholipase C-g. Phospholipase C-g induces calcium mobilization, whereas the GTP-binding proteins control a series of Ser/Thr kinase cascades (MAPK cascades). All these effectors act to regulate the function of transcription factors (e.g. NFAT, Jun, Fos). (From Alberola-Ila J, Takaki S, Kerner JD, et al. Differential signaling by lymphocyte antigen receptors. *Ann Rev Immunol* 1997;15:127, Fig. 1, with permission.)

differentiation status of the cell, the presence of antigen, and signals from cytokines themselves.

- The cytokine network is highly redundant, with different cytokines having similar actions. This property of multiple cytokines having the same functional effects is highly significant in the context of infectious disease. The redundancy significantly impedes the ability of microorganisms to evade immune responses by simply blocking or neutralizing a single cytokine or its receptor.
- Cytokines influence the production and action of other cytokines. The ability of one cytokine to induce the synthesis of other cytokines and cytokine receptors is critical to the ability of the innate and adaptive immune responses to respond rapidly to infectious agents. Exposing a cell to two or more cytokines may lead to mutual antagonism, an additive response, or synergistic effects.
- The action of cytokines can be autocrine (working on the same cell that produces it), paracrine (working on nearby cells), or endocrine (systemic, working at a distance) in nature. Typically, cytokines work in an autocrine or paracrine fashion.

RECEPTORS

A cell is rendered susceptible to the action of one or more cytokines by producing the appropriate receptors. Cytokine receptors consist of one or more transmembrane proteins whose extracellular domains contain a high-affinity binding site for the cytokine and whose intracellular portion is required for signal transduction. Cytokine receptors can be organized into five major classes based on the structural motifs found in their extracellular domains (Table 4.1). The class I cytokine receptors have structural similarities to the hematopoietin receptor and are composed of a unique ligand-binding chain and one or more signal-transducing chains, which are often shared by different receptors. This sharing of signal-transducing chains dictates the degree of redundancy in the cytokine repertoire. The class V receptors for the chemotactic cytokines (chemokines) span the cell membrane seven times and signal through G-protein–coupled mechanisms (99).

Different cytokine receptors activate distinct signaling pathways within the target cell (Table 4.1). In general, the signaling mechanism used by cytokines utilizes proteins that are constitutively associated with or recruited to the cytoplasmic tail of the receptor complex that, when triggered by docking of a cytokine in the receptor, activates a complex of signal transduction molecules. The best studied of the cytokine signaling pathways are the class I and class II receptors, which utilize the receptor-associated molecules in the Janus kinase (JAK/TYR) family of proteins and the cytoplasmic signaling molecules in the signal transducers and activators of transcription (STAT) family of proteins (100). The principal signal transduction molecules utilized by cytokines are outlined in Table 4.1.

The volume and complexity of information concerning the molecular and cell biology for each cytokine and for cytokine–cytokine interactions is formidable, and it is beyond the scope of this section to review. However, it is important to understand at some level the roles cytokines play in the

TABLE 4.1. Cytokine Receptors

	Designation of cytokine-specific chain	Common chain	Adaptor proteins	Signal transduction
Class I—hematopoietin receptors				
IL-2	CD122	γC (CD132)	JAK1/3	STAT5/3
IL-4	CD124	γC (CD132)	JAK1/3	STAT6
IL-7	CD127	γC (CD132)	JAK3	STAT5/3
IL-9	ND	γC (CD132)	JAK1/3	STAT5/3
IL-13	CD213	γC (CD132)	JAK1/3	STAT6/3
IL-15	ND	γC (CD132)	JAK1/3	STAT5/3
IL-21	ND	γC (CD132)	JAK1/3	STAT5/3/1
IL-6	CD126	gp130 (CD130)	JAK1/2	STAT3/1
IL-11	ND	gp130 (CD130)	JAK1	STAT3/1
IL-12	CD212	gp130 (CD130)	JAK2, TYK2	STAT4
G-CSF	ND	gp130 (CD130)	JAK1/2	STAT3
IL-3	CD123	gp140 (CD131)	JAK2	STAT5
IL-5	CD125	gp140 (CD131)	JAK2	STAT5
GM-CSF	CD116	gp140 (CD131)	JAK2	STAT5
Class II—interferon receptors				
IFN-α/β	CD118		JAK1, TYK2	STAT1/2/3/5
IFN-γ	CD119		JAK1/2	STAT1/5
IL-10	CD210		JAK1, TYK2	STAT1/3/5
IL-19	ND		?	STAT3
IL-20	ND		JAK1	STAT3
IL-22	ND		JAK1, TYK2	STAT1/3
IL-24/MDA-7	ND			STAT3
IL-26/AK156	ND			
Class III—TNF receptors				
TNF-α	CD120a (55 kd) CD120b (75 kd)		TRAF, FADD, TRADD, RIP, RAIDD	Caspases, phospholipases, kinases, AP-1, NF-κB
LT	CD120a (55 kd) CD120b (75 kd)		TRAF, FADD, TRADD, RIP, RAIDD	Caspases, phospholipases, kinases, AP-1, NF-κB
Class IV—immunoglobulin superfamily receptors				
IL-1	CD121		MyD88, IRAK, TRAF6	NFκB, JNK, p38 MAP kinase
IL-18	ND		MyD88, IRAK, TRAF6	NFκB, JNK, p38 MAP kinase
Class V—seven transmembrane-spanning receptors				
IL-8 (for other chemokines, see Table 4.2)	CD128		G proteins	MAPK, IP3K, PLC, PKC, Syc, ZAP-70, STATS

IL, interleukin; G-CSF, granulocyte colony-stimulating factor; GM-CSF, granulocyte-macrophage colony-stimulating factor; IFN, interferon; TNF, tumor necrosis factor; LT, lymphotoxin; ND, not determined.

induction, maintenance, and resolution of inflammatory responses mounted against pathogens. To facilitate this understanding, key cytokines will be discussed in the context of their roles in the innate (immediate, antigen-nonspecific) and the adaptive (delayed, antigen-specific) responses to pathogens. It is important to note that the innate and adaptive immune reactions are elements of an overall immune response with multiple induction and effector mechanisms, many of which overlap. Thus, cytokines that function in the innate response may have similar or additional roles in the context of a T-cell–controlled adaptive response.

Cytokines of Innate Immunity

Macrophages, dendritic cells, NK cells, endothelial cells, platelets, mast cells, and fibroblasts produce most of the cytokines released during the initial phases of the innate response. Initially, these cells recognize microbial pathogens with the pattern recognition receptors that have been mentioned previously (5). The consequences of engaging the pattern recognition receptors on these cells include cell activation and cytokine secretion. The principal cytokines produced during the innate phase of the immune response include tumor necrosis factor (TNF), IL-1, IL-6, IL-12, IL-15, IL-18, IL-10, and chemokines.

TUMOR NECROSIS FACTOR

TNF is a macrophage-derived mediator of acute inflammation induced by gram-negative bacteria and other microbes and is the cause of many of the systemic symptoms associated with severe infection. TNF is also referred to as TNF-α to distinguish it from the closely related TNF-β (also known as *lymphotoxin*). It was initially described as an activity in the serum of mice treated with LPS that caused hemorrhagic necrosis of implanted tumors and certain tumor cell lines (101,102). About the same time, it was identified as "cachectin" in the serum of rabbits with a wasting syndrome caused by the protozoan parasite *Trypanosoma brucei* (103). Subsequent studies showed that TNF and cachectin are the same molecule.

A potent stimulus for TNF production is LPS from gram-negative bacteria, and the major cellular sources of TNF are macrophages, T cells, and NK cells. TNF is initially produced as a homotrimeric membrane protein that is processed to yield a 51-kd homotrimeric secreted form of the cytokine. TNF has two distinct receptors of 55 kd (TNF-RI, CD120a) and 75 kd (TNF-RII, CD120b) that are found on nearly all cells. Binding of TNF to TNF-RI or TNF-RII can result in the initiation of two major pathways. First, binding can result in the recruitment of TNF receptor–associated factors (TRAFs) (104) that ultimately lead to cell activation. In contrast, binding of TNF to its receptors can lead to the recruitment of proteins that induce the cell to undergo programmed cell death (105). The specific mechanisms that dictate whether a cell undergoes activation or death are not known.

The primary functions of TNF are to induce the recruitment of monocytes and neutrophils to the site of infection and to activate these cells to eliminate the invading pathogens. TNF activates vascular endothelial cells to expressed adhesion molecules that are key to the recruitment of neutrophils and monocytes (and ultimately T cells) to locations of infection or damage. TNF-activated macrophages and endothelial cells produce chemokines that recruit more cells to the area of inflammation. TNF-activated macrophages also secrete IL-1, which has a number of overlapping functions with TNF (see later). TNF induces apoptosis in some cells (106), which may be significant in eliminating active or potential sites for the replication of intracellular pathogens.

When produced in large amounts, TNF has significant systemic consequences and is the source of many of the clinical and pathological outcomes of severe infection. TNF works directly on the hypothalamus to induce prostaglandin synthesis, resulting in fever. TNF acts on cells of the liver and results in the production of acute-phase proteins. Prolonged exposure to TNF due to chronic infections or tumors produces the metabolic changes that result in wasting of muscle cells and fat cells, which is characteristic of cachexia (107).

TNF is the primary mediator of endotoxin or septic shock, a severe complication of sepsis by gram-negative bacteria that is characterized by intravascular coagulation, vascular collapse, and metabolic imbalances (108). Septic shock is a direct result of exposure to large amounts of LPS that induces TNF as well as IL-1, IL-6, IL-12, and IFN-γ (109).

INTERLEUKIN-1

The actions of IL-1 that induce and control the initial inflammatory responses to infection overlap significantly with that of TNF. Similar to TNF, the main source of IL-1 is macrophages activated by exposure to microbial products, especially LPS. Unlike TNF, IL-1 is also produced by epithelial and endothelial cells (110). TNF is a potent inducer of IL-1.

The IL-1 family of proteins includes two agonists: IL-1α and IL-1β, both of which are synthesized as 31-kd precursors and then enzymatically cleaved to release the active mature 17-kd IL-1 forms. IL-1β is the main IL-1 found in the circulation. The third member of the IL-1 family is IL-1Ra, a 23-kd receptor antagonist that plays a key role in regulating the activity of IL-1 (111). The IL-1 receptor (CD121) is a transmembrane protein belonging to the immunoglobulin superfamily with similar affinity for IL-1α, IL-1β, and IL-1Ra. IL-1 receptor is found on T cells, fibroblasts, and epithelial and endothelial cells.

Many of the biologic activities of IL-1 are similar to those described for TNF. At low levels, IL-1 is a powerful regulator of local inflammation through activation of endothelial cells leading to an increase in expression of the adhesion proteins important for neutrophil migration (110). Systemic effects of IL-1 are fever, induction of acute-phase reactants, and promotion of cachexia. Unlike TNF, IL-1 does not induce apoptosis.

INTERLEUKIN-6

Like IL-1 and TNF, the function of IL-6 is to induce and regulate the initial inflammatory responses to infection. In the context of the innate immune response, the main cellular sources of IL-6 are macrophages, fibroblasts, and endothelial cells. IL-6 is 21 to 28 kd, depending on the cellular source. The heterogeneity is due to posttranslational modifications that include glycosylation and phosphorylation (112,113). IL-6 is readily induced by viral infection (114), LPS (115), and the cytokines TNF and IL-1 (116). The class I IL-6 receptor is found on a wide variety of cell types, including epithelial, fibroblastic, hematopoietic, and neuronal cells (117). IL-6 receptors are found on activated B cells, where they mediate the B-cell differentiation function of IL-6 (116). Like IL-1 and TNF, IL-6 induces the acute-phase response and fever (118).

INTERLEUKIN-12

IL-12 is a 70-kd heterodimeric molecule made up of two covalently linked glycoproteins of 35 and 40 kd. IL-12 is produced primarily by macrophages and dendritic cells in response to LPS, virus infection, and infection with a number of intracellular bacteria and protozoa. IFN-γ production by NK cells and T cells also induces macrophages to produce IL-12. The high-affinity IL-12 receptor (CD212), which is induced on T cells, NK cells by IFN-γ, and dendritic cells by IL-15 (119), is the only cytokine receptor known to signal through STAT4. IL-12 is critical for initiating the cell-mediated reactions necessary for elimination of intracellular pathogens. It does this through the stimulation of IFN-γ production by NK cells and T cells, which in turn activates macrophages and generates the effector responses required to kill microbes (120). In addition, IL-12 enhances the cytotoxic activity of NK cells during both innate and adaptive immune responses (121). Importantly, IL-12 acts as a differentiation factor that drives CD4$^+$ T cells to the T$_H$1 phenotype (122). Thus, IL-12 plays critical roles in the induction and regulation of cell-mediated immunity during both the innate and adaptive responses to intracellular pathogens.

INTERLEUKIN-18
IL-18 is an 18-kd glycoprotein derived by enzymatic cleavage of a 24-kd precursor protein (123). Although IL-18 is structurally homologous to IL-1, these two cytokines are only 12% to 19% identical to each other at the amino acid level. IL-18 is synthesized by a number of cell types, including macrophages, dendritic cells, keratinocytes, fibroblasts, T cells, and B cells (124), in response to LPS and infection with intracellular pathogens. The IL-18 receptor heterodimer is expressed on T cells, NK cells, macrophages, neutrophils, and chondrocytes (125). IL-18 functions in consort with IL-12 to induce IFN-γ production from T$_H$1 cells (126). Recently, it has been shown that NK cells, dendritic cells, nonpolarized T cells, and B cells also produce IFN-γ when exposed to IL-12 plus IL-18 (127). Thus, together with IL-12, IL-18 is a key molecule in the ontogeny of a cell-mediated immune response.

INTERLEUKIN-15
IL-15 is a 14- to 15-kd molecule produce by a broad range of cell types, including activated macrophages, dendritic cells, osteoblasts, and fibroblasts (128,129), in response to LPS and infection with intracellular pathogens. The production of active IL-15, which is structurally similar to IL-2, is posttranscriptionally regulated (130). IL-15 receptors are expressed by a variety of cell types, including T cells, NK cells, and antigen-presenting cells (119,131). A major biologic function of IL-15 is to promote the proliferation of NK cells during early responses to intracellular pathogens. Later, in the adaptive phase of the response, T-cell–derived IL-2 takes over as the cytokine that drives NK-cell proliferation. IL-15 also plays a role in the early activation of antigen-presenting cells (119) and in the generation of memory in CD8$^+$ T cells (132). IL-15 knockout mice have reduced numbers of NK cells, and their CD8$^+$ T-cell responses are compromised (132).

CHEMOKINES
The chemokines are a large family of small proteins that stimulate the migration and activation of cells, especially phagocytic cells and lymphocytes. Chemokines play key roles in the induction and maintenance of inflammatory responses by controlling the number, composition, and activation state of inflammatory infiltrates. All chemokines described to date are low-molecular-mass proteins (8 to 12 kd) that can be categorized into two main classes: the CXC or α chemokines and the CC or β chemokines. Nearly all chemokines are structurally related with four cysteines that are located in highly conserved positions. The CXC class has an amino acid positioned between the first and second cysteines. In the CC class of chemokines, the two cysteines are contiguous. Two minor classes of chemokines have been reported. One class, designated as C or γ chemokines, does not contain the first and third cysteines. The second minor class, the CX3C or δ chemokines, has three amino acids between the first two cysteines (Table 4.2). The main role that chemokines play in the innate phase of immunity is to direct cell movements necessary for the efficient initiation of a focused defense responses.

The specificity for various leukocyte subsets and their roles in cellular recruitment in inflammatory diseases (133), the circulation of memory T cells (134), and the regulation of the T$_H$1–T$_H$2 axis (135) have been extensively characterized for a large number of chemokines. In addition to their contributions to the regulation of inflammation, chemokines have also been shown to play more direct roles in host–pathogen interactions such as those described for HIV-1. The ability of certain chemokines to neutralize HIV-1 infection has led to the characterization of additional receptors for the virus, new insights into pathogenesis (136), and new targets for antiviral therapy (137).

INTERLEUKIN-10
Thus far, we have described cytokines that participate in the stimulation of innate immune responses. We are just beginning to understand the molecular mechanisms employed to down-regulate inflammation. IL-10 was discovered initially as an inhibitory factor for the induction of cell-mediated immunity (138) and has proved to be a key molecule in the homeostatic control of innate and cell-mediated reactions. Biologically active IL-10 is produced as a 36-kd homodimeric protein by a variety of cell types, including macrophages and T cells. The receptor (CD210) is found on monocytes, macrophages, dendritic cells, B cells and T cells. IL-10 controls cell-mediated and innate immune response through its ability to inhibit the functions of activated antigen-presenting cells. It inhibits the production of IL-12 and IFN-γ by activated macrophages. In addition, IL-10 inhibits the expression of class II MHC and co-stimulatory molecules on antigen-presenting cells, thus inhibiting T-cell activation and suppressing the induction of cell-mediated effector mechanisms (reviewed in reference 139). Although IL-10 is the best-described regulatory cytokine, it is highly likely that other cytokines also carry out this role. Indeed, the growing IL-10 family of proteins, which includes IL-19, IL-20, IL-22, IL-24, and IL-26, suggests a complex regulatory network (140).

The biologic importance of IL-10–mediated control of cell-mediated responses is underscored by adaptations that have evolved in a spectrum of viral species. To date, seven viruses, most notably Epstein-Barr virus (EBV) and human cytomegalovirus (CMV), have been shown to produce functional homologues of human IL-10 (reviewed in reference 140). These virus-derived proteins can act as IL-10 receptor agonists, leading to a dampening of the host's cell-mediated immune response and to enhanced virus survival. The importance of the control mechanisms mediated by IL-10 are further emphasized by the observation that mice deficient in the expression of IL-10 develop inflammatory bowel disease and are compromised in their ability to regulate the extent and duration of inflammatory responses (141,142).

CYTOKINES OF ADAPTIVE IMMUNITY
Cytokines regulate the differentiation and proliferation of antigen-specific lymphocytes after antigen exposure. Cytokines mediate the inductive phase of the antigen-specific response as well as the activation of the cells that carry out the effector functions of the adaptive immune response. T cells are the major source of cytokines in the adaptive immune response. As a consequence of the specific circumstances of antigen exposure and the qualitative aspects of the innate immune response, CD4$^+$ T cells differentiate along a T$_H$1 or T$_H$2 pathway, resulting in the production of characteristic mixtures of cytokines that support particular effector responses. The cytokines considered in this section are IL-2, IL-4, IL-5, IL-13, and IFN-γ.

Interleukin-2. IL-2 is a 14- to 17-kd glycoprotein produced predominantly by antigen-activated CD4$^+$ T cells. IL-2 production is typically short lived, with a peak 8 to 12 hours after

TABLE 4.2. Chemokines and Chemokine Receptors

Chemokine	Target cell	Receptor
CXC receptors—α chemokines		
IL-8	Neutrophils, basophils, T cells	CXCR1, 2
GROα	Neutrophils	CXCR2, 1
GROβ	Neutrophils	CXCR2
GROγ	Neutrophils	CXCR2
ENA-78	Neutrophils	CXCR2
LDGF-PBP	Neutrophils, fibroblasts	CXCR2
GPC-2	Neutrophils	CXCR2
PF4	Fibroblasts	Unknown
Mig	T cells (activated)	CXCR3
IP-10	T cells (activated)	CXCR3
SDF-1α/β	CD34$^+$ bone marrow cells, T cells, dendritic cells, B cells, T cells (activated)	CXCR4
BUNZO/STRC33	T cells, NK T cells	CXCR6
I-TAC	T cells (activated)	CXCR3
BLC/BCA-1	T cells (activated), B cells (naive)	CXCR5
CC receptors—β chemokines		
MIP-1α	Macrophages, monocytes, T cells, NK cells, basophils, immature dendritic cells,	CCR1, 5
MIP-1β	Macrophages, monocytes, T cells, NK cells, basophils, immature dendritic cells,	CCR1, 5
MDP	Immature dendritic cells, NK cells, T cells, thymocytes	CCR4
TECK	Macrophages, thymocytes, dendritic cells	CCR9
TARC	T cells, immature dendritic cells, NK cells, thymocytes	CCR4
RANTES	Macrophages, monocytes, T cells, NK cells, basophils, eosinophils, dendritic cells	CCR1, 3, 5
HHC-1	Monocytes	CCR1
HHC-4	Monocytes	CCR1
DC-CK1	T cells (naive)	Unknown
MIP-3α	T cells, peripheral blood mononuclear cells, dendritic cells	CCR6
MIP-3β	T cells (naive), dendritic cells, B cells	CCR7
MCP-1	T cells, monocytes, basophils	CCR2
MCP-2	T cells, monocytes, basophils, eosinophils	CCR2
MCP-3	T cells, monocytes, basophils, eosinophils, dendritic cells	CCR2
MCP-4	T cells, monocytes, basophils, eosinophils, dendritic cells	CCR2, 3
Eotaxin	Eosinophils	CCR3
I-309	Neutrophil, T cells	CCR8
CTACK	T cells	CCR10
MEC	T cells, eosinophils	CCR10, 3
C receptors—γ chemokines		
Lymphotactin	T cells, NK cells	XCR1
CX3C receptors—δ chemokines		
Fractalkine	T cells, monocytes	CX3CR1

activation. The class I, high-affinity IL-2 receptor is a heterotrimer that consists of an α chain, which is induced upon T-cell activation, a β-chain, and the common, signal-transducing γ chain (143). Although the high-affinity IL-2 receptor is found only on activated T cells, the lower-affinity $\beta\gamma$-chain IL-2 receptor is found on naive T cells, NK cells, and B cells (143). Because antigen stimulation induces the high-affinity receptor, T cells that are activated by the appropriate presentation of their cognate peptides are the cells that preferentially proliferate in response to physiological levels of IL-2. In addition to its role as an autocrine growth factor for T cells, IL-2 promotes the proliferation and differentiation of NK cells and expansion and antibody production by B cells (144). IL-2 also plays a role as a negative regulator of the adaptive immune response by mediating activation-induced cell death (145). Thus, IL-2 plays key roles in the activation and termination of antigen-specific adaptive immune responses.

Interleukin-4. Biologically active IL-4 is an 18-kd monomeric protein produced by antigen-activated CD4$^+$ T cells, activated mast cells, and basophils. The IL-4 receptor (CD124) is a class I molecule found primarily on B cells, macrophages, and T cells (146). IL-4 and IL-13 are the only cytokines that signal through STAT6 (147). IL-4 is responsible for the development and expansion of the T_H2 subset of T cells and functions as an autocrine growth factor for T cells of the T_H2 phenotype (148). Consistent with its role in promoting T_H2 phenotype, IL-4 blocks the macrophage-activating action of IFN-γ, thus inhibiting development of T_H1/cell-mediated responses. The IL-4 produced by T_H2 T cells is the principal factor that stimulates B cells to undergo class switching for the production of IgE and IgG4 in humans (149).

Interleukin-13. The gene for IL-13 encodes a 15-kd protein and is located only 25 kilobases upstream of the gene for IL-4, suggesting that these genes arose from a duplication event (150). A number of the redundant functions observed for these two cytokines can be accounted for by receptor usage. The functional IL-13 receptor is a heterodimer made up of the IL-4 α chain and an IL-13 α1 chain that can bind both IL-13 and IL-4 (151). Ligation of the IL-13 receptor, like the IL-4 receptor, results in signal transduction through JAK1/3 and STAT6 (151). Although they share a number of functions, it has become clear that IL-13 and IL-4 have distinct and unique actions *in vivo* (152,153). Studies in mice have identified IL-13 as a critical mediator of the effector phase in allergic asthma responses (154), and polymorphisms in the IL-13 gene in humans have been associated with the asthmatic phenotype (155,156).

Interleukin-5. IL-5 is a T-cell–derived cytokine whose active form is a homodimer of a 20-kd gene product. Along with IL-4, IL-5 is a signature cytokine produced by CD4$^+$ T cells of the T$_H$2 phenotype. The IL-5 receptor is a heterodimer composed of a chain that has affinity for IL-5 and a signal-transducing chain, CD130, which is shared with IL-3 and GM-CSF (157). A major biologic function of IL-5 is to stimulate the growth and differentiation of eosinophils (158). IL-5 also activates eosinophils to be more efficient effector cells. IL-5 receptors are also found on B cells, where they mediate class switching to IgA production (159).

Interferon-γ. IFN-γ is the signature cytokine of the T$_H$1 response. IFN-γ is a glycoprotein produced by CD4$^+$ T$_H$1 cells, CD8$^+$ T cells, and NK cells as a 50-kd homodimer. T cells produce IFN-γ in response to antigen, and production is enhanced by IL-12 (160). NK cells secrete IFN-γ in response to IL-12 and after exposure to pathogens. The T-cell–derived IFN-γ of the adaptive immune response has a number of proinflammatory properties (reviewed in reference 161). It activates macrophages, NK cells, and neutrophils to kill pathogens more efficiently. T-cell–derived IFN-γ also enhances antigen presentation through the induction of molecules that are important in T-cell recognition, including class I and II MHC, co-stimulation molecules, the transporters associated with antigen processing (TAP-1 and TAP-2), and components of the proteome. In addition, IFN-γ induces the production of the p40 subunit of IL-12 by mononuclear phagocytes, therefore indirectly promoting the generation of T$_H$1 responses. At the sites of pathogen invasion, IFN-γ functions along with TNF-α to stimulate vascular endothelial cells to express adhesion molecules, thus directing additional cells to the site of inflammation. Engaging IFN-γ receptors on B cells promotes class switching to IgG1 in humans and blocks IL-4–mediated induction of IgE and IgG4. Mice deficient in IFN-γ production or signaling through the IFN-γ receptor are highly susceptible to intracellular pathogens (162) and are defective in macrophage activation (163).

T-Cell Subsets Distinguished by Lymphokine Secretion Patterns

Cytokines are secreted in certain patterns, and the secretion of certain cytokines precludes the secretion of others. CD4$^+$ T cells differentiate into subpopulations that produce distinct "cocktails" of cytokines that influence their effector functions. Those CD4$^+$ T cells secreting primarily IL-2 and IFN-γ are referred to as T$_H$1 cells and those CD4$^+$ T cells secreting IL-4, IL-5, IL-13, and IL-10 are termed T$_H$2 cells (164). In addition to controlling effector functions, the cytokines produced by T$_H$1 and T$_H$2 cells are important for the development and expansion of the respective subsets. IFN-γ promotes additional T$_H$1 differentiation and inhibits the proliferation of T$_H$2 cells (165–167). Conversely, IL-4 promotes T$_H$2 expansion and, along with IL-10, blocks differentiation of T$_H$1 cells (168). The T$_H$1 and T$_H$2 subsets develop from the same naive precursors, with the fate of the cells being dic-

tated by the stimuli present early in the immune responses. The T$_H$1 developmental pathway is initiated by antigens or infections that activate macrophages and NK cells and is dependent on macrophage- and dendritic cell–derived IL-12 production early in the response (169–171). The differentiation to the T$_H$2 phenotype is dependent on IL-4 production early in the response. The source of IL-4 that drives the early events in T$_H$2 differentiation is still not clear but may be from eosinophils, mast cells, and a specialized CD4$^+$ cell called the NK 1.1$^+$ T cell (172).

The main function of T$_H$1 cells is to activate the cells that will eliminate intracellular pathogens. IFN-γ produced by T$_H$1 cells activates phagocytes to destroy microbes and induces B cells to produce the IgG isotypes most efficient in opsonization and complement fixation. In addition, IFN-γ and IL-2 work in consort to stimulate CD8$^+$ T cells to kill infected cells. The principal function of T$_H$2 cells, through the production of IL-4, IL-5, and IL-13, is to induce the production of IgE and mast cell/eosinophil–mediated immunity. T$_H$2 immunity is important in combating helminth parasites and in allergy. Another important action of T$_H$2 responses is in the control of magnitude and duration of T$_H$1 responses system.

CD8$^+$ T cells can also be stimulated to differentiate into subpopulations that produce characteristic sets of cytokines. The physiological importance of these CD8$^+$ subsets is not known.

Cell-Mediated Destruction of Intracellular Pathogens

Two major mechanisms of target cell killing have been described. First, a calcium-dependent mechanism involves secretion of two products, perforin and granzymes (173) (Fig. 4.3). Perforin is a complement-like secretory product that assembles on the surface of the target cell to form pores in the target cell's membrane (174). Other CTL granule proteins, termed *granzymes*, act in concert with perforin to enhance target cell killing. Granzymes may be taken into the target cells through the perforin-generated pores or by interaction with specific receptors (175). Once released from vesicles by the cytotoxic cell, the granzymes promote cell death through apoptosis (176,177).

Although the reduction in CTL activity observed in perforin-deficient mice clearly demonstrates the importance of this protein in normal CTL function, some residual CTL activity is observed in these mice. This activity results from the interaction of Fas ligand on T cells with Fas on target cells (178–182), the second major killing mechanism (Fig. 4.3). Fas, also called Apo-1, expressed on the surface of potential CTL targets binds to Fas ligand (FasL) on the cytotoxic cell, resulting in the activation of the apoptotic pathway in the target cell. Engagement of Fas activates a tightly regulated series of enzymes, termed *caspases*, within the target cell. Those target cells lacking Fas, such as epithelial cells, would therefore likely be killed through perforin-dependent mechanisms. Even among cells that express Fas, their susceptibility to Fas versus perforin-mediated lysis can be influenced by factors such as the stage of the cell cycle in which the target cell is found when contact with the CTL occurs (183), the level of antigen expression on the target cell (184), and the specific organism infecting that cell (185).

Immune Destruction of Intracellular and Extracellular Bacteria

The immune mechanisms by which bacteria, fungi, and parasites that survive and multiply within phagocytic cells can be destroyed have been shown to involve both CD4$^+$ and CD8$^+$ T cells.

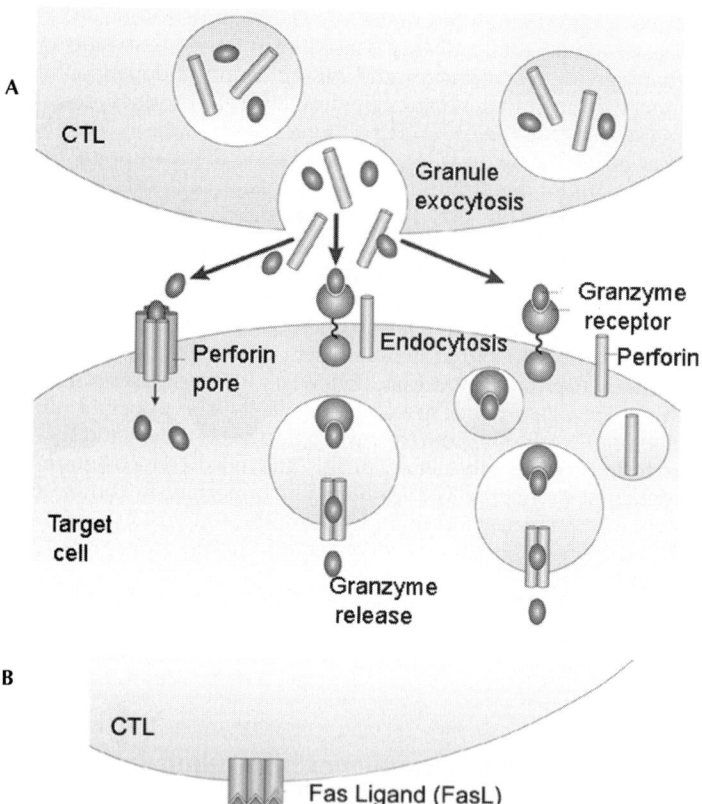

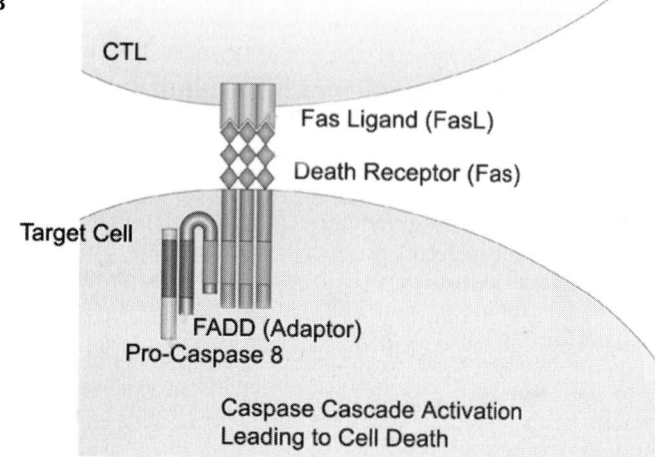

Figure 4.3. A: Pathways of entry for granzyme B. On interaction of a cytotoxic T lymphocyte (CTL) with a target cell, there is a directed exocytosis of the CTL granules into the extracellular space between the two cells. The original view was that perforin polymerized to form a pore in the target cell membrane through which granzymes could pass. More recently, the discovery of a receptor for granzyme B has indicated that granzymes might be taken up by receptor-mediated endocytosis and that perforin acts to release granzymes that are sequestered in endosomes into the cytosol of the target cell. In addition, granzymes might bind to the cell surface such that granzyme uptake is stimulated by perforin-mediated damage to the membrane. **B:** Engagement of Fas on a target cell with CTL-expressed Fas ligand results in apoptotic death. Stimulation of the Fas receptor results in recruitment of the initiator caspase, caspase-8, through interaction with the adaptor molecule Fas-associated death domain protein (FADD) by means of death domains and death effector domains. This results in the activation of other members of the caspase cascade, ultimately resulting in fragmentation of cellular DNA and cell death. (From Barry M, Bleackley RC. Cytotoxic T lymphocytes: all roads lead to death. *Nat Rev Immunol* 2002;402, Fig. 1, with permission.)

Early studies by Zinkernagel and colleagues (186) showed adaptive protection against infection with the intracellular pathogen, *Listeria monocytogenes*, to be class II restricted, indicating that cytotoxic mechanisms, which are predominantly class I restricted, were not involved. *Listeria* then became widely used in model systems for *in vitro* analysis of the basis for this protection (187).

Such *in vitro* studies with intracellular pathogens demonstrated that lymphokines produced by CD4$^+$ T cells that were exposed to microbial antigens could activate macrophages to kill organisms that were not killed by macrophages that had not been exposed to immune T cells. This activation was nonspecific in that, once activated, the macrophages showed increased ability to destroy unrelated organisms or even tumor cells (188). IFN-γ was subsequently identified as the primary T-cell product that activated macrophages to increase microbicidal activity (189).

More recent studies have indicated that CD8$^+$, as well as CD4$^+$, T cells may be important in resistance to *Listeria* (190,191). Like CD4$^+$ T cells, these cells can activate macrophages by secretion of IFN-γ (192). As indicated earlier, CD8$^+$ T cells are capable of being activated by unique bacterial components presented in association with class Ib MHC or CD1 (193,194). The mechanisms by which CTLs kill their targets can also be used to kill bacteria-infected cells. It is notable that a product of CD8$^+$ T cells, granulysin (195) is also capable of directly inhibiting the growth of a wide array of extracellular and intracellular microorganisms, including *Candida albicans*, *Cryptococcus neoformans*, *Salmonella typhimurium*, *Staphylococcus aureus*, and *Escherichia coli* (194). Thus, the simple paradigm that humoral immunity protects against extracellular microorganisms and T-cell–mediated immunity against intracellular microorganisms no longer appears valid. The *in vivo* relevance of granulysin is not yet established but can be considered in the context of earlier *in vivo* studies in animal model systems demonstrating protective T-cell immunity to extracellular bacteria (196–199).

The explosive growth in our understanding of T-lymphocyte biology has revealed a myriad of mechanisms by which this cell interacts with the microbial world. Populations of T lymphocytes that respond exclusively to bacterial glycolipids or to signature bacterial peptide sequences and the ability of T cells to kill both intracellular and extracellular microorganisms speak to the degree to which interactions with the microbial world have influenced T-cell evolution. Our success in combating the great infectious disease challenges of the twenty-first century may well depend on our ability to harness the remarkable functional plasticity of this cell to prevent and control those diseases for which direct antimicrobial therapy offers little hope.

REFERENCES

1. Gordon S. Macrophages and the immune response. In: Paul WE, ed. *Fundamental immunology* (4th ed). Philadelphia: Lippincott-Raven, 1999:533–545.
2. Ismail N, Olano JP, Feng HM, et al. Current status of immune mechanisms of killing of intracellular microorganisms. *FEMS Microbiol Lett* 2002;207:111–120.
3. Banchereau J, Briere F, Caux C, et al. Immunobiology of dendritic cells. *Annu Rev Immunol* 2000;18:767–811.
4. Pulendran B, Smith JL, Caspary G, et al. Distinct dendritic cell subsets differentially regulate the class of immune response in vivo. *Proc Natl Acad Sci USA* 1999;96:1036–1041.
5. Uthaisangsook S, Day NK, Bahna SL, et al. Innate immunity and its role against infections. *Ann Allergy Asthma Immunol* 2002;88:253–264.
6. Linehan SA, Martinez-Pomares L, Gordon S. Macrophage lectins in host defence. *Microbes Infect* 2000;2:279–288.
7. Hornung V, Rothenfusser S, Britsch S, et al. Quantitative expression of toll-like receptor 1-10 mRNA in cellular subsets of human peripheral blood mononuclear cells and sensitivity to CpG oligodeoxynucleotides. *J Immunol* 2002;168:4531–4537.
8. Takeuchi O, Sato S, Horiuchi T, et al. Cutting edge: role of toll-like receptor 1 in mediating immune response to microbial lipoproteins. *J Immunol* 2002;169:10–14.
9. Trinchieri G. Biology of natural killer cells. *Adv Immunol* 1989;47:187–376.
10. Carson WE, Giri JG, Lindemann MJ, et al. Interleukin (IL) 15 is a novel cytokine that activates human natural killer cells via components of the IL-2 receptor. *J Exp Med* 1994;180:1395–1403.
11. Zhang T, Kawakami K, Qureshi MH, et al. Interleukin-12 (IL-12) and IL-18 synergistically induce the fungicidal activity of murine peritoneal exudate

cells against *Cryptococcus neoformans* through production of gamma interferon by natural killer cells. *Infect Immun* 1997;65:3594–3599.

12. Rayner AA, Grimm EA, Lotze MT, et al. Lymphokine-activated killer (LAK) cells: analysis of factors relevant to the immunotherapy of human cancer. *Cancer* 1985;55:1327–1333.

13. Moretta A, Bottino C, Vitale M, et al. Activating receptors and coreceptors involved in human natural killer cell-mediated cytolysis. *Annu Rev Immunol* 2001;19:197–223.

14. Smyth MJ, Thia KY, Cretney E, et al. Perforin is a major contributor to NK cell control of tumor metastasis. *J Immunol* 1999;162:6658–6662.

15. Bauer S, Groh V, Wu J, et al. Activation of NK cells and T cells by NKG2D, a receptor for stress-inducible MICA. *Science* 1999;285:727–729.

16. Cosman D, Mullberg J, Sutherland CL, et al. ULBPs, novel MHC class I-related molecules, bind to CMV glycoprotein UL16 and stimulate NK cytotoxicity through the NKG2D receptor. *Immunity* 2001;14:123–133.

17. Auron PE, Webb AC, Rosenwasser LJ, et al. Nucleotide sequence of human monocyte interleukin 1 precursor cDNA. *Proc Natl Acad Sci USA* 1984;81:7907–7911.

18. Karlhofer FM, Ribaudo RK, Yokoyama WM. MHC class I alloantigen specificity of Ly-49+ IL-2-activated natural killer cells. *Nature* 1992;358:66–70.

19. Moretta A, Bottino C, Vitale M, et al. Receptors for HLA class-I molecules in human natural killer cells. *Annu Rev Immunol* 1996;14:619–648.

20. Lorenzo ME, Ploegh HL, Tirabassi RS. Viral immune evasion strategies and the underlying cell biology. *Semin Immunol* 2001;13:1–9.

21. Ploegh HL. Viral strategies of immune evasion. *Science* 1998;280:248–253.

22. Cerwenka A, Lanier LL. Natural killer cells, viruses and cancer. *Nat Rev Immunol* 2001;1:41–49.

23. Hu PF, Hultin LE, Hultin P, et al. Natural killer cell immunodeficiency in HIV disease is manifest by profoundly decreased numbers of CD16+CD56+ cells and expansion of a population of CD16dimCD56− cells with low lytic activity. *J Acquir Immune Defic Syndr Hum Retrovirol* 1995;10:331–340.

24. Peruzzi M, Azzari C, Rossi ME, et al. Inhibition of natural killer cell cytotoxicity and interferon gamma production by the envelope protein of HIV and prevention by vasoactive intestinal peptide. *AIDS Res Hum Retroviruses* 2000;16:1067–1073.

25. Albright JW, Hatcher FM, Albright JF. Interaction between murine natural killer cells and trypanosomes of different species. *Infect Immun* 1984;44:315–319.

26. Hauser WE Jr, Tsai V. Acute toxoplasma infection of mice induces spleen NK cells that are cytotoxic for T. gondii in vitro. *J Immunol* 1986;136:313–319.

27. Cantor H, Boyse EA. Functional subclasses of T-lymphocytes bearing different Ly antigens. I. The generation of functionally distinct T-cell subclasses is a differentiative process independent of antigen. *J Exp Med* 1975;141:1376–1389.

28. Townsend AR, Skehel JJ. The influenza A virus nucleoprotein gene controls the induction of both subtype specific and cross-reactive cytotoxic T cells. *J Exp Med* 1984;160:552–563.

29. Cantor H, Shen FW, Boyse EA. Separation of helper T cells from suppressor T cells expressing different Ly components. II. Activation by antigen: after immunization, antigen-specific suppressor and helper activities are mediated by distinct T-cell subclasses. *J Exp Med* 1976;143:1391–1340.

30. Silva RA, Florido M, Appelberg R. Interleukin-12 primes CD4+ T cells for interferon-gamma production and protective immunity during *Mycobacterium avium* infection. *Immunology* 2001;103:368–374.

31. Sun Q, Burton RL, Lucas KG. Cytokine production and cytolytic mechanism of CD4(+) cytotoxic T lymphocytes in ex vivo expanded therapeutic Epstein-Barr virus-specific T-cell cultures. *Blood* 2002;99:3302–3309.

32. Canaday DH, Wilkinson RJ, Li Q, et al. CD4(+) and CD8(+) T cells kill intracellular *Mycobacterium tuberculosis* by a perforin and Fas/Fas ligand-independent mechanism. *J Immunol* 2001;167:2734–2742.

33. Kagi D, Ledermann B, Burki K, et al. CD8+ T cell-mediated protection against an intracellular bacterium by perforin-dependent cytotoxicity. *Eur J Immunol* 1994;24:3068–3072.

34. Callan MF, Fazou C, Yang H, et al. CD8(+) T-cell selection, function, and death in the primary immune response in vivo. *J Clin Invest* 2000;106:1251–1261.

35. Medana IM, Gallimore A, Oxenius A, et al. MHC class I-restricted killing of neurons by virus-specific CD8+ T lymphocytes is effected through the Fas/FasL, but not the perforin pathway. *Eur J Immunol* 2000;30:3623–3633.

36. Littman DR, Thomas Y, Maddon PJ, et al. The isolation and sequence of the gene encoding T8: a molecule defining functional classes of T lymphocytes. *Cell* 1985;40:237–246.

37. Rosenthal AS, Shevach EM. Function of macrophages in antigen recognition by guinea pig T lymphocytes. I. Requirement for histocompatible macrophages and lymphocytes. *J Exp Med* 1973;138:1194–1212.

38. Katz DH, Hamaoka T, Benacerraf B. Cell interactions between histoincompatible T and B lymphocytes. II. Failure of physiologic cooperative interactions between T and B lymphocytes from allogeneic donor strains in humoral response to hapten- protein conjugates. *J Exp Med* 1973;137:1405–1418.

39. Zinkernagel RM, Doherty PC. Restriction of in vitro T cell-mediated cytotoxicity in lymphocytic choriomeningitis within a syngeneic or semiallogeneic system. *Nature* 1974;248:701–702.

40. Shearer GM, Rehn TG, Garbarino CA. Cell-mediated lympholysis of trinitrophenyl-modified autologous lymphocytes: effector cell specificity to modified cell surface components controlled by H-2K and H-2D serological regions of the murine major histocompatibility complex. *J Exp Med* 1975;141:1384–1364.

41. Srivastava R, Duceman BW, Biro PA, et al. Molecular organization of the class I genes of human major histocompatibility complex. *Immunol Rev* 1985;84:93–121.

42. Bell JI, Denny DW Jr, McDevitt HO. Structure and polymorphism of murine and human class II major histocompatibility antigens. *Immunol Rev* 1985;84:51–71.

43. Rouse BT, Norley S, Martin S. Antiviral cytotoxic T lymphocyte induction and vaccination. *Rev Infect Dis* 1988;10:16–33.

44. Harris HW, Gill TJ 3rd. Expression of class I transplantation antigens. *Transplantation* 1986;42:109–117.

45. Brooks CF, Moore M. Differential MHC class II expression on human peripheral blood monocytes and dendritic cells. *Immunology* 1988;63:303–311.

46. Krieger JI, Chesnut RW, Grey HM. Capacity of B cells to function as stimulators of a primary mixed leukocyte reaction. *J Immunol* 1986;137:3117–3123.

47. Kirkham BW, Pitzalis C, Kingsley GH, et al. Rheumatoid T lymphocyte MHC class II expression: in vitro stimulation produces normal MHC class II expression, independent of proliferation. *J Rheumatol* 1986;16:270–275.

48. Manyak CL, Tse H, Fischer P, et al. Regulation of class II MHC molecules on human endothelial cells: effects of IFN and dexamethasone. *J Immunol* 1988;140:3817–3821.

49. Dib SA, Vardi P, Bonner-Weir S, et al. Selective localization of factor VIII antigenicity to islet endothelial cells and expression of class II antigens by normal human pancreatic ductal epithelium. *Diabetes* 1988;37:482–487.

50. Allen PM, Unanue ER. Antigen processing and presentation at a molecular level. *Adv Exp Med Biol* 1987;225:147–154.

51. Grey HM, Chestnut R. Antigen processing and presentation to T cells. *Immunol Today* 1985;6:101.

52. Townsend AR, Gotch FM, Davey J. Cytotoxic T cells recognize fragments of the influenza nucleoprotein. *Cell* 1985;42:457–467.

53. Buus S, Sette A, Colon SM, et al. The relation between major histocompatibility complex (MHC) restriction and the capacity of Ia to bind immunogenic peptides. *Science* 1987;235:1353–1358.

54. Morrison LA, Lukacher AE, Braciale VL, et al. Differences in antigen presentation to MHC class I- and class II-restricted influenza virus-specific cytolytic T lymphocyte clones. *J Exp Med* 1986;163:903–921.

55. Spies T, DeMars R. Restored expression of major histocompatibility class I molecules by gene transfer of a putative peptide transporter. *Nature* 1991;351:323–324.

56. Spies T, Cerundolo V, Colonna M, et al. Presentation of viral antigen by MHC class I molecules is dependent on a putative peptide transporter heterodimer. *Nature* 1992;355:644–646.

57. Powis SJ, Townsend AR, Deverson EV, et al. Restoration of antigen presentation to the mutant cell line RMA-S by an MHC-linked transporter. *Nature* 1991;354:528–531.

58. Powis SJ, Deverson EV, Coadwell WJ, et al. Effect of polymorphism of an MHC-linked transporter on the peptides assembled in a class I molecule. *Nature* 1992;357:211–215.

59. Lapham CK, Bacik I, Yewdell JW, et al. Class I molecules retained in the endoplasmic reticulum bind antigenic peptides. *J Exp Med* 1993;177:1633–1641.

60. Degen E, Cohen-Doyle MF, Williams DB. Efficient dissociation of the p88 chaperone from major histocompatibility complex class I molecules requires both beta 2-microglobulin and peptide. *J Exp Med* 1992;175:1653–1661.

61. Shen Z, Reznikoff G, Dranoff G, et al. Cloned dendritic cells can present exogenous antigens on both MHC class I and class II molecules. *J Immunol* 1997;158:2723–2730.

62. Kurlander RJ, Shawar SM, Brown ML, et al. Specialized role for a murine class I-b MHC molecule in prokaryotic host defenses. *Science* 1992;257:678–679.

63. Sha WC, Nelson CA, Newberry RD, et al. Positive and negative selection of an antigen receptor on T cells in transgenic mice. *Nature* 1988;336:73–76.

64. Kappler JW, Roehm N, Marrack P. T cell tolerance by clonal elimination in the thymus. *Cell* 1987;49:273–280.

65. Davis MM, Bjorkman PJ. T-cell antigen receptor genes and T-cell recognition. *Nature* 1988;334:395–402.

66. Schwartz RH. Immune response (Ir) genes of the murine major histocompatibility complex. *Adv Immunol* 1986;38:31–201.

67. Saito H, Kranz DM, Takagaki Y, et al. Complete primary structure of a heterodimeric T-cell receptor deduced from cDNA sequences. *Nature* 1984;309:757–762.

68. Yague J, White J, Coleclough C, et al. The T cell receptor: the alpha and beta chains define idiotype, and antigen and MHC specificity. *Cell* 1985;42:81–87.

69. Dembic Z, Haas W, Weiss S, et al. Transfer of specificity by murine alpha and beta T-cell receptor genes. *Nature* 1986;320:232–238.

70. Saito T, Weiss A, Miller J, et al. Specific antigen-Ia activation of transfected human T cells expressing murine Ti alpha beta-human T3 receptor complexes. *Nature* 1987;325:125–130.

71. Clevers H, Alarcon B, Wileman T, et al. The T cell receptor/CD3 complex: a dynamic protein ensemble. *Annu Rev Immunol* 1988;6:629–662.

72. Weiss A, Imboden J, Hardy K, et al. The role of the T3/antigen receptor complex in T-cell activation. *Annu Rev Immunol* 1986;4:593–619.

73. Borst J, van Dongen JJ, Bolhuis RL, et al. Distinct molecular forms of human T cell receptor gamma/delta detected on viable T cells by a monoclonal antibody. *J Exp Med* 1988;167:1625–1644.

74. Lanier LL, Ruitenberg JJ, Phillips JH. Human CD3+ T lymphocytes that express neither CD4 nor CD8 antigens. *J Exp Med* 1986;164:339–344.

75. Holtmeier W, Pfander M, Hennemann A, et al. The TCR-delta repertoire in

normal human skin is restricted and distinct from the TCR-delta repertoire in the peripheral blood. *J Invest Dermatol* 2001;116:275–280.

76. Bank I, DePinho RA, Brenner MB, et al. A functional T3 molecule associated with a novel heterodimer on the surface of immature human thymocytes. *Nature* 1986;322:179–181.

77. Moingeon P, Ythier A, Goubin G, et al. A unique T-cell receptor complex expressed on human fetal lymphocytes displaying natural-killer-like activity. *Nature* 1986;323:638–640.

78. Moingeon P, Jitsukawa S, Faure F, et al. A gamma-chain complex forms a functional receptor on cloned human lymphocytes with natural killer-like activity. *Nature* 1987;325:723–726.

79. Bukowski JF, Morita CT, Brenner MB. Human gamma delta T cells recognize alkylamines derived from microbes, edible plants, and tea: implications for innate immunity. *Immunity* 1999;11:57–65.

80. Morita CT, Beckman EM, Bukowski JF, et al. Direct presentation of nonpeptide prenyl pyrophosphate antigens to human gamma delta T cells. *Immunity* 1995;3:495–507.

81. Tanaka Y, Morita CT, Nieves E, et al. Natural and synthetic non-peptide antigens recognized by human gamma delta T cells. *Nature* 1995;375:155–158.

82. Carreno BM, Collins M. The B7 family of ligands and its receptors: new pathways for costimulation and inhibition of immune responses. *Annu Rev Immunol* 2002;20:29–53.

83. Tivol EA, Borriello F, Schweitzer AN, et al. Loss of CTLA-4 leads to massive lymphoproliferation and fatal multiorgan tissue destruction, revealing a critical negative regulatory role of CTLA-4. *Immunity* 1995;3:541–547.

84. Gauen LK, Zhu Y, Letourneur F, et al. Interactions of p59fyn and ZAP-70 with T-cell receptor activation motifs: defining the nature of a signalling motif. *Mol Cell Biol* 1994;14:3729–3741.

85. Samelson LE, Klausner RD. Tyrosine kinases and tyrosine-based activation motifs: current research on activation via the T cell antigen receptor. *J Biol Chem* 1992;267:24913–24916.

86. Germain RN, Stefanova I. The dynamics of T cell receptor signaling: complex orchestration and the key roles of tempo and cooperation. *Annu Rev Immunol* 1999;17:467–522.

87. Weiss A. T cell antigen receptor signal transduction: a tale of tails and cytoplasmic protein-tyrosine kinases. *Cell* 1993;73:209–212.

88. Straus DB, Weiss A. Genetic evidence for the involvement of the lck tyrosine kinase in signal transduction through the T cell antigen receptor. *Cell* 1992;70:585–593.

89. Fraser JD, Straus D, Weiss A. Signal transduction events leading to T-cell lymphokine gene expression. *Immunol Today* 1993;14:357–362.

90. Straus DB, Chan AC, Patai B, et al. SH2 domain function is essential for the role of the Lck tyrosine kinase in T cell receptor signal transduction. *J Biol Chem* 1996;271:9976–9981.

91. Weiss A, Littman DR. Signal transduction by lymphocyte antigen receptors. *Cell* 1994;76:263–274.

92. Weil R, Cloutier JF, Fournel M, et al. Regulation of Zap-70 by Src family tyrosine protein kinases in an antigen-specific T-cell line. *J Biol Chem* 1995;270:2791–2799.

93. Iwashima M, Irving BA, et al. Sequential interactions of the TCR with two distinct cytoplasmic tyrosine kinases. *Science* 1996;263:1136.

94. Cooper JA. MAP kinase pathways: straight and narrow or tortuous and intersecting? *Curr Biol* 1994;4:1118–1121.

95. Simons K, Ikonen E. Functional rafts in cell membranes. *Nature* 1997;387:569–572.

96. Brown D. Structure and function of membrane rafts. *Int J Med Microbiol* 2002;291:433–437.

97. Zhang W, Sloan-Lancaster J, Kitchen J, et al. LAT: the ZAP-70 tyrosine kinase substrate that links T cell receptor to cellular activation. *Cell* 1998;92:83–92.

98. Abbas AK, Lichtman AH, Pober KS. *Cellular and molecular immunology* (4th ed). Philadelphia: WB Saunders, 2000.

99. Mellado M, Rodriguez-Frade JM, Manes S, et al. Chemokine signaling and functional responses: the role of receptor dimerization and TK pathway activation. *Annu Rev Immunol* 2001;19:397–421.

100. Kisseleva T, Bhattacharya S, Braunstein J, et al. Signaling through the JAK/STAT pathway, recent advances and future challenges. *Gene* 2002;285:1–24.

101. Carswell EA, Old LJ, Kassel RL, et al. An endotoxin-induced serum factor that causes necrosis of tumors. *Proc Natl Acad Sci USA* 1975;72:3666–3670.

102. Helson L, Green S, Carswell E, et al. Effect of tumour necrosis factor on cultured human melanoma cells. *Nature* 1975;258:731–732.

103. Rouzer CA, Cerami A. Hypertriglyceridemia associated with *Trypanosoma brucei brucei* infection in rabbits: role of defective triglyceride removal. *Mol Biochem Parasitol* 1980;2:31–38.

104. Pullen SS, Labadia ME, Ingraham RH, et al. High-affinity interactions of tumor necrosis factor receptor-associated factors (TRAFs) and CD40 require TRAF trimerization and CD40 multimerization. *Biochemistry* 1999;38:10168–10177.

105. Mak TW, Yeh WC. Signaling for survival and apoptosis in the immune system. *Arthritis Res* 2002;4:S243–252.

106. Maher S, Toomey D, Condron C, et al. Activation-induced cell death: the controversial role of Fas and Fas ligand in immune privilege and tumour counterattack. *Immunol Cell Biol* 2002;80:131–137.

107. Kawakami M, Murase T, Ogawa H, et al. Human recombinant TNF suppresses lipoprotein lipase activity and stimulates lipolysis in 3T3-L1 cells. *J Biochem (Tokyo)* 1987;101:331–338.

108. Karima R, Matsumoto S, Higashi H, et al. The molecular pathogenesis of endotoxic shock and organ failure. *Mol Med Today* 1999;5:123–132.

109. Kox WJ, Volk T, Kox SN, et al. Immunomodulatory therapies in sepsis. *Intensive Care Med* 2000;26:S124–128.

110. Apte RN, Voronov E. Interleukin-1-a major pleiotropic cytokine in tumor-host interactions. *Semin Cancer Biol* 2002;12:277–290.

111. Dayer JM. The saga of the discovery of IL-1 and TNF and their specific inhibitors in the pathogenesis and treatment of rheumatoid arthritis. *Joint Bone Spine* 2002;69:123–132.

112. May LT, Ghrayeb J, Santhanam U, et al. Synthesis and secretion of multiple forms of beta 2-interferon/B-cell differentiation factor 2/hepatocyte-stimulating factor by human fibroblasts and monocytes. *J Biol Chem* 1988;263:7760–7766.

113. May LT, Santhanam U, Tatter SB, et al. Phosphorylation of secreted forms of human beta 2-interferon/hepatocyte stimulating factor/interleukin-6. *Biochem Biophys Res Commun* 1988;152:1144–1150.

114. Cayphas S, Van Damme J, Vink A, et al. Identification of an interleukin HP1-like plasmacytoma growth factor produced by L cells in response to viral infection. *J Immunol* 1987;139:2965–2969.

115. Lee SW, Youn JW, Seong BL, et al. IL-6 induces long-term protective immunity against a lethal challenge of influenza virus. *Vaccine* 1999;17:490–496.

116. Van Snick J. Interleukin-6: an overview. *Annu Rev Immunol* 1990;8:253–278.

117. Lauta VM. Interleukin-6 and the network of several cytokines in multiple myeloma: an overview of clinical and experimental data. *Cytokine* 2001;16:79–86.

118. Ritchie DG, Fuller GM. Hepatocyte-stimulating factor: a monocyte-derived acute-phase regulatory protein. *Ann N Y Acad Sci* 1983;408:490–502.

119. Ohteki T, Suzue K, Maki C, et al. Critical role of IL-15-IL-15R for antigen-presenting cell functions in the innate immune response. *Nat Immunol* 2001;2:1138–1143.

120. Trinchieri G. Interleukin-12: a cytokine at the interface of inflammation and immunity. *Adv Immunol* 1998;70:83–243.

121. Hafner M, Falk W, Echtenacher B, et al. Interleukin-12 activates NK cells for IFN-gamma-dependent and NKT cells for IFN-gamma-independent antimetastatic activity. *Eur Cytokine Netw* 1999;10:541–548.

122. Ma X, Trinchieri G. Regulation of interleukin-12 production in antigen-presenting cells. *Adv Immunol* 2001;79:55–92.

123. Ghayur T, Banerjee S, Hugunin M, et al. Caspase-1 processes IFN-gamma-inducing factor and regulates LPS-induced IFN-gamma production. *Nature* 1997;386:619–623.

124. McInnes IB, Gracie JA, Leung BP, et al. Interleukin 18: a pleiotropic participant in chronic inflammation. *Immunol Today* 2000;21:312–315.

125. Liew FY, McInnes IB. The role of innate mediators in inflammatory response. *Mol Immunol* 2002;38:887–890.

126. Okamura H, Tsutsi H, Komatsu T, et al. Cloning of a new cytokine that induces IFN-gamma production by T cells. *Nature* 1995;378:88–91.

127. Tsutsui H, Matsui K, Okamura H, et al. Pathophysiological roles of interleukin-18 in inflammatory liver diseases. *Immunol Rev* 2000;174:192–209.

128. Grabstein KH, Eisenman J, Shanebeck K, et al. Cloning of a T cell growth factor that interacts with the beta chain of the interleukin-2 receptor. *Science* 1994;264:965–968.

129. Waldmann TA, Tagaya Y. The multifaceted regulation of interleukin-15 expression and the role of this cytokine in NK cell differentiation and host response to intracellular pathogens. *Annu Rev Immunol* 1999;17:19–49.

130. Waldmann T, Tagaya Y, Bamford R. Interleukin-2, interleukin-15, and their receptors. *Int Rev Immunol* 1998;16:205–226.

131. Lodolce JP, Boone DL, Chai S, et al. IL-15 receptor maintains lymphoid homeostasis by supporting lymphocyte homing and proliferation. *Immunity* 1998;9:669–676.

132. Kennedy MK, Glaccum M, Brown SN, et al. Reversible defects in natural killer and memory CD8 T cell lineages in interleukin 15-deficient mice. *J Exp Med* 2000;191:771–780.

133. Murdoch C, Finn A. Chemokine receptors and their role in inflammation and infectious diseases. *Blood* 2000;95:3032–3043.

134. Sallusto F, Mackay CR, Lanzavecchia A. The role of chemokine receptors in primary, effector, and memory immune responses. *Annu Rev Immunol* 2000;18:593–620.

135. Bonecchi R, Bianchi G, Bordignon PP, et al. Differential expression of chemokine receptors and chemotactic responsiveness of type 1 T helper cells (Th1s) and Th2s. *J Exp Med* 1998;187:129–134.

136. Poluektova L, Moran T, Zelivyanskaya M, et al. The regulation of alpha chemokines during HIV-1 infection and leukocyte activation: relevance for HIV-1-associated dementia. *J Neuroimmunol* 2001;120:112–128.

137. Murakami T, Yamamoto N. Roles of chemokines and chemokine receptors in HIV-1 infection. *Int J Hematol* 2000;72:412–417.

138. Fiorentino DF, Bond MW, Mosmann TR. Two types of mouse T helper cell. IV. Th2 clones secrete a factor that inhibits cytokine production by Th1 clones. *J Exp Med* 1989;170:2081–2095.

139. Moore KW, de Waal Malefyt R, Coffman RL, et al. Interleukin-10 and the interleukin-10 receptor. *Annu Rev Immunol* 2001;19:683–765.

140. Fickenscher H, Hor S, Kupers H, et al. The interleukin-10 family of cytokines. *Trends Immunol* 2002;23:89–96.

141. Chmiel JF, Konstan MW, Saadane A, et al. Prolonged inflammatory response to acute *Pseudomonas* challenge in interleukin-10 knockout mice. *Am J Respir Crit Care Med* 2002;165:1176–1181.

142. Takahashi I, Matsuda J, Gapin L, et al. Colitis-related public T cells are

selected in the colonic lamina propria of IL-10-deficient mice. *Clin Immunol* 2002;102:237–248.

143. Taniguchi T, Minami Y. The IL-2/IL-2 receptor system: a current overview. *Cell* 1993;73:5–8.

144. Minami Y, Kono T, Miyazaki T, et al. The IL-2 receptor complex: its structure, function, and target genes. *Annu Rev Immunol* 1993;11:245–268.

145. Wang R, Rogers AM, Rush BJ, et al. Induction of sensitivity to activation-induced death in primary CD4+ cells: a role for interleukin-2 in the negative regulation of responses by mature CD4+ T cells. *Eur J Immunol* 1996;26:2263–2270.

146. Hall IP: Interleukin-4 receptor alpha gene variants and allergic disease. *Respir Res* 2000;1:6–8.

147. Boothby M, Mora AL, Aronica MA, et al. IL-4 signaling, gene transcription regulation, and the control of effector T cells. *Immunol Res* 2001;23:179–191.

148. Fallon PG, Jolin HE, Smith P, et al. IL-4 induces characteristic Th2 responses even in the combined absence of IL-5, IL-9, and IL-13. *Immunity* 2002;17:7–17.

149. Oettgen HC. Regulation of the IgE isotype switch: new insights on cytokine signals and the functions of epsilon germline transcripts. *Curr Opin Immunol* 2000;12:618–623.

150. Smirnov DV, Smirnova MG, Korobko VG, et al. Tandem arrangement of human genes for interleukin-4 and interleukin-13: resemblance in their organization. *Gene* 1995;155:277–281.

151. David M, Ford D, Bertoglio J, et al. Induction of the IL-13 receptor alpha2-chain by IL-4 and IL-13 in human keratinocytes: involvement of STAT6, ERK and p38 MAPK pathways. *Oncogene* 2001;20:6660–6668.

152. Grunig G, Warnock M, Wakil AE, et al. Requirement for IL-13 independently of IL-4 in experimental asthma. *Science* 1998;282:2261–2263.

153. Wills-Karp M, Luyimbazi J, Xu X, et al. Interleukin-13: central mediator of allergic asthma. *Science* 1998;282:2258–2261.

154. Zhu Z, Homer RJ, Wang Z, et al. Pulmonary expression of interleukin-13 causes inflammation, mucus hypersecretion, subepithelial fibrosis, physiologic abnormalities, and eotaxin production. *J Clin Invest* 1999;103:779–788.

155. Graves PE, Kabesch M, Halonen M, et al. A cluster of seven tightly linked polymorphisms in the IL-13 gene is associated with total serum IgE levels in three populations of white children. *J Allergy Clin Immunol* 2000;105:506–513.

156. Heinzmann A, Mao XQ, Akaiwa M, et al. Genetic variants of IL-13 signalling and human asthma and atopy. *Hum Mol Genet* 2000;9:549–559.

157. Geijsen N, Koenderman L, Coffer PJ. Specificity in cytokine signal transduction: lessons learned from the IL-3/IL-5/GM-CSF receptor family. *Cytokine Growth Factor Rev* 2001;12:19–25.

158. Tomaki M, Zhao LL, Sjostrand M, et al. Comparison of effects of anti-IL-3, IL-5 and GM-CSF treatments on eosinophilopoiesis and airway eosinophilia induced by allergen. *Pulm Pharmacol Ther* 2002;15:161–168.

159. Hiroi T, Yanagita M, Iijima H, et al. Deficiency of IL-5 receptor alpha-chain selectively influences the development of the common mucosal immune system independent IgA-producing B-1 cell in mucosa-associated tissues. *J Immunol* 1999;162:821–828.

160. Robinson DS, O'Garra A. Further checkpoints in Th1 development. *Immunity* 2002;16:755–758.

161. Boehm U, Klamp T, Groot M, et al. Cellular responses to interferon-gamma. *Annu Rev Immunol* 1997;15:749–795.

162. van Schaik SM, Obot N, Enhorning G, et al. Role of interferon gamma in the pathogenesis of primary respiratory syncytial virus infection in BALB/c mice. *J Med Virol* 2000;62:257–266.

163. Nansen A, Christensen JP, Ropke C, et al. Role of interferon-gamma in the pathogenesis of LCMV-induced meningitis: unimpaired leucocyte recruitment, but deficient macrophage activation in interferon-gamma knock-out mice. *J Neuroimmunol* 1998;86:202–212.

164. Mosmann TR, Coffman RL. TH1 and TH2 cells: different patterns of lymphokine secretion lead to different functional properties. *Annu Rev Immunol* 1989;7:145–173.

165. Gajewski TF, Goldwasser E, Fitch FW. Anti-proliferative effect of IFN-gamma in immune regulation. II. IFN-gamma inhibits the proliferation of murine bone marrow cells stimulated with IL-3, IL-4, or granulocyte-macrophage colony-stimulating factor. *J Immunol* 1988;141:2635–2642.

166. Coffman RL, Seymour BW, Lebman DA, et al. The role of helper T cell products in mouse B cell differentiation and isotype regulation. *Immunol Rev* 1988;102:5–28.

167. Boom WH, Liano D, Abbas AK. Heterogeneity of helper/inducer T lymphocytes. II. Effects of interleukin 4- and interleukin 2-producing T cell clones on resting B lymphocytes. *J Exp Med* 1988;167:1350–1363.

168. Fiorentino DF, Zlotnik A, Vieira P, et al. IL-10 acts on the antigen-presenting cell to inhibit cytokine production by Th1 cells. *J Immunol* 1991;146:3444–3451.

169. Seder RA, Gazzinelli R, Sher A, et al. Interleukin 12 acts directly on CD4+ T cells to enhance priming for interferon gamma production and diminishes interleukin 4 inhibition of such priming. *Proc Natl Acad Sci USA* 1993;90:10188–10192.

170. Hsieh CS, Macatonia SE, Tripp CS, et al. Development of TH1 CD4+ T cells through IL-12 produced by Listeria-induced macrophages. *Science* 1993;260:547–549.

171. Hsieh CS, Macatonia SE, O'Garra A, et al. Pathogen-induced Th1 phenotype development in CD4+ alpha beta-TCR transgenic T cells is macrophage dependent. *Int Immunol* 1993;5:371–382.

172. Ho IC, Kaplan MH, Jackson-Grusby L, et al. Marking IL-4-producing cells by knock-in of the IL-4 gene. *Int Immunol* 1999;11:243–247.

173. Pinkoski MJ, Hobman M, Heibein JA, et al. Entry and trafficking of granzyme B in target cells during granzyme B-perforin-mediated apoptosis. *Blood* 1998;92:1044–1054.

174. Podack ER. Molecular mechanisms of cytolysis by complement and by cytolytic lymphocytes. *J Cell Biochem* 1986;30:133–170.

175. Motyka B, Korbutt G, Pinkoski MJ, et al. Mannose 6-phosphate/insulin-like growth factor II receptor is a death receptor for granzyme B during cytotoxic T cell-induced apoptosis. *Cell* 2000;103:491–500.

176. Alimonti JB, Shi L, Baijal PK, et al. Granzyme B induces BID-mediated cytochrome c release and mitochondrial permeability transition. *J Biol Chem* 2001;276:6974–6982.

177. MacDonald G, Shi L, Vande Velde C, et al. Mitochondria-dependent and -independent regulation of granzyme B-induced apoptosis. *J Exp Med* 1999;189:131–144.

178. Kagi D, Ledermann B, Burki K, et al. Cytotoxicity mediated by T cells and natural killer cells is greatly impaired in perforin-deficient mice. *Nature* 1994;369:31–37.

179. Kagi D, Vignaux F, Ledermann B, et al. Fas and perforin pathways as major mechanisms of T cell-mediated cytotoxicity. *Science* 1994;265:528–530.

180. Kojima H, Shinohara N, Hanaoka S, et al. Two distinct pathways of specific killing revealed by perforin mutant cytotoxic T lymphocytes. *Immunity* 1994;1:357–364.

181. Lowin B, Hahne M, Mattmann C, et al. Cytolytic T-cell cytotoxicity is mediated through perforin and Fas lytic pathways. *Nature* 1994;370:650–652.

182. Walsh CM, Matloubian M, Liu CC, et al. Immune function in mice lacking the perforin gene. *Proc Natl Acad Sci USA* 1994;91:10854–10858.

183. De Leon M, Jackson KM, Cavanaugh JR, et al. Arrest of the cell cycle reduces susceptibility of target cells to perforin-mediated lysis. *J Cell Biochem* 1998;69:425–435.

184. Kojima H, Toda M, Sitkovsky MV. Comparison of Fas- versus perforin-mediated pathways of cytotoxicity in TCR- and Thy-1-activated murine T cells. *Int Immunol* 2000;12:365–374.

185. Mullbacher A, Hla RT, Museteanu C, et al. Perforin is essential for control of ectromelia virus but not related poxviruses in mice. *J Virol* 1999;73:1665–1667.

186. Zinkernagel RM, Althage A, Adler B, et al. H-2 restriction of cell-mediated immunity to an intracellular bacterium: effector T cells are specific for Listeria antigen in association with H-21 region-coded self-markers. *J Exp Med* 1977;145:1353–1367.

187. Beller DI, Kiely JM, Unanue ER. Regulation of macrophage populations. I. Preferential induction of Ia-rich peritoneal exudates by immunologic stimuli. *J Immunol* 1980;124:1426–1432.

188. Ruco LP, Meltzer MS. Macrophage activation for tumor cytotoxicity: induction of tumoricidal macrophages by supernatants of PPD-stimulated Bacillus Calmette-Guérin-immune spleen cell cultures. *J Immunol* 1977;119:889–896.

189. Buchmeier NA, Schreiber RD. Requirement of endogenous interferon-gamma production for resolution of *Listeria monocytogenes* infection. *Proc Natl Acad Sci USA* 1985;82:7404–7408.

190. Kaufmann S. Possible role of helper and cytolytic T lymphocytes in antibacterial defense: conclusions based on a murine model of listeriosis. *Rev Infect Dis* 1987;9:S650.

191. Kaufmann SH. Which T cells are relevant to resistance against *Listeria monocytogenes* infection? *Adv Exp Med Biol* 1988;239:135–150.

192. Pawelec G, Schaudt K, Rehbein A, et al. Differential secretion of tumor necrosis factor-alpha and granulocyte/macrophage colony-stimulating factors but not interferon-gamma from CD4+ compared to CD8+ human T cell clones. *Eur J Immunol* 1989;19:197–200.

193. Lewinsohn DM, Alderson MR, Briden AL, et al. Characterization of human CD8+ T cells reactive with *Mycobacterium tuberculosis*-infected antigen-presenting cells. *J Exp Med* 1998;187:1633–1640.

194. Stenger S, Hanson DA, Teitelbaum R, et al. An antimicrobial activity of cytolytic T cells mediated by granulysin. *Science* 1998;282:121–125.

195. Pena SV, Hanson DA, Carr BA, et al. Processing, subcellular localization, and function of 519 (granulysin), a human late T cell activation molecule with homology to small, lytic, granule proteins. *J Immunol* 1997;158:2680–2688.

196. Markham RB, Goellner J, Pier GB. In vitro T cell-mediated killing of *Pseudomonas aeruginosa*. I. Evidence that a lymphokine mediates killing. *J Immunol* 1984;133:962–968.

197. Markham RB, Pier GB, Schreiber JR. The role of cytophilic IgG3 antibody in T cell-mediated resistance to infection with the extracellular bacterium, Pseudomonas aeruginosa. *J Immunol* 1991;146:316–320.

198. Powderly WG, Pier GB, Markham RB. T lymphocyte-mediated protection against *Pseudomonas aeruginosa* infection in granulocytopenic mice. *J Clin Invest* 1986;78:375–380.

199. Onderdonk AB, Markham RB, Zaleznik DF, et al. Evidence for T cell-dependent immunity to *Bacteroides fragilis* in an intraabdominal abscess model. *J Clin Invest* 1982;69:9–16.

CHAPTER 5
Clinical Approach to Fever

Burke A. Cunha

"If a physician is skilled enough to induce fever, it would be useless to search for another remedy against disease." *Rufus of Ephesus*

GENERAL CONCEPTS

Introduction

Fever usually indicates an inflammatory, infectious, or neoplastic disorder. The absence of fever does not rule out any of these conditions, but the abruptness of the onset of illness, appearance of the patient, fever magnitude and pattern, and associated clinical and laboratory findings usually provide sufficient information to assess the probable cause of the fever. Diseases behave biologically in a predictable manner even though the clinical presentation may be quite varied. The pattern of organ involvement and detached analysis of the key characteristic aspects of the fever determine the differential diagnosis of the cause of the fever.

For diagnostic purposes, fevers may be viewed as acute, subacute, or chronic, and with or without localizing signs. Febrile patients with localizing signs present few difficulties in diagnosis, but fever without localizing signs is a diagnostic challenge. In patients with fever only, careful analysis of the fever pattern may be the only way to arrive at a presumptive diagnosis. The most helpful localizing signs are hepatic or splenic enlargement, regular or generalized lymphadenopathy, and cutaneous findings such as rash. Clinically, fever should be viewed as an important clinical sign and as an essential host defense mechanism (1–4).

Thermoregulation

The daily temperature of each individual varies by a diurnal rhythm that peaks in late afternoon or evening and is at its lowest point in early morning. Fever may be defined as an increase in temperature above what is normal for a particular individual. The average temperature of individuals may be higher or lower by 1° to 2°F from what is considered normal (98°F). Temperature may increase with ovulation, hot weather, and eating and after physical exercise.

The febrile response is controlled by the preoptic nucleus of the anterior hypothalamus. Mononuclear cells excrete cytokines that enter the general circulation and reach the hypothalamus. Such cytokines may be mediated after mononuclear cells are stimulated by an allergic reaction, tumor cells (tumor necrosis factor [TNF]), or microorganisms, interleukins, and so on. The most important cytokines, clinically, are interleukin-1 (IL-1) and IL-6 elaborated by microorganisms, and TNF elaborated by neoplastic cells. The hypothalamus stimulates the thyroid by chemical mediators to increase its metabolic rate and increase the basal cell temperature. Chemical mediators also serve to induce peripheral vasoconstriction to conserve the heat generated by the increased activity of the thyroid. Together these reactions serve to increase body temperature as part of the febrile response. When the anterior hypothalamus is no longer stimulated by cytokines, the temperature falls because these febrile mechanisms are reversed. Body temperature is returned to normal as the febrile response is terminated (5–10).

Febrile Response

The febrile response is accompanied by a variety of signs and symptoms that are associated with fever. Headache, arthralgias, or myalgias may occur with fever, and mild confusion or delirium is common in elderly patients. Because fever is a manifestation of the inflammatory response to tissue injury, it is accompanied by a variety of nonspecific acute-phase reactions. In addition to fever, there may be leukocytosis or leukopenia, thrombocytosis or thrombocytopenia, a decrease in serum cations (iron, copper, and zinc), and many changes in serum proteins. Increases in C-reactive protein and erythrocyte sedimentation rate occur frequently along with modest increases of serum fibrinogen, haptoglobin, ceruloplasmin, α_1-antitrypsin, and the C3 component or complement. Serum albumin decreases as an acute-phase response. Thyroxine and glucocorticoid levels are also nonspecifically increased. Proteinuria, but not hematuria, frequently accompanies acute febrile infectious diseases (5,6,10).

CHARACTERISTICS OF FEVER

Definitions

Intermittent fevers are temperature elevations that return to normal at least once during most days. Sustained or continuing fevers do not vary more than 1°F per day. Remittent fevers are recurrent over days or weeks and may have any underlying fever pattern (e.g., intermittent, continuous, remittent). Biphasic illnesses are not truly recurrent and occur only once. Relapsing fevers should be differentiated from febrile diseases prone to relapse.

Fever patterns are of most help in diagnosing febrile illnesses without localizing signs and are of limited usefulness in nosocomial fevers. The classic fever patterns retain their usefulness and validity in many areas of the world where traditional infectious diseases are common and retain their importance (11,12).

Magnitude of Fever

Although temperature elevation does not correlate with disease severity, the height of the temperature elevation has important diagnostic significance at temperature extremes (e.g., hyperpyrexia or hypothermia). Temperature higher than 106°F is not due to infectious diseases, and a noninfectious etiology should be the focus of the diagnostic approach. Hypothermia or subnormal temperatures, if associated with bacteremia, are a bad prognostic sign. Slight hypothermia may be a normal variant in elderly people or may be due to overzealous antipyretic measures.

Most temperature elevations are encountered clinically between the extremes of hyperpyrexia and hypothermia. Temperatures between 98° and 102°F may be on an infectious basis but are usually due to noninfectious conditions common in hospitalized patients, especially in critical care units. For diagnostic purposes, it is clinically useful to divide fevers into those capable of temperature elevations to 102°F and those that nearly always remain below 102°F. The differential diagnosis of most commonly encountered causes of fever in the hospital and intensive care unit may be approached efficiently by applying this principle (12) (Table 5.1).

Fever Patterns

Fever spikes may be classified for diagnostic purposes as occurring once (quotidian) or more (double quotidian) daily, every

TABLE 5.1. Diagnostic Significance of Extreme Hyperpyrexia and Hypothermia

Extreme pyrexia (>106°F)	Hypothermia (<97°F)
Central fevers (neoplastic, trauma, or infection)	Elderly
Drug fever	Cold exposure
Heat stroke	Hypothyroidism
Human immunodeficiency virus	Overwhelming infection
Malignant hyperthermia	Sepsis in chronic renal failure
Malignant neuroleptic syndrome	Overzealous treatment with antipyretics

Adapted from Cunha BA. Clinical complications of fever. *Postgrad Med* 1989;85:188–200, with permission.

third (tertiary) or fourth (quartan) days. Fevers may also be described as intermittent, continuous or sustained, and remittent. Relapsing fevers recur at various intervals after the initial febrile episode. Isolated single fever spikes in a hospitalized patient running low-grade temperatures (102°F or less) for 1 to 2 weeks, who suddenly develops a single fever spike to 103°F that returns to normal without treatment by the next day, are probably not due to a systemic infectious disease. Single fever spikes are never due to infection and are commonly due to the transfusion of blood or blood products or to manipulation of a colonized or infected mucosal surface.

The most specific fever pattern is the double quotidian because only a few diseases are associated with two fever spikes a day (e.g., Still's disease, right-sided gonococcal endocarditis, visceral leishmaniasis [kala-azar]). A double quotidian fever is an important clue to the diagnosis of adult Still's disease because there are no other physical or laboratory findings to establish the diagnosis.

Most infectious diseases have no specific fever pattern. The classic fever curves are of limited diagnostic usefulness in hospitalized patients because most nosocomial fevers are not due to classic infectious diseases. The most important fever patterns are presented in Table 5.2 (11,12).

Pulse–Temperature Relationships

The relationship of the pulse to the temperature is often more useful than the fever pattern. If the pulse is elevated out of proportion to the temperature, the relationship is termed *relative tachycardia*. Relative tachycardia is associated with noninfectious conditions and toxin-mediated infections (e.g., gas gangrene). When the pulse is not elevated proportionately to the temperature elevation, then a pulse–temperature deficit exists (e.g., relative bradycardia). The finding of relative bradycardia has important diagnostic significance. For example, if a hospitalized patient presents with fevers and relative bradycardia, the differential diagnosis is limited to legionnaires' disease or drug fever. If the chest x-ray is negative, the workup should be focused on drug fever. Drug fever is usually accompanied by relative bradycardia; associated findings include negative blood cultures (excluding contaminants), slightly elevated serum transaminases, elevated erythrocyte sedimentation rate, and eosinophils present in the peripheral smear (eosinophilia is uncommon). Relative bradycardia is an early clue to malaria or typhoid fever in a traveler without localizing findings (Table 5.3).

High fever in patients looking inappropriately well suggests drug or factitious fever. Both drug and factitious fever are associated with relative bradycardia (2,13).

TABLE 5.2. Diagnostic Significance of Fever Patterns

Fever pattern	Usual causes
Single fever spike	Manipulation of a colonized/infected mucosal surface (not systemic infectious disease)
	Blood/blood products transfusion
	Infusion-related sepsis (contaminated infusate)
	Temperature error
Double quotidian fevers	Adult's Still's disease (adult juvenile rheumatoid arthritis)
	Visceral leishmaniasis
	Miliary tuberculosis
	Mixed malarial infections
	Right-sided gonococcal endocarditis
Tertian fevers	Malaria (*Plasmodium vivax*)
Quartan fevers	Malaria (*Plasmodium malariae*)
Intermittent fevers	Gram-negative/positive sepsis
	Abscesses (renal, abdominal, pelvic)
	Acute bacterial endocarditis
	Kawasaki disease
	Malaria
	Miliary tuberculosis
	Peritonitis
	Toxic shock syndrome
	Antipyretics
Remittent fevers	Viral upper respiratory infections
	Malaria (*Plasmodium falciparum*)
	Acute rheumatic fever
	Legionella species infection
	Mycoplasma species infection
	Tuberculosis
	Subacute bacterial endocarditis (SBE) (viridans streptococci)
Continuous/sustained fevers	Central fevers
	Roseola infantum (human herpesvirus-6)
	Brucellosis
	Kawasaki disease
	Psittacosis
	Rocky Mountain spotted fever
	Scarlet fever
	Enterococcal SBE (tularemia)
	Typhoid fever
	Drug fever
Biphasic ("camel back") fevers	Colorado tick fever
	Dengue fever
	Leptospirosis
	Brucellosis
	Lymphocytic choriomeningitis
	Yellow fever
	Poliomyelitis
	Smallpox
	Rat-bite fever (*Spirillum minus*)
	Chikungunya fever
	Rift Valley fever
	African hemorrhagic fevers (Marburg, Ebola, Lassa)
	Echovirus (Echo 9)

Duration of Fever

Most acute infectious diseases improve or worsen within 2 weeks. Not uncommonly, many infectious diseases cause persistent fever after clinical improvement, which may last 2 to 4 weeks. The diagnosis of the cause of such fevers is usually straightforward, but the cause of some remains obscure. These are best termed *prolonged fevers* to avoid confusing them with bona fide fevers of unknown origin. Fevers of unknown origin by definition include a temperature of 101°F or higher for at least

TABLE 5.3.   Diagnostic Significance of Temperature–Pulse Relationships

Relative bradycardia[a]

Dengue fever
Drug fever
Typhus
Legionnaires' disease
Leptospirosis
Lymphomas
Malaria
Psittacosis
Typhoid fever
Yellow fever
Central fevers
African hemorrhagic fevers (Marburg, Ebola, Lassa)
Factitious fever

Relative tachycardia

Anemia
Clostridial sepsis
Diphtheria
Hyperthyroidism
Pulmonary emboli
Supraventricular arrhythmias

Note: To determine the appropriate pulse rate for any temperature, take the temperature in °F, subtract 1 from the ones digit, multiply that number by 10, and add 100. For example, if the temperature is 104°F: 3 × 10 = 30 + 100 = 130. Therefore the appropriate pulse response for a temperature of 104°F is pulse rate of 130 beats/min., but ≤120 beats/min. signifies relative bradycardia.
[a]In immunocompetent adults (not on β-blockers) with temperature ≥102°F.
Adapted from Cunha BA. Clinical implications of fever. *Postgrad Med* 1989;85:188–200, with permission.

3 weeks and must remain undiagnosed after a week of inpatient or outpatient workup (2–4).

Fever Defervescence Patterns

Viral illnesses have a slow temperature defervescence, usually over a week. Febrile, noninfectious diseases will not resolve without specific therapy. Steroids and antipyretics will decrease temperatures nonspecifically, and this needs to be taken into account in assessing therapeutic responses. Clinicians may be misled into thinking an antibiotic is being effective as evidenced by a decrease in temperature, only to learn later that the patient was concomitantly receiving an antipyretic medication. For this and other reasons, fevers should not be eliminated without reason.

Bacterial infections usually manifest a prompt drop in temperature with appropriate treatment. However, infections respond at different rates, and this may be useful clinically. For example, enterococcal subacute bacterial endocarditis defervesces slowly over a week, in contrast to viridans streptococcal subacute bacterial endocarditis. Similarly, temperature from *Haemophilus influenzae* or *Klebsiella pneumoniae* decreases more slowly than if the patient had pneumococcal pneumonia. Pneumococcal and *H. influenzae* meningitis, in contrast, have a slower rate of temperature decrease than does meningococcal meningitis. Even the febrile response to antibiotic therapy may vary, as is the case with pneumococcal pneumonia, which has three patterns of febrile defervescence. The usual pattern of proven pneumonia is rapidly decreasing temperature during the first 24 to 36 hours of antibiotic therapy. The second pattern is a more gradual decrease over 3 to 4 days, usually seen in compromised hosts (e.g., alcoholic patients). Finally, after initial defervescence, a small group of patients will have another temperature spike on day 3 or 4 (3,4).

After an initial response to antimicrobial therapy, patients usually continue with low-grade or no fever until discharge.

Reappearance of fever during treatment suggests an infectious complication (septic emboli in a patient with subacute bacterial endocarditis). The reappearance of fever after an initial response is virtually never due to resistant organisms but may be due to superinfection. The diagnostic approach should be directed accordingly, and antibiotic therapy should not be changed because of the possibility of resistant organisms. Immunocompromised hosts, in general, defervesce more slowly than normal hosts (2,12).

Recurrent Fevers

Relapsing fevers may be due to a variety of infectious and noninfectious diseases. Multisystem disease characterized by exacerbation and remission may mimic infectious relapsing fever. Most temperature elevations occur at night as an exaggeration of our normal diurnal temperature variation, but the reversal of diurnal pattern occurs with few infectious diseases.

A biphasic fever is characterized by two fever spikes during the illness, usually over the course of a week or longer (e.g., African hemorrhagic fever). This is in contrast to relapsing fevers that are recurrent and not necessarily biphasic (Table 5.4).

TABLE 5.4.   Fevers Prone to Relapse

Infectious causes

Relapsing fever (*Borrelia recurrentis*)
Trench fever (*Rochalimaea quintana*)
Q fever
Typhoid fever
Vibrio fetus
Syphilis
Tuberculosis
Histoplasmosis
Coccidioidomycosis
Blastomycosis
Pseudomonas pseudomallei (melioidosis)
LCM
Dengue fever
Yellow fever
Chronic meningococcemia
Colorado tick fever
Leptospirosis
Brucellosis
Bartonellosis (Oroyo fever)
Acute rheumatic fever
Rat-bite fever (*Spirillum minus*)
Visceral leishmaniasis
Lyme disease
Malaria
Babesiosis
Noninfluenzal respiratory viruses
Epstein-Barr virus
Cytomegalovirus

Noninfectious causes

Beçhet's disease
Crohn's disease
Weber-Christian disease (panniculitis)
Leukoclastic angitis
Sweet's syndrome
Familial Mediterranean fever
[a]FAPA syndrome
Systemic lupus erythematosus
Hyper immunoglobulin D syndrome

[a]Fever, aphthous ulcers, pharyngitis, adenopathy.

CLINICAL APPROACH TO THE FEBRILE PATIENT

Fever without Localizing Signs

Fever can be approached from a diagnostic perspective as presenting with or without localizing signs. Infectious diseases presenting as acute febrile illnesses without localizing signs are the most difficult diagnostic problem (e.g., typhoid fever, malaria, ehrlichiosis, roseola infantum, typhoidal tularemia, Epstein-Barr virus mononucleosis, miliary tuberculosis). The preeruptive stages of Rocky Mountain spotted fever, viral hepatitis, and the childhood exanthems are further expanded. If no localizing signs are present, analysis of temperature and fever patterns are of clinical importance and may provide the only clue to guide further testing or suggest the diagnosis (Fig. 5.1).

Fever and Chills

Rigors, that is, true chills, often precede or accompany fever. True rigors (e.g., involuntary teeth-chattering chills) must be differentiated from the sensation of chilliness. Rigors, increasing muscle contractions that generate heat, have the effect of increasing core temperature. Rigors are commonly associated with bacterial infections and are not characteristic of viral (except viral influenza), chlamydial, or fungal infections.

Chills are characteristic of relatively few infectious diseases (e.g., bacteremia, cholangitis, abscesses, viral influenza, pyelonephritis, bacterial pneumonias, especially pneumococcal), typhoid fever, typhus, arthropod-borne viral infections, and plague. Single chills occur with viral influenza, pneumococcal pneumonia, leptospirosis, typhoid, typhus, or transient or sustained bacteremias. Recurrent chills are associated with persistent bacteremias, abscesses, septic thrombophlebitis, cholangitis, rat-bite fever, and brucellosis. Noninfectious diseases may have recurrent chills with fever (e.g., renal cell carcinoma, lymphomas, and overzealous antipyretic therapy) (2–4).

Fever Blisters

Fever blisters are perioral herpes simplex virus reactivation. Fever alone does not result in fever blisters. The common recurrent perioral vesicular lesions of herpes simplex virus are not associated with fever. Fever blisters are associated with pneumococcal meningitis, meningococcal meningitis, and malaria (2,3).

FEVER WITH LOCALIZING SIGNS

Fever and Rash

The approach to the acutely ill patient with rash and fever is to evaluate the location and character of the rash and the severity of the illness. There are many subacute or chronic rashes associated with temperature elevations, but the clinical challenge is to rapidly and accurately diagnose acutely ill patients with exanthems. Rash distribution may be viewed as primarily central or peripheral. If the rash involves the palms and soles, then diagnostic possibilities are narrowed considerably.

In addition to the location of the rash, its nature (i.e., predominantly petechial-hemorrhagic or maculopapular) is important. Associated clinical and laboratory findings then permit approaching both types of rash in acutely ill febrile patients. Miscellaneous cutaneous findings may provide diagnostic clues. For example, it may be difficult to distinguish acute malaria from typhoid fever early in the illness, but rose spots appearing late in the first week point to typhoid fever. Typhoid fever usually has few truncal rose spots, but the paratyphical enteric fevers and *Shigella sonnei* infection may be associated with many rose spots, so that even the number of rose spots has diagnostic value. Similarly, fever blisters are an important finding in patients with meningitis. Meningococcal and pneumococcal pneumonitis are associated with fever blisters, but herpes simplex meningoencephalitis is not. In herpes simplex meningoencephalitis, the fever blister precedes, but does not usually appear simultaneously with, the meningoencephalitis. Rash and fever usually occur together, but in some illnesses, the fever abates when the rash appears (e.g., roseola infantum due to human herpesvirus-6) (3,13–17) (Tables 5.5 to 5.7).

Fever and Erythema Nodosum or Erythema Multiforme

Erythema nodosum or erythema multiforme in a patient with or without fever can be a clue to an underlying condition. Diagnostic accuracy is enhanced if multiple variables (e.g., diagnostic findings) are combined to increase diagnostic specificity. If a patient with sore throat, diarrhea, and an ill-defined pulmonary infiltrate has erythema multiforme, the diagnosis of *Mycoplasma* species infection can confidently be made. Erythema nodosum has historically been due to systemic mycoses and tuberculosis and is associated with sarcoidosis, streptococcal infection, and inflammatory bowel disease(3,15) (Tables 5.8 and 5.9).

Fever and Jaundice

Jaundice may be considered a localizing sign in a febrile patient. Relatively few infectious diseases present with jaundice and fever. Many infectious and noninfectious diseases cause hyperbilirubinemia, but not jaundice. Bacteremias, not uncommonly, are accompanied by elevated bilirubin levels, but clinical jaundice is less common. Aside from disease primarily affecting the liver, several systemic infections may result in jaundice with fever (4,17) (Table 5.10).

Fever and Lymphadenopathy

Lymph node enlargement may be regional or general. Local lymph node enlargement suggests a regional or local cause for nodal enlargement. However, enlargement in certain regional lymph node groups may suggest a systemic illness (e.g.,

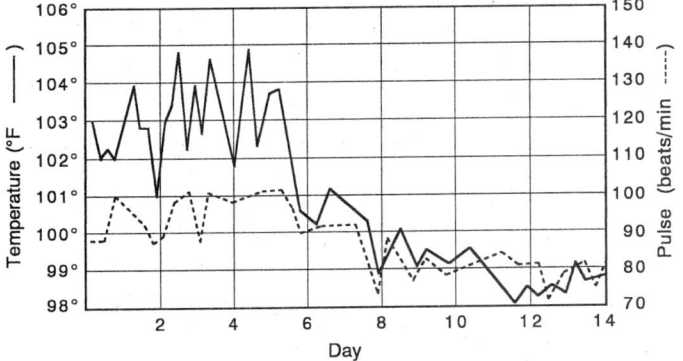

Figure 5.1. The pulse-temperature chart shows relative bradycardia in a patient with legionnaires' disease.

TABLE 5.5. Differential Diagnosis of Petechial/Hemorrhagic Rashes in the Acutely Ill Patient

Disease	Primary distribution of rash		Apperance of rash after fever	Associated features
	Central	Peripheral		
Acute meningococcemia	+	+	1–2 h	Bilateral conjunctivitis Irregular lesions/distribution Late winter/early spring Severe headache Herpes labialis (if meningitis) History of mild recent upper respiratory tract infection
Disseminated intravascular coagulation (DIC)	+	+	Variable	Source tumor or infection Thrombocytopenia Microangiopathic hemolytic anemia Bleeding from venipuncture sites Renal insufficiency
Overwhelming staphylococcal sepsis	–	+	Variable	Usually obvious staphylococcal focus or staph acute bacterial endocarditis Distal extremity hemorrhagic nodules/infarcts (asymmetrical)
Overwhelming pneumococcal sepsis	–	+	1–2 d	Asplenic patients (trauma, staging procedures for lymphoma, sickle cell anemia)
Typhus	+	–	3–6 d	Begins in axilla Severe headache, dry cough Relative bradycardia Gangrene of nose, earlobes, scrotum, vulva, fingers, toes Occasionally splenomegaly
Rocky Mountain spotted fever	–	+	2–3 d	Late spring/early fall Begins in wrists/ankles Severe headache, splenomegaly Periorbital/peripheral edema No lung involvement Positive OX-2, OX-19 serology Leukopenia, thrombocytopenia
Dengue fever	+	–	3–4 d	Appropriate travel history Begins in thorax/axilla Biphasic fever curve Severe headache/severe myalgias "Palpable pinpoint petechiae" Relative bradycardia Leukopenia
Toxic shock syndrome (TSS)	+	+	1–2 d	Persistent hypotension despite fluid replacement Conjunctivits Tampon user/surgical wound/menses Liver/renal dysfunction Maculopapular rash Periorbital/facial/extremity edema Sore throat/vagina (oral/vaginal erythema) Watery diarrhea Nausea/vomiting Headache/myalgias
Enteroviruses (Echo 4, 9, 11; Coxsackievirus A9, B3)	+	–	5–7 d	Rash may have maculopapular component Sore throat, diarrhea Aseptic meningitis, may resemble early meningococcemia
African hemorrhagic fevers (Marburg, Ebola virus)	+	–	1–2 d	Rash scarlatiniform/maculopapular before becoming petechial/purpuric Conjunctival suffusion Severe headache Dry cough/sore throat Nausea/vomiting/diarrhea Leukopenia; thrombocytopenia ↑ LFTs Biphasic fever pattern
Capnophagia canimorsus (DF-2)	–	+	Variable	Common splenectomized patients Associated with lymphomas, steroids Usually history of dog exposure/bite Acute renal failure Hypotension/shock Thrombocytopenia Purpura/eschar/gangrene may develop Buffy coat positive for DF-2

(continued)

TABLE 5.5.   (continued)

Disease	Primary distribution of rash		Apperance of rash after fever	Associated features
	Central	**Peripheral**		
Scarlet fever	−	+	1–2 d	Nausea/vomiting Circumoral pallor "Strawberry" tongue Pastia's lines on arms "Sandpaper" skin Pseudoappendicitis (right rectus syndrome) Abdominal pain Eosinophilia Wound/sore throat Secondary group A strep Palatal petechiae
Measles	+	−	2–3 d	Toxic appearance Deep red/purple/brown rash begins on face Cough Conjunctivitis Pneumonia (giant cell) Encephalitis Pseudoappendicitis Koplik's spots Desquamation late
Rubella	+	−	1–7 d	Postcervical/occipital adenopathy Palatal petechiae (Forscheimer's spots) No upper respiratory tract infection Face to feet in 3 days Conjunctivitis
Enteroviruses	+	−	5–7 d	Predilection for face Usually maculopapular Diarrhea/sore throat Aseptic meningitis
Atypical measles	−	+	2–3 d	History of "killed" measles vaccine (1963–1967) Begins on extremities, may be vesicular, urticarial, or petechial Always pneumonia/pulmonary infiltrate ↑ ESR ↑ Rheumatoid factors Eosinophilia
Kawasaki disease	+	−	Variable	Conjunctivitis Edema of hands/feet Erythema tongue/mouth Erythema multiforme–like lesions Thrombocytosis Nonspecific ECG changes <5 years of age Sustained high fever >1 week Negative strep. throat cultures
Drug fever	+	−	Variable	Negative blood cultures Looks "relatively well" unless coexistent infection ↑ LFTs, ESR Relative bradycardia
Spotted fevers	+	−	5–7 d	Rash maculopapular, may become petechial Severe headache Ankles/wrist rash spread to trunk Palms/soles rash
Leptospirosis	+	−	4–5 d	Morbilliform or scarlatiniform rash Biphasic fever Conjunctival suffusion ↑ LFTs/bilirubin Leukocytosis Jaundice (Weil's disease) Rose spots (rarely)
EBV infectious mononucleosis	+	−	Variable	Bilateral upper lid edema (Hoagland's sign) Bilateral posterior cervical adenopathy Exudative/nonexudative pharyngitis Palatal petechiae ↑ LFTs, ESR About 30% group A strep pharyngeal colonization (not infection)

LFTs, liver function tests; ESR, erythrocyte sedimentation rate; ECG, electrocardiogram; EBV, Epstein-Barr virus.

TABLE 5.6.   Rash and Fever Involving the Palms/Soles

Acute or subacute bacterial endocarditis
Scarlet fever
Toxic shock syndrome
Kawasaki disease
Ehrlichia species infection
Rocky Mountain spotted fever
Erythema multiforme
Secondary syphilis
Smallpox
Chickenpox
Overwhelming staphylococcal or pneumococcal sepsis
Hand, foot, and mouth disease
Dengue fever
Rubella
Orf
Capnocytophaga canimorsus (DF-2)
Measles
Gonococcemia
Meningococcemia
Milker's nodules
Drug fever
Atypical measles
Enterovirus (Echo 9)
Rat-bite fever *(Spirillum moniliformis)*
Epstein-Barr virus infectious mononucelosis

TABLE 5.7.   Fever and Miscellaneous Skin Findings

Rose spots

Salmonella enteric fever (few spots)
Nontyphi *Salmonella* enteric fevers (many spots)
Pseudomonas aeruginosa
Shigella sonnei
Leptospirosis

Horder's spots

Psittacosis

Eschars

All rickettsial infections (except Q fever and rickettsial pox)
Capnocytophaga canimorsus (DF-2)

Ecthyma gangrenosum

Pseudomonas aeruginosa
Aeromonas hydrophila
Serratia marcescens

Annular lesions

ECM (Lyme disease)
Erythema marginatum (ARF)
Tinea species
Erythema multiforme
Kawasaki disease
Yaws/pinta

Hemorrhagic bullae

Leukemias
Capnocytophaga canimorsus (DF-2)
Gas gangrene
Vibrio vulnificus
Necrotizing fasciitis
Aeromonas hydrophila
Invasive group A streptococci
Anthrax

Splinter hemorrhages

Severe anemia
Trauma
Acute/subacute bacterial endocarditis
Postpericardiotomy (Dressler's) syndrome
SLE

Fever blisters

Pneumococcal meningitis
Meningococcal meningitis
Nontyphoidal *Salmonella*
Malaria

Cellulitis-like lesions

Leukoclastic angitis
Sweet's syndrome
SLE
Cutaneous lymphoma

ECM, erythema chronica migrans; ARF, acute rheumatic fever; SLE, systemic lupus erythematosus.

preauricular nodes in tularemia, postoccipital nodes in rubella, postcervical nodes in Epstein-Barr virus infectious mononucleosis). Some diseases may present with either local or general node enlargement (e.g., Epstein-Barr virus infectious mononucleosis).

Generalized adenopathy usually signifies a systemic disorder that may be infectious or noninfectious. Adenopathy alone or with liver or spleen enlargement provides additional diagnostic information (3,15) (Table 5.11).

Fever and Hepatosplenomegaly

An enlarged liver or spleen is an important diagnostic finding. Relatively few infectious diseases cause isolated enlargement of the liver or spleen. This information can be used to diagnostic advantage in a febrile patient. Similarly, enlargement of both the liver and spleen (hepatosplenomegaly) has its own differential diagnosis (3,15) (Table 5.12).

FEVER IN AMBULATORY AND HOSPITALIZED PATIENTS

Fever in the Ambulatory Setting

Most ambulatory patients with noncritical infectious diseases have self-limited illnesses and become afebrile in 1 to 2 weeks. High fevers (temperature of 102°F or higher) in ambulatory patients are usually due to community-acquired pneumonia, pyelonephritis, intraabdominal and pelvic abscesses, pharyngitis, pelvic inflammatory disease, septic arthritis, acute osteomyelitis, and intravenous line infections from home intravenous therapy. Skin infections, urethritis, cystitis, prostatitis, subacute bacterial endocarditis (SBE), chlamydial infections, common respiratory viral infections (excluding viral influenza), viral hepatitis, and infectious diarrhea (excluding enteric fevers) usually present with temperatures of 102°F or higher. Many infections are not associated with much fever (e.g., sexually transmitted diseases [excluding disseminated gonococcal disease], Lymphogranuloma venereum, human immunodeficiency virus

TABLE 5.8. Differential Diagnosis of Erythema Nodosum

Infectious causes

Streptococci (β-hemolytic)
Mycobacteria
Lymphogranuloma venereum (LGV)
Coccidioidomycosis
Blastomycosis
Histoplamosis
Coxsackievirus (B5)
Psittacosis
Yersinia species
Campylobacter jejuni
Salmonella species
Cat-scratch disease
Tularemia
Hepatitis C
Epstein-Barr virus mononucleosis
Tuberculosis

Noninfectious causes

Ulcerative colitis
Crohn's disease
Systemic lupus erythematosus
Sulfonamides
Bromides
Barbiturates
Sarcoidosis
Leukemia
Lymphomas
Pregnancy
Behçet's disease
Oral contraceptives

TABLE 5.9. Differential Diagnosis of Erythema Multiforme

Infectious causes

Herpes simplex virus
Epstein-Barr virus
Vaccinia
Enterovirus
Adenovirus (7)
Hepatitis B virus
Influenza A
Coxsackievirus (B5, B16)
Mycoplasma pneumoniae
Francisella tularensis
Yersinia species
Vibrio parahaemolyticus
Tuberculosis
Treponema pallidum
Histoplasma capsulatum
Coccidioides immitis

Noninfectious causes

Neoplasms (leukemia, lymphoma, leiomyoma, pelvic tumor)
Systemic lupus erythematosus
Radiation therapy
Inflammatory bowel disease (regional enteritis, ulcerative colitis)
Sarcoidosis
Pregnancy
Sunlight
Immunization (diphtheria-pertussis, polio, typhoid, measles vaccine)
Drugs (especially sulfonamides, phenylbutazone, penicillin, diphenylhydantoin)

TABLE 5.10. Fever and Jaundice

Malaria	Human immunodeficiency virus (*Cryptosporidium* species)
Typhoid fever (rare)	
Ascending cholangitis	Hepatic abscesses (pyogenic, amebic)
Yersinia	Epstein-Barr virus infectious mononucleosis
Viral hepatitis (hepatitis A, B, C, etc.)	Leptospirosis (Weil's disease)
Biliary ascariasis	Yellow fever
Portal pyemia (typhilitis)	Dengue fever
Overwhelming gram-positive or -negative sepsis	*Pneumocystis carinii* pneumonia
	Toxic shock syndrome
Babesiosis	Relapsing fever (*Borrelia recurrentis*)

[HIV], Lyme disease, superficial and chronic skin infections, chronic or recurrent pharyngitis, chronic osteomyelitis) (3,4,11).

Fever in Hospitalized Patients

Fever in hospitalized patients may be due to many infectious and noninfectious diseases. Fever patterns help to eliminate diagnostic possibilities as often as providing diagnostically meaningful information. Medical diagnosis usually depends on assessing the significance of multiple clinical variables when combined to form a clinical syndrome. The syndromic approach permits the clinician to arrive rapidly at a working diagnosis upon which to base further tests and empirical therapy. The main clinical problem in practice is to differentiate infectious from noninfectious diseases (e.g., noninfectious pulmonary infiltrates from pneumonia). Once this diagnosis is narrowed to an organ system, then specific diagnostic tests can determine the definitive diagnosis (18–24) (Table 5.13).

TABLE 5.11. Differential Diagnosis of Lymphadenopathy

Regional adenopathy	Generalized adenopathy
Any local infection	Brucellosis
Tularemia (ulceroglandular)	Leptospirosis
Syphilis (primary)	Miliary tuberculosis
Tuberculosis (typical/atypical)	Histoplasmosis
Sporotrichosis	Epstein-Barr virus infectious mononucleosis
Herpes simplex virus	Cytomegalovirus infectious mononucleosis
Cat-scratch disease	
Scrub typhus	Dengue fever
Lymphogranuloma venereum (LGV)	Syphilis
Rat-bite fever (*Spirillum minus*)	Toxoplasmosis
	Rubella
Metastatic carcinoma	Waldenström's macroglobulinemia
Lymphomas	Lymphomas
Bubonic plague	Human immunodeficiency virus
Kawasaki disease	Serum sickness
Toxoplasmosis	Pseudolymphoma
Epstein-Barr virus infectious mononucleosis	Hyperthyroidism
	Systemic lupus erythematosus
	Rheumatoid arthritis
	Sarcoidosis
	Viral hepatitis
	Myeloid metaplasia
	Immunoblastic lymphadenopathy

TABLE 5.12. Fever and Hepatopmegaly, Splenomegaly, and Hepatosplenomegaly

Organ involvement	Usual causes
Hepatomegaly	Amebic liver abscess
	Brucellosis
	Chagas' disease
	Clonorchiasis
	Echinococcosis
	Fascioliasis
	Histoplasmosis
	Malaria
	Viral hepatitis
	Opisthorchiasis
	Schistosomiasis
	Toxocariasis
	Typhoid fever
	Visceral leishmaniasis
	Bartonella species infection
	Hydatid cysts
Splenomegaly	Typhus
	Chagas disease
	Malaria[a]
	Subacute bacterial endocarditis
	Schistosomiasis
	Typhoid fever
	Brucellosis
	Histoplasmosis
	Myelofibrosis[a]
	Systemic lupus erythematosus
	Visceral leishmaniasis[a]
	Leukemia[a]
	Lymphoma[a]
	Tuberculosis
	Epstein-Barr virus infectious mononucleosis
Hepatosplenomegaly	Typhoid fever
	Tularemia
	Brucellosis
	Hypernephroma
	Histoplasmosis
	Toxocara (visceral larva migrans) species infection
	Visceral leishmaniasis
	Schistosomiasis
	Relapsing fever
	Epstein-Barr virus infectious mononucleosis
	Cytomegalovirus infectious mononucleosis
	Psittacosis
	Malaria
	Syphilis
	Typhus
	Rocky Mountain spotted fever
	Tuberculosis
	Babesiosis

[a] Very large spleen: chronic myelocytic leukemia, myelofibrosis, malaria, visceral leishmaniasis, lymphoma.

TABLE 5.13. Differential Diagnosis of Fever in Hospitalized Patients Based on Temperature

Temperature < 102°F	Temperature ≥ 102°F
Acute cholecystitis	Cholangitis
Acute myocardial infarction	Pericarditis
Simple phlebitis	Suppurative thrombophlebitis
Pulmonary emboli/infarction	Septic pulmonary emboli
Acute pancreatitis	Pancreatic abscess/infected pseudocyst
Viral hepatitis (hepatitis A, B, C, etc.)	Nonhepatitis viral/liver disease (Epstein-Barr virus infectious mononucleosis, leptospirosis, drug fever)
Uncomplicated wound infections	Severe/complicated wound infections (e.g., invasive group A strep, *Vibrio vulnificus*)
	Abscess deep to wound
Gastrointestinal bleed	Bowel infarction
Catheter-associated bacteriuria cystitis	Pyelonephritis
Cystitis	

Adapted from Cunha BA. Clinical implications of fever. *Postgrad Med* 1989;85:188–200, with permission.

and arboviral and zoonotic infections are uncommon (3,25–27) (Table 5.14).

TREATMENT OF FEVER

Benefits of Fever

The febrile response is an important physiologic defense mechanism against invasion by various microorganisms. Fever is part of the acute-phase response, which is the primordial and primary defense by the body against microbial invasion. Elevated temperatures have an inhibitory effect on many organisms. There is also a direct effect of elevated temperatures on many microorganisms, and high temperature may inhibit the replication of many microorganisms (viral replication and gram-negative aerobic bacillary replication). Temperature elevation may cause lysis of certain microorganisms, such as gonococci and *Treponema pallidum*. Fever exerts a positive effect on the immune system, and increased temperatures optimize chemotaxis complement activity and phagocytosis. The serum iron concentration, an important virulence factor for bacterial pathogens, is decreased with fever. Similarly, lysis of phagolysosomes is increased at elevated temperatures, thereby eliminating intracellular pathogens (4,28).

ANTIPYRETIC THERAPY

Because fever is a major host defense mechanism, temperature should only be artificially decreased if the fever is a threat to the host. Extreme hyperpyrexia (temperature of 106°F or higher) may cause central nervous system damage. For this reason, very elevated temperatures should be brought down to the 102°F to 104°F level as soon as possible to avoid permanent neurological damage. Febrile patients with severe cardiopulmonary disease should not be allowed to have temperatures much higher than 102°F because 1°F of temperature elevation results in a commensurate increase of 10 beats/min in pulse rate. The excessive demands of temperature on the cardiorespiratory system may result in deleterious effects such as acute myocardial infarction or respiratory failure.

Fever and Recent Foreign Travel

Visitors or host country nationals returning from Latin America, Asia, or Africa with acute febrile illness or rash present a specific problem. Usually, returning travelers have common rather than exotic rare infections. Patients may be initially approached syndromally (e.g., acute diarrheal illness, pulmonary symptoms or pneumonia, jaundice) or with suspicion of an acute undifferentiated febrile illness. The conditions associated with traveler's diarrhea are well known. Lung findings point to a typical or atypical pneumonia or tuberculosis. Fever (less than 102°F) and jaundice point to viral hepatitis. Typhoid fever and malaria are then left as common diagnostic considerations,

TABLE 5.14. Fever and Recent Foreign Travel

	Incubation period		
	2 wk	2–3 wk	>3 wk
Common			
Malaria		•	•
Pneumonias			•
Viral hepatitis (hepatitis A, B, C, etc.)			•
Typhoid fever		•	
Diarrhea	•		
Toxigenic *Escherichia coli*			
Cholera			
Amebic dysentery			
Shigella species dysentery			
Campylobacter species infection			
Giardiasis			
Yersinia species infection			
Cryptosporidium species infection			
Cyclospora			
Uncommon			
Human immunodeficiency virus			•
Typhus	•		
Viral hemorrhagic fevers			
Asian		•	
African		•	
Latin American		•	
Leptospirosis		•	
Brucellosis		•	
Arboviral infections (dengue fever)	•		
Visceral leishmaniasis			•
Treponemiasis		•	

tipyretic measures are introduced when the temperature rises above 102°F, febrile seizures may be avoided. Adults do not have febrile seizures. If an adult is febrile and develops a seizure, a careful search must be made to determine the cause of the seizure, which is not due to the fever by itself. Aside from central nervous system infections, some infectious agents cause seizures in the absence of high temperature elevations, as is the case with *Shigella dysenteriae*, which may cause seizures with relatively low increases in temperature (29–37).

REFERENCES

1. Kluger MJ, ed. *Fever: Its biology, evolution, and function.* Princeton, NJ: Princeton University Press, 1979.
2. Cluff LE, Johnson JE, eds. *Clinical concepts of infectious diseases (3rd ed).* Boston: Williams & Wilkins, 1982:61–74.
3. Cunha BA. Infectious diseases. In: Samiy AH, Bardoness J, Douglas RG, eds. *Textbook of diagnostic medicine.* Philadelphia: Lea & Febiger 1987:131–166.
4. Cunha BA, ed. Fever. *Infect Dis Clin North Am* 1996;10:33–222.
5. Dinarello CA, Bunn PA Jr. Fever. *Semin Oncol* 1997;24:288–298.
6. Dinarello CA. Thermoregulation and the pathogenesis of fever. *Infect Dis Clin North Am* 1996;10:433–449.
7. Netea MG, Kullberg BJ, Van der Meer JW. Circulating cytokines as mediators of fever. *Clin Infect Dis* 2000;31(Suppl 5):S178–184.
8. Bodel P. Tumors and fever. *Ann N Y Acad Sci* 1974;230:6–13.
9. Kozak W, Kluger MJ, Tesfaigzi J, et al. Molecular mechanisms of fever and endogenous antipyresis. *Ann N Y Acad Sci* 2000;917:121–134.
10. Dinarello CA, Cannon JG, Wolff SM. New concepts on the pathogenesis of fever. *Rev Infect Dis* 1988;10:168–189.
11. Woodward TE. The fever pattern as diagnostic aid. In: Mackowiak PA ed. *Fever: Basic mechanisms and management (2nd ed).* Philadelphia: Lippincott-Raven, 1997:215–235.
12. Cunha BA. The clinical significance of fever patterns. *Infect Dis Clin North Am* 1996;10:12–44.
13. Cunha BA. Diagnostic significance of relative bradycardia. *Clin Microbiol Infect Dis* 2000;6:633–634.
14. Cunha BA. The diagnostic approach to rash and fever in the CCU. *Crit Care Clin* 1998;8:35–54.
15. Schlossberg D, Shulman JA, eds. *Differential diagnosis of infectious disease.* Baltimore: Williams & Wilkins, 1996.
16. Pankey GA, ed. Dermatologic manifestations of infectious diseases. *Infect Dis Clin North Am* 1994;8:677–688.
17. Schlossberg D. Fever and rash. *Infect Dis Clin North Am* 1996;10:101–110.
18. Cunha BA. Infections in acutely ill non-leukopenic compromised hosts with diabetes mellitus, SLE, asplenia, or on steroids. *Crit Care Clin* 1998;8:263–282.
19. Cunha BA. Infections in SLE. *Infect Dis Pract* 1997;21:41–45.
20. Johnson DH, Cunha BA. Infections in alcoholic cirrhosis. *Infect Dis Clin* 2001;16:363–372.
21. Cunha BA. Approach to fever in the CCU. *Crit Care Clin* 1998;8:1–14.
22. Mackowiak PA, LeMaistre CF. Drug fever: a critical appraisal of conventional concepts. *Ann Intern Med* 1987;106:728–733.
23. Johnson DH, Cunha BA. Drug fever. *Infect Dis Clin North Am* 1996;10:85–91.
24. Norman DC, Yoskikawa TT. Fever in the elderly. *Infect Dis Clin North Am* 1996;10:93–99.
25. Saxe SE, Gardner P. The returning traveler with fever. *Infect Dis Clin North Am* 1992;6:427–439.
26. Manson-Bahr PEC, Bell DR, eds. *Manson's tropical diseases (19th ed).* London: Balliere-Tindall, 1987.
27. Strickland GT, ed. *Hunter's tropical medicine and emerging infectious diseases (8th ed).* Philadelphia: WB Saunders, 2000:1–1122.
28. Kluger MJ, Kozak W, Conn C, et al. The adaptive value of fever. *Infect Dis Clin North Am* 1996;10:1–20.
29. Cunha BA. Antipyretic therapy in infectious diseases. *Antibiot Clinicians* 2000;4:60–62.
30. Axelrod P. External cooling in the management of fever. *Clin Infect Dis* 2000;31(Suppl 5):S224–229.
31. Richardson JD. Diagnosis and management of systemic infections and fever in neurological patients. *Semin Neurol* 2000;20:387–391.
32. Mayer S, Commichau C, Scarmeas N, et al. Clinical trial of an air-circulating cooling blanket for fever control in critically ill neurologic patients. *Neurology* 2001;56:292–298.
33. Mackowiak PA. Physiological rationale of suppression of fever. *Clin Infect Dis* 2000;31(Suppl 5):S185–189.
34. Mackowiak PA. Antipyretic therapy's future. *Clin Infect Dis* 2000;31(Suppl 5):S242–243.
35. Gozzoli V, Schottker P, Suter PM, et al. Is it worth treating fever in intensive care unit patients? Preliminary results from a randomized trial of the effect of external cooling. *Arch Intern Med* 2001;161:121–123.
36. Sawari AR, Mackowiak PA. The pharmacologic consequences of fever. *Infect Dis Clin North Am* 1996;10:21–32.
37. Klein NC, Cunha BA. Treatment of fever. *Infect Dis Clin North Am* 1996;10:211–216.

Fevers are well tolerated by most patients, even up to 106°F; however, some patients are made very uncomfortable by relatively low elevations of temperature (e.g., 99°F to 101°F). Antipyretic therapy in these patients may be given for symptomatic relief. Most patients who have clinically significant fevers have temperatures between 102°F and 106°F. If temperature decrease is necessary from a physiologic standpoint, the temperature should be lowered slowly to avoid wide swings in temperature that will result in chills. Wide temperature swings induced by antipyretics resemble a hectic-septic fever pattern and make the patient very uncomfortable. This leads the physician to believe that the patient is clinically deteriorating and is facing a septic process. From the patient's standpoint, the patient clearly feels worse with the introduction of antipyretics.

In addition to physiologic and patient comfort requirements, there are no data indicating that lowering of temperature is of any benefit to the host, and it may be detrimental. The use of antipyretics to lower the temperature of a patient should be accomplished by acetylsalicylic acid, acetaminophen, or sponge baths. If the patient is ambulatory, a cool shower or bath will rapidly lower the core temperature. Hypothermia blankets are an inefficient way to lower core body temperature; other antipyretic measures should be used in preference to hypothermia blanket application.

Rapid increases in temperature in children should be minimized because they may result in febrile seizures. The rapidity of the increase in temperature, rather than the absolute temperature elevation, predisposes children to febrile seizures. If an-

CHAPTER 6

The Role and Use of Cytokines in Infectious Diseases

Robert W. Finberg

INTRODUCTION: HISTORY AND NAMING OF CYTOKINES

Although viruses and bacteria carry virulence genes that are capable of causing the death of the host, it is clear that most of the symptoms we associate with infectious diseases (symptoms such as sore throat, myalgias, and malaise, or signs such as fever, rigors, and hypotension) are caused not by the organism but by the host response to the organism. This response is principally mediated through production of soluble protein mediators released by cells that come into contact with microbes that are recognized as foreign (1–4).

Both the innate immune response (the response that occurs without prior sensitization) and the acquired immune response (consisting of B cells and T cells) are important in the elimination of infectious agents. Both use soluble mediators to activate cells important in host defense. Cytokines are secreted proteins of various sizes and molecular families that are produced by cells and that have in common the property that they act on immunologically important cells.

Five different families of proteins fit this definition of cytokines: (a) the interferons, (b) the interleukins, (c) the chemokines, (d) the tumor necrosis factor (TNF) family, and (e) the hematopoietic cell growth factors (Table 6.1). The differentiations between the families of molecules are largely historical and, not surprisingly, considerable overlap exists. Interferons were first defined as proteins that functioned in viral "interference," the prevention of infection of a virally infected cell by a second virus (5–8). Interleukins were described as secreted proteins that explained the interactions between cells of the immune system (9,10). Chemokines, a family of small (8 to 14 kd), structurally related proteins were originally defined by their ability to affect the migration of polymorphonuclear leukocytes (11). The TNF family of proteins was described after the first description of TNF (now TNF-α) as a protein released by a variety of cells that is important in the clinical manifestations of sepsis (it causes fever, capillary leak syndrome, and shock) and that is capable of killing certain tumor cells (12–14). Because most secreted proteins have multiple effects, and because these proteins exert their effects through receptors that are widely distributed throughout the body, it would be surprising if these effects did not overlap and vary among different areas of the body. Similarly, because the definitions of the different families are historical, it is not surprising that these groupings (which we cite because they account for the naming of the proteins) are not really accurate descriptions of either their activities or their protein structure or expression. For example, the cytokine termed interleukin-8 (IL-8) is clearly a chemokine on the basis of its DNA sequence, protein structure, expression, and primary mode of activity; and interferon-γ (IFN-γ) can be said to be a classical interleukin because its principal activity appears to be to stimulate macrophage and T-cell activation and differentiation and because it is produced exclusively by cells of the immune system.

Historically, the interferons were described first, and because they were discovered on the basis of their antiviral activity, their potential as modulators of infectious diseases was recognized immediately. For this reason, the use of interferons as therapeutic agents occurred even before they were cloned and characterized (15).

The first cytokine described as an interleukin (IL-1) was initially found to be produced by macrophages and to have an effect on T cells (stimulating their antigen-specific proliferation). Interleukins, as the name indicates, act between white cells (macrophages, polymorphonuclear leukocytes, B and T lymphocytes, and natural killer [NK] cells—all of which would qualify as leukocytes). It is now recognized that IL-1 is produced by a number of different cell types and that it exerts effects on many others (9,10). IL-2, the second cytokine defined, is not only produced by T cells but also acts on T cells (it works in an "autocrine" manner) as well as on other cells (9,10). The list of cytokines has grown very long, and it has also been recognized over the past several years that proteins not thought to be important in immunity (like growth hormone) may affect immune cells and thus function as cytokines (16).

Several small proteins, termed *chemoattractant cytokines* (or *chemokines*) have been described on the basis of their ability to affect migration of neutrophils. Chemokines, which are produced by a variety of cells (including platelets, megakaryocytes, endothelial cells, and eosinophils, in addition to lymphocytes and macrophages), are divided into two different families of molecules based on their N-terminal amino acid sequences: C-C chemokines and CXC chemokines (17). Although originally described as mediators of neutrophil activity, it is clear that they have effects on many different cells, and their receptors are important as a route of viral infection, especially by human immunodeficiency virus type 1 (HIV-1) (11).

The hematopoietic growth factors are another group of soluble mediators that are important in the host response to infection. They will have a primary effect on host defense by virtue of their proliferative effects and are now used for that purpose clinically (to induce more rapid recovery of neutrophils in patients who have received chemotherapy). In addition, these cytokines have other effects on these same cells (and sometimes other cells) that may lead to their differentiation or activation. For example, whereas the primary activity of granulocyte colony-stimulating factor (G-CSF) and granulocyte-macrophage colony-stimulating factor (GM-CSF) is thought to be on the stimulation of the marrow to produce more granulocytes and macrophages, they have both been used "prophylactically" to prevent infections in neutropenic patients. At the same time, both of these agents can activate already grown neutrophils and macrophages to increase their phagocytic properties. Thus, both have been used clinically as adjuvants in cases in which the host is failing (18–25).

Because the immune system presumably evolved to prevent invasion of the body by infectious organisms, and the immune system is regulated by cytokines (as the endocrine system is regulated by hormones), the response to any infectious disease is regulated by cytokines (26). Although administration of cytokines can be shown to affect certain infectious diseases, assessing the role of a given cytokine by the inborn deficiencies that their absence would cause has not yet been possible (10). Thus, much of what we understand about the role of various cytokines comes from *in vitro* experiments or animal models. In a few cases, cytokines have begun to appear as human therapeutic agents. As we learn more about cytokine receptors and their activation, it is anticipated that small molecules that are able to activate cells or mimic the effects of cytokines will become preferable agents. At the same time, it is anticipated that substances that bind to

TABLE 6.1. Families of Human Cytokines

Cytokine family	Producing cells	Functions	Role in infectious diseases
Interferons	Nonimmune (type I) and immune (type II)	Antiviral, antiproliferative	Used to treat several chronic viruses; direct antiviral effects
Interleukins	Cells of the immune system	Regulate immune cells—stimulate and inhibit proliferation of immune cells	Function as immune stimulators
Chemokines	Endothelial and epithelial cells	Attraction of neutrophils and macrophages	Initiate movement of immune cells, activate immune cells
TNF family	Endothelial, epithelial, and immune cells	Inflammatory; initiate vascular permeability and migration of cells	Antibodies to TNF and TNF family receptors decrease inflammation; inhibitors used in control of sepsis syndrome
Hematopoietic growth factors	Multiple cells	Stimulate growth and differentiation of bone marrow–derived cells	Enhance production of polys; "arm" macrophages; may be important in immune stimulation

TNF, tumor necrosis factor.

PATHOPHYSIOLOGY OF CYTOKINES IN INFECTIOUS DISEASES

The initial engagement of a microbial antigen with the human immune system leads to interaction with macrophages and other cells that recognize the antigen as foreign through the stimulation of "pattern recognition" proteins (such as CD14 and the toll-like receptors). The interaction between the macrophage (or polymorphonuclear leukocyte) leads to production of "inflammatory cytokines." These cytokines (which include IL-1, TNF-α, and IL-6) have in common the property of increasing vascular permeability, thus leading to the local swelling and erythema that is associated with local invasion by infectious organisms. In addition, these cytokines act as "endogenous pyrogens," leading to the production of fever and (when present at high levels) hypotension (1–4). Although the interaction of lipopolysaccharide (LPS) of gram-negative bacilli has been well studied as an inducer of cytokines, other bacterial and even viral antigens (including proteins, lipids, and polysaccharides) may induce the same cytokines when they interact with cell surface proteins (27,28). The inflammatory cytokines up-regulate expression of vascular endothelial cell surface proteins called *selectins* (such as intercellular adhesion molecule 1 [ICAM-1] and E- and P-selectin), which are important in binding to neutrophils and lead to accumulation of neutrophils in the area. In addition, the inflammatory cytokines (particularly IL-1 and TNF) have direct effects on T cells, which in turn stimulate the release of immunomodulatory cytokines (such as IFN-γ). The production of IFN-γ in turn leads to migration of macrophages and activation of macrophages to become more phagocytic. Activated monocytes also release IL-8, a member of the chemokine family (see later), and this protein (initially termed *macrophage-derived neutrophil chemotactic factor*) is responsible for attracting neutrophils. The inflammatory cytokines have short half-lives, and their activities are in many cases inhibited by proteins such as thymus cell growth factor-β (TCGF-β) that are released by endothelial cells (29).

Stimulation of the T cells by inflammatory cytokines leads to antigen-driven expansion of T and B cells that are specific for the bacterial, viral, and parasitic proteins. These cells in turn release interleukins such as IL-2, which leads to growth of T cells, and IL-12, which not only leads to T-cell proliferation and differentiation but also activates NK cells, which in turn recognize virally infected cells. This feedback loop, which includes autocrine loops (IL-2 is not only released by T cells but also stimulates their growth), is presumably held in check by the elimination of antigen. The continued presence of antigen (an unnatural result) would lead to chronic inflammation and its associated abnormalities (including TNF-mediated weight loss, IL-1α, TNF, and IL-6–mediated fever and other systemic disturbances) (28,30).

USE OF CYTOKINES AS THERAPEUTIC AGENTS FOR INFECTIOUS DISEASES

Interferons

After it was determined that substances that prevented infections by virus could be produced either by the infected cell directly or by immune cells, the interferons were divided into two families. Type II interferons are produced by immune cells, and type I interferons are produced by cells that are not part of the immune system (5,31,32). Several different subgroups of type I interferons have been described. IFN-α, IFN-β, IFN-ω, and a remnant of the IFN-δ gene have been demonstrated in humans. IFN-τ is found in ruminants and is postulated to be important in pregnancy in sheep and cows. Interestingly, although it is not produced in humans, its antiviral effects are broad and include human cells (33).

A recently described type I interferon (IFN-κ) is selectively expressed in human keratinocytes. (34). The traditional type I family of interferons consists of 15 functional genes, 13 of which encode different IFN-α subtypes, one gene encodes IFN-β, and one encodes IFN-ω. IFN-γ is a type II interferon and is produced by T cells and NK cells (in contrast to the type I interferons, which are produced by all cells).

Because the interferons were discovered before the other cytokines, it is not surprising that they were the first to be tried as therapeutic agents. Four type I human interferons and human IFN-γ have been tested in clinical trials, and all are available commercially (Table 6.2).

One of the first uses of interferons was in the treatment of warts, a viral disease. A leukocyte-derived product (made from pooled human leukocytes stimulated with Sendai virus preparation (IFN-n3) is licensed for use against warts. Several recombinant interferon preparations are in clinical use. Because of their antiproliferative effects, interferons have been used in the treatment of a variety of cancers.

cytokine receptors will also be capable of preventing many of the harmful side effects of cytokines.

TABLE 6.2. Use of Interferons as Therapeutics for Infectious Diseases

Interferon	Type	Production	Brand name	Current use	Comments
α2a	rIFN-A	Recombinant protein produced in bacteria	Roferon-A	Chronic hepatitis C, AIDS-related KS, hairy cell leukemia, CML	Currently first-line therapy for hepatitis C when given with ribavirin
α2b	rIFN-α2	Recombinant protein produced in bacteria	Intron A	Chronic hepatitis C, condyloma acuminata, hairy cell leukemia, malignant melanoma, AID-related KS, follicular non-Hodgkin's lymphoma	Currently first-line therapy for hepatitis C when given with ribavirin
Peg-interferon α2b	rIFN-α2	Recombinant protein produced in bacteria coupled with polyethylene glycol	PEG-Intron	Chronic hepatitis C	Longer half life than conventional IFN
Alphacon	Synthetic gene representing several α types	Bacteria-produced synthetic gene product	Infergen	Chronic hepatitis C	
αn3		Derived from Sendai virus–stimulated leukocytes	Alferon	Condylomata accumunata	This is a noncloned product, derived from stimulated human cells
β1a	rIFN-β	Recombinant protein produced in bacteria	Avonex	Multiple sclerosis	Mechanism of action not well defined
β1b	rIFN-β	Recombinant protein produced in bacteria	Betaseron	Multiple sclerosis	Mechanism of action not well defined
γ1b	rIFN-γ	Recombinant protein produced in bacteria	Actimmune	Reduction of frequency and severity of infections in patients with chronic granulomatous disease	Data are suggestive as an activator of cells in the treatment of fungal infections, leishmania, viruses, including HIV-1, but it is not licensed for this use

rIFN, recombinant interferon; KS, Kaposi's sarcoma; CML, chronic myelogenous leukemia; HIV-1, human immunodeficiency virus type 1.

Current uses of IFN-α include treatment of chronic hepatitis B and C (35,36). The use of interferon complexed to polyethylene glycol (PEG interferon) has increased its half-life. IFN-β is licensed for use only in multiple sclerosis at this time.

The only type II interferon, IFN-γ, has multiple effects apart from its antiviral activity. It has been shown *in vitro* to activate both macrophages and polymorphonuclear leukocytes and has activity in several animal models of infections with intracellular pathogens, including *Cryptococcus*, *Leishmania*, and *Toxoplasma* species (37,38). Although recombinant IFN-γ has been used in humans in refractory fungal infections (as an activator of polys and macrophages) and in leishmaniasis (37,38), it is currently licensed for use only in patients with chronic granulomatous disease, in whom it can reverse the polymorphonuclear leukocyte defect and aids in preventing and treating bacterial illness.

Although interferons are licensed for treatment of certain leukemias and multiple sclerosis, their primary indications are for infectious diseases. The broad range of activity of interferons would appear to make them ideal therapeutics for illness caused by many different varieties of viruses (such as "cold" viruses). Early studies using nasal application of interferons do indicate that they could be used clinically to eliminate rhinoviruses. They clearly have antiviral activity. Unfortunately, the side effects of the preparations (which include nasal bleeding) limit the usefulness of locally administered interferons (39). Studies of systemic use of interferons for the treatment of serious viral infections, such as cytomegalovirus (CMV), were disappointing both for their lack of efficacy as well as for their side effects. The development of drugs (ganciclovir, foscarnet, and cidofovir) has supplanted the use of interferons for CMV. IFN-α is the mainstay therapy for both hepatitis B and C. However, its side effects (which include fever, myalgias, weakness, depression) and the need to give the drug chronically limit its use and make it very expensive to administer. Thus, despite their demonstrable antiviral effect, the poor therapeutic-to-toxic ratio of these drugs is likely to limit the future use of interferons for any viral illness as new antivirals become available.

Interleukins

The identification of IL-1 as an early mediator of the inflammatory events that result in septic shock made this cytokine an early target for inhibition with the hope that by inhibiting IL-1 activity bacterial septic shock could be avoided. Despite some animal data, human trials of IL-1 receptor antagonists as well as anti-TNF agents have been disappointing (40).

Because of their demonstrated ability to stimulate T cells, recombinant cytokines have been used in the treatment of HIV-1. Although early trials of IL-2 in patients with HIV infection were disappointing, more recent results suggest that chronic administration of low-dose IL-2 will increase CD4 counts (41–45). IL-12, another cytokine that potentiates T_H1 T-cell responses has been tested in patients with chronic hepatitis C (46). Animal experiments suggest a role for IL-17 in experimental models of pneumonia (47), and in vitro data indicate that IL-15 is important in the activity of natural killer cells (48). Experiments in animals suggest that IL-18 and IL-20 have activity in promoting the elimination of intracellular organisms (49–51).

Although many cytokines enhance elimination of bacteria or intracellular parasites in animal models, none of them have been shown to cure anything by themselves, so that all must be classified as adjuvants for antimicrobial agents. Their specific activities and cellular origins are both diverse and redundant (Table 6.3). A small number of cytokines are in use clinically (Table 6.4).

Chemokines

Chemokine is a term used to designate a family of closely related chemotactic (or chemoattractant) cytokines. Proteins in this family have in common a highly conserved N-terminal sequence. On the basis of this sequence, the superfamily has been divided into four different families: CXC, CC, C, and CX3C, where C is the N-terminal amino acid cysteine and X is a nonconserved amino acid residue. Most of the more than 40 known chemokines fall into the CC or CXC group (11,16). IL-8, the best characterized of the chemokines, is a CXC chemokine produced by a variety of cell types, including monocytes, macrophages, endothelial cells, fibroblasts, and neutrophils (11). It appears to play a major role in both neutrophil migration and activation. In general, the CXC chemokines are potent chemoattractants for neutrophils, whereas the CC chemokines recruit monocytes. Not surprisingly, chemokines are secreted in response to inflammatory stimuli, such as LPS, IL-1, TNF, and IFN-γ. In addition, as noted earlier, infection of cells induces production of several chemokines, which vary in both the cell infected and the infectious agent. Infection of microglial cells by herpes simplex virus induces the release of TNF-α, IL-1β, RANTES (regulated upon activation normal T-cell expressed and secreted), and interferon-induced protein-10 (IP-10) by human microglial cells (52). Hantavirus infection induces the expression of RANTES and IP-10 (but not TNF-α, IL-8, monocyte chemotactic protein 1 [MCP-1], macrophage inhibitory protein-1 α [MIP-1α], or MIP-1β) in human lung microvascular endothelial cells (53). Further work, now that the individual chemokines and their receptors have been defined, will be required to define the significance of these differences for the diseases produced.

The nomenclature for chemokines is based on the amino acid sequence followed by an L (for ligand) and serial numbers. IL-8 is the prototype for the CXC chemokine and 1 (MCP-1) is the prototypic CC chemokine (54,55). A full list of the described chemokines includes a separation of different families based on the presence or absence of the glutamic acid–leucine–arginine (ELR) motif immediately before the first cysteine residue. Chemokines have been demonstrated to bind to defined receptor proteins on the cell surface. Some of these receptor proteins are receptors for HIV-1. Chemokine receptor 4 (CCR-4) is a receptor for certain CXC chemokines and is important in entry of T-cell tropic strains of HIV-1. Chemokine receptor 5 (CCR-5), which serves as a binding protein for certain CC chemokines (including RANTES, MIP-1α, and MIP-1β), is a receptor for certain macrophage tropic strains of HIV-1. In

vitro, the addition of RANTES, MIP1-α, and MIP-1β will inhibit HIV-1 infection by certain M-tropic strains (11,16). Although the role for certain chemokines in infection has been documented, and others can be postulated based on their known ability to affect migration of polys or macrophages, in most cases, the exact role of a given chemokine has not been well defined. The fact that multiple chemokines use the same receptor (and therefore probably activate the same genes) in part explains their apparent redundancy. Experiments in knockout mice, which might ordinarily be expected to allow for a definition of the role of a given chemokine, do not reveal a clear phenotype, whereas antibody neutralization studies may demonstrate an effect of a chemokine. At this time, there are no chemokines in clinical use, but their role in local defense, their attraction of polys and macrophages, and the demonstration that they are secreted in lung, skin, and other cells suggest that they have important roles, and substances that stimulate or antagonize chemokines and their receptors will alter the response to infectious diseases (4,11,16,54–58) (Table 6.5).

Tumor Necrosis Factor Family of Proteins

TNF was cloned simultaneously as tumor necrosis factor, whose properties included the ability to kill tumor cells, and cachectin, a cytokine that caused appetite suppression and led to weight loss in mice. Although the use of TNF as an antineoplastic agent was limited by its toxicity, it has been found to be, along with IL-1 and IL-6, a major mediator of inflammation induced by infectious organisms (13,14,52). Its association with bacteria-induced septic shock and its ability to function as a mediator of acute immunologic reactions have led to the production of anti-TNF antibodies, which are currently in clinical use as treatment for severe autoimmune diseases such as otherwise unresponsive rheumatoid arthritis (see later) (13,59,60). Of interest is the fact that the use of this agent has been associated with activation of tuberculosis (59).

The TNF family of proteins is composed of both soluble proteins (such as TNF) and membrane-bound proteins. Some may exist in both forms. TNF receptors are membrane-spanning proteins that bind ligands such as CD30, CD40, and FAS in addition to TNF-α, TNF-β, and lymphotoxins. Table 6.6 is a partial list of the known human TNF superfamily members. In addition to those listed subsequently, a number of additional receptors and ligands have been recently defined (12).

Although antibodies to TNF were shown to be efficacious in preventing septic shock in some animal models, a large series of studies in humans did not demonstrate activity (14,40). These agents have been demonstrated to be useful in controlling autoimmune diseases, and their importance in preventing infection is underscored by the fact that patients treated with anti-TNF antibodies have a higher-than-normal incidence of infections.

Hematopoietic Growth Factors

The hematopoietic growth factors have a major role in regulation of immunity and immune response to infection. Not only are these proteins essential for the production of red cells, polys, platelets, and macrophages, many of them, including G-CSF, GM-CSF, and macrophage colony-stimulating factor (M-CSF), have been shown to activate polys or macrophages, making them natural choices for situations in which host defense may be marginal. Consequently, they have been used in this manner (18,19,23,26). Clinical studies support the use of G-CSF and GM-CSF in patients recovering from cytotoxic chemotherapy as

TABLE 6.3. Cytokines and Infectious Diseases

Cytokine	Type	Cell producing	Clinical data	Potential therapeutic uses	Reference
IL-1	Inflammatory	Macrophages, monocytes, others	Associated with fever, acute-phase reactants	Inhibitors (IL-1Ra) used in sepsis syndrome failed to improve mortality	40
IL-2	T-cell growth factor	T cells	Stimulates T-cell growth	Used to restore T cells in HIV-1	41–45
IL-3	Growth factor	T cells, NK cells, mast cells	Stimulates growth of platelets and macrophages	Not effective as in one study to prevent infections in BMT	62
IL-4	B-cell growth factor	T cells, mast cells	B-cell growth factor, stimulates IgG1, IgE	Potentiates T$_H$2 responses	63
IL-5	B-cell growth factor	T cells, mast cells	Stimulates B cells and differentiates eosinophils	Stimulates eosinophils	
IL-6	T-cell growth factor	T cells	Responsible for fever and induction of acute phase	Stimulates T cells and B cells	
IL-7	Pre–T- and Pre–B-cell growth factor	Marrow, thymus, some T cells			
IL-8	Chemokine	Macrophages, endothelial cells	Attracts neutrophils	Attracts and activates neutrophils; may be associated with inflammatory disease	54
IL-9	Mast cell activator	T cells	Activates mast cells	May affect intracellular parasites	63, 64
IL-10	Inhibits T-cell growth	T$_H$2 cells and macrophages	Inhibits T$_H$1 cells	Could be used as an antiinflammatory, anti–T-cell factor; inhibits HIV production in vitro	65
IL-11	Platelet growth factor	Fibroblasts	Stimulates megakaryocytes	Acts on mucous membranes to antagonize the effects of inflammatory cytokines; improves survival in animals	66, 67
IL-12	T-cell and NK-cell activator	B cells and macrophages	Stimulates T$_H$1 responses	Stimulates IFN-γ release; could be used to stimulate T$_H$1 cells; has been used to treat hepatitis C	46, 49, 58
IL-13	B-cell growth factor	T cells	Stimulates B cells to produce Ig	Stimulates Ig production; mouse studies suggest an inhibitor may prevent schistome induced responses	68
IL-14	B-cell growth factor	T cells	Stimulates B-cell memory		
IL-15	T-cell growth factor	T cells, epithelial cells	Stimulates neutrophils	May stimulate neutrophil function; in vitro activation of NK activity	48, 49
IL-16	T-cell growth factor		Stimulates T cells	May augment IL-2 activity	69
IL-17	Neutrophil growth and activation factor	T cells	Expression induces inflammatory cytokines	May activate neutrophils; animal model of Klebsiella pneumoniae	70, 71
IL-17C and IL-17F	Neutrophil growth and activation factor	T cells	Expression induces inflammatory cytokines	Members of the IL-17 family	82
IL-18		T cells, NK cells	Stimulates production of IFN-γ by NK cells	May activate NK cells to eliminate intracellular organisms; possible role in pneumonia	50, 72
IL-19			Homologous to IL-10		
IL-20			Homologous to IL-10	Mouse models suggest a role in skin disease	
IL-21		T cells, NK cells, B cells	Related to IL-12 and IL-15		73
IL-22			Reported to be involved in IL-10 signaling	Inhibits IL-4 production by T$_H$2 cells	74, 75
IL-23	T-cell activation factor	T cells	Combines with the p40 subunit of IL-12 to form a new factor that stimulates T cells to proliferate and produce IFN-γ	Could be used with IL-12 as a T-cell activator	76
IL-24	T$_H$1 stimulant	T cells and monocytes	Induces T$_H$1 cytokines in PBMCs	IL-10 family member formerly termed melanoma differentiation-associated gene 7	79, 80
IL-25	T-cell produced growth factor	T cells	Induces T$_H$2 cytokines		81
IL-26	IL-10 family	T$_H$2 cells and monocytes		IL-10 family member formerly termed AK155	83

IL, interleukin; NK, natural killer; Ig, immunoglobulin; HIV-1, human immunodeficiency virus type 1; BMT, bone marrow transplants; IFN-γ, interferon-γ; PBMC, peripheral blood mononuclear cell.

TABLE 6.4. Licensed Cytokines and Anticytokines in Clinical Use

Cytokine or anticytokine	Brand name	Preparation	Activity	Clinical uses	Reference
IL-2	Proleukin	Bacteria produced recombinant human protein	Stimulates T-cell growth	Currently licensed for treatment of metastatic renal cell cancer and melanoma; several studies suggest chronic administration will increase T-cell numbers in patients with HIV-1	41–45
Denileukin diftitox, IL-2 toxin conjugate	Ontak	Recombinant IL-2 diphetheria toxin protein	Kills T cells expressing IL-2 receptors	T-cell lymphomas expressing IL-2 receptors	77
Infliximab	Remicade	Monoclonal anti-TNF antibody	Inhibits TNF	Severe rheumatoid arthritis; colitis	59

IL-2, interleukin-2; TNF, tumor necrosis factor; HIV-1, human immunodeficiency virus type 1.

TABLE 6.5. Classification of Chemokines

Chemokine	Systematic name	Receptor	Role in infectious disease
CXC chemokine			Animal models suggest a role for CXCR2 ligands in *Nocardia* species infection
ELR Motif Chemokine			
Gro/MGSA-α	CXCL1	CXCR2	
Gro/MGSA-β	CXCL2	CXCR2	
Gro/MGSA-γ	CXCL3	CXCR2	
ENA-78	CXCL5	CXCR2	
GCP-2	CXCL6	CXCR1, CXCR2	
NAP-2	CXCL7	CXCR2	
IL-8	CXCL8	CXCR1, CXCR2	
Non-ELR motif chemokine			
PF-4	CXCL4	Not known	
Mig	CXCL9	CXCR3	
IP-10	CXCL10	CXCR3	Mouse experiments suggest a role in viral disease of the central nervous system
I-TAC	CXCL11	CXCR3	
SDF-1/PBSF	CXCL12	CXCR4	
BLC/BCA-1	CXCL13	CXCR5	
BRAK	CXCL14	Not known	
CXCL16	CXCL16	CXCR6	
CC chemokine			
I-309	CCL1	CCR8	
MCP-1	CCL2	CCR2	
MIP-1α	CCL3	CCR1, CCR5	
MIP-1β	CCL4	CCR5	
RANTES	CCL5	CCR1, CCR3, CCR5	
MCP-3	CCL7	CCR1, CCR2, CCR3	
Eotaxin	CCL11	CCR3	
MCP-4	CCL13	CCR2, CCR3	
HHC-1	CCL14	CCR1	
HHC-2/Leukotactin-1	CCL15	CCR1, CCR3	
HHC-4/LEC	CCL16	CCR1, CCR2, CCR5, CCR8	
TARC	CCL17	CCR4	
PARC/DC-CK1/AMAC-1	CCL18	Not known	
ELC/MIP-2b/Exodus-3	CCL19	CCR7	
LARC/MIP-3a/Exodus-1	CCL20	CCR6	
SLC/6Ckine/Exodus-2	CCL21	CCR7	
MDC/STCP-1	CCL22	CCR4	
MPIF-1	CCL23	CCR1	
MPIF-2/eotaxin-2	CCL24	CCR3	
TECK	CCL25	CCR9	
Eotaxin-3	CCL26	CCR3	
ILC/CTACK/Eskine	CCL27	CCR10	
MEC/CCL28	CCL28	CCR10, CCR3	

TABLE 6.6.   Classification of TNF Family Members

TNF family member	Receptor bound	Role in infection
TNF-α	TNFRI, TNFRII	Secretion stimulated by a variety of infectious agents; animal data suggest a use for TNF antagonists in infections, but human studies have been disappointing
TNF-β (Lta)	TNFRI, TNFRII, HVEM, LTβR	
OX40L	OX40	
CD40L	CD40	
FasL/CD95L/APOIL	Fas, DcR2	
CD27L	CD27	
CD30L	CD30	
4-IBBL	4-IBB	
TRAIL	DR4,DR5,DcR1, DcR2,OPG	
RANKL/TRANCE	RANK,OPG	
TWEAK	DR3/LARD/Apo3	
APRIL/TALL-2	Not known	
LIGHT/HVEML	HVEM,LT-bR,DcR3	
VEGI/TL-1	Not known	
THANK/BAFF/SlysS/TALL-1	TACI,BCMA	

TNF, tumor necrosis factor.

a means of increasing neutrophil counts. Clinical data thus far do not support their routine use as adjuvants (20) (Table 6.7).

CYTOKINE RECEPTORS AND THEIR FAMILIES

Five families of cytokine receptors are recognized: (a) immunoglobulin superfamily receptors (a group of cell surface proteins that resemble each other in having at least one immunoglobulin like extracellular domain), (b) class I (type I) cytokine receptor family, (c) class II (type II) cytokine receptor family, (d) TNF receptor (type III cytokine receptor) family, and (e) chemokine receptor family. IL-1 binds to an immunoglobulin superfamily member. A large number of cytokines bind to a dimeric receptor referred to as a *class I cytokine receptor*. Class I cytokine receptors are composed of a chain that is specific for the cytokine and an α, β, or γ chain, which transmits the cytokine initiated signal. Most cytokines appear to use class I receptors. The cytokines IL-2, IL-3, IL-4, IL-5, IL-6, IL-7, IL-9, IL-11, IL-12, IL-13, and IL-15 all bind to class I (type I) cytokine receptors, as

TABLE 6.7.   Mammalian Cell-Produced Growth Factors Used to Treat Infections

Growth factor	Preparation	Brand name	Activity	Clinical use	Reference
Erythropoietin	Recombinant protein	Epogen	Stimulates production of red cells	Used in patients with HIV and anemia	
G-CSF (filgastrim)	Bacteria-produced recombinant human protein	Neupogen	Stimulates proliferation of neutrophils	Shortens duration of neutropenia in patients receiving chemotherapy; animal experiments suggest a role in treatment of established infections	23, 25
GM-CSF (saugramostim)	Yeast-produced recombinant protein	Leukine	Stimulates proliferation of neutrophils; *in vitro* studies indicate augmentation of activity against intracellular pathogens	Shortens duration of neutropenia in patients receiving chemotherapy; has been used anecdotally to activate polys and macrophages; human studies do not support its routine use, but it may be warranted in selected settings	22, 24
IL-3			Stimulates proliferation of white cells and platelets	Unable to prevent infections in bone marrow transplant recipients	62
M-CSF			Stimulates proliferation and activation of monocytes and macrophages	Animal data suggest an effect on fungal infections	78

G-CSF, granulocyte colony-stimulating factor; GM-CSF, granulocyte-macrophage colony-stimulating factor; IL-3, interleukin-3; M-CSF, macrophage colony-stimulating factor; HIV, human immunodeficiency virus.

do the hematopoietic growth factors GM-CSF and G-CSF. The interferons (α, β, and γ) all bind to another family of cell surface proteins, which are the class II (type II) cytokine receptors. IFN-α, IFN-β, and IFN-γ all bind to this cell surface heterodimer (31). The TNF family (TNF-α, TNF-β, CD30, CD40, and Fas) may bind to membrane-spanning receptors or to soluble proteins. The TNF receptor family (type III cytokine receptor family) is a single transmembrane protein. The chemokines bind to a family of proteins that span the cell seven times (seven spanners) and signal through their association with G proteins (Table 6.5).

Interestingly, although sequence heterogeneity in the TNF-α gene has been described, its significance in terms of host defense is not clear (although heterogeneity in the TNF sequences has been associated with susceptibility to infections, this may be because of the close association of the TNF gene with the HLA locus) (26). On the whole, there is very little heterogeneity in cytokine sequences, and deficiency states have not been described. On the other hand, mutations that affect function have been described in both IFN-γ receptor chains and two of the IL-12 heterodimer chains. Patients with these mutations (usually found in consanguineous populations) have severe recurrent infections with intracellular parasites (including *Salmonella* species, nontuberculous mycobacteria, and *Listeria* species) (10,26,61).

PROSPECTS FOR THE FUTURE

Although several cytokines (including several classes of interferons and some hematopoietic growth factors) are used to treat a number of infectious diseases, the likelihood that these agents will continue to be used to treat specific infections in the future is small. They will be limited by their side effects, lack of specificity, and poor therapeutic-to-toxic ratios. On the other hand, until we better understand how to activate their receptor proteins directly, the hematopoietic growth factors will probably continue to be used to maintain granulocytes, red cells, and platelets counts in patients whose marrow is compromised by their disease or treatment (21). Advances in the use of small molecules to block interleukin or chemokine receptors may prevent infection-related host damage while avoiding the problems of the toxic side effects of proteins.

REFERENCES

1. Kaiser L, Fritz RS, Straus SE, Gubareva L, et al. Symptom pathogenesis during acute influenza: interleukin-6 and other cytokine responses. *J Med Virol* 2001;64:262–268.
2. Imanishi J. Expression of cytokines in bacterial and viral infections and their biochemical aspects. *J Biochem* 2000;127:525–530.
3. Wang, Z-M, Liu C, Dziarski R. Chemokines are the main proinflammatory mediators in human monocytes activated by *Staphylococcus aureus*, peptidoglycan, and endotoxin. *J Biol Chem* 2000;275:20260–20267.
4. Kampik D, Schulte R, Autenrieth IB. *Yersinia enterocolitica* invasin protein triggers differential production of interleukin-1, interleukin-8, monocyte chemoattractant protein 1, granulocyte-macrophage colony-stimulating factor, and tumor necrosis factor alpha in epithelial cells: implications for understanding the early cytokine network in *Yersinia* infections. *Infect Immun* 2000;68:2484–2492.
5. Tossing G. New developments in interferon therapy [Review] [104 refs]. *Eur J Med Res* 2001;6:47–65.
6. Meager A, Gaines Das R, Zoon K, et al. Establishment of new and replacement World Health Organization International Biological Standards for human interferon alpha and omega. *J Immunol Methods* 2001;257:17–33.
7. Oritani K, Kincade PW, Zhang C, et al. Type I interferons and limitin: a comparison of structures, receptors, and functions. [Review] [104 refs] *Cytokine Growth Factor Rev* 2001;12:337–348.
8. Sen GC. Viruses and interferons. *Ann Rev Microbiol* 2001;55:255–281.
9. Van der Meer JW, Vogels MT, Netea MG, et al. Proinflammatory cytokines and treatment of disease. [Review] [59 refs] *Ann N Y Acad Sci* 1998;856:243–251.
10. van Deventer SJH. Cytokine and cytokine receptor polymorphisms in infectious disease. *Intensive Care Med* 2000;26:S98–S102.
11. Yoshie O, Imai T, Nomiyama H. Chemokines in immunity. *Adv Immunol* 2001;78:57–110.
12. Zapata JM, Pawlowski K, Haas E, et al. A diverse family of proteins containing tumor necrosis factor receptor-associated factor domains. *J Biol Chem* 2001;276:24242–24252.
13. Aggarwal BB. Tumour necrosis factors receptor associated signaling molecules and their role in activation of apoptosis, JNK and NF-κB. *Ann Rheum Dis* 2000;59(Suppl I):I6–I16.
14. Reinhart K, Karzai W. Anti-tumor necrosis factor therapy in sepsis: update on clinical trials and lessons learned. *Crit Care Med* 2001;29(Suppl 1):S121–S125.
15. Pieters, Toine. Marketing medicines through randomized controlled trials: the case of interferon [Education and Debate]. *Br Med J* 1998;317:1231–1233.
16. Bagiolini M. Chemokines in pathology and medicine. *J Intern Med* 2001;250:91–104.
17. Onyeji CO, Nicolau DP, Nightingale CH, et al. Modulation of efficacies and pharmacokinetics of antibiotics by granulocyte colony-stimulating factor in neutropenic mice with multidrug-resistant *Enterococcus faecalis* infection. *J Antimicrob Chemother* 2000;46:429–436.
18. Bilgin K, Yaramis A, Haspolat K, et al. A randomized trial of granulocyte-macrophage colony-stimulating factor in neonates in sepsis and neutropenia. *Pediatrics* 2001;107:36–41.
19. Anaissie EJ, Vartivarian S, Bodey GP, et al. Randomized comparison between antibiotics alone and antibiotics plus granulocyte-macrophage colony-stimulating factor (Escherichia coli-derived in cancer patients with fever and neutropenia). *Am J Med* 1996;100:17–23.
20. Armstrong WS, Kazanjian P. Use of cytokines in human immunodeficiency virus-infected patients: colony-stimulating factors, erythropoietin, and interleukin-2 [Review] [85 refs]. *Clin Infect Dis* 2001;32:766–773.
21. Marodi L, Tournay C, Kaposzta R, et al. Augmentation of human macrophage candidacidal capacity by recombinant human myeloperoxidase and granulocyte-macrophage colony-stimulating factor. *Infect Immun* 1998;66:2750–2754.
22. Dallaire F, Ouellet N, Simared M, et al. Efficacy of recombinant human granulocyte colony-stimulating factor in a murine model of pneumococcal pneumonia: effects of lung inflammation and timing of treatment. *J Infect Dis* 2001;183:70–77.
23. Abu Jawdeh L, Haidar R, Bitar F, et al. *Aspergillus* vertebral osteomyelitis in a child with a primary monocyte killing defect: response to GM-CSF therapy. *J Infect* 2000;41:97–100.
24. Euler HH, Harten P, Zeuner RA, et al. Recombinant human granulocyte colony stimulating factor in patients with systemic lupus erythematosus associated neutropenia and refractory infections. *J Rheumatol* 1997;24:2153–2157.
25. Robinstein M, Dinarell CA, Oppenheim JJ, et al. Recent advances in cytokines, cytokine receptors, and signal transduction. *Cytokine Growth Factor Rev* 1999;9:175.
26. Lichtenauer-Kaligis EG, de Boer T, Verreck FA, et al. Severe Mycobacterium bovis BCG infections in a large series of novel IL-12 receptor beta 1 deficient patients and evidence for the existence of partial IL-12 receptor beta 1 deficiency. *Eur J Immunol* 2003;33:59–69.
27. Kurt-Jones, EA, Popova, L, Kwinn, L, et al. Pattern recognition receptors TLR4 and CD14 mediate response to respiratory syncytial virus. *Nat Immunol* 2000;1:398–401.
28. Guidotti LG, Chisari FV. Cytokine-mediated control of viral infections. *Virology* 2000;273:221–227.
29. Imai K, Takeshita A, Hanazawa S. Transforming growth factor-β inhibits lipopolysaccharide-stimulated expression of inflammatory cytokines in mouse macrophages through downregulation of activation protein 1 and CD14 receptor expression. *Infect Immun* 2000;68:2418–2423.
30. Poveda F, Camacho J, Arnalich F, et al. Circulating cytokine concentrations in tuberculosis and other chronic bacterial infections. *Infection* 1999;27:272–274.
31. Goodsell DS. The molecular perspective: interferons. *Stem Cells* 2001;19:467–468.
32. Siegal FP, Kodowaki N, Shodell M, et al. The nature of the principal type 1 interferon-producing cells in human blood. *Science* 1999;284:1835–1837.
33. Alexenko AP, Ealy AD, Roberts RM. The cross-species antiviral activities of different IFN-τ subtypes on bovine, murine, and human cells: contradictory evidence for therapeutic potential. *J Interferon Cytokine Res* 1999;19:1335–1341.
34. LaFleur DW, Nardelli B, Tsareva T, et al. Interferon-κ, a novel type 1 interferon expressed in human keratinocytes. *J Biol Chem* 2001;276:39765–39771.
35. Gross JB Jr. Clinician's guide to hepatitis C. *Mayo Clin Proc* 1998;73:355–361.
36. Keating MR. Antiviral agents for non-human immunodeficiency virus infections [Symposium on Antimicrobial Agents—Part XV]. *Mayo Clin Proc* 1999;74:1266–1283.
37. Murray HW. Interferon-gamma and host antimicrobial defense: current and future clinical applications [Review]. *Am J Med* 1994;97:459–467.
38. Gallin JI, Farber JM, Holland SM, et al. Interferon-gamma in the management of infectious diseases. *Ann Intern Med* 1995;123:216–224.
39. Hayden FG, Albrecht JK, Kaiser DL, et al. Prevention of natural colds by contact prophylaxis with intranasal alpha$_2$-interferon. *N Engl J Med* 1986;314:71–75.
40. Opal S, Fisher CJ, Dhainaut J-FA, et al. Confirmatory interleukin-1 receptor antagonist trial in severe sepsis: a phase III, randomized, double blind, placebo-controlled, multicenter trial. *Crit Care Med* 1997;25:1115–1124.
41. Smith KA. Low-dose daily interleukin-2 immunotherapy: accelerating immune restoration and expanding HIV-specific T-cell immunity without toxicity [Review] [49 refs]. *AIDS* 2001;(15 Suppl 2):S28–S35.
42. Ruxrungtham K, Suwanagool S, Tavel JA, et al. A randomized, controlled

24-week study of intermittent subcutaneous interleukin-2 in HIV-1 infected patients in Thailand. *AIDS* 2000;14:2509–2513.

43. Miller KD, Spooner K, Herpin BR, et al. Immunotherapy of HIV-infected patients with intermittent interleukin-2: effects of cycle frequency and cycle duration on degree of CD4(+) T-lymphocyte expansion. *Clin Immunol* 2001;99: 30–42.

44. Kovacs JA, Vogel S, Albert JM, et al. Controlled trial of interleukin-2 infusions in patients infected with the human immunodeficiency virus. *N Engl J Med* 1996;335:1350–1356.

45. Imami N, Hardy GA, Nelson MR, et al. Induction of HIV-1-specific T cell responses by administration of cytokines in late-stage patients receiving highly active anti-retroviral therapy. *Clin Exp Immunol* 1999;118:78–86.

46. O'Brien CB, Moonka DK, Henzel BS, et al. A pilot trial of recombinant interleukin-12 in patients with chronic hepatitis C who previously failed treatment with interferon-alpha. *Am J Gastroenterol* 2001;96:2473–2479.

47. Ye P, Garvey PB, Zhang P, et al. Interleukin-17 and lung host defense against *Klebsiella pneumoniae* infection. *Am J Respir Cell Mol Biol* 2001;25:335–340.

48. Mastroianni CM, d'Ettorre G, Forcina G, et al. Interleukin-15 enhances neutrophil functional activity in patients with human immunodeficiency virus infection. *Blood* 2000;96:1979–1984.

49. Kawakami K, Koguchi Y, Qureshi MH, et al. IL-18 contributes to host resistance against infection with *Cryptococcus neoformans* in mice with defective IL-12 synthesis through induction of IFN-gamma production by NK cells. *J Immunol* 2000;165:941–947.

50. Cai G, Kastelein R, Hunter CA. Interleukin-18 (IL-18) enhances innate IL-12-mediated resistance to Toxoplasma gondii. *Infect Immun* 2000;68:6932–6938.

51. Blumberg H, Conklin D, Xu WF, et al. Interleukin 20: discovery, receptor identification, and role in epidermal function. *Cell* 2001;104:9–19.

52. Lokensgard JR, Hu S, Sheng W, et al. Robust expression of TNF-alpha, IL-1beta, RANTES, and IP-10 by human microglial cells during nonproductive infection with herpes simplex virus. *J Neurovirol* 2001;7:208–219.

53. Sundstrom JB, McMullan LK, Spiropoulou CF, et al. Hantavirus infection induces the expression of RANTES and IP-10 without causing increased permeability in human lung microvascular endothelial cells. *J Virol* 2001;75: 6070–6085.

54. Grimm MC, Elsbury SKO, Pavli P, et al. Interleukin 8: cells of origin in inflammatory bowel disease. *Gut* 1996;38:90–98.

55. Belperio J, Keane MP, Burdick MD, et al. Critical role for the chemokine MCP-1/CCR2 in the pathogenesis of bronchiolitis obliterans syndrome. *J Clin Invest* 2001;108:547–556.

56. Moore TA, Newstead MW, Strieter RM, et al. Bacterial clearance and survival are dependent on CXC chemokine receptor-2 ligands in a murine model of pulmonary *Nocardia asteroides* infection. *J Immunol* 2000;164:908–915.

57. Liu MT, Chen BP, Oertel P, et al. The T cell chemoattractant IFN-inducible protein 10 is essential in host defense against viral-induced neurologic disease. *J Immunol* 2000;165:2327–2330.

58. Kawakami K, Shibuya K, Qureshi MH, et al. Chemokine responses and accumulation of inflammatory cells in the lungs of mice infected with highly virulent *Cryptococcus neoformans*: effects of interleukin-12. *FEMS Immunol Med Microbiol* 1999;25:391–402.

59. Keane J, Gershon S, Wise RP, et al. Tuberculosis associated with infliximab, a tumor necrosis factor alpha-neutralizing agent. *N Engl J Med* 2001;354:1098–1104.

60. Edwards, CK III. PEGylated recombinant human soluble tumour necrosis factor receptor type I (r-Hu-sTNF-RI): novel high affinity TNF receptor designed for chronic inflammatory diseases. *Ann Rheum Dis* 1999;58(Suppl I):I73–I81.

61. Holland SM. Treatment of infections in the patient with mendelian susceptibility to mycobacterial infection [Review] [100 refs]. *Microbes Infect* 2000;2:157–1590.

62. Brouwer RE, Vellenga E, Zwinderman KH. Phase III efficacy study of interleukin-3 after autologous bone marrow transplantation in patients with malignant lymphoma. *Br J Haematol* 1999;106:730–736.

63. Monteyne P, Renauld JC, Van Broeck J, et al. IL-4-independent regulation on in vivo IL-9 expression. *J Immunol* 1997;159:2616–2623.

64. Gessner A, Blum H, Rollinghoff M. Differential regulation if IL-9-expression after infection with *Leishmania major* in susceptible and resistant mice. *Immunobiology* 1993;189:419–435.

65. Shin HD, Winkler C, Stephens JC, et al. Genetic restriction of HIV-1 pathogenesis to AIDS by promoter alleles of IL-10. *Proc Natl Acad Sci USA* 2000;97:14467–14472.

66. Opal SM, Keith JC, Palardy JE, et al. Recombinant human interleukin-11 has anti-inflammatory actions yet does not exacerbate systemic *Listeria* infection. *J Infect Dis* 2000;181:754–756.

67. Opal SM, Jhung JW, Keith JC Jr, et al. Recombinant human interleukin-11 in experimental *Pseudomonas aeruginosa* sepsis in immunocompromised animals. *J Infect Dis* 1998;178:1205–1208.

68. Hein J, Sing A, Di Genaro MS, et al. Interleukin-12 and interleukin-18 are indispensable for protective immunity against enteropathogenic *Yersinia*. *Microb Pathog* 2001;31:195–199.

69. Kornfeld H, Cruikshank WW. Prospects for IL-16 in the treatment of AIDS [Review] [59 refs]. *Expert Opin Biol Ther* 2001;1:425–432.

70. Shellito JE, Quan Zheng M, Ye P, et al. Effect of alcohol consumption on host release of interleukin-17 during pulmonary infection with *Klebsiella pneumoniae*. *Alcoholism Clin Exp Res* 2001;25:872–881.

71. Ye P, Rodriguez FH, Kanaly S, et al. Requirement of interleukin-17 receptor

signaling for lung CXC chemokine and granulocyte colony-stimulating factor expression, neutrophil recruitment, and host defense. *J Exp Med* 2001;194:519–527.

72. Brombacher F. The role of interleukin-13 in infectious diseases and allergy [Review] [87 refs]. *Bioessays* 2000;22:646–656.

73. Parrish-Novak J, Dillon SR, Nelson A, et al. Interleukin 21 and its receptor are involved in NK cell expansion and regulation of lymphocyte function. *Nature* 2000;408:57–63.

74. Xie MH, Aggarwal S, Ho WH, et al. Interleukin (IL)-22, a novel human cytokine that signals through the interferon receptor-related proteins CRF2-4 and IL-22R. *J Biol Chem* 2000;275:31335–31339.

75. Xu W, Presnell SR, Parrish-Novak J, et al. A soluble class II cytokine receptor, IL-22RA2, is a naturally occurring IL-22 antagonist. *Proc Natl Acad Sci USA* 2001;98:9511–9516.

76. Oppmann B, Lesley R, Blom B, et al. Novel p19 protein engages IL-12p40 to form a cytokine, IL-23, with biological activities similar as well as distinct from IL-12. *Immunity* 2000;13:715–725.

77. Olsen E, Duvic M, Frankel A, et al. Pivotal phase III trial of two dose levels of denileukin diftitox for the treatment of cutaneous T-cell lymphoma. *J Clin Oncol* 2001;19:376–388.

78. Kuhara T, Uchida K, Yamaguchi H. Therapeutic efficacy of human macrophage colony-stimulating factor, used alone and in combination with antifungal agents, in mice with systemic *Candida albicans* infection. *Antimicrob Agents Chemother* 2000;44:19–23.

79. Caudell EG, Mumm JB, Poindexter N, et al. The protein product of the tumor suppressor gene, melanoma differentiation–associated gene 7, exhibits immunostimulatory activity and is designated IL-14. *J Immunol* 2002;168:6041–6046.

80. Wolk K, Kunz S, Asadulla K, et al. Cutting edge: immune cells as sources and targets of the IL-10 family members? *J Immunol* 2002;168:5397–5402.

81. Fort MM, Cheung J, Yen D, et al. IL-25 induces IL-4, IL-5, and IL-13 and T$_H$2-associated pathologies in vivo. *Immunity* 2001;15:985–995.

82. Hurst SD, Muchamuel T, Gorman DM, et al. New IL-17 family members promote T$_H$1 or T$_H$2 responses in the lung: in vivo function of the novel cytokine IL-25. *J Immunol* 2002;169:443–453.

83. Fickenscher H, Hor S, Kupers H, et al. *Trends Immunol* 2002;23:89–96.

Epidemiology

CHAPTER 7
Epidemiology of Community-Acquired Infections

Mitchell L. Cohen

Epidemiology involves the study of almost any aspect of a disease or condition and the populations it affects. For infectious diseases, such aspects include defining the occurrence of the disease, its clinical manifestations and management, characteristics of the affected population, the mechanisms of transmission, and the characteristics of the causative organism. The clinical aspects, microbiology, diagnostics, and management of specific diseases are discussed in other chapters. The purpose of this chapter is to examine general concepts of epidemiology and their application to community-acquired infections.

EPIDEMIOLOGICAL METHOD AND ITS LIMITATIONS

Epidemiology defines the who, what, when, where, how, and why of infectious diseases. The *who* is the populations at risk for infection. The *what* is the scope and impact of infections. The *when* is the temporal trends. The *where* is the geographic location of disease. The *how* defines the reservoirs of disease and the mechanisms of transmission. The *why* addresses the issue of risk factors or the reasons disease affects some persons but not others.

Descriptive and Analytic Epidemiology

The two most commonly used epidemiological methods for studying infectious diseases are descriptive and analytic epidemiology (1). Descriptive epidemiology involves the collection and analysis of all data that describe the disease in the population. Analysis of these data frequently leads to the development of hypotheses. Analytic epidemiology typically involves the testing of hypotheses—the comparison of characteristics of persons who are ill and those who are well. Using a combination of these two methods frequently leads to the identification of associations or risk factors for disease.

There are important limitations to both epidemiological approaches. One important limitation of descriptive epidemiology is underreporting or underascertainment of cases of a specific disease. For many diseases, calculated incidences are underestimates because many variables affect reporting. For example, for a case of an illness such as salmonellosis to be reported, a culture must be referred to the state health laboratory for serotyping. For many cases of salmonellosis, physicians are not consulted, or cultures are not obtained or sent for serotyping. One study has estimated that only 1 in 38 of the actual number of cases of salmonellosis in the United States is reported (2).

Analytic epidemiology is limited by several additional factors. Associations demonstrated by epidemiological studies do not necessarily ensure causation. A statistically significant association simply implies that the likelihood of the association occurring by chance alone is small. Inferring causation requires statistical and logical epidemiological associations (3), but proving it often requires results from animal studies to fulfill Koch's postulates. Analytic studies may be affected by confounding and by a variety of biases. Confounding is a spurious identification of a risk factor because it is associated with a true causative factor. In addition, bias can be introduced unsuspectedly during the collection or analysis of data (4). Comparison groups that are different in some systematic fashion may indicate a selection bias. Differences in how or what data are collected for different groups result in ascertainment bias. Sound epidemiological studies attempt to minimize such bias by appropriate design and analysis of findings.

Endemic and Epidemic Disease

Epidemiological methods may be used to study either endemic or epidemic disease. Illness occurs as sporadic or isolated cases or as parts of recognized outbreaks or epidemics. The term *endemic* is typically used for cases of an illness that are not connected with each other and that occur at an expected frequency. Several studies, however, have demonstrated that the distinction between endemic or sporadic disease and epidemic illness can be somewhat artificial. What is thought to be endemic disease may actually be miniepidemics in which the association between cases is not recognized (5).

An epidemic can be defined as an occurrence of disease at a rate greater than expected. Increased frequency of disease may not indicate a true increase but may be related to changes in recognition (i.e., better diagnosis or an increase in reporting). A real increase in the incidence of disease, however, usually indi-

cates changes in exposure, in the population at risk, or in the characteristics of the organism (e.g., antigens or pathogenicity). In practice, an increase in disease frequency often suggests increased exposure and therefore an opportunity for intervention and prevention.

Much epidemiological information is gathered by investigating epidemics, or outbreaks, of disease. The investigation of an outbreak requires an orderly approach of data collection, hypothesis generation and testing, and intervention (6). Outbreaks frequently provide sufficiently large numbers of ill persons to allow statistical analyses to determine risk factors for infection, mechanisms of transmission, and reservoirs of the agent organism. Such investigations can also lead to the identification of new pathogens. Investigations of bloody diarrhea outbreaks in Oregon and Michigan in 1982 led to the identification of *Escherichia coli* O157:H7 as a cause of hemorrhagic colitis (7). In this instance, the presence of the same serotype of *E. coli* in a number of ill persons suggested that the organism might be a pathogen despite the fact that it lacked any recognized toxin or other pathogenic characteristic.

Case Definition

For many epidemiological studies or epidemic investigations, it is necessary for the epidemiologist to develop a case definition. This definition may be based on the results of a laboratory test, such as a blood culture, or on the presence of certain signs and symptoms, such as for toxic shock syndrome, or some combination of clinical manifestations and laboratory tests. The case definition is an important step that can profoundly affect the outcome of the analysis. For example, a strict clinical case definition may limit the recognized spectrum of disease, whereas a loose clinical case definition may be likely to include persons whose illness has an entirely different cause.

In a sense, an epidemiologist can manipulate a case definition to achieve desired degrees of sensitivity and specificity. In case-control studies, a specific definition is usually desirable because including too many persons as cases who do not have the illness under study would reduce the likelihood of demonstrating associations between cases and risk factors. As with diagnostic tests in clinical medicine, it would be desirable in epidemiology to have a case definition that was 100% sensitive and 100% specific—a situation that is not realistic.

Different case definitions can easily affect the outcome of studies. A vaccine efficacy study that uses sputum cultures to define cases could misidentify pneumococci as the cause of a certain number of pneumonia cases because patients, regardless of the cause of their pneumonia, are commonly colonized with *Streptococcus pneumoniae*. Thus, this less specific case definition, which leads to the inclusion of false-positive pneumococcal cases, might falsely lower the values for vaccine efficacy. On the other hand, a study that uses a more specific case definition that requires isolation of the pneumococci from blood excludes the nonbacteremic cases of pneumococcal pneumonia and determines vaccine efficacy only for preventing the more severe, invasive disease. The impact of different case definitions may partially explain conflicting values for pneumococcal vaccine efficacy obtained in different studies (8,9).

Epidemiology and the Laboratory

Epidemiological studies have been much assisted by laboratory advances, particularly in molecular biology (10,11). In the past, many epidemiological investigations were stymied by the inability to distinguish between strains of common microorganisms and thus accurately define a case. When *Salmonella typhimurium* infection, which accounts for 25% of all *Salmonella* species serotypes, occurred in the community, the epidemiologist was unable to distinguish between strains unless they were carrying unusual antibiotic-resistant markers. Thus, epidemiological studies might be unable to show associations because the *S. typhimurium* isolates studied would include different strains transmitted by different vehicles (a classification error). With the advent of plasmid profile analysis, ribotyping, enzyme typing, deoxyribonucleic acid (DNA) probes, and most recently, pulsed field gel electrophoresis (PFGE), subtyping has become possible and practical (12–14), and the location of an outbreak-related strain can be more accurately determined. These methods, by allowing a greater degree of subtyping, have made possible many important epidemiological studies and are now being used in the development of networks of laboratories, such as PulseNet, to detect disease outbreaks rapidly (15).

EPIDEMIOLOGICAL CONCEPTS

Incidence

Epidemiology attempts to quantify the frequency of disease. Knowing the number of cases of disease and the number of persons in the population, one can calculate the incidence of an infectious disease. For the purposes of this chapter, an *incidence rate* is defined as the number of times an infection is noted in an observed population during the defined period divided by the number of persons observed in that time (16). For most infectious diseases, the incidence is reported as an annual rate. For a few infectious diseases that cause a chronic illness, it may be more appropriate to refer to the *prevalence* of disease, the proportion of the population ill in a defined time period (16). Because most infectious diseases have a short duration, however, the frequency of the illness is usually given as an annual rate.

The incidence of the disease can be determined by a variety of methods. Most commonly, an illness is declared reportable by state law, and a formal surveillance system is established. Programs at state and federal levels conduct surveillance for these diseases and tabulate the reported cases. A crude annual incidence can be calculated by dividing the number of reported cases by the size of the population. Some surveillance systems are passive, based on reports submitted to local and state health departments. Newer, active surveillance systems have been developed in which health officials seek cases of specific diseases by directly contacting laboratories or practitioners (17,18). Active systems have the potential for more rapid and complete ascertainment.

The incidence of a disease can provide important information. Observed over time, changes in incidence can identify an emerging problem or determine the effectiveness of prevention or control measures. Comparing incidence of different diseases can assist public health officials in allocating resources or the clinician in considering the most likely causes of a particular syndrome. Comparing the incidence of disease in different populations can provide clues to how the disease is being transmitted or indicate the presence of specific susceptibilities in the population.

Study Populations

Infectious disease epidemiology studies the occurrence and characteristics of specific infections in defined populations. A population may be defined by a specific geographic location, host characteristic, or exposure—for example, all residents of a county or state, participants in a church supper, children in a day care center, or patients in an intensive care unit. In

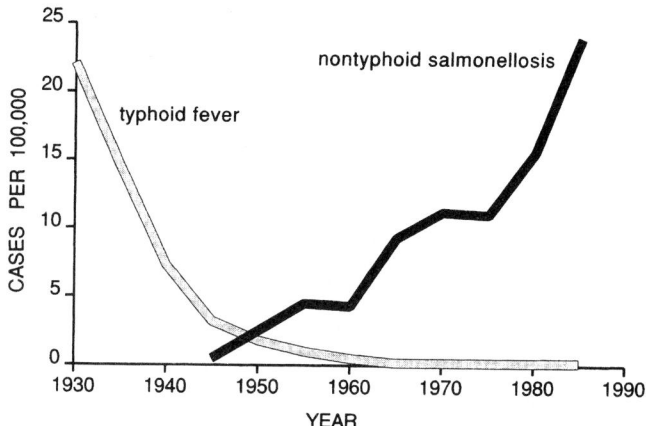

Figure 7.1. Reported incidence of typhoid fever and nontyphoid salmonellosis in the United States, 1930 to 1985.

different populations, the same infection may have different epidemiological characteristics. For example, salmonellosis in the developed world is often transmitted by food in the community, whereas in the developing world, it is often transmitted person to person in hospitals (19,20).

Temporal Characteristics

The incidence of many infectious diseases varies over time. A *secular trend* is a change in the incidence of disease over an extended period. Diseases that are transmitted by the fecal-oral route, such as typhoid, have decreased with improvements in sanitation, water treatment, and sewage disposal. On the other hand, the occurrence of diseases such as nontyphoid salmonellosis has increased as a result of changes in food production and distribution (Fig. 7.1). A *periodic trend* is a change in the secular trend that tends to recur at consistent intervals. Before the widespread use of vaccine, measles demonstrated a periodic trend in the United States, with peaks every 2 years. Most periodic trends have been attributed to either changes in the organism or changes in population immunity. A *seasonal trend* is a consistent pattern in the annual occurrence of a disease. Meningococcal meningitis has a clear late winter, early spring peak (21) (Fig. 7.2). Many of the bacterial enteric pathogens, such as *Salmonella*, *Shigella*, and

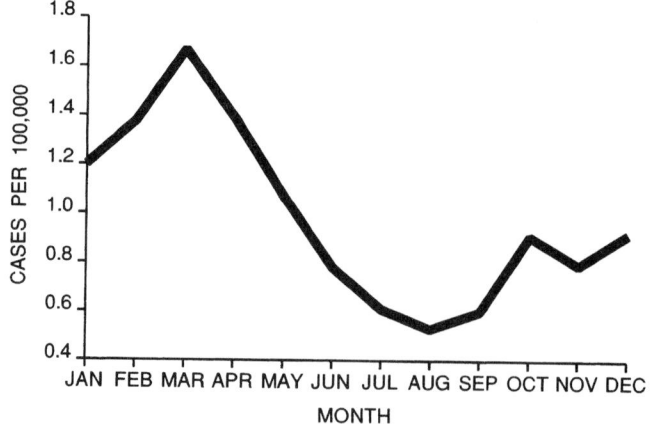

Figure 7.2. Distribution of meningococcal disease, by month, 1982 to 1984. (Adapted from Harrison LH, Broome CV. The epidemiology of meningococcal meningitis in the U.S. civilian population. In: Vedros NA [ed]. *Evolution of meningococcal disease.* Boca Raton, FL: CRC Press, 1987:27–45, with permission.)

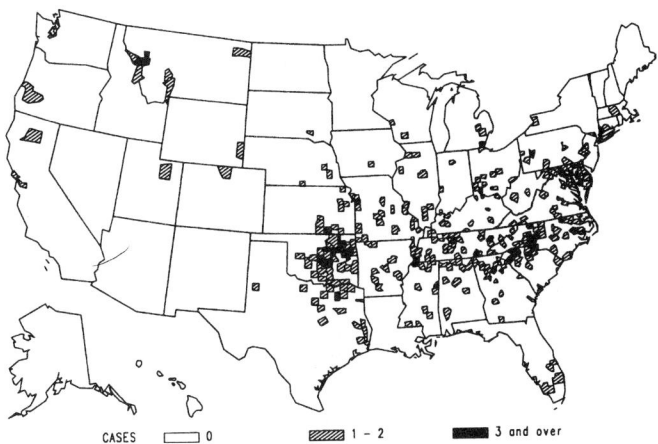

Figure 7.3. Reported cases of Rocky Mountain spotted fever, by county, in the United States, 1987.

Campylobacter species, have a seasonal peak in summer to fall. Another enteric pathogen, rotavirus, has a winter peak in the United States. The explanation for a seasonal trend is usually not known but is frequently the subject of speculation. For example, the greater occurrence of salmonellosis in the summer has been attributed to factors such as inadequate refrigeration during times when refrigeration is most critical.

Geographic Characteristics

Disease may occur with different frequencies in different geographic areas, as does Rocky Mountain spotted fever, the occurrence of which correlates with the distribution of its vectors (22) (Fig. 7.3). Other diseases may reflect differences in the demographic characteristics of the population, variation in exposures, or differences in reporting. One specific *Salmonella* serotype, *Salmonella newport*, peaks in the spring in rural areas and in the summer in both rural and urban areas (Fig. 7.4). The explanation for the additional spring peak in rural areas is unknown, but it may be related to humans having close contact with infected animals. The summer peak in both rural and urban areas is likely due to food-borne infections.

Reservoirs and Routes of Transmission

To prevent and control infectious diseases, public health officials devise intervention strategies by using both descriptive and an-

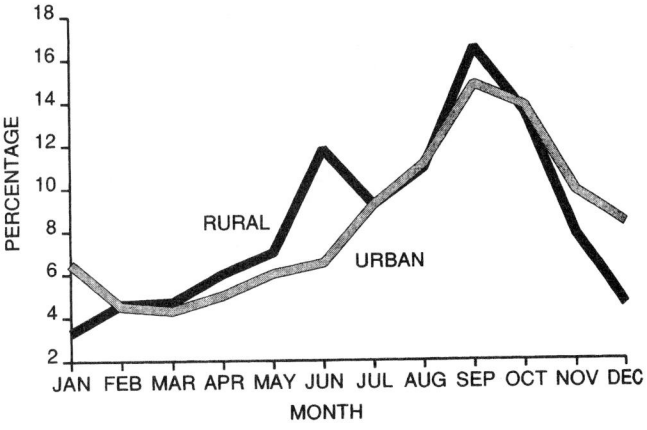

Figure 7.4. Distribution of *Salmonella newport* isolates from urban and rural counties in the United States, by month, 1968 to 1982.

alytic epidemiology to identify reservoirs for infectious agents and define the routes and mechanisms of transmission. For an organism to perpetuate itself, it must have an ecological niche, or reservoir, in the environment or in animal or human populations where it can replicate. These reservoirs can vary from the environment (*Legionella* species in cooling towers or hot-water systems) to animals (*Salmonella* species in food animals) to human populations (the agents of tuberculosis, smallpox, measles, or typhoid). Some organisms may be sustained in several reservoirs (*Giardia* species or influenza virus).

To be a successful pathogen, the organism must be transmitted from the reservoir to a susceptible host in sufficient numbers and in a site where it can persist and replicate. The precise route of transmission is determined by characteristics of both organism and host. In a healthy adult, salmonellae are transmitted primarily in food because infection requires relatively large numbers of organisms. In the more susceptible neonates, salmonellosis can be caused by the fewer organisms transmitted person to person by fecal-oral contact. On the other hand, shigellae, which require only a small dose for infection, are readily transmitted to both children and adults by person-to-person fecal-oral contact.

The routes of transmission can be straightforward: *Legionella* species may be transmitted in aerosol from a contaminated cooling tower or in shower water from a contaminated water-heating system. Hepatitis B virus and human immunodeficiency virus (HIV) may be transmitted by blood transfusion, parenteral drug abuse, or sexual contact with infected persons. Alternatively, the routes of transmission can be extremely convoluted. In one *Salmonella heidelberg* outbreak, the organism was transmitted from ill calves to a farmer's pregnant daughter, who subsequently transmitted the organism to her newborn infant. The organism was then transmitted in the hospital nursery from the infected newborn to two other infants, probably by direct contact with the hands of nurses (23).

Risk Factors

One of the purposes of analytic epidemiology is to identify the risk factors associated with disease. This is typically accomplished by case-control or cohort analysis that attempts to identify different frequencies of characteristics or exposures in ill (cases) and well (controls) persons. Risk factors are typically characteristics of the ill person, such as age, sex, race, socioeconomic status, area of residence, or exposures such as foods, smoking, medications, illicit drug use, travel history, day care attendance, or sexual activity. In perhaps the first example of analytic epidemiology, John Snow examined the occurrence of cholera in 1853 in two areas of London, which differed only in the source of their water. He was able to demonstrate that the death rate from cholera was 10 times higher in the houses supplied by a company whose source of water was a more sewage-contaminated area of the Thames River (24). Some factors, such as breast-feeding or immunization, may be associated with decreased risk for disease and be protective. Determining the risk factors that are associated with disease can lead to identification not only of the exposures and the vehicles or route of transmission but also of susceptibilities present in case patients that can allow targeting of specific control strategies to that portion of the population.

Prevention and Control

The ultimate goal of public health is control and prevention. Infectious disease prevention strategies operate in three general areas: (a) interruption or prevention of transmission, (b) prevention of colonization or infection, and (c) prevention of illness. The tools to implement these strategies include physical or chemical methods, immunology, and education.

A wide variety of physical and chemical interventions are available. Most attempt to prevent transmission of pathogenic microorganisms. Some of the most time-honored methods of prevention physically remove microorganisms, such as by hand washing, or provide barriers to transmission, such as use of quarantine, surgical masks, gloves, condoms, or protective environments. Other methods, such as adequate cooking, pasteurization, chlorination, and chemotherapy, prevent transmission by killing microorganisms. Immunological tools, such as vaccination, also can reduce transmission by reducing the number of persons susceptible to infection or illness. The elimination of susceptible persons from a population leads not only to the reduction of transmission but also to the real (smallpox) or potential (*Haemophilus influenzae* type b, measles, poliomyelitis) elimination of diseases that are restricted to a human reservoir. A final and important tool of prevention is education, which can influence all areas of prevention. Epidemiologists have long appreciated the importance of certain behaviors in increasing the risk for disease. Educational efforts may be directed at increasing use of other prevention strategies, such as immunization, hand washing, or safe food handling. Thus, recent educational efforts have targeted behaviors that increase risk for infectious disease, such as unprotected sexual activity or smoking.

The clinician plays an important role in the prevention of disease by ensuring appropriate immunization, treatment, prophylaxis, and education of patients and by recognizing and reporting public health problems. Unfortunately, preventive measures are not used to their maximum benefit. Low rates of immunization for many adult populations at high risk for certain vaccine-preventable diseases (25) and insufficient educational efforts in the prevention of disease indicate a need for more intensive prevention activities.

FREQUENCY AND IMPACT OF INFECTIOUS DISEASE IN THE UNITED STATES

Accurate estimates of the impact of infectious diseases or the relative importance of various syndromes or microbial infections are often lacking. Even for illnesses for which national surveillance systems exist, reporting is often incomplete or affected by variables that complicate comparisons. For example, data from isolates reported to the Centers for Disease Control and Prevention (CDC) show that the 1986 incidences of salmonellosis and campylobacteriosis were 18 and 4 per 100,000, respectively (26); however, a population-based study conducted in a large health maintenance organization in Seattle, Washington, between May 1985 and April 1986 showed rates for salmonellosis and campylobacteriosis of 21 and 50 per 100,000, respectively (27). Data from many of the surveillance systems are best used for following trends or changes in the descriptive epidemiology of a specific pathogen.

In 1984, a Carter Center report attempted to quantify the impact of various infectious diseases (28). The authors estimated that infectious diseases accounted for more than 740 million illnesses and 190,000 deaths each year in the United States. The cost of infectious diseases exceeded $17 billion and resulted in 1 billion disability days. Each year, infectious diseases accounted for more than 2 million of the 12 million (18%) years of life lost before age 65 years. The authors estimated that the four major pathogen groups accounted for about 290 million illnesses and 90,000 deaths (Table 7.1). As better data have been collected

TABLE 7.1. Estimated Impact of Infectious Diseases in the United States, by Pathogen Group

Pathogen group	Deaths	Incidence
Viral	17,000	207,329,000
Bacterial	68,200	36,026,000
Parasitic	1,800	26,620,000
Fungal	1,200	18,027,000

Adapted from Bennett JV, Holmberg SD, Rogers MF, et al. Infectious and parasitic diseases. In: Amler RW, Dull HB, eds. *Closing the gap. The burden of unnecessary illness.* New York: Oxford University Press, 1987:102–114, with permission.

through improved surveillance systems, some of these estimates have been revised. For example, the 1984 study suggested that 6 million cases of food-borne illness occurred each year in the United States; newer studies suggest that the figure is closer to 70 million (29).

Globally, the World Health Organization has estimated that in 1998, infectious diseases accounted for more than 13 million deaths (30), almost one fourth of total deaths. The most important specific causes of death were pneumonia, diarrheal disease, and AIDS (Table 7.2).

TRENDS IN COMMUNITY-ACQUIRED INFECTIONS

The twentieth century has witnessed major trends in infectious diseases that are strongly influenced by changes in society and technology. With increasing development, better nutrition, increasing emphasis on personal hygiene, better sewage disposal, and safer food and water, a number of diseases have become less frequent. Immunization has led to the eradication of smallpox and the control of many childhood diseases. Antimicrobial chemotherapy has reduced mortality rates for a number of diseases, such as typhoid fever, tuberculosis, meningitis, and endocarditis, and has reduced the incidence of complications of other infections.

On the other hand, societal and technological changes have also resulted in the emergence of new diseases and have altered the epidemiological character of old infections. In October 1992, the Institute of Medicine published a report entitled *Emerging Infections: Microbial Threats to Health in the United States* (31). The factors influencing the emergence of infectious diseases were placed into six categories (Table 7.3). The recurrent theme for

TABLE 7.2. Global Estimates of Infectious Causes of Death, 1998

Type of infection	Deaths (millions)
Pneumonia	3.5
Acquired immunodeficiency syndrome	2.3
Diarrheal disease	2.2
Tuberculosis	1.5
Malaria	1.1
Measles	1.0

From World Health Organization. *Removing obstacles to healthy development.* Geneva: World Health Organization, 1999, with permission.

TABLE 7.3. Factors Influencing the Emergence of Infectious Diseases

Changes in human demographics and behavior
Changes in technology and industry
Economic development and land use
International travel and commerce
Microbial adaption and change
Breakdown of public health measures

each factor is change—often societal, technologic, or microbial—that results in a frequently unanticipated impact on infectious diseases (32). Technological advances, for example, have facilitated travel and commerce. Today, a contaminated food can be rapidly distributed to wide geographic areas. This has converted food-borne outbreaks from events involving dozens at church suppers to interstate or international outbreaks involving hundreds of thousands of people. In 1985, a multistate outbreak of *S. typhimurium* infection caused by contaminated pasteurized milk affected an estimated 200,000 persons in the midwestern United States (33). In 1984, a food-borne outbreak aboard multiple planes of a British airline disseminated *Salmonella enteritidis* infections over at least four continents (34). Advances in transportation itself are changing the geographic distribution of diseases. The febrile patient in a U.S. emergency department can be a tourist returning from an African vacation with a case of malaria or trypanosomiasis. Immigration to the United States in the 1970s and 1980s after natural disasters or political change has increased the incidence of diseases such as leprosy and tuberculosis and produced patients infected with a variety of exotic parasitic diseases.

Technological advances have also provided new reservoirs of infection and mechanisms of transmission. Air conditioning, cooling towers, and hot-water systems have been associated with outbreaks of legionnaires' disease. Certain superabsorbent menstrual tampons with specific chemical compositions were associated with toxic shock syndrome.

New pathogens have gained prominence as a result of HIV infections, and technological advances in medical care have increased the population of immunocompromised persons. These persons are susceptible to a variety of bacterial, viral, fungal, and parasitic organisms that seldom cause illness in the immunocompetent person. Although many of these infections are nosocomial, several can be community acquired, particularly by patients infected with HIV. In addition, patients with HIV infection have a 100 to 200 times greater risk for developing infections that are not traditionally thought to be opportunistic, such as tuberculosis and pneumococcal pneumonia (35,36). The rapidly increasing rate of organ transplantation is an additional factor, creating exquisitely susceptible populations that are becoming infected with unique groups of uncommon pathogens (37).

The emergence of antimicrobial resistance is a trend of particular concern (38–40). By the early 1990s, strains of *Mycobacterium tuberculosis* and enterococci had become essentially untreatable with existing antibiotics. Strains of other organisms, including *Staphylococcus aureus* and *Streptococcus pneumoniae*, were susceptible to only one or two antimicrobial agents. The emergence of resistance was related to both the selective pressures of antimicrobial use in humans and animals and factors increasing the transmission of drug-resistant organisms.

Social changes can have similar impact on the epidemiology of community-acquired infections. The sexual revolution of the 1960s and 1970s provided opportunity for emergence of HIV and

for drug resistance in sexually transmitted diseases. The return of mothers to the workplace and the increase in single-parent households prompted a tremendous increase in the use of day care. By 1990, more than 6 million children younger than age 6 years were estimated to attend full- or part-time day care (41). The day care setting has been associated with increased rates of diarrheal diseases, hepatitis A, meningitis, and otitis media and has also played an important role in the emergence of antimicrobial resistance of *S. pneumoniae* (42).

The impact of technology and social change on infectious diseases is not new. In the Middle Ages, advances in agriculture, overpopulation, and urbanization were some of the factors in the emergence and transmission of the Black Death (43). With the current rate of technological and societal change, we should anticipate continued changes in the epidemiology of established community-acquired infections and the emergence of new pathogens as important causes of morbidity and mortality.

REFERENCES

1. Evans AS. Epidemiological concepts. In: Evans AS, Feldman HA, eds. *Bacterial infections of humans.* New York: Plenum Publishing, 1982:3–4.
2. Chalker R, Blaser M. A review of human salmonellosis. III. Magnitude of *Salmonella* infections in the United States. *Rev Infect Dis* 1988;10:111–124.
3. Rothman KJ. *Modern epidemiology.* Boston: Little, Brown, 1986.
4. Sackett DL. Bias in analytic research. *J Chronic Dis* 1979;32:51–63.
5. Riley LW, DiFerdinando GT Jr, DeMelfi TM, et al. Evaluation of isolated cases of salmonellosis by plasmid profile analysis: introduction and transmission of a bacterial clone by precooked roast beef. *J Infect Dis* 1983;148:12.
6. Gregg MB. The principles of an epidemic field investigation. In: Holland WW, Detels R, Knox G, eds. *Oxford textbook of public health.* Oxford: Oxford University Press, 1985:284.
7. Riley LW, Remis RS, Helgerson SD, et al. Hemorrhagic colitis associated with a rare *Escherichia coli* serotype. *N Engl J Med* 1983;308:681.
8. Simberkoff MS, Cross AP, Al-Ibrahim M, et al. Efficacy of pneumococcal vaccine in high-risk patients: results of a Veterans Administration cooperative study. *N Engl J Med* 1986;315:1318.
9. Bolan G, Broome CV, Facklam RR, et al. Pneumococcal vaccine efficacy in selected populations in the United States. *Ann Intern Med* 1986;104:1.
10. Mayer LW. Use of plasmid profiles in epidemiologic surveillance of disease outbreaks and in tracing the transmission of antibiotic resistance. *Clin Microbiol Rev* 1988;1:228.
11. Wachsmuth K. Molecular epidemiology of bacterial infections: examples of methodology and of investigations of outbreaks. *Rev Infect Dis* 1986;8:682.
12. Tompkins LS, Troup N, Labigne-Roussel A, et al. Cloned, random chromosomal sequences as probes to identify *Salmonella* species. *J Infect Dis* 1986;154:156.
13. Holmberg SD, Wachsmuth IK, Hickman-Brenner FW, et al. Comparison of plasmid profile analysis, phage typing, and antimicrobial susceptibility testing in characterizing *Salmonella typhimurium* isolates from outbreaks. *J Clin Microbiol* 1984;19:100.
14. Barrett TJ, Lior H, Green JH, et al. Laboratory investigation of a multistate foodborne outbreak of *Escherichia coli* O157:H7 by using pulsed-field gel electrophoresis and phage typing. *J Clin Microbiol* 1994;32:3013–3017.
15. Swaminathan B, Barrett TJ, Hunter SB, et al. PulseNet: the molecular subtyping network for foodborne bacterial disease surveillance, United States. *Emerg Infect Dis* 2001;7:382–389.
16. MacMahon B, Pugh TF. *Epidemiology: principles and methods.* Boston: Little, Brown, 1970.
17. Schuchat A, Hilger T, Zell E, et al. Active bacterial core surveillance of the emerging infections program network. *Emerg Infect Dis* 2001;7:92–99.
18. Angulo FJ, Voetsch AC, Vugia D, et al. Determining the burden of human illness from foodborne diseases. *Vet Clin North Am* 1998;14:165–172.
19. Riley LW, Ceballos BSO, Trabulsi LR, et al. The significance of hospitals as reservoirs for endemic multiresistant *Salmonella typhimurium* causing infection in urban Brazilian children. *J Infect Dis* 1984;150:236.
20. Holmberg SD, Osterholm MT, Senger KA, et al. Drug-resistant *Salmonella* from animals fed antimicrobials. *N Engl J Med* 1984;311:617.
21. Harrison LH, Broome CV. The epidemiology of meningococcal meningitis in the U.S. civilian population. In: Vedros NA, ed. *Evolution of meningococcal disease.* Boca Raton: CRC Press, 1987:27–45.
22. Centers for Disease Control. Summary of notifiable diseases, United States, 1987. *MMWR Morb Mortal Wkly Rep* 1988;36:48.
23. Lyons RW, Samples CL, DeSilva NN, et al. An epidemic of resistant *Salmonella* in a nursery: animal to human spread. *JAMA* 1980;243:546.
24. Fox JP, Hall CE, Elveback LR. *Epidemiology: man and disease.* London: Macmillan, 1970.
25. Williams WW, Hickson MA, Kane MA, et al. Immunization policies and vaccine coverage among adults. *Ann Intern Med* 1988;108:616.

26. Tauxe RV, Hargrett-Bean N, Patton CM, et al. *Campylobacter* isolates in the United States, 1982–1986. CDC Surveillance Summaries. *MMWR Morb Mortal Wkly Rep* 1988;37:SS-1.

27. MacDonald KL, O'Leary MJ, Cohen ML, et al. *Escherichia coli* O157:H7, an emerging gastrointestinal pathogen. *JAMA* 1988;259:3567.

28. Bennett JV, Holmberg SD, Rogers MF, et al. Infectious and parasitic diseases. In: Amler RW, Dull HB, eds. *Closing the gap: the burden of unnecessary illness*. New York: Oxford University Press, 1987.

29. Mead PS, Slutsker L, Dietz V, et al. Food-related illness and death in the United States. *Emerg Infect Di* ; 1999;5:607–625.

30. World Health Organization. *Removing obstacles to healthy development: report on infectious diseases*. Geneva: World Health Organization, 1999.

31. Institute of Medicine. *Emerging infections: microbial threats to health in the United States*. Washington DC: National Academy Press, 1992.

32. Cohen ML. Changing patterns of infectious disease. *Nature* 2000;406:762.

33. Ryan CA, Nickels MK, Hargrett-Bean NT, et al. Massive outbreak of antimicrobial-resistant salmonellosis traced to pasteurized milk. *JAMA* 1987;258:3269.

34. Tauxe RV, Tormey MP, Mascola L, et al. Salmonellosis outbreak on trans-Atlantic flights: foodborne illness on aircraft: 1947–1984. *Am J Epidemiol* 1987;125:150.

35. Redd SC, Rutherford GW, Sande MA, et al. The role of human immunodeficiency virus infection in pneumococcal bacteremia in San Francisco residents. *J Infect Dis* 1990;162:1012.

36. Castro KG. Tuberculosis as an opportunistic disease in persons infected with human immunodeficiency virus. *Clin Infect Dis* 1995;21:566.

37. Dixon DM, McNeil MM, Cohen ML, et al. Fungal infections: a growing threat. *Public Health Rep* 1996;111:226–239.

38. Cohen ML. Epidemiology of drug resistance: implications for a post-antimicrobial era. *Science* 1992;257:1050.

39. Cohen ML. Antimicrobial resistance: prognosis for public health. *Trends Microbiol* 1994;2:422.

40. Hofmann J, Cetron MS, Farley M, et al. The prevalence of drug-resistant *Streptococcus pneumoniae* in Atlanta. *N Engl J Med* 1995;333:481.

41. Haskins R, Kotch J. Day care and illness: evidence, costs, and public policy. *Pediatrics* 1986;77:951.

42. Reichler MR, Allphin AA, Breiman RF, et al. The spread of multiply resistant *Streptococcus pneumoniae* at a day care center in Ohio. *J Infect Dis* 1992;166:1346.

43. Gottfried RS. *The Black Death: natural and human disaster in Medieval Europe*. New York: The Free Press, 1983.

CHAPTER 8

Epidemiology and Prevention of Nosocomial Infections

Deborah S. Yokoe

The term *nosocomial* is defined as "denoting a new disorder (not the patient's original condition) associated with being treated in a hospital, such as a hospital-acquired infection" (1). Nosocomial infections impose a huge burden on the health-care system in the United States, both economically and in terms of adverse patient outcomes. The Centers for Disease Control and Prevention (CDC) estimates that nearly 2 million patients annually develop a nosocomial infection, and approximately 88,000 die as a direct or indirect result of their infection. Nosocomial infections often lead to increases in lengths of hospitalization, and result in about $4.5 billion in excess costs annually (2).

Because of the volume of medical procedures now performed in the ambulatory setting as well as the increased care provided in nonacute hospital settings, it is useful to expand this definition to also include health care–associated infections that occur outside of the acute care environment.

The central aim of hospital epidemiology is to prevent the acquisition of health care–associated infections. Health care–associated infections are included in the preventable adverse patient events described by the Institute of Medicine in the 1999

report "To Err is Human: Building a Safer Health System" (3), and efforts aimed at preventing health care–associated infections are an integral part of the national patient safety agenda.

SURVEILLANCE FOR HEALTH CARE–ASSOCIATED INFECTION

Nosocomial infections impose a significant burden on the healthcare system. Central to efforts aimed at reducing the rates of these infections is the development of efficient and accurate methods of surveillance. The goals of surveillance include establishing baseline rates of infections, identifying epidemics, enabling infection control personnel to present data accurately and convincingly, assessing control measures, reducing rates of nosocomial infections, and providing data for interhospital comparison (4).

The importance of surveillance for the prevention and control of nosocomially acquired infections is supported by a number of studies. The results of the Study on the Efficacy of Nosocomial Infection Control (SENIC) Project as well as several subsequent studies support the relationship between active surveillance programs and reduced rates of nosocomial infections (5). In addition, information obtained from surveillance is useful for accrediting and quality improvement/quality assurance organizations as indicators of the quality of patient care.

History of Surveillance

The use of surveillance for the prevention and control of nosocomial infections dates back at least to the work of Ignaz Semmelweis in the 1840s in which he demonstrated the role of person-to-person spread of puerperal sepsis and the effectiveness of hand disinfection for control of transmission (6). In the United States, surveillance techniques developed for public health efforts in the 1940s were gradually applied to surveillance of hospital infections (7).

During the late 1950s and early 1960s, hospitals voluntarily began to form infection control committees with the purpose of controlling hospital-acquired infections. These efforts were largely inspired by the epidemic of staphylococcal infections brought to light by early hospital surveillance efforts during that period of time (8–10). Investigators noted that the seriousness of a hospital's infection problems and the need for control efforts were often not apparent to medical staff and hospital administrators until quantitative measures obtained from surveillance data were made available to them (7).

In the late 1960s, the CDC recommended that hospitals conduct surveillance of nosocomial infections to obtain epidemiologic data on which to base control measures (10,11).

In 1964, the Joint Commission on Accreditation of Healthcare Organizations (JCAHCO) made infection surveillance a responsibility of the medical staff, and in 1976 incorporated a detailed surveillance system into their standards for accreditation (12).

An international conference on nosocomial infections was held in 1970, followed by a nationwide movement toward establishment of organized infection surveillance and control programs. By 1975, over half of U.S. hospitals had organized surveillance programs with infection control nurses (13).

In 1970, the CDC initiated the National Nosocomial Infections Study, later renamed the National Nosocomial Infections Surveillance (NNIS) system, in which selected hospitals contributed their nosocomial infection surveillance data to create the only source of national data on the epidemiology of nosocomial infections in the United States. Initially, all patients at participating hospitals were monitored for infections at all sites.

Since 1986, each hospital has been given the flexibility to select one or more standardized protocols, termed surveillance components, which include (a) hospital-wide, (b) adult and pediatric intensive care unit (ICU), (c) high-risk nursery, and (d) surgical surveillance (14).

In 1974, the Study on the Efficacy of Nosocomial Infection Control (SENIC) Project was established by the CDC with the objectives of estimating the magnitude of nosocomial infections in U.S. hospitals, describing the extent to which hospitals had adopted the infection surveillance and control program approach, and determining the effectiveness of this approach in reducing nosocomial infection risks. This study was motivated in large part by a growing concern over the cost effectiveness of infection control activities. The results of the SENIC Project were published in 1985 and suggested that the combination of ongoing surveillance of infections, active control efforts, and qualified staff could prevent up to one third of nosocomial infections (15).

Other studies have suggested that surveillance results in reduced rates of nosocomial infections, although the presence of confounding factors limits interpretation of these findings (15–17).

Surveillance data are now routinely used by hospitals to develop strategies for preventing and controlling the spread of health care–associated infections.

Surveillance Methods

Surveillance includes (a) defining as concisely as possible the events to be surveyed, (b) collecting the relevant data in a systematic way, (c) consolidating or tabulating the data into meaningful arrangements, and (d) analyzing and interpreting the data, with the goal of using this information to bring about change (18).

The utility of surveillance data depends on a number of factors, including use of meaningful definitions of infections, the ability to identify and count the infections accurately, and appropriate classification with respect to important risk factors, such as neutropenia, intubation, obesity, and diabetes. None of these requirements is straightforward and free from controversy. The most widely applied surveillance definitions are those used by the CDC for the NNIS system (19,20). These definitions include clinical and laboratory data as well as physician diagnosis.

The range of surveillance methods is broad, extending from self-reporting by patients and physicians to universal, prospective surveillance by trained personnel (16,21–24). Virtually all widely used surveillance systems depend on review of the medical record, which is labor intensive. The accuracy of such systems depends on the completeness of the medical record and the submission of cultures when infection is suspected. Additional surveillance methods include review of microbiology laboratory results and reports of chest radiography before they are returned to the medical records, review of nurses' records, interviews with the nursing staff, and interviews with and examinations of patients (25). In general, the more intensive the surveillance, the larger the number of infections identified but at a correspondingly greater cost. For example, review of nursing records, interviews with clinical staff, and examination of patients increase the yield but may place an unacceptable burden on the infection control program's resources. Striking a balance between exhaustive efforts to capture nearly every infection and targeted surveillance aimed at detecting the most important problems remains a difficult and controversial problem. For example, there is legitimate debate about the merits of identifying and reporting superficial postoperative wound infections. Although they rarely cause substantial morbidity, they may serve as indicators

for more serious events that occur so infrequently that they are difficult to study. Similar considerations apply to asymptomatic nosocomial urinary tract infections.

Several methods have been proposed to allow more efficient utilization of reviewer time, including review of laboratory data as a primary source to target patients for intensive review or to identify important colonization, for example, by methicillin-resistant *Staphylococcus aureus*, before infection occurs. Additional methods include prescreening of the nursing records and ICU checklists (26). Especially interesting are recent research endeavors that focus on methods for using automated data systems to identify patients who are likely to have nosocomial infections (27–29). These systems draw on data from the microbiology laboratory, the pharmacy, the radiology department, the operating room, coded medical record diagnoses, and admission diagnoses to identify patients with characteristics that suggest infection. Skilled personnel can then use this information to focus their efforts preferentially at assessing patients most likely to have infections (30–32).

The effectiveness of methods that use these data to identify health care–associated infections can be assessed by comparing several components of each method, including (a) informativeness of the data obtained, (b) accuracy and consistency of the information, (c) the resources needed to obtain the data, and (d) significance of the infections identified in terms of excess morbidity and cost. The accuracy and consistency of the data depend in part on the degree of objectivity with which the information can be obtained. Consistency also affects the feasibility of interhospital comparisons of nosocomial infection rates. The significance of the infections identified by various methods of surveillance may differ in terms of clinical status of the patients, their morbidity, and their resource utilization.

PREVENTING HEALTH CARE–ASSOCIATED INFECTIONS

Hand Hygiene

The importance of hand hygiene in preventing health care–associated infections has been recognized since the 19th century. The Hungarian obstetrician Ignaz Semmelweis, in the 1840s, dramatically lowered the maternal mortality rate in the First Clinic at the General Hospital of Vienna by requiring medical students and physicians to disinfect their hands with a chlorine solution between patients (6). Despite the intervening century and a half, published observations of health-care worker adherence to recommended hand hygiene practices continue to suggest that hand hygiene practice is frequently suboptimal (33–54).

Transmission of nosocomial pathogens from patient to patient can occur via the hands of health-care workers in the absence of adequate hand antisepsis. A number of studies have demonstrated that contamination of the hands of health-care workers can occur through a variety of patient care activities (55,56). Pittet et al. showed that more frequent hand antisepsis performed by health-care workers was associated with reduced acquisition of nosocomial pathogens (36). Larson et al. also showed that the prevalence of nosocomial infections decreased as adherence to recommended hand hygiene measures improved (57).

A number of guidelines outlining recommendations for hand washing in the health-care setting have been published by the CDC, the Association for Professionals in Infection Control (APIC), and the Hospital Infection Control Practices Advisory Committee (HICPAC) (58,59). Despite incorporation of the APIC and HICPAC recommendations into the infection control guidelines for most hospitals, observed adherence of health-care workers to recommended hand-washing practices has remained unacceptably low. Pittet et al. conducted a large observational study of adherence to hand hygiene recommendations during routine patient care (33). They found that of 2,834 observed opportunities for hand hygiene, the average adherence was 48%, with the highest rates of nonadherence in the ICUs during procedures with a high risk for bacterial contamination and when the intensity of patient care was high. These results suggest that adherence to guidelines may not be feasible during the periods when the risk for transmission of pathogens to patients is highest.

Based on this information, many health-care facilities are currently focusing on facilitating access to hand hygiene by providing products such as alcohol-based hand antisepsis agents as an alternative to traditional soap and water. Alcohol-based hand agents may be superior to soap and water because they require less time, act faster, are associated with less skin irritation (60–63), and are more effective (64–66). Sustained improvements in hand hygiene practice among health-care workers will likely require a combination of the availability of new products and system-wide changes that prioritize the importance of hand hygiene for patient safety.

Transmission Precautions

Published recommendations for isolation precautions have existed in the United States for over a century. In 1970, the CDC published a manual to assist hospitals with isolation precautions and revised the manual in 1975 (67,68). The original CDC guidelines recommended that hospitals adopt a category-specific isolation system. Diseases were grouped into categories of isolation based on their usual mode of transmission: strict isolation for diseases spread by both contact and the air (droplet nuclei); contact isolation for diseases spread by contact with the patient or the patient's contaminated environment; respiratory isolation for disease spread by close contact with large contaminated respiratory droplets; tuberculosis isolation for infections, such as tuberculosis, that are transmitted by airborne droplet nuclei; enteric precautions for diseases spread by the fecal-oral route; drainage-secretion precautions for infections spread by contact with purulent infective material; and blood and body fluid precautions for blood-borne diseases. By the mid-1970s, 93% of U.S. hospitals had adopted this isolation system (13). In 1983, the CDC published the "CDC Guideline for Isolation Precautions in Hospitals" (69). Changes from the previous manual included allowing hospital infection control committees to select either category-specific or disease-specific isolation precautions. In the disease-specific system, precautions were based on the known or suspected mode of transmission of individual infectious diseases, providing a more customized approach to isolation once the clinical picture or cultures suggested a specific diagnosis.

In 1985, universal precautions were introduced to protect health-care workers from blood-borne infectious agents, especially the human immunodeficiency virus and hepatitis B and C viruses. Universal precautions were originally designed to apply the CDC's previous blood and body fluid precautions universally to all patients, but the CDC (70) broadened the scope of these guidelines to apply to nonintact skin and mucosal surfaces and to many other body fluids, such as pleural, pericardial, and cerebrospinal fluids and any fluid that contains visible blood. Universal precautions rely on the use of barrier techniques. They have specifically been shown to decrease the risk for exposure to blood and body fluids (71). In 1991, the Occupational Safety and Health Administration (OSHA) published "Occupational

Exposure To Bloodborne Pathogens; Final Rule," thus federally mandating that health-care facilities provide education aimed at reducing the risk for occupational exposure to blood and body fluids and hepatitis B vaccine to all employees at risk.

Some infection control specialists believed that the CDC isolation precaution systems did not provide a mechanism for interrupting spread of pathogens from patients who did not have recognized infections or culture-demonstrated colonization. An alternative system of isolation, body substance isolation, was proposed in 1987 and represented a novel effort to cope with some of the difficulties presented by the traditional CDC systems (72). In the body substance isolation system, personnel are required to wear gloves when having contact with any potentially contaminated substance (e.g., excreta, secretions, fluids), as well as mucous membranes and nonintact skin of all hospitalized patients. Hand washing is still recommended after removal of the gloves but not after routine contacts with patients that do not require the use of gloves. If soiling of clothes is likely, a gown is also worn, and suitable barriers are used if a splash in the face seems possible.

In 1996, the CDC and HICPAC revised the "CDC Guidelines for Isolation Precautions in Hospitals" (73), and these recommendations are now widely used. The revised guidelines contain two tiers of precautions. The first tier consists of "standard precautions" that are the foundation of recommendations applicable for the care of all patients in hospitals, regardless of infection status. The second tier of precautions is focused on the care of patients known or suspected to be infected or colonized with infectious agents transmitted by airborne or droplet transmission or by contact with skin or contaminated surfaces.

Standard precautions combine universal precautions (aimed at preventing transmission of blood borne pathogens from patients to health-care workers) and the body substance isolation system (designed to prevent transmission of pathogens via moist body substances between patients) and are applied to all patients regardless of diagnosis or presumed infection status. Standard precautions include recommendations regarding hand washing; use of gloves when touching blood, body fluids, secretions, excretions, and contaminated items; use of a mask and eye protection or a face shield; and use of a gown during procedures and patient care activities likely to generate splashes or sprays of potentially infectious material; handling of soiled patient-care equipment; cleaning of environmental surfaces and linen; and prevention of occupational injuries associated with transmission of blood-borne pathogens from patients to health-care workers.

The three types of transmission-based precautions to be used in addition to standard precautions for patients with suspected or documented infection or colonization with epidemiologically important pathogens are airborne precautions, droplet precautions, and contact precautions (Table 8.1). These can be combined for diseases with multiple routes of transmission. Airborne precautions apply to patients known or suspected to be infected with infectious agents transmitted by airborne droplet nuclei ($\leq 5\ \mu$m) that remain suspended in air and that can be dispersed widely by air currents. These patients should ideally be placed in special negative pressure rooms. Special respiratory protective equipment is also recommended for infections such as tuberculosis. Droplet precautions apply to patients known or suspected to be infected with microorganisms transmitted by large particle droplets that are generated by coughing, sneezing, talking, or during procedures such as sputum induction, including *Bordetella pertussis* and *Neisseria meningitidis*. These patients should be placed in a private room or at least 3 feet away from other patients, and all hospital personnel working within 3 feet of the patient should wear a surgical mask. Contact precautions apply

TABLE 8.1. Summary of Indications for Transmission-Based Precautions

Precaution category	Mode of transmission	Major examples
Airborne	Droplet nuclei—long distances	Measles, smallpox Varicella-zoster virus (varicella) Tuberculosis
Droplet	Large-particle droplets—short distances	*Bordetella pertussis* Influenza *Neisseria meningitidis* Other important pathogens[a]
Contact	Direct contact with patient or fomites	Multidrug-resistant bacteria Selected enteric pathogens[b] Selected viral pathogens in children[c] Others[d]

[a]Including *Corynebacterium diphtheriae, Mycoplasma pneumoniae, Yersinia pestis* (pneumonic plague), mumps virus, and rubella virus.
[b]Including *Clostridium difficile;* for diapered or incontinent patients: enterohemorrhagic *Escherichia coli* O157:H7, *Shigella*, rotavirus, and hepatitis A virus.
[c]Respiratory syncytial virus, parainfluenza virus, enterovirus.
[d]Including highly contagious skin pathogens, viral conjunctivitis agents, hemorrhagic fever viruses.

to patients known or suspected to be colonized or infected with microorganisms that can be transmitted by direct contact with the patient or contact with environmental surfaces or patient care items in the patient's environment, including methicillin-resistant *Staphylococcus aureus* and vancomycin-resistant enterococci. These patients should ideally be placed in a private room and hospital personnel should wear gloves when entering the patient room and a gown if anticipating contact of clothing with the patient, the patient's environment, or contaminated patient care items.

Equipment and Environment

Approximately 27 million surgical procedures are performed each year in the United States (74). Large numbers of other invasive medical procedures such as gastrointestinal endoscopy and bronchoscopy are also performed (75). Adequate cleaning, disinfection, and sterilization of medical equipment used during these procedures are essential for preventing infections associated with person-to-person transmission and transmission of environmental pathogens. Inadequate disinfection and sterilization practices have been associated with a number of outbreaks of infection. In addition, it is important to be aware that adequate disinfection and sterilization can be difficult to achieve for many newly developed medical devices because of structural complexity (e.g., devices containing small lumens) and incompatibility with standard disinfection and sterilization methods (76).

Cleaning is defined as the removal of organic and inorganic material from objects and surfaces, usually through wiping or washing with detergents or enzymatic agents. Lack of thorough cleaning before disinfection and sterilization can interfere with the effectiveness of these processes. *Disinfection* is defined as a process that eliminates most pathogenic microorganisms, with the exception of bacterial spores, and includes the use of liquid chemicals or wet pasteurization. *Sterilization* is the complete elimination or destruction of all forms of microbial life. Sterilization methods include dry heat, steam under pressure, ethylene oxide gas, hydrogen peroxide gas plasma, and liquid chemicals.

The adequacy of both disinfection and sterilization depend on prior cleaning of the device, the level of contamination, the nature of the device, temperature and pH, presence of biofilms, and the concentration and exposure time to the germicidal agent. Detailed recommendations for disinfection and sterilization in the health-care setting have been published (75,77,78).

The health-care environment can also harbor organisms that can cause opportunistic infections among severely immunocompromised patients, including solid and hematopoietic stem cell transplant recipients. In particular, construction activities within hospitals have been associated with airborne and waterborne infections. Examples include outbreaks associated with *Aspergillus* species during periods of construction (79–82) and legionellosis associated with contamination of water systems with *Legionella* species (83,84). Preventing health care–associated infections among immunocompromised patients associated with environmental pathogens requires close collaboration between architects, engineers, and infection control professionals.

Occupational Health

Efforts to control the transmission of infections in the hospital must include the involvement and participation of health-care workers. The infection control aspects of occupational health encompass both protecting personnel from contagious disease encountered in the workplace and protecting patients from infections harbored by hospital personnel. Comprehensive reviews may be found in the general infection control textbooks and in guidelines issued by the CDC (85–89). Specific elements for the protection of employees are now often mandated by OSHA, particularly for preventing transmission of blood-borne pathogens (90). Important components of an effective occupational health program include screening of health-care workers for immunity to infections such as rubella and measles, offering vaccinations aimed at protecting health-care workers (e.g., hepatitis B and influenza vaccines), providing adequate engineering controls and personal protective equipment (e.g., negative air pressure rooms for patients with tuberculosis and needle devices with engineered sharps injury protection designed to reduce the risk for occupational exposure to blood), and educating health-care workers about methods to prevent occupational exposure to infectious agents.

EPIDEMIOLOGY AND PREVENTION OF SPECIFIC TYPES OF NOSOCOMIAL INFECTIONS

The four major types of health care–associated infection are bloodstream infection (BSI), pneumonia, urinary tract infection, and postoperative infection (Table 8.2), and intensive efforts have been directed toward preventing these device- and procedure-related problems. The CDC, through HICPAC, has developed a number of guidelines for the prevention and control of nosocomial infections based on extensive evaluation of published data (74,91,92).

Intravascular Catheter-Associated Bloodstream Infections

Intravascular catheters are ubiquitous in health care, particularly in the inpatient setting. Although peripheral venous catheters are the most frequently used intravascular devices and can be associated with local or systemic infections, the overall rate of BSI associated with peripheral venous catheters is very low in comparison with the BSI rates associated with central venous

TABLE 8.2. Device-Associated Infections

Site of nosocomial infection	Invasive device	Infected site	Extraluminal[a]	Intraluminal
Urinary tract	Bladder catheter	Bladder, kidney	Perineal flora	Catheter lumen from catheter junction, and drainage bag
Lower respiratory tract	Endotracheal tube	Trachea, lung	Pharynx or skin around tracheostomy tubing	Ventilator reservoir and tubing
Intravascular	Intravascular cannula	Blood vessel	Skin	Intravascular fluids, tubing connections, or catheter hubs
Surgical wound	Drains and wicks	Subcutaneous tissues	Skin	Lumen of drains

[a]Organisms may arise from the flora at that site or others that gain access to it.

catheters (CVCs) (91,93). A number of studies have estimated the morbidity and mortality associated with infectious complications of CVCs, particularly in the ICU setting (93–96). The attributable mortality rate for CVC-related BSIs has ranged from 12% to 25%, and attributable cost per infection has been estimated to be $3,700 to $40,000 (97,98), bringing the annual cost in the United States of caring for patients with CVC-associated BSIs to between $296 million and $2.3 billion.

The rate of CVC-associated BSIs depends in part on the definitions used. Although it is usually straightforward to identify patients with positive blood culture results, it is important to realize that the indications for obtaining these cultures may vary widely. A potential bias is also introduced by clinicians in attempts to distinguish "contaminants" from "true bacteremia" (99). Although the CDC's NNIS system definitions for laboratory-confirmed BSI are widely used, modifications have been proposed aimed at minimizing the potential for subjective interpretation of available data (100). Determining the attributable source of a BSI is also subject to variable interpretation of data. Most surveillance definitions, including the NNIS definition for catheter-associated BSI, include all nosocomial BSIs that occur among patients with CVCs, when other sites of infection have been excluded. These considerations are particularly important when attempting to compare CVC-associated BSIs rates over time or between health-care institutions. Several techniques aimed at identifying BSIs attributable to catheter infections include quantitative catheter culture methods (101,102), simultaneous quantitative blood cultures comparing blood obtained through a CVC and a peripheral vein (103), and comparing the differential time to positivity of simultaneous blood cultures drawn from the CVC and a peripheral vein (104,105).

The CDC and JCAHCO recommend expressing the rate of CVC-associated BSIs as the number of catheter-associated BSIs per 1,000 catheter-days (catheter-days are the total number of days that at least one CVC is in place) (106,107). This denominator adjusts for both the number of CVCs and the number of days the catheter is in place (108), two potentially modifiable risk factors, but is labor intensive to obtain for most hospitals.

Based on data from the CDC's NNIS system, most nosocomial BSIs are associated with the use of a CVC, and rates of CVC-associated BSIs vary by hospital size, hospital service/unit, and type of CVC. For January 1992 through June 2001, the NNIS hospitals reported ICU pooled mean rates of CVC-associated BSIs ranging from 2.9 (cardiothoracic ICU) to 9.7 (burn ICU) CVC-associated BSIs per 1,000 catheter-days (109).

The distribution of etiologic agents has evolved somewhat over time. Based on NNIS data obtained between 1986 and 1989, the most common organisms causing BSIs were coagulase-negative staphylococci (27%) and Staphylococcus au-

reus (16%) (110). Between 1992 and 1999, coagulase-negative staphylococci (37%) and enterococci (13.5%) were the organisms that most frequently caused BSIs, followed by S. aureus (12.6%) (106). Yeast, particularly Candida species, was associated with a substantial proportion of BSIs (8%) (106,110–113). The frequency of BSIs caused by organisms with resistance to conventional first-line antibiotics (e.g., methicillin-resistant S. aureus, vancomycin-resistant enterococci, extended spectrum β-lactamase–producing Enterobacteriaceae, fluconazole-resistant Candida) also has increased, particularly in the ICU setting (112–114). These changes are likely associated with an increased use of wide-spectrum antibiotics, more frequent use of invasive medical devices, and an increase in the severely immunocompromised patient population.

Most CVC-associated BSIs are thought to originate from migration of skin organisms at the catheter insertion site into the catheter tract with colonization of the catheter tip. Contamination of the catheter hub or the bell of the port leading to intraluminal colonization also can lead to BSIs. This mechanism may be particularly relevant for long-term catheters (115–117). These sites can become contaminated through the hands of health-care workers during manipulation of the catheter. Catheters also can become colonized through hematogenous spread from another infection site. Contamination of infusate is a rare source of BSIs (118).

Improvements in intravenous catheter design appear to have had a substantial impact on the risk for infections associated with intravenous devices. Catheters made of Teflon, silicone elastomer, or polyurethane are less likely to support adherence of microorganisms than materials such as polyvinyl chloride or polyethylene (119,120). Avoidance of thrombogenic catheter materials also may reduce the risk for subsequent CVC-associated BSIs (121,122).

The site of catheter insertion may influence the risk for infection. Because the higher density of skin flora at the internal jugular and femoral sites may increase the risk for subsequent infection, the CDC's HICPAC guidelines recommend placement of CVCs in a subclavian site (91). Although no randomized trials have compared infection rates associated with various catheter insertion sites, several studies have shown that infection rates were higher for catheters inserted into an internal jugular vein compared with infection rates for catheters inserted into a subclavian or femoral vein (115,123,124). In addition, femoral catheters are associated with a higher risk for deep venous thrombosis that may predispose the patient to infection (125–128). Preference for a subclavian site based on a decreased risk for infection must, however, be weighed against the increased risk for mechanical complications based on individual patient characteristics and the experience of the insertor.

HICPAC recommends the use of full barrier precautions for insertion of CVCs, including the use of a cap, mask, sterile gown, sterile gloves, and large sterile drapes based on studies that suggest a reduction of CVC-related BSI risk associated with use of full barrier precautions (93,129).

Adequate skin antisepsis prior to catheter insertion is recommended. A number of recent studies have compared the efficacy of povidone-iodine with that of chlorhexidine gluconate used for preparation of the central venous and arterial insertion sites for reducing catheter-associated BSIs (130–132). The results of a recent metanalysis suggest that the incidence of CVC-associated BSIs is significantly reduced in patients who receive chlorhexidine gluconate versus povidone-iodine for insertion site skin disinfection (133). Recent studies have not shown a difference in the risk for CVC-related BSIs between use of transparent dressing versus gauze dressing (134). A chlorhexidine-impregnated sponge placed over the catheter insertion site may reduce the risk for contamination of CVCs by skin flora in high-risk patients (135).

Antimicrobial- or antiseptic-impregnated or -coated catheters and cuffs may decrease the risk for CVC-associated BSIs in selected patient populations. A multicenter randomized trial showed that CVCs impregnated with minocycline-rifampin were associated with lower CVC-related BSI rates compared with chlorhexidine-silver sulfadiazine–impregnated catheters (136). The results of a metanalysis suggest that CVCs impregnated with chlorhexidine and silver sulfadiazine also appear to be effective (137). Although clarification of the clinical and economic impact of the use of these catheters will require additional studies, chlorhexidine-silver sulfadiazine– or minocycline-rifampin–impregnated catheters may be useful in select high-risk patient populations or in situations where the CVC-associated BSI rate is high (91,138).

There are no recommendations for routine CVC replacement at scheduled time intervals. Two studies have compared routine replacement for CVCs every 7 days and CVC replacement as needed, and found no significant difference in catheter-associated BSI rates (139,140). A number of studies have compared routine replacement of CVCs by guidewire exchange compared with replacement as needed. A metanalysis of 12 studies showed no significant benefit to routine replacement by guidewire exchange (141). Guidewire exchange should not be performed if CVC-associated BSI is suspected. Catheters inserted under emergency conditions when adherence to aseptic technique cannot be ensured should be replaced within 48 hours of insertion (91). Studies suggest that the risk for catheter-associated BSIs due to pulmonary artery catheters may increase after 5 days (142), but randomized trials have not been performed.

Ventilator-Associated Pneumonia

Based on NNIS data, pneumonias account for about 15% of all hospital-acquired infections and are the second most common type of nosocomial infection after urinary tract infections (143,144). Nosocomial pneumonia rates vary by type of institution (e.g., nonteaching vs. university-affiliated hospital). In addition, the rate of mechanical ventilator–associated pneumonia varies by type of ICU (NNIS), most likely reflecting differences in patient risks for nosocomial pneumonia (145). Nosocomial pneumonia has been associated with high attributable mortality rates, with reported rates ranging from 30% to 33% (146–154). Patients receiving mechanical ventilation have higher mortality rates than patient without ventilatory support. Several studies suggest that nosocomial pneumonia may prolong hospitalization by 4 to 9 days and that the direct costs of excess hospital stay due to pneumonia is in the range of $1.2 billion a year for the United States (153–156).

Surveillance definitions for nosocomial pneumonia are difficult to apply consistently. Most definitions, including the NNIS definition for lower respiratory tract infection, include the use of criteria that that can be variably documented (e.g., presence of cough or rales) or subjective and labor-intensive to consistently monitor (e.g., presence of infiltrates on chest radiography) (20).

In addition, methods for the diagnosis of nosocomial pneumonia have been difficult to standardize (157–166). Cultures of sputum or tracheal aspirates are highly nonspecific for the diagnosis of pneumonia, especially among patients on mechanical ventilation. Standardized methods for diagnosis of pneumonia for clinical research have been used that involve bronchoscopic techniques such as quantitative culture of protected-specimen brushings and protected bronchoalveolar lavage (167–169). Routine use of these methods for clinical surveillance, however, is not currently practical for many hospitals.

Most pneumonias are a result of aspiration of bacteria colonizing the oropharynx or upper gastrointestinal tract. The high incidence of pneumonias due to gram-negative bacilli among hospitalized patients is associated with increased oropharyngeal colonization by gram-negative bacteria among patients with a number of hospital-associated conditions, including endotracheal or nasogastric tubes and exposure to antibiotics (170–172). Gastric bacterial colonization, particularly in individuals without elevated gastric pH, also may lead to aspiration and resultant pneumonia (172–175).

A number of general categories of risk factors for nosocomial pneumonia have been identified, including (a) host factors such as immunosuppression; (b) factors that enhance colonization of the oropharynx or stomach by microorganisms, such as exposure to antibiotics, underlying chronic lung disease, or coma; (c) conditions that favor aspiration or reflux, such as endotracheal intubation, placement of a nasogastric tube, or supine position; (d) prolonged use of mechanical ventilatory support with potential exposure to contaminated or colonized hands of healthcare workers; and (e) factors that interfere with pulmonary toilet, such as surgical procedures involving the head, neck, thorax, or upper abdomen, or immobilization due to trauma or illness (92).

The role of gastric pH is controversial. The administration of antacids and histamine (H_2) blockers for prevention of stress ulcers has been associated with gastric bacterial overgrowth (174–181), but results of clinical trials are varied. Several randomized trials have found that sucralfate is associated with lower rates of ventilator-associated pneumonia than are antacids or H_2 blockers (182).

Selective decontamination of the digestive tract (SDD), aimed at preventing oropharyngeal and gastric colonization with gram-negative bacilli and *Candida* species, has not gained routine acceptance. Several recent studies have shown a lack of effect of SDD on patient mortality (183–185), and there are also concerns about the potential for increasing the risk for infections caused by antibiotic-resistant organisms. Additional studies are needed to evaluate the possible usefulness of SDD for selected patient populations.

Several preventative measures may decrease the risk for aspiration of oropharyngeal or gastric microorganisms. These include avoidance of large gastric volumes by minimizing use or pharmacologic agents that interfere with gastric emptying and monitoring of gastric residual volumes after intragastric feedings

(92). Placing patients in a semirecumbent position also may reduce the risk for aspiration (186).

The use of continuous, mechanically assisted ventilation should be minimized, because these patients have 6 to 21 times the risk for developing nosocomial pneumonia compared with patients not receiving ventilatory support (176,187–189), and the risk for developing ventilator-associated pneumonia increases by 1% per day (190).

Catheter-Associated Urinary Tract Infections

Catheter-associated urinary tract infections (CAUTIs) are the most common type of nosocomial infection in both acute and long-term health-care facilities (191,192). Although most CAUTIs are asymptomatic (193), several studies suggest that CAUTIs are associated with an increased risk for mortality among individuals in acute and long-term care facilities (194,195).

Most CAUTIs result from either extraluminal contamination during insertion of the urinary catheter or by microorganisms ascending from the perineum along the external catheter surface, or through intraluminal contamination from reflux of organisms resulting from a break in the closed drainage system or contamination of urine in the collection bag (196). The presence of a biofilm consisting of a matrix of host proteins and microbial exoglycocalyx is present intraluminally and extraluminally in most infected urinary catheters and is postulated to be important in the pathogenesis of CAUTIs (197).

Risk factors for CAUTI identified by prospective studies of catheterized patients include female gender, catheter inserted outside the operating room, other active sites of infection, and major preexisting chronic conditions such as diabetes, malnutrition, and renal insufficiency (196,198). The most important potentially modifiable risk factor is prolonged catheterization beyond 6 days. By the 30th day of catheterization, nearly all patients meet criteria for CAUTIs. Use of systemic antibiotics appears to decrease the risk for infections from catheters that stay in place for a small number of days but to increase the risk if the catheter is in place for more than 6 days. Moreover, the risk for infection with antibiotic-resistant organisms such as multidrug-resistant *Pseudomonas aeruginosa* and vancomycin-resistant enterococci is increased (198,199).

A number of recommendations for prevention of CAUTIs exist, although the utility of most of these practices has not been evaluated through randomized controlled trials. Recommendations include avoidance of unnecessary indwelling urinary catheterization and removal of catheters as soon as feasible; insertion of catheters using aseptic technique; use of suprapubic catherization or, for incontinent males without bladder obstruction, use of condom drainage; maintenance of a closed drainage system; and optimal positioning of the drainage system (i.e., collection tubing and bag below the level of the patient's bladder and drainage tubing above the level of the collection bag) (196,200–202).

Several technologic innovations aimed at decreasing the risk for CAUTIs have been evaluated, including the use of antimicrobial-impregnated catheters, and catheters coated with materials that inhibit adherence of microorganisms to the catheter surface (196).

Surgical Site Infections

Approximately 27 million surgical procedures are performed each year in the United States (203). Surgical site infections (SSIs) are the third most frequently reported nosocomial infection, accounting for 14% to 16% of all nosocomial infections among hospitalized patients, and is the most common type of nosocomial infection among surgical patients (144). Estimates of the extra length of hospitalization vary from 5 to 24 days (155,204–206). A study from 1992 estimated that the average SSI resulted in $3,152 in extra charges (207).

The reported rates of SSIs depend on both the definition of infection and the intensity and duration of surveillance (208,209). The CDC's NNIS system has developed standardized surveillance criteria for defining SSIs that are widely used (19). By these criteria, SSIs are classified as superficial incisional (involving only skin or subcutaneous tissue), deep incisional (involving deeper soft tissues), or organ/space (involving any part of the anatomy other than incised body wall layers that was opened or manipulated during an operation).

The duration of follow-up required depends in part on the type of procedure. As an example, SSIs involving orthopedic prostheses can occur many months after implantation. The NNIS system includes SSIs that occur within 30 days after the operation if no implant is left in place or within 1 year if an implant is in place and the infection is related to the operation (19,210).

Duration of surveillance is especially important given decreasing lengths of hospitalization following many procedures and the increasing proportion of procedures performed in the ambulatory setting in recent years. Between 12% and 84% of SSIs are detected after patients are discharged from the hospital (211–227). Decreases in the length of hospital stay may further compromise the completeness of SSI surveillance that depends on inpatient detection. There is currently no consensus regarding methods for performing postdischarge SSI surveillance. Surveillance based on surgeon and patient responses have been shown to lack both sensitivity and specificity (222,228). A recent study suggested that use of models based on diagnosis, testing, and pharmacy data routinely collected by managed care organizations can be used to identify individuals most likely to have had SSIs detected in the ambulatory setting (222).

The pathogenesis of SSIs involves microbial contamination of the surgical site, and the subsequent occurrence of SSIs is dependent on the dose of bacterial contamination, virulence of the causative organisms, and susceptibility of the host (229,230). The most common source of pathogens is the patient's endogenous skin, mucous membrane, or hollow viscera flora, with the spectrum of organisms dependent on the extent of surgery (231). Incision of skin or mucous membranes, for example, is usually associated with SSIs due to aerobic gram-positive organisms, whereas procedures involving gastrointestinal organs also can be associated with gram-negative or anaerobic organisms. Seeding of the surgical site from distant foci of infection can occur, particularly if the surgical procedure involves placement of an implant (232,233). In addition to endogenous pathogens, SSIs are less frequently associated with exogenous sources of contamination, including surgical personnel, the operating room environment, and surgical equipment (234–236).

The risk for infection depends on many factors. Procedure type is among the most important. One of the best known classification systems creates four categories of procedures (237), assigned on the basis of wound contamination. The classes are clean, clean-contaminated, contaminated, and infected. This scoring system allows separation of procedures into classes whose risks of infection are 2.9% for clean procedures, 3.9% for clean-contaminated procedures, 8.5% for procedures at a contaminated site, and 12.6% for procedures that involve an infected site (238).

A more sophisticated system developed by the CDC takes into account characteristics of the host as well as the procedure, thereby allowing a more accurate estimate of the underlying risk for postoperative SSIs (238,239). This scoring system assigns one point each for the following risk factors: Anesthesiology Society of America score of 3 or more, contaminated or dirty surgery, and procedure length greater than the 75th percentile for similar procedures in the NNIS data set. Although this risk stratification system reduces the risk for making misleading comparisons (e.g., between hospitals) because of differences in underlying severity of illness or case mix, it still does not account for much of the variability in infection risk. For instance, the risk can vary by nearly an order of magnitude among clean procedures for low-risk individuals, from less than 1% for orthopedic surgery to 5% to 10% for breast surgery. In addition, this scoring system shares the feature of many such systems in that it depends on the availability and accuracy of the clinical information recorded in medical records. In many hospitals, substantial effort is required to collect these data on a routine basis for all procedures (uninfected as well as infected); in addition, the accuracy of the classification is not known. Finally, risk factors such as duration of surgery are almost certainly approximations of the actual factors that increase risk. Other risk stratification methods, such as use of the chronic disease score based on ambulatory pharmacy dispensing information (240) and the use of procedure-specific risk indices (238,241,242), are the subjects of ongoing research.

A number of patient characteristics have been identified as risk factors for SSI, including diabetes, smoking, systemic steroid use, malnutrition, and obesity. Several nonrandomized studies have suggested that increased glucose levels in the immediate postoperative period were associated with increase risk for SSIs (243–245). Additional studies are needed to assess the usefulness of perioperative glucose control to prevent SSIs. Preoperative nares colonization with *Staphylococcus aureus* has been associated with subsequent development of SSIs. Perioperative use of nasal mupirocin for colonized patients may be a useful strategy for reducing the SSI risk in these patients. A large, randomized, placebo-controlled trial found that prophylactic intranasal application of mupirocin did not significantly reduce the rate of *S. aureus* SSIs overall, but did significantly decrease the rate of all nosocomial *S. aureus* infections among patients who were *S. aureus* carriers (246).

Surgical practice is particularly bound by tradition, and few of its rituals are supported by well-designed clinical trails. Nonetheless, a consensus has emerged regarding a number of control measures (74). Preoperative shaving of the surgical site has been associated with a higher SSI risk than depilatory agents or no hair removal, and may be due to microscopic cuts in the skin caused by shaving that later serve as the nidus of SSIs (229,247–252). Shaving or clipping of hair immediately before surgery has been associated with a lower risk for SSIs than hair removal by either method the night before surgery (248). Several agents can be used to disinfect skin at the operative site prior to surgery, including iodophors such as povidone-iodine, alcohol-containing agents, and chlorhexidine gluconate (74). The agent should be applied in concentric circles, starting in the area where the incision will be made, and the prepared area should be large enough to extend the incision or include drain sites, if needed. All members of the surgical team who have direct contact with the sterile operating field or sterile instruments or supplies used in the field should perform adequate hand and forearm disinfection using agents containing povidone-iodine, chlorhexidine gluconate, or alcohol (74,253,254). Although use of a brush to scrub preoperatively has been common practice for many years, this practice may damage skin and result in increased shedding of bacteria from hands (255,256). A number of reports have implicated long or artificial nails of surgical personnel and other healthcare workers colonized with bacterial or fungal pathogens as the source of outbreaks of nosocomial infections, and current rec-

ommendations are for surgical personnel to avoid wearing artificial fingernails or extenders when providing patient care and to keep nails 1/4 inch long (257,258). In addition, a number of intraoperative recommendations exist regarding operating room ventilation; cleaning of environmental surfaces; cleaning, disinfection, and sterilization of surgical instruments;, surgical attire; and the use of gowns and drapes (74,257,259). Surgical technique is believed to influence the risk for SSIs, including maintaining effective hemostasis, preventing hypothermia, removing devitalized tissue, and optimal placement and use of surgical drains (74,260,261).

For many procedures, the use (or lack of use) of appropriately timed perioperative antimicrobial prophylaxis is a major, modifiable, risk factor (262,263). Surgical antimicrobial prophylaxis is a brief course of antibiotics initiated before the surgical incision, and is aimed at reducing the microbial burden of intraoperative contamination. The HICPAC guidelines (74) describe four principles that must be followed to maximize the benefits of antimicrobial prophylaxis: (a) use for all operations or classes of operations in which its use has been shown to reduce SSI rates or for those operations in which an SSI would represent a catastrophe; (b) use of an agent that is safe, inexpensive, and bactericidal, with a spectrum of activity that covers the most probable intraoperative contaminants for the operation; (c) timing the infusion so that a bactericidal concentration of the drug is established in serum and tissues by the time the skin is incised; and (d) maintaining therapeutic levels in both serum and tissues throughout the operation. Cefazolin is widely used for many clean and clean-contaminated procedures, given its activity against common gram-positive skin flora. Second-generation cephalosporins that provide additional gram-negative and anaerobic coverage are often used for procedures that involve entering the gastrointestinal tract. Prophylactic antibiotics have been shown to be effective for a number of clean procedures and are almost always used when prosthetic materials and devices are implanted, cases in which wound infection would have catastrophic consequences. It is clear that the timing of the administration of prophylactic antibiotics is critical. Data on both animals and patients support the need to deliver antibiotics just before surgery (263). If antibiotics are delivered more than 2 hours before surgery or after the operation has commenced, the risk for infection is increased. Unfortunately, when carefully examined, many routine hospital systems do not ensure timely antibiotic administration; quality improvement efforts may be necessary to do so. In addition, intraoperative redosing of prophylactic antibiotics is recommended for prolonged surgical procedures. A recent retrospective study of patients who underwent cardiac surgery demonstrated that redosing was associated with a lower SSI rate for very long (≥6.5 hours) procedures (264).

CONTROL OF EPIDEMIC INFECTIONS

In addition to minimizing the risk for endemic infections associated with procedures or the use of invasive medical devices, infection control teams also must be prepared to respond to the occurrence of unusual health care–associated infections or unusual numbers of infections that may have a common source or be associated with a breach in practice. First, the infection control team must confirm that an outbreak exists. The next phase involves an intensification of routine procedures, including a review of current practices, clarification of existing recommendations, assessment of barriers to compliance, and correction of any immediately apparent problems. Concurrently, a case definition must be drafted and tested, then the extent of the outbreak gauged. Every effort should be made to identify as many cases as possible, which facilitates both epidemiologic investigation and outbreak control. For many pathogens, comprehensive case finding requires detection of carriers as well as infected individuals, and the hospital microbiologist should be consulted about the most efficient screening procedures. Published information concerning the usual mode of spread of the epidemic pathogen should help narrow the focus of the investigation. It is important to develop data in a systematic fashion while having an open dialogue with staff concerning alternative explanations for a problem.

Some outbreaks can be traced to a common source, such as a faulty air-handling system, an environmental reservoir, a carrier on the hospital staff, or a contaminated device or solution. Accordingly, review of new policies or procedures for new devices is important and may be particularly relevant for equipment (265). However, most outbreaks are attributable to a breakdown in routine aseptic procedures and person-to-person spread. When person-to-person transmission is thought to be the principal source of the problem, appropriate precautions should be instituted and barrier techniques intensified.

CONCLUSION

The work of preventing health care–associated infections has become increasingly challenging and exciting as patients have become more severely ill and susceptible to serious infection in the setting of increasing complexity of health-care delivery systems. Superimposed on this changing health-care environment, economic pressures have made it increasingly important for infection control teams to prove to hospitals that they "add value" in terms of improving the quality of care, reducing costs attributable to health care–associated infections, and enhancing the efficiency of patient care activities. Advances in preventing health care–associated infections will require ongoing support of innovative basic and applied research.

ACKNOWLEDGMENT

I thank Richard Platt, Donald A. Goldmann, and Cyrus C. Hopkins, the authors of the original chapters upon which this chapter is based, for their valuable advice and guidance. I also thank Susan Marino for her insightful comments and suggestions.

REFERENCES

1. Hensley WR. *Stedman's medical dictionary*. Baltimore: Williams & Wilkins, 1990.
2. Centers for Disease Control and Prevention. Public health focus: surveillance, prevention, and control of nosocomial infections. *MMWR* 1992;41:783–787.
3. Korn L, Corrigan J, Donaldson M. *To err is human: building a safer health system*. Washington, DC: Institute of Medicine, National Academy Press, 1999.
4. Gaynes RP, Horan T. Surveillance of nosocomial infections. In: Mayhall CG, ed. *Hospital epidemiology and infectio control*. Baltimore: Williams & Wilkins, 1996:1017–1031.
5. Haley R, Culver D, White J. The efficacy of infection surveillance and control programs in preventing nosocomial infections in US hospitals. *Am J Epidemiol* 1985;121:182.
6. Carter KC. *Ignaz Semmelweis. The etiology, concept, and prophylaxis of childbed fever*. Madison: University of Wisconsin Press, 1983.
7. Hughes JM. Nosocomial infection surveillance in the United States: historical perspective. *Infect Control* 1987;8:450–453.
8. Eickhoff TC, Brachman PW, Bennett JV, et al. Surveillance of nosocomial infections in community hospitals. I. Surveillance methods, effectiveness, and initial results. *J Infect Dis* 1969;120:305–317.
9. Berntsen C, McDermott W. Increased transmissibility of staphylococci to patients receiving an antimicrobial drug. *N Engl J Med* 1960;262:637–642.
10. Langmuir A. The surveillance of communicable diseases of national importance. *N Engl J Med* 1963;268:182–192.
11. Brachman PW. Surveillance of institutionally acquired infections. In: *Proceedings of the National Conference on Institutionally Acquired Infections, Minneapolis, University of Minnesota School of Public Health 1963*. Public Health Service publication no. 1188. Washington, DC: 1964:138–147.
12. Joint Commission on Accreditation of Hospitals. *Accreditation manual for hospitals*. Chicago: Joint Commission on Accreditation of Hospitals, 1976.
13. Haley RW, Shachtman RH. The emergence of infection surveillance and control programs in US hospitals: an assessment, 1976. *Am J Epidemiol* 1980;111:574–591.
14. Emori TG, Culver DH, Horan TC, et al. National nosocomial infections surveillance system (NNIS): description of surveillance methods. *Am J Infect Control* 1991;19:19–35.
15. Haley RW, Culver DH, White JW, et al. The efficacy of infection surveillance and control programs in preventing nosocomial infections in US hospitals. *Am J Epidemiol* 1985;121:182–205.
16. Cruse PJ, Foord R. The epidemiology of wound infection. A 10-year prospective study of 62,939 wounds. *Surg Clin North Am* 1980;60:27–40.
17. Condon RE, Schulte WJ, Malangoni MA, Anderson-Teschendorf MJ. Effectiveness of a surgical wound surveillance program. *Arch Surg* 1983;118:303–307.
18. Gaynes R, Culver D, Emori T. The national nosocomial infections surveillance system: plans for the 1990s and beyond. *Am J Med* 1991;91(suppl):116.
19. Horan TC, Gaynes RP, Martone WJ, et al. CDC definitions of nosocomial surgical site infections, 1992: a modification of CDC definitions of surgical wound infections. *Infect Control Hosp Epidemiol* 1992;13:606–608.
20. Garner JS, Jarvis WR, Emori TG, et al. CDC definitions for nosocomial infections, 1988. *Am J Infect Control* 1988;16:128–140.
21. Abrutyn E, Talbot GH. Surveillance strategies: a primer. *Infect Control* 1987;8:459–464.
22. Garvey JM, Buffenmyer C, Rycheck RR, et al. Surveillance for postoperative infections in outpatient gynecologic surgery. *Infect Control* 1986;7:54–58.
23. Simchen E, Wax Y, Pevsner B, et al. The Israeli Study of Surgical Infections (ISSI): I. Methods for developing a standardized surveillance system for a multicenter study of surgical infections. *Infect Control Hosp Epidemiol* 1988;9:232–240.
24. Birnbaum D. Nosocomial infection surveillance programs. *Infect Control* 1987;8:474–479.
25. Wenzel RP, Osterman CA, Hunting KJ, et al. Hospital-acquired infections. I. Surveillance in a university hospital. *Am J Epidemiol* 1976;103:251–260.
26. Milliken J, Tait GA, Ford-Jones EL, et al. Nosocomial infections in a pediatric intensive care unit. *Crit Care Med* 1988;16:233–237.
27. Burke JP, Classen DC, Pestotnik SL, et al. The HELP system and its application to infection control. *J Hosp Infect* 1991;18(suppl A):424–431.
28. Classen DC, Burke JP, Pestotnik SL, et al. Surveillance for quality assessment: IV. Surveillance using a hospital information system. *Infect Control Hosp Epidemiol* 1991;12:239–244.
29. Evans RS, Burke JP, Classen DC, et al. Computerized identification of patients at high risk for hospital-acquired infection. *Am J Infect Control* 1992;20:4–10.
30. Thornsberry C. Methicillin-resistant staphylococci. *Clin Lab Med* 1989;9:255–267.
31. Wenzel RP, Streed SA. Surveillance and use of computers in hospital infection control. *J Hosp Infect* 1989;13:217–229.
32. Yokoe DS, Platt R. Surveillance for surgical site infections: the uses of antibiotic exposure. *Infect Control Hosp Epidemiol* 1994;15:717–723.
33. Pittet D, Mourouga P, Perneger TV. Compliance with handwashing in a teaching hospital. Infection Control Program. *Ann Intern Med* 1999;130:126–130.
34. Boyce JM. It is time for action: improving hand hygiene in hospitals. *Ann Intern Med* 1999;130:153–155.
35. Doebbeling BN, Stanley GL, Sheetz CT, et al. Comparative efficacy of alternative hand-washing agents in reducing nosocomial infections in intensive care units. *N Engl J Med* 1992;327:88–93.
36. Pittet D, Hugonnet S, Harbarth S, et al. Effectiveness of a hospital-wide programme to improve compliance with hand hygiene. Infection Control Programme. *Lancet* 2000;356:1307–1312.
37. Sattar SA, Abebe M, Bueti AJ, et al. Activity of an alcohol-based hand gel against human adeno-, rhino-, and rotaviruses using the fingerpad method. *Infect Control Hosp Epidemiol* 2000;21:516–519.
38. Lund S, Jackson J, Leggett J, et al. Reality of glove use and handwashing in a community hospital. *Am J Infect Control* 1994;22:352–357.
39. Mayer JA, Dubbert PM, Miller M, et al. Increasing handwashing in an intensive care unit. *Infect Control* 1986;7:259–262.
40. Kaplan LM, McGuckin M. Increasing handwashing compliance with more accessible sinks. *Infect Control* 1986;7:408–410.
41. Bischoff WE, Reynolds TM, Sessler CN, et al. Handwashing compliance by health care workers: the impact of introducing an accessible, alcohol-based hand antiseptic. *Arch Intern Med* 2000;160:1017–1011.
42. Wurtz R, Moye G, Jovanovic B. Handwashing machines, handwashing compliance, and potential for cross-contamination. *Am J Infect Control* 1994;22:228–230.
43. Albert RK, Condie F. Hand-washing patterns in medical intensive-care units. *N Engl J Med* 1981;304:1465–1466.
44. Larson E. Compliance with isolation technique. *Am J Infect Control* 1983;11:221–225.
45. Graham M. Frequency and duration of handwashing in an intensive care unit. *Am J Infect Control* 1990;18:77–81.

46. Dubbert PM, Dolce J, Richter W, et al. Increasing ICU staff handwashing: effects of education and group feedback. *Infect Control Hosp Epidemiol* 1990;11:191–193.

47. Simmons B, Bryant J, Neiman K, et al. The role of handwashing in prevention of endemic intensive care unit infections. *Infect Control Hosp Epidemiol* 1990;11:589–594.

48. Raju TN, Kobler C. Improving handwashing habits in the newborn nurseries. *Am J Med Sci* 1991;302:355–358.

49. Shay DK, Maloney SA, Montecalvo M, et al. Epidemiology and mortality risk of vancomycin-resistant enterococcal bloodstream infections. *J Infect Dis* 1995;172:993–1000.

50. Slaughter S, Hayden MK, Nathan C, et al. A comparison of the effect of universal use of gloves and gowns with that of glove use alone on acquisition of vancomycin-resistant enterococci in a medical intensive care unit. *Ann Intern Med* 1996;125:448–456.

51. Watanakunakorn C, Wang C, Hazy J. An observational study of hand washing and infection control practices by healthcare workers. *Infect Control Hosp Epidemiol* 1998;19:858–860.

52. Avila-Aguero ML, Umana MA, Jimenez AL, et al. Handwashing practices in a tertiary-care, pediatric hospital and the effect on an educational program. *Clin Perform Qual Health Care* 1998;6:70–72.

53. Maury E, Alzieu M, Baudel JL, et al. Availability of an alcohol solution can improve hand disinfection compliance in an intensive care unit. *Am J Respir Crit Care Med* 2000;162:324–327.

54. Muto CA, Sistrom MG, Farr BM. Hand hygiene rates unaffected by installation of dispensers of a rapidly acting hand antiseptic. *Am J Infect Control* 2000;28:273–276.

55. Casewell M, Phillips I. Hands as route of transmission for *Klebsiella* species. *BMJ* 1977;2:1315–1317.

56. Ehrenkranz NJ, Alfonso BC. Failure of bland soap handwash to prevent hand transfer of patient bacteria to urethral catheters. *Infect Control Hosp Epidemiol* 1991;12:654–662.

57. Larson EL, Early E, Cloonan P, et al. An organizational climate intervention associated with increased handwashing and decreased nosocomial infections. *Behav Med* 2000;26:14–22.

58. Larson EL. APIC guideline for handwashing and hand antisepsis in health care settings. *Am J Infect Control* 1995;23:251–269.

59. Boyce JM, Pittet D. Guideline for hand hygiene in health-care settings. Recommendations of the Healthcare Infection Control Practices Advisory Committee and the HICPAC/SHEA/APIC/IDSA Hand Hygiene Task Force. *MMWR* 2002;51(RR-16):1–44.

60. Winnefeld M, Richard MA, Drancourt M, et al. Skin tolerance and effectiveness of two hand decontamination procedures in everyday hospital use. *Br J Dermatol* 2000;143:546–550.

61. Boyce JM, Kelliher S, Vallande N. Skin irritation and dryness associated with two hand-hygiene regimens: soap-and-water hand washing versus hand antisepsis with an alcoholic hand gel. *Infect Control Hosp Epidemiol* 2000;21:442–448.

62. Larson EL, Aiello AE, Bastyr J, et al. Assessment of two hand hygiene regimens for intensive care unit personnel. *Crit Care Med* 2001;29:944–951.

63. Larson EL, Aiello AE, Heilman JM, et al. Comparison of different regimens for surgical hand preparation. *AORN J* 2001;73:412–414, 417–418, 420 passim.

64. Casewell MW, Law MM, Desai N. A laboratory model for testing agents for hygienic hand disinfection: handwashing and chlorhexidine for the removal of *Klebsiella*. *J Hosp Infect* 1988;12:163–175.

65. Huang Y, Oie S, Kamiya A. Comparative effectiveness of hand-cleansing agents for removing methicillin-resistant *Staphylococcus aureus* from experimentally contaminated fingertips. *Am J Infect Control* 1994;22:224–227.

66. Wade JJ, Desai N, Casewell MW. Hygienic hand disinfection for the removal of epidemic vancomycin-resistant *Enterococcus faecium* and gentamicin-resistant *Enterobacter cloacae*. *J Hosp Infect* 1991;18:211–218.

67. National Communicable Disease Center. *Isolation techniques for use in hospitals*, 1st ed. Public Health Service publication no. 2054. Washington, DC: U.S. Government Printing Office, 1970.

68. Centers for Disease Control and Prevention. *Isolation techniques for use in hospitals*, 2nd ed. HHS publication no. (CDC) 80-8314. Washington, DC: U.S. Government Printing Office, 1975.

69. Garner JS, Simmons BP. Guideline for isolation precautions in hospitals. *Infect Control* 1983;4:245–325.

70. Centers for Disease Control. Update: universal precautions for prevention of transmission of human immunodeficiency virus, hepatitis B virus, and other bloodborne pathogens in health-care settings. *N Y State J Med* 1988;88:649–651.

71. Kristensen MS, Wernberg NM, Anker-Moller E. Healthcare workers' risk of contact with body fluids in a hospital: the effect of complying with the universal precautions policy. *Infect Control Hosp Epidemiol* 1992;13:719–724.

72. Lynch P, Jackson MM, Cummings MJ, et al. Rethinking the role of isolation practices in the prevention of nosocomial infections. *Ann Intern Med* 1987;107:243–246.

73. Garner JS. Guideline for isolation precautions in hospitals. The Hospital Infection Control Practices Advisory Committee. *Infect Control Hosp Epidemiol* 1996;17:53–80.

74. Mangram AJ, Horan TC, Pearson ML, et al. Guideline for prevention of surgical site infection, 1999. Hospital Infection Control Practices Advisory Committee. *Infect Control Hosp Epidemiol* 1999;20:250–278; quiz 279–280.

75. Alvarado CJ, Reichelderfer M. APIC guideline for infection prevention and control in flexible endoscopy. Association for Professionals in Infection Control. *Am J Infect Control* 2000;28:138–155.

76. Centers for Disease Control and Prevention. *Pseudomonas aeruginosa* infections associated with defective bronchoscopes. *MMWR* 2002;51:190.

77. Centers for Disease Control and Prevention. Recommendations for prevention of HIV transmission in health-care settings. *MMWR* 1987;36(suppl 2):1–18.

78. Rutala WA. APIC guideline for selection and use of disinfectants. 1994, 1995, and 1996 APIC Guidelines Committee. Association for Professionals in Infection Control and Epidemiology, Inc. *Am J Infect Control* 1996;24:313–342.

79. Sarubbi FA Jr, Kopf HB, Wilson MB, et al. Increased recovery of *Aspergillus flavus* from respiratory specimens during hospital construction. *Am Rev Respir Dis* 1982;125:33–38.

80. Arnow PM, Sadigh M, Costas C, et al. Endemic and epidemic aspergillosis associated with in-hospital replication of *Aspergillus* organisms. *J Infect Dis* 1991;164:998–1002.

81. Flynn PM, Williams BG, Hetherington SV, et al. *Aspergillus terreus* during hospital renovation. *Infect Control Hosp Epidemiol* 1993;14:363–365.

82. Streifel AJ, Stevens PP, Rhame FS. In-hospital source of airborne *Penicillium* species spores. *J Clin Microbiol* 1987;25:1–4.

83. Johnson JT, Yu VL, Best MG, et al. Nosocomial legionellosis in surgical patients with head-and-neck cancer: implications for epidemiological reservoir and mode of transmission. *Lancet* 1985;2:298–300.

84. Blatt SP, Parkinson MD, Pace E, et al. Nosocomial Legionnaires' disease: aspiration as a primary mode of disease acquisition. *Am J Med* 1993;95:16–22.

85. Williams WW. Guideline for infection control in hospital personnel. *Infect Control* 1983;4:326–349.

86. Bolyard EA, Tablan OC, Williams WW, et al. Guideline for infection control in healthcare personnel, 1998. Hospital Infection Control Practices Advisory Committee. *Infect Control Hosp Epidemiol* 1998;19:407–463.

87. Immunization of health-care workers: recommendations of the Advisory Committee on Immunization Practices (ACIP) and the Hospital Infection Control Practices Advisory Committee (HICPAC). *MMWR* 1997;46:1–42.

88. Guidelines for preventing the transmission of *Mycobacterium tuberculosis* in health-care facilities, 1994. Centers for Disease Control and Prevention. *MMWR* 1994;43:1–132.

89. Public Health Service guidelines for the management of health-care worker exposures to HIV and recommendations for postexposure prophylaxis. Centers for Disease Control and Prevention. *MMWR Recomm Rep* 1998;47:1-33.

90. Occupational exposure to bloodborne pathogens—OSHA. Final rule. *Fed Regist* 1991;56:64004-182.

91. O'Grady NP, Alexander M, Dellinger EP, et al. Guidelines for the prevention of intravascular catheter-related infections. *MMWR* 2002;51(RR-10):1–29.

92. Tablan OC, Anderson LJ, Arden NH, et al. Guideline for prevention of nosocomial pneumonia. The Hospital Infection Control Practices Advisory Committee, Centers for Disease Control and Prevention. *Infect Control Hosp Epidemiol* 1994;15:587–627.

93. Mermel LA. Prevention of intravascular catheter-related infections. *Ann Intern Med* 2000;132:391–402.

94. Collignon PJ. Intravascular catheter associated sepsis: a common problem. The Australian Study on Intravascular Catheter Associated Sepsis. *Med J Aust* 1994;161:374–378.

95. Heiselman D. Nosocomial bloodstream infections in the critically ill. *JAMA* 1994;272:1819–1820.

96. Arnow PM, Quimosing EM, Beach M. Consequences of intravascular catheter sepsis. *Clin Infect Dis* 1993;16:778–784.

97. Pittet D, Tarara D, Wenzel RP. Nosocomial bloodstream infection in critically ill patients. Excess length of stay, extra costs, and attributable mortality. *JAMA* 1994;271:1598–1601.

98. Digiovine B, Chenoweth C, Watts C, et al. The attributable mortality and costs of primary nosocomial bloodstream infections in the intensive care unit. *Am J Respir Crit Care Med* 1999;160:976–981.

99. Freeman J, Platt R, Sidebottom DG, et al. Coagulase-negative staphylococcal bacteremia in the changing neonatal intensive care unit population. Is there an epidemic? *JAMA* 1987;258:2548–2552.

100. Yokoe DS, Anderson J, Chambers R, et al. Simplified surveillance for nosocomial bloodstream infections. *Infect Control Hosp Epidemiol* 1998;19:657–660.

101. Sherertz RJ, Heard SO, Raad II. Diagnosis of triple-lumen catheter infection: comparison of roll plate, sonication, and flushing methodologies. *J Clin Microbiol* 1997;35:641–646.

102. Raad II, Sabbagh MF, Rand KH, et al. Quantitative tip culture methods and the diagnosis of central venous catheter–related infections. *Diagn Microbiol Infect Dis* 1992;15:13–20.

103. Capdevila JA, Planes AM, Palomar M, et al. Value of differential quantitative blood cultures in the diagnosis of catheter-related sepsis. *Eur J Clin Microbiol Infect Dis* 1992;11:403–407.

104. Blot F, Schmidt E, Nitenberg G, et al. Earlier positivity of central-venous- versus peripheral-blood cultures is highly predictive of catheter-related sepsis. *J Clin Microbiol* 1998;36:105–109.

105. Blot F, Nitenberg G, Chachaty E, et al. Diagnosis of catheter-related bacteraemia: a prospective comparison of the time to positivity of hub-blood versus peripheral-blood cultures. *Lancet* 1999;354:1071–1077.

106. National Nosocomial Infections Surveillance (NNIS) System report, data summary from January 1990–May 1999, issued June 1999. *Am J Infect Control* 1999;27:520–532.

107. Joint Commission on the Accreditation of Healthcare Organizations.

Accreditation manual for hospitals. In: *Organizations Joint Commission on the Accreditation of Healthcare Organizations.* Chicago, 1994:121–140.

108. Nosocomial infection rates for interhospital comparison: limitations and possible solutions. A Report from the National Nosocomial Infections Surveillance (NNIS) System. *Infect Control Hosp Epidemiol* 1991;12:609–621.

109. National Nosocomial Infections Surveillance (NNIS) System Report, Data Summary from January 1992–June 2001, issued August 2001. *Am J Infect Control* 2001;29:404–421.

110. Schaberg DR, Culver DH, Gaynes RP. Major trends in the microbial etiology of nosocomial infection. *Am J Med* 1991;91(suppl):72–75.

111. Banerjee SN, Emori TG, Culver DH, et al. Secular trends in nosocomial primary bloodstream infections in the United States, 1980–1989. National Nosocomial Infections Surveillance System. *Am J Med* 1991;91(suppl):86–89.

112. Pfaller MA, Jones RN, Messer SA, et al. National surveillance of nosocomial blood stream infection due to *Candida albicans*: frequency of occurrence and antifungal susceptibility in the SCOPE Program. *Diagn Microbiol Infect Dis* 1998;31:327–332.

113. Pfaller MA, Jones RN, Messer SA, et al. National surveillance of nosocomial blood stream infection due to species of *Candida* other than *Candida albicans*: frequency of occurrence and antifungal susceptibility in the SCOPE Program. SCOPE Participant Group. Surveillance and Control of Pathogens of Epidemiologic. *Diagn Microbiol Infect Dis* 1998;30:121–129.

114. Fridkin SK, Gaynes RP. Antimicrobial resistance in intensive care units. *Clin Chest Med* 1999;20:303–316, viii.

115. Mermel LA, McCormick RD, Springman SR, et al. The pathogenesis and epidemiology of catheter-related infection with pulmonary artery Swan-Ganz catheters: a prospective study utilizing molecular subtyping. *Am J Med* 1991;91(suppl):197–205.

116. Linares J, Sitges-Serra A, Garau J, et al. Pathogenesis of catheter sepsis: a prospective study with quantitative and semiquantitative cultures of catheter hub and segments. *J Clin Microbiol* 1985;21:357–360.

117. Raad I, Costerton W, Sabharwal U, et al. Ultrastructural analysis of indwelling vascular catheters: a quantitative relationship between luminal colonization and duration of placement. *J Infect Dis* 1993;168:400–407.

118. Maki DG. Infections associated with intravascular lines. In: Remington JS, ed. *Current clinical topics in infectious diseases.* New York: McGraw-Hill, 1982:309–363.

119. Sheth NK, Franson TR, Rose HD, et al. Colonization of bacteria on polyvinyl chloride and Teflon intravascular catheters in hospitalized patients. *J Clin Microbiol* 1983;18:1061–1063.

120. Ashkenazi S, Weiss E, Drucker MM. Bacterial adherence to intravenous catheters and needles and its influence by cannula type and bacterial surface hydrophobicity. *J Lab Clin Med* 1986;107:136–140.

121. Nachnani GH, Lessin LS, Motomiya T, et al. Scanning electron microscopy of thrombogenesis on vascular catheter surfaces. *N Engl J Med* 1972;286:139–140.

122. Stillman RM, Soliman F, Garcia L, et al. Etiology of catheter-associated sepsis. Correlation with thrombogenicity. *Arch Surg* 1977;112:1497–1499.

123. Heard SO, Wagle M, Vijayakumar E, et al. Influence of triple-lumen central venous catheters coated with chlorhexidine and silver sulfadiazine on the incidence of catheter-related bacteremia. *Arch Intern Med* 1998;158:81–87.

124. Richet H, Hubert B, Nitenberg G, et al. Prospective multicenter study of vascular-catheter-related complications and risk factors for positive central-catheter cultures in intensive care unit patients. *J Clin Microbiol* 1990;28:2520–2525.

125. Joynt GM, Kew J, Gomersall CD, et al. Deep venous thrombosis caused by femoral venous catheters in critically ill adult patients. *Chest* 2000;117:178–183.

126. Mian NZ, Bayly R, Schreck DM, et al. Incidence of deep venous thrombosis associated with femoral venous catheterization. *Acad Emerg Med* 1997;4:1118–1121.

127. Durbec O, Viviand X, Potie F, et al. A prospective evaluation of the use of femoral venous catheters in critically ill adults. *Crit Care Med* 1997;25:1986–1989.

128. Trottier SJ, Veremakis C, O'Brien J, et al. Femoral deep vein thrombosis associated with central venous catheterization: results from a prospective, randomized trial. *Crit Care Med* 1995;23:52–59.

129. Raad II, Hohn DC, Gilbreath BJ, et al. Prevention of central venous catheter-related infections by using maximal sterile barrier precautions during insertion. *Infect Control Hosp Epidemiol* 1994;15:231–238.

130. Maki DG, Ringer M, Alvarado CJ. Prospective randomised trial of povidone-iodine, alcohol, and chlorhexidine for prevention of infection associated with central venous and arterial catheters. *Lancet* 1991;338:339–343.

131. Mimoz O, Pieroni L, Lawrence C, et al. Prospective, randomized trial of two antiseptic solutions for prevention of central venous or arterial catheter colonization and infection in intensive care unit patients. *Crit Care Med* 1996;24:1818–1823.

132. Humar A, Ostromecki A, Direnfeld J, et al. Prospective randomized trial of 10% povidone-iodine versus 0.5% tincture of chlorhexidine as cutaneous antisepsis for prevention of central venous catheter infection. *Clin Infect Dis* 2000;31:1001–1007.

133. Chaiyakunapruk N, Veenstra DL, Lipsky BA, et al. Chlorhexidine compared with povidone-iodine solution for vascular catheter-site care: a meta-analysis. *Ann Intern Med* 2002;136:792–801.

134. Maki DG, Ringer M. Evaluation of dressing regimens for prevention of infection with peripheral intravenous catheters. Gauze, a transparent polyurethane dressing, and an iodophor-transparent dressing. *JAMA* 1987;258:2396–2403.

135. Maki DG, Mermel LA, Klugar D, et al. The efficacy of a chlorhexidine impregnated sponge (Biopatch) for the prevention of intravascular catheter-elated infection—a prospective randomized controlled multicenter study. Toronto, Ontario, Canada: Interscience Conference on Antimicrobial Agents and Chemotherapy (ICAAC), 2000.

136. Darouiche RO, Raad II, Heard SO, et al. A comparison of two antimicrobial-impregnated central venous catheters. Catheter Study Group. *N Engl J Med* 1999;340:1–8.

137. Veenstra DL, Saint S, Saha S, et al. Efficacy of antiseptic-impregnated central venous catheters in preventing catheter-related bloodstream infection: a meta-analysis. *JAMA* 1999;281:261–267.

138. Maki DG, Stolz SM, Wheeler S, et al. Prevention of central venous catheter-related bloodstream infection by use of an antiseptic-impregnated catheter. A randomized, controlled trial. *Ann Intern Med* 1997;127:257–266.

139. Eyer S, Brummitt C, Crossley K, et al. Catheter-related sepsis: prospective, randomized study of three methods of long-term catheter maintenance. *Crit Care Med* 1990;18:1073–1079.

140. Uldall PR, Merchant N, Woods F, et al. Changing subclavian haemodialysis cannulas to reduce infection. *Lancet* 1981;1:1373.

141. Cook D, Randolph A, Kernerman P, et al. Central venous catheter replacement strategies: a systematic review of the literature. *Crit Care Med* 1997;25:1417–1424.

142. Maki DG, Stolz SS, Wheeler S, et al. A prospective, randomized trial of gauze and two polyurethane dressings for site care of pulmonary artery catheters: implications for catheter management. *Crit Care Med* 1994;22:1729–1737.

143. Horan TC, White JW, Jarvis WR, et al. Nosocomial infection surveillance, 1984. *MMWR* 1986;35:17SS–29SS.

144. Emori TG, Gaynes RP. An overview of nosocomial infections, including the role of the microbiology laboratory. *Clin Microbiol Rev* 1993;6:428–442.

145. Jarvis WR, Edwards JR, Culver DH, et al. Nosocomial infection rates in adult and pediatric intensive care units in the United States. National Nosocomial Infections Surveillance System. *Am J Med* 1991;91(suppl):185–191.

146. Fagon JY, Chastre J, Hance AJ, et al. Nosocomial pneumonia in ventilated patients: a cohort study evaluating attributable mortality and hospital stay. *Am J Med* 1993;94:281–288.

147. Celis R, Torres A, Gatell JM, et al. Nosocomial pneumonia. A multivariate analysis of risk and prognosis. *Chest* 1988;93:318–324.

148. Kollef MH. Ventilator-associated pneumonia. A multivariate analysis. *JAMA* 1993;270:1965–1970.

149. Craven DE, Kunches LM, Lichtenberg DA, et al. Nosocomial infection and fatality in medical and surgical intensive care unit patients. *Arch Intern Med* 1988;148:1161–1168.

150. Graybill J, Marshall L, Charache P, et al. Nosocomial pneumonia—a continuing major problem. *Am Rev Respir Dis* 1973;108:1130–1140.

151. Gross P, VanAntwerpen C. Nosocomial infections and hospital deaths. *Am J Med* 1983;75:658–662.

152. Stevens RM, Teres D, Skillman JJ, et al. Pneumonia in an intensive care unit. A 30-month experience. *Arch Intern Med* 1974;134:106–111.

153. Craig CP, Connelly S. Effect of intensive care unit nosocomial pneumonia on duration of stay and mortality. *Am J Infect Control* 1984;12:233–238.

154. Leu HS, Kaiser DL, Mori M, et al. Hospital-acquired pneumonia. Attributable mortality and morbidity. *Am J Epidemiol* 1989;129:1258–1267.

155. Haley RW, Schaberg DR, Crossley KB, et al. Extra charges and prolongation of stay attributable to nosocomial infections: a prospective interhospital comparison. *Am J Med* 1981;70:51–58.

156. Freeman J, Rosner BA, McGowan JE Jr. Adverse effects of nosocomial infection. *J Infect Dis* 1979;140:732–740.

157. Chastre J, Fagon JY, Soler P, et al. Diagnosis of nosocomial bacterial pneumonia in intubated patients undergoing ventilation: comparison of the usefulness of bronchoalveolar lavage and the protected specimen brush. *Am J Med* 1988;85:499–506.

158. Fagon JY, Chastre J, Hance AJ, et al. Detection of nosocomial lung infection in ventilated patients. Use of a protected specimen brush and quantitative culture techniques in 147 patients. *Am Rev Respir Dis* 1988;138:110–116.

159. Davidson M, Tempest B, Palmer DL. Bacteriologic diagnosis of acute pneumonia. Comparison of sputum, transtracheal aspirates, and lung aspirates. *JAMA* 1976;235:158–163.

160. Berger R, Arango L. Etiologic diagnosis of bacterial nosocomial pneumonia in seriously ill patients. *Crit Care Med* 1985;13:833–836.

161. Salata RA, Lederman MM, Shlaes DM, et al. Diagnosis of nosocomial pneumonia in intubated, intensive care unit patients. *Am Rev Respir Dis* 1987;135:426–432.

162. Pham LH, Brun-Buisson C, Legrand P, et al. Diagnosis of nosocomial pneumonia in mechanically ventilated patients. Comparison of a plugged telescoping catheter with the protected specimen brush. *Am Rev Respir Dis* 1991;143:1055–1061.

163. Meduri GU. Ventilator-associated pneumonia in patients with respiratory failure. A diagnostic approach. *Chest* 1990;97:1208–1219.

164. Tobin MJ, Grenvik A. Nosocomial lung infection and its diagnosis. *Crit Care Med* 1984;12:191–199.

165. Villers D, Derriennic M, Raffi F, et al. Reliability of the bronchoscopic protected catheter brush in intubated and ventilated patients. *Chest* 1985;88:527–530.

166. Guckian JC, Christensen WD. Quantitative culture and Gram stain of sputum in pneumonia. *Am Rev Respir Dis* 1978;118:997–1005.

167. Meduri GU, Chastre J. The standardization of bronchoscopic techniques for ventilator-associated pneumonia. *Chest* 1992;102(suppl):557–564.

168. Baselski VS, el-Torky M, Coalson JJ, et al. The standardization of criteria for processing and interpreting laboratory specimens in patients with suspected ventilator-associated pneumonia. *Chest* 1992;102(suppl):571–579.
169. Wunderink RG, Mayhall CG, Gibert C. Methodology for clinical investigation of ventilator-associated pneumonia. Epidemiology and therapeutic intervention. *Chest* 1992;102(suppl):580–588.
170. Lowy FD, Carlisle PS, Adams A, et al. The incidence of nosocomial pneumonia following urgent endotracheal intubation. *Infect Control* 1987;8:245–248.
171. Mackowiak PA, Martin RM, Jones SR, Smith JW. Pharyngeal colonization by gram-negative bacilli in aspiration-prone persons. *Arch Intern Med* 1978;138:1224–1227.
172. Valenti WM, Trudell RG, Bentley DW. Factors predisposing to oropharyngeal colonization with gram-negative bacilli in the aged. *N Engl J Med* 1978;298:1108–1111.
173. Drasar BS, Shiner M, McLeod GM. Studies on the intestinal flora. I. The bacterial flora of the gastrointestinal tract in healthy and achlorhydric persons. *Gastroenterology* 1969;56:71–79.
174. Ruddell WS, Axon AT, Findlay JM, et al. Effect of cimetidine on the gastric bacterial flora. *Lancet* 1980;1:672–674.
175. Donowitz LG, Page MC, Mileur BL, et al. Alteration of normal gastric flora in critical care patients receiving antacid and cimetidine therapy. *Infect Control* 1986;7:23–26.
176. Craven DE, Kunches LM, Kilinsky V, et al. Risk factors for pneumonia and fatality in patients receiving continuous mechanical ventilation. *Am Rev Respir Dis* 1986;133:792–796.
177. Kappstein I, Schulgen G, Friedrich T, et al. Incidence of pneumonia in mechanically ventilated patients treated with sucralfate or cimetidine as prophylaxis for stress bleeding: bacterial colonization of the stomach. *Am J Med* 1991;91(suppl):125–131.
178. Daschner F, Kappstein I, Engels I, et al. Stress ulcer prophylaxis and ventilation pneumonia: prevention by antibacterial cytoprotective agents? *Infect Control Hosp Epidemiol* 1988;9:59–65.
179. Driks MR, Craven DE, Celli BR, et al. Nosocomial pneumonia in intubated patients given sucralfate as compared with antacids or histamine type 2 blockers. The role of gastric colonization. *N Engl J Med* 1987;317:1376–1382.
180. Daschner F. Stress ulcer prophylaxis and the risk of nosocomial pneumonia in artificially ventilated patients. *Eur J Clin Microbiol* 1987;6:129–131.
181. Prod'hom G, Leuenberger P, Koerfer J, et al. Nosocomial pneumonia in mechanically ventilated patients receiving antacid, ranitidine, or sucralfate as prophylaxis for stress ulcer. A randomized controlled trial. *Ann Intern Med* 1994;120:653–662.
182. Cook DJ, Reeve BK, Guyatt GH, et al. Stress ulcer prophylaxis in critically ill patients. Resolving discordant meta-analyses. *JAMA* 1996;275:308–314.
183. Gastinne H, Wolff M, Delatour F, et al. A controlled trial in intensive care units of selective decontamination of the digestive tract with nonabsorbable antibiotics. The French Study Group on Selective Decontamination of the Digestive Tract. *N Engl J Med* 1992;326:594–599.
184. Hammond JM, Potgieter PD, Saunders GL, et al. Double-blind study of selective decontamination of the digestive tract in intensive care. *Lancet* 1992;340:5–9.
185. Meta-analysis of randomised controlled trials of selective decontamination of the digestive tract. Selective Decontamination of the Digestive Tract Trialists' Collaborative Group. *BMJ* 1993;307:525–32.
186. Torres A, Serra-Batlles J, Ros E, et al. Pulmonary aspiration of gastric contents in patients receiving mechanical ventilation: the effect of body position. *Ann Intern Med* 1992;116:540–543.
187. Haley RW, Hooton TM, Culver DH, et al. Nosocomial infections in U.S. hospitals, 1975–1976: estimated frequency by selected characteristics of patients. *Am J Med* 1981;70:947–959.
188. Cross AS, Roup B. Role of respiratory assistance devices in endemic nosocomial pneumonia. *Am J Med* 1981;70:681–685.
189. Hanson LC, Weber DJ, Rutala WA. Risk factors for nosocomial pneumonia in the elderly. *Am J Med* 1992;92:161–166.
190. Fagon JY, Chastre J, Domart Y, et al. Nosocomial pneumonia in patients receiving continuous mechanical ventilation. Prospective analysis of 52 episodes with use of a protected specimen brush and quantitative culture techniques. *Am Rev Respir Dis* 1989;139:877–884.
191. Burke JP, Riley DK. Nosocomial urinary tract infection. In: Mayhall CG, ed. *Hospital epidemiology and infection control*. Baltimore: Williams & Wilkins, 1996:139–153.
192. Warren JW. Catheter-associated urinary tract infections. *Infect Dis Clin North Am* 1997;11:609–622.
193. Tambyah PA, Maki DG. Catheter-associated urinary tract infection is rarely symptomatic: a prospective study of 1,497 catheterized patients. *Arch Intern Med* 2000;160:678–682.
194. Platt R, Polk BF, Murdock B, et al. Mortality associated with nosocomial urinary-tract infection. *N Engl J Med* 1982;307:637–642.
195. Kunin CM, Douthitt S, Dancing J, et al. The association between the use of urinary catheters and morbidity and mortality among elderly patients in nursing homes. *Am J Epidemiol* 1992;135:291–301.
196. Maki DG, Tambyah PA. Engineering out the risk for infection with urinary catheters. *Emerg Infect Dis* 2001;7:342–347.
197. Nickel JC, Costerton JW, McLean RJ, et al. Bacterial biofilms: influence on the pathogenesis, diagnosis and treatment of urinary tract infections. *J Antimicrob Chemother* 1994;33(suppl A):31–41.
198. Platt R, Polk BF, Murdock B, et al. Risk factors for nosocomial urinary tract infection. *Am J Epidemiol* 1986;124:977–985.
199. Platt R, Polk BF, Murdock B, et al. Reduction of mortality associated with nosocomial urinary tract infection. *Lancet* 1983;1:893–897.
200. Rabkin DG, Stifelman MD, Birkhoff J, et al. Early catheter removal decreases incidence of urinary tract infections in renal transplant recipients. *Transplant Proc* 1998;30:4314–4316.
201. Warren JW. Urethral catheters, condom catheters, and nosocomial urinary tract infections. *Infect Control Hosp Epidemiol* 1996;17:212–214.
202. Kunin CM, McCormack RC. Prevention of catheter-induced urinary-tract infections by sterile closed drainage. *N Engl J Med* 1966;274:1155–1161.
203. Centers for Disease Control and Prevention, National Center for Health Statistics. *Vital and health statistics, detailed diagnoses and procedures. National Hospital Discharge Survey, 1994.* Vol. 127. Hyattsville, Maryland: Department of Health and Human Services, 1997.
204. Haley RW, Schaberg DR, Von Allmen SD, et al. Estimating the extra charges and prolongation of hospitalization due to nosocomial infections: a comparison of methods. *J Infect Dis* 1980;141:248–257.
205. Freeman J, McGowan JE Jr. Methodologic issues in hospital epidemiology. III. Investigating the modifying effects of time and severity of underlying illness on estimates of cost of nosocomial infection. *Rev Infect Dis* 1984;6:285–300.
206. Pinner RW, Haley RW, Blumenstein BA, et al. High cost nosocomial infections. *Infect Control* 1982;3:143–149.
207. Martone WJ, Jarvis WR, Culver DH, et al. Incidence and nature of endemic and epidemic nosocomial infections. In: Bennett JV, Brachman PS, eds. *Hospital infections.* Boston: Little, Brown, 1992:577–596.
208. Ehrenkranz NJ, Richter EI, Phillips PM, et al. An apparent excess of operative site infections: analyses to evaluate false-positive diagnoses. *Infect Control Hosp Epidemiol* 1995;16:712–716.
209. Taylor G, McKenzie M, Kirkland T, et al. Effect of surgeon's diagnosis on surgical wound infection rates. *Am J Infect Control* 1990;18:295–299.
210. Taylor S, Pearce P, McKenzie M, Taylor GD. Wound infection in total joint arthroplasty: effect of extended wound surveillance on wound infection rates. *Can J Surg* 1994;37:217–220.
211. Cruse PJ, Foord R. A five-year prospective study of 23,649 surgical wounds. *Arch Surg* 1973;107:206–210.
212. Olson MM, Lee JT Jr. Continuous, 10-year wound infection surveillance. Results, advantages, and unanswered questions. *Arch Surg* 1990;125:794–803.
213. Burns SJ, Dippe SE. Postoperative wound infections detected during hospitalization and after discharge in a community hospital. *Am J Infect Control* 1982;10:60–65.
214. Polk BF, Tager IB, Shapiro M, et al. Randomised clinical trial of perioperative cefazolin in preventing infection after hysterectomy. *Lancet* 1980;1:437–440.
215. Brown RB, Bradley S, Opitz E, et al. Surgical wound infections documented after hospital discharge. *Am J Infect Control* 1987;15:54–58.
216. Rosendorf LL, Octavio J, Estes JP. Effect of methods of postdischarge wound infection surveillance on reported infection rates. *Am J Infect Control* 1983;11:226–229.
217. Ferraz EM, Ferraz AA, Coelho HS, et al. Postdischarge surveillance for nosocomial wound infection: does judicious monitoring find cases? *Am J Infect Control* 1995;23:290–294.
218. Keeling NJ, Morgan MW. Inpatient and post-discharge wound infections in general surgery. *Ann R Coll Surg Engl* 1995;77:245–247.
219. Manian FA, Meyer L. Adjunctive use of monthly physician questionnaires for surveillance of surgical site infections after hospital discharge and in ambulatory surgical patients: report of a seven-year experience. *Am J Infect Control* 1997;25:390–394.
220. Manian FA, Meyer L. Comparison of patient telephone survey with traditional surveillance and monthly physician questionnaires in monitoring surgical wound infections. *Infect Control Hosp Epidemiol* 1993;14:216–218.
221. Reimer K, Gleed C, Nicolle LE. The impact of postdischarge infection on surgical wound infection rates. *Infect Control* 1987;8:237–240.
222. Sands K, Vineyard G, Platt R. Surgical site infections occurring after hospital discharge. *J Infect Dis* 1996;173:963–970.
223. Weigelt JA, Dryer D, Haley RW. The necessity and efficiency of wound surveillance after discharge. *Arch Surg* 1992;127:77–81; discussion 81–82.
224. Gravel-Tropper D, Oxley C, Memish Z, et al. Underestimation of surgical site infection rates in obstetrics and gynecology. *Am J Infect Control* 1995;23:22–26.
225. Hulton LJ, Olmsted RN, Treston-Aurand J, et al. Effect of postdischarge surveillance on rates of infectious complications after cesarean section. *Am J Infect Control* 1992;20:198–201.
226. Law DJ, Mishriki SF, Jeffery PJ. The importance of surveillance after discharge from hospital in the diagnosis of postoperative wound infection. *Ann R Coll Surg Engl* 1990;72:207–209.
227. Avato JL, Lai KK. Impact of postdischarge surveillance on surgical-site infection rates for coronary artery bypass procedures. *Infect Control Hosp Epidemiol* 2002;23:364–367.
228. Seaman M, Lammers R. Inability of patients to self-diagnose wound infections. *J Emerg Med* 1991;9:215–219.
229. Cruse PJ. Surgical wound infection. In: Wonsiewicz MJ, ed. *Infectious diseases.* Philadelphia: WB Saunders, 1992:758–764.
230. Krizek TJ, Robson MC. Evolution of quantitative bacteriology in wound management. *Am J Surg* 1975;130:579–584.
231. Altemeier WA, Culbertson WR, Hummel RP. Surgical considerations of endogenous infections—sources, types, and methods of control. *Surg Clin North Am* 1968;48:227–240.

232. Valentine RJ, Weigelt JA, Dryer D, et al. Effect of remote infections on clean wound infection rates. *Am J Infect Control* 1986;14:64–67.
233. Heggeness MH, Esses SI, Errico T, et al. Late infection of spinal instrumentation by hematogenous seeding. *Spine* 1993;18:492–496.
234. Calia FM, Wolinsky E, Mortimer EA Jr, et al. Importance of the carrier state as a source of *Staphylococcus aureus* in wound sepsis. *J Hyg (Lond)* 1969;67:49–57.
235. Dineen P, Drusin L. Epidemics of postoperative wound infections associated with hair carriers. *Lancet* 1973;2:1157–1159.
236. Mastro TD, Farley TA, Elliott JA, et al. An outbreak of surgical-wound infections due to group A *Streptococcus* carried on the scalp. *N Engl J Med* 1990;323:968–972.
237. Centers for Disease Control and Prevention. Guidelines for the prevention and control of nosocomial infections. Guidelines for prevention of surgical wound infections, 1985. *Am J Infect Control* 1986;14:71–82.
238. Haley RW, Culver DH, Morgan WM, et al. Identifying patients at high risk of surgical wound infection. A simple multivariate index of patient susceptibility and wound contamination. *Am J Epidemiol* 1985;121:206–215.
239. Culver DH, Horan TC, Gaynes RP, et al. Surgical wound infection rates by wound class, operative procedure, and patient risk index. National Nosocomial Infections Surveillance System. *Am J Med* 1991;91(suppl):152–157.
240. Kaye KS, Sands K, Donahue JG, et al. Preoperative drug dispensing as predictor of surgical site infection. *Emerg Infect Dis* 2001;7:57–65.
241. Roy MC, Herwaldt LA, Embrey R, et al. Does the Centers for Disease Control's NNIS system risk index stratify patients undergoing cardiothoracic operations by their risk of surgical-site infection? *Infect Control Hosp Epidemiol* 2000;21:186–190.
242. Horan T, et al. Results of a multicenter study on risk factors for surgical site infections (SSI) following C-section [Abstract]. *Am J Infect Control* 1996;24:84.
243. Latham R, Lancaster AD, Covington JF, et al. The association of diabetes and glucose control with surgical-site infections among cardiothoracic surgery patients. *Infect Control Hosp Epidemiol* 2001;22:607–612.
244. Furnary AP, Zerr KJ, Grunkemeier GL, et al. Continuous intravenous insulin infusion reduces the incidence of deep sternal wound infection in diabetic patients after cardiac surgical procedures. *Ann Thorac Surg* 1999;67:352–360; discussion 360–362.
245. Zerr KJ, Furnary AP, Grunkemeier GL, et al. Glucose control lowers the risk of wound infection in diabetics after open heart operations. *Ann Thorac Surg* 1997;63:356–361.
246. Perl TM, Cullen JJ, Wenzel RP, et al. Intranasal mupirocin to prevent postoperative *Staphylococcus aureus* infections. *N Engl J Med* 2002;346:1871–1877.
247. Mishriki SF, Law DJ, Jeffery PJ. Factors affecting the incidence of postoperative wound infection. *J Hosp Infect* 1990;16:223–230.
248. Seropian R, Reynolds BM. Wound infections after preoperative depilatory versus razor preparation. *Am J Surg* 1971;121:251–254.
249. Hamilton HW, Hamilton KR, Lone FJ. Preoperative hair removal. *Can J Surg* 1977;20:269–271, 274–275.
250. Olson MM, MacCallum J, McQuarrie DG. Preoperative hair removal with clippers does not increase infection rate in clean surgical wounds. *Surg Gynecol Obstet* 1986;162:181–182.
251. Moro ML, Carrieri MP, Tozzi AE, et al. Risk factors for surgical wound infections in clean surgery: a multicenter study. Italian PRINOS Study Group. *Ann Ital Chir* 1996;67:13–19.
252. Winston KR. Hair and neurosurgery. *Neurosurgery* 1992;31:320–329.
253. Boyce JM, Potter-Bynoe G, Opal SM, et al. A common-source outbreak of *Staphylococcus epidermidis* infections among patients undergoing cardiac surgery. *J Infect Dis* 1990;161:493–499.
254. Recommended practices for surgical hand scrubs. *AORN J* 1999;69:842, 845–850.
255. Meers PD, Yeo GA. Shedding of bacteria and skin squames after handwashing. *J Hyg (Lond)* 1978;81:99–105.
256. Kikuchi-Numagami K, Saishu T, Fukaya M, et al. Irritancy of scrubbing up for surgery with or without a brush. *Acta Derm Venereol* 1999;79:230–232.
257. Association of Operating Room Nurses. *Standards, recommended practices, guidelines*. Denver: Association of Operating Room Nurses, 1999.
258. Pottinger J, Burns S, Manske C. Bacterial carriage by artificial versus natural nails. *Am J Infect Control* 1989;17:340–344.
259. Lidwell OM. Clean air at operation and subsequent sepsis in the joint. *Clin Orthop* 1986;211:91–102.
260. Smilanich RP, Bonnet I, Kirkpatrick JR. Contaminated wounds: the effect of initial management on outcome. *Am Surg* 1995;61:427–430.
261. Dougherty SH, Simmons RL. The biology and practice of surgical drains. Part II. *Curr Probl Surg* 1992;29:633–730.
262. Dellinger EP, Gross PA, Barrett TL, et al. Quality standard for antimicrobial prophylaxis in surgical procedures. The Infectious Diseases Society of America. *Infect Control Hosp Epidemiol* 1994;15:182–188.
263. Classen DC, Evans RS, Pestotnik SL, et al. The timing of prophylactic administration of antibiotics and the risk of surgical-wound infection. *N Engl J Med* 1992;326:281–286.
264. Zanetti G, Giardina R, Platt P. Intraoperative redosing of cefazolin and risk for surgical site infection in cardiac surgery. *Emerg Infect Dis* 2001;7:828–831.
265. Flaherty JP, Garcia-Houchins S, Chudy R, et al. An outbreak of gram-negative bacteremia traced to contaminated O-rings in reprocessed dialyzers. *Ann Intern Med* 1993;119:1072–1078.

CHAPTER 9
The Pathogens of Hospital Infections

Stephanie R. Black and Robert A. Weinstein

Nosocomial infections are a leading cause of morbidity and mortality, costing an estimated $4.5 billion and contributing to over 80,000 deaths annually. Advances in medical technology—improvements in chemotherapy, intensive care support, and immunosuppression for transplantation and connective tissue disease—contribute to an enlarging population at risk for hospital-acquired infection.

This chapter reviews common nosocomial pathogens, their epidemiology, the commonly associated sites and clinical scenarios of nosocomial infections, and resultant infection control needs. Pathogens are divided into tables (Tables 9.1, 9.2, and 9.3) according to microbiologic characteristics, and the text highlights important and controversial concepts regarding epidemiology, types of infection, and infection control issues.

EPIDEMIOLOGY

Hospital infections follow epidemiologic patterns that are related to the infecting pathogens and clinical settings. Understanding these patterns is important because they are an important factor in guiding infection control measures.

Reservoirs and Sources

Common reservoirs for nosocomial pathogens include the animate environment—infected or colonized personnel, patients and hospital visitors—and the inanimate environment—such as hospital equipment, sinks, ventilators, and bedrails.

ANIMATE RESERVOIRS

The reservoirs and sources of nosocomial gram-positive organisms are usually personnel or patients; common sites of carriage are skin, nares, axillae, perineum, vagina, pharynx, or the gastrointestinal (GI) tract. Carriage of some organisms such as vancomycin-resistant enterococci (VRE) or *Streptococcus pyogenes* may persist for months (11,12). Nosocomial gram-negative organisms, such as *Pseudomonas* and *Enterobacter*, rapidly colonize the GI or respiratory tracts of hospitalized patients (13–16). Nosocomial gram-negative bacilli are associated with more transient colonization of health care workers (HCWs) and may be transmitted from patient to patient on unwashed hands of HCWs (17,18).

Patients in long-term care facilities are an important reservoir of nosocomial pathogens. Chronically ill patients who have received multiple courses of antibiotics are frequently colonized by resistant pathogens. These patients introduce and reintroduce resistant organisms with each hospital admission, providing a steady influx of pathogens, often to intensive care units (ICUs) (19–22).

INANIMATE RESERVOIRS

The inanimate environment has been implicated as a reservoir for hearty organisms, such as VRE (23,24), and for spore formers, such as *Clostridium difficile*, that may survive for long periods on inanimate surfaces (25–27; see also Chapter 74).

TABLE 9.1. Characteristics of and Control Measures for Common Nosocomial Gram-Positive Organisms

Organism	Epidemiology				Sites of nosocomial infection	Infection control measures beyond standard precautions[a]
	Reservoir	Transmission	Host risk factors	Special organism characteristics		
Coagulase negative staphylococcus	Skin commensal Gut of neutropenics	Contact	Hemodialysis Indwelling catheter Prosthetic material	Polysaccharide adhesions Extracellular glycocalyx—ability to adhere to artificial surfaces	11%[b] BSI SSI Endocarditis CNS shunt infection Endophthalmitis	Remove devices
Enterococcus	GI tract commensal Skin, wounds Chronic decubitus ulcers	Contact	Elderly Genitourinary pathology Immunocompromised Prior antibiotics (cephalosporin) Urinary tract instrumentation	—	10%[b] (includes VRE) UTI SSI BSI Endocarditis Hepatobiliary Pneumonia	Antibiotic restriction Remove urinary and i.v. catheters
Glycopeptide intermediate coagulase-negative staphylococci	Skin commensal	Contact	Critically ill with central venous catheter Extended use of vancomycin (>40 days)	Must use MIC method to detect (disc diffusion is too insensitive)	BSI Peritonitis	Follow GISA precautions (controversial)
Glycopeptide-intermediate *Staphylococcus aureus* (GISA)	Unknown	Unknown	Long-term vancomycin treatment	Must use MIC method to detect (disc diffusion is too insensitive)	BSI Peritonitis	Strict isolation, cohort; notify state health department and CDC (1,2) and SEARCH @ cdc.gov
Group A streptococcus	Patient or HCW: colonization of pharynx, rectum, vagina	Droplet Contact with contaminated secretions	Age extremes Alcoholics Chronic illness Diabetes mellitus HIV Malignancy Surgery or postpartum Varicella	Toxins	BSI Endometritis SSI Streptococcal toxic shock syndrome Postcesarian section	≥1 case = outbreak until proven otherwise
Group B streptococcus	Lower GI tract, vagina	Contact Vertical	Alcoholics Cardiovascular disease Diabetes mellitus Genitourinary disease Neonates Nonhematologic malignancy	—	1%[b] BSI Endocarditis Meningitis	Maternal screening or risk-based peripartum prophylaxis (3)
Methicillin-resistant *Staphylococcus aureus* (MRSA)	LTCF patients HCW carriers Environment blood pressure cuffs, bed linens, overbed tables, floors, clothes worn by HCWs	Contact	Colonization pressure ICU stay Increased severity of illness (e.g., high APACHE score) Intravascular device Prior antibiotics Transfer from LTCF Transfer units within hospital	Similar to MSSA	13%[b] (includes MSSA) See MSSA	Contact precautions until off antibiotics and culture negative (4) Masks (see text)
Methicillin-susceptible *Staphylococcus aureus* (MSSA)	Colonization of skin (≈30% of persons colonized at any one time) nares, axillae, perineum, denuded skin Infected patients Occasional HCW carriers Hospital environment	Contact Shedding "Cloud adult"	Diabetes mellitus Hemodialysis Immunodeficiency i.v. drug users Prior upper respiratory infections	Surface protein adhesins: bind fibronectin, collagen, or fibrinogen Enterotoxin TSST-1 Epidermolytic toxins Membrane damaging toxins	13%[b] (includes MRSA) SSI Pneumonia BSI: risk of dissemination with metastatic foci) Burns Prosthetic material Skin/soft tissue	Barrier precautions for major skin, wound, or burn (4) Perioperative prophylaxis Antibiotic-impregnated catheters (5)
Vancomycin-resistant enterococcus (VRE)	GI tract of LTCF patients Environment (6)	Contact	Abdominal surgery Cirrhosis Debilitated Dialysis Elderly History of nosocomial infection Severe underlying illness	Ability to grow in presence of bile and salt Resistant to heat and removal by washing with bland soap Colonization pressure Contamination of environment (more likely in patients with diarrhea)	10%[b] (includes enterococcus) UTI SSI BSI	Surveillance cultures with emphasis on barrier precautions Cohorting Less use of vancomycin and third-generation cephalosporins (7)

[a]See text for standard precautions. Additional infection control measures applicable to all antibiotic-resistant pathogens include antimicrobial audit program and barrier precautions including gloves and gown if contact with body fluids possible; cohort patients and staff if spread of resistant strains continues.
[b]Percentage distribution of nosocomial pathogens by infection site in NNIS system data, January 1990 to March 1996 (110).
HCW, health-care worker; SSI, surgical site infection; BSI, bloodstream infection; CNS, central nervous system; UTI, urinary tract infection; LTCF, long-term care facility; GI, gastrointestinal; MIC, minimum inhibitory concentration; HIV, human immunodeficiency virus.

TABLE 9.2. Characteristics of and Control Measures for Common Nosocomial Gram-Negative Organisms

Organism	Reservoir	Transmission	Host risk factors	Special organism characteristics	Sites of nosocomial infection	Infection control measures beyond standard precautions[a]
		Epidemiology				
Glucose nonfermenters						
Acinetobacter	Inanimate environment Skin commensal Colonized and infected patients	Contact Droplet Common source	ICU patient with multiple courses of broad-spectrum antibiotics	Survival for weeks on dry surfaces Seasonality: late summer	1%[b] Pneumonia BSI UTI Meningitis Wounds	During outbreak, perform surveillance cultures to direct isolation precautions and cohorting
Pseudomonas	Hospital environment Colonized and infected patients	Contact Common source	Severe underlying illness	Multiple mechanisms of resistance (including resistance to antiseptics) Survival in moist environment Lipopolysaccharide cell wall Lipid A endotoxin	9%[b] Pneumonia UTI SSI BSI Burns Endophthalmitis Keratitis Meningitis Biliary tract	Avoid standing water Avoid aqueous benzalkonium chloride Do not reuse single-use vials
Stenotrophomonas	Inanimate environment Water, soil, plants, food Colonized and infected patients	Contact Common source	i.v. or broad-spectrum antibiotics Neutropenia Prolonged intubation Severe underlying illness	Adhesion to Teflon (8)	BSI Endophthalmitis Meningitis Pneumonia UTI Skin/soft tissue	—
Glucose fermenters						
Citrobacter	GI tract Colonized and infected patients Colonized HCWs	Contact Vertical	—	Prolonged survival in hospital environment	≤1%[b] ("other Enterobacteriacae") UTI Brain abscess (C. diversus) BSI Meningitis Pneumonia	Nursery cohorting Employee surveillance for colonization during outbreaks
Enterobacter	GI tract Urinary/respiratory tract of hospitalized patients Contaminated infusate Multidose vials	Contact Common source	Immunosuppression Indwelling catheter or recent procedure Severe underlying illness	Antibiotic may increase adhesion capacities	6%[b] Pneumonia SSI UTI BSI Endophthalmitis Meningitis	—
Escherichia coli	Gut of hospitalized patients LTCF patients [may harbor extended-spectrum beta-lactamase (ESBL) positive strains] Environment Improperly disinfected cystoscopes Contaminated prep solutions	Contact Common source	Debilitating illness Elderly Female Instrumented genitourinary tract	KI antigen (virulence factor)	12%[b] UTI SSI BSI Pneumonia Diarrhea (O157:H7)	Limit urinary catheter use Aseptic technique during insertion and care Closed system Replace catheter only when obstructed or malfunctioning
Klebsiella	GI tract colonization of patients in LTCF patients (especially ESBL carriers)	Contact	Elderly Immunocompromised Infants Treatment with third-generation cephalosporin or aminoglycoside	Cell wall receptors Capsular polysaccharide Endotoxin	5%[b] UTI Pneumonia Neonatal Septic arthritis	Antibiotic restriction (ceftazidime/ third-generation cephalosporin)
Morganella	LTCF patients with urinary catheters or urinary incontinence	—	Elderly Nursing home residence Prior antibiotics Severe underlying illness Surgical patients	Biofilms on inner surface of catheter	≤1%[b] ("other Enterobacteriacae") BSI Pneumonia SSI UTI	Avoid indwelling urinary catheter
Proteus	LTCF patients Colonized and infected patients	Contact Common source	Genitourinary manipulation	Hemolysis Urease Catheter incrustation	3%[b] UTI SSI Pneumonia BSI Endophthalmitis	—

(continued)

TABLE 9.2. (*continued*)

Organism	Reservoir	Transmission	Host risk factors	Special organism characteristics	Sites of nosocomial infection	Infection control measures beyond standard precautions[a]
				Epidemiology		
Providencia	LTCF patients with urinary catheters or urinary incontinence	—	Long-term urinary catheterization Use of aminoglycosides	MR/K fimbriae promote adherence	≤1%[b] ("other Enterobacteriacae") Burns SSI UTI	—
Serratia	GI tract of neonates Respiratory tract of hospitalized patients Hospital equipment Leech-borne (associated with plastic surgery)	Contact Common source	Debilitated patients History of antibiotics or steroids Invasive procedures Ventilated patients	Pink/red color to abscess caused by prodigiosin Mulitply in nutrient poor medium Survive in wet environment, even in contact with disinfectant	1%[b] Pneumonia Arthritis BSI Endocarditis Keratitis Meningitis Skin/soft tissue SSI Transplant (heart) UTI	Avoid reuse of single-dose vials Avoid "topping off" soap dispensers

[a]See text for standard precautions. Additional infection control measures applicable to all antibiotic-resistant pathogens include antimicrobial audit program and barrier precautions including gloves and gown if contact with body fluids possible; cohort patients and staff if spread of resistant strains continues.
[b]Percentage distribution of nosocomial pathogens by infection site in NNIS system data, January 1990 to March 1996 (110).
HCW, health-care worker; SSI, surgical site infection; BSI, bloodstream infection; CNS, central nervous system; UTI, urinary tract infection; LTCF, long-term care facility; ICU, intensive care unit; GI, gastrointestinal; i.v., intravenous.

Aerobic gram-negative bacilli are the nosocomial bacteria most often associated with the environment. *Pseudomonas aeruginosa*, the quintessential nosocomial pathogen, is such a common problem in moist areas of the environment that it is often called a "water bug." Contamination of inadequately disinfected endoscopes (both GI and bronchoscopic) has led to outbreaks of *Pseudomonas* bacteremia and nosocomial respiratory tract colonization and infection (28,29). *Acinetobacter* may remain viable for several weeks on dry surfaces and has led to sporadic outbreaks in ICUs (30).

Transmission

Transmission of pathogens in health care facilities results most often from indirect contact, airborne, or droplet spread.

CROSS-CONTAMINATION AND COLONIZATION PRESSURE

Indirect contact or cross-contamination of nosocomial pathogens between patients occurs most often due to inadequate HCW hand hygiene. This problem is exacerbated when ill patients are seen by multiple consultants who, at teaching centers, are frequently accompanied by teams of residents and students. As the HCWs make their daily rounds, so do potential nosocomial pathogens (7,31).

Closely related to cross-contamination is the concept of "colonization pressure," defined as the proportion of other patients colonized with problem pathogens (11). In a study of VRE, colonization pressure was a more important variable than length of stay, personnel compliance with infection control measures, Acute Physiology and Chronic Health Evaluation (APACHE) scores, or the proportion of days that a patient received vancomycin, a third-generation cephalosporin, sucralfate, or enteral feeding. Once the VRE colonization pressure was greater than 50%, this became the major factor affecting VRE acquisition. Colonization pressure also has been recognized as an important independent risk factor for acquisition of methicillin-resistant *Staphylococcus aureus* (MRSA) in an ICU (32).

Although we think of ICUs as epicenters of nosocomial problems, many pathogens already colonize patients at the time of ICU admission. In a study of the epidemiology of *Pseudomonas aeruginosa* in the ICU, the admission of colonized patients contributed to the endemic persistence of *Pseudomonas*; 35% of all patients with positive respiratory tract cultures were already colonized by the time of ICU transfer or admission (33).

AIRBORNE, AEROSOL, AND VERTICAL TRANSMISSION

Airborne and droplet spread are less common means of transmission of nosocomial pathogens but may lead to HCW, as well as patient, risk. Airborne transmission is defined as the spread of pathogens by droplet nuclei that are 5.0 μm or smaller in size. This size allows the particles to remain suspended in the air and to be inhaled easily into the deep airways. In contrast, droplets per se are larger and more likely to settle, traveling about 3 feet, a distance often likened to the area of protection provided by an umbrella (concept courtesy of Jeff Nelson, M.D.). Organisms that have potential for airborne spread, include varicella (see also Chapter 234), tuberculosis (see also Chapter 265), and measles (see also Chapter 244). Pathogens that spread as droplets include influenza (see also Chapter 241), *Neisseria meningitidis* (see also Chapter 193), *Haemophilus influenzae* (see also Chapter 203), *Steptococcus pyogenes* (see also Chapter 183), mycoplasma (see also Chapter 223), parvovirus B19 (see also Chapter 236), and parainfluenza virus (34; see also Chapter 242).

Some nosocomial pathogens that are traditionally associated with contact transmission, such as staphylococci or group A streptococci (GAS), may become airborne when shed from colonized personnel who have concomitant viral upper respiratory tract infections (URIs). The term *cloud adult*—derived from the 1960 study of the "cloud baby" phenomenon (35)—was applied to a carrier of MRSA who shed *S. aureus* only in the presence of a viral URI. After experimental inoculation with rhinovirus, this individual's airborne dispersal of *S. aureus* increased 40-fold (36). An outbreak of MRSA infections affecting eight patients over 3 weeks in a surgical ICU was attributed to this mechanism of spread.

TABLE 9.3.   Characteristics of and Control Measures for Common Nosocomial Fungi

Organism	Epidemiology					Infection control measures beyond standard precautions[a]
	Reservoir	Transmission	Host risk factors	Special organism characteristics	Sites of nosocomial infection	
Aspergillus (9)	Ubiquitous: unfiltered air, ventilation systems, carpeting, plants, food Water	Airborne Ingestion Contact	Bone marrow transplant Contaminated dust during hospital construction Neutropenic Steroid therapy	—	CNS infection Pulmonary disease: fungal ball, invasive/infarct Sinusitis SSI/skin	Positive pressure room for neutropenic patients Special environmental precautions to minimize exposure of high-risk patients to construction (10) HCW should keep nails short and not wear artificial nails
Candida albicans	GI tract Subungual space of HCWs	Contact Common source Vertical	Acute pancreatitis Age extremes Antibiotic exposure Contaminated infusate Hyperalimentation Lack of fluconazole prophylaxis Liver failure Neutropenia Severe underlying illness Surgery	Proliferates in glucose-containing solutions	5%[b] UTI BSI SSI Endocarditis Endophthalmitis Pneumonia Hepatosplenic candidiasis Peritonitis Septic arthritis	
Candida krusei	GI tract	—	Fluconazole prophylaxis (controversial) Neutropenia	Resistant to azoles	BSI Endophthalmitis	—
Candida lusitaniae	GI tract Respiratory tract	Contact	—	Resistant to amphotericin B	BSI	
Candida parapsilosis	Hands of HCWs	Contact Common source	Cardiac surgery Contact lens wear Diabetes mellitus Immunosuppression Intravascular devices i.v. drug user Parenteral nutrition	Produces slime which adheres to prosthetic material	Arthritis BSI Endocarditis Endophthalmitis Peritonitis	—
Candida tropicalis	GI tract	Contact	Chronic indwelling urinary catheter Increased severity of illness Lack of fluconazole prophylaxis Neutropenia	—	BSI UTI	—
Candida/ Torulopsis glabrata	GI tract	Contact Common source	Fluconazole prophylaxis (controversial)	Variable resistance to azoles	UTI	—
Fusarium	Environment	Airborne Contact	Construction activity Diabetes mellitus Hematologic malignancy Myelosuppression Prior antibiotics Renal failure	—	BSI Endophthalmitis Nails Skin	—
Zygomycetes	Environment	Airborne Contact Ingestion	Construction activity Diabetes mellitus Hematologic malignancy High iron load Myelosuppression Prior antibiotics Renal failure	—	CNS GI tract Pneumonia Sinusitis Skin	—

[a]See text for standard precautions.
[b]Percentage distribution of nosocomial pathogens by infection site in NNIS system data, January 1990 to March 1996 (110).
HCW, health-care worker; SSI, surgical site infection; BSI, bloodstream infection; CNS, central nervous system; UTI, urinary tract infection; LTCF, long-term care facility; GI, gastrointestinal.

Acinetobacter bacteremia has been traced to contaminated aerosols. In an outbreak that affected eight infants in the Bahamas, bloodstream infections occurred more frequently during months of high humidity. Cultures from the drip pans and exhaust vents of air conditioners were positive, suggesting that environmental conditions that increased condensate on air conditioners may have predisposed to aerosol or droplet spread of *Acinetobacter* (37).

At the time of writing we are in the midst of a global epidemic of Severe Acute Respiratory Syndrome (SARS), due to a novel coronavirus; transmission to healthcare workers from hospitalized patients has been a major problem in some hos-

pitals. Spread appears to be via respiratory droplets, but because of the apparent occurrence of superspreaders (37a), airborne spread may be a mode of transmission in some settings. There is also concern that shedding of coronavirus in urine or stool may be related to some episodes of transmission. Recommended infection control measures include use of contact, droplet, and airborne precautions. Because of the evolving nature of the information and recommendations, readers are referred to the CDC (*www.cdc.gov/ncidod/sars*) and WHO (*www.who.int/csr/sars/en/*) websites for up-to-date information.

Vertical transmission of potential pathogens from mothers to newborns is an important mode of contact transmission for

Streptococcus agalactiae (group B streptococci), *Citrobacter* (38), and at times for *Candida* (39).

Risk Factors for Nosocomial Infections

Risk factors for nosocomial infections have been well described, particularly for patients in ICUs (40–42). Underlying illness, immunosuppression, malnutrition, and violation of normal mucosa and skin barriers by mechanical devices, surgery, or trauma are common risk factors for infection in ICU patients (40). Site-specific risk factors for infection are addressed in Chapter 8. Risk factors must be interpreted in light of the context in which they were studied; that is, the evaluation of risk may be confounded by a number of factors, particularly patients' severity of illness, hospital length of stay, and antibiotic use. Multivariate statistical analysis attempts to adjust for these potential confounders.

RISK FACTORS FOR SPECIFIC ORGANISMS

Analysis of risk factors depends on the availability of well-conducted epidemiologic studies. For example, although only six U.S. cases of glycopeptide-intermediate *S. aureus* (GISA) had been identified as of January 2001, similarities among these cases suggest potential risk factors. Implicated factors include hemo- or peritoneal dialysis, recurrent MRSA bacteremias from infected central venous catheters or prosthetic material, and resultant prolonged treatment with vancomycin (6–18 weeks) in the 3 to 6 months prior to GISA infection (1).

Colonization and infection with VRE have been associated with advanced age, severe underlying illness, hematologic malignancy, neutropenia, cirrhosis, recent abdominal surgery, renal dialysis, prior nosocomial infection, and decubitus ulcers (43–48).

Outbreaks in ICUs have led to several investigations to assess risk factors for nosocomial acquisition of *Acinetobacter* pneumonia, bacteremia, or urinary tract infections (49–57). Multivariate analyses have identified risk factors for *Acinetobacter* bloodstream infection, including prior antibiotic use, immunosuppression, respiratory failure at admission, number of invasive procedures before bacteremia, unscheduled admission to the hospital, and prior episode of bacteremia in the ICU (58). Male gender, length of stay, hyperalimentation, use of third-generation cephalosporins, and urinary catheterization were additional risk factors determined by multivariate analysis for colonization with multidrug-resistant *Acinetobacter* (59). The most common sites of infection in this study were the urinary tract and the bronchopulmonary tree. *Acinetobacter* has become endemic in many burn units. A case-control study with multivariate analysis demonstrated that in addition to prior antibiotics, other risk factors included female gender (in contrast to the prior study in 1995) (59), hydrotherapy, and burn covering greater than 50% of the total body surface area (51).

Stenotrophomonas maltophilia, another pathogen of increasing clinical significance, has been associated with prior antibiotic use in multiple studies and has affected various populations, including adults with and without malignancy and pediatric patients with cystic fibrosis (60–63). A small study in allogeneic bone marrow transplant patients demonstrated an association of *S. maltophilia* bacteremia with prolonged duration of neutropenia, severe mucositis, and total parenteral nutrition, although this study did not include a multivariate analysis (64).

RISK FACTORS IN SPECIFIC POPULATIONS: HUMAN IMMUNODEFICIENCY VIRUS AND NEONATES

Risk factors have been identified for nosocomial infection in a number of specific populations. We detail here the risk factors for patients infected with human immunodeficiency virus (HIV) (65–67) and for neonates (68,69) as examples of highly vulnerable populations.

Nosocomial infections in the HIV-infected population are clinically challenging due to the potential for atypical presentation of infections such as tuberculosis (70). In addition, confusion exists about nosocomial versus community acquisition of infection in patients who are often in the clinic and on inpatient wards. These challenges may lead to delay in diagnosis. Important nosocomial respiratory pathogens include *Mycobacterium tuberculosis* (71), gram-negative bacilli (especially *Klebsiella*, *Enterobacter*, and *Pseudomonas*) (72), and gram-positive cocci [primarily, *S. aureus* (73) and *Streptococcus pneumoniae* (74)]. In addition, a cluster of *Pneumocystis carinii* pneumonias on a renal transplant unit was attributed to nosocomial spread from patients with acquired immunodeficiency syndrome (AIDS) (75). Five renal transplant patients attended the same outpatient clinic as AIDS patients. In three cases, comparison of cases with matched controls demonstrated that cases had more encounters with AIDS patients who had or developed *Pneumocystis* pneumonia.

A number of nosocomial problems have emerged among AIDS patients. Indwelling central venous catheters have been frequent sources of *S. aureus* and *Pseudomonas* bacteremias (76,77). Antibiotic-associated diarrhea and colitis due to *C. difficile*, a common nosocomial pathogen, is especially prevalent on AIDS wards (78). Because of increased rates of hospitalization for community-acquired diarrheal infections, such as salmonellosis, patients on AIDS wards are at risk for nosocomial spread of a variety of enteric pathogens (79). Waterborne pathogens such as *Cryptosporidium*, *Legionella*, and *Mycobacterium avium-intracellulare* have led to nosocomial infection in AIDS patients. *Cryptosporidium* has been associated with a contaminated ice machine and subsequent person-to-person nosocomial transmission of infection (80,81). *M. avium intracellulare* colonization of potable water has been a source of nosocomial infection in AIDS patients (82,83). Norwegian scabies has been transmitted from AIDS patients to other hospitalized patients and HCWs (84).

Neonatal infections are divided into early (within 3–7 days of birth) and late-occurring infections. Prior to 3 days, infection is assumed to be vertically transmitted from the mother. After this time, neonatal infection is attributed to spread among neonates by HCWs or from the environment (68). Data from the Centers for Disease Control and Prevention's (CDC) National Nosocomial Infections Surveillance (NNIS) system from 1986 to 1994 reported on 13,179 nosocomial infections in neonatal ICUs. The most frequent nosocomial infection was bacteremia, followed by pneumonia, infection of the GI tract, and infections of the eye, ear, nose, and throat (85). Risk factors for neonatal nosocomial infection include low birth weight, respiratory illness, presence of vascular catheters, parenteral nutrition, and assisted ventilation (86).

Special Characteristics of Nosocomial Pathogens

Evaluation of the molecular basis for the pathophysiologic events that underlie hospital-acquired infections is an evolving area of study. At the simplest level, recognizing the growth requirements (or lack thereof) can provide epidemiologic clues to which pathogens are likely to occur in a certain setting. Pathogen tropisms also affect reservoirs and modes of transmission.

ADHERENCE

Adherence to host tissue is an essential step in the pathogenesis of *S. aureus* infections. *S. aureus* surface protein adhesins can bind host cellular fibronectin, collagen, or fibrinogen (87). These adhesin proteins are thought to play a role in the tenacity with which *S. aureus* adheres to prosthetic material (88). Such proteins are present in coagulase-negative staphylococci, but to a lesser extent than in *S. aureus* (88). Adhesin proteins may be a future target of antimicrobial therapy (89).

Several pathophysiologic events contribute to the persistence of nosocomial pathogens in patients with indwelling bladder catheters. *Proteus* species produce urease, which alkalinizes the urine and causes crystallization of struvite and apatite, which in turn can result in formation of an encrusted "sanctuary site" on the inside surface of urinary catheters (90). The associated biofilms have been shown to promote antimicrobial resistance. *Providencia stuartii* organisms have specific fimbriae (the MR/K fimbriae), which are finger-like projections that can promote adherence to urinary catheters (91). *Morganella* species also can form a biofilm on the inner surface of urinary catheters, aided by either fimbriae or urease (90).

TOLERANCE TO THE ENVIRONMENT

Several nosocomial pathogens are notable for their ability to survive in the animate and inanimate environments. An outbreak strain of *Enterococcus faecium* was shown to survive up to 30 minutes after inoculation on the fingertips of volunteers. In this study, hand washing with soap and water was the least effective method of disinfecting hands. Alcoholic chlorhexidine provided more rapid and persistent hand disinfection (92). In addition, *Enterococcus* is capable of growth in the presence of bile and salt (48), and strains of *E. faecium* have demonstrated ability to survive heat treatment of up to 68°C (93).

Pseudomonas and *Acinetobacter* are capable of prolonged survival—weeks to months—in the hospital environment. *Pseudomonas* has survived in dried sputum for up to 1 week and has been isolated from sinks, soaps, baths, toys, tables, brushes, and cloths (94). *Pseudomonas* survives and often grows in moist environmental reservoirs; such contamination creates a risk for common source outbreaks (28). Examples of contaminated reservoirs that have led to outbreaks in hospitals even include antiseptics and disinfectants, such as dilute aqueous benzalkonium chloride, biguanides, hexachloropene, and iodophors (95–100). Gram-negative contamination of inanimate sites that are directly related to patient care also has occurred; for example, contamination by *Pseudomonas pickettii* (other names *Burkholderia pickettii; Ralstonia pickettii*) of commercial respiratory therapy solutions (101).

The role of more "remote" environmental reservoirs of *Pseudomonas*, such as sink traps, has been questioned. Although they may be reservoirs for highly resistant *Pseudomonas* organisms, sinks are not usually the source of bacteria colonizing ICU patients (102). A study of the clinical significance of sink drain isolates used molecular typing to show that sinks were the source of at most two of five acquisitions of *P. aeruginosa* by patients over a 6-week period. A subsequent study that compared environmental *P. aeruginosa* strains with clinical isolates found little correspondence. Typing results showed that patient strains were more likely associated with each other, suggesting person-to-person spread (103).

The ability of *Acinetobacter* to survive desiccation facilitates its contamination of the inanimate environment. Point-source outbreaks have resulted from *Acinetobacter* contamination of mattresses (104), pillows (105), and even washcloths (despite 7 days of storage in dry conditions) (106).

UNIQUE TISSUE TROPISMS

Some organisms have striking but unexplained tissue tropisms. For example, nosocomial *Citrobacter diversus* is associated with brain abscess formation in neonates; 77% of *C. diversus* meningitis is complicated by development of brain abscesses (107). Most infants affected are under 6 weeks of age. Pathogenesis is thought to be via hematogenous spread from the leptomeninges to the ventricles, directly into brain tissue (108). The mortality rate is

34%, and most children suffer varying degrees of dysfunction if they recover. Less than 5% of children make a full recovery. Isolation of *C. diversus* from the meninges should prompt radiographic evaluation of the brain. Nosocomial transmission of *C. diversus* from HCWs' hands to neonates' umbilical areas in a nursery outbreak resulted in meningitis and sepsis in two of 128 infants cultured over a 1-month period. Nine additional infants had asymptomatic umbilical colonization (109).

SITES OF NOSOCOMIAL INFECTION

National estimates of the frequencies of nosocomial pathogens by site (Table 9.4) have been derived from a nonrandom sample of U.S. hospitals by the CDC's NNIS system. In January 1999 the NNIS hospital-wide component was discontinued. In part, it has been argued that the hospital-wide component did not yield data that were meaningful for interhospital comparisons because the NNIS rates were not risk adjusted (111). However, rates reported in the hospital-wide component are generally reflective of the relative frequencies of recovery of common isolates, such as coagulase-negative *Staphylococcus*, *S. aureus*, and *Enterococcus*, from nosocomial infections (111). The NNIS data also document and track the increasing antibiotic resistance of other important nosocomial pathogens, such as *Escherichia coli*, *Klebsiella*, *Enterobacter*, and *Pseudomonas*.

The etiologic role of some NNIS pathogens has been questioned. Nevertheless, such strains may be a concern because of their potential to spread among patients, even when the index infection is of low clinical significance. For example, *Candida*, which is isolated from 5% of nosocomial pneumonias in the NNIS system, is unlikely to cause clinically important lower respiratory tract infection, but may spread among colonized patients and lead to clinically significant intravenous catheter and bloodstream infection (112).

INFECTION CONTROL

Important components of an effective infection control program include surveillance, hand hygiene, isolation and barrier precautions, oversight of use of antibiotics and of invasive devices, and environmental (especially air and water quality) controls (113; see also Chapter 8).

General Infection Control Principles

High levels (in excess of 60%–80%) of hand hygiene adherence have been difficult to achieve in health care facilities. These failures have been attributed to HCW lack of time, inaccessibility of sinks, and the damaging effects on skin of repeated washing (114). To deal with this national problem, the CDC has recommended a move to universal use of sinkless alcohol hand rubs for hand hygiene, based on data from Europe and the United States that show increased compliance and improved hand conditions when these agents have been the focus of aggressive hospital campaigns (115).

HCWs should consider "universal gloving" (i.e., gloving when entering the room of any patient) as a potentially useful adjunct to hand hygiene (6,116,117). This approach is recommended because of the extensive "resistance iceberg" of hospital and nursing home patients who have unrecognized colonization by potential problem pathogens, such as VRE, MRSA, and antibiotic-resistant gram-negative bacilli (22,118–120). Of note, gloves must be changed between patients and hands should be cleaned with alcohol rub or washed after glove removal (116).

TABLE 9.4. Percentage Distribution of Nosocomial Pathogens, by Infection Site, Hospital-Wide Component of National Nosocomial Infections Surveillance System, January 1990 to March 1996

Pathogens	All sites (N = 101,821 isolates)	UTI (N = 35,079 isolates)	SSI (N = 17,671 isolates)	BSI (N = 14,424 isolates)	PNEU (N = 13,433 isolates)	Other (N = 21,214 isolates)
Staphylococcus aureus	13	2	20	16	19	18
Escherichia coli	12	24	8	5	4	4
Coagulase-negative staphylococci	11	4	14	31	2	14
Enterococcus species	10	16	12	9	2	5
Pseudomonas aeruginosa	9	11	8	3	17	7
Enterobacter species	6	5	7	4	11	4
Candida albicans	5	8	3	5	5	4
Klebsiella pneumoniae	5	8	3	5	8	3
Gram-positive anaerobes	4	0	1	1	0	19
Proteus mirabilis	3	5	3	1	2	2
Other *Streptococcus* species	2	1	3	3	1	2
Other *Candida* species	2	3	1	3	1	1
Other fungi	2	3	0	1	1	1
Acinetobacter species	1	1	1	2	4	1
Serratia marcescens	1	1	1	1	3	1
Citrobacter species	1	2	1	1	1	1
Other Nonenterobacteriaceae aerobes	1	0	1	1	4	1
Group D streptococcus	1	2	2	1	0	1
Group B streptococcus	1	1	1	2	1	1
Haemophilus influenza	1	0	0	0	5	1
Other *Klebsiella* species	1	1	1	1	1	1
Other Enterobacteriaceae aerobes	1	0	1	0	1	1
Other gram-positive aerobes	1	0	2	1	0	2
Viruses	1	0	0	0	1	0
Bacteroides fragilis	1	0	2	1	0	0

UTI, urinary tract infection; SSI, surgical site infection; BSI, bloodstream infection; PNEU, pneumonia.
Data from the CDC's National Nosocomial Infections Surveillance (NNIS) system; 231 hospitals including community and teaching institutions provided data on all sites of nosocomial infections for all patients. Infection rates were calculated by service using hospital discharges or patient-days as the denominator. Data are cumulative for all hospital units (110).

Isolation precautions (4) are based on modes of transmission. Standard precautions include use of hand hygiene and use of gloves, gowns, and/or mask or face shield as needed for protection from stool, blood, or other body fluids.

A current concern is the potential for introduction of agents of bioterrorism into health care facilities. All patients suspected or diagnosed as infected with an agent of bioterrorism should be placed on standard isolation precautions. Patients with pneumonic plague and smallpox require additional precautions (121,122). Pneumonic plague requires droplet precautions until the patient has completed 72 hours of antimicrobial therapy. Droplet precautions mandate HCW masking within 3 feet of the patient, placing the patient in a private room, cohorting patients with the same symptoms in the same room if private rooms are not available, maintaining patient spatial separation of at least 3 feet when cohorting is not achievable, and avoiding placement of a patient requiring droplet precautions in the same room as an immunocompromised patient. Special air handling is unnecessary and the door may remain open. Smallpox requires airborne and contact precaution (see also Chapter 8) in addition to standard precautions (123). Health care facilities without appropriate negative pressure isolation rooms need a plan to transfer suspected or confirmed cases of smallpox to facilities that have the appropriate isolation rooms. When tularemia is in the differential diagnosis, microbiology personnel should be alerted to this possibility because of the risk for spread in the laboratory, such as manipulations of cultures of *Pasteurella tularemia* that may involve aerosolization or droplet production require biosafety level 3 (124). However, patients with pneumonic tularemia do not require droplet or airborne precautions given the lack of proven human-to-human transmission (125).

Antibiotic control can be achieved by formulary restriction policies, decided on the basis of local needs and patterns of resistance. Antibiotic cycling has been proposed as a measure to avoid excessive pressure from any single class of antimicrobial. Studies to evaluate this approach in ICUs are in progress.

Surveillance

Surveillance is considered an integral component of infection control programs. The methods of surveillance for nosocomial infections vary and include monitoring culture results and monitoring antimicrobial use. Nosocomial infection rates are measured per 100 admissions, per 1,000 patient-days, or per 1,000 device-days. Studies of VRE and ceftazidime-resistant gram-negative bacilli have shown that clinical cultures detect only a fraction of the total patients colonized—the resistance iceberg (118). For example, studies of VRE demonstrate that only 10% to 20% of patients colonized with VRE are detected by clinical culture results (126).

An additional method of surveillance, especially for antimicrobial-resistant strains, is to screen all or selected hospital admissions for colonization. Routine screening for MRSA colonization on admission to a pediatric ICU and weekly screening thereafter was part of a program that resulted in a decrease in MRSA colonization from 34% to 2% and a decrease in infection rates from 5.9 to 0.8 per 1,000 patient-days (127). This decline in MRSA infections was attributed to improved adherence with infection control measures, as a result of increased awareness of the extent of MRSA. Selective screening for other populations at high risk for MRSA colonization has been shown to reduce

ICU-acquired cases from 5.8% to 2.6% and has been recommended for use in high-risk populations (128,129).

The benefit of surveillance cultures depends on the extent of endemicity of target organisms. If there is low prevalence of a particular organism, efforts to isolate patients who may introduce such organisms into the hospital environment may be more successful. However, once the target strain becomes highly endemic, elimination of carriage may be more difficult (129,130). In the latter case, efforts and resources may be better directed toward increased staffing. Because of the potential expense, more evidence is necessary to demonstrate the benefit of surveillance culture programs (e.g., improved patient outcomes) before such programs can be recommended as a routine control measure (113).

Pathogen-Specific Control Measures

STAPHYLOCOCCUS AUREUS

The use of intranasal mupirocin for decontamination of S. aureus colonization, in patients or HCWs, is a controversial issue. Potential advantages of intranasal mupirocin include reduced colonization and infection rates in patients at risk for staphylococcal infection. Disadvantages include the possible need for repeated courses of treatment and for active culture surveillance for recolonization and the risk for development of S. aureus resistance to mupirocin or of colonization with gram-negative organisms. Although mupirocin does not have many traditional therapeutic indications, it has been an important agent used to control MRSA epidemics. An outbreak of MRSA in a neonatal ICU was controlled effectively with nasal mupirocin when conventional measures were unsuccessful (131). Several sources have recommended using an agent such as mupirocin to treat epidemiologically implicated HCWs who have MRSA nasal carriage (130,132–134). A consensus statement from the American Society of Consultant Pharmacists, Society for Healthcare Epidemiology (SHEA), and the National Association of Nursing Administration has endorsed the use of nasal mupirocin for colonized patients to control this reservoir during MRSA outbreaks (135).

Nasal mupirocin ointment has been used to decrease the rate of S. aureus colonization and infection in several populations. Randomized, controlled trials have examined the role of mupirocin in HCWs, in patients with recurrent staphyloccocal skin infections, and in patients with HIV. Recent attention has focused on mupirocin prophylaxis in dialysis patients and those undergoing cardiovascular surgery (136–141).

In a recent study, 854 open heart surgery patients treated with nasal mupirocin the night prior to surgery, the morning of surgery, and twice daily for five days postoperatively were compared to 992 historical control patients who were not given mupirocin prophylaxis intranasally. The rate of sternal wound infections declined significantly from 2.7% to 0.9%; a benefit was seen in patients with and without diabetes. The use of mupirocin was described as highly cost effective (approximately $13 per patient) based on an estimated average cost of $81,018 ± $41,567 for deep wound infections (141).

In studies of patients on peritoneal dialysis who received intranasal mupirocin, there was a significant increase in the proportion of peritonitis episodes due to gram-negative pathogens, from 9.2% to 23.1%, despite a significant reduction in proportion of S. aureus catheter exit site infections, from 90% to 44%. Recolonization with S. aureus occurred by 4 months in 48% of patients after a single 7-day course of 2% mupirocin nasal ointment (142). A multicenter, randomized controlled trial in which peritoneal dialysis patients were treated with intranasal mupirocin showed significantly fewer exit site infections, but there was no statistically significant effect on the incidence of other staphylococcal infections, including peritonitis and tunnel catheter infections. The overall cost of antibiotic therapy was greater in those patients treated with mupirocin (138,143). Daily application of mupirocin to peritoneal dialysis catheter exit sites has been compared with the use of oral rifampin in a cohort of dialysis patients; there was an equally significant reduction in S. aureus catheter infections, S. aureus peritonitis, and catheter loss due to S. aureus infections, with both regimens compared with historical controls (144). Resistance was not addressed in this study.

Controversy about the use of prophylactic mupirocin also involves the recognized risk for plasmid-mediated mupirocin resistance (145) and the durability of clearing S. aureus. Two studies of hemodialysis patients, both with historical controls, demonstrated a decline in S. aureus bacteremia in patients treated with nasal mupirocin. In one study, there were no mupirocin-resistant isolates in 67 patients followed for up to 6 months (137). In the other study, one case of resistance to mupirocin occurred after treatment for 19 months in a group of 80 patients followed for a total of 108 patient-years (136). However, high-level resistance to mupirocin [minimum inhibitory concentration (MIC) >700 mg/L] has been described in patients treated with mupirocin on an as-needed basis for dermatologic conditions (146). Furthermore, a study attempting to eradicate nasal MRSA carriage in patients at a Veterans Affairs long-term care facility demonstrated the development of eight strains of MRSA resistant to mupirocin among 65 colonized patients; one of the eight strains demonstrated high-level mupirocin resistance (MIC >5,000 µg/mL) (147). In five patients, the mupirocin-resistant strain had the same phage type as the patient's prior mupirocin-sensitive isolate; in two patients, the resistant strains differed from previous strains and were presumed to represent cross-infection; one isolate was not typed. Of the 65 patients who were treated with weekly maintenance mupirocin, 40% became recolonized with MRSA.

Masks are another intervention thought to prevent transient carriage and colonization of MRSA by HCWs; 27 staff members on two dedicated MRSA units were screened for MRSA with nasal, throat, and hand swabs before and after each 8-hour duty period. Masks, capable of filtering 1.0-µm particles, were worn by HCWs for intensive patient contact and for activities involving close contact with infected body sites. In the first phase, when staff did not wear masks, 48% were culture positive for MRSA; however, in the masking phase, 26% were positive. The wearing of masks was found to significantly reduce the number of acquisitions of MRSA by HCWs (148). Masking also has decreased shedding of MRSA from an HCW carrier who shed when he had URIs (36).

STREPTOCOCCUS PYOGENES

The Working Group on Prevention of Invasive Group A Streptococcal Infections recommended enhanced surveillance and limited epidemiologic investigation following one episode of nosocomial GAS infection on a surgical or obstetric ward (149). Following identification of a patient with postoperative or postpartum infection due to GAS, medical and laboratory records should be reviewed for other infections, and isolates should be stored for further epidemiologic analysis (149). Because GAS is an unusual cause of postoperative or postpartum infections and because surgical and obstetric patients are particularly vulnerable to infection, we suggest aggressive investigation of even a single case. Such investigations often reveal the source of infection to be colonized operating room (OR) staff; sites of colonization have included the anus (150–152), vagina (153,154), skin (155), and pharynx (156). For example in Toronto, Ontario, Canada, three of eight investigations of nosocomial GAS infections following a single case identified an asymptomatic carrier

(157). The presumed mode of transmission from OR staff is by droplets or possibly droplet nuclei.

When a postpartum patient develops a nosocomial GAS infection, screening is recommended for all HCWs present at delivery as well as those who performed vaginal examinations prior to delivery. For cases in postsurgical patients, screening should include all HCWs present in the OR and staff who changed dressings. HCWs may return to work pending culture results. If culture results are positive for GAS, implicated HCWs should avoid patient care for 24 hours while initiating appropriate antibiotic therapy and until culture negative (149,150,152,153,158). Analysis of epidemiologic data and strain typing results are needed to establish causation. Surveillance cultures of implicated HCWs should be done for up to a year since colonization may recur (149).

Selective Decontamination of the Digestive Tract

The risks and benefits of selective decontamination of the digestive tract (SDD) to prevent nosocomial infections, especially ventilator-associated pneumonia, have been debated for over 20 years. As an example of studies that have supported SDD, a recent multicenter randomized, double-blind, placebo-controlled trial showed decreased episodes of ventilator-associated pneumonia in a cohort of severely ill ICU patients (mean APACHE score 26.6), decreased length of stay, and decreased cost in patients treated with SDD. The SDD regimen consisted of topical gentamicin, polymixin E, and amphotericin B. However, there was no significant difference in mortality between the treated and placebo group. The authors attributed this finding to a small sample number (271 patients) (159).

Against the practice of SDD is the concern for the development of antibiotic resistance in gram-negative pathogens and the colonization of critically ill patients with organisms "selected" by SDD therapy, including MRSA, VRE, and resistant enterobacteriacae (159–161). For example, in the study cited above (159), there were significantly more positive cultures for MRSA in the SDD patients (109) than in the placebo group (43). Another randomized controlled trial at a tertiary care center demonstrated the emergence of tobramycin-resistant enterobacteriacae, ofloxacin-resistant gram-negative nonfermenters, and MRSA in the SDD patients (160).

Several metanalyses of SDD have been published (162,163), and the use of SDD continues to be debated (164). At this time the concern for colonization and subsequent infection with resistant pathogens appears to outweigh the benefits reported in trials of SDD.

EMERGING NOSOCOMIAL PATHOGENS

Infection control strategies in the future will need to address emerging resistant pathogens and agents of bioterrorism in addition to the ongoing need to shore up the traditional, but unfortunately cracked, cornerstones of infection control, such as hand hygiene and antibiotic stewardship.

Gram-negative challenges in the future include the potential for increasing rates of, and antibiotic resistance in, *Acinetobacter* and for more extended-spectrum β-lactamases (ESBLs). ESBLs in *Klebsiella, E. coli, Proteus mirabilis,* and Amp C resistance in *Enterobacter* and *Citrobacter freundii* are of increasing importance (165). ESBLs are becoming more prevalent in nursing home facilities that serve as reservoirs for resistant pathogens that may be transferred to and from hospitals (166).

Among the emerging nosocomial pathogens, non-albicans *Candida* organisms are an increasing problem due to extensive use of azole antifungal agents and a growing population of immunocompromised and immunosuppressed patients. Infection with *Candida parapsilosis* has been associated with personnel carriers (167), administration of parenteral nutrition, and use of intravascular devices (168,169). *Candida tropicalis* is a common cause of bacteremia (170) and UTIs (171,172). Fungemia due to *Candida krusei*, which is intrinsically resistant to fluconazole, has been reported with increasing frequency in patients with hematologic malignancy (173), and compared with *Candida albicans* fungemia, it had higher mortality rates (48% vs. 28%, respectively). *Fusarium* species have been linked to a hospital water distribution system as a reservoir for nosocomial infection (174). *Aspergillosis* continues to be a threat to immunocompromised patients, necessitating infection control surveillance of air quality during periods of hospital construction (10).

Aggressive application of proven infection control strategies, judicious use of current antibiotics, and the development of new antibiotics and devices that minimize the risk for infection are strategies to cope with these challenges.

	Precautions	
APPENDIX. Type and Duration of Precautions Needed for Selected Infections and Conditions		
Infection/condition	**Type[a]**	**Duration[b]**
Abscess		
Draining, major[c]	C	DI
Draining, minor or limited[d]	S	
Acquired immunodeficiency syndrome	S	
Actinomycosis	S	
Adenovirus infection, in infants and young children	D,C	DI
Amebiasis	S	
Anthrax		
Cutaneous	S	
Pulmonary	S	
Antibiotic-associated colitis (see *Clostridium difficile*)		
Arthropod-borne viral encephalitides (eastern, western, Venezuelan equine encephalomyelitis; St Louis, California encephalitis)	S[e]	
Arthropod-borne viral fevers (dengue, yellow fever, Colorado tick fever)	S[e]	
Ascariasis	S	

(continued)

APPENDIX. (*continued*)

Infection/condition	Precautions Type[a]	Precautions Duration[b]
Aspergillosis	S	
Babesiosis	S	
Blastomycosis, North American, cutaneous or pulmonary	S	
Botulism	S	
Bronchiolitis (see Respiratory infectious disease in infants and young children)		
Brucellosis (undulant, Malta, Mediterranean fever)	S	
Campylobacter gastroenteritis (see Gastroenteritis)		
Candidiasis, all forms including mucocutaneous	S	
Cat-scratch fever (benign inoculation lymphoreticulosis)	S	
Cellulitis, uncontrolled drainage	C	DI
Chancroid (soft chancre)	S	
Chickenpox (varicella; see F[f] for varicella exposure)	A,C	F[f]
Chlamydia trachomatis		
Conjunctivitis	S	
Genital	S	
Respiratory	S	
Cholera (see gastroenteritis)		
Closed-cavity infection		
Draining, limited or minor	S	
Not draining	S	
Clostridium		
C. botulinum	S	
C. difficile	C	DI
C. perfringens	S	
Food poisoning	S	
Gas gangrene	S	
Coccidioidomycosis (valley fever)		
Draining lesions	S	
Pneumonia	S	
Colorado tick fever	S	
Congenital rubella	C	F[g]
Conjunctivitis		
Acute bacterial	S	
Chlamydia	S	
Gonococcal	S	
Acute viral (acute hemorrhagic)	C	DI
Coxsackievirus disease (see Enteroviral infections)		
Creutzfeldt-Jakob disease	S[h]	
Croup (see Respiratory infectious disease in infants and young children)		
Cryptococcosis	S	
Cryptosporidiosis (see Gastroenteritis)		
Cysticercosis	S	
Cytomegalovirus infection, neonatal, or immunosuppressed	S	
Decubitus ulcer, infected		
Major[c]	C	DI
Minor or limited[d]	S	
Dengue	S[e]	
Diarrhea, acute-infective etiology suspected (see Gastroenteritis)		
Diphtheria		
Cutaneous	C	CN[i]
Pharyngeal	D	CN[i]
Ebola viral hemorrhagic fever	C[j]	DI
Echinococcosis (hydatidosis)	S	
Echovirus (see enteroviral infection)		
Encephalitis or encephalomyelitis (see specific etiologic agents)		
Endometritis	S	
Enterobiasis (pinworm disease, oxyuriasis)	S	
Enterococcus species (see Multidrug-resistant organisms if epidemiologically significant or vancomycin resistant)		
Enterocolitis, *Clostridium difficile*	C	DI
Enteroviral infections		
Adults	S	
Infants and young children	C	DI
Epiglottitis, due to *Haemophilus influenzae*	D	U[24 h]
Epstein-Barr virus infection, including infectious mononucleosis	S	
Erythema infectiosum (also see parvovirus B19)	S	
Escherichia coli gastroenteritis (see Gastroenteritis)		

(continued)

APPENDIX. (*continued*)

Infection/condition	Precautions	
	Type[a]	Duration[b]
Food poisoning	S	
Botulism	S	
Clostridium perfringens or *welchii*	S	
Staphylococcal	S	
Furunculosis-staphylococcal	C	DI
Infants and young children	S	
Gangrene (gas gangrene)		
Gastroenteritis	S[k]	
Campylobacter species	S[k]	
Cholera	C	DI
Clostridium difficile	S[k]	
Crytosporidium species		
Escherichia coli	S[k]	
Enterohemorrhagic O157:H7	C	DI
Diapered or incontinent	S[k]	
Other species	S[k]	
Giardia lamblia	S[k]	
Rotavirus	C	DI
Diapered or incontinent	S[k]	
Salmonella species (including *S. typhi*)	S[k]	
Shigella species	C	DI
Diapered or incontinent	S[k]	
Vibrio parahaemolyticus	S[k]	
Viral (if not covered elsewhere)	S[k]	
Yersinia enterocolitica	D	F[l]
German measles (rubella)		
Giardiasis (see Gastroenteritis)		
Gonococcal ophthalmia neonatorum (gonorrheal ophthalmia, acute conjunctivitis of newborn)	S	
Gonorrhea	S	
Granuloma inguinale (donovanosis, granuloma venereum)	S	
Guillain-Barré syndrome	S	
Hand, foot, and mouth disease (see Enteroviral infections)		
Hantavirus pulmonary syndrome	S	
Helicobacter pylori	S	
Hemorrhagic fevers (e.g., Lassa and Ebola)	C[j]	DI
Hepatitis, viral	S	
Type A	C	F[m]
Diapered or incontinent patients	S	
Type B, HBsAg positive	S	
Type C and other unspecified non-A, non-B	S	
Type E		
Herpangina (see Enteroviral infections)		
Herpes simplex (*Herpesvirus* hominid)	S	
Encephalitis	C	DI
Neonatal (see F[n] for neonatal exposure)	C	DI
Mucocutaneous, disseminated or primary, severe	S	
Mucocutaneous, recurrent (skin, oral, genital)		
Herpes zoster (varicella-zoster)	A,C	DI[o]
Localized in immunocompromised patient, or disseminated	S[o]	
Localized in normal patient	S	
Histoplasmosis	S	
Hookworm disease (ancylostomiasis, uncinariasis)	S	
Human immunodeficiency virus (HIV) infection	C	U[24h]
Impetigo	S	
Infectious mononucleosis	D[p]	DI
Influenza	S	
Kawasaki syndrome	C[j]	DI
Lassa fever	S	
Legionnaires' disease	S	
Leprosy	S	
Leptospirosis	C	U[24h]
Lice (pediculosis)	S	
Listeriosis	S	
Lyme disease	S	
Lymphocytic choriomeningitis	S	
Lymphogranuloma venereum	S[e]	
Malaria	C[j]	DI
Marburg virus disease		

(*continued*)

APPENDIX. (*continued*)

Infection/condition	Type[a]	Duration[b]
Measles (rubeola), all presentations	A	DI
Melioidosis, all forms	S	
Meningitis	S	
Aseptic [nonbacterial or viral meningitis (also see Enteroviral infections)]	S	
Bacterial, gram-negative enteric, in neonates	S	
Fungal	S	
Haemophilus influenzae, known or suspected	D	U^{24h}
Listeria monocytogenes	S	
Neisseria meningitidis (meningococcal) known or suspected	D	U^{24h}
Pneumococcal	S	
Tuberculosis[q]	S	
Other diagnosed bacterial	S	
Meningococcal pneumonia	D	U^{24h}
Meningococcemia (meningococcal sepsis)	D	U^{24h}
Molluscum contagiosum	S	
Mucormycosis	S	
Multidrug-resistant organisms, infection or colonization[r]		
Gastrointestinal	C	CN
Respiratory	C	CN
Pneumococcal	S	
Skin, wound, or burn	C	CN
Mumps (infectious parotitis)	D	F[s]
Mycobacteria, nontuberculosis (atypical)		
Pulmonary	S	
Wound	S	
Mycoplasma pneumonia	D	DI
Necrotizing enterocolitis	S	
Nocardiosis, draining lesions or other presentations	S	
Norwalk agent gastroenteritis (see Gastroenteritis viral)		
Orf	S	
Parainfluenza virus infection, respiratory in infants and young children	C	DI
Parvovirus B19	D	F[t]
Pediculosis (lice)	C	U^{24h}
Pertussis (whooping cough)	D	F[u]
Pinworm infection	S	
Plague		
Bubonic	S	
Pneumonic	D	U^{72h}
Pleurodynia (see Enteroviral infections)		
Pneumonia		
Adenovirus	D,C	DI
Bacterial not listed elsewhere (including gram-negative bacterial)	S	
Burkholderia cepacia in cystic fibrosis patients, including respiratory tract colonization	S[v]	
Chlamydia	S	
Fungal	S	
Haemophilus influenzae		
Adults	S	
Infants and children (any age)	D	U^{24h}
Legionella	S	
Meningococcal	D	U^{24h}
Multidrug-resistant bacterial (see multidrug-resistant organisms)		
Mycoplasma (primary atypical pneumonia)	D	DI
Pneumococcal		
Multidrug-resistant (see multidrug-resistant organisms)		
Pneumocystis carinii	S[w]	
Pseudomonas cepacia (see *Burkholderia cepacia*)	S[v]	
Staphylococcus aureus	S	
Streptococcus, group A		
Adults	S	
Infants and young children	D	U^{24h}
Viral		
Adults	S	
Infants and young children (see Respiratory infectious disease, acute)		
Poliomyelitis	S	

(continued)

APPENDIX. (*continued*)

Infection/condition	Precautions	
	Type[a]	Duration[b]
Psittacosis (ornithosis)	S	
Q fever	S	
Rabies	S	
Rat-bite fever (*Streptobacillus moniliformis* disease, *Spidllum minus* disease)	S	
Relapsing fever	S	
Resistant bacterial infection or colonization (see multidrug-resistant organisms)		
Respiratory infectious disease, acute (if not covered elsewhere)		
Adults	S	
Infants and young children[e]	C	DI
Respiratory syncytial virus infection, in infants and young children, and immunocompromised adults	C	DI
Reye's syndrome	S	
Rheumatic fever	S	
Rickettsial fevers, tick-borne (Rocky Mountain spotted fever, tick-borne typhus fever)	S	
Rickettsialpox (vesicular rickettsiosis)	S	
Ringworm (dermatophytosis, dermatomycosis, tinea)	S	
Ritter's disease (staphylococcal scalded skin syndrome)	S	
Rocky Mountain spotted fever	S	
Roseola infantum (exanthem subitum)	S	
Rotavirus infection (see Gastroenteritis)		
Rubella (German measles; also see Congenital rubella)	D	F[l]
Salmonellosis (see Gastroenteritis)		
Scabies	C	U[24h]
Scalded skin syndrome, staphylococcal (Ritter's disease)	S	
Schistosomiasis (bilharziasis)	S	
Severe acute respiratory syndrome	A,C,S	F[y]
Shigellosis (see gastroenteritis)		
Sporotrichosis	S	
Spirillum minus disease (rat bite fever)	S	
Staphylococcal disease (*S. aureus*)		
Skin, wound, or burn		
Major[c]	C	DI
Minor or limited[d]	S	
Enterocolitis	S[k]	
Multidrug-resistant (see multidrug-resistant organisms)		
Pneumonia	S	
Scalded skin syndrome	S	
Toxic shock syndrome	S	
Streptobacillus moniliformis disease (rat bite fever)	S	
Streptococcal disease (group A streptococcus)		
Skin, wound, or burn		
Major[c]	C	U[24h]
Minor or limited[d]	S	
Endometritis (puerperal sepsis)	S	
Pharyngitis in infants and young children	D	U[24h]
Pneumonia in infants and young children	D	U[24h]
Scarlet fever in infants and young children	D	U[24h]
Streptococcal disease (group B streptococcus), neonatal	S	
Streptococcal disease (not group A or B) unless covered elsewhere	S	
Multidrug-resistant (see multidrug-resistant organisms)		
Strongyloidiasis	S	
Syphilis		
Skin and mucous membrane, including congenital, primary, secondary	S	
Latent (tertiary) and seropositivity without lesions	S	
Tapeworm disease		
Hymenolepis nana	S	
Taenia solium (pork)	S	
Other	S	
Tetanus	S	
Tinea (fungus infection dermatophytosis, dermatomycosis, ringworm)	S	
Toxoplasmosis	S	
Toxic shock syndrome (staphylococcal disease)	S	
Trachoma, acute	S	
Trench mouth (Vincent's angina)	S	
Trichinosis	S	
Trichomoniasis	S	
Trichuriasis (whipworm disease)	S	

(*continued*)

APPENDIX. (*continued*)

Infection/condition	Precautions Type[a]	Precautions Duration[b]
Tuberculosis		
Extrapulmonary, draining lesion (including scrofula)	S	
Extrapulmonary, meningitis[q]	S	
Pulmonary, confirmed or suspected or laryngeal disease	A	F[x]
Skin test positive with no evidence of current pulmonary disease	S	
Tularemia		
Draining lesion	S	
Pulmonary	S	
Typhoid (*Salmonella typhi*) fever (see Gastroenteritis)		
Typhus, endemic and epidemic	S	
Urinary tract infection (including pyelonephritis), with or without urinary catheter	S	
Varicella (chickenpox)	A,C	F[f]
Vibrio parahaemolyticus (see Gastroenteritis)		
Vincent's angina (trench mouth)	S	
Viral diseases		
Respiratory (if not covered elsewhere)		
Adults	S	
Infants and young children (see Respiratory infectious disease, acute)		
Whooping cough (pertussis)	D	F[u]
Wound infections		
Major[c]	C	DI
Minor or limited[d]	S	
Yersinia enterocolitica gastroenteritis (see Gastroenteritis)		
Localized in immunocompromised patient, disseminated	A,C	DI[o]
Localized in normal patient	S[o]	
Zygomycosis (phycomycosis, mucormycosis)	S	
Zoster (varicella-zoster) (see herpes zoster)		

[a] Type of precautions: A, airborne; C, contact; D, droplet; S, standard; when A, C, and D are specified, also use S.

[b] Duration of precautions: CN, until off antibiotics and culture-negative; DI, duration of illness (with wound lesions, DI means until they stop draining); U, until time specified in hours (h) after initiation of effective therapy; and F, see footnote letter.

[c] No dressing or dressing does not adequately contain drainage.

[d] Dressing covers and contains drainage adaquately.

[e] Install screens in windows and doors in endemic areas.

[f] Maintain precautions until all lesions are crusted. The average incubation period for varicella is 10 to 16 days, with a range of 10 to 21 days. After exposure, use varicella zoster immune globulin (VZIG) when appropriate, and discharge susceptible patients if possible. Place exposed susceptible patients on airborne precautions beginning 10 days after exposure and continuing until 21 days after last exposure (up to 28 days if VZIG has been given). Susceptible persons should not enter the room of patients on precautions if other immune caregivers are available.

[g] Place infant on precautions during any admission until 1 year of age, unless nasopharyngeal and urine cultures are negative for virus after age 3 months.

[h] Additional special precautions are necessary for handling and decontamination of blood, body fluids and tissues, and contaminated items from patients with confirmed or suspected disease. See latest College of American Pathologists (Northfield, IL) guidelines or other references.

[i] Until two cultures taken at least 24 hours apart are negative.

[j] Call state health department and CDC for specific advice about management of a suspected case.

[k] Use Contact Precautions for diapered or incontinent children <6 years of age for duration of illness.

[l] Until 7 days after onset of rash.

[m] Maintain precautions in infants and children <3 years of age for duration of hospitalization; in children 3 to 14 years of age, until 2 weeks after onset of symptoms; and in others, until 1 week after onset of symptoms.

[n] For infants delivered vaginally or by C-section and if mother has active infection and membranes have been ruptured for more than 4 to 6 hours.

[o] Persons susceptible to varicella are also at risk for developing varicella when exposed to patients with herpes zoster lesions; therefore, susceptible persons should not enter the room if other immune caregivers are available.

[p] Many hospitals encounter logistic difficulties and physical plant limitations when admitting multiple patients with suspected influenza during community outbreaks. If sufficient private rooms are unavailable, consider cohorting patients, or, at the very least, avoid room sharing with high-risk patients.

[q] Patient should be examined for evidence of current (active) pulmonary tuberculosis. If evidence exists, additional precautions are necessary (see tuberculosis).

[r] Resistant bacteria judged by the infection control program, based on current state, regional, or national recommendations, to be of special clinical and epidemiologic significance.

[s] For 9 days after onset of swelling.

[t] Maintain precautions for duration of hospitalization when chronic disease occurs in an immunodeficient patient. For patients with transient aplastic crisis or red-cell crisis, maintain precautions for 7 days.

[u] Maintain precautions until 5 days after patient is placed on effective therapy.

[v] Avoid cohorting or placement in the same room with a cystic fibrosis (CF) patient who is not infected or colonized with *B cepacia*. Persons with CF who visit or provide care and are not infected or colonized with *B cepacia* may elect to wear a mask when within 3 feet of a colonized or infected patient.

[w] Avoid placement in the same room with an immunocompromised patient.

[x] Discontinue precautions only when TB patient is on effective therapy, is improving clinically, and has three consecutive negative sputum smears collected on different days, or TB is ruled out.

[y] Discontinue precautions only 10 days after resolution of fever, provided respiratory symptoms are absent or improving. See SARS website for further information (*www.cdc.gov/ncidod/sars/*).

Table adapted from (1).

REFERENCES

1. Fridkin SK. Vancomycin-intermediate and -resistant *Staphylococcus aureus*: what the infectious disease specialist needs to know. *Clin Infect Dis* 2001;32:108–115.
2. *www.cdc.gov/ncidod/hip/default.htm*.
3. Prevention of perinatal group B streptococcal disease: a public health perspective. *MMWR* 1996;45:1–24.
4. Garner JS for the Hospital Infection Control Practices Advisory Committee. Guideline for isolation precautions in hospitals. *Infect Control Hosp Epidemiol* 1996;17:53–80.
5. Maki DG, Stolz SM, Wheeler S, et al. Prevention of central venous catheter-related bloodstream infection by use of an antiseptic-impregnated catheter. *Ann Intern Med* 1997;127:257–266.
6. Hayden MK, Blom DW, Lyle EA, et al. The risk of hand and glove contamination by healthcare workers (HCWs) after contact with a VRE (+) patient (pt) or the pt's environment (env) [Abstract K-1334]. 41st ICAAC Abstracts, Chicago, IL, September 22–25, 2001.
7. Austin DJ, Bonten MJM, Weinstein RA, et al. Vancomycin-resistant enterococci in intensive-care hospital settings: transmission dynamics, persistence, and the impact of infection control programs. *Proc Natl Acad Sci USA* 1999;96:6908–6913.
8. Jucker BA, Harms H, Zehnder AJB. Adhesion of the positively charged bacterium *Stenotrophomonas* (*Xanthomonas*) *maltophilia* 70401 to glass and Teflon. *J Bacteriol* 1996;178:5472–5479.
9. Anaissie EJ, Costa SF. Nosocomial *Aspergillosis* is waterborne. *Clin Infect Dis* 2001;33:1546–1548.
10. Cheng SM, Streifel AJ. Infection control considerations during construction activities: land excavation and demolition. *Am J Infect Control* 2001;29:321–328.
11. Bonten MJM, Slaughter S, Ambergen AW, et al. The role of "colonization pressure" in the spread of vancomycin-resistant enterococci. *Arch Intern Med* 1998;158:1127–1132.
12. Viglionese A, Nottebart VF, Bodman A, et al. Recurrent group A streptococcal carriage in a health care worker associated with widely separated nosocomial outbreaks. *Am J Med* 1991;91:3295–3335.
13. Griffith SJ, Nathan C, Selander RK, et al. The epidemiology of *Pseudomonas aeruginosa* in oncology patients in a general hospital. *J Infect Dis* 1989;160:1030–1036.
14. Flynn DM, Weinstein RA, Kabins SA. Infections with gram-negative bacilli in a cardiac surgery intensive care unit: the relative role of *Enterobacter*. *J Hosp Infect* 1988;11(suppl A):367–373.
15. Flynn DM, Weinstein RA, Nathan C, et al. Patients' endogenous flora as the source of "nosocomial" *Enterobacter* in cardiac surgery. *J Infect Dis* 1987;156:363–368.
16. Olson B, Weinstein RA, Nathan C, et al. Epidemiology of endemic *Pseudomonas aeruginosa*: why infection control efforts have failed. *J Infect Dis* 1984;150:808–816.
17. Turck M, Stamm W. Nosocomial infection of the urinary tract. *Am J Med* 1981;70:651–654.
18. Jarvis WR, Munn VP, Highsmith AK, et al. The epidemiology of nosocomial infections caused by *Klebsiella pneumoniae*. *Infect Control* 1985;6:68–74.
19. Gaynes RP, Weinstein RA, Chamberlin W, et al. Antibiotic-resistant flora in nursing home patients admitted to the hospital. *Arch Intern Med* 1985;145:1804–1807.
20. Garibaldi RA. Residential care and the elderly: the burden of infection. *J Hosp Infect* 1999;43(suppl):9–18.
21. Dennesen PJW, Bonten MJM, Weinstein RA. Multiresistant bacteria as a hospital epidemic problem. *Ann Med* 1998;30:176–185.
22. Trick WE, Weinstein RA, DeMarais PL, et al. Colonization of skilled-care facility residents with antimicrobial-resistant pathogens. *J Am Geriatr Soc* 2001;49:270–276.
23. Noskin GA, Stosor V, Cooper I, et al. Recovery of vancomycin-resistant enterococci on fingertips and environmental surfaces. *Infect Control Hosp Epidemiol* 1995;16:577–581.
24. Noskin GA, Bednarz P, Suriano T, et al. Persistent contamination of fabric-covered furniture by vancomycin-resistant enterococci: implications for upholstery selection in hospitals. *Am J Infect Control* 2000;28:311–313.
25. Wilcox MH, Fawley WN. Hospital disinfectants and spore formation by *Clostridium difficile*. *Lancet* 2000;356:2098–2099.
26. Worsley MA. Infection control and prevention of *Clostridium difficile* infection. *J Antimicrob Chemother* 1998;41:59–65.
27. Foulke GE, Silva J. *Clostridium difficile* in the intensive care unit: management problems and prevention issues. *Crit Care Med* 1989;17:822–826.
28. Merighi A, Contato E, Scagliarini R, et al. Quality improvement in gastrointestinal endoscopy: microbiologic surveillance of disinfection. *Gastrointest Endosc* 1996;43:457–462.
29. Spach DH, Silverstein FE, Stamm WE. Transmission of infection by gastrointestinal endoscopy and bronchoscopy. *Ann Intern Med* 1993;118:117–128.
30. Wendt C, Dietze B, Dietz E, et al. Survival of *Acinetobacter baumannii* on dry surfaces. *J Clin Microbiol* 1997;35:1394–1397.
31. Bonten MJM, Austin DJ, Lipsitch M. Understanding the spread of antibiotic resistant pathogens in hospitals: mathematical models as tools for control. *Clin Infect Dis* 2001;33:1739–1746.
32. Merrer J, Santoli F, Appere-De Vecchi C, et al. "Colonization pressure" and risk of acquisition of methicillin-resistant *Staphylococcus aureus* in a medical intensive care unit. *Infect Control Hosp Epidemiol* 2000;21:718–723.
33. Bonten MJM, Bergmans DCJJ, Speijer H, et al. Characteristics of polyclonal endemicity of *Pseudomonas aeruginosa* colonization in intensive care units. *Am J Respir Crit Care Med* 1999;160:1212–1219.
34. Zambon M, Bull T, Sadler CJ, et al. Molecular epidemiology of two consecutive outbreaks of parainfluenza 3 in a bone marrow transplant unit. *J Clin Microbiol* 1998;36:2289–2293.
35. Eichenwald H, Kotsevalov O, Fasso LA. The "cloud baby": an example of bacterial-viral interaction. *Am J Dis Child* 1960;100:161–173.
36. Sherertz RJ, Reagen DR, Hampton KD, et al. A cloud adult: the *Staphylococcus aureus*–virus interaction revisited. *Ann Intern Med* 1996;124:539–547.
37. McDonald LC, Walker M, Carson L, et al. Outbreaks of *Acinetobacter* spp. bloodstream infections in a nursery associated with contaminated aerosols and air conditioners. *Pediatr Infect Dis J* 1998;17:716–722.
37a. Centers for Disease Control and Prevention. Cluster of severe acute respiratory syndrome cases among protected health-care workers. *MMWR* 2003; 52(19):433–436.
38. Mastrobattista JM, Parisi VM. Vertical transmission of a *Citrobacter* infection. *Am J Perinatol* 1997;14:465–467.
39. Waggoner-Fountain LA, Walker MW, Hollis RJ, et al. Vertical and horizontal transmission of unique *Candida* species to premature newborns. *Clin Infect Dis* 1996;22:803–808.
40. Fridkin SK, Welbel SF, Weinstein RA. Magnitude and prevention of nosocomial infections in the intensive care unit. *Infect Dis Clin North Am* 1997;11:479–496.
41. Richards MJ, Edwards JR, Culver DH, et al. Nosocomial infections in medical intensive care units in the United States. *Crit Care Med* 1999;27:887–892.
42. Bonten MJM, Weinstein RA. Bird's-eye view of nosocomial infections in medical ICU: blue bugs, fungi, and device-days. *Crit Care Med* 1999;27:853–854.
43. Montecalvo MA, Horowitz H, Cedris C, et al. Outbreak of vancomycin, ampicillin, and aminoglycoside-resistant *Enterococcus faecium* bacteremia in an adult oncology unit. *Antimicrob Agents Chemother* 1994;38:1363–1367.
44. Edmond MB, Ober JF, Weinbaum DL. Vancomycin-resistant *Enterococcus faecium* bacteremia: risk factors for infection. *Clin Infect Dis* 1995;20:1126–1133.
45. Henning KJ, Delencastre H, Eagan J, et al. Vancomycin-resistant *Enterococcus faecium* on a pediatric oncology ward: duration of stool shedding and incidence of clinical infection. *Pediatr Infect Dis J* 1996;15:848–854.
46. Linden PK, Pasculle AW, Manez R, et al. Differences in outcomes for patients with bacteremia due to vancomycin-resistant *Enterococcus faecium* or vancomycin-susceptible *E. faecium*. *Clin Infect Dis* 1996;22:663–670.
47. Hayden MK. Insights into the epidemiology and control of infection with vancomycin-resistant enterococci. *Clin Infect Dis* 2000;31:1058–1065.
48. Hayden MK. Vancomycin-resistant enterococci: a threat for the ICU?—U.S. Perspective. In: Weinstein RA, Bonten MJM, eds. *Infection control in the ICU environment*. Boston: Kluwer Academic, 2002:33–56.
49. Fierobe L, Lucet JC, Decre D, et al. An outbreak of imipenem-resistant *Acinetobacter baumannii* in critically ill surgical patients. *Infect Control Hosp Epidemiol* 2001;22:35–40.
50. Husni RN, Goldstein LS, Arroliga AC, et al. Risk factors for an outbreak of multi-drug resistant *Acinetobacter* nosocomial pneumonia among intubated patients. *Chest* 1999;115:1378–1382.
51. Wisplinghoff H, Perbix W, Seifert H. Risk factors for nosocomial bloodstream infections due to *Acinetobacter baumannii*: a case-control study of adult burn patients. *Clin Infect Dis* 1999;28:59–66.
52. Baraibar J, Correa H, Mariscal D, et al. Risk factors for infection by *Acinetobacter baumannii* in intubated patients with nosocomial pneumonia. *Chest* 1997;112:1050–1054.
53. Koeleman JGM, Parlevliet GA, Dijkshoorn L, et al. Nosocomial outbreak of multi-resistant *Acinetobacter baumannii* on a surgical ward: epidemiology and risk factors for acquisition. *J Hosp Infect* 1997;37:113–123.
54. Kaul R, Burt JA, Cork L. Investigation of a multiyear multiple critical care unit outbreak due to relatively drug-sensitive *Acinetobacter baumannii*: risk factors and attributable mortality. *J Infect Dis* 1996;174:1279–1287.
55. Scerpella EG, Wanger AR, Armitige L, et al. Nosocomial outbreak caused by a multiresistant clone of *Acinetobacter baumannii*: results of the case-control and molecular epidemiologic investigations. *Infect Control Hosp Epidemiol* 1995;16:92–97.
56. Tilley PAG, Roberts FJ. Bacteremia with *Acinetobacter* species: risk factors and prognosis in different clinical settings. *Clin Infect Dis* 1994;18:896–900.
57. Gomez J, Simarro E, Banos V, et al. Six-year prospective study of risk and prognostic factors in patients with nosocomial sepsis caused by *Acinetobacter baumannii*. *Eur J Clin Microbiol Infect Dis* 1999;18:358–361.
58. Garcia-Garmendia JL, Ortiz-Leyba C, Garnacho-Montero J, et al. Risk factors for *Acinetobacter baumannii* nosocomial bacteremia in critically ill patients: a cohort study. *Clin Infect Dis* 2001;33:939–946.
59. Mulin B, Talon D, Viel JF, et al. Risk factors for nosocomial colonization with multiresistant *Acinetobacter baumannii*. *Eur J Clin Microbiol Infect Dis* 1995;14:569–576.
60. Krcmery V, Sykora P, Trupl J, et al. Antibiotic use and development of resistance in blood culture isolates: 8 years of experience from a cancer referral center. *J Chemother* 2001;13:133–142.
61. Talmaciu I, Varlotta L, Mortensen J, et al. Risk factors for emergence of *Stenotrophomonas maltophilia* in cystic fibrosis. *Pediatr Pulmonol* 2000;30:10–15.
62. Denton M, Kerrr KG. Microbiological and clinical aspects of infection associated with *Stenotrophomonas maltophilia*. *Clin Microbiol Rev* 1998;11:67–80.

63. VanCouwenberghe CJ, Farver TB, Cohen SH. Risks factors associated with isolation of *Stenotrophomonas* (*Xanthomonas*) *maltophilia* in clinical specimens. *Infect Control Hosp Epidemiol* 1997;18:316–321.

64. Labarca JA, Leber AL, Kern VL, et al. Outbreak of *Stenotrophomonas maltophilia* bacteremia in allogenic bone marrow transplant patients: role of severe neutropenia and mucositis. *Clin Infect Dis* 2000;30:195–197.

65. Duse AG. Nosocomial infections in HIV-infected/AIDS patients. *J Hosp Infect* 1999;43(suppl):191–201.

66. Craven DE, Steger KA, Hirschhorn LR. Nosocomial colonization and infection in persons infected with human immunodeficiency virus. *Infect Control Hosp Epidemiol* 1996;17:304–318.

67. DeMarais PL, Gertzen J, Weinstein RA. Nosocomial infections in human immunodeficiency virus–infected patients in a long-term-care setting. *Clin Infect Dis* 1997;25:1230–1232.

68. Baltimore RS. Neonatal nosocomial infections. *Semin Perinatol* 1998;22:25–32.

69. Laing RBS. Nosocomial infections in patients with HIV disease. *J Hosp Infect* 1999;43:179–185.

70. Barnes PF, Bloch AB, Davidson PT, et al. Tuberculosis in patients with human immunodeficiency virus infection. *N Engl J Med* 1991;324:1644–1650.

71. Couldwell DL, Dore GJ, Harkness JL, et al. Nosocomial outbreak of tuberculosis in an outpatient HIV treatment room. *AIDS* 1996;10:521–525.

72. Witt DJ, Craven DE, McCabe WR. Bacterial infections in adult patients with the acquired immune deficiency syndrome (AIDS) and AIDS-related complex. *Am J Med* 1987;82:900–906.

73. Goetz AM, Squier C, Wagener MM, et al. Nosocomial infections in the human immunodeficiency virus–infected patient: a two-year survey. *Am J Infect Control* 1994;23:334–339.

74. Blumberg HM, Rimland D. Nosocomial infection with penicillin-resistant pneumococci in patients with AIDS. *J Infect Dis* 1989;160:725–726.

75. Chave JP, David S, Wauters JP. Transmission of *Pneumocystis carinii* from AIDS patients to other immunosuppressed patients: a cluster of *Pneumocystis carinii* pneumonia in renal transplant recipients. *AIDS* 1991;5:927–932.

76. Jacobson MA, Gellerman H, Chambers H. *Staphylococcus aureus* bacteremia and recurrent staphylococcal infection in patients with acquired immunodeficiency syndrome and AIDS-related complex. *Am J Med* 1988;85:172–176.

77. Dropulic LK, Leslie JM, Eldred LJ, et al. Clinical manifestations and risk factors of *Pseudomonas aeruginosa* infection in patients with AIDS. *J Infect Dis* 1995;171:930–937.

78. Barbut F, Mario N, Meyhohas MC, et al. Investigation of a nosocomial outbreak of *Clostridium difficile*-associated diarrhoea among AIDS patients by random amplified polymorphic DNA (RAPD) assay. *J Hosp Infect* 1994;26:181–189.

79. Paton S, Nicolle L, Mwongera M, et al. *Salmonella* and *Shigella* gastroenteritis at public teaching hospital in Nairobi, Kenya. *Infect Control Hosp Epidemiol* 1991;12:710–717.

80. Ravn P, Lundgren JD, Kjaelgaard P, et al. Nosocomial outbreak of cryptosporidiosis in AIDS patients. *BMJ* 1991;302:277–280.

81. Koch KL, Phillips DJ, Aber RC, et al. Cryptosporidiosis in hospital personnel. *Ann Intern Med* 1985;102:593–596.

82. von Reyne CF, Maslow JN, Barber TW, et al. Persistent colonization of potable water as a source of *Mycobacterium avium* infection in AIDS. *Lancet* 1994;343:1137–1141.

83. Blatt SP, Dolan MJ, Hendrix CW. Legionnaires' disease in human immunodeficiency virus-infected patients: eight cases and review. *Clin Infect Dis* 1994;18:227–232.

84. Sirera G, Romeu J, Ribera M, et al. Hospital outbreak of scabies stemming from two AIDS patients with Norwegian Scabies. *Lancet* 1990;335:1227.

85. Gaynes RP, Edwards JR, Jarvis WR, et al. Nosocomial infections among neonates in high-risk nurseries in the United States. *Pediatrics* 1996;98:357–361.

86. Beck-Sague CM, Azimi P, Fonseca SN, et al. Bloodstream infections in neonatal intensive care unit patients: results of a multicenter study. *Pediatr Infect Dis J* 1994;13:1110–1116.

87. Foster TJ, Hook M. Surface protein adhesins of *Staphylococcus aureus*. *Trends Microbiol* 1998;6:484–488.

88. Herrmann M, Vaudaux PE, Pittet D, et al. Fibronectin, fibrinogen, and laminin act as mediators of adherence of clinical staphylococcal isolates to foreign material. *J Infect Dis* 1988;158:693–701.

89. John JF, Barg NL. *Staphylococcus aureus*. In: Mayhall CG, ed. *Hospital epidemiology and infection control.* Philadelphia: Lippincott Williams & Wilkins, 1999:325–345.

90. Stamm WE. Catheter-associated urinary tract infections: epidemiology, pathogenesis, and prevention. *Am J Med* 1991;91(suppl):65–71.

91. Mobley HLT, Chippendale GW, Tenney JH, et al. MR/K hemagglutination of *Providencia stuartii* correlates with adherence to catheters and with persistence in catheter-associated bacteriuria. *J Infect Dis* 1988;157:264–271.

92. Wade JJ, Desai N, Casewell MW. Hygienic hand disinfection for the removal of epidemic vancomycin-resistant *Enterococcus faecium* and gentamicin-resistant *Enterobacter cloacae*. *J Hosp Infect* 1991;18:211–218.

93. Gordon CLA, Ahmad MH. Thermal susceptibility of *Streptococcus faecium* strains isolated from frankfurters. *Can J Microbiol* 1991;37:609–612.

94. Zimakoff J, Hoiby N, Rosendal K, et al. Epidemiology of *Pseudomonas aeruginosa* infection and the role of contamination in a cystic fibrosis clinic. *J Hosp Infect* 1983;4:31–40.

95. Martone WJ, Tablan OC, Jarvis WR. The epidemiology of nosocomial epidemic *Pseudomonas cepacia* infections. *Eur J Epidemiol* 1987;3:222–232.

96. Arnow PM, Flaherty JP. Nonfermentative gram-negative bacilli. In: Mayhall CG, ed. *Hospital epidemiology and infection control.* Philadelphia: Lippincott Williams & Wilkins, 1999:431–451.

97. Dixon RE, Kaslow RA, Mackel DC, et al. Aqueous quaternary ammonium antiseptics and disinfectants. *JAMA* 1976;236:2415–2417.

98. Frank MJ, Schaffner W. Contaminated aqueous benzalkonium chloride. *JAMA* 1976;236:2418–2419.

99. Ovchinnikov AA, Dratvin SA, Pilavina LV. On the methods of disinfecting bronchofibroscopes. *J Hyg Epidemiol Microbiol Immunol* 1990;34:371–379.

100. Shiraishi T, Nakagawa Y. Review of disinfectant susceptibility of bacteria isolated in hospital to commonly used disinfectants. *Postgrad Med J* 1993;69(suppl):70–77.

101. Anderson RL, Bland LA, Favero MS, et al. Factors associated with *Pseudomonas pickettii* intrinsic contamination of commercial respiratory therapy solutions marketed as sterile. *Appl Environ Microbiol* 1985;50:1343–1348.

102. Levin MH, Olson B, Nathan C, et al. Pseudomonas in the sinks in an intensive care unit: relation to patients. *J Clin Pathol* 1984;37:424–427.

103. Orsi GB, Mansi A, Tomao P, et al. Lack of association between clinical and environmental isolates of *Pseudomonas aeruginosa* in hospital wards. *J Hosp Infect* 1994;27:49–60.

104. Sherertz RJ, Sullivan ML. An outbreak of infections with *Acinetobacter calcoaceticus* in burn patients: contamination of patients' mattresses. *J Infect Dis* 1985;151:252–258.

105. Weernink A, Severin WPJ, Tjernberg I, et al. Pillows, an unexpected source of *Acinetobacter*. *J Hosp Infect* 1995;29:189–199.

106. Buxton AE, Anderson RL, Werdegar D, et al. Nosocomial respiratory tract infection and colonization with *Acinetobacter calcoaceticus*. *Am J Med* 1978;65:507–513.

107. Graham DR, Band JD. *Citrobacter diversus* brain abscess and meningitis in neonates. *JAMA* 1981;245:1923–1925.

108. Kline MW, Kaplan SL, Hawkins EP, et al. Pathogenesis of brain abscess formation in an infant rat model of *Citrobacter diversus* bacteremia and meningitis. *J Infect Dis* 1988;157:106–112.

109. Parry MF, Hutchinson JH, Brown NA, et al. Gram-negative sepsis in neonates: a nursery outbreak due to hand carriage of *Citrobacter diversus*. *Pediatrics* 1980;65:1105–1109.

110. Hospital Infections Program, Centers for Disease Control. National Nosocomial Infections Surveillance (NNIS) report, data summary from October 1986–April 1996, issued May 1996. *Am J Infect Control* 1996;24:380–388.

111. National Nosocomial Infections Surveillance semiannual report. December 2000.

112. Treger TR, Visscher DW, Bartlett MS, et al. Diagnosis of pulmonary infection caused by *Aspergillus*: usefulness of respiratory cultures. *J Infect Dis* 1985;152:572–576.

113. Flaherty JP, Wiener J, Weinstein RA. Conventional infection control measures: value or ritual? In: Weinstein RA, Bonten MJM, eds. *Infection control in the ICU environment.* Boston: Kluwer Academic, 2002:195–211.

114. Larson E, Killien M. Factors influencing handwashing behavior of patient care personnel. *Am J Infect Control* 1982;10:93–99.

115. *www.cdc.gov/ncidod/hip/hhguide.htm*

116. Tenorio AR, Badri SM, Sahgal NB, et al. Effectiveness of gloves in the prevention of hand carriage of vancomycin-resistant *Enterococcus* species by health care workers after patient care. *Clin Infect Dis* 2001;32:826–829.

117. Trick WE, DeMarais PL, Jarvis WR, et al. Comparison of universal gloving to contact isolation precautions to prevent transmission of multidrug-resistant bacteria in a long-term care facility [Abstract S-M2-03]. Presented at the 4th Decennial International Conference on Nosocomial and Healthcare-Associated Infections, Atlanta, GA, March 2000.

118. Weinstein RA. Epidemiology and control of nosocomial infections in adult intensive care units. *Am J Med* 1991;3B(suppl):179–184.

119. Stamm WE, Weinstein RA, Dixon RE. Comparison of endemic and epidemic nosocomial infections. *Am J Med* 1981;70:393–397.

120. Weinstein RA. Controlling antimicrobial resistance in hospitals: infection control and use of antibiotics. *Emerg Infect Dis* 2001;7:1–5.

121. *www/bt/cdc/gov/*

122. *www.cdc.gov/ncidod/hip/Bio/13apr99APIC-CDCBioterrorism.PDF*

123. *www.bt.cdc.gov/DocumentsApp/smallpox/RPG/index.asp*

124. *www.cdc.gov/od/ohs/biosfty/biosafty.htm#GUIDELINES*

125. Dennis DT, Inglesby TV, Henderson DA, et al. Tularemia as a biological weapon. *JAMA* 2001;285:2763–2773.

126. Bonten MJM, Hayden MK, Nathan C, et al. Epidemiology of colonization of patients and environment with vancomycin-resistant enterococci. *Lancet* 1996;348:1615–1619.

127. Zerbib MC, Afonso AMR, Naas T, et al. A control programme for MRSA (methicillin-resistant *Staphylococcus aureus*) containment in a paediatric intensive care unit: evaluation and impact on infections caused by other microorganisms. *J Hosp Infect* 1998;40:225–235.

128. Girou E, Pujade G, Legrand P, et al. Selective screening of carriers for control of methicillin-resistant *Staphylococcus aureus* (MRSA) in high-risk hospital areas with a high level of endemic MRSA. *Clin Infect Dis* 1998;27:543–550.

129. Barrett SP, Mummery RV, Chattopadhyay B. Trying to control MRSA causes more problems than it solves. *J Hosp Infect* 1998;39:85–93.

130. Mulligan ME, Murray-Leisure KA, Ribner BS, et al. Methicillin-resistant *Staphylococcus aureus*: a consensus review of the microbiology, pathogenesis, and epidemiology with implications for prevention and management. *Am J Med* 1993;94:313–328.

131. Hitcomi S, Kubota M, Mori N, et al. Control of a methicillin-resistant *Staphylococcus aureus* outbreak in a neonatal intensive care unit by unselective use of nasal mupirocin ointment. *J Hosp Infect* 2000;45:123–129.
132. Boyce JM. Methicillin-resistant *Staphylococcus aureus:* is control necessary? U.S. Point of view. In Weinstein RA, Bonten MJM, eds. *Infection contol in the ICU environment.* Boston: Kluwer Academic, 2002:57–65.
133. Boyce JM, Jackson MM, Pugliese G, et al. Methicillin-resistant *Staphylococcus aureus* (MRSA): a briefing for acute care hospitals and nursing facilities. *Infect Control Hosp Epidemiol* 1994;15:105–115.
134. Herwaldt LA. Control of methicillin-resistant *Staphylococcus aureus* in the hospital setting. *Am J Med* 1999;106(suppl):11–18.
135. Wenzel RP, Reagan DR, Bertino JS, et al. Methicillin-resistant *Staphylococcus aureus* outbreak: a consensus panel's definition and management guidelines. *Am J Infect Control* 1998;26:102–110.
136. Boelaert JR, van Landuyt HW, Godard CA, et al. Nasal mupirocin ointment decreases the incidence of *Staphylococcus aureus* bacteraemias in haemodialysis patients. *Nephrol Dial Transplant* 1993;8:235–239.
137. Kluytmans JAJW, Manders MJ, van Bommel E, et al. Elimination of nasal carriage of *Staphylococcus aureus* in hemodialysis patients. *Infect Control Hosp Epidemiol* 1996;17:793–797.
138. The Mupirocin Study Group. Nasal mupirocin prevents *Staphylococcus aureus* exit-site infection during peritoneal dialysis. *J Am Soc Nephrol* 1996;7:2403–2408.
139. Herwaldt LA. Reduction of *Staphylococcus aureus* nasal carriage and infection in dialysis patients. *J Hosp Infect* 1998;40(suppl):13–23.
140. Kluytmans J. Reduction of surgical site infections in major surgery by elimination of nasal carriage of *Staphylococcus aureus. J Hosp Infect* 1998;40(suppl):25–29.
141. Cimochowski GE, Harostock MD, Brown R, et al. Intranasal mupirocin reduces sternal wound infection after open heart surgery in diabetics and nondiabetics. *Ann Thorac Surg* 2001;71:1572–1579.
142. Perez-Fontan M, Garcia-Falcon T, Rosales M, et al. Treatment of *Staphylococcus aureus* nasal carriers in continuous ambulatory peritoneal dialysis with mupirocin: long-term results. *Am J Kidney Dis* 1993;22:708–712.
143. Davey P, Craig AM, Hau C, et al. Cost-effectiveness of prophylactic nasal mupirocin in patients undergoing peritoneal dialysis based on a randomized, placebo-controlled trial. *J Antimicrob Chemother* 1999;43:105–112.
144. Bernardini J, Piraino B, Holley J, et al. A randomized trial of *Staphylococcus aureus* prophylaxis in peritoneal dialysis patients: mupirocin calcium ointment 2% applied to the exit site versus cyclic oral rifampin. *Am J Kidney Dis* 1996;27:695–700.
145. Perez-Roth E, Claverie-Martin F, Villar J, et al. Multiplex PCR for simultaneous identification of *Staphylococcus aureus* and detection of methicillin and mupirocin resistance. *J Clin Microbiol* 2001;39:4037–4041.
146. Reginald PW, Kooner JS, Samarage SU. Intravenous dihydroergotamine to relieve pelvic congestion with pain in young women. *Lancet* 1987;15:387–388.
147. Kauffman CA, Terpenning MS, He X, et al. Attempts to eradicate methicillin-resistant *Staphylococcus aureus* from a long-term-care facility with the use of mupirocin ointment. *Am J Med* 1993;94:371–378.
148. Lacey S, Flaxman D, Scales J, et al. The usefulness of masks in preventing transient carriage of epidemic methicillin-resistant *Staphylococcus aureus* by healthcare workers. *J Hosp Infect* 2001;48:308–311.
149. MMWR Report. Nosocomial group A streptococcal infections associated with asymptomatic health-care workers—Maryland and California, 1997. *MMWR* 1999;48:163–166.
150. Schaffner W, Lefkowitz LB, Goodman JS, et al. Hospital outbreak of infections with group A streptococci traced to an asymptomatic anal carrier. *N Engl J Med* 1969;280:1224–1225.
151. Viglionese A, Nottebart VF, Bodman HA, et al. Recurrent group A streptococcal carriage in a health care worker associated with widely separated nosocomial outbreaks. *Am J Med* 1991;91(suppl):329–333.
152. McKee WM, DiCaprio JM, Roberts CE, et al. Anal carriage as the probable source of a streptococcal epidemic. *Lancet* 1966;2:1007–1009.
153. Stamm WE, Feeley JC, Facklama RR. Wound infections due to group A streptococcus traced to a vaginal carrier. *J Infect Dis* 1978;138:287–292.
154. Berkelman RL, Martin D, Graham DR, et al. Streptococcal wound infections caused by a vaginal carrier. *JAMA* 1982;247:2680–2682.
155. Mastro TD, Farley TA, Elliott JA, et al. An outbreak of surgical-wound infections due to group A streptococcus carried on the scalp. *N Engl J Med* 1990;323:968–972.
156. Paul SM, Genese C, Spitalny K. Postoperative group A β-hemolytic streptococcus outbreak with the pathogen traced to a member of a healthcare worker's household. *Infect Control Hosp Epidemiol* 1990;11:643–646.
157. Green K, Low D, Schwartz B, et al. Prospective surveillance for nosocomial group A streptococcal infections in Ontario: do single cases warrant an investigation? [Abstract 1393]. Presented at the 33rd Interscience Conference on Antimicrobial Agents and Chemotherapy, New Orleans, LA, October 1993.
158. The Working Group on Prevention of Invasive Group A Streptococcal Infections. Prevention of invasive group A streptococcal disease among household contacts of case patients. *JAMA* 1998;279:1206–1210.
159. Garcia MS, Galache JAC, Diaz JL, et al. Effectiveness and cost of selective decontamination of the digestive tract in critically ill intubates patients. *Am J Respir Crit Care Med* 1998;158:908–916.
160. Verwaest C, Verhaegen J, Ferdinande P, et al. Randomized, controlled trial of selective digestive decontamination in 600 mechanically ventilated patients in a multidisciplinary intensive care unit. *Crit Care Med* 1997;25:63–71.
161. Daschner F. Emergence of resistance during selective decontamination of the digestive tract. *Eur J Clin Microbiol Infect Dis* 1992;11:1–3.
162. Kollef MH. The role of selective digestive tract decontamination on mortality and respiratory tract infections. *Chest* 1994;105:1101–1108.
163. Selective Decontamination of the Digestive Tract Trialists' Collaborative Group. Meta-analysis of randomized controlled trials of selective decontamination of the digestive tract. *BMJ* 1993;307:525–532.
164. Daschner F. Selective decontamination of the digestive tract. *J Hosp Infect* 2001;47:69–77.
165. Jones RN. Resistance patterns among nosocomial pathogens: trends over the past few years. *Chest* 2001;119(suppl):397–404.
166. Wiener J, Quinn JP, Bradford PA, et al. Multiple antibiotic-resistant *Klebsiella* and *Escherichia coli* in nursing homes. *JAMA* 1999;281:517–523.
167. Saiman L, Ludington E, Dawson JD, et al. Risk factors for *Candida* species colonization of neonatal intensive care unit patients. *Pediatr Infect Dis J* 2001;20:1119–1124.
168. Weems JJ. *Candida parapsilosis:* epidemiology, pathogenicity, clinical manifestations, and antimicrobial susceptibility. *Clin Infect Dis* 1992;14:756–766.
169. Solomon SL, Alexander H, Eley JW, et al. Nosocomial fungemia in neonates associated with intravascular pressure-monitoring devices. *Pediatr Infect Dis* 1986;5:680–685.
170. Komshian SV, Uwaydah AK, Sobel JD, et al. Fungemia caused by *Candida* species and *Torulopsis glabrata* in the hospitalized patient: frequency, characteristics, and evaluation of factors influencing outcome. *Rev Infect Dis* 1989;11:379–390.
171. Weinberger M, Sacks T, Sulkes J, et al. Increasing fungal isolation from clinical specimens: experience in a university hospital over a decade. *J Hosp Infect* 1997;35:185–195.
172. Lundstrom T, Sobel J. Nosocomial candiduria: a review. *Clin Infect Dis* 2001;32:1602–1607.
173. Abbas J, Bodey GP, Hanna HA, et al. *Candida krusei* fungemia. *Arch Intern Med* 2000;160:2659–2664.
174. Anaissie EJ, Kuchar RT, Rex JH. Fusariosis associated with pathogenic *Fusarium* species colonization of a hospital water system: a new paradigm for the epidemiology of opportunistic mold infections. *Clin Infect Dis* 2001;33:1871–1878.

CHAPTER 10
Emerging Infections

Larry J. Strausbaugh and Daniel B. Jernigan

Humankind and its pathogens have evolved over many millennia in ways that maintain both a complex and dynamic relationship. Human populations, microorganisms, and their environments continue to change, as do their interactions and the lens through which medical science views them. These changes underlie the diverse and fluctuating landscape of clinical infectious disease. These fundamental considerations and their ramifications have received renewed attention and appreciation during the past decade.

BACKGROUND

Pandemics exemplify the role that emerging and reemerging infectious diseases have played throughout history (1) (Table 10.1). But every age and geographic location witness noteworthy alterations in patterns of infectious morbidity and mortality. During any given temporal period, new or reemerging infectious diseases appear in many locales (Table 10.2). Similarly, in any given geographic region, new infectious diseases appear over time (2) (Table 10.3). Despite the seeming primacy of these principles, an unparalleled wave of optimism in the 1950s and 1960s obscured their importance and diminished respect for their relevance.

This optimism arose from the progress made against infectious diseases in the United States and Western Europe during the first half of the twentieth century. By mid-century, improved

TABLE 10.1. Noteworthy Pandemics in Human History

Plague of Athens in 430 B.C.
The Black Death in Asia and Europe during the 14th century
Syphilis in Europe during the 15th and 16th centuries
Smallpox in the Americas during the 16th century
Cholera in America and Europe during the 19th century
Tuberculosis in America and Europe during 19th century
Spanish influenza in 1918
Acquired immunodeficiency syndrome in the late 20th and
    21st centuries

TABLE 10.3. New Infectious Diseases—United States, 1980 to Present

Human immunodeficiency virus infections and acquired
    immunodeficiency syndrome
Staphylococcal toxic shock syndrome
Escherichia coli O157:H7 infections
Cyclosporiasis
Ehrlichiosis
Streptococcal toxic shock syndrome
Bacillary angiomatosis
Hantavirus cardiopulmonary syndrome
West Nile virus meningoencephalitis

Adapted from McDade JE, Hughes JM. New and emerging infectious diseases. In: Mandell GL, Bennett JE, Dolin R, eds. *Principles and practice of infectious diseases,* 5th ed. Philadelphia: Churchill Livingstone, 2000:178–183, with permission.

measures for sanitation and food production as well as the development of vaccines and antimicrobial agents reduced rates of morbidity and mortality from infection to all-time lows. A statement attributed to then Surgeon General William Stewart in 1967 captured the hubris of the period: "The time has come to close the book on infectious diseases. We have basically wiped out infection in the United States" (3). Similarly, Sir McFarland Burnet, an immunologist and Nobel laureate, declared in 1962, "One can think of the middle of the twentieth century as the end of one of the most important social revolutions in history, the virtual elimination of the infectious diseases as a significant factor in social life" (4).

The optimism of this era slowly faded during the next two decades as a series of events repudiated the notion that infectious diseases were no longer important (5). New pathogens and new infectious diseases appeared with regularity, e.g., Legionnaires' disease, toxic shock syndrome, acquired immunodeficiency syndrome (AIDS), Ebola hemorrhagic fever, etc. Certain chronic diseases (e.g., T-cell lymphoma-leukemia and peptic ulcer disease) became linked to previously unknown infectious agents—human T-cell lymphotropic virus and *Helicobacter pylori,* respectively. At the same time, malaria, often caused by drug-resistant strains, and dengue resurged in many parts of the world. Cholera reentered the Americas. Drug-resistant bacteria (e.g., methicillin-resistant *Staphylococcus aureus*) became increasingly prevalent in U.S. hospitals. Throughout this period, infectious diseases remained the leading cause of death in the world at large. Although much of this mortality occurs in developing countries, both the percentage of hospitalizations and mortality associated with infectious diseases increased in the United States during the 1980s (Fig. 10.1) (6–8). The cumulative effect of these events and advances in the fields of microbiology and

epidemiology set the stage for renewed attention to infectious diseases.

In 1991, the Institute of Medicine (IOM) convened a multi-disciplinary committee to study emerging microbial threats to health in the United States. The subsequent report, published in the following year, articulated a paradigm that has shaped most of the subsequent discussion about emerging and resurgent infectious diseases (5). The IOM report defined these diseases as "new, re-emerging, or drug-resistant infections whose incidence in humans has increased within the past two decades or whose incidence threatens to increase in the near future." Importantly, the IOM report delineated root causes that promote the emergence and resurgence of infectious diseases. These factors, which will likely remain operative for the foreseeable future, provide a framework for anticipating and combating challenges posed by new and reemerging infectious diseases.

FACTORS RESPONSIBLE FOR EMERGING INFECTIOUS DISEASES

Although the 1992 IOM report specified six factors underlying the emergence of infectious diseases, a more recent publication from the IOM's Forum on Emerging Infections expanded this number to 10, splitting off new categories from some of the original ones (9). The following discussion follows this later enumeration. Some of the newer divisions emphasize the importance of specific factors (e.g., separation of urbanization from the broader category of demographics). It should be noted also that all of these factors are highly interrelated.

Increased Human Intrusion into Tropical Forests

As the population of the world increases and the need for economic opportunities expands, more and more people come in contact with previously isolated places. Tropical rain forests and inaccessible wilderness have their own ecology with pathogens, vectors, and hosts that, heretofore, have not included humans. The chance that new human diseases will emerge from these "zoonotic pools" of infections increases as humans encroach on the great variety of microorganisms living in these environments (10).

Each day, an estimated 93,000 acres of tropical rain forest are cleared (11). People living on the fringes of the forest come in contact with natural reservoirs of zoonotic diseases that may infect them directly. Changes to the ecology also occur as pests and livestock exchange vectors and pathogens with their forest cousins, allowing infectious agents to expand their reach. In

TABLE 10.2. New Outbreaks Reported by the World Health Organization 2001

Measles in Republic of Korea
Meningococcal disease in the African meningitis belt, Angola, and
    Democratic Republic of Congo
Yellow fever in Brazil, Peru, Liberia, Guinea, and Cote d'Ivoire
Plague in Zambia
Isolation of influenza A (H5N1) from poultry in Hong Kong, Republic
    of China
Acute neurological syndrome in Bangladesh
Crimean-Congo hemorrhagic fever in Kosovo
Legionellosis in Spain and Norway
Cholera in United Republic of Tanzania, Chad, Afghanistan, India,
    West Africa, and Nigeria
Anthrax in the United States
Ebola hemorrhagic fever in Gabon

From *www.who.int/disease-outbreak-news/n2001/index.html*

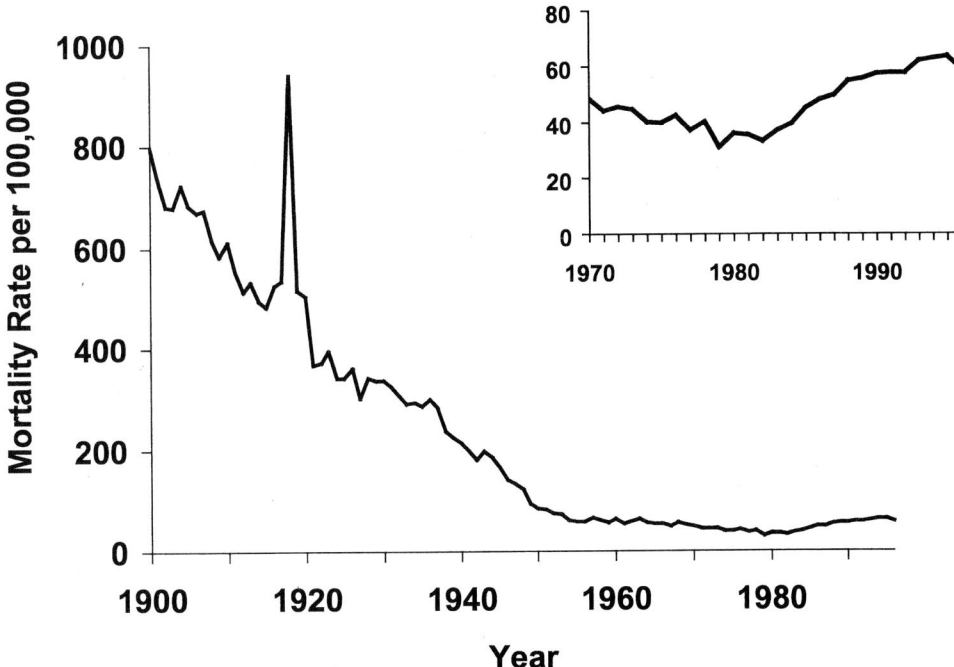

Figure 10.1. Crude infectious disease mortality rate in the United States from 1900 through 1996. The inset graphs the same data on a different scale for 1970 to 1996 (provided courtesy of Gregory L. Armstrong and Robert W. Pinner).

South America, epidemics of Brazilian hemorrhagic fever have been attributed to rodents living in the margin between the forest and harvested grasslands (12). Outbreaks of monkeypox, an illness similar to smallpox, have occurred in an increasing number of persons living in tropical rain forests in western and central African countries (13). Epidemics of leishmaniasis in Argentina have been associated with deforestation (9). Human illness due to the Australian alphavirus Barmah Forest virus has been recognized for about 15 years, and it appears to be extending its area of infectivity (14). Ebola virus has caused massive hemorrhagic fever epidemics in central Africa (15). Along with Marburg virus, another of the hemorrhagic filoviruses, Ebola has emerged in people living in or near tropical rain forests. Despite several ecologic investigations, the actual reservoir is unknown, although nonhuman primates appear to bridge the gap from a source in the forest to humans.

Although emerging infections can occur from encroachment of humans on the forest, newly recognized diseases also can occur from encroachment of the forest on humans. In the northeastern United States, lands previously cleared for farming have returned to forest, allowing deer and tick populations to proliferate. Increased residential development in suburban, wooded areas appears responsible for the rising incidence of Lyme disease and other tick-borne infections such as babesiosis and ehrlichiosis (16). Living or working in close proximity to wilderness areas also appears related to increasing numbers of plague and hantavirus cardiopulmonary syndrome cases in the southwestern United States (17,18).

Access to Health Care

The term *access* encompasses a number of considerations that make it possible for individuals and groups to receive needed medical services (19). Barriers to access may include structural factors (e.g., the number, type, or organizational configuration of health care providers); financial factors (e.g., the ability of patients to pay or the willingness of physicians to accept certain forms of payment); and personal or cultural factors that influence patient willingness to seek or accept treatment. In the United States, discussions about access usually focus on insurance coverage, which plays a major role in utilization of health care services (20). In developing nations, such concerns focus on numbers and quality of health care facilities, medical personnel, and supplies. In both settings, lack of access can impede efforts to recognize, track, control, and prevent infectious diseases. Accordingly, lack of access to health care services may permit emerging or resurgent infections to spread unchecked and allow their human reservoirs to persist or enlarge.

In the United States, approximately 43 million persons lack basic health insurance (21). Low-income persons and minorities account for a large percentage of this group. Negative outcomes associated with their lack of access to health care services include resurgence of congenital syphilis in the early 1990s as well as outbreaks of measles and other infections linked to inadequate immunization status (19,22). Lack of access also facilitates the continuing spread of human immunodeficiency virus (HIV) disease in these subpopulations (23).

Globally it is estimated that 1.5 billion individuals—the majority of whom reside in developing countries—lack access to basic health care (24). Their lack of access contributes not only to the staggering statistics of the HIV pandemic—25 million cases in sub-Saharan Africa (25)—but also to ongoing problems with infections that have been controlled or eradicated elsewhere (e.g., malaria, tuberculosis, and diarrheal disease in children) (9). Without recognition, surveillance, and education about preventive measures, the toll from ongoing HIV transmission will continue to mount as the experiences in Africa, India, and China demonstrate. Without timely diagnosis and adequate treatment, the reservoirs for malaria and tuberculosis will persist in developing countries, maintaining endemic disease levels in these countries and exporting resurgences to other countries via infected travelers, immigrants, and military personnel. Without adequate immunization services, the developing world will continue to struggle with vaccine-preventable infections and maintain reservoirs for poliomyelitis, measles, *Haemophilus influenzae* type B, and hepatitis B, among others. From such reservoirs, these ancient foes can arise to challenge lax policies and complacent health care systems in developed nations.

Population Growth and Changes in Demographics

The world's population continues to grow at an alarming rate. Over the past 75 years, it has increased from 2 billion to 6 billion persons (26). At its present rate, the world's population increases annually by almost 86 million persons. Estimates for the ultimate population of the planet range from a hopeful six to eight billion to a frightening 18 to 20 billion (27). The sheer magnitude of these increases, in concert with other factors described in this section (e.g., travel) establish substrates for ongoing problems with infectious diseases. Changes in demographics (e.g., trends toward greater urbanization) provide specific avenues for the emergence and resurgence of certain pathogens.

The aging of the population, especially in developed countries, illustrates an additional avenue. About 600 million persons in the world today are over age 60; by 2030, population projections place this number at 1.3 billion (27). At that time, more than 20% of Americans and Europeans will be over 65 and 5% will be over 80. Similar trends, albeit of smaller magnitude, are projected for Asia, Latin America, and Africa. This older segment of the population is especially vulnerable to infection. The age-related diminution of cell-mediated immunity renders elderly individuals susceptible to a variety of infections, including tuberculosis (28). Chronic medical conditions (e.g., cancer and obstructive pulmonary disease) occur more commonly in the elderly and predispose them to other types of infection such as pneumonia. Gross and colleagues have demonstrated that older individuals have significantly increased rates of nosocomial infection (29). They observed a decade-specific risk of 10 per 1,000 discharges from birth through the fifth decade. However, this risk of nosocomial infection steadily rose from the fifth decade onward, exceeding 100 infections per 1,000 discharges in patients at least 70 years of age. Accordingly, the susceptible elderly population offers a beachhead for emergent and resurgent pathogens that can later spread to the larger population.

Immunosuppressed individuals constitute another vulnerable subpopulation whose numbers are growing. The 36 million persons currently living with HIV infection constitute an important component of this group (25), as do recipients of allogeneic transplants of bone marrow or solid organs. In the United States, more than 20,000 persons enter this latter group each year (30). Use of radiation and immunosuppressive therapies for malignant and nonmalignant disease also adds thousands to this risk pool each year. In the United States and Europe, the medical literature continues to record the occurrence of new and reemerging infections, especially ones caused by drug-resistant microbes, in this large group of immunosuppressed individuals (30). Finally, malnutrition, which can impair cell-mediated immunity and other host defenses, deserves recognition. It likely renders a majority of the world's 2 billion persons who live in poverty more susceptible to emerging and resurgent infectious diseases (24).

Changes in Human Behavior

Changes in human behavior that influence the emergence of infectious diseases often focus on sexually transmitted diseases and those associated with injection drug use (5). In the United States, the sexual revolution, which began in the 1960s, set the stage for a resurgence of gonorrhea and syphilis and the rise of *Chlamydia trachomatis*, genital herpes, and HIV infection. Changing sexual mores in other parts of the world have played a role in the worldwide pandemic of HIV disease (25). Injection drug use, which has contributed to the spread of HIV disease, also has

facilitated the spread of hepatitis B, C, and D, and periodically, it foments outbreaks with unusual infectious agents like that caused by *Clostridium novyi* in Scotland, Ireland, and England during 2000 (31).

Changes in human behavior have impacted the epidemiology of infectious diseases in several other ways. The increasing utilization of day-care facilities by American parents has given rise to outbreaks caused by enteric and respiratory pathogens and promoted the dissemination of certain antimicrobial-resistant microbes (e.g., penicillin-resistant pneumococci) (2,32). Changing dietary practices have made their own contribution to the increasing prevalence of food-borne disease. For example, outbreaks of *Escherichia coli* O157:H7, salmonellosis caused by uncommon serotypes, and other emerging food-borne diseases have arisen from the increasing consumption of raw or unpasteurized food products (33). Likewise, the increasing choice of American families to eat in commercial establishments has spawned food-borne outbreaks caused by new and resurgent agents. Leisure time avocations, such as golfing and camping, have put humans in contact with the vectors of emerging infectious diseases such as Lyme borreliosis, ehrlichiosis, and babesiosis (16,34,35).

War and bioterrorism constitute other forms of human behavior that influence the emergence and resurgence of infectious diseases. For example, famine and civil war in Somalia resulted in outbreaks of measles and diarrheal disease in 1992, which killed an estimated 74% of children under 5 years of age (36). Dengue fever affected American military personnel serving in Haiti (37), viscerotropic leishmaniasis occurred in soldiers returning from Desert Storm (38), and spotted fever rickettsiosis caused an outbreak in soldiers participating in a training exercise in Botswana (39). The intentional mailing of anthrax spores to prominent Americans during the fall of 2001, which resulted in 10 cases of inhalation disease, testifies to potential effects of bioterrorism (40).

Inadequate and Deteriorating Public Health Infrastructure

Of all the factors contributing to emerging diseases, perhaps the most unfortunate has been the neglect or incomplete implementation of public health prevention and control activities. Effective vaccines, antimicrobial drugs, safe drinking water, and sanitation are all public health successes of the twentieth century. Burgeoning urban populations and diminishing resources, however, threaten to reverse these victories. This problem disproportionately affects developing nations where the per capita spending on health has been estimated to be $4 each year compared with $220 each year in developed countries (41).

This problem also affects more developed countries. In the former Soviet Union, childhood immunization levels began declining in the 1980s after a period of well-supported vaccination programs from the 1950s to 1970s (42). Deteriorating economic and political conditions, coupled with failed strategies to prevent diphtheria before and after the breakup of the union, produced a growing number of susceptible hosts. Not surprisingly, in 1990, an epidemic of diphtheria, mostly among adolescents and adults, began to spread through Russia and the newly independent states in central Asia (43). By 1994, the countries of the former Soviet Union accounted for almost 90% of reported diphtheria cases worldwide (9).

The tuberculosis prevention and control programs in Russia also suffered. Despite the presence of effective drugs and proven control strategies, the incidence of tuberculosis has continued to rise, especially multidrug-resistant tuberculosis (MDRTB) in Russian prisons (44). In affluent, developed countries, tuberculosis control programs have maintained small numbers of cases. In many developing countries, which are increasingly burdened with HIV disease and diminishing resources, MDRTB seems likely to emerge and spread.

Inadequate and deteriorating public health infrastructure has contributed to the emergence or reemergence of malaria, due to unsuccessful vector control; measles, due to ineffective vaccination; and, various hemorrhagic viruses, due to inadequate protection of workers in poorly supported health care settings. In Haiti and the Dominican Republic, poliomyelitis has resisted eradication, despite near elimination of the disease in the Western Hemisphere. Even in developed countries, failure to invest in basic public health infrastructure can promote emerging infectious diseases. Inadequate protection and treatment of a public water system contributed to a massive outbreak of cryptosporidiosis affecting an estimated 400,000 people in Milwaukee, Wisconsin, in 1993 (45).

Misuse of Antibiotics and Other Antimicrobial Drugs

Antimicrobial resistance evolves and spreads in response to selective pressures generated by the use of antiinfective agents. It has developed in all countries that have used antibacterial, antifungal, antiviral, and antiparasitic agents to any extent. Regrettably, a variety of studies have indicated that a large proportion of antimicrobial usage is inappropriate. Hence, misuse of these valuable agents accounts for a significant proportion of the emerging resistance, which is now a worldwide problem (46,47).

In developed countries, inappropriate use of antimicrobial agents occurs in all spheres of practice. An estimated 25% to 45% of the 190 million annually defined daily doses of antimicrobials used in U.S. hospitals represent overuse (46). Similarly, of the 145 million courses of antimicrobial agents prescribed in U.S. outpatient settings each year, 20% to 50% appear to represent overuse. Use for viral respiratory tract infections accounts for a sizable portion of these percentages. Data for a recent year indicate that 50% to 66% of physician visits for "colds," upper respiratory tract infections, and bronchitis culminated in an antibiotic prescription (48).

Of the 50 million pounds of antimicrobial agents produced annually in the United States, about half is used for therapeutic purposes and growth promotion in animals (46). The latter includes annual use of 147 pounds of antibiotics per acre of farmed salmon and 40,000 to 50,000 pounds of antibiotics sprayed on fruit trees to control bacterial infections. Forty percent to 80% of the animal usage has been deemed to represent overuse. The frequency of resistance in each of the clinical, animal, and agricultural settings tends to correlate with the type and amount of antimicrobials used.

Data on antimicrobial usage in developing countries are sparse; however, a variety of reports suggest that large volumes of antimicrobials are used and misused in these countries. The telltale sign of resistance points to this conclusion, as does the observation that many of the antimicrobial-resistant pathogens in the United States originated elsewhere (5,9,49). In developing countries, individuals may purchase these antibiotics and other antimicrobial agents without a prescription, and they often get their advice on the agent from a health assistant or pharmacy shopkeeper rather than a physician (50). Use of inappropriate or substandard agents and subtherapeutic doses in settings with poor infection control practices and warm climates

also promote the development and spread of resistance in these countries.

Microbial Adaptation

Microbial adaptation figures prominently in the emergence and resurgence of many infectious diseases. The development of resistance to antiinfective agents epitomizes the importance of this factor. The sequential appearance of resistance to one newly released agent after another punctuates the history of the antimicrobial era, beginning with penicillin-resistant *Staphylococcus aureus*, sulfonamide-resistant *Streptococcus pyogenes*, and streptomycin-resistant *Mycobacterium tuberculosis* in the 1940s and running through today's penicillin-resistant pneumococci, fluconazole-resistant *Candida* species, and antiretroviral-resistant HIV, among others (47,51). Some form of resistance has developed to virtually all of the antiinfective agents ever licensed. This history showcases the amazing adaptability of microbial pathogens, and the dissemination of resistant strains emphasizes the threat that they pose to medical progress.

Antigenic change also affects the emergence and resurgence of infectious diseases. Changes in the hemagglutinin and neuraminidase antigens of influenza A, for example, created the strains responsible for this century's major pandemics (5,52). The isolation of H5N1 and H9N2 strains in Hong Kong from poultry and humans in 1997 and 1999, respectively, highlights the ongoing potential of the natural interaction of avian, human, and porcine strains to create novel antigenic strains with pandemic potential (53,54). Antigenic variation appears to have played a role in the initiation of cholera pandemics (55). Finally, antigenic variation can enable pathogens to persist and thrive in humans after they cross the species barrier. For example, replication errors in RNA viruses such as HIV and hepatitis C virus have facilitated the spread of these and other viruses in human populations (32). The changing antigenicity of these viruses prevents the generation of neutralizing antibody, allowing both chronic infection and formation of a human reservoir. Antigenic variation plays a similar role in infections caused by *Borrelia* species, *Plasmodium falciparum*, *Trypanosoma brucei*, and other arthropod-borne infections (56).

Microbial adaptability also allows transfer of virulence properties, a process that may promote the emergence or resurgence of various infectious diseases. Transfer of toxin-producing capabilities and other virulence factors among strains of *E. coli* and other enteric pathogens underlies the emergence of some diarrheal diseases (57). Similar transfers may have contributed to the emergence of staphylococcal and streptococcal toxic shock syndrome during the past two decades (58,59). The capacity of some *S. aureus* strains to exploit new environments created by superabsorbent tampons also contributed to the emergence of staphylococcal toxic shock syndrome.

Urbanization and Crowding

During the twentieth century, the percentage of the world's population living in cities rose dramatically; most of that growth occurred in densely inhabited megacities in the developing world. Many of these cities have been unable to keep pace with the growing demand for water, sanitation, and health care. In addition, the size of the urban population living in absolute poverty is increasing, exceeding 50% in some cities (60).

The growth of the urban population partly reflects the influx of people from surrounding rural areas. On arrival, they often encounter conditions that are worse than those in their original setting. Squatter settlements and slums, which often lack sanitary supplies of potable water and facilities for disposal of human waste, facilitate the emergence of old and new infectious diseases. Conditions in slums constitute a challenge for the control of epidemic cholera, where contamination can occur both in poorly maintained water supplies as well as in vessels for carrying drinking water (61,62). Open water storage containers, drainage canals, and other sources of standing water have expedited the introduction and increase in various mosquito species with a resurgence of dengue/dengue hemorrhagic fever, yellow fever, malaria, and other vector-borne illnesses (63). For example, investigation of a 1999 outbreak in Malaysia that caused fever and arthralgias in more than 100 residents of a squatter settlement ultimately identified the causative agent as chikungunya virus, a pathogen not previously recognized in that country (14). In the United States and France, cases of "urban trench fever" due to *Bartonella quintana* have occurred among individuals in poor living conditions that favored exposure to body lice (64).

Crowding in urban settings is not restricted to humans. Companion animals, domesticated livestock, and pests also live in close proximity to each other and to humans, providing opportunities for the transmission of certain infections. For example, in 1997, 18 cases of influenza A virus subtype H5N1 occurred in Hong Kong; six individuals died (65). This particularly virulent strain was transmitted from bird to humans, likely during visits to poultry stalls at city markets. In some urban settings the concurrence of floods, increased population density, and presence of rats, cats, and dogs have increased the risk for leptospiral outbreaks. Outbreaks of leishmaniasis, campylobacteriosis, and Japanese encephalitis also have occurred in urban settings where humans live in close contact with animals (9).

Modern Travel and Mass Migration

Each year, an increasing number of people, and their microbes, travel great distances in a decreasing amount of time. Around the globe, an estimated 1.4 million people travel by air every day (66). Travelers can now reach almost anyplace in the world within 24 to 36 hours, rendering the travel time shorter than the incubation period of many infectious diseases. Detection of illness among travelers can be difficult because symptoms and signs may not develop until after the traveler has returned.

The introduction of infectious diseases from travelers is not new. Syphilis and smallpox followed travelers to the New World, and previously exotic illnesses like plague and cholera became worldwide with steamship travel. Modern travel, however, has added new dimensions to the potential problem, as the large numbers of travelers, the diversity of destinations, and the short duration required for long trips imply.

Dengue fever has had a recent dramatic resurgence in epidemic form in tropical areas of the world, including the emergence of the more fatal presentation of dengue hemorrhagic fever (63). The mosquito vector of dengue, *Aedes aegypti*, has returned to the tropics years after its elimination during campaigns to control yellow fever. Air travelers incubating the dengue virus have provided the ideal circumstances for transporting dengue between urban areas of the tropics, which has resulted in the reintroduction of the virus to the mosquito population. Humans are the only vertebrate host of dengue, and when an epidemic subsides, the virus can disappear. Travelers provide the means for constant exchange of dengue viruses and other pathogens.

The availability of rapid air travel has resulted in the importation of various diseases, including influenza, pneumonic plague, tuberculosis, malaria, and polio, among others. Notably,

cases of viral hemorrhagic fevers have occurred in air travelers. In 1990, an individual returning to the United States from Nigeria was found to have Lassa fever (67). Over 100 individuals were exposed prior to his death; all received ribavirin prophylaxis, and fortunately, no further cases occurred. In 1997, a patient with Ebola traveled from western Africa and subsequently transmitted the infection to a hospital nurse in southern Africa (68).

The movement of people around the world, both voluntary and involuntary, is occurring at an unprecedented level. The effects of war, natural disasters, drought, and other factors have contributed to these mass migrations, many of which are taking place in developing countries. At present, approximately 50 million persons in the world are either refugees outside their own countries' borders or internally displaced. They are often placed in camps where malnutrition, poor sanitation, inadequate drinking water, low levels of vaccination, and limited medical care contribute to the amplification of infectious diseases. Of considerable concern has been the emergence of hepatitis E, epidemic strains of *Neisseria meningitidis*, and multidrug-resistant strains of various pathogens, including *Shigella dysenteriae*, malaria, and cholera (69,70). For example, the displacement of 500,000 to 800,000 Rwandan refugees into Zaire in 1994 resulted in explosive outbreaks of diarrheal disease caused by *Vibrio cholerae* 01 and *Shigella dysenteriae* type 1 and the resurgence of typhus. Outbreaks of malaria, meningococcal meningitis, and hepatitis, among others diseases, continue to recur in such settings and account for mortality rates that are 20 to 30 times higher than those in either adjacent local communities or those in the countries of origination before the migration.

Animals, like people, migrate to new environments, and their pathogens can emerge as new infectious disease threats. In the summer of 1999, clinicians and public health officials in New York City investigated case reports of encephalitis due to West Nile virus (WNV), a member of the family Flaviviridae (71,72). WNV had been reported first in 1937 in the West Nile district of Uganda; the cases in New York City represented the first introduction in recent history of an Old World flavivirus into the New World. The outbreak of WNV infections in humans was accompanied by an epizootic in the New York City area, notably among American crows (*Corvus brachrhynchos*), but also in other birds, horses, and dogs (73). Virus has been found in 14 mosquito species, and is maintained through avian populations. In 2001, the virus had been identified in 12 states and the District of Columbia. Bird migrations are expected to allow the continued geographic expansion of WNV activity. WNV is widely distributed in Africa, Europe, the Middle East, and western Asia, and the potential now exists for wide distribution in the Americas as well.

Increased Trade and Expanded Markets for Imported Foods

We live in a global village, we shop in a global market, and now our infections can originate from anyplace on the globe. Since World War II, global trade has increased considerably. Trade facilitates emerging diseases by allowing for the transport of infectious agents and vectors of disease. Mosquitos infected with malaria and dengue have brought these infections to new areas aboard trading ships. Cholera, carried in contaminated ballast water of ships, has been emptied into harbors (74). Highways in central Africa used by cargo trucks facilitated the initial spread of HIV infection on that continent (75).

Global distribution of food, new processes for preparation, and consumer demand for more exotic and fresher foods have contributed to the emergence of new food-borne pathogens (76). *E. coli* O157:H7 was first identified in 1982 as the cause of a large outbreak of hemorrhagic colitis from contaminated hamburgers sold at a chain of fast-food restaurants (77). The bacterium has been associated with outbreaks from eating contaminated apple cider, unpasteurized milk, sprouts, and other food products. *Cyclospora cayetanensis* is a small parasite that has caused outbreaks of diarrhea due to eating imported Guatemalan raspberries; the contamination likely occurred from surface water carrying the parasite that was sprayed onto the berries (78). Outbreaks of diarrhea due to Norwalk-like virus have occurred from oysters contaminated from improper waste disposal on fishing boats. *Salmonella*, a common cause of food-borne illness, has acquired resistance and has emerged as the multi-resistant strain of *S. enteriditis* DT104.

Food-borne infections have been estimated to cause 76 million illnesses and 5,000 deaths in the United States each year (79). Among the various causes of food-borne illness are a number of newly described pathogens that have emerged. A number of factors have contributed to the appearance of these new agents, including global distribution of foods, new processes for preparation, and consumer demand for more exotic and fresher foods.

RESPONSES TO EMERGING INFECTIOUS DISEASES

Several groups have taken up the challenge posed by emerging infectious diseases. The IOM has continued to hold forums and workshops on issues that require a public health response (9,46,80–82). The Centers for Disease Control and Prevention (CDC) and the World Health Organization (WHO) have assumed major roles in planning, developing, and implementing the coordinated response necessary to combat a number of microbial threats.

Centers for Disease Control and Prevention

The CDC has a coordinated approach for addressing emerging infectious diseases using collaborations with health departments and other federal agencies in the United States, international public health organizations, and ministries of health in other countries. Since 1994, the CDC has followed a strategy to protect the public from infectious diseases by focusing on four major goals (83,84).

GOAL 1: IMPROVE DISEASE SURVEILLANCE AND OUTBREAK RESPONSE

The CDC has provided resources to state, territorial, and large local health departments through the Epidemiology and Laboratory Capacity (ELC) program to improve laboratory detection and reporting capabilities. These funds have permitted the development of core public health capacities and allowed creation of innovative systems for early detection and investigation of outbreaks. They also have facilitated monitoring of antimicrobial resistance patterns and ensured electronic reporting of surveillance data such as those derived from the national molecular subtyping network for food-borne disease surveillance known as PulseNet.

Emerging Infections Programs (EIPs) constitute another complementary program to improve surveillance and response. Through partnerships with health departments and academic centers, the EIPs conduct population-based surveillance and research that goes beyond the routine functions of local health departments. Examples of EIP surveillance activity include (a)

active bacterial core surveillance, which has focused on invasive infections caused by drug-resistant *S. pneumoniae*, *S. pyogenes*, *N. meningitidis*, and other pathogens; (b) Foodborne Diseases Active Surveillance Network (FoodNet), which has focused on *E. coli* O157, *Listeria*, *Salmonella*, *Cyptosporidium*, *Cyclospora*, and other enteric pathogens; and (c) Unexplained Deaths and Critical Illness Project, which has focused on the identification and characterization of agents responsible for serious illnesses that go undiagnosed. EIP activities have permitted monitoring of trends in antimicrobial-resistant pneumococcal disease and food-borne illness, evaluation of the impact from deployment of new vaccines, and assessment of prevention strategies for neonatal group B streptococcal disease (85).

The CDC has sought to improve surveillance and response efforts through development of provider-based sentinel networks to monitor syndromes and diseases. Through collaborations with professional societies, networks of specialists have been established to monitor and evaluate conditions that are not covered by health department surveillance. These networks include the Infectious Diseases Society of America Emerging Infections Network, the Emergency Department Sentinel Network for Emerging Infections, the Sentinel Network of Travel Medicine Clinics (GeoSentinel), and the Border Infectious Disease Surveillance Project. These networks help fill in the gaps in emerging infectious disease surveillance by monitoring and collating the observations of clinicians in key practice settings (86–88).

GOAL 2: SUPPORT RESEARCH TO UNDERSTAND AND COMBAT EMERGING INFECTIOUS THREATS

The CDC provides resources to develop, evaluate, and disseminate testing methods for infectious agents, particularly for "orphan" diseases—those for which the market for diagnostic testing is not great enough to stimulate research and development by private industry. In addition, the CDC supports research to assess the role of infectious agents in causing or exacerbating chronic diseases and syndromes for which the causative agents are unknown.

The CDC coordinates efforts to examine the potential role that genetic factors play in determining an individual's risk of contracting infectious diseases. It also collaborates with other organizations to develop and evaluate new antimicrobial drugs and prophylactic agents, new methods to control disease vectors and reservoirs, and new methods of disinfection.

GOAL 3: STRENGTHEN PUBLIC HEALTH INFRASTRUCTURE AND TRAINING

Given the primacy of microbiology laboratories in the detection of emerging infectious disease threats, the CDC has endeavored to enhance the nation's public health laboratory infrastructure by improving laboratories at the CDC and at state and local health departments. Such efforts have included dissemination of better tests for diagnosis, susceptibility determinations, and strain typing. The CDC has supported improvements in electronic communications to facilitate rapid sharing of laboratory and epidemiologic findings and to integrate various systems used for communicable disease surveillance. Working with state and local health departments, other federal agencies, organizations of first responders (such as firefighters and emergency medical workers), and international partners, the CDC has developed plans to maintain "surge" capacity and for management of large outbreaks, including those caused by the deliberate release of toxins or infectious agents. Through a CDC cooperative agreement program, health departments have received resources to improve their capacity to detect and respond to bioterrorist events. Finally, the CDC continues to provide training in applied public health through the Epidemic Intelligence Service, which assigns highly qualified epidemiologists to various activities at the CDC and at state health departments. Along with other laboratory and field programs, these training efforts ensure a ready force of well-trained public health practitioners to respond to emerging infectious disease problems.

GOAL 4: PREVENT INFECTIOUS DISEASES BY IMPLEMENTING DISEASE CONTROL PROGRAMS AND COMMUNICATING PUBLIC HEALTH INFORMATION

Prevention of emerging infectious diseases requires different approaches to control various pathogens. The CDC has expanded existing domestic and international community-based control programs for preventing infectious diseases, including dengue hemorrhagic fever in Puerto Rico, malaria in Kenya, and HIV in the United States. New prevention projects are being evaluated, including prevention of antimicrobial resistance, foodborne and waterborne illness, and others. A national action plan to combat antimicrobial resistance has either identified or initiated activities to prevent and control infections caused by resistant organisms. The CDC continues to promote vaccination programs to ensure that U.S. children and adults are appropriately immunized; some of these target drug-resistant pathogens (e.g., penicillin-resistant *S. pneumoniae*). The CDC continues to work with foreign governments, the WHO, and other organizations to promote global programs for the prevention and control of infectious diseases such as the WHO's Expanded Program on Immunization and programs to eradicate polio and Guinea worm disease. Finally, the CDC communicates information about prevention of emerging infectious diseases to professionals and the public through several channels, including (a) publication of the peer-reviewed journal *Emerging Infectious Diseases*; (b) live, interactive satellite and Internet broadcasts to rapidly inform clinicians and public health officials about specific topics (e.g., anthrax); and (c) publication of prevention guidelines such as those for infection control and HIV prevention.

World Health Organization

Given the global nature of the problem, the WHO has responded by expanding its surveillance and other operations to meet the challenge of emerging and resurgent infectious diseases. Three aspects are of note. First, the WHO has supported the monitoring and control of known problems such as measles, cholera, yellow fever, meningitis, and other infections. It has addressed these infections with disease-specific networks of national and international public health agencies to control outbreaks using established protocols and ensuring that appropriate vaccines and other supplies are available when needed.

Second, the WHO has responded to unexpected problems through heightened vigilance and rapid response to emerging infectious agents and agents used in acts of bioterrorism. Building on available electronic communications, the WHO through partnership with Health Canada, has used semiautomated methods to search various Internet sites and other news and information sources to identify outbreaks and other emerging infectious disease threats. Issues requiring response are evaluated by the WHO Global Outbreak Alert and Response Network, a collaboration with 72 agencies worldwide, including the CDC and the U.S. Department of Defense. When large-scale international assistance has been needed, the WHO has coordinated the response using partnerships with various national and international public health agencies. In addition, the WHO has developed a plan for combating antimicrobial resistance (89).

Third, the WHO continues to sponsor training for epidemiologists and laboratorians. In collaboration with the CDC and others, the WHO has formed the Training Programmes in Epidemiology and Public Health Interventions network to enhance the effectiveness of national training programs. In order to ensure that the short-term effects of a rapid response to an outbreak are translated into longer-term measures for disease control, the WHO has developed and coordinated an Early Warning and Response Network in partnership with nongovernmental organizations within specific countries. This effort intends to build capacity among local communities to ensure more rapid detection and containment of outbreaks using available local resources.

The WHO's capacity for alert and response efforts derives from its privileged access to various countries, widely distributed field offices and staff, over 250 laboratories participating as WHO Collaborating Centres, electronic surveillance networks (e.g., fluNet), and technical expertise available within the WHO or through collaborations with the CDC and other agencies.

FUTURE CONSIDERATIONS

In addition to the concerns for the future alluded to previously, other specters loom on the horizon. The predicted rise in the world's temperature over the next century raises concerns about the spread of arthropod-borne infections and other tropical diseases (24,27). If, according to current predictions, the earth's temperature rises by 1° to 4°C during the 21st century, anopheline and *Aedes* mosquitoes will transcend their customary ranges, spreading dengue, malaria, and other arboviral infections to new areas. Global warming also may increase the incidence of leishmaniasis, trypanosomiasis, and filariasis (90).

Variant Creutzfeldt-Jakob disease (vCJD), the human prion disease linked to bovine spongiform encephalopathy (BSE), raises another concern for the future. Popularly known as "mad cow disease," BSE first appeared in England during 1986 (91). By 1999, more than 175,000 cases had been recognized in England, and more than 1,000 cases had been recognized elsewhere in Europe. Japan reported cases in 2001 (92). Reports of vCJD cases appeared in 1996 (93). Since then more than 100 cases have arisen. Epidemiological evidence suggests that BSE arose from the feeding of scrapies-infected sheep to cattle and that vCJD arose from human ingestion of BSE-infected beef. Two pressing questions arise from these observations: How many cases of vCJD will occur ultimately and what other prion diseases might enter the human food chain? With regard to the first question, it is estimated that 136,000 cases of vCJD will occur by 2040 in the United Kingdom (94). Uncertainty surrounds this figure (91,95), and estimation of the likely global burden is not possible. With regard to the second question, three recent cases of CJD in deer hunters have raised concern; however, none of these hunters resided in areas where chronic wasting disease is known to be endemic in deer (91).

Two areas of current medical research arouse concerns about the possibility of new infectious diseases. The first is xenotransplantation. The perpetual shortage of solid organs for transplantation likely will continue to drive medicine toward the use of animal organs. Although the risk of xenozoonoses in humans is unknown, experience with human allografts suggests that the risk is not negligible (96). Borie and colleagues have described the numerous microbiological hazards associated with xenotransplantation of porcine organs (97). Other species pose similar risks. Not surprisingly, the CDC has issued revised guidelines to guard against infections from this source (98).

Gene therapy constitutes the other area of concern in medical research (99–102). Although the risks are poorly defined, the possibility that secondary infection could arise from engineered viral vectors—especially ones derived from replication-competent viruses like vaccinia—raise troubling issues. The highly publicized death of one gene therapy recipient in 2000, although not clearly due to infection, prompted the U.S. Food and Drug Administration to put a number of U.S. studies on hold (103). The publication of guidelines for infection control measures in gene therapy also signifies the concern raised by this topic (101).

The potential of these various threats to intrude on the future of human history underscore the need for watchfulness and anticipation. They apply not only to the CDC, WHO, and other public health entities, but also to clinicians in their individual practice settings where the next emerging infectious disease may be just around the corner.

REFERENCES

1. Garrett L. *The coming plague—newly emerging diseases in a world out of balance.* New York: Farrar, Straus & Giroux, 1994.
2. McDade JE, Hughes JM. New and emerging infectious diseases. In: Mandell GL, Bennett JE, Dolin R, eds. *Principles and practice of infectious diseases,* 5th ed. Philadelphia: Churchill Livingstone, 2000:178–183.
3. (As quoted by) Surowiecki J. The financial page—no profit, no cure. *The New Yorker* 2001;Nov 5:46.
4. Burnet FM. *Natural history of infectious diseases,* 3rd ed. Cambridge: Cambridge University Press, 1962:iii.
5. Institute of Medicine. Emerging infections: microbial threats to health in the United States. Washington, DC: National Academy Press, 1992.
6. Pinner RW, Teutsch SM, Simonsen L, et al. Trends in infectious diseases mortality in the United States. *JAMA* 1996;275:189–193.
7. Simonsen L, Conn LA, Pinner RW, et al. Trends in infectious diseases hospitalizations in the United States, 1980–1994. *Arch Intern Med* 1998;158:1923–1928.
8. Armstrong GL, Conn LA, Pinner RW. Trends in infectious disease mortality in the United States during the 20th century. *JAMA* 1999;281:61–66.
9. Institute of Medicine. *Emerging infectious diseases from the global to the local perspective. Workshop Report.* Washington, DC: National Academy Press, 2001.
10. Morse SS. Examining the origins of emerging viruses. In: Morse SS, ed. *Emerging viruses.* New York: Oxford University Press, 1993:15.
11. World Resources Institute, United Nations. Environment Programme, United Nations Development Programme and the World Bank. *1998–99 World resources: a guide to the global environment.* New York: Oxford University Press, 1998.
12. Peters CJ. Hemorrhagic fevers: how they wax and wane. In: Scheld WM, Armstrong D, Hughes JM, eds. *Emerging infections 1.* Washington, DC: American Society for Microbiology Press, 1998:15–25.
13. Heyman DL, Szczeniowski MV, Esteves K. Re-emergence of monkeypox in Africa: a review of the past six years. *Br Med Bull* 1998;54:693–702.
14. Mackenzie JS, Chua KB, Daniels PW, et al. Emerging viral diseases of Southeast Asia and the Western Pacific. *Emerg Infect Dis* 2001;7(3 suppl):497–504.
15. Khan AS, Tshioko FK, Heymann DL, et al. The reemergence of Ebola hemorrhagic fever, Democratic Republic of the Congo, 1995. *J Infect Dis* 1999;179(suppl 1):76–86.
16. Persing DH. The cold zone: a curious convergence of tick-transmitted diseases. *Clin Infect Dis* 1997:25(suppl 1):35–42.
17. Dennis DT. Plague as an emerging disease. In: Scheld WM, Craig WA, Hughes JM, eds. *Emerging infections 2.* Washington, DC: American Society for Microbiology Press, 1998:169–183.
18. Zeitz PS, Butler JC, Cheek JE, et al. A case-control study of hantavirus pulmonary syndrome during an outbreak in the southwestern United States. *J Infect Dis* 1995;171:864–870.
19. Institute of Medicine. *Access to health care in America.* Washington, DC: National Academy Press, 1993.
20. American College of Physicians. Access to health care. *Ann Intern Med* 1990;112:641–661.
21. Ayanian JZ, Weissman JS, Schneider EC, et al. Unmet health needs of uninsured adults in the United States. *JAMA* 2000;284:2061–2069.
22. Schulte JM, Brown GR, Zetzman MR, et al. Changing immunization referral patterns among pediatricians and family practice physicians, Dallas County, Texas, 1988. *Pediatrics* 1991;87:204–207.
23. Whitehead TL. Urban low-income African American men, HIV/AIDS, and gender identity. *Med Anthropol Q* 1997;11:411–447.
24. Louria DB, Carbon C. Emerging and re-emerging pathogens and disease. In: Armstrong D, Cohen J, eds. *Infectious diseases.* London: Harcourt, 1999:5.1–5.12.
25. Sepkowitz KA. AIDS—the first 20 years. *N Engl J Med* 2001;344:1764–1772.
26. United Nations Population Fund. *The state of the world population 1995.* New York: United Nations Population Fund, 1995.
27. Louria DB. Emerging and reemerging infections: the critical societal determinants, their mitigation, and our responsibilities. In: Scheld WM, Armstrong D, Hughes JM, eds. *Emerging infections 1.* Washington, DC: American Society for Microbiology Press, 1998:247–259.
28. Strausbaugh LJ. Emerging healthcare-associated infections in the geriatric population. *Emerg Infect Dis* 2001;7:268–271.
29. Gross PA, Rapuano C, Adrignolo A, et al. Nosocomial infections: decade-specific risk. *Infect Control* 1983;4:145–147.
30. Kaplan JE, Hanson DL, Jones JL, et al. Opportunistic infections (OIs) as emerging infectious diseases: challenges posed by OIs in the 1990s and beyond. In: Scheld WM, Craig WA, Hughes JM, eds. *Emerging infections 2.* Washington, DC: American Society for Microbiology Press, 1998:257–272.
31. Centers for Disease Control and Prevention. Update: *Clostridium novyi* and unexplained illness among injection-drug users—Scotland, Ireland, and England, April–June 2000. *MMWR* 2000;49:543–545.
32. Mahy BWJ, Murphy FA. Emergence and re-emergence of viral infections. In: Collier L, Mahy BWJ, eds. *Topley and Wilson's microbiology and microbial infections,* 9th ed. Vol. 1. New York: Oxford University Press, 1998:1011–1025.
33. Swerdlow DL, Altekruse SF. Food-borne diseases in the global village: what's on the plate for the 21st century. In: Scheld WM, Craig WA, Hughes JM, eds. *Emerging infections 2.* Washington, DC: American Society for Microbiology Press, 1998:273–294.
34. Walker DH. Emerging human ehrlichioses: recently recognized, widely distributed, life-threatening tick-borne diseases. In: Scheld WM, Armstrong D, Hughes JM, eds. *Emerging infections 1.* Washington, DC: American Society for Microbiology Press, 1998:81–91.
35. Kjemtrup AM, Conrad PA. Emerging perspectives on human babesiosis. In: Scheld WM, Craig WA, Hughes JM, eds. *Emerging infections 5.* Washington, DC: American Society for Microbiology Press, 2001:175–195.
36. Moore PS, Marfin AA, Quenemoen LE, et al. Mortality rates in displaced and resident populations of central Somalia during 1992 famine. *Lancet* 1993;341:935–938.
37. Howard MJ, Brillman JC, Burkle FM Jr. Infectious diseases emergencies in disasters. *Emerg Med Clin North Am* 1996;14:413–428.
38. Centers for Disease Control and Prevention. Viscerotropic leishmaniasis in persons returning from Operation Desert Storm: 1990–1991. *MMWR* 1992;41:131–134.
39. Smoak BL, McClain JB, Brundage JF, et al. An outbreak of spotted fever rickettsiosis in U.S. army troops deployed to Botswana. *Emerg Infect Dis* 1996;2:217–221.
40. Jernigan JA, Stephens DS, Ashford DA, et al. Bioterrorism-related inhalational anthrax: the first 10 cases reported in the United States. *Emerg Infect Dis* 2001;7:933–944.
41. Carballo M. Poverty, development, population movements and health. In: Whitman J, ed. *The politics of emerging and resurgent infectious diseases.* New York: St. Martin's Press, 2000:28.
42. Galazka AM, Robertson SE, Oblapenko GP. Resurgence of diphtheria. *Eur J Epidemiol* 1995;11:95–105.
43. Glinyenko VM, Abdikarimov ST, Firsova SN, et al. Epidemic diphtheria in the Kyrgyz Republic, 1994–1998. *J Infect Dis* 2000;181(suppl 1):98–103.
44. Kimerling ME, Kluge H, Vezhnina N, et al. Inadequacy of the current WHO retreatment regimen in a central Siberian prison: treatment failure and MDR-TB. *Int J Tuberc Lung Dis* 1999;3:451–453.
45. MacKenzie WR, Schell WL, Blair KA, et al. Massive outbreak of waterborne cryptosporidium infection in Milwaukee, Wisconsin: recurrence of illness and risk of secondary transmission. *Clin Infect Dis* 1995;21:57–62.
46. Institute of Medicine. *Antimicrobial resistance: issues and options. Workshop report.* Washington, DC: National Academy Press, 1998.
47. Levy SB. The challenge of antibiotic resistance. *Sci Am* 1998;278:46–53.
48. Avorn J, Solomon DH. Cultural and economic factors that (mis)shape antibiotic use: the nonpharmacologic basis of therapeutics. *Ann Intern Med* 2000;133:128–135.
49. Okeke IN, Edelman R. Dissemination of antibiotic-resistant bacteria across geographic borders. *Clin Infect Dis* 2001;33:364–369.
50. Okeke IN, Lamikanra A, Edelman R. Socioeconomic and behavioral factors leading to acquired bacterial resistance to antibiotics in developing countries. *Emerg Infect Dis* 1999;5:18–27.
51. Richman DD. Emergence of human immunodeficiency virus drug resistance. In: Scheld WM, Craig WA, Hughes JM, eds. *Emerging infections 4.* Washington, DC: American Society for Microbiology Press, 2000:17–21.
52. Cox NJ, Subbarao K. Influenza. *Lancet* 1999;354:1277–1282.
53. Yuen KY, Chan PKS, Peiris M, et al. Clinical features and rapid viral diagnosis of human disease associated with avian influenza A H5N1. *Lancet* 1998;351:467–471.
54. Uyeki TM, Chong Y-H, Katz JM, et al. Lack of evidence for human-to-human transmission of avian influenza A (H9N2) viruses in Hong Kong, China 1999. *Emerg Infect Dis* 2002;8:1–11.
55. Tauxe RV, Barrett TJ. Cholera and *Vibrio cholerae:* new challenges from a once and future pathogen. In: Scheld WM, Craig WA, Hughes JM, eds. *Emerging infections 2.* Washington, DC: American Society for Microbiology Press, 1998:125–144.
56. Barbour AG, Restrepo BI. Antigenic variation in vector-borne pathogens. *Emerg Infect Dis* 2000;6:449–457.

57. Whittam TS, McGraw EA, Reid SD. Pathogenic *Escherichia coli* O157:H7: A model for emerging infectious diseases. In: Krause RM, ed. *Emerging infections—biomedical research reports.* San Diego: Academic, 1998:163–183.

58. Musser JM, Krause RM. The revival of group A streptococcal diseases, with a commentary on staphylococcal toxic shock syndrome. In: Krause RM, ed. *Emerging infections—biomedical research reports.* San Diego: Academic, 1998: 185–218.

59. Low DE, Schwartz B, McGeer A. The re-emergence of severe group A streptococcal disease: an evolutionary perspective. In: Scheld WM, Armstrong D, Hughes JM, eds. Emerging infections 1. Washington, DC: American Society for Microbiology Press, 1998:93–123.

60. Harpham T, Stephens C. Urbanization and health in developing countries. *World Health Stat Q* 1991;44:62–69.

61. Tauxe RV, Mintz ED, Quick RE. Epidemic cholera in the New World: translating field epidemiology into new prevention strategies. *Emerg Infect Dis* 1995;1:141–146.

62. Mintz ED, Reiff FM, Tauxe RV. Safe water treatment and storage in the home; a practical new strategy to prevent waterborne disease. *JAMA* 1995;273:948–953.

63. Gubler DJ, Clark GG. Dengue/dengue hemorrhagic fever: the emergence of a global health problem. *Emerg Infect Dis* 1995;1:55–57.

64. Spach DH, Kanter AS, Dougherty MJ, et al. Bartonella (Rochalimaea) *quintana* bacteremia in inner-city patients with chronic alcoholism. *N Engl J Med* 1995;332:424–428.

65. Mounts AW, Kwong H, Izurieta HS, et al. Case-control study of risk factors for avian influenza A (H5N1) disease, Hong Kong, 1997. *J Infect Dis* 1999;180:505–508.

66. Cetron M, Keystone J, Schlim D, et al. Travelers' health. *Emerg Infect Dis* 1998;4:405–407.

67. Holmes GP, McCormick JB, Trock SC, et al. Lassa fever in the United States: investigation of a new case and guidelines for management. *N Engl J Med* 1990;323:1120–1123.

68. Richards GA, Murphy S, Jobson R, et al. Unexpected Ebola virus in a tertiary setting: clinical and epidemiologic aspects. *Crit Care Med* 2000;28:240–244.

69. Mast EE, Polish LB, Favorov MO, et al. Hepatitis E among refugees in Kenya: minimal apparent person-to-person transmission, evidence for age-dependent disease expression, and new serological assays. In: Kishioka K, Suzuki H, Mishiro S, et al., eds. *Viral hepatitis and liver disease.* Tokyo: Springer-Verlag, 1994:375–378.

70. Moore PS, Toole MJ, Nieburg P, et al. Surveillance and control of meningococcal meningitis epidemics in refugee populations. *Bull WHO* 1990;68:587–596.

71. Asnis DS, Conetta R, Teixeira AA, et al. The West Nile Virus outbreak of 1999 in New York: the Flushing Hospital experience. *Clin Infect Dis* 2000;30:413–418.

72. Nash D, Mostashari F, Fine A, et al. Outbreak of West Nile virus infection, New York City area, 1999. *N Engl J Med* 2001;344:1807–1814.

73. Petersen LR, Roehrig JT. West Nile Virus: a reemerging global pathogen. *Emerg Infect Dis* 2001;7:611–614.

74. Centers for Disease Control and Prevention. Isolation of *Vibrio cholerae* 01 from oysters—Mobile Bay, 1991–1992. *MMWR* 1992;42:91–93.

75. Bwayo J, Plummer F, Omari M, et al. Human immunodeficiency virus infection in long-distance truck drivers in east Africa. *Arch Intern Med* 1994;154:1391–1396.

76. Tauxe RV. Emerging foodborne diseases: an evolving public health challenge. *Emerg Infect Dis* 1997;3:425–434.

77. Riley LW, Remis RS, Helgerson SD, et al. Hemorrhagic colitis associated with a rare *Escherichia coli* serotype. *N Engl J Med* 1983;308:681–685.

78. Herwaldt BL. *Cyclospora cayetanensis*: a review, focusing on the outbreaks of cyclosporiasis in the 1990s. *Clin Infect Dis* 2000;31:1040–1057.

79. Mead PS, Slutsker L, Dietz V, et al. Food-related illness and death in the United States. *Emerg Infect Dis* 1999;5:607–625.

80. Institute of Medicine. *Orphans and incentives: Developing technologies to address emerging infectious diseases. Workshop report.* Washington, DC: National Academy Press, 1997.

81. Institute of Medicine. *Managed care systems and emerging infections: challenges and opportunities for strengthening surveillance, research and prevention. Workshop summary.* Washington, DC: National Academy Press, 2000.

82. Institute of Medicine. *Public health systems and emerging infections: assessing the capabilities of the public and private sectors. Workshop summary.* Washington, DC: National Academy Press, 2000.

83. Centers for Disease Control and Prevention. *Addressing emerging infectious disease threats: a preventive strategy for the United States.* Atlanta: Centers for Disease Control and Prevention, 1994.

84. Centers for Disease Control and Prevention. *Preventing emerging infectious diseases: a strategy for the 21st century.* Atlanta: Centers for Disease Control and Prevention, 1998.

85. Schuchat A. Group B streptococcal disease: from trials and tribulations to triumph and trepidation. *Clin Infect Dis* 2001;33:751–756.

86. Executive Committee of the Infectious Diseases Society of America Emerging Infections Network. The emerging infections network: a new venture for the Infectious Diseases Society of America. *Clin Infect Dis* 1997;25:34–36.

87. Talan DA, Moran, GJ, Mower WR, et al. EMERGEncy ID NET: an emergency department-based emerging infections sentinel network. *Ann Emerg Med* 1998;32:703–711.

88. Freedman DO, Kozarsky PE, Weld LH, et al. GeoSentinel: the global emerging infections sentinel network of the International Society of Travel Medicine. *J Travel Med* 1999;6:94–98.

89. World Health Organization. World Health Organization Global Strategy for the Containment of Antimicrobial Resistance. Published by World Health Organization, 2001. Document no. WHO/CDS/CSR/DRS/2001.2. (Available at URL *www.who.int/emc/amr.html*)

90. Patz JA, Epstein PR, Burke TA, et al. Global climate change and emerging infectious diseases. *JAMA* 1996;275:217–223.

91. MacKnight C. Clinical implications of bovine spongiform encephalopathy. *Clin Infect Dis* 2001;32:1726–1731.

92. Watts J. Bovine spongiform encephalopathy case found in Japan. *Lancet* 2001;358:991.

93. Will RG, Ironside JW, Zeidler M, et al. A new variant of Creutzfeldt-Jakob disease in UK. *Lancet* 1996;347:921–925.

94. Ghani AC, Ferguson NM, Donnelly CA, et al. Predicted vCJD mortality in Great Britain. *Nature* 2000;406:583–584.

95. Brown P, Will RG, Bradley R, et al. Bovine spongiform encephalopathy and variant Creutzfeldt-Jakob disease: background, evolution and current concerns. *Emerg Infect Dis* 2001;7:6–16.

96. Pearson ML, Jarvis WR, Folks TM, et al. Xenotransplantation: is the future upon us? *Infect Control Hosp Epidemiol* 1998;19:305–307.

97. Borie DC, Cramer DV, Phan-Thanh L, et al. Microbiological hazards related to xenotransplantation of porcine organs into man. *Infect Control Hosp Epidemiol* 1998;19:355–365.

98. Centers for Disease Control and Prevention. U.S. Public Health Service guidelines on infectious disease issues in xenotransplantation. *MMWR* 2001; 50(RR-15):1–48.

99. Evans ME, Lesnaw JA. Infection control in gene therapy. *Infect Control Hosp Epidemiol* 1999;20:568–576.

100. Weber DJ, Rutala WA. Gene therapy: a new challenge for infection control. *Infect Control Hosp Epidemiol* 1999;20:530–532.

101. Evans ME, Jordan CT, Chang SMW, et al. Clinical infection control in gene therapy: a multidisciplinary conference. *Infect Control Hosp Epidemiol* 2000;21:659–673.

102. Strausbaugh LJ. Gene therapy and infection control: more light on the way. *Infect Control Hosp Epidemiol* 2000;21:630–632.

103. McCarthy M. FDA puts US gene-therapy trial on hold. *Lancet* 2000;355:908–910.

CHAPTER 11
Bioterrorism

John G. Bartlett

Weapons of mass destruction are classified as biologic, chemical, or nuclear. Biologic weapons have a long and fascinating history, but only modest success in influencing world history. Nevertheless, at least 10 to 14 nation states and a large number of dissident groups have bioterrorism arsenals. A report by the U.S. Office of Technology Assessment reported in 1993 that a release of 100 kg of anthrax spores upwind of Washington, DC, would cause 130,000 to 3,000,000 deaths, thus matching the lethal potential of a hydrogen bomb (1). The reality of this risk was brought into sharp focus in 2001 with the epidemic of 22 cases of anthrax associated with contaminated letters (2). The United States responded with the establishment of the new Department of Homeland Security with 170,000 employees and a $40 billion budget in 2002. The goal of this chapter is to review the status of bioterrorism and bioterrorism defense.

HISTORY

Large-scale bioterrorism potential and application is largely limited to the last century (3). The initial large-scale attack in the twentieth century was directed against animals using *Burkholderia mallei* in World War I (4). During World War II the United States, Soviet Union, Japan, and Germany all had active bioweapon programs, but only Japan used it (plague) on a large scale. The U.S. bioterrorism effort was started at Camp Detrick in 1942, but in 1969 President Nixon ended the program (5). The Soviet Union bioweapon program was the largest and most scientifically advanced, with about 50 facilities and 60,000 employees, including some of their best scientists (6). In 1972, the Biologic and Toxin Weapons Convention was established to eliminate the threat of bioterrorism and was signed by 140 nations. In 1979, there was an accidental release of *Bacillus anthracis* from a Soviet weapon plant in Sverdlovsk, giving clear testimony to breaches of the 1972 document (7). Following the collapse of the Soviet Union, President Yeltsin issued a 1992 decree to disband the program.

Despite the efforts, 2002 estimates were that multiple nations harbor bioweapon programs, including Iraq, North Korea, Serbia, Sudan, and Libya. The most information was available for Iraq's bioweapon program, based on inspections through 1997 and defectors, which indicated that the program included 19,000 L of botulism toxin (10,000 L weaponized) and 8,500 L of anthrax spores (6,500 L weaponized) (8). There was also speculation that at least four nations have smallpox stores for potential use in bioterrorism.

The continuing threat of bioterrorism is exemplified by a 1984 attempt by a dissident religious cult to influence an election by contaminating restaurant salad bars with *Salmonella*; 751 persons developed salmonellosis, but the election was not disrupted (9). A subsequent effort was the use of sarin nerve gas in a Tokyo subway by a Japanese cult, the Aum Shinrykio; this resulted in 6,000 casualties and 12 deaths (10). In 2001, there were 22 cases of anthrax at four locations in the United States, representing the consequences of contaminated mail (2).

BIOTERRORISM PREPAREDNESS AND THE ANTHRAX EPIDEMIC OF 2001

In the year prior to the anthrax bioterrorism event, there were two large-scale bioterrorism simulations—one with plague in Denver ("TOPOFF") (11) and one of smallpox in Oklahoma ("Dark Winter") (12). Both were instructive in identifying major problems in preparedness with specific deficiencies in defining leadership, adequate health care capacity, and ability to contain contagion. These and other issues were put directly to test in the anthrax bioterrorism epidemic of 2001 (2,13–15).

The 2001 anthrax epidemic became apparent on October 4, 2001, with the announcement that a 63-year-old man was hospitalized in Palm Beach County, Florida, with inhalation anthrax (11,13). During the ensuing 2 months there were 22 cases of anthrax, 11 cutaneous and 11 inhalation, clustered in Boca Raton, Florida, New York City, New Jersey, and Washington, DC (2). There were several lessons from this experience that are potentially important for application in any subsequent episodes of bioterrorism that relate to epidemiology, management, and resource utilization.

Epidemiology

- Of the 22 cases, 20 had contact with contaminated mail through four letters (16).
- Fifteen cases associated with the National Broadcasting Company (NBC) suite were cutaneous, and the two Washington, DC cases were inhalational. This presumably reflects the milling, which produced small nearly single spore–sized particles in the letters to Senator Daschle and Senator Leahy versus the large particles sent to NBC. The difference was that the Washington letters produced widespread aerosolized spores as indicated by confluent growth of *B. anthracis* in the nasal

cultures of persons in Senator Daschle's office; by contrast, the NBC building had the largest portion of positive environment cultures, but large particle size, which limited aerosolization and inhalation (16,17).
- Molecular typing of *B. anthracis* strains from four contaminated letters, 12 cases, and over 100 environmental isolates showed a single strain, the Ames strain isolated in Texas in the 1960s. This finding linked all cases to a single source (16).
- Epidemiologic investigations identified about 10,000 persons considered to be at risk for inhalation anthrax; prophylactic antibiotics were recommended for these patients (16).

Medical Management

- The medical management was notably assisted by preemptive medical planning, which, in retrospect, covered all necessary facets of medical management designed for this and other category A agents by a consensus process involving representatives of anthrax experts, public health, and the health care system (17).
- Decisions were quickly made for treatment and prophylaxis based on the consensus document, *in vitro* sensitivity tests of the epidemic strain, and prior results of *in vivo* testing in the primate model (16).
- Of the 11 cases of inhalation anthrax, all received the recommended antimicrobial agents. An additional medical management issue learned and disseminated to clinical practitioners was the importance of chest computed tomography (CT) scans for the diagnosis and drainage of bloody pleural effusions (2).
- Prophylaxis was given using recommended antibiotics to an estimated 10,000 exposed persons, including several who had confluent growth of *B. anthracis* on nasal culture, an indication of heavy exposure; none of the 10,000 subsequently developed anthrax (16,18,19).
- The anthrax epidemic included only 22 cases, so surge capacity could not be tested.

Resource Utilization

- One of the most profound messages concerned the fact that only 22 cases were identified, but these cases nearly incapacitated the public health system (16).
- The Centers for Disease Control and Prevention (CDC) assigned over 1,000 personnel to this epidemic and still periodically seemed overwhelmed.
- In a 28-day period, the New York City Health Department managed 15,340 telephone inquiries.
- Prior to this event, there were over 200 mailed or telephoned threats of bioterrorism that resulted in the inappropriate management of 1,300 victims (20).
- Antibiotic prophylaxis was recommended for 10,000 individuals, but over 30,000 received at least some antibiotics, and over half reported side effects to doxycycline or ciprofloxacin (16). None had serious side effects.

CATEGORIZATION OF BIOLOGIC TERRORISM AGENTS

In 1999, there was a congressional initiative to develop a national public health response to acts of bioterrorism. This led to the establishment of the Bioterrorism Preparedness in Response Office. A subsequent meeting of national experts reviewed potential biologic agents to determine priority for public health preparedness based on their features as potential agents of bioterrorism acts (20). Results were based on (a) impact on public health in

TABLE 11.1.   Classification of Bioterrorism Agents

| Agent | Public health impact | | Dissemination[a] | | Public perception[b] | Special preparation[c] | Category |
	Disease	Death	Delivery potential	Person-to-person			
Smallpox	+	++	+	+++	+++	+++	A
Anthrax	++	+++	+++	0	+++	+++	A
Plague	++	+++	++	+++	++	+++	A
Botulism	++	+++	++	0	++	+++	A
Tularemia	++	+++	+	0	+	+++	A
Viral hemorrhagic fever	++	+++	+	+	+++	++	A
Viral encephalitis	++	+	+	0	++	++	B
Q fever	+	+	++	0	+	++	B
Brucella	+	+	++	0	+	++	B
Glanders	++	+++	++	0	0	++	B
Melioidosis	+	+	++	0	0	++	B
Psittacosis	+	+	++	0	0	+	B
Ricin toxin	++	++	++	0	0	++	B
Typhus	+	+	++	0	0	+	B
Cholera	+	+	++	+/−	+++	+	B
Shigellosis	+	+	++	+	+	+	B

+++, death for >50%; ++, 21%–49%; +, <20%.
[a]Potential for rapid large-scale dissemination.
[b]Number of media reports with +++ = >45 titles in surveying 233 newspapers and 70 TV/radio sources.
[c]Needs for therapeutics, surveillance, laboratory demands.

terms of illness and death; (b) delivery potential based on stability of agent, ability to mass produce and distribute, and the potential for person-to-person transmission; (c) the public perception in terms of potential for civil disruption; and (d) special needs for public health response. The agents were classified as A (greatest potential), B (less likely or important), or category C (not believed to be a high bioterrorism risk). The results of this assessment are summarized in Table 11.1.

CATEGORY A AGENTS

Anthrax

The features of anthrax are summarized in Table 11.2 (21).

HISTORY
Inhalation anthrax, along with smallpox, has always been the greatest concern for bioterrorism based on its properties of stability, ease of aerosolization, high rate of infection, and high mortality rate. In 1995, Iraq acknowledged producing and weaponizing *B. anthracis* (22), and a recent review indicates the probability that at least 13 countries are developing anthrax as a component of a biologic weapon program (21). Clinical experience with naturally occurring (zoonotic) inhalation anthrax is limited to 18 reported cases in the twentieth century, the accidental release of anthrax Sverdlovsk in 1979 (6), and the more recent experience with 22 cases of anthrax in the 2001 bioterrorism event in the United States (2). In 1970, the World Health Organization (WHO) estimated that 50 kg of *B. anthracis* released over an urban population of 5 million would cause disease in 250,000 and kill 100,000 (23). A more recent analysis by the U.S. Congressional Office of Technology estimated that a release of 100 kg would cause 130,000 to 3,000,000 deaths, thus matching the lethality of a hydrogen bomb (1).

PATHOGENESIS
Anthrax is acquired by three routes: inhalation, cutaneous contact, or ingestion, and symptoms reflect these three routes. The

major threat with bioterrorism is inhalation of spores milled to less than 5 μm to permit both aerosolization and inhalation. Following inhalation, the spores are taken by the alveolar macrophage to mediastinal lymph nodes, where they are converted to vegetative forms with production of protective antigen,

TABLE 11.2.   Inhalation Anthrax

Epidemiology	Last case naturally occurring inhalation anthrax in the United States was in 1976. Epidemic—sudden outbreak of severe acute febrile illness with fulminant course. No person-to-person spread. Illness in persons at defined risk.
Clinical features	Incubation period 4–5 days. Acute febrile illness with flu symptoms rapidly progressing to shock with mediastinitis, bloody pleural effusions, and positive blood cultures.
Diagnostic tests	Chest radiography and CT scan. Blood cultures: GPB
Pathology	Hemorrhagic mediastinitis, pleural effusions
Case fatality	45%–80%
Treatment (adults)	Ciprofloxacin 400 mg i.v. every 12 h or doxycycline 100 mg i.v. every 12 h, each with one or two additional drugs—imipenem, clindamycin, vancomycin penicillin, ampicillin, rifampin, chloramphenicol, or clarithromycin—for 10–14 days, then doxycycline p.o. 100 mg b.i.d. or ciprofloxacin p.o. 500 mg b.i.d. to complete 60-day course.
Postexposure	Candidates: defined by outbreak investigation
Prophylaxis (adults)	Preferred: ciprofloxacin (500 mg p.o. b.i.d.) or doxycycline (100 mg p.o. b.i.d.) for 60–100 days ± anthrax vaccine
Infection control	Isolation is not recommended.

CT, computed tomography; GPB, Gram-positive bacilli; i.v., intravenously; p.o., orally; b.i.d., twice daily.

lethal factor, and edema factor. The protective antigen combines with the other two to form two toxins, lethal toxin and edema toxin, that presumably account for clinical features (21,24). The result is a hemorrhagic thoracic lymphadenitis, hemorrhagic mediastinitis, pleural effusions, and shock. Cutaneous anthrax accounted for 11 of the cases in 2001 and reflects contact with the organism on surfaces. This is the common form of naturally occurring anthrax as a zoonotic disease. There are approximately 2,000 cases reported annually worldwide, 224 reported in the United States from 1944 through 1994 and one naturally occurring U.S. case in 2000 (25–27). Gastrointestinal (GI) anthrax results from ingestion of inadequately cooked contaminated meat; this is rare, but highly lethal (25,28).

EPIDEMIOLOGY

The ability to produce an epidemic of inhalation anthrax depends largely on milling of the organism to produce sufficiently small particles of spores for aerosolization and inhalation. The last case of naturally occurring inhalation anthrax in the United States was in 1976, implying that any case of inhalation anthrax should trigger a high suspicion of bioterrorism (21): Cutaneous anthrax may still be seen as a naturally occurring zoonosis in the United States, with one case reported in 2000 (27), but it should still be considered suspect, particularly if acquired in an urban area. An epidemic of inhalation anthrax would be characterized by the sudden outbreak of a severe, acute, febrile illness with a fulminant course. Cases would presumably have an epidemiologic link, as with the 2001 epidemic in which 20 of the 22 victims were postal workers, media personnel, or politicians or their staff (2,21). There is no person-to-person spread, so secondary cases are not seen.

CLINICAL FEATURES

Data from the Sverdlovsk epidemic following accidental cases of inhalation anthrax occurred 2 to 43 days after exposure (6), but the 2001 epidemic showed a relatively uniform time of 4 to 6 days from the time of predicted contact to the onset of clinical symptoms (2,10). The initial clinical features occur after germination with toxin release and result in a two-stage disease: initial symptoms are nonspecific and flu-like, with fever, malaise, headache, and GI complaints. Features that tend to distinguish this stage from influenza include the lack of coryza and prominent GI symptoms as well as the anticipated exposure history. The second stage is profound sepsis [without disseminated intravascular coagulation (DIC)] with chest pain, chest compression from large pleural effusions and mediastinal expansion, multiple organ failure, obtundation, cyanosis, and hypotension with death often occurring usually within hours (2,29–31). The mortality rate with antibiotic treatment was originally reported in the Sverdlovsk experience as 68 of 70 (87%) (6), but a more recent analysis suggests 100/250 (32). In the 2001 epidemic there were 5 deaths among 11 patients (45%). In fatal cases, the interval between the onset of symptoms and deaths averaged 3 to 4 days (21).

DIAGNOSIS

B. anthracis is an aerobic, gram-positive, spore-forming bacillus that is grown easily in routine media. In the 2001 epidemic, blood cultures were uniformly positive within 16 to 24 hours in all eight patients who had pretreatment blood cultures (21). The report from Sverdlovsk indicated positive blood cultures in all patients sampled within 21 hours of treatment, with quantitative cultures indicating concentrations as high as 10^8/mL blood (6). *B. anthracis* is suspected when the laboratory recovers a gram-positive, nonhemolytic, encapsulated, penicillin-sensitive, spore-forming bacillus. Confirmatory tests require referral to a Laboratory Response Network facility to perform definitive identification by immunohistochemical staining, gamma phage, and polymerase chain reaction (PCR) assays (for details see *www.bt.cdc.gov/LABISSUES/index.asp*). Other laboratory findings that support this diagnosis are the chest radiograph showing the characteristic wide mediastinum and a CT scan showing hyperdense hilar and mediastinal nodes with pleural effusions (2). A highly characteristic feature is bloody pleural effusions, which may be an important clinical clue to this diagnosis; in the Sverdlovsk outbreak, autopsies showed the average case had 1,700 mL of bloody pleural fluid collections (6).

TREATMENT

Recommendations for treatment are rapid institution of combination antibiotics (Table 11.1) and supportive care. Antibiotic selection is based on *in vitro* sensitivity tests of the epidemic strain. Three drugs are approved by the U.S. Food and Drug Administration (FDA) for anthrax based largely on the primate model in which monkeys had an aerosol challenge with eight 50% lethal dose (LD50) *B. anthracis* spores followed by treatment for 30 days with doxycycline, penicillin, or ciprofloxacin (32,33). All of these antibiotics worked, although 5 of 29 developed lethal inhalation anthrax after the drugs were discontinued at 30 days, suggesting that a longer course was necessary. In the 2001 epidemic, the recommended antibiotics were doxycycline or ciprofloxacin based on these animal experiments, FDA approval, and *in vitro* sensitivity tests of the epidemic strain. Penicillin was active *in vitro* at 0.06 μg/mL, but had an inducible β-lactamase of unknown significance, which accounts for its deletion as a preferred agent (21). (It should be noted that strains of *B. anthracis* recovered from the 1960s also had this inducible β-lactamase, indicating that the epidemic strain was not engineered for this resistance factor.) The recommendation was to combine one of the preferred agents with one or two additional antibiotics such as clindamycin due to its ability to shut down protein synthesis or an antibiotic that shows good penetration into the central nervous system. Particularly important in supportive care is the drainage of pleural effusions because chest compression appeared to be an important factor in morbidity and mortality, and the 2001 experience showed that many of the patients required chest tube drainage (2). There is no need to isolate patients because there is no person-to-person transmission.

PROPHYLAXIS

This is probably the most important facet of management because prophylaxis appears to be highly effective in preventing disease. In the 2001 epidemic, 10,000 patients were identified as being at risk and received prophylaxis with doxycycline or ciprofloxacin; none subsequently developed anthrax. The recommendation was initially for a 60-day course based on animal experiments of Friedlander (33) and Henderson (34) that showed *in vivo* persistence of spores for up to 100 days. The original recommendation was subsequently modified based on concern for very heavy exposures in some persons, resulting in the option of antibiotics for 60 days, antibiotics for 100 days, or a combination of antibiotics for 100 days combined with anthrax vaccine (35). Although there was concern and substantial publicity about adverse reactions to the prophylactic agents, the frequency of serious reactions was nil (36). Decisions about who should receive vaccine are a public health decision based on timing, location, and conditions of exposure (37).

Smallpox

Features of smallpox are summarized in Table 11.3 (38).

TABLE 11.3. Smallpox	
Epidemiology	Airborne spread; greatest risk is hospital personnel and household contacts; greatest risk is persons within 6–8 feet of patient after onset of fever to scab stage.
Clinical features	Incubation period 12–14 days. Initial symptoms: high fever, malaise, headache, then maculopapular rash → vesicular rash → pustular rash → scabs (14–21 days).
Diagnostic tests	Laboratory—requires BSL-4 facility with specimens collected by recently vaccinated person. Virus detected by electromyography of vesicular or postular fluid or scabs. Definitive microbial diagnosis: cell culture and polymerase chain reaction.
Case fatality	30%
Treatment	Smallpox vaccine within 4 days postexposure Cidofovir (experimental)
Prevention	Smallpox vaccination
Infection control	Negative pressure room with high-efficiency particulate air filtration Gowns, gloves, and masks

HISTORY

The global campaign to eradicate smallpox began in 1967, and the last case was reported in 1977 (39). In 1980, the WHO recommended that all laboratories destroy stocks of variola or transfer them to one of the two WHO reference laboratories in Moscow or at the CDC in Atlanta. These remaining supplies were to be destroyed, but a 1999 World Health Assembly agreed to retain these supplies through 2002 to permit further research, including development of a more attenuated vaccine and antiviral drugs (40). It is now believed that at least four countries harbor stocks of smallpox, although the true number is unknown. Persons in the United States born after 1972 have no immunity, and those who were vaccinated before that time have questionable protection (38,41). The mortality rate of smallpox is approximately 30% in unvaccinated persons, and person-to-person spread is highly efficient. This makes smallpox an ideal agent for bioterrorism.

EPIDEMIOLOGY

Smallpox is spread from person to person in droplets from the oral pharynx (38,39). The greatest risk is to persons within 6 to 8 feet of a case, and prior epidemics have consistently demonstrated that most cases occur in household members and by hospital contact. Because this disease was eradicated from the globe, any confirmed case of smallpox implies bioterrorism. The main challenge is not recognizing smallpox as an indicator of bioterrorism but distinction of smallpox from other rash-associated diseases.

CLINICAL FEATURES

The incubation period is generally 12 to 14 days, with a range of 7 to 17 days. Initial symptoms are high fever, malaise, prostration, headache, and backache (39). The rash first appears on day 3 as a maculopapular eruption that subsequently evolves to a vesicular and then postular rash that goes on to form scabs that separate and leave the characteristic pitted scars. The rash starts in the pharynx, face, and forearms, and then spreads to the trunk and legs. Transmission takes place primarily during the rash phase. The disease is lethal in about 30% of cases, with death occurring usually at day 5 or 6 of the rash and is presumed to reflect elaboration of cytokines (42). The course of this infection in patients with immune deficiency is unknown because smallpox was eradicated prior to organ transplantation, human

immunodeficiency virus, and chronic corticosteroid therapy, but it is assumed that those with defective cell-mediated immunity would have severe and progressive disease.

DIAGNOSIS

The laboratory diagnosis requires specimens collected by a recently vaccinated person with appropriate protection, usually with cotton swabs to obtain fluid from vesicular or pustular lesions. The laboratory examination requires a BL-4 (maximum containment) facility using growth on cell culture and strain characterization using PCR and restriction fragment-length polymorphisms (38,43,44). These studies can be completed within a few hours. For the clinician, the main differential is chickenpox, which is distinguished by lesions that evolve at different stages, lesions that are more superficial, and a centripetal distribution with more involvement of the trunk, face, and extremities.

TREATMENT

There is no therapy with established merit. Animal models suggest that cidofovir may be effective, but supporting clinical evidence is nil and the drug has substantial renal toxicity (45,46).

POSTEXPOSURE INFECTION CONTROL

Vaccination given within 4 days of exposure provides some protection against infection and significant protection against fatal outcome (38,39,45). The efficacy of preexposure preventive vaccination is 90% or more (39,48). Thus, the major goal will be to vaccinate those with anticipated risks such as military personnel and a hospital-based first response team. In the event of an outbreak, the highest priority will be household contacts and other face-to-face contacts of patients after the onset of fever (38). Health care workers with prior smallpox vaccinations should receive a high priority in this vaccination process (49). The vaccination has been associated with substantial risk, the most serious complications being (a) postvaccinial encephalitis with a rate of 1 per 300,000 vaccinations in primary vaccinees; (b) progressive vaccinia, which is a progressive and usually lethal complication of disseminated vaccinia in patients with cell-mediated immunity disorders; and (c) eczema vaccinatum in patients who have eczema or a history of eczema or atopic dermatitis (50–52). Vaccinia immune globulin may be used for the latter two complications, but the supply appears limited (51,53).

INFECTION CONTROL

Patients should be cared for at home or in a hospital room with a negative pressure and high-efficiency particulate air filtration system. Standard precautions include use of gloves, gowns, and masks. Laboratory testing requires a BL-4 facility.

Plague

Features of plague are summarized in Table 11.4 (54).

HISTORY

The plague pandemic that began in 1314 known as the "Black Death" killed 20 to 30 million people in Europe, about one third of the European population (55). This is the largest epidemic in the history of medicine in terms of deaths over a brief period of time. It is known that the Soviet scientists produce large quantities of Yersinia pestis for bioterrorism (56), but the United States never succeeded in producing large quantities when it had a bioweapon program, and relatively few scientists in the United States study the disease. It was estimated by the WHO that a 50-kg release of Y. pestis over an urban population of 5 million would result in 150,000 cases of plague pneumonia and 36,000

TABLE 11.4.	Plague
Epidemiology	Naturally occurring 8–10 cases/yr in the United States; 84% bubonic, 16% septicemic, and 2% pneumonic. Highly lethal outbreak of pneumonic illness due to aerosolized delivery with bioterrorism
Clinical features	Incubation period 1–6 days. Pneumonic symptoms with bloody sputum, fever, and prominent GI symptoms. Fulminant course with high fatality rate.
Diagnosis	Blood or sputum grain stain—bipolar (safety pin) GNB. Semiautomated bacterial ID systems may misidentify; up to 6 days required for ID. If suspected instruct laboratory to culture at 28°C as well as 37°C.
Treatment (adults)	Preferred: streptomycin (1 g i.m. b.i.d.) or gentamicin (5 gm/kg/day) for 10 days. Alternative: doxycycline (100 mg i.v. b.i.d.), ciprofloxacin (400 mg i.v. b.i.d.) or chloramphenicol (25 mg/kg i.v. q.i.d.) for 10 days.
Prophylaxis	Exposed persons defined by epidemic investigation. Household, hospital, and close contacts of patients. Doxycycline (100 mg p.o. b.i.d.) or ciprofloxacin (500 mg p.o. b.i.d.) for 7 days.
Infection control	Use disposable surgical masks. Patient isolation until treated 48 h.

GI, gastrointestinal; GNB, Gram-negative bacilli; ID, identification; i.m., intramuscularly; b.i.d., twice daily; i.v., intravenously; p.o., orally.

people would die (23). It was also calculated that the organism would remain viable in an aerosol for approximately 1 hour.

EPIDEMIOLOGY

There are approximately 50 to 80 cases of plague in the United States every year, but the great majority of these are bubonic plague, and only about 2% are pneumonic (54,57). Thus, any case of pneumonic plague, particularly cases acquired in urban areas, should raise the suspicion of bioterrorism. An outbreak of a pneumonic illness that is highly lethal reflects association with aerosol delivery, and severe cases of pneumonia with hemoptysis are clinical clues.

CLINICAL FEATURES

The incubation period is 1 to 6 days. An aerosol delivery would result in pneumonic plague with cough, fever, bloody sputum, and prominent GI symptoms, including nausea, vomiting, abdominal pain, and diarrhea (54,58–60). The course is rapidly progressive, with the sepsis syndrome and death at 2 to 6 days.

DIAGNOSIS

Y. pestis is a gram-negative coccobacillus with bipolar staining that resembles a safety pin. The diagnosis might be suspected on the basis of a Gram stain of sputum or blood that shows small gram-negative coccobacilli (58,61), but standard laboratory techniques may take an extended period of identification using standard automated identification methods. When this diagnosis is suspected, the laboratory should be warmed to split the culture with incubation at 28°C for rapid growth and a second with growth at 37°C for identification of the capsular (F1) antigen if available. Some rapid laboratory diagnostic tests are available from state health departments, the CDC, and some military laboratories (58).

TREATMENT

Pneumonic plague has a fatality rate exceeding 50%, but this is reduced to 5% to 14% with aminoglycoside treatment, which is the preferred class, primarily streptomycin and gentamycin (57,58). Treatment recommendations may require modification based on *in vitro* sensitivity testing for the epidemic strain, particularly when using alternative drugs such as doxycycline or fluoroquinolones (62). With regard to infection control, there are limited data regarding efficiency of person-to-person spread. In earlier epidemics, transmission could be prevented relatively easily by masks, which are recommended along with gowns, gloves, and eye protection (63–66). Isolation may be discontinued after 48 hours of antibiotic treatment and clinical improvement.

POSTEXPOSURE PROPHYLAXIS

Persons at risk of exposure from an aerosol distribution should receive prophylactic antibiotics for 7 days, usually with doxycycline, sulfonamides, chloramphenicol, or fluoroquinolones (63). This type of prophylaxis should also be provided for close contacts described as less than 2 m from a case who has not been treated for over 48 hours (64).

Botulism

Features of botulism are summarized in Table 11.5 (67).

HISTORY

After the Persian Gulf War, Iraq acknowledged production of 19,000 L of concentrated botulinum toxin, including 10,000 L that were weaponized (7). It is estimated that an aerosol release of botulinum toxin would kill or incapacitate 10% of persons within 0.5 km (23). Another possible mechanism of bioterrorism with botulinum toxin would be contamination of food.

EPIDEMIOLOGY

In the United States there are approximately 150 cases of botulism each year, most of which are food-borne or infant

TABLE 11.5.	Botulism
Epidemiology	United States—100 to 200 cases/year, nearly all infant and food-borne cases; bioterrorism—inhalation form.
Clinical features	Incubation period 2–4 days (inhalation). Acute, afebrile, symmetric, descending flaccid paralysis. Multiple cranial nerve palsies—diplopia, dysarthria, dysphagia, dysphonia.
Diagnosis	Microbiology availably only at the CDC and some state health laboratories. Specimens (blood, vomitus, stool, gastric aspirate) for mouse bioassay for toxin typed by type-specific antitoxin. Electromyography with repetitive nerve stimulation at 20–50 Hz supports this diagnosis.
Fatality	60%
Therapy	Treatment (ABE) or bivalent (AB) antitoxin in 10-mL vials containing 5,500–8,500 IU each. The vial is diluted 1:10 and given by slow i.v. Heptavalent antitoxin (ABCDE) (experimental, but necessary if type C or D used).
Prophylaxis	Antitoxin will prevent, but supply limited and risks may outweigh benefit. Botulism toxoid: not recommended due to limited supply and delayed response.
Infection control	Isolation is not recommended.

botulism (67,68). The greatest threat is aerosolized toxin producing inhalation botulism. Thus, large numbers of adult patients with typical neurologic findings without a food-borne source should suggest bioterrorism.

CLINICAL FEATURES

There are four forms of botulism (infant, food-borne, wound, and inhalation), and all show identical symptoms reflecting absorption of the toxin with distribution to peripheral cholinergic synapsis (67,69). Clinical features are an afebrile, symmetric descending flaccid paralysis with prominent cranial nerve involvement producing the four D's: diplopia, dysarthria, dysphonia, and dysphagia (67–74).

DIAGNOSIS

The microbial diagnosis can be made only with clinical specimens (blood, vomitus, stool, or gastric aspirates) for mouse bioassay provided at the CDC and some state health departments (67). The diagnosis is established by mouse inoculation with protection using type-specific antitoxin. This diagnosis also may be determined via electromyography using repetitive nerve stimulation at 20 to 50 Hz (74,75).

TREATMENT

Treatment consists of type-specific antitoxin using commercially available antitoxin for toxin type A, B, and E, the three forms of naturally occurring botulism. There is concern that other toxins might be used for bioterrorism, and an investigational heptavalent antitoxin to types A through G may be required (76). The antitoxin is available in 10-mL vials, with 5,500 to 8,500 IU of each type-specific antitoxin, which is diluted 1:10 with normal saline for slow intravenous (i.v.) infusion. This is an equine preparation that may cause serum sickness or anaphylaxis (77). The rest of the care is supportive, including placing the patient in the reverse Trendelenburg position to 20 to 25 degrees to facilitate airway protection. This is a toxin-mediated disease, and there is no person-to-person transmission, so no form of infection control is necessary.

PROPHYLAXIS

The only potential form of prophylaxis would be antitoxin, but this has inherent risks and the supply is too limited for widespread use.

Tularemia

Features of tularemia are summarized in Table 11.6 (78).

HISTORY

Francisella tularensis was one of several bioweapons developed by the U.S. military and was a part of the Soviet arsenal, including the production of strains claimed to be resistant to antibiotics and vaccines (56). The WHO estimated that an aerosol delivery of 50 kg of *F. tularensis* over a metropolitan area of 5 million people would cause 250,000 illnesses and 19,000 deaths (26). An average of 124 cases are reported annually in the United States, primarily from arthropod bites in the summer and handling of animal carcasses in the winter (79). Laboratory workers are especially vulnerable when accidentally exposed by inoculation or inhalation (80). Most naturally occurring cases are sporadic or occur in small clusters. With bioterrorism, the anticipation is that the disease would be acquired by inhalation and would involve large numbers. Outbreaks in urban areas would be particularly suspect.

TABLE 11.6. Tularemia	
Epidemiology	United States—100–200 cases/yr rural disease. Bioterrorism—large number of cases of acute nonspecific febrile illness with pleuropneumonitis. Urban, nonagricultural setting.
Clinical	Incubation period 3–5 days. Fever progressing to pharyngitis, bronchitis, pneumonitis, pleuritis, and hilar adenopathy.
Diagnostic tests	Respiratory secretions show gram-negative coccobacilli. Culture blood and sputum on cysteine-containing medium (warn laboratory). Direct immunofluorescence (DFA) and polymerase chain reaction for rapid identification. X-ray shows peribronchial infiltrates with pleural fluid and/or hilar adenopathy.
Fatality rate	1%–2%
Treatment (adults)	Preferred-streptomycin (1 g i.m. b.i.d.) or gentamycin (5 mg/kg/day i.v.) for 10 days. Alternative—doxycycline (100 mg i.v. b.i.d.), chloramphenicol (60 mg/kg/day i.v.) or ciprofloxacin (400 mg i.v. b.i.d.) for 14–21 days.
Prophylaxis (adults)	Recipients defined by outbreak Doxycycline (100 mg p.o. b.i.d.) or ciprofloxacin (500 mg p.o. b.i.d.) for 14 days
Infection control	Isolation is not recommended.

i.m., intramuscularly; b.i.d., twice daily; i.v., intravenously; p.o., orally.

CLINICAL FEATURES

The incubation period is 3 to 5 days. With inhalation tularemia, typical initial symptoms include fever, fatigue, headache, and chills (81–85). Chest symptoms are variable, and are most prominent with *F. tularensis* biovar tularensis (type A), which causes a more severe course (79). Nevertheless, many patients have minimal evidence of pneumonia by clinical features. Compared with plague or anthrax, inhalation tularemia is slower in progression and has a low fatality rate. It is much more like Q fever, which also may represent an agent of bioterrorism.

DIAGNOSTIC TESTS

Respiratory secretions show small gram-negative coccobacilli, but not the "safety pin" form of plague. Definitive diagnosis of the organism may be made by a direct immunofluorescent antibody (DFA) stain, but the reagents are available only in the Laboratory Response Network facilities (79). Growth on agar requires cystine-enriched media or chocolate. The laboratory must be warned to take appropriate precautions and to use the right media. Specialized laboratory tests include PCR, enzyme immunoassay (EIA), immunoblots, and pulsed-field gel electrophoresis, but these are only available in special reference laboratories (86–89). Radiography may be particularly helpful when it shows typical peribronchial infiltrates with pleural fluid or hilar adenopathy.

TREATMENT

The preferred treatment is aminoglycoside, primarily streptomycin or gentamycin. Isolation is not recommended because there is no human-to-human transmission. Thus, routine precautions are appropriate (90). However, laboratory personnel should be alerted as noted previously.

TABLE 11.7. Viral Hemorrhagic Fever

Virus	Clinical features	Person-to-person transmission	Mortality	Treatment	Distribution	Vector
Ebola	High fever, rash day 5, DIC	Yes	50%–90%	Supportive	Africa	?
Marburg	High fever, rash, DIC	Yes	23%–70%	Supportive	Africa	?
Lassa fever	Gradual onset, fever, conjunctivitis	Yes	15%–20%	Ribavirin	Africa	Rodent
New world Arenaviridae	Gradual onset, GI symptom, conjunctivitis, adenopathy	Yes	15%–30%	Ribavirin	South America	Rodent
Rift Valley	Fever, photophobia, jaundice	No	<1%	Ribavirin	Africa, Saudi Arabia	Mosquito
Yellow fever	Fever, conjunctivitis, jaundice, renal failure	No	20%	Supportive	Africa, Americas	Mosquito
Omsk hemorrhagic fever	Fever, cough, conjunctivitis, adenopathy	No	0.5%–10%	Supportive	Central Asia	Tick
Kyasanur forest disease	Biphasic illness, 50% meningoencephalitis	No	3%–10%	Supportive	India	Tick

DIC, disseminated intravascular coagulation; GI, gastrointestinal.

POSTEXPOSURE PROPHYLAXIS

Preferred antibiotics for postexposure prophylaxis are doxycycline or ciprofloxacin for 14 days.

Hemorrhagic Fever Viruses

Features of hemorrhagic fever viruses are summarized in Table 11.7 (91).

HISTORY

The hemorrhagic fever viruses include diverse agents that are not found in the United States, cause clinical illness characterized by fever and bleeding, and belong to one of four families: Filoviridae, Arenaviridae, Bunyaviridae, or Flaviviridae (91). The agents summarized in Table 11.7 are the members of this group that are most likely to be used in bioterrorism because of their features.

EPIDEMIOLOGY

These agents are transmitted by contact with infected animals or arthropod vectors, although the natural reservoir invectors of Ebola and Marburg viruses are unknown. None of these viruses are found endemically in the United States, and any case involving these agents occurring in a nonendemic area probably represents bioterrorism unless the patient was in the endemic area within the previous 2 to 22 days depending on the agent (Table 11.6).

CLINICAL FEATURES

The onset of illness is generally nonspecific and includes fever and myalgias, with frequent additional symptoms that are virus dependent, such as rash, encephalitis, pharyngitis, adenopathy, and GI symptoms (91–94). There is then progressive disease expressed with hemorrhage presenting with petechiae, hematuria, hematemesis, hemoptysis, or melena. This may be followed by DIC with shock, delirium, convulsions, and coma. Laboratory studies show leukopenia, anemia or hemoconcentration, thrombocytopenia, and elevated liver function tests. The mortality rate is highly variable for the various agents, ranging from 0.5% for Omsk hemorrhagic fever to 90% for Ebola virus (92,95).

DIAGNOSIS

The microbial diagnosis should be made in a BSL-4 for viral isolation (see *www.cdc.gov/od/ohs/biosfty/bmbl4/bmbl4s3.htm*). Other special diagnostic methods include EIA and reverse transcriptase PCR. In general, the diagnosis is made based on clinical criteria, and laboratory testing is used to confirm the diagnosis with appropriate care to handle specimens.

TREATMENT

Ribavirin given i.v. has been shown to reduce mortality with Lassa fever (96) and some New World arenaviruses (97–99). The drug is given i.v. in a dose of 30 mg/kg and then 16 mg/kg i.v. every 6 hours for 4 days and then 8 mg/kg i.v.; the main form of therapy for most patients is supportive care. With regard to infection control, there needs to be strict adherence to hand hygiene, double gloves, impermeable gowns, N-95 masks, shoe coverings, face shields, eye protection, and negative pressure rooms with high-efficiency particulate air filtration (99–101). Laboratory specimens require special handling, including double bagging with hand carriage to the laboratory at defined times when the specimen may be decontaminated using a detergent such as Triton X-100 for serum.

POSTEXPOSURE PROPHYLAXIS

There is no effective antiviral agent that can be used, including ribavirin (102,103).

ROLE OF THE INFECTIOUS DISEASE PHYSICIAN

The following are recommendations for preparedness and response:

- Accept bioterrorism as plausible with the implied need for planning.
- Support/participate in regional plans.
- Recognize the clinical and microbial clues to bioterrorism.
- Know the response plan.
- Support education efforts.

REFERENCES

1. Office of Technology Assessment, U.S. Congress. *Proliferation of weapons of mass destruction.* Publication no. OTA0ISC-599. Washington, DC: U.S. Government Printing Office, 1993:53.
2. Jernigan J, Stephens D, Ashford D, et al. Bioterrorism-related inhalation anthrax: the first 10 cases reported in the United States. *Emerg Infect Dis* 2001;7:933.
3. Tucker JB. Historical trends related to bioterrorism: an empirical analysis. *Emerg Infect Dis* 1999;5:498.

4. Christopher GW, Cieslak TJ, Pavlin JA, et al. Biological warfare. A historical perspective. *JAMA* 1997;278:412.

5. David CJ. Nuclear blindness: an overview of the biological weapons programs of the former Soviet Union and Iraq. *Emerg Infect Dis* 1999;5:509.

6. Alibek K, Handelman S. *Biohazard: the chilling true story of the largest covert biological weapons program in the world—told from inside by the man who ran it.* New York: Random House, 1999.

7. Meselson M, Guillermin J, Hugh-Jones M, et al. The Sverdlovsk anthrax outbreak of 1979. *Science* 1994;266:1202.

8. Stone R. Peering into the shadows: Iraq's bioweapons program. *Science* 2002;297:110.

9. Torok TJ, Tauxe RV, Wise RP, et al. A large community outbreak of salmonellosis caused by intentional contamination of restaurant salad bars. *JAMA* 1997;278:389.

10. Okumura T, Takasu N, Ishimatsu S, et al. Report on 640 victims of the Tokyo subway sarin attack. *Ann Emerg Med* 1996;28:129.

11. Inglesby TV, Grossman R, O'Toole T. a plague on your city: observations from TOPOFF. *Clin Infect Dis* 2001;32:436.

12. O'Toole T, Mair M, Inglesby TV. Shining light on "dark winter." *Clin Infect Dis* 2002;34:972.

13. Bush LM, Abrams BH, Beall A, et al. Index case of fatal inhalational anthrax due to bioterrorism in the United States. *N Engl J Med* 2001;345:1607.

14. Lane HC, Fauci AS. Bioterrorism on the home front: a new challenge for American medicine. *JAMA* 2001;286:2595.

15. Freedman A, Afonja O, Chang M, et al. Cutaneous anthrax associated with microangiopathic hemolytic anemia and coagulopathy in a 7-month-old infant. *JAMA* 2002;287:869.

16. Office of Public Health and Emergency Preparedness, National Institutes of Health and the Center for Disease Control and Prevention. *Strategies for optimizing post-exposure prophylaxis of inhalational anthrax.* National Academy of Sciences, December 12, 2001.

17. Inglesby TV, Henderson DA, Bartlett JG, et al. Anthrax as a biological weapon. *JAMA* 1999;281:1735.

18. Centers for Disease Control and Prevention. Update: investigation of bioterrorism-related anthrax and interim guidelines for clinical evaluation of persons with possible anthrax. *MMWR* 2001;50:941.

19. Centers for Disease Control and Prevention. Update: investigation of bioterrorism-related anthrax and interim guidelines for exposure management and antimicrobial therapy. *MMWR* 2001;50:909.

20. Rotz LD, Khan AS, Lillibridge SR. Public health assessment of potential biological terrorism agents. *Emerg Infect Dis* 2002;8:225.

21. Inglesby TV, O'Toole T, Henderson DA, et al. Anthrax as a biological weapon 2002: updated recommendations for management. *JAMA* 2002;287:2236.

22. Zillinskas RA. Iraq's biological weapons. *JAMA* 1997;278:418.

23. World Health Organization. *Health aspects of chemical and biological weapons.* Geneva, Switzerland: World Health Organization, 1970.

24. Hanna PC, Ireland JA. Understanding *Bacillus anthracis* pathogenesis. *Trends Microbiol* 1999;7:180.

25. Brachman P, Friedlander A. Anthrax. In: Plotkin S, Orenstein W, eds. *Vaccines,* 3rd ed. Philadelphia: WB Saunders, 1999:629.

26. Summary of notifiable diseases, 1945–1994. *MMWR* 1994;43:70.

27. Human anthrax associated with an epizootic among livestock. *MMWR* 2001;50:677.

28. Sirisanthana T, Navacharoen N, Tharavichitkul P, et al. Outbreak of oral-pharyngeal anthrax. *Am J Trop Med Hyg* 1984;33:144.

29. Friedlander A. Anthrax. In: Zajtchuk R, Bellamy R, eds. *Textbook of military medicine: medical aspects of chemical and biological warfare.* Washington, DC: Office of the Surgeon General, U.S. Department of the Army, 1997:467.

30. Brachman P, Friedlander A. Inhalation anthrax. *Ann NY Acad Sci* 1980; 353:83.

31. Vessal K, Yeganehdoust J, Dutz W, et al. Radiologic changes in inhalation anthrax. *Clin Radiol* 1975;26:471.

32. Brookmeyer R, Blades N, Hugh-Jones M, Henderson D. The statistical analysis of truncated data: application to the Sverdlovsk anthrax outbreak. *Biostatistics* 2001;2:233.

33. Friedlander AM, Welkos SL, Pitt ML, et al. Postexposure prophylaxis against experimental inhalation anthrax. *J Infect Dis* 1993;167:1239.

34. Henderson DW, Peacock S, Belton FC. Observations on the prophylaxis of experimental pulmonary anthrax in the monkey. *J Hyg* 1956;54:28.

35. Centers for Disease Control and Prevention. Additional options for preventive treatment for persons exposed to inhalation anthrax. *MMWR* 2001;50: 1142.

36. Update: adverse events associated with anthrax prophylaxis among postal employees: New Jersey, New York City, and the District of Columbia metropolitan area, 2001. *MMWR* 2001;50:1051.

37. Perkins WA. Public health implications of airborne infection. *Bacteriol Rev* 1961;25:347.

38. Henderson DA, Inglesby TV, Bartlett JG, et al. Smallpox as a biological weapon: medical and public health management. *JAMA* 1999;281:2127.

39. Fenner F, Henderson DA, Arita I, et al. *Smallpox and its eradication.* Geneva, Switzerland: World Health Organization, 1988:1460.

40. World Health Organization. Smallpox eradication: temporary retention of variola virus stocks. *Wkly Epidemiol Rec* 2001;76:142.

41. Centers for Disease Control and Prevention. Vaccinia (smallpox) vaccine recommendations of the immunization practices advisory committee. *MMWR* 2001;50(RR-10):1; 40(RR-14):445.

42. LuDuc JW, Damon I, Meegan JM, et al. Update on smallpox preparedness, 2001. *Emerg Infect Dis* 2002 (in press).

43. Ropp SL, Knight JC, Massung RF, et al. PCR strategy for identification and differentiation of smallpox and other orthopoxviruses. *J Clin Microbiol* 1995;33:2069.

44. Esposito JJ, Massung RF. Poxvirus infections in humans. In: Murray RP, Baron EJ, Pfaller MA, et al., eds. *Manual of clinical microbiology,* 6th ed. Washington, DC: American Society of Microbiology, 1995:1131.

45. DeClercq F. Cidofovir in the treatment of poxvirus infections. *Antivir Res* 2002;55:1.

46. McConnell J. Gearing up for smallpox. *Lancet Infect Dis* 2002;2:390.

47. Dixon CW. *Smallpox.* London: Churchill, 1962:1460.

48. Downie AW, McCarthy K. The antibody response to man following infection with viruses of the pox group, III: antibody response in smallpox. *J Hyg* 1958;56:479.

49. Centers for Disease Control and Prevention. Interim smallpox response plans and guidelines. Draft 21, November 2001. Available at *www.cdc.gov.*

50. Lane JM, Ruben FL, Neff JM, et al. Complications of smallpox vaccination, 1968: national surveillance in the United States. *N Engl J Med* 1969;281: 1201.

51. Goldstein VA, Neff JM, Lande JM, Koplan J. Smallpox vaccination reactions, prophylaxis and therapy of complications. *Pediatrics* 1975;55:342.

52. Neff JM, Lane JM, Fulginiti VA, Henderson DA. Contact vaccinia—transmission of vaccinia from smallpox vaccination. *JAMA* 2002;288:1901.

53. Kempe CH. Studies on smallpox and complications of smallpox vaccination. *Pediatrics* 1960;26:176.

54. Inglesby TV, Dennis DT, Henderson DA, et al. for the Working Group on Civilian Biodefense. Plague as a biological weapon. *JAMA* 2000;283:2281.

55. Slack P. the black death past and present. *Trans R Soc Trop Med Hyg* 1989;83: 461.

56. Alibek K, Handelman S. *Biohazard.* New York: Random House, 1999.

57. Centers for Disease Control and Prevention. Fatal human plague—Arizona and Colorado, 1996. *MMWR* 1997;46:617.

58. Butler T. *Yersinia* species (including plague). In: Mandell GL, Bennett JE, Dolin R, eds. *Principles and practice of infectious diseases.* New York: Churchill Livingstone, 1995:2070.

59. Crook LD, Tempest B. Plague: a clinical review of 27 cases. *Arch Intern Med* 1992;152:1253.

60. Dennis D, Meier F. Plague. In: Horsburgh CR, Nelson AM, eds. *Pathology of emerging infections.* Washington, DC: ASM Press, 1997:21.

61. Perry Rd, Fetherston JD. *Yersinia pestis*—etiologic agent of plague. *Clin Microbiol Rev* 1997;10:35.

62. Ryzhko IV, Shcherbaniuk AI, Samokhodkina ED, et al. Virulence of rifampicin and quinolone resistant mutants of strains of plague microbe with Fra$^+$ and Fra$^-$ phenotypes. *Antibiot Khimioter* 1994;39:32.

63. American Public Health Association. Plague. In: Benenson AS, ed. *Control of communicable diseases manual.* Washington, DC: American Public Health Association, 1995:353.

64. Centers for Disease Control and Prevention. Prevention of plague: recommendations of the Advisory Committee on Immunization Practice (ACIP). *MMWR* 1996;45(RR-14):1.

65. Mayer K. Pneumonic plague. *Bacteriol Rev* 1961;25:249.

66. Chernin E. Richard Pearson Strong and the Manchurian epidemic of pneumonic plague, 1910–1911. *J Hist Med Allied Sci* 1989;44:296.

67. Arnon SA, Schecter R, Inglesby TV, et al. Botulinum toxin as a biological weapon: medical and public health management. *JAMA* 2001;285:1059.

68. Hatheway CL, Johnson EA. *Clostridium:* the spore-bearing anaerobes. In: Collier L, Balows A, Sussman M, eds. Topley &Wilson's *Microbiology and microbial infections,* 9th ed. New York: Oxford University Press, 1998:731.

69. Shapiro RL, Hatheway C, Swerdlow DL. Botulism in the United States: a clinical and epidemiologic review. *Ann Intern Med* 1998;129:221.

70. Franz DR, Jahrling PB, Friedlander AM, et al. Clinical recognition and management of patients exposed to biological warfare agents. *JAMA* 1997;278: 399.

71. Hughes JM, Blumenthal JR, Merson MH, et al. Clinical features of types A and B food-borne botulism. *Ann Intern Med* 1981;95:442.

72. Duchen LW. Motor nerve growth induced by botulinum toxin as a regenerative phenomenon. *Proc R Soc Med* 1972;65:196.

73. Mann JM, Martin S, Hoffman R, Marrazzo S. Patient recovery from type A botulism: morbidity assessment following a large outbreak. *Am J Public Health* 1981;71:266.

74. Cherington M. Clinical spectrum of botulism. *Muscle Nerve* 1998;21:701.

75. Maselli RA, Bakshi N. American Association of Electrodiagnostic Medicine case report 16: botulism. *Muscle Nerve* 2000;23:1137.

76. Hibbs RG, Weber JT, Corwin A, et al. Experience with the use of an investigational F(ab^1)$_2$ heptavalent botulism immune globulin of equine origin during an outbreak of type E botulism in Egypt. *Clin Infect Dis* 1996;23:337.

77. Black RE, Gunn RA. Hypersensitivity reactions associated with botulinal antitoxin. *Am J Med* 1980;69:567.

78. Dennis DT, Inglesby TV, Henderson DA, et al, for the Working Group on Civilian Biodefense. Tularemia as a biological weapon. *JAMA* 2001;285: 2763.

79. Centers for Disease Control and Prevention. Tularemia—United States, 1990–2000. *MMWR* 2002;51:181.

80. Shapiro DS, Schwartz DR. Exposure of laboratory workers to *Francisella tularensis* despite a bioterrorism procedure. *J Clin Microbiol* 2002;40:2278.

81. Dahlstrand S, Ringertz O, Zetterberg B. Airborne tularemia in Sweden. *Scand J Infect Dis* 1971;3:7.

82. Ohara Y, Sato T, Homma M. Arthropod-borne tularemia in Japan: clinical analysis of 1,374 cases observed between 1924 and 1996. *J Med Entomol* 1998;35:471.

83. Perez-Castnillon J, Bachiller-Luque P, Mena-Martin FJ. An outbreak of primary pneumonic tularemia. *N Engl J Med* 2002;346:1027.

84. Young LS, Bicknell DS, Archer BG, et al. Tularemia epidemic, Vermont, 1968: forty-seven cased linked to contact with muskrats. *N Engl J Med* 1969;280:1253.

85. Evans ME, Gregory DW, Schaffner W, McGee ZA. Tularemia: a 30-year experience with 88 cases. *Medicine (Baltimore)* 1985;64:251.

86. Syrjaia H, Koskela P, Ripatti T, et al. Agglutination and ELISA methods in the diagnosis of tularemia in different clinical forms and severities of the disease. *J Infect Dis* 1986;153:142.

87. Bevanger L, Macland JA, Naess AI. Agglutinins and antibodies to *Francisella tularensis* outer membrane antigens in the early diagnosis of disease during an outbreak of tularemia. *J Clin Microbiol* 1988;26:433.

88. Grunow R, Splettstoesser W, McDonald S, et al. Detection of *Francisella tularensis* in biological specimens using a capture enzyme-linked immunosorbent assay, an immunochromatographic handheld assay, and a PCR. *Clin Diagn Lab Immunol* 2000;7:86.

89. Higgins JA, Hubalek Z, Halouzka J, et al. Detection of *Francisella tularensis* in infected mammals and vectors using a problem-based polymerase chain reaction. *Am J Trop Med Hyg* 2000;62:310.

90. Garner JS. Guideline for isolation precautions in hospitals. *Infect Control Hosp Epidemiol* 1996;17:53.

91. Borio L, Inglesby T, Peters CJ, et al. Hemorrhagic fever viruses as biological weapons: medical and public health management. *JAMA* 2002;287:2391.

92. Peters CJ, Jahrling PB, Khan AS. Patients infected with high-hazard viruses. *Arch Virol Suppl* 1996;11:141.

93. Colebunders R, Borchert M. Ebola haemorrhagic fever—a review. *J Infect* 2000;40:16.

94. White HA. Lassa fever: a study of 23 hospital cases. *Trans R Soc Trop Med Hyg* 1972;66:390.

95. Muyembe-Tamfum JJ, Kipasa M, Kiyungu C, et al. Ebola outbreak in Kikwit, Democratic Republic of the Congo: discovery and control measures. *J Infect Dis* 1999;179(suppl 1):259.

96. McCormick JB, King IJ, Webb PA, et al. Lassa fever: effective therapy with ribavirin. *N Engl J Med* 1986;314:20.

97. Update: management of patients with suspected viral hemorrhagic fever—United States. *MMWR* 1995;44:475.

98. Enria DA, Maizlegui JI. Antiviral treatment of Argentine hemorrhagic fever. *Antiviral Res* 1994;23:23.

99. Huggins JW. Prospects for treatment of viral hemorrhagic fevers with ribavirin, a broad-spectrum antiviral drug. *Rev Infect Dis* 1989;11(suppl 4):750.

100. LeDuc JW. Epidemiology of hemorrhagic fever viruses. *Rev Infect Dis* 1989;11(suppl 4):730.

101. Centers for Disease Control and Prevention/World Health Organization. *Infection control for viral hemorrhagic fevers in the African health care setting.* Atlanta, GA: Centers for Disease Control and Prevention. Available at *www.cdc.gov/ncidod/dvrd/spb/mnpages/vhfmanual.htm*

102. Kenyon RH, Canonico PG, Green De, Peters CJ. Effect of ribavirin and tributylribavirin on argentine hemorrhagic fever (Junin virus) in guinea pigs. *Antimicrob Agents Chemother* 1986;29:521.

103. Seiler P, Senn BM, Klenerman P, et al. Additive effect of neutralizing antibody and antiviral drug treatment in preventing virus escape and persistence. *J Virol* 2000;74:5896.

II

Diagnosis of Infectious Diseases

CHAPTER 12

Clinical Microbiology

Henry D. Isenberg and Stephen G. Jenkins

The most basic prerequisite for the successful treatment of a patient with an infectious disease is identification of the causative agent by the clinical microbiologist. Lacking such information makes diagnosis and therapy, at best, an educated guess. The clinical microbiology service directs all efforts to isolate, characterize, and identify infectious agents as well as assessing the host reactions and microbial responses to therapeutic agents using microscopic, cultural, biochemical, immunologic, and molecular approaches. Recent advances in molecular microbiology have made essentially all potentially harmful microbial and viral agents amenable to detection, identification, and quantification. In addition, the discipline of clinical microbiology addresses approaches for the evaluation of successful therapy while concerning itself with the safety of all patients, institutional employees, and the community whenever the potential for dissemination of a host-harmful isolate is recognized. This chapter's focus encompasses all of these parameters, except immunologic (serologic) diagnosis, which is the subject of another chapter.

SPECIMEN COLLECTION AND PROCESSING

General Principles

Proper specimen collection is the key to the accurate microbiologic diagnosis of infectious disease. The major challenge in collecting specimens is avoidance of contamination of the specimen with microorganisms that are indigenous to the skin and mucous membranes (Table 12.1). General approaches to address the problem of contamination include disinfecting the applicable body surface before aspiration or biopsy, bypassing the area with indigenous microbiota, using selective culture techniques, and performing quantitative cultures. Disinfection of the skin is reasonably successful provided that the skin surface is exposed to the disinfectant for a minimum of 30 seconds. Disinfection of mucous membranes is far less successful and contamination of specimens obtained through the surface of the oral cavity or the vagina is frequently unavoidable. Aspiration, such as transtracheal or suprapubic, is a method used to bypass an area that is heavily colonized by indigenous microbiota. Specimens for the culture of mycobacteria are decontaminated and then inoculated to media containing antimicrobial agents, which minimizes

contamination of cultures by other bacteria. Such selective techniques are also used for the culture of fungi, viruses, chlamydiae, and mycoplasmas. Quantification, often used to differentiate between indigenous microbiota and pathogens, has formed the basis for diagnosis of urinary tract infection for many years. This approach has also been applied to bronchoalveolar lavage specimens and protected brushes for the diagnosis of pneumonia and in efforts to distinguish colonizing from infecting microorganisms in wounds, vascular catheter tips, and burns. Repeated isolation of an alleged indigenous microorganism from the same body site suggests, however, its potential role in the pathogenesis of the symptom or lesion.

Swabs, especially cotton, are the most common devices used for the collection and transport of specimens for microbiologic analysis. Unfortunately, the amount of specimen provided in/on a swab is usually less than optimal for culture, let alone for culture and smear preparation. Cotton also contains substances injurious to a number of microorganisms, and cotton fiber mesh interferes with the recovery of some microorganisms. Some of the recently developed commercially available porous plastic fiber substitutes release most if not the entire clinical specimen, protect against desiccation, and maintain viability of almost all constituents of the population in the specimen. When submitted in duplicate, one swab can be used for smear preparation and the other for culture. The use of swabs should be restricted to lesions of the skin and mucous membranes. They are not an acceptable alternative to aspiration of fluid or pus from a body site. A variety of commercially available transport vials for accumulated body fluids and pus maintain the viability of anaerobic and aerobic bacteria, fungi, and viruses for a length of time usually adequate for carriage to the clinical microbiology laboratory for processing and analysis. Clinical material should be aspirated and injected into the vial for transport to the laboratory. If the amount of fluid or pus is limited, lesions may be irrigated with a small amount of bacteriostat-free saline or, preferably, lactated Ringer solution.

Invasive procedures for specimen collection must always be performed with constant attention to standard infection control precautions extending at all times to the maintenance of appropriate conditions of transport containers and requisitions. Microbiology laboratory personnel cannot be expected to handle grossly contaminated containers, lids, or, especially, syringes with needles attached. The surgeon obtaining tissue at operation should take a large enough sample to provide material for both histologic and microbiologic examination. Ideally, the tissue is divided at the operating table and a separate portion submitted for each of the two types of examination. If a single large lesion or abscess is present, several portions of the lesion or abscess wall should be collected for microbiologic examination. If, on the other hand, there are multiple smaller lesions or abscesses,

TABLE 12.1.   Bacteria Commonly Found on Healthy Human Body Surfaces[a]

Bacteria	Skin	Conjunctiva	Upper respiratory tract	Mouth	Lower intestine	External genitalia	Anterior urethra	Vagina
Aerobic and facultatively anaerobic								
Staphylococci	+	+	+	+	±	+	++	+
Streptococci								
Viridans	±	±	+	++	+	+	±	+
Group A			±	±				
Group D			+	+	+	+	+	+
Streptococcus pneumoniae		±	+	+				
Neisseriae		±	±	+			+	±
Corynebacteria	+	+	+	+	+	+	+	+
Haemophilus		±	+	+				
Enterobacteriaceae			±	±	++	+	+	±
Anaerobic								
Clostridia				±	++		±	±
Propionibacteria	++		+	±	±		±	
Actinomycetes			+	+	±			
Lactobacilli				+	+		±	++
Bifidobacteria				+	++			++
Bacteroides			+	++	++	+	+	+
Fusobacteria			+	++	+	+	+	±
Cocci								
Gram-positive	+		+	++	++	+	±	+
Gram-negative			+	++	+		±	+

[a] ±, Irregular; +, common; ++, prominent.
From Washington JA II. Medical bacteriology. In Henry JB, ed: *Clinical diagnosis and management by laboratory methods,* ed 18. Philadelphia: WB Saunders, 1991:1025–1073, with permission.

the surgeon should obtain specimens from a sufficient number of sites to assure that all potential pathogens are detected. Because the number of microorganisms diminishes with duration of infection, the more chronic the infection, the larger the portion of a lesion that should be obtained. Redundancy in reminding surgeons and operating room personnel that formalin is lethal for microorganisms should be encouraged.

Despite all efforts, the microbiology laboratory may still have difficulty establishing the pathogen in an infectious process. Technical problems may preclude collection of specimens that are representative of the disease process, or, in some cases, it may simply be impossible to obtain a specimen devoid of contamination with indigenous microbiota. Specimens, although appropriate, may be procured after effective initiation of antimicrobial therapy. In patients treated with antimicrobial agents, in substance abusers, and in those patients with compromised immune function, indigenous bacteria may be replaced by gram-negative members of the families *Enterobacteriaceae* and *Pseudomonadaceae*, further obfuscating the distinction between indigenous and pathogenic microbiota. Laboratories establish protocols to detect the most likely pathogens based on the site of origin of the specimen and may, therefore, not seek uncommon pathogens in the absence of a clinical impression or history. Related to all of the forgoing, laboratories are seldom if ever aware of the suspected diagnosis for a patient because such information is only rarely provided on the requisition form, as required by laboratory accrediting agencies (e.g., the College of American Pathology). Agents that are not cultivatable by usually employed laboratory techniques (e.g., *Coxiella burnetii*), will be routinely missed unless effective communication with the clinical microbiologist is established. Misunderstandings between clinicians and microbiologists result far more frequently from poor communication than from laboratory negligence. Finally, with the exception of those instances in which the identity of the pathogen can be established on the basis of direct specimen examination, definitive diagnosis depends on the recovery of the microorganism in culture, which may take from 1 day to 8 weeks or longer, depending on the nature of the microorganism involved and the degree of instrument sophistication in the specific laboratory.

The extent of microbiologic services provided varies considerably from one laboratory to the next. Most clinical microbiology laboratories provide a relatively full range of services in bacteriology, but their services in mycology, mycobacteriology, virology, parasitology, and molecular microbiology are variable. For example, many laboratories perform acid-fast stains and process specimens for mycobacterial culture but refer all mycobacterial isolates to a reference laboratory for further identification and susceptibility testing. Many laboratories provide services for the isolation of fungi and identification of yeasts, but filamentous molds that grow in culture may be forwarded to a reference facility for identification. Similarly, on special request, antifungal susceptibility testing of yeasts may be referred to a laboratory with appropriate expertise. Such differences in levels of service are recognized by national laboratory inspection and accrediting agencies and proficiency testing programs appropriate for the varied types of laboratory are offered and graded accordingly.

All clinical laboratories must provide medical and nursing personnel with instructions for the proper collection and transport of specimens (1) (Table 12.2). Microbiologists, moreover, must actively participate in in-service educational programs for nurses to whom physicians often relegate the responsibility for specimen collection and transport. Interns, residents, pathology and infectious disease fellows, and medical students all require detailed education because most have not been exposed to the rigorous requirements for asepsis, the collection kits

TABLE 12.2. **Specimen Collection and Transport for Bacteriology**

Specimen	Collection and transport	Comments
Blood	**Adults** 1. 10 mL into each of two 100-mL vacuum bottles (may include one bottle with SeptiChek™ attachment) or 2. 5 mL into each of two 50-mL vacuum bottles + 10 mL into ISOLATOR or 3. 10 mL into one 100-mL vacuum bottle + 10 mL into ISOLATOR tube or 4. 10 mL into each if two BACTEC high volume resin bottles **Infants** 1. 1–3 mL into each of two 10- or 100-mL vacuum bottles or 2. 0.5–1.5 mL into pediatric ISOLATOR tube and any remaining blood into 50- or 100-mL vacuum bottle	A minimum of two and a maximum of four cultures per septic episode are recommended
Intravascular catheter	Remove catheter aseptically, cut one (from 2- to 3-inch catheter) or two (from 8- to 24-inch catheter) 2-inch segments, and transfer into transport device	Catheter segments should be cultured semiquantitatively
Exudate (transudate, drainage, ulcer)	Swab or sterile, screw-capped tube	Such specimens are rarely suitable for anaerobic culture
Eye	See text of source book for table	
Feces	Freshly passed specimen in sealed container or rectal swab	Transport medium is recommended if delay is anticipated
Fluids Cerebrospinal	Sterile, screw-capped tube to be delivered to the laboratory immediately	Refrigeration may be harmful to some *Neisseria* or *Haemophilus* spp.
Peritoneal (including dialysate)	Inoculate 10 mL into ISOLATOR tube or into blood culture bottles	Direct inoculation of blood culture systems has increased yield of bacteria from patients with spontaneous peritonitis and continuous ambulatory peritoneal dialysis-associated peritonitis
Pleural	Inoculate a portion of the specimen into an anaerobic transport system	Pleural or empyema fluid is a major source of anaerobic bacteria causing pleuro- pulmonary infection
Genitourinary system For *Neisseria gonorrhoeae*	Send swab moistened with Stuart or Amies transport medium directly to the laboratory (4h maximal transport time) or directly inoculate modified Thayer-Martin medium in Transgrow or JEMBEC device	**Women** Cervix: Moisten speculum with water before inserting into vagina; insert swab into cervical canal. Anal swab: insert swab approximately 2 cm and move from side to side to sample crypts. Urethra or vagina: Cultures indicated when cervical not possible **Men** Urethra: Swab may be used when a discharge is present; otherwise, a sterile bacteriologic loop is inserted to obtain scrapings for smear and culture. Anal canal: As for women
Cervix, vagina for other bacteria	Swab	Specimens from these sites are not suitable for anaerobic culture
Urine Midstream Catheter	Collect in sterile screw-capped container which must be transported to the laboratory within 2 h of collection unless refrigerated	
Suprapubic aspirate	Inject protion of aspirate into an anaerobic transport tube or vial	This is the only type of urine specimen that is acceptable for anaerobic culture
Abscess, traumatic or post-	Aspirate pus with syringe and needle and transport to laboratory by injecting aspirate into an anaerobic transport vial or taking the syringe (needle removed) directly to laboratory	A swab provides too little material for Gram-stained smear or aerobic and anaerobic cultures. If the amount of pus is limited, one may inject the area with 0.5–1.0 mL of bacteriostat-free lactated Ringer's solution, and aspirate material
Respiratory tract for *Bordetella pertussis*	Use flexible wire calcium alginate–tipped swab or soft rubber catheter to obtain nasopharyngeal specimen	Cough plate is not recommended
Throat	Swab posterior pharynx, tonsils, and any areas of purulence or ulceration; a dry swab is acceptable if the specimen is cultured within 2 h of collection; otherwise, moisten the swab with Stuart or Amies transport medium	Avoid contamination with oral secretions. Ordinarily, testing for *Streptococcus pyogenes* is sufficient, but groups C and G β-hemolytic streptococci cause a pharyngitis clinically indistinguishable from that caused by Group A β-hemolytic streptococci and these organisms are reported to be associated with post-streptococcal glomerulonephritis as a sequela to infection. The laboratory must be notified in cases of suspected diphtheria, pertussis, or gonorrhea.

(continued)

TABLE 12.2. (*continued*)

Specimen	Collection and transport	Comments
Sputum	Obtain specimen by expectorating a deep cough into a sterile, screw-capped jar.	Specimens should be screened cytologically and another specimen requested when >25 squamous epithelial cells are observed per low-power field.
Transtracheal aspirate	Collect aspirate in a Lukens trap or inject into an anaerobic transport vial	Such specimens are suitable for anaerobic culture
Protected brush	The brush is served from the inner cannula and transported to the laboratory in 1 mL of bacteriostat-free lactated Ringer solution	Quantitative culture of the vortexed lactated Ringer solution helps differentiate upper from lower respiratory tract origin.
Bronchoalveolar lavage	Obtain at least 40 mL for complete microbiologic examination	Quantitative culture will help to differentiate upper from lower respiratory tract origin.
Tissue	Sterile, Screw-capped container	Sufficient amounts of tissue must be submitted separately for both histopathologic and microbiologic examination.

From Washington JA II. Medical microbiology. In Henry JB, ed: *Clinical diagnosis and management by laboratory methods,* ed 18. Philadelphia: WB Saunders, 1991:1025–1073, with permission.

available to them, and the essentiality for rapid delivery to the laboratory necessary to preserve the microbiologic integrity of each and every clinical specimen. Educational efforts on the part of microbiologists should alleviate this steadily escalating problem. Personnel in operating rooms, recovery areas, intensive and progressive care units, hematology and oncology services, and transplant units who collect or assist in procurement of specimens must continuously be exposed to in-service education programs to reinforce their expertise in accurate collection and transport of specimens for microbiologic analysis. The microbiologist is responsible for selecting the most appropriate specimen collection and transport devices and for ensuring that these devices are distributed to and available in all areas where they are needed. For example, operating rooms must have an inventory of sterile anaerobic transport devices on hand at all times. There are also situations in which the microbiologist must either be at the patient bedside to prepare smears and inoculate cultures or must train other medical personnel to perform these techniques effectively. Thus, in cases of corneal or intraocular infection yielding specimens so minute that the odds of loss in any transport system are extremely high, ophthalmologists, both in the outpatient setting and in the operating room, must be trained to optimally prepare smears and inoculate culture media. Although transport media may support the viability of some microorganisms for 24 hours, survival of many microorganisms during storage and transport is limited. Therefore, measures to ensure prompt delivery of all specimens to the microbiology laboratory are imperative. Special transport media that allow for delayed delivery to the microbiology laboratory are available for a growing number of pathogens. For example, some such devices contain fixatives that preserve parasites in fecal specimens for subsequent detection by tinctorial methods in the laboratory. Specimens for culture of *Chlamydia trachomatis* may be placed into a special transport medium; if transport is delayed, the medium can be frozen so that the specimen may be cultured on arrival in the microbiology laboratory.

SPECIFIC GUIDELINES

Septicemia

Prompt detection of septicemia is among the most important functions of the clinical microbiology laboratory. Certain principles are important to bear in mind for success with this process.

First, with the notable exception of intravascular infections such as endocarditis, most bacteremias are intermittent in nature. For this reason collection of a single blood culture is rarely, if ever, indicated. Two separate blood culture specimens are necessary, and usually sufficient, to rule out or establish a diagnosis of bacteremia. In cases in which the level of suspicion is high, three or four cultures may, however, be indicated for detection of bacteremia when either the anticipated pathogen is frequently interpreted as a skin contaminant (as in prosthetic valve endocarditis) or the patient has received antimicrobial therapy for possible endocarditis (1,2).

The second important principle for detection of septicemia is that the volume of blood per culture is the single most important determinant of yield. The difference in recovery between cultures of 10 and 20 mL of blood is often as great as 40%. The incremental yield is smaller (approximately 10% to 15%) for cultures of 30 versus 20 mL of blood. Regardless of the blood culture system in use by the laboratory, the microbiologist should use a protocol designed to accommodate 20 mL of blood per culture from adults. The volume of blood collected per culture is often of concern to nursing personnel and physicians in intensive care units and in hematology-oncology units, where patients are frequently subjected to multiple phlebotomies and blood loss may be a clinical factor; however, this concern must be tempered by the higher probability of yield with a 20-mL specimen than with 10 mL of blood or less and the greater likelihood of appropriate antimicrobial therapy. Blood is better collected by peripheral venipuncture than through an intravascular line because manipulation of the catheter increases the likelihood of contamination of both the line and the specimen. Culture specimens of blood obtained through intravascular lines have significantly greater yields of coagulase-negative staphylococci, the significance of which is frequently difficult to assess unless the same strain is isolated concurrently from a peripheral venipuncture sample. Some investigators have advocated concurrent quantitative culture of blood obtained through an intravascular line and by venipuncture to assist in the diagnosis of intravascular line-associated bacteremia (2). Others, however, have not noted line-related bacteremia to be consistently associated with larger numbers of bacteria per milliliter in blood taken through the intravascular line than in blood taken from a peripheral vein (2). Currently, quantification of organisms in blood is most practically accomplished with a lysis-centrifugation blood culture system.

The third important point regarding blood cultures entails the use of sterile techniques for their collection and manipulation. Disinfection of the skin can be performed with a variety of agents, including iodine, iodophor, chlorhexidine, and even 70% alcohol. The disinfectant should remain in contact with the skin surface for a minimum of 30 seconds before venipuncture. The vein should be palpated after skin preparation only with a sterile-gloved finger. The rubber diaphragms on blood culture bottles or devices must be similarly disinfected before blood is injected through them. Although experimental data suggest that the optimal time for blood culture collection is before the onset of fever and chills, in practicality the first blood culture specimen is usually obtained as soon as possible after recognition of such signs. Subsequent blood culture specimens should then be collected at intervals of 1 to 2 hours to enhance the probability of detecting intermittent bacteremia. It is routine practice in laboratories today to use blood culture systems that allow for the recovery of both aerobic and anaerobic bacteria as well as *Candida* species. For this purpose, it is necessary to inoculate blood into at least two separate devices. Usually bottles containing two different formulations of media are used, but in some centers a bottle along with a lysis-centrifugation tube, or some other acceptable combination, is used. The lysis-centrifugation tube is capable of detecting both aerobic bacteria and *Candida* spp., but has a reduced capacity for the detection of anaerobic bacteria. It, therefore, should only be used selectively (e.g., in children admitted from the outpatient setting) as a single device.

Blood culture collection from infants and small children is a problem in that the volume of blood that can be obtained is limited. A commonly posed question asks whether a limited 0.5- to 1.0-mL sample of blood should be inoculated into the aerobic or the anaerobic culture bottle. This dilemma may be addressed by the use of a pediatric lysis-centrifugation tube, which allows the user to distribute the lysed blood onto media as needed for aerobic and anaerobic culture.

Mycobacteremia due to *Mycobacterium avium* complex (and, to a lesser extent, *Mycobacterium tuberculosis*) has been noted with increasing frequency since the advent of the acquired immunodeficiency syndrome (AIDS) epidemic. There are two commonly used approaches to the detection of mycobacteremia: (a) lysis-centrifugation with culture of the lysed sediment onto mycobacterial isolation media; and (b) direct inoculation of blood into mycobacterial liquid medium.

Although *Candida* species are usually detected reasonably well in the aerobic bottle of blood culture systems, optimal detection of other yeasts and filamentous fungi requires the use of the lysis-centrifugation technique with culture of the lysed sediment on suitable fungus isolation media incubated at 25°C to 30°C for up to 6 weeks. Recent modifications of certain media now make select automated blood culture instruments efficient for the recovery of fungi. In most clinical laboratories, blood culture for viruses is restricted to the isolation of human cytomegalovirus from buffy coat preparations of blood collected from organ transplant recipients.

Leptospira spp. can be isolated only from cultures of blood taken during the first few days of illness. Requests for blood cultures for leptospires should be screened by the laboratory director to ascertain the duration of patient's symptoms. Cultures of urine may be indicated during the first 2 to 3 weeks of illness but are unrewarding thereafter. When leptospirosis is among the differential diagnoses, it is probably most important to obtain acute and convalescent-phase sera for antibody testing (1). When malaria is suspected, the optimal time for blood collection is midway between febrile paroxysms; the least optimal time is during or immediately after febrile paroxysms, when species differentiation is most difficult because infected erythrocytes have ruptured, releasing the parasites. *Wuchereria bancrofti*

and *Brugia malayi* have a nocturnal periodicity. Thus, the probability of microfilarial detection is highest when blood for preparation of smears is collected between 10:00 p.m. and 8:00 a.m. In contrast, because *Loa loa* has diurnal periodicity, the optimal time for collection of blood and preparation of smears is midday. Whereas anticoagulated blood is satisfactory for the preparation of smears for detection of microfilariae, anticoagulants may distort the morphologic features of erythrocytes. Smears for the diagnosis of malaria, therefore, (both thin and thick smears are necessary) should be prepared from a finger stick. The thin film should be prepared as for hematologic examination. For the thick film, a drop of blood should be applied to the slide and spread with the corner of another glass slide in a circular motion to form a film approximately the size of a dime. The film should be thin enough that newsprint can be read through it. If too thick, the film will simply peel off the slide during the staining procedure.

The purpose of the thick film is to facilitate more rapid screening of blood for the presence of parasites whereas the purpose of the thin film is to maintain the cellular detail required for identification of the malarial parasite (3).

Central Nervous System Infections

Central nervous system infections are caused by a variety of bacteria, mycobacteria, fungi, viruses, and parasites; the likelihood that a given agent is responsible varies with the patient's age and immune status, the season, environmental exposure, and a variety of other variables. Neonatal meningitis, for example, is most frequently caused by *Streptococcus agalactiae* or *Escherichia coli*; meningitis in children aged 4 months to 4 years immunized against *Haemophilus influenzae* type b is now most likely due to *Neisseria meningitidis* or *Streptococcus pneumoniae*. In non-immunized infants and children, *H. influenzae* serogroup b remains the primary scourge. The type of agent suspected may also be suggested by various cerebrospinal fluid (CSF) parameters, including glucose and protein concentrations, or by the differential leukocyte counts.

Culturing provides a definitive diagnosis in cases of bacterial, mycobacterial, and fungal meningitis. The isolation of viruses from CSF is highly variable, depending on the particular agent involved. For example, mumps virus is readily isolated from CSF whereas herpes simplex virus (HSV) is seldom recovered. Detection of HSV using molecular techniques (e.g., polymerase chain reaction; PCR) is far more sensitive than culture for diagnostic purposes. Such assays are at present, however, available in few routine clinical laboratories. Because HSV encephalitis is a medical emergency, specimens for molecular analysis should be forwarded to a reputable reference laboratory that guarantees rapid (within 24 hours) turnaround time from receipt of specimen. Similarly, the enteroviruses are isolated with moderate frequency from CSF but are readily detected using sensitive molecular techniques.

Viruses are, however, also frequently isolated from throat or stool specimens of infected patients (Table 12.3). Brain biopsy provides a definitive diagnosis for HSV encephalitis, but is a far more invasive technique to perform. In many instances of viral CNS infection, the diagnosis is based on serologic testing (see Table 12.3). A major impediment to the detection of infectious agents in CSF, particularly mycobacteria, fungi, and viruses, is the small volume of fluid frequently available for microbiologic examination. A minimum of 1 mL of fluid should be collected for each of these examinations.

A definitive diagnosis of bacterial meningitis may frequently be made on the basis of direct examination of the specimen. The gram-stained smear is positive, on average, in 80% of cases of

TABLE 12.3.   Appropriate Tests for Laboratory Diagnosis of Viral Agents of Central Nervous System Infections

Viral agent isolated	Throat	Stool	CSF	Urine	Other
Enteroviruses	+++	++++	+++	—	Autopsy tissue
Mumps Virus	++++	—	+++	+	—
Herpes simplex virus[b]					
Type 1	—	—		—	Brain biopsy (++++)
Type 2	—	—		—	Genital or rectal swabs (+++)
Arboviruses[c]	—	—	++	—	Blood (+), autopsy tissue(++)

Relative yield from source[a]

[a]Indicates relative frequency of positive yield in attempts at culture.
[b]Detection of Herpes simplex in CSF is best accomplished by DNA amplification.
[c]Because of the difficulty in isolating these agents from CNS specimens in cases of the disease in question, it is emphasized that serologic tests are important to improve opportunity for diagnosis.
CSF, cerebrospinal fluid.

H. influenzae meningitis and in a somewhat smaller proportion of cases caused by *N. meningitidis* or *S. pneumoniae*. The accuracy of the gram-stained smear depends to a large extent on the skill and experience of the microscopist. A variety of commercial products have become available that allow detection in CSF, blood, and/or urine of soluble antigens of *H. influenzae, N. meningitidis, S. pneumoniae, S. agalactiae,* and *Escherichia coli* K1. The sensitivity of these immunochemical tests approximates that of the gram-stained smear, varying directly with the amount of microbial polysaccharide in the specimen. The sensitivity, therefore, parallels the Gram stain in that it is a function of the number of bacteria present in the sample. In some previously treated patients, the immunochemical test results may be positive in the face of a negative culture result. Overall, when a CSF culture result is negative and the immunologic test result is positive, bacterial meningitis is present (4). False-positive immunochemical test results are most likely to occur when the tests are performed with concentrated urine specimens. Immunologic tests for bacterial pathogens in CSF are, in many institutions, significantly overused. These assays have limited clinical use because cultures are required for definitive diagnosis. Many hospital laboratories have eliminated immunologic screening of CSF unless warranted by atypical circumstances (5). In sharp contrast, the latex agglutination test for cryptococcal antigen is a highly sensitive and specific test for the diagnosis of *Cryptococcus neoformans* meningitis and should replace the traditional India ink preparation, which has less than 50% sensitivity. Material aspirated from brain abscesses should be examined for both aerobic and anaerobic bacteria. Such material should be transported to the microbiology laboratory either in the syringe (properly capped) used for the aspiration or, preferably, in an anaerobic transport vial. The sensitivity of the microscopic examination of Gram stain smears of CSF is significantly enhanced by the use of cytocentrifugation techniques. To improve sensitivity, CSF cultures for bacteria, mycobacteria, and fungi are frequently concentrated by either centrifugation or filtration. Viral cultures require the inoculation of a variety of cell lines. For more specific details on the media and the cell lines to be inoculated, the reader should consult the *Clinical microbiology procedures handbook* (1).

Upper Respiratory Tract Infections

The definitive approach to identification of the etiologic agent(s) in cases of sinusitis and acute otitis media (AOM) is direct aspiration of the site rather than performance of nasopharyngeal culture. Because the microbiology of these two syndromes is often predictable and amenable to empirical therapy, aspiration is generally limited to cases of more chronic disease. However, because of increasing antimicrobial resistance among strains of *S. pneumoniae* to agents frequently used for treatment of AOM (e.g., amoxicillin and the macrolides), ear taps (tympanocenteses) are increasingly being performed to recover the causative pathogens in order that antimicrobial susceptibility testing might be performed. By comparison, in chronic cases of otitis media and sinusitis, a greater variety of aerobic, facultatively anaerobic, and anaerobic bacteria as well as fungi may be involved. In such instances, it is critical that specimens be submitted in containers suitable for both aerobic and anaerobic culture.

The most common agents of pharyngitis are viruses and group A β-hemolytic streptococci. In epidemic situations, streptococci belonging to Lancefield groups C and G may be responsible for up to 17% of bacterial pharyngitis clinically indistinguishable from that caused by *Streptococcus pyogenes*. These serovars of streptococci, however, are not generally associated with nonsuppurative sequelae. Poststreptococcal glomerulonephritis has been reported following group C streptococcal pharyngitis and cases of acute glomerulonephritis in association with group G β-hemolytic streptococcal infection have been anecdotally reported, without definitive causality (6–10). Acute rheumatic fever is not, however, associated with either groups C or G streptococcal pharyngitis. Less common causes of pharyngitis include *Arcanobacterium haemolyticum* (especially in association with Epstein-Barr virus infection), *Neisseria gonorrhoeae, Corynebacterium diphtheriae,* and *Bordetella pertussis*. Because the colony morphology and the hemolysis produced by *A. haemolyticum* are very similar to that of *S. pyogenes* and other β-hemolytic streptococci, Gram stain from growth on solid media should be performed when attempting to detect this species. In practice, it is generally considered adequate to examine throat swabs for the presence or absence of group A β-hemolytic streptococci unless one of the other known causes of pharyngitis is specifically suspected. Rapid office tests for group A β-hemolytic streptococci may generate misleading results. Many small-colony forming β-hemolytic streptococci containing group A antigens may actually be strains of *Streptococcus anginosus* (previously *Streptococcus milleri*). Because these organisms do not warrant antimicrobial therapy, such isolates should be identified using other than serologic techniques to differentiate them from *S. pyogenes*. Efficiency in the recovery of group A streptococci in culture may be related to the vigor with which the throat is swabbed, including the posterior pharynx, areas of purulence in the tonsillar areas, and any other obvious areas of inflammation with exudate. Because there is considerable variation in this practice among physicians and allied health personnel, it is essentially impossible for the laboratorian to assign greater significance to a culture displaying many colonies of group A streptococci than to one yielding only a few colonies. Moreover, studies in children and in adults have demonstrated that seroconversion (antistreptolysin O and anti-DNAse B) occurs as frequently among patients with a light growth of group A streptococci in culture as in patients with a heavy growth of the organism (11,12). These observations are of some relevance to the use of rapid antigen tests for the detection of group A streptococci because the sensitivity of such tests is a direct function of the number of colonies present in the specimen. Consequently, it has been recommended by an American Heart Association Council on Cardiovascular Disease in the Young that negative rapid antigen test results be confirmed by culture because even sparse growth of group A streptococci, undetected by antigen detection methods, may indicate active infection, not just the presence of a carrier state (13).

Dry swabs are suitable for the isolation of group A streptococci if specimens are inoculated to appropriate culture media within 2 hours of collection. If longer storage and transport time is anticipated, swabs should be placed into a transport medium, such as Stuart, Amies, or one of the numerous modification thereof. Swabs of the Culturette EZ II system (Becton Dickinson Microbiology Systems) consist of porous polymers that permit microorganisms to survive for a minimum of 24 hours without the addition of transport media. Because the system contains two swabs, it can be used simultaneously for specimen collection, culture, smear, and/or antigen detection. Alternative swab transport systems, also acceptable for collection of pharyngeal specimens for viral culture, are now commercially available.

Lower Respiratory Tract Infections

Lower respiratory tract infections are caused by a variety of bacteria, mycobacteria, fungi, viruses, parasites, *Chlamydia trachomatis, Chlamydophila (Chlamydia) pneumoniae, Chlamydophila (Chlamydia) psittaci,* and *Mycoplasma pneumoniae.* The agent most likely responsible for an infection is a function of the patient's age, occupation, travel history, immune status, and a variety of environmental factors including the season. Diagnostic approaches vary based on the agent suspected as well as the patient's underlying disease, history, and clinical condition. Procedures may be broadly classified as noninvasive or invasive (14). The most frequently used noninvasive approach for the diagnosis of lower respiratory tract infection is the collection of expectorated sputum. Unfortunately, laboratories are actually far more likely to receive saliva than sputum and, therefore, all specimens labeled as "sputum" must be screened before culture to ascertain that they are, in fact, from the lower respiratory tract. A gram-stained smear of the sample submitted is examined under low-power (100×) magnification. Acceptability for culture is based on examination of 10 to 20 low-power microscopic fields. Specimens acceptable for culture should display: neutrophils, 1 to 9/field and squamous epithelial cells, none or few (greater than 9/field); or, neutrophils, 10 to 25/field and squamous epithelial cells, less than 25/field. Specimens that fail to meet these criteria should not be analyzed. Another specimen, actually representing lower respiratory tract secretions, should expeditiously be requested from the ordering clinician. When a sputum specimen is obtained from a truly neutropenic patient, the presence of ciliated epithelial cells can serve as an indicator of the lower respira-

tory tract origin of the specimen (15). Acceptable smears may be examined by oil immersion (1,000×) and the preponderance of any specific morphologic type of bacteria (e.g., pneumococcus-like, *Neisseria*-like, *Staphylococcus*-like, gram-negative bacilli) reported. The presence of *Haemophilus*-like or *Neisseria*-like bacteria in the gram-stained smear should prompt the laboratory to include a chocolate agar plate as a culture medium for the recovery of *Haemophilus influenzae* or *N. meningitidis* and to examine the culture plates carefully for *Moraxella catarrhalis.* Because *Haemophilus* and *Neisseria* species are often part of the indigenous microbiota of the oropharynx, isolation, of these organisms is indicated only when organisms resembling these genera are predominant in the gram-stained smear of a sputum containing pus cells.

Throat swabs are suitable for the isolation of *C. trachomatis* from infants with pneumonitis, *M. pneumoniae,* and a variety of respiratory viruses including influenza, parainfluenza, and adenovirus. The optimal specimen for respiratory syncytial virus (RSV) is obtained by nasal washing rather than by throat swab. RSV can be detected in specimens rapidly and accurately using immunofluorescence or immunoassay techniques. As noted previously, the recovery of RSV in culture can be successfully accomplished from throat swabs in Stuart or Amies transport medium as well as from viral transport medium. Swabs taken for isolation of *C. trachomatis,* on the other hand, must be placed into a sucrose-phosphate medium and, if not cultured shortly thereafter, frozen at −70°C. Sucrose-phosphate transport medium is also recommended for swabs collected for culture of *M. pneumoniae.*

For the diagnosis of pulmonary mycobacterial disease, it is recommended that a single, freshly expectorated sputum specimen be collected on each of 3 consecutive days. Pooled sputum specimens are unacceptable because heavy bacterial overgrowth occurs during specimen storage. In patients with suspected mycobacterial or fungal infection who do not have a productive cough, sputum may be induced using hypertonic sodium chloride aerosolization. There is no established role for sputum induction for the diagnosis of bacterial pneumonia. Induced sputum is, however, also useful for the diagnosis of *Pneumocystis carinii* pneumonia, both in patients with AIDS and in other immunocompromised patients (14,15).

A second major category of specimens from the lower respiratory tract include those obtained by invasive techniques. Today, the most frequently used methods are those based on fiberoptic bronchoscopy using bronchoalveolar lavage or a protected catheter brush (15). Bronchoalveolar lavage is performed by instilling 40 to 50 mL of a sterile, nonbacteriostatic saline solution into the affected lobe and then aspirating as much of the instilled fluid as possible for analysis. Because this process is repeated four or five times, the total volume of instilled saline approximates 250 mL. The aspirated lavage fluid is examined microscopically for cells and stained for bacteria, mycobacteria, fungi, and *P. carinii.* Cytologic stains are often concomitantly used to detect malignant cells or cells with characteristic viral inclusions. When possible, such smears should be prepared by cytocentrifugation. Aspirate specimens should be cultured quantitatively for the presence of bacteria. A second aliquot requires concentration for culture of mycobacteria, fungi, and viruses. An alternative approach for the diagnosis of lower respiratory tract infection in seriously ill patients is use of a protected catheter brush in which a double-lumen, distally occluded catheter is passed through the bronchoscope into an area of purulence. An inner brush is then used to sample the lesion. The brush is then withdrawn into its protective sheath and, after removal, is immersed in 1 mL of sterile lactated

Ringer's solution or nonbacteriostatic saline for transport to the microbiology laboratory. After resuspending cellular material with a vortex mixer or a mechanical stirrer, quantitative bacterial cultures are prepared from the fluid for the detection of aerobic and anaerobic bacteria. A colony count of greater than 10,000 colony-forming units (CFU)/mL of a single species is usually predictive of infection with that organism. Contaminating microorganisms are usually present in smaller numbers. Both procedures, used for the diagnosis of bacterial pneumonia in intubated, intensive care unit patients, have been found to provide complementary results.

In immunosuppressed patients, transbronchial biopsy may be performed for histologic and complete microbiologic analyses. Other invasive procedures include thoracentesis, transtracheal aspiration (TTA), and transthoracic needle aspiration. Thoracentesis may be useful for diagnosis of *H. influenzae* pneumonia in children and for the diagnosis of anaerobic pleuropulmonary disease in adults. In general, TTA should only be performed by experienced clinicians when a specific bacterial pathogen is suspected or is to be ruled out, the severity of the illness justifies the risk of the procedure, alternative specimens obtained by less invasive methods provide inconclusive results, and laboratory resources are available for prompt processing of the specimen (15). Moreover, there should be no contraindications to the procedure. One significant limitation of the technique is in the diagnosis of pneumonia for patients who have received antimicrobial therapy. Transthoracic needle aspiration is carried out principally for the diagnosis of malignant neoplasms and has relatively limited value, except in children, for the diagnosis of pneumonia. Open lung biopsy is primarily used for diagnosis of pneumonia in immunosuppressed patients when attempts at diagnosis have not been successful using the approaches previously described. These newer techniques have significantly diminished the need for open lung biopsies. Nonetheless, when the procedure is performed, a pre-existing protocol must be in place for both the histologic and microbiologic examination of the specimen. A freshly cut surface of the specimen is used for impression smears (touch preps) stained with Gram and Gomori methenamine silver and for direct immunofluorescence stains for *Legionella pneumophila*. After smear preparation, the specimen should be homogenized and the homogenate used for calcofluor white (detects both fungi and *Pneumocystis carinii*) examination and routine cultures for potential microbial and viral pathogens. Lung sections prepared histologically should be stained for bacteria, mycobacteria, and fungi.

Urinary Tract Infections

A variety of specimens may be submitted for the laboratory diagnosis of urinary tract infection (UTI), depending on the suspected site of infection or the etiologic agent, but the majority are clean-voided midstream urine samples (see Table 12.2). Proper instruction of patients by allied health personnel in the correct antiseptic approach for collection of urine from female patients is imperative to minimize specimen contamination by introital and periurethral flora. Because the urethra is normally colonized by diverse aerobic and anaerobic bacteria, it is customary to discard the first several milliliters of voided urine and to collect a midstream sample for culture (2,16). The goal of urethral catheterization is usually therapeutic, and the procedure should not be performed solely for the purpose of obtaining a specimen for culture. In such instances, urine should preferably be collected immediately after catheterization or, only when necessary, from chronic indwelling urethral catheters. Another procedure used

for collection of urine for culture, albeit less frequently, is suprapubic aspiration. This technique is particularly useful for obtaining specimens from infants and small children, and from adults when results of clean-voided midstream specimens are inconclusive, or when bacteriuria due to anaerobic or other fastidious bacteria is suspected. Infection due to fastidious microorganisms should be considered when the laboratory fails to propagate organisms on routine urine culture and a gram-stained specimen demonstrates bacteria. UTIs caused by anaerobic bacteria, relatively uncommon, can be accurately documented only by culture of urine obtained by suprapubic aspiration. *Gardnerella vaginalis*, for example, is not infrequently isolated from women's midstream clean-catch specimens, but its role in bacteriuria demands culture of urine collected by suprapubic aspiration. In another example, a variable number of colonies of a yeast, such as *Candida albicans*, may be isolated repeatedly from midstream urine specimens; again, their causative role can only be definitively established by culture of urine obtained by suprapubic aspiration. Less frequently, urine specimens are submitted to pinpoint the actual site affected. Because accurate assessment is based on the relative differences in the numbers of bacteria identified in specimens from each anatomic locus, these analyses require careful quantitation of each sample. When urine is to be cultured for mycobacteria or fungi, only a freshly voided specimen, not a pooled specimen, should be submitted. Urine culture is generally contraindicated for young, otherwise healthy women with uncomplicated UTIs and for asymptomatic patients with chronic, indwelling urethral catheters because antimicrobial therapy is typically empirical (17).

Urine specimens should be cultured within 2 hours of collection or, only when necessary, stored up to 24 hours at refrigeration temperature until inoculation of culture media can be accomplished. Because urine is an excellent culture medium, small, probably insignificant numbers of bacteria can rapidly proliferate in specimens stored at room temperature for longer than 2 hours. Commercially available urine transport devices may be useful for follow-up cultures of outpatients if they are received by the laboratory within 24 hours of specimen collection. A variety of marketed "mini-culture" devices use a small agar surface on a slide or paddle that is dipped into a voided urine specimen. The device is then forwarded to a laboratory for incubation and interpretation. Such devices are useful screening tools, but the small size of the agar surface makes isolation of colonies for organism identification and susceptibility testing difficult and often misleading. A variety of rapid detection methods for bacteriuria have been devised (18), among them gram-stained smears, filtration, photometry, bioluminescence, automation, detection of nitrite ions, and leukocyte esterase activity. A number of urine microscopy protocols for the detection of bacteriuria have also been used (19). Detection of at least two bacteria of the same morphotype in each of several oil-immersion fields (1,000×) by an experienced microscopist correlates 95% with bacteriuria of approximately 10^5 CFU/mL. By comparison, the sensitivity of the leukocyte esterase/nitrite ion dipstick is only approximately 85% for detection of the same level of bacteriuria. This increasingly popular method requires caution, especially in evaluating hospitalized patients with diminished cellular responses and patients infected with microorganisms that do not reduce nitrate. Dipsticks may be useful in community clinics, but dipstick use in tertiary care facilities in lieu of culture is unacceptable. The sensitivity of filtration and bioluminescence methods also approximates 95%. Both procedures can be carried out in 2 minutes or less per specimen; in contrast, photometric methods may require from 1 to 12 hours for completion. The negative predictive value for all of these tests is 95% or greater when the criterion for bacteriuria is 10^5 CFU/mL. If the diagnostic breakpoint is 10^4 CFU/mL, only Gram stain and bioluminescence demonstrate negative predictive values of 95% or greater. Therefore, depending on the criterion being used to define bacteriuria, the volume of specimen, the prevalence of bacteriuria, and the assay's cost, it may be both feasible and practical to screen urine samples as a prerequisite to culture. Because the prevalence of specimens with bacteriuria in a typical hospital, even employing a diagnostic cut-off value of 10^4 CFU/mL, is only approximately 10%, a test with a high negative predictive value may prove useful for rapid urine screening. Although culture is seldom, if ever, indicated for the diagnosis of acute dysuric syndrome in young women, bacteriuria as low as 100 CFU/mL may be significant in this setting. If cultures are requested in such cases, special techniques must be used and the laboratory staff informed of the specific purpose for the examination.

> The concept of significant bacteriuria and the criterion of 100,000 or more CFU/mL is a useful, but not absolute, criterion that has stood well the test of time . . .[SC] There have been efforts on the part of some workers to lower the criterion for significant bacteriuria in women with urethritis syndrome. This is a special group . . . In my view, it would be most unfortunate if findings in this group are projected to other individuals. It would be far better to single them out for special attention by the . . . laboratory (20).

This statement by Kunin is reassuring to many microbiologists because urine specimens usually constitute the single most frequently submitted specimen type to the clinical microbiology laboratory and because requisitions accompanying these specimens rarely contain the diagnostic information necessary to suggest to the laboratorian that special studies might be required to detect the lower levels of bacteriuria considered clinically significant under special circumstances. Cultures of urine from patients who have long-term indwelling urethral catheters are complicated by a number of factors. In a study by Warren and co-workers (21) of 605 consecutive weekly urine specimens from 20 such patients, 98% contained bacteria in high concentrations and 77% of the cultures were polymicrobial in nature (mean, 2.6 species per weekly specimen). Moreover, in a study by Tenney and Warren (22), significantly larger numbers of bacteria and more species were detected in urine specimens collected from persons with long-term indwelling catheters than from patients with replacement catheters. *Proteus mirabilis, Morganella morganii, Providencia* spp., *Pseudomonas aeruginosa,* and other gram-negative bacilli as well as enterococci were significantly more common in specimens from patients catheterized long term than from those whose catheter had been recently replaced. Thus, although culture of urine from indwelling catheters provides a sensitive method for detection of organisms associated with urosepsis and bacteremia, results of such cultures are highly nonspecific (22). For this reason, it is recommended that laboratories limit identification of isolates from urine of patients who have long-term indwelling catheters to specimens that contain no more than two species in concentrations of $\geq 10^5$ CFU/mL and to report the presence of larger numbers of species at high concentrations as "mixed," suggesting a repeat culture. Most clinical laboratories desist from analyzing catheter-obtained cultures unless there is a documented clinical need (16). Opposed to the situation with bacteria, colony counts of yeasts in cultures of urine have not proven to be useful diagnostic indicators of UTI; even a small number of colonies in immunocompromised individuals may be of import and their presence may be the only laboratory indicator of disseminated disease. Therefore, to prevent confusion on the part of the clinician who must interpret the results

of such cultures, the presence of yeasts in any amount should be reported routinely, without quantitation.

Gastroenteritis

The list of microorganisms implicated as causes of diarrheal diseases has increased considerably in recent years. To the list of traditional enteric bacterial pathogens—*Salmonella* spp., *Shigella* spp., *Yersinia enterocolitica* and *Vibrio cholerae*—have been added *Campylobacter* spp., *Plesiomonas shigelloides*, the *Aeromonas hydrophila* group, *Clostridium difficile, E. coli* (enterotoxigenic, enteroinvasive, enteropathogenic, enterohemorrhagic, and enteroadherent), a variety of additional *Vibrio* and *Yersinia* spp. *Giardia lamblia* and *Entamoeba histolytica* remain the major parasitic agents of diarrheal disease; however, the importance of *Cryptosporidium* species, the several microsporidia, and *Cyclospora* as causes of diarrhea in both immunosuppressed and immunocompetent patients has been appreciated only since the advent of AIDS. The list of viruses that have been associated with diarrhea includes not only rotaviruses and Norwalk-like viruses (small round viruses), but also enteric adenoviruses, caliciviruses, astroviruses, and coronaviruses. Many other infectious agents have been shown to infect the gastrointestinal tract of AIDS patients. These include *N. gonorrhoeae, C. trachomatis, M. avium* complex, *Treponema pallidum, Isospora belli,* human cytomegalovirus, and herpes simplex virus. Of this lengthy list, only the various pathogenic categories of *E. coli* and the viruses other than rotaviruses cannot be readily detected by most clinical laboratories today. The inability of *E. coli* 0157:H7 to rapidly ferment sorbitol provides a ready means for the microbiologist to screen for this bacterium with the use of sorbitol-MacConkey agar. However, other increasingly appreciated verotoxin-producing strains of *E. coli* will not be detected with this medium. Immunoassays for detection of verotoxin (Shiga-like toxin) directly in the stool of symptomatic patients improves diagnostic sensitivity by detecting toxin-producing, sorbitol-fermenting serovars of *E. coli.* Direct microscopic examination of fecal material and immunological-based methods have both been successfully used is for the diagnosis of parasitic infections. To achieve optimum sensitivity for the detection of parasites, a minimum of three stool specimens collected on separate days should be examined. When parasitic infection is suspected but the patient does not have diarrhea, it may be helpful to prescribe a saline purgative, such as magnesium sulfate (Epsom salts) or buffered sodium phosphate (Fleet Phospho-Soda), which should be ingested upon rising in the morning and followed by breakfast. Specimen collection may be performed at home or in another outpatient setting. To preserve the morphologic character and number of parasites and ova, stool specimens should be transferred to a commercially available two-vial transport system, one with 10% formalin and the other with polyvinyl alcohol. The polyvinyl alcohol-preserved specimens of diarrheal stools is smeared for trichrome staining for protozoa, acid-fast staining for cryptosporidia and *Cyclospora* spp., and for modified trichrome staining to detect microsporidia (*Nosema, Encephalitozoon, Enterocytozoon, Pleistophora,* and *Microsporidium* species) (3). Ova and larvae can be detected in direct or centrifuged aliquots of the formalin-fixed submission (3). When giardiasis is suspected and at least three separately collected stool specimen examination results have been negative, it may be necessary to obtain duodenal material by aspiration or using the enteric string technique. In addition, antigen detection methods including direct fluorescent antibody and enzyme-linked immunosorbent assay methods are now available for detection of *Giardia lamblia* and *Cryptosporidium parvum* in stool specimens. These methods, mandated by law in some states, have proven to be very sensitive and can reduce the time necessary to screen specimens for these parasitic agents.

Direct microscopic examination of fecal specimens is also useful in differentiating inflammatory processes due to organisms such as *Shigella, Campylobacter,* and enteroinvasive *E. coli* from noninflammatory processes, as seen with *V. cholerae,* enterotoxigenic *E. coli* and viral agents. Although some experts have advocated limiting stool culture to specimens that contain leukocytes (WBCs), the presence of WBCs in fecal specimens is highly variable with *Salmonella, Yersinia,* and *Aeromonas* infections. In addition, limiting the type of specimen that should be cultured on the basis of consistency of the specimen or the presence or absence of WBCs may preclude detection of carrier states of *Salmonella* and *Yersinia,* although the clinical significance of the carrier state with *Y. enterocolitica* remains unclear. Routine laboratory stool culture procedures should include methods optimized for recovery of *Salmonella, Shigella,* and *Campylobacter* species. Specimens should be submitted in appropriately buffered, commercially available stool preservative (e.g., buffered glycerol with indicator). The laboratory should be informed of any travel history and the types of foods consumed by the patient when unusual pathogens are suspected (1). Whether stool specimens should be routinely cultured for *Y. enterocolitica* remains a subject of debate because the frequency of yersiniosis demonstrates wide geographic variability. Laboratory procedures in coastal regions and for patients with a history of diarrhea after ingestion of shellfish should include culture for vibrios. The role of the *A. hydrophila* group in diarrheal disease remains controversial. As a result, the decision to examine specimens for these organisms is frequently based on local prejudice. If culture procedures include a selective medium for the recovery of *Yersinia* spp., in all likelihood organisms belonging to the *A. hydrophila* group will also be isolated. Routine stool cultures for *Salmonella, Shigella,* and *Campylobacter* species are among the most labor-intensive and expensive procedures carried out in the microbiology laboratory. Protocols characteristically include the inoculation of a variety of differential and selective media and, in most laboratories, use of enrichment broths that following overnight incubation are subcultured onto additional selective and differential media. Unlike salmonellae, shigellae are generally not recovered from subcultures of most enrichment broths. It is usual practice in most clinical microbiology laboratories to screen lactose-negative colonies recovered on enteric differential and selective media with a limited number of biochemical tests to rule out *Salmonella* or *Shigella* spp. Subsequently, the laboratory performs definitive identification of those isolates for which the biochemical test screening results are compatible for these species. The entire process of ruling out the presence of *Salmonella* or *Shigella* may, therefore, require 4 or 5 days to complete. Recently, antibody-based latex agglutination tests have become commercially available that allow laboratories to definitively identify suspect colonies of these two genera directly from primary plating media. This approach significantly reduces the turnaround time for this process, but at added material expense to the laboratory. Unless examination of stool specimens for vibrios is part of the laboratory's routine protocol, a specific request must be made of the microbiology lab whenever vibriosis is among the clinician's differential diagnoses.

The optimal approach to the laboratory diagnosis of *Clostridium difficile* diarrhea and antibiotic-associated pseudomembranous colitis is also controversial. Culture for the organism may be the most sensitive but is also the least specific approach because asymptomatic, healthy persons may be colonized with nontoxigenic strains of *C. difficile.* Cell culture assays for the detection of *C. difficile* toxin are considered the most specific, but are probably less sensitive than the time-consuming, slow, and nonspecific culture technique. Cytotoxic assays require a level of cell culture expertise that is characteristically unavailable in laboratories that do not perform tests for viral isolation. Enzyme immunoassays (EIA) that correspond well with cell culture results are now available commercially and can be used readily in most clinical laboratories. One frequently used latex agglutination assay does not actually detect either of the two toxins of *C. difficile,* but rather, a nonspecific toxin-associated protein. Rotaviruses and enteric adenoviruses can be detected by EIA or, in the case of rotaviruses, by latex agglutination. The sensitivity of latex agglutination assays for rotaviruses appears to be somewhat less than that of EIA. These assays do appear, however, to be as sensitive as EIA when applied to specimens collected within the first day or two of illness, but decrease in sensitivity on subsequent days.

Sexually Transmitted Diseases

The focus of sexually transmitted disease diagnosis has expanded substantially from gonorrhea, syphilis, and chancroid to include infections caused by *Chlamydia trachomatis,* herpes simplex virus, *Trichomonas vaginalis, Ureaplasma urealyticum,* scabies, and a variety of other agents capable of causing extragenital manifestations of disease such as those associated with AIDS. Microbiology laboratories however, primarily perform testing that assists in the diagnosis of gonorrhea, syphilis, chancroid, and infections caused by *C. trachomatis,* herpes simplex viruses, and *T. vaginalis.*

Swabs of the cervix, urethra, and anorectal region are most frequently submitted for testing, but in some cases, it may also be appropriate to collect and submit a pharyngeal swab. Culture for *N. gonorrhoeae* remains the standard against which other diagnostic tests are compared. For specimens collected from usually sterile sites, culture on chocolate agar medium incubated in an enriched CO_2 atmosphere is satisfactory; however, specimens from the urethra and cervix that are heavily colonized with indigenous microorganisms should be inoculated onto Thayer-Martin medium or one of its modifications. To facilitate direct inoculation of specimens onto media, Thayer-Martin medium is available both in a bottle containing carbon dioxide (Transgrow) or in an enclosed rectangular plate (JEMBEC). After inoculation onto the plate, a tablet of sodium bicarbonate is placed into the device and the entire system is sealed in a plastic bag. The humidity from the medium activates the sodium bicarbonate to produce CO_2 during incubation. Both Transgrow and JEMBEC facilitate the transport of cultures to laboratories for examination; however, because gonococci do not grow at room temperature, both systems require overnight incubation before shipment if a delay in transport is anticipated. If a delay of 6 hours or less between specimen collection and culture is expected, the use of a transport medium such as Stuart or Ames is satisfactory.

Presumptive identification of isolated colonies recovered from culture of an appropriate site may be based on results of a Gram stain and a positive oxidase reaction. Definitive confirmatory identification of *N. gonorrhoeae* can be made with carbohydrate utilization tests, immunoagglutination procedures, or by immunofluorescence.

The gram-stained smear remains the most accurate, rapid method for detection of *N. gonorrhoeae* in a urethral specimen collected from a symptomatic male. Both the sensitivity and specificity of this test are 95%, in contrast with gram-stained smears of urethral specimens from asymptomatic men (approximately 60% and 95%, respectively) (23). The sensitivity and specificity of gram-stained smears of cervical secretions from symptomatic females are 40% to 70% and 95%, respectively (23).

Most recently, commercially available molecular diagnostic techniques have become widely used for the diagnosis of gonorrhea. These include deoxyribonucleic acid (DNA) amplification procedures (polymerase chain reaction, ligase chain reaction, strand displacement amplification, and transcription-mediated amplification) and genetic probes using nucleic hybridization. The two-hour GenProbe PACE® assay, which utilizes a liquid-phase, nonisotopic ribosomal ribonucleic acid–directed DNA probe, has been found to be both highly sensitive and specific when compared to culture for the detection of *N. gonorrhoeae* in a high risk population (24). These DNA-based assays can be used to concomitantly detect both *N. gonorrhoeae* and *C. trachomatis* from a single patient sample. In addition, some of these molecular methods have been shown to be highly sensitive for the detection of these pathogens in urine samples of males, obviating the painful collection procedures otherwise required. If, however, gonococcal antimicrobial susceptibility studies are needed, a separate specimen must be submitted for culture.

Definitive diagnosis of *C. trachomatis* genitourinary tract infection is made using cell culture techniques. Culture, however, has been supplanted in most clinical microbiology laboratories by direct detection methods. Urethral specimens should be collected with a small cotton-tipped, aluminum-shafted swab; endocervical specimens may be collected with cotton- or Dacron-tipped, aluminum- or plastic-shafted swabs. To collect a urethral specimen, the swab must be inserted 3 to 5 cm into the urethra and withdrawn. For collection of an endocervical specimen, the cervix must first be cleaned of excess mucus; the swab used to collect the specimen should then be placed within the endocervical canal and rubbed vigorously against its wall. To enhance chances for recovery of the organism in culture or detection of chlamydial antigen it is essential that as much cellular material as possible is collected. While more elementary bodies are recovered with a cytobrush than with a swab or a cytologic scraper, experienced clinicians' use of the cytobrush does not appear to significantly increase the number of patients with positive immunofluorescence or EIA test results (25,26). Specimens, appropriately placed into a sucrose-phosphate medium for transport to the laboratory may be stored under refrigeration for up to 72 hours before being inoculated onto cell cultures. However, specimens requiring a longer period of storage should be frozen at −70°C immediately after collection (27). Using a temperature-controlled instrument, specimens are inoculated by low-speed centrifugation onto a monolayer of cycloheximide-treated McCoy cells cultivated on coverslips in 1-dram vials (27) or, alternatively, onto monolayers in microdilution plate wells. The later procedure facilitates the processing of large numbers of specimens but appears to demand more stringent techniques (27) to achieve results comparable to those of the shell vial methods. Because published reports often fail to analyze such technical variables, it is difficult to assess the relative sensitivities of differing culture methods and, consequently, also problematic to compare their sensitivity and specificity to nonculture methods. The presence of *C. trachomatis* antigens in the cell monolayers is detected by immunofluorescence or immunoperoxidase staining with genus-reactive monoclonal antibodies.

Nonculture methods are used extensively; in part, because cell culture techniques are often unavailable in laboratories that do not perform diagnostic virology. Two such methods are the direct immunofluorescence test and the EIA test (Chlamydiazyme™) (28). Fluorescein-labeled monoclonal antibodies are available from several commercial sources. The results of several published evaluations of both methods were reviewed by Stamm (26,29), who concluded that any analysis of published data must consider variations in specimen collection, culture technique, study populations, laboratory equipment, and the ex-

pertise of laboratorians. In his review of 15 published studies on the use of direct immunofluorescence tests, he reported that the test sensitivity in a population of symptomatic men averaged 92% (range, 90% to 100%) and the specificity 97% (range, 72% to 99%). The advantages of direct immunofluorescence (26,28) include the ability to assess the quality of the specimen on the basis of its cell content and its short turnaround time; its disadvantages include the need for a fluorescence microscope, expertise in immunofluorescence microscopy, and inefficiency when more than a few specimens must be examined. The advantages of the EIA method include greater technical simplicity, ease when examining multiple specimens, objective results, and economy in batch processing of specimens; its disadvantages include a 4-hour turnaround time and its expense when multiple specimens are not being batch processed. As described previously for *N. gonorrhoeae*, highly sensitive and specific DNA probes for *C. trachomatis* are also available commercially (26,28). The advantages and disadvantages of DNA probes in many ways are similar to those of EIA. Implementation of any of these techniques in the laboratory must be preceded by a careful analysis of advantages, disadvantages, and cost. When outcome measurements are used, DNA amplification systems for detection of *Chlamydia trachomatis* have been shown to be as or more cost-effective than DNA probes for detection of this pathogen (30).

Because syphilis is usually diagnosed serologically, the following discussion will be limited to darkfield examination for the diagnosis of primary syphilis. To prevent transmission of infection, clinicians collecting specimens from a chancre should wear surgical gloves. The lesion should first be abraded with a dry gauze sponge until it just begins to bleed. Excess blood should be blotted with a gauze sponge, and a coverslip applied to the base of the chancre. It may be necessary to apply pressure to the base of the chancre to increase the amount of serous exudate available for examination. The coverslip should be inverted onto a glass microscope slide and the edge sealed with Vaspar or Lanolin to prevent evaporation. The specimen must be examined immediately with a darkfield microscope at a magnification of 450×. Diagnosis is based upon observation of motile, tightly wound spirochetes. The person performing darkfield examinations for *T. pallidum* must be trained to perform this procedure; the untrained observer may confuse various artifacts with motile spirochetes (31).

Isolation of herpes simplex virus in cell culture remains the standard against which nonculture methods are compared. Isolation of the virus is optimized by obtaining material from intact vesicles by needle aspiration or on a Dacron- or cotton-tipped swab after unroofing the vesicle. Isolation rates are significantly lower when crusted lesions are sampled. Upon collection, swabs should be placed into a transport medium, such as Stuart or Ames. Swab extracts are inoculated onto cell culture monolayers that, in 24 to 96 hours, demonstrate typical cytopathic effects when virus is present. The time to detection of the virus may be reduced when specimens are inoculated using low speed centrifugation onto a monolayer of cells on a coverslip in a 1-dram vial. After approximately 15 hours incubation, the coverslip is stained with a fluorescent-labeled monoclonal antibody and examined by immunofluorescence microscopy. The sensitivity of this method is equivalent to that of conventional cell culture. A disadvantage of both methods is the requirement for cell culture. In cases of therapeutic failure, however, only culture techniques allow for referral of viral isolates to a qualified reference laboratory for antiviral susceptibility testing. The major nonculture methods currently in use are direct immunofluorescence and enzyme immunoassay. The sensitivity of direct immunofluorescence with monoclonal antibodies is 85% to 90%. As with culture, the rate of viral detection is diminished with progression of the lesion. Comparable levels of sensitivity have been reported with immunoperoxidase staining and with EIA (32–35).

Laboratory diagnosis of vaginitis and bacterial vaginosis remains a problem. Apparently least unreliable is the detection of *Trichomonas vaginalis* by direct microscopic examination of vaginal secretions. Some investigators, however, have found conventional wet mount examination to be insensitive when compared to culture (3). Microscopic detection of the organism appears to be improved through the use of direct immunofluorescence and monoclonal antibodies. The microbiologic diagnosis of vaginal candidiasis is complicated by the fact that vaginal cultures of up to 25% of healthy, asymptomatic women yield *Candida*. Laboratory diagnosis of *Candida* vaginitis is usually made by direct microscopic examination of vaginal secretions revealing budding yeasts and pseudohyphae. Compared with culture, though, direct microscopic examination demonstrates only approximately 75% sensitivity (36). The etiology of nonspecific vaginitis or bacterial vaginosis is incompletely resolved.

Originally believed to be caused by *Gardnerella vaginalis*, current thinking implicates a variety of *Bacteroides* spp., *Peptostreptococcus* spp., and anaerobic curved rods including *Mobiluncus* spp., with a concomitant reduction in numbers of lactobacilli (37,38). Although frequently present in cases of bacterial vaginosis, *G. vaginalis* may also be isolated from the vaginal secretions of from 20% to 50% of healthy, asymptomatic women. Due to the complexity of the microbiology and the culture techniques required, diagnosis is often made based on the character of the vaginal discharge; a pH above 4.5, a positive test result for amines, and the presence of clue cells (39). Krohn and colleagues studied the microbial populations of patients with bacterial vaginosis diagnosed by clinical signs, gas-liquid chromatography, and gram-stained vaginal smears to assess the predictive value of each method (38). *G. vaginalis*, *Bacteroides* spp., *Peptostreptococcus* spp., *Ureaplasma urealyticum*, and *Mycoplasma hominis* were more frequently observed in secretions of women who had bacterial vaginosis than in women who did not. *Mobiluncus* spp. were recovered from less than 50% of women with bacterial vaginosis. An abnormal discharge characterized by an amine odor, the presence of clue cells, and a pH of 4.7 or higher was less frequently noted in the pregnant women studied by Krohn and co-workers (38) than in previous studies of nonpregnant women (39).

Diagnostic sensitivity could be improved by using the following criteria: a gram-stained smear demonstrating fewer than five organisms morphologically similar to *Lactobacillus* species and the presence of curved gram-variable rods or fusiforms in each oil-immersion field. In summary, direct microscopic examination of vaginal secretions for the presence of *T. vaginalis,* budding yeast and pseudohyphae, reduced numbers of lactobacilli with increased numbers of gram-negative and gram-variable bacilli, and the presence of clue cells can provide rapid and useful diagnostic information. It may, however, have only moderate sensitivity relative to culture and, in the case of bacterial vaginosis, to gas-liquid chromatography, or a combination of any three of the following four test results: vaginal pH 4.7 or higher, the presence of clue cells, an amine odor, and a homogeneous character of the discharge. For *Candida* vaginitis, culture is highly sensitive but lacks specificity whereas for bacterial vaginosis, culture is expensive, time-consuming, and impractical for routine laboratory purposes.

Musculoskeletal Infections

Musculoskeletal infections may be caused by aerobic, facultatively anaerobic, and/or obligately anaerobic bacteria and, less frequently, by mycobacteria or fungi. In most cases, causative pathogens can be recovered from previously undrained and unopened abscesses, provided that specimens are properly collected and transported to the laboratory in a timely manner. Open wounds, ulcers, and sinus tracts are characteristically contaminated with cutaneous, mucosal, and/or environmental organisms. As a rule, swab specimens provide the laboratory with insufficient clinical material for adequate examination. Therefore, whenever possible, a generous quantity of material should be aspirated through a sterile needle into a syringe and the contents injected into an anaerobic transport vial for conveyance to the laboratory. Anaerobic transport media, available commercially, also support the recovery of facultatively or obligately aerobic bacteria. Many laboratories, by policy, do not accept swab specimens for anaerobic culture. The predictive value of a culture collected by swab at the orifice of a sinus tract, as frequently originates in bone secondary to chronic osteomyelitis, is poor compared with that of a surgically obtained specimen (40). Although difficult in cases of diabetic foot infections, every effort must be made to avoid contamination from ulcers or other open lesions when culture material is obtained from bullae, abscesses, necrotic soft tissue, or bone (41,42). The microbiologic etiology of musculoskeletal infections slowly changed with time from predominantly staphylococci, streptococci, and clostridia to an increased prevalence of gram-negative bacilli. This trend was observed for postoperative wound infections, chronic osteomyelitis, and posttraumatic wounds (43). However, these types of infections have undergone a recent shift back to gram-positive bacteria, many of which display broad resistance to commonly prescribed antimicrobial agents. Practical anaerobic bacteriology methods have increasingly facilitated laboratory recognition of musculoskeletal infections associated both with anaerobic bacilli and cocci (44).

Quantitative bacteriology of wound biopsy specimens has proven useful for the treatment of patients with acute open wounds, those for whom delayed wound closure is contemplated, and for those scheduled to receive skin grafts (45). Numerous studies have demonstrated a correlation between the presence of more than 10^5 CFU/g of tissue at the time of wound closure and subsequent development of wound sepsis (46–48). Essential for performance and interpretation of the results from quantitative culture of wounds are thorough cleansing and debridement of the wound before biopsy and collection of a tissue sample of at least 1 cm^3. Multiple specimens should be obtained when wounds are large. Tissue should be carefully weighed in a sterile vessel and homogenized for preparation of a quantitative gram-stained smear and for culture (45,48) (Fig. 12.1). For the gram-stained smear, 0.4 mL of the undiluted homogenate should be transferred to a clean glass microscope slide and spread over an area not greater than 15 mm in diameter. Drying is expedited by placing the slide in a 75°C oven for 15 minutes or on a slide warmer for methanol fixation before Gram stain. The entire smear should be examined under oil immersion (1,000×); the presence of any organisms constitutes a positive smear result, which correlates with the presence of l0^5 CFU/g or more of tissue.

Normally Sterile Body Fluids (except Cerebrospinal Fluid, Thoracentesis, and Urine)

Because the processing of thoracentesis and cerebrospinal fluid has already been discussed, this section focuses only on peritoneal, pericardial, and synovial fluids. Historically, small aliquots of peritoneal fluid or dialysate were cultured for bacteria and fungi using routine methods. More recently,

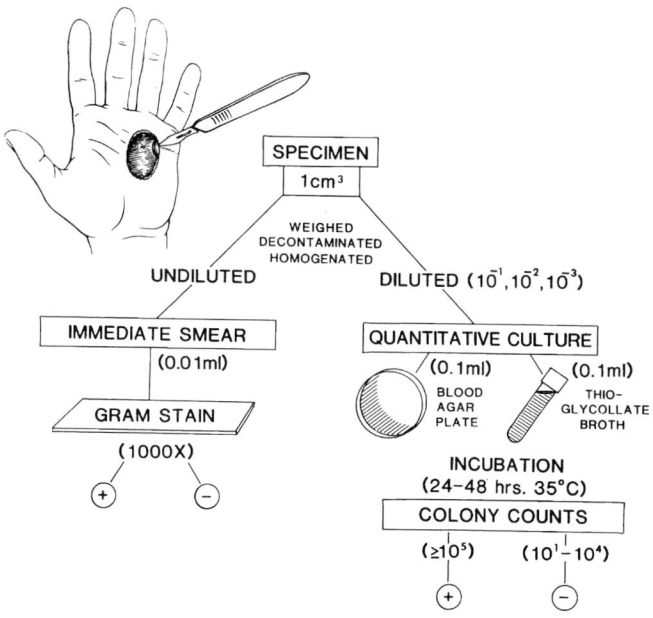

Figure 12.1. Procedure for quantitative smear and culture of tissue from traumatically acquired wounds after cleansing and débridement. (From Cooney WP III, Fitzgerald RH Jr, Dobyns JH, et al. Quantitative wound cultures in upper extremity trauma. *J Trauma* 1982;22:112–117, with permission.)

centrifugation or filtration concentrates of larger volumes of fluid have been used as inocula. With the advent of continuous ambulatory peritoneal dialysis (CAPD), increasing attention has been paid to the processing of peritoneal fluid. Approaches for the analysis of CAPD fluid are numerous. On the basis of results generated from several studies, however, lysis-centrifugation of 5 to 10 mL of well-mixed specimen is now considered superior to inoculation of CAPD fluid into blood culture bottles, which is deemed more effective than culture of the centrifugate from 50 mL of dialysate, for recovery of the wide range of pathogens associated with infection in these patients (49–52). The gram-stained smear, when positive, may still be contributory, helping to direct initial antimicrobial therapy. The etiology of purulent pericarditis is diverse and includes both aerobic and anaerobic gram-positive and gram-negative bacteria, *Nocardia* spp., mycobacteria, and fungi. Therefore, it is essential that specimens be cultured appropriately for this wide range of pathogenic microorganisms. Similar procedures must be used with synovial fluid, although anaerobes are rarely incriminated in septic arthritis unless preceded by open trauma. Particular attention, however, must be given to choosing procedures that optimize isolation of *N. gonorrhoeae* and *H. influenzae*. One must consider the possibility that potential pathogens may be missed when heparinized syringes are used for collection of pericardial or synovial fluid, because all commercially available heparin products contain a preservative that has been shown to interfere with microbial recovery.

METHODS FOR DETECTING MICROBES

Microscopy

Microscopic examination is often the single most rapid means for detection of microorganisms in clinical specimens. One must appreciate, though, that the sensitivity of microscopy is characteristically less than that of culture. Whenever feasible, submission of

specimens for both microscopic examination and cultural analysis should be routinely practiced. For example, visualization of at least two bacteria per each oil-immersion field (1,000×) in a urine specimen indicates the presence of at least 10^5 CFU/mL. The sensitivity of the gram-stained smear for this purpose approximates 95%. On the other hand, the sensitivity of a gram-stained smear of sputum for diagnosis of pneumococcal pneumonia is only approximately 50%, if a preponderance of lancet-shaped gram-positive diplococci is the criterion for positivity. Obviously, a less strict criterion increases the sensitivity of the gram-stained smear in this setting, but at the expense of specificity. The sensitivity of a gram-stained smear of CSF centrifugate from children with meningitis is approximately 75%, whereas that of a gram-stained smear of peritoneal or ascites fluid in patients with peritonitis is typically only about 30% but may be as high as 50%. Unlike urine, most normally sterile body fluids, such as CSF, are concentrated by centrifugation prior to microscopic examination for bacteria. Concentration procedures for normally sterile body fluids, as well as of bronchoalveolar lavage fluid, for the purpose of microscopic examination, are further enhanced by the use of cytocentrifugation (53,54). In many clinical laboratories, when compared to culture, the sensitivity of acid-fast smears of sputum for tubercle bacilli is only approximately 50%, although it varies considerably depending on the stage and extent of disease (55).

The traditional method for detecting *C. neoformans* in CSF has been the microscopic examination of an India ink wet mount preparation. However, because the sensitivity of this method is less than 50% when compared to culture, the latex agglutination test for cryptococcal antigen is now recommended. This test requires controls to detect the presence of rheumatoid factor (RF), which may interfere with the assay, causing false-positive reactions. When detected, RF may be inactivated with a proteolytic enzyme, thereby rendering the test interpretable. A potassium hydroxide wet mount preparation may be used to examine sputum and many other specimens for the presence of fungi including *Blastomyces dermatitidis* and *Coccidioides immitis*. Fluorescence microscopy using potassium hydroxide-calcofluor white further enhances their detection (56). Immunofluorescence microscopy, latex agglutination, EIA, genetic probes, and DNA amplification methods are all used to increase the frequency of detection for a wide variety of microorganisms. Specific applications of such techniques have been described in this book's section on specimen collection, transport, and processing. Although the decision to use any of these methods requires complex evaluation, these approaches represent the only means of detection and/or quantification of infectious agents in some instances (e.g., human papillomavirus, hepatitis viruses, and HIV). In other situations, these approaches increase the speed of detection for microorganisms with fastidious growth requirements.

Genetic probes and DNA amplification methods are now available for detection of a wide variety of antimicrobial resistance genes. These include mutations in the genome that typically encodes for topoisomerase IV (*parC*), DNA gyrase (*gyrA*), macrolide-lincosamide-streptogramin-B (MLS$_B$) (*erm*), erythromycin efflux (*mef*) (57), plasmid-mediated β-lactamases, and plasmid-mediated aminoglycoside-modifying enzymes. Such tests could, if amenable to use in the clinical laboratory, potentially be used to detect specific resistance mechanisms of microorganisms in clinical specimens, directing antimicrobial decisions. A number of problems are associated with such an approach. First, genotypic resistance may not reflect phenotypic resistance. Second, antimicrobial resistance may be caused by another mechanism; e.g., macrolide resistance resulting from mutations in the genome encoding for two ribosomal proteins, L4 and

L22. Third, direct specimen testing may detect a resistance gene in the indigenous microbiota that is not present in the pathogen of interest, a clinical false-positive result.

Microbial Identification

Microorganisms recovered in culture may be identified by a variety of methods, which are described in detail in standard clinical microbiology textbooks (1). Many bacteria and yeasts are identified by commercially available kits and devices, some of which are semi-automated or automated and combine identification with antimicrobial susceptibility testing as a single process. A major responsibility of the clinical microbiologist is to design and implement procedures that result in isolation of the most likely pathogens by specimen source or site of infection, while limiting identification of microorganisms to those of clinical import. The microbiologist must make every effort to differentiate indigenous microbiota and contaminating microbiota from true pathogens. Reporting indigenous microbiota, particularly with associated antimicrobial susceptibility test results, implies that the organisms are clinically important and often leads to the inappropriate or unnecessary use of antimicrobial agents. For example, only a limited number of bacterial species cause acute pharyngitis, and *H. influenzae, S. aureus*, viridans group streptococci, Enterobacteriaceae, *Neisseria* spp. other than *N. gonorrhoeae*, and *M. catarrhalis* are not among them. If any of these representatives of the indigenous oropharyngeal microbiota are reported, they be misinterpreted as being clinically significant, and unnecessary antimicrobial therapy may be initiated. To cite another example, the microbial causes of vaginosis/vaginitis are relatively few in number. Although the presence of *S. aureus* in increased numbers is unusual in vaginal secretions except in association with toxic shock syndrome, other microorganisms such as Enterobacteriaceae are not known to cause vaginitis, vaginosis, or cervicitis and the reporting of such species may, again, result in initiation of inappropriate antibiotic therapy. Identification and antimicrobial susceptibility testing of indigenous microbiota are also enormously labor-intensive and consume technologist time that might be better devoted to clinically relevant tests and procedures. However, when an organism not characteristically interpreted as pathogenic at a particular body site is recovered repeatedly in culture, in the absence of a typical pathogen, consultation with the patient's physician to assess its possible role in an infectious process is appropriate.

Clinical microbiologists must also establish priorities according to the severity of illness and the importance of microbial identification with susceptibility testing of a pathogen or pathogens in reducing the morbidity and/or preventing mortality due to an infectious process. These functions cannot be effectively accomplished unless pertinent clinical information and patient history is communicated to the microbiologist by the physician requesting the microbiologic analysis. There are few more critical functions of the clinical microbiology laboratory than optimal detection of the etiologic agents of septicemia and meningitis and no less important function than the identification of indigenous microbiota for purposes of reporting.

TESTS OF ANTIMICROBIAL ACTIVITY

Antimicrobial Susceptibility Testing

INDICATIONS FOR TESTING AND SELECTION OF ANTIMICROBIALS

Antimicrobial susceptibility testing should be considered when the response of a pathogen to commonly employed antimicrobial agents cannot be predicted based on its identity. Such is the case with staphylococci, the Enterobacteriaceae, pseudomonads, *Acinetobacter baumanii/haemolyticus, H. influenzae, S. pneumoniae, Enterococcus* spp., and many streptococci. *Streptococcus pyogenes*, by comparison, is predictably susceptible to penicillin. Antimicrobial susceptibility testing is, therefore, not necessary unless a patient is allergic to penicillins thereby requiring treatment with an alternative antibiotic such as a macrolide or tetracycline to which resistance occurs. The susceptibility of anaerobic bacteria to ampicillin-sulbactam, ticarcillin-clavulanate, imipenem, chloramphenicol, and metronidazole is sufficiently predictable that antimicrobial susceptibility testing of *Bacteroides* spp. and other anaerobes to these antimicrobials is not ordinarily indicated. Standardized procedures have been established by the National Committee for Clinical Laboratory Standards (NCCLS) for diffusion and dilution testing of bacteria that grow under aerobic conditions and for dilution testing of anaerobic bacteria (59–61). The E-test (AB BIODISK North America, Piscataway, NJ), a technique designed to determine antimicrobial susceptibility of aerobic and anaerobic microorganisms, utilizes a continuous gradient of antibiotic on plastic strips and is especially useful for performance of anaerobic minimal inhibitory concentration testing and for rapid detection of penicillin-tolerant or penicillin-resistant pneumococci (62).

Antimicrobial susceptibility testing should be limited to bacteria of presumed clinical importance. Whenever possible, laboratorians should minimize such testing on indigenous microorganisms. Regardless of the method used for testing, the term "susceptible" should be taken to mean that an infection caused by the microorganism tested may be treated with the recommended dosage of the antibiotic, unless the drug is otherwise contraindicated. The term "resistant" indicates either that the microorganism tested is not inhibited at safely achievable concentrations of the antimicrobial agent following usual recommended dosing or that the organism possesses or is likely to possess resistance mechanisms that may interfere with the activity of the compound and that therapy with the agent is unlikely to be clinically effective. Clearly, in addition to the *in vitro* susceptibility of an organism to the drug, antimicrobial activity *in vivo* depends on multiple additional factors. These include the absorption characteristics of the compound, its volume of distribution and its pharmacokinetics, its route of excretion; whether the patient suffers from renal or hepatic dysfunction; the extent of the drug's protein binding; its degree of post-antibiotic effect; whether the agent is administered in combination with another antimicrobial agent; and whether serious underlying diseases exist in the patient, including immunosuppression. In some instances, organisms are reported to be intermediate in their susceptibility to a particular antimicrobial agent. Such a report implies that the organism should be inhibited at concentrations of the drug that may be obtainable either by maximal dosing or due to concentration in a specific body compartment (such as the urinary tract). "Intermediate" results also serve as "buffer zones" that should prevent small, uncontrolled technical factors from causing major interpretive errors. The term is usually applied to antimicrobial agents with narrow toxic/therapeutic ratios (e.g., aminoglycosides) that cannot be administered in doses higher than those recommended without serious risk of toxicity. Clinicians should be aware of the fact that NCCLS-based changes in interpretation of susceptibility test results occur with some frequency, based on evolving clinical experience and other emerging issues.

The selection of antimicrobial agents for testing in the clinical microbiology laboratory is complex (63). In principle, agents to be tested should mirror those included in the hospital antibiotic formulary. Thus, it is essential that the microbiologist work in concert with the pharmacy and therapeutics committee of the medical staff. Unfortunately, the antibiotics on hospitals' formularies differ so greatly that it is often difficult or impossible for the microbiologist using commercially manufactured kits or devices for performance of susceptibility testing to achieve complete concordance between the institution's formulary and the drugs included in such commercially prepared panels. In some instances, equivalence of activity among agents in a particular category of antimicrobial agents is so great that the activity of one can be used to predict the activity of others. For example, susceptibility of staphylococci to oxacillin indicates susceptibility to methicillin, nafcillin, and other penicillinase-resistant penicillins. Susceptibility to cephalothin likewise serves as a surrogate for susceptibility to other first-generation parenteral and oral cephalosporins. Similarly, susceptibility of Enterobacteriaceae to cefotaxime implies susceptibility to ceftizoxime and ceftriaxone. Conversely, staphylococcal resistance to oxacillin indicates resistance to other penicillinase-resistant penicillins as well as to cephalosporins, carbapenems such as imipenem, and β-lactam/β-lactamase inhibitor combinations. Because occasional isolates of oxacillin-resistant staphylococci appear to be susceptible to some cephalosporins *in vitro*, clinical microbiologists must routinely report such isolates as resistant not only to oxacillin but also to all other β-lactams tested. Although cross-resistance and cross-susceptibility among aminoglycosides is not predictable, gram-negative enteric bacilli that are resistant to amikacin are also usually resistant to all other marketed aminoglycosides. Laboratories may elect to selectively report the activity *in vitro* of certain antimicrobial agents. For example, if a gram-negative bacillus is susceptible to cefazolin or cephalothin, the microbiologist may report this result while withholding the results for the susceptibility testing of second- and third-generation cephalosporins, which are clinically no more effective but characteristically more expensive. Likewise, if a gram-negative bacillus is susceptible to gentamicin, the clinical microbiologist may elect to withhold the susceptibility test results for tobramycin and amikacin. Algorithms for selective (cascade or suppression) reporting become much more difficult to use when microorganisms of differing susceptibilities are recovered in mixed culture. A guideline for selecting antimicrobial agents to be tested against various categories of bacteria that grow aerobically is presented in Table 12.4.

For clinically significant isolates of *H. influenzae*, the first and simplest test to perform is that for β-lactamase production. β-lactamase-negative isolates should be tested for susceptibility to ampicillin because chromosomally mediated β-lactamase-negative ampicillin-resistant (BLNAR) strains cannot be detected using a β-lactamase test. Therapy with ampicillin or amoxicillin may be appropriate if the β-lactamase test result is negative and the isolate is susceptible to ampicillin. If an isolate produces β-lactamase or is resistant to ampicillin, further susceptibility testing may or may not be indicated because β-lactamase–producing isolates of *H. influenzae* are uniformly susceptible to the β-lactam/β-lactamase inhibitor combinations and ampicillin-resistant isolates are universally susceptible to third-generation cephalosporins. Chloramphenicol-resistant isolates of *H.influenzae* remain rare in the United States; however, if therapy with chloramphenicol is contemplated, resistance may be determined by the disk diffusion method or more rapidly by a test for chloramphenicol acetyltransferase, the enzyme responsible for inactivating chloramphenicol. Susceptibility testing of the macrolides, amoxicillin-clavulanate, oral cephalosporins, and trimethoprim-sulfamethoxazole should be limited to isolates of *H. influenzae* recovered from localized, non-life threatening disease. Of particular concern today is the increasing incidence of

antimicrobial resistance among gonococci. The genome encoding for tetracycline and penicillin resistance may be located either on plasmids or on the organism's chromosome whereas resistance to the macrolides and spectinomycin is characteristically chromosomally mediated. Although nucleic acid probes have been developed for detection of plasmids that mediate penicillin resistance, none is, as yet, commercially available. Therefore, detection of penicillinase production by strains of *N. gonorrhoeae* (PPNG) necessitates the testing of isolated colonies with a rapid β-lactamase test. By comparison, detection of chromosomally mediated resistance to penicillins requires either disk diffusion or dilution testing of isolated colonies. Clinical microbiologists should consider routinely performing a β-lactamase test on all gonococcal isolates whereas they may wish to test isolates only from treatment failures for their susceptibility to penicillin by the disk diffusion or a dilution method. If the prevalence of chromosomally mediated penicillin resistance in the community is known to be on the order of at least 3% to 5%, susceptibility testing of β-lactamase-negative isolates should be considered. Because tetracyclines are no longer recommended as first-line agents for treatment of gonococcal infections, susceptibility testing of isolates to this class of compounds is probably not routinely necessary. Similarly, resistance to spectinomycin, a compound only rarely used in clinical practice, remains rare in the United States. In addition, because of limited resources and the to-date universal susceptibility of *N. gonorrhoeae* to ceftriaxone and cefotaxime, most clinical laboratories have now abandoned performance of any antimicrobial susceptibility testing on gonococcal isolates. If needed, susceptibility testing should be performed by either the disk diffusion or the agar dilution method using GC agar base, according to methods described by the NCCLS (59,60). Another confounding issue is the fact that many laboratories now diagnose gonorrhea using commercially available genetic probes rather than culture. Isolates, therefore, are not available for performance of any type of susceptibility testing. Consequently, the monitoring of isolates of *N. gonorrhoeae* by public health laboratories for emergence of resistance to fluoroquinolones, advanced generation cephalosporins, and other commonly prescribed compounds may, therefore, become critically important for this pathogen (64).

Anaerobic bacteria may be tested to determine patterns of susceptibility locally, regionally, and/or nationally; to monitor the emergence of resistance over time; and to assist in the antimicrobial management of patients with central nervous system infections, endocarditis, osteomyelitis, joint infections (extremely rare unless there is history of an open joint wound), prosthetic device infections, vascular graft infections, and refractory or recurrent bacteremia. Of significance is the reported change in the susceptibility patterns of members of the *Bacteroides fragilis* group over the past several years (65). *M. tuberculosis* isolates are only routinely tested for susceptibility to the primary drugs used for chemotherapy; isoniazid, streptomycin, rifampin, and ethambutol. In some instances, susceptibility testing may be reserved for isolates recovered from patients with life-threatening disease or who are at increased risk of harboring resistant strains. Whenever such selective testing algorithms are used, however, all isolates that were not initially tested should be stored in the event that susceptibility tests are required subsequently. Although the reference procedure for susceptibility testing of mycobacteria remains the agar proportion method, this technique is not practical for use in routine clinical laboratories. An alternative method for testing this pathogen is the radiometric method. Rapidly growing mycobacteria may be tested by a microdilution, a gradient agar (Etest®), or a disk diffusion method (66). The radiometric method is being adapted to provide accurate results with some

TABLE 12.4. Guidelines for Selection of Antibacterial Agents for Susceptibility Testing

Antimicrobial agent	Staphyhlococci	Enterococci	Nonentercoccal streptococci	Pseudomonads and other non-enterobacteriaceae	Enterobacteriaceae
Amikacin				S	S
Ampicillin		P	P		P
Amoxicillin-clavulanic acid or ampicillin sulbactam					S
Azithromycin or clarithromycin or eryhrthromycin	S	S	P		
Aztreonam				S	S
Carbenicillin				U	U
Cefamandole (or cefonicid or cefuroxime)					S
Cefazolin					P
Cefepime				S	S
Cefmetazole or cefotetan or cefoxitin			S		S
Cefoperazone				S	S
Cefotaxime or ceftriaxone			S	S	S
Ceftazidime				P	S
Ceftizoxime				U	S
Chloramphenicol	S	S	S	S	U
Cinoxacin					S
Ciprofloxacin	S	U		S	S
Clindamycin	S		S		
Gatifloxacin	S				U
Gentamicin	S	S[a]		P	P
Imipenem or meropenem				S	S
Kanamycin					S
Levofloxacin	S	U	S	U	S
Linezolid	S	S	S		
Lomefloxacin	U			U	U
Loracarbef					U
Mezlocillin (or piperacillin or ticarcillin)				P	S
Netilmicin				S	S
Nitrofurantoin	U	U		U	
Norfloxacin	U	U		U	U
Ofloxacin	S		S	U	U
Oxacillin (or methicillin or nafcillin)	P[b]				
Penicillin G	P	P	P		S
Piperacillin-tazobactam					
Quinupristin/dalfopristin		S	S		
Rifampin	S	S			
Sulfisoxazole	U			U	U
Tetracycline	S	S		U	S
Ticarcillin-clavulanic acid					S
Tobramycin				S	U
Trimethoprim	U				S
Trimethoprim-sulfamethoxazole	S			S[c]	S
Vancomycin	S	S	S		

[a] Gentamicin (high level resistance screen only). Gentamicin should be tested at a concentration of 500 μg/mL to detect highly resistant enterococci that are not synergistically affected by the combination of a penicillin and gentamicin.
[b] Oxacillin- (or nafcillin- or methicillin-) resistant staphylococci are resistant to all currently available beta-lactam antibiotics. Susceptibility or resistance to a wide range of beta-lactams can be deduced from testing only penicillin and oxacillin.
[c] Applies only to species other than *Pseudomonas aeruginosa.*
P, primary agents to be tested and reported routinely; S, secondary agents to be tested routinely but reported only selectively or to be tested only under special circumstances such as in institutions harboring epidemic or endemic strains of bacteria resistant to one or more of the primary agents, for treatment of patients who are allergic to one of the primary agents, or as an epidemiological tool; U, urinary tract–specific agents that should be reported only for isolates recovered from urinary tract culture specimens.

Mycobacterium spp. that grow more slowly than *M. tuberculosis*. However, it is important that data validating this procedure are available for specific species-antimicrobial combinations before testing is performed and results reported by the clinical laboratory.

Standards for antifungal susceptibility testing of both yeasts and filamentous fungi have also now been developed and published (67,68). Although some difficulties have historically been noted in correlating results *in vitro* with efficacy *in vivo*, recent work indicates that the results of antifungal susceptibility tests in some populations are at least as predictive as those for bacterial studies (69).

Antiviral susceptibility testing is assuming increasing importance with the recognition of acyclovir- and ganciclovir-resistant isolates of both herpes simplex virus and human cytomegalovirus. Of greater import is the use of these techniques for assessing the activity of compounds designed for treatment of patients with HIV. Although progress has recently been made in standardizing the procedures, antiviral susceptibility testing remains technically complex and will, therefore, continue in the domain of research and reference laboratories for the foreseeable future (70).

SUSCEPTIBILITY TESTING VARIABLES

Variations in inoculum size remain the major cause of day-to-day differences in susceptibility test results. Because an increasing number of clinical laboratories have implemented microdilution testing for routine purposes, it is essential that techniques be used that ensure an inoculum $\cong 5 \times 10^5$ CFU/mL. For quality assurance purposes, every laboratorian performing antimicrobial susceptibility testing must, on a regularly scheduled basis, enumerate organisms in the test-prepared inoculum to ensure accurate results. Failure to achieve the recommended 5×10^5 CFU/mL inoculum results in the false reporting of susceptibility for penicillinase-producing staphylococci, oxacillin-resistant staphylococci, and β-lactamase-producing gram-negative bacilli. The frequency of non-penicillinase–producing staphylococci is so small in the United States that any staphylococcal isolate for which the penicillin minimum inhibitory concentration (MIC) is 0.12 μg/mL or less mandates confirmatory β-lactamase testing because such MICs almost invariably reflect an inadequate inoculum size. Another clue that inadequate inocula are in use can be garnered from the review of ampicillin activity against Enterobacter cloacae. If greater than 5% of strains are susceptible, it is probable that the inoculum in use by the laboratory is too low (63).

Another variable of considerable significance is the cation content of the medium. The in vitro activity of aminoglycosides against P. aeruginosa is inversely proportional to the amount of calcium and magnesium in the test medium. To ensure reproducible test results, use of Mueller-Hinton media containing 20 to 25 mg/L of calcium and 10 to 12.5 mg/L of magnesium is recommended (59). Most commercially available Mueller-Hinton preparations are now so adjusted. Haemophilus Test Medium, an enriched formulation that supports the growth of H. influenzae, should be routinely used for antimicrobial susceptibility testing of this species. Periodically, for reference purpose, antimicrobial susceptibility testing of anaerobic bacteria should be by the agar dilution technique, using either Wilkins-Chalgren agar or Brucella blood agar. Because agar dilution is not practical for routine laboratory purposes, however, broth microdilution or Etest® procedures are recommended (61,62). Interpretive criteria for disk diffusion testing of rapidly growing aerobic bacteria must not be extrapolated to disk diffusion testing of anaerobic bacteria because necessary incubation conditions significantly impact zones of inhibition with these species.

Bactericidal Testing

There are several methods used for assessing the bactericidal activity of antimicrobial agents. These include determinations of the minimal bactericidal or lethal concentration (MBC or MLC), the serum bactericidal titer (Schlichter test), and the time-

kill curve. Standardized methods for determining the bactericidal activity of antimicrobial agents and for performance of the serum bactericidal test have been developed but are only infrequently used by clinical laboratories (71,72). Although useful for comparative investigations of new antimicrobial agents, the clinical utility of these assays remains limited due to problems related to reproducibility and the considerable difficulty experienced in interpreting test results. In general, the MBC of a drug is determined by subculturing the wells of a broth microdilution susceptibility testing plate that fail to exhibit macroscopically discernible growth after standard overnight incubation onto antibiotic-free media, which are again incubated overnight. The MBC is defined as the lowest concentration of an antimicrobial that kills $\geq$99.9% of the initial inoculum. The MBC is typically identical to or within one or two doubling dilutions of a drug's MIC when bactericidal activity exists. If, however, the MBC exceeds the MIC by a factor of 32 or more, the organism is considered tolerant to the drug. Although tolerant viridans group streptococci and pneumococci have been identified on the basis of autolytic defects, the clinical significance of such strains is incompletely understood. A considerable volume of information has been published on tolerant strains of S. aureus; nevertheless, variables such as the growth phase of the inoculum, the survival of organisms on the inside wall of the test tube above the meniscus, and the subculture volume can determine whether a strain of S. aureus appears to be tolerant; for example, the outcome of the test can be affected by the test method. Such issues render the clinical literature purporting to show that "tolerant" staphylococci are associated with more frequent complications and/or require more protracted therapy virtually impossible to interpret. Similarly, test variability, and lack of consensus on the optimal times for specimen collection as well as the minimum titers associated with treatment success or failure, make the clinical literature on the value of the serum bactericidal test difficult to interpret. In most published studies, the number of patients with low serum bactericidal titer is too small for statistical analysis. It would obviously be unethical to limit the antibiotic dose as would be required to perform the critical experiments needed to assess the true clinical value of the serum bactericidal titer. The time-kill curve is a research tool that assesses both how much of the original inoculum was killed and the rate of such killing. Because tolerance, particularly among staphylococci, is most accurately expressed by a slow rate of killing, it has been recommended that abbreviated time-kill studies be used to determine tolerance among staphylococci (73,74). Time-kill curves have also been used to study the interactions between combinations of antimicrobial agents, and, more specifically, to determine whether the interactions are synergistic, antagonistic, or indifferent. For example, it has been demonstrated that the combination of penicillin and gentamicin produces statistically significantly greater killing of enterococci than does either agent alone. This interaction is of considerable clinical import because serious enterococcal infections, particularly endocarditis, require such combinations for cure. A more practical approach to assess whether synergy will occur between penicillin and either streptomycin or gentamicin is to determine the enterococcal isolate's susceptibility to 2,000 ug/mL of streptomycin or 500 ug/mL of gentamicin. Inhibition of the organism by either of these concentrations of aminoglycosides is predictive of a synergistic interaction between that aminoglycoside and penicillin whereas failure of inhibition is predictive of lack of synergy between that aminoglycoside and penicillin. In this specific situation, the clinical laboratory can easily and routinely provide results that are analogous to those of time-kill studies. Unfortunately, similar simple alternatives to time-kill analyses are not available for other bacterial species (75–77).

Antibiotic Assays

The concentration of an antimicrobial agent that is achieved in the serum depends not only on the dose of drug administered, but also on its route of administration, the formulation of the agent, the patient's compliance and body weight, the extracellular fluid volume, the extent of protein binding of the antimicrobial agent, the agent's elimination or excretion rate, the patient's disease state, the interaction of the antimicrobial with other drugs being administered, the timing of blood sampling for assay, and the analytic method used. Patients for whom antimicrobial assays are usually indicated include those who are receiving prolonged (longer than 5 days) antimicrobial therapy, those who do not respond to antimicrobial therapy, those in whom signs or symptoms of ototoxicity or nephrotoxicity develop while receiving antimicrobial therapy, those with impaired or rapidly changing renal function, those undergoing dialysis, elderly persons, those with cystic fibrosis or burns, those who are obese or have expanded extracellular fluid volume, those with infections at sites where penetration of an antimicrobial may be uncertain or variable (e.g., CSF), those with malabsorption syndromes who are receiving oral antimicrobial agents, and those with normal renal function (to ensure that peak concentrations are in the recommended therapeutic range and that trough concentrations are not excessive).

In practice, antibiotic assays are most often performed to determine concentrations of antimicrobials that have a narrow toxic/therapeutic ratio, such as the aminoglycosides, 5-FC, and vancomycin. Chloramphenicol is another such drug, but the expanded-spectrum cephalosporins have largely replaced it in clinical settings. Consequently, relatively few assays for chloramphenicol are performed today. The usual doses, therapeutic ranges, and concentrations associated with potential toxicity of antimicrobials with narrow toxic/therapeutic ratios are listed in Table 12.5. Assays of antimicrobials with favorable toxic/therapeutic ratios (e.g., β-lactams) are rarely indicated unless the route of administration or presence of an underlying disease may cause serum levels to differ markedly from the usual range and/or the infection is in a tissue or body fluid into which penetration is variable or uncertain.

To assay for peak levels, blood should be collected 30 minutes after an intravenous dose, 60 minutes after an intramuscular dose, or 60 to 120 minutes after an oral dose. Trough levels, collected just before the next administration of drug are, however, more sensitive indicators of decreased clearance and accumulation of drugs. If assays cannot be performed immediately, it is recommended that serum specimens be frozen at −70°C or less or that a small volume of a β-lactamase be added to prevent inactivation of aminoglycosides by β-lactam antibiotics when both have been administered to a patient.

Today, immunoassays are usually used to determine serum concentrations of aminoglycosides and vancomycin. These assays are rapid, simple, sensitive, and specific. Quantification of other antimicrobial agents is generally performed by microbiologic assay or, if the equipment and expertise are available, high-performance liquid chromatography.

This cursory account of clinical microbiology represents an effort to underscore the essential role of this discipline in the diagnosis of infectious diseases. The paramount message of this chapter is the need for constant dialogue between clinicians and microbiologists. Such dialogue is essential if pertinent and accurate information is to be disseminated by the laboratory in an expeditious manner. During this era of decreased financial support for all health care functions, justification for analyses is often demanded, unfortunately, by individuals with little appreciation of the rationale for performance of the examinations requested. Simultaneously, a variety of heretofore rare or unknown microorganisms are intruding into the intimate biosphere of patients both within health care facilities as well as in the community, further complicating the processes of clinical microbiologists. Frequently exaggerated coverage by poorly informed television and printed media commentators of emerging or re-emerging pathogens succeeds in creating confusion, if not fear,

TABLE 12.5. Factors That Affect Monitoring of Selected Antimicrobial Agents[a]

Antimicrobial agent	Usual dose	Dosage interval (h)	Maximal dose (24 h)	Normal serum half-life (h)	Major route of elimination	Remove by dialysis Hemodialysis	Remove by dialysis Peritoneal dialysis	Peak	Trough	Recommendation basis for dosage adjustment
Amikacin	5–7.5 g/kg	8–12	15 mg/kg	2–3	Renal	Yes	Yes	20–25	5–10	P,T
Gentamicin	1.7 mg/kg	8	5 mg/kg	2–3	Renal	Yes	Yes	4–8	1–2	P,T
Kanamycin	5–7.5 g/kg	8–12	15 mg/kg	2–3	Renal	Yes	Yes	20–25	5–10	P,T
Netilmicin	2–2.5 mg/kg	8	7.5 mg/kg	2–3	Renal	Yes	Yes	6–10	0.5–2	P,T
Streptomycin	0.5–1 g	8–12	2g	2–3	Renal	—	—	5–20	<5	P,T
Tobramycin	1.7 mg/kg	8	5 mg/kg	2–3	Renal	Yes	Yes	4–8	1–2	P,T
Chloramphenicol	0.5–1 g	6	4g	4[b]	Hepatic/renal	No	No	15–25	8–10	T
Flucytosine	37.5 mg/kg	6	150 mg/kg	4	Renal	Yes	Yes	100	50	T
TMP-SMX[c]										
TMP	5 mg/kg	6	20 mg/kg	11	Renal	Yes	Yes	≥5	—	P
SMX	25 mg/kg	6	100 mg/kg	13	Renal	Yes	Yes	≥100	—	P
Vancomycin	0.5–1 g	8–12	2 g	6	Renal	No	No	20–40	5–10	T

P, peak level; T, trough level; TMP-SMX, trimethoprim-sulfamethoxazole. These recommendations are valid when dose interval is not greater than twice the usual. Blood for peak levels should be drawn 30 min after completion of an IV infusion, 1 h after an oral dose.
[a]Once daily dosing of aminoglycosides is recommended by many experts for patients with normal renal function; doses and peaks/troughs should be modified accordingly.
[b]Half-life in children younger than 4 wk can be much prolonged. Half-life is affected only slightly in renal failure but can be greatly prolonged with liver disease.
[c]Maximal dosages of trimethoprim-sulfamethoxazole (TMP-SMX) apply to treatment of *Pneumocystis carinii* infection. Serum half-life is shortened in adolescents and children. Measurement of either TMP or SMX alone is sufficient for dosage adjustment.
From Anhalt JP, Wilkowske CJ, Washington JA II. Manual of antimicrobial agents, ed 11. Philadelphia: RC Deulas, 1983. Reprinted by permission of Mayo Foundation.

among the public, increasing the demand for clinical and laboratory detection of such microorganisms. Only through collaboration between the clinician and the laboratorian can a perspective be maintained that reassures the public of our awareness of and efforts to control such microorganisms.

REFERENCES

1. Isenberg HD, ed. *Clinical microbiology procedures handbook.* Washington DC: American Society for Microbiology, 1992.
2. Baron EJ, Peterswon LR, Finegold SM. *Bailey & Scott's diagnostic microbiology,* 9th ed. St. Louis: Mosby, 1994.
3. Garcia LS, Bruckner DA. Diagnostic medical parasitology, 2nd ed. Washington DC: American Society for Microbiology, 1993.
4. Wilson CB, Smith AL. Rapid tests for the diagnosis of bacterial meningitis. *Clin Top Infect Dis* 1986;134:56.
5. Jenkins SG. Central nervous system specimens. In: Tilton RC, Balows A, Hohnadel D, et al, eds. *Clinical laboratory medicine.* St. Louis: Mosby, 1992.
6. Duca E, Teodorovici G, Radu C, et al. A new nephritogenic streptococcus. *J Hyg* 1969;67:691–698.
7. Barnham M, Thornton TJ, Lange K. Nephritis caused by *Streptococcus zooepidemicus* (Lancefield group C). *Lancet* 1983;1:945–948.
8. Rolston KVI. Group G streptococcal infections. *Arch Intern Med* 1986;146:857–858.
9. Poon-King T, Mohammed I, Cox R, et al. Recurrent epidemic nephritis in South Trinidad. *N Engl J Med* 1967;227:728–733.
10. Reid HF, Bassett DC, Poon-King T, et al. Group G streptococci in healthy schoolchildren and in patients with glomerulonephritis in Trinidad. *J Hyg* 1985;94:61–68.
11. Gerber MA, Randolph MF, Chanatry J, et al. Antigen detection tests for streptococcal pharyngitis: Evaluation of sensitivity with respect to true infections. *J Pediatr* 1986;108:654.
12. Komaroff A, Pas TM, Aronson MD, et al. The prediction of streptococcal pharyngitis in adults. *J Gen Intern Med* 1986;1:1.
13. Dajani AS, Bisno AL, Chung KJ, et al. Prevention of acute rheumatic fever: A statement for health professionals by the Committee on Rheumatic Fever, Endocarditis and Kawasaki Disease of the Council on Cardiovascular Disease in the Young, the American Heart Association. *Pediatr Infect Dis J* 1989;8:263.
14. Isenberg HD, Fritsche TR, Lancz G, et al. Lower respiratory tract specimens. In: Howanitz JH, Howanitz PJ, eds. *Laboratory medicine: test selection and interpretation.* New York: Churchill Livingstone, 1991:655–674.
15. Bartlett JG, Ryan KJ, Smith TF, et al. Laboratory diagnosis of lower respiratory tract infections. In: Washington JA, ed. *Cumitech 7A.* Washington DC: American Society for Microbiology, 1987:1–18.
16. Pezzlo M. Urine culture procedure. In: Isenberg HD, ed. *Clinical microbiology procedures handbook.* Washington DC: American Society for Microbiology, 1992:1.17.1–1.17.15.
17. Mobley HLT, Warren JW. *Urinary tract infections: molecular pathogenesis and clinical management.* Washington DC: American Society for Microbiology, 1995.
18. Pezzlo M. Detection of urinary tract infections by rapid methods. *Clin Microbiol Rev* 1988;1:268.
19. Jenkins RD, Fenn JP, Matsen JM. Review of urine microscopy for bacteriuria. *JAMA* 1986;255:3397.
20. Kunin C. *Detection, prevention, and management of urinary tract infections,* 4th ed. Philadelphia: Lea & Febiger, 1987:60.
21. Warren JW, Tenney JH, Hoopes JM, et al. Prospective microbiological study of bacteriuria in patients with chronic indwelling urethral catheters. *J Infect Dis* 1982;146:719.
22. Tenney JH, Warren JW. Bacteriuria in women with long-term catheters: comparison of indwelling and replacement catheters. *J Infect Dis* 1988;157:199.
23. Dallabetta G, Hook EW. Gonococcal infections. *Infect Dis Clin North Am* 1987;1:25.
24. Granato PA, Roefaro Franz MA. Evaluation of a prototype DNA probe test for the noncultural diagnosis of gonorrhea. *J Clin Microbiol* 1989;27:632.
25. Boyle JF. Laboratory diagnosis of chlamydial infections: introduction. In: Isenberg HD, ed. *Clinical microbiology procedures handbook.* Washington DC: American Society for Microbiology, 1992.
26. Schachter J, Stamm WE. *Chlamydia.* In: Murray PR, Baron EJ, Pfaller MA, et al., eds. *Manual of clinical microbiology,* 7th ed. Washington DC: ASM Press, 1999.
27. Peterson E. Isolation of *Chlamydia* spp. in cell culture. In: Isenberg HD, ed. *Clinical microbiology procedures handbook.* Washington DC: American Society for Microbiology, 1992.
28. Boyle JF, Clarke LM. Direct assays for the laboratory diagnosis of chlamydial infections. In: Isenberg HD, ed. *Clinical microbiology procedures handbook.* Washington DC: American Society for Microbiology, 1992.
29. Stamm WE. Diagnosis of *Chlamydia trachomatis* genitourinary infections. *Ann Intern Med* 1988;108:710.
30. Jenkins SG. Evaluation of new technology in the clinical microbiology laboratory. *Diagn Microbiol Infect Dis* 1995;23:53–60.
31. Larsen SA, Norris SJ, Pope V. Treponema and other host-associated spirochetes. In: Murray PR, Baron EJ, Pfaller MA, et al., eds. *Manual of clinical microbiology,* 7th ed. Washington DC: ASM Press, 1999:759–776.
32. Clarke LM. Laboratory diagnosis of viral and rickettsial infections: introduction. In: Isenberg HD, ed. *Clinical microbiology procedures handbook.* Washington DC: American Society for Microbiology, 1992:8.1.1–8.1.6.
33. Clarke LM, McPhee, JM, Cummings RV. Isolation of viruses in conventional tube culture: selection and inoculation of cell cultures. In: Isenberg HD, ed. Clinical microbiology procedures handbook. Washington DC: American Society for Microbiology, 1992:8.5.1–8.5.13.
34. Wold AD. Shell vial assay for the rapid detection of viral infections. In: Isenberg HD, ed. *Clinical microbiology procedures handbook.* Washington DC: American Society for Microbiology, 1992:8.6.1–8.6.10.
35. Keller EW. Detection and identification of viruses by immunofluorescence. In: Isenberg HD, ed. *Clinical microbiology procedures handbook.* Washington DC: American Society for Microbiology, 1992:8.9.1–8.9.10.
36. Fredericsson B, Frisk Å, Hagström B, et al. Vaginal mycoses: aspects on diagnosis and their treatment with econazole nitrate. *Curr Ther Res* 1980;27:309.
37. Holst E, Wathne B, Hovelius B, Mårdh P-A. Bacterial vaginosis: microbiological and clinical findings. *Eur J Clin Microbiol* 1987;6:536.
38. Krohn MA, Hillier SL, Eschenbach DA. Comparison of methods for diagnosing bacterial vaginosis among pregnant women. *J Clin Microbiol* 1989;27:1266.
39. Amsel R, Totten PA, Spiegel CA, et al. Nonspecific vaginitis: diagnostic criteria and microbial and epidemiologic associations. *Am J Med* 1983;74:14.
40. Mackowiak PA, Jones SR, Smith JW. Diagnostic value of sinus-tract cultures in chromic osteomyelitis. *JAMA* 1978;239:2772.
41. Wheat J, Allen SD, Henry M, et al. : Diabetic foot infections: bacteriologic analysis. *Arch Intern Med* 1986;146:1935.
42. Bamberger DM, Daus GP, Gerding DM. Osteomyelitis in the feet of diabetic patients: long-term results, prognostic factors, and the role of antimicrobial and surgical therapy. *Am J Med* 1987;83:653.
43. Washington JA II. The microbiology of musculoskeletal infection. *Orthop Clin North Am* 1975;6:115.
44. Summanen P, Baron EJ, Citron DM, et al. *Wadsworth anaerobic bacteriology manual,* 5th ed. Belmont, CA: Star Publishing, 1993.
45. Strain B. Quantitative bacteriology: tissues and aspirates: In: Isenberg HD, ed. *Clinical microbiology procedures handbook.* Washington DC: American Society for Microbiology, 1992:1.16a.1–1.16a.4.
46. Raahav D, Friis-Moller A, Bjerre-Jepsen K, et al. The infective dose of aerobic and anaerobic bacteria in postoperative wound sepsis. *Arch Surg* 1986;121:924.
47. Marshall KA, Edgerton MT, Rodheaver GT, et al. Quantitative microbiology: its application to hand injuries. *Am J Surg* 1976;131:730.
48. Cooney WP III, Fitzgerald RH Jr, Dobyns JH, et al. Quantitative wound cultures in upper extremity trauma. *J Trauma* 1982;22:112.
49. von Graevenitz A. Is there an optimal methodology for the microbiological analysis of effluent in CAPD peritonitis? *Zentralbl Bakteriol Mikrobiol Hyg* 1988;267:331.
50. Hächler H, Vogt K, Binswanger U, et al. Centrifugation of 50 ml of peritoneal fluid is sufficient for microbiological examination in continuous ambulatory peritoneal dialysis (CAPD) patients with peritonitis. *Infection* 1986;14:102.
51. Ludlam HA, Price TNC, Berry HA, et al. Laboratory diagnosis of peritonitis in patients on continuous ambulatory peritoneal dialysis. *J Clin Microbiol* 1988;26:1757.
52. Woods GS, Washington JA II. Comparison of methods for processing dialysate in suspected continuous ambulatory peritoneal dialysis-associated peritonitis. *Diagn Microbiol Infect Dis* 1987;7:155.
53. Shanholtzer CJ, Schaper PJ, Peterson LIZ. Concentrated gram stains prepared with a cytospin centrifuge. *J Clin Microbiol* 1982;16:1052.
54. Gill VJ, Nelson NA, Stock F, et al. Optimal use of the cytocentrifuge for recovery and diagnosis of *Pneumocystis carinii* in bronchoalveolar lavage and sputum specimens. *J Clin Microbiol* 1988;26:1641.
55. Kim TC, Lackman RS, Heatwole KN, et al. Acid-fast bacilli in sputum smears of patients with pulmonary tuberculosis: prevalence and significance of negative smears pretreatment and positive smears posttreatment. *Am Rev Respir Dis* 1984;129:264.
56. Pasareh L, Schell WA. Potassium hydroxide-calcofluor white procedure. In: Isenberg HD, ed. *Clinical microbiology procedures handbook.* Washington DC: American Society for Microbiology, 1992:6.4.1–6.4.2.
57. Farrell DJ, Morrissey I, Bakker S, et al. Detection of macrolide resistance mechanisms in *Streptococcus pneumoniae* and *Streptococcus pyogenes* using a multiplex rapid cycle PCR with microwell-format probe hybridization. *J Antimicrob Chemother* 2001;48:541.
58. National Committee for Clinical Laboratory Standards. *Performance standards for antimicrobial disk susceptibility tests; approved standard,* 7th ed. NCCLS document-M2-A7. Wayne, PA: NCCLS, 2000.
59. National Committee for Clinical Laboratory Standards. *Methods for dilution antimicrobial susceptibility tests for bacteria that grow aerobically; approved standard,* 5th ed. NCCLS document-M7-A5. Wayne, PA: NCCLS, 2000.
60. National Committee for Clinical Laboratory Standards. *Methods for antimicrobial susceptibility testing of anaerobic bacteria; approved standard,* 5th ed. NCCLS document-M11-A5. Wayne, PA: NCCLS, 2001.
61. Novak SM. E-test susceptibility testing. In: Isenberg HD, ed. *Clinical microbiology procedures handbook.* Washington DC: American Society for Microbiology, 1992:5.2a.1–5.2a.17.
62. Hindler J, Barriere SL. Selecting antimicrobial agents for testing and reporting. In: Isenberg HD, ed. *Clinical microbiology procedures handbook.* Washington DC: American Society for Microbiology, 1992:5.24.1–5.24.14.

63. Turnidge JD, Jorgensen JH. Antimicrobial susceptibility testing: general considerations. In: Murray PR, Baron EJ, Pfaller MA, et al., eds. *Manual of clinical microbiology*, 7th ed. Washington DC: ASM Press, 1999:1469–1473.

64. Aldridge KE, Ashcraft D, Cambre K, et al. Multicenter survey of the changing *in vitro* antimicrobial susceptibilities of clinical isolates of the *Bacteroides fragilis* group, *Prevotella, Fusobacterium, Porphyromonas*, and *Peptostreptococcus* species. *Antimicrob Agents Chemother* 2001;45:1238.

65. National Committee for Clinical Laboratory Standards. *Susceptibility testing of Mycobacteria, Nocardia, and other aerobic Actinomycetes; tentative standard*, 2nd ed. NCCLS document-M24-T2. Wayne, PA: NCCLS, 2000.

66. National Committee for Clinical Laboratory Standards. *Reference method for broth antifungal susceptibility testing of yeasts; approved standard*, 2nd ed. NCCLS document-M27-A2. Wayne, PA: NCCLS, 2002.

67. National Committee for Clinical Laboratory Standards. *Reference method for broth antifungal susceptibility testing of filamentous fungi; approved standard*. NCCLS document-M38-A. Wayne, PA: NCCLS, 2002.

68. Rex JH, Pfaller MA, Walsh TJ, et al. Antifungal susceptibility testing: practical aspects and current challenges. *Clin Microbiol Rev* 2001;14:643.

69. National Committee for Clinical Laboratory Standards. *Antiviral susceptibility testing; proposed standard*. NCCLS document-M33-P. Wayne, PA: NCCLS, 2000.

70. National Committee for Clinical Laboratory Standards. *Methodology for the serum bactericidal test; approved standard*. NCCLS document-M21-A. Wayne, PA: NCCLS, 1998.

71. National Committee for Clinical Laboratory Standards. *Method for determining bactericidal activity of antimicrobial agents; approved guideline*. NCCLS document-M26-A. Wayne, PA: NCCLS, 1998.

72. Handwerger S, Tomasz A. Antibiotic tolerance among isolates of bacteria. *Rev Infect Dis* 1985;7:368.

73. Sherris JC. Problems in in vitro determination of antibiotic tolerance in clinical isolates. *Antimicrob Agents Chemother* 1986;30:633.

74. Knapp C, Moody JA. Tests to assess bactericidal activity. In: Isenberg HD, ed. *Clinical microbiology procedures handbook*. Washington DC: American Society for Microbiology, 1992:5.16.1–5.16.33.

75. Griffin J. serum inhibitory and bactericidal titers: In: Isenberg HD, ed. *Clinical microbiology procedures handbook*. Washington DC: American Society for Microbiology, 1992:5.17.1–5.17.18.

76. Moody JH. Synergism testing: Broth microdilution checker board and broth macrodilution methods. In: Isenberg HD, ed. *Clinical microbiology procedures handbook*. Washington DC: American Society for Microbiology, 1992:5.18.1–5.18.28.

CHAPTER 13
Immunodiagnosis

Noel R. Rose

Since the remarkable specificity of antigen-antibody reactions was recognized at the end of the 19th century, a number of diagnostic tests based on immunologic specificity have been developed. We use the term immunodiagnosis as more appropriate than the older term serodiagnosis, because some of the most important procedures measure cell-mediated rather than humoral immunity. Immunodiagnosis implies evaluation of total immune response rather than simply the study of the antibody products of the immune response found in the serum. Two different approaches to the application of immunologic methods should be distinguished: (a) a known antigen is used to detect an immune response in patient's serum, and (b) an antibody of defined specificity serves as reagent for the identification of the corresponding pathogen. Both of these principal applications of immunologic methods are discussed in this chapter.

MEASUREMENT OF THE IMMUNE RESPONSE

Under favorable circumstances, the etiologic diagnosis of infectious disease is based on the isolation and identification of the causative agent. Frequently, we seek indirect evidence of infec-

tion by demonstrating an antibody response in the serum of a patient or by performing a skin test on the patient. For such a test for an infectious disease, it is necessary to make a reasonable speculation about the causative agent, based on either clinical or epidemiologic findings. The appropriate antigen or antigens can then be used as a reagent for measuring antibodies in serum or for eliciting skin test reactions.

Because of their outstanding sensitivity and specificity, antigen-antibody reactions lend themselves to diagnostic applications. In an immunochemical sense, *sensitivity* refers to the ability of an immunologic reagent to detect small amounts of antigen (or vice versa), whereas *specificity* describes the discriminating power of the selective reaction between antigen and its corresponding antibody. The great sensitivity of antibody-mediated reactions allows the detection of minuscule amounts of antibody, which is often useful for demonstrating a response early in the course of disease or a long time after an infection. The specificity of antibody reactions permits precise delineation of the antigen responsible for the immune response. It must be remembered, however, that a given antigen can be represented on a number of different organisms. Although the antigen-antibody reaction itself is specific, the identification of the antibody may sometimes be ambiguous.

The terms sensitivity and specificity are defined somewhat differently in a clinical or statistical context. Sensitivity is defined as the proportion of subjects with the disease who have a positive test result for the disease. Specificity is the proportion of subjects without the disease who have a negative test result. Equally important in evaluating a test is its *predictive value*. Positive predictive value is the probability of disease in a patient with a positive test result. Negative predictive value is the probability of not having the disease if the test result is negative or normal. The predictive value, therefore, is determined by the sensitivity and specificity of the test and the prevalence of disease in the population being studied.

In evaluating antibody-mediated reactions, the terms false negative and false positive are often used. *False negative* refers to the fact that antibody may not always be present in diagnostic quantities in cases of the disease. A false-negative result may represent a problem in sampling (for example, the serum specimen may have been taken too early in the course of infection) or a defect in the patient's immune response. The antigen preparation itself may not be appropriate for the individual case, because different patients recognize different antigenic determinants. False-negative results, therefore, limit the sensitivity of serologic methods.

A distinction is sometimes made between biologic false-positive and technical false-positive reactions. Technical false-positive results accrue from faults in the test procedure itself; for example, ill patients sometimes produce acute-phase reactants, such as C-reactive protein, that mimic in some respects the antigen-antibody reactions. Rheumatoid factors representing antibody to the immunoglobulin molecule may invalidate serologic tests. In fact, high levels of globulins themselves may result in a nonspecific interaction between a patient's serum and antigen. Biologic false-positive results, on the other hand, are not really false but reflect the fact that the same antigenic determinant may appear on a number of different pathogens. False-positive results, then, may compromise the specificity of serologic diagnosis.

Because the predictive value of a test depends on prevalence, it varies with the population to which it is applied. For example, even with a very specific test, positive results applied to a disease of low prevalence are more likely to be false-positive results. Conversely, negative results, even with a very sensitive test, are likely to be false-negative results when applied to a disease of higher prevalence. Thus, the interpretation of an immunodiagnostic test depends on the setting.

The first immunodiagnostic procedure based on the demonstration of an antibody response in patients' sera was described by Widal in 1896, when he showed that the serum of patients suffering from typhoid fever agglutinated typhoid bacilli. His test, which is still a cornerstone of the diagnosis of typhoid fever, depends on the fact that typhoid bacilli are antigenically homogeneous. Were there many different antigenic types of typhoid bacilli, it would be impractical to demonstrate antibody by such a test. Usually it is not feasible to perform a Widal-type test for other salmonelloses, because there are many different antigenic varieties of *Salmonella*. Unless there is information to suggest which species of *Salmonella* is likely involved in a particular case, all 1,500 serotypes would have to be tested. Sometimes an organism isolated from patients in an outbreak, or even from an individual patient, can be used as antigen in a Widal-type test for *Salmonella* infection. Another problem is that gram-negative bacilli share many somatic and flagellar antigens. Because so many antigens are shared among related or even unrelated microorganisms, normal persons have a low level of antibody to most pathogens. Therefore, antibody-based diagnosis generally depends on demonstrating a rise in antibody titer during the course of the disease. A comparison of titers of "acute" and "convalescent" serum specimens taken at least 2 weeks apart is a most important criterion for establishing the diagnosis. A fourfold increase in titer is usually indicative of current infection. If only a single sample is available, a high titer of antibody—well beyond the range found in normal persons—is required.

In addition to antigen specificity, the class of an antibody provides important clinical information. Immunoglobulin M (IgM) antibodies generally appear 7 to 10 days after infection and reach a peak after 2 or 3 weeks. The titer then drops, and immunoglobulin G (IgG) antibodies follow, which may persist in the patient's serum for long periods. IgM antibody, therefore, generally represents recent infection, whereas IgG antibody may reflect previous infection. IgG antibody is capable of crossing the placenta from mother to fetus, but IgM antibody is not. The presence of IgG antibody in cord serum, therefore, may be a reflection of antibody in the maternal serum. IgM antibody in the serum of a newborn is taken as evidence of antibody production by the infant.

There are other instances when the class of antibody is important; for example, the presence of immunoglobulin A (IgA) antibody in infections involving mucosal surfaces indicates a local response. IgA antibody in fecal specimens is sometimes useful in documenting intestinal infections such as cholera or poliomyelitis.

There are instances when the absence of antibody in the face of infection must be interpreted with caution. Infants, for example, are usually unable to produce antibody against carbohydrate antigens such as bacterial capsules. Patients receiving immunosuppressive drugs may also fail to produce antibody to a variety of antigenic stimuli. In fact, the absence of antibody to common antigens and the failure to produce antibody after appropriate stimuli are important clues for the diagnosis of immunodeficiency disease.

Immunodeficient patients often fail to produce antibodies when given a powerful antigenic stimulus, such as tetanus toxoid or pneumococcus polysaccharide. They may even lack the "natural" blood group antibodies, anti-A and anti-B. Infection with human immunodeficiency virus leads to a decrease in CD4+ T cells, which serve as helpers for antibody formation. Patients with acquired immunodeficiency syndrome often produce relatively weak IgM antibodies and fail to produce IgG antibodies on stimulation, because CD4+ T cells are needed for isotype class switching.

In addition to using antibody, it is possible to use skin test reactions for the indirect diagnosis of infectious disease. Two types of skin tests can be used. In the case of diseases such as diphtheria and scarlet fever, the symptoms are due to a discrete exotoxin. A toxin neutralization skin test can be performed. Microorganisms that are primarily intracellular in their habitat often induce cell-mediated responses. They can be measured by means of the delayed hypersensitivity skin test.

IDENTIFICATION OF MICROORGANISMS

Defined antisera are widely used in medical microbiology for the identification of microorganisms. Labeled antisera may be applied directly to specimens from the patient, including body fluids and tissue. Such methods are often of great value because they can provide an immediate diagnosis.

Another application of antibody reagents is the identification of microorganisms in culture. The identification of viral isolates, for example, frequently depends on the ability of an antiserum to neutralize some discernible effect of the cultured virus. An additional use of defined antibodies is in grouping and typing of microorganisms. Identification of the serotypes of *Salmonella* is possible only by the application of a panel of defined serologic reagents.

There has been a great effort to apply molecular methodology rather than antibody probes to the identification of microorganisms directly in specimens from patients. Molecular testing can be divided into two approaches: the use of deoxyribonucleic acid (DNA) probes to detect directly a specific target sequence, or nucleic acid amplification to detect specific target DNA or ribonucleic acid (RNA). The direct use of DNA probes is now widely accepted as a rapid approach to identifying certain specific pathogens in tissues or cultures. Amplification techniques are more sensitive but subject to false-positive results caused by contamination.

ANTIBODY RESPONSE

Neutralization

From a theoretical point of view, the antibodies most relevant to infectious diseases are those that neutralize the pathogenic effects of the microorganism. In the case of toxigenic diseases, such as tetanus, diphtheria, and *Clostridium difficile* gastroenteritis, direct tests of toxin neutralization are feasible in specially equipped laboratories. It has proved to be simpler and less expensive, however, to measure the toxin immunochemically, using one of the immunoassays to be discussed subsequently. In the past, mouse protection tests were the standard procedure for identifying type-specific antibodies to pneumococci, but this method has also been largely replaced by simpler immunochemical procedures *in vitro*. Viruses that produce obvious cytopathic effects in tissue culture, such as those of measles and mumps, lend themselves to neutralization tests, which are both sensitive and specific. They require, however, that stocks of living virus be available in the laboratory. Rather than by cytopathic effects, some viruses can be detected by their ability to produce hemagglutination. Hemagglutination inhibition reactions are used for measurement of antibodies to influenza virus, adenovirus, and rubella virus. *Mycoplasma* infection produces measurable metabolic changes in infected cells, so that metabolic inhibition tests can be performed for this group of organisms.

Neutralization tests can also be performed with major bacterial products that produce biologic effects. The β-hemolytic streptococcus is remarkable for the number of biologically active secretions it produces. Antibodies to streptolysin O, to DNase B, streptokinase, and hyaluronidase are conveniently measured in the diagnostic laboratory and are useful as evidence of current or recent streptococcal infection. Their greatest application is in the diagnosis of sequelae of streptococcal infection, such as glomerulonephritis and rheumatic fever.

Another approach is to measure the direct effect of antibody on the living microorganism. The original demonstration of antibody-directed, complement-mediated bacteriolysis was carried out by Pfeiffer using *Vibrio cholerae*, and this method is still used occasionally in specialized laboratories. Complement-mediated lysis of *Neisseria meningitidis* is sometimes a useful procedure, not only for demonstrating the presence of antibody but also for determining the integrity of the complement system in a patient's serum. Persons with deficiency in the later components of the complement cascade are inordinately susceptible to meningococcal infections. Opsonization followed by phagocytosis is mediated by antibody to the microbial surface and is a useful technique for measuring protective antibody to *Brucella*.

Agglutination

Agglutination occurs when antibody molecules combine with particulate antigens. The most commonly used particulate antigens are whole bacterial cells and red blood cells. The ready availability of standardized suspensions of killed bacteria enables the clinical laboratory to make an indirect diagnosis of an infectious disease even when the pathogen cannot be isolated from the patient. A rising titer of antibody during the progression and resolution of the illness is an indication of infection with that organism.

The febrile agglutination test uses a panel of possible pathogens to identify the microorganism against which there is the most marked immunologic response. The panel is made up of organisms that are appropriate for the patient's symptoms and correspond with local epidemiologic findings. A typical panel may be composed of suspensions of *Salmonella typhi* (both H and O antigen suspensions are usually included), other *Salmonella* species prevalent in the particular community, *Brucella*, *Yersinia pestis*, and *Francisella tularensis*. In addition, *Proteus vulgaris* suspensions are included because of their cross-reaction with certain rickettsiae, as represented by the Weil-Felix reaction to be described later. Similar agglutination reactions are sometimes performed with suspensions of *Bordetella pertussis*, *V. cholerae*, *Listeria monocytogenes*, and *Leptospira icterohaemorrhagiae* if there is clinical evidence of infection by one of these organisms.

The interpretation of the results of these diagnostic agglutination tests requires considerable knowledge and experience. Several points must be kept in mind:

1. Microorganisms, particularly gram-negative bacilli, share many antigens, so the presence of even a high titer of antibody is not necessarily indicative of infection by that particular species.
2. A test result usually does not become positive until 2 or 3 weeks after infection. Therefore, a negative test result early in disease does not exclude the diagnosis.
3. Antibodies may persist long after infection has subsided or may be produced by previous vaccination. A high titer of antibody, therefore, is not always indicative of current infection.

The interpretation of agglutination tests, therefore, depends much on the clinical situation and history of the patient.

Some of the most useful agglutination tests depend on the presence of shared antigens. Members of the typhus spotted fever and scrub typhus groups of *Rickettsia* share some antigens with certain strains of *Proteus*, providing the basis for the Weil-Felix reaction referred to before. Patients with *Mycoplasma pneumonia* generally produce high titers of cold hemagglutinins that act on normal human erythrocytes, and patients with infectious mononucleosis produce heterophil antibodies to sheep and ox erythrocytes.

Precipitation

When a soluble antigen comes in contact with its corresponding antibody in solution, antigen-antibody complexes result, which may become insoluble. Precipitation is highly dependent on the proportions of antibody and antigen, as well as the temperature, salt concentration, and pH of the solution. Therefore, precipitation reactions must be carried out under carefully controlled conditions. In particular, it must be remembered that precipitation can be inhibited by an excess of antigen, so a range of antigen concentrations must be tested. In addition, precipitation is relatively insensitive as a measure of antibody, although it may be quite sensitive as far as testing antigen is concerned.

Originally, precipitin reactions were carried out in fluid media. Under these conditions, however, it is not possible to distinguish different antigen-antibody combinations that occur simultaneously in the same tube. Therefore, precipitin reactions are now usually carried out in gelled media. An advantage of precipitation in agar, in addition to separating individual reactions, is that it is possible to relate an unknown antigen-antibody reaction with a known one. One can definitively identify antibodies to pathogenic fungi, such as *Blastomyces*, *Coccidioides*, and *Aspergillus*; and parasites, such as *Entamoeba*, *Trypanosoma*, *Trichinella*, and *Echinococcus*, by reactions of identity in agar. In addition, antibodies to important constituents of microorganisms, such as staphylococcal teichoic acid, can be precisely identified by precipitation in gel, because the patient's serum forms a single precipitin line of identity with the positive control serum and purified teichoic acid.

Counterimmunoelectrophoresis makes use of endosmotic flow to concentrate antigen and antibody at an interface. During electrophoresis, the slow-moving immunoglobulins migrate toward the cathode while most antigens move in a concentrated front toward the anode. By appropriate arrangement of wells, antigen and antibody can thus be made to collide, forming a precipitate between the two wells. The precipitation lines develop rapidly, usually giving maximum intensity within 30 to 90 minutes, depending on the strength of the reagents. This technique provides a sensitive measure of antigens of mycotic pathogens such as *Cryptococcus* and can be applied to cerebrospinal fluid. Bacterial antigens from *N. meningitides*, *Haemophilus influenzae* type b, and *Streptococcus pneumoniae* can also be demonstrated in cerebrospinal fluid by counterimmunoelectrophoresis.

Methodologically, flocculation tests resemble precipitin reactions. The Venereal Disease Research Laboratory (VDRL) test for syphilis contains as antigen cardiolipin fortified with cholesterol and lecithin. The test measures both IgG and IgM antibodies formed by the host in response to release of cardiolipin from damaged host cells during syphilitic infection as well as to the lipid of the treponeme itself. Antibody acts on this lipidic suspension to produce visible floccules, which can be seen either macroscopically or microscopically. Because of its sensitivity, the VDRL test is widely used as an exclusionary screening test. With cerebrospinal fluid, it is valuable in the diagnosis of neurosyphilis. For large-scale screening programs, the highly sensitive rapid plasma reagin test is widely used, but it is usually combined with a less sensitive confirmatory test.

Conditioned, Indirect, or Passive Agglutination

The greater sensitivity and convenience of agglutination testing rather than of precipitin reactions have encouraged the development of methods to convert precipitation to agglutination. This is done by attaching the soluble antigen to an inert particle. The most widely used carrier is the red blood cell, but latex, bentonite, and even collodion particles have been used. The red blood cells may be used in their native state or fixed. Fixation not only increases the life span of the red blood cell but sometimes removes native cell surface antigens to which the patient might have antibodies. Alternatively, when fresh red blood cells can be used, complement-mediated lysis with consequent release of hemoglobulin can be used as an indication of antigen-antibody interaction at the red blood cell surface.

The first requirement in developing a passive hemagglutination reaction is to coat the red blood cell. Some substances adhere to red blood cells spontaneously, but most require chemical coupling, which may be effected by treating the cells with tannic acid or chromic chloride or by covalently bonding the antigen with bisdiazotized benzene or some similar linker. Sometimes carbohydrates and lipopolysaccharides bind directly to red blood cells without chemical linkage. The coated cells must then be washed thoroughly to remove any soluble antigen and added to dilutions of serum. Antibody titers are determined exactly by agglutination.

Among the antigens that are often used in passive hemagglutination tests are pneumococcus and *Meningococcus* polysaccharides and capsular antigens of *Y. pestis* and *H. influenzae* type b. Protein antigens, such as diphtheria and tetanus toxins and the Vi antigen of the typhoid bacillus, lend themselves to passive hemagglutination. Antibodies to *Treponema pallidum* can be detected by using a microhemagglutination assay. Latex particles have proved useful carriers for a number of microbial antigens, including those of *Histoplasma*, *Cryptococcus*, and other systemic fungi; and *Entamoeba histolytica* and other parasitic protozoa.

A related method that has been exploited extensively is coagglutination. It uses selected strains of staphylococci that express protein A on their surface. This surface protein binds the Fc portion of an antibody molecule. Such antibody-coated staphylococcal organisms readily take up the corresponding antigen and provide an appropriate coated particle for agglutination reactions. The method has proved to be a useful adjunct for the diagnosis of gonorrhea.

Complement Fixation

The complement fixation reaction is valuable if the antigen is not present in a readily accessible or purified form. It represents a highly sensitive technique for measuring low concentrations of antibody. Because each antibody molecule may trigger the activation of hundreds of complement molecules, a considerable amplification of the antigen-antibody reaction can be achieved.

The test is performed in two stages. In the first, antigen-antibody mixtures are incubated with a measured amount of complement; in the second stage, a suspension of sheep red blood cells sensitized with rabbit antibody to sheep red blood cells is added as an indicator system to detect free or unfixed complement after the original antigen-antibody reaction. Complement can be measured most accurately by determining the quantity necessary to lyse 50% of a standard suspension of antibody-coated red blood cells. The test then can be quantitated by measuring the amount of complement actually consumed. Alternatively, the dilution of serum able to give 50% fixation of a standard quantity of complement with a previously determined optimal dilution of antigen can be determined.

The complement fixation test is rather intricate, because it depends on the standardization of a number of reagents; however, the indicator system is the same for all tests used. The only difference is in the antigen that is used. Therefore, once the complement fixation method has been established in a laboratory, it is readily applicable to a number of different tests. A major drawback of complement fixation is that certain human sera are anticomplementary, that is, they inactivate complement directly. Anticomplementarity may be due to the presence of circulating antigen-antibody complexes, to increased levels of immunoglobulin, or to unknown factors in the serum. In any case, it invalidates the complement fixation test.

Historically, the greatest application of complement fixation has been for serologic diagnosis of syphilis. The antigen used in the test is cardiolipin, which was originally obtained as an alcohol extract of beef heart. Complement fixation is particularly appropriate as a test for syphilis because the sensitivity and specificity are readily adjusted. For screening purposes it is often necessary to have a highly sensitive test, that is, one that detects all patients suffering from the disease. Such tests inevitably have a high proportion of false-positive results. For diagnosis, on the other hand, a more specific test may be advantageous to determine only the active cases of syphilis. It is important that both the immunologist and the clinician agree on the optimal sensitivity/specificity ratio of the test in particular circumstances.

The list of other pathogens to which the complement fixation method has been applied is lengthy. It includes bacteria such as *Bordetella*, *Listeria*, *Neisseria*, and *Nocardia*; fungi such as *Aspergillus*, *Blastomyces*, *Coccidioides*, and *Histoplasma*; *Chlamydia*; *Rickettsia*; and viruses, including herpes simplex virus, cytomegalovirus, respiratory syncytial virus, adenovirus, and influenza virus.

Immunofluorescence and Immunoenzyme Procedures

Antigen-antibody reactions can be visualized directly by labeling either antigen or antibody with an appropriate marker. Possible markers are fluorochromes, enzymes, and electron-opaque substances. In the diagnostic immunology laboratory, fluorescein isothiocyanate is the most commonly used reagent. Fluorochromes absorb radiation (e.g., ultraviolet light) and emit visible light. Immunofluorescence techniques, therefore, require a special microscope capable of admitting ultraviolet light. As a method for demonstrating antibodies, immunofluorescence is highly versatile. Indirect immunofluorescence is performed by adding a patient's serum to a slide containing the appropriate microorganism. The microorganism might be obtained from a pure culture specimen, a tissue culture specimen, or a tissue section. After the serum is incubated with this substrate, the slide is washed and a fluorescein-labeled antiglobulin reagent is added. The slide is washed again, mounted, and studied under an ultraviolet microscope. If antibodies are present in the serum, the microorganism will fluoresce.

Immunofluorescence is widely used for organisms that cannot be grown in pure culture. *Treponema pallidum* has yet to be cultured; however, the organism can be grown in the rabbit testis and films prepared on slides for an indirect immunofluorescence reaction, referred to as the fluorescent treponemal antigen test. A further refinement of the test is necessary because many human sera contain antibodies to treponemes, presumably induced by the common spirochetal inhabitants of the mouth. Therefore, the fluorescent treponemal antibody absorption test has been developed. In this procedure, the patient's serum is first absorbed with a suspension of nonpathogenic treponemes and then tested by the fluorescent antibody method. Because the method is rather complex and expensive, it is reserved for confirmatory testing when the clinical signs or history disagree with the rapid plasma reagin, VDRL, or other nontreponemal test results.

The indirect fluorescent antibody test is equally useful for the serologic diagnosis of many viral infections, such as infectious mononucleosis. The viral capsid antigen is present in cultured cells harboring Epstein-Barr virus. Smears of these cells are prepared, along with controls of uninfected cell lines; they are treated with the patient's serum and the reaction is developed with a fluorescein-labeled antiglobulin. The results are read under the fluorescence microscope. By using a class-specific antiglobulin, the isotype of the patient's antibody can be determined. The same procedure can be used for other Epstein-Barr virus antigens, such as Epstein-Barr nuclear antigen, which is localized in the cell nucleus.

Fluorescent methods have proved to be useful for many other pathogens that are most readily grown in tissue culture, such as *Chlamydia* and *Rickettsia*.

Radioimmunoassay and Enzyme Immunoassay

Immunoassays are performed by measuring direct binding of antibody to antigen. In the simplest test, a radiolabeled antigen is added to bind the antibody. The test can be carried out either in fluid medium or on a solid surface. In fluid, the antigen-antibody complex must be separated from free antibody, usually by addition of ammonium sulfate or antiglobulin. The radioactivity of the precipitate is then measured. A solid-phase test is carried out by attaching the antigen to a glass or plastic surface. In some cases, the attachment requires first putting down a layer of antibody and then adding the appropriate antigen. The patient's serum is then added, followed by the labeled antiglobulin. After washing, the reaction is quantitated by the amount of radioactivity attached to the surface. Because this method is highly sensitive as well as quantitative, it has been widely adopted in the diagnostic immunology laboratory. Radioimmunoassays are, for example, the most common method for measuring antibodies to the hepatitis viruses.

For immunodiagnostic purposes, enzyme immunoassays offer a number of important advantages. The enzyme-linked reagents have a long half-life, are free from the legal limitations surrounding radioisotopes, and are adaptable to single tests or to large-scale automation. Enzyme immunoassays can be divided into two major groups: homogeneous assays, in which the enzyme activity is altered during the immune reaction, and heterogeneous assays, in which the enzyme activity of the labeled reagent is not affected by precipitation in the immune reaction. In heterogeneous assays, there must be an additional step to separate the bound from the unreacted labeled reagent. Although homogeneous assays are simpler in principle, the enzyme-linked immunosorbent assay is most widely used in immunodiagnosis. In principle, it can be used for the measurement of antibody to virtually any infectious agent. A particular attraction of the method is that the same conjugate can be used in any application. Class-specific, enzyme-labeled antiglobulins permit recognition of the immunoglobulin class, if such information is desired. Anticomplement antibodies may provide a useful alternative if complement is added to the antigen-antibody

combination. The procedure calls for coating the wells of plastic microplates with the relevant antigen, adding the patient's serum in one or more dilutions, washing, and adding enzyme-labeled antihuman immunoglobulin conjugate. After further incubation, the enzyme substrate is added and incubated, and the degradation of a chromogenic substrate is measured by means of color intensity. The reaction can be stopped at a selected point in time, or kinetic measurements can be made of substrate breakdown. In this manner, a relationship can be calculated between the enzymatic activity and the amount of antibody in the serum.

The basic method can be modified in a number of ways. If the antigen is not present in reasonably purified form, the wells can be coated with specific antibody, either polyclonal or monoclonal antibody, followed by addition of crude antigen. These tests are referred to as capture assays. The test is then carried out in the usual manner. Enzyme-labeled staphylococcal protein A can be used instead of the antiglobulin reagent. This method is effective only to detect antibody classes IgG1, IgG2, and IgG4, which react with protein A. In the sandwich method, the well is coated with antigen and then the sample of serum to be tested is added, followed by enzyme-labeled antigen and substrate. It is obvious that the versatility of the enzyme-linked immunosorbent assay accounts for its broad applications in immunodiagnosis.

A number of fluorescent immunoassays have been widely adopted by clinical laboratories. These procedures are rapid and sensitive and lend themselves to automation. The fluorescent labels used are generally the same as in immunofluorescence, and the test procedures resemble enzyme immunoassays. Homogeneous assays are feasible when the antigen-antibody reaction leads to quenching of the fluorescence. As an example, such an assay was introduced for the serologic diagnosis of syphilis. Fluorescein-labeled liposomes containing cardiolipin antigen are added to a patient's serum. The antibody-antigen interaction sterically inhibits the reaction of the fluorescein-labeled cardiolipin with antifluorescein antibody. When reacted with fluorescein, the antifluorescein antibody will quench the fluorescence. The anticardiolipin antibody level correlates with the degree of fluorescence emitted.

WESTERN IMMUNOBLOT

A specialized application of enzyme immunoassays valuable for crude antigens is the Western immunoblot. A complex antigen mixture is first separated by electrophoresis in detergent-containing gel and then transferred to a nitrocellular membrane. The membrane is covered with the patient's serum, washed, and exposed to labeled antiglobulin reagent. The reactions, seen as colored bands, are localized according to the approximate molecular weight of the particular components. This method is widely used for confirmation of human immunodeficiency virus infection.

Skin Tests

TOXIN NEUTRALIZATION

The exotoxins of organisms such as *Corynebacterium diphtheriae* are potent antigens and regularly evoke neutralizing antibodies, which are protective against the disease in humans. The measurement of this immune response during the course of disease in an individual patient plays little role in diagnosis or management; however, information about the immune status of populations is valuable for epidemiologic studies. Antitoxin levels can be estimated by use of hemagglutination tests with toxin-coated red blood cells, but sometimes it is necessary to determine the levels of antibodies that actually neutralized the toxin. These studies use the Schick test for estimating diphtheria antitoxin levels. The Schick test is capable of dividing a population into susceptible and nonsusceptible groups based on their response to a standard dose of diphtheria toxin. Persons who have Schick-positive results possess a serum antitoxin level of more than 0.01 antitoxin units (AU) per milliliter, whereas most persons who have Schick-negative results have levels of less than 0.01 AU/mL. The test is performed by intracutaneous injection of an appropriate dilution of diphtheria toxin into the flexor surface of the arm and the same amount of heat-inactivated toxin in the other arm. This inactivated control serves to detect allergic reactions to the medium. The control is important because most toxin preparations used in the Schick test are not highly purified. This control material may give rise to an immediate wheal-and-flare reaction or to a delayed erythematous response that can be mistaken for a positive Schick test result.

In nonimmune persons, the toxin produces an area of redness in approximately 18 hours that grows in size and intensity in 3 to 5 days. A central area of necrosis may develop. With adequate levels of circulating antitoxin and no sensitivity to other corynebacterial antigens, no reaction will be seen at the site of either injection.

DELAYED HYPERSENSITIVITY

Delayed hypersensitivity skin tests are a cost-effective way to evaluate cellular immunity in patients with infectious diseases. Demonstration of cutaneous hypersensitivity reduces the need for costly studies of cellular immunity *in vitro*. Demonstration of the cellular response complements measurement of humoral immunity. The information may be useful diagnostically, especially in chronic intracellular infections produced by bacteria, viruses, and fungi. A positive skin test may also be useful in prognosis, because patients with delayed hypersensitivity sometimes have a better outlook than patients who lack such responses. Finally, tests of cell-mediated immunity are an important part of the evaluation of possible immunodeficiency.

The presence of hypersensitivity reactions accompanying an infection was first demonstrated in Robert Koch's description of local induration and swelling after subcutaneous reaction of tuberculin. The value of tuberculin tests for diagnosis was recognized by von Pirquet and Schick in 1903, using percutaneous skin tests, and Mantoux in 1910, using intradermal injections of tuberculin. The Mantoux test remains the standard method for clinical applications of delayed hypersensitivity assessment in infectious diseases.

It is critical to recognize the different types of cutaneous reactions that may follow injection of a microbial product into the skin. Immediate hypersensitivity reactions appear in the form of a wheal and erythema within a few minutes of the injection. They result from the interaction of cell-fixed antibodies, usually IgE, with the injected antigen. The Jones-Mote reaction begins within 2 to 4 hours of antigen challenge and reaches a maximum intensity in 24 to 72 hours. It is characterized by a basophil-rich cell infiltrate and is usually accompanied by the production of circulating IgG antibodies. The Arthus reaction, manifested by local erythema and edema and sometimes even necrosis, can occur 18 to 24 hours after challenge. This reaction is caused by the interaction of circulating complement-fixing antibodies (IgG or IgM) with locally deposited antigen. Delayed hypersensitivity reactions are usually maximal 48 to 72 hours after injection. Perivascular infiltrates of small and large lymphocytes develop by 4 to 6 hours, followed by a diffuse infiltrate composed of lymphocytes, monocytes, and basophils. Most of

the infiltrating cells bear the phenotypic markers of helper T lymphocytes. The induration of delayed hypersensitivity is believed to be due to the production of cytokines by these invading lymphocytes.

The application and reading of delayed hypersensitivity skin tests require considerable skill and experience. It is necessary first to ensure that the antigen is delivered intracutaneously. Next, the reaction must be evaluated carefully 48 and 72 hours after administration. A positive reaction is denoted by the presence of induration, defined as palpable thickening of the skin, and is independent of erythema and swelling.

The appearance of delayed hypersensitivity depends on previous contact with the microorganism. The interpretation of the test, therefore, depends on particular circumstances. A positive tuberculin test result in a child, for example, is probably indicative of infection. On the other hand, the absence of skin reaction to common microorganisms in adults can be used as evidence of immunodeficiency. Such deficiency may be general or antigen specific. General tests are usually performed by applying a panel of common microbial antigens, including streptococcal streptokinase, *Trichophyton*, *Candida*, and tetanus toxoid.

The tuberculin test is the classic method of detecting infection with *Mycobacterium tuberculosis*. The original tuberculin, old tuberculin, is made by cultivating a virulent strain of *M. tuberculosis* on liquid medium for several months, at which time the medium containing numerous bacterial products is filtered, sterilized, and concentrated. In 1934, Seibert developed the purified protein derivative as a way of isolating the principal antigen. For clinical purposes, the intradermal Mantoux test is indicated. The tine tests, in which the prongs of the tine are covered with dried tuberculin, are more feasible for extensive epidemiologic studies. The indications for a tuberculin test are suspected tuberculosis, evaluation of contacts, and exclusion of tuberculosis. The specificity of the test is sufficiently high that a positive result provides compelling evidence of past or present mycobacterial infection; however, because of extensive sharing of antigenic determinants within the genus, there is cross-reaction among the various mycobacteria. For instance, a patient infected with *Mycobacterium intracellulare* is more likely to develop a reaction to purified protein derivative. A positive reaction is also found in persons vaccinated with bacille Calmette-Guerin. False-negative reactions may be attributable to technical errors. More substantive causes of negative reactions are transient anergy associated with viral exanthemata (such as measles) and treatment with immunosuppressive drugs; particularly corticosteroids. Patients with early tuberculosis who are tested before the development of delayed hypersensitivity have a negative reaction. On the other hand, patients with extensive pulmonary or miliary tuberculosis are sometimes specifically anergic, and this represents a sign of poor prognosis.

Delayed hypersensitivity skin tests are available for a number of other infectious diseases—histoplasmosis, coccidioidomycosis, candidiasis, nocardiosis, and leprosy, among others. In general, their application and interpretation are similar to those for the tuberculin test; however, the test reagents are often poorly standardized. Some skin test reagents, such as that for histoplasma, may elicit production of antibodies. Blood samples for serologic tests, therefore, should be taken before the skin test reagent is applied.

Skin test reagents are difficult to apply in infants and older persons with atrophic skin. Additional contraindications may prevent the use of skin tests. In these instances, tests *in vitro* of cell-mediated immunity can be used. There are two major analogs *in vitro* of delayed hypersensitivity, lymphocyte transformation and production of lymphokines such as interleukin-2.

These tests are normally performed on peripheral blood lymphocytes, but lymph node and pleural fluid cells can sometimes be used. The validation of these tests depends on their correlation with skin tests in large-scale studies.

In some diseases, protective immunity seems to depend mainly on cytotoxic T cells. Tests in vitro of T-cell–mediated destruction of virus-infected target cells have been introduced for human immunodeficiency virus infection.

Identification of Microorganisms by Immunologic Methods

DIRECT APPLICATIONS

At times, it is advantageous to demonstrate the organism or antigenic products of the organism directly in clinical specimens. This approach does not require waiting for an antibody response; these tests are effective even in immuno-compromised individuals. The diagnosis of pneumococcal pneumonia, for example, can be made rapidly by demonstrating *S. pneumoniae* in sputum by means of the quellung capsular swelling test. The organism also releases copious amounts of polysaccharide that can be demonstrated in body fluids. Sputum samples can be tested for capsular antigens with pools of type-specific antisera using counterimmunoelectrophoresis or coagglutination. Serum is not as reliable a specimen as sputum for detection of pneumococcal antigen in pneumonia patients, although antigenemia is present in 20% to 40% of cases. Moreover, the detection of circulating antigen is a sign of poor prognosis. Urine does not yield as high an antigen positivity rate as sputum in cases of pneumococcal pneumonia; however, pneumococcal antigen can be detected by counterimmunoelectrophoresis in the cerebrospinal fluid of some patients with pneumococcal meningitis. A great advantage of these tests for antigen in cerebrospinal fluid is that an etiologic diagnosis can be made immediately without waiting for the results of culture.

Because meningitis can be considered a medical emergency, speed is important in the diagnosis. Therefore, latex reagents are available for the demonstration in cerebrospinal fluid of antigen from a number of different pathogens, including *S. pneumoniae*, *Streptococcus pyogenes*, *H. influenzae*, *Cryptococcus neoformans*, *Candida albicans*, and *N. meningitidis* as well as group B streptococci.

An alternative approach for etiologic diagnosis is to demonstrate the pathogen directly in the affected tissues. Biopsy and autopsy specimens are generally used for this purpose. If specific antisera are available, immunofluorescence and immunoperoxidase can often be applied successfully. For example, fluorescein-labeled antibodies can be used to demonstrate *T. pallidum* in tissue samples, replacing the more demanding darkfield method. DNA or RNA probes for particular organisms have been produced, which can be applied to tissue sections, using radioautography to develop the localized reaction. The polymerase chain reaction greatly amplifies the microbial nucleic acid and increases the sensitivity of the method considerably. The great sensitivity of the method requires special attention to technical details, because even trace contamination of specimens can produce false-positive reactions.

Because of their speed and cost-effectiveness, antigen detection methods are being used more often in clinical laboratories, as specific antisera become available. They are also applicable in previously treated patients when there is trouble isolating the pathogen in culture. Sometimes, in fact, they are the only means of identifying the agent of infection. The methods are, however, limited by the cross-reactions known to occur among microorganisms. Moreover, antigen detection methods do not permit assessment of antibiotic susceptibility. They are, therefore, likely to remain auxiliary techniques for the foreseeable future.

IDENTIFICATION OF MICROORGANISMS IN CULTURE

Because of their specificity, antibodies are ideal reagents for identification of microorganisms. The wide availability of monoclonal antibodies has greatly increased the specificity of immunologic methods of species identification. Many of the techniques described earlier in this chapter can be applied to antigen identification, including agglutination of bacterial cells, precipitation of microbial products, and neutralization of toxins or infectious virus. Immunofluorescent methods are widely used, as are enzyme immunoassays and radioimmunoassays. All of these methods depend on the specificity and potency of the antibody reagents. In the past, this goal required purification of the respective antigens before immunization and removal of unwanted antibodies by specific absorption. These steps are unnecessary if carefully selected monoclonal antibodies are used.

In addition to species identification, specific antibodies can be used for grouping and typing isolated microorganisms. The many serotypes of *Salmonella* are defined primarily by means of their antigenic specificity. The grouping of streptococci and the typing of pneumococci and of *H. influenzae* all depend on the availability of appropriate antisera. The information obtained is sometimes of clinical value but more often is needed for epidemiologic studies. Grouping and typing, therefore, are generally carried out in specialized central or reference laboratories.

SUMMARY

This chapter describes the application of immunologic methods to the diagnosis of infectious diseases. The major method of immunodiagnosis depends on the demonstration of an increasing titer of circulating antibodies to the particular pathogen in the serum of the patient. The method is of great value because serum is generally readily available and the tests are technically straightforward. Its usefulness is limited, however, by the fact that antibodies require time to appear in the bloodstream and may remain for a considerable period after infection. Moreover, related organisms may induce production of cross-reactive antibodies. In a few diseases, the presence of cell-mediated immunity to an organism has more diagnostic value than the presence of circulating antibody. In these cases, delayed hypersensitivity skin tests or their correlates *in vitro* are used. Finally, immunologic means and molecular hybridization can be used to aid in the identification of infectious microorganisms. Monoclonal and selected polyclonal antibodies and DNA and RNA probes can detect microorganisms in specimens from patients. The polymerase chain reaction greatly amplifies microbial nucleic acid and offers an extraordinarily sensitive technique for identifying pathogens directly in specimens. The tests may be carried out directly on body fluids or tissues from the patient, providing a relatively rapid means of identification. Antibody reagents are also used in the laboratory to assist in identification of cultured pathogens.

BIBLIOGRAPHY

Murray PR, Baron EJ, Haller MA, et al., eds. *Manual of clinical microbiology,* ed 7. Washington DC: American Society for Microbiology, 1999.
Rose NR, et al., eds. *Manual of clinical laboratory immunology,* ed 6. Washington DC: American Society for Microbiology, 2002.

CHAPTER 14

Molecular Techniques for the Detection, Identification, and Quantitation of Infectious Agents

Fred C. Tenover

Today, the emphasis in clinical microbiology is on rapid diagnostic techniques that will reduce the time required to identify the presence of pathogenic microorganisms in clinical samples. Rapid techniques can be divided into three major categories: microscopic methods, immunologic methods, and nucleic acid–based (i.e., molecular) methods. Whereas each has a role to play in the laboratory diagnosis of infectious diseases, nucleic acid–based methods have the greatest potential for increasing the sensitivity of detecting infectious agents directly in clinical samples while maintaining high specificity. Nucleic acid–based techniques also have the broadest diagnostic applications, including the ability to detect and identify infectious agents that cannot be cultured *in vitro*, and the ability to quantitate viral burden. Although the major strength of molecular methods is for organism identification, these nucleic acid–based techniques can also be adapted for (a) strain typing to aid epidemiologic investigations, (b) detection of antimicrobial resistance genes in bacteria to guide therapy early in the course of disease, and (c) detection of mutations associated with antiviral resistance. Nucleic acid amplification methods are based on simple deoxyribonucleic acid (DNA)-to-DNA or DNA-to-ribonucleic acid (RNA) hybridization reactions. In this chapter, the basic principles of nucleic acid hybridization, amplification, and quantitation are presented along with examples of how these molecular methods are applied to the diagnosis of infectious diseases.

TYPES OF NUCLEIC ACID–BASED METHODS

The three major formats of nucleic acid–based diagnostic testing are hybridization assays using nucleic acid probes, nucleic acid amplification assays, and DNA/RNA sequence analysis. The underlying premise of molecular diagnostic technologies is that each organism contains, within its genetic complement, sequences of either DNA or RNA that are unique to that species (1). The goal of the technology is to indicate the presence or absence of those unique sequences in clinical samples in lieu of culturing the organism *in vitro*. The hybridization assay is the simplest nucleic acid–based test. It involves 1) denaturing the target nucleic acid in the sample to single strands, usually by exposure to heat or sodium hydroxide; 2) adding the probe (which can be either DNA or RNA) to the reaction mixture and allowing it to bind to its complementary target sequences, thereby forming a stable double-stranded molecule; and 3) detecting the new double-stranded molecules. Most probes tend to be short molecules (40 bases in length or less) so that hybridization times require only minutes to an hour to complete. Detection systems range from chemiluminescent substrates that are chemically coupled to the probes, to molecular beacons that fluoresce as they bind to their targets (Fig. 14.1). Most commercial DNA probe

assays are homogeneous, that is, hybridization and detection of reaction products take place in a single tube, which simplifies assay conditions and reduces the problems of extrinsic contamination (2).

Nucleic acid–based diagnostic tests of the second broad class replace the biologic amplification step provided by traditional culture techniques, i.e., growing organisms on agar plates or in tissue culture lines before identification, with the enzymatic-based amplification of either nucleic acid substrates, or amplification of the signal after hybridization (3). The primary advantages of biochemical amplification of nucleic acids over biologic amplification or whole organisms are sensitivity and speed. New amplification technology and real-time monitoring of the accumulation of amplification products allow detection of organisms directly in clinical samples in as little as 45 minutes from the time of specimen receipt (4).

DNA/RNA sequence analysis has finally developed into a useful diagnostic tool. Several public and proprietary databases enable the identification of bacterial species based on 16S ribosomal RNA (rRNA) sequences. For example, Gingeras et al. used DNA microarrays to identify ten different *Mycobacterium* species (5), while Tang et al. demonstrated the utility of a commercial DNA sequencing system to identify a variety of unusual aerobic gram-negative pathogenic bacteria (6). Sequencing also plays a vital role in determining effective antiretroviral therapy for human immunodeficiency virus type 1 (HIV-1) infections (7).

Applications of DNA Probes

DNA probe assays can be used to identify organisms already available in pure culture (culture confirmation) or organisms directly in clinical samples, including organisms fixed in tissue sections. In culture confirmation assays, unique sequences of DNA or RNA are used to identify organisms in place of a set of biochemical or immunologic reactions. For slow-growing or fastidious organisms, this reduces the time to identification dramatically from that of conventional biochemical methods, particularly for *Mycobacterim* species (8). Ribosomal RNA sequences are often the targets of DNA probes. Identification of mycobacteria growing either on agar or in the liquid growth systems is the most common application of DNA probes for culture confirmation (8,9). Examples of commercially available culture confirmation probes are shown in Table 14.1. The combination of continuously monitored, nonradiometric liquid growth systems, such as the BACTEC[1] MGIT 960 (BD BioSciences, Sparks, MD) or MB/BacT (Organon Teknika, Raleigh, NC) plus DNA probes for *Mycobacterium tuberculosis, M. avium* complex, or *M. kansasii* often allows identification of these organisms in an average of 2 weeks or less from the time of specimen collection, in contrast to traditional culture and identification methods, which may take up to 6 weeks to complete. Sputum samples showing large numbers of organisms per high-power field can often be identified as containing *M. tuberculosis* using DNA probes in less than a week. Fluorescent-labeled peptide nucleic acids are an alternative method of identifying *Mycobacterium* species using in situ hybridization without the need for additional instrumentation (10). The hydrophobic nature of the peptides allows them to penetrate the lipophilic mycobacterial cell wall without sonication or treatment with glass beads, thus reducing the biohazard associated with traditional DNA probe technology. However, neither DNA nor PNA probes are sensitive enough to detect mycobacteria directly in clinical samples.

DNA probes can also be used to identify a number of yeasts and dimorphic molds, such as *Histoplasma capsulatum, Blastomyces dermatitidis, Cryptococcus neoformans*, and *Coccidiodies immitis* (Table 14.2). Probes are particularly effective in identifying

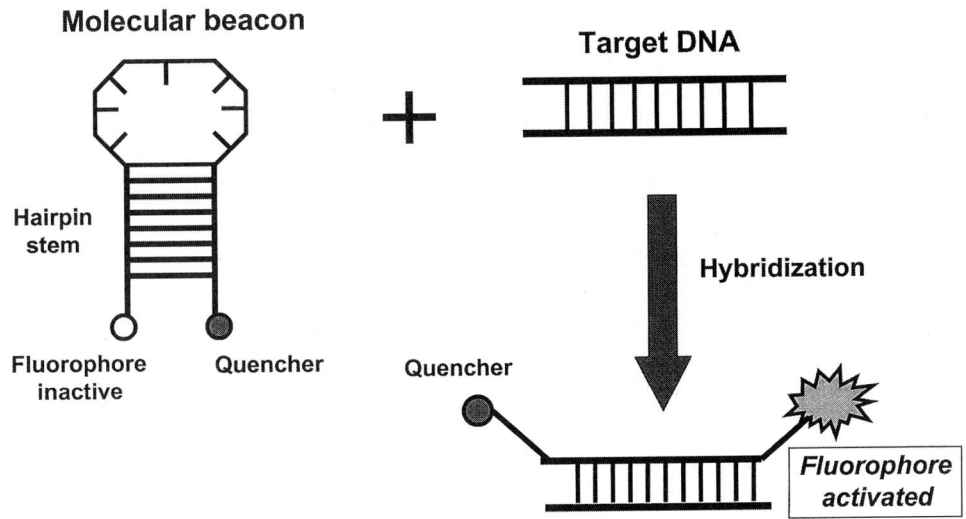

Figure 14.1. Molecular beacons are single-stranded deoxyribonucleic acid probes that form hairpin structures. They are labeled at one end with a fluorescent molecule and at the other with a substance that quenches the fluorescent signal. The binding of the probe to its target sequence moves the fluorescent moiety away from the quencher, allowing the fluorescent signal to be detected.

molds in the early stages of hyphal growth before diagnostic fruiting structures are apparent (11).

Probes for the Direct Detection of Infectious Agents in Clinical Samples

Commercial DNA probe assays to detect *Neisseria gonorrhoeae* and *Chlamydia trachomatis* in urethral and endocervical specimens continue to be marketed as alternatives to traditional culture and immunoenzyme assay techniques for these sexually transmitted pathogens (12). In many laboratories, however, the probe assays have been replaced by nucleic acid amplification methods that exhibit greater sensitivity (13,14). Another commercial probe test that continues to be used, albeit infrequently, is the assay for direct detection of *Streptococcus pyogenes* in throat swabs (Table 14.3). Although not yet commercially available, fluorescent-labeled DNA probes have been developed to identify a variety of bacterial and fungal organisms growing in blood culture systems. The technique uses fluorescence in situ hybridization and microscopy to identify organisms in blood films de-

posited on glass slides (15). Nucleic acid capture probes are also available for detection and typing of human papillomaviruses (Table 14.3).

Applications of Nucleic Acid Amplification Tests

Assays utilizing the polymerase chain reaction (PCR), strand displacement, transcription-mediated amplification, and nucleic acid sequence-based amplification (NASBA) are the most widely used amplification technologies for detection and identification of infectious agents. Probe amplification systems, including the ligase chain reaction (LCR) and cycling probe assays, and signal amplification systems, such as branched DNA and molecular beacons, are also available. Examples of commercially available amplification tests are shown in Table 14.4. The major applications of commercially prepared assays for detection and identification of bacterial pathogens are for *N. gonorrhoeae* and *C. trachomatis*, which can be detected in either urine specimens or vaginal or urethral swabs (14,16), or for *M. tuberculosis* from respiratory and other specimens (17,18). Commercial line probe assays, which use a reverse hybridization format, can be used in conjunction with amplification assays for identification of mycobacterial organisms growing in liquid media (19).

Commercial amplification assays for viral pathogens can be used for detection and quantitation of HIV-1 and cytomegalovirus (CMV) from plasma samples, detection of human T-cell leukemia virus-I/II, and quantitation of hepatitis B and hepatitis C viruses (20). Assays for quantitation of viral burden are now performed routinely in many laboratories, particularly to assess progression of HIV-1 infection (21,22).

TABLE 14.1. Culture Confirmation Assays for Bacterial Pathogens[a]

Organism	Commercial source
Enterococci	Gen-Probe
Group A streptococci	Gen-Probe
Group B streptococci	Gen-Probe
Haemophilus influenzae	Gen-Probe
Listeria monocytogenes	Gen-Probe
Mycobacterium tuberculosis complex	Gen-Probe
Mycobacterium avium	Gen-Probe
Mycobacterium avium complex	Gen-Probe
Mycobacterium gordonae	Gen-Probe
Mycobacterium intracellulare	Gen-Probe
Mycobacterium kansasii	Gen-Probe
Neisseria gonorrhoeae	Gen-Probe
Staphylococcus aureus	Gen-Probe
Streptococcus pneumoniae	Gen-Probe
Thermophilic campylobacters[b]	Gen-Probe

[a]All tests cited in the table have received clearance from the U.S. Food and Drug Administration.
[b]Includes *Campylobacter jejuni*, *Compylobacter coli*, and *Campylobacter lari*.

TABLE 14.2. Culture Confirmation Assays for Fungal Pathogens[a]

Organism	Commercial source
Blastomyces dermatiditis	Gen-Probe
Candida albicans	Gen-Probe
Coccidioides immitis	Gen-Probe
Cryptococcus neoformans	Gen-Probe
Histoplasma capsulatum	Gen-Probe

[a]All tests cited in the table have received clearance from the U.S. Food and Drug Administration.

TABLE 14.3. DNA Probes for Direct Detection of Organism in Clinical Samples[a]

Organism	Commercial source
Bacteria	
Chlamydia trachomatis	Gen-Probe
Chlamydia trachomatis	Digene
Group A streptococcus	Gen-Probe
Neisseria gonorrhoeae	Gen-Probe
Neisseria gonorrhoeae	Digene
Viruses	
Human papillomavirus	Digene
Cytomegalovirus	Digene

[a]All tests cited in the table have received clearance from the U.S. Food and Drug Administration.

Nucleic Acid Sequence Analysis

Nucleic acid sequencing technology is used to identify a variety of infectious agents in clinical laboratories throughout the world. Direct amplification and sequencing of ribosomal DNA (rDNA) enhance identification of nonculturable pathogens, such as *Tropherema whippleii* (23), and permit detection of bacterial agents from specimens from patients already started on antimicrobial chemotherapy (24). Commercial assays using DNA sequence analysis, such as the MicroSeq system (PE Applied Biosystems, Foster City, CA), have shown promise for identification of a variety of *Mycobacterium* species and other uncommon pathogens (6,25). However, this technology is expensive.

Another approach to sequencing uses oligonucleotide arrays, which increase the number of pathogens that can potentially be detected during a single assay (5,26). In addition to oligonucleotide arrays, microelectronic chip arrays have been shown to identify multiple genera of bacteria in addition to mutations associated with antimicrobial resistance (27). Sequence-based analysis is critical to viral susceptibility testing protocols, particularly for guiding therapy for HIV-1 infections (28). Several commercial assays are available for detecting mutations associated with resistance to reverse transcriptase inhibitors and protease inhibitors. These include traditional sequencing and oligonucleotide array–based technologies (29,30).

BRIEF REVIEW OF AMPLIFICATION METHODS

PCR requires a source of target nucleic acid, small DNA primers that are complementary to sequences at the 5' and 3' ends of the region of DNA to be amplified, an enzyme to synthesize DNA (i.e., the polymerase), and an instrument to modulate reaction temperatures during the various cycles. PCR usually consists of a three-step cycle of denaturing the DNA present in a sample; allowing the single-stranded DNA primers to bind (anneal) to the denatured DNA; and duplicating the target material between the primers by using DNA polymerase, which results in two double-stranded copies of the target DNA (Fig. 14.2). The cycle is initiated again with the denaturation of the newly created double-stranded DNA. The second cycle yields four copies of the target DNA; additional cycles increase the amount of target DNA exponentially. Thirty cycles yield approximately a millionfold amplification of the original target sequence. PCR can be adapted to the amplification of RNA targets by incorporating a reverse transcription step before the first amplification cycle. A single enzyme is now available that is capable of both reverse transcription and polymerization steps. The accumulation of amplification products can be measured in real time with use of fluorescently labeled probes or molecular beacons (31). By incorporating unique fluorophores on different probes, multiple pathogens can be assayed simultaneously. For example, molecular beacons have been used to identify four unique retroviral pathogens in blood (32). Instruments are now available that

TABLE 14.4. Examples of Commercially Available Target, Probe, and Signal Amplification Assays for Infectious Agents

Organism	Method	Commercial source
Bacteria		
Chlamydia trachomatis	PCR[a]	Roche Diagnostics
Chlamydia trachomatis/Neisseria gonorrhoeae	LCR[a]	Abbot Diagnostics
Chlamydia trachomatis/Neisseria gonorrhoeae	SDA	BD BioSciences
Chlamydia trachomatis/Neisseria gonorrhoeae	TMA[a]	Gen-Probe
Mycobacterium avium	PCR[b]	Roche Diagnostics
Mycobacterium intracellulare	PCR[b]	Roche Diagnostics
Mycobacterium tuberculosis	PCR[a]	Roche Diagnostics
Mycobacterium tuberculosis	LCR[c]	Abbott Diagnostics
Mycobacterium tuberculosis	TMA[c]	Gen-Probe
Mycobacterium tuberculosis	SDA[c]	Becton Dickinson
Neisseria gonorrhoeae	PCR[a]	Roche Diagnostics
Viruses		
Cytomegalovirus	PCR[c]	Roche Diagnostics
Human immunodeficiency virus	PCR[a]	Roche Diagnostics
Human immunodeficiency virus	Branched DNA[a]	Bayer
Hepatitis B virus	PCR[c]	Roche Diagnostics
Hepatitis B virus	Branched DNA[c]	Bayer
Hepatitis C virus	PCR[c]	Roche Diagnostics
Hepatitis C virus	Branched DNA[c]	Bayer

[a]Clearance received from the U.S. Food and Drug Administration.
[b]Research use only outside of United States.
[c]Research use only.
LCR, ligase chain reaction; PCR, polymerase chain reaction; SDA, strand displacement assay; TMA, transcription-mediated amplification.

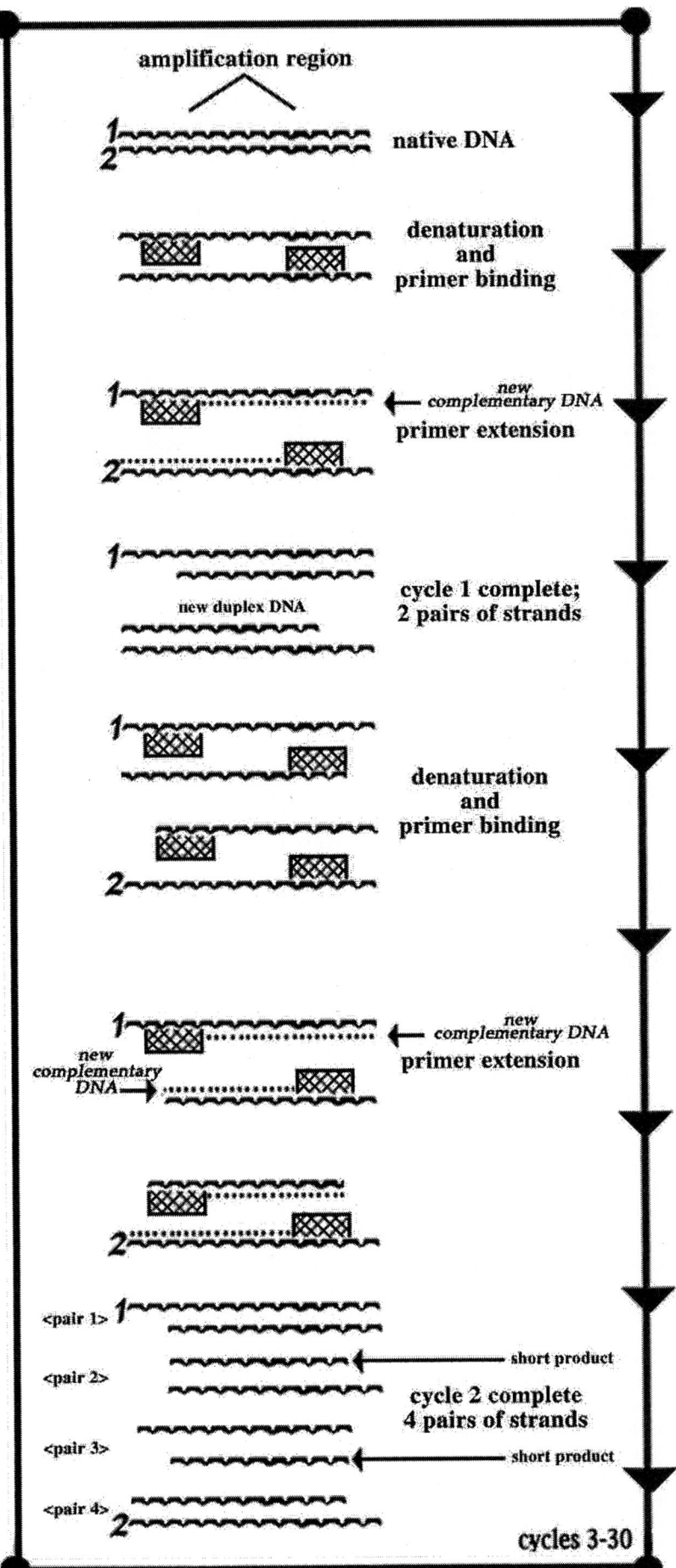

Figure 14.2. Polymerase chain reaction is a nucleic acid amplification method that targets specific sequences of deoxyribonucleic acid or ribonucleic acid for replication via binding of specific primer sequences.

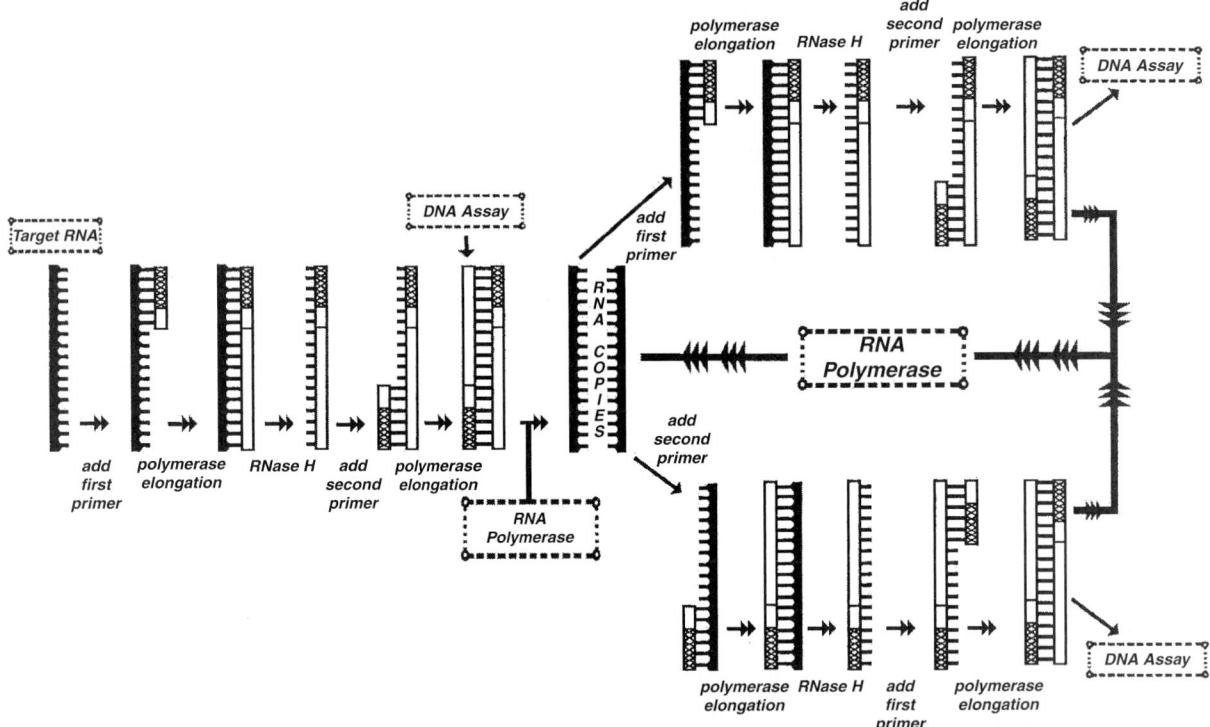

Figure 14.3. Transcription-mediated amplification is an isothermal process in which ribonucleic acid targets are converted to double-stranded deoxyribonucleic acid intermediates that in turn serve as additional templates for nucleic acid amplification.

allow assays of differing cycling temperatures and times to be run simultaneously, allowing flexibility in the types of pathogens sought.

The major drawback to PCR is the potential for contamination of samples by previously amplified material that strays into a clinical sample during specimen preparation. Such DNA may serve as a template for amplification, producing a false-positive result. Chemical approaches to prevent carryover contamination have been developed to alleviate this problem. The opposite problem, the presence of substances inhibitory to the PCR reaction, is also encountered in samples such as whole blood, stool, and urine (33,34). Controls to indicate the presence of inhibitors in samples should be incorporated into the assay format.

Transcription-mediated amplification is a target amplification method that, unlike PCR, is isothermal. It is a two-step process that begins with production of a double-stranded DNA molecule from target RNA (Fig. 14.3). In the second step, RNA copies are produced from the DNA strands in an exponential manner. These RNA copies then serve as templates for additional synthesis of DNA strands that can re-enter the amplification cycle. Commercial kits using this technology are available for the detection of *C. trachomatis* (35) and *M. tuberculosis*. NASBA assays, which use similar technology, are also available for detection of *C. trachomatis* and *N. gonorrhoeae* from genital tract specimens (36) and for quantitation of HIV-1.

Another target amplification system is the strand displacement assay, which is an isothermal process that uses a unique DNA polymerase and a complement of four probes to the sense and antisense strands of nucleic acid to effect sequence amplification. Tests for *M. tuberculosis, C. trachomatis*, and *N. gonorrhoeae* have been described using this technology (37).

A different approach to amplification, if the nucleotide sequence of the target is known, is LCR. This system uses two DNA probes that are complementary to contiguous pieces of DNA on the target nucleic acid. If the target nucleic acid is present in the sample, the two probes are joined by DNA ligase, and the newly ligated probe is replicated enzymatically in a continuous reaction. LCR methodology is available commercially for detection of *C. trachomatis* and *N. gonorrhoeae* (38).

Branched DNA is a true signal amplification system in which a DNA probe first captures a target molecule, and the DNA complex is then bound to a second DNA backbone on a solid support. A third DNA probe containing numerous reporter moieties is then allowed to bind to the complex, which dramatically increases the signal initiated by the binding of the first probe to the target. Either DNA or RNA sequences can be targeted in this method, which has found high acceptance as a means of quantitating HIV-1, hepatitis B, and hepatitis C viral loads (39).

Many of the above amplification technologies, including PCR and NASBA, can incorporate the use of molecular beacons to allow detection of organisms in real time.

Detection of Antimicrobial Resistance Genes

The goal of using molecular methods to identify bacteria directly in clinical samples is to speed identification and improve sensitivity, obviating the need for culture. However, by eliminating culture, the laboratory also eliminates its ability to perform antimicrobial susceptibility testing. Although this currently is not an issue for *C. trachomatis*, it is an important issue for drug-resistant *N. gonorrhoeae* and especially for *M. tuberculosis, Staphylococcus aureus*, and a multitude of other bacteria for which multidrug resistance has been described. Particularly for amplification-based methods, the loss of susceptibility results to guide therapy could be a major deficit. One approach to this problem is to use PCR, or other amplification methods, to detect key resistance determinants in the organism directly in the clinical sample. More than 100 PCR assays targeting resistance genes have been described (40). The utility of such an approach for detecting an organism and mutations associated with resistance, such as in *M. tuberculosis*, has been demonstrated (31). *Helicobacter pylori* is another organism for which multiplex amplification assays (i.e., multiple PCR primers in the same reaction tube) have been developed that indicate the presence of the organism in tissue biopsies (via detection of specific rDNA to *vacA* loci) and simultaneously identify up to three mutations in rRNA associated with clarithromycin resistance that are known to lead to treatment failure (41). Such multiplex assays linking organism identification and antimicrobial resistance detection are likely to become more common.

Although nucleic acid–based techniques are also used for bacterial, fungal, and viral strain typing (42), those applications will be covered elsewhere in this volume.

In summary, nucleic acid–based diagnostics have become a mainstay in the clinical microbiology laboratory, offering speed of detection, the ability to identify nonculturable organisms, and the ability to quantitate viral burdens.

REFERENCES

1. Tenover FC. DNA probes for infectious diseases. *Clin Microbiol Rev* 1988;1:82–101.
2. Arnold LJ, Jr., Hammond PW, Wiese WA, et al. Assay formats involving acridinium-ester-labeled DNA probes. *Clin Chem* 1989;35:1588–1594.
3. Persing DH. In vitro nucleic acid amplification techniques pp 51-87. In: Persing DH, Smith TF, Tenover FC, et al, eds. *Diagnostic molecular microbiology. Principles and applications.* Washington, DC: American Society for Microbiology, 1993.
4. Bergeron MG, Ke D, Menard C, et al. Rapid detection of group B streptococci in pregnant women at delivery. *N Engl J Med* 2000;343:175–179.
5. Gingeras TR, Ghandour G, Wang E, et al. Simultaneous genotyping and species identification using hybridization pattern recognition analysis of generic mycobacterium DNA arrays. *Genome Res* 1998;8:435–448.
6. Tang YW, Ellis NM, Hopins MK, et al. Comparison of phenotypic and genotypic techniques for identification of unusual aerobic pathogenic gram-negative bacilli. *J Clin Microbiol* 1998;36:3674–3679.
7. Hirsch MS, Brun-Vezinet F, D'Aquila RT, et al. Antiretroviral drug resistance testing in adult HIV-1 infection: recommendations of an international AIDS society-USA panel. *JAMA* 2000;283:2417–2426.
8. Peterson EM, Lu R, Floyd C, et al. Direct identification of *Mycobacterium tuberculosis, Mycobacterium avium,* and *Mycobacterium intracellulare* from amplified primary cultures in BACTEC media using DNA probes. *J Clin Microbiol* 1989;27:1543–1547.
9. Alcaide F, Benítez A, Escriba JM, et al. Evaluation of the BACTEC MGI 960 and the MB/MacTR Systems for recovery of mycobacteria from clinical specimens and for species identification by DNA AccuProbe. *J Clin Microbiol* 2000;398–401.
10. Stender H, Lund K, Petersen KH, et al. Fluorescence in situ hybridization assay using peptide nucleic acid probes for differentiation between tuberculous and nontuberculous mycobacterium species in smears of mycobacterium cultures. *J Clin Microbiol* 1999;37:2760–2765.
11. Stockman L, Clark KA, Hunt JM, et al. Evaluation of commercially available acridinium ester-labelled chemiluminescent DNA probes for culture identification of *Blastomyces dermatitides, Coccidioides immitis, Cryptococcus neoformans,* and *Histoplama capsulatum.* *J Clin Microbiol* 1993;31:845–850.
12. Limberger RJ, Biega R, Evancoe A, et al. Evaluation of culture and the Gen-Probe PACE-2 assay for detection of *Neisseria gonorrhoeae* and *Chlamydia trachomatis* in endocervical specimens transported to a state health laboratory. *J Clin Microbiol* 1992;30:1162–1166.
13. Wylie JL, Moses S, Babcock R, et al. Comparative evaluation of Chlamydiazyme, PACE 2, and AMP-CT assays for detection of *Chlamydia trachomatis* in endocervical specimens. *J Clin Microbiol* 1998;36:3488–3491.
14. Lauderdale TL, Landers L, Thorneycroft I, et al. Comparison of the PACE 2 assay, two amplification assays and Clearview EIA for detection of *Chlamydia trachomatis* in female endocervical and urine specimens. *J Clin Microbiol* 1999;37:2223–2229.
15. Kempf VA, Trebesius K, Autenrieth IB. Fluorescent in situ hybridization allows rapid identification of microorganisms in blood cultures. *J Clin Microbiol* 2000;38:830–838.
16. Goessens WHF, Mouton JW, vander Mejiden WI, et al. Comparison of three commercially available amplification assays AMP CT, LCx, and COBAS AMPLICOR, for detection of *Chlamydia trachomatis* in first-void urine. *J Clin Microbiol* 1997;35:2628–2633.
17. Della-Latta P, Whittier S. Comprehensive evaluation of performance, laboratory application, and clinical usefulness of two direct amplification technologies for the detection of *Mycobacterium tuberculosis* complex. *Am J Clin Pathol* 1998;110:301–310.

18. Brown TJ, Power EGM, French GL. Evaluation of three commercial detection systems for *Mycobacterium tuberculosis* where clinical diagnosis is difficult. *J Clin Pathol* 1999;52:193–197.
19. Miller N, Infante S, Cleary T. Evaluation of the LiPA Mycobacteria assay for identification of mycobacterial species from BACTEC 12B bottles. *J Clin Microbiol* 2000;38:1915–1919.
20. Berger A, Preiser W, Doerr HW. The role of viral load determination for the management of human immunodeficiency virus, hepatitis B virus, and hepatitis C virus infection. *J Clin Virol* 2001;20:23–30.
21. Nolte FS, Boysza J, Thurmond C, et al. Clinical comparison of an enhanced-sensitivity branched-DNA assay and reverse transcriptase-PCR for quantitation of human immunodeficiency virus type I RNA in plasma. *J Clin Microbiol* 1998;36:716–720.
22. Murphy DG, Cote L, Fauvel M, et al. Multicenter comparison of Roche COBAS AMPLICOR MONITOR version 1.5, Organon Teknika NucliSens QT with Extractor, and Bayer Quantiplex version 3.0 for quantification of human immunodeficiency virus type 1 RNA in plasma. *J Clin Microbiol* 2000;38:4034–4041.
23. Maiwald M, Relman D. Whipple's disease and *Tropheryma whippelii*: secrets slowly revealed. *Clin Infect Dis* 2001;32:457–463.
24. Rantakokko-Jalava K, Nikkari S, Jalava J, et al. Direct amplification of rRNA genes in the diagnosis of bacterial infections. *J Clin Microbiol* 2000;38:32–39.
25. Patel JB, Leonard DGB, Pan X, et al. Sequence-based identification of *Mycobacterium* species using the MicroSeq 500 16S rDNA bacterial identification system. *J Clin Microbiol* 2000;38:246–251.
26. Anthony RM, Brown TJ, French GL. Rapid diagnosis of bacteremia by universal amplification of 23S ribosomal DNA followed by hybridization to an oligonucleotide array. *J Clin Microbiol* 2000;38:781–788.
27. Westin L, Miller C, Vollmer D, et al. Antimicrobial resistance and bacterial identification using a microelectronic chip array. *J Clin Microbiol* 2001;39:1097–1104.
28. Kartsonis NA, D'Aquila RT. Clinical monitoring of HIV-1 infection in the era of antiretroviral resistance testing. *Infect Dis Clin North Am* 2000;14:879–899.
29. Wilson JW, Bean P, Robins T, et al. Comparative evaluation of three human immunodeficiency virus genotyping systems: the HIV-GenotypR method, the HIV PRT GeneChip assay, and the HIV-1 RT line probe assay. *J Clin Microbiol* 2000;38:3022–3028.
30. Fontaine E, Riva C, Peeters M, et al. Evaluation of two commercial kits for the detection of genotypic drug resistance on a panel of HIV type 1 subtypes A through J. *Am J Acquired Immune Defic Syndr* 2001;28:254–258.
31. Piatek AS, Telenti A, Murray MR, et al. Genotypic analysis of *Mycobacterium tuberculosis* in two distinct populations using molecular beacons: implications for rapid susceptibility testing. *Antimicrob Agents Chemother* 2000;44:103–110.
32. Vet JAM, Majithia AR, Marras SAE, et al. Multiplex detection of four pathogenic retroviruses using molecular beacons. *Proc Natl Acad Sci USA* 1999;96:6394–6399.
33. Tang YW, Persing DH. Molecular detection and identification of microorganisms. In: Murray P, Baron ES, Pfaller MA, et al, eds. *Manual of clinical microbiology,* 7th ed. Washington, DC: American Society for Microbiology, 1999:215–245.
34. Mahony J, Chong S, Jang D, et al. Urine specimens from pregnant and nonpregnant women inhibitory to amplification of *Chlamydia trachomatis* nucleic acid by PCR, ligase chain reaction and transcription-mediated amplification: identification of urinary substances associated with inhibition and removal of inhibitory activity. *J Clin Microbiol* 1998;36:3122–3126.
35. Ferrero DV, Meyers NH, Schultz DE, et al. Performance of the Gen-Probe AMPLIFIED *Chlamydia trachomatis* assay in detecting *Chlamydia trachomatis* in endocervical and urine specimens from women and urethral and urine specimens from men attending sexually transmitted disease and family planning clinics. *J Clin Microbiol* 1998;36:3230–3233.
36. Mahony JB, Song X, Chong S, et al. Evaluation of the NucliSens Basic Kit for detection of *Chlamydia trachomatis* and *Neisseria gonorrhoeae* in genital tract specimens using nucleic acid sequence-based amplification of 16S rRNA. *J Clin Microbiol* 2001;39:1429–1435.
37. van der Pol B, Ferrero DV, Buck-Barrington L, et al. Multicenter evaluation of the BDProbeTec ET system for detection of *Chlamydia trachomatis* and *Neisseria gonorrhoeae* in urine specimens, female endocervical swabs, and male urethral swabs. *J Clin Microbiol* 2001;39:1008–1016.
38. Carroll KC, Aldeen WE, Morrison M, et al. Evaluation of the Abbott ligase chain reaction assay for detection of *Chlamydia trachomatis* and *Neisseria gonorrhoeae* in urine and genital swab specimens from a sexually transmitted disease clinic population. *J Clin Microbiol* 1998;36:1630–1633.
39. Erice A, Brambilla D, Bremer J, et al. Performance characteristics of the QUANTIPLEX HIV-1 RNA 3.0 assay for detection and quantitation of human immunodeficiency virus type 1 RNA in plasma. *J Clin Microbiol* 2000;38:2837–2845.
40. Tenover FC, Rasheed JK. Genetic methods for detecting antimicrobial resistance genes. In: Murray P, Baron ES, Pfaller MA, et al, eds. *Manual of clinical microbiology,* 7th ed. Washington, DC: American Society for Microbiology, 1999:1578–1592.
41. Chisholm SA, Owen RJ, Teare EL, et al. PCR-based diagnosis of *Helicobacter pylori* infection and real-time determination of clarithromycin resistance directly from human gastric biopsy samples. *J Clin Microbiol* 2001;39:1217–1220.
42. Tenover FC, Arbeit RD, Goering RV and the Molecular Typing Working Group. How to select and interpret molecular strain typing methods for epidemiologic studies of bacterial infections: a review for health care epidemiologists. *Infect Control Hosp Epidemiol* 1997;18:426–439.

CHAPTER 15

Diagnostic Significance of Nonspecific Laboratory Abnormalities in Infectious Diseases

Burke A. Cunha

Antimicrobial therapy in infectious disease is based on the presumptive diagnosis. Presumptive diagnosis is based on the clinical working or syndromic presentation pending a definitive diagnosis. When body fluid or tissue specimens are not available for staining or rapid diagnostic tests, the clinician must rely on the clinical presentation based on history, physical examination, and nonspecific laboratory tests. Routine laboratory tests are not definitive, but may support or argue against the diagnosis. Nonspecific laboratory abnormalities may also suggest an otherwise unexpected diagnosis; e.g., the finding of atypical lymphocytes in the automated differential white blood cell count of the complete blood cell count with acute febrile illness in a returned traveler, with or without localizing signs, should suggest malaria and prompt the request for malarial smears. Nonspecific laboratory abnormalities, if consistent with the working diagnosis, may add additional support to the diagnosis being entertained. Conversely, the absence of a nonspecific laboratory abnormality that is characteristic of the diagnosis may make the infectious disease being considered a lesser diagnostic possibility. Some laboratory abnormalities are so characteristic that the absence of such abnormalities should lead the clinician to question the diagnosis or consider an alternate diagnosis; e.g., acute viral hepatitis accompanied by leukocytosis argues strongly against this diagnosis. The clinician should use routine laboratory tests as part of the diagnostic process in evaluating the presenting syndrome complex. Nonspecific laboratory tests may be useful in differentiating infectious disease from noninfectious diseases considered in the differential diagnosis. Nonspecific laboratory tests are rarely diagnostic themselves, and should always be interpreted in the clinical context. Isolated routine laboratory findings have an extensive differential diagnosis and should not be considered in a vacuum but rather evaluated in the clinical context. For example, hypophosphatemia in a patient without fever or pneumonia has little diagnostic significance in infectious disease, but otherwise unexplained hypophosphatemia in a patient with community-acquired pneumonia should suggest the possibility of Legionnaires' disease (1–10).

Not only should nonspecific laboratory abnormalities be considered in the appropriate clinical context, but the degree of the abnormality also confers diagnostic specificity. Many infectious diseases are associated with lymphocytosis, but greater than 60% lymphocytosis is usually limited to pertussis. Using atypical lymphocytes as an example, the absence of atypical lymphocytes in diseases or infections with which they are regularly associated, should prompt the clinician to question the diagnosis, e.g., malaria. If atypical lymphocytes are present in the peripheral smear, as in malaria, this has a different diagnostic significance than if there is atypical lymphocytosis. The diagnosis of atypical lymphocytosis depends on the relative percentage of atypical lymphocytes in the peripheral smear. Atypical lymphocytes should not be confused with abnormal lymphocytes, which are a sign of hematologic malignancy. Atypical lympho-cytes have a varied morphology whereas the morphology of abnormal lymphocytes is monotonous and unvarying. In terms of differential diagnosis, there is considerable difference between 5% or fewer atypical lymphocytes in the peripheral smear versus 20% or greater atypical lymphocytosis. Several infectious and noninfectious disease entities may be associated with few atypical lymphocytes in the peripheral smear. However, only usually Epstein-Barr virus (EBV) and cytomegalovirus (CMV) are associated with atypical lymphocytosis of 20% or more in the peripheral smear.

Clinicians should remember that laboratory abnormalities are snapshots of a dynamic process induced by the patient's illness. The trend of laboratory abnormalities from the normal to the abnormal range, or from the abnormal to the normal range, should also be considered. Clinicians should be particularly careful of near-normal values, i.e., either slightly abnormal or normal, but nearly abnormal values that may be more significant than initially appreciated. Serial testing may be helpful to determine whether test values were or soon will become abnormal. Laboratory abnormalities are usually printed on computerized forms indicating normal and abnormal values. Clinicians should carefully consider the abnormal potential of normal values that are close to the limits of normality. If the laboratory test is within the normal zone but increasing, subsequent testing may reveal this trend. Conversely, if values were borderline abnormal and the laboratory test has just returned to within the normal range, the patient may indeed have had significant abnormality before the previous test (1,11).

In summary, the clinician should be familiar with the characteristic laboratory abnormalities associated with key infectious disease entities, and their noninfectious counterparts in the differential diagnosis. Nonspecific laboratory abnormalities may serve as diagnostic clues in the process of evaluating the patient's clinical syndrome. Routine laboratory tests may be viewed as supporting or arguing against a particular diagnosis. The absence of characteristic laboratory abnormalities with certain infectious diseases should alert the clinician to consider an alternate diagnosis. Not only is the presence or absence of an abnormality important in selected infectious diseases, but the degree of the abnormality has additional diagnostic significance. Nonspecific laboratory abnormalities are unhelpful in many infectious diseases, but may be very helpful in selected infectious diseases. Nonspecific laboratory abnormalities are also useful in differentiating noninfectious disease disorders that mimic infectious diseases. Diagnostically, the key point is not to interpret laboratory abnormalities as isolated features but rather to evaluate their significance in the context of a clinical syndrome presentation. In this way, nonspecific laboratory abnormalities can increase diagnostic specificity. Laboratory abnormalities limited to relatively few possibilities, or those that are characteristic of various infectious disease disorders, are the most helpful diagnostically. The clinician should pay particular attention to uncommon findings, and combine nonspecific laboratory abnormalities to other specific clinical findings to increase diagnostic specificity (11).

NONSPECIFIC HEMATOLOGIC ABNORMALITIES

Leukocytosis

Leukocytosis is a nonspecific finding and is related to the demargination of white blood cells (WBCs) in blood vessels, which is influenced by many factors, including catecholamine release. Many acute noninfectious disease disorders are associated with leukocytosis. The degree of a left shift in a patient with leukocytosis is reflective of the degree of demargination of minute WBCs secondary to infections or non-infections to which the host is being subjected. This means that leukocytosis has very limited significance in infectious disease except in a negative sense; e.g., infectious diseases usually associated with leukopenia should be questioned if leukocytosis is present (typhoid fever). Otherwise, leukocytosis does not differentiate between inflammation (a noninfectious disease disorder) and infection, which greatly limits its diagnostic utility (4,12,13).

Leukopenia

Leukopenia is more specific than leukocytosis because fewer infectious and noninfectious disease entities are associated with leukopenia than leukocytosis. Leukopenia is characteristic of viral hepatitis and typhoid fever. Leukopenia is characteristic of a variety of viral infections, e.g., viral hepatitis, EBV, CMV, viral influenza, etc. Leukopenia may also be a feature of drug therapy, SLE, pre-leukemias, pernicious anemia, Felty's syndrome, Gaucher's disease, cyclic neutropenia, or may occur as the result of splenomegaly. Leukopenia is most useful diagnostically if it is not present in infectious diseases where leukopenia is characteristic, e.g., viral hepatitis, typhoid fever, etc. (8–10,13).

Lymphocytosis

Lymphocytosis is a nonspecific finding that is common during the convalescent period of many acute infectious diseases. Lymphocytosis is characteristic of tuberculosis, EBV, CMV, etc. Noninfectious diseases associated with lymphocytosis include rheumatoid arthritis, vasculitis, Hashimoto's thyroiditis, myxedema, hypopituitarism, and adrenal insufficiency. Lymphocytosis may accompany phenytoin therapy, PAS, or serum sickness. As with other laboratory abnormalities, the degree of lymphocytosis has diagnostic significance. Lymphocytosis of greater than 60% is characteristic of pertussis. Abnormal lymphocytosis is characterized by a monotonous and unvarying morphology, and is present in patients with lymphomas or lymphocytic leukemias (5,12,14).

Lymphopenia

Because fewer disorders are associated with lymphopenia, lymphopenia has more diagnostic specificity than lymphocytosis. Infectious diseases characterized by lymphopenia include human immunodeficiency virus (HIV) infection, tuberculosis, typhoid fever, malaria, and brucellosis. Noninfectious diseases associated with lymphopenia include cytotoxic drugs, alcohol, steroids, and radiation therapy. Other disorders, such as sarcoidosis, SLE, and rheumatoid arthritis, are also characterized by lymphopenia. Lymphopenia is a feature of Wiskott-Aldrich syndrome, ataxia-telangiectasia, Whipple's disease, severe combined immunodeficiency, cardiovascular immunodeficiency, CD_4 lymphocytopenia/CD_4 cytopenia syndrome, DiGeorge's syndrome, Anzelof's syndrome, or intestinal lymphangiectasia (7,10,15).

Monocytosis

Monocytosis is often associated with tuberculosis, SBE, Rocky Mountain spotted fever, diphtheria, histoplasmosis, brucellosis, kala-azar, and African trypanosomiasis. Monocytosis frequently follows recovery from a wide variety of infectious diseases and therefore is of limited diagnostic usefulness. Noninfectious diseases associated with monocytosis include myeloproliferative

disorders, lymphomas, Gaucher's disease, inflammatory bowel disease, and celiac disease. Rheumatoid arthritis, SLE, periarteritis nodosa, temporal arteritis, and sarcoidosis commonly have monocytosis as part of their hematologic profile. Monocytosis is a common occurrence after splenectomy (1,16).

Atypical Lymphocytosis

Atypical lymphocytosis is an important nonspecific diagnostic finding that has important exclusionary or inclusionary diagnostic significance. Atypical lymphocytes are not uncommon in the differential WBC count in drug fever among noninfectious disorders. Atypical lymphocytes, either present in the peripheral smear or sufficiently increased to result in atypical lymphocytosis, are characteristic of selected viral and parasitic infections. Some, but not all, viral infections are associated with atypical lymphocytes in the peripheral smear, but atypical lymphocytes are typically present with mumps, measles, rubella, and viral hepatitis. The degree of atypical lymphocytosis is useful if the differential diagnosis involves viruses. Although most viral infections are not accompanied by an atypical lymphocytic response, atypical lymphocytosis is characteristic of EBV, CMV, and human herpesvirus-6 (HHV-6). Among parasitic infections, atypical lymphocytes are commonly present in malaria, toxoplasmosis, and babesiosis. Atypical lymphocytes, not necessarily atypical lymphocytosis, are a regular feature of malaria, and the diagnosis should be questioned if atypical lymphocytes are not present in the peripheral smear in a patient with suspected acute malaria. An atypical lymphocytosis of less than 5% typically occurs with toxoplasmosis, drug fever, babesiosis, and malaria. A lymphocytosis between 5% and 10% would be characteristic of viral-induced atypical lymphocytosis, but atypical lymphocytosis of 20% or greater should suggest EBV or CMV, or HHV-6 (10,17,18).

Eosinophilia

Eosinophilia has wide differential diagnostic implications limiting its diagnostic usefulness. The degree of eosinophilia increases the diagnostic specificity of the eosinophilic response in peripheral blood. Eosinophilia usually accompanies the acute tissue migration phase of a wide variety of parasites. Gastrointestinal parasites associated with eosinophilia are usually located in the proximal gastrointestinal tract with the notable exception of giardiasis. Protozoa, in general, do not elicit an eosinophilic response with the notable exception of *Isospora belli*, where eosinophilia is characteristic. Noninfectious disorders associated with eosinophilia include drug reactions, allergic/rheumatic diseases, lymphomas, leukemias, malignancies, and myeloproliferative disorders. Other disorders frequently associated with eosinophilia include sarcoidosis, inflammatory bowel disease, Wiskott-Aldrich syndrome, IgA deficiency, hyper-IgE syndrome, and Sweet's syndrome. Eosinopenia is associated with steroid excess. Paradoxical eosinophilia following steroid therapy should suggest the possibility of SLE (19,22).

Basophilia

Basophilia is an uncommon but important diagnostic finding because the differential diagnosis of basophilia is limited. Basophilia usually suggests a noninfectious disorder, such as preleukemias, acute leukemias, lymphomas, malignancies, or myeloproliferative disorders. The infectious disease disorders associated with basophilia include chicken pox and smallpox (8–10).

Red Blood Cell Abnormalities

Schistocytes indicate a micro-enteropathic hemolytic anemia and are associated with a variety of noninfectious disorders, particularly disseminated intravascular coagulation (DIC). Schistocytes are present with DIC whether caused by a noninfectious disorder, e.g., malignancy, or an infectious basis, e.g., meningococcemia with DIC. Spherocytes are characteristic of gas gangrene but may also be found in various other disorders including autoimmune hemolytic anemias, cirrhosis, transfusion reactions, and severe burns. Howell-Jolly bodies are an indicator of impaired splenic function. Howell-Jolly bodies may be found in patients with otherwise unexplained severe pneumococcal pneumonia or fulminant pneumococcal sepsis (7,12,13).

Erythrophagocytosis

Erythrophagocytosis, e.g., the ingestion of red blood cells by phagocytic WBCs may be seen in a wide variety of infectious diseases. Erythrophagocytosis may occur in association with SBE, typhoid fever, syphilis, Listeria, leishmaniasis, histoplasmosis, toxoplasmosis, malaria, babesiosis, parvovirus B-19 infections, EBV, CMV, herpes simplex virus, leprosy, tuberculosis, brucellosis, Q fever, *Penicillium marneffii*, and HIV. Malignancies and myeloproliferative disorders are the most common causes of noninfectious-associated erythrophagocytosis (10,13,23).

Thrombocytopenia

Thrombocytopenia may be approached diagnostically as acute or chronic. Chronic thrombocytopenia suggests a noninfectious cause. Possibilities include fat emboli syndrome, thrombotic thrombocytopenic purpura, idiopathic thrombocytopenic purpura, hemolytic-uremic syndrome, acute leukemias, lymphomas, carcinomas, multiple myeloma, myeloproliferative disorders, Gaucher's disease, cirrhosis, and SLE, or may be drug-induced. The most common cause of hospital-acquired thrombocytopenia is drugs. Acute thrombocytopenia may accompany a variety of infectious disorders, including sepsis. Thrombocytopenia associated with sepsis is acute and short-lived, because the process rapidly improves or worsens, but does not persist for days. Thrombocytopenia accompanies a variety of viral infections including measles, rubella, dengue, the hemorrhagic fevers, EBV, CMV, varicella, mumps, and HIV. Thrombocytopenia is also characteristic of toxic shock syndrome, trypanosomiasis, malaria, ehrlichiosis, typhus, and Rocky Mountain spotted fever (10,12,24).

Thrombocytosis

Thrombocytosis also may be viewed as acute and chronic from a diagnostic perspective. Acute thrombocytosis suggests hemorrhage or Kawasaki's disease. Chronic thrombocytosis is associated with a variety of chronic disorders including myeloproliferative disorders, cirrhosis, or malignancies. Thrombocytosis may occur with chronic inflammatory disorders, including rheumatoid arthritis, Wegener's granulomatosis, vasculitis, temporal arteritis, and periarteritis nodosa. Thrombocytosis may occur after splenectomy (13,24).

Pancytopenia

Pancytopenia may be a feature of miliary tuberculosis, brucellosis, histoplasmosis, hepatitis B virus, or HIV. Noninfectious causes of pancytopenia include myeloproliferative disorders, malignancies with bone marrow invasion, Chédiak-Higashi syndrome, megaloblastic anemias, Gaucher's disease, hypersplenism, sarcoidosis, SLE, paroxysmal nocturnal hemoglobinuria, as well as leukemias and lymphomas. Pancytopenia may be drug-induced, e.g., chloramphenicol (12,13,25).

Erythrocyte Sedimentation Rate

The erythrocyte sedimentation rate (ESR) is a very sensitive, but nonspecific, test. Its diagnostic usefulness is enhanced if ESRs are very fast, i.e., very highly elevated, and it is combined with other findings in the appropriate clinical context. The ESR may be elevated acutely in both infectious and inflammatory diseases. The degree of ESR elevation may be helpful in differentiating lower from upper abdominal infectious diseases. In upper abdominal infections, e.g., gastritis, cholecystitis, duodenitis, etc., the ESR is usually moderately elevated, e.g., 20 to 40 mm/hour, but the ESR is usually more highly elevated, e.g., greater than 40 to less than 100 mm/hour in lower abdominal infectious conditions, e.g., appendicitis, diverticulitis, peritonitis, salpingitis, etc. The diagnostic specificity of the ESR is increased at the extremes of the ESR scale. ESRs approaching zero are characteristic of trichinosis or chronic fatigue syndrome (CFS). ESR may be applied clinically in patients with myositis because most causes of myositis are associated with an elevated ESR. A subnormal ESR approaching zero should suggest trichinosis as a diagnostic possibility. The ESR in CFS is also extremely low, approaching zero. Utilizing this point, if a patient is presumed to have CFS and the ESR is in the normal or elevated range, then an alternate diagnosis should be entertained. The ESR is also low in cachexia, severe anemia, massive hepatic necrosis, DIC, polycythemia vera, hypofibrinogenemia, and macroglobulinemia. If the ESR is very highly elevated, i.e., 100 mm/hour or higher, differential diagnostic possibilities are limited to relatively few entities. Among infectious diseases, an ESR of 100 mm/hr or higher should suggest SBE, osteomyelitis, or abscess. Noninfectious diseases associated with a very high ESR (100 mm/hour or higher) include rheumatic disorders, particularly collagen vascular diseases, polymyalgia rheumatica, giant cell arteritis, and vasculitis. Uremia and chronic renal failure will also increase the ESR. Malignancies and drug fevers are common causes of an ESR 100 mm/hour or higher. The ESR may be normal in disorders usually associated with an elevated ESR, e.g., malignancy, and if not elevated, has no diagnostic usefulness. The great value of the ESR is that it is elevated before other tests are diagnostic, e.g., occult malignancies.

An otherwise unexplained elevation of the ESR should prompt further appropriate diagnostic testing to determine the cause of the abnormality. The ESR is not helpful in differentiating cholangitis from cholecystitis, but may be useful in differentiating pancreatic abscess from pancreatic pseudocyst, or acute pancreatitis. The ESR will not help differentiate left atrial myxoma from endocarditis, but may be helpful in differentiating benign gammopathy of the elderly from myeloma. The clinician should use the degree of elevation of the ESR in conjunction with the clinical presentation for maximum diagnostic utility. The ESR should not be used to differentiate disorders with similar ranges of ESR elevation, e.g., rheumatoid arthritis versus SLE or left atrial myxoma from endocarditis, pulmonary tuberculosis from bronchogenic carcinoma. The ESR is most useful, if elevated, in differentiating dissimilar disorders,

TABLE 15.1. Erythrocyte Sedimentation Rate in Differential Diagnosis

Diagnostic problem	≥50 mm/hr	≤50 mm/hr
Cholangitis	+	
vs		
Cholecystitis		+
vs		
Pelvic inflammatory disease	+	
vs		
Ovarian cyst		+
vs		
Appendicitis	+	
vs		
Cholecystitis		+
vs		
Cystitis		+
vs		
Pyelonephritis	+	
vs		
Streptococcal pharyngitis		+
vs		
Infectious mononucleosis pharyngitis	+	
vs		
Trichinosis		+
vs		
Polymyositis	+	
vs		
Rheumatoid arthritis	+	
vs		
Osteoarthritis		+
vs		
Carcinoma	+	
vs		
Cachexia		+
vs		
Myeloma	+	
vs		
Benign monoclonal gammopathy		+
vs		
Malignant gastric ulcer	+	
vs		
Benign gastric ulcer		+
vs		
Angina		+
vs		
Myocardial infarction	+	
vs		
Synovitis		+
vs		
Septic arthritis (hip)	+	
vs		
Loose hip/knee prosthesis		+
vs		
Infected hip/knee prosthesis	+	

TABLE 15.2. Causes of an Extremely High Erythrocyte Sedimentation Rate (>100 mm/hr)

Infectious diseases
    Subacute bacterial endocarditis
    Abscesses
    Osteomyelitis
Collagen vascular disease
    Polymyalgia rheumatica/giant cell arteritis
    Rheumatoid arthritis
    Systemic lupus erythematosus
Malignancies
    Multiple myeloma
    Leukemias
    Lymphomas
    Carcinomas
Miscellaneous
    Drug hypersensitivity reactions (drug fevers)

gamma globulin fraction. Polyclonal gammopathy is associated with cirrhosis, SLE, chronic active/immune hepatitis, sarcoidosis, atrial myxoma, angioimmunoblastic lymphadenopathy with dysproteinemia, Takayasu's arteritis, and lymphomas among the noninfectious disorders. Polyclonal gammopathy is characteristic of HIV, African trypanosomiasis, kala-azar, and non-acute malaria (1,10,20,21).

Cold Agglutinins

Cold agglutinins are present in a variety of noninfectious disorders, including lymphomas, chronic lymphatic and myelogenous leukemia, multiple myeloma, Waldenström's macroglobulinemia, and cold agglutinin disease. The classical infectious disease associated with elevated cold agglutinins is *Mycoplasma pneumoniae*. Cold agglutinins have been reported with several infectious agents including EBV, CMV, mumps, syphilis, malaria, listeria, and SBE. Cold agglutinins may be elevated in a low titer in the infectious and noninfectious diseases mentioned, however high elevations of cold agglutinin titers are usually only associated with cold agglutinin disease among the noninfectious disorders, and *M. pneumoniae* among the infectious disorders. If a patient has a community-acquired pneumonia and a cold agglutinin titer of ≥1:64, it is most likely that the cold agglutinins are mycoplasmal in origin. Although cold agglutinins are not present in all patients with *M. pneumoniae* pneumonia, when they are elevated in high titer, they have the greatest diagnostic significance. Conversely, in a patient with community-acquired pneumonia, a cold agglutinin titer of 1:16 would not be diagnostic of *M. pneumoniae* and serial cold agglutinin determinations are necessary to determine the extent of the cold agglutinin titer rise. Alternately, a moderately elevated cold agglutinin titer in a patient with community-acquired pneumonia would argue strongly against other typical and atypical organisms as the etiology of the patient's community-acquired pneumonia (4,10,14).

NON-HEMATOLOGIC LABORATORY TESTS

Alkaline Phosphatase

Most disorders that increase the serum alkaline phosphatase concentration also increase the serum transaminase concentrations but differ in the relative proportion of each enzyme elevation. High levels of alkaline phosphatase, when not derived from bone, suggest biliary tract obstruction. Liver abscess is the

or those with different ESR elevations (7,10,26) (Tables 15.1 and 15.2).

Serum Protein Electrophoresis

Serum protein electrophoresis (SPEP) is most frequently utilized to identify monoclonal gammopathies, which range from benign monoclonal gammopathy in the elderly to multiple myeloma or Waldenström's macroglobulinemia. From the infectious disease perspective, the SPEP is most useful when polyclonal gammopathy is present. Polyclonal gammopathy occurs when there is B-lymphocyte hyperreactivity combined with impaired T-lymphocyte function, expressed as a polyclonal increase in the main cause of an isolated moderate-to-high increase in serum alkaline phosphatase concentration. Noninfectious diseases presenting with similar elevations of alkaline phosphatase include postnecrotic cirrhosis, Paget's disease, osteogenic sarcoma, posthepatic obstruction, and primary biliary cirrhosis. Mild elevations of the alkaline phosphatase concentration may occur with a variety of infectious diseases that are more commonly associated with increases in the serum transaminases, e.g., Legionnaires' disease, viral hepatitis, EBV, CMV, Q fever, secondary or tertiary syphilis involving the liver, toxic shock syndrome, hepatosplenic candidiasis, or clonorchiasis. There are many noninfectious disorders associated with mild elevations of the alkaline phosphatase that are often involved in infectious disease differential diagnosis, including cirrhosis, alcoholic hepatitis, hepatoma, hyperthyroidism, hyperparathyroidism, and ulcerative colitis. Uncommonly, an isolated elevation of the alkaline phosphatase may be a normal variant in elderly patients without an underlying pathologic condition (8,10).

Serum Transaminases

Elevation of the serum glutamic-oxaloacetic transaminase (SGOT) is reflective of hepatocellular liver involvement due to a variety of infectious and noninfectious agents affecting the liver. Because the liver receives the portal blood supply and is an important component of the reticular endothelial system, it is not surprising that many infectious diseases have liver involvement and are accompanied by increased serum transaminases. Among the atypical pneumonias, Legionnaires' disease, psittacosis, and Q fever are frequently associated with mild elevations of the serum transaminases. Early anicteric viral hepatitis also is associated with mild elevations of the serum transaminases. Other viruses that affect the liver include EBV, HHV-6, CMV, and adenovirus, and regularly cause serum transaminase elevations. Brucellosis, ehrlichiosis, Rocky Mountain spotted fever, malaria, shigellosis, toxic shock syndrome, and relapsing fever may also be accompanied by mild elevations of the serum transaminases. Myocardial, cerebral, or pulmonary infarcts are among the noninfectious causes of serum transaminase elevations. Intrahepatic cholestasis, pancreatitis, and ulcerative colitis may also be accompanied by mild increases in the SGOT. High elevations of the serum transaminases, i.e., 1,000 IU or greater, should suggest viral hepatitis, yellow fever, or one of the arboviral hemorrhagic fevers. The only noninfectious disorder associated with such high elevations of the serum transaminases is shock liver (2,8,10).

Serum Bilirubin

Increases in serum bilirubin are commonly associated with noninfectious disorders including hemolysis, Gilbert's syndrome, alcoholic hepatitis, and choledocholithiasis. Obstructive pancreatic or biliary carcinomas may also result in increased bilirubin levels. Among infectious diseases, gonococcemia, Legionnaires' disease, and pneumococcal bacteremia may be associated with mild increases in the total bilirubin. EBV, CMV, and liver abscess, depending upon the severity of infection and degree of biliary obstruction, may be associated with increases in the serum bilirubin.

Lactate Dehydrogenase

The enzyme lactate dehydrogenase (LDH) is present in red blood cells (RBCs) in high concentration; RBCs contain seven times more LDH than any other cell. Increased LDH in the serum may be caused by any process, infectious or noninfectious, related to hemolysis. Such disorders range from immune hemolytic anemia to "Waring Blender syndrome" associated with prosthetic valves. The serum LDH is increased in megaloblastic anemias, as well as pulmonary, myocardial, or renal infarction. LDH is also increased in hepatitis and other forms of liver injury. Malignancies may also be associated with an increased LDH. From an infectious disease perspective, malaria, babesiosis, and *Pneumocystis carinii* pneumonia (PCP) are the infectious diseases usually associated with increases in the serum LDH. With babesiosis and malaria, LDH levels are proportional to the degree of RBC hemolysis. In compromised hosts with community-acquired pneumonia presenting with hypoxemia and bilateral perihilar interstitial infiltrates, a highly elevated LDH should suggest PCP versus CMV or other interstitial pulmonary pathogens (10,13).

IgM Rheumatoid Factors

IgM rheumatoid factors are produced in the liver, and any acute disorder associated with acute liver inflammation may result in increased levels of IgM rheumatoid factors. Such entities include acute liver disease, cirrhosis, Waldenström's macroglobulinemia, sarcoidosis, rheumatoid arthritis, SLE, and cryoglobulinemia. Increased IgM rheumatoid factors are common in SBE, tuberculosis, kala-azar, leprosy, secondary syphilis, and HIV. Viral infections involving the liver, e.g., viral hepatitis, EBV, and CMV are often accompanied by some degree of IgM rheumatoid factor elaboration (2,10) (Table 15.3).

Diagnostic Usefulness of Nonspecific Laboratory Tests

If characteristic of an infectious disease disorder, nonspecific laboratory tests may be used to support certain diagnostic possibilities. The absence of a characteristic finding in an infectious disease argues against the diagnosis and should suggest an alternate diagnosis, e.g., Rocky Mountain spotted fever is unlikely without thrombocytopenia. The degree of the abnormality present also has diagnostic specificity, e.g., mild elevations of LDH may occur in pneumonias, but very high elevations should suggest the possibility of PCP in the appropriate clinical setting. The significance of the laboratory abnormality or the normality of the diagnostic laboratory value can be of assistance in differential diagnosis if properly applied to the clinical syndrome, while a severe, rapidly progressive hemolytic anemia is not necessary to suspect or confirm the diagnosis of clostridial myonecrosis. This information would be useful in evaluating a patient with clostridial bacteremia. The absence of rapid hemolysis a postoperative patient with a wound infection and positive clostridial blood culture results, without hemolytic anemia, unlikely to have gas gangrene. Nonspecific laboratory abnormalities are most useful when the differential diagnosis is limited to a few infectious or noninfectious conditions.

Diagnostic specificity is increased, not only when the abnormality is characteristic of the infectious disease, but also when multiple abnormalities are present. For example, normal WBC count, hypocholesteremia, decreased cholinesterase levels, thrombocytopenia, and atypical lymphocytes in the peripheral smear in an acute febrile illness without localizing signs, in a recently returned traveler, should suggest the diagnosis of malaria, not typhoid fever (27). While not helpful in all cases, clinicians applying these principles to nonspecific laboratory findings in the differential diagnosis of infectious diseases can eliminate, and can increase or decrease the possibilities of diagnoses. In many

TABLE 15.3.   Diagnostic Utility of Laboratory Tests

Infectious disease	Typical laboratory abnormalities	Laboratory abnormalities arguing against the diagnosis	Associated features/comments
Legionnaires' disease	↑SGOT/SGPT Hypophosphatemia ↑CPK Leukocytosis Microscopic hematuria Myoglobinemia ↑Bilirubin ↑CRP	Normal SGOT/SGPT Thrombocytopenia ↑Cold agglutinins (>1:64) Leukopenia Normal serum phosphorous Normal CRP	Diagnosis by culture/specific *Legionella* serology
Tularemia	Normal WBC count Normal SGOT/SGPT Normal ESR	Leukopenia Leukocytosis ↑SGOT/SGPT ↑Cold agglutinins (>1:64) Hypophosphatemia	Diagnosis by specific *Francisella tularensis* serology
Q Fever	↑SGOT/SGPT Normal WBC count	Hypophosphatemia ↑Cold agglutinins (>1:64) Normal serum transaminases	Diagnosis by specific *Coxiella burnetii* serology
Mycoplasma pneumoniae pneumonia	↑Cold agglutinins (>1:64) Normal SGOT/SGPT	↑SGOT/SGPT Hypophosphatemia ↑CPK	Diagnosis by culture/specific IgM *Mycoplasma* serology
Psittacosis	↑SGOT/SGPT Normal WBC count	Leukopenia Leukocytosis Normal SGOT/SGPT ↑Cold agglutinins (>1:64) Hypophosphatemia	Diagnosis by specific *Chlamydia psittaci* serology
Acute HIV	Anemia Thrombocytopenia Leukopenia ↓ CD$_4$ count ↓ Albumin Polycolonal gammopathy (SPEP) ↑SGOT (r/o co-existing HBV/HCV infection) Pancyctopenia	Normal platelet count Leukocytosis ↓C$_3$ Atypical lymphocytes Eosinophilia (unrelated to drugs)	Diagnosis by HIV serology/viral load
EBV infectious mononucleosis	↑ESR ↑SGOT/SGPT ↑Atypical lymphocytes Thrombocytopenia Erythrophagocytosis (+) Direct Coombs test ↑Cold agglutinins ↑ANA ↑ IgM rheumatoid factors ↑ BFP VDRL/FTA-ABS Polyclonal gammopathy	Normal ESR Normal SGOT/SGPT No lymphocytosis Leukocytosis ↑ASO titer Eosinophilia	Diagnosis by ↑ IgM EBV VCA 30% of EBV infectious mononucleosis patients have pharynx colonized by group A streptococci Gram stain of pharynx shows minimal/no inflammatory response in EBV vs grp A streptococcal pharyngitis.
CMV infectious mononucleosis	↑ Cold agglutinins ↑ IgM rheumatoid factors ↑ BFP VDRL/FTA-ABS ↑ SGOT/SGPT Erythrophagocytosis ↑ Cryoglobulins Polyclonal gammopathy (SPEP)	Normal SGOT/SGPT ↑ IgM EBV VCA titers ↑ IgM HHV-6 titers Eosinophilia	Diagnosis by culture/↑ IgM CMV titers
HHV-6 infectious mononucleosis	↑ Cold agglutinins ↑ SGOT/SGPT Polyclonal gammopathy (SPEP) Erythrophagocytosis	Leukocytosis Normal SGOT/SGPT ↑ IgM EBV VCA titers ↑ IgM CMV titers	Diagnosis by culture/↑ IgM HHV-6 titers
Ehrlichiosis	Leukopenia Anemia Thrombocytopenia ↑ SGOT/SGPT ↑ ESR ↑ CPK ↑ Creatinine	Normal platelet count Leukocytosis Eosinophilia Normal SGOT/SGPT	Diagnosis by specific *Ehrlichia* serology morula in HGE > HME

(continued)

TABLE 15.3. (*continued*)

Infectious disease	Typical laboratory abnormalities	Laboratory abnormalities arguing against the diagnosis	Associated features/comments
Rocky Mountain spotted fever	Leukopenia Lymphocytosis Thrombocytopenia ↑ ESR Microscopic hematuria Monocytosis ↑ CPK ↑ SGOT/SGPT	Normal platelet count Leukocytosis Eosinophilia Normal SGOT/SGPT ↑IgM HME/HGE titers	Diagnosis by specific *Rickettsiae* serology
Leptospirosis	Normal WBC count Anemia ↑ ESR ↑ SGOT/SGPT Microscopic hematuria ↑ CPK Myoglobinuria	Leukopenia Leukocytosis Eosinophilia	Diagnosis by demonstrating *Leptospira* in blood cultures early in infection ↑ CPK not a feature of viral hepatitis
Brucellosis	Leukopenia Lymphocytosis Atypical lymphocytes Monocytosis ↑ SGOT/SGPT Anemia ↑ ESR	Leukocytosis Lymphopenia Eosinophilia Anemia	Diagnosis by specific *Brucella* serology
Toxoplasmosis	Erythrophagocytosis Atypical lymphocytosis	Thrombocytopenia Eosinophilia	Diagnosis by lymph node histology/↑IgM *Toxoplasma* serology
Miliary tuberculosis	↑ ESR Monocytosis Lymphopenia Pancytopenia Granulocytic leukemoid reaction	Leukopenia Eosinophilia	AF smear/culture of *M. tuberculosis* from liver or bone marrow biopsy
Leprosy	↑ IgM rheumatoid factors Hypocalcemia Anemia ↓ ESR ↓ Cholesterol BFP VDRL/FTA-ABS Erythrophagocytosis Polyclonal gammopathy (SPEP)	Leukopenia Thrombocytopenia Eosinophilia	Diagnosis by smear/culture of *Mycobacterium leprae* from tissue specimens
African trypanosomiasis	Polyclonal gammopathy (SPEP) ↑ ESR Monocytosis ↑ SGOT/SGPT ↑ LDH ↑ Indirect bilirubin Thrombocytopenia	Eosinophilia Normal platelet count Normal SGOT/SGPT	Trypanosomiasis in blood, lymph nodes, or bone marrow
Visceral leishmaniasis (kala-azar)	Leukopenia Thrombocytopenia Monocytosis Polyclonal gammopathy (SPEP) Hematuria ↑ ESR ↑ SGOT/SGPT Anemia (secondary to hypersplenism) Erythrophagocytosis ↑ IgM rheumatoid factors	Normal platelet count Leukocytosis Normal WBC count Eosinophilia Normal SGOT/SGPT	*Leishmania* bodies in blood, bone marrow, liver biopsy
Typhoid fever	Leukopenia ↓ ESR Anemia ↑ SGOT/SGPT Lymphopenia Erythrophagocytosis	↑ ESR Thrombocytopenia Leukocytosis (suggests intestinal perforation) Eosinophilia	Diagnosis by culture of *Salmonella typhi* in blood, rose spots, liver biopsy, bone marrow biopsy, feces, or urine
Typhus	Leukopenia Lymphocytosis Thrombocytopenia ↑ ESR Microscopic hematuria	Leukocytosis May occur late/2° to congestion Normal platelet count	Specific rickettsial serologic diagnosis

(*continued*)

TABLE 15.3.   (*continued*)

Infectious disease	Typical laboratory abnormalities	Laboratory abnormalities arguing against the diagnosis	Associated features/comments
Malaria	Thrombocytopenia Anemia ↑ LDH Atypical lymphocytes Leukopenia Monocytosis Erythrophagocytosis Polyclonal gammopathy (SPEP) ↑ Cold agglutinins ↑ SGOT/SGPT ↑ ESR ↑ BFP VDRL/FTA-ABS ↑ Bilirubin ↑ Reticulocyte count ↓ Cholinesterase levels	Leukocytosis Eosinophilia Normal platelet count No atypical lymphocytes Normal LDH Normal bilirubin	*Plasmodia* in peripheral smear diagnostic. Do not confuse with Cabot's rings, Heinz, or Pappenheimer bodies.
Babesiosis	Thrombocytopenia Anemia ↓ Haptoglobin ↑ LDH Atypical lymphocytes Leukopenia Monocytosis Erythrophagocytosis Polyclonal gammopathy (SPEP) ↑ Cold agglutinins ↑ SGOT/SGPT ↑ ESR ↑ BFP VDRL/FTA-ABS ↑ Indirect bilirubin ↑ Reticulocyte count Hemoglobinuria	Eosinophilia Lymphocytosis Normal LDH levels Normal reticulocyte count No atypical lymphocytes Normal platelet count RBC pigment deposits (hemozoin)	Babesia in peripheral smear Tetrads of merozoites rare, but diagnostic RBC pigment deposits present in malaria are absent in babesiosis.
Gas gangrene	Leukocytosis Thrombocytopenia ↑ LDH ↑ Bilirubin Spherocytosis Hemoglobinuria Myoglobinuria	No hemolytic anemia Leukopenia Normal LDH	Clinical diagnosis/*Clostridia* (without spores) in areas of myonecrosis
Toxic Shock Syndrome (TSS)	Leukocytosis ↑ Bilirubin ↑ SGOT/SGPT ↑ CPK ↑ BUN/creatinine Sterile pyuria Thrombocytopenia Hypophosphatemia Hypocalcemia ↑ PT/PTT	↓ ESR Normal platelet count Leukopenia Normal SGOT/SGPT	Culture of *Staphylococcus aureus* (TSS-1) strain from patient

ANA, antinuclear antibody; BFP, biologic false-positive; BUN, blood urea nitrogen; CMV, cytomegalovirus; CPK, creatine phosphokinase; CRP, C-reactive protein; EBV, Epstein-Barr virus; ESR, erythrocyte sedimentation rate; FTA-ABS, fluorescent treponemal antibody absorption; HBV, hepatitis B virus; HCV, hepatitis C virus; HE, hemoglobin electrophoresis; HGE, human granulocytic ehrlichiosis; HHV, human herpesvirus; HME, human monocytic ehrlichiosis; LDH, lactate dehydrogenase; PT/PTT, prothrombin time/partial thromboplastin time; SGOT, serum glutamic-oxaloacetic transaminase; SGPT, serum glutamic pyruvic transaminase; SPEP, serum protein electrophoresis; VDRL, Venereal Disease Research Laboratories.

situations, nonspecific laboratory abnormalities are diagnostic clues to the presence of a previously unconsidered infectious or noninfectious disease.

REFERENCES

1. Bakerman S. *Bakerman's ABCs of interpretive laboratory data*, 3rd ed. Myrtle Beach, NC: Interpretive Laboratory Data, 1994:1–543.
2. Dufour DR. *Clinical use of laboratory data*. Philadelphia: Williams & Wilkins, 1998:1–599.
3. Balows A, Hausler WJ Jr., Ohashi M, et al., eds. *Laboratory diagnosis of infectious diseases—principles and practice*, vols. I and II. New York: Springer-Verlag, 1988: 1–1101.
4. Henry JB. *Clinical diagnosis and management by laboratory methods*, 19th ed. Philadelphia: WB Saunders, 1996:1–1556.
5. Ravel R. *Clinical laboratory medicine*, 6th ed. New York: Mosby, 1995:1–724.
6. Sacher RS, McPherson RA, Campos JM. *Widmann's clinical interpretation of laboratory tests*, 11th ed. Philadelphia: FA Davis, 2000:1–1092.
7. Schlossberg D, Shulman JA. *Differential diagnosis of infectious diseases*. Baltimore: Williams & Wilkins, 1996:1–339.
8. Tietz NW, ed. *Clinical guide to laboratory tests*, 3d ed. Philadelphia: WB Saunders, 1995:1–1096.
9. Tilton RC, Balows A, Hohnadel DC, et al., eds. *Clinical laboratory medicine*. St. Louis, Mosby YearBook, 1992:1–1207.
10. Wallach J. *Interpretation of diagnostic tests*, 7th ed. Philadelphia: Lippincott Williams & Wilkins, 2000:1–1026.
11. Cunha BA. Diagnostic reasoning in medicine. *Winthrop-University Hospital Medical Journal* 1999;21:115–117.

12. Humes HD, ed. *Kelley's textbook of internal medicine*, 4th ed. Philadelphia: Lippincott Williams & Wilkins, 2000:1–3131.
13. Isselbacher KJ, Braunwald E, Wilson JDs, et al., eds. *Harrison's principles of internal medicine*, 13th ed. New York: McGraw-Hill 1994:1–2496.
14. Christie AB. *Infectious diseases: epidemiology and clinical practice*, vols. I and II, 4th ed. Edinburgh: Churchill Livingstone, 1987:1–1317.
15. Shafiq M, Cunha BA. Diagnostic significance of lymphopenia. *Infect Dis Pract* 1999;23:81–82.
16. Cunha BA. Monocytosis. *Infect Dis Pract* 1995;19:62.
17. Cunha BA. Atypical lymphocytosis. *Infect Dis Pract* 1995;19:25.
18. Rosenbaum GS, Johnson DH, Cunha BA. Atypical lymphocytosis in babesiosis. *Clin Infect Dis* 1995;18:203–204.
19. Cunha BA. Diagnostic significance of eosinophilia in HIV. *Infect Dis Pract* 1997;21:109–110.
20. Garcia LS. *Diagnostic medical parasitology*, 4th ed. Washington DC: ASM Press, 2001:1–1092.
21. Guerrant RL, Walker DH, Weller PF, eds. *Essentials of tropical infectious diseases*. New York: Churchill Livingstone, 2001:1–637.
22. Sullivan CL, Cunha BA. The significance of eosinophilia in infectious disease. *Hosp Physician* 1989;25:21–27.
23. Qadir MT, Cunha BA. Differential diagnosis of erythrophagocytosis. *Infect Dis Pract* 1997;21:21.
24. Cunha BA. The significance of thrombocytosis and thrombocytopenia in infectious disease. *Infect Dis Pract* 1995;19:68.
25. Conn RB, Borer WZ, Snyder JW, eds. *Current diagnosis 9.* Philadelphia: WB Saunders, 1997:1–1241.
26. Cunha BA. The diagnostic significance of erythrocyte sedimentation rate. *Intern Med* 1992;13:48–51.
27. Cunha BA. The diagnosis of imported malaria. *Arch Intern Med* 2001;161:1926–1928.

CHAPTER 16
Skin Testing

George S. Deepe, Jr.

HISTORY

Skin testing originated in 1890 when Robert Koch described the inflammatory response induced by tubercle bacilli that were injected into the skin of *Mycobacterium tuberculosis*–infected guinea pigs (1). In the following year, he discovered that injected culture medium from growing tubercle bacilli also evoked an inflammatory response. The active constituent was called *old tuberculin* (2). Because this material, when injected into infected guinea pigs, appeared to inhibit growth of *M. tuberculosis*, Koch advocated its use as specific therapy for tuberculosis. Extensive clinical trials failed to demonstrate efficacy; nevertheless, the substance was useful as a skin test reagent to detect exposure to *M. tuberculosis*. Widespread application of skin testing in clinical medicine became possible after the introduction of two techniques, intracutaneous and contact testing, by Mantoux (3) and von Pirquet (4), respectively. Indeed, von Pirquet (5) was the first to recognize a cutaneous tuberculin reaction as an allergic phenomenon, and he also termed the lack of tuberculin reactivity in children with active measles anergy.

That cutaneous reactivity was mediated by specific cells was demonstrated by Landsteiner and Chase (6), who successfully transferred contact sensitivity to naive animals using peritoneal exudate cells from sensitized ones. Shortly thereafter, Chase (7) transferred tuberculin reactivity to naive animals and similar studies were performed in humans (8). Since that time, skin testing has provided a powerful and simple technique for detecting past or recent infection with certain pathogenic microbes (Table 16.1), for assessing the integrity of cellular immune responses, and for evaluating immediate hypersensitivity to antibiotics. In general, however, skin testing with antigens prepared from pathogenic microbes is not useful as a diagnostic procedure because it does not distinguish active *disease* from remote sensitization.

MORPHOLOGY AND HISTOLOGY

The delayed cutaneous hypersensitivity response should be considered a dynamic process involving the ingress and egress of immunocompetent cells. Much of what is known about the morphologic features of cutaneous reactivity to protein antigens is derived from studies of tuberculin hypersensitivity. Presumably, the response to other antigens is similar, if not identical. In humans, the earliest macroscopic finding is erythema, which is evident by 12 hours after intradermal challenge. Induration develops within 24 hours and peaks by 48 to 72 hours. Histologically, the erythema results from vasodilation that is induced by various cytokines, principally vasoactive amines; induration is accompanied by a vigorous influx of mononuclear cells, into the perivascular areas initially and then into the dermis and subcutaneous (9–11). Only a few scattered polymorphonuclear leukocytes are evident. Immunohistological studies have demonstrated that both CD4+ and CD8+ T cells are present in lesions, at ratios of 2:1 to 5:1 (11,12). A sizable proportion of T cells contain surface markers that suggest an activated state (e.g., anti–interleukin-2 receptor [anti–IL-2], CD71, and CD38)(13).

Within 12 hours of challenge, the number of Langerhans' cells in the epidermis increases. Subsequently, these cells are observed in the dermis, suggesting that they emigrate from the area of inflammation to distant organs. Because Langerhans' cells can function as antigen-presenting cells, it is possible that they also transport antigen during migration (11).

A second type of response to foreign antigen was discovered by Jones and Mote (14,15). This cutaneous reaction is characterized by a softened induration with a large area of erythema. Microscopically, basophils are a prominent cell population in the Jones-Mote reaction (16).

IMMUNOLOGY OF CUTANEOUS REACTIVITY

The skin test stands as one of the major hallmarks of the cell-mediated immune system. Although it is a relatively simple test to perform, expression of a positive skin response requires a complex series of cellular interactions culminating in induration (Fig. 16.1). Studies of experimental models of infection have indicated that with few exceptions the principal T-cell subset involved in elaborating cutaneous reactivity is the CD4+ T cell (17–19). Those exceptions are viral infections. Cells that mediate delayed-type hypersensitivity (DTH) responses have been referred to as T_{DTH}. The presence of DTH often correlates with the capacity of T cells to exert a protective immune response; thus, it was generally believed that these two cell subsets were one and the same. However, evidence exists that T_{DTH} cells and T cells that mediate protection are distinct functional subpopulations (18,20,21). The capacity to propagate cloned T cells offered a way to assess whether a monoclonal population of cells could both express DTH and provide protection, but these studies have been hampered by the finding that cloned T cells are unable to traffic normally in hosts (17,22,23).

The biochemical, molecular, and cellular events that lead to expression of DTH are currently under intense investigation. After intradermal inoculation of antigen, it is ingested by accessory cells that include macrophages, dendritic cells, and Langerhans' cells. With few exceptions, CD4+ T cells recognize native

TABLE 16.1.   Skin Tests That Are Useful in Human Infectious Disease

Infectious disease	Microbe	Skin-test reagent	Source of reagent
Coccidioidomycosis	*Coccidioides immitis*	Coccidioidin	Culture filtrate of mycelial-phase organisms
		Spherulin	Autolysate of spherules
Histoplasmosis	*Histoplasma capsulatum*	Histoplasmin	Culture filtrate from mycelial-phase organisms
Leishmaniasis	*Leishmania braziliensis*	Leishmanin	Phenol-treated promastigotes suspended in saline at concentration of 1-2 x 10⁶ per mL
	Leishmania mexicana		
	Leishmania donovani		
	Leishmania major		
	Leishmania tropica		
Leprosy	*Mycobacterium leprae*	Lepromin	Extract of organisms obtained from armadillo liver or from nodules of patients with lepromatous leprosy (bacilli suspended at 1.6 x 10⁸ per mL)
		Dharmendra antigen	Formalin and ether extract of *M. leprae*
Paracoccidioidomycosis	*Paracoccidioides brasiliensis*	Paracoccidioidin	Culture filtrate from mycelial-phase organisms
Tuberculosis	*Mycobacterium tuberculosis*	Purified protein derivative	Purified culture filtrate of *M. tuberculosis*

antigen that has been degraded or "processed" into immunogenic peptides that become associated with class II major histocompatibility complex (MHC) molecules (24–30). T cells become activated, expand, and release a number of cytokines, including IL-2, IL-3, and IL-4, interferon-γ (IFN-γ), and colony-stimulating factors.

CD4⁺ T cells can be separated into two functionally distinct subsets, termed T_H1 and T_H2 cells. The division is based on the profile of cytokines secreted by each subset. T_H1 cells produce IL-2 and IFN-γ, whereas T_H2 cells release IL-4, IL-5, and IL-10 (31,32). Both subsets elaborate tumor necrosis factor-β and colony-stimulating factors. T_H1 cells have been identified as the cells that mediate DTH reactivity (31,32).

Anergy signifies the failure to mount a response to an antigen (5). Although this obviously happens in nonsensitized persons, there are numerous ways, at the cellular and molecular levels, to explain unresponsiveness in previously sensitized subjects (Table 16.2). In infectious disease states, the highest prevalence of anergy is among persons with progressive disseminated infections, but nonresponsiveness may be found in those with limited infections (33–36) (Table 16.3). Moreover, experimental models of infection have suggested a direct correlation between the presence of anergy and the burden of microorganisms or microbial antigens (31–40). The significance of this has yet to be explained.

PHARMACOLOGIC MODULATION OF SKIN-TEST REACTIVITY

Human studies concerning the modification of skin-test reactivity by pharmacologic agents are sparse. Corticosteroids, when given at dosages of more than 15 mg per day for 3 weeks, inhibit expression of tuberculin hypersensitivity in humans (41,42). The mechanism of the inhibition has not been defined precisely, but it is presumably alterations in the number of T cells and

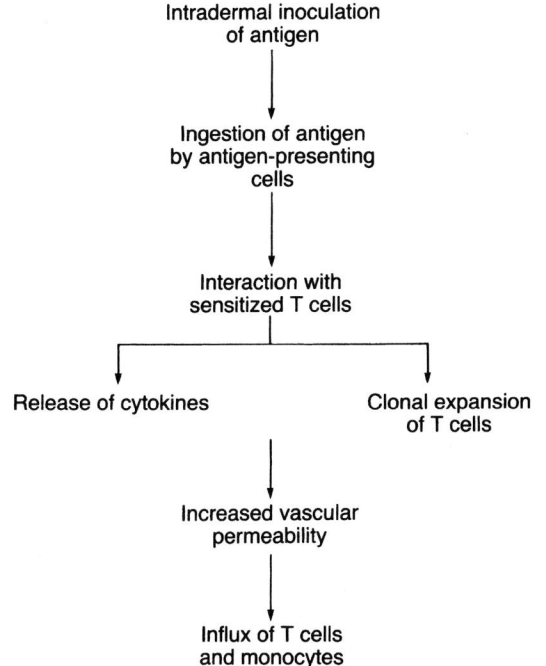

Figure 16.1. Schema for cellular events that lead to a positive skin-test result. After intradermal inoculation of antigen, the antigen is ingested by antigen-presenting cells and immunogenic peptides become bound to class II major histocompatibility complex molecules. Antigen-specific T cells (CD4⁺) recognize the bimolecular complex and become activated. Consequently, there is proliferation of T cells and release of cytokines. Vascular permeability is increased, and T cells and monocytes begin to infiltrate into the inflamed area.

TABLE 16.2.   Putative Cellular and Molecular Causes of Anergy in Infectious Diseases

Activation of suppressor T cells or suppressor macrophages
Production of suppressor factors
Defects in antigen presentation
Lack of antigen-reactive T cells
    Clonal deletion
    Human immunodeficiency virus–mediated destruction
    Pharmacological modulation
    Iatrogenic or idiopathic cytopenia
Defective cytokine production
Viral infections other than human immunodeficiency virus (e.g., measles)

TABLE 16.3.   Skin-test Anergy in Infectious Diseases

Microbe	Infectious disease state	Anergy to Specific Antigen[a] (%)
Coccidioides immitis	Acute pulmonary coccidioidomycosis	<10
	Chronic pulmonary coccidioidomycosis	30–75
	Disseminated coccidioidomycosis	30–70
Histoplasma capsulatum	Acute pulmonary histoplasmosis	<10
	Chronic pulmonary histoplasmosis	10–30
	Disseminated histoplasmosis	45–70
Leishmania tropica	Cutaneous leishmaniasis	<10
Leishmania major	Cutaneous leishmaniasis	<10
Leishmania mexicana	Cutaneous leishmaniasis	<10
	Diffuse cutaneous leishmaniasis	>90
Leishmania braziliensis	Cutaneous leishmaniasis	<10
	Mucocutaneous leishmaniasis	<10
Leishmania aethiopica	Diffuse cutaneous leishmaniasis	>90
Leishmania donovani	Visceral leishmaniasis	>90
Mycobacterium leprae	Tuberculoid leprosy	<20
	Borderline leprosy	40–100
	Lepromatous leprosy	>80
Mycobacterium tuberculosis	Pulmonary tuberculosis	10–20
	Disseminated tuberculosis	50–70
Paracoccidioides brasiliensis	Asymptomatic paracoccidioidomycosis	<10
	Progressive pulmonary paracoccidioidomycosis	30–55
	Disseminated paracoccidioidomycosis	>70

[a]Data from references 33–36, 50–62, 71, 83, 88, 93, 99, 112–122, with permission.

in biologic function. Short-term administration of large doses of methylprednisolone, on the other hand, does not render a subject anergic (43).

Prostaglandins can inhibit cellular immune responses *in vitro* (44). A single study has demonstrated that indomethacin, which irreversibly blocks prostaglandin synthesis, has improved skin-test responses in two patients with common variable immunodeficiency (45). This effect was not detected in normal hosts (46).

In experimental animals, the effects of various immunomodulators on DTH responses have been examined. Only a few are listed here. Amphotericin B can enhance contact sensitivity in mice, probably by inhibiting suppressor cell activity (47). Cyclophosphamide can also enhance DTH responses by the same mechanism (48). Other immunodepressants such as 6-mercaptopurine can cause depression of DTH (49), but in humans, it may be difficult to separate the effects of the drug and those of the underlying disease.

SKIN TESTS FOR SPECIFIC INFECTIOUS DISEASES

Mycobacterial Infections

TUBERCULOSIS

Two to four weeks after infection with *M. tuberculosis,* most immunocompetent persons mount a positive skin-test response to intermediate-strength (5 tuberculin units [TU]) purified protein derivative; this response mirrors the healing process exerted by cell-mediated immune mechanisms *in vivo*. Among persons with active pulmonary tuberculosis, up to 20% may manifest either antigen-specific anergy or a more generalized lack of reactivity to a battery of recall antigens (50–52). In disseminated tuberculosis, the incidence of anergy approaches 50% to 70%, especially in miliary disease and meningitis (53–60). Furthermore, the responsiveness to tuberculin may be diminished by immunosuppressive therapy or by certain underlying diseases such as chronic renal failure, hematologic disorders, and immun-

odeficiency syndromes (61–66). In normal hosts, cutaneous sensitivity usually recovers after weeks to months of antituberculous therapy. The cause of the immunoregulatory disturbance in those without known preexisting immunologic defects is incompletely understood. Studies *in vitro* have implicated circulating monocytes as mediators of antigen-specific suppression in anergic subjects who had pulmonary tuberculosis (67). Removal of these cells from peripheral mononuclear blood cells enhances responsiveness *in vitro* of T cells to tuberculin.

For clinical diagnosis and epidemiologic studies, the tuberculin skin test with 5 TU of purified protein derivative remains an important tool, although certain problems with this test are acknowledged. Because *M. tuberculosis* shares antigens with numerous nontuberculous mycobacteria, cross-reactivity may lead to a false-positive skin-test result. Moreover, persons vaccinated with bacille Calmette-Guérin may also show a positive tuberculin reaction. Another difficulty in construing the significance of a positive skin-test result arises with the so-called *booster phenomenon*. If reactivity to tuberculin in infected persons has waned over time, skin testing may produce either a small reaction or no reaction. Rechallenge, however, may prompt an amnestic response with an increase in the size of the tuberculin reaction (68). This problem is most often observed in situations of repeated testing in short periods and may lead to the false impression of conversion. The booster phenomenon may be overcome by retesting those with a response less than 10 mm within a week (69).

Exactly how long a skin-test result remains positive is not known. In general, it appears that tuberculin sensitivity is lifelong (70). As the population of many countries ages, the possibility of waning reactivity may become a significant clinical problem in elderly persons. Lack of hypersensitivity may be misinterpreted as indicating that tuberculosis cannot be the cause of a patient's illness.

LEPROSY

Both the clinical manifestations and the immunologic features of leprosy are spectral. Patients with the limited forms of infection, tuberculoid and borderline tuberculoid leprosy, exhibit a skin-test response to lepromin, a heat-killed suspension of bacilli prepared from infected armadillos or skin nodules of patients with lepromatous disease. At 48 to 72 hours after challenge, an area of induration becomes apparent (the Fernandez reaction). Subsequently, the response progresses to nodule formation and possibly ulceration (the Mitsuda reaction) during the 3 to 4 weeks after injection. Also, it is important to emphasize that many normal persons who have not been exposed to *Mycobacterium leprae* may manifest a reaction to lepromin. In contrast, untreated patients with borderline disease or lepromatous leprosy do not mount a response to lepromin; moreover, the anergy is frequently generalized (71). Responses to nonspecific antigens may be regained after antibiotic therapy in lepromatous patients, but unlike the situation with tuberculosis, the specific response to lepromin often remains negative (71).

The cutaneous reactivity to purified protein derivative of patients with untreated and treated lepromatous leprosy has been examined in detail. Fifty-eight percent of patients with lepromatous leprosy responded, and the percentage was higher in those treated longer than 18 months (72). The reaction was characterized by early onset of induration, which was maximal at 4 days and was observed for up to 21 days. T cells and circulating monocytes constituted the majority of cells in positive responders, and CD4$^+$ T cells were predominant. One interesting feature was the destruction of macrophages containing leprosy bacilli in areas of skin testing. This is reminiscent of Koch's original observation that skin testing with tuberculin reduced the number of tubercle bacilli in the skin of *M. tuberculosis*–infected guinea pigs.

Several reasons have been proposed to explain anergy in lepromatous leprosy, among them the existence of suppressor cells (73,74), defective production of cytokines (75,76), impaired expression of IL-2 receptors (77), and the presence of serum factors that depress cell-mediated immunity (78).

Fungal Infections

Useful skin-test reagents are available for *Candida, Histoplasma, Coccidioides,* and *Paracoccidioides.* The definition of a positive skin-test reaction in fungal diseases is a 5-mm area of induration (79). Approximately 50% to 90% of normal persons respond to *Candida* antigens as a result of colonization by this ubiquitous organism (80–82). Because such a large percentage of individuals demonstrate a positive response to the *Candida* antigen skin test, it is included in a battery of recall antigens to test for immunocompetence in an individual. This skin-test preparation is not useful in the detection of infection with *Candida* species.

It is presumed that between 90% and 100% of those who have convalesced from acute pulmonary histoplasmosis, coccidioidomycosis, or paracoccidioidomycosis manifest a positive skin-test reaction to the respective antigen (34,83). Cross-reactivity has been observed between histoplasmin and coccidioidin and between paracoccidioidin and histoplasmin. The time required for conversion to a positive skin-test result appears to be approximately 4 weeks (84,85). The persistence of a positive skin-test response to these fungal antigens in immunocompetent persons apparently is lifelong, although several studies have suggested that it may be short lived. Waning reactivity has been reported in persons residing in endemic areas (86,88). It has been argued that reversion of coccidioidin reactivity to negative suggests susceptibility to reactivation of infection (88).

In disseminated forms of histoplasmosis, coccidioidomycosis, paracoccidioidomycosis, and leishmaniasis, the percentage of positive responders drops to 30% to 50% (33,34,83,89). Anergy in histoplasmosis or coccidioidomycosis may have important prognostic value and may indicate progression of infection beyond the pulmonary system. In addition, the failure to detect a positive skin-test reaction in an ill patient may be misconstrued as an indication that the person is not infected with fungus. This incorrect assumption could lead to marked delay in diagnosis and treatment. Experimental evidence suggests that anergy in these diseases may be caused in part by suppressor cells (37,90,91) or deficient cytokine production (92).

Leishmaniasis

The vast majority of persons with cutaneous or mucocutaneous leishmaniasis manifest skin-test positivity to specific antigens (93,94). A positive skin-test response may provide indirect evidence of active infection but only in conjunction with the appropriate clinical findings. False-positive reactions may be seen in those exposed to nonpathogenic *Leishmania* species.

Skin-test responses to specific antigens are absent in a large proportion of persons with diffuse cutaneous leishmaniasis or visceral leishmaniasis (95–99). After treatment, most patients mount a skin-test response to antigen. One study of humans with diffuse cutaneous leishmaniasis has demonstrated that anergy is associated with a circulating population of adherent suppressor cells (35). Addition of indomethacin restored reactivity *in vitro* to *Leishmania* antigens by peripheral blood cells from infected patients (35). There are, however, no data to suggest that treatment with this pharmacologic agent *in vivo* restores cellular immune responses of such patients.

Studies of both humans and experimental animals infected with *Leishmania donovani* have described several mechanisms to account for the loss of DTH associated with visceral leishmaniasis: impaired production of IL-1 and IL-2 (100,101), generation of suppressor T cells and suppressor macrophages (102,103), and suppression of macrophage expression of class I and class II MHC molecules (104,105).

SKIN TESTING TO DETECT ANTIBIOTIC HYPERSENSITIVITY

Skin testing to assess antibiotic allergy is used to measure immediate (immunoglobulin E–mediated) hypersensitivity, but not DTH reactions (cell-mediated immune mechanisms). Among reactions to antibiotics, penicillin allergy has been studied most thoroughly, and it is the one antibiotic for which standard skin tests exist. Penicillin G forms antigenic determinants categorized as major and minor. The major determinant is benzylpenicilloyl, and some of the minor determinants are benzyl-D-penicilloate and benzyl-D-penicilloic acid (106). Testing with the major determinants detects many but not all patients at risk of anaphylaxis. The minor determinants, however, appear to be responsible for most of the severe immediate reactions to penicillin (107). Unfortunately, there is no adequate preparation of minor determinants. Some have used aged penicillin G, but studies have shown that this is not a reliable preparation for minor determinants (108).

The prevalence of a positive skin-test result is related to the time that has elapsed between clinical reaction and application of the skin test (108). A positive skin-test result is highly indicative of immediate hypersensitivity, and a negative skin-test result strongly suggests that no allergy exists (109). Approximately 1% to 2% of individuals who are skin-test negative for penicillin react to systemic administration of this antibiotic (108–111). In such cases, the symptoms are usually mild and develop several days after initiation of therapy; none of the reactions has been life threatening. Skin testing is, therefore, exceptionally safe, and only mild reactions have been noted in studies of several thousand subjects (109). The utility of testing with other antibiotics remains to be determined because of a lack of uniform preparations for skin testing.

REFERENCES

1. Koch R. Weitere mitteilung über ein heilmittel gegen tuberkulose. *Dtsch Med Wochenschr* 1890;16:1029.
2. Koch R. Weitere mitteilung über das tuberkulin. *Dtsch Med Wochenschr* 1891;17:1189.
3. Mantoux C. Uintradermal reaction a la tuberculine et son interpretation clinique. *Presse Med* 1910;18:10.
4. von Pirquet C. Quantitative experiments with cutaneous tuberculin reaction. *J Pharmacol Exp Ther* 1909;1:151.
5. von Pirquet C. Das verhalten der kutanen tuberkulinreaktion während der Maseru. *Dtsch Med Wochenschr* 1908;34:1297.
6. Landsteiner K, Chase MW. Experiments on transfer of cutaneous sensitivity to simple compounds. *Proc Soc Exp Biol Med* 1942;49:688.
7. Chase MW. The cellular transfer of cutaneous hypersensitivity to tuberculin. *Proc Soc Exp Biol Med* 1945;59:134.
8. Lawrence HS. The cellular transfer of cutaneous hypersensitivity to tuberculin in man. *Proc Soc Exp Biol Med* 1949;71:516.
9. Bosnan C, Feldman JD. Composition, morphology, and source of cells in delayed skin reactions. *Am J Pathol* 1970;58:201.
10. Dvorak HF, Mihm MC Jr, Dvorak AC, et al. Morphology of delayed-type hypersensitivity reactions in man, I: quantitative description of the inflammatory response. *Lab Invest* 1974;31:111.
11. Poulter LW, Seymour GJ, Duke O, et al. Immunohistological analysis of delayed-type hypersensitivity in man. *Cell Immunol* 1982;74:358.
12. Platt JL, Grant BW, Eddy AA, et al. Immune cell populations in cutaneous delayed-type hypersensitivity. *J Exp Med* 1983;158:1227.
13. Fullmer MA, Shen JY, Modlin RL, et al. Immunohistological evidence of lymphokine production and lymphocyte activation antigens in tuberculin reactions. *Clin Exp Immunol* 1987;67:383.
14. Jones TD, Mote JR. The phases of foreign protein sensitization in human beings. *N Engl J Med* 1934;210:120.
15. Mote JR, Jones TD. The development of foreign protein sensitization in human beings. *J Immunol* 1936;30:149.
16. Richerson HB, Dvorak HF, Leskowitz S. Cutaneous basophil hypersensitivity, I: a new look at the Jones-Mote reaction, general characteristics. *J Exp Med* 1970;132:546.
17. Deepe GS Jr. Protective immunity in murine histoplasmosis: functional comparison of adoptively transferred T-cell clones and splenic T cells. *Infect Immun* 1988;56:2350.
18. Hussein S, Curtis J, Akuffo H, et al. Dissociation between delayed-type hypersensitivity and resistance to pathogenic mycobacteria demonstrated by T-cell clones. *Infect Immun* 1987;55:564.
19. Czuprynski CJ, Brown JF, Young KM, et al. Administration of purified anti-L3T4 monoclonal antibody impairs the resistance of mice to *Listeria monocytogenes* infection. *Infect Immun* 1989;57:100.
20. Murphy JW. Effects of first-order *Cryptococcus*-specific T suppressor cells on induction of cells responsible for delayed-type hypersensitivity. *Infect Immun* 1985;48:439.
21. Orme IM. Induction of nonspecific acquired resistance and delayed-type hypersensitivity, but not specific acquired resistance in mice inoculated with killed mycobacterial vaccines. *Infect Immun* 1988;56:3310.
22. Dailey MO, Fathman CG, Butcher EC, et al. Abnormal migration of T-lymphocyte clones. *J Immunol* 1982;128:2134.
23. Dailey MO, Gallatin WM, Weissman IL. The *in vivo* behavior of T-cell clones: altered migration due to loss of the lymphocyte homing receptor. *J Mol Cell Immunol* 1985;2:27.
24. Ziegler HK, Unanue ER. Identification of a macrophage antigen-processing event required for I region-restricted antigen presentation to T lymphocytes. *J Immunol* 1981;127:1869.
25. Unanue ER. Antigen presenting function of the macrophage. *Annu Rev Immunol* 1984;2:395.
26. Allen PM, Beller DI, Braun J, et al. The handling of *Listeria monocytogenes* by macrophages: the search for an immunogenic molecule in antigen presentation. *J Immunol* 1984;132:323.
27. Babbitt BP, Allen PM, Matseuda G, et al. Binding of immunogenic peptides to Ia histocompatibility molecules. *Nature* 1985;316:359.
28. Unanue ER, Allen PM. The basis for the immunoregulatory role of macrophages and other accessory cells. *Science* 1987;236:551.
29. Marrack P, Kappler J. The antigen-specific, major histocompatibility complex–restricted receptor on T cells. *Adv Immunol* 1986;38:1.
30. Marrack P, Kappler J. The T-cell receptor. *Science* 1987;238:1073.
31. Sher A, Coffman RL. Regulation of immunity to parasites by T cells and T-cell derived cytokines. *Annu Rev Immunol* 1992;10:385.
32. Fitch FW, McKisic MD, Lancki DW, et al. Differential regulation of murine T lymphocyte subsets. *Annu Rev Immunol* 1993;11:29.
33. Furculow MF. Comparison of treated and untreated severe histoplasmosis. *JAMA* 1963;183:823.
34. Drutz DJ, Catanzaro A. Coccidioidomycosis. *Am Rev Respir Dis* 1978;117:559.
35. Petersen EA, Neva FA, Oster CN, et al. Specific inhibition of lymphocyte-proliferation by adherent suppressor cells in diffuse cutaneous leishmaniasis. *N Engl J Med* 1982;306:387.
36. Turk JL, Bryceson ADM. Immunological phenomena in leprosy and related diseases. *Adv Immunol* 1971;13:209.
37. Nickerson DA, Havens RA, Bullock WE. Immunoregulation in disseminated histoplasmosis. *Cell Immunol* 1981;60:287.
38. Cox RA, Kennell W. Suppression of T-lymphocyte response by *Coccidioides immitis* antigen. *Infect Immun* 1988;56:1424.
39. Murphy JW, Moorhead JW. Regulation of cell-mediated immunity in cryptococcosis, I: induction of specific afferent suppressor cells by cryptococcal antigen. *J Immunol* 1982;128:276.
40. Fahey JR, Herman R. Relationship between delayed hypersensitivity response and acquired cell-mediated immunity in C57BL/6J mice infected with *Leishmania donovani*. *Infect Immun* 1985;49:447.
41. Bovornkitti S, Kangsadal P, Sathirapat P, et al. Reversion and reconversion rate of tuberculin skin reactions in correlation with the use of prednisone. *Dis Chest* 1960;38:51.
42. Schatz M, Patterson R, Kloner R. The prevalence of tuberculin positive skin tests in a steroid-treated asthmatic population. *Ann Intern Med* 1976;84:261.
43. Fan PT, Yu DTY, Clements PJ, et al. Effects of corticosteroids on the human immune response: comparison of one and three daily 1 gm intravenous pulses of methylprednisolone. *J Lab Clin Med* 1978;91:625.
44. Goodwin JS, Webb DR. Regulation of the immune response by prostaglandins. *Clin Immunol Immunopathol* 1980;15:106.
45. Goodwin JS, Bankhurst AD, Murphy SA, et al. Partial reversal of the cellular immune defect in common variable immunodeficiency with indomethacin. *J Clin Lab Immunol* 1978;1:197.
46. Goodwin JS, Selinger DS, Messner RP, et al. Effect of indomethacin *in vivo* on humoral and cellular immunity in humans. *Infect Immun* 1978;19:430.
47. Shirley SF, Little JR. Immunopotentiating effects of amphotericin B, I: enhanced contact sensitivity in mice. *J Immunol* 1979;123:2878.
48. Askenase PW, Hayden BJ, Gershon RK. Augmentation of delayed-type hypersensitivity by doses of cyclophosphamide which do not affect antibody responses. *J Exp Med* 1975;141:697.
49. Phillips SM, Zweiman B. Mechanisms of the suppression of delayed hypersensitivity in the guinea pig by 6-mercaptopurine. *J Exp Med* 1973;137:149.
50. McMurray DN, Echeverri A. Cell-mediated immunity in anergic patients with pulmonary tuberculosis. *Am Rev Respir Dis* 1978;118:827.
51. Nash D, Douglass JE. Anergy in active pulmonary tuberculosis. A comparison between positive and negative reactors and an evaluation of 5 TU and 250 TU skin test doses. *Chest* 1980;77:1.
52. Daniel TM, Oxtoby MJ, Pinto EM, et al. The immune spectrum in patients with pulmonary tuberculosis. *Am Rev Respir Dis* 1981;123:556.
53. Proudfoot AT, Akhtar AJ, Douglas AC, et al. Miliary tuberculosis in adults. *Br Med J* 1969;2:273.
54. Munt PW. Miliary tuberculosis in the chemotherapy era: with a clinical review in 69 American adults. *Medicine* 1971;51:139.
55. Sahn SA, Neff TA. Miliary tuberculosis. *Am J Med* 1974;56:495.
56. Grieco MH, Chmel H. Acute disseminated tuberculosis as a diagnostic problem. A clinical study based on twenty-eight cases. *Am Rev Respir Dis* 1974;109:554.
57. Barrett-Connor E. Tuberculous meningitis in adults. *South Med J* 1969;60:1061.
58. Haas EJ, Madhavan T, Quinn EL. Tuberculous meningitis in an urban general hospital. *Arch Intern Med* 1977;137:1518.
59. Klein NC, Damsker B, Hirschman SZ. Mycobacterial meningitis. Retrospective analysis from 1970 to 1983. *Am J Med* 1985;79:29.
60. Ogawa SK, Smith MA, Brennessel DJ, et al. Tuberculous meningitis in an urban medical center. *Medicine (Baltimore)* 1987;66:317.
61. Andrew OT, Schoenfeld PY, Hopewell PC. Tuberculosis in patients with end-stage renal disease. *Am J Med* 1980;68:59.
62. Rutsky EA, Rostand SG. Mycobacteriosis in patients with chronic renal failure. *Arch Intern Med* 1980;140:57.
63. Navari RM, Sullivan KM, Springmeyer SC, et al. Mycobacterial infection in marrow transplant patients. *Transplantation* 1983;36:509.
64. Kaplan MH, Armstrong D, Rosen P. Tuberculosis complicating neoplastic disease. A review of 201 cases. *Cancer* 1974;33:850.
65. Pitchenik AE, Cole C, Russell BW, et al. Tuberculosis, atypical mycobacteriosis, and the acquired immunodeficiency syndrome among Haitian and non-Haitian patients in south Florida. *Ann Intern Med* 1984;101:641.
66. Centers for Disease Control and Prevention. Tuberculosis and human immunodeficiency virus infection: recommendations of the Advisory Committee for the Elimination of Tuberculosis (ACET). *MMWR Morb Mortal Wkly Rep* 1989;38:236.
67. Ellner JJ. Suppressor adherent cells in human tuberculosis. *J Immunol* 1978;121:2573.
68. Narain R, Nair SS, Rao GR, et al. Enhancing of tuberculin allergy by previous tuberculin testing. *Bull World Health Organ* 1966;34:623.

69. Thompson NJ, Glassroth JL, Snider DE Jr, et al. The booster phenomenon in serial tuberculin skin testing. *Am Rev Respir Dis* 1979;119:587.

70. Stead WW, To T. The significance of tuberculin skin testing in elderly persons. *Ann Intern Med* 1987;107:837.

71. Bullock WE. Studies on immune mechanisms in leprosy, I: depression of delayed allergic response to skin test antigens. *N Engl J Med* 1968;278:298.

72. Kaplan G, Laal S, Sheftel G, et al. The nature and kinetics of a delayed immune response to purified protein derivative of tuberculin in the skin of lepromatous leprosy patients. *J Exp Med* 1988;168:1811.

73. Mehra V, Mason LH, Rothman W, et al. Delineation of a human T-cell subset responsible for lepromin-induced suppression in leprosy patients. *J Immunol* 1980;125:1183.

74. Modlin RL, Kato H, Mehra V, et al. Genetically restricted suppressor T-cell clones derived from lepromatous leprosy lesions. *Nature* 1986;322:459.

75. Watson S, Bullock W, Nelson K, et al. Interleukin 1 production by peripheral blood mononuclear cells from leprosy patients. *Infect Immun* 1984;45:787.

76. Haregewoin A, Godal T, Mustafa AS, et al. T cell-conditioned media reverse T-cell unresponsiveness in lepromatous leprosy. *Nature* 1983;303:342.

77. Mohagheghpour N, Gelber RH, Larrick JW, et al. Defective cell-mediated immunity in leprosy: failure of T cells from lepromatous leprosy patients to respond to *Mycobacterium leprae* is associated with defective expression of interleukin 2 receptors and is not reconstituted by interleukin 2. *J Immunol* 1985;135:1443.

78. Bullock WE, Fasal P. Studies of immune mechanisms in leprosy, III: the role of cellular and humoral factors in impairment of the *in vitro* immune response. *J Immunol* 1971;106:888.

79. Sarosi GA, Catanzaro A, Daniel TM, et al. Clinical usefulness of skin testing in histoplasmosis, coccidioidomycosis, and blastomycosis. *Am Rev Respir Dis* 1988;138:1081.

80. Hassett AM, Woods RJ, Temperly IJ, et al. Cell-mediated immunity to recall antigens *in vivo* and *in vitro*. *Ir J Med Sci* 1977;146:167.

81. Ferguson AC, Kershar HE, Collin WK, et al. Correlation of cutaneous hypersensitivity with lymphocyte response to *Candida albicans*. *Am J Clin Pathol* 1977;68:499.

82. Shannon DC, Johnson G, Rosen F, et al. Cellular activity to *Candida albicans* antigen. *N Engl J Med* 1966;275:690.

83. Schwarz J. *Histoplasmosis*. New York: Praeger, 1981.

84. Loosli CG, Grayston JT, Alexander ER, et al. Epidemiological studies of pulmonary histoplasmosis in a farm family. *Am J Hyg* 1952;55:392.

85. Murray JF, Lurie HI, Kaye J, et al. Benign pulmonary histoplasmosis (cave disease) in South Africa. *S Afr Med J* 1957;31:245.

86. Zeidberg LD, Dillon A, Gass RS. Some factors in the epidemiology of histoplasmin sensitivity in Williamson County, Tennessee. *Am J Public Health* 1951;41:80.

87. Pappagianis D. Epidemiological aspects of respiratory mycotic infections. *Bacteriol Rev* 1967;31:25.

88. Sievers ML. Disseminated coccidioidomycosis among southwestern American Indians. *Am Rev Respir Dis* 1974;109:602.

89. Catanzaro A, Spitler LE, Moser KM. Cellular immune response in coccidioidomycosis. *Cell Immunol* 1975;15:360.

90. Catanzaro A: Suppressor cells in coccidioidomycosis. *Cell Immunol* 1981;64:235.

91. Stobo JD, Paul S, Van Scoy RE, et al. Suppressor thymus-derived lymphocytes in fungal infection. *J Clin Invest* 1976;57:319.

92. Watson SR, Schmitt SK, Hendricks DE, et al. Immunoregulation in disseminated murine histoplasmosis: disturbances in the production of interleukins 1 and 2. *J Immunol* 1985;135:3487.

93. Carvalho EM, Johnson WD, Barreto E, et al. Cell mediated immunity in American cutaneous and mucosal leishmaniasis. *J Immunol* 1985;135:4144.

94. Jones TC, Johnson WD Jr, Barretto AC, et al. Epidemiology of American cutaneous leishmaniasis due to *Leishmania braziliensis braziliensis*. *J Infect Dis* 1987;156:73.

95. Bryceson ADM. Diffuse cutaneous leishmaniasis in Ethiopia, III: immunological studies. *Trans R Soc Trop Med Hyg* 1970;64:380.

96. Convit J, Pinardi ME, Rondon A. Diffuse cutaneous leishmaniasis. A disease due to an immunological defect. *Trans R Soc Trop Med Hyg* 1972;66:603.

97. Rezai HR, Ardekalai SM, Amirhakimi G, et al. Immunological features of kala-azar. *Am J Trop Med Hyg* 1978;27:1079.

98. Carvalho EM, Teixeira RS, Johnson WD. Cell mediated immunity in American visceral leishmaniasis: reversible immunosuppression during acute infection. *Infect Immun* 1981;33:498.

99. Ho M, Koech DK, Iha DW, et al. Immunosuppression in Kenyan visceral leishmaniasis. *Clin Exp Immunol* 1983;51:207.

100. Crawford GD, Wyler DJ, Dinarello CA. Parasite-monocyte interactions in human leishmaniasis: production of interleukin 1 *in vitro*. *J Infect Dis* 1985;152:315.

101. Reiner N, Finke JH. Interleukin 2 deficiency in murine *Leishmania donovani* and its relationship to depressed spleen cell responses to phytohemagglutinin. *J Immunol* 1983;131:1487.

102. Nickol AD, Bonventre PF. Visceral Leishmaniasis in congenic mice of susceptible and resistant phenotypes: T lymphocyte–mediated immunosuppression. *Infect Immun* 1984;50:169.

103. Murray HW, Carriero SM, Donelly DM. Presence of a macrophage-mediated suppressor cell mechanism during cell-mediated immune response in experimental visceral leishmaniasis. *Infect Immun* 1986;54:487.

104. Reiner NE, Ng W, McMaster WR. Parasite-accessory cell interactions in murine leishmaniasis, II: *Leishmania donovani* suppresses macrophage expression of class I and class II major histocompatibility complex products. *J Immunol* 1987;138:1926.

105. Blatt SP, Hendrix CW, Butzin CA, et al. Delayed-type hypersensitivity skin testing predicts progression to AIDS in HIV-infected patients. *Ann Intern Med* 1994;119:177.

106. Ressler C, Mendelson LM. Skin test for diagnosis of penicillin allergy–current status. *Ann Allergy* 1987;59:167.

107. Levine RB, Redmond AP, Fellner MJ, et al. Penicillin allergy and the heterogeneous immune response to benzylpenicillin. *J Clin Invest* 1966;45:1895.

108. Ressler C, Neag PM, Mendelson LM. A liquid chromatographic study of stability of the minor determinants of penicillin allergy. A stable minor determinant mixture skin test preparation. *J Pharm Sci* 1985;74:448.

109. Sullivan TJ, Wedner HJ, Shatz GS, et al. Skin testing to detect penicillin allergy. *J Allergy Clin Immunol* 1981;68:171.

110. Green GR, Rosenblum AH, Sweet LC. Evaluation of penicillin hypersensitivity: value of clinical history and skin testing with penicilloyl-polylysine and penicillin G. *J Allergy Clin Immunol* 1977;60:339.

111. Sogn DD, Evans R 3rd, Shepherd GM, et al. Results of the National Institute of Allergy and Infectious Diseases Collaborative Clinical Trial to test the predictive value of skin testing with major and minor penicillin derivatives in hospitalized patients. *Arch Intern Med* 1992;152:1025.

112. Smith CE, Whiting EG, Baker EE, et al. The use of coccidioidin. *Am Rev Tuberc* 1955;57:330.

113. Smith CE, Beard RR, Saito MT. Pathogenesis of coccidioidomycosis with special reference to pulmonary cavitation. *Ann Intern Med* 1948;29:623.

114. Winn WA. A long term study of 300 patients with cavitary-abscess lesions of the lung of coccidioidal origin. An analytical study with special reference to treatment. *Dis Chest* 1968;54:268.

115. Hyde L. Coccidioidal pulmonary cavitation. *Dis Chest* 1968;54:273.

116. Wiant JR, Smith JW. Coccidioidin skin reactivity in pulmonary coccidioidomycosis. *Chest* 1973;63:100.

117. Myrvang V, Godal T, Ridley DS, et al. Immune responsiveness to *Mycobacterium leprae* and other mycobacterial antigens throughout the clinical and histopathological spectrum of leprosy. *Clin Exp Immunol* 1973;14:541.

118. Nath I Curtiss J, Sharma AK, et al. Circulating T-cell numbers and their mitogenic potential in leprosy–correlation with mycobacterial load. *Clin Exp Immunol* 1977;29:363.

119. Restrepo A. Immune response to *Paracoccidioides brasiliensis* in human and animal hosts. *Curr Top Med Mycol* 1988;2:239.

120. Mussatti C, Rezkallah-Iwasso MT, Mendes E, et al. *In vivo* and *in vitro* evaluation of cell-mediated immunity in patients with paracoccidioidomycosis. *Cell Immunol* 1978;24:365.

121. Mota NGS, Rezkallah-Iwasso MT, Peracoli MT, et al. Correlation between cell-mediated immunity and clinical forms of paracoccidioidomycosis. *Trans R Soc Trop Med Hyg* 1985;79:765.

122. Mok WY, Fava-Netto C. Paracoccidioidin and histoplasmin sensitivity in Coari (state of Amazonas), Brazil. *Am J Trop Med Hyg* 1978;27:808.

Treatment of Infectious Diseases

Principles of Treatment

CHAPTER 17
Pharmacologic Principles

Michael Barza

The physician must have a basic understanding of pharmacologic principles to use antimicrobial agents in the safest and most effective way. The purpose of this chapter is to outline the most important of these principles from the point of view of a clinical consultant in infectious diseases.

For most antimicrobial agents, the bulk of the pharmacokinetic information available deals with the concentrations of the drugs in plasma or serum. Data on the concentrations of drugs in peripheral sites are more scarce; furthermore, when the concentrations of drugs are monitored during treatment, it is generally serum concentrations that are studied, even when the primary focus of infection is extravascular, because serum is more accessible than other body fluids. Fortunately, measurements of concentrations in serum may provide a good guide to concentrations in peripheral sites, provided that a few basic principles are kept in mind. Accordingly, this chapter begins with a consideration of the determinants of the concentration profile in serum and goes on to discuss the relation between the concentrations in serum and those in peripheral sites. Data regarding the intracellular penetration of drugs are also reviewed.

ANTIBIOTIC CONCENTRATIONS IN SERUM

Serum Concentrations and Time for Equilibration

After a rapid intravenous injection (bolus injection) of an antibiotic, the concentration of drug in the serum promptly reaches a peak and then begins to decline (Fig. 17.1). The first portion of the decline, the α phase, is steep as a result of mixing of the bolus with the blood and distribution to rapidly equilibrating compartments. In the second portion, the β phase (or elimination phase), the decline is mainly the result of drug elimination. The β phase is used to determine the serum half-life ($t_{1/2}$) of the drug. For most drugs, diffusion between the tissues and the plasma occurs quickly enough that the serum half-life in the β phase not only is the time in which the serum concentration drops by half but also approximates the time in which the total amount of drug in the body is reduced by half. The serum half-life is related to the elimination rate as follows:

$$t_{1/2} = 0.693/K \qquad [17.1]$$

where K is the elimination rate constant. If $t_{1/2}$ is expressed in hours, then the units of K are hour^{-1}.

If a drug is administered at regular intervals without a loading dose, there will be a steady rise in the peak and trough concentrations in the serum until an equilibrium is reached, at which time, the rate of drug elimination is equal to the rate of administration (Fig. 17.2). The number of doses (N) required for the peak serum concentration to reach 95% of the equilibrium concentration can be determined by dividing the serum half-life by the dosing interval (t_i) and multiplying by 4.32. The time required for the peak concentrations to reach 95% of the equilibrium value (by definition, $N \times t_i$) can be calculated by multiplying the half-life of the drug by 4.32 (1). For example, if gentamicin has a serum half-life of 8 hours in a patient with renal impairment and is administered at a fixed dose every 24 hours, the number of doses required for the peak serum concentration to reach 95% of the equilibrium value is $4.32 \times 8/24$, or 1.44 dose, and the time to reach 95% of the equilibrium value is 34.6 hours.

Equilibrium can be achieved quickly if a loading dose is given initially (Fig. 17.2A). In general, a loading dose is about 1.5 to

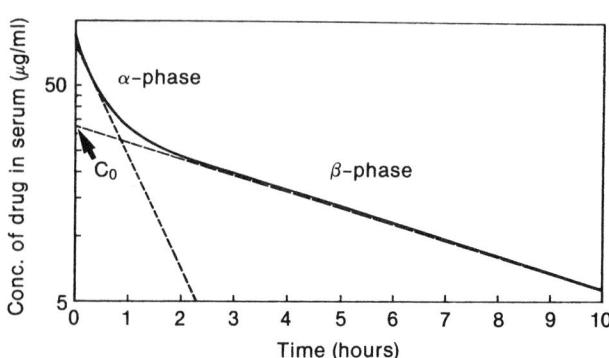

Figure 17.1. Concentration of a drug in the serum illustrating the α phase and the β phase of the serum concentration curve. Note that the ordinate scale is logarithmic. C_0 is the estimated peak concentration that would occur if equilibrium were immediate—that is, if there were no α phase. The apparent volume of distribution (V_d) after a single bolus injection can be calculated from C_0 (see Eq. 17.5).

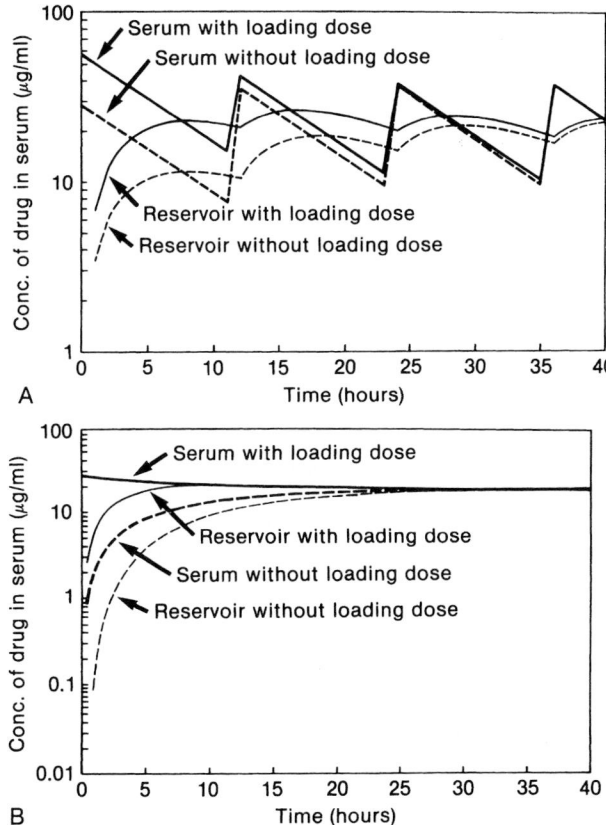

Figure 17.2. Concentrations of vancomycin in the serum and in a large reservoir (e.g., peritoneal fluid) during administration by intermittent infusion (**A**) or during continuous infusion (**B**) with or without a loading dose. The dose is 1 g every 12 hours, and the half-life is 6 hours. The initial dose (loading dose) is 1.5 g. Whether the drug is given by intermittent or continuous infusion, about four half-lives of the drug are required for the peak serum concentration to reach 95% of the equilibrium peak concentration in the absence of a loading dose. Equilibration is markedly hastened by the administration of a loading dose.

Area Under the Curve

A convenient way to consider the changes in concentration in a given site over time is to calculate the area under the curve (AUC) of time versus concentration for that interval. The units are concentration multiplied by time (e.g., micrograms per milliliter multiplied by minutes). The mean concentration of a drug in a site during the dosing interval can be calculated by dividing the AUC by the dosing interval. A simple method of calculating the AUC is shown in Equation 17.4 (see later). It has been suggested that the mean concentration in the serum of a patient receiving the drug by intermittent infusion can be estimated by plotting the peak and trough concentrations on a logarithmic scale and determining the midpoint between them (2), but this approach produces an underestimate (3).

Drug Absorption

The absorption of most antimicrobial agents after oral administration occurs primarily by passive diffusion and takes place in the small intestine. Overall, the determinants of the absorbability of antimicrobial agents are not well understood. Lipid solubility appears to be important for the oral absorption of penicillins in relatively acidic conditions but perhaps not at more neutral pH values (4). Among cephalosporins, the possession of an arylglycine side chain favors oral absorption. Despite these general observations, it is difficult to predict from the structure of a compound how well it will be absorbed by mouth, and the final determination rests on the results of clinical studies.

Some penicillins and cephalosporins have been formulated as prodrugs to facilitate absorption when they are taken orally. Many prodrugs are esters of the parent compound, with the ester being split off by enzymes in the intestinal mucosa or in the plasma to release the free drug into the serum.

The absorption of many antimicrobial agents is affected when they are ingested with food. The effect of food on most penicillins is to delay absorption but not to reduce the total amount absorbed; some other drugs, such as several cephalosporins, show reduced absorption when they are taken with food (4). For still other compounds, food has no effect or may even enhance absorption. There have been some variations in the results from study to study (5).

The coadministration of nonabsorbable antacids or histamine H_2 receptor blockers may diminish the absorption of some antimicrobial agents by at least two mechanisms: (a) reduction of gastric acidity and (b) in the case of antacids, chelation. For example, the absorption of ketoconazole requires an acid environment and is sharply diminished in patients with decreased gastric acidity. Tetracyclines are chelated by the divalent cations present in antacids and dairy products, The coadministration of antacids or zinc markedly reduces the oral absorption of fluoroquinolones.

Appreciable quantities of antibiotics may be absorbed from sites of topical application, as in lavage of joints or the peritoneum and irrigation of tissues. In the case of drugs such as the aminoglycosides, systemic toxic effects may occur, especially in patients with unsuspected renal impairment. Most such applications are unnecessary if a well-chosen antimicrobial agent is given by conventional routes. Indeed, the U.S. Food and Drug Administration has advised against using solutions containing neomycin for irrigation of wounds, joints, or body cavities (except the urinary bladder) because these treatments carry an appreciable risk of toxic effects without conferring a clear benefit.

2 times larger than the maintenance dose. For drugs that have a short serum half-life in relation to the dosing interval (e.g., most penicillins and cephalosporins), there is little or no accumulation between doses and there is no need for a loading dose; however, with agents that have a longer half-life and a relatively narrow therapeutic index (such as the aminoglycosides), it is common practice to administer a loading dose to patients with serious infections to achieve equilibrium concentrations quickly.

If a drug is given by continuous infusion (Fig. 17.2B) rather than by rapid intravenous injection, again the serum concentration rises slowly until equilibrium is reached. As with intermittent infusions, the time required to achieve 95% of the equilibrium concentration is the product of 4.32 and the half-life of the drug. Thus, the time required to achieve equilibrium is independent of whether the drug is given by intermittent or continuous infusion. As with intermittent dosing, equilibrium can be achieved much more quickly if a loading dose is given.

The analysis of serum concentration curves is more complicated when drugs are administered by the oral or intramuscular route than when they are given by the intravenous route because drug elimination and absorption occur simultaneously. The elimination half-life cannot be reliably determined until drug absorption is complete. Nevertheless, the underlying pharmacologic principles are the same for all routes.

Drug Elimination

There are three major routes of drug elimination. A fourth route, back-diffusion across the colonic epithelium, is important for only a few antibiotics.

KIDNEYS

The principal route of elimination of many antimicrobial agents, including the penicillins, cephalosporins, aminoglycosides, and vancomycin, is by the kidneys. Renal elimination may occur either by glomerular filtration or by tubular secretion. Glomerular filtration is a passive diffusional process. For drugs that are bound to serum proteins, only the unbound fraction is eliminated by glomerular filtration. The rate of elimination of free drug by glomerular filtration is roughly proportional to the rate of clearance of creatinine, but not precisely proportional because a small fraction of the creatinine is actively secreted into the urine. In contrast to glomerular filtration, tubular secretion is an active transport process that is not affected by serum protein binding. Tubular secretion is a more efficient excretory process than glomerular filtration; hence, drugs that are eliminated by tubular secretion have shorter serum half-lives than those that are eliminated by glomerular filtration alone. Probenecid inhibits the active transport pump for penicillins and many cephalosporins and prolongs the half-life of these agents.

LIVER AND GALLBLADDER

The hepatobiliary system is a dominant route of elimination for a few commonly used antimicrobial agents, notably cefoperazone, of which about 60% of an intravenous dose is eliminated in the bile, and ceftriaxone, of which about 40% is eliminated in the bile.

There are several consequences of a high degree of biliary elimination of an antibiotic. First, little dosage adjustment is necessary for patients with renal impairment. Second, depending on the antibacterial spectrum of the drug, there may be major alterations in the fecal flora and a tendency of the drug to produce diarrhea. By contrast, if biliary elimination is slight, alterations in the fecal flora will be minimal even if the drug has a broad spectrum; this is the case with imipenem. Although it might be speculated that there should be a direct relation between the extent of alterations in the fecal flora and the degree of colonization by resistant strains, this has not been shown experimentally (6). Most antimicrobial agents are excreted in appreciable concentrations in the bile if the biliary tract is unobstructed but are undetectable in the bile when there is high-grade biliary obstruction. An exception is cefoperazone, which achieves appreciable concentrations even with complete biliary obstruction.

Severe hepatobiliary disease is likely to alter the clearance rate of drugs that are eliminated mainly by hepatobiliary mechanisms. However, in contrast to the usefulness of the serum creatinine value for estimating the effect of renal failure on the half-life of drugs eliminated primarily by glomerular filtration, no simple clinical laboratory test is available to allow the physician to estimate changes in hepatic clearance and to make precise dosage adjustments in patients with hepatobiliary disease; as a consequence, the adjustments are generally crude.

METABOLISM

Metabolism is an important means of elimination for a number of antimicrobial agents, including many penicillins and cephalosporins, clindamycin, chloramphenicol, macrolides, metronidazole, rifampin, sulfonamides, isoniazid, and some tetracyclines. Metabolism generally occurs in the liver and results in a loss of antibacterial activity. In most instances, the metabolites are more polar and thus more water soluble than the parent compound, so they are more readily eliminated in urine or bile than the parent compound. The rate of acetylation

of isoniazid is genetically determined; subjects can be classified as rapid acetylators or slow acetylators. Dosages of drugs that are extensively metabolized do not have to be adjusted for patients with renal failure unless the metabolites have an adverse effect.

BACK-DIFFUSION

A fourth means of eliminating drugs from the circulation is by back-diffusion across the colonic epithelium and elimination in the feces. Although this is not an important route for most drugs, minocycline and ciprofloxacin are eliminated to some degree by this route.

Renal Failure

Drugs that are eliminated primarily by renal mechanisms accumulate in patients whose renal function is impaired. In general, the total daily dose must be reduced to about the same extent as renal function is reduced. The calculation is easiest for drugs that are eliminated mainly by glomerular filtration. For example, in a patient with stable renal impairment and a serum creatinine concentration (Cr_s) of 5.0 mg/dL, it may be inferred that the rate of glomerular filtration is about 20% of normal and that the total daily dose should be reduced by 80%. A more precise way of assessing renal function in men is to estimate the creatinine clearance rate as follows (7):

$$\text{creatinine clearance (mL/min)} = \frac{(140 - \text{age})(\text{weight})}{Cr_s \text{ (mg/dL)} \times 72} \quad [17.2]$$

where age is expressed in years and weight in kilograms. For women, the factor in the divisor is 85, rather than 72.

The daily dose may be reduced to compensate for the effects of renal failure by prolonging the interval between doses, by reducing the dose given at each administration, or by a combination of these approaches. The choice of whether to modify the dose or the dosing interval is a difficult one that touches on many controversial issues in antimicrobial chemotherapy. The issue has been debated extensively with respect to the aminoglycosides. On the one hand, giving the usual dose at longer intervals results in widely fluctuating serum concentrations (Fig. 17.3). The trough concentrations may be below the inhibitory threshold for the infecting microorganisms for substantial periods; however, the long postantibiotic effect of aminoglycosides should mitigate this consequence. On the other hand, decreasing the dose but

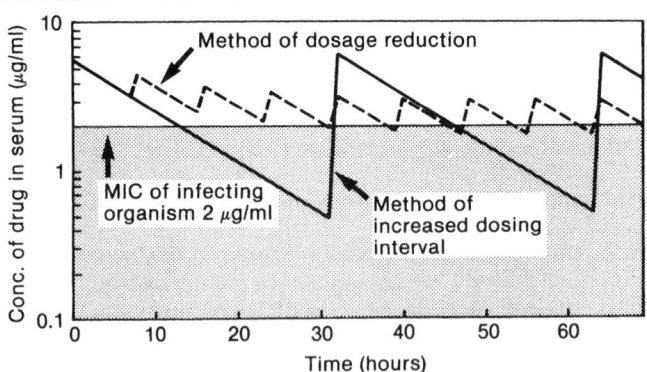

Figure 17.3. Dosage adjustment for gentamicin in renal failure. The serum creatinine concentration is 4.0 mg/dl, and the half-life of the drug is 8.5 hours. The method of increasing the dosing interval, shown here as the administration of 80 mg every 32 hours, results in low trough concentrations, which could be below the minimum inhibitory concentration (MIC) of the infecting organism for prolonged periods. The dosage reduction method, shown here as the administration of 20 mg every 8 hours, results in higher trough concentrations, which some believe could predispose to nephrotoxic effects.

maintaining the usual dosing interval produces higher trough concentrations. Some investigators believe that high trough concentrations are an important risk factor for the nephrotoxic effects of aminoglycosides. Nevertheless, others suggest that high trough concentrations are simply an early manifestation of renal impairment from infection or other conditions, rather than a cause of renal impairment. As a practical matter, if the aminoglycoside is being used as the principal antibacterial agent for treatment of the infection, I try to adopt a regimen that does not result in potentially subinhibitory concentrations for more than 6–8 hours at a time. The postantibiotic effect and the concentration-dependent bactericidal activity of aminoglycosides generally render such an interval tolerable without adverse consequences. By contrast, for serious infections being treated with β-lactam antibiotics, subinhibitory concentrations for this long an interval should be avoided because β-lactam antibiotics are inhibitory only as long as the concentrations are above the MIC and the postantibiotic effect against gram-negative organisms is short (8).

Removal of Drugs by Dialysis

Peritoneal dialysis removes little of most antimicrobial agents that accumulate in renal failure, but hemodialysis removes substantial amounts. This is not because the peritoneum is poorly permeable to antibiotics; on the contrary, drugs instilled into the peritoneal cavity are rapidly absorbed into the systemic circulation. In fact, a convenient means of maintaining serum concentrations at a specific level is to add the drug to the dialysis fluid at the desired concentration. The apparent paradox whereby the equilibrium between peritoneal fluid and the systemic circulation appears to occur more rapidly when drugs are placed in the peritoneal fluid than when they are placed in the systemic circulation may be explained by the fact that the peritoneal surface area is larger in relation to the peritoneal cavity than it is in relation to the total systemic circulation (see section "Estimating Concentration in Extravascular Sites ").

Sample Estimations of Serum Concentrations

Before we consider the distribution of antibiotics to extravascular sites, it may be useful to give some examples of calculations that allow clinicians to estimate peak and trough concentrations of antimicrobial agents using the information available from standard textbooks of pharmacology.

INTERMITTENT ADMINISTRATION

The *increase* in peak serum concentration from a dose of drug is equal to the intravenous dose (expressed in milligrams) divided by the apparent volume of distribution (V_d, expressed in liters). Values for V_d may be obtained from the literature. The concept of apparent V_d is discussed in the section "Apparent Volume of Distribution."

For a drug such as gentamicin, which is negligibly protein bound, a typical dose, given once daily might be 5 mg/kg. For a 70-kg patient with a calculated V_d of 20 L, the dose of about 350 mg would produce a peak serum concentration of 17.57 μg/mL.

The calculation of peak concentration applies to free drug in the serum. For an agent that is appreciably bound to serum protein, the total serum concentration (free plus bound drug) could be calculated by dividing the concentration of free drug by the fraction that is free. For example, if a drug is 70% protein bound and the concentration of free drug in the serum is 10 μg/mL, the total concentration can be estimated to be 33 μg/mL (i.e., 10 divided by 0.3).

Once the peak serum concentration is known, values at intervals after the peak can be estimated on the assumption that the concentration will decrease by half every half-life. In patients with stable renal impairment, the serum half-life of an aminoglycoside (hours) can be estimated roughly by multiplying the steady-state serum creatinine concentration by 4.0 (9,10). For example, if the serum creatinine concentration is 3.0 mg/dL, the serum half-life of gentamicin can be estimated as 12 hours. One way to adjust the dosage in a patient with renal impairment is to give a full initial dose, followed by half this dose every half-life. However, computer-based nomograms are now readily available and provide more accurate dosing schedules.

These formulas and nomograms are only a rough guide to the anticipated serum concentrations. It has been shown repeatedly that estimates of serum concentrations of aminoglycosides based on body weight and the serum creatinine concentration are imprecise. To verify the results, serum concentrations of drugs with a narrow therapeutic index (e.g., aminoglycosides) should be measured directly at regular intervals.

The formula for calculating the mean serum concentration (C_{mean}) during the dosing interval in a patient receiving the drug by intermittent infusions is as follows:

$$C_{mean} = \frac{dose}{V_d \times t_i \times K} = \frac{dose \times t_{1/2}}{V_d \times t_i \times 0.693} \qquad [17.3]$$

where V_d is the volume of distribution, t is the dosing interval, K is the elimination rate constant, and $t_{1/2}$ is the serum half-life of the drug. Because t_i multiplied by C_{mean} is the AUC during the dosing interval, or AUC_i, it can be calculated as follows:

$$AUC_1 = \frac{dose \times t_{1/2}}{V_d \times 0.693} \qquad [17.4]$$

CONTINUOUS INFUSION

The steady-state serum concentration (C_s) of free drug during continuous infusion can be calculated by varying Equation 17.3 so that dose divided by t_i is replaced by I, the infusion rate:

$$C_s = \frac{I}{V_d \times K} = \frac{I \times t_{1/2}}{V_d \times 0.693} \qquad [17.5]$$

Suppose that carbenicillin is being given at a rate of 1,000 mg per hour, that V_d (from the literature) is estimated to be 14 L, and that the serum half-life is estimated to be 1 hour. Then C_s is 1,000 mg per hour divided by (14 × 0.693), or 103 mg/L (μg/mL). Assuming that the drug is 50% bound to serum protein, the total serum concentration is 206 mg/L.

DISTRIBUTION TO PERIPHERAL SITES

Major Influences on Distribution

There are three major determinants of the distribution of drugs between the plasma (central compartment) and extravascular sites (peripheral compartment). The first is the nature of the capillary bed. In most tissues and organs, the capillary bed is fenestrated by small pores that permit the ready diffusion of substances with molecular masses up to about 1,000 daltons. This encompasses most antimicrobial agents. A few sites in the body, which may be termed specialized sites, possess unfenestrated capillaries. Because drugs must pass through the endothelial cells of the capillaries to reach the extravascular space in these specialized sites, the rate of diffusion is determined by the degree of lipid solubility of the drug.

The most clinically important specialized sites are the central nervous system (CNS), the retina, and the prostate gland. Drugs that are weakly lipid soluble, such as the β-lactams, aminoglycosides, some tetracyclines, and vancomycin, penetrate poorly into the brain and cerebrospinal fluid (CSF), the vitreous humor, and the secretions of the prostate gland. Weakly lipid-soluble drugs also penetrate poorly into most cells, an important consideration in the concept of V_d. Drugs that are more lipid soluble, such as metronidazole, rifampin, chloramphenicol, trimethoprim, doxycycline, minocycline, and the fluoroquinolones, penetrate more readily into these specialized sites and into cells.

A second major determinant of the distribution of drugs into the periphery is the degree of serum protein binding of the drug. Protein binding is a reversible process; however, at any moment, only the proportion of drug that is unbound (free drug) is available for diffusion across capillaries. Only free drug is antibacterially active. The major binding protein for most drugs is albumin. Accordingly, the extent of binding is greatest in the plasma. Nevertheless, there may be an appreciable degree of protein binding in extravascular sites. For example, in cellulitis, there may be extensive leakage of serum albumin into the extravascular compartment.

Active transport pumps are a third major determinant of distribution for certain agents. The best studied of these pumps act on organic anions and are located in the choroid plexus of the brain and the retina of the eye; the pumps transport β-lactam drugs out of the CNS and the vitreous humor. They are competitively inhibited by probenecid. Similar pumps in the cells of the proximal tubule of the kidney and in the biliary ducts are responsible for secretion of drugs into the urine and bile.

Estimating Concentration in Extravascular Sites

NONSPECIALIZED SITES

It is much easier to envision the relation between drug concentrations in serum and extravascular sites in a state of equilibrium than in nonequilibrium situations. At equilibrium, the average concentration of free drug in nonspecialized extravascular sites is equal to that in the serum during the dosing interval. This assumes that no drug is destroyed in the site. If there is rapid local destruction of the drug, as might occur in an abscess because of bacterial enzymes, the equilibrium concentration in the extravascular site will be lower than that in the serum.

The rapidity with which equilibrium is reached and the shape of the concentration curve in peripheral sites are related to the ratio of surface area to volume in the site (11,12), as described in the next two paragraphs. Examples of results for sites with large and small ratios of surface area to volume in a patient receiving antibiotic by intermittent intravenous injection are shown in Figure 17.4. Estimating the time required to reach the equilibrium concentration in the extravascular compartment is difficult because it requires knowledge of the permeability coefficient P for the site; P may vary strikingly from site to site (12).

Interstitial Fluid Model. In the thin layer of interstitial fluid that surrounds capillaries, the ratio of surface area to volume is great (i.e., diffusion distances are short) (see Fig 17.4A). There is a large area for exchange of drug between serum and site compared with the volume into which the drug must be distributed. Equilibration occurs promptly, and the concentration of drug in the interstitial fluid follows closely the concentration of free drug in the plasma.

Large Fluid Collections. In collections such as pleural or ascitic fluid, in which the ratio of surface area to volume is low and the diffusional distances are great, equilibration with serum occurs slowly and the concentration of drug in the center of the collection fluctuates much less than in the serum (see Fig. 17.4B). The mean concentration of free drug in the extravascular site at equilibrium can be easily inferred because it is equal to that in the serum. The serum value can be estimated by use of Equa-

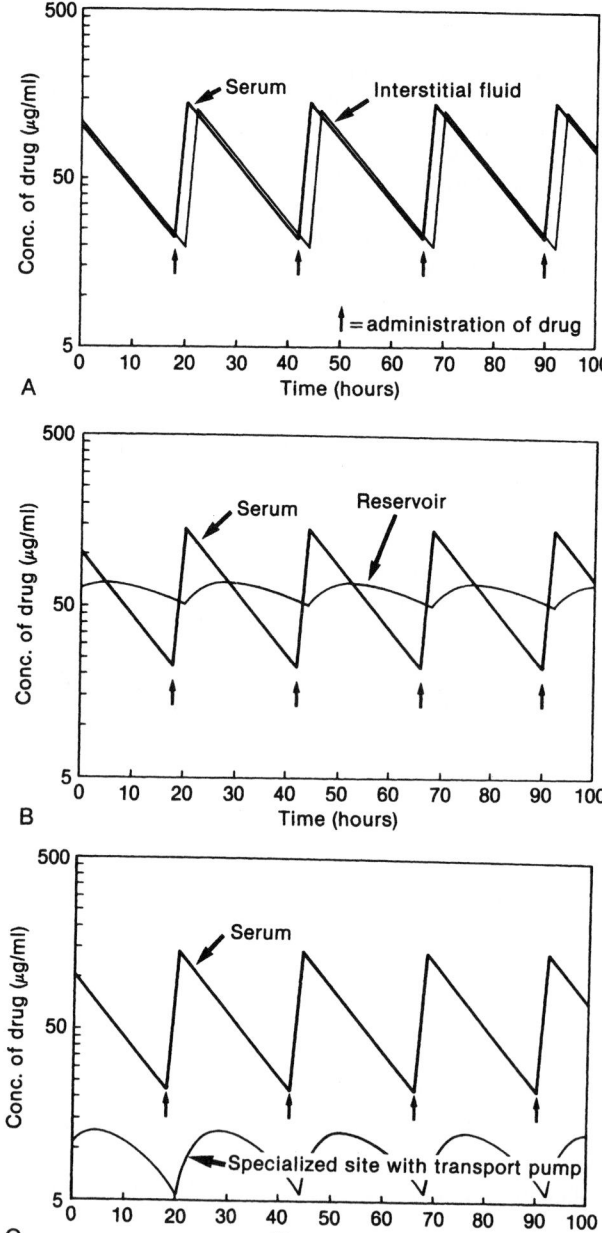

Figure 17.4. Concentration of drug in the serum and in three kinds of extravascular sites at equilibrium. **A:** In interstitial fluid, there is ready transport between the vascular and extravascular sites, and concentrations in the extravascular site closely mimic those in the serum. **B:** In a large reservoir, such as pleural fluid, equilibration between serum and the site occurs slowly, as shown in Figure 17.2. At equilibrium, the mean concentration in the large reservoir is equal to that in the serum, but the fluctuations in concentration are much less in the large reservoir than in the serum. **C:** In a specialized site, such as cerebrospinal fluid, there is a barrier to drug transport because the capillaries are nonfenestrated. The combination of a penetration barrier and active transport (e.g., of a β-lactam drug) results in concentrations that are much lower in the extravascular site than in the serum, even at equilibrium.

tion 17.3 if the drug is being given by intermittent infusion and by use of Equation 17.5 if the drug is being given by continuous infusion. For sites with intermediate ratios of surface area to volume, the curves lie between those shown in Fig. 17.4A and B.

Diffusion into abscesses may occur somewhat less readily than into interstitial fluid; however, the difficulty of sterilizing abscesses by chemotherapy probably is related not to impediments to drug penetration but to the large bacterial inoculum (inoculum effect), the degradation of drug by bacterial enzymes, and the adverse effect of the milieu (including the low pH level) on the activity of the drug. Bacteria that are dividing slowly (e.g., in an abscess) are much less susceptible than rapidly dividing bacteria to various antimicrobial agents, including not only drugs that act on the cell wall but also those that act on deoxyribonucleic acid and on protein synthesis. A related phenomenon is seen in the diminished susceptibility to antibiotics of bacteria growing in biofilms (13).

SPECIALIZED SITES

For specialized tissues with unfenestrated capillaries, primarily the brain, CSF, and vitreous humor, the situation is more complicated (see Fig. 17.4C). These sites behave like large reservoirs, not only because of their low ratios of surface area to volume but also because of the slowness of diffusion through the unfenestrated capillaries, especially for drugs that are not lipid soluble. Nevertheless, in the absence of drug destruction, the mean concentrations of drugs in these sites would be expected eventually to be equal to those in the plasma, were it not for the active transport pumps, principally those for β-lactam drugs. Although the transport pumps are relatively inefficient, their effect is exaggerated by the diffusional barriers. In evaluating clinical reports of the concentrations of antibiotics in these sites, we should keep in mind that equilibrium may not have been achieved even after prolonged periods of drug administration.

One other factor that may militate against the achievement of equilibrium concentrations in the CSF is that the fluid is continually being replaced. The volume of CSF in a normal adult is about 120 mL, and the rate of resorption and new formation is about 30 mL per hour. At this rate of CSF turnover, the half-life of a substance that is removed passively as the CSF is resorbed is 2.8 hours simply because of dilution.

Many reports indicate that the concentrations of antibiotics that are poorly lipid soluble are low in the brain and CSF, typically less than 10% of the corresponding serum concentration. In the case of the β-lactam drugs, this probably reflects the combined effects of serum protein binding, the poor permeability of the unfenestrated capillaries, and especially the active transport pump for organic anions in the choroid plexus.

Aminoglycosides also reach relatively low concentrations in the CNS. These drugs are negligibly bound to serum proteins. Local degradation of the drugs is unlikely to occur. There is a transport pump for aminoglycosides in the choroid plexus of animals, but it appears to be weak. Therefore, one would anticipate that with time, concentrations of aminoglycosides in the CNS would approach the mean serum concentration. The concentrations reported have been lower than this, perhaps because patients have been studied before equilibrium has been reached, because the pump has some effect, or because of the continual removal of the drug as CSF is resorbed.

For highly lipid-soluble drugs, one would anticipate that concentrations in specialized sites would approximate the mean serum concentration unless local degradation or active transport pumps are operating. Indeed, the CSF concentrations of metronidazole and chloramphenicol are reportedly similar to the serum concentrations of these agents. The somewhat lower concentrations of rifampin suggest that there may be an active transport pump for this agent (14).

PENETRATION INTO CELLS

Organisms that cause suppurative infections are found primarily in the interstitial fluid of tissues. In the treatment of such infections, it is presumably the extracellular concentration of drug that is important. By contrast, many species of organisms, such as *Listeria monocytogenes, Salmonella* species, *Legionella pneumophila,* and *Mycobacterium* species, survive and multiply within host cells, especially macrophages. The chemotherapy of infections caused by these species presumably depends on the intracellular concentration of drug. The pharmacologic principles relating to the intracellular penetration of antibiotics are far more complicated than those dealing with penetration into the extracellular space, and knowledge of these principles is rudimentary.

A significant issue in studying the intracellular penetration of antibiotics relates to the subcellular distribution of the drug. Many studies report the "average" intracellular concentration of drugs, but for most agents, it is unlikely that intracellular concentrations are homogeneous. For example, many drugs that are accumulated intracellularly, such as lincosamides, macrolides, and aminoglycosides, are weak bases and are found primarily in the acidic lysosomes. Paradoxically, in this location, their antibacterial activity may be diminished by the acidity of their environment. In some instances, the intracellular microorganism is found in a subcellular location different from that in which the antibiotic is accumulated. This appears to be the case with azithromycin and *Toxoplasma gondii* (15). Nevertheless, the drug has some activity against the parasite. To further complicate the issue, drug penetration may vary depending on the type of cell under study. Although many issues concerning the intracellular penetration and activity of drugs remain unclear, there is evidence to suggest that the most effective drugs for the treatment of infection by intracellular pathogens are those that are well accumulated within cells.

Table 17.1 summarizes the pharmacologic and pharmacodynamic properties of selected antibiotics as derived from extensive reviews (16–18). The experiments have been done in various cell types, polymorphonuclear leukocytes, macrophages, fibroblasts, and HeLa cells, with somewhat different results in the various cell types. For most drugs, entry is mainly by simple diffusion and distribution is in accord with pH partition. There is some suggestion of active transport of clindamycin and the macrolides. In general, the β-lactam drugs penetrate poorly into cells, even after prolonged exposure. Aminoglycosides are accumulated slowly to reach concentrations exceeding those in the extracellular fluid by twofold to fourfold. Clindamycin (but not lincomycin) and the macrolides, especially clarithromycin and azithromycin, reach much higher concentrations in cells than in the extracellular fluid; much of the accumulated drug is within lysosomes, where activity may not be optimal. The fluoroquinolones show moderate accumulation within cells, to about twofold to eightfold the extracellular concentration. Efflux from cells appears to be rapid for all agents except the aminoglycosides and azithromycin. This observation probably accounts for the finding of low levels of aminoglycosides in urine long after the end of treatment and for the efficacy of azithromycin in brief treatment courses, such as the single-dose treatment of chlamydial urethritis and cervicitis.

Intracellular drug not only may exert an effect against intracellular pathogens but could be slowly released into the interstitial fluid. In this manner, the intracellular space could serve as a "reservoir" or depot, leading to more sustained drug concentrations in interstitial fluid between doses. This may be the case with azithromycin. It has also been suggested that antibiotic-laden neutrophils could carry antibiotics to sites of infection with beneficial effects, but this is unclear.

Additional Considerations

As discussed, drugs that are weakly lipid soluble penetrate most types of cells poorly. For these agents, most of the drug in

TABLE 17.1. Intracellular Accumulation and Activity of Selected Antibiotics

Agent	Drug concentration[a]	Mechanism of cellular drug uptake	Localization in cell	Kinetics of influx and efflux	Activity in cells
β-Lactams	Intracellular/extracellular ratio of ≤0.7 in PMN leukocytes, macrophages, fibroblasts, and HeLa cells, even after prolonged incubation	Diffusion and pH partition	Free in cytoplasm	Rapid influx and efflux (half-life, 20–30 min)	Variable, from no activity (especially in PMN leukocytes) to some activity (especially in macrophages and monocytes); some activity evident by best methods
Aminoglycosides	Slow intracellular accumulation to 2–4 times extracellular level after 72 hr of incubation	Endocytosis and diffusion	50% in lysosomes, 50% in cytoplasm	Slow	Less activity than at same concentration extracellularly; possible reduction of activity as pH falls with phagosome–lysosome fusion; better activity in macrophages than in PMN leukocytes
Rifampin	Intracellular level 2–3 times extracellular level	Diffusion	In cytoplasm	Rapid	Activity in cells equal to activity in cell-free medium
Lincosamides	Intracellular versus extracellular level: clindamycin, 10- to 50-fold in PMN leukocytes and macrophages: lincomycin, ratio of ≤2	Diffusion and pH partition; clindamycin may use energy-requiring nucleoside transport system	50% in lysosomes, 50% in cytoplasm	Rapid	Despite high intracellular concentrations of clindamycin, intracellular no greater than extracellular activity
Macrolides	Intracellular versus extracellular level: erythromycin, 10- to 30-fold in PMN leukocytes and alveolar macrophages, lower in cultured human and HeLa cells; intracellular levels higher for newer macrolides	Diffusion and pH partition; active transport different from nucleoside transport of clindamycin	50% in lysosomes, 50% in cytoplasm	Rapid influx and efflux (half-life, 15–20 min) of all except azithromycin	Erythromycin potent against obligate intracellular organisms such as Legionella; no effect on Staphylococcus aureus in PMNs
Fluoroquinolones	Intracellular level 2–8 times extracellular level in macrophages and fibroblasts	Not known	In cytoplasm or loosely associated with organelles	Rapid	Active against S. aureus in PMNs

Note: PMN, Polymorphonuclear.
[a] Average concentration in whole cells.
Source: From Barza M. Tissue-directed antibiotic therapy: antibiotic dynamics in cells and tissue. Challenges to antibiotic activity in tissue. *Clin Infect Dis* 1994;19:910–915, with permission.

tissues lies in the interstitial fluid. Calculations based on the assumption that the total amount of drug detected in a sample of tissue is distributed evenly throughout cells and the interstitial fluid will lead to a marked underestimate of the interstitial fluid concentration.

The methods of homogenizing and assaying tissues may have a major impact on the results. For example, a number of studies purport to show that different cephalosporins penetrate bone to different degrees. In fact, these variations probably relate to differences in the methods used to extract the drug from the bone. Careful studies indicate that the concentrations of cephalosporins in the interstitial fluid of normal and osteomyelitic bone are similar to those in the serum (19,20).

There is still controversy about both theoretic and experimental aspects of drug penetration into the prostate gland. The capillary bed of the organ is unfenestrated, so drugs that are poorly lipid soluble penetrate with difficulty. The barrier appears to be maintained in all but the most acute states of inflammation.

The unique pharmacologic feature of the prostate gland relates to the issue of pH partition, or ion trapping. The prostatic secretions of the dog have a pH level of only 6.4. Most β-lactam drugs are anions, which are less ionized, and therefore are more lipid soluble, in the acidic secretions of the prostate gland than in the serum. Accordingly, they diffuse more readily out of the prostate gland than into it. At equilibrium, concentrations in the prostate are lower than those in the serum. In contrast, weak bases such as the aminoglycosides and erythromycin exhibit the reverse phenomenon; they are trapped in the prostate gland. However, the mean pH of prostatic secretions from normal men is 7.28, and from men with bacterial prostatitis it is 8.32—values that are strikingly different from those in the prostate gland of dogs. The alkaline pH level in patients with chronic prostatitis should favor the accumulation of weak acids such as penicillins, cephalosporins, sulfonamides, and rifampin. It is difficult to test the validity of these hypotheses clinically. Studies of the concentration of drugs in human prostatic secretions are complicated by the fact that contamination of ejaculate by even minute amounts of urine produces spurious results because of the high concentrations in the urine.

APPARENT VOLUME OF DISTRIBUTION

Drugs that are highly lipid soluble penetrate readily into most tissues and fluids of the body and are said to have a large V_d. By contrast, drugs that are weakly lipid soluble tend to be restricted to the extracellular fluid, which comprises about 20% to 30% of the body weight. For a given dose, the serum concentration of a highly lipid-soluble agent would be much lower than that of a weakly lipid-soluble agent because the highly lipid-soluble agent is distributed into a much larger volume. The V_d of a hydrophilic drug is much increased in a patient with a large "third space" (e.g., with abundant ascites). V_d values for a number of drugs are available from standard textbooks of pharmacology. In addition, the V_d can be estimated during continuous infusion by use of Equation 17.5 and during intermittent infusion by use of Equation 17.3. An even simpler way of estimating the V_d after a single rapid injection of a drug is to project the β-phase curve to time zero (see Fig. 17.1). This value is the peak concentration after correcting for the α phase. The dose divided by this concentration is the V_d.

Measurements of the V_d provide only a gross idea of the peripheral distribution of a drug. Peculiarities of a drug sometimes lead to spuriously low serum concentrations and therefore spuriously high V_d values, even if tissue penetration is not unusually good. For example, the apparent V_d of nafcillin is larger and the serum concentrations are lower than would be expected from the degree of lipid solubility or of penetration into peripheral sites because nafcillin is taken up extensively by the liver. Amphotericin B is not well distributed to the periphery, but its serum concentrations are low, resulting in a large estimated V_d value because the drug binds to cholesterol-containing membranes of cells. Thus, the V_d should be considered only as a rough guide to the actual penetration of drugs into cells and specialized sites.

CLINICAL RELEVANCE OF ANTIBIOTIC CONCENTRATIONS *IN VIVO*

The antimicrobial effect of a drug *in vivo* cannot be fully predicted by simple extrapolation from its pharmacokinetic behavior and its effects *in vitro*. This fact is not surprising. Aside from the important effects of host defenses, which are difficult to simulate *in vitro*, there are likely to be marked differences between the situations *in vitro* and *in vivo* in inoculum size and rate of growth of microbial cells, as well as in pH level and other aspects of the microenvironment. All of these factors may have a marked influence on the antibacterial efficacy of the drug.

For most infections, it is not necessary to maintain drug concentrations in the serum at an inhibitory level throughout the treatment period to have a good result. There are several explanations for this finding. One is that the antibacterial effect of the drug may persist up to several hours after the substance is no longer detectable in the environment. The duration of this "postantibiotic effect" depends on the particular species of bacterium and the drug (8). Another explanation is that drug concentrations in extravascular sites may fluctuate much less than in serum (see Fig. 17.4). A third reason is the protective effect of host defenses.

Many studies have attempted to relate the bactericidal titer of antibiotics in the serum to the outcome of infections (21). A few have shown a significant correlation between the serum bactericidal titer and cure of the infection (22–24); others have shown little correlation, again indicating the difficulties in extrapolating from the situation *in vitro* to that *in vivo*. Increased knowledge of the interaction between drugs and microbes *in vitro* and *in vivo* and greater sophistication in the application of computer models hopefully may render such extrapolations more useful. In the last analysis, the determination of the value of an antibiotic in the treatment of clinical infectious diseases must rest on carefully conducted trials in humans.

REFERENCES

1. Tallarida RJ, Murray RB. *Manual of pharmacologic calculations.* New York: Springer-Verlag New York, 1981:46–47.
2. Peterson LIZ, Gerding DN. Prediction of cefazolin penetration into high- and low-protein-containing fluid: new method for performing simultaneous studies. *Antimicrob Agents Chemother* 1978;14:533.
3. Gonda I. On predictions of free antibiotic (cefazolin) concentrations in extravascular fluids from "logarithmic mean serum concentrations." *J Antimicrob Chemother* 1982;9:53.
4. Tsuji A, Miyamoto E, Kubo O, et al. GI absorption of β-lactam antibiotics III. Kinetic evidence for in situ absorption of ionized species of monobasic penicillins and cefazolin from the rat small intestine and structure-absorption rate relationships. *J Pharm Sci* 1979;68:812.
5. Welling PG, Tse FLS. The influence of food on the absorption of antimicrobial agents. *J Antimicrob Chemother* 1982;9:7.
6. Barza M, Giuliano M, Jacobus NV, et al. Effect of broad-spectrum antibiotics on "colonization resistance" of intestinal microflora of humans. *Antimicrob Agents Chemother* 1987;31:723.
7. Cockcroft DW, Gault MH. Prediction of creatinine clearance from serum creatinine. *Nephron* 1976;16:31.
8. Vogelman B, Gudmundsson S, Turnidge J, et al. *In vivo* postantibiotic effect in a thigh infection in neutropenic mice. *J Infect Dis* 1988;157:287.
9. Cutler RE, Gyselynck AM, Fleet WP, et al. Correlation of serum creatinine concentration and gentamicin half-life. *JAMA* 1972;219:1037.
10. McHenry MC, Tavan TL, Gifford RW Jr. Gentamicin dosages for renal insufficiency. *Ann Intern Med* 1971;74:192.
11. Van Etta L, Peterson LIZ, Fasching CE, et al. Effect of the ratio of surface area to volume on the penetration of antibiotics into extravascular spaces in an in vitro model. *J Infect Dis* 1982;146:423.
12. Barza M, Cuchural G. General principles of antibiotic tissue penetration. *J Antimicrob Chemother* 1985;15[Suppl A]:59.
13. Stewart PS, Costerton JW. Antibiotic resistance of bacteria in biofilms. *Lancet* 2001;358:135.
14. Thea D, Barza M. Use of antibacterial agents in infections of the central nervous system. *Infect Dis Clin North Am* 1989;3:553.
15. Schwab JC, Cao Y, Slowik MR, et al. Localization of azithromycin in *Toxoplasma gondii*–infected cells. *Antimicrob Agents Chemother* 1994;38:1620.
16. Barza M. Challenges to antibiotic activity in tissue. *Clin Infect Dis* 1994;19:910.
17. Tulkens PM: Intracellular distribution and activity of antibiotics. *Eur J Clin Microbiol Infect Dis* 1991;10:100.
18. van den Broek PJ. Antimicrobial drugs, microorganisms, and phagocytes. *Rev Infect Dis* 1989;11:213.
19. Lunke RJ, Fitzgerald RH Jr, Washington JA II. Pharmacokinetics of cefamandole in osseous tissue. *Antimicrob Agents Chemother* 1981;19:851.
20. Daly RC, Fitzgerald RH Jr, Washington JA II. Penetration of cefazolin into normal and osteomyelitic canine cortical bone. *Antimicrob Agents Chemother* 1982;22:461.
21. Wolfson JS, Swartz MN. Serum bactericidal activity as a monitor of antibiotic therapy. *N Engl J Med* 1985;312:968.
22. Sculler JP, Klastersky J. Significance of serum bactericidal activity in gram-negative bacillary bacteremia in patients with and without granulocytopenia. *Am J Med* 1984;76:429.
23. Weinstein MP, Stratton CW, Ackley A, et al. Multicenter collaborative evaluation of a standardized serum bactericidal test as a prognostic indicator in infective endocarditis. *Am J Med* 1985;78:262.
24. Weinstein MP, Stratton CW, Hawley HB, et al. Multicenter collaborative evaluation of a standardized serum bactericidal test as a predictor of therapeutic efficacy in acute and chronic osteomyelitis. *Am J Med* 1987;83:218.

Antimicrobial Drugs

CHAPTER 18
Penicillins

William A. Craig

Although Fleming isolated penicillin from *Penicillium notatum* in 1928 (1), it took another decade for this discovery to achieve clinical utility. Investigators at Oxford University, including Florey, Chain, and Abraham, systematically studied the physical, chemical, and structural characteristics of penicillin. They solved its stability problems, determined its structure, and isolated sufficient quantities of the drug to begin clinical testing in 1941 (2,3). Trials in Great Britain and the United States demonstrated dramatic benefits (4,5). Production improvements brought about by deep fermentation procedures, use of cornsteep liquor, and a new strain, *Penicillium chrysogenum*, led to widespread availability of the drug by the end of the 1940s (6,7).

CHEMISTRY

The basic structure of the penicillins is a nucleus with fused β-lactam and thiazolidine rings and a side chain group (Fig.18.1). The penicillin nucleus, 6-aminopenicillanic acid, can be obtained from *P. chrysogenum* in a medium devoid of precursors for a side chain or after removal of the side chain by enzymatic treatment with an amidase (8). The biosynthesis of penicillins represents a combination of two amino acids, cysteine and valine (9). The presence of an intact β-lactam ring is essential for activity. Because a free carboxyl group is also required for activity, most penicillins are available as salts. Carboxyl ester formulations require hydrolysis by nonspecific esterases in serum and tissues for *in vivo* activity.

The side chain provides diversity in the physicochemical and biologic characteristics of the penicillins (10). Different side chains occur naturally (e.g., penicillins F and G), by addition of precursors to the fermentation medium (e.g., penicillin V), or by chemical attachment of specific structures to 6-aminopenicillanic acid. The last-named method has led to the development of many clinically useful semisynthetic penicillins.

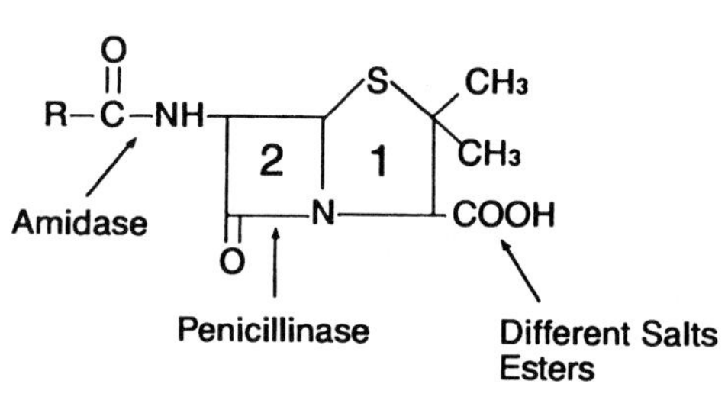

1 = Thiazolidine ring
2 = β-Lactam ring

Figure 18.1. Basic structure of penicillins and sites of β-lactamase inactivation, amidase removal of side chains in synthesis of semisynthetic analogs, and salt and ester formulations.

MECHANISM OF ACTION

Penicillins inhibit bacterial growth by interfering with the synthesis of the cell wall. The first two steps in cell wall synthesis (i.e., formation of an acetylmuramate pentapeptide followed by alternating linkage to acetylglucosamine to form peptidoglycan chains) are unaffected by penicillin. It is the final step in this process, in which strands of peptidoglycan are cross-linked by peptide side chains, that is inhibited by penicillin (11). This transpeptidation reaction occurs at the surface of the cell membrane. Penicillins, because of their structural similarity to the terminal D-alanine-D-alanine of the pentapeptide, bind covalently to the active site of the transpeptidase enzyme (12).

Although acylation of the transpeptidase enzyme is of major importance for the inhibitory effects of penicillin on bacterial growth, there are additional targets or proteins at the cell membrane that bind penicillins (13–15). These membrane components, with molecular weights from 35,000 to 120,000, are called penicillin-binding proteins (PBPs). They are numbered by convention in the order of decreasing molecular weight. PBPs with similar molecular weights are differentiated by letters. Gram-negative bacilli typically contain seven to ten PBPs; gram-positive and gram-negative cocci have three to five PBPs. In addition, some proteins are found in small amounts, whereas others are abundant. In *Escherichia coli*, PBPs 2 and 5 account for about 1% and 65%, respectively, of the binding of penicillin G to these proteins (16).

Some of the PBPs correspond to known enzymes (i.e., transpeptidases and carboxypeptidases) involved in cell wall synthesis. Others have not yet been identified. Binding to some PBPs is associated with bacterial cell death, whereas attachment to others changes bacterial morphologic characteristics. With *Escherichia coli*, binding to the PBP 1 complex correlates with the lethal activity of penicillin. Preferential binding to PBP 2 is associated with loss of rod shape and formation of large ovoid cells. High affinity for PBP 3 results in filament formation without septa (15,16).

Although penicillins are bactericidal drugs, the mechanisms by which they kill bacteria vary for different species. For pneumococci and *E. coli*, killing is caused by lysis resulting from deregulation of the autolytic enzyme system (i.e., peptidoglycan hydrolases) (17,18). Penicillin appears to trigger autolysis by causing the loss of normally present inhibitors (e.g., lipoteichoic acid) of peptidoglycan hydrolases (19). Penicillins may also directly enhance autolytic activity (20). For staphylococci, autolytic activity actually decreases during exposure to penicillin (21). Lysis of these organisms is apparently due to punching of a few minute holes into the cell wall, caused by the lytic activity of vesicular structures called murosomes (22,23). Under normal circumstances, murosomes initiate the separation of bacteria into daughter cells. For *Streptococcus pyogenes*, killing is due to penicillin-induced hydrolysis of cellular ribonucleic acid (24).

In general, the rate of killing of bacteria by penicillins exhibits minimal dependence on the concentration of drug (25). Maximal killing rates are usually observed at concentrations of four times the minimal inhibitory concentration (MIC). Although penicillins induce persistent suppression of bacterial growth (i.e., postantibiotic effect) of several hours' duration with staphylococci, extremely short or no postantibiotic effects are observed for these drugs with streptococci and gram-negative bacilli (26,27). The duration of time that concentrations exceed the MIC is the pharmacokinetic/pharmacodynamic (PK/PD) parameter determining the efficacy of penicillins (28). Durations of 40% to 50% of the dosing interval are associated with high rates of bacterial eradication and clinical success (29).

SPECTRUM OF ACTIVITY

The penicillins are active against a wide variety of aerobic and anaerobic bacteria (30–46) (Tables 18.1–18.3). Because the peptidoglycan cell wall of gram-negative bacteria lies within a lipid membrane, a penicillin must pass this outer barrier before reaching the site of action. Thus, penicillins are more active against gram-positive bacteria than against gram-negative bacteria. However, the presence of different side chains on the penicillin nucleus has significantly altered the spectrum of activity of some derivatives. This also provides a method for classification of the different penicillins. The *natural penicillins* (penicillin G and V) are highly active against streptococci, penicillinase-negative staphylococci, meningococci, anaerobic cocci, *Clostridium perfringens*, and spirochetes. However, penicillin G is 5 to 10 times more active than penicillin V against *Haemophilus influenzae* and gram-negative cocci. The *penicillinase-resistant penicillins* (methicillin, nafcillin, oxacillin, cloxacillin, dicloxacillin, and flucloxacillin) are active against most penicillinase-producing staphylococci. However, they are less potent than other penicillins against other organisms.

The *extended-spectrum penicillins* consist of three groups of drugs. The aminopenicillins (ampicillin and amoxicillin) have enhanced activity against *E. coli*, *Proteus mirabilis*, salmonellae, shigellae, *H. influenzae*, and enterococci. The carboxypenicillins (carbenicillin and ticarcillin) are active against *Pseudomonas aeruginosa* and *Proteus vulgaris* as well as *Providencia*, *Morganella*, and *Enterobacter* species. However, they are significantly less potent than ampicillin against streptococci and enterococci. The ureidopenicillins (mezlocillin, azlocillin, and piperacillin) combine characteristics of both of the other two groups of extended-spectrum penicillins. Some of these drugs are also active against most *Klebsiella* species.

RESISTANCE

The primary mechanism for resistance to the penicillins is enzymatic hydrolysis of the β-lactam ring by β-lactamases (47). Most penicillins are susceptible to inactivation by the penicillinase elaborated by most hospital strains and at least 80% of community isolates of *Staphylococcus aureus*. β-Lactamase production in gram-positive cocci is plasmid-mediated and inducible. When exposed to penicillins, such organisms secrete large amounts of enzyme into the surrounding environment to destroy all available drug. The development of penicillins with bulky side chains resulted in drugs that were more resistant to inactivation by these β-lactamases. However, some strains of *S. aureus* produce excessive amounts of the enzyme and can exhibit borderline susceptibility or resistance to the penicillinase-resistant penicillins (48).

In gram-negative bacilli, β-lactamases are located in the periplasmic space between the outer and inner cell membranes. Penicillin molecules that pass the outer membrane could come in contact with a β-lactamase before reaching the site of action. Although all gram-negative bacteria appear to contain β-lactamase, the type and amount can vary markedly (47). They can be chromosome- or plasmid-mediated, constitutive or inducible, and active against only certain classes of β-lactam drugs or against a broad spectrum of such drugs. The ability of penicillins to inhibit the growth of gram-negative bacilli is dependent on the rate of influx across the outer membrane being greater than the rate of hydrolysis by β-lactamases (49). Alterations in the penicillin side chain that governs gram-negative activity generally enhance penetration across the outer membrane rather than reduce the rate of hydrolysis (50).

The spread of plasmid-mediated β-lactamases such as TEM-1 among Enterobacteriaceae and to *H. influenzae* and *Neisseria gonorrhoeae* has greatly altered susceptibility to the penicillins (51,52). Penicillins are also inactivated by the newer extended-spectrum β-lactamases (ESBLs). Plasmid-mediated staphylococcal penicillinase has also apparently spread to *Enterococcus faecalis* (53). Selection of stable derepressed clones producing a chromosome-mediated β-lactamase has increased resistance to penicillins in *P. aeruginosa* and *Enterobacter* species (54).

Another mechanism of increasing importance for resistance to penicillins involves alteration of the target site. This form of resistance accounts for penicillin resistance in pneumococci, methicillin resistance in staphylococci, and non-β-lactamase resistance to penicillins in *Neisseria* species, *H. influenzae*, and some gram-negative bacilli (55–59). PBPs with reduced affinity for penicillin result from amino acid substitutions and insertions in PBPs. For example, penicillin-resistant isolates of *Streptococcus pneumoniae* have shown up to 38 amino acid substitutions in the sequence of PBP 2b (60). In *S. pneumoniae* and *Neisseria* species, altered PBPs can apparently result from replacement of part of the gene coding for PBP with corresponding genes from related species. For example, the deoxyribonucleic acid sequences of the gene coding for PBP of penicillin-resistant *S. pneumoniae* exhibit striking similarities with those from viridans streptococci (61). Likewise, the gene coding for PBP 2 in penicillin-resistant isolates of *Neisseria meningitidis* and *N. gonorrhoeae* contains part of the gene coding for PBP 2 from *Neisseria flavescens* (62). The chromosomal gene (i.e., *mecA* determinant) that encodes the low-affinity PBP 2a in methicillin-resistant staphylococci may be a fusion product of a regulatory region of the staphylococcal penicillinase gene and a gene coding for PBP of *E. coli* (63).

Altered permeability of the outer membrane of gram-negative bacilli provides another mechanism for resistance to the penicillins. Mutants with reduced or altered porin channels show twofold to 16-fold higher MICs to the broad-spectrum penicillins (64,65). Overexpression of efflux pumps, such as the MexAB-Opr in *P. aeruginosa*, can also produce resistance (66). However, in most resistant clinical isolates, decreased permeability or efflux has occurred jointly with altered PBPs or inducible β-lactamases (67,68).

Resistance to the bactericidal effects of penicillins is known as tolerance (69). This phenomenon is considered present when the minimal bactericidal concentration is significantly greater (usually more than 16-fold) than the MIC (70). It is observed primarily with staphylococci, streptococci, enterococci, and *Listeria monocytogenes* (70, 71). Organisms exhibiting tolerance appear to have reduced or altered autolytic activity with exposure to penicillin. Infections with tolerant bacteria may be associated with a reduced or slower response to penicillin therapy (70,72).

PHARMACOKINETIC PROPERTIES

Changes in the penicillin side chain alter pharmacokinetic properties as well as the spectrum of activity (73–90) (Table 18.4). Penicillin G, methicillin, the carboxypenicillins, and the ureidopenicillins are unstable in the acidic milieu of the stomach (i.e., half-life less than 30 minutes at pH 2) and are largely restricted to parenteral administration. Penicillin V, the isoxazolyl penicillins, the aminopenicillins, and the indanyl ester formulation of carbenicillin are acid stable with half-lives of 2 to 6 hours at pH 2; all are available for use as oral preparations. The acid stability of nafcillin is intermediate. Penicillins not inactivated by gastric acid are generally well absorbed and exhibit peak serum levels in 1 to 2 hours. Among the aminopenicillins, ampicillin exhibits

TABLE 18.1. Activity of Penicillins Against Aerobic Cocci, *Haemophilus influenzae*, and Gram-Positive Bacilli

Organism	Penicillin G	Penicillin V	Methicillin	Nafcillin, oxacillin cloxacillin, dicloxacillin, flucloxacillin	Ampicillin, amoxicillin	Carbenicillin, ticarcillin	Azlocillin, mezlocillin, piperacillin	Amdinocillin	Temocillin
	Mean minimal inhibitory concentration (mg/L)[a]								
Staphylococcus aureus	0.02 (>32)	0.02 (>32)	1 (2)	0.2 (0.4)	0.1 (>32)	1 (16)	1 (16)	2 (>128)	>128
Staphylococcus epidermidis	0.02 (>32)	0.02 (>32)	2 (2)	0.2 (0.4)	0.1 (>32)	2 (16)	0.2 (16)	4 (>128)	>128
Streptococcus pyogenes	0.005	0.01	0.2	0.02	0.01	0.2	0.02	2	128
Streptococcus agalactiae	0.05	0.05	2	0.1	0.2	1	0.2	2	>128
Streptococcus pneumoniae	0.01	0.02	0.1	0.05	0.02	0.4	0.02	2	>128
Penicillin intermediate	1	—	—	2	0.5	8	1	—	—
Penicillin resistant	4	—	—	8	2	64	4	—	—
Viridans group streptococci	0.05	0.05	1	0.2	0.05	0.4	0.2	4	>128
Enterococcus faecalis	2	4	>32	16	1	32	1	>128	>128
Neisseria gonorrhoeae	0.05 (>32)	0.2 (>32)	0.4 (1)	1 (2)	0.05 (>32)	0.1 (8)	0.05 (2)	0.1 (>32)	0.5 (1)
Neisseria meningitidis	0.05	0.2	0.5	4	0.05	0.05	0.01	1	—
Moraxella catarrhalis	0.1 (2)	—	—	—	0.01 (2)	0.1 (4)	0.1 (0.5)	—	—
Haemophilus influenzae	0.4 (>16)	4	2	16	0.4 (>16)	0.4 (4)	0.1 (0.5)	16	0.5 (0.5)
Listeria monocytogenes	0.4	—	>4	4	0.2	2	1	—	0.5 (0.5)
Corynebacterium diphtheriae	0.1	—	—	0.1	0.2	0.2	0.5	—	—

[a]Mean minimal inhibitory concentration for β-lactamase-positive strains is given in parentheses.
Data from references 30–42.

TABLE 18.2. Activity of Penicillins Against Enterobacteriaceae and Pseudomonas

Organism[a]	Mean minimal inhibitory concentration (mg/L)					
	Penicillin G	Ampicillin, amoxicillin	Carbenicillin (C), ticarcillin (T)	Azlocillin (A), mezlocillin (M), piperacillin (P)	Amdinocillin	Temocillin
Escherichia coli	64	4	4	8	1	4
Proteus mirabilis	32	4	2	0.5	4	1
Klebsiella pneumoniae	>128	>128	>128	M, P = 8; A = 32	2	2
Enterobacter sp.	>128	128	8	M, P = 4; A = 16	2	2
Citrobacter sp.	>128	32	8	4	2	4
Serratia sp.	>128	>128	128	32	64	16
Salmonella sp.	8	2; amox = 1	4	2	2	4
Shigella sp.	16	2; amox = 4	2	4	1	2
Morganella sp.	>128	128	16	8	8	2
Providencia sp.	>128	>128	16	8	128	1
Proteus vulgaris	>128	64	8	16	64	2
Acinetobacter sp.	>128	32	16	8	64	>128
Pseudomonas Aeruginosa	>128	>128	T = 32; C = 64	A, P = 8; M = 32	>128	>128

[a]Strains resistant to penicillins are frequently observed; 90% minimal inhibitory concentrations are listed for ampicillin, amoxicillin, ticarcillin, and piperacillin in Table 18.5.
Data from references 41–44.

only 30% to 60% absorption; amoxicillin and the carboxyl ester formulations of ampicillin are almost completely absorbed. Food delays absorption and reduces peak levels of most penicillins. Amoxicillin is affected less by food than ampicillin (82). The ampicillin esters show enhanced absorption when they are taken with food.

Absorption from intramuscular injection sites is also generally rapid, with peak serum levels occurring within 1 hour. Procaine and benzathine salts of penicillin G are relatively insoluble preparations that are absorbed slowly from intramuscular injection sites. The water solubility of procaine and benzathine penicillin G is fourfold and 60-fold less, respectively, than is observed with sodium and potassium salts of the drug (74). Intramuscular administration of these formulations results in lower but more sustained blood levels than those that result from penicillin G.

Distribution of the penicillins within the body is governed by the lipid solubility of the drug and the extent of protein binding. Although penicillins bind almost exclusively to albumin, the extent of binding can vary from 20% to 97% (75). Because only unbound drug can pass through capillary pores into interstitial fluid or across cell membranes into intracellular fluid, avidly bound penicillins tend to exhibit high serum concentrations and low tissue concentrations (91). Likewise, fetal serum and amniotic fluid concentrations of the penicillins tend to correlate with the unbound drug level in maternal serum, rather than the total drug level (92).

In general, the penicillins are largely confined to the extracellular compartment. Nafcillin and the isoxazolyl penicillins have the highest lipid solubility and the best potential for passage across cell membranes into intracellular fluid (93). However, these are the same penicillins that have the highest degree of protein binding (89% to 97%). Drug penetration ex vivo into human erythrocytes is higher for nafcillin and isoxazolyl penicillins than for ampicillin and penicillin G (94). However, the presence of albumin markedly reduces penetration of the highly bound drugs.

Concentrations of unbound drug in various tissues and inflammatory fluids are close to those in serum (77,95). In the absence of infection, concentrations in cerebrospinal fluid (CSF)

TABLE 18.3. Activity of Penicillins Against Anaerobic Bacteria

Organism	Minimal inhibitory concentration (mean/90%) (mg/L)					
	Penicillin G	Oxacillin	Amoxicillin, ampicillin	Carbenicillin ticarcillin	Azlocillin, mezlocillin, piperacillin	Temocillin
Clostridium perfringens	0.1/0.5	0.5/1	0.1/0.5	0.5/2	0.5/2	>128
Eubacterium sp.	0.5/2	2/16	0.2/1	2/16	2/16	—
Peptococcus sp.	0.1/0.5	0.5/4	0.1/0.5	0.1/1	0.1/0.5	128/>128
Peptostreptococcus sp.	0.1/1	0.4/8	0.2/1	0.5/4	0.5/2	16/>128
Propionibacterium sp.	0.1/0.5	0.5/1	0.1/0.5	0.2/1	0.2/1	—
Bacteroides fragilis	16/64	>128	16/64	32/128	32/128	32/64
Prevotella sp.	0.2/8	32	0.2/8	0.5/4	0.5/4	16/64
Fusobacterium sp.	0.1/2	>128	0.1/8	0.5/4	0.1/4	8/64
Veillonella sp.	0.2/1	8/32	0.2/1	2/8	4/32	—

Data from references 41, 42, 45, and 46.

TABLE 18.4. Pharmacokinetic Characteristics of the Penicillins

Drug	Acid stable	Protein binding (%)	Peak serum level (mg/L) Oral dose (500 mg)	Peak serum level (mg/L) Intravenous infusion (1 g)	Route of excretion	Half-life (h) Normal	Half-life (h) Creatinine clearance <10 mL/min
Penicillin G	No	60	2	60[a]	Renal	0.5	5
Penicillin V	Yes	78	5	—	Renal	0.5	4
Methicillin	No	37	—	100	Renal	0.5	4
Nafcillin	Slight	89	4	160	Renal + hepatic	0.5	1
Oxacillin	Yes	93	6	200	Renal + hepatic	0.5	1
Cloxacillin	Yes	94	12	200	Renal + hepatic	0.4	1
Dicloxacillin	Yes	97	15	—	Renal + hepatic	0.4	1
Flucloxacillin	Yes	96	16	180	Renal + hepatic	0.7	1.5
Ampicillin	Yes	18	3.5	100	Renal	0.8	1.6
Amoxicillin	Yes	17	8	100	Renal	1.0	10
Bacampicillin	Yes	—	10	—	Renal	0.9	10
Carbenicillin	No	47	5[b]	170	Renal		See ampicillin
Ticarcillin	No	45	—	170	Renal	1:1	15
Azlocillin	No	40	—	220	Renal	1.2	15
Mezlocillin	No	35	—	200	Renal + hepatic	1.0	5
Piperacillin	No	50	—	200	Renal + hepatic	1.0	4
Clavulanate	Yes	Low	3[c]	5[a]	Renal + hepatic	1.0	4
Sulbactam	No	Low	18[c]	100	Renal	0.8	10
Tazobactam	No	Low	—	26[a]	Renal	1	10
					Renal	1	7

[a]Based on a dose of 1 million units for penicillin G; 100 mg intravenously for clavulanate; and 375 mg intravenously for tazobactam.
[b]Administered as indanyl ester, which is stable to acid.
[c]Based on a dose of 125 mg orally for clavulanate and a dose of 590 mg for sulbactam administered as sultamicillin.
Data from references 74–90.

are less than 3% of the value in serum. The presence of an active transport system that transports penicillins from CSF back to serum contributes to the low drug levels in CSF (96). Infection results in higher, therapeutic levels in CSF, because inflammation enhances penetration and interferes with efflux by active transport (97). Probenecid also blocks active transport and elevates penicillin concentrations in CSF (98). Drug concentrations in human milk, aqueous humor, saliva, tears, respiratory secretions, and prostatic fluid are also lower than those in serum and further reflect the low penetration of penicillins across cell membranes (92,95).

Penicillins are eliminated primarily by the kidney; the major mechanism for renal excretion is tubular secretion. This active transport process is largely unaffected by protein binding and results in rapid excretion of the penicillins, with half-lives ranging from 30 to 80 minutes, and high urinary concentrations. Maximal tubular excretion rates can vary for different penicillins (e.g., 5.5 and 1.0 g/hour for penicillin G and cloxacillin, respectively) (99). Probenecid inhibits this organic acid transport system and prolongs the half-life of penicillins. A daily dose of 2 g gives maximal inhibition of tubular secretion of penicillin (100). Because tubule function is not fully developed until 1 or 2 months of age, renal excretion of penicillins in newborns is markedly slower than in older children, which necessitates dosage modification.

It has been shown that the rapid elimination of penicillin G is followed after several hours by a slow elimination phase with a half-life of about 3 hours (76) (Fig. 18.2). As a result, 1 million units of intravenous penicillin G will provide serum concentrations above the minimal inhibitory concentration for many streptococci for longer than 9 hours. Other penicillins may have a similar slow elimination phase. However, it would be of therapeutic importance only for susceptible organisms.

Penicillins are not extensively metabolized (101). However, breakdown products, such as penicilloic and penicillanic acids, are produced that can contribute to the development of hypersensitivity. Penicillins are excreted into bile, but only nafcillin,

the isoxazolyl penicillins, and the ureidopenicillins exhibit significant elimination (25% to 40%) by this route. Bile levels are two to ten times higher than serum concentrations for penicillin G and the aminopenicillins and 20 to 40 times higher than simultaneous serum levels for nafcillin and the ureidopenicillins (95).

The maximal daily dosages of many penicillins need to be reduced in renal impairment (90). However, significant

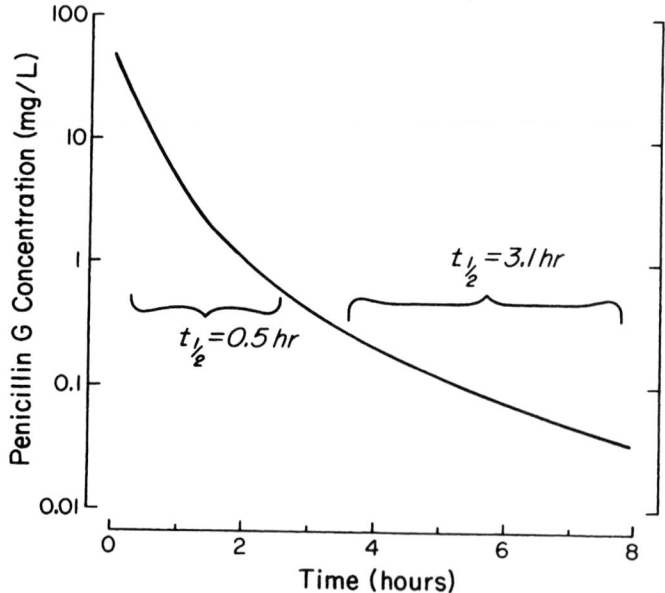

Figure 18.2. Mean serum concentrations for penicillin G in eight normal subjects. (Data from Ebert SC, Leggett J, Vogelman B, et al. Evidence for a slow elimination phase for penicillin G. *J Infect Dis* 1988;158:200, with permission.)

modification of the ureidopenicillins and the penicillinase-resistant penicillins is required only with creatinine clearances less than 10 mL/minute. Although longer half-lives of certain penicillins have been observed in patients with liver disease, the extent of impaired elimination does not require dosage modification unless there is concomitant renal disease (102).

CLINICAL USE OF SPECIFIC AGENTS

Natural Penicillin

PENICILLIN G

Benzylpenicillin, or penicillin G, is still a major drug for the treatment of streptococcal infections (Fig. 18.3). Although *S. pneumoniae* organisms resistant to penicillin have been found in various parts of the world, decreased efficacy of penicillin G has been observed primarily in meningitis (103). In pneumococcal pneumonia, there appears to be no difference with high-dose penicillin therapy in the mortality rates of patients infected by susceptible or resistant strains (104). Penicillin G is highly effective in treatment of *S. pyogenes* infections. It is the major agent for viridans streptococcal endocarditis. The drug is also useful for prophylaxis of bacterial endocarditis and to prevent recurrences of rheumatic fever.

Because nearly all *N. meningitidis* strains are still susceptible, penicillin G remains the drug of choice for meningococcal infections. However, the drug is ineffective in eliminating the meningococcal carrier state. Penicillin G is no longer the drug of choice for *N. gonorrhoeae* infections because a significant number of resistant strains have emerged. Treponemal infections, including all stages of syphilis, are best treated with penicillin G. Although penicillin G is beneficial in late Lyme disease, ceftriaxone may be a more effective agent (105). Penicillin G also reduces morbidity in severe leptospirosis (106).

Penicillin G is still the recommended drug for actinomycosis, rat-bite fever (due to *Streptobacillus moniliformis* or *Spirillum minus*), erysipeloid, fusospirochetal infections, gas gangrene, and periodontal infections (107). Although penicillin G in moderately high concentrations is effective in many anaerobic infections of the lung, clindamycin appears to be more effective in cases of lung abscess (108). While penicillin G appears to be quite effective in cutaneous anthrax, the drug is less effective than ciprofloxacin and doxycycline in animal models (109,110).

Because penicillin G is acid labile, it is generally given by intravenous injection in doses of 0.5 to 1 million units (equivalent to 300 to 600 mg) every 6 hours for many streptococcal infections. However, 12 million to 20 million units (7.2 to 12 g) per day is required for meningitis, endocarditis, and severe infections and for pneumonia caused by resistant strains. Procaine penicillin G, 600,000 units intramuscularly every 12 hours, is as effective as 20 million units of intravenous penicillin G for pneumococcal pneumonia caused by penicillin-susceptible strains (111). In areas where penicillin resistance is not a problem, treatment for gonorrhea includes a dose of 4.8 million units of procaine penicillin G, divided between two sites, injected after a 1-g oral dose of probenecid. Benzathine penicillin G (1.2 to 2.4 million units) provides low serum levels for 3 to 4 weeks. It is indicated for treatment of syphilis, group A β-hemolytic streptococcal pharyngitis, and skin infections and for prevention of streptococcal infections in patients with previous rheumatic fever. Both repository forms produce CSF levels that are too low and variable to be recommended for neurosyphilis, especially in patients infected with human immunodeficiency virus (112).

PENICILLIN V

The phenoxymethyl penicillin is stable in gastric acid and is thus suitable for oral dosing. It can substitute for penicillin G for mild-to-moderate streptococcal infections of the upper respiratory tract, skin, and soft tissues. Daily dosages of 0.5 to 2 g for adults and 25 to 50 mg/kg for children should be given in two to four divided doses. Once-daily dosing for streptococcal pharyngitis results in an unacceptable failure rate (113). Although penicillin V is effective in early Lyme disease, it may not be as effective as tetracycline in preventing late complications (114). Phenethicillin, the phenoxyethyl derivative of penicillin G, has pharmacologic properties similar to those of penicillin V but is not available in the United States.

Penicillinase-Resistant Penicillin

METHICILLIN

Methicillin was the first available penicillin that was resistant to the penicillinase of staphylococci (Fig. 18.4). Despite the

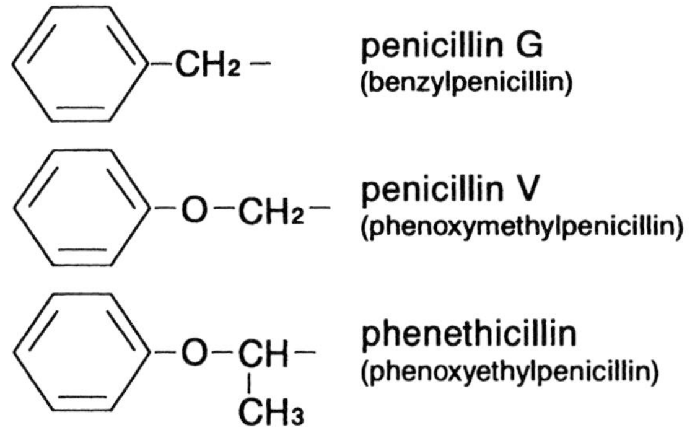

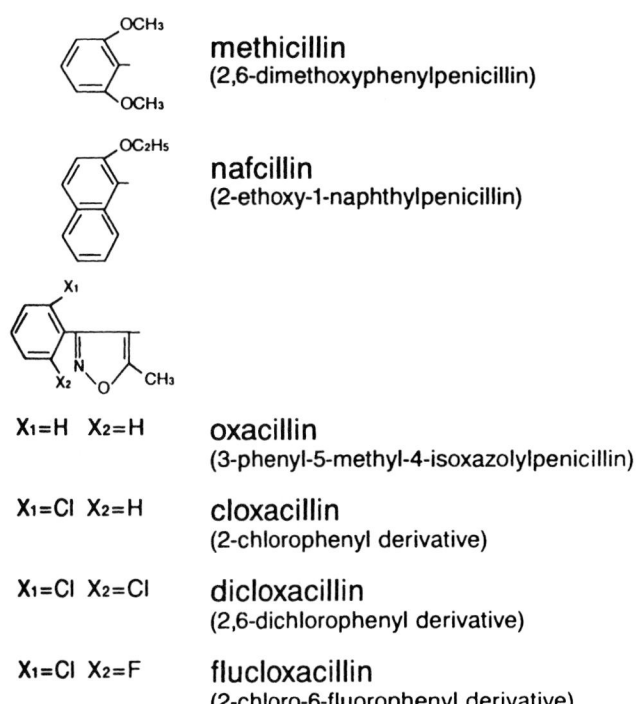

Figure 18.4. Structure of side chains for penicillinase-resistant penicillins.

Figure 18.3. Structure of side chains for natural and related penicillins.

increasing occurrence of methicillin-resistant strains (which are resistant to all penicillins), this drug and the other penicillinase-resistant penicillins remain the drugs of choice for most *S. aureus* infections. However, the high prevalence of methicillin resistance in coagulase-negative staphylococci has reduced the use of these drugs for these organisms (115). Because methicillin is rapidly destroyed by gastric acid, the drug is available only for parenteral administration. The usual daily dosage is 4 to 12 g for adults and 100 to 300 mg/kg for children, given in four to six divided doses.

NAFCILLIN

Nafcillin is approximately ten times more potent than methicillin against staphylococci and streptococci. It is, however, more highly protein bound than methicillin. When both binding and intrinsic antimicrobial activity are taken into consideration, the biologic activities of both drugs in serum are similar (116). Although the indications and dosage regimens for this drug are the same as those for methicillin, nafcillin may be the preferred agent for staphylococcal central nervous system infections because of enhanced CSF penetration (117). Nafcillin may also be associated with a lower frequency of adverse reactions than methicillin (118). The drug's high biliary excretion rate eliminates the need for dosage modification in renal impairment. Because nafcillin is not completely stable to acid, its absorption is erratic and results in variable serum levels.

ISOXAZOLYL PENICILLINS

These drugs are stable to gastric acid. Thus, they are used for oral therapy for less severe staphylococcal infections. Osteomyelitis and septic arthritis, in both children and adults, have been effectively treated with oral therapy (119,120). As with nafcillin, the avid protein binding of these drugs is compensated for by their high intrinsic activity. Cloxacillin and dicloxacillin yield higher total and unbound serum concentrations than does oxacillin (75). Flucloxacillin, which is not available in the United States, exhibits the best oral absorption. The usual oral daily dosage for these drugs is 1 to 4 g for adults and 50 to 100 mg/kg for children, given in four divided doses. Parenteral oxacillin is available and can be used at dosages similar to those of nafcillin and methicillin. Parenteral cloxacillin, which is also not available in the United States, has been shown to reduce perioperative infections after craniotomy (121). All of the isoxazolyl penicillins have extensive hepatic elimination and do not require modification with renal impairment.

Aminopenicillins

AMPICILLIN

Aminobenzylpenicillin or ampicillin provides effective therapy for many upper respiratory tract infections and exacerbations of chronic bronchitis due to *S. pneumoniae*, *Moraxella catarrhalis*, and *H. influenzae* (Fig. 18.5). However, the relatively high frequency of β-lactamase–positive strains of *H. influenzae* and *M. catarrhalis* in many locations has reduced empirical use of ampicillin in more severe infections. Its use for meningitis in children, *Salmonella* and *Shigella* infections, and urinary tract infections has also been curtailed by the appearance of resistant strains and the availability of effective alternatives. In pyelonephritis, ampicillin is less effective than trimethoprim-sulfamethoxazole (122). Ampicillin is preferred to penicillin G for enterococcal infections and those due to *L. monocytogenes*. Ampicillin plus an aminoglycoside is effective for many community-acquired gram-negative infections. This combination is also recommended for endocarditis

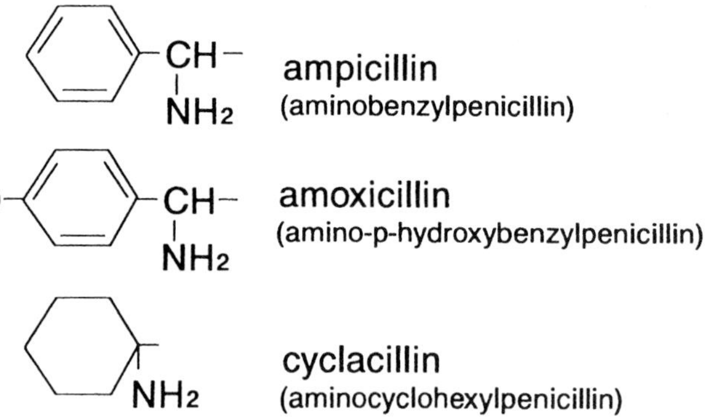

Figure 18.5. Structure of side chains for aminopenicillins.

prophylaxis for patients with high risk and for gastrointestinal and genitourinary procedures (123).

Although ampicillin is stable in gastric acid, oral absorption is incomplete. The usual daily dosage is 1 to 4 g for adults and 25 to 100 mg/kg for children, given in four or six divided doses. Daily doses as high as 8 to 16 g (200 to 400 mg/kg for children) are used for meningitis and other severe infections.

AMOXICILLIN

Amoxicillin is the p-hydroxy derivative of ampicillin. This change primarily enhances oral absorption, resulting in blood levels that are two to three times higher than those obtained with similar doses of ampicillin. Amoxicillin is also the most potent penicillin against penicillin-resistant pneumococci (34). Thus, it remains the drug of choice for initial treatment of otitis media in children. Amoxicillin, in combination with other antibiotics or antiulcer drugs, is also used in the treatment of *Helicobacter pylori* infections (124). Other indications for the use of amoxicillin parallel those for ampicillin. However, due to its greater absorption, less drug is left in the intestinal tract, which markedly reduces its efficacy in shigellosis. In the United States, amoxicillin is available only for oral administration. The usual daily dosage is 0.75 to 1.5 g for adults and 20 to 40 mg/kg for children, given in three divided doses. A single 3-g dose of amoxicillin has been effective in uncomplicated cystitis in women (125). Amoxicillin is also the recommended drug for oral prophylaxis against endocarditis; a single 2-g dose 1 hour before the procedure is now recommended (123). Cyclacillin, another well-absorbed analog of ampicillin, is no longer available in the United States.

AMPICILLIN ESTERS

Bacampicillin, pivampicillin, and talampicillin are 1-carboxyl esters of ampicillin. They are inactive until hydrolyzed to ampicillin by esterase enzymes present in the gastrointestinal epithelium and in serum (126). These ester formulations result in almost complete absorption of ampicillin. Only bacampicillin is available in the United States. It produces peak blood levels of ampicillin that are even slightly higher than those of amoxicillin (83). The indications for use are the same as for amoxicillin. The usual daily dosage is 0.8 to 1.6 g (equivalent to 0.56 to 1.12 g of ampicillin) for adults and 12.5 to 25 mg/kg for children, given in two divided doses.

Carboxypenicillins

CARBENICILLIN

Carbenicillin is the carboxybenzyl derivative of penicillin (Fig. 18.6). Although the main indications for its use are infections

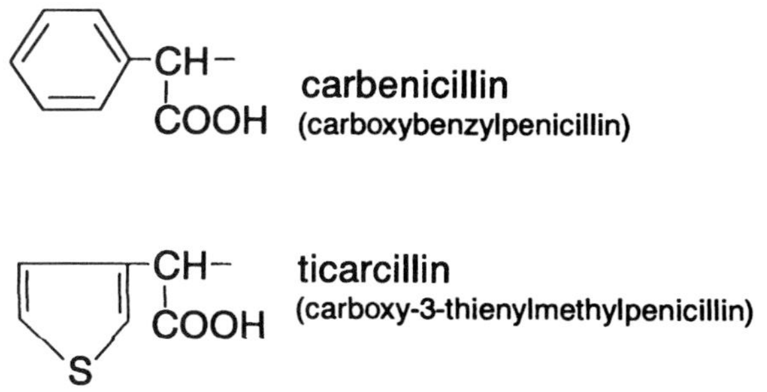

Figure 18.6. Structure of side chains for carboxypenicillins.

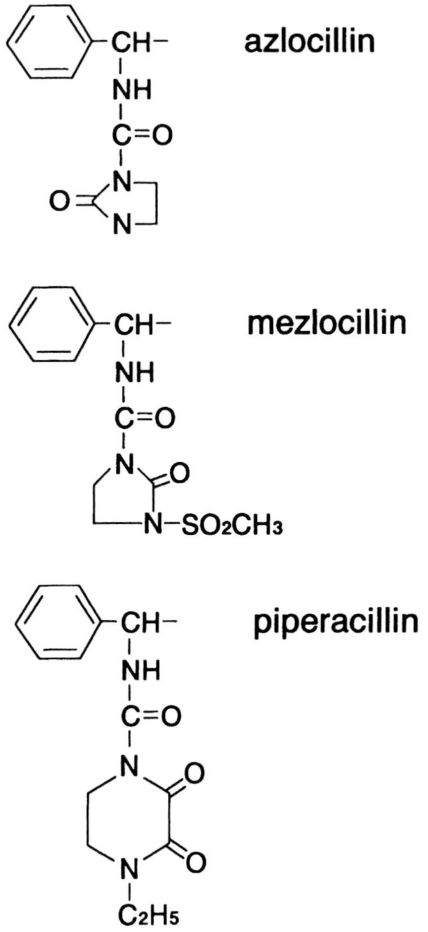

Figure 18.7. Structure of side chains for ureidopenicillins.

caused by *P. aeruginosa*, carbenicillin is active against other ampicillin-resistant gram-negative bacilli, such as *P. vulgaris* as well as *Enterobacter*, *Morganella*, and *Providencia* species (127). A daily intravenous dose of 30 to 40 g (400 to 600 mg/kg for children) is required for systemic pseudomonal infections. Because carbenicillin is a disodium salt, each gram contains 4.7 mEq of sodium; large doses can precipitate congestive heart failure as well as induce hypokalemia and inhibit platelet function. Parenteral carbenicillin is no longer available in the United States. Indanyl carbenicillin is an α-carboxyl ester of carbenicillin that is resistant to acid inactivation (128). This oral formulation is useful only for urinary tract infections, especially those due to *P. aeruginosa*. The daily dose is 1.5 to 3.0 g, given in four divided doses.

TICARCILLIN

Ticarcillin has replaced carbenicillin in the treatment of serious pseudomonal infections because it has similar pharmacologic properties but is twofold to fourfold more active against *P. aeruginosa* (129). This reduces the recommended daily dose to 4 g for urinary tract infections and 200 to 300 mg/kg (approximately 15 to 21 g) for systemic infections, given in four to six divided doses. The lower dose of ticarcillin also reduces the frequency of adverse reactions observed with carbenicillin (130).

Ureidopenicillins

PIPERACILLIN

The antimicrobial spectrum of iperacillin combines the activities of ampicillin and ticarcillin (Fig. 18.7). The drug is also active against many isolates of *Klebsiella* (131). Its pharmacologic properties are similar to those of the carboxypenicillins except that about a third of the drug is eliminated by biliary excretion. Thus, dosage modification is required only with severe renal impairment. The drug is used for the treatment of serious gram-negative infections, including those due to *P. aeruginosa* (132). Its high biliary excretion may enhance efficacy in the treatment of biliary tract infections. Its clearance with increasing concentrations is nonlinear because of saturation of biliary excretion. This allows less frequent dosing than with the carboxypenicillins (i.e., every 6 hours rather than every 4 hours). The usual daily dose is 4 to 8 g for urinary tract infections and 12 to 18 g (200 to 300 mg/kg) for systemic infections. Because the drug is a derivative of ampicillin, it is a monosodium salt and less likely to result in the adverse reactions associated with the carboxypenibcillins.

AZLOCILLIN

Azlocillin is similar in pharmacologic action and antimicrobial spectrum to piperacilliin, except that it is relatively inactive

against *Klebsiella* species (133). Dosage regimens are similar to those for piperacillin. It is no longer available in the United States.

MEZLOCILLIN

Mezlocillin is about fourfold less active than piperacillin and azlocillin against *P. aeruginosa*, but unlike azlocillin, it maintains its activity against *Klebsiella* species. Its pharmacologic properties, indications for use, and usual dosage regimens are similar to those for piperacillin (134).

β-Lactamase Inhibitors

Clavulanic acid, the first β-lactamase inhibitor, is produced by *Streptomyces clavuligerus* (133) (Fig. 18.8). Its structure differs from penicillin in that it has no side chain on the β-lactam ring, has an oxygen atom in place of the sulfur atom, and contains a hydroxyethylidene substitution on the oxazolidine ring. Sulbactam and tazobactam are semisynthetic penicillanic acid sulfones (134). All three compounds have weak antibacterial activity except for modest activity against *Neisseria* species. Sulbactam and tazobactam are also active against *Acinetobacter calcoaceticus*. They are irreversible "suicide" inhibitors of staphylococcal penicillinase and Richmond-Sykes class II to class V β-lactamases of gram-negative bacilli (135). This includes most of the plasmid-mediated β-lactamases (e.g., TEM-, SHV-, OXA-, and PSE-type

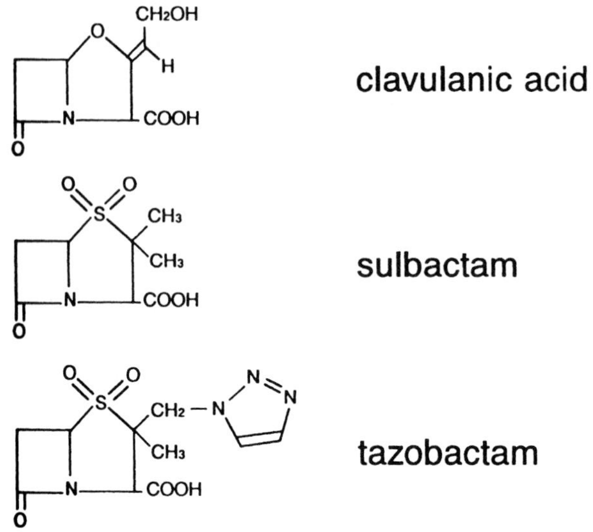

Figure 18.8. Structure of side chains for β-lactamase inhibitors.

enzymes) and the chromosomal β-lactamases of *Klebsiella* and *Bacteroides* species. However, the chromosomal class I enzymes present in many gram-negative bacilli are not inhibited by these drugs. Nevertheless, a β-lactamase inhibitor combined with amoxicillin, ampicillin, ticarcillin, and piperacillin enhances their activity against β-lactamase-producing strains of staphylococci, gonococci, *H. influenzae*, *M. catarrhalis*, *Bacteroides* and *Klebsiella* species, and *E. coli* (136–143) (Table 18.5). The activity against other gram-negative bacilli is largely unaffected by these β-lactamase inhibitors.

The pharmacokinetic profile of clavulanic acid is similar to that of amoxicillin (88). In contrast, sulbactam and tazobactam are poorly absorbed orally. With intravenous administration, the pharmacologic action of sulbactam and tazobactam is similar to that of ampicillin (89,144). All three β-lactamase inhibitors are eliminated predominantly by the kidney with a half-life of approximately 1 hour, have low protein binding, and distribute primarily to extracellular fluid.

AMOXICILLIN-CLAVULANATE

Only the oral formulation of amoxicillin-clavulanate is available in the United States. It has been especially useful for otitis media, sinusitis, and lower respiratory tract infections due to penicillin-resistant pneumococci and β-lactamase-producing *H. influenzae* and *M. catarrhalis* (145) It is effective in staphylococcal and streptococcal skin infections and is the recommended agent for infections after animal and human bites (146). The usual daily dose is 1.75 g of amoxicillin plus 0.275 g of clavulanate given in two divided doses or 0.75 to 1.5 g of amoxicillin plus 0.375 g of clavulanate given in three divided doses. Newer doses with 14:1 and 16:1 ratios of amoxicillin-clavulanate (90/6.4 mg/kg for pediatric use and 4.0/0.25 g for adult use, both given in two divided doses) are designed to enhance eradication of more resistant pneumococci with MICs of 2 to 4 μg/mL (147,148). Administration of more than 0.375 g of clavulanate per day is associated with a high frequency of diarrhea.

AMPICILLIN-SULBACTAM

Only the parenteral fixed 2:1 ratio of ampicillin-sulbactam is currently available in the United States. Its indications are similar to those for amoxicillin-clavulanate but include intraabdominal and gynecologic infections and more severe skin and soft tissue infections (149). The usual dose is 6 to 12 g/d (4 to 8 g of ampicillin), divided into four doses.

TICARCILLIN-CLAVULANATE

A fixed 30:1 ratio of ticarcillin-clavulanate is available for intravenous administration. Its broad spectrum of activity has resulted in successful treatment of nosocomial pneumonia, intraabdominal infections, and severe skin and soft tissue infections (150). This combination is also active against many *Stenotrophomonas* (formerly *Xanthomonas*) *maltophilia* strains (151). A dose of 3.1 g is given four to six times daily.

PIPERACILLIN-TAZOBACTAM

A fixed 8:1 mixture of piperacillin and tazobactam provides the broadest spectrum of activity of any of the β-lactamase inhibitor combinations (152). Its indications are similar to those for ticarcillin-clavulanate, except that this combination has weak

TABLE 18.5.   Effect of β-Lactamase Inhibitors on Activity of Amoxicillin, Ampicillin, Ticarcillin, and Piperacillin Against Gram-Positive and Gram-Negative Bacteria

| Organism | Minimal inhibitory concentration (mg/L) for 90% of strains | | | | | | |
	Amoxicillin, ampicillin	Amoxicillin-clavulanate	Ampicillin-sulbactam	Ticarcillin	Ticarcillin-clavulanate	Piperacillin	Piperacillin-tazobactam
Staphylococcus aureus	>128	0.5	2	16	2	32	2
Neisseria gonorrhoeae	128	1	1	32	0.5	—	—
Moraxella catarrhalis	16	0.2	0.25	4	0.5	8	1
Haemophilus influenzae	64	2	1	8	0.5	64	1
Bacteroides fragilis	128	2	2	>128	2	>128	4
Escherichia coli	>128	32	16	>128	32	>128	16
Proteus mirabilis	4	0.5	1	8	1	32	2
Proteus vulgaris	>128	8	16	32	1	32	2
Klebsiella pneumoniae	>128	8	16	>128	8	>128	16
Enterobacter sp.	>128	>128	16	128	128	>128	128
Serratia sp.	>128	>128	>128	128	64	>128	32
Acinetobacter sp.	64	64	4	32	32	64	16
Pseudomonas aeruginosa	>128	>128	>128	64	64	64	64

Data from references 138–143.

activity against *S. maltophilia*. The usual dose is 3.75 g every 4 to 6 hours.

Other Penicillins

AMDINOCILLIN

Amdinocillin, formerly named mecillinam, is active against many of the Enterobacteriaceae but has poor activity against gram-positive bacteria (153). Because it binds primarily to PBP 2, the drug acts synergistically with other β-lactams. It is not acid stable and must be given orally as a pivaloyl ester or parenterally. It has been used for urinary tract infections, but it is not currently available in the United States (154).

TEMOCILLIN

This 6-α-methoxy derivative of ticarcillin is resistant to inactivation by β-lactamases. It is active against most of the Enterobacteriaceae but has poor activity against gram-positive bacteria and *P. aeruginosa* (155). Because of its long half-life, it is administered twice daily. Although it has been effective in severe gram-negative infections, it is not available in the United States (156).

ADVERSE REACTIONS

Hypersensitivity reactions are the most common adverse effects associated with penicillin therapy. They are mediated by antibodies, whose production is induced by penicillin degradation products bound to protein (i.e., haptens). The penicilloyl derivative, which results from the opening of the β-lactam ring, accounts for the largest amount of protein bound degradation products and is known as the major determinant of penicillin allergy (157). Additional metabolites (e.g., penicilloate and penilloate derivatives) are present in smaller amounts and are called the minor determinants. Virtually everyone makes antibodies after exposure to penicillins, but these are primarily of the immunoglobulin M and immunoglobulin G classes. However, the rarer immunoglobulin E antibodies are associated with immediate hypersensitivity reactions. Anaphylaxis is seen in 0.004% to 0.015% of cases; urticaria occurs in 1% to 5% (158). Both determinants can mediate each reaction. However, minor determinants are associated more with anaphylaxis; the major determinant is involved more with urticarial reactions.

Immunoglobulin M and immunoglobulin G antibodies may be involved in non-urticarial skin reactions. Morbilliform rashes occur in 5% to 9% of individuals receiving ampicillin but in only 2% to 3% of those receiving penicillin G (159–161). The occurrence of ampicillin rashes is also enhanced by Epstein-Barr virus and cytomegalovirus infections and by concomitant use of allopurinol (162). Although erythema multiforme and exfoliative dermatitis are rare reactions to the penicillins, these β-lactams are the most common known cause of Stevens-Johnson syndrome (163). Serum sickness is an uncommon adverse effect of penicillins and results from deposition of immune complexes in tissue. Drug fever may have a similar mechanism.

Cytotoxic reactions from immunoglobulin G and immunoglobulin M antibodies can account for hematologic side effects observed with the penicillins. Coombs-positive hemolytic anemia usually results from antipenicillin antibodies reacting with drug already bound to red blood cell membranes (164). Complement is not activated, and intravascular hemolysis rarely occurs. Instead, these cells are removed extravascularly and de-

stroyed by the reticuloendothelial system. Similar mechanisms may cause the more commonly observed neutropenia, which appears to be enhanced by high-dose therapy (165,166). Although platelet dysfunction can also result from large doses, especially those of carbenicillin and ticarcillin, clinical bleeding is uncommon. By binding to platelet membranes, penicillins impair the interaction of agonists with receptors on the platelet surface (167,168).

The interstitial nephritis seen with penicillins is basically a cytotoxic hypersensitivity reaction. Penicilloyl metabolites initially bind to kidney tissue. Antipenicillin antibodies then react with the penicillin and complement is activated, resulting in cellular damage (169). Tubule basement membrane can be released in the process, and antibodies to this antigen may contribute to the kidney damage (170). Cell-mediated toxicity may also play a role in this adverse reaction (171). Although this complication has been reported with most penicillins, it is apparently most commonly observed with methicillin, prolonged therapy, and daily doses greater than 6 g (117).

High doses of penicillins, especially the carboxypenicillins, can produce fluid overload because of their sodium content. Hypokalemia results because large amounts of these drugs in the distal tubule act as nonreabsorbable anions, creating a favorable gradient for excessive excretion of potassium (172,173).

Myoclonic jerks, hyperreflexia, seizures, and coma have been associated with intrathecal instillations of various penicillins and with high-dose intravenous therapy, primarily in patients with renal impairment (174). Decreased protein binding and inhibition of active transport from the CSF occur in uremia and may contribute to enhanced toxicity in patients with renal impairment (175,176).

Gastrointestinal reactions, including enterocolitis due to *Clostridium difficile*, can occur with all penicillins. Diarrhea has been most common with oral ampicillin and combinations with β-lactamase inhibitors. Hepatotoxicity is uncommon and observed primarily with oxacillin and carbenicillin (177,178). The frequency of oxacillin hepatotoxicity appears to be increased in patients infected with human immunodeficiency virus (179).

Drug interactions with penicillins are uncommon. Nafcillin has resulted in a few cases of warfarin resistance and subtherapeutic cyclosporine levels (180,181). Penicillins, especially the carboxypenicillins and ureidopenicillins, can inactivate gentamicin and tobramycin (182). This inactivation is insignificant in patients with normal renal function. With renal impairment, concomitant administration of a penicillin can shorten aminoglycoside half-lives, necessitating more frequent dosing (183).

REFERENCES

1. Fleeting A. On antibacterial action of cultures on penicillium, with special reference to their use in isolation of *B. influenzae*. *Br J Exp Pathol* 1929;10: 226.
2. Chain E, Florey HW, Gardner AD, et al. Penicillin as chemotherapeutic agent. *Lancet* 1940;2:226.
3. Abraham EP, Chain E, Fletcher CM, et al. Further observations on penicillin. *Lancet* 1941;2:177.
4. Florey ME, Florey HW. General and local administration of penicillin. *Lancet* 1943;1:387.
5. Keefer CS, Blake FG, Marshall EK Jr, et al. Penicillin in the treatment of respiratory infections; a report of 500 cases; statement by committee on chemotherapeutic and other agents. *JAMA* 1943;122:1217.
6. Raper KB, Alexander DF, Coghill RD. Penicillin; natural variation and penicillin production in *Penicillium notatum* and allied species. *J Bacteriol* 1944;48:639.
7. Moyer AJ, Coghill RD. Penicillin; production of penicillin in surface cultures. *J Bacteriol* 1946;51:57.

8. Batchelor FR, Doyle FP, Naylor JHC, et al. Synthesis of penicillin: 6-aminoperucillanic acid in penicillin fermentations. *Nature* 1959;183:257.
9. Queener SW. Molecular biology of penicillin and cephalosporin biosynthesis. *Antimicrob Agents Chemother* 1990;34:943.
10. Hou JP, Poole JW. β-Lactam antibiotics; their physicochemical properties and biological activities in relation to structure. *J Pharm Sci* 1971;60:503.
11. Wise EM Jr, Park JT. Penicillin: its basic site of action as an inhibitor of a peptide cross-linking reaction in cell wall mucopeptide synthesis. *Proc Natl Acad Sci USA* 1965;54:75.
12. Tipper DJ, Strominger JL. Mechanism of action of penicillins: a proposal based on their structural similarity to aryl-D-alanyl-D-alanine. *Proc Natl Acad Sci USA* 1965;54:1133.
13. Tomasz A. Penicillin-binding proteins in bacteria. *Ann Intern Med* 1982; 96:502.
14. Waxman DJ, Strominger JL. Penicillin binding proteins and the mechanism of action of beta-lactam antibiotics. *Annu Rev Biochem* 1983;52:825.
15. Spratt BG. Distinct penicillin-binding proteins involved in the division, elongation and shape of *Escherichia coli* K12. *Proc Natl Acad Sci USA* 1975;72: 2999.
16. Suzuki H, Nishimura Y, Hirota Y. On the process of cellular division in *Escherichia coli*: a series of mutants of *E. coli* altered in the penicillin-binding proteins. *Proc Natl Acad Sci USA* 1978;75:664.
17. Tomasz A, Waks S. Mechanism of action of penicillin: triggering of the pneumococcal autolytic enzyme by inhibitors of cell wall synthesis. *Proc Natl Acad Sci USA* 1975;72:4162.
18. Kitano K, Tomasz A. *Escherichia coli* mutants tolerant to beta-lactam antibiotics. *J Bacteriol* 1979;140:955.
19. Höltje JV, Tomasz A. Lipoteichoic acid: a specific inhibitor of autolysin activity in pneumococcus. *Proc Natl Acad Sci USA* 1975;72:1690.
20. Fontana R, Satta G, Romanzi CA. Penicillins activate autolysins extracted from both *Escherichia coli* and *Klebsiella pneumoniae* envelopes. *Antimicrob Agents Chemother* 1977;12:745.
21. Reinicke B, Bhimel P, Labischinski H, et al. Neither an enhancement of autolytic wall degradation nor an inhibition of the incorporation of cell wall material are pre-requisites for penicillin-induced bacteriolysis in staphylococci. *Arch Microbiol* 1985;141:309.
22. Giesbrecht P, Labischinski H, Wecke J. A special morphogenetic wall defect and the subsequent activity of "murosomes" as the very reason for penicillin-induced bacteriolysis in staphylococci. *Arch Microbiol* 1985;141:315.
23. Maidhof H, Johannsen L, Labischinski H, et al. Onset of penicillin-induced bacteriolysis in staphylococci is cell cycle dependent. *J Bacteriol* 1989;171:2252.
24. McDowell TD, Reed KE. Mechanism of penicillin killing in the absence of bacterial lysis. *Antimicrob Agents Chemother* 1989;33:1680.
25. Vogelman B, Craig WA. Kinetics of antimicrobial activity. *J Pediatr* 1986; 108:835.
26. Craig WA, Gudmundsson S. Postantibiotic effect. In: Lorian V, ed. *Antibiotics in laboratory medicine*, 4th ed. Baltimore: Williams & Wilkins, 1996:296–329.
27. Vogelman B, Gudmundsson S, Turnidge J, et al. In-vivo postantibiotic effect in a thigh infection in neutropenic mice. *J Infect Dis* 1988;157:287.
28. Vogelman B, Gudmundsson S, Leggett J, et al. Correlation of antimicrobial pharmacokinetic parameters with therapeutic efficacy in an animal model. *J Infect Dis* 1987;158:831.
29. Craig WA. Pharmacokinetic/pharmacodynamic parameters: rationale for antibacterial dosing of mice and men. *Clin Infect Dis* 1998;26:1.
30. Sabath LD, Gamer C, Wilcox C, et al. Susceptibility of *Staphylococcus aureus* and *Staphylococcus epidermidis* to 65 antibiotics. *Antimicrob Agents Chemother* 1976;9:962.
31. Finland M, Garner C, Wilcox C, et al. Susceptibility of beta-hemolytic streptococci to 65 antibacterial agents. *Antimicrob Agents Chemother* 1976;9:11.
32. Persson KM-S, Forsgren A. Antimicrobial susceptibility of group B streptococci. *Eur J Clin Microbiol* 1986;5:165.
33. Linares J, Alonso T, Perez JL, et al. Decreased susceptibility of penicillin-resistant pneumococci to twenty-four β-lactam antibiotics. *J Antimicrob Chemother* 1992;30:279.
34. Butler DL, Gagnon RC, Miller LA, et al. Differences between the activity of penicillin, amoxicillin, and co-amoxyclav against 5,252 *Streptococcus pneumoniae* isolates tested in the Alexander Project 1992–1996. *J Antimicrob Chemother* 1999;43:777.
35. Pankuch GA, Jacobs MR, Appelbaum PC. Susceptibilities of 200 penicillin-susceptible and -resistant pneumococci to piperacillin, piperacillin-tazobactam, ticarcillin, ticarcillin-clavulanate, ampicillin, ampicillin-sulbactam, ceftazidime, and ceftriaxone. *Antimicrob Agents Chemother* 1994;38: 2905.
36. Cooksey RC, Swenson JM. In vitro antimicrobial inhibition patterns of nutritionally variant streptococci. *Antimicrob Agents Chemother* 1979;16:514.
37. Pérez JL, Riera L, Valls F, et al. A comparison of the in-vitro activity of seventeen antibiotics against *Streptococcus faecalis*. *J Antimicrob Chemother* 1987;20:357.
38. Hall WH, Schierl EA, Maccani JE. Comparative susceptibility of penicillinase-positive and -negative *Neisseria gonorrhoeae* to 30 antibiotics. *Antimicrob Agents Chemother* 1979;15:562.
39. Trallero EP, Arenzana JMG, Ayestaran I, et al. Comparative activity in vitro of 16 antimicrobial agents against penicillin susceptible meningococci and meningococci with diminished susceptibility to penicillin. *Antimicrob Agents Chemother* 1989;33:1622.

40. Doern GV, Tubert TA. In vitro activities of 39 antimicrobial agents for *Branhamella catarrhalis* and comparison of results with different quantitative susceptibility test methods. *Antimicrob Agents Chemother* 1988;32:259.
41. Wiedemann B, Grimm H. Susceptibility to antibiotics: species incidence and trends. In: Lorian V, ed. *Antibiotics in laboratory medicine*, 4th ed. Baltimore: Williams & Wilkins, 1996:900–1168.
42. Neu HC. Structure-activity relationships of new β-lactam compounds and in vitro activity against common bacteria. *Rev Infect Dis* 1983;5[Suppl 2]: S319.
43. Parry MF, Folta D. The in vitro activity of mezlocillin against community hospital isolates in comparison to other penicillins and cephalosporins. *J Antimicrob Chemother* 1983;11[Suppl C]:97.
44. Verbist L. Comparison of the activities of the new ureidopenicillins piperacillin, mezlocillin, azlocillin, and Bay k 4999 against gram-negative organisms. *Antimicrob Agents Chemother* 1979;16:115.
45. Suffer VL, Finegold SM. Susceptibility of anaerobic bacteria to 23 antimicrobial agents. *Antimicrob Agents Chemother* 1976;10:736.
46. Appelbaum PC, Chatterton SA. Susceptibility of anaerobic bacteria to ten antimicrobial agents. *Antimicrob Agents Chemother* 1978;14:371.
47. Livermore DM. β-Lactamases in laboratory and clinical resistance. *Clin Microbiol Rev* 1995;8:557.
48. McDougal LK, Thornsberry C. The role of β-lactamase in staphylococcal resistance to penicillinase-resistant penicillins and cephalosporins. *J Clin Microbiol* 1986;23:832.
49. Nikaido H. Outer membrane barrier as a mechanism of antimicrobial resistance. *Antimicrob Agents Chemother* 1989;33:1831.
50. Nikaido H. Role of permeability barriers in resistance to β-lactam antibiotics. *Pharmacol Ther* 1985;27:197.
51. Medeiros AA, O'Brien TF. Ampicillin-resistant *Haemophilus influenzae* type B possessing a TEM-type beta-lactamase but little permeability barrier to ampicillin. *Lancet* 1975;1:716.
52. Elwell LP, Roberts M, Mayer LW, et al. Plasmid-mediated β-lactamase production in *Neisseria gonorrhoeae*. *Antimicrob Agents Chemother* 1977;11: 528.
53. Murray BE, Mederski-Samoraj B, Foster SK, et al. In-vitro studies of plasmid-mediated penicillinase from *Streptococcus faecalis* suggest a staphylococcal origin. *J Clin Invest* 1986;77:289.
54. Sanders CC, Sanders WE Jr. Type 1 beta-lactamases of gram-negative bacteria: interactions with beta-lactam antibiotics. *J Infect Dis* 1986;154:792.
55. Malouin F, Bryan LE. Modification of penicillin-binding proteins as mechanisms of β-lactam resistance. *Antimicrob Agents Chemother* 1986;30:1.
56. Chambers HF. Methicillin-resistant staphylococci. *Clin Microbiol Rev* 1988; 1:173.
57. Jabes D, Nachman S, Tomasz A. Penicillin-binding protein families: evidence for the clonal nature of penicillin resistance in clinical isolates of pneumococci. *J Infect Dis* 1989;159:16.
58. Mendelman PM, Campos J, Chaffin DO, et al. Relative penicillin G resistance in *Neisseria meningitidis* and reduced affinity of penicillin-binding protein 3. *Antimicrob Agents Chemother* 1988;32:706.
59. Mendelman PM, Chaffin DO, Kalaitzoglou G. Penicillin-binding proteins and ampicillin resistance in *Haemophilus influenzae*. *J Antimicrob Chemother* 1990;25:525.
60. Smith AM, Klugman KP. Alterations in penicillin-binding protein 2B from penicillin-resistant wild-type strains of *Streptococcus pneumoniae*. *Antimicrob Agents Chemother* 1995;39:859.
61. Coffey TJ, Dowson CG, Daniels M, et al. Genetics and molecular biology of β-lactam-resistant pneumococci. *Microb Drug Resist* 1995;1:29.
62. Spratt BG, Zhang Q-Y, Jones DM, et al. Recruitment of a penicillin-binding protein gene from *Neisseria flavescens* during the emergence of penicillin resistance in *Neisseria meningitidis*. *Proc Natl Acad Sci USA* 1989;86: 8988.
63. Song MD, Wachi M, Doi M, et al. Evolution of an inducible penicillin-target protein in methicillin-resistant *Staphylococcus aureus* by gene fusion. *FEBS Lett* 1987;221:167.
64. Harder KJ, Nikaido H, Matsuhashi M. Mutants of *Escherichia coli* that are resistant to certain beta-lactam compounds lack the *ompF* porin. *Antimicrob Agents Chemother* 1981;20:549.
65. Jaffé A, Chabbert YA, Derlot E. Selection and characterization of β-lactam-resistant *Escherichia coli* K-12 mutants. *Antimicrob Agents Chemother* 1983;23:623.
66. Masuda N, Sakagawa E, Ohya S, et al. Substrate specificities of MexAB-OprM, MexCD-OprJ, and MexXY-OprM efflux pumps in *Pseudomonas aeruginosa*. *Antimicrob Agents Chemother* 2000;44:3322.
67. Hancock RE, Woodruff WA. Roles of porin and β-lactamase in β-lactam resistance in *Pseudomonas aeruginosa*. *Rev Infect Dis* 1988;10:770.
68. Rice LB, Carias LL, Hujer AM, et al. High level expression of chromosomally encoded SHV-1 beta-lactamase and an outer membrane protein change confer resistance to ceftazidime and piperacillin-tazobactam in a clinical isolate of *Klebsiella pneumoniae*. *Antimicrob Agents Chemother* 2000;44:362.
69. Tomasz A, Albino A, Zanati E. Multiple antibiotic resistance in a bacterium with suppressed autolytic system. *Nature* 1970;227:138.
70. Handwerger S, Tomasz A. Antibiotic tolerance among clinical isolates of bacteria. *Rev Infect Dis* 1985;7:368.
71. Sabath LD, Wheeler N, Laverdiere M, et al. A new type of penicillin resistance of *Staphylococcus aureus*. *Lancet* 1977;1:443.
72. Rajashekaraiah KR, Rice T, Rao VS, et al. Clinical significance of tolerant

strains of *Staphylococcus aureus* in patients with endocarditis. *Ann Intern Med* 1980;93:796.

73. McCarthy CG, Finland M. Absorption and excretion of four penicillins: penicillin G, penicillin V, phenethicillin and phenylmercaptomethyl penicillin. *N Engl J Med* 1960;263:315.

74. Bergan TB. Penicillins. *Antibiotic Chemother* 1978;25:1.

75. Craig WA, Suh B. Protein binding and the antimicrobial effects: methods for the determination of protein binding. In: Lonan V, ed. *Antibiotics in laboratory medicine*, 3d ed. Baltimore: Williams & Wilkins, 1991:367–402.

76. Ebert SC, Leggett J, Vogelman B, et al. Evidence for a slow elimination phase for penicillin G. *J Infect Dis* 1988;158:200.

77. Bryan CS, Stone WJ. "Comparable massive" penicillin G therapy in renal failure. *Ann Intern Med* 1975;82:189.

78. Bulger RJ, Lindholm DD, Murry JS, et al. Effect of uremia on methicillin and oxacillin blood levels: excretion and inactivation in renal failure and hemodialysis. *JAMA* 1964;187:319.

79. Nauta EH, Mattie H. Dicloxacillin and cloxacillin pharmacokinetics in healthy and hemodialysis patients. *Clin Pharmacol Ther* 1976;20:98.

80. Roder BL, Frimodt-Moller N, Espersen F, et al. Dicloxacillin and flucloxacillin: pharmacokinetics, protein binding and serum bactericidal titers in healthy subjects after oral administration. *Infection* 1995;23:107.

81. Spyker DA, Ruglowski RJ, Vann RL, et al. Pharmacokinetics of amoxicillin: dose dependence after intravenous, oral and intramuscular administration. *Antimicrob Agents Chemother* 1977;11:132.

82. Welling PG, Huang H, Koch PA, et al. Bioavailability of ampicillin and amoxicillin in fasted and nonfasted subjects. *J Pharm Sci* 1977;66:549.

83. Craig WA. Pharmacokinetics of bacampicillin tablets in adults. *Bull NY Acad Med* 1983;59:457.

84. Libke RD, Clarke JT, Ralph ED, et al. Ticarcillin vs carbenicillin: clinical pharmacokinetics. *Clin Pharmacol Ther* 1975;17:441.

85. Bergan T. Overview of acylureidopenicillin pharmacokinetics. *Scand J Infect Dis Suppl* 1981;29:33.

86. Neu HC, Srinivasan S, Francke EL, et al. Pharmacokinetics of amdinocillin and pivamdinocillin in normal volunteers. *Am J Med* 1983;75[Suppl 2A]:60.

87. Boelaert J, Daneels R, Schurgers M, et al. The pharmacokinetics of temocillin in patients with normal and impaired renal function. *J Antimicrob Chemother* 1983;11:349.

88. Adam D, De Visser I, Koeppe P. Pharmacokinetics of amoxicillin and clavulanic acid administered alone and in combination. *Antimicrob Agents Chemother* 1982;22:353.

89. Johnson CA, Halstenson CE, Kelloway JS, et al. Single-dose pharmacokinetics of piperacillin and tazobactam in patients with renal disease. *Clin Pharmacol Ther* 1992;51:32.

90. Gilbert DN, Bennett WM. Use of antimicrobial agents in renal failure. *Infect Dis Clin North Am* 1989;3:517.

91. Wise R, Gillet AP, Cadge B, et al. Influence of protein binding on the tissue levels of 6 β-lactams. *J Infect Dis* 1980;142:77.

92. Nau H. Clinical pharmacokinetics in pregnancy and perinatology. *Dev Pharmacol Ther* 1987;10:174.

93. Craig WA, Welling PG. Protein binding of antimicrobials: clinical, pharmacokinetic and therapeutic implications. *Clin Pharmacokinet* 1977;2:252.

94. Kornguth ML, Kunin CM. Uptake of antibiotics by human erythrocytes. *J Infect Dis* 1976;133:175.

95. Gerding DN, Hughes CE, Bamberger DM, et al. Extravascular antimicrobial distribution and the respective blood concentrations in humans. In: Lorian V, ed. *Antibiotics in laboratory medicine*, 4th ed. Baltimore: Williams & Wilkins, 1996:835–899.

96. Dixon RL, Owens ES, Rall DP. Evidence of active transport of benzyl-^{14}C-penicillin from cerebrospinal fluid to blood. *J Pharm Sci* 1969;58:1106.

97. Spector R, Lorenzo AV. Inhibition of penicillin transport from the cerebrospinal fluid after intracisternal inoculation of bacteria. *J Clin Invest* 1974;54:316.

98. Dacey RG, Sande MA. Effect of probenecid on cerebrospinal fluid concentration of penicillin and cephalosporin derivatives. *Antimicrob Agents Chemother* 1974;6:437.

99. Bins JW, Mattie H. Saturation of the tubular excretion of β-lactam antibiotics. *Br J Clin Pharmacol* 1988;25:41.

100. Overbosch D, Van Gulpen C, Hermans J, et al. The effect of probenecid on the renal tubular excretion of benzylpenicillin. *Br J Clin Pharmacol* 1988;25:51.

101. Cole M, Kenig MD, Hewitt VA. Metabolism of penicillins to penicilloic acids and 6-aminopenicillanic acid in man and its significance in assessing penicillin absorption. *Antimicrob Agents Chemother* 1973;3:463.

102. Turnidge JD, Craig WA. β-Lactam pharmacology in liver disease. *J Antimicrob Chemother* 1990;11:499.

103. Klugman KP. Pneumococcal resistance to antibiotics. *Clin Microbiol Rev* 1990;3:171.

104. Pallares R, Linares J, Vadillo M, et al. Resistance to penicillin and cephalosporin and mortality from severe pneumococcal pneumonia in Barcelona, Spain. *N Engl J Med* 1995;333:474.

105. Dattwyler RJ, Halperin JJ, Volkman DJ, et al. Treatment of late lyme borreliosis-randomised comparison of ceftriaxone and penicillin. *Lancet* 1988;1:1191.

106. Watt G, Padre LP, Tuazon ML, et al. Placebo-controlled trial of intravenous penicillin for severe and late leptospirosis. *Lancet* 1988;1:433.

107. MacGowan A. When is penicillin monotherapy the antibiotic treatment of choice? *J Antimicrob Chemother* 1992;29:239.

108. Levison ME, Mangura CT, Lorber B, et al. Clindamycin compared with penicillin for the treatment of anaerobic lung abscess. *Ann Intern Med* 1983;98:466.

109. Oncul O, Ozsoy MF, Gul HC, et al. Cutaneous anthrax in Turkey: a review of 32 cases. *Scand J Infect Dis* 2002;34:413.

110. Bryskier A. *Bacillus anthracis* and antibacterial agents. *Clin Microbiol Infect* 2002;8:467.

111. Brewin A, Arango L, Hadley WK, et al. High-dose penicillin therapy and pneumococcal pneumonia. *JAMA* 1974;230:409.

112. Musher DM, Hamill RJ, Baughn RE. Effect of human immunodeficiency virus (HIV) infection on the course of syphilis and on the response to treatment. *Ann Intern Med* 1990;113:872.

113. Gerber MA, Randolph MF, DeMeo K, et al. Failure of once daily penicillin V therapy for streptococcal pharyngitis. *Am J Dis Child* 1989;143:153.

114. Steere AC, Hutchinson GL, Rahn DW, et al. Treatment of the early manifestations of lyme disease. *Ann Intern Med* 1983;99:22.

115. Thornsberry C. The development of antimicrobial resistance in staphylococci. *J Antimicrob Chemother* 1988;21[Suppl C]:9.

116. Craig WA, Ebert SC. Protein binding and its significance in antibacterial therapy. *Infect Dis Clin North Am* 1989;3:407.

117. Kane JG, Parker RH, Jordan GW, et al. Nafcillin concentration in cerebrospinal fluid during treatment of staphylococcal infections. *Ann Intern Med* 1977;87:309.

118. Kancir LM, Tuazon CU, Cardella TA, et al. Adverse reactions to methicillin and nafcillin during treatment of serious *Staphylococcus aureus* infections. *Arch Intern Med* 1978;138:909.

119. Tetzlaff TR, McCracken GH, Nelson JD. Oral antibiotic therapy for skeletal infections of children. II. Therapy of osteomyelitis and suppurative arthritis. *J Pediatr* 1978;92:485.

120. Black J, Hunt TL, Godley PJ, et al. Oral antimicrobial therapy for adults with osteomyelitis or septic arthritis. *J Infect Dis* 1987;155:968.

121. Van Ek B, Dijkmans BAC, Van Dulken H, et al. Antibiotic prophylaxis in craniotomy: a prospective double-blind placebo controlled study. *Scand J Infect Dis* 1988;20:633.

122. Stamm WE, McKevitt M, Counts GW. Acute renal infection in women: treatment with trimethoprim-sulfamethoxazole or ampicillin for two or six weeks. A randomized trial. *Ann Intern Med* 1987;106:341.

123. Dajani AS, Taubert KA, Wilson W, et al. Prevention of bacterial endocarditis: recommendations by the American Heart Association. *JAMA* 1997;277:1794.

124. Bayerdorffer E, Miehlke S, Marines G, et al. Double-blind trial of omeprazole and amoxicillin to cure *Helicobacter pylori* infection in patients with duodenal ulcers. *Gastroenterology* 1995;108:1412.

125. Philbrick JT, Bracikowski JP. Single-dose antibiotic treatment for uncomplicated urinary tract infections. *Arch Intern Med* 1985;145:1672.

126. Swahn A. Gastrointestinal absorption and metabolism of two 35S-labelled ampicillin esters. *Eur J Clin Pharmacol* 1976;9:299.

127. Neu HC, Swarz H. Carbenicillin: clinical and laboratory experience with a parenterally administered penicillin for treatment of *Pseudomonas* infections. *Ann Intern Med* 1969;71:903.

128. Butler K, English AR, Briggs B, et al. Indanyl carbenicillin: chemistry and laboratory studies with a new semisynthetic penicillin. *J Infect Dis* 1973;127:S97.

129. Fuchs PC, Thornsberry C, Barry AL, et al. Ticarcillin: a collaborative in vitro comparison with carbenicillin against 9,000 clinical bacterial isolates. *Am J Med Sci* 1977;274:255.

130. Parry MF, Neu HC. A comparative study of ticarcillin plus tobramycin versus carbenicillin plus gentamicin for the treatment of serious infections due to gram-negative bacilli. *Am J Med* 1978;64:961.

131. Holmes B, Richard DM, Brodgen RN, et al. Piperacillin: a review of antibacterial activity, pharmacokinetic properties, and their therapeutic use. *Drugs* 1984;28:375.

132. Winston DJ, Murphy W, Young LS, et al. Piperacillin therapy for serious bacterial infections. *Am J Med* 1980;69:255.

133. Parry MF. The in-vitro activity of azlocillin: a community hospital study of 1900 clinical isolates. *J Antimicrob Chemother* 1983;11[Suppl B]:15.

134. Bergan T. Pharmacokinetics of mezlocillin in healthy volunteers. *Antimicrob Agents Chemother* 1978;14:801.

135. Reading C, Cole M. Clavulanic acid: a beta-lactamase-inhibiting beta-lactam from *Streptomyces clavuligerus*. *Antimicrob Agents Chemother* 1977;11:852.

136. Aronoff SC, Jacobs MR, Johenning S, et al. Comparative activities of the β-lactamase inhibitors YTR 830, sodium clavulanate, and sulbactam combined with amoxicillin or ampicillin. *Antimicrob Agents Chemother* 1984;26:580.

137. Bush K. β-Lactamase inhibitors from laboratory to clinic. *Clin Microbiol Rev* 1988;1:109.

138. Fuchs PC, Barry AL, Thornsberry C, et al. In vitro evaluation of augmentin by both microdilution and disk diffusion susceptibility testing: regression analysis, tentative interpretive criteria, and quality control limits. *Antimicrob Agents Chemother* 1983;24:31.

139. Jones RN. In vitro evaluations of aminopenicillin/β-lactamase inhibitor combinations. *Drugs* 1988;35[Suppl 7]:17.

140. Barry AL, Ayers LW, Gavan TL, et al. In vitro activity of ticarcillin plus clavulanic acid against bacteria isolated in three centers. *Eur J Clin Microbiol* 1984;3:203.

141. Fuchs PC, Barry AL, Thornsberry C, et al. In vitro activity of ticarcillin plus clavulanic acid against 632 clinical isolates. *Antimicrob Agents Chemother* 1984;25:392.

142. Kuck NA, Jacobus NV, Petersen PJ, et al. Comparative in vitro and in vivo activities of piperacillin combined with the β-lactamase inhibitors tazobactam, clavulanic acid, and sulbactam. *Antimicrob Agents Chemother* 1989;33:1964.

143. Murray P, Cantrell HF, Lankford RB, et al. Multicenter evaluation of the in vitro activity of piperacillin-tazobactam compared with eleven selected β-lactam antibiotics and ciprofloxacin against more than 42,000 aerobic gram-positive and gram-negative bacteria. *Diagn Microbiol Infect Dis* 1994;19:111.

144. Noguchi JK, Gill MA. Sulbactam: a β-lactamase inhibitor. *Clin Pharmacokinet* 1988;7:37.

145. Todd PA, Benfield P. Amoxicillin/clavulanic acid. An update of its antibacterial activity, pharmacokinetic properties and therapeutic use. *Drugs* 1990;39:264.

146. Goldstein EJC, Reihardt JF, Murray PM, et al. Outpatient therapy of bite wounds: demographic data, bacteriology, and a prospective, randomized trial of amoxicillin/clavulanic acid versus penicillin/dicloxacillin. *Int J Dermatol* 1987;26:123.

147. File TM Jr, Jacobs MR, Poole MD, et al. Outcome of treatment of respiratory tract infections due to Streptococcus pneumoniae, including drug-resistant strains, with pharmacokinetically enhanced amoxycillin/clavulanate. *Int J Antimicrob Agents* 2002;20:235.

148. Dagan R, Hoberman A, Johnson C, et al. Bacteriologic and clinical efficacy of high dose amoxicillin/clavulanate in children with acute otitis media. *Pediatr Infect Dis J* 2001;20:829.

149. Lees L, Milson JA, Knirsch AK, et al. Sulbactam plus ampicillin: interim review of efficacy and safety for therapeutic and prophylactic use. *Rev Infect Dis* 1986;8[Suppl 5]:S644.

150. Meylan PR, Calandra T, Casey PA, et al. Clinical experience with timentin in severe hospital infections. *J Antimicrob Chemother* 1986;17[Suppl C]:127.

151. Khardori N, Elting L, Wong E, et al. Nosocomial infections due to *Xanthomonas maltophilia* (*Pseudomonas maltophilia*) in patients with cancer. *Rev Infect Dis* 1990;12:997.

152. Bryson HM, Brogden RN. Piperacillin/tazobactam. A review of its antibacterial activity, pharmacokinetic properties and therapeutic potential. *Drugs* 1994;47:506.

153. Neu HC. Penicillin-binding proteins and role of amdinocillin in causing bacterial cell death. *Am J Med* 1983;75[Suppl 2A]:9.

154. Cox CE. Parenteral amdinocillin for treatment of complicated urinary tract infections. *Am J Med* 1983;75[Suppl 2A]:82.

155. Verbist L. In vitro activity of temocillin (BRL 17421), a novel beta-lactamase-stable penicillin. *Antimicrob Agents Chemother* 1982;22:157.

156. Lindsay G, Beattie AD, Taylor EW. Temocillin in the treatment of serious gram-negative infections. *Drugs* 1985;29[Suppl 5]:191.

157. Saxon A, Beall GN, Rohr AS, et al. Immediate hypersensitivity reactions to beta-lactam antibiotics. *Ann Intern Med* 1987;107:204.

158. Idsoe O, Guthe T, Wilcox RR, et al. Nature and extent of penicillin side reactions, with particular reference to fatalities from anaphylactic shock. *Bull World Health Organ* 1968;38:159.

159. Shapiro S, Siskin V, Slone D, et al. Drug rash with ampicillin and other penicillins. *Lancet* 1969;2:69.

160. Arndt KA, Jick H. Rates of cutaneous reactions to drugs. A report from the Boston Collaborative Drug Surveillance Program. *JAMA* 1976;235:918.

161. Ressler C, Mendelson LM. Skin test for diagnosis of penicillin allergy-current status. *Arm Allergy* 1987;59:167.

162. Kerns DL, Shira JE, Go S, et al. Ampicillin rash in children. Relationship to penicillin allergy and infectious mononucleosis. *Am J Dis Child* 1973;125:187.

163. Huff JC. Erythema multiforme. *Dermatol Clin* 1985;3:141.

164. Kerr RO, Cardamone J, Dalmasso AP, et al. Two mechanisms of erythrocyte destruction in penicillin-induced hemolytic anemia. *N Engl J Med* 1972;287:1322.

165. Olaison L, Alestig K. A prospective study of neutropenia induced by high doses of β-lactam antibiotics. *J Antimicrob Chemother* 1990;25:449.

166. Markowitz SM, Rothkopf M, Holden FD, et al. Nafcillin-induced agranulocytosis. *JAMA* 1975;232:1150.

167. Shattil SJ, Bennett JS, McDonough M, et al. Carbenicillin and penicillin G inhibit platelet function in vitro by impairing the interaction of agonists with the platelet surface. *J Clin Invest* 1980;71:619.

168. Burroughs SF, Johnson GJ. β-Lactam antibiotic-induced platelet dysfunction: evidence for irreversible inhibition of platelet activation in vitro and in vivo after prolonged exposure to penicillin. *Blood* 1990;75:1473.

169. Baldwin DS, Levine BB, McCluskey RT, et al. Renal failure and interstitial nephritis due to penicillin and methicillin. *N Engl J Med* 1968;279:1245.

170. Border WA, Lehman DH, Egan JD, et al. Antitubular basement membrane antibodies in methicillin-associated interstitial nephritis. *N Engl J Med* 1974;291:381.

171. Colvin RB, Burton JR, Hyslop NE Jr, et al. Penicillin-associated interstitial nephritis. *Ann Intern Med* 1974;81:404.

172. Brunner FP, Frick PG. Hypokalaemia, metabolic alkalosis and hypernatraemia due to "massive" sodium penicillin therapy. *BMJ* 1968;4:550.

173. Klastersky J, Vanderkelen B, Daneau D, et al. Carbenicillin and hypokalemia. *Ann Intern Med* 1973;78:774.

174. Martian FA, Stone WJ, Alford RH. Adverse antibiotic effects associated with renal insufficiency. *Rev Infect Dis* 1990;12:236.

175. Craig WA, Evenson MA, Sarver KP, et al. Correction of protein binding defect in uremic sera by charcoal treatment. *J Lab Clin Med* 1976;87:637.

176. Spector R, Snodgrass SR. The effect of uremia on penicillin flux between blood and cerebrospinal. fluid. *J Lab Clin Med* 1976;87:749.

177. Wilson FM, Belamavic J, Lauter CB, et al. Anicteric carbenicillin hepatitis. Eight episodes in four patients. *JAMA* 1967;232:818.

178. Onorato JM, Axelrod JM. Hepatitis from intravenous high-dose oxacillin therapy. *Ann Intern Med* 1978;89:497.

179. Saliba B. Oxacillin hepatotoxicity in HIV infected patients. *Ann Intern Med* 1994;120:1048.

180. Heilker GM, Fowler JW, Self TH. Possible nafcillin-warfarin interaction. *Arch Intern Med* 1994;154:822.

181. Vermis S, Maddux MS, Pollak R, et al. Subtherapeutic cyclosporin concentrations during nafcillin therapy. *Transplantation* 1987;43:913.

182. Wallace SM, Chart L-Y. In vitro interaction of aminoglycosides with β-lactam penicillins. *Antimicrob Agents Chemother* 1985;28:274.

183. Riff LJ, Jackson GG. Laboratory and clinical conditions for gentamicin inactivation by carbenicillin. *Arch Intern Med* 1972;130:887.

CHAPTER 19
Cephalosporins

Robert C. Moellering, Jr., Deborah E. Sentochnik, and John G. Bartlett

HISTORICAL BACKGROUND

The discovery of penicillin by Alexander Fleming in 1928 and its subsequent characterization a decade later by Howard Florey, Ernst Chain, Norman Heatley, E.P. Abraham, and others at Oxford University set the stage for the first clinical use of penicillin in the early 1940s. The success of this venture led numerous other investigators to search for antibiotic-producing microorganisms. The first microbial producer of a cephalosporin, *Cephalosporium acremonium* (now also known as *Acremonium chrysogenum*), was isolated from a sewage outlet in the harbor at Cagliari, Sardinia, by Giuseppi Brotzu, a professor of bacteriology at the University of Cagliari (1). Brotzu suspected that the occasional clearing of the waters surrounding the sewage outfall might be related to the presence of antibiotic-producing microorganisms, the search for which led to isolation of the initial strain of *C. acremonium*. Brotzu was able to make crude filtrates from his original isolate, which he used to treat various infections. He injected the material directly into boils and other skin infections with moderate success and even administered the filtrates intramuscularly and intravenously to Sardinian patients suffering from typhoid fever and brucellosis (2). Although the patients receiving these filtrates had severe febrile reactions, Brotzu thought that the material was instrumental in their recovery from the infections. This is ironic, because none of the early cephalosporins exhibited any useful clinical activity against either typhoid fever or brucellosis.

Brotzu was unable to carry out further studies on his antibiotic-producing microorganisms, and he was unable to interest the Italian pharmaceutical industry in his findings. Thus, in 1948, he sent a culture of his *C. acremonium* to Sir Howard Florey at Oxford. Initial studies there showed that Brotzu's microorganism produced a substance (named cephalosporin P) that had activity against gram-positive bacteria only. It seemed unlikely, however, that this compound could have accounted for the clinical activity noted by Brotzu. Further studies revealed that in the aqueous phase that remained after extraction of cephalosporin P, there remained another compound, initially called cephalosporin N. This compound was active against gram-negative bacilli (especially *Salmonella* species) and undoubtedly was the substance that was responsible for the original clinical activity reported by Brotzu. Subsequent studies, however, showed that this compound was actually a penicillin, not a cephalosporin, and it was renamed penicillin N and proved to be identical to another antibiotic isolated in the United States called synnematin B. In 1953, a third antibiotic was isolated from *C. acremonium*. This compound, named cephalosporin C, was only about one tenth as active against *Salmonella typhi* and staphylococci as penicillin N; however, unlike penicillin N, which was readily destroyed by penicillinase-producing strains of staphylococci and *Bacillus cereus*, cephalosporin C was noted to be active against microorganisms that produced these enzymes. Interest in this compound was heightened when it was noted to be relatively nontoxic and was effective in treating various infections in animal models (2).

CHEMISTRY AND NOMENCLATURE

Cephalosporin C was subsequently shown to be quite similar to penicillin N in that it had a D-α-aminoadipyl side chain attached to a β-lactam ring. However, in the case of cephalosporin C, the β-lactam ring was fused to a six-member dihydrothiazine (cephem) ring, rather than the five-member thiazolidine (penam) ring found in penicillin N (Figs. 19.1 and 19.2). This initial observation showed that the presence of a cephem ring, as opposed to a thiazolidine ring, conferred relative resistance to certain β-lactamases, including those produced by *Staphylococcus aureus* and *B. cereus*. Although cephalosporin C was used to treat a few urinary tract infections in children, it was not active enough for serious clinical development. The discovery that the nucleus of penicillin (6-aminopenicillanic acid) could be produced in pure crystalline form in 1958 led to the discovery of various new semisynthetic penicillins produced by chemically adding side chains at the 6 position of 6-aminopenicillanic acid (3). The subsequent production of 7-aminocephalosporanic acid set the

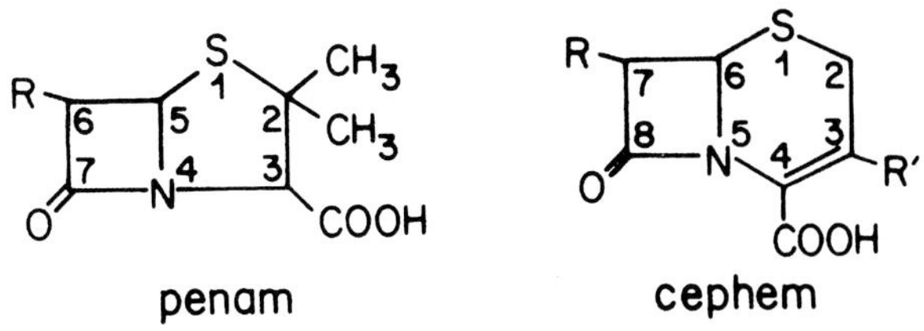

Figure 19.1. Nuclear structure of the penicillins (penam nucleus) and cephalosporins (cephem nucleus).

stage for the development of a number of new and potentially clinically useful cephalosporins. Unlike the penicillins, chemical modification can be made at both the 7 and the 3 positions of the cephalosporin molecule. The initial cephalosporins produced for clinical use (cephalothin, cephaloridine, and several years later, cefazolin) exhibited good activity against gram-positive organisms (with the exception of enterococci and methicillin-resistant staphylococci), and they showed activity against certain gram-negative bacilli, including *Escherichia coli*, *Proteus mirabilis*, and *Klebsiella pneumoniae*, as well as *Salmonella* and *Shigella* (see Fig. 19.2). Unfortunately, although these compounds were active *in vitro* against *Salmonella*, they were not effective for the treatment of systemic salmonellosis. Although the cephalosporins are relatively stable to the staphylococcal β-lactamases, there are a broad variety of other β-lactamases, particularly those produced by gram-negative bacilli, which are capable of destroying these compounds. The presence of a methoxy group at the 7 position markedly enhances the stability of cephalosporins to a broad variety of gram-negative cephalosporinases, especially those produced by *Bacteroides* species. Cefoxitin was the first compound with a 7-methoxy group to be developed for clinical use (Fig. 19.3). Technically, cefoxitin is not a true cephalosporin but a cephamycin, having been initially derived from a strain of *Streptomyces lactamdurams* (4). Despite this technicality, most

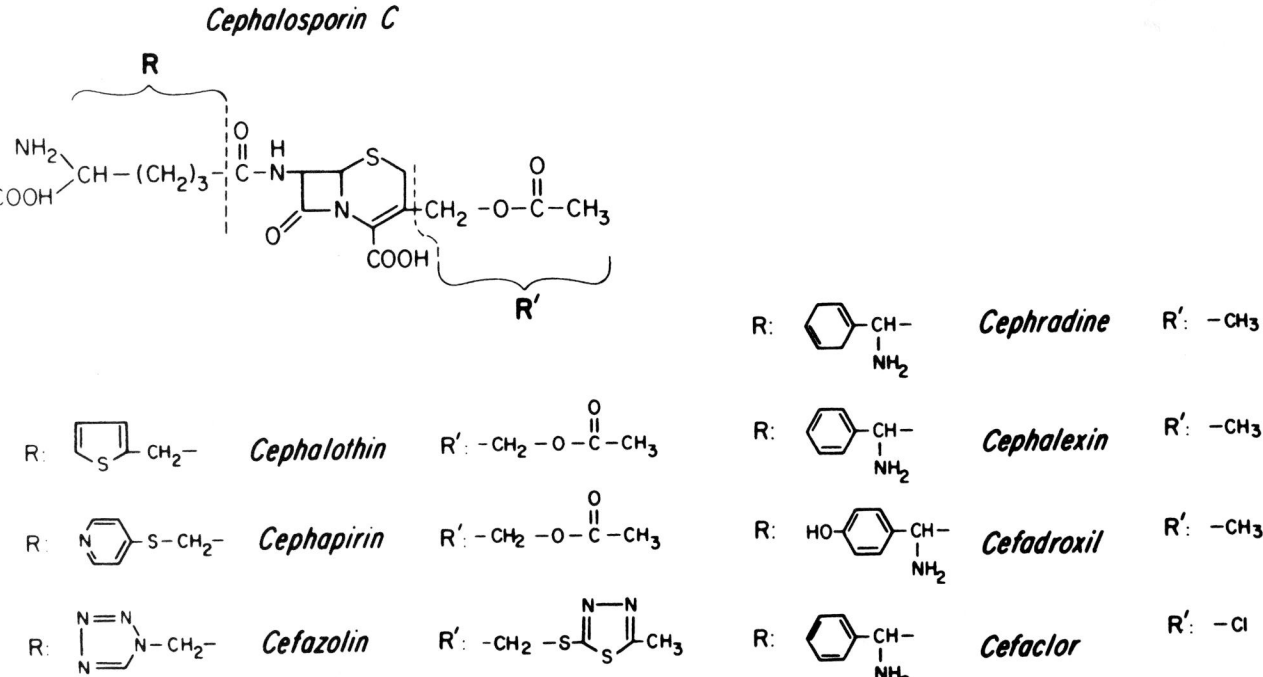

Figure 19.2. Structural formulae of cephalosporin C and the first-generation cephalosporins. (From Calderwood SB, Moellering RC Jr. Principles of anti-infective therapy. In: Stein JH, ed. *Internal medicine*, 3rd ed. Boston: Little, Brown and Company, 1990:1202–1218, with permission.)

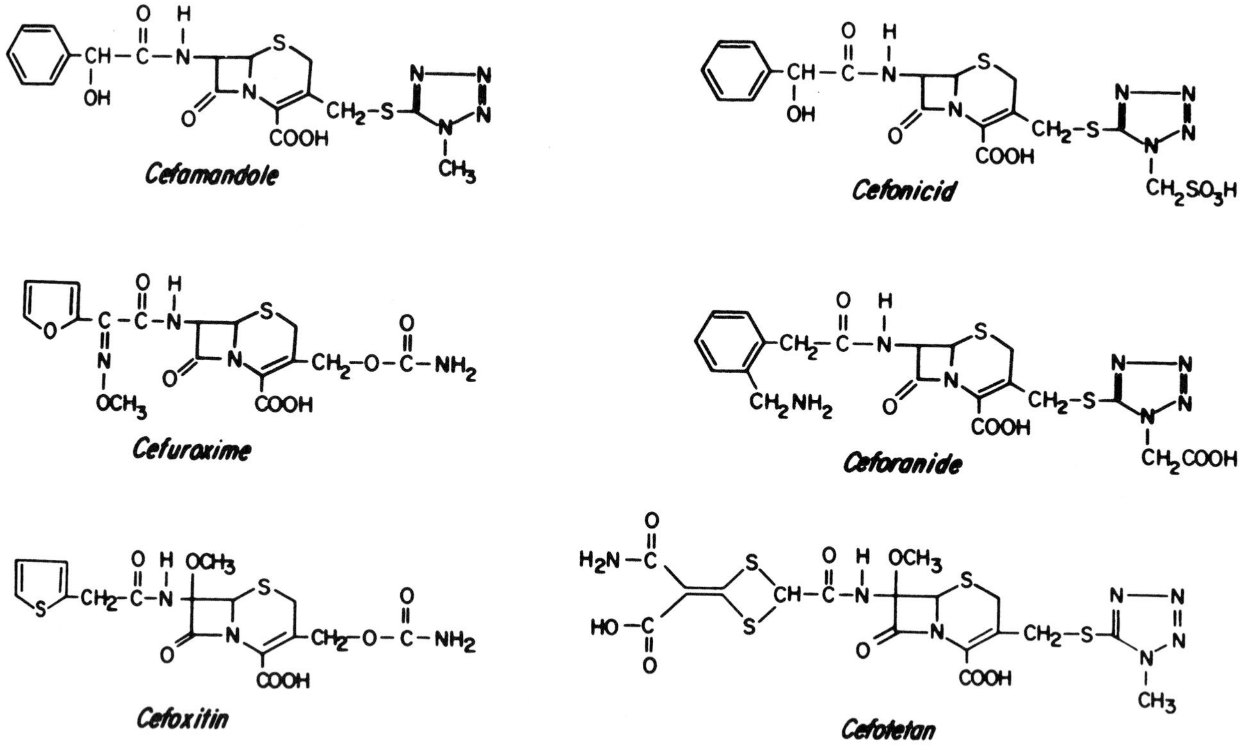

Figure 19.3. Structural formulas of the parenteral second-generation cephalosporins. (From Calderwood SB, Moellering RC Jr. Principles of anti-infective therapy. In: Stein JH, ed. *Internal medicine,* 3rd ed. Boston: Little, Brown and Company, 1990:1202–1218, with permission.)

authors have considered cefoxitin and other cephamycins to be cephalosporins, and these compounds are considered along with the true cephalosporins in this chapter. In general, cephalosporins containing a 7-methoxy group (such as cefoxitin, cefmetazole, cefotetan, and moxalactam) (Figs. 19.3 and 19.4) exhibit enhanced activity against β-lactamase–producing strains of *Bacteroides fragilis,* but this advantage is, to a degree, offset by a moderate loss of intrinsic activity against gram-positive organisms, including *S. aureus* (5). Various substitutions at both the 3 and the 7 position of the cephalosporin molecule have produced enhanced activity against gram-negative bacilli. One such substitution is the methylthiotetrazole (MTT) moiety that is present at the 3 position in compounds such as cefamandole, cefotetan, cefoperazone, moxalactam, and cefmetazole. As a result, each of these compounds exhibits enhanced activity against a broad range of gram-negative bacilli. Unfortunately, however, the MTT group is also associated with the disulfiram-like reactions and prolongation of prothrombin time that can accompany the use of cephalosporins containing this moiety (5). Another modification that has resulted in enhanced activity against gram-negative bacteria is the incorporation of an aminothiazolyl group in the acyl side chain at the 7 position of various cephalosporins (6). It is also possible to add a methoxy group directly to the oxime residue that abuts the aminothiazolyl portion of the side chain at the 7 position. The resultant aminothiazolylmethoxy group confers enhanced resistance to β-lactamase without the loss of activity against gram-positive organisms seen when the methoxy group is instead attached directly to the β-lactam ring at the 7 position (7). It appears that the presence of an aminothiazolyl group enhances the ability of the resulting cephalosporins to penetrate through the outer cell envelope of gram-negative bacilli and may enhance the affinity of these compounds for penicillin-binding proteins (PBPs) as well (5). Activity of cephalosporins against *Pseudomonas aeruginosa* can be enhanced by incorporating an acidic moiety on the 7 position side chain, as is seen in

ceftazidime and moxalactam. Moxalactam has a carboxyl group on its side chain that is similar to that found in carbenicillin. The carboxypropyl group on the acyl side chain of ceftazidime subserves a similar function (5).

Although substitutions at the 3 position can alter intrinsic activity of cephalosporins, most of the chemical changes at the 3 position have been effected to alter pharmacokinetic properties of these drugs. The presence of a bulky side chain at the 3 position markedly impairs oral absorption of these compounds. The true cephalosporins, which are absorbed orally, generally have a simple methyl group at the 3 position (e.g., cephalexin, cephradine, or cefadroxil). In the case of cefaclor, a chlorine atom replaces the methyl group at the 3 position. The side chain at position 3 in cefixime is a vinyl moiety. The bioavailability of even these compounds, however, is limited by the polarity of the carboxyl group at the 4 position. Because this moiety is crucial for activation of the β-lactam ring, it cannot be removed without destroying the activity of the entire molecule (5). However, esterification of this carboxyl group results in an inactive compound that is absorbed well from the gastrointestinal tract. Naturally occurring esterases in the intestinal tract and serum then hydrolyze the ester bond, releasing active drugs; cefuroxime axetil and cefpodoxime proxetil are the currently available esters of this type. Cefetamet pivoxil remains an investigational agent in the United States (8).

Finally, alterations in the side chain at the 3 position of the cephalosporin molecule can also have a striking influence on protein binding and renal excretion of these compounds. Cefamandole and cefonicid are structurally identical, except that the latter has a sulfomethyl instead of a methyl group at the 1 position of the MTT side chain at position 3 of the cephem nucleus. The net result is markedly enhanced serum protein binding for cefonicid (98%) compared with cefamandole (67% to 80%) and a serum half-life for cefonicid (4.5 hours) that is considerably greater than that of cefamandole (0.5 to 0.9 hours) (5). The side

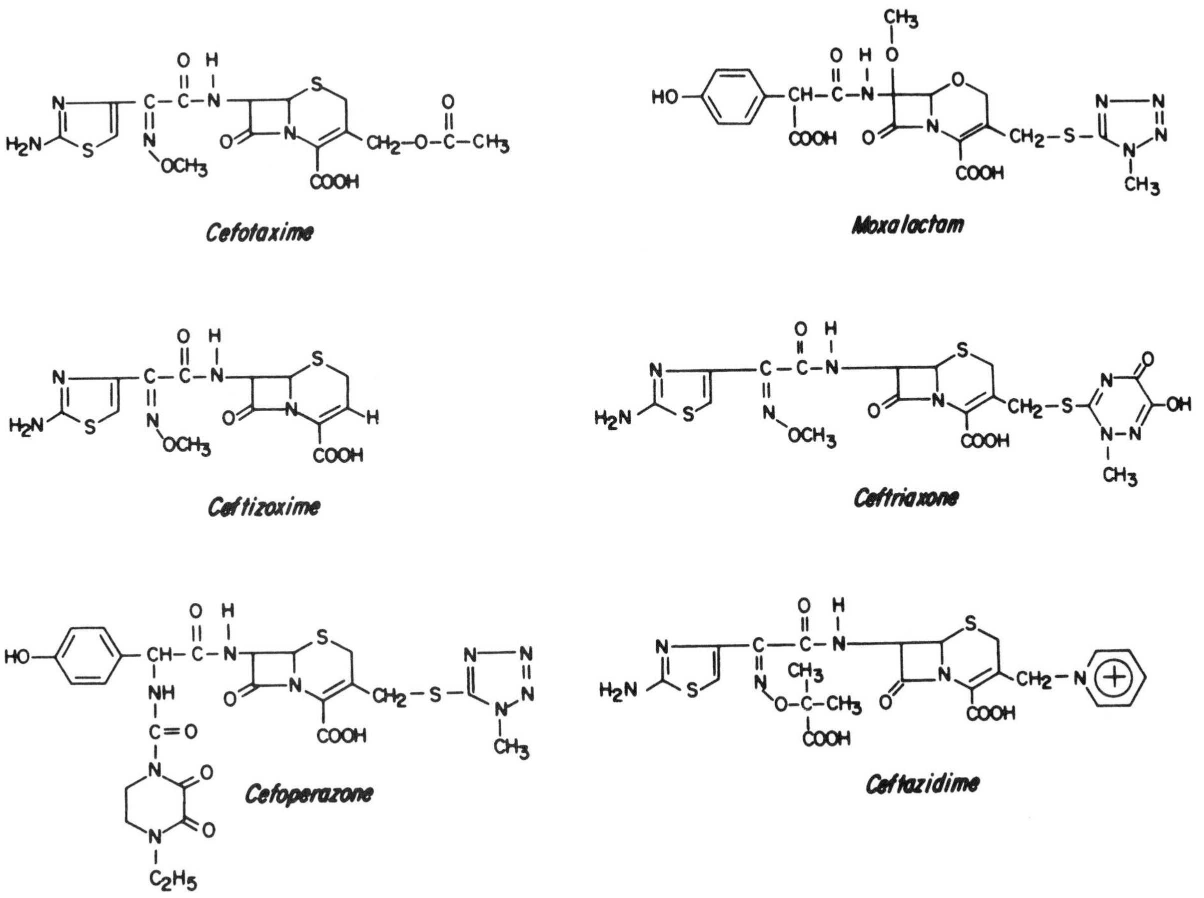

Figure 19.4. Structural formulas of the third-generation cephalosporins. (From Calderwood SB, Moellering RC Jr. Principles of anti-infective therapy. In: Stein JH, ed. *Internal medicine,* 3rd ed. Boston: Little, Brown and Company, 1990:1202–1218, with permission.)

chain at position 3 of ceftriaxone is responsible for its enhanced protein binding and prolonged serum half-life as well.

The carbacephems are a relatively new class of β-lactam antibiotic (9). They are chemically similar to cephalosporins, except that the sulfur atom in the dihydrothiazine ring of the cephalosporin is replaced by a methylene group in the tetrahydropyridine ring of the carbacephem nucleus, which lends increased stability to the molecule. Loracarbef is the cephem analog of cefaclor and is the first commercially available carbacephem.

Classification of the cephalosporins is an imprecise science at best. A number of classification schemes have been devised and all have certain shortcomings. The most widely used "system" involves the use of "generations" of cephalosporins. By current convention, the older narrower spectrum cephalosporins are considered to be first-generation cephalosporins (Table 19.1). In general, the second-generation cephalosporins consist of a group of both cephalosporins and cephamycins with enhanced gram-negative (and in some instances anaerobic) spectrums of activity compared with the first-generation cephalosporins. The third-generation cephalosporins in general have the greatest activity against gram-negative bacilli, although one of these compounds cefsulodin is not remarkably active against gram-negative bacilli other than *P. aeruginosa.* The fourth-generation cephalosporins such as cefepime comprise compounds that combine the expanded spectrum of the third-generation agents versus gram-negative bacilli and the activity of first-generation agents versus gram-positive cocci. Nevertheless, cefepime lacks activity against methicillin-resistant *S. aureus,* enterococci, and *B. fragilis.* The listing in Table 19.1 represents a classification

scheme based on generations, but it should be noted that other authors classify some of the compounds differently. For instance, cefaclor is sometimes called a first-generation cephalosporin, whereas cefotetan, cefmetazole, and cefixime have occasionally been classified as third-generation cephalosporins.

In an effort to avoid using the term *generation* in relationship to cephalosporins (because it is clearly imprecise), Williams

TABLE 19.1. Classification of the Cephalosporins

First generation	Third generation
Cephalothin	Cefotaxime
Cephapirin	Ceftizoxime
Cefazolin	Ceftriaxone
Cephradine	Cefoperazone
Cephalexin	Ceftazidime
Cephadroxil	Cefixime
Second generation	Cefpodoxime proxetil
Cefamandole	Ceftibuten
Cefuroxime	Cefdinir
Cefuroxime axetil	Fourth generation
Cefonicid	Cefepime
Ceforanide	
Cefaclor	
Cefprozil	
Loracarbef	
Cefamycins	
Cefoxitin	
Cefotetan	
Cefmetazole	

(10) has proposed a scheme based on microbiology, pharmacokinetic properties, and metabolic stability to classify the parenteral cephalosporins. Williams classified all of the orally absorbable cephalosporins separately and excluded them from the general classification. According to his scheme, group I consists of a group of parenteral cephalosporins with high activity against gram-positive bacteria. These agents include cephaloridine, cefazolin, cephalothin, and cephacetrile. Group II consists of cephalosporins with high activity against Enterobacteriaceae (cefamandole, cefuroxime, ceftizoxime, cefmenoxine, cefonicid, ceftriaxone, and cefotaxime). Included in group III are ceftazidime, cefsulodin, cefepime, and cefoperazone, which have "high activity against *Pseudomonas* and related species." Group IV consists of compounds with prominent activity against *Bacteroides,* including cefoxitin, cefmetazole, and cefotetan (10). Williams pointed out compounds that exhibit atypical pharmacodynamics, including three compounds with prolonged serum half-lives (cefonicid, ceftriaxone, cefotetan) and one with prominent biliary excretion (cefoperazone). Three of the compounds (cephalothin, cephacetrile, cefotaxime) are noted to be metabolically unstable in this classification scheme.

Overall, it is probably better to consider the cephalosporins in aggregate and to differentiate those properties that confer unique attributes on individual agents. Unfortunately, none of the available classification schemes is perfect and none provides an ideal shortcut to acquisition of knowledge about each of the individual agents.

MECHANISMS OF ACTIVITY

The cephalosporins exert their antimicrobial activity in the same manner as the penicillins, by interfering with the synthesis of the peptidoglycan component of the cell wall. The peptidoglycan is a heteropolysaccharide composed of alternating N-acetylglucosamine and N-acetylmuramic acid residues that are cross-linked by oligopeptide bridges, thus forming a lattice structure. After being formed in the cytoplasm and transported to the outer surface of the cell membrane, the new sugar residues are inserted into the existing cross-linked structure through the action of transpeptidases, carboxypeptidases, and endopeptidases. The highly stressed amide group of the β-lactam ring in β-lactam antibiotics is conformationally similar to the D-alanyl-D-alanine bond of the peptidoglycan pentapeptides, thereby causing the peptidases to "mistake" the drug for their natural substrate (11). Once bound to this site, the enzymes lose their catalytic activity. Such enzymes have become known as PBPs.

The precise makeup and number of PBPs in a cell vary among species. These enzymes differ in their affinity for various β-lactams and in the effect that their lack of appropriate participation in cell wall synthesis has on the cell. Inactivation of some PBPs affects cell wall growth; and of others, cell morphology. Precisely how the inhibition of PBPs results in an antibacterial effect is not yet clear (12). There may be more than one mechanism, even in one organism, depending on which PBP is bound to the β-lactam.

MECHANISMS OF RESISTANCE

Resistance to β-lactam antimicrobials, including cephalosporins (13), can occur by three mechanisms, which have a dynamic relationship: (a) alterations in target PBPs, (b) enzymatic destruction of the antibiotic, and (c) inability of the drug to reach its binding site in the cell. Resistance can occur intrinsically or as a result of selection of resistant subclones or mutants during exposure to cephalosporins (14). Target PBPs can be modified to have decreased affinity for a β-lactam antibiotic (15,16). Functional replacement of a sensitive PBP by one that is less sensitive to the antibiotic has also been documented (17).

To reach its target PBP, a cephalosporin must penetrate an organism's cell envelope. This is done relatively easily in the case of gram-positive organisms, as the peptidoglycan structure that makes up the cell wall routinely allows the passage of cephalosporin-sized particles. Gram-negative organisms possess a more formidable barrier, a complex structure composed of polysaccharides, lipids, and proteins. Materials penetrate this outer cell envelope through water-filled channels, or porins, produced by various outer membrane proteins (18). Passage by a cephalosporin depends on channel size, charge, and hydrophilic properties. There appears to be other pathways across the cell envelope, but they remain to be elucidated (19).

β-Lactamases (20) are enzymes produced by bacteria that can destroy β-lactams by hydrolyzing the bond between the carbon and nitrogen atom of the β-lactam ring. Their effectiveness in doing so depends on a combination of enzyme location and quantity, as well as target affinity. Gram-positive bacteria release large amounts of β-lactamases directly into their extracellular space. Growth of susceptible cells in an environment containing cephalosporins depends on their collective ability to decrease the amount of active drug present to tolerable levels. In gram-negative bacilli, β-lactamases are found in the periplasmic space and are not released "nonspecifically" into the surrounding environment. The ability of gram-negative bacilli to grow in the presence of a cephalosporin is thus a function of the individual cell. Several classification schemes for the β-lactamases exist based on characteristics such as amino acid sequences, molecular weight, or isoelectric point and are discussed further in Chapter 31. Genetic information for coding of the enzymes can be carried chromosomally or on transposons on plasmids, with production being inducible or constitutive (21,22). Of note is that in addition to the plasmid-mediated β-lactamases that have a broad spectrum of activity, a number of more cephalosporin-specific enzymes have been discovered. They have been found in some gram-negative bacteria and are active against the third-generation cephalosporins, and aztreonam in particular (23–25).

PHARMACOKINETICS

The pharmacokinetics of the cephalosporins (26–28) is summarized in Tables 19.2 and 19.3. Ceftriaxone is noteworthy for its prolonged half-life, which allows once- or twice-daily dosing (29). Cefotaxime is special because 20% to 40% of it is excreted as desacetyl cefotaxime, which may be synergistic with the parent compound in antibacterial activity against certain organisms (30). The primary mode of excretion for the cephalosporins is renal, with the exception of cefoperazone (31), which has a major degree of hepatic excretion. Ceftriaxone also has some hepatic secretion (about 40%) in humans. Dosing adjustments for the cephalosporins in renal failure are outlined in Table 19.4. Although tissue penetration by the cephalosporins is, in general, excellent, only the third-generation agents and cefuroxime reach clinically useful levels in cerebrospinal fluid (CSF) (32).

SPECTRUM OF ANTIMICROBIAL ACTIVITY

The cephalosporins are broad-spectrum agents (33). As a rule, gram-positive activity diminishes and gram-negative activity

TABLE 19.2. Pharmacokinetics of Parenteral Cephalosporins

Agent	Half-life (hr)	Standard dose (g)	Usual dose interval (hr)
Cephalothin	0.6	1–2	4
Cefazolin	1.9	0.5–1.5	8
Cephapirin	0.6	1–2	4–6
Cephradine	0.8	0.5–2	4–6
Cefamandole	0.7	1–2	4–6
Cefuroxime	1.2	0.75–1.5	6–8
Cefonicid	4.4	1–2	24
Cefoxitin	0.8	1–2	6–8
Cefotetan	3.5	1–2	12
Cefmetazole	1.1	2	6–8
Cefotaxime	1.0	1–2	6
Ceftizoxime	1.7	1–2	6–12
Ceftriaxone	6.4	1–2	12–24
Ceftazidime	2.0	1–3	8
Cefoperazone	2.1	1–3	8
Cefepime	2.0	0.5–2.0	12

TABLE 19.3. Pharmacokinetics of Oral Cephalosporins

Agent	Half-life (hr)	Standard dose (g)	Usual dose interval (hr)
Cephradine	0.8	0.5–1.0	6
Cephalexin	0.9	0.25–0.5	6
Cefadroxil	1.5	1	12
Cefaclor	0.6	0.25–0.5	8
Cefprozil	1.2	0.25–0.5	12–24
Loracarbef	1.1	0.2–0.4	12
Cefuroxime axetil	1.3	0.125–0.5	12
Cefixime	3.0	0.2–0.4	12–24
Cefpodoxime proxetil	2.2	0.2–0.4	12
Cefditroen	1.6	0.2–0.4	12
Ceftibutin	2.4	0.4	24
Cefdinir	1.7	300	12

improves as one progresses from first- to third-generation agents. Anaerobic coverage is best by the second-generation agents, specifically the cephamycins. None of the cephalosporins is active against enterococci, *Listeria monocytogenes,* or methicillin-resistant *S. aureus.* Disc-diffusion susceptibility tests may sometimes provide misleading results against methicillin-resistant *S. aureus,* but all such *S. aureus* should be considered cross-resistant to all cephalosporins (31). Ceftazidime and cefepime exhibit the most substantial anti–*P. aeruginosa* activity, but neither is particularly active against other *Pseudomonas* species.

The first-generation agents have excellent activity against gram-positive organisms such as methicillin-susceptible staphylococci and penicillin-susceptible streptococci. They have good activity against the large majority of community-acquired *E. coli, K. pneumoniae,* and *P. mirabilis,* but other gram-negative or-

ganisms should be considered resistant until proven otherwise. Although most oral anaerobes, especially those usually considered penicillin susceptible, are susceptible to these agents, *B. fragilis* is not. All the first-generation agents, both oral (35,36) and parenteral (37–40), have essentially the same antibacterial activity with a few minor exceptions. Although cephalothin has slightly better gram-positive coverage and cefazolin a slightly better gram-negative activity than the remaining drugs in the group, this is not clinically significant.

Cefuroxime (41,42) compares favorably with the first-generation cephalosporins for streptococcal coverage but is slightly less active against staphylococci and less active than cefotaxime or ceftriaxone against *S. pneumoniae* (43,44). It has enhanced gram-negative coverage; in addition to being active against *E. coli, K. pneumoniae,* and *P. mirabilis,* it has good activity against *Haemophilus influenzae,* including β-lactamase producers. Cefuroxime is active against about 30% more of the Enterobacteriaceae, including *Klebsiella oxytoca, Morganella morganii,* and *Citrobacter* species, than are the first-generation cephalosporins.

TABLE 19.4. Suggested Dosage of Cephalosporins in Patients in Renal Failure

Agent	GFR of >50	GFR of 10–50 mL/min	GFR of 10 mL/min	Removed by Hemodialysis	Peritoneal dialysis
Cephalothin	2/4	2/6	1/8	X	X
Cefazolin	1.5/8	1/12	1/24	X	
Cephapirin	2/6	2/6	1/8	X	X
Cephradine	0.5/6	0.25/6	0.25/12	X	
Cefadroxil	0.5/12	0.5/24	0.5/36	X	
Cephalexin	0.5/6	0.25/8	0.25/12	X	X
Cefuroxime	1.5/6	1.5/8	0.75/24	X	
Cefamandole	2/6	2/8	1/8	X	
Cefonicid	2/24	1/24	1/72		
Cefoxitin	2/6	2/8	1/12	X	
Cefotetan	2/12	2/24	1/24	X	?
Cefaclor	0.5/8	0.25/8	0.25/8	X	X
Cefotaxime	2/6	2/8	2/12	X	
Ceftizoxime	2/6	1/12	0.5/12	X	
Cefoperazone	3/8	3/8	3/8	X	X
Ceftazidime	2/8	2/12	1/24	X	
Ceftriaxone	2/12	2/12	2/12		
Cefepime	1/12	1/24	5/24	X	
Cefdinir	0.3/12	0.3/24	0.3/48	X	
Ceftibutin	0.4/24	0.2/24	0.1/24	X	

GFR, glomerular filtration rate.

Activity is not good against *Proteus vulgaris* or *Providencia* and *Serratia* species. The drug is fairly active *in vitro* against gastrointestinal pathogens such as *Yersinia*, *Salmonella*, and *Shigella*. Cefuroxime is also quite active against many isolates of *Neisseria* species. Anaerobic coverage is similar to that of the first-generation agents (45). The spectrum of activity of cefamandole is similar to that of cefuroxime, except that it shows more activity *in vitro* against coagulase-negative staphylococci and it is not as resistant as cefuroxime to certain gram-negative β-lactamases, including the plasmid-mediated (transmission electron microscopy [TEM]) β-lactamase found in ampicillin-resistant *H. influenzae*. Cefuroxime axetil (46) is an oral preparation of cefuroxime with more gram-negative coverage than that offered by the older second-generation oral agent cefaclor (47). The spectrum of activity of cefaclor is identical to that of the first-generation cephalosporins except that it also has good activity against *H. influenzae*, including some α-lactamase–producing strains. Loracarbef (48) has essentially the same coverage, although with further enhanced activity against *Moraxella catarrhalis* and *H. influenzae*, including β-lactamase–producing strains. The spectrum of activity of cefprozil is also similar to that of cefaclor but with gram-negative coverage approaching that of cefuroxime (49,50). Oral cephalosporins that are preferred for infections involving *S. pneumoniae* include cefprozil, cefpodoxime, cefdinir, and ceftibuten (51,52).

The cephamycins cefoxitin (53), cefotetan (54,55), and cefmetazole (56) are noteworthy for their anaerobic coverage. However, they are inferior to metronidazole and imipenem in their coverage of *B. fragilis* (57,58), generally being active against about 80% of isolates. More recent studies show modest increases in resistance of the *B. fragilis* group to cefoxitin, but the increase in resistance is much greater with clindamycin (59,60). Cefoxitin is significantly more active against anaerobic gram-negative bacilli than cefotetan (59,60). The cephamycins have good (though not outstanding) activity against *Neisseria gonorrhoeae*.

All of the third-generation agents (61–67) have excellent activity *in vitro* against gram-negative organisms. More than 80% of the Enterobacteriaceae are susceptible to the third-generation cephalosporins. Nonfermenters such as *Acinetobacter* and *Pseudomonas* species are less susceptible. Of note, resistance has been seen to develop during therapy of *Serratia marcescens*, *Citrobacter freundii*, *Enterobacter cloacae*, and *P. aeruginosa* and is due to the selection of mutants that are derepressed for the production of chromosomally mediated type I cephalosporinases, which can destroy the third-generation cephalosporins (13). Ceftazidime (68–70) has the greatest activity against *P. aeruginosa*. All the drugs, particularly ceftriaxone (71,72), are extremely active against *N. gonorrhoeae* (including penicillinase producers). The gram-positive coverage is slightly inferior to that of the second-generation agents.

Cefepime (73–75) is a parenteral cephalosporin with a broad range of coverage that is classified a "fourth-generation" cephalosporin because of its activity against *Streptococcus pneumoniae*, *Streptococcus pyogenes*, *H. influenzae*, *Neisseria* species, Enterobacteriaceae, and *P. aeruginosa*.

A spate of oral preparations marketed as third-generation cephalosporins include cefixime, cefpodoxime, ceftibutin, and cefdinir (51,52, 76–82).

CLINICAL APPLICATIONS

The dazzling array of oral and parenteral cephalosporins can be made comprehensible if physicians become familiar with the outstanding general features of several of the more useful agents and apply some of the basic tenets of proper antibiotic use. Empiric therapy should be aimed at the most likely responsible organisms, which depends on whether an infection is community acquired or nosocomial, the site of the infection, and specific host factors, such as immune status. Antimicrobial therapy should be as narrowly focused as possible, particularly when bacteriologic data become available. Although a cephalosporin is rarely a drug of first choice for an established infection, these antibiotics are important, especially for initial coverage, because of their low toxicity and broad-activity spectrums. They may be tolerated well by patients allergic to penicillins, provided the allergy is not of the immediate or anaphylactic type. In addition, aminoglycoside therapy can sometimes be avoided by substituting these agents for aminoglycosides in established infections and using them to replace β-lactam/aminoglycoside combinations for initial empiric coverage in some settings. Limitations of this class of antibiotics include lack of activity against enterococci, methicillin-resistant staphylococci, and *Listeria*; poor penetration into CSF by older agents; and undependable activity against *P. aeruginosa* except by ceftazidime.

In general, first-generation agents are reasonable choices for predominantly gram-positive infections, especially skin and soft tissue infections, if one is trying to avoid using a penicillin. The first-generation agents, especially cefazolin, are the mainstay of surgical prophylaxis (83). The second-generation agents can be thought of in two groups: the cephamycins, which are effective for community-acquired mixed aerobic and anaerobic infections of mild to moderate severity; and cefuroxime, with excellent activity against *H. influenzae*–related illnesses such as pneumonia and various head and neck infections. The importance of the third-generation agents lies in their coverage for gram-negative organisms, including many multiresistant Enterobacteriaceae. Because of their excellent penetration into CSF, these drugs (except cefoperazone) are agents of choice for gram-negative meningitis. They may need to be combined with other antibiotics to treat infections with a heavy gram-positive or anaerobic component. Ceftazidime has good activity against *P. aeruginosa* (84).

FIRST-GENERATION CEPHALOSPORINS

The first-generation parenteral cephalosporins, cephalothin, cephapirin, cephradine, and cefazolin (82), are essentially interchangeable in most clinical situations (2,85–89). The longer half-life of cefazolin has made it the most widely used agent in this category (88). These antibiotics are rational choices for infections caused by gram-positive organisms such as methicillin-sensitive staphylococci and nonenterococcal streptococci when one would like to avoid administration of penicillin (90,91). The first-generation agents have a unique role in surgical prophylaxis and remain the standard for cardiac, thoracic, orthopedic, vascular, and most abdominal and obstetric surgery (83). Cefazolin and its relatives should not be used when *Pseudomonas* species, enterococci, *H. influenzae*, or nonstreptococcal anaerobes are of primary concern. In addition, these drugs are useless in central nervous system infection, because they do not penetrate even into inflamed meninges.

Cephalexin, cephradine, and cefadroxil are the so-called first-generation oral cephalosporins (85). They are equivalent in clinical use, including applications for urinary tract and soft tissue infections. Although cefadroxil is promoted for once- or twice-daily dosing, it remains extremely expensive and without advantages other than serum half-life over the other two drugs in the group.

SECOND-GENERATION CEPHALOSPORINS

The extended anaerobic spectrum of the cephamycins renders them especially useful as single-agent therapy of mild to moderately severe community-acquired mixed aerobic and anaerobic infections (57–60): intraabdominal infections such as complications of diverticulitis, pelvic infections including therapy of pelvic inflammatory disease (92), and certain skin and soft tissue infections such as infected diabetic feet and sacral decubiti, in which multidrug-resistant gram-negative organisms are not of utmost concern. They are not appropriate monotherapy for empiric treatment of most nosocomial infections, including intraabdominal sepsis, because coverage in these situations is not predictable. These agents are also inappropriate for infections that are caused primarily by gram-positive organisms. They are popular as prophylactic agents in colorectal surgery, especially when oral agents cannot be used (6,93).

Cefuroxime and cefamandole have roughly comparable spectrums of activity, but cefuroxime (94) has assumed the role of cefamandole in many clinical situations because of its longer half-life and lack of an MTT side chain. Cefuroxime occupies a special niche in the treatment of infections such as certain pneumonias, epiglottitis, complicated sinusitis, and exacerbations of chronic bronchitis in which β-lactamase–producing *H. influenzae* is the major potential pathogen. Bacteremias, urinary tract infections, and soft tissue infections caused by susceptible organisms can also be treated with this agent; its initially promising role in the therapy of meningitis has largely been usurped by the third-generation agents. The same is true of empiric therapy of nosocomial infections or life-threatening gram-negative bacteremia.

The second-generation oral agents, including loracarbef, may be useful in a wide range of community-acquired infections of mild to moderate severity including sinusitis, bronchitis, skin and soft tissue infections, otitis media, and urinary tract infections. However, these agents are expensive and often provide a broader range of coverage than what is indicated. Cefuroxime axetil has been shown to have efficacy for the treatment of early Lyme disease (94,95).

THIRD-GENERATION CEPHALOSPORINS

The third-generation cephalosporins are important in clinical medicine because of their general characteristics of broad antibacterial, especially gram-negative, activity and their penetration into CSF. Particular agents in the group are outstanding because of their antipseudomonal activity (ceftazidime) or their long half-life (ceftriaxone).

Cefotaxime (96–99) and ceftizoxime (100) can be considered equivalent in terms of clinical use. They are especially useful for treating gram-negative nosocomial infections such as pneumonia, complicated urinary tract infections, osteomyelitis, and wound infections. For life-threatening infections, it is prudent to add an aminoglycoside until the infecting organisms and susceptibilities are known, to ensure coverage of organisms such as *Citrobacter, Enterobacter,* and *Serratia.* Better agents are available for treatment of primarily gram-positive or anaerobic infections. These relative gaps in coverage must be provided for by the use of additional drugs if resistant gram-positive or anaerobic bacteria are playing a significant role. These drugs are rarely necessary for community-acquired infections but may be reasonable empiric therapy for a severe illness, especially if *Klebsiella* might be responsible, until bacteriologic data are available. Cefotaxime has

an important role in the treatment of neurologic manifestations of Lyme disease (101,102).

Ceftriaxone can be categorized in the same way as the previous two agents for excellent coverage of many multidrug-resistant gram-negative organisms, with the same general indications (103,104). The newer agent has a unique role in several setting; for example, ceftriaxone is effective therapy for typhoid fever (105) as well as for focal *Salmonella* infection (106); ceftriaxone is used in the treatment of gonococcal disease and is recommended by the Centers for Disease Control and Prevention as one option for therapy of gonococcal disease (92,104–106); and ceftriaxone has gained prominence for the treatment of refractory acute Lyme disease, including meningitis and other neurologic complications (102,107). As the focus on home antibiotic therapy has increased, so has the interest in using ceftriaxone in this setting, because of its infrequent dosing and effectiveness as either an intravascular or an intramuscular agent (105,109). Twice-daily dosing is still preferred by many physicians for serious infections such as meningitis and endocarditis, but once-daily dosing is effective even in these settings (109–111).

The empiric use of ceftriaxone or cefotaxime is recommended for community-acquired meningitis typically caused by *N. meningitides* or *S. pneumoniae.* These agents can be useful in the treatment of meningitis caused by gram-negative organisms, but only ceftazidime can be used for the treatment of cases caused by *P. aeruginosa.* There have been reports of ceftriaxone failures in the treatment of meningitis caused by *S. pneumoniae* with relative and especially high-level resistance to penicillin (115,116). Recommendations, pending results of susceptibility testing, suggest preferential therapy with vancomycin plus cefotaxime or ceftriaxone in suspected cases of pneumococcal meningitis (117). None of the cephalosporins has a role in the treatment of *L. monocytogenes* meningitis.

Ceftazidime and cefepime are similar to the agents already discussed in general effectiveness for gram-negative infections and can be employed in the therapy of *P. aeruginosa*–related infection. Many studies have examined the role of these drugs, alone or in combination with an aminoglycoside, as empiric therapy for febrile neutropenic patients (118–122). Although controversy exists, it seems most prudent to use the combination in this setting as well as in treating most serious *P. aeruginosa* infections in normal hosts. Special clinical situations in which ceftazidime or cefepime can be considered the treatment of choice for *Pseudomonas* infections include *P. aeruginosa* meningitis (123,124) and cystic fibrosis pulmonary infections (125,126).

The third-generation cephalosporins have proven to be of great clinical importance, but their precise clinical roles are still being defined. Some of the evolving issues that need to be evaluated systematically include the problems of superinfection with enterococci (127,128) and the role of these drugs in promoting vancomycin-resistant enterococcus (129,130). The same concern applies to highly resistant gram-negative organisms including the likelihood of resistance developing during therapy, especially by extended-spectrum β-lactamase production (131,132). The prudent use of the broad-spectrum late-generation cephalosporins and stringent adherence to infection control measures appear to be the best available methods for containing emergence and nosocomial spread of organisms resistant to these agents. The precise role of the third-generation oral cephalosporins in the outpatient armamentarium remains to be defined. As is true of the second-generation agents, these oral cephalosporins are often expensive and may cover a broader range of organisms than is appropriate in the treatment of a specific outpatient infection.

TOXICITY

Local Reactions

The cephalosporins are quite safe; grave adverse effects are rare. As with any intravenous agent, the potential for phlebitis (133) exists. Prevalence rates from different studies vary from 1% to 5%, with no agent being more irritating than others. Cefoxitin and cephalothin are poorly tolerated when administered via the intramuscular route unless accompanied by a local anesthetic.

Hypersensitivity Reactions

Immediate hypersensitivity reactions to the cephalosporins rarely occur (134,135). More common but still infrequent are drug fever, eosinophilia, angioedema, and rash. The true incidence of these manifestations is not known, but a rash, the most common reaction, has been estimated to occur in 1% to 3% of patients (33,136) (Table 19.5).

The extent to which cross-allergy between the penicillins and cephalosporins exists has long been debated, but the largest review with analysis of 15,987 patients showed the reaction rate to cephalosporin in those with penicillin allergy was 8.1% compared with 1.9% in those with no such history. Thus, the risk is about fourfold. For patients with a positive skin-test result to penicillin, the reaction rate is 6 (4.4%) of 135 compared with 2 (0.6%) of 351 in those with negative penicillin skin-test results (137). The true incidence of cross-reactivity probably lies in the range of 3% to 7%. Based on these observations, the following recommendations are options for patients with penicillin allergy who are candidates for cephalosporin therapy:

1. Select an antibiotic that does not have a β-lactam ring.
2. Give a cephalosporin only if the risk of anaphylaxis is considered low enough to justify the risk.
3. Perform a skin test for penicillin allergy, preferably with both major and minor determinants because this defines the risk of cephalosporin allergy; about 80% to 90% of patients with a history of penicillin allergy have a negative test result and there is no useful skin test for cephalosporins. This strategy is particularly attractive when cephalosporin therapy is strongly indicated.
4. For those with a history of allergy to cephalosporin, cephalosporins should be avoided, including all drugs in this class. Desensitization to cephalosporins has been tried, but it has not been standardized and experience is limited.
5. It is important to establish the need for cephalosporin, in addition to a history of allergy to cephalosporins or a skin-test result positive for penicillin allergy; desensitization regimens should be done only by trained personnel.

TABLE 19.5.   Reactions to Cephalosporins

Reaction	Rate
Rash	1.0–2.8%
Coombs' positive	1.0–2.0%
Anaphylaxis	0.0001–0.1%
Fever	0.5–0.9%
Eosinophilia	2.7–8.2%

Source: From Kelkar PS, Li J T-C. Cephalosporin allergy. *N Engl J Med* 2001;345:804, with permission.

Serum sickness–like reactions can result from the tissue deposition of β-lactam–specific immunoglobulin G or immunoglobulin M antibodies and circulating β-lactam antigens (138). Although this occurs rarely with cephalosporin use overall, cefaclor use in children has been associated with serum sickness 15 times more frequently than ampicillin use (139).

Hepatic and Gastrointestinal Disturbances

Elevated transaminase levels have been reported in conjunction with use of almost all the cephalosporins, occurring at a frequency of 1% to 7%, but whether this is due to the antibiotic or to the underlying condition the antibiotic is treating is unclear (140). Profound hepatic injury has been reported but is quite rare (141).

The reported frequency of nonspecific antibiotic-associated diarrhea varies greatly among various studies but is usually reported in registration trials to be at 2% to 5% (142). Diarrhea caused by *Clostridium difficile* is more frequently attributed to cephalosporins than any other class of drugs, although this is due in part to heavy usage rates, especially in nosocomial *C. difficile*–associated diarrhea (142–145).

Ceftriaxone has been associated with formation of biliary sludge detectable by ultrasound examination. This is typically asymptomatic, but symptoms of cholecystitis can occur, leading to cholecystectomy (145–149). This complication is related to dose (>40 mg/kg per day) and duration of therapy and reflects the precipitation of calcium ceftriaxone (146). Sludge may present with rapid onset of biliary obstruction with biliary colic, acute pancreatitis, or acute cholecystitis, and it may disappear rapidly when the drug is discontinued (148,149).

Neurotoxicity

Although seizures have been associated with several of the cephalosporins, they have occurred generally in the setting of excessive doses (150,151). The neurotoxicity of these agents is quite low, and they have been used safely intraventricularly (150).

Disulfiram-like Reactions

Disulfiram-like reactions have occurred with the ingestion of alcohol several hours after administration of cephalosporins with 3-MTT side chains, such as are found on molecules of cefoperazone, cefotetan, cefonicid, and cefamandole (152,153). This is likely due to an accumulation of acetaldehyde, which is the result of the ability of the MTT metabolite to inhibit aldehyde dehydrogenase. This enzyme normally metabolizes the ethanol breakdown product acetaldehyde to water and carbon dioxide (150).

Nephrotoxicity

One of the older cephalosporins (33), cephaloridine, became renowned for its dose-dependent nephrotoxicity (154) and is no longer in clinical use. Cephalothin has, on rare occasion, been associated with renal failure, probably because of tubular injury (155). Although ceftazidime may cause a decrease in the glomerular filtration rate, tubule function is affected to only a small degree (156) and clinical problems are not apparent (157). Overall, the potential for nephrotoxicity by available agents is extremely low (158); interstitial nephritis can be seen as part of a hypersensitivity reaction to cephalosporins (140).

Hematologic Toxicity

Although development of a positive reaction to the Coombs' test is thought to be relatively frequent (3%) in patients receiving cephalosporins (159), most reports and reviews focus on the older drugs in this class. The actual incidence with use of the more recently developed members of the group is unclear (160,161). The incidence of hemolytic anemia is extremely low, even in patients with a positive Coombs' reaction, and is most often due to an immune complex–mediated process (162,163). Neutropenia is an unusual (1%) complication that reverses rapidly with cessation of therapy and typically occurs only after several weeks of treatment. Eosinophilia or thrombocytosis is frequently seen (5%), but these conditions are most likely results of the underlying infection. Isolated cases of immune-mediated platelet dysfunction have been reported for several cephalosporins.

The cephalosporins can affect hemostasis. Hypoprothrombinemia with the use of many antibiotics, including cephalosporins, has been thought to arise from depletion of vitamin K–processing intestinal flora (164,165). There is compelling evidence that those cephalosporins with an MTT side chain induce hypoprothrombinemia by inhibiting vitamin K metabolism and carboxylation of glutamic acid. Estimates of the prevalence of hypoprothrombinemia due to these agents range from 4% to 68% (167,168). The precise incidence of bleeding caused by cephalosporin use has been difficult to assess, because multiple confounding factors appear to be involved. Among agents in use, clinically apparent bleeding has been reported with cefoperazone (169) and cefotetan (170) and is more likely to occur in the setting of renal failure and debilitation. A single subcutaneous injection of vitamin K reverses hypoprothrombinemia, usually in a matter of hours unless the cephalosporin has an MTT side chain, in which case the prothrombin time may take 24 to 36 hours to normalize (168). If bleeding is present, fresh frozen plasma may be necessary.

CEPHALOSPORINS IN PERSPECTIVE

Cephalosporins are among the most frequently used drugs in medicine in large part because of its extraordinary record of clinical efficacy and safety. These agents are listed as preferred agents by the *Medical Letter* (113) for pneumococcal pneumonia (ceftriaxone or cefotaxime), for common forms of pyogenic meningitis (ceftriaxone or cefotaxime), for nosocomial pneumonia (cefepime or ceftazidime), for sepsis (cefotaxime, ceftizoxime, ceftriaxone, cefepime, or ceftazidime), for many anaerobic infections (cefoxitin, cefotetan, or cefmetazole), and for most surgical prophylaxis (cefazolin). For outpatients, they are frequently recommended for common bacterial respiratory tract infections (loracarbef, cefprozil, cefuroxime, cefpodoxime, ceftibuten, cefdinir, or cefditoren), infections involving methicillin-sensitive *S. aureus* (cephalexin or cephradine), and urinary tract infections (cefixime, cefpodoxime, cefdinir, and ceftibuten). This extensive use has not been without penalties and it now appears that the use and abuse of these drugs has contributed substantially to some of the greatest problems in the current practice of infectious diseases. Specific associations with cephalosporins are infections involving penicillin-resistant *S. pneumoniae*, coagulase-negative staphylococci, enterococci including vancomycin-resistant enterococci, methicillin-resistant *S. aureus*, *Candida albicans*, extended-spectrum β-lactam–producing bacteria, *P. aeruginosa*, and *C. difficile* (171). Policies that restrict use of cephalosporins appear to benefit in terms of reduced prevalence of resistant bacteria (172–175), although it is often unclear that such restriction should be applied to any single class (173).

REFERENCES

1. Abraham EP. Cephalosporins 1945–1986. In: Williams JD, ed. *The cephalosporin antibiotics.* Auckland, New Zealand: Adis Press, 1987:1–14.
2. Abraham EP, Loder PB. Cephalosporin C. In: Flynn EH, ed. *Cephalosporins and penicillins: chemistry and biology.* New York: Academic Press, 1972:2–26.
3. Rolinson GN. The influence of 6-aminopenicillanic acid on antibiotic development. *J Antimicrob Chemother* 1988;22:5.
4. Oniski HR, Daoust DR, Zimmerman SB, et al. Cefoxitin, a semisynthetic cephamycin antibiotic: resistance to β-lactamase inactivation. *Antimicrob Agents Chemother* 1974;5:38.
5. Allan JD, Eliopoulos GM, Moellering RC Jr. Antibiotics: future directions by understanding structure-function relationships. In: Root RK, Trunkey DD, Sande MA, eds. *Contemporary issues in infectious diseases,* vol 6. New York: Churchill Livingstone, 1987:263–284.
6. Dunn GL. Ceftizoxime and other third generation cephalosporins: structure-activity relationships. *J Antimicrob Chemother* 1982;10[Suppl C]:1.
7. Neu HC. Relation of structural properties of β-lactam antibiotics to antibacterial activity. *Am J Med* 1985;79:2.
8. Fassbender M, Lode H, Schaberg T, et al. Pharmacokinetics of new cephalosporins, including a new carbacephem. *Clin Infect Dis* 1993;16:646.
9. Cooper RD. The carbacephems: a new β-lactam antibiotic class. *Am J Med* 1992;92:25.
10. Williams JD. Classification of cephalosporins. In: Williams JD, ed. *The cephalosporin antibiotics.* Auckland, New Zealand: Adis Press, 1987:15–22.
11. Yocum RR, Rasmussin JR, Strominger SL. The mechanism of action of penicillin: penicillin activates the active site of *Bacillus stearothermophilus* D-alanine carboxypeptidase. *J Biol Chem* 1980;255:3977.
12. Tomasz A. Penicillin-binding proteins in bacteria. *Ann Intern Med* 1982;96:502.
13. Jacoby GA, Archer GL. New mechanisms of bacterial resistance to antimicrobial agents. *N Engl J Med* 1991;324:601.
14. Sanders CC, Sanders WE Jr. Microbial resistance to newer generation β-lactam antibiotics: clinical and laboratory implications. *J Infect Dis* 1985;151:399.
15. Fontano R, Grossato A, Rossi L, et al. Transition from resistance to hyper-susceptibility to β-lactam antibiotics associated with loss of a low-affinity penicillin-binding protein in a *Streptococcus faecium* mutant highly resistant to penicillin. *Antimicrob Agents Chemother* 1985;28:678.
16. Hartman BJ, Tomasz A. Low-affinity penicillin-binding protein associated with β-lactam resistance in *Staphylococcus aureus. J Bacteriol* 1984;158:513.
17. Handwerger S, Tomasz A. Alterations in the penicillin-binding proteins of clinical and laboratory isolates of *Streptococcus pneumoniae* with low levels of penicillin resistance. *J Infect Dis* 1986;153:83.
18. Gutmann L, Williamson R, Collatz E. The possible role of porins in antibiotic resistance. *Ann Intern Med* 1984;101:554.
19. Mitsuyama J, Hiruma R, Jagamuchi A, et al. Identification of porins in outer membrane of *Proteus, Morganella* and *Providencia* spp. and their role in outer membrane permeation of β-lactams. *Antimicrob Agents Chemother* 1987;31:379.
20. Sanders CC. Beta-lactamases of gram-negative bacteria: new challenges for new drugs. *Clin Infect Dis* 1992;14:1089.
21. Sanders WE, Sanders CC. Inducible β-lactamases: clinical and epidemiologic implications for use of newer cephalosporins. *Rev Infect Dis* 1988;10:830.
22. Cullmann W, Opferkuch W, Stieglitz M, et al. Influence of spontaneous and inducible β-lactamase production in the antimicrobial activity of recently developed β-lactam compounds. *Chemotherapy* 1984;30:175.
23. Medeiros AA. Nosocomial outbreaks of multiresistant bacteria: extended-spectrum beta-lactamases have arrived in North America. *Ann Intern Med* 1993;119:428.
24. Jacoby GA, Medeiros AA. More extended-spectrum β-lactamases. *Antimicrob Agents Chemother* 1991;35:1697.
25. Sanders CC. New beta-lactams: new problems for the internist. *Ann Intern Med* 1991;115:650.
26. Donowitz GR, Mandell GL. Beta-lactam antibiotics. *N Engl J Med* 1988;313:490.
27. Brogard JM, Conte F. Pharmacokinetics of the new cephalosporins. *Antimicrob Agents Chemother* 1982;21:592.
28. Bergan T. Pharmacokinetic properties of the cephalosporins. In: Williams JD, ed. *The cephalosporin antibiotics.* Auckland, New Zealand: Adis Press, 1987:89–104.
29. Patel IH, Kaplan SA. Pharmacokinetic profile of ceftriaxone in man. *Am J Med* 1984;77[Suppl 4G]:17.
30. Chin NX, Neu HC. Cefotaxime and desacetyl cefotaxime: an example of advantageous antimicrobial metabolism. *Diagn Microbiol Infect Dis* 1984;2:215.
31. Kemmerich B, Lode H, Borner K, et al. Biliary excretion and pharmacokinetics of cefoperazone in humans. *J Antimicrob Chemother* 1983;12:27.
32. Cherubin CE, Eng RH, Norrby R, et al. Penetration of newer cephalosporins into cerebrospinal fluid. *Rev Infect Dis* 1989;11:526.
33. Gustaferro CA, Steckelberg JM. Cephalosporin antimicrobial agents and related compounds. *Mayo Clin Proc* 1991;66:1064.
34. Basker MJ, Edmonson RA, Sutherland R. Comparative stabilities of penicillins and cephalosporins to staphylococcal β-lactamase and activities against *Staphylococcus aureus. J Antimicrob Chemother* 1980;6:333.

35. Hartstein AI, Patrick KE, Jones SR, et al. Comparison of pharmacologic and antimicrobial properties of cefadroxil and cephalexin. *Antimicrob Agents Chemother* 1977;12:93.

36. Silver MS, Counts GW, Zeleznik D, et al. Comparison of in vitro antibacterial activity of three oral cephalosporins: cefaclor, cephalexin and cephradine. *Antimicrob Agents Chemother* 1977;12:591.

37. Renzini G, Ravagnan G, Oliva B. *In vitro* and *in vivo* microbiological evaluation of cephapirin, a new antibiotic. *Chemotherapy* 1975;21:289.

38. Bergeron MG, Brusch JL, Barza M, et al. Bactericidal activity and pharmacology of cefazolin. *Antimicrob Agents Chemother* 1973;4:396.

39. Phair JP, Carlton J, Tan JS. Comparison of cefazolin, a new cephalosporin antibiotic, with cephalothin. *Antimicrob Agents Chemother* 1972;2:329.

40. Turck M, Anderson KN, Smith RH, et al. Laboratory and clinical evaluation of a new antibiotic: cephalothin. *Ann Intern Med* 1965;63:199.

41. Neu HC, Fu KP. Cefuroxime, a β-lactamase–resistant cephalosporin with a broad spectrum of gram-positive and -negative activity. *Antimicrob Agents Chemother* 1978;13:657.

42. O'Callaghan CH, Sykes RB, Griffiths A, et al. Cefuroxime, a new cephalosporin antibiotic: activity *in vitro*. *Antimicrob Agents Chemother* 1976;9:511.

43. Bartlett JG, Dowell SF, Mandell LA, et al. Practice guidelines for the management of community-acquired pneumonia in adults. *Clin Infect Dis* 2000;31:347.

44. Jones ME, Karlowsky JA, Blosser-Middleton R, et al. Longitudinal assessment of antipneumococcal susceptibility in the United States. *Antimicrob Agents Chemother* 2002;46:2651.

45. Rolfe D, Finegold SM. Comparative *in vitro* activity of new β-lactam antibiotics against anaerobic bacteria. *Antimicrob Agents Chemother* 1981;20:600.

46. Ginsburg CM. Pharmacokinetics and bactericidal activity of cefuroxime axetil. *Antimicrob Agents Chemother* 1985;28:504.

47. Medical Letter. Two new oral cephalosporins. *Med Lett Drugs Ther* 1979;31:85.

48. Brogden RN, McTavish D. Loracarbef: a review of its antimicrobial activity, pharmacokinetic properties and therapeutic efficacy. *Drugs* 1993;45:716.

49. Wiseman LR, Benfield P. Cefprozil: a review of its antibacterial activity, pharmacokinetic properties and therapeutic potential. *Drugs* 1993;45:295.

50. Thornsberry C. Review of the *in vitro* antibacterial activity of cefprozil, a new cephalosporin. *Clin Infect Dis* 1992;1:95.

51. Ross GH, Hovde LB, Ibrahim KH, et al. Comparison of once daily versus twice daily administration of cefdinir against typical bacterial respiratory tract pathogens. *Antimicrob Agents Chemother* 2001;45:2936.

52. Anonymous. Cefditoren (Spectracef)—a new oral cephalosporin. *The Medical Letter* 2002;44:5.

53. Birnbaum J, Stapley EO, Miller AK, et al. Cefoxitin, a semisynthetic cephamycin: a microbiologic overview. *J Antimicrob Chemother* 1978;4:15.

54. Ward A, Richards DM. Cefotetan: a review. *Drugs* 1985;30:382.

55. Ayres LW, Jones RN, Barry AL, et al. Cefotetan, a new cephamycin. *Antimicrob Agents Chemother* 1982;22:859.

56. Jones RN. Review of the *in-vitro* spectrum and characteristics of cefmetazole. *J Antimicrob Chemother* 1989;12[Suppl D]:1.

57. Goldstein EJC, Citron DM. Annual incidence, epidemiology and comparative *in vitro* susceptibilities to cefoxitin, cefotetan, cefmetazole and ceftizoxime of recent community-acquired isolates of the *Bacteroides fragilis* group. *J Antimicrob Chemother* 1988;26:2361.

58. Back VT, Roy I, Thadepalli H. Susceptibility of anaerobic bacteria to cefoxitin and related compounds. *Antimicrob Agents Chemother* 1977;11:912.

59. Snydman DR, Jacobus NW, McDermott LA, et al. National survey on the susceptibility of *Bacteroides fragilis* group: report and analysis of trends for 1997–2000. *Clin Infect Dis* 2002;35[Suppl 1]:S126.

60. Aldridge KE, Ashcraft D, Cambre K, et al. Multicenter survey of the changing in vitro antimicrobial susceptibilities of clinical isolates of *Bacteroides fragilis* group, *Prevotella*, *Fusobacterium*, *Porphyromonas* and *Peptostreptococcus*. *Antimicrob Agents Chemother* 2001;45:1238.

61. Neu HC. Pathophysiologic basis for the use of third-generation cephalosporins. *Am J Med* 1990;88[Suppl 4A]:35.

62. Goldberg DM. The cephalosporins. *Med Clin North Am* 1987;71:1113.

63. Thornsberry C. Review of *in vitro* activity of third-generation cephalosporins and other newer β-lactam antibiotics against clinically important bacteria. *Am J Med* 1985;79:14.

64. Carmine AA, Brogden RN, Heel RC, et al. Cefotaxime: a review of its antibacterial activity, pharmacological properties and therapeutic use. *Drugs* 1983;25:223.

65. Fass RJ. Comparative *in vitro* activities of third-generation cephalosporins. *Arch Intern Med* 1983;143:1743.

66. Jones RN, Thornsberry C. Cefotaxime: a review of *in vitro* antimicrobial properties and spectrum of activity. *Rev Infect Dis* 1982;4[Suppl]:5300.

67. Fu KP, Neu HC. Antibacterial activity of ceftizoxime, a β-lactamase stable cephalosporin. *Antimicrob Agents Chemother* 1980;17:583.

68. Neu HC, Labthavikul P. Antibacterial activity and β-lactamase stability of ceftazidime. *Antimicrob Agents Chemother* 1982;21:11.

69. Gozzard DJ, Geddes AM, Farrell ID, et al. Ceftazidime—a new extended-spectrum cephalosporin. *Lancet* 1982;1:1152.

70. Brogden RN, Carmine A, Heel RC, et al. Cefoperazone: a review of its *in vitro* antimicrobial activity, pharmacological properties and therapeutic efficacy. *Drugs* 1981;22:423.

71. Cleeland R, Squires E. Antimicrobial activity of ceftriaxone: a review. *Am J Med* 1984;77:3.

72. Center for Disease Control and Prevention. Sexually transmitted diseases treatment guidelines 2002. *MMWR Morb Mortal Wkly Rep* 2002;51(RR-6):1.

73. Barradell LB, Bryson HM. Cefepime: a review of its antibacterial activity, pharmacokinetic properties and therapeutic use. *Drugs* 1994;47:471.

74. Grassi GG, Grassi C. Cefepime: an overview of activity *in vitro* and *in vivo*. *J Antimicrob Chemother* 1993;32[Suppl B]:87.

75. Jones RN, Kirby JT, Beach ML, et al. Geographic variations in activity of broad-spectrum betalactams against *Pseudomonas aeruginosa*: summary of the worldwide SENTRY Antimicrobial Surveillance Program 1997–2000. *Diagn Microbiol Infect Dis* 2002;43:239.

76. Neu HC. Oral beta-lactam antibiotics from 1960–1993. *Infect Dis Clin Pract* 1993;6:394.

77. Bluestone CD. Review of cefixime in the treatment of otitis media in infants and children. *Pediatr Infect Dis J* 1993;12:75.

78. Leggett NJ, Caravaggio C, Rybak MJ. Cefixime. *DICP* 1990;24:489.

79. Chocas EC, Paap CM, Godley PJ. Cefpodoxime proxetil: a new, broad-spectrum oral cephalosporin. *Ann Pharmacother* 1993;27:1369.

80. Wiseman LR, Balfour JA. Ceftibuten. A review of its antibacterial activity, pharmacokinetic properties and clinical efficacy. *Drugs* 1994;47:784.

81. Darkes MJ, Plosker GL. Cefditoren pivoxil. *Drugs* 2002;62:319.

82. Sultan T, Baltch AL, Smith RF, et al. *In vitro* activity of cefdinir (FK482) and ten other antibiotics against gram-positive and gram-negative bacteria isolated from adult and pediatric patients. *Chemotherapy* 1994;40:80.

83. Geroulanos S, Marathias K, Kriaras J, et al. Cephalosporins in surgical prophylaxis. *J Chemother* 2001;13:23.

84. Ramphal R, Hoban DJ, Pfaller MA, et al. Comparison of the activity of two broad spectrum cephalosporins tested against 2,299 strains of *Pseudomonas aeruginosa* isolated at 38 North American medical centers participating in the SENTRY antimicrobial surveillance program 1997–98. *Diagn Microbiol Infect Dis* 2000;36:125.

85. Moellering RC Jr, Swartz MN. The newer cephalosporins. *N Engl J Med* 1976;294:24.

86. Van Scoy RE, Wilkowske CJ. Prophylactic use of anti-microbial agents in adult patients. *Mayo Clin Proc* 1992;67:288.

87. Perkins RL, Saslaw S. Experiences with cephalothin. *Ann Intern Med* 1966;64:13.

88. Quintiliani R, Nightingale CH. Cefazolin. *Ann Intern Med* 1978;89:650.

89. Perl B, Gottchrer NP, Raveh D, et al. Cost-effectiveness of blood cultures for adult patients with cellulitis. *Clin Infect Dis* 1999;29:1483.

90. Neu HC. The place of cephalosporins in antibacterial treatment of infectious diseases. *J Antimicrob Chemother* 1980;6[Suppl A]:1.

91. Quinn EL, Pohlod D, Madhavan T, et al. Clinical experience with cefazolin and other cephalosporins in bacterial endocarditis. *J Infect Dis* 1983;128[Suppl]:S386.

92. Behra-Miellet J, Dubreuil L, Jumas-Bilak E. Antianaerobic activity of moxifloxacin compared to that of ofloxacin, clindamycin, metronidazole and beta-lactams. *Int J Antimicrob Agents* 2002;20:366.

93. Gorbach SL. The role of cephalosporins in surgical prophylaxis. *J Antimicrob Chemother* 1989;23[Suppl D]:61.

94. Luger SW, Paparone P, Wormser GP, et al. Comparison of cefuroxime axetil and doxycycline in treatment of patients with early Lyme disease associated with erythema migrans. *Antimicrob Agents Chemother* 1995;39:661.

95. Wormser GP, Nadelman RB, Dennis DT, et al. Practice guidelines for the treatment of Lyme disease. *Clin Infect Dis* 2000;31[Suppl 1]:1.

96. Smith CR, Ambinder R, Lipsky JJ, et al. Cefotaxime compared with nafcillin plus tobramycin for serious bacterial infections: a randomized, double-blind trial. *Ann Intern Med* 1984;101:469.

97. Karakusis PH, Feczko JM, Goodman LJ, et al. Clinical efficacy of cefotaxime in serious infections. *Antimicrob Agents Chemother* 1982;21:119.

98. Francke EL, Neu HC. Use of cefotaxime, a β-lactamase stable cephalosporin in therapy of serious infection, including those due to multiresistant organisms. *Am J Med* 1981;71:435.

99. Young JPW, Hussan JM, Bruch K, et al. The evaluation of efficacy and safety of cefotaxime: a review of 2500 cases. *J Antimicrob Chemother* 1980;6[Suppl A]:293.

100. Scully BE, Neu HC. The use of ceftizoxime in the treatment of critically ill patients infected with multiply antibiotic resistant bacteria. *J Antimicrob Chemother* 1982;10:141.

101. Halperin JJ. Neuroborreliosis. *Am J Med* 1995;98[Suppl 4A]:53S.

102. Wormser GP. Treatment and prevention of Lyme disease, with emphasis on antimicrobial therapy for neuroborreliosis and vaccination. *Semin Neurol* 1997;17:45.

103. Klempner MS, Hu LT, Evans J, et al. Two controlled trials of antibiotic treatment in patients with persistent symptoms and a history of Lyme disease. *N Engl J Med* 2001;345:85.

104. Lind I. Antimicrobial resistance in *Neisseria gonorrhoeae*. *Clin Infect Dis* 1997;24:S93.

105. Judson FN, Ehret JM, Handsfield HH. Comparative study of ceftriaxone and spectinomycin for treatment of pharyngeal and anorectal gonorrhea. *JAMA* 1985;253:1417.

106. Laga M, Naamara W, Brunham RC, et al. Single-dose therapy of gonococcal ophthalmia neonatorum with ceftriaxone. *N Engl J Med* 1986;315:1382.

107. Dattwyler RJ, Halperin JJ, Volkman DJ, et al. Treatment of late Lyme borreliosis-randomised comparison of ceftriaxone and penicillin. *Lancet* 1988;1:1191.

108. Baumgartner JD, Glauser MP. Single daily dose treatment of severe refractory

infections with ceftriaxone: cost savings and possible outpatient treatment. *Arch Intern Med* 1983;143:1868.

109. Francioli PB. Ceftriaxone and outpatient treatment of infective endocarditis. *Infect Dis Clin* 1993;7:97.

110. Cabellos C, Viladrich PF, Verdaguer R, et al. A single daily dose of ceftriaxone for bacterial meningitis in adults. *Clin Infect Dis* 1995;20:1164.

111. Francioli P, Etienne J, Hoigne R, et al. Treatment of streptococcal endocarditis with a single daily dose of ceftriaxone sodium for four weeks. *JAMA* 1992;267:264.

112. Durand ML, Calderwood SB, Weber DJ, et al. Acute bacterial meningitis: a review of 493 episodes. *N Engl J Med* 1993;328:21.

113. Anonymous. The choice of antibacterial drugs. *Med Lett Drugs Ther* 2001;43:69.

114. Scholz H, Hofmann T, Noack R, et al. Prospective comparison of ceftriaxone and cefotaxime for the short term treatment of bacterial meningitis in children. *Chemotherapy* 1997;44:142.

115. John CC. Treatment failure with use of a third-generation cephalosporin for penicillin-resistant pneumococcal meningitis: case report and review. *Clin Infect Dis* 1994;18:188.

116. van der Beek D, de Gans J, Spanjaard L, et al. Antibiotic guidelines and antibiotic use in adult bacterial meningitis in The Netherlands. *J Antimicrob Chemother* 2002;49:661.

117. Moller K, Skinhoj P. Guidelines for managing acute bacterial meningitis. *BMJ* 2000;320:1290.

118. Bodey GP. Empirical antibiotic therapy for fever in neutropenic patients. *Clin Infect Dis* 1993;17[Suppl 2]:S378.

119. Hughes WT, Armstrong D, Bodey GP, et al. Guidelines for the use of antimicrobial agents in neutropenic patients with unexplained fever. *J Infect Dis* 1990;161:381.

120. EORTC International Antimicrobial Therapy. Cooperative group: ceftazidime combined with a short or long course of amikacin for empirical therapy of gram-negative bacteremia in cancer patients with granulocytopenia. *N Engl J Med* 1987;317:1692.

121. Tam VH, McKinnon PS, Akins RL, et al. Pharmacodynamics of cefepime in patients with gram-negative infections. *J Antimicrob Chemother* 2002;50:425.

122. Sanz MA, Lopez J, Lahuerta JJ, et al. Cefepime plus amikacin versus piperacillin-tazobactam plus amikacin for initial antibiotic therapy in haematology patients with febrile neutropenia: results of an open randomized, multicenter trial. *J Antimicrob Chemother* 2002;50:79.

123. Fong IW, Tomkins B. Review of *Pseudomonas aeruginosa* meningitis with special emphasis on treatment with ceftazidime. *Rev Infect Dis* 1985;7:604.

124. Blumer JL, Stern RC, Klinger JD, et al. Ceftazidime therapy in patients with cystic fibrosis and multiply, drug-resistant *Pseudomonas. Am J Med* 1985;79[Suppl 2A]:37.

125. Lyczak JB, Cannon CL, Pier GB. Lung infections associated with cystic fibrosis. *Clin Microbiol Rev* 2002;15:194.

126. Robinson CA, Kuhn RJ, Craigmyle J, et al. Susceptibility of *Pseudomonas aeruginosa* to cefepime vs. ceftazidime in patients with cystic fibrosis. *Pharmacotherapy* 2001;21:1320.

127. Pallares R, Pujol M, Pena C, et al. Cephalosporins as risk factor for nosocomial *Enterococcus faecalis* bacteremia. *Arch Intern Med* 1993;153:1581.

128. Moellering RC Jr. Enterococcal infections in patients treated with moxalactam. *Rev Infect Dis* 1982;4[Suppl]:S708.

129. Carmeli Y, Eliopoulos GM, Samore MH. Antecedent treatment with different antibiotic agents as a risk factor for vancomycin-resistant enterococcus. *Emerg Infect Dis* 2002;8:802.

130. Fridkin SK, Edwards JR, Courval JM, et al. The effect of vancomycin and third generation cephalosporins on the prevalence of vancomycin-resistant enterococci in 126 U.S. adult intensive care units. *Ann Intern Med* 2001;135:175.

131. Nordmann P, Guibert M. Extended spectrum betalactamases in *Pseudomonas aeruginosa. J Antimicrob Chemother* 1998;42:128.

132. Quale JM, Landman D, Bradford PA, et al. Molecular epidemiology of a citywide outbreak of extended-spectrum betalactamase–producing *Klebsiella pneumoniae* infection. *Clin Infect Dis* 2002;35:834.

133. Berger S, Ennst EC, Barza M. Comparative incidence of phlebitis due to buffered cephalothin, cephapirin, and cefamandole. *Antimicrob Agents Chemother* 1976;9:575.

134. Lin RY. A perspective on penicillin allergy. *Arch Intern Med* 1992;152:930.

135. Saxon A, Beall GN, Rohr AS, et al. Immediate hypersensitivity reactions to β-lactam antibiotics. *Ann Intern Med* 1987;107:204.

136. Kelkar PS, Li JT-C. Cephalosporin allergy. *N Engl J Med* 2001;345:804.

137. Lin RY. A perspective on penicillin allergy. *Arch Intern Med* 1992;152:930.

138. Wendel GD Jr, Stark BJ, Jamison RB, et al. Penicillin allergy and desensitization in serious infections during pregnancy. *N Engl J Med* 1985;312:1229.

139. Heckbert SR, Stryker WS, Coltin KL, et al. Serum sickness in children after antibiotic exposure. *Am J Epidemiol* 1990;132:336.

140. Norrby SR. Problems in evaluation of adverse reactions to β-lactam antibiotics. *Rev Infect Dis* 1986;8[Suppl 3]:S358.

141. Ammann R, Neftel K, Hardmeier TH, et al. Cephalosporin-induced cholestatic jaundice. *Lancet* 1982;2:336.

142. Bartlett JG. Antibiotic-associated diarrhea. *N Engl J Med* 2002;346:334.

143. Winstrom J, Norrby SR, Myhre EB, et al. Frequency of antibiotic-associated diarrhea in 2,462 antibiotic-treated hospitalized patients. *J Antimicrob Chemother* 2001;47:43.

144. Bartlett JG. Antimicrobial agents implicated in *Clostridium difficile* toxin-associated diarrhea or colitis. *Johns Hopkins Med J* 1981;149:6.

145. Lopez AJ, O'Keefe P, Morrissey M, et al. Ceftriaxone-induced cholelithiasis. *Ann Intern Med* 1991;115:712.

146. Park HZ, Lee SP, Schy AL. Ceftriaxone-associated gallbladder sludge: Identification of calcium-ceftriaxone salt as a major component of gallbladder precipitate. *Gastroenterology* 1991;100:1665.

147. Centers for Disease Control and Prevention. Ceftriaxone-associated biliary complications of treatment of suspected disseminated Lyme disease—New Jersey 1990–1992. *JAMA* 1993;269:979.

148. Kim YS, Kestell MF, Lee SP. Gallbladder sludge: lessons from ceftriaxone. *J Gastroenterol Hepatol* 1992;7:618.

149. Ko CW, Sekijima JH, Lee SP. Biliary sludge. *Ann Intern Med* 1999;130:301.

150. Klion AD, Kallsen J, Cowl CT, et al. Ceftazidime-related nonconvulsive status epilepticus. *Arch Intern Med* 1994;154:586.

151. Fekety FR. Safety of parenteral third-generation cephalosporins. *Am J Med* 1990;88[Suppl 4A]:38S.

152. Elenbaas RM, Ryan JL, Robinson WA, et al. On the disulfiram-like activity of moxalactam. *Clin Pharmacol Ther* 1982;32:347.

153. Buening MK, Wold JS, Israel KS, et al. Disulfiram-like reactions to β-lactams. *JAMA* 1981;245:2027.

154. Tune BM, Fravert D. Mechanisms of cephalosporin nephrotoxicity: a comparison of cephaloridine and cephaloglycin. *Kidney Int* 1980;18:591.

155. Barza M. Nephrotoxicity of cephalosporins: an overview. *J Infect Dis* 1978;137[Suppl]:S60.

156. Alestig K, Trollfors B, Andersson R, et al. Ceftazidime and renal function. *J Antimicrob Chemother* 1984;13:177.

157. Meyers BR. Comparative toxicities of third-generation cephalosporins. *Am J Med* 1985;79[Suppl 7A]:96.

158. Zhanel AA. Cephalosporin-induced nephrotoxicity: does it exist? *DICP* 1990;24:262.

159. Bang NA, Kammer RB. Hematologic complications associated with β-lactam antibiotics. *Rev Infect Dis* 1983;5[Suppl]:S380.

160. Spath P, Garratty A, Petz LD. Studies on the immune response to penicillin and cephalothin in humans, II: immunohematologic reactions to cephalothin administration. *J Immunol* 1971;107:860.

161. Kuwahara S, Miney L, Nishata M. Immunogenicity of cefazolin. *Antimicrob Agents Chemother* 1971;1:374.

162. Chenoweth CE, Judd WJ, Steiner EA, et al. Cefotetan-induced immune hemolytic anemia. *Clin Infect Dis* 1992;15:863.

163. Garratty G, Postoway N, Schwellenbach J, et al. A fatal case of ceftriaxone-induced hemolytic anemia associated with intravascular immune hemolysis. *Transfusion* 1991;31:176.

164. Nichols RL, Wikler MA, McDevitt JT, et al. Coagulopathy associated with extended-spectrum cephalosporins in patients with serious infections. *Antimicrob Agents Chemother* 1987;31:281.

165. Conly JM, Ramotark S, Chubb H. Hypoprothrombinemia in febrile, neutropenic patients with cancer association with antimicrobial suppression of intestinal flora. *J Infect Dis* 1984;150:202.

166. Lipsky JJ. Antibiotic associated hypoprothrombinemia. *J Antimicrob Chemother* 1988;21:281.

167. Shevchuk YM, Conly JM. Antibiotic-associated hypoprothrombinemia. A review of prospective studies, 1966–1988. *Rev Infect Dis* 1990;12:1109.

168. Sattler FR, Weitekamp MR, Ballard JO. Potential for bleeding with the new β-lactam antibiotics. *Ann Intern Med* 1986;105:924.

169. Sattler FR, Colao DJ, Caputo GM, et al. Cefoperazone for empiric therapy in patients with impaired renal function. *Am J Med* 1986;81:229.

170. Conjura A, Bell W, Lipsky JJ. Cefotetan and hypoprothrombinemia. *Ann Intern Med* 1988;108:643.

171. Dancer SJ. The problem with cephalosporins. *J Antimicrob Chemother* 2001;48:463.

172. Stone SP, Beric V, Quick A, et al. The effect of an enhanced infection control policy on the incidence of *Clostridium difficile* infection and methicillin-resistant *Staphylococcus aureus* colonization in acute elderly medical patients. *Age Ageing* 1998;27:561.

173. Ayliffe GAJ. The progressive intercontinental spread of MRSA. *Clin Infect Dis* 1997;24[Suppl 1]:S74.

174. Voss A. *Staphylococcus aureus.* Pan-European antibiotic resistance and infection control. *Chemotherapie J* 1996;5:5.

175. Voss A, Milatovic D, Wallrauch-Schwarz C, et al. Methicillin-resistant *Staphylococcus aureus* in Europe. *Eur J Clin Microbiol Infect Dis* 1994;13:50.

CHAPTER 20
Other β-Lactam Antibiotics

Kenneth S. Thomson and Philip D. Lister

The β-lactam antibiotics are a large family of diverse compounds, each of which contains a four-membered β-lactam ring (Fig. 20.1). The three major groups within this family differ from one another in the general nature of the substituent adjacent to the β-lactam ring (1). The first group contains compounds with a five-membered ring fused to the β-lactam ring (see Fig. 20.1). Included in this group are the penams (penicillins and the β-lactamase inhibitors sulbactam and tazobactam), the penems (several compounds under investigation), the clavams (β-lactamase inhibitor clavulanic acid), and the carbapenems (imipenem and meropenem). Similar structural variations are possible within the second major group of β-lactam antibiotics, which have a six-membered ring fused to the β-lactam ring (see Fig. 20.1). This group includes the cephems (cephalosporins and cephamycins), oxacephems (moxalactam), and carbacephems (loracarbef). Several other compounds within this second group are under investigation. The third group of β-lactam antibiotics contains the monocyclic compounds (see Fig. 20.1). This group includes the monobactams such as aztreonam and numerous related investigational compounds.

This chapter covers β-lactam antibiotics not dealt with elsewhere in this text: the carbapenems and the monocyclic β-lactam antibiotics.

MONOCYCLIC β-LACTAM ANTIBIOTICS

History and Development

Among the monocyclic β-lactam antibiotics, the monobactams have been studied the most intensively. The monobactams were discovered as naturally occurring compounds produced by gram-negative bacteria. They originally possessed only weak antibacterial activity, but intensive structure–activity relationship studies led to the development of the synthetic monobactams, which exhibit good antibacterial activity and stability to β-lactamases (2). Aztreonam has the same side chain as ceftazidime and a 4-α-methyl group. Although its activity is confined to gram-negative bacteria (3–5), aztreonam remains one of the most stable compounds in the presence of many β-lactamases produced by gram-negative bacteria (4–7).

The overall structure of the monobactams has also been modified to improve activity against *Pseudomonas aeruginosa*, and for some investigational agents, to provide good oral bioavailability. A number of investigational monobactam derivatives have been studied, but none has achieved clinical usefulness (8–10). One unique monobactam is the catechol-containing monobactam, BMS-180680 (11). This compound, like other catechol-containing β-lactams, is unique because the iron-chelating catecholic substituent provides more efficient penetration across the outer membrane of gram-negative bacteria through the TonB-dependent iron transport systems (11). Penetration through this iron transport system enhances the antibacterial activity of these compounds, including their potency against *P. aeruginosa*. BMS-180680 is 32-fold more potent than aztreonam and 8-fold more potent than imipenem against *P. aeruginosa* (11). The clinical future of this unique monobactam derivative is still unknown, despite its potent *in vitro* activity.

Aztreonam

SPECTRUM OF ACTIVITY AND RESISTANCE ISSUES

Aztreonam is the only monocyclic β-lactam antibiotic currently available for clinical use. It is a synthetic parenteral monobactam with clinically useful activity against gram-negative bacteria (12,13). Like other β-lactam antibiotics, it is bactericidal and interferes with cell wall biosynthesis. Aztreonam binds primarily to penicillin-binding protein-3 (PBP-3) of *Escherichia coli* (5,12). Among gram-negative bacteria, it is active *in vitro* against most Enterobacteriaceae, *Neisseria gonorrhoeae*, *Haemophilus influenzae*, *Aeromonas* species, and *P. aeruginosa* (4,5,14). It is not active *in vitro* against gram-positive bacteria, obligate anaerobes, and various nonfermentative gram-negative bacteria such as *Acinetobacter* species, *Alcaligenes denitrificans*, and *Achromobacter*, *Moraxella*, *Myroides* species (formerly *Flavobacterium odoratum*), and *Chryseobacterium* species (formerly *Flavobacterium meningosepticum*, *Flavobacterium balustinum*, *Flavobacterium indologenes*, and *Flavobacterium gleum*) (4,5,14).

Aztreonam is not readily hydrolyzed by many prevalent plasmid-mediated β-lactamases, including the older TEM-1, TEM-2, and SHV-1 enzymes found in many Enterobacteriaceae, *H. influenzae*, and *Neisseria* species (4,5,14). However, there are certain enzymes that can confer resistance to aztreonam. Although aztreonam is active against many Enterobacteriaceae and *P. aeruginosa* that produce low levels of their chromosomal AmpC cephalosporinases, high-level production of AmpC in derepressed mutants provides resistance to aztreonam and most other β-lactams (15). Creating a further resistance threat to aztreonam has been the movement of the chromosomal AmpC to plasmids and dissemination to *E. coli* and *Klebsiella pneumoniae*, as well as other members of the Enterobacteriaceae (16). Strains of bacteria that acquire these plasmid-encoded AmpCs can exhibit resistance to aztreonam and most other β-lactam antibiotics.

The evolution of extended-spectrum β-lactamases (ESBLs) has also provided an important resistance threat to the efficacy of aztreonam (16). Most ESBLs are derivatives of older plasmid-encoded enzymes that have mutated their active site to enhance hydrolysis of aztreonam and extended-spectrum cephalosporins like ceftazidime and cefotaxime. The most commonly identified ESBLs are derivatives of TEM-1 and SHV-1 (16) and are found primarily in *E. coli* and *K. pneumoniae*. However, these enzymes have also been identified in other genera of Enterobacteriaceae and in *P. aeruginosa*, *Burkholderia cepacia*, and *Capnocytophaga ochracea*. In addition to the TEM- and SHV-derived ESBLs, there are many other types of ESBLs, including those of the PER, OXA, and CTX-M families (16). Laboratory mutants less susceptible to aztreonam via nonenzymatic mechanisms have also been described. Most of these mutants exhibit a decrease in the permeability of the drug (17).

PHARMACOKINETICS

Therapeutic levels of aztreonam can be achieved via either intravenous or intramuscular injection but not via oral administration (12). The time to peak serum levels after an intramuscular dose is 1 hour, and the half-life in serum averages 1.7 hours after parenteral administration. Levels in the cerebrospinal fluid are significantly lower than those in serum, even in the presence of meningeal inflammation (12,18), and efficacy in meningitis has yet to be investigated thoroughly. Aztreonam is metabolized to a limited extent, and the major metabolite is the biologically inactive open ring structure (12). Two thirds of a dose is excreted unchanged in urine, and only 1% is excreted unchanged in feces. Twenty-six percent of a dose is excreted as inactive metabolites, half in urine and half in feces (12). Aztreonam is excreted equally by active tubular secretion and glomerular filtration in

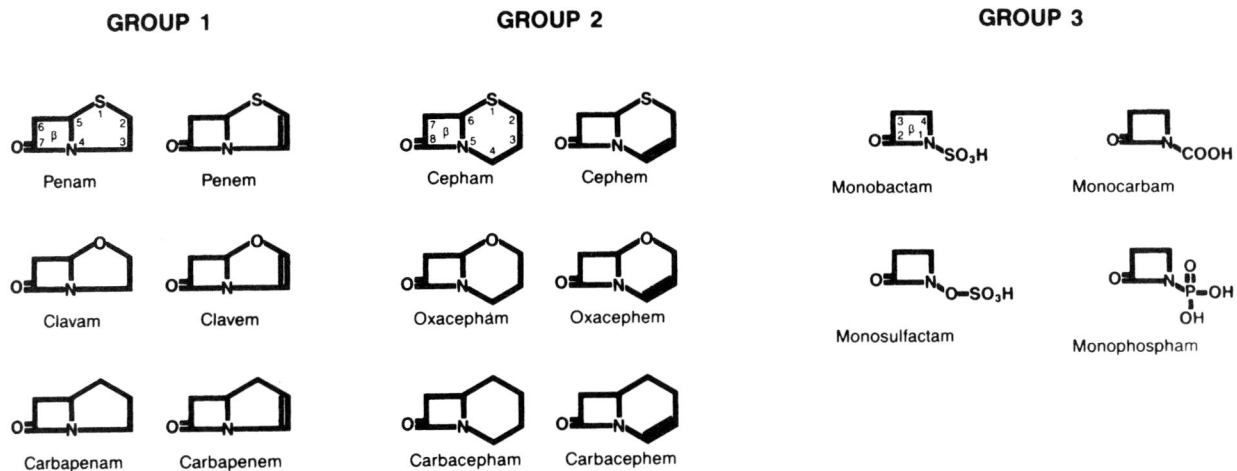

Figure 20.1. Major structures within the β-lactam family.

the kidneys, and probenecid and furosemide do not significantly increase serum levels of the drug. Aztreonam doses must be adjusted in patients with compromised renal function, and the drug is effectively removed by both hemodialysis and peritoneal dialysis (12). To date, there is no evidence for pharmacologic interactions with other antibiotics that might be used in combination with aztreonam (19).

ADVERSE REACTIONS
The safety profile of aztreonam seems to be similar to that of most other β-lactam antibiotics (20). The most commonly encountered side effects include local reaction at the infusion site (1.7%), rash (1.8%), nausea and vomiting (0.6%), and diarrhea (0.8%). Pseudomembranous colitis has been reported in patients receiving aztreonam, although its occurrence is quite low (20). Superinfections, when they occur, are often due to gram-positive bacteria, especially the enterococci (12,21). Cross-allergenicity between aztreonam and other β-lactam antibiotics is quite low (21,22). Thus, aztreonam may be a valuable therapeutic agent for patients with known allergy to penicillin or other β-lactam antibiotics.

CLINICAL USE
Clinical trials have shown aztreonam to be effective in the treatment of various infections with gram-negative bacteria. These include both complicated and uncomplicated urinary tract infections, lower respiratory tract infections, septicemia, skin and skin structure infections, intraabdominal infections, and gynecologic infections including endometritis and pelvic cellulitis (12). Because of its low cross-allergenicity with other β-lactam antibiotics, it is a useful therapeutic alternative for patients allergic to penicillins or cephalosporins. However, because aztreonam exhibits a limited spectrum of activity, it is not recommended for empiric therapy in clinical settings that might involve gram-positive bacteria or obligate anaerobes. Though not approved for use in children or neonates, aztreonam can be useful in certain pediatric settings (23). These include treatment of pyelonephritis, patients allergic to penicillins or cephalosporins (especially those with cystic fibrosis), and patients who cannot tolerate the disruption of the gastrointestinal tract flora that broader spectrum β-lactam antibiotics produce.

MONOBACTAM β-LACTAMASE INHIBITORS
In addition to exhibiting potent activity against gram-negative bacteria, aztreonam is also a potent competitive inhibitor of the chromosomal-encoded AmpC β-lactamases of Enterobacteriaceae and *P. aeruginosa* (6,7). Although aztreonam is eventually hydrolyzed by these enzymes, the half-lives of these reactions are long enough that the enzymes remain inactive through several generations of bacterial growth (6). The clinical potential of this inhibitory interaction was demonstrated in patients with cystic fibrosis who were being treated with various β-lactams for *P. aeruginosa* infections (24). Over 15 days of therapy, a significant increase in AmpC levels was observed in the sputum of patients treated with piperacillin, ceftazidime, and imipenem. In contrast, no cephalosporinase activity was detected in day 15 samples from 19 of 21 patients treated with aztreonam. However, when the samples were dialyzed overnight against buffer, hydrolysis of the aztreonam was completed and a significant amount of free AmpC enzyme was detected in these same samples, suggesting aztreonam was inhibiting the cephalosporinase activity *in situ* (24). The potential use of aztreonam against a β-lactamase inhibitor in the treatment of AmpC-producing Enterobacteriaceae has been difficult to evaluate due to the potent antibacterial activity of aztreonam alone. However, data from recent studies with a combination of cefepime-aztreonam against *P. aeruginosa* using an *in vitro* pharmacodynamic model have suggested that the β-lactamase inhibitory activity of aztreonam can significantly enhance the antibacterial activity of cefepime, even against fully depressed mutants of *P. aeruginosa* expressing high levels of AmpC and resistance to both drugs alone (25). In addition to aztreonam, other monobactam derivatives are being developed as inhibitors of AmpC cephalosporinases and non metallocarbapenemases (26,27).

CARBAPENEMS

The nucleus of the carbapenems resembles that of a penicillin except that a carbon atom has been substituted for the sulfur atom at position 1 in the five-membered ring and there is a double bond in that ring (see Fig. 20.1).

Imipenem and Meropenem

ACTIVITY RESISTANCE
Imipenem and meropenem are the only carbapenems available in Europe and the United States. They have the broadest antibacterial spectrum of currently available β-lactams, being highly active against a wide range of gram-positive and gram-negative

TABLE 20.1. Antibacterial Spectrum of Imipenem and Meropenem

Susceptible	Resistant	Resistance may emerge or be acquired
Gram positive		
Staphylococci	Methicillin-resistant staphylococci	
Streptococci		Pneumococci and viridans streptococci (meropenem)
Enterococcus faecalis	*E. faecium*	
Gram negative		
Enterobacteriaceae	*Stenotrophomonas maltophilia*	Enterobacteriaceae (rare strains)
Pseudomonas aeruginosa	*Burkholderia cepacia*	*P. aeruginosa*
Acinetobacter	*Chryseobacterium*	*Acinetobacter*
Haemophilus	*Myroides*	
Neisseria		
Anaerobes		
Bacteroides	*Bacteroides fragilis* (rare strains)	
Clostridium	*Clostridium difficile*	

bacteria, including obligate anaerobes, with the exceptions of *Clostridium difficile* and rare strains of *Bacteroides fragilis* (Table 20.1) (28–31). Like other β-lactam antibiotics, they are bactericidal and inhibit cell wall biosynthesis; however, unlike other β-lactams, their major lethal targets in *E. coli* are PBP-1 and PBP-2 (28,30,31). Their potency against gram-negative bacteria has been attributed to resistance to hydrolysis by β-lactamases, the relatively small number of lethal targets in the cell, and good penetration through the outer membrane. Good penetration into gram-negative bacteria has been attributed to the small size and the zwitterionic nature of the molecules (28,32). In *P. aeruginosa*, penetration appears to be further enhanced by a selective porin that permits carbapenem entry (33). Meropenem is slightly more active than imipenem against Enterobacteriaceae and *P. aeruginosa* but is less active against gram-positive cocci (30,31). Current major therapeutic issues are the potency of the carbapenems against gram-negative pathogens that produce ESBLs or high levels of AmpC β-lactamases, as well as emerging resistance (16).

Among gram-positive bacteria, *Corynebacterium jeikeium*, *Enterococcus faecium*, and methicillin-resistant staphylococci should be regarded as resistant. Other enterococci, *Listeria monocytogenes*, and *Clostridium* species exhibit tolerance (i.e., bactericidal activity is achieved only at concentrations much higher than the minimal inhibitory concentrations). Early clinical studies with imipenem suggested that carbapenems may not be effective if used as a single-agent therapy for serious infections such as endocarditis and meningitis caused by tolerant bacteria (34–36). Among gram-negative aerobes, carbapenems are not active against *Stenotrophomonas* (formerly *Xanthomonas*) *maltophilia*, most *Burkholderia* (formerly *Pseudomonas*) *cepacia*, *Chryseobacterium meningosepticum*, and *Myroides* species, an increasing number of strains of *P. aeruginosa* and *Acinetobacter*, and rare strains of *Proteus* species and *Serratia marcescens* (37–39).

There are three mechanisms of carbapenem resistance: altered target, drug hydrolysis, and decreased drug accumulation due to active efflux and/or diminished penetration across the outer membrane of gram-negative bacteria. In gram-positive bacteria, altered PBPs are responsible for carbapenem resistance and tolerance in strains of staphylococci, pneumococci, and enterococci (40,41).

Carbapenem-hydrolyzing enzymes are the most diverse of all β-lactamases. The most important carbapenem-hydrolyzing enzymes are the metallo-β-lactamases, which hydrolyze all

β-lactam agents, except aztreonam, are resistant to currently available β-lactamase inhibitors, and require zinc as a cofactor. Chromosomally encoded metallo-β-lactamases are produced by *Bacillus cereus*, *Stenotrophomonas maltophilia*, *Aeromonas* species, *C. meningosepticum*, *Myroides* species, *Sphingobacterium multivorum*, *Legionella gormanii*, and rare strains of *B. fragilis*. Of these organisms, *S. maltophilia* poses the greatest clinical threat because it is a pathogen of increasing clinical importance and it is invariably carbapenem resistant (16,42).

Of recent concern is the occurrence and spread of transmissible plasmid-mediated metallo-β-lactamases. These were first recognized in 1990 and have since been reported in rare clinical isolates of *B. fragilis*, *P. aeruginosa*, *Pseudomonas putida*, *Pseudomonas fluorescens*, *Alcaligenes xylosoxidans*, *Acinetobacter* species, *E. coli*, *Citrobacter freundii*, *Enterobacter aerogenes*, *E. cloacae*, *Proteus vulgaris*, *Providencia rettgeri*, *S. marcescens*, and *K. pneumoniae*, mostly from Japan, but also from Singapore, Italy, England, and Portugal. In addition to metallo-β-lactamases, there are rare non-metallo-carbapenem–hydrolyzing enzymes that have been detected in some strains of *Acinetobacter*, *E. cloacae*, *K. pneumoniae*, and *S. marcescens* (42–44).

P. aeruginosa possesses at least four active efflux systems, which if expressed at high levels, cause multiple antibiotic resistance. These systems are controlled by the MexAB-OprM, MexCD-OprJ, MexEF-OprN, and MexXY-OprM operons. None of the systems extrude imipenem, but meropenem is a substrate for the MexAB-OprM system (and possibly the MexCD-OprJ and MexXY-OprM systems) (45–47).

Resistance arising from diminished outer membrane permeability has emerged during carbapenem therapy of infections caused by *P. aeruginosa*, *Proteus* species, *E. cloacae*, and *S. marcescens* (30,40,48). Carbapenem resistance emerges more frequently in *P. aeruginosa* than in other organisms. Resistance to imipenem, and meropenem to a lesser extent, is associated with loss of the carbapenem-specific OprD porin in the outer membrane in combination with high-level AmpC expression (48–50). In rare strains of some members of the family Enterobacteriaceae, resistance to imipenem arises from diminished production of porins combined with production of high levels of AmpC β-lactamase.

Inhibition of β-lactamase activity is a feature of carbapenems that is due either to enzyme inactivation or to the formation of long-lived enzyme–drug complexes (40). Carbapenems are also strong inducers of the Bush group 1 enzymes and the chromosomal metallo-β-lactamases of *S. maltophilia* and *Aeromonas hydrophila* (51,52). This characteristic precludes use of carbapenems with other β-lactam antibiotics because of the potential for antagonism to occur.

PHARMACOKINETICS

Imipenem and meropenem are not absorbed orally. After intravenous administration, imipenem is readily hydrolyzed by the mammalian renal dipeptidase, dehydropeptidase-I (DHP-I), located on the luminal surface of proximal tubular cells. Degradation caused by DHP-I results in significant loss of antibacterial activity and the formation of a product that in animals exhibits nephrotoxicity similar to that of cephaloridine. This problem is overcome by coadministering imipenem in a 1:1 ratio with the DHP inhibitor cilastatin (30). Meropenem has greater stability to DHP-I and does not require the coadministration of a DHP inhibitor (53,54). Clinical trials conducted to date suggest that meropenem and imipenem are generally similar in overall efficacy. Potential advantages of meropenem include a lower incidence of seizures and efficacy in meningitis (53–58).

Hemodialysis removes meropenem, imipenem, and cilastatin (30,59). Intravenous meropenem and imipenem are well distributed in most tissues and fluids, with only 2% and 20% of each agent, respectively, binding to plasma proteins. Cerebrospinal fluid levels of imipenem are significantly lower than serum levels, even in the presence of inflamed meninges (30,59,60).

ADVERSE REACTIONS

The major adverse effects of intravenous imipenem-cilastatin and meropenem are similar, none of which occur in more than 3% of patient exposures. These include nausea and vomiting or diarrhea (approximately 2%), allergic reactions (1.3%), and phlebitis or erythema at the infusion site (1.2%). Imipenem-cilastatin is associated with a slightly higher incidence of drug-related seizures than meropenem (0.08% vs. 0.28% in patients with infections other than meningitis) (61). Seizures usually occur in elderly persons or in patients with underlying abnormalities of the central nervous system (CNS) (28,61,62). Other associated predisposing factors include renal impairment and long-term alcoholism (28,60). Anticonvulsant therapy and dosage adjustment or withdrawal of antibiotics is required if seizures occur (30). Dosage adjustment is also required for patients with diminished renal function (59,63). Colonization and superinfection—particularly by fungi, carbapenem-resistant pseudomonads, and acinetobacters—may occur in patients receiving carbapenems. Pseudomembranous colitis has also been reported (0.1%). There is no evidence of renal impairment or bleeding related to carbapenem therapy. Carbapenems are contraindicated for patients with a history of β-lactam allergy (30,59–61,64).

CLINICAL USE

In general, intravenous carbapenems should be regarded as reserve antibiotics for the treatment of hospital-acquired infections caused by multiple antibiotic-resistant bacteria and complicated polymicrobial infections caused by mixtures of aerobic and anaerobic bacteria. Clinical trials have demonstrated the efficacy of carbapenems in a range of infections of lower respiratory tract, CNS, abdomen, female reproductive tract, bones and joints, skin, and soft tissues, as well as in bacteremia. Outside the United States, imipenem and meropenem are approved for a wide range of infections, but in the United States, meropenem is approved for only two indications: intraabdominal infections and bacterial meningitis of patients 3 months and older. Imipenem is currently not approved for use in the treatment of infections of the CNS. Carbapenems are relatively expensive and should not be used when cheaper or narrower spectrum antibiotics would suf-

fice. Indiscriminate use escalates costs and promotes the emergence of resistant bacteria (30,60). Unfortunately in some centers, the increasing occurrence of multiple-antibiotic–resistant pathogens that produce ESBLs and/or plasmid-mediated AmpC β-lactamases leaves few, if any, alternatives for therapy of serious infections caused by gram-negative pathogens (65).

Carbapenems should not be used for therapy of infections caused by methicillin-resistant staphylococci or as monotherapy for serious *Pseudomonas* or *Enterococcus* infections. Because of their ability to induce certain chromosomal β-lactamases, they should not be combined with other β-lactams for therapy of infections caused by *P. aeruginosa*, *Enterobacter* species, *C. freundii*, *S. marcescens*, *Morganella morganii*, *P. vulgaris*, *Providencia* species, or *A. hydrophila*.

INTRAMUSCULAR IMIPENEM-CILASTATIN

An intramuscular preparation of imipenem-cilastatin has become available for use (64). Slow absorption of imipenem but not cilastatin from the intramuscular site results in peak plasma levels of imipenem by 2 hours and cilastatin by 1 hour. This slow absorption of imipenem prolongs the drug's plasma half-life to 2 to 3 hours and permits 12-hour dosing of the intramuscular formulation (66,67). The intramuscular preparation is approved for use only for mild to moderate infections (64).

REFERENCES

1. Brown AG. Beta-lactam nomenclature. *J Antimicrob Chemother* 1982;10(5):365–368.
2. Bonner DP, Sykes RB. Structure activity relationships among the monobactams. *J Antimicrob Chemother* 1984;14(4):313–327.
3. Sykes RB, Bonner DP. Discovery and development of the monobactams. *Rev Infect Dis* 1985;7[Suppl 4]:S579–S604.
4. Phillips I, King A, Shannon K, et al. SQ 26,776: in-vitro antibacterial activity and susceptibility to beta-lactamases. *J Antimicrob Chemother* 1981;8[Suppl E]:103–110.
5. Sykes RB, Bonner DP, Bush K, et al. Aztreonam (SQ 26,776), a synthetic monobactam specifically active against aerobic gram-negative bacteria. *Antimicrob Agents Chemother* 1982;21(1):85–92.
6. Bush K. β-Lactamase inhibitors from laboratory to clinic. *Clin Microbiol Rev* 1988;1:109–123.
7. Bush K, Freudenberger JS, Sykes RB. Interaction of aztreonam and related monobactams with β-lactamases from gram-negative bacteria. *Antimicrob Agents Chemother* 1982;22:414–420.
8. Tanaka SK, Summerill RA, Minassian BF, et al. In vitro evaluation of tigemonam, a novel oral monobactam. *Antimicrob Agents Chemother* 1987;31(2):219–225.
9. Imada A, Kondo M, Okonogi K, et al. In vitro and in vivo antibacterial activities of carumonam (AMA-1080), a new *N*-sulfonated monocyclic beta-lactam antibiotic. *Antimicrob Agents Chemother* 1985;27(5):821–827.
10. Zurenko GE, Truesdell SE, Yagi BH, et al. In vitro antibacterial activity and interactions with beta-lactamases and penicillin-binding proteins of the new monocarbam antibiotic U-78608. *Antimicrob Agents Chemother* 1990;34(5):884–888.
11. Fung-Tomc J, Bush K, Minassian B, et al. Antibacterial activity of BMS-180680, a new catechol-containing monobactam. *Antimicrob Agents Chemother* 1997;41(5):1010–1016.
12. Brogden RN, Heel RC. Aztreonam. A review of its antibacterial activity, pharmacokinetic properties and therapeutic use. *Drugs* 1986;31(2):96–130.
13. Brewer NS, Hellinger WC. The monobactams. *Mayo Clin Proc* 1991;66(11):1152–1157.
14. Neu HC, Labthavikul P. Antibacterial activity of a monocyclic beta-lactam SQ 26,776. *J Antimicrob Chemother* 1981;8[Suppl E]:111–122.
15. Sanders CC. Chromosomal cephalosporinases responsible for multiple resistance to newer β-lactam antibiotics. *Annu Rev Microbiol* 1987;41:573–593.
16. Thomson KS, Smith Moland E. Version 2000: the new beta-lactamases of gram-negative bacteria at the dawn of the new millennium. *Microbes Infect* 2000;2[11]:1225–1235.
17. Aggeler R, Then RL, Ghosh R. Reduced expression of outer-membrane proteins in beta-lactam–resistant mutants of *Enterobacter cloacae*. *J Gen Microbiol* 1987;133[Pt 12]:3383–3392.
18. Greenman RL, Arcey SM, Dickinson GM, et al. Penetration of aztreonam into human cerebrospinal fluid in the presence of meningeal inflammation. *J Antimicrob Chemother* 1985;15(5):637–640.

19. Creasey WA, Adamovics J, Dhruv R, et al. Pharmacokinetic interaction of aztreonam with other antibiotics. *J Clin Pharmacol* 1984;24(4):174–180.
20. Newman TJ, Dreslinski GR, Tadros SS. Safety profile of aztreonam in clinical trials. *Rev Infect Dis* 1985;7[Suppl 4]:S648–655.
21. Chandrasekar PH, Smith BR, LeFrock JL, et al. Enterococcal superinfection and colonization with aztreonam therapy. *Antimicrob Agents Chemother* 1984;26(2):280–282.
22. Adkinson NF Jr, Saxon A, Spence MR, et al. Cross-allergenicity and immunogenicity of aztreonam. *Rev Infect Dis* 1985;7[Suppl 4]:S613–S621.
23. Aronoff SC. Aztreonam: new developments in the treatment of gram-negative infections in children. Chicago, Illinois, November 17, 1988. Proceedings. *Pediatr Infect Dis J* 1989;8[Suppl 9]:S99–S132.
24. Giwercman B, Meyer C, Lambert PA, et al. High-level β-lactamase activity in sputum samples from cystic fibrosis patients during antipseudomonal treatment. *Antimicrob Agents Chemother* 1992;36:71–76.
25. Lister PD, Sanders WE Jr, Sanders CC. Cefepime-aztreonam: a unique double β-lactam combination for *Pseudomonas aeruginosa*. *Antimicrob Agents Chemother* 1998;42:1610–1619.
26. Nishida K, Kunugita C, Uji T, et al. *In vitro* and *in vivo* activities of Syn2190, a novel beta-lactamase inhibitor. *Antimicrob Agents Chemother* 1999;43(8):1895–1900.
27. Mourey L, Kotra LP, Bellettini J, et al. Inhibition of the broad spectrum non-metallocarbapenamase of class A (NMC-A) beta-lactamase from *Enterobacter cloacae* by monocyclic beta-lactams. *J Biol Chem* 1999;274(36):25260–25265.
28. Wise R. *In vitro* and pharmacokinetic properties of the carbapenems. *Antimicrob Agents Chemother* 1986;30(3):343–349.
29. Kahan FM, Kropp H, Sundelof JG, et al. Thienamycin: development of imipenem-cilastatin. *J Antimicrob Chemother* 1983;12[Suppl D]:1–35.
30. Barza M. Imipenem: first of a new class of beta-lactam antibiotics. *Ann Intern Med* 1985;103(4):552–560.
31. Edwards JR. Meropenem: a microbiological review. *J Antimicrob Chemother* 1995;36[Suppl A]:1–17.
32. Neu HC. Beta-lactam antibiotics: structural relationships affecting *in vitro* activity and pharmacologic properties. *Rev Infect Dis* 1986;8[Suppl 3]:S237–S259.
33. Studemeister AE, Quinn JP. Selective imipenem resistance in *Pseudomonas aeruginosa* associated with diminished outer membrane permeability. *Antimicrob Agents Chemother* 1988;32(8):1267–1268.
34. Chandrasekar PH, Levine DP, Price S, et al. Comparative efficacies of imipenem-cilastatin and vancomycin in experimental aortic valve endocarditis due to methicillin resistant *Staphylococcus aureus*. *J Antimicrob Chemother* 1988;21(4):461–469.
35. Chambers HF. Methicillin-resistant staphylococci. *Clin Microbiol Rev* 1988;1:173–186.
36. Auckenthaler R, Wilson WR, Wright AJ, et al. Lack of *in vivo* and *in vitro* bactericidal activity of N-formimidoyl thienamycin against enterococci. *Antimicrob Agents Chemother* 1982;22(3):448–452.
37. Carmeli Y, Troillet N, Eliopoulos GM, et al. Emergence of antibiotic-resistant Pseudomonas aeruginosa: comparison of risks associated with different antipseudomonal agents. *Antimicrob Agents Chemother* 1999;43(6):1379–1382.
38. Costa SF, Woodcock J, Gill M, et al. Outer-membrane proteins pattern and detection of beta-lactamases in clinical isolates of imipenem-resistant *Acinetobacter baumannii* from Brazil. *Int J Antimicrob Agents* 2000;13(3):175–182.
39. Fierobe L, Lucet JC, Decre D, et al. An outbreak of imipenem-resistant *Acinetobacter baumannii* in critically ill surgical patients. *Infect Control Hosp Epidemiol* 2001;22(1):35–40.
40. Neu HC. Carbapenems: special properties contributing to their activity. *Am J Med* 1985;78(6A):33–40.
41. Carsenti-Etesse H, Durant J, Salvador FD, et al. *In vitro* development of resistance of *Streptococcus pneumoniae* to β-lactam antibiotics. *Microb Drug Resist* 1995;1:85–94.
42. Bush K, Jacoby GA, Medeiros AA. A functional classification scheme for β-lactamases and its correlation with molecular structure. *Antimicrobial Agents Chemother* 1995;39:1211–1233.
43. Naas T, Livermore DM, Nordmann P. Characterization of an LysR family protein, SmeR from *Serratia marcescens* S6, its effect on expression of the carbapenem-hydrolyzing beta-lactamase Sme-1, and comparison of this regulator with other beta-lactamase regulators. *Antimicrob Agents Chemother* 1995;39(3):629–637.
44. Nordmann P, Mariotte S, Naas T, et al. Biochemical properties of a carbapenem-hydrolyzing β-lactamase from *Enterobacter cloacae* and cloning of the gene into *Escherichia coli*. *Antimicrob Agents Chemother* 1993;37:939–946.
45. Masuda N, Sakagawa E, Ohya S, et al. Substrate specificities of MexAB-OprM, MexCD-OprJ, and MexXY-oprM efflux pumps in *Pseudomonas aeruginosa*. *Antimicrob Agents Chemother* 2000;44(12):3322–3327.
46. Kohler T, Michea-Hamzehpour M, Plesiat P, et al. Differential selection of multidrug efflux systems by quinolones in *Pseudomonas aeruginosa*. *Antimicrob Agents Chemother* 1997;41:2540–2543.
47. Masuda N, Gotoh N, Ishii C, et al. Interplay between chromosomal beta-lactamase and the MexAB-OprM efflux system in intrinsic resistance to beta-lactams in *Pseudomonas aeruginosa*. *Antimicrob Agents Chemother* 1999;43(2):400–402.
48. Quinn JP, Studemeister AE, DiVincenzo CA, et al. Resistance to imipenem in *Pseudomonas aeruginosa*: clinical experience and biochemical mechanisms. *Rev Infect Dis* 1988;10:892–898.
49. Livermore DM. Interplay of impermeability and chromosomal beta-lactamase activity in imipenem-resistant *Pseudomonas aeruginosa*. *Antimicrob Agents Chemother* 1992;36(9):2046–2048.
50. Trias J, Nikaido H. Outer membrane protein D2 catalyzes facilitated diffusion of carbapenems and penems through the outer membrane of *Pseudomonas aeruginosa*. *Antimicrob Agents Chemother* 1990;34(1):52–57.
51. Braveny I. *In vitro* activity of imipenem—a review. *Eur J Clin Microbiol* 1984;3(5):456–462.
52. Sanders CC, Sanders WE Jr, Thomson KS, et al. Meropenem: activity against resistant gram-negative bacteria and interactions with beta-lactamases. *J Antimicrob Chemother* 1989;24[Suppl A]:187–196.
53. Pryka RD, Haig GM. Meropenem: a new carbapenem antimicrobial. *Ann Pharmacother* 1994;28(9):1045–1054.
54. Edwards JR, Turner PJ, Wannop C, et al. *In vitro* antibacterial activity of SM-7338, a carbapenem antibiotic with stability to dehydropeptidase I. *Antimicrob Agents Chemother* 1989;33(2):215–222.
55. Chmelik V, Gutvirth J. Meropenem treatment of post-traumatic meningitis due to *Pseudomonas aeruginosa*. *J Antimicrob Chemother* 1993;32(6):922–923.
56. Donnelly JP, Horrevorts AM, Sauerwein RW, et al. High-dose meropenem in meningitis due to *Pseudomonas aeruginosa*. *Lancet* 1992;339(8801):1117.
57. Klugman KP, Dagan R. Randomized comparison of meropenem with cefotaxime for treatment of bacterial meningitis. Meropenem Meningitis Study Group. *Antimicrob Agents Chemother* 1995;39(5):1140–1146.
58. Brismar B, Malmborg AS, Tunevall G, et al. Meropenem versus imipenem/cilastatin in the treatment of intra-abdominal infections. *J Antimicrob Chemother* 1995;35(1):139–148.
59. Merrem I.V. (meropenem for injection). In: Sifton DW, ed. *Physicians' desk reference*. Montvale, NJ: Medical Economics, 2001:629–633.
60. Canadian Infectious Disease Society Committee on Antimicrobial Agents. Imipenem: a new carbapenem. *Can Med Assoc J* 1988;139(6):505–506.
61. Norrby SR, Gildon KM. Safety profile of meropenem: a review of nearly 5,000 patients treated with meropenem. *Scand J Infect Dis* 1999;31(1):3–10.
62. Merck and Co. Primaxin I.V. (imipenem and cilastatin for injection) package insert. West Point PA, 1999.
63. Pestotnik SL, Classen DC, Evans RS, et al. Prospective surveillance of imipenem/cilastatin use and associated seizures using a hospital information system. *Ann Pharmacother* 1993;27(4):497–501.
64. Physicians Desk Reference. Primaxin I.M. (imipenem-cilastatin sodium for suspension). In: Sifton DW, ed. *Physicians' desk reference*, 55th ed. Montvale, NJ: Medical Economics, 2001:1196–1198.
65. Bradley JS, Garau J, Lode H, et al. Carbapenems in clinical practice: a guide to their use in serious infection. *Int J Antimicrob Agents* 1999;11(2):93–100.
66. Kahan FM, Rogers JD. Imipenem/cilastatin: evolution of the sustained-release intramuscular formulation. *Chemotherapy* 1991;37[Suppl 2]:21–25.
67. Onishi A, Otawa M, Hara K. A clinical phase I study on intramuscular imipenem/cilastatin sodium. *Jpn J Antibiot* 1991;44(8):860–876.

CHAPTER 21
Tetracyclines

David N. Williams

The tetracycline antibiotics were the first broad-spectrum antibiotics and were initially effective against a wide range of microorganisms. Although tetracyclines are now less generally used because of the development of antimicrobial resistance and the appearance of newer and more effective chemotherapeutic agents, they have special niches in our therapeutic armamentarium. For the most part, tetracyclines are used in the ambulatory setting. In the United States, a study by the National Center for Health Statistics of the antimicrobial drug–prescribing practices of office-based physicians from 1980 to 1992 found that although there was no trend in the rate of prescriptions for tetracyclines during the study period, tetracyclines ranked third (behind amoxicillin and erythromycin) among generic antimicrobial drugs in 1992 (1). In a comparison of nonhospital antibiotic use in countries of the European Union conducted in 1997, Cars et al. (2) noted that tetracyclines accounted for 14% of antibiotic sales overall (third, behind the broad-spectrum penicillins and macrolides and lincosamines). There was wide variation of antibiotics used between countries, and in Finland and Germany, tetracyclines were the most frequently prescribed antibiotics.

CLASSIFICATION

Tetracyclines can be divided into three groups, based on pharmacologic characteristics: (a) short-acting compounds such as chlortetracycline, oxytetracycline, and tetracycline; (b) an intermediate group, consisting of demeclocycline and methacycline; and (c) long-acting compounds such as doxycycline and minocycline. Novel analogs, the glycylcyclines, show promise *in vitro* against a wide range of organisms with characterized tetracycline-resistant determinants that have yet to be clinically studied (3).

STRUCTURE

The basic structure consists of a hydroxynaphthacene nucleus containing, as the name implies, four fused benzene rings. Substitution on the rings accounts for the number and diversity of tetracyclines. Chlortetracycline (1947) and oxytetracycline (1950) were the first to be discovered, as a result of an intensive screening of soil organisms for antimicrobial properties (from *Streptomyces aureofaciens* and *Streptomyces rimosus*, respectively). The parent compound, tetracycline, was produced by the catalytic dehalogenation of chlortetracycline in 1953. Doxycycline and minocycline are semisynthetic derivatives discovered in 1966 and 1972, respectively.

MECHANISMS OF ACTION

Tetracyclines are bacteriostatic drugs that act on the bacterial ribosome. Tetracycline penetration of the bacterial cell wall probably occurs as a result of both passive diffusion and active transport. Once the drug is within the bacterial cell, inhibition of protein synthesis occurs by binding to a specific domain on the 30S ribosomal subunit, to block the binding of aminoacyl-transfer ribonucleic acid (RNA) to the acceptor site on the messenger RNA ribosome complex. This prevents the addition of new amino acids to the growing peptide chain (4).

SPECTRUM OF ACTIVITY

Tetracyclines are now less active against various gram-positive and gram-negative organisms than they once were. Although tetracycline is the most representative congener and sensitivities for all tetracyclines are determined by using the standard 30-μg tetracycline antimicrobial disk, clinically, doxycycline is the most frequently prescribed congener. Differences in antimicrobial activities between the congeners do exist, with doxycycline and minocycline being the most active. The increased activity of doxycycline against *Streptococcus pneumoniae* may have clinical significance (5). Tetracyclines retain activity against a variety of microorganisms, including the three *Chlamydia* species (*Chlamydia trachomatis*, *Chlamydia pneumoniae*, and *Chlamydia psittaci*), *Mycoplasma* species, rickettsiae, *Ehrlichia* species, spirochetal organisms, and select mycobacterial, fungal, and protozoal organisms.

Resistance to tetracyclines is primarily genetically mediated. The genes usually reside in plasmids and/or transposons and are transferrable. There are two major mechanisms of resistance: (a) an active efflux mechanism (mediated by resistant proteins inserted into the bacterial cytoplasmic membrane), which results in a reduction of the intracellular accumulation of tetracycline, and (b) ribosomal protection (in which a cytoplasmic protein interacts with the ribosome, reducing its sensitivity to tetracycline) (4,6). There has also been concern that the use of tetracyclines in animal husbandry as a food additive for growth promotion and prophylaxis leads to increased microbial resistance.

CLINICAL PHARMACOLOGY

Ten tetracyclines are currently in clinical use, although not all are available in all countries. This discussion focuses on tetracycline (as a standard or parent drug), doxycycline, and minocycline. Tetracycline has a half-life of 10 hours, compared with 15 hours for minocycline and 18 hours for doxycycline. Tetracycline is traditionally given four times a day; doxycycline and minocycline are usually given on a once- and twice-daily basis, respectively. The reported degree of protein binding varies, depending on the methods used: Tetracycline is about 60% and doxycycline and minocycline are 80% to 90% protein bound.

After oral administration, drug absorption occurs in the stomach and proximal small intestine. The degree of absorption varies from 60% to 80% for tetracycline and reaches almost 100% for doxycycline and minocycline. Tetracycline absorption is impaired with the concomitant ingestion of milk, antacids, or food, although this is thought to be less of a problem with doxycycline, because it binds less avidly to calcium and magnesium ions. After oral administration of 500 mg of tetracycline, peak serum levels of about 3 to 4 μg/mL occur at approximately 1 to 3 hours, falling to about 2 μg/mL at 8 hours. Peak serum levels of about 2.5 μg/mL (after about 2 hours) occur after a 200-mg dose of oral doxycycline or minocycline. After oral absorption of tetracycline, there is an active enterohepatic circulation, resulting in biliary levels that are at least fivefold to tenfold higher than the corresponding serum levels. The peak serum level after a 200-mg intravenous dose of doxycycline or minocycline is approximately 4 μg/mL. Doxycycline is the best tolerated and thus most favored intravenous formulation; it should be administered over about 60 minutes, to reduce the likelihood of local thrombophlebitis. Intramuscular administration of tetracycline, doxycycline, and minocycline should be avoided because of local irritation and severe pain.

Minocycline and doxycycline are lipophilic and are thus more diffusible, resulting in excellent tissue penetration including the brain, eye, and prostate. Tetracyclines also penetrate the sebum and are excreted in perspiration, properties that attest to the usefulness of these drugs in the treatment of acne. The ability of tetracyclines to cross the placental barrier may lead to problems with dental and bone growth in the unborn child because of the avidity with which they bind to calcium.

The degree to which tetracyclines are excreted in the urine and feces varies. Urinary excretion depends on the glomerular filtration rate, and urinary recovery rates vary from 60% for tetracycline to 35% and 10% for doxycycline and minocycline (7). Tetracyclines should be avoided in renal insufficiency. Doxycycline is the exception, because in renal failure, it diffuses into the intestinal lumen, where it becomes chelated, and the chelated doxycycline cannot be reabsorbed (8).

TOXICITY

The use of tetracyclines may result in a number of adverse effects. True hypersensitivity is rare. Occasionally, rashes and even anaphylaxis can occur. During the treatment of spirochetal and other infections, a Jarisch-Herxheimer reaction can occur. Photosensitivity was classically described with demeclocycline.

Photosensitivity now appears to be a toxic rather than an allergic reaction, presumably related to drug accumulation in the skin. It occurs infrequently with doxycycline and minocycline. Minocycline has been associated with increased skin pigmentation.

Tetracycline use may cause unwanted dental staining. This reaction is most likely to occur between the fourth and sixth months of intrauterine life, but the threat of interference with dental and bone growth persists to the age of 8 years. Most authorities urge avoidance of tetracycline until the age of 12 years. Dental staining seems to be dose dependent and to some degree drug dependent. It is least likely to occur with doxycycline, presumably because of less avid chelation. Repeated courses of any tetracycline should be avoided in childhood.

Tetracyclines are acidic in solution and may cause esophageal irritation and ulceration, in part caused by local irritation (9). This may be of particular concern in elderly patients with preexisting esophageal disease. Patients should be encouraged to take tetracycline (and especially doxycycline) in an upright position with at least 100 mL of fluid an hour or so before retiring. Hepatotoxicity was classically described in pregnant women with preexisting renal insufficiency receiving more than 2 g per day of intravenous tetracycline and characterized histologically as microvesicular fatty change. A case-control study (10) using Medicaid billing data on patients hospitalized with acute liver disease found an adjusted odds ratio for acute hepatitis for tetracycline of 3.6. There have been case reports of acute liver failure associated with minocycline (11). Additionally, various hypersensitive reactions including drug-induced lupus erythematosus and pneumonitis have been described, albeit rarely, with minocycline (12–14).

Renal insufficiency may occur as a result of a tetracycline-induced reduction of protein synthesis, leading to increased azotemia from amino acid catabolism. Dizziness, vertigo, and ataxia are seen exclusively with minocycline, and these side effects seem to occur primarily in women (15). Vestibular symptoms appear to be related to concentration of the drug in the lipid-laden cells of the vestibular apparatus.

The reduced absorption of all tetracyclines due to the interaction with divalent metals (calcium, magnesium, and aluminium) is well known—hence, the admonition to avoid taking tetracyclines with milk, antacids, and iron preparations. Tetracyclines chelate divalent metals, and the resulting compound cannot be absorbed. A number of drugs, particularly the antiepileptic drugs carbamazepine, diphenylhydantoin, and barbiturates, induce the hepatic metabolism of tetracyclines, thus shortening their serum half-lives.

CLINICAL INDICATIONS

Tetracyclines are no longer used as initial single-drug therapy for unknown acute infections with the possible exception of tick-borne infections. They should be avoided in children younger than 12 years, in pregnant women, and in patients with liver or kidney disease. Tetracyclines are used in a number of specific situations, some of which are discussed in the following sections (Table 21.1).

Acne

In the National Ambulatory Medical Care Survey (1) of oral antimicrobial drug prescribing by office-based physicians in the United States, acne was the most frequently reported complaint associated with a tetracycline prescription. If the in-

flammatory response is severe enough to warrant systemic antibiotic therapy, many authorities believe that tetracyclines are the drugs of choice, based on effectiveness, toxicity, and cost.

Spirochetal Infections

Oral doxycycline at 100 mg twice daily for 14 to 21 days is one of the recommended regimens for the treatment of early Lyme disease (solitary erythema migrans or early disseminated infection in the absence of neurologic involvement or third-degree heart block) (16). For late Lyme disease (oligoarthritis, encephalopathy, neuropathy), oral doxycycline (or amoxicillin) for 28 days is recommended for patients with arthritis, whereas intravenous ceftriaxone at 2 g once daily for 2 to 4 weeks is the usually recommended regimen for patients with neurologic involvement (16).

Recent evidence suggests that patients with a known tick bite with *Ixodes scapularis* can prevent Lyme disease with a single 100-mg dose of doxycycline, if taken within 72 hours of the bite (17).

Tetracycline has also been used in the treatment of relapsing fever *(Borrelia recurrentis)* and for penicillin-allergic patients in the treatment of first, second, and early latent stages of syphilis. In those circumstances, doxycycline at 100 mg twice daily for 2 weeks is recommended. Note that for neurosyphilis, congenital syphilis, syphilis in pregnancy, and human immunodeficiency virus–infected patients, penicillin desensitization is recommended (18). Doxycycline is also effective in the treatment and prophylaxis of leptospirosis (19).

Tick-borne Infections

Although Lyme disease (see the section "Spirochetal Infections") remains the most common arthropod-borne infectious disease in the United States, a number of other infectious agents can be transmitted by various arthropod vectors. In the United States, human granulocytic ehrlichiosis (transmitted by *I. scapularis* and *Ixodes pacificus*), human monocytic ehrlichiosis (amblyomma americanum, *Dermatocentor variabilis*), Rocky Mountain spotted fever (*D. variabilis* and *Dermatocentor andersoni*) are important considerations. Infections transmitted by these agents respond promptly to treatment with doxycycline (100 mg twice daily for 7 days). African tick-bite fever (*Rickettsia africae*) and Mediterranean spotted fever (*Rickettsia conorii*) present with fever, flu-like symptoms and cutaneous eschar(s). A brief (1-day) course of doxycycline has been proposed as definitive treatment (20).

Genital Infections

C. trachomatis is an important pathogen in a number of genital infections, including nongonococcal urethritis, cervicitis, pelvic inflammatory disease (PID), epididymitis, and proctitis. Sequelae of chlamydial infections include PID, infertility, and ectopic pregnancy. Asymptomatic infection is common among sexually active men and women, and routine screening during annual examination is recommended for sexually active women 24 years or younger. Treatment of infected patients and their sexual partners with doxycycline at 100 mg orally twice daily for 7 days (or with a single 1-g dose of azithromycin) is recommended (18). Patients with PID should receive 14 days of doxycycline, in addition to a second- or third-generation cephalosporin or ampicillin sulbactam. The recommended treatment for both lymphogranuloma venereum (due to invasive serovars L1, L2, or L3

TABLE 21.1.   Some Uses of Tetracyclines

Prophylaxis
   Plasmodium falciparum malaria (doxycycline); leptospirosis (doxycycline); cholera
Therapy

Single drug	Combination

Bacterial
   Actinomyces israelii
   Bartonella species
   Borrelia burgdorferi (Lyme disease)
   Borrelia recurrentis (relapsing fever)
   Calymmatobacterium granulomatis
      (granuloma inguinale)
   Legionella species
   Pasturella multocida
   Vibrio cholera, parahaemolyticus,
      vulnificus
	Bacterial
	   Burkholderia pseudomallei (melioidosis) (with
	      chloramphenicol and sulfa-trimethoprim)
	   Brucellosis species (with streptomycin or rifampin)
	   Francisella tularensis (tularemia) (with streptomycin)
	   Helicobacter pylori (metronidazole, or
	      clarithromycin or amoxicillin, bismuth
	      subsalicylate, and a proton pump inhibitor)
	   Yersinia pestis (Plague) (with streptomycin)

Other microorganisms	Other microorganisms

Bacillus anthracis
Chlamydia pneumoniae
Chlamydia psittaci
Chlamydia trachomatis
Coxiella burnetii (Q fever)
Ehrlichiosis
   Human granulocytic *(Ehrlichia*
      phagocytophila, Ehrlichia equi)
   Human monocytic *(Ehrlichia*
      chaffeensis)
Mycobacterium marinum (minocycline)
Mycoplasma pneumoniae
Mycoplasma hominis
Rickettsial infections
   African tick-bite fever
   Endemic typhus
   Mediterranean spotted fever
   Rocky Mountain spotted fever
   Scrub typhus
   Trench fever
Ureaplasma urealyticum
Syndromes
   Acne vulgaris, acne rosacea
   Malabsorption syndromes (Whipple's
      disease; sprue and blind-loop
      syndromes)
   Chronic bronchitis
   Dysuria-frequency syndrome
   Prostatitis; epididymitis
   Pelvic inflammatory disease
   Periodontal disease (minocycline)
   ?Acute aphthous ulcers (topical
      tetracycline)
Noninfectious uses
   Rheumatoid arthritis (minocycline)
   Pleurodesis (minocycline and
      doxycycline)
	Mycobacterium fortuitum and *Mycobacterium*
	   chelonae (with amikacin)
	Mycobacterium leprae (minocycline and various
	   combinations)
	Entamoeba histolytica
	Plasmodium falciparum
	
	x

of *C. trachomatis*) is doxycycline at 100 mg orally twice daily for 21 days (18).

Respiratory Tract Infections

Doxycycline retains an important role in the treatment of community-acquired pneumonia largely because of its activity against various potential pathogens: *Mycoplasma pneumoniae, Legionella pneumophila, C. pneumoniae, C. psittaci, Coxiella burnetti,* and *Francisella tularensis.* In addition, doxycycline is one of the preferred agents for pneumonia in the context of bioterrorism. The agents most likely to be used as biological weapons that present as pneumonia include *Bacillus anthracis, Yersinia pestis,* and *F. tularensis* (21).

Although several authors (21–23) have emphasized the role of doxycycline in the treatment of community-acquired pneumonia, there is a paucity of supporting *in vitro* and *in vivo* data. Nonetheless, in the management of community-acquired pneumonia in a nonhospitalized patient, doxycycline (or a macrolide, or a fluoroquinolone with enhanced activity against *S. pneumoniae*) is listed as a preferred antimicrobial (21). There are studies showing the *in vitro* superiority of doxycycline over tetracycline versus *S. pneumoniae* (5). A recent survey (1999 to 2000) of sensitivity data on more than 15,000 clinical isolates of *S. pneumoniae* collected from 33 U.S. medical centers (24) showed a disturbing trend toward increased antimicrobial resistance over time. Tetracycline resistance increased from 7.6% in 1994 to 16.6% in 1999 to 2000. The precise therapeutic implication of this trend is unclear.

Malaria Prophylaxis and Treatment

Doxycycline is used as a causal prophylactic agent against *Plasmodium falciparum*. The need to take doxycycline daily raises concerns about compliance, thus limiting its use to travelers for whom mefloquine is contraindicated and those traveling to areas where mefloquine-resistant strains of *P. falciparum* have been documented (e.g., eastern Thailand, Thailand-Myanmar border, and Cambodia) (25). Doxycycline should be taken in a dose of 100 mg per day starting 1 day before and continuing during and for 4 weeks after leaving a malarious area. Doxycycline, in combination with quinine, can be used to treat chloroquine-resistant *P. falciparum*.

Bacillus anthracis

Tetracycline is one of three drugs approved by the U.S. Food and Drug Administration for the treatment and prevention of anthrax. This was historically an occupational disease associated with contact with anthrax-infected animals or anthrax-contaminated animal products. In the United States, there were 224 cases of cutaneous anthrax reported between 1944 and 1994 (26), but naturally occurring disease nearly disappeared in the 1990s (26). More recently, *B. anthracis* became the source of an epidemic of cutaneous and inhalation anthrax as a component of bioterrorism (27). Cutaneous anthrax occurs as a result of skin contact with *B. anthracis* and can easily be treated with a 7- to 10-day course of tetracycline or doxycycline. Far more concerning is the inhalation form of anthrax, which has a reported mortality rate of 80% to 90% (27). This form of disease is rare but has been studied extensively in a primate model using an aerosol challenge. Doxycycline is highly effective in preventing disease, but the drug must be given for 60 days because of relapses after more abbreviated courses that are attributed to the persistence of spores in mediastinal nodes (27,28). As a result of these observations, the Centers for Disease Control and Prevention has recommended doxycycline as a preferred agent for the treatment and prevention of anthrax (29). It is important to document susceptibility of the epidemic strain to tetracycline because there is a claim of genetic engineering to produce a tetracycline-resistant strain of *B. anthracis* by Russian bioterrorism scientists in the early 1990s (27). When tetracycline is given, the usual form is doxycycline in a dose of 100 mg intravenously or orally twice daily.

Other Infections

Tetracyclines retain an important role in the treatment of a diverse list of organisms either alone or in combination with other drugs (see Table 21.1). Tetracycline, usually in combination with chloramphenicol and trimethoprim-sulfamethoxazole, remains an important drug in the treatment of melioidosis (*Burkholderia pseudomallei*), but the combination of ceftazidime and trimethoprim-sulfamethoxazole is the current regimen of choice for patients with disseminated septicemia (30). Doxycycline for 45 days remains the drug of choice in the treatment of

brucellosis in combination with either streptomycin (14 days) or rifampin (45 days) (31).

In the treatment of *Mycobacterium fortuitum* infections, doxycycline plus amikacin is a useful combination, whereas doxycycline or minocycline alone for 12 weeks may be used for *Mycobacterium marinum* infection. Studies have shown bactericidal activity of minocycline, either alone or in combination with clarithromycin, against *Mycobacterium leprae* in lepromatous leprosy (32). Minocycline shows promise as a component in the multidrug treatment of this disease.

A double-blind placebo-controlled trial showed that minocycline (200 mg per day) was safe and effective for patients with mild to moderate rheumatoid arthritis (33). It should be emphasized that the benefit was modest but was statistically significant for joint swelling and joint tenderness and for several laboratory parameters. The mechanism of action is unclear.

REFERENCES

1. McCaig LF, Hughes JM. Trends in antimicrobial drug prescribing among office-based physicians in the United States. *JAMA* 1995;273:214–219.
2. Cars O, Molstad S, Melander A. Variation in the antibiotic use in the European Union. *Lancet* 2001;357:1851–1853.
3. Tally FT, Ellestad GA, Testa RT. Glycylcyclines: a new generation of tetracyclines. *J Antimicrob Chemother* 1995;35:449–452.
4. Chopra I, Hawkey PM, Hinton M. Tetracyclines, molecular and clinical aspects. *J Antimicrob Chemother* 1992;29:245–277.
5. Shea KW, Cunha BA, Ueno Y, et al. Doxycycline activity against streptococcus pneumoniae. *Chest* 1998;108:1775–1776.
6. Schnappinger D, Hillen W. Tetracyclines: antibiotic action, uptake, and resistance mechanisms. *Arch Microbiol* 1996;165:3459–369.
7. Fabre J, Milek E, Kalfopoulos P. The kinetics of tetracycline in man. Excretion, penetration in normal inflammatory tissues, behavior in renal insufficiency and hemodialysis. *Schweiz Med Wochenschr* 1971;101:625–633.
8. Whelton A, Schach von Wittenau M, et al. Doxycycline pharmacokinetics in the absence of renal function. *Kidney Int* 1974;5:365–371.
9. Morris TJ, Davis TP. Doxycycline-induced esophageal ulceration in the U.S. military service. *Mil Med* 2000;165:316–319.
10. Carson JL, Strom BL, Duff A, et al. Acute liver disease associated with erythromycins, sulfonamides, and tetracyclines. *Ann Intern Med* 1993;119:576–583.
11. Min DI, Burke PA, Lewis WD, et al. Acute hepatic failure associated with oral minocycline: a case report. *Pharmacotherapy* 1992;12:68–71.
12. Byrne PAC, Williams BD, Pritchard MH. Minocycline-related lupus. *Br J Rheumatol* 1994;33:674–676.
13. Guillon J, Joly P, Autran B, et al. Minocycline-induced cell-mediated hypersensitivity pneumonitis. *Ann Intern Med* 1992;117:476–481.
14. Shapiro LE, Knowles SR, Shear MH. Comparative safety of tetracycline, minocycline, and doxycycline. *Arch Dermatol* 1997;133:1224–1230.
15. Williams DN, Laughlin LW, Lee Y. Minocycline: possible vestibular side effects. *Lancet* 1974;2:744–746.
16. Wormser GP, Nadelman RB, Dattwyl RJ, et al. Practice guidelines for the treatment of Lyme disease. *Clin Infect Dis* 2000;31:1–14.
17. Nadelman RB, Nowakowski J, Fish D, et al. Prophylaxis with single-dose doxycycline for the prevention of Lyme disease after an *Ixodes scapularis* tick bite. *N Engl J Med* 2001;345:79–84.
18. Centers for Disease Control and Prevention. 1998 guidelines for treatment of sexually transmitted diseases. *MMWR Morb Mortal Wkly Rep* 1998;47(RR-1):1–116.
19. McLain JBL, Ballou WP, Harrison SM, et al. Doxycycline therapy for leptospirosis. *Ann Intern Med* 1984;100:696–698.
20. Raoult D, Fournier PE, Fenollar F, et al. *Rickettsia africae*, a tick-borne pathogen in travelers to Sub-Saharan Africa. *N Engl J Med* 2001;344:1504–1510.
21. Bartlett JG, Dowell SF, Mandell LA, et al. Practice guidelines for the management of community-acquired pneumonia in adults. *CID* 2000;31:347–382.
22. Joshi N, Miller DQ. Doxycycline revisited. *Arch Intern Med* 1997;157:1421–1428.
23. Ailani RK, Sgastya G, Ailani RK, et al. Doxycycline is a cost-effective therapy for hospitalized patients with community-acquired pneumonia. *Arch Intern Med* 1999;159:266–270.
24. Doern GV, Heilmann KP, Huynh HK, et al. Antimicrobial resistance among clinical isolates of *Streptococcus pneumoniae* in the Unites States during 1999–2000, including a comparison of resistance rates since 1994–1995. *Antimicrob Agents Chemother* 2001;45(6):1721–1729.
25. Wyler DJ. Malaria chemoprophylaxis for the traveler. *N Engl J Med* 1993;329:31–37.
26. Centers for Disease Control and Prevention. Summary of notifiable diseases, 1945–1994. *MMWR Morb Mortal Wkly Rep* 1994;43:70.

27. Inglesby TV, Henderson DA, Bartlett JG. Anthrax as a biological weapon: medical and public health management. *JAMA* 1999;281:1735.
28. Friedlander A, Welkos SL, Pitt ML, et al. Postexposure prophylaxis against experimental inhalation anthrax. *J Infect Dis* 1993;167:1239.
29. Centers for Disease Control and Prevention. Update: investigation of bioterrorism-related anthrax and interim guidelines for exposure management and antimicrobial therapy, October 2001. *MMWR Morb Mortal Wkly Rep* 2001;50:909.
30. Sookpranee M, Boonma P, Susaengrat W, et al. Multicenter prospective randomized trial comparing ceftazidime plus co-trimoxazole with chloramphenicol plus doxycycline and co-trimoxazole for treatment of severe melioidosis. *Antimicrob Agents Chemother* 1992;36,1:158–162.
31. Solera J, Martinez-Alfaro E, Espinosa A. Recognition and optimum treatment of brucellosis. *Drugs* 1997;53(2):245–256.
32. Ji B, Jamet P, Perani EG, et al. Powerful bactericidal activities of clarithromycin and minocycline against *Mycobacterium leprae* in lepromatous leprosy. *J Infect Dis* 1993;168:188–190.
33. Tilley BC, Alarcon GS, Heyse SP, et al. Minocycline in rheumatoid arthritis. A 48-week, double-blind, placebo-controlled trial. MIAA Trial Group. *Ann Intern Med* 1995;122:81–89.

CHAPTER 22
Macrolides and Clindamycin

Graeme N. Forrest and David W. Oldach

The macrolide (erythromycin, clarithromycin, and azithromycin) and lincosamide (clindamycin) antibiotics are structurally unrelated, but they have similarities in antimicrobial activity, mechanism of resistance, and action on bacteria. They have been available for many years and have been a useful alternative to penicillin. Erythromycin is the macrolide that has been the longest in clinical use and continues to be an inexpensive and effective therapy for many diseases. In the past decade, several newer macrolides have become available with broader spectrum and better tolerability and safety profile. Azithromycin (an azilide) and clarithromycin have better pharmacokinetics and fewer gastrointestinal (GI) side effects, and they are effective in the treatment of opportunistic infections, including intracellular pathogens. The ketolides are a new addition to the macrolide class and appear promising in overcoming gram-positive–resistant organisms. Telithromycin is likely to be the first ketolide approved for use in the United States.

Other macrolide products of the Actinomycetales such as cyclosporine, tacrolimus, and rapamycin have been developed to exploit their immunosuppressive properties and demonstrate varying degrees of antifungal and antibacterial activity.

Clindamycin remains important in gram-positive and anaerobic infections but is limited by its GI toxicity. Lincomycin is mostly of historical interest.

ERYTHROMYCIN

Derivation, Chemistry, and Formulations

Erythromycin is a macrolide consisting of a 14-membered, macrocyclic lactone ring attached to two sugar moieties (a neutral sugar cladinose and an amino sugar desosamine). (Fig. 22.1). It was isolated in 1952 from the *Streptomyces erythraeus*, a soil organism found in the Philippines (1). Erythromycin is poorly water soluble and has a pK$_a$ of 8.8. The bitter-tasting base is the biologically active form of the drug, and its activity increases as the pH level increases from 5.5 to 8.5 (2). Erythromycin is rapidly inactivated by gastric acid and has variable absorption after oral administration. Serum levels are higher if the drug is taken on an empty stomach (3). To prevent degradation by gastric acid and to improve absorption, the pharmaceutical industry has prepared acid-resistant enteric coatings. Three enteric-coated preparations are available: enteric-coated tablets (E-Mycin, Ery-Tab, and generics), enteric-coated pellets in capsules (Eryc), and "film"-coated tablets of the base (filmtab). Another strategy has been to alter the chemical structure of the base to improve absorption by forming a salt (the stearate), an ester (the ethylsuccinate), or the estolate (the lauryl sulfate salt of the propionyl ester). Preparations of these salts are ethylsuccinate ester (EES, EryPed), lauryl sulfate (Ilosone), and the stearate form (Erythrocin) (4). The salt and esters are more acid resistant, form a stable suspension in water, and are tasteless. Pediatric liquid suspensions depend on these characteristics. The stearate dissolves in the duodenum, releasing the base, which is subsequently absorbed in the upper small intestine (4). Absorption of the stearate form of erythromycin is improved when it is taken with a meal (5). The two ester derivatives are absorbed intact and must be partially hydrolyzed to the biologically active base systemically (6). The ester and estolate are less affected by gastric acid, but higher plasma levels are produced when they are taken in the fasting state (7). Intravenous preparations of erythromycin include gluceptate and lactobionate (8). Intramuscular erythromycin is painful, is irregularly absorbed, and causes sterile abscesses. This route of administration is not recommended.

Mechanism of Action

Erythromycin reversibly binds to a single high-affinity site on the 50S subunit of the 70S bacterial ribosome (9). The binding inhibits ribonucleic acid (RNA)–dependent protein synthesis by preventing transpeptidation and translocation of peptidyl transfer RNA (10). It has been suggested that the macrolide binds to the peptidyl donor site and competitively interferes with the translocation of the peptide chain from the acceptor of the donor site (11). Azithromycin and clarithromycin have a similar mechanism of action. In some bacterial systems, the macrolides interfere with the ribosomal binding of chloramphenicol, clindamycin, and other macrolide antimicrobials (12). As members of the group of drugs that inhibit bacterial protein synthesis, the macrolide antibiotics are considered bacteriostatic antimicrobials. In fact, each of these drugs may be bactericidal, depending on the species of organism, inoculum size, growth phase, and drug concentration tested (13–15).

Antimicrobial Action and Resistance Mechanisms

Erythromycin has a broad spectrum of activity against many gram-positive and some gram-negative bacteria, including *Actinomyces* and *Mycoplasma* species (Table 22.1). It also has activity against *Chlamydia* and *Rickettsia* species. Erythromycin is inactive against *Pseudomonas* species and the Enterobacteriaceae, except in an alkaline environment, because of its decreased ability to enter the cell (16,17). Only organisms rendered cell wall deficient are susceptible (10,12). Because erythromycin is a weak base, it is ionized in acidic environments but has to be in the un-ionized state to pass through the cell wall of Enterobacteriaceae (18,19). It works best against both gram-positive and gram-negative bacteria with an increasing pH level.

Erythromycin is active *in vitro* against many strains of streptococcal species, including groups A and B streptococci, *Streptococcus pneumoniae*, and *Streptococcus viridans* (16,20). However,

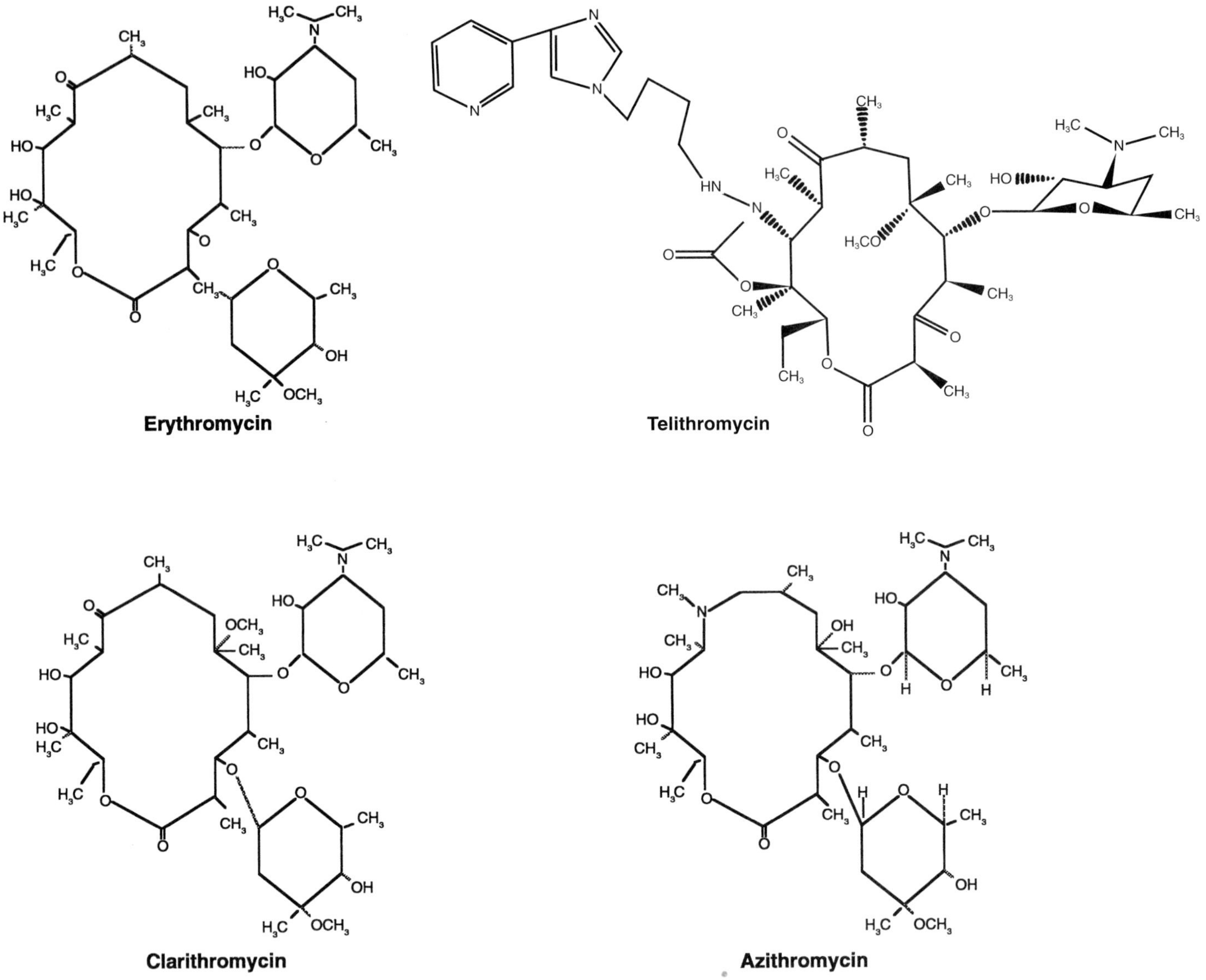

Figure 22.1. Chemical structures of erythromycin, clarithromycin, telithromycin (a ketolide antibiotic), and azithromycin (a 15-membered ring azalide antibiotic).

increasing resistance among all these species has been noted (21–28). Erythromycin resistance among *Streptococcus pyogenes* isolates is increasing globally and in the United States is now approaching 10% (24,26). In Asia, where macrolides are commonly used for respiratory tract infections, 60% of strains were highly resistant to erythromycin (22). In Finland, it was observed that erythromycin-resistant isolates had risen to 44% by the early 1990s, but the subsequent implementation by the government of a policy to reduce macrolide usage in respiratory tract and skin infections saw a decline in resistance from 16.2% in 1992 to 8.6% in 1996 (21,29). Group B streptococci are also showing increased antibiotic resistance with isolates collected from pregnant women and neonates showing macrolide resistance from 20% to 25% (30,31).

Erythromycin has historically been active against pneumococci, although just as with penicillin, macrolide resistance is increasing rapidly globally (32). Loss of this inexpensive and readily accessible drug for this indication is a worldwide problem. Reports examining isolates collected in the United States of invasive *S. pneumoniae* isolates from 1995 to 1998 demon-

strated that erythromycin resistance had increased to 16% from 11%. In some areas such as Georgia and Tennessee, penicillin-resistant strains had increased to 30% of isolates or more (33). The Spanish have reported *S. pneumoniae* isolates with 50% resistance to at least one antibiotic, with an overall high penicillin resistance rate of 33% and macrolide resistance of 27% (34). It appears that these resistant strains are carried in the nasopharynx of healthy children and adults (35). About 40% of strains of *S. pneumoniae* with penicillin-intermediate resistance (minimum inhibitory concentration [MIC] = 0.12 to 1.0 μg/mL) and 65% of penicillin-resistant strains (MIC > 2.9 μg/mL) are resistant to macrolides (23,32,36). *S. pneumoniae* strains demonstrate complete cross-resistance among the macrolides (35–39), but the resistance mechanism varies, so the decision to use erythromycin for the treatment of community-acquired pneumonia must be made in the context of the ongoing pandemic of antibiotic resistance (38–41). The "viridans" streptococci generally remain susceptible to erythromycin; however, in Spain, 39% of strains were macrolide resistant in neutropenic patients (42). Fewer than 50% of enterococcal isolates are sensitive (43).

TABLE 22.1. Mean Minimal Inhibitory Concentrations of Selected Pathogens to Macrolide Antibiotics

Pathogen	Minimal inhibitory concentration (μg/mL)			
	Erythromycin	Clarithromycin	Azithromycin	Telithromycin
Bacteroides spp. (including *Bacteroides fragilis*)	4–32	2–8	2–8	4–64
Bartonella spp. (*Bartonella quintana, Bartonella henselae*)	0.06–0.25	0.006–0.015	0.006–0.03	—
Bordetella pertussis	0.03	0.03	0.03	0.03
Borrelia burgdorferi	0.03–0.06	0.015	0.015	—
Campylobacter jejuni	1.0–2.0	2–4	0.24–0.5	—
Chlamydia pneumoniae	<0.125	<0.03	0.25	<0.02
Chlamydia trachomatis	0.064–>1.0	—	0.12	—
Clostridium perfringens	1.0–1.56	—	0.25–0.78	—
Eikenella corrodens	4.0	—	2.0–4.0	—
Enterococci—vancomycin sensitive	>50	>50	>50	0.15–4.0
Enterococci—vancomycin resistant	>50	>50	>50	>16
Fusobacterium spp.	16	—	4	2–64
Haemophilus ducreyi	0.03	0.01	<0.01	—
Haemophilus influenzae	4.0–8.0	4–16	0.5–2.0	2–4
Helicobacter pylori	0.22	0.03	<0.25	0.5–0.125
Legionella spp.	0.06–0.5	0.25	0.25–2.0	<0.25
Listeria monocytogenes	0.25	0.13	0.5	—
Moraxella catarrhalis	0.13–0.5	<0.25	<0.25–0.50	0.12
Mycobacterium avium complex (MAC)	16–>64	1.0–8.0	32–64	5–20
Mycobacterium abscessus	>8.0	0.50	8	—
Mycobacterium chelonae	8	0.25	2	—
Mycoplasma pneumoniae	—	—	0.002–0.01	—
Neisseria gonorrhoeae	2.0	0.25	0.25	—
Pasteurella spp.	1.56	—	0.1–2.0	—
Peptostreptococcus spp.	>8	2.6	2.3	0.03–4.0
Propionibacterium acnes	0.03	0.03	0.03	0.03
Rhodococcus equi	16	—	4–8	16
Salmonella enteritidis	128	—	4–8	—
Staphylococcus aureus				
Methicillin sensitive	0.41–1.76	0.06	0.8–1.6	0.03–0.12
Methicillin resistant	>128	>128	>128	>64
Staphylococcus epidermidis				
Methicillin sensitive	<0.05	0.06	<0.27	—
Methicillin resistant	>4	—	>4	—
Streptococcus pneumoniae				
Penicillin susceptible	<0.25	<0.25	<0.25	<0.25
Penicillin intermediate	<0.25	<0.25	<0.25	<0.25
Penicillin resistant	>128	>128	>128	0.25
Streptococcus pyogenes	<0.25	<0.25	0.1–0.5	<0.25
Streptococcus spp. (groups B, C, E)	0.06	0.06	0.13	<0.06
Streptococcus viridans	1.24	0.03	<2.0	—
Ureaplasma urealyticum	0.25–4.0	<0.25	0.064–2.0	—
Yersinia enterocolitica	>50	—	3.12	—
Yersinia pestis	—	—	32	—

Note: Data values are reported in referenced publications.

Methicillin-sensitive strains of *Staphylococcus aureus* are often sensitive to erythromycin, whereas methicillin-resistant strains of *S. aureus* are resistant to erythromycin (44). As with clindamycin, the possibility of emergence of resistance exists while patients are on therapy (45). Dissociated resistance may develop among isolates sensitive to erythromycin when not exposed to the antimicrobial but with rapid induction of resistance on exposure to the drug (46). Other sensitive gram-positive bacteria include *Actinomyces israelii, Bacillus anthracis, Listeria monocytogenes, Corynebacterium diphtheriae, Clostridium perfringens, Clostridium tetani,* and *Erysipelothrix rhusiopathiae* (16). Some strains of *C. perfringens* are only moderately sensitive (48). Susceptible gram-negative organisms include *Neisseria meningitidis, Neisseria gonorrhoeae, Moraxella catarrhalis, Bordetella pertussis, Legionella* species, *Haemophilus ducreyi,* and *Campylobacter jejuni* (18). The drug is active against *Haemophilus influenzae,* although strain sensitivity is variable (48). *Treponema pallidum, Borrelia*

burgdorferi, Bartonella species, *Chlamydia trachomatis, Mycoplasma pneumoniae,* and some *Ureaplasma urealyticum* isolates are also sensitive (13,16,49). Erythromycin is active against some gram-negative anaerobes, although *Bacteroides fragilis* is typically resistant (50).

Several mechanisms may result in bacterial resistance to the macrolide antibiotics, including impermeability of the bacterial cell wall (14), active efflux pumping of the antibiotic (51), target site alteration (52), and drug inactivation (53). As described already, the cell envelopes of the Enterobacteriaceae and *Pseudomonas* species are relatively impermeable to macrolides (14). However, the protoplast of these organisms, formed by stripping off the cell wall, is sensitive to erythromycin (19).

S. aureus, Staphylococcus epidermidis, and enterococci use plasmid-mediated, energy-dependent efflux pumps as a mechanism of resistance to allow them to actively export the macrolides from within themselves (51,54). This mechanism is encoded by the *msr*A/*msr*B gene, which codes for the transmembrane proteins to complete the transporter functions (55). An alternative mechanism for an efflux system is the M phenotype. It affects 14- and 15-membered macrolides, lincosamides, and streptogramin B and was elucidated in erythromycin-resistant *S. pneumoniae* and *S. pyogenes.* These efflux pumps are encoded by *mef*A in *S. pyogenes* and *mef* E in *S. pneumoniae* (24,38,39,41,56).

Another resistance mechanism is an alteration in a single amino acid in the 50S ribosomal protein that decreases the binding affinity of the macrolides (and lincosamide antimicrobials), rendering organisms resistant (57). This one-step, high-level resistance is the result of chromosomal mutation and has been described in some strains of *Escherichia coli, S. pyogenes, S. aureus,* and *Campylobacter* species. Resistance caused by chromosomal mutation is usually unstable and occurs at a low frequency (58). Posttranscriptional modification of the 23S ribosomal RNA of the 50S subunit by an adenine-specific *N*-methyltransferase is a common mechanism of resistance. The genes encoding for this methylase have been named *erm* (erythromycin ribosome methylation) (52). The *erm* genes have been identified in multiple gram-positive bacteria, including *Staphylococcus, Lactobacillus,* and *Bacillus,* as well as enterococcal, streptococcal, and enterobacteria species and some anaerobes (e.g., *Bacteroides, Clostridium*). Multiple *erm* genes have been isolated from *Streptomyces* species, the source organisms of most macrolide antibiotics (52). Adenosine methylation may also confer resistance to other macrolides, clindamycin, and the streptogramin antibiotics—thus the term *MLS resistance* (macrolides, lincosamides, and streptogramins). The *erm* genes are frequently plasmid associated. Expression may be constitutive (the entire bacterial population is resistant) or inducible by subinhibitory levels of drug (52). The latter mechanism probably accounts for the phenomenon of dissociated resistance found in some strains of staphylococci (46).

Enzymatic inactivation has been demonstrated in certain strains of *E. coli* and gram-positive organisms (53). A gene for an inducible macrolide 2′-phosphotransferase of *E. coli* that inactivates the 14-membered macrolides has been characterized (59). Macrolides can be inactivated by glycosylation (59). Some bacterial strains inactivate erythromycin with a plasmid-encoded esterase that cleaves the lactone ring (*ere*A and *ere*B genes) (54).

Pharmacology

All the macrolide antibiotics undergo enterohepatic circulation; after oral administration of such drugs, significant serum levels accumulate only after saturation of first-pass metabolism and biliary excretion has occurred. This fact complicates calculations of oral bioavailability (60). As a class, they are characterized by their ability to achieve higher tissue concentrations than plasma concentrations and the persistence of tissue concentrations. Each macrolide achieves a rapid and significant intracellular accumulation, with each varying to the amount they can accumulate both intracellularly and within tissues; however, the clinical significance of these differences remains unclear (60).

Erythromycin is rapidly inactivated by gastric acid and has variable absorption after oral administration (2). Serum levels are higher if the drug is taken on an empty stomach (3). The salt and esters are more acid resistant, form a stable suspension in water, and are tasteless. The stearate dissolves in the duodenum, releasing the base, which is subsequently absorbed in the upper small intestine (4). Absorption of the stearate form of erythromycin is improved when it is taken with a meal (5). After absorption, 45% of the ethylsuccinate preparation is present in the serum as the inactive ester and 55% as the active base (61). The absorption of base is variable and produces peak serum concentrations within 4 hours of ingestion (3–6,62–64) (Table 22.2). The stearate and ethylsuccinate preparations are more evenly absorbed, producing peak serum levels after 3 and 2 hours, respectively. Approximately 45% of the ethylsuccinate preparation reaches the serum as inactive ester and 55% as active base (6,7). The estolate is absorbed from the intestine as the propionate ester. More estolate is absorbed from the gut within 2 hours of ingestion than with the other erythromycin compounds. Although serum levels of total drug are higher, only 23% to 35% of the total is active base (6). Consequently, enteric-coated base tablets taken in the fasting state produce as high a plasma level of active erythromycin as estolate capsules (62).

TABLE 22.2. Serum Concentrations of Macrolide Antibiotics

Preparation	Dose (mg)	Route	Hours after dose	Peak serum concentration range (μg/mL) (at steady state)	Terminal half-life (hr)[a]
Erythromycin					
Base	250	p.o.	4	0.3–1.7	—
	500	p.o.	4	0.3–1.9	—
Stearate	250	p.o.	2–3	0.2–1.3	—
	500	p.o.	3	0.4–1.8	1.2–2.0
Ethylsuccinate	400	p.o.	0.5–2.5	0.6	—
Estolate	250	p.o.	2–4	1.2	—
	500	p.o.	2–4	3.0	—
Gluceptate	250	i.v.	1	2.6–3.5	—
	1,000	i.v.	1	9.9	—
Lactobionate	500	i.v.	1	9.9	—
Clarithromycin	250	p.o.	3	2.0	3–4
14-Hydroxydarithromycin	—	—	3	0.7	5–7
Extended Release	500	p.o.	4–8	2–3	5–7
Azithromycin	500	p.o.	3.2	0.24–0.4	68
	500	i.v.	1–1.13	3.63	68
Dirithromycin (erythromycylamine)	500	p.o.	4.1	0.48	45

Note: Data reported from reference publications. p.o., oral; i.v., intravenous.
[a] Terminal half-life, at the end of a 5- to 14-day course of therapy.

Erythromycin is distributed throughout the body water (64). Protein binding of active drug varies between 40% and 90% (65). It passes readily into ascitic and pleural fluid, reaching concentrations of approximately 50% of that in serum, and levels in prostatic fluid and semen are about one third those in blood (45). After a delay, erythromycin diffuses into middle ear fluid in concentrations therapeutic for group A streptococci and pneumococci but not for *H. influenzae* (66). The drug also passes into sinus fluid after a lag period similar to that observed with middle ear fluid (67). Erythromycin achieves higher levels that are sustained longer in pulmonary tissues and secretions than comparable doses of amoxicillin (68). Intravenous administration of erythromycin produces drug concentrations in sputum three to four times higher than those produced by oral administration (68). High concentrations of drug are also found in tonsillar and adenoidal tissue (69). Erythromycin does not achieve therapeutic levels in cerebrospinal fluid (CSF) or brain because it does not readily cross the meninges and blood–brain barrier, so it should not be used to treat infections of the central nervous system (CNS) (66). The drug is not recommended for septic arthritis because of inadequate penetration into synovial fluid (70). Orally administered base produces sufficient concentrations in stool to suppress most anaerobic bacteria (66). Erythromycin crosses transplacentally; fetal serum concentrations are about 2% of maternal blood concentrations, but higher concentrations accumulate in fetal tissue. The drug is excreted in breast milk (71). In more than four decades of use, there have been no reported cases of teratogenic effects (16).

Erythromycin is concentrated in the liver and may be partially inactivated by demethylation (72). The drug is mostly excreted unaltered in the bile, so high levels are found in the stool (73). Approximately 2.5% of an oral dose and 15% of an intravenous dose of erythromycin is excreted unchanged in the urine (3). The serum half-life of the drug is normally $1\frac{1}{2}$ hours but increases to 4 to 6 hours in anuric patients (63,64). Peritoneal dialysis and hemodialysis do not significantly reduce serum levels (79). The antibiotic remains longer in tissue than in serum, a characteristic shared by all of the macrolide antibiotics (15,60). Because the major site of elimination is the liver, changes in dosing are not recommended for most patients with renal failure (74); ototoxicity has been reported, however, in elderly patients with renal failure (75). It is recommended that patients with liver disease and renal failure have some dose reduction.

Erythromycin requires energy to be concentrated in neutrophils and macrophages (76,77). Alveolar macrophages and neutrophils achieve concentrations 9 to 23 times greater than extracellular fluid concentrations (76–78). These high intracellular concentrations may have clinical implications in the treatment of *Legionella* species (78). All the macrolides accumulate to high levels within cells, with prolonged intracellular half-lives. This enhances their activity against organisms that proliferate intracellularly. The mechanism of cellular accumulation and concentration is believed to be passive diffusion, with trapping through ribosomal binding and within cell lysosomes. They also demonstrate a postantibiotic effect by inhibiting bacterial growth of respiratory tract pathogens from 2 to 8 hours after exposure to the antibiotic (79). The postantibiotic effects of azithromycin and clarithromycin are extended in the presence of concentrations of the drugs lower than the MIC from the observed 2 to 8 hours for common respiratory tract pathogens up to 6 to 20 hours (79).

ADVERSE REACTIONS

Erythromycin has a reputation as a safe nontoxic antimicrobial. The most frequent side effects of oral therapy are abdominal cramps, nausea, vomiting, and mild diarrhea (66). GI upset is dose related and may be ameliorated by decreasing the dose.

Cases of hypertrophic pyloric stenosis have been attributed to erythromycin estolate (80). Enteric-coated erythromycin preparations do not reduce the common dose-related GI side effects seen with the base (81). The GI effects of erythromycin are attributed to the drug's agonist action at the GI receptor for the polypeptide hormone motilin (82). These effects have been exploited clinically in the treatment of diabetic gastroparesis (83).

Cholestatic jaundice, an uncommon complication accompanied by fever, abdominal pain, eosinophilia, hyperbilirubinemia, and elevated transaminase values, has been associated most often with erythromycin estolate and typically occurs 10 to 20 days after initiation of therapy (84,85). Cholestatic liver disease has an incidence of less than 1 in 1,000 treated patients and is more common in adults, especially pregnant women, than children (86). Jaundice is reversible in days to weeks after discontinuation of the medication, and chronic liver disease or death has not been described (87). Rechallenge in patients with erythromycin estolate–induced hepatitis has resulted in recurrent disease with a shorter incubation period, suggesting a hypersensitivity reaction, although direct hepatocyte toxicity of erythromycin propionate has been described (88). Interference of the estolate with colorimetric determinations of transaminase levels may result in artifactual elevations (89); this phenomenon should not be confused with drug-associated cholestasis. Because the estolate has no therapeutic advantage, it should not be given to adults, although it is probably safe for children and is better tolerated than the ethylsuccinate preparation.

Many reports of erythromycin-associated ototoxicity, including tinnitus, deafness, high-frequency hearing loss, and vertigo, have been described (90). Erythromycin-associated ototoxicity is reversible within 6 to 14 days and usually occurs in patients older than 60 years who were receiving 4 g per day of erythromycin or more (91).

Antibiotic-associated colitis has rarely been associated with macrolides, although they reduce anaerobic and aerobic flora of the gut (92). Superinfection of the vagina or gut with *Candida* species does occur, as with other antibiotics. Allergic reactions such as fever, rashes, and eosinophilia are uncommon (15,16). Torsade de pointes (polymorphic ventricular tachycardia with QT-interval prolongation) has been rarely reported with erythromycin, although it is more often seen in association with interactions with other drugs (93). Erythromycin has been shown to have a direct effect on repolarization in guinea pig models, where it blocked electrical current in the myocytes (94). Intravenous infusions of erythromycin lactobionate frequently produce side effects such as local pain at the infusion site and a feeling of lightheadedness. Diluting the drug and slowing the infusion rate can limit thrombophlebitis (63).

DRUG INTERACTIONS

Macrolide antibiotics interact with other drugs by interfering with hepatic metabolism through the cytochrome P450 (CYP) enzyme system, especially via the CYP 3A subclass (95,96). This competitive inhibition of metabolism of other medications by erythromycin may result in serious toxicities of these medications drug (96,97). Drugs metabolized by the CYP system, which may be significantly affected by the coadministration of erythromycin, are presented in Table 22.3. When coadministered with erythromycin, several drugs (such as cisapride and terfenadine) had elevated serum concentrations causing QT-interval prolongation and leading to ventricular arrhythmias. Similarly, benzodiazepines used with erythromycin could lead to prolonged unconsciousness (95). Therefore, the use of erythromycin with drugs metabolized by the CYP system should be done with attention to the potential for adverse interactions. Erythromycin may cause digoxin toxicity in some patients because it suppresses

TABLE 22.3.   Drugs with Potential Drug Interactions with the Macrolides

Macrolide	Interacting drug
Erythromycin	Astemizole, benzodiazepines, buspirone, carbamazepine, cisapride, cyclosporine, digoxin, diltiazem, dofetilide, ergot alkaloids, felodipine, halothane, HMG-CoA reductase inhibitors loratadine, oral contraceptives, pimozide, protease inhibitors, quinidine, silfandil, tacrolimus, theophyllines, valproate, warfarin.
Clarithromycin	Astemizole, benzodiazepines, carbamazepine, cisapride, cyclosporine, delavirdine, digoxin, efavirenz, HMG-CoA reductase inhibitors, protease inhibitors, quinidine, rifamycins, tacrolimus, thophyllines, vinca alkaloids, warfarin, zidovudine.
Azithromycin	Digoxin

Note: Erythromycin and clarithromycin generally cause an elevation of the interacted drug, because of interaction with CYP 3A enzyme system in the liver. Digoxin toxicity is from suppression of anaerobic flora. HMG-CoA, hydroxymethylglutocyl-coenzymes A.
Source: From references 98–100, 127, 155–161, 207, 208, with permission.

the gut flora that normally degrade digoxin allowing for improved absorption of digoxin (95–98).

Intravenous preparations of erythromycin are incompatible with certain other drugs, including vitamin B complex, vitamin C, chloramphenicol, cephalothin, colistin, heparin, tetracyclines, and phenytoin.

The interaction of erythromycin with other antimicrobials has been well studied. An important interaction is the combination of rifampin or penicillin and erythromycin, which may have antagonistic effects when treating *Listeria* infection (99).

Preparations and Dosing

Erythromycin is available in several oral and intravenous preparations, as described previously. Topical solutions and ointments of 1.5%, 2%, and 3% erythromycin base are used to treat acne vulgaris. Ophthalmic ointments of 0.5% are also available for the treatment of bacterial conjunctivitis and prophylaxis against neonatal chlamydial and gonococcal ophthalmic infections. Peak serum levels of erythromycin base depend on formulation, dose, and route (see Table 22.2). Available oral formulations yield comparable serum concentrations of active drug. The serum levels of erythromycin required to inhibit sensitive organisms (listed in Table 22.1) are clinically attainable. The recommended dose of drug for most indications varies between 250 and 500 mg four times daily. For moderate to severe infections, including those caused by *Legionella* species, the recommended dose of intravenous erythromycin is 4 g per day.

Uses of Erythromycin

With the advent of the newer macrolides, erythromycin's role as a front-line agent has declined. However, despite increasing resistance among many organisms, it is still an inexpensive and effective alternative, especially in the penicillin-allergic patient. Erythromycin is an effective agent for infections of the respiratory tract, especially by *Legionella* and *Mycoplasma* species, but with increasing erythromycin-resistant strains of *S. pneumoniae*, it should not be used as single-agent therapy and is recom-

mended with a third-generation cephalosporin in the treatment of community-acquired pneumonia (32). Erythromycin is considered a drug of choice for infection with *Legionella* species (100). In severe cases, the combination erythromycin-rifampin is now favored, although the newer macrolides and fluoroquinolones are more active than erythromycin *in vitro* and appear to be preferred clinically (101,102). With *Mycoplasma* infections, erythromycin has been shown to reduce the duration of fever and respiratory symptoms and hasten the resolution of pulmonary infiltrates, but it does not eliminate the organism from the nasopharynx (103,104). Erythromycin has proven clinical efficacy in the treatment of pneumonia caused by *Chlamydia pneumoniae* (105,106) and will treat *Chlamydia psittaci* and *Coxiella burnetii* infections (107,108).

Erythromycin remains effective treatment of mild to moderate cases of community-acquired pneumonia associated with *S. pneumoniae, M. catarrhalis, S. pyogenes,* or *H. influenzae* (2–108). However, as noted already, its effectiveness is being limited by the increasing incidence of penicillin-resistant *S. pneumoniae* infection, because such strains are usually resistant to erythromycin (28).

Erythromycin may have an antiinflammatory benefit in treating acute exacerbations of chronic bronchitis (109). *H. influenzae* has variable sensitivity to erythromycin, but treated patients have shown a decrease in symptom severity and duration (109). The newer macrolides are superior in treating *H. influenzae* infections. Streptococcal pharyngitis responds to erythromycin treatment, and the drug is as effective as the penicillins in preventing acute rheumatic fever (14,110). Early administration of erythromycin in the course of pertussis reduces the contagiousness but does not shorten the duration of clinical illness (111). It is effective prophylaxis for nonimmunized children who have been exposed to pertussis (111). Erythromycin effectively eliminates the acute and chronic carrier state of lysogenic *C. diphtheriae* in more than 90% of adults, but it does not alter the course of infection (112).

Skin and soft tissue infections with *S. pyogenes* have been treated successfully with erythromycin (3). Treatment failure suggests a mixed infection with erythromycin-resistant strains of *S. aureus* (16). Erythromycin should be avoided for deep-seated staphylococcal infections because of the potential for the emergence of resistant strains during therapy (14,15,45). Penicillinase-resistant penicillins, cephalosporins, or vancomycin may be required in this situation (113). Erythromycin is safe inexpensive therapy for chronic acne vulgaris; however, azithromycin is more active and tolerable (114).

Erythromycin has consistent activity against *C. jejuni* infection and has been demonstrated to reduce the duration of positive stool culture results and moderate symptoms of gastroenteritis related to this pathogen; however, fluorinated quinolones are active against this organism and are preferred therapy (115,116). Erythromycin is recommended for the treatment of *U. urealyticum, Chlamydia* infections including lymphogranuloma venereum, and chancroid (49,117,118).

DIRITHROMYCIN

Dirithromycin is a semisynthetic 14-membered macrolide antibiotic derived through the condensation of erythromycylamine and an aliphatic aldehyde (119). Erythromycylamine, the active moiety in the prodrug dirithromycin, in comparison with erythromycin, has a similar spectrum of activity and markedly prolonged half-life (119). The clinical efficacy, toxicity, and antimicrobial spectrum of dirithromycin appear to be similar to those of erythromycin, with the potential advantage of once-daily dosing. Dirithromycin is available only as 250-mg enteric-coated tablets. The antimicrobial activity of dirithromycin against gram-positive bacteria is about the same or half that of erythromycylamine, which is about fourfold less active than erythromycin against *S. pneumoniae, H. influenzae,* and *M. catarrhalis* infections (120,121). It is also less active against the atypical pneumonia organisms (119–121). There is complete cross-resistance between erythromycin and dirithromycin.

Dirithromycin is rapidly hydrolyzed to its primary metabolite after absorption. The active agent, erythromycylamine, reaches peak serum concentrations in 4 to 5 hours after a single dose. Absorption of dirithromycin is increased when taken with food; however, despite accumulating high tissue concentrations, serum concentrations are lower than those achieved by the other macrolides. The drug is excreted primarily in the bile and feces, with an elimination half-life of 30 to 44 hours, allowing use of single daily doses. After single dosing with dirithromycin, 62% to 81% of the drug (primarily as erythromycylamine) is excreted in feces; less than 3% is recovered from urine. Erythromycylamine is not cleared by hemodialysis (7,122).

The adverse reactions of dirithromycin have been limited to GI intolerance, similar to erythromycin. However, it does not interfere with the CYP hepatic enzyme system and has not been implicated in drug interactions (120). Although effective in treating some upper respiratory tract infections such as acute pharyngitis, bronchitis, and skin infections, its limited *in vitro* antimicrobial activity precludes recommending it for widespread use (121).

CLARITHROMYCIN

Clarithromycin is one of the newer macrolides, which has better oral absorption, longer half-life, fewer GI side effects, and a greater antimicrobial spectrum, especially against *Mycobacterium* species.

Chemistry and Preparations

Clarithromycin (see Fig. 22.1) has a 14-membered lactone ring but has substituted an *O*-methyl group at position C6 with resultant acid stability and improved antimicrobial and pharmacokinetic properties (13,123). In addition, the primary metabolite of clarithromycin (14-hydroxyclarithromycin) has significant antimicrobial activity. Clarithromycin is available as film-coated tablets and granules for oral suspension. Film-coated tablets contain 250 or 500 mg of clarithromycin. In the year 2000, an extended-release formulation of the film-coated tablet was released. When clarithromycin granules are resuspended, they result in drug concentrations of 125 or 250 mg per 5 mL in flavored preparations for pediatric use. No intravenous formulation of clarithromycin is available.

Mechanism of Action and Resistance

Clarithromycin binds to the same receptor on the bacterial 50S ribosomal subunit and inhibits RNA-dependent protein synthesis by the same mechanism as erythromycin (123). Clarithromycin appears to be more active against *H. influenzae* infection than erythromycin, but less so than azithromycin. It is considered a bacteriostatic antibiotic, although it is bactericidal against *S. pneumoniae, S. pyogenes,* and *H. influenzae* (125).

Organisms with acquired resistance to erythromycin, in particular through the acquisition of *erm* (the MLS phenotype) and *ere* genes, are generally resistant to clarithromycin (51,125). Resistance develops rapidly when clarithromycin is used as

monotherapy in the treatment of *Mycobacterium avium* complex (MAC) infections (126,127). The rate of acquisition of resistance by *M. avium* when clarithromycin was used alone is comparable to that found for *Mycobacterium tuberculosis* with rifampin, suggesting a single-step mutation mechanism (128). The resistance appears to be related to a point mutation in 23S ribosomal RNA and presumably alters the binding of drug to the ribosome (128). The same mechanism is seen when clarithromycin is used as monotherapy in *H. pylori* infections, with subsequent development of resistance (129).

Antimicrobial Activity

Clarithromycin, in conjunction with its primary metabolite, 14-hydroxyclarithromycin, has a broad range of activity that is similar to that of azithromycin and erythromycin. *In vitro,* the drug is comparable or superior to erythromycin (and azithromycin) in its activity against gram-positive organisms (13). Clarithromycin has about fourfold more activity than erythromycin against gram-positive bacteria, especially *S. pneumoniae, S. pyogenes,* and methicillin-sensitive *S. aureus* (124). Almost all methicillin-resistant strains of *S. aureus* are resistant to clarithromycin (126). Clarithromycin is as active as erythromycin against gram-negative bacteria, but the 14-hydroxyclarithromycin makes it more effective against *H. influenzae* (130,131). The drug is active *in vitro* against *M. catarrhalis, Legionella pneumophila, M. pneumoniae, C. pneumoniae,* and *C. trachomatis* (129–135). Clarithromycin is the most active of the macrolide antibiotics against *H. pylori,* nontuberculous *Mycobacterium* species including MAC infection, and *Mycobacterium leprae* (136–139). Against MAC infection, clarithromycin has about fourfold more activity and is more rapid in clearing bloodstream infection than azithromycin (140–142). Like azithromycin, clarithromycin suppresses *Toxoplasma gondii* tachyzoite replication (143).

Pharmacology

Clarithromycin is available in tablet form and in granules for oral suspension. The drug is rapidly absorbed from the GI tract and its bioavailability is approximately 50% after a single 250-mg dose. Peak clarithromycin plasma concentrations after a single dose of 250 or 500 mg of drug were achieved in 3 hours (0.62 to 0.84 μg/mL and 1.77 to 1.89 μg/mL, respectively) (13). In the liver, clarithromycin undergoes rapid biotransformation to the active metabolite 14-hydroxyclarithromycin (peak concentrations of 3.1 to 4.9 μg/mL and 6.1 to 6.9 μg/mL were measured after single doses of 250 and 500 mg, respectively) (13). Steady-state peak serum concentrations of the drug are achieved after four to six doses and are approximately 1 μg/mL (250 mg twice a day) and 2 to 3 μg/mL (500 mg twice a day). The drug is 42% to 70% protein bound at these concentrations (144–146). Coadministration of food does not appreciably alter clarithromycin pharmacokinetic parameters (13,146). The extended-release formulation provides lower and later steady-state peak plasma concentrations but equivalent area-under-the-curve (AUC) values for clarithromycin and its metabolite. The extended-release capsule has to be taken with food because its concentration declines 30% when taken in the fasted state (147). As with the other macrolide antibiotics, clarithromycin and its metabolites have exceptional tissue penetration and accumulation within cells (146,148). Concentrations of the drug within alveolar cells were 1,700-fold greater than those in plasma versus 0.01 μg/mL 48 hours after the fifth and final dose of a dosing regimen of 500 mg each 12 hours (148); at that time, lung epithelial lining fluid concentrations were 23.4 μg/mL (145). Clarithromycin and its metabolite achieve appreciable levels in the middle ear of children to exceed MIC of most strains of middle ear pathogens. Clarithromycin enters the CSF at concentrations that are insufficient to be therapeutic (149).

Approximately 50% of administered doses of clarithromycin is excreted by the kidneys, in the form of clarithromycin or its 14-hydroxy metabolite. In the setting of severe renal impairment, dosage adjustment is required. The elimination half-life of the drug is approximately 3 to 4 hours when given as 250 mg every 12 hours, increasing to 7 to 8 hours when given as 500 mg every 12 hours (148–152). In the setting of significant liver disease, there is diminished generation of the 14-hydroxy metabolite. Clarithromycin has demonstrated teratogenic effects in animal studies and is not safe for use in pregnancy.

ADVERSE REACTIONS AND DRUG INTERACTIONS

Clarithromycin side effects are mostly GI, with diarrhea, nausea, and abdominal pain, but discontinuation is rarely needed. A metallic taste disturbance, headaches, and dizziness are frequently reported (123,125). Rare other events include reversible ototoxicity and tinnitus when using high doses to treat MAC infection. Clarithromycin can inhibit the CYP 3A system in the liver and results in the elevations of many drug levels, which can lead to serious toxicity (150). Clarithromycin appears to interact with the same spectrum of drugs that erythromycin does (150–153). One drug interaction seen in clinical practice was alteration of rifabutin levels (when clarithromycin and rifabutin are used to treat MAC), resulting in neutropenia and uveitis (151–153). Clarithromycin has been associated with digoxin toxicity also (152). Clarithromycin may decrease zidovudine concentration and may affect protease inhibitor concentrations (154,155).

Uses of Clarithromycin

Clarithromycin effectively treats all infections erythromycin does (123). The recommended dose of clarithromycin for treatment of respiratory tract and skin and soft tissue infections in adults is 250 to 500 mg twice daily for 7 to 14 days. The new extended-release formulation is given as 1 g (two tablets) daily for 10 days and is approved only for respiratory tract infections (147). For prophylaxis against MAC infections in adults, 500 mg twice daily is recommended, whereas for therapy for established infection, multidrug regimens including clarithromycin at 500 to 1,000 mg twice daily are recommended (141,156,157); for children, the dosage is calculated as 7.5 mg/kg twice a day (13,156).

Clarithromycin has been proven effective in many clinical trials in treating otitis media, sinusitis, pharyngitis, and pneumonia. It also has been proven effective in treating skin and soft tissue infections (123,158,159). It shows excellent activity against *L. pneumophila, M. pneumoniae, Chlamydia* species, and *B. pertussis* (158,160). Clarithromycin is unique in having a lower MIC for gram-positive organisms, compared with azithromycin, and exceptional activity against *Mycobacterium*, especially MAC members. Also, the major metabolite of clarithromycin, 14-hydroxyclarithromycin, is active against *H. influenzae* (158). Therapy of MAC infection in patients with acquired immunodeficiency syndrome (AIDS) has been dramatically enhanced by the development of clarithromycin. When used as monotherapy for MAC disease, clarithromycin (500 mg twice daily) was associated with reduction or clearance of bacteremia and reduced fever and constitutional symptoms; however, recurrence of bacteremia with clarithromycin-resistant strains occurred frequently (127,161). It is recommended that treatment of disseminated MAC infection in patients with human immunodeficiency virus (HIV) infection includes clarithromycin in combination

with either ethambutol or rifabutin (142,162). However, the combination therapy has been associated with increased side effects (163). Clarithromycin given 500 mg twice daily is effective as MAC prophylaxis in the HIV-positive patient with CD4+ T-lymphocyte cell counts of less than 100 cells/mm³ and has shown increased survival (141).

Clarithromycin has been used effectively in the treatment of other mycobacterial infections including *Mycobacterium kansasii, Mycobacterium marinum,* and disseminated *Mycobacterium chelonae* (136–138). Clarithromycin monotherapy was associated with significant clinical improvement in patients with lepromatous leprosy, suggesting that the agent is bactericidal for *M. leprae,* and should have a significant role in the treatment of this disease (164).

Clarithromycin plays an important part in the treatment of *H. pylori* infections causing ulcers of the stomach and duodenum (165). Three-drug therapy is required to treat *H. pylori* infection, with about an 85% cure rate (165). Clarithromycin with a proton pump inhibitor plus either amoxicillin, tetracycline, or metronidazole given for 14 days appears to be the most effective (165). Failure of therapy is often associated with the emergence of secondary resistance, which usually results from the use of one antimicrobial in therapy (166,167). Clarithromycin in combination with minocycline has been used as effective salvage and/or maintenance treatment of cerebral toxoplasmosis in patients with AIDS (168).

AZITHROMYCIN

Azithromycin is an azalide antibiotic that differs from the other macrolides by the insertion of a methyl-substituted nitrogen in the lactone ring to generate a 15-membered macrolide (or azalide) (see Fig. 22.1) (125). This gives it a broad spectrum of activity against gram-negative organisms and other intracellular pathogens, diminished acid lability, and pharmacokinetics allowing for convenient daily dosing for shorter durations (13,123). Azithromycin is available in gelatin capsules containing 250 mg of the active ingredient azithromycin dihydrate; in tablets containing 600 mg of the active agent; in granules for oral suspension for pediatric use; and in 1,000-mg single-dose packets containing granules for oral suspension. The formulation for flavored pediatric oral suspension results in drug concentrations of 100 or 200 mg per 5 mL. The intravenous formulation of azithromycin is available as 500 mg taken daily (169).

Mechanism of Action and Resistance

Azithromycin has a similar mechanism of action as erythromycin by binding to the same receptor on the bacterial 50S ribosomal subunit and inhibiting RNA-dependent protein synthesis (123,124). Azithromycin differs significantly from the other macrolides by having a greatly enhanced activity against gram-negative organisms, in particular *H. influenzae* (130,170). Azithromycin has proven efficacy for treatment of *C. trachomatis* infections (171). Despite azithromycin being bactericidal to *S. aureus, S pneumoniae,* and *S. pyogenes,* it has about a twofold to tenfold lower MIC for the same susceptible gram-positive organisms than erythromycin and clarithromycin (123,130). Similarly, acquired resistance to erythromycin via the acquisition of *erm* (the MLS phenotype) and *ere* genes means resistance to azithromycin (47,117). The acquisition of resistance to azithromycin by *M. avium* and *H. pylori* is similar to clarithromycin with the development of a point mutation in 23S ribosomal RNA (128,172).

Antimicrobial Activity

Azithromycin is bactericidal against *S. pneumoniae, S. pyogenes,* and methicillin-sensitive *S. aureus.* Resistance of these species is the same as with erythromycin (123,125). Azithromycin is also active against gram-positive intracellular organisms such as *Rhodococcus equi* (173); however, *Enterococcus* species are mostly resistant (174). Azithromycin has activity against some anaerobes such as *Actinomyces* and *Propionibacterium* species, some *Bacteroides* species, *Prevotella,* and *Porphyromonas,* but not *Clostridium, Peptostreptococcus, Fusobacterium,* and *Veillonella* species (175,176). This antianaerobic activity may account for the development of *C. difficile* infection in patients while on therapy (123).

Azithromycin is highly active against a number of gram-negative pathogens *in vitro,* including *Haemophilus* species, *B. pertussis, M. catarrhalis, N. gonorrhoeae, N. meningitidis, Salmonella,* and *Campylobacter* species (15). *Actinobacillus, Brucella melitensis, Bartonella* species, and *H. pylori* are sensitive (124). *Yersinia enterocolitica* isolates are usually sensitive, although *Yersinia pestis* isolates are not (177). Azithromycin also has excellent gram-negative coverage against *Eikenella corrodens, Pasteurella,* and *Capnocytophaga* species (176). A role for azithromycin in the treatment of *Pseudomonas aeruginosa* pneumonia may emerge, because of the drug's ability to inhibit flagellin expression, altering biofilm metabolism and bacterial motility (178–181). Although azithromycin has no bactericidal effect at subinhibitory concentrations, the drug demonstrated reduced buccal adherence in patients with cystic fibrosis with significantly reduced episodes of pneumonia with *P. aeruginosa* (180). A similar effect has been reported in HIV-infected patients (181).

Azithromycin has comparable activity against *Chlamydia* species and *M. pneumoniae* and appears to be more active than erythromycin against *Mycoplasma hominis* and *U. urealyticum* (182). Azithromycin has activity against *T. gondii, Babesia microti, B. burgdorferi, Bartonella* species, some *Rickettsia* species, and all *Plasmodium* species (183–191). As with clarithromycin, azithromycin has been demonstrated to reduce bacteremia and relieve symptoms in patients with AIDS and MAC infection (192), and it can be used in combination therapy for the treatment of *H. pylori* infections. However, like clarithromycin, when given as monotherapy, it has been associated with the development of resistance (129,134). Azithromycin, like the other macrolides, has a strong antiinflammatory activity by interfering with the oxidant production within neutrophils, acceleration of neutrophil apoptosis, and suppression of postinflammatory cytokines (193–195).

Clinical Pharmacology

Oral azithromycin is available in multiple formulations for dosing and after ingestion is rapidly absorbed and distributed widely throughout the body. Food decreases drug bioavailability (peak concentrations drop by 50%, and AUC concentrations by 43%). Accordingly, the drug should be taken 1 hour before or 2 hours after meals. Approximately 37% of a single 500-mg dose is bioavailable. Aluminum- and magnesium-containing antacids should be avoided because they reduce peak serum levels. It is 50% protein bound at concentrations of 0.02 to 0.05 μg/mL, and as concentrations increase, the protein-bound fraction diminishes rapidly (at 1.0 μg/mL, 7% protein bound) (15,123). The intravenous formulation of azithromycin is given once a day and maintains peak concentrations up to 80% higher than the oral equivalent dose over 24 hours. It is also 50% bound to protein and accumulates in AUC concentrations by 61% during a 5-day course (169).

Drug concentrations in tissues are markedly higher than those in serum, and elimination is more gradual. Tissue concentrations after a single dose of 500 mg of azithromycin ranged from 1 to 10 μg/mL in gastric, muscle, fat, bone, prostate, lung, kidney, and tonsil tissues. Elimination half-life from tissues after a single dose was estimated to be 56 to 76 hours (196–199). After a single 500-mg dose of azithromycin, concentrations of the drug in bronchial mucosa, alveolar macrophages, cervical mucosa, and tonsils were 70 to 100 times greater than serum concentrations within 96 hours after the dose (199). Azithromycin concentrations in monocytes and neutrophils exceed plasma levels by 400- to 1,200-fold, respectively, after multiple doses (144). Accumulation of azithromycin in phagocytes does not affect their function, but the extraordinary levels of drug in cells and tissues allow once-daily therapy for 5 days for conditions such as community-acquired pneumonia and bronchitis (145). Azithromycin has poor penetration of CSF and aqueous humor of the eye (200). The drug has a slow release from tissues, with an average terminal half-life of 68 hours, and it has been estimated that it has significant antibacterial activity for at least 5 days after a 5-day course (123,125).

Azithromycin is excreted primarily in feces, with approximately 75% of excreted drug-related material being unchanged. Biliary concentrations are significantly higher than serum concentrations (123). Less than 6% of an oral dose of azithromycin is excreted in the urinary tract within 1 week of consumption (196). Caution should be used in liver disease, but there are no data for dosage adjustment in renal failure (123).

ADVERSE EFFECTS AND DRUG INTERACTIONS
Azithromycin is usually well tolerated, with GI complaints being the main adverse effect (150). Mild reversible transaminase elevations may occur during therapy (150). Reversible ototoxicity has also been reported with azithromycin, especially in those patients receiving long-term azithromycin in combination with ethambutol and clofazimine for *M. avium* infection (201). Intravenous azithromycin causes significantly less phlebitis than erythromycin but has been associated with ototoxicity (202). Azithromycin has very few drug interactions, because it does not inhibit the CYP system in human models (150). Caution is still advised though, particularly with warfarin, digoxin, and benzodiazepines (203,204).

Uses of Azithromycin

Azithromycin with its great pharmacokinetics and ease of administration has many indications where it can be used effectively. Azithromycin has been proven to be as effective as other selected antimicrobial agents in the treatment of sinusitis, pharyngitis, skin and soft tissue infections, bacterial exacerbations of chronic obstructive pulmonary disease, and for the treatment of community-acquired pneumonia including *C. pneumoniae* and *M. pneumonia* (123–125,205–208). The recommended dosage in the treatment of these conditions is 500 mg given on day 1 of therapy, followed by 250 mg given daily on days 2 through 5 of therapy. If the patient is unwell, then giving intravenous azithromycin on the first day, followed by the oral course, has also shown to be effective (205). The 5-day course is adequate because of the prolonged persistence of good tissue concentrations of azithromycin (123–125). With the empiric treatment of *S. pneumoniae* infection with azithromycin with increasing penicillin and erythromycin resistance in the community, the Drug-Resistant *S. pneumoniae* Therapeutic Working Group suggests that the concentrations obtained by azithromycin in the lung would allow its use alone in the outpatient setting. However, it was recommended that it be combined with another agent in serious pneumococcal infections requiring hospitalization (207). Ewig et al. (34) also showed that using azithromycin to treat drug-resistant strains of *S. pneumoniae* was not associated with an increase in mortality. Azithromycin has shown superior results in animal models, and recent reports demonstrate excellent intracellular killing of *L. pneumophila* (208) and its effectiveness in treating *Legionella* pneumonia (101,208). Depending on the severity of illness, oral or intravenous azithromycin can be used from 5 to 10 days. Azithromycin is effective in the treatment of otitis media in children and is dosed at 10 mg/kg of body weight on day 1, followed by 5 mg/kg for the next 4 days. Azithromycin taken three times a week is as effective as clindamycin or tetracycline taken daily for 4 weeks in treating acne (114).

Azithromycin has significant benefits in treating sexually transmitted diseases, with its one-time dosing making compliance better. Azithromycin in a single 1-g dose has become a mainstay in the treatment of uncomplicated genital tract infection with *C. trachomatis* because of high efficacy, ease of administration, and assurance of compliance (117,210). Acute nongonococcal urethritis (caused by *C. trachomatis* or *U. urealyticum*) and chancroid can be treated with a 1-g single oral dose in men (211). A single 2-g dose of azithromycin had efficacy comparable to that of a 7-day course of doxycycline or single-dose ceftriaxone in the treatment of uncomplicated *N. gonorrhoeae* infection (212,213); however, it is associated with more nausea and vomiting. However, in Hawaii, there are reports of azithromycin-resistant strains of gonorrhea (214). Azithromycin has *in vitro* activity against *T. pallidum*, and in a pilot study, a 10-day course of the drug was effective in the treatment of primary or secondary syphilis (215). The effectiveness of single-dose azithromycin for the eradication of incubating syphilis is unknown, and the drug is not yet recommended for treatment of syphilis (183,216).

Azithromycin prophylaxis at a dose of 1,200 mg given once a week is effective for prevention of MAC infection in patients with AIDS (157,217,218). A randomized trial comparing ethambutol with either 600 mg daily of azithromycin or 500 mg twice daily of clarithromycin in treating disseminated MAC infections demonstrated the azithromycin group had more rapid clearance of bloodstream infection and less resistance developed (192). Therefore, azithromycin with ethambutol is an alternative treatment of disseminated MAC infections.

Azithromycin in combination with omeprazole and metronidazole is as effective as clarithromycin-containing regimens in the treatment of *H. pylori*–induced peptic ulcer disease (129,134). Azithromycin shows comparable efficacy to ciprofloxacin in the treatment of *Campylobacter* enteritis (219). A 7-day course of azithromycin has been shown to completely eradicate *Salmonella typhi* infections in patients from both the bloodstream and the stool (220,221).

In the treatment of early Lyme disease, azithromycin is considered only second-line therapy compared with doxycycline (186). Azithromycin (500 mg on day 1 and 250 mg on days 2 through 7) with atovaquone has been demonstrated to be as effective with much less adverse effects than clindamycin and quinine in the treatment of babesiosis (185). Azithromycin has had reported effects in treating *Bartonella* species, including bacillary angiomatosis and some *Rickettsia* species (189,190). Trachoma is a common cause of blindness in Africa, and azithromycin given three times a week over 6 weeks resulted in less active infection, better clinical response to active disease, and less relapse than topical tetracycline (223). Single-dose azithromycin adequately treats active trachoma of the eyes but may be complicated by relapse (224).

Azithromycin appears to have a secondary role in the treatment and prophylaxis of malaria (191). It has been shown to have excellent protection against *Plasmodium vivax*, but only 70% of *Plasmodium falciparum* are sensitive (224). Azithromycin has some activity against the hepatic and trophozoite stage of *P. falciparum* but is ineffective against the gametocytes (225). Therefore, it should be reserved for patients who are unable to tolerate the standard regimens (226,227).

In patients with the AIDS, azithromycin has shown promise in combination with pyrimethamine for the treatment of acute *Pneumocystis carinii* pneumonia (228). Alone, it may also prevent the disease (228). Azithromycin has been used successfully in the treatment of AIDS-related bacillary angiomatosis (*Bartonella henselae* infection) (188). Azithromycin may have a role in the treatment of AIDS-associated cryptosporidiosis, although currently available data are limited to case reports (230,231).

Ongoing studies are addressing the hypothesis that azithromycin may alter the natural history of coronary artery disease through its effects on chronic infections, especially *C. pneumoniae*. The Azithromycin and Coronary Events Study (ACES) is evaluating whether azithromycin can reduce primary coronary events (231). Azithromycin is taken up in the coronary plaque, although there are data that suggest it may not kill *C. pneumoniae* within the plaques (233,234). Further long-term studies are required (235).

KETOLIDES

The ketolides are a new class of 14-membered ring macrolides (236). They are characterized by a keto group in position 3 of the erythronolide A ring, which replaces the cladinose moiety, a sugar long considered to be essential for antibacterial activity (236). The first drug of this new class of antibiotics is telithromycin (Ketek, Aventis Pharmaceuticals) and is one of several in development (see Fig. 22.1). The ketolides were developed because of the increasing resistance to the macrolides, especially by *S. pneumoniae*. In comparison to the other macrolides, they bind ten times more tightly to the 50S ribosome subunit. They also are not inducers of the *erm* methyltransferase gene and thus can kill bacteria that are normally macrolide resistant. This strong binding makes the ketolides an active agent in treating many gram-positive infections, especially *S. aureus*, *S. pneumoniae*, and *S. pyogenes*. They have better activity against some strains of enterococci (237,238). It is active against gram-negative organisms including *Legionella*, as well as atypical pathogens such as *C. pneumoniae* and *M. pneumoniae* (239). Its anaerobic activity is similar to that of azithromycin (175,176). When approved, telithromycin will be available in an oral formulation as an 800-mg tablet taken once a day. Adverse reactions in phase 3 trials included GI intolerance and elevated transaminase level. The drug interacts with CYP 3A in the liver and interferes with metabolism of many of the same drugs erythromycin does. It also is associated with QT-interval prolongation, like erythromycin (235). Its main benefit appears to be in the treatment of penicillin and erythromycin-resistant *S. pneumoniae* infections, where phase 3 data show efficacy similar to that of the quinolones (236). Other ketolides in development may offer more expansive therapy depending on their safety and cost.

Clindamycin

Two lincosamide antimicrobials are available in the United States: lincomycin and clindamycin. Lincomycin is of historical interest only, having been replaced by its versatile derivative, clindamycin. Lincomycin was found near Lincoln, Nebraska, and was isolated from a soil actinomycete, *Streptomyces lincolnensis* in 1962 by Mason, Dietz, and Deboer (240). It was modified to the 7-deoxy, 7-chloro derivative clindamycin (241), which resulted in improved GI absorption, increased activity against aerobic gram-positive cocci, and a broader spectrum of activity against anaerobic organisms and the protozoa *Toxoplasma* and *Plasmodium* (242–245). Clindamycin has largely replaced lincomycin because of these therapeutic advantages.

STRUCTURE AND MECHANISMS OF ACTION

Clindamycin is composed of the amino acid *trans*-L-4*n*-propylhygrinic acid, which is attached to a sulfur-containing derivative of an octose (Fig. 22.2). The lincosamides inhibit bacterial protein synthesis at the site of peptide bond formation (the peptidyltransferase loop) in the 23S ribosomal RNA of the 50S ribosomal subunit (246). They affect chain elongation by either interfering with the subsequent ribosomal binding of aminoacyl transfer RNAs or inducing their dissociation (247). Because the lincosamides, the macrolides, and chloramphenicol have similar or overlapping sites, each may interfere with the effect of the other. Lincomycin and clindamycin have equivalent affinities for their shared ribosomal target site, suggesting that the increased activity of clindamycin for gram-negative bacteria is due to more effective penetration of the bacterial membranes (246). Clindamycin is considered a bacteriostatic drug because it inhibits protein synthesis; however, it may be bactericidal in certain circumstances (248,249). Clindamycin may potentiate the opsonization and phagocytosis of bacteria at subinhibitory concentrations while consuming complement in the process (250,251). It may also inhibit bacterial protein synthesis by altering the bacterial cell surface, facilitating phagocytosis, and enhancing intracellular killing of the organism (252).

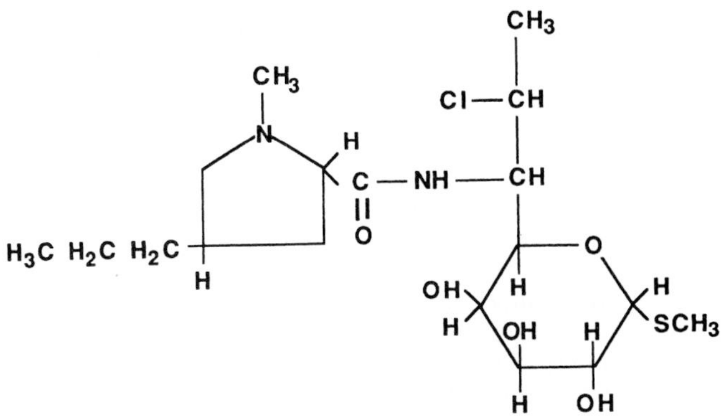

Figure 22.2. Chemical structure of clindamycin.

SPECTRUM OF ACTIVITY

The antimicrobial spectrum of clindamycin includes aerobic gram-positive cocci, gram-positive and gram-negative anaerobes, and certain protozoa. (Table 22.4) (242–257). Clindamycin is highly active and bactericidal against *S. pyogenes*, *S. pneumoniae*, *S. viridans*, *Streptococcus bovis*, and *S. aureus* (242,243,254,255). *Enterococcus* species are usually resistant (255). About 80% of *S. aureus* strains remain sensitive to clindamycin (242,243,258, 259); however, a significant level of the resistance has developed in *S. aureus* and *S. epidermidis* that necessitates sensitivity studies before initiation of therapy for serious infections (243,258–260). Some *S. aureus* strains, which are erythromycin resistant, may be sensitive to clindamycin, whereas others are cross-resistant (242,243,261). Clindamycin therapy of *S. aureus* infections due to erythromycin-resistant, clindamycin-sensitive strains may cause the emergence of clindamycin resistance (dissociated

TABLE 22.4.   In Vitro Susceptibility of Selected Organisms to Clindamycin and Percentage of Sensitive Isolates

Organism	Minimal inhibitory concentration (µg/mL)		Sensitive isolates (%)
	Median	Range	
Staphylococcus aureus[a]	0.1	0.05–1.5	70–90
Staphylococcus epidermidis[a]	0.1	0.1–1.5	35–75
Streptococcus pyogenes	0.04	0.02–0.1	Majority
Streptococcus pneumoniae[a]	0.01	0.002–0.05	Changing rapidly
Streptococcus viridans	0.02	0.005–0.05	Majority
Enterococcus faecalis, Enterococcus faecium	100	12.5≥100	<10–20
Corynebacterium diphtheriae	0.2		Majority
Neisseria gonorrhoeae	3.1	0.01–6.3	N/A
Neisseria meningitidis	12.5	6.3–25	N/A
Haemophilus influenzae	12.5	1.6–25	N/A
Clostridium difficile	4	0.06>128	<10
Clostridium perfringens	0.12–1.0	0.06–8.0	80–100
Clostridium spp. (other)	1.0–4.0	0.06≥128.0	70–90
Bacteroides fragilis group	0.25–1.0	0.125≥256	75–90
Bacteroides thetaiotaomicron	1.0–8.0	0.5–128	44–88
Prevotella/Porphyromonas spp.	0.06–4.0	0.06≥128	93–100
Fusobacterium spp.[a]	0.06–16.0	0.06≥128	97–100
Peptococcus spp.	0.25	0.06≥128	78–100
Mobiluncus spp.	0.25–1.0	0.5	100
Gardnerella vaginalis	0.5	<0.12–1.0	100
Propionibacterium spp.	0.03	0.03	100
Mycoplasma pneumoniae	3.1	1.6–3.1	N/A
Chlamydia trachomatis	1	0.25–2.0	N/A

Note: Data from referenced publications. N/A, not available.
[a] Some strains are markedly more resistant.

cross-resistance) (260–263). Most methicillin-resistant strains of *S. aureus* are resistant to clindamycin (44). Clindamycin may have an advantage over the penicillin groups in the treatment of *S. pyogenes* and *S. aureus* because of the suppression of the exotoxins secreted by these organisms in severe infections (264,265). Clindamycin in subtherapeutic concentrations appear to diminish M protein, exotoxin, and opsonically activate *S. pyogenes* for phagocytosis (265). In a mouse model of pyomyositis using *S. pyogenes*, clindamycin administration was more effective than penicillin in limiting bacterial growth and improving survival. This may be due to the long postantibiotic effect of the drug (264). Also, clindamycin may inhibit protein synthesis at the ribosomal level and subsequent inhibition of toxin synthesis. Indeed, clindamycin is known to inhibit synthesis of *C. perfringens* α toxin, and of *S. aureus* TSST-1 (265). The Enterobacteriaceae, *Acinetobacter* and *Pseudomonas* species, are resistant as a rule, apparently because of poor permeability of the outer envelope of the drug (242,243,254). At clinically achievable concentrations, clindamycin is mostly inactive against *H. influenzae*, *N. meningitidis*, and *N. gonorrhoeae* (242,243,256).

Clindamycin has a major clinical role against anaerobic organisms, especially the clinically important *B. fragilis* group (244,266). Although most species and strains are sensitive, clindamycin resistance has significantly increased in many the *Bacteroides* subspecies. A multicenter survey of 501 strains of the *B. fragilis* group in the United States in 1999 indicated that the prevalence of clindamycin resistance had rapidly increased in all species. Rates were as follows: *Bacteroides vulgates*, 26.8%; *Bacteroides ovatus*, 20.7%; *Bacteroides thetaiotaomicron*, 20%; *B. fragilis*, 14%; and *Bacteroides distasonis*, 11% (267). *Bacteroides* species resistance to clindamycin is increasing worldwide and can vary from region to region, from rates of 20% in Canada to 49% in Spain (268,269). As a result, the role of clindamycin in the treatment of intraabdominal anaerobic infections is diminished. Clindamycin remains active against anaerobic streptococci, peptococci, *Veillonella*, *Prevotella melaninogenica*, *C. perfringens*, *Actinomyces* species, *C. tetani*, and *Fusobacterium* (268–271). About 10% to 20% of non–*C. perfringens* clostridia, *Fusobacterium*, and peptostreptococci are resistant (269–272). Clindamycin is active against *C. trachomatis* and has been a cornerstone in regimens for the treatment of pelvic inflammatory disease (260,273). The drug also has activity against anaerobic vaginal flora and *Gardnerella vaginalis* and is effective for the treatment of bacterial vaginosis (274).

Clindamycin is active against both chloroquine-sensitive and chloroquine-resistant strains of *P. falciparum* (275–278). *P. vivax* is also sensitive, but the extraerythrocytic phase is resistant (275). The drug is also active against *T. gondii* and *P. carinii* (247,279–282). Although clindamycin resembles erythromycin in mechanism of action, it is ineffective against *M. pneumoniae* and *T. pallidum* (283,284).

MECHANISMS OF RESISTANCE

Clindamycin resistance can develop during therapy, and this has been documented for many organisms, especially strains of *S. aureus*, *S. pyogenes*, and *S. pneumoniae* (263,285–291). The best example is the exposure of subcultures of *S. aureus* daily to clindamycin, leading to slow incremental emergence of resistance (254,292). This phenomenon may occur via chromosomal mutations or plasmid transfer (292–294).

Several mechanisms can lead to clindamycin resistance. The first is caused by changes in the ribosomal binding site, which overlaps that of the macrolide antibiotics (294). The second has been attributed to methylation of the 23S ribosomal RNA of the 50S ribosome subunit, preventing attachment of antimicrobials (260). This resistance occurs in staphylococci and *Bacteroides* species. The expression of the methylase responsible for this alteration can be constitutive (resulting in the full macrolide-lincosamide-streptogramin–resistance phenotype) or inducible. Erythromycin is a greater inducer of the expression of this gene, which results in the *in vitro* erythromycin-resistant, clindamycin-sensitive phenotype (dissociated cross-resistance) (260,263). Inducible clindamycin resistance during therapy has been demonstrated in both gram-positive and gram-negative anaerobic species (294,295). Third, resistance can be conferred through plasmids that code for clindamycin resistance and are transferable within the genus *Bacteroides* (293,294). The transfer of clindamycin and tetracycline resistance from one strain of *B. fragilis* to another has been demonstrated in an experimental abscess model (295). Also, resistance transference has been shown to occur in the intestinal tracts of humans (296). These observations suggest that in polymicrobial infections, resistance may be transferred between strains and species of varying antibiotic susceptibility (297). Fourth, enzymatic inactivation of clindamycin is rare and probably not clinically important.

CLINICAL PHARMACOLOGY

One parenteral preparation and two oral formulations are available for clindamycin. The hydrochloride salt tastes bitter and comes in capsules. The water-soluble palmitate ester, which is not bitter tasting, is used in the oral suspension. Clindamycin phosphate is the water-soluble ester of clindamycin and phosphoric acid used for parenteral administration. The palmitate and phosphate esters must be hydrolyzed systemically to be biologically active (298,299). Absorption of clindamycin is 90% from the GI tract; however, food delays but does not decrease absorption (299–302). Absorption of the hydrochloride is rapid, producing peak serum levels in 45 minutes (300–302). Slightly higher levels are produced by the palmitate (303) (Table 22.5). A trivial amount of the drug is absorbed dermally after topical application (304). The phosphate ester, which causes little pain on intramuscular injection, is well absorbed and reaches a peak serum level in 1 hour in children and 3 hours in adults (298–301). Intravenously administered drug produces a peak serum level at the end of infusion (305,306).

Clindamycin achieves high concentrations in many tissues but does not cross the blood–brain barrier, precluding its use in meningitis (307). The drug achieves excellent levels in dental alveolar serum, and the bone–tissue concentration is approximately one third that of serum (308–312). In pregnant patients, clindamycin readily crosses the placenta and enters the fetal tissues (71). (Safety in pregnancy has not been fully established.)

Clindamycin is actively transported into macrophages and polymorphonuclear leukocytes. The concentrations in neutrophils and pulmonary macrophages in experimental abscesses are up to 50 times the peak serum levels. These intracellular concentrations may be therapeutically important (77,314). Clindamycin is 60% to 95% protein bound and its half-life varies from 2 to 2½ hours (298,315,316). In adults, 6% to 10% of the administered dose is excreted in the urine (303,306), and infants and children excrete twice as much (305).

Clindamycin is metabolized in the liver to the biologically active *N*-dimethyl derivative and sulfoxide (300). Its metabolites are mainly eliminated in the bile, where high concentrations are achieved in the absence of biliary tract obstruction (287,298,300). These metabolites are found in bile and urine but not in serum (298,301). Levels in the bile are two to five times those in serum and peak in 2 hours (298,302). The bile has negligible amounts in the presence of biliary obstruction even though it is elevated in liver tissue (316). High concentrations of its metabolites are found in the stool even after parenteral administration

TABLE 22.5. Serum Concentration of Clindamycin in Adults

Preparation	Dose (mg)	Route	Time (hr)	Peak concentration (μg/mL)
Clindamycin hydrochloride	150	p.o.	0.75	2.55 ± 0.92[a]
Clindamycin hydrochloride	300	p.o.	1	3.6
Clindamycin palmitate	150	p.o.	0.75	3.8
Clindamycin phosphate	300	i.m.	3	5
Clindamycin phosphate	300	i.m.	End of infusion	2.6–26
Clindamycin phosphate	600	i.v.	End of infusion	6.0–30

Note: See reference publications. p.o., oral; i.m., intramuscular; i.v., intravenous.
[a]With renal failure 3.39 ± 0.68 μg/mL.

(298). Active liver disease can prolong the serum half-life to 8 to 12 hours and requires a dose adjustment (287,317). The percentage excreted by the kidneys is increased with liver disease and markedly decreased with renal failure (79,318). Because clindamycin is hepatically eliminated, no dosage adjustment is required for renal dysfunction, but some suggest that the dosage be halved in the face of severe renal failure (318,319). In the presence of combined renal and liver disease, the dosage should be reduced significantly and serum clindamycin levels be monitored (287). Neither peritoneal dialysis nor hemodialysis can remove clindamycin (79,319). Clindamycin and its active bile metabolite, N-dimethyl derivative, cause suppression of anaerobic flora in the gut, leading to one of its major complications, antibiotic-associated colitis (320). Antimicrobial activity persists in the stool for 5 days after a 48-hour course of parenteral drug and causes a major reduction of numbers of susceptible bacteria in the colon (321). This alteration of gut flora may last up to 14 days after the drug is discontinued.

TOXICITY AND ADVERSE EFFECTS

The most significant adverse effect is diarrhea, which may progress to life-threatening antibiotic-associated colitis (320–326). About 20% of patients develop diarrhea while taking oral clindamycin. Most suffer from simple diarrhea, with fewer than 10% of persons developing colitis. Antibiotic-associated diarrhea is self-limited and abates when the drug is discontinued (326,327). It is not related to dose or route of administration, because it may also occur with parenteral administration. These complications have been encountered with the other antimicrobials, as well as with immunosuppressive and antitumor drugs, but to a lesser extent than clindamycin (320,328). Antibiotic-associated colitis should be viewed as a superinfection of the bowel with C. difficile, which is commonly found in the hospital environment (329). Restriction of clindamycin usage may curtail nosocomial epidemics of C. difficile–associated diarrhea (330). C. difficile colitis usually presents with loose stool, fever, and cramps. C. difficile toxin can be readily detected in the stool of many patients, and in some patients, this condition can be fatal. Oral metronidazole or vancomycin is the main treatment of C. difficile (320–330).

Hypersensitivity reactions—including morbilliform rashes, urticaria, erythema multiforme (Stevens-Johnson syndrome), drug-related fever, eosinophilia, and anaphylactoid reactions—have been attributed to clindamycin (331). Contact dermatitis with burning, itching, and peeling may occur with topical use (332). Local irritation is rare with intramuscular injection or intravenous infusion.

Hypotension, electrocardiographic changes, and cardiovascular collapse have been described after bolus administration of lincomycin (331). Infusion durations of 10 to 60 minutes prevent this complication. There are rare reports of hematopoietic effects, including neutropenia, agranulocytosis, and thrombocytopenia (331). Reversible liver function abnormalities, such as elevations of serum transaminase levels (aspartate transaminase, alanine transaminase), have been associated with clindamycin (306). These represent false-positive elevations due to drug interference with the colorimetric measurement (242). True hepatotoxicity with hepatocellular damage and jaundice has been reported; in one case, it was attributed to the vanishing bile duct syndrome (333,334).

DRUG INTERACTIONS

Clindamycin may potentiate the action of neuromuscular blocking drugs, including pancuronium and D-tubocurarine chloride (335,336). In solution, clindamycin phosphate is physically incompatible with ampicillin, aminophylline, barbiturates, calcium gluconate, magnesium sulfate, and phenytoin sodium.

There are mixed reports about synergy between clindamycin and gentamicin for E. coli, Proteus mirabilis, and P. aeruginosa (331,337). The combination of clindamycin and trimethoprim-sulfamethoxazole has an additive effect for S. aureus, S. pyogenes, E. coli, Klebsiella and Enterobacter species, and H. influenzae (256).

PREPARATIONS AND DOSING RECOMMENDATIONS

Clindamycin is available as the hydrochloride salt in 75-, 150-, and 300-mg capsules; the palmitate hydrochloride, a water-soluble salt of the ester in flavored granules for reconstitution in suspension (75 mg per 5 mL); and the phosphate ester (150 mg/mL) for intramuscular and intravenous use. Clindamycin phosphate is also prepared as a topical solution and topical gel (10 mg/mL) for external use in the treatment of acne vulgaris.

Peak serum levels depend on formulation, dose, and route (see Table 22.5). The recommended oral dosage for children is 8 to 16 mg/kg per day in three or four equal doses; for severe infections, it is 16 to 20 mg/kg per day in three or four doses. For adults, the usual oral dosage is 150 to 300 mg every 6 hours; for more severe infections, it is 300 to 450 mg every 6 hours. As parenteral therapy in more severe infections, especially when B. fragilis or C. perfringens is suspected, the adult dosage is 1,200 to 2,700 mg per day in three or four doses. Dose reduction is indicated in patients with active liver disease and to a small extent in those with renal failure (287,317–319, 338).

CLINICAL INDICATIONS

The unique antimicrobial spectrum and pharmacokinetics of clindamycin make it a good agent for the following conditions: serious gram-positive coccal infections, especially of the bone, occurring in penicillin-allergic patients, and infections in the

TABLE 22.6. Clinical Uses of Clindamycin

Mixed anaerobic and aerobic infections
  Intraabdominal,[a] for example, ruptured or gangrenous appendix, diverticulitis, penetrating trauma, perforated ulcer, intestinal fistula, ischemic bowel, hepatic and pancreatic abscess
  Pelvic,[a] for example, ovarian abscess, chronic salpingitis, septic abortion, endometritis, posthysterectomy vaginal cuff infections
  Bartholin's gland abscess
  Pulmonary, for example, aspiration pneumonia, necrotizing pneumonia, empyema, putrid lung abscess
  Odontogenic
  Upper respiratory tract,[a] for example, chronic sinusitis, chronic otitis
  Diabetic foot ulcers[a]
  Decubitus ulcers[a]
  Soft tissue,[b] for example, clostridial infections, necrotizing fasciitis, synergistic gangrene
Gram-positive infections
  Group A streptococcus pharyngeal carriers
  Recurrent tonsillitis
  Staphylococcal infections
  Corynebacterium diphtheriae carrier state
  Acne vulgaris (topical)
Osteomyelitis
  Staphylococcal
  Anaerobic
Toxoplasma
  Chorioretinitis
  Encephalitis
Malaria
  Plasmodium falciparum (chloroquine sensitive and resistant)
Pneumocystis carinii pneumonia
  Treatment

[a]Plus an aminoglycoside or aztreonam.
[b]Gram-negative aerobic coverage may be necessary.

abdomen, pelvis, and lung involving anaerobes, particularly *B. fragilis* (Table 22.6). Fear of antibiotic-associated colitis has caused many clinicians to substitute other antimicrobials in situations in which clindamycin would have been used. The drug remains a relatively safe antibiotic if patients are monitored closely.

Clindamycin is useful in treating infections caused by polymicrobial flora including anaerobes: intraabdominal sepsis, pelvic infections in women, diabetic foot ulcers, decubitus ulcers, and certain respiratory tract infections (339–345). In animal models, the drug prevented intraabdominal abscess formation due to fecal organisms like *B. fragilis* (339,340). Clindamycin is not as pH sensitive (e.g., like aminoglycosides) and can enter polymorphonuclear cells and be more active within abscesses (314,315).

Clindamycin has a proven role in the treatment of intraabdominal sepsis; however, because of the likely presence of Enterobacteriaceae also, they are used in combination with a β-lactam antibiotic or aminoglycoside to achieve this goal. Clindamycin appears to prevent morbidity from intraabdominal abscess and appears superior to β-lactams and aminoglycosides (346–352). With the increasing prevalence of resistant *Bacteroides* isolates to clindamycin (267–270,348–350), there is a need for complete antimicrobial sensitivity data because antimicrobial susceptibility of isolates from abdominal and pulmonary infections has been statistically correlated with clinical outcomes (353,354). Alternative drugs recommended for intraabdominal infection include cefotetan, cefoxitin, ampicillin-sulbactam, ticarcillin-clavulanate, piperacillin-tazobactam, imipenem-cilastatin, and

meropenem. Clindamycin-containing regimens are clearly effective for severe intraabdominal sepsis; however, depending on local clindamycin resistance, alternative regimens (e.g., imipenem-cilastatin) should be considered (355–357).

Infections of the female genital tract—ovarian abscess, chronic salpingitis, endometritis, septic abortion, posthysterectomy vaginal cuff infection, and Bartholin's gland abscess—typically contain mixed flora (343,352). Clindamycin-aminoglycoside and clindamycin–β-lactam combinations in conjunction with appropriate surgical intervention have been shown repeatedly to decrease morbidity and mortality (340,343,347,352). For the treatment of pelvic inflammatory disease, the Centers for Disease Control and Prevention (CDC) has recommended that antibiotic therapy target *N. gonorrhoeae*, *C. trachomatis*, and common genital tract flora such as *E. coli*, *Prevotella* and *Bacteroides* species, and anaerobic streptococci (358). The CDC recommends intravenous therapy with clindamycin-gentamicin as an option in severe infection, but there are now many options from third generation cephalosporins, metronidazole, and newer quinolones (349–357). Although clindamycin is active against *C. trachomatis*, either azithromycin, doxycycline, or a quinolone is a better choice (257). However, clindamycin has proven efficacy in the treatment of *C. trachomatis* infection (273). Topical and systemic clindamycin therapy has been found to be effective in the treatment of bacterial vaginosis as metronidazole (274).

Clindamycin is effective therapy for pulmonary infections involving anaerobes, including aspiration pneumonia, necrotizing pneumonia, empyema, and putrid lung abscesses (351,359–361). Up to 35% of isolates are β-lactamase producers, including such common pathogens as *Fusobacterium* species, *Prevotella* species, *Peptostreptococcus*, and *B. fragilis* (361).This may explain the superiority of clindamycin to penicillin in controlled trials for these infections (361–363). Concerns of increasing clindamycin resistance among *Bacteroides* species have some advocating alternative treatment regimens such as β-lactam/β-lactamase inhibitors, imipenem, or penicillin plus metronidazole (361).

Anaerobes play a major role in pyogenic orofacial infections. They may arise from a dental source and cause suppurative complications including maxillary sinusitis, mediastinitis, retropharyngeal abscess, infection of the floor of the mouth (Ludwig's angina), cavernous sinus thrombosis, pleuropulmonary abscess, and hematogenously disseminated abscesses of brain, liver, kidneys, and bone (364). Penicillin-resistant organisms, including *Prevotella* and *Bacteroides* species, are frequently isolated. Also, human and animal bites contain the same oral flora, making clindamycin an effective therapy. Caution is advised because some human bites transmit *Eikenella corrodens* and cat bites transmit *Pasteurella multocida*, both of which are resistant to clindamycin (365). Infected diabetic foot ulcers and decubitus ulcers commonly contain anaerobic and aerobic gram-positive and gram-negative flora. Clindamycin combined with a quinolone, an aminoglycoside, aztreonam, or a β-lactam antibiotic provides appropriate antibacterial activity (339,366–369). In necrotizing fasciitis and mixed soft tissue infections, clindamycin may have an important therapeutic role in their treatment (264,265,370–372). As discussed earlier, a mouse model showed clindamycin was superior to penicillin and metronidazole for *S. pyogenes* infections and this has been shown with *C. perfringens* gas gangrene. It has been related to clindamycin having a rapid effect on bacterial toxin production (370–372). There have been no clinical trials to demonstrate this theoretical benefit in human disease. Also, with *C. perfringens* infection, combination therapy is required because some strains are clindamycin resistant (372).

Clindamycin poorly penetrates the blood–brain barrier and is not indicated for the treatment of brain abscess, although it has a role in CNS toxoplasmosis (307).

Chronic pharyngeal carriage of β-hemolytic streptococci that fails to respond to penicillin has been treated successfully with clindamycin; in one trial, a 10-day course of oral clindamycin was demonstrated to be superior to intramuscular benzathine penicillin plus oral rifampin for the treatment of chronic carriers (373,374). Carriers of group A streptococci harbor various organisms in the pharynx, including *S. aureus* and *Bacteroides* and *Prevotella* species, which may produce sufficient β-lactamase to inactivate penicillin (374). Clindamycin, by eliminating the carrier state, can terminate recurrent tonsillitis (375). Clindamycin may be used in the penicillin-allergic patient in the treatment of staphylococcal infections other than endocarditis (263); however, susceptibilities should be obtained before initiating therapy. Clindamycin has been recommended as an appropriate alternative agent for endocarditis prophylaxis for patients with penicillin allergy and erythromycin intolerance (376). Clindamycin has been proven to be valuable in the treatment of staphylococcal and anaerobic osteomyelitis (368,377,378). It is unique in that it is bactericidal against *S. aureus* and many strains of *Bacteroides*, an important virtue in the treatment of osteomyelitis (242,249). Both of these species elaborate a glycocalyx, which in experimental models plays a major role in the adherence of bacteria to bone and in protection from phagocytosis, antibodies, and the effect of antibiotics (379–381). Clindamycin interferes with the production of this glycocalyx (379,380). Oral clindamycin achieves therapeutic levels, making treatment of osteomyelitis feasible on an outpatient basis (378).

Topical clindamycin is superior to tetracycline in the treatment of acne vulgaris (382). However, *C. difficile* colitis has been associated with topical clindamycin (328). Oral clindamycin is effective therapy for severe pustular acne (383).

Intravenous clindamycin plus oral pyrimethamine has been demonstrated to be effective in the treatment of *Toxoplasma* encephalitis in patients with AIDS when compared with pyrimethamine plus sulfadiazine (279,280); however, it should be reserved for patients with sulfa allergy, as a randomized controlled trial showed that this regimen was less effective in preventing relapses (280). In the presence of inflammation, clindamycin has sufficient penetration to cross the blood–brain barrier but requires higher daily dosages. The high relapse rates after initial therapy may be due to lessening of the inflammation and less penetration of the drug into the CNS. Clindamycin is not appropriate for primary prophylaxis because of a high toxicity rate (280). Ocular toxoplasmosis has been treated successfully with oral clindamycin (245). Subconjunctival and retrobulbar injections of the drug have also been used for *Toxoplasma* chorioretinitis; however, injections may cause diplopia and papillitis (245). Clindamycin in combination with primaquine has been shown to be safe and effective (compared with trimethoprim-sulfamethoxazole) in the treatment of mild to moderately severe *P. carinii* pneumonia in patients with AIDS (281,384). In addition, this regimen is effective as salvage therapy for patients unable to tolerate primary therapy with trimethoprim-sulfamethoxazole or pentamidine (384). Rash and methemoglobinemia were frequent side effects of the combination of clindamycin and primaquine. Clindamycin does not have a role in *P. carinii* pneumonia prophylaxis because of its GI side effects. Clindamycin has been used alone and in combination with quinine to treat chloroquine-sensitive and chloroquine-resistant falciparum malaria (275–278). In addition, clindamycin with oral quinine has been recommended for the treatment of *Babesia* infections (385).

REFERENCES

1. McGuire JM, Bunch RL, Anderson RC, et al. "Ilotycin" a new antibiotic. *Antibiot Chemother* 1952;2:281.
2. Haight TH, Finland M. The antibacterial action of erythromycin. *Proc Soc Exp Biol Med* 1952;81:175–183.
3. Nicholas P. Erythromycin: clinical review 1. Clinical pharmacology. *N Y State J Med* 1977;77:2088–2094.
4. Fraser DG. Selection of an oral erythromycin product. *Am J Hosp Pharm* 1980;37:1199–1205.
5. Mahnborg AS. Effect of food on absorption of erythromycin. A study of two derivatives, the stearate and the base. *J Antimicrob Chemother* 1979;5:591.
6. Bechtol LD, Stephens VC, Pugh CT, et al. Erythromycin esters—comparative *in vivo* hydrolysis and bioavailability. *Curr Ther Res* 1976;20:610.
7. Thompson PJ, Burgess KR, Marlin GE. Influence of food on absorption of erythromycin ethylsuccinate. *Antimicrob Agents Chemother* 1980;18:829–831.
8. Austin KL, Mather LE, Philpot CR, et al. Intersubject and dose-related variability after intravenous administration of erythromycin. *Br J Clin Pharmacol* 1980;10:273–279.
9. Pestka S. Binding of ^{14}C-erythromycin to *Escherichia coli* ribosomes. *Antimicrob Agents Chemother* 1974;6:474–478.
10. Otaka T, Kaji A. Release of (oligo) peptidyl-tRNA from ribosomes by erythromycin. *Proc Natl Acad Sci U S A* 1975;72:2649–2652.
11. Chittum HS, Champney WS. Erythromycin inhibits the assembly of the large ribosomal subunit in growing *Escherichia coli* cells. *Curr Microbiol* 1995;30:273–279.
12. Oleinick NL, Wilhelm JM, Corcoran JW. Nonidentity of the site of action of erythromycin A and chloramphenicol on *Bacillus subtilis* ribosomes. *Biochim Biophys Acta* 1968;155:290–292.
13. Peters DH, Clissold SP. Clarithromycin: a review of its antimicrobial activity, pharmacokinetic properties, and therapeutic potential. *Drugs* 1992;44:117–164.
14. Haight TH, Finland M. Observations on mode of action of erythromycin. *Proc Soc Exp Biol Med* 1952;81:188–193.
15. Peters DH, Friedel HA, McTavish D. Azithromycin. A review of its antimicrobial activity, pharmacokinetic properties and clinical efficacy. *Drugs* 1992;44:750–799.
16. Washington JA II, Wilson WR. Erythromycin: a microbial and clinical perspective after 30 years of clinical use. *Mayo Clin Proc* 1985;60:189–203.
17. Sabath LD, Gerstein PA, Loder PB, et al. Excretion of erythromycin and its enhanced activity in urine against gram-negative bacilli with alkalinization. *J Lab Clin Med* 1968;72:916–923.
18. Mao JCH, Futterman M. Accumulation in gram-positive and gram-negative bacteria as a mechanism of resistance to erythromycin. *J Bacteriol* 1968;95:1111.
19. Taybeneck U. Susceptibility of *Proteus mirabilis* and its stable L forms to erythromycin and other macrolides. *Nature* 1962;196:195.
20. Finland M. Changing patterns of susceptibility of common bacterial pathogens to antimicrobial agents. *Ann Intern Med* 1972;76:1009–1036.
21. Seppala H, Nissinen A, Jarvinen H, et al. Resistance to erythromycin in group A streptococci. *N Engl J Med* 1992;326:292–297.
22. Hsueh PR, Chen HM, Huang AH, et al. Decreased activity of erythromycin against *Streptococcus pyogenes* in Taiwan. *Antimicrob Agents Chemother* 1995;39:2239–2242.
23. Hofmann J, Cetron MS, Farley MM, et al. The prevalence of drug-resistant *Streptococcus pneumoniae* in Atlanta. *N Engl J Med* 1995;333:481–486.
24. Kataja J, Huovinen P, Seppala H. Erythromycin resistance genes in group A streptococci of different geographical origins. The Macrolide Resistance Study Group. *J Antimicrob Chemother* 2000;46:789–792.
25. Schmitz FJ, Petridou J, Fluit AC, et al. Distribution of macrolide-resistance genes in *Staphylococcus aureus* blood-culture isolates from fifteen German university hospitals. M.A.R.S. Study Group. Multicentre Study on Antibiotic Resistance in Staphylococci. *Eur J Clin Microbiol Infect Dis* 2000;19:385–387.
26. De Mouy D, Cavallo JD, Leclercq R, et al. Antibiotic susceptibility and mechanisms of erythromycin resistance in clinical isolates of *Streptococcus agalactiae*: French multicenter study. *Antimicob Agents Chemother* 2001;45:2400–2402.
27. Oster P, Zanchi A, Cresti S. Patterns of macrolide resistance determinants among community-acquired *Streptococcus pneumoniae* isolates over a 5-year period of decreased macrolide susceptibility rates. *Antimicrob Agents Chemother* 1999;43:2510–2512.
28. Amsden GW. Pneumococcal macrolide resistance—myth or reality? *J Antimicrob Chemother* 1999;44:1–6.
29. Seppala H, Klaukka T, Vuopio-Varkila J, et al. The effect of changes in the consumption of macrolide antibiotics on erythromycin resistance in group A streptococci in Finland. Finnish Study Group for Antimicrobial Resistance. *N Engl J Med* 1997;337:441–446.
30. Andrews JI, Diekema DJ, Hunter SK, et al. Group B streptococci causing neonatal bloodstream infection: antimicrobial susceptibility and serotyping results from SENTRY centers in the Western Hemisphere. *Am J Obstet Gynecol* 2000;183:859–862.
31. Fitoussi F, Loukil C, Gros I, et al. Mechanisms of macrolide resistance in clinical group B streptococci isolated in France. *Antimicrob Agents Chemother* 2001;45:1889–1891.

32. Bartlett JG, Breiman RF, Mandell LA, et al. Community-acquired pneumonia in adults: guidelines for management. The Infectious Diseases Society of America. *Clin Infect Dis* 1998;26:811–838.
33. Doern GV, Heilmann KP, Huynh HK, et al. Antimicrobial resistance among clinical isolates of streptococcus pneumoniae in the United States during 1999–2000, including a comparison of resistance rates since 1994–1995. *Antimicrob Agents Chemother* 2001;45:1721–1729.
34. Ewig S, Ruiz M, Torres A, et al. Pneumonia acquired in the community through drug-resistant *Streptococcus pneumoniae*. *Am J Respir Crit Care Med* 1999;159:1835–1842.
35. Sa-Leao R, Tomasz A, Sanches IS, et al. Carriage of internationally spread clones of *Streptococcus pneumoniae* with unusual drug resistance patterns in children attending day care centers in Lisbon, Portugal. *J Infect Dis* 2000;182:1153–1160.
36. Thornsberry C, Jones ME, Hickey ML, et al. Resistance surveillance of *Streptococcus pneumoniae, Haemophilus influenzae* and *Moraxella catarrhalis* isolated in the United States, 1997–1998. *J Antimicrob Chemother* 1999;44:749–759.
37. Ednie LM, Visalli MA, Jacobs MR, et al. Comparative activities of clarithromycin, erythromycin, and azithromycin against penicillin-susceptible and penicillin-resistant pneumococci. *Antimicrob Agents Chemother* 1996;40:1950–1952.
38. Sutcliffe J, Tait-Kamradt A, Wondrack L, et al. *Streptococcus pneumoniae* and *Streptococcus pyogenes* resistant to macrolides but sensitive to clindamycin: a common resistance pattern mediated by an efflux system. *Antimicrob Agents Chemother* 1996;40:1817–1824.
39. Tait-Kamradt A, Clancy J, Cronan M, et al. mefE is necessary for the erythromycin-resistant M phenotype in *Streptococcus pneumoniae*. *Antimicrob Agents Chemother* 1997;41:2251–2255.
40. Jones RN, Cormican MG, Wanger A. Clindamycin resistance among erythromycin-resistant *Streptococcus pneumoniae*. *Diagn Microbiol Infect Dis* 1996;25:201–204.
41. Widdowson CA, Klugman KP. Emergence of the M phenotype of erythromycin-resistant pneumococci in South Africa. *Emerg Infect Dis* 1998;4:277–281.
42. Alcaide F, Carratala J, Linares J, et al. In vitro activities of eight macrolide antibiotics and RP-59500 (quinupristin-dalfopristin) against viridans group streptococci isolated from blood of neutropenic cancer patients. *Antimicrob Agents Chemother* 1996;40:2117–2120.
43. Toala P, McDonald A, Wilcox C, et al. Susceptibility of group D streptococcus (enterococcus) to 21 antibiotics in vitro, with special reference to species differences. *Am J Med Sci* 1969;258:416.
44. Maple PA, Hamilton-Miller JM, Brumfitt W. World-wide antibiotic resistance in methicillin-resistant *Staphylococcus aureus*. *Lancet* 1989;1:537–540.
45. Griffith RS, Black HR. Erythromycin. *Med Clin North Am* 1970;54:1199–1215.
46. Garrod LP. The erythromycin group of antibiotics. *Br Med J* 1957;2:57–63.
47. Martin WJ, Gardner M, Washington JA II. In vitro antimicrobial susceptibility of anaerobic bacteria isolated from clinical specimens. *Antimicrob Agents Chemother* 1972;1:148–158.
48. Finland M, Garner C, Wilcox C, et al. Susceptibility of pneumococci and *Haemophilus influenzae* to antibacterial agents. *Antimicrob Agents Chemother* 1976;9:274–287.
49. Spaepen MS, Kundsin RB. Simple, direct broth-disk method for antibiotic susceptibility testing of *Ureaplasma urealyticum*. *Antimicrob Agents Chemother* 1977;11:267–270.
50. Tally FP, Cuchural GJ, Jacobus NV, et al. Susceptibility of the *Bacteroides* group in the United States in 1981. *Antimicrob Agents Chemother* 1983;23:536–540.
51. Goldman RC, Capobianco JO. Role of an energy-dependent efflux pump in plasmid pNE24-mediated resistance to 14- and 15-membered macrolides in *Staphylococcus epidermidis*. *Antimicrob Agents Chemother* 1990;34:1973–1980.
52. Weisblum B. Erythromycin resistance by ribosome modification. *Antimicrob Agents Chemother* 1995;39:577–585.
53. Barthelemy P, Autissier D, Gerbaud G, et al. Enzymic hydrolysis of erythromycin by a strain of *Escherichia coli*. *J Antibiot (Tokyo)* 1984;37:1692–1696.
54. Leclerq R, Courvalin P. Intrinsic and unusual resistance to macrolide, lincosamide and streptogramin antibiotics in bacteria. *Antimicrob Agents Chemother* 1991;35:1273–1276.
55. Ross JI, Eady EA, Cove JH, et al. Minimal functional system required for expression of erythromycin resistance by msrA in *Staphylococcus aureus* RN4220. *Gene* 1996;183:143–148.
56. Clancy J, Petitpas J, Dib-Hajj F, et al. Molecular cloning and functional analysis of a novel macrolide-resistance determinant, mefA, from *Streptococcus pyogenes*. *Mol Microbiol* 1996;22:867–879.
57. Oleinick NL. The erythromycins. In: Corcoran JW, Hahn FE, eds. *Mechanisms of action of antimicrobial and antitumor agents*. New York: Springer-Verlag, 1975:396.
58. Lacey RW. Lack of evidence for mutation to erythromycin resistance in clinical strains of *Staphylococcus aureus*. *J Clin Pathol* 1977;30:602–605.
59. Jenkins G, Cundliffe E. Cloning and characterization of two genes from *Streptomyces lividans* that confer inducible resistance to lincomycin and macrolide antibiotics. *Gene* 1991;108:55–62.
60. Williams JD, Sefton AM. Comparison of macrolide antibiotics. *J Antimicrob Chemother* 1993;31[Suppl C]:11–26.
61. Malmborg AS. Effect of food on absorption of erythromycin. A study of two derivatives, the stearate and the base. *J Antimicrob Chemother* 1979;5:591–599.
62. DiSanto AR, Tserng KY, Chodos DJ, et al. Comparative bioavailability evaluation of erythromycin base and its salts and esters, I: erythromycin estolate capsules versus enteric-coated erythromycin base tablets. *J Clin Pharmacol* 1980;20:437–443.
63. Austin KL, Mather LE, Philpot CR, et al. Intersubject and dose-related variability after intravenous administration of erythromycin. *Br J Clin Pharmacol* 1980;10:273–279.
64. Houin G, Tillement JP, Lhoste F, et al. Erythromycin pharmacokinetics in man. *J Int Med Res* 1980;8[Suppl 2]:9–14.
65. Prandota J, Tillement JP, d'Athis P, et al. Binding of erythromycin base to human plasma proteins. *J Int Med Res* 1980;8[Suppl 2]:1–8.
66. Bass JW, Steele RW, Wiebe RA, et al. Erythromycin concentrations in middle ear exudates. *Pediatrics* 1971;48:417–422.
67. Paavolainen M, Kohonen A, Palva T, et al. Penetration of erythromycin stearate into maxillary sinus mucosa and secretions in chronic maxillary sinusitis. *Acta Otolaryngol (Stockh)* 1977;84:292–295.
68. Wollmer P, Rhodes CG, Pike VW, et al. Measurement of pulmonary erythromycin concentrations in patients with lobar pneumonia by means of positron tomography. *Lancet* 1982;2:1361–1364.
69. Ginsburg CM, McCracken GH, Culbertson MC. Concentrations of erythromycin in serum and tonsils. Comparisons of the estolate and ethylsuccinate suspensions. *J Pediatr* 1976;89:1011–1013.
70. Rapp GF, Griffith RS, Hebble WM. The permeability of traumatically inflamed synovial membrane to commonly used antibiotics. *J Bone Joint Surg Am* 1966;48:1534.
71. Philipson A, Sabath LD, Charles D. Transplacental passage of erythromycin and clindamycin. *N Engl J Med* 1973;288:1219–1221.
72. Mao JCH, Tardrew PL. Demethylation of erythromycins by rabbit tissue *in vitro*. *Biochem Pharmacol* 1965;14:1049.
73. Chelvan P, Hamilton-Miller JMT, Brumfitt W. Biliary excretion of erythromycin after parenteral administration. *Br J Clin Pharmacol* 1979;8:233–235.
74. Bennett WM, Muther RS, Parker RA, et al. Drug therapy in renal failure: dosing guidelines for adults, part I: antimicrobial agents, analgesics. *Ann Intern Med* 1980;93:62–89.
75. Mery JP, Kanfer A. Ototoxicity of erythromycin in patients with renal insufficiency. *N Engl J Med* 1979;301:944.
76. Johnson JD, Hand WL, Francis JB, et al. Antibiotic uptake by alveolar macrophages. *J Lab Clin Med* 1980;95:429–436.
77. Prokesch RC, Hand WL. Antibiotic entry into human polymorphonuclear leukocytes. *Antimicrob Agents Chemother* 1982;21:373–380.
78. Miller MF, Martin JR, Johnson P, et al. Erythromycin uptake and accumulation by human polymorphonuclear leukocytes and efficacy of erythromycin in killing ingested *Legionella pneumophila*. *J Infect Dis* 1984;119:714–718.
79. Odenholt-Tornqvist I, Lowdin E, Cars O. Postantibiotic effects and postantibiotic sub-MIC effects of roxithromycin, clarithromycin and azithromycin on respiratory tract pathogens. *Antimicrob Agents Chemother* 1995;39:221–226.
80. Filippo JA. Infantile hypertrophic pyloric stenosis related to ingestions of erythromycin estolate. A report of five cases. *J Pediatr Surg* 1976;11:177.
81. Ellsworth AJ, Christensen DB, Volpone-McMahon MT. Prospective comparison of patient tolerance to enteric-coated vs. nonenteric-coated erythromycin. *J Fam Pract* 1990;31:265–270.
82. Itoh Z, Suzuki T, Nakaya M, et al. Gastrointestinal motor-stimulating activity of macrolide antibiotics and analysis of their side effects on the canine gut. *Antimicrob Agents Chemother* 1984;26:863–869.
83. Janssens J, Peeters TL, Vantrappen G, et al. Improvement of gastric emptying in diabetic gastroparesis by erythromycin. *N Engl J Med* 1990;322:1028–1031.
84. Sullivan D, Csuka ME, Blanchard B. Erythromycin ethylsuccinate hepatotoxicity. *JAMA* 1980;243:1074.
85. Derby LE, Jick H, Henry DA, et al. Erythromycin-associated cholestatic hepatitis. *Med J Aust* 1993;158:600–602.
86. McCormack WM, George H, Donner A, et al. Hepatotoxicity of erythromycin estolate during pregnancy. *Antimicrob Agents Chemother* 1977;12:630–635.
87. Hopkins S. Clinical toleration and safety of azithromycin. *Am J Med* 1991;91(3A):40A–45A.
88. Dujovne CA, Shoeman D, Bianchine J, et al. Experimental bases for the different hepatotoxicity of erythromycin preparations in man. *J Lab Clin Med* 1972;70:832–844.
89. Sabath LD, Gerstein DA, Finland M. Serum glutamic oxalacetic transaminase: false elevation during administration of erythromycin. *N Engl J Med* 1968;279:1137–1139.
90. Brummett RE. Ototoxic liability of erythromycin and analogues. *Otolaryngol Clin North Am* 1993;26:811–819.
91. Swanson DJ, Sung RJ, Fine MJ, et al. Erythromycin ototoxicity: prospective assessment with serum concentrations and audiograms in a study of patients with pneumonia. *Am J Med* 1992;92:61–68.
92. Gantz NM, Zawacki JK, Dickerson WJ, et al. Pseudomembranous colitis associated with erythromycin. *Ann Intern Med* 1979;91:866–867.
93. Chennareddy SB, Siddique M, Karim MY, et al. Erythromycin-induced polymorphous ventricular tachycardia with normal QT interval. *Am Heart J* 1996;132:691–694.
94. Daleau P, Lessard E, Groleau MF, et al. Erythromycin blocks the rapid component of the delayed rectifier potassium current and lengthens repolarization of guinea pig ventricular myocytes. *Circulation* 1995;91(12):3010–3016.
95. Ludden TM. Pharmacokinetic interactions of the macrolide antibiotics. *Clin Pharmacokinet* 1985;10:63–79.

96. Nahata M. Drug interactions with azithromycin and the macrolides: an overview. *J Antimicrob Chemother* 1996;37[Suppl C]:133–142.

97. Periti P, Mazzei T, Mini E, et al. Pharmacokinetic drug interactions of macrolides. *Clin Pharmacokinet* 1992;23:106–131.

98. Saha JR, Butler VP, Neu HC, et al. Digoxin-inactivating bacteria: identification in human gut flora. *Science* 1983;220:325–327.

99. Penn RL, Ward TT, Steigbigel RT. Effects of erythromycin in combination with penicillin, ampicillin or gentamicin on the growth of *Listeria monocytogenes*. *Antimicrob Agents Chemother* 1982;22:289–294.

100. Swartz MN. Clinical aspects of legionnaire's disease. *Ann Intern Med* 1979;90:492–495.

101. Edelstein PH. Antimicrobial chemotherapy for legionnaires' disease: a review. *Clin Infect Dis* 1995;21[Suppl 3]:S265–S276.

102. Stout JE, Arnold B, Yu VL. Comparative activity of ciprofloxacin, ofloxacin, levofloxacin, and erythromycin against *Legionella* species by broth microdilution and intracellular susceptibility testing in HL-60 cells. *Diagn Microbiol Infect Dis* 1998;30:37–43.

103. Rasch JR, Mogabgab WJ. Therapeutic effect of erythromycin on *Mycoplasma pneumoniae* pneumonia. *Antimicrob Agents Chemother* 1965;5:693.

104. Smith CB, Friedewald WT, Chanock RM. Shedding of *Mycoplasma pneumoniae* after tetracycline and erythromycin. *N Engl J Med* 1967;276:1172.

105. Chirwin K, Roblin PM, Hammerschlag MR. In vitro susceptibilities of *Chlamydia pneumoniae* (*Chlamydia* sp. strain TWAR). *Antimicrob Agents Chemother* 1989;33:1634–1635.

106. Schonwald S, Gunjaca M, Kolacny L, et al. Comparison of azithromycin and erythromycin in the treatment of atypical pneumonias. *J Antimicrob Chemother* 1990;25[Suppl A]:123–126.

107. Covelli HD, Husky DL, Dolphin RE. Psittacosis. Clinical presentations and therapeutic observations. *West J Med* 1980;132:242–245.

108. D'Angelo LJ, Hetherington R. Q fever treated with erythromycin. *Br Med J* 1979;2:305–306.

109. Fraschini F, Avallon R, Copponi V, et al. Bactericidal action of an average dose of erythromycin in the bronchi. *Curr Med Res Opin* 1979;6:111–117.

110. Ginsburg CM, McCracken GH, Crow SD, et al. Erythromycin therapy for group A streptococcal pharyngitis. Results of a comparative study of the estolate and ethylsuccinate formulations. *Am J Dis Child* 1984;138:536–539.

111. Lambert H. Antimicrobial drugs in the treatment and prevention of pertussis. *J Antimicrob Chemother* 1979;5:329–331.

112. Miller LW, Bickham S, Jones WL, et al. Diphtheria carriers and the effect of erythromycin therapy. *Antimicrob Agents Chemother* 1974;6:166.

113. Dagan R, Bar-David Y. Double-blind study comparing erythromycin and mupirocin for treatment of impetigo in children: implications of a high prevalence of erythromycin-resistant *Staphylococcus aureus* strains. *Antimicrob Agents Chemother* 1992;36:287–290.

114. Fernandez-Obregon AC. Azithromycin for the treatment of acne. *Int J Dermatol* 2000;39:45–50.

115. Mandal BK, Ellis ME, Dunbar EM, et al. Double-blind placebo controlled trial of erythromycin in the treatment of clinical *Campylobacter infection*. *J Antimicrob Chemother* 1984;13:619–623.

116. DuPont HL, Ericsson CD, Robinson A, et al. Current problems in antimicrobial therapy for bacterial enteric infection. *Am J Med* 1987;82[Suppl 4A]:324–328.

117. Weber JT, Johnson RE. New treatments for *Chlamydia trachomatis* genital infection. *Clin Infect Dis* 1995;20[Suppl 1]:566–571.

118. Schulte JM, Schmid GP. Recommendations for treatment of chancroid, 1993. *Clin Infect Dis* 1995;20[Suppl 1]:539.

119. Brogden R, Peters D. Dirithromycin. A review of its antimicrobial activity, pharmacokinetic properties, and therapeutic efficacy. *Drugs* 1994;48:599–616.

120. Dirithromycin. *Med Lett Drugs Ther* 1995;37:109–110.

121. Stout JE, Arnold B, Yu VL. Activity of azithromycin, clarithromycin, roxithromycin, dirithromycin, quinupristin/dalfopristin and erythromycin against *Legionella* species by intracellular susceptibility testing in HL-60 cells. *J Antimicrob Chemother* 1998;41:289–291.

122. Sides GD, Cerimele BJ, Black HR, et al. Pharmacokinetics of dirithromycin. *J Antimicrob Chemother* 1993;31[Suppl C]:65–75.

123. Zuckerman JM. The newer macrolides: azithromycin and clarithromycin. *Infect Dis Clin North Am* 2000;14(2):449–462

124. Retsema J, Girard A, Schelkly W, et al. Spectrum and mode of action of azithromycin (CP-62,993), a new 15-membered ring macrolide with improved potency against gram-negative organisms. *Antimicrob Agents Chemother* 1987;31:1939–1947.

125. Piscitelli SC, Danziger LH, Rodvold KA. Clarithromycin and azithromycin: new macrolide antibiotics. *Clin Pharm* 1992;11:137–152.

126. Young LS, Wiviott L, Wu M, et al. Azithromycin for treatment of *Mycobacterium avium-intracellulare* complex infection in patients with AIDS. *Lancet* 1991;338:1107–1109.

127. Chaisson RE, Benson CA, Dube MP, et al. Clarithromycin therapy for bacteremic *Mycobacterium avium* complex disease in patients with AIDS. A randomized double-blind dose-ranging study in patients with AIDS. *Ann Intern Med* 1994;121:905–911.

128. Doucet-Populaire F, Truffot-Pernot C, Grosset J, et al. Acquired resistance in *Mycobacterium avium* complex strains isolated from AIDS patients and beige mice during treatment with clarithromycin. *J Antimicrob Chemother* 1995;36:129–136.

129. Glupczynski Y, Burette A. Failure of azithromycin to eradicate *Campylobacter pylori* from the stomach because of acquired resistance during treatment. *Am J Gastroenterol* 1990;85:98–99.

130. Barry AL, Jones RN, Thornsberry C. In vitro activities of azithromycin (CP 63,993), clarithromycin (A-56268; TE-031), erythromycin, roxithromycin, and clindamycin. *Antimicrob Agents Chemother* 1988;32:752–754.

131. Olsson-Liljequist B, Hoffman BM. In vitro activity of clarithromycin combined with its 14-hydroxy metabolite A-62671 against *H. influenzae*. *J Antimicrob Chemother* 1991;27[Suppl A]:11–17.

132. Cassell GH, Drnec J, Waites KB, et al. Efficacy of clarithromycin against *Mycoplasma pneumoniae*. *J Antimicrob Chemother* 1991;27[Suppl A]:47–59.

133. Edelstein PM, Meyer RD. Susceptibility of *Legionella pneumophila* to twenty antimicrobial agents. *Antimicrob Agents Chemother* 1980;18:403–408.

134. McNulty CA, Dent JC. Susceptibility of clinical isolates of *Campylobacter pylori* to twenty-one antimicrobial agents. *Eur J Clin Microbiol Infect Dis* 1988;7:566–569.

135. Ridgway GL, Mumtaz G, Fenelon L. The in vitro activity of clarithromycin and other macrolides in the type strain of *Chlamydia pneumoniae*. *J Antimicrob Chemother* 1991;27[Suppl A]:43–45.

136. Yew WW, Piddock LJ, Li MS, et al. In-vitro activity of quinolones and macrolides against mycobacteria. *J Antimicrob Chemother* 1994;34:343–351.

137. Brown BA, Wallace RJ Jr, Onyi GO. Activities of clarithromycin against eight slowly growing species of nontuberculous mycobacteria, determined by using a broth microdilution MIC system. *Antimicrob Agents Chemother* 1992;36:1987–1990.

138. Klemens SP, Cynamon MH. Activities of azithromycin and clarithromycin against nontuberculous mycobacteria in beige mice. *Antimicrob Agents Chemother* 1994;38:1455–1459.

139. Gornyski E, Gutman S, Allen W. Comparative antimycobacterial activities of difloxacin, temafloxacin, enoxacin, pefloxacin, reference fluoroquinolones, and a new macrolide, clarithromycin. *Antimicrob Agents Chemother* 1989;33:591–592.

140. Wallace RJ Jr, Brown BA, Griffith DE, et al. Initial clarithromycin monotherapy for *Mycobacterium avium-intracellulare* complex lung disease. *Am J Respir Crit Care Med* 1994;149:1335–1341.

141. Pierce M, Crampton S, Henry D, et al. A randomized trial of clarithromycin as prophylaxis against disseminated *Mycobacterium avium* complex infection in patients with advanced acquired immunodeficiency syndrome. *N Engl J Med* 1996;335:384–911.

142. Gordin FM, Sullam PM, Shafran SD, et al. A randomized, placebo-controlled study of rifabutin added to a regimen of clarithromycin and ethambutol for treatment of disseminated infection with *Mycobacterium avium* complex. *Clin Infect Dis* 1999;28:1080–1085.

143. Araujo F, Prokocimer P, Lin T, et al. Activity of clarithromycin alone or in combination with other drugs for treatment of murine toxoplasmosis. *Antimicrob Agents Chemother* 1992;36:2454–2457.

144. Honeybourne D, Kees F, Andrews JM, et al. The levels of clarithromycin and its 14-hydroxy metabolite in the lung. *Eur Respir J* 1994;7:1275–1280.

145. Conte JR Jr, Golden JA, Duncan S, et al. Intrapulmonary pharmacokinetics of clarithromycin and of erythromycin. *Antimicrob Agents Chemother* 1995;39:334–338.

146. Chu S, Park B, Locke C, et al. Drug–food interaction potential of clarithromycin, a new macrolide antimicrobial. *J Clin Pharmacol* 1992;32:32–36.

147. Guay DR, Gustavson LE, Devcich KJ, et al. Pharmacokinetics and tolerability of extended-release clarithromycin. *Clin Ther* 2001;23:566–577.

148. Fraschini F, Scaglione F, Pintucci G, et al. The diffusion of clarithromycin and roxithromycin into nasal mucosa, tonsil and lung in humans. *J Antimicrob Chemother* 1991;27[Suppl A]:61–65.

149. Schmidt T, Froula J, Tauber MG. Clarithromycin lacks bactericidal activity in cerebrospinal fluid in experimental pneumococcal meningitis. *J Antimicrob Chemother* 1993;32:627–632.

150. Pai MP, Graci DM, Amsden GW. Macrolide drug interactions: an update. *Ann Pharmacother* 2000;34:495–513.

151. Kuper JI, D'Aprile M. Drug–Drug interactions of clinical significance in the treatment of patients with *Mycobacterium avium* complex disease. *Clin Pharmacokinet* 2000;39:203–214.

152. Gooderham MJ, Bolli P, Fernandez PG. Concomitant digoxin toxicity and warfarin interaction in a patient receiving clarithromycin. *Ann Pharmacother* 1999;33:796–799.

153. Jewelewicz DA, Schiff WM, Brown S, et al. Rifabutin-associated uveitis in an immunosuppressed pediatric patient without acquired immunodeficiency syndrome. *Am J Ophthalmol* 1998;125:872–873.

154. Polis MA, Piscitelli SC, Vogel S, et al. Clarithromycin lowers plasma zidovudine levels in persons with human immunodeficiency virus infection. *Antimicrob Agents Chemother* 1997;41:1709–1714.

155. Malaty LI, Kuper JJ. Drug interactions of HIV protease inhibitors. *Drug Saf* 1999;20:147–169.

156. Clarithromycin and azithromycin. *Med Lett Drugs Ther* 1992;34:45.

157. Shafran SD, Singer J, Zarowny DP, et al. A comparison of two regimens for the treatment of *Mycobacterium avium* complex bacteremia in AIDS: rifabutin, ethambutol and clarithromycin versus rifampin, ethambutol, clofazimine, and ciprofloxacin. *N Engl J Med* 1996;335:337–383.

158. McCarty JM. Clarithromycin in the management of community-acquired pneumonia. *Clin Ther* 2000;22:281–294, 265.

159. Genne D, Siegrist HH, Humair L, et al. Clarithromycin versus amoxicillin-clavulanic acid in the treatment of community-acquired pneumonia. *Eur J Clin Microbiol Infect Dis* 1997;16:783–788.

160. Aoyama T, Sunakawa K, Iwata S, et al. Efficacy of short-term treatment of pertussis with clarithromycin and azithromycin. *J Pediatr* 1996;129(5):761–764.

161. Taylor DE. Pathophysiology of antibiotic resistance: clarithromycin. *Can J Gastroenterol* 2000;14:891–894.

162. Masur H, US Public Health Service Task Force on Prophylaxis and Therapy for *Mycobacterium avium* complex. Recommendations on the prophylaxis and therapy for disseminated *Mycobacterium avium* complex disease in patients infected with the human immunodeficiency virus. *N Engl J Med* 1993;329:898–904.

163. Cohn DL, Fisher EJ, Peng GT, et al. A prospective randomized trial of four three-drug regimens in the treatment of disseminated *Mycobacterium avium* complex disease in AIDS patients: excess mortality associated with high-dose clarithromycin. Terry Beirn Community Programs for Clinical Research on AIDS. *Clin Infect Dis* 1999;29:125–133.

164. Chan GP, Garcia-Ignacio BYY, Chavez VE, et al. Clinical trial of clarithromycin for lepromatous leprosy. *Antimicrob Agents Chemother* 1994;38:515–517.

165. Walsh JH, Peterson WL. Drug therapy: the treatment of *Helicobacter pylori* infection in the management of peptic ulcer disease. *N Engl J Med* 1995;333:984–991.

166. Osato MS, Reddy R, Reddy SG, et al. Pattern of primary resistance of *Helicobacter pylori* to metronidazole or clarithromycin in the United States. *Arch Intern Med* 2001;161:1217–1220.

167. Buckley MJ, Xia HX, Hyde DM, et al. Metronidazole resistance reduces efficacy of triple therapy and leads to secondary clarithromycin resistance. *Dig Dis Sci* 1997;42:2111–115.

168. Lacassin F, Schaffo D, Perronne C, et al. Clarithromycin-minocycline combination as salvage therapy for toxoplasmosis in patients infected with human immunodeficiency virus. *Antimicrob Agents Chemother* 1995;39:276–277.

169. Garey KW, Amsden GW. Intravenous azithromycin. *Ann Pharmacother* 1999;33:218–228.

170. Goldstein FW, Emirian MF, Coutrot A, et al. Bacteriostatic and bactericidal activity of azithromycin against *Haemophilus influenzae*. *J Antimicrob Chemother* 1990;25[Suppl A]:25–28.

171. Scieux C, Bianchi A, Chappey B, et al. In-vitro activity of azithromycin against *Chlamydia trachomatis*. *J Antimicrob Chemother* 1990;25[Suppl A]:7–10.

172. Wang G, Wilson TJ, Jiang Q, et al. Spontaneous mutations that confer antibiotic resistance in *Helicobacter pylori*. *Antimicrob Agents Chemother* 2001;45:727–733.

173. Giacometti A, Cirioni O, Ancarani F, et al. In vitro activities of polycationic peptides alone and in combination with clinically used antimicrobial agents against *Rhodococcus equi*. *Antimicrob Agents Chemother* 1999;43:2093–2096.

174. Chang SC, Chen YC, Luh KT, et al. Macrolides resistance of common bacteria isolated from Taiwan. *Diagn Microbiol Infect Dis* 1995;23:147–154.

175. Goldstein EJ, Citron DM, Merriam CV, et al. Activities of telithromycin (HMR 3647, RU 66647) compared to those of erythromycin, azithromycin, clarithromycin, roxithromycin, and other antimicrobial agents against unusual anaerobes. *Antimicrob Agents Chemother* 1999;43:2801–2805.

176. Goldstein EJ, Citron DM, Merriam CV, et al. Comparative in vitro activities of ABT-773 against aerobic and anaerobic pathogens isolated from skin and soft-tissue animal and human bite wound infections. *Antimicrob Agents Chemother* 2000;44:2525–2529.

177. Smith MD, Vinh DX, Hoa NTT, et al. In vitro antimicrobial susceptibilities of strains of *Yersinia pestis*. *Antimicrob Agents Chemother* 1995;39:2153–2154.

178. Kawamura-Sato K, Iinuma Y, Hasegawa T, et al. Effect of subinhibitory concentrations of macrolides on expression of flagellin in *Pseudomonas aeruginosa* and *Proteus mirabilis*. *Antimicrob Agents Chemother* 2000;44:2869–2872.

179. Vranes J. Effect of subminimal inhibitory concentrations of azithromycin on adherence of *Pseudomonas aeruginosa* to polystyrene. *J Chemother* 2000;12:280–285.

180. Baumann U, Fischer J, Gudowuis P, et al. Buccal adherence of *Pseudomonas aeruginosa* in patients with cystic fibrosis under long-term therapy with azithromycin. *Infection* 2001;29:7–11.

181. Sorvillo F, Beall G, Turner P, et al. incidence and determinants of *Pseudomonas aeruginosa* infection among persons with HIV: association with hospital exposure. *Am J Infect Control* 2001;29:79–84.

182. Renaudin H, Bebear C. Comparative in vitro activity of azithromycin, clarithromycin, erythromycin, and lomefloxacin against *Mycoplasma pneumoniae*, *Mycoplasma hominis* and *Ureaplasma urealyticum*. *Eur J Clin Microbiol Infect Dis* 1990;9:838–841.

183. Hook EW III, Stephens J, Ennis DM. Azithromycin compared with penicillin G benzathine for treatment of incubating syphilis. *Ann Intern Med* 1999;131:434–437.

184. Barsic B, Maretic T, Majerus L, et al. Comparison of azithromycin and doxycycline in the treatment of erythema migrans. *Infection* 2000;28:153–156.

185. Krause PJ, Lepore T, Sikand VK, et al. Atovaquone and azithromycin for the treatment of babesiosis. *N Engl J Med* 2000;343:1454–1458.

186. Luft BJ, Dattwyler RJ, Johnson RC, et al. Azithromycin compared with amoxicillin in the treatment of erythema migrans. A double-blind, randomized, controlled trial. *Ann Intern Med* 1996;124:785–791.

187. Blais J, Beauchamp D, Chamberland S. Azithromycin uptake and intracellular accumulation by *Toxoplasma gondii*–infected macrophages. *J Antimicrob Chemother* 1994;34:371–382.

188. Conrad DA. Treatment of cat-scratch disease. *Curr Opin Pediatr* 2001;13:56–59.

189. Bass JW, Freitas BC, Freitas AD, et al. Prospective randomized double blind placebo-controlled evaluation of azithromycin for treatment of cat-scratch disease. *Pediatr Infect Dis J* 1998;17:447–452.

190. Ives TJ, Manzewitsch P, Regnery RL, et al. In vitro susceptibilities of *Bartonella henselae*, *B. quintana*, *B. elizabethae*, *Rickettsia rickettsii*, *R. conorii*, *R. akari*, and

191. *R. prowazekii* to macrolide antibiotics as determined by immunofluorescent-antibody analysis of infected Vero cell monolayers. *Antimicrob Agents Chemother* 1997;41:578–582.

191. Andersen SL, Ager A, McGreevy P, et al. Activity of azithromycin as a blood schizonticide against rodent and human plasmodia in vivo. *Am J Trop Med Hyg* 1995;52:159.

192. Dunne M, Fessel J, Kumar P, et al. A randomized, double-blind trial comparing azithromycin and clarithromycin in the treatment of disseminated *Mycobacterium avium* infection in patients with human immunodeficiency virus. *Clin Infect Dis* 2000;31:1245–1252.

193. Koch CC, Esteban DJ, Chin AC, et al. Apoptosis, oxidative metabolism and interleukin-8 production in human neutrophils exposed to azithromycin: effects of *Streptococcus pneumoniae*. *J Antimicrob Chemother* 2000;46:19–26.

194. Ianaro A, Ialenti A, Maffia P, et al. Anti-inflammatory activity of macrolide antibiotics. *J Pharmacol Exp Ther* 2000;292:156–163.

195. Girard AE, Cimochowski CR, Faiella JA. Correlation of increased azithromycin concentrations with phagocyte infiltration into sites of localized infection. *J Antimicrob Chemother* 1996;37[Suppl C]:9–19.

196. Foulds G, Shepard RM, Johnson RB. The pharmacokinetics of azithromycin in human serum and tissues. *J Antimicrob Chemother* 1990;25[Suppl A]:73–82.

197. Glaudue RP, Snider ME. Intracellular accumulation of azithromycin by cultured human fibroblasts. *Antimicrob Agents Chemother* 1990;34:1056–1060.

198. Nahata MC, Koranyi KI, Gadgil SD, et al. Pharmacokinetics of azithromycin in pediatric patients after oral administration of multiple doses of suspension. *Antimicrob Agents Chemother* 1993;37:314–316.

199. Baldwin DR, Wise R, Andrews JM, et al. Azithromycin concentrations at the sites of pulmonary infections. *Eur Respir J* 1990;3:886–890.

200. Jaruratanasirikul S, Hortiwakul R, Tantisarasart T, et al. Distribution of azithromycin into brain tissue, cerebrospinal fluid, and aqueous humor of the eye. *Antimicrob Agents Chemother* 1996;40:825–826.

201. Wallace RM, Miller LK, Nguyen M, et al. Ototoxicity with azithromycin. *Lancet* 1994;343:241.

202. Bizjak ED, Haug MT III, Schilz RJ. Intravenous azithromycin-induced ototoxicity. *Pharmacotherapy* 1999;19:245–248.

203. Amsden GW, Nafziger AN, Foulds G, et al. A study of the pharmacokinetics of azithromycin and nelfinavir when coadministered in healthy volunteers. *J Clin Pharmacol* 2000;40:1522–1527.

204. Beckey NP, Parra D, Colon A. Retrospective evaluation of a potential interaction between azithromycine and warfarin in patients stabilized on warfarin. *Pharmacotherapy* 2000;20:1055–1059.

205. Plouffe J, Schwartz DB, Kolokathis A, et al. Clinical efficacy of intravenous followed by oral azithromycin monotherapy in hospitalized patients with community-acquired pneumonia. The Azithromycin Intravenous Clinical Trials Group. *Antimicrob Agents Chemother* 2000;44:1796–1802.

206. Vergis EN, Indorf A, File TM Jr, et al. Azithromycin vs cefuroxime plus erythromycin for empirical treatment of community-acquired pneumonia in hospitalized patients: a prospective, randomized, multicenter trial. *Arch Intern Med* 2000;160:1294–1300.

207. Heffelfinger JD, Dowell SF, Jorgensen JH, et al. Management of community-acquired pneumonia in the era of pneumococcal resistance: a report from the Drug-Resistant *Streptococcus pneumoniae* Therapeutic Working Group. *Arch Intern Med* 2000;160:1399–1408.

208. Jonas D, Engels I, Daschner FD, et al. The effect of azithromycin on intracellular *Legionella pneumophila* in the Mono Mac 6 cell line at serum concentrations attainable in vivo. *J Antimicrob Chemother* 2000;46:385–390.

209. McLinn S. Double blind and open label studies of azithromycin in the management of acute otitis media in children: a review. *Pediatr Infect Dis J* 1996;15[Suppl]:S20–S23.

210. Jacobson GF, Autry AM, Kirby RS, et al. A randomized controlled trial comparing amoxicillin and azithromycin for the treatment of *Chlamydia trachomatis* in pregnancy. *Am J Obstet Gynecol* 2001;184:1352–1354, 1354–1356.

211. Stamm WE, Hicks CB, Martin DH, et al. Azithromycin for empirical treatment of the nongonococcal urethritis syndrome in men. A randomized double-blind study. *JAMA* 1995;274:545–549.

212. Handsfield HH. Azithromycin in gonorrhea. *Int J STD AIDS* 1997;8:472–473.

213. Handsfield HH, Dalv ZA, Martin DA, et al. Multicenter trial of single-dose azithromycin vs ceftriaxone in the treatment of uncomplicated gonorrhea. *Sex Transm Dis* 1994;21:107–111.

214. Zarantonelli L, Borthagaray G, Lee EH, et al. Decreased susceptibility to azithromycin and erythromycin mediated by a novel mtr(R) promoter mutation in *Neisseria gonorrhoeae*. *J Antimicrob Chemother* 2001;47:651–654.

215. Verdon MS, Handsfield HH, Johnson RB. Pilot study of azithromycin for the treatment of primary and secondary syphilis. *Clin Infect Dis* 1994;19:486–488.

216. Rolfs RT. Treatment of syphilis, 1993. *Clin Infect Dis* 1995;20[Suppl 1]:S23–S28.

217. Oldfield EC III, Fessel WJ, Dunne MW, et al. Once weekly azithromycin therapy for prevention of *Mycobacterium avium* complex infection in patients with AIDS: a randomized, double-blind, placebo-controlled multicenter trial. *Clin Infect Dis* 1998;26:611–619.

218. Havlir DV, Dube MP, Sattler FR, et al. Prophylaxis against disseminated Mycobacterium avium complex with weekly azithromycin, daily rifabutin, or both. California Collaborative Treatment Group. *N Engl J Med* 1996;335:392–398.

219. Kuschner RA, Trofa AF, Thomas RJ, et al. Use of azithromycin for the treatment of *Campylobacter* enteritis in travelers to Thailand, an area where ciprofloxacin resistance is prevalent. *Clin Infect Dis* 1995;21:536–541.

220. Frenck RW Jr, Nakhla I, Sultan Y, et al. Azithromycin versus ceftriaxone for the treatment of uncomplicated typhoid fever in children. *Clin Infect Dis* 2000;31:1134–1138.
221. Butler T, Sridhar CB, Daga MK, et al. Treatment of typhoid fever with azithromycin versus chloramphenicol in a randomized multicentre trial in India. *J Antimicrob Chemother* 1999;44:243–250.
222. Weber K, Wilske B, Preac-Mursic V, et al. Azithromycin versus penicillin V for the treatment of early Lyme borreliosis. *Infection* 1993;21:367–372.
223. Tabbara KF. Trachoma: a review. *J Chemother* 2001;13[Suppl 1]:18–22.
224. Bregani ER, Tien TV, Monzani V, et al. Azithromycin in the treatment of *Plasmodium falciparum* gametocytes. Preliminary observation. *Panminerva Med* 2000;42:197–199.
225. Taylor WR, Richie TL, Fryauff DJ, et al. Malaria prophylaxis using azithromycin: a double-blind, placebo-controlled trial in Irian Jaya, Indonesia. *Clin Infect Dis* 1999;28:74–81.
226. Anderson SL, Berman J, Kuschner R, et al. Prophylaxis of *Plasmodium falciparum* malaria with azithromycin administered to volunteers. *Ann Intern Med* 1995;123:771–773.
227. Kuschner RA, Heppner DG, Andersen SL, et al. Azithromycin prophylaxis against a chloroquine-resistant strain of *Plasmodium falciparum*. *Lancet* 1994;343:1396–1397.
228. Dunne MW, Bozzette S, McCutchan JA, et al. Efficacy of azithromycin in prevention of *Pneumocystis carinii* pneumonia: a randomised trial. California Collaborative Treatment Group. *Lancet* 1999;354:891–895.
229. Giacometti A, Cirioni O, Barchiesi F, et al. Activity of nitazoxanide alone and in combination with azithromycin and rifabutin against *Cryptosporidium parvum* in cell culture. *J Antimicrob Chemother* 2000;45:453–461.
230. Smith NH, Cron S, Valdez LM, et al. Combination drug therapy for cryptosporidiosis in AIDS. *J Infect Dis* 1998;178:900–903.
231. Jackson LA. Description and status of the azithromycin and coronary events study (ACES). *J Infect Dis* 2000;181[Suppl 3]:S579–S581.
232. Schneider CA, Diedrichs H, Riedel KD, et al. In vivo uptake of azithromycin in human coronary plaques. *Am J Cardiol* 2000;86:789–791.
233. Semaan HB, Gurbel PA, Anderson JL, et al. The effect of chronic azithromycin therapy on soluble endothelium-derived adhesion molecules in patients with coronary artery disease. *J Cardiovasc Pharmacol* 2000;36:533–537.
234. Muhlestein JB, Anderson JL, Carlquist JF, et al. Randomized secondary prevention trial of azithromycin in patients with coronary artery disease: primary clinical results of the ACADEMIC study. *Circulation* 2000;102:1755–1760.
235. Champney WS, Tober CL. Structure-activity relationships for six ketolide antibiotics. *Curr Microbiol* 2001;42:203–210.
236. Johnson AP, Henwood CJ, Tysall L, et al. Activity of the ketolide telithromycin (HMR-3647) against erythromycin-susceptible and -resistant pneumococci isolated in the UK. *Int J Antimicrob Agents* 2001;18:73–76.
237. Guitton M, Delachaume C, Le Priol P, et al. In vitro and in vivo efficacy of a novel fluoro-ketolide HMR 3562 against enterococci. *J Antimicrob Chemother* 2001;48:131–135.
238. Malathum K, Coque TM, Singh KV, et al. In vitro activities of two ketolides, HMR 3647 and HMR 3004, against gram-positive bacteria. *Antimicrob Agents Chemother* 1999;43:930–936.
239. Baltch AL, Smith RP, Ritz WJ, et al. Antibacterial effect of telithromycin (HMR 3647) and comparative antibiotics against intracellular *Legionella pneumophila*. *J Antimicrob Chemother* 2000;46:51–55.
240. Mason KJ, Dietz A, Deboer C. Lincomycin, a new antibiotic, I: discovery and biologic properties. *Antimicrob Agents Chemother* 1963;1962:555.
241. Magerlein BJ, Birkenmeyer RD, Kagan F. Clinical modification of lincomycin. *Antimicrob Agents Chemother* 1967;1966:727–736.
242. McGehee RF Jr, Smith CB, Wilcox C, et al. Comparative studies of antibacterial activity in vitro and absorption and excretion of lincomycin and clindamycin. *Am J Med Sci* 1968;256:279–292.
243. Garrison DW, DeHaan RM, Lawson JB. Comparison in vitro antibacterial activities of 7-chloro-7-deoxylincomycin, lincomycin and erythromycin. *Antimicrob Agents Chemother* 1968;1967:397–400.
244. Bartlett JG. Anti-anaerobic antibacterial agents. *Lancet* 1982;2:478–481.
245. Tabbara KF, O'Connor GR. Treatment of ocular toxoplasmosis with clindamycin and sulfadiazine. *Ophthalmology* 1980;87:129–134.
246. Douthwaite S. Interaction of the antibiotics clindamycin and lincomycin with E. coli 23S ribosomal RNA. *Nucleic Acids Res* 1992;20:4717–4720.
247. Menninger JR, Coleman RA. Lincosamide antibiotics stimulate dissociation of peptidyl-tRNA from ribosomes. *Antimicrob Agents Chemother* 1993;37:2027–2029.
248. Sande MA, Johnson ML. Antimicrobial therapy of experimental endocarditis caused by Staphylococcus aureus. *J Infect Dis* 1975;131:367–375.
249. Nastro LJ, Finegold SM. Bactericidal activity of five antimicrobial agents against Bacteroides fragilis. *J Infect Dis* 1972;126:104–107.
250. Gemmell CG, Peterson PK, Schmeling D, et al. Potentiation of opsonization and phagocytosis of *Streptococcus pyogenes* following growth in the presence of clindamycin. *J Clin Invest* 1981;67:1249–1256.
251. Milatovic D, Braveny I, Verhoef J. Clindamycin enhances opsonization of *Staphylococcus aureus*. *Antimicrob Agents Chemother* 1983;24:413–417.
252. Proctor RA, Olbrantz PJ, Mosher DF. Subinhibitory concentrations of antibiotics alter fibronectin binding to *Staphylococcus aureus*. *Antimicrob Agents Chemother* 1983;24:823–826.
253. Leigh DA. Antibacterial activity and pharmacokinetics of clindamycin. *J Antimicrob Chemother* 1981;7[Suppl A]:A3–A9.
254. Meyers BR, Kaplan K, Weistein L. Microbiological and pharmacological behavior of 7-chlorolincomycin. *Appl Microbiol* 1969;17:653–657.
255. Karchmer AW, Moellering RC Jr, Watson BK. Susceptibility of various serogroups of streptococci to clindamycin and lincomycin. *Antimicrob Agents Chemother* 1975;7:164–167.
256. Marks MI. In vitro activity of clindamycin and other antimicrobials against gram-positive bacteria and *Haemophilus influenzae*. *Can Med Assoc J* 1975;112:170–173.
257. Harrison HR, Riggins RM, Alexander ER, et al. In vitro activity of clindamycin against strains of *Chlamydia trachomatis*, *Mycoplasma hominis* and *Ureaplasma urealyticum* isolated from pregnant women. *Am J Obstet Gynecol* 1984;149:477–480.
258. Reeves DS, Holt HA, Phillips I, et al. Activity of clindamycin against *Staphylococcus aureus* and *Staphylococcus epidermidis* from four UK centers. *J Antimicrob Chemother* 1991;27:469–474.
259. Lemmen S, Kropec A, Engels I, et al. MIC and serum bactericidal activity of clindamycin against methicillin-resistant and -sensitive staphylococci. *Infection* 1993;21:407–409.
260. Barrett FF, McGehee RF Jr, Finland M. Methicillin-resistant *Staphylococcus aureus* at Boston City Hospital. *N Engl J Med* 1968;279:441–448.
261. Desmyter J, Reybrouck G. Lincomycin sensitivity of erythromycin-resistant staphylococci. *Chemotherapia* 1964;9:183–189.
262. Duncan IBR. Development of lincomycin resistance by staphylococci. *Antimicrob Agents Chemother* 1968;1967:723–729.
263. Watanakunakorn C. Clindamycin therapy of *Staphylococcus aureus* endocarditis. Clinical relapse and development of resistance to clindamycin, lincomycin and erythromycin. *Am J Med* 1976;60:419–425.
264. Russell NE, Pachorek RE. Clindamycin in the treatment of streptococcal and staphylococcal toxic shock syndromes. *Ann of Pharmcother* 2000;34:936–939.
265. Sriskandan S, McKee A, Hall L, et al. Comparative effects of clindamycin and ampicillin on superantigenic activity of *Streptococcus pyogenes*. *J Antimicrob Chemother* 1997;40:275–277.
266. Chow AW, Montgomerie JZ, Guze LB. Parenteral clindamycin therapy for severe anaerobic infections. *Arch Intern Med* 1974;134:78–82.
267. Snydman DR, Jacobus NV, McDermott LA, et al. Multicenter survey of in vitro susceptibility of *Bacteroides fragilis* group, 1995 to1996, with comparison of trends from 1990 to 1996. *Antimicrob Agents Chemother* 1999;43:2417–2422.
268. Oteo J, Aracil B, Alos JI, et al. High prevalence of resistance to clindamycin in *Bacteroides fragilis* group. *J Antimicrob Chemother* 2000;45:691–693.
269. Labbe AC, Bourgault AM, Vincellette J, et al. Trends in antimicrobial resistance among clinical isolates of the *Bacteroides fragilis* group from 1992 to 1997 in Montreal, Canada. *Antimicob Agents Chemother* 1999;43:2517–2519.
270. Horn R, Robson HG. Susceptibility of the *Bacteroides fragilis* group to newer quinolones and other standard anti-anaerobic agents. *J Antimicrob Chemother* 2001;48:127–130.
271. Aldridge KE, Ashcraft D, Cambre K, et al. Multicenter survey of the changing in vitro antimicrobial susceptibilities of clinical isolates of *Bacteroides fragilis* group, *Prevotella*, *Fusobacterium*, *Porphyromonas*, and *Peptostreptococcus* species. *Antimicob Agents Chemother* 2001;45:1238–1243.
272. Bartlett JG, Sutter VL, Finegold SM. Treatment of anaerobic infections with lincomycin and clindamycin. *N Engl J Med* 1972;287:1006–1010.
273. Alger LS, Lovchik JC. Comparative efficacy of clindamycin versus erythromycin in eradication of antenatal *Chlamydia trachomatis*. *Am J Obstet Gynecol* 1991;165:375–381.
274. Sweet RL. New approaches for the treatment of bacterial vaginosis. *Am J Obstet Gynecol* 1993;169:479–482.
275. Kremsner PG, Winkler S, Brandts C, et al. Curing of chloroquine-resistant malaria with clindamycin. *Am J Trop Med Hyg* 1993;49:650–654.
276. Kremsner PG, Winkler S, Brandts C, et al. Clindamycin in combination with chloroquine or quinine is an effective therapy for uncomplicated *Plasmodium falciparum* malaria in children from Gabon. *J Infect Dis* 1994;169:467–470.
277. Kremsner PG, Radloff P, Metzer W, et al. Quinine plus clindamycin improves chemotherapy of severe malaria in children. *Antimicrob Agents Chemother* 1995;39:1603–1605.
278. Parola P, Ranque S, Badagia S, et al. Controlled trial of 3-day quinine-clindamycin treatment versus 7-day quinine treatment for adult travelers with uncomplicated falciparum malaria imported from the tropics. *Antimicrob Agents Chemother* 2001;45:932–935.
279. Blais J, Tardif C, Chamberland S. Effect of clindamycin on intracellular replication, protein synthesis, and infectivity of *Toxoplasma gondii*. *Antimicrob Agents Chemother* 1993;37:2571–2577.
280. Dannemann B, McCutchan A, Israelski D, et al. Treatment of toxoplasma encephalitis in patients with AIDS. A randomized trial comparing pyrimethamine plus clindamycin to pyrimethamine plus sulfadiazine. *Ann Intern Med* 1992;116:33–43.
281. Toma E, Fournier S, Dumont M, et al. Clindamycin/primaquine versus trimethoprim-sulfamethoxazole as primary therapy for *Pneumocystis carinii* pneumonia in AIDS: a randomized, double-blind pilot trial. *Clin Infect Dis* 1993;17:178–184.
282. Black JR, Feinberg J, Murphy RL, et al. Clindamycin and primaquine therapy for mild-to-moderate episodes of *Pneumocystic carinii* pneumonia in patients with AIDS. AIDS Clinical Trials Group 044. *Clin Infect Dis* 1994;18:905–913.
283. Smilack JD, Burgin WW Jr, Moore WL Jr, et al. *Mycoplasma pneumoniae* pneumonia and clindamycin therapy. Failure to demonstrate efficacy. *JAMA* 1974;228:729–731.

284. Brause BD, Borges JS, Roberts RB. Relative efficacy of clindamycin, erythromycin and penicillin in treatment of *Treponema pallidum* in skin syphilomas of rabbits. *J Infect Dis* 1976;134:93–96.

285. Santos Sanches I, Mato R, de Lencastre H, et al. Patterns of multidrug resistance among methicillin-resistant hospital isolates of coagulase positive and coagulase negative staphylococci collected in the international multicenter study RESIST in 1997–1998. *Microb Drug Resist* 2000;6:199–211.

286. Semel JD, Trenholme GM, Levin S. Gentamicin and clindamycin-resistant *Staphylococcus aureus. Am J Med Sci* 1980;280:4–9.

287. Williams DN, Crossley K, Hoffman C, et al. Parenteral clindamycin phosphate: pharmacology with normal and abnormal liver function and effect on nasal staphylococci. *Antimicrob Agents Chemother* 1975;7:153–158.

288. Bartlett J. Treatment of community acquired pneumonia. *Chemotherapy* 2000;46[Suppl 1]:24–31.

289. Nelson CT, Mason EO, Kaplan SL. Activity of oral antibiotics in middle ear and sinus infections caused by penicillin-resistant *Streptococcus pneumoniae:* implications for treatment. *Pediatr Infect Dis* 1994;13:585–589.

290. Brook I, Gober AE, Leyva F. *In vitro* and *in vivo* effects of penicillin and clindamycin on expression of group A beta-hemolytic streptococcal capsule. *Antimicrob Agents Chemother* 1995;39:1565–1568.

291. Doern GV, Heilmann KP, Hutnh HK, et al. Antimicrobial resistance among clinical isolates of *Streptococcus pneumoniae* in the United States during 1999–2000, including a comparison of resistance rates since 1994–1995. *Antimicrob Agents Chemother* 2001;45:1721–1729.

292. Tally FP, Snydman DR, Gorbach SL, et al. Plasmid-mediated transferable resistance to clindamycin and erythromycin in *Bacteroides fragilis. J Infect Dis* 1979;139:83–88.

293. Tally FP, Cuchural GJ Jr, Malamy MH. Mechanisms of resistance and resistance transfer in anaerobic bacteria: factors influencing antimicrobial resistance. *Rev Infect Dis* 1984;6[Suppl 1]:S260–S269.

294. Lai CJ, Weisblum B, Fahnestock SR, et al. Alteration of 23S ribosomal RNA and erythromycin-induced resistance to lincomycin and spiramycin in *Staphylococcus aureus. J Mol Biol* 1973;74:67–72.

295. Reig M, Moreno A, Baquero F. Resistance of *Peptostreptococcus* species to macrolides and lincosamides: inducible and constitutive phenotypes. *Antimicrob Agents Chemother* 1992;36:662–664.

296. Reig M, Fernandez MC, Ballesta JPG, et al. Inducible expression of ribosomal clindamycin resistance in *Bacteroides vulgatus. Antimicrob Agents Chemother* 1992;36:639–642.

297. Smith HW. Transfer of antibiotic resistance from animal and human strains of *Escherichia coli* to resident *E. coli* in the alimentary tract of man. *Lancet* 1969;1:1174–1176.

298. DeHaan RM, Metzler CM, Schnellenberg D. Pharmacokinetic studies of clindamycin phosphate. *J Clin Pharmacol* 1973;13:190–209.

299. Forist AA, DeHaan RM, Metzler CM. Clindamycin bioavailability from clindamycin-2 palmitate and clindamycin-2 hexadecylcarbonate in man. *J Pharmacokinet Biopharmacol* 1973;1:89–98.

300. Wagner JG, Novak E, Patel NC, et al. Absorption, excretion and half-life of clindamycin in normal adult males. *Am J Med Sci* 1968;256:25–37.

301. DeHaan RM, Metzler CM, Schellenberg D, et al. Pharmacokinetic studies of clindamycin hydrochloride in human. *J Clin Pharmacol Ther Toxicol* 1972;6:105–119.

302. DeHaan RM, Vanden Bosch WD, Metzler CM, et al. Clindamycin serum concentrations after administration of clindamycin palmitate with food. *J Clin Pharmacol* 1972;12:205–209.

303. Cambell IW, Hossack DJN, Munro JF. Absorption and urinary excretion of clindamycin palmitate in the elderly. *Curr Med Res Opin* 1973;1:369–375.

304. Algra RJ, Rosen T, Waisman M. Topical clindamycin in acne vulgaris. Safety and stability. *Arch Dermatol* 1977;113:1390–1391.

305. Kauffman RE, Shoeman DW, Wan SH, et al. Absorption and excretion of clindamycin-2-phosphate in children after intramuscular injection. *Clin Pharmacol Ther* 1972;13:704–709.

306. Fass RJ, Saslaw S. Clindamycin. Clinical and laboratory induction of parenteral therapy. *Am J Med Sci* 1972;263:369–382.

307. Rodriguez W, Ross S, Khan W, et al. Clindamycin in the treatment of osteomyelitis in children. A report of 29 cases. *Am J Dis Child* 1977;131:1088–1093.

308. Picardi JL, Lewis HP, Tan JS, et al. Clindamycin concentrations in the central nervous system in primates before and after head trauma. *J Neurosurg* 1975;43:717–720.

309. Panzer JD, Brown DC, Epstein WL, et al. Clindamycin levels in various body tissue and fluids. *J Clin Pharmacol* 1972;12:259–262.

310. Bystedt H, Dahlback A, Nord CE. Concentration of azidocillin, erythromycin, doxycycline and clindamycin in dental alveolar serum after single oral dose. *Int J Oral Surg* 1977;6:65–74.

311. Nicholas P, Meyers PB, Levy RN, et al. Concentration of clindamycin in human bone. *Antimicrob Agents Chemother* 1975;8:220–221.

312. Smilack JD, Flittie WH, Williams TW Jr. Bone concentrations of antimicrobial agents after parenteral administration. *Antimicrob Agents Chemother* 1976;9:169–171.

313. Baird P, Sullivan M, Hughes S, et al. Penetration into bone and tissues of clindamycin phosphate. *Postgrad Med J* 1978;54:65–67.

314. Johnson JD, Hand WL, Francis JB, et al. Antibiotic uptake by alveolar macrophages. *J Lab Clin Med* 1980;95:429–439.

315. Joiner KA, Lowe BR, Dzink JL, et al. Antibiotic levels in infected and sterile abscesses in mice. *J Infect Dis* 1981;143:487–494.

316. Brown RB, Martyak SN, Barza M, et al. Penetration of clindamycin phosphate into the abnormal human biliary tract. *Ann Intern Med* 1976;84:168–170.

317. Hinthorn DR, Baker LH, Romig DA, et al. Use of clindamycin in patients with liver disease. *Antimicrob Agents Chemother* 1976;9:498–501.

318. Peddie BA, Dann E, Bailey RR. The effect of impairment of renal function and dialysis on the serum and urine levels of clindamycin. *Aust N Z J Med* 1975;5:198–202.

319. Van Scoy RE, Wilson WR. Antimicrobial agents in patients with renal insufficiency. *Mayo Clin Proc* 1977;52:704–706.

320. Kelly CP, LaMont JT. *Clostridium difficile* infection. *Annu Rev Med* 1998;49:375–390.

321. Kager L, Liljequist L, Malmborg AS, et al. Effect of clindamycin prophylaxis on the colonic microflora in patients undergoing colorectal surgery. *Antimicrob Agents Chemother* 1981;20:736–740.

322. Tedesco FJ, Barton RW, Alpers DH. Clindamycin-associated colitis: a prospective study. *Ann Intern Med* 1974;81:429–433.

323. Condon RE, Anderson MJ. Diarrhea and colitis in clindamycin treated surgical patients. *Arch Surg* 1978;113:794–797.

324. Swartzberg JE, Maresca RM, Remington JS. Clinical study of gastrointestinal complications associated with clindamycin therapy. *J Infect Dis* 1977;135[Suppl]:S99–S103.

325. Lusk RH, Fekety FR Jr, Silva J Jr, et al. Gastrointestinal side effects of clindamycin and ampicillin therapy. *J Infect Dis* 1977;135[Suppl]:S111–S119.

326. Neu HC, Prince A, Neu CO, et al. Incidence of diarrhea and colitis associated with clindamycin therapy. *J Infect Dis* 1977;135[Suppl]:S120–S125.

327. Brause BD, Romankiewick JA, Gotz V, et al. Comparative study of diarrhea associated with clindamycin and ampicillin therapy. *Am J Gastroenterol* 1980;73:244–248.

328. Mylonakis E, Ryan ET, Calderwood SB. *Clostridium difficile*–associated diarrhea: a review. *Arch Intern Med* 2001;161:525–533.

329. McFarland LV, Mulligan ME, Kwok MS, et al. Nosocomial acquisition of *Clostridium difficile* infections. *N Engl J Med* 1989;320:204–210.

330. Pear SM, Williamson TH, Bettink K, et al. Decrease in nosocomial *Clostridium difficile*–associated diarrhea by restricting clindamycin use. *Ann Intern Med* 1994;120:272–277.

331. Dhawan VK, Thadepalli H. Clindamycin. A review of fifteen years of experience. *Rev Infect Dis* 1982;4:1133–1153.

332. Thomsen RJ, Stranieri A, Knutson D, et al. Topical clindamycin treatment of acne. Clinical, surface lipid composition and quantitative surface microscopy response. *Arch Dermatol* 1980;1116:1031–1034.

333. Elmore M, Rissing JP, Rink L, et al. Clindamycin-associated hepatotoxicity. *Am J Med* 1974;57:627–630.

334. Altraif I, Lilly L, Wanless IR, et al. Cholestatic liver disease with ductopenia (vanishing bile duct syndrome) after administration of clindamycin and trimethoprim-sulfamethoxazole. *Am J Gastroenterol* 1994;89:1230–1234.

335. Fogdall RP, Miller RD. Prolongation of a pancuronium-induced neuromuscular blockage by clindamycin. *Anesthesiology* 1974;41:407–408.

336. Becker LD, Miller RD. Clindamycin enhances a nondepolarizing neuromuscular blockade. *Anesthesiology* 1976;45:84–87.

337. Zinner SH, Provonchee RB, Elias K, et al. Effect of clindamycin on the *in vitro* activity of amikacin and gentamicin against gram-negative bacilli. *Antimicrob Agents Chemother* 1976;9:661–664.

338. Joshi A, Stein R. Altered serum clearance of intravenously administered clindamycin phosphate in patients with uremia. *J Clin Pharmacol* 1974;14:140–144.

339. Berger SA, Barza M, Haher J, et al. Penetration of clindamycin into decubitus ulcers. *Antimicrob Agents Chemother* 1978;14:498–499.

340. Weinstein WM, Onderdonk AB, Bartlett JG, et al. Antimicrobial therapy of experimental intraabdominal sepsis. *J Infect Dis* 1975;132:282–286.

341. Louie TJ, Onderdonk AB, Gorbach SL, et al. Therapy, for experimental intraabdominal sepsis: comparison of four cephalosporins with clindamycin plus gentamicin. *J Infect Dis* 1977;135[Suppl]:S18–S22.

342. Gorbach SL, Thadepalli H. Clindamycin in pure and mixed anaerobic infections. *Arch Intern Med* 1974;134:87–92.

343. Leigh DA, Simmons K, Williams S. The treatment of abdominal and gynecological infections with parenteral clindamycin phosphate. *J Antimicrob Chemother* 1977;3:493–500.

344. Nichols RL. Intraabdominal sepsis. Characterization and treatment. *J Infect Dis* 1977;135[Suppl]:S54–S57.

345. Thadepalli H, Gorbach SL, Broido PW, et al. Abdominal trauma, anaerobes and antibiotics. *Surg Gynecol Obstet* 1973;137:270–276.

346. Pitkin D, Sheikh W, Wilson S, et al. Comparison of the activity of meropenem with that of other agents in the treatment of intraabdominal, obstetric/gynecological, and skin and soft tissue infections. *Clin Infect Dis* 1995;20[Suppl 2]:S372–S375.

347. deGroot AGW, Hustinx PA, Lampe AS, et al. Comparison of imipenem/cilastatin with the combination of aztreonam and clindamycin in the treatment of intraabdominal infections. *J Antimicrob Chemother* 1993;32:491–500.

348. Giamarellou H. Anaerobic infection therapy. *Int J Antimicrob Agents* 2000; 16:341–346.

349. Bartlett J. Intra-abdominal sepsis. *Med Clin North Am* 1995;79:599–617.

350. McClean KL, Sheehan GJ, Harding GKM. Intraabdominal infections: a review. *Clin Infect Dis* 1994;19:100–116.

351. Levison ME, Santoro J, Bran JL, et al. *In vitro* activity and clinical efficacy of clindamycin in the treatment of infections due to anaerobic bacteria. *J Infect Dis* 1977;135[Suppl]:S49–S53.

352. Harding GKM, Buckwold FJ, Ronald AR, et al. Prospective, randomized comparative study of clindamycin, chloramphenicol, and ticarcillin each in combination with gentamicin in therapy for intraabdominal and female genital tract sepsis. *J Infect Dis* 1980;142:384–393.

353. Wilson SE, Hopkins JA. Clinical correlates of anaerobic bacteriology in peritonitis. *Clin Infect Dis* 1995;20[Suppl 2]:S251–S256.

354. Hopkins JA, Lee JCH, Wilson SE. Susceptibility of intraabdominal isolates at operation. A predictor of post-operative infection. *Ann Surg* 1993;59:791–796.

355. Younes Z, Johnson DA. New developments and concepts in antimicrobial therapy for intra-abdominal infections. *Curr Gastroenterol Res* 2000;2:277–288.

356. de Lalla F. Antimicrobial chemotherapy in control of surgical infectious complications. *J Chemother* 1999;11:440–445.

357. Larsen JW, Gold-Hughes K, Kreter B, et al. The clinical efficacy and tolerability of imipenem-cilastatin versus clindamycin-gentamicin for serious pelvic infections. *Clin Ther* 1992;14:90–96.

358. Centers for Disease Control and Prevention. Sexually transmitted diseases treatment guidelines. *MMWR Morb Mortal Wkly Rep* 1998;47:1–118.

359. Bartlett JG, Gorbach SL. Treatment of aspiration pneumonia and primary lung abscess. *JAMA* 1975;234:935–937.

360. Brook I. Clindamycin in treatment of aspiration pneumonia in children. *Antimicrob Agents Chemother* 1979;15:342–345.

361. Civen R, Somer HJ, Marina M, et al. A retrospective review of cases of anaerobic empyema and update of bacteriology. *Clin Infect Dis* 1995;20[Suppl 2]:S224–S229.

362. Levison ME. Anaerobic pleuropulmonary infection. *Curr Opin Infect Dis* 2001;14:187–191.

363. Bartlett JG, Gorbach SL. Penicillin or clindamycin for primary lung abscess? An editorial. *Ann Intern Med* 1983;98:546–548.

364. Chow AW, Roser SM, Brady FA. Orofacial odontogenic infections. *Ann Intern Med* 1978;88:392–402.

365. Malinowski RW, Strate RG, Perry JF, et al. Management of human bite injuries of the hand. *J Trauma* 1979;19:655–659.

366. Louie TJ, Bartlett JG, Tally FP, et al. Aerobic and anaerobic bacteria in diabetic foot ulcers. *Ann Intern Med* 1976;85:461–463.

367. Chow AW, Galpin JE, Guze LB. Clindamycin for treatment of sepsis caused by decubitus ulcers. *J Infect Dis* 1977;135[Suppl]:S65–S68.

368. Lipsky BA, Berendt AR. Principles and practice of antibiotic therapy of diabetic foot infections. *Diabetes Metab Res Rev* 2000;16[Suppl 1]:S42–S44.

369. Gerding D. Foot infections in diabetic patients. The role of anaerobes. *Clin Infect Dis* 1995;20[Suppl 2]:S283–S288.

370. Stevens DL, Gibbons AE, Bergstrom R, et al. The Eagle effect revisited: efficacy of clindamycin, erythromycin, and penicillin in the treatment of streptococcal myositis. *J Infect Dis* 1988;158:23–28.

371. Stevens DL, Laine BM, Mitten JE. Comparison of single and combination antimicrobial agents for prevention of experimental gas gangrene caused by *Clostridium perfringens*. *Antimicrob Agents Chemother* 1987;31:312–316.

372. Stevens DL, Bryant AE, Hackett SP. Antibiotic effects on bacterial viability, toxin production, and host response. *Clin Infect Dis* 1995;20[Suppl 2]:S154–S157.

373. Brook I, Leyva F. The treatment of the carrier state of group A β-hemolytic streptococci with clindamycin. *Chemotherapy* 1981;27:360.

374. Brook I, Yocum P, Friedman EM. Aerobic and anaerobic bacteria in tonsils of children with recurrent tonsillitis. *Ann Otol Rhinol Laryngol* 1981;90:261–263.

375. Brook I, Hirokawa S. Treatment of patients with a history of recurrent tonsillitis due to group A β-hemolytic streptococci. *Clin Pediatr* 1985;24:331–336.

376. Dajani AS, Taubert KA, Wilson W, et al. Prevention of bacterial endocarditis: guidelines by American Heart Association. *Clin Infect Dis* 1997;25:6448–6458.

377. Feigin RD, Pickering LK, Anderson D, et al. Clindamycin treatment of osteomyelitis and septic arthritis in children. *Pediatrics* 1975;55:213–223.

378. Norden CW, Shinners E, Niederriter K. Clindamycin treatment of experimental chronic osteomyelitis due to *Staphylococcus aureus*. *J Infect Dis* 1986;153:956–959.

379. Mayberry-Carson KJ, Tober-Meyer B, Lambe DW Jr, et al. An electron microscopic study of the effect of clindamycin therapy on bacterial adherence and glycocalyx formation in experimental *Staphylococcus aureus* osteomyelitis. *Microbios* 1986;43:189–206.

380. Mayberry-Carson KJ, Tober-Meyer B, Smith JK, et al. Bacterial adherence and glycocalyx formation in osteomyelitis experimentally induced with *Staphylococcus aureus*. *Infect Immun* 1984;43:825–833.

381. Lambe DW Jr, Mayberry-Carson KJ, Ferguson KP. Morphological stabilization of the glycocalyces of 23 strains of five *Bacteroides* species using specific antisera. *Can J Microbiol* 1984;30:809–819.

382. Stoughton RB, Cornell RC, Gange RW, et al. Double-blind comparison of topical 1 percent clindamycin phosphate (Cleocin T) and oral tetracycline 500 mg/day in the treatment of acne vulgaris. *Cutis* 1980;26:424–425.

383. Basler RSW. Clindamycin for tetracycline-resistant acne. *Cutis* 1980;25:527–528.

384. Smego R, Nagar S, Maloba B, et al. A meta-analysis of salvage therapy for *Pneumocystis carinii* pneumonia. *Arch Intern Med* 2001;161:1529–1533.

385. Hecht DW, Lederer L, Osmolski JR, et al. Susceptibility results for the *Bacteroides fragilis* group: comparison of the broth microdilution and agar dilution methods. *Clin Infect Dis* 1995;20[Suppl 2]:S342.

CHAPTER 23
Vancomycin and Teicoplanin

Raul E. Davaro and Richard H. Glew

Vancomycin is a glycopeptide antibiotic directed primarily against gram-positive bacteria. It acts by inhibiting the biosynthesis of the major structural polymer of the bacteria cell wall. Clinically introduced in 1958, it enjoyed widespread use in the treatment of infections caused by penicillin-resistant gram-positive bacteria, particularly *Staphylococcus aureus* (1,2). After the introduction of the bactericidal antistaphylococcal penicillins and cephalosporins methicillin and cephalothin, vancomycin was relegated to the role of alternative therapy in patients allergic to β-lactam antibiotics, largely because of the perception that vancomycin was more toxic. Vancomycin was resurrected in the late 1970s in response to the spread of methicillin-resistant *S. aureus* strains (MRSA) and coagulase-negative staphylococcal infections in association with vascular catheters and indwelling medical devices and for treatment of antibiotic-associated colitis. With increased use has come the epidemic spread of vancomycin-resistant organisms, particularly among enterococci, and the emergence of vancomycin-resistant *S. aureus* (3–9). Strategies to treat and contain these organisms are problematic and continue to evolve (10–13).

MICROBIOLOGY

Mode of Antimicrobial Action

Vancomycin accomplishes its bactericidal activity by inhibiting bacterial cell wall synthesis in dividing organisms. During the second stage of cell wall synthesis, vancomycin prevents polymerization of UDP-N-acetylmuramyl pentapeptide and N-acetylglucosamine into peptidoglycan via tight binding of D-alanyl-D-alanine at the free carboxyl end of the cross-linking pentapeptide to the cleft in the chlorine-bearing face of vancomycin, thereby preventing binding of the peptide to the enzyme peptidoglycan synthetase (14). Because penicillins and cephalosporins inhibit the subsequent cross-linkage of the pentapeptide side chains of peptidoglycan, there is no cross-resistance between vancomycin and the β-lactams. The large molecular size of vancomycin prevents it from crossing the outer cell membrane of gram-negative bacteria, thus restricting its activity to gram-positive species.

Antimicrobial Spectrum

The antibacterial activity spectrum of vancomycin is limited chiefly to aerobic and anaerobic gram-positive organisms. Virtually all strains of *S. aureus*, including those that are β-lactam resistant, are susceptible to vancomycin in low concentrations, with minimal inhibitory concentrations (MICs) less than 5 mg/L. Vancomycin susceptibility is noted with most of the non-*aureus* *Staphylococcus* species, including *S. epidermidis*, *S. saprophyticus*, *S. haemolyticus*, *S. hominis*, and *S. warneri*, and unspeciated coagulase-negative staphylococci (15).

Although most strains of *Streptococcus pneumoniae*, including penicillin-resistant isolates, have been susceptible to vancomycin, tolerance of *Streptococcus pneumoniae* to vancomycin has recently emerged as a problem of significant concern and may serve as a marker for eventual resistance (16–19).

Vancomycin is bactericidal for all strains of *Streptococcus pyogenes* (group A streptococci), group C and group G streptococci, viridans streptococci, and *Streptococcus bovis* but is only bacteriostatic against most strains of enterococci, with minimal bactericidal concentrations (MBCs) usually more than 32 times higher than MICs (20). Occasional isolates of group B streptococci (*Streptococcus agalactiae*) appear resistant to vancomycin, although most isolates exhibit MICs less than 4.0 mg/L. In addition, vancomycin may have relatively high MBCs for occasional strains of viridans streptococci, *S. bovis*, and group B streptococci (20–23). Most strains of *Listeria monocytogenes* are inhibited by clinically achievable levels of vancomycin, but MBCs are much higher than MICs and generally exceed achievable serum levels (24). All strains of diphtheroids (nondiphtheria *Corynebacterium* species, including *Corynebacterium jeikeium* and *Corynebacterium D2*) appear to be susceptible to modest concentrations (MICs lower than 1 mg/L) of vancomycin (25–28).

The susceptibility of lactobacilli is variable. *Bacillus* species usually are susceptible to vancomycin (29,30).

Among anaerobes, vancomycin is active against most clostridial isolates, including *Clostridium perfringens* and *Clostridium difficile;* most isolates are inhibited by less than 1 mg/L (31,32). On the other hand, no more than half of *Actinomyces* species appear susceptible to vancomycin (33). Microaerophilic and anaerobic streptococci usually are susceptible, whereas *Bacteroides* species and other gram-negative anaerobes are not.

Vancomycin exhibits no significant activity against most gram-negative bacteria, including the Enterobacteriaceae and Pseudomonadaceae as well as *Legionella* species (34). Rickettsiae, chlamydiae, and mycobacteria are resistant as well (34). Some strains of *Neisseria* appear susceptible *in vitro*, but the clinical significance of these findings is unknown (35).

Resistance

Vancomycin enjoyed consistent activity against virtually all gram-positive species for the first 30 years of its clinical use, but subsequent years have witnessed a dramatic increase in the prevalence of vancomycin-resistant enterococci (VRE) (3–6,36–40). Among the members of the National Nosocomial Infection Survey, hospitals reporting any isolates of VRE rose from 0.3% to 7.9% of facilities from 1989 to 1993 (10). In 1999, 25.2% of enterococci associated with nosocomial infections in intensive care unit patients were vancomycin resistant (41). Clinical infection with VRE occurs in the setting of prolonged length of hospital stay, prior antibiotic use, and renal failure requiring hemodialysis or peritoneal dialysis (37–39).

The majority of VRE isolates from U.S. hospitals (67% in one series) bear the VanA phenotype (5,6). This is characterized by high-level resistance to vancomycin (MIC, 64 μg/mL or higher) and teicoplanin (MIC, 16 to 128 μg/mL, or higher). The *vanA* is a nine-gene complex that alters the usual target of vancomycin, the terminal D-alanyl-D-alanine of the muramyl pentapeptide, substituting instead D-alanyl-D-lactate (42,43). It is located on a transposable genetic element, transposon 1546, which may be plasmid associated. VanA has been observed in *Enterococcus faecium*, *Enterococcus faecalis*, and *Enterococcus avium*. The VanB phenotype usually displays lower-level vancomycin resistance (MIC, 16 to 1,024 μg/mL), with preservation of teicoplanin susceptibility (MIC, 2 μg/mL, or lower), and is seen in both *E. faecium* and *E. faecalis* (6,40). The VanC pattern, isolated from *Enterococcus gallinarum*, has low-level resistance to vancomycin (MIC, 4 to 16 μg/mL) with teicoplanin susceptibility. VanC-like pheno-

types have also been observed in *Enterococcus casseliflavus* and *Enterococcus raffinosus* (6). The low-level resistance that characterizes the VanB and VanC isolates may be missed by some short-incubation automated susceptibility systems (44). There have been reports of enterococci that have evolved from the VanB phenotype to require the presence of vancomycin for growth (45,46).

No clear consensus has emerged regarding the therapy for VanA isolates, many of which are β-lactam resistant as well as glycopeptide resistant; suggestions have included use of β-lactam-aminoglycoside combinations, chloramphenicol, and newer agents such as quinupristin-dalfopristin and linezolid (11,12,47–50). VRE with low-level resistance have been treated with teicoplanin, although acquired resistance to this agent has been observed (47,49).

The Centers for Disease Control and Prevention have issued guidelines designed to limit the epidemic spread of VRE, detailing educational efforts, isolation procedures, laboratory screening methods, and survey techniques to detect asymptomatic colonization (10). In an attempt to reduce the impact of VRE, medical facilities are advised to (a) establish methods for screening for VRE, (b) use barrier methods (gowns, gloves) to prevent transmission from known cases, and (c) curtail the use of vancomycin (especially enteral) when reasonable therapeutic alternatives exist or when cultures fail to document β-lactam–resistant gram-positive infection (10,51,52).

Other gram-positive species have manifested vancomycin resistance, including less frequently encountered genera such as *Leuconostoc, Pediococcus,* group G streptococci, *Lactobacillus,* and *Erysipelothrix* (9,53–56). Strains of coagulase-negative staphylococcus, including *S. epidermidis* and *S. haemolyticus,* have been found to demonstrate vancomycin resistance, often in an incremental fashion after drug exposure (56–58). In 1997, the first strain of *S. aureus* with reduced susceptibility to vancomycin and teicoplanin was reported from Japan. To date, six clinical infections with vancomycin-intermediate *S. aureus* (VISA) have been reported in the United States. Intermediate resistance appears to develop from preexisting strains of MRSA in the presence of vancomycin (59).

Antibiotic Combinations

Evaluation *in vitro* of the interaction between various antibiotics in combination with vancomycin may produce conflicting results, probably owing to differences in testing methods (checkerboard titrations versus time–kill curves), end points (bacteriostatic versus bactericidal), size and growth phase of the starting inoculum, and sampling times. Results must be interpreted with caution in the absence of data *in vivo*. Vancomycin and gentamicin are synergistic against most sensitive strains of enterococci, viridans streptococci, *S. bovis*, methicillin-sensitive and methicillin-resistant *S. aureus,* and one third to one half of strains of *S. epidermidis* (60–63). The combination of vancomycin plus rifampin generally has produced less favorable and conflicting results. Against *S. epidermidis,* the combination of vancomycin plus rifampin commonly is synergistic and rarely demonstrates antagonism (63,64). However, vancomycin–rifampin synergism has been demonstrated against only one fifth to one third of *S. aureus* isolates, and antagonism is noted frequently (65–70). Furthermore, clinical experience with the combination of vancomycin plus rifampin in the treatment of serious *S. aureus* infections has been inconsistent. Against enterococci, the combination of vancomycin plus rifampin is not synergistic and occasionally is antagonistic (62). In summary, the most predictable situations for obtaining synergism with vancomycin combinations are (a) vancomycin plus gentamicin against enterococci, *S. bovis,* and viridans streptococci; (b) vancomycin plus gentamicin against methicillin-sensitive and methicillin-resistant *S. aureus;* and (c) vancomycin plus rifampin against non-*aureus* staphylococci.

PHARMACOKINETICS

Absorption

Vancomycin absorption from the gastrointestinal tract is minimal, although occasional reports have documented therapeutic (and, rarely, potentially toxic) serum concentrations during administration of oral or intracolonic vancomycin to patients with pseudomembranous colitis and marked renal impairment (71–73). Intramuscular injection of vancomycin produces severe pain and tissue necrosis, and only the intravenous (IV) route is employed. To minimize phlebitis and infusion-related reactions, it is recommended that the IV dose be reconstituted in 100 to 250 mL of dextrose or normal saline solution and infused at a rate not exceeding 1 g per hour (74).

Distribution

The distribution of vancomycin after IV administration is a biphasic process and fits a three-compartment, open pharmacokinetic model (75,76). The distribution half-life, about 8 minutes, is followed by an intermediate half-life of 30 to 90 minutes, then an elimination half-life that is long and highly variable, ranging from 3 to 13 hours (average, 6 hours) in persons with normal renal function (75–79).

Peak serum levels of vancomycin after IV infusion are proportional to the administered dose. Serum levels of vancomycin measured 2 hours after single-dose IV infusion are 2 to 10 mg/L after a dose of 500 mg, 25 mg/L after 1 g, and 45 mg/L after 2 g (76).

With multiple-dose administration, penetration of vancomycin is good (more than 75% of serum levels) into ascitic, pericardial, and synovial fluids and moderately good (more than 50% of serum levels) into pleural fluid; therapeutic concentrations (more than 2.5 mg/L) are obtained in all these fluids after IV administration of one or more doses (74,80). Penetration of vancomycin from serum into peritoneal dialysis fluid is variable and unpredictable (81).

Penetration of vancomycin into the cerebrospinal fluid (CSF) is variable in general and poor in patients with uninflamed meninges but fair to moderately good (1% to 37% of serum levels) in patients with inflamed meninges; many patients with meningitis are likely to have therapeutic CSF concentrations with IV therapy alone (74,76). In one case series of pneumococcal meningitis, an initial response to vancomycin was seen in all 11 patients, but subsequent clinical failure occurred in 4 patients on days 4 to 8, associated with falling levels of vancomycin in the CSF (82). In cases of meningitis associated with neurosurgical devices, coagulase-negative staphylococci and corynebacteria are encountered commonly (83). The CSF levels achieved with administration of intrathecal or intraventricular vancomycin are variable, and therapeutic drug levels in the CSF may need to be monitored (84,85). Continuous infusion of vancomycin in patients with meningitis achieves therapeutic concentrations in the CSF (86).

Although biliary levels are about 30% to 50% of serum levels and may be therapeutic *in vitro* against streptococci (including enterococci), the drug should not be considered first-line treatment for gram-positive biliary tract infection. Like many other antibiotics, vancomycin does not penetrate well into ocular tissues (87).

Limited data for humans indicate tissue levels higher than serum levels in heart, aorta, kidney, liver, and lung (88). Penetration of vancomycin into abscess fluid is good, with levels about equal to those in serum (88). Penetration of vancomycin into bone is variable and generally is modest; higher concentrations are achieved in medullary bone than in cortical bone. About 3 hours after infusion of a single IV dose of 15 mg/kg vancomycin into normal subjects, Graziani and associates noted cancellous bone levels of vancomycin of less than 2 μg/g in most patients; the mean bone-to-serum ratio was 13% for cancellous bone and 7% for cortical bone (89). In patients with osteomyelitis, vancomycin therapy resulted in cancellous bone concentrations of 3.6 μg/g (21% of serum level) in one patient; cortical bone levels were 3.5 and 8.5 μg/g (21% to 38% of serum levels) in two specimens and were undetectable in three (84). In another study, penetration into uninfected sternal bone was 30% to 70% of serum levels, with mean osseous concentrations of 9.3 μg/g (90).

Elimination

Vancomycin is excreted almost entirely by the kidneys, primarily by glomerular filtration, and there is no evidence of tubular secretion or reabsorption (74). There is a linear relationship between vancomycin clearance (C_{vanc}) and creatinine clearance (C_{cr}) (75). The ratio of C_{vanc} to C_{cr} is about 70% in all patients, and the difference between the two clearance rates is explained by the about 55% binding of vancomycin to serum proteins (75).

Administration and Dosing

In adults with normal renal function, dosing of vancomycin is simple: administration of 30 mg/kg per day (i.e., 2 g per day to the average adult) in two to four divided doses generally results in trough and peak serum concentrations in the desired therapeutic range. Traditional therapeutic drug monitoring requires (a) that a trough serum value be obtained just before (and not more than 1 hour before) a dose, with a target of 5 to 10 mg/L for patients receiving vancomycin at 12-hour intervals and 10 to 15 mg/L for 6-hour dosing intervals; and (b) that a peak serum level be measured 1 to 2 hours after completion of an IV infusion, with the desired range 25 to 40 mg/L, depending on the infecting organism and the site and severity of infection (74,76,78). Some authors have argued that vancomycin dosing without determination of therapeutic drug levels should be adopted into common practice, based on the lack of clear data linking drug concentrations to clinical efficacy and the relative rarity of ototoxic and nephrotoxic effects caused by modern preparations of vancomycin when used alone. However, we continue to advocate therapeutic drug monitoring in critically ill patients, those receiving higher-than-usual doses, anephric patients undergoing hemodialysis and receiving infrequent doses of vancomycin for serious systemic infections, patients with rapidly changing renal function, those receiving concomitant nephrotoxins (especially aminoglycosides), and those undergoing prolonged therapy.

Vancomycin dosing should be individualized on the basis of pharmacokinetic data derived from measured concentrations in serum. Because the kidney is the only significant route of excretion of vancomycin, the dosage must be reduced for patients with impaired renal function and for elderly patients. To avoid potentially toxic serum levels of vancomycin, C_{cr} can be used to determine the appropriate dosing schedule for these patients.

C_{cr} can be estimated with reasonable accuracy using the patient's age, gender, weight, and serum creatinine value:

$$C_{cr} = \frac{(140 - \text{age}) \times (1.00 \text{ [males]}; 0.85 \text{ [females]}) \times \text{wt (kg)}}{72 \times \text{serum creatinine}}$$

where C_{cr} is in milliliters per minute, weight is in kilograms, and the serum creatinine value is in milligrams per deciliter (91).

This formula can not be used to calculate the glomerular filtration rate (GFR) in patients with changing renal function.

Several dosing methods have been proposed to sustain appropriate serum vancomycin concentrations in patients with varying degrees of renal insufficiency, but results of studies designed to evaluate the comparative predictability and reliability of various nomograms have been inconclusive (78,92–96). Regardless of the dosing nomogram employed, serum vancomycin concentrations, together with serum creatinine concentrations, should be monitored at least once weekly for patients with renal insufficiency because there is substantial interpatient variation in vancomycin clearance.

The oral administration of vancomycin produces negligible serum and tissue concentrations and is used exclusively for the treatment of *C. difficile* colitis (97,98).

Dialysis

Vancomycin commonly is used to treat gram-positive infections in hemodialysis patients; traditionally, a dosage of 1 g per week has been employed. The use of high-flux dialyzer membranes has been associated with an abrupt drop in vancomycin concentration (by up to 40%) after treatment, followed by a reequilibration between serum and tissue levels of the drug (99,100). The net effect was a reduction by 16% of serum levels with each treatment or removal of one third of the dose in a typical week with three dialysis treatments (99).

Vancomycin commonly is used in the treatment of peritonitis associated with continuous ambulatory peritoneal dialysis (CAPD) (101,102). IV administration of vancomycin to CAPD patients results in intraperitoneal (IP) levels that are 20% to 25% of serum levels, or about 1 to 5 mg/L (103,104). IP dosing of vancomycin is therapeutically equivalent to IV administration and is complicated by fewer side effects (104,105). Both intermittent (30 mg/kg per week) and continuous (15 mg/kg initially, followed by 30 mg/L dialysate) IP dosing regimens produce therapeutic serum levels and are effective clinically (104,106). Reports of chemical peritonitis after IP administration of a particular formulation of vancomycin have not been common in recent years (107).

Pharmacokinetics of vancomycin can be affected by patient-related factors other than renal function. As with aminoglycosides, the half-life of vancomycin appears to be shorter and the dose requirements higher in burn patients (108). Obese patients exhibit a relatively large volume of distribution for vancomycin, which indicates that vancomycin dosage should be calculated on total body weight rather than lean body weight (unlike aminoglycosides) (109). Vancomycin clearance appears to be delayed in patients with liver impairment (110).

Pediatric Dosing

Schaad and associates recommended that dosing of vancomycin for children be based on age: for neonates younger than 1 week, 15 mg/kg every 12 hours; for neonates 8 to 30 days, 15 mg/kg every 8 hours; and for older infants and children, 10 mg/kg every 6 hours (110a). Considerably higher doses were required to achieve therapeutic concentrations of vancomycin among a group of pediatric cancer patients (111). In this group, accelerated drug clearance was predictable from elevated creatinine clearance.

In preterm infants, James and co-workers (112) offered recommendations for administering vancomycin on the basis of postconceptional age and using lower total doses than those recommended by Schaad: for premature infants of gestational age younger than 27 weeks, 27 mg/kg every 36 hours; for gestational age 27 to 30 weeks, 24 mg/kg every 24 hours; for gestational age 31 to 36 weeks, 18 mg/kg every 12 hours; and for gestational age older than 37 weeks, 22.5 mg/kg every 12 hours. Longer drug half-lives requiring lower dosages among critically ill neonates who had low urine output or who required dopamine were noted by Seay and colleagues (113).

The report of the Committee on Infectious Diseases of the American College of Pediatrics recommends dosage on the basis of postnatal age and birth weight. For newborns younger than 1 week old and weight between 1,200 and 2,000 g, the dose is 10 to 15 mg/kg every 12 to 18 hours. For newborns younger than 1 week old and weight more than 2,000 g, the dose is 10 to 15 mg/kg every 8 to 12 hours. In children older than 1 week old and weight less than 2,000 g the dose is 10 to 15 mg/kg every 8 to 12 hours; for children with weight more than 2,000 g, the dose is 10 to 15 mg/kg every 6 to 8 hours (114).

Adverse Effects

Clinical experience with purified formulations of vancomycin indicates that in general, it is a relatively safe antibiotic (115).

INFUSION-RELATED REACTIONS

The most frequent adverse reactions associated with vancomycin therapy are those related to IV administration. The red man syndrome is an infusion rate–dependent, nonimmunological reaction to vancomycin related to histamine release (116–119). It consists of pruritus and erythematous flushing of the head, face, neck, and upper torso, often with hypotension (occasionally profound and dangerous, particularly during surgery); these effects usually subside within minutes when the infusion is terminated. This reaction occurred in 35% to 90% of volunteers receiving 1,000 mg of vancomycin during 1 hour and in up to 10% of patients receiving 500 mg during 1 hour (116–127). In patients manifesting the reaction effects can be minimized by infusing 500 mg in 1 hour or 1,000 mg in 2 hours (118). Pretreatment with antihistamines also reduces the likelihood of the reaction (119,120). Concomitant administration of narcotics may potentiate the red man syndrome (121). Although early preparations of vancomycin were associated with high rates of chemical thrombophlebitis, the frequency with modern formulations has been in the range of 5% to 13% (74,123).

ALLERGIC REACTIONS

Hypersensitivity reactions, including skin eruptions (typically an erythematous, maculopapular rash and less often urticaria) as well as medication-associated fevers, have been noted in about 1% to 8% of patients receiving vancomycin (115,124).

HEMATOPOIETIC COMPLICATIONS

Adverse hematopoietic reactions associated with vancomycin therapy appear to be uncommon (115). Thrombocytopenia has been reported rarely and eosinophilia sporadically (126). Vancomycin-associated neutropenia has been reported occasionally, usually about 2 to 3 weeks into therapy, and appears unrelated to vancomycin serum levels (115,127,128). An immune mechanism probably is involved because some of these patients exhibit concomitant fever or rash. Periodic monitoring of the neutrophil count is recommended in patients receiving IV vancomycin therapy.

OTOTOXICITY

Impairment of auditory function caused by vancomycin therapy is extremely uncommon; most cases have been reported in patients who are receiving other ototoxic medications (particularly aminoglycosides) concurrently (129,130). Sorrell and Collignon evaluated 54 patients prospectively, 11 with serial audiograms; 1 patient (also receiving gentamicin) was noted to have unilateral mild hearing impairment (124). Vancomycin does not appear to produce ototoxic effects in experimental animals (126,129,131).

NEPHROTOXICITY

Studies suggest that nephrotoxic effects associated with vancomycin occur occasionally and are most common in certain clinical settings: (a) elderly patients; (b) concomitant administration of an aminoglycoside; (c) patients receiving higher than usual doses of vancomycin; (d) changing renal function; (e) elevated serum concentrations of vancomycin; (f) hemodynamic instability. Farber and Moellering noted nephrotoxic reactions in 35% of patients receiving vancomycin plus an aminoglycoside and in only 5% of patients receiving vancomycin alone (115). Sorrell and Collignon reported nephrotoxic reactions in 14% of patients who received vancomycin plus an aminoglycoside and in no patients who received vancomycin alone (124). In a study of older patients, Downs and associates reported nephrotoxic reactions in 27% of patients who had received recent or concurrent aminoglycoside therapy; of elderly individuals who received vancomycin alone, 7% exhibited diminished renal function, a rate not significantly different from the frequency noted in age-matched patients being treated with nonnephrotoxic antibiotics (132).

CLINICAL APPLICATIONS

Staphylococcus aureus

Vancomycin is the treatment of choice in β-lactam–intolerant patients who have serious infections due to *S. aureus*, including bacteremia, endocarditis, skin and soft tissue infections, pneumonia, and septic arthritis (133–135). The relatively slow rate of sterilization of blood cultures by vancomycin as compared with β-lactam antibiotics in cases of *S. aureus* endocarditis has led some investigators to suggest that the drug is inferior to traditional β-lactams for this indication and should be used with caution for serious *S. aureus* infections in nonallergic individuals solely for convenience of dosing (136,137). Vancomycin is indicated for the treatment of staphylococcal osteomyelitis in patients allergic to penicillins, although the variable and modest penetration of vancomycin into bone suggests that first-generation cephalosporins and clindamycin probably are superior. Vancomycin is the drug of choice for the treatment of methicillin-resistant *S. aureus* infections (88,89,135–139).

The emergence of *S. aureus* with intermediate resistance to glycopeptides (VIRSA), as defined by a minimal inhibitory concentration to vancomycin of 8 to 16 μg/mL, threatens to return us to the preantibiotic era. Therapeutic alternatives in the treatment of infections due to VIRSA may include minocycline, oxazolidinones, quinupristin-dalfopristin, and gentamicin (50,59,140,141).

Coagulase-negative Staphylococci

Vancomycin is the mainstay of therapy for infections due to coagulase-negative staphylococci (142). Indeed, the most common setting for vancomycin use is the empirical or directed therapy of infection caused by these organisms involving indwelling medical devices, including bacteremia associated with vascular catheters, prosthetic valve endocarditis, vascular graft infections, prosthetic joint infections, and central nervous system shunt infections (83,142–146). In general, the device must be removed to achieve cure of most staphylococcal infections associated with a foreign body, this is probably due to the ability of coagulase-negative staphylococci to form biofilms, which impair the killing power of vancomycin *in vitro* (147–149). However, vancomycin therapy without removal of the device often is successful in CAPD-associated peritonitis and in postoperative endophthalmitis in recipients of intraocular lens implants and occasionally in prosthetic valve endocarditis, bacteremia associated with tunneled central venous catheters (Hickman or Broviac), and meningitis due to CSF shunts (101,144–148,150,151). Combination therapy (vancomycin plus rifampin and gentamicin) often is employed in prosthetic valve endocarditis due to staphylococci (144).

Streptococci

Vancomycin is an effective antibiotic for treatment of serious infections caused by streptococci in patients allergic to β-lactam antibiotics and can be used successfully to treat endocarditis due to viridans streptococci or *S. bovis* (134,152). Vancomycin is an alternative for penicillin-allergic patients with serious infections due to enterococci but must be used in combination with an aminoglycoside (gentamicin) for endocarditis (134).

Pneumococcal Meningitis

Inclusion of vancomycin in patients with meningitis in areas where penicillin-resistant pneumococci (MIC above 2.0 μg/mL) are prevalent must be considered. Vancomycin must be used with either ceftriaxone or cefotaxime. This combination was more effective than either agent alone against penicillin-resistant strains in animal studies (16,17,82,153,154).

Diphtheroids

Vancomycin is the antibiotic of choice for treatment of infections due to diphtheroids, a group of gram positive, nonsporulating, nondiphtheria corynebacteria that are pathogens in patients with underlying malignant disease and neutropenia or with prosthetic devices (150,155,156).

Other Clinical Settings

Orally administered vancomycin in doses of 125 mg four times daily is as effective as metronidazole for treating antibiotic-associated colitis (97,98). IV administration of vancomycin produces low fecal concentrations of drug, probably owing to minimal biliary excretion, and is not effective in the treatment or prevention of antibiotic-associated colitis (157). Vancomycin has often been part of antibiotic therapy for fever in the neutropenic host. However, Rubin and co-workers found that outcomes for patients were not affected adversely by omitting vancomycin from the treatment regimen until β-lactam–resistant gram-positive infection had been documented by culture (53). The empirical use of vancomycin should be considered when febrile neutropenic patients show clinical signs of gram-positive infection (e.g., inflammation near vascular catheters) or in those treated prophylactically with fluoroquinolones, in whom infection more frequently involves gram-positive infection (158,159).

The agents of bacterial peritonitis in patients receiving CAPD are commonly gram-positive organisms, particularly *S. aureus* and non-*aureus* staphylococci, against which vancomycin is highly effective. Although continuous IP administration of vancomycin at a concentration of 25 to 50 mg/L in the dialysate (often with an initial IV loading dose) has been the most common mode of treatment, studies suggest that intermittent IP administration alone can be employed for CAPD-associated peritonitis. Studies have demonstrated that once-weekly IP administration of vancomycin (30 mg/kg in 2 L of dialysate with 6-hour dwell time) results in prolonged, effective peritoneal concentrations of vancomycin, and two IP doses (30 mg/kg in 2 L 1 week apart) can be as effective and safe as continuous IP vancomycin therapy in managing CAPD-associated peritonitis (104,106).

Vancomycin has been used successfully to treat bacterial meningitis and central nervous system shunt infections caused by susceptible organisms, especially coagulase-negative staphylococci (145–160). Usually, the shunt is removed completely, with a ventriculostomy device used for drainage and intrathecal drug administration. Acceptable cure rates have also been achieved with exteriorization of the distal end of the shunt alone. The usual intrathecal doses of vancomycin range from 5 to 10 mg in infants to 10 to 20 mg in children and adults. Vancomycin has also been used in the treatment of nonneurosurgical meningitis due to susceptible organisms in patients with severe (e.g., anaphylactic) penicillin allergy, or in patients infected with penicillin-resistant pneumococci, but experience with this therapy is limited (16,17,82,161).

Vancomycin can be employed for surgical prophylaxis in procedures involving implantation of a prosthesis in β-lactam–allergic patients. It is also the drug of choice for endocarditis prophylaxis in β-lactam–allergic, high-risk individuals (162).

The widespread use of vancomycin and other antimicrobials has resulted in a dramatic increase in the prevalence of vancomycin-resistant enterococci infections and may lead to a similar increase in the prevalence of *S. aureus* with intermediate resistance. The Hospital Infection Control Practices Advisory Committee has issued guidelines in an attempt to reduce the overall use of antimicrobials (163,164).

TEICOPLANIN

Teicoplanin (formerly known as teichomycin A₂) is a newer glycopeptide antibiotic similar to vancomycin but with novel structural and pharmacological properties. It is used widely in Europe but is investigational in the United States (162). Derived from fermentation products of *Actinoplanes teichomyceticus*, teicoplanin differs chemically from vancomycin in that its carbohydrate moieties are D-glycosamine and D-mannose instead of D-glucose and vancosamine, and two dihydroxyphenyglycines are present instead of aspartic acid and *N*-methylleucine; it is distinct from all other glycopeptides in having an acyl substituent, which is a fatty acid (165,166). It is larger than vancomycin, with a molecular weight of about 2,000. As with vancomycin, its mechanism of action is the inhibition of polymerization of peptidoglycan by interacting with the D-alanyl-D-alanine terminus of the muramyl pentapeptide, which fits into a cleft inside the antibiotic molecule (162). Owing to the presence of the fatty acid moiety, teicoplanin is far more lipophilic than vancomycin, which probably accounts for its greater tissue and cellular penetration (162,166). Teicoplanin exhibits a much higher degree of protein binding than does vancomycin (about 90% versus 55%), and it is likely that this feature and strong tissue binding explain its delayed clearance and much longer half-life (33 to 48 hours, compared with about 6 hours for vancomycin) (167,168).

Teicoplanin has excellent activity against gram-positive organisms, including *S. pyogenes*, *E. faecalis*, *S. aureus* (even MRSA), *S. pneumoniae*, *Clostridium* species, *C. jeikeium*, *Propionibacterium acnes* and *L. monocytogenes*. It is about as active as vancomycin against staphylococci but generally four to eight times more active against streptococci and clostridia (168–171). Like vancomycin, teicoplanin is bactericidal against growing cells; the MBC typically is no more than two to four times the MIC for most organisms (165,170). Although teicoplanin has greater inhibitory activity than vancomycin against enterococci, each is only bacteriostatic; the MBC is usually above achievable serum concentrations and more than 32 times the MIC (171). Teicoplanin and vancomycin exhibit similar bactericidal synergism in combination with gentamicin against sensitive strains of enterococci. Teicoplanin is active against vancomycin-resistant enterococci bearing the VanB phenotype, but the *in vivo* development of teicoplanin resistance has been observed (6,40,172). It has no activity against VanA isolates, nor does it demonstrate synergistic killing with β-lactams against these isolates (44). Like vancomycin, teicoplanin is bacteriostatic for *L. monocytogenes* (171).

Because of its long terminal half-life, teicoplanin can be administered less frequently than vancomycin. Many early studies indicated clinical success with teicoplanin administered in a loading dose of about 6 mg/kg (about 400 to 600 mg) followed by a maintenance regimen of 2 to 3 mg/kg (about 200 mg) once daily (173–175). However, subsequent studies with serious staphylococcal infections suggested that more aggressive loading therapy is needed to obtain adequate serum levels rapidly (176,177). A high loading dose, or administration of two or three initial maintenance doses at 12-hour intervals after the loading dose, may be necessary to establish adequate serum levels promptly (trough concentration of 5 to 10 mg/L and peak serum levels of 25 to 30 mg/L) in seriously ill patients. Bibler and associates recommended that teicoplanin treatment of patients with grampositive bacteremia should begin with three IV doses of 6 to 7 mg/kg at 12-hour intervals followed by single daily doses of the same amount (176). However, Fortún and colleagues noted breakthrough bacteremia at doses of 7 mg/kg per day in cases of *S. aureus* endocarditis, suggesting that the optimal dosage of teicoplanin for this disease remains to be defined (179).

At doses of 6 mg/kg per day, teicoplanin was as effective as and less toxic than vancomycin for treatment of gram-positive infections in neutropenic hosts (179,180). The drug has also been employed in the treatment of infections caused by sensitive strains of enterococci, although its role in serious infection and endocarditis remains uncertain (181). Teicoplanin has been used in oral form to treat *C. docile* colitis (182–184).

It appears that adverse reactions are less common with teicoplanin than with vancomycin. Intramuscular injection is tolerated well except for mild pain at the injection site and results in excellent absorption (90% bioavailability) (162,169). Phlebitis is uncommon with IV administration of teicoplanin, and infusion-related red man syndrome does not seem to occur (169,174,175). Occasional allergic reactions (rash, eosinophilia) have been noted with teicoplanin. Transient elevations and liver chemistries have been noted to occur occasionally. Renal and otic toxic effects are uncommon (162,173–175).

REFERENCES

1. Wilhelm MP, Estes L. Vancomycin. *Mayo Clin Proc* 1999;74:928.
2. Geraci JE, Heilman FR, Wellman WE, et al. Some laboratory and clinical experiences with a new antibiotic, vancomycin. *Proc Staff Meet Mayo Clin* 1956;31:564.
3. Leclercq R, Derlot E, Duval J, et al. Plasmid-mediated resistance to vancomycin and teicoplanin in *Enterococcus faecium*. *N Engl J Med* 1988;319:157.
4. Shlaes DM, Bouvet A, Devine C, et al. Inducible, transferable resistance

to vancomycin in *Enterococcus faecalis* A256. *Antimicrob Agents Chemother* 1989;33:198.

5. Leclercq R, Derlot E, Weber M, et al. Transferable vancomycin and teicoplanin resistance in *Enterococcus faecium*. *Antimicrob Agents Chemother* 1989;33:10.

6. Clark NC, Cooksey RC, Hill BC, et al. Characterization of glycopeptide-resistant enterococci from U.S. hospitals. *Antimicrob Agents Chemother* 1993;37:2311.

7. Handwerger S, Raucher B, Altarac D, et al. Nosocomial outbreak due to *Enterococcus faecium* highly resistant to vancomycin, penicillin, and gentamicin. *Clin Infect Dis* 1993;16:750.

8. Livomese LL, Dias SD, Samel C, et al. Hospital-acquired infection with vancomycin-resistant *Enterococcus faecium* transmitted by electronic thermometers. *Ann Intern Med* 1992;117:112.

9. Johnson AP, Uttley AH, Woodford N, et al. Resistance to vancomycin and teicoplanin: an emerging clinical problem. *Clin Microbiol Rev* 1990;3:280.

10. Centers for Disease Control and Prevention. Preventing the spread of vancomycin resistance: a report from the Hospital Infection Control Practices Advisory Committee prepared by the Subcommittee on Prevention and Control of Antimicrobial Resistant Microorganisms in Hospitals. *Fed Regist* 1994;59:25758.

11. Caron F, Pestel M, Kitzis MD, et al. Comparison of different β-lactam-glycopeptide-gentamicin combinations for an experimental endocarditis caused by a highly β-lactam-resistant and highly glycopeptide-resistant isolates of *Enterococcus faecium*. *J Infect Dis* 1995;171:106.

12. Green M, Binczewski B, Pasculle AW, et al. Constitutively vancomycin-resistant *Enterococcus faecium* resistant to synergistic β-lactam combinations. *Antimicrob Agents Chemother* 1993;37:1238.

13. Murray BE. Editorial response: what can we do about vancomycin-resistant enterococci? *Clin Infect Dis* 1995;20:1134.

14. Sheldrick GM, Jones PG, Kennard O, et al. Structure of vancomycin and its complex with acetyl-D-alanyl-D-alanine. *Nature* 1978;271:223.

15. Kloos WE, Bannerman TL. Update on clinical significance of coagulase-negative staphylococci. *Clin Microbiol Rev* 1994;7:117.

16. Jacobs MR. Treatment and diagnosis of infections caused by drug-resistant *Streptococcus pneumoniae*. *Clin Infect Dis* 1992;15:119.

17. Friedland IR, McCracken GH Jr. Management of infections caused by antibiotic-resistant *Streptococcus pneumoniae*. *N Engl J Med* 1994;331:377.

18. Normark BH, Novak R, Ortqvist A, et al. Clinical isolates of *Streptococcus pneumoniae* that exhibit tolerance of vancomycin. *Clin Infect Dis* 2001;32:552.

19. Atkinson RM, Mitchell LS, Tuomanen E. Mechanism of tolerance to vancomycin I *Streptococcus pneumoniae*. *Infect Med* 2000;17:793.

20. Krogstad DJ, Parquette AR. Defective killing of enterococci: a common property of antimicrobial agents acting on the cell wall. *Antimicrob Agents Chemother* 1980;17:965.

21. Watanakunakorn C. Mode of action and in vitro activity of vancomycin. *J Antimicrob Chemother* 1984;14(Suppl):7.

22. Stratton CW, Liu C, Ratner HB, et al. Bactericidal activity of daptomycin (LY 146032) compared with those of ciprofloxacin, vancomycin and ampicillin against enterococci as determined by kill-kinetic studies. *Antimicrob Agents Chemother* 1987;31:1014.

23. Kim MJ, Weiser M, Gottschall S, et al. Identification of *Streptococcus faecalis* and *Streptococcus faecium* and susceptibility studies with newly developed antimicrobial agents. *J Clin Microbiol* 1987;25:787.

24. Tuazon CU, Shamsuddin D, Miller H. Antibiotic susceptibility and synergy of clinical isolates of *Listeria monocytogenes*. *Antimicrob Agents Chemother* 1982;21:525.

25. Jadeja L, Fainstein V, LeBlanc B, et al. Comparative in vitro activities of teichomycin and other antibiotics against JK diphtheroids. *Antimicrob Agents Chemother* 1983;24:145.

26. Riley PS, Hollis DG, Utter GB, et al. Characterization and identification of 95 diphtheroid (group JK) cultures isolated from clinical specimens. *J Clin Microbiol* 1979;9:418.

27. Gill VJ, Manning C, Lamson M, et al. Antibiotic-resistant group JK bacteria in hospitals. *J Clin Microbiol* 1981;13:472.

28. Santamaria M, Ponte C, Wilhelmi I, et al. Antimicrobial susceptibility of *Corynebacterium* group D2. *Antimicrob Agents Chemother* 1985;28:845.

29. Bayer AS, Chow AW, Betts D, et al. Lactobacillemia: report of nine cases. *Am J Med* 1978;4:808.

30. Holliman RE, Bone GP. Vancomycin resistance of clinical isolates of lactobacilli. *J Infect* 1988;16:279.

31. Sapico FL, Kwok Y-Y, Sutter VI, et al. Standardized antimicrobial disc susceptibility testing of anaerobic bacteria. In vitro susceptibility of *Clostridium perfringens* to nine antibiotics. *Antimicrob Agents Chemother* 1972;2:320.

32. George WL, Sutter VL, Finegold SM. Toxigenicity and antimicrobial susceptibility of *Clostridium difficile*, a cause of antimicrobial agent-associated colitis. *Curr Microbiol* 1978;1:55.

33. Lerner PI. Susceptibility of pathogenic actinomycetes to antimicrobial compounds. *Antimicrob Agents Chemother* 1974;5:302.

34. Cheung RPF, DiPiro JT. Vancomycin: an update. *Pharmacotherapy* 1986;6:153.

35. Jaffe HW, Lewis JS, Wiesner PJ. Vancomycin-sensitive *Neisseria gonorrhoeae*. *J Infect Dis* 1981;144:198.

36. Uttley AH, Collins CH, Naidoo J, et al. Vancomycin-resistant enterococci [Letter]. *Lancet* 1988;1:57.

37. Edmond MB, Ober JF, Weinbaum DL, et al. Vancomycin-resistant *Enterococcus faecium* bacteremia: risk factors for infection. *Clin Infect Dis* 1995;20:1126.

38. Herman DJ, Gerding DN. Minireview: antimicrobial resistance among enterococci. *Antimicrob Agents Chemother* 1991;35:1.

39. Courvalin P. Minireview: resistance of enterococci to glycopeptides. *Antimicrob Agents Chemother* 1990;34:2291.

40. Quintiliani R Jr, Evers S, Courvalin P. The *vanB* gene confers various levels of self-transferable resistance to vancomycin in enterococci. *J Infect Dis* 1993;167:1220.

41. Gold HS. Vancomycin-resistant enterococci: mechanism and clinical observations. *Clin Infect Dis* 2001;33:210.

42. Walsh CT. Vancomycin resistance: decoding the molecular logic. *Science* 1993;261:308.

43. Fan C, Moews PC, Walsh CT, et al. Vancomycin resistance: structure of D-alanine:D-alanine ligase at 2.3 Å resolution. *Science* 1994;266:439.

44. Tenover FC, Tokars J, Swenson J, et al. Ability of clinical laboratories to detect antimicrobial agent-resistant enterococci. *J Clin Microbiol* 1993;31:1695.

45. Fraimow HS, Jungkind DL, Lander DW, et al. Urinary tract infection with an *Enterococcus faecalis* isolate that requires vancomycin for growth. *Ann Intern Med* 1994;121:22.

46. Green M, Shlaes JH, Barbadora K, et al. Bacteremia due to vancomycin-dependent *Enterococcus faecium*. *Clin Infect Dis* 1995;20:712.

47. Hayden MK, Koenig GI, Trenholme GM. Bactericidal activities of antibiotics against vancomycin-resistant *Enterococcus faecium* blood isolates and synergistic activities of combinations. *Antimicrob Agents Chemother* 1994;38:1225.

48. Norris AH, Reilly JP, Edelstein PH, et al. Chloramphenicol for the treatment of vancomycin-resistant enterococcal infections. *Clin Infect Dis* 1995;20:1137.

49. Lynn WA, Clutterbuck E, Want S, et al. Treatment of CAPD-peritonitis due to glycopeptide-resistant *Enterococcus faecium* with quinupristin/dalfopristin. *Lancet* 1994;344:1025.

50. Waldvogel FA. New resistance in *Staphylococcus aureus*. *N Engl J Med* 1999;340:556.

51. Edberg SC, Hardalo CJ, Kontnick C, et al. Rapid detection of vancomycin-resistant enterococci. *J Clin Microbiol* 1994;32:2182.

52. Boyce JM, Opal SM, Chow JW, et al. Outbreak of multidrug resistant *Enterococcus faecium* with transferable *vanB* class vancomycin resistance. *J Clin Microbiol* 1994;32:1148.

53. Rubin LG, Vellozzi E, Shapiro J, et al. Infection with vancomycin-resistant "streptococci" due to *Leuconostoc* species. *J Infect Dis* 1988;157:216.

54. Swenson JM, Facklam RR, Thornsberry C. Antimicrobial susceptibility of vancomycin-resistant *Leuconostoc*, *Pediococcus*, and *Lactobacillus* species. *Antimicrob Agents Chemother* 1990;34:543.

55. Noble JT, Tyburski MB, Berman M. Antimicrobial tolerance in group G streptococci. *Lancet* 1980;2:982.

56. Ruoff KL, Kuritzkes DR, Wolfson JS, et al. Vancomycin resistant gram-positive bacteria isolated from human sources. *J Clin Microbiol* 1988;26:2064.

57. Schwalbe RS, Stapleton JT, Gilligan PH. Emergence of vancomycin resistance in coagulase-negative staphylococci. *N Engl J Med* 1987;316:927.

58. Archer GL, Climo MW. Mini-review: antimicrobial susceptibility of coagulase-negative staphylococci. *Antimicrob Agents Chemother* 1994;38:2231.

59. Smith TL, Pearson ML, Wilcox KR, et al. Emergence of vancomycin resistance in *Staphylococcus aureus*. *N Engl J Med* 1999;340:493.

60. Mandell GL, Lindsey E, Hook EW. Synergism of vancomycin and streptomycin for enterococci. *Am J Med Sci* 1970;259:346.

61. Harwick HB, Kalmanson GM, Guze LB. In vitro activity of ampicillin or vancomycin combined with gentamicin or streptomycin against enterococci. *Antimicrob Agents Chemother* 1973;4:383.

62. Watanakunakorn C, Tisone JC. Synergism between vancomycin and gentamicin or tobramycin for methicillin-susceptible and methicillin-resistant *Staphylococcus aureus* strains. *Antimicrob Agents Chemother* 1982;22:903.

63. Ein ME, Smith NJ, Aruffo JF, et al. Susceptibility and synergy studies of methicillin-resistant *Staphylococcus epidermidis*. *Antimicrob Agents Chemother* 1979;16:655.

64. Lowy F, Wexler MA, Steigbigel NH. Therapy of methicillin-resistant *Staphylococcus epidermidis* experimental endocarditis. *J Lab Clin Med* 1982;100:94.

65. Tuazon CU, Lin MYC, Sheagren JN. In vitro activity of rifampin alone and in combination with nafcillin and vancomycin against pathogenic strains of *Staphylococcus aureus*. *Antimicrob Agents Chemother* 1978;13:759.

66. Tuazon CU, Miller H. Comparative in vitro activities of teichomycin and vancomycin alone and in combination with rifampin and aminoglycosides against staphylococci and enterococci. *Antimicrob Agents Chemother* 1984;25:411.

67. Bayer AS, Morrison JO. Disparity between time-kill and checkerboard methods for determination of in vitro bactericidal interactions of vancomycin plus rifampin versus methicillin-susceptible and -resistant *Staphylococcus aureus*. *Antimicrob Agents Chemother* 1984;26:220.

68. Zinner SH, Lagast H, Klastersky J. Antistaphylococcal activity of rifampin with other antibiotics. *J Infect Dis* 1981;144:365.

69. Watanakunakorn C, Guerriero JC. Interaction between vancomycin and rifampin against *Staphylococcus aureus*. *Antimicrob Agents Chemother* 1981;19:1089.

70. Hackbarth CJ, Chambers HF. Methicillin-resistant staphylococci: genetics and mechanisms of resistance. *Antimicrob Agents Chemother* 1989;33:991.

71. Bryan CS, White WL. Safety of oral vancomycin in functionally anephric patients. *Antimicrob Agents Chemother* 1978;14:634.

72. Spitzer PG, Eliopoulos GM. Systemic absorption of enteral vancomycin in a patient with pseudomembranous colitis. *Ann Intern Med* 1984;100:533.

73. Pasic M, Carrel T, Opravil M, et al. Systemic absorption after local intracolonic vancomycin in pseudomembranous colitis. *Lancet* 1993;342:443.

74. Matzke GR, Zhanel GG, Guay DRP. Clinical pharmacokinetics of vancomycin. *Clin Pharmacol* 1986;11:257.

75. Krogstad DJ, Moellering RC Jr, Greenblatt DJ. Single-dose kinetics of intravenous vancomycin. *J Clin Pharmacol* 1980;20:197.

76. Moellering RC Jr. Pharmacokinetics of vancomycin. *J Antimicrob Chemother* 1984;14:43.

77. Cunha BA, Quintiliani R, Deglin JM, et al. Pharmacokinetics of vancomycin in anuria. *Rev Infect Dis* 1981;3:S269.

78. Healy DP, Polk RE, Garson ML, et al. Comparison of steady state pharmacokinetics of two dosage regimens of vancomycin in normal volunteers. *Antimicrob Agents Chemother* 1987;31:393.

79. Rotschafer JC, Crossley K, Zaske DE, et al. Pharmacokinetics of vancomycin: observations in 28 patients and dosage recommendations. *Antimicrob Agents Chemother* 1982;22:391.

80. Geraci JE, Heilman FR, Nichols DR, et al. Some laboratory and clinical experiences with a new antibiotic, vancomycin. *Antibiot Ann* 1957;1956–1957:90.

81. Glew RH, Pavuk RA, Hennick K. *Vancomycin pharmacokinetics and toxicity.* Presented at the 13th International Congress of Chemotherapy, August 28–September 2, 1983, Vienna, Austria.

82. Viladrich PF, Gudiol F, Linares J, et al. Evaluation of vancomycin for therapy of adult pneumococcal meningitis. *Antimicrob Agents Chemother* 1991;35: 2467.

83. Morris A, Low DE. Nosocomial bacterial meningitis, including central nervous system shunt infections. *Infect Dis Clin North Am* 1999;13:735.

84. Krontz DP, Strausbaugh LJ. Effect of meningitis and probenecid on the penetration of vancomycin into cerebrospinal fluid in rabbits. *Antimicrob Agents Chemother* 1980;18:882.

85. Luer MS, Hatton J. Vancomycin administration into the cerebrospinal fluid: a review. *Ann Pharmacother* 1995;27:912.

86. Albanese J, Leone M, Bruguerolle B, et al. Cerebrospinal fluid penetration and pharmacokinetics of vancomycin administered by continuous infusion to mechanically ventilated patients in an intensive care unit. *Antimicrob Agents Chemother* 2000;44:1356.

87. MacIlwaine WA, Sande MA, Mandell GL. Penetration of antistaphylococcal antibiotics into the human eye. *Am J Ophthalmol* 1974;77:589.

88. Torres JR, Sanders CV, Lewis AC. Vancomycin concentration in human tissues: preliminary report. *J Antimicrob Chemother* 1979;5:475.

89. Graziani AL, Lawson LA, Gibson GA, et al. Vancomycin concentrations in infected and noninfected human bone. *Antimicrob Agents Chemother* 1988;32:1320.

90. Massias L, Dubois C, de Lentdecker P, et al. Penetration of vancomycin in uninfected sternal bone. *Antimicrob Agents Chemother* 1992;36:2539.

91. Cockcroft DW, Gault MH. Prediction of creatinine clearance from serum creatinine. *Nephron* 1976;16:31.

92. Nielsen HE, Hansen HE, Korsager B, et al. Renal excretion of vancomycin in kidney disease. *Acta Med Scand* 1975;197:261.

93. Leonard AE, Boro MS. Vancomycin pharmacokinetics in middle-aged and elderly men. *Am J Hosp Pharm* 1994;51:798.

94. Rodvold KA, Blum RA, Fischer JH, et al. Vancomycin pharmacokinetics in patients with various degrees of renal function. *Antimicrob Agents Chemother* 1988;32:848.

95. Rybak MJ, Boike SC. Monitoring vancomycin therapy. *Drug Intell Clin Pharm* 1986;20:757.

96. Musa DM, Pauly DJ. Evaluation of a new vancomycin dosing method. *Pharmacotherapy* 1987;7:69.

97. Teasley DG, Gerding DN, Olson MM, et al. Prospective randomised trial of metronidazole versus vancomycin for *Clostridium difficile*-associated diarrhoea and colitis. *Lancet* 1983;2:1043.

98. Fekety R, Silva J, Kaufman C, et al. Treatment of antibiotic-associated *Clostridium difficile* colitis with oral vancomycin: comparison of two dosage regimens. *Am J Med* 1989;86:15.

99. Böhler J, Reetze-Bonorden P, Keller E, et al. Rebound of plasma vancomycin levels after haemodialysis with highly permeable membranes. *Eur J Clin Pharmacol* 1992;42:635.

100. Quale JM, O'Halloran JJ, DeVincenzo N, et al. Removal of vancomycin by high-flux hemodialysis membranes. *Antimicrob Agents Chemother* 1992;36:1424.

101. Keane WF, Everett ED, Fine RN, et al. Continuous ambulatory peritoneal dialysis (CAPD) peritonitis treatment recommendations: 1989 update. *Perit Dial Int* 1989;9:247.

102. Peterson PK, Matzke G, Keane WF. Current concepts in the management of peritonitis in patients undergoing continuous ambulatory peritoneal dialysis. *Rev Infect Dis* 1987;9:604.

103. Blevins RD, Halstenson CE, Salem NG, et al. Pharmacokinetics of vancomycin in patients undergoing continuous ambulatory peritoneal dialysis. *Antimicrob Agents Chemother* 1984;25:603.

104. Morse GD, Farolino DF, Apicella MA, et al. Comparative study of intraperitoneal and intravenous vancomycin pharmacokinetics during continuous ambulatory peritoneal dialysis. *Antimicrob Agents Chemother* 1987;31:173.

105. Bailie GR, Morton R, Ganguli L, et al. Intravenous or intraperitoneal vancomycin for the treatment of continuous ambulatory peritoneal dialysis-associated gram-positive peritonitis? *Nephron* 1987;46:316.

106. Boyce NW, Wood C, Thompson NM, et al. Intraperitoneal (IP) vancomycin therapy for CAPD peritonitis: a prospective, randomized comparison of intermittent versus continuous therapy. *Am J Kidney Dis* 1988;4:304.

107. Freiman JP, Graham DJ, Reed TG, et al. Chemical peritonitis following the intraperitoneal administration of vancomycin. *Perit Dial Int* 1992;12:57.

108. Garrelts JC, Peterie JD. Altered vancomycin dose vs. serum concentration relationship in burn patients. *Clin Pharmacol Ther* 1988;44:9.

109. Blouin RA, Bauer LA, Miller DD, et al. Vancomycin pharmacokinetics in normal and morbidly obese subjects. *Antimicrob Agents Chemother* 1982;21: 575.

110. Brown N, Ho DHW, Fong K-LL, et al. Effects of hepatic function on vancomycin clinical pharmacology. *Antimicrob Agents Chemother* 1983;23:603.

110a. Schaad UB, Nelson JD, McCracker GH Jr. Pharmacology and efficacy of vancomycin for staphylococcal infections in children. *Rev Infect Dis* 1981;3:S282.

111. Chang D, Liem L, Malogolowkin M. A prospective study of vancomycin pharmacokinetics and dosage requirements in pediatric cancer patients. *Pediatr Infect Dis* 1994;13:969.

112. James A, Koren G, Milliken J, et al. Vancomycin pharmacokinetics and dose recommendations for preterm infants. *Antimicrob Agents Chemother* 1987;31:52.

113. Seay RE, Brundage RC, Jensen PD, et al. Population pharmacokinetics of vancomycin in neonates. *Clin Pharmacol Ther* 1994;56:169.

114. American Academy of Pediatrics. Antibacterial drugs for newborn infants. In: Pickering LK, ed. 2000 *Red book: report of the Committee of Infectious Diseases* (25th ed.). Elk Grove Village, IL: American Academy of Pediatrics, 2000: 652.

115. Farber BF, Moellering RC Jr. Retrospective study of the toxicity of preparations of vancomycin from 1974 to 1981. *Antimicrob Agents Chemother* 1983;23:138.

116. Polk RE, Healy DP, Schwartz LB, et al. Vancomycin and the red-man syndrome: pharmacodynamics of histamine release. *J Infect Dis* 1988;157:502.

117. Newfield P, Roizen MF. Hazards of rapid administration of vancomycin. *Ann Intern Med* 1979;91:581.

118. Healy DP, Sahai JV, Fuller SH, et al. Vancomycin-induced histamine release and "red man syndrome": comparison of land 2-hour infusions. *Antimicrob Agents Chemother* 1990;34:550.

119. Wallace MR, Mascola JR, Oldfield EC. Red man syndrome: incidence, etiology, and prophylaxis. *J Infect Dis* 1991;164:1180.

120. Sahai J, Healy DP, Garris R, et al. Influence of antihistamine pretreatment on vancomycin-induced red man syndrome. *J Infect Dis* 1989;160:876.

121. Wong JT, Ripple RE, MacLean JA, et al. Vancomycin hypersensitivity: synergism with narcotics and "desensitization" by a rapid continuous intravenous protocol. *J Allergy Clin Immunol* 1994;94:189.

122. Bergeron L, Boucher FD. Possible red-man syndrome associated with systemic absorption of oral vancomycin in a child with normal renal function. *Ann Pharmacother* 1994;28:581.

123. Griffith RS. Introduction to vancomycin. *Rev Infect Dis* 1981;3:S200.

124. Sorrell TC, Collignon PJ. A prospective study of adverse reactions associated with vancomycin therapy. *J Antimicrob Chemother* 1985;16:235.

125. Markman M, Lim HW, Bluestein HG. Vancomycin-induced vasculitis. *South Med J* 1986;79:382.

126. Zenon GJ, Cadle RM, Hamill RJ. Vancomycin-induced thrombocytopenia. *Arch Intern Med* 1991;151:995.

127. Kesarwala HH, Rahill WJ, Amaram N. Vancomycin-induced neutropenia [Letter]. *Lancet* 1981;1:1423.

128. Farwell AP, Kendall LG Jr, Vakil RD, et al. Delayed appearance of vancomycin-induced neutropenia in a patient with chronic renal failure. *South Med J* 1984;77:664.

129. Brummet RE, Fox KE. Vancomycin- and erythromycin-induced hearing loss in humans. *Antimicrob Agents Chemother* 1989;33:791.

130. Bailie GR, Neal D. Vancomycin ototoxicity and nephrotoxicity: a review. *Med Toxicol* 1988;3:376.

131. Wold JS, Turnipseed SA. Toxicology of vancomycin in laboratory animals. *Rev Infect Dis* 1981;3:S224.

132. Downs NJ, Niehart RE, Dolezal JM, et al. Mild nephrotoxicity associated with vancomycin use. *Arch Intern Med* 1989;149:1777.

133. Kirby WMM. Vancomycin therapy in severe staphylococcal infections. *Rev Infect Dis* 1981;3:S236.

134. Geraci JE, Wilson WR. Vancomycin therapy for infective endocarditis. *Rev Infect Dis* 1981;3:S250.

135. Lowy FD. *Staphylococcus aureus* infections. *N Engl J Med* 1998;339:520.

136. Levine DP, Fromm BS, Reddy BR. Slow response to vancomycin or vancomycin plus rifampin in methicillin-resistant Staphylococcus aureus endocarditis. *Ann Intern Med* 1991;115:674.

137. Small PM, Chambers HF. Vancomycin for *Staphylococcus aureus* endocarditis in intravenous drug users. *Antimicrob Agents Chemother* 1990;34:1227.

138. Myers JP, Linnemann CC Jr. Bacteremia due to methicillin-resistant *Staphylococcus aureus*. *J Infect Dis* 1982;145:532.

139. Cafferkey MT, Hone R, Keane CT. Antimicrobial chemotherapy of septicemia due to methicillin-resistant Staphylococcus aureus. *Antimicrob Agents Chemother* 1985;28:819.

140. Sieradzki K, Roberts EB, Haber SW, et al. The development of vancomycin resistance in a patient with methicillin-resistant *Staphylococcus aureus* infection. *N Engl J Med* 1999;340:517.

141. Ford C, Hamel JS, Moerman J, et al. Oxazolidinones: a new class of antimicrobials. *Infect Med* 1999;16:435.

142. Rupp ME, Archer GL. Coagulase-negative staphylococci: pathogens associated with medical progress. *Clin Infect Dis* 1994;19:231.

143. Wade JC, Schimpff SC, Newman KA, et al. *Staphylococcus epidermidis:* an increasing cause of infection in patients with granulocytopenia. *Ann Intern Med* 1982;97:503.

144. Karchmer AW, Archer GL, Dismukes WE. *Staphylococcus epidermidis*

causing prosthetic valve endocarditis: microbiology and clinical observation as guides to therapy. *Ann Intern Med* 1983;98:447.

145. Swayne R, Rampling A, Newsom SWB. Intraventricular vancomycin for treatment of shunt-associated ventriculitis. *J Antimicrob Chemother* 1987;19:249.

146. Gillespie WJ. Prevention and management of infection after total joint replacement. *Clin Infect Dis* 1997;25:1310.

147. Mermel LA, Farr BM, Sherertz RJ, et al. Guidelines for the management of intravascular catheter-related infections. *Clin Infect Dis* 2001;32:1249.

148. Dickinson GM, Bisno AL. Infections associated with indwelling devices: infections related to extravascular devices. *Antimicrob Agents Chemother* 1989;33:602.

149. Evans RC, Holmes CJ. Effect of vancomycin hydrochloride on *Staphylococcus epidermidis* biofilm associated with silicone elastomer. *Antimicrob Agents Chemother* 1987;31:889.

150. Weber DJ, Hoffman KL, Thoft RA, et al. Endophthalmitis following intraocular lens implantation: report of 30 cases and review of the literature. *Rev Infect Dis* 1986;8:12.

151. Press OW, Ramsey PG, Larson EB, et al. Hickman catheter infections in patients with malignancies. *Medicine* (Baltimore)1984;63:189.

152. Wilson WR, Karchmer AW, Dajani AS, et al. Antibiotic treatment of adults with infective endocarditis due to streptococci, enterococci, staphylococci, and HACEK microorganisms. *JAMA* 1995;274;1706.

153. Leggiadro RJ. The clinical impact of resistance in the management of pneumococcal disease. *Infect Dis Clin North Am* 1997;11:867.

154. Whitney CG, Farley MN, Hadler J, et al. Increasing prevalence of multidrug-resistant Streptococcus pneumoniae in the United States. *N Engl J Med* 2000;343:1917.

155. Lipsky BA, Goldberger AC, Tompkins LS, et al. Infections caused by nondiphtheria corynebacteria. *Rev Infect Dis* 1982;4:1220.

156. Riebel W, Frantz N, Adelstein D, et al. *Corynebacterium* JK: a cause of nosocomial device-related infection. *Rev Infect Dis* 1986;8:42.

157. Oliva SL, Guglielmo BJ, Jacobs R, et al. Failure of intravenous vancomycin and intravenous metronidazole to prevent or treat antibiotic-associated pseudomembranous colitis. *J Infect Dis* 1989;159:1154.

158. Hughes WT, Armstrong DJ, Bodey GP, et al. Guidelines for the use of antimicrobial agents in neutropenic patients with unexplained fever. *Clin Infect Dis* 1997;25:551.

159. Bow EJ, Loewen R, Vaughan D. Reduced requirement for antibiotic therapy targeting gram-negative organisms in febrile, neutropenic patients with cancer who are receiving antibacterial chemoprophylaxis with oral quinolones. *Clin Infect Dis* 1995;20:907.

160. McLaurin RL, Frame PT. Treatment of infections of cerebrospinal fluid shunts. *Rev Infect Dis* 1987;9:595.

161. Gump DW. Vancomycin for treatment of bacterial meningitis. *Rev Infect Dis* 1981;3:S289.

162. Durack DT. Prevention of infective endocarditis. *N Engl J Med* 1995;332:38.

163. Murray BE. Vancomycin-resistant enterococcal infections. *N Engl J Med* 2000;342:710.

164. Hayden MK. Insights into the epidemiology and control of infection with vancomycin-resistant enterococci. *Clin Infect Dis* 2000;31:1058.

165. Brogden RN, Peters DH. Teicoplanin: a reappraisal of its antimicrobial activity, pharmacokinetic properties and therapeutic efficacy. *Drugs* 1994;47:823.

166. Somma S, Gastaldo L, Corti A. Teicoplanin, a new antibiotic from *Actinoplanes teichomyceticus* nov. sp. *Antimicrob Agents Chemother* 1984;26:917.

167. Parenti F. Structure and mechanism of action of teicoplanin. *J Hosp Infect* 1986;7(Suppl):79.

168. Parenti F. Glycopeptide antibiotics. *J Clin Pharmacol* 1988;28:136.

169. Lagast H, Dodion P, Klastersky J. Comparison of pharmacokinetics and bactericidal activity of teicoplanin and vancomycin. *J Antimicrob Chemother* 1986;18:513.

170. Verbist L, Tjandramaga B, Hendrickx B, et al. In vitro activity and human pharmacokinetics of teicoplanin. *Antimicrob Agents Chemother* 1984;26:881.

171. Williams AH, Gruneberg RN. Teicoplanin. *J Antimicrob Chemother* 1984;14:441.

172. Hayden MK, Trenholme GM, Schultz JE, et al. In vivo development of teicoplanin resistance in a VanB *Enterococcus faecium* isolate. *J Infect Dis* 1993;167:1224.

173. Pallanza R, Berti M, Goldstein BP, et al. Teicoplanin: in vitro and in vivo evaluation and comparison to other antibiotics. *J Antimicrob Chemother* 1983;11:419.

174. Drabu YJ, Walsh B, Blakemore PH, et al. Teicoplanin in infections caused by methicillin-resistant staphylococci. *J Antimicrob Chemother* 1987;21(Suppl):89.

175. Stille W, Sietzen W, Dieterich H-A, et al. Clinical efficacy and safety of teicoplanin. *J Antimicrob Chemother* 1988;21(Suppl):69.

176. Bibler MR, Frame PT, Hagler DN, et al. Clinical evaluation of efficacy, pharmacokinetics, and safety of teicoplanin for serious gram-positive infections. *Antimicrob Agents Chemother* 1987;31:207.

177. Calain P, Krause K-H, Vaudaux P, et al. Early termination of a prospective, randomized trial comparing teicoplanin and flucloxacillin for treating severe staphylococcal infections. *J Infect Dis* 1987;155:187.

178. Galanakis N, Giamarellou H, Vlachogiannis N, et al. Poor efficacy of teicoplanin in treatment of deep-seated staphylococcal infections. *Eur J Clin Microbiol Infect Dis* 1988;7:130.

179. Fortún J, Pérez-Molina JA, Añón MT, et al. Right-sided endocarditis caused by *Staphylococcus aureus* in drug abusers. *Antimicrob Agents Chemother* 1995;39:525.

180. Rolston KVI, Nguyen H, Amos G, et al. A randomized double blind trial of vancomycin versus teicoplanin for the treatment of gram-positive bacteremia in patients with cancer. *J Infect Dis* 1994;169:350.

181. Menichetti F, Martino P, Bucaneve G, et al. Effects of teicoplanin and those of vancomycin in initial empirical antibiotic regimen for febrile, neutropenic patients with hematologic malignancies. *Antimicrob Agents Chemother* 1994;38:2041.

182. Schmit JL. Efficacy of teicoplanin for enterococcal infections: 63 cases and review. *Clin Infect Dis* 1992;15:302.

183. De Lalla F, Privitera G, Rinaldi E, et al. Treatment of *Clostridium docile*-associated disease with teicoplanin. *Antimicrob Agents Chemother* 1989;33:1125.

184. Fridkin SK. Vancomycin-intermediate and resistant *Staphylococcus aureus*: what the infectious disease specialist needs to know. *Clin Infect Dis* 2001;32:108.

CHAPTER 24
Oxazolidinones, Quinupristin-Dalfopristin, and Daptomycin

Raul E. Davaro, Richard H. Glew, and Jennifer S. Daly

OXAZOLIDINONES

The oxazolidinones are a chemically distinct class of synthetic antibiotics initially developed in the 1980s by E. I. DuPont de Nemours and Company for control of bacterial and fungal foliage diseases of plants. This new class of antimicrobials inhibits bacterial protein synthesis by preventing formation of the initiation complex. Linezolid (Zyvox), the first oxazolidinone approved by the U.S. Food and Drug Administration (FDA) for use in humans, was developed by Pharmacia and Upjohn in the 1990s by modifying the oxazolidinone molecule to improve toxicity profile. The oxazolidinones have activity against gram-positive organisms, including methicillin-resistant *Staphylococcus aureus* (MRSA), glycopeptide-intermediate *Staphylococcus aureus* (GISA), vancomycin-resistant enterococci (VRE), and penicillin-resistant *Streptococcus pneumoniae* (PRSP). Linezolid exhibits bacteriostatic activity against staphylococci and enterococci and bactericidal activity against streptococci. Linezolid is approved for the treatment of nosocomial pneumonia caused by *S. pneumoniae* (penicillin-susceptible strains only) or *S. aureus* (methicillin-susceptible *Staphylococcus aureus* [MSSA] and MRSA strains), community acquired pneumonia due to penicillin-susceptible *S. pneumoniae* or *S. aureus* (MRSA only), skin and skin structure infection, including those due to MRSA, and infections due to vancomycin resistant *Enterococcus faecium* (1–5).

Mechanism of Action

Oxazolidinones, as a group, target protein synthesis at an early stage. Although the precise mechanism of action has not been established conclusively, linezolid and its closely related analog, eperezolid, inhibit protein synthesis by binding to the 50S subunit within domain V of the 23S ribosomal ribonucleic acid RNA (rRNA) during formation of the preinitiation complex. By virtue of this unique mechanism of action, cross-resistance of oxazolidinones with other currently available antimicrobial agents is unlikely and has not been reported in the literature. As seen with other agents that inhibit protein synthesis (chloramphenicol, clindamycin, and macrolides), combinations of these agents with each other or with bactericidal antibiotics may be antagonistic (6–8).

Spectrum of Activity

Linezolid is active against clinically important gram-positive pathogens, including *S. aureus* (MSSA, MRSA, and GISA), enterococci (both vancomycin susceptible and VRE), coagulase-negative staphylococci, penicillin and cephalosporin-resistant *S. pneumoniae*, *Streptococcus agalactiae*, and *Streptococcus pyogenes* (minimal inhibitory concentration [MIC_{90}] of 2 to 4 mg/L). Linezolid exhibits concentration-dependent postantibiotic effect against *S. aureus*, *Staphylococcus epidermidis*, *E. faecalis*, and *S. pneumoniae* (7,8) a fact that helps support twice-daily dosing (9–11). The spectrum of activity extends to other gram-positive organisms: *Corynebacterium* species, *Listeria monocytogenes*, *Rhodococcus equi*, and *Bacillus* species (MIC_{90} less than 2 mg/L). Linezolid shows *in vitro* activity against some anaerobes, including *Clostridium perfringens* (MIC_{90} of 1 to 4 mg/L), *Clostridium difficile* (MIC_{90} of 1 to 2 mg/L), *Bacteroides fragilis* (MIC_{90} of 2 to 4 mg/L), and *Fusobacterium nucleatum* (MIC_{90} less than 0.03 to 1 mg/L) and against the pigmented nonfermentive gram-negative rod, *Flavobacterium meningosepticum* (MIC_{90} of 2 to 4 mg/L). Linezolid shows activity against *Mycobacterium tuberculosis*, *Mycobacterium avium* complex, *Legionella* and *Borrelia* species, and the rapidly growing atypical mycobacteria. Anecdotal clinical success has been reported against *Mycobacterium chelonei*, and the oxazolidinones have potential in the treatment of mycobacterial disease. Linezolid has only moderate *in vitro* activity against *Haemophilus influenzae* and is inactive against Enterobacteriaceae and *Pseudomonas aeruginosa* (1,4,12,13).

Clinical Pharmacology

Absorption of linezolid is rapid and complete (bioavailability 100%) following oral administration, with a time to peak plasma concentration of 1 to 2 hours. Linezolid absorption is unaffected by food. The volume of distribution is about 40 to 50 L. In individuals receiving multiple oral doses of 600 mg of linezolid given every 12 hours, steady-state concentration is achieved after two to four doses, and the average steady-state minimum and maximum plasma concentrations were 6.2 and 21.2 mg/L, respectively. The corresponding values for linezolid, 600 mg given every 12 hours intravenously, were 3.7 and 15.1 mg/mL. Plasma protein binding is about 30%. Linezolid is metabolized primarily in the liver by oxidation and, because the oxidation is independent of hepatic cytochrome P450 (CYP450), the drug does not induce or inhibit human CYP isoforms (cytochrome P).

The pharmacokinetics of linezolid remains unaffected in patients with mild to moderate liver disease, and dosage adjustment is unwarranted in this patient group. It appears that linezolid dosage does not need to be modified in patients with mild (40 to 79 mL minute) to moderate (creatinine clearance 10 to 39 mL per minute) renal impairment; hemodialysis removes about 38% of the administered dose (and removes the metabolites), indicating that patients on dialysis should receive the dose after the dialysis session. Metabolites of the drug may accumulate in patients with severe renal failure not yet on dialysis, but toxicity data for the metabolites is not available. If dosage adjustments are made in patients with severe renal failure serum, concentrations can be measured by high-performance liquid chromatography (HPLC). Given *in vitro* and animal data, full dosages should be used to prevent development of resistance. If serum levels fall below the MIC for the infecting organism, linezolid may not be efficacious or resistance may be expected, making underdosing a problem (14–16).

Toxicity

Short courses of linezolid in general are well tolerated. The most common adverse effects involve the gastrointestinal tract: diarrhea (8% of treated patients), nausea (6%), vomiting (4%), constipation (2%), tongue discoloration (1%), and oral moniliasis (1%). Headache (2%), rash (2%), insomnia (1%), and dizziness (1%) have been also reported. With short-course therapy in the early studies, thrombocytopenia was observed to occur at a rate of 2.4%. With therapy duration greater than 10 days, 32% of patients in one study developed thrombocytopenia (platelet count less than 100,000), and 4 required platelet transfusions. Platelet counts should be monitored in patients with preexisting thrombocytopenia and in those who receive more than 10 days of treatment. This adverse effect is usually reversible. A reversible enhancement of the vasopressor response of either pseudoephedrine hydrochloride or phenylpropanolamine is observed when linezolid is administered to healthy normotensive subjects. The oxazolidinones are weak monoamine oxidase inhibitors and have the potential for interaction with adrenergic agents used to support blood pressure in the intensive care unit or foods with a high tyramine content (1,4,16,17).

Clinical Indications

There are few comparative data in patients with endocarditis or osteomyelitis, although cures have been reported in individual cases in patients infected with organisms resistant to other agents. The advantage over older agents is the excellent oral bioavailability, but the disadvantages are cost and potential development of resistance. Until more information becomes available, linezolid should be reserved for patients with infection due to organisms resistant to older, traditional antimicrobials. Susceptibility testing against staphylococcal species is relatively easy, but laboratories should be aware that incubation of *S. pneumoniae* in carbon dioxide depresses the activity of linezolid, and testing may not be reliable given current breakpoint criteria for susceptibility (18,19).

Vancomycin-resistant Enterococcal Infections

Since first emerging in 1988, the prevalence of VRE has increased rapidly. Most clinically important VRE infections are caused by *E. faecium*, with *E. faecalis* accounting for only a small proportion. The treatment of VRE infections poses a unique set of challenges. Linezolid has been used with an efficacy of about 67% in patients with VRE urinary tract infections, pneumonia, peritonitis, bacteremia, febrile neutropenia, endocarditis, and meningitis. Infections with vancomycin-resistant *E. faecium* resistant to linezolid have been described recently in patients receiving linezolid. *In vitro*, resistance of *E. faecalis* and *E. faecium* to linezolid due to a single base-pair mutation in the 23S ribosomal RNA gene can be induced by passage in subinhibitory concentrations of the compound. There are four to six copies of the gene in enterococci, and mutations in multiple copies may cause a stepwise increase in MICs (20–26).

Staphylococcus aureus

Linezolid has been used in skin and soft-tissue infections, community- and nosocomial-acquired pneumonia, and surgical wound infections due to MSSA and MRSA (25,27–30). A strain of MRSA resistant to linezolid has been recovered in a patient receiving treatment with this agent for dialysis-associated peritonitis (31). Given the bacteriostatic activity of this class of agents, potential of thrombocytopenia, and lack of data on the treatment of endocarditis and osteomyelitis, the oxazolidinones should not replace agents such as oxacillin or vancomycin given intravenously, even though oral administration could simplify care of patients with *S. aureus*, including MRSA infections in bone or bloodstream. Linezolid has been compared against *S. aureus* (oxacillin-susceptible) with no treatment or treatment of animals with cefazolin in a dog model of osteomyelitis. Cefazolin was superior, and quantitative cultures from linezolid-treated animals were equivalent to control. In models using higher doses of linezolid, comparable efficacy to other agents was observed. When prolonged therapy is needed for difficult-to-treat infections such as endocarditis or osteomyelitis, physicians should continue to use conventional agents for susceptible strains until human clinical data are available.

Dosage

Linezolid is available in a ready-to-use sterile isotonic solution for intravenous infusion. Each mL contains 2 mg of linezolid. Linezolid is available also in tablets for oral administration containing 600 mg of linezolid and as an oral flavored granule-powder for reconstitution into a suspension for oral administration. In patients with infections caused by MRSA or VRE, the recommended dosage of linezolid (intravenous or oral) is 600 mg every 12 hours. When switching from intravenous to oral administration, there is no need for dosage adjustment. The appropriate dose of linezolid in infants and children has not been established. Linezolid has been used safely and with good tolerance and efficacy in pediatric patients as young as 12 months of age at 10 mg/kg every 12 hours (maximum, 600 mg twice daily) (30).

Linezolid has been shown to be secreted into the breast milk of lactating animals; the clinical implications of this for humans is unknown (32). There are no adequate and well-controlled studies in pregnant women.

QUINUPRISTIN-DALFOPRISTIN

Quinupristin-dalfopristin (Synercid) is a combination of two synergistic antibiotics from the streptogramin class that is part of the macrolide-lincosamide streptogramin group of agents. Quinupristin and dalfopristin have inhibitory activity against gram-positive bacteria, including difficult-to-treat organisms such as MRSA and coagulase-negative staphylococci, GISA, vancomycin-resistant *E. faecium* (VREF), penicillin-resistant and macrolide-resistant pneumococci, other streptococci, *C. perfringens*, and *Peptostreptococcus* species. The combination is bactericidal against staphylococci and streptococci that are susceptible to both of the components and bacteriostatic against *E. faecium*. Quinupristin-dalfopristin has been approved for intravenous treatment of bacteremia and life-threatening infection caused by VREF and for treatment of complicated skin and skin structure infections caused by *S. aureus* and *S. pyogenes* (33–35).

Mechanism of Action

Quinupristin and dalfopristin bind to sequential sites located on the 50S subunit of the bacterial ribosome, causing a confor-

mational change in the ribosome that subsequently increases the binding of quinupristin, thereby creating a stable drug–ribosome complex that inhibits the protein synthesis (36,37).

Spectrum of Activity

Quinupristin-dalfopristin exhibits consistently good activity against staphylococci (MIC_{90} of 0.5 to 1 mg/L for MSSA and MRSA, respectively). The *S. epidermidis* MIC_{90} ranged between 0.25 and 0.75 mg/L. Most isolates of *E. faecium* are susceptible, including vancomycin-resistant strains. The median MIC_{90} values for *E. faecium* and VREF are 2 and 1 mg/L, respectively. The combination has similar activity against *E. faecium* exhibiting VanA and VanB resistance. *E. faecalis* typically is resistant to quinupristin-dalfopristin with an MIC_{90} of greater than 8 mg/L. Quinupristin-dalfopristin has excellent activity against *S. pneumoniae*, including penicillin- and macrolide-resistant strains (MIC_{90} of 0.5 to 1 mg/L), and other streptococci, including *S. pyogenes*, *S. agalactiae*, and viridans streptococci (MIC_{90} of 0.25 mg/L, 0.12 mg/L, and 1 mg/L, respectively). The activity of the combination is variable against *Corynebacterium jeikeium* (MIC_{90} of 0.2 to 2 mg/L), *L. monocytogenes* (MIC_{90} of 0.25 to 2 mg/L), and *Leuconostoc* species (MIC_{90} of 0.25 to 8 mg/L), suggesting that other agents are preferable to treat patients with these organisms. Quinupristin-dalfopristin displays good activity against *C. perfringens* (MIC_{90} of 0.125 to 1 mg/L) and *Peptostreptococcus* species (MIC_{90} of 0.25 to 1 mg/L) and little activity against *B. fragilis* (MIC_{90} of 2 to 16 mg/L) and generally is not used to treat anaerobic infections given the availability of more active antimicrobials. Quinupristin-dalfopristin has good activity against *Moraxella catarrhalis* (MIC_{90} of 0.5 mg/L), *Mycoplasma pneumoniae* (MIC_{90} of 0.0625 mg/L), *Legionella pneumophila* (MIC_{90} of 0.12 to 1 mg/L), *Neisseria meningitidis* (MIC_{90} of 0.12 to 0.5 mg/L), and *Neisseria gonorrhoeae* (MIC_{90} of 0.5 to 2 mg/L), but clinical data are not available. Quinupristin-dalfopristin possess significant postantibiotic effect against *S. aureus* and *S. pneumoniae*. Enterobacteriaceae, *Pseudomonas aeruginosa*, and *Acinetobacter* species are inherently resistant because of cell wall impermeability (34–38).

Clinical Pharmacology

Quinupristin-dalfopristin is composed of two synthetic pristinamycin derivatives in a 30:70 (wt/wt) ratio. The combination is given by intravenous route only and undergoes hepatic metabolism by a system that is independent of CYP450 to active compounds that contribute to the antibacterial activity. The metabolites of quinupristin have MIC that is twofold higher than that of the parent compound. Based on current data, an adjustment in dosage to 5 mg/kg is warranted in patients with Child-Pugh-Turcot class A and B liver failure scores. Renal elimination plays a secondary role, and dosage adjustments are unnecessary in patients with renal failure, including those undergoing peritoneal dialysis and hemodialysis. Protein binding of quinupristin is between 55% to 78% and that of dalfopristin is between 11% to 26%, and this is not considered significant. The elimination half-lives of quinupristin and dalfopristin are about 0.85 and 0.7 hours, respectively. Age, gender, and obesity appear to have no clinical impact on the pharmacokinetics of quinupristin-dalfopristin (39–42).

Mechanism of Resistance

Three mechanisms of resistance have been described for streptogramins: modification of drug target, drug inactivation, and active efflux. Modification of drug target implies a change in residues within domain V of the 23S rRNA that are involved in the action of streptogramin antibiotics. This target modification results in an isolate resistant to quinupristin and resistant to macrolide-lincosamide-streptogramin B (MLSB) antibiotics, but not to dalfopristin, a streptogramin A derivative. Most MRSA strains in the clinical environment have constitutive (*C-MLSB*) resistance. Among MLS-resistant staphylococci, the activity of the individual agents was variable, but the combination remains active owing to the activity of the dalfopristin component (34,35).

Drug inactivation has been described in some staphylococcal and enterococcal species, mediated by production of a quinupristin-dalfopristin hydrolase or a dalfopristin-acetyltransferase. Treatment failure in some cases has been linked to the development of resistance on therapy (43). Genes involved in streptogramin efflux have been found in staphylococci (44–46).

Toxicity

Infusion site–related reactions (e.g., inflammation, burning, pain, and edema), thrombophlebitis, and nonspecific reactions are common administration-related adverse effects. Administration in a large volume of fluid, or through a central or peripherally inserted central venous catheter, minimizes these problems. Myalgias and arthralgias are the most common side effects, occur in up to 33% to 47% of patients, and appear to be dose related (47). The mechanism of arthralgias and myalgias is unknown. In severely ill patients with multiple comorbidities, the incidence of arthralgias or myalgias led to discontinuation of the treatment in 4% of the cases. Other side effects include nausea (4.6%), vomiting and diarrhea (2.5%), and skin rash (2.5%). Less common side effects (incidence less than 1%) include stomatitis, pancreatitis, pseudomembranous colitis, insomnia, anxiety, dizziness, confusion, urticaria, and maculopapular rash. Elevations in liver enzymes (2% to 7%) or total and direct bilirubin (1% to 5%), thrombocytopenia (3%), and anemia (2.6%) are the most common laboratory abnormalities found in patients receiving quinupristin-dalfopristin (35,39,40,48).

Drug Interactions

Because quinupristin-dalfopristin is an inhibitor of the CYP450 3A4 enzyme pathway, caution is warranted with the concomitant use of other medications that undergo metabolism by this system. Careful monitoring of cyclosporine levels to avoid renal toxicity is recommended in patients receiving that agent. Medications whose serum concentrations are predicted to be enhanced by quinupristin-dalfopristin include astemizole, terfenadine, delavirdine, nevirapine, ritonavir, indinavir, diazepam, midazolam, cisapride, lovastatin, tacrolimus, carbamazepine, lidocaine, disopyramide, verapamil, diltiazem, paclitaxel, docetaxel and methylprednisolone (34–36).

Clinical Indications

The greatest benefit of quinupristin-dalfopristin is likely to be in the management of patients with infections caused by multidrug vancomycin-resistant *E. faecium* or methicillin-resistant *S. aureus* (49,50). Use in these patients should be based on susceptibility results because resistance has been found in wild-type strains (51,52).

Vancomycin-resistant *Enterococcus faecium* Infections

Quinupristin-dalfopristin is highly active against VREF. VREF infections are problematic because these organisms frequently are resistant to most currently available antibiotics. The clinical efficacy of this combination is lower for intraabdominal infections and bacteremia of unknown origin (59% and 52%, respectively) than for treatment of urinary tract infections (90%), skin and soft tissue infections (73%), and central catheter–related bacteremia (84%). One of the caveats with studies of these infections is that they often resolve without specific treatment and that infection is sometimes hard to distinguish from colonization. Emergence of resistance to quinupristin-dalfopristin during treatment has been observed to occur at a rate of 4%. Therapy with quinupristin-dalfopristin may favor *E. faecalis* superinfection (43,53–56).

Quinupristin-dalfopristin shows synergy *in vitro* with doxycycline and with ampicillin-sulbactam against VREF. *In vivo* synergy using a triple combination of quinupristin-dalfopristin, doxycycline, and rifampin has been shown by kill-time assays (57,58).

Methicillin-resistant Staphylococcal Infection

Vancomycin remains the treatment of choice in patients with MRSA infections, and quinupristin-dalfopristin should be considered when others regimens have failed or caused unacceptable side effects. Intravenous quinupristin-dalfopristin has a consistent response rate more than 60% in patients with MRSA infections, but it is lower in patients with endocarditis (55% to 60%) or respiratory tract infections (30% to 58%) (59–63).

Other Uses

Quinupristin-dalfopristin has been used successfully to treat infections in an outpatient setting or step-down units, including infections such as cellulitis, wound infections, peritonitis, empyema, community- and nosocomial-acquired pneumonia, and septic arthritis, but given its need for intravenous administration, other drugs are preferable if the pathogen is susceptible (64).

Dosage

The recommended adult dosage of quinupristin-dalfopristin is 7.5 mg/kg intravenously every 8 hours (for nosocomial infections and VREF infections) or every 12 hours (for complicated skin and soft tissue infections); the dose should be infused over 60 minutes. Quinupristin-dalfopristin is supplied in a 500-mg (150-mg quinupristin, 350-mg dalfopristin) preparation for intravenous use. If venous irritation occurs following peripheral venous administration, consideration should be given to increasing the infusion volume to 500 or 750 mL, changing the infusion site, or infusing using a peripherally inserted central catheter (PICC) or a central venous catheter.

Experience in pediatric patients is limited. Children treated with quinupristin-dalfopristin have received 7.5 mg/kg two or three times daily. Anecdotal observations have been published describing the use of quinupristin-dalfopristin intrathecally and in peritoneal dialysis patients. Quinupristin is excreted in the milk of lactating rats. Caution should be exercised when considering this drug in nursing women. No studies have been done in pregnant women, and it should be used only if the benefits outweigh the potential risks in this group (39–42).

DAPTOMYCIN

Daptomycin is a cyclic lipopeptide derived from *Streptomyces roseosporus*. Daptomycin exhibits rapid, concentration-dependent bactericidal activity *in vitro* against a broad range of susceptible and resistant gram-positive bacterial pathogens, including MRSA, VRE, PRSP, and GISA strains. Daptomycin is inactive against gram-negative bacteria. The mechanism of action of daptomycin, although not yet fully elucidated, is unique, killing by disrupting multiple aspects of bacterial plasma membrane function without penetrating the cytoplasm. It has a prolonged postantibiotic effect. The drug is excreted primarily through the kidney, with low potential for interference with hepatically metabolized drugs (65,66).

Doses of 6 mg/kg of body weight have been shown to be potentially effective against some type of infections. Higher doses of 8 mg/kg of body weight, divided in two doses administered every 12 hours, resulted in reversible myopathy of the skeletal muscle. Once-a-day dosing seems to optimize daptomycin safety (66–68).

REFERENCES

1. Bung H, Kirshenbaum H, Batatunde O. Linezolid: an oxazolidinone antimicrobial agent. *Clin Ther* 2001;23:356.
2. Daly JS, Eliopoulos GM, Willey S, et al. Mechanism of action and in vitro and in vivo activities of s-6123, a new oxazolidinone compound. *Antimicrob Agents Chemother* 1988;32:1341.
3. Daly JS, Eliopoulos GM, Reiszner E, et al. Activity and mechanism of action of dup 105 and dup 721, new oxazolidinone compounds. *J Antimicrob Chemother* 1988;21:721.
4. Perry CM, Jarvis B. Linezolid: a review of its use in the management of serious gram-positive infections. *Drugs* 2001;61:525.
5. Anonymous. Linezolid (Zyvox). *Med Lett Drugs Ther* 2000;42:45.
6. Lin AH, Murray RW, Vidmar TJ, et al. The oxazolidinone eperezolid binds to the 50s ribosomal subunit and competes with binding of chloramphenicol and lincomycin. *Antimicrob Agents Chemother* 1997;41:2127.
7. Shinabarger DL, Marotti KR, Murray RW, et al. Mechanism of action of oxazolidinones: effects of linezolid and eperezolid on translation reactions. *Antimicrob Agents Chemother* 1997;41:2132.
8. Swaney SM, Aoki H, Ganoza MC, et al. The oxazolidinone linezolid inhibits initiation of protein synthesis in bacteria. *Antimicrob Agents Chemother* 1998;42:3251.
9. Cercenado E, Garcia-Garrote F, Bouza E. In vitro activity of linezolid against multiply resistant gram-positive clinical isolates. *J Antimicrob Chemother* 2001; 47:77.
10. Gemmell CG. Susceptibility of a variety of clinical isolates to linezolid: A European inter-country comparison. *J Antimicrob Chemother* 2001;48:47.
11. Munckhof WJ, Giles C, Turnidge JD. Post-antibiotic growth suppression of linezolid against gram-positive bacteria. *J Antimicrob Chemother* 2001;47: 879.
12. Brown-Elliott BA, Wallace RJ Jr, Blinkhorn R, et al. Successful treatment of disseminated *Mycobacterium chelonei* infection with linezolid. *Clin Infect Dis* 2001;33:1433.
13. Cynamon MH, Klemens SP, Sharpe CA, et al. Activities of several novel oxazolidinones against mycobacterium tuberculosis in a murine model. *Antimicrob Agents Chemother* 1999;43:1189.
14. Slatter JG, Stalker DJ, Feenstra KL, et al. Pharmacokinetics, metabolism, and excretion of linezolid following an oral dose of [(14)C]linezolid to healthy human subjects. *Drug Metab Dispos* 2001;29:1136.
15. Gee T, Ellis R, Marshall G, et al. Pharmacokinetics and tissue penetration of linezolid following multiple oral doses. *Antimicrob Agents Chemother* 2001;45: 1843.
16. Dresser LD, Rybak MJ. The pharmacologic and bacteriologic properties of oxazolidinones, a new class of synthetic antimicrobials. *Pharmacotherapy* 1998; 18:456.
17. Attassi K, Hershberger E, Alam R, et al. Thrombocytopenia associated with linezolid therapy. *Clin Infect Dis* 2002;34:695.
18. Hamilton-Miller JM, Shah S. Susceptibility testing of linezolid by two standard methods. *Eur J Clin Microbiol Infect Dis* 1999;18:225.
19. Biedenbach DJ, Jones RN. In vitro activity of linezolid (u-100766) against *Haemophilus influenzae* measured by three different susceptibility testing methods. *Diagn Microbiol Infect Dis* 2001;39:49.
20. Bailey EM, Faber MD, Nafziger DA. Linezolid for treatment of vancomycin-resistant enterococcal peritonitis. *Am J Kidney Dis* 2001;38:E20.
21. Chien JW, Kucia ML, Salata RA. Use of linezolid, an oxazolidinone, in the treatment of multidrug-resistant gram-positive bacterial infections. *Clin Infect Dis* 2000;30:146.
22. Babcock HM, Ritchie DJ, Christiansen E, et al. Successful treatment of vancomycin-resistant enterococcus endocarditis with oral linezolid. *Clin Infect Dis* 2001;32:1373.
23. Prystowsky J, Siddiqui F, Chosay J, et al. Resistance to linezolid: characterization of mutations in rRNA and comparison of their occurrences in vancomycin-resistant enterococci. *Antimicrob Agents Chemother* 2001;45:2154.
24. Gonzales RD, Schreckenberger PC, Graham MB, et al. Infections due to vancomycin-resistant *Enterococcus faecium* resistant to linezolid. *Lancet* 2001; 357:1179.
25. Zeana C, Kubin CJ, Della-Latta P, et al. Vancomycin-resistant *Enterococcus faecium* meningitis successfully managed with linezolid: case report and review of the literature. *Clin Infect Dis* 2001;33:477.
26. Rice LB. Resistance mutations to linezolid. In press.
27. Li Z, Willke RJ, Pinto LA, et al. Comparison of length of hospital stay for patients with known or suspected methicillin-resistant staphylococcus species infections treated with linezolid or vancomycin: A randomized, multicenter trial. *Pharmacotherapy* 2001;21:263.
28. Melzer M, Goldsmith D, Gransden W. Successful treatment of vertebral osteomyelitis with linezolid in a patient receiving hemodialysis and with persistent methicillin-resistant *Staphylococcus aureus* and vancomycin-resistant *Enterococcus* bacteremias. *Clin Infect Dis* 2000;31:208.
29. Stevens DL, Smith LG, Bruss JB, et al. Randomized comparison of linezolid (pnu-100766) versus oxacillin-dicloxacillin for treatment of complicated skin and soft tissue infections. *Antimicrob Agents Chemother* 2000;44:3408.
30. Rubinstein E, Cammarata S, Oliphant T, et al. Linezolid (pnu-100766) versus vancomycin in the treatment of hospitalized patients with nosocomial pneumonia: a randomized, double-blind, multicenter study. *Clin Infect Dis* 2001;32: 402.
31. Tsiodras S, Gold HS, Sakoulas G, et al. Linezolid resistance in a clinical isolate of *Staphylococcus aureus*. *Lancet* 2001;358:207.
32. Chin KG, Mactal-Haaf C, McPherson CE. Use of anti-infective agents during lactation: Part 1—β-Lactam antibiotics, vancomycin, quinupristin-dalfopristin, and linezolid. *J Hum Lact* 2000;16:351.
33. Anonymous. Quinupristin/dalfopristin. *Med Lett Drugs Ther* 1999;41:109.
34. Delgado G Jr, Neuhauser MM, Bearden DT, et al. Quinupristin-dalfopristin: an overview. *Pharmacotherapy* 2000;20:1469.
35. Lamb HM, Figgitt DP, Faulds D. Quinupristin/dalfopristin: a review of its use in the management of serious gram-positive infections. *Drugs* 1999;58:1061.
36. Allington DR, Rivey MP. Quinupristin/dalfopristin: a therapeutic review. *Clin Ther* 2001;23:24.
37. Bonfiglio G, Furneri PM. Novel streptogramin antibiotics. *Expert Opin Investig Drugs* 2001;10:185.
38. Ling TK, Fung KS, Cheng AF. In vitro activity and post-antibiotic effect of quinupristin/dalfopristin (Synercid). *Chemotherapy* 2001;47:243.
39. Rubinstein E, Prokocimer P, Talbot GH. Safety and tolerability of quinupristin/dalfopristin: administration guidelines. *J Antimicrob Chemother* 1999;44[Suppl A]:37.
40. Rotschafer JC, Wright DH, Brown GH. Gram-positive infections: pharmacy issues and strategy for quinupristin/dalfopristin. *Diagn Microbiol Infect Dis* 1999;33:95.
41. Chevalier P, Rey J, Pasquier O, et al. Pharmacokinetics of quinupristin/dalfopristin in patients with severe chronic renal insufficiency. *Clin Pharmacokinet* 2000;39:77.
42. Johnson CA, Taylor CA 3rd, Zimmerman SW, et al. Pharmacokinetics of quinupristin-dalfopristin in continuous ambulatory peritoneal dialysis patients. *Antimicrob Agents Chemother* 1999;43:152.
43. Winston DJ, Emmanouilides C, Kroeber A, et al. Quinupristin/dalfopristin therapy for infections due to vancomycin-resistant enterococcus faecium. *Clin Infect Dis* 2000;30:790.
44. Bozdogan B, Leclercq R. Effects of genes encoding resistance to streptogramins a and b on the activity of quinupristin-dalfopristin against *Enterococcus faecium*. *Antimicrob Agents Chemother* 1999;43:2720.
45. Dowzicky M, Talbot GH, Feger C, et al. Characterization of isolates associated with emerging resistance to quinupristin/dalfopristin (Synercid) during a worldwide clinical program. *Diagn Microbiol Infect Dis* 2000;37:57.
46. Soltani M, Beighton D, Philpott-Howard J, et al. Mechanisms of resistance to quinupristin-dalfopristin among isolates of enterococcus faecium from animals, raw meat, and hospital patients in Western Europe. *Antimicrob Agents Chemother* 2000;44:433.
47. Olsen KM, Rebuck JA, Rupp ME. Arthralgias and myalgias related to quinupristin-dalfopristin administration. *Clin Infect Dis* 2001;32:e83.
48. Dodge RA, Daly JS, Davaro R, et al. High-dose ampicillin plus streptomycin for treatment of a patient with severe infection due to multiresistant enterococci. *Clin Infect Dis* 1997;25:1269.
49. Jones RN, Low DE, Pfaller MA. Epidemiologic trends in nosocomial and community-acquired infections due to antibiotic-resistant gram-positive bacteria: the role of streptogramins and other newer compounds. *Diagn Microbiol Infect Dis* 1999;33:101.
50. Livermore DM. Quinupristin/dalfopristin and linezolid: where, when, which and whether to use? *J Antimicrob Chemother* 2000;46:347.
51. Werner G, Klare I, Heier H, et al. Quinupristin/dalfopristin-resistant enterococci of the sata (vatd) and satg (vate) genotypes from different ecological origins in Germany. *Microb Drug Resist* 2000;6:37.

52. Werner G, Cuny C, Schmitz FJ, et al. Methicillin-resistant, quinupristin-dalfopristin-resistant *Staphylococcus aureus* with reduced sensitivity to glycopeptides. *J Clin Microbiol* 2001;39:3586.

53. Linden PK, Moellering RC Jr, Wood CA, et al. Treatment of vancomycin-resistant *Enterococcus faecium* infections with quinupristin/dalfopristin. *Clin Infect Dis* 2001;33:1816.

54. Moellering RC. Quinupristin/dalfopristin: therapeutic potential for vancomycin-resistant enterococcal infections. *J Antimicrob Chemother* 1999; 44[Suppl A]:25.

55. Moellering RC, Linden PK, Reinhardt J, et al., for the Synercid Emergency-Use Study Group. The efficacy and safety of quinupristin/dalfopristin for the treatment of infections caused by vancomycin-resistant enterococcus faecium. *J Antimicrob Chemother* 1999;44:251.

56. Murray BE. Vancomycin-resistant enterococcal infections. *N Engl J Med* 2000; 342:710.

57. Matsumura SO, Louie L, Louie M, et al. Synergy testing of vancomycin-resistant *Enterococcus faecium* against quinupristin-dalfopristin in combination with other antimicrobial agents. *Antimicrob Agents Chemother* 1999;43:2776.

58. Matsumura S, Simor AE. Treatment of endocarditis due to vancomycin-resistant *Enterococcus faecium* with quinupristin/dalfopristin, doxycycline, and rifampin: a synergistic drug combination. *Clin Infect Dis* 1998;27:1554.

59. Pechere JC. Current and future management of infections due to methicillin-resistant staphylococci infections: the role of quinupristin/dalfopristin. *J Antimicrob Chemother* 1999;44[Suppl A]:11.

60. Drew RH, Perfect JR, Srinath L, et al., for the Synercid Emergency-Use Study Group. Treatment of methicillin-resistant *Staphylococcus aureus* infections with quinupristin-dalfopristin in patients intolerant of or failing prior therapy. *J Antimicrob Chemother* 2000;46:775.

61. Raad I, Bompart F, Hachem R. Prospective, randomized dose-ranging open phase ii pilot study of quinupristin/dalfopristin versus vancomycin in the treatment of catheter-related staphylococcal bacteremia. *Eur J Clin Microbiol Infect Dis* 1999;18:199.

62. Fagon J, Patrick H, Haas DW, et al., for the Nosocomial Pneumonia Group. Treatment of gram-positive nosocomial pneumonia: prospective randomized comparison of quinupristin/dalfopristin versus vancomycin. *Am J Respir Crit Care Med* 2000;161:753.

63. Nichols RL, Graham DR, Barriere SL, et al., for the Synercid Skin and Skin Structure Infection Group. Treatment of hospitalized patients with complicated gram-positive skin and skin structure infections: two randomized, multicentre studies of quinupristin/dalfopristin versus cefazolin, oxacillin or vancomycin. *J Antimicrob Chemother* 1999;44:263.

64. Rehm SJ, Graham DR, Srinath L, et al. Successful administration of quinupristin/dalfopristin in the outpatient setting. *J Antimicrob Chemother* 2001; 47:639.

65. Rybak MJ, Hershberger E, Moldovan T, et al. In vitro activities of daptomycin, vancomycin, linezolid, and quinupristin-dalfopristin against staphylococci and enterococci, including vancomycin-intermediate and -resistant strains. *Antimicrob Agents Chemother* 2000;44:1062.

66. Tally FP, DeBruin MF. Development of daptomycin for gram-positive infections. *J Antimicrob Chemother* 2000;46:523.

67. Oleson FB Jr, Berman CL, Kirkpatrick JB, et al. Once-daily dosing in dogs optimizes daptomycin safety. *Antimicrob Agents Chemother* 2000;44: 2948.

68. Muangsiri W, Kirsch LE. The kinetics of the alkaline degradation of daptomycin. *J Pharm Sci* 2001;90:1066.

CHAPTER 25

Trimethoprim-Sulfamethoxazole

Richard Gleckman and Claudia Altschuller-Felberg

Trimethoprim-sulfamethoxazole (TMP-SMX) is a fixed-dose combination chemotherapeutic agent that became available in the United States in oral form in 1973. The parenteral preparation was released in 1981. The drug is marketed in the United States under the trade names Bactrim and Septra and is known in numerous countries as co-trimoxazole. Standard-dose oral tablets have 80 mg of TMP and 400 mg of SMX. The liquid form has 40 mg of TMP and 200 mg of SMX per 5 mL. Each 5-mL vial of parenteral TMP-SMX for infusion contains 80 mg of TMP and 400 mg of SMX.

MECHANISM OF ACTION

Sulfamethoxazole, a bacteriostatic synthetic compound and structural analog of paraaminobenzoic acid, competitively inhibits the incorporation of paraaminobenzoic acid into tetrahydropteric acid. As a member of the sulfonamide family of drugs, sulfamethoxazole inhibits the microbial enzyme dihydropteroate synthetase. TMP, a dihydrofolate reductase inhibitor, impedes the conversion of dihydrofolate to tetrahydrofolate (1). In essence, these compounds, sulfamethoxazole and TMP, produce a sequential blockade of folic acid synthesis in microorganisms.

PHARMACOKINETICS

For most susceptible bacteria, maximal synergistic inhibition occurs at a serum ratio for TMP-SMX of 1:20. By preparing the drugs in a fixed 1:5 ratio, peak serum concentrations of TMP and SMX of about 1:20 are achieved by administration of the oral and parenteral compounds.

ORAL ADMINISTRATION

Both TMP and SMX are absorbed well from the gastrointestinal tract, even by patients with enteritis. Peak serum levels average about 1.75 μg/mL for TMP and 37.5 μg/mL for non–protein-bound SMX after a single double-strength tablet is ingested by patients with normal renal function. The peak serum levels of TMP and SMX occur at 2 and 4 hours, respectively. TMP is 45% bound to plasma protein, and SMX is 66% plasma bound.

PARENTERAL ADMINISTRATION

After intravenous infusion, peak concentrations of TMP and SMX are more predictable and occur more rapidly—in about 1 to 1.5 hours. When intravenous doses are infused at 8-hour intervals, the mean plasma peak and trough concentrations of TMP are 8.8 μg/mL and 5.6 μg/mL, and the mean peak and trough concentrations of SMX are 105.6 μg/mL and 70.7 μg/mL, respectively.

Penetration of TMP and SMX into tissues and body fluids is not identical, often resulting in a therapeutic ratio that deviates from the presumed ideal serum ratio of 1:20. TMP and SMX are metabolized primarily through hepatic mechanisms. Five to 30% of TMP is metabolized to oxide and hydroxylated metabolites, and about 20% of SMX is metabolized, by glucuronidation, but predominantly by N-acetylation. About half of each drug's dose is excreted in the urine; however, nearly all the TMP is excreted in an active, nonmetabolized form, whereas only 20% of SMX is excreted intact.

Tissue concentrations of SMX are generally less than the corresponding serum or plasma concentrations. TMP concentrations in saliva, breast milk, uninflamed prostatic tissue, seminal fluid, inflamed lung tissue, and bile often exceed those measured in the serum. Penetration of TMP-SMX into cerebrospinal fluid (CSF) is variable; concentration ranges of TMP vary from 20% to 60% of the levels obtained in the serum and those of SMX from 12% to 50%.

In patients with normal renal function, the half-life of TMP is 11 hours, and that of SMX is 9 hours. The usual adult parenteral dosage is 2 to 3 vials every 8 hours administered intravenously; the typical oral dose is one single- or double-strength tablet every 12 hours. Dosage of TMP-SMX in children is based on the severity of the infectious process and on body weight: the usual oral dose is 8 mg/kg per day for TMP and 40 mg/kg per day for SMX given at 12-hour intervals; daily parenteral doses are based on 10 mg/kg for TMP and 50 mg/kg for SMX divided into three doses. The dose of TMP-SMX must be adjusted for patients with renal insufficiency, particularly when the creatinine clearance rate approaches 30 mL minute. For both oral and parenteral use, a single loading dose of TMP-SMX is given as if no renal impairment existed, followed by one half to one third of the usual amount administered at the same dose interval for the duration of therapy. Urinary concentrations of TMP and SMX are reduced in patients with severely compromised renal function, but the levels achieved appear adequate to treat patients harboring traditional bacterial uropathogens, including *Escherichia coli* and indole-negative *Proteus* species (2).

Serum drug concentrations should be monitored in patients undergoing hemodialysis to help adjust the dosage. After a loading dose, follow-up doses (one half or one third of the original dose) are administered every 24 to 48 hours to patients undergoing dialysis.

Minimal data exist as to the proper dose of TMP-SMX for patients who require chronic peritoneal dialysis (3). Peritoneal losses contribute insignificantly to TMP-SMX elimination during continuous ambulatory peritoneal dialysis. The consensus is that these patients should receive one double-strength tablet administered every 48 hours.

ADVERSE REACTIONS

Adverse drug reactions occur in 6% to 8% of patients who do not have acquired immunodeficiency syndrome (AIDS). Nearly half of the adverse reactions develop within 72 hours of drug administration. Discontinuation of the medication almost always results in the resolution of the drug-associated adverse reaction. The most common adverse reactions include gastrointestinal distress (particularly nausea and vomiting) and cutaneous events (morbilliform, maculopapular, urticarial eruptions) (4). Less commonly, additional gastrointestinal reactions (diarrhea, pseudomembranous colitis, altered taste, stomatitis, glossitis, pancreatitis, and hepatocellular or cholestatic liver injury) and cutaneous reactions (photosensitivity rash, drug eruption, erythema multiforme, and toxic epidermal necrolysis) have been attributed to TMP-SMX.

The central nervous system is, on occasion, the target for drug-induced adverse reactions, as manifested by headache, insomnia, vertigo, confusion, tremor, acute psychosis, and a syndrome consistent with "septic meningitis" (5,6).

Patients receiving TMP-SMX have experienced anaphylaxis, serum sickness with polyarthritis, pruritus or fever unassociated with rash, acute interstitial nephritis, and vasculitis (7). A wide range of hematological abnormalities (leukopenia, thrombocytopenia, agranulocytosis, hemolytic anemia, aplastic anemia) and metabolic derangements (hyperkalemia, very rarely hypoglycemia) have been ascribed to TMP-SMX (8–10). Individuals with glucose-6-phosphate dehydrogenase deficiency are at risk for hemolytic anemia when prescribed TMP-SMX. Isolated case reports suggest an association between the administration of TMP-SMX and the development of uveitis, torsades de pointes, and acute febrile neutrophilic dermatosis (Sweet's syndrome) (11,12).

TMP-SMX is the preferred medication for both the primary or secondary prophylaxis and definitive treatment of disease caused by *Pneumocystis carinii* for patients with human immunodeficiency virus (HIV) infection. These patients have not tolerated TMP-SMX well, however, and often this medication must be prematurely discontinued. Some researchers have suggested that pharmacokinetic monitoring of the serum concentrations of TMP and SMX can be helpful to reduce adverse reactions when patients with AIDS receive TMP-SMX to manage *Pneumocystis carinii* pneumonia (PCP) (13,14). This approach to drug administration has not become the standard of care, however. Limited data also suggest that gradual initiation of TMP-SMX for primary PCP prophylaxis reduced the incidence and severity of treatment-limiting toxicity compared with routine initiation (15).

Two forms of systemic hypersensitivity reactions have been observed in HIV-infected patients who receive TMP-SMX (16,17). The first, a rare event, resembles septic shock and is characterized by the sudden onset of fever, rash, hypotension, and diffuse pulmonary infiltrates experienced by patients who had previously (usually within the previous few weeks) received TMP-SMX. The mechanism of this severe, unusual reaction to TMP-SMX is not known, but it has features of both immunoglobulin E (IgE)-mediated anaphylaxis and tumor necrosis–mediated effects. Fortunately, with discontinuation of the TMP-SMX and supportive therapies, patients experience resolution of these severe hypersensitivity reactions.

A much more common drug hypersensitivity syndrome consists of a combination of any of the following features: fever, skin reactions, transaminase elevations, and hematological abnormalities. These adverse drug reactions are noted after a week of TMP-SMX therapy. Many patients experiencing this hypersensitivity syndrome can safely continue to receive TMP-SMX and experience resolution of their adverse reactions either spontaneously or with the assistance of adjunctive measures, such as an antihistamine, antipyretic, or corticosteroid (18).

There have been extensive research efforts to understand the pathogenesis of TMP-SMX–induced hypersensitivity reactions. Although the precise mechanisms remain unknown, the available data suggest that the SMX-hydroxylamine metabolite and the slow acetylation phenotype are risk factors involved in the pathogenesis of hypersensitivity to TMP-SMX in HIV-infected patients (19).

The clinician has a number of options to consider when an HIV-infected patient experiences an adverse reaction attributed to TMP-SMX: continuing the treatment (which has been safe for most patients who have experienced minor adverse reactions); discontinuing the treatment and offering an alternative medication; or, after the adverse reactions have subsided, either rechallenging the patient (rarely followed by a severe hypersensitivity reaction) or offering a program of incremental administration, known as *desensitization* (rarely causing a severe hypersensitivity reaction or toxic epidermal necrolysis) (20). No evidence-based research has been conducted to offer the clinician meaningful guidelines. One study suggests that comparable effectiveness occurs when desensitization is compared with rechallenge for patients who have experienced a previous, non–life-threatening adverse reaction to TMP-SMX (21).

DRUG INTERACTIONS

TMP-SMX has the potential to enhance the anticoagulant effect of warfarin, and, when there is coadministration, predispose to adverse drug reactions caused by phenytoin, methotrexate, cyclosporine, and the oral sulfonylurea-hypoglycemic compounds. Elderly patients who receive both TMP-SMX and a thiazide diuretic are at risk for thrombocytopenia. TMP has the ability to increase serum digoxin concentrations in elderly patients, presumably owing to decreased renal tubular secretion of digoxin. Coadministration of lamivudine with TMP-SMX results in an increased area under the concentration–time curve and decrease in renal clearance of lamivudine, but it is unlikely that these alterations have clinical significance (22).

Pharmacodynamic interactions are of concern for the HIV-infected patient when TMP-SMX is administered concomitantly with those compounds that have the potential to cause similar toxicities. Examples include the following: pancreatitis (when didanosine, zalcitabine, pentamidine, or hydroxyurea is administered); rash/hypersensitivity events (when nevirapine or abacavir is administered); and neutropenia (when ganciclovir or zidovudine is administered).

ANTIMICROBIAL SPECTRUM

Introduced in the United States 28 years ago, TMP-SMX was heralded as an inexpensive, broad-spectrum, fixed-dose combination agent, which was considered to exert synergistic effect and capable of inhibiting resistance to each of the component medications. It was initially viewed as an antimicrobial with an ability to inhibit the growth of those bacterial pathogens that commonly contribute to respiratory tract infections (*Streptococcus pneumoniae, Haemophilus influenzae, Moraxella catarrhalis*), skin infections (*Staphylococcus aureus*), urinary tract infections (*E. coli*; *Klebsiella, Enterobacter*, and *Proteus* species), infectious enterocolitis (*Shigella* and *Salmonella* species, enterotoxigenic *E. coli*) and sexually transmitted diseases (*Neisseria gonorrhoeae, Haemophilus ducreyi*). Subsequently, it was appreciated that TMP-SMX possessed inhibitory activity, as well as clinical efficacy for infections caused by *Serratia* and *Brucella* species, *Yersinia enterocolitica, Stenotrophomonas maltophilia, Burkholderia cepacia, Nocardia asteroides, Listeria monocytogenes, Mycobacterium marinum*, fungi (*P. carinii*), and coccidian parasites (*Isospora belli, Cyclospora cayetanensis*). *In vitro* susceptibility to *Enterococcus* species has not translated into *in vivo* activity (23).

During the past two decades, however, there has been a dramatic increase in resistance to TMP-SMX. The SENTRY antimicrobial surveillance program has identified high rates of resistant *S. pneumoniae* and *H. influenzae* in the United States as well as resistant extended-spectrum β-lactamase–producing *E. coli, Proteus mirabilis*, and *Salmonella* species (24). In a nationwide study of the susceptibility pattern of *E. coli* isolates recovered from the urine of adult female outpatients, the resistance ranged from 10% in the Northeast to 22% in western United States (25). Extensive resistance to *Shigella* species, enterotoxigenic *E. coli, Salmonella* species, methicillin-resistant *S. aureus, N. gonorrhoeae*, and *H. ducrei* has reduced the value of TMP-SMX in the management of infections caused by these organisms. Resistance to TMP-SMX has been associated with treatment failure for patients with acute, bacterial, community-acquired pyelonephritis and AIDS patients with PCP (caused by organisms demonstrating a mutation in dihydropteroate synthase gene) (26,27).

Bacterial resistance to TMP-SMX is mediated by permeability barrier and efflux pumps, naturally insensitive target enzymes, regulational changes in the target enzymes, recombinational changes in the target enzymes, and acquired resistance by drug-resistant target enzymes (28).

PREGNANCY

TMP-SMX has been accorded a pregnancy category C by the U.S. Food and Drug Administration (FDA). There is a concern that TMP inhibits folate metabolism and that a decrease in the concentration of folate in red blood cells is associated with an increased risk for neural tube defects in genetically disposed individuals. There is also the concern that during the third trimester, SMX administration could contribute to kernicterus. Limited data, derived retrospectively from women who received TMP-SMX to manage urinary tract infections, during pregnancy, failed to reveal increased evidence of congenital abnormalities. More recently, however, researchers have reported that HIV-infected pregnant women, who were administered combination antiretroviral therapy with TMP-SMX, did have fetuses with severe spinal malformations (29).

THERAPEUTIC INDICATIONS

The clinical indications for TMP-SMX have declined because of the rapid spread of resistance to this compound, the potential of the drug to cause unexpected and serious hypersensitivity reactions, and the recent introduction of newer fluoroquinolones as well as novel antimicrobial compounds. In addition, researchers have noted that a number of the therapeutic indications for TMP-SMX can be managed as effectively with less risk for adverse reactions by prescribing TMP as monotherapy (30,31).

PREVENTION

Pneumocystis carinii Pneumonia

Primary TMP-SMX chemoprophylaxis against PCP is recommended for those adults (including those pregnant women and those on HAART) who are HIV-infected and have a CD4$^+$ T-lymphocyte count of less than $200/\mu$L or a history of oropharyngeal candidiasis (32). Secondary chemoprophylaxis is indicated for those adult patients who have previously experienced PCP and are unable through HAART to sustain a T-lymphocyte count of more than $200/\mu$L. The TMP-SMX is administered as one double-strength tablet per day; however, one single-strength tablet per day is effective and better tolerated. The prophylaxis can be discontinued when the patient manifests a sustained increase in CD4$^+$ T-lymphocyte counts to more than 200 cells/μL. Prophylaxis with TMP-SMX should not be discontinued when the HIV-infected patient has a concomitant disorder that causes immunodeficiency (e.g., non-Hodgkin's lymphoma) or the patient receives immunosuppressive medication (a corticosteroid). This prophylaxis appears to offer an additional benefit, namely, prevention of disease caused by *Listeria* species, *Nocardia* species, *Toxoplasma gondii, Salmonella* species, or *H. influenzae* (33).

In addition to specific HIV-infected patients, there are selective immunocompromised hosts who are candidates for *P. carinii* prophylaxis with TMP-SMX. These are patients who are not allergic to the medication and have received an allogeneic bone marrow transplantation or a solid organ transplantation, or who have autoimmune disorders and are receiving a daily glucocorticosteroid combined with a cytotoxic agent, such as cyclophosphamide, azathioprine, or methotrexate (34). Transplant recipients should receive prophylaxis with one single-strength (80 mg TMP, 400 SMX) tablet for the first 6 months after transplantation. This prophylaxis appears to offer an additional benefit, namely, prevention of urinary tract infections, as well as disease caused by *Listeria* species, *Nocardia* species, and *T. gondii*.

Prophylaxis beyond 6 months is indicated for those individuals who have persistent risk factors for the development of PCP. This includes patients who have experienced multiple episodes of rejection treated with OKT3 monoclonal antibodies and patients with persistent allograft dysfunction, particularly when they receive augmented immunosuppressive treatment.

Neutropenic Patient

Prophylactic TMP-SMX administration, as one tablet containing 160 mg TMP and 800 mg SMX every 12 hours, to selective patients (those with acute myelogenous leukemia, recipients of marrow transplantation) who had profound (less than 100 absolute neutrophils) and prolonged neutropenia (1 week or greater) has, in some clinical trials, resulted in a reduction in febrile episodes (presumably infectious) and the need to administer antibiotics as well as a diminution of serious invasive bacterial infections. These potential advantages of prophylactic TMP-SMX are, to some extent, counterbalanced by the ability of TMP-SMX to cause toxicity, including myelosuppression; to foster the emergence of resistant bacteria; and to produce suprainfection from bacteria and fungi.

Enterocolitis

TMP-SMX, administered as one double-strength tablet each day, is one of many drugs that have been used for the prevention of the clinical syndrome known as traveler's diarrhea. Unfortunately, however, with the worldwide increasing resistance of enterotoxigenic *E. coli*, as well as other bacterial enteropathogens commonly causing traveler's diarrhea, TMP-SMX is no longer considered an optimum prophylactic or therapeutic agent for this disorder (35).

In addition to its historical role as a safe, inexpensive, and effective prophylactic agent to prevent acute symptomatic bacterial cystitis in young women who experience more than three episodes per year, TMP-SMX has an established prophylactic value to prevent spontaneous bacterial peritonitis in patients with alcoholic cirrhosis complicated with ascites, to reduce relapses in patients with Wegener's granulomatosis in remission, and in patients with AIDS, to offer secondary prophylaxis for intestinal disease caused by the protozoa *I. belli* (36–37).

TREATMENT OF ESTABLISHED INFECTIONS

Respiratory Infections

TMP-SMX has been effective therapy to treat patients with community-acquired acute maxillary sinusitis, otitis media, an exacerbation of chronic bronchitis, and pneumonia caused by susceptible strains of *S. pneumoniae, H. influenzae,* and *Branhamalla catarrhalis,* as well as patients with nosocomial pneumonia caused by susceptible strains of Enterobacteriaceae.

TMP-SMX is the agent of choice to treat pulmonary and extrapulmonary disease caused by *P. carinii.* Prednisone is added to the treatment when the PaO$_2$ is less than 70 mm Hg or the A-a gradient is more than 35 mm Hg.

Urinary Infections

TMP-SMX has an established track record for the management of women with acute bacterial cystitis and pyelonephritis; men with acute and chronic bacterial prostatitis; and men with asymptomatic bacterial invasive infections, when caused by susceptible Enterobacteriaceae.

Enterocolitis

TMP-SMX is the preferred drug treatment for patients with enterocolitis caused by *I. belli* or *C. cayetanensis* (38). TMP-SMX has been an effective compound for the patient with disease caused by *Y. enterocolitica* and drug-susceptible *Shigella* species.

Meningitis and Encephalitis

TMP-SMX is a therapeutic consideration for the patient with a known history of significant penicillin allergy who develops meningitis caused by *L. monocytogenes,* and it appears to be an effective treatment of cerebral toxoplasmosis in patients with AIDS (39).

Miscellaneous

TMP-SMX has an established therapeutic niche for the treatment of patients with infections caused by unusual susceptible organisms, including *Stenotrophomonas maltophilia, Burkholderia (Pseudomonas) cepacia, Chryseobacterium meningosepticum, Ochrobactrum anthropi,* and *Achromobacter xylosoxidans,* as well as *Mycobacterium fortuitum* and *Mycobacterium marinum.* TMP-SMX is an appropriate drug selection with or without additional compounds to treat patients with invasive disease caused by *Nocardia asteroides* and *Pseudomonas pseudomallei,* patients with Whipple's disease, and patients with Wegener's granulomatosis. TMP-SMX, when combined with gentamicin, is one of the recommended therapies for patients with brucellosis and is a medication to be considered for the patient with "complicated" cat-scratch disease.

TMP-SMX is one of the suggested alternative oral agents to treat diabetic patients with foot infections regarded as mild or moderate in severity, when these patients are intolerant of or allergic to clindamycin or β-lactam antibiotics (40).

TMP-SMX is also an alternative to vancomycin, linezolid, and quinupristin-dalfopristin to treat patients with methicillin-resistant *S. aureus*-related infections (41).

REFERENCES

1. Burchall JJ. Mechanism of action of trimethoprim-sulfamethoxazole. *J Infect Dis* 1973;128[Suppl]:437–444.
2. Craig WA, Kunin CM. Trimethoprim-sulfamethoxazole: pharmacodynamic effects of urinary pH and impaired renal function. *Ann Intern Med* 1973;78:491–497.
3. Walker SE, Paton DN, Churchill B, et al. Trimethoprim-sulfamethoxazole pharmacokinetics during continuous ambulatory peritoneal dialysis (CAPD). *Perit Dial Int* 1989;9:51–55.
4. Cribb AE, Lee BL, Trepanier LA, et al. Adverse reactions to sulphonamide and sulphonamide-trimethoprim antimicrobials: clinical syndromes and pathogenesis. *Adverse Drug React Toxicol Rev* 1996;15:9–50.
5. Patterson RG, Couchenour RL. Trimethoprim-sulfamethoxazole-induced tremor in an immunocompetent patient. *Pharmacotherapy* 1999;19:1456–1458.
6. Muller MP, Richardson DC, Walmsley SL. Trimethoprim-sulfamethoxazole induced aseptic meningitis in a renal transplant patient. *Clin Nephrol* 2001;55:80–84.
7. Sen Sait, Bayrak R, Ok E, et al. Drug-induced acute interstitial nephritis and vasculitis or vascular rejection in renal allografts. *Am J Kidney Dis* 2001;37:1–4.
8. Keisu M, Viholm BE, Palmblad J. Trimethoprim-sulphamethoxazole-associated blood dyscrasias: ten years' experience of the Swedish spontaneous reporting system. *J Intern Med* 1990;228:353–360.
9. George JN, Raskob GE, Shah SR, et al. Drug-induced thrombocytopenia: a systematic review of published case reports. *Ann Intern Med* 1998;129:886–890.
10. Alappan R, Perazella MA, Buller GK. Hyperkalemia in hospitalized patients treated with trimethoprim-sulfamethoxazole. *Ann Intern Med* 1996;124:316–320.
11. Lopez JA, Harold JG, Rosenthal MC, et al. QT prolongation and torsades de pointes after administration of trimethoprim-sulfamethoxazole. *Am J Cardiol* 1987;59:376–377.
12. Walker DC, Cohen PR. Trimethoprim-sulfamethoxazole-associated acute febrile neutrophilic dermatosis: case report and review of drug-induced Sweet's syndrome. *J Am Acad Dermatol* 1996;34:918–923.
13. Sattler FR, Cowan R, Nielsen DM, et al. Trimethoprim-sulfamethoxazole compared with pentamidine for treatment of Pneumocystis carinii pneumonia in the acquired immunodeficiency syndrome. *Ann Intern Med* 1988;109:280–287.
14. Klinker H, Langmann P, Zully M, et al. Drug monitoring during the treatment of AIDS-associated *Pneumocystis carinii* pneumonia with trimethoprim-sulfamethoxazole. *J Clin Pharm Ther* 1998;23:149–154.

15. Para MF, Finkelstein D, Becker S, et al. Reduced toxicity with gradual initiation of trimethoprim-sulfamethoxazole as primary prophylaxis for *Pneumocystis carinii* pneumonia: AIDS clinical trials group 268. *J AIDS* 2000;24:337–343.

16. Kelly JW, Dooley DP, Lattuada CP, et al. A severe, unusual reaction to trimethoprim-sulfamethoxazole in patients infected with human immunodeficiency virus. *Clin Infect Dis* 1992;14:1034–1039.

17. Martin GJ, Paparello SF, Docker CF. A severe systemic reaction to trimethoprim-sulfamethoxazole in a patient infected with the human immunodeficiency virus. *Clin Infect Dis* 1993;16:175–176.

18. Gordin FM, Simon GL, Wofsy CB, et al. Adverse reactions to trimethoprim-sulfamethoxazole in patients with the acquired immunodeficiency syndrome. *Ann Intern Med* 1984;100:495–499.

19. Koopmans PP, van der Ven AJ, Vree TB, et al. Pathogenesis of hypersensitivity reactions to drugs in patients with HIV infection: allergic or toxic? *AIDS* 1995;9:217–222.

20. Jung AC, Paauw DS. Management of adverse reactions to trimethoprim-sulfamethoxazole in human immunodeficiency virus-infected patients. *Arch Intern Med* 1994;154:2402–2406.

21. Bonfanti P, Pusterla L, Parazzini F, et al. The effectiveness of desensitization versus rechallenge treatment in HIV-positive patients with previous hypersensitivity to TMP-SMX: a randomized multicentric study. *Biomed Pharmacother* 2000;54:45–49.

22. Moore KHP, Yuen GJ, Raasch RH, et al. Pharmacokinetics of lamivudine administered alone and with trimethoprim-sulfamethoxazole. *Clin Pharmacol Ther* 1996;59:550–558.

23. Goodhart GL. In vivo v in vitro susceptibility of enterococcus to trimethoprim-sulfamethoxazole *JAMA* 1984;252:2748–2749.

24. Hoban DJ, Doern GV, Fluit AC, et al. Worldwide prevalence of antimicrobial resistance in *Streptococcus pneumoniae, Haemophilus influenzae*, and *Moraxella catarrhalis* in the SENTRY antimicrobial surveillance program, 1997–1999. *Clin Infect Dis* 2001;32[Suppl 2]:581–593.

25. Gupta K, Sahm DF, Mayfield D, et al. Antimicrobial resistance among uropathogens that cause community-acquired urinary tract infections in women: a nationwide analysis. *Clin Infect Dis* 2001;33:89–94.

26. Talan DA, Stamm WE, Hooton TM, et al. Comparison of ciprofloxacin (7 days) and trimethoprim-sulfamethoxazole (14 days) for acute uncomplicated pyelonephritis in women: a randomized trial. *JAMA* 2000;283:1583–1590.

27. Mei Q, Gurunathan S, Masur H, et al. Failure of co-trimoxazole in *Pneumocystis carinii* infection and mutations in dihydropteroate synthase gene. *Lancet* 1998;351:1631–1632.

28. Huovinen P. Resistance to trimethoprim-sulfamethoxazole. *Clin Infect Dis* 2001;32:1608–1614.

29. Richardson MP, Osrin D, Donaghy S, et al. Spinal malformations in the fetuses of HIV infected women receiving combination antiretroviral therapy and co-trimoxazole. *Eur J Obstet Gynecol Reprod Biol* 2000;93:215–217.

30. Brumfitt W, Hamilton-Miller JMT. Limitations of and indications for the use of co-trimoxazole. *J Chemother* 1994;6:3–11.

31. Howe RA, Spencer RC. Cotrimoxazole: rationale for re-examining its indications for use. *Drug Safety* 1996;14:213–218.

32. 1999 USPHS/IDSA guidelines for the prevention of opportunistic infections in persons infected with human immunodeficiency virus. *MMWR Morb Mortal Wkly Rep* 1999;48[RR-10]:1–70.

33. Dworkin MS, Williamson J, Jones JL, et al. Prophylaxis with trimethoprim-sulfamethoxazole for human immunodeficiency virus infected patients: impact on risk for infectious diseases. *Clin Infect Dis* 2001;33:393–398.

34. CDD: CDC/IDSA/ASBMT guidelines for the prevention of opportunistic infection (OIs) in hematopoietic stem cell transplantation (HSCT) recipients. *MMWR Morb Mortal Wkly Rep* 2000;49[RR10]:1–128.

35. Ryan ET, Kain KC. Health advice and immunization for travelers. *N Engl J Med* 2000;343:1045–1046.

36. Singh N, Gaywoski T, Yu VL, et al. Trimethoprim-sulfamethoxazole for the prevention of spontaneous bacterial peritonitis in cirrhosis: a randomized trial. *Ann Intern Med* 1995;122:595–598.

37. Stegeman CA, Tervaert JWC, de Jong PE, et al. Trimethoprim-sulfamethoxazole (co-trimoxazole) for the prevention of relapses of Wegener's granulomatosis. *N Engl J Med* 1996;335:16–20.

38. Verdier RI, Fitzgerald DW, Johnson WD, et al. Trimethoprim-sulfamethoxazole compared with ciprofloxacin treatment and prophylaxis of *Isospora belli* and *Cyclospora cayetanensis* infection in HIV-infected patients: a randomized, controlled trial. *Ann Intern Med* 2000;132:885–888.

39. Torre D, Speranza F, Martegani R, et al. A retrospective study of treatment of cerebral toxoplasmosis in AIDS patients with trimethoprim-sulphamethoxazole. *J Infect* 1998;37:15–18.

40. Lipsky BA. Evidence-based antibiotic therapy of diabetic foot infections. *FEMS Immunol Med Microbiol* 1999;26:267–276.

41. Markowitz N, Quinn EL, Saravolatz LD. Trimethoprim-sulfamethoxazole compared with vancomycin for the treatment of Staphylococcus aureus infection. *Ann Intern Med* 1992;117:390–398.

CHAPTER 26
Quinolones

Vincent T. Andriole

The first of the quinolone antibacterial agents, nalidixic acid, was introduced in 1962 (1). Oxolinic acid and cinoxacin were introduced in the 1970s. These compounds had limited clinical use. Shortly thereafter, several key discoveries led to better compounds with superior properties: addition of a fluorine atom at C-6 enhanced antibacterial potency; a piperazine group at C-7 improved activity against aerobic gram-negative bacteria and staphylococci; a second fluorine group at C-8 increased absorption and half-life, but also increased phototoxicity; ring alkylation improved anti–gram-positive activity and half-life; a cyclopropyl group at N-1, an amino group at C-5, and a fluorine at C-8 increased activity against mycoplasmas and chlamydiae; and addition of a methoxy group at C-8 targeted both topoisomerase II and IV and probably decreased development of quinolone resistance. These changes led to the development of numerous new compounds of clinical importance because of their broad antibacterial spectrum, unique mechanism of action, good absorption from the gastrointestinal tract after oral or intravenous administration, excellent tissue distribution, and low incidence of adverse reactions (2,3).

CHEMISTRY AND CLASSIFICATION

The quinolone antibacterial agents, although structurally similar, can be divided into four general groups: naphthyridines, cinnolines, pyridopyrimidines, and quinolines (Fig. 26.1). A common skeleton, 4-oxo-1,4-dihydroquinolone (4-quinolone), is produced by adding an oxygen molecule at the 4 position in the basic nucleus (2). The naphthyridines (nalidixic acid, enoxacin, tosufloxacin, trovafloxacin, and gemifloxacin), with an additional nitrogen in the 8 position, are 8-aza-4-quinolones. The cinnolines (cinoxacin), with a second nitrogen in the 2 position, are 2-aza-4-quinolones. The pyridopyrimidines (pipemidic and piromidic acids), with additional nitrogens in the 6 and 8 positions, are 6,8-diaza-4-quinolones (Fig. 26.2). All of the other highly active agents are classified as 4-quinolones (2,3). Numerous additional compounds have been synthesized, and some are undergoing development (3).

The 1,8-naphthyridine derivatives include nalidixic acid (1-ethyl-7-methyl-1, 8-naphthyridin-4-one-3-carboxylic acid),

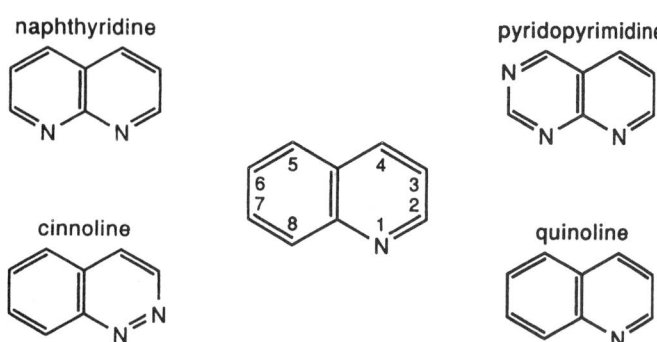

Figure 26.1. Chemical structure of the four general groups of the quinolones and the system of ring numbering.

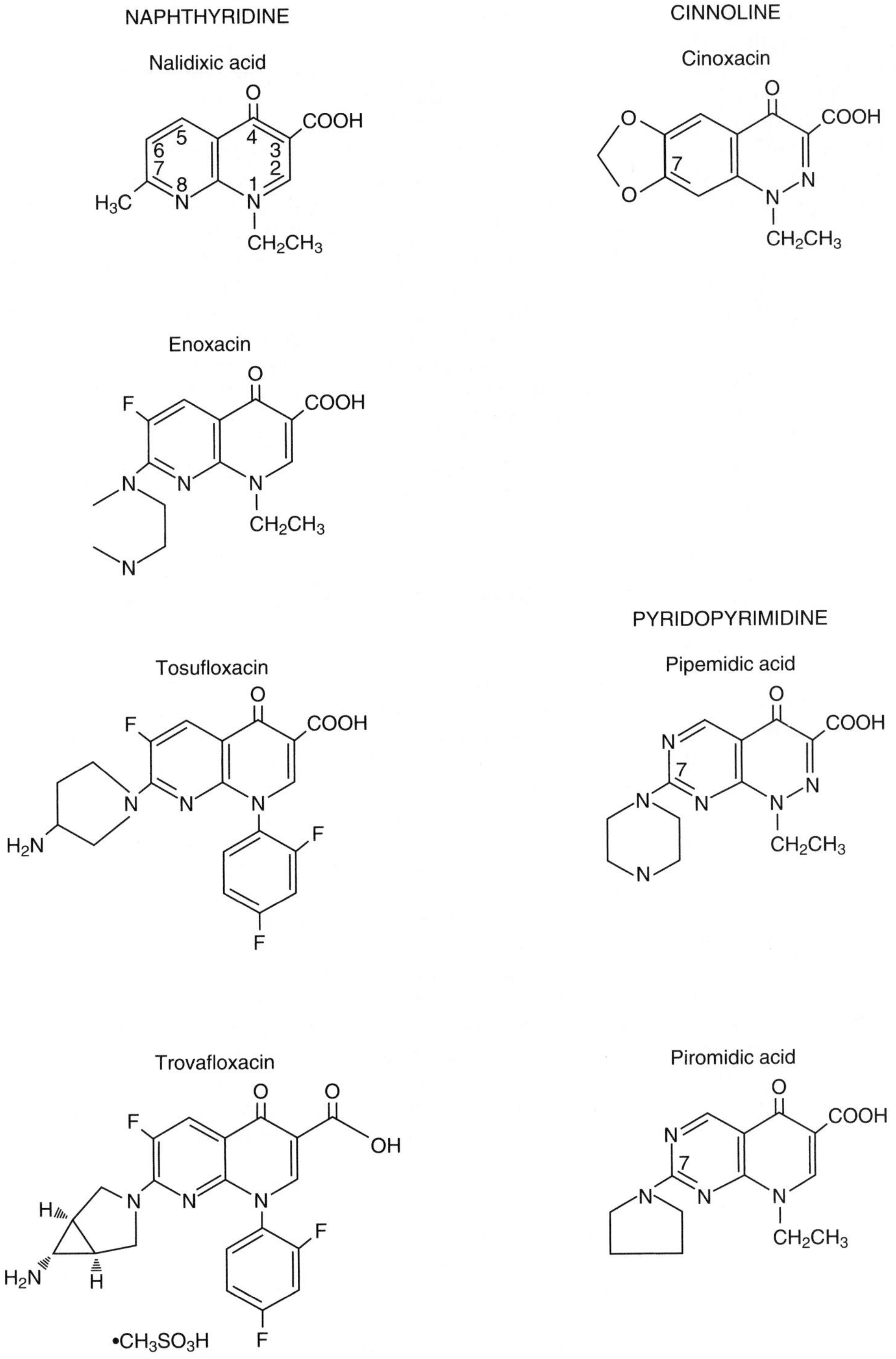

NAPHTHYRIDINE

Nalidixic acid

CINNOLINE

Cinoxacin

Enoxacin

PYRIDOPYRIMIDINE

Pipemidic acid

Tosufloxacin

Trovafloxacin

Piromidic acid

Figure 26.2. Structures of naphthyridine, cinnoline, and pyridopyrimidine derivatives.

enoxacin [1-ethyl-6-fluoro-1,4-dihydro-4-oxo-7-(1-piperazinyl) 1,8-naphthyridine-3-carboxylic acid], tosufloxacin [7-(3-amino-1-pyrrolidinyl)-1-(2,4-difluo-rophenyl)-6-fluoro-1,4-dihydro-4-oxo-1,8-naphthyridine-3-carboxylic acid], trovafloxacin [7-(1a, 5a,6a)-6-amino-3-azabicyclo[3.1.0]hex-3-yl)-6-fluoro-l-(2,4-difluorophenyl)-1, 4-dihydro-4-oxo-1,8-naphthyridine-3-carboxylic acid], and gemifloxacin [(R,S)-7-(3-aminomethyl-4-*syn*-methoxyamino-1-pyrrolidinyl)-1-cyclopropyl-6-fluoro-1,4-dihydro-4-oxo-1,8-napthyridine-3-carboxylic acid methanesulfonate]. Cinoxacin and oxolinic acid are no longer in use. The quinoline derivatives include norfloxacin [1-ethyl-6-fluoro-1,4-dihydro-4-oxo-7-(1-piperazinyl)-3-quinoline-carboxylic acid] (3,4), ciprofloxacin [1-cyclopropyl-6-fluoro-1,4-dihydro-4-oxo-7-(1-piper-

azinyl)-3-quinoline-carboxylic acid hydrochloride (2,5), ofloxacin [9-fluoro-2,3-dihydro-3-methyl-10-(4-methyl-l-piperazinyl)-7-oxo-7H-pyrido [1,2,3-*de*]-1,4-benzoxazine-6-carboxylic acid], fleroxacin [6,8-difluoro-l-(2-fluoroethyl)-1,4-dihydro-7-(4-methyl-l-piperazinyl)-4-oxo-3-quinohnecarboxylic acid], lomefloxacin [1-ethyl-6,8-difluoro-1,4-dihydro-7-(3-methyl-l-piperazinyl)-4-oxo-3-quinolinecarboxylic acid], pefloxacin [1-ethyl-6-fluoro-1,4-dihydro-7-(4-methyl-l-piperazinyl)-4-oxo-3-quinolinecarboxylic acid], sparfloxacin [5-amino-1-cyclopropyl-7-(*cis*-3,5-dimethyl-1-piperazinyl)-6,8-difluoro-1,4-dihydro-4-oxo-3-quinolinecarboxylic acid] (6), levofloxacin [(−)-(S)-9-fluoro-2,3-dihydro-3-methyl-10-(4-methyl-l-piperazinyl)-7-oxo-7H-pyrido[1,2,3, *de*] [1,4] benzoxazine-6-carboxylic acid] (2,3,6), gatifloxacin (+)-1-cyclopropyl-6-fluoro-1,4-dihydro-8-methoxy-7-(3 methyl-1-piperazinyl)-4-oxo-3-quinolinecarboxylic acid sesquihydrate, and moxifloxacin (1-cyclopropyl-7-([S,S]-2,8-diazabicyclo[4.3.0]-non-8-yl)-6-fluoro-1,4-dihydro-8-methoxy-4-oxo-3-quinoline carboxylic acid. Other newer quinolone compounds are undergoing clinical investigation (3,6,7). Some promising compounds (temafloxacin, grepafloxacin, and clinafloxacin) have been withdrawn from clinical use because of toxicity.

MECHANISM OF ACTION

Quinolones rapidly inhibit bacterial DNA synthesis, resulting in rapid cell death (2). Quinolones inhibit DNA gyrase (topoisomerase II), of which four subunits (two A and two B monomers, products of gyrA and gyrB genes) have been defined, and topoisomerase IV (2,8,9). Topoisomerase II supercoils strands of bacterial DNA into the bacterial cell and transiently nicks each chromosomal domain during supercoiling. When supercoiling is completed, this enzyme seals the nicked DNA (2,10,11). Topoisomerase IV separates the linked daughter DNA molecules after replication is complete (2,12). These two topoisomerases are essential in permitting successful replication and cell partitioning of DNA molecules (2,12–15). Quinolones bind to these two topoisomerases and effectively inhibit their normal function in the bacterial cell, which has helped us to understand the bactericidal mechanism of action of the quinolones (2,15,16). Recent evidence also suggests that the new C-8 methoxy quinolones, moxifloxacin and gatifloxacin, are more likely to kill nongrowing bacterial cells and to have enhanced activity against resistant mutants than compounds without a C-8 methoxy side chain. This observation may have important clinical effects because it may delay the emergence of resistant organisms. However, the bactericidal activity of the quinolones is reduced significantly if RNA or protein synthesis is inhibited (17). These drugs have a single most bactericidal concentration and in greater or lesser concentrations kill fewer bacteria (18). This paradoxical effect of decreased killing at higher concentrations is most likely the result of dose-dependent inhibition of RNA synthesis (18). Also, some quinolones may kill by more than one mechanism (19).

ANTIMICROBIAL ACTIVITY

Table 26.1 presents an overview of the antimicrobial activity of selected quinolones in vitro. The newer quinolones are quite active against enteric gram-negative aerobic bacteria and against other aerobic gram-negative organisms, including gram-negative cocci, that is, Moraxella catarrhalis and Neisseria species (2,20,21). Ciprofloxacin is the most active presently available quinolone against aerobic gram-negative bacteria. The newer quinolones also have activity against staphylococci (20,22). They have moderate activity against Pseudomonas aeruginosa, and ciprofloxacin is the most active. The earlier quinolones have variable activity against streptococci and poor activity against anaerobes (2,20,22). However, the newest agents, such as trovafloxacin, sparfloxacin, gatifloxacin, moxifloxacin, and gemifloxacin, do have significant activity against streptococci and anaerobes, although trovafloxacin is the most potent against the Bacteroides fragilis group (20). The quinolones have excellent activity against Legionella pneumophila, and trovafloxacin is the most active (20,23). The quinolones are active against Mycoplasma pneumoniae and Chlamydia pneumoniae, and the newest quinolones are the most active (20). The quinolones are also active against Chlamydia trachomatis, Mycoplasma hominis, and Ureaplasma urealyticum (20,24).

The quinolones have variable activity against Mycobacterium species. In general, they are not so active against Mycobacterium avium-intracellulare, whereas some newer quinolones are active against Mycobacterium tuberculosis, Mycobacterium kansasii, and Mycobacterium fortuitum but have less activity against Mycobacterium chelonei (20,25). Sparfloxacin and ofloxacin have activity against Mycobacterium leprae and have also shown efficacy in patients with lepromatous leprosy (26,27).

Combinations of other classes of antimicrobial agents with the quinolones generally show an additive or indifferent effect, occasionally show a synergistic effect but only in a few strains, and rarely show antagonism (28). The bactericidal activity of quinolones is reduced during the postantibiotic effect by rifampin (29).

MECHANISMS OF BACTERIAL RESISTANCE

The frequency with which bacteria develop resistance to the quinolones is lower for the fluoroquinolones (10^{-12}) than for nonfluorinated compounds (10^{-8}). Also, gram-positive bacteria mutate to quinolone resistance at higher frequencies than gram-negative organisms (2,30). Reduced susceptibility to the quinolones has occurred after serial exposure of bacteria to subinhibitory drug concentrations (20,30). Bacteria become resistant to quinolones by mutations in the target molecules, that is, the topoisomerases II and IV or by active efflux, although the latter is responsible for low-level resistance that might act as a first step in resistance selection (30). Mutations that result in diminished production of outer membrane proteins, particularly OmpF, may also contribute to resistance by reducing uptake of quinolones in some species. Relative resistance to nonquinolone antibiotics has been observed when reduced susceptibility to the quinolones is caused by reduced outer membrane protein activity (31). However, the role of outer membrane proteins in acquired resistance is not well defined because protein mutations do not significantly alter quinolone minimal inhibitory concentrations (MICs) (30,32).

In gram-negative bacteria, topoisomerase II is the primary target for the quinolones, particularly the gyrA subunit (30). Mutations in topoisomerase IV can further increase the level of resistance. In gram-positive bacteria, both topoisomerase II and IV can be the primary targets. Mutations in these topoisomerases result in reduced quinolone affinity and binding to the target enzyme (30,32,33). Single-step mutations generally lead to a twofold to eightfold increase in MICs, and mutational resistance to one quinolone may confer some degree of resistance to all other drugs in the group. Organisms that are likely to develop resistance after a single-step mutation are those that have borderline susceptibility, whereas organisms that are highly susceptible usually remain within the susceptible range after single-step mutations and require multiple mutations before resistance develops (30,32).

Because quinolones interfere with DNA gyrase activity, which is necessary for plasmid replication, quinolones were expected to promote loss of plasmids and to inhibit transfer of R-factor–mediated resistance (34); however, although plasmid-mediated resistance may be possible, it has not yet been observed in clinical isolates (35,36).

PHARMACOKINETICS

The currently available quinolones are well absorbed from the gastrointestinal tract after oral administration and have excellent bioavailability. Most of the quinolones are excreted by the kidney into the urine, although some are metabolized in the liver (37). The pharmacokinetic properties of some of the newer quinolones are summarized in Table 26.2. An intravenous preparation is also available for ciprofloxacin, fleroxacin, ofloxacin, pefloxacin, levofloxacin, trovafloxacin, gatifloxacin, and moxifloxacin. However, the use of ofloxacin, sparfloxacin, pefloxacin, lomefloxacin, enoxacin, fleroxacin, and trovafloxacin has declined because of either their toxicity profile or their lack of expanded microbiologic activity compared with other more commonly used fluoroquinolones (ciprofloxacin, levofloxacin, gatifloxacin, and moxifloxacin). In general, the newer quinolones exhibit linear pharmacokinetics. Peak serum concentrations occur 1 to 3 hours after oral administration. Food and histamine-2 (H_2) blockers (ranitidine) delay absorption, so that serum peaks appear later and are moderately lower (37).

Absorption is also reduced by concurrent administration of magnesium hydroxide or aluminum hydroxide antacids containing divalent metals, with which they form insoluble chelates, and by other drugs that decrease peristalsis or delay gastric emptying time (37). The pharmacokinetics of intravenous fluoroquinolones are similar to those following oral administration. Cerebrospinal concentrations of the quinolones are about one third to one half of corresponding plasma levels; the presence of inflammation appears to enhance penetration significantly (37,38). The newer quinolones are not extensively bound to serum proteins, and they have large volumes of distribution. Their long serum half-life allows twice-daily or once-daily dosing. The newer quinolones are metabolized in the kidneys and liver. Ciprofloxacin, levofloxacin, gatifloxacin, and gemifloxacin are highly dependent on renal elimination, which is by glomerular filtration and active tubular secretion and which is blocked by probenecid (except for fleroxacin). These renally eliminated quinolones have significantly longer half-lives in patients with reduced renal function, and dosing should be adjusted appropriately. Moxifloxacin, pefloxacin, nalidixic acid, sparfloxacin, and trovafloxacin are not dependent on renal elimination but are metabolized to varying degrees by the liver (37). The antibacterial activity of the quinolones is reduced at lower urinary pH values (pH of 5.5 to 6.0 vs. pH 7.4) (37). Changes in pharmacokinetics in elderly patients are usually small; thus, dosage adjustments are not usually needed because of age alone. Biliary concentrations of some quinolones are two to eight times the serum concentrations, and high concentrations are found in the feces.

Quinolones provide good tissue distribution, with excellent interstitial fluid levels, entry into phagocytic cells, and high urinary concentrations after oral administration (37). Quinolones, except for nalidixic acid, accumulate in the prostate gland, and concentrations in prostatic tissue, prostatic fluid, and seminal fluid are higher than those in plasma (39,40). Ciprofloxacin, ofloxacin, nalidixic acid, and pefloxacin are excreted into breast milk of lactating women (41).

DOSAGE ADJUSTMENTS FOR RENAL OR HEPATIC INSUFFICIENCY

For patients whose creatinine clearance rate is below 50 mL per minute, dosage adjustments of ofloxacin, fleroxacin, and lomefloxacin are suggested because these drugs are excreted largely unchanged in the urine and undergo minimal hepatic metabolism (37,42,43). The suggested adjustment for ofloxacin is a standard dose and for fleroxacin and lomefloxacin is an initial standard dose followed by one half a standard dose at 24-hour intervals for patients with creatinine clearance rates of 10 to 50 mL per minute; the suggested adjustment for ofloxacin, fleroxacin, and lomefloxacin is one half the standard dose every 24 hours for patients with creatinine clearance rates less than 10 mL per minute (42,43). Dosage adjustments for ciprofloxacin, levofloxacin, gatifloxacin, sparfloxacin, gemifloxacin, enoxacin, and norfloxacin may be necessary for patients with moderate renal insufficiency but only when the creatinine clearance rate is substantially depressed, that is, less than 30 mL per minute, when maintenance doses can be given at 18- to 24-hour intervals (37,42,44). Dosage adjustments are not required for trovafloxacin, moxifloxacin, pefloxacin, and nalidixic acid. Hemodialysis has a minimal effect on the clearance of the newer quinolones (i.e., ciprofloxacin, enoxacin, fleroxacin, lomefloxacin, norfloxacin, and ofloxacin) and a slightly higher effect on the clearance of pefloxacin (42–44). Peritoneal dialysis has no substantial effect on the clearance of ciprofloxacin, fleroxacin, and ofloxacin (43,44). Nevertheless, a maintenance dose for ciprofloxacin is recommended after hemodialysis or peritoneal dialysis and for fleroxacin, but only after hemodialysis. Dosage recommendations based on renal function are summarized in Table 26.3.

For patients with hepatic disease without concomitant renal insufficiency, no dosage adjustment is needed for currently used quinolones except for trovafloxacin (37,45). However, the dosage of pefloxacin and possibly of enoxacin may have to be adjusted in patients with hepatic disease (42,45).

TOXICITY AND ADVERSE REACTIONS

The frequency of adverse events in patients receiving quinolones is rather low when compared with those seen with other antimicrobial agents; they are considered relatively safe (3,31,46,47). Overall rates of 6% to 11% have been reported, but less than 1% have been serious. Although the type of adverse events is similar for all quinolones, the frequency and severity vary among individual quinolones.

Gastrointestinal disturbances (anorexia, nausea, diarrhea, vomiting, dyspepsia, and abdominal discomfort) are the adverse reactions reported most frequently (2% to 11%). Antibiotic-associated colitis has been seen but rarely (48). Central nervous system (CNS) reactions (1% to 7%) may occur in the form of headache, dizziness, tiredness, vertigo, syncope, restlessness, insomnia, tinnitus, abnormal vision, and sensory changes (31,46). Severe neurotoxic reactions are rare (less than 0.5%) and include psychotic reactions, hallucinations, depression, and grand mal seizures, which are reversible with cessation of therapy. Thus, the quinolones should be used with caution in patients with known or suspected CNS disorders (e.g., epilepsy) or other conditions that predispose to seizures. These direct CNS effects correlate roughly with quinolone binding at the γ-aminobutyric acid (GABA) type A receptors in the brain, blocking GABA and leading to CNS stimulation (46). Hypersensitivity reactions are also rare (0.4% to 2%) and include erythema, pruritus, urticaria, and rash. Equally rare are anaphylactoid reactions, including hypotension, bronchospasm, and angioedema. Patients with human immunodeficiency virus (HIV) infection seem to be prone to these reactions (31). Thrombocytopenia, leukopenia, and anemia have also been rarely described, as have rare cases of

TABLE 26.1. *In Vitro* Antimicrobial Activity of Selected Quinolones

Organism	Nalidixic acid	Ciprofloxocin	Enoxacin	Norfloxacin	Ofloxacin	Pefloxacin	Lomefloxacin
			MIC$_{90}$ (Range) (μg/mL)				
Gram-negative aerobes							
Escherichia coli	8 (4–128)	0.03 (0.015–0.06)	0.5 (0.25–1)	0.125 (0.06–0.5)	0.125 (0.06–0.25)	0.125 (0.125–0.25)	0.2 (0.06–1.0)
Klebsiella pneumoniae	8 (1–128)	0.125 (0.06–0.25)	0.5	0.25 (0.125–1)	0.25 (0.03–0.25)	0.5	1 (0.2–0.25)
Enterobacter species	32 (4–128)	0.125 (0.03–0.5)	0.5 (0.25–4)	0.5 (0.125–2)	0.5 (0.115–1)	0.5 (0.25–1)	0.5 (≤0.25–1)
Citrobacter species	8 (4–>100)	0.03 (0.03–0.06)	0.5	0.25 (0.125–0.5)	0.5 (0.03–2)	0.5	0.5 (0.12–25)
Serratia marcescens	>128 (16–>256)	0.25 (0.06–0.5)	2 (0.5–4)	1 (0.5–8)	1 (0.25–2)	1 (0.2.5–2)	2 (0.25–25)
Shigella species	4	0.03 (0.015–0.06)	0.125	0.06 (0.03–0.125)	0.125 (0.06–0.12)	0.125	(0.06–0.25)
Salmonella species	8 (4–8)	0.015 (≤0.015–0.03)	0.25 (0.125–0.25)	0.125 (0.06–0.125)	0.125 (0.06–0.12)	0.125	0.25
Proteus mirabilis	16 (4–32)	0.06 (0.03–0.125)	0.5 (0.25–1)	0.25 (0.125–0.5)	0.25 (0.25–0.5)	0.125 (0.06–0.25)	0.5–1
Proteus vulgaris	8 (4–16)	0.12 (0.03–0.25)	0.25 (0.25–0.5)	0.125 (0.06–0.125)	0.12 (0.03–1)	0.5 (0.25–1)	0.5 (0.25–1)
Morganella morganii	8 (2–8)	0.015 (0.015–0.03)	0.125 (0.03–0.25)	0.125 (0.03–0.25)	0.125 (0.125–0.2)	0.25 (0.25–0.5)	0.25 (0.25–12.5)
Brucella melitensis	—	0.5 (0.25–0.5)	—	—	2	—	—
Legionella species	0.25 (0.12–0.25)	(0.03–0.125)	0.2	(0.125–0.5)	0.015 (0.008–0.1)	—	≤0.06
Pseudomonas cepacia	16	0.5 (0.12–2)	25 (16–25)	8 (8–50)	3.1 (3–32)	4 (2–8)	4 (4–>60)
Pseudomonas aeruginosa	>128	0.5 (0.25–1)	4 (2–8)	2 (0.06–8)	4 (0.5–4)	—	16
Haemophilus influenzae	1 (1–2)	0.03 (0.007–0.06)	0.125 (0.06–0.25)	0.06 (0.03–0.125)	0.03 (0.03–0.06)	0.06 (0.03–0.06)	(≤0.06–0.12)
Neisseria gonorrhoeae	1 (1–2)	≤0.015 (≤0.015)	0.03 (0.015–0.06)	0.06 (0.015–0.125)	0.03 (0.015–0.06)	0.06 (0.03–0.06)	0.12
Neisseria meningitidis	2	0.004	0.06	0.03	0.015	0.03	(≤0.06–0.42)
Acinetobacter species	32–256	0.5 (0.015–1)	1–2	8–64	1 (0.12–2)	(1–8)	4
Aeromonas species	0.5	≤0.008 (≤0.008–0.05)	—	0.06	0.03–0.5 (0.003–10)	0.03	0.12
Campylobacter jejuni	8	(0.12–0.78)	(1–32)	(0.25–2)	(0.12–2)	0.5	(0.125–1)
Moraxella catarrhalis	2	0.06 (0.007–0.06)	0.06	0.4	(0.06–0.50)	0.25	(≤0.1–1)
Providencia rettgeri	16	1 (≤0.008–2)	1 (0.5–0.25)	2 (0.25–3.1)	1 (0.25–2)	0.5	4 (1.6–6.2)
Providencia stuartii	32	0.25 (≤0.008–1)	1–2	2 (≤0.25–2)	1 (0.6–1)	4	1 (1–4)
Stenotrophomonas	16	4 (1–4)	8 (3–16)	4 (4–>64)	4 (0.5–4)	4.0	8 (8–25)
Yersinia enterocolitica	4 (1–8)	0.06 (0.015–0.06)	0.12–0.25	≤0.12	(0.06–0.25)	0.25	(≤0.06–0.25)
Hafnia alvei	—	0.03 (0.015–0.06)	—	—	0.12 (0.15–0.25)	—	—
Helicobacter pylori	—	0.31 (0.039–0.31)	—	—	—	—	—
Gram-positive aerobes							
Enterococcus faecalis	>128 (>128)	4 (0.5–4)	8 (8–16)	8 (4–32)	4 (2–6.2)	4–8	8 (4–16)
Enterococcus faecium	>64	4 (2–8)	32	≥12.5	6.2 (2–16)	—	8
Staphylococci (coag neg)	128 (32–256)	0.5 (0.06–0.5)	1 (0.5–1)	1 (0.25–2)	0.5 (0.25–0.5)	0.5 (0.25–1)	1 (0.5–1)
Staphylococci (coag neg/meth res)	>128 (16–>128)	64 (0.12–>64)	—	—	64 (0.12–>64)	—	—
Staphylococcus aureus	64 (32–128)	0.5 (0.12–2)	2 (0.5–2)	2 (0.5–4)	0.5 (0.12–1)	0.5 (0.25–1)	1 (0.5–2)
Staphylococcus aureus (meth susc)	64 (8–64)	1 (0.25–2)	—	—	0.5 (0.25–32)	—	—
Staphylococcus aureus (meth res)	>128 (32–>28)	64 (0.25–>64)	—	—	32 (0.25–>128)	—	—
Streptococcus (viridans group)	>128 (128–>28)	4 (0.12–8)	—	—	4 (1–8)	—	—
Streptococcus pyogenes	>100	1 (0.25–2)	>8	4 (2–16)	2 (0.05–4)	8 (8–16)	8 (4–12.5)
Streptococcus agalactiae	>128	2 (0.5–4)	>8	16 (4–16)	2 (1–4)	32	16 (8–32)
Streptococcus pneumoniae	>128 (128–>28)	4 (0.5–1)	16 (8–16)	16 (4–>16)	4 (0.05–4)	12 (8–16)	8 (2–16)
Listeria monocytogenes	>64	2 (0.5–4)	8–16	8 (4–16)	2 (1–4)	6–8	(6.2–8)
Corynebacterium species	0.06 (0.03–0.12)	1 (0.05–128)	8 (4–>128)	4 (4–>28)	1 (0.5–64)	8 (8–>28)	>12.5
Anaerobic bacteria and other organisms							
Peptostreptococcus species	>128 (64–128)	4 (0.25–16)	—	—	8 (0.25–32)	—	—
Clostridium species	>128 (4–>28)	0.5 (0.25–2)	(16–32)	(2–8)	8 (0.25–16)	(1–8)	(2–16)
Clostridium difficile	>128 (64–>28)	12.5 (8–25)	128	128	8 (8–16)	64	≥32
Prevotella species	128 (64–128)	16 (0.25–16)	—	—	16 (0.5–16)	—	—
Mycobacterium fortuitum	—	0.3	—	2	(1–3.1)	2	—
Mycobacterium tuberculosis	128 (16–128)	1	>5	8	1 (0.12–4)	8	4
Mycobacterium avium complex	>256 (128≥256)	16	>256	≥16	32 (4–64)	>64	—
Mycobacterium chelonae	—	8	—	>16	>20	>64	—
Mycobacterium kansasii	—	1	25	8	(1–3.1)	4	—
Bacteriodes species	512	16 (4–>16)	16	128	(2–32)	—	(8–32)
Bacteroides fragilis	128 (128–>128)	16 (4–>16)	32	>128	(2–12.5)	16	(8–04)
Fusobacterium species	128 (32–>128)	8 (2–8)	32	16	4 (0.5–8)	32	16
Anaerobic Gram-positive cocci	(256–512)	(2–6.25)	(2–8)	(16–64)	(2–8)	16	(4–25)
Chlamydia pneumoniae	(>64)	(1–2)	—	—	0.25	—	4
Chlamydia psittaci	—	1	—	—	0.5	—	—
Chlamydia trachomatis	(>64)	(1–1.56)	6.3	≥16	(1–1.56)	—	(2–3.1)
Mycoplasma hominis	>256	(0.5–2)	8	(8–16)	(1–2)	4	2
Mycoplasma pneumoniae	—	(0.78–2)	8	12	(0.78–2)	4	(4–8)
Ureaplasma urealyticum	—	4	—	—	(2–4)	—	—

MIC$_{90}$, minimal inhibitory concentration for 90% of strains; coag neg, coagulase negative; meth res, methicillin resistant; meth susc, methicillin susceptible.

nephrotoxic reactions, resulting from crystalluria with elevated serum creatinine levels. All resolve when therapy is discontinued (31,46).

Moderate to severe phototoxicity, manifested by an exaggerated sunburn reaction, has been observed in patients who are exposed to direct sunlight while receiving some members of the quinolone class of drugs, especially lomefloxacin, pefloxacin, fleroxacin, and sparfloxacin. Quinolones that accumulate in high concentrations in skin have a higher risk for producing phototoxicity (46,47).

Arthralgia has been observed in 1.5% of treatment courses in children with cystic fibrosis treated with ciprofloxacin and in 14% of adolescents receiving pefloxacin; the joint damage seen in young dogs does not occur in children, and the arthralgia resolves when therapy is stopped. Tendonitis and Achilles tendon rupture have been associated most frequently with pefloxacin

TABLE 26.1. (*continued*)

MIC$_{90}$ (Range) (μg/mL) *continued*

Fleroxacin	Sparfloxacin	Trovafloxacin	Clinafloxacin	Levofloxacin	Gatifloxacin	Moxifloxacin	Gemifloxacin
0.1 (0.03–2)	0.03 (≤0.015–0.12)	0.06 (≤0.008–0.12)	≤0.03 (0.03–0.06)	0.10	0.06 (0.013–6.25)	0.06	0.015 (0.004–32)
0.5 (0.12–0.25)	0.012 (≤0.008–0.25)	0.05 (0.05–1)	0.13 (≤0.03–0.13)	0.25	0.1 (0.013–1.56)	0.5	0.25 (0.008–32)
(0.12–0.25)	0.06–.25 (0.015–1)	0.05	0.13 (≤0.03–0.25)	(0.18–0.39)	0.1 (0.025–0.20)	0.2–1.0	0.25 (0.008–16)
0.12 (≤0.06–25)	0.06–0.5 (≤0.015–1)	0.1 (0.06–0.25)	—	(0.03–0.78)	0.39 (0.025–1.56)	1.0	2.0 (0.004–16)
0.5 (0.25–25)	1 (0.25–1)	0.5 (0.05–2)	—	3.13	12.5 (0.05–25.0)	0.3–8.0	0.25 (0.008–4)
≤0.125	0.06 (0.015–0.12)	0.06 (0.03–0.12)	—	—	0.03–0.06	0.02	0.008
(≤0.12–0.25)	0.06 (0.015–0.12)	0.05	≤0.03 (≤0.03)	0.12	0.12	0.18–0.74	0.015
0.5 (≤0.12–0.5)	0.5 (0.06–0.5)	(0.2–2)	≤0.03 (≤0.03)	0.19	0.25 (0.10–1.56)	0.2	0.25 (0.016–0.5)
0.12 (≤0.12–0.25)	0.5 (0.12–1)	0.5	—	0.20	0.25 (0.05–1.56)	0.5	0.125 (0.016–0.125)
0.12 (<0.06–12.5)	0.25 (≤0.015–0.5)	0.25	≤0.03 (≤0.03)	0.12	0.25 (0.025–12.5)	0.13	0.125 (0.008–8)
—	0.25	—	0.06 (0.03–0.06)	—	—	—	0.016 (0008–0.06)
≤0.06	≤0.06	—	—	(0.05–0.12)	0.06 (0.016–0.06)	0.06–0.12	0.5 (0.008–0.5)
2 (2–>50)	1 (1–8)	3 (0.5–32)	0.25 (≤0.03–0.25)	5.12	256 (0.03–256)	256 (0.03–512)	4.0 (0.125–32)
4 (4–16)	1 (0.12–2)	.25	0.25 (≤0.03–0.12)	3.13	32.0 (0.25–128)	8.0 (0.25–64)	0.016 (0.001–0.06)
(≤0.06–1)	≤0.015 (≤0.015–0.03)	0.03 (0.03–0.12)	≤0.03 (≤0.03)	0.02	0.016 (0.008–0.03)	0.06 (0.001–0.25)	0.06 (0.001–0.06)
0.2	≤0.015 (0.015–0.03)	0.25 (≤0.001–0.25)	—	0.02	0.016 (0.002–.03)	0.016 (0.001–0.016)	0.006
(0.03–0.25)	≤0.06	0.008 (0.004–0.015)	—	—	0.008	0.015	0.125 (0.001–0.25)
0.5–4 (0.5–32)	0.25 (0.015–0.5)	8	—	—	0.125 (0.002–2)	0.125 (0.001–0.25)	0.03 (0.001–0.06)
0.12–0.25 (0.12–1)	0.12 (≤0.015–0.25)	0.03	—	—	0.03 (0.008–0.06)	0.06 (0.016–0.125)	
0.5	(0.1–0.12)	—	—	—	0.25 (0.06–0.25)	0.125 (0.03–0.125)	
(0.25–2)	(0.01–0.12)	0.03 (0.007–0.03)	(≤0.03)	0.10	0.03 (0.004–0.03)	0.25 (0.016–0.125)	0.03 (0.004–0.03)
0.5 (0.12–1)	0.5 (0.12–1)	0.5	—	—	1.56 (0.025–6.25)	0.5	8.0
1 (0.5–2)	2 (0.12–8)	2	—	0.39	0.39 (0.025–0.78)	0.5	>8
3 (3–25)	0.5 (0.03–1)	2 (0.2–2)	—	3.13	4.0 (0.06–32)	1.0 (0.03–2)	4.0 (0.016–16)
(≤0.06–2)	0.06 (≤0.015–0.25)	(0.03–0.05)	≤0.03 (≤0.03)	—	—	—	0.015
—	0.25 (0.015–0.25)	0.06 (0.008–0.06)	—	—	—	—	>0.3
	(0.25–4)	0.25 (0.031–0.25)	—	—	0.25 (0.125–0.25)	0.125 (0.06–0.125)	—
8 (8–>16)	0.5 (0.25–0.5)	2	0.25 (0.01–1)	1.56	2.0	1.0 (0.125–1.0)	2.0 (0.03–16)
8	1 (0.5–1)	2	0.5 (0.5–0.5)	3.13	4.0 (0.20–50)	4.0	64 (0.12–64)
1 (0.25–8)	0.125 (0.03–8)	1–4 (0.015–16)	0.03 (≤0.007–0.25)	0.78	2.0 (0.06–2)	0.06 (0.03–0.125)	0.03 (0.004–0.06)
4 (0.5–64)	4 (0.06–>16)	4 (0.015–16)	—	2.12	0.25 (0.05–12.5)	0.13	(0.25–4)
1 (0.25–1)	0.06 (0.03–2)	—	0.03 (≤0.007–0.125)	—	0.125 (0.03–0.25)	0.06 (0.016–0.06)	0.06 (0.004–0.06)
32 (0.2–64)	0.25 (0.03–0.25)	0.06 (0.015–4)	—	0.39	0.13 (0.025–6.25)	0.06 (0.016–0.06)	0.03 (0.008–16)
64 (32–64)	0.25 (0.03–1)	2 (0.015–8)	—	0.78	16 (0.025–25)	4.0	8 (0.016–16)
—	0.25 (0.03–0.5)	0.25 (0.015–0.25)	0.06 (0.06–0.13)	(≤0.007–0.06)	0.5 (0.125–0.5)	0.25 (0.25–0.5)	0.12 (0.004–4)
8 (4–12.5)	0.5 (0.12–0.5)	0.12	(≤0.03–0.06)	1.56	0.5 (0.10–1.56)	0.5 (0.06–0.5)	0.03 (0.008–0.06)
8 (≥8)	0.5 (0.12–0.5)	0.25	(≤0.06–0.13)	2 (0.5–2)	0.5 (0.06–1)	0.5 (0.06–0.5)	0.03 (0.016–1)
8 (8–25)	0.5 (0.064–0.5)	0.25 (0.064–0.5)	0.06 (≤0.008–0.06)	1.56	1.0 (0.06–1)	0.25 (0.125–0.25)	0.016 (0.008–0.06)
8 (4–>16)	2 (0.12–2)	0.25 (0.12–0.25)	—	—	0.5	0.5	0.125
2 (1–32)	0.25 (0.25–64)	(0.03–>32)	—	—	—	—	16.0
—	4 (0.25–4)	1 (0.06–2)	0.5 (0.015–0.5)	5.56	1.56 (0.06–8)	0.25 (0.016–0.25)	0.06 (0.004–0.06)
(2–32)	0.25 (0.015–2)	(<0.06–4)	0.12 (0.06–0.12)	0.78	1.0 (0.06–1)	8.0 (0.26–16)	1 (0.008–1)
(16–32)	6.25	4 (0.5–4)	0.5 (0.03–1)	6.25	1.56 (0.78–1.56)	1.0	1 (0.008–1)
—	(8–16)	2 (0.06–4)	—	8.0	8.0	2.0	2 (0.06–16)
≤0.05	1.56	—	—	2.78	0.78	1.0	
≤0.05	0.2	32 (2–64)	—	0.32	0.2	0.25–1.0	>4.0
16	12.5	64 (4–64)	—	16.50	0.39–16.0	0.5–16.0	
>32	(6.25–>100)	—	—	—	6.25	—	—
≥0.5	—	—	—	2.39	1.56	0.06	—
(2–64)	2	0.5 (0.5–2)	—	5.12	0.39–1.56	0.5 (0.5–8)	16 (—)
≥16	2 (1–2)	0.5 (0.12–4)	—	4.0	1.0 (0.25–8)	2.0 (0.5–8)	2.0 (0.25–16)
16	2	2 (0.12–2)	—	—	0.39 (0.05–0.39)	1.0 (0.06–1)	0.25 (0.03–0.5)
(8–12.5)	—	—	—	—	0.39	0.25 (0.016–0.25)	0.06 (0.004–0.06)
2	(0.01–0.25)	0.12	—	0.5	0.12 (0.06–0.5)	0.12	—(0.06–0.125)
—	0.03	—	—	—	—	—	—
(1.5–6.3)	(0.05–0.063)	0.06	—	—	0.06–0.25	0.03–0.125	—(0.03–0.06)
2	≤0.06 (0.01–0.06)	—	—	—	—	0.06	<0.008 (<0.008)
4	(0.1–0.25)	—	—	0.50	0.12	0.12	0.125 (<0.008–0.125)
—	0.5	—	—	2.0	—	0.12	0.250 (<0.008–0.5)

therapy and are more likely to occur in hypomagnesemic patients (46). Although there is limited experience with the use of quinolones in children, to date there is little evidence of quinolone-induced arthropathy in humans (49).

Some quinolones (ciprofloxacin, ofloxacin, nalidixic acid, and pefloxacin) are excreted into breast milk, and quinolones, in general, should not be given to nursing mothers (41). Quinolones should also be avoided during pregnancy because their safety has not been established. However, ciprofloxacin has been recommended in pregnant women for the prevention and treatment of anthrax.

Transient elevations in liver enzymes have been observed rarely with quinolones (3,46,50). The most noteworthy hepatotoxicity data was observed in the postmarketing surveillance of trovofloxacin. A serious hepatic adverse event incidence rate of 0.00585 was observed. Jaundice developed in 65 patients; an incidence of 0.0025 in jaundiced patients. Toxicity occurred either as a hypersensitivity hepatitis with eosinophilia and eosinophilic

TABLE 26.2. Pharmacokinetic Properties of Selected Newer Quinolones

Quinolone	Dose (mg)	Peak serum concentration (mg/L)	Half-life (h)	Protein binding (%)	Bioavailability (%)	Volume of distribution (L)	Urinary excretion Unchanged (%)	Urinary excretion Metabolites (%)
Ciprofloxacin	500	2–3	3–4.5	35	85	250	30–60	10
Enoxacin	400	2–3	4–6	43	90	190	50–55	15
Fleroxacin	400	4–6	10	23	96	100	60–70	10
Levofloxacin	500	5.7	7.6	—	—	102	—	—
Lomefloxacin	400	3	8	14–25	>95	190	70	10
Norfloxacin	400	1.5	3–4.5	15	80	225	20–40	20
Ofloxacin	400	3.5–5	5–6	8–30	85–95	100	70–90	5–10
Pefloxacin	400	4–5	10–11	25	90	110	5–15	55
Sparfloxacin	400	1.2–1.6	15.2–20.6	45	>60	322	<15	25
Trovafloxacin	100–300	1.4–4.3	7.1–9.6	70	60–85	90–110	8.8	—
Gatifloxacin	400	3.4–3.8	7–8	20	96–98	150–200	79–88	<0.1
Moxifloxacin	400	3.1–4.5	12–13	20–50	86–92	184	15–21	10
Gemifloxacin	320	1.0–1.5	6–8	70	70	350	20–40	—

infiltration in the liver that resolved with discontinuation of trovafloxacin, or as direct hepatotoxicity with hepatic necrosis, which appeared to occur in patients treated for 14 days or longer. Minimal elevations in liver function tests have occurred in less than 1% of patients treated with moxifloxacin or gatifloxacin and have been inconsequential (3,46,50).

Recently, the cardiovascular effects of the quinolones, particularly the newer agents, have been closely evaluated during clinical trials and during postmarketing surveillance studies. The cardiotoxic potential of these agents varies. Dose-related prolongation of the QTc interval, a new potential side effect of fluoroquinolones, was noted during clinical trials of sparfloxacin and was related to the maximum peak serum concentration (3,50). Rare cases of significant arrhythmias including torsades de pointes were reported in patients taking sparfloxacin and to a lesser extent in those treated with grepafloxacin. Such complications have also been described infrequently in patients treated with levofloxacin or ofloxacin and rarely in patients treated with gatifloxacin. There was no confirmed case of torsades de pointes in 6 million patients treated with moxifloxacin (3,50,51). Fluoroquinolones, however, are not recommended for use in patients receiving class IA drugs that have class III properties (e.g. quinidine, procainamide) or class III (e.g. amiodarone, sotalol) antiarrhythmic agents (3).

DRUG INTERACTIONS

The quinolones are known to interact with a variety of other compounds. Specifically, bioavailability of some quinolones is reduced after oral administration with alkaline earth and transition metal cations because quinolones form chelates with several polyvalent cations, such as calcium, magnesium, iron, and aluminum (37,46,47,50). Therefore, administration of quinolones with antacids containing calcium, aluminum, or magnesium; with sucralfate; with divalent or trivalent cations, such as iron; or with multivitamins containing zinc may substantially interfere with the absorption of the quinolones, resulting in low systemic levels, so that simultaneous oral administration should be avoided. These agents should not be taken within the 2-hour period before or after quinolone administration. Even then, there is sufficient variability between patients to warrant avoidance of these compounds during oral quinolone therapy. Also, the absorption of some quinolones may be affected minimally by food.

Other quinolone drug interactions are those with either theophylline or caffeine and those with certain nonsteroidal antiinflammatory drugs (NSAIDs), such as fenbufen or its metabolite biphenylacetic acid (37,46,50,52,53). These are important interactions because they may result in significant CNS toxicity. Data

TABLE 26.3. Dosage Guide for Adult Patients Based on Renal Function

Drug	Doses for creatinine clearance (mL/min) >50	50–10	<10	Dose after dialysis
Ciprofloxacin	250–500 mg q12h	250–500 mg q18h	250–500 mg q24h	250–500 mg Hemodialysis + peritoneal
Enoxacin	200–400 mg q12h	100–200 mg q12h	100–200 mg q24h	None
Fleroxacin	400 mg q24h	200 mg q24h*	200 mg q24h*	400 mg Hemodialysis
Lomefloxacin	400 mg q24h	200 mg q24h*	200 mg q24h*	None
Nalidixic acid	0.5–1.0 g q6h	0.5–1.0 g q6h	0.5–1.0 g q6h	—
Norfloxacin	400 mg q12h	400 mg q24h	400 mg q24h	None
Ofloxacin	200–400 mg q12h	200–400 mg q24h	100–200 mg q24h	None
Pefloxacin	400 mg q12h	400 mg q12h	400 mg q12h	None
Levofloxacin	500 mg q24h	250 mg q24h	250 mg q48h	None
Trovafloxacin	200–300 mg q24h	200–300 mg q24h	200–300 mg q24h	None
Moxifloxacin	400 mg q24h	400 mg q24h	400 mg q24h	None

*Daily maintenance dose after initial 400 mg loading dose.

have shown that some quinolones strongly inhibit the hepatic cytochrome P450 (isoform CYP1A2) enzymes that metabolize theophylline and caffeine, thereby reducing their clearance and leading to their accumulation and toxicity (37,46,50,54). These studies have shown a structure–side-effect profile for theophylline interactions that is controlled primarily by the R_7 side chain, somewhat by the R_1 substituent, and to a lesser extent by X_8 (46,47,54), and not by the oxo metabolites of the side chains as was suggested previously (55). The highest interactions occur for small nonbulky R_7 substituents, whereas bulkier R_7 side chains diminish the interaction. Also, a nitrogen in the X_8 position (naphthyridines) is the least preferred, although a bulky R_7 substituent can compensate for a nitrogen at X_8 (2,47). These data explain prior observations that enoxacin (a naphthyridine compound) has the greatest effect on theophylline metabolism, with significant increases in theophylline plasma concentrations (111%) and reduced clearance. In contrast, theophylline plasma concentrations are increased by ciprofloxacin (23%), ofloxacin (12%), and minimally by norfloxacin, fleroxacin, and lomefloxacin. Pefloxacin reduces theophylline clearance by 30% (52). Theophylline doses should probably be halved for patients receiving enoxacin, and theophylline serum levels should be monitored for patients receiving enoxacin or ciprofloxacin. No routine reduction in theophylline dose is recommended for patients receiving norfloxacin, ofloxacin, fleroxacin, or lomefloxacin. Caffeine clearance is interfered with by the newer quinolones. Enoxacin increases the plasma concentration of caffeine by 41% and reduces the clearance by 78%. Ciprofloxacin increases the half-life of caffeine only modestly (15%), and ofloxacin and lomefloxacin do so only minimally (53).

The quinolones may interact to varying degrees with other drugs, including warfarin, H_2-receptor antagonists, cyclosporine, rifampin, and NSAIDs. However, the interaction of the newer quinolones with H_2 blockers, proton pump inhibitors, and cyclosporine is clinically insignificant (37). Concomitant administration of an NSAID with a quinolone may increase the risk for CNS stimulation and convulsive seizures. Quinolones at high concentrations inhibit GABA receptor binding, which leads to CNS stimulation, but the inhibitory concentrations are not therapeutically relevant unless these quinolones are combined with certain NSAIDs, which potentiate quinolone GABA receptor binding by 100- to 3,000-fold. This brings the inhibitory concentration into the therapeutic range. Again, the R_7 group has the greatest influence on the NSAID-potentiated CNS effects of the quinolones. However, the real clinical importance of the effects of NSAIDs and quinolones remains to be determined because of the low incidence of NSAID-induced CNS effects (47,56).

Disturbances of blood glucose, including symptomatic hyperglycemia and hypoglycemia, have been reported, usually in diabetic patients receiving concomitant treatment with an oral hypoglycemia agent or insulin. For these patients, careful monitoring of blood glucose is recommended, and the quinolone should be discontinued if a hypoglycemic reaction occurs. Nalidixic acid-glucuronide conjugates may produce a false-positive reaction for urine glucose when tested with Benedict solution but not with glucose oxidase strips. Nitrofurantoin interferes with the therapeutic action of nalidixic acid.

CLINICAL APPLICATIONS

Many infectious diseases can be treated successfully with both oral and parenteral fluoroquinolones, and most can be treated with oral therapy. Specifically, clinical efficacy with the fluoroquinolones has been demonstrated in respiratory infections (i.e.,

acute bacterial exacerbations of chronic bronchitis, community-acquired pneumonia, and sinusitis); uncomplicated and some complicated urinary tract infections; bacterial prostatitis; skin and soft tissue infections; bone and joint infections; and gastrointestinal infections, especially infectious diarrhea caused by toxigenic *Escherichia coli, Salmonella* (including typhoid and paratyphoid fevers, salmonella sepsis, and the chronic salmonella carrier state), *Shigella, Campylobacter, Aeromonas, Vibrio* species, and *Plesiomonas shigelloides*. They have also been effective in treating some sexually transmitted diseases (gonococcal and chlamydia infections, as well as chancroid) and pelvic infections. Also, prophylaxis can be given orally, particularly for immunocompromised patients (6,7,32). Adequate evidence of efficacy with the newer quinolones, particularly ciprofloxacin, levofloxacin, gatifloxacin, grepafloxacin, trovafloxacin, and moxifloxacin, has been demonstrated by clinical investigation.

It is imperative to emphasize that all fluoroquinolones have *not* been approved for use in all of these infections. Unfortunately, many physicians use fluoroquinolones interchangeably (i.e., for unapproved indications) because they do not realize that there is no scientific evidence of efficacy in a specific infection unless the drug has been approved by our regulatory agency for use in that specific infection (3). Quinolones approved for use in the United States include nalidixic acid, norfloxacin, ciprofloxacin, ofloxacin, enoxacin, temafloxacin (withdrawn in 1992), lomefloxacin, sparfloxacin, levofloxacin, grepafloxacin (withdrawn in 1999), trovafloxacin (restricted use in United States), gatifloxacin, and moxifloxacin. Quinolones available outside the United States include pefloxacin, fleroxacin, and tosufloxacin (3). Indications approved by our regulatory agency for the four most frequently used oral and intravenous fluoroquinolones, that is, ciprofloxacin, levofloxacin, gatifloxacin, and moxifloxacin, are shown in Table 26.4.

Urinary Tract Infections

Ciprofloxacin has had the most clinical experience in the treatment of uncomplicated and complicated urinary tract infections, including acute pyelonephritis. However, nalidixic acid, norfloxacin, ciprofloxacin, ofloxacin, enoxacin, fleroxacin, lomefloxacin, pefloxacin, levofloxacin, trovafloxacin, and gatifloxacin have been approved for use in treating urinary tract infections (40,57). Nalidixic acid (adults, 1 g four times daily for 1 to 2 weeks, thereafter, if needed, 0.5 g; children, 55 mg/kg per day in four divided doses for 1 to 2 weeks, thereafter, if needed, 33 mg/kg) has been used in acute and recurrent uncomplicated urinary infections with susceptible organisms. Nalidixic acid has also been used as long-term therapy for frequent recurrent bacteriuria, but cure rates have not been optimal, and resistance commonly emerges during treatments (3,40,57).

The newer quinolones are as effective as other well-established nonquinolone agents for treating *uncomplicated* urinary infections (40,57). Although single doses of norfloxacin (800 mg), ciprofloxacin (100 or 250 mg), fleroxacin (400 mg), and ofloxacin (200 mg) are often curative in patients with uncomplicated lower tract infections caused by Enterobacteriaceae, 3-day regimens result in higher cure rates (3,40,57–60). Also, failure of single-dose quinolone therapy for *Staphylococcus saprophyticus* infection, the second most frequently isolated pathogen in acute cystitis, is critical evidence against the recommendation of single-dose quinolone therapy for acute cystitis (40,57).

Quinolone therapy with norfloxacin, ciprofloxacin, or levofloxacin, for 10 to 14 days, is effective in the treatment of acute uncomplicated *pyelonephritis*. Ofloxacin, levofloxacin, enoxacin,

---

TABLE 26.4. Approved Indications for the Four Most Frequently Used Fluoroquinolones

Ciprofloxacin (oral, IV)
- Urinary tract infections—uncomplicated and complicated, including cystitis and pyelonephritis (especially pathogens resistant to standard agents)
- Chronic bacterial prostatitis
- Uncomplicated urogenital and rectal gonorrhea
- Skin and soft tissue infections
- Bone and joint infections
- Infectious diarrhea
- Typhoid fever
- Intraabdominal infections (used with metronidazole)
- Sinusitis
- Lower respiratory tract infections, including acute bacterial exacerbations of chronic bronchitis, pneumonia (other than pneumococcal pneumonia), and *Legionella* species infections
- Anthrax

Ciprofloxacin IV has also been approved for all of the above indications as well as for nosocomial pneumonia and as empirical therapy in febrile neutropenic patients.

Levofloxacin (oral, IV)
- Urinary tract infections, including uncomplicated and complicated and pyelonephritis
- Uncomplicated skin and skin structure infections
- Sinusitis
- Community-acquired pneumonia
- Acute bacterial exacerbations of chronic bronchitis

Gatifloxacin (oral, IV)
- Urinary tract infections, including uncomplicated and complicated and pyelonephritis
- Uncomplicated urogenital gonorrhea
- Sinusitis
- Acute bacterial exacerbations of chronic bronchitis
- Community-acquired pneumonia

Moxifloxacin (oral, IV)
- Sinusitis
- Acute bacterial exacerbations of chronic bronchitis
- Community-acquired pneumonia
- Uncomplicated skin and soft tissue infections

---

fleroxacin, pefloxacin, and gemifloxacin are also likely to be effective in the treatment of acute uncomplicated pyelonephritis (57). Quinolones, for 7 to 14 days, are effective for treatment of *complicated* urinary tract infections caused by susceptible organisms. Relapse rates remain high, almost 50% by 6 weeks, primarily because the underlying genitourinary abnormalities that lead to infection have not been reversed (40,57,61). Acceptable cure rates have been observed when norfloxacin, ciprofloxacin, ofloxacin, fleroxacin, lomefloxacin, enoxacin, pefloxacin, sparfloxacin, gatifloxacin, and gemifloxacin were given for 7 to 14 days to patients with *nosocomial* urinary infections (40,57,62,63).

Ciprofloxacin (1,000 mg per day), ofloxacin (300 to 600 mg per day), pefloxacin (800 mg per day), and norfloxacin (800 mg per day), given to patients with either acute or chronic *prostatitis* for 28 (range, 5 to 84) days, cured 63% to 92% of patients (40,57).

Respiratory Tract Infections

The earlier quinolones have excellent *in vitro* activity (except for *Streptococcus pneumoniae* and other streptococcal species) against the respiratory tract pathogens responsible for community-acquired pneumonia, including the agents responsible for atypical pneumonia, such as *L. pneumophila*, *M. pneumoniae*, and *C. pneumoniae* (Table 26.1). The quinolones are also effective against most organisms responsible for acute bacterial exacerbations of chronic bronchitis and for nosocomial respiratory tract infections

(Table 26.1). Therefore, because of their antimicrobial spectrum of activity and pharmacokinetic advantages that include excellent penetration into respiratory tissue and high bioavailability with oral therapy, quinolones are extremely effective for the therapy of common respiratory infections, including community-acquired pneumonia, acute bacterial exacerbations of chronic bronchitis, and bacterial sinusitis. Most patients with purulent bronchitis, acute exacerbations of chronic bronchitis, or pneumonia treated for 10 (range, 7 to 15) days with ciprofloxacin, ofloxacin, enoxacin, fleroxacin, lomefloxacin, or pefloxacin experienced clinical cure or improvement (76% to 95%) and bacterial cure (68% to 96%) (64–66). Bacterial persistence, relapse, or treatment failure occurred in 49% of *P. aeruginosa* infections, in 39% of *S. pneumoniae* infections, and in 33% of *Staphylococcus aureus* infections (64,66).

The newest members of the quinolone class, moxifloxacin and gatifloxacin, have significant advantages over their older counterparts because they have the most potent activity against *S. pneumoniae,* including penicillin-resistant, penicillin-sensitive, and macrolide-resistant strains, as well as excellent activity against other gram-positive, gram-negative, and atypical pathogens (64,67). They also have two bacterial targets (topoisomerase II and IV) that impede resistance development, improved activity against anaerobes, metabolism that does not rely on the cytochrome P450 system, and dosage that need not be altered in the setting of renal or hepatic impairment (moxifloxacin) or hepatic impairment (gatifloxacin) (37). However, only moxifloxacin has been approved for 5 days of treatment for acute bacterial exacerbations of chronic bronchitis. Furthermore, recent studies have shown that patients treated with moxifloxacin experience faster resolution of symptoms, fewer work hours missed, and higher work productivity than patients treated with earlier-generation quinolones or β-lactam antibiotics or macrolides (67).

Ciprofloxacin and ofloxacin have been used successfully to treat patients with community-acquired pneumonias caused by *M. catarrhalis, Haemophilus influenzae, M. pneumoniae, Legionella* species, and *C. pneumoniae* (64,68). Although some patients with pneumococcal pneumonia have been cured with intravenous ciprofloxacin or ofloxacin, treatment failures have occurred. Because the newer quinolones have improved activity against *S. pneumoniae,* three (levofloxacin, gatifloxacin, and moxifloxacin) are currently used frequently in the treatment of community-acquired pneumonia (64,67). Of these, moxifloxacin is the most potent against the pneumococcus regardless of whether it is penicillin resistant or sensitive (20,64,67). Gatifloxacin also has excellent antipneumococcal activity, whereas levofloxacin is four to eight times less active, so that pneumococcal quinolone resistance is more likely to occur when levofloxacin is used. In fact, high-level levofloxacin resistance to pneumococci is being reported with increasing frequency, as is resistance to gram-negative aerobic rods (64,67,69). All three quinolones have excellent activity against other respiratory pathogens, including *Legionella, Chlamydia,* and *Mycoplasma* species (64,67,68).

Clinical data indicate that intravenous ciprofloxacin, ofloxacin, pefloxacin, and fleroxacin have been used successfully in hospital-acquired pneumonia caused by aerobic gram-negative bacteria, although the bacteriological eradication rate for *P. aeruginosa* is lower (64,70,71). However, of the most frequently used fluoroquinolones, only **ciprofloxacin** has been approved for use in the treatment of nosocomial pneumonia (67). Ciprofloxacin, levofloxacin, gatifloxacin, and moxifloxacin have also been approved for the treatment of acute bacterial sinusitis (67).

Exacerbations of acute pulmonary infections in patients with cystic fibrosis who have *P. aeruginosa* in their sputum have responded to ciprofloxacin (750 mg twice daily orally) or ofloxacin

(400 mg twice daily orally), although resistant organisms may emerge (3,72,73). Malignant external otitis caused by *P. aeruginosa* may also respond to ciprofloxacin therapy (750 mg twice daily orally) given for 1 to 6 months (74).

Gastrointestinal Infections

The bacterial pathogens that cause diarrheal disease, including toxigenic *E. coli, Salmonella, Shigella, Campylobacter,* and *Vibrio* species, are highly susceptible to the newer quinolones. These agents also provide high drug concentrations in the lumen of the gut and the mucosa, which contribute to eradication of these pathogens from the intestine within 48 hours of initiation of therapy (75,76). Ciprofloxacin, 500 mg twice daily, and norfloxacin, 400 mg twice daily, for 3 to 5 days or a single oral 400-mg dose of fleroxacin cures more than 90% of cases of acute bacterial diarrhea and acute traveler's diarrhea, and these are comparable to trimethoprim-sulfamethoxazole (3,75–78). Single-dose fleroxacin was as effective as 2 or 3 days of therapy in patients with cholera, shigellosis, and *Vibrio parahaemolyticus* infections (75,78). Single-dose therapy with 800 mg of norfloxacin (75,79) or 1 g of ciprofloxacin (80) was also effective in treating shigellosis, except for patients infected with *Shigella dysenteriae* type 1 (75,80). Quinolones are not routinely recommended as prophylaxis against acute traveler's diarrhea because the disease responds promptly to treatment when symptoms develop and because resistance may develop more rapidly with indiscriminate use of the newer quinolones. However, prophylaxis is recommended for patients with impaired health, and daily doses of 400 mg of norfloxacin, 500 mg of ciprofloxacin, 300 mg of ofloxacin, or 400 mg of fleroxacin have been highly effective in preventing traveler's diarrhea (75,80).

Patients with typhoid fever have responded to ciprofloxacin, 500 mg twice daily, or fleroxacin, 400 mg daily, for 7 days or to ofloxacin, 200 mg twice daily, with greater than 90% cure rates (3,75,81–84). Also, ciprofloxacin, 500 to 750 mg twice daily for 4 weeks, eliminated the chronic *Salmonella* carrier state in 86% of patients followed up for 10 to 12 months (3,75).

Currently, of the four most frequently used quinolones, ciprofloxacin is the only fluoroquinolone that has been approved for use in the treatment of infectious diarrhea and typhoid and paratyphoid fevers.

Although the newer quinolones inhibit *Helicobacter pylori,* these agents have not been effective in the treatment of *H. pylori*–associated gastritis, and treatment has resulted in quinolone resistance (85–87). Ciprofloxacin may have some value in *Clostridium difficile* enterocolitis (88). Relapses have been reported in patients with *Brucella* species infection who have been treated with quinolones (89).

Skin and Soft Tissue Infections

Many fluoroquinolones are highly effective and appropriate therapy in cellulitis, subcutaneous abscesses, postoperative and posttraumatic wound infections, infected decubitus, ischemic and diabetic ulcers, and infected burns caused by facultative gram-negative bacilli or these organisms in combination with aerobic gram-positive cocci. Ciprofloxacin, ofloxacin, enoxacin, fleroxacin, levofloxacin, trovafloxacin, and moxifloxacin have been very effective in the treatment of complex skin and soft tissue infections (32,90–92). The antibacterial activity of newer quinolones and the poor activity of earlier compounds against anaerobic gram-negative bacilli suggest that quinolones should not be used alone to treat severe anaerobic infections (90,91). Also, quinolones should not be used as first-line therapy for

complex skin and soft tissue infections caused by methicillin-resistant *Staphylococcus aureus* (MRSA) because quinolone treatment has resulted in low rates of eradication, high rates of recolonization, and frequent emergence of quinolone-resistant strains (32,90). The earlier quinolones are not optimally active against β-hemolytic streptococci and should not be used to treat necrotizing (streptococcal) fasciitis (32,90). Experience with the newer quinolones, which are more active against streptococci, is not available, so that they cannot be recommended for treatment of this severe infection (90).

Colonization with MRSA has been eradicated in 50% to 79% of evaluable patients with ciprofloxacin, 750 mg orally twice daily for 7 to 28 days (93,94). When rifampin was combined with ciprofloxacin, the eradication rate was 100% when the isolates were susceptible to both agents, and these patients remained free of MRSA for at least 1 month (93). Although ciprofloxacin may eradicate MRSA colonization or cure MRSA infection, resistant strains have rapidly emerged (3,95,96).

Osteomyelitis

The oral quinolones (ciprofloxacin, pefloxacin, ofloxacin, and fleroxacin) have been effective as monotherapy for osteomyelitis, particularly when it is caused by gram-negative aerobic organisms (3,90,97,98). Most patients with acute or chronic osteomyelitis, either in native bone or complicating a foreign body, have been treated with ciprofloxacin, ofloxacin, fleroxacin, or pefloxacin for 6 to 8 weeks (range, 4 days to 6 months). Clinical cure or improvement occurred in about 80% of patients treated with ciprofloxacin with adequate follow-up of at least 6 months to more than 1 year. Treatment failures occurred in 15% to 20%, and a few patients developed recurrent infection. Resistant strains developed in some patients, principally those with *P. aeruginosa* infections (90,97,98). Ciprofloxacin, ofloxacin, and fleroxacin have had modest success in a small number of patients with septic arthritis (90).

Sexually Transmitted Diseases

Most quinolones are extremely active *in vitro* against *Neisseria gonorrhoeae,* including penicillinase-producing strains, and against *Haemophilus ducreyi* (20,99). *C. trachomatis* isolates are most susceptible to sparfloxacin, grepafloxacin, trovafloxacin, gatifloxacin, lomefloxacin, ofloxacin, and ciprofloxacin but are resistant to fleroxacin, pefloxacin, enoxacin, and norfloxacin (99). Although *Gardnerella vaginalis* and *U. urealyticum* are relatively resistant to these agents, ciprofloxacin is active against the latter about 50% of the time (99). Thus, quinolones have been used to treat a variety of sexually transmitted diseases but are not effective against *Treponema pallidum,* and there is currently no role for these drugs in the treatment of syphilis (99).

Gonococcal Infections

The lowest effective single oral doses are 100 mg of ciprofloxacin; 200 mg of enoxacin, ofloxacin, or sparfloxacin; 400 mg of norfloxacin, pefloxacin, fleroxacin, or gatifloxacin. These doses cured 95% to 100% of uncomplicated gonococcal infections in both men and women, including infections with penicillinase-producing *N. gonorrhoeae.* Thus, 100 mg of ciprofloxacin, the lowest effective oral single dose of the newer quinolones, has cured almost 100% of patients with urethral as well as rectal gonorrhea and is probably effective for pharyngeal gonococcal infections (99). As quinolone use for the treatment of gonorrhea has increased, resistance to these agents has become more widespread. There is little experience with the quinolones in the treatment of disseminated gonococcal infections.

Chlamydial Urethritis and Postgonococcal and Nongonococcal Urethritis

None of the current quinolones is effective as single-dose therapy for *C. trachomatis* urethritis, nor do they prevent postgonococcal urethritis when used as single-dose therapy for gonococcal infections. Although ciprofloxacin at 750 mg orally twice daily for 4 days eradicated *C. trachomatis* in 60% of co-infected patients and reduced the incidence of postgonococcal urethritis from 35% to 12.8%, the response rates with 7 days of therapy with ciprofloxacin or norfloxacin were not optimal (99). Ofloxacin (300 mg twice daily) for 7 days was as effective as doxycycline in patients with nongonococcal urethritis or *C. trachomatis* cervicitis (99,100). Clinical studies have also shown that fleroxacin, grepafloxacin, trovafloxacin, tosufloxacin, and sparfloxacin, when used for 7 to 14 days, are effective in the treatment of chlamydial infections (99). The quinolones are less effective than doxycycline or azithromycin for nongonococcal urethritis regardless of the presence or absence of *Chlamydia* or *Ureaplasma* species infection (99,101).

Chancroid

The most active quinolones against *H. ducreyi*, in decreasing potency, are ciprofloxacin, sparfloxacin, ofloxacin, fleroxacin, norfloxacin, pefloxacin, and enoxacin (99). Patients with chancroid (*H. ducreyi*) infections have responded successfully to a single 500-mg oral dose of ciprofloxacin (95% cure rate); however, 500 mg of ciprofloxacin twice daily for 3 days cured 100% of patients with chancroid. Fleroxacin, at a single dose of 400 mg in HIV-negative men or at 400 mg daily for 5 days in HIV-positive men, cured more than 90% of these patients with chancroid (102). Currently, ciprofloxacin, 550 mg twice daily for 3 days, is the only quinolone regimen recommended for chancroid in the Centers for Disease Control and Prevention sexually transmitted diseases treatment guidelines (99).

Donovanosis, caused by *Calymmatobacterium granulomatis*, is a major cause of genital ulcer disease in Asia, Africa, and some parts of the Caribbean. Results in a few patients treated with either ciprofloxacin or norfloxacin suggest that these two quinolones may be effective for this disease (99).

Other Infections

IMMUNOCOMPROMISED HOST

In neutropenic patients receiving cytotoxic therapy, prophylactic administration of some of the earlier quinolones has been associated with reductions in bacteremias caused by enterobacteria, but not those infections caused by gram-positive bacteria. Quinolones have contributed to the emergence of these latter organisms as important pathogens in the neutropenic patient (32,103). Ciprofloxacin (500 mg twice daily), norfloxacin (400 mg twice or three times daily), ofloxacin (300 mg twice daily), and pefloxacin (400 mg twice daily) given orally have been used successfully for prophylaxis in granulocytopenic patients. The incidence of bacteremia and colonization with gram-negative bacilli and the amount and duration of antibiotic therapy directed against gram-negative bacilli were significantly reduced in febrile neutropenic patients (103–105), which was most effectively accomplished with ciprofloxacin (103,104). However, they do not have a significant impact on fever-related morbidity or infection related mortality (103). Also, the emergence of

quinolone-resistant gram-negative organisms has been observed in neutropenic cancer patients who received quinolone prophylaxis (103–106). For this reason, guidelines from the Infectious Diseases Society of America do not recommend routine use of quinolone prophylaxis, but suggest that they be used in high-risk patients with profound and prolonged neutropenia, for as short a period as possible, in order to limit the emergence of resistance (103). Monotherapy with the quinolones for febrile neutropenic patients is not recommended. Combining quinolones with agents such as rifampin, penicillins, or macrolides significantly reduces the incidence of gram-positive (particularly streptococcal) infections (103). The newest quinolones, which have more potent activity against gram-positive bacteria, especially against streptococci, have not been fully evaluated in neutropenic patients.

CENTRAL NERVOUS SYSTEM INFECTIONS

The newer quinolones have specific advantages that make them potentially useful in the therapy of bacterial meningitis. They have excellent *in vitro* activity against gram-negative aerobic bacteria as well as against penicillin- and cephalosporin-resistant and penicillin- and cephalosporin-sensitive pneumococci (38). Although ciprofloxacin, ofloxacin, and pefloxacin penetrate into the cerebrospinal fluid and brain tissue, higher concentrations are achieved with the newer quinolones (38). Clinical experience with the quinolones as therapeutic agents for CNS bacterial infections is limited (107,108), except for a comparative clinical trial of trovafloxacin versus ceftriaxone in patients with meningococcal meningitis, in which trovafloxacin orally or intravenously was as effective as ceftriaxone (38). In nasopharyngeal carriers of *Meningococcus* species infection, oral ciprofloxacin, 500 mg twice daily for 5 days, 250 mg twice daily for 2 days, or at a 750-mg single dose (15 mg/kg single dose for 2- to 18-year-old patients) eradicated the organism in more than 90% of patients (109–112). Similar results were observed in a small study using a single dose of 400 mg of ofloxacin (38).

MISCELLANEOUS INFECTIONS

Ciprofloxacin and ofloxacin have been used with some success, in combination with other drugs, to treat multidrug-resistant pulmonary tuberculosis (ciprofloxacin and ofloxacin) and *M. avium-intracellulare* bacteremia in patients with acquired immunodeficiency syndrome (ciprofloxacin) (103,113–115). In general, the current quinolones are, at best, second-line agents to be used in combination for treating mycobacterial disease, except for *M. leprae*. Sparfloxacin, pefloxacin, and ofloxacin have shown efficacy in patients with lepromatous leprosy (26,27).

Ciprofloxacin (intravenously for 1 week and then orally for 3 weeks) plus oral rifampin (4 weeks) cured 10 patients who were intravenous drug abusers with right-sided *S. aureus* endocarditis who completed 4 weeks of therapy (116). Nineteen patients with Mediterranean spotted fever caused by *Rickettsia conorii* were cured with oral ciprofloxacin (500 mg twice daily for 2 days) (117), and five patients with cat-scratch disease experienced rapid improvement when treated with oral ciprofloxacin at 500 mg twice daily (118).

OTHER NOVEL QUINOLONES

Current interest in quinolones continues to be great, so that many other compounds are in various stages of development. Those in late stages of development include gemifloxacin, nadifloxacin, pazufloxacin, and sitafloxacin. In addition, a new class of compounds, the des-fluorinated quinolones, is under development. These compounds do not have a fluorine group in the C-6 position of the basic quinolone molecule, yet they do have great potency against gram-negative as well as gram-positive bacteria (119). New insights into structure–activity relationships suggest that newer compounds will continue to be made.

REFERENCES

1. Lesher GY, Froelich EJ, Gruett MD, et al. 1,8-Naphthyridine derivatives: a new class of chemotherapeutic agents. *J Med Pharm Chem* 1962;5:1063.
2. Brighty KE, Gootz TD. Chemistry and mechanism of action of the quinolone antibacterials. In: Andriole VT, ed. *The quinolones.* San Diego: Academic Press, 2000:33–97.
3. Andriole VT. The quinolones: prospects. In: Andriole VT, ed. *The quinolones.* San Diego: Academic Press, 2000:477–495.
4. Downs J, Andriole VT, Ryan JL. In vitro activity of MK-0366 against clinical urinary pathogens including gentamicin-resistant *Pseudomonas aeruginosa. Antimicrob Agents Chemother* 1982;21:670.
5. Wise R, Andrew JM, Edwards LJ. In vitro activity of Bay 09867, a new quinolone derivative, compared with those of other antimicrobial agents. *Antimicrob Agents Chemother* 1983;23:559.
6. Andriole VT. The future of the quinolones. *Drugs* 1993;45(3):1.
7. Andriole VT. The future of the quinolones. Proceedings of the 6th International Symposium on New Quinolones, Denver, CO, 1998. *Drugs* 1999;[Suppl 2]:1–5.
8. Higgins NP, Peebles CL, Sugino A, et al. Purification of subunits of *Escherichia coli,* DNA gyrase and reconstitution of enzymic activity. *Proc Natl Acad Sci USA* 1978;75:1773.
9. Pedrini A. Nalidixic acid. In: Hahn FE, ed. *Antibiotics,* Vol 5. Berlin: Springer-Verlag, 1979.
10. Wang JC. Interactions between DNAs and enzymes: the effect of superhelical turns. *J Mol Biol* 1974;87:797.
11. Wang JC. DNA topoisomerases. *Annu Rev Biochem* 1985;54:665.
12. Kato J, Nishimura Y, Imamura R, et al. New topoisomerase essential for chromosome segregation in *E. coli. Cell* 1990;63:393–404.
13. Marians KJ. Replication fork progression. In: Neidhartdt FC, ed. E. coli *and* Salmonella *cellular and molecular biology,* 2nd ed, Vol 1. Washington DC: American Society for Microbiology, 1996:749–763.
14. Kornberg A, Baker TA. *DNA replication.* New York: WH Freeman, 1992.
15. Shen LL, Chu DTW. Type II DNA topoisomerases as antibacterial targets. *Curr Pharmaceut Design* 1996;2:195–208.
16. Lewis RJ, Tsai FTF, Wigley DB. Molecular mechanisms of drug inhibition of DNA gyrase. *Bioessays* 1996;18:661–671.
17. Bauernfeind A. Comparative in vitro activities of the new quinolone, BAY y 3118, and ciprofloxacin, sparfloxacin, tosufloxacin, CI-960 and CI-990. *J Antimicrob Chemother* 1993;31:505–522.
18. Hong CY, Kim YK, Chang JH, et al. Novel fluoroquinolone antibacterial agents containing oxime-substituted (aminomethyl) pyrrolidines: synthesis and antibacterial activity of 7-(4-)aminomethyl)-3-(methoxyimino)pyrrolidin-1-yl)-1-cyclopropyl-6-fluoro-4-oxo-1,4dihydro[1,8]naphthyridine-3-carboxylic acid (LB20304). *J Med Chem* 1997;40:3584–3593.
19. Akasaka T, Kurosaka S, Uchida Y, et al. Antibacterial activities and inhibitory effects of sitafloxacin (DU-6859a) and its optical isomers against type II topoisomerases. *Antimicrob Agents Chemother* 1998;42:1284–1287.
20. Phillips I, King A, Shannon K. Comparative in vitro properties of the quinolones. In: Andriole VT, ed. *The quinolones,* 3rd ed. San Diego: Academic Press, 2000:99–137.
21. Garcia-Rodriguez JA, Garcia Sanchez JE, Trujillano I, et al. Susceptibilities of *Brucella melitensis* isolates to clinafloxacin and four other new fluoroquinolones. *Antimicrob Agents Chemother* 1995;39:1194.
22. Piddock LJV. New quinolones and gram-positive bacteria. *Antimicrob Agents Chemother* 1994;38:163.
23. Dubois J, St. Pierre C. Comparative in vitro activity and postantibiotic effect of gemifloxacin against *Legionella* spp. *J Antimicrob Chemother* 999;44[Suppl A]:136.
24. Felmingham D, Robbins M, Dencer C, et al. In vitro activity of gemifloxacin against *Streptococcus pneumoniae, Haemophilus influenzae, Neisseria catarrhalis, Legionella pneumophila* and *Chlamydia* spp. *J Antimicrob Chemother* 1999;44[Suppl A]:131.
25. Ruiz-Serrano MJ, Alcala L, Martinez L, et al. In vitro activity of six quinolones against clinical isolates of *Mycobacterium* tuberculosis susceptible and resistant to first-line antituberculosis drugs. Abstract of the 39th Interscience Conference on Antimicrobial Agents of Chemotherapy, San Francisco, #P1492, 1999.
26. Chan GP, Garcia-Ignacio BY, Chavez VE, et al. Clinical trial of sparfloxacin for lepromatous leprosy. *Antimicrob Agents Chemother* 1994;38:61.
27. Ji B, Perani EG, Petinom C, et al. Clinical trial of ofloxacin alone and in combination with dapsone plus clofazimine for treatment of lepromatous leprosy. *Antimicrob Agents Chemother* 1994;38:662.
28. Neu HC. Synergy and antagonism of combinations with quinolones. *Eur J Clin Microbiol Infect Dis* 1991;10:255.
29. Meng X, Nightingale CH, Sweeney KR, et al. Loss of bactericidal activities of quinolones during the post-antibiotic effect induced by rifampicin. *J Antimicrob Chemother* 1994;33:721.
30. Kohler T, Pechere JC. Bacterial resistance to quinolones. In: Andriole VT, ed. *The quinolones.* San Diego: Academic Press, 2000:139–167.
31. Sanders CC, Sanders WE Jr, Goering RV, et al. Selection of multiple antibiotic resistance by quinolones, β-lactams, and aminoglycosides with special reference to cross-resistance between unrelated drug classes. *Antimicrob Agents Chemother* 1984;26:797.
32. Andriole VT. Quinolones. In: Finch RG, Greenwood D, Norrby SR, et al., eds. *Antibiotic and chemotherapy,* 8th ed. New York: Elsevier Science, 2003:351–375.
33. Willmott CJR, Maxwell A. A single point mutation in the DNA gyrase A protein greatly reduces binding of fluoroquinolones to the gyrase-DNA complex. *Antimicrob Agents Chemother* 1993;37:126.
34. Hirai K, Irikura T, Iyobe S, et al. Inhibition of conjugal transfer of R plasmids by norfloxacin in *Pseudomonas aeruginosa. Chemotherapy* 1984;32:471.
35. Crumplin GC. Plasmid-mediated resistance to nalidixic acid and new 4-quinolones? *Lancet* 1987;2:854.
36. Munshi MH, Sack DA, Haider K, et al. Plasmid-mediated resistance to nalidixic acid in *Shigella dysenteriae* type I. *Lancet* 1987;2:419.
37. Kim MK, Nightingale CH. Pharmacokinetics and pharmacodynamics of the fluoroquinolones. In: Andriole VT, ed. *The quinolones.* San Diego: Academic Press, 2000:169–202.
38. Hasbun R, Quagliarello VJ. Use of the quinolones in treatment of bacterial meningitis. In: Andriole VT, ed. *The quinolones,* 3rd ed. San Diego: Academic Press, 2000:325–343.
39. Sorgel F, Kinzig M. Pharmacokinetics of gyrase inhibitors. Part 1. Basic chemistry and gastrointestinal disposition. *Am J Med* 1993;94[Suppl 3A]:44.
40. Andriole VT. Use of quinolones in treatment of prostatitis and lower urinary tract infections. *Eur J Clin Microbiol Infect Dis* 1991;10:342.
41. Giamarellou H, Kilokythas E, Petrikkos G, et al. Pharmacokinetics of three newer quinolones in pregnant and lactating women. *Am J Med* 1989;87[Suppl 5A]:49.
42. Lode H, Hoffken G, Olschewski P, et al. Pharmacokinetics of ofloxacin after parenteral and oral administration. *Antimicrob Agents Chemother* 1987;31:1338.
43. Weidekamm E. Pharmacokinetics of fleroxacin in renal impairment. *Am J Med* 1993;94[Suppl 3A]:70.
44. Fillastre JP, Leroy A, Moulin B, et al. Pharmacokinetics of quinolones in renal insufficiency. *J Antimicrob Chemother* 1990;26[Suppl B]:51.
45. Montay G, Gaillot J. Pharmacokinetics of fluoroquinolones in hepatic failure. *J Antimicrob Chemother* 1990;26[Suppl B]:61.
46. Stahlmann R, Lode H. Safety overview: toxicity, adverse effects, and drug interactions. In: Andriole VT, ed. *The quinolones,* 3rd ed. San Diego: Academic Press, 2000:397–453.
47. Domagala JM. Structure-activity and structure-side-effect relationships for the quinolone antibacterials. *J Antimicrob Chemother* 1994;33:685.
48. Adam D, Syndrassy K, Christ W, et al. Arbeitsgemeinschaft "Arzneimittelsicherheit" der Paul Ehrlich Gesellschaft fur Chemotherapie. Vertraglichkeit der Gyrase Hemmer. *Muench Med Wochenschr* 1987;129:45.
49. Schaad UB. Use of quinolones in pediatrics. In: Andriole CT, ed. *The quinolones,* 3rd ed. San Diego: Academic Press, 2000:455–475.
50. Dembry, LM, Farrington JM, Andriole, VT. Fluoroquinolone antibiotics: adverse effects and safety profiles. *Infect Dis Clin Pract* 1999;8:421–428.
51. Iannini PB, Andriole VT. Moxifloxacin: a review of its worldwide safety profile in more than six million patients. *Clin Ther* (In press.)
52. Robson RA. The effects of quinolone on xanthine pharmacokinetics. *Am J Med* 1992;92[Suppl 4A]:22.
53. Stille W, Harder S, Mieke S, et al. Decrease of caffeine elimination in man during co-administration of 4 quinolones. *J Antimicrob Chemother* 1987;20:729.
54. Fuhr U, Strobl G, Manaut F, et al. Quinolone antibacterial agents: relationship between structure and in vitro inhibition of human cytochrome P-450 isoform CYP1A2. *Mol Pharmacol* 1993;43:191.
55. Hasegawa T, Nadai M, Kuzuya T, et al. The possible mechanism of interaction between xanthines and quinolones. *J Pharm Pharmacol* 1990;42:767.
56. Janknegt R: Drug interactions with quinolones. *J Antimicrob Chemother* 1990;26[Suppl D]:7.
57. Nicolle LE. Use of quinolones in urinary tract infection and prostatitis. In: Andriole VT, ed. *The quinolones,* 3rd ed. San Diego: Academic Press, 2000:203–225.
58. Iravani A. Multicenter study of single-dose and multiple-dose fleroxacin versus ciprofloxacin in the treatment of uncomplicated urinary tract infections. *Am J Med* 1993;94[Suppl 3A]:89.
59. Saginur R, Nicolle LE. Single dose compared with 3-day norfloxacin treatment of uncomplicated urinary tract infection in women. *Arch Intern Med* 1992;152:1233.
60. Nicolle LE, DuBois J, Martel AY, et al. Treatment of acute uncomplicated urinary tract infections with 3 days of lomefloxacin compared with treatment with 3 days of norfloxacin. *Antimicrob Agents Chemother* 1993;37:574.
61. Rubin RH, Shapiro ED, Andriole VT, et al. Evaluation of new anti-infective drugs for the treatment of urinary tract infection. *Clin Infect Dis* 1992;15[Suppl 1]:S216–S227.
62. Pittman W, Moon JO, Hamrick LC, et al. Randomized doubleblind trial of high- and low-dose fleroxacin versus norfloxacin for complicated urinary tract infection. *Am J Med* 1993;94[Suppl 3A]:101.

63. Cox CE. A comparison of the safety and efficacy of lomefloxacin and ciprofloxacin in the treatment of complicated or recurrent urinary tract infections. *Am J Med* 1992;92[Suppl 4A]:82.

64. Iannini PB, Niederman MS, Andriole VT. Treatment of respiratory infections with quinolones. In: Andriole VT, ed. *The quinolones,* 3rd ed. San Diego: Academic Press, 2000:255–284.

65. Chodosh S. Efficacy of fleroxacin versus amoxicillin in acute exacerbations of chronic bronchitis. *Am J Med* 1993;94[Suppl 3A]:131.

66. Andriole VT. *The use of quinolones in respiratory tract infections: summary.* Proceedings of the 17th International Congress of Chemotherapy, Berlin, Germany, 1991. *Infection* 1991;19[Suppl 7]:391.

67. Andriole CL, Andriole VT. Are all quinolones created equal? In: Andriole VT, ed. *Mediguide to infectious diseases* 2002;21:1–5.

68. Lipsky BA, Tack KJ, Kuo C, et al. Ofloxacin treatment of *Chlamydia pneumoniae* (strain TWAR) lower respiratory tract infections. *Am J Med* 1990;89:722.

69. Glatz K, Szabo D, Szabo G, et al. Emergence of extremely high penicillin and cefotaxime resistance and high-level levofloxacin resistance in clinical isolates of *Streptococcus pneumoniae* in Hungary. *J Antimicrob Chemother* 2001;48:731–734.

70. Peloquin CA, Cumbo TJ, Nix DE, et al. Evaluation of intravenous ciprofloxacin in patients with nosocomial lower respiratory tract infections: impact of plasma concentrations, organism, minimum inhibitory concentration, and clinical condition on bacterial eradication. *Arch Intern Med* 1989;149:2269.

71. Gentry LO, Rodriguez-Gomez G, Kohler RB, et al. Parenteral followed by oral ofloxacin for nosocomial pneumonia and community-acquired pneumonia requiring hospitalization. *Am Rev Respir Dis* 1992;145:31.

72. Bosso JA, Black PG, Matsen JM. Ciprofloxacin versus tobramycin plus azlocillin in pulmonary exacerbations in adult patients with cystic fibrosis. *Am J Med* 1987;82[Suppl]:180.

73. Scully BE, Nakatomi M, Ores C, et al. Ciprofloxacin therapy in cystic fibrosis. *Am J Med* 1987;82[Suppl]:196.

74. Giamarellou H. Use of quinolones in malignant otitis externa. *Quinolone Bull* 1993;10:19.

75. Hamer DH, Gorbach SL. Use of quinolones for treatment and prophylaxis of bacterial gastrointestinal infections. In: Andriole VT, ed. *The quinolones,* 3rd ed. San Diego: Academic Press, 2000:303–323.

76. DuPont HL, Ericsson CD. Prevention and treatment of traveler's diarrhea. *N Engl J Med* 1993;328:1821.

77. Steffen R, Jori R, DuPont HL, et al. Efficacy and toxicity of fleroxacin in the treatment of traveler's diarrhea. *Am J Med* 1993;94[Suppl 3A]:182.

78. Butler T, Lolekha S, Rasidi C, et al. Treatment of acute bacterial diarrhea: a multicenter international trial comparing placebo with fleroxacin given as a single dose or once daily for three days. *Am J Med* 1993;94[Suppl 3A]:187.

79. Gotuzzo E, Oberhelman RA, Maguina C, et al. Comparison of single-dose treatment with norfloxacin and standard 5-day treatment with trimethoprim-sulfamethoxazole for acute shigellosis in adults. *Antimicrob Agents Chemother* 1989;33:1101.

80. Bennish ML, Salam MA, Khan WA, et al. Treatment of shigellosis. III. Comparison of one- and two-dose ciprofloxacin with standard 5-day treatment. A randomized, blinded trial. *Ann Intern Med* 1992;117:7278.

81. Uwaydah AK, Al Soub H, Matar I. Randomized prospective study comparing two dosage regimens of ciprofloxacin for treatment of typhoid fever. *J Antimicrob Chemother* 1992;30:707.

82. Wang F, Gu X-J, Zhang M-F, et al. Treatment of typhoid fever with ofloxacin. *J Antimicrob Chemother* 1989;23:785.

83. Arnold K, Hong CS, Nelwan R, et al. Randomized comparative study of fleroxacin and chloramphenicol in typhoid fever. *Am J Med* 1993;94[Suppl 3A]:195.

84. Gotuzzo E, Guerra JG, Benavente L, et al. Use of norfloxacin to treat chronic typhoid carriers. *J Infect Dis* 1988;157:1221.

85. Simor AE, Ferro S, Low DE. Comparative in vitro activities of six new fluoroquinolones and other oral antimicrobial agents against *Campylobacter pylori. Antimicrob Agents Chemother* 1989;33:108.

86. Glupczynski Y, Labbe M, Burette A, et al. Treatment failure of ofloxacin in *Campylobacter pylori* infection. *Lancet* 1987;2:1096.

87. Mertens JCC, Dekker W, Ligtvoet EEJ, et al. Treatment failure of norfloxacin against *Campylobacter pylori* and chronic gastritis in patients with nonulcerative dyspepsia. *Antimicrob Agents Chemother* 1989;33:245.

88. Lettau LA. Oral fluoroquinolone therapy in *Clostridium difficile* enterocolitis. *JAMA* 1988;260:2216.

89. Lang R, Rubinstein E. Quinolones for the treatment of brucellosis. *J Antimicrob Chemother* 1992;29:1063.

90. Karchmer AW. Use of quinolones in skin and skin structure (osteomyelitis) and other infections. In: Andriole VT, eds. *The quinolones,* 3rd ed. San Diego: Academic Press, 2000:371–395.

91. Goldstein EJC. Possible role for the new fluoroquinolones (levofloxacin, grepafloxacin, trovafloxacin, clinafloxacin, sparfloxacin, and DU-6859a) in the treatment of anaerobic infections: review of current information on efficacy and safety. *Clin Infect Dis* 1996;23[Suppl 1]:S25–S30.

92. Gentry LO. Review of quinolones in treatment of infections of the skin and skin structure. *J Antimicrob Chemother* 1991;28[Suppl C]:97.

93. Mulligan ME, Ruane PJ, Johnston L, et al. Ciprofloxacin for eradication of methicillin-resistant *Staphylococcus aureus* colonization. *Am J Med* 1987;82[Suppl]:215.

94. Smith SM, Eng RHK, Tecson-Tumang F. Ciprofloxacin therapy for methicillin-resistant *Staphylococcus aureus* infections or colonizations. *Antimicrob Agents Chemother* 1989;33:181.

95. Piercy EA, Barbaro D, Luby JP, et al. Ciprofloxacin for methicillin-resistant *Staphylococcus aureus* infections. *Antimicrob Agents Chemother* 1989;33:128.

96. Trucksis M, Hooper DC, Wolfson JS. Emerging resistance to fluoroquinolones in staphylococci: an alert. *Ann Intern Med* 1991;114:424.

97. Andriole VT. Treatment of osteomyelitis with quinolones. *Quinolone Bull* 1987;3:15.

98. Gentry LO. Oral antimicrobial therapy for osteomyelitis [Editorial]. *Ann Intern Med* 1991;114:986.

99. DiCarlo RP, Martin DH. Use of quinolones in sexually transmitted diseases. In: Andriole VT, ed. *The quinolones,* 3rd ed. San Diego: Academic Press, 2000:227–254.

100. Hooton TM, Batteiger BE, Judson FN, et al. Ofloxacin versus doxycycline for treatment of cervical infection with *Chlamydia trachomatis. Antimicrob Agents Chemother* 1992;36:1144.

101. Stamm WE, Hicks CB, Martin DH, et al. Azithromycin for empirical treatment of the nongonococcal urethritis syndrome in men: a randomized double-blind study. *JAMA* 1995;274:545.

102. Tyndall MW, Plourde PJ, Agoki E, et al. Fleroxacin in the treatment of chancroid: an open study in men seropositive or seronegative for the human immunodeficiency virus type I. *Am J Med* 1993;94[Suppl 3A]:85.

103. Ralston KVI. Use of the quinolones in immunocompromised patients. In: Andriole VT, ed. *The quinolones,* 3rd ed. San Diego: Academic Press, 2000:343–369.

104. D'Antonio D, Piccolomini R, Iacone A, et al. Comparison of ciprofloxacin, ofloxacin and pefloxacin for the prevention of the bacterial infection in neutropenic patients with haematological malignancies. *J Antimicrob Chemother* 1994;33:837.

105. Bow EJ, Loewen R, Vaughan D. Reduced requirement for antibiotic therapy targeting gram-negative organisms in febrile, neutropenic patients with cancer who are receiving antibacterial chemoprophylaxis with oral quinolones. *Clin Infect Dis* 1995;20:907.

106. Kern WV, Andriof E, Oethinger M, et al. Emergence of fluoroquinolone-resistant *Escherichia coli* at a cancer center. *Antimicrob Agents Chemother* 1994;38:681.

107. Segev S, Barzilai A, Rosen N, et al. Pefloxacin treatment of meningitis caused by gram-negative bacteria. *Arch Intern Med* 1989;149:1314.

108. Schonwald S, Beus I, Lisic M, et al. Brief report: ciprofloxacin in the treatment of gram-negative bacillary meningitis. *Am J Med* 1989;87[Suppl 5A]:248.

109. Renkonen OV, Sivonen A, Visakorpi R. Effect of ciprofloxacin on carrier rate of *Neisseria meningitidis* in army recruits in Finland. *Antimicrob Agents Chemother* 1987;31:962.

110. Pugsley MP, Dworzack DL, Horowitz EA, et al. Efficacy of ciprofloxacin in the treatment of nasopharyngeal carriers of *Neisseria meningitidis. J Infect Dis* 1987;156:211.

111. Dworzack DL, Sanders CC, Horowitz EA, et al. Evaluation of single-dose ciprofloxacin in the eradication of *Neisseria meningitidis* from nasopharyngeal carriers. *Antimicrob Agents Chemother* 1988;21:1740.

112. Cuevas LE, Kazembe P, Mughogho GK, et al. Eradication of nasopharyngeal carriage of *Neisseria meningitidis* in children and adults in rural Africa: a comparison of ciprofloxacin and rifampicin. *J Infect Dis* 1995;171:728.

113. Yew WW, Kwan SY, Ma WK, et al. In vitro activity of ofloxacin against *Mycobacterium tuberculosis* and its clinical efficacy in multiply resistant pulmonary tuberculosis. *J Antimicrob Chemother* 1990;26:227.

114. de Lalla F, Maserati R, Scarpellini P, et al. Clarithromycinciprofloxacin-amikacin for therapy of *Mycobacterium avium–Mycobacterium intracellulare* bacteremia in patients with AIDS. *Antimicrob Agents Chemother* 1992;36:1567.

115. Kemper CA, Meng T-C, Nussbaum J, et al. Treatment of *Mycobacterium avium* complex bacteremia in AIDS with a four-drug oral regimen. *Ann Intern Med* 1992;116:466.

116. Dworkin RJ, Sande MA, Lee BL, et al. Treatment of right-sided *Staphylococcus aureus* endocarditis in intravenous drug abusers with ciprofloxacin and rifampicin. *Lancet* 1989;2:1071.

117. Gudiol F, Pallares R, Carratala J, et al. Randomized double-blind evaluation of ciprofloxacin and doxycycline for Mediterranean spotted fever. *Antimicrob Agents Chemother* 1989;33:987.

118. Holley HP. Successful treatment of cat-scratch disease with ciprofloxacin. *JAMA* 1991;265:1563.

119. Bassetti M, Dembry LM, Farrel PA, et al. Antimicrobial activities of BMS-284756 compared with those of fluoroquinolones and β-lactams against gram-positive clinical isolates. *Antimicrob Agents Chemother* 2002;46:234–238.

CHAPTER 27
Chloramphenicol

Graeme N. Forrest and David W. Oldach

For several decades, chloramphenicol proved to be efficacious in the treatment of infections caused by gram-positive and gram-negative bacteria, including anaerobes and *Rickettsia* species. It once was the only antimicrobial available that was consistently active against *Salmonella* species, including *Salmonella typhi* (1). However, the recognition of life-threatening toxic effects (i.e., gray syndrome and aplastic anemia) caused clinicians to restrict the use of this drug (2,3). Less toxic antimicrobials have since replaced the drug in treating many of these diseases. However, chloramphenicol is still widely used in developing countries because it is inexpensive and readily available over the counter for the treatment of enteric fever. Many of the previously treatable organisms are resistant to chloramphenicol, making its use less reliable in these countries. The use of chloramphenicol should be limited to well-defined clinical situations for seriously ill patients because of its potential toxicity.

DERIVATION, STRUCTURE, AND PREPARATIONS

After the discovery and manufacture of penicillin in the 1940s, soil organisms were actively screened for antimicrobial production. Chloramphenicol was isolated from the organism *Streptomyces venezuelae*, which was discovered in a field near Caracas, Venezuela (4,5).

Chloramphenicol has a simple structure and is easily mass produced by chemical synthesis (6). It is composed of a *p*-nitrobenzene ring attached to a propanediol moiety with a dichloracetamide side chain (Fig. 27.1). The antimicrobial activity depends on the integrity of the propanediol moiety and dichloracetamide side chain. The aromatic ring and the acyl side chain may be substituted without loss of bacteriostasis (7). In addition to chloramphenicol base, two esters of the drug are commercially available: chloramphenicol succinate and chloramphenicol palmitate (8,9). The esters must be hydrolyzed to chloramphenicol to be biologically active. Preparations of chloramphenicol are listed in Table 27.1 and dosing in Table 27.2. Oral chloramphenicol is well absorbed from the gastrointestinal tract where the intravenous ester formulation must be hydrolyzed systemically. Oral and parenteral dosing recommendations are similar (10,11).

Triamphenical, a chloramphenicol analogue available in Europe and Japan but not in the United States, has a methylsulfonyl group, which has replaced the *p*-nitro group on the benzene ring. It has been associated with reversible bone marrow depression but not aplastic anemia (12).

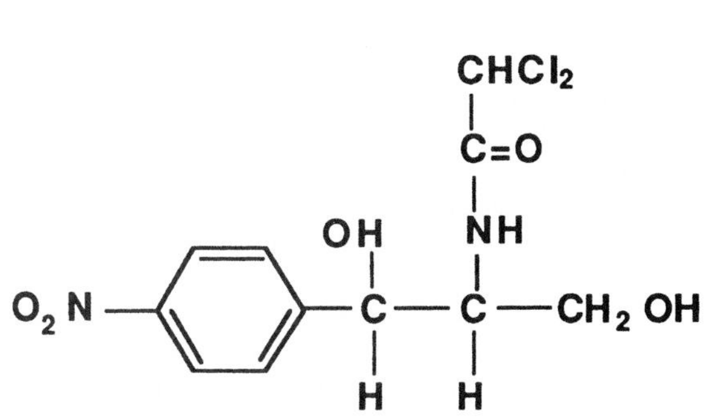

MECHANISM OF ACTION

Chloramphenicol inhibits protein synthesis in bacteria, but nucleic acid synthesis is unaffected (13). The drug binds reversibly to the larger 50S subunit of the 70S ribosome. It inhibits protein synthesis by preventing the attachment of aminoacyl-transfer RNA to the 50S binding site (14). This makes the amino acid substrate unavailable to the peptidyl transferase and prevents the formation of the peptide bond (15). With protein synthesis affected, there is subsequent bacteriostasis of most sensitive organisms (16). However, chloramphenicol is bactericidal for some organisms, including *Streptococcus pneumoniae*, *Haemophilus influenzae*, and *Neisseria meningitidis* (17,18). The killing mechanism has not been elucidated. Most protein synthesis occurs on 80S ribosomes in mammals; however, their mitochondria contain 70S ribosomes (19). Therefore, chloramphenicol-induced inhibition of mammalian mitochondrial protein synthesis may account for some of the significant toxicity encountered with this agent.

SPECTRUM OF ACTIVITY

Chloramphenicol is the prototype of the broad-spectrum antimicrobial. The drug demonstrates activity against bacteria, rickettsiae, ehrlichiae, chlamydiae, and spirochetes (20,21). Sensitive organisms are susceptible to serum levels that are easily achieved clinically. The drug is active against most aerobic and anaerobic gram-positive bacteria, with the exception of *Nocardia* species, group D streptococci, and methicillin-resistant *Staphylococcus aureus* (22). Many of the Enterobacteriaceae, especially *Escherichia coli* and *Proteus mirabilis*, are sensitive to chloramphenicol, whereas *Klebsiella*, *Enterobacter*, *Serratia*, and indole-positive *Proteus* species have varying sensitivities (23). *Pseudomonas* species and *Acinetobacter* species are mostly resistant, with the exception of *Burkholderia pseudomallei* (24). Other gram-negative organisms, including *N. meningitidis*, *Neisseria gonorrhoeae*, *H. influenzae* (β-lactamase–positive and β-lactamase–negative strains), *Vibrio cholerae*, *Brucella* species, and *Bordetella pertussis*, are usually sensitive (22). Chloramphenicol is active *in vitro* against most anaerobes, including *Bacteroides fragilis* (25). New β-lactam antibiotics and fluoroquinolones have replaced chloramphenicol in treating the Enterobacteriaceae and many *Pseudomonas* species. The drugs metronidazole, clindamycin, and the β-lactam/β-lactamase inhibitor combinations are generally safer and have largely replaced chloramphenicol for therapy of *B. fragilis* infections (26,27).

In the United States, childhood vaccination against *H. influenzae* type B has almost eradicated this organism as a cause of meningitis and other severe infections in children. The third-generation cephalosporins are the preferred agents used for the empirical treatment of bacterial meningitis (28,29). However, in many developing countries, chloramphenicol is still the main treatment of penicillin-allergic patients with meningitis (30). The drug obtains high cerebrospinal fluid levels, giving it excellent bactericidal activity against *N. meningitidis* and most *S. pneumoniae* isolates, including β-lactamase–producing strains. However, the drug cannot be relied on to treat these serious infections because isolates are showing increasing chloramphenicol resistance (31–36).

Figure 27.1. Chloramphenicol chemical structure.

TABLE 27.1. Preparations of Chloramphenicol

Oral	
Chloramphenicol capsules[a]	250 mg
	500 mg
Chloramphenicol palmitate suspension[a]	150 mg/5 mL
Intravenous	
Chloramphenicol sodium succinate	1 g/vial
Ophthalmic	
Chloramphenicol ophthalmic solution	25 mg/vial
Chloramphenicol ophthalmic cream	1%
Otic	
Chloramphenicol otic solution	5 mg/mL

[a]Not available in the United States (see text).

TABLE 27.3. Mechanisms of Resistance to Chloramphenicol by Organisms

Resistance mechanism	Organisms (reference)
Nitroreduction	*Bacteroides* and *Clostridium* species (59)
Altered 50S binding	*Bacillus subtilis* (60)
Altered cell wall permeability	*Escherichia coli, Pseudomonas aeruginosa, Serratia, Haemophilus influenzae* (61–63)
Transposon mediated (plasmid)	*Pseudomonas* species (64)
Chromosomally mediated (gene)	*Haemophilus influenzae* (65)
Efflux pump	*Pseudomonas* species (66)

Penicillin-resistant strains of *S. pneumoniae* are also resistant to chloramphenicol, with elevated minimal inhibitory concentrations (MICs) for the drug. The toxicity of chloramphenicol outweighs the benefit of using higher doses of the drug to overcome intermediate resistance. In addition, *in vitro* antagonism between chloramphenicol and β-lactam antibiotics has been observed repeatedly (35–38), although the clinical significance of this effect remains uncertain.

Worldwide, *Salmonella* species, including *Salmonella typhi*, are showing increasing chloramphenicol resistance (39,40). In a Spanish survey of isolates collected through 1994, 78% were shown to be chloramphenicol resistant (41). In the United States, imported cases are likely to be resistant (42,43), and quinolones are now considered first-line agents for the treatment of typhoid fever. Importantly, increasing resistance to the quinolone class of antibiotics is also being observed around the world at this time (44–49). *Shigella* species isolates resistant to multiple antibiotics, including chloramphenicol, are common in developing countries and are showing similar resistance patterns as *Salmonella* species (47). The use of chloramphenicol in the treatment of this disease is limited, and the quinolones are more effective substitutes (48,49).

Chloramphenicol is active against most clinically important ricksettsiae, ehrlichiae, chlamydiae, spirochetes, and mycoplasmas; however, other less toxic therapeutic alternatives, such as the tetracyclines, are often recommended (50,51).

MECHANISMS OF RESISTANCE

The six mechanisms of resistance to chloramphenicol are shown in Table 27.3.

The most significant of these mechanisms is the plasmid-mediated production of chloramphenicol acetyltransferase (52). The R factors carrying this gene may confer simultaneous resis-

TABLE 27.2. Dosing of Chloramphenicol

Age	Dose	Comments
Newborn younger than 2 wk and premature infants	25 mg/kg/d in 6-h intervals	Assay of serum levels mandatory
Infants 1–2 wk old	25 mg/kg q12h	
Older children and adults	50 mg/kg/d in 6-h intervals	
Older children and adults with meningitis	100 mg/kg/d in 6-h intervals	

tance to multiple antibiotics (43). Outbreaks of chloramphenicol-resistant typhoid fever and shigella dysentery have been associated with these plasmids (42,53,54). In the United States, outbreaks of plasmid-mediated chloramphenicol-resistant *S. enteritidis* serotype *Newport* infections have been reported in humans (55,56). Other *Salmonella* outbreaks have been linked to either contaminated hamburger meat or raw-milk cheese prepared from cattle raised on dairy farms where the use of chloramphenicol was common (57,58).

PHARMACOLOGY

Serum concentrations of chloramphenicol are determined by dose, route of administration, and product form. Chloramphenicol is well absorbed from the gastrointestinal tract after oral administration and produces peak serum levels within 1 to 2 hours (67). The drug is only slightly water-soluble and bitter tasting. Consequently, the oral suspension used in children is the more soluble tasteless palmitate ester. The intravenous formulation is a 3-monosuccinate ester, which must be hydrolyzed either in the gastrointestinal tract by pancreatic lipase or systemically by the liver, kidneys, and lungs to the active chloramphenicol base (8,68). Hydrolysis is variable, and serum levels of active drug after palmitate administration are usually less than levels achieved after comparable doses of the base drug (69). Chloramphenicol succinate is rapidly cleared from the plasma during intravenous administration (70). The renal clearance of prodrug is 27% in adults and 41% in children (10). About 70% of intravenously administered succinate ester undergoes hydrolysis to the active base, and the resulting serum levels are about 70% of those achieved after a similar oral dose of nonester (11). Chloramphenicol palmitate produces lower levels than chloramphenicol base but higher levels than intravenous chloramphenicol succinate (10). Serum levels of active drug after an intramuscular dose are about one half to two thirds of a comparable intravenous dose because of delayed absorption of the ester from the injection site resulting in less hemolysis of the succinate (71). A comparison of intramuscular therapy with oral or intravenous treatment in typhoid fever and Rocky Mountain spotted fever demonstrated delayed therapeutic responses and an increased frequency of relapse (72). Use of intramuscular chloramphenicol is therefore not recommended.

Chloramphenicol in ophthalmic ointments and solutions is absorbed into the aqueous humor, producing bacteriostatic concentrations of the drug (73). Subconjunctival injections do not produce adequate levels in the aqueous humor, and systemic therapy is required for panophthalmitis (74). Topical drug should not be used to treat bacterial conjunctivitis (75).

Chloramphenicol enters most body fluid compartments, including cerebrospinal, pleural, pericardial, peritoneal, and joint fluids (9,76,77). A plasma concentration of 40% to 65% is achieved in cerebrospinal fluid in the presence or absence of inflamed meninges (9,78,79). The drug is highly lipophilic, achieving concentrations in brain tissue up to nine times that of serum (80). Only small concentrations of active drug are found in the bile (81). Its metabolism is primarily by the liver, where it is conjugated to glucuronic acid and excreted in this inactive form by the kidney. Only 5% to 10% of the drug is excreted in the active form by glomerular filtration (81). Probenecid increases serum concentrations of inactive glucuronide without affecting levels of active drug. Chloramphenicol achieves adequate urine concentrations, which are sufficient to treat urinary tract infections in patients with normal renal function but are inadequate in patients with renal failure (82). In patients with poor renal function (e.g., those undergoing dialysis, hemodialysis, or peritoneal dialysis), there is little dose modification required because the glucuronide is nontoxic, and the glomerular filtration rate does not affect the serum half-life of the active drug (83,84).

In adults with normal liver function, chloramphenicol has a half-life of 3 to 4 hours and is 25% to 50% protein bound (81–86). Recommended doses usually produce serum concentrations of 5 to 25 μg/mL. Susceptible bacteria are defined as organisms inhibited by a concentration of 16 μg/mL or less (87). Caution is required in patients with significant parenchymal liver disease. Chloramphenicol is metabolized slowly in patients with hepatic insufficiency, and bone marrow depression may ensue because of increased levels of the active compound (85). The dose should be reduced in such patients, and the course of therapy should be as brief as possible. The hydrolysis of chloramphenicol succinate in children is variable, especially during the neonatal period (86). Newborns have a deficiency of the glucuronide-conjugating mechanism as well as a reduced glomerular filtration rate (87). The low rate of conjugation and reduction in renal clearance produces higher levels of drug per dose than in older infants (88). Reduced dosing and careful monitoring of serum levels of drug are required in this age group (86). The drug crosses the placenta and is also found in breast milk. Caution is advised in treating pregnant or lactating women (89).

TOXICITY AND ADVERSE REACTIONS

Gray Syndrome

A symptom complex of vomiting, abdominal distention, lethargy, cyanosis, hypotension, irregular respirations, hypothermia, and death have been described in full-term neonates and premature infants treated with chloramphenicol (3,90–92). This syndrome develops because the neonate is unable to conjugate and excrete chloramphenicol, resulting in toxic accumulation of the drug (86). As chloramphenicol levels elevate, the mitochondrial cytochrome system is affected, resulting in reduced oxidative phosphorylation. As drug concentrations rise to higher than 100 μg/mL, chloramphenicol inhibits electron transport in the NADPH oxidase portion of the mitochondrial respiratory chain. The heart, liver, kidneys, and skeletal muscle have high oxygen consumption and are particularly susceptible to these toxic effects (93–95). Gray syndrome begins typically 3 to 4 days after the initiation of therapy, and concentrations of serum chloramphenicol are usually greater than 50 μg/mL (3). Accumulation of lactic acid results in a metabolic acidosis, which does not respond to bicarbonate therapy. Subsequent cardiovascular collapse occurs within 6 to 12 hours from onset of symptoms (95). Hypoperfusion causes the peculiar pallor and cyanosis that result in the characteristic gray color of the skin. A vicious circle ensues with continuing tissue hypoperfusion leading to lactic acid accumulation, impaired hepatocyte metabolism, and drug conjugation, resulting in still higher serum levels of chloramphenicol (96). The syndrome is reversible if the drug is terminated immediately after the onset of symptoms. About 40% of affected infants die within 2 to 3 days. Exchange transfusions and charcoal-column hemoperfusion have been used successfully (97). Although most cases occur in infants younger than 30 days, the syndrome has been described in children 25 months of age and older who have elevated serum levels of drug and in adults who have accidentally ingested excessive quantities of chloramphenicol (98).

Hematologic Toxicity

Chloramphenicol may affect the hematopoietic system in several ways. Two potentially life-threatening toxic effects involving the bone marrow are well described (2,59,89,99).

A dose-related, reversible depression of the marrow is a direct toxic effect. Chloramphenicol inhibits mitochondrial enzymes at serum concentrations of 10 μg/mL or higher, including the enzyme ferrochelatase, which catalyzes the final step in heme synthesis (100). A reduction of serum iron use and incorporation into red blood cell precursors results from this inhibition (101). The earliest sign of toxicity is reticulocytopenia, which occurs after 5 to 7 days of drug therapy (102). Serum iron concentrations may double within 6 to 10 days. At chloramphenicol serum concentrations of 30 μg/mL or greater, the bone marrow develops morphologic changes, producing vacuolization in erythroid and myeloid precursors (103,104). The vacuolization of precursors is not specific for chloramphenicol intoxication; similar changes have been described in alcoholism, DiGuglielmo's syndrome, phenylketonuria, and riboflavin deficiency (105).

Bone marrow depression may cause anemia, granulocytopenia, and thrombocytopenia, with the latter developing later in the course of treatment, about day 16 or later (102). Patients deficient in folic acid and vitamin B$_{12}$ do not respond to replacement therapy if they are given chloramphenicol concurrently (102). Factors commonly associated with marrow depression are doses in excess of 4 g per day, liver disease, and serum concentrations in excess of 25 μg/mL (85,102). Marrow depression is reversible with discontinuation of the antibiotic, and failure to recognize this complication in time may result in terminal infection or hemorrhage.

The second type of bone marrow toxicity, thought to be idiosyncratic, is usually fatal (2). Data suggest that chloramphenicol produces this irreversible aplastic anemia in 1 in 25,000 to 45,000 patients exposed to the drug, with about 26% of all cases attributable to chloramphenicol (106). The majority of cases occur 3 to 12 weeks after chloramphenicol therapy is initiated, although aplasia may develop months and, according to some anecdotal case reports, even years, after therapy (89,106–108). The aplastic anemia is not dose related; indeed, there have been reported cases occurring after the administration of chloramphenicol eye drops (109). The exact mechanism producing aplasia is not clearly defined. A genetic predisposition is suggested by concordance studies in identical twins (110). Aplastic anemia was first described only after oral administration and toxic bacterial degradation products of chloramphenicol absorbed from the gut were implicated (111). This view was supported by the observation that bacterial degradation products of the drug were shown to cause damage to human bone marrow cells and lymphocytes in culture (112,113). Subsequently, aplasia has been reported in patients treated with parenteral drug only or in conjunction with cimetidine (114). Thus, aplasia is a risk regardless of route of administration (115). Therefore, a complete blood count performed at least twice weekly is recommended during chloramphenicol administration to monitor for the development of leukopenia, anemia, or thrombocytopenia, and this would signal immediate discontinuation of the drug. Frequent monitoring may not predict most cases of aplastic anemia, but dose-related marrow depression can be identified earlier this way (115). Bone marrow transplantation is the treatment of choice for aplasia; without it, all patients died within 18 months of the diagnosis (87–117).

Acute myeloblastic leukemia has developed in some patients who developed bone marrow hypoplasia attributable to chloramphenicol (118). In China, children who received more than 10 days of chloramphenicol were found to have a greater risk for acute nonlymphocytic and acute lymphocytic leukemia than were control subjects. Acute nonlymphocytic leukemia developed more frequently than acute lymphocytic leukemia (119). Chloramphenicol and several metabolites have been demonstrated to induce chromosomal aberrations and DNA strand breakage in cultured rat and human cell lines (113,120,121). It is classified as a probable carcinogen by the International Agency for Research on Cancer (122).

Chloramphenicol may induce acute hemolysis in patients with the Mediterranean form of glucose-6-phosphate dehydrogenase deficiency. Hemolysis has not been reported in black persons, who have the milder a type of this deficiency (123,124).

Optic Neuritis

Optic neuritis resulting in decreases in vision, central scotoma, and alterations in red-green color discrimination has been reported in patients receiving prolonged courses of chloramphenicol (125–127). These changes are reversible, but permanent changes have also been described (126). Other neurological syndromes observed include ophthalmoplegia, peripheral neuropathy, acute encephalopathy, depression, and headache (127).

Other Types of Reactions

Hypersensitivity reactions associated with chloramphenicol are uncommon but include drug fever and various dermatological reactions (128). Jarisch-Herxheimer reactions have been reported in patients with relapsing fever, brucellosis, typhoid fever, and syphilis who were treated with chloramphenicol. Gastrointestinal complaints, such as nausea, vomiting, and diarrhea, have been noted, and glossitis has been produced by high doses of the drug (129). Chloramphenicol has been demonstrated to suppress the primary immune response and cell-mediated immunity in animal models. The clinical significance of this immunosuppression is not known (130,131).

Drug Interactions

Chloramphenicol irreversibly inhibits the hepatic, drug-metabolizing microsomal enzymes, and the cytochrome P450 complex (132). The drug prolongs the half-life of warfarin, phenytoin, cyclosporine, tolbutamide, and chlorpropamide by this mechanism (133,134). Similar caution with tacrolimus is warranted. Phenytoin, rifampin, and phenobarbital induce hepatic microsomal enzymes and may decrease the serum concentration and increase clearance of chloramphenicol (134). Acetaminophen has been reported to block hepatic uptake of chloramphenicol and prolong clearance of the drug (135). The occurrence of aplasia in patients receiving concurrent chloramphenicol and cimetidine or acetazolamide may indicate additional important drug interactions (114).

ASSAY

Monitoring of serum levels of chloramphenicol is important in patients with high risk for toxicity. Serum levels of chloramphenicol should be monitored in newborns, premature infants, patients with liver disease, and those receiving drugs that interfere with the metabolism of the antibiotic (85,86,132). Serum concentrations should range between 10 and 25 μg/mL. Bone marrow depression occurs at concentrations greater than 25 μg/mL (102). Currently available methods include microbiologic and radioenzymatic assays and high-performance liquid chromatography.

TABLE 27.4. Indications for Chloramphenicol Use

Disease process	Initial antimicrobial therapy	Chloramphenicol indication and comments
Bacterial meningitis	Ceftriaxone	Useful in penicillin allergic
Streptococcus pneumonia	Vancomycin for penicillin-	patient; no benefit with
Neisseria meningitides	resistant pneumococcal	penicillin-resistant
Haemophilus influenzae	strains	pneumococcal strains
Brain abscess	Metronidazole and ceftriaxone	Useful alternative
Burkholderia mallei (Glanders)	Ceftazidime, quinolones	Use with streptomycin
Burkholderia pseudomallei (melioidosis)	Ceftazidime	Use with doxycycline
Ehrlichiosis	Doxycycline	As with rickettsial infection
Francisella tularensis	Streptomycin	Not a first-line agent
Rickettsial infections	Doxycycline	Where patient is pregnant,
—Rocky Mountain spotted fever		breast-feeding, or <9
—Typhus		year old
—Scrub typhus		
—Q fever		
Salmonella typhi	Quinolones, ceftriaxone	Most strains resistant
Vancomycin-resistant enterococci	Linezolid, Quinupristin-dalfopristin	Often used with doxycycline or quinupristin-dalfopristin
Vibrio vulnificus	Quinolones, doxycyline	Possible alternative agent
Yersinia pestis	Streptomycin	Not a first-line agent

Information from references 17, 20, 22–40, 139–150.

Bioassays are specific but not sensitive and require an appropriate test organism, which may be confounded when other antibiotics are given concurrently (136,137). Radioenzymatic assays using chloramphenicol acetyltransferase are rapid and specific but require expensive equipment (137). High-performance liquid chromatography has all the advantages of the radioenzymatic assay and can distinguish among prodrug, active drug, and conjugate (138).

CLINICAL INDICATIONS

Chloramphenicol is no longer the primary therapy for any specific infection. Table 27.4 summarizes the clinical indications when the primary treatment is unavailable.

Chloramphenicol is beneficial in the treatment of ricksettsial or ehrlichial infections in pregnancy, in the setting of tetracycline allergy, and in children younger than 9 years of age (139). Some pediatricians avoid using chloramphenicol to treat children with Rocky Mountain spotted fever and prefer to use a short course of doxycycline because of its lower calcium-binding avidity to avoid tooth discoloration (in comparison with tetracycline) (140,141). Chloramphenicol is an effective alternative to the penicillins and cephalosporins in treating older children and adults with meningitis who have severe penicillin allergy (19,34,142). During the 1990s, vancomycin-resistant enterococcus (VRE) emerged as a nosocomial pathogen especially affecting the immunocompromised and intensive care unit patient. Chloramphenicol and doxycycline were often combined for the treatment of serious infections (143,144). Its efficacy has never been demonstrated in controlled trials, and resistance developed rapidly to both drugs. However, the development of new antimicrobial agents against VRE, such as linezolid and quinupristin-dalfopristin, has returned chloramphenicol to a third-line agent (144).

The disease melioidosis (*B. pseudomallei* infection), once an indication for chloramphenicol therapy, is now preferably treated with cetazidime-containing regimens because of the lower mortality and relapse rates associated with these regimens (146–148). Chloramphenicol is bacteriostatic for *Francisella tularensis* and *Yersinia pestis*, and intramuscular streptomycin is the preferred therapy, but in extraordinary circumstances such as those currently created by the threat of bioterrorism, chloramphenicol may be considered for treatment of clinical disease due to these pathogens (149,150).

REFERENCES

1. Kucers A. Current position of chloramphenicol chemotherapy. *J Antimicrob Chemother* 1980;6:1–4.
2. Rich ML, Ritterhof RJ, Hoffman RJ. A fatal case of aplastic anemia following chloramphenicol (Chloromycetin) therapy. *Ann Intern Med* 1950;33:1459.
3. Burns LE, Hodgman JE, Cass AB. Fatal circulatory collapse in premature infants receiving chloramphenicol. *N Engl J Med* 1959;261:1318.
4. Ehrlich J, Bartz QR, Smith RM, et al. Chloromycetin, a new antibiotic from a soil actinomycete. *Science* 1947;106:417.
5. Ehrlich J, Gottlieb D, Burkholder RR, et al. *Streptomyces venezuelae:* N. sp., the source of Chloromycetin. *J Bacteriol* 1948;56:467.
6. Malik VS. Chloramphenicol. *Adv Appl Microbiol* 1972;15:297–336.
7. Hahn FE, Gund P. A structured model of chloramphenicol receptor site. In: Drews J, Hahn FE, eds. *Drug receptor interactions in antimicrobial chemotherapy.* New York: Springer-Verlag, 1975:245–266.
8. Glazko AJ, Edgerton WH, Dill WA, et al. Chloromycetin palmitate: a synthetic ester of Chloromycetin. *Antibiot Chemother* 1952;2:234.
9. McCrumb FR Jr, Snyder MJ, Hicken WJ. The use of chloramphenicol acid succinate in the treatment of acute infections. In: *Antibiotics annual 1957–1958.* New York: Medical Encyclopedia, 1958:837–841.
10. Smith AL, Weber A. Pharmacology of chloramphenicol. *Pediatr Clin North Am* 1983;30:209–236.
11. Glazko AJ, Dill AW, Kinkel JR, et al. Absorption and excretion of parenteral doses of chloramphenicol sodium succinate in comparison with perioral doses of chloramphenicol. *Clin Pharmacol Ther* 1977;21:104.
12. Yunis AA: Chloramphenicol toxicity: 25 years of research [Review]. *Am J Med* 1989;87:44N–48N.
13. Wisseman CL, Smadel JE, Hahn FE, et al. Mode of action of chloramphenicol.1. Action of chloramphenicol on assimilation of ammonia and on synthesis of proteins and nucleic acids in *Escherichia coli. J Bacteriol* 1954;67:662.
14. Pestka S. Studies on the formation of transfer ribonucleic acid-ribosome complexes. XI. Antibiotic effects on phenylalanyl-oligonucleotide binding to ribosomes. *Proc Natl Acad Sci USA* 1969;64:709–714.
15. Vazquez D, Barbacid M, Fernandez-Munoz R. Antibiotic action on the ribosomal peptidyl transferase center. In: Drews J, Hahn FE, eds. *Drug receptor interactions in antimicrobial chemotherapy.* New York: Springer-Verlag, 1975:193–216.
16. Vazquez D. Uptake and binding of chloramphenicol by sensitive and resistant organisms. *Nature* 1964;203:257.
17. Wehrle PF, Mathies AW, Leedom JM, et al. Bacterial meningitis. *Ann N Y Acad Sci* 1967;145:488–498.
18. Rahal JJ Jr, Simberkoff MS. Bactericidal and bacteriostatic action of chloramphenicol against meningeal pathogens. *Antimicrob Agents Chemother* 1979;16:13–18.
19. Freeman KB. Inhibition of mitochondrial and bacterial protein synthesis by chloramphenicol. *Can J Biochem* 1970;48:479–485.
20. Feder HM Jr, Osier C, Maderazo EG. Chloramphenicol: a review of its use in clinical practice. *Rev Infect Dis* 1981;3:479–491.
21. Barry AL, Thornsberry C. Susceptibility testing: appendix 2. In: Lennette EH, ed. *Manual of clinical microbiology,* 3rd ed. Washington, DC: American Society for Microbiology, 1980:498–499.
22. Finland M. Changing patterns of susceptibility of common bacterial pathogens to antimicrobial agents. *Ann Intern Med* 1972;76:1009–1036.
23. Finland M, Garner C, Wilcox C, et al. Susceptibility of "Enterobacteria" to aminoglycoside antibiotics: comparisons with tetracyclines, polymyxins, chloramphenicol and spectinomycin. *J Infect Dis* 1976;134[Suppl]:S57–74.
24. Eickhoff TC, Bennett JV, Hayes PS, et al. *Pseudomonas pseudomallei* susceptibility to chemotherapeutic agents. *J Infect Dis* 1970;121:95–102.
25. Robertson RP, Wahab MFA, Rasch FO. Evaluation of chloramphenicol and ampicillin in *Salmonella* enteric fever. *N Engl J Med* 1968;278:171–176.
26. Rubinstein E, Shamberg B. In vitro activity of cinoxacin, ampicillin, and chloramphenicol against *Shigella* and non-typhoid *Salmonella. Antimicrob Agents Chemother* 1977;11:577.
27. Kasten MJ. Clindamycin, metronidazole, and chloramphenicol. *Mayo Clin Proc* 1999;74:825–833.
28. Harding GKM, Buckwald FJ, Ronald AR, et al. Prospective, randomized comparative study of clindamycin, chloramphenicol, and ticarcillin, each and in combination with gentamicin, in therapy for intraabdominal and female genital tract sepsis. *J Infect Dis* 1980;142:384–393.
29. Cuchural GJ Jr, Tally FP, Jacobus NV, et al. Susceptibility of the *Bacteroides fragilis* group in the United States: analysis by site of infection. *Antimicrob Agents Chemother* 1988;32:717–722.
30. McCracken GH Jr, Nelson JD, Kaplan SL, et al. Consensus report: antimicrobial therapy for bacterial meningitis in infants and children. *Pediatr Infect Dis J* 1987;6:501–505.
31. Strandberg DA, Jorgensen JH, Drutz DJ. Activities of newer beta-lactam antibiotics against ampicillin, chloramphenicol, or multiply-resistant *Haemophilus influenzae. Diagn Microbiol Infect Dis* 1984;2:333–337.
32. Westenfeld GO, Paterson PY. Life-threatening infections: choice of alternate drugs when penicillin cannot be given. *JAMA* 1969;210:845.
33. Lee HJ, Park JY, Jang SH, et al. High incidence of resistance to multiple antimicrobials in clinical isolates of *Streptococcus pneumoniae* from a University Hospital in Korea. *Clin Infect Dis* 1995;20:826–827.
34. Ostroff SM, Harrison LH, Khallaf N, et al. Resistant patterns of *Streptococcus pneumoniae* and *Haemophilus influenzae* isolates recovered in Egypt from children with pneumonia. *Clin Infect Dis* 1997;23:1069–1074.
35. Doern GV, Heilmann KP, Huynh PR, et al. Antimicrobial resistance among clinical isolates of *Streptococcus pneumoniae* in the United States during 1999–2000, including a comparison of resistance rates since 1994–1995. *Antimicrob Agents Chemother* 2001;45:1721–1729.
36. Galimand M, Gerbaud G, Guibourdenche M, et al. High-level chloramphenicol resistance in *Neisseria meningitidis. N Engl J Med* 1998;339:868–874.
37. Friedland IR, Shelton S, McCracken GH. Chloramphenicol in penicillin-resistant pneumococcal meningitis. *Lancet* 1993;342:240–241.
38. Friedland IR, Klugman KP. Failure of chloramphenicol therapy in penicillin-resistant pneumococcal meningitis. *Lancet* 1992;339:405–408.
39. Wallace JF, Smith RH, Arcia M, et al. Studies on the pathogenesis of meningitis: antagonism between penicillin and chloramphenicol in experimental pneumococcal meningitis. *J Clin Lab Med* 1967;70:408–418.
40. Kenny JF, Isburg CD, Michaels RH. Meningitis due to *Haemophilus influenzae* type b resistant to both ampicillin and chloramphenicol. *Pediatrics* 1980;66:14–16.
41. Smith SM, Palumbo PE, Edelson PJ. *Salmonella* strains resistant to multiple antibiotics: therapeutic implications. *Pediatr Infect Dis* 1984;3:455–460.
42. Goldstein FW, Chumpitaz JC, Guevara JM, et al. Plasmid-mediated resistance to multiple antibiotics in *Salmonella typhi. J Infect Dis* 1986;153:261–266.
43. Gallardo F, Ruiz J, Marco F, et al. Increase in incidence of resistance to ampicillin, chloramphenicol and trimethoprim in clinical isolates of *Salmonella*

serotype typhimurium: an investigation of molecular epidemiology and mechanisms of resistance. *J Med Microbiol* 1999;48:367–374.

44. DuPont HL. Quinolones in *Salmonella typhi* infection. *Drugs* 1993;45[Suppl 3]:119–124.

45. Lasserre R, Sangalang RP, Santiago L. Three-day treatment of typhoid fever with two different doses of ceftriaxone, compared to a 14-day therapy with chloramphenicol: A randomized trial. *J Antimicrob Chemother* 1991;28:765–772.

46. Islam A, Butler T, Kabir I, et al. Treatment of typhoid fever with ceftriaxone for 5 days or chloramphenicol for 14 days: a randomized clinical trial. *Antimicrob Agents Chemother* 1993;37:1572–1575.

47. Murray BE. Resistance of *Shigella, Salmonella* and other selected enteric pathogens to antimicrobial agents. *Rev Infect Dis* 1986;8[Suppl]:S172–S181.

48. Molbak K, Baggesen DL, Aarestrup MF, et al. An outbreak of multidrug-resistant, quinolone resistant *Salmonella enterica* serotype typhimurium DT 104. *N Engl J Med* 1999;341:1420–1435.

49. Olsen SJ, DeBess EE, McGivern TE, et al. A nosocomial outbreak of fluoroquinolone-resistant salmonella infection. *N Engl J Med* 2001;344:1572–1579.

50. Harrel GT. Treatment of Rocky Mountain spotted fever with antibiotics. *Ann N Y Acad Sci* 1952;55:1027.

51. Romansky MJ, Olansky S, Taggart SR, et al. The antitreponemal effect of oral chloromycetin in 23 cases of early syphilis in man: a preliminary report. *Science* 1949;110:639.

52. Benveniste R, Davies J. Mechanisms of antibiotic resistance in bacteria. *Annu Rev Biochem* 1973;42:471–506.

53. Datta N, Richards H, Datta C. *Salmonella typhi* in vivo acquires resistance to both chloramphenicol and co-trimoxazole. *Lancet* 1981;1:1181–1183.

54. Cherubin CE, Neu HC, Rahal JJ, et al. Emergence of resistance to chloramphenicol in *Salmonella*. *J Infect Dis* 1977;135:807.

55. Tacket CO, Dominguez LB, Fisher HJ, et al. An outbreak of multiple-drug-resistant *Salmonella* enteritis from raw milk. *JAMA* 1985;253:2058–2060.

56. Spika JS, Waterman SH, Soo Hoo GW, et al. Chloramphenicol resistant *Salmonella newport* traced through hamburger to dairy farms. *N Engl J Med* 1987;316:565–570.

57. Cody SH, Abbott SL, Marfin AA, et al. Two outbreaks of multidrug-resistant *Salmonella* serotype typhimurium DT 104 infections linked to raw-milk cheese in Northern California. *JAMA* 1999;281:1805–1810.

58. Villar RG, Macek MD, Simons S, et al. Investigation of multidrug-resistant *Salmonella* serotype typhimurium DT 104 infections linked to raw-milk cheese in Washington State. *JAMA* 1999;281:1811–1815.

59. Yunis A. Chloramphenicol: relation of structure to activity and toxicity. *Annu Rev Pharmacol Toxicol* 1988;28:83–100.

60. Osawa S, Takata R, Tanaka K, et al. Chloramphenicol resistant mutants of *Bacillus subtilis*. *Mol Gen Genet* 1973;127:163–173.

61. Gaffney DF, Cundliffe E, Foster TJ. Chloramphenicol resistance that does not involve chloramphenicol acetyltransferase encoded by plasmids from gram negative bacteria. *J Gen Microbiol* 1981;125:113–121.

62. Irvin JE, Ingram JM. Chloramphenicol-resistant variants of *Pseudomonas aeruginosa* defective in amino acid transport. *Can J Biochem* 1980;58:1165–1171.

63. Traub WH, Fukushima PI. Nonspecific resistance of *Serratia marcescens* against antimicrobial drugs. *Chemotherapy* 1979;25:196–203.

64. Burns JL, Rubens CE, Mendelman PM, et al. Cloning and expression in *Escherichia coli* of a gene encoding nonenzymatic chloramphenicol resistance from *Pseudomonas aeruginosa*. *Antimicrob Agents Chemother* 1986;29:445–450.

65. Bums JL, Mendelman PM, Levy J, et al. A permeability barrier as a mechanism of chloramphenicol resistance in *Haemophilus influenzae*. *Antimicrob Agents Chemother* 1985;27:46–54.

66. Li XZ, Livermans DM, Nikaido H. Role of efflux pump(s) in intrinsic resistance of *Pseudomonas aeruginosa*: resistance to tetracycline, chloramphenicol, and norfloxacin. *Antimicrob Agents Chemother* 1994;38:1732–1741.

67. Bartelloni PJ, Calia FM, Minchew BH, et al. Absorption and excretion of two chloramphenicol products in humans after oral administration. *Am J Med Sci* 1969;258:203–208.

68. Kaufman RE, Miceli JN, Strebel L, et al. Pharmacokinetics of chloramphenicol and chloramphenicol succinate in infants and children. *J Pediatr* 1981;98:315.

69. Sack CM, Koup JR, Smith AL. Chloramphenicol pharmacokinetics in infants and young children. *Pediatrics* 1980;66:579–584.

70. Pickering LK, Hoecker JL, Kramer WG, et al. Clinical pharmacology of two chloramphenicol preparations in children: sodium succinate (IV) and palmitate (oral) esters. *J Pediatr* 1980;96:757–761.

71. Shah PN, D'Souza J, Dathani KK. Absorption of chloramphenicol by various routes of administration. *Indian J Med Res* 1977;65:549–553.

72. DuPont HL, Hornick RB, Weiss RB, et al. Evaluation of chloramphenicol acid succinate therapy of induced typhoid fever and Rocky Mountain spotted fever. *N Engl J Med* 1970;282:53–57.

73. George FJ, Hanna C. Ocular penetration of chloramphenicol. *Arch Ophthalmol* 1977;93:184.

74. McPherson SD Jr, Presley GD, Crawford JR. Aqueous humor assays of subconjunctival antibiotics. *Am J Ophthalmol* 1968;66:430–435.

75. Jarudi N. Comparison of antibiotic therapy in presumptive bacterial conjunctivitis. *Am J Ophthalmol* 1975;79:790–794.

76. Bennett WM, Singer L, Golper T, et al. Guidelines for drug therapy in renal failure. *Ann Intern Med* 1977;86:754–783.

77. Rapp GF, Griffith RS, Hebble WM. The permeability of traumatically inflamed synovial membrane to commonly used antibiotics. *J Bone Joint Surg Am* 1966;48:1534.

78. Friedman CA, Lovejoy FC, Smith AL. Chloramphenicol disposition in infants and children. *J Pediatr* 1979;95:1071–1077.

79. Rensimer ER, Pickering LK, Ericsson C, et al. Sequential CSF concentration of chloramphenicol after administration of oral chloramphenicol palmitate. *Lancet* 1981;1:165.

80. Kramer PW, Griffith RS, Campbell RL. Antibiotic penetration of the brain. *J Neurosurg* 1969;31:295–302.

81. Glazko AJ, Wolf LM, Dill WA, et al. Biochemical studies on chloramphenicol (Chloromycetin). *J Pharmacol Exp Ther* 1949;96:445.

82. Lindberg AA, Nilsson LH, Bucht H, et al. Concentrations of chloramphenicol in the urine and blood in relation to renal function. *Br Med J* 1966;2:724.

83. Kunin CM, Glazko AJ, Finland M. Persistence of antibiotics in blood of patients with acute renal failure. II. Chloramphenicol and its metabolism products in the blood of patients with severe renal disease or hepatic cirrhosis. *J Clin Invest* 1959;38:1498.

84. Kunin CM. A guide to use of antibiotics in patients with renal disease. *Ann Intern Med* 1967;67:151–158.

85. Suhrland LG, Weisberger AS. Chloramphenicol toxicity in liver and renal disease. *Arch Intern Med* 1963;112:161.

86. Weiss CF, Glazko AJ, Weston JK. Chloramphenicol in the newborn infant: a physiologic explanation of its toxicity when given in excessive doses. *N Engl J Med* 1960;262:787.

87. National Committee for Clinical Laboratory Standards. *Methods for antimicrobial susceptibility testing of anaerobic bacteria*, 2nd ed, approved standard. Villanova, PA: National Committee for Clinical Laboratory Standards, 1990. NCCLS publication M11–A2.

88. Grafnetterova J, Grafnetter D, Schuck O, et al. The effect of endogenous compounds isolated from sera of uremic patients on chloramphenicol binding to proteins. *Biochem Pharmacol* 1979;28:2923–2928.

89. Havelka J, Hejzlar M, Popov V, et al. Excretion of chloramphenicol in human milk. *Chemotherapy* 1968;13:204–211.

90. Christiansen LK, Skovsted L. Inhibition of drug metabolism by chloramphenicol. *Lancet* 1969;2:1397.

91. Adams HR, Isaacson EL, Masters BS. Inhibition of hepatic microsomal enzymes by chloramphenicol. *J Pharmacol Exp Ther* 1977;203:388–396.

92. Sutherland JM. Fatal cardiovascular collapse of infants receiving large amount of chloramphenicol. *Am J Dis Child* 1959;97:761.

93. Abou-Khalil S, Abou-Khalil WH, Yunis AA. Differential effects of chloramphenicol and its nitrosoanalogue on protein synthesis and oxidative phosphorylation in rat liver mitochondria. *Biochem Pharmacol* 1980;29:2605–2609.

94. Freeman KB, Halder D. The inhibition of mammalian mitochondrial NADPH oxidation by chloramphenicol and its isomer and analogues. *Can J Biochem* 1968;46:1003–1008.

95. Freeman KB. Effects of chloramphenicol and its isomers and analogues on the mitochondrial respiratory chain. *Can J Biochem* 1970;48:469–478.

96. Evans LS, Kleiman MB. Acidosis as a presenting feature of chloramphenicol toxicity. *J Pediatr* 1986;108:475–477.

97. Kessler DL, Smith AL, Woodrum DE. Chloramphenicol toxicity in a neonate treated with exchange transfusion. *J Pediatr* 1980;96:140–141.

98. Thompson WL, Anderson SE Jr, Lipsky JJ, et al. Overdoses of chloramphenicol [Letter]. *JAMA* 1975;243:149.

99. Holt D, Harvey D, Harvey R. Chloramphenicol toxicity. *Adverse Drug React Toxicol Rev* 1993;12:83–95.

100. Mangan DR, Arimura GK, Yunis AA. Chloramphenicol-induced erythroid suppression and bone marrow ferrochelatase in dogs. *J Lab Clin Med* 1972;79:137–144.

101. Rubin D, Weisberger AS, Botti RE, et al. Changes in iron metabolism in early chloramphenicol toxicity. *J Clin Invest* 1958;37:1286.

102. Saidi P, Wallerstein RO, Aggeler PM. Effect of chloramphenicol on erythropoiesis. *J Lab Clin Med* 1961;57:247.

103. Scott JL, Finegold SM, Belkin GA, et al. A controlled double blind study of the hematologic toxicity of chloramphenicol. *N Engl J Med* 1965;272:1137.

104. Yunis AA, Smith US, Restrepo A. Reversible bone marrow suppression from chloramphenicol: a consequence of mitochondrial injury. *Arch Intern Med* 1970;126:272–275.

105. Meissner HC, Smith AL. The current status of chloramphenicol. *Pediatrics* 1979;64:348–356.

106. Wallerstein RO, Condit PK, Kasper CK, et al. Statewide study of chloramphenicol therapy and fatal aplastic anemia. *JAMA* 1969;208:2045–2050.

107. Best WK. Chloramphenicol-associated blood dyscrasias. *JAMA* 1967;201:181.

108. Clarke WTW. Fatal aplastic anemia and chloramphenicol. *Can Med Assoc J* 1967;97:815.

109. Lancaster T, Stewart AM, Jick H. Risk of serious hematological toxicity with use of chloramphenicol eye drops in a British general practitioner database. *BMJ* 1998;316:667.

110. Nagao T, Mauer AM. Concordance for drug induced aplastic anemia in identical twins. *N Engl J Med* 1969;281:7–11.

111. Holt R. The bacterial degradation of chloramphenicol. *Lancet* 1967;1:1259–1260.

112. Jiminez JJ, Arimura GK, Abou-Khalil WH, et al. Chloramphenicol-induced bone marrow injury: possible role of bacterial metabolites of chloramphenicol. *Blood* 1987;70:1180–1185.

113. Frayssinet CL, Robba NA, Barnat S, et al. Cytotoxicity and DNA damaging potency of chloramphenicol and six metabolites: a new evaluation in human lymphocytes and Raji cells. *Mutat Res* 1994;320:207–215.

114. Fink TJ, Gump DW. Chloramphenicol: an inpatient study of use and abuse. *J Infect Dis* 1978;138:690–694.
115. West BC, DeVault GA Jr, Clement JC, et al. Aplastic anemia associated with parenteral chloramphenicol: review of 10 cases, including the second case of possible increased risk with cimetidine. *Rev Infect Dis* 1988;10:1048–1051.
116. Plaut ME, Best WR. Aplastic anemia after parenteral chloramphenicol: warning reviewed [Letter]. *N Engl J Med* 1982;306:1486.
117. Daum RS, Cohen DL, Smith AL. Fatal aplastic anemia following apparent dose-related chloramphenicol toxicity. *J Pediatr* 1979;94:403–406.
118. Pillow PR, Epstein RB, Buckner CD. Treatment of bone marrow failure by isogenic marrow infusion. *N Engl J Med* 1966;275:94.
119. Adamson RH, Seiber SM. Clinically induced leukemia in humans. *Environ Health Res* 1981;39:93–103.
120. Shu XO, Gao YT, Linet MS, et al. Chloramphenicol use and childhood leukaemia in Shanghai. *Lancet* 1987;2:934–937.
121. Sbrana I, Caretto S, Rainaldi G, et al. Induction of chromosomal aberrations and sister-chromatid exchanges by chloramphenicol. *Mutat Res* 1991;248:145–153.
122. Martelli A, Mattioli F, Pastorino G, et al. Genotoxicity testing of chloramphenicol in rodent and human cells. *Mutat Res* 1991;260:65–72.
123. International Agency for Research on Cancer. *Monograph on the evaluation of carcinogenic risks to humans*, Vol 50. Lyon, France: International Agency for Research on Cancer, 1990:169–173.
124. McCaffrey RP, Halsted CH, Wahab MFA, et al. Chloramphenicol-induced hemolysis in Caucasian glucose-6-phosphate dehydrogenase deficiency. *Ann Intern Med* 1971;74:722–26.
125. Wallenstein L, Snyder J. Neurotoxic reactions to chloromycetin. *Ann Intern Med* 1952;36:1526.
126. Huang NN, Harley RD, Promadhattavedi V, et al. Visual disturbances in cystic fibrosis following chloramphenicol administration. *J Pediatr* 1966;68:32.
127. Cocke JG, Brown RE, Geppert LJ. Optic neuritis with prolonged use of chloramphenicol. *J Pediatr* 1966;68:27–31.
128. Levine PH, Regelson W, Holland JF. Chloramphenicol associated encephalopathy. *Clin Pharmacol Ther* 1970;11:194–199.
129. Woodward TE, Wisseman CL Jr. *Chloromycetin (chloramphenicol)*. New York: Medical Encyclopedia, 1958:24–28.
130. Weisberger AS, Daniel TM. Suppression of antibody synthesis by chloramphenicol analogs. *Proc Soc Exp Biol Med* 1969;131:570–575.
131. DaMert GJ, Sohle PG. Effect, of chloramphenicol on in vitro function of lymphocytes. *J Infect Dis* 1979;139:220–224.
132. Halpert J. Further studies of the suicide inactivation of purified rat liver cytochrome P-450 by chloramphenicol. *Mol Pharmacol* 1982;21:166–172.
133. Serino F, Grevel J, Napoli KL, et al. Oxygen radical formation by the cytochrome P450 system as a cellular mechanism for cyclosporine toxicity. *Transplant Proc* 1994;26:2916–2917.
134. Krasinski K, Kusmiez H, Nelson JD. Pharmacologic interactions among chloramphenicol, phenytoin and phenobarbital. *Pediatr Infect Dis* 1982;1:232–235.
135. Buchanan M, Moodley GP. Interaction between chloramphenicol and paracetamol. *Br Med J* 1979;2:307.
136. Bannatyne RM, Cheung R. Chloramphenicol bioassay. *Antimicrob Agents Chemother* 1979;16:43–45.
137. Jorgensen JH, Alexander GA. Rapid bioassay for chloramphenicol in the presence of other antibiotics. *Am J Clin Pathol* 1981;4:472–475.
138. Velagapudi R, Smith RV, Ludden TM, et al. Simultaneous determination of chloramphenicol and chloramphenicol succinate in plasma using high-performance liquid chromatography. *J Chromatogr* 1982;228:423–428.
139. Kelsey DS. Rocky Mountain spotted fever. *Pediatr Clin North Am* 1979;26:367–376.
140. Ford G, Benincari C. Doxycycline and the teeth [Letter]. *Lancet* 1969;1:78.
141. Abramson JS, Givner LB. Should tetracycline be contraindicated for therapy of presumed Rocky Mountain spotted fever in children less than 9 years of age? *Pediatrics* 1990;86:123.
142. Brewer NS, MacCarty CS, Wellman WE. Brain abscess: a review of recent experience. *Ann Intern Med* 1975;82:571–576.
143. Norris AH, Reilly JP, Edelstein PA, et al. Chloramphenicol for the treatment of vancomycin-resistant enterococcal infections. *Clin Infect Dis* 1995;20:1137–1144.
144. Murray BE. Drug therapy: vancomycin-resistant enterococal infections. *N Engl Med J* 2000;342:710–720.
145. Fishbein DB, Dawson JE, Robinson LE. Human ehrlichiosis in the United States, 1985 to 1990. *Ann Intern Med* 1994;120:736–743.
146. Sookpranee M, Boonma P, Susaengut W, et al. Multicenter prospective randomized trial comparing ceftazidime plus co-trimoxazole with chloramphenicol plus doxycycline and co-trimoxazole for treatment of severe melioidosis. *Antimicrob Agents Chemother* 1992;36:158–162.
147. Samuel M, Ti TY. Interventions for treating melioidosis [Cochrane Review]. *Cochrane Database Syst Rev* 2001;2:CD1263.
148. Heine HS, England MJ, Wang DM, et al. In vitro antibiotic susceptibility of *Burkholderia mallei* (causative agent of Glanders). Determined by broth microdilution and E-test. *Antimicrob Agents Chemother* 2001;45:2119–2121.
149. McCrumb FR, Mercier S, Robic G, et al. Chloramphenicol and Terramycin in the treatment of pneumonic plague. *Am J Med* 1953;14:284.
150. McCrumb FR, Snyder MJ, Woodward TE. Studies on human infection with *Pasteurella tularensis*: comparison of streptomycin and chloramphenicol in the prophylaxis of clinical disease. *Trans Assoc Am Physicians* 1957;70:74.

CHAPTER 28
Metronidazole and Other Nitroimidazoles

Glenn E. Mathisen

METRONIDAZOLE

Metronidazole, an antimicrobial agent that has excellent activity against strict anaerobic bacteria and certain parasites, has become an important agent in the treatment of a wide variety of anaerobic infections. Its excellent penetration into all tissues (including the central nervous system) and bactericidal activity against strict anaerobes have made it especially useful for treatment of certain deep-seated infections, such as brain abscess and anaerobic osteomyelitis. Although questions about the mutagenicity of the drug have been raised, increasing experience suggests that it is a safe, well-tolerated drug that has few major side effects when used properly.

Mode of Action

The mode of action of metronidazole can be thought of as involving four successive steps: (a) entry of the drug into the bacterial cell, (b) reductive activation, (c) toxic effect of the reduced intermediate product(s), and (d) release of inactive end products. Reductive activation occurs when the nitro group of the drug (which acts as a preferential electron acceptor) is reduced by low-redox potential electron transport proteins. This reduces the intracellular concentration of unchanged drug and produces a gradient that promotes further entry of the unchanged drug into the cell. Short-lived intermediate compounds or free radicals are believed to damage the cell through interaction with DNA or other macromolecular compounds. The metabolic products of metronidazole include a hydroxy derivative that also has significant anaerobic activity (1) and other breakdown products (e.g., acid derivative) that have considerably less activity or may not be taken up by the target organism (2). Susceptible organisms have low-redox potential and carry out reductive activation of the drug either in cytoplasm or specialized intracellular organelles; aerobic cells lack sufficiently low redox potential to accomplish this activation (3). Although the mechanism is not completely clear, organisms that develop clinical resistance to the metronidazole have alterations in the proteins involved in reductive activation of the drug. Metronidazole acts as a potent bactericidal agent; organisms are typically killed at the same concentration as or within a twofold dilution of that required for inhibition (4).

Spectrum of Activity and Resistance

The activity of metronidazole against 793 strains of anaerobic and microaerophilic bacteria is summarized in Table 28.1 (3). Metronidazole demonstrated excellent activity against strict anaerobic organisms such as *Bacteroides fragilis*—virtually all the organisms were inhibited by 16 μg/mL or less, the breakpoint for the drug. Despite widespread use of metronidazole, most susceptibility surveys suggest that *B. fragilis* and related organisms remain almost uniformly susceptible to metronidazole (5,6). Nevertheless, resistance has been reported among isolated strains of *B. fragilis*, *Bacteroides distasonis*, *Prevotella*

TABLE 28.1. Activity of Metronidazole Against Anaerobic and Microaerophilic Bacteria

Bacteria	No. of strains	Cumulative percentage susceptible to indicated concentration (μg/mL)			
		4	8	16	32
Bacteroides fragilis[a]	161	90	99	100	—
Prevotella melaninogenica[b]	60	98	100	—	—
Other Bacteroides and Selenomonas species	154	95	98	100	—
Fusobacterium species	65	100	—	—	—
Anaerobic gram-negative cocci	24	92	96	100	—
Anaerobic gram-positive cocci	124	98	—	—	—
Clostridium perfringens	18	94	100	—	—
Other Clostridium species	73	97	99	—	100
Gram-positive nonsporulating bacilli	87	57	60	62	66
Capnocytophaga species	27	52	70	93	—

[a]Includes all species of the *B. fragilis* group.
[b]Includes *P. melaninogenica* (formerly *Bacteroides melaninogenicus*) and *Porphyromonas asaccharolytica* (formerly *Bacteroides asaccharolyticus*).
From Sutter VL *In vitro* susceptibility of anaerobic and microaerophilic bacteria to metronidazole and its hydroxy metabolite. In: Finegold SM, George WL; Rolfe RD, eds. *Proceedings of the First United States Metronidazole Conference.* Tarpon Springs, FL, February 1982. New York: Biomedical Information, 1982:61, with permission.

melaninogenica (formerly *Bacteroides melaninogenicus*), and *Bacteroides bivius*—especially after prolonged usage of the drug (7,8). Metronidazole is much less active against gram-positive non-spore-forming anaerobes; only 25% of *Actinomyces* and *Arachnia* strains are susceptible to metronidazole at achievable levels. *Propionibacterium acnes* is often resistant, with some strains requiring greater than 100 μg/mL for inhibition (9,10). *In vitro* studies have also indicated the drug's poor activity against facultative anaerobes and microaerophilic streptococci-organisms frequently found in mixed aerobic-anaerobic infections. In these infections, metronidazole alone is inadequate, and antimicrobial agents active against microaerophilic streptococci (e.g., penicillin G) and gram-negative facultative anaerobes should also be administered.

Metronidazole also has activity against a variety of other organisms such as *Treponema pallidum*, oral spirochetes, *Campylobacter fetus, Helicobacter pylori, Trichomonas vaginalis* and *Gardnerella vaginalis*.

Pharmacology

Metronidazole is almost completely absorbed after oral administration (11). Serum levels are similar after equivalent oral and intravenous doses. The drug is generally given in an intravenous loading dose of 15 mg/kg followed by a maintenance dose of 7.5 mg/kg every 6 hours. This results in peak and trough steady-state plasma levels averaging 25 and 18 μg/mL; serum half-life is approximately 8 hours, so dosage at longer intervals is certainly feasible. Although total absorption of the drug is not affected by administration with food, peak serum levels are markedly delayed. Metronidazole is well absorbed via the rectal route, with peak levels occurring approximately 3 hours after administration. Metronidazole is absorbed after vaginal administration, although peak levels (mean 1.2 μg/mL) and bioavailability (20%) are lower than after administration via the oral or intravenous route (12,13). Metronidazole readily crosses the placenta; intravenous administration to pregnant women produces equivalent fetal serum levels (14).

Metronidazole has excellent penetration at almost all sites and has been shown to achieve therapeutic levels in the following tissues and fluids: alveolar bone, amniotic fluid, unobstructed biliary tract, cerebrospinal fluid and brain abscess contents, cord

blood, pleural empyema fluid, hepatic abscesses, middle-ear discharge, middle-ear mucosa, breast milk, pelvic tissues, saliva, seminal fluid, and vaginal secretions. Penetration into aqueous humor results in levels one half to one third those of serum levels (15). Metronidazole has little protein binding, and its volume of distribution is approximately 80% of body weight.

Metronidazole is metabolized in the liver with the formation of five major metabolic products: the hydroxy derivative, an acid metabolite, acetylmetronidazole, metronidazole glucuronide, and the glucuronide conjugate of hydroxymetronidazole. Metronidazole and its metabolites are eliminated primarily in the urine (60% to 80%); 6% to 15% is excreted in the feces. In patients with severe renal failure, the hydroxy metabolite of metronidazole accumulates; this is not generally a problem, and dose adjustment is not required unless there is concomitant hepatic failure. Metronidazole is rapidly eliminated during hemodialysis, which reduces the elimination half-life of the drug to 2.6 hours. The drug is also eliminated during peritoneal dialysis, and dose reduction is generally not recommended during chronic ambulatory peritoneal dialysis (16). Serum clearance of metronidazole is delayed in patients with impaired hepatic function. Although data are limited, a dose reduction of 50% has been recommended in patients with severe hepatic dysfunction regardless of the presence of renal failure (17,18).

Administration and Dosage

Current recommended dosing schedules for metronidazole are shown in Table 28.2. Intravenous administration is recommended for seriously ill patients, although the excellent serum levels after oral administration allow this route to be used as conditions warrant. The manufacturer recommends intravenous administration during a 1-hour period, although a number of investigators have administered the drug in as little as 20 minutes without any apparent adverse effects.

After reconstitution, metronidazole hydrochloride should be diluted with intravenous fluid to a concentration not exceeding 8 μg/mL and should be neutralized to a pH of 6.0 to 7.0 with sodium bicarbonate before administration. The drug is also available from the manufacturer in a premixed, ready-to-use isotonic solution that does not require dilution or buffering before infusion.

TABLE 28.2.   Major Indications for Metronidazole: Administration and Dosage

Indication	Route of administration	Dosage
Susceptible anaerobic infections	i.v.	Loading dose of 15 mg/kg, then 7.5 mg/kg every 6 h
	p.o.	1–2 g/d in 2–4 doses every 6–12 h
Nonspecific vaginitis	p.o.	500 mg b.i.d. for 7 days
	Intravaginally	5 g 0.75% metronidazole gel b.i.d. for 5 days
Trichomonas vaginitis	p.o.	250 mg t.i.d. for 7 days or 500 mg b.i.d. for 5 days or 2 g in a single dose
Amebiasis (intestinal or extraintestinal)	i.v. or p.o.	750 mg t.i.d. for 10 days
Giardiasis	p.o.	250 mg b.i.d. or t.i.d. for 5–7 days or 2 g/d for 3 days
Pseudomembranous enterocolitis	p.o.	500 mg every 6–12 h for 7–10 days
	i.v.[a]	500 mg every 6–8 h

[a]For use in patients unable to take oral therapy. The optimal drug and dose in this situation have not been determined. See references 35, 36, 37.
i.v., intravenous; p.o., oral; b.i.d., twice daily; t.i.d., three times daily.

The recommended duration of therapy in various situations is noted in Table 28.2. For serious infections, 2 to 4 weeks of therapy is recommended; certain patients may require more prolonged therapy depending on the clinical situation and the physician's judgment.

Dosage adjustment for patients with severe hepatic dysfunction was discussed in a previous section.

Adverse Reactions

Metronidazole is well tolerated, and major adverse reactions are uncommon when the drug is used properly. Table 28.3 lists the most common major and minor adverse reactions. The most serious adverse reactions involve the central nervous system and include seizures, encephalopathy, cerebellar ataxia, and peripheral neuropathy. These reactions are rare and generally occur in patients who are receiving high doses of the drug for a prolonged period. Caution should be exercised when the drug is administered to patients with a history of seizures or neurologic problems; administration of the drug should be discontinued

TABLE 28.3.   Adverse Effects Related to Metronidazole Therapy

Major adverse reactions (rare)
  Seizures, encephalopathy
  Cerebellar dysfunction, ataxia
  Peripheral neuropathy
  Disulfiram reaction with alcohol
  Potentiation of effects of warfarin
  Pseudomembranous colitis
  Pancreatitis
  Aseptic meningitis
  Hepatotoxicity
Minor adverse reactions
  Minor gastrointestinal disturbances
  Reversible neutropenia
  Metallic taste
  Dark or red-brown urine
  Maculopapular rash, urticaria
  Urethral, vaginal burning
  Gynecomastia

immediately if any of these toxic effects develop. Gastrointestinal side effects include nausea, anorexia, and epigastric distress; diarrhea and vomiting are less common. Although metronidazole is used to treat pseudomembranous colitis, metronidazole-resistant *Clostridium difficile* has been reported and it has rarely been reported to cause the condition. This possibility should be considered in patients who develop diarrhea while receiving the drug. In addition to these side effects, other reactions such as stomatitis, dry mouth, furring of the tongue, glossitis, headache, fever, dizziness, pneumonitis, syncope, aseptic meningitis, and oral or vaginal candidiasis may be seen.

Concerns have been raised about the potential mutagenicity of the drug on the basis of tests in the Ames *Salmonella* mutant system and the evidence of possible carcinogenicity of metronidazole in some animal models (19). It is believed that antibacterial activity and mutagenic activity are related to nitroreduction of the drug. The fact that little nitroreduction takes place in eukaryotic cells suggests that mutagenicity is less likely to occur in humans. Indeed, when metronidazole was studied for mutagenic potential in eukaryotic test systems, no evidence of mutagenicity could be detected (20,21). Results of animal carcinogenicity and human studies are confusing. Although prolonged administration of metronidazole has resulted in increased tumor rates in some animal models, other studies have been negative or even suggested that metronidazole reduced the effect of some carcinogens (22,23). In humans, a study in volunteers demonstrated transient DNA breakage in lymphocytes from those taking the drug (24), and one report (25) raised the possibility of carcinogenicity in patients with Crohn's disease who received prolonged therapy. On the other hand, long-term follow-up of a cohort of 771 women who received metronidazole therapy for the treatment of vaginal trichomoniasis during the 1960s has not shown an increased incidence of malignancy (26). In general, metronidazole appears safe when used in standard doses for limited periods of time (e.g., 2–3 weeks); prolonged (e.g., months) use of the drug should be avoided unless absolutely necessary.

Metronidazole crosses the placental barrier, and concerns have been raised about possible teratogenicity. However, a study of pregnant women who had received metronidazole during pregnancy uncovered no evidence of an increased incidence of birth defects or adverse events in infants born after the exposure (27). Animal studies (28) and one anecdotal human case (29) have suggested the possibility of teratogenicity, but it is difficult to extrapolate from these few data. A metaanalysis reviewed 32 published studies referring to the use of metronidazole in pregnancy; no excess of teratogenicity was demonstrated in the 7 evaluable studies (1,336 patients) (30). Although use of metronidazole appears to be safe during the latter part of pregnancy, it should be restricted to situations in which it is clearly needed. Metronidazole should probably not be given during the first trimester unless clearly necessary.

Clinical Use

ANAEROBIC INFECTIONS

Metronidazole is used for treatment of a wide variety of anaerobic infections. An important caveat is that the microbial flora of anaerobic infections is frequently mixed and often includes microaerophilic streptococci and other organisms resistant to metronidazole (e.g., anaerobic non–spore-forming gram-positive rods). In these situations, the addition of penicillin G or ampicillin (erythromycin for the penicillin-allergic patient) is necessary for optimal antimicrobial coverage. The presence of facultative anaerobic gram-negative rods would also require an additional drug for adequate coverage. These considerations help to explain the suboptimal response described when metronidazole alone is used in the treatment of anaerobic pleuropulmonary infection (31).

Metronidazole's excellent tissue penetration and bactericidal activity make it a useful agent for deep-seated infections that are difficult to treat, such as anaerobic central nervous system infections (e.g., brain abscess), endocarditis caused by susceptible anaerobes, and anaerobic infection in the immunocompromised host. For example, metronidazole (in combination with penicillin) has become the agent of choice for anaerobic brain abscess and is probably one factor that has enhanced survival of these patients. Metronidazole has been found to be useful in the treatment of a number of other anaerobic infections, including bacteremia, infections of bones and joints, soft tissue infections, oral and dental infections, intraabdominal infections, intravaginal infections, and head and neck infections. Metronidazole is useful for therapy of nonspecific vaginitis, a condition in which various anaerobes (and G. vaginalis) may play a role (32–34). Metronidazole's role in the therapy of pseudomembranous colitis has already been mentioned; several studies suggest that metronidazole may even be effective as parenteral therapy when oral agents cannot be taken because of ileus or toxic megacolon (35–37). Metronidazole is an important component of combination regimens for treatment of duodenal ulcer disease; however its efficacy depends on the local prevalence of metronidazole-resistant Helicobacter pylori (38). In the treatment of tetanus, a clinical study suggests that metronidazole may be more effective than procaine penicillin (39).

PARASITIC INFECTIONS

Metronidazole is quite useful in the therapy of a number of parasitic infections with single-cell parasites such as Entamoeba histolytica, Giardia lamblia, and T. vaginalis. Metronidazole is the treatment of choice for amebic liver abscess and invasive intestinal amebiasis; data even suggest that it effectively eradicates cysts in the asymptomatic intestinal carrier. Vaginitis caused by T. vaginalis can be successfully treated with any one of a number of regimens utilizing metronidazole (Table 28.2). Treatment failures resulting from resistant strains have been described; however, highly resistant strains are uncommon and can be overcome with higher doses of metronidazole or therapy with other agents such as tinidazole, paromomycin, and clindamycin

(40–42). Metronidazole is quite useful in the therapy of giardiasis, although occasional treatment failures may require alternative therapy. Metronidazole may have some value in therapy for cutaneous leishmaniasis; however, it appears to be less effective than other agents (43).

Other Therapeutic Uses

Metronidazole is helpful in the treatment of a number of syndromes believed related to overgrowth of intestinal bacterial flora. These conditions include the complications of jejunoileal bypass for obesity (44) and dysfunction of the continent ileostomy (45). It can also be used to prevent intrahepatic cholestasis associated with total parenteral nutrition (46). Although use in Crohn's disease is controversial, some studies have suggested that metronidazole may have a beneficial effect in this condition (47). It appears to be able to lessen the diarrhea and may be effective for other complications such as perianal fistula, erythema nodosum, and metastatic skin lesions (48,49). Unfortunately, prolonged therapy is necessary in this situation, and concerns about peripheral neuropathy (50) and potential carcinogenicity may limit its usefulness.

Metronidazole may be used for surgical prophylaxis in abdominal and gynecologic surgery; however, some studies have shown it to be less effective as a single agent when compared with other regimens (51,52).

Tinidazole

Tinidazole is a nitroimidazole compound that is similar to metronidazole in its mechanism of action, antimicrobial spectrum, and toxicity. Although there is far less clinical experience with tinidazole, its longer half-life suggests that it may have some advantages in certain clinical situations. Oral absorption of the drug is almost complete, and serum levels are comparable with those seen after intravenous administration; after the standard oral dose of 2 g, serum levels between 40 and 60 μg/mL are reached (53). The prolonged serum half-life (12.5 hours) allows therapeutic levels (10 μg/mL) to be present 24 hours after oral administration.

Because of the drug's pharmacokinetics, single-dose regimens are effective for treatment of trichomoniasis in both men and women (54). Several studies have shown that single-dose tinidazole is as effective as (or more effective than) various single- and multiple-dose regimens of metronidazole in the treatment of giardiasis (55). Tinidazole is also active against E. histolytica; relatively short courses (3 days) of therapy appear to be as effective as longer courses of metronidazole in the therapy of intestinal amebiasis (56). Tinidazole appears to be as effective as metronidazole in the treatment of amebic liver abscess, although treatment may occasionally fail if other adjunctive measures (i.e., needle aspiration and drainage) are not used for more seriously ill patients.

The single-dose regimens of tinidazole offer definite advantages in clinical situations where cost and compliance are an issue. Although it would be reasonable to assume that tinidazole would be as effective as metronidazole in the therapy of serious intraabdominal infection, there are relatively few clinical data at this time.

OTHER NITROIMIDAZOLE COMPOUNDS

Several other agents are closely related to metronidazole, but these remain investigational for the most part. Secnidazole has an antianaerobe spectrum similar to that of metronidazole and appears equally efficacious in the treatment of amebiasis (57,58). Nimorazole is comparable with metronidazole and tinidazole in the treatment of giardiasis and trichomoniasis; however, it appears to be far less active against obligately anaerobic gram-negative bacilli (59). Ornidazole is similar to tinidazole and metronidazole and has been used successfully to treat a variety of bacterial and parasitic infections; one potential drawback is its increased incidence of side effects. There are limited data on carnidazole; however, it has been used as a single-dose treatment for vaginal trichomoniasis (60).

REFERENCES

1. Suffer VL. *In vitro* susceptibility of anaerobic and microaerophilic bacteria to metronidazole and its hydroxy metabolite. In: Finegold SM, George WL, Rolfe RD, eds. *Proceedings of the First United States Metronidazole Conference.* Tarpon Springs, FL, February 1982. New York: Biomedical Information, 1982: 61.
2. Müller M. Mode of action of metronidazole on anaerobic bacteria and protozoa. *Surgery* 1983;93:165.
3. Land KM, Johnson PJ. Molecular basis of metronidazole resistance in pathogenic bacteria and protozoa. *Drug Resist Updates* 1999;2:289–294.
4. Nastro LJ, Finegold SM. Bacterial activity of five antimicrobial agents against *Bacteroides fragilis. J Infect Dis* 1972;136:104.
5. Turgeon P, Turgeon V, Gourdeau M, et al. Longitudinal study of susceptibilities of species of the *Bacteroides fragilis* group to five antimicrobial agents in three medical centers. *Antimicrob Agents Chemother* 1994;38:2276.
6. Horn R, Robson HG. Susceptibility of the *Bacteroides fragilis* group to newer quinolones and other standard anti-anaerobic agents. *J Antimicrob Chemother* 2001;48:127–130.
7. Ingham HR, Eaton S, Venables CW, et al. *Bacteroides fragilis* resistant to metronidazole after long-term therapy. *Lancet* 1978;1:214.
8. Sprott MS, Ingham HR, Hickman JE, et al. Metronidazole-resistant anaerobes. *Lancet* 1983;1:1220.
9. Wust J. Susceptibility of anaerobic bacteria to metronidazole, omidazole, and tinidazole and routine susceptibility testing by standardized methods. *Antimicrob Agents Chemother* 1977;11:631.
10. Rosenblatt JE, Edson RS. Metronidazole. *Mayo Clin Proc* 1983;58:154.
11. Lamp KC, Freeman CD, Klutman NE, et al. Pharmacokinetics and pharmacodynamics of the nitroimidazole antimicrobials. *Clin Pharmacokinet* 1999;36:353–373.
12. Fredricsson B, Hagstrom B, Nord C-E, et al. Systemic concentrations of metronidazole and its main metabolites after intravenous, oral and vaginal administration. *Gynecol Obstet Invest* 1987;24:200.
13. Cunningham E, Kraus DM, Brubaker L, et al. Pharmacokinetics of intravaginal metronidazole gel. *J Clin Pharmacol* 1994;34:1060.
14. Visser AA, Hundt HKL. The pharmacokinetics of a single intravenous dose of metronidazole in pregnant patients. *J Antimicrob Chemother* 1984;13:279.
15. Mattila J, Nerdrum K, Rouhiainen H, et al. Penetration of metronidazole and tinidazole into the aqueous humor in man. *Chemotherapy* 1983;29:188.
16. Guay DR, Meatherall RC, Baxter H, et al. Pharmacokinetics of metronidazole in patients undergoing continuous ambulatory peritoneal dialysis. *Antimicrob Agents Chemother* 1984;25:306.
17. Lau AH, Evans R. Chang C-W, et al. Pharmacokinetics of metronidazole in patients with alcoholic liver disease. *Antimicrob Agents Chemother* 1987;31: 1662.
18. Loft S, Sonne J, Dossing M, et al. Metronidazole pharmacokinetics in patients with hepatic encephalopathy. *Scand J Gastroenterol* 1987;22:117.
19. Dobias L, Cerna M, Rossner P, et al. Genotoxicity and carcinogenicity of metronidazole. *Mutat Res* 1994;317:177.
20. Lambert B, Lindblad A, Lindsten H, et al. Genotoxic effects of metronidazole in human lymphocytes *in vitro* and *in vivo*. In: Phillips I, Collier J, eds. Metronidazole: *Proceedings of the Second International Symposium on Anaerobic Infections.* Geneva, April 1979. New York: Grune & Stratton, 1979:229.
21. Hartley-Asp AB. Chromosomal studies on human lymphocytes exposed to metronidazole *in vivo* and *in vitro*. In Phillips I, Collier J, eds. *Metronidazole: Proceedings of the Second International Symposium on Anaerobic Infections.* Geneva, April 1979. New York: Grune & Stratton, 1979:237.
22. Finegold SM. Metronidazole. *Ann Intern Med* 1980;93:585.
23. Rainey JB, Maeda M, Williams C, et al. The carcinogenic effect of intrarectal deoxycholate in rats is reduced by oral metronidazole. *Br J Cancer* 1984;49: 631.
24. Menendez D, Rojas E, Herrera LA, et al. DNA breakage due to metronidazole treatment. *Mutat Res* 2001;478:153–158.
25. Krause JR, Ayuyang HQ, Ellis LD. Occurrence of three cases of carcinoma in individuals with Crohn's disease treated with metronidazole. *Am J Gastroenterol* 1985;80:978.
26. Beard CM, Noller KL, O'Fallon WM, et al. Cancer after exposure to metronidazole. *Mayo Clin Proc* 1988;63:147.
27. Robbie MO, Sweet RL. Metronidazole use in obstetrics and gynecology: a review. *Am J Obstet Gynecol* 1983;145:865.
28. Garry VF, Nelson RL. Host-mediated transformation: metronidazole. *Mutat Res* 1987;190:289.
29. Cantu JM, Garcia-Cruz D. Midline facial defect as a teratogenic effect of metronidazole. *Birth Defects* 1982;18:85.
30. Burtin P, Taddio A, Ariburnu O, et al. Safety of metronidazole in pregnancy: a meta-analysis. *Am J Obstet Gynecol* 1995;172:525.
31. Sanders CV, Hanna BJ, Lewis AC, et al. The use of metronidazole in the treatment of anaerobic pleuropulmonary infections. In: Phillips I, Collier J, eds. *Metronidazole: Proceedings of the Second International Symposium on Anaerobic Infections.* Geneva, April 1979. New York: Grune & Stratton, 1979: 83.
32. Swedberg J, Steiner JD, Deiss F, et al. Comparison of single-dose vs one-week course of metronidazole for symptomatic bacterial vaginosis. *JAMA* 1985;254:1046.
33. Livengood CH 3rd, McGregor JA, Soper DE, et al. Bacterial vaginosis: efficacy and safety of intravaginal metronidazole treatment. *Am J Obstet Gynecol* 1994;170:759.
34. Mikamo H, Izumi K, Ito K, et al. Study on treatment of bacterial vaginosis with oral administration of metronidazole or cefdinir. *Chemotherapy* 1994;40: 362.
35. Kleinfeld DI, Sharpe RJ, Donta ST. Parenteral therapy for antibiotic-associated pseudomembranous colitis. *J Infect Dis* 1988;157:389.
36. Bolton RP, Culshaw MA. Faecal metronidazole concentrations during oral and intravenous therapy for antibiotic associated colitis due to *Clostridium difficile. Gut* 1986;27:1169.
37. Friedenberg F, Fernandez A, Kaul V, et al. Intravenous metronidazole for the treatment of *Clostridium difficile* colitis. *Dis Colon Rectum* 2001;44:1176–1180.
38. Gisbert JP, Parjares JM. *Helicobacter pylori* therapy: first-line options and rescue regimen. *Dig Dis* 2001;19:134–143.
39. Ahmadsyah I, Salim A. Treatment of tetanus: an open study to compare the efficacy of procaine penicillin and metronidazole. *BMJ* 1985;291:648.
40. Robertson DHH, Heyworth R, Harrison C, et al. Treatment failure in *Trichomonas vaginalis* infections in females. I. Concentrations of metronidazole in plasma and vaginal content during normal and high dosage. *J Antimicrob Chemother* 1988;21:373.
41. Midler M, Lossick JG, Gorrell TE. *In vitro* susceptibility of *Trichomonas vaginalis* to metronidazole and treatment outcome in vaginal trichomoniasis. *Sex Transm Dis* 1988;15:17.
42. Sobel JD, Nyirjesy P, Brown W. Tinidazole therapy for metronidazole-resistant vaginal trichomoniasis. *Clin Infect Dis* 2001;33:1341–1346.
43. Chong H. Oriental sore: a look at trends in and approaches to the treatment of leishmaniasis. *Int J Dermatol* 1986;25:615.
44. Drenick E. Extraintestinal complications of jejunoileal bypass for obesity. In: Finegold SM, George WL, Rolfe RD, eds. *Proceedings of the First United States Metronidazole Conference.* Tarpon Springs, FL, February 1982. New York: Biomedical Information, 1982:371.
45. Kelly DG, Phillips SF, Kelly KA, et al. Dysfunction of the continent ileostomy: clinical features and bacteriology. *Gut* 1983;24:193.
46. Capron J-P, Herve M-A, Gineston J-L, et al. Metronidazole in prevention of cholestasis associated with total parenteral nutrition. *Lancet* 1983;1:446.
47. Prantera C, Zannoni F, Scribano ML, et al. An antibiotic regimen for the treatment of active Crohn's disease: a randomized, controlled clinical trial of metronidazole plus ciprofloxacin. *Am J Gastroenterol* 1996;91:328–332.
48. Gilat T. Metronidazole in Crohn's disease [Editorial]. *Gastroenterology* 1982;83:702.
49. Duhra P, Paul CJ. Metastatic Crohn's disease responding to metronidazole. *Br J Dermatol* 1988;119:87.
50. Duffy LF, Daum F, Fisher SE, et al. Peripheral neuropathy in Crohn's disease patients treated with metronidazole. *Gastroenterology* 1985;88:681.
51. Vinceletto J, Finkelstein F, Aoki FY, et al. Double-blind trial of perioperative intravenous metronidazole prophylaxis for abdominal and vaginal hysterectomy. *Surgery* 1983;93:185.
52. Keiser TA, MacKenzie RL, Feld R, et al. Prophylactic metronidazole in appendectomy: a double-blind controlled trial. *Surgery* 1983;93:201.
53. Wood BA, Faulkner JK, Monro AM. The pharmacokinetics, metabolism and tissue distribution of tinidazole. *J Antimicrob Chemother* 1982;10(suppl):43.
54. Jones R, Enders P. An evaluation of tinidazole as single-dose therapy for the treatment of *Trichomonas vaginalis. Med J Aust* 1977;2:679.
55. Levi GC, De Avila CA, Neto VA. Efficacy of various drugs for treatment of giardiasis: a comparative study. *Am J Trop Med Hyg* 1977;26:564.
56. Swami B, Lavakusulu D, Sitha Devi C. Tinidazole and metronidazole in the treatment of intestinal amoebiasis. *Curr Med Res Opin* 1977;5:152.
57. Gillis JC, Wiseman LR. Secnidazole. A review of its antimicrobial activity, pharmacokinetic properties and therapeutic use in the management of protozoal infections and bacterial vaginosis. *Drugs* 1996;51:621–638.
58. Bhatia S, Karnad DR, Oak JL. Randomized double-blind trial of metronidazole versus secnidazole in amebic liver abscess. *Ind J Gastroenterol* 1998;17:53–54.
59. Reynolds AV, Hamilton-Miller JMT, Brumfitt W. A comparison of the *in vitro* activity of metronidazole, tinidazole, and nimorazole against gram-negative anaerobic bacilli. *J Clin Pathol* 1975;28:775.
60. Notowicz A, Stolz E, DeKoning GAJ. First experiences with single-dose treatment of vaginal trichomoniasis with carnidazole (R25831). *Br J Vener Dis* 1977;53:129.

BIBLIOGRAPHY

Finegold SM. Metronidazole. *Ann Intern Med* 1980;93:585.

Finegold SM, George WL, eds. *Anaerobic infections in humans.* San Diego: Academic Press, 1989.

Finegold SM, George WL, Rolfe RD, eds. *Proceedings of the First United States Metronidazole Conference.* Tarpon Springs, FL, February 1982. New York: Biomedical Information, 1982.

Finegold SM, McFadzean JA, Roe FJC, eds. *Metronidazole: Proceedings of the International Metronidazole Conference.* Montreal, May 1, 1976. Princeton, NJ: Excerpta Medica, 1977.

"Flagyl" (Metronidazole) in anaerobic infections. Essex, England: May & Baker, 1979.

Kucers A, Bennett NM, Kemp RJ, eds. Metronidazole. In: *The use of antibiotics.* Philadelphia: JB Lippincott, 1987:1290–1329.

Phillips I, Collier J, eds. *Metronidazole: Proceedings of the Second International Symposium on Anaerobic Infections.* Geneva, April 1979. New York: Grune & Stratton, 1979.

Proceedings of the North American Metronidazole Symposium on Anaerobic Infections, Scottsdale, AZ. *Surgery* 1983;93:123.

Rosenblatt JE, Edson RS. Metronidazole. *Mayo Clin Proc* 1987;62:1013.

Stanz MH, Bradley WE. Metronidazole (Flagyl IV, Searle). *Drug Intell Clin Pharm* 1981;15:838.

CHAPTER 29

Rifampin and Related Drugs

William A. Craig

The rifamycin antibiotics were first isolated in 1957 as fermentation products from *Streptomyces mediterranei* (1). Rifamycin SV and rifamide were the first clinically released semisynthetic compounds, but both were poorly absorbed when taken by mouth. Rifampin (also called rifampicin) was discovered in 1965 and found to be the most active derivative after oral administration (2). More recent semisynthetic derivatives with increased activity against mycobacteria include rifabutin (ansamycin), rifapentine, rifaximin, and the benzoxazinorifamycins (3–6).

CHEMISTRY

The rifamycins consist of a naphthalenic ring that is spanned by a long aliphatic loop or "ansa" (Fig. 29.1). Changes primarily in the 3 and 4 positions of the naphthalenic ring have led to the different semisynthetic derivatives. Alterations in the aliphatic loop result in loss of activity (6). They are lipid-soluble compounds, display their best aqueous solubility at acidic pH, and behave like zwitterions in solution.

MECHANISM OF ACTION

The rifamycins inhibit DNA-dependent RNA polymerase by binding to the β subunit of the enzyme in susceptible microorganisms (7). This interferes with protein synthesis by preventing chain initiation but not elongation. Inhibition of mammalian enzymes requires concentrations more than 1,000 times greater than that active against bacterial enzymes (8). The drugs are bactericidal. Intermittent exposure to rifampin results in some of the longest durations of persistent suppression of bacterial growth (i.e., postantibiotic effect) observed with any antimicrobial (9).

SPECTRUM OF ACTIVITY

Rifampin is active against a large variety of aerobic and anaerobic bacteria (10–21). Among the gram-positive bacteria (Table 29.1), rifampin is most active against staphylococci. Minimal inhibitory concentrations (MICs) for methicillin-resistant strains are similar to those for methicillin-susceptible staphylococci (10). Except for *Enterococcus faecalis*, most gram-positive bacteria have MICs of 1.0 mg/L or less. Against *Clostridium difficile*, rifampin is as active as metronidazole and vancomycin (12).

With gram-negative bacteria (Table 29.2), rifampin exhibits excellent activity against *Neisseria gonorrhoeae*, *Neisseria meningitidis*, *Moraxella catarrhalis*, *Haemophilus influenzae*, *Haemophilus ducreyi*, and *Rochalimaea* species (13–19). It is one of the most active antimicrobials against all of the *Legionella* species (14,20). Most strains of *Brucella* are also susceptible to rifampin (21). Although Enterobacteriaceae and *Pseudomonas* species have minimal inhibitory concentrations for rifampin that are greater than 2 mg/L, the RNA polymerase enzymes from these organisms are only slightly less sensitive to the drug than those from staphylococci. Rifampin has demonstrated *in vitro* synergy with aminoglycoside and β-lactam antibiotics against *Pseudomonas aeruginosa* (22).

The rifamycins vary markedly in their activity against different mycobacteria (23–26) (Table 29.3). Rifampin is active against *Mycobacterium tuberculosis*, *Mycobacterium kansasii*, and *Mycobacterium marinum*; intermediate against *Mycobacterium avium-intracellulare*; and inactive against *Mycobacterium fortuitum* and *Mycobacterium chelonei*. *Mycobacterium leprae* is also susceptible to rifampin (27).

Chlamydia trachomatis (including lymphogranuloma venereum strains), *Chlamydia psittaci*, and *Coxiella burnetii* are also quite susceptible to rifampin (28,29). The drug even exhibits activity against all erythrocytic forms of *Plasmodium vivax* and against several fungi in the presence of other drugs such as amphotericin B (30,31).

RESISTANCE

The rapid emergence of resistant bacteria has been a common problem for monotherapy with the rifamycins. Susceptible bacteria develop resistance to these drugs by insertion, deletion, or point mutations in the gene (*rpoB*) encoding the β subunit of the RNA polymerase enzyme (32). These mutations, which result in extra, missing, or substituted amino acids in the enzyme, can occur (a) at various sites in the *rpoB* gene, but primarily at codons 531 and 526 and (b) at frequencies ranging from 1 per 10^6 to 1 per 10^9 bacteria (32,33).

Except for short-term use for prophylaxis, the rifamycins should not be used alone. A variety of antituberculous drugs

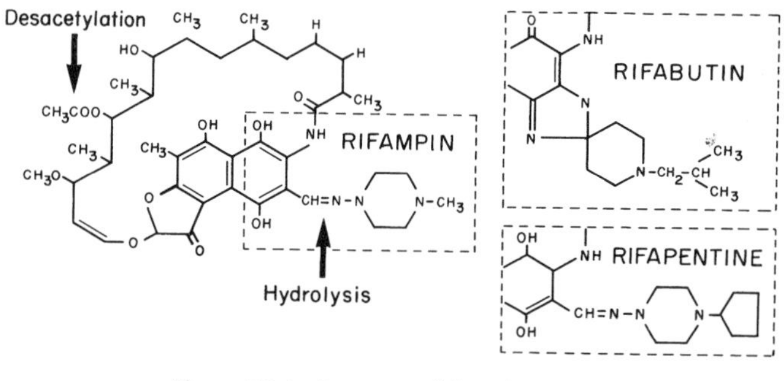

Figure 29.1. Structure of the rifamycins.

TABLE 29.1. Activity of Rifampin against Gram-Positive Bacteria

Organism	Minimal inhibitory concentration (mg/L)	
	MIC$_{50}$	MIC$_{90}$
Staphylococcus aureus	0.015	0.015
Staphylococcus epidermidis	0.015	0.015
Streptococcus pyogenes	0.12	0.12
Streptococcus agalactiae	1.0	1.0
Streptococcus pneumoniae	0.12	4.0
Viridans group streptococci	0.06	0.12
Enterococcus faecalis	4.0	16.0
Corynebacterium jeikei	0.05	0.05
Listeria monocytogenes	≤0.12	0.25
Clostridium difficile	≤0.2	≤0.2
Clostridium perfringens	≤0.1	≤0.1
Eubacterium species	≤0.1	0.4
Peptococcus species	0.2	1.6
Peptostreptococcus species	≤0.1	1.6
Propionibacterium acnes	≤0.1	≤0.1

Data from references 10–14.

TABLE 29.2. Activity of Rifampin against Gram-Negative Bacteria

Organism	Minimal inhibitory concentration (mg/L)	
	MIC$_{50}$	MIC$_{90}$
Neisseria gonorrhoeae	0.25	0.5
Neisseria meningitidis	≤0.03	0.12
Moraxella catarrhalis	0.03	0.03
Haemophilus influenzae	0.25	0.5
Haemophilus ducreyi	0.004	0.03
Legionella pneumophila	0.03	0.03
Brucella species	2.5	4.0
Rochalimaea species	≤0.125	≤0.125
Escherichia coli	8	16
Klebsiella pneumoniae	32	32
Proteus mirabilis	4	8
Enterobacter species	32	64
Citrobacter species	32	32
Serratia marcescens	64	64
Providencia species	8	32
Acinetobacter species	8	8
Pseudomonas aeruginosa	32	64
Bacteroides fragilis	0.4	0.8
Prevotella species	≤0.1	0.2
Fusobacterium species	0.2	1.6
Veillonella species	1.6	1.6

Data from references 13–21.

are effective in preventing the emergence of rifampin-resistant tubercle bacilli. Primary resistance of *M. tuberculosis* to rifampin occurs in about 3.5% of newly diagnosed patients in the United States (34). With staphylococci, β-lactam antibiotics appear to be more effective than vancomycin in preventing the emergence of rifampin-resistant organisms with combined use (35,36).

PHARMACOKINETIC PROPERTIES

Rifampin is rapidly and virtually completely absorbed after oral dosing, resulting in serum concentrations similar to those after intravenous administration (37,38) (Fig. 29.2). The drug is cleared from the circulation primarily by hepatic metabolism and biliary excretion; its half-life is 2 to 5 hours. Because the excretory capacity of the liver for rifampin tends to saturate at doses of 300 to 450 mg, larger amounts result in a disproportionate increase in maximal serum levels and area under the curve (37). Peak serum concentrations after ingestion of 600 mg or 10 mg/kg usually fall in the range of 7 to 15 mg/L (37–39). Lower levels can be observed in patients with human immunodeficiency virus (HIV) infections (40). About 80% of the drug is bound to serum proteins.

Rifampin and other rifamycins are metabolized in the liver by desacetylation to a less active metabolite (38) (Fig. 29.1). The desacetyl derivative accounts for most of the drug in bile. Hydrolysis of rifampin to the inactive 3-formylrifampin apparently occurs only in the urine. Because rifampin is a potent inducer of hepatic microsomal cytochrome P450 enzymes, it stimulates its own metabolism. Repeated administration increases clearance of the drug and decreases peak serum concentrations and area under the curve about 30% to 40%. Because only 6% to 25% of rifampin is excreted in the urine, dosage modification is not required in patients with renal impairment. Although use of rifampin in patients with liver disease is not recommended except in case of necessity, hepatic dysfunction only doubles the drug's half-life (41). The pharmacokinetics of rifampin in children and in elderly patients is similar to that in adults (42,43).

TABLE 29.3. Activity of Rifampin, Rifabutin, and Rifapentine against *Mycobacterium* Species

Organism	Minimal inhibitory concentration (mg/L)					
	Rifampin		Rifabutin		Rifapentine	
	MIC$_{50}$	MIC$_{90}$	MIC$_{50}$	MIC$_{90}$	MIC$_{50}$	MIC$_{90}$
M. tuberculosis	0.3	0.6	0.06	0.06	0.08	0.16
M. avium-intracellulare	2.0	4.0	0.25	1.0	0.5	2.0
M. kansasii	0.6	2.5	≤0.5	≤0.5	≤0.5	—
M. marinum	1.25	2.5	≤0.5	≤0.5	—	—
M. fortuitum	>20	>20	>2	>2	>2	>2
M. chelonae	>20	>20	>2	>2	>2	>2

Data from references 3,4, 23–26.

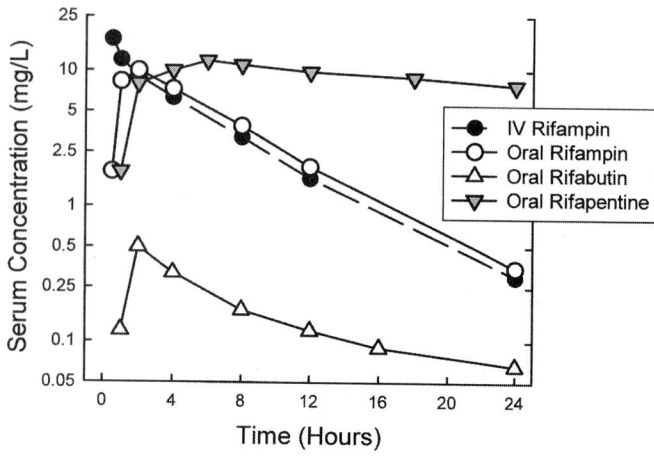

Figure 29.2. Serum concentrations of rifampin after oral and intravenous (IV) administration of 600 mg and of rifabutin and rifapentine after oral dosing of 600 mg.

The high lipid solubility of rifampin results in tissue concentrations similar to those observed in serum (38). Therapeutic concentrations are obtained in saliva, tears, sputum, pancreatic juice, bone, cardiac valve tissue, and pleural, ascitic, blister, and tubercle cavitary fluids (38,39,44). Intravenous infusions of 20 mg/kg in children and 600 mg in adults with uninflamed meninges produces cerebrospinal fluid concentrations of 0.1 to 3.0 mg/L (45,46). Higher concentrations up to 2.4 mg/L are observed in patients with meningitis (47). Oral doses of 600 mg produce concentrations of 0.2 to 1.3 mg/L in the aqueous humor (48). The drug also readily enters phagocytic cells and is capable of killing intracellular bacteria and sterilizing abscesses (49).

Rifampin is available for both oral and intravenous administration. The intravenous preparation should not be administered by the intramuscular or subcutaneous route. The recommended dosage is 600 mg in adults and 10 to 20 mg/kg, not to exceed 600 mg, in children. A 1% suspension can be prepared by adding the powder from four 300-mg capsules to 120 mL of syrup (50).

CLINICAL USE

Mycobacterial Infections

Since its introduction into clinical medicine in 1968, rifampin has joined isoniazid as one of the cornerstones in the chemotherapy of tuberculosis. Drug combinations including rifampin have produced cure rates after 6 to 9 months of therapy equivalent to those obtained with 18 months of therapy with regimens lacking rifampin (51,52). Currently recommended regimens include 6 months of treatment with a combination of rifampin at 15 mg/kg per day (maximum, 600 mg), isoniazid at 10 mg/kg per day (maximum, 300 mg), and pyrazinamide at 15 to 30 mg/kg per day (maximum, 2 g) during the first 2 months of therapy(53). A fourth drug (ethambutol or streptomycin) is usually recommended until susceptibility results are known. Rifampin is effective for preventive therapy (54). Four months of rifampin or 2 months of rifampin plus pyrazinamide is the recommended regimen for prophylactic therapy of latent infection (55). Rifampin, in combination with other drugs, is also useful in the treatment of infections due to *M. kansasii, M. marinum, Mycobacterium xenopi,* and *M. avium-intracellulare* (56–61).

Rifampin is currently the major drug for the treatment of leprosy. Once-monthly therapy with rifampin is highly bactericidal against *M. leprae* but is used in combination with dapsone to prevent the emergence of resistant strains (62).

Prophylaxis

Rifampin can eradicate a variety of organisms from the nasopharynx of carriers and is therefore useful in the prophylaxis of infection. For prophylaxis of close contacts of patients with severe meningococcal infections, a single daily dose of 10 mg/kg or 600 mg for 2 or 4 days has reduced the carriage of *N. meningitidis* by 75% to 95%. (63,64). The drug is also effective in eradicating carriage of *H. influenzae* type b. A single daily dose of rifampin at 20 mg/kg (maximum, 600 mg) for 2 or 4 days reduces carriage of *H. influenzae* in more than 90% of children (65). A 4-day course of rifampin, 10 mg/kg twice daily, plus benzathine penicillin G is highly effective in eradicating carriage of *Streptococcus pyogenes,* but such therapy is rarely indicated (66).

A 5- to 10-day course of rifampin can reduce the carriage of *Staphylococcus aureus* by 73% to 95% (67–70). Five-day courses of rifampin repeated every 3 months reduce the frequency of shunt infections in patients undergoing hemodialysis and decrease the episodes of catheter site infection and peritonitis in patients undergoing peritoneal dialysis (69,70). Rifampin, in combination with trimethoprim or minocycline, has good efficacy in eradicating the nasal carriage of methicillin-resistant *S. aureus* in hospitalized patients (71,72). However, these regimens have had less success in eliminating the organism from extranasal sites.

Staphylococcal Infections

The absence of adequate controlled clinical trials makes the use of rifampin in the treatment of staphylococcal infections a controversial topic. The addition of rifampin to standard therapy has resulted in some dramatic responses in patients with serious infections due to *S. aureus* (73–75). However, one of the concerns with the use of rifampin in serious staphylococcal infections is the reported *in vitro* antagonism by rifampin of the killing of staphylococci by β-lactam drugs and vancomycin (76). Animal studies, on the other hand, usually demonstrate similar or enhanced activity of drug combinations containing rifampin (77). Although an unblinded, prospective clinical trial suggested that the addition of rifampin to oxacillin improved clinical outcome in patients with serious staphylococcal infections, a subsequent double-blind, placebo-controlled trial by the same investigators showed no major benefit (74,78). In general, the addition of rifampin is recommended for cases of staphylococcal infection associated with myocardial and metastatic abscesses. Rifampin has been combined with a fluoroquinolone to provide an entirely oral regimen for the treatment of right-sided *S. aureus* endocarditis in intravenous drug abusers (79).

Rifampin, in combination with vancomycin and gentamicin, is recommended for the treatment of prosthetic valve endocarditis due to *Staphylococcus epidermidis.* In the only prospective trial, the three-drug regimen was as effective as the combination of rifampin and vancomycin but resulted in a lower frequency of rifampin resistance during therapy (80,81).

Osteomyelitis is another infection caused by *S. aureus* in which the use of rifampin has been studied. In animal models, the best efficacy is observed with antimicrobial regimens containing rifampin (82). The only controlled clinical trial in patients with chronic staphylococcal osteomyelitis demonstrated a trend toward better response (80% vs. 50%) with the nafcillin plus rifampin regimen than with nafcillin alone (83), although the small number of patients in the study made it impossible to demonstrate statistical significance. Rifampin combinations have also been useful in the treatment of orthopedic implant-related infections caused by gram-positive cocci (84).

Brucella Species Infections

Rifampin appears to have an increasing role in the treatment of brucellosis. Treatment for 45 days with doxycycline plus rifampin exhibits a clinical response similar to that seen with tetracycline plus streptomycin (85). In another study, rifampin combined with ofloxacin was equally effective as rifampin plus doxycycline (86). Rifampin has also been successful in the treatment of *Brucella* species endocarditis (87).

Other Infections

Despite limited clinical experience, a combination of rifampin, vancomycin, and a third-generation cephalosporin has been recommended by some physicians for meningitis caused by penicillin-resistant pneumococci (88). Although rifampin has been added when *Legionella* species infection responded poorly to erythromycin, no clinical trials have demonstrated enhanced activity of combined therapy. The addition of rifampin to ticarcillin plus tobramycin resulted in a dramatic improvement in a few cases of infection due to *P. aeruginosa* that were failing to respond to combination therapy (89). In a prospective, randomized trial, the addition of rifampin to combination therapy of an antipseudomonal penicillin and aminoglycoside significantly increased the frequency of bacteriological cure, but this did not reduce mortality (90). Rifampin has also demonstrated clinical efficacy in cases of chancroid, cutaneous leishmaniasis, Buruli ulcer, Mediterranean spotted fever, Q fever, bartonellosis, pulmonary actinomycosis, *Rhodococcus* infections, relapsing *C. difficile*–associated diarrhea, central nervous system–shunt infections, and meningitis due to *Chryseobacterium meningosepticum* (91–96).

SIDE EFFECTS

The most common side effect observed with rifampin is an orange-red discoloration of the urine. Permanent staining of soft contact lenses can also occur during rifampin therapy. Two- to 4-day courses of rifampin for prophylaxis are associated with a variety of mild, reversible side effects, such as abdominal pain or diarrhea, nausea and vomiting, headache or visual change, dizziness or drowsiness, and pruritus or rash (97).

Important side effects with more prolonged therapy include hepatitis, interstitial nephritis, influenza-like syndrome, thrombocytopenia, anemia, and leukopenia (98–100). Although elevated liver enzyme activities are observed in about 5% to 10% of patients, hepatitis occurs in only 0.15% to 0.43% of patients treated with rifampin alone (98). The frequency of hepatitis rises to 2.5% in patients receiving multiple-drug therapy for tuberculosis; however, most studies suggest that rifampin does not enhance the hepatotoxicity of isoniazid. In one study, the frequency of hepatotoxicity during prophylaxis was 7 times higher with 2 months of rifampin plus pyrazinamide than with 6 months of isoniazid alone (101).

Interstitial nephritis is a rare complication of rifampin and occurs primarily with intermittent dosing. Renal failure due to massive hemolysis, glomerulonephritis, and the tubular precipitation of light-chain proteins produced by rifampin have also been reported (98,102).

An influenza-like syndrome, with fever, chills, malaise, and headache, has also been associated with intermittent dosing of

TABLE 29.4. Drugs that Exhibit Increased Clearance with Concomitant Rifampin Therapy

Aprenavir	Haloperidol	Quinidine
Barbiturates	Indinavir	Repaglinide
Buspirone	Itraconazole	Ritonavir
Chloramphenicol	Ketoconazole	Saquinavir
Cimetidine	Lorcainide	Sertraline
Clarithromycin	Losartan	Simvastatin
Clofibrate	Medazolam	Sulfasalazine
Contraceptives (oral)	Methadone	Sulfonylureas
Cyclosporine	Metoprolol	Tacrolimus
Dapsone	Metronidazole	Tamoxifen
Delavirdine	Mexiletine	Theophylline
Diazepam	Nelfinavir	Thyroxine
Digitoxin	Nevirapine	Tocainide
Digoxin	Nifedipine	Triazolam
Diltiazem	Nilvadipine	Verapamil
Disopyramide	Nitrazepam	Voriconazole
Doxycycline	Nortriptyline	Warfarin
Efavirenz	Ondansetron	Zidovudine
Estrogens	Opiates	Zolpidem
Fluconazole	Phenytoin	Zopiclone
Glucocorticoids	Propafenone	
Glyburide	Propranolol	

Data from references 104–108.

rifampin. It rarely occurs with daily dosing and is most common with intermittent dosing less than twice weekly and with doses greater than 900 mg (98). It most likely represents an immunologic reaction due to the formation of rifampin antibody complexes. Most hematologic toxic effects also appear to be immunologic reactions related to rifampin-induced antibodies. In healthy subjects, rifampin did not produce any detectable effect on immunoglobulin levels, antigen responsiveness, and skin test reactivity (103).

Because the rifamycins are potent inducers of the hepatic microsomal cytochrome P450 (CYP) enzymes, especially CYP3A4, and the P-glycoprotein (P-gp) transport system, their use with other drugs may result in clinically significant drug interactions. Rifamycins have been shown to increase the rate of elimination of a large number of drugs (104,105) (Table 29.4). This can result in decreased efficacy of concomitant drug therapy with rifampin therapy or in concomitant drug toxicity after rifampin is stopped. The complications resulting from rifampin therapy have been failure of oral contraceptive therapy, relapse of asthma and Addison's disease in patients receiving glucocorticoid therapy, relapse of arrhythmia in patients taking quinidine or verapamil, exacerbation of diabetes in individuals receiving oral hypoglycemic agents, and acute rejection in transplant recipients taking cyclosporine. Rifampin can also reduce the concentrations of clarithromycin, doxycycline, fluconazole, itraconazole, most protease inhibitors, some nonnucleoside reverse transcriptase inhibitors (NNTRIs), and zidovudine, which may have therapeutic consequences (106–108).

Because the rifamycins are lipid soluble, they readily penetrate the placenta. Large doses of rifampin can produce teratogenic effects in rodents. Although similar effects have not been observed in humans, rifampin should be given to pregnant women only to treat active cases of tuberculosis (53).

RIFABUTIN

Rifabutin is a semisynthetic derivative of rifamycin S that is 4 to 10 times more active than rifampin against *M. tuberculosis* and

M. avium-intracellulare (109,110) (Table 29.3). The drug is primarily used for the treatment and prevention of *M. avium-intracellulare* infections. In patients with acquired immunodeficiency syndrome (AIDS) and CD4+ cell counts less than $200/mm^3$, daily doses of 300 mg of rifabutin reduce acquisition of *M. avium-intracellulare* bacteremia by about 50% (111). Rifabutin prophylaxis is recommended for AIDS patients with CD4+ cell counts less than $100/mm^3$ (112). Rifabutin use for treatment of *M. avium-intracellulare* infections in HIV-infected patients has produced variable results (113–115).

Although rifabutin is rapidly absorbed, oral bioavailability is only 12% to 20% (116). The drug has a larger volume of distribution than rifampin does, so that serum concentrations of rifabutin are much less than those of rifampin (Fig. 29.2). With oral doses of 300 to 600 mg, peak serum concentrations of rifabutin range from 0.3 to 0.9 mg/L (116–118). About 70% of the drug is bound to serum proteins. The concentrations of rifabutin in cerebrospinal fluid are 30% to 70% of those in serum (119). The drug is eliminated from the circulation like rifampin, with only 10% recovered in the urine.

Side effects with rifabutin therapy differ from those observed with rifampin. Uveitis and an arthralgia-arthritis syndrome have been the major toxic effects observed with long-term prophylaxis with rifabutin (120,121). The drug also induces CYP3A enzymes to a lesser degree than rifampin does (122,123). Thus, rifabutin is recommended for treatment and prevention of mycobacterial infections in patients on highly active antiretroviral therapy (HAART). However, most protease inhibitors and some NNTRIs are inhibitors of CYP3A as well as substrates and can result in higher and potentially toxic levels of rifabutin (104). Guidelines recommend a modified dose of rifabutin at 150 mg daily or 300 mg two or three times per week in these situations (124). A similar increase in rifabutin serum concentrations is observed with concomitant use of clarithromycin and fluconazole (104,125).

RIFAPENTINE

Rifapentine is two to three times more active than rifampin against *M. avium-intracellulare* and *M. tuberculosis* (4,26) (Table 29.3). Rifapentine exhibits good oral bioavailability and results in mean peak serum concentrations of 8 to 15 mg/L after ingestion of 600 mg or a dose of 8 mg/kg (126,127). However, 97% of the drug is bound to serum proteins. This may contribute to the longer serum half-life of rifapentine (14 to 20 hours) than is observed with rifampin and rifabutin. The extensive hepatic metabolism, high biliary excretion, low renal elimination, and wide tissue distribution of the drug are similar to those of rifampin.

Rifapentine is approved for the treatment of tuberculosis. The initial dosage of 600 mg twice weekly for the first 2 months (along with daily isoniazid, pyrizinamide, and ethambutol) is followed by 600 mg once weekly for the last 4 months (along with once-weekly isoniazid). This regimen was equivalent to short-course therapy daily rifampin (along with daily isoniazid, pyrazinamide, and ethambutol) for the first 2 months and twice-weekly rifampin and isoniazid for the last 4 months (128). Although the relapse rate was higher in the rifapentine arm, most were associated with noncompliance. A trial in HIV-infected patients, comparing once-weekly rifapentine-isoniazid with twice weekly rifampin-isoniazid for the consolidation phase of short-course therapy, observed relapse with monoresistance to rifamycin only in patients receiving once-weekly rifapentine-isoniazid (129).

OTHER RIFAMYCINS

Rifaximin is a poorly absorbed rifamycin derivative that is used primarily to reduce bacterial numbers within the gastrointestinal tract (130). In initial clinical trials, it has demonstrated efficacy in hepatic encephalopathy, acute diverticulitis, and surgical prophylaxis. The more recently developed benzoxazinorifamycin KRM-1648 is 16 to 64 times more potent than rifampin against most mycobacteria (5,131,132). It is even active against some rifampin-resistant strains of *M. tuberculosis* and *M. avium-intracellulare*.

REFERENCES

1. Sensi P. History of the development of rifampin. *Rev Infect Dis* 1983;5[Suppl 3]:5402.
2. Maggi N, Pasqualucci CR, Ballotta R, et al. Rifampicin: a new orally active rifamycin. *Chemotherapy* 1966;11:285.
3. Della Bruna C, Schioppacassi G, Ungheri D, et al. LM 427, a new spiropiperidylrifamycin: in vitro and in vivo studies. *J Antibiot* (Tokyo) 1983;36:1502.
4. Arioli V, Berti M, Carniti G, et al. Antibacterial activity of DL 473, a new semisynthetic rifamycin derivative. *J Antibiot* (Tokyo) 1981;34:1026.
5. Saito H, Tomioka H, Emori M, et al. In vitro antimycobacterial activities of newly synthesized benzoxazinorifamycins. *Antimicrob Agents Chemother* 1991;35:542.
6. Wehrli W, Staehelin M. The rifamycins: relation of chemical structure and action on RNA polymerase. *Biochim Biophys Acta* 1969;182:24.
7. Hartman G, Honikel KO, Knusel F. The specific inhibition of the DNA-directed RNA synthesis by rifamycin. *Biochim Biophys Acta* 1967;145:843.
8. Buss WC, Morgan R, Guttmann J, et al. Rifampicin inhibition of protein synthesis in mammalian cells. *Science* 1978;200:432.
9. Bundtzen RW, Gerber AU, Cohn DL, et al. Postantibiotic suppression of bacterial growth. *Rev Infect Dis* 1981;3:28.
10. Pohlod DJ, Saravolatz LD, Somerville MM. In-vitro susceptibility of gram-positive cocci to LY146032 teicoplanin, sodium fusidate, vancomycin, and rifampicin. *J Antimicrob Chemother* 1987;20:197.
11. Púrez JL, Riera L, Valls F, et al. A comparison of the in-vitro activity of seventeen antibiotics against *Streptococcus faecalis*. *J Antimicrob Chemother* 1987;20:357.
12. Fekety R, Silva J, Toshniwal R, et al. Antibiotic-associated colitis: effects of antibiotics on *Clostridium difficile* and the disease in hamsters. *Rev Infect Dis* 1979;1:386.
13. Martin WJ, Gardner M, Washington JA II. In vitro antimicrobial susceptibility of anaerobic bacteria isolated from clinical specimens. *Antimicrob Agents Chemother* 1972;2:148.
14. Thornsberry C, Hill BC, Swenson JM, et al. Rifampin: spectrum of antibacterial activity. *Rev Infect Dis* 1983;5[Suppl 3]:5412.
15. Trallero EP, Arenzana JMG, Ayestaran I, et al. Comparative activity in vitro of 16 antimicrobial agents against penicillin-susceptible meningococci and meningococci with diminished susceptibility to penicillin. *Antimicrob Agents Chemother* 1989;33:1622.
16. Doern GV, Jorgensen JH, Thornsberry C, et al. National collaborative study of the prevalence of antimicrobial resistance among clinical isolates of *Haemophilus influenzae*. *Antimicrob Agents Chemother* 1988;32:180.
17. Doem GV, Tubert TA. In vitro activities of 39 antimicrobial agents for *Branhamella catarrhalis* and comparison of results with different quantitative susceptibility test methods. *Antimicrob Agents Chemother* 1988;32:259.
18. Dangor Y, Miller SD, Exposto FDL, et al. Antimicrobial susceptibilities of southern African isolates of *Haemophilus ducreyi*. *Antimicrob Agents Chemother* 1988;32:1458.
19. Maurin M, Raoult D. Antimicrobial susceptibility of *Rochalimaea quintana*, *Rochalimaea vinsonii*, and the newly recognized *Rochalimaea henselae*. *J Antimicrob Chemother* 1993;32:587.
20. Schulin T, Wennersten CB, Ferraro MJ, et al. Susceptibilities of Legionella spp. to newer antimicrobials in vitro. *Antimicrob Agents Chemother* 1998;42:1520.
21. Rubinstein E, Lang R, Shasha B, et al. In vitro susceptibility of *Brucella melitensis* to antibiotics. *Antimicrob Agents Chemother* 1991;35:1925.
22. Valdes JM, Baltch AL, Smith RP, et al. The effect of rifampicin on the in-vitro activity of cefpirome or ceftazidime in combination with aminoglycosides against *Pseudomonas aeruginosa*. *J Antimicrob Chemother* 1990;25:575.
23. Lorian V, Finland M. In vivo effect of rifampin on mycobacteria. *Appl Microbiol* 1969;17:202.
24. Rynearson TK, Shronts JS, Wolinsky E. Rifampin: in vitro effect on atypical mycobacteria. *Am Rev Respir Dis* 1971;104:272.
25. Heifets LB, Lindholm-Levy PJ, Iseman MD. Rifabutine: minimal inhibitory and bactericidal concentrations for *Mycobacterium tuberculosis*. *Am Rev Respir Dis* 1988;137:719.
26. Cynamon MH. Comparative in vitro activities of MDL 473, rifampin, and

Ansamycin against *Mycobacterium intracellulare*. *Antimicrob Agents Chemother* 1985;28:440.

27. Rees RJW. Rifampicin: the investigation of a bactericidal antileprosy drug. *Lepr Rev* 1975;46[Suppl 1]:121.

28. Schachter J. Rifampin in chlamydial infections. *Rev Infect Dis* 1983;5[Suppl 3]:S562.

29. Yeaman MR, Mitscher LA, Baca OG. In vitro susceptibility of *Coxiella burnetti* to antibiotics including several quinolones. *Antimicrob Agents Chemother* 1987;31:1079.

30. Pukrittayakamee S, Viravan C, Charoenlarp P, et al. Antimalarial effects of rifampin in *Plasmodium vivax* malaria. *Antimicrob Agents Chemother* 1994;38:511.

31. Medoff G. Antifungal action of rifampin. *Rev Infect Dis* 1983;5[Suppl 3]:S614.

32. Wehrli W. Rifampin: mechanisms of action and resistance. *Rev Infect Dis* 1983;5[Suppl 3]:S407.

33. Garcia L, Alonzo-Sanz M, Rebello MJ, et al. Mutations in the rpoB gene of rifampin-resistant *Mycobacterium tuberculosis* in Spain and their rapid detection by PCR-enzyme-linked immunosorbent assay. *J Clin Microbiol* 2001; 39:1813.

34. Bloch AB, Cauthen GM, Onorato IM, et al. Nationwide survey of drug-resistant tuberculosis in the United States. *JAMA* 1994;271:665.

35. Simon GL, Smith RH, Sande MA. Emergence of rifampin-resistant strains of *Staphylococcus aureus* during combination therapy with vancomycin and rifampin: a report of two cases. *Rev Infect Dis* 1983;5[Suppl 3]:S507.

36. Eng RHK, Smith SM, Buccini FJ, et al. Differences in ability of cell-wall antibiotics to suppress emergence of rifampicin resistance in *Staphylococcus aureus*. *J Antimicrob Chemother* 1985;15:201.

37. Acocella G. Clinical pharmacokinetics of rifampicin. *Clin Pharmacokinet* 1978; 3:108.

38. Kenny MT, Strates B. Metabolism and pharmacokinetics of the antibiotic rifampin. *Drug Metab Rev* 1981;12:159.

39. Archer GL, Armstrong BC, Kline BJ. Rifampin blood and tissue levels in patients undergoing cardiac valve surgery. *Antimicrob Agents Chemother* 1982;21:800.

40. Sahai J, Gallicanto K, Swick L, et al. Reduced plasma concentrations of antituberculous drugs in patients with HIV infections. *Ann Intern Med* 1997;127:289.

41. Acocella G, Bonollo L, Garimoldi M, et al. Kinetics of rifampicin and isoniazid administered alone and in combination to normal subjects and patients with liver disease. *Gut* 1972;13:47.

42. Koup JR, Williams-Warren J, Weber A, et al. Pharmacokinetics of rifampin in children. I. Multiple dose intravenous infusion. *Ther Drug Monit* 1986;8:11.

43. Advenier C, Gobert C, Houin G, et al. Pharmacokinetic studies of rifampicin in the elderly. *Ther Drug Monit* 1983;5:61.

44. Solberg CO, Halstensen A, Digranes A, et al. Penetration of antibiotics into human leukocytes and dermal suction blisters. *Rev Infect Dis* 1983;5[Suppl 3]:S468.

45. Nahata MC, Fan-Havard P, Barson WJ, et al. Pharmacokinetics, cerebrospinal fluid concentration, and safety of intravenous rifampin in pediatric patients undergoing shunt placements. *Eur J Clin Pharmacol* 1990;38:515.

46. Nau R, Prange HW, Menck S, et al. Penetration of rifampicin into the cerebrospinal fluid of adults with uninflamed meninges. *J Antimicrob Chemother* 1992;29:719.

47. D'Oliveira JJG. Cerebrospinal fluid concentrations of rifampin in meningeal tuberculosis. *Am Rev Respir Dis* 1972;106:432.

48. Outman WR, Levitz RE, Hill DA, et al. Intraocular penetration of rifampin in humans. *Antimicrob Agents Chemother* 1992;36:1575.

49. Mandell GL, Vest TK. Killing of intraleukocytic *Staphylococcus aureus* by rifampin: in vitro and in vivo studies. *Rev Infect Dis* 1983;5[Suppl 3]:S463.

50. Krukenberg CC, Mischler PG, Massad EN, et al. Stability of 1% rifampin suspensions prepared in five syrups. *Am J Hosp Pharm* 1986;43:2225.

51. British Thoracic and Tuberculosis Association. Short-course chemotherapy in pulmonary tuberculosis: a controlled trial by the British Thoracic and Tuberculosis Association. *Lancet* 1976;2:1102.

52. British Thoracic Association. A controlled trial of six months chemotherapy in pulmonary tuberculosis. Second report: results during the 24 months after the end of chemotherapy. *Am Rev Respir Dis* 1982;126:460.

53. American Thoracic Society. Treatment of tuberculosis and tuberculosis infection in adults and children. *Am J Respir Crit Care Med* 1994;149:1359.

54. Polesky A, Farber HW, Gottlieb DJ, et al. Rifampin preventive therapy for tuberculosis in Boston's homeless. *Am J Respir Crit Care Med* 1996;154:1473.

55. American Thoracic Society and Centers for Disease Control and Prevention. Targeted tuberculin testing and treatment of latent tuberculosis infection. *Am J Respir Crit Care Med* 2000;161:S221.

56. Alm CH, Lowell JR, Ahn SS, et al. Chemotherapy for pulmonary disease due to *Mycobacterium kansasii*: efficacies of some individual drugs. *Rev Infect Dis* 1981;3:1028.

57. Donta ST, Smith PW, Levitz RE, et al. Therapy of *Mycobacterium marinum* infections. *Arch Intern Med* 1986;146:902.

58. Bogaerts Y, Elinck W, van Renterghem D, et al. Pulmonary disease due to *Mycobacterium xenopi*: report of two cases. *Eur J Respir Dis* 1982;63:298.

59. Kemper CA, Meng TC, Nussbaum J, et al. Treatment of *Mycobacterium avium* complex bacteremia in AIDS with a four-drug oral regimen: rifampin, ethambutol, clofazimine, and ciprofloxacin. *Ann Intern Med* 1992;116:466.

60. Jacobson MA, Yajko D, Northfelt D, et al. Randomized, placebo controlled trial of rifampin, ethambutol, and ciprofloxacin for AIDS patients with disseminated *Mycobacterium avium* complex infection. *Ann Intern Med* 1993;168:112.

61. Research Committee of the British Thoracic Society. First randomized trial of treatments for pulmonary disease caused by *M. avium intracellulare, M. malmoense*, and *M. xenopi* in HIV negative patients: rifampicin, ethambutol and isoniazid versus rifampicin and ethambutol. *Thorax* 2001;56:167.

62. Gilbody JS. Impact of multidrug therapy on the treatment and control of leprosy. *Int J Leprosy* 1991;59:458.

63. Beam WE Jr, Newberg NR, Devine LF, et al. The effect of rifampin on the nasopharyngeal carriage of *Neisseria meningitidis* in a military population. *J Infect Dis* 1971;124:39.

64. Schwartz B, Al-Tobaiqi A, Al-Ruwais A, et al. Comparative efficacy of ceftriaxone and rifampin in eradicating pharyngeal carriage of group A *Neisseria meningitidis*. *Lancet* 1988;1:1239.

65. Green M, Li KI, Wald ER, et al. Duration of rifampin chemoprophylaxis for contacts of patients infected with *Haemophilus influenzae* type B. *Antimicrob Agents Chemother* 1992;36:545.

66. Tanz RR, Shulman ST, Barthel MJ, et al. Penicillin plus rifampin eradicates pharyngeal carriage of group A streptococci. *J Pediatr* 1985;106:876.

67. Wheat LJ, Kohler RB, White AL, et al. Effect of rifampin on nasal carriage of coagulase-positive staphylococci. *J Infect Dis* 1981;144:177.

68. McAnally TP, Lewis MR, Brown DR. Effect of rifampin and bacitracin on nasal carriage of *Staphylococcus aureus*. *Antimicrob Agents Chemother* 1984;25:422.

69. Yu VL, Goetz A, Wagener M, et al. *Staphylococcus aureus* nasal carriage and infection in patients on hemodialysis: efficacy of antibiotic prophylaxis. *N Engl J Med* 1986;315:91.

70. Zimmerman SW, Ahrens E, Johnson CA, et al. Randomized, controlled trial of prophylactic rifampin for peritoneal dialysis catheter-related infections and peritonitis. *Kidney Int* 1990;37:335.

71. Roccaforte JS, Bittner MJ, Stumpf LA, et al. Attempts to eradicate methicillin-resistant *Staphylococcus aureus* colonization with the use of trimethoprim-sulfamethoxazole, rifampin, and bacitracin. *Am J Infect Control* 1988;16:141.

72. Darouiche R, Wright C, Hamill R, et al. Eradication of colonization by methicillin-resistant *Staphylococcus aureus* by using oral minocycline-rifampin and topical mupirocin. *Antimicrob Agents Chemother* 1991;35:1612.

73. Acar JF, Goldstein FW, Duval J. Use of rifampin for the treatment of serious staphylococcal and gram-negative bacillary infections. *Rev Infect Dis* 1983;5[Suppl 3]:502.

74. Van Der Auwera P, Meunier-Carpentier F, Klatersky J. Clinical study of combination therapy with oxacillin and rifampin for staphylococcal infections. *Rev Infect Dis* 1983;5[Suppl 3]:S515.

75. Faville RJ, Zaske DE, Kaplan EL, et al. *Staphylococcus aureus* endocarditis: combined therapy with vancomycin and rifampin. *JAMA* 1978;240:1963.

76. Watanakunakorn C, Tisone JC. Antagonism between nafcillin or oxacillin and rifampin against *Staphylococcus aureus*. *Antimicrob Agents Chemother* 1982;22:920.

77. Zak O, Scheld WM, Sande MA. Rifampin in experimental endocarditis due to *Staphylococcus aureus* in rabbits. *J Infect Dis* 1983;5[Suppl 3]:S481.

78. Van der Auwera P, Klastersky J, Thys JP, et al. Double-blind, placebo-controlled study of oxacillin combined with rifampin in the treatment of staphylococcal infections. *Antimicrob Agents Chemother* 1985;28:467.

79. Dworkin RJ, Lee BL, Sande MA, et al. Treatment of right-sided *Staphylococcus aureus* endocarditis in intravenous drug users with ciprofloxacin and rifampicin. *Lancet* 1989;2:1071.

80. Heldman AW, Hartert TV, Ray SC, et al. Oral antibiotic treatment of right-sided staphylococcal endocarditis in injection drug users: prospective randomized comparison with parenteral therapy. *Am J Med* 1996;101:68.

81. Karchmer AW, Archer GA. *Methicillin-resistant* Staphylococcus epidermidis (SE) prosthetic valve (PV) endocarditis (E): a therapeutic trial. In: Program and Abstracts of the 24th Interscience Conference on Antimicrobial Agents and Chemotherapy, October 8–10, 1984. Abstract 476.

82. Norden CW. Experimental chronic staphylococcal osteomyelitis in rabbits: treatment with rifampin alone and in combination with other antimicrobial agents. *Rev Infect Dis* 1983;5[Suppl 3]:S491.

83. Norden CW, Bryant R, Palmer D, et al. Chronic osteomyelitis caused by *Staphylococcus aureus*: controlled clinical trial of nafcillin therapy and nafcillin-rifampin therapy. *South Med J* 1986;79:947.

84. Widmer AF, Gaechter A, Ochsner PE, et al. Antimicrobial treatment of orthopedic implant-related infections with rifampin combinations. *Clin Infect Dis* 1992;14:1251.

85. Ariza J, Gudiol F, Pallares R, et al. Treatment of human brucellosis with doxycycline plus rifampin or doxycycline plus streptomycin: a randomized, double-blind study. *Ann Intern Med* 1992;117:25.

86. Akova M, Uzum O, Akalin HE, et al. Quinolones in treatment of brucellosis: comparative trial of ofloxacin-rifampin versus doxycycline-rifampin. *Antimicrob Agents Chemother* 1993;37:1831.

87. Jacobs F, Abramowicz D, Vereerstraeten P, et al. *Brucella* endocarditis: the role of combined medical and surgical treatment. *Rev Infect Dis* 1990;12:740.

88. Catalan MJ, Fernandez JM, Varquez A, et al. Failure of cefotaxime in the treatment of meningitis due to relatively resistant *Streptococcus pneumoniae*. *Clin Infect Dis* 1994;18:766.

89. Yu VL, Zuravleff JJ, Peacock JE, et al. Addition of rifampin to carboxypenicillin-aminoglycoside combination for the treatment of *Pseudomonas aeruginosa* infection: clinical experience with four patients. *Antimicrob Agents Chemother* 1984;26:575.

90. Korvick JA, Peacock JE Jr, Muder RR, et al. Addition of rifampin to combination antibiotic therapy for *Pseudomonas aeruginosa* bacteremia: prospective trial using the Zelen protocol. *Antimicrob Agents Chemother* 1992;36:620.

91. Morris AB, Brown RB, Sands M. Use of rifampin in nonstaphylococcal, non-mycobacterial disease. *Antimicrob Agents Chemother* 1993;37:1.

92. Plummer PA, Nsanze H, D'Costa LJ, et al. Short-course and single-dose antimicrobial therapy for chancroid in Kenya: studies with rifampin alone and in combination with trimethoprim. *Rev Infect Dis* 1983;5[Suppl 3]:565.

93. Bella F, Espejo E, Uriz S, et al. Randomized 5-day rifampin versus 1-day doxycycline therapy in Mediterranean spotted fever. *J Infect Dis* 1991;164:433.

94. Espey DK, Djomand G, Diomande I, et al. A pilot study of treatment with Buruli ulcer with rifampin and dapsone. *Int J Infect Dis* 2002;6:60.

95. Maguina C, Garcia PJ, Gotuzzo E, et al. Bartonellosis (Carrion's disease) in the modern era. *Clin Infect Dis* 2001;33:772.

96. Levy PY, Drancourt M, Etienne J, et al. Comparison of different antibiotic regimens for therapy of 32 cases of Q fever endocarditis. *Antimicrob Agents Chemother* 1991;35:533.

97. Band JD, Fraser DW. Adverse effects of two rifampicin dosage regimens for the prevention of meningococcal infection. *Lancet* 1984;1:101.

98. Girlin DJ. Adverse reactions to rifampicin in antituberculosis regimens. *J Antimicrob Chemother* 1977;3:115.

99. Van Assendelft AHW. Leucopenia in rifampicin chemotherapy. *J Antimicrob Chemother* 1985;16:407.

100. Grosset J, Leventis S. Adverse effects of rifampin. *Rev Infect Dis* 1983;5[Suppl 3]:5440.

101. Jasmer RM, Saukkonen JJ, Blumberg HM, et al. Short-course rifampin and pyrazinamide compared with isoniazid for latent tuberculosis infection: a multicenter clinical trial. *Ann Intern Med* 2002;137:640.

102. Soffer O, Nassar VH, Campbell WG Jr. Light chain cast nephropathy and acute renal failure associated with rifampin therapy. *Am J Med* 1987;82:1052.

103. Humber DP, Nsanzumuhire H, Aluoch HA, et al. Controlled double-blind study of the effect of rifampin on humoral and cellular immune responses in patients with pulmonary tuberculosis and in tuberculosis contacts. *Am Rev Respir Dis* 1980;122:425.

104. Finch CK, Christman CR, Baciewicz AM, et al. Rifampin and rifabutin drug interactions: an update. *Arch Intern Med* 2002;162:985.

105. Venkatesan K. Pharmacokinetic drug interactions with rifampicin. *Clin Pharmacokinet* 1992;22:47.

106. Burger DM, Meenhorst PL, Koks CHW, et al. Pharmacokinetic interaction between rifampin and zidovudine. *Antimicrob Agents Chemother* 1993;37:1426.

107. Colmenero JD, Fernandez-Gallardo LC, Agundez JAG, et al. Possible implications of doxycycline-rifampin interaction for treatment of brucellosis. *Antimicrob Agents Chemother* 1994;38:2798.

108. Wallace RJ Jr, Brown BA, Griffith DE, et al. Reduced serum levels of clarithromycin in patients treated with multidrug regimens including rifampin or rifabutin for *Mycobacterium avium-M. intracellulare* infection. *J Infect Dis* 1995;171:747.

109. Heifets LB, Iseman MD. Determination of in vitro susceptibility of mycobacteria to Ansamycin. *Am Rev Respir Dis* 1985;132:710.

110. Heifets LB, Iseman MD, Lindholm-Levy PJ, et al. Determination of Ansamycin MICs for *Mycobacterium avium* complex in liquid medium by radiometric and conventional methods. *Antimicrob Agents Chemother* 1985;28:570.

111. Nightingale SD, Cameron DW, Gordin FM, et al. Two controlled trials of rifabutin prophylaxis against *Mycobacterium avium* complex infection in AIDS. *N Engl J Med* 1993;329:828.

112. U.S. Public Health Service Task Force on Prophylaxis and Therapy for *Mycobacterium avium* Complex. Recommendations on prophylaxis and therapy for disseminated *Mycobacterium avium* complex for adults and adolescents infected with human immunodeficiency virus. *MMWR Morb Mortal Wkly Rep* 1993;42(RR-9):14.

113. Agins BD, Berman DS, Spicehandler D, et al. Effect of combined therapy with Ansamycin, clofazimine, ethambutol, and isoniazid for *Mycobacterium avium* infection in patients with AIDS. *J Infect Dis* 1989;159:784.

114. Hoy J, Mijch A, Sandland M, et al. Quadruple-drug therapy for *Mycobacterium avium-intracellulare* bacteremia in AIDS patients. *J Infect Dis* 1990;161:801.

115. Sullam PM, Gordin FM, Wynne BA, et al. Efficacy of rifabutin in the treatment of disseminated infection due to *Mycobacterium avium* complex. *Clin Infect Dis* 1994;19:84.

116. Skinner MH, Hsieh M, Torseth J, et al. Pharmacokinetics of rifabutin. *Antimicrob Agents Chemother* 1989;33:1237.

117. Narang PK, Lewis RC, Bianchine JR. Rifabutin absorption in humans: relative bioavailability and food effect. *Clin Pharmacol Ther* 1992;52:335.

118. Battaglia R, Pianezzola E, Salgarollo G, et al. Absorption, disposition and preliminary metabolic pathway of ^{14}C-rifabutin in animals and man. *J Antimicrob Chemother* 1990;26:813.

119. Brogden RN, Fitton A. Rifabutin: a review of its antimicrobial activity, pharmacokinetic properties and therapeutic efficacy. *Drugs* 1994;47:983.

120. Havlir D, Torriani F, Dube M. Uveitis associated with rifabutin prophylaxis. *Ann Intern Med* 1994;121:510.

121. Siegel FP, Eilbott D, Burger H, et al. Dose-limiting toxicity of rifabutin in AIDS-related complex: syndrome of arthralgia/arthritis. *AIDS* 1990;4:433.

122. Perucca E, Grimaldi R, Frigo GM, et al. Comparative effects of rifabutin and rifampicin on hepatic microsomal enzyme activity in normal subjects. *Eur J Clin Pharmacol* 1988;34:595.

123. Gallicano K, Sahai J, Swick L, et al. Effect of rifabutin on the pharmacokinetics of zidovudine in patients infected with human immunodeficiency virus. *Clin Infect Dis* 1995;21:1008.

124. Centers for Disease Control and Prevention. Updated guidelines for the use of rifabutin or rifampin for the treatment and prevention of tuberculosis among HIV-infected patients taking protease inhibitors or nonnucleoside reverse transcriptase inhibitors. *MMWR Morb Mortal Wkly Rep* 2000;49:185.

125. Griffith DE, Brown BA, Girard WM, et al. Adverse events associated with high-dose rifabutin in macrolide-containing regimens for the treatment of *Mycobacterium avium* complex lung disease. *Clin Infect Dis* 1995;21:594.

126. Keung AC-F, Owens RC Jr, Eller MG, et al. Pharmacokinetics of rifapentine in subjects seropositive for the human immunodeficiency virus: a phase I study. *Antimicrob Agents Chemother* 1999;43:1230.

127. Keung A, Eller MC, McKenzie KA, et al. Single and multiple dose pharmacokinetics of rifapentine in man: part II. *Int J Tuberculosis Lung Dis* 1999;3:437.

128. Benator D, Bhattacharya M, Bozeman L, et al. Rifapentine and isoniazid once a week versus rifapicin and isoniazid twice a week for treatment of drug-susceptible pulmonary tuberculosis in HIV-negative patients: a randomized clinical trial. *Lancet* 2002;360:528.

129. Vernon A, Burman W, Benator D, et al. Acquired rifamycin monoresistance in patients with HIV-related tuberculosis treated with once-weekly rifapentine and isoniazid. *Lancet* 1999;353:1843.

130. Gillis JC, Brogden RN. Rifaximin: a review of its antibacterial activity, pharmacokinetic properties and therapeutic potential in conditions mediated by gastrointestinal bacteria. *Drugs* 1995;49:467.

131. Luna-Herrera J, Reddy MV, Gangadharam PRJ. In vitro activity of the benzoxazinorifamycin KRM-1648 against drug-susceptible and multidrug-resistant tubercle bacilli. *Antimicrob Agents Chemother* 1995;39:440.

132. Moghazeh SL, Pan X, Arain T, et al. Comparative antimycobacterial activities of rifampin, rifapentine, and KRM-1648 against a collection of rifampin-resistant *Mycobacterium tuberculosis* isolates with known *rpoB* mutations. *Antimicrob Agents Chemother* 1996;40:2655.

CHAPTER 30
Miscellaneous Drugs

Burt R. Meyers, Fernando Borrego, and Alejandra C. Gurtman

POLYMYXIN B/COLISTIN

The polymyxins are a group of polypeptide antibiotics isolated from a soil bacillus (*Bacillus polymyxa*); a number of these compounds (A, B, C, D, E) are isolated from different strains of the bacillus. Colistin, produced by *Bacillus colistinus*, was originally thought to be different but was soon found to be identical to polymyxin E. All of these drugs have molecular weights of approximately 1,000 kDa. Of the five polymyxins, only two are currently in clinical use: polymyxins B and E (colistin).

Mode of Action and Antibiotic Activity

All the polymyxins act on bacterial membranes, interacting with phospholipids; their lipophobic groups disrupt the membranes, changing their permeability. Polymyxins act like cationic detergents that bind to the lipids of the bacterial cytoplasmic membrane and cause damage that results in alteration of the osmotic barrier of the membrane and causes leakage of essential intracellular metabolites and nucleosides. Antibiotic sensitivity of these compounds is probably related to the phospholipid content of the cell wall. Damage to this structure breaks the osmotic barrier and leads to a leaking of intracellular materials and perhaps allows entry of other agents. Toxic effects due to this binding have been postulated (1). Binding to phospholipids may explain some of the biologic activity of polymyxin B, which has been found to block the biologic effect of endotoxin lipopolysaccharide (LPS). Polymyxin B inhibits pyrogenicity from LPS (2) and

LPS-induced interleukin-1 release by monocytes (3). It also inhibits the endotoxin effect of decreasing natural killer cell activity in burn patients (4). Mortality in experimentally induced endotoxemia in animals was reduced. Polymyxin B also protected against gram-negative septicemia (5–8). It was demonstrated in an *Escherichia coli* sepsis rabbit model that polymyxin B moderated acidosis and decreased hypotension compared with control subjects, whereas corticosteroids and antibodies to LPS failed (9). Polymyxin B also prevents LPS release of tumor necrosis factor-α from alveolar macrophages (10). Further studies have shown that incubation of polymyxin B with LPS inhibits the tumoricidal action of these macrophages (11). Polymyxin B decreases endotoxin concentrations in experimental animals with meningitis due to *E. coli* after treatment with antibiotics (12).

Antibacterial Activity

Both polymyxin B and colistin are active against gram-negative organisms, including *E. coli*, *Klebsiella* spp., *Enterobacter* spp., *Salmonella* spp., *Shigella* spp., and *Pseudomonas aeruginosa*. In vitro, polymyxin B is more active than colistin against *P. aeruginosa* (13–15). Minimal inhibitory concentrations (MICs) vary between 0.02 and 2.0 μg/mL; the MICs for *P. aeruginosa* are somewhat higher. Species of *Pseudomonas* other than *P. aeruginosa* (i.e., *B. cepacia*, *S. maltophilia*, and so forth) are usually resistant. These agents have less activity against *Serratia marcescens* and are inactive against *Proteus* spp. Other sensitive gram-negative bacteria include *Haemophilus influenzae*, *Bordetella pertussis*, *Neisseria meningitidis*, *Neisseria gonorrhoeae*, *Brucella* spp., and cholera strains excluding *Vibrio cholerae* (biotype *eltor*). Although some strains of *Bacteroides* spp. and *Fusobacterium* spp. are sensitive, *Bacteroides fragilis* is resistant. All gram-positive organisms are resistant. Bacterial resistance of previously sensitive organisms is not commonly acquired. There is cross-resistance between polymyxin B and colistin for all strains, but there is no cross-resistance with other antimicrobial agents, and resistance rarely develops during treatment (16). Resistance is most likely due to decreased permeability across the outer membrane (17). In vitro synergy has been demonstrated with sulfa compounds for resistant strains of *P. aeruginosa*, *Proteus* spp., and *S. marcescens*. Synergy with trimethoprim and polymyxin B has been demonstrated in vitro for *Serratia* spp. Combinations of sulfamethoxazole, trimethoprim, and colistin have also demonstrated synergy. (18,19) Colistin has also shown *in vitro* activity against the highly resistant (e.g., imipenem-resistant) *Acinetobacter baumannii* (19a).

In vitro, polymyxin B may affect the cell membranes of certain fungi, increasing permeability to tetracycline with inhibition of the growth (20). Other studies have shown polymyxin B to enhance amphotericin B activity against *Coccidioides immitis* (21). Synergy with bacitracin and miconazole and polymyxin B against *Staphylococcus aureus* and *Staphylococcus epidermidis* suggests that entry of these agents occurs because of membrane perturbation (1). Colistin has activity against strains of *Mycobacterium* including *M. tuberculosis*, *M. intracellulare*, *M. xenopi*, and *M. fortuitum* (15, 23).

The antibacterial effect of the polymyxins can be prevented by the divalent cations magnesium and calcium and by ethylenediaminetetraacetic acid (24); they stabilize membranes, preventing polymyxin B from competitively displacing these ions on negatively charged phosphate groups on membrane lipids. This may be clinically significant because physiologic concentrations of calcium affect polymyxin, suggesting less activity *in vivo* than could be predicted by susceptibility *in vitro* (25). Polymyxin B exerts an anti-insulin effect (26); it is a protein kinase C inhibitor, and this has the effect on glucose metabolism of decreasing glucose-stimulated insulin secretion (27–29).

Pharmacokinetics

Polymyxin B and colistin are not absorbed when given orally. After intramuscular injection of polymyxin B, peak serum levels of 2 to 8 μg/mL are observed. The half-life ($t_{1/2}$) in serum is 6 hours (30,31). Serum levels decline slowly during 8 to 12 hours. Accumulation has been reported in patients given 2.5 mg/kg per day, with peak levels reported 7 days later of 15 μg/mL. When colistin methane sulfonate (polymyxin E) is given intramuscularly at a dose of 2.5 mg/kg to adults, peak serum levels of 5 to 7 μg/mL occur between 1 and 2 hours; the $t_{1/2}$ is 1.6 to 2.7 hours. Drug accumulation was found, with peak levels of 12 μg/mL. When given intravenously by bolus and then by slow infusion, serum levels of 5 to 6 μg/mL are maintained. Excretion of polymyxin B is mainly renal via glomerular filtration, although only a small amount of polymyxin B is recovered in the first 12 hours; 60% of the injected dose of polymyxin B sulfate can be found in the urine for days. Urinary concentration varies between 20 and 100 μg/mL after parenteral therapy. Colistin is excreted more rapidly by the kidney, with 40% excretion in the first 8 hours; a high fluid intake decreases urinary concentrations to 20 μg/mL (33) from the usual level of 200 μg/mL. In the presence of renal insufficiency, the $t_{1/2}$ is 48 to 72 hours (30,34). Polymyxins are not found in the biliary tract and do not enter the cerebrospinal fluid even in the presence of inflammation.

Others have found a shorter $t_{1/2}$ (35). In animals, the drug is distributed to liver, kidney, brain, heart, muscle, and lung, and persists up to 72 hours after a single injection. Protein binding is low with both of these compounds. The exact method of inactivation is not known.

Administration and Dosage

Both agents can be given by the intramuscular and intravenous routes. The usual dose of polymyxin is 15,000 to 25,000 units/kg per day (1.5 to 2.5 mg/kg per day) (1 mg polymyxin B = 10,000 units). The intramuscular dose of polymyxin B is 2.5 to 5 mg/kg per day every 4 or 6 hours. In patients with normal renal function, the usual intravenous dosage of polymyxin is 50 mg/500 mL infused during 8 hours (not to exceed 25,000 units/kg per day). The same dose can be added to 100 mL and infused during 30 minutes; rapid intravenous injection should be avoided. For colistimethate, the intramuscular and intravenous dosage is 2.5 to 5.0 mg/kg per day in two to four divided doses; the higher dosage is reserved for severe infections. Because both these agents accumulate in renal failure, the doses should be modified. (31,35–39) Regimens include giving the standard dose 150 mg polymyxin B or 120 mg colistin at adjusted intervals according to renal function (37). Colistin at 2 to 3 mg/kg may be given after each session of hemodialysis (40).

Polymyxin B can be administered intrathecally. The usual dosage for adults is 5 to 10 mg given daily for 3 days and then on alternate days. Treatment is continued for at least 3 days after the cerebrospinal fluid is sterile, usually more than 2 weeks. The dosage in children younger than 2 years of age is 2.0 mg daily for 3 or 4 days, then 2.5 mg every other day. This drug should be delivered in sterile saline (not procaine) to obviate toxic effects. Polymyxin B can be given orally in doses of 100 to 200 mg, three or four times daily. A dose of 800 mg daily has been used for intestinal decontamination in patients with leukemia or to prevent infection in the intensive care unit (41). Colistin sulfate can be administered orally at a dosage of 5 to 15 mg/kg per day in three equally divided doses, but the oral preparation is no longer available in the United States.

Adverse Effects

Nephrotoxicity is commonly seen with polymyxin B and, less frequently, with colistin; this may be because methane sulfonate is used and believed to be less toxic than the sulfate derivative used in polymyxin E. Toxicity is manifested by proteinuria, hematuria, and casts. Renal dysfunction is manifested by an elevated serum creatinine level. Nephrotoxicity is usually noted in the first few days of therapy but may be found after the drug is stopped. In one study, nephrotoxicity occurred in 20% of patients (42); oliguric renal failure and tubular necrosis were reported, although usually at higher dosages. These agents are poorly dialyzed during hemodialysis; colistin is only partially cleared by peritoneal dialysis (43). Great caution is necessary when these drugs are used in the presence of renal dysfunction. Serum levels reach high concentrations and may further increase nephrotoxicity. Administration with cephalothin increases toxicity.

Numbness, paresthesias (often perioral), peripheral neuropathy, slurred speech, dyphasia, and ataxia have been noted, usually in the first 4 days. More serious events, including psychosis, convulsions, coma, and ataxia, may occur. Facial flushing and dizziness are more commonly seen in those with renal insufficiency.

Neuromuscular blockade manifested as respiratory paralysis may occur, even after the first dose of either drug; it is more common in renal failure with high serum concentrations. Restlessness and dyspnea may be the first signs. In most cases, other factors—including anesthesia, sedation, hypoxia, and hypocalcemia—are noted. The neuromuscular blockade is different than that seen with aminoglycosides, which can be reversed by neostigmine. However, with polymyxin B, a noncompetitive blockade occurs that is not reversible by drugs. Treatment requires support of respiratory function usually for 24 hours until the drug has dissipated. Because aminoglycosides may interfere with nerve conduction, they should not usually be administered concomitantly.

After oral administration, nausea, vomiting, and diarrhea often occur. The polymyxins are not absorbed through denuded skin, and side effects are rarely noted with topical administration. Hypersensitivities such as rash and pruritus are found infrequently.

Clinical Applications

Polymyxin B and colistin should be considered only as second-line drugs in the treatment of gram-negative infections, unless treating highly resistant organisms. Experimental P. aeruginosa infection in animals revealed that other agents such as gentamicin and tobramycin were more effective and less toxic than colistin and polymyxin B (44). Polymyxin B and colistin have been used in the past to treat infections caused by P. aeruginosa, including bacteremia, pneumonia, burns, meningitis, and urinary tract infections (14,43). In the early 1960s, Pseudomonas septicemia was treated with polymyxin (45). Other infections treated included Pseudomonas meningitis, in which the agents were used parenterally and intrathecally, and infected burns, in which the agents were used both parenterally and topically. Polymyxin B has been used parenterally in the treatment of pulmonary infections with some success and was effective in six of seven patients with septicemia (43). It has also been aerosolized and given prophylactically into the respiratory tract for critically ill patients in an attempt to prevent pneumonia due to P. aeruginosa; in this study, however, pneumonia developed with polymyxin B–resistant organisms (i.e., S. maltophilia and B. cepacia) (46). Investigators have attempted to prevent colonization and subsequent respiratory tract infections with local antimicrobial prophylaxis. This prophylaxis consisted of polymyxin B administered orally, either alone or in combination with gentamicin, parenteral cefotaxime, nalidixic acid, and neomycin. Colistin has been substituted for polymyxin B with these agents (47–49). Intestinal decontamination has been used to control nosocomial infections with multidrug-resistant gram-negative bacilli (50). When polymyxin B and gentamicin were administered as a paste to the nose or oral pharynx and orally in patients in an intensive care unit, there were decreased colonization of the oral pharynx and trachea and decreased cases of pneumonia compared with control patients (51). Emergence of bacterial resistance was studied in a surgical intensive care unit in patients receiving parenteral cefotaxime and oral polymyxin during a 30-month period. There was an 8% increase in strains of Proteus and Morganella spp.; 10% of the patients were colonized by cefotaxime-resistant strains, which were eliminated with the nonabsorbable oral therapy (52).

In one study, 600 mg daily of polymyxin B orally or intravenously suppressed intestinal microflora but was associated in half the volunteers with severe gastrointestinal side effects (53). Polymyxin B and colistin have been used orally as prophylaxis of infection of leukopenic patients. These agents have been combined with neomycin, gentamicin, trimethoprim-sulfamethoxazole, ofloxacin, and nalidixic acid (54–60); in some cases, however, candidal overgrowth was seen when amphotericin B was not included. When used alone, the dose of polymyxin for decontamination was 800 mg daily (41). Polymyxin B is moderately inactivated by food and feces (28). So in combination with tobramycin, inactivation of polymyxin was reduced; the dose could be decreased to 400 mg daily to prevent infection in trauma patients.

In a prospective but nonblinded or controlled study using polymixin B lozenges at 2 mg, tobramycin at 1.8 mg, and amphotericin B at 10 mg four times daily to patients undergoing radiation therapy for head and neck cancer, the incidence of mucositis was decreased compared with historical control subjects. Colonization by gram-negative bacilli was decreased, and no oral fungal infections occurred (61). Polymyxin B may offer an alternative for the treatment of infections due to gram-negative bacilli that are resistant to commonly used antibiotics; ceftazidime-resistant Klebsiella pneumoniae, Enterobacter spp., and P. aeruginosa infections have been treated successfully. It has been combined with rifampin to treat resistant S. marcescens infection and with trimethoprim-sulfamethoxazole to treat infections with P. cepacia and S. marcescens. Urinary tract infections caused by P. aeruginosa have been treated with these agents; colistin may be a better choice of therapy because higher urinary concentrations are more rapidly obtained than with polymyxin B.

In patients with central nervous system infections, polymyxin B may have a role in the treatment of multidrug resistant gram-negative bacilli, including P. aeruginosa; because levels are not obtained after systemic administration, intrathecal therapy is required. A patient has been treated successfully with colistin and piperacillin (62).

Colistin has been combined with trimethoprim-sulfamethoxazole for the prevention of infection in patients with acute nonlymphocytic leukemia. The authors concluded that combination therapy was better than trimethoprim-sulfamethoxazole alone (60). In another study, polymyxin was included in a regimen of oral nonabsorbable antibiotics used to prevent infection in cirrhotic patients with gastrointestinal hemorrhage; infections with enteric bacteria occurred less frequently in patients given this prophylaxis (63). It has also been suggested that polymyxin B be studied as adjuvant therapy for severe gram-negative infection (9). Although it has been demonstrated that serum endotoxin levels are increased in patients with obstructive jaundice, polymyxin B had no effect on endotoxemia and outcome after operation to relieve jaundice (64). Others have recommended that this agent be used as preoperative bowel decontamination to prevent infection after orthotopic liver transplantation (65).

Polymyxin B sulfate has been prepared for topical and ophthalmic use, usually in combination with other compounds such as neomycin and bacitracin. These preparations include creams, ointments, drops, and sprays. When these drugs are used topically, bacterial resistance and allergic reactions are uncommon. Absorption through denuded burn surfaces and mucous membranes is poor; thus, infections of the external ear canal, skin, eyes, and mucous membranes are often treated with these agents. Corneal ulcers caused by *P. aeruginosa* have been treated both topically and with subconjunctival injection of polymyxin B; the mupirocin-polymyxin B combination was effective in treating keratitis with *P. aeruginosa*, *S. aureus* and *Serratia* (65a); the drug has been used topically in the eye to treat *Acanthamoeba* spp. infections associated with contact lens wear (66).

Colistin sulfate (Coly-Mycin) has been used to treat diarrheal infections in infants and children caused by susceptible strains of enteropathogenic *E. coli*; the usual dosage is 5 to 15 mg/kg per day in three divided doses. Others believe that these agents are of no clinical efficacy for treating gastroenteritis caused by gram-negative bacilli (67,68).

Future Use of Polymyxin

The association of circulating endotoxin with the development of adult respiratory distress syndrome and sepsis (particularly gram-negative septic shock) has been demonstrated and it is actively investigated (69,69a). Polymyxin B obviates the effects of endotoxin, as demonstrated in multiple models that use more selective absorption techniques (e.g., apheresis, direct hemoperfusion), by blocking the effect of cytokines that are liberated from cellular elements and suppressing of further secretion of those cytokines. This is achieved by using polymyxin as an absorbent, lowering the concentration of toxins and cytokines in the blood through plasma filtration, and effectively reducing mortality by improving hyperdynamic circulation. Other techniques, such as nonselective plasma exchange, which mixes centrifugation and plasma replacement, had shown encouraging results further lowering mortality, and their role in these clinical situations (e.g., adult respiratory distress syndrome, septic shock) is being evaluated (69b–69d).

Polymyxin E paste (2%) can be combined with tobramycin and applied to the buccal mucosa and oral cavity in intensive care units as prophylaxis for nosocomial pneumonia (70). No infections occurred in 27 patients who were studied this way.

METHENAMINE

Methenamine was discovered in 1894. It is a cyclic hydrocarbon condensation product of ammonia and formaldehyde with properties of a monoacidic base; it is soluble in water and forms a weak basic solution at a pH of 8.0 to 8.5. It is available in three different forms: alone as a pure base, or combined with either mandelic acid or hippuric acid.

Mode of Action

In acidic urine, methenamine is hydrolyzed to formaldehyde and ammonia by the following reaction:

$$N_4(CH_2)_6 + 6H_2O + 4H^+ = 4NH_4^+ + 6HCHO$$

Because the release of formaldehyde occurs only in an acidic medium, the antimicrobial activity of methenamine is related to the urinary pH; however, there is no documentation that acidification of the urine enhances methenamine's therapeutic activity (70a).

Antibacterial Activity

Methenamine is active against all gram-negative and gram-positive bacteria, even fungi, except for urea-splitting organisms such as *Proteus* spp. (71). Bacterial resistance to formaldehyde does not develop, and no cross-resistance with any other antibiotic has been reported (72).

Pharmacokinetics

After oral ingestion, methenamine is well absorbed and circulates unchanged. Approximately 10% to 30% is hydrolyzed by gastric fluid. After a single (1-g) dose, approximately 82% of methenamine is recovered in urine in 24 hours, and 90% is recovered during continuous administration. The peak serum level is 35 μg/mL at 1 hour; 20% of methenamine is converted to formaldehyde in the urine. Concentrations of formaldehyde of 10 to 15 μg/mL have bacteriostatic activity; concentrations greater than 28 μg/mL are bactericidal (73). A urinary pH less than 6.0 is necessary to achieve the bactericidal effect; the addition of hippurate or mandelic acid ensures the acidity of the urine. The mean half-life is 4.3 hours (74).

Renal clearance of methenamine approximates creatinine clearance; caution is required in patients with renal insufficiency (75). Methenamine is widely distributed throughout the body fluids (e.g., cerebrospinal fluid, aqueous humor, and pericardial and synovial fluids).

Dosage

For adults, the oral dose is 1 g every 6 hours for methenamine mandelate and 1 g every 12 hours for the hippurate form. In children, half the adult dose is recommended.

Adverse Effects

This drug is well tolerated; gastrointestinal disturbances such as nausea, vomiting, and diarrhea have occasionally been reported (76). Skin reactions, bladder irritation, and inflammation accompanied by dysuria, hematuria, and proteinuria may occur (77). It has been associated with bilateral anterior uveitis (78). Methenamine should not be administered in conjunction with sulfonamides, which may precipitate when formaldehyde is released (79). It is contraindicated in patients with gout, because urate crystals may precipitate in urine (80).

Clinical Applications

Methenamine is indicated only for treatment of lower urinary tract infections, and even this is controversial (81,82). It is effective as preoperative prophylaxis in bacteriuric patients undergoing transurethral prostatic resection (83), cystoscopy, and vaginal surgery (84). Use with urinary acidifying agents in combination (e.g., hemiacidrin) is recommended. In patients receiving methenamine, bacteriuria is reduced in those requiring intermittent catheterization (85,86); however, relapses or reinfections in patients with spinal cord injuries who have neurogenic bladders have been reported (87). Methenamine mandelate and hippurate are effective in the prevention of recurrent urinary tract infections except in patients with Foley catheters or who require intermittent catheterization (70a).

Methenamine is not more effective than trimethoprim alone; its failure may be due to the drug's inability to alter the periurethral flora (88). A potential use for methenamine is in the treatment of calcium stone disease because renal secretion of oxalate is decreased (89). Further clinical trials are necessary to confirm this activity.

FUSIDIC ACID

Fusidic acid, available since 1962, was isolated from the fungus *Fusidium coccineum*; it has a steroid-like structure and is related chemically to cephalosporin P. It is poorly soluble in water and thus is prepared as a sodium salt for oral administration and as a diethanolamine salt for intravenous administration. It is a weak acid (pH 5.7) that, is largely ionized at the pH values of the blood (90).

Mode of Action

Fusidic acid inhibits bacterial protein synthesis by interacting with the ribosome and interfering with the polypeptide chain elongation. It inhibits the elongation factor G and guanosine diphosphate, decreasing guanosine triphosphate hydrolysis. This inhibition leads to less protein A on the surface of gram-positive bacteria (*S. aureus*), increasing susceptibility to phagocytosis (91).

Antibacterial Activity

Fusidic acid is highly effective against staphylococci, including penicillin-sensitive *S. aureus*, β-lactamase-producing strains, methicillin-resistant strains (92,93), and *S. epidermidis* (94). The MIC for *S. aureus* is between 0.063 and 1.0 mg/L (median, 0.125 mg/L); the minimal bactericidal concentration is between 0.25 and 16 mg/dL (median, 8 mg/dL) (95). Synergy with rifampin and dicloxacillin has been demonstrated (96) and antagonism between fusidic acid and rifampin reported. (97) Other gram-positive bacteria, such as streptococci, are much less susceptible to fusidic acid, with MIC values of 8.6 μg/mL for *S. pneumoniae*, 6.8 μg/mL for *Streptococcus pyogenes*, and 1.6 μg/mL for *Streptococcus viridans*; in vitro synergism with gentamicin against enterococcus has been demonstrated (98). Gram-positive anaerobes such as *Clostridium tetani* (MIC of 0.016 μg/mL) and *Clostridium perfringens* are sensitive. The MIC of fusidic acid for *B. fragilis* is 0.25 to 4.0 μg/mL. (99) All gram-negative bacilli are resistant; but some gram-negative cocci (i.e., *N. meningitidis* and *N. gonorrhoeae*) with MIC values of 0.56 and 0.66 μg/mL, respectively (100), are susceptible. Other sensitive organisms include *Nocardia asteroides* (MIC of 2.5 mg/mL) (101) and *M. tuberculosis* (MIC of 1.0 μg/mL).

Fusidic acid resistance in *Staphylococcus aureus* results from point mutations within the chromosomal *fusA* gene encoding EF-G (102).

Pharmacokinetics

After oral dosing of 500 mg of fusidic acid, the peak serum level of 20 mg/mL was achieved in 2 hours, although the variation for the rate of absorption is variable among subjects. The $t_{1/2}$ is 5 to 6 hours (90); some accumulation may occur when the drug is administered every 8 hours. After 96 hours of therapy, a plasma concentration between 21 and 71 μg/mL was obtained. With the oral suspension, a faster peak but lower mean peak concentration is observed than with the tablets (90). After intravenous administration, an initial high level of 20 mg/L is noted (mean, 44 μg/mL) after a 2-hour infusion (103).

Excretion

Fusidic acid is metabolized in the liver and probably undergoes enterohepatic circulation. At least seven different metabolites have been found in bile (104), some of them with microbiologic activity. Approximately 2% of fusidic acid is found in the feces, probably due to biliary excretion, as well as a small quantity of nonabsorbed drug. Small amounts of fusidic acid are renally excreted, and less than 1% of the drug can be recovered from the urine (105). Fusidic acid is not renally excreted, so patients with renal failure or undergoing hemodialysis do not need dose adjustments (106). The drug should be avoided in patients with hepatic failure, because it competes with bilirubin for albumin binding sites.

Distribution

Fusidic acid is strongly protein bound (99%) (107); it is well distributed throughout the body, with good diffusion into different cell types including lymphocytes, macrophages, and fibroblasts (108). Fusidic acid penetrates the synovial fluid of inflamed joints with levels that approach those of plasma. In bone, concentrations that exceed the MIC for most strains of *S. aureus* have been observed. Some of these levels may exceed the MIC by a factor of 100 (109). Heart tissue levels are one third those of plasma, and the drug penetrates better into atrial appendages than do cephalosporins. It is not affected by cardiopulmonary bypass (110). Fusidic acid enters purulent collections, prostatic fluid, and aqueous humor. Cerebrospinal fluid concentrations are quite low, although in cerebral abscesses levels approach the serum concentrations (111). Fusidic acid passes through the placenta and can be detected in fetal tissue.

The usual oral dose for adults is 500 mg given three times daily, but the dose can be doubled in severe infections. A suspension of 250 mg of fusidic acid hemihydrate per 5 mL is available but has less bioavailability than the enteric-coated tablets with 250 mg of fusidic acid. For children younger than 1 year of age, the recommended dose is 50 mg/kg per day. The intravenous preparation contains, per vial, 580 mg of diethanolamine salt, equivalent to 500 mg of fusidic acid. The dose is diluted in saline and should be infused during 6 hours. The dosage for adults is 580 mg diethanolamine fusidate three times daily; it is 10 mg/kg for children. A 2% ointment for topical administration is available.

Adverse Effects

After oral administration, nausea, vomiting, and diarrhea may occur. Ingestion of food decreases dyspepsia without affecting blood levels. After intravenous administration, severe local pain may occur, as well as venospasm and thrombophlebitis (112) resulting from an irritant effect on the vein wall. This effect can be minimized with slow infusions in a large peripheral vein. Because fusidic acid is highly protein bound, it competes with bilirubin for albumin binding sites, reversibly increasing free bilirubin concentrations (113). Fusidic acid should be used cautiously in patients with liver impairment, especially in neonates, because of the potential for brain damage (107). Neutropenia and rashes have rarely been reported (114).

Clinical Applications

Fusidic acid in its oral, parenteral, and topical forms has been used to treat staphylococcal infections of skin and soft tissue (e.g., abscesses, furunculosis, and infected burns). It is an alternative therapy to penicillinase-resistant penicillins and cephalosporins for osteomyelitis, septic arthritis, endocarditis, sepsis, and pneumonia when *S. aureus* is isolated or suspected (115). Children with cystic fibrosis have been treated for *S. aureus* infections (116). Because of the development of drug resistance, fusidic acid is not recommended as monotherapy but should be given with other antistaphylococcal agents (e.g., β-lactamase–resistant penicillins or cephalosporins) (96). Fusidic acid has been added to bone cement for prophylaxis of infections before hip replacement. Fusidic acid has been used to treat nasal carriers of methicillin-resistant *S. aureus* (117); pseudomembranous colitis due to *Clostridium difficile* may benefit from fusidic acid therapy (118). It appears to be a weak bactericidal antileprosy agent, which may have a role in the multidrug treatment of leprosy (119). A case of successfully treated legionellosis has been reported (120). Fusidic acid is active *in vitro* against many methicillin-resistant *S. aureus* strains, so it should be considered for use with other agents such as vancomycin, rifampin, and possibly ciprofloxacin in refractory cases (93). There are few reports in the literature suggesting that fusidic acid may be a promising candidate for prophylaxis in neurosurgery (121,122). Fusidic acid is excreted into the bile and discharged into the small intestine where the colonization with *Giardia* organisms is maximal; thus, a potential use in combination with metronidazole can be considered in refractory cases of giardiasis (123). It has also been used as self-administration prophylaxis before cataract surgery with significant reduction of *S. aureus* and *S. epidermidis* infection and attainment of a sterile eye field (124). Finally, because fusidic acid penetrates lymphocytes and macrophages, an attempt was made to treat patients with human immunodeficiency virus infection; no response of p24 antigen or increase in CD4$^+$ cells was detected (125). Recently, fusidic acid was shown to be effective in the treatment of impetigo in children younger than 12 years (126).

NITROFURANTOIN

Nitrofurantoin has been available since 1953 and is one of the nitrofuran compounds, which consist of a primary nitro group joined to a heterocycle ring. It is poorly soluble in water and is available in crystalline and macrocrystalline forms.

Mode of Action

The precise mechanism of action is unknown; it is probably due to inhibition of bacterial enzymes and may also interfere with DNA. Drug activity is increased in acidic urine.

Antibacterial Activity

Nitrofurantoin is active against most gram-negative bacteria that cause urinary tract infection. *E. coli* strains are sensitive, with an MIC of 16 μg/mL; other gram-negative bacilli with an MIC of 32 μg/mL or less are considered susceptible to the drug. *Enterobacter* spp. and *Klebsiella* spp. are less susceptible, with MIC

values usually greater than 100 μg/mL, whereas *Proteus* spp. and *P. aeruginosa* are almost always resistant, with MIC values greater than 200 μg/mL (127).

Nitrofurantoin is also active against gram-positive bacteria that sometimes produce urinary tract infections, such as *Enterococcus*, *S. aureus*, *S. epidermidis*, and *Staphylococcus saprophyticus*. The MIC values for gram-positive cocci are lower: 4 μg/mL for *S. aureus* and 25 μg/mL for *Enterococcus*.

Other microorganisms, such as *S. pyogenes*, *S. pneumoniae*, *Corynebacterium* spp., *Salmonella* spp., *Shigella* spp., and *B. fragilis*, are sensitive *in vitro*. Organisms usually do not develop resistance to nitrofurantoin, but cross-resistance with aminoglycosides with *E. coli* has been reported (128). Nitrofurantoin has been an alternative drug for Escherichia coli isolates from the urinary tract from female outpatients that are resistant to trimethoprim-sulfamethoxazole. Among these isolates tested in U.S. laboratories from 1998 through 2001, 9.5% were resistant to ciprofloxacin and 1.9% were resistant to nitrofurantoin; 10.4% of ciprofloxacin-resistant isolates were resistant to nitrofurantoin (129).

Pharmacokinetics

The standard crystalline form is more rapidly absorbed than the macrocrystalline form. Nitrofurantoin has an extremely short half-life ($t_{1/2} = 20$ minutes) (130). Serum levels are low, with peak concentrations in plasma near 0.72 mg/L detected after 2 hours (131).

Excretion

About one third of the dose appears in urine as active drug, with urine levels of 50 to 250 μg/mL. Recovery from the urine is related to creatinine clearance. The drug tends, however, to accumulate in patients with abnormal renal function (132). Nitrofurantoin also penetrates the interstitial tissue of the renal medulla (133). Some drug is excreted into the bile; it is inactivated in all body tissues, but hepatic degradation may be the most significant.

Administration

Nitrofurantoin is available for oral use but not for intravenous administration in the United States. Sustained-release nitrofurantoin in the form of microcapsules may decrease the severity of side effects (134,135). Oral dosage for adults is 50 to 100 mg every 6 hours.

Adverse Effects

Adverse reactions to nitrofurantoin are quite common, varying from mild, reversible effects to severe reactions with long-term sequelae. The most common side effects include gastrointestinal reactions (e.g., nausea and vomiting), usually dose-related. These reactions tend to occur during the first week of therapy and are more frequent in women. The macrocrystalline form, which is more slowly absorbed, has fewer gastrointestinal side effects (136,137). Diarrhea, abdominal pain, and gastrointestinal bleeding are rare complications (130).

Three different types of hepatic toxicity may occur: (a) acute hepatocellular damage; (b) cholestatic jaundice, more common in elderly patients and sometimes associated with rash and eosinophilia (138); and (c) chronic active hepatitis with severe necroinflammatory disease associated with hypergammaglobulinemia and high titers of antinuclear antibodies, usually seen in women (139). There is a possible association between particular human leukocyte antigen (HLA) molecules and immunoallergic hepatitis; HLA-DRG and HLA-DRS have been linked to nitrofurantoin-associated hepatitis (140). Discontinuation of the drug often results in clinical and laboratory improvement. However, in one report, a patient required orthotopic liver transplantation after chronic therapy with low-dose nitrofurantoin (141). Pancreatitis and parotitis have been reported, sometimes associated with fever and increased serum amylase level (142,143); thyroid inflammation has also been noted.

Pulmonary Reactions

Nitrofurantoin can produce different types of adverse pulmonary effects. The first type is acute bronchitis, asthma, and pneumonitis (144); these usually occur 5 to 10 days after therapy is initiated. Cough, dyspnea, and fever with or without infiltrates on the chest radiograph may be observed; eosinophilia has been seen. This reaction is believed to be allergic and usually resolves with discontinuation of the drug. The two other types of pulmonary effect are subacute pneumonitis and chronic lung involvement with interstitial fibrosis producing chronic cough and dyspnea (145,146). The chronic form is more common in women; hypergammaglobulinemia and antinuclear antibodies may be found. Pathologic examination reveals interstitial inflammation and fibrosis. It is believed that nitrofurantoin generates toxic oxygen radicals that produce this lung injury. Indirect damage resulting from nitrofurantoin may have the ability to recruit neutrophils to the lung tissue (147) and produce an inflammatory response. Clinical and radiographic resolution of this severe side effect is unpredictable.

Hematologic Reactions

There are different types of blood dyscrasia: acute hemolytic anemia in patients with glucose-6-phosphate dehydrogenase deficiency and red cell enzyme deficiencies such as enolase and glutathione peroxidase deficiencies (148,149).

Megaloblastic anemia, probably due to folic acid deficiency; leukopenia (l50); thrombocytopenia; agranulocytosis; and aplastic anemia have been described (130).

Neurologic Reactions

Polyneuropathy with a stocking-glove distribution is one of the most severe side effects. It is seen more frequently in patients with renal insufficiency. Although the clinical presentation is variable, sensory loss, pain, and motor weakness occur. Nitrofurantoin has also been associated with retrobulbar neuritis (151), seventh cranial nerve palsy (152), and pseudotumor cerebri (153). The mechanism is believed to be related to a direct toxic effect of the drug.

Hypersensitivity Reactions

Eosinophilia, rashes, and drug fever have been reported, as has drug-induced lupus erythematosus (154).

Clinical Applications

Today the only indication for nitrofurantoin is the treatment of urinary tract infections involving the upper and lower genitourinary tract. It has also been used for prostatitis, in prophylaxis of recurrent urinary tract infection, and in prevention of bacteriuria after prostatectomy (155). Suppressive therapy with nitrofurantoin has the advantage that resistance does not usually occur.

BACITRACIN

Bacitracin was isolated in 1943 from a strain of *Bacillus subtilis*, today known as *Bacillus licheniformis*. It is a polypeptide composed of peptide-linked amino acids containing a thiazolidine ring and is highly soluble in water. The commercial preparation is a mixture of at least nine bacitracins with bacitracin A as the major constituent. The activity of bacitracin is expressed in a unit that represents 26 jig of a standard preparation.

Mode of Action

Bacitracin acts at stage 2 in cell wall synthesis, inhibiting conversion of phospholipid pyrophosphate to phospholipid, which is an essential reaction for the regeneration of the lipid carrier involved in cell wall synthesis (156).

Antibacterial Activity

Bacitracin is active at low concentrations against gram-positive cocci and bacilli, particularly *S. aureus* and *S. pyogenes*; groups C and G are less susceptible, whereas group B strains are resistant. *Neisseria* spp., *H. influenzae*, *Treponema pallidum*, *Actinomyces* spp., and *Fusobacterium* spp. are also sensitive. Gram-negative bacilli are usually highly resistant (157). The development of resistance to bacitracin is uncommon in patients treated with this compound.

Pharmacokinetics

After oral administration of 25,000 or 50,000 units of intramuscular bacitracin, the serum concentration varied between 0.006 and 1.0 unit/mL at 2 hours (158,159). Bacitracin penetrates pleural and ascitic fluid well; extremely small concentrations can be detected in cerebrospinal fluid. Most of the drug is inactivated, low protein binding, and 30% can be found in a 24-hour urine sample in the active form (117).

Adverse Effects

When used parenterally, bacitracin is highly nephrotoxic, producing dose-related renal failure due to tubular and glomerular necrosis (156). When bacitracin is used as a topical preparation, skin irritation and allergic reactions are unusual (160). Anaphylaxis after intraoperative irrigation in patients previously sensitized (161) or after topical therapy when the drug can penetrate the systemic circulation through ulcerated skin or open cancellous bone has been reported (162).

Clinical Applications

Bacitracin is available in a variety of different topical forms as creams, ointments, sprays, powders, and irrigating solutions for treatment of staphylococcal infections of the skin and soft tissue, including furunculosis, impetigo, pyoderma, and abscesses (157). It has also been used for intraoperative irrigation in neurosurgery and orthopedic surgery, which has decreased the incidence of postoperative wound infection (163,164). Bacitracin alone or a bacitracin-zinc combination has been used to treat patients infected with *Giardia lamblia*. Cure rates were higher than 86% (165). Colonization with methicillin-resistant *S. aureus* may be treated with a combination of bacitracin, rifampin, and trimethoprim-sulfamethoxazole. This causes short-term eradication of the microorganism, although relapse or reinfection may be seen (166). Bacitracin 25,000 units every 6 hours is a cost-effective alternative to oral vancomycin or metronidazole in the treatment of *C. difficile*, but has not been as well studied as either drug (167). Finally, strategies to suppress or eradicate the vancomycin-resistant enterococci intestinal reservoir have been reported for the combination of oral doxycycline plus bacitracin and oral ramoplanin (a novel glycolipodepsipeptide). If successful, a likely application of such an approach is the reduction of VRE infection during high risk periods in high risk patient groups such as the post-chemotherapy neutropenic nadir or early post-solid abdominal organ transplantation (168,169).

REFERENCES

1. Kunin CM, Bugg A. Binding of polymyxin antibratus to tissue: the major determinant of distribution and persistence in the body. *J Infect Dis* 1971;124:394.
2. Warner SJ, Mitchell D, Savage N, et al. Dose-dependent reduction of lipopolysaccharide pyrogenicity by polymyxin B. *Biochem Pharmacol* 1985;34:3995.
3. Cavaillon JM, Haeffner-Cavaillon N. Polymyxin-B inhibition of LPS-induced interleukin-1 secretion by human monocytes is dependent upon the LPS origin. *Mol Immunol* 1986;23:965.
4. Bender BS, Winchurch RA, Thupari JN, et al. Depressed natural killer cell function in thermally injured adults: successful in vivo and in vitro immunomodulation and the role of endotoxin. *Clin Exp Immunol* 1988;71:120–125.
5. Rifkind D. Prevention by polymyxin B of endotoxin lethality in mice. *J Bacteriol* 1966;93:1463.
6. From AHL, Fong JSC, Good RA. Polymyxin B sulfate modification of bacterial endotoxin: effects on the development of endotoxin shock in dogs. *Infect Immun* 1979;23:660.
7. Hughes B, Madan BR, Parratt JR. Polymyxin B sulphate protects cats against the haemodynamic and metabolic effects of *E. coli* endotoxin. *Br J Pharmacol* 1981;74:701.
8. Craig WA, Turner JH, Kunin CM. Prevention of generalized Shwartzman reaction and endotoxin lethality by polymyxin B localized in tissues. *Infect Immun* 1974;10:287.
9. Flynn PM, Shenep JL, Stokes DC, et al. Polymyxin B moderates acidosis and hypotension in established, experimental gram negative septicemia. *J Infect Dis* 1987;156:706.
10. Stokes DC, Shenep JL, Fishman M, et al. Polymyxin B prevents lipopolysaccharide-induced release of tumor necrosis factors from alveolar macrophages. *J Infect Dis* 1989;160:52.
11. Cameron DJ, Churchill MH. Cytotoxicity of human macrophages for tumor cells: enhancement mycobacterial lipopolysaccarides (LPS). *J Immunol* 1980;124:708.
12. Tauber MG, Shibl AM, Hackbarth CJ, et al. Antibiotic therapy, endotoxin concentration in cerebrospinal fluid, and brain edema in experimental *Escherichia coli* meningitis in rabbits. *J Infect Dis* 1987;156:456.
13. Duncan IB. Susceptibility of 1500 isolates of *Pseudomonas aeruginosa* to gentamicin, carbenicillin colistin and polymyxin B. *Antimicrob Agents Chemother* 1974;5:9.
14. Nord NM, Hoeprich PD. Polymyxin B and colistin. *N Engl J Med* 1965;270:1030.
15. Rastogi N, Potar MC, David HL. Antimycobacterial spectrum of colistin (polymixin E). *Ann Inst Pasteur Microbiol* 1986;137A:45.
16. Moore RA, Hancock RE. Involvement of outer membrane of *Pseudomonas cepacia* in aminoglycoside and polymyxin resistance. *Antimicrob Agents Chemother* 1986;30:923.
17. Peterson AA, Fesik SW, McGroarty EJ. Decreased binding of antibiotics to lipopolysaccharides from polymyxin-resistant strains of *Escherichia coli* and *Salmonella typhimurium*. *Antimicrob Agents Chemother* 1987;31:230.
18. Nord C-E, Wadstrom T, Wretlind B. Synergistic effect of combinations of sulfamethoxazole, trimethoprim, and colistin against *Pseudomonas maltophilia* and *Pseudomonas cepacia*. *Antimicrob Agents Chemother* 1974;6:521.
19. Rosenblatt JE, Stewart PR. Combined activity of sulfamethoxazole, trimethoprim, and polymyxin B against gram-negative bacilli. *Antimicrob Agents Chemother* 1974;6:84.
19a. Kim M-N, et al. In vitro antimicrobial synergy against imipenem resistant *Acinetobacter baumannii*. Presented at the 102nd General Meeting of the American Society of Microbiology (ASM), May 19–23, 2002, Salt Lake City, Utah.
20. Schwartz SN, Medoff G, Kobayashi GS, et al. Antifungal properties of polymyxin B and its potentiation of tetracycline as an antifungal agent. *Antimicrob Agents Chemother* 1972;2:36.
21. Collins MS, Pappagagionis D. Inhibition of *Coccidiodes immitis* in vitro and enhancement of amphotericin B by polymyxin B. *Antimicrob Agents Chemother* 1975;7:781.
22. Cornelissen F, Van de Bossche H. Synergism of the antimicrobial agents miconazole, bacitracin and polymyxin B. *Chemotherapy* 1983;29:419.
23. Rastogi N, Henrotte JG, David HL. Colistin (polymyxin E)-induced cell leakage in *Mycobacterium aurum*. *Zentralbl Bakteriol Mikrobiol Hyg (A)* 1987;263:548.
24. Nicas TI, Hancock RE. Alteration of susceptibility to EDTA, polymyxin B and gentamicin in *Pseudomonas aeruginosa* by divalent cation regulation of outer membrane protein H1. *J Gen Microbiol* 1983;129:509.
25. Davis SD, Ianetta A, Wedgwood RJ. Activity of colistin against *Pseudomonas aeruginosa*: inhibition by calcium. *J Infect Dis* 1971;124:610.
26. Gremeaux T, Tanti JF, Van Obberghen E, et al. Polymyxin B selectively inhibits insulin effects on transport in isolated muscle. *Am J Physiol* 1987;252:13248.
27. Strutchfield J, Jones PM, Howell SL. The effects of polymyxin B, a protein kinase C inhibitor, on insulin secretion from intact and permeabilized islets of Langerhans. *Biochem Biophys Res Commun* 1986;136:1001.
28. Henriksen EJ, Sleeper MD, Zierath JR, et al. Polymyxin B inhibits stimulation of glucose transport in muscle by hypoxia or contractions. *Am J Physiol* 1989;256:13662.
29. Amir S, Sasson S, Kaiser N, et al. Polymyxin B is an inhibitor of insulin-induced hypoglycemia in the whole animal model: studies on the mode of inhibitory action. *J Biol Chem* 1987;262:6663.
30. Kunin CM. A guide to the use of antibiotics in patients with renal disease. *Ann Intern Med* 1967;67:151.
31. Fekety R. Polymyxin. In: Mandell G, Douglas RC, Bennett JE, eds. *Principles and practices of infectious diseases*, 2nd ed. New York: John Wiley & Sons, 1985:235.
32. Cox CE, Harrison LH. Intravenous sodium colistimethate therapy of urinary-tract infections: pharmacological and bacteriological studies. *Antimicrob Agents Chemother* 1970;10:296.
33. McMillar M, Price TML, MacLaren DM, et al. *Pseudomonas pyocyanea* infection treated with colistin methane sulphonate. *Lancet* 1962;2:737.
34. Kunin CM. More on antimicrobials in renal failure. *Ann Intern Med* 1968;69:397.
35. Goodwin NJ, Fredman EA. The effects of renal compartment, peritoneal dialysis and hemodialysis on serum colistimethate levels. *Ann Intern Med* 1968;68:984.
36. Appel GB, Neu HC. The nephrotoxicity of antimicrobial agents. *N Engl J Med* 1977;296:663.
37. Bennett WM, Muther RS, Parker RA, et al. Drug therapy in renal failure: dosing guidelines for adults. Part 1. Antimicrobial agents. *Ann Intern Med* 1980;93:62.
38. Froman J, Gross L, Curatala S. Serum and urine levels following parenteral administration of sodium colistimethate to normal individuals. *J Urol* 1970;103:210.
39. MacKay D, Kaye D. Serum concentrations of colistin in patients with normal and impaired renal function. *N Engl J Med* 1964;270:394.
40. Curtis JR, Eastwood JB. Colistimethate sodium administration during hemodialysis and peritoneal dialysis. *BMJ* 1968;1:484.
41. Slejjfer DTh, Mulder NH, deVries-Hospens HG, et al. Infection prevention in granulocytopenic patients by selective decontamination of the digestive tract. *Eur J Cancer* 1980;16:859.
42. Koch-Weser J, Sidel VW, Federman EB, et al. Adverse effects of sodium colistimethate: manifestations and specific reaction rates during 317 courses of therapy. *Ann Intern Med* 1970;72:857.
43. Fekety Jr FR, Norman PS, Cluff LE. The treatment of gramnegative bacillary infections with colistin. *Ann Intern Med* 1962;57:214.
44. Pedersen MF, Pederson JF, Madsen PO. A clinical and experimental comparative study of sodium colistimethate and polymyxin B sulfate. *Invest Urol* 1971;9:234.
45. Murdock J MCC. The treatment of severe *Pseudomonas pyocyanea* infections with colistin. In: Proceedings of the Third International Congress of Chemotherapy, Stuttgart, Germany; 1964:319.
46. Feeley TW, DuMoulin GC, Hedley-Whyte J, et al. Aerosol polymyxin and pneumonia in seriously ill patients. *N Engl J Med* 1975;193:471.
47. Klastersky J, Hensgens C, Noterman J, et al. Endotracheal antibiotics for the prevention of tracheo-bronchial infections in tracheotomized unconscious patients: a comparative study of gentamicin and aminosidin-polymyxin B combination. *Chest* 1975;68:302.
48. Ledingham IM, Alcock SR, Eastaway AT, et al. Triple regimen of selective decontamination of the digestive tract, systemic cefotaxime, and microbiological surveillance for prevention of acquired infection in intensive care. *Lancet* 1988;1:785.
49. Johanson WG Jr, Seidenfeld JJ, de los Santos R, et al. Prevention of nosocomial pneumonia using topical and parenteral antimicrobial agents. *Am Rev Respir Dis* 1988;137:265.
50. Hazenberg MP, Pennock-Schroder AM, van de Merwe JP. Reversible binding of polymyxin B and neomycin to the solid part of faeces. *J Antimicrob Chemother* 1986;17:333.
51. Unertl K, Ruckdeschel G, Selbmann HK, et al. Prevention of colonization and respiratory infections in long-term ventilated patients by local antimicrobial prophylaxis. *Intensive Care Med* 1987;13:106.
52. VanSaene HK, Stontenbeck CP, Zandstra DF. Cefotaxime combined with selective decontamination in intensive care unit patients: virtual absence of emergence of resistance. *Drugs* 1988;35:29.
53. Van Saene JJ, van Saene HK, Tarko-Smit NJ, et al. Enterobacteriaceae suppression by three different oral doses of polymyxin E in human volunteers. *Epidemiol Infect* 1988;100:407.
54. Clasener HAL, Yollaard EJ, van Saene HKF. Long-term prophylaxis of infection by selective decontamination in leukopenia and in mechanical ventilation. *Rev Infect Dis* 1987;9:295.
55. de Vries-Hospers H, Sleijfer DT, Mulder NH, et al. Bacteriological aspects of selective decontamination of the digestive tract as a method of infection prevention in granulocytopenic patients. *Antimicrob Agents Chemother* 1981;19:813.

56. Storring RA, Jameson B, McElwain TJ, et al. Oral nonabsorbed antibiotics prevent infection in acute non-lymphoblastic leukaemia. *Lancet* 1977;2:837.

57. Dekker AW, Rozenberg-Arska M, Verhoef J. Infection prophylaxis in acute leukemia: a comparison of ciprofloxacin with trimethoprim-sulfamethoxazole and colistin. *Ann Intern Med* 1987;106:7.

58. Manan P, Kibbler CC, Noone P. Activity of ciprofloxacin and colistin against *Pseudomonas aeruginosa* isolates from neutropenic patients: a possible approach to prophylaxis (letter). *J Antimicrob Chemother* 1988;22:953.

59. Kurrle E, DeKiler AW, Gaus W, et al. Prevention of infection in acute leukemia: a prospective randomized study of two different drug regimens for antimicrobial prophylaxis. *Infection* 1986;14:226.

60. Rosenberg-Arska M, Dekker AW, Berhoef J. Colistin and trimethoprim-sulfamethoxazole for the prevention of infection in patients with acute non-lymphocytic leukaemia: disease in emergence of resistant bacteria. *Infection* 1983;11:167.

61. Spijkervet FKL, van Saene HKF, van Saene JJM, et al. Effect of selective elimination of the oral flora on mucositis in irradiated head and neck cancer patients. *J Surg Oncol* 1991;46:167.

62. Karpuch J, Schiffer J, Boldur I, et al. Purulent meningitis due to *Pseudomonas aeruginosa* successfully treated with colistin and piperacillin. *J Infect* 1985;11:272.

63. Rimola A, Bory F, Teres J, et al. Oral non-absorbable antibiotics to prevent infection in cirrhotics with gastrointestinal hemorrhage. *Hepatology* 1985;5:463.

64. Ingoldby CJ, McPherson GA, Blumgart LH. Endotoxemia in human obstructive jaundice: Effect of polymyxin B. *Am J Surg* 1984;147:766.

65. Wiesner RH, Hermans P, Rakela J, et al. Selective bowel decontamination to prevent gram-negative bacterial and fungal infection following orthotopic liver transplantation. *Transplant Proc* 1987;19:2420.

65a. Moreau JM, Conerly LL, Hume EB, et al. Effectiveness of mupirocin and polymyxin B in experimental *Staphylococcus aureus, Pseudomonas aeruginosa,* and *Serratia marcescens* keratitis. *Cornea* 2002;21:807–811.

66. Moore MB, McCulley JP. Acanthamobea keratitis associated with contact lenses: six consecutive cases of successful management. *Br J Ophthalmol* 1989;73:271.

67. Marsden HB, Hyde WA. Colistin methane sulphonate in childhood infections. *Lancet* 1962;2:144.

68. Gotoff SP, Lepper MH. Treatment of *Salmonella* carriers with colistin sulfate. *Am J Med Sci* 1965;249:399.

69. Parsons P, Worthen GS, Moore EE, et al. The association of circulating endotoxin with the development of the adult respiratory distress syndrome. *Am Rev Respir Dis* 1989;140:294.

69a. Nemoto H, Nakamoto H, Okada H, et al. Newly developed immobilized polymyxin B fibers improve the survival of patients with sepsis. *Blood Purif* 2001;19:361–368; discussion 368–369.

69b. Stegmary BG. Apheresis as therapy for patients with severe sepsis and multiorgan dysfunction syndrome. *Ther Apher* 2001;5:123–127.

69c. Uriu K, Osajima A, Hiroshige K, et al. Endotoxin removal by direct hemoperfusion with an absorvent column using polymixing B-immobilized fiber ameliorates systemic circulatory disturbance in patients with septic shock. *Am J Kidney Dis* 2002;39:937–947.

69d. Tsuzuki H, Tani T, Ueyama H, et al. Lipopolysaccharide: neutralization by polymyxin B shuts down the signaling pathway of nuclear factor kappaB in peripheral blood mononuclear cells, even during activation. *J Surg Res* 2001;100:127–134.

70. vanUffenen R, Rommes JH, vanSawne HK. Preventing lower airway colonization and infection in mechanically ventilated patients. *Crit Care Med* 1987;15:99.

70a. Gleckman R, Alvarez S, Joubert DW, et al. Drug therapy reviews: methenamine mandelate and methenamine hippurate. *Am J Hosp Pharmacol* 1979;36:1509–1512.

71. Kucers A. Fusidate sodium. In: Kucers A, Bennett NM, eds. *The use of antibiotics,* 4th ed. London: William Heinemann Medical Books, 1987:808–818.

72. Scudi JV, Duca CJ. Some antibacterial properties of Mandelamine (methenamine mandelate). *J Urol* 1949;61:459.

73. Pearman JW, Peterson GJ, Nash JB. The antimicrobial activity of urine of paraplegic patients receiving methenamine mandelate. *Invest Urol* 1978;16:91.

74. Klinge E, Mannisto P, Mantyla R, et al. Pharmacokinetics of methenamine in healthy volunteers. *J Antimicrob Chemother* 1982;9:209.

75. Bennett WM, Singer I, Coggins CM. A practical guide to drug usage in adult patients with impaired renal function. *JAMA* 1970;214:1468.

76. Gleckman R, Alvarez S, Joubert DW, et al. Drug therapy reviews: methenamine mandelate and methenamine hippurate. *Am J Hosp Pharmacol* 1979;36:1509.

77. Elo J, Sarna S, Ahava K, et al. Methenamine hippurate in urinary tract infections in children: prophylaxis, treatment and side effects. *J Antimicrob Chemother* 1978;4:355.

78. Kolker RJ. Medication-induced bilateral anterior uveitis. *Arch Ophthalmol* 1991;109:1343.

79. Lipton JH. Incompatibility between sulfamethizole and methenamine mandelate. *N Engl J Med* 1963;268:92.

80. U.S. Public Health Service Cooperative Study. Prevention of recurrent bacteriuria with continuous chemotherapy. *Ann Intern Med* 1968;69:655.

81. Cronberg S, Welin CD, Henriksson L, et al: Prevention of recurrent acute cystitis by methenamine hippurate: double blind controlled crossover long term study. *BMJ* 1987;294:1507.

82. Vainrub B, Musher DM. Lack of effect of methenamine in suppression of, or prophylaxis against, chronic urinary infection. *Antimicrob Agents Chemother* 1977;12:625.

83. Olsen JM, Friss-Moller A, Jensen SK, et al. Cefotaxime for prevention of infectious complications in bacteriuric men undergoing transurethral prostatic resection: a controlled comparison with methenamine. *Scand J Urol Nephrol* 1983;17:299.

84. Tyreman NO, Andersson PO, Kroon L, et al. Urinary tract infection after vaginal surgery: effect of prophylactic treatment with methenamine hippurate. *Acta Obstet Gynecol Scand* 1986;65:731.

85. Kevorkian CG, Merritt JL, Ilstrup DM. Methenamine mandelate with acidification: an effective urinary antiseptic in patients with neurogenic bladder. *Mayo Clin Proc* 1984;59:523.

86. Krebs M, Halvorsen RB, Fishman IJ, et al. Prevention of urinary tract infection during intermittent catheterization. *J Urol* 1984;131:82.

87. Kuhlemeier KV, Stover SL, Lloyd LK. Prophylactic antibacterial therapy for preventing urinary tract infections in spinal cord injury patients. *J Urol* 1985;134:514.

88. Brumfitt W, Hamilton-Miller JMT, Gargan RA, et al. Long-term prophylaxis of urinary infections in women: comparative trial of trimethoprim, methenamine hippurate and topical povidone-iodine. *J Urol* 1983;130:1110.

89. Fellstrom B, Butz M, Bo G, et al. The effects of methenaminehippurate upon urinary risk factors for renal stone formation. *Scand J Urol Nephrol* 1985;19:125.

90. Reeves DS. The pharmacokinetics of fusidic acid. *J Antimicrob Chemother* 1987;20:467.

91. Kucers A. Methenamine mandelate and methenamine hippurate. In: Kucers A, Bennett NM, eds. *The use of antibiotics,* 4th ed. London: William Heinemann Medical Books, 1987:1344–1348.

92. Moorhouse EC, Mulvihill TE, Jones L, et al. The in vitro activity of some antimicrobial agents against methicillin-resistant *Staphylococcus aureus. J Antimicrob Chemother* 1985;15:291.

93. Foldes M, Munro R, Sorell TC, et al. In vitro effects of vancomycin, rifampicin, and fusidic acid, alone and in combination against methicillin-resistant *Staphylococcus aureus. J Antimicrob Chemother* 1983;77:21.

94. Yu VL, Zuravleff JJ, Bornholm J, et al. In vitro synergy testing of triple antibiotic combination against *Staphylococcus epidermidis* isolates from patients with endocarditis. *J Antimicrob Chemother* 1984;14:359.

95. McDonald M, Hurse A, Sim KN. Methicillin-resistant *Staphylococcus aureus* bacteremia. *Med J Aust* 1981;2:191.

96. Jensen K, Lassen HC. Combined treatment with antibacterial chemotherapeutical agents in staphylococcal infections. *Q J Med* 1969;38:91.

97. Zinner SH, Lagast H, Klastersky J. Antistaphylococcal activity of rifampicin with other antibiotics. *J Infect Dis* 1981;144:365.

98. Traub WH, Spohr M, Bauer D. *Streptococcus faecalis:* in vitro susceptibility to antimicrobial drugs, single and combined, with and without defibrinated human blood. *Chemotherapy* 1986;32:270.

99. Stirling J, Goodwin S. Susceptibility of *Bacteroides fragilis* to fusidic acid. *J Antimicrob Chemother* 1977;3:522.

100. Miles RS, Moyes A. Comparison of susceptibility of *Neisseria meningitidis* to sodium sulphadiazine and sodium fusidate in vitro. *J Clin Pathol* 1978;31:355.

101. Black WA, McNellis DA. Comparative in vitro sensitivity of *Nocardia* species to fusidic acid and sulphonamides. *J Med Microbiol* 1971;4:293.

102. Besier S, Ludwig A, Brade V, et al. Molecular analysis of fusidic acid resistance in *Staphylococcus aureus. Mol Microbiol* 2003;47:463–469.

103. Copperman IJ. The prolonged use of intravenous fusidic acid in severe staphylococcal infection. *Br J Clin Pract* 1972;26:83.

104. Godtfredsen WO, Vangedal S. On the metabolism of fusidic acid in man. *Acta Chem Scand* 1966;20:1599.

105. Wise R, Pippard M, Mitchard M. The disposition of sodium fusidate in man. *Br J Clin Pharmacol* 1977;4:615.

106. Hobby JA. Fucidin in patients on hemodialysis. *J Clin Pathol* 1970;23:484.

107. Brodersen R. Fusidic acid binding to serum albumin and interaction with binding of bilirubin. *Acta Paediatr Scand* 1985;74:874.

108. Brown KN, Percival A. Penetration of antimicrobials into tissue culture cells and leukocytes. *Scand J Infect Dis Suppl* 1978;14:251.

109. Sattar MA, Barrett SP, Cawley ID. Concentrations of some antibiotics in synovial fluid after oral administration, with special reference to antistaphylococcal activity. *Ann Rheum Dis* 1983;42:67.

110. Bergeron MG, Desaulniers D, Lessard C, et al. Concentrations of fusidic acid, cloxacillin and cefamandole in sera and atrial appendages of patients undergoing cardiac surgery. *Antimicrob Agents Chemother* 1985;27:928.

111. Louvois J, Gortvai P, Hurley R. Antibiotic treatment of abscess of the central nervous system. *BMJ* 1977;2:985.

112. Iwarson S, Fasth S, Olaison L, et al. Adverse reactions to intravenous administration of fusidic acid. *Scand J Infect Dis* 1981;13:65.

113. Humble MW, Eykyn S, Phillips I. Staphylococcal bacteraemia, fusidic acid, and jaundice. *BMJ* 1980;280:1495.

114. Evans DI. Granulocytopenia due to fusidic acid (letter). *Lancet* 1988;2:851.

115. Anderson JD. Fusidic acid: new opportunities with an old antibiotic. *Can Med Assoc J* 1980;122:765.

116. Kraemer R. Sputum penetration of fusidic acid in patients with cystic fibrosis. *Eur J Pediatr* 1982;138:172.

117. Guenthner SH, Wenzel RP. In vitro activities of teichomycin, fusidic acid, flucloxacillin, fosfomycin and vancomycin against methicillin-resistant *Staphyloccus aureus. Antimicrob Agents Chemother* 1984;26:268.

118. Cronberg S, Castor B, Thoren A. Fusidic acid for the treatment of antibiotic-associated colitis induced by *Clostridium difficile*. *Infections* 1984;12:276.

119. Franzblau SG, Chan GP, Garcia-Ignacio BG, et al. Clinical trial of fusidic acid for lepromatous leprosy. *Antimicrob Agents Chemother* 1994;38:1651.

120. Friis-Moller A, Rechnitzer C, Nielsen L, et al. Treatment of *Legionella* lung abscess in a renal transplant recipient with erythromycin and fusidic acid (letter). *Eur J Clin Microbiol* 1985;4:513.

121. Mindermann T, Zimmerli W, Gratzl O. Randomized placebo controlled trial of single-dose antibiotic prophylaxis with fusidic acid in neurosurgery. *Acta Neurochir* 1993;121:9.

122. Mindermann T, Zimmerli W, Rajacic Z, et al. Penetration of fusidic acid into human brain tissue and cerobrospinal fluid. *Acta Neurochir* 1993;121:12.

123. Farthing MJ, Inge MG. Antigiardial activity of the bile salt-like antibiotic sodium fusidate. *J Antimicrob Chemother* 1986;17:165.

124. Gray TB, Keenan JI, Clemett RS, et al. Fusidic acid prophylaxis before cataract surgery: patient self-administration. *Aust NZ J Ophthalmol* 1993;21:99.

125. Youle MS, Hawkins DA, Lawrence AG, et al. Clinical, immunological, and virological effects of sodium fusidate in patients with AIDS or AIDS-related complex (ARC): an open study. *J Acquir Immune Defic Syndr* 1989;2:59.

126. Koning S, van Suijlekom-Smit LW, Nouwen JL, et al. Fusidic acid cream in the treatment of impetigo in general practice: double blind randomised placebo controlled trial. *BMJ* 2002;324:203–206.

127. Kucers A. Nitrofurans. In: Kucers A, Bennett NM, eds. *The use of antibiotics*, 4th ed. London: William Heinemann Medical Books, 1987:1276–1289.

128. Obaseiki-Ebor EE. Cross resistance to nitrofurans of aminoglycoside-aminocyclitol resistant strains of *Escherichia coli*. *J Antimicrob Chemother* 1983;11:485.

129. Karlowsky JA, Thornsberry C, Jones ME, et al. Susceptibility of antimicrobial-resistant urinary *Escherichia coli* isolates to fluoroquinolones and nitrofurantoin. *Clin Infect Dis* 2003;36:183–187.

130. D'Arcy PF. Nitrofurantoin. *Drug Intell Clin Pharmacol* 1985;19:540.

131. Mannisto PT, Lammingsivu U. Nitrofurantoin is highly bound to plasma protein. *J Antimicrob Chemother* 1982;9:327.

132. Sachs J, Geer T, Noell P, et al. Effect of renal function on urinary recovery of orally administered nitrofurantoin. *N Engl J Med* 1968;278:1032.

133. Currie GA, Little PJ, McDonald SJ. The localization of cephaloridine and nitrofurantoin in the kidney. *Nephron* 1966;3:282.

134. Spencer RC, Moseley DJ, Greensmith MJ. Nitrofurantoin modified release versus trimethoprim or co-trimoxazole in the treatment of uncomplicated urinary tract infection in general practice. *J Antimicrob Chemother* 1994;33[Suppl A]:121.

135. Ertan G, Karasulu E, Abou-nada M, et al. Sustained-release dosage form of nitrofurantoin. Part 2. In vivo urinary excretion in man. *J Microencaps* 1994;11:137.

136. Hailey FJ, Glascock HW Jr. Gastrointestinal tolerance to a new form of nitrofurantoin: a collaborative study. *Curr Ther Res* 1967;9:600.

137. Kalowski S, Radford N, Kincaid-Smith P. Crystalline and macrocrystalline nitrofurantoin in the treatment of urinary tract infection. *N Engl J Med* 1974;290:385.

138. Ernaelsteen D, Williams R. Jaundice due to nitrofurantoin. *Gastroenterology* 1961;41:590.

139. Black M, Rabin L, Schatz N. Nitrofurantoin-induced chronic active hepatitis. *Ann Intern Med* 1980;92:62.

140. Berson A, Freneaux E, Larrey D, et al. Possible role of HLA in hepatotoxicity. An exploratory study in 71 patients with drug-induced idiosyncratic hepatitis. *J Hepatol* 1994;20:336.

141. Hebert MF, Roberts JP. Endstage liver disease associated with nitrofurantoin requiring liver transplantation. *Ann Pharmacother* 1993;27:1193.

142. Nelis GF. Nitrofurantoin-induced pancreatitis: report of a case. *Gastroenterology* 1983;84:1032.

143. Christophe JL. Pancreatitis induced by nitrofurantoin. *Gut* 1994;35:712.

144. Pineura RF, Hartnett JS. Acute pulmonary reaction to nitrofurantoin. *Thorax* 1974;29:599.

145. Sovijari AR, Lemola M, Stenius B, et al. Nitrofurantoin induced acute subacute and chronic pulmonary reactions. *Scand J Respir Dis* 1977;58:41.

146. Holmberg L, Boman G, Bottiger LE, et al. Adverse reactions to nitrofurantoin: analysis of 921 reports. *Am J Med* 1980;69:733.

147. Martin WJ. Nitrofurantoin: potential direct and indirect mechanisms of lung injury. *Chest* 1983;83:51S.

148. Stefanin M. Chronic hemolytic anemia associated with erythrocyte deficiency exacerbated by ingestion of nitrofurantoin. *Am J Clin Pathol* 1972;58:408.

149. Steinberg M, Brauer MJ, Necheles TF. Acute hemolytic anemia associated with erythrocyte glutathione-peroxidase deficiency. *Arch Intern Med* 1970;125:302.

150. Levy S, Meyers BR, Mellin H. Reversible granulocytopenia in a patient with polycythemia vera taking nitrofurantoin. *J Mt Sinai Hosp* 1969;36:26.

151. Hakamies L. Die Nitrofurantoin-Polyneuropathie. *Schweiz Med Wochenschr* 1970;100:2212.

152. Thomson RG, James OF. Seventh-nerve palsy and hepatitis associated with nitrofurantoin. *Hum Toxicol* 1986;5:387.

153. Korzets A, Rathaus M, Chen B, et al. Pseudotumor cerebrii and nitrofurantoin (letter). *Drug Intell Clin Pharmacol* 1988;22:345.

154. Chapman JA. An unusual nitrofurantoin-induced drug reaction. *Ann Allergy* 1986;56:16.

155. Weiss J, Wein A, Jacobs J, et al. Use of nitrofurantoin macrocrystals after transurethral prostatectomy. *J Urol* 1983;130:479.

156. Harshberger SE, ed. *Medical pharmacology*. St. Louis: CV Mosby, 1984:605.

157. Kucers A. Bacitracin and gramicidin. In: Kucers A, Bennett NM, eds. *The use of antibiotics*, 4th ed. London: William Heinemann Medical Books, 1987:751–753.

158. Dudley MN, McLaughlin JC, Carrington G, et al. Oral bacitracin vs vancomycin therapy for *Clostridium difficile*-induced diarrhea. *Arch Intern Med* 1986;146:1101.

159. Zintel HA, Ma RA, Nicholas AC, et al. The absorption, distribution, excretion and toxicity of bacitracin in man. *Am J Med Sci* 1949;218:439.

160. Fischer AA. Adverse reactions to bacitracin, polymyxin and gentamicin sulfate. *Cutis* 1983;32:510.

161. Netland PA, Baumgartner JE, Andrews BT. Intraoperative anaphylaxis after irrigation with bacitracin: case report. *Neurosurgery* 1987;21:927.

162. Schechter JF, Wilkinson RD, DelCarpia J. Anaphylaxis following the use of bacitracin ointment. *Arch Dermatol* 1984;120:909.

163. Benjamin JB, Volz RG. Efficacy of a topical antibiotic irrigant in decreasing or eliminating bacterial contamination in surgical wounds. *Clin Orthop* 1984;184:114.

164. Cannon SC, Graham MD, Bojrab DI, et al. Use of bacitracin for neurotologic surgery. *Laryngoscope* 1988;98:1050.

165. Andrews BJ, Panitescu D, Jipa GH, et al. Chemotherapy for giardiasis: randomized clinical trial of acitretin, bacitracin zinc, and a combination of bacitracin zinc with neomycin. *Am J Trop Med Hyg* 1995;52:318.

166. Roccaforte JS, Bitner MJ, Stumpf CA, et al. Attempts to eradicate methicillin-resistant *Staphylococcus aureus* colonization with the use of trimethoprim-sulfamethoxazole, rifampin, and bacitracin. *Am J Infect Control* 1988;16:141.

167. Yu VL, Goetz A, Wagener M, et al. *Staphylococcus aureus* nasal carriage and infection in patients on hemodialysis. *N Engl J Med* 1986;315:91.

168. O'Donovan CA, Fan-Havard P, Tecson-Tumang FT, et al. Enteric eradication of vancomycin-resistant *Enterococcus faecium* with oral bacitracin. *Diagn Microbiol Infect Dis* 1994;18:105.

169. Linden PK. Treatment options for vancomycin-resistant enterococcal infections. *Drugs* 2002;62:425–441.

CHAPTER 31

Mechanisms of Bacterial Resistance to Antimicrobial Drugs

George M. Eliopoulos and Howard S. Gold

In response to the ongoing evolution of bacterial resistance traits, an impressive variety of antimicrobial compounds have been developed and introduced into clinical practice over the past several decades. Nevertheless, the continued emergence of increasingly resistant bacteria challenges both the ingenuity of medicinal chemists who seek to develop more effective agents and the skill of clinicians who wish to apply available antimicrobials to the best effect. To this end, a general understanding of microbial resistance mechanisms will assist the clinician in identifying situations in which standard laboratory methods may not reveal the full potential of drug resistance, in anticipating circumstances that favor the emergence of resistant strains during therapy, and in assessing the likelihood that alternative antimicrobials would prove useful against resistant bacterial isolates.

REQUIREMENTS FOR ANTIMICROBIAL ACTIVITY AND GENERAL MECHANISMS OF RESISTANCE

To understand bacterial resistance mechanisms, it is useful first to consider the properties of an antibiotic required for efficacy. Simply stated, the antibiotic must be able to (a) penetrate to the site of its normal molecular target in adequate amounts; (b) encounter

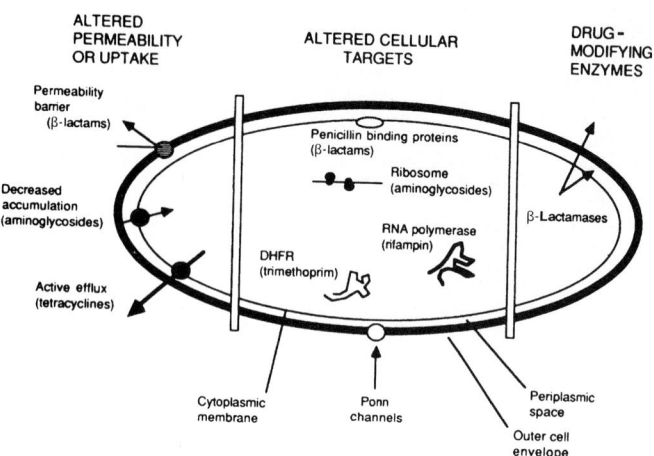

Figure 31.1. General mechanisms of bacterial resistance to antimicrobials. Examples are given of resistance mechanisms against representative antimicrobials (in parentheses) that may be encountered in gram-negative bacilli.

target molecules capable of interacting with the drug in such a manner as to initiate the desired antimicrobial effect; and (c) escape inactivation by intracellular or extracellular bacterial enzymes. Bacterial resistance mechanisms have evolved that can impede antibiotic efficacy at any of these steps (Fig. 31.1). First, because the principal targets of most antibiotics lie deep to the external surface of bacteria, any barrier to penetration of the drug through the bacterial cell wall can reduce activity. In some cases, intracellular accumulation of the antibiotic is reduced by efflux

TABLE 31.1. Antimicrobial Compounds and Their Resistance Mechanisms

Drug class	Resistance mechanism
β-lactams	Altered penicillin-binding proteins
	Reduced permeability
	β-lactamases
	Efflux
Glycopeptides	Altered peptidoglycan precursors
Aminoglycosides	Decreased ribosomal binding
	Reduced permeability or uptake
	Aminoglycoside-modifying enzymes
	Efflux
Macrolide-lincosamide	Decreased ribosomal binding
	Reduced permeability
	Enzymatic modification (various)
	Efflux
Chloramphenicol	Decreased ribosomal binding
	Reduced permeability
	Chloramphenicol acetyltransferase
	Efflux
Tetracyclines	Target (ribosome) protection
	Efflux
	Drug detoxification
Quinolones	Target (DNA gyrase and/or topoisomerase IV) resistance
	Reduced permeability
	Efflux
Rifampin	Reduced RNA polymerase binding
	Modification of drug
Inhibitors of folate synthesis	Dihydropteroate synthase or dihydrofolate reductase target resistance
	Reduced permeability
	Efflux

pumps, which actually remove drug that has already entered the cell. Second, the natural molecular targets may be altered in a way that reduces effective interaction with the antibiotic yet does not interfere with normal physiologic functions of the target molecules. Bacteria may also use alternative biochemical pathways, insensitive to drug action, that bypass the functions of the primary target. Finally, inactivating or modifying enzymes may act on the antimicrobial agent, rendering it ineffective. Frequently, interactions between two or more of these mechanisms may result in levels of resistance substantially greater than any one mechanism alone would achieve. These mechanisms of resistance are examined in detail as they relate to antimicrobial compounds in common use (Table 31.1).

RESISTANCE DUE TO ALTERED TARGET MOLECULES

β-Lactam Antibiotics

The targets of β-lactam antibiotics are penicillin binding proteins (PBPs) associated with the bacterial cytoplasmic membrane. The number (generally four to eight) and molecular sizes of PBPs vary with individual species (1,2). These proteins are involved in cell wall synthesis and remodeling. Individual β-lactams display differential binding to specific PBPs. Binding by β-lactams to essential PBP targets results in inhibition of cell growth and may culminate in cell death and lysis (2,3). Alterations of PBP targets have been implicated in resistance to β-lactam antibiotics in a number of important pathogens.

Resistance or relative resistance to penicillin among pneumococci is an important problem in the United States and elsewhere (4–8). In 1980 it was shown that stepwise transformation of DNA from a penicillin-resistant South African strain of *Streptococcus pneumoniae* [penicillin minimum inhibitory concentration (MIC) of 6.2 μg/mL] into a susceptible recipient pneumococcus (penicillin MIC of 0.06 μg/mL) resulted in a series of organisms with incremental increases in penicillin resistance associated with changes in PBP patterns to progressively resemble those of the donor strain (9). Multiple changes in PBPs resulting in reduced binding of penicillin thus account for penicillin resistance in pneumococci (2). Genes mediating production of reduced-affinity PBPs may have been acquired from other bacterial species by recombinational events (10). Reduced-affinity PBPs are also responsible for resistance to third-generation cephalosporins in some strains (11).

Methicillin resistance in *Staphylococcus aureus* results from a new PBP, termed PBP 2′ or PBP 2a, with markedly reduced binding affinities for β-lactams (12,13). Synthesis of this PBP is inducible in the presence of β-lactams (14–16). In the presence of β-lactams at concentrations fully inactivating other PBPs, PBP 2a retains critical synthetic functions necessary for cell survival. The structural gene for PBP 2a, *mecA*, is necessary but not sufficient to produce homogeneous high-level resistance to antistaphylococcal penicillins; auxiliary factors contribute to resistance (17–20). The *mecA* gene and low-affinity PBP 2a it specifies also account for the high rate of methicillin resistance among nosocomial isolates of coagulase-negative staphylococci (21–24).

Low-affinity PBP target molecules result in resistance to β-lactams among enterococci (25,26). Markedly reduced affinity of PBP 5 accounts for particularly high levels of resistance to penicillin encountered in *Enterococcus faecium*, with MICs sometimes reaching 500 μg/mL (25–29). The amino acid sequence of an enterococcal low-affinity PBP showed considerable similarity with the sequence of PBP 2a (30). β-Lactam resistance in various gram-negative bacteria, including *Neisseria gonorrhoeae*,

Neisseria meningitidis, Haemophilus influenzae, and *Pseudomonas aeruginosa,* has been related to altered PBP targets (2,31–35). The contribution of target site modifications to β-lactam resistance is more difficult to assess in gram-negative bacteria because β-lactamases, permeability barriers, and efflux mechanisms are common.

Glycopeptide Antibiotics

Vancomycin-resistant enterococci have emerged as a major clinical problem (36). The normal molecular target of this antibiotic is the D-alanine-D-alanine component of peptidoglycan precursors. In resistant strains, altered peptidoglycan target terminating in D-alanine-D-lactate or D-alanine-D-serine demonstrates substantially reduced binding affinity for vancomycin (37). In strains of *S. aureus* with reduced susceptibility to vancomycin, the target appears to be intact, but less accessible to glycopeptide by virtue of altered cell wall structure (38).

Aminoglycosides

Mutations or modification of ribosomal targets can result in resistance to aminoglycosides. For example, mutation in the *rpsL* gene results in alteration of a protein (S12) that controls binding of streptomycin to the 30S ribosomal subunit (39,40). Other mutations affecting a 16S ribosomal RNA gene confer resistance to streptomycin (41,42). Ribosomal resistance to streptomycin has been documented in clinical isolates of various species, including *N. gonorrhoeae* (43), *S. aureus* (44), *P. aeruginosa* (45), *Enterococcus faecalis* (46), and *Mycobacterium tuberculosis* (42,47). Ribosomal resistance to deoxystreptamine aminoglycosides (e.g., kanamycin or gentamicin) has been described but is probably uncommon among clinical isolates (48–52).

Macrolide-Lincosamide Antibiotics

Although barriers to penetration contribute to the intrinsic resistance of Enterobacteriaceae to erythromycin (53), macrolide resistance in gram-positive organisms results from alteration of the 50S ribosomal subunit target (or from efflux mechanisms). Target resistance commonly involves not only macrolides (erythromycin) but also antibiotics of the lincosamide (clindamycin, lincomycin) and streptogramin B classes and is thus referred to as MLS$_B$ resistance. The responsible *erm* genes are commonly found on transposons and plasmids (54–56). These resistance genes mediate production of methylase enzymes, which methylate adenine residues on 23S rRNA, thus rendering the ribosome resistant to the antibiotics (55,57). Resistance may be inducible or constitutive. Bacteria with inducible resistance often demonstrate dissociated resistance, appearing to be resistant to erythromycin (a good inducer) but susceptible to clindamycin; once resistance is induced, cells generally demonstrate resistance to other members of the MLS$_B$ class (58). The mechanism by which exposure to erythromycin results in methylase induction is termed translational attenuation. In the absence of erythromycin, the relevant mRNA is sequestered in a form not available for translation. Association of erythromycin with the ribosome complex induces a conformational change that yields a translationally active form of mRNA (58).

Mutations affecting 23S rRNA can result in resistance to macrolides and lincosamides alone or with streptogramins (59). Ribosomal resistance to lincosamides alone has been described (60). Rarely, alterations in ribosomal proteins lead to macrolide or macrolide-streptogramin B resistance (61).

Chloramphenicol

Resistance to chloramphenicol because of decreased binding of drug to bacterial 50S ribosomal subunits has been reported in laboratory mutants, but target site resistance does not appear to be common among clinical isolates (62).

Tetracyclines

Resistance to tetracycline at the level of ribosomal protein synthesis is associated with acquisition of any of several genes such as *tet* (M) (63). The presence of this gene product protects ribosomal protein synthesis from inhibition by tetracyclines (64). The *tet* (M) gene has been found in various gram-positive and gram-negative bacteria and confers resistance to tetracycline in *Ureaplasma urealyticum* and *Mycoplasma hominis* as well (65–67).

Quinolones

The principal targets of quinolone antimicrobials are the enzymes DNA gyrase (topoisomerase II) and topoisomerase IV (68). Mutations in genes coding for these proteins confer resistance to inhibition by quinolones (69). Efflux pumps or permeability barriers may contribute to levels of resistance seen; in *S. aureus*, inhibitory activities of various quinolones on partially purified gyrase parallel growth-inhibitory activities of the drugs (70). With the introduction of fluoroquinolones into hospital environments, resistance in *S. aureus*, especially among methicillin-resistant strains, emerged in a large proportion of isolates (71–73).

Rifampin

Antimicrobial activity of rifampin requires binding of the drug to the β subunit of RNA polymerase. Single-step mutations resulting in single amino acid substitutions occur with moderate frequency (approximately 10^{-8} in *Escherichia coli*). Resulting polymerases vary in degree of sensitivity to rifampin and in levels of resistance conferred (74).

Folate Pathway Inhibitors

Target alterations confer resistance to sulfonamides and trimethoprim. Resistance typically results from acquisition of genes mediating drug-resistant enzymes rather than from mutations affecting chromosomal genes. Low-affinity dihydropteroate synthases mediate sulfonamide resistance. Genetic determinants for these occur on transposons and plasmids with a broad host range, which permits efficient dissemination among bacteria (75).

Several dihydrofolate reductases with reduced sensitivity to inhibition by trimethoprim have been described, genes for which can also be acquired via resistance plasmids and transposons (76–78). In some species (e.g., *Bacteroides, Clostridium, Neisseria, Moraxella,* and *Nocardia*), intrinsic insensitivity of the native dihydrofolate reductase to trimethoprim contributes to drug resistance (76). Trimethoprim resistance due to overproduction of structurally altered chromosomal enzyme has been described in laboratory mutants and some clinical isolates (76,79,80). Mutational loss of thymidylate synthase activity, with the resulting requirement for exogenous thymine or thymidine, can uncommonly result in trimethoprim resistance (80).

RESISTANCE DUE TO PERMEABILITY BARRIERS OR DIMINISHED DRUG UPTAKE OR ACCUMULATION

β-Lactams

Studies with *E. coli* demonstrated that water-filled transmembrane pores created by outer membrane proteins (especially those designated OmpF and OmpC) serve as a major route by which β-lactams, and cephalosporins in particular, traverse the lipid-rich outer membrane of gram-negative bacteria (81). The rate of antibiotic penetration through these porin protein channels depends on the physical characteristics of each drug (82). Laboratory mutants of Enterobacteriaceae selected for β-lactam resistance may demonstrate diminished amounts of OmpF or other putative porin proteins. Such permeability mutants often demonstrate small increases in resistance to other antibiotics as well; higher levels of resistance to other antimicrobials such as aminoglycosides, chloramphenicol, tetracyclines, trimethoprim, or quinolones most likely reflect pleiotropic mutations rather than porin deficiency alone (83–85).

The activity of imipenem is often preserved against porin-deficient mutants, probably because its compact zwitterionic structure permits rapid penetration, it is inherently β-lactamase stable, and the limited number of primary targets PBP 2 require that only a few drug molecules penetrate (86). Because defects in cell permeability retard but do not prevent penetration of β-lactams, significant increases in resistance typically require the contribution of additional resistance mechanisms such as periplasmic β-lactamases, efflux, or target alterations (87). Diminished permeability through the outer membrane contributes to intrinsic and acquired β-lactam resistance in *P. aeruginosa* (82,88,89). Imipenem resistance emerges relatively commonly when this antibiotic is used alone to treat *P. aeruginosa* infections (90). Impaired penetration of the carbapenem is associated with loss of specific outer membrane channels consisting of trimers of a protein termed OprD, which is selective for small zwitterionic compounds (82,91–93). Active efflux mechanisms also contribute to β-lactam resistance in this species (94).

Aminoglycosides

Factors impeding penetration of aminoglycosides to their ribosomal target sites are complex. Resistance to multiple aminoglycosides has been associated with loss or reduction of outer membrane proteins in Enterobacteriaceae (95) or even with the appearance of new outer membrane proteins in *P. aeruginosa* (96). In the latter species, alterations in surface lipopolysaccharide composition may affect intracellular uptake of aminoglycosides (97). Amikacin-resistant strains of *P. aeruginosa* arising during treatment with this aminoglycoside demonstrate impaired intracellular uptake of the drug (98). Studies with "small colony variant" strains of aminoglycoside-resistant *P. aeruginosa* recovered from experimental animals failing to respond to therapy reveal defective aminoglycoside uptake like that seen in normal cells poisoned with cyanide (99). Such strains generate inadequate transmembrane electrical potentials compared with normal isolates of *P. aeruginosa*. Generation of transmembrane electrical gradients is also important for the uptake of aminoglycosides in *S. aureus* (100); small colony variants of this species also show defective uptake of aminoglycosides (101). One strain of *E. faecalis* has been described that displayed a specific transport defect for gentamicin (but not tobramycin), resulting in failure of penicillin-gentamicin synergism (102).

Macrolides

Intrinsic low-level resistance to erythromycin in Enterobacteriaceae can be attributed to limited drug permeability. Enhanced penetration of nonionized drugs at alkaline pH results in greater antimicrobial activity under these conditions (53,54). Active efflux is now recognized as a major mechanism of resistance to macrolides in a wide variety of organisms, including pneumococci, group A streptococci, enterococci, and some staphylococci (103–105).

Chloramphenicol

Reduced intracellular penetration of chloramphenicol has been described in several bacterial species, sometimes associated with loss of specific outer membrane proteins or altered lipopolysaccharide patterns (62,106,107). Efflux systems for removal of chloramphenicol from the cell have been demonstrated in both gram-positive and gram-negative bacteria (64,108,109).

Tetracyclines

Although mutations affecting outer membrane (porin) proteins or surface lipopolysaccharides of gram-negative bacteria have been associated with reduced activities of hydrophilic (tetracycline) or lipophilic (minocycline) tetracycline analogs, respectively, efflux systems are important in determining ultimate levels of intracellular accumulation of tetracyclines (63,110–112). Tetracycline efflux systems may be either chromosomal or plasmid mediated (104).

Quinolones

Resistance to fluoroquinolones in gram-negative bacteria can result from decreased expression of major outer membrane proteins (e.g., ompF) and by active efflux (113–121). Inhibition of a *P. aeruginosa* multidrug-resistance efflux pump not only enhances fluoroquinolone activity against test strains, but also decreases the frequency at which resistant mutants are selected (120). Active efflux also contributes to fluoroquinolone resistance in gram-positive organisms, including *S. aureus* and *S. pneumoniae* (69,121). When expressed in *B. subtilis*, the NorA membrane efflux protein of *S. aureus* conferred resistance to fluoroquinolones and unrelated antibiotics including chloramphenicol and puromycin (121).

Folate Pathway Inhibitors

Permeability barriers to trimethoprim occur intrinsically in *P. aeruginosa*. This may result from overexpression of multidrug efflux systems such as MexEF-OprN (117). In Enterobacteriaceae, resistance is associated with diminished levels of putative porin proteins and pleiotropic resistance to drugs of other antimicrobial classes (76,84,95). Intrinsic or acquired resistance to sulfonamides in gram-negative organisms may also result from decreased intracellular penetration (122).

Resistance to Multiple Antibiotics

In some cases, mutations affecting a single genetic locus may result in changes in susceptibility to several unrelated antimicrobials. One such locus, termed *mar* (multiple antibiotic resistance), appears to control expression of resistance to multiple antibiotics, including chloramphenicol, tetracycline, fluoroquinolones, and β-lactams (123). With such mutations, evidence of both increased efflux and decreased drug penetration (reduced OmpF) can be observed (124). When *E. coli mar* mutants selected on exposure to low concentrations of chloramphenicol or tetracycline were subsequently exposed to norfloxacin, substantially higher frequencies of resistance to norfloxacin were observed (approximately 10^{-7}) as compared with exposure of the initial wild-type isolate to the fluoroquinolone, in which case resistant mutants were rarely observed (less than 10^{-9}) (125). Such phenomena, involving simultaneous activation of multiple resistance determinants with cross-resistance to unrelated classes of antimicrobials, illustrates the enormous complexity of antibiotic resistance mechanisms in gram-negative bacteria.

RESISTANCE DUE TO INACTIVATION OF ANTIMICROBIALS

β-Lactam Antibiotics

Inactivation of β-lactams by enzymatic hydrolysis of the β-lactam ring is the most common and best-understood mechanism of resistance to this class of drugs. By a recent count, 340 of these enzymes have been described, produced by various bacteria, differing in substrate profiles, potential for inhibition, and physical characteristics (126,127). Several classification schemes have been proposed, the most recent and comprehensive of which was developed by Bush, Jacoby, and Medeiros (126,128). This method divides β-lactamases into four major groups based largely on their antibiotic substrates and inhibition profiles (Table 31.2). The relationships between these enzymes are further elucidated using phylogenetic trees based on amino acid and nucleotide sequences (128).

GRAM-POSITIVE BACTERIA

β-lactamase–mediated resistance to penicillins among gram-positive cocci (Bush-Jacoby-Medeiros group 2a) is exemplified by the exoenzymes of *S. aureus* (129,130). These enzymes and those of coagulase-negative staphylococci are less active against cephalosporins and antistaphylococcal penicillins than they are against penicillin G, and they are inhibited by β-lactamase inhibitors such as clavulanic acid, sulbactam, and tazobactam. Al-

though penicillinase-producing enterococci were first described in 1983, they remain exceedingly uncommon (131,132). Molecular studies suggest that genetic determinants of this enzyme arose in staphylococci (133). Other β-lactamases have been described in various gram-positive bacilli, but such stains are relatively uncommon human pathogens.

GRAM-NEGATIVE BACTERIA

Numerous β-lactamases have been described in gram-negative organisms, including plasmid-encoded and chromosomally determined enzymes. The former are important because of their potential for dissemination, whereas the latter have contributed to β-lactam resistance among troublesome nosocomial pathogens such as *P. aeruginosa* and *Enterobacter* species.

Inducible, Chromosomally Mediated Enzymes. In most clinical isolates of *P. aeruginosa, Enterobacter, Citrobacter, Serratia*, and several other species of gram-negative bacilli, chromosomally mediated β-lactamases (primarily cephalosporinases, designated group 1) are produced at extremely low levels unless organisms are exposed to β-lactams. Alternatively, selection of stably derepressed mutant hyperproducers of β-lactamase can occur. The activity of a particular antimicrobial agent reflects its capacity to induce enzyme production, its vulnerability to hydrolysis by that β-lactamase, and its ability to penetrate to its target. At the extremely low antibiotic concentrations calculated to exist in the periplasmic space of organisms with intact permeability barriers, these β-lactamases can effectively hydrolyze relatively stable third-generation cephalosporins, hence the incrementally superior activity of the even more stable and rapidly penetrating fourth-generation agents like cefepime (134,135). The emergence of resistance to third-generation cephalosporins among gram-negative species with inducible chromosomal β-lactamases is a significant clinical problem.

Plasmid-Mediated β-Lactamases. Plasmid-mediated penicillin-hydrolyzing enzymes of the type designated TEM have long been recognized as a common cause of resistance to ampicillin among various gram-negative bacteria, including *E. coli, H. influenzae*, and *N. gonorrhoeae*. Also common are the SHV

TABLE 31.2. Classification of β-Lactamases

Enzyme class	Characteristics	Examples
Group 1	Cephalosporinases not inhibited by clavulanic acid or EDTA	Chromosomal enzymes of *Pseudomonas aeruginosa, Enterobacter cloacae*, plasmid-encoded AmpC enzymes
Groups 2a–2f	Penicillinases and/or cephalosporinases inhibited by clavulanic acid[a], but not by EDTA	Plasmid-mediated TEM type including ESBLs; staphylococcal penicillinase and *Klebsiella oxytoca* chromosomal enzyme
Group 3a–c	Metalloenzymes, inhibited by EDTA, but not by clavulanic acid	Imipenem-hydrolyzing enzyme of *Stenotrophomonas maltophilia*, plasmid-encoded carbapenemases of *Bacteroides fragilis*
Group 4	Penicillinases not inhibited by clavulanic acid	Chromosomal enzyme of *Burkholderia cepacia*

[a]Some representatives are resistant to inhibition by clavulanate, such as Bush-Jacoby-Medeiros group 2br (IRT) and group 2d (OXA).
EDTA, ethylenediamine tetraacetic acid; ESBL, extended-spectrum β-lactamase.
Data from references 126 and 128.

β-lactamases, derived from the chromosomally-mediated enzyme of *Klebsiella pneumoniae*. Both TEM and SHV are members of group 2. The development of β-lactamase–stable second- and third-generation cephalosporins, as well as the β-lactam/β-lactamase inhibitor combinations offered alternatives against strains bearing common plasmid-mediated enzymes. However, an ever-growing number of plasmid-encoded β-lactamases can confer resistance to these agents (136).

Extended-Spectrum β-Lactamases.

Beginning in the early 1980s, several plasmid-mediated β-lactamases were recognized that conferred resistance to third-generation cephalosporins (137). For the most part, these enzymes belong to the TEM or SHV families, with as little as a single nucleotide mutation producing minor alterations in amino acid sequences that confer marked changes in substrate specificity (138,139).

Currently more than 100 such enzymes, classified as group 2be, have been identified (*www.lahey.org/studies/webt.htm*). Genes mediating their production tend to occur on large plasmids (encoding additional resistance determinants) that are often transferable (140). Numerous outbreaks of infection or colonization with such organisms have occurred in the United States and abroad (141–146). Of note, there is marked geographic variability in prevalence of strains, and isolates from non-ICU areas tend to show less resistance than those from ICUs (*www.cdc.gov/ncidod/hip/NNIS/DEC2000SAR.PDF*).

Resistance to β-Lactamase Inhibitors.

In the late 1980s, several isolates of *E. coli* were encountered that produced TEM-1 β-lactamase (which should have been susceptible to inhibition by β-lactamase inhibitors) that were resistant to the combination of amoxicillin-clavulanate. These isolates were found to produce the enzyme at levels up to 30-fold greater than those of typical enzyme-producing strains, mediated by genes localized on small, multicopy plasmids (147). Porin mutations, when combined with production of TEM-1, contribute to resistance to inhibitor combinations as well (148). Subsequently, strains of *E. coli* were identified that produced a TEM-related enzyme that was relatively insensitive to inhibition by β-lactamase inhibitors. Like the TEM- and SHV-derived extended-spectrum β-lactamases, these inhibitor-resistant TEM enzymes are the result of a relatively limited number of mutations (149).

Plasmid-Mediated "Chromosomal" β-Lactamases.

An extremely broad-spectrum enzyme that was plasmid mediated and insensitive to inhibition by the standard β-lactamase inhibitors was identified in *K. pneumoniae* and designated MIR-1 (150). Partial sequencing of the responsible gene demonstrated approximately 90% identity to the chromosomal *ampC* cephalosporinase of *E. cloacae*. In addition to those that show similarity to *Enterobacter* β-lactamases, other plasmid-encoded group 1 enzymes bear marked homology to *Citrobacter freundii*, *Morganella morganii*, and *Hafnia alvei* chromosomal enzymes, and lesser degrees of homology to other gram-negative bacilli (*www.rochester.edu/College/BIO/labs/HallLab*). As a group, they exemplify the transfer of chromosomal resistance genes into plasmids, increasing the possibility of subsequent dissemination. Plasmid-encoded AmpC β-lactamases represent an emerging mechanism of resistance with an expanding list of enzymes in this family. It is of particular concern that Enterobacteriaceae producing these enzymes in the presence of porin mutations may manifest resistance even to carbapenems (151).

Other Cephalosporinases.

In addition to those mentioned above, a variety of other enzymes hydrolyze cephalosporins. The CTX-M β-lactamases (in group 2be), so-named for their efficient hydrolysis of cefotaxime, are primarily found in *Salmonella enterica* and *E. coli* in South America and Europe (136). OXA enzymes (group 2d) comprise a somewhat heterogeneous group of inhibitor-resistant β-lactamases that preferentially hydrolyze oxacillin. Some of these also confer cephalosporin resistance in *E. coli* and *Klebsiella pneumoniae*, as well as other Enterobacteriaceae (136).

Carbapenemases.

Chromosomal β-lactamases of *P. aeruginosa* and possibly *Enterobacter* species contribute only to a slight degree to carbapenem resistance. In contrast, zinc metalloenzymes (group 3) found in *Stenotrophomonas* (formerly *Xanthomonas*) *maltophilia* and *Aeromonas* species contribute substantially to resistance (152). Chromosomal carbapenem-hydrolyzing enzymes have been encountered in rare isolates of *Serratia marcescens* and *E. cloacae* (153–155). These group 2f enzymes share considerable amino acid sequence identity and have a serine active site type. Carbapenem-hydrolyzing metalloenzymes resembling those of *Aeromonas*, *Bacillus cereus*, and *Bacteroides fragilis* have been found to be encoded by plasmids in isolates of *P. aeruginosa*, *S. marcescens*, and *K. pneumoniae* (153,156,157).

Aminoglycosides

Enzymatic modification of aminoglycosides is achieved by acetylation of vulnerable amino groups or by adenylylation or phosphorylation of hydroxyl groups on these compounds (158). Differences in susceptibilities of various aminoglycosides to modifying enzymes depend on the presence or absence of such vulnerable groups and whether these are accessible to the enzyme in three-dimensional conformation. Genetic elements mediating production of aminoglycoside-modifying enzymes are usually plasmid mediated but may exist on the bacterial chromosome as well. Several genes are transposon mediated (159-161). Enzymes are produced constitutively, although multiplication of gene copy number, with increased levels of resistance, can occur. Several distinct modifying enzymes have been described (162–164). For example, at least nine genes have been identified to date yielding enzymes that acetylate 2-deoxystreptamine aminoglycosides at the 6' position alone (165). Production of an aminoglycoside-modifying enzyme does not necessarily render bacteria resistant to a modifiable drug. For example, *E. coli* producing 2″-adenylyltransferase and *S. aureus* producing 3'-phosphotransferase may remain susceptible *in vitro* to netilmicin and amikacin, respectively, despite the ability to demonstrate modification of the aminoglycoside in each case (164,166). Susceptibility appears to depend on a balance of opposing forces: the efficiency of drug inactivation versus the effectiveness of inhibitory or bactericidal drug activity. Other bacterial cell factors, such as the level of drug accumulation, can markedly affect phenotypic expression of plasmid-mediated aminoglycoside-resistance determinants (167). In enterococci, the presence of aminoglycoside-modifying enzymes may confer resistance to penicillin-aminoglycoside bactericidal synergism even when levels of enzyme activity are not sufficient to raise minimal inhibitory concentrations above those for strains lacking enzyme activity (168).

Several aminoglycoside-modifying enzymes may be present simultaneously within a single organism. For example, among recent isolates of *E. faecium*, it would not be uncommon to encounter high-level streptomycin resistance based on nucleotidyl-transferase, chromosomal 6'-acetyltransferase inherent to the species, plasmid (transposon)-mediated resistance to gentamicin and other deoxystreptamine aminoglycosides based on the bifunctional 6'-acetyltransferase-2''-phosphotransferase enzyme, and additional kanamycin- and amikacin-modifying activity due to a 3'-phosphotransferase (165,169).

It may not always be possible to deduce susceptibility to aminoglycoside-modifying enzymes based on the presence or absence of groups vulnerable to modification. In one example, overproduction of a 3'-phosphotransferase in *E. coli* led to low-level tobramycin resistance despite the absence of a vulnerable 3'-hydroxyl group on tobramycin (170). It was postulated that resistance resulted from sequestration of the aminoglycoside due to formation of a heat-labile complex between the enzyme and aminoglycoside.

MLS Antimicrobials

Inactivation of MLS class antimicrobials has been reported in both gram-positive and gram-negative organisms (54,105). Erythromycin esterases, which hydrolyze the antibiotic lactone ring, have been encountered among clinical isolates of *E. coli, K. pneumoniae,* and *Enterobacter agglomerans*. Genetic determinants of these enzymes are plasmid borne. Presence of the enzymes confers levels of resistance that are substantially higher than can be attributed to the intrinsic low-level resistance to erythromycin among Enterobacteriaceae (51,171,172). Erythromycin esterase genes may coexist with ribosome modification (ribosomal RNA methylase) genes in enteric bacteria (173). A macrolide 2'-phosphotransferase has also been detected in *E. coli* (174). Staphylococcal lincosamide-modifying enzymes (4-lincosamide -O-nucleotidyltransferases) have been described that fully inactivate lincomycin but confer only relative resistance to clindamycin. The latter is manifested only by high minimum bactericidal concentrations or decreased inhibitory activity when tested against high bacterial inocula (175). Genetic elements mediating enzymes that inactivate streptogramin A and B drugs have been encountered in gram-positive bacteria (105,173,176).

Chloramphenicol

Drug inactivation is the major mechanism of resistance to chloramphenicol among gram-positive organisms. Chloramphenicol acetyltransferase production is plasmid mediated and inducible in *S. aureus* (62). Similar enzymes are found in enterococci, pneumococci and other streptococci, clostridia, and *Bacillus* species. In gram-negative organisms, chloramphenicol acetyltransferase genes are often plasmid borne and located on transposable elements. Studies in enterococci have shown that acetylation occurs at the 3-hydroxyl position. Nonenzymatic transfer of the acetyl group to the 1 position follows, and the resulting 1-acetyl-chloramphenicol is subject to repeated acetylation at the 3 position (177). Fluorinated chloramphenicol analogs, which resist enzymatic inactivation, have been synthesized but not further developed because of the limited practical utility of such compounds (178).

Tetracycline and Rifampin

A *B. fragilis* transposon has been encountered that mediates tetracycline resistance both by promoting active drug efflux and by drug detoxification (179). Detoxification occurs via an NADP-requiring oxidoreductase (180). Minocycline, doxycycline, and other tetracycline analogs are subject to the detoxification pathway described. The clinical significance of such resistance mechanisms, if any, is unknown (181). Modification of rifampin to yield inactive compounds has been reported in *Nocardia* species and several *Mycobacterium* isolates (182).

ANTIMICROBIAL CROSS-RESISTANCE

Because members of any one antimicrobial class often share common targets and similar susceptibilities to inactivation, it is not surprising that bacteria often demonstrate extensive cross-resistance to several agents of a class. In some situations, cross-resistance may not be apparent by routine susceptibility testing. For example methicillin resistance in staphylococci may not be detected by standard susceptibility tests with cephalosporins (183). In other cases, resistance to one antimicrobial agent may signal decreased susceptibility but not absolute resistance to other members of the class. For example, compared with strains that are fully susceptible to nalidixic acid, nalidixic acid–resistant Enterobacteriaceae tend to display higher MICs against newer fluoroquinolones even though these often remain within the susceptible range (184).

Cross-resistance also occurs between antibiotics of different classes. In gram-negative bacteria, permeability or efflux mutants sometimes demonstrate resistance to diverse agents such as quinolones, trimethoprim, and chloramphenicol (117,123,124,185).

Simultaneous resistance to two or more drug classes can result from acquisition of multiple resistance elements or of a single transmissible element with multiple resistance genes. Genes encoding β-lactamases and aminoglycoside-modifying enzymes may coexist on plasmids or transposons (141,186). Mostly studied in Enterobacteriaceae, integrons represent another system by which organisms accumulate multiple resistance genes. These elements can contain one or more resistance gene cassettes under control of a common promoter. A broad variety of genes mediating resistance to β-lactams, aminoglycosides, chloramphenicol, trimethoprim, and other agents have been detected on such elements (187). As exemplified by *M. tuberculosis*, multiple drug resistance in individual isolates can result from the accumulation of chromosomal mutations, each affecting a specific antibiotic resistance gene. Multiple drug resistance can also occur through a combination of chromosomal mutational events and acquisition of exogenous resistance genes as seen in penicillin-resistant pneumococci, many isolates of which also demonstrate resistance to trimethoprim-sulfamethoxazole, chloramphenicol, and tetracycline. As a result, selective pressure based on extensive use of one antimicrobial may promote continued resistance to drugs of other classes, even if use of those is restricted.

STRATEGIES TO REDUCE ANTIMICROBIAL RESISTANCE

Antibiotic Combinations

The use of two or more antimicrobials in combination to prevent bacterial resistance and clinical treatment failure is exemplified by multidrug regimens in the treatment of tuberculosis. Such combinations have proved highly effective, even though resistance to individual components of the regimens develops rapidly when they are used as single agents (188,189). The success of this approach rests on the mathematic improbability that mutational resistance to two or more drugs would develop simultaneously in a single bacterial colony.

Rifampin is a drug with excellent activity against a variety of bacterial pathogens but to which resistance develops rapidly.

Rifampin has been used in combination with other agents against nonmycobacterial infections. For example, rifampin-vancomycin combinations have proved effective in the treatment of prosthetic valve endocarditis due to coagulase-negative staphylococci (190). It is now clear, however, that coadministration of a second antimicrobial may not completely prevent the development of rifampin resistance. This incomplete protection may result from differential penetration of the antibiotics deeply into tissues or into phagocytic cells that harbor viable bacteria (168).

Antibiotic combinations, particularly β-lactams plus aminoglycosides, have been widely used in the treatment of serious gram-negative bacillary infections, at least in part in an attempt to minimize the development of resistance to either component (168). This approach is supported by animal studies and some but not all clinical trials (191). The value of adding an aminoglycoside (with its attendant cost and toxicities) to a highly potent β-lactam would be difficult to demonstrate unequivocally in most clinical situations. Still, many clinicians strongly favor the use of such combinations in treating serious gram-negative infections, especially in neutropenic or otherwise immunocompromised patients and particularly when infection is due to *P. aeruginosa* (168). In such cases, any benefits might result from synergistic bactericidal activity rather than prevention of resistance.

The strategy of using antimicrobial combinations to delay the emergence of resistance to individual agents is predicated on the assumption that resistance to one agent occurs with a probability independent of resistance to the other. As discussed in the preceding section, this is often not the case. Acquisition of resistance to two or more drugs simultaneously can arise in a number of ways, limiting the usefulness of this strategy.

Minimization of Selective Pressure

Although for the individual patient appropriately aggressive use of antibiotic therapy targeted at a specific pathogen is likely to reduce the risk of microbial drug resistance, there is substantial evidence that extensive antibiotic use promotes the selection, propagation, and maintenance of drug-resistant microorganisms, especially in the hospital environment (145,192–194). Particularly striking in this regard has been the experience with the liberal use of topical aminoglycoside (gentamicin) in burn units, which has resulted in outbreaks of colonization with gentamicin-resistant strains of *P. aeruginosa* (195). In this and other examples, restricted use of the antimicrobial has dramatically decreased isolation rates of resistant microorganisms (195). It is important to note, however, that the recognition of a serious institutional problem with antibiotic-resistant pathogens, leading to severe restrictions on the use of antimicrobials, is also likely to enhance awareness of and compliance with other infection control measures. The appropriate use of measures such as barrier precautions has been demonstrated to be effective in decreasing colonization of patients with nosocomial pathogens (196) and would contribute substantially to any beneficial effect of antibiotic restriction alone.

Given that the use of antibiotics for surgical prophylaxis accounts for a significant fraction of total antibiotic use in many hospitals, prophylactic regimens should adhere to accepted standards relating to antimicrobial spectrum (i.e., avoiding overly broad regimens) and duration of administration (197).

REFERENCES

1. Eliopoulos GM, Wennersten C, Moellering RC Jr. Resistance to β-lactam antibiotics in *Streptococcus faecium*. *Antimicrob Agents Chemother* 1982;22:295.
2. Georgopapadakou NH. Penicillin-binding proteins and bacterial resistance to β-lactams. *Antimicrob Agents Chemother* 1993;37:2045.
3. Malouin F, Bryan LE. Modification of penicillin-binding proteins as mechanisms of β-lactam resistance. *Antimicrob Agents Chemother* 1986;30:1, 1986.
4. Haglund LA, Istre GR, Pickett DA, et al. Invasive pneumococcal disease in central Oklahoma: emergence of high-level penicillin resistance and multiple antibiotic resistance. *J Infect Dis* 1993;168:1532.
5. Doern GV, Heilmann KP, Huynh HK, et al. Antimicrobial resistance among clinical isolates of *Streptococcus pneumoniae* in the United States during 1999–2000, including a comparison of resistance rates since 1994–1995. *Antimicrob Agents Chemother* 2001;45:1721.
6. Scares S, Kristinsson KG, Musser JM, et al. Evidence for the introduction of a multiresistant clone of serotype 6B *Streptococcus pneumoniae* from Spain to Iceland in the late 1980s. *J Infect Dis* 1993;168:158.
7. Muñoz R, Coffey TJ, Daniels M, et al. Intercontinental spread of a multiresistant clone of serotype 23F *Streptococcus pneumoniae*. *J Infect Dis* 1991;164:302.
8. Marton A, Gulyas M, Muñoz R, et al. Extremely high incidence of antibiotic resistance in clinical isolates of *Streptococcus pneumoniae* in Hungary. *J Infect Dis* 1991;163:542.
9. Zighelboim S, Tomasz A. Penicillin-binding proteins of multiply antibiotic-resistant South African strains of *Streptococcus pneumoniae*. *Antimicrob Agents Chemother* 1980;17:434.
10. Spratt BG. Resistance to antibiotics mediated by target alterations. *Science* 1994;264:388.
11. Figueiredo AMS, Connor JD, Severin A, et al. A pneumococcal clinical isolate with high-level resistance to cefotaxime and ceftriaxone. *Antimicrob Agents Chemother* 1992;36:886.
12. Hartman BJ, Tomasz A. Low-affinity penicillin-binding protein associated with β-lactam resistance in *Staphylococcus aureus*. *J Bacteriol* 1984;158:513.
13. Chambers HF, Sachdeva M. Binding of β-lactam antibiotics to penicillin-binding proteins in methicillin-resistant *Staphylococcus aureus*. *J Infect Dis* 1990;161:1170.
14. Ubukata K, Yamashita N, Konno M. Occurrence of a β-lactam–inducible penicillin-binding protein in methicillin-resistant staphylococci. *Antimicrob Agents Chemother* 1985;27:851.
15. Chambers HF, Hartman BJ, Tomasz A. Increased amounts of a novel penicillin-binding protein in a strain of methicillin-resistant *Staphylococcus aureus* exposed to nafcillin. *J Clin Invest* 1985;76:325.
16. Hackbarth CJ, Chambers HF. blal and blaR1 regulate β-lactamase and PBP 2a production in methicillin-resistant *Staphylococcus aureus*. *Antimicrob Agents Chemother* 1993;37:1144.
17. Murakami K, Tomasz A. Involvement of multiple genetic determinants in high-level methicillin resistance in *Staphylococcus aureus*. *J Bacteriol* 1989;171:874.
18. Hackbarth CJ, Miick C, Chambers HF. Altered production of penicillin-binding protein 2a can affect phenotypic expression of methicillin-resistance in *Staphylococcus aureus*. *Antimicrob Agents Chemother* 1994;38:2568.
19. Gustafson J, Strässle A, Hächler H, et al. The femC locus of *Staphylococcus aureus* required for methicillin resistance includes the glutamine synthetase operon. *J Bacteriol* 1994;176:1460.
20. Chambers HF. Methicillin resistance in staphylococci: molecular and biochemical basis and clinical implications. *Clin Microbiol Rev* 1997;10:781.
21. Trees DL, Iandolo JJ. Identification of a *Staphylococcus aureus* transposon (Tn4291) that carries the methicillin resistance gene(s). *J Bacteriol* 1988;170:149.
22. Chambers HF. Coagulase-negative staphylococci resistant to β-lactam antibiotics *in vivo* produce penicillin-binding protein 2A. *Antimicrob Agents Chemother* 1987;31:1919.
23. Tesch W, Strässle A, Berger-Bachi B, et al. Cloning and expression of methicillin resistance from *Staphylococcus epidermidis* in *Staphylococcus carnosus*. *Antimicrob Agents Chemother* 1988;32:1494.
24. Archer GL, Climo MW. Antimicrobial susceptibility of coagulase-negative staphylococci. *Antimicrob Agents Chemother* 1994;38:2231.
25. Fontana R, Cerini R, Longoni P, et al. Identification of a streptococcal penicillin-binding protein that reacts very slowly with penicillin. *J Bacteriol* 1983;155:1343.
26. Williamson R, LeBouguenec C, Gutmann L, et al. One or two low affinity penicillin-binding proteins may be responsible for the range of susceptibility of *Enterococcus faecium* to benzylpenicillin. *J Gen Microbiol* 1985;131:1933.
27. Grayson ML, Eliopoulos GM, Wennersten CB, et al. Increasing resistance to β-lactam antibiotics among clinical isolates of *Enterococcus faecium*: a 22-year review of one institution. *Antimicrob Agents Chemother* 1991;35:2180.
28. Klare I, Rodloff AC, Wagner J, et al. Overproduction of a penicillin-binding protein is not the only mechanism of penicillin resistance in *Enterococcus faecium*. *Antimicrob Agents Chemother* 1992;36:783.
29. Fontana R, Aldegheri M. Ligozzi M, et al. Overproduction of a low-affinity penicillin-binding protein and high-level ampicillin resistance in *Enterococcus faecium*. *Antimicrob Agents Chemother* 1994;38:1980.
30. Piras G, El Kharroubi A, van Beeumen J, et al. Characterization of an *Enterococcus hirae* penicillin-binding protein 3 with low penicillin affinity. *J Bacteriol* 1990;172:6856.
31. Godfrey AJ, Bryan LE, Rabin HR. β-Lactam-resistant *Pseudomonas aeruginosa* with modified penicillin-binding proteins emerging during cystic fibrosis treatment. *Antimicrob Agents Chemother* 1981;19:705.
32. Dougherty TJ. Involvement of a change in penicillin target and peptidoglycan structure in low-level resistance to β-lactam antibiotics in *Neisseria gonorrhoeae*. *Antimicrob Agents Chemother* 1985;28:90.

33. Mendelman PM, Chaffin DO, Stull TL, et al. Characterization of non-β-lactamase–mediated ampicillin resistance in *Haemophilus influenzae*. *Antimicrob Agents Chemother* 1984;26:235.

34. Parr TR Jr, Bryan LE. Mechanisms of resistance of an ampicillin-resistant, β-lactamase-negative clinical isolate of *Haemophilus influenzae* type b to β-lactam antibiotics. *Antimicrob Agents Chemother* 1984;25:747.

35. Spratt BG, Cromie KD. Penicillin-binding proteins of gram-negative bacteria. *Rev Infect Dis* 1988;10:699.

36. Gold HS. Vancomycin-resistant enterococci: mechanisms and clinical observations. *Clin Infect Dis* 2001;33:210.

37. Arthur M, Courvalin P. Genetics and mechanisms of glycopeptide resistance in enterococci. *Antimicrob Agents Chemother* 1993;37:1563.

38. Tenover FC, Biddle JW, Lancaster MV. Increasing resistance to vancomycin and other glycopeptides in *Staphylococcus aureus*. *Emerg Infect Dis* 2001;7:327.

39. Hancock REW. Aminoglycoside uptake and mode of action with special reference to streptomycin and gentamicin. *J Antimicrob Chemother* 1981;8:249.

40. Bryan LE. General mechanisms of resistance to antibiotics. *J Antimicrob Chemother* 1988;22(suppl A):1.

41. Honor N, Cole ST. Streptomycin resistance in mycobacteria. *Antimicrob Agents Chemother* 1994;38:238.

42. Morris S, Han Bai G, Suffys P, et al. Molecular mechanisms of multiple drug resistance in clinical isolates of *Mycobacterium tuberculosis*. *J Infect Dis* 1995;171:954.

43. Maness MJ, Foster GC, Sparling PF. Ribosomal resistance to streptomycin and spectinomycin in *Neisseria gonorrhoeae*. *J Bacteriol* 1974;120:1293.

44. Lacey RW, Chopra I. Evidence for mutation to streptomycin resistance in clinical strains of *Staphylococcus aureus*. *J Gen Microbiol* 1972;73:175.

45. Tseng JT, Bryan LE, Van den Elzen HM. Mechanisms and spectrum of streptomycin resistance in a natural population of *Pseudomonas aeruginosa*. *Antimicrob Agents Chemother* 1972;2:136.

46. Eliopoulos GM, Farber, BF, Murray B, et al. Ribosomal resistance of clinical enterococcal isolates to streptomycin. *Antimicrob Agents Chemother* 1984;25:398.

47. Shaila MS, Gopinathan KP, Ramakrishnan T. Protein synthesis in *Mycobacterium tuberculosis* H37Rv and the effect of streptomycin in streptomycin-susceptible and resistant strains. *Antimicrob Agents Chemother* 1973;4:205.

48. Yamada T, Nagata A, Ono Y, et al. Alteration of ribosomes and RNA polymerase in drug-resistant clinical isolates of *Mycobacterium tuberculosis*. *Antimicrob Agents Chemother* 1985;27:921.

49. Ahmad MH, Rechenmacher A, Bock A. Interaction between aminoglycoside uptake and ribosomal resistance mutations. *Antimicrob Agents Chemother* 1980;18:798.

50. Holmes DJ, Cundliffe E. Analysis of a ribosomal RNA methylase gene from *Streptomyces tenebrarius* which confers resistance to gentamicin. *Mol Gen Genet* 1991;229:229.

51. Davies C, Bussiere DE, Golden BL, et al. Ribosomal proteins S5 and L6: high-resolution crystal structures and roles in protein synthesis and antibiotic resistance. *J Mol Biol* 1998;279:873.

52. Jacoby GA, Archer GL. New mechanisms of bacterial resistance to antimicrobial agents. *N Engl J Med* 1991;324:601.

53. Arthur M, Andremont A, Courvalin P. Distribution of erythromycin esterase and rRNA methylase genes in members of the family Enterobacteriaceae highly resistant to erythromycin. *Antimicrob Agents Chemother* 1987;31:404.

54. Auckenthaler RW, Zwahlen A, Waldvogel FA. Macrolides. In: Peterson PK, Verhoef J, eds. *Antimicrobial agents annual 1*. Amsterdam: Elsevier Science, 1986:115–126.

55. Weisblum B. Erythromycin resistance by ribosomal modification. *Antimicrob Agents Chemother* 1995;39:577.

56. Weisblum B. Inducible resistance to macrolides, lincosamides and streptogramin type B antibiotics: The resistance phenotype, its biological diversity, and structural elements that regulate expression-A review. *J Antimicrob Chemother* 1985;16(suppl A):63.

57. Mitsuhashi S, Inoue M. Resistance to macrolides and lincomycins. In: Bryan LE, ed. *Antimicrobial drug resistance*. Orlando, FL: Academic, 1984:279–291.

58. Weisblum B. Insights into erythromycin action from studies of its activity as inducer of resistance. *Antimicrob Agents Chemother* 1995;39:797.

59. Vester B, Douthwaite S. Macrolide resistance conferred by base substitutions in 23S rRNA. *Antimicrob Agents Chemother* 2001;45:1.

60. Quiros LM, Fidalgo S, Mendez FJ, et al. Novel mechanisms of resistance to lincosamides in *Staphylococcus* and *Arthrobacter* spp. *Antimicrob Agents Chemother* 1988;32:420.

61. Tait-Kamradt A, Davies T, Appelbaum PC, et al. Two new mechanisms of macrolide resistance in clinical strains of *Streptococcus pneumoniae* from Eastern Europe and North America. *Antimicrob Agents Chemother* 2000;44:3395.

62. Smith AL, Burns JL. Resistance to chloramphenicol and fusidic acid. In: Bryan LE, ed. *Antimicrobial drug resistance*. Orlando, FL: Academic, 1984:293.

63. Levy SB, McMurry LM, Barbosa TM, et al. Nomenclature for new tetracycline resistance determinants. *Antimicrob Agents Chemother* 1999;43:1523.

64. Taylor DE, Chau A. Tetracycline resistance mediated by ribosomal protection. *Antimicrob Agents Chemother* 1996;40:1.

65. Morse SA, Johnson SR, Biddle JW, et al. High-level resistance in *Neisseria gonorrhoeae* is result of acquisition of streptococcal *tetM* determinant. *Antimicrob Agents Chemother* 1986;30:664.

66. Knapp JS, Johnson SR, Zenilman JM, et al. High-level tetracycline resistance resulting from TetM in strains of *Neisseria* spp., *Kingella denitrificans*, and *Eikenella corrodens*. *Antimicrob Agents Chemother* 1988;32:765.

67. Brown JT, Roberts MC. Cloning and characterization of *tetM* gene from a *Ureaplasma urealyticum* strain. *Antimicrob Agents Chemother* 1987;31:1852.

68. Hooper DC. Mechanisms of action of antimicrobials: focus on fluoroquinolones. *Clin Infect* 2001;32(suppl 1):9.

69. Hooper DC. Emerging mechanisms of fluoroquinolone resistance. *Emerg Infect Dis* 2001;7:337.

70. Takahata M, Nishino T. DNA gyrase of *Staphylococcus aureus* and inhibitory effect of quinolones on its activity. *Antimicrob Agents Chemother* 1988;32:1192.

71. Isaacs RD, Kunke PJ, Cohen RL, et al. Ciprofloxacin resistance in epidemic methicillin-resistant *Staphylococcus aureus*. *Lancet* 1988;2:843.

72. Shalit I, Berger SA, Gorea A, et al. Widespread quinolone resistance among methicillin-resistant *Staphylococcus aureus* isolates in a general hospital. *Antimicrob Agents Chemother* 1989;33:593.

73. Blumberg HM, Rimland D, Carroll DJ, et al. Rapid development of ciprofloxacin resistance in methicillin-susceptible and -resistant *Staphylococcus aureus*. *J Infect Dis* 1991;163:1279.

74. Wehrli W. Rifampin: mechanisms of action and resistance. *Rev Infect Dis* 1983;5(suppl 3):S407.

75. Radstrom P, Swedberg G. RSF1010 and a conjugative plasmid contain *sulII*, one of two known genes for plasmid-borne sulfonamide resistance dihydropteroate synthase. *Antimicrob Agents Chemother* 1988;32:1684.

76. Huovinen P, Sundström L, Swedberg G, et al. Trimethoprim and sulfonamide resistance. *Antimicrob Agents Chemother* 1995;39:279.

77. Galetto DW, Johnston JL, Archer GL. Molecular epidemiology of trimethoprim resistance among coagulase-negative staphylococci. *Antimicrob Agents Chemother* 1987;31:1683.

78. Huovinen P. Resistance to trimethoprim-sulfamethoxazole. *Clin Infect Dis* 2001;32:1608.

79. DeGroot R, Campos J, Moseley SL, et al. Molecular cloning and mechanisms of trimethoprim resistance in *Haemophilus influenzae*. *Antimicrob Agents Chemother* 1988;32:477.

80. Hamilton-Miller JMT. Resistance to antibacterial agents acting on antifolate metabolism. In: Bryan LE, ed. *Antimicrobial drug resistance*. Orlando, FL: Academic, 1984:173.

81. Yoshimura F, Nikaido H. Diffusion of β-lactam antibiotics through the porin channels of *Escherichia coli* K-12. *Antimicrob Agents Chemother* 1985;27:84.

82. Nikaido H. Outer membrane barrier as a mechanism of antibiotic resistance. *Antimicrob Agents Chemother* 1989;33:1831.

83. Sanders CC, Sanders WE Jr, Goering RV, et al. Selection of multiple antibiotic resistance by quinolones, β-lactams, and aminoglycosides with special reference to cross-resistance between unrelated drug classes. *Antimicrob Agents Chemother* 1984;26:797.

84. Gutmann L, Billot-Klein D, Williamson R, et al. Mutation of *Salmonella paratyphi* A conferring cross-resistance to several groups of antibiotics by decreased permeability and loss of invasiveness. *Antimicrob Agents Chemother* 1988;32:195.

85. Hooper DC, Wolfson JS, Souza KS, et al. Genetic and biochemical characterization of norfloxacin resistance in *Escherichia coli*. *Antimicrob Agents Chemother* 1986;29:639.

86. Sanders CC, Sanders WE Jr. Type I beta-lactamase of gram-negative bacteria: interactions with beta-lactam antibiotics. *J Infect Dis* 1986;154:792.

87. Hancock REW. Role of porins in outer membrane permeability. *J Bacteriol* 1987;169:929.

88. Hancock REW, Woodruff WA. Roles of porin and β-lactamase in β-lactam resistance of *Pseudomonas aeruginosa*. *Rev Infect Dis* 1988;10:770.

89. Godfrey AJ, Bryan LE. Penetration of β-lactams through *Pseudomonas aeruginosa* porin channels. *Antimicrob Agents Chemother* 1987;31:1216.

90. Carmeli Y, Troillet N, Eliopoulos GM, et al. Emergence of antibiotic-resistant *Pseudomonas aeruginosa*: comparison of risks associated with different antipseudomonal agents. *Antimicrob Agents Chemother* 1999;43:1379.

91. Lynch MJ, Drusano GL, Mobley HTL. Emergence of resistance to imipenem in *Pseudomonas aeruginosa*. *Antimicrob Agents Chemother* 1987;31:1892.

92. Buscher K, Cullman W, Dick W, et al. Imipenem resistance in *Pseudomonas aeruginosa* resulting from diminished expression of an outer membrane protein. *Antimicrob Agents Chemother* 1987;31:703.

93. Nikaido H. Antibiotic resistance caused by gram-negative multidrug efflux pumps. *Clin Infect Dis* 1998;27(suppl 1):32.

94. Li X-Z, Ma D, Livermore DM, et al. Role of efflux pump(s) in intrinsic resistance of *Pseudomonas aeruginosa*: active efflux as a contributing factor to β-lactam resistance. *Antimicrob Agents Chemother* 1994;38:1742.

95. Collatz E, Gutmann L. Bacterial porins as mediators of antibiotic susceptibility. In: Peterson PK, Verhoef J, eds. *Antimicrobial agents annual 2*. Amsterdam: Elsevier Science, 1987:442.

96. Norris SA, Sciortino CV. Monoclonal antibody to an aminoglycoside-resistance factor from *Pseudomonas aeruginosa*. *J Infect Dis* 1988;158:1324.

97. Bryan LE, O'Hara K, Wong S. Lipopolysaccharide changes in impermeability-type aminoglycoside resistance in *Pseudomonas aeruginosa*. *Antimicrob Agents Chemother* 1984;26:250.

98. Maloney J, RimLand D, Stephens DS, et al. Analysis of amikacin-resistant *Pseudomonas aeruginosa* developing in patients receiving amikacin. *Arch Intern Med* 1989;149:630.

99. Parr TR Jr, Bayer AS. Mechanisms of aminoglycoside resistance in variants of

Pseudomonas aeruginosa isolated during treatment of experimental endocarditis in rabbits. *J Infect Dis* 1988;158:1003.

100. Mates SM, Patel L, Kaback HR, et al. Membrane potential in anaerobically growing *Staphylococcus aureus* and its relationship to gentamicin uptake. *Antimicrob Agents Chemother* 1983;23:526.

101. Miller MH, Edberg SC, Mandel LJ, et al. Gentamicin uptake in wild-type and aminoglycoside-resistant small-colony mutants of *Staphylococcus aureus*. *Antimicrob Agents Chemother* 1980;18:722.

102. Moellering RC Jr, Murray BE, Schoenbaum SC, et al. A novel mechanism of resistance to penicillin-gentamicin synergism in *Streptococcus faecalis*. *J Infect Dis* 1980;141:81.

103. Singh KV, Malathum K, Murray BE. Disruption of an *Enterococcus faecium* species-specific gene, a homologue of acquired macrolide resistance genes of staphylococci, is associated with an increase in macrolide susceptibility. *Antimicrob Agents Chemother* 2001;45:263.

104. Levy SB. Active efflux mechanisms for antimicrobial resistance. *Antimicrob Agents Chemother* 1992;36:695.

105. Roberts MC, Sutcliffe J, Courvalin P, et al. Nomenclature for macrolide and macrolide-lincosamide-streptogramin B resistance determinants. *Antimicrob Agents Chemother* 1999;43:2823.

106. Bums JL, Rubens CE, Mendelman PM, et al. Cloning and expression in *Escherichia coli* of a gene encoding nonenzymatic chloramphenicol resistance from *Pseudomonas aeruginosa*. *Antimicrob Agents Chemother* 1986;29:445.

107. Bums JL, Hedin LA, Lien DM. Chloramphenicol resistance in *Pseudomonas cepacia* because of decreased permeability. *Antimicrob Agents Chemother* 1989;33:131.

108. McMurry LM, George AM, Levy SB. Active efflux of chloramphenicol in susceptible *Escherichia coli* strains and in multiple antibiotic-resistant (Mar) mutants. *Antimicrob Agents Chemother* 1994;38:542.

109. Li X-Z, Livermore DM, Nikaido H. Role of efflux pump(s) in intrinsic resistance of *Pseudomonas aeruginosa*: resistance to tetracycline, chloramphenicol, and norfloxacin. *Antimicrob Agents Chemother* 1994;38:1732.

110. Levy SB. Resistance to the tetracyclines. In: Bryan LE, ed. *Antimicrobial drug resistance*. Orlando, FL: Academic, 1984:191.

111. McMurray L, Petrucci RE Jr, Levy SB. Active efflux of tetracycline encoded by four genetically different tetracycline resistance determinants in *Escherichia coli*. *Proc Natl Acad Sci USA* 1980;77:3974.

112. Thanassi DG, Suh GSB, Nikaido H. Role of outer membrane barrier in efflux-mediated tetracycline resistance of *Escherichia coli*. *J Bacteriol* 1995;177:998.

113. Diver J. The mode of action of the 4-quinolones: an update. *Quinolone Bull* 1988;4:25.

114. Hirai K, Aoyama H, Irikura T, et al. Differences in susceptibility to quinolones of outer membrane mutants of *Salmonella typhimurium* and *Escherichia coli*. *Antimicrob Agents Chemother* 1986;29:535.

115. Robillard NJ, Scarpa AL. Genetic and physiological characterization of ciprofloxacin resistance in *Pseudomonas aeruginosa* PAO. *Antimicrob Agents Chemother* 1988;32:535.

116. Daikos GI, Lolans VT, Jackson GG. Alterations in outer membrane proteins of *Pseudomonas aeruginosa* associated with selective resistance to quinolones. *Antimicrob Agents Chemother* 1988;32:785.

117. Kohler T, Epp SF, Curty LK, et al. Characterization of MexT, the regulator of the MexE-MexF-OprN multidrug efflux system of *Pseudomonas aeruginosa*. *J Bacteriol* 1999;181:6300.

118. Masuda N, Sakagawa E, Ohya S. Outer membrane proteins responsible for multiple drug resistance in *Pseudomonas aeruginosa*. *Antimicrob Agents Chemother* 1995;39:645.

119. Zhanel GG, Karlowsky JA, Saunders MH, et al. Development of multiple-antibiotic-resistant (Mar) mutants of *Pseudomonas aeruginosa* after serial exposure to fluoroquinolones. *Antimicrob Agents Chemother* 1995;39:489.

120. Lomovskaya O, Warren MS, Lee A, et al. Identification and characterization of inhibitors of multidrug resistance efflux pumps in *Pseudomonas aeruginosa*: novel agents for combination therapy. *Antimicrob Agents Chemother* 2001;45:105.

121. Neyfakh AA, Borsch CM, Kaatz GW. Fluoroquinolone resistance protein NorA of *Staphylococcus aureus* is a multidrug efflux transporter. *Antimicrob Agents Chemother* 1993;37:128.

122. Then RL. Mechanisms of resistance to trimethoprim, the sulfonamides, and trimethoprim-sulfamethoxazole. *Rev Infect Dis* 1982;4:261.

123. Cohen SP, Yan W, Levy SB. A multidrug resistance regulatory chromosomal locus is widespread among enteric bacteria. *J Infect Dis* 1993;168:484.

124. Ariza RR, Li Z, Ringstad N, et al. Activation of multiple antibiotic resistance and binding of stress-inducible promoters by *Escherichia coli* Rob protein. *J Bacteriol* 1995;177:1655.

125. Cohen SP, McMurry LM, Hooper DC, et al. Cross-resistance to fluoroquinolones in multiple-antibiotic resistant (Mar) *Escherichia coli* selected by tetracycline or chloramphenicol: decreased drug accumulation associated with membrane changes in addition to OmpF reduction. *Antimicrob Agents Chemother* 1989;33:1318.

126. Bush K. New beta-lactamases in gram-negative bacteria: diversity and impact on the selection of antimicrobial therapy. *Clin Infect Dis* 2001;32:1085.

127. Livermore DM. Beta-lactamases in laboratory and clinical resistance. *Clin Microbiol Rev* 1995;8:557.

128. Bush K, Jacoby GA, Medeiros AA. A functional classification scheme for beta-lactamases and its correlation with molecular structure. *Antimicrob Agents Chemother* 1995;39:1211.

129. Zygmunt DJ, Stratton CW, Kernodle DS. Characterization of four beta-lactamases produced by *Staphylococcus aureus*. *Antimicrob Agents Chemother* 1992;36:440.

130. McDougal LK, Thornsberry C. The role of β-lactamase in staphylococcal resistance to penicillinase-resistant penicillin and cephalosporin. *J Clin Microbiol* 1986;23:832.

131. Murray BE, Mederski-Samoraj B. Transferable β-lactamase: a new mechanism for *in vitro* penicillin resistance in *Streptococcus faecalis*. *J Clin Invest* 1983;72:1168.

132. Eliopoulos GM. Increasing problems in the therapy of enterococcal infections. *Eur J Clin Microbiol Infect Dis* 1993;12:409.

133. Murray BE, Mederski-Samoraj B, Foster SK, et al. *In vitro* studies of plasmid-mediated penicillinase from *Streptococcus faecalis* suggest a staphylococcal origin. *J Clin Invest* 1986;77:289.

134. Sanders CC. Cefepime: the next generation? *Clin Infect Dis* 1993;17:369.

135. Vu H, Nikaido H. Role of beta-lactam hydrolysis in the mechanism of resistance of a beta-lactamase-constitutive *Enterobacter cloacae* strain to expanded spectrum beta-lactams. *Antimicrob Agents Chemother* 1985;27:393.

136. Bradford PA. Extended-spectrum beta-lactamases in the 21st century: characterization, epidemiology, and detection of this important resistance threat. *Clin Microbiol Rev* 2001;14:933.

137. Sirot J, Chanal C, Petit A, et al. *Klebsiella pneumoniae* and other Enterobacteriaceae producing novel plasmid-mediated β-lactamases markedly active against third-generation cephalosporins. Epidemiologic studies. *Rev Infect Dis* 1988;10:850.

138. Philippon A, Labia R, Jacoby G. Extended-spectrum β-lactamases. *Antimicrob Agents Chemother* 1989;33:1131.

139. Du Bois SK, Marriott MS, Amyes SGB. TEM- and SHV-derived extended-spectrum β-lactamases: relationship between selection, structure and function. *J Antimicrob Chemother* 1995;35:7.

140. Jacoby GA, Medeiros AA. More extended-spectrum β-lactamases. *Antimicrob Agents Chemother* 1991;35:1697.

141. Rice LB, Eckstein EC, DeVente J, et al. Ceftazidime-resistant *Klebsiella pneumoniae* isolates recovered at the Cleveland Department of Veteran Affairs Medical Center. *Clin Infect Dis* 1996;23:118.

142. Wiener J, Quinn JP, Bradford PA, et al. Multiple antibiotic-resistant *Klebsiella* and *Escherichia coli* in nursing homes. *JAMA* 1999;28:517.

143. Gaillot O, Maruejouls C, Abachin E, et al. Nosocomial outbreak of *Klebsiella pneumoniae* producing SHV-5 extended-spectrum beta-lactamase, originating from a contaminated ultrasonography coupling gel. *J Clin Microbiol* 1998;36:1357.

144. Urban C, Meyer KS, Mariano N, et al. Identification to TEM-26 beta-lactamase responsible for a major outbreak of ceftazidime-resistant *Klebsiella pneumoniae*. *Antimicrob Agents Chemother* 1994;38:392.

145. Rice KB, Willey SH, Papanicolaou GA, et al. Outbreak of ceftazidime resistance caused by extended-spectrum beta-lactamases at a Massachusetts chronic-care facility. *Antimicrob Agents Chemother* 1990;34:2193.

146. Burwen DR, Banerjee SN, Gaynes RP, et al. Ceftazidime resistance among selected nonsocomial gram-negative bacilli in the United States. *J Infect Dis* 1994;170:1622.

147. Martinez JL, Vincente MF, Delgado-Iribarren A, et al. Small plasmids are involved in amoxicillin-clavulanate resistance in *Escherichia coli*. *Antimicrob Agents Chemother* 1989;33:595.

148. Reguera JA, Baquero F, Perez-Diaz JC, et al. Factors determining resistance to beta-lactam combined with beta-lactamase inhibitors in *Escherichia coli*. *J Antimicrob Chemother* 1991;27:569.

149. Vedel G, Belaaouaj A, Gilly L, et al. Clinical isolates of *Escherichia coli* producing TRI β-lactamases: novel TEM-enzymes conferring resistance to β-lactamase inhibitors. *J Antimicrob Chemother* 1992;30:449.

150. Papanicolaou GA, Medeiros AA, Jacoby GA. Novel plasmid-mediated β-lactamase (MIR-1) conferring resistance to oxyimino- and α-hydroxy-β-lactams in clinical isolates of *Klebsiella pneumoniae*. *Antimicrob Agents Chemother* 1990;34:2200.

151. Bradford PA, Urban C, Mariano N, et al. Imipenem resistance in *Klebsiella pneumoniae* is associated with the combination of ACT-1, a plasmid-mediated AmpC beta-lactamase, and the loss of an outer membrane protein. *Antimicrob Agents Chemother* 1997;41:563.

152. Livingstone D, Gill MJ, Wise R. Mechanisms of resistance to the carbapenems. *J Antimicrob Chemother* 1995;35:1.

153. Rasmussen BA, Bush K. Carbapenem-hydrolyzing beta-lactamases. *Antimicrob Agents Chemother* 1997;41:223.

154. Naas T, Vandel L. Sougakoff W, et al. Cloning and sequence analysis of the gene for a carbapenem-hydrolyzing class A β-lactamase, Sme-1; from *Serratia marcescens* S6. *Antimicrob Agents Chemother* 1994;38:1262.

155. Queenan AM, Torres-Viera C, Gold HS, et al. SME-type carbapenem-hydrolyzing class A beta-lactamases from geographically diverse *Serratia marcescens* strains. *Antimicrob Agents Chemother* 2000;44:3035.

156. Ito H, Arakawa Y, Ohsuka S, et al. Plasmid-mediated dissemination of the metallo-β-lactamase gene bla$_{IMP}$ among clinically isolated strains of *Serratia marcescens*. *Antimicrob Agents Chemother* 1995;39:824.

157. Watanabe M, Iyobe S, Inoue M, et al. Transferable imipenem resistance in *Pseudomonas aeruginosa*. *Antimicrob Agents Chemother* 1991;35:147.

158. Eliopoulos GM, Moellering RC Jr. A critical comparison of the newer aminoglycosidic aminocyclitol antibiotics. In: Remington JS, Swartz MN, eds. *Current clinical topics in infectious diseases*. Vol. 4. New York: McGraw-Hill, 1983:378.

159. Storrs MJ, Courvalin P, Foster TJ. Genetic analysis of gentamicin resistance in methicillin- and gentamicin-resistant strains of *Staphylococcus aureus* isolated in Dublin hospitals. *Antimicrob Agents Chemother* 1988;32:1174.

160. Tomalsky ME, Chamorro RM, Crosa JH, et al. Transposon-mediated amikacin resistance in *Klebsiella pneumoniae. Antimicrob Agents Chemother* 1988;32:1416.

161. Hodel-Christian SL, Murray BE. Characterization of the gentamicin resistance transposon Tn5281 from *Enterococcus faecalis* and comparison to staphylococcal transposons Tn4001 and Tn4031. *Antimicrob Agents Chemother* 1991;35:1147.

162. Mitsuhashi S, Kawabe H. Aminoglycoside antibiotic resistance in bacteria. In: Whelton A, Neu HC, eds. *The aminoglycosides: microbiology, clinical use and toxicology.* New York: Marcel Dekker, 1982:97.

163. Cartier C, Courvalin P. Resistance of streptococci to aminoglycoside-aminocyclitol antibiotics. In: Schlessinger D, ed. *Microbiology: 1982.* Washington, DC: American Society for Microbiology, 1982:162.

164. Shannon K, Phillips I. Mechanisms of resistance to aminoglycosides in clinical isolates. *J Antimicrob Chemother* 1982;9:91.

165. Costa Y, Galimand M, Leclercq R, et al. Characterization of the chromosomal acc(6')-Ii gene specific for *Enterococcus faecium. Antimicrob Agents Chemother* 1993;37:1896.

166. Bongaerts GPA, Molendijk L. Relation between aminoglycoside 2''-O-nucleotidyl transferase activity and aminoglycoside resistance. *Antimicrob Agents Chemother* 1984;25:234.

167. Perlin MH, Lerner SA. High-level amikacin resistance in *Escherichia coli* due to phosphorylation and impaired aminoglycoside uptake. *Antimicrob Agents Chemother* 1986;29:216.

168. Eliopoulos GM, Eliopoulos CT. Antibiotic combinations: should they be tested? *Clin Microbiol Rev* 1988;1:139.

169. Ferretti JJ, Gilmore KS, Courvalin P. Nucleotide sequence analysis of the gene specifying bifunctional 6'-aminoglycoside acetyltransferase 2''-aminoglycoside phosphotransferase enzyme in *Streptococcus faecalis* and identification. and cloning of. gene regions specifying the two activities. *J Bacteriol* 1986;167:631.

170. Menard R, Molinas C, Arthur M, et al. Overproduction of 3'-aminoglycoside phosphotransferase type I confers resistance totobramycin in *Escherichia coli. Antimicrob Agents Chemother* 1993;37:78.

171. Courvalin P, Ounissi H, Arthur M. Multiplicity of macrolide-lincosamide-streptogramin antibiotic resistance determinants. *J Antimicrob Chemother* 1985;16(suppl A):91.

172. Andremont A, Gerbaud G, Courvalin P. Plasmid-mediated high-level resistance to erythromycin in *Escherichia coli. Antimicrob Agents Chemother* 1986;29:515.

173. Leclercq R, Courvalin P. Intrinsic and unusual resistance to macrolide, lincosamide, and streptogramin antibiotics in bacteria. *Antimicrob Agents Chemother* 1991;35:1273.

174. O'Hara K, Kanda T, Ohmiya K, et al. Purification and characterization of macrolide 2'-phosphotransferase from a strain of *Escherichia coli* that is highly resistant to erythromycin. *Antimicrob Agents Chemother* 1989;33:1354.

175. Leclercq R, Brisson-Noel A, Duval J, et al. Phenotypic expression and genetic heterogeneity of lincosamide inactivations in *Staphylococcus* spp. *Antimicrob Agents Chemother* 1987;31:1887.

176. Rende-Fournier R, Leclercq R, Galimand M, et al. Identification of the *satA* gene encoding a streptogramin A acetyltransferase in *Enterococcus faecium* BM4145. *Antimicrob Agents Chemother* 1993;37:2119.

177. Nakagawa Y, Nitahara Y, Miyamura S. Kinetic studies on enzymatic acetylation of chloramphenicol in *Streptococcus faecalis. Antimicrob Agents Chemother* 1979;16:719.

178. Neu HC, Fu KP. *In vitro* activity of chloramphenicol and thiamphenicol analogs. *Antimicrob Agents Chemother* 1980;18:311.

179. Park BH, Levy SB. The cryptic tetracycline resistance determinants on Tn4400 mediates tetracycline degradation as well as tetracycline efflux. *Antimicrob Agents Chemother* 1988;32:1797.

180. Speer BS, Bedzyk L, Salyers AA. Evidence that a novel tetracycline resistance gene found on two *Bacteroides* transposons encodes an NADP-requiring oxidoreductase. *J Bacteriol* 1991;173:176.

181. Speer BS, Shoemaker NB, Salyers AA. Bacterial resistance to tetracycline: mechanisms, transfers, and clinical significance. *Clin Microbiol Rev* 1992;5:387.

182. Dabbs ER, Yazawa K, Mikami Y, et al. Ribosylation by mycobacterial strains as a new mechanism of rifampin inactivation. *Antimicrob Agents Chemother* 1995;39:1007.

183. Archer GL. Antimicrobial susceptibility and selection of resistance among *Staphylococcus epidermidis* isolates recovered from patients with infections of indwelling foreign devices. *Antimicrob Agents Chemother* 1978;14:353.

184. Thabaut A, Durosoir J-L. Comparative *in vitro* antibacterial activity of pefloxacin (1589RB), nalidixic acid, pipemidic acid and flumequin. *Drugs Exp Clin Res* 1983;9:229.

185. Gutmann L, Williamson R, Moreau N, et al. Cross-resistance to nalidixic acid, trimethoprim, and chloramphenicol associated with alterations in outer membrane proteins of *Klebsiella, Enterobacter,* and *Serratia. J Infect Dis* 1985;151:501.

186. Martin P, Gomez-Lus R, Ortiz JM, et al. Structure and mobility of an ampicillin and gentamicin resistance determinant. *Antimicrob Agents Chemother* 1987;31:1266.

187. Fluit AC, Schmitz FJ. Class 1 integrons, gene cassettes, mobility, and epidemiology. *Eur J Clin Microbiol Infect Dis* 1999;18:761.

188. Tuberculosis Chemotherapy Trials Committee of the Medical Research Council. The treatment of pulmonary tuberculosis with isoniazid. *BMJ* 1952;2:735.

189. Cohn ML, Middlebrook G, Russell WF Jr. Combined drug treatment of tuberculosis. I. Prevention of emergence of mutant populations of tubercle bacilli resistant to both streptomycin and isoniazid. *J Clin Invest* 1959;38:1349.

190. Karchmer AW, Archer GL, Dismukes WE Jr. Rifampin treatment of prosthetic valve endocarditis due to *Staphylococcus epidermidis. Am J Med* 1983;75(suppl 2A):90.

191. Eliopoulos GM, Moellering RC Jr. Antimicrobial combinations. In: Lorian V, ed. *Antibiotics in laboratory medicine,* 4th ed. Baltimore: Williams & Wilkins, 1996:330.

192. Goldmann DA, Weinstein RA, Wenzel RP, et al. Strategies to prevent and control the emergence and spread of antimicrobial-resistant microorganisms in hospitals. A challenge to hospital leadership. *JAMA* 1996;275:234.

193. O'Brien TF, Acar JF. Antibiotic resistance worldwide. In: Peterson PK, Verhoef J, eds. *Antimicrobial agents annual 2.* Amsterdam: Elsevier Science, 1987:457.

194. Murray BE. Can antibiotic resistance be controlled? *N Engl J Med* 1994;330:1229.

195. Shulman JA, Terry PM, Hough CE. Colonization with gentamicin-resistant *Pseudomonas aeruginosa,* pyocin type 5, in a burn unit. *J Infect Dis* 1971;124(suppl):18.

196. Klein BS, Perloff WH, Maki DG. Reduction of nosocomial infection during pediatric intensive care by protective isolation. *N Engl J Med* 1989;320:1714.

197. Anonymous. Antimicrobial prophylaxis in surgery. *Med Lett Drugs Ther* 1999;41(1060):75–79.

CHAPTER 32
Antiviral Therapy

Richard J. Whitley

Spurred by the increasing need for therapy of such chronic infections as hepatitis B and C and human immunodeficiency virus (HIV), antiviral chemotherapy has achieved remarkable success in the past decade. Nevertheless, further improvements are essential for improved human health. Unique problems are associated with the development of antiviral agents. First, viruses are obligate intracellular parasites that use many biochemical pathways of the infected host cell. Historically, clinically useful antiviral activity was difficult to achieve without also adversely affecting normal host cell metabolism, causing toxic effects in uninfected cells. Second, early diagnosis of viral infection is crucial for effective antiviral therapy, because by the time symptoms appear, several cycles of viral multiplication have occurred and replication is waning. Precise diagnosis is difficult for many viral infections because of the lack of specificity of many viral syndromes, for example, coryza and cough for rhinovirus infection or the encephalopathy associated with herpes simplex encephalitis. As a consequence, effective antiviral therapy is dependent on rapid, sensitive, specific, and practical means of diagnosing viral diseases. Nevertheless, there are some viral infections, such as herpes zoster or genital herpes, for which a clinical diagnosis is usually routine. Third, because many of the disease syndromes caused by viruses are common, relatively benign, and self-limiting, the therapeutic index, or ratio of efficacy to toxicity, must be extremely high for therapy to be acceptable. Obviously, there are exceptions to this observation, as encountered with herpes simplex encephalitis or cytomegalovirus (CMV) retinitis. Fortunately, molecular biology is helping solve two of these problems. Enzymes unique to viral replication have been identified that distinguish between virus and host cell functions. Unique events in viral replication serve as targets for antiviral agents, such as thymidine kinase (TK) of herpes simplex virus (HSV) and reverse transcriptase of HIV. Second, improved diagnostic methods have been made possible by recombinant DNA technology that uses monoclonal antibodies, DNA hybridization, and the polymerase chain reaction (PCR).

As with all infectious diseases, the effectiveness of therapy often depends on host defenses, and this principle is of paramount importance when discussing antiviral agents. Immunocompromised patients are at increased risk for the development of symptomatic herpesvirus infections and deserve special note. All herpesviruses become latent, and reactivation results in an extremely high incidence of both infection and disease. In renal transplant recipients, for example, 40% to 70% reactivate latent HSV; 80% to 100% reactivate CMV; and 5% to 35% reactivate varicella-zoster virus (VZV) within 1 year, as summarized by Zaia (1). Not only is the incidence of reactivation high, but these infections are often more severe in the immunocompromised host, for example, varicella in children with leukemia, HSV and CMV infections in transplant recipients, and patients with acquired immunodeficiency syndrome (AIDS).

This chapter summarizes specific antiviral drugs, as well as supportive measures and other interventions often not considered as drug therapy, including immunoglobulin therapy. Similarly, the use of interferon (IFN) deserves mention.

NONSPECIFIC MANAGEMENT OF VIRAL INFECTIONS

Supportive Care

Because chemotherapeutic approaches are limited, symptomatic and supportive treatments, including bed rest, hydration, and analgesics, remain the management of choice for many viral diseases, particularly acute upper respiratory infections. Animal model data elucidate this principle. Severe, repetitive, and exhausting exercise in mice infected with coxsackievirus B3 prolongs infection and results in a delay in the appearance of both circulating IFN and type-specific serum neutralizing antibodies. Virologically, there is a marked increase in the quantity of virus detected in the myocardium, which is associated with higher mortality (2).

Immunoglobulin Therapy

Efficacy has been established for prophylactic immunoglobulin administration for several viral infections. More recently, a monoclonal antibody (palivizumab; Synagis, MedImmune, Inc., Gaithersburg, Maryland) has been licensed for the prevention of respiratory syncytial virus (RSV) infection in high-risk infants. (3) The use of immunoglobulin therapy for established disease has not been proved unequivocally beneficial for any viral infection. This approach has been tried for the treatment of echovirus meningoencephalitis associated with agammaglobulinemia, chronic Epstein-Barr virus (EBV) infection in adolescents and adults, CMV pneumonia in transplant recipients, and RSV disease in hospitalized children (4–8). Clinical benefit has been suggested from small underpowered clinical trials for the administration of intravenous CMV hyperimmune globulin if combined with ganciclovir for the treatment of CMV pneumonia in bone marrow transplant recipients. Survival increased to 52% to 79% (9,10). This survival rate is significantly better than that of historical controls treated with either agent alone.

THERAPY OF HERPESVIRUS INFECTIONS

Acyclovir and Valaciclovir

Acyclovir is one of the most widely prescribed and clinically effective antiviral drugs available to date. Valaciclovir, the L-valine ester oral prodrug of acyclovir, was developed to improve the oral bioavailability of acyclovir.

CHEMISTRY, MECHANISM OF ACTION, AND ANTIVIRAL ACTIVITY

Acyclovir, 9-[2-(hydroxyethoxy)methyl]guanine, a synthetic acyclic purine nucleoside analog, is a selective inhibitor of replication of HSV types 1 and 2 and VZV (11,12). Acyclovir is converted by virus-encoded TK to its monophosphate (MP) derivative, an event that does not occur to any significant extent in uninfected cells (13). Subsequent di- and triphosphorylation are catalyzed by cellular enzymes, resulting in acyclovir triphosphate (TP) concentrations 40 to 100 times higher in HSV-infected than in uninfected cells. Acyclovir-TP inhibits viral DNA synthesis by competing with deoxyguanosine-TP as a substrate for viral DNA polymerase (14). Because acyclovir-TP lacks the 3'-hydroxyl group required for DNA chain elongation, viral DNA synthesis is terminated. Viral DNA polymerase is tightly associated with the terminated DNA chain and is functionally inactivated (15). Also, the viral polymerase has greater affinity for acyclovir-TP than does cellular DNA polymerase, resulting in little incorporation of acyclovir into cellular DNA. *In vitro*, acyclovir is most active against HSV-1 (average median effective concentration 0.04 μg/mL), HSV-2 (0.10 μg/mL), and VZV (0.50 μg/mL) (16). EBV requires higher acyclovir concentrations for inhibition, and CMV, which lacks a virus-specific TK, is resistant (17).

Valaciclovir (2-[2-amino-1,6-dihydro-6-oxo-9h-purin-9-yl-methoxy]ethyl-L valinate hydrochloride) is cleaved by valine hydrolase to acyclovir, which is then metabolized in infected cells to acyclovir-TP. Because it is metabolized to acyclovir, it has same spectrum of activity (17,18).

ABSORPTION, DISTRIBUTION, AND ELIMINATION

Acyclovir is available in topical, oral, and intravenous preparations. An ophthalmic preparation is available in some countries of the world. The topical preparation is 5% acyclovir in a polyethylene glycol ointment base. Oral formulations include a 200-mg capsule, an 800-mg tablet, and a suspension (200 mg per 5 mL). Absorption of acyclovir after oral administration is slow and incomplete, with oral bioavailability of about 15% to 30% (19). After multidose oral administration of 200 or 800 mg of acyclovir, the mean steady-state peak levels are about 0.57 and 1.57 μg/mL, respectively (20). Much higher plasma acyclovir levels can be achieved with intravenous administration. Steady-state peak acyclovir concentrations after intravenous doses of 5 or 10 mg/kg every 8 hours are about 9.9 and 20.0 μg/mL, respectively. Acyclovir penetrates most body tissues well, including the brain. The terminal plasma half-life is 2 to 3 hours in adults with normal renal function. Acyclovir is minimally metabolized, and about 85% is excreted unchanged in the urine via renal tubular secretion and glomerular filtration. Acyclovir dosage adjustment is required for patients with impaired renal function. In patients with creatinine clearance (C_{cr}) greater than 50 mL/min, 100% of the recommended intravenous dose is given at 8-hour intervals. For a C_{cr} of 25 to 50 or 10 to 25 mL/min, the dosing interval is extended to 12 or 24 hours, respectively. If the C_{cr} is less than 10 mL/min, the standard intravenous dose is reduced by 50% and is given every 24 hours. Recommendations for use in renal impairment appear in Table 32.1. For patients with severe renal failure (C_{cr} <10 mL/min), the dose of oral acyclovir should be reduced to 200 mg (for HSV) or 800 mg (for VZV) every 12 hours. Acyclovir is readily removed by hemodialysis but not by peritoneal dialysis.

Valaciclovir is available only as a tablet formulation (500 mg or 1 g). It is metabolized nearly completely to acyclovir within

TABLE 32.1. Dosage Adjustment for Intravenous Acyclovir in Patients with Impaired Renal Function (204)

Creatinine clearance (mL/min/1.73 m^2)	% of standard dose	Dosing interval (h)
>50	100	8
25–50	100	12
10–25	100	24
0–10[a]	50	24

[a] Administered after hemodialysis.

minutes after absorption. Notably, plasma levels of acyclovir that are achieved after 2 g of valaciclovir given by mouth three times a day approximate those achieved with 5 mg/kg administered every 8 hours intravenously. Dosage adjustments are not required unless the C$_{cr}$ is less than 25 mL/min, at which time the dosing frequency is decreased to twice daily (21).

CLINICAL INDICATIONS

Herpes Simplex Virus Infections

Genital Herpes. Initial genital HSV infection can be treated with topical, oral, or intravenous acyclovir; however, topical application should not be considered for therapy in spite of accelerated events of healing (22). Intravenous acyclovir is the most effective treatment for first-episode genital herpes and results in a significant reduction in the median duration of virus shedding, pain, and time to complete healing (8 vs. 14 days) (23,24). Because intravenous acyclovir therapy usually requires hospitalization, drug should be reserved for patients with systemic complications. Oral therapy (200 mg five times daily) is nearly as effective as intravenous acyclovir for initial genital herpes (25,26) and is a standard treatment. Neither intravenous nor oral acyclovir treatment of acute HSV infection alters the frequency of subsequent recurrences (24,26).

Recurrent genital herpes is less severe and resolves more rapidly than primary infection, offering a shorter time interval for successful antiviral chemotherapy. Orally administered acyclovir shortens the duration of virus shedding and time to healing (6 vs. 7 days) when initiated within 24 hours of onset, but the duration of pain and itching and the time to subsequent recurrence are not affected (27,28). Nevertheless, some physicians recommend episodic therapy of recurrences at a dosage of 200 mg five times daily or 400 mg three times daily.

Oral acyclovir is effective for suppression of frequently recurring genital herpes (29–31). Daily administration of acyclovir reduced the frequency of recurrences by up to 80%, and 25% to 30% of patients have no further clinical recurrences while taking acyclovir (30,32). Successful suppression for up to 10 years has been reported with no evidence of significant adverse effects (32). Titration of acyclovir (400 mg twice daily or 200 mg two to five times daily) may be required to establish the minimal acyclovir dose that is most effective and economic. Acyclovir treatment should be interrupted at 12-month intervals to reassess the need for continued suppression (33). Emergence of acyclovir-resistant HSV rarely occurs in immunologically normal individuals, although it has been documented (34). Asymptomatic virus shedding occurs despite clinical suppression, resulting in the possibility of person-to-person transmission (35).

Valaciclovir has been studied for the treatment of primary and recurrent genital herpes at dosages ranging from 500 mg twice daily to 1 g three times daily (3–7 days). Therapeutic benefit is equivalent to that of acyclovir administered at 200 mg three times

daily or five times daily; however, the ease of administration favors valaciclovir (21,36).

Herpes Labialis. Orally administered acyclovir at a dose of 200 mg five times daily for 5 days reduces the time to loss of crust by approximately 1 day (7 vs. 8 days) but did not alter the duration of pain or time to complete healing (37). If the dose is increased to 400 mg five times daily for 5 days, treatment started during prodrome or erythema stages reduces the mean duration of pain by 36% and time to loss of crust by 27% (38). Thus, oral acyclovir has modest clinical benefit only if initiated early after recurrence (18).

Short-term prophylactic acyclovir may benefit some patients with recurrent herpes labialis who anticipate high-risk activity (e.g., intense exposure to sunlight) (39). Intermittent acyclovir administration does not alter the frequency of subsequent recurrences.

Valaciclovir treatment of herpes labialis provides similar benefit to acyclovir administration. The standard dose is 500 mg twice daily (18).

Mucocutaneous Herpes Simplex Virus Infections in Immunocompromised Patients. HSV infections of the lip, mouth, skin, perianal area, or genitals may be more severe in immunocompromised patients than in normal hosts. Lesions tend to be more invasive, slower to heal, and associated with prolonged virus shedding. Clinical benefit from intravenous acyclovir is well documented (40). Acyclovir recipients have a significantly shorter duration of virus shedding and accelerated lesion healing (41). Oral acyclovir therapy is also effective for these conditions (42).

Acyclovir prophylaxis of HSV infections is of significant clinical value in severely immunocompromised patients, especially those undergoing induction chemotherapy or organ transplantation. Administration of intravenous or oral acyclovir reduced the incidence of symptomatic HSV infection from about 70% to between 5% and 20% (43,44). A sequential regimen of intravenous acyclovir followed by oral acyclovir for 3 to 6 months can virtually eliminate symptomatic HSV infections in transplant recipients. Various oral dosing regimens, ranging from 200 mg three times daily to 800 mg twice daily, have been used successfully. Among bone marrow transplant recipients, acyclovir-resistant HSV isolates have been identified more frequently after therapeutic acyclovir administration than during prophylaxis (45). Acyclovir is a therapeutic mainstay for physicians in treating and suppressing herpesvirus infections in immunocompromised patients.

Herpes Simplex Encephalitis. Herpes simplex encephalitis is associated with significant morbidity and mortality despite antiviral therapy (46,47). Acyclovir therapy at 10 mg/kg every 8 hours for 14 to 21 days reduces mortality at 3 months to 19% as compared with approximately 50% among vidarabine recipients (46). Furthermore, 38% of acyclovir recipients returned to normal function. These data stress the need for improved therapeutic regimens for herpes simplex encephalitis.

Neonatal Herpes Simplex Virus Infections. Newborns with HSV infections can be classified as having disease (a) localized to skin, eye, and mouth; (b) of the central nervous system (CNS); or (c) disseminated (multiorgan). Acyclovir is the only medication available to treat this disease. Kimberlin et al. reported that in their studies, no infant with disease localized to the skin, eye, or mouth died, whereas 5% and 25% of infants with CNS or disseminated infection, respectively, died (48,49). Among infants with HSV localized to the skin, eye, and mouth, and PCR negative in the cerebrospinal fluid (CSF) at presentation, all developed normally 2 years after infection. Among infants who survived encephalitis, 50% developed normally; for those with disseminated infection, 60% were developing normally. Clearance of virus from infants who received acyclovir is slower than from immunocompromised adults, implying a requirement for host defense. To improve outcome, therapy must prevent progression of infection to the CNS or to disseminated disease. The safety and ease of administration of acyclovir prompt its recommendation as the treatment of choice for neonatal HSV infections. The currently recommended intravenous dose is 20 mg/kg every 8 hours for 14 to 21 days.

Other Herpes Simplex Virus Infections. Case reports have described the successful use of acyclovir in the treatment of HSV causing hepatitis, pneumonia, herpetic esophagitis, proctitis, eczema herpeticum, erythema multiforme, and herpetic whitlow.

Varicella-Zoster Virus Infections

Varicella. Oral acyclovir therapy of chickenpox shortens the duration of new lesion formation by about 1 day, reduces total lesion count, and improves constitutional symptoms (50–53). Therapy of older patients with chickenpox is indicated, but treatment of children must be decided on a case-by-case basis. In uncontrolled studies, intravenous acyclovir may improve the outcome of varicella pneumonia in adults, including pregnant women (54).

Acyclovir therapy of chickenpox in immunocompromised children substantially reduces morbidity and mortality. In placebo-controlled trials, treatment with intravenous acyclovir improved the outcome, as evidenced by a reduction of VZV pneumonitis from 45% to less than 5% (55,56). The treatment of choice is intravenous acyclovir at a dosage of 500 mg/m^2 every 8 hours for 7 to 10 days; oral acyclovir therapy is not indicated for immunocompromised children with chickenpox.

Herpes Zoster. Intravenous acyclovir therapy of herpes zoster in the normal host produces some acceleration of cutaneous healing (57,58). Oral acyclovir administration (800 mg five times a day) results in accelerated cutaneous healing and reduction in the severity of acute neuritis (59,60). In placebo-controlled trials, acyclovir therapy accelerates cessation of new vesicle formation from 7.4 to 6.2 days and time to crusting from 10.1 to 8.4 days (59). Clinical benefits of therapy are most evident when drug administration is initiated within 48 hours of disease onset. Oral acyclovir treatment of herpes zoster ophthalmicus reduces the incidence of serious ocular complications such as keratitis and uveitis. If therapy can be initiated within 48 hours of the onset of rash, oral acyclovir (800 mg five times per day) is one treatment choice for immunocompetent patients with localized herpes zoster. Of note, a metaanalysis of the acyclovir placebo-controlled data indicate statistically significant benefit for reduction of postherpetic neuralgia (61).

Valaciclovir has been extensively evaluated for the treatment of herpes zoster in the immunocompetent host at 1 g three times daily for 7 days. These studies indicate that valaciclovir is superior to acyclovir for the reduction of pain associated with shingles. Treatment with valaciclovir is one of two preferred drugs recommended for the normal host suffering from shingles (62,63).

The increased frequency of significant morbidity in immunocompromised patients with herpes zoster highlights the need for effective antiviral chemotherapy. Intravenous acyclovir significantly reduces the frequency of cutaneous dissemination and visceral complications of herpes zoster in immunocompromised adults (64,65). While acyclovir is the standard therapy for hospitalized patients at a dose of 10 mg/kg or 500 mg/m^2 every 8 hours for 7 to 10 days, valaciclovir and famciclovir are being used on an ambulatory care basis despite the absence of any controlled studies.

RESISTANCE

Resistance of HSV to acyclovir can develop through mutations in the viral gene encoding TK via generation of TK-deficient mutants or the selection of mutants possessing a TK that is unable to phosphorylate acyclovir (66,67). Clinical isolates resistant to acyclovir are almost uniformly deficient in TK, although DNA polymerase mutants have been recovered from HSV-infected patients (68,69). Drug resistance was considered rare, and resistant isolates were thought to be less pathogenic until a series of acyclovir-resistant HSV isolates from patients with AIDS were characterized (45,70). These resistant mutants were deficient in TK but remained sensitive to vidarabine and foscarnet, drugs that do not require viral TK for activation (71,72). Acyclovir-resistant HSV isolates have been identified as the cause of pneumonia (73), encephalitis (74), esophagitis (68), and mucocutaneous infections (75,76), all occurring in immunocompromised patients. Acyclovir-resistant mutants have been described in the normal host (34,69). Acyclovir-resistant isolates of VZV have been identified much less frequently than acyclovir-resistant HSV but have been recovered from bone marrow transplant recipients and patients with AIDS (77,78). Acyclovir-resistant VZV isolates all have altered or absent TK function but remain susceptible to vidarabine and foscarnet (79).

Valaciclovir, because it is metabolized to acyclovir, has the same sensitivity patterns as the parent compound. Thus, cross-resistance can be anticipated.

ADVERSE EFFECTS

Acyclovir and valaciclovir therapies are associated with few adverse effects. Renal dysfunction induced by acyclovir has been reported but appears to be relatively uncommon and is usually reversible (80,81). Creatinine elevations have been noted in patients given large doses of acyclovir by rapid intravenous infusion and have been attributed to crystallization of drug in the renal tubules and collecting ducts, resulting in a transient nephropathy (82). The risk for nephrotoxicity can be minimized by administering acyclovir by slow infusion over 1 hour and ensuring adequate hydration. Neither oral acyclovir nor valaciclovir therapy has been associated with renal dysfunction. A few reports have linked high-dose intravenous acyclovir use with CNS disturbances, including agitation, hallucinations, disorientation, tremors, and myoclonus (83).

The Acyclovir in Pregnancy Registry has gathered data on prenatal acyclovir exposures. Although no significant risk to the mother or fetus has been documented, the total number of monitored pregnancies remains too small to detect any low-frequency events (84). Because acyclovir crosses the placenta and can concentrate in amniotic fluid, there is concern about the potential for fetal nephrotoxicity, although none has been observed (85).

CONCLUSIONS ON ACYCLOVIR AND VALACICLOVIR

The synthesis of acyclovir was a true milestone in the development of selective and specific inhibitors of viral replication. Many carefully conducted clinical trials have clearly established acyclovir and valaciclovir as drugs of choice for a wide range of infections caused by HSV and VZV. Because of the enhanced plasma concentrations of acyclovir that are achieved after valaciclovir administration, the latter drug is the preferred treatment for shingles and genital herpes. The appearance of isolates resistant to acyclovir underscores the necessity for continued development of new agents with alternative mechanisms of action.

Cidofovir

Cidofovir is the first of a class of nucleotide analogs licensed for the treatment of viral diseases. Other nucleotides include adefovir and tenfovir. Currently, adefovir remains investigational for therapy of chronic hepatitis B; tenfovir was recently licensed for the treatment of AIDS.

CHEMISTRY, MECHANISM OF ACTION, AND ANTIVIRAL ACTIVITY

(S)-1-(3-hydroxy-2-phosphonylmethoxypropyl) cytosine (HPM-PC) or cidofovir, a novel acyclic nucleotide analog, was developed primarily for the treatment of CMV retinitis but can be used to treat cases of acyclovir- and foscarnet-resistant HSV infection as well. Beta herpesviruses, including CMV human herpesviruses (HHV)-6 and -7, are particularly susceptible to the drug. The 50% inhibitory concentrations (IC_{50}) are in the range of 0.1 μg/mL for CMV (86). The drug also has *in vitro* activity against adenoviruses, human papillomaviruses, poxviruses, and JC virus.

The drug has a mechanism of action similar to that of nucleoside analogs but only employs cellular kinases to produce the active diphosphate form of the drug. Activated cidofovir has higher affinity for viral DNA polymerase and therefore selectively inhibits viral replication (87). The drug is less potent than acyclovir *in vitro*.

ABSORPTION, DISTRIBUTION, AND ELIMINATION

Cidofovir has demonstrated limited and variable oral bioavailability (2%–26%) when tested in rats and therefore is administered intravenously or by ocular implant (87). Peak plasma concentrations of 3.1 to 23.6 μg/mL are achieved with doses of 1.0 to 10.0 mg/kg, respectively. The terminal plasma half-life is 2.6 hours, and 90% of the drug is excreted in the urine.

In vivo, cidofovir persists in cells for prolonged periods (more than 48 hours), increasing drug activity (88). In addition, cidofovir produces active metabolites with long half-lives (17–48 hours), permitting once-weekly dosing (89). Unfortunately, drug concentrates in kidney cells at a rate 100 times greater than in other tissues and produces severe proximal convoluted tubule nephrotoxicity when administered systemically (90). Attempts to limit the drug's nephrotoxicity include coadministration of probenecid with intravenous hydration, and use of topical formulations (90).

CLINICAL INDICATIONS

Cidofovir is licensed for the treatment of CMV retinitis in patients with AIDS. The drug has been studied in patients who have failed ganciclovir or foscarnet. A treatment regimen of 5 mg/kg per week for 2 weeks followed by the same dose once weekly provided superior benefit over lower maintenance doses. Probenecid and liberal intravenous hydration have been added to intravenously administered cidofovir to prevent significant nephrotoxicity. Because of the nephrotoxicity, this regimen is much less attractive than oral valganciclovir therapy (87,91).

RESISTANCE

The development of resistance to cidofovir is uncommon. Altered susceptibility of CMV isolates has been reported after prolonged drug treatment. Thus, this finding suggests the possibility of mutations in the CMV DNA polymerase gene (92).

ADVERSE EFFECTS

The major side effect of cidofovir is nephrotoxicity that results in renal tubular damage. Two of five patients with HIV and asymptomatic CMV infection treated with cidofovir (3.0 mg/kg) experienced increased creatinine levels after 6 to 14 doses (87). Patients receiving higher doses (10 mg/kg) experienced nephrotoxicity after two doses. One case report documented systemic treatment of an acyclovir-resistant HSV infection; however, the drug was discontinued because of decreased renal function in this patient (87). Additionally, hypotony and iritis have been ascribed to cidofovir therapy.

CONCLUSIONS ON CIDOFOVIR

Cidofovir represents the first of a new class of medications licensed to treat viral diseases. Unfortunately, nephrotoxicity and hypotony are rate-limiting toxicities that limit drug use. As noted, cidofovir does have activity *in vitro* against pox viruses and therefore may provide the only available therapeutic solution should smallpox be used in a bioterrorist event.

Fomivirsen

Fomivirsen is the first antisense oligonucleotide licensed for the treatment of a viral disease.

CHEMISTRY, MECHANISM OF ACTION, AND ANTIVIRAL ACTIVITY

Fomivirsen (5'-GCG TTT GCT CTT CTT GCG-3'0) is approved for the treatment of CMV retinitis. The IC_{50} against laboratory strains of CMV is about 0.37 μM. Drug binds to the mRNA of the immediate early 2 gene of CMV.

ABSORPTION, DISTRIBUTION, AND ELIMINATION

Fomivirsen can only be administered by intravitreal injection. The pharmacokinetics of drug administration to the rabbit eye indicates a half-life of 62 hours (93,94).

CLINICAL INDICATIONS

Fomivirsen delays progression of CMV retinitis when administered at a dosage of 330 μg every other week on three occasions, followed by the same dose monthly. Drug is approved for patients intolerant to other medications (93,94).

RESISTANCE

Albeit of limited clinical experience, no isolates from humans have been reported as resistant to fomivirsen.

ADVERSE EFFECTS

Increased intraocular pressure and inflammation have been reported as the major side effects of fomivirsen therapy, occurring in as many as 20% of patients.

CONCLUSIONS ON FOMIVIRSEN

While fomivirsen is the first antisense oligonucleotide licensed for therapy, the route of administration and requirement for frequent administration limit its clinical utility.

Foscarnet

CHEMISTRY, MECHANISM OF ACTION, AND ANTIVIRAL ACTIVITY

Foscarnet, a pyrophosphate analog of phosphonoacetic acid, has potent *in vitro* and *in vivo* activity against herpesviruses. Drug inhibits the DNA polymerase of all human herpesviruses by blocking the pyrophosphate binding site, thus inhibiting the formation of the 3'-5' phosphodiester bond between primer and substrate and preventing chain elongation. Unlike acyclovir, which requires activation by a virus-specific TK, foscarnet acts directly on the virus DNA polymerase. TK-deficient, acyclovir-resistant herpesviruses remain sensitive to foscarnet. Foscarnet has been used successfully to treat severe mucocutaneous HSV infections caused by acyclovir-resistant HSV-2 (95). Foscarnet also inhibits influenza A RNA-dependent RNA polymerase and the reverse transcriptase of several other animal and human retroviruses, including HIV.

ABSORPTION, DISTRIBUTION, AND ELIMINATION

The oral bioavailability of foscarnet is extremely poor; thus, administration is by the intravenous route. An intravenous infusion of 60 mg/kg every 8 hours results in peak and trough plasma concentrations of approximately 450 to 575 and 80 to 150 μM, respectively. The CSF concentration of foscarnet is approximately two thirds that of the plasma level.

Renal excretion is the primary route of foscarnet clearance; more than 80% of the dose appears in the urine. Bone sequestration also occurs, resulting in complex plasma elimination.

CLINICAL INDICATIONS

Foscarnet is licensed for the treatment of CMV retinitis in individuals with HIV infection as well HSV and VZV diseases that are resistant to acyclovir or penciclovir in immunocompromised hosts. In the management of CMV retinitis, administration of foscarnet at 60 mg/kg every 8 hours for 14 to 21 days followed by maintenance therapy at 90 to 120 mg/kg per day results in stabilization of retinal disease in approximately 90% of patients (96). However, as is the case with ganciclovir therapy of CMV retinitis, relapse occurs (97).

Interestingly, foscarnet therapy resulted in improved overall survival in HIV infected patients with CMV retinitis as compared with the ganciclovir recipients (98). However, there was no difference between drugs in the outcome from CMV retinitis (99).

Mucocutaneous infections caused by HSV and those caused by VZV in immunocompromised hosts can be treated with foscarnet at dosages lower than that for the management of CMV retinitis. Foscarnet dosages of 40 mg/kg administered every 8 hours for 7 days or longer resulted in cessation of virus shedding and healing of lesions in the majority of patients (72). Relapses will occur that may or may not be amenable to acyclovir therapy.

RESISTANCE

Isolates of HSV, CMV, and VZV all can develop resistance to foscarnet in both laboratory and clinical settings (100,101). Isolates of HSV that are resistant to foscarnet have median effective concentrations greater than 100 $\mu g/mL$. These isolates are all DNA polymerase mutants.

ADVERSE EFFECTS

Toxicity is a major problem with foscarnet administration. Significant nephrotoxicity, including acute tubular necrosis and interstitial nephritis, can occur with administration, resulting in limited clinical use of drug. In addition, metabolic aberrations of calcium, magnesium, phosphate, and other electrolytes are associated with foscarnet administration and therefore warrant careful monitoring. Symptomatic hypocalcemia is the most common metabolic abnormality. Seizures, secondary to hypocalcemia, have been associated with foscarnet therapy but usually in patients with an underlying CNS disease. Drug interactions have been encountered with nephrotoxic agents, such as pentamidine, and zidovudine. Increases in serum creatinine develop in one half of treated patients but are usually reversible after dis-

continuation. Other CNS side effects include headache (25% of patients), tremor, irritability, and hallucinations.

CONCLUSIONS ON FOSCARNET

Foscarnet has a role in the physician's armamentarium for the management of CMV infections in high-risk populations, particularly patients with AIDS who have CMV retinitis. The utilization of this compound requires vigilance for potential untoward affects.

Ganciclovir/Valganciclovir

CHEMISTRY, MECHANISM OF ACTION, AND ANTIVIRAL ACTIVITY

CMV infections are a major cause of morbidity and mortality in immunocompromised patients. CMV retinitis occurs in 15% to 46% of patients with AIDS who fail highly active antiretroviral therapy (HAART) (102). Infection rates in transplant recipients average 50% to 60% and higher (103–105). CMV pneumonia can occur at a frequency as high as 17% in bone marrow transplant recipients and has an associated mortality rate as high as 85%, even with therapy (106).

Ganciclovir, 9-[1,3-dihydroxy-2-propoxy)methyl]guanine (Cytovene, Roche Laboratories, Nutley, NJ, U.S.A.), has enhanced *in vitro* activity against all herpesviruses compared with acyclovir, including 8 to 20 times greater antiviral activity against CMV (0.2–3.0 $\mu g/mL$) (107,108). HSV-1 and -2 are inhibited by 0.2 to 8.0 μM (0.05–2.0 $\mu g/mL$). Its activity is similar to that of acyclovir against HSV-1 *in vitro*, but is slightly superior against HSV-2. The 50% inhibitory dose for CMV ranges from 0.5 to 11 μM (0.125–2.75 $\mu g/mL$). EBV is inhibited by 1 to 4 μM and VZV by 4 to 40 μM.

As with acyclovir, the activity of ganciclovir in herpesvirus-infected cells depends on phosphorylation by virus-induced TK. Ganciclovir-MP is converted to its di- and triphosphate derivatives by cellular kinases. In cells infected by HSV-1 or HSV-2, ganciclovir-TP competitively inhibits the incorporation of guanosine-TP into viral DNA. Ganciclovir-TP is incorporated at internal and terminal sites of viral DNA and inhibits DNA synthesis. The mode of action of ganciclovir against CMV is mediated by a protein kinase, UL-97, that efficiently promotes the obligatory initial phosphorylation of ganciclovir to its monophosphate (108–112).

Valganciclovir, L-valine, 2-[2-amino-1,6-dihydro-6-oxo-9H-purin-9-yl)methoxy]-3-hydroxypropyl ester, is metabolized completely to ganciclovir; thus, it has the same spectrum of activity and mechanism of activity as the parent compound (113).

ABSORPTION, DISTRIBUTION, AND ELIMINATION

Ganciclovir is available as both intravenous and oral formulations. It can also be injected into the vitreous; an implantable ocular device is available. The oral bioavailability of ganciclovir is poor, approximately 5% to 7% (114,115). Peak and trough plasma levels are approximately 1 and 0.5 $\mu g/mL$, respectively, after administration of 1 g every 6 hours. Intravenous administration of a standard dose of 5 mg/kg results in peak and trough plasma concentrations of 8 to 11 $\mu g/mL$ and 0.5 to 1.2 $\mu g/mL$, respectively. Concentrations of ganciclovir in critical biologic fluids, including the aqueous humor and cerebrospinal fluid, tend to be less than those in the plasma. The levels of the drug in CSF are estimated to be 24% to 67% of those in plasma. Mean intravitreal ganciclovir levels of 14 μM were reported for samples taken a mean of 12 hours after therapy with a mean dose of 6 mg/kg daily. However, no significant correlations are noted between time after the last dose and intravitreal concentration.

The observed mean value in the eye is below the concentration of GCV required to achieve 50% or 90% inhibition of CMV plaque formation by clinical isolates, which may explain the difficulty in controlling CMV retinitis.

The plasma elimination half-life is 2 to 4 hours for individuals with normal renal function. The kidney is the major route of clearance of the drug; therefore, impaired renal function requires adjustment of dosage. Plasma levels of the drug can be reduced by approximately 50% to 90% with hemodialysis. The half-life on dialysis is approximately 4 hours. Patients undergoing dialysis should be given 1.25 mg/kg daily; therapy should also be administered after dialysis.

Ganciclovir is only 1% to 2% bound to plasma proteins, and drug interactions involving binding site displacement have not been defined. No significant pharmacokinetic interaction occurs when ganciclovir and foscarnet are given as concomitant or daily alternate therapy.

Valganciclovir is cleaved to ganciclovir by intracellular esterases of the gastrointestinal tract. Valganciclovir has an oral bioavailability of about 60%. Following the administration of 360 mg of valganciclovir, peak plasma levels of ganciclovir are achieved at 2.98 μg/mL as compared with 9.36 μg/mL with a 5 mg/kg dose (116).

CLINICAL INDICATIONS

Human Immunodeficiency Virus–Infected Patients
In the absence of therapy, CMV retinitis in patients with AIDS is progressive and eventually causes blindness. Ganciclovir has been administered to large number of AIDS patients with CMV retinitis. Most patients (78%) experience either improvement or stabilization of their retinitis as shown by fundoscopic examinations (117). Induction therapy is usually at a dosage of 5.0 mg/kg twice daily given intravenously for 14 to 21 days and is followed by maintenance therapy administered daily at the same dose. Median time to relapse for patients receiving no maintenance therapy averages 47 days. Maintenance therapy significantly lengthens the median time to relapse to 105 days (118,119). Virtually every patient treated experiences either a cessation or reduction of plasma viremia (119,120). Cultures of urine and blood usually become negative after 7 to 10 days of treatment (119). Visual acuity usually stabilizes at pretreatment levels but rarely improves dramatically. Initial response rates are 75% to 85%. Relapse occurs quickly in the absence of maintenance therapy, but usually occurs, eventually, even in patients receiving maintenance therapy. The optimal dosing schedule for maintenance therapy is unknown, but doses of 5 mg/kg for 5 to 7 days week are currently recommended. The significance of bone marrow toxicity must be taken into consideration as well, because 30% to 40% of patients develop neutropenia (118).

Similar reports of benefit have appeared for ganciclovir treatment of other CMV infections in patients with AIDS, particularly those involving the gastrointestinal tract: 85% of patients showed improvement or stabilization of disease (121). CMV infections in patients with AIDS recur after discontinuation of therapy.

Oral administration of ganciclovir—an adjunct to the treatment for CMV retinitis in patients with AIDS as well as the prevention of CMV end-organ disease in the same population—has been replaced by the use of valganciclovir (120).

Valganciclovir (Valcyte) was recently licensed in the United States for the treatment of CMV retinitis in patients with AIDS. Valganciclovir is considered comparable to ganciclovir for the treatment of CMV retinitis. The dose is 900 mg twice daily for 3 weeks followed by 900 mg once daily (122,123).

Organ Transplant Recipients
Therapy of opportunistic CMV infections in organ transplant recipients is complicated by the fact that decreasing immunosuppressive therapy is usually impossible; hence, elimination of CMV infection is uncommon. Nonetheless, CMV infections are extremely common and the cause of significant morbidity and mortality in these patients. The lung is among the most common sites of serious CMV disease for which therapy has been reported to be beneficial (124,125). Importantly, the routine monitoring of transplant recipients for evidence of CMV antigenemia allows early intervention with ganciclovir in order to prevent end-organ disease. As a consequence, CMV disease in high-risk patient populations is much less common.

Bone Marrow Transplant Patients
CMV infections in bone marrow transplant recipients are more devastating than in most other patient populations. CMV pneumonia can occur in as many as 17% of these patients and, if untreated, has a mortality rate as high as 85%. Ganciclovir combined with intravenous immunoglobulin adds benefit in the treatment of bone marrow transplant recipients with CMV pneumonia (9,10).

Ganciclovir has been administered in anticipation of CMV disease to bone marrow transplant recipients, as noted above. Several clinical trials utilizing different designs (e.g., initiation of ganciclovir after engraftment (i.e., prophylactic) versus initiation at the time of demonstration of antigen in blood or bronchial alveolar lavage but in the absence of clinical symptoms (i.e., preemptive therapy) have established the effectiveness of ganciclovir in preventing CMV pneumonia and reducing mortality during the period of treatment (126–128). The use of ganciclovir under these circumstances is gaining enhanced support among transplant physicians; however, long-term survival benefit (more than 120 days) is not apparent.

The use of valganciclovir in organ transplant populations is under investigation.

RESISTANCE
Clinical resistance to CMV can become evident by persistent CMV viremia and a deteriorating clinical course (129). With prolonged ganciclovir treatment, many AIDS and transplant patients acquire drug resistance (130). Two mechanisms of resistance to ganciclovir have been documented. First, the alteration of a protein kinase gene, identified as UL97, reduces the intracellular phosphorylation of ganciclovir, thereby rendering it inactive. The second mechanism of resistance is that of point mutations in the viral DNA polymerase gene (131–133). Resistance is associated with decreased sensitivity by a factor of up to 20. Should resistance develop, foscarnet is the treatment of choice.

ADVERSE EFFECTS
Hematologic toxicity is the most important adverse reaction following ganciclovir or valganciclovir administration whether intravenous or oral, occurring in 25% to 35% of patients. The IC_{50} for human bone marrow colony-forming cells is 39 ± 73 μM; for other cell lines it ranges from 110 to 2,900 μM. Toxicity frequently limits therapy. Marrow suppression develops at 5 mg/kg on alternate days. Neutropenia of less than 1,000/mm^3 occurs in nearly 40% of recipients and less than 500/mm^3 in upward of 30% for those given induction therapy of 10 mg/kg daily for 14 days, followed by 5 mg/kg daily. Neutropenia is reversible and develops during the early treatment or maintenance phase, but may occur later. Thrombocytopenia of less than 20,000/mm^3 and less than 50,000/mm^3 develops in about 10% and 19% of patients, respectively. Frequent monitoring of the full blood count is recommended (117).

Adverse effects on the CNS, including confusion, convulsions, psychosis, hallucinations, tremor, ataxia, coma, dizziness, headaches, and somnolence occur in approximately 5%. Liver function abnormalities, fever, and rash occur in about 2%. Intraocular injection of ganciclovir is associated with intense pain, and occasionally amaurosis lasting for 1 to 10 minutes afterward.

Animal studies indicate that inhibition of spermatogenesis and suppression of female fertility occurs. It is also potentially embryolethal, mutagenic, and teratogenic, and is contraindicated during pregnancy or lactation. Ganciclovir can cause local tissue damage and should not be administered intramuscularly or subcutaneously; patients should be adequately hydrated during treatment.

Valganciclovir, because it is metabolized to ganciclovir, has the same toxicity profile as the parent drug.

CONCLUSIONS ON GANCICLOVIR/VALGANCICLOVIR

Ganciclovir has been the most widely tested drug for the treatment of CMV infections. There is support for clinical use in patients with AIDS who have CMV retinitis and gastrointestinal infection. Benefit is suggested for CMV pneumonia in immunocompromised hosts. Because of the requirement for intravenous ganciclovir administration, the availability of valganciclovir offers a more patient-friendly approach to the management of CMV retinitis (93).

Idoxuridine and Trifluorothymidine

CHEMISTRY, MECHANISM OF ACTION, AND ANTIVIRAL ACTIVITY

Idoxuridine (5-iodo-2'-deoxyuridine, Stoxil) and trifluorothymidine (trifluridine; Viroptic, Monarch Pharmaceuticals, Bristol, TN, U.S.A.) are analogs of thymidine. When administered systemically, these nucleosides are phosphorylated by both viral and cellular TK to active TP derivatives that inhibit both viral and cellular DNA synthesis. The result is antiviral activity but also sufficient host cytotoxicity to prevent the systemic use of these drugs. These compounds are toxic when applied topically to the eye in the treatment of HSV keratitis. Both idoxuridine and trifluorothymidine are effective and licensed for treatment of HSV keratitis.

ABSORPTION, DISTRIBUTION, AND ELIMINATION

Topically applied idoxuridine or trifluorothymidine penetrates cells of the cornea. Low levels of drugs can be detected in the aqueous humor. Systemic concentrations of drug in the plasma are not detected after topical therapy of ocular disease.

CLINICAL INDICATIONS

Trifluorothymidine is the more efficacious compound (134). These agents are not of proven value in the treatment of stromal keratitis or uveitis, although trifluridine is more likely to penetrate the cornea and, ultimately, may prove beneficial. Some forms of stromal keratitis and uveitis are thought to be caused by immune mechanisms and thus would not respond to antiviral therapy, suggesting that topical corticosteroids may be of value in the treatment of these conditions (134).

RESISTANCE

Little effort has been directed to evaluating HSV isolates obtained from the eye, in large part because of the difficulty in accomplishing this task. As a consequence, clinical resistance to idoxuridine has not attracted attention from the biomedical community.

ADVERSE EFFECTS

The ophthalmic preparation of idoxuridine and trifluridine causes local irritation, photophobia, edema of the eyelids and cornea, punctual occlusion, and superficial punctate keratopathy (134).

Penciclovir and Famciclovir

CHEMISTRY, MECHANISM OF ACTION, AND ANTIVIRAL ACTIVITY

A new member of the guanine nucleoside family of drugs is famciclovir [9-(4-hydroxy-3-hydroxymethylbut-1-yl)guanine; Famvir, SmithKline Beecham, Pittsburgh, PA, U.S.A.], the prodrug of penciclovir [9-(4-hydroxy-3-hydroxy-3-hydroxymethylbut-1-yl)guanine], which is approved worldwide. Penciclovir does not have significant oral bioavailability (less than 5%). However, famciclovir provides excellent oral bioavailability (approximately 77%) and appears to have a good therapeutic index for therapy of both HSV and VZV infections (135). Famciclovir is the diacetylester of 6-deoxypenciclovir.

Penciclovir inhibits HSV-1, HSV-2, and VZV in vitro at IC_{50} of 0.4, 1.5, and 5.0 μg/mL. Activity against a variety of acyclovir-resistant strains has been examined. TK-negative strains are resistant to both penciclovir and acyclovir. The majority of acyclovir-resistant HSV and VZV clinical isolates are also cross-resistant to penciclovir; however, a few acyclovir-resistant strains are sensitive to penciclovir. Foscarnet-resistant HSV isolates are susceptible to both penciclovir and acyclovir.

Penciclovir is phosphorylated more efficiently than acyclovir in HSV- and VZV-infected cells. Host cell kinases phosphorylate both penciclovir and acyclovir to a small but comparable extent. The preferential metabolism in HSV- and VZV-infected cells is the major determinant of antiviral activity. Penciclovir-TP has, on the average, a 10-fold longer intracellular half-life than acyclovir-TP in HSV-1–, HSV-2–, and VZV-infected cells after drug removal. Penciclovir-TP is formed at concentrations sufficient to be an effective inhibitor of viral DNA polymerase, albeit at a lower inhibition constant (K_i) than that of acyclovir-TP. Penciclovir, like acyclovir, is relatively inactive against CMV and EBV. Penciclovir is also active against hepatitis B virus.

Cytotoxicity assays of uninfected cells for both penciclovir and acyclovir are in excess of the value of 100 μg/mL for most cell lines. Such values contribute to the conclusion that there is a high in vitro therapeutic index.

ABSORPTION, DISTRIBUTION, AND ELIMINATION

Conversion of famciclovir to penciclovir occurs at two levels. The major metabolic route of famciclovir is deacetylation of one ester group as the prodrug crosses the duodenal barrier of the gastrointestinal tract. The drug is transported to the liver via the portal vein, where the remaining ester group is removed and oxidation occurs at the sixth position of the side chain, resulting in penciclovir, the active drug. In humans, famciclovir is absorbed rapidly and extensively after oral administration. The first metabolite that appears in the plasma is almost entirely the deacetylated compound with little or no parent drug detected. Thus, the major metabolite of famciclovir is penciclovir. Maximal plasma concentrations of penciclovir indicate oral bioavailability of approximately 77% of famciclovir. Pharmacokinetic parameters for penciclovir are linear for famciclovir oral dose ranges of 125 to 750 mg. Penciclovir is eliminated rapidly and almost unchanged by active tubular secretion and glomerular filtration by the kidneys (135). The elimination half-life in healthy subjects is approximately 2 hours. Food appears to slow the rate of conversion of famciclovir to penciclovir but has no effect on the ultimate extent of availability of penciclovir (136). Dosages selected for human investigation include 125, 250, 500, and 750 mg per dose administered two or three times per day.

CLINICAL INDICATIONS

Herpes Zoster
In studies of shingles in individuals of all ages, more than 1,200 patients have been evaluated in studies using either placebo-controlled designs or administration of acyclovir as a control (137,138). Initial trials of famciclovir (250, 500, or 750 mg three times daily) indicated that it is equivalent to the standard acyclovir treatment of herpes zoster for cutaneous healing and, in a subgroup analysis, accelerated resolution of pain (zoster-associated pain) (137). A placebo-controlled study of famciclovir at a dosage of 500 or 250 mg three times daily shows acceleration of cutaneous healing and a two- to threefold reduction of time to resolution of postherpetic neuralgia, the latter being most evident in patients older than 50 years. The interpretation of these studies has been questioned because of definitions and subgroup analyses, but the apparent finding of accelerated resolution of postherpetic neuralgia is important and warrants clarification.

Genital Herpes Simplex Virus Infection
Studies of patients with recurrent genital HSV infection (with either intravenous penciclovir or oral famciclovir therapy) demonstrate clinical improvement (e.g., pain, virus shedding, duration). Famciclovir given twice daily (125, 250, or 500 mg twice daily for 5 days) (139) is effective therapy for recurrent genital herpes. Similarly, studies of the impact of famciclovir therapy on recurring HSV infections in immunocompromised hosts or effectiveness in suppressive therapy, particularly asymptomatic excretion of virus, also demonstrate clinical benefit (139,140).

RESISTANCE
HSV and VZV isolates resistant to penciclovir have been identified in the laboratory. These isolates have similar patterns of resistance, as compared with acyclovir. Namely, resistance variance is attributed to alterations or deficiencies of TK and DNA polymerase. Acyclovir-resistant viruses share resistance, for the most part, with penciclovir.

ADVERSE EFFECTS
Therapy with oral famciclovir is well tolerated, being associated only with headache, diarrhea, and nausea, common findings with other orally bioavailable antiviral agents (140,141). Preclinical studies of famciclovir found that chronic administration was tumorigenic (murine mammary tumors) and caused testicular toxicity in other rodents (142). The implications of these findings for humans are unknown. Famciclovir also interacts with digoxin, resulting in increased plasma concentrations of this medication (143).

CONCLUSIONS ON FAMCICLOVIR AND PENCICLOVIR
Famciclovir has significant activity in the treatment of herpes zoster in the elderly. The ease of administration three times daily compared with acyclovir (five times daily) provides a distinct advantage for famciclovir. Direct comparisons between valaciclovir and famciclovir do not provide a therapeutic advantage of one drug versus the other for the treatment of either herpes zoster or genital herpes (144).

Vidarabine
Vidarabine is a purine nucleoside analog with activity against HSV-1, HSV-2, and VZV. Drug is phosphorylated intracellularly to its mono-, di-, and triphosphate derivatives. The TP derivative competitively inhibits DNA-dependent DNA polymerases of some DNA viruses approximately 40 times more than those of host cells. In addition, vidarabine is incorporated into terminal positions of both cellular and viral DNA and thus inhibits elongation. Viral DNA synthesis is blocked at lower doses of drug than is host cell DNA synthesis, resulting in a relatively selective antiviral effect. However, large doses of vidarabine are cytotoxic to dividing host cells.

The benefit demonstrated in initial placebo-controlled clinical trials of this drug was a major impetus for the development of antiviral therapies. However, because of poor solubility and some toxicity, vidarabine was quickly replaced by acyclovir in the physician's armamentarium. Today it is no longer available as an intravenous formulation. Vidarabine should be recognized historically as the first drug licensed for systemic use in the treatment of a viral infection.

THERAPY OF RESPIRATORY VIRUS INFECTIONS

Background
The impact of respiratory viral illnesses on human health cannot be overestimated. Almost 90% of the population experience one of these illnesses each year, resulting in a staggering number of days lost from work and school and of visits to physicians, as well as in significant potential for serious morbidity and even death (145). Nonetheless, because these conditions in most populations of patients are self-limited and rarely fatal, the requirements for new drugs are stringent: an extreme degree of safety, moderate to high effectiveness, ease of administration, and low cost.

Amantadine and Rimantadine

CHEMISTRY, MECHANISM OF ACTION, AND ANTIVIRAL ACTIVITY
Amantadine was identified as effective against influenza A viruses and was soon shown to be effective against all type A variants (146–149). Amantadine was first reported to be effective for the prophylaxis of influenza A more than three decades ago, being approved for this indication in the United States in 1966. At concentrations achievable in humans, amantadine is useful only against influenza A (147). Influenza A viruses differ in their susceptibility to amantadine, and the drug may have different actions depending on the concentration and virus strain. Amantadine acts early in the replicative cycle of influenza A by interfering with the function of the M2 protein. The M2 protein acts as an ion channel, facilitating the hydrogen-mediated dissociation of the matrix protein from the nucleocapsid. By interfering with the function of the M2 protein, amantadine and rimantadine inhibit the acid-mediated association of the matrix protein from the ribonuclear protein complex within endosomes. The consequences are the potentiation of acidic pH-induced conformational changes in the hemagglutinin during its intracellular transport (150).

Rimantadine is the a-methyl derivative of amantadine (amethyl-l-adamantanemethylamine hydrochloride). Rimantadine is 5- to 10-fold more active than amantadine and has the same spectrum of activity, mechanism of action, and clinical indications.

ABSORPTION, DISTRIBUTION, AND ELIMINATION
There are differences in the absorption, distribution, and elimination of rimantadine and amantadine (151). Absorption of rimantadine is delayed compared with that of amantadine, and

equivalent doses of rimantadine produce lower plasma levels than amantadine, presumably because of a larger volume of distribution (151,152). Lower plasma levels may explain the lower incidence of side effects at similar doses. The side effects of rimantadine are similar to but less than those of amantadine and include gastrointestinal and CNS effects (153,154). Rimantadine has similar CNS side effects even though, unlike amantadine, this drug does not affect CNS catecholamine release and is not effective in the treatment of Parkinson's disease. The efficacy of rimantadine in both the prophylaxis and the treatment of influenza is similar to that of amantadine. Both amantadine and rimantadine are well absorbed after oral administration.

Amantadine is excreted in the urine by glomerular filtration and probably tubular secretion. It is not metabolized. The plasma elimination half-life is approximately 12 to 18 hours in individuals with normal renal function. However, the elimination half-life increases in elderly patients with impaired C_{cr}. Rimantadine is extensively metabolized by the liver after oral administration, having an elimination half-life that averages 24 to 36 hours. Approximately 15% of the dose is excreted unchanged in the urine.

CLINICAL INDICATIONS

As antiviral agents, amantadine and rimantadine are licensed for both chemoprophylaxis and treatment of influenza A infections. Because of a lower incidence of side effects associated with rimantadine compared with amantadine, it is used preferentially. Rimantadine can be given to any nonimmunized member of the general population who wishes to avoid influenza A, but prophylaxis is especially recommended for control of presumed influenza outbreaks in institutions housing high-risk persons. High-risk individuals include adults and children with chronic disorders of the cardiovascular or pulmonary system requiring regular follow-up or hospitalization during the preceding year, as well as residents of nursing homes and other chronic care facilities housing patients of any age with chronic medical conditions. In these instances, drug can be administered to all residents of the institution, whether or not they received an influenza vaccination the previous fall. To reduce the spread of virus and to minimize disruption of patients' care, prophylaxis should be offered to nonvaccinated staff who care for high-risk residents in chronic care institutions or hospitals experiencing a presumed influenza A outbreak. Rimantadine prophylaxis, as is the case with the neuraminidase inhibitors, is also recommended in the following situations:

1. As an adjunct to late immunization of high-risk individuals. Rimantadine does not interfere with antibody response to the vaccine.
2. For persons who have not been immunized and who care for high-risk persons in home settings, both to reduce the spread of virus and to allow persons to maintain care for high-risk persons in the home setting.
3. For immunodeficient persons, who may be expected to have a poor antibody response to vaccine.
4. For persons in whom influenza vaccine is contraindicated, such as those hypersensitive to egg protein.

There is general agreement that the efficacy of amantadine and rimantadine when used prophylactically for influenza A averages 70% to 80% (range 0%–100%), approximately the same as with influenza vaccines. In general, efficacy is about 66% for infections and about 75% for infection-related illnesses (145). Effectiveness has been demonstrated for prevention of both experimental (i.e., artificial challenge) and naturally oc-

curring infections for all three major subtypes of influenza A virus.

These drugs are also presumed to be effective for the treatment of influenza A. All studies showed a beneficial effect on the signs and symptoms of acute influenza, as well as a significant reduction in quantity of virus in respiratory secretions at some time during the course of infection. Because of the short duration of disease, therapy must be administered within 48 hours of symptom onset to show benefit. Aerosol administration of amantadine and rimantadine has been reported, but this route of administration needs further testing (148).

With the recent licensure of the neuraminidase inhibitors, alternatives for prophylaxis and treatment exist.

RESISTANCE

Rimantadine-resistant strains of influenza virus have been isolated from children treated for 5 days. Rimantadine-resistant strains are transmitted from person to person, resulting in clinical influenza (155,156). Development of resistance lends further support to the importance of vaccination in appropriate populations of patients.

Development of resistance of influenza A viruses is mediated by single nucleotide changes in RNA segment 7 that results in amino acid substitutions in the transmembrane of the M2 protein (155,157,158). Obviously, amantadine and rimantadine share cross-resistance.

ADVERSE EFFECTS

Amantadine causes side effects in 5% to 10% of healthy young adults who receive a dose of 200 mg per day (145,159). These side effects are usually mild and cease soon after amantadine is discontinued, although they often disappear with continued use of the drug as well (154). CNS side effects—5% to 33% in older individuals—are common and include difficulty thinking, confusion, lightheadedness, hallucinations, anxiety, and insomnia. Activities requiring mental alertness (e.g., driving) should be avoided until it is reasonable to assume that these symptoms will not occur. More severe adverse effects, such as mental depression and psychosis, are usually associated with doses exceeding 200 mg per day. About 5% of patients complain of nausea, vomiting, or anorexia. Older individuals are more likely to experience side effects. Rimantadine appears better tolerated (151,153).

Patients with renal disease should receive amantadine doses based on their C_{cr} values (Table 32.2). Doses for older people and children are usually lower as well. Persons with an active seizure

TABLE 32.2. Dosage Adjustment for Oral Amantadine in Patients with Impaired Renal Function

Creatinine clearance (mL/min/1.73 m²)	Suggested oral maintenance regimen after 200 mg (100 mg b.i.d.) on the first day
≥80	100 mg b.i.d.
60–80	100 mg b.i.d. alternating with 100 mg daily
40–60	100 mg daily
30–40	200 mg (100 mg b.i.d.) twice weekly
20–30	100 mg three times each week
10–20	200 mg (100 mg b.i.d.) alternating with 100 mg every 7 days
<10	100 mg every 7 days

b.i.d., twice daily.
Data from Whitley RJ. Antiviral therapy. In: Gorbach SL, Bartlett JG, Blacklow NR, eds. *Infectious diseases*, 2nd ed. Philadelphia: WB Saunders, 1998:330–350.

disorder may be at increased risk for seizures when amantadine is given at standard doses.

Side effects associated with rimantadine administration are significantly less than those encountered with amantadine, particularly those of the CNS. Rimantadine has been associated with exacerbations of underlying seizure disorders.

CONCLUSIONS ON AMANTADINE AND RIMANTADINE
Amantadine and rimantadine are efficacious for prevention and treatment of influenza A. Because of the high incidence of adverse effects associated with amantadine administration, rimantadine has replaced this compound for the most part. Because the newer neuraminidase inhibitors have activity against both influenza A and B, they will likely replace amantadine and rimantadine.

Oseltamivir

CHEMISTRY, MECHANISM OF ACTION, AND ANTIVIRAL ACTIVITY
Oseltamivir [ethyl(3R,4R,5S)-4-acetomido-5-amino-3-(1-ethylpropoxy)-1cyclohexene-1-carboxylate] is a selective neuraminidase inhibitor. Oseltamivir inhibits both influenza A and B virus at concentrations of 2 nM. Drug inhibits viral replication by targeting the neuraminidase protein via binding in a competitive fashion to the enzyme, rendering the virus incapable of reproducing. Because it has activity against influenza B, like zanamivir, it has an advantage over the adamantadines. It has no activity against any other virus (160).

ABSORPTION, DISTRIBUTION, AND METABOLISM
Oseltamivir is converted by oseltamivir carboxylate, the active compound, through hydrolysis by hepatic esterases. Oral bioavailability is about 75%. The active metabolite appears in the plasma in 30 minutes and peaks at 350 to 550 ng/mL within 4 hours of a standard dose. Drug is excreted as the caboxylate in the urine. Bronchoalveolar fluid drug levels are approximately 50% that of the plasma. The active metabolite is cleared by active tubular excretion—unchanged—in the urine. The plasma half-life is 8 to 10 hours in healthy adults (161,162).

CLINICAL INDICATIONS
Drug is licensed for the treatment and prevention of influenza A and B infections. In the United States it is licensed for individuals 2 years of age and older. Clinical trials indicate 30% acceleration in resolution of clinical symptoms. Of note, in pediatric studies, treatment accelerates disease resolution and is associated with a significantly decreased incidence of otitis media and antibiotic usage by 30% to 40%. Prophylactic efficacy is reported to be 75% to 85% (160,163–166).

RESISTANCE
Mutations in the neuraminidase have been detected rarely in patients exposed to medication. In clinical studies, 1.3% to 8.6% of posttreatment isolates have altered susceptibility to oseltamivir. *In vitro*, the emergence of a resistant variant occurs with the substitution of a lysine for the conserved arginine at amino acid 292 of the neuraminidase. Cross-resistance with zanamivir has been described *in vitro* (167,168).

ADVERSE EFFECTS
Oseltamivir is generally well tolerated. Adverse events relate to the gastrointestinal tract; the most common is nausea with or without vomiting in 10% of patients. Food alleviates side effects.

CONCLUSIONS ON OSELTAMIVIR
Because of oral bioavailability, oseltamivir is the choice for prevention and treatment of both influenza A and B viruses.

Zanamivir

CHEMISTRY, MECHANISM OF ACTION, AND ANTIVIRAL ACTIVITY
Zanamivir (5-acetylamino-4-[aminoiminomethyl-amino]-2,6-anhydro-3,4,5-trideoxy-D-glycero-D-galacto-non-2-enonic acid) is a neuraminidase inhibitor. Zanamivir, like oseltamivir, binds competitively to influenza neuraminidase, inhibiting both influenza A and B. The IC_{50} for influenza viruses is 0.9 ng/mL.

Influenza neuraminidase catalyzes the cleavage of the terminal sialic acid attached to glycolipids and glycoproteins. Drug binds to the conserved region of the neuraminidase.

ABSORPTION, DISTRIBUTION, AND ELIMINATION
Unlike oseltamivir, the oral bioavailability of zanamivir is poor, about 2%; thus, it is only available as an inhaled medication. Inhaled zanamivir provides local respiratory mucosal concentrations that greatly exceed those that are inhibitory for influenza A and B replication. The median concentrations exceed 1,000 ng/mL in the sputum 6 hours after inhalation and remain detectable for 24 hours. Inhalation results in 20% systemic absorption.

CLINICAL INDICATIONS
Zanamivir is licensed for the treatment and prevention of influenza A and B infections in patients over 7 years of age. In clinical trials, treatment reduced the duration of symptoms from 6 to 5 days and symptom scores by about 44%. The prophylactic efficacy of zanamivir is about 80% (169–171).

RESISTANCE
Resistance to zanamivir is an uncommon occurrence in clinical trials, occurring no more frequently than in 1% of exposed patients. As would be predicted, the site of mutation is that where drug binds the neuraminidase.

ADVERSE EFFECTS
Since medication is administered by inhalation, most adverse effects are related to the respiratory tree. These include rhinorrhea and, rarely, bronchospasm. Nausea and vomiting have been reported at low incidence (less than 3%).

CONCLUSIONS ON ZANAMIVIR
Zanamivir offers an alternative management for both the prevention and treatment of influenza A and B infections. However, the route of administration poses problems for ease of administration.

Ribavirin

CHEMISTRY, MECHANISM OF ACTION, AND ANTIVIRAL ACTIVITY
Ribavirin has antiviral activity against a variety of RNA- and DNA-containing viruses (172,173). Ribavirin has been evaluated most as a therapy for respiratory and hepatitis C virus infections, but its broad spectrum of activity has resulted in clinical trials for a number of viral infections (17).

Ribavirin is a nucleoside analog whose mechanisms of action are poorly understood and probably not the same for all viruses; however, its ability to alter nucleotide pools and the packaging of messenger RNA (mRNA) appears important (172–174). This process is not totally virus specific, but there is certain selectivity in that infected cells produce more mRNA than noninfected cells. A major action is the inhibition by ribavirin-5'-MP of inosine-MP dehydrogenase, an enzyme essential for DNA synthesis. This inhibition may have direct effects on the intracellular level of guanosine-MP; other nucleotide levels may be altered, but the mechanisms are at present unknown. Also, the 5'-TP of ribavirin inhibits the formation of the 5'-guanylation capping on the mRNA of vaccinia and Venezuelan equine encephalitis viruses. In addition, the TP is a potent inhibitor of viral mRNA (guanine-7) methyltransferase of vaccinia virus. The capacity of viral mRNA to support protein synthesis is markedly reduced by ribavirin. Of note, high concentrations of ribavirin also inhibit cellular protein synthesis. Ribavirin may inhibit RNA-dependent RNA polymerase of influenza A virus (145).

ABSORPTION, DISTRIBUTION, AND ELIMINATION

Ribavirin can be administered orally (bioavailability of approximately 40% to 45%), by aerosol, or intravenously (175). Aerosol administration was the standard for the treatment of RSV infections in children; however, it is no longer routinely used.

Oral doses of 600 and 1,200 mg result in peak plasma concentrations of 1.3 and 2.5 μg/mL, respectively. Intravenous doses of 500 and 1,000 mg result in plasma concentrations of 17 and 24 μg/mL, respectively. Aerosol administration of ribavirin results in plasma levels that are a function of the duration of exposure. Whereas respiratory secretions contain milligram quantities of drug, only microgram quantities (0.5–3.5 μg/mL) can be detected in the plasma.

The kidney is the major route of clearance of drug, accounting for approximately 40%. Hepatic metabolism also contributes to the clearance of ribavirin. Notably, ribavirin-TP concentrates in erythrocytes and persists for a month or longer. The persistence of ribavirin in erythrocytes probably contributes to its hematopoietic toxicity.

CLINICAL INDICATIONS

While ribavirin is licensed for the treatment of carefully selected, hospitalized infants with severe lower respiratory tract infections caused by RSV, for the vast majority of infants and children with RSV it is no longer used.

Ribavirin is a fundamental component of hepatitis C therapy in combination with IFN-α or pegylated IFN. When given in combination for 6 months, significant improvement in virologic and histologic response has been documented. Persistent response rates have been documented in 50% of patients (176,177). When given intravenously or orally, it has been reported to reduce mortality significantly in patients with Lassa fever (178). Of perhaps greater interest for Eastern countries, ribavirin was demonstrated to be useful for epidemic hemorrhagic fever (179). Combined ribavirin and pegylated IFN therapy are also discussed in Chapter 87.

RESISTANCE

Emergence of viruses resistant to ribavirin has not been documented.

ADVERSE EFFECTS

No adverse effect has been clearly attributable to aerosol therapy with ribavirin, although reports of adverse effects during or after therapy of infants with RSV have included bronchospasm, changes in pulmonary function tests, pneumothorax in ventilated patients, apnea, cardiac arrest, hypotension, and

concomitant digitalis toxicity. Changes in pulmonary function tests after ribavirin therapy in adults with chronic obstructive pulmonary disease have been noted as well, but one study reported no change in respiratory symptoms even though small changes in pulmonary function tests were demonstrated (182).

Precipitation of drug within the ventilatory apparatus of patients receiving mechanical ventilation can be a serious problem but is not a contraindication for its use. Reticulocytosis, rash, and conjunctivitis have been associated with the use of ribavirin aerosol. When the drug was given orally or intravenously, transient elevations of serum bilirubin values and mild anemia are reported. Although there are no pertinent human data, ribavirin is teratogenic and mutagenic in nearly all species in which it has been tested. This drug is therefore contraindicated for women who are or may become pregnant during exposure to the drug.

Some concern has been expressed about the risk to persons in the room with infants being treated with ribavirin aerosol, particularly women of childbearing age. Although this risk seems to be minimal with limited exposure, awareness and caution on the part of personnel are warranted, and continued evaluation is important (183,184). Furthermore, the use of a drug salvage hood is considered mandatory.

CONCLUSIONS ON RIBAVIRIN

Ribavirin has significant broad-spectrum antiviral activity. Its principal use is in the management of hepatitis C with an IFN-α product (185).

MISCELLANEOUS THERAPEUTICS

Interferons

CHEMISTRY, MECHANISM OF ACTION, AND ANTIVIRAL ACTIVITY

IFNs are glycoprotein cytokines (intracellular messengers) with a complex array of immunomodulating, antineoplastic, and antiviral properties. The name *interferon* was derived from landmark experiments by Isaacs and Lindemann in 1957 demonstrating the existence of a biologic substance that interfered with viral replication in infected cells. IFNs are classified as α, β, or γ; natural sources being leukocytes, fibroblasts, and lymphocytes, respectively. Each type of IFN can be produced via recombinant DNA technology.

Binding of IFN to the intact cell membrane is the first step in establishing an antiviral effect (186). IFN binds to specific cell surface receptors; IFN-γ appears to have a different receptor from either IFN-α or IFN-β, which may explain the purported synergistic antiviral and antitumor effects sometimes observed when IFN-γ is given with either of the other two IFN species.

A prevalent view of IFN action is that, after binding, there is synthesis of new cellular RNAs and proteins, which mediate the antiviral effect. Chromosome 21 is required for this antiviral state in humans no matter which species of IFN is used. At least three of the newly synthesized proteins in IFN-treated cells appear to be associated with the development of an antiviral state: 2',5'-oligoadenylate synthetase, a protein kinase, and an endonuclease. The antiviral state is not fully expressed until these primed cells are infected with virus. In addition to their antiviral effect, IFNs have a number of other biologic activities, both useful and potentially deleterious, including inhibition of cell proliferation and enhancement of the cytotoxic activities of lymphocytes, the expression of cell surface antigens, and the phagocytic and tumoricidal activities of macrophages. These properties may play an important role in the *in vivo* antiviral and antitumor effects of the IFNs (186,187).

ABSORPTION, DISTRIBUTION, AND ELIMINATION

IFN is administered intramuscularly or subcutaneously (including into a lesion, such as a wart). Plasma levels are dose dependent, peaking 4 to 8 hours after intramuscular administration and returning to baseline after 18 to 36 hours. There appears to be some variability in absorption in the three classes of IFN and in resultant plasma levels. Leukocyte IFN-α appears to have an elimination half-life of 2 to 4 hours. IFN is inactivated by various organs of the body in an as yet undefined method.

A long-acting, slow-release formulation of IFN has recently been licensed in which IFN is combined with polyethylene glycol. In contrast to the other IFN products that are administered three times weekly, pegylated IFN is given once a week.

CLINICAL INDICATIONS

IFN is licensed as an antiviral for therapy of hepatitis B and C and intralesional administration in the treatment of condyloma acuminatum, or genital wart, which is caused by human papillomaviruses.

Condyloma Acuminatum

Several large controlled trials have demonstrated the clinical benefit of IFN alfa therapy of condyloma acuminatum that was refractory to cytodestructive therapies. Benefit accrues as demonstrated by complete clearing of treated lesions (36% vs. 17% of placebo recipients), as well as by reduction in mean wart area (40% reduction vs. 46% increase) (188). In other well-controlled studies, either a similar (46%) or higher (62%) rate of clearance was reported. Notably, clearing responses of placebo recipients averaged 21% to 22% (189,190). When IFN is administered parenterally, the outcome is poorer (191).

Respiratory Papillomatosis

Recurrent respiratory papillomatosis is a disease in which squamous papillomas recur relentlessly within the larynx and trachea of both children and young adults. Standard management consists of careful microendoscopic excision, usually with a carbon dioxide laser. Numerous case reports and uncontrolled studies have indicated benefit from the use of IFN as an adjunct to surgical treatment. Results of placebo-controlled trials also have suggested benefit (192,193).

Hepatitis

The inhibitory effect of human leukocyte IFN-α on hepatitis B virus replication was documented by a reduction in hepatitis B DNA polymerase. Although this study and others are encouraging, the response rates are low, namely 30% to 40% (194–196).

The activity of IFN in the treatment of hepatitis C has been extensively evaluated (197). IFN dosages ranges from 1×10^6 subcutaneously three times weekly for 1 to 18 months. Only 2.6% of the placebo control subjects had normalized serum alanine aminotransferase values. In contrast, treatment led to serum alanine aminotransferase normalization in 33% to 45% of patients. Unfortunately 50% to 80% of patients had relapses. IFN-α therapy induced remission, but relapse is common, as reviewed (198).

RESISTANCE

Resistance to administered IFN has not been documented, although neutralizing antibodies to recombinant IFNs have been reported. The clinical importance of the latter observation is unknown.

ADVERSE EFFECTS

Side effects are frequent with IFN administration and are usually dose limiting. Influenza-like symptoms—fever, chills, headache, and malaise—commonly occur, but these symptoms usually become less severe with repeated treatments. At doses used in the treatment of condyloma acuminatum, these side effects rarely cause termination of treatment. For local treatment (intralesional administration), pain at the injection site does not differ significantly from that experienced by placebo-treated patients and is short lived. Leukopenia is the most common hematologic abnormality, occurring in up to 26% of patients treated for condyloma. Leukopenia is usually not clinically relevant and is reversible on discontinuation of therapy (199). Increased alanine aminotransferase levels also occur, as does nausea, vomiting, and diarrhea.

At higher doses of IFN, neurotoxicity is encountered, as manifested by personality changes, confusion, loss of attention, disorientation, and paranoid ideation. Early studies with IFN-γ show side effects similar to those with IFN-α and -β but with the addition of dose-limiting hypotension and a marked increase in triglyceride levels.

The amino acid sequences and differences in expression systems of IFN that are produced by recombinant DNA technology may lead to the development of neutralizing antibodies. The biologic significance of these antibodies is unknown.

CONCLUSIONS ON INTERFERONS

IFNs have a role in the treatment of viral and other diseases. At present, they remain one of the mainstays in the treatment of genital warts and hepatitis B and C.

PROMISING NEW COMPOUNDS

Four other antiviral compounds warrant brief note. One is licensed for the treatment of hepatitis B and three compounds are being considered for licensure in various countries of the world. The former compound is discussed in Chapter 86.

Lamivudine, 2'-deoxy-3'-thiacytidine, is the levorotatory enantiomer of a cytosine dideoxy-nucleoside analog. Lamivudine has been identified as a potent inhibitor of HIV-1 and HIV-2 *in vitro* as well as of hepatitis B virus and duck hepatitis B virus (17).

Lamivudine is licensed for the therapy of chronic hepatitis B. Treatment for 1 year normalizes serum alanine aminotransferase and improves histologic inflammatory scores in 50% to 70% of patients. Loss of hepatitis B e antigen (HBeAg) occurs in 30% of treated patients. Its use is limited by the rapid development of resistance to medication. Within 1 year as many as 25% of patients will have developed resistance to medication. Likely, it will be used with other drugs in the treatment of hepatitis B in the future (200–202).

Pleconaril, 3-[3,3-dimethyl-4[3-(3-methyl-5-isoxazolyl)propyl]oly]-5-(trifluoromethyl)-1,2,4-oxadiazole, is a broad spectrum antipicornaviral agent. It is currently being assessed for the treatment of rhinovirus infections in phase III trials. This medication binds to the hydrophobic pocket of the virus capsid protein VP1. By binding to this pocket, pleconaril induces conformational changes in the viral capsid that lead to altered receptor binding and viral uncoating. It is active against most enteroviruses and rhinoviruses. The current regulatory applications demonstrate antiviral activity for rhinovirus colds and chronic enterovirus infections of the CNS in patients with agammaglobulinemia.

TABLE 32.3. Antiviral Therapy for Specific Clinical Syndromes with Pediatric and Adult (Maximum) Doses and Alternatives

Virus	Clinical syndrome	Antiviral agent of choice	Alternative agents
Influenza A	Influenza, treatment	Oseltamivir; 2 mg/kg/d p.o. ÷ 2; maximum (>1 yr of age)	Rimantadine; 5 mg/kg/day p.o., adult maximum 200 mg p.o. daily or divided b.i.d. duration 5–7 days Amantadine: 5 mg/kg/d p.o., adult maximum 200 mg p.o. divided b.i.d.; duration 5–7 days
	Influenza, prophylaxis	Oseltamivir: 2 mg/kg/d p.o. ÷ 2; maximum (>1 yr of age)	Rimantadine: 5 mg/kg/d p.o., adult maximum 100–200 mg p.o. daily divided or b.i.d.; duration up to 6 wk Amantadine: 5 mg/kg/d p.o., adult maximum 100–200 mg p.o. daily divided or b.i.d.; duration up to 6 wk Zanamavir: inhaled, 10 mg b.i.d.
Influenza B	Influenza, treatment	Oseltamivir: 2 mg/kg/day p.o. ÷ 2; maximum (>1 yr of age)	Zanamavir, inhaled, 10 mg b.i.d.
Cytomegalovirus (CMV)	Retinitis in AIDS patients	Ganciclovir: Induction: 5 mg/kg per dose i.v. every 12 h for 14–21 days Maintenance: 6 mg/kg/d i.v. 5 times per week or oral at either 1,000 mg t.i.d. or 500 mg 6 times per day; duration indefinite or Valganciclovir: adult dosage 450 mg b.i.d. for 2 wk, 450 mg daily	Foscarnet: Induction: 60 mg/kg per dose i.v. every 8 h for 14–21 days Maintenance: 90 mg/kg/d i.v. daily; duration indefinite or Ganciclovir ocular insert Cidofovir: Induction: 5 mg/kg per dose once a week for two doses Maintenance: 3 mg/kg per dose once every other week
	Pneumonitis, colitis; esophagitis in immunocompromised patients	Ganciclovir: Induction: 2.5 mg/kg per dose i.v. every 8 h for 20 days (possibly with CMVIG or IVIG) Maintenance: 5 mg/kg/d 3–5 times per week for 20 doses ± CMVIG or IVIG	Foscarnet: Induction: 60 mg/kg per dose i.v. every 8 h for 14–21 days Maintenance: 90 mg/kg/d i.v. daily; duration 4–6 wk Cidofovir: Induction: 5 mg/kg per dose once a week for two doses Maintenance: 5 mg/kg per dose once every other week Valganciclovir, 900 mg once daily
Herpes simplex virus (HSV)	Neonatal herpes	Acyclovir: 60 mg/kg/d i.v. divided every 8 h; duration 14–21 days	
	HSV encephalitis	Acyclovir: 30 mg/kg/d i.v. divided every 8 h; duration 14–21 days	
	HSV gingivostomatitis	Supportive care	Acyclovir: 10 mg/kg per dose p.o. 5 times per day, adult maximum 200 mg p.o. 5 times per day; duration 7–10 days Acyclovir: 15 mg/kg/d i.v. divided every 8 h; duration until able to switch to oral therapy
	First episode of genital infection	Valaciclovir: 1,000 mg p.o. b.i.d.; duration 10 days or Famciclovir: 500 mg p.o. b.i.d.; duration 10 days	Acyclovir: 200 mg p.o. 5 times per day or 400 mg p.o. t.i.d.; duration 10 days Acyclovir: 15 mg/kg/d i.v. divided every 8 h; duration until able to switch to oral therapy
	Recurrent genital herpes	Valaciclovir: 500 mg p.o. b.i.d.; duration 5 days Famciclovir: 250 mg p.o. b.i.d.; duration 5 days	Acyclovir: 200 mg p.o. 5 times per day or 400 mg p.o. b.i.d.; duration 5 days
	Suppression of genital infection	Valaciclovir: 500 or 1,000 mg/d Famciclovir: 125 mg p.o. b.i.d.	Acyclovir: 200 mg p.o. t.i.d. or q.i.d. or 400 mg b.i.d. or t.i.d., duration 6–12 mo
	Whitlow	Famciclovir: 125 mg/b.i.d.	Acyclovir: 200 mg p.o. 5 times per day; duration 10 days
	Eczema herpeticum	Valaciclovir: 1,000 mg p.o. b.i.d.; duration 10 days Famciclovir: 500 mg p.o. b.i.d.; duration 10 days	Acyclovir: 10 mg/kg per dose p.o. 3–5 times per day, adult maximum 200 mg p.o. 5 times per day; duration 5–7 days
	Mucocutaneous in immunocompromised hosts: Mild	Acyclovir: 15 mg/kg/d i.v., divided every 8 h; duration until able to switch to oral therapy Valaciclovir: 1,000 mg p.o. b.i.d.; duration 10 days Famciclovir: 500 mg p.o. b.i.d.; duration 10 days	Acyclovir: 10–20 mg/kg per dose p.o. 5 times per day, adult maximum 200–400 mg p.o. 5 times per day; duration 10–21 days
	Moderate-severe	Acyclovir: 15 mg/kg per dose or 750 mg/m²/d i.v. divided every 8 h; duration 10–21 days	

(continued)

TABLE 32.3. (*continued*)

Virus	Clinical syndrome	Antiviral agent of choice	Alternative agents
HSV (*cont.*)	Prophylaxis in bone marrow	Acyclovir: 200 mg p.o. 3–5 times per day or 15 mg/kg/d i.v. divided every 8 h or 750 mg/m^2/d i.v., divided every 8 h; duration until no longer immunocompromised	Valaciclovir: 1,000 mg p.o. daily or Famciclovir: 500 mg p.o. b.i.d. until no longer immunosuppressed
	Acyclovir-resistant HSV	Foscarnet: 40 mg/kg per dose i.v. every 8 h; duration until lesion is completely healed	Cidofovir: 5 mg/kg per dose once weekly until symptoms resolved
	Keratitis or keratoconjunctivitis	Trifluridine: one drop every 2 h (maximum nine drops per day) until cornea is reepithelialized, then every 4 h for an additional 7 days (maximum 21 days)	Vidarabine: a thick strip of ointment (1.25 cm) every 3 h until cornea is completely reepithelialized, then b.i.d. for an additional 7 days
Varicella-zoster virus (VZV)	Chickenpox, healthy child	Supportive care	Acyclovir: 20 mg/kg per dose p.o. q.i.d., adult maximum 800 mg p.o. q.i.d. (start within 24 h of rash); duration 5 days (>14 years of age) or Valaciclovir: 1 gm p.o. t.i.d., duration 7 days or Famciclovir: 500 mg p.o. t.i.d., duration 7 days
	Chickenpox, immunocompromised child	Acyclovir: 1,500 mg/m^2/d i.v. divided every 8 h; duration 5–7 days	
	Zoster (shingles), healthy child	Supportive care	Acyclovir: 20 mg/kg per dose p.o. q.i.d., adult maximum 800 mg p.o. q.i.d.; duration 7–10 days or Famciclovir: 500 mg p.o. t.i.d.; duration 7 days or Valaciclovir: 1,000 mg t.i.d.; duration 7–14 days
	Zoster (shingles), immunocompromised child	Acyclovir: 1,500 mg/m^2/d i.v. every 8 h; duration 7 days Valaciclovir: 1,000 mg p.o. t.i.d. for 7 days	
	Zoster	Valaciclovir: 1 g p.o. t.i.d. for 7 days	Acyclovir: 800 mg p.o. every 4 h for 5 days
	Normal adult	Famciclovir: 500 mg p.o. every 8 h for 7 days	

^{a}If immunocompromised host.

p.o., orally; b.i.d., twice daily; i.v., intravenously; t.i.d., three times daily; CMVIG, CMV immune globulin; IVIG, intravenous immune globulin; q.i.d., four times daily.

Adefovir dipivoxil, bis-pivaloyloxymethyl-9-(2-phosphonylmethoxyethyl)adenine, is the orally bioavailable prodrug of adefovir. This drug has activity against both herpes and hepadnaviruses. It is in the nucleotide class of medications. Treatment of chronic hepatitis B at 10 mg daily significantly decreases HBV DNA polymerase (3.56 logs compared with 0.55 logs in placebo recipients), improves hepatitic histopathology scores, and induces loss of HBeAg (203).

Entecavir, [1S-(1α,3α,4β)]-2-amino-1,9-dihydro-9[4-hydroxymethyl0-2-methylenecyclopentyl]-6H-purin-6-one, is a nucleoside analog that is orally bioavailable for the treatment of chronic hepatitis B. Phase III trials are in progress.

CONCLUSION

Although relatively few antiviral drugs are licensed for use at this time, there is significant interest in the development of antiviral compounds. Table 32.3 summarizes the use of currently available antivirals for indications other than therapy of HIV infections. Systematic approaches have revealed a number of promising new drugs that are in various stages of evaluation. A better understanding of the molecular biology of virus replication and pathogenesis should elucidate drugs with enhanced virus-specific activity.

ACKNOWLEDGMENTS

Work that was performed and reported by the author was supported by contracts NO1-AI-15113, NO1-AI-62554, and NO1-AI-12667 from the Antiviral Research Branch of the National Institute of Allergy and Infectious Diseases, a grant from the Division of Research Resources (RR-032) from the National Institutes of Health, and a grant from the state of Alabama.

REFERENCES

1. Zaia JA. Infections in organ transplant recipients. In: Richmond DD, Whitley RJ, Hayden FG, eds. *Clinical virology.* Washington, DC: ASM Press, 2002:79–100.
2. Diamond C, Tilles JG. Myositis and myocarditis. In: Richmond DD, Whitley RJ, Hayden FG, eds. *Clinical virology.* Washington, DC: ASM Press, 2002:101–116.
3. Impact-RSV Study Group. Palivizumab, a humanized respiratory syncytial virus monoclonal antibody, reduces hospitalization from respiratory syncytial virus infection in high-risk infants. *Pediatrics* 1998;102:531–537.
4. Groothuis JR, Simoes EA, Levin MJ, et al. Prophylactic administration of respiratory syncytial virus immune globulin to high-risk infants and young children. The respiratory syncytial immune globulin study group. *N Engl J Med* 1993;329:1524–1530.
5. Winston DJ, Ho WG, Lin CH, et al. Intravenous immune globulin for prevention of cytomegalovirus infection and interstitial pneumonia after bone marrow transplantation. *Ann Intern Med* 1987;106:12–18.
6. Meyers JD, Leszczynski J, Zaia JA, et al. Prevention of cytomegalovirus

infection by cytomegalovirus immune globulin after marrow transplantation. *Ann Intern Med* 1983;98:442–446.

7. O'Reilly RJ, Reich L, Gold J. A randomized trial of intravenous hyper-immune globulin for the prevention of cytomegalovirus infections following marrow transplantation: preliminary results. *Transplant Proc* 1983;15:1405–1413.

8. Bowden RA, Sayers M, Flournoy N, et al. Cytomegalovirus immune globulin and seronegative blood products to prevent primary cytomegalovirus infection after marrow transplantation. *N Engl J Med* 1986;314:1006–1110.

9. Emanuel D, Cunningham I, Jules-Elysee K, et al. Cytomegalovirus pneumonia after bone marrow transplantation successfully treated with the combination of ganciclovir and high-dose intravenous immune globulin. *Ann Intern Med* 1988;109:777–782.

10. Reed EC, Bowden RA, Dandliker PS, et al. Treatment of cytomegalovirus pneumonia with ganciclovir and intravenous cytomegalovirus immunoglobulin in patients with bone marrow transplants. *Ann Intern Med* 1988;109:783–788.

11. Elion GB, Furman PA, Fyfe JA, et al. Selectivity of action of an antiherpetic agent, 9-(2-hydroxyethoxymethyl) guanine. *Proc Natl Acad Sci USA* 1977;74:5716–5720.

12. Schaeffer HJ, Beauchamp L, deMiranda P, et al. 9-(2-hydroxyethoxymethyl) guanine activity against viruses of the herpes group. *Nature* 1978;272:583–585.

13. Fyfe JA, Keller PM, Furman PA, et al. Thymidine kinase from herpes simplex virus phosphorylates the new antiviral compound, 9-(2-hydroxyethoxymethyl)guanine. *J Biol Chem* 1978;253:8721–8727.

14. Derse D, Chang Y-C, Furman PA, et al. Inhibition of purified human and herpes simplex virus-induced DNA polymerase by 9-(2-hydroxyethoxy methyl)guanine [acyclovir] triphosphate: effect on primer-template function. *J Biol Chem* 1981;256:11447–11451.

15. Furman PA, St. Clair MH, Spector T. Acyclovir triphosphate is a suicide inactivator of the herpes simplex virus DNA polymerase. *J Biol Chem* 1984;259:9575–9579.

16. Collins P, Bauer DJ. The activity *in vitro* against herpes virus of 9-(2-hydroxyethoxymethyl) guanine (acycloguanosine), a new antiviral agent. *J Antimicrob Chemother* 1979;5:432–436.

17. Balfour HH Jr. Antiviral drugs. *N Engl J Med* 1999;340:1255–1268.

18. Beutner KR. Valacyclovir: a review of its antiviral activity, pharmacokinetic properties, and clinical efficacy. *Antiviral Res* 1995;28:281–290.

19. deMiranda P, Blum MR. Pharmacokinetics of acyclovir after intravenous and oral administration. *J Antimicrob Chemother* 1983;12:29–37.

20. Laskin OL. Acyclovir: pharmacology and clinical experience. *Arch Intern Med* 1984;144:1241–1246.

21. Ormrod D, Scott LJ, Perry CM. Valaciclovir: a review of its long term utility in the management of genital herpes simplex virus and cytomegalovirus infections. *Drugs* 2000;59:839–863.

22. Corey L, Benedetti J, Critchlow C, et al. Treatment of primary first episode genital herpes simplex virus infections with acyclovir: results of topical, intravenous, and oral therapy. *J Antimicrob Chemother* 1983;12:79–88.

23. Corey L, Fife KH, Benedetti JK, et al. Intravenous acyclovir for the treatment of primary genital herpes. *Ann Intern Med* 1983;98:914–921.

24. Peacock JE, Kaplowitz LG, Sparling PF, et al. Intravenous acyclovir therapy of first episodes of genital herpes: a multicenter double-blind, placebo-controlled trial. *Am J Med* 1988;85:301–306.

25. Bryson YJ, Dillon M, Lovett M, et al. Treatment of first episodes of genital herpes simplex virus infection with oral acyclovir: a randomized double-blind controlled trial in normal subjects. *N Engl J Med* 1983;308:916–921.

26. Mertz GJ, Critchlow CW, Benedetti J, et al. Double-blind placebo-controlled trial of oral acyclovir in first-episode genital herpes simplex virus infection. *JAMA* 1984;252:1147–1151.

27. Reichman RC, Badger GJ, Mertz GJ, et al. Treatment of recurrent genital herpes simplex infection with oral acyclovir. Controlled trial. *JAMA* 1984;251:2103–2107.

28. Nilsen AE, Aasen T, Halsos AM, et al. Efficacy of oral acyclovir in the treatment of initial and recurrent genital herpes. *Lancet* 1982;2:571–573.

29. Douglas JM, Critchlow C, Benedetti J, et al. A double-blind study of oral acyclovir for suppression of recurrences of genital herpes simplex virus infection. *N Engl J Med* 1984;310:1551–1556.

30. Mertz GJ, Jones CC, Mills J, et al. Long-term acyclovir suppression of frequently recurring genital herpes simplex virus infection. *JAMA* 1988;260:201–206.

31. Straus SE, Takiff HE, Seidlin M, et al. Suppression of frequently recurring genital herpes: placebo-controlled double-blind trial of oral acyclovir. *N Engl J Med* 1984;310:1545–1550.

32. Kaplowitz LG, Baker D, Gelb L, et al., the Acyclovir Group. Prolonged continuous acyclovir treatment of normal adults with frequently recurring genital herpes simplex virus infections. *JAMA* 1991;265:747–751.

33. Straus SE, Croen KD, Sawyer MH, et al. Acyclovir suppression of frequently recurring genital herpes. Efficacy and diminishing need during successive years of treatment. *JAMA* 1988;260:2227–2230.

34. Kost RG, Hill EL, Tigges M, et al. Brief report: recurrent acyclovir resistant genital herpes in an immunocompetent host. *N Engl J Med* 1993;329:1777–1781.

35. Straus SE, Seidlin M, Takiff HE, et al. Effect of oral acyclovir treatment on symptomatic and asymptomatic shedding in recurrent genital herpes. *Sex Transm Dis* 1989;16:107–113.

36. Reitano M, Tyring SK, Lang W, et al. Valaciclovir for the suppression of recurrent genital herpes simplex virus infection: a large-scale dose range-finding

37. Raborn GW, McGaw WT, et al. Oral acyclovir and herpes labialis: a randomized, double-blind, placebo-controlled study. *J Am Dent Assoc* 1987;115:38–42.

38. Spruance SL, Stewart JCB, Rowe NH, et al. Treatment of recurrent herpes simplex labialis with oral acyclovir. *J Infect Dis* 1990;161:185–190.

39. Spruance SL, Hamill ML, Hoge WS, et al. Acyclovir prevents reactivation of herpes simplex labialis in skiers. *JAMA* 1988;260:1597–1599.

40. Wade JC, Newton B, McLaren C, et al. Intravenous acyclovir to treat mucocutaneous herpes simplex virus infection after marrow transplantation: double-blind trial. *Ann Intern Med* 1982;96:265–269.

41. Meyers JD, Wade JC, Mitchell CD, et al. Multicenter collaborative trial of intravenous acyclovir for treatment of mucocutaneous herpes simplex virus infection in immunocompromised host. *Am J Med* 1982;73:229–235.

42. Shepp DH, Newton BA, Dandliker PS, et al. Oral acyclovir therapy for mucocutaneous herpes simplex virus infections in immunocompromised marrow transplant recipients. *Ann Intern Med* 1985;102:783–785.

43. Saral R, Burns WH, Laskin OL, et al. Acyclovir prophylaxis of herpes simplex virus infections: a randomized, double-blind, controlled trial in bone-marrow-transplant recipients. *N Engl J Med* 1981;305:63–67.

44. Wade JC, Newton B, Flournoy N. Acyclovir for prevention of herpes simplex virus reactivation after marrow transplantation. *Ann Intern Med* 1984;100:823–828.

45. Wade JC, McLaren C, Meyers JD. Frequency and significance of acyclovir-resistant herpes simplex virus isolated from marrow transplant patients receiving multiple courses of treatment with acyclovir. *J Infect Dis* 1983;148:1077–1082.

46. Whitley RJ, Alford CA Jr, Hirsch MS, et al., the National Institute of Allergy and Infectious Diseases Collaborative Antiviral Study Group. Vidarabine versus acyclovir therapy in herpes simplex encephalitis. *N Engl J Med* 1986;314:144–149.

47. Skoldenberg B, Forsgren M, Alestig K, et al. Acyclovir versus vidarabine in herpes simplex encephalitis: a randomized multicentre study in consecutive Swedish patients. *Lancet* 1984;2:707–711.

48. Kimberlin DW, Lin C-Y, Jacobs RF, et al. The safety and efficacy of high-dose intravenous acyclovir in the management of neonatal herpes simplex virus infections. *Pediatrics* 2001;108:230–238.

49. Kimberlin DW, Lin C-Y, Jacobs RF, et al., and the National Institute of Allergy and Infectious Diseases Collaborative Antiviral Study Group. Natural history of neonatal herpes simplex virus infections in the acyclovir era. *Pedatrics* 2001;108:223–229.

50. Balfour HH Jr, Rotbart HA, Feldman S, et al., Collaborative Acyclovir Varicella Study Group. Acyclovir treatment of varicella in otherwise healthy adolescents. *J Pediatr* 1992;120:627–633.

51. Balfour HH, Kelly JM, Suarez CS, et al. Acyclovir treatment of varicella in otherwise healthy children. *J Pediatr* 1990;116:633–639.

52. Feder BM. Treatment of adult chickenpox with oral acyclovir. *Arch Intern Med* 1990;150:2061–2065.

53. Dunkle LM, Arvin AM, Whitley RJ, et al. A controlled trial of acyclovir for chickenpox in normal children. *N Engl J Med* 1991;325:1539–1544.

54. Haake DA, Zakowski PC, Haake DC, et al. Early treatment with acyclovir for varicella pneumonia in otherwise healthy adults: retrospective controlled study and review. *Rev Infect Dis* 1990;12:788–798.

55. Prober CG, Kirk LE, Keeney RE. Acyclovir therapy of chickenpox in immunosuppressed children—a collaborative study. *J Pediatr* 1982;101:622–625.

56. Nyerges G, Meszner Z, Gyarmati E, et al. Acyclovir prevents dissemination of varicella in immunocompromised children. *J Infect Dis* 1988;157:309–313.

57. Bean B, Braun C, Balfour HH Jr. Acyclovir therapy for acute herpes zoster. *Lancet* 1982;2:118–121.

58. McGill J, MacDonad DR, Fall C, et al. Intravenous acyclovir in acute herpes zoster infection. *J Infect Dis* 1983;6:157–161.

59. Wood MJ, Ogan PH, McKendrick MW, et al. Efficacy of oral acyclovir treatment of acute herpes zoster. *Am J Med* 1988;85:79–83.

60. Morton P, Thomson AN. Oral acyclovir in the treatment of herpes zoster in general practice. *N Z Med J* 1989;102:93–95.

61. Wood MJ, Kay R, Dworkin RH, et al. Oral acyclovir accelerates pain resolution in herpes zoster: a meta-analysis of placebo-controlled trials. *Clin Infect Dis* 1996;22:341–347.

62. Beutner KR, Friedman DJ, Forszpaniak C, et al. Valaciclovir compared with acyclovir for improved therapy for herpes zoster in immunocompetent adults. *Antimicrob Agents Chemother* 1995;39:1546–1553.

63. Ormrod D, Goa K. Valaciclovir: a review of its use in the management of herpes zoster. *Drugs* 2000;59:1317–1340.

64. Balfour HH Jr, Bean B, Laskin O, et al., the Burroughs Wellcome Collaborative Acyclovir Study Group. Acyclovir halts progression of herpes zoster in immunocompromised patients. *N Engl J Med* 1983;308:1448–1453.

65. Shepp D, Dandliker PS, Meyers JD. Treatment of varicella-zoster virus in severely immunocompromised patients: a randomized comparison of acyclovir and vidarabine. *N Engl J Med* 1987;314:208–212.

66. Crumpacker CS, Schnipper LE, Marlowe SI, et al. Resistance to antiviral drugs of herpes simplex virus isolated from a patient treated with acyclovir. *N Engl J Med* 1982;306:343–346.

67. Kimberlin DW, Coen DM, Biron KK, et al. Molecular mechanisms of antiviral resistance. *Antiviral Res* 1995;26:369–401.

study. International Valaciclovir HSV Study Group. *J Infect Dis* 1998;178:603–610.

68. Sacks SL, Wanklin RJ, Reece DE, et al. Progressive esophagitis from acyclovir-resistant herpes simplex. Clinical roles for DNA polymerase mutants and viral heterogeneity. *Ann Intern Med* 1989;111:893–899.
69. Kimberlin DW, Kern ER, Sidwell RW, et al. Models of antiviral resistance. *Antiviral Res* 1995;26:415–422.
70. Erlich KS, Mills J, Chatis P, et al. Acyclovir-resistant herpes simplex virus infections in patients with the acquired immunodeficiency syndrome. *N Engl J Med* 1989;320:293–296.
71. Safrin S, Crumpacker C, Chatis P, et al, other members of the Aids Clinical Trials Group. A controlled trial comparing foscarnet with vidarabine for acyclovir-resistant mucocutaneous herpes simplex in the acquired immunodeficiency syndrome. *N Engl J Med* 1991;325:551–555.
72. Erlich KS, Jacobson MA, Koehler JE, et al. Foscarnet therapy for severe acyclovir-resistant herpes simplex virus type-2 infections in patients with the acquired immunodeficiency syndrome (AIDS). *Ann Intern Med* 1989;110:710–713.
73. Ljungman P, Ellis MN, Hackman RC, et al. Acyclovir-resistant herpes simplex virus causing pneumonia after marrow transplantation. *J Infect Dis* 1990;162:244–248.
74. Gateley A, Gander RM, Jonson PC, et al. Herpes simplex virus type 2 meningoencephalitis resistant to acyclovir in a patient with AIDS. *J Infect Dis* 1990;161:711–715.
75. Englund JA, Zimmerman ME, Swierkosz EU, et al. Herpes simplex virus resistant to acyclovir. A study in a tertiary care center. *Ann Intern Med* 1990;112:416–422.
76. Marks GL, Nolen PE, Erlich KS, et al. Mucocutaneous dissemination of acyclovir-resistant herpes simplex virus in a patient with AIDS. *Rev Infect Dis* 1989;11:474–476.
77. Pahwa S, Biron K, Lim W, et al. Continuous varicella-zoster infection associated with acyclovir resistance in a child with AIDS. *JAMA* 1988;260:2879–2882.
78. Jacobson MA, Berger TC, Fikrig S, et al. Acyclovir-resistant varicella zoster virus infection after chronic oral acyclovir therapy in patients with the acquired immunodeficiency syndrome (AIDS). *Ann Intern Med* 1990;112:187–191.
79. Safrin S, Berger TG, Gilson I. Foscarnet therapy in five patients with AIDS and acyclovir-resistant varicella zoster virus infection. *Ann Intern Med* 1991;115:19–21.
80. Speigal DM, Lau K. Acute renal failure and coma secondary to acyclovir therapy. *JAMA* 1986;155:1882–1883.
81. Bianchetti MG, Roduit C, Oetliker OH. Acyclovir induced renal failure: course and risk factors. *Pediatr Nephrol* 1991;5:238–239.
82. Brigden D, Rosling AE, Woods NC. Renal function after acyclovir intravenous injection. *Am J Med* 1982;73:182–185.
83. Wade KC, Meyers JD. Neurologic symptoms associated with parenteral acyclovir treatment after bone marrow transplantation. *Ann Intern Med* 1983;98:921–925.
84. Andrews EB, Tilson HH, Hurin BA, et al. Acyclovir in Pregnancy Registry. An observational epidemiological approach. *Am J Med* 1988;85(suppl 2A):123–128.
85. Frenkel LM, Brown ZA, Bryson YJ, et al. Pharmacokinetics of acyclovir in the term human pregnancy and neonate. *Am J Obstet Gynecol* 1991;164:569–576.
86. Kendle JB, Fan-Havard P. Cidofovir in the treatment of cytomegaloviral disease. *Ann Pharmacother* 1999;33:752–753.
87. Plosker GL, Noble S. Cidofovir: a review of its use in cytomegalovirus retinitis in patients with AIDS. *Drugs* 1999;58:325–345.
88. Bronson JJ, Ferrara LM, Hitchcock MJ, et al. (S)-1-(3-hydroxy-2-(phosphonylmethoxy)propyl)cytosine (HPMPC): a potent antiherpesvirus agent. *Adv Exp Med Biol* 1990;278:277–283.
89. Yang H, Datema R. Prolonged and potent therapeutic and prophylactic effects of (S)-1-[(3-hydroxy-2-phosphonylmethoxy)propyl]cytosine against herpes simplex virus type 2 infections in mice. *Antimicrob Agents Chemother* 1991;35:1596–1600.
90. Lalezari JP, Drew WL, Glutzer E, et al. Treatment with intravenous (S)-1-[3-hydroxy-2-(phosphonylmethoxy)propyl)-cytosine of acyclovir-resistant mucocutaneous infection with herpes simplex virus in a patient with AIDS. *J Infect Dis* 1994;170:570–572.
91. The Ganciclovir Cidofovir Cytomegalovirus Retinitis Trial. The ganciclovir implant plus oral ganciclovir versus parenteral cidofovir for the treatment of cytomegalovirus retinitis in patients with acquired immunodeficiency syndrome. *Am J Ophthalmol* 2001;131:457–467.
92. Erice A. Resistance of human cytomegalovirus to antiviral drugs. *Clin Microbiol Rev* 1999;12:286–297.
93. Nichols WG, Boeckh M. Recent advances in the therapy and prevention of CMV infections. *J Clin Virol* 2000;16:25–40.
94. Perry CM, Balfour JA. Fomivirsen. *Drugs* 1999;57:375–380.
95. Chatis PA, Miller CH, Schrager LE, et al. Successful treatment with foscarnet of an acyclovir-resistant mucocutaneous infection with herpes simplex virus in a patient with acquired immunodeficiency syndrome. *N Engl J Med* 1989;320:297–300.
96. Palestine AG, Polis MA, DeSmet MD, et al. A randomized controlled trial of foscarnet in the treatment of cytomegalovirus retinitis in patients with AIDS. *Ann Intern Med* 1991;115:665–673.
97. Jacobson MA, Drew WL, Feinberg J, et al. Foscarnet therapy for ganciclovir-resistant cytomegalovirus retinitis in patients with AIDS. *J Infect Dis* 1991;163:1348–1351.
98. AIDS Clinical Trials Group. Mortality in patients with the acquired immunodeficiency syndrome treated with either foscarnet or ganciclovir for cytomegalovirus retinitis. Studies of ocular complications of AIDS research group. *N Engl J Med* 1992;326:213–220.
99. Wagstaff AJ, Bryson HM. Foscarnet: a reappraisal of its antiviral activity, pharmacokinetic properties and therapeutic use in immunocompromised patients with viral infectious. *Drugs* 1994;48:199–226.
100. Birch CJ, Tachedjian G, Doherty RR, et al. Altered sensitivity to antiviral drugs of herpes simplex virus isolates from a patient with the acquired immunodeficiency syndrome. *J Infect Dis* 1990;162:731–734.
101. Safrin S, Kemmerly S, Plotkin B, et al. Foscarnet-resistant herpes simplex virus infection in patients with AIDS. *J Infect Dis* 1994;169:193–196.
102. Palestine AG. Clinical aspects of cytomegalovirus retinitis. *Rev Infect Dis* 1988;10(suppl 3):515–521.
103. Griffiths PD, Emery VC. Cytomegalovirus. *Clinical virology.* Washington, DC: ASM Press (in press).
104. Gorensek MJ, Stewart RW, Keys TF, et al. A multivariate analysis of the risk of cytomegalovirus infection in heart transplant recipients. *J Infect Dis* 1988;157:515–522.
105. Zaia JA, Kovacs A, Forman SJ. Human cytomegalovirus-associated pneumonitis: pathogenesis, prevention, and treatment. *Transplant Proc* 1987;19:125–131.
106. Meyers JD. Cytomegalovirus infection following marrow transplantation: risk, treatment and prevention. In: Plotkin SA, Michelson S, Pagano JS, et al., eds. *CMV pathogenesis and prevention of human infection.* New York: Alan R. Liss, 1984:101–117.
107. Matthews T, Boehme R. Antiviral activity and mechanism of action of ganciclovir. *Rev Infect Dis* 1988;10:490–494.
108. Mar E-C, Cheng YC, Huang ES. Effect of 9-(1,3 dihydroxy-2-propoxymethyl) guanine on human cytomegalovirus replication *in vitro. Antimicrob Agents Chemother* 1983;24:518–521.
109. Frank KB, Chiou JF, Cheng YC. Interaction of herpes simplex virus–induced DNA polymerase with 9-(1,3-dihydroxy-2-propoxymethyl) guanine triphosphate. *J Biol Chem* 1984;259:1566–1569.
110. Biron KK, Stanat SC, Sorrell JB, et al. Metabolic activation of the nucleoside analog 9-[(2-hydroxy-1-(hydroxymethyl)ethyoxy]methyl) guanine in human diploid fibroblasts infected with human cytomegalovirus. *Proc Nat Acad Sci USA* 1985;82:2473–2477.
111. Biron KK, Stenbuck PJ, Sorrell JB. Inhibition of the DNA polymerases of varicella-zoster virus and human cytomegalovirus by the nucleoside analogs ACV and BW795U. *J Cell Biochem* 1984;8B:207.
112. Smee DF, Bochme R, Chernow M, et al. Intracellular metabolism and enzymatic phosphorylation of 9-(1,3, dihydroxy-2-propoxymethyl) guanine and acyclovir in herpes simplex virus-infected and uninfected cells. *Biochem Pharmacol* 1985;34:1049–1056.
113. Brown F, Banken L, Saywell K, et al. Pharmacokinetics of valganciclovir and ganciclovir following multiple oral dosages of valganciclovir in HIV- and CMV-seropositive volunteers. *Clin Pharmacokinet* 1999;37:167–176.
114. Jacobson MA, De Miranda P, Cederberg DM, et al. Human pharmacokinetics and tolerance of oral ganciclovir. *Antimicrob Agents Chemother* 1987;31:1251–1254.
115. Fletcher C, Sawchuk R, Chinnock B, et al. Human pharmacokinetics of the antiviral drug DHPG. *Clin Pharm Ther* 1986;1:281–286.
116. Cymeval RO. Valganciclovir. *Drugs Res Dev* 1999;5:318–319.
117. Crumpacker CS. Ganciclovir. *N Engl J Med* 1996;335:721–728.
118. Holland GN, Sidikaro Y, Kreiger AE, et al. Treatment of cytomegalovirus retinopathy with ganciclovir. *Ophthalmology* 1987;94:815–823.
119. Mills J, Jacobson MA, O'Donnell JJ, et al. Treatment of cytomegalovirus retinitis in patients with AIDS. *Rev Infect Dis* 1988;10:522–526.
120. Drew WL, Ives D, Lalezari JP, et al. Oral ganciclovir as maintenance treatment for cytomegalovirus retinitis in patients with AIDS. Syntex Cooperative Oral Ganciclovir Study Group. *N Engl J Med* 1995;333:615–620.
121. Dieterich DT, Chachoua A, Lafleur F, et al. Ganciclovir treatment of gastrointestinal infections caused by cytomegalovirus in patients with AIDS. *Rev Infect Dis* 1988;10:532–537.
122. Hoffman VF, Skiest DJ. Therapeutic developments in cytomegalovirus retinitis. *Expert Opin Invest Drugs* 2000;9:207–220.
123. Pescovitz MD, Rabkin J, Merion RM, et al. Valganciclovir results in improved oral absorption of ganciclovir in liver transplant recipients. *Antimicrob Agents Chemother* 2000;10:2811–2815.
124. Sydman DR. Ganciclovir therapy for cytomegalovirus disease associated with renal transplants. *Rev Infect Dis* 1988;10:554–560.
125. Keay S, Petersen E, Icenogle T, et al. Ganciclovir treatment of serious cytomegalovirus infection in heart and heart-lung transplant recipients. *Rev Infect Dis* 1988;10:563–572.
126. Schmidt GM, Horak DA, Niland JC, et al., City of Hope-Stanford-Syntex CMV Study Group. A randomized, controlled trial of prophylactic ganciclovir for cytomegalovirus pulmonary infection in recipients of allogeneic bone marrow transplants. *N Engl J Med* 1991;324:1005–1011.
127. Goodrich JM, Mori M, Gleaves CA, et al. Early treatment with ganciclovir to prevent cytomegalovirus disease after allogeneic bone marrow transplantation. *N Engl J Med* 1991;325:1601–1607.
128. Winston DJ, Ho WG, Bartoni K, et al. Ganciclovir prophylaxis of cytomegalovirus infection and disease in bone marrow transplant recipients. Results of a placebo-controlled, double-blind trial. *Ann Intern Med* 1993;118:179.
129. Erice A, Chou S, Biron KK, et al. Progressive disease due to ganciclovir-resistant cytomegalovirus in immunocompromised patients. *N Engl J Med* 1989;320:289–293.

130. Limaye AP, Corey L, Koelle DM, et al. Emergence of ganciclovir-resistant cytomegalovirus disease among recipients of solid-organ transplants. *Lancet* 2000;356:645–649.

131. Biron KK, Fyfe JA, Stanat SC, et al. A human cytomegalovirus mutant resistant to the nucleoside analog 9-([2-hydroxy-1-(hydroxymethyl) ethoxymethyl] ethoxy]methyl) guanine (BW B759U) induces reduced levels of BW B759U triphosphate. *Proc Natl Acad Sci USA* 1986;83:8769–8773.

132. Stanat SC, Reardon JE, Erice A, et al. Ganciclovir-resistant cytomegalovirus clinical isolates: mode of resistance to ganciclovir. *Antimicrob Agents Chemother* 1991;35:2191–2197.

133. Littler E, Stuart AD, Chee MS. Human cytomegalovirus UL97 open reading frame encodes a protein that phosphorylates the antiviral nucleoside analogue ganciclovir. *Nature* 1992;358:160–162.

134. Shuttleworth G, Shimeld C, Easty D. Viral disease of the eye. In: Richmond DD, Whitley RJ, Hayden FG, eds. *Clinical virology*. Washington, DC: ASM Press, 2002:145–169.

135. Fowles SE, Pue MA, Pierce D, et al. Pharmacokinetics of penciclovir in healthy elderly subjects following a single oral administration of 750 mg famciclovir. *Br J Clin Pharmacol* 1992;34(suppl 1):450P.

136. Pue MA, Pratt SK, Fairless AJ, et al. Linear pharmacokinetics of penciclovir following administration of single oral doses of famciclovir 125, 250, 500 and 750 mg to healthy volunteers. *J Antimicrob Chemother* 1994;33:119–127.

137. de Greef H, Famciclovir Herpes Zoster Clinical Study Group. Famciclovir, a new oral antiherpes drug: results of the first controlled clinical study demonstrating its efficacy and safety in the treatment of uncomplicated herpes zoster in immunocompetent patients. *Int J Antimicrob Agents* 1994;4:241–246.

138. Tyring S, Barbarash RA, Nahlik JE, et al., the Collaborative Famciclovir Herpes Zoster Study Group. Famciclovir for the treatment of acute herpes zoster. Effects on acute disease and postherpetic neuralgia: a randomized, double-blind, placebo-controlled trial. *Ann Intern Med* 1995;123:89–96.

139. Mertz GJ, Loveless MO, Levin MJ, et al. Oral famciclovir for suppression of recurrent genital herpes simplex virus infection in women. A multicenter, double-blind, placebo-controlled trial. Collaborative Famciclovir Genital Herpes Research Group. *Arch Intern Med* 1997;157:343–349.

140. Cirelli R, Heme K, McCrary M, et al. Famciclovir: review of clinical efficacy and safety. *Antiviral Res* 1996;29:141–151.

141. Saltzman R, Jurewicz R, Boon R. Safety of famciclovir in patients with herpes zoster and genital herpes. *Antimicrob Agents Chemother* 1994;38:2454–2457.

142. SmithKline Beecham Pharmaceuticals. Famvir (famciclovir) package insert. King of Prussia, PA, 1994.

143. Daniels S, Schentag JJ. Drug interaction studies and safety of famciclovir in healthy volunteers: a review. *Antiviral Chem Chemother* 1993;4(suppl 1):57–64.

144. Tyring SK, Beutner KR, Tucker BA, et al. Antiviral therapy for herpes zoster: randomized, controlled clinical trial of valacyclovir and famciclovir therapy in immunocompetent patients 50 years and older. *Arch Fam Med* 2000;9:863–869.

145. Couch RB. Respiratory diseases. In: Galasso G, Whitley R, Merigan TC, eds. *Antiviral agents and viral diseases of man,* 4th ed. New York: Lippincott-Raven, 1997:369–413.

146. Davies WL, Grunert RR, Haff RF, et al. Antiviral activity of 1-adamantanamine (amantadine). *Science* 1964;144:862–863.

147. Hoffman CE. Amantadine HCl and related compounds. In: Carter WA, ed. *Selective inhibitors of viral functions.* Cleveland: CRC Press, 1973:199–211.

148. Sears SD, Clements ML. Protective efficacy of low-dose amantadine in adults challenged with wild-type influenza A virus. *Antimicrob Agents Chemother* 1987;31:1470–1473.

149. Couch RB. Prevention and treatment of influenza. *N Engl J Med* 2000;343:1778–1787.

150. Hayden FG. Amantadine and rimantadine resistance in influenza A viruses. *Curr Opin Infect Dis* 1994;7:674–677.

151. Tominack RL, Hayden FG. Rimantadine hydrochlorida and amantadine hydrochloride use in influenza A virus infections. *Antiviral Chemother Infect Dis Clin North Am* 1987;1:459–478.

152. Hayden FG, Palese P. Influenza virus. In: Richmond DD, Whitley RJ, Hayden FG, eds. *Clinical virology.* Washington, DC: ASM Press, 2002:891–920.

153. Dolin R, Reichman RC, Madone HP, et al. A controlled trial of amantadine and rimantadine in the prophylaxis of influenza A infection. *N Engl J Med* 1982;307:580–584.

154. Mostow SR. Prevention, management, and control of influenza. *Am J Med* 1987;82:35–40.

155. Belshe RB, Burk B, Newman F. Resistance of influenza A virus to amantadine and rimantadine: results of one decade of surveillance. *J Infect Dis* 1989;159:430–435.

156. Hayden FG, Belshe RB, Clover RD, et al. Emergence and apparent transmission of rimantadine-resistant influenza A virus in families. *N Engl J Med* 1989;321:1696–1702.

157. Hay AJ. The action of adamantanamines against influenza A viruses: inhibition of the M2 ion channel protein. *Semin Virol* 1992;3:21–30.

158. Belshe RB, Smith MH, Hall CB, et al. Genetic basis of resistance to rimantadine emerging during treatment of influenza virus infection. *J Virol* 1988;62:1508–1512.

159. Hayden FG, Gwaltney JM Jr, Van de Castle RL, et al. Comparative toxicity of amantadine hydrochloride and rimantadine hydrochloride in healthy adults. *Antimicrob Agents Chemother* 1981;19:226–233.

160. Hayden FG, Atmar RL, Schilling M, et al., the Oseltamivir Study Group. Use

161. of the selective oral neuraminidase inhibitor oseltamivir to prevent influenza. *N Engl J Med* 1999;341:1336–1343.

161. He G, Massarella J, Ward P. Clinical pharmacokinetics of the prodrug oseltamivir and its active metabolite Ro 64-0802. *Clin Pharmacokinet* 1999;37:471–484.

162. Bardsley-Elliot A, Noble S. Oseltamivir. *Drugs* 1999;58:851–860.

163. Treanor JJ, Hayden FG, Vrooman PS, et al. Efficacy and safety of the oral neuraminidase inhibitor oseltamivir in treating acute influenza. *JAMA* 2000;283:1016–1024.

164. Whitley RJ, Hayden FG, Reisinger KS, et al. Oral oseltamivir treatment of influenza in children. *Pediatr Infect Dis J* 2001;20:127–133.

165. Nicholson KG, Aoki FY, Osterhause A, et al. Treatment of acute influenza: efficacy and safety of the oral neuraminidase inhibitor oseltamivir. *Lancet* 2000;355:1845–1850.

166. Welliver R, Monto AS, Carewicz O, et al., Oseltamivir Post Exposure Prophylaxis Investigator Group. Effectiveness of oseltamivir in preventing influenza in household contacts: a randomized controlled trial. *JAMA* 2001;285:748–754.

167. Gubareva LV, Kaiser L, Hayden FG. Influenza virus neuraminidase inhibitors. *Lancet* 2000;355:827–835.

168. Gubareva LV, Kaiser L, Matrosovich MN, et al. Selection of influenza virus mutants in experimentally infected volunteers treated with oseltamivir. *J Infect Dis* 2001;183:523–531.

169. Hayden FG, Osterhaus AD, et al. Efficacy and safety of the neuraminidase inhibitor zanamivir in the treatment of influenza virus. *N Engl J Med* 1997;337:874–880.

170. Hayden FG, Gubareva LV, Monto AS, et al., Zanamivir Family Study Group. Inhaled zanamivir for the prevention of influenza in families. *N Engl J Med* 2000;343:1282–1289.

171. Monto AS, Robinson DP, Herlocher ML, et al. Zanamivir in the prevention of influenza among healthy adults: a randomized controlled trial. *JAMA* 1999;282:31–35.

172. Sidwell RW, Huffman JH, Khare GP, et al. Broad-spectrum antiviral activity of Virazole: 1-B-D-ribofuranosyl-1, 2, 4-triazole-3-carboxamide. *Science* 1972;177:705–706.

173. Wray SK, Gilbert BE, Noall MW, et al. Mode of action or ribavirin: effect of nucleotide pool alterations on influenza virus ribonucleoprotein synthesis. *Antiviral Res* 1985;5:29–37.

174. Eriksson B, Helgstrand E, Johansson NG, et al. Inhibition of influenza virus ribonucleic acid polymerase by ribavirin triphosphate. *Antimicrob Agents Chemother* 1977;11:946–951.

175. Laskin OL, Longstreth JA, Hart CC, et al. Ribavirin disposition in high-risk patients for acquired immunodeficiency syndrome. *Clin Pharmacol Ther* 1987;41:546–555.

176. Heathcote EJ, Shiffman ML, Cooksley GE, et al. Peginterferon alfa-2a in patients with chronic hepatitis C and cirrhosis. *N Engl J Med* 2000;343:1673–1680.

177. Zeuzem S, Feinman SV, Rasenack J, et al. Peginterferon alpha-2a in patients with chronic hepatitis C. *N Engl J Med* 2000;343:1666–1672.

178. McCormick JB, King IJ, Webb PA, et al. Lassa fever: effective therapy with ribavirin. *N Engl J Med* 1986;314:20–26.

179. Huggins JW. Prospects for treatment of viral ribavirin, a broad spectrum of antiviral drug. *Rev Infect Dis* 1989;11(suppl):750–761.

180. Chapman LE, Khabbaz RF. Etiology and epidemiology of the four corners hantavirus outbreak. *Infect Agents Dis* 1994;3:234–244.

181. McHutchison JG, Gordon SC, Schiff ER, et al. Interferon alfa-2b alone or in combination with ribavirin as initial treatment for chronic hepatitis C. Hepatitis Interventional Therapy Group. *N Engl J Med* 1998;339:1485–1492.

182. Liss HP, Bernstien J. Ribavirin aerosol in the elderly. *Chest* 1988;93:1239–1240.

183. Rodriguez WJ, Bui RH, Conner JD, et al. Environmental exposure of primary care personnel to ribavirin aerosol when supervising treatment of infants with respiratory syncytial virus infections. *Antimicrob Agents Chemother* 1987;31:1143–1146.

184. Centers for Disease Control and Prevention. Assessing exposures of healthcare personnel to aerosols of ribavirin—California. *JAMA* 1988;260:1844–1845.

185. Davis GL, Esteban-Mur R, Rustgi V, et al. Interferon alfa-2b alone or in combination with ribavirin for the treatment of relapse of chronic hepatitis C. International Hepatitis Interventional Therapy Group. *N Engl J Med* 1998;339:1493–1499.

186. Cunningham T. Pathogenesis of viral infections. In: Galasso GJ, Whitley RJ, Merigan TC, eds. *Antiviral agents and viral diseases of man,* 4th ed. New York: Lippincott-Raven, 1997:45–78.

187. Ho M. Interferon for the treatment of infections. *Ann Rev Med* 1987;38:51–59.

188. Eron LJ, Judson F, Tucker S, et al. Interferon therapy for condylomata acuminata. *N Engl J Med* 1986;315:1059–1064.

189. Friedman-Kien A, Eron LJ, Conant M, et al. Natural interferon alpha for treatment of condylomata acuminata. *JAMA* 1988;259:533–538.

190. Reichman RC, Oakes D, Bonnez W, et al. Treatment of condyloma acuminatum with three different interferons administered intralesionally: a multicentered, placebo-controlled trial. *Ann Intern Med* 1988;108:675–679.

191. Reichman RC, Oakes D, Bonnez W, et al. Treatment of condyloma acuminatum with three different alpha interferon preparations administered parenterally: a double-blind, placebo-controlled trial. *J Infect Dis* 1990;162:248–258.

192. Haglund S, Jundquist P, Cantell K, et al. Interferon therapy in juvenile laryngeal papillomatosis. *Arch Otolaryngol* 1981;107:327–332.

193. Goepfert H, Gutterman J, Dichtel W, et al. Leukocyte interferon in patients with juvenile papillomatosis. *Ann Otol Rhinol Laryngol* 1982;91:431–436.
194. Greenberg HB, Pollard RB, Lutwick LI, et al. Effect of human leukocyte interferon on hepatitis B virus infection in patients with chronic active hepatitis. *N Engl J Med* 1976;295:517–522.
195. Alexander GJM, Brahm J, Fagan EA. Loss of HBsAg with interferon therapy in chronic hepatitis B virus infection. *Lancet* 1987;1:66–68.
196. Hoofnagle JH. Antiviral treatment of chronic type B hepatitis. *Ann Intern Med* 1987;107:414–415.
197. Davis GL, Balart LA, Schiff ER, et al., the Hepatitis Interventional Therapy Group. Treatment of chronic hepatitis C with recombinant interferon alfa: a multicenter randomized, controlled trial. *N Engl J Med* 1989;321:1501–1506.
198. Davis GL, Lim H. Current status of interferon therapy for chronic hepatitis C: a hepatologist's perspective. *Infect Agents Dis* 1993;2:150–154.
199. Petersen CS, Bjerring P, Larsen J, et al. Systemic interferon alpha-2b increases the cure rate in laser treated patients with multiple persistent genital warts: a placebo-controlled study. *Genitourin Med* 1991;67:99–102.
200. Dienstag JL, Schiff ER, Wright TL, et al. Lamivudine as initial treatment for chronic hepatitis B in the United States. *N Engl J Med* 1999;341:1256–1263.
201. Lai CL, Chien RN, Leung NW, et al. A one-year trial of lamivudine for chronic hepatitis B. Asia Hepatitis Lamivudine Study Group. *N Engl J Med* 1998;339:61–68.
202. Perrillo R, Schiff E, Yoshida E, et al. Adefovir dipivoxil for the treatment of lamivudine-resistant hepatitis B mutants. *Hepatology* 2000;32:129–134.
203. Gilson RJ, Chopra KB, Newell AM, et al. A placebo-controlled phase I/II study of adefovir dipivoxil in patients with chronic hepatitis B virus infection. *J Viral Hepatol* 1999;6:387–395.
204. Whitley RJ. Antiviral therapy. In: Gorbach SL, Bartlett JG, Blacklow NR, eds. *Infectious diseases*, 2nd ed. Philadelphia: WB Saunders, 1998:330–350.

CHAPTER 33
Antifungal Drugs

John W. Baddley and William E. Dismukes

The systemic mycoses are among the most difficult infectious diseases to treat. Long-term therapy for weeks to months is often necessary, as is close monitoring of the patient for potentially serious side effects of the antifungal agents. AMBd, lipid formulations of amphotericin B, flucytosine, ketoconazole, fluconazole, itraconazole, voriconazole, and caspofungin are among the drugs currently available for the therapy of systemic fungal diseases. Although there is growing evidence that the azole antifungal drugs (which have minimal toxicity and can be given orally) are appropriate alternatives in many clinical situations, the fungicidal agent amphotericin B, available since 1958, is the traditional drug of choice for severe systemic infections caused by common fungal pathogens such as *Aspergillus* species, *Blastomyces dermatitidis*, *Candida* species, *Coccidioides immitis*, *Cryptococcus neoformans*, and *Histoplasma capsulatum*. Here, the currently available drugs are discussed in detail, and investigational agents are described briefly.

AMPHOTERICIN B

Amphotericin B desoxycholate (tradename Fungizone, Apothecon), hereafter referred to as AMBd, is a polyene antibiotic and a bacterial by-product of *Streptomyces nodosus* (1). The name is derived from the ability of the drug to act as both an acid and a base. The drug is unstable at high or low pH and must be formulated in a neutral suspension of 5% dextrose and water (D₅W). Conventional amphotericin B, which is complexed with desoxycholate, a bile salt, in order to improve its solubility in water, is marketed in 50-mg vials for intravenous use.

Amphotericin B has a lipophilic structure and binds to cholesterol in mammalian cell membranes and more avidly to ergosterol, the principal sterol in fungal cytoplasmic membranes, resulting in a disruption of membrane integrity with subsequent leakage of intracellular contents and, ultimately, cell death (2). Fungi may rarely become resistant to AMBd and other polyene agents by decreasing membrane ergosterol or by altering the binding characteristics of ergosterol to AMBd (3). However, recent observations suggest that outcomes in immunocompromised hosts may be worse among patients with infections caused by yeasts that are more resistant to AMBd (4,5). In addition, several studies have suggested that the effectiveness of AMBd may be due in part to favorable immunomodulatory effects such as increased macrophage activation (2,6). Some of the enhanced fungicidal activity of monocytes and macrophages in the presence of AMBd may be attributable to accumulation of the drug within these cells rather than immunomodulation (7).

Absorption of AMBd after oral administration is minimal; therefore, intravenous dosing for treatment of systemic mycoses is required (8). Peak serum concentrations are approximately 0.5 to 2.0 μg/mL after a 50-mg dose. Following administration, the desoxycholate salt separates from the complex and amphotericin B becomes highly bound (91%–95%) by plasma proteins. Amphotericin B is distributed principally into the liver, spleen, lungs, kidneys, and to a lesser extent into aqueous humor, and pleural, peritoneal, and synovial fluids (1). Distribution into the central nervous system, vitreous humor, and amniotic fluid is minimal. Because of slow release from tissue stores, the drug can be detected in the serum for 7 to 8 weeks after treatment ceases.

AMBd is infused in 5% dextrose over a 2- to 4-hour interval, usually at a dose of 0.5 to 1.0 mg/kg per day. Vital signs should be monitored closely during the first hour of infusion. For patients with neutropenia and rapidly progressive infection (e.g., invasive aspergillosis) the daily dose may be rapidly escalated from 0.75 to 1.5 mg/kg, administered over a period of 2 to 6 hours, depending on patient tolerance. For patients who have significant infusion-related side effects, poor cardiopulmonary function, or more indolent fungal disease, AMBd may be administered in a slower, more cautious approach. Because of concern for adverse effects, a test dose of 1.0 mg AMBd in 50 to 100 mL D₅W infused over 15 to 30 minutes has been used to assess potential for reactions. Whether or not a test dose is given, patients with rapidly progressive infection should receive a full therapeutic dose within 24 hours. In the majority of patients, rapid infusions of AMBd (over 1 or 2 hours) are generally well tolerated (9), although more infusion-related adverse events, including rigors, tachycardia, nausea, and vomiting, were reported in patients given a 45-minute infusion compared with those given the standard 4-hour infusion (10). Because AMBd is degraded *in situ* and only small amounts are excreted as unchanged drug in the urine and feces, downward dosage adjustments are not necessary for patients with preexisting renal or hepatic impairment. Patients receiving hemodialysis or peritoneal dialysis require no additional dose of AMBd after dialysis, owing to the extensive plasma protein binding and the wide volume of distribution of the drug. Routine measurement of AMBd concentrations in body fluids is not indicated (1).

AMBd has traditionally been the mainstay of systemic antifungal therapy (1) (Table 33.1), and has been the drug of choice for patients with progressive life-threatening mold diseases such as invasive aspergillosis and zygomycosis. While AMBd, alone or in combination, is effective therapy for candidemia and other forms of disseminated candidiasis, azole compounds provide comparable efficacy with less toxicity in non-neutropenic hosts, especially those with catheter-associated uncomplicated

TABLE 33.1. Currently Available Therapy for Selected Systemic Mycoses

Disease	Recommended therapy	Alternatives
Aspergillosis	Voriconazole or amphotericin B or a lipid amphotericin B	Caspofungin Itraconazole
Blastomycosis	Itraconazole or amphotericin B	Ketoconazole Fluconazole
Candidiasis (invasive or disseminated)	Amphotericin B ± flucytosine or fluconazole	Caspofungin Voriconazole Itraconazole
Coccidioidomycosis	Fluconazole or itraconazole	Amphotericin B
Cryptococcosis	Amphotericin B + flucytosine or fluconazole	Itraconazole
Histoplasmosis	Itraconazole or amphotericin B	Ketoconazole Fluconazole
Zygomycosis	Amphotericin B or a lipid amphotericin B	None
Paracoccidioidomycosis	Itraconazole or amphotericin B	Ketoconazole Sulfonamides
Sporotrichosis	Itraconazole	Amphotericin B Fluconazole Terbinafine
Fusariosis	Amphotericin B + fluconazole or voriconazole	None
Scedosporiosis	Voriconazole	Itraconazole
Penicilliosis	Itraconazole + amphotericin B	

candidemia (11,12). Although available data support the effectiveness of fluconazole for hepatosplenic candidiasis (13,14), AMBd is often chosen for candidal syndromes, including meningitis, endocarditis, endophthalmitis, and hepatosplenic disease (15,16). The combination of AMBd and flucytosine is recommended in most patients with cryptococcal meningitis, and is usually given as "induction" therapy for a minimum of 2 weeks (17–19); induction therapy is usually followed by "consolidation" therapy with fluconazole for an additional 8 to 10 weeks. Fluconazole alone may be a reasonable alternative as initial therapy for patients with acquired immunodeficiency syndrome (AIDS) presenting with uncomplicated cryptococcal meningitis (20). The azole drugs provide effective alternative therapy for patients with mild to moderately severe blastomycosis, histoplasmosis, and coccidioidomycosis (21–26), but AMBd should be administered initially to all patients with serious, life-threatening forms of these diseases.

Amphotericin B has been the preferred agent for empiric therapy in the persistently febrile, neutropenic host (27,28), although recently, liposomal amphotericin B has been shown to have similar efficacy and increased tolerance when compared with AMBd (29). The role of AMBd for antifungal prophylaxis, in contrast to empiric therapy, in immunocompromised hosts is less clear. Patients undergoing bone marrow transplantation have less fungal colonization (30) and fewer invasive *Aspergillus* infections (31) when given prophylactic low-dose AMBd, but the overall risk:benefit ratio of this intervention is not known. In the setting of prophylaxis against fungal infection in the bone marrow or stem cell transplant recipient, fluconazole is currently the preferred agent (32,33), although fluconazole has less activity

than AMBd against several fungal pathogens of emerging importance, such as *Aspergillus* species, non-albicans *Candida* species, and the dematiaceous fungi.

Amphotericin B is associated with a variety of infusion-related events and organ toxicities (Table 33.2). Anaphylactic-type reactions manifested as hypotension, bronchospasm, arrhythmias, and even cardiac arrest are rare but have occurred during initial exposure to the drug. Infusion of AMBd frequently is accompanied by headache, nausea, chills, and fever, which in general tend to subside or decrease after several days to several weeks of therapy. Premedication with aspirin, acetaminophen, indomethacin, and diphenhydramine have been used to minimize these infusion-related reactions. If these measures are ineffective, intravenous hydrocortisone or meperidine may be given before the infusion or added to the infusion solution in an attempt to control the symptoms. Thrombophlebitis, which is associated with intravenous infusion of AMBd, may be minimized by coadministration of heparin (500–1,000 units), prolonging the period of infusion, frequently changing infusion sites, or utilizing a central venous catheter.

The kidneys and bone marrow are the organ targets of the major toxic effects of AMBd. Some degree of nephrotoxicity occurs in most patients, often in the form of azotemia, decreased urinary concentrating ability, and hypokalemia. Clinically significant renal tubular acidosis and hypomagnesemia may develop. Renal damage is, in part, dose related and is reversible up to a total dose of 2.0 to 5.0 g (34). The daily dose of AMBd should be decreased or the drug temporarily discontinued when a patient's serum creatinine rises above 2.5 to 3.0 mg/dL. If significant renal dysfunction persists or worsens, a change to a lipid formulation of AMBd should be considered. Efforts to prevent renal toxicity primarily involve the avoidance of other nephrotoxic agents and diuretics, and maintenance of an adequate intravascular volume. Renal toxicity can be reversed and may be prevented with adequate sodium loading and maintenance sodium intake, which interfere with tubuloglomerular feedback (35). A mild to moderate normocytic, normochromic anemia secondary to decreased production of erythropoietin occurs in most patients who receive more than 2 to 3 weeks of AMBd therapy and is usually reversible upon discontinuation of drug. Neutropenia and thrombocytopenia are rare adverse effects. Arachnoiditis and myelopathy are potential complications of intrathecal infusion.

LIPID FORMULATIONS OF AMPHOTERICIN B

Although AMBd continues to have an important role in the treatment of systemic mycoses, a narrow therapeutic index has limited its use. Novel approaches have been developed to improve the delivery of amphotericin B and to reduce toxicities. Theoretically, lipid formulations of the drug allow for selective transfer of amphotericin B to fungal as opposed to mammalian cells, resulting in reduced toxicity (36). With the lipid preparations, higher doses of amphotericin B can be administered safely in most patients. Preparations differ in their configuration, size, amphotericin B content, and lipid component (Table 33.3). Commercially available lipid formulations and approved dosages include amphotericin B lipid complex (ABLC; Abelcet, Enzon, Inc.), 5 mg/kg per day; amphotericin B colloidal dispersion (ABCD; Amphotec or Amphocil, Intermune, Inc.), 3 to 4 mg/kg per day; and liposomal amphotericin B (L-AmB; AmBisome, Fujisawa Healthcare), 3 to 5 mg/kg per day (37,38).

The pharmacokinetics and pharmacodynamics of lipid formulations of amphotericin B also differ greatly from those of AMBd; each lipid formulation has distinct properties,

TABLE 33.2. Adverse Effects of Currently Available Systemic Antifungal Agents

	Amphotericin B	Flucytosine	Ketoconazole	Fluconazole	Itraconazole	Voriconazole	Caspofungin
Acute, life-threatening	Hypotension, anaphylaxis, bronchospasm, arrhythmias						
Gastrointestinal tract	Anorexia, nausea, vomiting	Abdominal pain, diarrhea, nausea, vomiting	Abdominal pain, anorexia, nausea, vomiting	Anorexia, nausea, vomiting	Anorexia, nausea, vomiting	Nausea, vomiting	Anorexia, nausea, vomiting
Skin		Rash	Pruritus ± rash	Rash	Rash	Rash Photosensitivity	Flushing
Kidney	Azotemia, renal tubular acidosis, hypokalemia, hypomagnesemia						Proteinuria
Liver		Hepatitis[a]	Hepatitis[a]	Hepatitis[a]	Hepatitis[a]	Hepatitis[a]	Hepatitis[a]
Bone marrow	Anemia	Anemia leukopenia, thrombocytopenia					
Endocrine			Decreased libido, impotence, oligospermia, gynecomastia, menstrual irregularities				
Other	Headache, fever, chills, weight loss	Confusion, headache	Photophobia, somnolence, headache	Alopecia	Hypokalemia, pedal edema, hypertension, heart failure	Blurry vision, fever	Thrombophlebitis, fever, headache

[a]Usually asymptomatic elevations of transaminases.

TABLE 33.3.   Selected Characteristics of Amphotericin B Formulations

Factor	AMBd	L-AmB	ABCD	ABLC
Brand name	Fungizone	Ambisome	Amphotec/Amphocil	Abelcet
FDA approval	1958	1997	1996	1995
Configuration	Micelle	Unilamellar vesicle (liposome)	Disc	Ribbon, sheet
Size (nm)	<25	90	120–140	1,600–11,000
AmB content (mol%)	—	10	50	33
Lipid component	Deoxycholate	Distearoylphosphatidylglycerol Hydrogenated phosphatidylcholine cholesterol	Cholesteryl sulfate	Dimyristoylphosphatidylglycerol dimyristoylphosphatidylcholine
Cmax (μg/mL)	1.1 ± 0.2 (0.6 mg/kg)	83.0 ± 35.2 (5 mg/kg)	3.1 (5 mg/kg)	1.7 ± 0.8 (5 mg/kg)
AUC (μg/mL · hr)	17.1 ± 5 (0.6 mg/kg)	555 ± 311 (5 mg/kg)	43 (5 mg/kg)	14 ± 7 (5 mg/kg)
Usual dosage	0.5–1 mg/kg	3–5 mg/kg/d	3–4 mg/kg	5 mg/kg
Cost per day[a]	$18–$36	$942–$1319	$414–$480	$825

[a] 2001 average wholesale price at dosage indicated based on a 70-kg person.
AMBd, amphotericin B desoxycholate; L-AmB, liposomal amphotericin B; ABCD, amphotericin B colloidal dispersion; ABLC, amphotericin B lipid complex; FDA, U.S. Food and Drug Administration; Cmax, highest measured plasma concentration; AUC, area under the concentration-time curve.
Data from ref. 37–40.

particularly with respect to volume of distribution, clearance, and area under the concentration-time curve (AUC) (39) (Table 33.3). Generally, for all lipid preparations, kidney tissue concentrations are substantially lower than those with AMBd; in addition, clearance of the lipid preparations is lower than that of AMBd. These formulations allow amphotericin B to selectively bypass the kidneys and concentrate in the reticuloendothelial system or macrophages associated with fungal-induced inflammation (40). Among the lipid formulations, infusion of L-AmB results in greater AUC and maximal plasma concentration (Cmax) than other preparations (Table 33.3); conversely, the apparent volumes of distribution for ABCD and ABLC are much greater than that of L-AmB. Penetration of the lipid preparations into cerebrospinal fluid (CSF) is minimal, although clinical efficacy of lipid formulations has been demonstrated in the treatment of cryptococcal meningitis (41,42).

While approved indications for the lipid formulations are somewhat restricted, these drugs are increasingly used for the treatment of systemic mycoses. Superiority in clinical efficacy, with regard to one lipid preparation versus another, or a lipid preparation versus AMBd, has yet to be established in clinical trials (29,41–46). Important data on the efficacy of ABLC come from an open-label, emergency-use study of patients refractory to or intolerant of conventional therapies (43). Among 291 mycologically confirmed cases evaluable for therapeutic response, when all mycoses were combined, a complete or partial response was seen in 167 (57%) patients (43). In a more recent trial evaluating the safety of ABLC versus L-AmB in the empiric treatment of febrile neutropenic patients, therapeutic success was similar with both drugs, although the study was not designed primarily to evaluate efficacy (44). The efficacy of ABCD for the treatment of documented or suspected invasive aspergillosis was compared with AMBd in a historical cohort of patients with the same disease (45). Overall response was significantly greater in the group that received ABCD ($p < 0.001$); however, 85% of patients in the ABCD group had previously received AMBd, which may have contributed to the good response (45). In a recent trial comparing ABCD versus AMBd in the empiric treatment of febrile neutropenia, therapeutic success was similar with the two study drugs (46); ABCD was associated with decreased renal toxicity, but more frequent infusion-related events (46). In contrast to ABLC and ABCD, the efficacy of L-AmB has been evaluated in a greater number of patients (37). In a comparative trial of

L-AmB at 4 mg/kg with AMBd at 0.7 mg/kg for the treatment of cryptococcal meningitis in HIV-infected patients, a significantly greater number of patients who received L-AmB had CSF culture conversion to negative when evaluated at day 14 of therapy (42). Time to clinical response and failure rate did not differ between the two groups. In a recent study of L-AmB versus AMBd as empiric therapy for patients with persistent fever and neutropenia (29), the overall efficacy according to composite score was 50% for L-AmB and 49% for AMBd. However, there were fewer breakthrough fungal infections in patients who received L-AmB (3.2%) when compared with AMBd (7.8%, $p = 0.009$). In addition, patients who received L-AmB had significantly fewer infusion-related and nephrotoxic effects (29).

As a general rule, lipid formulations should not be used as first-line therapy for most patients with candidiasis, cryptococcosis, or the endemic mycoses, unless the patient has preexisting renal dysfunction (serum creatinine ≥ 2.5–3.0 mg/dL), or is refractory to or intolerant of AMBd or azole therapy. However, initial therapy with a lipid formulation should be considered when treating a patient with severe invasive mold disease, such as aspergillosis or zygomycosis, especially if the patient is already receiving nephrotoxic drugs (47). All three lipid formulations currently are indicated in patients with systemic mycoses, particularly aspergillosis, who are refractory to or intolerant of AMBd. In addition, L-AmB is approved as empiric therapy for the neutropenic patient with persistent fever, despite broad-spectrum antibiotics (29). Cost is an important consideration when considering these agents for use; lipid formulations are substantially more expensive than AMBd (Table 33.3).

The frequency of adverse events with lipid preparations of amphotericin B are difficult to estimate, largely because of lack of comparability among studies regarding dosing, premedications prior to dosing, and standardized definitions of adverse events and toxicity. Similar to AMBd, primary adverse events are infusion-related events (e.g., fever, chills, nausea, vomiting) and nephrotoxicity (Table 33.2). Infusion-related events associated with L-AmB appear to occur less frequently than those with ABLC, ABCD, or AMBd. In a recent trial evaluating the safety of L-AmB versus ABLC in the empiric treatment of febrile neutropenic patients, those receiving L-AmB experienced significantly less fever and chills/rigors than those receiving ABLC (44). Other important infusion-related events include hypoxia, hyper- or hypotension, and tachycardia. As with

AMBd, frequency and severity of infusion-related events may decrease with subsequent doses, and premedications are useful to ameliorate or prevent symptoms and events. Nephrotoxicity associated with the lipid preparations is less common than with AMBd. Although comparative studies are lacking, approximate rates of nephrotoxicity, defined as twice baseline serum creatinine, are as follows: ABCD approximately 25%; L-AmB approximately 20%; ABLC approximately 25%; and AMBd approximately 30% to 50% (37). The utility of measures such as volume expansion and sodium loading to reduce nephrotoxicity in patients receiving lipid preparations has not been clearly defined, although these measures are commonly used in clinical practice.

FLUCYTOSINE

Flucytosine (5-fluorocytosine, 5-FC; tradename Ancobon, ICN Pharmaceuticals, Costa Mesa, CA, U.S.A.) is an orally administered antifungal agent used principally in combination with AMBd for the treatment of cryptococcal meningitis and disseminated or invasive forms of candidiasis (2,48). The antifungal activity of this fluorine analog of cytosine results from its antimetabolite properties. After uptake by fungi, flucytosine is converted by intracellular deamination to 5-fluorouracil, which is incorporated into fungal RNA and inhibits protein synthesis. Flucytosine is also converted to fluorodeoxyuridine monophosphate, which interferes with DNA synthesis by inhibiting thymidylate synthetase.

Flucytosine is available in 250- and 500-mg capsules. Approximately 90% of an orally administered dose is absorbed (8). Minimal plasma protein binding and tissue accumulation result in a short half-life of 3 to 5 hours. Flucytosine concentrations in cerebrospinal, peritoneal, and synovial fluids, as well as in bronchial secretions, are approximately 75% of simultaneous plasma concentrations. Approximately 90% of a dose is excreted in unchanged, active form in the urine; consequently the urine concentration may be 100-fold higher than in plasma. For patients with normal renal function, the recommended dosage of flucytosine is 50 to 100 mg/kg per day divided into four doses. For patients with renal dysfunction, the daily dose must be adjusted. Patients receiving hemodialysis require an additional 37.5 mg/kg dose after dialysis. In addition, plasma levels of flucytosine should be monitored to maintain peak concentration between 50 and 100 μg/mL, because myelosuppression and other toxicities correlate with higher plasma levels of the drug.

Flucytosine is indicated for selected patients with fungal disease, especially cryptococcosis and invasive forms of candidiasis (Table 33.1). Flucytosine should not be administered as monotherapy, because of the potential development of drug resistance. Combination therapy with flucytosine and AMBd is aimed at achieving a synergistic effect and preventing the emergence of resistant fungi. Combination therapy has been well studied in the treatment of cryptococcal meningitis in both human immunodeficiency virus (HIV)-negative patients, and in patients with HIV/AIDS, and is highly effective (17–19). Combination therapy may also be indicated for patients with serious, life-threatening candidal syndromes such as meningitis, endocarditis, endophthalmitis, and hepatosplenic disease (15,16,48).

As shown in Table 33.2, the toxicities of flucytosine principally involve the gastrointestinal tract, liver, and bone marrow. These adverse effects most often are dose related and can be prevented or minimized by maintaining plasma levels below 100 μg/mL. In addition, the metabolite, fluorouracil, may

exert a toxic effect. Close monitoring of hepatic, renal, and hematopoietic function is essential. If a patient develops abdominal pain, nausea, vomiting, or diarrhea, flucytosine should be withdrawn or the dose reduced until these symptoms subside or improve. Approximately 5% of patients develop asymptomatic elevations in hepatocellular enzymes. Clinically significant hepatitis is rare, but deaths have been attributed to flucytosine-induced hepatic disease. About 10% to 15% of patients develop leukopenia, thrombocytopenia, or both; anemia is much less common. Although flucytosine-induced blood dyscrasias are usually reversible upon discontinuation of drug, fatal bone marrow suppression has been reported. Skin rash occurs but is uncommon.

THE AZOLES

Since the introduction of miconazole in 1978 and ketoconazole in 1981, the azole compounds have been used increasingly as effective and less toxic alternatives to AMBd and flucytosine for the treatment of superficial and systemic fungal infections (49). The azole compounds inhibit cytochrome P450–dependent 14-α-demethylase, thereby interrupting the conversion of lanosterol to ergosterol, the major component of the fungal cell membrane, and resulting in increased membrane permeability, leakage of intracellular contents, and, eventually, cell death. Fungicidal activity, likely secondary to direct membrane damage, may occur at higher concentrations. The imidazoles (miconazole and ketoconazole) contain two nitrogen atoms in the five-membered azole ring, while the triazoles (fluconazole, itraconazole, and voriconazole) contain three. The triazoles have a more selective affinity for fungal as compared with mammalian cytochrome P450 enzymes, resulting in fewer potential adverse effects of the triazoles compared with the imidazoles. Miconazole, in its parenteral formulation, is no longer commercially available.

KETOCONAZOLE

Ketoconazole (tradename Nizoral; Ortho Biotech) is an orally and topically administered imidazole compound that has a broad spectrum of activity, especially against yeasts and dimorphic fungi. However, the improved pharmacologic characteristics and better tolerability of the newer triazole compounds have made these agents superior alternatives to ketoconazole, especially for therapy of systemic fungal disease (49). As shown in Table 33.4, ketoconazole is highly protein bound. While the drug is distributed fairly extensively to most tissues and body fluids, CSF levels are negligible (50). Ketoconazole is metabolized in the liver and excreted principally as inactive drug in the bile; less than 5% of active drug is eliminated by the kidneys.

Ketoconazole, available as a 200-mg tablet, is absorbed fairly well: peak plasma concentrations 1 to 4 hours after a 200-mg dose are 2 to 4 μg/mL. An increase in the dosage results in a nearly linear increase in corresponding plasma levels; however, there is marked patient-to-patient variation. Because ketoconazole is weakly dibasic, gastric acidity must be normal for optimal absorption of the drug. As shown in Table 33.5, patients taking antacids, histamine-2 (H$_2$) receptor antagonists, or proton-pump inhibitors, and patients with achlorhydria or HIV-associated gastropathy, may not absorb ketoconazole adequately (51,52). Clinically significant interactions of ketoconazole with other drugs concomitantly administered have also been documented

TABLE 33.4. Pharmacologic Properties of Selected Antifungal Azole Drugs

Property	Ketoconazole	Itraconazole	Fluconazole	Voriconazole
Molecular weight	531	706	305	349
Water solubility	Poor	Poor	Good	Poor
Protein binding (%)	99	>99	11	58
Relative oral bioavailability (%)	75	>70	>80	96
Urinary excretion of active drug (%)	<5	<1	80	<2
Terminal elimination half-life (h)	7–10	24–42	22–31	6–9
CSF/plasma concentration (%)	<10	<1	>70	>50

Adapted from Como JA, Dismukes WE. Oral azole drugs as systemic antifungal therapy. *N Engl J Med* 1994;330:263–272.

(Table 33.5), and appear secondary to cytochrome P450 3A4 isoform interactions (53). Ketoconazole may enhance the effects of oral anticoagulants and sulfonylureas; decrease the clearance of cyclosporine, theophylline, and chlordiazepoxide; and variably interact with phenytoin, rifampin, and isoniazid (Table 33.5) (49).

Ketoconazole can be used to treat mucosal and cutaneous infections caused by *Candida* species and the dermatophytoses caused by *Epidermophyton*, *Trichosporon*, and *Microsporum* species (54). While ketoconazole is an effective therapy for many systemic mycoses (Table 33.1), one of the newer triazoles, fluconazole or itraconazole, is often preferred because of lesser toxicity and in some cases greater efficacy. Ketoconazole may be chosen for patients with indolent, non–life-threatening, nonmeningeal infections requiring prolonged treatment, such as mucosal candidiasis, blastomycosis, histoplasmosis, coccidioidomycosis, paracoccidioidomycosis, chromomycosis, penicilliosis, or pseudallescheriasis (21,55–59). Ketoconazole is also less expensive than the triazoles. In general, the dose of ketoconazole should be 400 mg per day initially and then 200 mg per day as

chronic maintenance therapy. For patients who demonstrate no response after 4 to 6 weeks, the dosage should be increased by 200-mg increments at monthly intervals up to a total dose of 800 mg per day, or other appropriate antifungal therapy should be substituted.

As shown in Table 33.2, the most common adverse effects of ketoconazole are dose-dependent anorexia, vomiting, and abdominal pain, which rarely necessitate discontinuation of drug provided the dosage is less than 600 to 800 mg per day (21). These gastrointestinal side effects may be minimized or prevented by administering the drug with food. Asymptomatic elevation of serum transaminase levels is seen in 2% to 10% of patients. While symptomatic hepatotoxicity is rare, fatal hepatitis attributed to ketoconazole has been reported (60). Rash, pruritus, and headache are occasional side effects. At dosages in excess of 400 mg per day, ketoconazole may interfere with steroidogenesis, resulting in endocrine abnormalities (61). Suppression of testosterone synthesis may cause gynecomastia, oligospermia, decreased libido, and impotence. Because of the effect of androgen suppression, ketoconazole has been used to treat refractory

TABLE 33.5. Drug Interactions Involving Azole Antifungals

Effect of interaction	Ketoconazole	Fluconazole	Itraconazole	Voriconazole
Decreased absorption of azoles	Antacids H$_2$ receptor antagonists Proton pump inhibitors Sucralfate		Antacids H$_2$ receptor antagonists Proton pump inhibitors	
Decreased plasma concentration of azole due to metabolism	Rifampin Rifabutin Phenytoin Isoniazid Carbamazepine	Rifampin	Rifampin Rifabutin Phenytoin Isoniazid Carbamazepine Nevirapine Phenobarbital	Rifampin Rifabutin Phenytoin
Increased plasma concentration of coadministered drug	Warfarin Sulfonylureas Cyclosporine Tacrolimus Phenytoin Midazolam Triazolam Alprazolam Corticosteroids Theophylline Ritonavir Saquinavir	Warfarin Sulfonylureas Cyclosporine Tacrolimus Phenytoin Midazolam Triazolam Alprazolam Theophylline Zidovudine Rifabutin	Warfarin Sulfonylureas Cyclosporine Tacrolimus Phenytoin Midazolam Triazolam Alprazolam Felodipine Verapamil Pimozide Statins Ritonavir Saquinavir Indinavir Digoxin	Warfarin Sulfonylureas Cyclosporine Tacrolimus Phenytoin Midazolam Triazolam Alprazolam Statins Omeprazole Vinca alkaloids

prostate cancer (62). Menstrual irregularities and alopecia may also occur, but the underlying mechanisms are unclear (63). Clinically significant adrenal insufficiency secondary to ketoconazole suppression of corticosteroid synthesis is rare and usually reversible (64).

FLUCONAZOLE

Fluconazole (tradename Diflucan, Pfizer), approved in 1990, is a triazole available in intravenous, tablet, or solution form. Fluconazole differs pharmacologically from ketoconazole and itraconazole (Table 33.4) in that it is highly water soluble, penetrates well into CSF (more than 70% CSF:plasma ratio), has a longer half-life (about 30 hours), is weakly protein-bound (11%), is evenly distributed throughout body fluids and tissues, and is excreted in the urine as active drug (80%) (49,65). Dose adjustment is required for patients with renal insufficiency.

As with other antifungal azoles, drug interactions must be considered (Table 33.5). Current data suggest no interaction with H_2 receptor antagonists; some potentiation of the effects of oral anticoagulants and sulfonylureas; and elevation of plasma levels of cyclosporine, phenytoin, and theophylline (49,65,66). Rifampin decreases serum concentrations of fluconazole; conversely, fluconazole therapy may increase levels of the closely related compound rifabutin.

Fluconazole has activity against a broad range of fungal pathogens and is useful in a diversity of clinical settings (49,65) (Table 35.1). Fluconazole is effective therapy for mucocutaneous forms of candidiasis. A single 150-mg oral dose produces a high cure rate in uncomplicated vaginal candidiasis (67). In prospective, double-blind studies of oropharyngeal candidiasis, fluconazole was shown to have superior efficacy and be better tolerated than oral ketoconazole and clotrimazole troches (68,69). In AIDS patients with esophageal candidiasis, fluconazole at 100 to 200 mg per day resulted in endoscopic cure in 91% of patients, compared with only 52% of cases treated with 200 to 400 mg per day of ketoconazole (55).

The treatment of invasive candidiasis has been simplified since the introduction of the azole antifungals. Two large randomized studies have demonstrated that fluconazole at 400 mg per day and AMBd at 0.5 to 0.6 mg/kg per day are similarly effective therapy for the treatment of candidemia in non-neutropenic patients, primarily with catheter-related infections (11,12). In both trials, there was substantially less toxicity associated with fluconazole when compared with AMBd. The results of two additional studies, which included neutropenic patients, suggest that fluconazole and AMBd are similarly effective in the treatment of candidemia in this subset of patients (70,71). While AMBd is considered to be standard therapy for hepatosplenic candidiasis, a number of patients with this entity have been successfully treated with fluconazole (13,14).

The use of fluconazole for cryptococcosis has been studied primarily in AIDS patients with cryptococcal meningitis. A randomized, multicenter comparison of fluconazole (200–400 mg per day) and AMBd (at least 0.3 mg/kg per day) with or without flucytosine as primary treatment of cryptococcal meningitis in patients with AIDS demonstrated that fluconazole is an effective, less toxic alternative for this disease (20). Among 194 evaluable patients, the rates of favorable response (including quiescent disease) were similar for the two groups (fluconazole 60%, and AMBd 64%). Mortality rates also were similar. However, more early deaths occurred in fluconazole-treated patients, and conversion of CSF cultures to negative was less rapid in these

patients (20). A subsequent prospective multicenter trial in patients treated with 14 days of induction therapy with AMBd with or without flucytosine followed by consolidation treatment with fluconazole 400 mg per day versus itraconazole 400 mg per day for 8 weeks showed that at the end of the 10-week treatment period, 68% and 70% of fluconazole- and itraconazole-treated patients, respectively, were free of symptoms (19). Negative CSF cultures were observed in 78% of patients who received fluconazole, compared with 60% of patients who received itraconazole (19). Finally, all AIDS patients with cryptococcal meningitis who survive the initial illness require some form of lifetime maintenance therapy. Results of two prospective, multicenter trials indicate that fluconazole (200 mg per day) is more effective as maintenance therapy than either AMBd (1.0 mg/kg per week) (72) or itraconazole (200 mg per day) (73).

Oral azole drugs have replaced AMBd for the management of most non–life-threatening *Coccidioides immitis* infections (24–26). Fluconazole is also effective therapy for coccidioidal meningitis and provides a welcome alternative to previous regimens involving prolonged intravenous or intrathecal AMBd (23). For other endemic mycoses, including blastomycosis, histoplasmosis, and sporotrichosis (Table 33.1), itraconazole is the azole drug of choice, since higher doses (more than 400 mg per day) of fluconazole appear necessary for cure (49).

In addition, fluconazole has been effectively used for antifungal prophylaxis in bone marrow transplant recipients, and currently is standard therapy at many institutions. Placebo-controlled trials of fluconazole at 400 mg per day as prophylaxis in patients undergoing bone marrow transplantation have demonstrated a reduction in the rate of fungal-associated deaths (32,33,74,75). The utility of prophylaxis with fluconazole in asymptomatic at-risk individuals, including neutropenic cancer patients, patients with AIDS, and non-neutropenic patients in intensive care units, is less clear (76–78). Although prophylaxis with fluconazole in many at-risk groups results in a decreased incidence of fungal infections, more studies are needed to evaluate survival benefit and cost-effectiveness before routine prophylaxis in these groups is warranted. Concern also exists over azole-resistant fungal isolates, including *Candida krusei* and *Candida glabrata*, which have become more frequent under the selective pressure of routine fluconazole prophylaxis in some clinical settings (79,80).

Fluconazole is well tolerated in dosages up to 400 mg per day. The most common adverse effects are nausea, vomiting, and skin rash (Table 33.2). Asymptomatic elevations in hepatocellular enzymes occasionally occur; severe and even fatal hepatotoxicity has been reported (81). In contrast to the toxicity profile of ketoconazole, there is no evidence of suppression of steroidogenesis by fluconazole in animals or humans. Alopecia has been associated with fluconazole and is usually reversible upon discontinuation of the drug (82).

ITRACONAZOLE

Itraconazole (tradename Sporanox, Ortho Biotech) is an orally (capsule or solution) or parentally administered antifungal triazole that was approved for treatment of both superficial and systemic mycoses in 1992. When taken with meals, oral itraconazole has greater than 70% bioavailability, is more than 99% protein bound, and has a half-life of greater than 24 hours (49) (Table 33.4). Concentrations of itraconazole in the lungs, kidneys, and epidermis are five times greater than simultaneous plasma concentrations. Because of its lipophilic properties, penetration into CSF is less than 1% of plasma concentration; however, itraconazole is effective in the treatment of fungal meningitis, probably as a result of excellent drug levels in the meninges and brain tissue (83). Less than 1% of active drug is excreted into the urine. Dose adjustment is required for the intravenous formulation in patients with renal dysfunction. No dose adjustment is required for patients with hepatic dysfunction.

The interactions between itraconazole and other drugs can be problematic in patients with complicated medical conditions (Table 33.5). Like ketoconazole, the absorption of itraconazole can be affected by drugs that alter gastric acidity. In addition, several other important itraconazole–drug interactions necessitate close monitoring of drug levels (phenytoin, cyclosporine) or avoidance altogether of certain drugs (lovastatin, midazolam) (49) (Table 33.5).

As shown in Table 33.1, itraconazole is considered the drug of choice for several endemic dimorphic fungal infections. For example, itraconazole is the currently recommended treatment for patients with mild or moderately severe blastomycosis (22). While life-threatening histoplasmosis should be treated with AMBd, itraconazole is indicated for most patients with or without AIDS who have less severe *Histoplasma* infection (22). In one study of AIDS patients with mild to moderately severe disseminated histoplasmosis, 85% of patients responded to itraconazole 300 mg orally twice daily for 3 days followed by 400 mg per day (84). In addition, itraconazole 200 to 400 mg per day is the preferred maintenance agent to prevent relapse of disseminated histoplasmosis in patients with AIDS (85). Itraconazole is also the drug of choice for most patients with lymphocutaneous or osteoarticular forms of sporotrichosis (86). In a comparative trial of itraconazole versus fluconazole for the treatment of patients with nonmeningeal coccidioidomycosis, there was a trend toward greater efficacy with itraconazole (24). Moreover, in a subgroup of patients with skeletal infections, by 12 months 37% of patients had responded to fluconazole and 70% had responded to itraconazole ($p = 0.03$) (24). In addition, open-labeled, noncomparative clinical trials in humans indicate that itraconazole is effective therapy for onychomycosis, chromomycosis, paracoccidioidomycosis, and penicilliosis when administered in daily doses of 50 to 600 mg for at least 3 to 6 months (87–89).

Although no randomized trials have compared itraconazole to AMBd in the treatment of invasive aspergillosis, open-label, noncomparative trials involving patients with invasive aspergillosis suggest that itraconazole is sometimes effective, and is associated with less toxicity than AMBd (90,91). Most authorities recommend itraconazole as consolidation therapy for patients who have had good responses to initial therapy with amphotericin B (either conventional or lipid formulations) for invasive aspergillosis. When compared with fluconazole as consolidation therapy for cryptococcal infections with AIDS after initial therapy with AMBd with or without flucytosine, mycologic response was similar with both drugs (19). However, when fluconazole and itraconazole were compared as maintenance therapy for cryptococcal meningitis in AIDS patients, fluconazole-treated patients were significantly less likely to relapse (73).

The most common adverse effects with itraconazole include nausea, anorexia, flatulence, headache, transient elevation of hepatocellular enzymes, and hypokalemia with or without pedal edema and increased blood pressure (49) (Table 33.2). Because of transient decreases in left ventricular ejection fraction seen in healthy volunteers receiving intravenous itraconazole, physicians should carefully review the risks and benefits of itraconazole therapy in patients with underlying cardiac disease.

VORICONAZOLE

Voriconazole (tradename Vfend; Pfizer, New York, New York, U.S.A.) is an orally and parentally active second-generation triazole that is derived through synthetic modification of the structure of fluconazole. Voriconazole, the newest triazole, was recently approved by the U.S. Food and Drug Administration for the treatment of invasive aspergillosis. The oral bioavailability is approximately 96%, and significant plasma protein binding occurs (Table 33.4). Voriconazole is distributed widely in tissues throughout the body, including the CSF. The drug is extensively metabolized in the liver, and approximately 2% of the drug is excreted unchanged in the urine. Administration of a loading dose results in a plasma concentration close to steady state within 24 hours.

Compared with the older azole drugs ketoconazole, fluconazole, and itraconazole, voriconazole has a broader spectrum of antifungal activity, including *Aspergillus* species, endemic fungi, azole-resistant *Candida* species, and a variety of other pathogenic opportunistic fungi such as *Fusarium* species, *Pseudallescheria boydii*, *Scedosporium* species, and dematiaceous fungi. Voriconazole has shown efficacy equal to that of fluconazole in the treatment of esophageal candidiasis in immunocompromised adults (92). In a comparative open-label trial for the treatment of invasive aspergillosis, voriconazole showed superior efficacy and tolerability when compared with AMBd (93). In a randomized trial of voriconazole versus L-AmB as empiric therapy for persistently febrile neutropenic patients, voriconazole was comparable with L-AmB in composite success score, clinically superior in reducing proven breakthrough fungal infections, and better tolerated (94). Studies evaluating voriconazole for the treatment of candidemia are currently underway.

The most common adverse events attributed to voriconazole are abnormal vision and mild hepatotoxicity (Table 33.2). Abnormal vision, described as altered visual perception or blurry vision, is transient, reversible, and tends to decline or disappear with continued therapy. Other less common adverse events include fever, rash, including photosensitivity, and nausea and vomiting. As with other azole agents, drug interactions with coadministration of voriconazole (Table 33.5) are important to consider, and include potentiation of the effects of warfarin, and elevation of plasma levels of cyclosporine, sulfonylureas, and phenytoin.

ECHINOCANDINS

The echinocandin class of antifungals was discovered in the 1970s as naturally occurring metabolites of fungal fermentation (95). Echinocandins act as inhibitors of β-(1,3)-D-glucan synthesis at the plasma membrane, leading to depletion of cell wall glucan, osmotic instability, and lysis of the fungal cell wall (96). Glucans are essential components of the cell wall in susceptible fungi, but are not present in mammalian cells. Echinocandins are active primarily against *Aspergillus* species, *Candida* species, and *Pneumocystis carinii*. Because of poor oral absorption (less than 5%), only intravenous formulations are available. Currently, caspofungin is the only commercially available echinocandin.

CASPOFUNGIN

Caspofungin (tradename Cancidas; Merck & Co., Inc.), a semisynthetic lipopeptide, is a water-soluble, parenterally administered antifungal that was approved for use in 2001 for the treatment of invasive aspergillosis in patients who are refractory to or intolerant of other antifungal therapies. Caspofungin is available as a 50- or 70-mg lypholized powder/cake for reconstitution and intravenous infusion. After administration, the drug is extensively bound to albumin (97%), and 92% of the initial dose is distributed into tissues by 36 to 48 hours. Plasma concentrations decline in a polyphasic manner, and β-phase half-life is 9 to 11 hours, allowing for once-daily dosing. Less than 5% of the drug is excreted unchanged in the urine. The recommended dose is 70 mg initially as a loading dose, followed by a 50-mg dose per day. In patients with moderate hepatic insufficiency (Child-Pugh score of 7–9), a decrease in the daily maintenance dose from 50 to 35 mg per day is recommended. No dosage adjustment is necessary in patients with renal insufficiency.

In vitro and *in vivo* animal studies have shown that caspofungin has excellent activity against *Candida* species (including non-albicans species and azole-resistant species), as well as *Aspergillus* species and *Pneumocystis carinii*. Caspofungin has moderate activity against dimorphic fungi, but poor activity against *Cryptococcus neoformans* and opportunistic molds (e.g., *Fusarium* species and *Rhizopus* species). In comparative trials of HIV-infected patients with esophageal candidiasis, caspofungin showed similar efficacy to AMBd, and fewer side effects (97). In an open-label, compassionate use trial of 69 patients with invasive aspergillosis refractory to or intolerant of other antifungal therapies, a favorable response was seen in 26 (41%) of 63 evaluable patients with caspofungin therapy (98). In a recent trial of caspofungin compared with AMBd for treatment of invasive candidiasis, caspofungin showed similar efficacy to AMBd, and fewer drug-related adverse events (99). Caspofungin may be useful for aspergillosis and various forms of candidiasis in patients who are refractory to or intolerant of other antifungal therapy. However, more data are needed to determine the appropriate therapeutic roles for caspofungin, especially as initial therapy.

In general, caspofungin is well tolerated. The most common adverse events experienced with caspofungin include fever, headache, thrombophlebitis, nausea and vomiting, and flushing; mild abnormalities of liver function tests have also been observed. Caspofungin is a poor substrate of the cytochrome P450 enzyme system. However, increases in maintenance dosing from 50 to 70 mg per day may be needed in patients concomitantly receiving efavirenz, nelfinavir, nevirapine, rifampin, dexamethasone, phenytoin, or carbamazepine, which induce clearance of caspofungin. The mechanism of these caspofungin–other drug interactions are not currently understood. In two clinical studies in patients receiving both caspofungin and cyclosporine, transient increases in liver function tests were seen, and the AUC of caspofungin was increased by approximately 35%. In addition, caspofungin may decrease the plasma concentration of tacrolimus. The pharmacokinetics of caspofungin are not altered with coadministration of itraconazole, AMBd, or mycophenolate.

TERBINAFINE

Terbinafine (tradename Lamisil, Novartis Consumer Health), a synthetic allylamine derivative that is available in oral and topical formulation, exerts its antifungal effect by inhibiting squalene epoxidase, a key enzyme involved in the synthesis of membrane ergosterol. Upon oral administration, terbinafine is 99% protein bound, and has an initial half-life of 12 hours. Terbinafine accumulates in skin, nails, and fat, and fungicidal levels may persist in plasma 4 to 8 weeks after dosing (100). Terbinafine has been used primarily in the United States as therapy for superficial dermatophyte infections, especially onychomycosis. Clinical studies with the oral formulation for the treatment of refractory oropharyngeal candidiasis, cutaneous sporotrichosis, and blastomycosis are ongoing. Terbinafine has been well tolerated at oral doses of 250 or 500 mg daily. The drug's main adverse effects are nausea and vomiting, diarrhea, rash, taste disturbance, and mild increases in liver enzymes.

NYSTATIN

A liposomal formulation of nystatin (tradename Nyotran; Antigenics, Inc.) is currently under investigation. The original compound, nystatin, licensed for use in 1954, is a polyene antifungal agent closely related in structure to AMBd. Intravenous use of nystatin was abandoned early on because of significant toxicities and insolubility. Topical formulations of nystatin are now used primarily in the treatment of oral, cutaneous, and vaginal fungal infections. Investigational intravenous liposomal nystatin has demonstrated *in vitro* activity against a wide spectrum of yeasts and molds, and is currently under evaluation in patients with refractory candidemia, cryptococcosis, and aspergillosis.

TABLE 33.6.   Selected Investigational Antifungal Agents

Class	Specific drugs	Site: mechanism of action	Spectrum of activity
Azoles	Posaconazole (SCH 56592) Ravuconazole (BMS 207147)	Plasma membrane: inhibit conversion of lanosterol to ergosterol	*Candida* species, *Aspergillus* species, *Cryptococcus neoformans*, Endemic fungi, dermatophytes, opportunistic molds
Echinocandins	Micafungin (FK 463) Anidulafungin (VER 002, LY 303366)	Cell wall: inhibit glucan synthesis	*Candida* species, *Aspergillus* species, *Pneumocystis carinii*
Nikkomycins	Nikkomycin Z	Cell wall: inhibit chitin synthesis	*Coccidioides immitis, Blastomyces dermatiditis*
Sordarins	GM 222712, GM 237354	Cytoplasm: inhibit protein synthesis by binding elongation factor 2	*Candida* species, *Aspergillus* species, *C. neoformans*
Cationic peptides	Histatins, cecropins, dermaseptins, indolicin, bacterial permeability–increasing factor	Plasma membrane: bind to ergosterol and cholesterol	*Aspergillus* species, *Candida* species, *C. neoformans*, and *Fusarium* species

Data from refs. 101 and 102.

OTHER SELECTED INVESTIGATIONAL THERAPIES

Other investigational compounds, including newer triazoles, echinocandins, nikkomycins, sordarins, and cationic peptides, are currently undergoing evaluation (101,102). These agents, sites and mechanisms of action, and antifungal activities are listed in Table 33.6.

In addition to currently used combination therapy with AMBd and flucytosine for the treatment of cryptococcosis and candidiasis, various combinations of antifungals are being evaluated for synergy *in vitro,* and in animal models, especially for aspergillosis. Several combinations under investigation include azoles plus terbinafine, azoles plus AMBd, azoles plus echinocandins, and echinocandins plus AMBd (including lipid-based formulations).

The addition of cytokines and other immunomodulatory approaches to antifungal therapy are actively being explored (103,104). Particularly intriguing are recombinant human gene products such as interferon-γ and colony-stimulating factors (CSFs; including granulocyte CSF and granulocyte-macrophage CSF), which are currently used in specific clinical settings to aid in the prevention or treatment of bacterial infections. Other immunomodulatory approaches to prophylaxis and adjunctive therapy under investigation include the use of interleukins (IL-12 and others) and monoclonal antibodies directed against specific fungal pathogens (104).

REFERENCES

1. Gallis HA, Drew RH, Pickard WW. Amphotericin B: 30 years of clinical experience. *Rev Infect Dis* 1990;12:308–329.
2. Medoff G, Kobayashi GS. Strategies in the treatment of systemic fungal infections. *N Engl J Med* 1980;302:145–155.
3. Dick JD, Merz WG, Saral R. Incidence of polyene-resistant yeasts recovered from clinical specimens. *Antimicrob Agents Chemother* 1980;18:158–163.
4. Dick JD, Rosengar BR, Merz WG, et al. Fatal disseminated candidiasis due to amphotericin B-resistant *Candida guilliermondii. Ann Intern Med* 1985;102:67–68.
5. Powderly WG, Kobayashi GS, Herzig GP, et al. Amphotericin B-resistant yeast infection in severely immunocompromised patients. *Am J Med* 1988;84:826–832.
6. Wilson E, Thorson L, Speert DP. Enhancement of macrophage superoxide anion production by amphotericin B. *Antimicrob Agents Chemother* 1991;35:796–800.
7. Martin E, Stuben A, Gorz A, et al. Novel aspect of amphotericin B action: accumulation in human monocytes potentiates killing of phagocytosed *Candida albicans. Antimicrob Agents Chemother* 1994;38:13–22.
8. Daneshmend TK, Warnock DW. Clinical pharmacokinetics of systemic antifungal drugs. *Clin Pharmacokinet* 1983;8:17–42.
9. Cruz JM, Peacock JE Jr, Loomer L, et al. Rapid intravenous infusion of amphotericin B: a pilot study. *Am J Med* 1992;93:123–130.
10. Ellis ME, al-Hokail AA, Clink HM, et al. Double-blind randomized study of the effect of infusion rates on toxicity of amphotericin B. *Antimicrob Agents Chemother* 1992;36:172–179.
11. Rex JH, Bennett JE, Sugar AM, et al. A randomized trial comparing fluconazole with amphotericin B for the treatment of candidemia in patients without neutropenia. *N Engl J Med* 1994;331:1325–1330.
12. Phillips P, Shafran S, Garber G, et al. Multienter randomized trial of fluconazole versus amphotericin B for treatment of candidemia in non-neutropenic patients. *Eur J Clin Microbiol Infect Dis* 1997;16:337–345.
13. Kauffman CA, Bradley SF, Ross SC, Weber DR. Hepatosplenic candidiasis: successful treatment with fluconazole. *Am J Med* 1991;91:137–141.
14. Anaissie E, Bodey GP, Kantargian H, et al. Fluconazole therapy for chronic disseminated candidiasis in patients with leukemia and prior amphotericin B therapy. *Am J Med* 1991;91:142–150.
15. Smego RA Jr, Perfect JR, Durack DT. Combined therapy with amphotericin B and 5-fluorocytosine for *Candida* meningitis. *Rev Infect Dis* 1984;6:791–801.
16. Thaler M, Pastakia B, Shawker TH, et al. Hepatic candidiasis in cancer patients: the evolving picture of the syndrome. *Ann Intern Med* 1988;108:88–100.
17. Bennett JE, Dismukes WE, Duma RG, et al. A comparison of amphotericin B alone and combined with flucytosine in the treatment of cryptococcal meningitis. *N Engl J Med* 1979;301:126–131.
18. Dismukes WE, Cloud G, Gallis HA, et al. Treatment of cryptococcal meningitis with combination amphotericin B and flucytosine for four as compared to six weeks. *N Engl J Med* 1987;317:334–341.
19. van der Horst CM, Saag MS, Cloud GA, et al. Treatment of cryptococcal meningitis associated with the acquired immunodeficiency syndrome. *N Engl J Med* 1997;337:15–21.
20. Saag MS, Powderly WG, Cloud GA, et al. Comparison of amphotericin B with fluconazole in the treatment of acute AIDS-associated cryptococcal meningitis. The NIAID Mycoses Study Group and the AIDS Clinical Trials Group. *N Engl J Med* 1992;326:83–89.
21. Dismukes WE, Cloud G, Bowles C, et al. Treatment of blastomycosis and histoplasmosis with ketoconazole. Results of a prospective randomized clinical trial. *Ann Intern Med* 1985;103:861–872.
22. Dismukes WE, Bradsher RW Jr, Cloud GC, et al. Itraconazole therapy for blastomycosis and histoplasmosis: NIAID Mycoses Study Group. *Am J Med* 1992;93:489–497.
23. Galgiani JN, Catanzaro A, Cloud GA, et al. Fluconazole therapy for coccidioidal meningitis. *Ann Intern Med* 1993;119:28–35.
24. Galgiani JN, Catanzaro A, Cloud GA, et al. Comparison of oral fluconazole and itraconazole for progressive, non-meningeal coccidioidomycosis. A randomized, double-blind trial. *Ann Intern Med* 2000;133:676–686.
25. Graybill JR, Stevens DA, Galgiani JN, et al. Itraconazole treatment of coccidioidomycosis. *Am J Med* 1990;89:282–290.
26. Catanzaro A, Galgiani JN, Levine BE, et al. Fluconazole in the treatment of chronic pulmonary and nonmeningeal disseminated coccidioidomycosis. *Am J Med* 1995;249–256.
27. Pizzo PA, Robichaud KJ, Gill FA, et al. Empiric antibiotic and antifungal therapy for cancer patients with prolonged fever and granulocytopenia. *Am J Med* 1982;72:101–111.
28. EORTC International Antimicrobial Therapy Cooperative Group. Empiric antifungal therapy in febrile granulocytopenic patients. *Am J Med* 1989;86:668–672.
29. Walsh TJ, Finberg RW, Arndt C, et al. Liposomal amphotericin B for empirical therapy in patients with persistent fever and neutropenia. *N Engl J Med* 1999;340:764–771.
30. Perfect JR, Klotman ME, Gilbert CC, et al. Prophylactic intravenous amphotericin B in neutropenic autologous bone marrow transplant recipients. *J Infect Dis* 1992;165:891–897.
31. Rousey SR, Russler S, Gottlieb M, Ash RC. Low-dose amphotericin B prophylaxis against invasive *Aspergillus* infections in allogeneic marrow transplantation. *Am J Med* 1991;91:484–492.
32. Goodman JL, Winston DJ, Greenfield RA, et al. A controlled trial of fluconazole to prevent fungal infections in patients undergoing bone marrow transplantation. *N Engl J Med* 1992;326:845–851.
33. Dykewicz CA. Summary of the guidelines for preventing opportunistic infections among hematopoietic stem cell transplant recipients. *Clin Infect Dis* 2001;33:139–144.
34. Bates DW, Su L, Yu DT, et al. Mortality and costs of acute renal failure associated with amphotericin B therapy. *Clin Infect Dis* 2001;32:686–693.
35. Branch RA. Prevention of amphotericin B-induced renal impairment: review on the use of sodium supplementation. *Arch Intern Med* 1988;148:2389–2394.
36. Hartsel S, Bolard J. Amphotericin B: new life for an old drug. *Trends Pharmacol Sci* 1996;17:445–449.
37. Wong-Beringer A, Jacobs RA, Guglielmo BJ. Lipid formulations of amphotericin B: clinical efficacy and toxicities. *Clin Infect Dis* 1998;27:603–618.
38. Patel R. Antifungal agents. Part I. Amphotericin B preparations and flucytosine. *Mayo Clin Proc* 1998;73:1205–1225.
39. Hiemenz JW, Walsh TJ. Lipid formulations of amphotericin B: recent progress and future directions. *Clin Infect Dis* 1996;22(suppl 2):133–144.
40. Janknegt R, deMarie S, Bakker-Woudenberg IA, et al. Liposomal and lipid formulations of amphotericin B. Clinical pharmacokinetics. *Clin Pharmacokinet* 1992;23:279–291.
41. Sharkey PK, Graybill JR, Johnson ES, et al. Amphotericin B lipid complex compared with amphotericin B in the treatment of cryptococcal meningitis in patients with AIDS. *Clin Infect Dis* 1996;22:315–321.
42. Leenders AC, Reiss P, Portegies P, et al. Liposomal amphotericin B (AmBisome) compared with amphotericin B both followed by oral fluconazole in the treatment of AIDS-associated cryptococcal meningitis. *AIDS* 1997;11:1463–1471.
43. Walsh TJ, Hiemenz JW, Seibel NL, et al. Amphotericin B lipid complex for invasive fungal infections: analysis of safety and efficacy in 556 cases. *Clin Infect Dis* 1998;26:1383–1396.
44. Wingard JR, White MH, Anaissie E, et al. A randomized, double-blind comparative trial evaluating the safety of liposomal amphotericin B versus amphotericin B lipid complex in the empirical treatment of febrile neutropenia. *Clin Infect Dis* 2000;31:1155–1163.
45. White MH, Anaissie EJ, Kusne S, et al. Amphotericin B colloidal dispersion vs. amphotericin B as therapy for invasive aspergillosis. *Clin Infect Dis* 1997;24:635–642.
46. White MH, Bowden RA, Sandler ES, et al. Randomized, double-blind clinical trial of amphotericin B colloidal dispersion vs. amphotericin B in the empirical treatment of fever and neutropenia. *Clin Infect Dis* 1998;27:296–302.
47. Graybill JR. Lipid formulations of amphotericin B: does the emperor need new clothes? *Ann Intern Med* 1996;124:921–922.
48. Rex JH, Walsh TJ, Sobel JD, et al. Practice guidelines for the treatment of candidiasis. *Clin Infect Dis* 2000;30:662–678.
49. Como JA, Dismukes WE. Oral azole drugs as systemic antifungal therapy. *N Engl J Med* 1994;330:263–272.

50. Daneshmend TK, Warnock DW, Turner A, et al. Pharmacokinetics of ketoconazole in normal subjects. *J Antimicrob Chemother* 1981;8:299–304.

51. Lelawongs P, Barone JA, Colaizzi JL, et al. Effect of food and gastric acidity on absorption of orally administered ketoconazole. *Clin Pharm* 1988;7:228–235.

52. Lake-Bakaar G, Tom W, Lake-Bakaar D, et al. Gastropathy and ketoconazole malabsorption in the acquired immunodeficiency syndrome (AIDS). *Ann Intern Med* 1988;109:471–473.

53. Piscitelli SC, Gallicano KD. Interactions among drugs for HIV and opportunistic infections. *N Engl J Med* 2001;344:984–996.

54. Cox FW, Stiller RL, South DA, et al. Oral ketoconazole for dermatophyte infections. *J Am Acad Dermatol* 1982;6:455–462.

55. Laine L, Dretler RH, Conteas CN, et al. Fluconazole compared with ketoconazole for the treatment of *Candida* esophagitis in AIDS: a randomized trial. *Ann Intern Med* 1992;117:655–660.

56. Negroni R, Robles AM, Arechavala A, et al. Ketoconazole in the treatment of paracoccidioidomycosis and histoplasmosis. *Rev Infect Dis* 1980;2:643–649.

57. Dismukes WE, Stamm AM, Graybill JR. Treatment of systemic mycosis with ketoconazole: emphasis on toxicity and clinical response in 52 patients. *Ann Intern Med* 1983;98:13–20.

58. Galgiani JN, Stevens DA, Graybill JR, et al. *Pseudallescheria boydii* infections treated with ketoconazole. *Chest* 1984;86:219–224.

59. Supparatpinyo K, Nelson KE, Merz WG, et al. Response to antifungal therapy by human immunodeficiency virus-infected patients with disseminated *Penicillium marneffei* infections and *in vitro* susceptibilities of isolates from clinical specimens. *Antimicrob Agents Chemother* 1993;37:2407–2411.

60. Lewis JH, Zimmerman HJ, Benson GD, et al. Hepatic injury associated with ketoconazole therapy: analysis of 33 cases. *Gastroenterology* 1984;86:503–513.

61. Sonino N. The use of ketoconazole as an inhibitor of steroid production. *N Engl J Med* 1987;317:812–818.

62. Reese DM, Small EJ. Secondary hormonal manipulations in hormone refractory prostate cancer. *Urol Clin North Am* 1999;26:311–321.

63. Sugar AM, Alsip SG, Galgiani JN, et al. Pharmacology and toxicity of high-dose ketoconazole. *Antimicrob Agents Chemother* 1987;31:1874–1878.

64. Pont A, Graybill JR, Craven PC, et al. High-dose ketoconazole therapy and adrenal and testicular function in humans. *Arch Intern Med* 1984;144:2150–2153.

65. Grant SM, Clissold SP. Fluconazole: a review of its pharmacodynamic and pharmacokinetic properties, and therapeutic potential in superficial and systemic mycoses. *Drugs* 1990;39:877–916.

66. Lazar JD, Wilner KD. Drug interactions with fluconazole. *Rev Infect Dis* 1990;12(suppl 3):327–333.

67. Kinghorn GR. Vulvovaginal candidiasis. *J Antimicrob Chemother* 1991;28(suppl A):59–66.

68. De Wit S, Weerts D, Goossens H, et al. Comparison of fluconazole and ketoconazole for oropharyngeal candidiasis in AIDS. *Lancet* 1989;1:746–748.

69. Koletar SL, Russell JA, Fass RJ, et al. Comparison of oral fluconazole and clotrimazole troches as treatment for oral candidiasis in patients infected with human immunodeficiency virus. *Antimicrob Agents Chemother* 1990;34:2267–2268.

70. Anaissie EJ, Vartivarian SE, Abi-Said D, et al. Fluconazole versus amphotericin B in the treatment of hematogenous candidiasis: a matched cohort study. *Am J Med* 1996;101:170–176.

71. Nguyen MH, Peacock JE Jr, Tanner DC, et al. Therapeutic approaches in patients with candidemia: evaluation in a multicenter, prospective, observational study. *Arch Intern Med* 1995;155:2429–2243.

72. Powderly WG, Saag MS, Cloud GA, et al. A controlled trial of fluconazole or amphotericin B to prevent relapse of cryptococcal meningitis in patients with the acquired immunodeficiency syndrome. The NIAID AIDS Clinical Trials Group and Mycoses Study Group. *N Engl J Med* 1992;326:793–798.

73. Saag MS, Cloud G, Graybill JR, et al. A comparison of itraconazole versus fluconazole as maintenance therapy for AIDS-associated cryptococcal meningitis. *Clin Infect Dis* 1999;28:291–296.

74. Slavin MA, Osborne B, Adams R, et al. Efficacy and safety of fluconazole prophylaxis for fungal infections after bone marrow transplantation: a prospective, randomized, double-blind study. *J Infect Dis* 1995;171:1545–1552.

75. Marr KA, Seidel K, Slavin MA, et al. Prolonged fluconazole prophylaxis is associated with persistent protection against candida-related death in allogeneic marrow transplant recipients: long-term follow-up of a randomized, placebo-controlled trial. *Blood* 2000;96:2055–2061.

76. Winston DJ, Chandrasekar PH, Lazarus HM, et al. Fluconazole prophylaxis of fungal infections in patients with acute leukemia: results of a randomized placebo-controlled, double-blind, multicenter trial. *Ann Intern Med* 1993;118:495–503.

77. Powderly WG, Finkelstein DM, Feinberg J, et al. A randomized trial comparing fluconazole with clotrimazole troches for the prevention of fungal infections in patients with advanced human immunodeficiency virus infection. *N Engl J Med* 1995;700–705.

78. Pelz RK, Hendrix CW, Swoboda SM, et al. Double-blind placebo controlled trial of fluconazole to prevent candidal infections in critically ill surgical patients. *Ann Surg* 2001;233:542–548.

79. Wingard JR, Merz WG, Rinaldi MG, et al. Association of *Torulopsis glabrata* infections with fluconazole prophylaxis in neutropenic bone marrow transplant patients. *Antimicrob Agents Chemother* 1993;37:1847–1849.

80. Wingard JR, Merz WG, Rinaldi MG. Increase in *Candida krusei* infection among patients with bone marrow transplantation and neutropenia treated prophylactically with fluconazole. *N Engl J Med* 1991;325:1274–1277.

81. Jacobson MA, Hanks DK, Ferrell LD. Fatal hepatic necrosis due to fluconazole. *Am J Med* 1994;96:188–190.

82. Pappas PG, Kauffman CA, Perfect J, et al. Alopecia associated with fluconazole therapy. *Ann Intern Med* 1995;123:354–357.

83. Terrell CL. Antifungal agents. Part II. The azoles. *Mayo Clin Proc* 1999;74:78–100.

84. Wheat J, Hafner R, Korzun A, et al. Itraconazole treatment of disseminated histoplasmosis in patients with the acquired immunodeficiency syndrome. *Am J Med* 1995;98:336–342.

85. Wheat J, Hafner R, Wulfsohn M, et al. Prevention of relapse of histoplasmosis with itraconazole in patients with the acquired immunodeficiency syndrome. The NIAID AIDS Clinical Trials Group and Mycoses Study Group Collaborators. *Ann Intern Med* 1993;118:610–616.

86. Sharkey-Mathis PK, Kauffman CA, Graybill JR, et al. Treatment of sporotrichosis with itraconazole. NIAID Mycoses Study Group. *Am J Med* 1993;95:279–285.

87. Piepponen T, Blomqvist K, Brandt H, et al. Efficacy and safety of itraconazole in the long-term treatment of onychomycosis. *J Antimicrob Chemother* 1992;29:195

88. Cauwenbergh G, De Doncker P, Stoops K, et al. Itraconazole in the treatment of human mycoses: review of three years of clinical experience. *Rev Infect Dis* 1987;9(suppl 1):146–152.

89. Sirisanthana T, Supparatpinyo K, Perriens J, et al. Amphotericin B and itraconazole for treatment of disseminated penicillium marneffei infection in human immunodeficiency virus-infected patients. *Clin Infect Dis* 1998;26:107–1110.

90. Denning DW, Lee JY, Hostetler JS, et al. NIAID Mycoses Study Group Multicenter Trial of oral itraconazole therapy for invasive aspergillosis. *Am J Med* 1994;97:135–144.

91. Dupont B. Itraconazole therapy in aspergillosis: study in 49 patients. *J Am Acad Dermatol* 1990;23:607–614.

92. Ally R, Shurmann D, Kreisel W, et al. A randomized, double-blind, double-dummy, multicenter trial of voriconazole and fluconazole in the treatment of esophageal candidiasis in immunocompromised patients. *Clin Infect Dis* 2001;33:1447–1454.

93. Herbrecht R, Denning DW, Patterson TF, et al. Voriconazole versus amphotericin B for primary therapy of invasive aspergillosis. *N Engl J Med* 2002;347:408–415.

94. Walsh TJ, Pappas PG, Winston DJ, et al. Voriconazole compared with liposomal amphotericin B for empirical antifungal therapy in patients with neutropenia and persistent fever. *N Engl J Med* 2002;346:225–234.

95. Hector RF. Compounds active against cell walls of medically important fungi. *Clin Microbiol Rev* 1993;6:1–21.

96. De Bono M, Gordee RS. Antibiotics that inhibit fungal cell wall development. *Ann Rev Microbiol* 1994;48:471–477.

97. Arathoon EG, Gotuzzo E, Noriega LM, et al. Randomized, double-blind, multicenter study of caspofungin versus amphotericin B for treatment of oropharyngeal and esophageal candidiases. *Antimicrob Agents Chemother* 2002;46:451–457.

98. Maertens J, Raad I, Sable CA, et al. Multicenter, noncomparative study to evaluate safety and efficacy of caspofungin in adults with invasive aspergillosis refractory to or intolerant of amphotericin B, amphotericin B lipid formulations, or azoles [Abstract 1103]. Presented at the 40th Interscience Conference on Antimicrobial Agents and Chemotherapy, September 2000, Toronto, Ontario, Canada.

99. Mora-Duarte J, Betts J, Rotstein C, et al. Comparison of caspofungin and amphotericin B for invasive candidiasis. *N Engl J Med* 2002;347:2020–2029.

100. Kovarik JM, Mueller EA, Zehender H, et al. Multiple-dose pharmacokinetics and distribution in tissue of terbinafine and metabolites. *Antimicrob Agents Chemother* 1995;39:2378–2741.

101. Groll AH, Piscitelli SC, Walsh TJ. Clinical pharmacology of systemic antifungal agents: a comprehensive review of agents in clinical use, current investigational compounds, and putative targets for antifungal drug development. *Adv Pharmacol* 1999;44:343–500.

102. Andriole VT. The 1998 Garrod lecture. Current and future antifungal therapy: new targets for antifungal agents. *J Antimicrob Chemother* 1999;44:151–162.

103. Stevens DA. Combination immunotherapy and antifungal chemotherapy. *Clin Infect Dis* 1998;26:1266–1269.

104. Casadevall A, Pirofski LA. Adjunctive immune therapy for fungal infections. *Clin Infect Dis* 2001;33:1048–1056.

CHAPTER 34

Antimycobacterial Drugs

Venkatarama Rao Koppaka,
C. Robert Horsburgh, Jr., and Kenneth G. Castro

INTRODUCTION

There are currently more than 58 recognized species of mycobacteria, most of which are not human pathogens, but are saprophytic organisms that occur naturally in soil and water (1,2). Bacteria in the *Mycobacterium tuberculosis* complex are the most common cause of disease affecting the pulmonary, lymphatic, meningeal, osteoarticular, and renal systems. In addition, they can cause disseminated disease. Nontuberculous mycobacteria have been described as causative of pulmonary disease, lymphadenitis, cutaneous ulcers, and disseminated disease (3). This chapter provides an overview of the available therapeutic agents for human disease caused by the various mycobacteria.

TUBERCULOSIS

Treatment for Active Disease

Tuberculosis (TB) is an ancient and deadly disease. In the 1800s, remedies such as bloodletting and cupping were replaced by regimens of bed rest and fresh air in sanatoria in the mountains or by the sea (4). Effective treatment for tuberculosis became possible with the discovery of streptomycin in the 1940s. It was soon realized, however, that the initial therapeutic response to streptomycin was quickly followed by a clinical deterioration as streptomycin resistance developed (5,6). Further investigation revealed that the development of resistance could be prevented by the use of two or more drugs in combination and standard regimens consisting of more than one drug (e.g., streptomycin, isoniazid, and para-aminosalicylic acid [PAS]) given for 18-24 months were adopted (7–11). These early regimens were effective but were poorly tolerated and their long duration made them impractical. As tuberculosis patients were moved out of sanatoria, the problem of patient nonadherence leading to treatment failure and drug resistance emerged. The introduction of rifampin in the 1970s revolutionized the treatment of tuberculosis, allowing the disease to be cured in less than 12 months (short-course chemotherapy). Highly effective regimens of only 6 months are the standard of care (12). Finally, the demonstration that short-course regimens dosed intermittently were effective made fully supervised therapy (directly observed therapy [DOT]) for adherence and prevent emergence of drug resistance, feasible (13).

General Principles of Antituberculosis Therapy

The patient with disease due to *Mycobacterium tuberculosis* is believed to harbor three distinct subpopulations of organisms (14). The largest of these subpopulations consists of rapidly growing tubercle bacilli that are predominantly extracellular. This subpopulation is likely to include drug-resistant mutants that arise spontaneously at a predictable frequency. The organisms that comprise the second subpopulation grow more slowly perhaps due to the acidic environment within the areas of necrosis in which they are found. The third subpopulation exists in a semidormant state, the organisms dividing only sporadically.

An effective treatment regimen relies on a combination of agents, whose activities are complementary and which together accomplish three therapeutic goals (Table 34.1): (a) rapid killing of the population of dividing extracellular tubercle bacilli (early bactericidal activity); (b) killing of drug-resistant mutant organisms to prevent their selection; and (c) prevention of long-term relapse by eliminating persisting semidormant bacilli (sterilizing activity) (15). Early bactericidal activity is observed clinically as a decrease in the number of bacilli in the sputum during the initial period of therapy, rapidly leading to improvement in symptoms and reduction in infectiousness (16,17). Preventing the selection of drug-resistant mutants prevents treatment failure due to acquired (secondary) drug resistance. Finally, sterilizing activity is important for determining the duration of therapy required to prevent long-term relapse.

Each of the antituberculosis drugs exerts a differential effect on these three subpopulations. Of the available antituberculosis drugs, isoniazid is the most bactericidal. Rifampin also has powerful bactericidal activity and like isoniazid, is effective at preventing the emergence of drug resistance. Compared with isoniazid and rifampin, ethambutol has moderate ability to prevent resistance and possesses intermediate bactericidal activity, particularly at the high doses used for intermittent therapy. In contrast, pyrazinamide has poor bactericidal activity and because it is active against only a subpopulation of organisms, it is poor at preventing the emergence of drug resistance. However, pyrazinamide plays a critical role in treatment regimens as a potent sterilizing agent and along with rifampin, which also has sterilizing activity, accounts for the low relapse rate seen with short course regimens (14,18).

Practical Application of Antituberculosis Therapy

One of the most important considerations in the treatment of patients with tuberculosis is adherence to therapy. Shortened treatment durations were a key development in improving adherence to therapy, thereby helping to prevent failure, relapse, further transmission, and the development of drug resistance (19). However, the most effective method of ensuring adherence is DOT (20,21). With DOT, a health care provider or other designated, non-family member observes the patient swallow each dose of antituberculosis medications. DOT is cost-effective when intermittent regimens are used (22), and has resulted in significant reductions in the rates of primary and acquired drug resistance and relapse when broadly applied (23). Clinicians caring for patients who have TB should contact their local health department tuberculosis control program for information about available DOT services.

Preventing the emergence of drug resistance during therapy (acquired drug resistance) is a second critical consideration in the management of patients with TB. All treatment regimens for TB disease must include two or more drugs to which the *M. tuberculosis* isolate is susceptible and which are able to prevent drug resistance (see Table 34.1). The susceptibility pattern of the isolate is usually not known when the initial regimen is chosen. Therefore, if preexisting (primary) resistance is not initially suspected, the standard initial treatment regimen may result inadequate (e.g., including only one drug to which the organism is susceptible). Because pyrazinamide is ineffective at preventing drug resistance, another agent (e.g., ethambutol or streptomycin) must be included to prevent emergence of resistance to rifampin when primary resistance to isoniazid is a possibility. On this basis and the fact that most areas in the United States have a rate of isoniazid resistant TB disease that exceeds 4%, an initial regimen consisting of four drugs (isoniazid, rifampin, pyrazinamide, and either ethambutol or streptomycin) is recommended for all

TABLE 34.1. Relative Activities of Antituberculosis Medications

Early bactericidal activity		Preventing drug resistance	Sterilizing activity	Activity
in vitro	*in vivo*			
INH	INH	INH	RIF	HIGH
RIF		RIF	PZA	
SM				
	EMB	SM	INH	
EMB	RIF			
PZA		EMB	SM	
	SM	THA	EMB	
	PZA			
THA	THA			
PAS	PAS	PZA	THA	LOW

INH, isoniazid; RIF, rifampin; PZA, pyrazinamide; EMB, ethambutol; THA, ethionamide.

patients (24). Drug susceptibility tests should be obtained on all initial *M. tuberculosis* isolates obtained from patients with active TB disease and the treatment modified based on these results.

Patients who are receiving antituberculosis therapy must be monitored closely for treatment response. The most important and objective marker of treatment success and noninfectiousness is the conversion of sputum cultures from positive to negative. With regimens containing both isoniazid and rifampin, sputum culture conversion occurs within the first 2 to 3 months of therapy in more than 80% of patients with drug-susceptible disease. Im-

provement in clinical signs and symptoms is an important early marker of a positive response to treatment and may occur in as little as 1 to 2 weeks after initiation of effective therapy. Conversion of sputum smear results from positive to negative, an important surrogate marker of non-infectiousness, can also indicate treatment efficacy, but is a less reliable indicator because it may occur either before or after culture conversion. Treatment failure is confirmed by failure of sputum cultures to convert to negative despite 4 to 5 months of chemotherapy. However, if early signs of treatment failure are present, clinicians should not wait for confirmation before evaluating the patient carefully for possible causes, which include nonadherence, drug resistance, or rarely malabsorption (25). Once treatment failure is confirmed or strongly suspected, use of DOT should be confirmed and at least two or three new drugs to which the isolate is susceptible should be added to the regimen. Suspected or confirmed treatment failure should never be managed by addition of a single drug. Doing so may have the same effect as treating active TB with a single drug and leads predictably to the emergence of additional drug resistance (26).

For practical considerations outlined below that include drug interactions and overlapping toxicities, physicians should avoid the simultaneous initiation of complex antiretroviral therapy and multidrug therapy for TB when treating patients infected with human immunodeficiency virus (HIV) with active TB (USPHS/IDSA Draft Guidelines for the Therapy of HIV-associated Opportunistic Infections. April 2002). Treatment of active pulmonary tuberculosis should never be delayed because of the risk of extended aerosol *Mycobacterium tuberculosis* transmission. However, initiation of antiretroviral therapy may be postponed for 4 to 8 weeks to facilitate patient adherence, and help identify the potential causes of side-effects. These decisions

TABLE 34.2. Drug Regimens for Culture-Positive Pulmonary Tuberculosis Caused by Drug-Susceptible Organisms

	Initial phase			Continuation phase				Rating[a] (Evidence)[b]	
Regimen	Drugs	Interval and doses[c] (*minimal duration*)	Regimen	Drugs	Interval and doses[c,d] (*minimal duration*)	Range of total doses (*minimal duration*)	HIV⁻	HIV⁺
1	INH RIF PZA EMB	Seven days per week for 56 doses (8 wk) *or* 5 d/wk for 40 doses (8 wk)[e]	1a	INH/RIF	Seven days per week for 126 doses (18 wk) *or* 5 d/wk for 90 doses (18 wk)[e]	182–130 (26 wk)	A (I)	A (II)
			1b	INH/RIF	Twice weekly for 36 doses (18 wk)	92–76 (26 wk)	A (I)	A (II)[f]
			1c[g]	INH/RPT	Once weekly for 18 doses (18 wk)	74–58 (26 wk)	B (I)	E (I)
2	INH RIF PZA EMB	Seven days per week for 14 doses (2 wk), *then* twice weekly for 12 doses (6 wk) *or* 5 d/wk for 10 doses (2 wk),[e] *then* twice weekly for 12 doses (6 wk)	2a	INH/RIF	Twice weekly for 36 doses (18 wk)	62–58 (26 wk)	A (II)	B (II)[f]
			2b[g]	INH/RPT	Once weekly for 18 doses (18 wk)	44–40 (26 wk)	B (I)	E (I)
3	INH RIF PZA EMB	Three times weekly for 24 doses (8 wk)	3a	INH/RIF	Three times weekly for 54 doses (18 wk)	78 (26 wk)	B (I)	B (II)
4	INH RIF EMB	Seven days per week for 56 doses (8 wk) *or* 5 d/wk for 40 doses (8 wk)[e]	4a	INH/RIF	Seven days per week for 217 doses (31 wk) *or* 5 d/wk for 155 doses (31 wk)[e]	273–195 (39 wk)	C (I)	C (II)
			4b	INH/RIF	Twice weekly for 62 doses (31 wk)	118–102 (39 wk)	C (I)	C (II)

EMB = Ethambutol; INH = isoniazid; PZA = pyrazinamide; RIF = rifampin; RPT = rifapentine.
[a] *Definitions of evidence ratings:* A = preferred; B = acceptable alternative; C = offer when A and B cannot be given; E = should never be given.
[b] *Definitions of evidence ratings:* I = randomized clinical trial; II = data from clinical trials that were not randomized or were conducted in other populations; III = expert opinion.
[c] When DOT is used, drugs may be given 5 days/week and the necessary number of doses adjusted accordingly. Although there are no studies that compare five with seven daily doses, extensive experience indicates this would be an effective practice.
[d] Patients with cavitation on initial chest radiograph and positive cultures at completion of 2 months of therapy should receive a 7-month (31-week; either 217 doses [daily] or 62 doses [twice weekly]) continuation phase.
[e] Five-day-a-week administration is always given by DOT. Rating for 5 day/week regimens is AIII.
[f] Not recommended for HIV-infected patients with CD4⁺ cell counts < 100 cells/ml.
[g] Options 1c and 2b should be used only in HIV-negative patients who have negative sputum smears at the time of completion of 2 months of therapy and who do not have cavitation on the initial chest radiograph. For patients started on this regimen and found to have a positive culture from the 2-month specimen, treatment should be extended an extra 3 months.
From American Thoracic Society, Infectious Diseases Society of America, Centers for Disease Control and Prevention. Treatment of tuberculosis. *Am J Resp Crit Care Med* 2003;167:603–662.

should be individualized and always include consultation with experts in the treatment of TB and HIV.

Currently Recommended Drug Regimens

The duration of therapy for tuberculosis depends on the drugs used, the drug susceptibility test results, and the patient's response to therapy (Table 34.2). Modern antituberculosis treatment for most patients with active TB consists of a 6-month multidrug regimen, divided into an initial phase (e.g., isoniazid, rifampin, pyrazinamide, and streptomycin or ethambutol) that lasts 2 months, followed by a continuation or sterilizing phase (isoniazid and rifampin) for a minimum of an additional 4 months. Because isoniazid resistance has been recently documented in nearly 10% of patients with TB nationwide, (27) ethambutol or streptomycin should be included in all initial treatment regimens. As soon as the results of drug susceptibility testing demonstrate that the isolate is susceptible to isoniazid and rifampin, the initial 2-month regimen can be limited to isoniazid, rifampin, and pyrazinamide. There are several highly-effective 6-month regimens that may be used (12,28–30) (see Table 34.2). Medications may be dosed intermittently (twice- or thrice-weekly) if treatment is directly observed. In patients who cannot tolerate or should not take pyrazinamide, the initial phase of treatment should consist of isoniazid, rifampin, and ethambutol or streptomycin daily for 2 months, and the continuation phase with isoniazid and rifampin should be extended for 7 months, for a total of 9 months of treatment (24). Also, the continuation phase of treatment should be extended to 7 months for patients with drug-susceptible, cavitary pulmonary tuberculosis whose sputum cultures remain positive after two months of treatment. These patients may receive isoniazid and rifampin daily, twice- or thrice-weekly by DOT. HIV-seronegative patients with non-cavitary pulmonary tuberculosis whose sputum culture is negative at two months of therapy may be offered isoniazid and rifapentine once-weekly by DOT for 4 months during the continuation phase, for a total of 6 months of treatment (24,31,32).

HIV INFECTION

HIV infected patients with active TB appear to respond adequately to standard antituberculosis treatment regimens and should be treated for a minimum of 6 months (33,34). However, it is critically important to monitor the clinical and bacteriologic response closely. If the response is slow or otherwise suboptimal, the patient should be reevaluated, and the continuation phase of therapy should be prolonged to 7 months (24).

Other special considerations are necessary to anticipate and avoid common problems during the coadministration of highly active antiretroviral therapy and antituberculosis therapy in HIV-infected persons with active TB. The use of rifampin is contraindicated in patients receiving most protease inhibitors (PIs) and nonnucleoside reverse transcriptase inhibitors (NNRTIs) due to unacceptable drug-drug interactions resulting in alterations in the metabolism of these antiretroviral drugs or rifampin from induction or inhibition of the hepatic cytochrome P-450 enzyme system (35,36). In contrast, available nucleoside reverse transcriptase inhibitors (NRTIs) have no significant clinical drug interactions with the rifamycins.

Rifampin can be used with the NNRTI efavirenz, in combination with two other NRTI drugs. Alternatively, rifampin may also be used in combination with adjusted doses of the PI ritonavir ($\geq$400 mg twice daily) when given alone or in combination with a second PI (37). Rifampin should not be used with the PIs nelfinavir, saquinavir, indinavir, amprenavir, lopinavir/ritonavir,

or other dual PI combinations requiring low-dose ritonavir ($\leq$200 mg daily).

Rifabutin is a rifamycin analogue of rifampin that is similar in efficacy in the treatment of tuberculosis, but has less of an impact on the metabolism of other antiretroviral drugs (38). In general, rifabutin can be used with PIs or NNRTIs and has fewer drug interactions than rifampin (35,36). When rifabutin is combined with antiretroviral agents, its dose and the dose of antiretroviral drugs may require adjustments (35). New information on drug-drug interactions related to use of rifamycins becomes available regularly and clinicians are advised to consult their state or local TB control programs or an expert in the management of HIV-related TB for the latest recommendations.

Clinicians must remain alert to the possibility of paradoxical, or immune reconstitution, reactions after antiretroviral regimens are used in patients undergoing treatment for active TB. Signs and symptoms are varied, and may include fever, temporary worsening of radiographic findings or symptoms, and enlarging lymphadenopathy (39,40). Less severe reactions can be treated symptomatically with nonsteroidal anti-inflammatory agents, and more severe reactions may be treated with corticosteroids.

EXTRAPULMONARY TUBERCULOSIS, PREGNANCY, AND LACTATION

Standard short-course regimens are also effective for the treatment of extrapulmonary tuberculosis. In adults, most forms of extrapulmonary TB can be cured with 6 months of chemotherapy, although clinical response should guide decisions on treatment duration, particularly for more serious forms of disease such as TB meningitis. Children who have miliary TB or TB meningitis should receive 9 to 12 months of therapy (24). Corticosteroids have also been recommended as adjunctive therapy for patients with TB pericarditis and TB meningitis.

The preferred treatment for pregnant or lactating women who have TB is isoniazid and rifampin for a minimum of 9 months (41,42). Ethambutol should be included until susceptibility to isoniazid and rifampin is confirmed. Streptomycin should be avoided during pregnancy because it interferes with fetal ear development and may cause congenital deafness. In the United States, pyrazinamide is not recommended for use during pregnancy because of inadequate data on its potential teratogenicity.

SPUTUM SMEAR-NEGATIVE AND CULTURE-NEGATIVE TUBERCULOSIS RESULTS

Patients with clinical and radiographic evidence of tuberculosis in whom all bacteriologic test results are negative may be diagnosed with smear negative, culture negative tuberculosis if a response (clinical and/or radiographic) to antituberculosis therapy can be demonstrated. Because the burden of organisms is much lower in these patients, a shorter duration of therapy is effective (43,44). Patients should be started on a standard combination of drugs (e.g., isoniazid, rifampin, pyrazinamide, and ethambutol). If follow-up after 2 months of treatment indicates radiographic and clinical improvement, but all culture results are negative, the patient should receive two additional months of isoniazid and rifampin to complete the 4-month total course.

DRUG-RESISTANT TUBERCULOSIS

For persons with TB whose isolates are resistant only to isoniazid, 6-month regimens containing rifampin, pyrazinamide, and either ethambutol or streptomycin have been shown to be effective (45). When isolated isoniazid resistance is documented after a four-drug regimen has been initiated, the isoniazid should be discontinued and the other three drugs continued for the entire 6 months (24). If pyrazinamide is not used initially, a minimum of

12 months of rifampin and ethambutol is an effective treatment alternative (46,47).

The treatment of tuberculosis resistant to both isoniazid and rifampin, also known as multidrug-resistant tuberculosis (MDR TB), is not standardized and is less successful than treatment of drug-sensitive disease (48). The keys to successful treatment are prompt recognition of drug resistance and rapid initiation of at least two drugs to which the *M. tuberculosis* isolate is susceptible *in vitro* (49–51). In general, the medications used to treat MDR TB are less potent and more toxic and require much longer administration (18 to 24 months) than standard antituberculosis therapy. Ideally, therapy for MDR TB should therefore consist of at least four drugs to which the isolate has documented *in vitro* susceptibility (52). The regimen should consist of "new" medications (ones that the patient has not received before), including one injectable medication. Ensuring adherence through the use of DOT is essential (53). Surgical resection of affected lung tissue has been used as an adjunct to medical therapy in selected cases of MDR TB, with improved outcome (54,55).

Treatment of Latent Tuberculosis Infection (Preventive Therapy)

The treatment of patients infected with *M. tuberculosis* is intended to prevent progression of latent TB infection (LTBI) to active TB disease. Although the terms "preventive therapy" and "chemoprophylaxis" have been applied to this strategy for many years, it is only rarely used to prevent initial infection in persons who have been exposed to patients with active pulmonary or laryngeal TB but who are not yet infected with *M. tuberculosis* (true primary prophylaxis). Therefore the term, "treatment of latent tuberculosis infection" is considered more accurate. The most common medication used in the treatment of LTBI is isoniazid. Several large randomized, placebo-controlled clinical trials have demonstrated the efficacy of isoniazid in preventing TB disease among those with LTBI (56–58). More recently, results of human clinical trials of "short-course" treatment of LTBI, predominantly involving patients co-infected with HIV, have become available. However, the efficacy of any regimen for treatment of LTBI is highly dependent on patient adherence (56).

Candidates for Treatment of Latent Tuberculosis Infection

LTBI is defined as the presence of a positive tuberculin skin test (TST—Mantoux method, 0.1 cc = 5 TU) in a patient with no evidence of active disease. Although all individuals with LTBI carry some risk of developing active tuberculosis, certain factors or characteristics increase this risk. Among these are HIV infection, other underlying medical conditions, and having recent infection (Table 34.3).

Previous recommendations for treatment of LTBI were based not only on the risk of development of TB disease, but also on the age of the infected person. The current recommendations do not provide an age limitation, focusing instead on screening for LTBI targeted exclusively toward those persons who would most benefit from treatment, that is, patients with risk of progression to TB once infected (59). Because patients diagnosed with LTBI through targeted screening would derive significant benefit from treatment, they should all be offered therapy regardless of age. As with treatment of any condition, in decisions to treat LTBI, the potential benefit of therapy must always be carefully weighed against the risk of adverse drug reactions. The most serious adverse reaction associated with therapy for LTBI using either isoniazid or the combination of rifampin and

TABLE 34.3. Priority Candidates for Targeted Tuberculin Testing and Treatment of Latent TB Infection

Indication for testing and treatment	Criteria for tuberculin skin testing positivity (mm induration)
Risk factors associated with recent infection	
Recent contact with a TB patient	≥5 mm
Recent skin-test conversion	≥10 mm increase in induration
Foreign-born persons in the US for less than 5 yr	≥10 mm
Medical conditions that increase risk of progression	
HIV infection	≥5 mm
Radiographic evidence of prior, untreated TB	≥5 mm
Organ transplantation	≥5 mm
Immunosuppression (≥15 mg prednisone for ≥1 mo)	≥5 mm
Injection drug use	≥10 mm
Silicosis	≥10 mm
Diabetes mellitus	≥10 mm
Chronic renal failure	≥10 mm
Hematologic disorders (e.g., leukemias, lymphomas)	≥10 mm
Selected malignancies (e.g., head and neck or lung carcinoma)	≥10 mm
Weight ≥10% below ideal body weight	≥10 mm
Gastrectomy	≥10 mm
Jejunoileal bypass	≥10 mm
Malabosrption/malnutrition	≥10 mm

pyrazinamide is drug-induced hepatitis (60,61). Asymptomatic increases in hepatic enzyme concentrations are common, but occasionally serious, even fatal hepatitis, may occur.

Recommended Regimens for Treatment of Latent Tuberculosis Infection

A 9-month course of isoniazid, alone in a single daily dose of 300 mg in adults and 10 to 15 mg/kg in children (300 mg maximum dose), is the preferred regimen for adults and children with LTBI, including those with HIV-coinfection (Table 34.4). Isoniazid may be given twice weekly to high-risk infected persons in institutions and facilities where preventive therapy can be directly observed by a staff member, although data on the efficacy of twice-weekly preventive therapy are limited.

Alternatively, rifampin (10 mg/kg) given daily for 4 months is recommended for persons who cannot tolerate isoniazid or for close contacts of infectious patients with active TB due to isoniazid-resistant strains (62,63). Rifampin alone is also recommended for persons with LTBI and in whom isoniazid and pyrazinamide are contraindicated.

A third alternative, rifampin (10 mg/kg) and pyrazinamide (15 to 20 mg/kg) given daily for 2 months has been studied in adult patients co-infected with HIV and shown to be of equivalent efficacy to 12 months of isoniazid in reducing the risk of progression to active TB disease (64). However, subsequent reports of severe liver injuries and deaths resulted in issuance of interim revised recommendations limiting the circumstances in which rifampin and pyrazinamide (along with careful monitoring for adverse effects) may be used (65).

For those likely to be infected with isoniazid- and rifampin-resistant TB, observation without therapy is usually recommended because the efficacy of other drugs has not been

TABLE 34.4. Recommended Drug Regimens for Treatment of Latent Tuberculosis Infection

Drug	Course and interval (maximum duration)	Comments	Rating (evidence) HIV−	HIV+
Isoniazid Isoniazid	270 daily doses (12 mo) 76 twice weekly doses (12 mo)	Preferred regimen for adults and children, including those with HIV co-infection May be administered with PIs and NNRTIs Intermittent regimen must be directly administered Use with caution in patients with risk of liver disease or in those who abuse alcohol or are taking medications associated with liver injury	A (II) B (II)	A (II) B (II)
Rifampin Pyrazinamide	60 daily doses (3 mo)	Efficacy and safety based on studies in adults co-infected with HIV Not recommended for use in children	B (II)	B (I)
Rifampin Pyrazinamide	16–24 twice-weekly doses (2–3 mo)	Not recommended for patients with underlying liver disease or with history of INH-associated hepatitis Use with caution in patients with risk of liver disease or in those who abuse alcohol or are taking medications associated with liver injury Evaluate clinically and measure AT/Bilirubin at 2, 4, and 6 wk of treatment	C (II)	C (I)
Rifampin	120 daily doses (12 mo)	Substitute rifabutin for rifampin in patients taking most PIs and NNRTIs. Recommended for infected contacts of patients with INH-resistant, rifampin-susceptible TB disease If appropriate clinical and laboratory monitoring can be provided, may be an acceptable alternative in patients with INH-associated hepatitis Efficacy has not been studied in patients co-infected with HIV	B (II)	B (III)

A, preferred; B, acceptable alternative; C, offer when A and B cannot be given; I, randomized clinical trial; II, data from clinical trials that were not randomized or were conducted in other populations; III, expert opinion.

evaluated. However, for persons likely to be infected with MDR TB who have a very high risk for the development of active TB (e.g., HIV-infected persons), alternative treatment regimens for LTBI have been recommended (66). Any such regimen should include at least two drugs to which the infecting organism has documented *in vitro* susceptibility. These patients should be monitored closely for the occurrence of side effects and for development of active TB (67).

Specific Antituberculosis Drugs

These drugs have been divided into "first-line" and "second-line" drugs based on their antibacterial activity, relative safety, and studied efficacy. First-line drugs are generally more effective and have fewer side effects than second line drugs. Unlike first

line drugs, second line drugs have not been studied for use in intermittent regimens. Second-line drugs are reserved for cases of drug resistance or drug intolerance.

First-Line Drugs

ISONIAZID

Isoniazid (INH) is highly active against *M. tuberculosis* and is the cornerstone of TB therapy (Tables 34.5, 34.6). It has profound early bactericidal activity, with efficacy against both intracellular and extracellular organisms, particularly those that are actively dividing. Isoniazid is well-absorbed from the gastrointestinal tract, although its bioavailability may be reduced by antacids and high carbohydrate foods. Peak blood

TABLE 34.5. First-Line Antituberculosis Drugs: Dosages

Drug	Route	Dose (mg/kg)[a] Daily Children	Adults	Twice weekly[b] Children	Adults	Thrice weekly[b] Children	Adults	Once weekly[b] Adults
Isoniazid	Oral	10–15 (300 mg)	5 (300 mg)	20–30 (900 mg)	15 (900 mg)	—	15 (900 mg)	15 (900 mg)
Rifampin	Oral	10–20 (600 mg)	10 (600 mg)	10–20 (600 mg)	10 (600 mg)	—	10 (600 mg)	—
Rifabutin	Oral	—	5 (300 mg)	—	5 (300 mg)	—	—	—
Rifapentine	Oral	—	—	—	—	—	—	10 (600 mg)
Pyrazinamide	Oral	15–30 (2 g)	15–30 (2 g)	50–70 (4 g)	50–70 (4 g)	—	50–70 (3 g)	—
Ethambutol	Oral	15–25	15–25	50	50	—	25–30	—

[a]Maximal dose is given in parentheses. Doses are for children under 12 y. Adjust weight-based doses as weight changes.
[b]All regimens administered two or three times a week should be used with directly observed therapy.
Adapted from Davis AL. A historical perspective on tuberculosis and its control. In: Reichman LB, Herschfield ES, eds. *Tuberculosis: a comprehensive international approach,* 2nd ed. New York: Marcel Dekker, 2003:1–54.

TABLE 34.6. First-Line Antituberculosis Drugs: Adverse Reactions

Drug	Adverse reactions	Monitoring	Comments

Isoniazid	Hepatic enzyme elevation
	Hepatitis
	Peripheral neuropathy
	Mild effects on central
	  nervous system
	Drug interactions
	Rash
		Baseline measurements of hepatic enzymes for
		  adults
		Repeat measurements
		  If baseline results are abnormal
		  If patient is at high risk for adverse reactions
		  If patient has symptoms of adverse reactions
			Hepatitis risk increases with age and alcohol
			  consumption
			Pyridoxine can prevent peripheral
			  neuropathy

Rifampin	Gastrointestinal upset
	Drug interactions
	Hepatitis
	Thrombocytopenia
	Influenza-like symptoms
	Rash
	Interstitial nephritis
		Baseline measurements for adults
		  Complete blood count and platelets
		  Hepatic enzymes
		Repeat measurements
		  If baseline results are abnormal
		  If patient has symptoms of adverse reactions
			Colors body fluids orange
			May permanently discolor soft contact lenses

Rifabutin	Rash
	Gastrointestinal upset
	Drug interactions
	hepatitis
	Neutropenia
	Joint pain
		Baseline measurements for adults
		  Complete blood count and platelets
		  Hepatic enzymes
		Repeat measurements
		  If baseline results are abnormal
		  If patient has symptoms of adverse reactions
			Colors body fluids orange
			May permanently discolor soft contact lenses

Rifapentine	Rash
	Gastrointestinal upset
	Drug interactions
	Hepatitis
	Neutropenia
	Joint pain
		Baseline measurements for adults
		  Complete blood count and platelets
		  Hepatic enzymes
		Repeat measurements
		  If baseline results are abnormal
		  If patient has symptoms of adverse reactions
			Colors body fluids orange
			May permanently discolor soft contact lenses

Pyrazinamide	Hepatitis
	Rash
	Gastrointestinal upset
	Joint aches
	Hyperuricemia
	Gout (rare)
		Baseline measurements for adults
		  Uric acid
		  Hepatic enzymes
		Repeat measurements
		  If baseline results are abnormal
		  If patient has sumptoms of adverse reactions
			Treat hyperuricemia only if patient has
			  symptoms

Ethambutol	Optic neuritis	Baseline and monthly tests
		  Visual activity
		  Color vision
			Not recommended for children too young to
			  be monitored for changes in vision unless
			  tuberculosis is drug resistant

concentrations of 3 to 7 μg/mL are achieved 1 to 2 hours after oral administration of the daily dose. A preparation for parenteral administration is available. No dosage adjustment is necessary in renal failure.

Hepatotoxicity associated with isoniazid administration may be manifested as asymptomatic elevation of the hepatic enzyme levels, overt hepatitis requiring cessation of therapy, fulminant hepatitis requiring liver transplantation, (68) or fatal hepatitis (69). The risk of clinically apparent hepatitis is relatively low, occurring in 0.10% to 0.15% of 11,141 receiving INH alone for LTBI in a recent study (70). The risk is increased in older age groups and in persons with underlying liver disease. Isoniazid may also cause neurotoxicity by interfering with pyridoxine metabolism. Peripheral neuropathy is the most common manifestation and occurs most frequently in persons who may be mildly pyridoxine deficient, such as pregnant women, alcohol abusers, and malnourished patients. Peripheral neuropathy can be prevented with as little as 10 mg of pyridoxine (vitamin B$_6$) daily. Antinuclear antibodies develop in approximately 20% of patients on prolonged isoniazid therapy (72) although overt systemic lupus erythematosus develops in a few (73). Hypersensitivity reactions, pancreatitis, gynecomastia, arthralgias, and arthritis have been rarely reported in association with isoniazid administration. Isoniazid may produce a monoamine oxidase inhibitor-like effect when foods such as cheese or red wine are ingested (74) or histidine reactions after ingestion of certain types of fish (75). Isoniazid inhibits the metabolism of some an-

ticonvulsants medications (76,77) and may reduce ketoconazole serum levels.

RIFAMPIN (RIFAMPICIN)

Rifampin (rifampicin) has a marked bactericidal effect on intracellular and extracellular *M. tuberculosis*, including a unique effect against semidormant organisms. It inhibits deoxyribonucleic acid (DNA)–dependent ribonucleic acid (RNA) polymerase, blocking RNA transcription. In addition, rifampin has a very potent sterilizing activity. The drug is well absorbed from the gastrointestinal tract, although concomitant food intake may interfere with absorption (78). Peak blood concentrations of 7 to 10 μg/mL are achieved 2 to 4 hours after oral administration of a 600-mg dose. An intravenous preparation is also available. No dosage adjustment is necessary in renal failure.

Rifampin is relatively nontoxic. It causes a harmless reddish or orange discoloration of the urine and other body fluids. Patients should be warned about this and about the possibility that contact lenses may become permanently discolored. The most common adverse reaction is gastrointestinal upset such as anorexia, nausea, and abdominal discomfort. Hepatitis occurs less frequently with rifampin than isoniazid, although there are some reports of an increased risk of hepatitis when the two medications are given concurrently (79). Some adverse reactions occur more frequently with intermittent rather than daily administration of rifampin. Thrombocytopenia, flu-like syndromes, and renal failure have all been reported, particularly with intermittent administration. As a potent inhibitor of hepatic cytochrome P-450 oxidative enzymes, rifampin accelerates the metabolism of many drugs, including anticoagulants, antiarrhythmics, anticonvulsants, glucocorticoids, cyclosporine, methadone, theophylline, ketoconazole, oral hypoglycemic agents, estrogens, and oral contraceptives (80). Rifampin can be used with the NNRTI efavirenz in combination with two other NRTIs, and may be used with adjusted doses of the PIs ritonavir (≥400 mg twice daily) when given alone or with a second PI (35). Because of unacceptable drug-drug interactions, the use of rifampin is contraindicated in patients also taking most other PIs or NNRTIs. Rifabutin, a rifamycin analogue of rifampin (see below), with appropriate dosage adjustment, may be given with selected PIs and NNRTIs and may be substituted for rifampin in standard treatment regimens.

RIFABUTIN

Rifabutin is an analogue of rifampin, belonging to the general class of rifamycins. It has a mechanism of action identical to that of rifampin and can substitute for rifampin in treatment of all forms of tuberculosis. The principal indication for rifabutin is in treatment of TB disease and LTBI in patients receiving any medication having an unacceptable interaction with rifampin (e.g., PIs or NNRTIs). Cross-resistance between rifabutin and rifampin is nearly complete. Although some rifampin-resistant strains exhibit *in vitro* sensitivity to rifabutin, its clinical efficacy in these situations is unclear and alternative agents should be employed in designing a treatment regimen. Rifabutin is typically administered at dosage of 5 mg/kg given daily, or thrice or twice weekly. The dose may have to be adjusted in patients receiving PIs or NNRTIs concomitantly. As with rifampin, no dosage adjustment is necessary for use in patients with renal insufficiency.

Rifabutin is relatively nontoxic at recommended doses. Uveitis, observed when higher doses were used, is rare at standard (300 mg) doses. The risk of uveitis is increased when rifabutin in used in combination with drugs that reduce its clearance (PIs, NNRTIs, azole antifungal agents) (81).

RIFAPENTINE

Rifapentine is a long-acting analog of rifampin recently approved for use in the United States by the Food and Drug Administration. Like other rifamycins, it inhibits DNA-dependent RNA polymerase and blocks RNA transcription. It is well absorbed from the gastrointestinal tract, reaching peak concentrations of 10 to 18 μg/mL 5 to 6 hours after ingestion of the recommended 600-mg dose (82,83). When taken with food, peak concentrations increase by approximately 40% of the fasting values. It is excreted partly in urine and mostly in feces. Its metabolite, 25-desacetyl rifapentine, is microbiologically active and contributes to some of the drug's activity. Both the drug and its metabolite have an elimination half-life of 13 to 35 hours.

Because of the observed occurrence of relapses due to rifamycin-resistant strains among HIV-infected study participants receiving rifapentine once weekly, it is contraindicated in persons with HIV infection (31). The principal indication for rifapentine is in the treatment of persons without HIV infection who have active TB but do not have pulmonary cavitary disease and whose sputum smear result has converted to negative (24). These persons can receive isoniazid and rifapentine once-weekly by DOT during the continuation phase of anti-tuberculosis therapy. Ongoing trials will evaluate the usefulness of rifapentine for the treatment of LTBI.

Rifapentine is relatively non-toxic at the recommended dose. Like other rifamyins, it causes the characteristic reddish or orange discoloration of body fluids and may permanently discolor contact lenses. Asymptomatic increases in aminotransferase levels were seen in 5% of study participants, and hyperuricemia has been described in persons receiving the drug twice weekly.

Compared with rifampin, rifapentine is a less potent inducer of the hepatic cytochrome P-450. However, such induction capacity can increase the metabolism and lower the concentrations of other drugs metabolized by this enzyme pathway.

ETHAMBUTOL

Ethambutol appears to inhibit incorporation of mycolic acids into the cell wall, and is effective only against actively growing bacteria. It is used as part of an initial four-drug regimen as a supplement to isoniazid and rifampin when primary resistance is suspected or in combination with other drugs when either isoniazid or rifampin or both cannot be used due to documented drug resistance or drug intolerance. Peak serum concentrations of 2 to 5 μg/mL are achieved 2 to 4 hours after the administration of a dose of 15 mg/kg. Ethambutol is administered by the oral route at a daily adult and pediatric dosage of 15 to 25 mg/kg. In retreatment cases, the higher dose is generally used for the first 2 months, after which the dose is decreased to 15 mg/kg/day after the first 2 months. The dosage should be reduced in renal failure (84). In patients with end-stage renal disease, ethambutol should be administered at a dose of 15 to 25 mg/kg three times a week after dialysis.

The main adverse reaction associated with ethambutol administration is optic neuritis. Signs and symptoms include blurry vision, central scotomata, and color blindness. These are usually completely reversible if the drug is stopped promptly. The ocular toxicity appears to be dose related, occurring in approximately 5% of persons who receive 25 mg/kg/day for longer than 2 months but only rarely in those getting 15 mg/kg per day. Ethambutol has been used safely in children, although should be used with caution in children younger than 5 years of age in whom visual acuity cannot be easily monitored (85). Other side effects include hypersensitivity reactions, elevated uric acid levels, and rarely, peripheral neuropathy.

PYRAZINAMIDE

Pyrazinamide (PZA) is a bactericidal drug in acid environments, and its potent sterilizing activity has enabled treatment regimens to be shortened to 6 months without an increase in relapse rate (86). There is rapid absorption from the gastrointestinal tract after oral administration with peak plasma concentrations of 33 to 65 μg/mL, 1 to 2 hours after oral administration of 1.5 g. Dosage should be adjusted in patients with renal insufficiency with a dose of 25 to 35 mg/kg administered three times weekly following dialysis.

Hepatotoxicity was fairly common when pyrazinamide was first used, but the risk is quite low at the currently recommended dosages. Elevated uric acid levels are common and do not require discontinuation of the drug unless associated with acute gout. Hypersensitivity reactions and gastrointestinal upset may occur.

Fixed-Dose Combinations

Because drug resistance may develop when patients with TB disease take a single drug, use of fixed-dose combination tablets containing more than one antituberculosis drug has been recommended for patients not on directly observed therapy (24,87,88). In the United States, a combination of isoniazid plus rifampin (Rifamate7) and isoniazid plus rifampin and pyrazinamide (Rifater7) are available. Two tablets of Rifamate provide the conventional dose of 300 mg of isoniazid and 600 mg of rifampin. Rifater, on the other hand, has 50 mg of isoniazid, 120 mg of rifampin, and 300 mg of pyrazinamide. The recommended dosage is five tablets a day for persons weighing less than 55 kg and six tablets a day for those weighing 55 kg or more. The six-tablet dosage provides a 720-mg dose of rifampin (which exceeds the usual maximum recommended dose) to compensate for the lower bioavailability of rifampin when given in the combination form. The use of fixed-dose combination tablets theoretically reduces the risk of medication errors by patients, makes the administration easier, and eliminates the possibility of monotherapy. Because of similarities between existing trade names, physicians must exercise caution when prescribing fixed-dose combination tablets to avoid confusion.

Second-Line Drugs

CYCLOSERINE
In susceptible bacteria, cycloserine interferes with cell wall synthesis; depending on serum concentrations, it may exert bactericidal or bacteriostatic activity against *M. tuberculosis* (Table 34.7). Cycloserine is readily absorbed from the gastrointestinal tract after the administration of 250 mg twice daily. Peak serum levels are 25 to 30 μm/mL at 4 to 8 hours. The drug is excreted mainly by the kidneys and should be used with caution in patients with renal insufficiency and should be avoided in patients having a creatinine clearance less than 50 mL/min. Because of a narrow therapeutic window, serum drug levels should be used to adjust the dose to achieve a peak serum concentration between 20 and 35 μg/mL.

Cycloserine frequently causes neurological or psychiatric disturbances, ranging from headache and drowsiness to convulsions or psychosis. Peripheral neuritis has also been described. These effects appear to be dose related and are exacerbated in renal insufficiency, but they generally disappear when the medication is discontinued. Concomitant use of pyridoxine may help prevent most serious reactions.

ETHIONAMIDE
Ethionamide appears to interfere with bacterial protein synthesis. Depending on the serum concentration, ethionamide may exert either bacteriostatic or bactericidal activity. It is an oral medication that may be given in single or divided doses. Peak serum concentrations of 9 μg/mL are reached between 1.8 and 3.0 hours after a single dose of 1 g.

TABLE 34.7.   Second-Line Antituberculosis Drugs: Dosages and Adverse Reactions

Drug[a]	Daily dose[b] {maximal dose} (usual dose)	Adverse reactions	Monitoring	Comments
Cycloserine	15–20 mg/kg PO in divided doses {1 g} (250–500 mg bid)	Psychosis Convulsions Depression Headaches Rash Drug interactions	Assess mental status Measure serum drug levels	Start with low dosage and increase as tolerated Pyridoxine may decrease central nervous system effects.
Ethionamide	15–20 mg/kg PO in divided doses {1 g} (250–500 mg bid)	Gastrointestinal upset Hepatoxicity Hypersensitivity Metallic taste Bloating	Measure hapatic enzyme levels	Start with low dosage and increase as tolerated May cause hypothyroid condition, especially if used with p-amino-salicylic acid
p-Aminosaliclic acid	150 mg/kg PO in divided doses {12 g} (4 g bid)	Gastrointestinal upset Hypersensitivity Hepatotoxicity Sodium load	Measure hepatic enzyme levels Assess volume status	Start with low dosage and increase as tolerated Monitor cardiac patients for sodium load
Capreomycin	15–30 mg/kg[c] IM or IV qd {1 g}	Toxicity Auditory Vestibular Renal	Assess Vestibular function Hearing function Measure Blood urea nitrogen Creatinine level	After bacteriologic conversion, dosage may be reduced to 2 or 3 times/wk
Kanamycin and amikacin	15–30 mg/kg[c] IM or IV qd {1 g}	Toxicity Auditory Vestibular Renal	Assess Vestibular function Hearing function Measure Blood urea nitrogen Creatinine level	After bacteriologic conversion, dosage may be reduced to 2 or 3 times/wk
Streptomycin	Adults: 15 mg/kg[c] IM or IV qd {1 g} Children: 40 mg/kg IM {1 g}	Toxicity Auditory Vestibular Renal	Assess Vestibular function Hearing function Measure Blood urea nitrogen Creatinine level	After bacteriologic conversion, dosage may be reduced to 2 or 3 times/wk
Levofloxacin	500 mg/d PO	Gastrointestinal upset Dizziness Hypersensitivity Drug interactions Headaches Restlessness	Drug interactions	Should not be used in children Avoid Antacids Iron Zinc Sucralfate

[a]Use these drugs only in consultation with a clinician experienced in the management of drug-resistant tuberculosis. Adjust weight-based dosages as weight changes.
[b]Doses for children are the same as those for adults, except where indicated.
[c]Reduce dose to 10 mg/kg in persons of more than 59 years of age.
PO, oral; IM, intramuscular; IV, intravenous; bid, twice daily; tid, three times daily; qd, every day.

Because of its toxicity, ethionamide is usually reserved for treatment of MDR TB. It frequently causes nausea, vomiting, anorexia, and abdominal pain. Gradually increasing to a full dose or administering the drug with meals or at bedtime, or with an antiemetic, may improve tolerance. Hypersensitivity reactions, hepatitis, and various forms of neurotoxicity may occur. Endocrinological disturbances, such as hypothyroidism, menstrual irregularities, impotence, and gynecomastia have been reported.

PARA-AMINOSALICYLIC ACID (PASER®)

PAS was a standard first-line drug, but now it is reserved for use in the treatment of MDR TB. Its exact mechanism of action is unknown, although it is thought to interfere with formation of folic acid. It is available in the United States as a granular formulation that is readily absorbed from the gastrointestinal tract, achieving a concentration of 25 to 26 μg/mL 4 hours after oral administration of a 4-g dose (89).

The most commonly reported side effect with PAS use is gastrointestinal irritation, although the granular formulation is better tolerated. Hypersensitivity reactions may occur in 5% to 10% of patients. Other reported adverse effects include acute pulmonary eosinophilia (Loeffler's syndrome), hepatitis (thought to result from a hypersensitivity reaction), thyroid dysfunction, crystalluria, hemolytic anemia, and a mononucleosis-like syndrome.

CAPREOMYCIN

Capreomycin is a polypeptide antibiotic with a mechanism of action similar to the aminoglycosides. It approaches streptomycin in its therapeutic effect against susceptible M. tuberculosis isolates and can only be administered parenterally due to poor absorption from the gastrointestinal tract. In adults, peak serum levels of 30 μg/mL occur 1 to 2 hours after the intramuscular administration of 1 g.

The most common side effect described with capreomycin is nephrotoxicity. Renal function should be closely monitored and the drug discontinued if nephrotoxicity develops. Capreomycin also may cause auditory and vestibular toxicity; audiometry should be performed monthly during therapy. Capreomycin's safety for use in pregnancy or lactation has not been established.

KANAMYCIN AND AMIKACIN

Kanamycin and amikacin are aminoglycoside antibiotics active against M. tuberculosis. There is complete cross-resistance between kanamycin and amikacin, and cross-resistance may also occur with capreomycin. Many strains resistant to streptomycin remain sensitive to amikacin or kanamycin. These agents are available in parenteral form for intramuscular or intravenous use. Side effects and precautions are similar to those related to the use of capreomycin. The most commonly reported toxic effects are auditory, renal, and vestibular. Therefore, patients taking these drugs should have undergo audiometry, vestibular function testing, and renal function should be monitored closely.

STREPTOMYCIN

Streptomycin is an aminoglycoside antibiotic, and was the first drug shown to be effective for treatment of TB (6). Streptomycin interferes with bacterial protein synthesis and is bactericidal against M. tuberculosis. It is most active in an alkaline environment and is usually given by intramuscular injection but may also be given intravenously. The mean plasma half life is 2.4 to 2.7 hours in adults 40 years or younger, but can be as long as 7 to 9 hours in newborn and elderly persons. The drug is cleared by the kidney and the dose should be reduced in persons with impaired renal function. The drug should be avoided in pregnancy because it may produce auditory damage in the fetus.

The most important adverse effects of streptomycin are ototoxicity and nephrotoxicity, and both occur more frequently in older patients. Vestibular disturbances are more common than auditory damage. The risk of ototoxicity is related to the total dose and the peak serum levels. Concomitant administration of other ototoxic drugs increases the risk. Hypersensitivity reactions, neuromuscular blockade, and hematologic effects have been reported.

LEVOFLOXACIN

The fluoroquinolones (e.g., levofloxacin, moxifloxacin, gatifloxacin, ofloxacin, and ciprofloxacin) are DNA gyrase inhibitors that have significant in vitro activity against M. tuberculosis. Based on cumulative experience, of the available agents in this class, levofloxacin offers the best balance between efficacy and patient tolerance. Cross-resistance exists among all member of this class currently in common use (e.g., ciprofloxacin, ofloxacin, and levofloxacin). These agents are not licensed for the treatment of tuberculosis and controlled trials demonstrating their effectiveness are lacking, but they have been used extensively in recent years for treatment of multidrug-resistant tuberculosis.

The recommended dose of levofloxacin is 500 to 1,000 mg daily. Available preparations include 250-mg, 500-mg, and 750-mg tablets and aqueous solution (500 mg) for intravenous administration. Levofloxacin and other fluoroquinolones are relatively nontoxic (90), hypersensitivity reactions and gastrointestinal complaints (e.g., bloating) reported most commonly. Other side effects reported in 0.5% of patients include confusion, dizziness, insomnia, tremulousness, and headaches. Rash, pruritus, and photosensitivity have also been reported. Antacids interfere with the absorption of fluoroquinolones and should therefore be avoided within 2 hours of administration. Fluoroquinolones should not be used in children or during pregnancy because of possible effect on bone and cartilage development.

NONTUBERCULOUS MYCOBACTERIA

The nontuberculous mycobacteria comprise a diverse group of microorganisms that can cause a variety of clinical syndromes. Regimens for treatment of these diseases are less well-studied and, in general, less effective than those available for treatment of tuberculosis disease. In this section, commonly accepted regimens are presented and discussed by causative organism and clinical syndrome. Antimycobacterial agents effective against these organisms and in addition to those used for treatment of tuberculosis are also described (Table 34.8).

TABLE 34.8. Agents Used in the Treatment of Nontuberculous Mycobacteria

Drug	Route	Adult dosage	Frequency
Azithromycin	PO	250–500 mg	once daily
Cefoxitin	IV	2 g	every 4 h
Clarithromycin	PO	500 mg	twice daily
Clofazimine	PO	100 mg	once daily
Dapsone	PO	100 mg	once daily
Sulfisoxazole	PO	2 g	four times daily
Cotrimoxazole	PO	DS	twice daily
Imipenem	IV	1 g	every 6 h
Doxycycline	PO	100 mg	twice daily
Minocycline	PO	100 mg	twice daily
Amikacin	IV	15 mg/kg	once daily

IV, intravenous; PO, oral.

M. avium Complex

The *M. avium* complex (MAC) comprises organisms of over 40 serotypes. These organisms are broadly divided into two groups, *M. avium* and *M. intracellulare*. These groups differ in their *in vitro* susceptibility to antimycobacterial agents; however, such differences do not appear to be clinically meaningful, and the two groups can be considered together.

DISSEMINATED *M. AVIUM* COMPLEX DISEASE

Disseminated disease due to MAC was uncommon before the AIDS epidemic, but is now seen in about 10% of patients with AIDS, making it the most common bacterial infection of AIDS patients (91). Early studies showed poor response to therapy, but the introduction of the macrolide/azalide antibiotics has resulted in suppression of bacteremia and substantial clinical improvement in patients with this disease. However, monotherapy with either agent leads to rapid development of resistance; thus, these drugs should never be given without another antimycobacterial agent. Combination regimens including either clarithromycin or azithromycin have been shown effective in trials (92,93). Resistance to clarithromycin and azithromycin is reciprocal, so that the two should not be used together, nor should one be substituted for the other when resistance is suspected.

A consensus committee of experts has suggested that at least one, and possibly two other antimycobacterial agents be used in conjunction with a macrolide/azalide when treating disseminated MAC disease (94). The optimal second drug is not known, but most experts prefer ethambutol, since it has *in vitro* activity against MAC, can be taken orally, and is well tolerated. Rifampin and rifabutin are also effective agents *in vitro* and could be used in combination with a macrolide to prevent the emergence of resistance. Triple antibiotic therapy with clarithromycin, ethambutol, and rifabutin did not have a clear benefit over therapy with clarithromycin and ethambutol (95). Fluoroquinolones show *in vitro* activity, but this is marginal, (96, 97) and maximal oral doses of ciprofloxacin or ofloxacin are not well tolerated by patients with AIDS (77, 98). Amikacin also has activity against MAC *in vitro*, and may be useful in salvage regimens.

The usefulness of antimicrobial susceptibility testing of MAC isolates is unproven, and such tests should not be routinely obtained. The only such tests with generally agreed upon usefulness are those for azithromycin and clarithromycin. Since nearly all MAC isolates from patients who have not received therapy with these agents are susceptible to both agents, initial testing has little value. However, when patients do not respond clinically or microbiologically (after 4 to 6 weeks of therapy) or appear to relapse (usually after 12 weeks of therapy), susceptibility testing is indicated. Such testing, if it reveals resistance, will allow discontinuation of expensive and potentially toxic medications.

Treatment of disseminated MAC in patients with AIDS should be continued until culture results have been negative for 12 months. If the patient's immunologic status has been improved on antiretroviral therapy, antimycobacterial therapy may be discontinued (99).

MYCOBACTERIUM-AVIUM INTRACELLULARE PULMONARY DISEASE

MAC pulmonary disease in the HIV-uninfected host was the most common form of MAC disease in man before AIDS. It accounts for roughly 3,000 cases annually in the United States (100). Treatment of this disease has also been improved by the advent of the azalide/macrolide drugs, and most experts recommend two- or three-drug oral regimens, at similar doses to those used

for disseminated disease (3). The optimal duration of therapy has not been established, but 12 months appears adequate in most cases. Both clarithromycin- and azithromycin-containing regimens are effective (101,102) and intermittent dosing can also be used (103,104). Elderly patients may not tolerate usual adult doses and may require reduced dosing or intermittent administration.

Patients who have resistance or intolerance to azalide/macrolides will have a more difficult course. Such patients should be treated with a regimen containing rifampin or rifabutin, ethambutol and amikacin (or streptomycin) (3).

The utility of *in vitro* susceptibility testing of isolates in designing therapeutic regimens for pulmonary MAC disease is also limited. As with disseminated disease, initial testing is not warranted. Patients who do not respond or who appear to relapse while on an azalide/macrolide containing regimen should have their isolate tested against azalide/macrolides (3).

M. AVIUM COMPLEX LYMPHADENITIS

Isolated MAC lymphadenitis is largely a disease of children, with over 60% of cases in children less than 3 years of age. The preponderance of cases are cervical nodes, usually a single node, but less often multiple contiguous nodes. It is estimated that 500 cases a year occur in the United States (100). Therapy has largely been surgical, with excision of the node(s) the treatment of choice (105). However, a recent report of cure with clarithromycin/ethambutol therapy in a case where excision was not possible suggests that antimycobacterial therapy may be an alternative to surgery (106).

M. AVIUM COMPLEX PROPHYLAXIS

Patients with AIDS and less than 50 CD4+ T-cells/mm^3 should receive rifabutin 300 mg orally per day, clarithromycin prophylaxis 500 mg orally twice daily, or azithromycin 1,200 mg once weekly (94). The azithromycin and clarithromycin regimens prevent 59% to 69% of disseminated MAC disease (107,108). Prophylaxis may be discontinued when the CD4+ T-cell count increases above 100 cells/mm^3 (109,110).

M. kansasii

M. kansasii causes disseminated disease in persons with AIDS and pulmonary disease in persons with or without HIV infection. All presentations are relatively uncommon, and data on therapeutic regimens are sparse. Early studies of therapy for *M. kansasii* pulmonary disease showed equivalent response rates with drug regimens of isoniazid, rifampin, and ethambutol; or isoniazid, rifampin, and streptomycin (111). Rifampin is an essential part of any treatment regimen for *M. kansasii* (112); therapy should be continued for 18 months (3).

There is no clear role for *in vitro* susceptibility testing in selecting initial therapeutic regimens, as isolates are routinely resistant to isoniazid at the doses tested, despite the usefulness of this drug in therapy. It is thought that the isolates are susceptible at levels slightly higher than those tested (3). However, in patients who have had previous treatment with rifampin, resistance to this drug may have arisen, and susceptibility testing should be performed. One study has reported success with treatment of rifampin-resistant *M. kansasii* disease using regimens selected on the basis of *in vitro* susceptibility (113). *M. kansasii* is susceptible to clarithromycin *in vitro*, suggesting a role for this drug in treatment of disease due to *M. kansasii* (114).

Therapy for disseminated disease should follow the same general principles. Case series of disseminated disease in patients with AIDS have reported limited success with regimens containing isoniazid, rifampin, ethambutol, and in some cases, trimethoprim/sulfamethoxazole (115,116). Clarithromycin may also be a useful addition in these patients. However, clarithromycin resistance may occur and limit therapeutic usefulness (117).

M. fortuitum Biovar Fortuitum

This organism has been reported largely as a cause of skin and soft tissue disease, although disseminated disease, pulmonary infection, endocarditis, and keratitis have been reported (118). Most isolates are susceptible to sulfamethoxazole, ciprofloxacin, cefoxitin, imipenem, and amikacin, but not clarithromycin (119,120). Initial therapy should include two of these agents; subsequent modifications should be made on the basis of *in vitro* susceptibility testing, which is a reliable predictor of therapeutic outcome (121). Therapy for uncomplicated skin lesions may require only 3 months; invasive disease in the HIV-uninfected host should receive 3 to 6 months of therapy, while disseminated disease in the HIV-infected host should continue for the life of the patient.

M. fortuitum Biovar Peregrinum

This organism is an uncommon cause of skin and soft tissue infections. Invasive disease has not been reported (116). Most isolates are susceptible to sulfamethoxazole, cefoxitin, amikacin, clarithromycin, and azithromycin (117,118). Initial therapy should include two of these agents; subsequent modifications should be made on the basis of in vitro susceptibility testing, which is a reliable predictor of therapeutic outcome (119).

M. fortuitum Third Biovar

This organism is also an uncommon cause of skin and soft tissue infections. Invasive disease has not been reported (116). Most isolates are susceptible to sulfamethoxazole, cefoxitin, and amikacin, but not clarithromycin or azithromycin (117,118). Initial therapy should include two of these agents; subsequent modifications should be made on the basis of *in vitro* susceptibility testing, which is a reliable predictor of therapeutic outcome (119).

M. chelonae (formerly M. chelonae ss chelonae)

This organism has been reported as a cause of skin and soft tissue infection. Disseminated disease and keratitis have been seen, but are rare (116). Isolates are routinely susceptible to clarithromycin, azithromycin, and amikacin (117); clarithromycin appears to be the therapy of choice for this infection (122); however, resistance may develop on monotherapy (123)). Invasive infection may require combination chemotherapy based on *in vitro* susceptibility testing (119). Therapy for uncomplicated skin lesions may require only 3 months; invasive disease in the HIV-uninfected host should receive 3 to 6 months of therapy.

M. abscessus (formerly M. chelonae ss abscessus)

This organisms has been reported to cause pulmonary disease, skin and soft tissue infections, and disseminated disease (116). Most isolates are susceptible to cefoxitin, amikacin, clarithromycin, and azithromycin (117,118). Initial therapy for serious infection should include amikacin and cefoxitin; (124) subsequent modifications should be made on the basis of *in vitro*

susceptibility testing, which is a reliable predictor of therapeutic outcome (119).

M. chelonae-Like Organisms

These organisms have been reported as causes of wound infection and catheter-related sepsis, and rarely as pathogens in patients with AIDS (125). These organisms are quite susceptible to most antibiotics, including amikacin, imipenem, cefoxitin, ciprofloxacin, and ofloxacin (120). Initial therapy should include two of these agents; subsequent modifications should be made on the basis of *in vitro* susceptibility testing, which is a reliable predictor of therapeutic outcome (119). Linazolid is active *in vitro* and may prove clinically useful (126).

M. marinum

This organism causes skin and soft tissue infections in nonimmunocompromised persons. Occasional cases of invasive arthritis and disseminated disease have been reported. *In vitro* susceptibilities are variable and a relationship between such results and responses to therapy has not been demonstrated (127–129). Most patients are treated with at least two of the following: rifampin, ethambutol, doxycycline, minocycline, or cotrimoxazole. *In vitro* studies suggest that clarithromycin may also be effective (130), and cures have been reported with clarithromycin plus ethambutol (131). Surgical removal of involved lymph nodes has improved outcomes in some series. Therapy is continued for a minimum of 3 months (3).

M. ulcerans

This organism causes necrotic skin ulcers (Buruli ulcer), largely in Africa, Australia, and New Guinea. The mycobacteria secrete a potent cytotoxin that is responsible for the tissue damage. Antimycobacterial agents are not effective (132,133), presumably because they are not given until the toxin has been secreted; penetration to the site of infection may also be impaired by the extensive necrosis. Surgical excision of early lesions and skin grafting for extensive lesions are recommended (130).

M. leprae

Hansen's disease, or leprosy, affects over 5 million persons worldwide, but is uncommon in the United States (134,135). Dapsone, rifampin, clofazimine, and ethionamide are useful agents. Multidrug regimens are usually used, both to prevent emergence of drug resistance, and to eliminate persistent organisms. However, a recent study showed that long term outcomes of dapsone monotherapy were also satisfactory as long as dapsone resistant organisms were not present (136).

For paucibacillary leprosy, dapsone is given daily and rifampin 10 mg/kg monthly, both for 6 months. For multibacillary forms, daily dapsone, monthly rifampin and clofazimine 300 mg monthly and 50 mg daily are given for 2 years (137). Directly observed therapy of the monthly doses is strongly recommended. *In vitro* susceptibility testing is not available. Recent animal studies suggest that minocycline, ofloxacin, and clarithromycin may also be useful in treatment of leprosy (138,139).

M. hemophilum

This organism is an infrequent cause of skin lesions; nearly all cases occur in immunocompromised patients, and dissemination can occur in the HIV-infected host (140–142). *In vitro* susceptibility testing suggests that most isolates are susceptible to clarithromycin, ciprofloxacin, cycloserine, and rifabutin; use of these agents for therapy appeared to be associated with an improved clinical outcome, but only 13 patients were reported. Others have recommended a regimen of amikacin, ciprofloxacin, and rifampin (143). The optimal duration of therapy and the role of *in vitro* susceptibility testing in guiding management are unknown.

M. xenopi

M. xenopi is a cause of pulmonary disease in both immunologically normal and immunosuppressed hosts; disseminated disease in patients with AIDS has also been reported (144). The organism is routinely susceptible to isoniazid and streptomycin, but intermediate to rifampin and resistant to ethambutol (146); most isolates are susceptible to clarithromycin but combination therapy with clarithromycin-containing regimens appears promising (3,147,148). Those failing medical therapy may benefit from surgical resection (149). Disseminated disease in AIDS has also shown a variable response to therapy.

M. szulgai

M. szulgai is a rare cause of pulmonary disease; cutaneous infection and olecranon bursitis have also been reported (150). Isolates of *M. szulgai* are usually susceptible to isoniazid, streptomycin, and rifampin; susceptibility to ethambutol is variable (147). Another report also showed susceptibility to clarithromycin (130). Therapy with three of these drugs is recommended (3); at least 12 months of treatment would appear prudent.

M. malmoense

This organism is similar in clinical presentation to MAC; it causes pulmonary disease in normal hosts, cervical lymphadenitis in children, and disseminated disease in patients with AIDS (151–153). It is common in Europe but rare in the United States. Most authors recommend 18 to 24 months of therapy with isoniazid, rifampin, and ethambutol, with an initial period of streptomycin for pulmonary or disseminated disease (3,154). The value of *in vitro* susceptibility testing as a guide to selection of drugs is unknown. Clarithromycin has not been clinically evaluated, but may prove useful.

M. genavense

This organism is biochemically and genetically related to *M. simiae*, but produces a clinical picture more similar to that of MAC, with disseminated disease in AIDS patients the dominant clinical presentation (155,156). Susceptibility studies are limited by the failure of growth on solid media; limited experience suggests that three drug regimens containing clarithromycin (such as those recommended for MAC) are effective (157).

M. simiae

This organism is a rare cause of pulmonary disease, and also a rare cause of disseminated disease in patients with AIDS (158–161). Most isolates are resistant to the majority of antimycobacterial agents, including clarithromycin (130), and therapeutic results are poor (158). An expert panel has recommended initiation of therapy with isoniazid, rifampin, ethambutol, and streptomycin, and adjusting the regimen on the basis of results of *in vitro* susceptibility tests (3).

M. scrofulaceum

This organism was a common cause of cervical lymphadenitis in children in the United States until the 1970s, but is rare today (105); it is also rarely seen as a cause of pulmonary disease (162) and as disseminated disease in AIDS (163). Treatment of isolated lymphadenitis should continue to be surgical. *M. scrofulaceum* is very susceptible *in vitro* to clarithromycin (130), and multidrug regimens containing clarithromycin have been advocated. Susceptibility to ethambutol and rifampin are variable, but these drugs might be useful additional drugs for initial therapy until susceptibility results are available. Duration of therapy is unknown, but should be lifelong in patients with AIDS.

M. celatum

This newly described pathogen is closely related to MAC and *M. xenopi*. The clinical spectrum includes pneumonia and disseminated disease in patients with AIDS (164,165). Isolates may be susceptible to clarithromycin, azithromycin, amikacin, ciprofloxacin, ofloxacin, clofazimine, rifampin, and rifabutin. We recommend a therapeutic strategy similar to that for MAC.

M. smegmatis

This organism is rarely reported to cause skin and soft tissue infection, especially after inoculation (166). Isolates are usually susceptible to amikacin, imipenem, ethambutol, ciprofloxacin, doxycycline, and sulfamethoxazole. Results of *in vitro* susceptibility testing are recommended as a guide to therapy, and clinical outcomes are, on the whole, favorable (167). Superficial infection may be cured by excision, without antibiotics (168).

M. gordonae

This organism is a common saprophyte and almost never a pathogen; only a handful of well-documented cases of human infection have been reported (169). Susceptibility *in vitro* to ethambutol, clarithromycin, rifampin, and amikacin have been reported (130,169). Few isolates have been tested against quinolones or trimethoprim sulfa. Results of treatment are mixed; the paucity of cases precludes conclusions about therapy.

M. terrae Complex

These organisms cause tenosynovitis, bone and joint infection, pneumonia, and disseminated disease (170). Isolates are usually susceptible to azithromycin, clarithromycin, ethambutol, and aminoglycosides (170). Clinical experience is limited but combination regimens have proven effective in some cases (170).

Specific Antimycobacterial Drugs for Nontuberculous Mycobacteria

AZITHROMYCIN

Azithromycin is a macrolide antibiotic with a 15-membered macrolide ring, known as an azalide (see Table 34.8). It inhibits bacterial protein synthesis by binding to the 50S ribosomal subunit; this is thought to be the mechanism of action in mycobacteria as well. Azithromycin is active *in vitro* against MAC and other nontuberculous mycobacteria, but is not active against *M. tuberculosis*. The drug is well absorbed orally and is concentrated in tissues, where levels ten to 100 times higher than serum levels may be achieved (171,172). The half-life is nearly 5 days, so that dosing may be at intervals greater than daily, although for convenience daily dosing is usually used. The drug is metabolized and excreted in the liver; it should be used with caution in persons with potential hepatic impairment. As with other macrolides, gastrointestinal (GI) toxicity can occur, although azithromycin appears to have less GI toxicity than either erythromycin or clarithromycin. This toxicity is dose related and may be circumvented by dividing or reducing doses (104,173). Diarrhea and nausea, as well as frank abdominal pain, are seen. Skin rashes or other evidence of hypersensitivity are rare. More worrisome is hearing loss, which has been reported in patients receiving therapy for MAC with high doses of the drug (174). While this is reversible if the drug is discontinued early, continuation may result in permanent loss. There appear to be few interactions with rifamycins or antiretroviral agents. When the drug is given with rifabutin, uveitis appears to be rare, in contrast with the experience when clarithromycin is given with rifabutin.

CEFOXITIN

Cefoxitin is a beta-lactam antibiotic that interferes with cell wall synthesis of gram-negative and gram-positive bacteria; its mode of action against mycobacteria is unknown but may be similar. Cefoxitin is active against all biovars of *M. fortuitum*, *M. abscessus*, and *M. chelonae*–like mycobacteria, and it is used primarily for invasive infections with these organisms. The drug is poorly absorbed orally must be given by the intramuscular or intravenous route, with the latter being preferred. The half life in the serum is 1 hour; 85% of the drug is excreted in the urine, so dose adjustment should be made when used in patients with altered renal function. High doses are recommended when treating mycobacterial infections with cefoxitin (12 g/day) (120). Toxicities include rash, fever, eosinophilia, and mild leukopenia and elevations in liver function tests. All are uncommon (<3%).

CLARITHROMYCIN

Clarithromycin is a macrolide antibiotic that is closely related to erythromycin. It inhibits bacterial protein synthesis by binding to the 50S ribosomal subunit; this is thought to be the mechanism of action in mycobacteria as well. Clarithromycin is active in vitro against MAC and other nontuberculous mycobacteria, but is not active against *M. tuberculosis*. The drug is well absorbed orally and is concentrated in tissues, where levels two to six times higher than in serum may be achieved (175). The half life is 2.6 to 4.4 hours; this has led to twice-daily dosing, although the slow growth rate of mycobacteria would undoubtedly allow daily dosing; however, GI intolerance of the correspondingly larger single dose has effectively limited this strategy. The drug is metabolized and excreted in the liver, but 30% is also excreted in the urine, and dose adjustment is needed in persons with impaired renal function. As with other macrolides, GI toxicity can occur, but clarithromycin has substantially less GI toxicity than erythromycin. Toxicity is dose-related; persons unable to tolerate 500 mg twice daily (the highest recommended dose) may successfully tolerate 250 mg four times daily or may require dose reduction to 250 mg orally twice daily (104). Moreover, those who do not tolerate clarithromycin may tolerate azithromycin without difficulty. Diarrhea and nausea, as well as abdominal pain or dyspepsia, are the most common manifestations, occurring in 11% of patients. Skin rashes or other evidence of hypersensitivity are rare. Hearing loss appears to be less common than with azithromycin. As with other macrolides, hepatic toxicity may

occur with use of clarithromycin (176). There is a bidirectional interaction between clarithromycin and rifabutin, with increased levels of rifabutin and decreased levels of clarithromycin when the drugs are taken concurrently (177–179). This interaction may be responsible for the occurrence of uveitis when clarithromycin is used in conjunction with 600 mg per day of rifabutin (180). Uveitis appears uncommon, however, if the rifabutin dose does not exceed 300 mg per day. This uveitis resolves when rifabutin doses are lowered or the drug is discontinued. Oral doses greater than 500 mg bid have been associated with shortened survival and should not be used (181).

CLOFAZIMINE

Clofazimine is riminophenazine dye that binds to DNA, but its mechanism of antimycobacterial action is unknown. It has activity against MAC and *M. leprae* and is primarily used in treatment of infections with these organisms. Clofazimine has variable absorption, but is effective when given orally. It is extremely fat-soluble, with a large volume of distribution; consequently, the drug is not detectable in the serum for up to 3 months after initiation of oral therapy, and the half-life is 70 days. It is excreted in the stool, with less than 1% of drug found in the urine. Toxicity is minimal, with an orange-bronze discoloration of the skin the most common effect in light-skinned individuals. This pigmentation gradually resolves if the drug is discontinued. Dry skin and scaling can also be bothersome to the patient. GI disturbances, including nausea, vomiting, and diarrhea, are uncommon when doses of 100 mg daily are used, but become more frequent as higher doses are used.

DAPSONE

Dapsone is a long-acting sulfa compound that is effective against *M. leprae*, for which it is the major antimycobacterial agent. Its mechanism of action is presumed to be inhibition of mycobacterial synthesis of folic acid, by analogy with its activity in other bacteria. The drug is well absorbed orally and has a mean plasma half-life of 28 hours. Excretion occurs in the stool after hepatic metabolism, and enterohepatic circulation occurs, leading to prolongation of the drug in the body. The major toxicity is hemolytic anemia, occurring in persons with glucose-6-phosphate dehydrogenase deficiency, and patients should be screened for this defect before beginning dapsone therapy. Rare individuals will have a hypersensitivity syndrome comprising fever, jaundice, anemia, and exfoliative dermatitis; this syndrome resolves with discontinuation of the drug.

SULFISOXAZOLE

Sulfisoxazole is a sulfa drug with activity against all biovars of *M. fortuitum*. Its mechanism of antimycobacterial action is presumed to be inhibition of bacterial synthesis of folic acid, by analogy with its activity in other bacteria. The drug is absorbed well from the GI tract and can be given orally. The half-life is 5 to 6 hours, and over 95% of the drug is excreted in the urine; thus dose adjustment must be made for patients with impaired renal function. Toxicities include rash, fever, photosensitization, anemia, and (rarely) Stevens-Johnson syndrome.

COTRIMOXAZOLE

Cotrimoxazole is a fixed combination of sulfamethoxazole and trimethoprim. The combination has activity against *M. marinum*, and this is the only mycobacterial species for which it is used. Its mechanism of antimycobacterial action is presumed to be inhibition of bacterial synthesis of folic acid, by analogy with its activity in other bacteria. The drug is absorbed well from the GI tract and can be given orally. The half-life of the sulfa portion is 10 to 12 hours, and most of the drug is excreted in the urine;

thus, dose adjustment must be made for patients with impaired renal function. The half-life of the trimethoprim moiety is 9 to 11 hours and it is also excreted in the urine. Toxicities include rash, fever, photosensitization, anemia, leukopenia, and (rarely) Stevens-Johnson syndrome.

IMIPENEM

Imipenem is a beta-lactam antibiotic that is given with cilastin to counter enzymatic breakdown of imipenem in the kidney. Imipenem acts by binding to penicillin binding proteins of many bacteria; the antimycobacterial activity is also thought to result from such binding. The drug is active against *M. fortuitum* bv fortuitum and *M. chelonae*–like organisms. It is an alternative agent for treatment of invasive infections with these organisms. Imipenem is given intravenously and has a half-life of 1 hour. Seventy percent of the drug is excreted in the urine; thus dose reduction is required in persons with impaired renal function. Toxicities include rash and fever, nausea, and vomiting. Diarrhea and local thrombophlebitis at the site of infusion are also seen. Seizures have also been reported, but are uncommon.

DOXYCYCLINE

Doxycycline is a long-acting tetracycline analogue that is active against *M. marinum* and is used in treatment of infection with this organism. Tetracyclines inhibit protein synthesis by interfering with attachment of RNA to the ribosome, primarily at the 30S ribosomal subunit; presumably its activity against *M. marinum* involves such a mechanism. Doxycycline is well absorbed from the gut and is given orally. The serum half-life is 18 hours, and somewhat less than half of the drug appears in the urine. Dose adjustment in renal failure is not required. Toxicities include nausea and photosensitivity, but these are uncommon.

MINOCYCLINE

Minocycline is also a long-acting tetracycline analogue that is active against *M. leprae* and *M. marinum* and is used as an alternative therapy in treatment of infections with these organisms. Tetracyclines inhibit protein synthesis by interfering with attachment of RNA to the ribosome, primarily at the 30S ribosomal subunit; presumably its activity against mycobacteria involves such a mechanism. Minocycline is well absorbed from the gut and is given orally. The serum half-life is 16 hours, and less than 10% of the drug appears in the urine. Dose adjustment in renal failure is therefore not required. Toxicities include nausea and photosensitivity, but these are uncommon. Vertigo and ataxia may result from this tetracycline and limit its use in some patients.

AMIKACIN

Amikacin is an aminoglycoside antibiotic that is presumed to act by interfering with the bacterial ribosome to prevent accurate protein synthesis, although the exact mechanism of its action in mycobacteria has not been elucidated. Amikacin is active against MAC, *M. fortuitum* (all biovars), *M. chelonae*, *M. chelonae*–like organisms, *M. abscessus*, and *M. hemophilum*. However, its use is generally restricted to invasive infections with isolates that are not susceptible to oral agents. Amikacin is not absorbed from the GI tract and is generally given intravenously, although intramuscular injections can also be given. The serum half-life is 8 hours; because of the slow growth of mycobacteria, once daily dosing is sufficient. The drug is excreted by the kidney, and doses must be adjusted in patients with impaired renal function. Monitoring of serum drug levels is recommended. Amikacin has considerable ototoxicity and nephrotoxicity. Ototoxicity can be either cochlear or vestibular, and increases with the duration of therapy. This poses a particular problem in treatment of mycobacterial infections, where months to years of treatment are often desir-

able. In practice, amikacin is given only for a brief period of 1 to 3 months; treatment for over 3 months with full-dose amikacin almost guarantees ototoxicity. Hearing loss is reversible if the drug is stopped promptly, but onset can be insidious and disability permanent. Nephrotoxicity is more easily monitored, but likewise common. Biweekly serum creatinine determinations and weekly gentamicin levels should be obtained while the patient is on therapy; doses must be adjusted if renal function impairment occurs.

REFERENCES

1. Good RC, Mastro TD. The modern mycobacteriology laboratory: how it can help the clinician. *Clin Chest Med* 1989;10:315–322.
2. Wolinsky E, Rynearson TK. Mycobacteria in soil and their relation to disease-associated strains. *Am Rev Resp Dis* 1968;97:1032–1037.
3. Wallace RJ Jr, Glassroth J, Griffith DE, Olivier KN, Cook JL, Gordin F, American Thoracic Society. Diagnosis and treatment of disease caused by nontuberculous mycobacteria. *Am J Resp Crit Care Med* 1997;156[Suppl. 2]:S1–S25.
4. Davis AL. A historical perspective on tuberculosis and its control. In: Reichman LB, Herschfield ES, eds. *Tuberculosis: a comprehensive international approach*, 2nd ed. New York: Marcel Dekker, 2003:1–54.
5. Medical Research Council. A Medical Research Council Investigation. Streptomycin treatment of pulmonary tuberculosis. *BMJ* 1948;ii:769–782.
6. Hinshaw HC, Feldman WH, Pfuetze KH. Treatment of tuberculosis with streptomycin. A summary of observation in one hundred cases. *JAMA* 1946;13:778–782.
7. Medical Research Council. A Medical Research Council Investigation. Treatment of pulmonary tuberculosis with streptomycin and para-aminosalicylic acid. *BMJ* 1950;ii:1073–1085.
8. Medical Research Council. The treatment of pulmonary tuberculosis with isoniazid, and interim report to the Medical Research Council by their Tuberculosis Chemotherapy Trials Committee. *BMJ* 1953;ii:735–746.
9. Medical Research Council. Various combinations of isoniazid with streptomycin or with PAS in the treatment of pulmonary tuberculosis. Seventh report to the Medical Research Council by their Tuberculosis Chemotherapy Trials Committee. *BMJ* 1955;i:434–445.
10. Crofton J. Drug treatment of tuberculosis. Standard chemotherapy. *BMJ* 1960;ii:370–373.
11. Medical Research Council-Tuberculosis Chemotherapy Trials Committee. Long-term chemotherapy in the treatment of chronic pulmonary tuberculosis with cavitation. *Tubercle* 1962;43:201–267.
12. Combs DL, O'Brien RJ, Geiter LJ. USPHS short-course chemotherapy trial 21: effectiveness, toxicity, and acceptability. The report of final results. *Ann Intern Med* 1990;112:397–406.
13. Fox W. General considerations in intermittent drug therapy of pulmonary tuberculosis. *Postgrad Med* 1971;47:729–736.
14. Mitchison DA. The action of antituberculosis drugs in short-course chemotherapy. *Tubercle* 1985;66:219–226.
15. Mitchison DA. Basic mechanisms of chemotherapy. *Chest* 1979;6:771–781.
16. Jindani A, Aber VR, Edwards EA, Mitchison DA. The early bactericidal activity of drugs in patients with pulmonary tuberculosis. *Am Rev Respir Dis* 1980;121:939–949.
17. Dickinson JM, Aber VR, Mitchison DA. Bactericidal activity of streptomycin, isoniazid, rifampin, ethambutol and pyrazinamide alone and in combination against *Mycobacterium tuberculosis*. *Am Rev Respir Dis* 1977;116:627–635.
18. Grosset J. The sterilizing value of rifampicin and pyrazinamide in experimental short-course chemotherapy. *Tubercle* 1978;59:287–297.
19. Fox W. The problem of self-administration of drugs; with particular reference to pulmonary tuberculosis. *Tubercle* 1958;39:269–274.
20. McDonald RJ, Memon AM, Reichman LB. Successful supervised ambulatory management of tuberculosis treatment failures. *Ann Intern Med* 1982;96:297–302.
21. Sbarbaro JA. Of pride and program planning—a lesson in reality. *Chest* 1998;114:1229–1230.
22. Chaulk CP, Kazandjian VA. Directly observed therapy for treatment of tuberculosis: consensus statement of the Public Health Tuberculosis Guidelines Panel. *JAMA* 1998;279:943–948.
23. Weis SE, Slocum PC, Blais FX, et al. The effect of directly observed therapy on the rates of drug resistance and relapse in tuberculosis. *N Engl J Med* 1994;330:1179–1184.
24. American Thoracic Society, Infectious Diseases Society of America, Centers for Disease Control and Prevention. Treatment of tuberculosis. *Am J Resp Crit Care Med* 2003;167:603–662.
25. Patel KB, Belmonte R, Crowe HM. Drug malabsorption and resistant tuberculosis in HIV-infected patients. *N Engl J Med* 1995;332:336–337.
26. Mahmoudi A, Iseman MD. Pitfalls in the care of patients with tuberculosis. *JAMA* 1993;270:65–68.
27. Centers for Disease Control and Prevention. Reported tuberculosis in the United States, 2000. Atlanta, GA: US Department of Health and Human Services, CDC; August 13, 2001.

28. Cohn DL, Catlin BJ, Peterson KL, Judson FN, Sbarbaro JA. A 62-dose 6-month therapy for pulmonary and extrapulmonary TB. A twice-weekly, directly observed, and cost-effective regimen. *Ann Intern Med* 1990;112:407–415.

29. Hong Kong Chest Service/British Medical Research Council. Controlled trial of 4 three-times-weekly regimens and a daily regimen given for 6 months for pulmonary TB. Second report: the results up to 24 months. *Tubercle* 1982;63:89–98.

30. Hong Kong Chest Service/British Medical Research Council. Five-year follow-up of a controlled trial of five 6-month regimens of chemotherapy for pulmonary tuberculosis. *Am Rev Respir Dis* 1987;136:1339–1342.

31. Vernon A, Burman W, Benator D, Khan A, Bozeman L. Acquired rifamycin monoresistance in patients with HIV-related tuberculosis treated with once-weekly rifapentine and isoniazid. *Lancet* 1999;353:1843–1847.

32. Tuberculosis Trials Consortium. Once-weekly rifapentine and isoniazid versus twice-weekly rifampin and isoniazid in the continuation phase of therapy for drug susceptible pulmonary tuberculosis. *Lancet* 2002 (in press).

33. Small PM, Schechter GF, Goodman PC, Sande MA, Chaisson RE, Hopewell PC. Treatment of tuberculosis in patients with advanced human immunodeficiency virus infection. *N Engl J Med* 1991;324:289–294.

34. Perriens JH, St Louis ME, Mukadi YB, et al. Pulmonary tuberculosis in HIV-infected patients in Zaire: a controlled trial of treatment for either 6 or 12 months. *N Engl J Med* 1995;332:779–784.

35. Centers for Disease Control and Prevention. Updated guidelines for the use of rifabutin or rifampin for the treatment and prevention of HIV-infected patients taking protease inhibitors or nonnucleoside reverse transcriptase inhibitors. *MMWR* 2000;49:185–189.

36. Munsiff S, Fujiwara P. Treatment of tuberculosis in patients taking antiretrovirals. *AIDS Read* 2000;10:102–108.

37. Veldkamp AI, Hoetelmans MW, Beijnen JH, Mulder JW, Meenhorst PL. Ritonavir enables combined therapy with rifampin and saquinavir. *Clin Infect Dis* 1999;29:1586.

38. Gonzalez-Montaner LJ, Natal S, Yongchaiyud P, Olliaro P. Rifabutin for the treatment of newly diagnosed pulmonary tuberculosis: a multinational, randomized, comparative study versus rifampicin. *Tuberc Lung Dis* 1994;75:341–347.

39. Narita M. Ashkin D, Hollender ES, Pitchenick AE. Paradoxical worsening of tuberculosis following antiretroviral therapy in patients with AIDS. *Am J Resp Crit Care Med* 1998;158:157–161.

40. De Simone JA, Pomerantz RJ, Babichack TJ. Inflammatory reactions in HIV-1 infected persons after intitaion of highly active antiretroviral therapy. *Ann Intern Med* 2000;133:447–454.

41. Snider DE Jr. Should women taking antituberculosis drugs breast-feed? *Arch Intern Med* 1984;144:589–590.

42. Snider DE Jr, Layde PM, Johnson MW, Lyle MA. Treatment of tuberculosis during pregnancy. *Am Rev Resp Dis* 1980;122:65–79.

43. Dutt AK, Moers D, Stead WW. Smear- and culture-negative pulmonary tuberculosis: Four-month short-course chemotherapy. *Am Rev Respir Dis* 1989;139:867–870.

44. Hong Kong Chest Service/Tuberculosis Research Centre, Madras/British Medical Research Council. A controlled trial of 3-month, 4-month, and 6-month regimens of chemotherapy for sputum-smear-negative pulmonary tuberculosis. Results at 5 years. *Am Rev Respir Dis* 1989;139:871–876.

45. Mitchison DA, Nunn AJ. Influence of initial drug resistance on the response to short-course chemotherapy of pulmonary tuberculosis. *Am Rev Respir Dis* 1986;133:423–430.

46. Babu Swai O, Aluoch JA, Githui WA, et al. Controlled clinical trial of a regimen of two durations for the treatment of isoniazid resistant pulmonary tuberculosis. *Tubercle* 1988;69:5–14.

47. Hong Kong Tuberculosis Treatment Service/British Medical Research Council. Controlled trial of 6-month and 9-month regimens of daily and intermittent streptomycin plus isoniazid plus pyrazinamide for pulmonary tuberculosis in Hong Kong: the results up to 30 months. *Am Rev Respir Dis* 1977;115:727–735.

48. Goble M, Iseman MD, Madsen LA, Waite D, Ackerson L, Horsburgh CR. Treatment of 171 patients with pulmonary tuberculosis resistant to isoniazid and rifampin. *N Engl J Med* 1993;328:527–532.

49. Salomon N, Perlman DC, Friedmann P, Buchstein S, Kreisworth BN, Mildvan D. Predictors and outcome of multidrug-resistant tuberculosis. *Clin Infect Dis* 1995;21:1245–1252.

50. Telzak EE, Sepkowitz K, Alpert P, et al. Multidrug-resistant tuberculosis in patients without HIV infection. *N Engl J Med* 1995;333:907–911.

51. Turett GS, Telzak EE, Torian LV, et al. Improved outcomes for patients with multidrug-resistant tuberculosis. *Clin Infect Dis* 1995;21:1238–1244.

52. Iseman MD. Treatment of multidrug-resistant tuberculosis. *N Engl J Med* 1993;329:784–791.

53. Centers for Disease Control and Prevention. *Improving patient adherence to tuberculosis treatment.* Atlanta: US Department of Health and Human Services, Public Health Service, CDC, 1994.

54. Iseman MD, Madsen L, Goble M, Pomerantz M. Surgical intervention in the treatment of pulmonary disease caused by drug-resistant *M. tuberculosis. Am Rev Respir Dis* 1990;141:623–625.

55. Treasure RL, Seaworth BJ. Current role of surgery in *Mycobacterium tuberculosis. Ann Thorac Surg* 1995;59:1405–1409.

56. Ferebee SH. Controlled chemoprophylaxis trials in tuberculosis: a general review. *Adv Tuberc Res* 1969;17:28–106.

57. Hsu KH. Thirty years after isoniazid: its impact on tuberculosis in children and adolescents. *JAMA* 1984;251:1283–1285.

58. International Union Against Tuberculosis Committee on Prophylaxis. Efficacy of various durations of isoniazid preventive therapy for tuberculosis: five years of follow-up in the IUAT trial. *Bull WHO* 1982;60:555–564.

59. Centers for Disease Control and Prevention. Targeted tuberculin testing and treatment of latent tuberculosis infection. *MMWR* 2000;49(no. RR-6).

60. Kopanoff DE, Snider DE Jr, Caras GJ. Isoniazid-related hepatitis: a U.S. Public health service cooperative surveillance study. *Am Rev Respir Dis* 1978;117:991–1001.

61. Hong Kong Chest Service, Tuberculosis Research Centre, Madras, and British Medical Research Council. A double blind placebo controlled clinical trial of three antituberculosis chemoprophylaxis regimens in patients with silicosis in Hong Kong. *Am Rev Respir Dis* 1992;145:36–41.

62. Ormerod LP. Rifampicin and isoniazid prophylactic chemotherapy for tuberculosis. *Arch Dis Child* 1998;78:169–171.

63. Villarino ME, Ridzon R, Weismuller PC, et al. Rifampin preventive therapy for tuberculosis infection: experience with 157 adolescents. *Am J Resp Crit Care Med* 1997;155:1735–1738.

64. Gordin FM, Chaison RE, Matts JP, et al. An international, randomized trial of rifampin and pyrazinamide versus isoniazid for prevention of tuberculosis in HIV-infected persons. *JAMA* 2000;283:1445–1450.

65. Centers for Disease Control and Prevention. Update: fatal and severe liver injuries associated with rifampin and pyrazinamide for latent tuberculosis infection, and revisions in American Thoracic Society/CDC recommendations—United States, 2001. *MMWR* 2001;50:733–735.

66. Centers for Disease Control. Management of persons exposed to multidrug-resistant tuberculosis. *MMWR* 1992;41:59–71.

67. Horn DL, Hewlett D, Alfalla C. Limited tolerance of ofloxacin and pyrazinamide prophylaxis against tuberculosis [letter]. *N Engl J Med* 1994;330:1241.

68. Centers for Disease Control and Prevention. Severe isoniazid-associated hepatitis—New York, 1991–1993. *MMWR* 1993;42:545–547.

69. Moulding TS, Redeker AG, Kanel GC. Twenty isoniazid-associated deaths in one state. *Am Rev Respir Dis* 1989;140:700–705.

70. Nolan CM, Goldberg SV, Buskin SE. Hepatotoxicity associated with isoniazid preventive therapy. *JAMA* 1999;281:1014–1018.

71. Snider DE. Pyridoxine supplementation during isoniazid therapy. *Tubercle* 1980;61:191–196.

72. Rothfield NF, Bierer MF, Garfield JW. Isoniazid induction of antinuclear antibodies. *Ann Intern Med* 1978;88:650–652.

73. Alarcon-Segovia D, Fishbein E, Betancourt VM. Antibodies to nucleoprotein in tuberculous patients receiving isoniazid. *Clin Exp Immunol* 1969;5:429–437.

74. Smith CK, Durack DT. Isoniazid and reaction to cheese. *Ann Intern Med* 1978;88:520–521.

75. Uragoda CG. Histamine poisoning in tuberculous patients after ingestion of tuna fish. *Am Rev Respir Dis* 1980;121:157–159.

76. Block SH. Carbemezepine-isoniazid interaction. *Pediatrics* 1982;69:494.

77. Kutt H, Brennan R, Dehejia H, Verebely K. Diphenylhydantoin intoxication. A complication of isoniazid therapy. *Am Rev Resp Dis* 1970;101:377.

78. Zent C, Smith P. Study of the effect of concomitant food on the bioavailability of rifampicin, isoniazid, and pyrazinamide. *Tubercle* 1995;76:109–113.

79. Steele MA, Burk RF, DesPrez RM. Toxic hepatitis with isoniazid and rifampin. *Chest* 1991;99:465–471.

80. Borcherding SM, Baciewicz AM, Self TH. Update on rifampin drug interactions II. *Arch Intern Med* 1992;152:711–716.

81. Tseng AL, Walmsley SL. Rifabutin-associated uveitis. *Ann Pharmacol* 1995;29:1149–1155.

82. Marshall JD, Abdel-Rahman S, Johnson K, Kauffman RE, Kearns GL. Rifapentine pharmacokinetics in adolescents. *Pediatr Infect Dis J* 1999;18:882–888.

83. Burman WJ, Gallicano K, Pelloquin C. Comparative pharmacokinetics of the rifamycin antibacterials. *Clin Pharmacokinet* 2001;40:327–341.

84. Varughese A, Brater DC, Benet LZ, Lee CS. Ethambutol kinetics in patients with impaired renal function. *Am Rev Respir Dis* 1986;134:34–38.

85. Trebucq A. Should ethambutol be recommended for routine treatment of tuberculosis in children? A review of the literature. *Int J Tuberc Lung Dis* 1997;1:12–15.

86. Steele MA, Des Prez RM. The role of pyrazinamide in tuberculosis chemotherapy. *Chest* 1988;94:842–844.

87. Drugs for tuberculosis. *Med Lett* 1995;37:67–70.

88. Moulding T, Dutt AK, Reichman LB. Fixed-dose combinations of antituberculous medications to prevent drug resistance. *Ann Intern Med* 1995;122:951–954.

89. Peloquin CA, Berning SE, Huitt GA, et al. Once daily and twice-daily dosing of p-aminosalicylic acid granules. *Am J Respir Crit Care Med* 1999;159:932–934.

90. Berning SL, Madsen L, Iseman MD, Peloquin CA. Long-term safety of ofloxacin and ciprofloxacin in the treatment of mycobacterial infections. *Am J Respir Crit Care Med* 1995;151:2006–2009.

91. Horsburgh CR. *Mycobacterium avium* complex infection in the acquired immunodeficiency syndrome. *N Engl J Med* 1991;324:1332–1338.

92. Shafran SD, Singer J, Zarowny DP, et al. A comparison of two regimens for the treatment of *Mycobacterium avium* complex bacteremia in in AIDS: rifabutin, ethambutol, and clarithromycin versus rifampin, ethambutol, clofazimine, and ciprofloxacin. *N Engl J Med* 1996;335:377–383.

93. Koletar SL, Berry AJ, Cynamon MH, et al. Azithromycin as treatment for disseminated *Mycobacterium avium* complex in AIDS patients. *Antimicrob Agents Chemother* 1999;43:2869–2872.

94. Centers for Disease Control and Prevention. 1999 USPHS/IDSA guidelines for the prevention of opportunistic infections in persons infected with human immunodeficiency virus. *MMWR* 1993;48(RR-10):1–59.

95. Gordin FM, Sullam PM, Shafran SD, et al. A randomized, placebo-controlled study of rifabutin added to a regimen of clarithromycin and ethambutol for treatment of disseminated infection with *Mycobacterium avium* complex. *Clin Infect Dis* 1999;28:1080–1085.

96. Heifets LB, Lindholm-Levy PJ. Bacteriostatic and bactericidal activity of ciprofloxacin and floxacin against *Mycobacterium tuberculosis* and *Mycobacterium avium* complex. *Tubercle* 1987;68:267–276.

97. Young LS, Berlin OGW, Inderlied CD. Activity of ciprofloxacin and other fluorinated quinolones against mycobacteria. *Am J Med* 1987;82(SA):23–26.

98. Gordon SM, Horsburgh CR, Peloquin CA, et al. Low serum levels of oral antimycobacterial agents in patients with disseminated *Mycobacterium avium* complex disease. *J Infect Dis* 1993;168:1559–1562.

99. Aberg JA, Yajko DM, Jacobson MA. Eradication of AIDS-related disseminated mycobacterium avium complex infection after 12 months of antimycobacterial therapy combined with highly active antiretroviral therapy. *J Infect Dis* 1998;178:1446–1449.

100. O'Brien RJ, Geiter LJ, Snider DE. The epidemiology of nontuberculous mycobacterial diseases in the United States. Results from a national survey. *Am Rev Respir Dis* 1987;135:1007–1014.

101. Wallace RJ, Brown BA, Griffith DE, Girard WM, Murphy DT. Clarithromycin regimens for pulmonary *Mycobacterium avium* complex. The first 50 patients. *Am J Resp Crit Care Med* 1996;153:1766–1772.

102. Griffith DE, Brown BA, Girard WM, et al. Azithromycin-containing regimens for treatment of *Mycobacterium avium* complex lung disease. *Clin Infect Dis* 2001;32:1547–1553.

103. Griffith DE, Brown BA, Cegieski P, Murphy DT, Wallace RJ Jr. Early results (at 6 months) with intermittent clarithromycin-inducing regimens for lung disease due to *Mycobacterium avium* complex. *Clin Infect Dis* 2000;30:288–292.

104. Griffith DE, Brown BA, Murphy DT, et al. Initial (6 month) results of three-times weekly azithromycin in treatment regimens for *Mycobacterium avium* complex lung disease in human immunodeficiency virus-negative patients. *J Infect Dis* 1998;178:121–126.

105. Wolinsky E. Mycobacterial lymphadenitis in children: a prospective study of 105 nontuberculous cases with long-term follow-up. *Clin Infect Dis* 1995;10:954–963.

106. Green PA, von Reyn CF, Smith RP. *Mycobacterium avium* complex parotid lymphadenitis: successful therapy with clarithromycin and ethambutol. *Pediatr Infect Dis J* 1993;12:615–616.

107. Pierce M, Crampton S, Henry D, et al. A randomized trial of clarithromycin as prophylaxis against disseminated *Mycobacterium avium* complex infection in AIDS. *N Engl J Med* 1996;335:384–391.

108. Havlir DV, Dube MP, Sattler FR, et al. Prophylaxis against disseminated *Mycobacterium avium* complex with weekly azithromycin, daily rifabutin, or both. *N Engl J Med* 1996;335:392–398.

109. El-Sadr WM, Burman WJ, Brant LB, et al. Discontinuation of prophylaxis against *Mycobacterium avium* complex disease in HIV-infected patients who have a response to antiretroviral therapy. *N Engl J Med* 2000;342:1085–1092.

110. Currier JS, Williams PL, Koletar SL, et al. Discontinuation of *Mycobacterium avium* complex prophylaxis in patients with antiretroviral therapy-induced increases in CD4+ cell count. *Ann Intern Med* 2000;133:493–503.

111. Ahn CH, Hurst GA. The treatment of disease due to *Mycobacterium kansasii*. *Semin Resp Med* 1981;2:228–232.

112. Lillo M, Orengo S, Cernoch P, et al. Pulmonary and disseminated infection due to *Mycobacterium kansasii*: a decade of experience. *Rev Infect Dis* 1990;12:760–767.

113. Wallace RJ, Dunbar D, Brown BA, et al. Rifampin-resistant *Mycobacterium kansasii*. *Clin Infect Dis* 1994;18:736–743.

114. Biehle J, Cavalieri SJ. In vitro susceptibility of *Mycobacterium kansasii* to clarithromycin. *Antimicrob Agents Chemother* 1992;36:2039–2041.

115. Levine B, Chaisson RE. *Mycobacterium kansasii*: a cause of treatable pulmonary disease associated with advanced human immunodeficiency virus (HIV) infection. *Ann Intern Med* 1991;114:861–868.

116. Carpenter JL, Parks JM. *Mycobacterium kansasii* infections in patients positive for human immunodeficiency virus. *Rev Infect Dis* 1991;13:789–796.

117. Burman WJ, Stone BL, Brown BA, Wallace RJ Jr, Bottger EC. AIDS-related *Mycobacterium kansasii* infection with initial resistance to clarithromycin. *Diagn Microbiol Infect Dis* 1998;31:369–371.

118. Wallace RJ, Swenson JM, Silcox VA, et al. Spectrum of disease due to rapidly growing mycobacteria. *Rev Infect Dis* 1983;5:657–679.

119. Brown BA, Wallace RJ, Onyi GO. Activities of four macrolides, including clarithromycin, against *Mycobacterium fortuitum*, *Mycobacterium chelonae*, and *M. chelonae*-like organisms. *Antimicrob Agents Chemother* 1992;36:180–184.

120. Wallace RJ. The clinical presentation, diagnosis, and therapy of cutaneous and pulmonary infections due to the rapidly growing mycobacteria, *M. fortuitum* and *M. chelonae*. *Clin Chest Med* 1989;10:419–429.

121. Wallace RJ, Swenson JM, Silcox VA, et al. Treatment of nonpulmonary infections due to *Mycobacterium fortuitum* and *Mycobacterium chelonei* on the basis of in vitro susceptibilities. *J Infect Dis* 1985;151:500–513.

122. Wallace RJ, Tanner D, Brennan PJ, et al. Clinical trial of clarithromycin for cutaneous (disseminated) infection due to *Mycobacterium chelonae*. *Ann Intern Med* 1993;119:482–486.

123. Tebas P, Sultan F, Wallace RJ, et al. Rapid development of resistance to clarithromycin following monotherapy for disseminated *Mycobacterium chelonae* infection in a heart transplant patient. *Clin Infect Dis* 1995;20:443–444.

124. Muschatt DM, Witzig RS. Successful treatment of *Mycobacterium abscessus* infections with multidrug regimens containing clarithromycin. *Clin Infect Dis* 1995;20:1441–1442.

125. Wallace RJ, Silcox VA, Tsukamura M, et al. Clinical significance, biochemical features, and susceptibility patterns of sporadic isolates of the *Mycobacterium chelonae*-like organism. *J Clin Microbiol* 1993;31:3231–3239.

126. Wallace RJ Jr, Brown-Elliot BA, Ward SC, et al. Activities of linezolid against rapidly growing mycobacteria. *Antimicrob Agents Chemother* 2001;45:764–767.

127. Iredell J, Whitby M, Blacklock Z. *Mycobacterium marinum* infection: epidemiology and presentation in Queensland 1971–1990. *Med J Aust* 1992;157:596–598.

128. Donta ST, Smith PW, Levitz RE, et al. Therapy of *Mycobacterium marinum* infections. *Arch Intern Med* 1986;146:902–904.

129. Kullavanijaya P, Sirimachan S, Bhuddhavudhikrai P. *Mycobacterium marinum* cutaneous infections acquired from occupations and hobbies. *Int J Dermatol* 1993;32:504–507.

130. Brown BA, Wallace RJ, Onyi GO. Activities of clarithromycin against eight slowly growing species of nontuberculous mycobacteria, determined by using a broth microdilution MIC system. *Antimicrob Agents Chemother* 1992;36:1987–1990.

131. Bonnet E, Debat-Zoguereh D, Petit N, et al. Clarithromycin: a potent agent against infections due to *Mycobacterium marinum*. *Clin Infect Dis* 1994;18:664–666.

132. Revil WDL, Pike MC, Morrow RH, Ateng J. A controlled trial of the treatment of *Mycobacterium ulcerans* infection with clofazimine. *Lancet* 1973;2:873–877.

133. Hayman J. *Mycobacterium ulcerans* infection. *Lancet* 1991;337:124.

134. Noordeen SK, Lopez Bravo L, Sundaresan TK. Estimated number of leprosy cases in the world. *Bull WHO* 1992;70:7–10.

135. Mastro TD, Redd SC, Breiman RF. Imported leprosy in the United States, 1978 through 1988: an epidemic without secondary transmission. *Am J Publ Health* 1992;82:1127–1130.

136. Dietrich M, Gaus W, Kern P, et al. An international randomized study with long-term follow-up of single versus combination chemotherapy of multibacillary leprosy. *Antimicrob Agents Chemother* 1994;38:2249–2257.

137. World Health Organization. *Chemotherapy of leprosy for control programmes*. WHO Technical Report Series no. 675, Geneva, 1982.

138. Gelber RH. Hansen's disease. *West J Med* 1993;158:583–590.

139. Miller RA. Hansen's disease-A time for cautious optimism. *West J Med* 1993;158:631–633.

140. Dever LL, Martin JW, Seaworth B, et al. Varied presentations and responses to treatment of infections caused by *Mycobacterium haemophilum* in patients with AIDS. *Clin Infect Dis* 1992;14:1195–1200.

141. Rogers PL, Walker RE, Lane HC, et al. Disseminated *Mycobacterium haemophilum* infection in two patients with the acquired immunodeficiency syndrome. *Am J Med* 1988;84:640–642.

142. Straus WL, Ostroff SM, Jernigan DB, et al. Clinical and epidemiologic characteristics of *Mycobacterium haemophilum*, an emerging pathogen in immunocompromised patients. *Ann Intern Med* 1994;120:118–125.

143. Kiehn TE, White M, Pursell KJ, et al. A cluster of four cases of *Mycobacterium haemophilum* infection. *Eur J Clin Microbiol Infect Dis* 1993;12:114–118.

144. Eng RH, Forrester C, Smith SM, et al. *Mycobacterium xenopi* infection in a patient with acquired immunodeficiency syndrome. *Chest* 1984;86:145–147.

145. Tecson-Tumang FT, Bright JL. *Mycobacterium xenopi* and the acquired immunodeficiency syndrome. *Ann Intern Med* 1984;100:461–462.

146. Costrini AM, Mahler DA, Gross WM, et al. Clinical and roentgenographic features of nosocomial pulmonary disease due to *Mycobacterium xenopi*. *Am Rev Respir Dis* 1981;123:104–109.

147. Banks J, Jenkins PA. Combined versus single antituberculosis drugs on the in vitro sensitivity patterns of non-tuberculous mycobacteria. *Thorax* 1987;42:838–842.

148. Banks J, Hunter AM, Campbell IA, et al. Pulmonary infection with *Mycobacterium xenopi*: review of treatment and response. *Thorax* 1984;39:376–382.

149. Parrot RG, Grosset JH. Post-surgical outcome of 57 patients with *Mycobacterium xenopi* pulmonary infection. *Tubercle* 1988;69:47–55.

150. Maloney JM, Gregg CR, Stephens DS, et al. Infections caused by *Mycobacterium szulgai* in humans. *Rev Infect Dis* 1987;9:1120–1126.

151. Henriques B, Hoffner SE, Petrini B, et al. Infection with *Mycobacterium malmoense* in Sweden: report of 221 cases. *Clin Infect Dis* 1994;18:595–600.

152. Chocarro A, Gonzalez Lopez A, Breznes MF, et al. Disseminated infection due to *Mycobacterium malmoense* in a patient infected with human immunodeficiency virus. *Clin Infect Dis* 1994;19:203–204.

153. Claydon EJ, Coker RJ, Harris JRW. *Mycobacterium malmoense* infection in HIV positive patients. *J Infect* 1991;23:191–194.

154. Zaugg M, Salfinger M, Opravil M, et al. Extrapulmonary and disseminated infections due to *Mycobacterium malmoense*: case report and review. *Clin Infect Dis* 1993;16:540–549.

155. Bottger EC, Teske A, Kirschner P, et al. Disseminated "*Mycobacterium genavense*" infection in patients with AIDS. *Lancet* 1992;340:76–80.

156. Pechère M, Opravil M, Wald A, et al. Clinical and epidemiologic features of infection with *Mycobacterium genavense*. *Arch Intern Med* 1995;155:400–404.

157. Bessesen MT, Shlay J, Stone-Venohr B, et al. Disseminated *Mycobacterium genavense* infection: clinical and microbiological features and response to therapy. *AIDS* 1993;7:1357–1361.

158. Bell RC, Higuchi JH, Donovan WN, et al. *Mycobacterium simiae*. Clinical features and follow-up of twenty four patients. *Am Rev Respir Dis* 1983;127:35–38.

159. Huminer D, Dux S, Samra Z, et al. *Mycobacterium simiae* infection in Israeli patients with AIDS. *Clin Infect Dis* 1993;17:508–509.

160. Torres RA, Nord J, Feldman R, LaBombardi V, Barr M. Disseminated mixed *Mycobacterium simiae-Mycobacterium avium* complex infection in acquired immunodeficiency syndrome. *J Infect Dis* 1991;164:432–433.

161. Levy-Frebault V, Pangon B, Bure A, et al. *Mycobacterium simiae* and *Mycobacterium avium-M. intracellulare* mixed infection in acquired immune deficiency syndrome. *J Clin Microbiol* 1987;25:154–157.

162. Wolinsky E. Nontuberculous mycobacteria and associated diseases. *Am Rev Respir Dis* 1979;119:107–159.

163. Sanders JW, Walsh A, Snider RL, et al. Disseminated *Mycobacterium scrofulaceum* infection: a potentially treatable complication of AIDS. *Clin Infect Dis* 1995;20:54–56.

164. Tortoli E, Piersimoni C, Bacosi D. Isolation of the newly described species *Mycobacterium celatum* from AIDS patients. *J Clin Microbiol* 1995;33:137–140.

165. Butler WR, O'Connor SP, Yakrus MA. *Mycobacterium celatum* sp. nov. *Int J Syst Bacteriol* 1993;43:539–548.

166. Wallace RJ, Nash DR, Tsukamura M, et al. Human disease due to *Mycobacterium smegmatis*. *J Infect Dis* 1988;158:52–59.

167. Newton JA, Weiss PJ, Bowler WA, et al. Soft-tissue infection due to *Mycobacterium smegmatis*: report of two cases. *Clin Infect Dis* 1993;16:531–533.

168. Plaus WJ, Hermann G. The surgical management of superficial infections caused by atypical mycobacteria. *Surgery* 1991;110:99–103.

169. Weinberger M, Berg SL, Feuerstein IM, et al. Disseminated infection with *Mycobacterium gordonae*: report of a case and critical review of the literature. *Clin Infect Dis* 1992;14:1229–1239.

170. Smith DS, Lindholm-Levy P, Huitt GA, Heifets LB, Cook JL. Mycobacterium terrae: case reports, literature review, and in vitro antibiotic susceptibility testing. *Clin Infect Dis* 2000;30:444–453.

171. Foulds G, Shepard RM, Johnson RB. The pharmocokinetics of azithromycin in human serum and tissues. *J Antimicrob Chemother* 1990;25:S73–S82.

172. Gladue RP, Bright GM, Isaacson RE, et al. In vitro and in vivo uptake of azithromycin by phagocytic cells: possible mechanism of delivery and release at sites of infection. *Antimicrob Agents Chemother* 1989;33:277–282.

173. Brown BA, Griffith DE, Girard W, Levin J, Wallace RJ Jr. Relationship of adverse events to serum drug levels in patients receiving high-dose azithromycin for myocbacterial lung disease. *Clin Infect Dis* 1997;24:958–964.

174. Wallace MR, Miller LK, Nguyen M, et al. Ototoxicity with azithromycin. *Lancet* 1994;343:241.

175. Barradell LB, Plosker GL, McTavish D. Clarithromycin: a review of its pharmacological properties and therapeutic use in *Mycobacterium avium-intracellulare* complex infection in patients with acquired immune deficiency syndrome. *Drugs* 1993;46:289–312.

176. Brown BA, Wallace RJ, Griffith DE, et al. Clarithromycin-induced hepatotoxicity. *Clin Infect Dis* 1995;20:1073–1074.

177. DATRI 001 Study Group. *Clarithromycin plus rifabutin for MAC prophylaxis: evidence for a drug interaction (abstract 291).* Abstracts of the first national conference on human retroviruses. Washington DC: American Society of Microbiology, 1993:106.

178. DATRI 001 Study Group. *Coadministration of clarithromycin alters the concentration-time profile of rifabutin (abstract A2).* Abstracts of the 34th ICAAC. Washington DC: American Society of Microbiology, 1994:3.

179. Wallace RJ, Brown BA, Griffith DE, et al. Reduced serum levels of clarithromycin in patients on multidrug regimens including rifampin or rifabutin for treatment of *Mycobacterium avium-intracellulare* (abstract M59). Abstracts of the 34th ICAAC. Washington DC: American Society of Microbiology, 1994:246.

180. Shafran SD, Deschenes J, Miller M, et al. Uveitis and pseudojaundice during a regimen of clarithromycin, rifabutin, and ethambutol. *N Engl J Med* 1994;330:438–439.

181. Cohn DL, Fisher EJ, Peng GT, et al. A prospective randomized trial of four three-drug regimens in the treatment of disseminated *Mycobacterium avium* complex disease in AIDS patients: excess mortality associated with high-dose clarithromycin. *Clin infect Dis* 1999;29:125–133.

CHAPTER 35
Antiparasitic Drugs

Martin S. Wolfe

Antiparasitic drugs are used in the treatment of protozoa, helminths, and parasitic arthropods. The drugs described in this chapter are for the most part those approved and available in the United States. Some of these available drugs are considered investigational for certain purposes in the United States.[1] Particular unavailable drugs may be obtained from the Centers for Disease Control and Prevention.[2]

The safety during pregnancy of many of the drugs listed has not been determined with certainty, and they are often contraindicated unless the benefit is thought to outweigh their potential hazard to the fetus.

For each drug, listed generically in alphabetic order, the following information is generally provided: brand name; major indications; mechanism of action when known; side effects, contraindications, and significant drug interactions; and doses for adults and children. Table 35.1 summarizes the drug's availability (brand name, manufacturer, formulation) and doses for adults and children for various parasites.

ALBENDAZOLE (ALBENZA)

Albendazole is a benzimidazole broad-spectrum anthelmintic. Studies have shown a single 400-mg adult dose to be effective and well tolerated for treatment of ascariasis, hookworm infections, enterobiasis, and most cases of trichuriasis (1). The same dose repeated for three consecutive days was effective against strongyloidiasis, cestodiasis, heavy trichuriasis (1), and cutaneous larva migrans (2). In these doses, albendazole appeared to be nearly devoid of significant side effects. Safety has not been established in pregnancy or in children younger than 2 years. Albendazole has been used in hydatid disease. Indications include inoperable lesions, disseminated disease, and prophylaxis before surgery. A large proportion of cysts were affected beneficially by a treatment regimen of 800 mg per day for three 28-day cycles with 14 days' rest between cycles (3). The frequency of clinical side effects was low. Albendazole has also been used against cerebral cysticercosis. In a comparative evaluation versus praziquantel for this condition, both appeared to be effective at the doses used (15 mg/kg per day for 30 days with albendazole); albendazole showed a slightly better overall response (4). Albendazole has also been found to be an effective therapy for gnathostomiasis in Thailand (5). Preliminary data suggest that albendazole has good clinical and antiparasitic efficacy in treating the intestinal microsporidian *Septata intestinalis* in patients with the acquired immunodeficiency syndrome (AIDS), but is less effective in treating another intestinal microsporidian, *Enterocytozoon bieneusi* (6). Albendazole is approved by the U.S. Food and Drug Administration (FDA) for treatment of *Echinococcus granulosis* infection and parenchymal neurocysticercosis caused by *Taenia solium*. Albendazole in a 5- to 7-day course has been effective against *Giardia lamblia*, and can be considered as an alternative treatment (7). In

---

[1] These investigational drugs and some others described that are not available in the United States and are also considered investigational are marked with a single asterisk in the text.

[2] Unavailable drugs that may be obtained from the CDC Drug Service, Centers for Disease Control and Prevention, Atlanta, GA 30333 (telephone 404-639-3670) are marked with a dagger in the text.

TABLE 35.1.   Drug Treatment of Parasitic Infections

Parasite and disease	Drug	Adult dosage	Pediatric dosage	Proprietary name, form (manufacturer)
Intestinal protozoa				
Entamoeba histolytica				
Amebic dysentery	**Drug of choice**			
	Metronidazole	750 mg tid × 10 d	50 mg/kg/d in 3 doses × 10 d	Flagyl tablets, IV (Searle)
	followed by			
	Paromomycin	500 mg tid × 7 d	30 mg/kg/d in 3 doses × 7d	Humatin tablets (Parke-Davis)
	or			
	Iodoquinol	650 mg tid × 20 d	40 mg/kg/d in 3 doses × 20 d	Yodoxin tablets (Glenwood)
	or			
	Diloxanide furoate	500 mg tid × 10 d	20 mg/kg/d in 3 doses × 10 d	Furamide tablets (Boots, England)
	Alternatives			
	Tinidazole[a] followed by paromomycin, iodoquinol, or diloxanide furoate as for amebic dysentery	600 mg bid × 5–10 d	50 mg/kg/d (max 2 g) in 1 dose for 5–10 d	Fasigyn[a] tablets (Pfizer)
Moderately severe Nondysenteric amebiasis	**Drug of choice**			
	Metronidazole	500 mg tid × 10 d	35 mg/kg/d in 3 doses × 10 d	
	Alternatives			
	Tinidazole[a] followed by paromomycin, iodoquinol, or diloxanide furoate as for amebic dysentery	600 mg bid × 5 d	50 mg/kg/d (max 2 g) in 1 dose × 5 d	
Mildly symptomatic Nondysenteric amebiasis	**Drug of choice**			
	Paromomycin	500 mg tid × 7 d	30 mg/kg/d in 3 doses × 7d	
	Alternative			
	Diloxanide furoate	500 mg tid × 10 d	20 mg/kg/d in 3 doses × 10 d	
Asymptomatic cyst-passing state	Paromomycin	500 mg tid × 7 d	30 mg/kg/d in 3 doses × 7 d	
	or			
	Iodoquinol	650 mg tid × 20 d	40 mg/kg/d in 3 doses × 20 d	
	or			
	Diloxanide furoate	500 mg tid × 10 d	20 mg/kg/d in 3 doses × 10 d	
Amebic liver abscess	**Drug of choice**			
	Metronidazole followed by paromomycin, iodoquinol, or diloxanide furoate as for amebic dysentery	750 mg tid × 10 d	50 mg/kg/d in 3 doses × 10 d	
	Alternative			
	Tinidazole (alone)[a] followed by paromomycin, iodoquinol, or diloxanide furoate as for amebic dysentery	800 mg tid × 5 d	50 mg/kg/d (max 2 g) in 1 dose × 3 d	
Giardia lamblia	Metronidazole[a]	250 mg tid × 7 d	5 mg/kg tid × 7 d	
	or			
	Quinacrine	100 mg tid × 5 d	2 mg/kg tid × 5 d	
	or			
	Furazolidone	100 mg (tablet) qid × 7–10 d	1.25 mg/kg (suspension) qid × 7–10 d	Furoxone tablets and suspension (Roberts)
	or			
	Tinidazole[a]	One 2-g dose	One 50 mg/kg dose	Fasigyn[a] tablets (Pfizer)
	or			
	Nitazoxanide	500 mg bid × 3 d	Age 12–47 mos: 100 mg (5 ml) bid × 3 d Age 4–11 y: 200 mg (10 ml) bid × 3 d	Alinia liquid (Romark)
Dientamoeba fragilis	Paromomycin[a]	500 mg tid × 7 d	30 mg/kg/d in 3 doses × 7 d	Humatin capsules (Parke-Davis)
	or			
	Iodoquinol	650 mg tid × 20 d	40 mg/kg/d in 3 doses × 20 d	Yodoxin tablets (Glenwood)
	or			
	Tetracycline[a]	500 mg qid × 10 d	Not recommended for children younger than 8 y	

(*continued*)

TABLE 35.1. (*continued*)

Parasite and disease	Drug	Adult dosage	Pediatric dosage	Proprietary name, form (manufacturer)
Intestinal protozoa (*continued*)				
Balantidium coli	Iodoquinol[a] or	As for *D. fragilis*	As for *D. fragilis*	
	Tetracycline[a]	As for *D. fragilis*	As for *D. fragilis*	
Isospora belli	Trimethoprim-sulfamethoxazole (TMP-SMX)	TMP 160 mg + SMX 800 mg qid × 10 d, then bid × 3 wk	TMP 5 mg/kg + SMX 25 mg/kg bid ×10 d	Bactrim tablets (Roche) Septra tablets (Burroughs Wellcome)
Cryptosporidium sp.	Nitazoxamide	500 mg bid × 3 d	100–200 mg bid × 3 d	Alinia (Romark)
Cyclospora	Trimethoprim-sulfamethoxazole (TMP-SMX)	As for *I. belli* for 7 d	As for *I. belli* for 7 d	
Other protozoan infections				
Naegleria sp. (primary amebic meningoence-phalitis)	Amphotericin B[a]	1 mg/kg/d IV, for indefinite period	As for adults	Fungizone[a] injection (Apothecon)
Leishmania braziliensis, L. mexicana (American cutaneous and mucocutaneous leishmaniasis)	**Drug of choice** Stibogluconate sodium[b]	20 mg/kg/d IV or IM × 28 d (may be repeated or continued until there is a response)	As for adults	Pentostam[b] injection (Glaxo-Wellcome, England)
	Alternative Amphotericin B[a]	0.25–1 mg/kg by slow infusion daily or every 2 d for up to 8 wk	As for adults	
Leishmania donovani (kala-azar, visceral leishmaniasis)	**Drug of choice** Stibogluconate sodium[b]	20 mg/kg/d IM or IV × 28 d (may be repeated)	As for adults	
	Alternative Pentamidine isethionate	2–4 mg/kg/d IV or IM for up to 15 doses (may be repeated)	As for adults	Pentam 300 injection (Fujisawa)
Leishmania tropica, L. major (oriental sore, cutaneous leishmaniasis)	**Drug of choice** Stibogluconate sodium[b]	20 mg/kg/d IM or IV × 20 d (may be repeated)	As for adults	
Pneumocystis carinii	**Drug of choice** Trimethoprim-sulfamethoxazole (TMP-SMX)	TMP 15 mg/kg/d + SMX 75 mg/kg/d PO or IV in 4 doses × 14–21 d	As for adults	Bactrim tablets (Roche) Septra tablets (Burroughs Wellcome)
	Alternative Pentamidine isethionate	3–4 mg/kg/d IM × 14–21 d	As for adults	
Toxoplasma gondii (toxoplasmosis)	**Drug of choice** Pyrimethamine plus	25–100 mg/d × 3–4 wk	2 mg/kg/d × 3 d, then 1 mg/kg/d (max 25 mg/d) × 4 wk	Daraprim tablets (Glaxo-Wellcome)
	Sulfadiazine	1–1.5 g/d × 3–4 wk	100–200 mg/kg/d × 3–4 wk	
	Alternative Spiramycin[a]	3–4 g/d × 3–4 wk	50–100 mg/kg/d × 3–4 wk	Rovamycine[a] tablets (Aventis)
Trichomonas vaginalis (trichomoniasis)	**Drug of choice** Metronidazole	2 g once or 250 mg tid PO × 7 d	15 mg/kg/d PO in 3 doses × 7 d	Flagyl tablets (Searle)
Trypanosoma cruzi (South American trypanosomiasis, Chagas' disease)	**Drug of choice** Nifurtimox[b]	8–10 mg/kg/d PO in 4 doses × 30–90 d	Age 1–10 y: 15–20 mg/kg/d in 4 doses qod × 30–90 d Age 11–16 y: 12.5–15 mg/kg/d in 4 doses qod × 30–90 d	Lampit[b] tablets (Bayer, Germany)
	Alternative Benznidazole[a]	5–7 mg/kg × 30–120 d	up to 12 yrs: 10 mg/kg/d in 2 doses × 30–120 d	Rochagan[a] tablets (Roche, Brazil)
Trypanosoma brucei gambiense, T. brucei rhodesiense (African trypanosomiasis, sleeping sickness) Hemolymphatic stage	**Drug of choice** Suramin[b]	100–200 mg (test dose) IV, then 1 g IV on days 1, 3, 7, 14, and 21	20 mg/kg on days 1, 3, 7, 14, and 21, after a test dose	Germanin[b] injection (Bayer, Germany)

(continued)

TABLE 35.1. (*continued*)

Parasite and disease	Drug	Adult dosage	Pediatric dosage	Proprietary name, form (manufacturer)
Other protozoan infections (*continued*)	**Alternative** Pentamidine isethionate	4 mg/kg/d IM × 10 d	4 mg/kg/d IM × 10 d	Pentam 300 injection (Fujisawa)
Late disease with central nervous system involvement	**Drug of choice** Melarsoprol[b]	2–3.6 mg/kg/d IV × 3 d; after 1 wk, 3.6 mg/kg/d IV × 3 d; repeat again after 10–21 d	18–25 mg/kg total over 1 mo: initial dose, 0.36 mg/kg IV, increasing gradually to max 3.6 mg/kg at intervals of 1–5 d for total of 9–10 doses	Arsobalt injection (Aventis)
T. b. gambiense (both stages) (variable effectiveness with *T. b. rhodesiense*)	Eflornithine	100 mg/kg q 6 h IV for 14 d	—	Ornidyl (Ilex-Oncology, Inc.)
Malaria treatment regimens *Plasmodium falciparum* acquired where chloroquine resistance does not occur and *P. malariae, P. ovale,* and *P. vivax* (non-chloroquine-resistant)	Chloroquine phosphate or	600 mg base PO stat then 300 mg after 6 h, then 300 mg/d for 2 d (total 1500 mg base)	10 mg/kg base PO stat, 5 mg/kg after 6 h, then 5 mg/kg for 2 d	Aralen tablets (Sanofi)
	Chloroquine hydrochloride	If patient is vomiting, give 200 mg IM every 6 h until oral ingestion is possible (max 800 mg/d)	IM chloroquine not recommended	Aralen hydrochloride injection (Sanofi)
P. falciparum acquired in areas with chloroquine-resistant strains	Quinine sulfate (salt) plus	650 mg PO tid × 3 d	25 mg/kg/d in 3 doses × 3 d	Quinine sulfate capsules (various manufacturers)
	Pyrimethamine-sulfadoxine **Alternatives** For chloroquine resistance or where resistance occurs to pyrimethamine-sulfadoxine:	One 3-tablet dose on last day of quinine	<1 yr: ¼ tab 1–3 yr: ½ tab 4–8 yr: 1 tab 9–14 yr: 2 tabs	Fansidar tablets (Roche)
	Quinine sulfate (salt) plus	650 mg PO tid × 3 d	25 mg/kg/d in 3 doses × 3 d	
	Tetracycline or	250 mg qid × 7 d	Above age 8 y: 5 mg/kg qid × 7 d	Tetracycline tablets (various manufacturers)
	Mefloquine alone or	One 1,250-mg dose PO	Children weighing <45 kg: one 25-mg/kg dose; ≥45 kg: as for adults	Lariam tablets (Roche)
	Atovaquone	1,000 mg/d × 3 d	As Malarone Ped Tab 11–20 kg: 1 tab/d × 3 d	Malarone tablets (Glaxo-Smith Kline)
	Plus Proguanil	400 mg/d × 3 d	21–30 kg: 2 tabs/d × 3 d 31–40 kg: 3 tabs/d × 3 d	
P. falciparum (severe or complicated infection)	Quinine dihydrochloride (salt IV) or	20 mg/kg loading dose over 4 h, followed by 10 mg/kg over 2 to 4 h; repeat every 8 h until oral treatment can be started (max 1,800 mg/d)	Same as for adults	Quinine dihydrochloride (Not available in U.S.A)
	Quinidine gluconate (IV) followed by either quinidine or quinine orally (for total of 3 d) plus	See quinidine in text	See quinidine in text	Quinidine gluconate injection (Lilly)
	Tetracycline	250 mg qid × 7 d	Above age 8 y: 5 mg/kg qid × 7 d	
Plasmodium vivax and *P. ovale*	Chloroquine phosphate followed by	As for nonresistant *P. falciparum* and *P. malariae*	As for nonresistant *P. falciparum* and *P. malariae*	
	Primaquine phosphate	15 mg base/d × 14 d	0.3 mg base/kg/d × 14 d	Primaquine tablets (Sanofi)

(*continued*)

TABLE 35.1. (*continued*)

Parasite and disease	Drug	Adult dosage	Pediatric dosage	Proprietary name, form (manufacturer)
Malaria Prophylaxis				
In areas with chloroquine-sensitive strains	Chloroquine phosphate	300 mg base/wk (500 mg salt) continue for 4 wk after leaving malarial area	5 mg base/kg/wk	Aralen tablets (Sanofi)
In areas with chloroquine-resistant strains	Mefloquine	250 mg once weekly and for 4 wk after leaving malarial area	Children weighing <15 kg: ¼ tablet/wk 15–19 kg: ¼ tablet/wk 20–30 kg: ½ tablet/wk 31–45 kg: ¾ tablet/wk >45 kg: 1 tablet/wk	
	or			
	Doxycycline	100 mg/d during exposure and 4 wk thereafter	Contraindicated for children younger than 8 yr After age 8 y: 2 mg/kg/d (max 100 mg/d)	Vibramycin tablets (Pfizer)
	Atovaquone/Proguanil	250/100 mg (1 tablet daily)	Children weighing 11–20 kg: 62.5/25 mg daily 21–30 kg: 125/50 mg daily 31–40 kg: 187.5/75 mg daily	
Against later relapses	Primaquine phosphate	15 mg base/d × 14 d	0.3 mg base/kg/d × 14 d	Primaquine tablets (Sanofi)
Intestinal helminths **Nematoda**				
Ascaris lumbricoides	**Drug of choice** Mebendazole	100 mg bid × 3 d	For children aged >2 yrs, as for adults	Vermox tablets (Mc Neil)
	or Albendazole[a]	400 mg once	400 mg once	Albenza (Glaxo-Smith Kline)
Trichuris trichiura	Mebendazole	100 mg bid × 3 d	As for *A. lumbricoides*	
	or Albendazole[a]	400 mg once	400 mg once	
Necator americanus, Ancylostoma duodenale (hookworm)	**Drug of choice** Mebendazole	100 mg bid × 3 d	As for *A. lumbricoides*	
	or Albendazole[a]	400 mg once	400 mg once	
Enterobius vermicularis	**Drug of choice** Mebendazole	One 100-mg dose; repeat in 2 wk	As for adults	
	or **Alternative** Albendazole[a]	400 mg once; repeat in 2 wk	As for adults	
Strongyloides stercoralis	**Drug of choice** Ivermectin[a]	200 μg/kg daily for 2d	As for adults	Stromectol (Merck)
	Alternative Thiabendazole	25 mg/kg bid × 2 d (max 3 g/d)	As for adults	Mintezol suspension (Merck)
Trichostrongylus sp.	Albendazole[a]	400 mg once	400 mg once	
	or Pyrantel pamoate[a]	11 mg/kg once	11 mg/kg once	Antiminth (Pfizer)
	or Mebendazole[a]	100 mg bid × 3 d	100 mg bid × 3 d	
Cestoda				
Taenia saginata, Taenia solium, Diphyllobothrium latum, Dipylidium caninum	**Drug of choice** Praziquantel[a]	5–10 mg/kg once	As for adults	Biltricide[a] tablets (Miles)
Hymenolepis nana and *H. diminuta*	**Drug of choice** Praziquantel[a]	One 25 mg/kg dose	As for adults	
Cerebral cysticercosis cellulosae	Praziquantel[a]	50–100 mg/kg/d in 3 doses × 30 d	As for adults	
	or Albendazole	400 mg bid for 30 d	15 mg/kg/d in 2 doses × 8–30 d	Albenza (Glaxo-Smith Kline)
Echinococcus granulosus	Albendazole or Praziquantel	As per text and prescribing information	As per prescribing information	

(*continued*)

TABLE 35.1. (*continued*)

Parasite and disease	Drug	Adult dosage	Pediatric dosage	Proprietary name, form (manufacturer)
Trematoda				
Schistosoma mansoni	**Drug of choice**			
	Praziquantel	40 mg/kg/d in 2 doses for 1 d	As for adults	Biltricide tablets (Miles)
	Alternative			
	Oxamniquine	Caribbean and S. American strains: one 15 mg/kg dose African strains: 40–60 mg/kg/d over 2–3 d	As for adults	Vansil tablets (Pfizer)
Schistosoma japonicum	Praziquantel	60 mg/kg/d in 3 doses × 1 d	As for adults	
Schistosoma mekongi	Praziquantel	As for *S. japonicum*	As for *S. japonicum*	
Schistosoma intercalatum	Praziquantel	As for *S. mansoni*	As for *S. mansoni*	
Schistosoma haematobium	Praziquantel	40 mg/kg/d in 2 doses for 1 d	As for adults	
Fasciolopsis buski	Praziquantel[a]	25 mg/kg tid × 1 d	As for adults	Biltricide[a] tablets (Miles)
Heterophyes heterophyes	Praziquantel[a]	25 mg/kg tid × 1 d	As for adults	
Metagonimus yokogawai	Praziquantel[a]	25 mg/kg tid × 1 d	As for adults	
Liver and lung flukes				
Paragonimus westermani	Praziquantel[a]	25 mg/kg tid × 2 d	As for adults	
Opisthorchis viverrini, Clonorchis sinensis	Praziquantel[a]	25 mg/kg tid × 1 d	As for adults	
Fasciola hepatica	Bithionol[b]	30–50 mg/kg on alternate days × 10–15 doses (max 2 g/d)	As for adults	Bitin[b] capsule (Tanabe, Japan)
Other helminths				
Filarioidea				
Wuchereria bancrofti	Diethylcarbamazine[b]	Day 1, 50 mg PO	Day 1, 25–50 mg	Hetrazan[b] tablets
Brugia malayi		Day 2, 50 mg tid	Day 2, 25–50 mg tid	
Loa loa		Day 3, 100 mg tid	Day 3, 50–100 mg tid	
Mansonella perstans		Days 4–28, 2 mg/kg tid	Days 4–28, 2 mg/kg tid	
Tropical pulmonary eosinophilia	Diethylcarbamazine[b]	2 mg/kg tid × 14 d	As for adults	
Onchocerca volvulus	Ivermectin	150 μg/kg PO once; repeat at approximately 1-y intervals until asymptomatic	As for adults	Stromectol tablets (Merck)
Miscellaneous helminths				
Cutaneous larva migrans	Albendazole[a]	400 mg daily × 3 d	400 mg daily × 3 d	
	or			
	Ivermectin[a]	200 μg/kg daily × 2 d	200 μg/kg daily × 2 d	
	or			
	Thiabendazole	25 mg/kg bid PO or topically (max 3 g/d) × 2–5 d		Mintezol suspension (Merck)
Visceral larva migrans	Albendazole[a]	400 mg bid × 5 d	As for adults	
	or			
	Mebendazole[a]	100–200 mg bid × 5 d	As for adults	
Parasitic arthropoda				
Pediculus humanus, P. humanus capitis, Phthirus pubis, Sarcoptes scabiei (scabies)	Permethrin			
	Lice	1% rinse, single application	As for adults	Nix Creme Rinse (Glaxo-Wellcome)
	Scabies	5% cream, single application	As for adults	Elimite Cream (Allergan)

[a]Considered an investigational drug for this purpose in the United States.
[b]In the United States, this drug is available from the CDC Drug Service, Centers for Disease Control and Prevention, Atlanta, GA 30333, telephone 404-639-3670.
IM, intramuscular; IV, intravenous; PO, oral; bid, twice daily; qid, four times a day; qod, every other day; tid, three times a day; max, maximum.

a cohort of 20 metronidazole-resistant *Giardia* cases, a combined albendazole-metronidazole course was effective in all cases (7).

AMPHOTERICIN B (FUNGIZONE)*

Amphotericin B is an antifungal antibiotic used for amebic meningoencephalitis caused by *Naegleria* species (8) and as an alternative treatment for American mucocutaneous leishmaniasis (9) (see also Chapter 280). It is poorly absorbed from the gastrointestinal tract and for these infections is given intravenously (IV).

A large number and variety of side effects have been described. Amphotericin B is considered an investigational drug for both these indications.

ARTEMISININ*

Artemisinin is the active principle of the Chinese herb qinghaosu, used in traditional Chinese medicine for treatment of febrile illnesses. Derivatives of artemisinins used for treatment of multidrug resistant *Plasmodium falciparum* malaria include artesunate, artemether, and arteether. Administration varies for these derivatives, and they can be given orally, intravenously, intramuscularly, and as a suppository. These derivatives are inexpensive, are rapidly and highly effective, and well tolerated (10,11). Artemisinin derivatives are often given with mefloquine, a particularly useful combination for severe malaria (11). A combination of artemether and lumefantrine (co-artemether) was found to be better tolerated than, and as effective as artesunate-mefloquine (12). Although available in many malarious areas of Asia and Africa, artemisinin derivatives are not yet approved or available in the United States.

ATOVAQUONE (MEPRON)

Atovaquone is a hydroxynaphthoquinolone used alone for treatment and prophylaxis of *Pneumocystis* pneumonia (13). Combined with pyrimethamine, it is an alternative in sulfa-intolerant patients infected with human immunodeficiency virus (HIV) and central nervous system (CNS) toxoplasmosis (13). Given with azithromycin, atovaquone is an alternative treatment for babesiosis (14). A combination of atovaquone 250 mg plus proguanil 100 mg (Malarone™) has been approved in the United States for oral treatment and prophylaxis of chloroquine-resistant *P. falciparum* malaria. Both components have causal prophylactic activity against the liver stage of this parasite. It is thus necessary to only take Malarone beginning 1 day before, while in, and for 7 days after departing the malarious area, making it particularly useful for short-term exposure. Studies have shown Malarone to be highly efficacious and well-tolerated against *P. falciparum* (15). Insufficient data are presently available to confirm efficacy against the other three species of malaria. The adult treatment regimen is four tablets as a single dose daily for 3 days. Pediatric Malarone tablets are also available, containing 62.5-mg atovaquone and 25-mg proguanil. Pediatric doses for prophylaxis and treatment are given in Table 35.1. Malarone does not act against persisting liver forms of *P. vivax* and *P. ovale*, acting only as a suppressive agent against these species. A terminal course of primaquine is therefore required to prevent relapse with these species (16). In a study in Thailand, Malarone was well tolerated and more effective than mefloquine in the treatment of acute uncomplicated multidrug-resistant *P. falciparum* (17).

BENZNIDAZOLE (ROCHAGAN)*

Benznidazole is a nitroimidazole drug available in South America for the treatment of the acute phase of *Trypanosoma cruzi* infection (Chagas' disease). The efficacy of this drug in chronic Chagas' disease has not been established (18). It has been shown in only limited use to be effective in reducing the severity and duration of the acute phase. It remains controversial whether benznidazole is curative (19). Side effects include rash, gastrointestinal symptoms, headache, weight loss, and polyneuritis. The regimen used in adults and children is 5 to 7 mg/kg by mouth daily for 30 to 120 days.

BITHIONOL (BITIN)†

Bithionol is used in the treatment of *Fasciola hepatica* (20) and *Paragonimus westermani* infections (21). It is manufactured in Japan. The anthelmintic effect of oral bithionol is poorly understood. Side effects include photosensitivity, skin reactions, ur-

ticaria, and gastrointestinal disturbances. For treatment of fascioliasis and paragonimiasis, the dose for both adults and children is 30 to 50 mg/kg on alternate days for 10 to 15 doses. Maximal dosage is 2 g per day.

CHLOROQUINE PHOSPHATE (ARALEN)

Chloroquine is a 4-aminoquinoline used primarily for the suppression and treatment of susceptible strains of malaria. In the United States, chloroquine is marketed only as oral Aralen phosphate in 500-mg salt tablets (equal to 300 mg of base). In Europe and Africa, chloroquine sulfate is marketed as Nivaquine in tablet, liquid, and injectable forms. A chloroquine hydrochloride salt, Aralen hydrochloride, is a parenteral solution for intramuscular (IM) use (each milliliter contains 50 mg of the salt, equal to 40 mg of base), which can be substituted for the oral phosphate salt when severe nausea or vomiting is present, when oral absorption is in question, or when an infection is particularly severe. Chloroquine's action is on the asexual erythrocytic forms of malaria parasites, but it does not affect the liver stages of plasmodia and therefore will not prevent relapses of malaria caused by species that have a liver stage in their life cycle. Chloroquine is almost completely absorbed from the gastrointestinal tract, is deposited in the tissues in considerable amounts, and is excreted slowly. Frequent side effects with suppressive use include gastrointestinal upset, headache, dizziness, and blurred vision. Less common side effects include rash, pruritus, partial alopecia, myopathy, and CNS stimulation. Irreversible retinal damage, seen when chloroquine is used in large daily doses for prolonged periods for collagen diseases, is virtually unheard of in the usual doses recommended for malaria suppression and treatment (22,23). Chloroquine should not be given to patients with psoriasis or porphyria or in the presence of retinal changes of any cause. Chloroquine is considered safe in recommended doses for infants and pregnant women at risk for malaria (24). Strains of *P. falciparum* in most malarious areas have developed resistance to chloroquine, and an alternative drug should be used in areas of known chloroquine resistance for both suppression and treatment of malaria with these strains (16). In recent years, chloroquine-resistant *Plasmodium vivax* malaria has been documented in Indonesia, Papua New Guinea, South America and Myanmar (25). For malaria suppression in adults, 300 mg of base is taken weekly, beginning 1 week before entering a malarious area and continuing while in the malarious area and for 4 weeks after leaving. For infants and children, a weekly dose of 5 mg/kg base is given, not to exceed the adult dose regardless of weight. For oral treatment of chloroquine-sensitive *P. falciparum* infection as well as the other three species of malaria, adults receive 600 mg of base initially, followed by 300 mg 6 hours later, and 300 mg 24 and 48 hours thereafter. For children, 10 mg/kg base is given initially, followed by 5 mg/kg in 6 hours, and 5 mg/kg 24 and 48 hours thereafter. When Aralen hydrochloride is used to treat acute malaria, adults should receive an initial IM dose of 200 mg of base, repeated every 6 hours until oral chloroquine can be taken. The total parenteral dosage in the first 24 hours should not exceed 800 mg of base.

DIETHYLCARBAMAZINE CITRATE (HETRAZAN)†

Diethylcarbamazine is a piperazine derivative used to treat filariasis (26). Although licensed, it is not presently available commercially in the United States and must be obtained from the CDC Parasitic Disease Drug Service. Abroad it is available as

Banocide and Notezine. Diethylcarbamazine is readily absorbed from the gastrointestinal tract and kills microfilariae of most species of filariae found in humans. There is presumptive evidence that it kills adult worms of *Wuchereria bancrofti* and *Brugia malayi*. Repeated courses are often necessary to kill *Loa loa* and *Mansonella perstans* adult worms. It has relatively little action on adult *Onchocerca volvulus* worms. Diethylcarbamazine has no effect on *Mansonella ozzardi* (27). A 50- to 100-mg dose of diethylcarbamazine is used as a provocative test for onchocerciasis (the Mazzotti reaction) (28), and a 200-mg dose has been used to increase the number of circulating microfilariae of *W. bancrofti* for diagnosis (29). Common side effects include headache, dizziness, nausea, and fever. Rapid destruction of microfilariae in the initial days of treatment may cause allergic reactions, including exacerbation of rash and pruritus in onchocerciasis and lymphadenopathy and nodular swellings along the course of lymphatics in bancroftian and malayan filariasis (30). In patients with heavy *L. loa* infections, encephalopathy has occurred (31). To attempt to decrease these early allergic reactions, particularly in onchocerciasis with ocular involvement, the initial daily dose of diethylcarbamazine should be small and the dose should be increased gradually to the maximal daily recommended dose. An initial 50-mg dose is gradually increased until a maximum of 2 mg/kg three times daily is reached; this dose is given for 28 days. For bloodborne filariasis, 2 mg/kg three times a day for 28 days is given to both adults and children. For tropical pulmonary eosinophilia, the same dose is given for 21 days. Antihistamines or corticosteroids may be required to control allergic reactions to diethylcarbamazine, particularly in onchocerciasis and bancroftian filariasis (30). Diethylcarbamazine has been shown to be effective in preventing loiasis in long-term residents in endemic areas, in a dose of 300 mg weekly (32).

DILOXANIDE FUROATE (FURAMIDE)

Diloxanide furoate is used in the treatment of amebiasis. Its mode of action is unknown. It is poorly absorbed and is most effective in the asymptomatic cyst-passing state and in mild noninvasive amebiasis (33). The most frequently observed side effect is excessive flatulence; mild gastrointestinal side effects occasionally occur. For asymptomatic and mildly symptomatic intestinal amebiasis in adults, it is used alone in a dose of 500 mg three times a day for 10 days. Children receive 20 mg/kg per day in three divided doses for 10 days. The same dose can be used in follow-up luminal treatment of more severe amebiasis. In the United States, diloxanide furoate is not commercially available and can be obtained only from certain compounding pharmacists.

EFLORNITHINE (ORNIDYL)

Eflornithine is highly effective in both CNS and non-CNS infections with *Trypanosoma brucei gambiense*. Eflornithine is much less effective against *Trypanosoma brucei rhodesiense* (9). Side effects, including diarrhea, anemia, and hair loss, are common but tolerable and reversible. The usual treatment regimen is 100 mg/kg every 6 hours infused IV in 1 hour for 14 days (34). Eflornithine is not marketed and is currently difficult to obtain.

FURAZOLIDONE (FUROXONE)

Furazolidone is a nitrofuran derivative used in the treatment of giardiasis (35). It is marketed in tablets and as a liquid. The liquid form is particularly useful in treating infants and young children. Furazolidone can produce a disulfiram-type reaction when it is taken with alcohol, and it is also a monoamine oxidase inhibitor. Occasional hypersensitivity reactions may occur, including hypotension, urticaria, fever, and arthralgia, as may nausea, vomiting, and headache. Furazolidone may cause mild hemolysis in glucose-6-phosphate dehydrogenase–deficient persons. Metabolic degradation products may produce brown urine. The dosage for adults is 100 mg four times daily for 7 to 10 days. Children should receive 6 mg/kg per day in four divided doses for 7 to 10 days, but the drug should not be given to infants younger than 1 month. Furazolidone is less effective than other anti-*Giardia* drugs.

HALOFANTRINE (HALFAN)

Halofantrine is used in the treatment of chloroquine-resistant *P. falciparum* (CRPF) malaria. In some areas of mefloquine-resistant *P. falciparum*, there is also cross-resistance to halofantrine. Halofantrine is not recommended for malaria chemoprophylaxis. The drug is available in 500-mg tablets, and although it was approved in the United States, it is not being marketed. The adult treatment dosage is 500 mg every 6 hours for three doses in a 1-day course. Children's dosage is 8 mg/kg every 6 hours for three doses. The manufacturer recommends that a second full course be taken by nonimmune individuals 1 week after completion of the first course. Side effects have included abdominal pain, diarrhea, and nausea. The drug is contraindicated in pregnancy and during breast-feeding (36). Halofantrine has been found to cause dose-related lengthening of the PR and QTc intervals (37). It should not be taken 1 hour before to 3 hours after meals and should not be used for patients with known cardiac conduction defects. Cardiac monitoring is recommended.

IODOQUINOL (YODOXIN)

Iodoquinol is a halogenated oxyquinoline used in the treatment of amebiasis, *Dientamoeba fragilis* infection, and *Balantidium coli* infection (38). It was formerly produced as Diodoquin, but this brand has been removed from the U.S. market. Iodoquinol acts against amoebae primarily in the intestinal lumen and is ineffective against invasive amebiasis. Because so little of the drug is absorbed, it has relatively little toxicity. It rarely causes abdominal pain, diarrhea, or rash. It is contraindicated in persons with iodine intolerance. In doses recommended for intestinal protozoa, iodoquinol has not been shown to cause the optic atrophy occasionally seen with long-term administration to children in large doses for acrodermatitis enteropathica and nonspecific diarrhea. In the treatment of asymptomatic intestinal amebiasis by itself, or used as a follow-up luminal drug, the dosage for adults is 650 mg three times a day for 20 days. Children receive 40 mg/kg per day in three doses for 20 days. Similar doses have been used for *Dientamoeba fragilis* and *B. coli* infections.

IVERMECTIN (STROMECTOL)

Ivermectin is now the drug of choice for the treatment of onchocerciasis. It has also been used as a wide-spectrum antihelmintic in humans against intestinal helminths, including strongyloidiasis, and against blood-stage filariasis (39). In onchocerciasis, ivermectin acts against microfilariae by paralyzing them and allowing them to be removed by the reticuloendothelial system. Intrauterine microfilariae are damaged and degenerate and are reduced in number. The drug has no effect against adult worms, and treatment must be repeated with buildup of microfilariae at approximately yearly intervals for the duration of the adult worms' lives (approximately 10 to 15 years). Side effects with the required single oral dose have generally been mild and include fever, pruritus, and rash. The dose for onchocerciasis for both adults and children is 150 μg/kg, once orally, with repeated doses at approximately yearly intervals. A randomized trial comparing ivermectin and thiabendazole for treatment of chronic infection with *Strongyloides stercoralis* showed that ivermectin in a course of 200 μg/kg daily for 2 days had equal efficacy and was better tolerated (40). Ivermectin is also highly effective against cutaneous larva migrans. In one noncomparative study, a single dose of ivermectin, 200 μg/kg, cured 57 of 58 subjects (41).

MEBENDAZOLE (VERMOX)

Mebendazole is a synthetic benzimidazole; broad-spectrum anthelmintic used in the treatment of trichuriasis (42), ascariasis (42), enterobiasis (43), and hookworm disease (43). Mebendazole is also used in treating hydatid cysts when surgery is contraindicated or cysts rupture spontaneously during surgery (44). It acts by blocking glucose uptake by the susceptible helminths and is poorly absorbed from the gastrointestinal tract. Mebendazole is well tolerated and only rarely causes abdominal pain, nausea, and diarrhea. It is contraindicated in pregnant women and in children younger than 2 years of age. For trichuriasis, ascariasis, and hookworm infections, both adults and children receive 100 mg twice daily for 3 days. For enterobiasis, a single 100-mg tablet is taken and the dose repeated 2 weeks later. Mebendazole has also been experimentally used, along with steroids, in the treatment of severe trichinosis (45).

MEFLOQUINE (LARIAM)

Mefloquine is used in the chemoprophylaxis and treatment of CRPF and *P. vivax* malaria (46,47). Mefloquine acts by destroying the asexual blood forms of the parasites. Side effects include vomiting and dizziness. Cases of CNS toxic effects have been seen after treatment doses and much less frequently with prophylactic use (47–49). Mefloquine should not be used for self-treatment because of these potential side effects. Because mefloquine has occasionally been associated with cardiac problems, it should not be used by persons with cardiac conduction abnormalities. Ordinarily, mefloquine should not be given concurrently with quinine or quinidine; if these drugs are to be used in the initial treatment of severe malaria, mefloquine administration should be deferred until at least 12 hours after the last dose. Mefloquine is not recommended in persons with a history of epilepsy or psychiatric disorder. A review of mefloquine use in pregnancy suggests that it is not associated with adverse effects and it can be considered for use in women who are pregnant or likely to become so when exposure to multidrug-resistant *P. falciparum* is unavoidable (46,50). For curative treatment of malaria, the total dose of mefloquine for adults and children weighing more than 45 kg is 1,250 mg administered as a single dose. Alternatively, for possible better tolerance, it can be given as 750 mg followed 6 to 8 hours later by 500 mg. A lower total dose of 750 to 1,000 mg is sufficient for patients with partial immunity living in malarious areas. Children who weigh less than 45 kg (regardless of immunity status) receive 25 mg/kg in a single dose. For chemoprophylaxis, adults and children who weigh more than 45 kg receive 250 mg once weekly while exposed to malaria and for 4 weeks afterward. Doses for children weighing less than 45 kg are given in Table 35.1. *P. falciparum* strains resistant to mefloquine are reported (46). Mefloquine has a long half-life in humans, with a range of 6 to 23 days, and a mean of 14 days.

MELARSOPROL (ARSOBAL)†

Melarsoprol is a trivalent arsenic compound. It is the drug of choice for late-stage *T. brucei rhodesiense* and *T. gambiense* infection with CNS involvement (51). It is manufactured in France in a clear sterile solution. After IV administration, a small but therapeutically significant amount of the drug penetrates the cerebrospinal fluid and has a lethal effect on trypanosomes infecting the CNS. During administration, care must be taken to prevent leakage into the tissues. Side effects are common during treatment: these can include encephalopathy, myocardial damage, albuminuria, hypertension, Jarisch-Herxheimer-type reaction, vomiting, and peripheral neuropathy (51). Because of its toxicity, melarsoprol should not be used for early, untreated hemolymphatic trypanosomiasis. For adults, 2 to 3.6 mg/kg per day IV is given for three doses; this course is repeated after 7 days and again after 10 to 21 days. Children should receive 18 to 25 mg/kg total dose during 1 month; an initial dose of 0.36 mg/kg IV is given, increasing gradually to a maximum of 3.6 mg/kg at intervals of 1 to 5 days for a total of nine to ten doses.

METRONIDAZOLE (FLAGYL)

Metronidazole is a nitroimidazole compound used in the treatment of vaginal trichomoniasis, amebiasis, and giardiasis (52). It is trichomonacidal and giardicidal; it is amebicidal at both intestinal and extraintestinal sites. It is absorbed well and is more effective for symptomatic or invasive amebiasis than for the asymptomatic cyst-passing state (53). Common side effects are nausea, headache, and a metallic taste. Dizziness, vomiting, abdominal cramps, diarrhea, and peripheral neuropathy are less common. *Candida* overgrowth may occur. Dark urine may develop from a metabolite of the drug. Metronidazole should not be used with alcohol because it can give a disulfiram-like reaction. Metronidazole has caused lung tumors in mice but not in hamsters and is mutagenic to some bacteria. The risk to humans of carcinogenicity and mutagenicity is considered to be low, if not negligible (54). Metronidazole is the drug of choice for *Trichomonas vaginalis* in a standard dose of 250 mg three times a day for 7 days. An alternative is a single 2-g dose, which has been found to have comparable efficacy and side effects (55). For symptomatic nondysenteric intestinal amebiasis, adults should receive 500 mg three times a day and children 50 mg/kg per day in three divided doses for 10 days. For acute amebic dysentery and amebic liver abscess, adults should receive 750 mg three times a day and children 50 mg/kg per day in three divided doses, both for 10 days. Metronidazole is available as an IV preparation for use in severe infections. When used for amebiasis, metronidazole should always be followed by a luminal active drug. Metronidazole has never been approved by the FDA for treatment of giardiasis, but it is regularly used for this infection. Dosage is 250 mg tid for adults and 5 mg/kg tid for children, both for 7 days.

NIFURTIMOX (LAMPIT)[†]

Nifurtimox is used in the treatment of *T. cruzi* infection (Chagas' disease). It has been useful in the treatment of the acute phase of infection, but there is no evidence that it alters the development of the established lesions of chronic Chagas disease (9). Side effects are common and can be severe, including nervousness (and rarely hallucinations and convulsions), weight loss, and peripheral neuritis. It is tolerated better by younger than older patients and is not recommended during pregnancy. The adult dose is 8 to 10 mg/kg per day orally in four divided doses for 30 to 90 days. Children's doses are given in Table 35.1.

NITAZOXANIDE (ALINIA)

Nitazoxanide is a newly FDA-approved drug in liquid form for the treatment of giardiasis (in children aged 1 to 11 years) and cryptosporidiasis; a tablet formulation for use in adults is under review (55a). Nitazoxanide is also effective against *Ascaris lumbricoides*, *Trichuris trichiura*, and *Hymenolepsis nana* (55b). The drug is a nitrothiazolyl-salicylamide derivative and its mechanism may be related to the inhibition of reactions essential to anaerobic energy cell metabolism. For treatment of cryptosporidiasis in HIV-negative patients, a 3-day course of 100 mg or 200 mg bid in children and 500 mg bid in adults led to marked symptomatic and parasitologic improvement. In HIV-positive children and adults, particularly those with low CD4 counts, similar doses were less successful. For treatment of giardiasis, a 3-day course of 100 or 200 mg bid gave cure rates of 85% of patients, comparable to an 80% cure rate with metronidazole. The dose for children 12 to 47 months old is 100 mg (5 ml) bid for 3 days, and for children 4 to 11 years old 200 mg (10 ml) bid. The doses should be taken with food. A trial in Egypt in HIV-negative adults cured 91% with a dose of 500 mg bid for 3 days. Nitazonamide is well tolerated, and in studies adverse effects were similar to those in patients given a placebo (55a).

OXAMNIQUINE (VANSIL)

Oxamniquine is an alternative to praziquantel in the treatment of *Schistosoma mansoni* infection (56). Rare side effects include dizziness, drowsiness, neuropsychiatric disturbances, and gastrointestinal symptoms. For South American and Caribbean strains of *S. mansoni*, a single 15 mg/kg oral dose is effective. Some experts recommend 40 to 60 mg/kg per day for 2 to 3 days in parts of Africa (57).

PAROMOMYCIN (HUMATIN)

Paromomycin is a broad-spectrum, poorly absorbed antibiotic used in the treatment of amebiasis (58) and *D. fragilis* infection. It should be given with caution to persons with ulcerative lesions of the bowel, to avoid renal toxic effects through inadvertent absorption. Because it is poorly absorbed, it is most effective for asymptomatic and mildly symptomatic intestinal amebiasis and should not be used by itself to treat invasive amebiasis. It can also be used as a follow-up luminal active drug for invasive amebiasis. The adult dose for amebiasis and *D. fragilis* infection is 500 mg bid for 7 days; children should receive 30 mg/kg per day in three divided doses, also for 7 days. IV paromomycin has been found to be effective against visceral and cutaneous leishmaniasis and in a topical formulation against cutaneous leishmaniasis

(59). Oral paromomycin treatment has resulted in improvement of both clinical and parasitologic parameters in cryptosporidiosis in patients with AIDS (60).

PENTAMIDINE ISETHIONATE (PENTAM 300)

Pentamidine isethionate is an aromatic diamidine used as an alternative treatment of early Gambian sleeping sickness without CNS involvement, leishmaniasis, and *Pneumocystis carinii* pneumonia (61). The mode of action of the diamidines is not completely understood, but they may act by interfering with nuclear metabolism. Side effects can include hypotension, ventricular arrhythmias, vomiting, blood dyscrasias, renal damage, and pain or sterile abscess at the injection site. Both hypoglycemia and hyperglycemia may occur. Pentamidine should be used with caution in patients with hypertension, diabetes, malnutrition, or hepatic or renal disease. Experience with Rhodesian sleeping sickness is more limited, and because of the associated early CNS involvement, pentamidine is not usually recommended (61). Pentamidine should be freshly prepared by dissolving the powder in sterile distilled water, not saline solution. The dose for African trypanosomiasis for both adults and children is 4 mg/kg per day IM for 10 days. Pentamidine is an alternative treatment for leishmaniasis (9); the dose is 2 to 4 mg/kg per day IV or IM for up to 15 days. Formerly, pentamidine, in a dose of 3 to 4 mg/kg per day IM for 14 to 21 days, was the only available treatment for *P. carinii* pneumonia for both adults and children. However, trimethoprim-sulfamethoxazole is at least as effective and less toxic and is presently considered the drug of choice for initial therapy (62). Pentamidine is recommended for persons who have a severe allergy to a sulfonamide or are unable to tolerate or fail to respond to trimethoprim-sulfamethoxazole. Aerosolized pentamidine has been found effective for primary and secondary prophylaxis of *P. carinii* pneumonia (62).

PERMETHRIN

Permethrin is a synthetic pyrethroid used to impregnate clothing and mosquito nets for protection against mosquitoes and ticks. A 1% permethrin product (Nix Creme Rinse) is used for treatment of head lice (63), and a 5% product (Elimite Cream) is used against scabies infestation (64), both in single-dose treatments. Itching and burning may occur as side effects. No systemic reactions have been reported.

PRAZIQUANTEL (BILTRICIDE)

Praziquantel is the drug of choice for most fluke infections, including schistosomiasis (65,66). It is also used for the treatment of intestinal tapeworms and cysticercosis (67). Side effects are mild and include dizziness and drowsiness. The only specific contraindication is ocular cysticercosis, because destruction of parasites in the eye may cause serious damage. For *Schistosoma mansoni*, *Schistosoma hematobium* and *Schistosoma intercalatum*, the dose for adults and children is 40 mg/kg per day in two doses for 1 day. For *Schistosoma japonicum* and *Schistosoma mekongi*, the dose for adults and children is 60 mg/kg per day in three doses for 1 day. For *Paragonimus westermani*, 25 mg/kg three times a day is given for 2 days. The same regimen for 1 day is given for *Clonorchis sinensis*, *Opisthorchis* species, *Fasciolopsis buski*, *Heterophyes heterophyes*, and *Metagonimus yokogawai*. *Fasciola hepatica* infections do not respond well to praziquantel (68). For the tapeworms, *D. latum*, *T. saginata*, *T. solium*, and *D. caninum*, 5 to 10 mg/kg in a single dose has been effective. For *H. nana*, 25 mg/kg in a single dose is effective. Praziquantel is useful in the treatment of neurocysticercosis (4,69,70). The regimen currently used is 50 to 100 mg/kg per day in three divided doses for 30 days. To decrease cerebral edema from dying parasites, corticosteroids should be administered concurrently, beginning 2 days before and continued during the 30-day course of praziquantel (70).

PRIMAQUINE PHOSPHATE

Primaquine phosphate is an 8-aminoquinoline used to prevent relapses and to provide radical cure of *P. vivax* and *P. ovale* malaria by acting on hypnozoites of these species in the liver. It also has a gametocidal effect against *P. falciparum* malaria parasites (71). It is marketed as primaquine phosphate in 26.3-mg salt (15-mg base) tablets. Minor side effects include nausea, abdominal discomfort, and headache. Acute hemolytic anemia occurs in persons with glucose-6-phosphate dehydrogenase deficiency (72). Primaquine should not be given to patients who are simultaneously receiving other potentially hemolytic drugs, or agents capable of depressing the myeloid elements of the bone marrow. Primaquine is contraindicated in pregnancy. For radical cure of acute *P. vivax* or *P. ovale* malaria to prevent relapses, adults receive 15 mg of base daily for 14 days, after completing initial schizonticidal therapy, usually with chloroquine. Children receive 0.3 mg/kg base daily for 14 days in broken-up tablets because there is no liquid preparation and the tablets do not go into solution. Primaquine is also recommended to prevent relapses after travelers with prolonged exposure leave malarious areas where *P. vivax* or *P. ovale* occurs. This is best taken after completing the usual 4-week terminal doses of the chemosuppressive drug. A daily dose of 30 mg of base for 14 days may be required for adults exposed to primaquine-resistant *P. vivax* malaria, particularly in parts of the Southwest Pacific and Southeast and South Asia (73). Primaquine alone has been found to be effective prophylaxis against falciparum malaria in a number of studies (74). Primaquine plus clindamycin is used as an alternative treatment for *Pneumocystis* pneumonia in patients who have failed to respond to or are intolerant of standard therapy (75).

PROGUANIL HYDROCHLORIDE (PALUDRINE)*

Proguanil hydrochloride is used for the chemoprophylaxis of malaria. In combination with atovaquone it is marketed as Malarone™ (see under atovaquone, p. 350). Proguanil acts by slowly arresting the development of maturing schizonts and is effective against the primary liver phase of *P. falciparum*. It also renders gametocytes incapable of developing in the mosquito. It is rapidly absorbed, is readily excreted, does not accumulate in the body when given in therapeutic doses, and must be taken daily. Proguanil by itself is not licensed for use in the United States, but it is widely available in Europe and Africa. It is tolerated well but can cause gastrointestinal side effects and occasionally mouth ulcers. It can be used as an alternative drug in persons intolerant of chloroquine in areas where *P. falciparum* is sensitive to chloroquine. In areas of CRPF malaria, proguanil can be given daily and chloroquine weekly. The adult proguanil dosage is 200 mg daily during exposure and for 4 weeks afterward. Children's doses are given in Table 35.1. Proguanil used with chloroquine has been found to be most useful in East Africa, but is less effective than in combination with atovaquone (as Malarone) or other prophylactic drugs used in CRPF areas (76).

PYRANTEL PAMOATE (ANTIMINTH ORAL SUSPENSION)

Pyrantel pamoate is a broad-spectrum anthelmintic used in the treatment of hookworm, ascariasis, and enterobiasis (77,78). It has also been used against *Trichostrongylus* species, with varying results in different parts of the world (78). The anthelmintic activity is probably due to its neuromuscular blocking property. Pyrantel pamoate is tolerated well and only rarely causes gastrointestinal disturbances, headaches, dizziness, and rash. For treatment of ascariasis, enterobiasis, and trichostrongyliasis, both adults and children receive 11 mg/kg (maximum 1 g) in a single dose. For enterobiasis, the dose is repeated after 2 weeks. For hookworms, the same single oral dose is given for 3 consecutive days.

PYRIMETHAMINE (DARAPRIM)

Pyrimethamine is an aminopyrimidine derivative, formerly used alone for the suppression of susceptible strains of malaria, and for treatment of toxoplasmosis (79). Pyrimethamine, 25 mg, combined with 500 mg sulfadoxine (a long-acting sulfonamide) is marketed as Fansidar and used for treatment of susceptible strains of CRPF (80). Pyrimethamine, 12.5 mg, is also combined with dapsone, 100 mg, as Maloprim, an antimalarial manufactured in England (80,81). Pyrimethamine is a folic acid antagonist, and its therapeutic action is based on the differential requirement between host and parasite for nucleic acid precursors involved in growth. This activity is highly selective against plasmodia and *Toxoplasma gondii*. In the recommended dosage of 25 mg weekly used for malaria suppression, side effects are uncommon. Excessive or prolonged doses required for toxoplasmosis may produce a macrocytic anemia because of interference with folic acid metabolism, and it is advisable to administer 10 mg of folinic acid per day in this situation (79). There is widespread resistance by malaria parasites to pyrimethamine. Although it is available in the United States, it is probably the least effective antimalarial and is seldom recommended by itself. Fansidar is no longer recommended for chemoprophylaxis of CRPF malaria because of the high risk of death from Stevens-Johnson syndrome. A single three-tablet adult dose of Fansidar can be used for self-treatment of a febrile illness thought to be CRPF malaria when medical care is not immediately available (80). Children's emergency treatment doses are given in Table 35.1. *P. falciparum* is also resistant to Fansidar in many malarious areas. Fansidar is contraindicated for persons allergic to sulfonamides, in pregnancy at term, and for infants younger than 2 months. Maloprim is not approved in the United States, and there is concern about the risk for toxic effects to bone marrow and resistance to CRPF malaria (82). For treatment of toxoplasmosis in adults, 25 to 100 mg per day of pyrimethamine along with 1 to 1.5 g of sulfadiazine qid is taken for 3 to 4 weeks. For children, 2 mg/kg per day (maximum, 25 mg per day) of pyrimethamine along with 100 to 200 mg/kg per day of sulfadiazine is also taken for 3 to 4 weeks. In immunocompromised persons, including those with AIDS, with CNS toxoplasmosis, therapy with high doses of pyrimethamine and sulfonamides or clindamycin is recommended for prolonged periods (83).

QUINACRINE (ATABRINE)

Quinacrine was originally used as an antimalarial, but has been supplanted by other drugs for this purpose. Quinacrine is effective against *Giardia lamblia*, with an efficacy of 90% or more (84). Since 1992, it has not been commercially available in the United States, but can be obtained in capsule form from certain compounding pharmacists. Quinacrine acts against *G. lamblia* by causing an inhibition of nucleic acid synthesis. Although somewhat more effective than metronidazole, quinacrine may cause toxic psychosis (84). The dosage for adults is 100 mg three times a day and for children 2 mg/kg three times a day, for 5 days.

QUINIDINE GLUCONATE

Quinidine gluconate, an isomer of quinine, is used for IV treatment of severe *P. falciparum* malaria where there is quinine resistance (in Thailand) or where IV quinine is not available (in the United States) (85). Adults and children receive an initial loading dose of 10 mg/kg salt (6.2 mg/kg base) administered in an hour, followed by a continuous infusion of 0.02 mg/kg salt (0.0125 mg/kg base) per minute (85,86). With both regimens, oral quinidine sulfate or quinine is substituted when patients can swallow and retain oral medications. Quinidine treatment should be continued for 72 hours total. During IV quinidine use, infusion speed must be carefully monitored, and the blood pressure and electrocardiogram should be monitored closely for evidence of toxic reactions.

QUININE

Quinine is an alkaloid extracted from the bark of the cinchona tree used for the treatment of CRPF malaria and of severe *P. falciparum* malaria (11). It is available as oral quinine sulfate in 650-mg and 325-mg tablets and as quinine dihydrochloride for IV use. The IV preparation is not available in the United States. Quinine's primary action is schizonticidal, and no lethal effect is exerted on sporozoites or preerythrocytic tissue forms. Usual therapeutic doses of quinine frequently cause some degree of cinchonism (tinnitus, headache, nausea, abdominal pain, blurred vision, and altered auditory acuity), but these symptoms are usually not severe enough to require cessation of treatment. Blood dyscrasias rarely occur, as may urticaria, asthma, drug fever, and hypoglycemia. IV administration of quinine dihydrochloride may lead to arrhythmias, hypotension, and acute circulatory failure. It must be given slowly in dilute solutions with constant monitoring of the pulse and blood pressure, and oral quinine sulfate should be substituted when possible. For oral treatment of CRPF malaria in adults, quinine sulfate, 650 mg three times a day, is given for 3 days, followed by either tetracycline, 250 mg four times a day, for 7 days or three tablets of pyrimethamine-sulfadoxine (Fansidar). For children, 25 mg/kg per day is given in three divided doses for 3 days, followed by pyrimethamine-sulfadoxine in reduced doses. For IV treatment of severe *P. falciparum* malaria in adults, quinine dihydrochloride is administered as a 20 mg/kg loading dose over 4 hours, followed by 10 mg/kg in 2 to 8 hours, repeated every 8 hours until oral quinine therapy can be started (11,86). For children, the same dose as for adults is used (maximum, 1800 mg/d for children and adults). Pyrimethamine-sulfadoxine or clindamycin should then be given to ensure total cure.

SPIRAMYCIN (ROVAMYCINE)*

Spiramycin is used as an alternative treatment for toxoplasmosis and has also proved safe in pregnant women with this condition

(87). Gastrointestinal symptoms and allergic reactions have occurred. For toxoplasmosis in adults, 3 to 4 g per day is given and in pregnancy is continued until delivery. The FDA has not approved spiramycin for routine use, and it is not commercially available in the United States.

STIBOGLUCONATE SODIUM; SODIUM ANTIMONY GLUCONATE (PENTOSTAM)†

Pentostam is a solution containing 30% to 34% pentavalent antimony. It is the drug of choice for visceral, cutaneous, and mucocutaneous leishmaniasis (59,88,89). A related antimony drug, meglumine antimonate (Glucantime*) is manufactured in France but is not available in the United States (88,89). The mechanism of action of these pentavalent antimony compounds is unknown. Drug reactions, as a rule, are not severe, due in part to rapid excretion of the drugs. Side effects can include gastrointestinal symptoms, muscle pain and joint stiffness, bradycardia and electrocardiographic changes, and rash. This drug should be used cautiously in those patients who have received antimony therapy within 2 months; it should be withheld from those who manifest toxic reactions to the drug; and is best not given to patients with heart, liver, or kidney disease. For visceral and mucocutaneous leishmaniasis, the dose for both adults and children is 20 mg/kg per day IM or IV for 28 days. For cutaneous leishmaniasis, the standard treatment is 20 mg/kg per day for 20 days for adults and children. This is usually given IV but can be given IM (89). Some types of visceral, cutaneous, and mucocutaneous leishmaniasis are more difficult to treat and may require higher doses, more prolonged treatment, or alternative drugs (59).

SURAMIN (GERMANIN)†

Suramin is a synthetic urea compound and the drug of choice for therapy of early bloodstage Rhodesian (*T. brucei rhodesiense*) and Gambian (*T. brucei gambiense*) trypanosomiasis (51). Suramin has also been used to kill adult worms in onchocerciasis (90). The exact mechanism of action is uncertain, although it is known to inhibit numerous enzyme systems. Suramin clears the blood of trypanosomes, and a full course cures nearly all early cases. It does not cross the blood-brain barrier and does not cure the infection if CNS invasion has occurred. Suramin can cause a variety of side effects, including vomiting, pruritus, urticaria, fever, paresthesias, and hyperesthesia of the palms and soles. A moderate degree of albuminuria is usual, but if casts appear, indicating more severe kidney damage, treatment should be discontinued. It should not be used when renal or hepatic disease is present. Idiosyncrasy may lead to circulatory collapse, and deaths have occurred from immediate hypersensitivity. The drug powder must be mixed into a 10% solution with 5 mL of distilled water immediately before use, and this should not be stored for more than 0.5 hour. A 100- to 200-mg IV dose to test for sensitivity should be given initially. In trypanosomiasis, 1 g is then given slowly IV on days 1, 3, 7, 14, and 21. Children receive 20 mg/kg on the same schedule. A second course of treatment should not be given earlier than 3 months after the first course. Ivermectin has replaced suramin for most onchocerciasis infections.

TETRACYCLINE HYDROCHLORIDE

Tetracycline is an antibiotic used in the treatment of certain intestinal protozoa, including *D. fragilis* and *B. coli* (38). Tetracycline is also used after quinine or quinidine, in treatment of CRPF malaria (11). A long-acting form of tetracycline, doxycycline, can be used for chemoprophylaxis against multidrug-resistant *P. falciparum* malaria (91). Tetracyclines have a relatively slow-acting schizonticidal effect against *P. falciparum* and cannot be relied on alone to treat acute attacks in nonimmune persons. (See Chapter XX for a discussion of the side effects of tetracycline hydrochloride.) Tetracycline is contraindicated in pregnant women and children younger than 8 years of age. Clindamycin can be substituted for treatment of young children and pregnant women. A dose of 500 mg tetracycline four times a day for 10 days has been used for *D. fragilis* and *B. coli* infections in adults. For treatment of CRPF malaria, tetracycline, 250 mg four times a day, or doxycycline 100 mg twice a day for 7 days is given after quinine or quinidine. For chemoprophylaxis of multidrug-resistant *P. falciparum* malaria, 100 mg of doxycycline daily is taken during exposure and for 4 weeks thereafter. Photosensitivity is a potential hazard with doxycycline.

THIABENDAZOLE (MINTEZOL)

Thiabendazole is a broad-spectrum benzimidazole anthelmintic used as an alternative treatment of strongyloidiasis (92) and cutaneous larva migrans (93). It has been used experimentally against *Capillaria* species (94), *Dracunculus medinensis* (95), and *Trichinella spiralis* infections (96). Thiabendazole is thought to act on parasites by interfering with microtubule aggregation and through inhibition of the enzyme fumarate reductase. It also has anti-inflammatory properties, which may explain its usefulness in dracunculiasis and trichinosis. The most frequently encountered side effects are nausea, vomiting, headache, and dizziness, which occur more in adults than in children. Rare side effects include liver damage, hypotension, angioneurotic edema, and Stevens-Johnson syndrome. Because CNS side effects may occur, activities requiring mental alertness should be avoided, and it should be used with caution in patients with liver disease. The drug should be taken after meals. For strongyloidiasis the dose for both adults and children is 25 mg/kg twice daily (maximum, 3 g per day) for 2 days. For disseminated strongyloidiasis, treatment should be continued for at least 5 days. For cutaneous larva migrans, similar oral doses are taken for 2 days. Alternatively, thiabendazole suspension may be applied topically to lesions (93). Thiabendazole, 25 mg/kg bid for 5 days, has been used in trichinosis, but its effect on larvae in muscle is thought to be more anti-inflammatory than lethal (96), and it is less effective than mebendazole.

TINIDAZOLE (FASIGYN)*

Tinidazole is a nitroimidazole used outside the United States for giardiasis, amebiasis, and vaginal trichomoniasis (97). In comparative trials with the related nitroimidazole metronidazole, tinidazole has been as effective in shorter, better tolerated courses (98.) About 10% of patients experience mild gastrointestinal side effects and headache. For giardiasis, adults are given a single 2-g oral dose, and children receive a single 50-mg/kg dose (maximum 2 g per day). Symptomatic intestinal amebiasis has been treated with 600 mg twice daily for 5 to 10 days for adults. Single daily doses of 2 g have been used for 3 days. For amebic liver abscess, the more successful regimens have been 800 mg three times a day for 5 days or a single daily dose of 2 g for 3 days. Children's doses are given in Table 35.1. As with metronidazole in treating amebiasis, tinidazole should always be followed with a luminal amebicide to decrease the possibility of relapse. For vaginal trichomoniasis, a single 2-g dose is given.

TRIMETHOPRIM-SULFAMETHOXAZOLE (BACTRIM, SEPTRA)

Trimethoprim-sulfamethoxazole is a synthetic antibacterial combination used as treatment of choice for *P. carinii* (62), *Isospora belli* infections (99), and *Cyclospora* infection (100). Available evidence suggests that trimethoprim is relatively nontoxic to humans. Reactions to sulfamethoxazole are similar to those caused by other short- and medium-acting sulfonamides. For *P. carinii* infection, the dose for both children and adults is trimethoprim 15 mg/kg per day and sulfamethoxazole 75 mg/kg per day, orally or IV, in four divided doses for 14 to 21 days. Patients with AIDS should be treated for 21 days, and they may have exaggerated reactions to the drug, including fever, rash, granulocytopenia, and bone marrow depression (62). This drug is also used for prophylaxis of *P. carinii* infection (62). For *I. belli* infection in adults, trimethoprim, 160 mg, and sulfamethoxazole, 800 mg, are given two times a day for 10 days. The high rate of recurrence in HIV patients suggests that an initial shorter 1- to 2-week course followed by an indefinite period of daily doses prophylactically may be a better approach. For *Cyclospora* infection in adults, trimethoprim, 160 mg, plus sulfamethoxazole, 800 mg twice daily, is given for 7 days. Children receive trimethoprim, 5 mg/kg, plus sulfamethoxazole, 25 mg/kg twice daily, for 7 days. (See Chapter 25 for a more detailed discussion of this agent.)

REFERENCES

1. Rossignol JF, Maisonneuve H. Albendazole: placebo-controlled study in 870 patients with intestinal helminths. *Trans R Soc Trop Med Hyg* 1983;7:707.
2. Jones SK, Reynolds NJ, Oliewicki S, et al. Oral albendazole for treatment of cutaneous larva migrans. *Br J Dermatol* 1990;22:9.
3. Horton RJ. Chemotherapy of echinococcus infection in man with albendazole. *Trans R Soc Trop Med Hyg* 1989;83:97.
4. Cruz M, Cruz I, Horton J. Albendazole versus praziquantel in the treatment of cerebral cysticercosis: clinical evaluation. *Trans R Soc Trop Med Hyg* 1991;85:244.
5. Kraivichian P, Kulkumthorn M, Yingyourd P, et al. Albendazole for the treatment of human gnathostomiasis. *Trans R Soc Trop Med Hyg* 1992;86:418.
6. Molina JM, Oksenhendler E, Beauvais B, et al. Disseminated microsporidiosis due to *Septata intestinalis* in patients with AIDS: clinical features and response to albendazole therapy. *J Infect Dis* 1995;171:245.
7. Gardner TB, Hill DB. Treatment of giardiasis. *Clin Microbiol Rev* 2001;14:114.
8. Duma R. Disease caused by free-living amebae. *Infect Dis Newslett* 1989;8:25.
9. Jernigan JA, Pearson RD: Chemotherapy of leishmaniasis, chagas' disease and african trypanosomiasis. *Curr Opin Infect Dis* 1993;6:794.
10. Nosten F. Artemisinin: large community studies. *Trans Roy Soc Trop Med Hyg* 1994;88[suppl 1].
11. World Health Organization. Severe falciparum malaria. *Trans R Soc Trop Med Hyg* 2000;94[suppl 1].
12. van Vugt M, Looareesuwan S, Wilairatana P, et al. Artemether-lumefantrine for the treatment of multidrug resistant falciparum malaria. *Trans Roy Soc Trop Med Hyg* 2000;94:545.
13. Spencer CM, Goa KL. Atovaquone. A review of its pharmacological properties and therapeutic efficacy in opportunistic infections. *Drugs* 1995;50:176.
14. Krause PJ, Telford S, Spielman A, et al. Treatment of babesiosis: comparison of atovaquone and azithromycin with clindamycin and quinine, abstract 430. *Am J Trop Med Hyg* 1997;46:247.
15. Overbosch D, Schilthuis H, Bienzle U, et al. Atovaquone-proguanil versus mefloquine for malaria prophylaxis in nonimmune travelers: results from a randomized double-blind study. *Clin Infect Dis* 2001;33:1015.
16. Kain KC, Shanks GD, Keystone JS. Malaria chemoprophylaxis in the age of drug resistance. I. Currently recommended drug regimens. *Clin Infect Dis* 2001;33:226.
17. Looareesuwan S, Wilairatana P, Chlalermrut K, et al. Efficacy and safety of atovaquone/proguanil compared with mefloquine for treatment of acute *Plasmodium falciparum* malaria in Thailand. *Am J Trop Med Hyg* 1999;60:526.
18. Marr JJ, Docampo R. Chemotherapy for Chagas' disease. A perspective of current therapy and considerations for future research. *Rev Infect Dis* 1986;8:884.
19. de Andrade AL, Zicker E, Oliveira RM, et al. Randomized trial of efficacy of benznidazole in the treatment of early *Trypanosomiasis cruzi* infections. *Lancet* 1996;348:1407.
20. Ariona R, Riancho JA, Aguado JM, et al. Fascioliasis in developed countries: a review of classic and aberrant forms of the disease. *Medicine* 1995;74:13.
21. Singh TS, Mutum SS, Razaque MA. Pulmonary paragonimiasis: clinical features, diagnosis and treatment of 39 cases in Manipur. *Trans R Soc Trop Med Hyg* 1986;80:967.

22. Appleton B, Wolfe MS, Mishtowt GI. Chloroquine as a malarial suppressive: absence of visual effects. *Milit Med* 1973;138:225.

23. Lange WR, Frankenfield DL, Moriarty-Sheehan M, et al. No evidence for chloroquine-associated retinopathy among missionaries on long-term malaria chemoprophylaxis. *Am J Trop Med Hyg* 1994;51:392.

24. Wolfe MS, Cordero JF. Safety of chloroquine in chemosuppresion of malaria during pregnancy. *BMJ* 1985;290:1496.

25. Baird JK, Leksana B, Masbar S, et al. Diagnosis of resistance to chloroquine by *Plasmodium vivax*: timing of recurrence and whole blood chloroquine levels. *Am J Trop Med Hyg* 1997;56:621.

26. Mackenzie CD, Kron MA. Diethylcarbamazine: a review of its action in onchocerciasis, lymphatic filariasis, and inflammation. *Trop Dis Bull* 1985;82:81.

27. Weller PF, Simon HB, Parkhurst BH, et al. Tourism-acquired *Mansonella ozzardi* microfilaremia in a regular blood donor. *JAMA* 1978;240:858.

28. Keystone JS, Davies D. Single-blind Mazzotti test for onchocerciasis. *Lancet* 1992;339:678.

29. Sullivan TJ, Hembree SC. Enhancement of the density of circulating microfilariae with diethylcarbamazine. *Trans R Soc Trop Med Hyg* 1970;64:787.

30. Ottesen EA. Description, mechanisms, and control of reactions to treatment in the human filariases. *Ciba Found Symp* 1987;127:265.

31. Carme B, Boulesteix J, Boutes H, et al. Five cases of encephalitis during treatment of loiasis with diethylcarbamazine. *Am J Trop Med Hyg* 1991;44:684.

32. Nutman TB, Miller KB, Mulligan M, et al. Diethylcarbamazine prophylaxis for human loiasis. Results of a double blind study. *N Engl J Med* 1988;319:752.

33. Wolfe MS. Nondysenteric intestinal amebiasis: treatment with diloxanide furoate. *JAMA* 1973;224:1601.

34. Milord F, Pepin J, Loko L, et al. Efficacy and toxicity of eflornithine for treatment of *Trypanosoma brucei gambiense* sleeping sickness. *Lancet* 1992;340:652.

35. Murphy TV, Nelson JD. Five versus ten days' therapy with furazolidone for giardiasis. *Am J Dis Child* 1983;137:267.

36. Bryson HM, Goa KL. Halofantrine. A review of its antimalarial activity, pharmacokinetic properties and therapeutic potential. *Drugs* 1992;43:236.

37. Monlun E, LeMetayer P, Szwant S, et al. Cardiac complications of halofantrine: a prospective study of 20 patients. *Trans Roy Soc Trop Med Hyg* 1995;89:430.

38. Wolfe MS. The treatment of intestinal protozoan infections. *Med Clin North Am* 1982;66:707.

39. Campbell WC. Ivermectin as an antiparasitic agent for use in humans. *Annu Rev Microbiol* 1991;45:445.

40. Gann PH, Neva FA, Gam AA. A randomized trial of single- and two-dose ivermectin versus thiabendazole for treatment of strongyloidiasis. *J Infect Dis* 1994;169:1076.

41. Caumes E, Carriere J, Guermonprez G, et al. Dermatoses associated with travel to tropical countries: a prospective study of the diagnosis and management of 269 patients presenting to a tropical disease unit. *Clin Infect Dis* 1995;20:542.

42. Wolfe MS, Wershing JM. Mebendazole: treatment of trichuriasis and ascariasis in Bahamian children. *JAMA* 1974;230:1408.

43. Keystone JS, Murdock JK. Mebendazole. *Ann Intern Med* 1979;91:582.

44. Bartoloni C, Tricerri A, Guidi L, et al. The efficacy of chemotherapy with mebendazole in human cystic echinococcosis: long-term followup of 52 patients. *Ann Trop Med Parasitol* 1992;86:249.

45. Levin ML. Treatment of trichinosis with mebendazole. *Am J Trop Med Hyg* 1983;32:980.

46. Schlagenhauf P. Mefloquine for malaria chemoprophylaxis 1992–1998: a review. *J Travel Med* 1999;6:122.

47. White NJ. Mefloquine in the prophylaxis and treatment of falciparum malaria. *BMJ* 1994;308:286.

48. Petersen E, Ronne T, Ronn A, et al. Reported side effects to chloroquine, chloroquine plus proguanil, and mefloquine as chemoprophylaxis against malaria in Danish travelers. *J Travel Med* 2000;7:79.

49. Barrett PJ, Emmins PD, Clark PD, et al. Comparison of adverse events associated with use of mefloquine and combination of chloroquine and proguanil as antimalarial prophylaxis: Postal and telephone survey of travellers. *BMJ* 1996;313:525.

50. Phillips-Howard PA, Steffen R, Kerr L, et al. Safety of mefloquine and other antimalarial agents in the first trimester of pregnancy. *J Travel Med* 1998;5:121.

51. Apted FIC. Present status of chemotherapy and chemoprophylaxis of human trypanosomiasis in the Eastern hemisphere. *Pharmacol Ther* 1980;11:391.

52. Rosenblatt JE, Edson RS. Metronidazole. *Mayo Clin Proc* 1987;62:1013.

53. Spillman R, Ayala S, DeSanchez CE. Double-blind test of metronidazole and tinidazole in the treatment of asymptomatic *Entamoeba histolytica* and *Entamoeba hartmanni* carriers. *Am J Trop Med Hyg* 1976;25:549.

54. Goldman P. Metronidazole: proven benefits and potential risks. *Johns Hopkins Med J* 1980;147:1.

55. Hager WD, Brown ST, Kraus SJ, et al. Metronidazole for vaginal trichomoniasis: seven day vs single dose regimens. *JAMA* 1980;244:1219.

55a. Nitazoxanide (Alinia)—a new antiprotozoal agent. *Med Lett Drugs Ther* 2003;45:29.

55b. White AC. Nitazoxanide: an important advance in anti-parasitic therapy (editorial). *Am J Trop Med Hyg* 2003;68:382.

56. Foster R. A review of clinical experience with oxamniquine. *Trans R Soc Trop Med Hyg* 1987;81:55.

57. Shekhar KC. Schistosomiasis drug therapy and treatment considerations. *Drugs* 1991;42:379.

58. Sullam PM, Slutkin G, Gottlieb AB, et al. Paromomycin therapy of endemic amebiasis in homosexual men. *Sex Transm Dis* 1986;13:151.

59. Berman JD. Human leishmaniasis: clinical diagnostic and chemotherapeutic developments in the last 10 years. *Clin Infect Dis* 1997;24:684.

60. White CA, Chappell CL, Hayat CS, et al. Paromomycin for cryptosporidiosis in AIDS: a prospective double-blind trial. *J Infect Dis* 1994;170:419.

61. Sands M, Kron MA, Brown RB: Pentamidine: a review. *Rev Infect Dis* 1985;7:625.

62. Masur H. Prevention and treatment of *Pneumocystis* pneumonia. *N Engl J Med* 1992;327:1853.

63. Permethrin for head lice. *Med Lett Drugs Ther* 1986;28:89.

64. Permethrin for scabies. *Med Lett Drugs Ther* 1990;32:21.

65. Pearson RD, Guerrant RC. Praziquantel: a major advance in anthelminthic therapy. *Ann Intern Med* 1983;99:195.

66. King CH, Mahmoud AAF. Drugs five years later: praziquantel. *Ann Intern Med* 1989;110:290.

67. Groll E. Praziquantel for cestode infections in man. *Acta Trop* 1980;37:293.

68. Farid Z, Trabolsi B, Boctor F, et al. Unsuccessful use of praziquantel to treat acute fascioliasis in children. *J Infect Dis* 1986;154:920.

69. Vasconcelos D, Cruz-Segura H, Mateos-Gomez H, et al. Selective indications for the use of praziquantel in the treatment of brain cysticercosis. *J Neurol Neurosurg Psychiatry* 1987;50:383.

70. Rikus van Dellen J, McKeown CP. Praziquantel in active cerebral cysticercosis. *Neurosurgery* 1988;22:92.

71. Grewal RS. Pharmacology of 8-amino-quinolines. *Bull WHO* 1981;59:397.

72. Clyde DF. Clinical problems associated with the use of primaquine as a tissue schizonticidal and gametocytocidal drug. *Bull WHO* 1981;59:391.

73. Doherty JF, Day JH, Warhurst DC, et al. Treatment of *Plasmodium vivax*-time for a change? *Trans Roy Soc Trop Med Hyg* 1997;91:76.

74. Shanks GD, Kain K, Keystone JS. Malaria chemoprophylaxis in the age of drug resistance. II. Drugs that may be available in the future. *Clin Infect Dis* 2001;33:381.

75. Ruf B, Pohle HD. Clindamycin/primaquine for *Pneumocystis carinii* pneumonia. *Lancet* 1989;2:626.

76. Hogh B, Clarke PD, Camus D, et al. Atovaquone-proguanil versus chloroquine-proguanil for malaria prophylaxis in non-immune travelers: a randomized double-blind study. *Lancet* 2000;356:1888.

77. Seah SKK. Pyrantel pamoate in treatment of helminthiasis in a nonendemic area. *Southeast Asian J Trop Med Public Health* 1973;4:534.

78. Farahmandian I, Saliba GH, Arfaa F, et al. A comparative evaluation of the therapeutic effect of pyrantel pamoate and bephenium hydroxynaphthoate on *Ancylostoma duodenale* and other intestinal helminths. *J Trop Med Hyg* 1972;75:205.

79. McCabe RE, Remington JS. The diagnosis and treatment of toxoplasmosis. *Eur J Clin Microbiol* 1983;2:95.

80. Brown GV. Chemoprophylaxis of malaria. *Med J Aust* 1993;159:187.

81. Cook IF. Inadequate prophylaxis of malaria with dapsone-pyrimethamine. *Med J Aust* 1985;142:340.

82. Bruce-Chwatt L, ed. Essential malariology, 2nd ed. London: Heinemann, 1985:226–227.

83. Luft BJ, Hafner R, Korzum AH, et al. Toxoplasmic encephalitis in patients with the acquired immunodeficiency syndrome. *N Engl J Med* 1993;329:995.

84. Wolfe MS. Giardiasis. *JAMA* 1975;233:1362.

85. Centers for Disease Control and Prevention: Treatment with quinidine gluconate of persons with severe *Plasmodium falciparum* malaria: discontinuation of parenteral quinine from CDC Drug Service. *MMWR* 1991;40(RR-4):21.

86. White NJ. The treatment of malaria. *N Engl J Med* 1996;335:800.

87. Desmonts G, Couvseur J. Congenital toxoplasmosis: a prospective study of 378 pregnancies. *N Engl J Med* 1974;290:1110.

88. Berman JD. Chemotherapy for leishmaniasis: biochemical mechanisms, clinical efficacy, and future strategies. *Rev Infect Dis* 1988;10:560.

89. Herwaldt BL, Berman JD. Recommendations for treating leishmaniasis with sodium stibogluconate (pentostam) and review of pertinent clinical studies. *Am J Trop Med Hyg* 1992;46:296.

90. Hawking F. Suramin: with special reference to onchocerciasis. *Adv Pharmacol Chemother* 1978;15:289.

91. Pang LW, Limsomwong N, Singharaj P. Prophylactic treatment of vivax and falciparum malaria with low dose doxycycline. *J Infect Dis* 1988;158:1124.

92. Grove DI. Treatment of strongyloidiasis with thiabendazole: an analysis of toxicity and effectiveness. *Trans R Soc Trop Med Hyg* 1982;76:114.

93. Davies HD, Sakuls P, Keystone JS. Creeping eruption. A review of clinical presentation and management of 60 cases presenting to a tropical disease unit. *Arch Dermatol* 1993;129:558.

94. Campbell WC, Cuckler AC. Thiabendazole in the treatment and control of parasitic infections in man. *Tex Rep Biol Med* 1969;27[suppl 2]:665.

95. Kale OO, Elemile T, Enahoro F. Controlled comparative trial of thiabendazole and metronidazole in the treatment. of dracontiasis. *Ann Trop Med Parasitol* 1983;77:151.

96. Campbell WC, Blair LS. Chemotherapy of *Trichinella spiralis* infections (a review). *Exp Parasitol* 1974;35:304.

97. Sawyer PP, Brogden RN, Pinder RM, et al. Tinidazole: a review of its antiprotozoal activity and therapeutic efficacy. *Drugs* 1976;11:423.

98. Bassily S, Farid Z, El-Masry A, et al. Treatment of intestinal *E. histolytica* and *G. lamblia* with metronidazole, tinidazole, and ornidazole: a comparative study. *J Trop Med Hyg* 1987;90:9.

99. Pape JW, Verdier R-I, Johnson WD. Treatment and prophylaxis of *Isospora belli* infection in patients with the acquired immunodeficiency syndrome. *N Engl J Med* 1989;320:1044.

100. Hoge CW, Shlim DR, Ghimire M, et al. Placebo-controlled trial of co-trimoxazole for cyclospora infections among traveler's and foreign residents in Nepal. *Lancet* 1995;345:691.

CHAPTER 36

Immune Globulin Therapy (Passive Immunization) for Augmentation of the Host Response

Jeffrey K. Griffiths and David R. Snydman

OVERVIEW AND HISTORY

Products of serum can treat, ameliorate, and prevent many infectious diseases, including many of major public health importance. These preparations are used in therapy when the patient is unable to mount an early or adequate humoral response to a pathogen or its toxins. Most beneficial properties of serum lie in the immunoglobulin fraction, which has been used for many decades in the prevention of infectious diseases. Serum therapy has a unique place in medicine, as the administration of serum and its products predated the antibiotic era.

Intravenous (IVIG) and intramuscular immunoglobulin has proved beneficial in a number of specific circumstances, such as the replacement of immunoglobulin in the permanently or transiently deficient host. Those with congenital agammaglobulinemia or immunoglobulin G (IgG) subclass deficiency with recurrent infections fit into this group. Another major role for immunoglobulin is in the administration of specific antibody for a specific infection. This is especially useful if no specific drug therapy exists, such as with rabies exposure or parvovirus infection. An evolving role for IVIG is for combination therapy of viral infections, such as cytomegalovirus (CMV) pneumonia after transplantation, with concurrent high-titer hyperimmune antibody and antiviral drugs.

The modern era of serum therapy began with three of Robert Koch's students (1). Emil Behring and Shibasaburo Kitasato developed a sheep antiserum to diphtheria toxin, which was given in 1891 to a girl dying of diphtheria who recovered within hours and survived (2). Paul Ehrlich produced and used horse antisera to tetanus toxin in 1897 (3). In the 1920s and 1930s, Maxwell Finland and colleagues demonstrated that early, specific treatment with animal immune sera was efficacious in conditions such as pneumococcal pneumonia (4,5). Serum preparations derived from human placentas (6) were shown to prevent and treat measles in 1935 (7). Cohn and colleagues (8) fractionated serum using cold ethanol and produced fractions highly enriched in γ-globulins. It was used in World War II to prevent hepatitis A and measles (9). This preparation was used by Bruton (10) to treat a child with recurrent sepsis and agammaglobulinemia in 1951, beginning the era of replacement therapy for the immunodeficient host.

From this collective experience, central observations about immunotherapy (first enunciated in Finland) were made. These included the realization that immunotherapy reduces the mortality and morbidity related to infection, as long as early and specific diagnosis of the infection was made and early administration of immunoglobulins was accomplished. At that time, toxicity was common with animal preparations, such as horse hyperimmune sera to *Streptococcus pneumoniae*. These principles have meaning today.

Intravenous (IV) use of early gamma globulin preparations was limited because of the risk of cardiovascular collapse and death. Intramuscular (IM) or subcutaneous injections were used, although these methods were limited by volumes that could be given, pain at the site of injection, and abscess formation. Moreover, in immunoglobulin A (IgA)-deficient patients, antiallotypic IgA antibody reactions limited the use of gamma globulin, which contains IgA. Plasma infusions were used by some, but many difficulties (hepatitis transmission, large volumes needed) remained (11). IVIG administration was reinvestigated in the 1960s, and reactions were found to be related to protein aggregates and complement activation (12). Technology developed in the late 1970s and 1980s to prevent complement activation by aggregates has rendered current human IV preparations relatively free of these problems and resulted in a rebirth of the use of IVIG.

We review the inherent characteristics and pharmacology of immune globulins (IGs), their potential side effects, and their uses in normal and immunodeficient hosts and address a number of miscellaneous states in which IGs may be salubrious.

IMMUNE GLOBULIN CHARACTERISTICS: PREPARATION, PHARMACOLOGY, AND SIDE EFFECTS

IG is a preparation of human IGs pooled from blood donors or plasmapheresis patients. Unselected immune serum globulin contains antibodies to various viruses and microorganisms as reflected in the plasma pool of the population sampled. IG that has not been denatured has been shown to exhibit good opsonic activity against a large number of gram-negative and gram-positive bacterial species. In addition, antibody to a wide variety of viral and fungal organisms can be found.

Incremental advances have led to preparations that are safe for IV use (Table 36.1). This goal has been attained by a variety of means, including chemical treatment, pepsin digestion, diethylaminoethyl (DEAE) column chromatography, acidification, ultracentrifugation, and ultrafiltration (13,14). Ideally, immunoglobulin for IV use should be composed of the native molecules (IgG subclasses) in proportion to that found in serum, with full biologic properties, a pharmacokinetic profile similar to that seen with other gamma globulins, and no impurities. Theoretically, minimal alteration of the immunoglobulin molecule should protect maximal biologic activity. Because 1 in 600 people are IgA deficient (15), immunoglobulin preparations should have minimal IgA to reduce the risk of antiallotypic allergic reactions. Some currently available gamma globulin is nearly pure monomeric IgG, with little or no IgA and without complement-activating properties. However, variations exist in chemical properties, antibody titers to specific pathogens, IgA, and IgG subclasses in commercial products (14,16–19).

Virus inactivation steps, such as a solvent-detergent step, need not alter the function of IVIG, as measured by *in vitro* assays of Fc functional activity (20). A variety of steps, such as ethanol fractionation, polyethylene glycol (PEG) precipitation, solvent-detergent treatment, and pasteurization, have been tested against a variety of viral pathogens, such as human immunodeficiency virus (HIV), hepatitis C virus (HCV), mumps virus, vaccinia virus, chikungunya virus, vesicular stomatitis virus, Sindbis virus, and echovirus. In some circumstances, multiple steps are required to inactivate infectious virus particles (21). For example, Louie and colleagues (22) have shown that coupling the cold ethanol Cohn-Oncley process with formulation at pH 4.25 caused a 10,000-fold decrease in bovine viral diarrhea virus intentionally added to the plasma pool and complete inactivation of 1,000 chimpanzee infectious doses per milliliter of HCV.

When IG is given intravenously to IgG-deficient individuals, peak serum levels are proportional to the doses administered.

TABLE 36.1. Characteristics of Commercially Available Intravenous Immunoglobulin

Product	Method of preparation	IgG subclasses as a percentage of total IgG				
		IgG1	IgG2	IgG3	IgG4	IgA (μq/mL)
IVIG preparations						
Gammagard S/D (Baxter/Hyland); Also marketed as Polygam S/D (American Red Cross/Hyland)	Cohn fractionation, DEAE-Sephadex adsorption and ultrafiltration, and detergent treatment; stabilization with 2% glucose, 0.22% glycine, 0.2% PEG, 0.3% albumin	72.1	22	5.5	0.4	<3.7 (<10)
Gammar-P IV (Armour)	Cohn fractionation, filtration, pasteurization (60°C for 10 h), sterile filtration; stabilized with albumin and sucrose	69	23	6	2	25
Gamimune N, 5% (Miles Biologics)	Cohn fractionation-effluent III ultrafiltration, followed by formulation at pH 4.5 in 10% maltose	58.7	29.3	6.3	5.1	270
Gamimune N, 10% (Miles Biologics)	Cohn fractionation-effluent III ultrafiltration, followed by formulation at pH 4.5 in 0.16-0.24 M glycine	71.1	22.2	5.3	1.4	113
Iveegam (Immuno AG)	Cohn fractionation, immobilized trypsin treatment, followed by PEG fractionation; stabilized in 5% glucose	60–70 (64.1)	30–40 (29.4)	0 (4.0)	2 (1.5)	<100 (<10)
Sandoglobulin	Cohn fractionation, pepsin treatment at pH 4; stabilization in 5% sucrose	60.5	30.2	6.6	2.6	720
Venoglobulin-I	Cohn fractionation, followed by PEG fractionation and DEAE-Sephadex treatment; stabilized with 2% mannitol and 1% albumin	60.9	29.4	5.3	4.4	20–24
Venoglobulin-S	Cohn fractionation, followed by PEG fractionation and DEAE-Sephadex treatment, treatment with tri-n-butyl phosphate (TNBP) and polysorbate 80, and stabilization with 5% sorbitol	65.7–67.2	23.7–25.3	5.7–5.9	3.0–3.4	11–14
Reference IgG (World Health Organization)		60.0	29.4	6.5	4.1	
CMV hyperimmune globulin (CMVIg; CytoGam) (Massachusetts State Biological Laboratories; MedImmune)	Cohn fractionation, ultrafiltration, stabilization with sucrose and albumin, 0.22-μm filter filtration, solvent detergent	65–66	27–28	5.2	1.7–1.8	30–200
Respiratory syncytial virus hyperimmune globulin (RSVIg; RespiGam) (Massachusetts State Biological Laboratories and MedImmune)	Cohn fractionation, ultrafiltration, stabilization with sucrose and albumin, 0.22-μm filter filtration, solvent detergent	65–66	27–28	5.2	1.7–1.8	30–200

Data are from manufacturers and published comparisons (published values are in parentheses). As preparations change, the reader is urged to review the specific manufacturer's package insert information before use. The most biologically relevant characteristics of IG preparations may be the specific neutralizing titers to specific pathogens, not the distribution of IgG subclasses.

A doses of 200 mg/kg leads to an increase of approximately 100 mg/dL and a dose of 1 g/kg to an increase of approximately 500 mg/dL. Serum IgG levels peak and fall rapidly, but 3 to 7 days after infusion the levels stabilize at 35% to 50% of the peak serum level (23–25). Thereafter, serum IgG levels decrease slowly in an exponential fashion, reaching baseline levels in 3 to 4 weeks. This has been interpreted as meaning that IgG redistributes from the vascular compartment into the extravascular space, accounting for the rapid fall, and is then eliminated at a slower pace from all compartments in a terminal elimination phase. Other reasons for a rapid initial fall include elimination of denatured IgG, immune complex formation, high catabolic states, steroid administration before transplant surgery, and binding of target antigens. When given IM, immune serum globulin results in an increment in peak serum levels of IgG that is about half that of IVIG and also has a half-life of 21 to 28 days. Greater increases of serum levels occur with IV than with IM administration when identical amounts of globulin are given.

Elimination of administered IgG is rapid in protein-losing states, such as after burns (26,27). Some but not all premature neonates eliminate IgG quickly (25). In bone marrow transplant recipients, the half-life of immune serum globulin, as measured by CMV antibody determination, may be as short as hours (28). Half-lives between 6 and 15 days have been observed for CMV hyperimmune globulin in kidney and liver transplantation (29). After liver or kidney transplantation, the CMV antibody half-life is approximately 7 to 8 days during the first 2 months and increases to 16 to 18 days in the third month (30). It is thought that infection with a specific agent leads to depletion of specific antibody, accounting for the shortened half-life noted during CMV and pneumococcal infections (31).

It is believed that the mechanism of action of exogenous IG is the same as that of endogenously produced antibody. This has been reviewed by Schiff (31) and others (32). Immunoglobulins are discussed comprehensively in Chapter 2. The specific activity of a lot of IVIG against a certain pathogen appears to be most related to the donor pool and not to the method of manufacture. It has been suggested that clinicians may want to select IVIG on the basis of pathogen-specific antibody (33), which may vary from lot to lot. Alas, this information is rarely available in the clinical setting. Current U.S. Food and Drug Administration (FDA) regulations specify that IGs have a minimal titer only against diphtheria, poliomyelitis, measles, and hepatitis B.

High-dose IVIG (600 mg/kg per month) does not appear to substantially improve phagocytic function (phagocytosis, intracellular bactericidal activity, chemotaxis, superoxide production) over that seen with lower dose IVIG (200 mg/kg per month) (34). Meissner and colleagues (35) have discussed the functional properties of IVIG, with particular attention to its use in Kawasaki syndrome and respiratory syncytial virus (RSV) prophylaxis.

Our understanding of the effects of IVIG on the immune system is incomplete. Aukrust and co-workers (36) documented striking changes in plasma cytokine and interleukin (IL)-1 receptor antagonist levels after the administration of 400 mg/kg IVIG to 12 individuals with primary agammaglobulinemia. These included rapid increases in IL-6, IL-8, and tumor necrosis factor-α (TNF-α), which are proinflammatory. Subsequently, there were prolonged increases in soluble TNF receptors and in IL-1 receptor antagonist, suggestive of a counter-regulatory response. These compounds regulate the inflammatory response, and thus these findings may be relevant to the effects of IVIG in immunologically mediated disorders.

Serious side effects of IVIG are rare (19). More common, minor side effects of IVIG, such as mild fever, mild headache, chills, fatigue, and diarrhea, are reported in approximately one third to one half of all IVIG recipients. Immediate severe reactions related to intact IgG appear to be vanishingly rare. IVIG should be administered cautiously to individuals with high levels of serum IgG, to decrease the risk of hyperviscosity syndromes, or to those with immune complex disease. It has been suggested that IVIG, given to increase platelet counts in patients with idiopathic thrombocytopenic purpura, could lead to thrombosis in individuals with severe atherosclerosis; the evidence for this is slight. Fears that high-dose IVIG, by blocking reticuloendothelial system clearance, could lead to decreased opsonization of bacterial or fungal pathogens also do not appear substantiated. As alluded to previously, a reaction after IVIG administration in IgA-deficient individuals may occur, although it is unusual, and IVIG preparations with little IgA can be chosen for use in this circumstance. Aseptic meningitis, secondary to high-dose IVIG (2 g/kg) for the treatment of various immune-related neuromuscular diseases, has been reported to be more common in those with a history of migraine (37). It can rarely occur after use of IVIG at normal doses (38). Acute renal failure has been described as a rare complication of IVIG, with no evidence to date of immune complex-mediated, or inflammatory, renal disease (39). This complication varies from asymptomatic decreases in glomerular filtration rates to anuric renal failure, usually with rapid recovery of function after cessation of therapy. As with any other manufactured product given intravenously, there is a risk of contamination or of infusion of infected material. It appears that IVIG is not supportive of bacterial growth but does support the growth of yeast at 25°C or 37°C *in vitro* (40).

A major theoretical concern has been the potential transmission of bloodborne pathogens, such as HIV, hepatitis B virus, and HCV (41). Before the advent of blood product screening for HIV, there were reports of false-positive HIV antibody test results after the administration of IVIG, representing passive transfer of antibody in the immunoglobulin. It has been demonstrated that HIV is inactivated by the Cohn-Oncley fractionation method for preparing IVIG, with an estimated reduction in HIV titer during IVIG manufacture on the order of 10^{15} (42, 43). The use of screening for HIV antibody in blood donors and the use of the Cohn-Oncley procedure render the risk of HIV transmission essentially zero.

However, hepatitis C transmission has been documented in patients with primary hypogammaglobulinemia after treatment with IG (44). Several commercial and experimental lots of IVIG from one manufacturer have been found to contain HCV ribonucleic acid (RNA) by polymerase chain reaction detection. Ethanol, which is used in the manufacture of IVIG by the Cohn-Oncley process, does not affect HCV RNA at concentrations up to 25% (45). This finding may help explain why HCV, unlike some other viruses such as HIV, may be found in some commercial preparations.

Paradoxically, lots of IVIG that lack antibody to HCV may be more likely to transmit HCV than lots with anti-HCV antibody. Yu and co-workers reported the detection of infectious HCV RNA in lots of IVIG manufactured by Baxter Healthcare, which withdrew its IVIG preparation Gammagard in February 1994 because of reports of HCV transmission (46). Of lots of plasma that had been screened and found negative for anti-HCV antibody, 20 of 24 were positive for HCV RNA by polymerase chain reaction assays. It has been suggested that this finding indicates that the presence of anti-HCV antibody in the IVIG plasma pools may assist in partitioning the infectious virus during the manufacturing process. Others have concluded on the basis of HCV RNA polymerase chain reaction testing that the reason for the Gammagard-associated HCV infections was probably the use of HCV-contaminated plasma and the lack of a potent HCV-inactivating step during production (47). Consistent with this line of reasoning was the finding that chimpanzees that received unprocessed plasma from a pool of 2,887 HCV sero-negative donors contracted HCV, but chimpanzees that received IVIG processed from the same plasma pool did not contract HCV. These studies suggest that withholding plasma that is HCV seropositive does not render a plasma pool noninfectious and that the safety of IVIG manufactured from such pools is not compromised by withholding the seropositive units. Previous experience with hepatitis B suggests that antibody to hepatitis B surface antigen may assist in inactivating or precipitating the hepatitis B particle during manufacture (48,49). Thus, screening of donors may decrease the viral burden in plasma pools used for IVIG manufacture but may exclude antibody useful in inactivating infectious viruses.

Between 1983 and 1994, there were at least 17 reports of transmission of non-A, non-B hepatitis or transaminitis connected with the use of six different IVIG preparations. The latter were produced without including a validated virus inactivation method during manufacture. Key elements of safe IVIG production and safety from viral transmission must include minimization of virus contamination in the source plasma, good manufacturing practices, and the use of a rigorous virus inactivation procedure (50). As a result of the outbreaks of hepatitis C, the FDA now requires evidence of HCV inactivation with a virus inactivation step, typically use of a solvent, detergent or acidic pH, or evidence that no HCV RNA can be detected by the polymerase chain reaction.

Commercial lots of IVIG contain detectable levels of antibody to pathogens such as hepatitis B virus and CMV, and these passively transferred antibodies may confound the interpretation of laboratory studies (51).

COST

The cost of IG preparations varies widely, from only a dollar or so per milliliter of IG for IM administration to thousands of dollars for a monthly course of IVIG. Lifelong dependence on IVIG replacement is expensive. Thus, the current cost of IVIG alone, at a dose of 400 mg/kg per month for a 70-kg individual, approaches $8,640 wholesale per year.

Home IV therapy has been touted as an inexpensive alternative to in-hospital therapy (52). Hyperimmune preparations are usually far more potent than unselected preparations and may be less costly overall than larger amounts of less potent preparations. Use of some hyperimmune globulins, such as CMV hyperimmune globulin after transplantation, has been shown to be cost-effective (53).

PROPHYLAXIS AND TREATMENT IN THE NORMAL HOST

The normal host has relatively little need for immune serum globulin or IVIG, and there is little indication for its use. For example, IM immune serum globulin does not appear to reduce the frequency of otitis media in children with normal levels of IgG and recurrent episodes of otitis media (54). There is no indication for serum product use in normal hosts without exposure to a specific pathogen. It was found decades ago that IM immune serum globulin prevented clinical illness caused by a number of specific pathogens such as diphtheria, tetanus, and measles in closed populations (such as army recruits or asylum residents) during an epidemic with the same pathogen. Indeed, this concept of specific pre- or postexposure prophylaxis has led to the development of hyperimmune globulin preparations.

USE OF UNSELECTED INTRAMUSCULAR IMMUNE SERUM GLOBULIN

Traditionally, unselected IM immune serum globulin has been used for hepatitis A prophylaxis (55) as outlined in Table 36.2. Despite the availability of hepatitis A vaccine, IM globulin remains an attractive option for prophylaxis after exposure to hepatitis A because of its rapidity of action, low cost, and wide availability. Similarly, immune serum globulin can prevent or ameliorate

TABLE 36.2. Indications for Unselected Immune Globulins and Hyperimmune Globulins in the Prevention of Specific Infectious Diseases

Infection	Indication	Globulin preparation and dose
Botulism	Treatment and prevention of botulism in ingestor of botulinus toxin	Trivalent (types A, B, and E) specific equine antibody; call CDC (404-639-3670). Does not reverse toxin already bound to nerve endings but neutralizes circulating unbound toxin. Serum sickness seen in ~10% of treated patients.
Cytomegalovirus infection	Prophylaxis and treatment of CMV in CMV seronegative kidney transplant recipients of CMV seropositive donors	See package insert; hyperimmune anti-CMV IVIG is given IV.
Diphtheria	Respiratory diphtheria-probably no role in cutaneous diphtheria	Call CDC at 404-639-3670[a]
Hepatitis A	Postexposure prophylaxis: family contacts; sexual contacts; institutional or daycare center outbreaks	Unselected IG; 0.02 mL/kg, up to 2 mL total for defined exposures. Administration more than 2 wk after exposure is not likely to be beneficial.
	Preexposure prophylaxis in travelers	0.06 mL/kg up to 5 mL for long-term travel, with repeated doses at intervals of 4–6 mo. Hepatitis A vaccine may replace IG in most preexposure situations. IG use does not replace avoidance behaviors, such as careful selection of safe food and water.
Hepatitis B	Percutaneous or mucosal exposure	Hepatitis B IG (HBIG); hyperimmune preparation; 0.06 mL/kg. Vaccinate with hepatitis B vaccine if repeated exposure (e.g., health care worker) is likely[a]
	Newborns of hepatitis B surface antigen-positive mothers	HBIG, 0.5 ml at birth, and vaccinate with hepatitis B vaccine.
	Sexual contacts of persons with acute or chronic hepatitis B	HBIG, 0.06 mL/kg, and vaccinate with hepatitis B vaccine.[a]
Measles	Nonimmune contacts of acute cases exposed fewer than 6 d previously	Unselected IG 0.25 mL/kg up to 15 mL for normal hosts, 0.5 mL/kg up to 15 mL for immunocompromised persons.
Rabies	Exposure to rabid or potentially rabid animals, such as a bite injury, salivary contact, or aerosol	Hyperimmune rabies immune globulin, HRIG, 20 IU/kg IM, with half given in the region of the exposure.
Respiratory syncytial virus (RSV) infection	Prophylaxis of RSV infection in children with bronchopulmonary dysplasia or prematurity	Hyperimmune, monthly administration to susceptible children and neonates during the RSV transmission season.
Tetanus	Contaminated wound injury and either an uncertain tetanus toxoid vaccination history or a history of less than three doses of tetanus toxoid	Tetanus (hyper)immune globulin (TIG); 250 units IM if tetanus immunization history is unknown or if less than three doses of tetanus toxoid have been administered and if the wound is contaminated, for example, by feces, saliva, or dirt, or is a puncture wound, or is the result of a crush, burn, frostbite, or missile injury[a]
Vaccinia	Severe reaction to vaccinia vaccination	Hyperimmune preparation, available from CDC (404-639-3670).
Varicella-zoster	Substantial exposure by immunosuppressed or newborn contacts, such as household contacts of the index case; close indoor contact lasting more than 1 h; sharing the same hospital room with an infected person; prolonged face-to-face contact with an infected person, such as occurs with nurses and physicians	Hyperimmune preparation; varicella-zoster IG (VZIG); 125 units/10 kg up to a maximum of 625 units. Higher doses in immunosuppressed adults may be necessary (insufficient data available). Fractional doses are not recommended (e.g., given in aliquots of 125 units). Pregnant women and infants born to mothers in whom varicella develops within 5 d or before 48 h after delivery should also receive VZIG. VZIG does not prevent infection but ameliorates the disease.[a]

[a]If hyperimmune preparations are not available and administration of VZIG, TIG, HBIG, or equine antidiphtheria globulins is indicated, unselected IG or IVIG may be given although the efficacy of unselected preparations is probably less than that of hyperimmune globulins. HIBG should be given at a dose of 0.06 mL/kg in this circumstance.

measles in the normal host. Unselected IG may also be used when hyperimmune globulin preparations are not available for exposures to tetanus or hepatitis B, although hyperimmune globulin is preferable.

USE OF HYPERIMMUNE GLOBULINS

Hyperimmune globulins derived from donor pools of individuals immunized to, or selected for, specific pathogens with high titer to the pathogen or its toxin have been useful (see Table 36.2) (55). The rationale for the production of hyperimmune globulins is to ensure lot-to-lot consistency of antibody titers with enriched preparations that may have some in vitro consistency as well. The incremental antibody titers of these hyperimmune preparations can be large. For example, unselected immune serum globulin has an anti-hepatitis B titer of 1:100, whereas the hepatitis B Ig has an anti-hepatitis B surface antigen titer of 1:100,000 (56). For varicella-zoster and tetanus immune globulins, the hyperimmune antibody titers are approximately fourfold to eightfold higher than in the unselected preparations. Specific indications exist for the use of these hyperimmune globulin preparations for normal and immunodeficient hosts at risk of acquiring certain disease (57,58) (see Table 36.2). Diseases included in this category are hepatitis B, measles, rabies, varicella, vaccinia, tetanus, CMV infection, and pertusis. An RSV hyperimmune globulin preparation as well as a humanized monoclonal antibody have also been licensed for use in neonates with bronchopulmonary dysplasia and those children with cardiopulmonary disorders (59) and are discussed later in this chapter.

Animal preparations of hyperimmune globulins are available in the developing world and the developed world for the treatment of some infectious diseases, such as rabies, diphtheria, botulism, and tetanus (60). Being efficacious, they are preferable to no treatment at all, but they have more side effects. Equine antibody preparations are available in the United States from the Centers for Disease Control and Prevention (CDC; telephone 401-639-3670, 24 hours a day) against types A, B, and E botulism; diphtheria; tetanus; Western equine encephalitis; and vaccinia.

There is no intellectual reason why hyperimmune serum has to be limited to a single antigen or pathogen. For example, immunization and subsequent plasmapheresis of volunteers against a number of bacterial polysaccharide antigens (*S. pneumoniae*, *Haemophilus influenzae*, and *Neisseria meningitidis*) have been used to manufacture a polyvalent hyperimmune globulin termed bacterial polysaccharide IG. In studies of Apache Indian infants, a group at high risk of developing *H. influenzae* type b and pneumococcal infections, protection against serious *H. influenzae* type b or pneumococcal disease could be demonstrated after prophylaxis with bacterial polysaccharide IG (61).

AUGMENTATION OF THE NORMAL RESPONSE: GRAM-NEGATIVE BACTERIAL SEPSIS

There continues to be interest in the use of IVIG or other similar products in gram-negative sepsis because there is high mortality despite aggressive use of antimicrobial agents and intravascular volume expanders (62). Many studies have investigated the relative contributions of bacterial products (e.g., endotoxin) and host mediators (e.g., cytokines) in the sepsis syndrome, with the hope that antibody binding of these products will increase survival during sepsis (63). Immune plasma from volunteers immunized with the J-5 *Escherichia coli* mutant prevented death in patients with gram-negative sepsis (64) and reduced infectious

complications (but not overall mortality) in high-risk surgical patients (65). Results of subsequent studies using plasma and IV gamma globulin were not as favorable (66,67), whereas somewhat positive results were found with the use of a human or murine monoclonal IgM antiendotoxin antibody in a subset of patients with the sepsis syndrome caused by gram-negative organisms (68,69). These differences may be explained by the relatively low capacity of unselected IgG, and the relatively high capacity of hyperimmune or monoclonal IgM, to bind endotoxin and thus possibly to prevent shock related to endotoxin release. The treatment of sepsis with unselected IVIG or with antibody to endotoxin components has not proved statistically beneficial in individual trials; however, a meta-analysis of all trials by the Cochrane Collaborative has recently concluded that the use of intravenous immune globulin has been shown to be effective in reducing mortality but given the number of patients studied, such use should be considered experimental (70–72). Discussion of mediators other than antibody can be found in Chapters 6 and 61.

PROPHYLAXIS AND TREATMENT OF THE DEFICIENT HOST: REPLACEMENT THERAPY OF THE CONGENITALLY DEFICIENT HOST

Bruton's original description of agammaglobulinemia and recurrent sepsis, controlled by IM gamma globulin, was of a child with X-linked hypogammaglobulinemia (10). Given the obvious benefit of IM IG, no controlled trial comparing Ig with placebo was ever conducted, but few doubt the lifesaving consequences of IG in this situation. Subsequent randomized trials have demonstrated the superiority of IVIG over the IM product in the treatment of congenital hypogammaglobulinemia (Table 36.3). High-dose IV therapy (i.e., 200 to 500 mg/kg per month) has been shown to be associated with fewer infections and decreased use of antibiotics compared with lower doses (73). Other primary humoral deficiency states warrant IVIG prophylaxis. These include transient hypogammaglobulinemia of infancy, especially if accompanied by symptomatic infections; common variable immunodeficiency, especially if IgG levels fall below 250 mg/dL; X-linked hyper-IgM syndrome; and selective deficiency of IgG subclasses (74,75). Although total IgG may not be decreased in the last condition, replacement therapy is indicated (76). Selective immunoglobulin deficiencies are being recognized as part of other syndromes, such as congenital heart disease and Down syndrome (77–79), and replacement therapy may become part of standard management in these diseases. IgA deficiency is regarded as a contraindication to IVIG treatment, given the possibility of anti-IgA–mediated anaphylaxis, although some individuals with IgA and IgG subclass deficiency may benefit from IVIG (80).

Another set of indications for the use of IVIG includes combined immunodeficiencies, in which abnormal T-lymphocyte function is associated with antibody production defects. Thus, individuals with ataxia-telangiectasia, Wiskott-Aldrich syndrome, hyper-IgE syndrome, or DiGeorge syndrome benefit from IVIG. Individuals with X-linked lymphoproliferative syndromes or Chédiak-Higashi disease may also reasonably receive IVIG (81,82).

REPLACEMENT THERAPY AND PROPHYLAXIS OF THE TRANSIENTLY DEFICIENT HOST

Neonatal Sepsis

Premature neonates are deficient in antibody and are at great risk of serious infection. Most maternal antibody crosses the placenta

TABLE 36.3. Recommended and Probably or Possibly Beneficial (Investigational) Uses of Intravenous Immunoglobulin in the Augmentation of the Host Response

Primary immunodeficiency syndromes
  Recommended use
    Agammaglobulinemia
    Ataxia-telangiectasia
    Common variable immunodeficiency
    DiGeorge syndrome
    Selective antibody deficiency (e.g., subclass deficiency) with a
      history of recurrent infections
    Severe combined immunodeficiency
    Short-limbed dwarfism
    Wiskott-Aldrich syndrome
    X-linked lymphoproliferative syndrome
    X-linked hyper-IgM syndrome
    X-linked agammaglobulinemia
  Possible use[a]
    Congenital heart disease
    Down syndrome
Acquired immunodeficiency syndromes
  Recommended
    Transplantation
  Possible use[a]
    After surgery or trauma
    Protein-losing nephropathy if total serum IgG < 600 mg/dL
    HIV seropositive children
    Chronic lymphocytic leukemia[b]
    Multiple myeloma[b]
  Recommended
    Hemorrhagic virus infections (immune plasma) such as Lassa
      fever or Argentinian hemorrhagic fever
    Kawasaki disease (mucocutaneous lymph node syndrome)
    Parovirus B19 infection
    RSV infection prevention in children and neonates with either
      bronchopulmonary dysplasia, congenital heart disease, or
      prematurity
    Toxic shock syndrome
  Possible use[a]
    Enteric infections with agents such as *Clostridium difficile* or
      Cryptosporidium using hyperimmune preparations
    Prevention of necrotizing enterocolitis in premature neonates

[a]As yet unproved. Routine use of IVIG is not recommended at this time.
[b]May not be cost-effective; selection of patients is urged.
HIV, human immunodeficiency virus; RSV, respiratory syncitial virus.

only after 34 weeks of gestation, and IgG2 subclass molecules are poorly transferred, as are IgM and IgA. Moreover, premature neonates have decreased complement and fibronectin levels, impaired phagocyte function, low levels of cytokine production, and small marrow reserves of neutrophils (83–86). Although the indications for the use of IVIG in neonatal sepsis are still unclear, both fresh-frozen plasma and IVIG are sometimes used for prophylaxis against, and treatment for, neonatal infections (see Table 36.3).

A large multicenter placebo-controlled double-blind study of 587 infants weighing 500 to 1,750 g at birth revealed that IVIG at 500 mg/kg given periodically led to a significant decrease (approximately 30%) in the risk of a first nosocomial infection and, in infants with an infection, a decrease in the mean number of hospital days (from 101 to 80 days) (87). Another study of 753 neonates who were randomized to receive either IVIG at 500 mg/kg with high opsonic activity to group B streptococci or albumin found that survival during the first 7 days was higher in septic infants receiving IVIG, but by 8 weeks of age no significant difference in mortality was present (88). A comparison of granulocyte transfusions versus 1,000 mg/kg per day for the first 3 days of sepsis in neutropenic premature neonates showed

higher survival in the group given granulocytes, but the dose of IVIG was so high that Fc receptor blockade may have occurred in the IVIG treatment group (89).

Although some studies have suggested that prophylactic IVIG is useful in the prevention of infections in neonatal intensive care units, especially in the developing world, others have failed to show any efficacy, including those in the developing world (90). One potential explanation for this contradictory set of data is the increase in infections caused by nosocomial (and otherwise unusual) pathogens such as *Staphylococcus epidermidis* in neonatal intensive care units. A Cochrane database meta-analysis concludes that intravenous immune globulin results in a 3% reduction in sepsis without any reduction in hospital mortality or length of stay (91). Furthermore, it concludes that there is no justification for the use of IVIG for suspected or proven infections in neonates (92).

Viral infections are also of major importance in neonates. CMV hyperimmune globulin (CMVIG) given to prevent CMV disease in multiply transfused premature neonates showed a trend toward benefit with fewer clinical CMV syndromes (14% vs. 4%, $p = 0.18$), fewer ventilator days, and shorter hospital stay compared with neonates given albumin (93). A conclusive answer to the benefit of CMVIG in premature neonates requires a larger cohort of infants.

Burns

In thermal burns, the major cause of death is sepsis resulting from opportunistic bacteria, such as *P. aeruginosa* (94). Serum immunoglobulin levels fall rapidly after burns, and the size of the decrement is related to the size of the burn (95). IG enriched in antibody to *P. aeruginosa* was protective when burned mice were inoculated with *Pseudomonas* (96). Studies with IM IG in burn patients have produced contradictory results (97,98). One study found an antipseudomonal polyvalent vaccine or IM hyperimmune IG, in conjunction with antimicrobial agents, to be superior than antimicrobial agents alone for preventing death of burned patients (99). However, a prospective, randomized, double-blind placebo-controlled study of IVIG (500 mg/kg) given twice weekly to 50 seriously burned patients found no difference in outcome (100); similarly, a trial of IVIG at 500 mg/kg for 1 week versus albumin showed no difference in mortality (101). Further studies are needed before IG can be recommended for burn patients.

Major Surgery and Trauma

Surgery results in a temporary immunodeficiency state, called by some the postsurgery or posttraumatic immunodeficiency syndrome. This syndrome is characterized by elevations in serum acute-phase reactants, IL-2 receptors, and neopterin, concurrent with declines in serum immunoglobulins, complement components, circulating T cells, and natural killer cells (102). The use of IVIG has been investigated in this syndrome both to replace antibody and to modulate the inflammatory changes (103). In a multicenter double-blind study of 329 patients comparing placebo, IVIG, and IVIG high in antibody to endotoxin, a subset of patients who had undergone major surgical procedures appeared to have benefited from standard IVIG but not the hyperimmune preparation (104). In another study of patients with gastrointestinal cancer, 159 patients were given either 15 g of IVIG on days 1 and 5 after surgery or placebo. Patients who had undergone colon surgery but not others appeared to have benefited from IVIG, although there was a trend toward benefit in the group overall (105). These studies point out the need to conduct large randomized studies to evaluate any potential benefit of IVIG therapy and to identify subgroups in whom efforts should be concentrated.

Chronic Lymphocytic Leukemia, Multiple Myeloma, and Chemotherapy

Much of the γ-globulin produced by people with chronic lymphocytic leukemia (CLL), multiple myeloma (MM), or Waldenström macroglobulinemia is nonfunctional, and infection becomes increasingly common as the disease progresses (106,107). IVIG is known to reduce the number of bacterial infections in B-cell CLL, in which hypogammaglobulinemia is common. IVIG, 400 mg/kg given every 3 weeks, decreased by half the number of bacterial infections in people with CLL (108,109). In an attempt to determine the amount of IVIG needed to prevent infectious complications, Jurlander and colleagues (110) in Denmark gave 15 patients with CLL 10 g of IVIG every 3 weeks, which stabilized serum immunoglobulin levels just above the lower limit of normal after 11 doses. The number of hospitalizations and febrile episodes during therapy fell by 69% and 51%, respectively, compared with the pretherapy period. Similarly, Gamm and co-workers (111) found that doses of IVIG as low as 250 mg/kg per 4 weeks decreased the rate of infection in CLL. In a cautionary note, one study of patients with CLL has suggested that IVIG replacement is not cost-effective because its benefits do not lead to reduced mortality despite reductions in infections (112).

The benefit of IG in MM has been less clear. One early study with IM IG showed no benefit (113); in contrast, evidence has been reported from a prospective, crossover study that higher doses of IVIG are beneficial (114). IVIG does appear to decrease the incidence of severe bacterial infections in people with stable-phase MM. A double-blind, randomized, placebo-controlled multicenter study has shown a major impact of IVIG on infections in those with plateau-phase MM (115). Eighty-two patients with stable plateau-phase MM received IVIG at 400 mg/kg per month or placebo during 1 year. Concurrent chemotherapy was not altered, and no one received prophylactic antibiotics. There were major decreases in the incidence of pneumonia or sepsis and the overall incidence of infections in the group given IVIG. This protective effect was most marked in patients with a poor (less than twofold increase) response to pneumococcal vaccine (Pneumovax), suggesting that a subpopulation of those with MM and altered humoral immunity can be identified and treated with IVIG. On the basis of this information, prophylactic IVIG is likely to be beneficial for patients with advanced CLL or MM, although more information is needed.

Nephrosis and Protein-Losing Enteropathies

Infection has long been recognized as a complication of the nephrotic syndrome. People with these conditions are frequently hypogammaglobulinemic and individuals may benefit from IG therapy (116), but few controlled studies have been conducted from which to generalize. Among 86 consecutive adults with nephrotic syndrome and no diabetes, the relative risk of infection in individuals with a serum IgG level below 600 mg/dL was 6.74 times higher than in individuals with a serum IgG concentration above 600 mg/dL (117). This risk of infection was independent of the increased risk (5.31-fold) seen in those with creatinine values above 2.0 mg/dL. When IVIG was administered prospectively to patients with serum IgG levels below 600 mg/dL to raise it above that level, the rate of infection was reduced to that seen in those whose unmanipulated serum level was higher than

600 mg/dL. We believe that further studies in this area are warranted given these encouraging results.

PROPHYLAXIS AND TREATMENT IN TRANSPLANTATION

The major risk of death in transplantation is from infection related to immunosuppression. The most common and significant infection is that with CMV (118). CMV infection is associated with graft rejection, superinfections with both bacterial and fungal pathogens, serious morbidity, and death. Antirejection therapy, especially with OKT3 antibody or antilymphocyte serum, may increase the likelihood of infectious complications (119). In those who undergo bone marrow transplantation, an additional risk is graft-versus-host disease. High doses of IVIG or CMVIG attenuate the severity of CMV disease and appear to significantly improve survival in kidney and bone marrow transplantation (120,121). The benefit of IG therapy is most marked in CMV seronegative kidney transplant recipients whose donors are seropositive.

In a series of prospective studies of CMV seronegative recipients of kidney transplants from seropositive donors, using CMVIG given within 72 hours of transplantation and then at 2, 4, 6, 8, 12, and 16 weeks, highly significant reductions in CMV-associated syndromes (from 60% in control subjects to 31% in CMVIG recipients) were seen, as well as decreases of approximately 50% in graft loss and overall death. Fungal and parasitic superinfections were markedly reduced in CMVIG recipients, with an overall reduction in incidence from 20% to 4%. It appears that CMV induced immunosuppression, which when combined with transplantation provides the milieu for opportunistic fungal and protozoan infections, may be prevented by CMVIG. This appears true despite the fact that CMVIG does not appear to significantly alter infection rates in transplant recipients (122–124). Allograft rejection is often linked to CMV infection, and reducing the rate of symptomatic CMV disease with CMVIG may protect the allograft from damage. Furthermore, prophylaxis with CMVIG appears to be cost-effective (53).

Two studies examining IVIG use in liver transplant recipients suggested trends in reduction of CMV disease (125,126). In a randomized, double-blind, placebo-controlled trial of CMVIG in liver transplantation, globulin reduced the rate of CMV disease from 31% in the placebo group to 19% in the treated group, although, as might be expected, the infection rate was similar (61% and 57%) (126). A retrospective analysis of 39 primary orthotopic liver transplants revealed no symptomatic CMV disease or deaths after prophylaxis with CMVIG and ganciclovir. In this study, ganciclovir alone was reported to be ineffective as CMV prophylaxis (127); in a study of ganciclovir or acyclovir intravenous prophylaxis, ganciclovir alone reduced the CMV disease rate to 9%, but the effect was limited to CMV-seropositive recipients (128). Studies of combination ganciclovir and CMVIG prophylaxis in liver transplant recipients show some benefit of the combination over CMV immune globulin alone for the highest risk group, the CMV donor positive to CMV recipient group (129).

In heart transplant recipients, CMV hyperimmune IG may reduce the severity of CMV disease (130). New studies using combined CMV hyperimmune globulin and ganciclovir prophylaxis suggest that the combination reduces the likelihood of coronary intimal thickening in the transplanted heart and reduces the likelihood of coronary atherosclerosis (131). Prospective studies are needed to substantiate these data.

In a review of clinical uses for IVIG during marrow transplantation (120), Berkman and colleagues pooled the results of six controlled trials of prophylactic IgG for CMV infections in bone marrow transplantation (120) and concluded that prophylactic IgG decreases the incidence of CMV infection proceeding to interstitial pneumonia and of acute graft-versus-host (GVH) disease. A study of IVIG in bone marrow transplantation patients showed, in patients who received IVIG, a marked diminution in interstitial pneumonia; a decreased relative risk of gram-negative sepsis and local infections; and, in patients 20 years of age or older, a reduction in the incidence of acute GVH disease and a decrease in deaths in some human leukocyte antigen-identical subgroups (132). Several intravenous IGs have licensed indications for prevention of graft-versus-host disease. However, when shortages of IVIG occurred in 1999 to 2001, many centers abandoned use of IVIG to prevent GVHD.

There are some data that the use of high dose intravenous immune globulin or cytomegalovirus immune globulin combined with ganciclovir may improve the outcome of treatment for CMV interstitial pneumonia in bone marrow transplantation (133–135). The exact dose, timing, and duration have not been fully examined but many groups use a dose of 100 mg/kg of CMV immune globulin given intravenously every other day combined with intravenous ganciclovir. Animal models of lethal CMV infection support the concept that combination immunoglobulin and an antiviral are synergistic (136).

The use of intravenous immune globulin to prevent CMV disease in bone marrow transplantation has generally been abandoned with the advent of effective antiviral prophylaxis.

ACQUIRED IMMUNODEFICIENCY SYNDROME AND INTRAVENOUS IMMUNE GLOBULIN

Polyclonal hypergammaglobulinemia is common in HIV disease, and it is associated with a decreased response to neoantigens and immunizations. The data on the role of IVIG in individuals with HIV infection are confusing. It is helpful to remember that some trials have been done with unselected IVIG administration and others with hyperimmune anti-HIV plasma and to think of them separately.

Children with congenital HIV infection appear to have more profound humoral deficits than do adults with HIV, presumably because adults have a pool of memory cells that predates the HIV infection (137). Recurrent bacterial infection is a major problem in this group of children (138). A number of studies, some of which had crossover designs (none of which were prospective and randomized), have shown major benefits of IVIG therapy in pediatric HIV infection, with decreased episodes of infection, resolution of intractable diarrhea, and fewer hospital days (139–144).

Spector and colleagues (144) conducted a controlled trial of IVIG in children receiving azidothymidine for advanced HIV infection. They found a beneficial effect in children between the ages of 3 months and 12 years who received IVIG at 400 mg/kg every 28 days, compared with children who received a 0.1% albumin control solution. This decrease in the rate of infection of approximately 40% was most evident in children who were not receiving trimethoprim-sulfamethoxazole (TMP-SMX) prophylaxis for *Pneumocystis carinii* pneumonia. Paradoxically, the children who were receiving TMP-SMX prophylaxis and received IVIG had a higher rate of bacterial infection than did the control subgroup that was receiving TMP-SMX. In contrast, Mofenson and co-workers (145) found that IVIG was an effective prophylactic agent against bacterial infections in children. In an open-label study conducted as a follow-up to their randomized placebo-controlled study, they found that in the children who crossed over from placebo to IVIG, the rate of serious and of minor bacterial infections was significantly lower after the change. This decreased rate of infection was observed independently of the use of TMP-SMX. In contrast, in the group that had received IVIG during the first trial, there was no significant change in the rate of infection when IVIG was continued. We believe that there is a role for IVIG in children with AIDS, but that the exact indications are not yet understood and that prophylaxis with TMP-SMX probably independently diminishes the benefit of IVIG.

Lambert and Stiehm have reviewed the protective role of passive immunity in the prevention of maternal-fetal HIV transmission (146). There is no current indication for the use of IVIG during the pregnancy of HIV seropositive women, except perhaps for thrombocytopenia (147).

Yap (148) has summarized the current indications for IVIG for AIDS patients as the prevention or treatment of respiratory and other infections in children with AIDS, potentially infections in adults, idiopathic thrombocytopenic purpura, severe parvovirus B19 infection or measles, or autoimmune disorders in which IVIG is helpful. What subgroups of people with AIDS will benefit from IVIG is still unresolved. A common problem in HIV infection is thrombocytopenia. As in HIV-seronegative people, high-dose IVIG may produce a rise in platelet counts. It is unclear how long the benefit of IVIG lasts in this situation (149).

Because of improved enhancement of immunity through the use of highly active antiretroviral regimens, current practice does not generally include the use of intravenous immune globulin to prevent bacterial infections in HIV-infected individuals except for some of the indications noted below such as thrombocytopenia and parvovirus B19 infection.

MISCELLANEOUS CONDITIONS AND INDICATIONS FOR THERAPY

A number of other specific circumstances exist that clearly do, or may, benefit from IG, IVIG, or hyperimmune IVIG therapy (150). These include Kawasaki disease; the toxic shock syndrome; infections with parvovirus B19, RSV, and the hemorrhagic fever viruses; some enteric infections; and malaria (see Table 36.3).

Kawasaki Disease (Mucocutaneous Lymph Node Syndrome)

It is controversial whether there is an infectious agent in the mucocutaneous lymph node syndrome, or Kawasaki disease, but it is clear that IVIG is helpful in treatment of the disease. The current treatment of choice in Kawasaki disease is IVIG and aspirin (151,152). IVIG at a dose of 400 mg/kg per day for 5 days in conjunction with aspirin prevented more coronary artery lesions than did a lower dose of 100 or 200 mg/kg per day for the same period, and it has been noted that alkylated IVIG was less effective than native unaltered IVIG (153). Trials have shown that single-treatment, high-dose IVIG is also efficacious (154–156). Some authors have pointed out that a delay in treatment during the presentation of Kawasaki disease often leads to high incidence of coronary lesions, and given the safety of IVIG, have recommended the early use of IVIG when a child presents with a syndrome consistent with early Kawasaki disease. Recurrence of Kawasaki disease does not appear to be related to the use of IVIG during the primary episode. Possible mechanisms of action of intravenous immune globulin in Kawasaki syndrome include inhibition of cytokine induced endothelial activation, anti-idiotypic antibody inhibition of anti-endothelial antibodies, reduction of cytokine production, or the presence of antigen-specific antibodies which neutralize the causative microbe or toxin yet to be discovered. The mechanisms of action of IVIG in Kawasaki disease have been reviewed (35).

Toxic Shock Syndrome

Toxic shock syndrome (TSS), a syndrome mediated by a toxin that can be produced by either *S. aureus* or group A *Streptococcus*, can be prevented in experimental rabbit models using monoclonal antibodies to the toxin (157). Killing the invading bacteria with antimicrobial agents does not eliminate the toxic shock toxin, but the use of appropriately selected antibodies may. There is increasing evidence that the toxic shock syndrome is the result of superantigenic stimulation by the toxin, which is thought to bind to the major histocompatibility complex class II receptors of monocytes and macrophages outside the classic antigen groove. This toxin-receptor complex is then recognized nonspecifically by a broad variety of T lymphocytes, leading to nonspecific and disordered systemic release of IL1, TNF, and INF-γ (158). Experimental evidence supports the notion that IVIG inhibits superantigenic stimulation by staphylococcal toxins (159,160). Although no randomized trial of IVIG in toxic shock syndrome has been reported, the evidence suggests that adjunctive therapy with IVIG improves survival in patients with streptococcal TSS (161,162).

Parvovirus B19 Infection

Parvovirus B19, the ubiquitous causative agent of fifth disease (erythema infectiosum), can also cause persistent anemia in children with sickle cell disease (aplastic crisis), individuals with aplastic anemia, or individuals with immunosuppression such as those with AIDS or malignancies. In addition, parvovirus B19 appears to be a rare cause of fetal hydrops. Usually, development of specific antibody to the virus leads to termination of the infection. IVIG has been reported to be curative in all of these circumstances because resolution of the infection appears to be due to a neutralizing antibody response (163–165). There is no other known treatment besides IVIG for serious parvovirus B19 infection. Kurtzman and colleagues (165) have described a young man with aplastic anemia of 10 years' duration related to persistent parvovirus B19 infection. He had no IgG specific for a viral capsid protein and had high levels of immunoglobulin M. He was cured of the infection with IVIG that contained parvovirus-neutralizing IgG. In addition, it appears that superficially unrelated symptoms or syndromes may also resolve with IVIG. For example, Nigro and co-workers reported the successful use of IVIG in hypogammaglobulinemic infant with anemia and neurologic disorders (166). Finkel and colleagues (167) reported that three patients with a systemic necrotizing vasculitis and chronic parvovirus B19 infection had resolution of both the chronic infection and the vasculitis with IVIG after corticosteroids and cyclophosphamide failed to control the vasculitis.

Respiratory Syncytial Virus Infection

The FDA approved the licensure of hyperimmune anti-RSV IVIG in January 1996 (RespiGam, manufactured by the Massachusetts State Biological Laboratories) to prevent RSV disease in neonates and children younger than 24 months with bronchopulmonary dysplasia or a history of prematurity. RSV has been shown to be a major cause of death and morbidity in children with bronchopulmonary dysplasia, congenital heart disease, and immunodeficiency such as in AIDS or cancer (168–170). Adults undergoing bone marrow transplantation are also at risk of death resulting from RSV (171). Attempts to prevent RSV disease with vaccines in the 1960s resulted in an immunogenic product that

paradoxically exacerbated naturally acquired disease in vaccinated children. Epidemiologic studies in the 1970s found that infants with serum anti-RSV titers higher than 1:200 were at significantly less risk of bronchiolitis and pneumonia than children with lower antibody levels (172). Clinical trials with unselected IVIG and hyperimmune anti-RSV IVIG were conducted. Despite encouraging early results, unselected IVIG was not shown to be efficacious in reducing RSV morbidity and mortality in a series of trials, principally because commercial lots of IVIG did not contain sufficient amounts of RSV neutralizing antibody and could not achieve a 1:400 target titer after infusion (173–175). Siber and colleagues at the Massachusetts State Biological Laboratories then selected lots of IVIG for high anti-RSV activity by microneutralization techniques (176). This product was used in a randomized prospective trial in which RespiGam was given at a dose of 750 mg/kg monthly during three RSV transmission seasons to 274 infants and children at high risk of RSV disease because of chronic pulmonary disease (principally bronchopulmonary dysplasia), congenital heart disease, or premature birth (35 weeks of gestation or less). RespiGam reduced the frequency of RSV lower respiratory tract infection by 62%, and hospitalization was decreased by 57%; moreover, the need for the number of intensive care unit hospitalizations was nearly eliminated with a 97% decrease, and mechanical ventilation was completely eliminated (177). These benefits were not seen with a lower dose of 150 mg/kg. Efficacy of RSVIG in other groups, such as older children with congenital heart disease or cystic fibrosis, has not been established.

There have been several attempts to develop a monoclonal antibody against RSV. Two humanized monoclonal IgG antibodies directed against the F glycoprotein have evaluated the use of monthly intramuscular injections in high risk infants to prevent RSV disease. Interestingly only one of the two preparations demonstrated an effect (178). The monoclonal antibody that proved to be effective was palivizumab, Synagis (MedImmune). Studies showed that administration monthly in a dosage of 15 mg/kg reduced the incidence of RSV-associated hospitalization by 55% compared to placebo recipients (179). The use of the intramuscular product was well tolerated and the frequency and types of adverse events was no different from placebo. Current recommendations include use in infants less than 24 months of age with chronic lung disease who have required medical therapy within the past 6 months, neonates born at greater than 28 and less than 32 weeks' gestation without chronic lung disease who are less than 6 months of age at the start of RSV season, neonates born at 28 weeks' gestation or less without chronic lung disease who are less than 12 months of age at the start of RSV season, and neonates born between 32 and 35 weeks' gestation without chronic lung disease who are less than 6 months of age who have additional high risk factors including school age siblings, crowding in the home, day care attendance, exposure to tobacco smoke in the home, or multiple births. Recent data suggest that palivizumab will prevent RSV disease requiring hospitalization in infants with congenital cardiac disease (180). The use of palivizumab IM has generally superceded the use of intravenous RSVIG on the basis of ease of administration. There is insufficient data on use of palivizumab for therapy of RSV pneumonia in either children or adults with bone marrow transplantation.

Enteric Infections

This chapter has focused on the use of parenteral IGs, but gut mucosal immunity is increasingly recognized for its central role in host immunity. It is estimated that 70% to 80% of the IG-producing cells in humans are located in the intestinal mucosa, and the majority of antibodies produced daily are excreted into the gut (181). Many studies have shown the protective effects of breast milk (182). Eibl and colleagues (183,184) administered an oral IG preparation enriched in IgA to low-birth-weight neonates and found that it significantly decreased the incidence of necrotizing enterocolitis. This study was not "blinded" and had no control treatment group, yet necrotizing enterocolitis did not develop in 88 neonates given the supplement, but the disease developed in six of 91 control infants given standard feedings ($p = 0.0143$). It is likely that orally administered IG will be investigated for enteric diseases caused by enteric viruses, bacteria, and protozoa in high-risk or immunodeficient populations. Trials investigating hyperimmune antitoxin globulin preparations given enterically for refractory *Clostridium difficile* colitis are under way. *Cryptosporidium parvum*, which causes cholera-like watery diarrhea in immunocompromised people with cancer or AIDS, has occasionally been controlled if not cured after the administration of bovine hyperimmune anti-*Cryptosporidium* colostrum (185,186).

Hepatitis B Prevention

Hepatitis B hyperimmune globulin (HBIG) is derived from plasma donors who have been stimulated by immunization with hepatitis B vaccine and have high titers of antibody to hepatitis B surface antigen (HBsAg) (187). As an IM agent, HBIG is useful as postexposure prophylaxis to hepatitis B virus (HBV) and is always given in combination with HBV vaccine. The use of hepatitis B hyperimmune globulin has become common in prevention of hepatitis B in many settings where hepatitis B immunity is insufficient, and when hepatitis B vaccine may not be efficacious due to timing of exposure for prevention or lack of efficacy due to immunosuppression (188). For example, hepatitis B immune globulin may be given after a needle stick or birth to a hepatitis B carrier mother.

IV HBIG has been used to prevent recurrent HBV infection in HBsAg-positive patients who receive an orthotopic liver transplant. In Europe, frequent, long-term therapy with high doses of IV HBIG appears to reduce the recurrence of HBV infection (36%) compared to short term (3 month) therapy (74%) or no therapy (75%) at 2 years follow-up (189).

A recent U.S. study also demonstrated a benefit of IV HBIG prophylaxis in HBsAg positive liver transplant recipients (190). IV HBIG (10,000 IU) was given daily during the first 7 days post-transplantation and monthly thereafter. The 2-year recurrence rate of HBsAg was 19% with treatment compared to 76% in historical controls given no immunoprophylaxis. HBIG has been given intravenously (off label and not approved yet by the FDA) with the intramuscular solvent detergent treated and filtered HBIG preparation by NABI. This has become one of the modalities to prevent the recurrence of hepatitis B in orthotopic liver transplantation. Doses and protocols vary among institutions. Typically doses of 10,000 units are given during the an-hepatic phase of surgery and then daily for the first week after transplant, then weekly or every other week after transplant. Doses are given to maintain a level of anti-HBs at 500 milli-international units per milliliter (191). There are protocols to add the use of antiviral drugs as well to prevent the recurrence of hepatitis B after liver transplantation (192). The optimal regimen to prevent hepatitis B recurrence in this setting has not yet been determined.

Hemorrhagic Fever and Other Hemorrhagic Virus Infections

Lassa virus and other viruses such as Bolivian and Argentinian hemorrhagic fever viruses are arenaviruses transmitted from peridomestic rodents. Survival after Lassa fever is directly dependent on the development of neutralizing antibody (193). Infections with Lassa virus have been treated with immune plasma as well as ribavirin (193). It appears that either agent is efficacious if given within the first week of illness, and the agents are especially effective if given together. This finding is analogous to the finding that CMVIG and ganciclovir are more effective given together than alone in the treatment of CMV pneumonia after bone marrow transplantation. In view of the prohibitive cost of antiviral agents in the developing world, hyperimmune plasma pools may be the most reasonable way to treat symptomatic disease, especially if plasma can be screened for HIV and other blood-borne infectious agents.

Argentinian hemorrhagic fever is caused by Junin virus, which is closely related to Machupo virus, the causative agent of Bolivian hemorrhagic fever. In the 1960s, empirical therapy with convalescent plasma was found to be therapeutic during Argentinian hemorrhagic fever, and in a controlled trial of Argentinian hemorrhagic fever plasma mortality was reduced from 16% to 1% compared with the placebo group (194). Death usually occurs only in those given plasma after 8 days of illness or those given plasma with inadequate levels of neutralizing antibody (195). Other hemorrhagic fever viruses, such as *Nairovirus*, which causes Crimean-Congo hemorrhagic fever, and *Hantavirus*, are global in distribution. They may be candidates for hyperimmune preparations.

The thread that binds these diverse viral illnesses together would appear to be the ability of neutralizing antibody to prevent death. It can be argued that small lots of hyperimmune plasma should be available to public health authorities should outbreaks of these disease occur (195).

Malaria

Malaria is rapidly becoming resistant to drug therapy, and in some regions such as the Myanmar (Burma)-Thailand border region, *Plasmodium falciparum* resistance to mefloquine and other agents has been documented. An antimalarial IVIG preparation made from plasma donated in a malaria hyperendemic region of the Ivory Coast in Africa was administered to eight Thai patients with falciparum malaria. Asexual parasitemia was reduced by a mean of 728-fold, as fast as or faster than with drugs, and the effect was consistent in all eight patients (196). This study demonstrated that protective antibody is not geographically limited and, although not curative, it is quite beneficial. As therapeutic options become more limited for the treatment of malaria, it is possible that a low-volume hyperimmune antimalaria preparation of IVIG may have a treatment role in selected circumstances. We are anecdotally aware of clinicians in Africa treating cerebral malaria in children with chloroquine-resistant falciparum malaria with plasma, but to our knowledge no prospective trials have been conducted.

REFERENCES

1. Rousell RH, Pennington JE. An historical overview of immunoglobulin therapy. In: Yap PL, ed. *Clinical applications of intravenous immunoglobulin therapy.* Edinburgh: Churchill Livingstone, 1992:1–15.
2. Behring E. Zur Behandlung der Diphtherie mit Diptherie Heilserum. *Dtsch Med Wochenschr* 1893;19:543.
3. Ehrlich P. Die Wertbemessung des Diphtherieheilserums und deren theoretische Grundlagen. *Klin Jahrb* 1897;6:299.
4. Finland M. The serum treatment of lobar pneumonia. *N Engl J Med* 1930;202:1244.
5. Finland M. Adequate dosage in the specific serum treatment of pneumococcus type I pneumonia. *Am J Med Sci* 1936;192:849.
6. McKhann CF, Chu FT. Antibodies in placental extracts. *J Infect Dis* 1933;52:268.

7. McKhann CF, Greene AA, Coady H. Factors influencing the effectiveness of placental extract in the prevention and modification of measles. *J Pediatr* 1935;6:603.

8. Cohn EJ, Oncley JL, Strong LE, et al. Chemical, clinical and immunological studies on the products of human plasma fractionation. I. The characterization of protein fractions of human plasma. *J Clin Invest* 1944;23:417.

9. Ordman CW, Jenning CG, Janeway CA. Chemical, clinical, and immunological studies on the products of human plasma fractionation. XII. The use of concentrated normal human serum gammaglobulin (human immune serum globulin) in the prevention and attenuation of measles. *J Clin Invest* 1944;23:541.

10. Bruton OC. Agammaglobulinemia. *Pediatrics* 1952;9:722.

11. Dwyer JM. Thirty years of supplying the missing link. *Am J Med* 1984;73[Suppl 3A]:46.

12. Barandun S, Kistler P, Jeunet F, Isliker H. Intravenous administration of human gammaglobulin. *Vox Sang* 1962;7:157.

13. Lundblad JL, Londeree N. The effect of processing methods on intravenous immune globulin preparation. *J Hosp Infect* 1988;12[Suppl D]:3.

14. McIver J, Grady GF. Immunoglobulin preparations. In: Churchill WH, Kurtz SR, eds. *Transfusion medicine.* Boston: Blackwell Scientific, 1988:189–209.

15. Burks AW, Steele RW. Selective IgA deficiency. *Ann Allergy* 1986;57:3.

16. Apfelzeig R, Piskiewicz D, Hooper JA. Immunoglobulin A concentrations in commercial immune globulins. *J Clin Immunol* 1987;7:46.

17. Lewis RB, Matzke DS, Albrecht TB, Pollard RB. Assessment of the presence of cytomegalovirus-neutralizing antibody by a plaque-reduction assay. *Rev Infect Dis* 1986;8[Suppl 4]:S434.

18. Lundblad JL, Mitra G, Sternberg MM, Schroeder DD. Comparative studies of impurities in intravenous immunoglobulin preparations. *Rev Infect Dis* 1986;8[Suppl 4]:S382.

19. Yap PL, Williams PE. The safety of IVIG preparations. In: Yap PL, ed. *Clinical applications of intravenous immunoglobulin therapy.* Edinburgh: Churchill Livingstone, 1992:43–62.

20. Yang YH, Ngo C, Yeh IN, Uemura Y. Antibody Fc functional activity of intravenous immunoglobulin preparations treated with solvent-detergent for virus inactivation. *Vox Sang* 1994;67:337.

21. Uemura Y, Yang YH, Heldebrant CM, et al. Inactivation and elimination of viruses during preparation of human intravenous immunoglobulin. *Vox Sang* 1994;67:246.

22. Louie RE, Galloway CJ, Dumas ML, et al. Inactivation of hepatitis C virus in low pH intravenous immunoglobulin. *Biologicals* 1994;22:13.

23. Schiff RI. Half-life and clearance of pH 6.8 and pH 4.25 immunoglobulin G intravenous preparations in patients with primary disorders of humoral immunity. *Rev Infect Dis* 1986;8[Suppl 4]:5449.

24. Pirofsky B. Safety and toxicity of a new serum immunoglobulin G intravenous preparation, IGIV pH 4.25. *Rev Infect Dis* 1986;8[Suppl 4]:5457.

25. Weisman LE, Fischer GW, Hemming VG, Peck CC. Pharmacokinetics of intravenous immunoglobulin (Sandoglobulin) in neonates. *Pediatr Infect Dis* 1986;5[Suppl 3]:5185.

26. Arturson G, Hogman CF, Johansson SGO, Killander J. Changes in immunoglobulin levels in severely burned patients. *Lancet* 1969;1:546.

27. Munster AM, Hoagland HC, Pruitt BA Jr. The effect of thermal injury on serum immunoglobulins. *Ann Surg* 1970;172:965.

28. Hagenbeek A, Brummelhuis HGJ, Donkers A, et al. Rapid clearance of cytomegalovirus-specific IgG after repeated intravenous infusions of human immunoglobulin into allogeneic bone marrow transplant recipients. *J Infect Dis* 1987;155:897.

29. Snydman DR, McIver J, Leszczynski J, et al. A pilot trial of a novel cytomegalovirus immune globulin in renal transplant recipients. *Transplantation* 1984;38:553.

30. Snydman DR. Prevention of cytomegalovirus-associated diseases with immunoglobulin. *Transplant Proc* 1991;23[Suppl 1]:131.

31. Schiff RI. Intravenous gammaglobulin: pharmacology, clinical uses and mechanisms of action. *Pediatr Allergy Immunol* 1994;5:63.

32. Ballow M. Mechanisms of action of intravenous immune serum globulin therapy. *Pediatr Infect Dis J* 1994;13:806.

33. Weisman LE, Cruess DF, Fischer GW. Opsonic activity of commercially available standard intravenous immunoglobulin preparations. *Pediatr Infect Dis J* 1994;13:1122.

34. Van T, Sussman G, Pruzanski W. Impact of intravenous infusion of low and high doses of gamma globulins (IVIG) on phagocytic functions in adults with primary humoral immunodeficiency. *Inflammation* 1994;18:419.

35. Meissner HC, Schlievert PM, Leung DY. Mechanisms of immunoglobulin action: observations on Kawasaki syndrome and RSV prophylaxis. *Immunol Rev* 1994;139:109.

36. Aukrust P, Froland SS, Liabakk NB, et al. Release of cytokines, soluble cytokine receptors, and interleukin-1 receptor antagonist after intravenous immunoglobulin administration in vivo. *Blood* 1994;84:2136.

37. Sekul EA, Cupler EJ, Dalakas MC. Aseptic meningitis associated with high-dose intravenous immunoglobulin therapy: frequency and risk factors. *Ann Intern Med* 1994;121:259.

38. De Vlieghere FC, Peetermans WE, Vermylen J. Aseptic granulocytic meningitis following treatment with intravenous immunoglobulin. *Clin Infect Dis* 1994;18:1008.

39. Cantu TG, Hoehn-Saric EW, Burgess KM, et al. Acute renal failure associated with immunoglobulin therapy. *Am J Kidney Dis* 1995;25:228.

40. Pfeiffer RW, Siegel J, Ayers LW. Assessment of microbial growth in intravenous immune globulin preparations. *Am J Hosp Pharm* 1994;51:1676.

41. Schiff RI. Transmission of viral infections through intravenous immune globulin [Editorial]. *N Engl J Med* 1994;331:1649.

42. Mitra G, Wong MF, Mozen MM, et al. Elimination of infectious retroviruses during preparation of immunoglobulins. *Transfusion* 1986;26:394.

43. Wells MA, Wittek AE, Epstein JS, et al. Inactivation and partition of human T-cell lymphotrophic virus, type III, during ethanol fractionation of plasma. *Transfusion* 1986;26:210.

44. Bjoro K, Froland SS, Yun Z, et al. Hepatitis C infection in patients with primary hypogammaglobulinemia after treatment with contaminated immune globulin. *N Engl J Med* 1994;331:1607.

45. Yu MY, Mason BL, Tankersley DL. Detection and characterization of hepatitis C virus RNA in immune globulins. *Transfusion* 1994;34:596.

46. Yu MW, Mason BL, Guo ZP, et al. Hepatitis C transmission associated with intravenous immunoglobulins [Letter]. *Lancet* 1995;345:1173.

47. Nübling CM, Willkommen H, Löwer J. Hepatitis C transmission associated with intravenous immunoglobulins [Letter]. *Lancet* 1995;345:1174.

48. Tabor E, Gerety RJ. Transmission of hepatitis B by immune serum globulin. *Lancet* 1979;2:1293.

49. Tabor E, Aronson DL, Gerety RJ. Removal of hepatitis B virus infectivity from factor IX complex by hepatitis B immune globulin. Experiments in chimpanzees. *Lancet* 1980;2:69.

50. Hellstem P. Clinical experience with the viral safety of immunoglobulins. *Blood Coagul Fibrinol* 1994;5[Suppl 3]:531.

51. Kama P, Murray DL, Valduss D, et al. Passive transfer of hepatitis antibodies during intravenous administration of immune globulin. *J Pediatr* 1995;125:463.

52. Bielory L, Long GC. Home health care costs: intravenous immunoglobulin home infusion therapy. *Ann Allergy Asthma Immunol* 1995;74:265.

53. Tsevat J, Snydman DR, Pauker SG, et al. Which renal transplant patients should receive cytomegalovirus immune globulin? A cost-effectiveness analysis. *Transplantation* 1991;52:259.

54. Jorgensen F, Andersson B, Hanson LA, et al. Gamma-globulin treatment of recurrent acute otitis media in children. *Pediatr Infect Dis J* 1990;9:389.

55. Committee on Infectious Diseases, American Academy of Pediatrics. *The report of the committee on infectious diseases,* 25th ed. Elk Grove Village, IL: American Academy of Pediatrics, 2000.

56. Centers for Disease Control. Recommendations of the Immunization Practices Advisory Committee (ACIP): recommendations for prevention against viral hepatitis. *MMWR* 1985;34:313, 329.

57. ACP Task Force on Adult Immunization and Infectious Diseases Society of America. *Guide for adult immunizations,* 2nd ed. Philadelphia: American College of Physicians, 1990.

58. Gershon AA, Steinberg S, Brunnell PA. Zoster immune globulin: a further assessment. *N Engl J Med* 1974;290:243.

59. Respiratory syncytial virus hyperimmune globulin (RespiGam) package insert. Jamaica Plain, MA: Massachusetts State Biological Laboratories and MedImmune.

60. Wilde H, Chutivongse S. Equine rabies immune globulin: a product with an undeserved poor reputation. *Am J Trop Med Hyg* 1990;42:175.

61. Santosham M, Reid R, Ambrosino DM, et al. Prevention of *Haemophilus influenzae* type b infections in high-risk infants treated with bacterial polysaccharide immune globulin. *N Engl J Med* 1987;317:923.

62. Cohen J. Intravenous immunoglobulin (IVIG) for gram-negative infection-A critical review. *J Hosp Infect* 1988;12[Suppl D]:47.

63. Natanson C, Hoffman WD, Suffredini AF, et al. Selected treatment strategies for septic shock based on proposed mechanisms of pathogenesis. *Ann Intern Med* 1994;120:771.

64. Ziegler EJ, McCutchan JA, Fierer J, et al. Treatment of gram-negative bacteremia and shock with human antiserum to a mutant UDP-GAL epimerase deficient mutant *Escherichia coli. N Engl J Med* 1982;307:1225.

65. Baumgartner JD, Gauser MP, McCutcheon JA, et al. Prevention of gram-negative shock and death in surgical patients by antibody to endotoxin core glycolipid. *Lancet* 1985;2:59.

66. Greisman SE, Johnston CA. Failure of antisera to J5 and 8595 rough mutants to reduce endotoxemic lethality. *J Infect Dis* 1988;157:54.

67. Ziegler EJ. Protective antibody to endotoxin core: the emperor's new clothes? *J Infect Dis* 1988;158:286.

68. Ziegler EJ, Fisher CJ Jr, Sprung CL, et al, for The HA-1A Sepsis Study Group. Treatment of gram-negative bacteremia and septic shock with HA-1A human monoclonal antibody against endotoxin: a randomized, double-blind placebo-controlled trial. *N Engl J Med* 1991;324:429.

69. Greenman R, Schein R, Martin M, et al. A controlled clinical trial of E5 murine monoclonal IgM antibody to endotoxin in the treatment of gram-negative sepsis. *JAMA* 1991;266:1097.

70. McCloskey RV, Straube RC, Sanders C, et al. Treatment of septic shock with human monoclonal antibody HA-1A. *Ann Intern Med* 1994;121:1.

71. Cross AS. Antiendotoxin antibodies: a dead end? [Editorial]. *Ann Intern Med* 1994;121:58–59.

72. Alejandria MM, Lansang MA, Dans LF, Mantaring JB. Intravenous immunoglobulin for treating sepsis and septic shock. *Cochrane Database Syst Rev* 2002;(1):CD001090.

73. Roifman CM, Levison H, Gelfand EW. High-dose versus low-dose intravenous immunoglobulin in hypogammaglobulinaemia and chronic lung disease. *Lancet* 1987;1:1075.

74. Rosen FS, Cooper MD, Wedgwood RJP. The primary immunodeficiencies (1). *N Engl J Med* 1984;311:235.

75. Rosen FS, Cooper MD, Wedgwood RJ. The primary immunodeficiencies (2). *N Engl J Med* 1984;311:300.

76. Beard LJ, Ferrante A. Aspects of immunoglobulin replacement therapy. *Pediatr Infect Dis J* 1990;9[Suppl 8]:554.

77. Radford DJ, Thong YH. The association between immunodeficiency and congenital heart disease: a review. *Pediatr Cardiol* 1988;9:103.

78. Loh RKS, Harth SC, Thong YH, Ferrante A. Immunoglobulin G subclass deficiency and predisposition to infection in Down's syndrome. *Pediatr Infect Dis J* 1990;9:547.

79. Thong YH. Clinical value of IgG subclass investigations in pediatric practice. *Pediatr Infect Dis J* 1990;9:S36.

80. Björkander J, Bengtsson U, Oxelius V, Hanson LA. Symptoms in patients with lowered levels of IgG subclasses, with or without IgA deficiency, and effects of immunoglobulin prophylaxis. *Monogr Allergy* 1986;20:157.

81. Schiff RI. Intravenous gammaglobulin: pharmacology, clinical uses and mechanisms of action. *Pediatr Allergy Immunol* 1994;5:63.

82. Schiff RI. Intravenous gammaglobulin, 2: pharmacology, clinical uses and mechanisms of action. *Pediatr Allergy Immunol* 1994;5:127.

83. Gonzalez LA, Hill HR. The current status of intravenous gammaglobulin use in neonates. *Pediatr Infect Dis J* 1989;8:315.

84. Edwards MS. Complement in neonatal infections: an overview. *Pediatr Infect Dis* 1986;5[Suppl 3]:S168.

85. Wilson CB, Lewis DB. Basis and implications of selectively diminished cytokine production in neonatal susceptibility to infection. *Rev Infect Dis* 1990;12[Suppl 4]:S410.

86. Berger M. Complement deficiency and neutrophil dysfunction as risk factors for bacterial infection in newborns and the role of granulocyte transfusion in therapy. *Rev Infect Dis* 1990;12[Suppl 4]:401.

87. Baker CJ, Melish ME, Hall RT, et al. Intravenous immune globulin for the prevention of nosocomial infection in low-birth-weight neonates. *N Engl J Med* 1992;327:213.

88. Weisman LE, Stoll BJ, Kueser TJ, et al. Intravenous immune globulin therapy for early-onset sepsis in premature neonates. *J Pediatr* 1992;121:434.

89. Cairo MS, Worcester CC, Rucker RW, et al. Randomized trial of granulocyte transfusions versus intravenous immune globulin therapy for neonatal neutropenia and sepsis. *J Pediatr* 1992;120:281.

90. Paul V. Immunoglobulin prophylaxis does not prevent nosocomial infections in very low birth weight neonates. *Natl Med J India* 1995;8:24.

91. Ohlsson A, Lacy JB. Intravenous immunoglobulin for preventing infection in preterm and/or low-birth-weight infants. *Cochrane Database System Rev* 2001;(2):CD000361.

92. Ohlsson A, Lacy JB. Intravenous immunoglobulin for suspected or subsequently proven infection in neonates. *Cochrane Database System Rev* 2001;(2):CD001239.

93. Snydman DR, Werner BG, Meissner HC, et al. Use of cytomegalovirus immunoglobulin in multiply transfused, premature neonates. *Pediatr Infect Dis J* 1995;14:34.

94. Pruitt BA, McManus AT. Opportunistic infections in severely burned patients. *Am J Med* 1984;76[Suppl 3A]:146.

95. Liljedahl S-O, Olhagen B, Plantin L-O, Birke G. Studies on burns. VII. The problem of infection, with special reference to gammaglobulin. *Acta Chir Scand* 1963;309[Suppl]:3.

96. Collins MS, Roby RE. Protective activity of an intravenous immune globulin (human) enriched in antibody against lipopolysaccharide antigens of *Pseudomonas aeruginosa*. *Am J Med* 1984;76[Suppl 3A]:168.

97. Stone HH, Graber CD, Martin JD Jr, Kolb L. Evaluation of gamma globulin for prophylaxis against burn sepsis. *Surgery* 1965;58:810.

98. Wesley J, Fisher A, Fisher MW. Immunization against *Pseudomonas* in infection after thermal injury. *J Infect Dis* 1974;130[Nov Suppl]:S152.

99. Jones RJ, Roe EA, Gupta JL. Controlled trial of *Pseudomonas* immunoglobulin and vaccine in burn patients. *Lancet* 1980;2:1263.

100. Waymack JP, Jenkins ME, Alexander JW, et al. A prospective trail of prophylactic intravenous immune globulin for the prevention of infections in severely burned patients. *Burns* 1989;15:71.

101. Munster AM, Moran KT, Thupari J, et al. Prophylactic intravenous immunoglobulin replacement in high-risk burn patients. *J Burn Care Rehabil* 1987;8:376.

102. Grob P, Holch M, Fierz W, et al. Immunodeficiency after major trauma and selective surgery. *Pediatr Infect Dis J* 1988;7:537.

103. Zanetti G, Glauser MP, Baumgartner J-D. Use of immunoglobulins in prevention and treatment of infection in critically ill patients: review and critique. *Rev Infect Dis* 1991;13:985.

104. Cometta A, Baumgartner J-D, Lee ML, et al. Prophylactic intravenous administration of standard immune globulin as compared with core-lipopolysaccharide immune globulin in patients at high risk of postsurgical infection. *N Engl J Med* 1992;327:234.

105. Gipponi M, Canova G, Bonalumi U, et al. Immunoprophylaxis in "septic risk" patients undergoing surgery for gastrointestinal cancer. Results of a randomized, multicenter clinical trial. *Int Surg* 1993;78:63.

106. Broder S, Humphrey R, Durm M, et al. Impaired synthesis of polyclonal (nonparaprotein) immunoglobulins by circulating lymphocytes from patients with multiple myeloma. *N Engl J Med* 1975;293:887.

107. Besa EC. Recent advances in the treatment of chronic lymphocytic leukemia: defining the role of intravenous gammaglobulin. *Semin Hematol* 1992;29:14.

108. Cooperative Group for the Study of Immunoglobulin in Chronic Lymphocytic Leukemia. Intravenous immunoglobulin for the prevention of infection in chronic lymphocytic leukemia. A randomized, controlled clinical trial. *N Engl J Med* 1988;319:902.

109. Griffiths H, Brennan V, Lea J, et al. Crossover study of immunoglobulin replacement therapy in patients with low-grade B-cell tumors. *Blood* 1989;73:366.

110. Jurlander J, Geisler CH, Hansen MM. Treatment of hypogammaglobulinaemia in chronic lymphocytic leukaemia by low-dose intravenous gammaglobulin. *Eur J Haematol* 1994;53:114.

111. Gamm H, Huber C, Chapel H, et al. Intravenous immune globulin in chronic lymphocytic leukaemia. *Clin Exp Immunol* 1994;97[Suppl 1]:17.

112. Weeks JC, Tierney MR, Weinstein MC. Cost effectiveness of prophylactic intravenous immune globulin in chronic lymphocytic leukemia. *N Engl J Med* 1991;325:81.

113. Salmon SE, Samal BA, Hayes DM, et al. Role of gammaglobulin for immunoprophylaxis in multiple myeloma. *N Engl J Med* 1967;277:1336.

114. Schedel I. Application of immunoglobulin preparations in multiple myeloma. In: Morrell A, Nydegger UE, eds. *Clinical uses of intravenous immunoglobulins.* London: Academic Press, 1986:123–132.

115. Chapel HM, Lee M, Hargreaves R, et al, for The UK Group for Immunoglobulin Replacement Therapy in Multiple Myeloma. Randomised trial of intravenous immunoglobulin as prophylaxis against infection in plateau-phase multiple myeloma. *Lancet* 1994;343:1059.

116. Wilfert CM, Katz SL. Etiology of bacterial sepsis in nephrotic children, 1963-1967. *Pediatrics* 1968;42:840.

117. Ogi M, Yokoyama H, Tomosugi N, et al. Risk factors for infection and immunoglobulin replacement therapy in adult nephrotic syndrome. *Am J Kidney Dis* 1994;24:427.

118. Emmanuel D. Treatment of cytomegalovirus disease. *Semin Hematol* 1990;27:22–27.

119. Snydman DR. Prevention of cytomegalovirus disease with intravenous immune globulin. *Transplant Proc* 1991;23[Suppl 1]:20.

120. Berkman SA, Lee ML, Gale RP. Clinical uses of intravenous immunoglobulins. *Ann Intern Med* 1990;112:278.

121. Champlin RE, Ho WG, Winston DJ. Acute graft-vs.-host disease and interstitial pneumonitis interrelated problems following allogeneic bone marrow transplantation: effects of intravenous immune globulin and other interventions. *J Hosp Infect* 1988;12[Suppl D]:29.

122. Snydman DR, Werner BG, Heinze-Lacey B, et al. Use of cytomegalovirus immune globulin to prevent cytomegalovirus disease in renal-transplant recipients. *N Engl J Med* 1987;317:1049.

123. Snydman DR, Werner BG, Tilney NL, et al. A final analysis of primary cytomegalovirus disease prevention in renal transplant recipients with a cytomegalovirus immune globulin: comparison of randomized and open-label trials. *Transplant Proc* 1991;23:1357.

124. Werner BG, Snydman DR, Freeman R, et al. Cytomegalovirus immune globulin for the prevention of primary CMV disease in renal transplant patients: analysis of usage under treatment IND status. *Transplant Proc* 1993;25:1442.

125. Saliba F, Arulnaden JL, Gugenheim J, et al. CMV hyperimmune globulin prophylaxis after liver transplantation: a prospective randomized controlled study. *Transplant Proc* 1989;21:2260.

126. Snydman DR, Werner BG, Dougherty NN, et al. Cytomegalovirus immune globulin prophylaxis in liver transplantation. A randomized, double-blind, placebo-controlled trial. *Ann Intern Med* 1993;119:984.

127. Prian GW, Koep LJ. Elimination of cytomegalovirus disease in liver transplant patients treated prophylactically with combination cytomegalovirus hyperimmune globulin and ganciclovir. *Transplant Proc* 1994;26[Suppl 1]:54.

128. Winston DJ, Wirin D, Shaked A, Busuttil RW. Randomised comparison of ganciclovir and high-dose acyclovir for long-term cytomegalovirus prophylaxis in liver-transplant recipients. *Lancet* 1995;346:69.

129. Snydman DR, Falagas ME, Avery R, et al. Use of combination cytomegalovirus immune globulin plus ganciclovir for prophylaxis. *Transplant Proc* 2001;33(4):2571–2575.

130. Schafers HJ, Wahlers T, Jurmann M, et al. Hyperimmunoglobulin for cytomegalovirus prophylaxis following heart transplantation. *J Hosp Infect* 1998;12[Suppl D]:61.

131. Valantine HA, Luikart H, Doyle R, et al. Impact of cytomegalovirus hyperimmune globulin on outcome after cardiothoracic transplantation: a comparative study of combined prophylaxis with CMV hyperimmune globulin plus ganciclovir versus ganciclovir alone. *Transplantation* 2001;72:1647–1652.

132. Sullivan KM, Kopecky KJ, Jocom J, et al. Immunomodulatory and antimicrobial efficacy of intravenous immunoglobulin in bone marrow transplantation. *N Engl J Med* 1990;323:705.

133. Emmanuel D, Cunningham I, Jules-Elysee K, et al. Cytomegalovirus pneumonia after bone marrow transplantation successfully treated with the combination of ganciclovir and high-dose intravenous immune globulin. *Ann Intern Med* 1988;109:777.

134. Reed EC, Bowden RA, Dandliker PS, et al. Treatment of cytomegalovirus pneumonia with ganciclovir and intravenous cytomegalovirus immunoglobulin in patients with bone marrow transplants. *Ann Intern Med* 1988;109:783.

135. Schmidt GM, Horak DA, Niland JC, et al. A randomized, controlled trial of prophylactic ganciclovir for cytomegalovirus pulmonary infection in recipients of allogeneic bone marrow transplants. *N Engl J Med* 1991;324:1005.

136. Rubin RH, Lynch P, Pasternack MS, Schoenfeld D, Medearis DN Jr. Combined antibody and ganciclovir treatment of murine cytomegalovirus-infected normal and immunosuppressed BALB/c mice. *Antimicrob Agents Chemother* 1989;133:1975–1979.

137. Bernstein LJ, Ochs HD, Wedgwood RJ, Rubinstein A. Defective humoral immunity in pediatric acquired immune deficiency syndrome. *J Pediatr* 1985;107:352.

138. Krasinski K, Borkowsky W, Bonk S, et al. Bacterial infections in human immunodeficiency virus-infected children. *Pediatr Infect Dis J* 1988;7:323.

139. Calvelli TA, Rubinstein A. Intravenous gammaglobulin in infant acquired immunodeficiency syndrome. *Pediatr Infect Dis* 1986;5[Suppl 3]:S207.

140. Oleske JM, Connor EM, Bobila R, et al. The use of IVIG in children with AIDS. *Vox Sang* 1987;52:172.

141. Schaad UB, Gianella-Borradori A, Perret B, et al. Intravenous immune globulin in symptomatic pediatric human immunodeficiency virus infection. *Eur J Pediatr* 1988;147:300.

142. Williams PE, Hague RA, Yap PL, et al. Treatment of human immunodeficiency virus antibody positive children with intravenous immunoglobulin. *J Hosp Infect* 1988;12[Suppl D]:67.

143. Hague RA, Yap PL, Mok JYQ, et al. Intravenous immunoglobulin in HIV infection: Evidence for the efficacy of treatment. *Arch Dis Child* 1989;64:1146.

144. Spector SA, Gelber RD, McGrath N, et al. A controlled trial of intravenous immune globulin for the prevention of serious bacterial infections in children receiving zidovudine for advanced human immunodeficiency virus infection. *N Engl J Med* 1994;331:1181.

145. Mofenson LM, Moye J Jr, Korelitz J, et al, for The National Institute of Child Health and Human Development Intravenous Immunoglobulin Clinical Trial Study Group. Crossover of placebo patients to intravenous immunoglobulin confirms efficacy for prophylaxis of bacterial infections and reduction of hospitalization in human immunodeficiency virus-infected children. *Pediatr Infect Dis J* 1994;13:477.

146. Lambert JS, Stiehm ER. Passive immunity in the prevention of maternal-fetal transmission of human immunodeficiency virus infection. *Ann NY Acad Sci* 1993;693:186.

147. Mandelbrot L, Schlienger I, Bongain A, et al. Thrombocytopenia in pregnant women infected with human immunodeficiency virus: maternal and neonatal outcome. *Am J Obstet Gynecol* 1994;171:252.

148. Yap PL. Does intravenous immune globulin have a role in HIV-infected patients? *Clin Exp Immunol* 1994;97[Suppl 1]:59.

149. Pollak AN, Janinis J, Green D. Successful intravenous immune globulin therapy for human immunodeficiency virus-associated thrombocytopenia. *Arch Intern Med* 1988;148:695.

150. Ratko TA, Burnett DA, Foulke GE, et al. Consensus statement. Recommendations for off-label use of intravenously administered immunoglobulin preparations. *JAMA* 1995;273:1865.

151. Plotkin SA, Daum RS, Giebink GS, et al. Intravenous *y*-globulin use in children with acute Kawasaki disease. *Pediatrics* 1988;82:122.

152. Rowley AH, Schulman ST. What is the status of intravenous gamma-globulin for Kawasaki syndrome in the United States and Canada? *Pediatr Infect Dis J* 1988;7:463.

153. Onouchi Z, Yanagisawa M, Hirayama T, et al. Optimal dosage and differences in therapeutic efficacy of IGIV in Kawasaki disease. *Acta Paediatr Jpn* 1995;37:40.

154. Engle MA, Fatica NS, Bussel JB, et al. Clinical trial of singledose intravenous gamma globulin in acute Kawasaki disease. *Am J Dis Child* 1989;143:1300.

155. Barron KS, Murphy DJ, Silverman ED, et al. Treatment of Kawasaki syndrome: a comparison of two dosage regimens of intravenously administered immune globulin. *J Pediatr* 1990;117:638.

156. Newburger JW, Takahashi M, Beiser AS, et al. A single intravenous infusion of gamma globulin as compared with four infusions in the treatment of acute Kawasaki syndrome. *N Engl J Med* 1991;324:1633.

157. Best GK, Scott DF, Kling JM, et al. Protection of rabbits in an infection model of toxic shock syndrome (TSS) by a TSS toxin-1-specific monoclonal antibody. *Infect Immun* 1988;56:998.

158. Zumla A. Superantigens, T cells, and microbes. *Clin Infect Dis* 1992;15:313.

159. Takei S, Arora YK, Walker SM. Intravenous immunoglobulin contains specific antibodies inhibitory to activation of T cells by staphylococcal toxin superantigens. *J Clin Invest* 1993;91:602.

160. Dwyer JM. Manipulating the immune system with immune globulin. *N Engl J Med* 1992;326:107.

161. Kaul R, McGeer A, Norrby-Teglund A, et al, for The Canadian Streptococcal Study Group. Intravenous immunoglobulin therapy for streptococcal toxic shock syndrome—a comparative observational study. *Clin Infect Dis* 1999;28:800–807.

162. Schlievert PM. Use of intravenous immunoglobulin in the treatment of staphylococcus and streptococcal toxic shock syndromes and related illnesses. *J Allergy Clin Immunol* 2001;108[4 Suppl]:S107–S110.

163. Pattison JR, Jones SE, Hodgson J, et al. Parvovirus infections and hypoplastic crisis in sickle-cell anaemia. *Lancet* 1981;1:664.

164. Kurtzman GJ, Frickhofen N, Kimball J, et al. Pure red cell aplasia of ten years' duration due to B19 parvovirus infection and its cure with immunoglobulin therapy. *N Engl J Med* 1989;321:519.

165. Frickhofen N, Abkowitz JL, Safford M, et al. Persistent B19 parvovirus infection in patients infected with human immunodeficiency virus-1: a treatable cause of anemia in AIDS. *Ann Intern Med* 1990;113:926.

166. Nigro G, D'Eufemia P, Zerbini M, et al. Parvovirus B19 infection in a hypogammaglobulinemic infant with neurologic disorders and anemia: successful immunoglobulin therapy. *Pediatr Infect Dis J* 1994;13:1019.

167. Finkel TH, Torok TJ, Ferguson PJ, et al. Chronic parvovirus B19 infection and systemic necrotising vasculitis: opportunistic infection or aetiological agent? *Lancet* 1994;343:1255.

168. Groothuis JR, Gutierrez KM, Lauer BA. Respiratory syncytial virus infections in children with bronchopulmonary dysplasia. *Pediatrics* 1988;82:199.

169. MacDonald NE, Hall CB, Suffin SC, et al. Respiratory syncytial viral infection in infants with congenital heart disease. *N Engl J Med* 1982;307:397.

170. Hall CB, Powell KR, MacDonald NE, et al. Respiratory syncytial virus infection in children with compromised immune function. *N Engl J Med* 1986;315:77.

171. Hertz MI, Englund JA, Snover D, et al. Respiratory syncytial virus-induced acute lung injury in adult patients with bone marrow transplants: a clinical approach and review of the literature. *Medicine (Baltimore)* 1989;68:269.

172. Parrot RH, Kim HK Arrobio JOP, et al. Epidemiology of respiratory syncytial virus in Washington DC. II. Infection and disease with respect to age, immunologic status, race, and sex. *Am J Epidemiol* 1973;98:289.

173. Hemming VG, Rodriguez W, Kim HW, et al. Intravenous immunoglobulin treatment of respiratory syncytial virus infections in infants and young children. *Antimicrob Agents Chemother* 1987;31:1882.

174. Groothuis JR, Levin MJ, Rodriguez W, et al. Use of intravenous gamma globulin to passively immunize high-risk children against respiratory syncytial virus: safety and pharmacokinetics. *Antimicrob Agents Chemother* 1991;35:1469.

175. Meissner HC, Fulton DR, Groothuis JR, et al. Controlled trial to evaluate protection of high risk infants against respiratory syncytial virus disease by using standard intravenous immune globulin. *Antimicrob Agents Chemother* 1993;37:1655.

176. Siber GR, Leszczynski J, Pena-Cruz V, et al. Protective antibody of a human respiratory syncytial virus immune globulin prepared from donors screened by microneutralization assay. *J Infect Dis* 1992;165:456.

177. Groothuis JR, Simoes EAF, Levin ML, et al. Prophylactic administration of respiratory syncytial virus immune globulin to high-risk infants and young children. *N Engl J Med* 1993;329:1524.

178. The IMPACT Study Group. Reduction of respiratory syncytial virus hospitalization among premature infants and infants with bronchopulmonary dysplasia using respiratory syncytial virus monoclonal antibody prophylaxis. *Pediatrics* 1998;102:531–537.

179. Meissner HC, Welliver RC, Chartrand SA, et al. Immunoprophylaxis with palivizumab, a humanized respiratory syncytial virus monoclonal antibody, for prevention of respiratory syncytial virus infection in high risk infants: a consensus opinion. *Pediatr Infect Dis J* 1999;18:223–231.

180. Sondheimer HM, Cabalka AK, Feltes TF, Piazza FM, Connor EM, and the Cardiac Synagis Study Group. Palivizumab (PV) reduces hospitalization due to respiratory syncytial virus (RSV) in young children with serious congenital heart disease (CHD). *Pediatr Cardiol* 2002;23:664.

181. Brandtzaeg P. Overview of the mucosal immune system. *Curr Top Microbiol Immunol* 1989;146:13.

182. Welsh JK, May JT. Anti-infective properties of breast milk. *J Pediatr* 1979;94:1.

183. Eibl MM, Wolf HM, Fumkranz H, Rosenkranz A. Prevention of necrotizing enterocolitis in low-birth-weight infants by IgA-IgM. *N Engl J Med* 1988;319:1.

184. Eibl MM, Wolf HM, Furnkranz H, Rosenkranz A. Prophylaxis of necrotizing enterocolitis by oral IgA-IgG: review of a clinical study in low birth weight infants and discussion of the pathogenic role of infection. *J Clin Immunol* 1990;10[Nov Suppl]:S72.

185. Tzipori S, Robertson D, Cooper DA, et al. Chronic cryptosporidial diarrhoea and hyperimmune cow colostrum. *Lancet* 1987;2:344.

186. Ungar BLP, Ward DJ, Fayer RF, et al. Cessation of cryptosporidium-associated diarrhea in an acquired immunodeficiency patient after treatment with hyperimmune bovine colostrum. *Gastroenterology* 1990;98:486.

187. Samuel D, Muller R, Alexander G, et al. Liver transplantation in european patients with the hepatitis B surface antigen. *N Engl J Med* 1993;329:1842–1847.

188. McGory RW, Ishitani MB, Oliveira WM, et al. Improved outcome of orthotopic liver transplantation for chronic hepatitis B cirrhosis with aggressive passive immunization. *Transplantation* 1996;61:1358–1364.

189. Terrault NA, Zhou S, Combs C, et al. Prophylaxis in liver transplant recipients using a fixed dosing schedule of hepatitis B immunoglobulin. *Hepatology* 1996;24:1327–1333.

190. Rosenau J, Bahr MJ, Tillmann HL, et al. Lamivudine and low-dose hepatitis B immune globulin for prophylaxis of hepatitis B reinfection after liver transplantation possible role of mutations in the YMDD motif prior to transplantation as a risk factor for reinfection. *J Hepatol* 2001;34:943–945.

191. Marzan A, Salizzoni M, Debernardi-Venon W, et al. Prevention of hepatitis B virus recurrence after liver transplantation in cirrhotic patients treated with lamivudine and passive immunoprophylaxis. *J Hepatol* 2001;34:903–910.

192. Jahrling PB, Peters CJ. Passive antibody therapy of lassa fever in cynomolgus monkeys: importance of neutralizing antibody and lassa virus strain. *Infect Immun* 1984;44:528.

193. Jahring PB, Frame JD, Rhoderick JB, Monson MH. Endemic lassa fever in liberia. IV. Selection of optimally effective plasma for treatment by passive immunization. *Trans R Soc Trop Med Hyg* 1985;79:380.

194. Maiztegui JI, Fernandez N, Damilano A. Efficacy of immune plasma in treatment of Argentine haemorrhagic fever and association between treatment and a late neurological syndrome. *Lancet* 1979;2:1216.

195. Griffiths JK, Snydman DR. The use of intravenous immunoglobulin in viral infections. In: Yap PL, ed. *Clinical applications of intravenous immunoglobulin therapy.* Edinburgh: Churchill Livingstone, 1992:167–202.

196. Sabchareon A, Burnouf T, Ouattara D, et al. Parasitologic and clinical human response to immunoglobulin administration in falciparum malaria. *Am J Trop Med Hyg* 1991;45:297.

IV

Prevention of Infectious Diseases

CHAPTER 37
Immunization of Children and Adults

Jerome O. Klein

Immunization may be achieved by active or passive means. Active immunity is achieved when an appropriate antigen stimulates immune cells to produce protective antibodies. Passive immunity is achieved by introduction of preformed protective antibodies.

The vaccine products available in the United States (as of March 2002) are listed in Table 37.1. Eleven products are considered for universal immunization of children, including diphtheria and tetanus toxoids and acellular pertussis vaccine (DTaP); live measles, mumps, and rubella virus vaccines (MMR); inactivated poliovirus vaccine (IPV); hepatitis B virus (HBV) vaccine; varicella virus vaccine; and conjugate *Haemophilus influenzae* type B (Hib) vaccine and heptavalent conjugate pneumococcal polysaccharide vaccine (PCV-7). Fourteen vaccines are available for special circumstances: (a) six virus vaccines, including Japanese B encephalitis, hepatitis A, influenza, rabies, yellow fever vaccines, and vaccinia; and (b) eight bacterial vaccines, including anthrax, bacille Calmette-Guérin (BCG), cholera, Lyme disease, meningococcal polysaccharide, plague, pneumococcal polysaccharide, and typhoid vaccines. Combined products include DTaP, MMR, and Hib vaccine plus DTaP or HBV, Hib plus HBV and IPV, and a recently approved HBV and hepatitis A virus (HAV) vaccine.

Products available in 2002 for protection by passive immunization include immune globulin (IG) prepared from pooled plasma of adults and used for replacement therapy in antibody-deficiency disorders, HAV prophylaxis, and measles prophylaxis. Specific IGs are prepared from blood of donors with high titers of the desired antibodies. Current specific IGs include hepatitis B IG (HBIG), rabies IG (RIG), tetanus IG (TIG), varicella-zoster IG (VZIG), and respiratory syncytial virus IG (RSVIG). In addition, palivizumab, a humanized mouse monoclonal antibody that is administered intramuscularly, is available for children younger than 24 months at high risk of respiratory syncytial virus (RSV) infection.

Recommendations for use of new vaccines and use of modified old ones are frequent, so health care personnel must be alert for changes. Important sources of vaccine information include *Morbidity and Mortality Weekly Reports (MMWR)*, which is published weekly by the Centers for Disease Control and Prevention (CDC), which also publishes regular and special recommendations of the Advisory Committee on Immunization Practices (ACIP) of the U.S. Public Health Service. Guidelines for use of vaccines in children and adults are published at regular intervals by the American Academy of Pediatrics (AAP) *(Report of the Committee on Infectious Diseases)*, the American College of Physicians *(Guide for Adult Immunization)*, the American Academy of Family Physicians, the American College of Obstetricians and Gynecologists (technical bulletins), state and local health departments, and the Division of Immunization of the CDC. Addresses and telephone numbers for these sources are provided in the *MMWR* (1989;38:205). A textbook by Plotkin and Orenstein provides extensive discussions of available vaccines (1). In addition, there are a number of web sites of value including the CDC *(www.cdc.gov)*, the National Network for Immunization Information *(www.immunizationinfo.org)*, and the Vaccine Page *(www.unisci.com)*.

GENERAL ISSUES OF ADMINISTRATION OF VACCINES

Constituents of Vaccines

Vaccines consist of an antigen that elicits production of protective antibody; a suspending fluid, which may include materials derived from the system used to produce the vaccine; preservatives to prevent bacterial contamination or stabilize the antigen; and sometimes adjuvants that amplify the immunogenic effect. The most effective and frequently used preservative, thimerosal, is an ethyl mercury and has been eliminated from most pediatric vaccines because of concern for mercury toxicity. Patients may have allergic reactions to a constituent of the vaccine: Egg proteins are present in measles, mumps, influenza, and yellow fever vaccines, and patients who have demonstrated severe allergy to eggs should not receive these products; trace amounts of antibiotics present in oral poliovirus vaccine (OPV) (streptomycin and neomycin) and MMR (neomycin) vaccines may provoke reactions in persons allergic to the drugs.

Route and Schedule of Immunization

The package insert should be consulted to determine the optimal site for administration of the vaccine (see Table 37.1). Vaccine schedules (Table 37.2) are constructed to take into account the earliest time a person can respond to the antigen and the time of life when protection is needed (i.e., age at highest incidence and morbidity of the disease). For some vaccines, a compromise is necessary to provide maximal protection for most persons; pertussis vaccine is less immunogenic in early infancy, but young

TABLE 37.1. Vaccine Products Available in the United States, by Type and Recommended Routes of Administration

Vaccine	Type	Route
Anthrax	Inactivated bacteria	Subcutaneous
BCG (bacille Calmette-Guérin)	Live bacteria	Intradermal or subcutaneous
Cholera	Inactivated bacteria	Subcutaneous or intradermal[a]
DTaP (diphtheria, tetanus, and acellular pertussis)	Toxoids and bacterial products	Intramuscular
DTP (diphtheria, tetanus, pertussis)	Toxoids and inactivated bacteria	Intramuscular
HB (hepatitis B)	Inactive viral antigen	Intramuscular
Haemophilus influenzae b Polysaccharide (HbPV) or conjugate (HbCV) (Hib)	Bacterial polysaccharide or polysaccharide conjugate	Subcutaneous or intramuscular[b]
HbCV + DTP	Combined product	Intramuscular
HbCV + DTaP[c]	Combined product	Intramuscular
HB + HbCV	Combined product	Intramuscular
Hepatitis A	Inactivated virus	Intramuscular
Influenza	Inactivated virus or viral components	Intramuscular
IPV (inactivated poliovirus vaccine)	Inactivated viruses of all three serotypes	Subcutaneous
Japanese encephalitis	Inactivated virus	Subcutaneous
Lyme disease	Recombinant outer surface protein	Intramuscular
Measles	Live virus	Subcutaneous
Meningococcal	Bacterial polysaccharides of serotypes A/C/Y/W-135	Subcutaneous
MMR (measles, mumps, rubella)	Live viruses	Subcutaneous
Mumps	Live virus	Subcutaneous
OPV (oral poliovirus vaccine)	Live viruses of all three serotypes	Oral
Pertussis, acellular	Bacterial products	Intramuscular
Plague	Inactivated bacteria	Intramuscular
Pneumococcal	Bacterial polysaccharides of 23 pneumococcal types or polysaccharide conjugate for 7 serotypes	Intramuscular or subcutaneous
Rabies	Inactivated virus	Subcutaneous or intradermal[d]
Rubella	Live virus	Subcutaneous
Smallpox (vaccinia)	Live animal poxvirus	Multiple puncture
Tetanus	Inactivated toxin (toxoid)	Intramuscular[e]
Td or DT[f] (tetanus, diphtheria)	Inactivated toxins (toxoids)	Intramuscular[e]
Typhoid, oral	Live bacteria	Oral
Typhoid, parenteral	Inactivated bacteria	Subcutaneous[g]
Typhoid polysaccharide	Capsular polysaccharide	Intramuscular
Varicella	Live virus	Subcutaneous
Yellow fever	Live virus	Subcutaneous

[a]The intradermal dose is lower.
[b]Route depends on the manufacturer; consult package insert for recommendation for specific product used.
[c]Available only for administration as the fourth dose in the DTaP series for children 15 months or older.
[d]Intradermal dose is lower and used only for preexposure vaccination.
[e]Preparations with adjuvants should be given intramuscularly.
[f]DT, tetanus, and diphtheria toxoids for use in children younger than 7 years; Td, tetanus, and diphtheria toxoids for use in persons 7 years or older. Td contains the same amount of tetanus toxoids as DTP or DT, but a reduced dose of diphtheria toxoid.
[g]Boosters may be given intradermally unless acetone-killed and dried vaccine is used.

infants are the group at greatest risk of natural infection. Other schedules need to be considered for children not immunized in the first year of life or for children living in developing countries with limited medical facilities.

Vaccine schedules are changed periodically; the interested reader should consult current reports from the ACIP published in *MMWR* and the reports of the Committee on Infectious Diseases of the AAP The two advisory groups work together to develop uniform recommendations. The current recommended childhood immunization schedules were published in January 2002 (2).

Adverse Reactions

No vaccine is completely safe. Adverse reactions of varying severity, both local and systemic, are relatively frequent with some vaccines (pertussis, parenteral typhoid) and infrequent

with others (polysaccharide vaccines). Contraindications to the first or subsequent immunization are identified in the reports of the Committee on Infectious Diseases of the AAP and in statements of the ACIP in *MMWR* and are outlined later in the sections on special populations and in discussions of the vaccines. Because of misconceptions about reasons to withhold vaccines, the ACIP included a review (3) of conditions that were not contraindications to immunization, including mild acute illness, current antimicrobial therapy, premature exposure to an infectious disease, breast-feeding, history of non–vaccine-associated allergies, and family history of convulsions or sudden infant death. Reporting of specific adverse events is mandated by the National Childhood Vaccine Injury Act, which became effective in March 1988.

Allergy to egg or egg products should be considered when administering measles, mumps, influenza, or yellow fever vaccines. Severe reactions to egg antigens are rare after administration of these vaccines, but the products should be avoided in

TABLE 37.2. Recommended Schedule for Active Immunization of Normal Infants and Children: 2003

Recommended age	Immunizations	Comments
Birth	HBV	Birth is the preferred age for the first dose; infants born Hb$_s$Ag-positive mothers should receive HBIG
1–2 mo	HBV	Antigen-negative mothers at 0–2 mo, dose 2 at 4 mo, and dose 3 at 6–18 mo.
2 mo	DTaP, Hib, PCV-7, IPV	
4 mo	DTaP, Hib, PCV-7, IPV	
6 mo	DTaP, Hib, PCV-7, IPV	Third dose of IPV can be given between 6 and 18 mo
12–15 mo	Hib, PCV-7	
12–18 mo	Varicella	
15–18 mo	DTaP	I
12–15 mo	MMR	
4–6 yr	DTaP, IPV	
11–12 yr	MMR	MMR alternatively may be administered at 4–6 yr
	Td	

Note: Approved by the Advisory Committee on Immunization Practices, American Academy of Pediatrics, and the American Academy of Family Physicians. For all products used, consult manufacturer's package insert for instructions for storage, handling, dosage, and administration. Biologics prepared by different manufacturers may vary, and package inserts of the same manufacturer may change from time to time. Therefore, the physician should be aware of the contents of the current package insert.
DTaP, diphtheria and tetanus toxoids with acellular pertussis vaccine; HBV, hepatitis B virus vaccine; IPV, inactivated poliovirus vaccine containing poliovirus types 1, 2, and 3; MMR, live measles, mumps, and rubella viruses in a combined vaccine (see text for discussion of single vaccines versus combination); Hib, *Haemophilus infuenzae* type b conjugate vaccine; PCV-7, heptavalent pneumococcal conjugate polysaccharide vaccine; Td, adult tetanus toxoid (full dose) and diphtheria toxoid (reduced dose) for adult use.

patients with histories of anaphylactic reactions to egg or egg products.

Simultaneous Administration of Vaccines

Use of multiple products in a single-dose form and simultaneous administration of vaccines is the rule (see Table 37.2). For infants who may not return for well-child care and for those who have not received vaccines or are behind schedule, administration of all vaccines appropriate for age is warranted and appears to be satisfactory in terms of immune response. For example, DTaP, MMR, Hib vaccine, PCV-7/HBV, and IPV may be administered at the same visit.

Combination Vaccines

The increased number of new and improved vaccines to prevent childhood diseases has lead to more combination vaccines to reduce the number of injections during single clinic visits (4). Combination vaccines available for many years include diphtheria toxoid, tetanus toxoid, and pertussis (DTP) and MMR. Combinations licensed recently include DTaP, DTaP-Hib, and Hib-HBV. A bivalent vaccine containing yeast-derived recombinant hepatitis B surface antigen (HBsAg) and inactivated HAV was introduced in 2001 in the United States for use in adults but has not been approved for use in children. Limitations to further combinations include chemical incompatibility or immunologic interference when different antigens are combined. Vaccine combinations that require different schedules may cause confusion. Nevertheless, fewer shots because of increased use of combination vaccines should increase compliance with approved vaccine schedules in children.

Immunization after Exposure to Disease

Because of the prolonged incubation period, immunization may be valuable for unimmunized patients after exposure to rabies, measles (within 3 days of exposure), HBV, and tetanus (if the primary series was incomplete). Administration of rabies and hepatitis vaccines and tetanus toxoids should be accompanied by the specific IG. Rubella and mumps vaccines are ineffective when given after the exposure.

Special Patients

PREGNANT WOMEN

Because of the paucity of data about effects of vaccines on the fetus, pregnant women should receive immunizing products only for approved indications. Live-virus vaccines are contraindicated except for yellow fever vaccine, which may be administered to susceptible women who must travel to endemic areas. In the United States, tetanus and diphtheria vaccines are recommended for unimmunized pregnant women. Influenza vaccine should be considered for women who have a cardiorespiratory disorder that would place them at risk if infected.

IMMUNODEFICIENT PATIENTS

Live-virus vaccines are contraindicated for patients who are immunodeficient. Inactivated vaccines may be used for immunodeficient patients, although their efficacy varies with the stage of the disease. Patients with asymptomatic or symptomatic human immunodeficiency virus (HIV) infection should receive inactivated vaccines on schedule (5). Children aged 2 years and older with HIV infection should receive, in addition, pneumococcal, meningococcal, and Hib vaccines. Live vaccines with the exception of MMR are contraindicated for children with symptomatic

HIV infection. Because measles in children with acquired immunodeficiency syndrome (AIDS) tends to be severe, the ACIP suggests that both symptomatic and asymptomatic children with HIV infection be given MMR.

ADOLESCENTS AND COLLEGE STUDENTS

Adolescents and young adults may be incompletely protected from diseases for which vaccines are available because vaccines were never provided, were ineffective, or were administered at inappropriate ages or by inappropriate routes, or because protection has waned over time. Outbreaks of measles, mumps, rubella, and pertussis in high schools and colleges have underlined the need for systems to identify appropriate vaccine histories and to initiate primary or repeated immunization. Single cases and clusters of invasive meningococcal disease in high schools and colleges have lead to recommendations for students living in dormitories (particularly the first year of dormitory life). Adolescent immunization is part of a program of comprehensive health services for adolescents. The vaccine initiative is directed to those who are 11 to 12 years of age and includes booster doses of MMR, tetanus and diphtheria toxoids, and HBV immunization for those who have not completed the series previously, and varicella vaccine for those who do not have protective antibody from immunization or prior infection.

HEALTH CARE PROFESSIONALS

For adults whose occupations place them in contact with patients with contagious diseases, protection by immunization is important to them and to their patients. Hospitals, clinics, and private offices should have policies for immunizing health care workers against measles, rubella, influenza, HBV, and varicella.

REFUGEES

Refugees' vaccine histories usually are unavailable. In addition, vaccines used in the home country may not have been adequate for durable protection. Vaccines may be administered in camps or at the sites of embarkation before arrival in the United States. In the absence of documentation, the physician must assume that the patient received no prior immunization. Patients may be given multiple vaccines simultaneously to bring them up to standard schedules for age.

FOREIGN TRAVELERS

Because endemic and epidemic disease may vary in time and place, travelers must be provided with information and appropriate vaccines by the responsible physician. Current information available from the CDC is published in the annual booklet *Health Information for International Travel* (available from the Superintendent of Documents, U.S. Government Printing Office, Washington, DC 20402).

DIPHTHERIA AND TETANUS TOXOIDS AND ACELLULAR PERTUSSIS VACCINES

DTP vaccine (now DTaP) has been used widely for routine immunization of children in the United States since about 1945. The primary series of DTaP is administered at 2, 4, and 6 months, with a booster dose administered at 18 months and between 4 and 6 years. Outbreaks of pertussis and diphtheria and decreased protective levels of antibody to DTP in adolescents and adults indicate the need for repeated immunization. After the child's seventh birthday, primary immunization should consist of adult-type tetanus toxoid and a reduced dose of diphtheria toxoid (Td); boosters should be administered every 10 years throughout life at mid-decade ages (15 years, 25 years, and so on).

Diphtheria Toxoid

Diphtheria toxoid is prepared from a strain of *Corynebacterium diphtheriae* that is known to produce large amounts of toxin and grown in a liquid medium to enhance toxin production. The toxin is incubated with formalin to prepare the toxoid and is subsequently adsorbed onto an aluminum salt.

Although no controlled trials have been performed to evaluate the efficacy of diphtheria toxoid in preventing disease, efficacy is believed to be more than 80% and disease is milder in immunized patients. Universal immunization likely contributes to the low incidence of disease now in the United States; fewer than five cases of diphtheria per year have been reported since 1980 (6) However, many adults lack protective antibody. A serologic survey in north London showed that 25% of those aged 20 to 29 years were susceptible and 52.8% of those aged 50 to 59 years (7).

Epidemic diphtheria began in 1990 in the New Independent States of the former Soviet Union. More than 140,000 cases and more than 4,000 deaths occurred from 1990 to 1998. An important factor in the outbreak was the presence of a large number of susceptible children and adults, which enabled the spread of toxigenic strains of *C. diphtheriae* (8). Since the epidemic began, cases of diphtheria associated with the outbreak have been reported in patients in Eastern and Western Europe and in U.S. citizens working in or visiting the former Soviet Union. The epidemic underlines the need for renewed efforts to maintain diphtheria immunization schedules throughout life.

Tetanus Toxoid

Like diphtheria toxoid, tetanus toxoid is prepared by formalin inactivation of the toxin. Although tetanus is a completely preventable disease, 70 to 100 cases occur in the United States each year (9), principally in older adults. A population-based serologic survey of immunity to tetanus in the United States identified decreased protective levels of tetanus antibodies in adolescents and adults; the rate decreased from 87.7% among those 6 to 11 years of age to 27.8% among those 70 years or older (10). After the primary series, protection against tetanus (and diphtheria) is sustained by scheduling booster doses routinely every 10 years.

Postexposure wound management includes consideration of both tetanus toxoid (administered as DTP or DTaP for children younger than 7 years and Td to older persons) and TIG. If the wound occurs within 10 years of the third of a series of doses of tetanus toxoid, neither toxoid nor TIG is necessary. If more than 10 years has elapsed since the last dose, or if the immunization history is unknown or consisted of fewer than three doses, tetanus toxoid is administered for both clean minor wounds and contaminated severe wounds. In patients with unknown or incomplete history of tetanus toxoid immunization, TIG is added for contaminated wounds.

Pertussis Vaccines

A whole-cell pertussis vaccine has been documented to be 80% to 90% effective in preventing disease and to reduce the morbidity of disease in vaccinees who develop whooping cough. The major concern has been local and systemic reactions. Neurologic reactions include brief seizures that occur in association with approximately 1 in 1,750 doses administered, usually within 12 to 24 hours of immunization and frequently associated with fever (11); it is estimated that the association of acute encephalopathy with permanent neurologic sequelae is 1 in 310,000 doses (12).

To maintain the immunogenicity of the whole-cell vaccine but limit reactivity, investigators have sought a safe and effective acellular, or subunit, vaccine. Pertussis antigens have been identified that are believed to contribute to the development of antibodies for pertussis protection: Lymphocytosis-promoting factor (LPF) or pertussis toxoid (PT) play a role in attachment of the organism to ciliated respiratory cells and in propagation of the infection; filamentous hemagglutinin (FHA) is associated with attachment of organisms to the host cell; agglutinogens induce agglutinating antibodies, which correlate with clinical protection; and pertactin (P), a 69-kd outer membrane protein, is immunogenic in humans. Four products incorporating one or more pertussis antigens are now available in combination with DT: Tripedia (PT, FHA); Acel-Imune (PT, FHA, P and fimbria 2); Infanrix (PT, FHA, P); and Certiva (PT). In clinical trials, the acellular pertussis vaccines were equivalent to or more effective than the whole-cell vaccines. Significantly fewer local and systemic reactions occurred after the acellular pertussis vaccines compared with the whole-cell vaccines. Because of the lesser reactivity and comparable efficacy, acellular pertussis vaccines have replaced whole-cell vaccines for primary series and boosters (13).

Outbreaks of pertussis in junior and senior high schools and colleges suggest waning immunity to pertussis in adolescents and young adults and the need to reconsider booster doses with the acellular pertussis vaccines in this population. From 1989 to 1998, the incidence of pertussis increased in Massachusetts adolescents and adults; by 1998, 92% of cases occurred in adolescents and adults (14). The increased incidence may be due in part to availability of a specific serologic test and active surveillance in Massachusetts. Although the disease is usually relatively mild in adults, with the major sign being persistent cough, adults serve as a reservoir for spread of infection to infants and young children.

Studies of the safety of acellular vaccines in adolescents and young adults are in progress. Booster doses in adolescent and adult groups may prevent or diminish morbidity of the disease and reduce transmission of infection to infants and young children (15).

MEASLES, MUMPS, AND RUBELLA VACCINES

The MMR live-virus vaccines are administered in one preparation at 15 months of age. A second dose of vaccine is now recommended for measles only but is for practical purposes administered as MMR. Contraindications to MMR include known pregnancy, anaphylaxis to egg ingestion, anaphylactic allergy to neomycin, compromised immunity (except for HIV infection), and recent administration of IG. Suggested intervals between IG and administration of MMR depend on the indication for IG, varying between 3 months after intramuscular IG for HAV prophylaxis to 11 months for intravenous IG administered for idiopathic thrombocytopenia or Kawasaki's disease.

Measles Vaccine

Live attenuated measles vaccine is prepared by multiple passage in chick embryos. The vaccine was introduced in the United States in 1966 and has been responsible for a decline in cases of more than 98%. An increase in incidence of measles was apparent beginning in 1986, when measles cases were reported from 46 states. Although most cases occurred in preschool-aged children who had not been immunized, many of those affected were immunized teenagers and young adults who contracted the disease in outbreaks in high schools and colleges. The increased incidence of measles in persons who had been properly immunized prompted the AAP and ACIP to recommend a second dose

of vaccine (16). Their recommendations include the following measures:

1. Two doses of measles vaccine for all children after the first birthday, with the first dose administered as MMR at 12 to 15 months of age and the second on entrance to grade or junior high school. Age for initial vaccination should be lowered to 6 months in outbreak areas if cases are occurring in children younger than 1 year.
2. Colleges and other institutions beyond high school should require documentation of two doses of measles-containing vaccines before entry of students.
3. Health care workers born after January 1, 1957, should receive two doses of MMR or measles vaccine (if there is no history of measles or laboratory evidence of measles immunity). The 1957 date was chosen because of the assumption that virtually all children born before that date had had natural measles.

In contrast to those with other disorders that are accompanied by immunologic defects, children with HIV infection should receive live measles vaccine. The live vaccine is suggested for these patients because of reports of severe and often fatal natural measles in children with HIV infection and disease and the lack of complications from the live-virus vaccine in these patients.

A purported association of MMR vaccine and autistic-spectrum disorder has received much public and political attention. However, there is no credible evidence that supports the hypothesis that MMR vaccine causes autism or associated disorders (17).

Mumps Vaccine

Live mumps virus vaccine is prepared in chick embryo cell cultures. The vaccine was licensed in 1967 and is believed to be more than 98% effective in providing durable protection. An increase in the number of mumps cases has been noted since 1986 by the CDC (18). The relative increase in mumps cases is believed to be due to failure to vaccinate susceptible persons, particularly teenagers.

Rubella Vaccine

Live rubella virus vaccine was licensed in 1969. The current product in the United States is produced in human diploid cell culture. Serum antibody is produced in almost all recipients and provides durable, perhaps lifelong, immunity. Viremia occurs after immunization, and virus has been recovered from placental and fetal tissues. To investigate potential teratogenicity, the CDC in 1971 established a registry of women who had received a rubella vaccine within 3 months before or after conception. None of 212 live-born infants of susceptible women who received the currently used (human diploid) rubella vaccine had signs of congenital rubella syndrome (19). Because of the theoretic risk of teratogenicity, the CDC continues to recommend that rubella vaccine not be given to pregnant women, but it is not necessary to screen for pregnancy before administering the vaccine.

Susceptible postpubertal girls and women in the childbearing years should be encouraged to receive rubella vaccine (when not pregnant). Both male and female college students, day care personnel, health care workers, and military recruits should be immunized for their protection and to limit spread of infection to contacts.

Arthritis (usually of small peripheral joints) has been reported in up to 15% of susceptible postpubertal women who were immunized with the human diploid vaccine. Chronic arthritis and neuropathies have been reported after vaccination of adult women. Other side effects include a mild rubella-like illness with rash, fever, and lymphadenopathy.

LIVE ORAL AND KILLED PARENTERAL POLIO VACCINES

IPV was introduced in the United States in 1955 and was used extensively until OPV was licensed in 1961; OPV became the standard material for primary immunization of all but immuno-compromised patients, and IPV use rapidly declined to a level of less than 1% of polio vaccines used in the United States. Extensive use of OPV has been extraordinarily successful. The Western Hemisphere is now free of paralytic polio caused by wild poliovirus; the last case of paralytic disease occurred in 1991 in Peru. Poliovirus infection remains endemic in central and West Africa and in Southeast Asia. Because of the continued incidence of OPV-associated paralytic disease, the AAP now recommends a four-dose all-IPV vaccine schedule for routine immunization of infants and children in the United States (20).

Although the immunization policy in the United States resulted in elimination of endemic poliomyelitis, cases of paralytic poliomyelitis were associated with administration of OPV. The approximate risk of vaccine-associated paralytic disease in the United States was 1 case per 2.4 million doses of OPV vaccine distributed. The rate after the first dose was approximately 1 case per 750,000 doses, including vaccine recipient and contact cases (20). A more potent IPV was licensed by the U.S. Food and Drug Administration (FDA) in April 1988. The new IPV is produced in a human diploid cell line grown on microcarriers in suspension culture and has been termed *enhanced-potency IPV*. No serious adverse events, including vaccine-associated paralytic disease, have been associated with IPV.

The current recommendation in the United States to use only IPV is based on the absence of wild poliovirus in the Western Hemisphere and the concern that the only paralytic polio disease likely to be encountered by children and contacts in the United States was due to OPV. Although OPV continues to be used in developing countries to complete the program for worldwide eradication of poliovirus disease, the continued burden of OPV vaccine–associated paralytic polio can no longer be justified in areas where wild polio is no longer present.

VARICELLA VACCINE

In March 1995, the FDA approved a live attenuated varicella virus vaccine for individuals 12 months and older who have not had varicella. The OKA strain of virus used in the vaccine is attenuated by passage in human and embryonic guinea pig cell cultures. More than 2 million doses had been given in Japan and Korea before approval by the FDA in the United States. The development of the live attenuated varicella vaccine and current recommendations for vaccine use were reviewed by the Committee on Infectious Diseases of the AAP (21).

A single dose of the vaccine resulted in seroconversion in more than 95% of children 1 to 12 years of age. Seroconversion in 13- to 17-year-olds was 79% and in adults was 82% after one dose and 94% after two doses. In children, the vaccine was approximately 70% effective in prevention of disease but more than 95% effective against more severe disease. Approximately 70% of adults who converted after immunization are protected against varicella; the remaining 30% of these adults may developed attenuated disease after close exposure.

Adverse events are minimal. Maculopapular rash or vesicular lesions may occur in 7% of susceptible children and 8% of susceptible adolescents and adults. The frequency of zoster is less in vaccinated individuals than after natural infection. Transmission of the vaccine virus from healthy vaccinees to susceptible contacts is possible, because virus has been recovered from skin lesions of vaccinees, but no clinical cases of varicella from contact with healthy vaccinees have been reported.

A single subcutaneous dose is recommended for healthy children between 1 and 12 years of age. Two doses of varicella vaccine 4 to 8 weeks apart are recommended for healthy adolescents and adults with no history of varicella. The vaccine should not be given routinely to patients who are immunocompromised or patients in households with potentially immunocompromised contacts. Pregnant women should not receive this live-virus vaccine because the effects on fetal development are unknown.

POLYSACCHARIDE AND POLYSACCHARIDE CONJUGATE VACCINES: PNEUMOCOCCAL, MENINGOCOCCAL, AND *HAEMOPHILUS INFLUENZAE* TYPE B VACCINES

The capsular polysaccharides of Hib, *Streptococcus pneumoniae*, and *Neisseria meningitidis* produce protective antibodies in patients older than 2 years. Because the highest age-specific attack rates for invasive disease due to these three encapsulated species occur in infants younger than 2 years, a more effective immunogen was needed to provide consistent concentrations of protective antibody. Conjugated polysaccharide vaccines using proteins to amplify the immune response stimulated protective levels of antibody in infants as young as 2 months. Coupling the polysaccharide to protein carriers stimulates a T-cell–dependent response. Conjugate Hib vaccine was introduced in October 1990 and has virtually eliminated invasive disease due to *H. influenzae* type B in areas where the vaccine has been extensively used. Conjugate pneumococcal vaccine (PCV-7) was introduced in the United States in the spring of 2000. A meningococcal group C conjugate vaccine was approved for use in the United Kingdom as a response to a widespread outbreak but is not yet approved in the United States.

Pneumococcal Vaccines

A 23-type vaccine composed of capsular polysaccharide antigens was licensed in the United States in 1983, replacing a 14-type vaccine licensed in 1977. Each polysaccharide antigen is prepared separately and stimulates a type-specific immune response. Currently, there are two licensed pneumococcal polysaccharide vaccines available in the United States. Each contains 23 purified pneumococcal capsular polysaccharide serotypes: 1, 2, 3, 4, 5, 6B, 7F, 8, 9V, 10A, 11A, 12F, 14, 15B, 17A (Wyeth-Lederle vaccines) or 17F (Merck Vaccines), 18C, 19A, 19F, 20, 22F, 23F, and 33F. The current vaccine includes capsular antigens for approximately 90% of the types responsible for bacteremic pneumococcal disease in the United States. Protective levels of antibody are available for 5 to 10 years in adults. However, the polysaccharide vaccine is not immunogenic for infants 2 years and younger. In children older than 2 years who received the polysaccharide vaccine, concentrations of antibody will fall to unprotective levels in 3 to 5 years. Based on these serologic data, the AAP recommends reimmunization after 3 to 5 years for children and adults who remain at high risk of invasive pneumococcal disease.

The first pneumococcal vaccine capable of eliciting protective antibodies in infants—a conjugate heptavalent pneumococcal vaccine (PCV-7)—was approved by the FDA in February 2000. The vaccine contains the polysaccharides of *S. pneumoniae* serotypes 4, 6B, 9V, 14, 18C, 19F, and 23 F conjugated to a non-toxic diphtheria protein CRM 197. About 80% of cases of invasive pneumococcal disease and more than 60% of episodes of acute otitis media in the United States are due to serotypes included in the vaccine. In a clinical trial involving approximately 38,000 infants in northern California, the conjugate vaccine was 97.4% effective in preventing pneumococcal invasive disease caused by vaccine serotypes (22). The vaccine was less effective in reducing the incidence of acute otitis media; children who received PCV-7 had approximately 7% fewer episodes than children who received the control vaccine (22,23). The vaccine elicits an antibody response to all seven serotypes after primary immunization and produces an amnestic response after a booster dose. The conjugate vaccine is recommended for universal immunization of infants 2 years and younger and for selected children with risk features who are 2 to 5 years of age. The polysaccharide vaccine should be used in conjunction with the conjugate vaccine in children 2 to 5 years of age who are high risk including patients with sickle cell disease, functional or anatomic asplenia, HIV infection, or nephrotic syndrome; those about to have cytoreduction therapy for Hodgkin's disease; and those who have cerebrospinal fluid leaks.

Meningococcal Vaccines

With the success of the *H. influenzae* type B conjugate vaccine, *N. meningitidis*, and *S. pneumoniae* are the leading causes of bacterial meningitis in all age-groups. In the United Sates, most invasive meningococcal disease is caused by serogroups B, C, and Y. A quadrivalent vaccine against groups A, C, Y, and W-135 is available. No vaccine is available for group B. Development of an immunogenic group B vaccine is of particular importance because this group remains a major cause of meningococcal disease throughout the world including the United States. Group A vaccine is immunogenic in children as young as 5 months, but the other meningococcal group vaccines are poor immunogens in children younger than 2 years. Efficacy of a meningococcal serogroup C conjugate vaccine in toddlers and teenagers led to approval of the product in Great Britain in 2000 (24). The incidence of invasive meningococcal disease in adolescents and young adults of high school and college age has recently increased in the United States (25). This has led to recommendations that meningococcal polysaccharide vaccine be offered to the group at highest risk: college freshman who are dormitory residents. The vaccine is given to all U.S. military personnel and has significantly reduced the incidence of endemic and epidemic disease at military bases.

Current applications of meningococcal vaccine include the following:

1. Immunoincompetent children and adults, including those with functional or anatomic asplenia and those with terminal complement deficiencies
2. Contacts of a patient with invasive meningococcal disease (secondary cases may occur several weeks after the index case)
3. Travelers to countries with epidemic disease
4. College students

Haemophilus influenzae Type B Vaccines

In April 1985, the FDA licensed a polysaccharide vaccine for Hib infections. Because it was a poor immunogen in children 2 years and younger (the age-group with the highest attack rate for invasive Hib disease), the vaccine was of limited value (26). In October 1990, the FDA approved use of a conjugate vaccine; an oligosaccharide nontoxic mutant diphtheria toxin protein vaccine for infants at 2, 4, and 6 months of age, with a booster at 12 to 15 months. The approval was based on the results of a single study in northern California that enrolled more than 30,000 children and identified a decrease in invasive disease of more than 90% in those who received two or more doses (27). Subsequent approval was given also for a conjugate vaccine incorporating an outer membrane protein of group B meningococcus to be administered on a schedule of 2, 4, and 12 months of age. The conjugate vaccines have been extraordinarily successful; in areas with high rates of immunization, invasive disease caused by Hib is now a rare occurrence. The success of the vaccine in populations with partial immunization was believed to be due to reduction in nasopharyngeal carriage of Hib, thereby interrupting transmission of infection (28).

VIRUS VACCINES FOR SPECIFIC POPULATIONS OR SPECIAL INDICATIONS

Influenza Virus Vaccines

Influenza virus vaccines are prepared in embryonated eggs and are subsequently inactivated. The vaccines contain different viral subtypes; the types are chosen each spring in anticipation of the expected strains the following winter. The optimal time for immunization is the fall of the year, but immunization is effective to the end of the influenza season.

Three preparations are used in the United States: a whole-virus vaccine prepared from intact, purified virus particles; a "split-virus" vaccine prepared by an additional step of disrupting the lipid-containing membrane of the virus; and a purified surface antigen vaccine. Only the split-virus and purified surface antigen formulations are to be used in children to age 13 years. After vaccination, most young adults develop hemagglutination inhibition titers that are likely to protect them against infection. Children who have not had experience with influenza virus infection or vaccine require two doses of vaccine administered 1 month apart. Annual vaccination is recommended because immunity is limited in duration and infectious strains vary from year to year. Because influenza vaccine is prepared in eggs, it should not be administered to patients with a history of significant allergy to eggs.

Vaccination is directed toward persons who are likely to suffer severe morbidity if infected with influenza virus or who are at high or moderate risk of infection (29). Patients at high risk if they contract influenza include children (6 months or older), adults with chronic respiratory tract or cardiovascular disease (defined as requiring regular medical follow-up or hospitalization during the previous year), and residents (of any age) of nursing homes and other long-term care facilities who have chronic medical conditions.

Patients at modest risk if they contract influenza include healthy persons older than 65 years, adults and children who have had regular medical follow-up or hospitalization during the previous year because of chronic metabolic diseases (including diabetes mellitus), renal disease, hemoglobinopathies, or immunosuppression; also children and teenagers who are receiving long-term aspirin therapy and therefore may be at risk of contracting Reye's syndrome after influenza.

Health care workers and personnel in nursing homes and long-term care facilities should also be immunized against influenza to prevent nosocomial transmission to patients at risk.

Hepatitis B Vaccine

In 1982, a safe and effective HBV vaccine derived from plasma of infected patients and subsequently inactivated was licensed in the United States; this vaccine is no longer available in the United States but is available in other countries. In 1986, the first of two currently available genetically engineered HBV vaccines was licensed in the United States; its immunogenicity was comparable to that of the plasma-derived vaccine. The recombinant vaccine is produced in *Saccharomyces cerevisiae* (baker's yeast) into which a plasmid containing the gene for the HBsAg has been inserted. When it is administered in a three-dose series, protective antibodies develop in more than 95% of healthy young adults. The schedule of administration includes an interval of 1 month between the first two doses and 5 months after the second.

Candidates to receive HBV vaccine include health care workers who were exposed through blood or needlesticks, patients and staff in institutions for developmentally disabled persons, patients undergoing hemodialysis, homosexually active men, users of illicit injectable drugs, recipients of certain blood products, and household members and sexual contacts of HBV carriers. Vaccination should be considered for prisoners, heterosexually active persons, and international travelers to HBV-endemic areas.

In November 1991, the ACIP determined that routine infant HBV vaccination would be the most effective means to prevent HBV spread in the United States (30). HBV vaccine is recommended for all infants born to HBsAg-negative mothers. Three doses of vaccine before 18 months of age are recommended: The first dose is given between birth and 2 months of age; the second, 1 to 2 months later; and the third, at 6 to 18 months of age. Vaccination is recommended for all 11- to 12-year-old children who have not previously received HBV vaccine.

A combination HBIG-HBV vaccine provides immediate and durable protection for exposed persons. Transmission of perinatal HBV infection can be prevented in infants born to HBV surface antigen–positive mothers if HBIG is given within 12 hours after birth followed by HBV vaccine shortly after birth. A combination HBIG-HBV vaccine should be administered to previously unvaccinated persons who have percutaneous exposure to blood that contains or might contain this antigen.

Hepatitis A Vaccine

HAV vaccine was approved by the FDA in February 1995. The vaccine is prepared in human cell culture, purified, and inactivated with formalin. The adult schedule is an initial intramuscular injection, followed by a booster 6 to 12 months later. The pediatric formulation recommended for children 2 to 18 years of age is two intramuscular doses 1 month apart, followed by a booster dose 6 to 12 months after the first dose. In clinical trials in Thailand and the United States, the vaccine was 90% and 100% effective, respectively (31). Local reactions may occur, but systemic reactions are rare. The vaccine is indicated for military personnel, travelers to endemic areas, groups in endemic areas or communities with consistently elevated HAV rates, homosexual and bisexual men, intravenous drug users, patients with clotting factor disorders, day care center employees, health care personnel, food handlers, workers at institutions for people with mental retardation, and possibly other workers in high-risk areas such as prisons, sewerage, and dietary professions. If immediate protection is needed against HAV, intramuscular IG (0.02 mL/kg) should be administered. Use of IG is recommended after contact with a case for household, day care and sexual contacts, and newborn infants of HAV-infected mothers. The vaccine should displace the periodic use of IG for travelers and military personnel who spend variable periods in endemic areas.

Rabies Vaccine

Although the number of human rabies cases in the United States has ranged from zero to five per year, approximately 25,000 persons receive rabies prophylaxis. The rabies vaccine available in the United States is prepared by growing fixed rabies virus in human diploid cell cultures and subsequently inactivating it. Vaccine induces an active immune response that requires about 7 to 10 days to develop and persists for a year or more. Postexposure prophylaxis consists of local treatment of wounds, vaccination, and use of rabies-specific IG.

Physicians should consult local or state public health officials for current information about endemic rabies in the area. Use of rabies vaccine depends on the species of biting animal, the circumstances of the bite (penetration of the skin), and the type of exposure (provoked or not). In the United States, carnivorous wild animals (skunks, raccoons, foxes, and coyotes) are the animals most often infected. The chance of a domestic dog or cat being infected varies by region. Rodents (squirrels, hamsters, guinea pigs, gerbils, rats, and mice) are rarely infected and have not been known to cause human rabies in the United States. Rabies vaccine is used prophylactically by members of high-risk populations such as veterinarians. Because of the long incubation period, rabies vaccine is also effective when given after exposure.

Yellow Fever Vaccine

Yellow fever is enzootic in some sylvatic areas in South America, and virus has been isolated from mosquitoes on Trinidad. Yellow fever vaccine is recommended for travelers 9 months or older who are likely to visit endemic areas. The vaccine is prepared in eggs; precautions noted before for measles, mumps, and influenza virus vaccines should be considered for patients with egg allergy.

Smallpox Vaccine (Vaccinia)

Concern for the potential of smallpox as a weapon of bioterrorism has heightened since the events of September 2001. New stockpiles of smallpox vaccine have been ordered as a contingency for protection of civilian and military personnel and plans are in progress to immunize first responders. The currently available smallpox vaccine consists of a lyophilized live poxvirus (vaccinia) that was grown on the skin of calves. Vaccinia vaccine does not contain smallpox (variola) virus. The vaccine is administered using the multiple-puncture technique with a bifurcated needle (32).

Vaccinia is a highly effective vaccine that enabled global eradication of smallpox. The last naturally occurring case of smallpox occurred in Somalia in 1977. In the United States, recommendations for routine smallpox vaccination ended in 1971. Immunization of military personnel ended in 1990. Since the end of routine use of vaccinia, immunization has been recommended only to protect laboratory workers for possible infection while working with nonvariola orthopoxviruses (e.g., vaccinia and monkeypox). Vaccines prepared from highly attenuated poxvirus strains are used for recombinant vaccine development.

Severe adverse reactions occur, including eczema vaccinatum, generalized vaccinia, progressive vaccinia, postvaccinial encephalitis, and vaccinial keratitis. Vaccinia immunoglobulin is available and may be indicated in severe cases of eczema vaccinatum and may be effective for progressive vaccinia. Overall rates of complications are approximately 1,200 per 1 million following primary vaccination and 108 per 1 million after revaccination.

The intent of the federal government is to stockpile sufficient doses of smallpox vaccine to immunize all Americans. The purpose of this large number of doses is to act as a deterrent against bioterrorism. At present, vaccine is being administered to selected first responders only. Plans for wider distribution to health care workers are under consideration.

BACTERIAL VACCINES FOR SPECIAL POPULATIONS AND SPECIAL INDICATIONS

Anthrax Vaccine

The events of the fall of 2001 have heightened awareness and concern about anthrax as a mode of bioterrorism. A cell-free vaccine produced by the BioPort Corporation in Lansing, Michigan, is the only licensed product in the United States. The vaccine is prepared from sterile filtrates of cultures of an attenuated unencapsulated strain of *Bacillus anthracis*. The current product induces an immune response in more than 90% of those who receive two doses, but the duration of immunity is relatively brief; three boosters at 6-month intervals followed by annual boosters is recommended. Routine immunization is recommended for workers who handle potentially contaminated animal products, including wool, goat hair, hides, and bones from countries in which animal anthrax is present. Laboratory workers who come in contact with *B. anthracis* should be immunized. The recommended vaccination schedule includes subcutaneous injections at 0, 2, and 4 weeks then 6, 12, and 18 months. Annual booster injections are necessary if immunity is to be maintained.

Bacille Calmette-Guérin

BCG prepared from a strain of *Mycobacterium bovis* attenuated through serial passage in culture was first administered to humans in 1921. Current vaccines vary because of changes in the bacterial strains and different methods of production. Vaccines available in the United States have been evaluated only for their ability to produce delayed hypersensitivity. Vaccine efficacy remains a subject of controversy. A large controlled trial in Madras, India, with a 15-year follow-up failed to identify any difference in the rate of pulmonary tuberculosis among persons who were immunized with BCG and those who received placebo (34).

In the United States, the ACIP recommends that tuberculosis is best controlled by effective case detection, chemotherapy, and preventive therapy. Although in prior years, BCG had been recommended for health care workers in endemic areas, current policy is to provide protection by periodic skin testing, rather than BCG. BCG should be considered for certain infants and children whose skin-test results are negative and who are likely to be exposed to infectious contacts who may not have received adequate therapy. In addition, BCG should be considered for infants and children of groups in which the rate of new infection exceeds 1% per year and for whom usual surveillance and treatment programs have limited efficacy. Because rare complications of osteomyelitis and disseminated BCG infection have been reported in patients with HIV and other forms of immunodeficiency, BCG should be administered to these patients.

Cholera Vaccine

Cholera vaccines prepared from classic or *eltor* strains provide limited protection. Current vaccines provide only about 50% efficacy in reducing the incidence of clinical illness, and protection is limited to 3 to 6 months after immunization. Immunization does not prevent transmission of infection.

Because of its minimal efficacy, the World Health Organization no longer recommends cholera vaccination for travelers to or from cholera-affected areas. Some countries still require cholera vaccination for entry though.

Plague Vaccine

A plague vaccine was prepared before 1900. Today, an inactivated whole-cell bacterial vaccine is used in persons whose vocations (geologist, laboratory worker) are likely to bring them into contact with infected rodents or their fleas, and it is recommended for travelers to areas where plague is occurring and domestic rats are known to be infected.

Salmonella typhi Vaccines

Three typhoid vaccines are available for use in the United States. A phenol-inactivated whole-cell *Salmonella typhi* vaccine (initially developed in the 1890s) produces protective serum antibodies when administered subcutaneously in two doses. An orally administered live attenuated vaccine is available for children 6 years and older (data about efficacy in children younger than 6 years are unavailable) and adults. The oral vaccine is derived from a stable mutant of the Ty21a strain of *S. typhi*, induces both intestinal and serum antibodies to *S. typhi* lipopolysaccharide, and requires four doses. The third vaccine is a capsular polysaccharide vaccine for intramuscular administration and is effective in a single dose.

The vaccines produce a comparable but limited degree of protection, which can be overcome by the ingestion of a large inoculum of *S. typhi*. For example, two trials of the oral vaccine in Chilean school children resulted in reduction of infection by 66% during 5 years in one trial but only 33% during 3 years in a second trial (35).

Side effects of the heat-inactivated parenteral vaccine, including fever, local pain, and swelling, are frequent, and the efficacy is not greater than that of the oral vaccine or the vaccine prepared from capsular polysaccharide. Thus, the latter two products with fewer reported side effects are the more acceptable ones. Indications for vaccination include travel to areas where typhoid fever is endemic and a recognized risk of exposure will occur, intimate exposure to a documented typhoid fever carrier, and frequent contact with the organism in laboratory work.

The schedule for the oral vaccine is one capsule taken four times on alternate days. The primary vaccination with the polysaccharide vaccine is one dose intramuscularly. The vaccine is not recommended for children younger than 2 years. The schedule for the parenteral inactivated vaccine consists of two subcutaneous injections separated by 4 weeks. Thus, for travelers who are leaving for endemic areas, the schedule for the oral vaccine and the parenteral polysaccharide vaccine is more useful. Because the oral vaccine is prepared with live bacteria, it is not recommended for persons who are immune deficient.

Lyme Disease Vaccine

In 1999 a recombinant outer surface protein A Lyme disease vaccine was approved for persons aged 15 to 70 years in the United States. Approval of the vaccine was based on clinical trials identifying safety and efficacy of the vaccine in residents in the northeastern and north central United States (36). The vaccine is administered in a three-dose schedule of 0, 1, and 12 months. The vaccine is recommended for persons who reside, work, or play in areas of high or moderate risk including those who perform activities that result in frequent or prolonged exposure to tick-infested areas. The vaccine should be considered an adjunct to, not a replacement for, the practice of personal protective measures against tick exposure including measures against tick exposure and early diagnosis and treatment of Lyme disease.

IMMUNE GLOBULINS

Intramuscular Immune Globulin

IG is derived from the pooled plasma of adults and consists principally of immunoglobulin G with trace amounts of immunoglobulins A and M. At least 1,000 donors contribute to the final product, and the specific antibodies of each lot reflect the infectious and immunization experience of the donors. IG is administered by intramuscularly and achieves peak serum levels within 72 hours after inoculation. The half-life of IG is about 23 days. It has demonstrated efficacy when used early enough to prevent infection or ameliorate disease caused by measles and HAV and for replacement therapy in patients with antibody-deficiency disorders.

Intravenous Immune Globulin

Intravenous IG is prepared from pooled adult plasma and is modified to make it suitable for intravenous use. Current indications include replacement therapy in antibody-deficiency disorders, idiopathic thrombocytopenic purpura, Guillain-Barré disease, and Kawasaki's disease, as well as for prophylaxis in patients with chronic lymphocytic leukemia and bone marrow transplantation. Conflicting or incomplete data for prophylactic use of intravenous IG are available for neonates, pediatric patients with AIDS, and critical care and surgical patients (37).

Specific Immune Globulins

Specific IGs are prepared from donors known to have high titers of the desired antibody. Available specific IGs are HBIG, RIG, TIG, VZIG, and RSVIG.

HBIG is administered as soon as possible after birth to infants of mothers who are HB antigen positive. Simultaneous administration of HBIG and hepatitis vaccine does not diminish the infant's response to the vaccine. Other uses of HBIG include percutaneous (needlestick) inoculation of a susceptible individual from a known carrier.

RIG is administered with rabies vaccine as soon as possible after exposure (regardless of the interval between exposure and treatment). One dose is administered to provide immediate antibodies until the patient responds to the vaccine.

TIG is used to manage severe and contaminated wounds of patients whose primary immunization series with tetanus toxoid is either unknown or incomplete.

Administration of VZIG is recommended after significant exposure: household contact, playmate contact of more than 1 hour indoors, hospital exposure of prolonged face-to-face contact, or newborn infant of mother with onset of varicella 5 days or less before delivery or within 48 hours after delivery. Its use should be considered after such exposures for the following groups: immunodeficient children, normal susceptible adolescents and adults, newborn infants of mothers who had onset of varicella within 5 days of delivery or within 4 hours after delivery, premature infants of more than 28 weeks of gestation whose mothers lack a history of varicella, and premature infants of less than 28 weeks of gestation regardless of maternal history.

RSVIG has been demonstrated to be valuable for prophylaxis of, but not therapy for, RSV disease. Children who received RSVIG monthly during the RSV season had fewer infections, hospitalizations, and hospital days (38). Because of the difficulty of monthly administration of the IG, monoclonal antibodies with neutralizing activity against RSV (palivizumab), which could be administered intramuscularly, were developed and are now the preferred product for prevention of RSV disease in infants. Palivizumab is recommended for infants and children younger than 2 years with chronic lung disease and for very low birth weight and premature infants. Monthly doses are given during the RSV season.

REFERENCES

1. Plotkin SA, Orenstein WA, eds. *Vaccines*, 3rd ed. Philadelphia: WB Saunders, 1999.
2. Committee on Infectious Diseases, American Academy of Pediatrics. 2002 recommended childhood immunization schedule. *Pediatrics* 2002;109:162.
3. Immunization Practices Advisory Committee. General recommendations on immunization. *MMWR Morbid Mortal Wkly Rep* 1989;38:223.
4. Centers for Disease Control and Prevention. Combination vaccines for childhood immunization: recommendations of the Advisory Committee on Immunization Practices, the American Academy of Pediatrics, and the American Academy of Family Physicians. *MMWR Morb Mortal Wkly Rep* 1999;48(RR-5):1–15.
5. Immunization Practices Advisory Committee. Immunization of children infected with human immunodeficiency virus—supplementary ACID statement. *MMWR Morbid Mortal Wkly Rep* 1988;37:181–183.
6. Centers for Disease Control and Prevention. Summary of notifiable diseases, United States, 1987. *MMWR Morbid Mortal Wkly Rep* 1989;36:5–59.
7. Maple PA, Efstratiou A, George RC, et al. Diphtheria immunity in UK blood donors. *Lancet* 1995;345:936–965.
8. Vitek CR and Wharton M. Diphtheria in the former Soviet Union: reemergence of a pandemic disease. *Emerg Infect Dis* 1998;4:539–550.
9. Centers for Disease Control and Prevention. Tetanus—United States, 1985–1986. *MMWR Morbid Mortal Wkly Rep* 1987;36:477–481.
10. Gergen PJ, McQuillan GM, Kiely M, et al. A population-based serologic survey of immunity to tetanus in the United States. *N Engl J Med* 1995;332:761–766.
11. Cody CL, Baraff LJ, Cherry JD, et al. Nature and rates of adverse reactions associated with DTP and DT immunizations in infants and children. *Pediatrics* 1981;68:650–660.
12. Edwards KM, Decker MD, Mortimer EA Jr. Pertussis vaccine. In: Plotkin SA, Orenstein WA, eds. Vaccine, 3rd ed. Philadelphia: WB Saunders, 1999:293–344.
13. Committee on Infectious Diseases. Acellular pertussis vaccine: recommendations for use as the initial series in infants and children. *Pediatrics* 1997;99:282–288.
14. Yih WK, Lett SM, des Vignes FN, et al. The increasing incidence of pertussis in Massachusetts adolescents and adults, 1989–1998. *J Infect Dis* 2000;182:1409–1416.
15. Edwards KM, Decker MD, Graham BS, et al. Adult immunization with acellular pertussis vaccine. *JAMA* 1993;269:53–56.
16. Immunization Practices Advisory Committee. Measles prevention: recommendations of the Immunization Practices Advisory Committee (ACIP). *MMWR Morbid Mortal Wkly Rep* 1989;38[Suppl 9]:1–18.
17. Halsey NA, Hyman SL, and the Conference Writing Panel. Measles-mumps-rubella vaccine and autistic spectrum disorder: report from the new challenges in Childhood Immunizations Conference convened in Oak Brook, IL June 12–13, 2000. *Pediatrics* 2001;107:1–23.
18. Cochi SL, Preblud SR, Orenstein WA. Perspectives on the relative resurgence of mumps in, the United States. *Am J Dis Child* 1988;142:499–507.
19. Centers for Disease Control and Prevention. Rubella vaccination during pregnancy—United States, 1971–1988. *MMWR Morb Mortal Wkly Rep* 1989;38:289–293.
20. American Academy of Pediatrics. Poliovirus infections. In Pickering LK, ed. 2000 red book. Report of the Committee on Infectious Diseases, 25th ed. Elk Grove Village, IL: American Academy of Pediatrics, 2000:465–470.
21. Committee on Infectious Disease. Recommendations for the use of live attenuated varicella vaccine. *Pediatrics* 1995;95:791–796.
22. Black S, Shinefield H, Fireman B, et al. Efficacy, safety and immunogenicity of heptavalent pneumococcal conjugate vaccine in children. *Pediatr Infect Dis J* 2000;19:187–195.
23. Eskola J, Kilpi T, Palmu A, et al. Efficacy of a pneumococcal conjugate vaccine against acute otitis media. *N Engl J Med* 2001;344:403–409.
24. Ramsey ME, Andrews N, Kaczmarski EB, et al. Efficacy of meningococcal serogroup C conjugate vaccine in teenagers and toddlers in England. *Lancet* 2001;357:195–196.
25. Bruce MG, Rosenstein NE, Capparella JM, et al. Risk factors for meningococcal disease in college students. *JAMA* 2001;286:688–693.

26. Mortimer EA. Efficacy of *Haemophilus* b polysaccharide vaccine: an enigma. *JAMA* 1988;260:1454–1455.
27. Black SB, Shinefield HR, Fireman B, et al. Efficacy in infancy of oligosaccharide conjugate *Haemophilus influenzae* type b vaccine in a United States populations of 61,080 children. *Pedatr Infect Dis J* 1991;10:97–104.
28. Mohle-Boetani JC, Ajello G, Breneman E, et al. Carriage of *Haemophilus influenzae* type b in children after widespread vaccination with conjugate *Haemophilus influenzae* type b vaccines. *Pediatr Infect Dis J* 1993;12:589–593.
29. Centers for Disease Control and Prevention. Prevention and control of influenza: recommendations of the Advisory Committee on Immunization Practices (ACIP). *MMWR Morb Mortal Wkly Rep* 1995;44(RR-3):1–22.
30. Advisory Committee on Immunization Practices. Hepatitis B virus: a comprehensive strategy for eliminating transmission in the United States through universal childhood vaccination. *MMWR Morb Mortal Wkly Rep* 1991;40(RR-13):1–19.
31. Innis BL, Snitbhan R, Kunasol P, et al. Protection against hepatitis A by an inactivated vaccine. *JAMA* 1994;271:1328–1334.
32. Centers for Disease Control and Prevention. Vaccinia (smallpox) vaccine: recommendations of the Advisory Committee on Immunization Practices. *MMWR Morb Mortal Wkly Rep* 2001;50(RR-10):1–25.
33. Centers for Disease Control and Prevention. Use of anthrax vaccine in the United States; recommendations of the Advisory Committee on Immunization Practices. *MMWR Morb Mortal Wkly Rep* 2001;49:(RR-15).
34. Tripathy SP. Fifteen-year follow-up of the Indian BCG prevention trial. Proceedings of the XXVIth IUAT World Conference on Tuberculosis and Respiratory Diseases. Singapore, Professional Postgraduate Services, International, 1987 [cited in *MMWR Morbid Mortal Wkly Rep* 1988;37:674].
35. Levine MM, Ferreccio C, Black RE, et al. Large-scale field trial of Ty21a live oral typhoid vaccine in enteric-coated capsule formulation. *Lancet* 1987;329:1049–1052.
36. Centers for Disease Control and Prevention. Recommendations for the use of Lyme disease vaccine: recommendations of the Advisory Committee on Immunization Practices. *MMWR Morb Mortal Wkly Rep* 1999;48(RR-7)1.
37. Pennington JE. Newer uses of intravenous immunoglobulins as anti-infective agents. *Antimicrob Agents Chemother* 1990;34:1463–1466.
38. Prober CG, Sullender WM. Advances in prevention of respiratory syncytial virus infections. *J Pediatr* 1999;135:546–558.

CHAPTER 38

Management of Urinary Catheters

Calvin M. Kunin

Urinary catheters are an essential part of medical care. They are widely used to provide temporary relief of anatomic or physiologic obstruction, to facilitate surgical repair of the urethra and surrounding structures, to provide a dry environment for a comatose or incontinent patient, and to permit accurate measurement of urine output in severely ill patients. Unfortunately, when used inappropriately or left in place too long, they can present a hazard to the very patients they are designed to protect. They are the leading cause of nosocomial urinary tract infections (UTIs) and the most common predisposing factor for preventable gram-negative sepsis in hospitals (1).

RISKS OF CATHETERIZATION

The risk of acquisition of UTI from catheterization depends on host factors, how long the catheter is left in place, and how well it is managed once in place.

SINGLE CATHETERIZATION

Indications

1. To relieve temporary obstruction or inability to void
2. To obtain urine from patients who cannot provide a clean

voided specimen because of weakness, obesity, or major medical problems

3. To determine the volume of residual urine (other methods include postvoiding films after intravenous urograms and bladder ultrasonography)

The rate of acquisition of UTIs in healthy persons after a single catheterization is relatively low, on the order of 1% to 2% (2). There may be several reasons: (a) the enteric gram-negative bacteria that produce UTIs are not ordinarily present in the periurethral area (3); (b) the few organisms that are introduced at the time of catheterization are washed out by the flow of urine; and (c) a foreign body is not left in place. Certain groups seem to be more susceptible to infection. The rate of infection may exceed 20% in women postpartum (4,5). Other high-risk groups include men with prostatic obstruction, diabetics, elderly and debilitated persons, and those who retain significant residual urine in the bladder.

Antimicrobial Prophylaxis

Prophylactic antimicrobial therapy to prevent acquisition of infection after single catheterizations in high-risk patients appears to be reasonable, although proof of efficacy is difficult to find in the literature. A single dose of an effective agent such as trimethoprim, trimethoprim-sulfamethoxazole (TMP-SMX), nitrofurantoin, or a quinolone may be useful in high-risk patients. Another approach is to irrigate the bladder with an antimicrobial solution such as neomycin-polymyxin or chlorhexidine (5). *The most important message, however, is to avoid unnecessary instrumentation.*

INTERMITTENT CATHETERIZATION

About 40 years ago, Sir Ludwig Guttmann introduced the concept of intermittent catheterization for the early treatment of patients with traumatic paraplegia (6). Guttmann reasoned that aseptic intermittent catheterization would eliminate the foreign body and mimic the normal cycle of bladder emptying. This technique was a major advance in long-term care, markedly reducing the incidence of UTIs and morbidity among paraplegic patients. These observations led Lapides et al. (7) to introduce clean, but not necessarily aseptic, "self-catheterization" as an effective measure for children with neurogenic disorders of bladder function. Urinary diversion procedures are needed much less often now. Advantages and disadvantages of intermittent catheterization are described in Table 38.1.

The frequency of UTIs is decreased but not eliminated by intermittent catheterization. Nevertheless, infection is much more readily treated. Methods to prevent acquisition of bacteriuria in patients should be individualized because patients are highly variable. Some may develop infection rarely, and each infection may be treated with a brief course of antimicrobial therapy. Others may develop persistent symptomatic infection and may require long-term prophylaxis with an effective agent. Various methods have been claimed to be effective for paraplegic patients: instillation of a solution of neomycin-polymyxin into the bladder at the termination of each catheterization (8), oral prophylaxis with nitrofurantoin (9), and methenamine mandelate combined with ammonium chloride to acidify the urine (10). Bladder irrigations with polymyxin-neomycin may be complicated by superinfection with yeasts and enterococci. Bleeding and development of urethral strictures, false urethral passages, and epididymitis may complicate intermittent catheterization in men. These problems may be overcome in patients with detrusor-external sphincter dyssynergia by

---

TABLE 38.1.   Advantages and Disadvantages of Intermittent Catheterization

Advantages
  Mimics normal emptying of the bladder
  Eliminates a persistent foreign body
  Prevents overflow incontinence
  Improves patients' self-esteem
  Allows antimicrobial therapy to be more effective
  Decreases complications of catheter care (fewer episodes of sepsis,
    less stone formation), protects the upper tract, and decreases the
    need for urinary diversion procedures
Disadvantages
  Requires more nursing time in hospitals
  Requires cooperation of patients or assistance at home
  May produce strictures and false passages
  May ultimately require bladder neck surgery for males
Unresolved issues
  Do antimicrobial irrigation solutions decrease infections?
  Should asymptomatic bacteriuria be treated?

Source: From Kunin CM. Urinary tract infections: detection, prevention, and management, 5th ed. Baltimore: Williams & Wilkins, 1997, with permission.

performing a sphincterotomy (11) or inserting an endoluminal urethral stent. The patient is then placed on external condom drainage. An alternative approach is to insert a suprapubic catheter. Long-term placement of a suprapubic catheter in men is useful for preventing urethral strictures, epididymitis, and orchitis, but it does not prevent acquisition of UTIs.

POSTOPERATIVE URINARY CATHETERIZATION

Catheterization need not be used routinely in postoperative patients who have difficulty voiding. It is not uncommon for a male patient to trace the onset of recurrent prostatitis or a female patient to relate recurrent UTIs to postoperative or postpartum catheterization. The patient should be given adequate time, placed in a comfortable position to void, and most important allowed privacy to relieve inhibitions. A single or several intermittent catheterizations may suffice for the patient who cannot void after several hours. The surgeon may elect to use an indwelling catheter for 1 or 2 days instead of intermittent catheterization. In one study (12), short-term use of the indwelling catheter reduced the occurrence of urine retention and bladder distention without increasing the rate of UTI.

Regardless of the method used to relieve postoperative urinary retention, it is recommended that microscopic examination of the urine or culture be done after the catheter is removed, and that infection be eradicated by a short course of antimicrobial therapy.

INDWELLING URINARY CATHETER

The urethral indwelling catheter is one of the most commonly used instruments in hospitals. It is inserted in about 10% of all patients admitted to general hospitals and is used commonly in the care of elderly incontinent women in nursing homes. The risk of infection and its sequelae depend on the duration of catheterization, age, sex, type of service, and the presence of associated diseases. Women tend to acquire induced infections more readily than men (13,14). Men more frequently suffer from local suppurative complications.

According to the National Nosocomial Infections Study, 40% of the 2 million hospital-acquired infections arise from the urinary tract each year in the United States. About 800,000 of these patients per year develop nosocomial UTIs, mainly from indwelling catheters. It is estimated that at least 50,000 cases of nosocomial UTIs per year are associated with bacteremia and potentially life-threatening illness (1,15). Givens and Wenzel (16) estimated that Foley catheter–associated UTIs after five common surgical procedures extended hospital stays an average of 2.4 days. Rubinstein et al. (17) found that UTIs from catheters used in general and orthopedic surgery prolonged the average length of stay to 5.1 days. Platt et al. (18), working in a short-term care general hospital, reported a threefold increase in mortality among catheterized patients who became infected. It is not uncommon to encounter patients with severe sepsis and gram-negative bacteremia who are admitted with an indwelling urinary catheter from long-term care facilities. These are usually elderly female patients transferred from nursing homes or paraplegic patients. We noted in a study of elderly patients in nursing homes that there was a stepwise increase in mortality with duration of catheterization (19). This was independent of other risk factors for death. Patients who were catheterized for 76% or more of their days in the nursing homes were three times more likely to die within a year. The number of hospitalizations, duration of hospitalization, and use of antimicrobial drugs were three times greater among catheterized patients. In a randomized, prospective clinical trial comparing catheterization with incontinence pads among elderly female patients, McMurdo et al. (20) found that asymptomatic bacteriuria was common between both groups, but 73% of catheterized patients received treatment for clinical signs of infection, compared with 40% of patients managed with pads. Catheterized patients required less nursing time, but costs for catheter care were greater. Nordqvist et al. (21) compared catheter and noncatheter care in two wards and found no differences in mortality at 4 years. Nevertheless, they were favorably impressed by the advantages of noncatheter care: the relative ease of removing catheters from most patients, the spontaneous disappearance of bacteriuria and ease of eradicating infection with oral antimicrobial agents, improved contact with the staff, decrease in odors, absence of pressure sores, reduction in the number of gram-negative nosocomial strains of bacteria, and marked reduction in the use of antibiotics. Use of catheters may be less costly in the short run, but the long-term complications are unacceptable (22).

Effect of Catheters on the Voiding Mechanism

The bladder is a smooth-walled, distensible structure that contracts once the internal pressure exerted by the expanding volume of urine reaches a critical point. This detrusor activity is synchronized with a combination of voluntary and involuntary relaxation of the external sphincter. The flow of urine then distends the normally collapsed urethral passage, allowing virtually complete emptying of the bladder (23). This cyclic process is the bladder's chief mechanical defense against infection (24). The indwelling catheter violates this defense altogether. With the catheter, the cycle of filling, expansion, and emptying of the bladder is altered to produce continuous flow. The bladder cannot empty completely because of the presence of the retention balloon, pressure from which erodes the smooth mucosal surface. The urethra is distended, its blood supply is attenuated by lateral pressure, and the lubricating periurethral glands are blocked. There is a continuous open channel that permits microorganisms to flow upstream into the bladder and a stressed periurethral surface that offers a second channel for bacterial colonization around the urethra. In essence, the catheter converts a dynamic system to a static state.

Antimicrobial Prophylaxis

Antimicrobial prophylaxis may temporarily delay the onset of bacteriuria in patients with indwelling catheters, but it predisposes to superinfection with resistant microorganisms. Excessive use of fluoroquinolones in catheterized patients is associated with the emergence of ciprofloxacin-resistant *Escherichia coli* (25). The rate of nosocomial UTI at a university medical center doubled between 1982 and 1991 (26); this was associated with an increase in infections caused by yeasts, *Klebsiella pneumoniae,* and group B streptococci because of the selective pressure of antibiotic use. The breakdown of urea to ammonia by urease-producing *Proteus* and *Providencia* species produces alkaline urine and causes precipitation of struvite crystals (27). The crystals aggregate to form encrustations that block the channel and lead to obstruction and septic episodes.

Treatment after Removal of the Catheter

Harding et al. (28) found that bacteriuria resolved spontaneously in about one third of women after an indwelling catheter had been removed. Those who remained bacteriuric often developed symptomatic infection. A single dose of TMP-SMX, given to those who were still bacteriuric at 48 hours after removal of the catheter, was as effective as a 10-day course. It is recommended that prophylactic antibiotics not be used in catheterized patients; treatment should be reserved for documented infection after the catheter is removed.

Management of Sepsis in Patients with an Indwelling Catheter

Patients with indwelling catheters are usually afebrile and asymptomatic but may suffer acute episodes of fever and chill, sometimes accompanied by septic shock. Detecting sepsis may be difficult in elderly patients. They may have only low-grade fever, appear to be dehydrated, and develop mental confusion. The first step should be to remove the catheter, which may be kinked or blocked. The urine should be examined by Gram stain to obtain a preliminary assessment of the possible causative organisms. Gram-negative bacteria are usually suspected, but gram-positive bacteria (staphylococci and enterococci) or yeasts may be responsible. Blood cultures and standard laboratory tests should be conducted and attention directed at managing hypotension and repletion of fluids and electrolytes. Although antibiotics are customarily administered, how long they should be given is not known. Bacteremia is often transient and rarely metastatic.

Advances in Management of Indwelling Urinary Catheters

CLOSED DRAINAGE

Progress in this field has been remarkably slow. It took more than 30 years before Miller et al. (29) reintroduced the work of Dukes (30) on closed drainage. The use of closed drainage bags was not adopted widely in the United States until almost 10 years later (13,31). Attempts to improve indwelling catheter care are summarized in Table 38.2. All indwelling catheters should be attached to closed drainage. This delays colonization of the bladder in most patients by about 1 to 2 weeks. Thereafter, microbes ascend around the catheter in the periurethral

TABLE 38.2.   Attempts to Improve Indwelling Catheter Care

Site	Method
Urethra	Aseptic method of insertion[a]
	Antimicrobial lubricants[b]
	Washing the perineum[b]
	Applications of antimicrobial ointments[b]
	Chlorhexidine-soaked sponges[c]
Bladder	Irrigation with antimicrobial solutions[d]
Catheter	New materials (silicone versus latex)[e]
	Hydrophilic catheters[b]
	Conformable catheters[f]
	Impregnation with antimicrobial agents[b]
	The "silver" catheter (see text)
	Vented catheters[b]
Drainage tube junction	Preattached collecting systems[a]
	Construction (hanging characteristics,[c] leg bands,[c] vents,[g] drip chambers, valves, spigots[b])
Drainage bag	Antimicrobial additives[b] (povidone-iodine, hydrogen peroxide, chlorhexidine)
Systemic	Antimicrobial prophylaxis or therapy[b]
Epidemiologic	Geographic separation, sterilization of urine outflow from bags[g]
	Washing hands between patients[c]
	Sterilization of urine drained from bags[c]
	Measures that restrict use of common devices and irrigation syringes[g]
General	Proper positioning of the drainage system[g]
	Avoidance of breaking the closed system[g]

[a]Possibly effective.
[b]Not effective.
[c]Probably effective.
[d]Effective, but not more than closed drainage.
[e]Effective because silicone catheters tend to become less encrusted during long-term use.
[f]Appear to be more comfortable, but there is no evidence that the rate of infection is altered.
[g]Effective.
Source: From Kunin CM. *Urinary tract infections: detection, prevention, and management,* 5th ed. Baltimore: Williams & Wilkins, 1997, with permission.

space (32). This is not prevented by using antimicrobial lubricants or povidone-iodine ointment at the time of insertion (32) or by applying silver sulfadiazine cream twice daily to the urethral meatus (33). Even washing the periurethral area has not been shown to be beneficial. Continuous irrigation of the bladder with neomycin-polymyxin solutions is no more effective than closed drainage and does not provide additional benefit. Care must be taken to avoid breaking the junction between the catheter and drainage tube. Sealed joints are preferred by some workers (34), but use of a tape seal applied to the catheter–drainage tubing junction within 24 hours of catheter insertion was not associated with significantly lower rates of bacteriuria or mortality in patients undergoing short-term catheterization (35).

Several studies (36,37) have shown no difference in the time of onset and incidence of nosocomial UTI in patients managed with a simple drainage system compared with a more complex system that included a preconnected, coated catheter, a tamper seal at the catheter–drainage junction, a drip chamber, an antireflux valve, a hydrophobic drainage vent, and a povidone-iodine–releasing cartridge in line with the outlet tube of the urine collection bag. Adding an antimicrobial agent such as hydrogen peroxide or chlorhexidine to the drainage bag is not beneficial (38,39).

CATHETER MATERIALS

Latex catheters are less expensive than silicone or silicone-coated catheters but are no longer used because of fear of allergy in some patients. Silicone catheters tend to become encrusted less frequently than latex (40). Catheters need not be changed routinely unless they become blocked by encrustations. Patients who form encrustations ("blockers") may be managed effectively by changing the catheter at 1- to 2-week intervals (41). Although prevention of biofilms is of considerable interest, it is easier and more cost-effective to simply change to a fresh catheter or remove it as soon as possible.

Attempts to block the periurethral route by coating catheters with antimicrobial agents are currently receiving considerable attention (42). These include silver oxide (43,44), silver hydrogel (silver alloy) (45–49), nitrofurazone (50,51), and combinations of minocycline and rifampin (52,53). Current favorites are the silver alloy–coated and nitrofurazone-coated catheters. Nitrofurazone has been shown to be superior to silver hydrogel according to *in vitro* studies of their activity against microorganisms that commonly cause catheter-associated infection (50).

It is difficult to assess the clinical efficacy of silver alloy–coated catheters in preventing acquisition of bacteriuria despite enthusiastic proponents. The literature is somewhat contradictory, many of the abstracts remain unpublished as full articles, and which patients will benefit the most needs to be defined (54). Some clinical trials are well-designed prospective studies that determine the daily rate of acquisition of bacteriuria. Others are crossover studies that use clinical criteria to identify patients with infections. The crossover studies are usually not blinded and do not provide daily end points. For example, a preliminary account of a double-blind prospective study of a silver hydrogel–coated catheter reported a decrease in infections caused by enterococci, coagulase-negative staphylococci, and *Candida* but showed little effect against gram-negative bacilli (49). The same authors reported a fivefold reduction of acquisition of bacteriuria with a nitrofurazone-impregnated catheter but overall did not reach statistical significance (51). Two trials using clinical end points report reductions in the incidence of symptomatic UTIs of 47% (46) and 21% (47), but a more recent prospective sequential cohort study conducted over two consecutive 6-month periods, using a standard definition of nosocomial UTIs, found no significant difference between a silver hydrogel–coated and a regular urinary catheter (48). A clinical trial of the minocycline-rifampin–coated catheters found a significantly reduced rate of gram-positive, but not gram-negative, bacteriuria (53).

Several points must be considered before hospitals decide to purchase impregnated catheters. These include greater cost and lack of efficacy once bacteriuria is acquired. It does not seem appropriate to use these more expensive catheters in medical or surgical patients who require only a few days of drainage or in long-term care facilities where virtually all of the patients are already infected. Allocation of catheters can become a logistical nightmare. Often it is difficult to predict how long a catheter will be needed. Determination of bacteriuria on admission and acquisition of bacteriuria requires periodic cultures and increases costs. Although silver-coated and nitrofurazone-coated catheters have been reported to be safe in clinical trials, allergy or other adverse effects may occur with more widespread use. Until recently, latex was considered safe, and all latex products had to be removed from hospitals because of a few important allergic reactions. Argyria is a potential problem for long-term care patients. Furthermore, silver-resistant mutants of *E. coli* can be selected by stepwise exposure (55). Enthusiastic marketing of coated catheters may lead to a false sense of security and prolong unnecessary use. Sterilizing the periurethral space might delay acquisition of infection in some patients but will not eradicate infection within the bladder.

NEW CATHETER DESIGNS

These include a conformable catheter constructed with a flexible, thin rubber urethral portion (56). It is reported to be more comfortable, to stay in place several days longer, and to be less often obstructed by struvite crystals, but it has not been shown to prevent acquisition of infection.

USE OF BLADDER SCANS AS AN INDICATION FOR CATHETERIZATION

Portable bladder-scanning devices are now available to determine residual urine volume at the bedside. They can help determine noninvasively whether catheters are needed for initial management and when they are no longer needed (57).

FUTURE DEVELOPMENTS

The challenge is to produce an instrument that matches as closely as possible the normal physiologic and mechanical characteristics of the voiding system. It seems to me that this will require the construction of a thin-walled, continuously lubricated collapsible catheter to restore the integrity of the urethra; a system to hold the catheter in place without a balloon; and one that imitates the intermittent washing of the bladder urine. The efficacy of each component of the system will need to be evaluated in carefully conducted and controlled clinical trials. Catheters of the future may be more expensive but should be well worth the investment.

REFERENCES

1. Kunin CM. *Urinary tract infections: detection, prevention, and management*, 5th ed. Baltimore: Williams & Wilkins, 1997.
2. Turck M, Goffe B, Pertersdorf RG. The urethral catheter and urinary tract infection. *J Urol* 1962;88:834.
3. Daifuku R, Stamm WE. Bacterial adherence to bladder uroepithelial cells in catheter-associated urinary tract infection. *N Engl J Med* 1986;314:1208.
4. Brumfitt W, Davies BI, Rosser E. Urethral catheter as a cause of urinary tract infection in pregnancy and puerperium. *Lancet* 1961;2:1059.
5. Gillespie WA, Lennon GG, Linton KB, et al. Prevention of urinary infection in gynaecology. *Br Med J* 1964;2:423.
6. Guttmann L, Frankel H. The value of intermittent catheterization in the early management of traumatic paraplegia and tetraplegia. *Paraplegia* 1966;4:63.
7. Lapides J, Diokno AC, Silber SJ, et al. Clean, intermittent self-catheterization in the treatment of urinary tract disease. *J Urol* 1972;107:458.
8. Rhame FS, Perkash I. Urinary tract infections occurring in recent spinal cord injury patients on intermittent catheterization. *J Urol* 1979;122:669.
9. Anderson R. Prophylaxis of bacteriuria during intermittent catheterization of the acute neurogenic bladder. *J Urol* 1980;123:364.
10. Kevorkian CG, Merritt JL, Ilstrup DM. Methenamine mandelate with acidification: An effective urinary antiseptic in patients with neurogenic bladder. *Mayo Clin Proc* 1984;59:523.
11. Vapnek JM, Couillard DR, Stone AR. Is sphincterotomy the best management of the spinal cord injured bladder? *J Urol* 1994;151:961.
12. Michelson JD, Lotke PA, Steinberg ME. Urinary bladder management after total joint surgery. *N Engl J Med* 1988;319:321.
13. Kunin CM, McCormack RC. Prevention of catheter-induced urinary tract infections by sterile closed drainage. *N Engl J Med* 1966;274:1155.
14. Garibaldi RA, Burke JP, Britt MR, et al. Meatal colonization and catheter-associated bacteriuria. *N Engl J Med* 1980;303:316.
15. Pittet D, Wenzel RP. Nosocomial blood stream infections. Secular trends in rates, mortality, and contributions to hospital deaths. *Arch Intern Med* 1995;155:1177.
16. Givens CD, Wenzel RP. Catheter-associated urinary tract infections in surgical patients: a controlled study on the excess morbidity and costs. *J Urol* 1980;124:546.
17. Rubinstein E, Green M, Modan M, et al. The effects of nosocomial infection on the length of stay and hospital costs. *J Antimicrob Chemother* 1982;9[Suppl A]:93.
18. Platt R, Polk F, Murdock B, et al. Mortality associated with nosocomial urinary tract infection. *N Engl J Med* 1982;307:637.

19. Kunin CM, Douthitt S, Dancing J, et al. The association between the use of urinary catheters and morbidity and mortality among elderly patients in nursing homes. *Am J Epidemiol* 1992;135:291.

20. McMurdo ME, Davey PG, Elder MA, et al. The cost-effectiveness of the management of intractable urinary incontinence by urinary catheterization or incontinence pads. *J Epidemiol Commun Health* 1992;46:222.

21. Nordqvist P, Ekelund P, Edouard L, et al. Catheter-free geriatric care. Routines and consequences for clinical infection, care and economy. *J Hosp Infect* 1984;5:298.

22. Ouslander JG, Kane RL. The costs of urinary incontinence in nursing homes. *Med Care* 1984;22:69.

23. Kunin CM. Can we build a better urinary catheter? *N Engl J Med* 1988;319:365.

24. O'Grady F, Cattell WR. Kinetics of urinary infection, II: the bladder. *Br J Urol* 1966;38:156.

25. Ena J, Amador C Martinez C, et al. Risk factors for acquisition of urinary tract infections caused by ciprofloxacin resistant *Escherichia coli*. *J Urol* 1995;153:117.

26. Bronsema DA, Adams JR, Pallares R, et al. Secular trends in rates and etiology of nosocomial urinary tract infections at a university hospital. *J Urol* 1993;150:414.

27. Warren JW. *Providencia stuartii*: A common cause of antibiotic-resistant bacteriuria in patients with long-term indwelling catheters. *Rev Infect Dis* 1986;8:61.

28. Harding GKM, Nicolle LE, Ronald AR, et al. How long should catheter-acquired urinary tract infection in women be treated? *Ann Intern Med* 1991;114:713.

29. Miller A, Gillespie WA, Linton KB, et al. Prevention of urinary infection after prostatectomy. *Lancet* 1960;2:886.

30. Dukes C. Urinary tract infections after excision of the rectum: their causes and prevention. *Proc R Soc Med* 1928;22:1.

31. Desautels RE, Walter CW, Graves RC, et al. Technical advances in the prevention of urinary tract infection. *J Urol* 1962;87:487.

32. Burke JP, Jacobson JA, Garibaldi RA, et al. Evaluation of daily meatal care with poly-antibiotic ointment in prevention of urinary catheter–associated bacteriuria. *J Urol* 1983;129:331.

33. Huth TS, Burke JP, Larsen RA, et al. Randomized trial of meatal care with silver sulfadiazine cream for the prevention of catheter-associated bacteriuria. *J Infect Dis* 1992;165:14.

34. Platt R, Murdock B, Polk BF, et al. Reduction of mortality associated with nosocomial urinary tract infection. *Lancet* 1983;1:893.

35. Huth TS, Burke JP, Larsen RA, et al. Clinical trial of junction seals for the prevention of urinary catheter–associated bacteriuria. *Arch Intern Med* 1992;152:807.

36. Wille JC, Blusse van Oud Alblas A, Thewessen EA. Nosocomial catheter-associated bacteriuria: a clinical trial comparing two closed urinary drainage systems. *J Hosp Infect* 1993;25:191.

37. Leone M, Garnier F, Dubuc M, et al. Prevention of nosocomial urinary tract infection in ICU patients. Comparisons of effectiveness of two urinary drainage systems. *Chest* 2001;120:220–224.

38. Thompson RL, Haley CE, Searcy MA, et al. Catheter-associated bacteriuria. Failure to reduce attack rates using periodic instillations of a disinfectant into urinary drainage systems. *JAMA* 1984;151:747.

39. Gillespie WA, Simpson RA, Jones JE, et al. Does the addition of disinfectant to urine drainage bags prevent infection in catheterised patients? *Lancet* 1983;1:1037.

40. Kunin CM, Chin QF, Chambers ST. Formation of encrustations on indwelling catheters in the elderly: a comparison of different types of catheter materials in "blockers" and 'nonblockers." *J Urol* 1987;138:899.

41. Kunin CM, Chin QF, Chambers ST. Indwelling urinary catheters in the elderly. Relation of "catheter life" to formation of encrustations in patients with and without blocked catheters. *Am J Med* 1987;82:405.

42. Maki DG, Tambyah. Engineering out the risk of infection with urinary catheters. *Emerg Infect Dis* 2001;7:342–347.

43. Johnson JR, Roberts PL, Olsen RJ, et al. Prevention of catheter-associated urinary tract infection with a silver oxide–coated urinary catheter: clinical and microbiologic correlates. *J Infect Dis* 1990;162:1145–1150.

44. Riley DK, Classen DC, Stevens LE, et al. A large randomized clinical trial of a silver-impregnated urinary catheter: lack of efficacy and staphylococcal superinfection. *Am J Med* 1995;98:349–356.

45. Saint S, Elmore JG, Sullivan SD, et al. The efficacy of silver-coated urinary catheters in preventing urinary tract infections: a meta-analysis. *Am J Med* 1998;105:236–241.

46. Saint S, Veenstra DL, Sullivan SD, et al. The potential clinical and economic benefits of silver alloy urinary catheters in preventing urinary tract infection. *Arch Intern Med* 2000;160:2670–2675.

47. Karchmer TB, Giannetta ET, Muto CA, et al. A randomized crossover study of silver-coated urinary catheters in hospitalized patients. *Arch Intern Med* 2000;160:3294–3298.

48. Jandourek A, Nafziger D. Evaluation of a silver hydrogel catheter for prevention of nosocomial urinary tract infections [abstract 237]. In: Program and abstracts of the 39th annual meeting of the Infectious Diseases Society of America; San Francisco, CA; October 2001.

49. Maki DG, Knasinski V, Halvorson K, et al. *A novel silver-hydrogel–impregnated urinary catheter reduces CAUTIs: a prospective, randomized, double blind trial [abstract 10]. Program of the 8th annual meeting of the Society for Healthcare Epidemiology of America; Orlando, FL. Mt. Roay, NJ: Society for Healthcare Epidemiology of America*, 1998:27.

50. Johnson JR, Delavari P, Azar M. Activities of a nitrofurazone-containing urinary catheter and a sliver hydrogel catheter against multidrug-resistant bacteria characteristic of catheter-associated urinary tract infection. *Antimicrob Agents Chemother* 1999;43:2990–2995.

51. Maki DG, Knasinski V, Tambyah PA. A prospective investigator-blinded trial of a novel nitrofurazone-impregnated indwelling urinary catheter. *Infect Control Hosp Epidemiol* 1997;18[Pt 2]:50(abst M49).

52. Darouiche RO, Safar H, Raad II. *In vitro* efficacy of antimicrobial-coated bladder catheters in inhibiting bacterial migration along catheter surfaces. *J Infect Dis* 1997;176:1109–1112.

53. Darouiche RO, Smith JA Jr, Hanna H, et al. Efficacy of antimicrobial-impregnated bladder catheters in reducing catheter-associated bacteriuria: a prospective, randomized, multicenter clinical trial. *Urology* 1999;54:976–981.

54. Kunin CM. Nosocomial urinary tract infections and the indwelling catheter: what's new and what's true? *Chest* 2001;120:10–12.

55. Li X-Z, Nikaido H, Williams KE. Silver-resistant mutants of *Escherichia coli* display efflux of Ag+ and are deficient in porins. *J Bacteriol* 1997;179:6127–6132.

56. Brocklehurst C, Hickey DS, Davies I, et al. A new urethral catheter. *Br Med J* 1988;296:1691.

57. Slappendel R, Weber EW. Non-invasive measurement of bladder volume as an indication for bladder catheterization after orthopedic surgery and its effect on urinary tract infections. *Eur J Anaesthesiol* 1999;16:503–506.

CHAPTER 39
Prophylaxis for Surgical Infections

Ronald Lee Nichols

Postoperative wound infection remains the major source of infectious morbidity in the surgical patient (1). In a nationwide study conducted during a 12-month period, reported in 1985, it was estimated that wound infections accounted for about one fourth of all nosocomial infections (2). This number represented more than 500,000 wound infections, or about 2.8 per 100 operations performed. Many perioperative techniques have been shown to influence the development of surgical wound infection, including the use of antibiotic prophylaxis (3,4).

CLASSIFICATION OF SURGICAL WOUNDS

The best predictor of wound infection was previously thought to be the type of operative procedure. A description of the widely accepted classification of operative procedures follows.

Clean wounds: Clean wounds are uninfected operative wounds in which no inflammation is encountered and the respiratory, alimentary, genital, and uninfected urinary tracts have not been entered.

Clean-contaminated wounds: Clean-contaminated wounds are those from operations in which the respiratory, alimentary, genital, or urinary tract is entered under controlled conditions and without unusual contamination.

Contaminated wounds: Contaminated wounds include open, fresh, accidental wounds; those produced during operations in which there is a major break in sterile technique or gross spillage from the gastrointestinal (GI) tract; and incisions marked by acute, acute nonpurulent inflammation.

Dirty or infected wounds: Dirty wounds include old trauma wounds in which devitalized tissue is retained and those that involve existing clinical infection or perforated viscera.

The wound infection in clean operations by definition is due to airborne exogenous or skin microorganisms such as

Staphylococcus aureus, whereas in the other categories of surgery, the agent or agents usually originate from the endogenous polymicrobial aerobic and facultative anaerobic flora.

PATIENT AS A RISK OF INFECTION

Although this observation is unproved, the greatest risk factor for postoperative infection appears to be the patient's physical status. Haley et al. (5) were the first to publish on the importance of identifying individual patients who are at high risk of surgical wound infection for each category of operative procedure. To predict the likelihood of surgical wound infection from several risk factors, the authors used information collected from 58,498 patients undergoing operations in 1970 to develop a simple multivariate risk index. Analyzing ten possible risk factors by stepwise multiple logistic regression techniques, they developed a model containing four risk factors: (a) abdominal operation, (b) operation lasting longer than 2 hours, (c) contaminated or dirty infected operation by traditional wound classification system, and (d) patient having three or more different diagnoses. They used the resulting formula to predict an individual patient's probability of developing a postoperative wound infection. When this approach was tested on another group of 59,352 surgical patients admitted in 1975 and 1976, it was found to be a valid predictor of surgical wound infection. The authors concluded that their simplified index predicts surgical wound infection risk about twice as well as the traditional classification of wound contamination. Using this model, low-, medium-, and high-risk factors for developing wound infection were identified in the different categories of the traditional wound classification. In this study, the overall wound infection rate progressively increased from clean (2.9%), to clean contaminated (3.9%), to contaminated (8.5%), and to dirty or infected (12.6%). The range of infection risk in patients in each category was wide: in clean operations, 1.1% in persons at low risk to 15.8% in those at high risk; in clean-contaminated operations, 0.6% to 17.7%; in contaminated operations, 4.5% (medium risk) to 23.9%; and in dirty or infected operations, 6.7% (medium risk) to 27.4%. For contaminated and dirty or infected operations, no patients at low risk were identified.

The Centers for Disease Control and Prevention investigators have reported on a composite risk index used in the National Nosocomial Infections Surveillance System (6). This index uses a dichotomization of the American Society of Anesthesiology score to identify host factors as a risk for infection instead of three or more discharge diagnoses (7). This change facilitates data collection and apparently increases objectivity. Second, in the new risk index, "prolonged surgery" is defined individually for each procedure, rather than being 2 hours for all operations. For some procedures, such as cesarean section, the cutoff point is 1 hour; for others, such as coronary artery bypass graft operation, it is 5 hours. This adjustment makes the index more discriminating.

FACTORS OTHER THAN ANTIBIOTICS THAT HELP CONTROL THE INCIDENCE OF SURGICAL WOUND INFECTION

Many perioperative factors have been proven to have a significant influence on the development of postoperative wound infection, especially in clean surgical procedures, in which the infection rate is generally expected to be lower than 3%, because only airborne exogenous microorganisms are involved (8). These perioperative measures are aimed at preventing microbial contamination of the wound at the onset of the operation and during the period of operative manipulation.

Preoperative Stay in Hospital

A direct correlation is seen in the relationship between the duration of preoperative hospitalization and the development of postoperative wound infections. Cruse and Foord (8) reported that the overall infection rate was 1.1% for patients whose preoperative stay was 1 day; this rate doubled with each week the patient remained in the hospital before surgery. Most patients who undergo elective operation today are admitted to the hospital on the morning of surgery or on the day before the operation; this greatly decreases the chance for colonization with hospital bacteria and the chance of subsequent infection. Patients admitted for other medical problems should not undergo elective operations later in the same hospital stay because they are at a significant risk of infection by hospital-acquired bacteria.

Preoperative Shave

Preoperative razor shaving 1 day before surgery is associated with significantly higher wound infection rates (9). Seropian and Reynolds (9) documented an infection rate of 0.6% when a depilatory agent was used for hair removal and a rate of 5.6% for razor shaving done the day before surgery. It was postulated that even skillful razor preparation causes microscopic injury, which provides portals of exit from and entry to injured tissue, which in turn serves as a substrate for bacterial growth. Although the lowest infection rate found by Cruse and Foord (8) was in patients who had not been shaved, all surgeons prefer to operate in a "deforested" field. The investigators proposed the alternative of hair clipping, which has an acceptably low infection rate of 1.7%. Subsequently, this approach was found to be a viable alternative to shaving (10).

Preoperative Cleansing

Preoperative showering or bathing with a hexachlorophene antiseptic on the evening before surgery is associated with a lower rate of postoperative wound infection than bathing with regular soap (8). Today, many other antiseptic soaps are available that appear to offer similar protection. One large multihospital study of clean operative procedures showed no fewer wound infections when patients bathed twice preoperatively with chlorhexidine detergent than when they used detergent alone (11).

Presence of Remote Infections

The presence of an active remote infection at the time of elective operation has been shown to greatly influence the development of subsequent postoperative wound infections (12,13). In order of frequency, these infections occur in the urinary tract, skin, and respiratory tract. Antibiotic prophylaxis or surgical incision of a skin abscess on the night before surgery does not reduce the incidence of subsequent wound infections, but preoperative treatment (>24 hours before surgery) has been shown to reduce it significantly to a level similar to that for patients who have no remote infection (13).

Length of Operation

With each hour of operation, the infection rate almost doubles. Shapiro et al. (14) reported that an increasing duration of hysterectomy was associated with a decreasing effect of antibiotic prophylaxis in preventing infection at the operative site. This finding undoubtedly relates to the pharmacokinetics of the antibiotic prophylaxis and to the greater bacterial wound contamination that occurs in lengthy complicated operative procedures.

This study has undoubtedly influenced the current practice of repeating the dose of prophylactic antibiotics when adults' operations exceed 2 to 3 hours, although the exact risk associated with the duration of operation differs from procedure to procedure (6,15).

Use of Prophylactic Abdominal Drainage

Nora, Vanecko, and Bransfield (16) reported both clinical and experimental studies of the dangers of using prophylactic drains in abdominal surgery. On the basis of their frequent findings of skin bacteria in the interior of the abdominal drains, these investigators stressed the "two-way street" concept. Magee (17) demonstrated that the presence of either Silastic or latex Penrose drains in experimental wounds dramatically enhanced the wound infection rate, even in the presence of subinfective doses of bacteria. On the basis of these experimental and clinical studies, it appears safe to conclude that the prophylactic use of abdominal drains is unwarranted and indeed may be a dangerous practice. When drains are required to empty localized collections, they should be placed through sites other than the primary surgical incision, to decrease the incidence of subsequent wound infection. Closed suction drainage, as suggested by Alexander, Koorelitz, and Alexander (18), is the method of choice when abdominal drainage is indicated.

Operating Suite Design and Ventilation Systems

It appears that in most operative procedures, the patient and personnel are the chief factors in the control of wound infections, but architectural design concepts have evolved that also play a role in modern operating suites. I (19) reviewed the key features of design. These include the isolation of the surgical suite from the mainstream of common corridor traffic and the development of the "clean central core," which serves as the supply center and supposedly offers the cleanest environment. The inner corridors that surround the clean core are designed for use by clean traffic, which includes the preoperative patient, nurses, and surgeons. The peripheral corridors are designated for traffic that includes the postoperative patient, surgeons, and nurses after the operation or between cases. Infected patients should be transferred through the peripheral corridors before and after operation. Floors in the operating room should be nonporous, and other surfaces as dirt resistant as possible. The use of tacky or antiseptic mats at the entrance of the operating room is contraindicated.

The optimum size for most routine operating rooms is 20 by 20 feet with 10-foot ceilings, which allows for easy gowning, draping, circulation of personnel, and the use of equipment without the risk of contact contamination. The door of each operating room should be kept closed except to allow passage of equipment, personnel, and the patient. The number of personnel allowed to enter each operating room should be kept to an absolute minimum, because the origin of infecting bacteria can sometimes be traced to shedding that occurs during their movement in the operating room. Limiting the number of people in attendance, excessive conversation, and the number of times the doors are opened and monitoring the pattern of antibiotic prophylaxis have reduced the infection rate after implant surgery (20).

Today, most conventional operating rooms in the United States are ventilated with 20 to 25 changes per hour of high-efficiency filtered air delivered in unidirectional vertical flow (21). The most common system is high-efficiency particulate air filtration, which removes most bacteria that measure 0.5 to 5.0 μm. Therefore, the first air downstream from the high-efficiency particulate air filter is virtually bacteria free. Bacteria released in the operating room environment remain unaffected by the filter system. At least 20% of the air changes each hour should be fresh air. The air delivered should be at temperatures between 18°C and 24°C (65°F and 75°F) and at 50% to 55% humidity. Inlets should be located as high above the floor as possible and remote from the active exhaust outlets, which are located low on the walls. This arrangement allows for the unidirectional airflow. The operating room also should be under higher pressure than the surrounding corridors, to minimize the flow into the operating room when the doors are opened. Careful maintenance of such a ventilation system offers an environment that is virtually as clean as more costly special chambers unless abuses by personnel occur (19). The use of this type of air-handling system is clearly indicated for most clean surgical procedures and for all procedures where the patient's endogenous microflora are released during the surgical procedure. The debate continues about whether additional highly specialized laminar flow ventilation systems are advantageous when major implant surgery is to be undertaken (22).

Other Factors

Many other factors have been thought to influence postoperative wound infection—preoperative scrub technique, surgical glove damage, barrier materials—but there is no convincing evidence. Anecdotal experience and commercial interests, rather than scientific studies, usually account for these associations.

ANTIBIOTIC PROPHYLAXIS

Great strides have been accomplished in the last decade in the rational use of antibiotic prophylaxis (4,23–25). To better understand the current state of this art, it appears necessary to review a few of the historical milestones of the last three decades.

Historical Considerations

Confusing and heated debate concerning the efficacy of prophylactic antibiotics in surgery followed the publication of clinical trial results during the 1950s. Errors in study design of these early efforts included nonrandomization, lack of "blinding," faulty timing of initial antibiotic administration, prolonged antibiotic use, and incorrect choices of antimicrobial agents.

Experimental studies published during the early 1960s helped to clarify many of these problems and resulted in a more scientifically accurate approach to antimicrobial prophylaxis. Most significant was the report by Burke (26) that demonstrated the crucial relationship between timing of antibiotic administration and its prophylactic efficacy. His experimental studies showed that to greatly reduce experimental skin infection produced by penicillin-sensitive *S. aureus*, the penicillin must be in the skin shortly before or at the time of bacterial inoculation. Critical delays in antibiotic administration after bacterial inoculation of just 3 to 4 hours resulted in infected lesions that were indistinguishable in size and histologic appearance from those of animals that had received no prophylaxis. This study and others that followed helped to develop the attitude that to prevent subsequent infection, the antibiotic must be in the tissues before or at the time of bacterial contamination. This important change in strategy avoided the common error of administering the first prophylactic antibiotic in the recovery room after the operation was completed.

As early as 1964, Bernard and Cole (27) were the first to report on the successful use of prophylactic antibiotics in a randomized, prospective, placebo-controlled clinical study of GI tract operations. Their study design used three intramuscular doses of antibiotics of appropriate size given shortly before, during, and shortly after operation. Sixty-six patients who received the antibiotics had a significantly reduced postoperative infection rate of 8%, compared with the 27% infection rate observed in 79 placebo-treated patients. The success of antibiotic prophylaxis noted in this early study was clearly due to the investigators' appropriate selection of patients and wise choice of available agents, as well as to appropriate timing of their administration.

Further advances in our understanding of antibiotic prophylaxis in abdominal surgery occurred in the 1970s, when the qualitative and quantitative nature of the endogenous GI flora in health and in disease was accurately defined (28).

Principles of Antibiotic Prophylaxis

Authoritative reviews of countless clinical studies of surgical prophylaxis have identified which patients may be expected to benefit from perioperative antibiotics (29). Heretofore, prophylactic antibiotics were clearly indicated for *clean* operations that involved a foreign body implant and for all *clean-contaminated* procedures, but certain data suggest that prophylactic antibiotics are of value for some patients undergoing clean procedures *without* foreign implants, such as inguinal hernia repair or breast surgery (30). For patients with established infection (*dirty* cases), the use of antibiotics is considered to be therapeutic and is not discussed in this chapter.

Choice of Agents

No single antibiotic agent or combination should be relied on for effective prophylaxis in all operations. The agent or agents should be chosen principally on the basis of their efficacy against the usual exogenous and endogenous microorganisms known to cause infectious complications in each clinical setting, as well as on their safety profile and cost. When several drugs or regimens are equally efficacious and safe, local hospital cost analyses and utilization studies may result in use of the agent that is least expensive overall (31). Usual infecting microorganisms and antibiotic recommendations for each surgical procedure are listed in Table 39.1. Worldwide, the cephalosporins are the most widely used antibiotics for surgical prophylaxis (25). It has been stressed that antibiotic coverage for all the potential pathogens is not a desired feature of a prophylactic regimen. Nevertheless, it is important to maintain an up-to-date local hospital analysis of the antimicrobial susceptibilities of wound isolates to detect important shifts in patterns of resistance (32). Routine use of second- or third-generation cephalosporins has not improved the clinical results over those achieved with first-generation cephalosporins (33). Until there is evidence of their superiority, these agents should be reserved for procedures that require special coverage, such as the anaerobic coverage required in appendectomy and in other colon procedures (4).

Timing of Prophylaxis

The effective use of prophylactic antibiotics depends to a great extent on the appropriate timing of their administration. Historically, the most common errors in prophylaxis, which undoubtedly dulled the luster of this technique, were the faulty timing of the initial administration and the common practice of continuing to administer the antibiotic beyond 72 hours (34).

Current recommendations call for the parenteral antibiotic used in prophylaxis to be given in a sufficient dose within 2 hours of incision (4). This can be facilitated by having the anesthesiologist administer the drug in the operating room shortly before operative incision when the intravenous lines are started. The former practice of giving the antibiotic "on call" to the operating room frequently meant that it was given 3 to 4 hours before the incision was made, with the result that levels of antibiotic in tissue and serum at the time of operation were low or undetectable. Starting the antibiotic agent within 30 to 120 minutes of incision results in therapeutic drug levels in the wound and surrounding tissues during the operation. Evidence from clinical trials is mounting that supports the assertion that this single preoperative dose of antibiotic is as efficacious as multiple doses of prophylactic antibiotics given during the perioperative course (35). Advocates of single-dose prophylaxis generally recommend that another dose be given when the operation lasts longer than 2 or 3 hours. It also appears that no additional benefit can be derived from longer courses of antibiotic prophylaxis (>24 hours), even for immunosuppressed patients (29).

For oral preoperative antibiotic preparations commonly used before elective colon resection, the chosen agents should be given during the 24 hours before operation to attain significant intraluminal (local) and serum (systemic) levels (36,37). With oral neomycin and erythromycin base, it is necessary to give only three doses of each agent during the 19 hours before operative incision to accomplish these ends (38). Longer periods of preoperative preparation are unnecessary and have been associated with the isolation of resistant organisms within the colon lumen at the time of resection.

Route of Administration

Intravenous administration of the prophylactic antibiotic is preferred for most operative procedures. When this is accomplished in a relatively small volume over a short period (20 to 30 minutes), high serum and tissue levels are the rule. The pharmacokinetics of each individual antibiotic largely determine how long efficacious serum levels will be sustained. Doses of agents with short half-lives (<1 hour) should be repeated every 2 to 3 hours during the operation. The study of agents with different half-lives in surgical antibiotic prophylaxis in long-duration procedures has not been done. At this time, orally administered antibiotics have a major role only in the preparation of patients for elective colon operations (36).

Antibiotic Prophylaxis in Specific Surgical Procedures

There appears to be a clear consensus that antibiotic prophylaxis is necessary and helpful in clean-contaminated procedures that involve mucous membranes harboring an endogenous microflora and in clean procedures that involve the implantation of grafts or prosthetic devices. When infection is presumed to be present at the time of surgery, as in contaminated or dirty procedures, antibiotics are given with therapeutic intent. Perforation of the GI tract, whether by penetrating trauma or a disease

TABLE 39.1. Infecting Microorganisms Usually Associated with Certain Operative Procedures and Prophylactic Antibiotic Recommendations

Surgical procedure	Infecting microorganisms		Recommended agents	Route[a]	Dose (g)[b]	Alternative
	Facultative	Anaerobic				
Clean[c]	Staphylococcus Staphylococcus epidermidis	—	First-generation[d] cephalosporin (Cefazolin)	i.v.	1–2	2nd- or 3rd-generation cephalosporin (i.v.)[e] or vancomycin (i.v.)[f]
Gastroduodenal	Streptococci Coliforms	Bacteroides (other than B. fragilis) Peptostreptococci	Cefazolin	i.v.	1–2	2nd- or 3rd-generation cephalosporin (i.v.)
Cholecystectomy	Coliforms Enterococci	Clostridia	Cefazolin	i.v.	1–2	2nd- or 3rd-generation cephalosporin (i.v.)
Elective colon resection	Coliforms	B. fragilis Peptostreptococci Clostridia	Neomycin-erythromycin base[g]	p.o.	1 each x 3[h]	Aminoglycoside (p.o.) + metronidazole (p.o.) or tetracycline (p.o.)
Small intestine resection	Coliforms	B. fragilis Peptostreptococci	Neomycin-erythromycin base[g]	p.o.	1 each x 3	i.v. antibiotic with aerobic and anaerobic coverage[i]
Appendectomy	Coliforms	B. fragilis Peptostreptococci	Cefoxitin or ceftizoxime	i.v.	1–2	Other i.v. agents[g]
Penetrating abdominal trauma	Coliforms[j]	B. fragilis[j] Clostridia Peptostreptococci	Cefoxitin	i.v.	2[k]	Other i.v. agents[g]
Vaginal or abdominal hysterectomy	Coliforms Enterococci Group B streptococci	B. fragilis Clostridia	Cefazolin	i.v.	1	Other i.v. agents[g]
Cesarean section		Same as hysterectomy	Cefazolin	i.v.	1[l]	Other i.v. agents[g]
Abortion		Same as hysterectomy	Cefazolin[m]	i.v.	1	Other i.v. agents[g]
Prostatectomy[n]	Coliforms	—	Cefazolin[o]	i.v.	1	Based on sensitivity of infecting microorganisms
Traumatic hemopneumothorax[p]	S. aureus Streptococci	— —	Cefazolin or cefonicid	i.v.	0.5–1.0[q]	—

[a]i.v., intravenous; p.o., oral.
[b]Single-dose prophylaxis is preferred unless operative time is longer than 2 hr, in which case an additional intraoperative dose is indicated.
[c]Includes cardiac, vascular, and orthopedic procedures that utilize a prosthetic implant or device. Some recommend same approach in clean procedures such as hernia repair or breast surgery (30).
[d]Cephalothin and cephapirin are alternatives to cefazolin, but cefazolin is preferred because of its longer half-life and higher tissue levels.
[e]Some prefer agents such as cefuroxime, cefamandole, or ceftriaxone.
[f]Vancomycin is used in patients allergic to penicillins or cephalosporins or in hospitals where methicillin-resistant S. aureus and S. epidermidis frequently cause wound infection.
[g]Most also use an additional i.v. dose of antibiotic at time of operation with efficacy against facultative coliforms and anaerobic Bacteroides.
[h]Mechanical cleansing (see Table 40.2) precedes oral antibiotic intake. Timing of oral antibiotics also noted in Table 40.2.
[i]In nonelective small intestine surgery (bleeding or obstruction), systemic antibiotics alone are used.
[j]Intestinal flora expected in cases with observed leakage. If no perforation is noted, infecting flora is usually facultative gram-positive cocci (staphylococci).
[k]Single preoperative dose suffices when no intestinal leakage is observed at operation. When intestinal leakage is present, dosing continues 2–5 days.
[l]In high-risk sections only; to be given after cord is clamped.
[m]i.v. cefazolin is used in second-trimester abortions. In first-trimester abortions in patients with previous pelvic inflammatory disease, aqueous penicillin, 1 million units i.v., or doxycycline, 300 mg p.o., is recommended.
[n]In the presence of infected urine in the patient undergoing transurethral prostatic resection.
[o]If preoperative urine culture shows sensitive microorganism.
[p]Requiring placement of closed tube thoracostomy.
[q]Regimens vary from dosing every 8 hr for 24 hr to 1 g daily until chest-tube removal.

process (e.g., ruptured appendix, perforated colonic diverticulum), permits the escape of endogenous microflora, resulting in direct contamination of the peritoneal cavity and the operative incision at the time of operation. These clinical settings constitute high-risk situations for the development of postoperative infection; however, the use of perioperative antibiotic prophylaxis within a few hours of perforation appears to be efficacious. Longer delays, which are associated with the development of systemic sepsis or severe intraabdominal infections including abscess formation or diffuse peritonitis, require therapeutic antibiotic and surgical approaches. Operative procedures not specified in this chapter include ocular, neurosurgical, and head and neck operations and pulmonary resection. Few data are available on the efficacy of antibiotic prophylaxis in these clinical settings, and some recommendations have been made (29).

CLEAN SURGICAL PROCEDURES

Currently, antibiotic prophylaxis is indicated in clean surgical procedures that use a foreign material, grafts, or prosthetic devices—many vascular, cardiac, and orthopedic operations, among others (23,29). In these settings, the prophylactic drug regimen is often continued as long as 24 to 48 hours postoperatively despite lack of clear evidence that this practice is effective (29). Continuing the prophylactic antibiotic regimen beyond the immediate perioperative period dramatically increases the cost (39) and has been associated with the development of *Clostridium difficile* colitis (40) and with a high level of colonization with methicillin-resistant *Staphylococcus epidermidis* (41). Although the experience with single-dose prophylaxis in cardiovascular surgery is somewhat limited, it appears this approach is effective when a long-acting drug such as ceftriaxone is used (42).

When infection does occur postoperatively in these procedures, the pathogen is usually *S. aureus* (antibiotic recommendations are offered in Table 39.1). Several cephalosporin agents of different generations have been used, but none shows clear evidence of superiority (25). Vancomycin may be employed instead of the cephalosporin agents if a high degree of methicillin resistance has been noted in the individual hospital centers or in postoperative infections or in patients allergic to penicillin. The routine use of vancomycin prophylaxis in these cases is clearly not necessary and if done will lead to increasing bacterial resistance.

The use of antibiotic prophylaxis for clean surgical procedures that do not involve prostheses or other foreign materials is presently under debate. Future studies will undoubtedly indicate which groups of patients are at high risk of infection in other clean procedures in which a synthetic material is not implanted. These studies will also reveal whether antibiotic prophylaxis proves efficacious for patients at such high risk.

GASTRODUODENAL PROCEDURES

The most common indication for gastroduodenal operation before 1975 was for the treatment of chronic nonobstructing duodenal ulcer (43). The rarity of associated postoperative infectious complications fostered the belief that the stomach contents were often sterile and that antibiotic prophylaxis was not indicated. With the advent of modern medical treatment for chronic duodenal ulcer, surgeons are called on less frequently to operate for this indication. Gastroduodenal operations are now frequently performed for the complications of duodenal ulcer, gastric ulcer, and malignancy. The frequency of postoperative infection in such cases prompted a reappraisal of the role of antibiotic prophylaxis for gastroduodenal surgery.

Risk of Infection. Published studies have defined two risk groups for infections after gastric surgery (43). Patients at low risk (<5%) are those who undergo operation for chronic nonobstructing duodenal ulcer and have high or normal levels of gastric acid and normal motility These patients have few microorganisms, if any, in the gastric lumen at the time of resection. Another low-risk category includes patients operated on for perforating duodenal ulcer disease (44). The peritonitis encountered at operation in these cases is largely chemical, and a bacterial pathogen is found only if surgical intervention is long delayed.

Patients at high risk (>10%) of postoperative infection are those who undergo operation for bleeding or obstructing duodenal ulcer, gastric ulcer, or malignancy. Gastric colonization with organisms entering the stomach from saliva or refluxing through the pylorus is routinely observed in these cases.

Prophylactic Antibiotic Recommendations. Antibiotic prophylaxis is indicated for every patient at high risk (see Table 39.1). Prospective randomized clinical trials have shown the benefit to these patients of prophylaxis with a parenteral first- or second-generation cephalosporin (45). The optimal regimen would use a 1- to 2-g dose of the cephalosporin given intravenously within 30 minutes of incision. The administration of additional doses during the 24 hours after the start of operation appears to be unnecessary unless the operative procedure is quite complex and protracted.

ELECTIVE CHOLECYSTECTOMY

Cholecystectomy for chronic calculous cholecystitis is the only biliary tract operation for which antibiotic prophylaxis is employed. Operations for acute cholecystitis, empyema of the gallbladder, ascending cholangitis, or liver abscess require antibiotic treatment rather than prophylaxis.

The healthy human biliary tract rarely harbors significant concentrations of bacteria. In the presence of chronic calculous cholecystitis, bacteria have been isolated from bile in 15% to 30% of cases. The bacteria isolated are predominantly gram-negative bacilli. *Escherichia coli*, alone or mixed with another organism, is present in 50% of cultures that propagate an organism. Other coliforms—*Klebsiella, Enterobacter, Proteus*—are isolated less often. Anaerobic microorganisms are isolated in fewer than 20% of the cases, with *Clostridium perfringens* and *Bacteroides fragilis* being the most common. A polymicrobial infection by both facultative aerobes and anaerobes may be associated with liver abscess or long-standing common duct obstruction caused by choledocholithiasis.

Risk of Infection. Propagation in cultures of organisms collected at the time of cholecystectomy are associated with a high risk of postoperative infection. Several studies have defined the clinical factors that favor bactibilia and therefore a correspondingly greater risk of postoperative infection: age older than 70 years; history or presence of jaundice; previous biliary tract surgery; chills or fever within 1 week of operation; common duct disease; operations done within 1 month of an acute attack of cholecystitis; and diabetes mellitus (46).

Prophylactic Antibiotic Recommendations. Placebo-controlled studies have shown decreased rates of postoperative infection when antibiotic prophylaxis is used for cholecystectomy in high-risk patients (those who have one or more clinical risk factors) (46).

The principal controversy is whether only patients who have a clinical risk factor or positive intraoperative Gram stain examination should receive antibiotic prophylaxis before elective cholecystectomy. One clinical study recommended a single dose of cephalosporin for all patients undergoing cholecystectomy, regardless of clinical risk factors or Gram stain results (47). This study revealed a high wound infection rate (18%) after intraoperative administration of antibiotics when organisms were seen in Gram-stained preparations of bile from patients who had no clinical risk factors.

ELECTIVE COLON RESECTION

The human colon and distal small intestine contain an enormous reservoir of facultative aerobic and anaerobic bacteria that are sequestered from the rest of the body by the mucous membrane. When the mucous membrane barrier is disturbed by disease or trauma, or if the colon is opened to the peritoneal cavity during surgery, escape of bacteria into adjacent tissues may result in a serious infection. For this reason, finding a reliable method of sterilizing the colonic contents has been a goal of surgeons throughout this century. In the past 20 years, results of clinical trials have clearly shown that to significantly reduce septic complications after elective colon surgery, it is necessary to employ antibiotics that are active against both colonic facultative aerobes (e.g., *E. coli*) and anaerobes (e.g., *B. fragilis*). Controversy exists, however, over the optimal antibiotic regimen and route of administration.

Before the 1970s, most surgeons used mechanical cleansing alone before elective colon surgery (48). The oral antibiotics that had been used before that time (neomycin, kanamycin, streptomycin, sulfonamides) most often suppressed only the facultative aerobic colon flora and were associated with high rates of clinical failure. In addition, use of these oral antibiotics for 3 to 5 days before elective colon resection was frequently associated with overgrowth of staphylococci and yeast in the patient's GI tract, a development that rarely follows a 1-day course of oral antibiotic operative preparation.

Risk of Infection. All patients undergoing elective colon resection are at significant risk of developing postoperative infection because of the great number of bacteria in the colon microflora, which increases in protracted operations and in those done on the extraperitoneal rectum (37).

Kaiser et al. (49) studied different approaches to preoperative antibiotic prophylaxis for elective colon resection and showed a direct correlation between the duration of operation and the postoperative infection rate. In operations lasting fewer than 3 hours, no infections were identified when antibiotic prophylaxis was accomplished with a parenteral agent alone or a combination of oral and parenteral agents; however, in operations lasting more than 4 hours, significantly fewer infections were observed in patients who received the combination prophylactic regimen. In a similar study of elective colon resection, Coppa and Eng (50) stressed that postoperative wound infections are associated with the duration of operation and the location of the colon resection (intraperitoneal vs. rectal). These authors showed that the wound infection rate for high-risk patients who have operations lasting more than 215 minutes that involve rectal resection could benefit significantly from the use of a combination of oral and parenteral prophylactic antibiotics.

Mechanical Preparation. Mechanical cleansing of the colon lumen before elective colon resection is a time-tested procedure that when done properly, reduces the total fecal luminal mass, allowing easier operative manipulation of the colon. The cleansing also facilitates the action of oral antibiotics. Vigorous mechanical cleaning alone, using either lavage techniques or the classic approach of dietary restriction, enemas, and cathartics, has not significantly reduced the number of microorganisms in the residual colonic material. This microbiologic failure of mechanical cleansing alone also equates with clinical failure. In two large prospective, randomized, double-blind clinical trials investigating the efficacy of oral antibiotic prophylaxis, more than 40% of patients undergoing elective colon resection who were given mechanical cleansing alone developed septic complications (51,52).

Today, approaches to mechanical cleansing vary considerably (36). The time-honored 5-day preoperative preparation using dietary restriction, enemas, and cathartics was long ago abandoned, for many good reasons. At the top of this list were the severe iatrogenically induced metabolic abnormalities that were reported more than 20 years ago. Modern approaches include standard mechanical cleansing using dietary restriction, cathartics, and enemas for 2 days, or on the day before operation, whole-gut lavage with an electrolyte solution, sodium phosphate solution, or polyethylene glycol. A suggested schema for mechanical preparation is offered in Table 39.2 and Figure 39.1.

Antibiotic Preparation. Today the vast majority of surgeons employ both antibiotics and mechanical cleansing as preparation for elective colon resection (36). The chosen antibiotics should be effective in suppressing colonic facultative aerobes and anaerobes (53,54). Debate continues over which agents are ideal and which route of administration is preferred. Investigators who

---

TABLE 39.2.   Suggested Approach to Preoperative Preparation for Elective Colon Resection

Two days before surgery (at home):
1. Low residue or liquid diet *plus*
   sodium phosphate (Phosphosoda), 1½ oz p.o. at 8 p.m.
   Or
2. Nothing additional until next day

One day before surgery (at home or in hospital if necessary)
   Admit in morning (if necessary and allowed)
1. Continue clear liquid diet, i.v. fluids as needed *plus*
   Sodium phosphate (Phosphosoda), 1½ oz p.o. at 8 a.m.
   Or
2. Start clear liquid diet *plus*
   Whole-gut lavage with polyethylene glycol, 1 L/hr p.o. starting at 8 a.m. until diarrhea is clear (no longer than 3–4 hr)

No enemas

All patients receive 1 g neomycin and 1 g erythromycin base p.o. at 1 p.m., 2 p.m., and 11 p.m.

Day of surgery
   Operation at 8 a.m.
   A single dose of antibiotic with broad-spectrum aerobic/anaerobic activity given i.v. by anesthesia personnel in the operating room just before incision; repeat dosage if operation lasts more than 2 hr.

Note: p.o., orally; i.v., intravenously.

---

advocate oral antibiotics generally stress the importance of reducing the number of microorganisms in the colon lumen before opening the colon; those who rely on parenteral agents stress the importance of adequate tissue levels of antibiotics.

Oral Antibiotic Agents. At the present time, three regimens of oral agents are used, which combine neomycin with either erythromycin base, metronidazole, or tetracycline (36,37). The greatest experience in the United States has been with the neomycin-erythromycin base preparation, which was introduced in 1972 (53), whereas metronidazole plus either kanamycin or neomycin is popular in Great Britain (37). Authoritative reviews of antibiotic prophylaxis for colon surgery continue to support the value of oral neomycin-erythromycin base in preventing infections after elective colon resection (4,29,36,55). No convincing data are available to recommend the use of metronidazole over erythromycin base in this clinical setting. The pharmacokinetics of the oral neomycin-erythromycin base bowel preparation has been studied in healthy volunteers (38). The studies suggest that

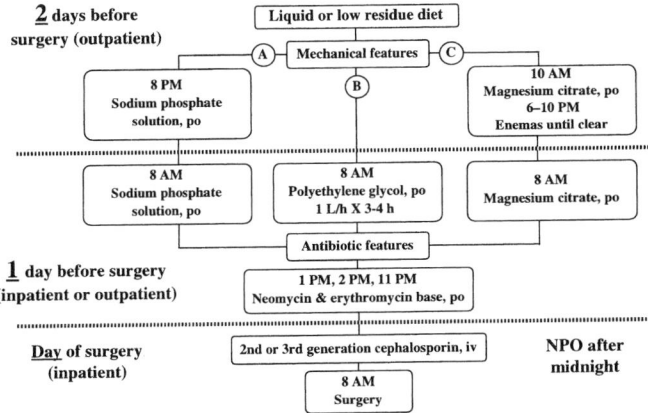

Figure 39.1. Preoperative bowel preparation.

when adequate mechanical preparation is used, both intraluminal (local) levels of antibiotics and the serum (systemic) level of erythromycin are significant, and that both mechanisms may play a role in preventing infection after colon surgery. The timing of administration of these oral agents appears to be critical. It is recommended that only 1 g of each agent, neomycin and erythromycin base, be given at 1:00 p.m., 2:00 p.m., and 11:00 p.m. on the day before surgery (6 g total; see Table 39.2). Surgery should be planned for about 8:00 a.m. when this schedule is followed. If the operation is scheduled for later in the day, the timing of the doses should be adjusted to preserve the 19 hours' preparation.

Parenteral Antibiotic Agents. The first prospective, randomized, double-blind study on parenteral antibiotic prophylaxis in elective colon resection (published in 1969) used perioperative intramuscular cephaloridine (56). This study revealed a significant reduction in postoperative infections (7% vs. 30%) in the group of patients who received antibiotics in addition to mechanical preparation as compared with those who had mechanical preparation alone, but other clinical studies using the same or similar first-generation cephalosporins for prophylaxis failed to show the superiority of this approach over placebo (mechanical preparation alone) or oral neomycin-erythromycin base (37). Clinical studies comparing parenteral cephalosporin alone in this setting showed a lack of efficacy unless the antibiotic was active against facultative aerobic and anaerobic organisms (57). Parenteral agents that have shown efficacy alone or in combination with an aminoglycoside include cefoxitin, cefotetan, metronidazole, and doxycycline (37). Most investigators recommend perioperative administration of one to five doses of parenteral agent during a 24-hour period starting shortly before operation; however, one multicenter study showed that a single intravenous dose of cefotetan resulted in a 14% infection rate, which was thought to be comparable to an 11% rate among patients who received multiple doses of intravenous cefoxitin (58). It should be noted, however, that the total infection rates in this study were higher than those reported in the Veterans Administration study using oral neomycin and erythromycin alone (6% to 9%) (51,59). In my opinion, potent therapeutic antibiotic agents such as imipenem, which was advocated, have no place in prophylactic antibiotic regimens used before elective colon resection (60).

Combination of Parenteral and Oral Antibiotic Agents. Most surgeons presently use both oral and parenteral antibiotic agents and mechanical cleansing as preoperative preparation before elective colon resection in the hope of reducing the postoperative infection rate. In a survey of more than 450 colorectal surgeons, reported in 1997, only 11% used systemic antibiotics alone before colon surgery, whereas 87% used a combination of oral and parenteral antibiotics (36). Parenteral antibiotics that are active against both facultative aerobic and anaerobic organisms (e.g., cefotetan, cefoxitin, and ceftizoxime) given in addition to oral neomycin-erythromycin base have been shown to be associated with a low incidence of infection (37). It appears at this time that the addition of one dose of parenteral antibiotic such as that already mentioned, given within 30 minutes of incision to the oral and mechanical bowel preparation, may be beneficial (see Table 39.2).

SMALL INTESTINAL OPERATIONS

Because the contents of the small intestine are liquid and transit time is rapid, extensive preoperative mechanical preparation for elective surgery is unnecessary. There are no antibiotic prophylaxis studies on surgery of the ileum, the site of most apparent risk of infection, because of the complex intestinal flora

present at this level (61). It seems prudent, however, to use the neomycin-erythromycin base oral bowel preparation for such elective procedures. Parenteral agents effective against fecal facultative aerobes and anaerobes are recommended for emergency procedures such as that for small bowel obstruction.

APPENDECTOMY

The bacteriology of perforated and gangrenous appendicitis is extremely complex. Bennion et al. (62) have isolated in these cases an average of 11 different bacteria from each specimen, including 3 facultative aerobes and 8 anaerobes. As in the other post–colonic resection infections, *B. fragilis* was the most commonly isolated anaerobe and *E. coli* the most common facultative aerobe.

Risk of Infection. The pathologic state of the appendix is the most important determinant of postoperative infection (63–65). The wound infection rate after appendectomy for perforated or gangrenous appendicitis is four to five times higher than that for early disease. A prospective study of nonperforated appendicitis that used a logistic regression analysis of risk factors has shown that the risk of postoperative wound infection is related only to failure to use perioperative antibiotics and the surgeon's determination of the appendix as being gangrenous (64). The highest rate of infection (77%) was predicted for patients who received placebo and had a gangrenous appendix, and the lowest rate (2%) for those who received an antibiotic perioperatively and did not have a gangrenous appendix at surgery. Perioperative antibiotic prophylaxis had a beneficial effect in decreasing hospital stay.

Antibiotic Recommendations. Because it is often impossible to determine the pathologic state of the appendix before or even during operation (64), it is recommended that a parenteral antibiotic agent be given prophylactically in all cases. Agents that are active against both aerobic gram-negative bacilli and anaerobes are more effective than those that are active only against the anaerobes. It appears that the prophylactic regimen can be a single dose (65) or three doses (64). For perforated appendicitis with evidence of local or general peritonitis or intraabdominal abscess, the use of antimicrobials should be considered therapeutic, not prophylactic.

PENETRATING ABDOMINAL TRAUMA

Risk of Infection. Hollow viscus damage with the associated escape of endogenous microorganisms is the principal risk factor for the development of postoperative infectious complications after exploratory laparotomy for penetrating abdominal trauma (66). Using a logistic regression analysis of such patients, we showed that a statistically higher risk of infection was also associated with increasing age of the patient, associated injury to the left colon necessitating colostomy, many units of blood or blood products administered at surgery, and a large number of injured organs identified at operation (66). Leaving the operative wound packed open with saline-soaked gauze decreases the frequency of postoperative wound infection in high-risk patients (67).

Antibiotic Recommendations. The use of one parenteral dose of antibiotic alone, given just before abdominal exploration for penetrating abdominal trauma, has been associated with a low postoperative infection rate in patients with no observed GI tract leakage (66). If GI tract leakage is identified at operation, it is usually recommended that the antibiotic agents be given for 1 to 3 days. In this clinical setting, it is important to use agents that have both facultative aerobic and anaerobic activity. Use of agents that do not provide adequate anaerobic coverage has been associated with a high rate of clinical failure.

TRAUMATIC CHEST INJURIES
Certain published studies (68,69) have shown the value of parenteral antibiotic prophylaxis in the prevention of pneumonia or empyema after the placement of a chest tube to correct the hemopneumothorax associated with chest trauma. In one study (68), 500 mg of cefazolin was given intravenously every 8 hours for 24 hours. In the other study (69), 1 g of cefonicid was administered every 24 hours until the time of chest tube removal. Significantly reduced infection rates were observed in both studies in the patients receiving antibiotics compared with the patients receiving placebo.

GYNECOLOGIC AND OBSTETRIC INFECTIONS
Parenteral antibiotic prophylaxis has been shown to decrease significantly the incidence of postoperative infections after vaginal hysterectomy and after emergency cesarean section and may be of benefit in abdominal hysterectomy (29).

Risk of Infection. In 1982, Shapiro et al. (14) were the first to use logistic regression analysis to identify the risk factors for operative site infections after abdominal or vaginal hysterectomy. They observed that increasing duration of operative time was associated with a decreasing effect of antibiotic prophylaxis for operative site infection. The statistically significant benefit of antibiotic prophylaxis in procedures that lasted 1 hour or less was lost in operations that lasted more than 3.3 hours.

In one large single hospital study of post–cesarean section wound infections, significantly higher rates of infections were observed among clinic patients (15.8%) than among private patients (6.0%) (70). All the significant individual risk factors for infection—including emergency versus elective operation, number of vaginal examinations before operation, duration of operation, vertical skin incision, and category of surgeon—were overrepresented in the clinic group.

Antibiotic Recommendations. A single intravenous dose of parenteral cefazolin given shortly before incision for abdominal or vaginal hysterectomy or after cord clamping in high-risk cesarean section is currently recommended (29). Many other second- or third-generation cephalosporin agents have also been proven efficacious in a single-dose regimen; however, evidence of their clinical superiority is lacking.

UROLOGIC PROCEDURES
Antimicrobial prophylaxis is not recommended before urologic operations if the patient has sterile urine (29). If culture of urine propagates organisms, the patient should be treated with appropriate antimicrobial agents before operation to sterilize the urine. Before prostatectomy, a single dose of intravenous prophylactic antibiotic is used immediately before operation if the urine in *not* sterile (29).

Overview of Antibiotic Prophylaxis in Surgery

Improvements in antibiotic prophylaxis, including the timing of initial administration, appropriate choice of antibiotic agents in each clinical setting, and short duration of administration, have proved the value of the use of prophylactic antibiotics and are currently recommended by authoritative groups (4,29). A computer-generated reminder of appropriate perioperative antibiotic treatment, placed in the patient's chart before operation, has been shown to improve prescribing habits and to

produce a concurrent decline in the number of postoperative wound infections (71). Future studies of antibiotic prophylaxis should strongly consider risk factors for the individual patient in addition to testing new antibiotic agents and administration approaches.

REFERENCES

1. Nichols RL. Postoperative wound infection. *N Engl J Med* 1982;307:1701.
2. Haley RW, Culver DH, White JW, et al. The nationwide nosocomial infection rate: a new need for vital statistics. *Am J Epidemiol* 1985;121:159.
3. Nichols RL. Techniques known to prevent postoperative wound infection. *Infect Control* 1982;3:34.
4. Nichols RL. Preventing surgical site infections: a surgeon's perspective. *Emerg Infect Dis* 2001;7:220.
5. Haley RW, Culver DH, Morgan WM, et al. Identifying patients at high risk of surgical wound infection. *Am J Epidemiol* 1985;121:206.
6. Culver DH, Horan TC, Gaynes RP, and the National Nosocomial Infections Surveillance Systems (NNIS). Surgical wound infection rates by wound class, operation, and risk index in U.S. hospitals. *Am J Med* 1991;91[Suppl 3B]:152S.
7. Keats AS. The ASA classifications of physical status—a recapitulation. *Anesthesiology* 1978;49:233.
8. Cruse PJE, Foord R. A five-year prospective study of 23,649 surgical wounds. *Arch Surg* 1973;107:206.
9. Seropian R, Reynolds BM. Wound infections after preoperative depilatory versus razor preparation. *Am J Surg* 1971;121:251.
10. Balthazar ER, Colt J, Nichols RL. Preoperative hair removal: a random, prospective study. *South Med J* 1982;75:799.
11. Rotter ML, Larsen SO, Cooke EM, et al. A comparison of the effects of preoperative whole-body bathing with detergent alone and with detergent containing chlorhexidine gluconate on the frequency of wound infections after clean surgery. *J Hosp Infect* 1988;11:310.
12. Edwards LD. The epidemiology of 2056 remote site infections and 1966 surgical wound infections occurring in 1865 patients: a four-year study of 40,923 operations at Rush-Presbyterian-St. Luke's Hospital, Chicago. *Ann Surg* 1976;184:758.
13. Valentine RJ, Weigelt JA, Dryer D, et al. Effect of remote infections on clean wound infection rates. *Am J Infect Control* 1986;14:64.
14. Shapiro M, Munoz A, Tager IB, et al. Risk factors for infection at the operative site after abdominal or vaginal hysterectomy. *N Engl J Med* 1982;307:1661.
15. Gorbach SL, Condon RE, Conte JE Jr, et al. Evaluation of new anti-infective drugs for surgical prophylaxis. *Clin Infect Dis* 1992;15[Suppl 1]:5313.
16. Nora PF, Vanecko RM, Bransfield JJ. Prophylactic abdominal drains. *Arch Surg* 1972;106:173.
17. Magee C. Potentiation of wound infection by surgical drains. *Am J Surg* 1976;131:547.
18. Alexander JW, Koorelitz J, Alexander NS. Prevention of wound infections: a case for closed suction drainage to remove wound fluids deficient in opsonic proteins. *Am J Surg* 1976;132:59.
19. Nichols RL. The operating room. In: Bennett JV, Brachman PS, eds. *Hospital infections*, 3rd ed. Boston: Little, Brown and Company, 1992:461–473.
20. Borst M, Collier C, Miller D. Operating room surveillance: a new approach in reducing hip and knee prosthetic wound infections. *Am J Infect Control* 1986;14:161.
21. LoCicero III J, Quebbeman EJ, Nichols RL. Health hazards in the operating room: An update. *Bull Am Coli Surg* 1987;72:4.
22. Lidwell OM, Lowbury EJL, Whyte W, et al. Effect of ultraclean air in operating rooms on deep sepsis in the joint after total hip or knee replacement: a randomised study. *Br Med J* 1982;285:10.
23. Nichols RL. Current approaches to antibiotic prophylaxis in surgery. *Infect Dis Clin Pract* 1993;2:149.
24. Nichols RL. Antibiotic prophylaxis in surgery. *Curr Opin Infect Dis* 1994;7:647.
25. Gorbach SL. The role of cephalosporins in surgical prophylaxis. *J Antimicrob Chemother* 1989;23[Suppl D]:61.
26. Burke JF. The effective period of preventive antibiotic action in experimental incision and dermal lesions. *Surgery* 1961;50:161.
27. Bernard HR, Cole WR. The prophylaxis of surgical infection: the effect of prophylactic antimicrobial drugs on the incidence of infection following potentially contaminated operations. *Surgery* 1964;56:151.
28. Nichols RL. Surgical bacteriology: an overview. In: Nyhus LM, ed. *Surgery annual*, vol 13. New York: Appleton-Century-Crofts, 1981:205–238.
29. Antimicrobial prophylaxis in surgery. *Med Lett* 2001;43:91.
30. Platt R, Zaleznik DF, Hopkins CC, et al. Perioperative antibiotic prophylaxis for herniorrhaphy and breast surgery. *N Engl J Med* 1990;322:153.
31. Westererman EL. Antibiotic prophylaxis in surgery. Historical background, rationale, and relationship to prospective payment. *Am J Infect Control* 1984;12:339.
32. Kernodle DS, Classen DC, Burke JP, et al. Failure of cephalosporins to prevent *Staphylococcus aureus* surgical wound infections. *JAMA* 1990;263:961.
33. DiPiro JT, Bowden TA Jr, Hooks VH III. Prophylactic parenteral cephalosporins in surgery: are the newer agents better? *JAMA* 1984;252:3277.

34. Shapiro M, Townsend TR, Rosner B, et al. Use of antimicrobial drugs in general hospitals: patterns of prophylaxis. *N Engl J Med* 1979;301:351.
35. DiPiro JT, Cheung RPF, Bowden TA Jr, et al. Single dose systemic antibiotic prophylaxis of surgical wound infections. *Am J Surg* 1986;152:552.
36. Nichols RL, Smith JW, Garcia RY, et al. Current practices of preoperative bowel preparation among North American colorectal surgeons. *Clin Infect Dis* 1997;24:609.
37. Nichols RL. Bowel preparations. In: Meakins J, ed. *Care of the surgical patient*, 2nd ed. New York: Scientific American, 1990:1–10.
38. Nichols RL, Condon RE, DiSanto AR. Preoperative bowel preparation. *Arch Surg* 1977;112:1493.
39. Moleski RJ, Andriole VT. Role of the infectious disease specialist in containing costs of antibiotics in the hospital. *Rev Infect Dis* 1986;8:488.
40. Cannon SR, Dyson PH, Sanderson PJ. Pseudomembranous colitis associated with antibiotic prophylaxis in orthopedic surgery. *J Bone Joint Surg Br* 1988;70:600.
41. Kernodle DS, Barg NL, Kaiser AB. Low-level colonization of hospitalized patients with methicillin-resistant coagulase-negative staphylococci and emergence of the organisms during surgical antimicrobial prophylaxis. *Antimicrob Agents Chemother* 1988;32:202.
42. Hall JC, Christiansen K, Carter MJ, et al. Antibiotic prophylaxis in cardiac operations. *Ann Thorac Surg* 1993;56:916.
43. Nichols RL, Smith JW. Intragastric microbial colonization in common disease states of the stomach and duodenum. *Ann Surg* 1975;182:557.
44. LoCicero J, Nichols RL. Sepsis after gastroduodenal operations: relationship to gastric acid, motility, and endogenous microflora. *South Med J* 1980;73:878.
45. Nichols RL, Webb WR, Jones JW, et al. Efficacy of antibiotic prophylaxis in high risk gastroduodenal operations. *Am J Surg* 1982;143:94.
46. Keighley MRB, Flinn R, Alexander-Williams J. Multivariate analysis of clinical and operative findings associated with biliary sepsis. *Br J Surg* 1976;63:528.
47. Murray WR, Bradley JA. Antibiotic prophylaxis in elective biliary surgery. *Res Clin Forums* 1983;5:97.
48. Nichols RL, Condon RE. Preoperative preparations of the colon. *Surg Gynecol Obstet* 1971;132:323.
49. Kaiser AB, Herrington JL Jr, Jacobs JK, et al. Cefoxitin versus erythromycin, neomycin, and cefazolin in colorectal operations. *Ann Surg* 1983;198:525.
50. Coppa GF, Eng K. Factors involved in antibiotic selection in elective colon and rectal surgery. *Surgery* 1988;104:853.
51. Clarke JS, Condon RE, Bartlett JG, et al. Preoperative oral antibiotics reduce septic complications of colon operations: results of prospective, randomized, double-blind clinical study. *Ann Surg* 1977;186:251.
52. Washington JA II, Dearing WH, Judd ES, et al. Effect of preoperative antibiotic regimen on development of infection after intestinal surgery: prospective, randomized, double-blind study. *Ann Surg* 1974;180:567.
53. Nichols RL, Condon RE, Gorbach SL, et al. Efficacy of preoperative antimicrobial preparation of the bowel. *Ann Surg* 1972;176:227.
54. Nichols RL, Broido P, Condon RE, et al. The effect of preoperative neomycin-erythromycin intestinal preparation on the incidence of infectious complications following colon surgery. *Ann Surg* 1973;178:453.
55. Mangram AJ, Horan TC, Pearson ML, et al. Guidelines for prevention of surgical site infection, 1999. *Infect Control Hosp Epidemiol* 1999;20:247.
56. Polk HC Jr, Lopez-Mayor JF. Postoperative wound infections. A prospective study of determinant factors and prevention. *Surgery* 1969;66:97.
57. Slama TG, Carey LC, Fass RJ. Comparative efficacy of prophylactic cephalothin and cefamandole for elective colon surgery. *Am J Surg* 1979;137:593.
58. Jagelman PG, Fabian TC, Nichols RL, et al. Single-dose cefoxitin versus multiple dose cefoxitin as prophylaxis in colorectal surgery. *Am J Surg* 1988;155(5A):71.
59. Condon RE, Bartlett JG, Greenlee H, et al. Efficacy of oral and systemic antibiotic prophylaxis in colorectal operations. *Arch Surg* 1983;118:496.
60. Karran SJ, Sutton G, Gartell P, et al. Imipenem prophylaxis in elective colorectal surgery. *Br J Surg* 1993;80:1196.
61. Nichols RL, Condon RE, Bentley DW, et al. Real microflora in surgical patients. *J Urol* 1971;105:351.
62. Bennion RS, Thompson JE, Baron EJ, et al. Gangrenous and perforated appendicitis with peritonitis: treatment and bacteriology. *Clin Ther* 1990;12:1.
63. Krukowski ZH. Preventing wound infection after appendectomy: a review. *Br J Surg* 1988;75:1023.
64. Browder W, Smith JW, Vivoda L, et al. Nonperforative appendicitis: a continuing surgical dilemma. *J Infect Dis* 1989;159:1088.
65. Bauer T, Vennits BO, Holm B, et al. Antibiotic prophylaxis in acute nonperforated appendicitis. *Ann Surg* 1989;209:307.
66. Nichols RL, Smith JW, Klein DB, et al. Risk of infection after penetrating abdominal trauma. *N Engl J Med* 1984;311:1065.
67. Nichols RL, Smith JW, Robertson GD, et al. Prospective alterations in therapy in penetrating abdominal trauma. *Arch Surg* 1993;128:55.
68. Cant PJ, Smyth S, Smart DO. Antibiotic prophylaxis is indicated for chest stab wounds requiring closed tube thoracostomy. *Br J Surg* 1993;80:464.
69. Nichols, RL, Smith JW, Muzik AC, et al. Preventive antibiotic usage in traumatic thoracic injuries requiring closed tube thoracostomy. *Chest* 1994;106:1493.
70. Webster J. Post-caesarean wound infection: a review of the risk factors. *Aust N Z J Obstet Gynaecol* 1988;28:201.
71. Larsen RA, Evans RS, Burke JP, et al. Improved perioperative antibiotic use and reduced surgical wound infection through use of computer decision analysis. *Infect Control Hosp Epidemiol* 1989;10:316.

CHAPTER 40
Antimicrobial Prophylaxis for Nonsurgical Infections

Jan V. Hirschmann

Physicians have applied the term *antimicrobial prophylaxis* to four different situations:

1. *Preventing infection by exogenous pathogens:* The target organisms are not members of the host's normal flora, and the antimicrobial agent, given before exposure, promptly eradicates the pathogens when they enter the bloodstream or tissues. An example of this type of prophylaxis is the continuous administration of penicillin to prevent streptococcal pharyngeal infections in patients with rheumatic heart disease.
2. *Preventing the host's resident flora from infecting a normally sterile site:* The antimicrobial agent, present in the tissues or body fluids, prevents infection in these sites caused by the host's own organisms, usually colonizing a contiguous cutaneous or mucosal surface. An example is the use of antimicrobials in predisposed women to prevent recurrent urinary tract infections by bacteria that originate from adjacent vaginal or fecal flora.
3. *Preventing disease by a dormant pathogen that is already infecting the host:* The infection occurred long ago, and the organism remains alive but dormant in the asymptomatic host. An example is the use of isoniazid to prevent reactivation of tuberculosis in a previously infected but untreated patient. Because infection has already occurred, the term *treatment of asymptomatic infection* may be more accurate than *prophylaxis* in this setting.
4. *Preventing disease by pathogens that recently infected the host who does not yet exhibit clinical manifestations:* An example is the use of antimicrobial agents shortly after an animal bite, but before clinical signs of infection have emerged. Because the organisms have already entered normally sterile tissues before the administration of the antimicrobials, *early therapy* is probably a more accurate term than *prophylaxis*.

This chapter discusses oral or parenteral antimicrobial prophylaxis used in the first two senses just mentioned in nonsurgical settings; it is organized by the anatomic sites at which the prophylaxis is directed. It is confined to prophylaxis against bacterial infections and summarizes some important examples demonstrating both the benefits and the problems of using antimicrobials for this purpose. Other chapters provide more detailed information about some of these and descriptions of antimicrobial prophylaxis in other settings, including in patients with infection with human immunodeficiency virus (HIV).

In general, antimicrobial prophylaxis is most likely to be successful if the target organisms have a stable pattern of susceptibility and the duration of use is short. Otherwise, resistance to the administered agent may develop. Demonstrating the efficacy of prophylaxis requires carefully controlled trials with clearly defined outcomes. Even when these studies show that prophylaxis is effective, however, the benefits should clearly exceed the liabilities, which include costs, adverse effects, and the potential for the emergence of antimicrobial-resistant organisms, both in the individual recipients and in the environment at large. Widespread use of antibiotics to prevent otitis media in children has probably contributed significantly to the increasing antimicrobial resistance of *Streptococcus pneumoniae* and *Haemophilus influenzae*, for example, and substantial use of prophylactic antibiotics in intensive care unit settings may cause the emergence of infections caused by multidrug-resistant bacteria. Clinicians, therefore, must be cautious in using antimicrobials to prevent infections.

RESPIRATORY TRACT

Group A Streptococcal Pharyngitis in Patients with Previous Rheumatic Fever

Group A streptococcus, *Streptococcus pyogenes*, remains sensitive to penicillin and continues to be effective in preventing streptococcal pharyngeal infections in patients with previous rheumatic fever. These infections, often asymptomatic, may provoke recurrences of rheumatic fever, the consequences of which are particularly serious for those with previous carditis, because each episode can cause further heart damage. A carefully controlled trial in patients with prior rheumatic fever has convincingly demonstrated that a monthly intramuscular dose of benzathine penicillin is superior to daily oral doses of penicillin or sulfadiazine in reducing the frequency of recurrent streptococcal infections and subsequent attacks of rheumatic fever in these patients (1). The advantage of benzathine penicillin arises partly because of greater compliance with a single monthly injection than with daily oral doses.

Streptococcal Pharyngitis in Military Recruits

In the mid-1940s, a controlled trial demonstrated that oral sulfadiazine substantially reduced the incidence of streptococcal infections in military recruits in whom large outbreaks of pharyngitis occurred. The emergence of sulfadiazine-resistant strains, however, rendered prophylaxis ineffective. Later programs administering benzathine penicillin to all recruits at centers with previous high rates of streptococcal infections markedly diminished their frequency. When routine prophylaxis ended, outbreaks of streptococcal disease recurred (2). In this setting, the long-acting penicillin presumably eradicated pharyngeal infection in those already infected (treatment of asymptomatic carriers) and prevented acquisition of the organism by those who were not (prophylaxis).

All members of the group require prophylaxis, however, because those who do not receive it may serve as reservoirs for transmitting the organism to the penicillin recipients as their drug levels fall and protection wanes (3). For penicillin-allergic recruits, oral erythromycin, which appears to be as effective as benzathine penicillin, should be used to ensure prophylaxis throughout the population (4). Another option is azithromycin (5).

Meningococcal Infection and *Haemophilus influenzae* Infection

Epidemics of meningococcal disease in military installations in World War II also led to trials of sulfadiazine prophylaxis, which was quite effective (6). The subsequent development of sulfadiazine resistance has made that agent useful only when the epidemic strain is known to be susceptible. Antimicrobial prophylaxis is now directed mainly at household contacts of patients with meningococcal disease, in whom the medication used functions principally to eradicate asymptomatic colonization already present rather than to prevent acquisition of the organism. The

agents used include oral agents—rifampin or ciprofloxacin–or parenteral ceftriaxone.

Administering antibiotics to contacts in households or day care centers of children with invasive *H. influenzae* type B infections serves the same purpose of eradicating the organism from asymptomatic carriers who are at increased risk of developing serious disease (7), although widespread use of a vaccine against *H. influenzae* had markedly reduced the incidence of childhood infections from this organism.

Otitis Media

Controlled trials have shown that sulfisoxazole (8,9), ampicillin (10), or amoxicillin (11) reduces the incidence of recurrent episodes of acute otitis media in children. Although the criteria for the studies differed, prophylaxis is probably most effective for those who have had at least three episodes in 6 months or four in 1 year (12), The emergence of penicillin-resistant *S. pneumoniae*, however, has caused experts to discourage use of antibiotics for this purpose.

Bacterial Superinfections of Viral Respiratory Diseases

Several studies have shown no benefit for antimicrobials in preventing bacterial superinfections of viral upper respiratory tract diseases. These include colds, influenza, and measles (13).

Bacterial Pneumonia

Administration of antibiotics to unconscious patients (14) or those with acute heart failures (15) does not diminish the incidence of bacterial pneumonia. Similarly, prophylactic tetracycline or minocycline given to Air Force trainees with nonbacterial pneumonia did not reduce the incidence of bacterial pneumonias (superinfections) (16).

To decrease the frequency of bacterial pneumonia and possibly other infections in critically ill patients, several studies have evaluated "selective decontamination" of the digestive tract. The goal is to prevent potential pathogens, primarily facultative gram-negative bacilli and yeasts, from colonizing the oropharynx and gastrointestinal (GI) tract, the presumed sites of origin from which these organisms migrate to cause pneumonias and other infections. Most trials have included patients in intensive care units receiving mechanical ventilation and have employed three types of antibiotics applied as a topical oropharyngeal paste and administered orally: polymyxin E or colistin, tobramycin, or gentamicin, and amphotericin B. Most have also given a parenteral cephalosporin, usually cefotaxime, for the first 3 to 5 days, based on the assumption that achieving decontamination takes several days and the systemic agents should prevent infection during that period of inadequate protection. The quality of the studies has varied; most of the rigorously performed trials show a dramatic reduction in the occurrence of pneumonia, especially from gram-negative bacilli (17). The diagnosis of pneumonia in ventilated patients is difficult, however, and definitions have varied. The studies with the most stringent criteria have shown significant but less impressive effects (18). Overall, the trials have demonstrated no decreased mortality, length of hospital stay, or costs. Because of the expense and adverse effects, particularly the emergence of antibiotic-resistant organisms, selective decontamination does not seem prudent unless more convincing evidence demonstrates that its benefits clearly outweigh its liabilities, even when used on a long-term basis (18).

URINARY TRACT

Daily doses of nitrofurantoin (19,20), methenamine mandelate with ascorbic acid (21), trimethoprim-sulfamethoxazole (TMP-SMX) (20,21), or TMP alone (20,22) reduce the frequency of urinary tract infections in women with recurrent episodes. Mandelamine, however, seems less effective than the other agents (21). TMP-SMX used thrice weekly works as well as daily doses (23) and continues to be effective for at least as long as 5 years of uninterrupted administration (24). An analysis of costs suggests that continuous antimicrobial prophylaxis is worthwhile for women who have three or more urinary tract infections per year (25). Other suggested agents include norfloxacin, cephalexin, cefaclor, and cephradine (26). For those with infections temporally related to intercourse, postcoital administration of TMP-SMX is an alternative to thrice-weekly doses (27).

Patients with neurogenic bladder dysfunction pursuing a bladder retraining program with intermittent urethral catheterization had significantly fewer episodes of bacteriuria when given methenamine mandelate and ammonium chloride for 21 days than a group who received placebo (28). Another study demonstrated that TMP-SMX delayed the onset of bacteriuria, decreased its frequency, and reduced symptomatic episodes. Subsequent bacteriuria with resistant organisms was common though, seriously limiting the usefulness of this approach (29).

GASTROINTESTINAL TRACT

Traveler's Diarrhea

Controlled trials have demonstrated the efficacy of doxycycline (30,31), TMP-SMX (32,33), TMP alone (33), norfloxacin (33), ciprofloxacin (34), and bicozamycin (35) in reducing the frequency of traveler's diarrhea by 50% to 85% in persons visiting high-risk areas. The common pathogen is apparently enterotoxigenic *Escherichia coli*, but many cases are due to viruses, parasites, or other bacteria. Some have argued that antimicrobial prophylaxis is more cost-effective than treating the diarrhea when it occurs (36); others have asserted that antimicrobial prophylaxis is not warranted for any group because of the possible (though rare) adverse effects, the infrequency of moderate to severe disease (<30%), and the prompt response to antimicrobial treatment (37). Prophylaxis is probably most appropriate for patients in whom diarrhea exacts a heavy toll: those with significant underlying disorders, such as inflammatory bowel disease, insulin-dependent diabetes mellitus, acquired immunodeficiency syndrome, and serious cardiac disorders (38).

Acute Pancreatitis

Two studies, one of 58 patients (39) and another of 86 patients (40), failed to show that prophylactic ampicillin reduced infectious complications of acute pancreatitis. The duration of fever or hospitalization was not diminished, and the frequency of pancreatic abscess in both the treated and the control group was quite low, but most of the patients had mild to moderately severe pancreatitis.

Antimicrobial prophylaxis, however, may be effective in patients with severe pancreatitis complicated by necrosis defined by computed tomographic (CT) criteria. In a randomized study, a 14-day course of imipenem significantly reduced the incidence of pancreatic sepsis from 30% in the 33 patients in the control group to 12% in the 41 antibiotic recipients (41). The frequency of extrapancreatic infections (e.g., pneumonia and urinary tract infections) was also significantly lower, but surgical intervention

and the mortality rates did not differ significantly between the two groups. Another randomized study of necrotizing pancreatitis compared imipenem in 30 patients with pefloxacin in 30 patients for 2 weeks (42). Pancreatic infection was 34% in the pefloxacin recipients and 10% in the imipenem group, a statistically significant difference, but there was no significant difference in extrapancreatic infections or mortality. A further study randomized 30 patients to cefuroxime and 30 to no prophylaxis (43). The frequency of pancreatic infection was similar, but the overall infection rate (including extrapancreatic sites) was significantly lower in the cefuroxime group, as was the mortality rate. Two smaller studies yielded conflicting results (44). One of 23 patients with alcoholic pancreatitis showed that a combination of ceftazidime, amikacin, and metronidazole for 10 days significantly decreased severe sepsis. The other of 26 patients with necrotizing pancreatitis primarily of biliary origin showed no benefit to ofloxacin and metronidazole.

Another approach is to employ selective bowel decontamination—the use of antimicrobials to decrease certain members of the bowel flora, from which the organisms responsible for pancreatic abscesses presumably originate. In a randomized trial of severe pancreatitis, but not necessarily with necrosis, 50 patients received oral and rectal nonabsorbable antibiotics (colistin, amphotericin, and norfloxacin), in addition to systemic cefotaxime, and 52 were in the control group (45). Pancreatic infections occurred in 18% of the antibiotic group compared with 37% in the controls, a significant difference primarily related to a decrease of infections with gram-negative bacilli. The mortality rate was also significantly lower.

Although the studies are not uniform in their findings, the evidence suggests that a 2-week course of imipenem may be worthwhile in patients with pancreatitis and CT-demonstrated necrosis.

SKIN

Recurrent Cellulitis and Staphylococcal Abscesses

In patients with lymphedema and recurrent episodes of cellulitis, monthly intramuscular doses of benzathine penicillin or daily oral doses of either penicillin or erythromycin for 1 week each month reduce the frequency of subsequent attacks (46). A study of patients with two or more episodes of erysipelas or cellulitis in the previous year demonstrated that daily erythromycin or penicillin prevented any recurrences, compared with a frequency of 50% in the control group (47). In a trial involving 22 patients with a history of recurrent staphylococcal skin abscesses, oral daily clindamycin for 3 months significantly reduced the frequency of this infection when compared with placebo (48).

MISCELLANEOUS INFECTIONS

Infections with Granulocytopenia

Attempts to prevent infections in patients with neutropenia from an underlying disease or from cancer chemotherapy have included antimicrobial agents aimed at "total decontamination" of the alimentary tract and a more selective regimen directed primarily at enteric gram-negative bacilli. The underlying assumption is that organisms that cause infection in granulocytopenic patients usually originate from their GI tract. The total decontamination program uses broad-spectrum oral nonabsorbable agents like vancomycin, nystatin, polymyxin B, and gentamicin, often in conjunction with protective isolation in units that employ laminar flow ventilation. Results of the studies are conflicting but in general suggest that the combination of prophylactic antimicrobials and strict isolation reduces the frequency of infections compared with antimicrobials alone, isolation alone, or neither (49). Overall, the survival rates and the incidence of complete remission in those with acute leukemia did not increase, despite the reduction in frequency of infections.

Because of the great expense of protective isolation, the high cost of the antimicrobial agents, and their frequent GI side effects, selective decontamination, which is directed predominantly at enteric gram-negative bacilli, has replaced the total decontamination program. This approach, which employs no protective isolation, assumes that anaerobic bowel flora help prevent colonization by potential pathogens and should not be eradicated. The agents most frequently used have been TMP-SMX and the quinolones.

When compared with placebo recipients or untreated control subjects, patients receiving TMP-SMX have consistently had a marked reduction in the number of enteric gram-negative bacilli in stool cultures (50–55), but sometimes colonization with resistant gram-positive (48) or gram-negative (52,56) organisms has occurred. In general, fungi have not increased. The clinical outcome of prophylaxis, however, has varied strikingly in these studies: Some have shown a significant reduction in the incidence of fever (50,51,57,58), whereas others have not (52,53,56,59); in most (51,53,55,56,59,60), but not all (50,52), TMP-SMX has reduced the frequency of documented infections. It usually has not diminished the number of deaths due to infection (51,52,54,58,59) and an equal number of studies have reported a decrease (51,53,54) or no difference (52,56,60) in intravenous antibiotic use in those receiving TMP-SMX. In some trials, the infections in those receiving TMP-SMX have often been from resistant organisms (51,55), and this agent has sometimes significantly prolonged the duration of granulocytopenia (51,58). Antimicrobial prophylaxis does not seem to be effective when the neutropenia is short lived (52); in nearly all studies that show any benefit, the average duration of granulocytopenia has been at least 3 weeks.

The remarkable diversity in the reported efficacy of TMP-SMX probably relates to several factors: differences in doses, bacterial susceptibility at the sites of the trials, definitions of criteria for outcomes, number of patients studied, and populations of patients enrolled. Many studies are small, some include patients with granulocytopenia associated with both malignant and benign conditions, some involve only one type of cancer (e.g., leukemia and small cell carcinoma), and many fail to report certain important details (e.g., intravenous antibiotic use and antimicrobial susceptibility of the infecting organisms). One consistent finding, however, is that antimicrobial prophylaxis does not decrease the *overall fatality* rate, even in those studies in which it reduces *infectious* mortality. Furthermore, although many trials show a diminution in infections among those who receive cancer chemotherapy, this benefit does not translate into an increased remission rate for the underlying malignancy.

Compared with oral nonabsorbable antimicrobials, TMP-SMX was better than neomycin and colistin in reducing fever and the use of other antibiotics (61); it was equivalent to oral gentamicin in reducing infection rates but was tolerated better (62). The addition of oral nonabsorbable antibiotics (framycetin and colistin) to TMP-SMX had no advantage over TMP-SMX alone (63). Compared with oral nalidixic acid, TMP-SMX caused more protracted neutropenia but also significantly delayed the appearance of infection (64). Granulocytopenia was also more prolonged with TMP-SMX than with TMP alone, although the infection rates were similar and colonization with resistant gram-negative bacilli was greater with TMP (65).

One study has compared the quinolone norfloxacin with placebo in patients with acute leukemia and granulocytopenia (66) Norfloxacin significantly delayed the onset and decreased the duration of fever, diminished the frequency of gram-negative bacillary infections, and reduced the colonization of the stool with aerobic organisms. Mortality due to infections was not affected. Other trials have compared the quinolones with other forms of prophylaxis. Norfloxacin was tolerated better than oral vancomycin and polymyxin; it was also effective in reducing documented infections, including gram-negative bacteremia, and in decreasing the acquisition of resistant gram-negative organisms in the stool (67). When compared with TMP-SMX, norfloxacin was better at preventing acquisition of resistant gram-negative bacilli in stool cultures; there was no difference in infection rates, but gram-positive bacteremias were significantly more frequent with norfloxacin (68). Another quinolone, ciprofloxacin, was superior to TMP-SMX plus colistin at reducing bacteriologically documented infections, including those due to gram-negative bacilli, and at preventing colonization by resistant gram-negative bacilli (69). When compared to TMP-SMX, ofloxacin was better tolerated and shortened the duration of fever and of parenteral antimicrobial therapy more. The superiority derived from decreased infections by gram-negative bacilli (70). A study comparing norfloxacin with ciprofloxacin showed that the latter was more effective (71). Experience with these agents is limited, however, and the emergence of resistant organisms because of overuse could easily destroy their potential as both therapeutic and prophylactic agents (72).

In summary, the efficacy of antimicrobial prophylaxis for patients with granulocytopenia remains unclear. Certainly, it does not seem worthwhile unless the neutropenia is prolonged (at least 3 weeks). Its utility is probably also related in part to the nature of the nosocomial flora of the medical center where the patients receive treatment. Because antibiotic prophylaxis does not decrease mortality or improve response to cancer chemotherapy, and because resistant organisms may develop, the risks of giving these agents probably exceed their benefits in most circumstances.

Group B Streptococcal Infection in Neonates

Colonization of neonates with group B streptococci acquired from the mother during birth can cause sepsis and meningitis. Antibiotic therapy of colonized women in the third trimester of pregnancy before delivery—even when their male partners are treated concurrently—is not always effective in eradicating the organism, which usually returns shortly after the antimicrobial drug is discontinued (73,74). When benzathine penicillin is used, however, colonization at delivery is diminished (75). Two alternative approaches are to treat the mother at delivery or to give antibiotics to the infant afterward. The effect of intrapartum antibiotics may be to reduce the number of organisms in the mother's genital tract at birth and by crossing the placenta to protect the child against invasive disease *in utero* and during the first hours of life. When given at delivery, intravenous ampicillin (76,77) and penicillin or erythromycin, either intramuscular (78) or oral (79), markedly reduce the frequency of colonization of the infant at birth. The effect is sustained throughout hospitalization, but colonization of the infants at 6 weeks is common (78).

In one trial in which all neonates received penicillin shortly after birth, the frequency of early onset group B streptococcal infection decreased, but disease from penicillin-resistant organisms increased, and the overall mortality rate from infection did not differ in penicillin recipients and untreated control subjects (80). In another study, infants weighing 2,000 g or less given penicillin did not have fewer early onset group B streptococcal infections (81). In most cases, the infants were symptomatic at birth or within 4 hours afterward, and results of their initial blood cultures were positive, suggesting that infection had occurred *in utero* or during birth before penicillin administration. These studies indicate that intrapartum antibiotics are the most effective regimen for decreasing group B streptococcal colonization in the neonate.

One recommended approach to decreasing the frequency of group B streptococcal perinatal infections is to screen all pregnant women at 26 to 28 weeks of gestation for anogenital colonization and to give intrapartum antibiotics to all those with positive culture results and one or more of the following: (a) intrapartum temperature of 37.5°C or higher that is not attributable to an extrauterine source; (b) membrane rupture or onset of labor before 37 weeks of gestation; and (c) membrane rupture for more than 24 hours. Prophylactic antibiotics would also be given to women with any of the aforementioned characteristics who did not have prenatal cultures and to all with a history of giving birth to an infant with early onset group B streptococcal disease (82).

Staphylococcus aureus Infections with Hemodialysis

Patients undergoing hemodialysis who were nasal carriers of *S. aureus* were randomly assigned to receive no treatment or topical bacitracin four times a day for 7 days and oral rifampin for 5 days every 3 months if results of the nasal culture were positive. (83) The frequency of *S. aureus* infections, including bacteremia, access site infections, and cutaneous abscesses, during the

---

TABLE 40.1.   Regimens for Recommended Medical Antimicrobial Prophylaxis: Adult Doses Except Where Indicated

Condition	Indication	Regimen
Streptococcal pharyngitis (and rheumatic fever)	Military recruits	Benzathine penicillin G i.m. 1.2 million units about day 14 of training, repeat in 30 days or Erythromycin p.o. 250 mg b.i.d. for 60 days
Streptococcal pharyngitis (and rheumatic fever) recurrence	Recent rheumatic fever or rheumatic heart disease	Benzathine penicillin G i.m. 1.2 million units every 4 wk or Penicillin V p.o. 250 mg b.i.d. or Erythromycin p.o. 250 mg b.i.d.
Meningococcal disease	Household contact with meningococcal disease	Rifampin p.o.: 600 mg b.i.d. for 2 days; Ciprofloxacin 500 mg (one dose); ceftriaxone 250 mg i.m. (one dose)
Haemophilus influenzae disease	Household or day-care center contact with patient younger than 2 yr with *H. influenzae* type b disease	Rifampin p.o. 20 mg/kg q.d. for 4 days (maximal daily dose 600 mg)
Recurrent urinary tract infections in women	At least three infections per year	TMP-SMX 200 mg; 40 mg three times a week or nitrofurantoin p.o. 100 mg q.h.s.
	Related to coitus	TMP-SMX p.o. 200 mg/40 mg after coitus
Neurogenic bladder	Intermittent catheterization; bladder retraining	Methenamine mandelate p.o. 1 g q6h
Traveler's diarrhea	Serious underlying diseases	Doxycycline p.o., 100 mg q.d. or TMP-SMX p.o. (800 mg; 160 mg) q.d. or Norfloxacin p.o. 400 mg q.d. or Ciprofloxacin 500 mg q.d.
Recurrent cellulitis	Multiple episodes	Benzathine penicillin i.m. 1.2 million units/mo or Erythromycin or penicillin V 250 mg b.i.d.
Recurrent staphylococcal skin infections	Multiple episodes	Clindamycin p.o. 150 mg q.d. for 3 mo
Group B streptococcal disease in neonates	See text	Aqueous penicillin G i.v. 5 million units q6h or ampicillin i.v. 2 g initially, then q6h until delivery or Clindamycin i.v. 600 mg q8h until delivery if penicillin allergic
Staphylococcus aureus infection in patients undergoing long-term hemodialysis	Recurrent infection and nasal colonization	Rifampin p.o. 600 mg b.i.d. for 5 days plus topical bacitracin to nares q.d. for 7 days every 3 mo if positive nasal cultures for *S. aureus*
Acute pancreatitis	Necrosis on computed tomography	Imipenem 500 mg t.i.d. 14 days
Cirrhosis with ascites	Previous spontaneous bacterial peritonitis or ascites protein <1.5 g/dL	Ciprofloxacin 750 mg every week
Streptococcus pneumoniae infections	Children with sickle-cell anemia	Penicillin V p.o. 250 mg b.i.d.

Note: i.m., Intramuscularly; p.o., orally; i.v., intravenously; b.i.d., twice daily; q.d. daily; q.h.s. every day at bedtime; TMP-SMX, Trimethoprim-sulfamethoxazole; t.i.d, three times a day; i.m., intra.

3.5 years of study was significantly lower in those receiving prophylaxis. Rifampin-resistant *S. aureus*, however, did emerge, although these organisms neither persisted in the nares nor caused infection.

Skull fractures with Cerebrospinal Fluid Leak

A trial of penicillin in patients with skull fractures and cerebrospinal fluid rhinorrhea or otorrhea failed to demonstrate that the antibiotic prevented meningitis, although the incidence of this infection was quite low in both treated and untreated patients (84). A study including both open and basilar skull fractures also failed to demonstrate a reduction in meningitis when patients received 3 days of ceftriaxone or combined ampicillin-sulfadiazine (85).

Pneumococcal Infections in Sickle Cell Anemia

A trial of daily oral penicillin in children younger than 3 years with sickle cell anemia demonstrated a significant reduction in the frequency of pneumococcal septicemia compared with a placebo group (86). In another trial, monthly benzathine penicillin was markedly superior to the pneumococcal vaccine in preventing bacteremia and meningitis (87).

Infections in Cirrhosis

In hospitalized patients with cirrhosis and GI tract hemorrhage, oral nonabsorbable antibiotics, consisting of gentamicin-nystatin or neomycin-colistin-nystatin, decreased the frequency of spontaneous bacteremia or peritonitis from about 21% to about 9% when given until 48 hours after the hemorrhage ceased (88). Although infectious mortality significantly diminished, the mortality rate for the whole hospitalization was unaffected. Another trial confined antimicrobial prophylaxis to patients with rebleeding or Child-Pugh class C disease, who were considered at high risk for infection (89). Those randomly assigned to a combination of ciprofloxacin and amoxicillin-clavulanate for 3 days had significantly fewer bacterial infections than the control group, but mortality was not significantly affected. A similar trial randomized patients with cirrhosis and bleeding esophageal varices to ofloxacin for 10 days or no antibiotic (90). The ofloxacin recipients had significantly fewer infections than the controls, but death rates were similar. A trial of oral norfloxacin for 7 days also showed a significant reduction in infections, but no change in mortality (91). A study of oral norfloxacin alone or combined with intravenous cefotaxime showed no benefit to adding the parenteral agent (92).

Cirrhotic patients with ascites are at risk of developing spontaneous bacterial peritonitis. In one investigation, patients with cirrhosis and a total protein concentration of less than 1.5 g/dL in the ascitic fluid received norfloxacin throughout their hospitalization, which averaged nearly 1 month in duration. Spontaneous bacterial peritonitis decreased from about 40% to about 3%, but no difference in mortality occurred in this study of 63 patients (93). Routine use of intravenous cefotaxime before emergency endoscopic variceal sclerotherapy for variceal bleeding did not reduce the frequency of peritonitis (94).

Other studies have evaluated long-term prophylaxis in outpatients with cirrhosis and ascites. In patients with a previous episode of spontaneous bacterial peritonitis, oral norfloxacin (400 mg every day), when compared to placebo, reduced the recurrence rate during 6 months of follow-up from 35% to 12% (95). Among patients with ascitic fluid protein levels less than 1.5 g/dL, ciprofloxacin (750 mg once weekly), compared with placebo, reduced the rate of spontaneous bacterial peritonitis from 22% to 6% during the 6 months of follow-up (96). TMP-SMX given five times a week showed similar results in patients with ascites irrespective of whether they had previous episodes or low ascitic protein (97). Another study examined patients without previous episodes who had low ascitic protein or serum bilirubin levels higher than 2.5 mg/dL. The use of oral norfloxacin reduced the incidence of spontaneous bacterial peritonitis from 17% to 2% during 43 weeks of antibiotic prophylaxis. Norfloxacin-resistant infections, however, began to develop in those receiving the antibiotic (98). In patients with low-protein ascites, norfloxacin for 6 months reduced the incidence of severe infections from 17% to 2% (99). The long-term use of norfloxacin prophylaxis, however, increased the risk of severe hospitalized staphylococcal infections (100) and norfloxacin-resistant *E. coli* (101). To gain the benefit of prophylaxis and minimize the risk of antimicrobial resistance, the best approach might be to confine its use to patients with previous episodes of spontaneous bacterial peritonitis or those with low-protein ascites.

SUMMARY

Table 40.1 summarizes the situations in which studies have demonstrated the efficacy of antibacterial prophylaxis with systemic antimicrobial agents and delineates the doses employed. Some of the indications, particularly for traveler's diarrhea and granulocytopenia, are controversial. Physicians considering the use of prophylaxis in these circumstances should carefully evaluate the original articles and thoughtfully weigh both the potential benefits and the liabilities involved.

REFERENCES

1. Wood HF, Feinstein AR, Taranta A, et al. Rheumatic fever in children and adolescents, III: comparative effectiveness of three prophylaxis regimens in preventing streptococcal infections and rheumatic recurrences. *Ann Intern Med* 1964;60[Suppl 5]:31.
2. Thomas RJ, Conwill DE, Morton DE, et al. Penicillin prophylaxis for streptococcal infections in United States Navy and Marine Corps Recruit Camps, 1951–1985. *Rev Infect Dis* 1988;10:125.
3. Gray GC, Escamilla J, Hyams KC, et al: Hyperendemic *Streptococcus pyogenes* infection despite prophylaxis with penicillin G benzathine. *N Engl J Med* 1991;325:92.
4. Fujikawa J, Struewing JP, Hyams KC, et al. Oral erythromycin prophylaxis against *Streptococcus pyogenes* infection in penicillin-allergic military recruits: a randomized clinical trial. *J Infect Dis* 1992;166:162.
5. Gray GC, McPhate DC, Leinonen M, et al. Weekly oral azithromycin as prophylaxis for agents causing acute respiratory disease. *Clin Infect Dis* 1998;26:103.
6. Kuhns DM, Nelson CT, Feldman HA, et al. Prophylactic value of sulfadiazine in control of meningococci meningitis. *JAMA* 1943;123:335.
7. Broome CV, Mortimer EA, Katz SL, et al. Use of chemoprophylaxis to prevent the spread of *Haemophilus influenzae* b in day care facilities. *N Engl J Med* 1987;316:1226.
8. Perrin JM, Charney E, MacWhinney TK, et al. Sulfisoxazole as chemoprophylaxis for recurrent otitis media. A double-blind crossover study in pediatric practice. *N Engl J Med* 1974;291:644.
9. Liston TE, Foshee WS, Pierson WD. Sulfisoxazole chemoprophylaxis for frequent otitis media. *Pediatrics* 1983;71:524.
10. Maynard JE, Fleshman JK, Tschopp CF. Otitis media in Alaskan Eskimo children: prospective evaluation of chemoprophylaxis. *JAMA* 1972;219:597.
11. Casselbrant ML, Kaleida PH, Rockette HE, et al. Efficacy of antimicrobial prophylaxis and of tympanostomy tube insertion for prevention of recurrent otitis media: results of a randomized clinical trial. *Pediatr Infect Dis* 1992;11:278.
12. Klein JO. Otitis media. *Clin Infect Dis* 1994;19:823.
13. Davis SD, Wedgwood RJ. Antibiotic prophylaxis in acute viral respiratory diseases. *Am J Dis Child* 1965;109:544.
14. Petersdorf RG, Curtin JA, Hoeprich PD, et al. A study of antibiotic prophylaxis in unconscious patients. *N Engl J Med* 1957;257:1001.
15. Petersdorf RG, Merchant RK. Study of antibiotic prophylaxis in patients with acute heart failure. *N Engl J Med* 1959;260:565.
16. Ellenbogen C, Graybill JR, Silva J, et al. Bacterial pneumonia complicating adenoviral pneumonia. A comparison of respiratory bacterial culture sources

and effectiveness of chemoprophylaxis against bacterial pneumonia. *Am J Med* 1974;56:169.

17. Heyland DC, Cook DJ, Jaeschke R, et al. Selective decontamination of the digestive tract. An overview. *Chest* 1994;105:1221.

18. Brun-Buisson C. Selective decontamination in critical care. Interpreting the synthesized evidence. *Chest* 1994;105:978.

19. Bailey RR, Roberts AP, Gower PE, et al. Prevention of urinary tract infection with low-dose nitrofurantoin. *Lancet* 1971;2:1112.

20. Stamm WE, Counts GW, Wagner KF, et al. Antimicrobial prophylaxis of recurrent urinary tract infections. A double-blind, placebo-controlled trial. *Ann Intern Med* 1980;92:770.

21. Harding GKM, Ronald AR. A controlled study of antimicrobial prophylaxis of recurrent urinary infection in women. *N Engl J Med* 1974;291:597.

22. Light RB, Ronald AR, Harding GKM, et al. Trimethoprim alone in the treatment and prophylaxis of urinary tract infection. *Arch Intern Med* 1981;141:1807.

23. Harding GKM, Buckwold FJ, Marrie TJ, et al. Prophylaxis of recurrent urinary tract infection in female patients. Efficacy of low-dose, thrice-weekly therapy with trimethoprim-sulfamethoxazole. *JAMA* 1979;242:1975.

24. Nicolle LE, Harding GKM, Thomson M, et al. Efficacy of five years of continuous low-dose trimethoprim-sulfamethoxazole prophylaxis for urinary tract infection. *J Infect Dis* 1988;157:1239.

25. Stamm WE, McKevitt M, Counts GW, et al. Is antimicrobial prophylaxis of urinary tract infections cost effective? *Ann Intern Med* 1981;94:251.

26. Stapleton A, Stamm WE. Prevention of urinary tract infection. *Infect Dis Clin North Am* 1997;11:719.

27. Stapleton A, Latham RH, Johnson C, et al. Postcoital antimicrobial prophylaxis for recurrent urinary tract infection. A randomized, double-blind, placebo-controlled trial. *JAMA* 1990;264:703.

28. Kevorkian CG, Merritt JL, Ilstrup DM. Methenamine mandelate with acidification: an effective urinary antiseptic in patients with neurogenic bladder. *Mayo Clin Proc* 1984;59:523.

29. Gribble MJ, Puterman ML. Prophylaxis of urinary tract infection in persons with recent spinal cord injury: a prospective, randomized, double-blind, placebo-controlled study of trimethoprim-sulfamethoxazole. *Am J Med* 1993;95:141.

30. Sack DA, Kaminsky DC, Sack RB, et al. Prophylactic doxycycline for travelers' diarrhea. Results of a prospective double-blind study of Peace Corps volunteers in Kenya. *N Engl J Med* 1978;298:758.

31. Sack RB, Froehich JL, Zulich AW, et al. Prophylactic doxycycline for travelers' diarrhea. Results of a prospective double-blind study of Peace Corps volunteers in Morocco. *Gastroenterology* 1979;76:1368.

32. DuPont HL, Evans DG, Rios N, et al. Prevention of travelers' diarrhea with trimethoprim-sulfamethoxazole. *Rev Infect Dis* 1982;4:533.

33. DuPont HL, Galindo E, Evans DG, et al. Prevention of travelers' diarrhea with trimethoprim-sulfamethoxazole and trimethoprim alone. *Gastroenterology* 1983;84:75.

34. Rademaker CM, Hoepelman IM, Wolfhagen MJ, et al. Results of a double-blind placebo-controlled study using ciprofloxacin for prevention of traveler's diarrhea. *Eur J Clin Microbiol Infect Dis* 1989;8:690.

35. Ericsson CD, DuPont HL, Galindo E, et al. Efficacy of bicozamycin in preventing travelers' diarrhea. *Gastroenterology* 1985;88:473.

36. Reves RR, Johnson PC, Ericsson CD, et al. A cost-effectiveness comparison of the use of antimicrobial agents for treatment or prophylaxis of travelers' diarrhea. *Arch Intern Med* 1988;148:2421.

37. Gorbach SL, Carpenter CCJ, Grayson R, et al. Consensus development conference statement. *Rev Infect Dis* 1986;2[Suppl]:S227.

38. DuPont HL, Ericsson CD. Prevention and treatment of traveler's diarrhea. *N Engl J Med* 1993;328:1821.

39. Finch WT, Sawyers JL, Schencker S. A prospective study to determine the efficacy of antibiotics in acute pancreatitis. *Ann Surg* 1976;183:667.

40. Howes R, Zuidema GD, Cameron JL. Evaluation of prophylactic antibiotics in acute pancreatitis. *J Surg Res* 1975;18:197.

41. Pederzoli P, Bassi C, Vesentini S, et al. A randomized multicenter clinical trial of antibiotic prophylaxis of septic complications in acute necrotizing pancreatitis with imipenem. *Surg Gynecol Obstet* 1993;176:480.

42. Bassi C, Falconi M, Talamini G, et al. Controlled clinical trial of pefloxacin versus imipenem in severe acute pancreatitis. *Gastroenterology* 1998;115:1513.

43. Sainio V, Kemppainen E, Puolakkainen PK, et al. Early antibiotic treatment in acute necrotizing pancreatitis. *Lancet* 1995;346:663.

44. Ratschko M, Fenner T, Lankisch PG. The role of antibiotic prophylaxis in the treatment of acute pancreatitis. *Gastroenterol Clin North Am* 1999;28:641.

45. Luiten EJT, Hop WCJ, Lange JF, et al. Differential prognosis of gram-negative versus gram-positive infected and sterile pancreatic necrosis: results of a randomized trial in patients with severe acute pancreatitis treated with adjuvant selective decontamination. *Clin Infect Dis* 1997;25:811.

46. Babb RR, Spittell JA, Martin WJ, et al. Prophylaxis of recurrent lymphangitis complicating lymphedema. *JAMA* 1966;195:871.

47. Kremer M, Zuckerman R, Avraham Z, et al. Long-term antimicrobial therapy in the prevention of recurrent soft-tissue infections. *J Infect* 1991;22:37.

48. Klempner MS, Styrt B. Prevention of recurrent staphylococcal skin infections with low-dose oral clindamycin therapy. *JAMA* 1988;260:2682.

49. Henry SA. Chemoprophylaxis of bacterial infections in granulocytopenic patients. *Am J Med* 1984;76:645.

50. Gurwith MJ, Brunton JL, Lank BA, et al. A prospective controlled investigation of prophylactic trimethoprim-sulfamethoxazole in hospitalized granulocytopenic patients. *Am J Med* 1979;66:248.

51. Dekker AW, Rozenberg-Arska M, Sixma JJ, et al. Prevention of infection by trimethoprim-sulfamethoxazole plus amphotericin B in patients with acute nonlymphocytic leukemia. *Ann Intern Med* 1981;95:555.

52. Weiser B, Lange M, Fialk MA, et al. Prophylactic trimethoprim-sulfamethoxazole during consolidation chemotherapy for acute leukemia: a controlled trial. *Ann Intern Med* 1981;95:436.

53. Kauffman CA, Liepman MK, Bergman AG, et al. Trimethoprim-sulfamethoxazole prophylaxis in neutropenic patients. *Am J Med* 1983;74:599.

54. DeJongh CA, Wade JC, Finley RS, et al. Trimethoprim-sulfamethoxazole versus placebo: A double-blind comparison of infection prophylaxis in patients with small cell carcinoma of the lung. *J Clin Oncol* 1983;1:302.

55. EORTC International Antimicrobial Therapy Project Group. Trimethoprim-sulfamethoxazole in the prevention of infection in neutropenic patients. *J Infect Dis* 1984;150:372.

56. Gualtieri RJ, Donowitz GR, Kaiser DL, et al. Double-blind randomized study of prophylactic trimethoprim-sulfamethoxazole in granulocytopenic patients with hematologic malignancies. *Am J Med* 1983;74:934.

57. Martino P, Venditti M, Petti MC, et al. Co-trimoxazole prophylaxis in patients with leukemia and prolonged granulocytopenia. *Am J Med Sci* 1984;287:7.

58. Kovatch AL, Wald ER, Albo VC, et al. Oral trimethoprim-sulfamethoxazole for protection of bacterial infection during the induction phase of cancer chemotherapy in children. *Pediatrics* 1985;76:754.

59. Henry SA, Armstrong D, Kempin S, et al. Oral trimethoprim-sulfamethoxazole in attempt to prevent infection after induction chemotherapy for acute leukemia. *Am J Med* 1984;77:663.

60. Estey E, Maksymiuk A, Smith T, et al. Infection prophylaxis in acute leukemia—comparative effectiveness of sulfamethoxazole and trimethoprim, ketoconazole, and a combination of the two. *Arch Intern Med* 1984;144:1562.

61. Watson JG, Powles RL, Lason DN, et al. Co-trimoxazole versus nonabsorbable antibiotics in acute leukaemia. *Lancet* 1982;1:6.

62. Wade JC, Schimpff SC, Hargadon MT, et al. A comparison of trimethoprim-sulfamethoxazole plus nystatin with gentamicin plus nystatin in the prevention of infections in acute leukemia. *N Engl J Med* 1981;304:1057.

63. Starke ID, Catovsky D, Johnson SA, et al. Co-trimoxazole alone for prevention of bacterial infection in patients with acute leukaemia. *Lancet* 1982;1:5.

64. Wade JC, deJongh CA, Newman KA, et al. Selective antimicrobial modulation as prophylaxis against infection during granulocytopenia: trimethoprim-sulfamethoxazole vs nalidixic acid. *J Infect Dis* 1983;147:624.

65. Bow EJ, Louie TJ, Riben PD, et al. Randomized controlled trial comparing trimethoprim-sulfamethoxazole and trimethoprim for infection prophylaxis in hospitalized granulocytopenic patients. *Am J Med* 1984;76:223.

66. Karp JE, Merz WG, Hendricksen C, et al. Oral norfloxacin for prevention of gram-negative bacterial infections in patients with acute leukemia and granulocytopenia. A randomized, double-blind, placebo-controlled trial. *Ann Intern Med* 1987;106:1.

67. Winston DJ, Ho WG, Nakao SL, et al. Norfloxacin versus vancomycin/polymyxin for prevention of infections in granulocytopenic patients. *Am J Med* 1986;80:884.

68. Bow EJ, Raynor E, Louie TJ. Comparison of norfloxacin with co-trimoxazole for infection prophylaxis in acute leukemia. The trade-off for reduced gram-negative sepsis. *Am J Med* 1988;84:847.

69. Dekker AW, Rozenberg-Arska M, Verhoef J. Infection prophylaxis in acute leukemia: A comparison of ciprofloxacin with trimethoprim-sulfamethoxazole and colistin. *Ann Intern Med* 1987;106:7.

70. Kern W, Kurrie E. Ofloxacin versus trimethoprim-sulfamethoxazole for prevention of infection in patients with acute leukemia and granulocytopenia. *Infection* 1991;19:73.

71. GIMEMA Infection Program. Prevention of bacterial infections in neutropenic patients with hematologic malignancies. A randomized, multicenter trial comparing norfloxacin with ciprofloxacin. *Ann Intern Med* 1991;115:7.

72. Young LS. The new fluorinated quinolones for infection prevention in acute leukemia. *Ann Intern Med* 1987;106:144.

73. Gardner SE, Yow MD, Leeds LJ, et al. Failure of penicillin to eradicate group B streptococcal colonization in the pregnant woman: a couple study. *Am J Obstet Gynecol* 1979;135:1062.

74. Hall RT, Barnes W, Krishnan L, et al. Antibiotic treatment of parturient women colonized with group B streptococci. *Am J Obstet Gynecol* 1976;124:630.

75. Lewin EB, Amstey MS. Natural history of group B streptococcus colonization and its therapy during pregnancy. *Am J Obstet Gynecol* 1981;139:512.

76. Yow MD, Mason EO, Leeds LJ, et al. Ampicillin prevents intrapartum transmission of group B streptococci. *JAMA* 1979;241:1245.

77. Boyer KM, Gadzala CA, Kelly PD, et al. Selective intrapartum chemoprophylaxis of neonatal group B streptococcal early onset disease, III: interruption of mother-to-infant transmission. *J Infect Dis* 1983;148:810.

78. Easmon CSF, Hastings MJG, Deeley J, et al. The effect of intrapartum chemoprophylaxis on the vertical transmission of group B streptococci. *Br J Obstet Gynecol* 1983;90:633.

79. Merenstein GB, Todd WA, Brown G, et al. Group B β-hemolytic streptococcus: randomized controlled treatment study at birth. *Obstet Gynecol* 1980;55:315.

80. Siegel JD, McCracken GH, Threlkeld N, et al. Single-dose penicillin prophylaxis of neonatal group B streptococcal disease. Conclusion of a 41-month controlled trial. *Lancet* 1982;1:1426.

81. Pyati SP, Pildes RS, Jacobs NM, et al. Penicillin in infants weighing 2 kilograms or less with early-onset group B streptococcal disease. *N Engl J Med* 1983;308:1383.
82. Centers for Disease Control and Prevention. Prevention of group B streptococcal diseases: a public health perspective. *Fed Reg* 1994;59:64764.
83. Yu VL, Goetz A, Wagener M, et al. *Staphylococcus aureus* nasal carriage and infection in patients on hemodialysis. Efficacy of antibiotic prophylaxis. *N Engl J Med* 1986;315:91.
84. Klastersky J, Sadeghi M, Brihaye J. Antimicrobial prophylaxis in patients with rhinorrhea or otorrhea. A double-blind study. *Surg Neurol* 1976;6:111.
85. Demetriades D, Charalambides D, Lakhoo M, et al. Role of prophylactic antibiotics in open and basilar fractures of the skull: a randomized study. *Injury* 1992;23:377.
86. Gaston MH, Verter JI, Woods G, et al. Prophylaxis with oral penicillin in children with sickle cell anemia. A randomized trial. *N Engl J Med* 1986;314:1593.
87. John AB, Ramlal A, Jackson H, et al. Prevention of pneumococcal infection in children with homozygous sickle cell disease. *Br Med J* 1984;288:1567.
88. Romola A, Bory F, Teres J, et al. Oral, nonabsorbable antibiotics prevent infection in cirrhotics with gastrointestinal hemorrhage. *Hepatology* 1985;5:463.
89. Pauwels A, Mostefa-Kara N, Debenes B, et al. Systemic antibiotic prophylaxis after gastrointestinal hemorrhage in cirrhotic patients with a high risk of infection. *Hepatology* 1996;24:802.
90. Blaise M, Pateron D, Trinchet JC, et al. Systemic antibiotic therapy prevents bacterial infection in cirrhotic patients with gastrointestinal hemorrhage. *Hepatology* 1994;20:34.
91. Soriano G, Guarner C, Tomas A, et al. Norfloxacin prevents bacterial infection in cirrhotics with gastrointestinal hemorrhage. *Gastroenterology* 1992;103:1267.
92. Sabat M, Kolle L, Soriano G, et al. Parenteral antibiotic prophylaxis of bacterial infections does not improve cost-efficacy of oral norfloxacin in cirrhotic patients with gastrointestinal bleeding. *Am J Gastroenterol* 1998;93:2457.
93. Soriano G, Guarner C, Teixido M, et al. Selective intestinal decontamination prevents spontaneous bacterial peritonitis. *Gastroenterology* 1991;100:477.
94. Selby WS, Norton ID, Pokorny CS, et al. Bacteremia and bacterascites after endoscopic sclerotherapy for bleeding esophageal varices and prevention by intravenous cefotaxime: a randomized trial. *Gastrointest Endosc* 1994;40:680.
95. Gines P, Rimola A, Planas R, et al. Norfloxacin prevents spontaneous bacterial peritonitis recurrence in cirrhosis: results of a double-blind, placebo-controlled trial. *Hepatology* 1990;12:716.
96. Rolachon A, Cordier L, Bacz Y, et al. Ciprofloxacin and long-term prevention of spontaneous bacterial peritonitis: results of a prospective controlled trial. *Hepatology* 1995;22:1171.
97. Singh N, Gayowski T, Yu VL, et al. Trimethoprim-sulfamethoxazole for the prevention of spontaneous bacterial peritonitis in cirrhosis: a randomized trial. *Ann Intern Med* 1995;122:595.
98. Novella M, Sola R, Soriano G, et al. Continuous versus inpatient prophylaxis of the first episode of spontaneous bacterial peritonitis with norfloxacin. *Hepatology* 1997;25:532.
99. Grange JD, Roulot D, Pelletier G, et al. Norfloxacin primary prophylaxis of bacterial infections in cirrhotic patients with ascites: a double-blind randomized trial. *J Hepatol* 1998;29:430.
100. Campillo B, Dupeyron C, Richardet JP, et al. Epidemiology of severe hospital-acquired infections in patients with liver cirrhosis: effect of long-term administration of norfloxacin. *Clin Infect Dis* 1998;26:1066.
101. Ortiz J, Vila MC, Soriano G, et al. Infections caused by *Escherichia coli* resistant to norfloxacin in hospitalized cirrhotic patients. *Hepatology* 1999;29:1064.

CHAPTER 41
Advice to Travelers

Mary E. Wilson

EPIDEMIOLOGY OF TRAVEL-ASSOCIATED INFECTIONS

Travel has become fast and frequent. In the early 1990s, more than 500 million persons annually crossed international borders on commercial airplane flights (World Tourism Organization, Madrid, unpublished data). Each year approximately 25 million North Americans travel to developing countries. Persons entering a new environment often encounter threats to health that differ from those at home (1). The risk profile of an area has many dimensions; some risks are typically greater and others are less than at home. The act of travel itself poses other risks. This chapter reviews the epidemiology of illnesses in travelers, describes various strategies to reduce risk, discusses briefly the evaluation of the sick returned traveler, and identifies key sources for information and assistance. Although many psychological and medical problems beset travelers, the main focus of this section is on infectious diseases related to travel.

Overview

The thought of travel to remote areas conjures up images of exotic, sometimes lethal infections such as African sleeping sickness, Lassa fever, and tsutsugamushi fever. It may come as a surprise to learn that infections are a rare cause of travel-related death and that most infections acquired during travel are caused by pathogens that are widely distributed but are more commonly encountered in tropical and developing areas of the world. Numerous studies have assessed the epidemiology of illness in travelers (2–4). Results vary by destination and other circumstances, although common findings emerge. Among the largest and most informative studies of travel-related illness were those done in Swiss travelers (2). Figure 41.1 depicts quantitative estimates of many problems encountered by travelers (3). The incidence rate is calculated per month of stay in developing countries. As has been confirmed by multiple studies in many areas of the world, diarrhea is the most common illness leading to disruption during travel. A study of 3,049 travelers from the United Kingdom who became ill during travel found that 1% required hospitalization on return home and 14% consulted a physician (5). A surveillance system that collected information about health problems in Peace Corps workers in Africa in 1990 found that the most commonly reported health problems were diarrhea, skin problems, amebiasis, injuries, dental problems, emotional problems, fevers, malaria, and giardiasis (6).

Other Risks during Travel

Preparation for travel frequently focuses on preventing infectious diseases. As a consequence, travelers often seek assistance from infectious disease physicians. Physicians and travelers should recognize the wide range of risks incurred by travelers, including many noninfectious diseases. Physicians should inquire about anticipated activities such as hiking at high altitudes (7) and spending time in extreme environments (e.g., heat, cold, and deep-sea diving) that may require special preparation (8). Sunburns and phototoxic skin reactions are especially common among travelers from northern latitudes who visit tropical areas during winter months.

Although infection is a common cause of disruption during travel, it rarely kills. In young adults, injury is by far the most common cause of death during travel (9). Rates of death from injury are higher in developing countries than in the United States (10). The majority of deaths in young travelers are a result of motor-vehicle crashes, drownings, aircraft crashes, homicides, and burns. For most destinations, injuries are the most common cause of travel-related death and the most common reason for air medical evacuation (11).

Diarrhea

Diarrhea occurs in 20% to 40% or more of short-term travelers from industrialized countries who visit developing countries (2,12,13). Studies that have analyzed data by age have found that younger persons experience higher rates of gastrointestinal (GI) tract illness. The term *traveler's diarrhea* describes

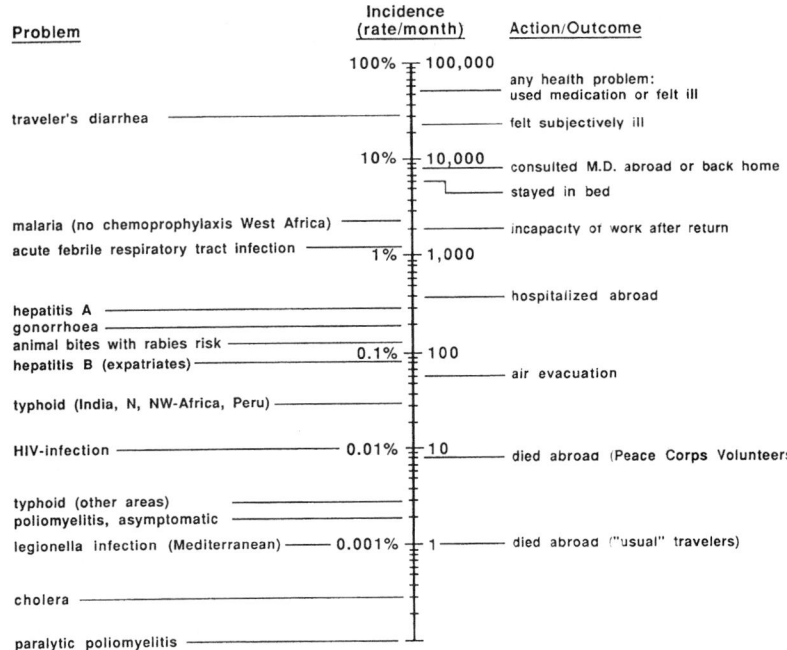

Figure 41.1. Epidemiology of travel-related infections. Incidence rate per month of health problems during a stay in developing countries. (From Steffen R, DuPont HL. Travel medicine: what's that? *J Travel Med* 1994;1:1–3, with permission.)

the circumstances of acquisition rather than the etiology. Although most often caused by toxigenic *Escherichia coli* (14), traveler's diarrhea has been associated with a wide range of organisms, including bacteria, viruses, and protozoa (12). Bacterial enteropathogens cause about 80% of traveler's diarrhea. The incidence of disease and relative proportion of disease caused by each pathogen vary by geographic region, by season, and over time and to some extent are influenced by host factors (15). The principal agents in most areas are enterotoxigenic *E. coli*, *Shigella* species, *Campylobacter jejuni*, *Aeromonas* species, *Plesiomonas shigelloides*, *Salmonella* species, and noncholera vibrios (12). Norovirus and rotavirus may cause up to 10% of diarrhea in some areas. *Giardia* and *Cryptosporidium* are the most commonly diagnosed protozoa causing diarrhea in travelers, although *Cyclospora cayetanensis* has been an important cause of diarrhea in Nepal (16). Recent studies show that *Cyclospora* is widely distributed around the world, and risk may vary with the season (17). Diarrhea caused by *Entamoeba histolytica* (amebic colitis or dysentery) is rare among short-term travelers.

Factors that have been associated with increased risk of traveler's diarrhea include living close to local residents during the travel, failure to adhere to strict principles in choosing food and drink, young age, reduced gastric acidity, underlying GI tract disease, and immunodeficiency disorders (12). For a more complete discussion of traveler's diarrhea, see Chapter 76.

Malaria

Malaria remains a threat to travelers in tropical regions (18). Approximately 30 million persons from nonendemic areas visit malarious countries each year. Risk of infection varies widely by geographic region, season of year, activities, and duration of stay. The malaria attack rate exceeded 1% in travelers to West Africa in the early 1990s (19). The relative risk for infection increases with longer stays. For example, for British travelers returning from West Africa, the attack rates per 100,000 travelers for malaria were 61 after a 1-week stay but reached almost 4,899 after visits of 6 months to 1 year (an 80-fold increase in the relative risk) (19). (Malaria is discussed in detail in Chapter 279.)

Hepatitis

Viral hepatitis has been an important cause of morbidity and mortality in travelers. Among Swiss travelers, hepatitis accounted for more days of inability to work (mean of 33 days) than any other travel-related infection (2). Well-documented agents include hepatitis viruses A, B, C, D, and E. Swiss travelers returning from Africa, Latin America, and Asia with acute hepatitis, studied at a time when only tests for hepatitis A and B were available, were found to have predominantly hepatitis A (60%) (20) Only 15% were found to have hepatitis B, and the remaining 25% were categorized as non-A, non-B hepatitis or unclassified. Hepatitis E has been documented in travelers now that diagnostic tests to detect hepatitis E virus are available (21). The estimated risk of symptomatic hepatitis A for a nonimmune person per month of travel in a developing country is 3 per 1,000, although it may be as high as 20 per 1,000 per month for backpackers and persons who eat and drink under poor hygienic conditions (20). Other infections that can cause prominent hepatic dysfunction (e.g., leptospirosis, yellow fever, typhoid fever, *Hantavirus* infections, dengue, rickettsial infections, and Q fever, among others) (1) are also seen in travelers but typically after a shorter incubation period than for most hepatitis viruses.

Sexually Transmitted Diseases

Sexual activity is common during travel, and sexually transmitted infections have been prominent among travel-related infections (22,23). Tours arranged specifically to facilitate sexual contacts (sexual tourism) are popular in some areas. Among short-term Swiss tourists traveling to tropical Africa, Asia, and Latin America, almost 60% of those identified in a high-risk group reported casual sexual contacts during their trip (24). Among Danish Volunteer Service personnel who worked in Kenya, Tanzania, and Zambia for 11 to 41 months, 48% (53/110) of the men and 29% (32/112) of the women reported heterosexual contact with local residents (25). In the mid-1980s, of American college students who traveled in the tropics (mean duration 74 days), 29% reported contact with a new partner, 44% without the use of condoms (26).

Systemic infections, such as hepatitis B, human immunodeficiency virus (HIV) infection, and cytomegalovirus infection, as well as infections causing only or primarily genital lesions, follow sexual contact. Although sexually transmitted diseases have a worldwide distribution, the incidence, locally prevalent infections, and antimicrobial resistance patterns vary by geographic regions. For example, chancroid, an uncommon or rare sexually transmitted disease in the United States, is the cause of more than half of genital ulcers in parts of Southeast Asia and Africa (27). Serologic studies found that 6% of U.S. troops stationed in Korea for 4 to 12 months became infected with hepatitis B. Although unrecognized intravenous drug use may have accounted for some of the transmission, 83% of those with acute hepatitis B infection gave a history of Korean sexual partners, each reporting a mean number of 6.32 partners (28).

Host Factors and Risk of Infection

Short-term travelers infrequently acquire helminthic infections, such as cysticercosis, strongyloidiasis, hookworm disease, and filarial infections (such as onchocerciasis, loiasis, and bancroftian filariasis). Although schistosomiasis is much more common in persons with prolonged exposures, many cases and clusters have occurred in short-term travelers. Among 30 Dutch travelers returning from Mali, West Africa, 28 of 29 who swam in freshwater pools became ill with schistosomiasis (29). The duration of exposure to freshwater ranged from a few minutes to hours. African trypanosomiasis, which can result from a single bite of an infective tsetse fly, is occasionally seen in persons who have been on safaris in Africa. Although in the United States between 1968 and 1985, only 13 cases of African trypanosomiasis were reported to the Centers for Disease Control and Prevention (CDC), a recent increase in cases reported in travelers requires heightened awareness of this generally unfamiliar infection (30).

Characteristics of the human host affect the risk of exposure to pathogens and expression of infection. Most of the relevant host factors can be broadly categorized as behavioral, immunologic, and genetic. Factors that are associated with increased risk of exposure to many infections during travel include prolonged duration of stay; travel to remote and rural areas; living under poor hygienic conditions; close contact with animals, water, and soil as might occur during field work; sexual contacts with local residents; and consumption of food from street vendors. At the

---

TABLE 41.1. Key Concepts: Travel-related Illness and Death

Injuries are an important cause of travel-related deaths.

Most infections acquired during travel to tropical and developing countries are caused by pathogens that are widely distributed.

Risk of infection from exposure to many widely distributed pathogens (e.g., hepatitis A, typhoid fever, salmonellosis) is substantially higher during travel to developing countries than during life at home.

Unusual infections can be found in temperate and industrialized countries, including the United States.

Recreational activities (e.g., swimming, hiking) facilitate exposure to many pathogens.

Activities that pose no risk at home may be hazardous in another environment (e.g., eating raw foods, swimming in fresh water, going barefooted, sustaining mosquito bites, petting stray animals).

Expensive hotels and posh restaurants are no guarantee of safe food and beverages.

Disease during and immediately after travel may be unrelated to exposures during travel (e.g., acute appendicitis, pyelonephritis).

Infections can be acquired en route and on brief layovers.

Travel-associated diseases include noninfectious diseases (e.g., pulmonary emboli related to prolonged sitting, drug reactions).

---

same time, it is important to recognize that persons who stay entirely in first-class or deluxe hotels and sleep in screened or air-conditioned rooms can acquire infections. Food- and waterborne infections still spread in sumptuous surroundings.

Immunologic and genetic factors may determine susceptibility to infection and expression of disease. Immunity to infection may come from past infection or from active or passive immunization. Persons who have always lived under good hygienic conditions lack immunity to pathogens that commonly contaminate food and water in developing countries (e.g., hepatitis A virus). Several key concepts about travel-related illness are summarized in Table 41.1.

SOURCES AND ACQUISITION OF INFECTION DURING TRAVEL

The major sources of pathogens during travel are food and drink, soil and water, animals and arthropods, and other humans. A few comments about each will help inform thinking about risks during travel.

Food and Drink

Fecally contaminated food and drink are the sources of traveler's diarrhea, hepatitis A, typhoid fever, poliomyelitis, cholera, and many other infections. Foods can also harbor parasites (e.g., eggs, larvae, or other forms) and pathogens from animals (e.g., *Brucella*, *Salmonella*). Contaminated water can be hidden in many forms, such as in ice cubes (31), reconstituted orange juice and other beverages, shower water (ingested while showering), and water sprayed on fresh produce. Produce may be contaminated in the fields (night soil or fecally contaminated water used on crops) or during shipping and processing. In many areas, refrigeration is unavailable or erratic. A warm, humid environment provides a milieu conducive to the rapid proliferation of bacteria that contaminate foods. In some places, bottled water consists of bottles refilled with water from sources of questionable purity.

Soil and Water

Sandy beaches may be contaminated with parasites from feces of humans and animals. Going barefoot or having direct skin contact with sand or soil places persons at risk of cutaneous larva migrans (32), hookworm, and other parasites that can penetrate the skin. The soil-associated fungus, *Histoplasma capsulatum*, which is acquired by inhalation, caused a large outbreak of respiratory tract infections in 2001 in college students visiting Mexico during spring break (33).

Recreational water can be a source of outbreaks of enteric infections such as shigellosis, hemorrhagic colitis, and cryptosporidiosis (34,35). Polluted marine bathing water can be a source of pathogens that cause acute gastroenteritis and conjunctivitis (36). Cercarial dermatitis (caused by animal schistosomes unable to complete their life cycle in humans) can result from exposures to freshwater and salt water in many areas of the world. Of greater importance is schistosomiasis, transmitted by contact with freshwater infested with cercariae that can penetrate intact human skin in 30 seconds to 10 minutes and mature in the human host. Exposures during bathing, wading, boating, and rafting have been associated with transmission of schistosomiasis. Leptospirosis, more common in tropical areas, can be acquired by contact with water, including during recreational activities such as rafting and swimming (37). Larvae of coelenterates, such as jellyfish and sea anemones, can penetrate intact skin during swimming and cause an annoying pruritic skin eruption known as seabather's eruption (38,39).

Animals and Arthropods

Animals can transmit infection by biting the human host. An underappreciated threat during travel is rabies, which is common in animals (especially dogs) in many parts of Asia, Africa, and Central and South America. For example, studies in Thailand have found rabies virus in 3% to 6% of stray dogs. In India, an estimated 40,000 to 50,000 persons die annually of rabies (40,41). More often animals play a role in human disease through indirect means. Humans eat animal flesh or animal products that contain pathogens, including parasites. Animal excreta and tissues contain pathogens (e.g., *Hantavirus*, Lassa virus) that can reach humans by various routes. Animals may be the site of an essential developmental step in the life cycle of the pathogen or serve as the reservoir host from which an arthropod vector carries the pathogen to humans. Many arthropods important for human disease are closely associated with animals. Among the most important infections in travelers, many are arthropod borne (e.g., malaria, dengue, rickettsial infections, leishmaniasis, Japanese encephalitis, yellow fever, and many others).

Other Humans

Humans are a source of infections that are transmitted by aerosols and droplets, sexual and other close contact, and fecal-oral spread. In many parts of the world, sterile needles and syringes are often unavailable, and blood and blood products used for transfusion may not be screened (42). Contact with needles or sharps (including tattooing, acupuncture, shaving, manicures), medical and dental care, and transfusions can be a source of infection. Blood transfusion can be a source of malaria, *Trypanosoma cruzi* infection, and other parasitic infections in some regions of the world, in addition to the more familiar risks, such as HIV infection, hepatitis B, hepatitis C, human T-cell lymphotropic virus infection, and syphilis (1).

Air Travel

The immobility associated with prolonged travel can predispose to venous thrombosis and pulmonary emboli (43). Several features of air travel predispose to respiratory tract illness: low humidity of air in aircraft, crowding of persons in a closed space with limited infusions of fresh air, and changes in air pressure with ascent and descent. Moreover, aircraft cabins are pressurized to the equivalent of 6,000 to 8,000 feet above sea level (44). Persons with underlying chronic lung disease who are marginally compensated at sea level may suffer from reduced partial pressure of oxygen while flying. Changes in air pressure associated with flying may exacerbate chronic ear and sinus problems or precipitate acute problems.

Although most of the reports of respiratory tract infections after air travel are anecdotal, transmission of infections, such as influenza, aboard aircraft has been well documented (45). Epidemiologic studies suggest that tuberculosis may occasionally be transmitted on aircraft (46).

Infections Acquired En Route

Although preparation for travel tends to focus on the destination, the vehicle of transportation can be the site for transmission of infection. Influenza has caused outbreaks on cruise ships (47); an outbreak of rubella occurred among crew members of commer-

TABLE 41.2. Geographically Focal Infections in Temperate and Industrialized Areas (Examples)

United States
  Colorado tick fever
  Relapsing fever
  Plague
  Babesiosis
  Eastern equine encephalitis
  Coccidioidomycosis
  Lyme disease
  Histoplasmosis
  Hantavirus pulmonary syndrome
Western and Southern Europe
  Lyme disease
  Hemorrhagic fever with renal syndrome
  Nephropathica hemorrhagica
  Visceral leishmaniasis
  Spotted fever due to *Rickettsia conorii* (boutonneuse fever)
Australia
  Angiostrongyliasis due to *Angiostrongylus cantonensis*
  Dengue fever
  Murray Valley encephalitis (Australian encephalitis)
  Ross River fever
  Spotted fever due to *Rickettsia australis* (north Queensland tick typhus)

cial cruise ships (48). Other infections acquired en route include norovirus and legionellosis transmitted on cruise ships (49), cholera on aircraft, shigellosis from food served on multiple flights (50), malaria thought to have been transmitted by a "commuter mosquito," and many other infections transmitted primarily by food or drink. Food and ice served on aircraft and ships generally come from the port of departure and may reflect conditions in that country.

Infections Acquired in Temperate and Industrialized Areas

Whereas tropical and developing countries may have a greater array and abundance of exotic pathogens, temperate and industrialized countries, including the United States, can also be the site for transmission of unfamiliar infections with geographically focal distributions. Some examples are listed in Table 41.2 and are a reminder that travel to a seemingly familiar place can result in unusual infections.

PREVENTIVE STRATEGIES

Preparation for travel should include a review of the entire itinerary, including intermediate stops. Persons planning prolonged stays in developing countries should undergo a complete medical evaluation and dental checkup. The pretravel evaluation is the time to identify specific geographic regions, planned activities, and host factors that require special attention.

Overview

Approaches used to reduce the risk of disruption and death related to travel generally fall into three broad categories: education that leads to a change in behavior, chemoprophylaxis or empiric or standby treatment, and immunization. Although immunizations have an important role in the prevention of travel-related infections, most infections acquired during travel are not vaccine preventable (with currently available vaccines), and vaccines are not the only means available to prevent vaccine-preventable infections (51). Several interventions are disease specific (e.g., yellow fever vaccine), and many others are more broadly applicable (e.g., insect repellents).

The burden of disease can be reduced by interventions at three points: preventing exposure to the pathogen, preventing infection after exposure has occurred (e.g., through protective immunity of host; preventive chemotherapy or immunoprophylaxis), and limiting the impact or severity of infection (e.g., by partial immunity to infection; early diagnosis and treatment; prevention of spread to others). Prevention of exposure is typically accomplished by specific behavior (e.g., avoiding person, place, or activity) or by use of physical (barrier) or chemical protection. Table 41.3 lists general recommendations that can protect against multiple diseases.

Medical Kit

Travelers should carry basic medical supplies with them. The composition of their personal medical kit will vary depending on duration of travel, destination, and planned activities. Prescription drugs should be kept in their original labeled containers and packed in carry-on bags. Sunscreens and insect repellents are essential for many destinations. Depending on destination and circumstances, the traveler may be advised to take materials for water purification, oral rehydration salts, bed nets, sterile needles and syringes, and permethrin-impregnated clothing. References advise about how to put together a personal medical kit (52).

Insurance

Before departure, travelers should determine whether their medical insurance would cover them if they become ill abroad. If it does not, they should obtain special trip insurance. Persons planning stays in remote areas and those with underlying diseases should obtain insurance that will cover medical evacuation, should that be necessary.

Injury

Many think of injury as unpredictable, hence not preventable. Although it is impossible to avoid all injuries, it is possible to anticipate many risks and to find ways to reduce them. This involves actions taken before and during the travel. Strategies include selecting cars that are in good repair and are equipped with seat belts, driving during daylight hours, avoiding driving and swimming when fatigued or after drinking, avoiding use of mopeds (use helmets to ride mopeds, bicycles, and motorcycles), arranging for a driver familiar with the roads in some instances, and obtaining good road maps of areas to be visited. Injury is the leading reason for blood transfusion in travelers visiting developing countries.

Prevention of Traveler's Diarrhea

Paying strict attention to choice of food and drink during travel can reduce but does not eliminate the risk of traveler's diarrhea (53). Thus, it is recommended that travelers to developing countries take medications with them to use for early therapy should diarrhea develop. Prophylactic antimicrobials against traveler's diarrhea are not routinely advised. Circumstances that might lead to the consideration of prophylactic antimicrobials include underlying diseases (such as insulin-dependent diabetes mellitus, active inflammatory bowel disease, acquired immunodeficiency syndrome, others) or extreme inconvenience if the trip were interrupted by traveler's diarrhea (12). Prophylactic agents that have been shown

TABLE 41.3. General Recommendations for Travelers

Mode of transmission	Preventive strategy	Supplemental protection
Sexually transmitted	Avoid sexual contact	Use condoms; see also Vaccines for Specific Diseases

Vector borne	Varies with vector; multiple possible interventions include
	  Stay in screened or air-conditioned rooms
	  Use bed nets (preferably impregnated with repellents) in malarious areas
	  Avoid outdoor exposure at biting time for vectors
	  Use insect repellents on skin and permethrin on clothing
	  Wear protective clothing (some insects can bite through clothing)
	  Inspect skin for ticks in areas with tick-borne infections
	  Avoid scented soaps, perfumes
		See also Vaccines (Yellow Fever and Japanese Encephalitis) and Chemoprophylaxis Against Malaria

Food and beverage borne	Choose foods and fluids that are generally safe, for example, steaming hot food, coffee and tea, wine and beer, bottled carbonated water or beverages, fruits that can be peeled by the consumer, bread (without fillings) Avoid raw and undercooked seafood and animal flesh Avoid raw fruits and vegetables (unless peeled by consumer) Avoid ice, tap water and beverages made with it Avoid buffets and foods held in open areas especially if abundant flies Avoid foods, ices, and beverages sold by street vendors Avoid unpasteurized milk and milk products	See also vaccines See also Prevention of Traveler's Diarrhea
Water and soil associated	Avoid skin contact with fresh water in schistosomiasis-endemic areas Avoid direct skin contact with soil and sand contaminated with feces Avoid going barefooted Avoid swimming in beaches near sewage outflow tracts Avoid swimming in ponds near where animals graze and wade Avoid ingesting water while swimming	

Note: These recommendations protect against multiple diseases, although the specific diseases may vary from one geographical area to another. How carefully the recommendations need to be followed will vary with the geographical region and the host.

effective in clinical studies include bismuth subsalicylate, the fluoroquinolones, trimethoprim-sulfamethoxazole (TMP-SMX) (160 mg of trimethoprim and 800 mg of sulfamethoxazole once daily), and doxycycline (100 mg daily) (54,55). Enteric pathogens in many parts of the world are now resistant to doxycycline and increasingly to TMP-SMX (56).

The approach preferred by most travelers to developing countries is to carry an antimotility agent and antimicrobials to take for self-therapy for specified symptoms. Travelers who develop acute diarrhea usually have good response to an antibacterial agent (e.g., quinolone, azithromycin, or TMP-SMX) plus loperamide (57,58). Travelers with fever or bloody stools should avoid taking an antimotility agent alone. Bismuth subsalicylate is a reasonable choice for mild disease (e.g., mild diarrhea with no fever or bloody stools) (59). Travelers should be reminded to maintain adequate hydration for any diarrheal illness and be cautioned to seek medical attention if diarrhea persists despite treatment or is associated with high fevers. This is especially important advice to persons traveling to malaria-endemic regions, because malaria can cause GI symptoms that can be misinterpreted as an enteric infection.

Chemoprophylaxis against Malaria

Chemoprophylaxis should be provided for persons traveling to malaria-endemic regions, along with instructions for personal protective measures to reduce the risk of mosquito bites (60–62). Malaria persists in many tropical regions, and it remains an important cause of potentially lethal infection in travelers (18). Travelers should be reminded that symptoms of malaria may first appear many months, and occasionally more than 1 year, after travel. Its protean clinical manifestations can delay recognition and treatment.

Immunoprophylaxis

Preparation for travel provides an opportunity to review and update routine vaccines and to assess the need for special vaccines (63). Vaccines fall into three general groups: those that are required for entry into the country; those that are prudent, given the risks the person will undergo; and routine vaccines that should be updated. Vaccines commonly used for adult travelers are listed in Table 41.4.

Vaccines used to prevent many common childhood infections save more money than they cost (e.g., measles, mumps, rubella, pertussis, *Haemophilus influenzae* infection) (64–67). In contrast, many vaccines used to prevent infections in travelers are extremely expensive per death averted or case prevented (68,69). Travelers have special characteristics that are pertinent in making decisions about vaccines (51). The cost of travel is high and the value placed on a day during a trip may greatly exceed the value of a day at home. Disruption during travel can be expensive and inconvenient, especially if it involves a change in itinerary or hospitalization. The availability and quality of medical treatment in many parts of the world are uncertain; treatment in a local facility may subject the traveler to risk of contact with needles and syringes or other equipment or materials that could be contaminated with HIV, hepatitis B, hepatitis C, or other pathogens. Most vaccines given before travel also have benefit that extends beyond the individual trip. Preventing infection in the traveler may also eliminate a potential source of spread of infection to family and friends on return (e.g., hepatitis A, typhoid fever).

TABLE 41.4. Vaccines for Adult Travelers

Routine
  Update as needed
    Diphtheria-tetanus
    Measles-mumps-rubella
  Routine for Defined Groups
    Influenza
    Hepatitis B
    Pneumococcal
    Varicella
Required by some countries (check current requirements)
  Yellow fever
  Meningococcal
Recommended for travelers to developing countries
  Standard for travelers to developing countries
    Hepatitis A vaccine (or immune globulin)
    Typhoid
    Poliovirus
  Special for travelers to developing countries
    Cholera (currently unavailable in the United States)
    Hepatitis B
    Meningococcal
    Japanese encephalitis
    Plague
    Rabies

ROUTINE VACCINES

Travelers to developing countries are at risk of exposure to many infections that have been largely controlled in the United States. These include poliomyelitis, pertussis, diphtheria, tetanus, measles, rubella, and mumps. Persons who are not up-to-date on any of these should receive the appropriate boosters (currently pertussis vaccine is not recommended in adults) (70). Many persons born between 1957 and 1980 never had natural measles, never received a second dose of measles vaccine, and may be susceptible to measles. Tetanus boosters should be updated so that travelers will not run the risk of needing a tetanus booster during travel. Many persons, particularly older adults, lack immunity to vaccine-preventable infections. A study of serum levels of antibody against tetanus in a representative noninstitutionalized population in the United States found that only 69.7% had protective levels of antibodies. Among persons 70 years or older, only 27.8% had protective levels of antibodies (71). A study of London blood donors done in 1993 found that 37.6% were susceptible to diphtheria according to internationally accepted definitions of immunity. More than half of those in the 50- to 59-year-old age-group were susceptible to diphtheria (72). The risk from waning levels of immunity to diphtheria is reinforced by events since the early 1990s in the New Independent States of the former Soviet Union where outbreaks of diphtheria occurred, reaching almost 50,000 reported cases in 1994 (73). Throughout the epidemic, about 70% of the cases were in persons 15 years or older.

The initial history should include review of varicella immunity. Those with no history of varicella should be tested for varicella antibodies, and those who are antibody negative should receive the vaccine before departure, if feasible (74). Varicella can be extremely disruptive if it occurs during travel.

The elderly population constitutes a growing percentage of the traveling public. In elderly persons, response to vaccines may be slower and less vigorous and immunity may wane more rapidly (75). Persons in risk groups for which pneumococcal and influenza vaccines are advised should receive these vaccines. Influenza occurs in all months of the year in tropical areas and appears mainly from May to August in the Southern Hemisphere. Recently summertime outbreaks have appeared in travelers. Passengers on cruise ships and persons on package tours to Alaska have experienced outbreaks of influenza (47). A recent study of healthy elderly Canadians found no additional benefit from a second dose of influenza vaccine given to travelers 12 weeks after the first dose. Antibody levels remained high at 24 weeks in both travelers and controls (76).

YELLOW FEVER VACCINE

Yellow fever vaccine is required for entry into many countries (77,78). The certificate of vaccination becomes valid 10 days after receipt of the vaccine. Decisions about the yellow fever vaccine must take into account the risk of infection, immunogenicity and potential side effects from this live-virus vaccine, and requirements of the countries to be visited. To be valid, the vaccine must be given at an official Yellow Fever Vaccination Center and recorded on the International Certificate of Vaccination, signed by a licensed physician or by a person designated by the physician. Persons without a valid certificate who try to enter a country requiring yellow fever vaccination may be denied entry, quarantined, or revaccinated at that site.

Several cases of severe multiorgan system failure and death following yellow fever vaccination (recovery of yellow fever vaccine virus from liver, other tissues) have led to careful review of indications for the use of the vaccine (79–82). These reports of adverse events come at a time of increased yellow fever activity and threats of yellow fever to large urban areas in South America. These multisystem adverse events following vaccination appear to be extremely rare, occurring in about 1 in 400,000 distributed doses from 1990 to 1998 (82). Risk factors are not well defined, although one study found increased risk in elderly travelers (83). Yellow fever vaccine should continue to be used but should be limited to persons who will be visiting endemic areas or regions reporting yellow fever activity. A letter of waiver can be given to persons who may be asked to show proof of vaccination but who should not receive the vaccine because of risk of adverse events or because they have no risk of exposure.

Information about individual country requirements is updated regularly in the booklets published by the World Health Organization and the CDC (77,78). Current information can be found on their web sites and is also published on the CDC blue sheets every 2 weeks. The country codes should be reviewed with care; some countries outside of the yellow fever–endemic zones require the yellow fever vaccine, and some countries within the endemic zone do not require travelers to be immunized.

Because it is a live-virus vaccine, there are concerns about use of yellow fever vaccine in young infants, pregnant women, and persons who are immunocompromised. Pregnant women and infants younger than 9 months should not be given the vaccine unless risk of infection is high. Yellow fever vaccine virus can infect the developing fetus, although the magnitude of risk for congenital defects from vaccine-associated infection is unknown (84). HIV-infected persons may be at increased risk of complications from the vaccine (although a few data suggest it is safe if CD4 count is > 200) and may not develop protective levels of antibodies. Vaccine-induced immunity may wane faster than in persons with normal immune status. If risk of infection is high, it may be useful to check serum antibody titers.

MENINGOCOCCAL VACCINE

Meningococcal vaccine has been required recently by Saudi Arabia for pilgrims to Mecca for the annual Hajj. Only the polysaccharide vaccine, available as a quadrivalent vaccine against A, C, Y, and W-135, should be used (monovalent and bivalent vaccines are available in other countries, but at present, only the quadrivalent is available in the United States) because recent outbreaks related to the Hajj have involved W-135 (85). Meningococcal vaccine is sometimes recommended for other travelers, such as those visiting the meningitis belt of Africa and other areas experiencing meningitis outbreaks.

CHOLERA VACCINE

Although no country has a formal requirement for cholera vaccine, travelers report occasional demands for vaccine documentation when international borders are crossed. The vaccine licensed in the United States has limited efficacy (50% to 60%) of brief duration. Risk of cholera to travelers on usual itineraries is extremely low. Cholera vaccine is no longer available in the United States. If another vaccine becomes available, recommendations for its use will have to be developed based on its safety, immunogenicity, efficacy, cost, and duration of activity.

HEPATITIS A PREVENTION

The hepatitis A vaccine, which is safe and highly effective, has largely replaced the use of immune globulin (IG) for the prevention of hepatitis A infection (86). IG provides immediate protection and is relatively inexpensive but protects for only 3 to 5 months. The hepatitis A vaccine series (two or three doses, depending on vaccine formulation) is projected to provide protection for 15 years or longer. Although official recommendations suggest that a dose should be given 2 to 4 weeks before departure, accumulated experience would suggest that administration just before departure is generally effective, given the relatively long incubation period of hepatitis A (87). The single-antigen hepatitis A vaccine is given at 0 and 6 to 12 months. A pediatric formulation with half the amount of antigen is also available. Because immune response develops more slowly in persons who are elderly, obese, or immunocompromised, it may be prudent to schedule the first dose of vaccine at least 4 weeks before departure in those persons or to use IG. The hepatitis A vaccine is well tolerated and has been given simultaneously with other vaccines without apparent adverse effect on immunogenicity. Because it is an inactivated vaccine, it can be given safely to immunocompromised persons.

A number of papers have analyzed use of the vaccine versus IG (69). Persons who have antibodies to hepatitis A because of prior natural infection will derive no benefit from the vaccine (but also experience no apparent harm from the vaccine). Travelers for whom the vaccine is most cost-effective are persons who have frequent or prolonged travel to developing countries. Testing for hepatitis A antibodies before administration should be considered for persons who have history of hepatitis (type unknown), have resided many years in a developing country, or are older than 60 years. Antibodies from prior infection, even if infection was clinically inapparent, should provide lifelong immunity. Antibody testing is not recommended after hepatitis A vaccination. Response to vaccine is almost universal, and the sensitivity of commercial tests is insufficient to pick up vaccine-induced antibodies in most instances. IG available in the United States does not protect against hepatitis E.

A combined hepatitis A–hepatitis B vaccine is now licensed in the United States (88) and is given in a three-dose schedule. For persons who are candidates for both hepatitis A and hepatitis B vaccines, use of the combination vaccine will reduce the number of required injections to complete both series from five to three. Each dose of the combination, marketed as TwinRix (Glaxo-SmithKline Biologicals), contains 720 enzyme-linked immunosorbent assay units of inactivated hepatitis A vaccine (half that included in the monovalent hepatitis A vaccine, Havrix) and 20 μg of recombinant hepatitis B surface antigen protein. The three doses are given at 0, 1, and 6 months. Immunogenicity appears excellent for both antigens. Two doses of vaccine (given a month apart) must be given before travel to provide reliable protection against hepatitis A.

TYPHOID FEVER VACCINES

Two typhoid vaccines are now available in the United States: an oral live attenuated vaccine made from the Ty21a strain of *Salmonella typhi* and capsular polysaccharide vaccine for parenteral use (Typhim Vi) (89). A parenteral heat-phenol–inactivated vaccine used for many years is no longer available. No direct comparative studies have assessed relative efficacy of the three. All have shown efficacy in field trials, typically in the range of 50% to 75%. The oral live vaccine requires careful attention to handling and administration (e.g., requires refrigeration and cannot be given with antibiotics). Four doses are taken in a period of 6 days. The polysaccharide vaccine has the advantage of requiring a single injected dose with recommendation for a booster every 2 years. Geographic areas reporting the highest frequency of typhoid fever in travelers are the Indian subcontinent including Nepal, parts of South America, Asia, and Africa. Persons who plan extended low-budget trips in remote and rural areas are at greatest risk. Increasing incidence of typhoid fever caused by multidrug-resistant bacteria may shift the threshold at which the vaccine is recommended (90). A new conjugate typhoid vaccine, not licensed in the United States, looks promising in field trials (91).

JAPANESE ENCEPHALITIS VACCINE

The Japanese encephalitis vaccine available in the United States is an inactivated vaccine (virus grown in mouse brain) manufactured by Biken, Japan, and distributed by Aventis Pasteur. Because symptomatic infections have been rare in travelers and adverse reactions to the vaccine, sometimes severe, occur in 1 to 104 per 10,000 vaccinees, use of the vaccine is recommended only for persons planning prolonged stays in rural areas during the transmission season. The vaccine is not recommended for short-term travelers (trips lasting <30 days) unless their itineraries place them at especially high risk (92). The vaccine series is given in three doses over 30 days. The last dose should be given at least 10 days before departure so adverse reactions can be handled before travel. Efficacy of the vaccine in children in endemic areas has been 80% to 90%.

RABIES VACCINE

Decisions about use of rabies vaccines can be difficult for several reasons: Vaccine is extremely expensive; rabies in travelers is rare; infection is lethal; and postexposure treatment in developing countries varies greatly in accessibility, efficacy, and safety (93). Rabies IG (RIG) is in short supply or is unavailable in many countries. Risk of exposure in many areas is much higher than that in the United States but is still low relative to the risk for other infections, such as malaria and typhoid fever. Whether the rabies vaccine is given, the prospective traveler needs to be educated about the risk from animal bites and licks. Dogs are the most important reservoir of rabies in most countries and are the source of about 90% of the human cases. Monkeys and other animals can also carry rabies. Travelers must be informed about the need to seek care if a bite occurs. Persons for whom preexposure vaccine should be considered are those spending prolonged periods in developing countries where animal rabies is common (especially if safe effective vaccines and RIG will be unavailable locally), particularly if the person will be biking, working with animals, or traveling to remote areas where access to medical care will be difficult (94). Children should also be targeted for vaccine because they are at increased risk of being bitten by a dog (which is more likely to be severe in children) and may not report it to caregivers.

HEPATITIS B VACCINE

A growing segment of the population has received the hepatitis B vaccine. The primary modes of transmission of hepatitis B are through sex and percutaneous injuries. Rates of chronic hepatitis B infection reach 8% to 15% or higher in parts of China, Southeast Asia, Africa, the Pacific Islands, and the Amazon Basin in South America. Persons planning prolonged stays in areas where infection is highly endemic should receive the vaccine. It is particularly important for persons who plan to work in a health care setting or plan to have sexual contact with local residents. Accelerated schedules that provide three doses initially (and fourth dose at 6 to 12 months) should be used for persons at high risk who will be departing in 1 to 2 months. (See the section "Hepatitis A Prevention" for a discussion of the combination hepatitis A–hepatitis B vaccine.)

Integrating Multiple Vaccines

Integration of multiple vaccines requires careful planning. Administration of antimicrobials and antimalarials influences the timing or route of administration of some vaccines. For example, persons taking chloroquine have a lower antibody response to the rabies vaccine than those who are not receiving the drug, so they should be given vaccine via the intramuscular route, which produces higher antibody levels (94). Most inactivated vaccines do not interfere with the immune response to other vaccines (inactivated or live), so these vaccines can be given simultaneously or before or after other vaccines. IG can impair antibody response to some live-virus vaccines (e.g., measles-mumps-rubella, varicella) but does not affect response to either oral live poliovirus or yellow fever vaccines. Measles-mumps-rubella vaccination should be delayed at least 3 months (recommended delay is dose dependent) after administration of IG, and varicella vaccination should be delayed for 5 months after receipt of IG or other antibody-containing blood products. IG should be deferred until at least 14 days after the measles-mumps-rubella vaccine is given and for 3 weeks after varicella vaccination. Physicians should also review the history for any other sources of antibodies (e.g., in blood or blood products, hepatitis B IG, RIG) because these will also interfere with immune response. The CDC *Yellow Book* (77) provides details about these intervals.

Special Groups

LONG-TERM TRAVELERS

Decisions about many vaccines are linked to duration of stay in a risky area (see above). Persons planning to spend more than 1 to 3 months in areas where rates of tuberculosis are substantially higher than those in the United States (95) should have a baseline tuberculin skin test placed before travel (if not already done within 3 to 6 months of travel). Skin testing should be repeated 2 to 3 months after return. Risk of tuberculin conversion is highest for health care workers with direct patient contact (96).

HIV-INFECTED TRAVELERS

Pretravel preparation for HIV-infected travelers requires special attention for several reasons: Travel-related infections may be more common and more severe; manifestations of infection may be atypical; usual forms of therapy may fail to cure infections; reactions to drugs are common and may mimic infectious diseases;

immune response to vaccines may be diminished; informed treatment and special drugs may be difficult to obtain should illness develop during travel; and legal and social issues may inhibit free movement of HIV-infected persons across international borders (97). In addition, HIV-infected persons may be taking multiple medications that must be considered when immunization and chemoprophylactic regimens are planned (98). A study in California found that travel was common in HIV-infected persons, despite advanced disease. Destinations included tropical and developing countries (99). Physicians must be able to identify risks, assess their magnitude, and review options to reduce the risk to HIV-infected persons who wish to travel.

PREGNANT WOMEN

Pregnant women require special attention. Some vaccines and chemoprophylactic agents are contraindicated during pregnancy. Reviews have outlined approaches to management (100,101) and the CDC *Yellow Book* has a section with recommendations for pregnancy and travel (77).

CHRONIC MEDICAL PROBLEMS

The expanding population traveling includes many persons with chronic medical conditions, such as diabetes mellitus and cardiac disease; those who are confined to wheelchairs; and persons on chronic renal dialysis. Various organizations, newsletters, books, and other resources, including web sites, are available to help such persons arrange their travel (102,103).

EVALUATION OF THE RETURNED TRAVELER

Evaluation of the patient after travel should begin with a consideration of what is possible had the person not traveled. The differential diagnosis should then be expanded to include diseases that may have been acquired during travel. Patients with fever need immediate attention (104). Initial focus should be on infections that are treatable, transmissible, or both. The geographic areas of travel, the types of exposures, and the time elapsed since the exposures along with the clinical findings are all key bits of data that allow construction of an informed differential diagnosis. It is essential to evaluate for malaria in persons who have visited malaria-endemic regions (105). Malaria can occur even if persons take malaria prophylaxis as prescribed. Dengue fever is spreading in tropical areas and occurs in urban areas frequently visited by tourists (106). Dengue, typhoid fever, malaria, and rickettsial infections share some clinical and laboratory features. Specific laboratory studies must be carried out to make a specific diagnosis so that appropriate therapy can be given.

Skin lesions are common in returned travelers. Although skin diseases rarely lead to hospitalization, they are a common reason for medical attention after travel (107). Many reflect superficial infections, reactions to insect bites, or other easily managed problems. Skin findings can also provide important clues to systemic infections or processes that may cause late complications (e.g., leishmaniasis) (108).

The distribution of diseases changes over time, making it important to obtain current information about what diseases occur in which geographic areas. Many web sites can now assist that search (103). Resistance patterns to antimicrobials and serotypes of pathogens may vary from one region to another. Table 41.5 lists several sources of information that are regularly updated. Although this chapter focuses on helping the traveler avoid disease and disruption, we should also recognize that the massive movement of humans today affects the distribution of infectious diseases and their impact on populations (109).

TABLE 41.5. Sources of Information

Centers for Disease Control and Prevention: Health Information for International Travel. (The Yellow Book) Revised regularly. Can be purchased from the Public Health Foundation, tel 877-252-1200 or at http://bookstore.phf.org

CDC Yellow Book 2001–2002 www.cdc.gov/travel/yellowbook.pdf

CDC Home Travel Information www.cdc.gov/travel/

CDC Travelers' Health Hotline: 877-FYI-TRIP

CDC fax information (toll free): 888-232-3299

CDC MMWR www.cdc.gov/mmwr

CDC *Emerging Infectious Diseases* (journal) available electronically

CDC WebServer http://www.cdc.gov

WHO International Travel and Health www.who.int/ith/

WHO disease surveillance www.who/int/wer/

EuroSurveillance www.eurosurveillance.org

ProMED-mail www.promedmail.org

Health Canada Travel Medicine www.TravelHealth.gc.ca

International Association for Medical Assistance to Travellers (IAMAT), 40 Regal Road, Guelph, Ontario N1K 1B5F. Publishes regularly updated summaries on immunizations, malaria prophylaxis, schistosomiasis, and American trypanosomiasis. World climate charts are also available. www.sentex.net/~iamat

Travel Medicine Advisor, published by American Health Consultants, Inc. Uses loose-leaf format to allow regular updating of sections. Provides newsletter every 2 months. Telephone 1-800-688-2421.

World Health Organization: International Travel and Health. Vaccination Requirements and Health Advice. World Health Organization, 1211 Geneva, Switzerland. Revised annually.

In addition to the Infectious Diseases Society of America and the American Society for Microbiology, the following organizations have regular scientific meetings that focus at least in part on infections in travelers:

International Society of Travel Medicine (publishes *Journal of Travel Medicine*) www.istm.org/jtm.html

Wilderness Medical Society (publishes a journal, *Wilderness and Environmental Medicine*) www.wms.org

American Committee on Clinical Tropical Medicine and Traveler's Health, within the American Society of Tropical Medicine and Hygiene (*American Journal of Tropical Medicine and Hygiene*) www.astmh.org. Directory of physicians certified by ASTMH in tropical and travel medicine www.astmh.org/clinics/clinindex.html

Current information can also be accessed at websites. See also reference Travelhealth, On-Line (consumer oriented) www.tripprep.com.

REFERENCES

1. Wilson ME. *A world guide to infections: diseases, distribution, diagnosis.* New York: Oxford University Press, 1991.
2. Steffen R, Rickenbach M, Wilhelm U, et al. Health problems after travel to developing countries. *J Infect Dis* 1987;156:84–91.
3. Steffen R, DuPont HL. Travel medicine: what's that? *J Travel Med* 1994;1:1–3.
4. Steffen R. Travel medicine—prevention based on epidemiologic data. *Trans R Soc Trop Med Hyg* 1991;85:156–162.
5. Reid D, Cossar JH. Epidemiology of travel. *Br Med Bull* 1993;49:257–268.
6. Eng TR, Bernard KW, Banks D, et al. Epidemiologic surveillance of health conditions among temporary residents of developing countries: the Peace Corps experience. In: Lobel HO, Steffen R, Kozarsky PE, eds. *Travel medicine*, 2nd ed. Atlanta: International Society of Travel Medicine, 1991:16–19.
7. Hackett PH, Roach RC. High-altitude illness. *N Engl J Med* 2001;345:107–114.
8. Auerbach PS. Marine envenomations. *N Engl J Med* 1991;325:486–493.
9. Guptill KS, Hargarten SW, Baker TD. American travel deaths in Mexico. Causes and prevention strategies. *West Med J* 1991;154:169–171.
10. Baker TD, Hargarten SW, Guptill KS. The uncounted dead—American civilians dying overseas. *Public Health Rep* 1992;107:155–160.
11. Hargarten SW. Injury prevention: a crucial aspect of travel medicine. *J Travel Med* 1994;1:48–50.
12. DuPont HL, Ericsson CD. Prevention and treatment of traveler's diarrhea. *N Engl J Med* 1993;328:1821–1827.
13. Ericsson CD, DuPont HL. Travelers' diarrhea: approaches to prevention and treatment. *Clin Infect Dis* 1993;16:616–626.
14. Gorbach SL, Kean BH, Evans DG, et al. Travelers' diarrhea and toxigenic *Escherichia coli. N Engl J Med* 1975;292:933–937.

15. Mattila L, Siitonen A, Kyronseppa H, et al. Seasonal variation in etiology of travelers' diarrhea. *J Infect Dis* 1992;165:383–388.

16. Hoge CW, Shlim DR, Rajah R, et al. Epidemiology of diarrheal illness associated with coccidian-like organism among travellers and foreign residents in Nepal. *Lancet* 1993;341:1175–1179.

17. Soave R, Herwaldt BL, Relman DA. Cyclospora. *Infect Dis Clin North Am* 1998;12:1–12.

18. Lackritz EM, Lobel HO, Howell JB, et al. Imported *Plasmodium falciparum* malaria in American travelers to Africa—implications for prevention strategies. *JAMA* 1991;265:383–385.

19. Phillips-Howard PA, Radalowicz J, Mitchell J, et al. Risk of malaria in British residents returning from malarious areas. *BMJ* 1990;300:499–503.

20. Steffen R, Kane MA, Shapiro CN, et al. Epidemiology and prevention of hepatitis A in travelers. *JAMA* 1994;272:885–889.

21. Centers for Disease Control and Prevention. Hepatitis E among U.S. travelers, 1989–1992. *MMWR Morb Mortal Wkly Rep* 1993;42:1–4.

22. De Schryver A, Meheus A. International travel and sexually transmitted diseases. *World Health Stat Q* 1989;42:90–99.

23. Mulhall BP. Sexually transmissible diseases and travel. *Br Med Bull* 1993;49:394–411.

24. Stricker M, Steffen R, Gutzwiller F, et al. Casual sexual contacts of Swiss tourist in tropical Africa, the Far East and Latin America. In: Lobel HO, Steffen R, Kozarsky PE, eds. *Travel medicine,* 2nd ed. Atlanta: International Society of Travel Medicine, 1991:220–221.

25. Nielsen NJ, Lindhardt BO, Ulrich K. HIV antibodies in Danish Volunteer Service personnel in Kenya, Tanzania and Zambia. *Trans R Soc Trop Med Hyg* 1987;81:680.

26. Smith RP, Smith D, Bern K, et al. Health risks of international travel among United States college students. In: Steffen R, Lobel HO, Bradley DJ, eds. *Travel medicine.* Berlin: Springer-Verlag, 1989:67–80.

27. Taylor DN, Duangmani C, Suvongse C, et al. The role of *Haemophilus ducreyi* in penile ulcers in Bangkok, Thailand. *Sex Transm Dis* 1984;11:148–151.

28. Aronson NE, Palmer BF. Acute viral hepatitis in American soldiers in Korea. *South Med J* 1988;81:949–951.

29. Visser LG, Polderman AM, Stuiver PC. Outbreak of schistosomiasis among travelers returning from Mali, West Africa. *Clin Infect Dis* 1995;20:280–285.

30. Moore DAJ, Edwards M, Escombe R, et al. African trypanosomiasis in travelers returning to the United Kingdom. *Emerg Infect Dis* 2002;8:74–76.

31. Dickens DL, DuPont HL, Johnson PC. Survival of bacterial enteropathogens in the ice of popular drinks. *JAMA* 1985;253:3141–3143.

32. Davies HD, Sakuls P, Keystone JS. Creeping eruption. A review of clinical presentation and management of 60 cases presenting to a tropical disease unit. *Arch Dermatol* 1993;129:588–591.

33. Centers for Disease Control and Prevention. Outbreak of acute respiratory febrile illness among college students—Acapulco, Mexico, March 2001. *MMWR Morb Mortal Wkly Rep* 2001;50:261–262.

34. Keene WE, McAnulty JM, Hoesly RC, et al. A swimming-associated outbreak of hemorrhagic colitis caused by *Escherichia coli* O157:H7 and *Shigella sonnei. N Engl J Med* 1994;331:579–584.

35. McAnulty JM, Fleming DW, Gonzalez AH. A community-wide outbreak of cryptosporidiosis associated with swimming at a wave pool. *JAMA* 1994;272:1597–1600.

36. Cabelli VJ, Dufour AP, McCabe LJ, et al. Swimming-associated gastroenteritis and water quality. *Am J Epidemiol* 1982;115:606–616.

37. Van Crevel R, Speelman P, Gravekamp C, et al. Leptospirosis in travelers. *Clin Infect Dis* 1994;19:132–134.

38. Tomchik RS, Russell MT, Szmant AM, et al. Clinical perspectives on seabather's eruption, also known as "sea lice." *JAMA* 1993;269:1669–1672.

39. Freudenthal AR, Joseph PR. Seabather's eruption. *N Engl J Med* 1993;329:542–544.

40. World Health Organization, Veterinary Public Health Unit. *World survey of rabies 25 (for year 1989).* Geneva: World Health Organization, 1992. Rabies/92.203.

41. Wilkerson JA. Rabies: epidemiology, diagnosis, prevention, and prospects for worldwide control. *Wilderness Environ Med* 1995;6:48–96.

42. Moore A, Herrera G, Nyamongo J, et al. Estimated risk of HIV transmission by blood transfusion in Kenya. *Lancet* 2001;358:657–660.

43. Lapostolle F, Surget V, Borron SW, et al. Severe pulmonary embolism associated with air travel. *N Engl J Med* 2001;345:779–783.

44. Dillard TA, Berg BW, Rajagopal KR, et al. Hypoxemia during air travel in patients with chronic obstructive pulmonary disease. *Ann Intern Med* 1989;111:362–367.

45. Moser MR, Bender TR, Margolis HS, et al. An outbreak of influenza aboard a commercial airliner. *Am J Epidemiol* 1979;110:1101–1106.

46. Driver CR, Valway SE, Margan WM, et al. Transmission of *Mycobacterium tuberculosis* associated with air travel. *JAMA* 1994;272:1031–1035.

47. Centers for Disease Control and Prevention. Update: outbreak of influenza A infection—Alaska and the Yukon Territory, July-August 1998. *MMWR Morb Mortal Wkly Rep* 1998;47:685–688.

48. Centers for Disease Control and Prevention. Rubella among crew members of commercial cruise ships—Florida, 1997. *MMWR Morb Mort Wkly Rep* 1998;46:1247–1250.

49. Jernigan DB, Hoffman J, Cetron MS, et al. Outbreak of legionnaires' disease among cruise ship passengers exposed to a contaminated whirlpool spa. *Lancet* 1996;347:494–499.

50. Hedberg CW, Levine WC, White KE, et al. An international foodborne outbreak of shigellosis associated with a commercial airline. *JAMA* 1992;268:3208–3212.

51. Wilson ME. Critical evaluation of vaccines for travelers. *J Travel Med* 1996;2:239–243.

52. Jong EC. Health concerns of international travelers. In: Jong EC, McMullen R, eds. *The travel and tropical medicine manual,* 3rd ed. Philadelphia: Saunders, 2003:3–17.

53. Blaser MJ. Environmental interventions for the prevention of travelers' diarrhea. *Rev Infect Dis* 1986;8:S142–S150.

54. Sack DA, Kaminsky DC, Sack RB, et al. Prophylactic doxycycline for travelers' diarrhea: results of a prospective double-blind study of Peace Corps volunteers in Kenya. *N Engl J Med* 1978;298:758–763.

55. DuPont HL, Ericsson CD, Johnson PC, et al. Prevention of travelers' diarrhea by the tablet formulation of bismuth subsalicylate. *JAMA* 1987;257:1347–1350.

56. Tauxe RV, Tuhr ND, Wells JG, et al. Antimicrobial resistance of *Shigella* isolates in the USA: the importance of international travelers. *J Infect Dis* 1990;162:1107–1111.

57. Murphy GS, Bodhidatta L, Echeverria P, et al. Ciprofloxacin and loperamide in the treatment of bacillary dysentery. *Ann Intern Med* 1993;118:582–586.

58. Taylor DN, Sanchez JL, Candler W, et al. Treatment of travelers' diarrhea: ciprofloxacin plus loperamide versus ciprofloxacin alone. A placebo-controlled, randomized trial. *Ann Intern Med* 1991;114:731–734.

59. Johnson PC, Ericsson CD, DuPont HL, et al. Comparison of loperamide with bismuth subsalicylate for the treatment of acute travelers' diarrhea. *JAMA* 1986;255:757–760.

60. Lobel HO, Kozarsky PE. Update on prevention of malaria for travelers. *JAMA* 1997;278:1767–1771.

61. Overbosch D, Schilthuis H, Bienzle U, et al. Atovaquone-proguanil versus mefloquine for malaria prophylaxis in nonimmune travelers: results from a randomized, double-blind study. *Clin Infect Dis* 2001;33:1015–1021.

62. Steffen R, Heusser R, Machler R, et al. Malaria chemoprophylaxis among European tourists in tropical Africa: use, adverse reactions, and efficacy. *Bull World Health Org* 1990;68:313–322.

63. Hilton E, Singer C, Kozarsky P, et al. Status of immunity to tetanus, measles, mumps, rubella, and polio among U.S. travelers. *Ann Intern Med* 1991;115:32–33.

64. White CC, Koplan JP, Orenstein WA. Benefits, risks and costs of immunization for measles, mumps and rubella. *Am J Public Health* 1985;75:739–744.

65. Koplan JP, Schoenbaum SC, Weinstein MC, et al. Pertussis vaccine—analysis of benefits, risks and costs. *N Engl J Med* 1979;301:906–911.

66. Hinman AR, Koplan JP. Pertussis and pertussis vaccine—reanalysis of benefits, risks and costs. *JAMA* 1984;251:3109–3113.

67. Hay JW, Daum RS. Economic analysis of *Haemophilus influenzae* type b vaccination. *Pediatr Infect Dis J* 1990;9:246–252.

68. Wilson ME, Fineberg HV. Rabies vaccine in travelers: a decision analysis. *Am J Trop Med Hyg* 1991;45[Suppl]:95(abstr 4).

69. Behrens RH, Roberts JA. Is travel prophylaxis worthwhile: economic appraisal of prophylactic measures against malaria, hepatitis A, and typhoid in travellers. *BMJ* 1994;309:918–922.

70. Herwaldt LA. Pertussis and pertussis vaccines in adults. *JAMA* 1993;269:93–94.

71. Gergen PJ, McQuillan GM, Kiely M, et al. A population-based serologic survey of immunity to tetanus in the United States. *N Engl J Med* 1995;332:761–766.

72. Maple PA, Efstratiou A, George RC, et al. Diphtheria immunity in UK blood donors. *Lancet* 1995;345:963–965.

73. Vitek CR, Wharton M. Diphtheria in the former Soviet Union: reemergence of a pandemic disease. *Emerg Infect Dis* 1998;4:539–550.

74. Centers for Disease Control and Prevention. Prevention of varicella. Updated recommendations of the Advisory Committee on Immunization Practices. *MMWR Morb Mortal Wkly Rep* 1999;48:1–5.

75. Leder K, Weller PF, Wilson ME. Travel vaccines and elderly persons: review of vaccines available in the United States. *Clin Infect Dis* 2001;33:1553–1566.

76. Buxton JA, Skowronski DM, Ng H. Influenza revaccination of elderly travelers: antibody response to single influenza vaccination and revaccination at 12 weeks. *J Infect Dis* 2001;184:188–191.

77. Centers for Disease Control and Prevention. *Health information for international travel, 2003–2004.* Atlanta: US Department of Health and Human Services, Public Health Service, 2003.

78. World Health Organization. *International travel and health.* Geneva: World Health Organization, 2003.

79. Martin M, Tsai TF, Cropp B, et al. Fever and multisystem organ failure associated with 17D-204 yellow fever vaccination: a report of four cases. *Lancet* 2001;358:98–104.

80. Vasconcelos PFC, Luna EJ, Galler R, et al. Serious adverse events associated with yellow fever 17DD vaccine in Brazil: a report of two cases. *Lancet* 2001;358:91–97.

81. Chan RC, Penney DJ, Little D, et al. Hepatitis and death following vaccination with 17D-204 yellow fever vaccine. *Lancet* 2001;358:121–122.

82. Centers for Disease Control and Prevention. Fever, jaundice, and multiple organ system failure associated with 17D-derived yellow fever vaccine, 1996–2001. *MMWR Morb Mortal Wkly Rep* 2001;50:643–645.

83. Martin M, Letteau L, Steele S, et al. Advanced age as a risk factor for illness temporally associated with yellow fever vaccination. *Emerg Infect Dis* 2001;7:945–951.

84. Tsai T, Paul R, Lynberg MC, et al. Congenital yellow fever virus infection after immunization in pregnancy. *J Infect Dis* 1993;168:1520–1523.
85. Centers for Disease Control and Prevention. Serogroup W-135 meningococcal disease among travelers returning from Saudi Arabia—United States, 2000. *MMWR Morb Mortal Wkly Rep* 2000;49:345–346.
86. Centers for Disease Control and Prevention. Prevention of hepatitis A through active or passive immunization. Recommendations of the Advisory Committee on Immunization Practices. *MMWR Morb Mortal Wkly Rep* 1999;48:1–37.
87. Wilson ME. Travel-related vaccines. *Infect Dis Clin North Am* 2001;15(1):231–251.
88. Centers for Disease Control and Prevention. FDA approval for a combined hepatitis A and B vaccine. *MMWR Morb Mortal Wkly Rep* 2001;50:806–807.
89. Centers for Disease Control and Prevention. Typhoid immunization—recommendations of the Advisory Committee on Immunization Practices (ACIP). *MMWR Morb Mortal Wkly Rep* 1994;43(RR-14):1–7.
90. Rowe B, Ward LR, Threlfall EJ. Multidrug-resistant *Salmonella typhi:* a worldwide epidemic. *Clin Infect Dis* 1995;24[Suppl 1]:S106–S109.
91. Lin FYC, Ho VA, Khiem HB, et al. The efficacy of a *Salmonella typhi* Vi conjugate vaccine in two-to-five-year-old children. *N Engl J Med* 2001;344:1263–1269.
92. Centers for Disease Control and Prevention. Inactivated Japanese encephalitis virus vaccine. Recommendations of the Advisory Committee on Immunization Practices (ACIP). *MMWR Morb Mortal Wkly Rep* 1993;42(RR-1):1–15.
93. Wilson ME. Rabies realities. *Infect Dis Clin Pract* 1998;7:31–33.
94. Centers for Disease Control: Human rabies prevention—United States. Recommendations of the Advisory Committee on Immunization Practices (ACIP). *MMWR Morb Mortal Wkly Rep* 1999;48(RR-1):1–48.
95. Dye C, Scheele S, Dolin P, et al. Consensus statement: global burden of tuberculosis: estimated incidence prevalence, and mortality by country: WHO Global Surveillance and Monitoring Project. *JAMA* 1999;282:677–686.
96. Cobelens FGJ, van Deutekom H, Draayer-Jansen IWE, et al. Risk of infection with *Mycobacterium tuberculosis* in travellers to areas of high tuberculosis endemicity. *Lancet* 2000;356:461–465.

97. Wilson ME, Iacoviello VR. Travel and HIV infection. In: Jong EC, McMullen R, eds. *The travel and tropical medicine manual,* 3rd ed. Philadelphia: Saunders, 2003:220–233.
98. Wilson ME, von Reyn CF, Fineberg HV. Infections in HIV-infected travelers: risks and prevention. *Ann Intern Med* 1991;114:582–592.
99. Klemper CA, Linett A, Kane C, et al. Frequency of travel of adults infected with HIV. *J Travel Med* 1995;2:85–88.
100. Samuel BU, Barry M. The pregnant traveler. *Infect Dis Clin North Am* 1998;12:325–354.
101. Munoz FM, Englund JA. Vaccines in pregnancy. *Infect Dis Clin North Am* 2001;15:253–271.
102. Sullivan MC, Jong EC. Travel with chronic medical conditions. In: Jong EC, McMullen R, eds. *The travel and tropical medicine manual,* 3rd edition. Philadelphia: Saunders, 2003:234–245.
103. Keystone JS, Kozarsky PE, Freedman DO. Internet and computer-based resources for travel medicine practitioners. *Clin Infect Dis* 2001;32:757–765.
104. Wilson ME, Pearson R. Fever and systemic systems. In: Guerrant RL, Walker DH, Weller PF, eds. *Tropical infectious diseases. Principles, pathogens, and practice.* Philadelphia: Churchill Livingstone, 1999:1381–1399.
105. Ryan ET, Wilson ME, Kain KC. Illness after international travel. *N Engl J Med* 2003;347:505–516.
106. Centers for Disease Control and Prevention. Imported dengue—United States, 1997 and 1998. *MMWR Morb Mortal Wkly Rep* 2000;49(12):248–253.
107. Caumes E, Carriere J, Guermonprez G, et al. Dermatoses associated with travel to tropical countries: a prospective study of the diagnosis and management of 269 patients presenting to a tropical disease unit. *Clin Infect Dis* 1995;20:542–548.
108. Wilson ME. Skin problems in the traveler. *Infect Dis Clin North Am* 1998;12:471–488.
109. Wilson ME. Travel and the emergence of infectious diseases. *Emerg Infect Dis* 1995;1:39–46.

Head and Neck

CHAPTER 42
Dental Infections

Walter J. Loesche

Dental infections such as dental caries and periodontal disease occur in and around the teeth. Dental caries or dental decay is unique among human infections because it involves the destruction of hard acellular tissue, the enamel and dentine of the tooth, and does not provoke an inflammatory response until the decay impinges on the pulp. Among the estimated 500 bacterial species that colonize the tooth surface in bacterial communities known as *dental plaque*, only the mutans streptococci, lactobacilli, and possibly yeast have been etiologically associated with dental decay. A different group of bacteria comprising mainly gram-negative anaerobes is associated with periodontal disease. These anaerobes accumulate in the plaque that forms at the gingival margin (Fig. 42.1) and produce an array of biologically active products that diffuse into and provoke an inflammatory response in the adjacent host tissue. These responses result in a loss of periodontal fibers that attach the tooth to the bone; a defect, known as a *periodontal pocket*, forms between the root surface of the tooth and the surrounding host tissue and becomes filled with more than 10^8 bacterial colony-forming units.

POSSIBLE ASSOCIATION OF DENTAL INFECTIONS WITH CARDIOVASCULAR DISEASE

Dental caries and periodontal disease have been the domain of the dentist and have been mostly ignored by the medical community. This may change if observations showing a statistically significant positive association between dental infections and cardiovascular disease (1–7) and premature births (8) can be confirmed.

In 1989, Finnish investigators reported that poor dental health could be associated with both an acute myocardial infarction (1) and a cerebrovascular accident (2). These investigators developed a measurement of dental disease, called the *total dental index*, that documented the number of missing, decayed, or periodontally involved teeth. Subsequently, in a 7-year prospective study, the total dental index ($p = 0.007$) and the number of pre-

vious myocardial infarctions ($p = 0.003$) were associated with a risk for developing a new and often fatal myocardial infarction (3). Traditional risk factors such as diabetes, hypertension, smoking, total cholesterol levels, high-density lipoprotein cholesterol levels, triglyceride levels, socioeconomic status, gender, and age were not significant predictors of a coronary event.

Other studies have confirmed this link between dental disease and coronary heart disease. A prospective cohort design study involving data for 9760 U.S. men examined three times between 1971 and 1987 found a slight but significant relationship between either periodontitis or edentulism (missing all teeth) and coronary heart disease, after adjusting for 13 known risk factors (4). A representative sample of 1,384 Finnish men, 45 to 64 years old, showed that the number of missing teeth, along with hypertension, geographical area, and educational level, were independent explanatory factors for the presence of ischemic heart disease (5). Among U.S. veterans, a significant association between periodontal disease and coronary heart disease and stroke could be demonstrated after adjusting for various cardiovascular risk factors (6).

Collectively, these studies imply that dental infections may be important contributors to cardiovascular pathology.

Although no causal link between dental disease and cardiovascular pathology has been demonstrated, several hypotheses have been proposed (6,7). The ones most relevant in the present context are those related to dental infections causing asymptomatic bacteremias; a generalized increase in white cell counts in the normal range; a generalized increase in inflammatory mediators, such as C-reactive protein (9); and possibly, specific effects on coagulation. These hypotheses are not discussed further in this chapter, but they should alert the physician to the possibility that dental caries and periodontal disease are potential risk factors for cardiovascular disease.

DENTAL CARIES

History

Dental caries is both an ancient and a modern infection. Fossil records of teeth from ancient humans have been used to describe the lineage of dental decay in the English from the Iron Age to modern times (10). The modern era of dental caries can be traced to the repeal by Parliament of the Corn Laws in 1850, which allowed the duty-free entry of cane sugar into the United Kingdom. Within 15 years, there was a sudden increase in dental caries, a phenomenon that has been observed in many cultures, including the African Bushmen, the Eskimos, the Tahitians, and currently the Nigerians, soon after the introduction of sugar (11).

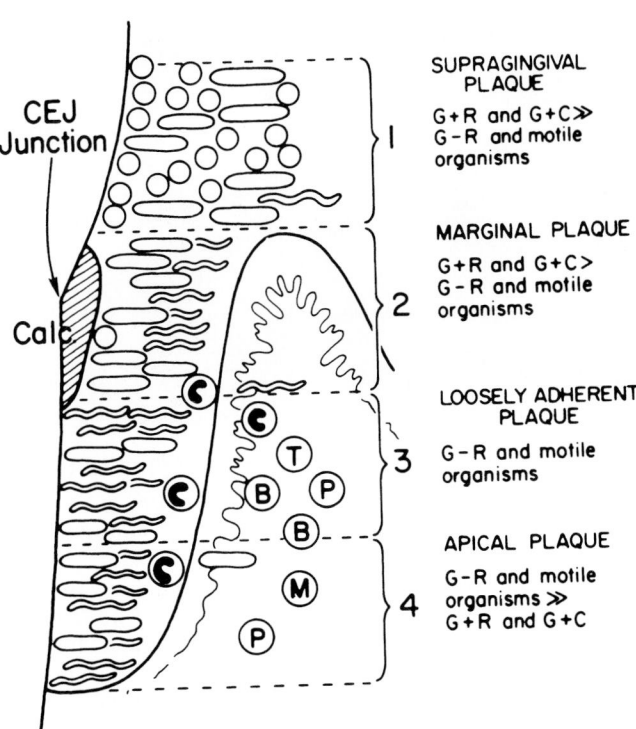

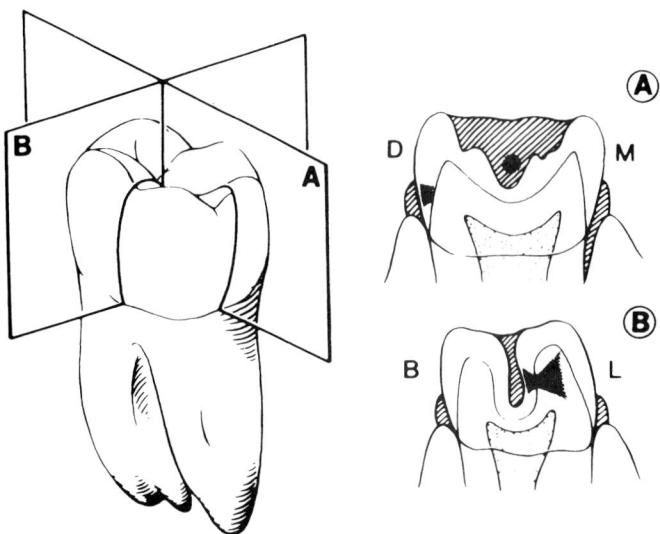

Figure 42.2. Sagittal (**A**) and cross-sectional (**B**) sections through a permanent molar. D, distal; M, mesial; B, buccal; L, lingual surfaces. Note fissure decay (*shaded area* midway down in fissure) and approximal decay (*subsurface shaded area* on distal surface). Note also supragingival plaque accumulations on mesial, distal, buccal, and lingual surfaces and the extension of the plaque subgingivally in the mesial surface.

Figure 42.1. Schematic diagram showing supragingival plaque colonized by gram-positive rods and cocci and the subgingival plaque colonized mostly by spirochetes and gram-negative rods. T cells, B cells, plasma (*P*) cells, macrophages (*M*), and neutrophils are shown in the gingival tissue. Neutrophils are shown in the subgingival environment, and an occasional spirochete and rod are shown invading the gingival tissue. The cementum–enamel junction (*CEJ*) is where the enamel ends and the root surface covered by the cementum begins. Calculus (*Calc*) is calcified plaque or tartar that forms on the teeth where stagnant conditions exist.

The connection between dietary carbohydrates and bacteria was the basis of a nineteenth century theory developed by Miller that was known as the chemoparasitic theory on the causation of caries (12). Miller was unable to find any consistent microbial association and concluded that decay was bacteriologically nonspecific. He noted that decay occurred almost uniformly in the retentive areas of the tooth, such as the occlusal fissures on the tops of the teeth and the approximal surfaces where the teeth made contact with each other (Fig. 42.2). He advocated keeping these areas clean of bacterial or plaque accumulations, which was translated to tooth brushing with abrasive powders and dentifrices and to frequent dental cleanings. No preventive benefit of this approach was ever shown until the 1960s, when fluoride was added to dentifrices (11).

The lack of a viable preventive procedure for dental caries led to an alarming dental morbidity among U.S. citizens. Dental caries and tooth loss were the most common cause of rejection for military service in World War I, World War II, the Korean War, and the early days of the Vietnam War. In 1960, about 60% of adults older than 65 years of age were without teeth. The cost of dental treatment, which was given mostly in response to symptoms, was enormous. In 1998, the cost of treatment in the United States was estimated to be more than $40 billion, with about 85% of this cost related to dental caries. Despite these staggering costs, this dental morbidity has been contained by the use of fluoride in drinking water, salt, and dentifrices. In the future, further cost containment should follow from the elucidation of the specific role of the mutans streptococci in dental caries that was first shown in animal models (13–15).

Characteristics of Odontopathogens: Mutans Streptococci

The mutans streptococci ferment mannitol and sorbitol, produce extracellular glucans (glucose polymers) from sucrose, and are cariogenic in animal models. In 1924, Clarke (16) isolated such organisms from human carious lesions and called them *Streptococcus mutans* because their pleomorphic coccal shape suggested a mutant form of a streptococcus. When *S. mutans* strains were collected from different sources, it became apparent that considerable serological and genetic heterogenicity existed. Eight serotypes could be recognized on the basis of carbohydrate antigens (17), and deoxyribonucleic acid (DNA) hybridization studies revealed four genetic groups (18). These genetic groups were given species names that reflected their original mammalian source of isolation (18). *S. mutans* was assigned to the predominant human isolates, whereas other human isolates were called *Streptococcus sobrinus*. *Streptococcus rattus* and *Streptococcus cricetus* were assigned to the mutans streptococci isolated from laboratory-bred rats and hamsters, respectively. Subsequently, new species of mutans streptococci were isolated from wild rats (*Streptococcus ferus*) and the macaque monkey (*Streptococcus macacae*). Thus, six distinct species have been identified as mutans streptococci, but only two species, *S. mutans* and *S. sobrinus*, have been associated with human caries.

BIOLOGIC AND BIOCHEMICAL PROPERTIES

For *S. mutans* and *S. sobrinus* to be uniquely associated with dental caries, there would need to be a special relationship between these species and sucrose. This would have to be something other than the ability to ferment sucrose because many of the other species that can be isolated from plaque can also ferment sucrose. In fact, when germ-free rats were monoassociated with various saccharolytic species and fed high-sucrose diets, there was usually no decay (19).

This means that something besides acid production per se was needed for decay to occur.

A clue to what one of these factors was came from hamster studies in which these animals were fed, at weaning, a diet containing either 56% sucrose or 56% glucose and then were inoculated with a streptomycin-resistant strain of *S. mutans* (20). In the sucrose-fed animals, *S. mutans* established on the teeth in high numbers, and the animals developed extensive decay. In the glucose-fed animals, *S. mutans* was recovered in low numbers, and the level of decay was similar to that found in the uninoculated control animals.

Studies soon showed that in the presence of sucrose, *S. mutans* and *S. sobrinus* formed adhesive colonies that stuck to the surfaces of culture vessels (21). Chemical analysis indicated that the adhesive material was a glucose homopolymer or glucan composed of two classes of compounds, an α-1,6 core-linked polymer classified as a dextran and a unique α-1,3–rich polymer classified as a mutan. The α-1,3–rich polymer was water insoluble and cell associated and was involved in smooth-surface decay, whereas the α-1,6–rich polymer was water soluble and was not associated with smooth-surface decay (11). These glucans apparently provided a mechanism by which the mutans streptococci extended their niche from the retentive fissure site to the nonretentive smooth tooth surface. However, these studies did not explain why *S. mutans* was cariogenic in retentive sites such as the fissure.

Insight into this mechanism was provided by a mutant of *S. mutans* that exhibited less decay than the wild type on both smooth and occlusal fissures and that possessed reduced aciduricity or the ability to grow in a low-pH environment (22). The pH in plaque can drop below 5.0 for 30 to 120 minutes after exposure to a fermentable dietary carbohydrate (23). *S. mutans* and, to a lesser extent, *S. sobrinus* have a pH optimum at about 5.0 to 5.5 (24) and can survive and actually grow at these low pH values found in plaque during and after eating. Because of this aciduricity, these mutans streptococci become dominant in the plaques, and because of their acid production, they lead to the demineralization of the tooth that, if unchecked, results in dental decay.

Pathogenesis of Decay

The saliva is a remarkably protective fluid for the tooth surface because it contains buffers and is supersaturated with calcium and phosphate ions, which favor remineralization of the tooth surface (25). When the plaque is exposed to fermentable dietary carbohydrates, there is an immediate and persistent drop in the pH. At a pH of about 5.0 to 5.5, known as the *critical pH*, the salivary buffers are overwhelmed; but the hydroxyapatite of the tooth acts as a buffer so that further pH drops are not encountered. But why would the tooth act as a buffer to maintain the pH in the vicinity of 5.0? If the pH dropped to 3 or 4, the enamel surface layer would be irreversibly lost, as occurs when a tooth is exposed to acid *in vitro*. However, at pH 5.0, the mineral is lost from the subsurface layers in such a way that repair, in the form of remineralization, can proceed once the pH returns to values above the critical pH. It is in this situation that the supersaturated levels of calcium and phosphate diffuse into the teeth and promote remineralization.

This remarkable dissolution pattern has great significance with regard to the development of dental decay. Whenever a fermentable dietary substrate diffuses into the plaque and is converted to acid end products, some degree of subsurface demineralization occurs. Then, between meals or snacks, the pH in the plaque returns to neutrality, and the supersaturated levels

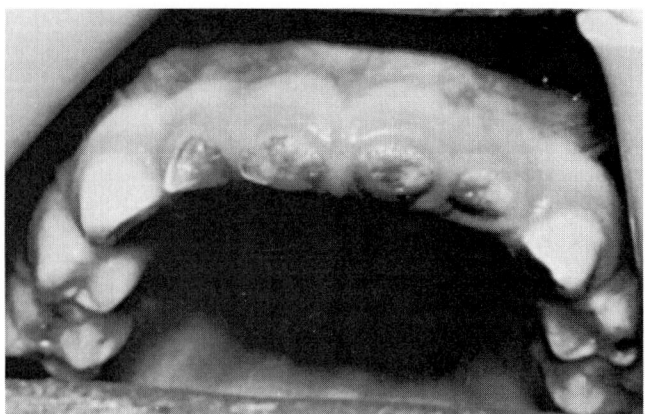

Figure 42.3. Nursing-bottle caries. Note that the crowns of the four maxillary anterior teeth are completely decayed, whereas the adjacent teeth are intact.

of calcium and phosphate ions promote remineralization. Demineralization that progresses to cavitation occurs if the frequency and magnitude of acid production overwhelm the repair process. This occurs with frequent eating (26) or if the repair process is compromised by xerostomia (27). In both situations, there would be a selection for aciduric organisms such as *S. mutans* and lactobacilli. This sequence of events can be illustrated by a situation in which sucrose availability is frequent, as in nursing-bottle caries, and by one in which salivary flow is reduced, as in postradiation xerostomia.

Nursing-bottle caries is extensive decay of the maxillary anterior teeth (Fig. 42.3) that is associated with prolonged and frequent bottle-feeding or breast-feeding (28). Liquid from the mother's breast or nursing bottle bathe all of the teeth except the lower incisors. The bacteria on these teeth have prolonged access to any fermentable substrates such as lactose or sucrose in the liquid. In one study, *S. mutans* accounted for more than 50% and lactobacilli for 5% of the flora on the teeth (29). These are the highest values for *S. mutans* and lactobacilli that have been reported for human teeth.

Rampant decay in patients receiving radiation treatment for head and neck cancer is so predictable that these individuals have been studied in a prospective fashion. In one such study, during the development of decay, a pronounced shift to *S. mutans* and lactobacilli occurred at the expense of noncariogenic organisms such as *Streptococcus sanguis* and *Bacteroides, Fusobacterium,* and *Neisseria* species. Three to four months after radiation therapy, the proportions of *S. mutans* peaked at 18% of the plaque flora, and five new carious lesions were present. Thereafter, the lactobacilli became the dominant aciduric species coincident with the lesions' becoming larger and more numerous (30).

This sequence of events indicated that *S. mutans* was involved with the initiation of decay, whereas the lactobacilli were associated with progression of the lesion. This was also suggested by a study in which the incipient lesion was monitored to determine whether it would progress to the stage of cavitation (31). *S. mutans* was the numerically dominant organism in the plaques but was isolated with equal frequency from progressive and nonprogressive lesions. *Lactobacillus casei* was present in 85% of the progressive lesions before the clinical diagnosis of progression was made and was never isolated from nonprogressive lesions. These findings indicate that dental decay is a two-stage process in which *S. mutans* is associated with the initial lesion and lactobacilli, especially *L. casei*, are associated with its progression.

Epidemiology

Epidemiological surveys indicate that dental decay is mainly a disease of youth, occurs in teeth shortly after their eruption, does not occur uniformly on all teeth or tooth surfaces, and tends to be symmetrical (11). The prevalence of decay is highest on the occlusal (or chewing) surfaces of first and second molars and lowest on the lingual surfaces of mandibular anterior teeth. Decay was and is the chief cause of tooth loss in populations consuming a sucrose-containing diet, resulting in edentulousness for more than 50% of the population older than 65 years. This pattern is changing: now many children younger than 10 years of age are caries free, and only 12% to 14% of Americans between 55 and 64 years of age were edentulous in 1985 (32). This means that more older individuals have more teeth and require more dental health care than previously. These teeth may be at increased risk for decay because so many medications that are prescribed by physicians, such as antidepressants, antihistamines, antihypertensives, and diuretics, cause as a side effect a reduction in salivary flow (33). When this reduction is combined with a tendency to snack and a reduced ability to perform oral hygiene, dental caries manifests itself as a disease of elderly people.

Diagnosis

Diagnosis of dental decay is usually a *post facto* event and devoid of any bacteriological testing. Any procedure that is intended to show an *S. mutans* infection is complicated by the fact that most individuals harbor *S. mutans* on their teeth. However, the level and persistence of the *S. mutans* colonization seem to determine the risk for decay (34,35). This level has been empirically determined for the saliva: individuals with salivary *S. mutans* levels above 10^6 colony-forming units per milliliter of saliva are at a high caries risk (36). The ability to detect *S. mutans* in saliva is dependent on the use of a selective medium that employs bacitracin and 20% sucrose (37). Various kits for office use employing this medium have been developed (38), as have tests for the detection of lactobacilli in saliva (39).

Treatment

The treatment of dental caries has been mechanical and symptomatic. The decayed tooth substance is completely removed and replaced with a metal or plastic material that is strong, has thermal characteristics similar to those of the tooth itself, and is aesthetically acceptable to the patient. The most common filling material is amalgam, so called because it is an amalgamation of silver, tin, and mercury, with lesser amounts of zinc and copper being present. The amalgam has a half-life of about 4 to 7 years in a caries-active mouth, with the main reason for failure being decay around the margin of the filling (40).

The tooth surface is the natural habitat of *S. mutans*. This has important implications for antimicrobial therapy because the agent need only be applied to the teeth; if it eliminates *S. mutans* from the tooth, there may be a prolonged period before a reinfection with *S. mutans* can occur. Also, the occlusal fissure that appears to be the preferential niche for *S. mutans* on the tooth (Fig. 42.2) is available for colonization in its depth only during a finite time period after the tooth erupts. These considerations have led to the development of two strategies to prevent an *S. mutans* infection from occurring or recurring: namely, to interrupt or delay the acquisition of *S. mutans* by infants and to suppress an existing *S. mutans* infection once it has been diagnosed.

INTERFERENCE WITH TRANSMISSION

Colonization by *S. mutans* occurs at about the time that teeth erupt in infants (41). Early colonization may be a reliable predictor of subsequent caries activity. In one study, children who harbored *S. mutans* by age 2 years developed 10.6 decayed surfaces by age 4 years. In contrast, children in whom *S. mutans* was detected between 2 and 4 years developed 3.4 decayed surfaces; and children in whom *S. mutans* could not be detected had 0.3 decayed surfaces by age 4 (42). Several investigators have demonstrated a significant relationship between maternal salivary levels of *S. mutans* and the salivary levels of *S. mutans* in their children (43). This suggested that treatment of the mothers could interfere with or delay the bacterial colonization of the children.

Kohler and associates (44,45) have interrupted this passage of *S. mutans* from mother to child by aggressively treating mothers who had salivary *S. mutans* levels above 10^6 colony-forming units per milliliter of saliva and whose infants had no erupted teeth. An intensive preventive program involving dietary counseling, professional tooth cleaning with a fluoride paste, topical fluoride treatments, and excavation of carious lesions was employed to get the mother's salivary levels of *S. mutans* below 2.5×10^5 colony-forming units per milliliter of saliva. In 60% of the mothers, this goal was achieved. In the remaining mothers, a topical gel containing 1% chlorhexidine (Hibitane) used once a day for 2 weeks was able to reduce the *S. mutans* organisms to this level. At 3 years of age, only 16% of the children of the treated mothers had decay, compared with 43% of the children of the untreated mothers. There was also a comparable decrease in the prevalence of *S. mutans* among the children of the treated mothers. These findings show that intensive measures directed toward the mother can delay or prevent the acquisition of *S. mutans* in the child, and that this can be associated with a reduced incidence of decay.

SUPPRESSION OF AN EXISTING INFECTION

Many agents, such as iodine, fluoride, chlorhexidine, vancomycin, and kanamycin, have reduced for a finite period the plaque and saliva proportions or levels of *S. mutans*. The universality of the response pattern, that is, decline in *S. mutans* followed by its eventual return, suggested that the antimicrobial agents used were unable to penetrate all the niches in which *S. mutans* exists on the tooth. Paramount among these would be the depths of the fissure and the incipient carious lesions. Stannous fluoride and chlorhexidine appear to penetrate the fissure, and fluoride penetrates the incipient lesion (11). Both fluoride and chlorhexidine exhibit substantivity on the tooth surfaces, where there is a persistent antimicrobial activity. The fluoride effect can come about as the plaque pH drop after ingestion of the food can release bound fluoride from the enamel. The chlorhexidine effect comes from the calcium ions in the saliva eluting any bound chlorhexidine from the tooth surface. The effectiveness of both antimicrobials can be enhanced by the use of slow-release delivery systems, in which the agents are painted onto the tooth surface as a varnish (46).

PERIODONTAL DISEASE

History

The treatment of periodontal disease has generally been neglected by the dental profession. As recently as 1977, dentists in general practice reported that less than 1% of their income was derived from the treatment of periodontal disease (47). Microbial specificity in periodontal disease has taken longer to demonstrate because most investigators focused their attention on supragingival plaque, which is the plaque above the gingival margin, and did not examine the subgingival plaque, which is below the gingival margin (Fig. 42.1). The subgingival flora is composed mainly of anaerobic species, most of which could not be cultured and, when cultured, could not be assigned to known species. The use of quantitative anaerobic culturing procedures has led to the isolation of many new species, and DNA technology indicates that more than 500 species may be present (48).

Characteristics of Putative Periodontal Pathogens

SPIROCHETES

Many spirochetes considered to be *Treponema* species are evident in subgingival plaque samples taken from periodontal pockets. They are easily recognizable because of their helical shape (Fig. 42.4) and vigorous motility when observed by either dark-field or phase-contrast microscopy. Many spirochetes are less than 0.2 μm in diameter and have been shown to invade the soft tissue adjacent to the plaque (49). A few spirochetes are cultivable, and of these, *Treponema denticola* possesses a wide array of proteolytic enzymes, which makes it a prime suspect in periodontal pathogenesis (50). Spirochetes are usually not detected or are present in low number in plaques removed from healthy periodontal sites. They increase in numbers and proportions in plaque associated with gingivitis and reach their highest absolute and relative values in plaques removed from sites with periodontitis, where they can constitute almost half the total flora.

BLACK-PIGMENTED SPECIES

Black-pigmented colonies isolated from dental plaque were initially called *Bacteroides melaninogenicus* (now *Prevotella melaninogenica*). DNA analysis has shown that these black-pigmented isolates are composed of at least nine species and are different from intestinal *Bacteroides* (51). Three black-pigmented species have been associated with dental infections. *Porphyromonas gingivalis* is frequently isolated in high proportions from the more aggressive forms of periodontitis, such as early-onset forms (52) and those refractory to treatment (52). *Porphyromonas endodontalis* is frequently isolated from infections of the dental pulp. *Prevotella intermedia* is uniquely associated with acute necrotizing ulcerative gingivitis and with pregnancy gingivitis (53) (Table 42.1). These black-pigmented species could contribute to periodontal

TABLE 42.1.   Relationship between Clinical Forms of Periodontal Disease and Various Bacterial Species

Clinical entity	Bacterial factor
Gingivitis	
Experimental	Plaque accumulation, streptococci, actinomycetes
Pregnancy	*Prevotella intermedia*
Puberty	*P. intermedia* (?)
Stress (acute necrotizing ulcerative gingivitis)	*P. intermedia*, spirochetes
Simple	Plaque accumulation, spirochetes
Generalized severe	Spirochetes
Periodontitis	
Prepuberty	Spirochetes, black-pigmented species
Localized juvenile	*Actinobacillus actinomycetemcomitans*, spirochetes
Early onset	Spirochetes, *Porphyromonas gingivalis*, *Bacteroides forsythus*, *Treponema denticola*
Adult	Spirochetes, *P. gingivalis*, *B. forsythus*, *T. denticola*
Progressive	Spirochetes, *P. gingivalis*, *B. forsythus*, *T. denticola*

disease by releasing endotoxin, various organic acids such as butyric acid, and low-molecular-weight compounds such as hydrogen sulfide and ammonia into the pocket microenvironment.

BACTEROIDES FORSYTHUS

B. forsythus is an anaerobic, gram-negative, pleomorphic, nonmotile, long, thin rod (54) that has been isolated from some but not all lesions that are actually breaking down (55).

BANA-POSITIVE SPECIES

T. denticola, *B. forsythus*, and *P. gingivalis* possess an arginine hydrolase that can be readily measured in plaque samples by hydrolysis of the synthetic trypsin substrate, benzoyl-DL arginine naphthylamide (BANA) (56). These BANA-positive species were the only species of 40 tested that were significantly associated with periodontal disease in more than 13,000 plaque species that were tested using DNA probes (57). BANA hydrolysis can be used to diagnose an anaerobic periodontal infection, resulting in successful treatment with the antianaerobic agent metronidazole (58).

ACTINOBACILLUS ACTINOMYCETEMCOMITANS

A. actinomycetemcomitans is a small, gram-negative, microaerophilic coccobacillus that has been associated with localized juvenile periodontitis, a unique clinical entity that presents with localized bone loss around the first molars and incisor teeth of teenagers (59). What is particularly supportive of the etiological role of *A. actinomycetemcomitans* is the production of a leukotoxin that inhibits neutrophils *in vitro* (60). If the leukotoxin is produced *in vivo*, as is likely given the presence of antibodies to this toxin in the patient's serum (61), it could locally disarm the neutrophils in the pocket. The host's main protective barrier would thereby be compromised (62), allowing *A. actinomycetemcomitans* to penetrate into the connective tissue (63), causing destruction of the periodontal attachment.

Epidemiology

The precise epidemiology of periodontal disease is not known, primarily because the disease is so chronic and insidious that

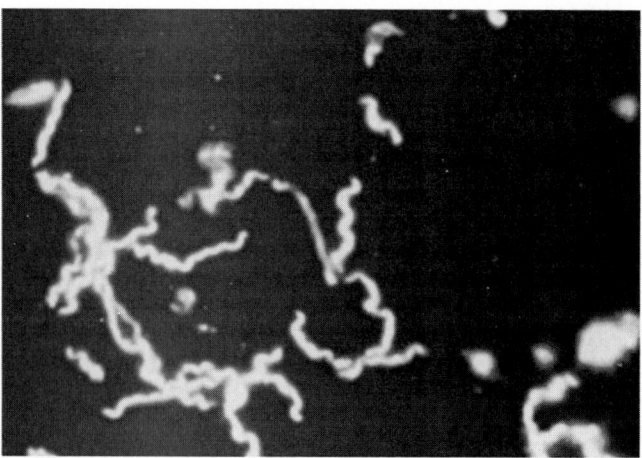

Figure 42.4. Dark-field microscopic examination of plaque showing small spirochetes.

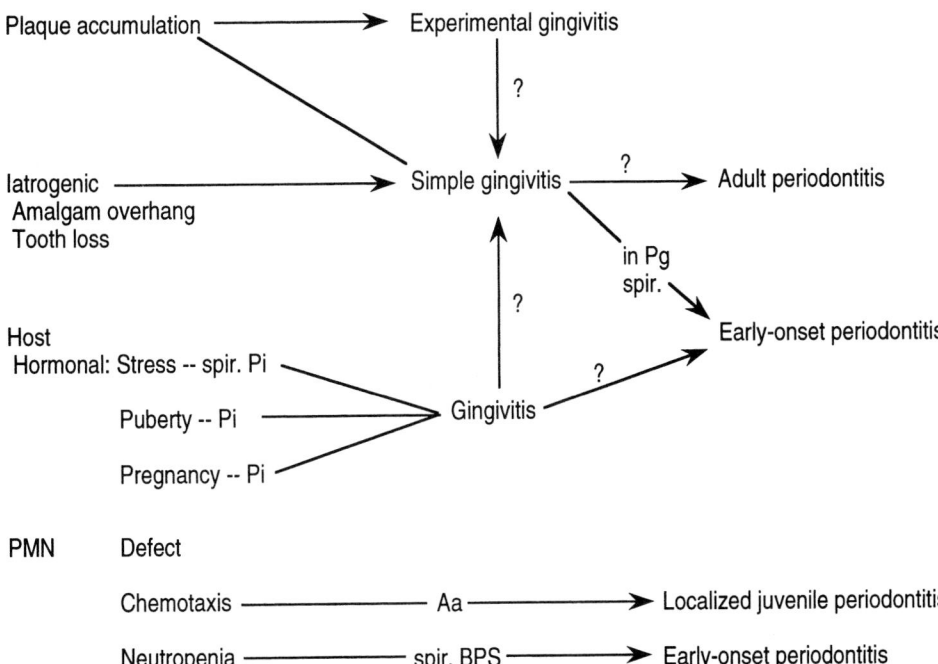

Figure 42.5. Possible sequence of events in periodontal disease. ?, Pathway not known; Bf, *Bacteroides forsythus*; spir., spirochetes; Pg, *Porphyromonas gingivalis*; Pi, *Prevotella intermedia*; Aa, *Actinobacillus actinomycetemcomitans*.

long-term studies are not practical (Fig. 42.5). The traditional view, based on cross-sectional epidemiological surveys, has been that gingivitis and periodontitis are a continuum, with periodontal attachment and bone loss occurring slowly with age. Longitudinal studies in Sri Lanka suggested that, at least in some individuals, attachment loss began in adolescence and proceeded at a rapid rate, whereas in most of the subjects, the loss of attachment occurred slowly (64). In other studies, patients with advanced periodontal disease were examined at 2-month intervals but were otherwise left untreated (65). During the monitoring period, about 5% of the sites showed attachment loss of 2 mm or more that occurred within 2 months, whereas most sites exhibited no change. This suggested that in a few sites, periodontal destruction could be acute and episodic.

Pathogenesis

The bacterial species associated with the disease (Table 42.1) are considered to be members of the normal plaque flora; thus, the mere presence of these organisms has no diagnostic implications. Each of these putative periodontal pathogens produces such a large array of biologically active molecules that it is surprising that so many teeth are retained by the host. This implies that under normal circumstances, the host's defensive barriers to bacterial invasion and inflammatory response to biologically active molecules are more than adequate to retain the teeth in the mouth. When these defenses are compromised, and especially when there are neutrophil defects, periodontal disease is severe and generalized (66). In fact, symptoms related to periodontal problems can be one of the chief complaints given by patients with cyclic neutropenia and chronic granulomatous disease. Not surprisingly, individuals with human immunodeficiency virus infection often present with aggressive forms of periodontal disease (67). However, nowhere is the relationship between neutrophils and plaque microbes better understood than in localized juvenile periodontitis.

Localized juvenile periodontitis occurs with a prevalence of about 0.1% in young subjects (68). Because the degree of bone loss around the molars and incisors occurred in the absence of gingivitis or calculus (tartar or mineralized plaque), this entity

was called periodontosis, and an unidentified host factor was believed to be involved. Subsequently, a neutrophil defect in chemotaxis was found (69) that appeared to be due to a reduced number of available binding sites for chemotactic peptides (70). This would lead *in vivo* to fewer neutrophils being recruited to the gingival and periodontal tissue in response to the chemotactic molecules produced by the plaque flora. However, this phenomenon should affect all teeth and not just the molars and incisors. Clearly, something else was needed to explain the localization to these teeth.

The missing element appears to be the involvement of *A. actinomycetemcomitans* and especially its leukotoxin. If *A. actinomycetemcomitans* overgrows in the pockets of molars and incisors, the resulting production of leukotoxin negates the protective effects of the neutrophils that eventually migrate to these sites. With time, *A. actinomycetemcomitans* invades the tissue, releasing its complement of cytotoxic factors, including the leukotoxin. The host mounts a containing response, including the production of antibodies to the leukotoxin. The amount of antibody formed to the leukotoxin is so great that it can easily be detected in the peripheral circulation (58) and most likely would be present in the gingival crevicular fluid around the teeth. If *A. actinomycetemcomitans* had not yet colonized a sulcus or overgrown in a site, this antibody could protect that site from subsequent colonization or infection. Hence, the *A. actinomycetemcomitans* infection is confined to the original sites of colonization or infection, which in most instances are the molars and incisors. Although the pathogenesis of the more typical forms of periodontal disease is not this apparent, most investigators suspect that this type of neutrophil–microbe interaction is responsible for tissue loss.

Clinical Manifestations

Periodontal disease is usually asymptomatic until the late stages, when frank periodontal abscesses cause pain and discomfort. Bleeding while brushing the teeth is the most common indicator of an underlying problem and one that usually brings an individual to the dentist. Halitosis is a less common reason for the patient's seeking treatment. Most dentists examine

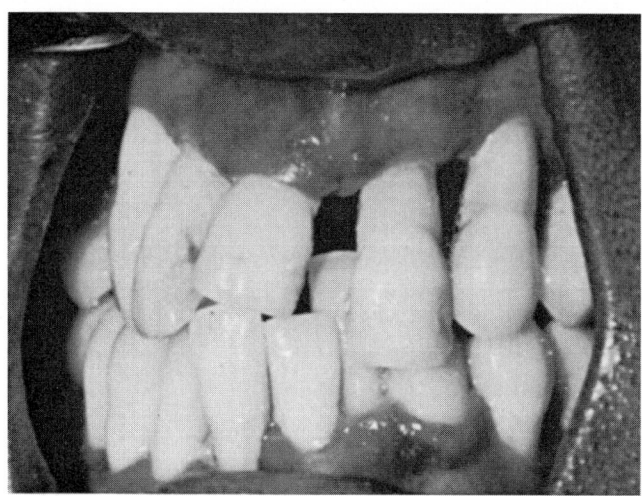

Figure 42.6. Early-onset periodontitis in a young adult. Note that teeth are separated because of bone loss.

for the degree of periodontal pocketing around the teeth and, when depths are consistently greater than 4 mm, recommend some form of mechanical débridement. Radiographs taken over time can document the amount and rate of bone loss. On some occasions, the patient seeks treatment because the teeth have shifted, with spacing being apparent between the anterior teeth (Fig. 42.6).

Diagnosis

Diagnosis is usually made by documenting the probing depths around the teeth and by the amount of bone support that has been lost. Probing depths greater than 6 mm are always indicative of disease, but whether it is an active process of attachment loss or loss that occurred years ago cannot be ascertained without some sort of longitudinal measurements or radiographs. It is in this situation that microbiologic monitors can be helpful. The simplest procedure would be to remove the subgingival plaque and examine it under the phase-contrast or dark-field microscope for the presence of motile organisms, including spirochetes (71). In healthy sites, the plaques are usually devoid of spirochetes, whereas in diseased sites, these organisms are abundant (72) (Fig. 42.4).

DNA probes to 40 distinct species have shown that only *P. gingivalis*, *B. forsythus*, and *T. denticola* are significantly elevated in diseased plaques (57). Others have shown with immunological reagents that these species are significantly associated with probing depth and bone loss (72). Because these species appear to be unique among the plaque flora in possessing the BANA enzyme (73), and because all are anaerobes, the presence of this enzyme could be used as a marker for diagnosis of an anaerobic infection. The BANA test has a diagnostic accuracy comparable to that obtained with either DNA probes or immunological reagents to *P. gingivalis*, *T. denticola*, or *B. forsythus* (74). However, because these species are members of the normal flora, the BANA test has low specificity and should not be used as a screening instrument because it often gives a positive reaction in plaque samples removed from healthy tooth sites (75).

Treatment

Treatment of periodontal disease has relied almost exclusively on mechanical débridement of the tooth surfaces. This involves labor-intensive débridement with hand instruments and, if access to these surfaces is difficult, various forms of periodontal surgery. With the evidence of bacterial specificity in periodontal disease, it is possible to conceive of a treatment protocol that would include short-term use of systemic and local antimicrobial agents. Shinn (76) reported in 1962 that metronidazole quickly improves cases of acute necrotizing ulcerative gingivitis, which eventuated in the demonstration that metronidazole is a specific inhibitor of anaerobic bacteria (77). Subsequently, metronidazole was shown to reduce the plaque levels of spirochetes and *P. intermedia* in cases of acute necrotizing ulcerative gingivitis (53). The similarity of the anaerobic flora in acute necrotizing ulcerative gingivitis to the anaerobic flora found in adult periodontitis suggested that metronidazole could be effective in the treatment of adult periodontitis.

Three double-blind studies have shown that metronidazole was effective in reducing probing depths in increasing attachment levels around the most severely involved teeth and in reducing the need for periodontal surgery and extractions (78–81). In a fourth double-blind study, if patients were treated with systemic and locally delivered antimicrobials, about 88% of the initially recommended surgical needs, including tooth extractions, could be avoided (82). There was no relapse in surgical needs for at least 5 years after the initial treatment (83). These studies indicated that most forms of periodontal disease that are diagnosed as anaerobic infections (about 90% in our experience) could be treated with short-term use of antimicrobial agents, such as metronidazole.

Treatment with metronidazole is compromised by noncompliance of patients, especially with a label attached to the bottle warning not to drink alcoholic beverages. When noncompliance is suspected, comparable results may be achieved with doxycycline, which needs to be taken only once per day. An alternative approach is to use devices that deliver the antimicrobial agent directly to the periodontal pocket. A variety of devices, including a cord that can be wrapped around the tooth (84), gels that can be placed into the pocket (85), or films that can be attached to the tooth (86), have been approved by the U.S. Food and Drug Administration.

These studies with metronidazole, doxycycline, and slow-release delivery devices suggest that in the future, periodontal disease can be controlled by the judicious usage of short-term antimicrobial therapy combined with the traditional débriding procedures. The use of the systemic antimicrobials should be based on the microbiologic diagnosis of either an anaerobic or a microaerophilic infection.

Prevention

The prevention of periodontal disease would be based on the control of gingivitis, on the assumption that most gingivitis leads to periodontitis. This is done by practicing good home oral hygiene and by the judicious use of antigingivitis agents such as chlorhexidine.

SUMMARY

Dental caries and periodontal disease are the two most common infections in humans. Although they represent a collection of infections, it is apparent that most can be treated as if they are specific *mutans streptococci* infections in the case of dental caries and as anaerobic infections in the case of adult periodontitis. This recognition provides the clinician, for the first time, with the ability to control the severity of the morbidity in patients; if patients present before morbidity occurs, the clinician may be able to keep them caries free and periodontally healthy for a lifetime. This in turn may have profound implications for the medical health of the individual, especially cardiovascular health.

REFERENCES

1. Mattila KJ, Nieminen MS, Valtonen VV, et al. Association between dental health and acute myocardial infarction. *BMJ* 1989;298:779–781.
2. Syrjänen J, Peltola J, Valtonen V, et al. Dental infections in association with cerebral infarction in young and middle-aged men. *J Intern Med* 1989;225:179–184.
3. Mattila KJ, Valtonen VV, Nieminen M, et al. Dental infection and the risk of new coronary events: prospective study of patients with documented coronary artery disease. *Clin Infect Dis* 1995;20:588–592.
4. DeStefano F, Anda RF, Kahn HS, et al. Dental disease and risk of coronary heart disease and mortality. *BMJ* 1993;306:688–691.
5. Paunio K, Impivaara O, Tiekso J, et al. Missing teeth and ischaemic heart disease in men aged 45-64 years. *Eur Heart J* 1993;14(Suppl K):54–56.
6. Beck JD, Offenbacher S, Williams R, et al. Periodontitis: a risk factor for coronary heart disease. *Ann Periodontol* 1998;3:127–141.
7. Loesche WJ. Periodontal disease: link to cardiovascular disease. *Compend Contin Educ Dent* 2000;21:463–448.
8. Offenbacher S, Jared HL, O'Reilly PG, et al. Potential pathogenic mechanisms of periodontitis associated pregnancy complications. *Ann Periodontol* 1998;3:233–250.
9. Slade GD, Offenbacher S, Beck JD, et al. Acute phase inflammatory response to periodontal disease in the US. *J Dent Res* 2000;79:49–57.
10. Corbett ME, Moore WJ. Distribution of dental caries in ancient British populations. IV. 19th century. *Caries Res* 1976;10:401–414.
11. Loesche WJ. *Dental caries: a treatable infection.* Grand Haven, MI: ADQ Publications, 1993.
12. Miller WD. *The micro-organisms of the human mouth.* Philadelphia: SS White Manufacturing, 1890.
13. Keyes PH. The infectious and transmissible nature of experimental dental caries: findings and implications. *Arch Oral Biol* 1960;1:304–320.
14. Fitzgerald RJ, Keyes PH. Demonstration of the etiologic role of streptococci in experimental caries in the hamster. *J Am Dent Assoc* 1960;61:9–19.
15. Loesche WJ. Chemotherapy of dental plaque infections. *Oral Sci Rev* 1976;9:65–107.
16. Clarke JK. On the bacterial factor in the aetiology of dental caries. *Br J Exp Pathol* 1924;5:141–146.
17. Perch B, Kjems E, Ravn T. Biochemical and serological properties of *Streptococcus mutans* from various human and animal sources. *Acta Pathol Microbiol Scand [B] Microbiol Immunol* 1974;82:357–370.
18. Coykendall AL. Proposal to elevate the subspecies of *Streptococcus mutans* to species status, based on their molecular composition. *Int J Syst Bacteriol* 1977;27:26–30.
19. Fitzgerald RJ. Dental caries research in gnotobiotic animals. *Caries Res* 1968;2:139–146.
20. Krasse B. Human streptococci and experimental caries in hamsters. *Arch Oral Biol* 1966;11:429–436.
21. Gibbons RJ, Berman KS, Knoettner P, et al. Dental caries and alveolar bone loss in gnotobiotic rats infected with capsule-forming streptococci of human origin. *Arch Oral Biol* 1966;11:549–560.
22. Donoghue HD, Newman NH. Effect of glucose and sucrose on survival in batch culture of *Streptococcus mutans* C67-25. *Infect Immun* 1976;13:16–21.
23. Stephan RM. Intra-oral hydrogen-ion concentrations associated with dental caries activity. *J Dent Res* 1944;23:257–266.
24. Harper DS, Loesche WJ. Growth and acid tolerance of human dental plaque bacteria. *Arch Oral Biol* 1984;29:843–848.
25. Hay DI, Moreno EC. Macromolecular inhibitors of calcium phosphate precipitation in human saliva: their roles in providing a protective environment for the teeth. In: Kleinberg I, Ellison SA, Mandel ID, eds. *Saliva and dental caries.* Washington, DC: Information Retrieval, 1979:45–58, Special Supplement Microbiology Abstracts.
26. Gustafsson BE, Quensel CE, Lanke LS, et al. The Vipeholm dental caries study: the effect of different levels of carbohydrate intake on caries activity in 436 individuals observed for five years. *Acta Odontol Scand* 1954;11:232–364.
27. Mandel ID, Ellison SA. Naturally occurring defense mechanisms in saliva. In: Tanzer JM, ed. *Animal models in cariology.* Washington, DC: Information Retrieval, 1981:367–379, Special Supplement Microbiology Abstracts.
28. Ripa LW. Nursing habits and dental decay in infants: "nursing bottle caries" *J Dent Child* 1978;45:274–275.
29. Berkowitz RJ, Turner J, Hughes C. Microbial characteristics of the human dental caries associated with prolonged bottle feeding. *Arch Oral Biol* 1984;29:949–951.
30. Brown LIZ, Dreizen S, Handler S. Effects of selected caries preventive regimens on microbial changes following irradiation-induced xerostomia in cancer patients. In Stiles M, Loesche WJ, O'Brien T, eds. *Proceedings of the microbial aspects of dental caries,* Vol 1. Washington, DC: Information Retrieval, 1976:275–290, Special Supplement Microbiology Abstracts.
31. Boyar RM, Bowden GH. The microflora associated with the progression of incipient carious lesions in teeth of children living in a water-fluoridated area. *Caries Res* 1985;19:298–306.
32. Miller AJ, Brunelle JA, Carlos JP. *Oral health of United States adults.* DHHS publication 87-2868. Bethesda, MD: National Institutes of Health, 1987.
33. Fox PC, van der Ven PF, Sorties BC, et al. Xerostomia: evaluation of a symptom with increasing significance. *J Am Dent Assoc* 1985;110:519–525.
34. Zickert I, Emilson CG, Krasse B. Correlation of level and duration of *Streptococcus mutans* infection with incidence of dental caries. *Infect Immun* 1983;39:982–985.
35. Loesche WJ. Role of *Streptococcus mutans* in human dental decay. *Microbiol Rev* 1986;50:353–380.
36. Krasse B. *Caries risk: a practical guide for assessment and control.* Chicago: Quintessence Publishing, 1985.
37. Gold OC, Jordan HV, van Houte J. A selective medium for *Streptococcus mutans. Arch Oral Biol* 1973;18:1356–1364.
38. Jensen B, Bratthall D. A new method for the estimation of mutans streptococci in human saliva. *J Dent Res* 1989;68:468–471.
39. Larmas M. A new dip-slide method for the counting of salivary lactobacilli. *Proc Finn Dent Soc* 1975;71:31–35.
40. Thylstrup A, Qvist V. Is health promotion the main issue of preventive dentistry? In Guggenheim B, ed. *Cariology today.* Basel: S Karger, 1984:321.
41. Berkowitz R, Jordan H, White G. The early establishment of *Streptococcus mutans* in the mouths of infants. *Arch Oral Biol* 1975;20:171–174.
42. Alaluusua S. *Streptococcus mutans* establishment and changes in salivary IgA in young children with reference to dental caries: longitudinal studies and studies on associated methods. *Proc Finn Dent Soc* 1983;79(Suppl 3):1–55.
43. Kohler B, Bratthall D. Intrafamilial levels of *Streptococcus mutans* and some aspects of the bacterial transmission. *Scand J Dent Res* 1978;86:35–42.
44. Kohler B, Bratthall D, Krasse B. Preventive measures in mothers influences the establishment of the bacterium *Streptococcus mutans* in their infants. *Arch Oral Biol* 1983;28:225–231.
45. Kohler B, Andreen I, Jonsson B. The effect of caries-preventive measures in mothers on dental caries and the oral presence of the bacteria *Streptococcus mutans* and lactobacilli in their children. *Arch Oral Biol* 1984;29:879–883.
46. Sandham HJ, Brown J, Phillips HI, et al. A preliminary report of long-term elimination of detectable mutans streptococci in man. *J Dent Res* 1988;67:9–14.
47. Douglas CW, Day JM. Cost and payment of dental services in the United States. *J Dent Educ* 1979;43:330–348.
48. Paster BJ, Boches SK, Galvin JL, et al. Bacterial diversity in subgingival plaque. *J Bacteriol* 2001;183:3770–3783.
49. Saglie R, Newman MG, Carranza FA Jr, et al. Bacterial invasion of gingiva in advanced periodontitis in humans. *J Periodontol* 1982;53:217–222.
50. Loesche WJ. The role of spirochetes in periodontal disease. *Adv Dent Res* 1988;2:275–283.
51. Shah HN, Collins DM. *Prevotella,* a new genus to include *Bacteroides melaninogenicus* and related species formerly classified in the genus *Bacteroides. Int J Syst Bacteriol* 1990;40:205–208.
52. Loesche WJ, Syed SA, Schmidt E, et al. Bacterial profiles of subgingival plaques in periodontitis. *J Periodontol* 1985;56:447–456.
53. Loesche WJ, Syed SA, Laughon B, et al. The bacteriology of acute necrotizing ulcerative gingivitis. *J Periodontol* 1982;53:223–230.
54. Tanner ACR, Listgarten MA, Ebersole JL, et al. *Bacteroides forsythus* sp. nov., a slow-growing, fusiform *Bacteroides* sp. from the human oral cavity. *J Syst Bacteriol* 1986;36:213–221.
55. Dzink JL, Socransky SS, Haffajee AD. The predominant cultivable microbiota of active and inactive lesions of destructive periodontal diseases. *J Clin Periodontol* 1988;15:316–323.
56. Loesche WJ, Lopatin DE, Giordano J, et al. Comparison of the benzoyl-DL-arginine-naphthylamide (BANA) test, DNA probes and immunological reagents for ability to detect anaerobic periodontal infections due to *Porphyromonas gingivalis, Treponema denticola,* and *Bacteroides forsythus. J Clin Microbial* 1992;30:417–433.
57. Socransky SS, Haffajee AD, Smith C, et al. Microbial complexes in subgingival plaque. *J Clin Periodontol* 1998;25:134–144.
58. Loesche WJ. The antimicrobial treatment of periodontal disease: changing the treatment paradigm. *Crit Rev Oral Biol Med* 1999;10:245–275.
59. Zambon JJ. *Actinobacillus actinomycetemcomitans* in human periodontal disease. *J Clin Periodontol* 1985;12:1–20.
60. Baehni P, Tsai CC, McArthur W, et al. Interaction of inflammatory cells and oral microorganisms. VIII. Detection of leukotoxic activity of a plaque-derived gram negative microorganism. *Infect Immun* 1979;24:233–243.
61. Tsai CC, McArthur WP, Baehni PC, et al. Serum neutralizing activity against *Actinobacillus actinomycetemcomitans* leukotoxin in juvenile periodontitis. *J Clin Periodontol* 1981;8:338–348.
62. Page RC, Schroeder HE. *Periodontitis in man and other animals: a comparative review.* Basel: S Karger, 1982.
63. Christersson LA, Albini B, Zambon J, et al. Demonstration of *Actinobacillus actinomycetemcomitans* in gingiva of localized periodontitis lesions. *J Dent Res* 1983;62:198–204.
64. Löe H, Anerud A, Boysen H, et al. Natural history of periodontal disease in man: rapid, moderate and no loss of attachment in Sri Lankan laborers 14 to 46 years of age. *J Clin Periodontol* 1986;13:431–440.
65. Goodson JM, Tanner ACR, Haffajee AD, et al. Patterns of progression and regression of advanced destructive periodontal disease. *J Clin Periodontol* 1982;9:472–481.
66. Genco RJ, Van Dyke TE, Levine MJ, et al. 1985 Kreshover lecture: molecular factors influencing neutrophil defects in periodontal disease. *J Dent Res* 1986;65:1379–1391.

67. Masouredis CM, Katz MH, Greenspan D, et al. Prevalence of HIV associated periodontitis and gingivitis in HIV infected patients attending an AIDS clinic. *J Acquir Immune Defic Syndr* 1992;5:479–483.

68. Saxen L, Murtomas H. Age-related expression of juvenile periodontitis. *J Clin Periodontol* 1985;12:21–26.

69. Van Dyke TE, Horoszewicz HU, Genco RJ. The polymorphonuclear leukocyte (PMNL) locomotor defect in juvenile periodontitis: study of random migration, chemokinesis and chemotaxis. *J Periodontol* 1982;53:682–687.

70. Van Dyke TE, Levine MJ, Tabak LA, et al. Reduced chemotaxic peptide binding in juvenile periodontitis: a method for neutrophil function. *Biochem Biophys Res Commun* 1981;100:1278–1284.

71. Keyes PH, Rams TE. A rationale for the management of periodontal diseases: rapid identification of microbial "therapeutic targets" with phase-contrast microscopy. *J Am Dent Assoc* 1983;106:803–812.

72. Grossi SG, Genco RJ, Marthei EE, et al. Assessment of risk for periodontal disease. II. Risk indicators for alveolar bone loss. *J Periodontol* 1995;66:23–29.

73. Loesche WJ, Bretz WA, Kerschensteiner D, et al. Development of a diagnostic test for anaerobic periodontal infections based on plaque hydrolysis of benzoyl-DL-arginine naphthylamide. *J Clin Microbiol* 1990;28:1551–1559.

74. Loesche WJ, Lopatin DE, Giordano J, et al. Comparison of the BANA test, DNA probes and immunological reagents for their ability to detect anaerobic periodontal infections due to *Porphyromonas gingivalis, Treponema denticola* and *Bacteroides forsythus. J Clin Microbiol* 1992;30:427–433.

75. Amalfitano J, de Fillippo AB, Bretz WA, et al. The effects of incubation length and temperature on the specificity and sensitivity of the BANA (N-benzoyl-DL-arginine-naphthylamide) test. *J Periodontol* 1993;64:848–852.

76. Shinn DLS. Metronidazole in acute ulcerative gingivitis. *Lancet* 1962;1:1191–1193.

77. Tally FP, Sutter VL, Finegold SM. Metronidazole versus anaerobes: in vitro data and initial clinical observations. *Calif Med* 1972;117:22–26.

78. Loesche WJ, Syed SA, Morrison EC, et al. Metronidazole in periodontitis. I. Clinical and bacteriological results after 15 to 30 weeks. *J Periodontol* 1984;55:325–335.

79. Joyston-Bechal S, Smales FC, Duckworth R. Effect of metronidazole on chronic periodontal disease in subjects using a topically applied chlorhexidine gel. *J Clin Periodontol* 1984;11:53–62.

80. Loesche WJ, Schmidt E, Smith BA, et al. Effect of metronidazole on periodontal treatment needs. *J Periodontol* 1991;62:247–257.

81. Loesche WJ, Giordano JR, Hujoel P, et al. Metronidazole in periodontitis. III. Reduced need for surgery. *J Clin Periodontol* 1992;19:103–112.

82. Loesche WJ, Giordano J, Soehren S, et al. The non-surgical treatment of periodontal patients. *Oral Surg Oral Med Oral Pathol* 1996;81:533–543.

83. Loesche WJ, Giordano J, Kariocoti N, et al. The non-surgical treatment of periodontal patients: results after five years. *J Am Dent Assoc* 2002;133:311–320.

84. Goodson JM, Tanner A, McArdle S, et al. Multicenter evaluation of tetracycline fiber therapy. III. Microbiological response. *J Periodontol* 1991;62:440–451.

85. Ainamo J, Lie T, Ellingsen BH, et al. Clinical response to subgingival application of a metronidazole 25% gel compared to the effect of subgingival scaling in adult periodontitis. *J Clin Periodontol* 1992;19:723–729.

86. Soskolne A, Heasman PA, Stabholz A, et al. Sustained local delivery of chlorhexidine in the treatment of periodontitis: a multi-center study. *J Periodontol* 1997;68:32–38.

CHAPTER 43
Infections of Head and Neck Spaces and Salivary Glands

Ann Sullivan Baker* and Anthony W. Chow

Deep neck infections are most often secondary to contiguous spread of local pharyngeal or dental foci. If not recognized and drained, they have the potential for life-threatening complications (1).

ANATOMY

Knowledge of the cervical compartments and interfascial spaces is essential to an understanding of the pathogenesis of infections in these spaces (Fig. 43.1).

*deceased

Cervical Fascia

The muscles, vessels, and visceral structures of the neck are enveloped in fascia; interfascial spaces are potential areas between fascial compartments. Two layers, superficial and deep, constitute the cervical fascia. The superficial fascia consists of the subcutaneous tissues of the neck, which completely enclose it and are continuous with the platysma anteriorly. The deep cervical fascia can be thought of as defining a series of cylindrical compartments that extend longitudinally from the base of the skull to the mediastinum. The superficial or investing layer of the deep cervical fascia encloses all the deeper parts of the neck. It begins at the nuchal line and extends anteriorly, dividing to enclose the trapezius, sternocleidomastoid, and strap muscles as well as the submaxillary and parotid glands. The middle or pretracheal fascia encloses the cervical viscera, including the pharynx, esophagus, larynx, trachea, and thyroid and parathyroid glands. The deep or prevertebral fascia arises from the nuchal ligament and encloses the vertebral column and muscles of the spine. It is continuous inferiorly with the posterior mediastinum. All three layers of the deep cervical fascia contribute to the carotid sheath, which forms a neurovascular compartment that encloses the carotid artery, the internal jugular vein, and the vagus nerve (Fig. 43.1B).

Fascial Spaces

Three major spaces of clinical importance lie between the planes of deep cervical fascia (2). The parapharyngeal (or lateral pharyngeal) or pharyngomaxillary space is located in the upper portion of the neck above the hyoid bone between the pretracheal fascia of the visceral compartment medially and the superficial fascia, which invests the parotid gland, internal pterygoid muscle, and mandible laterally (Fig. 43.1A). Its shape is an inverted cone, the base bounded superiorly by the skull and the apex directed inferiorly toward the hyoid bone. The carotid sheath, which runs in the posterior aspect of the parapharyngeal space, pierces the cone at its apex to enter the mediastinum.

The second space lies within the submental and submandibular triangles between the mucosa of the floor of the mouth and the superficial layer of deep fascia of these regions. This space is subdivided by the mylohyoid muscle into the submandibular space (which contains the submandibular salivary gland and lymph nodes) and the sublingual space (which contains sublingual gland, hypoglossal nerve, part of the submandibular gland, and loose connective tissue). The two divisions communicate around the mylohyoid muscle.

The third clinically important space is the retropharyngeal space, which runs longitudinally from the base of the skull to the posterior mediastinum between the prevertebral fascia posteriorly and the posterior aspect of the pretracheal fascia anteriorly (Fig. 43.1A and B). It communicates with the parapharyngeal space laterally, where it is bounded by the carotid sheaths. The retropharyngeal space is the most important communication between the neck and the chest.

Potential spaces such as the masticator, pterygopalatine, temporal, and prevertebral spaces are discussed in relation to clinical infections in those areas.

Lymph Nodes

The lymph nodes of the head and neck may be divided into 10 principal groups. Six groups (occipital, mastoid, parotid, facial, submandibular, and submental nodes) form a collar at the junction of the head and neck. Within this collar near the base of the tongue lie the sublingual and retropharyngeal nodes. The

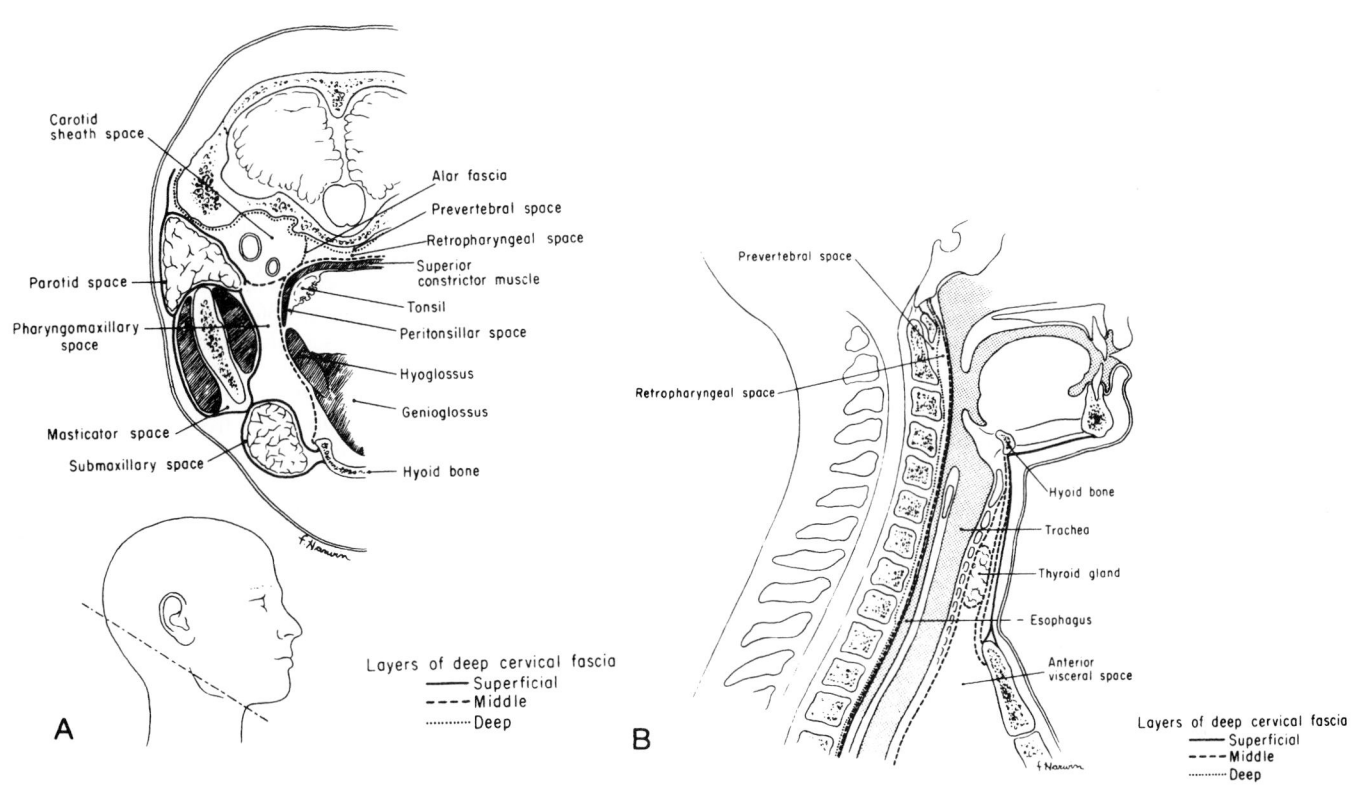

Figure 43.1. A: Oblique section through the head. **B:** Midsagittal section of the neck illustrating the anterior visceral space, retropharyngeal space, and prevertebral space. (**A** from Langenbrunner DJ, Dajani S. Pharyngomaxillary space abscess with carotid artery erosion. *Arch Otolaryngol* 1971;94:447–457, copyright 1971, American Medical Association, with permission; **B** from Levitt GW. Cervical fascia and deep neck infections. *Laryngoscope* 1970;80:409–435, with permission.)

anterior and lateral cervical nodes form a chain along the front and side of the neck, respectively. The lateral cervical chain serves as a common root for drainage. The final conduit from all lymphatics in the head and neck is the large deep chain situated along the carotid sheath. When inflamed, these nodes become adherent to the fascial sheath of the vessels, and it is understandable that the bloodstream is frequently infected by contiguous spread.

RADIOLOGICAL INVESTIGATION OF THE HEAD AND NECK

The most valuable plain radiograph for detecting soft tissue swelling in the neck is the lateral cervical view exposed for soft tissue detail. The soft tissues of the posterior wall of the hypopharynx are about 5 mm deep, less than one third the diameter of the fourth cervical vertebra (C-4). The retrolaryngeal soft tissues should be about two thirds the width of C-4, and the retrotracheal space slightly less. Dental films are indicated when a periapical abscess is suspected.

The axial imaging format of computed tomography (CT) is particularly well suited to the head and neck. CT allows the critical evaluation of soft tissues and especially bone from a single exposure. Because CT can localize a process and define its extent, particularly extension into the mediastinum or into the cranial vault, it is an invaluable tool for planning and guiding aspiration for culture or open drainage.

Magnetic resonance imaging (MRI) has assumed the premier role in the radiological evaluation of head and neck infection. MRI is more sensitive than CT and probably the bone scan in

detecting bone involvement. T2-weighted images may identify and localize areas of pus for drainage or aspiration. Gadolinium enhancement is important to define accurately the soft tissue component. Finally, MRI is useful for imaging vascular lesions, such as jugular thrombophlebitis (3,4).

MICROBIOLOGY

The bacteriology of head and neck infections reflects the normal oropharyngeal flora. The flora of the pharynx, tongue, buccal mucosa, tooth surfaces, and gingival crevices is unique. *Streptococcus pyogenes*, for example, adheres well to oral epithelial cells. *Streptococcus salivarius* and *Veillonella* species colonize the tongue and buccal mucosa; *Streptococcus mutans*, *Streptococcus mitis*, and *Actinomyces viscosus* colonize tooth surfaces (5).

The upper airway harbors large numbers of anaerobic bacteria. These bacteria have limited virulence unless they are allowed ingress to usually sterile areas (6,7). Although as many as 50 to 100 bacterial species may be present on the mucosal surface, the typical deep neck infection derived from the oral flora includes on the average only five or six bacterial types (8,9).

The major anaerobic pathogens include *Fusobacterium nucleatum*; pigmented *Prevotella* species, including *Prevotella melaninogenica* (formerly *Bacteroides melaninogenicus*), and anaerobic streptococci. Fusobacteria are considered normal flora of the oropharynx, saliva, and gingival crevice. *F. nucleatum* is an anaerobic, gram-negative, spindle-shaped bacillus with pointed ends. Anaerobic streptococci or *Peptostreptococcus* species predominate in the upper airways and account for about 13% of the bacteria in saliva (10). *Prevotella* species and anaerobic spirochetes are concentrated in the gingival crevice and become established residents after puberty. *Eikenella corrodens*, a facultative gram-negative anaerobe, is also part of the usual oral flora. A combination of aerobic streptococci and gram-negative organisms such as *Proteus* species may produce synergistic necrotizing cellulitis (11).

Actinomyces species are filamentous, branching gram-positive coccobacilli that live on dental plaque. *Actinomyces israelii* is the most common pathogen; less common are *Arachnia propionica*, *Actinomyces naeslundii*, *Actinomyces viscosus*, and *Actinomyces odontolyticus* (12,13). All of these organisms are part of the oral flora and produce similar infections. *Actinobacillus actinomycetemcomitans*, a fastidious capnophilic gram-negative coccobacillus, is commonly associated with the actinomyces (14). Other commonly associated bacteria include streptococci and many gram-negative bacilli such as *Bacteroides urealyticus*.

The bacteriological diagnosis of particular space infections may be anticipated from the microbial flora of the originating focus. Thus, most abscesses originating around the teeth harbor four or five organisms, mainly oral anaerobes, whereas infections arising from the pharynx contain oral anaerobes and *S. pyogenes* (15).

CLINICAL MANIFESTATIONS

Symptoms

In general, patients with peritonsillar, parotid, parapharyngeal, and submandibular abscesses complain of sore throat or pain and trismus. Trismus, the inability to open the jaw, indicates pressure or infection of the muscles of mastication (the masseter and the pterygoids) or involvement of the motor branch of the trigeminal nerve.

Dysphagia and odynophagia are secondary to inflammation around the cricoarytenoid joints. Dysphonia and hoarseness are late findings in neck infections and may indicate involvement of the tenth cranial nerve; unilateral tongue paresis indicates involvement of the twelfth cranial nerve. Stridor and dyspnea may be manifestations of local pressure or spread of infection to the mediastinum.

Physical Findings

In patients with peritonsillar, parotid, parapharyngeal, or submandibular abscess, findings include swelling of the face and neck, erythema, and purulent oral discharge. There may be pooling of saliva in the mouth and asymmetry of the oropharynx. Lymphadenopathy is usually present. Because of the dense superficial layer of the deep cervical fascia and its musculofascial planes, a fluctuant mass is not readily appreciated in deep neck infections. The characteristic signs of deep pus are pitting or a doughy feeling on firm deep palpation.

DEEP FASCIAL SPACE INFECTIONS

Peritonsillar Abscess (Quinsy)

A peritonsillar abscess is the most common deep infection of the head and neck. It is principally a disease of adolescents and adults; cases in children younger than 12 years of age are rare (16). The abscess is thought to occur as a complication of bacterial tonsillitis when infection breaks through the tonsillar capsule into the potential space between the tonsil and the superior constrictor muscle. Passy (17) has questioned abscess formation of the Weber salivary glands in the supratonsillar fossa as the cause. Peritonsillar abscess may occasionally occur in the setting of infectious mononucleosis (18,19).

Most peritonsillar abscesses are polymicrobial infections. Jousimies-Somer and colleagues (19) aspirated pus samples from 124 patients, which included 143 aerobes and 407 anaerobes. Aerobes were isolated from 86% of patients alone in 20 cases and together with anaerobes in 87 cases. *S. pyogenes* was most prominent (45%), followed by *Streptococcus milleri* (27%), *Haemophilus influenzae* (11%), and viridans streptococci (11%). Anaerobes were isolated from 82% of the samples and were the sole finding in 15 abscesses. *Fusobacterium necrophorum* and *P. melaninogenica* were both isolated from 38% of patients, *Prevotella intermedia* from 32%, *Peptostreptococcus micros* from 27%, *F. nucleatum* from 26%, and *A. odontolyticus* from 23%. Recurrences were more common with *F. necrophorum*.

The classic clinical presentation of peritonsillar abscess is gradually increasing pharyngeal discomfort and ipsilateral otalgia followed by trismus and dysarthria. Dysphagia is less common but is often accompanied by drooling (20). Edema and pain produce characteristic muffled or "hot potato in the mouth" speech. The patient is usually in a mildly toxic condition; a temperature above 39°C suggests bacteremia or extension of the abscess into the parapharyngeal space.

Physical examination reveals a tender, exudative peritonsillar mass with edema of the soft palate and uvula. Displacement of the soft palate medially and of the uvula to the opposite side differentiates peritonsillar abscess from other pharyngeal abscesses. Sloughing in the crypts of the tonsil or large necrotic ulcers of the tonsil may occasionally occur. Ipsilateral tender anterior cervical adenopathy is usually present.

Treatment with needle aspiration, combined with administration of parenteral antibiotics, is the simplest, most cost-effective therapy for peritonsillar abscess (21). Intravenous antibiotic therapy (penicillin, 1 to 2 million units every 4 hours, plus metronidazole, 500 mg every 6 hours; or clindamycin, 600 mg every 8 hours) should be followed by a total of 10 to 14 days of oral therapy (penicillin plus metronidazole; or clindamycin) (22). Interval tonsillectomy is indicated only when there is a history of recurrent tonsillitis or of peritonsillar abscess (20).

Complications result from extension beyond the peritonsillar space. As soon as the infection penetrates the muscle bed of the tonsillar fossa, it becomes a parapharyngeal space infection (see later). A peritonsillar abscess frequently spreads by this route. Necrotizing fasciitis has been described as a rare but lethal complication of peritonsillar abscess (23).

Submandibular Space Infections

LUDWIG'S ANGINA

The process first described in 1836 by Frederick Wilhelm von Ludwig (24) is a rapidly spreading phlegmon or cellulitis—not an abscess—involving the floor of the mouth and the loose areolar tissue above the mylohyoid diaphragm. The disease usually occurs in patients between the ages of 20 and 50 years who have abscessed teeth or pyorrhea (25), but pediatric cases have been reported (26). Apical infection from incisors, canines, and third molars perforates this sublingual space above the mylohyoid muscle. Inflammation from the tongue and the floor of the mouth, lingual tonsillitis, and local tonsillectomy are other, less likely causes.

Ludwig's angina begins as a localized cellulitis of the loose areolar tissue of the floor of the mouth. The patient may complain of a foul taste in the mouth, crepitus in the temporomandibular joint, or unilateral pharyngitis. A history of recent tooth extraction should be sought. Later, necrosis and pus formation accompany local lymphadenitis. A fulminating swelling develops, with pouting of the tissue over the edges of the lower teeth. At this time, manifestations of sepsis are evident. With the full-blown syndrome, the patient is in acute distress. Edema and induration elevate the floor of the mouth, thrusting the tongue upward and backward toward the palate (Fig. 43.2A). There is trismus as well as brawny induration of the submandibular area. Pain, redness, heat, and swelling—the classic picture of a phlegmon—are followed by dysphagia, dyspnea, and spiking fevers. The infection may break through the deep cervical fascia to produce a cellulitis that extends from the clavicle up over the face.

Oral bacteria, in particular streptococci and anaerobic organisms, are the predominant bacterial pathogens in Ludwig's angina. The peripheral white cell count is usually elevated, with a predominance of polymorphonuclear leukocytes. CT often illustrates increased soft tissue swelling or, rarely, an accumulation of pus in the sublingual-submandibular area (Fig. 43.2B). Pan-radiographic views of the teeth and jaws should be obtained to look for an apical abscess.

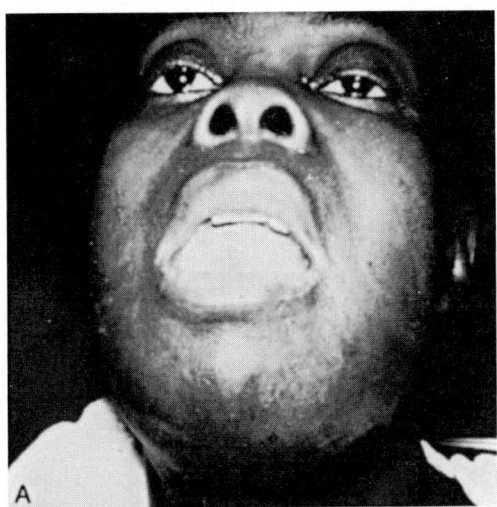

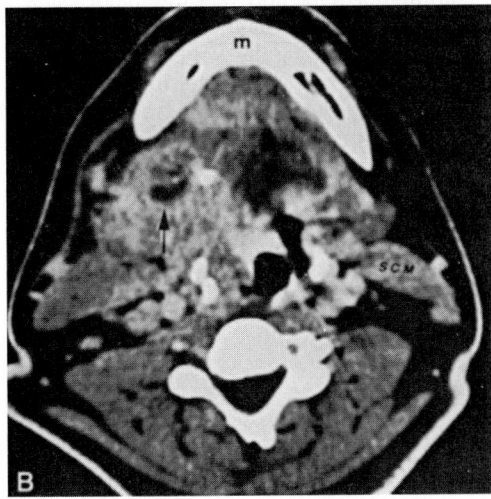

Figure 43.2. A: Patient with Ludwig's angina revealing massive sublingual swelling with upward protrusion of the tongue and bilateral neck swelling. **B:** Axial computed tomography view of patient with Ludwig's angina revealing lucent zone (*arrow*) in submandibular space posterior to mylohyoid muscle. m, Mandible; SCM, sternocleidomastoid muscle. (**A, B** courtesy of Dr. A. Weber, Massachusetts Eye and Ear Infirmary, Boston, MA.)

Treatment is aimed first at securing the airway and then at controlling the infection (27,28). Equipment for emergency endotracheal intubation or tracheostomy should be available at the bedside. Penicillin G and metronidazole, clindamycin, or ampicillin-sulbactam should be administered intravenously. If sepsis and respiratory compromise are both present, endotracheal intubation or tracheostomy should be performed, followed by surgical decompression. If sepsis is not present, a more conservative approach may be used (27,25).

Complications of Ludwig's angina include spread of infection into the parapharyngeal and retropharyngeal spaces and on into the superior mediastinum. In addition, submucosal swelling in the floor of the mouth has the added danger of producing asphyxiation.

SUBMANDIBULAR AND SUBMENTAL ABSCESSES

A submandibular abscess can develop after suppuration of the submandibular lymph nodes, an infection of the submandibular salivary gland, or apical infections of second and third molar teeth below the mylohyoid muscle. The fluctuant quality is more apt to be appreciated here than in other deep neck infections because there is no overlying musculature and the fascia is not so dense. Submental abscesses usually result from spread of an apical abscess of the lower incisors through the thin buccolabial areolar plate and below the mylohyoid muscle. Suppuration of a submental lymph node may be another source of infection. There may be moderate elevation of the floor of the mouth, but the exuberant swelling of the soft tissues of the mouth, as seen in Ludwig's angina, is lacking. Abscesses in submandibular or submental spaces are treated by incision and drainage.

Masticator Space Infections

The masticator space lies between the subperiosteal region of the mandible and the fascial sling containing the masseter and pterygoid muscles. Infection of this space usually follows extraction of a lower second or an impacted third molar tooth or curettage of an infected dental socket. Patients present with pain and fever of acute onset. There is broad induration over the angle and ramus of the mandible. The swelling often extends down the neck and occasionally across the midline. Marked trismus develops because of the muscles involved. There is pharyngeal swelling over the medial aspect of the involved mandible. The tonsils are pushed toward the midline, but the lateral pharyngeal wall posterior to the tonsil is not swollen (in contrast to parapharyngeal space infections).

Radiography of the involved mandible and teeth is helpful to reveal a hidden initiating focus. Treatment is the same as for other submandibular space infections.

Pterygopalatine, Infratemporal, and Temporal Fossa Infections

The pterygopalatine fossa is behind the maxillary antrum and below the orbital apex. It contains three important structures: the maxillary nerve and branches, the sphenopalatine ganglion, and the internal maxillary artery and branches. The abducens nerve, the inferior branch of the oculomotor nerve, and the maxillary nerves are in close relationship here and are often involved together in infection of the maxillary and sphenoid sinuses.

Infections of the pterygopalatine fossa and adjacent spaces usually follow extraction of a maxillary molar tooth or result from introduction of infection during local anesthesia of the superior alveolar nerve. A fulminating cellulitis develops,

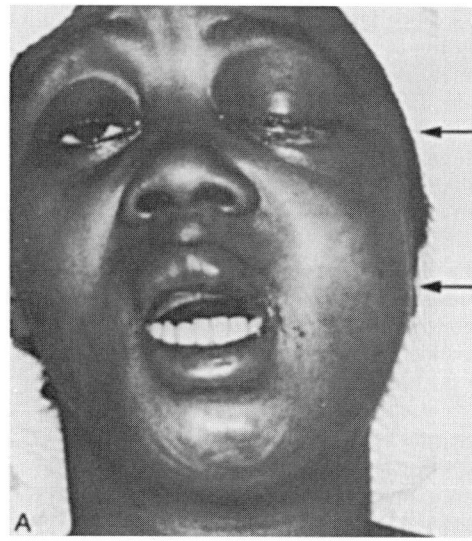

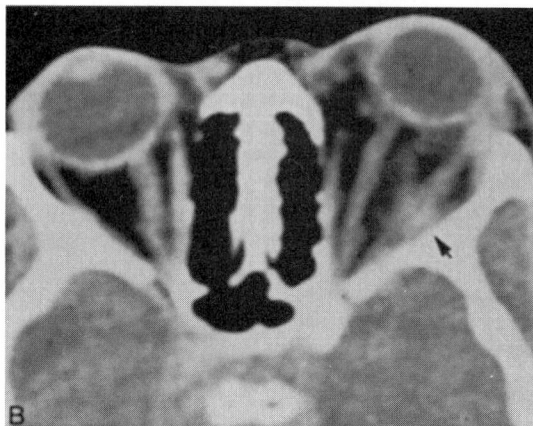

Figure 43.3. A: Pterygopalatine space and temporal space infection with an orbital abscess in a patient with an upper molar tooth abscess. **B:** Extension of pterygopalatine space infection into the left orbit; soft tissue mass is evident (*arrow*). (**A, B** courtesy of Dr. A. Weber, Massachusetts Eye and Ear Infirmary, Boston, MA.)

progressively involving the upper molar gingiva and the pterygopalatine, infratemporal, and temporal fossae; abscess formation in these spaces ensues.

On clinical presentation, there is painful swelling of the maxillary gingival tissues that spreads in a few days to involve the cheek (Fig. 43.3). Unchecked, the cellulitis progresses to involve the entire side of the head, including the nose, ear, and upper part of the neck. Proptosis of the globe may result from extension of infection into the orbit through the inferior orbital fissure. Vision may be threatened by the development of optic neuritis. If osteomyelitis of the maxilla is present, the maxillary sinus may become secondarily infected. CT or MRI of the pterygopalatine fossa and the orbit is crucial in the evaluation and localization of the cellulitis or abscess. If diagnostic evaluation reveals a mass, surgical drainage of both the pterygopalatine abscess and any orbital abscess should be initiated immediately. Intravenous penicillin remains the antibiotic of choice for treating deep oropharyngeal infections of odontogenic origin. Metronidazole (500 mg every 6 hours) is added or intravenous clindamycin (600 mg every 8 hours) or ampicillin-sulbactam is substituted in place of penicillin to cover mixed anaerobic infections, β-lactamase–producing anaerobes such as *Prevotella* species, gram-negative organisms, and *H. influenzae*.

Parapharyngeal Abscess

Parapharyngeal abscess most often arises as a complication of a peritonsillar abscess, but infections of the parotid gland, dental roots, and petrous pyramid or infections secondary to dental or pharyngeal surgery may extend into the parapharyngeal space. A cause is not always apparent, however, despite a detailed evaluation (29). Before the advent of antimicrobial chemotherapy, 50% of neck infections occurred in the parapharyngeal space; the most frequent cause was infection from the tonsils and pharynx (adenoids) (30). Antibiotic therapy has reduced the frequency dramatically such that parapharyngeal abscesses are currently a relatively rare cause of deep neck infections in both adults and children (31).

The triad of (a) tonsillar prolapse with swelling of the lateral pharyngeal wall, (b) trismus, and (c) parotid swelling indicates an abscess in the parapharyngeal space (Fig. 43.4). The first clinical symptoms and signs are fever and painful swallowing. If the abscess is located in the anterior muscle compartment of the parapharyngeal space, inflammation of the internal pterygoid muscles results in trismus. Dyspnea is a consequence of invasion of the pretracheal fascia; otalgia and odynophagia may also be present. Inflammation of the lymph nodes under the sternocleidomastoid muscle produces torticollis toward the side opposite the abscess. Continued signs of sepsis after drainage of the peritonsillar space usually indicate concomitant undrained parapharyngeal space infection.

An abscess localized to the posterior neurovascular compartment of the parapharyngeal space is manifested by sepsis and cranial nerve involvement (e.g., Horner's syndrome, hoarseness, unilateral tongue paresis) but with minimal trismus. The posterior tonsillar pillar is displaced. Swelling and displacement of the parotid gland usually occur with infection in either the anterior or posterior parapharyngeal space. Upper airway bleeding, secondary to erosion of the great vessels, is a late finding in untreated cases.

The site and extent of infection are best evaluated by CT or MRI; external drainage is mandatory for frank abscess. Internal drainage is contraindicated owing to the proximity of the great vessels.

Infection of the carotid sheath is a frequent complication of parapharyngeal abscess. Erosion of the internal carotid artery can cause fatal hemorrhage and was the major cause of death from infection of this space in the preantibiotic era. Thrombophlebitis of the internal jugular vein with intracranial extension is another vascular complication. Intracranial involvement may also occur by superior extension of the abscess to the base of the skull. Inferior extension to the piriform sinus may result in upper airway obstruction. Mediastinitis may occur by extension from the retropharyngeal space or carotid sheath.

Retropharyngeal Abscess

An acute retropharyngeal abscess may involve the space between the pharyngeal wall and the visceral fascia, the space between the visceral and alar fasciae, or the space between the alar and prevertebral fasciae (the danger space) (Fig. 43.1A and B). A retropharyngeal space infection often results from lymphatic spread of infection in the pharynx or sinuses to the retropharyngeal lymph nodes. The lymph nodes usually suppurate, which leads to abscess development. Retropharyngeal infections are most common in children because the lymph nodes atrophy by age 3 or 4 years (32). In children or adults, infections in this space may be secondary to accidental perforation of the pharynx or esophagus, for example, by a lollipop stick or other foreign body, by endoscopic trauma, or by surgery (33). Alternatively,

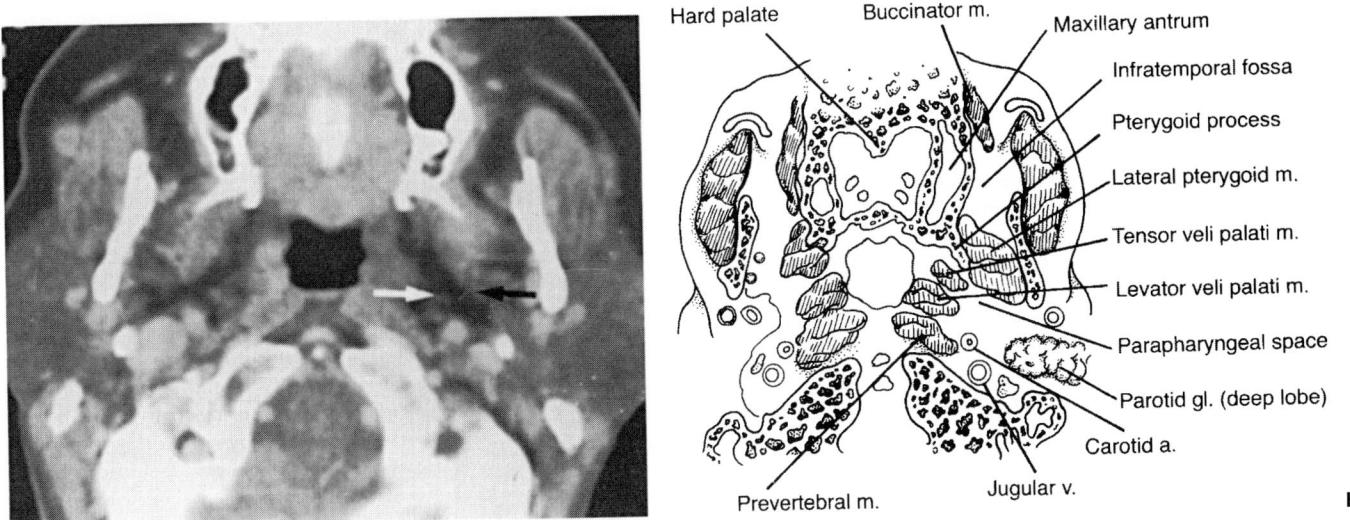

Figure 43.4. Parapharyngeal space. **A:** Computed tomography view (*arrows*). **B:** Anatomy.

a retropharyngeal abscess may extend from cervical vertebral osteomyelitis (34,35). Infections of the retropharyngeal space are usually polymicrobial, with anaerobes, streptococci, and staphylococci predominating (36).

The classic presentation of retropharyngeal abscess is chills and fever after pharyngitis, but no antecedent illness is identified in many patients (32). Adults may complain of dysphagia, neck pain, dyspnea, and regurgitation. In the child, the onset may be insidious, manifested primarily by irritability and refusal to eat. On physical examination, the neck may be rigidly hyperextended with local tenderness. As swelling increases, a muffled voice (dysphonia) and drooling are followed by tachypnea and stridor. The oropharynx should be examined carefully by indirect (mirror) hypopharyngeal inspection and gentle digital palpation. Bulging of the posterior pharyngeal wall may be noted, usually to one side of the midline. Cervical lymphadenopathy is usually present.

Differential diagnosis of retropharyngeal abscess includes cervical osteomyelitis, Pott's disease, meningitis, and calcific tendinitis of the long muscle of the neck (33). A lateral radiograph is the most important diagnostic procedure in the initial evaluation of a patient with suspected retropharyngeal abscess (Fig. 43.5). The neck should be fully extended during deep inspiration while the film is taken. The radiograph should be evaluated for increased thickness of the prevertebral soft tissues, air or air-fluid levels in the soft tissues, and the presence of foreign bodies. A chest radiograph should be obtained to identify mediastinal extension.

Treatment consists of expeditious drainage of the abscess and intravenous high-dose penicillin (2 to 4 million units every

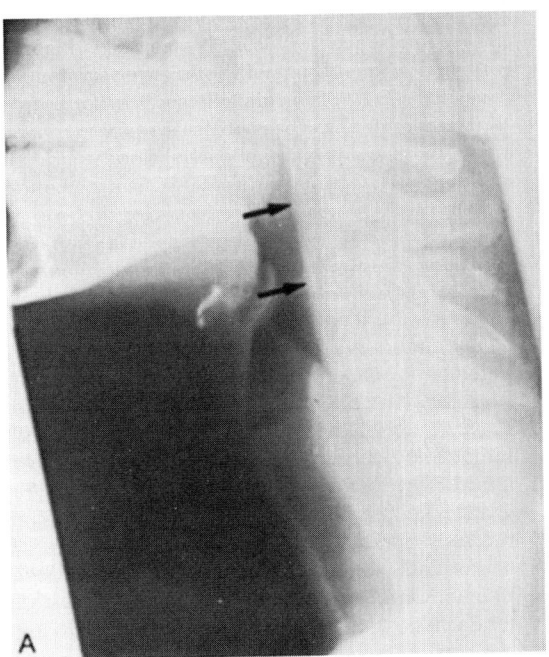
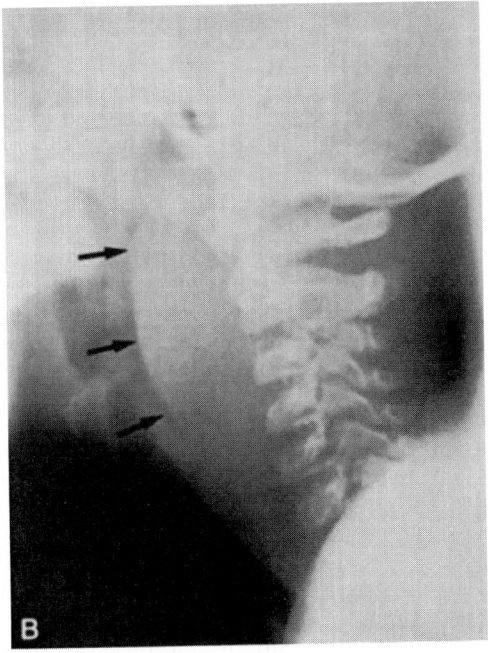

Figure 43.5. Retropharyngeal space. **A:** Normal lateral cervical view. **B:** Expansion of prevertebral soft tissues by retropharyngeal abscess. (**A, B** courtesy of Dr. A. Weber, Massachusetts Eye and Ear Infirmary, Boston, MA.)

4 hours) and metronidazole (500 mg every 6 hours) or ampicillin-sulbactam (2 g intravenously every 4 hours) for a minimum of 5 days. Antibiotics should be adjusted as culture data become available, and oral therapy is continued to complete at least a 14-day course.

Untreated retropharyngeal abscess may rupture spontaneously into the pharynx. Aspiration of the purulent drainage can lead to pneumonia and empyema. An abscess in the danger space between the alar and prevertebral fasciae may drain by gravity into the posterior mediastinum, resulting in mediastinitis that may include empyema (37). In the past, 70% of cases of mediastinitis were the result of infection spread in this manner. With the introduction of antibiotics, mediastinal extension has become uncommon, and most cases of mediastinitis result from esophageal perforation (38). Extension of infection into the mediastinum is characterized by chest pain, dyspnea, persistent fever, and radiographic evidence of a widened mediastinum. In children, stridor is suggestive of airway compromise from physical obstruction and is evidence of later-stage disease.

Hemorrhage in the setting of retropharyngeal infection suggests involvement of the major vessels in the neck (39). Another important vascular complication is phlebitis or thrombosis of the internal jugular vein (Lemierre's syndrome), which should be suspected when retropharyngeal abscess is associated with a septic clinical course (40) (see the next section).

VASCULAR COMPLICATIONS OF DEEP NECK INFECTIONS

Carotid Sheath Infections

The carotid sheath abuts all three layers of deep cervical fascia. Infection may therefore arise by spread from the parapharyngeal space, Ludwig's angina, or suppuration of deep cervical nodes (39). There are no characteristic symptoms or signs of carotid sheath infections. In some patients, there is diffuse swelling along the sternocleidomastoid muscle with marked tenderness and torticollis to the opposite side. Erosion of the carotid artery may be heralded by minor episodes of oral bleeding. Ligation of the carotid artery may be necessary in cases of major hemorrhage, but the mortality rate remains high, and the risk for stroke is significant (1,41).

Septic Jugular Thrombophlebitis (Postanginal Sepsis or Lamierre's Syndrome)

Postanginal sepsis was first described by Long (42) in 1912 and Mosher (43) in 1920. Also known as *Lemierre's syndrome*, the condition refers to septic thrombophlebitis of the internal jugular vein after an oropharyngeal infection and is complicated by spread to the parapharyngeal space (44). Symptoms of jugular vein thrombosis include pain in the neck made worse by turning the head away from the involved side. This motion causes the sternocleidomastoid muscle to compress the inflamed mass. Dysphagia and dysphonia may also occur. On examination, the tonsil is displaced medially. Vocal cord paralysis on the same side occurs together with edema of the lateral pharyngeal wall. Chills and sweats may indicate bloodstream infection. Septic emboli from the jugular venous system travel to the lung, followed by blood-borne dissemination of infection to other organs (45). Diagnosis and treatment of postanginal sepsis may be delayed because of the lack of an obvious source for the infection. In the absence of a demonstrable cause for sepsis, careful efforts should be made to elicit a history of pharyngitis. Contrast-enhanced CT may show the normal carotid artery and an enlarged jugu-

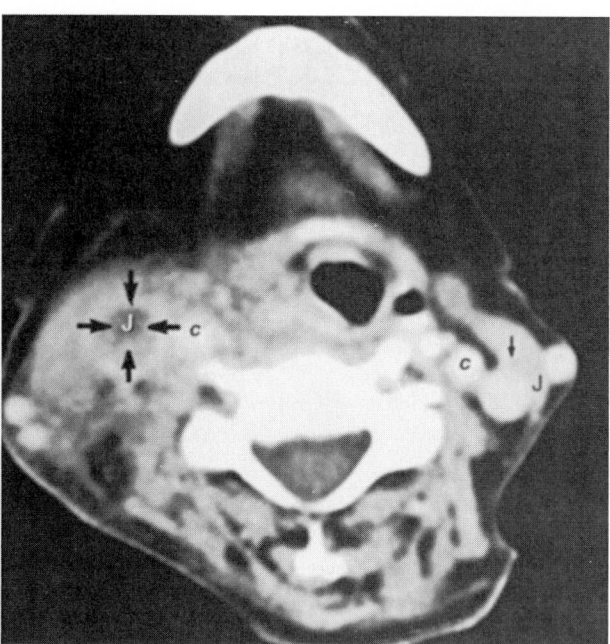

Figure 43.6. Jugular venous thrombosis. **A:** Contrast-enhanced axial computed tomography scan at C-3 shows the normal left carotid (*c*) and jugular (*J*) vessels (*arrow*). **B:** The right common carotid is normal, but the jugular vein is enlarged with a dense or enhancing wall (*arrows*) that surrounds the more lucent intraluminal clot. (Courtesy of Dr. A. Weber, Massachusetts Eye and Ear Infirmary, Boston, MA.)

lar venous wall surrounding a more lucent intraluminal clot (Fig. 43.6). Thrombosis of the jugular vein can also be demonstrated by magnetic resonance angiography.

The organisms most frequently involved in postanginal sepsis are anaerobic streptococci and *Bacteroides* (now including *Prevotella*) species and *Fusobacterium* species (40). Less common are α-hemolytic and group A β-hemolytic streptococci, the pneumococci, *Staphylococcus aureus*, and *E. corrodens*. Treatment usually consists of external drainage of the lateral pharyngeal space.

INFECTIONS OF THE SALIVARY GLANDS

Suppurative Parotitis

Acute bacterial parotitis typically occurs in an elderly, dehydrated, intubated, or postoperative inpatient, although this condition is also commonly seen in outpatients (46,47). Other predisposing factors include recent intensive teeth cleaning, use of anticholinergic drugs, and salivary calculi with obstruction. Salivary stasis permits retrograde seeding of the duct of Stensen with virulent oral flora (47). Raad and colleagues (48) found *S. aureus* to be the most common pathogen, followed by viridans streptococci, with only one gram-negative isolate in their study. However, acute parotitis resulting from anaerobes, enteric gram-negative bacilli, *Pseudomonas aeruginosa*, and *E. corrodens* has been documented (46,49).

Patients present with complaints of pain, swelling, and dysphagia. On examination, tense swelling over the parotid area, tenderness, and pain on opening the mouth are seen. A fluctuant quality is generally not appreciated because of the dense parotid fascia that overlies the gland. Purulent material may be expressed from the orifice of the Stensen duct and should be examined by Gram stain and culture. Treatment includes hydration and intravenous antibiotics directed against staphylococci and mouth flora, with coverage adjusted in response to culture results.

Viral Parotitis

In the prevaccine era, mumps virus was the most common cause of viral parotitis. Other viruses that are associated with parotitis include coxsackievirus, influenza virus, parainfluenza virus types 1 and 3, lymphocytic choriomeningitis virus, and cytomegalovirus (5,50). Parotitis is associated with human immunodeficiency virus (HIV) infection, both in children and in seropositive, asymptomatic adults (51). Patients with viral parotitis present with tender swelling of the parotid glands bilaterally along with fever, headache, and myalgias. Swelling is occasionally unilateral. The extreme parotid tenderness and systemic toxic effects of suppurative infection are absent in viral parotitis. For infections not related to HIV, symptoms usually resolve within 5 to 10 days, and treatment—hydration and relief of pain and fever—is directed at the symptoms. Specific therapy for HIV-related infections is dictated by the diagnosis.

Chronic Parotitis

Recurrent or persistent swellings of the parotid gland, which may or may not be painful, are loosely grouped as chronic parotitis. Whereas noninfectious entities such as Sjögren's syndrome, sarcoidosis, and even hyperuricemia should be considered, obstruction and abnormal duct architecture can lead to recurrent infections (52,53). Chronic pyogenic infections have bacteriologic diagnoses similar to those of acute infections; Iko (54) found *S. aureus*, viridans streptococci, *Streptococcus pneumoniae*, and *Klebsiella* species to be the most common etiologic agents in a group of patients with chronic pyogenic parotitis. *Mycobacterium tuberculosis*, *A. actinomycetemcomitans*, and actinomycosis can also cause chronic parotid swelling that can be confused with a parotid tumor (52,55,56). HIV infection has also been associated with chronic parotid swelling. The evaluation of chronic parotitis should include a search for parotid stones, ductal strictures, or other predisposing factors. Antimicrobials should be directed at the causative organism. Subtotal or total parotidectomy has been advocated for intractable recurrent infections (57).

REFERENCES

1. Chow AW. Life-threatening infections of the head, neck, and upper respiratory tract. In: Hall JB, Schmidt GA, Wood LDH, eds. *Principles of critical care*. New York: McGraw-Hill, 1998:887–902.
2. Grodinsky M. Ludwig's angina, retropharyngeal abscess, and other deep abscesses of the head and neck. *JAMA* 1940;114:18.
3. Latchaw RE, Hirsch WL Jr, Yock DH Jr. Imaging of intracranial infection. *Neurosurg Clin North Am* 1992;3:303–322.
4. Medlock MD, Olivero WC, Hanigan WC, et al. Children with cerebral venous thrombosis diagnosed with magnetic resonance imaging and magnetic resonance angiography. *Neurosurgery* 1992;31:870–876.
5. Chow AW. Infections of the oral cavity, neck and head. In: Mandell GL, Bennett JE, Dolin R, eds. *Principles and practice of infectious diseases*. New York: Churchill Livingstone, 2000:689–702.
6. Brook I. Aerobic and anaerobic bacteriology of intracranial abscesses. *Pediatr Neurol* 1992;8:210–214.
7. Sutter VL. Anaerobes as normal oral flora. *Rev Infect Dis* 1984;6:S62–S66.
8. Tanner A, Stillman N. Oral and dental infections with anaerobic bacteria: clinical features, predominant pathogens, and treatment. *Clin Infect Dis* 1993;16(Suppl 4):S304.
9. Chow AW, Roser SM, Brady FA. Orofacial odontogenic infections. *Ann Intern Med* 1978;88:392–402.
10. Roscoe DL, Chow AW. Normal flora and mucosal immunity of the head and neck. *Infect Dis Clin North Am* 1988;2:1–19.
11. Fliss DM, Tovi F, Zirkin HJ. Necrotizing soft-tissue infections of dental origin. *J Oral Maxillofac Surg* 1990;48:1104–1108.
12. Newman MG. Anaerobic oral and dental infection. *Rev Infect Dis* 1983.
13. Nithyanandam S, D'Souza O, Rao SS, et al. Rhinoorbitocerebral actinomycosis. *Ophthal Plast Reconstr Surg* 2001;17:134–136.
14. Slots J, Reynolds HS, Genco RJ. *Actinobacillus actinomycetemcomitans* in human periodontal disease: a cross-sectional microbiological investigation. *Infect Immun* 1980;29:1013–1020.
15. Matto J, Asikainen S, Vaisanen ML, et al. Role of *Porphyromonas gingivalis*, *Prevotella intermedia*, and *Prevotella nigrescens* in extraoral and some odontogenic infections. *Clin Infect Dis* 1997;25(Suppl 2):S194–S198.
16. Baker AS, Montgomery WW. Oropharyngeal space infections. *Curr Clin Topic Infect Dis* 1987;8:227–265.
17. Passy V. Pathogenesis of peritonsillar abscess. *Laryngoscope* 1994;104:185.
18. Portman M, Ingall D, Westenfelder G, et al. Peritonsillar abscess complicating infectious mononucleosis. *J Pediatr* 1984;104:742.
19. Jousimies-Somer H, Savolainen S, Ylikoski J. Bacteriologic findings in peritonsillar abscess. *Clin Infect Dis* 1993;16(Suppl 4):S292.
20. Schraff S, McGinn JD, Derkay CS. Peritonsillar abscess in children: a 10-year review of diagnosis and management. *Int J Pediatr Otorhinolaryngol* 2001;57:213–218.
21. Herzon FS, Nicklaus P. Pediatric peritonsillar abscess: management guidelines. *Curr Probl Pediatr* 1996;26:270–278.
22. Savolainen S, Jousimies-Somer H, Makitie AA, et al. Peritonsillar abscess: clinical and microbiologic aspects and treatment regimens. *Arch Otolaryngol Head Neck Surg* 1993;119:521.
23. Hadfield PJ, Motamed M, Glover GW. Synergistic necrotizing cellulitis resulting from peri-tonsillar abscess. *J Laryngol Otol* 1996;110:887–890.
24. von Ludwig FW. Eine neure Art von Halsentzuendung. *Med Correspond Blatt Wurtemberg Arztl Ver* 1836;6:1836.
25. Bramwell KJ, Davis DP. Ludwig's angina. *J Emerg Med* 1998;16:481.
26. Britt JC, Josephson GD, Gross CW. Ludwig's angina in the pediatric population: report of a case and review of the literature. *Int J Pediatr Otorhinolaryngol* 2000;52:79–87.
27. Barakate MS, Jensen MJ, Hemli JM, et al. Ludwig's angina: report of a case and review of management issues. *Ann Otol Rhinol Laryngol* 2001;110:453–456.
28. Busch RF. Ludwig angina: early aggressive therapy. *Arch Otolaryngol Head Neck Surg* 1999;125:1283–1284.
29. Har-El G, Aroesty JH, Shaha A, et al. Changing trends in deep neck abscess: a retrospective study of 110 patients. *Oral Surg Oral Med Oral Pathol* 1994;77:446–450.
30. Beck AL. Deep neck infections. *Ann Otol Rhinol Laryngol* 1947;56:439.
31. Sethi DS, Stanley RE. Parapharyngeal abscesses. *J Laryngol Otol* 1991;105:1025–1030.
32. Sakaguchi M, Sato S, Ishiyama T et al. Characterization and management of deep neck infections. *Int J Oral Maxillofac Surg* 1997;26:131–134.
33. Haug RH, Picard U, Indresano AT. Diagnosis and treatment of the retropharyngeal abscess in adults. *Br J Oral Max Surg* 1990;28:34–38.
34. Jang YJ, Rhee CK. Retropharyngeal abscess associated with vertebral osteomyelitis and spinal epidural abscess. *Otolaryngol Head Neck Surg* 1998;119: 705–708.
35. Faidas A, Ferguson JV, Nelson JE et al. Cervical vertebral osteomyelitis presenting as retropharyngeal abscess. *Clin Infect Dis* 1994;18:992.
36. Brook I. Microbiology of retropharynbgeal abscess in children. *Am J Dis Child* 1987;141:202.
37. Takao M, Ido M, Hamaguchi K, et al. Descending necrotizing mediastinitis secondary to retropharyngeal abscess. *Eur Respir J* 1994;7:1716.
38. Brook I, Frazier EH. Microbiology of mediastinitis. *Arch Intern Med* 1996; 156:333–336.
39. Alexander DW, Leonard JR, Trail ML. Vascular complications of deep neck abscesses. *Laryngoscope* 1968;78:361.
40. Sinave CP, Hardy GJ, Fardy PW. The Lemierre syndrome: suppurative thrombophlebitis of the internal jugular vein secondary to oropharyngeal infection. *Medicine (Baltimore)* 1989;68:85–94.
41. Kono T, Kohno A, Kuwashima S, et al. CT findings of descending necrotising mediastinitis via the carotid space ("Lincoln highway"). *Pediatr Radiol* 2001;31:84–86.
42. Long JW. Excision of internal jugular vein for streptococci: thrombosis of vein and cavernous sinus causing paralysis of orbital muscles. *Surg Gynecol Obstet* 1912;14:86.
43. Mosher HP. Deep cervical abscess and thrombosis of the internal jugular vein. *Laryngoscope* 1920;30:365.
44. Singhal A, Kerstein MD. Lemierre's syndrome. *South Med J* 2001;94:886–887.
45. Gowan RT, Mehran RJ, Cardinal P, et al. Thoracic complications of Lemierre syndrome. *Can Respir J* 2000;7:481–485.
46. Brook I. The swollen neck: cervical lymphadenitis, parotitis, thyroiditis and infected cysts. *Infect Dis Clin North Am* 1988;2:221–236.
47. Cohen MA, Docktor JW. Acute suppurative parotitis with spread to the deep neck spaces. *Am J Emerg Med* 1999;17:46–49.
48. Raad II, Sabbagh MF, Caranasos GJ. Acute bacterial sialadenitis: a study of 29 cases and review. *Rev Infect Dis* 1990;12:591.
49. Sherman JA. Pseudomonas parotid abscess. *J Oral Maxillofac Surg* 2001;59:833–835.
50. McQuone SJ. Acute viral and bacterial infections of the salivary glands. *Otolaryngol Clin North Am* 1999;32:793–811.
51. Colebunders R, Francis H, Mann JM, et al. Parotid swelling during human immunodeficiency virus infection. *Arch Otolaryngol Head Neck Surg* 1988;114: 330.

52. Williams HK, Connor R, Edmondson H. Chronic sclerosing sialadenitis of the submandibular and parotid glands: a report of a case and review of the literature. *Oral Surg Oral Med Oral Pathol Oral Radiol Endod* 2000;89:720–723.
53. Eilon A, Deutsch E, Zelig S. Hyperuricemia: a possible etiologic factor in chronic recurrent parotitis. *Laryngoscope* 1982;92:1181.
54. Iko BO. Computed tomography and sialography of chronic pyogenic parotitis. *Br J Radiol* 1984;57:1083.
55. O'Connell JE, George MK, Speculand B, et al. Mycobacterial infection of the parotid gland: an unusual cause of parotid swelling. *J Laryngol Otol* 1993;107:561.
56. Patel PK, Seitchik MW. *Actinobacillus actinomycetemcomitans*: a new cause for granuloma of the parotid gland and buccal space. *Plast Reconstr Surg* 1986;77:476.
57. Arriaga MA, Myers EN. The surgical management of chronic parotitis. *Laryngoscope* 1990;100:1270.

CHAPTER 44
Infections of the Sinuses and Parameningeal Structures

Anthony W. Chow

SINUS INFECTIONS

Sinusitis, an inflammation of the mucosal lining of the paranasal sinuses, is one of the most common complaints resulting in physician visits in the United States. It was the fifth leading indication for antibiotic prescriptions among office-based physicians (1), and total direct costs for treatment sinusitis approached $5.8 billion in 1996 (2). Yet, many symptoms suggestive of sinus infection are nonspecific, and it is often difficult to differentiate between bacterial sinusitis and viral upper respiratory infections, with the potential for misuse of antibiotics, contributing to widespread drug resistance and increasing health care costs. On the other hand, both acute and chronic sinusitis can lead to life-threatening complications, such as parameningeal and intracranial infections. A clear understanding of the anatomy, pathophysiology, predisposing conditions, clinical manifestations, and microbial etiology is essential for cost-effective diagnosis and treatment of this common condition.

Anatomical Considerations and Pathophysiology

The paranasal sinuses (maxillary, ethmoid, frontal, and sphenoid) are air-filled cavities lined by pseudostratified, ciliated columnar epithelium. They are interconnected through small tubular openings, the sinus ostia, which drain into various regions of the nasal cavity (Fig. 44.1). The frontal, anterior ethmoid, and maxillary sinuses open into the middle meatus; the posterior ethmoid and sphenoid sinuses open into the superior meatus. The osteomeatal complex, an area between the middle and inferior turbinates representing the confluence of the drainage areas from the paranasal sinuses, is a particularly important anatomical site because of the potential for mucosal thickening and retention of secretions, leading to infection even without mechanical obstruction of the ostia (3).

The maxillary sinuses are the most frequently infected, either alone or in combination with the ethmoid or frontal sinuses. The ostium of the maxillary sinus lies at an obtuse angle toward the roof (Fig. 44.1); thus, the maxillary sinus does not empty well in the erect posture but rather drains best when the patient is lying on the side opposite the affected sinus. The floor of the maxillary sinus directly adjoins the maxillary bone in which reside the apices of the first, second, and third molar teeth; hence, extraction or root infection of these teeth is a frequent cause of maxillary sinusitis. Furthermore, because the superior alveolar nerves (branches of the maxillary nerve) supply both the molar teeth and the mucous membranes of the sinus, maxillary sinusitis may frequently present as a toothache. Extension of infection from the maxillary sinus into the adjacent structures may result in osteomyelitis of the facial bones, including prolapse of the orbital antral wall with retroorbital cellulitis, proptosis, and ophthalmoplegia. Direct intracranial extension from the maxillary sinus is rare, except in rhinocerebral mucormycosis and other invasive fungal sinusitides.

The frontal sinus is not a frequent site of infection but may be a focus for spread of infection to the orbit or the central nervous system. The frontal sinus is supplied by the supraorbital branch of the ophthalmic division of the trigeminal nerve. Thus, headache is a prominent symptom of frontal sinusitis. Owing to the rich vascular supply in this area, infection may readily extend intracranially by the diploic veins to result in epidural or subdural empyema, brain abscess, meningitis, or cavernous sinus thrombosis (Fig. 44.2). Frontal sinusitis may also result in thrombosis of the superior sagittal sinus, which arises in the roof of the frontal air sinuses. Extension of infection into bone can lead to "Pott's puffy tumor," whereas orbital extension may lead to periorbital cellulitis.

The ethmoid sinus is composed of multiple air cells, which are separated by thin bony partitions, and each air cell drains by an independent ostium. The ethmoid sinuses are separated from the orbit by a paper-thin orbital plate. Perforation of the plate allows direct spread of infection into the retroorbital space. Ethmoid sinusitis can also spread to the superior sagittal vein, or the cavernous venous sinus (Fig. 44.2).

The sphenoid sinus also drains through an opening at an obtuse angle anteriorly (Fig. 44.2). Thus, this sinus empties only when the head is bent forward and does not drain well in the erect posture. The sphenoid sinus occupies the body of the sphenoid bone in proximity to the pituitary gland above; the optic nerve and optic chiasma in front; and the internal carotids, the cavernous sinuses, and the temporal lobes of the brain on each side (Fig. 44.2). Thus, sphenoid sinusitis can spread locally to cause cavernous sinus thrombosis, meningitis, temporal lobe abscess, and orbital fissure syndromes. The superior orbital fissure syndrome, characterized by orbital pain, exophthalmos, and ophthalmoplegia, is due to involvement of the abducens, oculomotor, and trochlear nerves and the ophthalmic division of the trigeminal nerve as they pass through the orbital fissure. Isolated acute sphenoid sinusitis is rare; however, chronic granulomatous infections of the sphenoid sinus, such as tuberculosis, can cause local destruction of the pituitary gland and lead to panhypopituitarism.

The paranasal sinuses are generally considered to be sterile, although transient colonization may occur (4). Because the upper respiratory tract, the oral cavity, and certain parts of the eyes and ears are closely related anatomically and are normally heavily populated by a resident flora, microbial access to the paranasal sinuses is easily attained (Fig. 44.3). Transient colonization would also seem to be supported by the observation that both acute and chronic sinusitis are caused by organisms that normally populate the upper airway (5,6).

A patent osteomeatal complex and normal mucociliary function are the key factors in maintaining aeration and mucosal defenses of the paranasal sinuses. The ciliated epithelium of the sinuses is contiguous with the nasal cavity and is covered with a fine layer of mucus. The cilia beat toward the ostia, propelling sinus contents toward this opening and clearing the sinus. The presence of secretory immunoglobulin A (s-IgA), lysozyme, and

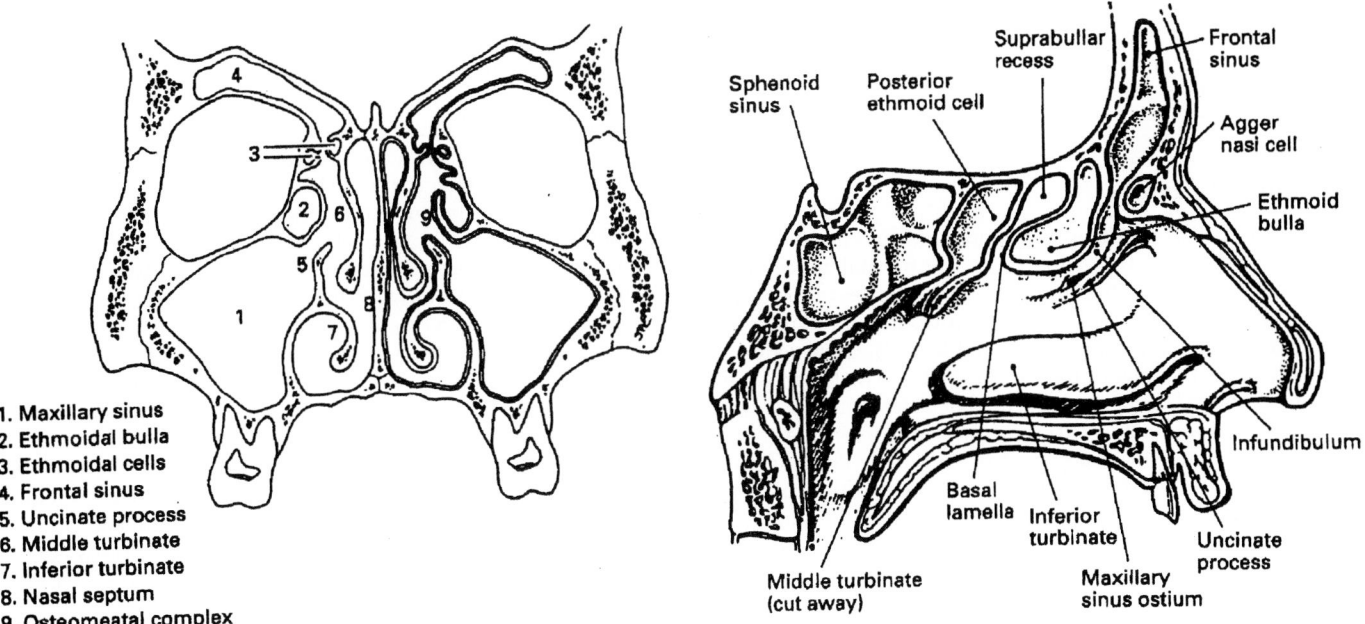

1. Maxillary sinus
2. Ethmoidal bulla
3. Ethmoidal cells
4. Frontal sinus
5. Uncinate process
6. Middle turbinate
7. Inferior turbinate
8. Nasal septum
9. Osteomeatal complex

A

B

Figure 44.1. Anatomic relationships of the paranasal sinuses. **A:** Coronal view. **B:** Sagittal view. The frontal, anterior ethmoidal, and maxillary sinuses drain into the middle meatus; the posterior ethmoidal and sphenoidal sinuses open into the superior meatus. Note that the ostium of the maxillary sinus drains at an obtuse angle toward the roof. The floor of the maxillary sinus is close to the superior alveolar ridge. (From Noye KA, Brodovsky D, Coyle S, et al. Classification, diagnosis and treatment of sinusitis: evidence-based clinical practice guidelines. *Can J Infect Dis* 1998;9(Suppl B):3B–24B, with permission.)

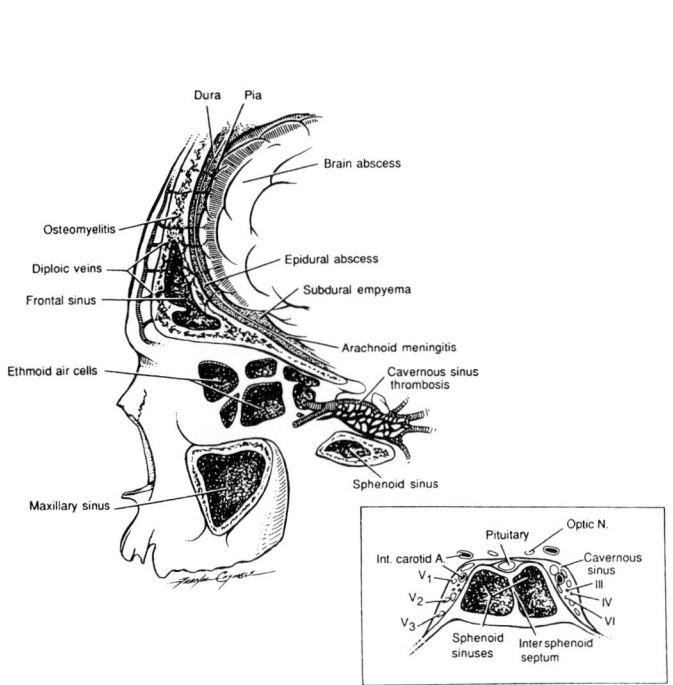

Figure 44.2. Intracranial complications of sinusitis. The sagittal section shows the major routes for intracranial extension of infection either directly or by the vascular supply. Note the proximity of the diploic veins to the frontal sinus and of the cavernous sinuses to the sphenoidal sinus. The coronal section demonstrates the structures adjoining the sphenoidal sinus.

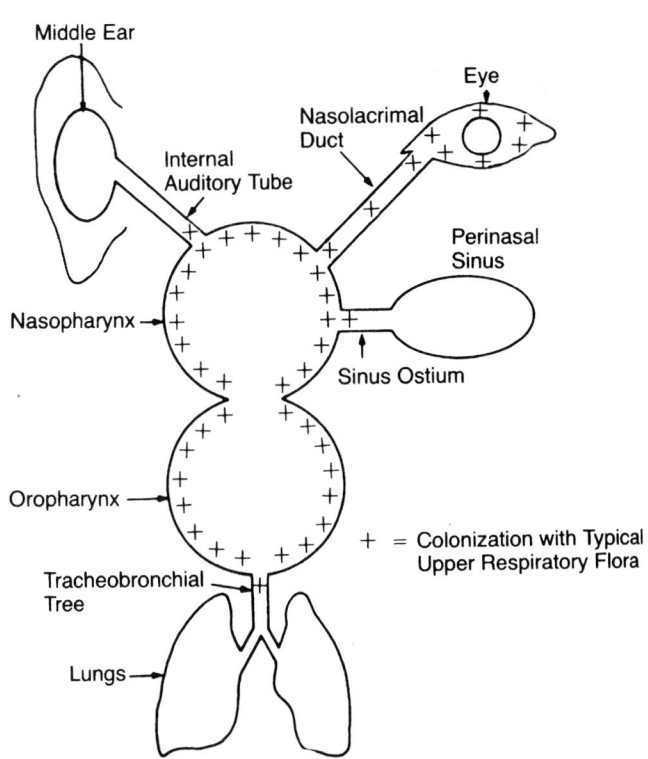

Figure 44.3. Diagrammatic illustration of the anatomic relationship of head and neck structures and distribution of the indigenous flora. (From Todd JK. Bacteriology and clinical relevance of nasopharyngeal and oropharyngeal cultures. *Pediatr Infect Dis* 1984;3:159–163, with permission.)

lactoferrin in normal sinus secretions serve as additional barriers to infection (7). Even if microorganisms have adhered to and penetrated the epithelium, continuous shedding of the epithelial cells serves to deter microbial invasion and contributes to mucosal self-cleaning.

Predisposing Factors

The conditions that predispose to sinus infection are those that affect the patency of the sinus ostia, the normal mucociliary function of the sinus epithelium, immune defenses of the upper airways, or events that facilitate direct introduction of microorganisms into the paranasal sinuses (Table 44.1). Obstruction or reduction in the patency of the ostia appears to be the most important predisposing factor for acute bacterial sinusitis. This is supported by evidence in experimental sinusitis in the rabbit, in which inoculation of a sinus cavity with a virulent microorganism in the absence of obstruction is insufficient to produce sinusitis (8). Gas exchange and oxygen content of the sinus cavity are dependent on the patency and size of the ostium (9). With obstruction of the ostia, ventilation and drainage are impaired, the oxygen tension falls, and there is a concomitant rise in carbon dioxide tension. Growth of anaerobic and facultative bacteria is favored under these conditions, and polymorphonuclear and phagocytic cell function is impaired. The retained secretions provide an ideal environment for microbial replication. Furthermore, various proinflammatory cytokines, especially IL-1, IL-6, and IL-8, are elevated within the sinus mucosa during acute sinusitis (10). These proinflammatory cytokines, as well as other proteolytic products released by granulocytes, lead to mucosal destruction and further disrupt the normal epithelial barrier.

The most common precipitating cause of acute bacterial sinusitis is a viral upper respiratory infection, the common cold (11). Adults develop two to three colds per year, and children have six to eight episodes per year—up to 2% of these cases become complicated by acute bacterial infection of the sinuses (5). Allergic rhinitis has also been considered an important predisposing factor to sinusitis, particularly chronic sinusitis both

in children (12) and adults (13). It has also been suggested that the abnormal production of proinflammatory cytokines among patients with allergic rhinitis may lead to a self-perpetuating inflammatory response that can cause symptoms indistinguishable from infectious sinusitis (7). Similarly, an association between asthma and sinusitis has long been appreciated, but a causal relationship has not been found (14).

Mild and selective immune deficiencies have been frequently demonstrated in children and adults with recurrent or persistent symptoms of sinus disease (15). In one study, 52% of more than 500 patients from four different centers had selective immunoglobulin deficiencies (IgG2 and IgG4 subclass, or IgA) or poor responsiveness to some polysaccharide antigens (16).

Certain activities or events may repeatedly traumatize the nasal mucosa and facilitate microbial invasion of the paranasal sinuses. These include head trauma, swimming and diving, cocaine sniffing, and nasotracheal or nasopharyngeal intubation. Transnasal intubation is an important cause of nosocomial sinusitis (17). Dental extraction and periapical infections of the maxillary molar teeth are particularly important causes of maxillary sinusitis. Odontogenic sources may account for 5% to 10% of acute maxillary sinusitis and more than 40% of chronic maxillary sinusitis (5,18).

Chronic or recurrent sinusitis is an important source of morbidity in patients with cystic fibrosis (19) and among human immunodeficiency virus (HIV)-infected patients (20).

Clinical Manifestations

Because sinusitis is often preceded by rhinitis, and because abnormalities of the nose and the sinus cavity are demonstrated simultaneously by computed tomography (CT) during the common cold (21), it has been proposed that "rhinosinusitis" may be a more appropriate term for this condition (22). The clinical manifestations of rhinosinusitis vary greatly, depending on the duration of infection (acute, subacute, chronic, or recurrent) and age of the patient (i.e., child or adult) (23).

- *Acute sinusitis* has a sudden onset, and symptoms last for up to 4 weeks with complete resolution of infection.
- *Subacute sinusitis* persists beyond 4 weeks and up to 12 weeks.
- *Chronic sinusitis* lasts longer than 12 weeks, during which there may be episodes of acute exacerbations.
- *Recurrent sinusitis* involves four or more episodes within a 1-year period, each lasting at least 7 days.

ACUTE SINUSITIS

Symptoms of acute sinusitis are often difficult to distinguish from those of the common cold or allergic (vasomotor) rhinitis. The two hallmarks, which suggest bacterial infection rather than viral or allergic rhinosinusitis, are the persistence (i.e., more than 10 days) and severity of respiratory symptoms. There is often a "double sickening" or biphasic illness in which symptoms suggestive of a common cold begin to improve, but the congestion and discomfort returns several days later. In children, the most common manifestations are cough (80%), nasal discharge (76%), and fever (63%) (24). Parents of preschoolers often report malodorous breath. Headache, facial pain, and swelling are rare. In adults, purulent postnasal discharge and facial pain over the affected sinus that worsens with movement or percussion are the cardinal symptoms (5). Fever occurs in less than 50% of cases. The combination of certain clinical findings, particularly history of maxillary toothache, colored nasal discharge, poor response to decongestants, and physical signs of purulent nasal secretions and abnormal transillumination, greatly enhance the diagnostic probability of acute sinusitis (25). Hyposmia, jaw pain with

---

TABLE 44.1.   Factors that Predispose to Sinusitis

Impaired mucociliary function
  Viral upper respiratory tract infection
  Allergic rhinitis
  Cold or dry air
  Chemicals, drugs (rhinitis medicamentosa)
  Human immunodeficiency virus infection
  Cystic fibrosis
  Ciliary dysmotility syndrome
Obstruction of sinus ostia
  Viral upper respiratory tract infection
  Allergic rhinitis
  Anatomic abnormalities (e.g., nasal polyps, deviated nasal septum, choanal atresia, foreign body, tumors)
Immune defects
  Immunoglobulin A deficiency
  Immunoglobulin G subclass deficiency (IgG2, IgG3 or IgG4)
  Acquired immunodeficiency syndrome
  Wegener's granulomatosis
  Diabetes mellitus
Increased risk for microbial invasion of the sinuses
  Odontogenic infections
  Nasotracheal or nasogastric intubation
  Head trauma
  Swimming or diving
  Cocaine sniffing

mastication, nasal congestion, and a history of recent upper respiratory tract infection are other manifestations. Pain on percussion of all the molar teeth of the upper jaw is characteristic of maxillary sinusitis, whereas more localized tooth tenderness points to an odontogenic source of infection.

In ethmoid sinusitis, edema of the eyelids and excessive tearing may be a prominent feature. Retroorbital pain and proptosis indicate extension of infection into the orbit. Anterior rhinoscopy may reveal hyperemic and edematous nasal turbinates, often with purulent discharge from the middle meatus, where the orifices of the maxillary, frontal, and anterior ethmoid sinuses enter the intranasal cavity. Severe intractable headache is dominant in sphenoid sinusitis and can mimic ophthalmic migraine or trigeminal neuralgia. Neurological deficit with hypoesthesia or hyperesthesia of the ophthalmic or maxillary dermatomes of the trigeminal nerve may be detected in one third of the patients (26). A depression of the mental status accompanied by clinical signs of meningeal irritation, ptosis, chemosis, proptosis, and paralysis of the third, fourth, and sixth cranial nerves suggests that the infection has extended to the cavernous sinus.

In patients with nosocomial sinusitis secondary to prolonged nasotracheal intubation, the clinical features may be relatively silent apart from unexplained fever. The presence of purulent rhinorrhea or a middle-ear effusion, as determined by pneumatic otoscopy, may be the only physical finding. A high index of suspicion and appropriate diagnostic procedures are required for early recognition of this entity (17). Immunocompromised patients with acquired immunodeficiency syndrome (AIDS) or malignancy are particularly susceptible to infection involving multiple sinuses that responds incompletely to antibiotic therapy, often resulting in chronic or recurrent sinusitis (27).

SUBACUTE AND CHRONIC SINUSITIS

Symptoms associated with subacute or chronic sinusitis are usually less intense but more protracted than are those of acute sinusitis. Fever is uncommon. Fatigue, general malaise, and an ill-defined feeling of unwellness and irritability can be more prominent than local symptoms of nasal congestion, facial pain, or postnasal drip. Chronic sinusitis may mimic asthma, allergic rhinitis, or chronic bronchitis. Physical findings may be subtle. Results of anterior rhinoscopy and mirror examination may be normal, although often there is evidence of posterior nasal discharge. Melen and colleagues (28) observed that 40% of 198 patients with chronic maxillary sinusitis had a dental cause. Marginal periodontitis and periapical granuloma together accounted for 83% of their cases of chronic odontogenic sinusitis. Nasal polyps were found in 16% of all patients with chronic maxillary sinusitis.

Diagnostic Approaches

HISTORY AND PHYSICAL EXAMINATION

In the primary care setting, diagnosis of acute sinusitis is primarily based on the history and physical examination. The goal is to detect clinical findings that may predict the presence of acute bacterial sinusitis without actually performing a sinus puncture. The nostrils may be examined using a short, wide speculum mounted on a handheld otoscope. Purulent secretion from the middle meatus has a high sensitivity (72%), but its specificity is only moderate (52%) (25). A topical vasoconstrictive spray may be needed to shrink the nasal mucosa to inspect this area. Direct inspection of the posterior pharynx or use of a pharyngeal mirror may also reveal purulent secretions. Fiberoptic rhinopharyngoscopy is performed in offices by otolaryngologists, allergists and many primary care physicians in cases of chronic or recurrent sinusitis. This technique permits a detailed examination of the nasopharynx, including the middle meatus and the sphenoethmoid recess into which the sinuses drain. It is particularly useful for identifying anatomical variations, polyps, and other abnormalities that may predispose to recurrent sinusitis.

Facial tenderness is best assessed by applying digital pressure over the maxillary and frontal sinuses and any areas of facial edema or erythema. Areas to be palpated should include (a) maxillary floor—palpated from the palate; (b) anterior maxillary wall—palpated from the cheeks; (c) lateral ethmoid wall—palpated from the medial canthus; (d) frontal floor—palpated from the roof of the orbit; and (e) anterior frontal wall—palpated from the supraorbital skull. Percussion of the maxillary teeth with a tongue depressor may reveal tenderness associated with a dental infection. This finding has a high specificity for acute maxillary sinusitis (93%), but its sensitivity is low (18%) (25).

Transillumination can be used to assess retained fluid in the sinuses. Transillumination should be performed in a completely darkened room. The finding of complete opacity is highly indicative of infection. Conversely, normal light transmission indicates that no infection is present. The finding of reduced or "dull" transmission is less helpful because only one fourth of such patients have bacterial infection as determined by sinus puncture (5). Transillumination is less useful for chronic sinusitis because of persistent mucosal abnormalities. Transillumination is also less informative in children younger than 6 years of age (24).

The utility of various clinical findings in diagnosing acute sinusitis has been prospectively evaluated using either four-view radiographs or CT as the gold standard (25,29). Five clinical findings, including four symptoms (maxillary toothache, history of colored nasal discharge, poor response to decongestants, double sickening [biphasic illness]) and two signs (purulent nasal secretion, abnormal transillumination) were identified by logistic regression analysis to be independent predictors of sinusitis. The presence of four or more of these signs and symptoms markedly increases the likelihood of acute sinusitis (likelihood ratio, 6.4). Conversely, when fewer than two of the above signs and symptoms are present, acute sinusitis can be ruled out. The diagnosis of sinusitis is less clear if only two or three signs and symptoms are present and other diagnostic procedures such as imaging studies may be helpful.

IMAGING STUDIES

In the primary care setting, imaging studies are not cost-effective and should not be used routinely in the initial assessment of patients with suspected sinusitis (30). However, when clinical findings are unclear or empirical therapy fails, imaging studies such as CT, sinus radiographs, ultrasonography, or magnetic resonance imaging (MRI) may be helpful (Fig. 44.4).

Computed Tomography

A coronal CT is the most cost-efficient study for the diagnosis of acute sinusitis compared with standard sinus radiographs and other imaging methods (31). Compared with plain radiographs, CT provides greater definition of the sinus cavity and its contents and offers better visualization of the ethmoid and sphenoid sinuses. CT is able to clarify anatomical variations that may play a role in recurrent or chronic sinusitis and is invaluable for assessing complications involving the orbit and intracranial spaces. CT also provides more accuracy than four-view sinus radiographs for demonstrating and localizing disease before endoscopic sinus surgery. However, although CT is very sensitive for detecting sinus abnormalities, it lacks specificity for bacterial infection because abnormalities of the sinus cavity can be demonstrated in more than 80% of patients with the common cold (21). Although the specificity of CT for bacterial infection

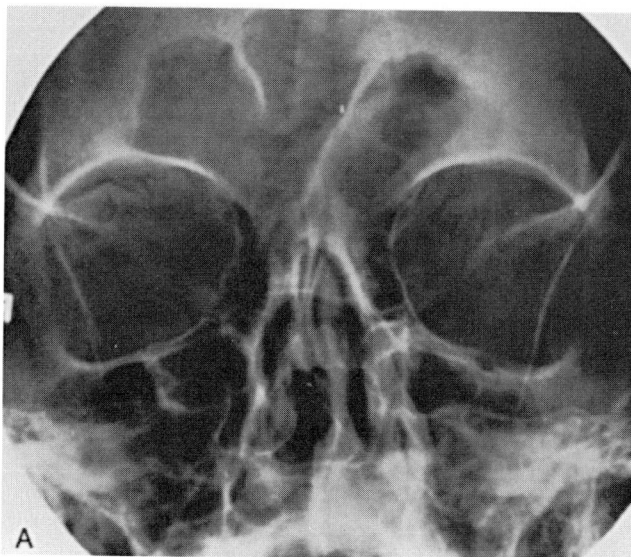
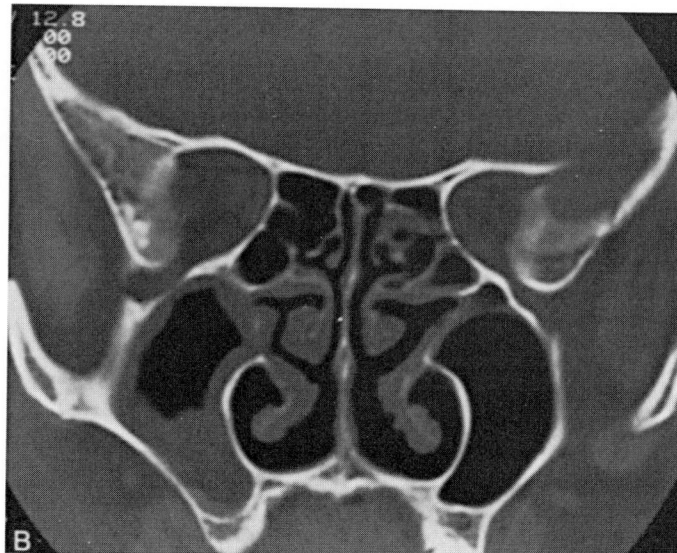

Figure 44.4. Imaging studies of sinusitis. **A:** Caldwell view of the frontal and ethmoidal sinuses. Note partial opacification of both frontal sinuses with mucosal thickening in the left frontal sinus and associated sclerosis in the left frontal bone. **B:** Coronal computed tomography view of the ethmoidal and maxillary sinuses. Note mucosal thickening in the right maxillary sinus. (**A, B** courtesy of Dr. W. D. Robertson.)

can be improved by the finding of a classic air-fluid level, its sensitivity is low (38%) when compared with positive aspirate-cultures (5). Thus, CT findings should not be interpreted in the absence of additional clinical information.

Sinus Radiography

Sinus radiographs are now largely superceded by CT for evaluating the sinonasal cavity. Sinus radiography may be indicated in elderly patients or young children who cannot tolerate a coronal CT examination. A single Waters' view should suffice rather than the standard four-view series: occipitomental (Waters') view to visualize the maxillary and frontal sinuses, occipitofrontal (Caldwell's) view to visualize the frontal and ethmoid sinuses, lateral view to evaluate the sphenoid sinuses, and submentovertex or oblique (Rhese's) view to evaluate the ethmoid and sphenoid sinuses. Radiographic changes in acute sinusitis may include a thickened (more than 6 mm) sinus mucosal membrane, an air-fluid level, or complete opacification of the involved sinuses. The presence of such findings is predictive for bacterial infection in 75% of cases as determined by sinus puncture, although its sensitivity is low (60%) (5). Plain radiographs of the sinuses can assist in excluding sinus disease when the clinical manifestations are unclear (a normal radiograph correlates with a negative aspirate in 80% of cases) (5). Radiographic examination is less useful in chronic sinusitis because of persistent abnormalities and in infants before the age of 1 year because of redundant sinus mucosa and asymmetry of facial bone or sinus development. An orthopantomogram is indicated if an odontogenic infection is suspected.

Ultrasonography

Ultrasonography can demonstrate the presence of retained fluid or thickened mucosa in the sinus, but the accuracy of this technique is highly operator dependent, and false-positive examinations are common (32). Despite a sensitivity of about 70%, its specificity for detecting sinusitis is low (11). Furthermore, young children present technical and diagnostic difficulties. Thus, the routine use of ultrasonography is not recommended except for individuals in whom radiography is not feasible, or to follow the response to therapy in patients in whom the presence of sinusitis has been documented by another method.

Magnetic Resonance Imaging

MRI is used rarely because of its cost and limitations in assessing cortical bone. Although MRI provides better visualization of soft tissues than CT, it is best reserved for the investigation of intracranial suppurative complications and for the delineation of the anatomical relationships between the intraorbital and extraorbital compartments.

SINUS PUNCTURE AND QUANTITATIVE CULTURES

Surface cultures of the nasal vestibule or the nasopharynx are unreliable for the microbiologic diagnosis of sinusitis owing to regular contamination by the resident microflora. Cultures obtained directly from the middle meatus during sinus endoscopy also have a low positive predictive value (38%) and overall accuracy (49%) as compared with sinus aspiration and are inadequate to guide antimicrobial therapy (33). Sinus puncture with aspiration remains the gold standard for establishing the microbial etiology in sinusitis and is a relatively painless and safe procedure when performed by an experienced operator. With the appropriate technique, more than 76% of such specimens yield positive cultures in acute maxillary sinusitis (34). Quantitative cultures demonstrating bacterial counts of at least 10^4 colony-forming units per milliliter are useful for distinguishing between colonization and contamination from true infection. However, this procedure is invasive and impractical in most primary care situations. In addition, it is not necessary in every patient because the microbial etiology of sinusitis is well characterized and relatively predictable in most immunocompetent persons (Table 44.2). Thus, sinus puncture should be considered only in the case of failure of empirical therapy, severe illness, suppurative complications especially with orbital or intracranial extension, nosocomial sinusitis, the immunocompromised host, or in the presence of diagnostic uncertainty (e.g., opacification of sinus in a patient with fever of undetermined origin and no other findings).

ENDOSCOPIC SINOSCOPY

Sinoscopy allows direct visualization of the sinonasal tract as well as the sinus mucosa and offers the added advantage of accessibility to mucosal biopsy specimens for microbiologic and histopathological investigation. It is particularly useful in

TABLE 44.2. Microbial Causes of Acute and Chronic Sinusitis Determined by Antral Sinus Aspirate or Sinus Surgery Specimens

Microbial agent	Prevalence mean (range)	
	Adults (%)	Children (%)
Acute sinusitis		
Streptococcus pneumoniae	34–43	37
Haemophilus influenzae	31–35	25
Anaerobes (*Bacteroides, Fusobacterium, Peptostreptococcus, Veillonella*)	7–12	—
Moraxella catarrhalis	4–5	25
Streptococcus pyogenes	2–7	—
Staphylococcus aureus	2–3	—
Rhinovirus	15	—
Influenza virus	5	—
Parainfluenza virus	3	2
Adenovirus	—	2
Chronic sinusitis		
Aerobes	29–43	20
Streptococcus species	9–14	6
Staphylococcus species	5–14	6
Haemophilus influenzae	1–6	3
Anaerobes	57–88	80
Peptostreptococcus species	25–38	23
Bacteroides species	14–27	29
Fusobacterium species	3–4	5

Adapted from Chow AW. Acute sinusitis: current status of etiologies, diagnosis and treatment. In: Remington JS, Swartz MN (eds). *Current clinical topics in infectious diseases*, Vol 21. Oxford, UK: Blackwell Science, 2001;90:31–63, with permission.

recurrent and chronic sinusitis when employed in conjunction with functional endoscopic sinus surgery (FESS) (see later).

Microbial Etiology

The precise microbial etiology of sinusitis can be determined only by direct aspiration of injection wash of the sinus cavity. Based on such studies, *Streptococcus pneumoniae* and nonencapsulated *Haemophilus influenzae* are responsible for about 70% of cases of acute sinusitis in adults (35), whereas *Moraxella catarrhalis*, in addition to *S. pneumoniae* and *H. influenzae*, accounts for 80% of cases in children (36) (Table 44.2). It should be noted that about 25% of patients with the clinical diagnosis of acute community-acquired sinusitis do not have bacterial growth from specimens collected by antral sinus puncture. Anaerobes are uncommonly isolated in acute sinusitis but are the predominant flora in chronic sinusitis. The isolation of anaerobes during acute sinusitis suggests an odontogenic source (37). *Staphylococcus aureus* is a common nasal contaminant and an infrequent cause of acute maxillary sinusitis. In contrast, *S. aureus*, viridans streptococci, and *S. pneumoniae* are the predominant isolates in acute sphenoid sinusitis. Rarely, paranasal sinuses can serve as a cryptic focus of *S. aureus* infection causing toxic shock syndrome.

The role of *Chlamydia pneumoniae* (TWAR agent) in acute sinusitis is unclear but appears to account for only a very small proportion of purulent maxillary sinusitis cases (38). More information is needed to determine the role of *C. pneumoniae* in sinus disease, particularly because it does not respond to currently recommended antimicrobial treatment for acute bacterial sinusitis. Similarly, *Mycoplasma pneumoniae* appears to be an uncommon pathogen in acute sinusitis. In contrast, serological evidence of respiratory viruses can be demonstrated in one third of young adults with acute maxillary sinusitis (39). Nevertheless, direct

isolation of respiratory viruses from antral aspirates has been relatively uncommon, with rhinovirus, influenza A, parainfluenza virus, and adenovirus occasionally isolated from the antrum in patients with acute maxillary sinusitis (35). The availability of polymerase chain reaction (PCR) techniques has allowed improved detection of rhinoviruses as well as respiratory syncytial virus and adenovirus from maxillary sinus brushings or mucosal biopsies in patients with acute community-acquired sinusitis (40).

Nosocomial sinusitis secondary to prolonged nasotracheal intubation is commonly a polymicrobial infection caused by gram-negative bacteria, *S. aureus*, and anaerobes (41). In patients with cystic fibrosis, *Pseudomonas aeruginosa* and nontypable *H. influenzae* are the most frequent pathogens. Sinusitis in HIV-infected patients is often due to gram-negative bacilli such as *P. aeruginosa* and unusual pathogens such as *Aspergillus* species and cytomegalovirus. These infections are frequently recurrent or chronic and difficult to eradicate (42,43).

The microbiology of chronic sinusitis differs from that of acute sinusitis and is typically polymicrobial. Viridans streptococci and nonencapsulated *H. influenzae* are the major facultative isolates, whereas *Bacteroides, Peptostreptococcus*, and *Fusobacterium* species are the most predominant anaerobes. Fungal sinusitis is rare, but *Aspergillus, Mucor*, and *Candida* species, *Pseudoallescheria boydii*, and other saprophytic fungi can cause invasive disease in the debilitated host (44).

Treatment

The goals of therapy for sinusitis are to eradicate the causative pathogens, restore and improve sinus function, provide symptomatic relief, and prevent intracranial complications and chronic sequelae. Thus, management options include antimicrobial therapy, symptomatic and supportive measures, and surgical adjunctive treatment (Table 44.3). Unfortunately, there have been very few randomized, placebo-controlled clinical trials to

TABLE 44.3. Management Options for Sinusitis

Medical

Antimicrobials (oral and parenteral)
Decongestants (topical and systemic)
Mucolytic agents
Analgesics
Antihistamines
Cromolyn sodium
Intranasal glucocorticosteroids
Humidification and hydration
Sinus irrigation (Poretz's procedure)

Surgical (functional endoscopic sinus surgery, FESS)

Promote drainage
  Intranasal antrostomy
  Ethmoidotomy
  Frontal sinus trephination
Remove diseased tissue
  Caldwell-Luc operation
  Ethmoidectomy
  Frontal sinus obliteration
  Sphenoidectomy
Correct intranasal, ostial, or other abnormalities
  Turbinectomy
  Septal surgery
  Polypectomy
  Adenoidectomy
  Tonsillectomy

evaluate rigorously the benefit and contribution of each modality of treatment in acute sinusitis. The quandary is compounded by the viral-bacterial dual etiology of infection, its self-limited natural history, and practical difficulties in obtaining pretreatment and posttreatment sinus puncture cultures for confirmation of the microbial etiology and response to therapy. Several placebo-controlled studies have indicated that 40% to 79% of patients with acute sinusitis recover within 10 to 14 days without antibiotic therapy (45–47). Contrariwise, the few placebo-controlled studies that did show a benefit for antibiotic treatment either enrolled patients with relatively high clinical severity scores (48,49) or demonstrated benefit only in the subgroup of patients with positive nasopharyngeal cultures (50). Because nasopharyngeal cultures require several days to process and do not accurately reflect the bacterial flora in the sinus, until more advanced diagnostic techniques become available, current recommendations of initial management have emphasized the use of clinical or radiographic features to guide antimicrobial therapy. The U.S. Department of Health Agency for Health Care Policy and Research (AHCPR) recently conducted a decision analysis from the patient's perspective to evaluate several treatment strategies for managing acute bacterial rhinosinusitis (30,51). The literature indexed in the Medline database between 1966 and 1998 was reviewed, and only randomized controlled trials were used to assess treatment efficacy. Four strategies in the initial management were assessed: (a) use of clinical criteria to guide treatment; (b) sinus radiography–directed approach; (c) initial symptomatic (ancillary) treatment; and (d) empirical use of antibiotics with either amoxicillin or a folate inhibitor. In terms of symptom days, the results are essentially equivalent between empirical, radiography-guided, and clinically guided treatments. Symptomatic treatment alone provided fewer symptom-free days but the very lowest prevalence of acute bacterial rhinosinusitis. In terms of cost, radiography is the most exorbitant at any prevalence, whereas the use of clinical criteria and initial symptomatic treatment are equivalent. Initial symptomatic treatment is the most cost-effective strategy at prevalence of up to 25%; the use of clinical criteria is most cost-effective for a prevalence between 25% and 83%. Empirical antibiotic treatment is cost-effective as an initial management strategy only at prevalence of greater than 83%. Thus, whereas antimicrobial therapy is clearly important in patients with complicated or severe illness, empirical antibiotic treatment in uncomplicated acute sinusitis need not be initiated unless the clinical findings, including the severity and duration of symptoms, strongly suggest that a bacterial rather than viral rhinosinusitis is present.

ANTIMICROBIAL THERAPY

Since 1996, there have been seven placebo-controlled, double-blind trials in adults and one trial in children. The benefit of antibiotic therapy was demonstrated in three of these studies, and in two others only among the subset of patients with positive nasopharyngeal cultures for putative respiratory pathogens (*S. pneumoniae, H. influenzae, M. catarrhalis*). From these placebo-controlled studies, it is clear that patients with more severe illness may benefit from antibiotics, whereas those with mild or uncomplicated disease do not require antibiotics. In fact, 40% to 79% of patients enrolled in the placebo arm recovered with symptomatic treatment alone without antibiotic therapy. It is also notable that none of the recent placebo-controlled trials employed pretreatment and posttreatment sinus aspiration for confirmation of microbiologic eradication in acute bacterial sinusitis. It is possible that many of the patients enrolled in the trials had viral rhinosinusitis without secondary bacterial infection and therefore would not be expected to benefit from antibiotic treatment.

In this regard, the recent report by Kaiser and associates (50), who obtained nasopharyngeal cultures from 265 patients with acute sinusitis or the common cold, is particularly illuminating. These authors found that nasopharyngeal cultures were positive for *S. pneumoniae, H. influenzae,* or *M. catarrhalis* in 29%, and radiographically confirmed sinusitis in 31% of patients. The median duration of symptoms was significantly longer among patients with positive nasopharyngeal cultures (4.7 versus 3.9 days). Furthermore, multiple logistic regression analysis revealed that only a history of colored nasal discharge at rhinoscopy (56% versus 23%) and the presence of radiologically confirmed sinusitis (51% versus 23%) were significantly associated with the presence of putative respiratory pathogens in nasopharyngeal cultures. Finally, antibiotic treatment was of clinical benefit only in the subset of patients with positive nasopharyngeal cultures. These data suggest that, compared with clinical examinations, culture of nasopharyngeal secretions can better identify those patients who benefit from antibiotic treatment and thus may prevent the inappropriate administration of antimicrobial agents to patients with presumed acute bacterial sinusitis. Based on the available evidence, the following recommendations for the antibiotic treatment of community-acquired bacterial sinusitis can be made:

- *When should empirical antimicrobial therapy be initiated?* A strategy of either initial symptomatic management or the use of clinical criteria to guide antibiotic treatment would appear to be the most cost-effective approach for the management of patients with uncomplicated acute sinusitis. Empirical antibiotic therapy need not be initiated unless the clinical findings, including the severity and duration of symptoms, strongly suggest that a bacterial rather than viral rhinosinusitis is present. A 7- to 10-day course of watchful waiting before prescribing antibiotics would appear reasonable. This is the general approach recommended by the AHCPR and adopted both by the Health Partners Program and the Mayo Clinic (52).

- *Which antimicrobial regimens should be used as first-line therapy?* The initial choice of antibiotic treatment should be selected on an empirical basis because routine sinus aspiration for culture and susceptibility testing is neither practical nor necessary. In adults, antibiotic therapy is primarily directed against *H. influenzae* and *S. pneumoniae*, whereas in children, therapy should be directed against *M. catarrhalis* in addition. A 10- to 14-day course of amoxicillin has remained effective and is generally recommended as the first choice for uncomplicated acute sinusitis because of its low cost and excellent tolerance (53). Trimethoprim-sulfamethoxazole (TMP-SMX) and erythromycin-sulfisoxazole are suitable alternatives for penicillin-allergic patients. Penicillin, cephalexin, erythromycin, and tetracycline do not cover all the major organisms in acute bacterial sinusitis, and their use is not recommended.

- Because β-lactamase production among respiratory pathogens is increasing in the United States and Canada (up to 40% of *H. influenzae*, 80% of *M. catarrhalis*, and 30% of respiratory tract anaerobes) (54), a case may be made for choosing a β-lactamase–resistant antibiotic (such as amoxicillin-clavulanate) for initial empirical therapy. However, randomized controlled trials of β-lactamase–resistant antibiotic regimens, including amoxicillin-clavulanate, cefaclor, cefuroxime-axetil, cefdinir, cefpodoxime proxetil, ceftibuten, cefcanel, and loracarbef, have not demonstrated added benefit. Therefore, until the need is clearly demonstrated by further controlled clinical trials, amoxicillin has remained the most commonly prescribed antimicrobial agent during initial therapy of presumed acute bacterial sinusitis in North America.

TABLE 44.4. Antimicrobial Regimens for Acute Sinusitis[a]

Agent	Adults (oral dose)	Children (oral dose)
Amoxicillin	500 mg q.i.d.	60–90 mg/kg/day b.i.d.
Amoxicillin-clavulanate	500/125 mg t.i.d.	45/10 mg/kg/day b.i.d.
Trimethoprim (80 mg)- sulfamethoxazole (40 mg)	160–800 mg b.i.d.	8–40 mg/kg/day b.i.d.
Erythromycin-sulfisoxazole		50/150 mg/kg/day q.i.d.
Doxycycline	200 mg q.d. on day 1 then, 100 mg q.d.	
Cefuroxime axetil	250 mg b.i.d.	45–60 mg/kg/day b.i.d.
Cefprozil	500 mg b.i.d.	30 mg/kg/day b.i.d.
Cefpodoxime proxetil	200 mg b.i.d.	10 mg/kg/day b.i.d.
Ceftibuten	400 mg o.d.	9 mg/kg/day q.d.
Cefixime	400 mg b.i.d.	8 mg/kg/day q.d.
Loracarbef	400 mg b.i.d.	30 mg/kg/day b.i.d.
Clarithromycin	500 mg b.i.d.	15 mg/kg/day b.i.d.
Azithromycin	500 mg q.d. on day 1 then, 250 mg q.d.	10 mg/kg/day q.d. on day 1 then, 5 mg/kg/day q.d.
Ciprofloxacin	500 mg b.i.d.	
Levofloxacin	500 mg q.d.	
Moxifloxacin	400 mg q.d.	
Gatifloxacin	400 mg q.d.	

[a]Cefaclor is associated with suboptimal response rates and is not recommended for the empirical treatment of acute bacterial sinusitis.

β-Lactamase–resistant antibiotics should be reserved for patients with severe symptoms and those who are immunocompromised or have failed to respond to first-line agents despite 48 to 72 hours of antimicrobial therapy. In patients with acute maxillary sinusitis of dental origin, treatment should be directed at mixed anaerobes and streptococci, which are the most common causative organisms (55); penicillin and clindamycin are suitable agents. The dosing regimens of selected antimicrobial agents commonly used in the treatment of acute bacterial sinusitis are summarized in Table 44.4.

- *How long should antimicrobials be administered?* The optimal length of antibiotic therapy has not been established, but a 10- to 14-day course is usually recommended in acute bacterial sinusitis. One study has shown equivalent effectiveness comparing 3 days and 10 days of TMP-SMX (56), but the standard practice is to continue therapy for the longer duration. Improvement is usually observed by day 3 of treatment.
- *How should sinusitis caused by penicillin-resistant* Streptococcus pneumoniae *be treated?* Whereas penicillin resistance in *H. influenzae* and *M. catarrhalis* is due to β-lactamase production, resistance to penicillin in *S. pneumoniae* is due to altered β-lactam target sites (penicillin-binding proteins) and hence cannot be overcome by the addition of a β-lactamase inhibitor. Furthermore, penicillin resistance in *S. pneumoniae* is often a marker for a multidrug-resistant (MDR) phenotype (57). Thus, *S. pneumoniae* isolates with intermediate- or high-level penicillin resistance often exhibit reduced susceptibility to oral cephalosporins, and in many instances to macrolides, TMP-SMX, and tetracyclines. However, even though the prevalence of penicillin-resistant *S. pneumoniae* is increasing in North America, ranging from 4% to 48% of isolates in various regions of the United States and Canada (58,59), high-level resistance (i.e., MIC ≥ 2 μg/mL penicillin) is relatively rare. Furthermore, treatment failure due to high-dose amoxicillin (500 mg three times daily), amoxicillin-clavulanate (500/125 mg three times daily), or cefuroxime (500 mg twice daily) is uncommon. Nevertheless, there is mounting concern that empirical treatment of acute bacterial sinusitis with first-line agents may be ill advised in regions known to have a high endemic

rate of penicillin- and cephalosporin-resistant pneumococci (24). Therapeutic options include amoxicillin-clavulanate, cefuroxime, cefpodoxime, or cefprozil (for intermediate-level penicillin-resistant pneumococci) as well as azithromycin and the newer fluoroquinolones (e.g., levofloxacin, gatifloxacin, and moxifloxacin). However, the optimal empirical therapy is still not known, and antibiotic selection should be guided by susceptibility results whenever possible. Seriously ill patients with evidence of orbital or intracranial extension should be treated intravenously with vancomycin, quinupristin-dalfopristin, a third-generation cephalosporin, or a combination of these.

- *What is the role of the newer macrolides and fluoroquinolones in acute bacterial sinusitis?* Both clarithromycin and azithromycin have been shown to be as effective as amoxicillin and amoxicillin-clavulanate in controlled clinical trials. However, macrolide-resistant strains of *H. influenzae* and *S. pneumoniae* are isolated with increasing frequency from the respiratory tract (54), even though the clinical significance of these isolates in acute bacterial sinusitis remains unclear (60). Ciprofloxacin is active against *H. influenzae* and *M. catarrhalis*, but its *in vitro* activity against *S. pneumoniae* is suboptimal and has been associated with a lower clinical success rate compared with clarithromycin (84% versus 91%; $p < 0.05$; relative risk [RR], 0.49; 95% confidence interval [CI], 0.45–0.55) (61). Thus, ciprofloxacin is not recommended as empirical treatment of community-acquired bacterial sinusitis but may be more useful in nosocomial sinusitis. The newer fluoroquinolones, such as levofloxacin, gatifloxacin, and moxifloxacin, have improved activity compared with ciprofloxacin against *S. pneumoniae*, including penicillin-resistant strains. These agents are also effective against other respiratory pathogens, such as *C. pneumoniae*, *M. pneumoniae*, and facultative gram-negative bacilli. The fourth-generation fluoroquinolones (gatifloxacin and moxifloxacin) are also highly active against respiratory anaerobes. Similar to the macrolides, the fluoroquinolones readily penetrate the sinus mucosa and achieve high concentrations within sinus secretions. Thus, the newer fluoroquinolones are attractive agents for the treatment of complicated acute bacterial sinusitis. However, a major concern is the potential for the development of resistance to fluoroquinolones, especially in *S. pneumoniae* (62). Thus, these agents should be reserved for complicated infections, such as for the treatment of acute bacterial sinusitis caused by high-level penicillin-resistant *S. pneumoniae* or suppurative infection with orbital or central nervous system invasion.

- *What should be done if the patient fails an initial course of antibiotics?* Patients in whom symptoms persist despite a 10- to 14-day course of first-line antibiotic therapy should receive an additional course of treatment with a β-lactamase–resistant agent. If this regimen fails, a sinus aspirate should be obtained, and further antimicrobial therapy should be guided by culture and sensitivity data. Patients with subacute or recurrent symptoms that fail to respond to the above approach should be investigated for predisposing conditions, such as cystic fibrosis, Wegener's granulomatosis, immunodeficiency syndromes, and possible underlying structural abnormalities should be excluded by endoscopic sinoscopy. Repeated antral lavage in addition to antibiotics may be required before consideration for a surgical approach.

- *How should nosocomial sinusitis be treated?* Nosocomial sinusitis should be strongly suspected in patients with prolonged transnasal intubation. It should be presumed to be present if there is also concurrent purulent rhinorrhea or otitis media (63). In such patients, the nasal tube should be removed and nasal decongestants as well as broad-spectrum antibiotics initiated to cover facultative gram-negative bacilli, *S. aureus*, and anaerobes (e.g., ceftazidime, imipenem, piperacillin-tazobactam, or an antipseudomonal fluoroquinolone such as ciprofloxacin) while continuing the search for other causes of fever. If fever persists and no other cause is found, CT of the paranasal sinuses or ultrasonography should be performed. If fluid is detected, maxillary sinus aspiration should be performed and additional antibiotic therapy tailored according to culture results.

- *When should antifungal agents be initiated?* Antimicrobial therapy for fungal sinusitis is required only if the disease is invasive or if the patient is severely immunocompromised and the risk for progressive disease is high. Noninvasive disease usually responds to surgical débridement alone (64). Most immunocompromised patients with invasive fungal infection should be treated with amphotericin B in cumulative doses exceeding 2 g (43). The role of azole antifungal agents, such as fluconazole or itraconazole, for invasive fungal sinusitis remains unclear at present.

- *How should patients with recurrent or chronic sinusitis be managed?* Antibiotic therapy alone is of questionable effectiveness in chronic sinusitis, and surgical procedures to relieve obstruction of the osteomeatal complex is often required (65). In choosing an antibiotic for chronic sinusitis, the initial coverage should include *S. aureus* and β-lactamase–producing organisms, including anaerobic species. Subsequent antimicrobial selection (including antifungal agents) should be guided by sinus culture results. Many of the second-line antibiotics used for acute bacterial sinusitis (Table 44.4) are also effective in chronic sinusitis, but the course of treatment is generally prolonged to 4 to 6 weeks. Clindamycin or metronidazole may be added if an anaerobic organism is suspected (e.g., dental source of infection).

SUPPORTIVE AND SYMPTOMATIC MANAGEMENT

Decongestants and Mucoevacuants. Few randomized, controlled trials have been conducted to investigate the use of these agents in sinusitis. Rather, their inherent value has been extrapolated from the large body of clinical trial evidence establishing their value in allergic rhinitis (66). Despite the lack of demonstrated effectiveness, mucolytic agents (e.g., guaiphenesin), which thin nasal secretions and therefore may promote drainage are frequently prescribed, often in over-the-counter preparations in combination with oral or nasal decongestants. Nasal decongestant sprays (e.g., 0.5% phenylephrine hydrochloride or 0.05% oxymetazoline hydrochloride), and oral decongestants to a lesser extent (e.g., pseudoephedrine and phenylpropanolamine), are α-adrenergic agonists that rapidly shrink the erectile vascular tissue of the turbinates, thus helping to relieve osteomeatal and nasal obstruction. However, there is conflicting evidence whether these agents functionally improve aeration of the sinuses. Prolonged use of nasal decongestants beyond 3 or 4 days in patients is also known to cause rebound vasodilation (rhinitis medicamentosa) (67). Thus, there is little evidence to support the use of decongestants in the management of community-acquired acute sinusitis or the common cold in the absence of concurrent allergic rhinosinusitis. If these agents are to be used, the oral route is preferred, but inappropriate usage may cause considerable adverse effects, including nervousness, insomnia, tachycardia, and hypertension.

Antihistamines. There are theoretical concerns that antihistamines might dry the mucous membrane and thicken nasal secretions, thereby impeding mucociliary clearance. However, Gwatlney and colleagues (68) demonstrated in double-blind, controlled trials that the use of clemastine fumarate, a first-generation antihistamine, resulted in significant improvement in sneezing and rhinorrhea both in human volunteers with experimental rhinovirus colds and in patients with naturally occurring common colds. The underlying mechanism for the salutary effect of this antihistamine remains unclear, but it has been suggested that this may be due to the anticholinergic rather than antihistamine effects of this agent. More work is required to clarify the role of antihistamines, if any, in the symptomatic management of common colds and acute sinusitis.

Intranasal Glucocorticosteroids. Although they are widely prescribed in acute sinusitis, there has been little evidence to support the use of intranasal glucocorticosteroids outside of allergic rhinosinusitis (69). However, two recent double-blind, placebo-controlled, randomized trials have indicated that the addition of intranasal steroids (flunisolide or budesonide nasal spray) as an adjunct to antibiotic therapy (amoxicillin-clavulanate) significantly improves the symptom scores of acute sinusitis (cough or rhinorrhea) in both adults (70) and children (71). Several studies have also demonstrated that intranasal steroids (e.g., beclomethasone or flunisolide, 1 to 2 sprays to each nostril three times daily) are useful in chronic or recurrent sinusitis (72).

Sinus Irrigation. Saline irrigation and drainage of the nasal cavity may result in dramatic relief of pain and prevent otherwise irreversible mucosal damage. Repeated sinus irrigation by Poretz's procedure is useful for subacute or chronic sinusitis. The intent is to irrigate sinuses with partially patent ostia. It is not recommended for untreated acute disease because there is a potential risk for hematogenous spread of infection. Hypertonic saline has been found to be more effective than normal saline for sinus irrigation of children with chronic sinusitis (73).

Other Miscellaneous Measures. The importance of adequate hydration, warm facial packs, steam baths, analgesic, and avoidance of irritants such as smoke and extreme cold air for comfort and pain relief is self-evident. In addition, the treatment of

TABLE 44.5. Clinical Spectrum and Investigation of Intracranial Complications of Sinusitis

Complication	Clinical signs	Cerebrospinal fluid findings	Computed tomography	
			Plain	Contrast enhanced
Meningitis	Headache, fever + + Stiff neck, lethargy + + Rapid death + +	High PMN count and protein; low glucose	Normal	Diffusely enhanced
Osteomyelitis	Pott's puffy tumor ±	Normal	Bone defect	Bone defect
Epidural abscess or mucocele	Headache ± Fever ±	Normal	Lucent area	Biconvex capsule
Subdural empyema	Headache + + Convulsions + + Hemiplegia + + Rapid death + +	High PMN count and protein; normal glucose	Lucent area	Crescent-shaped enhancement
Cerebral abscess	Convulsions + Headache + Personality change +	Lymphocytosis; normal glucose	Lucency with mass effect	Capsule
Venous sinus thrombosis (cavernous)	"Picket-fence" fever + + Rapid death + + (orbital edema + +, ocular palsies + +)	Normal or high PMN count	Nonspecific	Enhancing lesion

± May or may not be seen; + seen frequently; ++ seen characteristically; PMN, polymorphonuclear leukocyte.
Modified from Fairbanks DNF, Milmoe GJ. Complications and sequelae: an otolaryngologist's perspective. *Pediatr Infect Dis* 1985; 4(Suppl 6):575, with permission.

uncomplicated common cold has been the subject of a series of metaanalyses by the Cochrane group. However, the potential benefit of heated humidification (74), zinc lozenges (75), or Echinacea preparations (76) remains unclear.

SURGICAL MANAGEMENT

The surgical treatment of sinusitis is directed toward restoring sinus drainage and removing diseased tissue. It should be reserved for patients who have failed medical therapy, patients with chronic sinusitis, and patients with threatening or established complications. The absolute indications for surgery in rhinosinusitis include acute complicated sinusitis, obstruction of the osteomeatal complex due to nasal polyposis or mucopyoceles, and fungal infections. The wide spectrum of surgical procedures available includes intranasal antrostomy, Caldwell-Luc operation, intranasal sphenoethmoidectomy, transantral ethmoidectomy, frontal sinus trephination and obliteration, and functional endoscopic sinus surgery (FESS) (Table 44.3). The introduction of FESS in the past two decades has revolutionized surgery for sinus disease. It allows improved visualization of the sinuses, including relatively inaccessible areas such as the infundibulum of the anterior ethmoid sinus. The primary goal is to facilitate sinus drainage by removing any inflamed tissues near the osteomeatal complex in order to reestablish sinus ventilation and improve mucociliary clearance. Surgery is performed almost exclusively intranasally, with no external incisions. It can be performed under local anesthesia as an outpatient procedure and is particularly useful to correct intranasal pathology such as septal deviation and polyposis. Between 80% and 90% of patients undergoing FESS experience significant improvement in sinusitis symptoms, and complication rates are low (less than 1%) (77).

Complications and Prevention

Fortunately, the suppurative and life-threatening complications of acute and chronic sinusitis have become relatively infrequent in the postantibiotic era (78). Owing to the different anatomical locations that may be involved (Fig. 44.2), the clinical spectrum of such complications can be quite varied (Table 44.5). Diagnosis and management of these suppurative complications requires an aggressive and multidisciplinary approach, including specialists in radiology, otolaryngology, neurology, and neurosurgery (see later section "Infections of Parameningeal Structures"). Apart from pneumococcal and *H. influenzae* vaccines, there are currently no effective preventive measures for acute or chronic sinusitis. Efforts should be directed to early and aggressive treatment of acute sinusitis, surgical correction of anatomical deformities of the sinus ostia and intranasal structures, promotion of good dental hygiene, and effective control of underlying allergic manifestations.

INFECTIONS OF PARAMENINGEAL STRUCTURES

Infections of the parameningeal structures include subdural empyema, cranial and spinal epidural abscess, and cranial septic venous thrombosis. These infections most frequently arise by direct extension from a pericranial focus, such as chronic sinusitis, otitis media, mastoiditis, or petrous osteomyelitis (78,79). Hematogenous infection is more common with spinal epidural abscess, although contiguous spread from vertebral osteomyelitis, infection after epidural anesthesia or laminectomy, and extension of pressure sores are not uncommon (80). These suppurative infections carry a high rate of mortality and morbidity and should be considered both medical and surgical emergencies. Early diagnosis and effective therapy are the only means of preventing death and long-term neurological sequelae, yet the necessary diagnostic measures and therapeutic interventions are often delayed. This may be related in part to the complexity of the clinical problem: key and important medical history may be unobtainable in a comatose patient, and the differential diagnoses may be uncertain if the primary source of infection is unrecognized. A systematic approach with rapid mobilization and assistance from various specialists (such as neurologist, neurosurgeon, neuroradiologist, infectious disease specialist, and microbiologist) is essential for optimal management.

Anatomical Considerations

SUBARACHNOID AND DURA MATER

The cranial dura mater adheres tightly to the periosteum of the skull except where it invaginates into the cranial cavity to form the falx cerebri, falx cerebelli, tentorium cerebelli, and diaphragma sellae (Fig. 44.5). Infection in the extradural space, therefore, tends to be localized. Loculation of infection between the arachnoid and dura mater results in a subdural empyema. Because the arachnoid and dura are only loosely attached, subdural infection can spread rapidly over the surface of the cerebral hemisphere. This infection is usually unilateral because further spread is restricted medially by the falx cerebri and inferiorly by the tentorium cerebelli. In contrast to the cranial dura, the spinal dura mater and periosteum are separated by a fat-filled epidural space from the foramen magnum to the level of the seventh cervical vertebra. Thus, both spinal subdural empyema and spinal epidural abscess may

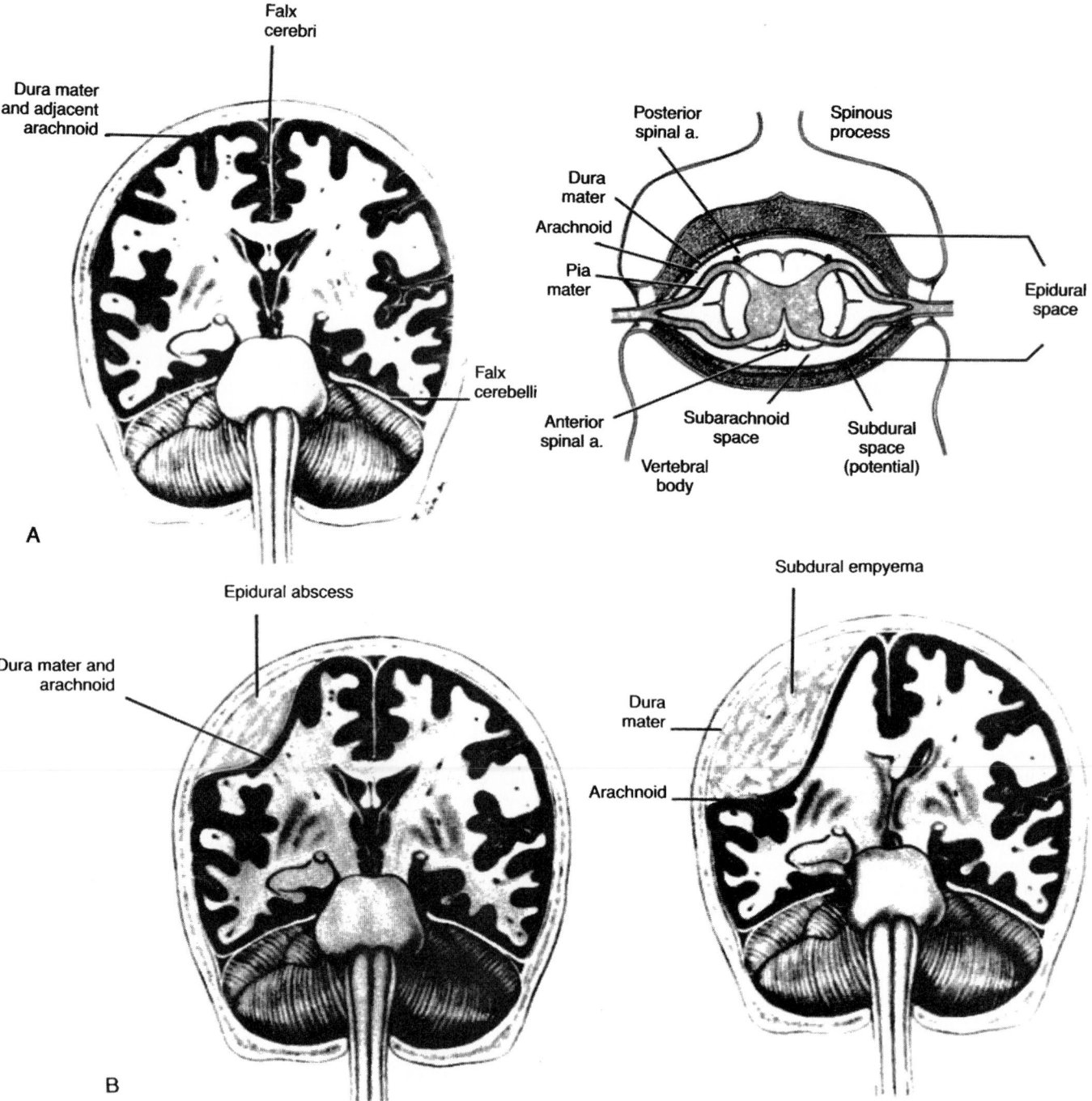

Figure 44.5. Anatomic relationships of normal cranial and spinal meninges (**A**) and cranial epidural abscess and subdural empyema (**B**). (Adapted from Greenlee JE. Anatomic considerations in central nervous system infections. In Mandell GL, Douglas RG Jr, Bennett JE, eds. *Principles and practice of infectious diseases*, 4th ed. New York: Churchill Livingstone, 1994:821–831, with permission; drawing in **A** modified from Baker AS, Ojeman RG, Swartz MN, et al. Spinal epidural abscess. *N Engl J Med* 1975;293:463–468, with permission. Copyright © 1975 Massachusetts Medical Society. All rights reserved.)

extend over many vertebral segments and are usually posterior to the cord.

CRANIAL VENOUS SINUSES AND ARTERIES

The cranium is drained by a network of superficial veins (external portions of the cerebrum and brainstem), deep veins (central white matter, basal ganglia, and thalamus), and venous sinuses within the dura mater. The intracranial venous system communicates extensively with the extracranial venous system through numerous emissary veins that cross the skull and meninges. The cortical venous sinuses also resorb cerebrospinal fluid through the arachnoid villi, most of which are located along the anterior third of the superior sagittal sinus. Thus, obstruction of venous outflow caused either by thrombosis of the superior sagittal sinus or by occlusion of both lateral sinuses may result in communicating hydrocephalus. The intracranial venous system and sinuses lack valves and allow bidirectional blood flow. Because of extensive anastomosis, cortical venous thrombosis or occlusion of venous sinuses often produces only transient neurologic manifestations and at times may be silent if collateral venous drainage is adequate. If the thrombus outstrips collateral flow, however, progressive neurological deficits will lead to impairment of consciousness, focal or generalized seizures, and increased intracranial pressure. Septic embolization of intracranial arteries may lead to necrosis in the arterial wall, resulting in dilation and possible rupture (mycotic aneurysm). Because the middle cerebral arteries receive the greatest volume of blood, they are more frequently involved in infectious processes, such as septic embolization or mycotic aneurysm, compared with other branches of the anterior and posterior circulation. The spinal arteries are seldom involved in infections.

CRANIUM AND CONTIGUOUS STRUCTURES

The understructures of the brain rest within the anterior, middle, and posterior cranial fossae. The anterior fossa forms the roof of the frontal and ethmoidal sinuses; thus, infection within either sinus may produce a frontal epidural abscess, a subdural empyema, or a frontal lobe brain abscess (Fig. 44.2). The sphenoidal sinus occupies the body of the sphenoid bone close to the pituitary gland above, with the optic nerve and optic chiasma in front, and the internal carotids, the cavernous sinuses, and the temporal lobes of the brain on each side (Fig. 44.2). Thus, infection originating from the sphenoidal sinus may extend locally to cause cavernous sinus thrombosis, anteriorly to involve the frontal lobe, and posteriorly to involve the temporal lobe. Similarly, infections of the middle ear or the mastoid within the petrous bone may extend into the middle fossa to involve the temporal lobe or into the posterior fossa to involve the cerebellum or brainstem. The skull overlying the dura of the cerebrum is covered extracranially by the galea aponeurotica. Thus, pericranial infections secondary to head trauma or a craniotomy may result in subgaleal abscess and cranial osteomyelitis, with possible retrograde spread through the emissary veins to the epidural, subdural, and subarachnoid spaces. Both cranial and spinal nerve roots may be involved either directly by contiguous infection or indirectly from increased intracranial pressure. Of particular importance is the close relationship of the third cranial nerve to the tentorium (uncal herniation of the temporal lobe); the third, fourth, fifth, and sixth cranial nerves to the cavernous sinus (septic cavernous sinus thrombosis); the fifth and sixth cranial nerves to the petrous portion of the temporal bone (chronic otitis media and petrous osteomyelitis); and the ninth and eleventh cranial nerves to the jugular foramen (septic jugular thrombophlebitis). The spinal dura mater and the periosteum are separated by a fat-filled epidural space from the foramen magnum to the level of C-7. Thus, both spinal subdural empyema and spinal epidural abscess may extend over many vertebral segments and are usually posterior to the cord.

Clinical Syndromes and Diagnosis

SUBDURAL EMPYEMA

The source of this parameningeal infection is usually in the frontal or ethmoid sinuses. The infection gains entry by direct extension or as a result of thrombophlebitis involving the venous sinuses (Fig. 44.2). An acute flare-up of local pain, increase in purulent nasal or aural discharge, generalized headache, and high fevers are the first indications of intracranial spread. These clinical features are followed within days by the appearance of focal neurological findings such as unilateral motor seizures, hemiplegia, hemianesthesia or aphasia, and signs of increased intracranial pressure with progressive lethargy and coma (79). The neck is stiff, but cerebrospinal fluid examination is more consistent with an aseptic meningitis syndrome. In infants and young children, however, an intracranial subdural empyema is almost invariably a complication of bacterial meningitis. Early signs such as irritability, poor feeding, and increased head size are nonspecific, but hemiparesis, convulsions, stupor, and coma may ensue rapidly (81). Plain radiographs and tomograms of the paranasal sinuses, mastoids, and petrous portion of the temporal bone may provide invaluable clues to contiguous foci of suppurative infection. However, CT is the procedure of choice for the diagnosis of subdural empyema and usually reveals a crescent-shaped area of low density directly between the inner table of the skull and the cerebral cortex or adjacent to the falx cerebri (82). With contrast, there is fine, irregular enhancement of the peripheral margins of the subdural empyema. Occasionally, CT may be inconclusive because density of the lesion may be similar to that of cerebral tissue, and the decreased attenuation may not be evident. MRI may offer an advantage over CT in such cases. Angiography is recommended on an emergency basis if CT results are normal and facilities for MRI are not available. As with brain abscess, lumbar puncture should be avoided in patients suspected of having a subdural empyema.

CRANIAL EPIDURAL ABSCESS

Intracranial epidural abscess is usually associated with a postcraniotomy infection or a cranial osteomyelitis secondary to chronic sinusitis or middle ear infection (83,84). The onset of symptoms may be insidious and overshadowed by the localized inflammatory process. Focal neurological findings are less common than in subdural empyema. Rarely, a fifth and sixth cranial nerve palsy may develop in association with infections of the petrous portion of the temporal bone (Gradenigo's syndrome). CT demonstrates a thick and circumscribed area of diminished density associated with extracerebral displacement and contiguous cranial osteomyelitis. As with subdural empyema, angiography may occasionally be required in highly suggestive cases when CT results are normal. The possibility of a coexistent intracranial suppurative process must be evaluated carefully.

SEPTIC INTRACRANIAL THROMBOPHLEBITIS AND MYCOTIC ANEURYSM

Intracranial suppurative thrombophlebitis most frequently follows infection of the paranasal sinuses, middle ear, mastoid, or oropharynx (79). Fortunately, this complication is relatively rare in the postantibiotic era. The clinical findings vary with the location of cortical veins or dural sinuses involved. *Cavernous sinus thrombosis* is characterized by abrupt onset with diplopia, photophobia, orbital edema, and progressive exophthalmos (85).

Involvement of the third, fourth, fifth, and sixth cranial nerves produces ophthalmoplegia, a midposition fixed pupil, loss of corneal reflex, and diminished sensation over the upper face. Obstruction of venous return from the retina results in papilledema, retinal hemorrhage, and visual loss. *Thrombosis of the superior sagittal sinus* produces bilateral leg weakness and may cause communicating hydrocephalus. *Occlusion of the lateral sinus* produces pain over the ear and mastoid and may cause edema over the mastoid (Griesinger's sign). Involvement of the fifth and sixth cranial nerves produces ipsilateral facial pain and lateral rectus weakness (Gradenigo's syndrome). The danger of septic pulmonary embolization is always present. *Intracranial mycotic aneurysm* usually results from septic embolization as a complication of infective endocarditis. The early clinical manifestations are similar to those of cerebral emboli and infarction. The funduscopic examination is particularly useful for the detection of an embolic source of infection because the ophthalmic artery is a branch of the internal carotid artery, and septic embolization within the anterior circulation may produce characteristic visual field defects and retinal lesions. In suppurative cranial thrombophlebitis, skull radiographs may show a pineal shift and evidence of sinusitis or mastoiditis. Lumbar puncture reveals increased intracranial pressure, a slight lymphocytic pleocytosis, and slightly elevated protein. The cerebrospinal fluid is usually sterile. MRI with angiography is the procedure of choice for the diagnosis of intracranial suppurative thrombophlebitis and mycotic aneurysm because of its ability to distinguish between flowing blood and thrombus. Angiography with close attention to the venous phase for evidence of nonfilling should be considered if venous sinus thrombophlebitis is suspected despite negative CT or MRI. Radionuclide scans may also be helpful. Abscess can be excluded by either CT or MRI. Cavernous sinus thrombosis is readily detected by CT. The definitive diagnosis of mycotic aneurysm requires the combination of both CT or MRI and angiography. The weakened vessel may be seen to increase in size progressively on serial angiograms.

SPINAL EPIDURAL ABSCESS

Spinal epidural abscess usually arises hematogenously or by contiguous spread from vertebral osteomyelitis, extension of pressure sores, or infection after epidural anesthesia or penetrating injury (86). Distant sources of infection include infective endocarditis, pneumonia, intraabdominal or pelvic sepsis, and urinary tract infection with entry of organisms through the paravertebral venous plexus. Spinal epidural abscess may span several vertebrae and may be inadvertently entered during a lumbar puncture. The abscess may develop acutely or follow a more chronic course. Four stages in the clinical presentation can be recognized. The first phase is usually accompanied by fever and back pain, and the second phase involves progression to root pain. Symptoms developing in the cervical or lumbar area suggest nerve root compression due to a ruptured disk. In the third phase, there is progression to motor weakness, sensory changes, and bowel or bladder dysfunction, signaling spinal cord compression. The fourth phase involves total paralysis, which may occur within hours after the onset of motor weakness. If the cervical cord is involved, respiratory function may be impaired. MRI is the diagnostic method of choice because it can visualize the cord and epidural space in both sagittal and transverse sections and can also identify an associated vertebral osteomyelitis or joint space infection. Myelography should be employed if MRI is not available or cannot be performed. CT with contrast enhancement may be helpful in differentiating subdural from epidural infection or in identifying osteomyelitis. Analysis of cerebrospinal fluid is usually nondiagnostic unless the abscess has ruptured into the subarachnoid space or the spinal needle

has inadvertently entered the epidural abscess during the lumbar puncture.

Antimicrobial and Adjunctive Therapy

SUBDURAL EMPYEMA AND CRANIAL EPIDURAL ABSCESS

Early surgical evacuation is the cornerstone of therapy for both subdural empyema and cranial epidural abscess. The incidence of mortality and neurological sequelae varies directly with the time elapsed before surgical drainage. In addition, the primary focus of infection, such as chronic sinusitis, mastoiditis, or petrous osteomyelitis, should be explored and débrided. The choice of initial empirical antimicrobial therapy is based on the suspected source of infection, the immunological status of the patient, and the most likely causative organisms (Table 44.6). In rhinogenic causes associated with chronic sinusitis, anaerobic or microaerophilic streptococci (*Peptostreptococcus* species, viridans streptococci, *Streptococcus anginosus*) and *Bacteroides* and *Prevotella* species predominate, often as mixed infections (79,87). In otogenic infection associated with chronic otitis media or mastoiditis, enteric gram-negative bacilli, such as *Pseudomonas aeruginosa* and *Proteus mirabilis*, as well as anaerobic organisms, are most common (78). Epidural abscesses secondary to penetrating cranial trauma or postoperative infection are most commonly caused by *S. aureus* and enteric gram-negative bacilli (84).

When anaerobes and microaerophilic streptococci are implicated, penicillin G remains the antibiotic of first choice even though β-lactamase–producing organisms are increasingly isolated in such infections. Chloramphenicol and metronidazole are useful alternatives in the penicillin-allergic patient and have the advantage of more effective coverage against β-lactamase–producing anaerobes. Metronidazole is particularly active against *Bacteroides* and *Fusobacterium*. However, its lack of activity against gram-positive anaerobic cocci, such as *Peptostreptococcus*, and facultative organisms, such as streptococci, is a disadvantage that precludes monotherapy of otogenic or odontogenic intracranial suppuration with metronidazole alone. Combination of penicillin with metronidazole or chloramphenicol is recommended. Clindamycin penetrates the blood–brain barrier poorly and is not usually recommended in central nervous system infections. For immunocompromised and critically ill patients, broad coverage with extended-spectrum β-lactams (e.g., cefotaxime, ceftizoxime, imipenem) for aerobic gram-negative bacilli, *S. aureus*, and anaerobes is indicated (Table 44.6). The fluoroquinolones (ciprofloxacin, levofloxacin, gatifloxacin, moxifloxacin) have excellent central nervous system penetration and antibacterial activity against gram-negative bacilli. If *S. aureus* is suspected, nafcillin or methicillin may be added. If the *S. aureus* strain is resistant to methicillin, vancomycin is the agent of choice. The final antibiotic selection should be guided by culture results and susceptibility data.

Maximal doses of systemic antimicrobials are required for the treatment of subdural empyema and epidural abscess. Therapy should generally be continued for at least 4 to 6 weeks. Patients should be carefully monitored both clinically and by repeated CT. Follow-up for up to 1 year is required to ensure against recurrence. In addition to antibiotic therapy, corticosteroids or osmotic diuretics are used frequently to decrease intracranial edema and pressure. External or ventriculoperitoneal shunting may be required if hydrocephalus is present.

SEPTIC CRANIAL VENOUS SINUS THROMBOSIS AND MYCOTIC ANEURYSM

Treatment of septic cranial thrombophlebitis requires maximum dosages of intravenous antibiotics and surgical decompression

TABLE 44.6. Empirical Antimicrobial Regimens for Suppurative Parameningeal Infections

Source or associated infection	Antimicrobial regimens	
	Normal host	**Compromised host**
Cranial parameningeal infections[a]		
Otogenic	Penicillin G, 2–4 MU i.v. q4–6h *or* Ciprofloxacin, 0.2 g q12h, *plus* Metronidazole, 0.5 g i.v. q6h *or* Chloramphenicol 0.5 g i.v. q6h	Cefotaxime, 2 g i.v. q6h *or* Ceftizoxime, 4 g i.v. q8h *or* Imipenem, 500 mg i.v. q6h
Rhinogenic	Penicillin G, 2–4 MU i.v. q4–6h, *plus* Metronidazole, 0.5 g i.v. q6h *or* Chloramphenicol, 0.5 g i.v. q6h	Same as for otogenic
Odontogenic	Same as for rhinogenic	Same as for otogenic
After cranial surgery	Nafcillin, 1.5 g IV q4–6h, *plus* Tobramycin, 2 mg/kg i.v. q8h *or* Ciprofloxacin, 0.2 g q12h	Vancomycin, 0.5 g i.v. q6h, *plus* cefotaxime, cefizoxime, *or* imipenem
Hematogenous from distant site	Choice based on suspected organism from primary site	
Spinal epidural abscess		
Extension of osteomyelitis or paravertebral infection	Nafcillin, 1.5 g i.v. q4–6h, *plus* Tobramycin, 2 mg/kg q8h *or* Ciprofloxacin, 0.2 g q12h	Vancomycin, 0.5 g i.v. q6h, *plus* cefotaxime, cefizoxime, *or* imipenem

[a]Includes subdural empyema, cranial epidural abscess, and septic venous thrombosis.

of the underlying predisposing infection. The choice of antimicrobial regimens is similar to that for subdural empyema (Table 44.6). Anticoagulation is controversial, and glucocorticoids or osmotic diuretics may be required to control intracranial hypertension. Internal jugular vein ligation has been used in lateral sinus thrombosis, and in a few instances, thrombectomy has been successful. Antimicrobial therapy of mycotic aneurysm is directed at the causative organism of the underlying endarteritis, often associated with positive blood cultures. Prolonged treatment with high-dose intravenous antibiotics for at least 6 to 8 weeks is required. Because the clinical course of a mycotic aneurysm is quite variable, and the risk for rupture with catastrophic cerebral hemorrhage cannot be predicted even after successful therapy of the underlying endocarditis, early surgical intervention is advised. Fortunately, these vascular lesions tend to occur in the distal branches of the middle or anterior cerebral arteries and hence are relatively accessible for surgical ligation or resection.

SPINAL EPIDURAL ABSCESS

Discovery of a spinal epidural abscess is an indication for immediate intravenous antibiotic therapy and surgical evacuation unless the abscess is located below the spinal cord (86). In selected cases, CT-guided needle aspiration may be used in place of laminectomy; if localized pain or radicular symptoms are present without neurological deficit, antibiotic therapy alone, with meticulous serial neurological examinations and repeated MRI or CT studies, may be considered (88). The appearance of neurologic deficit, worsening pain, and increasing temperature and leukocytosis while the patient is receiving antibiotic therapy are indications for surgery (89). The initial empirical antimicrobial therapy should be directed at both *S. aureus* (found in

about 50% of cases) and enteric gram-negative bacilli (Table 44.6). Thus, oxacillin or nafcillin plus an aminoglycoside, a third-generation cephalosporin (e.g., cefotaxime, ceftizoxime, ceftriaxone, or ceftazidime), or a systemic quinolone may be suitable. If infection with *S. aureus* is suspected, nafcillin or methicillin, 2 g every 4 hours, may be added. If the *S. aureus* strain is methicillin resistant, nafcillin should be replaced by vancomycin. An extended-spectrum penicillin (e.g., piperacillin-tazobactam, ticarcillin-clavulanate, imipenem or meropenem) plus an aminoglycoside or an antipseudomonal quinolone (e.g., ciprofloxacin) may be considered if *P. aeruginosa* is suspected. Intravenous therapy should be continued for 4 to 6 weeks after surgical drainage.

Prevention

Parameningeal infections can be prevented only by early and appropriate treatment of the underlying conditions, such as sinusitis, otitis media, mastoiditis, and vertebral osteomyelitis.

REFERENCES

1. McCaig LF, Hughes JM. Trends in antimicrobial drug prescribing among office-based physicians in the United States. *JAMA* 1995;273:214–219.
2. Ray NF, Baraniuk JN, Thamer M, et al. Healthcare expenditures for sinusitis in 1996: contributions of asthma, rhinitis, and other airway disorders. *J Allergy Clin Immunol* 1999;103:408–414.
3. Stammberger HR, Kennedy DW. Paranasal sinuses: anatomic terminology and nomenclature. *Ann Otol Rhinol Laryngol* 1995;167(Suppl):7–16.
4. Sobin J, Engquist S, Nord CE. Bacteriology of the maxillary sinus in healthy volunteers. *Scand J Infect Dis* 1992;24:633–635.
5. Gwaltney JM Jr. Acute community-acquired sinusitis. *Clin Infect Dis* 1996;23:1209–1225.
6. Gwaltney JM Jr, et al. Nose blowing propels nasal fluid into the paranasal sinuses. *Clin Infect Dis* 2000;30:387–391.

7. Kaliner MA, Osguthorpe JD, Fireman P, et al. Sinusitis: bench to bedside. Current findings, future directions. *J Allergy Clin Immunol* 1997;99:S829–S848.

8. Gnoy AR, Gannon PJ, Ganjian E, et al. A potential role for nasal obstruction in development of acute sinusitis: an infection study in rabbits. *Am J Rhinol* 1998;12:399–404.

9. Wagenmann M, Naclerio RM. Anatomic and physiologic considerations in sinusitis. *J Allergy Clin Immunol* 1992;90:419–423.

10. Rudack C, Stoll W, Bachert C. Cytokines in nasal polyposis, acute and chronic sinusitis. *Am J Rhinol* 1998;12:383–388.

11. Grant JA. Sinusitis and associated conditions. *Curr Pract Med* 1999;2:1767–1773.

12. Huang SW. The risk of sinusitis in children with allergic rhinitis. *Allergy Asthma Proc* 2000;21:85–88.

13. Berrettini S, Carabelli A, Sellari-Franceschini S, et al. Perennial allergic rhinitis and chronic sinusitis: correlation with rhinologic risk factors. *Allergy* 1999;54:242–248.

14. Annesi-Maesano I. Epidemiological evidence of the occurrence of rhinitis and sinusitis in asthmatics. *Allergy* 1999;54(Suppl 57):7–13.

15. Armenaka M, Grizzanti J, Rosenstreich DL. Serum immunoglobulins and IgG subclass levels in adults with chronic sinusitis: evidence for decreased IgG3 levels. *Ann Allergy* 1994;72:507–514.

16. Herrod GH. Immunologic considerations in the child with recurrent or persistent sinusitis. *Allergy Asthma Proc* 1997;18:145–148.

17. George DL, Falk PS, Umberto MG, et al. Nosocomial sinusitis in patients in the medical intensive care unit: a prospective epidemiological study. *Clin Infect Dis* 1998;27:463–470.

18. Bertrand B, Rombaux P, Eloy P, et al. Sinusitis of dental origin. *Acta Otorhinolaryngol Belg* 1997;51:315–322.

19. Isaacson G, Yanagisawa E. Cystic fibrosis and sinusitis. *Ear Nose Throat J* 1998;77:886–888.

20. Castillo L, Roger PM, Haddad A, et al. Chronic sinusitis in patients infected by HIV: therapeutic strategies. *Ann Otolaryngol Chir Cervicofac* 1999;116:162–166.

21. Gwaltney J Jr, Phillips CD, Miller RD, et al. Computed tomographic study of the common cold. *N Engl J Med* 1994;330:25–30.

22. Anon JB. Report of the Rhinosinusitis Task Force Committee meeting. *Otolaryngol Head Neck Surg* 1996;117(Suppl):S1–S57.

23. Lanza DC, Kennedy DW. Adult rhinosinusitis defined. *Otolaryngol Head Neck Surg* 1997;117 (Suppl):S1–S7.

24. Wald ER. Sinusitis. *Pediatr Ann* 1998;27:811–818.

25. Williams JW Jr, Simel DL, Roberts L, et al. Clinical evaluation for sinusitis: making the diagnosis by history and physical examination. *Ann Intern Med* 1992;117:705–710.

26. Lew D, Southwick FS, Montgomery WW, et al. Sphenoid sinusitis: a review of 30 cases. *N Engl J Med* 1983;309:1149–1154.

27. Rombaux P, Bertrand B, Eloy P. Sinusitis in the immunocompromised host. *Acta Otorhinolaryngol Belg* 1997;51:305–313.

28. Melen I, Lindahl L, Andreasson L et al. Chronic maxillary sinusitis: definition, diagnosis and relation to dental infections and nasal polyposis. *Acta Otolaryngol* 1986;101:320–327.

29. Lindbaek M, Hjortdahl P, Johnsen UL. Use of symptoms, signs, and blood tests to diagnose acute sinus infections in primary care: comparison with computed tomography. *Fam Med* 1996;28:183–188.

30. Benninger MS, Sedory Holzer SE, Lau J. Diagnosis and treatment of uncomplicated acute bacterial rhinosinusitis: summary of the Agency for Health Care Policy and Research evidence-based report. *Otolaryngol Head Neck Surg* 2000;122:1–7.

31. Cascade PN. ACR appropriateness criteria project. *Radiology* 2000;214(Suppl):21–25.

32. Laine K, Maatta T, Varonen H, et al. Diagnosing acute maxillary sinusitis in primary care: a comparison of ultrasound, clinical examination and radiography. *Rhinology* 1998;36:2–6.

33. Talbot G, Kennedy D, Scheld WM, et al. *Correlation of sinus endoscopy vs. sinus aspiration for microbiologic documentation of acute maxillary sinusitis* [Abstract]. Presented at the 35th International Conference on Antimicrobial Agents and Chemotherapy, San Francisco, September 17–20, 1995.

34. Jousimies-Somer HR, Savolainen S, Ylikoski JS. Bacteriological findings of acute maxillary sinusitis in young adults. *J Clin Microbiol* 1988;26:1919–1925.

35. Gwaltney J Jr. Microbiology of sinusitis. In: Druce HM, ed. *Sinusitis: pathophysiology and treatment.* New York: Marcel Decker, 1994:41–56.

36. Wald ER. Microbiology of acute and chronic sinusitis in children and adults. *Am J Med Sci* 1998;316:13–20.

37. Maresch G, Ulm C, Solar P et al. Etiology of odontogenic maxillary sinusitis. *Head Neck Otolaryngol* 1999;47:748–755.

38. Hammerschlag MR. The role of *Chlamydia* in upper respiratory tract infections. *Curr Infect Dis Rep* 2000;2:115–120.

39. Savolainen S, Jousimies-Somer H, Kleemola M, et al. Serological evidence of viral or *Mycoplasma pneumoniae* infection in acute maxillary sinusitis. *Eur J Clin Microbiol Infect Dis* 1989;8:131–135.

40. Pitkaranta A, Starck M, Savolainen S, et al. Rhinovirus RNA in the maxillary sinus epithelium of adult patients with acute sinusitis. *Clin Infect Dis* 2001;33:909–911.

41. Bert F, Lambert-Zechovsky N. Sinusitis in mechanically ventilated patients and its role in the pathogenesis of nosocomial pneumonia. *Eur J Clin Microbiol Infect Dis* 1996;15:533–544.

42. Del Borgo C, Del Forno A, Ottaviani F, et al. Sinusitis in HIV-infected patients. *J Chemother* 1997;9:83–88.

43. Hunt SM, Miyamoto RC, Cornelius RS, et al. Invasive fungal sinusitis in the acquired immunodeficiency syndrome. *Otolaryngol Clin North Am* 2000;33:335–347.

44. deShazo RD. Fungal sinusitis. *Am J Med Sci* 1998;316:39–45.

45. Stalman W, van Essen GA, van der GY, et al. Maxillary sinusitis in adults: an evaluation of placebo-controlled double-blind trials. *Fam Pract* 1997;14:124–129.

46. van Buchem FL, Knottnerus JA, Schrijnemaekers VJ, et al. Primary-care–based randomised placebo-controlled trial of antibiotic treatment in acute maxillary sinusitis. *Lancet* 1997;349:683–687.

47. Garbutt JM, Goldstein M, Gellman E, et al. A randomized, placebo-controlled trial of antimicrobial treatment for children with clinically diagnosed acute sinusitis. *Pediatrics* 2001;107:619–625.

48. Lindbaek M, Hjortdahl P, Johnsen ULH. Randomised, double-blind, placebo controlled trial of penicillin V and amoxycillin in treatment acute sinus infections in adults. *BMJ* 1996;313:325–329.

49. Hansen JG, Schmidt H, Grinsted P. Randomised, double blind, placebo controlled trial of penicillin V in the treatment of acute maxillary sinusitis in adults in general practice. *Scand J Prim Health Care* 2000;18:44–47.

50. Kaiser L, Morabia A, Stalder H, et al. Role of nasopharyngeal culture in antibiotic prescription for patients with common cold or acute sinusitis. *Eur J Clin Microbiol Infect Dis* 2001;20:445–451.

51. Agency for Health Care Policy and Research (AHCPR). Diagnosis and treatment of acute bacterial rhinosinusitis. *Evidence Report/Technology Assessment: Number 9.* Rockville, MD: AHCPR, US Department of Health and Human Services, 1999:1–7.

52. Institute for Clinical Systems Integration. Acute sinusitis in adults. *Postgraduate Med* 1998;103:154–168.

53. Williams JW Jr, Aguilar C, Makela M, et al. Antibiotics for acute maxillary sinusitis. *Cochrane Database Syst Rev* 2000;CD000243.

54. Thornsberry C, Ogilvie P, Kahn J, et al. Surveillance of antimicrobial resistance in *Streptococcus pneumoniae, Haemophilus influenzae,* and *Moraxella catarrhalis* in the United States in 1996–1997 respiratory season. *Diagn Microbiol Infect Dis* 1997;29:249–257.

55. Chow AW. Infections of the oral cavity, neck and head. In: Mandell GL, Bennett JE, Dolin R, eds. *Principles and practice of infectious diseases.* New York: Churchill Livingstone, 2000:689–702.

56. Williams JW Jr, Holleman DR Jr, Samsa GP, et al. Randomized controlled trial of 3 vs 10 days of trimethoprim/sulfamethoxazole for acute maxillary sinusitis. *JAMA* 1995;273:1015–1021.

57. Murray BE. The growing threat of penicillin-resistant *Streptococcus pneumoniae. Infect Dis Clin Pract* 1997;6(Suppl 2):S21–S27.

58. Doern GV, Pfaller MA, Kugler K, et al. Prevalence of antimicrobial resistance among respiratory tract isolates of *Streptococcus pneumoniae* in North America: 1977 results from the SENTRY Antimicrobial Surveillance Program. *Clin Infect Dis* 1998;27:764–770.

59. Zhanel GG, Karlowsky JA, Palatnick L, et al. Prevalence of antimicrobial resistance in respiratory tract isolates of *Streptococcus pneumoniae:* results of a Canadian national surveillance study. The Canadian Respiratory Infection Study Group. *Antimicrob Agents Chemother* 1999;43:2504–2509.

60. Low DE. Resistance issues and treatment implications: *Pneumococcus, Staphylococcus aureus* and gram negative rods. *Infect Dis Clin North Am* 1998;12:613–630.

61. Clifford K, Huck W, Shan M, et al. Double-blind comparative trial of ciprofloxacin versus clarithromycin in the treatment of acute bacterial sinusitis. Sinusitis Infection Study Group. *Ann Otol Rhinol Laryngol* 1998;108:360–367.

62. Chen DK, McGeer A, de Azavedo JC, et al. Decreased susceptibility of *Streptococcus pneumoniae* to fluoroquinolones in Canada. Canadian Bacterial Surveillance Network. *N Engl J Med* 1999;341:233–239.

63. Holzapfel L, Chastang C, Demingeon G, et al. A randomized study assessing the systematic search for maxillary sinusitis in nasotracheally mechanically ventilated patients: influence of nosocomial maxillary sinusitis on the occurrence of ventilator-associated pneumonia. *Am J Respir Crit Care Med* 1999;159:695–701.

64. Rizk SS, Kraus DH, Gerresheim G, et al. Aggressive combination treatment for invasive fungal sinusitis in immunocompromised patients. *Ear Nose Throat J* 2000;79:278–285.

65. Beste DJ, Capper DT, Shaffer K, et al. Antimicrobial effect on rabbit sinusitis after temporary ostial occlusion. *Am J Rhinol* 1997;11:485–489.

66. Noye KA, Brodovsky D, Coyle S, et al. Classification, diagnosis and treatment of sinusitis: evidence-based clinical practice guidelines. *Can J Infect Dis* 1998;9 (Suppl B):3B–24B.

67. Toohill RJ, Lehman RH, Grossman TW, et al. Rhinitis medicamentasa. *Laryngoscope* 1981;91:1614–1621.

68. Turner RB, Sperber SJ, Sorrentino JV, et al. Effectiveness of clemastine fumarate for treatment of rhinorrhea and sneezing associated with the common cold. *Clin Infect Dis* 1997;25:824–830.

69. Low DE, Desrosiers M, McSherry J, et al. A practical guide for the diagnosis and treatment of acute sinusitis [see comments]. *CMAJ* 1997;156(Suppl 6):S1–14.

70. Meltzer EO, Orgel HA, Backhaus JW, et al. Intranasal flunisolide spray as an adjunct to oral antibiotic therapy for sinusitis. *J Allergy Clin Immunol* 1993;92:812–823.

71. Barlan IB, Erkan E, Bakir M, et al. Intranasal budesonide spray as an adjunct to oral antibiotic therapy for acute sinusitis in children. *Ann Allergy Asthma Immunol* 1997;78:598–601.

72. Benninger MS, Anon J, Mabry RL. The medical management of rhinosinusitis. *Otolaryngol Head Neck Surg* 1997;117:S41–S49.
73. Shoseyov D, Bibi H, Shai P, et al. Treatment with hypertonic saline versus normal saline nasal wash of pediatric chronic sinusitis. *J Allergy Clin Immunol* 1998;101:602–605.
74. Singh M. Heated, humidified air for the common cold. *Cochrane Database Syst Rev* 2000;CD001728.
75. Marshall I. Zinc for the common cold. *Cochrane Database Syst Rev* 2000; CD001364.
76. Melchart D, Linde K, Fischer P, et al. Echinacea for preventing and treating the common cold. *Cochrane Database Syst Rev* 2000;CD000530.
77. Sobol SE, Wright ED, Frenkiel S. One-year outcome analysis of functional endoscopic sinus surgery for chronic sinusitis. *J Otolaryngol* 1998;27:252–257.
78. Chow AW. Life-threatening infections of the head, neck, and upper respiratory tract. In: Hall JB, Schmidt GA, Wood LDH, eds. *Principles of critical care.* New York: McGraw-Hill, 1998;887–902.
79. Gallagher RM, Gross CW, Phillips CD. Suppurative intracranial complications of sinusitis. *Laryngoscope* 1998;108:1635–1642.
80. Nussbaum ES, Rigamonti D, Standiford H, et al. Spinal epidural abscess: a report of 40 cases and review. *Surg Neurol* 1992;38:225–231.
81. Giannoni C, Sulek M, Friedman EM. Intracranial complications of sinusitis: a pediatric series. *Am J Rhinol* 1998;12:173–178.
82. Latchaw RE, Hirsch WL Jr, Yock DH Jr. Imaging of intracranial infection. *Neurosurg Clin North Am* 1992;3:303–322.
83. Ueberall MA, Wunsiedler U, Renner C, et al. Epidural and pericranial abscesses complicating frontal sinusitis in a comatose child. *Pediatr Neurol* 1998;19:385–387.
84. Koivunen P, Löppönen H, Syrjälä H. Epidural abscess due to deep-neck infection. *Clin Infect Dis* 1998;26:1461–1462.
85. Odabasi AO, Akgul A. Cavernous sinus thrombosis: a rare complication of sinusitis. *Int J Pediatr Otorhinolaryngol* 1997;39:77–83.
86. Mackenzie AR, Laing RBS, Smith CC, et al. Spinal epidural abscess: the importance of early diagnosis and treatment. *J Neurol Neurosurg Psychiatry* 1998;65:209–212.
87. Rosenfeld EA, Rowley AH. Infectious intracranial complications of sinusitis, other than meningitis, in children: 12 year review. *Clin Infect Dis* 1994;18:750–754.
88. Wheeler D, Keiser P, Rigamonti D, et al. Medical management of spinal epidural abscesses: case report and review. *Clin Infect Dis* 1992;15:22–27.
89. Rea GL, McGregor JM, Miller CA, et al. Surgical treatment of the spontaneous spinal epidural abscess. *Surg Neurol* 1992;37:274–279.
90. Chow AW. Acute sinusitis: current status of etiologies, diagnosis, and treatment. *Curr Clin Top Infect Dis* 2001;21:31–63.

CHAPTER 45
Ear and Mastoid Infections

Charles D. Bluestone

Otitis media is the most common diagnosis today for office visits to physicians in the United States. This finding was reported by the National Center for Health Statistics (1), which also found that the diagnosis had increased from about 10 million visits in 1975 to 25 million in 1990. Most likely, even more patients have the diagnosis in this new century. Although common in adults, the disease affects primarily infants and children. As reported by the National Center for Health Statistics, the annual visit rate for children younger than 2 years of age statistically increased by 224% during the period of the study, and significant increases occurred in older children, but not as dramatically. In Boston, a survey of about 17,000 office visits during the first year of life revealed that otitis media was the diagnosis in about one third of visits for illness and one fifth of all office visits (2). In a prospective study of newborns followed monthly from birth to their second birthday in Pittsburgh, Casselbrant and colleagues (3) reported that almost 90% had at least one episode of otitis media. It is likely that the increase in day care attendance, a known risk factor, during this same period is related to this rise in the disease in infants and young children.

It is estimated that more than $5 billion is spent annually for the care of otitis media in the United States (4). Of the estimated 120 million prescriptions written for oral antimicrobial agents each year in this country, more than one fourth are for the treatment of otitis media (5). Myringotomy with insertion of tympanostomy tube is the most common surgical procedure performed in children for which a general anesthetic is required, and tonsillectomy and adenoidectomy are still the most common major surgical procedures performed in children, many of which are for the prevention of otitis media. Otitis media is, indeed, a major health problem.

ACUTE OTITIS MEDIA

Diagnosis

The rapid, brief onset of signs and symptoms of infection in the middle ear is termed *acute otitis media*. Synonyms such as *acute suppurative* and *purulent otitis media* are acceptable. One or more of the following are present: otalgia (or pulling of the ear in the young infant), fever, or irritability of recent onset. The tympanic membrane is full or bulging and opaque, and it has limited or no mobility to pneumatic otoscopy, all of which are indicative of a middle ear effusion. The acute onset of ear pain, fever, and a purulent discharge (otorrhea) through a perforation of the tympanic membrane or tympanostomy tube would also be evidence of acute otitis media.

In this era of antibiotic-resistant bacterial pathogens causing acute otitis media, it is important to distinguish between acute otitis media and otitis media with effusion because the latter disease does not routinely require treatment unless it is chronic (6). The major difference between the diseases is that otitis media with effusion is relatively asymptomatic, whereas acute otitis media is associated with the signs and symptoms of acute infection, such as otalgia and fever.

When the diagnosis of acute otitis media is in doubt or when determination of the etiologic agent is desirable, aspiration of the middle ear should be performed by the clinician. If he or she is not skilled in this procedure, the patient can be referred to an otolaryngologist (7). Today, with the emergence of resistant bacterial organisms causing otitis media, such as β-lactamase–producing *Haemophilus influenzae* and *Moraxella catarrhalis*, and the more recent troublesome rise in penicillin- and multidrug-resistant pneumococcus (8,9), tympanocentesis is an important diagnostic procedure (10). Indications for tympanocentesis (or myringotomy) include the following:

- Otitis media in patients who have severe otalgia, are seriously ill, or appear toxic
- Unsatisfactory response to antimicrobial therapy
- Onset of otitis media in a child who is receiving appropriate and adequate antimicrobial therapy
- Otitis media associated with a confirmed or potential suppurative complication
- Otitis media in a newborn infant, an ill neonate, or an immunologically deficient patient, any of whom might harbor an unusual organism (11)

Unfortunately, nasopharyngeal cultures do not accurately identify the causative organism in children with acute otitis media.

Characteristics of the Pathogens

Effective treatment of acute otitis media in infants, children, and adults should be based on knowledge of the bacterial etiology. Figure 45.1 shows the distribution of bacteria from

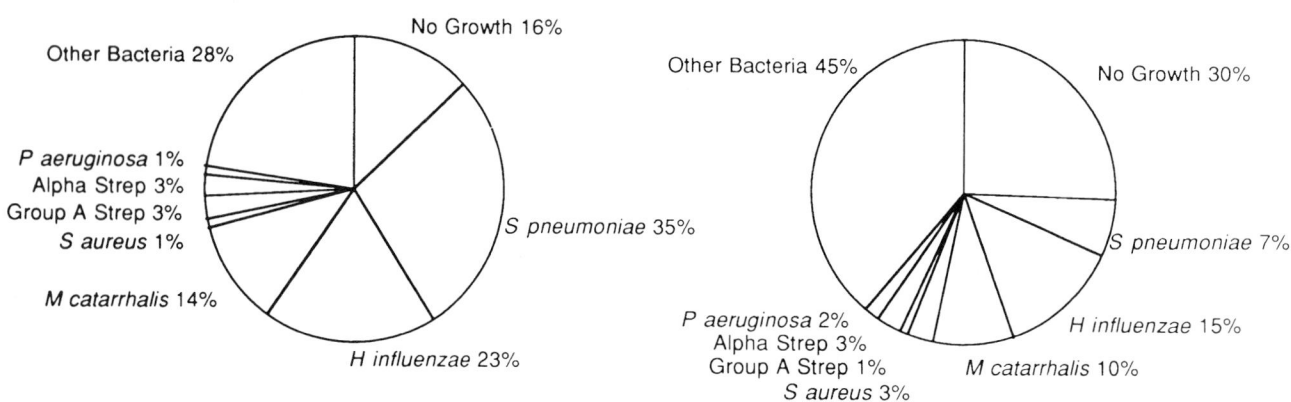

Figure 45.1. Comparison of bacteria from middle ear aspirates obtained by tympanocentesis in infants and children with acute otitis media (*AOM*) or otitis media with effusion (*OME*), the latter immediately before insertion of tympanostomy tubes. Totals may add up to more than 100% because of the presence of multiple pathogens. (From Bluestone CD, Stephenson JS, Martin LM. Ten-year review of otitis media pathogens. *Pediatr Infect Dis J* 1992;11:S7–S11, with permission.)

middle ear aspirates isolated from 1980 to 1989 at our Otitis Media Research Center (12). *Streptococcus pneumoniae* was the predominant pathogen cultured (35%) from aspirates of patients who had acute otitis media during this 10-year period; however, this rate significantly increased from 29% in 1980 to 44% in 1989 (Fig. 45.2). *H. influenzae* was the second most common pathogen isolated in acute ear infections (23%). Before 1980, the frequency of *M. catarrhalis* was less than 10%, but it is now present in 14% of acute effusions. Group A β-hemolytic streptococcus, *Staphylococcus aureus*, anaerobic bacteria, and viruses were infrequently cultured from middle ear aspirates of these children.

Figure 45.3 shows that the percentage of β-lactamase–producing *H. influenzae* (primarily nontypable in otitis media) is now more than 30% in the Pittsburgh area. This percentage has increased during the 1980s, as has that for *M. catarrhalis*. Currently, most if not all strains of *M. catarrhalis* produce β-lactamase. Mason and colleagues (13) reported that the middle ear was the most common site in which resistant pneumococcus was isolated at their children's hospital in Houston. Reichler and colleagues (14) reported a high rate of resistant pneumococcus

in day care centers. Jacobs and co-workers (15) reported that the incidence of penicillin-resistant strains varied between 36% and 62%. The Centers for Disease Control and Prevention (CDC) recently reported that the prevalence of multidrug-resistant pneumococcus has progressively increased in the United States in the 1990s. In 1993, we isolated resistant *S. pneumoniae* in fewer than 30% of isolates at the Children's Hospital of Pittsburgh, but in 2000, the rate of these resistant pneumococci was about 45% (unpublished data). The increase in the frequency of these antibiotic-resistant pathogens has an important impact on management of otitis media in children today.

Many have thought that *H. influenzae* is an uncommon etiologic agent in acute otitis media in adults. However, in a study conducted at our center that involved 34 adults who had an episode of acute otitis media, we found that 26% of acute middle ear effusions demonstrated isolates of this organism and that 22.5% of *H. influenzae* produced β-lactamase (16). *S. pneumoniae* was recovered in only 21% of the aspirates; both *M. catarrhalis* (β-lactamase–producing) and *Streptococcus pyogenes* were isolated in 3%. Overall, 9% of the subjects had β-lactamase–producing organisms.

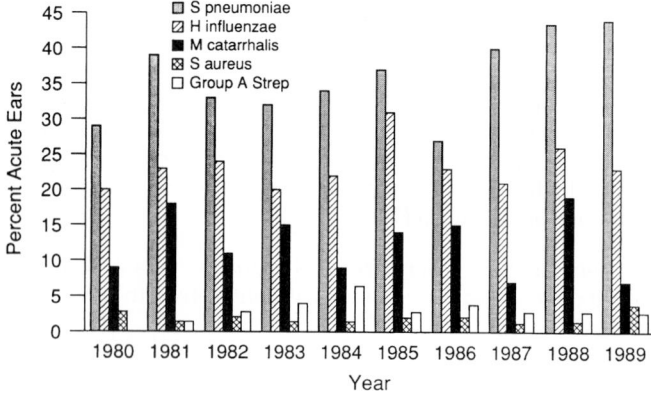

Figure 45.2. Frequency of the most common pathogens causing acute otitis media during the 1980s. (From Bluestone CD, Stephenson JS, Martin LM. Ten-year review of otitis media pathogens. *Pediatr Infect Dis J* 1992;11:S7–S11, with permission.)

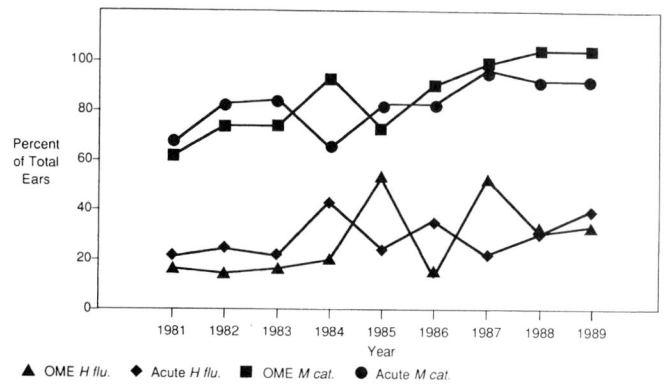

Figure 45.3. Percentage of β-lactamase–producing *H. influenzae* and *M. catarrhalis* in acute otitis media (*AOM*) and otitis media with effusion (*OME*), 1981 to 1989. (From Bluestone CD, Stephenson JS, Martin LM. Ten-year review of otitis media pathogens. *Pediatr Infect Dis J* 1992;11:S7–S11, with permission.)

Management

Most experts in the United States agree that patients who have the signs and symptoms of acute otitis media should receive antimicrobial therapy (6). However, several reports have questioned the need for antimicrobial agents in all cases (17–19). Nevertheless, in a clinical trial by Howie and Ploussard (20), antimicrobial agents were shown to be superior to placebo in "sterilizing" the middle ear effusion. In addition, a large clinical trial by Kaleida and colleagues (21) found that subjects who had "severe" acute otitis media and who had been randomized to receive myringotomy without antibiotics had statistically more initial treatment failures than those children who received an antimicrobial agent with or without the adjunctive use of a myringotomy. As part of that trial, another group of children who had "nonsevere" acute otitis media were randomized to receive either antibiotic or placebo, and those in the placebo group also had more treatment failures as well as more time with middle ear effusion than those in the antibiotic group.

An even more compelling reason to administer antimicrobials is that the rate of suppurative complications has decreased in the antibiotic era (22). Two important, large clinical trials conducted in Scandinavia in the 1950s, in which either patients were treated with an antibiotic or the agents were withheld, demonstrated that the suppurative complications of otitis media, such as mastoiditis and meningitis, occurred almost exclusively in those children who did not receive antimicrobial agents (23,24). Withholding antimicrobial therapy today will most likely result in an increase in complications. Indeed, Hoppe and colleagues (25) reported that the rate of acute mastoiditis has statistically increased in their children's hospital in Germany, which they attributed in some cases to withholding antimicrobial agents. However, Bahadori and colleagues (26) reported that the rate of acute mastoiditis has recently increased dramatically in a suburban children's hospital in Northern Virginia, which could be attributed neither to lack of antimicrobial treatment nor to penicillin-resistant pneumococcus. Another report from eight children's hospitals in the United States revealed that the rate of acute mastoiditis due to pneumococcus has not increased during the recent past despite the increase in antibiotic-resistant *S. pneumococcus* (27).

Amoxicillin is the drug currently preferred for initial empirical therapy of acute otitis media (6). It is active both *in vitro* and *in vivo* against most strains of *S. pneumoniae* and *H. influenzae*, and it is relatively inexpensive in the United States; 40 mg/kg/day in three divided doses for 10 days is recommended. If the patient is allergic to the penicillins, one of the newer macrolides, azithromycin or clarithromycin, is advocated; as an alternative, one of the cephalosporins (e.g., cefuroxime axetil, cefdinir, or cefpodoxime) could be used if the patient does not have hypersensitivity to these agents and does not have an immediate hypersensitivity reaction to the penicillins. If β-lactamase–producing *H. influenzae* or *M. catarrhalis* organisms are isolated by tympanocentesis or from otorrhea fluid—in which case amoxicillin would not be appropriate—then the choices would also be these antimicrobials or amoxicillin-clavulanate. Eight cephalosporins are currently approved for treatment of acute otitis media: the second-generation agents cefaclor, loracarbef, cefuroxime axetil, cefprozil, and cefdinir, and the third-generation drugs cefpodoxime, cefixime, and ceftriaxone (available only in the parenteral form). Trimethoprim-sulfamethoxazole would also be a possible alternative, but it is associated with adverse reactions. Antimicrobial agents currently approved by the Food and Drug Administration (FDA) in the United States for acute otitis media are listed in Table 45.1.

TABLE 45.1. Antimicrobial Agents Approved for Therapy of Acute Otitis Media: United States, 2001

Drug	Trade name
Amoxicillin	Amoxil
Amoxicillin-clavulanate	Augmentin
Cephalexin	Keflex
Cefaclor	Ceclor
Loracarbef	Lorabid
Cefixime	Suprax
Ceftibuten	Cedax
Cefprozil	Cefzil
Cefpodoxime	Vantin
Cefuroxime axetil	Ceftin
Cefdinir	Omnicef
Ceftriaxone IM	Rocephin
Erythromycin plus sulfisoxazole	Pediazole
Azithromycin	Zithromax
Clarithromycin	Biaxin
Trimethoprim-sulfamethoxazole	Bactrim, Septra
Ofloxacin otic	Floxin Otic

Even though no data are available on the efficacy of these antimicrobial agents for treatment of adults with acute otitis media, the recommendations discussed earlier should be applied to adults as well because the causative organisms are similar in adults and children. Thus, empirical use of such agents as the tetracyclines, penicillin V, erythromycin, or cephalexin is not recommended as monotherapy. The quinolones, such as ciprofloxacin, are not indicated in children younger than 17 years, and efficacy of these antimicrobial agents has not been reported in adults with acute otitis media.

If there is a high rate of penicillin-resistant *S. pneumoniae* in the community, the dose of amoxicillin should be increased to 80 mg/kg/day, which can now be administered in two divided doses per day. If a multidrug-resistant pneumococcus is isolated from the middle ear, the choice of agent should be selected according to the results of the susceptibility testing. Parenteral vancomycin is the drug of choice today when the patient is seriously ill and in a toxic condition because of to multidrug-resistant pneumococcus.

With appropriate antimicrobial therapy, most cases of acute bacterial otitis media improve significantly within 48 to 72 hours. If signs and symptoms of infection progress despite initial therapy, the patient should be reevaluated within 24 hours; a suppurative complication may have developed, or there may be a concurrent serious infection (e.g., an infant may have meningitis). Persistent or recurrent pain or fever, or both, during treatment would signal the need for tympanocentesis and myringotomy (for Gram stain, culture, and susceptibility testing), selection of another antimicrobial agent, or both. As stated before, tympanocentesis should be more frequently employed when appropriate and when adequate antimicrobial therapy fails because resistant organisms may be the cause of the antibiotic treatment failure.

If a middle ear aspirate is not obtained for culture and susceptibility testing, the agent chosen should be effective against whatever resistant bacteria have been found to be in the community that have been associated with symptomatic treatment failures. The new antimicrobial agent should be effective against penicillin-resistant pneumococcus and β-lactamase–producing bacteria, such as *H. influenzae* or *M. catarrhalis*. If amoxicillin was given initially in the standard dose, then the dose should be increased and given in combination with amoxicillin-clavulanate at this stage. An alternative would be either cefuroxime axetil or cefdinir. Also, a single parenteral dose of ceftriaxone (50 mg/kg) can be given, in which case the child should be reexamined in 48 hours and, if still symptomatic, another dose administered; a third dose in 48 to 72 hours may also be required. Also, ceftriaxone is an ideal agent when the child has severe symptoms, compliance with taking oral antimicrobials is doubtful, or the patient is vomiting.

Patients who have relatively severe acute otitis media, especially infants, should probably be reexamined at the end of the course of antibiotic therapy (i.e., after 10 to 14 days), at which time some patients (about 50%) will have a persistent middle ear effusion. The presence of persistent effusion after a 10-day trial of an antimicrobial agent is common, and it is usually asymptomatic in infants and children. However, Mandel and colleagues (28) conducted a clinical trial in children in which 20-day therapy was compared with the traditional 10-day course. They recommended having children who are asymptomatic return for their first follow-up visit in 4 weeks because further treatment with antimicrobial therapy immediately after 10-day treatment in the trial provided no long-term advantage. However, patients who still have any signs or symptoms of acute infection should be reevaluated during or at the end of the initial course of treatment and managed as a treatment failure (discussed earlier).

Additional supportive therapy, such as analgesics or antipyretics, may be helpful at the onset of the illness. An oral decongestant, such as pseudoephedrine hydrochloride, may relieve nasal congestion, and antihistamines may help patients with known or suspected nasal allergy; however, the use of antihistamines for treatment of upper respiratory tract infections is not recommended (29). Administration of antihistamines and decongestants in the treatment of acute otitis media has not been shown to be effective in children.

If complete resolution has occurred and the episode represents the only known attack, the patient may be discharged; however, periodic follow-up is indicated for infants and children who have had recurrent episodes.

PERSISTENT MIDDLE EAR EFFUSION

If the middle ear effusion, which is asymptomatic, persists after the initial 10 days of antimicrobial therapy, further treatment with an antimicrobial agent is not recommended (6). As described before, Mandel and coworkers (28) found no long-term advantage in retreating asymptomatic children with an antimicrobial agent at this stage. Also, two Pittsburgh studies demonstrated inefficacy of a combination of an oral decongestant and antihistamine, with and without amoxicillin, in eliminating persistent middle ear effusion that involved more than 1,000 infants and children, although these studies did not test the efficacy of this combination in patients older than 12 years or in those children who had documented nasal allergy (30,31). Thus, for this stage of otitis media, clinicians do not have to treat patients who have asymptomatic (except for hearing loss) persistent middle ear effusion still present after initial therapy with an antimicrobial agent because most patients will be effusion free at the end of 3 or 4 months without further treatment (32). However, the patient should be reexamined during this period to determine whether the effusion has persisted for 3 months or longer, at which point the effusion is chronic and should be treated as described later for otitis media with effusion. Also, some patients may benefit from further treatment at an earlier time. This is also described later.

RECURRENT ACUTE OTITIS MEDIA

Recurrent acute otitis media is a common problem of infants and young children. The child with recurrent acute otitis media whose infection clears completely between episodes may be treated as outlined previously. The bacteriology of middle ear infection in children who have recurrent episodes of acute otitis media separated by a month or more is similar to that found in first episodes: the predominant pathogens are *S. pneumoniae* and *H. influenzae*. When patients initially receive amoxicillin and then develop a recurrence soon after the course of amoxicillin is completed, resistant organisms are more frequently present. Such patients might benefit from a broader-spectrum antimicrobial agent (33).

If the episodes of acute otitis media are frequent and close together, which is common in infants, prevention of further attacks is desirable. When this occurs, the child requires further evaluation. Several avenues of investigation are open: a search for respiratory allergy may prove fruitful; roentgenograms of the paranasal sinuses may reveal sinusitis; immunological studies may be of value in the infant and young child if other organs are involved (i.e., the lung); but if the child is 5 or 6 years of age or older, an evaluation of immune function might be helpful even if recurrent or chronic ear disease is the only apparent problem. If none of these conditions is present, one or more of the popular methods of prevention may be attempted. For infants and children who have frequent episodes of acute otitis media, without middle ear effusion between the bouts, the most common nonsurgical and surgical methods employed for prevention are (a) vaccines; (b) chemoprophylaxis with an antimicrobial agent; (c) myringotomy with insertion of a tympanostomy tube; and (d) adenoidectomy. Also, the parents can aid in prevention by eliminating passive smoke exposure in the household, avoiding placing the child in a day care facility or choosing one in which there are the fewest number of children possible, keeping the infant in a supine position while sleeping, and taking the pacifier away from infants after the age of 1 year (7).

Vaccines

Since the advent of the widespread administration of the conjugate polysaccharide vaccine for *H. influenzae* type b, the rate of acute otitis media caused by this bacterium has been dramatically reduced, but it only caused about 2% of all attacks before the introduction of the vaccine. However, there are other vaccines that are potentially beneficial for prevention of acute middle ear infections.

Pneumococcal Vaccines. In February 2000, the new sevenvalent pneumococcal polysaccharide-protein conjugate vaccine (PCV7) (Prevnar, Wyeth Lederle Vaccines, St. Davids, Pennsylvania) was approved by the FDA for prevention of invasive pneumococcal disease (e.g., meningitis, bacteremia) in infants and young children. The CDC Advisory Committee on Immunization Practices (ACIP) recommends that the vaccine be given to all infants aged 2 to 23 months and for children aged 24 to 59 months who are at increased risk for pneumococcal disease, such as those children who have sickle cell disease, human immunodeficiency virus infection, and other immunocompromising or chronic medical conditions (34). The ACIP also recommends the vaccine be considered for all other children aged 24 to 59 months, with a priority given to (a) children 24 to 35 months of age; (b) children who are of Alaska Native, Native American, and African American descent; and (c) children who attend group day care centers. Even though this vaccine has been demonstrated to be safe and effective in preventing invasive pneumococcal infections, prevention of otitis media is another potential advantage.

Two large-scale randomized clinical trials were conducted in California and Finland during the past several years, and their outcomes have recently been reported. Black and colleagues

(35) conducted a double-blind trial in Northern California. The serotypes in the pneumococcal conjugate were 4, 6B, 9V, 14, 18C, 19F, and 23F, which are the most common serotypes causing invasive disease in the United States. The primary outcome of the trial was invasive pneumococcal disease caused by vaccine serotypes, but secondary outcome measures included effectiveness against clinical acute otitis media visits and episodes and impact against frequent and severe otitis media and tympanostomy tube placement. Although the vaccine substantially reduced the episodes of acute otitis media, the impact on the middle ear disease was less impressive than for invasive infections. Nevertheless, there was a significant overall decrease in the number of episodes (7.0% per protocol) and of otitis media visits (8.9%) in those who received the vaccine compared with controls. The beneficial impact of the vaccine appeared to favor those children who had recurrent acute otitis media; the need for tympanostomy tube placement was 20% less in those who received the pneumococcal vaccine compared with those who were in the control group.

In contrast to the Northern California trial, otitis media was the primary outcome measure in the clinical trial recently reported (in abstracts) from Finland that also evaluated the efficacy of PCV7 (36). The investigators randomly assigned infants to receive either PCV7 or hepatitis B (control) vaccine. Myringotomy was performed to confirm the presence of acute otitis media, and the middle ear effusion was aspirated to identify the causative bacterial pathogen and serotype pneumococci when isolated. The reduction in the rate of number of episodes was 57% against culture-confirmed vaccine serotypes, 34% against culture-confirmed pneumococcal acute otitis media, irrespective of serotype, and 6% of all acute otitis media, irrespective of etiology.

Thus, all infants in the United States receive the conjugated pneumococcal vaccine, but acute otitis media caused by this bacterium will still be a problem in some children. The vaccine may also benefit children who are older than 2 years of age, have recurrent attacks of acute otitis media, and have not received the vaccine in the past (37).

Viral Vaccines. In anticipation of epidemic influenzal disease, influenza A vaccine administered to infants in Finland attending day care centers reduced the incidence of upper respiratory tract infection, including acute otitis media (38). Also, influenza A vaccine reduced the incidence of acute otitis media in infants in North Carolina who were in day care centers during the influenza season (39). Thus, recommending the influenza vaccine in the fall for infants and children who have had recurrent episodes of acute otitis media appears to have merit.

Antimicrobial Prophylaxis

Several clinical trials conducted in the past have shown antimicrobial prophylaxis to be effective (40–42). A metaanalysis confirmed the beneficial effect of antibiotic prophylaxis (43). For the child who has repeated episodes of otitis media (e.g., three episodes in 6 months or four or five episodes in 12 months, with at least one episode being present during the preceding 6 months), it seems reasonable to recommend amoxicillin at 20 mg/kg in one dose (given at bedtime) (44). If the child is allergic to the penicillins, a daily dose of sulfisoxazole at 50 mg/kg may be substituted. This prophylactic regimen should be continued during the respiratory season. As a note of caution, trimethoprim-sulfamethoxazole is not recommended for prophylaxis of otitis media for any age group because of its possible serious side effects.

Children receiving prophylaxis should be examined at frequent and regular intervals (every 6 to 8 weeks) to be certain that unapparent middle ear effusion, which might become chronic,

does not occur. Prolonged antimicrobial prophylaxis is inappropriate if longstanding persistent middle ear effusion is present. In this case, surgical intervention should be considered, such as myringotomy and tympanostomy tube insertion, with or without adenoidectomy (see later section "Otitis Media with Effusion"). Today, with the emergence of resistant bacteria, myringotomy and tympanostomy tube insertion may be a reasonable alternative to antimicrobial prophylaxis (6,45).

There is no evidence that a topical or systemic nasal decongestant or antihistamine, either alone or in combination, administered daily or at the onset of an upper respiratory tract infection, prevents recurrent acute otitis media. Therefore, the use of such medications for prophylaxis is not recommended until their efficacy is proved.

Surgical Treatment

Because studies reported in the past have shown that some children still have recurrent episodes of acute otitis media despite use of the preventive dose of an antibiotic, myringotomy and tympanostomy tube placement should be considered for patients whose prophylaxis fails. Myringotomy with tympanostomy tube insertion has been shown to be effective for prevention of recurrent acute otitis media in otitis-prone infants compared with nonsurgical control groups (46,47). A clinical trial reported by Casselbrant and coworkers (44) has shown that both amoxicillin prophylaxis and myringotomy with tympanostomy tube insertion were more effective than placebo in the prevention of recurrent acute otitis media; antimicrobial prophylaxis was recommended as the initial method, and for those children in whom prophylaxis failed, tubes were then suggested as an alternative (Table 45.2). Adenoidectomy, with or without tonsillectomy, is frequently advocated for the prevention of recurrent acute otitis media, but only one randomized, controlled study has been reported that has shown the efficacy of adenoidectomy, albeit limited, for this condition. Paradise and co-workers (48) did demonstrate a significant difference in the attack rate of acute otitis media in children who had been randomized to receive adenoidectomy compared with those who did not receive this operation; all subjects in this clinical trial had at least one myringotomy and tympanostomy tube insertion before random assignment (Table 45.3). In a second clinical trial conducted by Paradise and colleagues (49), children who had not had tympanostomy tube placement in the past were randomly assigned to either adenoidectomy, adenotonsillectomy, or control, but in contrast to the first trial, no long-term efficacy in prevention of recurrent acute otitis media was found. However, as a note of caution, adenoidectomy in infants should be recommended only selectively (such as in those who also have severe nasal obstruction due to obstructive adenoids) because the operation carries some degree of increased risk in this age group.

In cases of recurrent otitis media, the decision should be between administering an antibiotic in a prophylactic dose and performing myringotomy with insertion of a tympanostomy tube, with adenoidectomy in selected patients. Today, a surgical option is more desirable than long-term antibiotic prophylaxis, given the antibiotic-resistance problem; antimicrobial prophylaxis is reserved for children who are anesthetic risks or are immunocompromised. My own preference is to insert tympanostomy tubes as the initial procedure, and if the patient continues to have recurrent attacks of acute middle ear infection following extrusion of the tubes, I recommend an adenoidectomy, irrespective of the size of the adenoids, and a reinsertion of the tympanostomy tubes.

In some patients, insertion of tympanostomy tubes prevents the severe symptoms of acute otitis media, but recurrent episodes of otorrhea still occur (44,50). A systemic antimicrobial agent,

TABLE 45.2.   Outcome of Randomized 2-Year Clinical Trial of Amoxicillin Prophylaxis and of Tympanostomy Tube Insertion Versus Placebo for Prevention of Recurrent Acute Otitis Media in 264 Pittsburgh Children, 7 to 35 Months of Age

	Treatment groups			p Value groups		
	1	2	3	1 vs. 2	3 vs. 2	1 vs. 3
Outcome measure	Amoxicillin	Placebo	Tympanostomy tube			
Rates of AOM or AOM-otorrhea (child-years)	0.60	1.08	1.02	<0.001	NS	0.001
Mean percentage of time with OM	10.0	15.0	6.6	0.03	<0.001	NS
Median time to first episode of AOM-otorrhea (months)	22.1	8.2	11.2	0.002	NS	—

AOM, acute otitis media; OM, otitis media; NS, not significant.
Adapted from Casselbrant ML, Kaleida PH, Rockette HE, et al. Efficacy of antimicrobial prophylaxis and of tympanostomy tube insertion for prevention of recurrent acute otitis media: results of a randomized clinical trial. *Pediatr Infect Dis J* 1992;11:278–286, with permission.

an ototopical antibiotic-cortisone medication, or both is usually effective in resolving the otitis media. Currently, the only FDA-approved ototopical agent when acute otorrhea develops following tympanostomy tube placement is ofloxacin (51).

For the rare child whose tympanostomy tubes fail to prevent frequently recurrent acute otitis media (who have otorrhea through the tube), the combination of antimicrobial prophylaxis and tympanostomy tube insertion is usually effective in preventing the recurrent episodes.

These management options should be offered only to children who do not have chronic middle ear effusion. If recurrent bouts of acute otitis media are superimposed on the chronic condition, the child should be treated as described in the following section on management of chronic otitis media with effusion.

OTITIS MEDIA WITH EFFUSION

Diagnosis

The presence of a relatively asymptomatic middle ear effusion has many synonyms, such as *secretory*, *nonsuppurative*, and *serous* otitis media, but the most acceptable term is *otitis media with effusion*. Pneumatic otoscopy frequently reveals either a retracted or concave tympanic membrane whose mobility is limited or absent. However, fullness or even bulging may be visualized. In addition, an air-fluid level, bubbles, or both may be observed through a translucent tympanic membrane. The duration (not the severity) of the effusion can be classified as acute (less than 3 weeks), subacute (3 weeks to 3 months), or chronic (longer than 3 months). The most important distinction between this type of

disease and acute otitis media is that the signs and symptoms of acute infection are lacking in otitis media with effusion (e.g., otalgia, fever), but hearing loss is usually present in both conditions.

Microbiology

For decades, otitis media with effusion was assumed to be sterile because several reports described unsuccessful attempts to culture bacteria (52,53). However, studies reported during the past 15 years identified bacteria by means of smears and cultures (54–57). A study was conducted in Pittsburgh by Riding and co-workers (57) of 179 children aged 1 to 16 years who had chronic middle ear effusions. Of 179 ears, bacteria were cultured from 86 (48%) chronic middle ear effusions. Bacteria were present in serous and mucoid effusions as well as in the purulent type.

More recent findings from our center (Fig. 45.1) showed that of middle ear aspirates from ears with chronic otitis media with effusion, about two thirds had bacteria isolated; of the one third that were considered to be pathogens, the most common bacteria were *H. influenzae*, *M. catarrhalis*, and *S. pneumoniae*, which are the common pathogens found in middle ear aspirates from children with acute otitis media. In addition, *Staphylococcus epidermidis* was cultured from many middle ears when it was not cultured from the external canal of the same ear. (A culture preceded sterilization and tympanocentesis.) β-Lactamase activity was similar to that reported for isolates from ears with acute otitis media; anaerobic bacteria were also isolated in about 10%. Currently, the antibiotic-resistance rates of three major pathogens are similar to those found in middle ear aspirates from acute effusions.

TABLE 45.3.   Efficacy of Adenoidectomy for Recurrent Otitis Media in Children Previously Treated with Tympanostomy Tube Placement

	Treatment group	No. of subjects	Mean no. episodes of otitis media	p Value[a]	Proportion of days otitis media present	p Value[a]
First year	Adenoidectomy	48	1.06	0.51	15.0	0.04
	Control	38	1.45		28.5	
Second year	Adenoidectomy	45	1.09	0.01	17.8	0.005
	Control	27	1.67		28.4	

[a]p Values by χ^2 test.
Adapted from Paradise JL, Bluestone CD, Rogers KD, et al. Efficacy of adenoidectomy for recurrent otitis media in children previously treated with tympanostomy-tube placement: results of parallel randomized and nonrandomized trials. *JAMA* 1990;263:2066–2073, with permission. Copyright 1900, American Medical Association.

Haddad and colleagues (58) recently reported that nonsusceptible *S. pneumoniae* was present in 52% of isolates from chronic effusions in children in New York.

Post and colleagues (59) found that 78% of middle ear effusions had evidence of the three major organisms (i.e., *H. influenzae*, *M. catarrhalis*, and *S. pneumoniae*) by polymerase chain reaction, whereas only 28% of the aspirates were culture positive. From this study, and a subsequent one by Rayner and co-workers (60), the investigators postulated that bacteria may have a larger role in the inflammatory process than previously believed.

Unfortunately, information concerning the microbiology of otitis media with effusion that occurs in adults is not available.

Infants and children who have otitis media with effusion most likely have a condition that is an extension of an upper respiratory tract infection, which should resolve spontaneously without active treatment (61). Casselbrant and coworkers (62) reported that about 80% of preschool-aged children who developed otitis media with effusion while attending a day care center in a Pittsburgh suburb had their effusions clear without treatment within 2 months. Treatment may be indicated in some children, however, because there are possible complications and sequelae associated with this condition. Because little information is presently available regarding the frequency of these complications and sequelae, some clinicians advocate taking a watch-and-wait position and not actively treating such a child (63). However, hearing loss of some degree usually accompanies a middle ear effusion (64). Although the significance of this hearing loss is still uncertain, such a loss may impair cognitive and language function and result in disturbances in psychosocial adjustment (65). Recently, Paradise and co-workers (66) were not able to find any differences in developmental outcomes between those children who had chronic otitis media with effusion and early placement of tympanostomy tubes and those whose tubes were delayed. Using a similar design, Maw and colleagues (67) did detect developmental differences between those children who had tube placement late and those who had early insertion. Nevertheless, there are other potential sequelae of longstanding middle ear effusion, such as structural damage to the middle ear structures and balance disturbance (68). With these uncertainties in mind, the clinician should decide whether to treat or to watch and, if treatment is decided on, which treatment options appear to be most appropriate in eliminating the middle ear effusion in the individual child.

Important factors other than hearing loss that should be considered in deciding whether to treat (and which treatment) include (a) occurrence in infants because they are unable to communicate about their symptoms and may have suppurative disease; (b) an associated acute purulent upper respiratory tract infection; (c) concurrent permanent conductive, sensorineural hearing loss, or both; (d) vertigo or tinnitus; (e) alterations of the tympanic membrane, such as severe atelectasis, especially a deep retraction pocket in the posterosuperior quadrant, the pars flaccida, or both; (f) middle ear changes, such as adhesive otitis or ossicular involvement; (g) effusion that persists for 3 months or longer (i.e., chronic otitis media with effusion); or (h) when the episodes recur frequently, such as in 6 of the preceding 12 months. The most common reason for treating the effusion would be its becoming chronic (6,61).

Management

Before the clinician embarks on a nonsurgical or surgical method of management of children with frequently recurrent or chronic effusions, a thorough search for an underlying cause should be attempted. Probably the most popular method of management—a trial with an orally administered combination of a decongestant and antihistamine—was shown to be ineffective in the Pittsburgh study of infants and children with acute, subacute, and chronic otitis media with effusion (30). The efficacy of systemic corticosteroid therapy for treatment of otitis media with effusion has not been established in clinical trials. We recently reported the lack of efficacy of this form of treatment (69). In addition, some clinicians consider the risks of corticosteroid therapy for otitis media with effusion in children to outweigh its possible benefits (61). As of yet, clinical trials have not been reported that have tested the efficacy of topical nasal treatment, immunotherapy, and control of allergy in children who have nasal allergy and middle ear disease. However, this method of management seems reasonable in children who have frequently recurrent or chronic otitis media with effusion and evidence of upper respiratory tract allergy. Inflation of the eustachian tube–middle ear by use of Politzer's method or Valsalva's maneuver has been advocated for more than a century for this condition. However, a randomized controlled trial by Chan and Bluestone (70) found a lack of efficacy of middle ear inflation for chronic otitis media with effusion, and therefore it is not recommended in children. However, inflation may be effective for adults and all age groups for the management of middle ear effusion that follows barotrauma (e.g., by air travel or scuba diving).

ANTIMICROBIAL TREATMENT

Of all the medical treatments that have been advocated, a trial of an antimicrobial agent would appear to be most appropriate in those children who have not received an antibiotic recently. Because bacteria similar to those found in acute otitis media have been isolated from a significant proportion of middle ear aspirates in children with chronic otitis media with effusion, the antibiotic chosen for treatment should be the same as that recommended for children who have acute otitis media. As in acute otitis media, amoxicillin is a reasonable choice for treating otitis media with effusion because a study reported by Mandel and associates (31) demonstrated its efficacy for some, although not all, of the 518 infants and children with otitis media with effusion who participated in the study. If the effusion is chronic and unresponsive to amoxicillin therapy, a trial with an antimicrobial agent effective against ampicillin-resistant bacteria may be helpful before surgery is considered.

Of the other possible antimicrobial agents currently available, such as erythromycin-sulfisoxazole, trimethoprim-sulfamethoxazole, cefaclor, cefuroxime axetil, cefixime, or amoxicillin-clavulanate, only amoxicillin-clavulanate, given for 10 days, has been shown to be marginally more effective than a 10-day course of amoxicillin for otitis media with effusion (71). Thomsen and colleagues (72) also demonstrated the efficacy of amoxicillin-clavulanate in a placebo-controlled study of children who had chronic otitis media with effusion, but both the drug and its placebo were given for 30 days in this trial. Mandel and colleagues (73) compared a 2-week course of cefaclor and erythromycin-sulfisoxazole with amoxicillin and failed to demonstrate an increased effect of these other agents over amoxicillin. Although no trial has been reported in which the efficacy of a course of amoxicillin longer than 10 days has been tested for chronic otitis media with effusion, it is possible that longer therapy is more effective than shorter therapy. A metaanalysis of the effect of antimicrobial agents in the treatment of otitis media with effusion was reported by Rosenfeld and Post (74), which confirmed the efficacy of this treatment. Another metaanalysis also confirmed the short-term effect in otitis media and tympanostomy tubes (43). Other strategies, such as antimicrobial prophylaxis (75), or more preferably surgery, are required for long-term control of this disease because the disease frequently recurs owing to repeated exposure to upper respiratory tract infections, especially in those who attend day care centers.

SURGICAL TREATMENT

If nonsurgical methods of management fail and the effusion is chronic, surgical intervention should be considered, and referral of the patient to an otolaryngologist is appropriate. In 109 Pittsburgh children with chronic otitis media with effusion that was unresponsive to amoxicillin, myringotomy with tympanostomy tube insertion was shown to be more effective than myringotomy without tube insertion or no surgery (76). After spontaneous extubation of the tympanostomy tube, reinsertion for recurrent effusion is indicated only after antimicrobial therapy has failed and the effusion has persisted for 3 months or longer. The outcome of this study was confirmed in a clinical trial conducted by the same group, which was similar in design to the first one and involved 111 subjects who were also observed monthly for 3 years (77) (Table 45.4). In some children, the procedure must be repeated for several years until the child grows older; the occurrence of otitis media with effusion is less frequent after 5 years of age (78).

Table 45.5 shows the current indications for insertion of tympanostomy tubes in children (79). These indications are derived from clinical trials as well as from long experience with otitis media in children, in whom the occurrence is vastly more common than in adults. Unfortunately, no similar published clinical trials have been conducted in adults, but the clinician can use the outcomes of the studies in children as a guide to treating adults. However, there are some important differences, such as the usual intolerance of adults when even relatively asymptomatic middle ear effusion of short duration is present and the feasibility of performing myringotomy, with or without tympanostomy tube insertion, by use of local anesthesia in teenagers and adults. Thus, surgical intervention should be considered at a much earlier stage in the natural history of acute otitis media, persistent middle ear effusion, recurrent acute otitis media, and otitis media with effusion in older patients.

Adenoidectomy, in conjunction with myringotomy and tympanostomy tube insertion or myringotomy alone, can benefit some children. However, others improve without removal of the adenoids, and still others have persistent disease despite adenoidectomy (48,80,81) (Table 45.3). Table 45.6 shows the outcomes of the clinical trial conducted by Gates and colleagues (81). Because the effectiveness of adenoidectomy for chronic oti-

tis media with effusion is apparently unrelated to adenoid size (48,82,83), the selection of children who might benefit from adenoidectomy at present must be based on the potential benefits weighed against the costs and potential risks. For children who have recurrent or chronic otitis media with effusion and who have had one or more myringotomy and tympanostomy tube operations in the past, adenoidectomy is a reasonable option. The presence of upper airway obstruction (due to obstructive adenoids), recurrent acute or chronic adenoiditis, or both conditions would also be a more compelling indication to consider adenoidectomy.

MASTOIDITIS

Mastoiditis can be classified into acute, subacute, and chronic; chronic mastoiditis is almost always associated with chronic suppurative otitis media (see later section "Chronic Suppurative Otitis Media [and Chronic Mastoiditis]").

TABLE 45.5. Indications for Tympanostomy Tube Insertion in Children

Chronic otitis media with effusion unresponsive to medical management, 3 months or more bilateral or 6 months or more unilateral; earlier when significant hearing loss (e.g., >25 dB), speech language delay, severe retraction pocket, disequilibrium-vertigo, or tinnitus is present
Recurrent episodes of middle ear effusion not meeting criteria for chronic disease, but cumulative duration excessive, e.g., 6 of 12 months
Recurrent acute otitis media, especially when antimicrobial prophylaxis fails to reduce frequency, severity, and duration of attacks; minimal frequency: three or more episodes in 6 months or four or more in 12 months, with one recent
Eustachian tube dysfunction (with or without effusion) or when persistent or recurrent signs and symptoms, e.g., hearing loss (usually fluctuating) or disequilibrium—vertigo, tinnitus, or a severe retraction pocket—are not relieved by medical treatment
Tympanoplasty when eustachian tube function is poor, e.g., surgery for cholesteatoma
Suppurative complication present or suspected

Adapted from Bluestone CD, Klein JO, Gates GA. "Appropriateness" of tympanostomy tubes: setting the record straight. *Arch Otolaryngol Head Neck Surg* 1994;120:1051–1053, with permission. Copyright 1994, American Medical Association.

TABLE 45.4. Morbidity for First Year of Randomized Trial of Myringotomy, Myringotomy and Tympanostomy Tube, and Surgery (Control) in 111 Pittsburgh Infants and Children with Chronic Otitis Media with Effusion

| | Treatment groups | | | |
Outcome measure	1 No surgery (n = 35)	2 Myringotomy (n = 38)	3 Myringotomy and tympanostomy tube (n = 36)	Statistically significant difference
Treatment failure (proportion of subjects)	0.56	0.70	0.06	Yes[a]
Acute otitis media (episodes/person-year)	0.95	0.81	0.23	p < 0.001[b]
Middle ear effusion (proportion of time)	0.64	0.61	0.17	p < 0.001[b]

[a]Actuarial rate; 90% confidence intervals for group 1–group 2 (−0.33, 0.05); group 1–group 3 (0.35, 0.66); group 2–group 3 (0.50, 0.78).
[b]For groups 1 versus 2 versus 3.
Adapted from Mandel EM, Rockette HE, Bluestone CD, et al. Efficacy of myringotomy with and without tympanostomy tubes for chronic otitis media with effusion. *Pediatr Infect Dis J* 1992;11:270–277, with permission.

TABLE 45.6.   Effectiveness of Various Treatments in 578 Children with Chronic Otitis Media with Effusion

Outcome[a]	Myringotomy	Myringotomy and tube insertion	Adenoidectomy and myringotomy	Adenoidectomy, myringotomy, and tube insertion
Percentage of time with effusion	49.1	34.9	30.2	25.8
Percentage of time with hearing loss[b]	37.5	30.4	22.0	22.4
Median time to first recurrence (days)	54	222	92	240
Number of surgical retreatments	66	36	17	17

[a]During 2-year follow-up.
[b]Hearing loss equal to or greater than 20 dB.
Adapted from Gates GA, Avery CA, Prihoda TJ, et al. Effectiveness of adenoidectomy and tympanostomy tubes in the treatment of chronic otitis media with effusion. *N Engl J Med* 1987;317:1444–1451, with permission. Copyright 1987, Massachusetts Medical Society. All rights reserved.

Acute Mastoiditis

Acute mastoiditis can be classified into its stages: acute mastoiditis without periosteitis or osteitis, acute mastoiditis with periosteitis, and acute mastoid osteitis (7).

ACUTE MASTOIDITIS WITHOUT PERIOSTEITIS OR OSTEITIS

Acute mastoiditis can be a natural extension and part of the pathological process of acute middle ear infection, in which instance periosteitis and osteitis are absent. Most likely the mastoid gas cells are involved in almost all children who have acute otitis media. No specific signs or symptoms of mastoid infection (e.g., protrusion of the pinna, postauricular swelling, tenderness, pain, and erythema) are present in this most common stage of mastoiditis. Computed tomography (CT) scans are not indicated when the process is self-limited, but when obtained—usually for other reasons—the mastoid area is frequently read as "cloudy mastoids," which is indicative of inflammation; no mastoid *osteitis* (i.e., bony erosion of the mastoid gas cells) is evident.

The process is usually reversible as the middle ear–mastoid infection resolves, either as a natural process or as a result of medical management (i.e., antimicrobial therapy with or without myringotomy). Thus, in the absence of osteitis of the mastoid, periosteal involvement of the postauricular region, and subperiosteal abscess, this first stage of acute mastoiditis is *not* a suppurative complication of otitis media.

When acute infection in the mastoid (and usually middle ear) does not resolve at this stage, the disease can rapidly progress to *acute mastoiditis with periosteitis*, with the next stage being *acute mastoid osteitis*, which can occur with or without the presence of a *subperiosteal abscess*.

ACUTE MASTOIDITIS WITH PERIOSTEITIS

When infection within the mastoid spreads to the periosteum covering the mastoid process, periosteitis can develop. The route of infection from the mastoid cells to the periosteum is by venous channels, usually the mastoid emissary vein. The condition should not be confused with the presence of a subperiosteal abscess because management of the latter condition usually requires a mastoidectomy, whereas the former frequently responds to medical treatment and tympanocentesis-myringotomy.

In the antibiotic era, the frequency of mastoidectomy for acute mastoiditis has decreased dramatically, but we still encounter a substantial number of children, especially infants, who develop this complication of acute otitis media (27,84). The rate has been reported to be increasing in one children's hospital in Northern Virginia (26). At the Children's Hospital of Pittsburgh, there were only 18 mastoidectomies performed between 1980 and 1995 for acute mastoiditis (85). The growing enthusiasm for withholding

antimicrobial therapy today in some countries may result in an increase in this suppurative complication (25,86).

Diagnosis and Microbiology

Clinically, the child will have the classic signs and symptoms of acute otitis media, such as fever and otalgia, but will also have postauricular erythema, mild tenderness, and some edema in the postauricular area. The pinna may or may not be displaced inferiorly and anteriorly, with loss of the postauricular crease. Subperiosteal abscess is absent. Examination of the eardrum typically reveals evidence of an acute middle ear infection. However, the middle ear may be effusion free in the presence of acute mastoiditis if there is an obstruction of the narrow passageway from the middle ear to the mastoid gas cell system (i.e., the *aditus ad antrum*); the middle ear effusion drains down the eustachian tube, but the infection in the mastoid cannot drain into the middle ear.

For this stage of acute mastoiditis, CT scans of the temporal bones (and intracranial cavity) should be obtained to determine whether osteitis of the mastoid is present. CT scans are not mandatory, however, if the infection is limited to the middle ear and mastoid, the child is not severely ill or toxic, and the child rapidly improves after tympanocentesis-myringotomy and antimicrobial therapy.

Middle ear aspirates reveal similar bacterial pathogens isolated from children's ears that have uncomplicated acute middle ear infection, such as *S. pneumoniae*, *S. pyogenes*, or *H. influenzae*, but there may be other organisms, such as *Pseudomonas aeruginosa*, if there has been otorrhea.

Management

The patient may be managed on an ambulatory basis if the infection is not severe. However, hospitalization is usually necessary because parenteral antimicrobial therapy is frequently needed and most patients require an immediate tympanocentesis (for aspiration and microbiological assessment of the middle ear–mastoid effusion) and myringotomy for drainage of the middle ear, which, in the absence of an *aditus-ad-antrum block*, should also drain the mastoid. If the child has had recurrent attacks of acute otitis media in the past, or if the episode of acute middle ear infection is superimposed on preexisting chronic otitis media with effusion, insertion of a tympanostomy tube is indicated. Placement of a tympanostomy tube is desirable because it will enhance drainage over a longer period of time than myringotomy alone. Even though reports have revealed that antibiotic treatment was successful in curing some children without the benefit of tympanocentesis or myringotomy, aspiration of the middle ear is an important diagnostic (and therapeutic) procedure today because an antibiotic-resistant bacterial pathogen such as multidrug-resistant pneumococcus may be the causative organism requiring an antimicrobial agent not frequently used for acute otitis media–mastoiditis, such as vancomycin (9,85,87,88).

Cultures for bacteria from the middle ear are required to identify the causative organisms. Antimicrobial susceptibility studies are important for selection of the most effective antibiotic agent. For empirical parenteral antimicrobial therapy, cefuroxime sodium, ticarcillin disodium with clavulanate potassium, or ampicillin-sulbactam can be initiated until the Gram stain, culture, and susceptibility studies of the middle ear aspirate are available. If a penicillin-resistant *S. pneumoniae* is the possible pathogen, some clinicians would also add vancomycin while awaiting the culture and susceptibly report.

The periosteal involvement should resolve within 24 to 48 hours after the tympanic membrane has been opened for drainage and adequate and appropriate antimicrobial therapy has begun. A mastoidectomy should be performed if (a) the symptoms of the acute infection, such as fever and otalgia, persist; (b) the postauricular involvement does not progressively improve; or (c) a subperiosteal abscess develops. CT scans can be helpful in the decision whether to intervene surgically. A mastoidectomy is also indicated if another intratemporal (extracranial) suppurative complication of otitis media is present, such as facial paralysis, labyrinthitis, petrous apicitis, or intracranial complication (e.g., meningitis, lateral sinus thrombosis, or abscess of the epidural or subdural space or brain).

In the review by Goldstein and colleagues (85), cited earlier, of the 72 infants and children with acute mastoiditis at the Children's Hospital of Pittsburgh, 54 (75%) were managed conservatively with broad-spectrum intravenous antibiotics and myringotomy, with and without tympanostomy tube insertion, whereas the other 18 (25%) required mastoidectomy; of these 18 children, 14 (78%) had one or more of the following: mastoid osteitis, subperiosteal abscess, cholesteatoma, or another suppurative complication, such as facial paralysis. In a recent review from Australia, Harley and associates (88) reported nearly the same experience as that in Pittsburgh. Between 1982 and 1993, 58 infants and children were admitted to the Royal Children's Hospital of Melbourne, and of these, 45 (78%) were treated conservatively with intravenous antimicrobial therapy, with and without tympanostomy tube insertion; the remaining 13 patients required mastoidectomy. Others have also reported that most children with acute mastoiditis can be managed conservatively, but other centers have reported that most of their patients required a mastoidectomy (89–92). Most likely the reasons for these conflicting reports are the lack of uniform definition of the disease, dissimilarity in presentation of the cases, and variation in management. In my opinion, most patients with acute mastoiditis with only periosteitis recover without the need for mastoidectomy.

Immediate treatment at this stage of acute mastoiditis is mandatory because failure to treat may result in the development of acute mastoid osteitis (with or without a subperiosteal abscess) or another suppurative complication such as meningitis or brain abscess, which may be potentially more life-threatening to the child.

In the absence of mastoid osteitis (with or without subperiosteal abscess), the primary care physician or infectious disease specialist can provide the initial medical care for patients with acute mastoiditis with periosteitis. However, tympanocentesis-myringotomy is required, and an otolaryngologist will be needed if the medical specialists are untrained in this procedure. Referral to an otolaryngologist is appropriate if a mastoidectomy is indicated, as described earlier. Also, immediate referral for surgical evaluation and management is indicated when acute mastoid infection develops in a child with chronic suppurative otitis media, cholesteatoma, or both.

ACUTE MASTOID OSTEITIS

Acute mastoid osteitis has also been called acute "coalescent" mastoiditis or acute surgical mastoiditis, but in reality, the pathological process is *osteitis*. A subperiosteal abscess may or may not be present. When infection within the mastoid progresses, rarefying osteitis can cause destruction of the bony trabeculae that separate the mastoid cells so that there is a "coalescence" of the cells. At this stage, a mastoid empyema is present. The pus may spread in one or more of the following directions: (a) anterior to the middle ear through the *aditus-ad-antrum*, in which case spontaneous resolution usually occurs; (b) lateral to the surface of the mastoid process, resulting in a postauricular subperiosteal abscess; (c) anterior into the zygomatic cells, developing into an abscess in the anterior and superior portion of the pinna and preauricular area; (d) inferior through the tip of the mastoid, burrowing beneath the skin to form a soft tissue abscess below the pinna or behind the attachment of the sternocleidomastoid muscle in the neck, which is known as *Bezold's abscess* (93,94); (e) medial to the petrous air cells, resulting in petrositis; or (f) posterior to the occipital bone, which can result in osteomyelitis of the calvarium or *Citelli's abscess*.

Infection may also spread medial to the labyrinth, involve the facial nerve, or extend into the intracranial cavity, causing one or more suppurative complications such as meningitis or brain abscess.

Clinical Presentation and Diagnosis

The child usually has the same signs and symptoms as those associated with acute otitis media, such as fever and otalgia, although the fever may be low grade with occasional temperature spikes. Some patients may have toxic symptoms. The signs and symptoms referable to the mastoid infection are (a) swelling, erythema, and tenderness to touch over the mastoid bone; (b) displacement of the pinna outward and downward; and (c) swelling or sagging of the posterosuperior external auditory canal wall. A fluctuant subperiosteal abscess or even a draining fistula from the mastoid to the postauricular area may be present. The subperiosteal abscess can be in any of the anatomical sites described previously.

Examination of the tympanic membrane usually reveals the presence of a middle ear effusion, or a purulent discharge and a perforation can be observed. Conversely, the tympanic membrane and middle ear may appear almost normal for the reasons described earlier when mastoiditis with periosteitis occurs; the middle ear disease resolves, but the infection remains in the mastoid. Acute mastoid osteitis (without otitis media) may also be the focus of infection when a child has a fever of unknown origin.

The diagnosis should be suspected on the basis of clinical signs and symptoms. CT scans of the mastoid area usually reveal one or more of the following: (a) haziness, distortion, or destruction of the mastoid outline; (b) loss of sharpness of the shadows of cellular walls due to demineralization, atrophy, and ischemia of the bony septa; (c) decrease in density and cloudiness of the areas of pneumatization due to inflammatory swelling of the air cells; or (d) in longstanding cases, a chronic osteoblastic inflammatory reaction that may obliterate the cellular structure. Small abscess cavities in sclerotic bone may be confused with pneumatic cells.

Management

An otolaryngologist should be consulted if a child has a diagnosis of acute mastoid osteitis. Parenteral antimicrobial therapy should be instituted as described previously for acute mastoiditis with periosteitis. To ensure that drainage of the middle ear and mastoid is adequate, in the absence of a large perforation and otorrhea, a wide-field large myringotomy should be done immediately. Insertion of a tympanostomy tube, in addition to a large myringotomy incision, can provide more prolonged drainage from the middle ear–mastoid than myringotomy alone. Also, the tympanostomy tube placement will help prevent recurrence of acute otitis media (and mastoiditis).

A complete, simple ("cortical") mastoidectomy will usually be required when there is evidence of acute mastoid osteitis, especially when the mastoid empyema has extended outside the mastoid bone and a subperiosteal abscess is present. The procedure should be considered an emergency, but the timing of the operation must be dependent on the status of the child. Ideally, sepsis should be under control, and the patient must be able to tolerate a general anesthetic. The principle is to clean out the mastoid infection, to drain the mastoid gas cell system into the middle ear by eliminating any obstruction that is caused by edema or granulation tissue in the *aditus-ad-antrum*, and to provide external drainage (95). If a suppurative intratemporal or intracranial complication is also present, surgical intervention for these conditions may also be required.

Subacute Mastoiditis (Masked Mastoiditis)

Although relatively uncommon, when the acute middle ear and mastoid infection does not totally resolve within the usual 10 to 14 days, subacute mastoiditis may develop, which has also been termed *masked mastoiditis* (96). The infection in the mastoid at this stage can even develop into an intratemporal or intracranial complication. Typically, the patient lacks the classic signs and symptoms of acute otitis media (and mastoiditis) but can have recurrent low-grade or no fever and mild otalgia. Also, the child may have persistent or recurrent mild to moderate postauricular pain. Examination of the tympanic membrane may reveal a middle ear effusion, although it can appear to be disease free if the middle ear infection has resolved but there is persistent mastoid infection due to an *aditus-ad-antrum* block.

The diagnosis is usually made by CT scans of the temporal bones or by obtaining a bone scan (97). Children who have an intratemporal or intracranial suppurative infection, which could possibly be due to mastoid infection, should have CT scans of the temporal bones included in the workup, even though there is no evidence of middle ear disease on otoscopy. Although unusual, a child who has a fever of unknown origin may have subacute mastoiditis.

Management of this stage of mastoiditis is the same as described earlier for acute mastoiditis with periosteitis, which is much more commonly encountered. Although some clinicians have recommended mastoidectomy for this condition, less aggressive management is usually successful, such as tympanocentesis (and possible myringotomy) to identify the causative organism and culture-directed antimicrobial therapy. In my experience, these children usually have persistent middle ear–mastoid infection, that is, subacute otitis media that is unresponsive to commonly prescribed antibiotics, and therefore, the offending bacterium should be identified and the appropriate antibiotic administered (98). Indications for consultation with the otolaryngologist and for possible mastoidectomy are similar to those described when acute mastoiditis is present.

Chronic Mastoiditis

Chronic mastoiditis is most commonly associated with chronic suppurative otitis media (see later). Occasionally, however, a child will develop acute mastoiditis that is either untreated or inappropriately treated, or the child is neglected, and the infection will progress into a chronic stage. These children may present with a fever of unknown origin or chronic otalgia and tenderness over the mastoid process. Examination reveals an intact tympanic membrane with evidence of middle ear effusion, but middle ear effusion can be absent if the chronic infection is localized only to the mastoid. CT scans should be obtained. The mastoid may be poorly pneumatized or sclerotic, or there may be evidence of bone destruction, with opacification of the mastoid.

The chronic infection at this stage may be brought under control by medical treatment with antimicrobial agents (similar to those recommended previously for acute mastoiditis). Tympanocentesis (for Gram stain, culture, and susceptibility studies) and myringotomy (for drainage) should be performed. When there are extensive amounts of granulation tissue and osteitis in the mastoid, or if the child fails to improve on medical therapy, a tympanomastoidectomy is required to eliminate the chronic mastoid osteitis.

Chronic mastoiditis can also be caused by a cholesteatoma, which is usually manifested by chronic otorrhea through a defect in the tympanic membrane and requires definitive surgical treatment.

Chronic Suppurative Otitis Media (and Chronic Mastoiditis)

Chronic suppurative otitis media is a sequela of otitis media in which there is chronic infection of the middle ear and mastoid and in which a perforation of the tympanic membrane (or a patent tympanostomy tube) is present; a discharge (otorrhea) may or may not be present; mastoiditis is invariably a part of the pathological process. Cholesteatoma may or may not be associated with chronic suppurative otitis media.

TERMINOLOGY

The most commonly accepted terminology for this stage of ear disease is *chronic suppurative otitis media*; chronic mastoiditis is assumed to be present. It has been called *chronic otitis media*, but this term can be confused with *chronic otitis media with effusion*, which is not characterized by perforation. It is also called *chronic suppurative otitis media and mastoiditis*, *chronic purulent otitis media*, and *chronic otomastoiditis*. When a cholesteatoma is also present, the term *chronic suppurative otitis media with cholesteatoma* is used; however, an acquired aural cholesteatoma does not have to be associated with chronic suppurative otitis media.

EPIDEMIOLOGY

Chronic suppurative otitis media is a major health problem in many populations around the world, affecting diverse racial and cultural groups living not only in temperate climates but also in climate extremes ranging from the Arctic Circle to the equator (99). Populations that have chronic suppurative otitis media associated with chronic perforations at highest rates are the Inuits of Alaska, Canada, and Greenland; Australian Aborigines; and certain Native Americans, including Apache and Navajo tribes. Populations with moderately high rates are certain natives of the South Pacific islands, such as natives of the Solomon Islands and the Maori of New Zealand. With the widespread use of tympanostomy tube placement in the developed nations of the world, however, chronic suppurative otitis media is not an uncommon complication (100). Despite advances in management of otitis media (e.g., tympanostomy tube placement to prevent middle ear negative pressure and subsequent atelectasis-retraction pocket), cholesteatoma is still a relatively common sequela of middle ear disease worldwide.

MICROBIOLOGY

Chronic suppurative otitis media develops from a chronic bacterial infection; however, the bacteria that caused the initial episode of acute otitis media with perforation and otorrhea may not be those that are isolated from the discharge when there is chronic infection in the middle ear and mastoid. In fact, Mandel and associates (101) reported that infants and young children who had the acute onset of otorrhea through a tympanostomy tube usually had the common organisms that cause acute otitis media when the tympanic membrane is intact, whereas in older children, especially in the summer, the predominant organism was frequently *Pseudomonas* species, presumably as a result of contamination of the middle ear during swimming. Thus, the antimicrobial therapy recommended for acute otitis media may not be effective for most cases of chronic suppurative otitis media. The microbiology of chronic suppurative otitis media without cholesteatoma in children has been reported by Kenna and co-workers (102). From 51 ear cultures obtained from 36 children, 23 microbiologic species were isolated. One organism was isolated from 18 ears, two from 20 ears, three from 3 ears, four from 4 ears, and five from 2 ears. The most common bacterial species isolated was *P. aeruginosa*, which was present in 34 ears (67%) and was the only isolate in 16 ears (31%). Of the 15 children who had bilateral otorrhea, 11 (73%) had the same organism identified in both middle ears: 7 children had *P. aeruginosa* isolated; 4 had *S. aureus*; and 1 each had *S. epidermidis, Candida albicans,* and diphtheroids.

The bacteriology of chronic suppurative otitis media with cholesteatoma in children and adults has been reported. The most common aerobic microbiologic organisms isolated were *P. aeruginosa* and *S. aureus;* the most frequent anaerobic organisms were *Bacteroides, Peptostreptococcus,* and *Peptococcus* species. It is important to make the distinction between chronic suppurative otitis media with and without cholesteatoma; tympanomastoid surgery is indicated when cholesteatoma is present, whereas medical management may be effective when it is not.

ETIOLOGY AND PATHOGENESIS

Chronic suppurative otitis media begins with an episode of acute otitis media. Thus, the factors that have been associated with acute otitis media may be initially involved, such as upper respiratory tract infection; anatomical factors, such as eustachian tube dysfunction; host factors, such as young age; immature or impaired immunological status; presence of upper respiratory allergy; familial predisposition; presence of older siblings in the household; male sex; race; method of feeding (bottle versus breast); environmental factors, such as smoking in the household; and social factors. Probably the most important factors related to the onset of acute otitis media in infants and young children are immaturity of the structure and function of the eustachian tube and immaturity of the immune system (103).

Acute otitis media with perforation (or when a tympanostomy tube is present) usually *precedes* chronic suppurative otitis media, and the process, if longstanding, results in *chronic osteitis* of the middle ear and mastoid gas cells (104). Because a spontaneous perforation commonly accompanies an episode of acute otitis media that is untreated with an antimicrobial agent, and less commonly despite adequate treatment, it may be part of the natural history of the disease process rather than a complication. Once a perforation develops and acute otorrhea persists, the perforation can become chronic, but the otitis media (with or without otorrhea) may or may not become chronic. A chronic perforation that is uninfected can be become reinfected if the middle ear becomes contaminated with water (e.g., bathing, swimming) from the external ear canal or from reflux of bacteria from the nasopharynx into the middle ear during an upper respiratory tract infection (105).

MANAGEMENT

Treatment of chronic suppurative otitis media is initially medical and directed toward eliminating the infection from the middle ear and mastoid. Because the bacteria most frequently cultured are gram negative, antimicrobial agents should be selected to be effective against these organisms. Management of cholesteatoma in children and adults is surgical, which is usually accomplished by performing a tympanomastoidectomy.

Ototopical Agents

Some experts advocate the use of ototopical agents as first-line treatment for chronic suppurative otitis media (106). Currently, the only FDA-approved ototopical agent is ofloxacin (Floxin Otic) for use in children when acute otitis media with otorrhea occurs when a tympanostomy tube is in place. At present, it is the only topical antimicrobial agent that has been demonstrated to be safe and effective (51,107) and approved for this indication in children. It is also approved for adults who have chronic suppurative otitis media, but it is not approved for this indication in children (108), even though it has been reported to be effective in this age group (109). Topical ofloxacin has been shown to be more effective than the combination of neomycin-polymyxin B-hydrocortisone otic drops in adults with chronic suppurative otitis media (110). Thus, the lack of reported clinical trials in children notwithstanding, it seems reasonable to use ofloxacin initially in children and adults who have uncomplicated chronic suppurative otitis media (111).

Ciprofloxacin with hydrocortisone (Cipro HC) has also been approved to treat otitis externa in both children and adults. Even though ciprofloxacin is not currently approved for treatment of chronic suppurative otitis media, it appears to be effective (112–115). One study showed that topical ciprofloxacin was more effective than topical gentamicin for chronic suppurative otitis media in adults (116), and another showed that this antibiotic was equally effective as tobramycin in adults with this infection (117). No apparent ototoxicity has occurred after using this ototopical agent in patients with chronic suppurative otitis media (118). In addition, topical ciprofloxacin did not cause ototoxicity in the monkey model of chronic suppurative otitis media (119). There is still no consensus about the potential efficacy of adding a corticosteroid component to the antimicrobial agent, but steroids may hasten resolution of the inflammation (120).

As an alternative to an antibiotic topical agent, some clinicians recommend antiseptic drops. An antiseptic ototopical agent (aluminum acetate) was found to be as effective as topical gentamicin sulfate for otorrhea in a randomized clinical trial reported from the United Kingdom (121). Thorp and colleagues (122) evaluated the *in vitro* activity of acetic acid and aluminum subacetate (Burow's solution) and found both to be effective against the major pathogens causing chronic suppurative otitis media. Burow's solution was somewhat more effective than acetic acid. Antiseptic drops (e.g., acetic acid) are commonly used in underdeveloped countries and are reputed to be effective. Because of cost and availability, antibiotic ototopical agents are used when antiseptic drops are ineffective.

If ototopical medication is elected, the patient should return to the outpatient facility periodically, even daily, so that the discharge can be aspirated thoroughly (i.e., aural toilet). Frequently, the discharge resolves within 1 to 2 weeks with this type of treatment.

Systemic Antimicrobial Agents

In children, orally administered antibiotics are usually not effective unless an organism is seen on Gram stain or is cultured from the discharge that will be susceptible, such as *S. aureus*. Oral antibiotics are also effective against the organisms that commonly cause acute otitis media, such as pneumococcus and *H. influenzae*; ciprofloxacin, an oral antimicrobial agent with activity against most of the organisms that cause chronic suppurative disease, may be effective, although randomized clinical trials demonstrating efficacy for this infection have not been reported. However, treatment of adults who have chronic suppurative otitis media with the quinolones when the causative organism is *Pseudomonas* seems reasonable; currently, these drugs are not indicated for patients younger than 17 years of age.

When the chronic middle ear infection fails to respond to ototopical medications (with or without orally administered antibiotics), we hospitalize the child and administer a parenteral β-lactam antipseudomonal drug, such as ticarcillin or piperacillin. The external ear canal and middle ear (if possible) are aspirated (aural toilet), and ototopical drops are instilled daily. In most children, the middle ear will be free of discharge within 7 to 10 days, and the signs of otitis media will be greatly improved or absent.

Surgery

When the chronic infection fails to respond to intensive medical therapy (including intravenous antimicrobial therapy in children), surgery on the middle ear and mastoid is indicated. In the Kenna and colleagues study (102) of 36 pediatric patients with chronic suppurative otitis media, all of whom received parenteral antimicrobial therapy and daily otic toilet, 32 children (89%) experienced resolution of their initial infection with medical therapy alone; 4 children required tympanomastoidectomy.

In a follow-up of that study, 51 of the original 66 were evaluated for their long-term outcomes (123). Of these 51 children, 40 (78%) had resolution of their initial or recurrent infection after medical treatment; 11 (22%) had to have mastoid surgery eventually. Failure was associated with older children and an early recurrence. Even though similar large-scale clinical trials of parenteral antimicrobial therapy have not been reported for adults, this management option also seems reasonable before mastoid surgery is performed in this age group.

PREVENTION

If the infection can be eliminated by the methods described, recurrence can usually be prevented by one of the following measures: prompt and appropriate antibiotic treatment of future attacks of acute otitis media, removal of the tympanostomy tube, surgical repair of the tympanic membrane defect, or antimicrobial prophylaxis when repair of the tympanic membrane perforation or removal of the tympanostomy tube is not feasible. The choice depends on several factors, such as the age of the patient and the function of the eustachian tube (95).

When the chronic infection developed following an episode of acute otitis media in which the tympanic membrane spontaneously ruptured, but the infection resolved and eardrum healed, treatment with an antimicrobial agent at the onset of a recurrent attack should prevent a similar chronic infection. When there have been frequently recurrent attacks of acute otitis media in the past, however, antimicrobial prophylaxis or tympanostomy tube placement are options because antibiotic-resistant bacteria can occur after prophylaxis. Surgery is more desirable today (124) (see earlier). If a chronic perforation of the tympanic membrane or tympanostomy tube is present, repair of the eardrum or removal of the tube should restore the normal physiology of the middle ear and prevent reflux of nasopharyngeal secretions and water contamination of the middle ear from the external ear canal (7).

When chronic suppurative otitis media is present with cholesteatoma, tympanomastoid surgery is indicated to eradicate the cholesteatoma (95). Preoperative antimicrobial therapy,

and possibly perioperative prophylaxis, may be helpful in reducing postoperative infection and should promote better healing.

ACKNOWLEDGMENT

Ms. Maria B. Bluestone helped with the preparation of this manuscript.

REFERENCES

1. Shappert SM. Office visits for otitis media: United States, 1975–90. *Vital Health Stat* 1992;214:1–18.
2. Teele DW, Klein JO, Rosner B, et al. Middle ear disease and the practice of pediatrics: Burden during the first 5 years of life. *JAMA* 1983;249:1026–1029.
3. Casselbrant ML, Mandel EM, Kurs-Lasky M, et al. Otitis media in black American and white American infants, 0 to 2 years of age. *Int J Pediatr Otorhinolaryngol* 1995;33:11–16.
4. Gates GA. Cost benefit analysis for otitis media. In: Lim DJ, Bluestone CD, Casselbrant ML, et al., eds. *Recent advances in otitis media: proceedings of the Sixth International Symposium.* Hamilton, Ontario: BC Decker, 1996:1–4.
5. Nelson WL, Kuritsky JN, Kennedy DL, et al. Outpatient pediatric antibiotic use in the U.S.: trends and therapy for otitis media, 1977–1986. In: *Program and abstracts of the 27th Interscience Conference on Antimicrobial Agents and Chemotherapy.* Washington, DC: American Society for Microbiology, 1987.
6. Dowell SF, Butler JC, Giebink GS, et al. Acute otitis media: management and surveillance in an era of pneumococcal resistance—a report from the Drug-Resistant Streptococcus pneumoniae Therapeutic Working Group. *Pediatr Infect Dis J* 1999;18:1–9.
7. Bluestone CD, Klein JO. *Otitis media in infants and children,* 3rd ed. Philadelphia: WB Saunders, 2001.
8. Spika JS, Facklam RR, Plikaytis BD, et al. Antimicrobial resistance of *Streptococcus pneumoniae* in the United States, 1979–1987. *J Infect Dis* 1991;163:1273–1278.
9. Welby PL, Keller DS, Cromien JL, et al. Resistance to penicillin and non-beta-lactam antibiotics of *Streptococcus pneumoniae* at a children's hospital. *Pediatr Infect Dis J* 1994;13:281–287.
10. Bluestone CD. Role of surgery for otitis media in the era of resistant bacteria. *Pediatr Infect Dis J* 1998;17:1090–1098.
11. Bluestone CD, Klein JO. Otitis media, atelectasis, and eustachian tube dysfunction. In: Bluestone CD, Stool SE, Kenna MA, eds. *Pediatric otolaryngology,* 3rd ed. Philadelphia: WB Saunders, 1996:470.
12. Bluestone CD, Stephenson JS, Martin LM. Ten-year review of otitis media pathogens. *Pediatr Infect Dis J* 1992;11:S7–S11.
13. Mason EO, Kaplan SL, Lamberth LB, et al. Increased rate of isolation of penicillin-resistant *Streptococcus pneumoniae* in a children's hospital and in vitro susceptibilities to antibiotics of potential use. *Antimicrob Agents Chemother* 1992;36:1703–1707.
14. Reichler MR, Allphin AA, Breiman RF, et al. The spread of multiple resistant *Streptococcus pneumoniae* at a day care center in Ohio. *J Infect Dis* 1992;166:1346–1353.
15. Jacobs MR, Bajaksouzian S, Zilles A, et al. Susceptibilities of *Streptococcus pneumoniae* and *Haemophilus influenzae* to 10 antimicrobial agents based on pharmakodynamic parameters: 1997 U. S. surveillance study. *Antimicrob Agent Chemother* 1999;43:1901–1908.
16. Celin SE, Bluestone CD, Stephenson J, et al. Bacteriology of acute otitis media in adults. *JAMA* 1991;266:2249–2252.
17. Diamant M, Diamant B. Abuse and timing of use of antibiotics in acute otitis media. *Arch Otolaryngol Head Neck Surg* 1974;100:226–232.
18. van Buchem FL, Dunk JHM, van't Hof MA. Therapy of acute otitis media: myringotomy, antibiotics, or neither? A double-blind study in children. *Lancet* 1981;2:883–887.
19. van Buchem FL, Peeters MF, van't Hof MA. Acute otitis media: a new treatment strategy. *BMJ* 1985;290:1033–1037.
20. Howie VM, Ploussard JH. Efficacy of fixed combination antibiotics versus separate components in otitis media. *Clin Pediatr* 1972;11:205–214.
21. Kaleida PH, Casselbrant ML, Rockette HE, et al. Amoxicillin or myringotomy or both for acute otitis media: results of a randomized clinical trial. *Pediatrics* 1991;87:466–474.
22. Sorensen H. Antibiotics in suppurative otitis media. *Otolaryngol Clin North Am* 1977;10:45–50.
23. Rudberg RD. Acute otitis media: comparative therapeutic results of sulfonamide and penicillin administered in various forms. *Acta Otolaryngol (Stockholm)* 1954;113:1.
24. Lahikainen EA. Clinico-bacteriologic studies on acute media: aspiration of tympanum as diagnostic and therapeutic method. *Acta Otolaryngol (Stockholm)* 1953;107(Suppl):1.
25. Hoppe JE, Koster S, Bootz F, et al. Acute mastoiditis: relevant once again. *Infection* 1994;22:178–182.
26. Bahadori RS, Schwartz RH, Ziai M. Acute mastoiditis in children: an increase in frequency in Northern Virginia. *Pediatr Infect Dis J* 2000;19:212–215.
27. Kaplan SL, Mason EO, Wald ER, et al. Pneumococcal mastoiditis in children. *Pediatrics* 2000;106:695–699.

28. Mandel EM, Casselbrant ML, Rockette HE, et al. Efficacy of 20- vs. 10-day antimicrobial treatment for acute otitis media. *Pediatrics* 1995;96:5–13.

29. Bluestone CD, Connell JT, Doyle WJ, et al. Symposium: questioning the efficacy and safety of antihistamines in the treatment of upper respiratory infection. *Pediatr Infect Dis J* 1988;7:239.

30. Cantekin EI, Mandel EM, Bluestone CD, et al. Lack of efficacy of a decongestant-antihistamine combination for otitis media with effusion ("secretory" otitis media) in children. *N Engl J Med* 1983;308:297–301.

31. Mandel EM, Rockette HE, Bluestone CD, et al. Efficacy of amoxicillin with and without decongestant-antihistamine for otitis media with effusion in children. *N Engl J Med* 1987;316:432–437.

32. Kaleida PH, Bluestone CD, Rockette HE, et al. Amoxicillin-clavulanate potassium compared with cefaclor for acute otitis media in infants and children. *Pediatr Infect Dis J* 1987;6:265–271.

33. Harrison CJ, Marks MI, Welch PF. Microbiology of recently treated acute otitis media compared with previously untreated acute otitis media. *Pediatr Infect Dis J* 1985;4:641–646.

34. Centers for Disease Control and Prevention. Preventing pneumococcal disease among infants and young children: recommendations of the Advisory Committee on Immunization Practices (ACIP). *MMWR Morb Mortal Wkly Rep* 2000;49:1–35.

35. Black S, Shinefield H, Fireman B, et al. Efficacy, safety and immunogenicity of heptavalent pneumococcal conjugate vaccine in children. *Pediatr Infect Dis J* 2000;19:187–195.

36. Eskola J, Kilpi T, Palmu A, et al. Efficacy of a pneumococcal conjugate vaccine against acute otitis media. *N Engl J Med* 2001;344:403–409.

37. Bluestone CD. Pneumococcal conjugate vaccine. *Arch Otolaryngol Head Neck Surg* 2001;127:464–467.

38. Heikkinen T, Ruuskanen O, Waris M, et al. Influenza vaccination in the prevention of acute otitis media in children. *Am J Dis Child* 1991;145:445–448.

39. Clements DA, Langdon L, Bland C, et al. Influenza A vaccine decreases the incidence of otitis media in 6- to 30-month children in day care. *Arch Pediatr Adolesc Med* 1995;149:1113–1117.

40. Liston TE, Foshee WS, Pierson WD. Sulfisoxazole chemoprophylaxis for frequent otitis media. *Pediatrics* 1983;71:524–530.

41. Maynard JE, Fleshman JK, Tschopp CF. Otitis media in Alaskan Eskimo children: prospective evaluation of chemoprophylaxis. *JAMA* 1972;219:597–599.

42. Perrin JM, Charney E, MacWhinney JB Jr, et al. Sulfisoxazole as chemoprophylaxis for recurrent otitis media: a double-blind crossover study in pediatric practice. *N Engl J Med* 1974;291:664–667.

43. Williams RL, Chalmers TC, Stange KC, et al. Use of antibiotics in preventing recurrent acute otitis media and in treating otitis media with effusion. *JAMA* 1993;270:1344–1351.

44. Casselbrant ML, Kaleida PH, Rockette HE, et al. Efficacy of antimicrobial prophylaxis and of tympanostomy tube insertion for prevention of recurrent acute otitis media: results of a randomized clinical trial. *Pediatr Infect Dis J* 1992;11:278–286.

45. Bluestone CD. Surgical management of otitis media: current indications and role related to increasing bacterial resistance. *Pediatr Infect Dis J* 1994;13:1058–1063.

46. Gebhart DE. Tympanostomy tubes in the otitis media prone child. *Laryngoscope* 1981;91:849–866.

47. Gonzalez C, Arnold JE, Woody EA, et al. Prevention of recurrent acute otitis media: chemoprophylaxis versus tympanostomy tubes. *Laryngoscope* 1986;96:1330–1334.

48. Paradise JL, Bluestone CD, Rogers KD, et al. Efficacy of adenoidectomy for recurrent otitis media in children previously treated with tympanostomy-tube placement: results of parallel randomized and nonrandomized trials. *JAMA* 1990;263:2066–2073.

49. Paradise JL, Bluestone CD, Colborn DK, et al. Adenoidectomy and adenotonsillectomy for recurrent acute otitis media: parallel randomized clinical trials in children not previously treated with tympanostomy tubes. *JAMA* 1999;282:945–953.

50. Ah-Tye C, Paradise JL, Colburn DK. Otorrhea in young children after tympanostomy-tube placement for persistent middle-ear effusion: prevalence, incidence, and duration. *Pediatrics* 2001;107:1251–1258.

51. Dohar JE, Garner ET, Nielsen RW, et al. Topical ofloxacin treatment of otorrhea in children with tympanostomy tubes. *Arch Otolaryngol Head Neck Surg* 1999;125:537–545.

52. Harcourt FL, Brown AK. Hydrotympanum (secretory otitis media). *Arch Otolaryngol Head Neck Surg* 1953;57:12.

53. Robinson JM, Nicholas HO. Catarrhal otitis media with effusion: a disease of a retropharyngeal and lymphatic system. *South Med J* 1951;44:777.

54. Healy GB, Teele DW. The microbiology of chronic middle ear effusions in young children. *Laryngoscope* 1977;87:1472–1478.

55. Liu YS, Lim DJ, Lang R, et al. Microorganisms in chronic otitis media with effusion. *Ann Otol Rhinol Laryngol* 1976;85:245–249.

56. Senturia BH, Gessert CF, Carr CD, et al. Studies concerned with tubotympanitis. *Ann Otol Rhinol Laryngol* 1958;67:440.

57. Riding KH, Bluestone CD, Michaels RH, et al. Microbiology of recurrent and chronic otitis media with effusion. *J Pediatr* 1978;93:739–743.

58. Haddad J, Saiman L, Gabriel PS, et al. Nonsusceptible *Streptococcus pneumoniae* in children with chronic otitis media with effusion and recurrent otitis media undergoing ventilating tube placement. *Pediatr Infect Dis J* 2000;19:432–437.

59. Post JC, Preston RA, Aul JJ, et al. Molecular analysis of bacterial pathogens in otitis media with effusion. *JAMA* 1995;273:1598–1604.

60. Rayner MG, Zhang Y, Gorry MC, et al. Evidence of bacterial metabolic activity in culture-negative otitis media with effusion. *JAMA* 1998;279:296–299.

61. Stool SE, Berg AO, Carney CJ, et al. *Otitis media with effusion in young children.* Clinical Practice Guideline 12. Rockville, MD: Agency for Health Care Policy and Research, Public Health Service, U.S. Department of Health and Human Services, July 1994. AHCPR publication 94–0622.

62. Casselbrant ML, Brostoff LM, Cantekin EI, et al. Otitis media with effusion in preschool children. *Laryngoscope* 1985;95:428–436.

63. Bluestone CD. Otitis media in children: to treat or not to treat? *N Engl J Med* 1982;306:1399–1404.

64. Fria TH, Cantekin EI, Eichler JA. Hearing acuity of children with otitis media with effusion. *Arch Otolaryngol Head Neck Surg* 1985;111:10–16.

65. Teele DW, Klein JO, Rosner BA, et al. Otitis media with effusion during the first three years of life and development of speech and language. *Pediatrics* 1984;74:282–287.

66. Paradise JL, Feldman HM, Campbell TF, et al. Effect of early or delayed insertion of tympanostomy tubes for persistent otitis media on developmental outcomes at the age of three years. *N Engl J Med* 2001;344:1179–1187.

67. Maw R, Wilks J, Harvey I, et al. Early surgery compared with watchful waiting for glue ear and effect on language development in preschool children: a randomized trial. *Lancet* 1999;353:960–963.

68. Casselbrant ML, Furman JM, Mandel EM, et al. Past history of otitis media and balance in four-year old children. *Laryngoscope* 2000;110:773–779.

69. Mandel EM, Casselbrant ML, Rockette HE, et al. Corticosteroid and 10- vs. 20-day therapy with amoxicillin for chronic otitis media with effusion. In: Lim DJ, Bluestone CD, Casselbrant ML, et al., eds. *Recent advances in otitis media: proceedings of the Seventh International Symposium.* Hamilton, Ontario: BC Decker, 2002 (CD-ROM).

70. Chan KH, Bluestone CD. Lack of efficacy of middle-ear inflation: treatment of otitis media with effusion in children. *Otolaryngol Head Neck Surg* 1989;100:317–323.

71. Chan KH, Mandel EM, Rockette HE, et al. A comparative study of amoxicillin-clavulanate and amoxicillin. *Arch Otolaryngol Head Neck Surg* 1988;114:142–146.

72. Thomsen J, Sederberg-Olsen J, Balle V, et al. Antibiotic treatment of children with secretory otitis media. *Arch Otolaryngol Head Neck Surg* 1989;115:447–451.

73. Mandel EM, Rockette HE, Paradise JL, et al. Comparative efficacy of erythromycin-sulfisoxazole, cefaclor, amoxicillin or placebo for otitis media with effusion in children. *Pediatr Infect Dis J* 1991;10:899–906.

74. Rosenfeld RM, Post JC. Meta-analysis of antibiotics for the treatment of otitis media with effusion. *Otolaryngol Head Neck Surg* 1992;106:378–386.

75. Mandel EM, Casselbrant ML, Rockette HE, et al. Efficacy of antimicrobial prophylaxis for recurrent middle ear effusion. *Pediatr Infect Dis J* 1996;15:1074–1082.

76. Mandel EM, Rockette HE, Bluestone CD, et al. Myringotomy with and without tympanostomy tubes for chronic otitis media with effusion. *Arch Otolaryngol Head Neck Surg* 1989;115:1217–1224.

77. Mandel EM, Rockette HE, Bluestone CD, et al. Efficacy of myringotomy with and without tympanostomy tubes for chronic otitis media with effusion. *Pediatr Infect Dis J* 1992;11:270–277.

78. Casselbrant ML, Brostoff LM, Cantekin EI, et al. Otitis media in children in the United States. In: Sade J, ed. *Proceedings of the International Conference on Acute and Secretory Otitis Media.* Amsterdam: Kugler Publications, 1986:161–164.

79. Bluestone CD, Klein JO, Gates GA. "Appropriateness" of tympanostomy tubes: setting the record straight. *Arch Otolaryngol Head Neck Surg* 1994;120:1051–1053.

80. Maw AR. Chronic otitis media with effusion (glue ear) and adenotonsillectomy: prospective randomized controlled study. *BMJ* 1983;287:1586–1588.

81. Gates GA, Avery CA, Prihoda TJ, et al. Effectiveness of adenoidectomy and tympanostomy tubes in the treatment of chronic otitis media with effusion. *N Engl J Med* 1987;317:1444–1451.

82. Maw AR. Age and adenoid size in relation to adenoidectomy in otitis media with effusion. *Am J Otolaryngol* 1985;6:245–248.

83. Gates GA, Avery CA, Prihoda TJ. Effect of adenoidectomy upon children with chronic otitis media with effusion. *Laryngoscope* 1988;98:58–63.

84. Ghaffer FA, Wordemann M, Mccracken GH. Acute mastoiditis in children: a seventeen-year experience in Dallas, Texas. *Pediatr Infect Dis J* 2001;20:376–380.

85. Goldstein NA, Casselbrant ML, Bluestone CD, et al. Intratemporal complications of acute otitis media in infants and children. *Otolaryngol Head Neck Surg* 1998;119:444–454.

86. Van Zuijlen DA, Schilder AGM, Van Balen FAM, et al. National differences in incidences of acute mastoiditis: relationship to prescribing patterns of antibiotics for acute otitis media. *Pediatr Infect Dis J* 2001;20:140–144.

87. Breiman RF, Butler JC, Tenover FC, et al. Emergence of drug-resistant pneumococcal infections in the United States. *JAMA* 1994;271:1831–1835.

88. Harley EH, Sdralis T, Berkowitz RG. Acute mastoiditis in children: a 12-year retrospective study. *Otolaryngol Head Neck Surg* 1997;116:26–30.

89. Hawkins DB, Dru D, House JW, et al. Acute mastoiditis in children: a review of 54 cases. *Laryngoscope* 1983;93:568–572.

90. Nadol D, Herrmann P, Baumann A, Fanconi A. Acute mastoiditis: clinical, microbiological, and therapeutic aspects. *Eur J Pediatr* 1990;149:560–564.

91. Luntz M, Keren G, Nusem S, et al. Acute mastoiditis—revisited. *Ear Nose Throat J* 1994;73:648–654.

92. Gliklich RE, Eavey RD, Iannuzzi RA, et al. A contemporary analysis of acute mastoiditis. *Arch Otolaryngol Head Neck Surg* 1996;122:135–139.

93. Bezold F, Siebenmann F. *Text-book of otology*. [Holinger J, translator]. Chicago: EH Cosgrove, 1908:179–185.

94. Smouha EE, Levenson MJ, Anand VK, et al. Modern presentations of Bezold's abscess. *Arch Otolaryngol Head Neck Surg* 1989;115:1126–1129.

95. Bluestone CD. Otologic surgical procedures. In: Bluestone CD, Stool SE, eds. *Atlas of pediatric otolaryngology*. Philadelphia: WB Saunders, 1995:27–128.

96. Mawson SR, Ludman H. *Diseases of the ear: a textbook of otology*. Chicago: Year Book Medical Publishers, 1979.

97. Tovi F, Gatot A. Bone scan diagnosis of masked mastoiditis. *Ann Otol Rhinol Laryngol* 1992;101:707–709.

98. Bluestone CD. Acute and chronic mastoiditis and chronic suppurative otitis media. *Semin Pediatr Infect Dis* 1998;9:12–26.

99. Bluestone CD. Epidemiology and pathogenesis of chronic suppurative otitis media: implications for prevention and treatment. *Int J Pediatr Otolrhinolaryngol* 1998;42:207–223.

100. Dohar JE, Kenna MA, Wadowsky RM. In vitro susceptibility of aural isolates of *P. aeruginosa* to commonly used ototopical antibiotics. *Am J Otol* 1996,17:207–209.

101. Mandel EM, Casselbrant ML, Kurs-Lasky M. Acute otorrhea: bacteriology of a common complication of tympanostomy tubes. *Ann Otol Rhinol Laryngol* 1994;103:713–718.

102. Kenna MA, Bluestone CD, Reilly JS, et al. Medical management of chronic suppurative otitis media without cholesteatoma in children. *Laryngoscope* 1986;96:146–151.

103. Bluestone CD. Pathogenesis of otitis media: role of eustachian tube. *Pediatr Infect Dis J* 1996;14:281–291.

104. Kenna MA, Bluestone CD. Medical management of chronic suppurative otitis media without cholesteatoma. In: Lim DJ, Bluestone CD, Klein JO, et al., eds. *Recent advances in otitis media: proceedings of the Fourth International Symposium*. Burlington, Ontario: BC Decker, 1988:222–226.

105. Bluestone CD. Clinical course, complications and sequelae of acute otitis media. *Pediatr Infect Dis J* 2000;19:S37–S46.

106. Hannley MT, Denneny JC 3rd, Holzer SS. Use of ototopical antibiotics in treating three common ear diseases. *Otolaryngol Head Neck Surg* 2000;122:934–940.

107. Goldblatt EL, Dohar J, Nozza RJ, et al. Topic ofloxacin versus systemic amoxicillin/clavulanate in purulent otorrhea in children with tympanostomy tubes. *Int J Pediatr Otorhinolaryngol* 1998;46:91–101.

108. Agro AS, Garner ET, Wright JW 3rd, et al. Clinical trial of ototopical ofloxacin for treatment of chronic suppurative otitis media. *Clin Ther* 1998;20:744–759.

109. Kaga K, Ichimura K. A preliminary report: clinical effects of otic solution of ofloxacin in infantile myringitis and chronic otitis media. *Int J Pediatr Otorhinolaryngol* 1998;42:199–205.

110. Tong MCF, Woo JKS, van Hasslet CA. A double-blind comparative study of ofloxicin otic drops versus neomycin-polymyxin B-hydrocortisone otic drops in the medical treatment of chronic suppurative otitis media. *J Laryngol Otol* 1996;110:309–314.

111. Bluestone, CD. Efficacy of ofloxacin and other ototopical preparations for chronic suppurative otitis media in children. *Pediatr Infect Dis J* 2001;20:111–118.

112. Dohar JE, Alper CM, Bluestone CD, et al. Treatment of chronic suppurative otitis media with topical ciprofloxacin. In: Lim DJ, Bluestone CD, Casselbrant ML, et al., eds. *Recent advances in otitis media: proceedings of the Sixth International Symposium*. Hamilton, Ontario: BC Decker, 1996:525–528.

113. Esposito S, D'Errico G, Montanaro C. Topical and oral treatment of chronic otitis media with ciprofloxacin. *Arch Otolaryngol Head Neck Surg* 1990;116:557–559.

114. Esposito S, Noviello S, D'Errico G, et al. Topical ciprofloxacin vs. intramuscular gentamicin for chronic otitis media. *Arch Otolaryngol Head Neck Surg* 1992;118:842–844.

115. Aslan A, Altuntas A, Titiz A, et al. A new dosage regimen for topical application of ciprofloxacin in the management of chronic suppurative otitis media. *Otolaryngol Head Neck Surg* 1998;118:883–885.

116. Tutkun A, Ozagar A, Koc A, et al. Treatment of chronic ear disease: topical ciprofloxacin vs. topical gentamicin. *Arch Otolaryngol Head Neck Surg* 1995;121:1414–1416.

117. Fradis M, Brodsky A, Ben-David J, et al. Chronic otitis media treated topically with ciprofloxacin or tobramycin. *Arch Otolaryngol Head Neck Surg* 1997;123:1057–1060.

118. Ozagar A, Koc A, Ciprut A, et al. Effects of topical otic preparation on hearing in chronic otitis media. *Otolaryngol Head Neck Surg* 1997;117:405–408.

119. Alper CM, Doyle WJ. Repeated inflation does not prevent otitis media with effusion in a monkey model. *Laryngoscope* 1999;109:1074–1080.

120. Crowther JA, Simpson D. Medical treatment of chronic otitis media: steroid or antibiotic with steroid ear-drops? *Clin Otolaryngol* 1991;16:142–144.

121. Clayton MI, Osborne JE, Rutherford D, et al. A double-blind, randomized, prospective trial of a topical antiseptic versus a topical antibiotic in the treatment of otorrhea. *J Otolaryngol* 1990;15:7–10.

122. Thorp MA, Kruger J, Oliver S, et al. The antibacterial acidity of acetic acid and Burow's solution as topical otological preparations. *J Laryngol Otol* 1998;112:925–928.

123. Kenna MA, Rosane BA, Bluestone CD. Medical management of chronic suppurative otitis media without cholesteatoma in children-Update 1992. *Am J Otol* 1993;14:469–4733.

124. Bluestone CD. Otitis media: management in the era of resistant bacteria. Summary and conclusions of the meeting. *Pediatr Infect Dis J* 1998;17:1099–1100.

CHAPTER 46
Infections of the Pharynx, Larynx, Epiglottis, Trachea, and Thyroid

Irmgard Behlau

PHARYNGITIS

Pharyngitis or pharyngotonsillitis is defined as an inflammation in the area of the posterior oral cavity involving lymphoid tissues of the posterior pharynx and lateral pharyngeal bands. Scarlatina anginosa, or sore throat, was described by James Sims in Boston and London in 1803 (1).

Etiology and Pathophysiology

The lymphoid tissues of the nasopharynx and pharynx, known as the Waldeyer ring, include the adenoid, palatine, and lingual tonsils (2). The lymphoid tissues are present at birth, enlarge in infancy and childhood, and undergo atrophy shortly after puberty. The adenoid, known as the pharyngeal tonsil or Luschka tonsil, is lymphoid tissue of the nasopharynx. It drains into the lymphatics of the retropharyngeal and pharyngomaxillary spaces and from there into the neck. The faucial or palatine tonsil is a cryptic, subepithelial encapsulated lymph node that lies in the tonsillar fossa. The fossa is formed by three muscles: the palatoglossus forms the anterior pillar, the palatopharyngeal forms the posterior pillar, and the superior pharyngeal constrictor forms the bed. The lingual tonsil covers the base of the tongue; it is located behind the circumvallate papillae and may extend to the base of the epiglottis. The lymphatics of the lingual tonsil drain into the suprahyoid, submaxillary, and deep cervical lymphatic chains. Whereas the other lymphoid tissue becomes atrophic after puberty, the lingual tonsil often becomes hypertrophic. The cervical lymph nodes effectively drain and filter microorganisms from the structures of the Waldeyer ring. The two potential spaces important in the spread of infection from the lymphatic structures of the Waldeyer ring are the pharyngomaxillary fossa and the retropharyngeal space (see Chapter 43).

Organisms responsible for acute pharyngitis and tonsillitis include viruses, bacteria, and less often mycoplasmas, spirochetes, and chlamydiae.

The most common viral agents of sore throat are rhinovirus, coronavirus, adenovirus, influenza A and B viruses, and parainfluenza viruses (3–7). Coronavirus and adenovirus may invade the pharyngeal mucosa directly. Other viruses associated with pharyngitis include herpes simplex virus (types 1 and 2), coxsackievirus A (types 2, 4, 5, 6, 8, and 10), Epstein-Barr virus (EBV), cytomegalovirus, and human immunodeficiency virus (8,9).

Of the bacterial organisms, group A β-hemolytic streptococci are estimated to cause approximately 15% of all cases of pharyngitis or pharyngotonsillitis. *Streptococcus pyogenes* is important to diagnose as an agent of pharyngitis because of the possibility of serious suppurative and nonsuppurative sequelae. *S. pyogenes* elaborates several factors—streptokinase, hemolysins, erythrogenic toxin, deoxyribonuclease, proteinase, and hyaluronidase—that may play a role in invasion (10). Less often, groups C and G β-hemolytic streptococci are responsible for sore throat (7,11–17). Group C streptococci have been associated with endemic pharyngitis among adults (12,13). Corynebacteria, including *Corynebacterium diphtheriae* and *Corynebacterium ulcerans, Arcanobacterium haemolyticum* (formerly *Corynebacterium haemolyticum*), *Yersinia enterocolitica, Neisseria gonorrhoeae*, mixed anaerobic infection (Vincent's angina), and *Treponema pallidum* are less common causes of pharyngitis (18–31). *C. diphtheriae* may in addition cause a fibrinous membrane of leukocytes, necrotic cells, and bacteria. Increased adherence of *S. aureus, Streptococcus pneumoniae* type I, and *H. influenzae* to pharyngeal cells early during experimental infection with influenza virus suggests that mucosal cell changes leading to increased adherence of selected bacteria also may contribute to the pathogenesis of these secondary infections (10,47). In patients with recurrent pharyngotonsillitis, the possibility of β-lactamase–producing bacteria [*Staphylococcus aureus, Haemophilus influenzae, Moraxella (Branhamella) catarrhalis, Bacteroides* species, *Prevotella, Porphyromonas,* and *Fusobacterium*] should be considered. Anaerobes are a major component of tonsil surface and core bacterial flora in patients with recurrent tonsillitis (32).

Mycoplasma pneumoniae may cause up to 10% of pharyngitis in adults (7,33). A less common cause of pharyngitis is *Mycoplasma hominis*. It has been shown to cause pharyngitis in 50% of human volunteers under experimental conditions (34,35), but it is a rare cause of naturally occurring pharyngitis (36,37). The role of *Chlamydia trachomatis* is even less firmly established (38–41). It may be a cause of pharyngitis in the sexually active population seen in sexually transmitted disease clinics, although data are conflicting (42). *Chlamydia pneumoniae*, previously a TWAR strain of *Chlamydia psittaci,* is associated with cases of pharyngitis, bronchitis, and pneumonia (43–46).

In temperate climates, pharyngitis occurs during colder months of the year. The peak prevalence of rhinoviruses is during spring and fall, of coronaviruses and adenoviruses (acute respiratory disease) mainly during the colder months, and of other adenoviruses (pharyngoconjunctival fever) in the early summer. Streptococcal pharyngitis occurs during the colder months of the year in temperate climates, and infection rates are higher in late winter and early spring. Fifteen percent to 20% of school children carry group A streptococci in their throats, but less than 10% have a sore throat. The disease is ordinarily spread by direct person-to-person contact, most likely by droplets of saliva or nasal secretions. Patients who do not receive antibiotic therapy develop type-specific antibodies that are detectable in serum between 4 and 8 weeks after infection; these opsonic antibodies protect against later infection.

Clinical Manifestations

Adenoviral pharyngitis is marked by severe sore throat, malaise, headache, chills, myalgia, and fever. On examination, pharyngeal erythema and inflammatory exudate are present; conjunctivitis (follicular) also may be present in 25% to 50% of cases. With influenzal pharyngitis, severe sore throat is present with myalgia, headache, cough, coryza, and temperature elevation, but erythema of the pharynx is mild. Only mild pharyngeal irritation is found with rhinovirus infection (common cold); on examination, the pharynx is only slightly inflamed. Primary infection with herpes simplex virus may present as acute painful pharyngitis with erythema and exudate; vesicles and shallow ulcers of both posterior (buccal) and anterior (labial) mucosa are helpful in the diagnosis if associated with gingival stomatitis. Chronic herpes simplex infection in immunocompromised hosts is characterized by progressive large, shallow, and painful ulcers.

Herpangina (coxsackievirus A) is more common in children and may present as severe sore throat; small vesicles (1–2 mm) are typically seen in the posterior pharynx only (soft palate, uvula, and anterior tonsillar pillars). Pharyngitis or exudative tonsillitis occurs in half of patients with infectious mononucleosis (EBV); usually fatigue, malaise, headache, adenopathy, and fever are all present. Pharyngitis with fever, myalgia, lethargy, and truncal maculopapular rash is characteristic of primary infection with human immunodeficiency virus (9,48).

The clinical pattern of pharyngitis with *S. pyogenes* ranges from abrupt onset of marked pain, headache, malaise, dysphagia, and fever (temperature higher than 39.4°C) with pharyngeal inflammation, edema, and gray-white tonsillar exudate and tender submandibular lymph nodes to only mild sore throat; pharyngitis due to strains of groups C and G streptococci may present in a similar fashion. The disease is self-limited; all acute signs subside within a week. Rare cases of toxic shock syndrome have been described with noninvasive streptococcal pharyngitis (49). Sore throat, diffuse maculopapular rash, and pharyngeal exudate and erythema may be seen in children and young adults with *A. haemolyticum* infection (24,25). *M. pneumoniae* usually produces mild pharyngitis, which may be associated with bronchitis or pneumonia (50). *C. pneumoniae* may be associated with chronic pharyngitis (45,46).

Diagnosis

A definitive diagnosis of pharyngitis may be difficult to make on clinical grounds alone, although the presence of pharyngeal or tonsillar exudate, tender lymph nodes at the angle of the mandible, rash, or conjunctivitis is helpful. Pharyngeal exudate is usually present with group A, C, or G streptococci, *C. diphtheriae, A. haemolyticum, Y. enterocolitica*, anaerobic bacteria, adenovirus, herpes simplex virus, and EBV. Pharyngeal exudate is not usually present with influenza or rhinovirus. Rash may suggest infection with *S. pyogenes, A. haemolyticum*, human immunodeficiency virus, or EBV. The presence of conjunctivitis suggests adenovirus infection or less commonly diphtheria or chlamydia infections. Diagnosis of group A streptococcal infections depends on recognizing the clinical syndrome and culturing the bacterium from a deep throat culture onto a blood agar plate. Tests are available that allow rapid diagnosis of streptococcal pharyngitis by detecting group A streptococcal antigen on throat swab specimens. Latex agglutination and other rapid systems are highly specific (95%–99%) and moderately sensitive (70%–90%) compared with throat cultures. Throat cultures should be obtained in clinically suspected cases with negative antigen test results (51). Most strains of group C and G are β-hemolytic and some are bacitracin sensitive; bacteria in both groups can produce many of the same enzymes and toxins produced by group A streptococci. Serologic tests are also useful in documenting recent streptococcal infection. The most widely used is the anti-streptolysin O titer, which is elevated after most respiratory tract infections. Anti-DNAse titers are also elevated after streptococcal pharyngitis.

A throat culture plated on Loeffler medium is necessary for any suspected case of diphtheria. The hemolysis associated with *A. haemolyticum* is maximal at 48 to 72 hours and is more prominent on rabbit and human blood agar (24). Diagnosis of *Mycoplasma* infection depends either on isolation of the organism in culture or on demonstration of an increase in antibody titer (39). Throat or sputum cultures are placed on SP-4 medium. Polymerase chain reaction tests for *Mycoplasma* and *Chlamydia* are in use in selected centers. The diagnosis of *Chlamydia* infections in the acute phase, especially by culture (43), is often difficult.

Serologic methods, particularly for *C. pneumoniae,* are helpful in retrospect (39–43).

Therapy

Group A streptococci continue to be uniformly sensitive to penicillin V potassium, which remains the drug of choice (52,53). Adults receive 10 days of oral therapy (500 mg every 6–8 hours), and children receive 25 to 50 mg/kg per day in three or four equal doses (53–55). A single intramuscular dose of 1.2 million units of benzathine penicillin is an excellent form of therapy because it does not require the patient's compliance. For penicillin-allergic patients, erythromycin, 500 mg four times daily for 10 days, is a good alternative. Optimal treatment should prevent acute rheumatic fever, reduce acute morbidity, and prevent suppurative complications such as peritonsillar abscess, bacteremia, and rarely postangina sepsis (56–59). Instituting treatment within 9 days of the onset of streptococcal pharyngitis prevents subsequent acute rheumatic fever (56,57). In addition to proven efficacy, the treatment of choice should be safe, have a narrow spectrum of activity, and be low in cost. Waiting for the results of throat culture before starting treatment or beginning therapy and discontinuing it if the culture is negative are both reasonable approaches. Multiple M types, most belonging to Fischetti "class I" proteins, have been implicated in acute rheumatic fever (60,61). Whether mucoid strains, especially M Fischetti "class I" type (18), are responsible for the resurgence of acute rheumatic fever remains to be evaluated (62,63). Studies have documented failure rates of 25% or more in patients treated with penicillin for acute tonsillitis and even higher for chronic tonsillitis (64). Factors include reinfection, noncompliance, carrier state (65,66), and possible selection of β-lactamase–producing bacteria. In the case of recurrent streptococcal tonsillitis, clindamycin, amoxicillin-clavulanate, or penicillin and metronidazole or a macrolide and metronidazole are reasonable. *Mycoplasma* and *Chlamydia* upper respiratory tract infections respond to macrolides such as erythromycin, 500 mg orally four times daily, or tetracycline, 500 mg orally four times daily for 14 days. Viral pharyngitis or chronic oral pharyngeal herpetic infection in an immunosuppressed patient should be treated with acyclovir; therapy is not necessary for acute herpetic pharyngitis in normal hosts. Symptomatic therapy is directed at relieving pharyngeal discomfort. Warm saline gargles, rest, acetaminophen, aspirin, and liquids are sufficient in most cases of viral pharyngitis.

VINCENT'S ANGINA

Vincent's angina is an acute pseudomembranous involvement of the pharynx or tonsils. Acute necrotizing ulcerative gingivitis, or trench mouth, is an ulcerative necrosis of the interdental papillae in the marginal gingivae. If the disease spreads to other oral structures, the term *acute necrotizing ulcerative mucositis,* or *Vincent's stomatitis,* is used. Acute necrotizing ulcerative gingivitis, acute necrotizing ulcerative mucositis, and Vincent's angina are all classified as Vincent's disease or Vincent's infection.

Etiology and Pathophysiology

Vincent's angina may start as aseptic necrosis secondary to capillary stasis due to poor oral hygiene, local irritation from food impaction, smoking, trauma, stress, and endocrine or metabolic disturbances. Poor oral hygiene may contribute to stasis by releasing bacterial products from the accumulating dental plaque

(67–69). The disease is most likely secondary to a combination of fusospirochetal organisms (most often *Fusobacterium nucleatum* and *Treponema vincentii*) and gram-negative anaerobic organisms (*Bacteroides* species, *Prevotella intermedius,* and *Prevotella melaninogenica*) (70–72).

Clinical Manifestations

The disease begins abruptly with pain, fetid odor of the breath, and gingival or tonsillar bleeding. There is necrosis, pseudomembrane, lymphadenopathy, and excessive salivation; fever and anorexia also may occur. The disease may spread to other mucosa and may lead to noma, a gangrenous stomatitis, beginning in the corner of the mouth or cheek and rapidly involving the entire thickness of the lips and cheeks with necrosis and tissue sloughing (73). Transient bacteremia or septicemia may develop from the massive bacterial flora at bleeding sites.

Diagnosis

Gram-stained specimens of the affected mucosa should be examined for gram-positive cocci, gram-negative bacilli, and fusospirochetal gram-negative organisms. Debrided material is optimal for anaerobic culture.

Therapy

Oral penicillin at 500 mg four times daily, metronidazole at 500 mg three times daily, and clindamycin at 600 mg three times daily are reasonable therapeutic options.

LARYNGITIS

The larynx rests in the hypopharynx anterior to the fourth, fifth, and sixth cervical vertebrae. The supraglottic larynx includes the laryngeal inlet formed by the epiglottis anteriorly and the arytenoepiglottic folds bilaterally, all merging inferiorly into false cords. The glottic larynx consists of the true vocal folds; the space between the folds is termed the glottis.

Etiology and Pathophysiology

Respiratory viruses such as influenza virus, parainfluenza virus, rhinovirus, and adenovirus are most often isolated in cases of laryngitis (74,75). *M. catarrhalis* has been recovered from the nasopharynx of 50% to 55% and *H. influenzae* from 8% to 15% of adults with acute laryngitis; whether these represent secondary bacterial invasion is not clear (76). Group A and G streptococci, *C. pneumoniae,* and *M. pneumoniae* also have been associated with acute laryngitis. Laryngeal diphtheria is rare and usually results from extension of pharyngeal involvement; it may occur in previously immunized persons. *M. hominis* is an uncommon but important pathogen as a cause of granulomatous laryngitis (77). Other causes of granulomatous laryngitis include fungal infections such as histoplasmosis, coccidioidomycosis, blastomycosis, and candidiasis (78–82). *Candida* infection commonly accompanies esophageal infection in compromised hosts. Laryngeal tuberculosis is rarely seen in the United States; it is associated with a large tuberculous load, and patients frequently have very active pulmonary involvement (83). Wegener's granulomatosis, sarcoidosis, and rhinoscleroma also should be considered (77). *T. pallidum,* herpes simplex virus, and herpes zoster virus may be isolated from the larynx (84).

Clinical Manifestations

Symptoms of acute laryngitis include hoarseness, odynophagia, and localized pain, which may be referred to other branches of the vagus and manifested by otalgia. Examination of the larynx reveals inflammation, edema, and secretions; there may be superficial mucosal ulcerations. The presence of an exudate or membrane on the pharyngeal or laryngeal mucosa should raise the suspicion of streptococcal infection, mononucleosis, or diphtheria; granulomatous infiltration is compatible with tuberculosis, fungal infection, sarcoidosis, and syphilis. Hoarseness in the patient with pulmonary lesions and productive cough should prompt biopsy of the larynx.

Therapy

Treatment consists of resting the voice and inhaling moistened air. Because acute laryngitis in adults is self-limiting and subjective symptoms spontaneously diminish after 1 week in most cases, empiric antibiotic treatment does not seem warranted as a general policy. Antimicrobial therapy is only indicated in those patients with a bacterial superinfection, and treatment is directed toward the causative agents. The usual duration of therapy is 10 to 14 days.

ACUTE SUPRAGLOTTITIS (EPIGLOTTITIS)

Supraglottitis (epiglottitis), first described in 1900 by Theisen (85), is characterized by a severe upper respiratory tract infection with fever, sore throat, hoarseness, dysphagia, and drooling that may rapidly progress to fatal airway obstruction. Although LeMierre and co-workers described the association of adult epiglottitis with *H. influenzae* infection in 1936 (86), it was not until the late 1960s with reports by Johnstone and Lawy (87) and Gorfinkel and colleagues (88) that supraglottitis was increasingly recognized in adults.

Epiglottitis, which most commonly affected children 2 to 7 years of age, continues to undergo a dramatic and changing epidemiologic pattern since the introduction of the *H. influenzae* type B (Hib) vaccines in the middle to late 1980s. With continued widespread vaccination of younger children with the conjugate Hib vaccines, Hib epiglottitis in young children is becoming a vanishing entity. Epiglottitis has become a disease of older children and adults, and it will be due predominantly to microbial pathogens other than Hib.

Etiology and Pathophysiology

Acute supraglottitis in children has been predominantly due to Hib, but other pathogens such as *S. pneumoniae, S. aureus,* other streptococci, *H. influenzae* type non-b, and *Haemophilus parainfluenzae* are becoming the predominant organisms, without an increase in the incidence of these other agents (89). In addition, the pharyngeal carriage rate of Hib in children has declined without an increase in the carriage of other pathogens (90,91). When Hib is the causative agent, the isolation rate for *H. influenzae* from blood cultures is between 80% and 100% (89,92). The bacteriology of adult epiglottitis is less well defined, but Hib is a principal agent, in some reports accounting for 26% of cases (93). The presence of *H. influenzae* bacteremia is associated with a more fulminant course, with the development of respiratory obstruction (93,94). In adults, infection also may occur with organisms other than Hib, including *S. pneumoniae, β*-hemolytic streptococci, *H. influenzae* type non-b, *H. parainfluenzae, S. aureus,* and *Pasteurella multocida* (95–97). The role of respiratory tract viruses

as pathogens in adults and children remains unclear. In many adult cases, an agent is not found (96).

Supraglottitis is characterized by inflammation and edema of the supraglottic structures, including the epiglottis, arytenoepiglottic folds, arytenoids, and false vocal cords; paradoxically, the epiglottis may be spared. The mechanism of supraglottic infection is unknown. Supraglottitis may arise from direct invasion by *H. influenzae* or other pathogens. It is possible that mucosal surface trauma secondary to eating or to an antecedent viral infection may lead to a secondary bacterial infection, but the role of viruses as primary pathogens has rarely been demonstrated (98,99). It is also not clear whether bacteremia, which is seen frequently in children, may be a primary event, with seeding of the supraglottis, or a secondary event.

Clinical Manifestations

In children, acute supraglottitis is typically characterized by a fulminating course of severe sore throat, high fever, dysphagia, drooling, and airway obstruction, which if left untreated, leads to death. Low-pitched inspiratory stridor is due to the approximation of the swollen supraglottic structures. On physical examination, the child looks toxic and apprehensive and frequently assumes an airway-preserving posture: sitting upright, with the jaw protruding forward, while drooling. Respirations are deliberate without marked tachypnea. Tachycardia out of proportion to the amount of pyrexia is a reflection of the hypoxia. Should stridor be absent, an unwary physician might underestimate the severity and rapidity of progression of the patient's worsening air exchange, which may result in cardiopulmonary arrest if left untreated.

The presentation of acute supraglottitis in adults is more variable; most adults have mild illness with a prolonged prodrome (96). Some may not seek medical attention or may be treated for presumed pharyngitis. This does not mean that the disease is any less serious; in some studies, it carries a mortality risk of 7.1% (96). In immunocompromised hosts, the clinical presentation may be less typical. In a report of five patients with acquired immunodeficiency syndrome (AIDS) (100), the clinical presentation was notable for a paucity of physical findings. Laryngoscopy revealed a large, pale, boggy epiglottis with an edematous supraglottis and cervical adenopathy coupled with rapidly progressing airway obstruction. Local complications of supraglottitis include spread into the retropharyngeal area and epiglottic abscess formation; systemic complications include bacteremia, pneumonia (in up to 25% of cases) (101), meningitis, arthritis, and cellulitis.

Diagnosis

Definitive diagnosis is made by examination of the epiglottis and supraglottic structures. No attempt should be made to visualize the epiglottis in an awake young child, so a severely ill child must often be examined in the operating room at the time of control of the airway. In adults, awake indirect laryngoscopy is usually sufficient to make the diagnosis. This examination should be performed only when it is possible to establish an artificial airway if necessary. In children, the epiglottis is typically fiery red and extremely swollen, but occasionally the major inflammation involves the ventricular bands and arytenoepiglottic folds, and the epiglottis appears relatively normal. In adults, the supraglottic structures may appear pale with watery edema.

Leukocytosis is a characteristic laboratory finding. Blood and supraglottic specimens should be obtained for culture; serum and urine samples for Hib antigen may be useful. Lateral soft

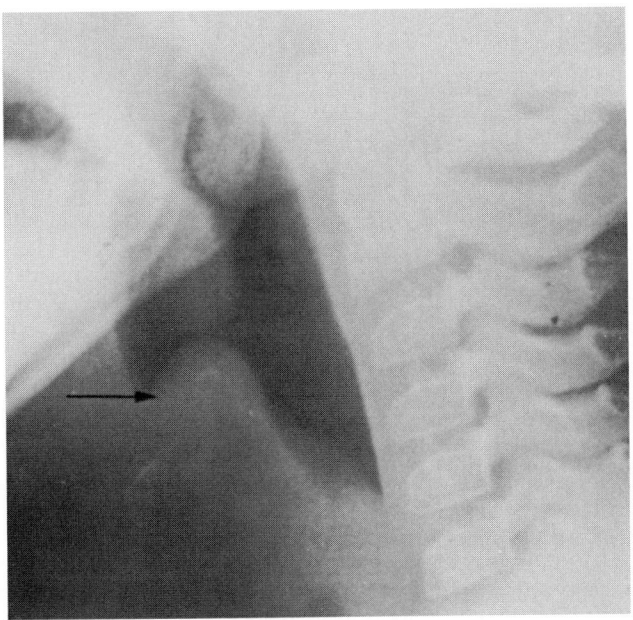

Figure 46.1. Thickened epiglottis (*arrow*) in a patient with epiglottitis. (Courtesy of Dr. A. Weber, Massachusetts Eye and Ear Infirmary, Boston, MA.)

tissue radiographs may reveal the classic thumb sign (Fig. 46.1) and, in some, swelling of the arytenoepiglottic folds and arytenoids, with a sensitivity of approximately 79% (89,94,102).

Major causes of upper airway obstruction can be classified by the anatomic level of involvement, using the glottis as the dividing line. Other supraglottic conditions are peritonsillar and retropharyngeal abscesses, severe tonsillitis, and adenotonsillar hypertrophy associated with infectious mononucleosis. Subglottic obstruction may be from croup (laryngotracheitis), laryngotracheobronchitis, diphtheria, angioedema (allergic laryngeal edema), foreign body aspiration, or neoplasm.

Therapy

Treatment of acute supraglottitis is directed at establishment of an airway and administration of appropriate antibiotics. The mortality rates of supraglottitis vary greatly; most deaths occur within the first few hours after arrival at a hospital. Children with epiglottitis should routinely have an artificial airway established; observation cannot be recommended because the associated mortality rate is 6% to 25%, and it increases to 33% to 80% for those who develop obstruction (103,104). The use of a "prophylactic airway" has reduced mortality in children from 6% to less than 1% (105). An endotracheal tube is preferred by most clinicians over a tracheotomy for provision of the artificial airway (105–107). Advantages of nasotracheal intubation are (a) the ease of removal of the tube 2 or 3 days after edema has subsided, thereby shortening hospitalization (106,107); (b) no surgery; and (c) mortality and complication rates equal to or lower than those for tracheotomy. If accidental extubation should occur, there is a grace period of 30 to 60 minutes caused by the ballooning effect of the endotracheal tube (106,108), which is not afforded by tracheotomy. Once the tube is in place, accidental extubation is uncommon (9%) (106). The management of airway in adult epiglottitis reflects the greater variability of clinical presentation and course; the range of mortality rates is 10% to 32% (92,94,109–112). Vigilant airway monitoring and continuous staging with uniform management protocols are needed for adults, whose

disease may progress to respiratory compromise requiring intubation (113–115).

Despite the changing epidemiology, antibiotics are still directed against *H. influenzae* as the predominant organism and antibiotic coverage should include *S. pneumoniae*, other streptococci, and *H. parainfluenzae*. Due to the risk for infection with ampicillin-resistant *H. influenzae* (89,116), intravenous cefuroxime, 50 mg/kg every 8 hours, ceftriaxone 50 to 100 mg/kg per day, or ampicillin-sulbactam 50 mg/kg every 6 hours are reasonable initial therapy for children. For adults, intravenous cefuroxime 0.75 to 1.5 g every 8 hours, ceftriaxone 2 g per day, or ampicillin-sulbactam are reasonable choices. The condition of most patients improves by 48 hours, but antibiotic therapy should be continued for 10 to 14 days.

The artificial airway can usually be removed by 48 hours. Criteria for safe removal of the airway are clinical response and either a leak around the endotracheal tube or evidence of resolution on direct visualization with a fiberoptic laryngoscope. An air leak has proved to be a reliable indicator of the extent of laryngeal inflammation, making direct visualization less crucial (108).

Prevention

Rifampin prophylaxis, a single daily dose for 4 days (20 mg/kg, not to exceed 600 mg per day) is recommended for (a) all household contacts when there are susceptible members under 4 years of age, (b) day care and nursery school classroom contacts (including adults), and (c) the patient, who should receive rifampin in the same dosage before discharge to prevent reintroduction of the organism into the household (117).

In Finland, large-scale vaccination of 94% to 98% of infants with the Hib conjugate vaccine was begun in 1986 (118). In the next 5 years, the incidence of Hib epiglottitis decreased from 50 to 60 cases annually in 1985 and 1986 to 2 cases in 1992. There was no increase in the occurrence of epiglottitis caused by other pathogens. In limited U.S. population studies, the incidence of epiglottitis appears to have also declined dramatically. In one larger study, Gorelick and Baker (119) reported an 84% decline in the incidence of epiglottitis from 10.9 per 10,000 admissions to the Children's Hospital of Philadelphia from 1979 to 1989 to an average annual incidence of 1.8 per 10,000 during 1990 to 1992. A more recent large-scale study of the reported incidence of all Hib invasive diseases has shown a decline of 98% (120). The vaccine appears to also decrease the carriage rates in most, but not all population groups. Despite vaccination coverage of Alaskan native children 6 years or younger of greater than 90%, a carriage rate of 8% has persisted. This same group has a fivefold greater risk for invasive disease. In addition, areas of poor vaccination coverage, such as inner city "pockets of need," require improvement for near-eradication of Hib epiglottitis and other forms of invasive Hib in children.

TRACHEITIS

Whether George Washington died of bacterial laryngotracheitis, supraglottitis, or peritonsillar abscess is unclear; his physician's description was that of "cynanche trachealis" (121). The classic description of "angina suffocativa" fits well with the entity described as bacterial tracheitis (122). Cases of probable bacterial tracheitis (laryngotracheobronchitis) with marked exudate were described in the 1940s by Orton and co-workers (123) and Neffson (124). This entity affects both children and adults. The syndrome develops as a sequela of injury to the trachea, as from a viral infection (most commonly parainfluenza) or intubation (125–128). The acute onset is marked by high fever, stridor, and dyspnea, with copious amounts of purulent sputum. The clinical picture may resemble that of epiglottitis and may progress rapidly, requiring endotracheal intubation.

The organisms most commonly recovered from the tracheal exudate are S. aureus, group A β-hemolytic streptococci, and Hib (129).

The rapidly progressive course demands prompt diagnosis and differentiation from epiglottitis and croup. Relapsing polychondritis develops more slowly. Endoscopic examination demonstrates a normal glottic larynx with purulent debris, ulceration, and edema of the subglottis and trachea. The lateral soft tissue radiograph of the neck characteristically reveals a normal epiglottis with subglottic narrowing (pencil sign). Gram stain examination and culture of the tracheal secretions are necessary to identify the pathogen. Initial antibiotic therapy should cover streptococci, S. aureus, and H. influenzae; ampicillin-sulbactam or nafcillin and cefuroxime are reasonable antibiotics.

THYROID INFECTIONS

Infections of the thyroid gland are rare, but may be life threatening. Thyroid infections (130) are divided into the rare acute suppurative thyroiditis, which is primarily bacterial, uncommonly fungal or parasitic, and subacute granulomatous thyroiditis (de Quervain's disease), which is a viral infection. Subacute granulomatous thyroiditis is the most common cause of a painful thyroid gland. Both chronic lymphocytic thyroiditis (Hashimoto's thyroiditis) and subacute lymphocytic thyroiditis are autoimmune conditions and not associated with an active infection.

Etiology and Pathophysiology

The thyroid gland sits in the anterior neck and consists of two lobes connected by the isthmus. It is in proximity to the trachea, parathyroid glands, esophagus, recurrent laryngeal nerve, and blood vessels. Accessory thyroid tissue may be found in the tongue and mediastinum. Lingual thyroid tissue is a remnant of embryonal median tubular diverticulum as it moves downward and bifurcates to form the thyroid. Remnants of this tube persist in the form of a thyroglossal duct. In addition, fistulae arising from the pyriform laryngeal sinuses may extend to the thyroid gland. Many children with acute suppurative thyroiditis appear to have a fistulous tract between the left piriform sinus and the left lobe of the thyroid gland (131–138). This congenital anomaly from a persistent thyroglossal duct or a third or fourth branchial arch is an important causative factor in many cases of thyroiditis and accounts for the high recurrence rate observed in the absence of appropriate surgical therapy. Hematogenous or lymphogenous spread from an upper respiratory illness, blunt trauma, and contiguous infection from adjacent structures is more common in adults than children. Two thirds of adult patients who present with a bacterial infection of the thyroid have a preexisting thyroid disorder, usually a goiter (139). The rarity of acute suppurative thyroiditis, even in the preantibiotic era, reflects the relative resistance of the thyroid gland to bacterial infection. The thyroid gland is completely encapsulated, has a rich blood supply and lymphatic drainage, and has a high iodide content (139,140).

Acute suppurative thyroiditis is usually caused by S. aureus, S. pyogenes, S. pneumonia, and other oral anaerobes found either alone or as part of a mixed infection (139). S. aureus is the most frequently observed and is found in one third of cultures.

Rarely Clostridia species, Salmonella species, and Actinomyces are identified (139). Most fungal infections are opportunistic infections in immunocompromised hosts, particularly those due to Aspergillus. Seeding of the thyroid gland should be considered in a patient with a history of disseminated Aspergillus infection and recurrent relapses despite therapy (139,141). Virtually all P. carinii infections have occurred in patients with AIDS, usually on pentamidine therapy (142,143). Rarely, mycobacterial infections occur.

Subacute granulomatous thyroiditis is caused by a recent viral infection, occurs three- to fivefold more often in women than men, and the average age of onset is 30 to 50 years (144–146); it has a seasonal occurrence, most often in the summer and fall. Numerous etiologic agents have been implicated, including mumps, measles, Coxsackie virus, influenzae, echovirus, adenovirus, and EBV. Cytomegalovirus infection usually occurs in immunocompromised hosts (147).

Clinical Manifestations

The classic presentation of acute suppurative thyroiditis with the acute onset of fever, anterior neck pain and tenderness, dysphagia, sweating, and dermal erythema was noted as early as 1903 (148). Fluctuance is notable in one third of cases and signifies the presence of an abscess. Tachycardia is also common; only in rare cases does thyroid storm occur. Most patients have a preexisting thyroid disorder. Of note, mycobacterial, fungal, or actinomycosis infection of the thyroid may present less commonly with fever, pain, tenderness, and warmth; the onset tends to be more gradual and the duration prolonged.

Subacute granulomatous thyroiditis presents with the subacute onset of pain in the thyroid region, exacerbated by head turning or swallowing with possible radiation to the jaw, ear, or chest. The thyroid is firm, nodular, and tender to palpation. In contrast, subacute lymphocytic thyroiditis is a painless enlargement of the thyroid (130).

Diagnosis

Acute suppurative thyroiditis may be diagnosed on the clinical presentation of pain, fever, swelling, dysphagia, tenderness, tachycardia, and possibly fluctuance. Leukocytosis and an elevated erythrocyte sedimentation rate (ESR) are common laboratory findings (149). The thyroid-stimulating hormone, thyroxine (T_4), and triiodothyronine (T_3) levels are usually normal. Thyroid nuclear imaging usually demonstrates diminished or no uptake in the involved lobe or pole and cold nodules in areas of abscess formation (150). Fine-needle aspiration (151) should be performed for Gram stain and culture; if negative, then biopsy may be needed. In addition, due to congenital anomalies, thyroid disorders, and frequent recurrences, a barium swallow to evaluate for a persistent thyroglossal duct or piriform sinus anomaly should be performed (151).

Subacute granulomatous thyroiditis is suggested by a painful, tender, firm, and nodular neck mass, usually preceded by an upper respiratory tract infection. The ESR is usually elevated. Thyrotoxicosis is present in 50% patients in the acute phase, and the serum T_4 concentration is disproportionately elevated compared with the serum T_3 concentration. Serum T_3 levels are low to undetectable. Thyroglobulin is elevated. The radioactive iodine uptake (RAIU) is notably low, often less than 2% at 24 hours. Therefore, the physical examination, elevated ESR, increased thyroglobulin, and depressed RAIU suggest the diagnosis (150,151). A needle biopsy should be considered to rule out other causes (151).

The differential diagnosis of thyroid pain and swelling includes thyroid malignancy, lymphoma, intracystic hemorrhage, cervical adenitis, Ludwig's angina, perichondritis of the laryngeal cartilage, cellulitis of the anterior neck, indolent fungal, actinomyces, and mycobacterial infection, and atypical Hashimoto's thyroiditis.

Therapy

For acute suppurative thyroiditis, initial empiric therapy should include coverage for S. aureus, streptococci, and anaerobic organisms. Patients with abscess formation require surgical drainage and possibly a thyroid lobectomy. If gas formation is present, then a more aggressive surgical approach and antibiotic coverage for Clostridia species is indicated. In patients with recurrent disease and demonstration of fistulas by barium swallow, extirpation of the abscess cavity and a fistulectomy is indicated along with antibiotic therapy (136–138,151).

Patients with subacute granulomatous thyroiditis may find symptomatic relief with antiinflammatory agents beneficial. The natural history involves four phases that unfold over 4 to 6 months. The acute phase of thyroid pain and thyrotoxicosis may last 3 to 6 weeks or longer. Transient asymptomatic euthyroidism follows. Hypothyroidism often ensues, which may last weeks to months and is transient in the vast majority of patients. The final phase is a recovery period during which thyroid function tests normalize.

REFERENCES

1. Sims J. Scarlatina anginosa, commonly called sore throat. In: *Observations*, 3rd ed. London: Hall & Hiller, 1803.
2. Pratt LW. Infections of the lymphoid tissue. *Otolaryngology* 1990;3:27.
3. MacMillan JA, Sandstrom C, Weiner LB, et al. Viral and bacterial organisms associated with acute pharyngitis in a school-aged population. *J Pediatr* 1986;109:747.
4. Hendley JO, Fishburne HB, Gwaltney JM Jr. Coronavirus infections in working adults. *Am Rev Respir Dis* 1972;105:805.
5. Wenzel RP, Hendley JO, Davies JA, et al. Coronavirus infections in military recruits. Three-year study with coronavirus strains OC43 and 229E. *Am Rev Respir Dis* 1974;109:621.
6. Evans AS, Dick EC. Acute pharyngitis and tonsillitis in University of Wisconsin students. *JAMA* 1964;190:699.
7. Glezen WP, Clyde WA Jr, Senior RJ, et al. Group A streptococci, mycoplasmas, and viruses associated with acute pharyngitis. *JAMA* 1967;202:455.
8. Glezen WP, Fernald GW, Lohr JA. Acute respiratory disease of university students with special reference to the etiologic role of *Herpesvirus hominis*. *Am J Epidemiol* 1975;101:111.
9. Valle SOL. Febrile pharyngitis as the primary sign of HIV infection in a cluster of cases linked by sexual contact. *Scand J Infect Dis* 1987;19:13.
10. Paradise JL. Etiology, diagnosis and antimicrobial treatment of pharyngitis and pharyngotonsillitis. *Ann Otol Rhinol Laryngol* 1981;90(suppl):75.
11. Meier FA, Centor RM, Graham L Jr, et al. Clinical and microbiological evidence for endemic pharyngitis among adults due to group C streptococci. *Arch Intern Med* 1990;150:825.
12. Turner JC, Hayden GF, Kiselica D, et al. Association of group C β-hemolytic streptococci with endemic pharyngitis among college students. *JAMA* 1990;264:2644.
13. Turner JC, Fox A, Fox K, et al. Role of group C beta-hemolytic streptococci in pharyngitis: epidemiologic study of clinical features associated with isolation of group C streptococci. *J Clin Microbiol* 1993;31:808.
14. Stryker WS, Fraser DW, Facklam RR. Food-borne outbreak of group G streptococcal pharyngitis. *Am J Epidemiol* 1982;116:533.
15. Cohen D, Ferne M, Rouach T, et al. Food-borne outbreak of group G streptococcal sore throat in an Israeli military base. *Epidemiol Infect* 1987;99:249.
16. Gerber MA, Randolph MF, Martin NJ, et al. Community-wide outbreak of group G streptococcal pharyngitis. *Pediatrics* 1991;87:598.
17. Tacket CO, Davis BR, Carter GP, et al. *Yersinia enterocolitica* pharyngitis. *Ann Intern Med* 1983;99:40.
18. Harnisch JP, Tronca E, Nolan CM, et al. Diphtheria among alcoholic urban adults. *Ann Intern Med* 1989;111:71.
19. Seidenfeld SM, Sutker WL, Luby JP. *Fusobacterium necrophorum* septicemia following oropharyngeal infection. *JAMA* 1982;248:1348.
20. Hutt DM, Judson FN. Epidemiology and treatment of oropharyngeal gonorrhea. *Ann Intern Med* 1986;105:655.
21. Green SL, LaPeter KS. Pseudodiphtheritic membranous pharyngitis caused by *Corynebacterium hemolyticum*. *JAMA* 1981;245:2330.
22. Kovatch AL, Schuit KE, Michaels RH. *Corynebacterium hemolyticum* peritonsillar abscess mimicking diphtheria. *JAMA* 1983;249:1757.
23. Miller RA, Brancato F, Holmes KK. *Corynebacterium hemolyticum* as a cause of pharyngitis and scarlatiniform rash in young adults. *Ann Intern Med* 1986;105:867.
24. Karpathios T, Drakonaki S, Zervoudaki A, et al. *Arcanobacterium haemolyticum* in children with presumed streptococcal pharyngotonsillitis or scarlet fever. *J Pediatr* 1992;12:735.
25. Greenman JL. *Corynebacterium hemolyticum* and pharyngitis. *Ann Intern Med* 1987;106:633.
26. Hart RJC. *Corynebacterium ulcerans* in humans and cattle in North Devon. *J Hyg* 1984;92:161.
27. Banck G, Nyman M. Tonsillitis and rash associated with *Corynebacterium haemolyticum*. *J Infect Dis* 1986;154:1037.
28. Carlson P, Renkonen OV, Kontiainen S. *Arcanobacterium haemolyticum* and streptococcal pharyngitis. *Scand J Infect Dis* 1994;26:283.
29. Rose FB, Camp CJ, Antes EJ. Family outbreak of fatal *Yersinia enterocolitica* pharyngitis. *Am J Med* 1987;82:636.
30. Shimizu H, Shinogi J, Majima Y, et al. Secondary syphilis of the tonsil. *Arch Otorhinolaryngol* 1989;246:117.
31. Mitchelmore IJ, Reilly PG, Hay AJ, et al. Tonsil surface and core cultures in recurrent tonsillitis: prevalence of anaerobes and beta-lactamase producing organisms. *Eur J Clin Microbiol Infect Dis* 1994;13:542.
32. Foy HM, Grayston JR, Kenny GE, et al. Epidemiology of *Mycoplasma pneumoniae* infections in families. *JAMA* 1966;197:859.
33. Mufson MA, Ludwig WM, Purcell RH, et al. Exudative pharyngitis following experimental *Mycoplasma hominis* type I infection. *JAMA* 1965;192:1146.
34. Mufson MA. *Mycoplasma hominis*: a review of its role as a respiratory tract pathogen of humans. *Sex Transm Dis* 1983;10:335.
35. Powell DA, Miller K, Clyde WA Jr. Submandibular adenitis in a newborn caused by *Mycoplasma hominis*. *Pediatrics* 1979;63:798.
36. Glezen WP, Clyde WA Jr, Senior RJ, et al. Group A streptococci, mycoplasmas, and viruses associated with pharyngitis. *JAMA* 1967;202(6):119.
37. Reed BD, Huck W, Lutz LJ, et al. Prevalence of *Chlamydia trachomatis* and *Mycoplasma pneumoniae* in children with and without pharyngitis. *J Fam Pract* 1988;26:387.
38. Komaroff AL, Aronson MD, Pass TM, et al. Serologic evidence of chlamydial and mycoplasmal pharyngitis in adults. *Science* 1983;222:927.
39. Gerber MA, Ryan RW, Tilton RC, et al. Role of *Chlamydia trachomatis* in acute pharyngitis in adults. *J Clin Microbiol* 1984;20:993.
40. Huss H, Jungkind D, Amadio P, et al. Frequency of *Chlamydia trachomatis* as the cause of pharyngitis. *J Clin Microbiol* 1985;22:858.
41. Jones RB, Rabinovitch RA, Katz BP, et al. *Chlamydia trachomatis* in the pharynx and rectum of heterosexual patients at risk of genital infection. *Ann Intern Med* 1985;102:757.
42. Grayston JT, Juo C-C, Wan S-P, et al. A new *Chlamydia psittaci* strain, TWAR, isolated at acute respiratory tract infections. *N Engl J Med* 1986;315:161.
43. Grayston JT. Infections caused by *Chlamydia pneumoniae* strain TWAR. *Clin Infect Dis* 1992;15:757.
44. Hammerschlag WR, Chirgwin K, Roblin PW, et al. Persistent infection with *Chlamydia pneumoniae* following acute respiratory illness. *Clin Infect Dis* 1992;14:178.
45. Falck G, Heyman L, Gnarpe J, et al. *Chlamydia pneumoniae* and chronic pharyngitis. *Scand J Infect Dis* 1995;27:179.
46. Cunningham MW. Pathogenesis of group A streptococcal infection. *Clin Microbiol Rev* 2000;13(3):470.
47. Fainstein V, Musher DM, Cate TR. Bacterial adherence to pharyngeal cells during viral infection. *J Infect Dis* 1980;141:2.
48. Kessler HA, Blaauw B, Spear J, et al. Diagnosis of human immunodeficiency virus infection in seronegative homosexuals presenting with an acute viral syndrome. *JAMA* 1987;258:1196.
49. Chapnick EK, Gradon JO, Lutwick LL et al. Streptococcal toxic shock syndrome due to noninvasive pharyngitis. *Clin Infect Dis* 1992;14:1074.
50. Murray HW, Masur H, Senterfit L, et al. The protean manifestations of *Mycoplasma pneumoniae* in adults. *Am J Med* 1975;58:229.
51. Centor RM, Meier FA, Dalton HP. Throat cultures and rapid tests for diagnosis of group A streptococcal pharyngitis. *Ann Intern Med* 1986;105:892.
52. Denny FW, Wanamaker LW, Brink WR, et al. Prevention of rheumatic fever. Treatment of the preceding streptococcal infection. *JAMA* 1950;143:151.
53. Bisno AL, Gerber MA, Gwaltney JM Jr, et al. Diagnosis and management of group A streptococcal pharyngitis: a practice guideline. *Clin Infect Dis* 1997;25:574.
54. Denny FW. Current management of streptococcal pharyngitis. *J Fam Pract* 1992;35:619.
55. Peter G. Streptococcal pharyngitis: current therapy and criteria for evaluation of new agents. *Clin Infect Dis* 1992;14(suppl):218, 231.
56. Catanzaro FJ, Stetson CA, Morris AJ, et al. Symposium on rheumatic fever and rheumatic heart disease: the role of the streptococcus in the pathogenesis of rheumatic fever. *Am J Med* 1954:17:749.
57. Massell BF. Prophylaxis of streptococcal infections and rheumatic fever. *JAMA* 1979;241:1589.
58. Shapiro J, Strome M, Fried MP. Postanginal sepsis. *Head Neck Surg* 1989;11:164.

59. Alvarez A, Schreiber JR. Lemierre's syndrome in adolescent children—anaerobic sepsis with internal jugular vein thrombophlebitis following pharyngitis. *Pediatrics* 1995;96(part 1):354.

60. Bessen D, Jones KF, Fischetti VA. Evidence for two distinct classes of streptococcal M proteins and their relationship to rheumatic fever. *J Exp Med* 1989;169:269.

61. Bessen DE, Veasy LG, Hill HR, et al. Serologic evidence for a class I group A streptococcal infection among rheumatic fever patients. *J Infect Dis* 1995;172:1608.

62. Veasy LG, Wiedmeier SE, Orsmond GS, et al. Resurgence of acute rheumatic fever in the intermountain area of the United States. *N Engl J Med* 1987;316:421.

63. Stollerman GH. Rheumatogenic group A streptococci and the return of rheumatic fever. *Adv Intern Med* 1990;35:1.

64. Orrling A, Stjernquist-Desatnik A, Schalen C, et al. Clindamycin in persisting streptococcal pharyngotonsillitis after penicillin treatment. *Scand J Infect Dis* 1994;26:535.

65. Osterlund A, Popa R, Nikkila T, et al. Intracellular reservoir of *Streptococcus pyogenes in vivo*: a possible explanation for recurrent pharyngotonsillitis. *Laryngoscope* 1997;107:640.

66. Neeman R, Keller N, Barzilai A, et al. Prevalence of the internalization-associated gene, *prtF1*, among persisting group A streptococcus strains isolated from asymptomatic carriers. *Lancet* 1998;352:1974.

67. Barnes PB, Bowles WF III, Carter HG. Acute necrotizing ulcerative gingivitis: a survey of 218 cases. *J Periodontol* 1973;44:35.

68. Russell AL. Epidemiology of periodontal disease. *Int Dent J* 1967;17:282.

69. Cardocci BJ, Clarke NG. Aetiology of acute necrotizing ulcerative gingivitis: a hypothetical explanation. *J Periodontol* 1974;45:830.

70. Uohara GI, Knapp MJ. Oral fusospirochetosis and associated lesions. *Oral Surg Oral Med Oral Pathol* 1967;24:113.

71. Listgarten MA, Lewis DW. The distribution of spirochetes in the lesion of acute necrotizing ulcerative gingivitis. An electron microscopic and statistical survey. *J Periodontol* 1967;38:379.

72. Loesche WJ, Syed SA, Laughon BE, et al. The bacteriology of acute necrotizing ulcerative gingivitis. *J Periodontol* 1982;53:223.

73. Ryan ME, Hopkins K, Wilbur RB. Acute necrotizing ulcerative gingivitis in children with cancer. *Am J Dis Child* 1983;137:592.

74. Dingle JH, Badger GF, Jordan WS Jr. *Illness in the home. A study of 25,000 illnesses in a group of Cleveland families.* Cleveland: Press of Western Reserve University, 1964:66.

75. McNamara MJ, Pierce WE, Crawford YE, et al. Patterns of adenovirus infection in the respiratory diseases of naval recruits, a longitudinal study of two companies of naval recruits. *Am Rev Respir Dis* 1962;86:485.

76. Schalen L, Christensen P, Kamme C, et al. High isolation rate of *Branhamella catarrhalis* from the nasopharynx in adults with acute laryngitis. *Scand J Infect Dis* 1980;12:277.

77. Case records of the Massachusetts General Hospital. *N Engl J Med* 1983;309:1569.

78. Dudley JP, Byrne WJ, Kobayashi R, et al. *Candida* laryngitis in chronic mucocutaneous candidiasis. Its association with *Candida* esophagitis. *Ann Otol Rhinol Laryngol* 1980;89:574.

79. Lawson R, Bodey G, Luna M: *Candida* infection presenting as laryngitis. *Am J Med Sci* 1980;280:173.

80. Donegan JO, Wood MD. Histoplasmosis of the larynx. *Laryngoscope* 1984;94:206.

81. Platt M. Laryngeal coccidioidomycosis. *JAMA* 1977;237:1234.

82. Suen JY, Wetmore SJ, Wetzel WJ,et al: Blastomycosis of the larynx. *Ann Otol Rhinol Laryngol* 1980;89:563.

83. Thaller SR, Gross JR, Pilch BZ, et al. Laryngeal tuberculosis as manifested in the decades 1963–1983. *Laryngoscope* 1987;97:848.

84. Karnauchow PN, Kaul WH. Chronic herpetic laryngitis with oropharyngitis. *Ann Otol Rhinol Laryngol* 1988;97:286.

85. Theisen CF. Angina epiglottidea anterior: report of 3 cases. *Albany Med Ann* 1900;21:395.

86. LeMierre A, Meyer A, Laplone R. Les septicimies a bacille de Pfeiffer. *Ann Med* 1936;39:97.

87. Johnstone JM, Lawy HS. Acute epiglottitis in adults due to infection with *Haemophilus influenzae* type B. *Lancet* 1967;2:134.

88. Gorfinkel HJ, Brown R, Kabin SA. Acute infectious epiglottitis in adults. *Ann Intern Med* 1969;70:289.

89. Crysdale WS, Sendi K. Evolution in the management of acute epiglottitis: a 10-year experience with 242 children. *Int Anesthesiol Clin* 1988;26:32.

90. Madore DV. Impact of immunization on *Haemophilus influenzae* type B disease. *Infect Agents Dis* 1996;5(1):8.

91. Mohle-Boetani JC, Ajello G, Breneman E, et al. Carriage of *Haemophilus influenzae* type B in children after widespread vaccination with conjugate *Haemophilus influenzae* type B vaccines. *Pediatr Infect Dis J* 1993;12:589.

92. Butt W, Shann F, Walker C, et al. Acute epiglottitis: a different approach to management. *Crit Care Med* 1988;16:43.

93. Mustoe T, Strome M. Adult epiglottitis. *Am J Otolaryngol* 1983;4:393.

94. Mayosmith MF, Hirsch PJ, Wodzinski SF, et al. Acute epiglottitis in adults: an eight-year experience in the state of Rhode Island. *N Engl J Med* 1986;314:1133.

95. Carenfelt C. Etiology of acute infectious epiglottitis in adults: septic vs. local infection. *Scand J Infect Dis* 1989;21:53.

96. Shapiro J, Eavey RD, Baker AS. Adult supraglottitis: a prospective analysis. *JAMA* 1988;259:563.

97. Wine N, Lim Y, Fierer J. *Pasteurella multocida* epiglottitis. *Arch Otolaryngol Head Neck Surg* 1997;123:759.

98. Musharrafieti UM, Araj GF, Fuleihan NS. Viral supraglottitis in an adult: a case presentation and literature update. *J Infect* 1999;39(2):157.

99. Slack CL, Allen GC, Morrison JE, et al. Post-varicella epiglottitis and necrotizing fasciitis. *Pediatrics* 2000;105:e13.

100. Rothstein SG, Persky MS, Edelman BA, et al. Epiglottitis in AIDS patients. *Laryngoscope* 1989;99:389.

101. Molteni RA. Epiglottitis: incidence of extraepiglottic infection. Report of 72 cases and review of the literature. *Pediatrics* 1976;58:526.

102. Nemzek WR, Katzberg RW, Van Slyke MA, et al. A reappraisal of the radiologic findings of acute inflammations of the epiglottis and supraglottic structures in adults. *Am J Neuroradiol* 1995;16:495.

103. Bass JW, Steele RW, Weibe RA. Acute epiglottitis: a surgical emergency. *JAMA* 1974;229:671.

104. Baines DB, Wark H, Overton JH. Acute epiglottitis in children. *Anaesth Intens Care* 1984;13:25.

105. Cantrell RW, Bell RA, Morioka WT. Acute epiglottitis: intubation versus tracheotomy. *Laryngoscope* 1978;88:994.

106. Crockett DM, Healy GB, McGill TJ, et al. Airway management of acute supraglottitis at the Children's Hospital, Boston: 1980–1985. *Ann Otol Rhinol Laryngol* 1988;97:114.

107. Oh TH, Motoyama ED. Comparisons of nasotracheal intubation and tracheotomy in management of acute epiglottitis. *Anesthesiology* 1983;46:214.

108. Arndal H, Andreassen UK. Acute epiglottitis in children and adults. Nasotracheal intubation, tracheostomy or careful observation. Current status in Scandinavia. *J Laryngol Otol* 1988;102:1012.

109. Robbins JP, Fitz-Hugh GS. Epiglottitis in the adult. *Laryngoscope* 1971;81:700.

110. Hawkins DB, Miller AH, Sachs GB, et al. Acute epiglottitis in adults. *Laryngoscope* 1973;83:1211.

111. Khilanam U, Khatib R. Acute epiglottitis in adults. *Am J Med Sci* 1984;287:65.

112. Baker AS, Eavey R. Adult supraglottitis (epiglottitis). *N Engl J Med* 1986;314:1185.

113. Stanley RE, Liang TS. Acute epiglottitis in adults (the Singapore experience). *J Laryngol Otol* 1988;102:1017.

114. Shih L, Hawkins DB, Stanley RB. Acute epiglottitis in adults. A review of 48 cases. *Ann Otol Rhinol Laryngol* 1988;97:527.

115. Friedman M, Toriumi DM, Grybauskas V, et al. A plea for uniformity in the staging and management of adult epiglottitis. *Ear Nose Throat J* 1988;67:873.

116. Kessler A, Wetmore RF, Marsh RR. Childhood epiglottitis in recent years. *Int J Pediatr Otorhinolaryngol* 1993;25:155.

117. Committee on Infectious Disease, American Academy of Pediatrics. *Redbook report.* Evanston, IL: American Academy of Pediatrics, 1988:11.

118. Takala AK, Peltola H, Eskola J. Disappearance of epiglottitis during large-scale vaccination with *Haemophilus influenzae* type B conjugate vaccine among children in Finland. *Laryngoscope* 1994;104:73.

119. Gorelick MH, Baker D: Epiglottitis in children, 1979 through 1992: Effects of *Haemophilus influenzae* type B immunization. *Arch Pediatr Adolesc Med* 1994;148:47.

120. Bisgard KM, Kao A, Leake J, et al. *Hemophilus influenzae* invasive disease in the United States, 1994–1995: near disappearance of a vaccine-preventable childhood disease. *Emerg Infect Dis* 1998;4:1.

121. Reece R. George Washington: his death and his doctors. *Minn Med* 1966;49:1185.

122. Bard S. *An enquiry into the nature, cause and cure of the angina suffocativa, or, sore throat distemper.* New York: S. Inslee & A. Car, 1771.

123. Orton HB, Smith EL, Bell HO. Acute laryngotracheobronchitis: analysis of sixty-two cases with report of autopsies in eight cases. *Arch Otolaryngol* 1941;33:926.

124. Neffson AL. Acute laryngotracheobronchitis: a 25 year review. *Am J Med Sci* 1944;208:524.

125. Nelson WE. Bacterial croup: a historical perspective. *J Pediatr* 1984;105:52.

126. Liston SL, Gehrz RC, Jarvis CW. Bacterial tracheitis. *Arch Otolaryngol* 1981;107:561.

127. Johnson JT, Liston SL. Bacterial tracheitis in adults. *Arch Otolaryngol Head Neck Surg* 1987;113:204.

128. Miller BP, Arthur JD, Parry WH, et al. Atypical croup and *Chlamydia trachomatis* [Letter]. *Lancet* 1982;1:1022.

129. Donnelly BW, McMillan JA, Weiner LB. Bacterial tracheitis: report of eight new cases and review. *Rev Infect Dis* 1990;12:729.

130. Hamburger JI. The various presentations of thyroiditis. Diagnostic considerations. *Ann Intern Med* 1986;104:219.

131. Abe K, Taguchi T, Okano A, et al. Acute suppurative thyroiditis in children. *J Pediatr* 1979;94:912.

132. Tayler WE, Myer CM, Hays LL, et al. Acute suppurative thyroiditis in children. *Laryngoscope* 1982;92:1269.

133. Ueda J, Kobayashi Y, Harra K, et al. Routes of infection of acute suppurative thyroiditis diagnosed by barium examination. *Acta Radiol Diagn* 1986;27:209.

134. DeLozier H. Pyriform sinus fistula: an unusual cause of recurrent retropharyngeal abscess and cellulitis. *Ann Otol Rhinol Laryngol* 1986;95:377.

135. Miyauchi A, Matsuzuka F, Kuma K, et al. Piriform sinus fistula: an underlying abnormality common in patients with acute suppurative thyroiditis. *World J Surg* 1990;14:400.

136. Skuza K, Rapaport R, Fieldman R, et al. Recurrent acute suppurative thyroiditis. *J Otolaryngol* 1991;20:126.

137. Nonomura N, Ikarashi F, Fujisaki T, et al. Surgical approach to pyriform sinus fistula. *Am J Otolaryngol* 1993;14:111.
138. Schneider U, Birnbacher R, Schick S, et al. Recurrent suppurative thyroiditis due to pyriform sinus fistulae: a case report. *Eur J Pediatr* 1995;154:640.
139. Berger SA, Zonszein J, Villamena P, et al. Infectious diseases of the thyroid gland. *Rev Infect Dis* 1983;5:108.
140. Burhans EC. Acute thyroiditis. A study of sixty-seven cases. *Surg Gynecol Obstet* 1928;47:478.
141. Myer RD, Young LS, Armstrong D, et al. Aspergillosis complicating neoplastic disease. *Am J Med* 1973;54:6.
142. Guttler R, Singer PA, Axline SG, et al. *Pneumocystis carinii* thyroiditis. Report of three cases and review of the literature. *Arch Intern Med* 1993;153:1002.
143. Danahey DG, Kelly DR, Forrest LA. HIV-related *Pneumocystic carinii* thyroiditis: a unique case and literature review. *Otolaryngol Head Neck Surg* 1996;114:158.
144. Volpe R, Row VV, Ezrin C. Circulating viral and thyroid antibodies in subacute thyroiditis. *J Clin Endocrinol Metab* 1967;27:1275.
145. Volpe R. Thyroiditis: current views of pathogenesis. *Med Clin North Am* 1975;59:1163.
146. Srinivasappa J, Garrelli C, Orodera T, et al. Virus-induced thyroiditis. *Endocrinology* 1988;122:563.
147. Frank TS, LiVolsi VA, Conner AM. Cytomegalovirus infection of the thyroid gland in immunocompromised adults. *Yale J Biol Med* 1987;60:1.
148. McArthur LL. Acute suppurative thyroiditis. *Chicago Med Recorder* 1903;25:363.
149. Singer PA. Thyroiditis: acute, subacute and chronic. *Med Clin North Am* 1991;75:61.
150. Shah SS, Baum SG. Diagnosis and management of infectious thyroiditis. *Curr Infect Dis Rep* 2000;2:147.
151. Szabo SM, Allen DB. Thyroiditis. Differentiation of acute suppurative and subacute. Case report and review of the literature. *Clin Pediatr* 1989;28:171.

CHAPTER 47
The Common Cold

W. Paul Glezen

The common cold is aptly named because it is one of the most common human maladies, and it is the common clinical manifestation of infection of the upper respiratory tract with many different viruses. Contributing to its commonness is the fact that there is no specific therapy for most of its causes, and there are no specific preventive measures.

HISTORY

The common cold has received notice since earliest recorded history (1). In the search for an etiological agent reported in 1914, volunteers who were inoculated with filtered nasal secretions from patients with colds developed colds themselves (2). The nasal secretions had been passed through filters that excluded bacteria, leading to the theory that an organism other than a bacterium, one small enough to pass through a bacterial filter, was the etiological agent of the common cold. Systematic studies of experimental colds in human volunteers were carried out by Andrewes (3) at the Common Cold Research Unit at Harvard Hospital in Salisbury, England, beginning in 1946. In the United States, Jackson and co-workers (4) used student volunteers to attack the problem during the next decade. These studies were all performed without knowledge of the specific agents; although several respiratory viruses including influenza viruses and adenoviruses were known at the time, the requirements for cultivating rhinoviruses and other agents of the common cold had not yet been described. It was subsequently learned that many of the filtered nasal secretions used to inoculate volunteers contained rhinoviruses.

These studies were also important for describing some of the conditions that favored the transmission of cold viruses and for determining some host factors related to susceptibility and resistance. Specifically, they showed that immunity to reinfection with the same secretion pool was acquired by primary infection (5), that moderate exposure to cold and dampness did not increase the risk for infection (6), and that women in the middle third of the menstrual cycle were more susceptible to infection (7).

VIROLOGY

More than 200 viruses have been associated with the common cold syndrome. These include specific serotypes of all of the respiratory virus groups listed in Table 47.1. Without question, the rhinoviruses of the Picornaviridae family are the most important etiological agents of the common cold, but even these are not associated with the majority of colds in most studies. To date, 100 distinct serotypes have been accepted, but more than 100 have been described, and others await discovery. The evidence suggests that antigenic variation is driven by immunity, which leads to the emergence of new strains (8). The important biologic characteristic that separates rhinoviruses from enteroviruses is acid lability; rhinoviruses are inactivated rapidly at pH 3.0, whereas enteroviruses are not. Rhinoviruses are relatively stable in the environment and will survive for long periods on surfaces and fomites. This stability is important for the dissemination of these viruses in human populations, as seen in the next section.

Human coronaviruses are also important causes of the common cold, but much less is known about their role because of the difficulty of isolating these viruses from clinical specimens and preparing reagents for diagnostic tests (9). Some new technologies have been brought to bear on the problem, and these will provide new information. At least two distinct serotypes cause upper respiratory illnesses (URIs) in humans, and reinfections—some of which are symptomatic—are common. These viruses have lipid envelopes and are less stable in the environment than are rhinoviruses.

Adenoviruses, parainfluenza viruses, respiratory syncytial viruses (RSVs), and influenza viruses also contribute to the burden of URI. Adenovirus types 1, 2, 5, and 6 are common causes of febrile, undifferentiated URI in children. The other adenovirus types are more specialized in their manifestations and settings. Types 3 and 7 cause pharyngoconjunctival fever in civilian

TABLE 47.1. Viruses Associated with the Common Cold

Virus type	No. of serotypes
Adenoviridae	
Adenoviruses	41
Coronaviridae	
Coronaviruses	2
Orthomyxoviridae	
Influenza viruses	3
Paramyxoviridae	
Parainfluenza viruses	4
Respiratory syncytial virus	1
Human metapneumovirus	1
Picornaviridae	
Rhinoviruses	100 +
Enteroviruses	60 +

populations; types 4, 7, and 21 cause particular problems for military recruits. Type 8 has been associated with epidemic keratoconjunctivitis.

Parainfluenza virus and RSV belong to the Paramyxoviridae family. They are noted more for their propensity to cause lower respiratory tract illness in infants and young children but are also important etiological agents of URI. For instance, virtually all children have been infected with parainfluenza virus type 3 and RSV by 3 years of age, and at least half of these infections involve only the upper tract. A new virus, human metapneumovirus, has been described that infects most children by age 5 years (10). Infections with parainfluenza virus types 1 and 2 occur at a slightly later age when an even higher proportion of infections may involve the upper tract. Less is known about type 4, but most documented infections have involved the upper tract. Reinfections with paramyxoviruses continue to occur throughout life, producing the common cold syndrome.

Influenza viruses must also be considered important causes of the common cold. Influenza C virus, the orthomyxovirus about which we know the least, infects most persons by adulthood and has usually been associated with URI. This virus grows in embryonated eggs, but it has different growth requirements than A and B viruses, and it is not as mutable as influenza viruses A and B. Our understanding of influenza C virus is incomplete, but it probably is an important cause of colds.

Primary infection with any of the three influenza virus A subtypes or with influenza B virus usually produces an influenza-like illness with appreciable systemic symptoms as well as upper or even lower tract findings. However, after the first infection, subsequent reinfection with the same virus or related variants may result in an afebrile URI. Longitudinal observations of the Houston Family Study revealed that about 30% of influenza virus infections were manifested by afebrile URI (11,12). Afebrile URI may be an important mechanism for spread of influenza because persons so affected usually do not limit their activity and therefore may have many contacts. Afebrile URI may not only be the result of infection confronting partial immunity, it may also have to do with the site of inoculation. An appreciable proportion of volunteers with low or undetectable specific antibodies developed colds after being inoculated with influenza virus by nose drops (13). The dose of virus required to infect volunteers by this route is relatively large, usually at least 300 $TCID_{50}$ (median tissue culture infective dose units). In contrast, less than 10 $TCID_{50}$ administered by small-particle aerosol and deposited in the lower respiratory tract may produce an influenza-like illness with tracheitis (14). Therefore, URI caused by influenza-like viruses may result from direct contact inoculation, whereas influenza-like illness may occur more frequently after exposure to natural aerosol.

By the sheer weight of their numbers, the picornaviruses are the most important causes of colds; however, adenoviruses, coronaviruses, and especially reinfection with myxoviruses and paramyxoviruses contribute out of proportion to their small numbers. Table 47.2 shows the proportions by which each of the virus groups contributed to the cause of acute respiratory illnesses of persons in three different studies carried out during several years in different geographical areas. The Tecumseh study provided data that are most representative of the general population (15). The Chapel Hill data are derived from intensive surveillance of children in day care (16), and the Cirencester study was carried out in the setting of a general practice in the United Kingdom (17). The proportions reflect the structure of the study and the populations involved; the contribution of coronaviruses is underestimated because of the difficulty in diagnosing infection with these viruses.

TABLE 47.2. Frequency of Association of Respiratory Agents with Acute Respiratory Illnesses in Ambulatory Settings

Agents	Percentage of total agents		
	Tecumseh[a]	Chapel Hill daycare[b]	Cirencester[c]
Rhinovirus	38.5	9.5	26.2
Parainfluenza virus	16.9	24.1	7.8
Influenza virus	11.9	4.7	24.4
Respiratory syncytial virus	5.9	9.5	2.6
Adenovirus	4.5	22.0	6.3
Enterovirus	4.3	13.6	7.3
Coronavirus	c. 4.0[d]	NT	0.4[e]
Other viruses	4.7	6.1	9.6
Streptococci	13.3	8.8	15.4[f]

[a]Data from ref. 14.
[b]Data from ref. 15.
[c]Data from ref. 16.
[d]Serologic test only.
[e]Virus isolation only.
[f]Includes groups C and G in addition to group A.
NT, not tested.

EPIDEMIOLOGY

Incidence

Respiratory infections are the most common acute conditions experienced by persons in the United States. Monto and Ullman (15) found that a representative population living in a small town reported an average of three acute respiratory illnesses a year, with a range of six per year for infants and about one per year for persons older than 60 years. Illnesses were more common among boys younger than 3 years of age, but for older persons, females had higher rates. Only a portion of these illnesses would be classified as colds.

In the National Health Survey, about one third of acute respiratory conditions reported by a representative sample of respondents are classified as common cold (18). In 1996, about one fourth of the population reported a common cold that altered their usual activities or caused them to seek medical care (Table 47.3). It was estimated that about 62 million colds met that definition. Less than half of these colds were reported for

TABLE 47.3. Frequency of Acute Respiratory Conditions that Alter Unusual Activities, United States, 1996

Type of condition	No. of patients	Rate per 100 persons
Common cold	62,251,000	23.6
Other upper respiratory illness	29,866,000	11.3
Influenza	95,049,000	36.0
Bronchitis	12,116,000	4.6
Pneumonia	4,791,000	1.8
Ear infections	26,766,000	8.2
Other	4,550,000	1.7
TOTAL	230,389,000	87.2

Data from the National Center for Health Statistics. *Current estimates from the National Health Interview Survey, United States, 1996.* No. 200. Washington, DC: U.S. Department of Health and Human Services, 1999, with permission.

children, and more than 13 million were reported by older adults (45 years and older). The 62 million colds resulted in 148 million days of restricted activity, and more than 27 million episodes were medically attended. As a result, about 20 million days were lost from work, and 21 million school days were missed by students 5 to 17 years of age. From these statistics, it can be seen that the economic burden imposed by colds is more than $1 billion each year.

The contribution of rhinoviruses to total acute respiratory illness is considerable. For children younger than 10 years, about one illness per year can be attributed to rhinovirus infection; however, because young children have high total illness rates, the rhinovirus infections account for only about one fourth or one fifth of their URIs. For employed young adults and mothers of young children who experience about one illness per year, rhinoviruses may be responsible for about half of their URIs.

Transmission

Most respiratory infections are spread by direct contact with the respiratory secretions of infected persons (19). This usually results from hand-to-hand transmission or transmission from hand to environmental surface to hand, with inoculation of the recipient's eye or nose. Inoculation by mouth is usually a less effective route. Direct contact spread explains the high secondary infection rates within households. Spread by aerosol has been documented for influenza viruses (20), and some experimental evidence for this has been reported for enteroviruses (21) and rhinoviruses (22); however, most studies favor spread by direct contact. The stability of rhinoviruses facilitates contact spread because the virus may remain infectious on environmental surfaces for hours or even days.

In temperate climates, the spread of respiratory viruses increases during the cooler months of the year. Some of the major groups of viruses have relatively distinct seasonal niches. As enterovirus activity is declining in the autumn, rhinovirus activity increases. Parainfluenza virus types 1 and 2 produce outbreaks in the autumn but only every other year. RSVs and influenza viruses usually constitute the midwinter peak. Coronaviruses are active in late winter and spring. Rhinoviruses and parainfluenza virus type 3 also have increased activity in the spring. The pattern of seasonal occurrence, illustrated in Figure 47.1, suggests an interference phenomenon, but there is no complete explanation for the seasonality of the various respiratory viruses (23).

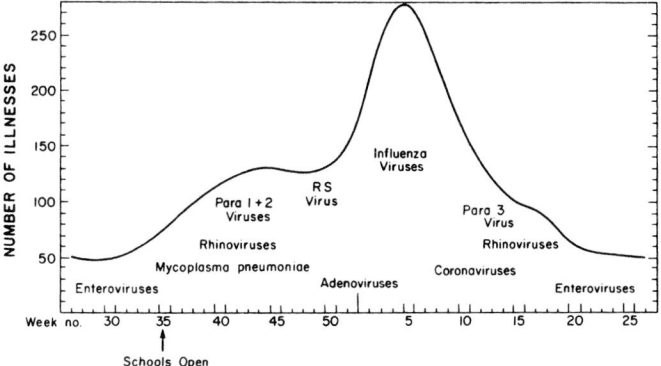

Figure 47.1. The 5-week running average of visits for acute respiratory illnesses to sentinel primary care facilities in Houston, 1975 to 1981. Superimposed are the respiratory agents contributing to illness during different seasons. Para, parainfluenza; RS, respiratory syncytial.

Increasing virus activity always accompanies the return of children to school. Many studies have demonstrated the importance of schoolchildren in the spread of respiratory viruses in the community and in the introduction of these viruses into the home (24). The increasing proportion of preschool-aged children in group day care also increases the opportunity for spread of respiratory viruses and increases the number of agents to which young children are exposed.

The role of climate and temperature change is not understood; lower temperature may increase congregation of persons indoors, resulting in more effective contact. Changes in the relative humidity may also be important. Viability of rhinoviruses may be favored by relative humidities in the range of 40% to 50%, which are common in the autumn and spring (19). Influenza and parainfluenza viruses remain viable in aerosol for longer periods in low relative humidity such as occurs in midwinter (25).

PATHOGENESIS

The incubation period for most respiratory viruses ranges from 1 to 4 days. The site of virus replication is the ciliated epithelium of the nasal turbinates and the nasopharynx. Viremia is not a regular feature of respiratory virus infection other than for enteroviruses; if it occurs with other viruses, it is transient and is not an important pathogenic feature. Systemic symptoms that accompany colds result from the inflammatory response to the surface infection, which produces variable destruction of the cells of the epithelium. Infection usually commences in the posterior pharynx and progresses toward the nose and glottis. Virus shedding usually peaks on the third or fourth day and may be undetectable by the fifth to the seventh day; virus excretion tends to be longer in children than in adults. Infection is limited by endogenous production of interferon and by mobilization of cytotoxic cells—both nonspecific natural killer cells and specific T lymphocytes.

Although there is some destruction of epithelial cells, the more impressive histopathological picture consists of edema of the submucosa accompanied by hyperemia with some subepithelial infiltration of inflammatory cells. The airways are narrowed by the swelling of the mucosa and filled by exudation of seromucinous fluid. Chemical mediators of inflammation can be detected in the nasal secretions, including interleukin-1 (26), kinins (27), the vasoactive peptides, and—especially in atopic individuals—histamine (28) and leukotrienes (29). Symptoms usually peak within 5 days, and recovery usually requires another 5 days.

CLINICAL MANIFESTATIONS

Some colds are preceded by a prodrome consisting of chilly sensations and some vague symptoms of non–well-being. (This prodrome is probably the source of the strong belief that chilling causes a cold.) The first symptom is usually a dry, scratchy sore throat, and this is soon followed by sneezing, nasal stuffiness, and rhinorrhea. Some systemic symptoms may occur, such as feverishness, malaise, myalgias, and headache, but temperature elevation is not common, and if it occurs, it is low grade. Hoarseness and cough may also occur; the cough, which is dry and annoying, results from irritation in the glottic region.

Complications

From the previous description of the pathological factors, it is logical to propose that the inflammation produced by common cold viruses will occlude the ostia of the paranasal sinuses and cause dysfunction of the eustachian tubes, leading to acute sinusitis and otitis media (30). This obstruction may trap bacteria in the closed space, resulting in suppuration. Sinusitis and otitis media are the most common complications of URIs. Children average about one episode of otitis media per year during the early years of life. These complications should be suspected if the patient develops fever 3 to 5 days after onset of a cold. Children with otitis media may complain of ear pain, and patients with sinusitis will have facial pain over the involved sinus. *Streptococcus pneumoniae* is the most common secondary invader. *Haemophilus influenzae,* usually nontypable, is the next most frequent cause, followed by *Branhamella (Moraxella) catarrhalis.*

Less common complications include bacteremias, bacterial meningitis, pneumonia, and other systemic bacterial infections (31,32). It is assumed that the inflammation in the upper respiratory tract allows the bacterial pathogens in the nasopharynx to invade the bloodstream, resulting in systemic infections at distant sites. URIs also appear to be a common triggering event for Guillain-Barré syndrome (33).

For children with reactive airway disease, respiratory virus infections are common initiators of asthma attacks (34). Welliver and colleagues (35) have found that young children with wheezing may have immunoglobulin E antibodies specific for RSV or parainfluenza virus in their nasal secretions. Rhinovirus and influenza virus infections commonly precede asthma attacks in older children. Many studies have found evidence that these virus infections may stimulate the production of chemical mediators of bronchospasm in atopic children. Because the frequency of severe asthma resulting in hospitalization and death of children is increasing, this may be one of the most urgent reasons for searching for methods to prevent colds.

DIAGNOSIS

The diagnosis is presumed from the clinical presentation. Specific etiological diagnosis is usually not warranted. For patients with sore throat, it is important to rule out the presence of group A streptococcus by culture or a rapid antigen detection test. This is the only uncomplicated upper respiratory infection that requires specific therapy.

Knowledge of the seasonal occurrence of the major virus groups provides a basis for assigning the presumptive etiological diagnosis. Rhinoviruses usually predominate in the autumn and early spring. Parainfluenza virus types 1 and 2 have been epidemic in the autumn of odd-numbered years since 1973 (23). Reinfection colds caused by parainfluenza viruses may include hoarseness; the signal illness for the presence of these viruses is croup, or laryngotracheobronchitis, which occurs with primary infection of young children. RSV and influenza viruses are epidemic in midwinter. RSV produces annual epidemics, which are clinically evident by the occurrence of bronchiolitis and pneumonia in infants. During this time, many of the URIs of older children and adults may be caused by RSV. The arrival of influenza in the community is heralded by the sudden appearance at primary care facilities of school-aged children with febrile respiratory illnesses. During influenza epidemics, many afebrile URIs will occur in partially immune schoolchildren and adults.

Rapid diagnosis of the causes of URIs during midwinter epidemics may be indicated under certain circumstances for epidemiological reasons. Influenza A infections can be aborted by early treatment with specific antiviral drugs, which has been shown to reduce virus shedding and therefore the risk for spreading the infection to vulnerable contacts. RSV, as well as influenza

virus, may produce life-threatening infections in chronically ill or immunocompromised patients. Therefore, timely information about their occurrence may be important.

Differential Diagnosis

Allergic rhinitis, or hay fever, may be confused with the common cold. A nasal smear may aid in differentiating allergic rhinitis from URIs. Eosinophils may be present in the nasal secretions of patients with allergic rhinitis. As mentioned before, group A streptococcal infection must be ruled out by throat culture or an antigen detection test for patients with sore throat. The clinical finding of hoarseness is negatively correlated with group A streptococcal infection. A reminder that continuous rhinorrhea (which may soak the pillow at night) may be the result of a spontaneous leak of cerebrospinal fluid is in order. In this situation, the nasal secretions should be tested for glucose, which is present in cerebrospinal fluid.

TREATMENT

There is no specific treatment for the common cold. Treatment of colds with specific antiviral drugs should be considered for certain persons during influenza epidemics (see Chapter 241).

Persons recommended for treatment are members of the health care team and those who are household contacts of high-risk patients. The purpose is to abort influenza infections and reduce the risk that vulnerable patients will be exposed to infection.

Several drugs have been tested for effect against rhinoviruses. The structure of rhinoviruses has been described, and antiviral drugs have been designed that block the attachment site of rhinoviruses *in vitro,* but clinical studies of most have been disappointing (36). One exception is pleconaril, which has shown some promise in clinical trials (37); an important obstacle is rapid identification of patients with picornavirus colds who will respond to treatment.

The use of antibiotics is not warranted for viral URIs (38). Double-blind studies have shown no benefit for treated subjects. Antibiotics do not reduce the frequency of bacterial complications but may alter the bacterial flora of the nasopharynx, allowing the emergence of resistant organisms.

Nonspecific Therapy

Relief of some symptoms of a cold can be achieved by administration of over-the-counter remedies. Aspirin may relieve some of the systemic symptoms, but its use should be limited; one study demonstrated prolonged excretion of rhinoviruses from persons who were given aspirin (39). Experimental studies of influenza virus infection have shown similar results (40). Aspirin is contraindicated for influenza infections in children because its use has been associated with increased risk for Reye's syndrome (41). Acetaminophen is probably a better choice for this purpose but should be used judiciously and only as necessary because the antipyretic effect probably does not favor recovery from infection.

Oral decongestants may relieve nasal stuffiness; pseudoephedrine is effective. Use of topical decongestants may be helpful also, but frequent use can lead to a distressing rebound phenomenon. Antihistamines have a drying effect on secretions and may be helpful if used in combination with decongestants. Newer antihistamines are available that do not produce the drowsiness that accompanied many of the earlier products.

A persistent dry cough may be troublesome and can be relieved by administration of a cough suppressant such as dextromethorphan. Caution should be used in administering such preparations to young children, for whom cough may be important for keeping the airways clear of upper tract secretions.

PREVENTION

The only vaccines available for respiratory viruses are influenza vaccines. In addition to the recommendation for patients with chronic underlying conditions, influenza vaccine is recommended for all members of the health care team and for household contacts of high-risk patients to reduce the risk for exposing vulnerable patients to influenza virus infection.

The large number of rhinovirus serotypes and the fact that no effective cross-protection is evident after infection with a given serotype make it unlikely that immunoprophylaxis will work. Furthermore, it appears that antigenic variation and the emergence of new types are driven by immunity. This makes it even less likely that vaccine development would be practical.

Endogenous interferon production appears to be the important limiting factor for rhinovirus infection. Experimental studies with human volunteers have demonstrated that nasal instillation of interferon will prevent rhinovirus colds (42,43). Studies have also shown that secondary rhinovirus infections can be prevented in household contacts of persons with natural rhinovirus colds by intranasal administration of recombinant interferon (44,45). The problem is that regular use of the interferon spray excites an inflammatory response in the nose, which results in a nasal obstruction and bloody nasal discharge. Therefore, the treatment is almost as annoying as the disease. Furthermore, interferon does not prevent infections with the other viruses associated with the common cold. At this juncture, the most promising prospect for cure (or prevention) of the common cold lies with development of more effective antiviral therapy. An antiviral preparation combined with products that block the mediators of inflammation may be the treatment of the future (46).

REFERENCES

1. Gwaltney JM Jr. Rhinoviruses. In: Evans AS, ed. *Viral infections of humans,* 2nd ed. New York: Plenum, 1982:491–517.
2. Kruse W. Die Erregen von Husten and Schupfen [the etiology of cough and nasal catarrh]. *Munch Med Wochenschr* 1914;61:1574.
3. Andrewes C. *In Pursuit of the common cold.* London: William Heinemann Medical Books, 1973.
4. Jackson GG, Dowling HF, Spiesman EG, et al. Transmission of the common cold to volunteers under controlled conditions. I. The common cold as a clinical entity. *Arch Intern Med* 1958;101:267.
5. Jackson GG, Dowling HF. Transmission of the common cold to volunteers under controlled conditions. IV. Specific immunity to the common cold. *J Clin Invest* 1959;38:762.
6. Dowling HF, Jackson GG, Spiesman IG, et al. Transmission of the common cold to volunteers under controlled conditions. III. The effect of chilling of the subjects upon susceptibility. *Am J Hyg* 1958;68:59.
7. Dowling HF, Jackson GG, Inouye T. Transmission of the experimental common cold in volunteers. II. The effect of certain host factors upon susceptibility. *J Lab Clin Med* 1957;50:516.
8. Couch RB. Rhinoviruses. In: Fields BN, Knipe DM, eds. *Fields virology,* 2nd ed. New York: Raven, 1990:607–629.
9. Monto AS. Coronaviruses. In: Evans AS, ed. *Viral infections of humans,* 2nd ed. New York: Plenum, 1982:151–165.
10. Van den Hoogen BG, DeJong JC, Groen J, et al. A newly discovered human pneumovirus isolated from young children with respiratory tract disease. *Nature Med* 2001;7:719–724.
11. Frank AL, Taber LH, Glezen WP, et al. Influenza B virus infections in the community and the family. *Am J Epidemiol* 1983;118:313.
12. Frank AL, Taber LH, Wells JM. Comparison of infection rates and severity of illness for influenza A subtypes H1N1 and H3N2. *J Infect Dis* 1985;151:73.
13. Douglas RG Jr. Influenza in man. In: Kilbourne ED, ed. The influenza viruses and influenza. New York: Academic Press, 1975:395–447.
14. Alford RH, Kasel JA, Geron PJ, et al. Human influenza resulting from aerosol inhalation. *Proc Soc Exp Biol Med* 1966;122:800.
15. Monto AS, Ullman BM. Acute respiratory illness in an American community. *JAMA* 1974;227:264.
16. Denny FW. Acute respiratory infections in children: etiology and epidemiology. *Pediatr Rev* 1987;9:135.
17. Higgins PG. Viruses associated with acute respiratory infections 1961–71. *J Hyg* (Camb) 1974;72:425.
18. National Center for Health Statistics. *Current estimates from the National Health Interview Survey, United States, 1996,* No. 200. Washington, DC: U.S. Department of Health and Human Services, 1999.
19. Hendley JO, Gwaltney JM Jr. Mechanisms of transmission of rhinovirus infections. *Epidemiol Rev* 1988;10:242.
20. Glezen WP, Couch RB. Influenza viruses. In: Evans AS, ed. *Viral infections of humans,* 3rd ed. New York: Plenum, 1989.
21. Couch RB, Douglas RG Jr, Lindgren KM, et al. Airborne transmission of respiratory infection with coxsackie virus A type 21. *Am J Epidemiol* 1970;91:78.
22. Dick EC, Jennings LC, Mink KA, et al. Aerosol transmission of rhinovirus colds. *J Infect Dis* 1987;156:442.
23. Glezen WP, Frank AL, Taber LH, et al. Parainfluenza virus type 3: seasonality and risk of infection and reinfection in young children. *J Infect Dis* 1984;150:851.
24. Glezen WP. Consideration of the risk of influenza in children and indications for prophylaxis. *Rev Infect Dis* 1980;2:408.
25. Glezen WP, Loda FA, Denny FW. Parainfluenza viruses. In: Evans AS, ed. *Viral infections of humans,* 3rd ed. New York: Plenum, 1989.
26. Proud D, Gwaltney JM Jr, Hendley JO, et al. Increased levels of interleukin-1 are detected in nasal secretions of volunteers during experimental rhinovirus colds. *J Infect Dis* 1994;169:1007.
27. Naclerio RM, Proud D, Lichtenstein LM, et al. Kinins are generated during experimental rhinovirus cold. *J Infect Dis* 1988;157:133.
28. Smith TF, Remigio LK. Histamine in nasal secretions and serum may be elevated during viral respiratory tract infections. *Int Arch Allergy Appl Immunol* 1982;67:380.
29. Volovitz B, Faden H, Ogra PL. Release of leukotriene C4 in respiratory tract during acute viral infection. *J Pediatr* 1988;112:218.
30. Buchman CA, Doyle WJ, Skoner D, et al. Otologic manifestations of experimental rhinovirus infection. *Laryngoscope* 1994;104:1295.
31. Kaplan SL, Taber LH, Frank AL, et al. Nasopharyngeal viral isolates in children with *Haemophilus influenzae* type b meningitis. *J Pediatr* 1981;99:591.
32. El-Sahly HM, Atmar RL, Glezen WP, et al. Spectrum of clinical illness in hospitalized patients with "common cold" virus infections. *Clin Infect Dis* 2000;31:96–100.
33. Leneman F. The Guillain-Barré syndrome. *Arch Intern Med* 1966;118:139.
34. Glezen WP. Reactive airway disorders in children: role of respiratory virus infections. *Clin Chest Med* 1984;5:635.
35. Welliver RC, Wong DT, Middleton E Jr, et al. Role of parainfluenza virus-specific IgE in pathogenesis of croup and wheezing subsequent to infection. *J Pediatr* 1982;101:889m.
36. McKinlay MA, Pevear DC, Rossman MG. Treatment of the picornavirus common cold by inhibitors of viral uncoating and attachment. *Annu Rev Microbiol* 1992;46:635.
37. Munoz FM, Galasso GJ, Gwaltney JM Jr, et al. Current research on influenza and other respiratory viruses. II. International Symposium. *Antiviral Res* 2000;46:91–124.
38. Soyka LF, Robinson DS, Lachant N, et al. The misuse of antibiotics for treatment of upper respiratory tract infections in children. *Pediatrics* 1975;55:552.
39. Stanley ED, Jackson GG, Panusarn C, et al. Increased virus shedding with aspirin treatment of rhinovirus infection. *JAMA* 1975;231:1247.
40. Husseini RH, Sweet C, Collie MH, et al. Elevation of nasal viral levels in suppression of fever in ferrets infected with influenza viruses of different virulence. *J Infect Dis* 1982;145:520.
41. Hurwitz ES, Barrett MJ, Bregman D, et al. Public Health Service Study on Reye's syndrome and medications. *N Engl J Med* 1985;313:849.
42. Samo TC, Greenberg SB, Couch RB, et al. Efficacy and tolerance of intranasally applied recombinant leukocyte A interferon in normal volunteers. *J Infect Dis* 1983;148:535.
43. Santo TC, Greenberg SB, Palmer JM, et al. Intranasally applied recombinant leukocyte A interferon in normal volunteers. II. Determination of minimal effective dose and tolerable dose. *J Infect Dis* 1984;150:181.
44. Douglas RM, Moore BW, Miles HB, et al. Prophylactic efficacy of intranasal alpha-interferon against rhinovirus infections in the family setting. *N Engl J Med* 1986;314:65.
45. Hayden FG, Albrecht JK, Kaiser DL, et al. Prevention of natural colds by contact prophylaxis with intranasal alpha interferon. *N Engl J Med* 1986;314:71.
46. Gwaltney JM Jr. Combined antiviral and antimediator treatment of rhinovirus colds. *J Infect Dis* 1992;166:776.

Pleuropulmonary

CHAPTER 48
Approach to the Patient with Pneumonia

John G. Bartlett

It is estimated that pneumonia accounts for 2 to 3 million cases, 10 million patient visits, 500,000 hospitalizations, and 45,000 deaths each year in the United States (1–3). Pneumonia also accounts for about 15% of all nosocomial infections. The total cost of these infections is estimated at about $4 billion per year or about $7,500 per case in hospitalized patients (4,5). Pneumonia is the sixth most common cause of death in the United States, accounting for approximately 30 deaths per 100,000 population (6). This represents 3.5% of all deaths in the United States and 46% of those directly due to infectious disease (6). Comparative data for the prepenicillin era are summarized in Table 48.1 (6–8). One of the most striking changes noted is the frequency with which the pneumococcus is implicated. There have been substantial additional changes relating to the other implicated pathogens, the host, and the treatment options. The purpose of this chapter is to provide a guideline for the approach to the patient with suspected pneumonia.

DEFINITIONS AND TERMS

Pneumonia indicates inflammation of the lung parenchyma that is usually caused by a microbial agent. In many cases, the term is modified to indicate a specific clinical setting, such as community-acquired pneumonia, nursing home pneumonia, nosocomial pneumonia, pneumonia in the immunocompromised host, and aspiration pneumonia, among others. These terms are important because of differences in likely microbial agents, prognosis, and diagnostic evaluation. Other classifications are based on the tempo of the disease, such as acute, subacute, or chronic pneumonia. Classification also may be based on observations with radiographs or scans to characterize the changes as lobar pneumonia, bronchopneumonia, interstitial pneumonia, or lung abscess, as well as accompanying findings, such as hilar adenopathy, pleural fluid, or atelectasis.

DIAGNOSIS

Clinical Features

Symptoms suggesting pneumonia include fever combined with respiratory complaints, including cough, dyspnea, sputum production, and pleurisy. Patients with chronic pneumonia often complain of unintentional weight loss, chronic fatigue, and night sweats. Physical examinations in patients with pneumonia show fever in the great majority; crackles are heard by auscultation in 60% to 80%, but this is regarded as an unreliable sign of pneumonia when compared with chest radiography (9).

Chest Radiography

An important diagnostic test is the chest radiograph, because this is usually necessary for a confirmed diagnosis. The distinction between bronchitis and pneumonia may be difficult on the basis of clinical observations. The issue is not trivial because most patients with pneumonias are treated with antimicrobial agents, whereas those with bronchitis generally derive no benefit from antimicrobial agents. Indications for chest radiography in the patient with a respiratory tract infection with cough according to the CDC guidelines are abnormal vital signs (temperature >38°C, respiratory rate >24 breaths/min, pulse >100 beats/min) or rales on physical examination (10).

False-positive results on radiographic examination may be noted with pulmonary infarct, congestive heart failure, carcinoma, sarcoidosis, interstitial lung disease, atelectasis, vasculitis, Wegener's granulomatosis, and others. False-negative radiographic results may occur rarely with dehydration, neutropenia, or early disease; false-negative radiographic findings are common only with *Pneumocystis carinii*, where in up to 30% of cases no infiltrates are seen (11). It is generally thought that radiographs do not distinguish bacterial from nonbacterial infection. Nevertheless, some findings on chest radiography strongly support selected diagnoses (Table 48.2). Changes on the chest film also may indicate the severity of the illness and guide management decisions.

Laboratory Tests

Laboratory tests that are commonly advocated in patients who are candidates for hospitalization are summarized in Table 48.3 (1). The goal is to determine the severity of illness, possible complications, and the status of underlying or associated conditions. Results, coupled with clinical observations, often dictate the need for hospitalization in community-acquired cases or may indicate the need for care in the intensive care unit. The data correlating clinical and laboratory findings with mortality have been systematically analyzed by the Patient Outcomes Research Team pneumonia study, including a validation study based on analysis of over 38,000 pneumonia patients (12). The results are a complicated point system that represents the "prediction rule" for outcome. Although intended to predict mortality, this system has subsequently been used to define guidelines for site of care, meaning the decision for hospitalization. This prediction rule is summarized in Table 48.4.

ETIOLOGIC DIAGNOSIS

The management of pneumonia is notably simplified if the etiologic agent is accurately identified. A probable pathogen is detected in 40% to 50% of cases in published reports that use an aggressive diagnostic menu that includes conventional bacteria, atypical agents, and viruses (13–17). Relatively poor yield may exaggerate the number with an etiologic diagnosis because of false-positive cultures of expectorated sputum by inconsistent or unacceptable serologic criteria used for detection of *Legionella*, *Chlamydia pneumoniae*, and *Mycoplasma pneumoniae*. Relatively few patients have a clearly documented pathogen as defined by the following:

1. A likely pulmonary pathogen is recovered from uncontaminated sources such as blood, pleural fluid, metastatic sites, or transtracheal aspirates.
2. The organism is considered pathogenic regardless of the

TABLE 48.1.   Pneumonia: Comparison of Data for the Prepenicillin Era and the Modern Era

Parameter	Prepenicillin era (annual, United States)[a]	Current era (annual, United States)[b]
Incidence (hospitalized patients/ 1,000 population)	3/1,000	2.5/1,000
Mortality rate (hospitalized patients)	33%	13.7%
Mortality (incidence/100,000 population)	90–110/100,000	25–30/100,000
Mortality as percentage of all deaths	8.5%	3.5%
Cases due to *Streptococcus pneumoniae*	81%	15%–20%

[a]Data for prepenicillin era from Heffron R. *Pneumonia.* Cambridge, MA: Harvard University Press, 1939. Mortality data are based on metanalysis of 18,540 cases reported from 1905 to 1937 (pp. 656–663); recovery rate of *S. pneumoniae* is based on experience of Bullowa with 4,416 cases from 1928 to 1936 (p. 2); rates are for major metropolitan areas from 1931 to 1933 (p. 276).
[b]Data for mortality from Pinner RW, Teutsch SM, Simonsen L, et al. Trends in infectious diseases mortality in the United States. *JAMA* 1996;275:189–193; based on analysis of tapes from National Center for Health Statistics for 1980 to 1992. Data for mortality rate and bacteriology are from Fine MJ, Smith MA, Carson CA, et al. Prognosis and outcomes of patients with community-acquired pneumonia. *JAMA* 1995;274:134–141; based on metanalysis of 33,148 patients reported in 122 English language reports published from 1966 to 1995.

specimen source because it does not colonize the respiratory tract in the absence of disease. Microbes in this category are summarized in Table 48.5 (1).

3. There is positive serology by well-standardized criteria for selected pathogens.

TABLE 48.2.   Chest Radiography: Differential Diagnosis

Immunocompetent	Immunosuppressed (acquired immunodeficiency syndrome)
Focal opacity	Focal opacity
Streptococcus pneumoniae	Pyogenic bacteria (as with
Haemophilus influenzae	immunocompetent)
Mycoplasma pneumoniae	*Cryptococcus neoformans*
Legionella	*Nocardia*
Chlamydia pneumoniae	*Mycobacterium tuberculosis*
Staphylococcus aureus	Kaposi's sarcoma
Mycobacterium tuberculosis	
Gram-negative bacteria	
Anaerobes	
Interstitial-miliary	Interstitial-miliary
Viruses	*Pneumocystis carinii*
Mycoplasma pneumoniae	*Mycobacterium tuberculosis*
Mycobacterium tuberculosis	Endemic fungi[a]
Endemic fungi[a]	*Leishmania donovani*
	Cytomegalovirus
Hilar adenopathy ± infiltrate	Hilar adenopathy
Epstein-Barr virus	*Mycobacterium tuberculosis*
Francisella tularensis	*Cryptococcus neoformans*
Chlamydia psittaci	Pathogenic fungi[a]
Mycoplasma pneumoniae	Lymphoma
Mycobacterium tuberculosis	Kaposi's sarcoma
Endemic fungi[a]	
Atypical rubella	
Cavitation	Cavitation
Anaerobes	Gram-negative bacilli
Mycobacterium tuberculosis	*Mycobacterium tuberculosis*
M. avium complex,	*M. kansasii*
M. kansasii	*Cryptococcus neoformans*
Endemic fungi[a]	Endemic fungi[a]
Gram-negative bacilli	*Rhodococcus equi*
Staphylococcus aureus	*Staphylococcus aureus* (injection drug use)

[a]*Histoplasma capsulatum, Coccidioides immitis,* and *Blastomyces dermatitidis.*

In practice, the physician is usually required to interpret the results of less definitive studies, most commonly the results of Gram stain and culture of expectorated sputum or to simply treat empirically. Alternative specimen sources, such as transtracheal aspiration, transthoracic needle aspiration, or bronchoscopy, are usually reserved for patients who have atypical presentation, severe disease, or disease in a specific host setting, as well as for patients who fail to respond to treatment. Diagnostic tests of choice by microbial pathogen are summarized in Table 48.6. The diagnostic yield from any specimen source is notably reduced by antecedent antibiotic use; fragile organisms such as *Streptococcus pneumoniae, Haemophilus influenzae,* and anaerobes are especially a problem.

Expectorated Sputum

The diagnostic utility of expectorated sputum and culture has been debated for decades. In the late 1960s and early 1970s, multiple studies showed that the yield of *S. pneumoniae* in expectorated sputum from patients with bacteremic pneumonia was only about 50% (18,19). The conclusion was that the usual specimen source for detecting *S. pneumoniae*, the most common identifiable agent of lower respiratory tract infections, was complicated by a high frequency of false-negative results, and the outcome was an intensive effort in the 1970s to deal more effectively with

TABLE 48.3.   Routine Tests in Hospitalized Patients with Community-Acquired Pneumonia

Chest radiograph
Arterial blood gas analysis
Complete blood count
Chemistry profile including kidney and liver function tests and electrolyte determinations
Human immunodeficiency virus serology (age 15–54 yr)
Blood culture twice (pretreatment)
Sputum Gram stain and culture ± acid-fast stain and culture, *Legionella* test (culture and/or urinary antigen assay)
Pleural fluid analysis (if present): white blood cell count and differential, lactate dehydrogenase, pH, protein, glucose; Gram stain, acid-fast stain; and culture for bacteria (aerobes and anaerobes), fungi, and mycobacteria

TABLE 48.4. Indications for Hospitalization Based on PORT Point Criteria

Demographic factors		Physical examination	
Age: Male	Age	RR >30 breaths/min,	20 each
Female	Age - 10	BP <90 mm Hg	
		Temp >40°C <35°C	15
Nursing home	10	Pulse >125 beats/min	10
Comorbidities		Laboratory	
Cancer	30	Arterial pH <7.35	30
Liver disease	20	BUN >30 mg/dL	20
Heart failure	10	Sodium <130 mEq/L	20
Cardiovascular disease	10	Glucose >250, Hct	
Renal failure	10	<30%, P_{O_2} <60, effusion	10 each

Site of care and mortality

Class	Points	Mortality	Site of care
I	Nil	0.1%	Home
II	<70	0.6%	Home
III	71–90	2.8%	Home or brief hospitalization
IV	91–130	8.2%	Hospital
V	>130	29.2%	Hospital, some ICU

RR, respiratory rate; BP, blood pressure; Temp, temperature; BUN, blood urea nitrogen; Hct, hematocrit; P_{O_2}, partial pressure of oxygen; ICU, intensive care unit.
Data from Fine MJ, Auble TE, Yealy DM, et al. A prediction rule to identify low-risk patients with community-acquired pneumonia. *N Engl J Med* 1997;336:243.

pathogen detection by using two approaches. The first was an attempt to obtain specimens that were not contaminated by the upper airway flora with use of transtracheal aspiration, transthoracic needle aspiration, or bronchoscopy. The second tactic was fostered by the impression that the only practical specimen was the expectorated sputum, and the need was to deal with the problem of contamination during passage through the upper airways by use of alternative methods to process sputum: wash procedures, quantitation of bacteria, and cytologic screening. From these studies, the only technique that has withstood the test of time and has subsequently been incorporated into standard laboratory practice is cytologic screening of expectorated sputum (20–23).

Many authorities (1) now believe that Gram stain and culture of expectorated sputum are important diagnostic tests for patients hospitalized with pneumonia because the yield, while low, may provide critical information in 20% to 30% of cases at a cost of less than 1% of hospital charges. Quality control criteria include the following: (a) the specimen must be obtained before antibiotic treatment; (b) there needs to be good effort in quality control for specimen procurement, expeditious transport to the laboratory, and proper processing; and (c) there needs to be cytologic screening to demonstrate the presence of secretions from the lower airway with limited upper airway contamination. The "classic" criterion for the last is a low-power examination (×100) showing more than 25 polymorphonuclear leukocytes per field or less than 10 epithelial cells per field (20), but most laboratories require simply a predominance of polymorphonuclear leukocytes or sparse epithelial cells (21,22). Cytologic screening is not necessary for detection of *Mycobacterium tuberculosis* and *Legionella*. Interpretation of Gram stain and culture must be based on clinical correlations. Specialized tests are required for detection of mycobacteria, chlamydiae, mycoplasma, fungi, and viruses, and some laboratories offer specialized tests for detection of pneumococci such as the Quellung stain or other antigen detection tests for pneumococcal capsular polysaccharide.

TABLE 48.5. Microbial Pathogens Recovered from Respiratory Secretions

Diagnostic of pathogenic role regardless of specimen source	Nondiagnostic if recovered from usual respiratory specimens[a]
Bacteria	
Legionella	Virtually all other bacteria
Mycobacteria	
Mycobacterium tuberculosis	Mycobacteria other than tuberculosis
Viruses	
Influenza virus	Cytomegalovirus
Respiratory syncytial virus	Herpes simplex virus
Parainfluenza virus	
Adenovirus	
Coxsackievirus	
Parasites	
Strongyloides	
Toxoplasma gondii	
Fungi	
Pneumocystis carinii	*Candida* species
Histoplasma capsulatum	*Cryptococcus neoformans*
Coccidioides immitis	*Aspergillus* species
Blastomyces dermatitidis	

[a]Sputum, bronchoscopy, nasotracheal suction, and others.

TRANSTRACHEAL ASPIRATION

This technique was originally reported in 1963 (23) and subsequently became popular between 1968 and 1980 (24). During this time, there were many large series using transtracheal aspiration in diverse settings, but there were also several reports of complications (24). The technique consists of a catheter inserted through

TABLE 48.6. Pulmonary Infections: Specimens and Tests for Detection of Lower Respiratory Tract Pathogens

Organism	Pulmonary specimen	Microscopy	Culture	Serology	Other
Bacteria					
Aerobic and facultatively anaerobic	Expectorated sputum, quant bronch, blood, TTA, empyema fluid	Grain stain	X	—	Urinary antigen for *S. pneumoniae*
Anaerobic	TTA, empyema fluid, quant bronch	Gram stain	X	—	
Legionella species	Sputum, pleural fluid TTA, bronch, blood	FA (*L. pneumophila*)	X	IFA, EIA	Urinary antigen (*L. pneumophila* serogroup 1)[a]
Nocardia species	Expectorated sputum, TTA, lung biopsy, BAL	Gram stain and modified carbolfuchsin stain	X	—	
Chlamydia species	Nasopharyngeal swab, expectorated sputum, bronch	Negative	X[a]	CF for *C. psittaci* MIF for *C. pneumoniae*[a]	PCR for *C. pneumoniae*[a] (experimental)
Mycoplasma species	Expectorated sputum, nasopharyngeal swab	Negative	X[a]	CF, EIA	PCR[a] (experimental) Cold agglutinins (titer ≥1:32)
Mycobacteria	Expectorated or induced sputum, TTA, bronch	Fluorochrome stain or carbolfuchsin stain	X	—	PPD skin test PCR[a]
Fungi			X		
Deep-seated					
Blastomyces species	Expectorated or induced sputum, bronch, biopsy	Potassium hydroxide with phase contrast, Calcofluor stain	X		
Coccidioides species				CF	
Histoplasma species			X	CF, ID	Antigen assay: BAL, blood, urine[a]
Opportunistic					
Pneumocystis carinii	Induced sputum or bronch	Giemsa, FA, or GMS stain	—	—	
Aspergillus species		H&E, GMS stain	X	ID[a]	Computed tomography
Candida species	Lung biopsy	H&E, GMS stain	X	—	
Cryptococcus species	Expectorated sputum, serum, transbronchial biopsy, or BAL	H&E, GMS stain, calcofluor white	X	—	Serum, or BAL antigen assay
Zygomycetes	Expectorated sputum, tissue	H&E, GMS stain	X	—	
Viruses					
Influenza virus, parainfluenza virus, respiratory syncytial virus, cytomegalovirus	Nasal washings, nasopharyngeal aspirate or swab, bronch	FA: influenza and respiratory syncytial viruses	X[a]	CF, EIA, LA, FA	Cytomegalovirus: shell viral culture, FA stain of BAL or biopsy specimen
Hantavirus		Negative	—	EIA for immunoglobulins G and M[a]	PCR[a] (experimental) complete blood count: thrombocytopenia, leukocytosis, left shift, and >10% immunoblasts

[a]Few clinical microbiology laboratories offer these tests.
BAL, bronchoalveolar lavage; bronch, bronchoscopy specimen including aspirate, brushing, BAL, or biopsy; quant bronch, quantitative bronchoscopy culture including quantitative brush catheter or BAL; TTA, transtracheal aspirate or transthoracic aspirate; biopsy, transbronchial, transthoracic, or open lung biopsy; CF, complement fixation; CIE, counterimmunoelectrophoresis; EIA, enzyme immunoassay; FA, fluorescent antibody stain; GMS, Gomori methenamine-silver nitrate; H&E, hematoxylin and eosin; ID, immunodiffusion; IFA, indirect fluorescent antibody; LA, latex agglutination; MIF, microimmunofluorescence test; PCR, polymerase chain reaction; PPD, purified protein derivative.

the cricoid membrane to the carina with suction aspiration to obtain specimens from the level of the carina. This procedure is now almost never executed owing to the lack of physicians trained in the technique, concern for side effects, and decreased emphasis on microbial diagnoses.

TRANSTHORACIC NEEDLE ASPIRATION

The most extensive experience with this technique was in the prepenicillin era when the major indication was to recover

S. pneumoniae to provide the necessary information for administration of type-specific antisera, which was the only therapy available at the time (25). More recently, this procedure has been undertaken primarily for cytologic evaluation in suspected malignant disease and in occasional patients for a microbial diagnosis. In brief, the area of involvement is determined radiographically, and this site is sampled by percutaneous insertion of an 18- to 22-gauge, thin-walled spinal needle or the "skinny" 25-gauge needle (24,26). A review of 19 reported series showed that the diagnostic yield with suspected bacterial pneumonia is 35% to 50% (24). Possibly the most accurate definition of the frequency of false-negative cultures is the experience with 211 patients with bacteremic pneumococcal pneumonia by Bullowa (25) in the prepenicillin era, which showed positive results for this organism in 165 (78%). The presumed explanation is improper placement of the needle or nonviable organisms. The most common complication is pneumothorax in 20% to 30%, but a chest tube is required in only 1% to 10% (19). A review of 105 institutions with transthoracic needle aspiration in 1,562 patients showed a mortality rate of 0.1%, major hemorrhage in 0.2%, and pneumothorax requiring a chest tube in 7% (27). At present, transthoracic needle aspiration is generally restricted to tertiary medical centers with appropriate expertise for use in selected clinical settings, primarily immunocompromised patients or patients with atypical presentation in which the usual diagnostic specimen sources are either contraindicated or negative.

BRONCHOSCOPY SPECIMENS

Bronchoscopy with the rigid bronchoscope was developed in the late 1930s, and fiberoptic techniques were introduced in the late 1960s. Cultures obtained by suction aspiration through the inner channel for the usual bacteria are generally no better than the results with expectorated sputum (28). The reason is that the inner channel becomes filled with saliva during instrument passage through the upper airways. The result is that bronchoscopy is now generally reserved for the recovery of specific microbes (*M. tuberculosis* in patients who do not expectorate or *P. carinii*), for a lung biopsy, or for the detection of common bacterial pathogens by use of quantitative techniques to distinguish colonization and infection. With regard to results with tuberculosis, the yield for both acid-fast stain and culture is superior with expectorated sputum.

The utility of bronchoscopy for detecting the usual bacterial pathogens in the lower airways has been pursued by adding quantitation to the analysis. Theoretical support for quantitative cultures is based on the assumption that bacterial pathogens are invariably present in concentrations exceeding 10^5/dL at the infected site; contaminants or colonizing bacteria are generally present in lower concentrations. This principle applies to specimens obtained at virtually any anatomic site, including expectorated sputum after liquefaction (30). The usual techniques for obtaining bronchoscopic specimens for quantitative culture are with bronchoalveolar lavage or a double-lumen catheter with a distal occluding plug (24,31,32). Brush specimens must be placed in a diluent, and serial dilutions are performed for quantitative culture. Specific techniques are described elsewhere, but they are critically important for accurate results. This requires a commitment to follow precise methodology by the bronchoscopist for specimen procurement and by the microbiologist for performing cultures. Major uses of this technique are for nosocomial pneumonia, particularly pneumonia in the intensive care unit and in intubated patients (24,33,34).

COMMUNITY-ACQUIRED PNEUMONIA

Microbiology

Major pathogens encountered in community-acquired pneumonia are summarized in Table 48.7. These results are based on three analyses: the researcher's review of 17 publications dealing with community-acquired pneumonia (13–17,35–47), primarily from the United States; a metaanalysis of 7 of 122 reports of community-acquired pneumonia in the English language literature from 1966 to 1996; and estimates by the British Thoracic Society (48) based on their study involving 25 hospitals in England in the early 1980s. There is a notable bias in all three analyses because most of the patients are from hospital-based experiences in academic centers. Studies in outpatients tend to show higher yields of *M. pneumoniae* and viruses (49). In addition, there is a substantial variation in attempts to recover some microbes, especially those requiring nonroutine microbiologic techniques with arbitrary serologic criteria for *Legionella*, *Chlamydia pneumoniae*, and *Mycoplasma pneumoniae*. The relatively low yield with expectorated sputum in many studies and skepticism about results

TABLE 48.7. Microbiology of Community-Acquired Pneumonia

Microbial agents	Literature review[a] (%)	British thoracic society[b] (%)	Metaanalysis[c] Cases (%)	Metaanalysis[c] Deaths (%)
Bacteria				
Streptococcus pneumoniae	20–60	60–75	65	66
Haemophilus influenzae	3–10	4–5	12	7
Staphylococcus aureus	3–5	1–5	2	6
Gram-negative bacilli	3–10	Rare	1	3
Miscellaneous agents	3–5	Not included	4	9
Atypical agents	10–20	—	12	6
Legionella species	2–8	2–5	4	5
Mycoplasma pneumoniae	1–6	5–18	7	1
Chlamydia pneumoniae	4–6	Not included	1	<1
Viral	2–15	8–16	3	<1
Aspiration pneumonia	6–10	Not included	—	—
No diagnosis	30–60	—	—	—

[a]Based on 15 published reports from North America. Low and high values are deleted (13–17, 35–47).
[b]Estimates are based on analysis of 453 adults in prospective study of community-acquired pneumonia in 25 British hospitals (45).
[c]Metaanalysis of 122 published studies of community-acquired pneumonia in the English language literature 1966 to 1995; data are limited to 7,057 patients who had an etiologic diagnosis (7). Percentage in death column refers to percentage of all deaths attributed to the designated pathogen.
[d]Includes *Branhamella* (formerly *Moraxella*) *catarrhalis*, group A streptococcus, and *Neisseria meningitidis* (each 1%–2%).

have prompted vigorous debate about the value of these specimens for stain and culture. The American Thoracic Society position paper opposes any diagnostic studies other than blood cultures (50). Others are much more proactive for pretreatment diagnostic studies to simplify antibiotic decisions and help track the epidemiology of selected agents, such as penicillin-resistant *S. pneumoniae*, *S. aureus*, and *Legionella* (1,22).

A historical perspective on studies of community-acquired pneumonia is of particular interest with regard to *S. pneumoniae*. In the prepenicillin era, *S. pneumoniae* accounted for more than 80% of pneumonias and 96% of lobar pneumonias (8,25). There has subsequently been a gradual reduction of the yield in various series so that nearly all studies reported during the past decade indicate a yield of only 10% to 22%. The implication is that this organism is disappearing, other agents are becoming more prevalent, or laboratory techniques for its recovery are now relatively poor. The truth is probably some combination of these observations. Many think that *S. pneumoniae* may account for a substantial portion of these enigmatic cases on the basis of the following: (a) studies using more aggressive methods to obtain uncontaminated specimens, such as transtracheal aspiration, show much higher yields (24,51–53); (b) multiple studies show that the frequency of *S. pneumoniae* from sputum culture in patients with bacteremic pneumococcal pneumonia is only 40% to 50% (18,19), suggesting that the yield in most studies should be at least doubled; and (c) an analysis by the British Thoracic Society Pneumonia Research Committee based on a review of 148 patients with no identifiable pathogens concluded that most of these cases were probably due to *S. pneumoniae* (54).

Anaerobic bacteria are an additional category of organisms that have been conspicuously absent in virtually all studies since 1980. This reflects the fact that transtracheal aspirations are no longer done. Studies using transtracheal aspiration indicated that anaerobic bacterial pneumonitis could not be easily distinguished from other common forms of bacterial pneumonia on the basis of clinical observations (55). In addition, studies by Ries and colleagues (56) using transtracheal aspiration in unselected patients with community-acquired pneumonia showed anaerobic bacteria in 29 of 89 patients (33%). A similar yield was found by Pollock and colleagues (57) using quantitative cultures of fiberoptic bronchoscopy aspirates; here the yield was 38 of 172 patients (22%). These observations suggest that anaerobic bacteria probably account for a significant number of enigmatic pneumonias.

The term *atypical agents* was initially used to indicate *M. pneumoniae* (58,59), but it subsequently came to include *Legionella* and *C. pneumoniae* as well. These three organisms collectively account for 10% to 20% of all cases according to most studies that use aggressive techniques for their detection. Recommended methods to detect *Legionella* include culture and urinary antigen assay. Urinary antigen assays are technically easy but are limited to the detection of *Legionella pneumophila* serogroup 1, which accounts for about 50% to 70% of cases (60). *M. pneumoniae* has been found in 1% to 8% of patients with community-acquired pneumonia who require hospitalization; the rates are much higher for young adults with "walking pneumonia"; some report *Mycoplasma* species in up to 10% of elderly patients who require hospitalization (17). The problem with *Mycoplasma* diagnostic studies is the lack of a consensus regarding diagnostic tests and the limited availability of these assays in most hospital laboratories. Measurement of cold agglutinins is somewhat nonspecific, but may support this diagnosis in patients with a compatible clinical illness and a titer of 1:64 or higher. The same problem with diagnostic testing previously applied to *C. pneumoniae*, which allegedly accounts for 5% to 10% of cases of community-acquired

pneumonia (1,13–17,61), but the problems with erratic diagnostic criteria have been fixed by a consensus statement requiring a fourfold increase in titer using microimmunofluorescence serology or one of four adequately tested polymerase chain reaction techniques (62).

Viral agents are detected in 2% to 15% of cases, most frequently influenza virus and less commonly parainfluenza virus and respiratory syncytial virus. Viruses probably account for a substantial number of pneumonia cases in young, otherwise healthy adults and most children. Influenza virus is a major cause of epidemics associated with an increase of at least 20,000 pneumonia deaths per year for most years (6,63). Viral respiratory tract infections are now recognized as a major cause of serious disease often requiring hospitalization due to complications, which include asthma, exacerbations of chronic bronchitis, sinusitis, otitis, and pneumonia (63).

Diagnostic Evaluation

There is consensus that outpatients do not require diagnostic testing for an etiologic agent and that hospitalized patients should have two pretreatment blood cultures (1,50). Most studies report the blood culture yield to be 5% to 20%; the mean for all reported cases is 12%, and *S. pneumoniae* accounts for two thirds of these (7). The Infectious Diseases Society of America (IDSA) guidelines for pneumonia recommend Gram stain and culture of expectorated secretions. If done properly, a likely microbial pathogen can be detected with Gram stain of expectorated sputum in about 50% of cases; the organism identified by Gram stain can be cultured in approximately 90% of cases (1,15,53,47). The yield with posttreatment specimens will be reduced by 50%, and the yield with delayed transport and processing and lack of cytologic screening will be much less as well.

Therapy

Decisions regarding the selection of antibiotics are obviously simplified if a microbial diagnosis is strongly suspected or established by stains and culture. Guidelines for the empirical treatment of pneumonia have been provided by the American Thoracic Society (50) and the IDSA (1) (Table 48.8).

TABLE 48.8. Recommendations for Empiric Treatment of Community-Acquired Pneumonia in Immunocompetent Adults

Outpatients
  Doxycycline
  Macrolide[a]
  Fluoroquinolone[b]
Hospitalized patients
  General medical ward
    Cephalosporin[c] + macrolide[a]
    Fluoroquinolone[c]
  Intensive care unit
    Cephalosporin[c] + macrolide[a]
    Cephalosporin[c] + fluoroquinolone[b]
  Exceptions[d]

---

[a]Macrolide: azithromycin, clarithromycin, and erythromycin.
[b]Fluoroquinolone: levofloxacin, moxifloxacin, and gatifloxacin.
[c]Cephalosporin: ceftriaxone and cefotaxime.
[d]Structural disease of lung: antipseudomonal agents. β-lactam allergy: fluoroquinolone + clindamycin. Aspiration: fluoroquinolone ± clindamycin, metronidazole, or β-lactam–β-lactamase inhibitor.

NOSOCOMIAL PNEUMONIA

Risk Factors and Rates

Risks for nosocomial pneumonia may be considered patient related, infection control related, or intervention related. Patient-related risks are associated with underlying disease that predisposes to upper airway colonization by gram-negative bacilli (discussed later), predisposition to aspiration, and predisposition to opportunistic infection (immunocompromised). Infection control–related risks are transmissible airborne pathogens (such as in tuberculosis, legionellosis, aspergillosis, and influenza) and contact transmission (as with *Staphylococcus aureus,* Enterobacteriaceae, *P. aeruginosa,* and *Acinetobacter*). The third risk is intervention related, such as surgery (especially thoracoabdominal surgery), medications (antibiotics, gastric pH neutralization, immunosuppressive agents, and sedatives), and tubes (nasogastric intubation, tracheostomy, and endotracheal intubation).

The rate of nosocomial pneumonia is 0.5% to 1.0% of all hospitalized persons. For intensive care units, the rate is reported at 15% to 20%; for mechanically ventilated patients, it is 18% to 60% (65). Fagon and colleagues (66) have challenged some of these incidence data by showing that over half of these patients who satisfy standard criteria (radiographic evidence of infiltrate combined with cough and fever) do not appear to have bacterial pneumonia on the basis of quantitative cultures of bronchoscopic aspirates. This report is now well accepted on the basis of confirmatory reports (67,68).

Pathophysiology

The dominant organisms in nosocomial pneumonia are gram-negative bacteria, which presumably reach the lower airways by aspiration of gastric contents or by "microaspiration" of upper airway secretions. This microbiologic pattern is distinctly different from that of community-acquired pneumonia, in which gram-negative bacteria play essentially no role except for precisely defined and unusual settings (69–75). The presumed explanation for the distinction is the high rates of colonization of the upper airways by gram-negative bacteria as a reflection of serious illness. The classic study to examine this association used throat cultures to determine the rate of asymptomatic carriage of gram-negative bacilli in various populations (75). Healthy persons, physicians, medical students, and psychiatric patients, all exposed to a common hospital environment, had colonization rates of 2% to 3%. The rate in patients who were moderately ill was 30% to 40%; in the intensive care unit, it was 60% to 70%. These studies were conducted in patients who were not receiving antibiotics, but this type of treatment would also favor colonization by gram-negative bacilli. The presumed source of bacteria is the patient's own colonic flora. Thus, the postulated mechanism is colonization of the upper airways in a patient rendered vulnerable by severe disease with microaspiration as the mechanism for seeding of the lower airways. Aspiration and airway entry are promoted by violations of airway integrity, such as tracheostomy or intubation. Other pathophysiologic mechanisms for nosocomial pneumonia involve inhalation of selected pathogens responsible for epidemic or sporadic cases, including tuberculosis, legionellosis, and aspergillosis.

Bacteriology

Studies of nosocomial pneumonia indicate that gram-negative bacteria account for 50% to 70% of cases (Table 48.9) (69–74). The most common is *P. aeruginosa,* followed by a diverse array

TABLE 48.9. Nosocomial Pneumonia: Microbiology

Microbial agent	%
Bacterial	
Gram-negative bacilli	50–70
Pseudomonas aeruginosa[a]	
Enterobacteriaceae[a]	
Staphylococcus aureus[a]	15–30
Anaerobic bacteria	10–30
Haemophilus influenzae	10–20
Streptococcus pneumoniae	10–20
Legionella[a]	4
Viral	
Cytomegalovirus	10–20
Influenza virus[a]	
Respiratory syncytial virus[a]	
Fungal	
Aspergillus[a]	<1

[a]May cause nosocomial epidemics.

of Enterobacteriaceae. *S. aureus* is second to gram-negative bacteria in most studies and accounts for 15% to 30%. Anaerobic bacteria may be found in up to 10% to 30% of cases but are not generally sought with the use of appropriate diagnostic specimen sources (70). When they are found, there is usually the concurrent presence of aerobic gram-negative bacilli or *S. aureus,* and the role of anaerobes is somewhat unclear. Other organisms found in 5% to 20% of cases include *S. pneumoniae, H. influenzae,* and possibly *C. pneumoniae. Legionella* has been responsible for about 4% of all lethal nosocomial infections, but there have been multiple large outbreaks of legionnaires' disease in hospitals that are usually traced to water supplies with distribution through cooling systems of air conditioners or showerheads (76–78). Tuberculosis accounts for a relatively small number of nosocomial infections, but obviously represents an important public health problem (79). Aspergillosis may occur in epidemics among patients who are vulnerable, usually those who have suppressed cell-mediated immunity or neutropenia. This infection should be suspected when a patient at risk develops a pleura-based lesion that shows characteristic features at computed tomography.

Diagnosis

Pulmonary infection is usually suspected in hospitalized patients with fever, respiratory symptoms, and a new infiltrate on chest radiography. However, studies by Fagon and co-workers (66) suggested that most of these patients have alternative diagnoses. These investigators used quantitative culture of fiberoptic bronchoscopy aspirates in patients with the characteristic clinical features and found positive results with quantitative cultures in only about 40%; the majority of patients with negative results were not treated with antibiotics and subsequently recovered.

The usual specimen for a microbiologic diagnosis is expectorated sputum for Gram stain and culture. This usually yields gram-negative bacilli and *S. aureus* in large concentrations if they are involved in the pulmonary infection. The most frequent problem here is false-positive cultures for these microbes. Patients with pneumonia in the intensive care unit, and especially those who are intubated, often undergo fiberoptic bronchoscopy with quantitative culture (24,31–34). This is regarded as a controversial issue among pulmonary physicians, who appear divided over the role of bronchoscopy to evaluate pneumonia in the intensive care unit (73).

Therapy

The predominant organisms are gram-negative bacteria and *S. aureus*. These organisms require *in vitro* sensitivity tests to define optimal therapy and are readily recovered from most patients with expectorated sputum, nasotracheal suction, or endotracheal tube aspiration. Empirical treatment decisions should be based on Gram stains of these specimens pending culture and *in vitro* sensitivity test results. Guidelines for empirical antibiotic selection from the *Medical Letter* (80) are an aminoglycoside plus one of the following: cefotaxime, ceftriaxone, cefepime, ticarcillin-clavulanate, piperacillin-tazobactam, meropenem, or imipenem (80). Vancomycin should be considered in hospitals where methicillin-resistant *S. aureus* is present.

Prevention

The high risk for pneumonia in intensive care units has prompted aggressive methods to prevent this complication (Table 48.10). The most important recommendations are the use of the semiupright position to reduce the risk for aspiration (81) and the use of appropriate precautions to prevent secondary cases by airborne spread or contact. It is common practice in intensive care units to give prophylaxis to prevent peptic ulceration, but neutralization of gastric acid eliminates the gastric barrier, the acid defense mechanism that prevents colonization of the stomach by various bacteria including gram-negative bacilli. Sucralfate is advocated as a substitute for histamine (H^2) blockers or antacids, and preliminary evidence suggests efficacy (82). Selective decontamination has been a popular method to interrupt the cycle of colonization of the colon by gram-negative bacilli followed by colonization of the pharynx with subsequent aspiration from either an upper airway source or gastric contents. The goal of selective decontamination is to eliminate or reduce gram-negative bacilli (and sometimes *S. aureus* and *Candida*) in the gastrointestinal tract with antibiotics that select for these organisms but preserve the anaerobic bacteria that appear critical for population control of flora in the colon. An extensive experience with this technique including 12 controlled trials with more than 4,000 participants showed that this tactic effectively reduces the frequency of pneumonia in intensive care units, but

there is no substantial impact on mortality rates (84,85). Major concerns are the failure to reduce mortality, excessive costs of the regimens, and the concern of antibiotic abuse with its impact on bacterial resistance. Most authorities consequently no longer recommend selective decontamination in this setting.

Topical antibiotics also have been tested by instillation of drugs through tracheostomies or endotracheal tubes or by aerosolization. Drugs that are usually given by these routes are polymyxin or aminoglycosides, although multiple different agents have been used (86). The most extensive experience is by Feeley and colleagues (87) using polymyxin in an attempt to prevent nosocomial infections with *P. aeruginosa*. They were able to reduce the frequency of *P. aeruginosa*, but there was no impact on mortality rates, and there was an associated risk for infection involving resistant strains, primarily *Proteus* infections. Most authorities discourage the use of topical agents except for cystic fibrosis and cases where there are no alternatives based on *in vitro* sensitivity tests (86).

PNEUMONIA IN THE IMMUNOCOMPROMISED HOST

The immunocompromised host now represents an enlarging component of the population of hospitalized patients and outpatients. A review of 385 consecutive patients hospitalized at Johns Hopkins Hospital with community-acquired pneumonia in 1991 showed that 56% were considered immunocompromised (15). The majority of these were patients with human immunodeficiency virus infection, but there were also a large number who were receiving immunosuppressive therapy for organ transplantation or cancer chemotherapy. Etiologic agents are highly variable and largely dependent on the nature of the host defect. The reader is referred to Chapters 53–55 for the approach to the immunocompromised host with suspected pneumonia; pneumonia in patients with human immunodeficiency virus infection is discussed in Chapter 115.

RESPONSE TO THERAPY

The response and outcome of patients with community-acquired pneumonia depend to a large extent on the microbial agent involved and the host status. Factors suggesting poor prognosis based on host status, clinical features, laboratory findings, and microbial pathogens for community-acquired pneumonia are summarized in Table 48.4. According to a metaanalysis of 25,629 patients from 80 cohort studies reported from 1966 to 1995, the overall mortality of patients hospitalized with community-acquired pneumonia was 13.6%; it was 17.6% for elderly patients, 19.6% for bacteremic patients, and 36.5% for patients hospitalized in the intensive care unit (7).

With regard to response by microbial pathogens, the greatest experience is with pneumococcal pneumonia. After initiation of penicillin treatment for penicillin-sensitive *S. pneumoniae*, most patients show clinical improvement within 24 to 48 hours with a decrease in temperature and reduction in systemic toxic effects (88). The mean duration of fever in bacteremic pneumococcal pneumonia is approximately 6 days (7). The time to resolution of changes on the chest film depends largely on the host (89). Young and previously healthy adults show a mean time to radiographic clearing of 3 weeks; older patients and those with complicated infections show an average of 12 weeks to radiographic clearing. A subset of pneumococcal pneumonia patients does poorly. Features of poor prognosis include multiple lobe

---

TABLE 48.10.   Prevention of Nosocomial Pneumonia

Strongly recommended
  Semiupright position to reduce risk of aspiration
  Contact precautions with mask for the following respiratory tract pathogens
    Bacteria: *Staphylococcus aureus*, group A streptococci, *Neisseria meningitidis*, *Bordetella pertussis*, *Yersinia pestis* (plague), penicillin-resistant *Streptococcus pneumoniae*, multidrug-resistant gram-negative bacilli
    Bacteria-like: *Mycoplasma pneumoniae*
    Mycobacteria: *Mycobacterium tuberculosis*
    Viruses: viral exanthems (measles, rubella, chickenpox, mumps), influenza virus, enterovirus
    Fungi: none
Encouraged
  Use of sucralfate in place of histamine (H_2) agonists or antacids to preserve the gastric barrier
Experimental
  Continuous aspiration of subglottic secretions in ventilated patients
Not recommended
  Selective decontamination of gastrointestinal tract
  Topical administration (intratracheal instillations or aerosolized administration) of antimicrobial agents

involvement, bacteremia, age older than 60 years, concomitant disease, and neutropenia (8). Studies since the introduction of penicillin have shown that this drug has obviously had a notable impact on outcome; nevertheless, there is also good evidence that penicillin and other antibiotics have had little impact on the mortality rate during the first 5 days of treatment in patients with bacteremic pneumococcal pneumonia. The overall mortality rate of pneumococcal pneumonia among 4,432 patients hospitalized with this diagnosis was 12.3%; for 1,145 patients with bacteremic pneumococcal pneumonia it was 19% (7).

Patients with *Mycoplasma* pneumonia usually become afebrile within 1 to 2 days after treatment with tetracycline or a macrolide. Extrapulmonary signs and symptoms usually respond more slowly, and the role of antibiotics for these complications is unclear. The mortality rate is virtually nil, although some patients with sickle cell disease and some elderly patients may have relatively severe disease (7,59). The prognosis also appears generally good for pneumonia caused by *C. pneumoniae* (61). *Legionella* pneumonia has a high mortality rate, usually reported at 10% to 20% for community-acquired cases and 20% to 40% for nosocomial cases (7,77).

Patients with persistent fever and progressive symptoms after 3 to 5 days of treatment must be considered possible therapeutic failures if no etiologic diagnosis was established. Diagnostic considerations in this clinical setting are summarized in Table 48.11. In many instances, the infection has progressed too far by the time treatment is initiated, or else the patient is an inadequate host because of debility, immunosuppression, or associated diseases that preclude clinical response. Nevertheless, a diagnostic evaluation is necessary to exclude alternative treatable conditions. This evaluation often consists of sequential cultures of expectorated sputum or some other specimen from the respiratory tract, but these cultures are likely to be misleading because of the inherent problem of the antibiotic effect on fragile, susceptible microbes and the probability of "sputum superinfection" reflecting colonization of the airways. Most studies show that the yield of gram-negative bacilli of *S. aureus* is 25% to 50% when specimens are collected after common forms of antibiotic treatment. Unfortunately, it is often difficult for physicians to resist the temptation to add new antibiotics with each new organism that represents a potential pathogen in the lower airways.

A diagnostic study that may be useful is fiberoptic bronchoscopy, which may detect conditions other than infections by conventional pathogens (such as *M. tuberculosis*, pathogenic fungal, and *P. carinii* infections) and noninfectious conditions (such as bronchogenic neoplasms, atelectasis, chemical pneumonitis, interstitial lung disease, and sarcoidosis). An additional diagnostic test to consider is computed tomography to detect pleural effusions, cavitary lung disease, adenopathy, and other anatomic changes that may alter the differential diagnosis. If pulmonary embolism is a diagnostic consideration, a reasonable next step is a lung scan or pulmonary angiography.

For nosocomial pneumonia, especially for cases in the intensive care unit, the mortality rate is often reported at 20% to 30% (73). In many cases, there are multiple contributing factors in addition to the pulmonary infection. Nevertheless, nosocomial pneumonia is regarded as a devastating disease associated with an extraordinarily high mortality rate, primarily in the intensive care unit and in intubated patients. The definition of severe nosocomial pneumonia is summarized in Table 48.12 (73).

TABLE 48.12.   Definition of Severe Hospital-Acquired Pneumonia

Admission to the intensive care unit
Respiratory failure, defined as the need for mechanical ventilation or the need for >35% oxygen to maintain an arterial oxygen saturation at >90%
Rapid radiographic progression, multilobar pneumonia, or cavitation of a lung infiltrate
Evidence of severe sepsis with hypotension or end-organ dysfunction
   Shock (systolic blood pressure <90 mm Hg, or diastolic blood pressure <60 mm Hg)
   Requirement for vasopressors for more than 4 h
   Urine output <20 mL/h or total urine output <80 mL in 4 h (unless another explanation is available)
Acute renal failure requiring dialysis

TABLE 48.11.   Causes of Failure to Respond to Treatment

Disease is too far advanced at time of treatment or treatment is delayed too long: most common with pneumonia due to *Streptococcus pneumoniae, Legionella,* or gram-negative bacilli
Wrong antibiotic selection: uncommon
Inadequate dose of antibiotic: most common with aminoglycosides owing to failure to use adequate dose or to monitor serum levels
Wrong diagnosis: noninfectious disease such as pulmonary embolism with infarction, congestive failure, Wegener's granulomatosis, sarcoidosis, atelectasis, chemical pneumonitis
Wrong microbial diagnosis
Inadequate host: debilitated, severe associated disease, immunosuppressed
Complicated pneumonia with undrained empyema, metastatic site of infection (meningitis), or bronchial obstruction (foreign body, carcinoma)
Pulmonary superinfection: most patients respond and then deteriorate with new fever

---

REFERENCES

1. Bartlett JG, Dowell SF, Mandell LA, et al. Practice guidelines for the management of community-acquired pneumonia in adults. *Clin Infect Dis* 2000;31:347.
2. Centers for Disease Control and Prevention. Premature deaths, monthly mortality, and monthly physician contacts: United States. *MMWR* 1997;46:556.
3. Marston BJ, Plouffe JF, File TM, et al. Incidence of community-acquired pneumonia requiring hospitalizations: results of a population-based active surveillance study in Ohio. Community-Based Pneumonia Incidence Study Group. *Arch Intern Med* 1997;157:1709.
4. Dixon RE. Economic costs of respiratory tract infections in the United States. *Am J Med* 1985;78(suppl 6B):45.
5. Lave JR, Lin CC, Fine MJ. The cost of treating patients with community-acquired pneumonia. *Semin Respir Crit Care Med* 1999;20:189.
6. Pinner RW, Teutsch SM, Simonsen L, et al. Trends in infectious diseases mortality in the United States. *JAMA* 1996;275:189.
7. Fine MJ, Smith MA, Carson CA, et al. Prognosis and outcomes of patients with community-acquired pneumonia. *JAMA* 1995;274:134.
8. Heffron R. *Pneumonia.* Cambridge, MA: Harvard University Press, 1939:302.
9. Wipf JE, Lipsky BA, Hirschmann JV, et al. Diagnosing pneumonia by physical examination: relevant or relic? *Arch Intern Med* 1999;159:1082.
10. Gonzales R, Bartlett JG, Besser RE, et al. Principles for appropriate antibiotic use for treatment of uncomplicated acute bronchitis. *Ann Intern Med* 2001;134:521.
11. Opravil M, Marincek B, Fuchs WA, et al. Shortcomings of chest radiography in detecting *Pneumocystis carinii* pneumonia. *J AIDS* 1994;7:39.
12. Fine MJ, Auble TE, Yealy DM, et al. A prediction rule to identify low-risk patients with community-acquired pneumonia. *N Engl J Med* 1997;336:243.
13. Marrie TJ, Durant H, Yates L. Community-acquired pneumonia requiring hospitalization: 5 year prospective study. *Rev Infect Dis* 1989;11:586.
14. Fang GD, Fine M, Orloff J, et al. New and emerging etiologies for community-acquired pneumonia with implication for therapy: a prospective multicenter study of 359 cases. *Medicine (Baltimore)* 1990;69:307.
15. Mundy LM, Auwaerter PG, Oldach D, et al. Community-acquired pneumonia: impact of immune status. *Am J Respir Crit Care Med* 1995;152:1309.
16. Jokinen C, Heiskanen L, Juvonen H, et al. Microbial etiology of community-acquired pneumonia in the adult population of four municipalities in Eastern Finland. *Clin Infect Dis* 2001;32:1141.

17. Fine TM, Segreti J, Dunbar L, et al. A multicenter, randomized study comparing the efficacy and safety of intravenous and/or oral levofloxacin versus ceftriaxone and/or cefuroxime axetil in treatment of adults with community-acquired pneumonia. *Antimicrob Agents Chemother* 1997;41:1965.

18. Barrett-Conner E. The nonvalue of sputum culture in the diagnosis of pneumococcal pneumonia. *Am Rev Respir Dis* 1971;103:845.

19. Mufson MA, Chang V, Gill V, et al. The role of viruses, mycoplasmas and bacteria in acute pneumonia in civilian adults. *Am J Epidemiol* 1967;86:526.

20. Murray PR, Washington JA II. Microscopic and bacteriologic analysis of expectorated sputum. *Mayo Clin Proc* 1975;50:339.

21. Van Scoy RE. Bacterial sputum cultures: a clinician's viewpoint. *Mayo Clin Proc* 1977;52:39.

22. Rein MF, Gwaltney JM Jr, O'Brien WM, et al. Accuracy of Gram's stain in identifying pneumococci in sputum. *JAMA* 1978;239:2671.

23. Pecora DV. A comparison of transtracheal aspiration with other methods of determining the bacterial flora of the lower respiratory tract. *N Engl J Med* 1963;296:664.

24. Bartlett JG. Invasive diagnostic techniques in pulmonary infections. In: Pennington JE, ed. *Respiratory infections: diagnosis and management*, 3rd ed. New York: Raven, 1994:73.

25. Bullowa JGM. The reliability of sputum typing and its relation to serum therapy. *JAMA* 1935;105:1512.

26. American Thoracic Society. Guidelines for percutaneous transthoracic needle aspiration. *Am Rev Respir Dis* 1989;140:255.

27. Herman PG, Hessel SJ. The diagnostic accuracy and complications of closed lung biopsies. *Radiology* 1977;125:11.

28. Bartlett JG, Alexander J, Mayhew J, et al. Should fiberoptic bronchoscopy aspirates be cultured? *Am Rev Respir Dis* 1976;114:73.

29. Jett JR, Cortese DA, Dines DE. The value of bronchoscopy in the diagnosis of mycobacterial disease. *Chest* 1981;80:575.

30. Bartlett JG, Finegold SM. Bacteriology of expectorated sputum with quantitative culture and wash technique compared to transtracheal aspirates. *Am Rev Respir Dis* 1978;117:1010.

31. Wimberly N, Faling J, Bartlett JG. A fiberoptic bronchoscopy technique to obtain uncontaminated lower airway secretions for bacterial culture. *Am Rev Respir Dis* 1979;119:337.

32. Wimberly NW, Bass JB, Boyd BS, et al. Use of a bronchoscopic protected catheter brush for the diagnosis of pulmonary infections. *Chest* 1982;81:556.

33. Papazian L, Thomas P, Garbe L, et al. Bronchoscopic or blind sampling techniques for the diagnosis of ventilator-associated pneumonia. *Am J Respir Crit Care Med* 1995;152:1982.

34. Chastre J, Fagon JY, Lamer CH. Procedures for the diagnosis of pneumonia in ICU patients. *Intens Care Med* 1992;18(suppl):10.

35. Fekety FR Jr, Caldwell J, Gump D, et al. Bacteria, viruses and mycoplasmas in acute pneumonia in adults. *Am Rev Respir Dis* 1971;104:499.

36. Sullivan RJ Jr, Dowdle WR, Marine WM, et al. Adult pneumonia in a general hospital: etiology and host risk factors. *Arch Intern Med* 1972;129:935.

37. Bisno AL, Griffin JR, Van Epps KA, et al. Pneumonia and Hong Kong influenza: a prospective study of the 1968–1969 epidemic. *Am J Med Sci* 1971;261:251.

38. Dorff GJ, Rytel MW, Farmer SG, et al. Etiologies and characteristic features of pneumonias in a municipal hospital. *Am J Med Sci* 1973;266:349.

39. Fick RB Jr, Reynolds HY. Changing spectrum of pneumonia—news media creation or clinical reality? *Am J Med* 1983;74:1.

40. Larsen RA, Jacobson JA. Diagnosis of community-acquired pneumonia: experience at a community hospital. *Compr Ther* 1984;10:20.

41. Farr BM, Sloman AJ, Fisch MJ. Predicting death in patients hospitalized for community-acquired pneumonia. *Ann Intern Med* 1991;115:428.

42. Bates JH, Campbell GD, Barron AL, et al. Microbial etiology of acute pneumonia in hospitalized patients. *Chest* 1992;101:1005.

43. Dans P, Charache PC, Fahey M, et al. Management of pneumonia in the prospective payment era. *Arch Intern Med* 1984;144:1392.

44. Marston BJ, Plouffe JF, Breiman RF, et al. Preliminary findings in a community-based pneumonia incidence study. In: Barbaree JM, Breiman RF, Dufour AP, eds. *Legionella*. Washington, DC: American Society for Microbiology, 1993:36.

45. Research Committee of the British Thoracic Society and the Public Health Laboratory Service. Community-acquired pneumonia in adults in British hospitals in 1982–1983: a survey of aetiology, mortality, prognostic factors and outcome. *Q J Med* 1987;239:195–220.

46. Lim I, Shaw DR, Stanley DP, et al. A prospective hospital study of the aetiology of community-acquired pneumonia. *Med J Aust* 1989;151:87–91.

47. Bartlett JG, Mundy LM. Community-acquired pneumonia. *N Engl J Med* 1995;333:1618.

48. The British Thoracic Society. Guidelines for the management of community-acquired pneumonia in adults admitted to hospital. *Br J Hosp Med* 1993;49:346.

49. Falguera M, Sacristan O, Nogues A, et al. Nonsevere community-acquired pneumonia: correlation between cause and severity or comorbidity. *Arch Intern Med* 2001;161:1866.

50. American Thoracic Society. Guidelines for the initial management of adults with community-acquired pneumonia: diagnosis, assessment of severity antimicrobial therapy and prevention. *Am J Respir Crit Care Med* 2001;163:1730.

51. Kalinske RW, Parker RH, Brandt E: Diagnostic usefulness and safety of transtracheal aspiration. *N Engl J Med* 1970;276:604.

52. Hoeprich PD. Etiologic diagnosis of lower respiratory tract infections. *Calif Med* 1970;112:1.

53. Bartlett JG. Diagnostic accuracy of transtracheal aspiration bacteriology. *Am Rev Respir Dis* 1977;115:777.

54. Farr BM, Kaiser DL, Harrison BDW, et al. Prediction of microbial aetiology at admission to hospital for pneumonia from the presenting clinical features. *Thorax* 1989;44:1031.

55. Bartlett JG. Anaerobic bacterial pneumonitis. *Am Rev Respir Dis* 1979;119:19–23.

56. Ries K, Levison ME, Kaye D. Transtracheal aspiration in pulmonary infection. *Arch Intern Med* 1974;133:453.

57. Pollock HM, Hawkins EL, Bonner JR, et al. Diagnosis of bacterial pulmonary infections during quantitative protected catheter cultures obtained during bronchoscopy. *J Clin Microbiol* 1983;17:255.

58. Chanock RM, Mufson MA, Bloom HH, et al. Eaton agent pneumonia. *JAMA* 1961;175:213.

59. Foy HM. Infections caused by *Mycoplasma pneumoniae* and possible carrier state in a different population of patients. *Clin Infect Dis* 1993;17(suppl):37.

60. Marston BJ, Lipman HB, Breiman RF. Surveillance for Legionnaires' disease. Risk factors for morbidity and mortality. *Arch Intern Med* 1994;154:2417.

61. Grayston JT, Campbell LA, Kuo CC, et al. A new respiratory tract pathogen: *Chlamydia pneumoniae*, strain TWAR. *J Infect Dis* 1990;161:618.

62. Dowell SF, Peeling RW, Boman J, et al. Standardizing *Chlamydia pneumoniae* assays: recommendations from the CDC and Laboratory Centre for Disease Control (Canada). *Clin Infect Dis* 2001;33:492.

63. Simonsen L, Fukudak, Schonberger LB, Cox NJ. The impact of influenza epidemics on hospitalization. *J Infect Dis* 2000;181:831.

64. Sullivan KM, Monto AS, Longini IM Jr. Estimates of the U.S. health impact of influenza. *Am J Public Health* 1993;83:1712.

65. Morehead RS, Pinto SJ. Ventilator-associated pneumonia. *Arch Intern Med* 2000;160:1926.

66. Fagon JY, Chastre J, Hance AJ, et al. Detection of nosocomial lung infection in ventilated patients: use of a protected specimen brush and quantitative culture techniques in 147 patients. *Am Rev Respir Dis* 1988;138:110.

67. Pillet D, Boten MJM. Towards invasive diagnostic techniques as a standard management of ventilator-associated pneumonia. *Lancet* 2000;356:874.

68. Fagon JY, Chastre J, Wolff M, et al. Invasive and noninvasive strategies for management of suspected ventilator-associated pneumonia. *Ann Intern Med* 2000;132:621.

69. Jones RN, Croco MAT, Kugler KC. Respiratory tract pathogens isolated from patients hospitalized with suspected pneumonia: frequency of occurrence & antimicrobial susceptibility patterns from the SENTRY Antimicrobial Surveillance. *Diagn Micro Infect Dis* 2000;37:115.

70. Bartlett JG, O'Keefe P, Tally FP, et al. Bacteriology of hospital-acquired pneumonia. *Arch Intern Med* 1986;146:868.

71. Rouby JJ, Martin De Lassale E, et al. Nosocomial bronchopneumonia in the critically ill: histologic and bacteriologic aspects. *Am Rev Respir Dis* 1992;146:1059.

72. Horan TC, White JW, Jarvis WR, et al. Nosocomial infection surveillance, 1984. *MMWR* 1986;35:17SS.

73. Schleupner CJ, Cobb DK. A study of the etiologies and treatment of nosocomial pneumonia in a community-based teaching hospital. *Infect Control Hosp Epidemiol* 1992;13:515.

74. American Thoracic Society. Hospital-acquired pneumonia in adults: diagnosis, assessment of severity, initial antimicrobial therapy and preventative strategies. A consensus statement. *Am Rev Respir Crit Care Med* 1996;153:1711.

75. Johanson WG, Pierce AK, Sanford JP. Changing pharyngeal bacterial flora of hospitalized patients: emergence of gram-negative bacilli. *N Engl J Med* 1969;281:1137.

76. Stout JE, Yu VL. Legionellosis. *N Engl J Med* 1997;337:682.

77. Edelstein PH. Legionnaires' disease. *Clin Infect Dis* 1993;16:741.

78. Carratala J, Gudiol F, Pallares R, et al. Risk factors for nosocomial *Legionella pneumophila* pneumonia. *Am J Respir Crit Care Med* 1994;149:625.

79. McGowan JE Jr. Nosocomial tuberculosis: new progress in control and prevention. *Clin Infect Dis* 1995;21:489.

80. Consultants of Medical Letter. The choice of antibacterial drugs. *Med Lett* 2001;43:69.

81. Torres A, Serra-Batlles J, Ros E, et al. Pulmonary aspiration of gastric contents in patients receiving mechanical ventilation: the effect of body position. *Ann Intern Med* 1992;116:540.

82. Driks MR, Craven DE, Celli BR, et al. Nosocomial pneumonia in intubated patients given sucralfate as compared with antacids or histamine type 2 blockers: the role of gastric colonization. *N Engl J Med* 1987;317:1376.

83. Prod'hom G, Leuenberger P, Koerfer J, et al. Nosocomial pneumonia in mechanically ventilated patients receiving antacid, ranitidine, or sucralfate as prophylaxis for stress ulcer: a randomized controlled trial. *Ann Intern Med* 1994;120:653.

84. Gastinne H, Wolff M, Delatour F, et al. A controlled trial in intensive care units of selective decontamination of the digestive tract with nonabsorbable antibiotics. *N Engl J Med* 1992;326:594.

85. Selective Decontamination of the Digestive Tract Trialists' Collaborative Group. Meta-analysis of randomised controlled trials of selective decontamination of the digestive tract. *BMJ* 1993;307:525.

86. Hamer DH. Treatment of nosocomial pneumonia and tracheobronchitis caused by multidrug resistant *Pseudomonas aeruginosa* with aerosolized colistin. *Am J Respir Crit Care Med* 2000;162:328.

87. Feeley TW, Du Moulin GC, Hedley-Whyte J, et al. Aerosol polymyxin and pneumonia in seriously ill patients. *N Engl J Med* 1975;293:471.

88. Austrian R, Winston AL. The efficacy of penicillin V in the treatment of mild or moderately severe pneumococcal pneumonia. *Am J Med Sci* 1956;232:624.

89. Jay SJ, Johanson WG, Pierce AK. The radiographic resolution of *Streptococcus pneumoniae* pneumonia. *N Engl J Med* 1975;293:798.

CHAPTER 49
Bacterial Pneumonia

John G. Bartlett

Lower respiratory tract infections are the major cause of death due to infectious diseases in the world. Current estimates are 395,000,000 infections annually with 4,400,000 deaths, accounting for approximately 8% of all deaths. In the United States, the death rate per 100,000 population was 30 in 1992, and this represented a 20% increase from 1980 (1). The most common identifiable cause of pneumonia is bacterial infection. This chapter reviews bacterial pneumonia by microbe for the most frequently implicated bacterial agents. Other related topics discussed elsewhere include the approach to the patient with pneumonia (Chapter 48), pneumonia in immunocompromised hosts (Chapters 53–55), viral pneumonia (Chapter 51), *Mycoplasma* pneumonia (Chapter 52), aspiration pneumonia (Chapter 57), legionnaires' disease (Chapter 55), *Chlamydia* pneumonia (Chapter 56), *Streptococcus pneumoniae* (Chapter 184), *Haemophilus influenzae* (Chapter 203), *Branhamella* (Chapter 194), and pulmonary infections in patients with human immunodeficiency virus (HIV) infection (Chapter 115).

HISTORY

S. pneumoniae plays a prominent role in the history of microbiology and pneumonia. It was originally described in 1881 by Pasteur in France and Sternberg in the United States, and both showed its pathogenic potential by injection of saliva into rabbits (2). The organism was subsequently referred to as pneumococcus in 1886, reflecting its role in pulmonary infections (3), and was named *Diplococcus pneumoniae* in 1920 in reference to the Gram stain appearance (4); it was renamed as a *Streptococcus* in 1974 (5). The organism was one of the first to be described in the development of the Gram stain in 1884 (6). Capsular serotypes and the role of type-specific antibody in opsonization were reported at the turn of the century by Neufeld and Haendel (7). The prominent role of *S. pneumoniae* in pulmonary infection was recognized by Frankel in 1884 (8). A classic description of pneumococcal pneumonia in these early reviews was provided by Lord (9):

> Pneumonia due to the pneumococcus differs from pulmonary infection with other organisms in that it has an explosive onset, usual massive lung involvement, short course, abrupt termination, and relatively rapid restoration of the involved area to normal.

Serotherapy with type-specific antisera from sensitized horses became a popular method of treatment in the 1930s (10); this prompted a period in history when microbiology studies were at their finest, reflecting that treatment required retrieval of the pathogen to permit serotyping. The role of penicillin therapy was reported in 1941 (11), and dramatic results in 500 cases were reported by Keefer and co-workers (12) in 1943.

PNEUMOCOCCAL PNEUMONIA

Frequency

S. pneumoniae is the major identifiable cause of pneumonia in virtually all studies of community-acquired pneumonia in patients who require hospitalization. In the prepenicillin era, this organism accounted for approximately 80% of all pneumonias and 96% of lobar pneumonias (13). During the ensuing decades, there has been a gradual decline in the frequency of recovery of *S. pneumoniae* that most studies in the 1990s showed a yield of only 10% to 20% (14–19). This decline is ascribed to multiple factors, including the impact of antecedent antibiotic treatment on recovery in respiratory secretions, failure to produce sputum, recognition of alternative agents of pneumonia, and sloppy microbiology. A metaanalysis of 122 reports in the English-language literature of community-acquired pneumonia from 1966 through 1995 showed that approximately 6,000 had a bacterial pathogen defined; *S. pneumoniae* accounted for 73% of all cases in this category and also accounted for 66% of those with a lethal outcome (Table 49.1) (14). The estimated annual rate of pneumococcal pneumonia is 1 to 10 per 1,000 in the United States, with an annual total of about 500,000 (20–23).

Microbiology

S. pneumoniae is a gram-positive coccus that usually appears in pairs with tapered ends referred to as lancet shaped. It is relatively fastidious and easily overgrown by other bacteria or overlooked because of confusion with other α-hemolytic streptococci. Identification is by susceptibility to ethylhydrocupreine hydrochloride (Optochin). Pathogenicity is related to the polysaccharide capsule with at least 84 identified serotypes. The capsular polysaccharide may be used for detection in the Quellung reaction or by antigen detection with use of blood, urine, or respiratory secretions. Most laboratories rely on conventional Gram stain and culture. The individual serotypes show differences in frequency, pathogenicity, and susceptibility to penicillin (24). The major use of serotyping is for epidemiologic investigation and for implementing strategies for disease control with pneumococcal vaccine, which contains polysaccharides of the 23 serotypes that account for 89% of invasive infections caused by *S. pneumoniae*.

Pathogenesis

The usual mechanism of pneumonia is by aspiration of *S. pneumoniae* that is harbored in the nasopharynx. Colonization rates are highly variable but usually reported at 5% to 10% among healthy adults (25). Antibody is type-specific and appears to play an important role in susceptibility to infection but does not prevent colonization. Virtually all patients are susceptible, and *S. pneumoniae* is clearly the most common identified

---

TABLE 49.1. Bacteriology of Community-Acquired Pneumonia: Metanalysis of 59 Reports, 1966 to 1995

Total number of cases with bacterial pathogen	6,104
Streptococcus pneumoniae	4,432 (73%)
Haemophilus influenzae	833 (14%)
Legionella	272 (4%)
Staphylococcus aureus	157 (3%)
Gram-negative bacilli	103 (2%)
Klebsiella	56
Pseudomonas aeruginosa	18

Analysis is restricted to cases with a bacterial pathogen. No likely etiologic agent was detected in 11,229 cases.
Data from Fine MJ, Smith MA, Carson CA, et al. Prognosis and outcomes of patients with community-acquired pneumonia: a meta-analysis. *JAMA* 1996;275:134–141.

pathogen in previously healthy adults requiring hospitalization for community-acquired pneumonia (14). Nevertheless, a variety of risk factors have been identified for both frequency and severity of pneumococcal pneumonia. The most well-established risks are advanced age, African-American race, chronic lung disease, cigarette use, congestive heart failure, neurologic conditions that predispose to aspiration, and alcoholism (20,26–28). Patients with compromised B-cell function have high rates of pneumococcal pneumonia, including conditions such as common variable immunodeficiency, X-linked agammaglobulinemia, multiple myeloma, and chronic lymphocytic leukemia. The rate of pneumococcal pneumonia is at least 100-fold greater among patients with HIV infection (29,30). Clustering also may be a factor with high rates of pneumococcal pneumonia, sometimes in epidemic form, in South African miners, in military personnel in closed quarters, or in association with day care centers, jails, and homeless shelters (31). Miscellaneous risks are found in patients who have undergone splenectomy, in Native Americans living on reservations, and with people in selected occupations, such as painters and welders.

Clinical Features

The classic presentation of pneumococcal pneumonia is a dramatic illness characterized by abrupt onset with a rigor followed by high fever, cough productive of sputum that is purulent and often rust colored, dyspnea, and in most cases pleuritic pain (32). In the absence of treatment, the classic description includes high fever, tachypnea, and severe toxic effects for 7 to 10 days (9,12,13,26). The development of antibody is accompanied by abrupt lysis of fever with dramatic clinical recovery despite the persistence of consolidation on chest radiographs. Many patients with pneumococcal pneumonia as seen in current practice have a less dramatic evolution of disease, and most have intervening antibiotic treatment that alters the natural course. Laboratory studies usually show leukocytosis with a leftward shift, mild to moderate hypoxemia, and characteristic changes on chest radiographs. There is a direct correlation between the extent of leukocytosis and mortality, although leukopenia is also viewed as a finding related to poor prognosis (26). The classic chest film finding is lobar consolidation, and the majority of patients with lobar consolidation have *S. pneumoniae* as the putative agent (13–21). Nevertheless, many or most patients show changes described as bronchopneumonic or even interstitial (33).

Diagnosis

An established diagnosis requires recovery of *S. pneumoniae* from an uncontaminated specimen source, including blood, pleural fluid, transtracheal aspirate, or transthoracic needle aspirate. *S. pneumoniae* accounts for 65% of bacteremic pneumonias, and 5% to 12% of hospitalized patients with community-acquired pneumonia have *S. pneumoniae* bacteremia (14). For the majority of patients, the diagnosis is established with Gram stain and culture of expectorated sputum (32). Culture of sputum is fraught with problems for both false-positive and false-negative results. False-positive results reflect contamination of the specimen in the 5% to 10% of adult patients who are colonized with *S. pneumoniae* in the nasopharynx. The rate of false-negative cultures based on studies of bacteremic pneumonia is estimated at approximately 50% (34,35). That is, *S. pneumoniae* is recovered in expectorated sputum cultures from about 50% of patients who have positive blood cultures accompanied by a pulmonary infiltrate on chest radiographs. The low yield of only 10% to 20% for *S. pneumoniae* in expectorated sputum cultures among all hospital-

ized patients with community-acquired pneumonia is ascribed to (a) absence of productive cough in 20% to 30% of patients; (b) antecedent antibiotic exposure, which usually precludes recovery of this fastidious pathogen in 20% to 30%; (c) delays in transport of specimens to the laboratory for prompt microbiologic processing; and (d) reduced competence or commitment of laboratory personnel for detection with routine methods of processing specimens. An analysis of cases of enigmatic pneumonia by the British Thoracic Society suggested that the majority were due to this pathogen (36). Alternative methods that have been used to increase the yield, include the Quellung reaction with expectorated sputum and detection of pneumococcal polysaccharide by latex agglutination or counterimmunoelectrophoresis in urine or respiratory secretions (37–40). Antigen detection is routinely used in many laboratories in Europe and Scandinavia, which presumably accounts for higher yields of the pneumococcus in studies of community-acquired pneumonia in those areas; many authorities think that these antigen detection techniques lack sufficient specificity for routine laboratory use.

Treatment

Penicillin has generally been regarded as the drug of choice for pneumococcal infections, and the standard dose for uncomplicated cases was 600,000 units of aqueous procaine penicillin given intramuscularly every 12 hours or oral penicillin V in a dose of 1 to 2 g per day (41). In the 1960s, this therapy was successful in the majority of uncomplicated cases of pneumococcal pneumonia. Patients with bacteremia or more complicated cases were generally treated with intravenous aqueous penicillin G in a daily dose of 2 million units, and higher doses were of no therapeutic benefit (42). These recommendations are now antiquated because of the evolution of penicillin resistance (43–46). Studies of *S. pneumoniae* in 1997 from multiple centers in the United States showed that approximately 15% of strains were resistant to penicillin (minimum inhibitory concentration >2 μg/mL) (Table 49.2) (35). Furthermore, strains of *S. pneumoniae* resistant to penicillin were often resistant to multiple other antimicrobial agents as well (Table 49.1). The result is increased emphasis on recovery of the pathogen, routine susceptibility testing of

TABLE 49.2. Antimicrobial Susceptibility of *Streptococcus pneumoniae*: Analysis of 1,527 Strains from 30 Medical Centers, United States, 1994 to 1995

Agent	% Resistant
Penicillin G	24
Intermediate	14
High level	10
Cephalosporins[a]	
Cefuroxime	12
Ceftriaxone	5
Cefotaxime	3
Erythromycin	10
Tetracycline	8
Chloramphenicol	4
Vancomycin	0

[a]Rank order of cephalosporins was cefotaxime = ceftriaxone ≥ cefpodoxime ≥ cefuroxime > cefprozil ≥ cefixime > cefaclor = loracarbef > cefadroxil = cephalexin.
Adapted from Doern GV, Brueggemann A, Holley HP Jr, et al. Antimicrobial resistance of *Streptococcus pneumoniae* recovered from outpatients in the United States during the winter months of 1994 to 1995: results of a 30-center national surveillance study. *Antimicrob Agents Chemother* 1996;40:1209–1213.

all clinically significant isolates of *S. pneumoniae*, knowledge of sensitivity profiles within the community, restraint in antibiotic abuse to reduce the problem, and use of pneumococcal vaccine (46). The probability of penicillin resistance is increased in children and in patients who have recently been hospitalized, those exposed to day care centers, those extensively exposed to antibiotics, and those who reside in or have recently traveled to areas that have high rates of resistance. Penicillin is regarded as the preferred agent for penicillin-sensitive strains, and this drug may be used in higher concentrations (10 to 12 million units per day intravenously) for strains showing intermediate susceptibility (47). Alternative drugs that are usually active include cefotaxime, ceftriaxone, macrolides, doxycycline, carbapenems, and fluoroquinolones (43–46). For highly penicillin-resistant strains, the most predictably active drugs are fluoroquinolones, vancomycin, and linezolid (43–47). Macrolides have usually been considered the standard alternative agent for patients with contraindications to β-lactams (48), but this option is confounded by high rates of reduced susceptibility, primarily in penicillin-resistant strains. Among the oral cephalosporins, the most active *in vitro* are cefpodoxime, cefprozil, and cefuroxime (32,43). Particularly promising for penicillin-resistant strains are the fluoroquinolones (32,43,44). Advantages of these drugs include the excellent track record in clinical trials, the availability of oral and parenteral formulations, the paucity of side effects, and the excellent activity not only against most penicillin-resistant *S. pneumoniae*, but also atypical strains (16,32,49,50). The main concern is the potential abuse of fluoroquinolones with the evolution of resistance (51).

Complications and Response to Therapy

The major complications of patients hospitalized with pneumococcal pneumonia are bacteremia in 12% of cases, empyema in 0.5% to 1%, and meningitis in 0.3% to 0.5% (14,26). Other infrequent complications include purulent pericarditis and septic arthritis. The overall mortality rate in hospitalized patients is 12% (14). Factors associated with a poor prognosis include age extremes, multilobar involvement, bacteremia, neutropenia, selected serotypes, alcoholism, and asplenia. The impact of age was well studied in the prepenicillin era, when it was noted that pneumococcal pneumonia was lethal in 24% of patients 20 to 39 years of age, in 36% of those 40 to 49 years of age, in 50% of persons 50 to 59 years of age, and in 72% of those who were over 60 years of age (26). It was also observed that the mortality rate was 13% without bacteremia and increased to 62% in those with bacteremia. Currently reported mortality rates for bacteremic pneumococcal pneumonia range from 6% to 20% depending largely on associated risks (52). More recent studies have also shown that the mortality rate of pneumococcal pneumonia has been substantially reduced by the impact of antibiotics, but there has been no significant decrease during the first 5 days of treatment (53). The mean time to resolution of fever is 3 to 5 days among patients who respond to antibiotics and 6 to 7 days in those with bacteremic pneumonia. Chest radiographs may normalize within 3 to 4 weeks in young, previously healthy adults, but this clearing is delayed to a mean of 13 weeks in older patients and in patients who have pneumococcal bacteremia, structural abnormalities of the lung, or coexisting medical conditions (54,55).

Prevention

The major preventive measure is the polyvalent pneumococcal vaccine, which includes 23 serotypes of *S. pneumoniae* that account for about 89% of cases of pneumococcal disease. This vaccine is recommended for persons over 50 years of age or in the presence of HIV infection, a cerebrospinal fluid leak, chronic renal failure, alcoholism, asplenia, diabetes, malignant neoplasia, chronic obstructive lung disease, and chronic cardiovascular disease. Revaccination is recommended at 5 years in those at high risk. Many clinicians recommend routine pneumococcal vaccine at the time of hospitalization for vaccine candidates because most patients with serious pneumococcal infections have been hospitalized within the prior 5 years (21,56). A major limitation is the lack of demonstrated efficacy in immunocompromised patients (21).

HAEMOPHILUS INFLUENZAE PNEUMONIA

History

H. influenzae was initially described in 1892 by Pfeiffer (57), who erroneously thought this to be the agent responsible for influenza. Support for this notion was based on high recovery rates in expectorated sputum as well as on experimental animal studies showing that intratracheal challenge to monkeys produced tracheobronchitis, bronchiolitis, or bronchopneumonia (58,59). The etiology of influenza became clarified with the description of a filterable virus in 1933 (60); the role of "the influenza bacillus" as a pulmonary pathogen was then disputed because most patients with lobar pneumonia or bronchopneumonia had other bacterial pathogens recovered concurrently in expectorated sputum (26). In 1931, Pittman (61) described encapsulated and unencapsulated forms and identified the six encapsulated types of *H. influenzae* on the basis of antigenically distinct capsular polysaccharides. It was noted that type B was the most virulent pathogen and the organism responsible for serious infections, including pneumonia, in young children. The role of *H. influenzae* as a cause of pneumonia in adults was clearly established in 1942 by Keefer and Rammelkamp (62), who described the recovery of *H. influenzae* from both blood and sputum cultures of a 30-year-old patient with lobar pneumonia. Since that time, *H. influenzae* has been implicated in 10% to 20% of bacterial pneumonias (14,15,32,35). The best established cases have been type B infections in children, but this form of *H. influenzae* disease has nearly disappeared since the implementation of the protective vaccine. *H. influenzae* disease with nontypeable and type B strains has been much more difficult to define in adults. This organism is second only to the pneumococcus as a pathogen recovered in expectorated sputum samples in adults with pneumonia, and it is a particularly prevalent isolate in patients with chronic bronchitis. Nevertheless, the number of well-confirmed cases of *H. influenzae* pneumonia in adults based on recovery from uncontaminated specimen sources is relatively sparse.

Frequency

H. influenzae is implicated in approximately 10% of all patients with a likely etiologic agent of community-acquired pneumonia sufficiently severe to require hospitalization, according to a review of 122 reports published from 1966 to 1995 (14). Because the yield of any pathogen is only 30% to 50% in most series, the overall recovery rate is 3% to 5% among all patients, and it is 10% to 15% in those with an identified bacterial pathogen (Table 49.1). This figure is confounded by the lack of diagnostic precision because of frequent false-positive and false-negative results. Bacteremia and recovery from extrapulmonary sites reflecting disseminated disease are unusual.

Microbiology

The organism is a small, somewhat pleomorphic gram-negative bacillus with fastidious growth requirements. An outer membrane polysaccharide provides the basis for grouping into serotypes designated A to F (61). Most cases complicated by bacteremia or empyema in the past were due to serotype B, but this is now virtually eliminated owing to widespread use of the vaccines (63–65). Most uncomplicated infections involving the respiratory tract are due to "rough" strains that are unencapsulated or nontypeable. The organism is difficult to recover, and only 30% to 50% of patients with bacteremic pneumonia have positive sputum cultures (66–71). Growth is optimal on enriched media such as chocolate agar. Colonization rates are variable but are higher in young persons and may reach rates of 25% to 85% in healthy adults (72,73). Only 4% to 10% of these are typeable strains. This organism must be distinguished from *Haemophilus parainfluenzae*, which is regarded as a nonpathogen when it is recovered in respiratory secretions.

Clinical Features

Analysis of *H. influenzae* pneumonia in reported cases in adults is confusing because of concerns about improper diagnosis based on reliance on expectorated sputum cultures. Clinical features of 151 cases reported in four series (66,67,70,73) are summarized in Table 49.3. The role of *H. influenzae* in most of these cases was verified by recovery in uncontaminated specimen sources; this will bias the findings but also limits analysis to patients with well-confirmed bacteriologic findings. The results showed that pneumonia ascribed to *H. influenzae* is not unique but resembles pneumonia due to multiple other bacterial pathogens. Some patients have a preceding upper respiratory tract infection, but this is unusual. Pneumonia due to *H. influenzae* appears to occur more frequently in patients with chronic obstructive lung disease or chronic bronchitis. Patients with HIV infection are predisposed to *H. influenzae* pulmonary infections (74,75), predominantly with nontypeable strains. Patients with humoral immune defects are predisposed to *H. influenzae* infections with type B strains. The usual findings with either type B or nontypeable strains are fever, cough, sputum production, and dyspnea. The chest radiograph usually shows bronchopneumonia, but lobar consolidation is reported in 23% to 37% of cases. As noted, *H. influenzae* pneumonia complicated by bacteremia, abscess formation, or empyema has historically been most commonly observed in children under 5 years of age and usually due to type B strains. These complications are unusual in adults.

Diagnosis

The usual diagnosis is based on Gram stain and culture of expectorated sputum. The difficulties encountered are the high rates of false-positive cultures, reflecting the high rates of colonization of *H. influenzae* in the upper airways (72,73,76) and high rates of false-negative cultures due to the fastidious growth requirements. There is also difficulty in recognition on Gram stain even with transtracheal aspirates (67). Complicated disease with bacteremia, meningitis, empyema, or lung abscess previously associated with type B strains has now become infrequent in clinical practice. The majority of reported cases are based on presumptive diagnoses with expectorated sputum, a tenuous conclusion. As noted, colonization by nontypeable strains in the upper airways is common in healthy adults; *H. influenzae* is also commonly found in large concentrations in the expectorated sputum of patients with chronic bronchitis (10^5 organisms per mL or higher) during periods of stability and during exacerbations (77). Again, the majority are nontypeable. In my experience with 488 transtracheal aspirates in patients with acute community-acquired pneumonia, *H. influenzae* was recovered in 28 (5.5%) (78). Even this figure is possibly too high because patients with chronic lung disease often have *H. influenzae* colonization of the lower airways (79).

Treatment

Ampicillin was generally considered the preferred drug for infections involving *H. influenzae* until the early 1970s, when β-lactamase production complicated this treatment. At present, approximately 35% to 40% of strains of both typeable and nontypeable *H. influenzae* strains are resistant to ampicillin (80). Alternative drugs that are active *in vitro* against most strains include second- and third-generation cephalosporins, trimethoprim-sulfamethoxazole, doxycycline, carbapenems, fluoroquinolones, any combination of a β-lactam and a β-lactamase inhibitor, clarithromycin, and azithromycin; drugs that are usually inactive include erythromycin, clindamycin, and vancomycin.

STAPHYLOCOCCUS AUREUS PNEUMONIA

History

S. aureus has been a recognized pulmonary pathogen since the beginning of the 20th century, when it was responsible for a fulminant pneumonia that occurred in influenza epidemics (81,82). The classic description is ascribed to Chickering and Park (83), who reported 153 cases during the influenza pandemic of 1918 at Camp Jackson. During this outbreak, there were 151 cases with only 2 survivors. Autopsy examinations showed circumscribed abscesses of 1 to 10 mm scattered throughout congested lung tissue. Subsequent reports also emphasized the association between influenza A and staphylococcal pneumonia during the Asian influenza epidemic in 1957 to 1958 (84) and the Hong Kong influenza epidemic in 1968 to 1969 (85). In 1933, Relman (86) implicated *S. aureus* in approximately 9% of atypical pneumonias that occurred sporadically in the absence of influenza. The initial and classic studies of staphylococcal pneumonia fostered a prevalent opinion that this usually occurs in association with

TABLE 49.3. Clinical Features of Pneumonia Caused by *Haemophilus influenzae* in Adults

Clinical feature	Four reports[a]	Range[a]
Age (mean yr)	53	50–55
Associated conditions		
Alcoholism	42/133 (32%)	27%–37%
Chronic lung disease	91/151 (60%)	44%–80%
Temperature >37.5°C	81/92 (88%)	87%–90%
Peripheral leukocyte count >10,000/mm^3	63/110 (57%)	30%–69%
Radiographic changes		
Consolidated	30/92 (33%)	23%–37%
More than one lobe involved	85/121 (70%)	39%–74%
Abscess formation	1/121 (1%)	0%–2%
Pleural effusion	32/121 (26%)	10%–49%
Mortality rate	31/151 (20%)	0%–37%

[a]Analysis of 151 cases in four reports (66, 67, 70, 73) with 18 to 62 cases each. The majority were established with bacteriologic confirmation based on positive cultures of blood, pleural fluid, or transtracheal aspirate. The denominator varies because of variation in the data reported.

influenza epidemics, follows a fulminant course, is usually complicated by tissue necrosis with abscess formation, and carries an extraordinary mortality rate even with appropriate antibiotic treatment. Subsequent reports have shown considerable variations from this pattern. In some of the settings in which staphylococcal pneumonia is likely to occur, the course shows substantial variation, and the mortality rate ranges from 0% to 65%, depending to a large extent on the host's status.

Frequency

S. aureus is recovered from respiratory secretions of about 1% of all patients with community-acquired pneumonia, 3% of patients with a bacteriologic diagnosis (Table 49.1) (14), and 10% to 30% of patients with nosocomial pneumonia. Staphylococcal pneumonia is rare in adults without specifically defined defects, as follows:

1. Nosocomial pneumonia, in which this organism is second only to gram-negative bacilli in frequency (74–76); *S. aureus* is especially common in ventilator-associated pneumonia, where it accounts for 10% to 30% of cases (87,88).
2. Postinfluenza pneumonia, in which this organism is second only to *S. pneumoniae* in frequency (83–85).
3. Septic pulmonary emboli, especially with tricuspid valve endocarditis associated with parenteral drug abuse (89).
4. Structural disease of the lung, including cystic fibrosis and bronchiectasis (90).
5. Specific defects in host defenses such as chronic granulomatous disease.
6. Pneumonia with empyema following thoracic surgery or traumatic hemothorax (91).
7. Other associations that are less clearly established, including corticosteroid administration, HIV infection, laryngeal or bronchogenic carcinoma, trauma, chronic bronchitis, central nervous system disease, and age over 50 years (92).

Microbiology

This organism grows readily on standard laboratory media such as blood agar and on selective agar such as mannitol salt agar. It is easily recovered and identified in common clinical specimens, including sputum, bronchoscopy specimens, pleural fluid, and blood.

Pathogenesis

Nasal cultures show colonization by *S. aureus* in 25% to 40% of healthy adults, but pharyngeal cultures show this organism in only 5% to 10% (93,94). The colonization rate is increased in injection drug users, insulin-dependent diabetic individuals, and hemodialysis patients. Colonization of the pharynx is promoted by viral pharyngitis, which may be a contributing factor in the association with influenza (95). The usual route of transmission is by aspiration of the organism in the upper airways. A less common mechanism is by the hematogenous route, as with staphylococcal pneumonia occurring in association with tricuspid valve endocarditis, pelvic vein septic thrombophlebitis, hemodialysis access site infection, and rare cases of intravenous catheter-associated septicemia (96–98). According to the mouse model, the likelihood of pneumonia is directly related to the inoculum size of the organism; on experimental challenge, 10^5 organisms are easily cleared, 10^6 are cleared slowly, and 10^7 or more generally result in pneumonia (99).

TABLE 49.4.   Clinical Features of Staphylococcal Pneumonia in Adults (29 Cases)[a]

Age (yr)	
Mean	61.3
Range	28–83
Associated major underlying conditions	29 (100%)
Hospital acquired	20 (69%)
Peak temperature	
Mean	102.9°F
Range	100°–105.6°F
Peripheral leukocyte count (mean)	18,900/mm³
Radiographic changes	
Abscess	3 (10%)
Effusion	14 (48%)
Multiple lobe involvement	14 (48%)
Bilateral	11 (38%)
Mortality rate	10 (34%)

[a]Etiologic diagnosis is based on recovery of *S. aureus* in pure culture from transtracheal aspirate (13 cases), pleural fluid (7 cases), lung aspirate (2 cases), and blood culture (9 cases) (102).

Clinical Features

The classic studies of staphylococcal pneumonia (83–85) suggested a distinctive clinical syndrome characterized by fulminant onset, high rates of tissue necrosis, and high fatality rates. Later studies suggested great variation in both the initial presentation and the subsequent course (91,100–102). Pneumonia due to *S. aureus* may be acute or chronic (102,103). The usual features are cough and fever that may be abrupt in onset or more subtle with a slowly evolving clinical presentation (Table 49.4). Most patients produce purulent sputum. The frequency of this infection among all patients with postinfluenza bacterial pneumonia is 6% to 20% (85). The illness classically occurs in two phases: there is the initial influenza syndrome with respiratory symptoms and constitutional complaints followed by improvement and then deterioration with the features of staphylococcal pneumonia after 1 to 2 weeks. Patients with tricuspid valve endocarditis generally present with a background of injection drug use combined with fever, chest radiographic evidence of embolic lesions in multiple noncontiguous areas of the lung, echocardiographic evidence of tricuspid valve endocarditis, and *S. aureus* bacteria (89,104). The lung is also a common site of secondary infection in patients with *S. aureus* bacteremia, but this may present with diverse changes on chest radiographs (96–98). In these cases, it is often difficult to determine whether the pneumonia is the primary event or a secondary feature of bacteremia. Reviews of *S. aureus* bacteremia showed that the lung is considered the primary portal of entry for 5% to 10% (98). The most common setting for staphylococcal pneumonia in more recent years has been with nosocomial acquisition, for which risk factors include antimicrobial exposure, advanced age, chronic lung disease, mechanical ventilation, and recent surgical procedures (87,88). Many of these same risk factors apply to the nursing home setting, where *S. aureus* is also relatively common as a cause of pneumonia (105,106). Chest radiographs in nonembolic staphylococcal pneumonia in both the nosocomial and the postinfluenza settings show a bronchopneumonic pattern. Lobar consolidation is relatively rare, and cavitation, contrary to popular opinion, is also a relatively unusual complication (103). Empyema was once reported as a complication in 8% to 30% of cases (100,101,107–109), but this is now less frequently observed, presumably reflecting the impact of effective antimicrobial treatment (102). *S. aureus* now accounts for 10% to 40% of all empyemas; it is most commonly seen in the settings described, and this is the most common pathogen encountered in empyema as a complication of thoracic surgery (see Table 66.1) (92,102). Pneumatocele is a characteristic feature of staphylococcal pneumonia in children but is an unusual feature in adults.

Diagnosis

The diagnosis is best established by the usual clinical features of pneumonia accompanied by recovery of *S. aureus* in an uncontaminated specimen source such as blood or pleural fluid. With expectorated sputum or bronchoscopic aspirates, there should be a compatible Gram stain showing typical gram-positive cocci in "bowling pin" arrangements combined with recovery of *S. aureus* in moderate to heavy growth or, with quantitative bronchoscopic cultures, concentrations exceeding 10^3 to 10^4 organisms per milliliter, depending on laboratory standards. False-positive cultures are common owing to the frequency of colonization of *S. aureus* in the upper airways, especially in hospitalized patients and those who have received prior antibiotic treatment (105,106). False-negative cultures of respiratory secretions are unusual, so the failure to recover *S. aureus* with standard microbiology techniques is strong evidence against the role of these organisms in the pulmonary infection.

Complications and Course

Staphylococcal pneumonia is regarded as a serious infection; mortality rates as high as 67% are reported even in the antibiotic era (100). This is highly variable and depends to a large extent on the setting and the host's health status (101,102). The prognosis for injection drug users with tricuspid valve endocarditis is usually good, with mortality rates of less than 5% in most series (89,104). Postinfluenza staphylococcal pneumonia shows a relatively high mortality rate in young, previously healthy adults when this complication is accompanied by the clinical features of toxic shock syndrome (110). With nosocomial pneumonia, the mortality rate is high; when it is accompanied by bacteremia, the mortality rate is often reported at 30% to 50% (87,88). Complications include toxic shock syndrome, extension to contiguous sites with purulent pericarditis, and, more commonly, pulmonary necrosis with abscess formation or a bronchopleural fistula leading to empyema. Chronic pneumonitis with a slowly evolving course is a feature in occasional cases (103).

Treatment

The standard treatment is based on *in vitro* sensitivity tests. For methicillin-sensitive strains the usual regimen is oxacillin or nafcillin in doses up to 12 g per day intravenously or first-generation cephalosporins with or without augmentation using rifampin or aminoglycosides. Patients with β-lactam allergy and those with methicillin-resistant strains should receive vancomycin, linezolid, or another agent based on *in vitro* test results. Other agents that are sometimes used include clindamycin, trimethoprim, sulfamethoxazole, or fluoroquinolones. The duration of treatment is arbitrary and depends to a large extent on complications and course. Most authorities recommend 2 to 4 weeks of treatment, some of which can be accomplished with oral agents on an outpatient basis.

NEISSERIA MENINGITIDIS PNEUMONIA

History

N. meningitidis became well established as a pulmonary pathogen when these organisms were recovered from lung tissue at autopsy during the 1918 to 1919 influenza pandemic (111–113). The majority of cases involved military personnel. Since World War II, fewer than 50 cases of meningococcal pneumonia have been reported, and only about 11 have involved civilians (14,114–123). The earlier studies emphasized the role of the meningococcus as a superinfecting organism in patients with viral respiratory tract infections, especially influenza (111–113); the more recent work has also emphasized the role of this organism as a transmissible agent in the hospital setting (120–123). Although the number of reported cases is relatively sparse, the true frequency of the disease is unknown.

Microbiology

N. meningitidis is subdivided into polysaccharide-specific serogroups designated A, B, C, D, X, Y, Z, 29E, and W135. Meningococcal disease, including pneumonia, often occurs in epidemics in military populations, and occurrence of the pathogen is more likely to be sporadic in civilians. Organisms belonging to group Y have become the major cause of meningococcal disease, including pneumonia among military personnel (118,119). These organisms replaced group C as the major cause of meningococcal disease in military recruits in the early 1970s, a shift ascribed to routine vaccination of basic trainees against *N. meningitidis* groups A and C (124). In civilians, group Y strains are the usual cause of pulmonary infections.

Clinical Features

Most reports, especially those from military populations, emphasize the predisposing role of respiratory tract infections, the most common being influenza (111,113,124), measles (112), and adenovirus infection (125). Experimental support for this association is available from a mouse model in which the rodent was rendered susceptible to an aerosol containing *N. meningitidis* after exposure to an avirulent encephalomyocarditis virus (126). Occasional cases occur in the context of an outbreak of meningococcal disease without a preceding viral infection. Nosocomial acquisition is occasionally suggested (120,122,123). There is nothing particularly distinctive about meningococcal pneumonia. Most patients do not have evidence of extrapulmonary involvement, such as meningitis or clinical signs of meningococcemia. Usual findings are cough, sputum production, fever, and leukocytosis. Chest radiographs typically show bronchial pneumonia or lobar consolidation; empyema is unusual, and lung abscess has not been reported. The prognosis is excellent. Although meningococcal pneumonia superimposed on influenza was often lethal in the early reports from military hospitals, nearly all patients described during the antibiotic era have survived.

Diagnosis

Expectorated sputum, the usual specimen source in patients with bacterial pneumonia, has proved to be particularly unrewarding in the detection of meningococcal pneumonia. In only 5 of 39 cases reported since 1970 were expectorated sputum cultures used for diagnosis (117–125,127–131). One problem is that *N. meningitidis* may be easily overgrown by the normal respiratory tract flora, so false-negative cultures are common. Some researchers have suggested that selective media, such as Thayer-Martin media, be used to facilitate recovery and identification (128). The problem is the potential for false-positive cultures as a result of asymptomatic carriage of *N. meningitidis*, which has been found in throat cultures from 5% to 15% of healthy persons (130,131). Using selective media for sputum cultures, Putsch and colleagues (130) recovered this organism from 30% of patients with acute pneumonia, but the recovery rate was approximately the same using sputum from patients without pneumonia. Lewis and co-workers (130) cultivated 2,604 sputum samples on Thayer-Martin media, recovered meningococci in 48, and concluded that 6 of these were consistent with meningococcal pneumonia. Laboratory detection is further complicated because most authorities do not recommend speciation of *Neisseria* isolates that are recovered in expectorated sputum samples and do not endorse the routine use of Thayer-Martin or other selected media. Thus, the usual method to establish diagnosis is by recovering the organism from uncontaminated specimens such as transtracheal aspirate, transthoracic aspirate, blood, pleural fluid, or extrapulmonary sources such as cerebrospinal fluid. Gram stain of expectorated sputum shows typical large gram-negative cocci that are often within leukocytes, providing an important clue. A review of 58 cases reported in 2000 showed that 79% were established with positive blood cultures (129). Other *Neisseria* species and *Moraxella* have nearly identical morphologic characteristics and are far more common pulmonary pathogens. The distinction is important because *M. catarrhalis* is usually resistant to penicillin.

Treatment

N. meningitidis is susceptible to a variety of antibiotics, including penicillin, cephalosporins, tetracycline, erythromycin, and chloramphenicol. Penicillin G, cefotaxime, or ceftriaxone are generally regarded as the preferred drug since resistance is nil. Respiratory precautions should be prescribed for patients with meningococcal pneumonia when the diagnosis is either established or strongly suspected. This should be continued until the organism has been eradicated from the respiratory tract or after treatment for 24 hours. Prophylaxis is recommended for close contacts, primarily those with exposure to respiratory secretions, using a fluoroquinolone or rifampin. This includes hospital personnel with the usual types of airborne exposure. One report of 58 cases noted secondary infections in 2 patients (129).

PULMONARY INFECTIONS INVOLVING OTHER SPECIES OF *NEISSERIA*

Neisseria gonorrhoeae is not generally regarded as a pulmonary pathogen, although a case of lobar pneumonia with empyema involving this organism has been reported (132). Other species of *Neisseria* are generally regarded as components of the normal flora of the upper airways. Occasional cases of pulmonary infection involve *Neisseria sicca*. *Moraxella catarrhalis* has been reported in up to 2% to 3% of community-acquired pneumonias (133,134). About 95% of strains produce β-lactamase, so penicillin and amoxicillin should be avoided (80), but nearly all antibiotics are active, including cephalosporins, macrolides, tetracyclines, trimethoprim-sulfamethoxazole, and fluoroquinolones.

GRAM-NEGATIVE BACILLARY PNEUMONIA

History

The history of gram-negative bacillary pneumonia in the prepenicillin era is largely restricted to the studies of *Klebsiella pneumoniae*. This organism was initially described in 1882 by Friedländer, who believed it to be the exclusive cause of pneumonia (135). The proposal was subsequently rejected with the discovery of the pneumococcus, although *Klebsiella* remained a well-established if infrequent cause of pneumonia in the preantibiotic era. Two forms of the disease were recognized. An acute form known as Friedländer's pneumonia resembled pneumococcal lobar pneumonia except for its occurrence almost exclusively in debilitated subjects and a possibly more fulminant course (136–138). The second form of the disease was a chronic infection that persisted for weeks or months and was, at times, confused with pulmonary tuberculosis (139). Both the acute and the chronic forms of the disease showed a distinct propensity for tissue necrosis with abscess formation (140). *Klebsiella* was never a common cause of pneumonia in the preantibiotic era, accounting for about 0.6% to 1.1% of cases reported at that time (26,138,141,142). This organism continues to be a rare cause of community-acquired pneumonia, still accounting for about 1% of cases (Table 49.1); cases conforming to the classic clinical descriptions are especially rare. Gram-negative bacillary pneumonia involving organisms other than *K. pneumoniae* is largely a product of the antibiotic era. These organisms were occasionally encountered in community-acquired pneumonia, but rates of recovery were always low; even when they were found, the source was usually respiratory secretions, raising questions about the validity of the results. In the 1960s, Tillotson and Lerner (143) published a series of reports on pneumonia caused by various gram-negative bacilli. The scientific community was divided on the validity of these studies, and many remained skeptical despite the authors' claim of stringent diagnostic criteria requiring the same gram-negative bacillus as the dominant potential pathogen in at least two expectorated sputum samples. Problems included the lack of confirmation with uncontaminated specimen sources such as blood or pleural fluid. Also, transtracheal aspiration that was commonly performed at that time almost never yielded gram-negative bacilli to the exclusion of other well-recognized pulmonary pathogens (78). The notable exception was the evolution of gram-negative bacteria as the major cause of hospital-acquired pneumonia, especially when it was acquired in intensive care units and in patients receiving mechanical ventilation (87,88). Another new setting in which these organisms play a prominent role is the compromised host, including transplant recipients, patients receiving chemotherapy, and patients with advanced acquired immunodeficiency syndrome.

Frequency

Gram-negative bacteria (Enterobacteriaceae and *Pseudomonas* species) are rare causes of community-acquired pneumonia. A metaanalysis of 122 reports of community-acquired pneumonia in the English-language medical literature from 1966 through 1995 showed that this category of bacteria accounted for only about 103 of the approximately 6,100 cases (2%) in which a microbial etiology was defined (Table 49.1) (14). By contrast, these organisms are the major causes of nosocomial pneumonia, accounting for 30% to 60% of cases in most series (87,88,144–147). Confirmation of their etiologic role based on specimen source is the high yield of these organisms in bacteremic patients (147), in transtracheal aspirates (145), and by quantitative cultures of bronchoscopic aspirates (146,148). In addition to nosocomial acquisition, other predisposing factors for infection involving gram-negative bacilli include neutropenia, structural disease of the lung such as bronchiectasis and cystic fibrosis, prior antibiotic treatment with pulmonary superinfection, and advanced acquired immunodeficiency syndrome. Gram-negative bacilli are also frequently encountered in "nursing home pneumonia."

Pathogenesis

Gram-negative bacillary pneumonia usually follows aspiration of these organisms when they reside in the upper airways or stomach (149–151). Previous studies indicated that colonization rates are highly variable, depending on the host's health status (149). Thus, patients classified as moderately ill show colonization rates of 30% to 40%, and those who are categorized as severely ill requiring placement in intensive care units have colonization rates that often exceed 60% (149,151). These associations are independent of antibiotic exposure, although antibiotic exposure favors this type of colonization as well (151). The conditions that are associated with increased colonization include advanced age, neutropenia, coma, renal failure, hypotension, ketoacidosis, physical impairment for daily living activities, alcoholism, diabetes mellitus, and viral respiratory tract infections. The usual source of gram-negative bacilli in the pharynx is the patient's colon, although these organisms are occasionally transmitted from patient to patient or through hospital personnel.

Microbiology

Enterobacteriaceae species that are frequently implicated in pneumonia, primarily nosocomial pneumonia, are *Klebsiella* species (primarily *K. pneumoniae* and, less frequently, *Klebsiella oxytoca*), *Enterobacter* species (*Enterobacter aerogenes*, *Enterobacter cloacae*, and *Enterobacter agglomerans*), *Escherichia coli*, *Serratia marcescens*, and *Proteus mirabilis* (87,88). *K. pneumoniae* has been the most frequently observed pathogen in this category, isolated in both community-acquired pneumonia (14) and nosocomial pulmonary infection (87,88). These organisms may be serotyped on the basis of composition of the capsular or K antigen (152,153). At least 77 different K serotypes have been identified. The classic studies of *K. pneumoniae* in the prepenicillin era showed that capsular serotypes K1 through K6 were most frequently seen, especially K2 (140–142,154). An attractive thesis is that this organism demonstrated unique pathogenic potential for the lung by virtue of the capsule of these specific serotypes. The gene encoding the K2 serotype polysaccharide has been cloned and transformed to unencapsulated strains, but this did not confer unique virulence properties, casting doubt on the thesis (155). *Klebsiella* also produced fimbriae that may account for unique pathogenic potential, including adherence to respiratory epithelium (156), but this has not been clearly demonstrated. Although older studies showed that serotypes K1 to K6 predominated, these serotypes have become far less common, and the classic features of *Klebsiella* pulmonary infections also appear to occur much less frequently. In fact, it has become difficult to define clinical features that distinguish pneumonia due to different members of Enterobacteriaceae and difficult to implicate organism-specific differences in virulence factors. Of particular importance is the resistance profile of these microbes, which will obviously influence recovery rates among patients who develop pneumonia in the presence of antibiotic exposure.

Pseudomonads resemble Enterobacteriaceae species morphologically but are found most frequently in extraintestinal sources, including water habitats. They are strict aerobes that will not grow anaerobically; they have only polar flagella; and, with few exceptions, they are oxidase positive. These organisms cannot be distinguished from Enterobacteriaceae species by Gram stain, and they also contain endotoxin as a major identifiable virulence factor. Other virulence factors include a polysaccharide capsule, fimbriae, exotoxin A, and leukocidin (157) (see Chapter 195). The mucoexopolysaccharide capsule may serve as an important virulence factor predisposing to colonization and infection because of binding to surface epithelial cells (158,159). *Pseudomonas aeruginosa* is uniquely associated with pulmonary infections in patients with cystic fibrosis (mucoid strains), bronchiectasis, advanced acquired immunodeficiency syndrome, and neutropenia. In 2001, Hatchette published a case report and review of 11 reported cases of *P. aeruginosa* pneumonia in previously healthy adults; this is testimony to the infrequency of this organism in the healthy host (160).

Clinical Features

Gram-negative bacillary pneumonia was classically described by Friedländer in 1882 and subsequent researchers in the prepenicillin era, as summarized earlier (135). Classic features included an abrupt onset with high fever and cough productive of copious amounts of bloody sputum that had the appearance of currant jelly. Chest radiography typically showed lobar consolidation, often with a bulging interlobar fissure (bulging fissure sign), indicating an expanding necrotic lesion with abscess formation usually involving an upper lobe (135–142). This classic presentation is infrequently encountered in the current era, possibly reflecting involvement of different serotypes of *K. pneumoniae*, as summarized before. Instead, gram-negative bacillary pneumonia usually presents with no unique clinical features that would easily distinguish this infection from pneumonia caused by other microbial pathogens, and no clinical features distinguish gram-negative bacillary pneumonia due to different species of Enterobacteriaceae or pseudomonads. The most common form is nosocomial pneumonia, most of the patients are severely compromised by associated medical conditions, most have antecedent colonization of the respiratory tract by the same species of gram-negative bacilli, the prognosis is often poor owing to both the pneumonia and the associated condition, and the mortality rates are high.

Diagnosis

The etiologic diagnosis is established by recovery of gram-negative bacilli from an uncontaminated specimen source (blood, pleural fluid, transtracheal aspirate) in association with a compatible clinical illness. This diagnosis is supported by the demonstration of gram-negative bacilli with the characteristic morphologic features on Gram stain combined with recovery of these organisms in moderate or heavy growth in culture from respiratory secretions. Gram-negative bacilli are easily detected in respiratory secretions because they grow readily on selective and nonselective media that are routinely used in microbiology laboratories. Thus, false-negative cultures with adequate specimens are rare. The main problem is false-positive cultures, especially in patients with prior antibiotic exposure. It is important in such cases to distinguish "sputum superinfection" from superinfection of the patient.

Treatment

Treatment of gram-negative bacillary pneumonia consists of supportive measures and an antibiotic directed against the implicated pathogens based on *in vitro* sensitivity testing. Recommendations for empirical use (161) in patients who are seriously ill are directed toward relatively resistant agents commonly encountered in the hospital environment and include a carbapenem (imipenem or meropenem), a third-generation cephalosporin, cefepime, and piperacillin-tazobactam, often in combination with an aminoglycoside. Any of these may be given in combination with an aminoglycoside, usually gentamicin or tobramycin.

REFERENCES

1. Pinner RW, Teutsch SM, Simonsen L, et al. Trends in infectious diseases mortality in the United States. *JAMA* 1996;275:189.
2. Watson DA, Musher DM, Jacobson JW, et al. A brief history of the pneumococcus in biomedical research: a panoply of scientific discovery. *Clin Infect Dis* 1993;17:913.
3. Fraenkel A. Weitere Beitrage Our Lecher von den Mikrococcen der genuinen fibrinosen Pneumonie. *Z Klin Med* 1886;11:437.
4. Winslow CIA, Broadhurst J, Buchanan RE, et al. The families and genera of the bacteria: final report of the committee of the Society of American Bacteriologists on characterization and classification of bacterial types. *J Bacteriol* 1920;5:191.
5. Deibel RH, Seeley HW Jr. Family II. Streptococcaceae fain now. In: Buchanan RE, Gibbons NE, eds. *Bergey's manual of determinative bacteriology*, 8th ed. Baltimore: Williams & Wilkins, 1974:490.
6. Gram C. Über die isolierte farbung der schizomyceten in schnittund trockenpraparaten. *Fortschr Med* 1884;2:185.
7. Neufeld F, Haendel L. Weitere untersuchungen über pneumokokken-Heilsera. III. Mitteilung. *Arb Kaiserlich Gesundh* 1910;34:293.
8. White B, with the collaboration of Robinson ES, Barnes LA. The biology of pneumococcus: the bacteriological, biochemical, and immunological characters and activities of *Diplococcus pneumoniae*. New York: Commonwealth Fund, 1937.
9. Lord FT. Immunity factors in recovery from lobar pneumonia and results of specific treatment in type I pneumococcus pneumonia. *N Engl J Med* 1931;205:854.
10. Finland M, Sutliff WD. Specific cutaneous reactions and circulating antibodies in the course of lobar pneumonia. II. Cases treated with antipneumococcic sera. *J Exp Med* 1931;54:653.
11. Abraham EP, Gardner AD, Chain E, et al. Further observations on penicillin. *Lancet* 1941;2:177.
12. Keefer CS, Blake FG, Marshall EK Jr, et al. Penicillin in the treatment of infections: a report of 500 cases. *JAMA* 1943;122:1217.
13. Bullowa JGM. The reliability of sputum typing and its relation to serum therapy. *JAMA* 1935;105:1512.
14. Fine MJ, Smith MA, Carson CA, et al. Prognosis and outcomes of patients with community-acquired pneumonia: a meta-analysis. *JAMA* 1996;275:134.
15. Mundy LM, Auwaerter PG, Oldach D, et al. Community-acquired pneumonia: impact of immune status. *Am J Respir Crit Care Med* 1995;152:1309.
16. File TM, Segreti J, Dunbar L, et al. A multicenter, randomized study comparing the efficacy and safety of intravenous and/or oral levofloxacin versus ceftriaxone and/or cefuroxime axetil in treatment of adults with CAP. *Antimicrob Agents Chemother* 1997;41:1965.
17. Ruiz M, Ewig S, Marcos MA, et al. Etiology of community-acquired pneumonia: impact of age, comorbidity, and severity. *Am J Respir Crit Care Med* 1999;160:397.
18. Fang GD, Fine M, Orloff J, et al. New and emerging etiologies for community-acquired pneumonia with implication for therapy: a prospective multicenter study of 359 cases. *Medicine* 1990;69:307.
19. Bartlett JG, Mundy LM. Current concepts: community-acquired pneumonia. *N Engl J Med* 1995;333:1618.
20. Nuorti JP, Butler JC, Farley MM, et al. Cigarette smoking and invasive pneumococcal disease. *N Engl J Med* 2000;342:681.
21. Centers for Disease Control and Prevention. Prevention of pneumococcal disease. *MMWR* 1997;46RR-8:424.
22. Mufson MA, Oley G, Hughey D. Pneumococcal disease in a medium-sized community in the United States. *JAMA* 1982;248:1486.
23. Austrian R. Some observations on the pneumococcus and on the current status of pneumococcal disease and its prevention. *Rev Infect Dis* 1981;3(suppl):1.
24. Scott JAG, Hall AJ, Dagan R, et al. Serogroup-specific epidemiology of *Streptococcus pneumoniae*: associations with age, sex, and geography in 7,000 episodes of invasive disease. *Clin Infect Dis* 1996;22:973.
25. Hendley JO, Sande MA, Steward PM, et al. Spread of *Streptococcus pneumoniae* in families. I. Carriage rates and distribution of types. *J Infect Dis* 1975;132:55.
26. Heffron R. *Pneumonia with special reference to pneumococcus lobar pneumonia*. New York: Commonwealth Fund, 1939.
27. Lipsky BA, Boyko EJ, Inui TS, et al. Risk factors for acquiring pneumococcal infections. *Arch Intern Med* 1986;146:2179.
28. Grandsden WR, Eykyn SJ, Phillips I. Pneumococcal bacteremia: 325 episodes diagnosed at St. Thomas' Hospital. *BMJ* 1985;290:505.
29. Janoff EN, Breiman RF, Daley CL, et al. Pneumococcal disease during HIV infection: epidemiologic, clinical, and immunologic perspectives. *Ann Intern Med* 1992;117:314.
30. Dworkin MS, Ward JW, Hanson DL, et al. Pneumococcal disease among HIV-infected persons: incidence, risk factors, and impact of vaccination. *Clin Infect Dis* 2001;32:794.
31. Hoge CW, Reichler MR, Dominguez EA, et al. An epidemic of pneumococcal disease in an overcrowded, inadequately ventilated jail. *N Engl J Med* 1994;331:643.
32. Bartlett JG, Dowell SF, Mandell LA, et al. Community-acquired pneumonia in adults: guidelines for management. *Clin Infect Dis* 2000;31:347.
33. Kantor HG. The many radiologic faces of pneumococcal pneumonia. *Am J Radiol* 1981;13:1213.
34. Barrett-Connor E. The nonvalue of sputum culture in the diagnosis of pneumococcal pneumonia. *Am Rev Respir Dis* 1971;103:845.
35. Bartlett JG, Mundy LM. Community-acquired pneumonia. *N Engl J Med* 1995;333:1618.
36. Farr BM, Kaiser DL, Harrison BDW, et al. Prediction of microbial aetiology at admission to hospital for pneumonia from the presenting clinical features. *Thorax* 1989;44:1031.
37. Levy M, Dromer F, Brion N, et al. Community-acquired pneumonia: importance of initial noninvasive bacteriologic and radiographic investigations. *Chest* 1988;92:43.
38. Merrill CW, Gwaltney JM, Hendley JO, et al. Rapid identification of pneumococci. *N Engl J Med* 1973;288:510.
39. Perlino CA. Laboratory diagnosis of pneumonia due to *Streptococcus pneumoniae*. *J Infect Dis* 1984;150:139.
40. Dans P, Charache PC, Fahey M, et al. Management of pneumonia in the prospective payment era. *Arch Intern Med* 1984;144:1392.
41. Austrian R, Winston AL. The efficacy of penicillin V (phenoxymethyl penicillin) in the treatment of mild and moderately severe pneumococcal pneumonia. *Am J Med Sci* 1958;232:624.
42. Brewin A, Arango L, Hadley WK, et al. High-dose penicillin therapy and pneumococcal pneumonia. *JAMA* 1974;230:409.
43. Whitney CG, Farley MM, Hadler J, et al. Increasing prevalence of multi-drug-resistant *Streptococcus pneumoniae* in the U.S. *N Engl J Med* 2000;343:1917.
44. Hobar DJ, Doern GV, Fluit AC, et al. Worldwide prevalence of antimicrobial resistance in *Streptococcus pneumoniae*, *Haemophilus influenzae*, and *Moraxella catarrhalis* in the SENTRY antimicrobial surveillance program, 1997–1999. *Clin Infect Dis* 2001;32(suppl 2):581.
45. Hofmann J, Cetron MS, Farley MM, et al. The prevalence of drug-resistant *Streptococcus pneumoniae* in Atlanta. *N Engl J Med* 1995;333:481.
46. Gold HS, Moellering RC Jr: Antimicrobial drug resistance. *N Engl J Med* 1996;335:1445.
47. Pallares R, Linares J, Vadillo M, et al. Resistance to penicillin and cephalosporin and mortality from severe pneumococcal pneumonia in Barcelona, Spain. *N Engl J Med* 1995;333:474.
48. Amsden GW. Pneumococcal macrolide resistance: myth or reality? *J Antimicrob Chemother* 1999;44:1.
49. Neiderman MS, Mandell LA, Anzueto A, et al. Guidelines for the management of adults with community-acquired pneumonia. *Am J Respir Crit Care Med* 2001;163:1730.
50. Marrie TJ, Lau CY, Wheeler SL, et al. A controlled trial of a critical pathway for treatment of community-acquired pneumonia. *JAMA* 2000;283:749.
51. Chea DK, Megeer A, DeAzavedo JC, et al: Decreased susceptibility of *Streptococcus pneumoniae* to fluoroquinolones in Canada. *N Engl J Med* 1999;341:233.
52. Kalin M, Ortgvist A, Almela M, et al. Prospective study of prognostic factors in community-acquired bacteremic pneumococcal disease in five countries. *J Infect Dis* 2000;132:840.
53. Austrian R, Gold J. Pneumococcal bacteremia with especial reference to bacteremic pneumococcal pneumonia. *Ann Intern Med* 1964;60:759.
54. Marrie TJ. Normal resolution of community-acquired pneumonia. *Semin Respir Infect* 1992;7:256.
55. Meeker DP, Longworth DL. Community-acquired pneumonia: an update. *Cleve Clin J Med* 1996;63:16.
56. Fedson DS. Improving the use of pneumococcal vaccine through a strategy of hospital based immunization. *J Am Geriatr Soc* 1985;33:142.
57. Pfeiffer R. Vorlaufige mitteilungen über die effeger der influenza. *Dtsch Med Wochenschr* 1892;18:28.
58. Blake FG, Cecil RL. Studies on experimental pneumonia. *J Exp Med* 1920;32:691.
59. Cecil RL, Blake FG. Studies on experimental pneumonia: pathology of experimental influenza and of *Bacillus influenzae* pneumonia in monkeys. *J Exp Med* 1920;32:719.
60. Smith W, Andrews CH, Laidlaw PP. A virus obtained from influenza patients. *Lancet* 1933;2:66.
61. Pittman M. Variation and type specificity in the bacterial species *Hemophilus influenzae*. *J Exp Med* 1931;53:471.
62. Keefer CS, Rammelkamp CH. *Hemophilus influenzae* bacteremia. *Ann Intern Med* 1942;51:1221.
63. Ginsberg CM, Howard JB, Nelson JD. Report of 65 cases of *Haemophilus influenzae* B pneumonia. *Pediatrics* 1979;64:283.
64. Jacobs NM, Harris VJ. Acute *Haemophilus* pneumonia in childhood. *Am J Dis Child* 1979;133:603.
65. Centers for Disease Control and Prevention. Progress toward elimination of *Haemophilus influenzae* type B disease among infants and children—United States, 1987–1995. *MMWR* 1996;45:901.
66. Wallace RJ Jr, Musher DM, Martin RR. *Hemophilus influenzae* pneumonia in adults. *Am J Med* 1978;64:87.
67. Everett ED, Rahm AE, Aaniya MR, et al. *Haemophilus influenzae* pneumonia in adults. *JAMA* 1977;238:319.
68. Goldstein E, Daly AK, Seamans C. *Haemophilus influenzae* as a cause of adult pneumonia. *Ann Intern Med* 1967;66:35.
69. Johnson WD, Kaye D, Hook EW. *Hemophilus influenzae* pneumonia in adults: report of five cases and review of the literature. *Am Rev Respir Dis* 1968;97:1112.
70. Levin DC, Schwarz MI, Matthay RA, et al. Bacteremic *Hemophilus influenzae* pneumonia in adults: a report of 24 cases and a review of the literature. *Am J Med* 1977;62:219.

71. Weinstein L. Type b *Haemophilus influenzae* infections in adults. *N Engl J Med* 1970;282:221.

72. Austrian R. The bacterial flora of the respiratory tract: some knowns and unknowns. *Yale J Biol Med* 1968;40:400.

73. Holdaway MD, Turk DC. Capsulated *Haemophilus influenzae* and respiratory tract disease. *Lancet* 1967;1:358.

74. Steinhart R, Reingold AL, Taylor F, et al. Invasive *Haemophilus influenzae* infections in men with HIV infection. *JAMA* 1992;268:3350.

75. Cordero E, Pachon J, Giron JA, et al. *Haemophilus influenzae* pneumonia in HIV-infected patients. *Clin Infect Dis* 2000;30:461.

76. Mulder J, Goslings WRO, Van der Plas MC, et al. Studies on the treatment with antibacterial drugs of acute and chronic mucopurulent bronchitis caused by *Haemophilus influenzae*. *Acta Med Scand* 1952;143:32.

77. Gump DW, Phillips CA, McIntosh K, et al. Role of infection in chronic bronchitis. *Am Rev Respir Dis* 1976;113:465.

78. Bartlett J. Diagnostic accuracy of transtracheal aspiration bacteriologic studies. *Am Rev Respir Dis* 1977;115:777.

79. Bjerkestrand G, Digranes A, Schreiner A. Bacteriological findings in transtracheal aspirates from patients with chronic bronchitis and bronchiectasis. *Scand J Respir Dis* 1975;56:201.

80. Blondeau JM, Vaughan D, Laskowski R, et al. Susceptibility of Canadian isolates of *Haemophilus influenzae*, *Moraxella catarrhalis*, and *Streptococcus pneumoniae* to oral agents. *Int J Antimicrob Agents* 2001;17:457.

81. Fraenkel A. *Spezielle pathologie and therapie der lungenkrankheiten*. Berlin: Urban & Schwarzenberg, 1904.

82. Netter R. Etude bacteriologique de la bronchopneumonie chez l'adulte et chez l'enfant. *Arch Med Exp* 1882;4:28.

83. Chickering HT, Park JH Jr. *Staphylococcus aureus* pneumonia. *JAMA* 1919;72:617.

84. Martin CM, Kunin CM, Gottleib LS, et al. Asian influenza A in Boston, 1957–1958. *Arch Intern Med* 1959;103:532.

85. Schwarzmann SW, Adler JL, Sullivan RJ, et al. Bacterial pneumonia during the Hong Kong influenza epidemic of 1968–1969. *Arch Intern Med* 1971;127:1037.

86. Relman HA. Primary staphylococcus pneumonia. *JAMA* 1933;101:514.

87. Pujol M, Corbella X, Pena C, et al. Clinical and epidemiological findings in mechanically-ventilated patients with methicillin-resistant *Staphylococcus aureus* pneumonia. *Eur J Clin Microbiol Infect Dis* 1998;17:622.

88. Rello J, Paiva JA, Baraibar J, et al. International conference for the development of consensus on the diagnosis and treatment of ventilator-associated pneumonia. *Chest* 2001;120:955.

89. Heldman AW, Hartert TV, Ray SC, et al. Oral antibiotic treatment of right-sided staphylococcal endocarditis in injection drug users: prospective randomized comparison with parenteral therapy. *Am J Med* 1996;101:68.

90. Smyth A, Walters S. Prophylactic antibiotics for cystic fibrosis. *Cochrane Database Syst Rev* 2000;2:CD001912.

91. Hirschtick RE, Glassroth J. *Staphylococcus aureus* pneumonia: when to suspect—how to treat. *J Crit Illness* 1992;7:1576.

92. Mandel AK, Thadepalli H, Mandal AK, et al. Posttraumatic empyema thoracis: a 24-year experience at a major trauma center. *J Trauma* 1997;43:764.

93. Kirmani N, Tuazon CU, Murray HW, et al. *Staphylococcus aureus* carriage rate of patients receiving long-term hemodialysis. *Arch Intern Med* 1978;138:1657.

94. Tuazon CU, Sheagren JN. Increased rate of carriage of *Staphylococcus aureus* among narcotic addicts. *J Infect Dis* 1974;129:725.

95. Fainstein V, Musher DM, Cate TR. Bacterial adherence to pharyngeal cells during viral infection. *J Infect Dis* 1980;141:172.

96. Narqi S, McDonnell G. Hematogenous staphylococcal pneumonia secondary to soft tissue infection. *Chest* 1981;79:173.

97. Tsao TCY, Tsai YH, Lan RS, et al. Pulmonary manifestations of *Staphylococcus aureus* septicemia. *Chest* 1992;101:574.

98. Mylotte JM, McDermott C, Spooner JA. Prospective study of 114 consecutive episodes of *Staphylococcus aureus* bacteremia. *Rev Infect Dis* 1987;9:891.

99. Onofrio JM, Toews GB, Lipscomb MF, et al. Granulocyte-alveolar-macrophage interaction in the pulmonary clearance of *Staphylococcus aureus*. *Am Rev Respir Dis* 1983;127:335.

100. Fisher AM, Trever RT, Curtin JA, et al. Staphylococcal pneumonia: a review of 21 cases in adults. *N Engl J Med* 1958;258:919.

101. Rebhan AW, Edwards HE. Staphylococcal pneumonia: a review of 329 cases. *Can Med Assoc J* 1960;82:513.

102. Kaye MG, Fox MJ, Bartlett JG, et al. The clinical spectrum of *Staphylococcus aureus* pulmonary infection. *Chest* 1990;97:788.

103. Kuberman AS, Fernandez RB. Subacute staphylococcal pneumonia. *Am Rev Respir Dis* 1970;101:95.

104. Frontera JA, Gradon JD. Right sided endocarditis in injection drug users: review of proposed mechanisms of pathogenesis. *Clin Infect Dis* 2000;30:374.

105. Garb JL, Brown RB, Garb JR, et al. Differences in the etiology of pneumonias in nursing home and community patients. *JAMA* 1978;240:2169.

106. Loeb M, McGeer A, McArthur M, et al. Risk factors for pneumonia and other lower respiratory tract infections in elderly residents of long term care facilities. *Arch Intern Med* 1999;159:2058.

107. Weese WC, Shindler ER, Smith IM, et al. Empyema of the thorax then and now. *Arch Intern Med* 1973;131:516.

108. Ede S, Davis GM, Holmes FH. Staphylococcic pneumonia. *JAMA* 1959;170:638.

109. Bartlett JG. Bacterial infections of the pleural space. *Semin Respir Infect* 1988;3:308.

110. Kain KC, Schulzer M, Chow AW. Clinical spectrum of nonmenstrual toxic shock syndrome (TSS): comparison with menstrual TSS by multivariate discriminant analysis. *Clin Infect Dis* 1993;16:100.

111. Fletcher W. Meningococcus broncho-pneumonia in influenza. *Lancet* 1919;1:104.

112. Herrick WW. Extra-meningeal meningococcus infections. *Arch Intern Med* 1919;23:409.

113. Holm ML, Davidson WC. Meningococcus pneumonia. *Bull Hopkins Hosp* 1919;30:324.

114. Brick IB. Meningococcal pneumonia. Report of two cases with meningococcal effusion in one. *N Engl J Med* 1948;238:289.

115. Meltzer JI, Kneeland Y Jr. Primary meningococcal lobar pneumonia without meningitis. *Ann Intern Med* 1959;46:183.

116. Paine TF Jr, Garrard CL, Walker PJ. Meningococcal pneumonia. *Arch Intern Med* 1967;119:111.

117. Ball JH, Young DA. Primary meningococcal pneumonia. *Am Rev Respir Dis* 1974;109:480.

118. Irwin RS, Woelk WK, Coudon WL III. Primary meningococcal pneumonia. *Ann Intern Med* 1975;82:493.

119. Reinecke ME. Group-Y meningococcal disease. *Ann Intern Med* 1975;82:719.

120. Barnes RV, Dopp AC, Gelberg HJ, et al. *Neisseria meningitidis*: a cause of nosocomial pneumonia. *Am Rev Respir Dis* 1975;111:229.

121. Galpin JE, Chow AW, Yoshikawa TT. Meningococcal pneumonia. *Am J Med Sci* 1975;269:247.

122. Cohen MS, Steere AC, Baltimore R, et al. Possible nosocomial transmission of group Y *Neisseria meningitidis* among oncology patients. *Ann Intern Med* 1979;91:7.

123. Rose HD, Lenz IE, Sheth NK. Meningococcal pneumonia: a source of nosocomial infection. *Arch Intern Med* 1981;141:575.

124. Young LS. A simultaneous outbreak of meningococcal and influenza infections. *N Engl J Med* 1972;287:5.

125. Reinarz TA, Sande MA, Silva J Jr. Bacterial pneumonia complicating adenoviral pneumonia. *Am J Med* 1974;56:169.

126. Goldstein E. Murine resistance to inhaled *Neisseria meningitidis* after infection with an encephalomyocarditis virus. *Infect Immun* 1972;6:398.

127. Nikoskelainen J, Leino A, Lahtonen E, et al. Is group specific meningococcal vaccination resulting in epidemics caused by groups of virulent meningococci? *Lancet* 1978;2:403.

128. Jacobs SA, Norden CW. Pneumonia caused by *Neisseria meningitidis*. *JAMA* 1974;227:67–68.

129. Winstead JM, McKinsey DS, Taylor S, et al. Meningococcal pneumonia: characterization and review of cases seen over the past 25 years. *Clin Infect Dis* 2000;30:87.

130. Putsch RW, Hamilton JD, Wolinsky E. *Neisseria meningitidis*, a respiratory pathogen? *J Infect Dis* 1970;121:48.

131. Farrell DG, Dahl EV. Nasopharyngeal carriers of *Neisseria meningitidis*: studies among Air Force recruits. *JAMA* 1966;198:1189.

132. Enos WF, Beyer JC, Zimmet SM, et al. Unilateral lobar pneumonia with empyema caused by *Neisseria gonorrhoeae*. *S Med J* 1980;73:266.

133. Johnson MA, Drew WL, Roberts M. *Branhamella* (*Neisseria*) *catarrhalis*—a lower respiratory tract pathogen? *J Clin Microbiol* 1981;13:1066.

134. Srinivasan G, Raff MJ, Templeton WC, et al. *Branhamella catarrhalis* pneumonia: report of two cases and review of the literature. *Am Rev Respir Dis* 1981;123:553.

135. Friedländer C. Ober die schizomyceter bei der acuten fibrosen pneumonie. *Virchows Arch Pathol Anat* 1882;87:319.

136. Belk WP. Pulmonary infections by Friedländer's bacillus. *J Infect Dis* 1926;38:115.

137. Fremmel F, Henrichsen KJ, Sweany HC. Pulmonary infections by Friedländer's bacillus. *Ann Intern Med* 1932;5:886.

138. Bullowa JGM, Chess J, Friedman NB. Pneumonia due to *Bacillus friedländeri*. *Arch Intern Med* 1937;9:735.

139. Collins LH Jr. Chronic pulmonary infection due to the Friedländer's bacillus. *Arch Intern Med* 1936;58:235.

140. Olcott CT. Pneumonia due to Friedländer's bacillus. *Arch Pathol* 1933;16:471.

141. Solomon S. Primary Friedländer pneumonia. *JAMA* 1937;108:937.

142. Bullowa JGM. *Management of the pneumonias*. New York: Oxford University Press, 1937:508.

143. Tillotson JR, Lerner AM. Pneumonias: caused by gram-negative bacilli. *Medicine (Baltimore)* 1966;45:65.

144. American Thoracic Society. Hospital-acquired pneumonia in adults: diagnosis, assessment of severity, initial antimicrobial therapy and preventative strategies. *Am J Respir Crit Care Med* 1995;153:1711.

145. Bartlett JG, O'Keefe P, Tally FP, et al. Bacteriology of hospital-acquired pneumonia. *Arch Intern Med* 1986;146:868.

146. Fagon JY, Chastre J, Hance A, et al. Nosocomial pneumonia in ventilated patients: a cohort study evaluating attributable mortality and hospital stay. *Am J Med* 1993;94:281.

147. Bryan CS Reynolds KL. Bacteremic nosocomial pneumonia. *Am Rev Respir Dis* 1984;129:668.

148. Torres A, Puig de la Bellacasa JP, Xaubet A, et al. Diagnostic value of quantitative cultures of bronchoalveolar lavage and telescoping plugged catheters in mechanically ventilated patients with bacterial pneumonia. *Am Rev Respir Dis* 1989;140:306.

149. Johanson WG, Pierce AK, Sanford JP. Changing pharyngeal bacterial flora of hospitalized patients: emergence of gram-negative bacilli. *N Engl J Med* 1969;281:1137.

150. Montgomerie JZ. Epidemiology of *Klebsiella* and hospital-associated infections. *Rev Infect Dis* 1979;1:736.

151. Tillotson JR, Finland M. Bacterial colonization and clinical superinfection of the respiratory tract complicating antibiotic treatment of pneumonia. *J Infect Dis* 1969;119:597.

152. Edwards PP, Fife MA. Capsule types of *Klebsiella*. *J Infect Dis* 1952;91:92.

153. Benge GR. Bactericidal, activity of human serum against strains of *Klebsiella* from different sources. *J Med Microbiol* 1988;27:11.

154. Julianelle LA. Biological classification of *Encapsulatus pneumoniae* (Friedländer's bacillus). *J Exp Med* 1926;44:113.

155. Arakawa Y, Ohta M, Wacharotayankun R, et al. Biosynthesis of *Klebsiella* K2 capsular polysaccharide in *Escherichia coli* HB101 requires the functions of rmpA and the chromosomal cps gene cluster of the virulent strain *Klebsiella pneumoniae* Chedid (O1:K2). *Infect Immun* 1991;59:2043.

156. Fader RC, Gondesen K, Tolley B, et al. Evidence that *in vitro* adherence of *Klebsiella pneumoniae* to ciliated hamster tracheal cells is mediated by type 1 fimbriae. *J Bacteriol* 1988;56:3011.

157. Hata JS, Fick RB. Airway adherence of *Pseudomonas aeruginosa*: mucoexopolysaccharide binding to human and bovine airway proteins. *J Lab Clin Med* 1991;117:410.

158. Ramphal R, Pier GB. Role of *Pseudomonas aeruginosa* mucoid exopolysaccharide in adherence to tracheal cells. *Infect Immun* 1985;47:1.

159. Woods DE, Straus DC, Johanson WG Jr, et al. Role of salivary protease activity in adherence of gram-negative bacilli to mammalian buccal epithelial cells *in vivo*. *J Clin Invest* 1981;68:1435.

160. Hatchette TF, Gupta R, Marrie TJ. *Pseudomonas aeruginosa* community-acquired pneumonia in previously healthy adults: case report and review of the literature. *Clin Infect Dis* 2000;31:1349.

161. Med Letter Consultants. Choice of antibacterial drugs. *Med Lett* 2001;43:69.

CHAPTER 50
Bronchitis

John G. Bartlett

Bronchitis is one of the most common conditions encountered in clinical practice. In general, there are two main categories in which acute infection is common: acute bronchitis and exacerbations of chronic bronchitis. Related syndromes based on the common clinical feature of cough include "postnasal drip syndrome," asthma, gastroesophageal reflux, chronic bronchitis, bronchiectasis, and selected miscellaneous conditions such as sarcoidosis, lung cancer, heart failure, and Zenker's diverticulum (1). This review deals with the guidelines for management of acute bronchitis and exacerbations of chronic bronchitis.

ACUTE BRONCHITIS

Incidence

Acute bronchitis accounts for about 70% of office visits for a cough illness. The estimated total is 30 million office visits per year (2). It most commonly occurs during acute respiratory tract infections, especially during winter months (3). Approximately 30% to 50% of all cases of common upper respiratory tract infections are accompanied by cough (4,5).

Definition

Acute bronchitis is defined as an upper respiratory tract infection of less than 3 weeks duration (1,2). Cough is commonly accompanied by sputum production, and there may be associated fever and constitutional complaints, especially with influenza or parainfluenza infections. Studies of pulmonary function show an increase in airway resistance and reactivity (6,7). A major consideration in the differential diagnosis is pneumonia, which can be distinguished with a chest radiograph.

Etiology

Infectious causes of acute bronchitis are primarily viral and include influenza A and B viruses, parainfluenza virus, rhinovirus, coronavirus, adenovirus, and respiratory syncytial virus (Table 50.1). Potentially treatable causes of acute bronchitis are *Mycoplasma pneumoniae*, *Chlamydia pneumoniae*, influenza virus, and *Bordetella pertussis* (1,2,8–14).

M. pneumoniae infection is common in young adults, with clinical features that include pharyngitis, fever, constitutional symptoms, and relatively high rates of extrapulmonary complications (16). The course is self-limited, usually with recovery in 1 to 2 weeks, but occasional cases are relatively chronic, with persistent symptoms for up to 4 to 6 weeks. The cough is usually accompanied by production of mucoid sputum. The diagnosis may be established by recovery of *M. pneumoniae*, serial serologic studies showing a fourfold increase in titer, an elevated serum immunoglobulin M titer, or gene amplification with polymerase chain reaction (15,16). None of these tests have consensus agreements regarding utility.

C. pneumoniae is a relatively newly recognized agent of respiratory tract infections that is most common in young adults (8,16). Common clinical features include pharyngitis, laryngitis, and bronchitis expressed with hoarseness, low-grade fever, and a cough that may persist for several weeks. This agent has been implicated in new-onset asthma and asthmatic bronchitis (10). Diagnostic studies include serology, microimmunofluorescence serology with demonstration of a fourfold increase in titer, or polymerase chain reaction using reagents with established validity (17).

Pertussis is a disease with substantial potential morbidity and mortality that has been notably reduced since the vaccine was introduced in the 1940s. The epidemiology of this disease since the early 1980s shows periodic increases in reported cases. Current rates in the United States are 1.5 to 3.0 cases per 100,000 population (18,19). This is primarily a disease of children, but about 30% of pertussis cases are reported in persons over 10 years of age.

TABLE 50.1. Acute Bronchitis: Infectious Agents and Treatment

Agent	Antimicrobial treatment
Viral	
Influenza A virus	Amantadine, rimantadine, zanamivir, oseltamivir
Influenza B virus	Zanamivir, oseltamivir
Parainfluenza virus	—
Coronavirus	—
Respiratory syncytial virus	Ribavirin (pediatrics only)
Rhinovirus	—
Adenovirus	—
Bacterial and bacteria-like	
Mycoplasma pneumoniae	Doxycycline or macrolide[a] (no proof of efficacy)
Chlamydia pneumoniae	Doxycycline or macrolide[a] (no proof of efficacy)
Bordetella pertussis	Erythromycin; alternatives—other macrolides or trimethoprims-sulfamethoxazole

[a]Macrolides are erythromycin, azithromycin, and clarithromycin.

The experience with the current vaccine shows 64% protection against mild disease and 95% protection against serious disease (20). The major clinical feature in adults is a barking cough that is often so prominent and severe that the patient has difficulty completing a sentence. Another common feature is the persistence of this cough for more than 3 weeks, which applies to 80% of adults with pertussis (19,21). Diagnosis is established with the traditional cough plate in which the agar plate appropriate for culture of *B. pertussis* is held before the patient's mouth for aerosolized inoculation during a typical coughing bout. Alternatives are nasopharyngeal aspirate for culture, polymerase chain reaction, and serology (22,23).

Influenza is another potentially treatable cause of bronchitis. The usual clinical features are respiratory tract complaints accompanied by bronchitis; the production of mucoid or purulent sputum; and constitutional symptoms that may be profound and include fever, fatigue, and malaise. Many patients have prolonged periods in which there is reduced pulmonary function after apparent clinical recovery (24,25). The diagnosis is established by viral culture, fluorescent stain of respiratory secretion, or demonstration of seroconversion. For practical purposes, the diagnosis is generally based on the observation of typical symptoms, including fever and malaise during an influenza epidemic. The specificities of these clinical criteria are as good as those of the rapid diagnostic methods (26,27).

Clinical Presentation

Cough is the prominent feature in patients with acute bronchitis. This is noted in 70% to 90% of patients with influenza and 30% to 50% of patients with other common viral infections of the upper airways. The cough is usually nonproductive initially and then becomes productive of mucoid or purulent sputum. The cough resolves spontaneously within 2 weeks in approximately half of patients. Prolonged cough often suggests *C. pneumoniae* infection or pertussis, but cough may last 3 weeks or longer in patients with common viral infections of the upper airways, including rhinovirus infection (28). A review by Kaiser Permanente in San Francisco from 1994 to 1995 showed that 12% of 154 adult patients complaining of cough persisting longer than 2 weeks had serologic evidence of pertussis (29). The diagnosis of pertussis was not suspected by the clinician in any of these cases. Other reports have shown similar findings (12). Dyspnea is unusual with acute bronchitis, except in patients with chronic obstructive lung disease. Fever is common in patients with influenza virus, parainfluenza virus, *M. pneumoniae*, and *C. pneumoniae* infections; fever is unusual with common viral infections of the upper airways. Physical examination often reveals rhonchi but no rales or signs of consolidation. Wheezing is relatively common in patients with asthma.

Most patients with bronchitis do not and should not undergo diagnostic studies except for a possible chest radiograph to exclude pneumonia, which is best justified in patients with rales, abnormal vital signs (temperature >38°C, respiratory rate >24 breaths/min, pulse >100 beats/min) or cough lasting more than 2 to 3 weeks (2,30). The physical examination alone is inadequate to exclude pneumonia (31–33). Diagnostic studies may be conducted for detection of influenza virus, although this may be a presumed diagnosis on clinical grounds in patients who have typical symptoms in an influenza epidemic (26,27).

Cough is defined as chronic when it persists for 3 weeks. For nonsmoking patients with normal findings on a chest radiograph, the most common cause is the postnasal drip syndrome followed by asthma and gastroesophageal reflux (Table 50.2) (32,33). Chronic bronchitis ascribed to smoking or to environmental pollutants ("industrial asthma") is the most common cause of chronic cough. Other causes are tuberculosis, bronchiectasis, angiotensin-converting enzyme inhibitors, congestive heart failure, sarcoidosis, Zenker's diverticulum, and carcinoma. The postnasal drip syndrome is an unscientific term referring to a number of clinical conditions of the upper respiratory tract characterized by postnasal drainage. Most of these patients describe the sensation of postnasal drainage with chronic cough or a perceived need to clear the throat. The usual causes include the common cold, allergic rhinitis, vasomotor rhinitis, postinfectious rhinitis, sinusitis, drug-induced conditions (primarily angiotensin-converting enzyme inhibitors), and environmental irritants. A diagnosis may be established in more than 90% of

TABLE 50.2. Major Causes of Chronic Cough in Nonsmoking Patients with Normal Findings on Chest Radiography

Condition	Frequency (%)	Presumptive diagnosis
Postnasal drip syndrome	41	Sensation of posterior drainage Frequent clearing of throat Examination of nasopharynx shows mucoid or mucopurulent secretions Radiography shows sinusitis
Asthma	24	Episodic wheezing, dyspnea with cough Physical examination shows wheezing Pulmonary function tests show reversible airway obstruction
Gastroesophageal reflux	21	Heartburn or sour taste in mouth Demonstration of reflux with radiography, endoscopy, or esophageal monitoring
Chronic bronchitis	5	Satisfy definition Pulmonary function tests show irreversible airway obstruction
Bronchiectasis	4	Cough with >30 mL, discolored sputum per day Radiography or high-resolution computed tomography shows typical changes

Adapted from Irwin RS, Curley FJ, French CL. Chronic cough. The spectrum and frequency of causes, key components of the diagnostic evaluation, and outcome of specific therapy. *Am Rev Respir Dis* 1990;141:640–647, with permission.

these patients (32). The usual diagnostic evaluation includes a history, physical examination, and chest radiography; this evaluation is followed by appropriate tests based on initial observations in terms of probabilities. With identification of the cause, therapy successfully eliminates the cough in more than 90% of patients.

Treatment

Most patients with acute bronchitis are best managed symptomatically based on symptoms and etiology as summarized in Table 50.3 (30,32,34).

The main controversy in these cases is the use of antibiotics. There is little or no evidence that chronic bronchitis is caused by bacterial pathogens; multiple controlled trials have shown that antibiotics are not effective (35–39), and numerous authorities have admonished physicians to avoid this unnecessary use of antibiotics (2,30,33). Despite these data, office surveys repeatedly show that 60% to 80% of patients who seek medical care for acute bronchitis are treated with these drugs (1,2,40,41). Exceptions to the general rule include the following:

- *Influenza:* This infection can be treated with antiviral agents directed against influenza if treatment is started within 48 hours of the onset of symptoms (42–45).
- *Pertussis:* Pertussis accounts for 10% to 15% of acute bronchitis cases in adults characterized by cough that persists over 3 weeks (11,12,18–21,29). The most characteristic features in adults with waning or absent immunity are the epidemiologic association and typical clinical features (barking cough in paroxysms, often with posttussive vomiting). The clinical features are often atypical due to partial immunity, and diagnostic tests are relatively insensitive and cumbersome (22). The preferred treatment is erythromycin 2 g per day for 14 days. Alternative agents for those who cannot tolerate erythromycin are trimethoprim-sulfamethoxazole, clarithromycin, and azithromycin.
- *M. pneumoniae and C. pneumoniae:* These pathogens are implicated in up to 10% of cases, but there is no evidence that

they require specific antibiotic therapy based on clinical trials (2,30,35–39).
- *Acute exacerbations of chronic bronchitis:* Discussed below.

EXACERBATIONS OF CHRONIC BRONCHITIS

Definition

Chronic bronchitis is characterized by cough and sputum production for an extended time. The standard definition is arbitrarily a productive cough and sputum production for at least 3 months per year for at least 2 years that is not caused by other conditions such as tuberculosis or bronchiectasis (34,46). Many patients have emphysema, and the two conditions are commonly combined with the appellation "chronic obstructive lung disease with bronchitis and emphysema." Chronic bronchitis associated with wheezing is often referred to as chronic or recurrent asthmatic bronchitis.

Incidence

Chronic bronchitis is noted in 10% to 25% of the adult population, is more common in men than in women, and is most common in persons over 40 years of age. Chronic obstructive lung disease represents the fifth leading cause of death in the United States.

Etiology

The major contributing factors in chronic bronchitis are cigarette smoking, infection, and environmental pollution. Industrial bronchitis is the term commonly used for bronchitis resulting from occupational exposure to dust, gas, or fumes (47,48). A small subset of these patients have congenital defects or immunodeficiency syndromes, such as cystic fibrosis, immunoglobulin A or selective immunoglobulin G subclass deficiency, abnormal polymorphonuclear function, primary ciliary dyskinesia, or α_1-globulin deficiency. The major culprit is cigarette smoking, and the frequency depends on the extent of smoking exposure. For patients with a history of 40 to 60 packs per year, the frequency of chronic bronchitis approaches 50% (49). The usual pathologic change noted in the lungs of patients with chronic bronchitis is an increase in the number of goblet cells on the surface epithelium of the bronchi with an increase in mucous glands (50,51).

Clinical Presentation

The hallmark of chronic bronchitis is the chronic cough, which is often accompanied by tenacious, mucoid sputum. Exacerbation may be ascribed to any of the following: smoking, air pollution, allergens, occupational exposure, and preclinical or subclinical asthma. Infection is thought to be an important cause, but this has been difficult to prove on the basis of microbiologic studies or with clinical trials. The organisms most commonly implicated are viral agents that cause upper respiratory tract infections and two commonly found bacterial species: *S. pneumoniae* and *H. influenzae*. Exacerbation of chronic bronchitis is one of the conditions in medicine that has been most extensively studied, but the role of infection as a major cause or as a factor in promoting progression of the underlying condition remains inconclusive. The following conclusions can be made on the basis of multiple studies:

1. Viral infections are found in association with exacerbations in 7% to 64% of cases (46,52–56). Perhaps the best studies have been conducted by Gump and colleagues (53), who found

TABLE 50.3.   Treatment of Acute Bronchitis

Cause	Treatment
Common cold	Dexbrompheniramine and sedating antihistamine (over-the-counter preparations)
	Neproxen and/or itraproporium
Cough	Medications containing codeine or dextromethorphan
Allergic rhinitis	Nonsedating (second-generation) antihistamine
Sinusitis	Treat for common cold and antibiotic if sinusitis symptoms are severe or >7 days
Asthma	Inhaled bronchodilator
Pertussis	Erythromycin, 500 mg q.i.d. for 14 days
Influenza	Rimantadine, zanamivir, or oseltamivir; selected by influenza virus type, cost, and side effect; must start <48 h of onset of symptoms
Exacerbations of chronic bronchitis	Inhaled bronchodilator and/or ipratropium Hospitalized patients: judicious use of systemic steroids and O_2 Antibiotics for severe exacerbations

q.i.d., four times daily.

viral infections in 32% of patients during exacerbations compared with 1% during remissions. Most commonly implicated are influenza A or B virus, parainfluenza virus, coronavirus, and rhinovirus (13,52–55).

2. The role of bacterial infection in exacerbations and in progression of chronic obstructive lung disease has been examined with sequential cultures, response rates to antibiotics in controlled trials, and sputum cytology. Sputum cytology is based on quantitative assessment of expectorated secretions obtained sequentially for a period of years during exacerbations and during periods of relative quiescence (56,57). Results indicate high concentrations of polymorphonuclear cells throughout the course of chronic bronchitis without notable changes during exacerbations. Thus, the perception of increased purulence cannot be confirmed by the concentration of leukocytes. Biopsies of bronchi show increased mucosal and mural inflammation with increased numbers of macrophages, CD4+ lymphocytes, and CD8+ lymphocytes (57,58).

3. Bacterial cultures of expectorated sputum in patients with chronic bronchitis show a high yield of potential respiratory tract pathogens during both exacerbations and remissions. One of the most comprehensive studies was by Gump and co-workers (53), who periodically obtained sputum from patients with chronic bronchitis for a period of years and performed quantitative cultures using serial dilutions. This work showed high counts of potential pathogens, primarily *S. pneumoniae* and *H. influenzae*, during both exacerbations and remissions; the mean count was about 10^7 per milliliter. The yield of *S. pneumoniae* in culture is 15% to 50%, but it is no higher during exacerbations than in remissions (53,59,60). Similar data apply to *H. influenzae* (53,59–61). Nearly all strains of *H. influenzae* are nontypeable (61). Transtracheal aspirates from many patients with chronic obstructive lung disease and chronic bronchitis show high rates of lower airway colonization by bacteria that are not seen in healthy control subjects; the dominant organisms are *S. pneumoniae, H. influenzae,* and nonpathogens such as α-hemolytic streptococci and *Haemophilus parainfluenzae* (59,62,63). These studies show that patients with chronic bronchitis have high rates of colonization by multiple bacteria that extends to the tracheobronchial tract below the level of the larynx. Furthermore, this work suggests that exacerbations cannot be distinguished from relatively quiescent periods in patients with chronic bronchitis by bacteriology studies using transtracheal aspirates or quantitative cultures of expectorated sputum.

4. There are multiple studies of antibiotics given for the treatment of exacerbations of chronic bronchitis, but relatively few have an appropriate study format with a placebo control (34,64–72). Antibiotics used in the studies that are considered optimal in terms of trial design include amoxicillin, tetracyclines, trimethoprim-sulfamethoxazole, and chloramphenicol. One of the largest and most frequently quoted studies was a double-blind, placebo-controlled trial of 173 patients with 362 exacerbations by Anthonisen et al. (71). This study showed an accelerated clinical recovery in 68% of antibiotic recipients compared with 55% in the placebo group, a difference that was statistically significant. Saint and colleagues (69) provided a metaanalysis of published trials to address this issue. A review of published reports from 1955 to 1994 showed that only 9 of 214 reports satisfied the selection criteria for a randomized trial with antibiotic treatment versus placebo (Table 50.4). The outcome parameters were diverse and included days of illness, symptom score, physician's evaluation, and peak expiratory flow rates. Results were variable, but seven of the nine studies showed a benefit of treatment, and the overall results demonstrated a small but statistically significant improvement. Analysis of six studies that measured peak expiratory flow rates showed an improvement of 10.75 L/min, favoring antibiotic treatment. This benefit is tiny, but statistically significant.

Diagnosis

Patients with exacerbations of bronchitis need to be evaluated for the severity of symptoms to determine the need for hospitalization, supportive care, and possible antibiotic treatment. A chest radiograph is often required to evaluate for pneumonitis or other complications such as atelectasis, heart failure, or carcinoma. Gram stains and culture of expectorated sputum are not recommended (64). Pulmonary function tests and blood gas analysis may indicate the severity of illness.

Treatment

The major treatment modality in patients who are seriously ill is respiratory support using bronchodilators, systemic corticosteroids, and oxygen therapy. The use of aminophylline and positive pressure ventilation is controversial (34).

The utility of short-term antibiotic treatment is controversial, although most clinicians use these agents. The best justification is severe exacerbations with increased cough, dyspnea,

TABLE 50.4. Antibiotics for Exacerbations of Chronic Obstructive Lung Disease: Metaanalysis

Study	Number	Setting	Antibiotic	Outcome	Result[a]
Elmes et al. (64)	113	Outpatients	Tetracycline	Days of illness	Benefit; NS
Berry et al. (65)	33	Outpatients	Tetracycline	Symptom score	Benefit; Sig
Fear and Edwards (66)	119	Outpatients	Tetracycline	Symptom score	Benefit; NS
Elmes et al. (67)	56	Hospitalized patients	Ampicillin	PEFR	Benefit; NS
Peterson et al. (68)	19	Hospitalized patients	Chloramphenicol	PEFR	No benefit; NS
Saint et al. (69)	149	Hospitalized patients	Tetracycline	Symptom score, PEFR	Benefit; Sig
Nicotra et al. (70)	40	Hospitalized patients	Tetracycline	Days of illness, PEFR	Benefit; NS
Anthonisen et al. (71)	310	Outpatients	TMP-SMX, amoxicillin, or doxycycline	Days of illness, PEFR	Benefit; Sig
Jorgensen et al. (72)	262	Outpatients	Amoxicillin	Symptom score, PEFR	No benefit; NS

[a]Results show benefit favoring antibiotic treatment. Individual studies evaluated for significance of difference for outcome measured. NS, not statistically significant; Sig, statistically significant. The overall results showed a small but statistically significant benefit with antibiotic treatment.
PEFR, peak expiratory flow rates; TMP-SMX, trimethoprim-sulfamethoxazole.

and sputum purulence (34). The usual treatment is a 7- to 10-day course of trimethoprim-sulfamethoxazole, amoxicillin, or doxycycline based on controlled trials as summarized earlier (Table 50.4) (34,64–72). Owing to the evolution of resistance, some clinicians now favor oral cephalosporins, fluoroquinolone, or a macrolide directed at *S. pneumoniae* and *H. influenzae* (65). Potential disadvantages of these newer agents are cost and the lack of adequately controlled studies to demonstrate superiority over the alternatives suggested (73).

REFERENCES

1. Gonzales R, Sande MA. Uncomplicated acute bronchitis. *Ann Intern Med* 2000;133:981.
2. Snow V, Mottur-Pilson C, Gonzales R. Principles of appropriate antibiotic use for treatment of acute bronchitis in adults. *Ann Intern Med* 2001;134:518.
3. Ayres JG. Seasonal pattern of acute bronchitis in general practice in the United Kingdom. *Thorax* 1986;41:107.
4. Dingle JH, Badger GF, Jordon WS Jr. *Illness in the home: a study of 25,000 illnesses in a group of Cleveland families.* Cleveland, OH: Press of Western Reserve University, 1964:68.
5. Hendley JO, Fishburne HB, Gwaltney JM Jr. Coronavirus infections in working adults: eight-year study with 229E and OC43. *Am Rev Respir Dis* 1972;105:805.
6. Hall WJ, Hall CB, Speers DM. Respiratory syncytial virus infection in adults: clinical, virologic, and serial pulmonary function studies. *Ann Intern Med* 1978;88:203.
7. Boldy DAR, Skidmore SJ, Ayres JG. Acute bronchitis in the community: clinical features, infective factors, changes in pulmonary function, and bronchial reactivity to histamine. *Respir Med* 1990;84:377.
8. Denny FW, Clyde WA, Glenzen WP. *Mycoplasma pneumoniae* disease. Clinical spectrum, pathophysiology, epidemiology and control. *J Infect Dis* 1971;123:74.
9. Grayston JT, Kuo C-C, Wang S-P, et al. A new *Chlamydia psittaci* strain, TWAR, isolated in acute respiratory tract infections. *N Engl J Med* 1986;315:161.
10. Hahn DL, Dodge RW, Golubjatnikov R. Association of *Chlamydia pneumoniae* (strain TWAR) infection with wheezing, asthmatic bronchitis, and acute onset asthma. *JAMA* 1991;266:225.
11. Herwaldt LA. Pertussis in adults: what physicians need to know. *Arch Intern Med* 1991;151:1510.
12. Strebel P, Nordin J, Edwards K, et al. Population-based incidence of pertussis among adolescents and adults, Minnesota, 1995–96. *J Infect Dis* 2001;183:1353.
13. Hall CB. Respiratory syncytial virus and parainfluenza virus. *N Engl J Med* 2001;344:1917.
14. Wright SW, Edwards KM, Decker MD, et al. Prevalence of positive serology for acute *Chlamydia pneumoniae* infection in emergency department patients with persistent cough. *Acad Emerg Med* 1997;4:179.
15. Uldum SA, Jensen JS, Sondergard-Anderson J, et al. Enzyme immunoassay for detection of immunoglobulin M (IgM) and IgG antibodies to *Mycoplasma pneumoniae*. *J Clin Microbiol* 1992;30:1198.
16. Bartlett JG, Dowell SF, Mandell LA, et al. Practice guidelines for the management of community-acquired pneumonia in adults. *Clin Infect Dis* 2000;31:347.
17. Dowell SF, Peeling RW, Bowman, et al. Standardizing *Chlamydia pneumoniae* assays: recommendations from the CDC (USA) and the Laboratory Centre for Disease Control (Canada). *Clin Infect Dis* 2001;33:492.
18. Christie CDC, Marx ML, Marchant CD, et al. The 1993 epidemic of pertussis in Cincinnati. *N Engl J Med* 1994;331:16.
19. Pasternack MS. Pertussis in the 1990s: diagnosis, treatment, and prevention. *Curr Clin Top Infect Dis* 1997;17:24.
20. Jenkinson D. Duration of effectiveness of pertussis vaccine: evidence from a 10-year community study. *BMJ* 1988;296:612.
21. Postels-Multani S, Schmitt HJ, Wirsing von Konig CH, et al. Symptoms and complications of pertussis in adults. *Infection* 1995;23:139.
22. Hoppe JE. Methods for isolation of *Bordetella pertussis* from patients with whooping cough. *Eur J Clin Microbiol Infect Dis* 1988;7:616.
23. Meade BD, Bollen A. Recommendations for use of the polymerase chain reaction in the diagnosis of *Bordetella pertussis* infections. *J Med Microbiol* 1994;41:51.
24. Little JW, Hall WJ, Douglas RG Jr, et al. Airway hyperactivity and peripheral airway dysfunction in influenza A infection. *Am Rev Respir Dis* 1978;118:295.
25. Homer GJ, Gray FD Jr. Effect of uncomplicated presumptive influenza on the diffusing capacity of the lung. *Am Rev Respir Dis* 1973;108:866.
26. Monto AS, Gravenstein S, Elliott M, et al. Clinical signs and symptoms predicting influenza infections. *Arch Intern Med* 2000;160:3243.
27. Medical Letter Consultants. Rapid diagnostic tests for influenza. *Med Lett* 1999;41:121.
28. Gwaltney JM Jr, Hendley JO, Simon G, et al. Rhinovirus infections in an industrial population. II. Characteristics of illness and antibody response. *JAMA* 1967;202:494.
29. Nennig ME, Shinefield HR, Edwards KM, et al. Prevalence and incidence of adult pertussis in an urban population. *JAMA* 1996;275:1672.
30. Gonzales R, Bartlett JG, Besser RE, et al. Principles for appropriate antibiotic use for treatment of uncomplicated acute bronchitis: background. *Ann Intern Med* 2001;134:521.
31. Wipf JE, Lipsley BA, Hirschmann JV. Diagnosing pneumonia by physical examination: relevant or relic? *Arch Intern Med* 1999;159:1082.
32. Irwin RS, Curley FJ, French CL. Chronic cough: the spectrum and frequency of causes, key components of the diagnostic evaluation, and outcome of specific therapy. *Am Rev Respir Dis* 1990;141:640.
33. Irwin R, Madison JM. The diagnosis and treatment of cough. *N Engl J Med* 2000;343:1715.
34. Snow V, Lascher S, Mottur-Pilson C. Evidence base for management of acute exacerbations of chronic obstructive pulmonary disease. *Ann Intern Med* 2001;134:595.
35. Hueston WJ. A comparison of albuterol and erythromycin for the treatment of acute bronchitis. *J Fam Pract* 1991;33:476.
36. Stott NCH, West RR. Randomised controlled trial of antibiotics in patients with a cough and purulent sputum. *BMJ* 1976;2:556.
37. Orr PH, Scherer K, MacDonald A, et al. Randomized placebo-controlled trials of antibiotics for acute bronchitis: a critical review of the literature. *J Fam Pract* 1993;36:507.
38. Fahey T, Stocks N, Thomas T. Quantitative systemic review of randomized controlled trials comparing antibiotic with placebo for acute cough in adults. *BMJ* 1998;316:906.
39. Bent S, Saint S, Vittinghoff E, et al. Antibiotics in acute bronchitis: a meta-analysis. *Am J Med* 1999;107:62.
40. Gonzales R, Sande M. What will it take to stop physicians from prescribing antibiotics in acute bronchitis? *Lancet* 1995;345:665.
41. Gonzales R, Wilson A, Crane LA, et al. What's in a name? Public knowledge, attitudes, and experiences with antibiotic use for acute bronchitis. *Am J Med* 2000;108:83.
42. Kaiser L, Keene ON, Hammond JM, et al. Impact of zanamivir on antibiotic use for respiratory events following acute influenza in adolescents and adults. *Arch Intern Med* 2000;160:3234.
43. Couch RB. Prevention and treatment of influenza. *N Engl J Med* 2000;343:1778.
44. Lalezari J, Campion K, Keene O, et al. Zanamivir for the treatment of influenza A & B infection in high-risk patients: a pooled analysis of randomized controlled trials. *Arch Intern Med* 2001;161:212.
45. Treanor JJ, Hayden FG, Vrooman PS, et al. Efficacy and safety of the oral neuraminidase inhibitor oseltamivir in treating acute influenza: a randomized controlled trial. *JAMA* 2000;283:1016.
46. Dantzker DR, Pingleton SK, Pierce JA, and other Task Force Members. Standards for the diagnosis and care of patients with chronic obstructive pulmonary disease and asthma—American Thoracic Society. *Am Rev Respir Dis* 1987;136:225.
47. Minette A. Is chronic bronchitis also an industrial disease? *Eur J Respir Dis* 1986;69(suppl 146):87.
48. Speizer FE, Tager B. Epidemiology of chronic mucus hypersecretion and obstructive airways disease. *Epidemiol Rev* 1979;1:124.
49. Linden M, Rasmussen JB, Piitulainen E, et al. Airway inflammation in smokers with nonobstructive and obstructive chronic bronchitis. *Am Rev Respir Dis* 1993;148:1226.
50. Gail DB, Lenfant CJM. Cells of the lung: biology and clinical implications. *Am Rev Respir Dis* 1983;127:366.
51. Reid L. Measurement of the bronchial mucous gland layer: a diagnostic yardstick in chronic bronchitis. *Thorax* 1960;15:132.
52. Eadie MB, Stott EJ, Grist NR. Virological studies in chronic bronchitis. *BMJ* 1966;2:671.
53. Gump DW, Phillips CA, Forsyth BR, et al. Role of infection in chronic bronchitis. *Am Rev Respir Dis* 1976;113:465.
54. Lamy ME, Pouthier-Simon F, Debacker-Willame E. Respiratory viral infections in hospital patients with chronic bronchitis. *Chest* 1973;63:336.
55. Stark JE, Heath RB, Curwen MP. Infection with parainfluenza viruses in chronic bronchitis. *Thorax* 1965;20:124.
56. Chodosh S. Examination of sputum cells. *N Engl J Med* 1970;282:854.
57. Fournier M, Lebargy F, Leroy Ladurie F, et al. Intraepithelial T-lymphocyte subsets in the airways of normal subjects and/or patients with chronic bronchitis. *Am Rev Respir Dis* 1989;140:737.
58. Saetta M, DiStefano A, Maestrelli P, et al. Activated T-lymphocytes and macrophages in bronchia mucosa of subjects with chronic bronchitis. *Am Rev Respir Dis* 1993;147:301.
59. Lees AW, McNaught W. Bacteriology of lower respiratory tract secretions, sputum, and upper respiratory tract secretions in "normals" and chronic bronchitis. *Lancet* 1959;2:1112.
60. Miller DL, Jones R. The bacterial flora of the upper respiratory tract and sputum of working men. *J Pathol Bacteriol* 1964;87:182.
61. Murphy TF, Apicella MA. Nontypable *Hemophilus influenzae*: a review of clinical aspects, surface antigens, and the human immune response to infection. *Rev Infect Dis* 1987;9:1.
62. Bjerkestrand G, Digranes A, Schreiner A. Bacteriological findings in transtracheal aspirates from patients with chronic bronchitis and bronchiectasis. *Scand J Respir Dis* 1975;56:201.
63. Bartlett J. Diagnostic accuracy of transtracheal aspiration bacteriologic studies. *Am Rev Respir Dis* 1977;115:777.
64. Elmes PC, Fletcher CM, Dutton AAC. Prophylactic use of oxytetracycline for exacerbations of chronic bronchitis. *BMJ* 1957;2:1272.

65. Berry DG, Fry J, Hindley CP, et al. Exacerbations of chronic bronchitis treatment with oxytetracycline. *Lancet* 1960;1:137.
66. Fear EC, Edwards G. Antibiotic regimes in chronic bronchitis. *Br J Dis Chest* 1962;56:153.
67. Elmes PC, King TKC, Langlands JHM, et al. Value of ampicillin in the hospital treatment of exacerbations of chronic bronchitis. *BMJ* 1965;2:904.
68. Petersen ES, Esmann V, Honcke P, et al. A controlled study of the effect of treatment on chronic bronchitis: an evaluation using pulmonary function tests. *Acta Med Scand* 1967;182:293.
69. Saint S, Bent S, Vittinghoff E, et al. Antibiotics in chronic obstructive pulmonary disease exacerbations: a meta-analysis. *JAMA* 1995;273:957.
70. Nicotra MB, Rivera M, Awe RJ. Antibiotic therapy of acute exacerbations of chronic bronchitis. *Ann Intern Med* 1982;97:18.
71. Anthonisen NR, Manfreda J, Warren CPW, et al. Antibiotic therapy in exacerbations of chronic obstructive pulmonary disease. *Ann Intern Med* 1987;106:196.
72. Jorgensen AF, Coolidge J, Pedersen PA, et al. Amoxicillin in treatment of acute uncomplicated exacerbations of chronic bronchitis. a double-blind, placebo-controlled multicentre study in general practice. *Scand J Prim Health Care* 1992;10:7.
73. Destache C, Dewan N, O'Donohue, WJ, et al. Clinical and economic considerations in the treatment of acute exacerbations of chronic bronchitis. *J Antimicrob Chemother* 1999;43(suppl A):107.

CHAPTER 51
Viral Pneumonia

Stephen G. Baum and David C. Perlman

Viral pneumonia is a subset of those pneumonitides that were previously referred to as atypical pneumonia. This term arose at the beginning of the antibiotic era to describe a group of lower respiratory tract infections in which no bacterial pathogen could be identified by Gram stain or culture and that did not respond to the antibiotics then available. With the advent of cell culture techniques, it became possible to isolate viruses and thereby establish the viral etiology of many of these infections.

Numerous viruses are capable of causing pneumonia. Some, such as influenza virus, respiratory syncytial virus (RSV), and adenovirus, do so as their primary disease manifestation; some, such as paramyxovirus (measles) and varicella-zoster virus, do so as only one aspect of a multisystem disease syndrome. Although viral respiratory syndromes are generally thought to be mild and self-limited, some (such as influenza) are responsible for thousands of deaths annually and, under epidemic conditions, can kill millions of people throughout the world in a matter of a few years. An increase in the number of people who are immunocompromised by virtue of age, cancer chemotherapy, organ transplantation, and acquired immunodeficiency syndrome (AIDS) has resulted in a corresponding increase in the incidence, severity, and diversity of viral pneumonias. On the other hand, effective vaccines are available to protect against several pneumotropic viruses, and only the incomplete implementation of vaccine programs prevents widespread use and the resultant reduction of morbidity, mortality, and financial cost.

PATHOGENS

The viruses to be discussed that are primary causes of the atypical pneumonia syndrome are influenza virus, adenovirus, RSV, parainfluenza viruses (PIVs), hantaviruses, and cytomegalovirus (CMV). Influenza virus, RSV, PIVs, and hantaviruses are single-stranded RNA viruses; adenovirus and CMV are double-stranded DNA viruses. Both adenovirus and CMV are capable of establishing latent infections that can undergo reactivation to a cellulytic cycle. Chapters on the individual viruses should be consulted for more detailed information.

EPIDEMIOLOGY

The epidemiology of the various pneumotropic viruses is varied, and knowledge of the epidemiology can provide the best clue as to the specific cause of the atypical pneumonia syndrome in a given patient.

Many if not all of the viruses discussed in this chapter can cause an influenza-like syndrome consisting of fever, malaise, cough, and myalgia. In fact, it is often difficult to differentiate disease caused by one virus from another on clinical grounds alone. Of all the agents, however, only influenza virus is known to cause widespread epidemics and pandemics, which in turn can produce excess mortality of tens of thousands of people (1).

There are three serologic types of influenza virus (A, B, and C), and these serotypes have different propensities for causing major outbreaks. Type A is the cause of most epidemic disease; type B causes clusters of infection in relatively closed populations, such as boarding schools; and type C is far less common and seems to cause primarily isolated cases. Type A epidemics have historically occurred in triennial cycles, with major pandemics occurring about once every decade or two (2). Between epidemics, this agent is also the cause of most sporadic cases of influenza throughout the world. The ability of type A virus to alter its surface antigens (hemagglutinin and neuraminidase) and its ability to infect agricultural animals, providing a reservoir of infection (3), appears to be responsible for the periodicity of epidemics. The alteration of surface antigens is known as antigenic drift when minor changes occur and antigenic shift when these changes are more pronounced. These phenomena and the molecular biologic basis for them are described more fully in Chapter 241.

The PIVs are second in frequency only to rhinoviruses as causes of respiratory tract illnesses in humans. After RSV, PIVs are the most common cause of lower respiratory tract disease in infants throughout the world (4). Outbreaks due to PIVs are associated with increased emergency department visits, hospitalizations, and substantial cost (5,6).

There are four major PIV serotypes, designated types 1 to 4, that are delineated by neutralization assays. Shared antigens, however, result in heterotypic *in vivo* antibody responses. PIV-4 has two major antigenic subtypes (A and B), but antigenic and genetic heterogeneity has been increasingly recognized among all four PIVs (7–10). Antigenic drift, such as is seen with influenza A virus, has not been observed with the PIVs (7,8).

The PIVs have a worldwide distribution (4). Although they are related to several animal paramyxoviruses, there are no known animal reservoirs for the human PIVs. PIV-1 and PIV-2 cause epidemics that occur in alternate years in the fall (5,6,11). Activity of PIV-1 and PIV-2 often declines as activity of RSV increases in the late fall (5). PIV-3 occurs throughout the year, but epidemics occurring in the spring have been observed in the United States (5,11,12). The epidemiology of PIV-4 is less well characterized, in part because of technical difficulties with viral isolation, weak hemadsorption, and the lack, until recently, of a rapid immunofluorescence method (13). Passively acquired antibody probably provides some protection to PIV-1 and PIV-2, because most severe disease is seen in children after 6 months of age (6,7,9). PIV-3 resembles RSV in its capacity to cause severe disease at a time when maternally acquired antibody is present (7,11,12). Seroprevalence data suggest that PIV-4 infection is common but disease is usually mild (13). By age 8 years, the majority of children have serologic evidence of prior infection with PIV types 1, 2, 3, and 4 (4,9).

The mode of transmission appears to be primarily by person-to-person aerosol droplet spread. However, transfer from environmental surface to fingers is readily accomplished, supporting a role for fomites in transmission (14). Nosocomial transmission has been reported, most commonly with PIV-3, but outbreaks due to PIV-1 and PIV-2 also have been reported (11,15). RSV is the most common cause of pneumonia in infants and children both in the United States and throughout the world (4,16). In this population, it causes approximately 90,000 hospitalizations and 4,500 deaths annually from lower respiratory tract disease in the United States (17). RSV outbreaks occur annually with seasonal periodicity. In the United States, RSV activity increases in the late fall, peaks in the winter, and returns to baseline levels in the spring (16,17). RSV outbreaks are associated with excess deaths related to lower respiratory tract disease in infants (18). Both strains A and B usually cocirculate in an outbreak, although their relative proportions may vary (19). There is often a decline in PIV-1 and PIV-2 activity as RSV activity increases (5). Influenza virus activity may increase during or subsequent to peak RSV activity. Infection with RSV is nearly universal. Peak attack rates occur in children under 6 months of age, at a time when they still have specific maternally derived antibody. Immunity from natural infection is incomplete, and reinfections with both heterologous and homologous strains occur (20,21). Attack rates and the severity of disease decrease with subsequent infections; however, attack rates among normal children for second and third infections are 75% and 65%, respectively (20). Comparable attack rates are seen among the institutionalized elderly (22); rates among older children and adults are between 38% and 47% (23). Transmission of RSV is by inoculation of virus, from secretions or fomites, through nasal or ocular mucosa. Virus may survive on hands for up to half an hour, on gloves for up to 2 hours, and on environmental surfaces for up to 7 hours (24).

Primary infection with adenoviruses most often occurs in childhood (25). Although there are about 50 adenovirus serotypes, types 1 to 7 cause the majority of respiratory infection, and three types (3, 4, and 7) cause most cases of adenoviral pneumonia. These three serotypes affect young adults, and there have been numerous outbreaks among military recruits (26). Spread is from person to person by aerosols. In immunocompromised patients, especially renal or bone marrow transplant recipients, types 31, 34, and 35 have caused overwhelming pneumonia (27,28). CMV is transmitted transplacentally, during delivery in vaginal and cervical secretions, and postnatally in breast milk. It is transmitted among young children in day care, where CMV has been shown to persist on toys and environmental surfaces for up to 30 minutes (29). CMV is found in high concentrations in semen and vaginal secretions, and sexual transmission is an important mode of spread. CMV may be transmitted by blood products and organ transplants. The prevalence of CMV infection continues to increase throughout life, and 80% to 100% of the U.S. population is infected by age 60 years (29,30). The hantavirus pulmonary syndrome (HPS) was recognized in 1993 as a clinically distinct form of hantavirus disease, caused by several previously unrecognized viruses of the *Hantavirus* genus (31). Illness associated with previously isolated hantaviruses (Hantaan, Seoul, Puumula) consists of various degrees of fever, renal disease, and hemorrhage without prominent pulmonary involvement. HPS differs from other *Hantavirus* illnesses in that it causes disease with primarily respiratory manifestations and with a higher mortality rate.

Sin Nombre virus is the primary agent of HPS, responsible for 95% of cases in North America (32). The agent was initially implicated by finding immunoglobulin M or G antibodies in patients with HPS that cross-reacted with previously recognized hantaviruses. Later, the agent was detected in tissue by immunohistochemical testing and by reverse transcriptase polymerase chain reaction amplification of the viral genome. The virus subsequently has been isolated in cell culture (33). The natural reservoir for Sin Nombre virus is the deer mouse, *Peromyscus maniculatus,* an indigenous North American species (34). This rodent has a broad geographic range throughout North America. In Arizona, New Mexico, and Colorado, 29% to 33% of *P. maniculatus* have serologic evidence of Sin Nombre virus infection (34). The majority of cases of HPS have occurred in the southwestern and western United States. Infrequent cases have been seen in other states, outside the usual range of the deer mouse, and can be due to several *Hantavirus* variants genetically distinct from Sin Nombre virus. This and other hantaviruses can produce lifelong asymptomatic infection in reservoir rodents, which shed virus in urine, feces, and saliva. Increased domestic rodent infestation and activities such as cleaning of barns and other outdoor structures, cleaning food storage areas, and plowing with hand tools, which increase the likelihood of exposure to infected rodents and their secretions or excreta, may be associated with acquisition of disease (35). Transmission is thought to occur primarily through the inhalation of infected excreta, although the presence of virus in saliva allows transmission by rodent bites. Neither arthropod vectors nor person-to-person transmission has been implicated in HPS or in illnesses caused by related hantaviruses. Serologic data suggest that clinically mild or asymptomatic disease is uncommon, but rare cases have been reported (36). The syndrome is probably not new; retrospective cases have been identified from stored serum. When pneumonia occurs as a complication of other systemic virus infections, such as varicella or rubeola, the epidemiology is that of the underlying infection.

PATHOPHYSIOLOGY

The viruses described in this chapter gain access to the body through the respiratory route. In addition, they have evolved receptors that have primary affinity for respiratory epithelial cells. In the case of influenza, the virus adsorbs to ciliated epithelial cells using the hemagglutinin glycoprotein on the virus surface (37). This results first in cessation of ciliary motility and later in desquamation of cells, thereby triggering cough. If the lower respiratory tract is involved, hyperemia and invasion by both polymorphonuclear and mononuclear cells occur. The alveoli may become involved, and formation of a hyaline membrane lining alveoli has been noted. This may be responsible for the profound hypoxemia that can result and this, in turn, for the relatively high morbidity and mortality in otherwise healthy adults.

PIVs enter through the mucosa of the nose and mouth. The incubation period is 2 to 6 days (7). PIVs may have a tropism for the epithelial cells of the subglottic region (4,12). Cell damage results from both direct viral effects and effects of the host immune response (7,9). Humoral immunity appears to play some role in host defense as evidenced by the general protection against PIV-1 and PIV-2 afforded by maternal antibody and by the fact that infants with high titers of passively acquired antibody to PIV-3 also have relative protection (7). However, the immunity conferred by homologous virus is incomplete, and as with RSV, reinfection with PIVs can occur, albeit with decreased frequency and severity (12). After initial RSV infection of the respiratory epithelium, there is an average incubation of 5 days. Spread of virus to the lower respiratory tract results in a lymphocytic peribronchiolar infiltration and edema, which may be followed by bronchiolar epithelial proliferation and necrosis. The resultant impedance of airflow, especially on expiration, results in the air trapping and hyperinflation seen in bronchiolitis. Pneumonia, with a mononuclear cell interstitial infiltration, edema, and necrosis with alveolar space filling, frequently coexists with pathologic findings of bronchiolitis.

The occurrence of lower respiratory tract RSV disease at a time when maternal antibody is still present and the exaggerated disease that was seen in recipients of a candidate inactivated RSV vaccine have led to the hypothesis that the host immunologic response may contribute to disease pathogenesis (38). Local production of immunoglobulin E, leukotriene C_4, and eosinophilic cationic protein may play an important role in virus-induced airway obstruction (38,39). The occurrence of severe RSV disease in patients with defects in host defenses due to either respiratory tract anatomic abnormalities or defects in cellular immunity suggests that these factors are important in the host's ability to resolve RSV infection (40). Adenoviruses are spread by the respiratory route as well, but can establish latency in oropharyngeal lymphoid tissue (41). The adenovirus pneumonia that typically occurs in young healthy adults is probably the result of primary infection, but adenovirus pneumonia in the immunocompromised patient is almost certainly the result of activation of latent infection (27,28). Adenoviruses adsorb to cells using the fiber protein that extends from the 12 corners of the capsid coat (see Chapter 229) (25).

The pathogenic potential and specific pathogenic mechanisms of CMV disease differ in different hosts and settings. Furthermore, given the ubiquitous nature of CMV infection, the distinction between disease and infection without pathogenicity is sometimes difficult (42,43). Higher rates of CMV infection among CMV-seropositive organ recipients than among -seronegative organ recipients suggest that the reactivation of latent infection is an important process (30,43,44). However, substantial rates of infection also occur among seronegative recipients of seropositive organs, and reinfections of seropositive recipients of seropositive organs has been documented. Each of these pathways to active CMV disease has been documented (45). The response of CMV pneumonia in renal transplant recipients and in infants with congenital CMV disease to antiviral therapy has been taken to suggest a prime role for direct viral replication in pathogenesis (43). Among recipients of allogeneic bone marrow transplants, the clinical response of CMV pneumonia to antiviral therapy has been limited, despite a clear impact on quantitative measures of viral burden, implicating an immunopathogenic mechanism. The higher rate of CMV pneumonitis among allogeneic bone marrow recipients than among autologous recipients, despite comparable CMV infection rates and comparable immunosuppression (46), and the identification of graft-versus-host disease as a significant risk factor for CMV pneumonia, suggest a role for transplanted allogeneic cells in disease pathogenesis (43,44). A T cell–mediated response to a virally induced antigen in the lung has been implicated (4,30). The primary sites of CMV latency are not completely known. Peripheral blood mononuclear cells have been shown to harbor latent virus; bone marrow, spleen, and lung are potential organ reservoirs of latent virus (30,42). In HPS, there is a tropism of Sin Nombre virus for capillary endothelial cells in general, and for the pulmonary capillary endothelium in particular, as detected by immunohistochemical staining for viral antigens. In fatal cases, most of the cells of the pulmonary microcirculation may contain Sin Nombre virus antigen (33). Lung specimens reveal variable degrees of edema, congestion, focal hyaline membranes, and a mononuclear cell infiltrate consisting of small and enlarged mononuclear cells and immunoblasts. Hantaviral inclusions have been demonstrated in pulmonary endothelial cells by electron microscopy. However, despite the high viral load in the pulmonary microvasculature, there is a paucity of necrosis, and pneumocytes and endothelial cells usually appear morphologically intact. These findings have led to the hypothesis that local immune responses to viral antigen may induce a functional derangement of the vascular

endothelium that contributes to the severe pulmonary edema observed clinically (33). High numbers of cytokine-producing T-lymphocytes and monocytes have been identified in lung tissue of patients with fatal hantavirus pulmonary syndrome, suggesting that HPS is in part an immunopathologic response to hantavirus infection (47). Each of the respiratory viruses also has evolved a special mechanism to permit infection of neighboring cells. Influenza virus uses its other main surface glycoprotein, neuraminidase, to cleave the budding virus from the cell surface, allowing the daughter virions to infect other cells (48). RSV and PIVs form syncytia, which facilitate cell-to-cell spread. Adenovirus replicates by a lytic cycle in which the infected cell bursts at the end of replication with the production of free daughter virions (25).

CLINICAL MANIFESTATIONS

Influenza Virus

Clearly, disease caused by influenza virus is the paradigm for so-called influenza-like illness. After an incubation period of 1 to 3 days, there is the rapid onset of chills, fever, cough, and prominent malaise and myalgia. These last two symptoms have given rise to the concept that the patient is experiencing viremia, but with rare exception (49,50), attempts to isolate influenza virus from the bloodstream at any stage of the disease have been unsuccessful. Experience using the interferons as therapeutic agents has shown that they produce similar symptoms, and it may be the induction of endogenous interferon in the course of influenza and other viral infections that is the cause of these symptoms.

Influenza upper respiratory infection, which takes the form of tracheobronchitis, is far more common than is pneumonia. This is a self-limited disease with a 5- to 7-day duration. During the severe epidemic of Asian (A2) influenza in 1957 to 1958, Louria and colleagues (51) described several distinct clinical patterns of disease. The first and most common was influenza upper respiratory infection. The virus was culturable from the sputum during the week-long illness. Most of these patients were adults with no underlying illness, and most recovered with no sequelae. In a second group of patients, pneumonia supervened, the patients' conditions worsened about the third day, and severe hypoxia and obtundation occurred. This group had influenza viral pneumonia, and virus could also be cultured from their sputum. This pattern of the disease was more common among patients with underlying cardiopulmonary disease, including those with rheumatic disease and mitral stenosis, especially in late pregnancy. A third group, while in the throws of influenza, developed a superinfecting bacterial pneumonia. This syndrome again was seen predominantly in patients with underlying disease and carried with it a high mortality. The fourth group of patients identified had influenza and, after a period of 1 to 2 weeks when they appeared to be recovering, developed bacterial pneumonia. This occurred primarily in the oldest of the patients. In the last two groups, influenza virus could not be isolated at the time that bacterial superinfection was occurring. The total number of patients in this study was small, but evidence from subsequent epidemics substantiates these patterns (52). Numerous studies have elucidated the mechanisms whereby influenza virus infection predisposes to bacterial superinfection of the lung. These include interruption of ciliary motility, denudation of mucosa, decrease in polymorphonuclear leukocyte and macrophage chemotaxis, and impaired humoral and cellular immunity.

These studies have further emphasized the need to be aware that *Staphylococcus aureus* can cause postinfluenzal bacterial pneumonia. Staphylococcal pneumonia is far more common after outbreaks of influenza than it is in years of low influenza prevalence (50,51). However, the most common cause of postinfluenzal pneumonia is *Streptococcus pneumoniae*, followed in frequency by *Haemophilus influenzae*, as is the case in patients who have not had recent influenza. The primary life-threatening aspect of influenza pneumonia is the development of diffuse alveolar involvement leading to the adult respiratory distress syndrome (ARDS). Other organ systems can be affected during influenza pneumonia, including the heart and pericardium (53), brain (54), and spinal cord (Guillain-Barré syndrome) (55). The pathophysiologic mechanisms of these complications are unclear. If the attendant bacterial pneumonia is due to toxigenic *S. aureus*, the toxic shock syndrome may supervene (56). One fascinating complication of influenza as well as of varicella-zoster virus infection is Reye's syndrome. After recovery from influenza or chickenpox, some children develop encephalopathy and coma complicated by hepatic failure. Although mortality is high, some children spontaneously recover. Hepatic enzyme levels are elevated, as are the serum ammonia and creatine kinase levels; jaundice is unusual. Examination of the cerebrospinal fluid shows few mononuclear cells and a striking hypoglycorrhachia, sometimes as low as 0 mg/dL. Influenza type B has most often been reported as the preceding event, and the chances of developing Reye's syndrome seem to be enhanced by treatment of the antecedent viral infection with salicylates (see Chapters 155 and 241 for further description) (57,58).

Parainfluenza Viruses

All the PIVs cause upper respiratory tract illnesses, including rhinitis, pharyngitis, and bronchitis. PIV-1, PIV-2, and PIV-3 are important causes of croup (6,9,12). PIV-3 is the second leading cause of hospitalization for acute respiratory infection and pneumonia in infants (4,9,12). PIV-4A and PIV-4B can cause severe lower respiratory tract disease but appear to do so infrequently (13). Syndromes caused by PIVs and RSV can be difficult to distinguish clinically. No characteristic radiographic pattern has been noted in PIV pneumonia. In the normal host, secondary bacterial infection after PIV infection is unusual (4). PIVs are rare causes of pneumonia in immunocompetent adults (59). Severe PIV disease manifestations, including giant cell pneumonia, respiratory failure, and death, have been reported in immunocompromised children and adults, including patients with severe combined immunodeficiency, solid organ transplants, and leukemia (60–62). Prolonged virus shedding also has been reported in immunocompromised hosts, including children with human immunodeficiency virus (HIV) infection (62,63). PIV-3 is the type most frequently isolated from immunocompromised hosts with lower respiratory tract disease.

Lower respiratory tract PIV disease is usually preceded by upper respiratory tract signs and symptoms, such as nasal congestion and pharyngitis. Fever and cough are usually present. Rales, rhonchi, wheezing, and intercostal muscle retractions may be present on physical examination. Chest radiographs may reveal interstitial infiltrates and hyperinflation, with consolidation present in up to 25% of cases, usually in the right upper or middle lobe. Severe hypoxemia may be present, often without cyanosis.

Respiratory Syncytial Virus

The most common manifestations of RSV infection occur in the upper respiratory tract, and the most serious in the lower respiratory tract. Lower respiratory tract involvement may occur in 30% to 70% of initial infections. Bronchiolitis accounts for a greater proportion of lower respiratory tract RSV involvement in children than does pneumonia. However, pneumonia may occur in 5% to 40%, and the two may be difficult to differentiate and may coexist (41).

Children with bronchopulmonary dysplasia, cystic fibrosis, prematurity, cyanotic or complicated congenital heart disease, congenital combined immunodeficiencies, and malignant neoplasms are at increased risk for severe RSV lower respiratory tract disease (64). Children receiving steroid therapy for other chronic conditions may not have more severe disease, but they have more prolonged virus shedding than do normal children. Children with HIV-1 infection may have prolonged virus shedding and may be at increased risk for lower respiratory tract disease, particularly pneumonia (65,66). In the otherwise healthy child with RSV pneumonia, early bacterial superinfection may occur, but late bacterial secondary infections are unusual (4). RSV infections in adults, by virtue of the near universality of childhood infection, are essentially all reinfections. These reinfections are more often limited to the upper respiratory tract. However, lower respiratory tract involvement, usually tracheobronchitis or pneumonia rather than bronchiolitis, may occur in both healthy and immunocompromised adolescents and adults (22,23,67). Outbreaks in the elderly have been associated with particularly high rates of bronchopneumonia with substantial morbidity and mortality (22). Bone marrow transplant recipients are at high risk for severe disease, with mortality rates up to 78% reported (68,69). RSV upper respiratory tract disease may be under-recognized in immunocompromised patients. Adults with leukemia also may be at high risk, particularly during times of increased RSV prevalence in the community, with mortality rates of 83% reported (70). Therefore, it may be important to consider RSV early in immunocompromised hosts who present with upper respiratory tract symptoms (41,68,69).

Adenovirus

Adult pneumonia caused by adenovirus has no particular distinguishing features. The clinical picture is much like that of influenza, and diagnosis would rest on the epidemiologic setting of a young adult entering a new closed population group. In children, in whom the adenoviruses are the single most common cause of upper respiratory infection, adenoviruses should always be suspected. One of the more common syndromes in this age group is pharyngoconjunctival fever due to infection with type 3 adenovirus. This often occurs in small epidemics in summer camps, where swimming pool water is the probable reservoir. Keratoconjunctivitis is another common adenovirus syndrome but is not associated with adenovirus pneumonia.

Cytomegalovirus

CMV pneumonia is rare in immunocompetent adults (71), but may occur in up to 6% of cases of CMV-induced mononucleosis (72). Patients may be asymptomatic or symptomatic. Radiographic findings and symptoms, when present, usually resolve spontaneously. CMV pneumonia develops in 50% of infants with CMV inclusion disease. Up to 20% of episodes of hospitalized pneumonia in infants 1 to 3 months of age may be due to CMV (73). Interstitial pneumonia is a common and important complication of organ transplantation, particularly bone marrow transplantation. It presents with tachypnea, hypoxemia, fever, and interstitial infiltrates on chest radiography. Specific microbiologic diagnosis usually requires bronchoscopy or surgical lung biopsy. Fifteen percent to 40% of allogeneic marrow transplant recipients develop interstitial pneumonitis (30,45,74).

CMV accounts for approximately one half of transplant interstitial pneumonitis cases, with the other half being due to *Pneumocystis carinii*, adenovirus, other viruses, or toxic effects of radiation or chemotherapeutic agents. The mortality rate from CMV pneumonia in this setting has been as high as 80% to 90%.

Heart-lung transplant recipients, particularly seronegative recipients of donor-positive organs, are at greater risk for CMV pneumonia than are other solid organ recipients (30,75). However, as previously mentioned, disease may occur in seropositive recipients through either reactivation of latent CMV strains or reinfection with a new strain.

Patients with AIDS are at substantial risk for the development of CMV disease, especially when CD4+ lymphocyte counts fall below 100/mm (3). Patients with AIDS and advanced immunosuppression frequently shed CMV in urine and semen and frequently have viremia without clinically apparent end-organ disease. The most common sites of CMV disease in persons with AIDS are the retina and the gastrointestinal tract. Disease may be due to both viral reactivation and reinfection, and coinfections with multiple strains have been reported. The response of CMV retinitis in AIDS to antiviral therapy is consistent with viral replication as the pathogenetic mechanism in these hosts (43). Despite the clear clinical significance of CMV retinitis and gastrointestinal disease among HIV-infected persons, the importance of CMV as a pulmonary pathogen in HIV-infected persons has been less clear (76,77). Among AIDS patients with symptomatic pneumonitis, in most instances in which CMV is identified ante mortem by culture or by characteristic cytopathic effects in bronchoscopic washings, coexistent pathogens such as *P. carinii* are also found (76). The presence of culturable CMV from bronchoscopy specimens has been shown not to affect the short-term morbidity or mortality of patients with first-episode *P. carinii* pneumonia (77). However, evidence of CMV pneumonia with viral inclusions may be found at autopsy (78), and there are reports of CMV pneumonia with CMV identified as a sole pathogen by the presence of numerous viral inclusions in alveolar cells in transbronchial biopsy specimens (79,80).

Hantavirus Pulmonary Syndrome

HPS begins, after an incubation period of 9 to 33 days (median approximately 14 days), with a prodromal illness consisting primarily of fever (in 98%–100%) and myalgias (in 57%–100%) (33,35,81). Cough, nausea, vomiting, headache, and other symptoms are variably present initially.

As the illness proceeds, patients develop progressive cough, dyspnea, tachypnea, tachycardia, and hypotension. Laboratory findings include hemoconcentration, thrombocytopenia, a prolonged partial thromboplastin time, and elevated serum lactate dehydrogenase levels. A marked leukocytosis is common, frequently with an increased proportion of immature forms and a mild atypical lymphocytosis (81). Initial chest radiographs frequently reveal interstitial edema with Kerly B lines and peribronchial cuffing (such as seen in cardiogenic pulmonary edema and not ARDS) but with a normal heart size (such as seen in ARDS and not cardiogenic pulmonary edema). Pleural effusions and airspace disease may develop rapidly, and the airspace disease may lack the peripheral distribution typical of ARDS (81,82). The mortality rate may be as high as 52% (36). Increases in the hematocrit, lactate dehydrogenase level, partial thromboplastin time, and white blood cell count are poor prognostic indicators (81).

DIAGNOSIS

The etiologic diagnosis of viral pneumonia on clinical grounds alone is inaccurate. During an epidemic, influenza etiology is probably overdiagnosed; at other times, sporadic cases of true influenza are often unrecognized. Much of the influenza-like illness that is seen in nonepidemic periods may be caused by some of the other viruses discussed in this chapter as well as by *Mycoplasma pneumoniae*, *Chlamydia psittaci*, *Chlamydia pneumoniae*, *Legionella pneumophila*, and *P. carinii*. Although adenovirus pneumonia can evolve into ARDS (26), this is relatively uncommon in immunocompetent patients. If ARDS occurs in the course of an influenza-like illness in an adult, the likely viral causes are influenza virus or hantavirus. The differentiation would be made acutely by lack of a history of rodent exposure in influenza. Clinical factors that may aid in establishing the etiology in a case of atypical pneumonia syndrome are shown in Table 51.1.

Diagnosis can be confirmed in a reference laboratory by viral culture enhanced by immunofluorescence assays of the infected cell culture and by demonstrating an increase in titer of complement-fixing or other antibodies. None of these tests is performed routinely. For adenovirus and PIV, the importance of a specific diagnosis is primarily in documenting the start of an outbreak. For influenza virus, RSV, CMV, and hantavirus, arriving at a specific etiologic diagnosis is important both because of the severity of disease that may prevail in these infections and because therapeutic modalities (with variable efficacy) may be required.

A presumptive diagnosis of lower respiratory tract RSV disease can often be made clinically in children in the RSV season,

TABLE 51.1. Clinical Aids to the Etiologic Diagnosis of the Atypical Pneumonia Syndrome

Pathogen	Symptoms	Signs	History	Laboratory
Influenza virus	Myalgia, severe respiratory distress	ARDS	Epidemic	↓ Po₂
Respiratory syncytial virus	Wheezing, persistent cough	Bronchospasm	—	—
Hantavirus	Severe respiratory distress	ARDS	Exposure to rodents or their excreta	Hemoconcentration, ↑ LDH ↓ platelets
Adenovirus	—	—	Military, school, AIDS, transplant	—
Cytomegalovirus	—	Retinitis, colitis	AIDS, transplant	—
Chlamydia psittaci	—	—	Bird exposure	
Mycoplasma pneumoniae	Insidious onset, cough	Negative chest examination findings	School, military	Cold agglutinins
Pneumocystis carinii	—	—	AIDS risk activity	↓ Po₂, ↑ LDH

ARDS, adult respiratory distress syndrome; AIDS, acquired immunodeficiency syndrome; LDH, lactate dehydrogenase; Po₂, oxygen tension.

with or without subsequent laboratory confirmation. The diagnosis in adolescents and adults, in whom the role of RSV as a pathogen is not as well recognized, usually requires specific laboratory methods. Nasal washes are superior to swabs of the throat and nasopharynx for viral isolation in cell culture (38,40). The two most widely used methods for rapid diagnosis with nasal washings are immunofluorescence staining for RSV antigen and enzyme-linked immunosorbent assays (38). Immunofluorescence assays of washings are sensitive, rapid, and may allow simultaneous screening for other respiratory pathogens, but require a trained technician, labile reagents, and a fluorescence microscope. Enzyme-linked immunosorbent assays may be slightly less sensitive than immunofluorescence techniques but are considered sensitive enough to be used in the clinical laboratory, are less operator dependent, and require no special equipment (38,82). Given the high prevalence of CMV infection in the population, serologic testing is of limited value in the diagnosis of CMV disease in adults. CMV can be identified in culture, but this finding correlates poorly with the presence of CMV disease (30,43,44,45,83). The definitive diagnosis of CMV end-organ disease usually requires the presence of the characteristic intranuclear ("owl's eye") viral inclusion bodies on tissue specimens. A presumptive diagnosis of CMV pneumonitis is frequently made based on the presence of a compatible clinical picture and either high titers of various CMV antigens in blood or tissue, or high levels of CMV DNA by quantitative PCR assays.

Among HIV-infected persons, the presence of CMV viruria or viremia suggests an increased likelihood of developing CMV end-organ disease. However, the positive predictive values for CMV viremia (35%) and CMV viruria (28%) in predicting CMV end-organ disease occurring within 6 months are low. In addition, the costs associated with surveillance viral cultures are not insignificant, and CD4$^+$ lymphocyte counts ($\leq$100 cells per mm^3) are more potent predictors of CMV disease risk (83). The distinction between situations in which evidence of active CMV infection reflects nonpathogenic virus shedding and those in which it reflects a pathogenic process can be difficult and has obvious therapeutic implications. The presence and abundance of CMV viral inclusions on lung biopsy specimens and the finding of CMV as a sole pathogen may suggest a role for antiviral therapy; the decision can occasionally be simplified by the identification of other concomitant CMV end-organ diseases (e.g., retinitis) that clearly require therapy.

The diagnosis of HPS may be difficult because of the lack of specificity of the initial symptoms (35). The diagnosis should be considered when severe respiratory symptoms follow a nonspecific febrile prodrome, especially if there is reason to suspect rodent exposure. Subsequently, the radiographic and laboratory findings may suggest the diagnosis.

Confirmatory enzyme-linked immunosorbent assays and Western blot assays have been developed (35,84). Diagnosis may be made by detecting immunoglobulin M antibody to Sin Nombre virus or a fourfold or greater increase in immunoglobulin G antibody in serum. Immunohistochemical staining has been used to identify Sin Nombre virus antigens in tissue, and reverse transcriptase polymerase chain reaction amplification has been used to identify the viral genome in tissue (33,35).

TREATMENT

Faced with a patient with apparent viral pneumonia, the physician's first task would be to attempt to identify and exclude some of the more readily treatable etiologic agents that can cause the syndrome. These include *M. pneumoniae* and *L. pneumophila*, which respond to treatment with a macrolide antibiotic such as erythromycin; *C. psittaci*, which can be treated with a tetracy-

cline; and *P. carinii*, which should be treated with trimethoprim-sulfamethoxazole or pentamidine. Guidelines for the evaluation and empiric treatment of community-acquired pneumonia have been published and are updated periodically (85,86). The therapy for most cases of influenza is supportive. Milder cases are treated with bed rest, high intake of oral fluids, and antipyretic analgesic medications such as acetaminophen. Aspirin should be avoided.

Amantadine has been licensed for use as a prophylactic agent to prevent infection with influenza type A virus. It appears to act at an early step in viral replication, probably uncoating of the RNA genome (87). Rimantadine, more recently licensed in the United States, has the same therapeutic effect as amantadine with a lower rate of side effects such as drowsiness and confusion (88,89). Amantadine has been used to treat influenza A, with resultant shortening and decreased severity of symptoms (90). Because viral syndromes probably result from multiple rounds of virus replication, it would be reasonable to expect that a drug that interferes with an early replication step would curtail the syndrome. Therefore, in patients at high risk for serious complications of influenza who have not been immunized, not only prophylaxis but also therapy with amantadine or rimantadine should be contemplated (90). Zanamivir and oceltamivir are neuraminidase inhibitors and block the release of newly budding virus from infected cells. They are about 75% effective in preventing influenza in susceptible hosts, and have been shown to truncate clinical symptoms by 1 to 2 days when used therapeutically. Zanamivir is administered as an inhaled powder and oceltamivir is an oral drug (91–93). Treatment of PIV infection is generally supportive, particularly in healthy hosts. There are currently no antiviral agents with documented clinical efficacy in the treatment of PIV infection. Ribavirin, a synthetic nucleoside analog that appears to inhibit viral messenger RNA formation and to alter cellular nucleotide pools, has *in vitro* activity against PIVs. There are anecdotal reports of clinical benefit of aerosolized ribavirin for PIV infection in infants with severe combined immunodeficiency (60,61). In an uncontrolled series, use of aerosolized ribavirin did not alter mortality among bone marrow transplant recipients with PIV infection, although delayed diagnoses and treatment may have contributed to this outcome (62). Ribavirin also has *in vitro* activity against RSV (94). Ribavirin is administered by an oxygen mask or in a hood or tent. A small-particle generator is used to create aerosols with a median diameter of 1 to 2 μm to allow distribution to the lower respiratory tract. Controlled studies have documented some beneficial effects on clinical signs, such as retractions and rales, and some significant improvements in arterial oxygen saturation. Treatment is indicated both for infants with severe lower respiratory tract RSV disease and for those with milder disease and coexisting medical conditions that increase the risk for severe disease. Ribavirin infrequently may cause reversible irritation of mucous membranes of hospital staff exposed during its aerosol administration. Reproductive and teratogenic toxic reactions have been observed in rodents but not in baboons and have not been reported in humans. Ribavirin has rarely been detected in the urine of exposed staff (94). Despite the lack of any clear suggestion of toxicity in humans, but because of the embryopathy observed in nonprimate animals, it has been recommended that pregnant women not care directly for patients receiving aerosolized ribavirin, that it be administered in a well-ventilated room, and that its administration be interrupted when the hood or tent is opened. Uncontrolled studies in immunocompromised patients suggest a potential role for RSV hyperimmune globulin or monoclonal antibody, particularly when combined with ribavirin (40).

Acyclovir and famciclovir have limited activity against CMV. Ganciclovir, foscarnet, and cidofovir have *in vitro* activity, and ganciclovir-resistant isolates generally retain susceptibility to foscarnet and cidofovir. Ganciclovir, foscarnet and cidofovir are effective in the treatment of CMV retinitis in persons with AIDS (95). Valganciclovir, a valine ester of ganciclovir with enhanced oral bioavailability, is also effective in the induction treatment for CMV retinitis and has the potential to play a role in the treatment of CMV pneumonia in immunocompromised hosts. Significant cumulative, uncontrolled experience with ganciclovir speaks for efficacy in renal transplant recipients with CMV pneumonia. However, the response of CMV pneumonia to ganciclovir among bone marrow transplant recipients has been more limited and appears to be enhanced by the addition of high-dose intravenous immunoglobulin (96). The duration of therapy required for CMV pneumonia in patients with AIDS and in transplant recipients is not well delineated. To prevent relapse, HIV-infected patients with significant immunosuppression who have CMV retinitis (and presumably those with CMV pneumonia) require ongoing, often parenteral antiviral therapy. In situations in which long-term intravenous access is a problem, they can be treated with oral ganciclovir, and potentially valganciclovir. It may be possible to discontinue anti-CMV therapy if antiretroviral therapy results in significant immune reconstitution.

The treatment of HPS is primarily supportive, with measures appropriate for noncardiogenic pulmonary edema (35,81). Both Sin Nombre virus and the related Hantaan virus, the cause of hemorrhagic fever with renal syndrome, are sensitive in cell culture to ribavirin. Intravenous ribavirin has a beneficial effect on the manifestations and mortality of hemorrhagic fever with renal syndrome (97). Corticosteroids also may diminish some of the morbidity of hemorrhagic fever with renal syndrome (98). However, in an open-label trial there were no clearly beneficial effects of intravenous ribavirin on outcomes in HPS (99). No data regarding the effect of corticosteroids on outcomes of HPS exist.

There is no specific antiviral therapy for adenovirus infection.

PREVENTION

One of the greatest advances in public health is the development of influenza vaccination. One of the greatest failures in public health is that only about one fifth of the people who should receive influenza vaccine get it (100). The U.S. Public Health Service recommends that all people over 55 years of age should be vaccinated. In addition, patients with cardiopulmonary disease, diabetes, chronic renal disease, or requirements for ongoing salicylate therapy and residents of nursing homes and chronic care facilities as well as all health-care workers should be vaccinated.

Influenza virus was isolated in 1933, and by the 1950s, vaccine virus had been produced by inoculation of embryonated hen eggs. This remains the most productive method of growing the virus, but fragmentation and purification procedures have been introduced to decrease the amount of egg protein in the vaccine. The most commonly used vaccine is a subvirion or split-virus product that has been enriched for the hemagglutinin and neuraminidase antigens. The vaccine is trivalent, containing two strains of type A and one strain of type B influenza virus chosen each year on the basis of those strains that emerge as the most prevalent at the end of the previous year. The vaccine must be given annually because of the phenomena of antigenic shift and drift and because immunity conferred by this killed subunit vaccine is short-lived. The optimal time for vaccination is in the late fall, and protection is in the range of 70%. The vaccine is safe for pregnant and immunocompromised patients, but the immunocompromised patient may not mount a protective antibody response. The only specific contraindication is allergy to egg protein (101). Amantadine, rimantadine, zanamivir and oceltamivir are about 70% effective in preventing influenza type A infections. In the face of an impending influenza A outbreak, one of these drugs should be given to any member of the high-risk populations named before who were not vaccinated in that year. Prophylaxis should be continued for the duration of the outbreak. If it is early in the influenza season, vaccination can be performed at the same time, because these drugs do not interfere with the normal antibody response (101). There are currently no effective vaccines for the PIVs. Inactivated vaccines were poorly immunogenic, and no protection was afforded. Live attenuated and subunit vaccines are being evaluated (7,9). Prevention of RSV infection in nosocomial settings requires adherence to infection control measures intended to reduce contact with infectious secretions and contaminated fomites. There is currently no vaccine available to prevent RSV. Trials of an inactivated RSV vaccine were conducted in the 1960s. Despite high antigenicity and the production of complement-fixing and neutralizing antibodies, many vaccinated children exposed to natural RSV infection developed enhanced disease, presumably owing to formation of antigen-antibody complexes on alveolar membranes (102). Alternative vaccine strategies including the use of specific viral proteins and adjuvant systems are being evaluated (103). Breast-feeding may provide infants some protection against severe RSV disease (104). Epidemiologic data suggest that breast-fed infants may have a lower risk of hospitalization for lower respiratory tract RSV infection. However, the risk reduction is by no means complete, and the specific mechanism through which protection may be conferred is uncertain.

The prophylactic monthly administration of intravenous immune globulin with high titers of RSV neutralizing antibody has been shown to reduce the frequency and severity of lower respiratory tract RSV disease among premature infants and young children with congenital heart disease or bronchopulmonary dysplasia (105). Transmission of RSV in the nosocomial setting may be diminished through implementation of and compliance with infection control measures designed to deter spread of virus from patient to patient, visitor to patient, and staff to patient. Such measures may include glove and gown precautions, the use of eye-nose goggles, the isolation or grouping of infected patients, and the use of cohort nursing (106–108). The potential for spread by gloves or hands contaminated by touching infectious secretions or environmental surfaces makes changing gloves and hand washing key means of interrupting nosocomial transmission.

Effective vaccines to prevent adenovirus infection with types 3, 4, and 7 were developed 40 years ago for use in the military population, where they are still used (26). They have not been licensed for use in the general population.

The prevention of CMV pneumonia in transplant recipients has been the focus of substantial investigation. Acyclovir, despite its limited therapeutic activity against CMV, when given intravenously or at high oral doses, reduces the frequency of CMV disease among bone marrow and renal transplant recipients but not among liver or lung transplant patients (109–110). CMV immune globulin can reduce the rate of severe CMV disease among renal, bone marrow, and liver transplant recipients but not among seronegative recipients of seropositive liver transplants (30,43,111). Prophylactic intravenous ganciclovir has been shown to significantly reduce the occurrence of CMV disease among allogeneic bone marrow transplant recipients, but neutropenia is a frequent complication (112). Oral ganciclovir has been shown to be effective in preventing CMV disease in recipients of seropositive liver or kidney transplants (113–114), and is commonly employed by many transplant centers (115). The role of valganciclovir prophylaxis is under evaluation. Among

HIV-infected persons with CD4$^+$ lymphocyte counts less than 100 per mm^3, oral ganciclovir reduces the frequency of CMV disease (116), but given issues of cost, pill burden, adherence, and the facts that CMV disease can be successfully detected early and treated and that effective anti-HIV therapy can promote immune reconstitution and reduce CMV disease risk, it is generally not used. The frequency with which prophylactic antiviral therapy may select for resistant CMV isolates is not fully known, and the potential for its doing so remains a significant concern. The strategy of limiting CMV prophylaxis to transplant patients with signs of active CMV replication detected by screening periodically for CMV antigenemia or for quantitative measures of CMV DNA in blood by PCR surveillance and instituting "preemptive" antiviral agents if screening tests are positive appears to be effective and well tolerated (110). However, whether routine prophylaxis of transplant patients or periodic screening with targeted antiviral therapy represents a more effective strategy remains unresolved (117). Measures to prevent HPS consist of rodent control and of attempts to reduce the likelihood of exposure to infected rodents and their secretions (35). Rodent infestation may be prevented or eliminated through the use of traps and rodenticides and by altering potential rodent habitats to make them less accessible. The risk to those potentially exposed during occupational and leisure activities may be diminished through avoiding rodent burrows, infested shelters, or potentially contaminated water; by using masks with high-efficiency particulate air filters when cleaning out potentially rodent-infested areas; and by burying, burning, or disposing of all trash in sealed containers to limit rodent food sources. There is no hantavirus vaccine, and there is no information on post-exposure prophylaxis. Universal precautions are appropriate in handling specimens from potentially infected patients.

A wide range of viruses are newly or increasingly recognized as rare or occasional causes of pneumonia, particularly in highly immunocompromised patients, such as transplant recipients or those with HIV infection or leukemia, including enteroviruses, rhinoviruses, herpes simplex, human metapneumovirus, and human herpesvirus 6, 7, and 8 (122).

SEVERE ACUTE RESPIRATORY SYNDROME

In late 2002 and early 2003, cases of severe, life threatening pneumonia not attributable to any previously recognized pathogens appeared in Southeast Asia and, shortly thereafter, in numerous countries throughout the world. The term "severe acute respiratory syndrome" (SARS) was adopted and a novel coronavirus was implicated as the pathogen (118). The clinical presentation includes fever, headache, malaise, rigors, and myalgias followed by a dry cough, shifting radiographic infiltrates, and dyspnea that may progress to hypoxemia and respiratory failure (119–121). The mortality may be 4% to 7% (119–121). SARS is spread person-to-person by droplets, but roles for contact, and in some circumstances airborne, transmission have not been excluded. Use of surgical or N95 masks (rather than paper masks) and contact precautions (masks, gowns, and handwashing) appear to be effective in reducing the risk of transmission (122). Further updated information is available on the Centers for Disease Control and Prevention and World Health Organization websites (*www.cdc.gov/ncidod/sars* and *www.who.int/ed/*, respectively).

REFERENCES

1. Choi K, Thacker SB. Mortality influenza epidemics in the United States, 1967–1978. *Am J Public Health* 1982;72:1280–1283.
2. Kilbourne ED. Epidemiology of influenza. In: Kilbourne ED, ed. *Influenza viruses and influenza.* New York: Academic, 1975:483.
3. Wells DL, Hopfensperger DJ, Arden NH, et al. Swine influenza virus infections. Transmission from ill pigs to humans at a Wisconsin agricultural fair and subsequent probable person-to-person transmission. *JAMA* 1991;265:478–481.
4. McIntosh K. Pathogenesis of severe acute respiratory infections in the developing world: respiratory syncytial virus and parainfluenza viruses. *Rev Infect Dis* 1991;131(suppl 6):492–500.
5. Centers for Disease Control and Prevention. Respiratory syncytial virus and parainfluenza virus surveillance—United States, 1989–90. *MMWR* 1990;39:832–833, 839.
6. Henrickson KJ, Kuhn SM, Savatski LM. Epidemiology and cost of infection with human parainfluenza virus types 1 and 2 in young children. *Clin Infect Dis* 1994;18:770–779.
7. Vainionpaa R, Hyypia T. Biology of parainfluenza viruses. *Clin Microbiol Rev* 1994;7:265–275.
8. Warner JL. Parainfluenza viruses. In: Balows A, Hausler WJ, Herrmann KL, et al., eds. *Manual of clinical microbiology,* 5th ed. Washington, DC: American Society for Microbiology, 1991:878–882.
9. Henrickson K, Ray R, Belshe R. Parainfluenza viruses. In: Mandell GL, Bennett JE, Dolin R, eds. *Mandell, Douglas and Bennett's principles and practice of infectious diseases,* 4th ed. New York: Churchill Livingstone, 1995:1489–1496.
10. Henrickson KJ, Savtski LL. Genetic variation and evolution of human parainfluenza virus type 1 hemagglutinin neuraminidase: analysis of 12 clinical isolates. *J Infect Dis* 1992;166:995–1005.
11. Knott AM, Long CE, Hall CB. Parainfluenza viral infections in pediatric outpatients: seasonal patterns and clinical characteristics. *Pediatr Infect Dis J* 1993;13:269–273.
12. Glezen WP, Frank AL, Taber LH, et al. Parainfluenza virus type 3: seasonality and risk of infection and reinfection in young children. *J Infect Dis* 1984;150:851–857.
13. Rubin EE, Quennec P, McDonald JC. Infections due to parainfluenza virus type 4 in children. *Clin Infect Dis* 1993;17:998–1002.
14. Ansari SA, Springthorpe VS, Sattar SA, et al. Potential role of hands in the spread of respiratory viral infections: studies with human parainfluenza virus 3 and rhinovirus 14. *J Clin Microbiol* 1991;29:2115–2119.
15. Karron RA, O'Brien KL, Froehlich JL, et al. Molecular epidemiology of a parainfluenza type 3 virus outbreak on a pediatric ward. *J Infect Dis* 1993;167:1441–1445.
16. Gilchrist S, Torok TJ, Gary HE, et al. National surveillance for respiratory syncytial virus, United States, 1985–1990. *J Infect Dis* 1994;170:986–990.
17. Centers for Disease Control and Prevention. Update: respiratory syncytial virus activity—United States, 1994–1995 season. *MMWR* 1994;43:920–922.
18. Anderson LJ, Parker RA, Strikas RL. Association between respiratory syncytial virus outbreaks and lower respiratory tract deaths of infants and young children. *J Infect Dis* 1990;161:640–646.
19. Anderson LJ, Hendry RM, Pierik LT, et al. Multicenter study of strains of respiratory syncytial virus. *J Infect Dis* 1991;163:687–692.
20. Henderson FW, Collier AM, Clyde WA, et al. Respiratory-syncytial-virus infections, reinfections and immunity: a prospective, longitudinal study in young children. *N Engl J Med* 1979;300:530–534.
21. Glezen WP, Taber LH, Frank AL, et al. Risk of primary infection and reinfection with respiratory syncytial virus. *Am J Dis Child* 1986;140:543–546.
22. Agius G, Dindinaud G, Biggar RJ, et al. An epidemic of respiratory syncytial virus (RSV) in elderly people: clinical and serologic findings. *J Med Virol* 1990;30:117–127.
23. Hall CB, Geiman JM, Biggar R, et al. Respiratory syncytial virus infections within families. *N Engl J Med* 1976;294:414–419.
24. Hall CB, Douglas RG Jr, Geiman JM. Possible transmission by fomites of respiratory syncytial virus. *J Infect Dis* 1980;141:98–102.
25. Baum SG. Adenovirus. In: Mandell GL, Bennett JE, Dolin R, eds. *Mandell, Douglas and Bennett's principles and practice of infectious diseases,* 4th ed. New York: Churchill Livingstone, 1995:1382–1387.
26. Dudding BA, Top FH Jr, Winter PE, et al. Acute respiratory disease in military trainees: the adenovirus surveillance program 1966–1971. *Am J Epidemiol* 1973;97:187–198.
27. Stalder H, Hierholzer JC, Oxman MN. New human adenovirus (candidate adenovirus type 35) causing fatal disseminated infection in a renal transplant recipient. *J Clin Microbiol* 1977;6:257–265.
28. Hierholzer JC, Wigand R, Anderson LJ. Adenoviruses from patients with AIDS: a plethora of serotypes and a description of five new serotypes of subgenus D (types 43–47). *J Infect Dis* 1988;158:804–813.
29. Forbes BA. Acquisition of cytomegalovirus infection: an update. *Clin Microbiol Rev* 1989;2:204–216.
30. Ho M. Cytomegalovirus. In: Mandell GL, Bennett JE, Dolin R, eds. *Mandell, Douglas and Bennett's principles and practice of infectious diseases,* 4th ed. New York: Churchill Livingstone, 1995:1351–1364.
31. Centers for Disease Control and Prevention. Outbreak of acute illness—Southwestern United States, 1993. *MMWR* 1993;42:421–424.
32. Nichol ST, Spiropoulou CF, Morzunov S, et al. Genetic identification of a hantavirus associated with an outbreak of acute respiratory illness. *Science* 1993;262:914–917.
33. Zaki SR, Greer PW, Coffield LM, et al. Hantavirus pulmonary syndrome: pathogenesis of an emerging infectious disease. *Am J Pathol* 1995;146:552–579.

34. Childs JE, Ksiazek TG, Spiropoulou CF, et al. Serologic and genetic identification of *Peromyscus maniculatus* as the primary rodent reservoir for a new hantavirus in the Southwestern United States. *J Infect Dis* 1994;169:1271–1280.
35. Butler JC, Peters CJ. Hantaviruses and hantavirus pulmonary syndrome. *Clin Infect Dis* 1994;19:387–395.
36. Kitsutani PT, Denton RW, Curtis CL, et al. Acute sin nombre hantavirus infection without pulmonary syndrome, United States. *Emerg Infect Dis* 1999;5:701–705.
37. Schulze IT. The biologically active proteins of influenza virus: the hemagglutinin. In: Kilbourne ED, ed. *The influenza viruses and influenza.* New York: Academic, 1975:53.
38. Welliver RC. Detection, pathogenesis, and therapy of respiratory syncytial virus infections. *Clin Microbiol Rev* 1988;1:27–39.
39. Garofalo R, Kimpen JLL, Welliver RC, et al. Eosinophil degranulation in the respiratory tract during naturally acquired respiratory syncytial virus infection. *J Pediatr* 1992;120:28–32.
40. Hall CB. Respiratory syncytial virus and parainfluenza virus. *N Engl J Med* 2001;344:1917–1928.
41. Rowe WP, Huebner RJ, Gillmore LK, et al. Isolation of a cytopathogenic human adenoids undergoing spontaneous degeneration in tissue culture. *Proc Soc Exp Biol Med* 1953;84:570–573.
42. Balthesen M, Meesserle M, Reddehase MJ. Lungs are a major organ site of cytomegalovirus latency. *J Virol* 1993;67:5360–5366.
43. Grundy JE. Virologic and pathogenic aspects of cytomegalovirus infection. *Rev Infect Dis* 1990;12(suppl 7):711–719.
44. Meyers JD, Flournoy N, Thomas ED. Risk factors for cytomegalovirus infection after human bone marrow transplantation. *J Infect Dis* 1986;153:478–488.
45. Chou S. Acquisition of donor strains of cytomegalovirus by renal-transplant recipients. *N Engl J Med* 1986;314:1418–1423.
46. Wingard JR, Mellitis ED, Sostrin MB, et al. Interstitial pneumonitis after allogeneic bone marrow transplantation. Nine year experience at a single institution. *Medicine (Baltimore)* 1988;67:175–186.
47. Mori M, Rothman AL, Kurane I, et al. High levels of cytokine-producing cells in the lung tissues of patients with fatal hantavirus pulmonary syndrome. *J Infect Dis* 1999;179:295–302.
48. Palese P, Tobita K, Ueda M, et al. Characterization of temperature sensitive influenza virus mutants defective in neuraminidase. *Virology* 1974;61:397–410.
49. Naficy K. Human influenza with proved viremia. *N Engl J Med* 1963;269:964–966.
50. Stanley ED, Jackson GG. Viremia in Asian influenza. *Trans Assoc Am Physicians* 1966;79:376–387.
51. Louria DB, Blumenfield HL, Ellis JT, et al. Studies on influenza in the pandemic of 1957–1958. II. Pulmonary complications of influenza. *J Clin Invest* 1959;38:213–265.
52. Schwarzmann SW, Adler JL Sullivan RF Jr, et al. Bacterial pneumonia during the Hong Kong influenza epidemic of 1968–1969. *Arch Intern Med* 1971;127:1037–1041.
53. Proby CM, Hackett D, Gupta S, et al. Acute myopericarditis in influenza A infection. *Q J Med* 1986;60:887–892.
54. Flewett TH, Hoult JG. Influenzal encephalopathy and postinfluenzal encephalitis. *Lancet* 1958;2:11–15.
55. Wells CEC, James WRL, Evans AD. Guillain-Barré syndrome and virus of influenza A (Asian strain). *Arch Neurol Psychiatry* 1959;81:699–705.
56. Sperber SJ, Francis JB. Toxic shock syndrome during an influenza outbreak. *JAMA* 1987;257:1086–1087.
57. Forsyth BW, Horwitz RI, Acampora D, et al. New epidemiologic evidence confirming that bias does not explain the aspirin–Reye's syndrome association. *JAMA* 1989;261:2517–2524.
58. Hurwitz ES, Nelson DB, Davis C, et al. National surveillance for Reye syndrome: a five-year review. *Pediatrics* 1982;6:895–900.
59. Wenzel RP, McCormick DP, Beam WE. Parainfluenza pneumonia in adults. *JAMA* 1971;221:294–295.
60. Gelfand EW, McCurdy D, Rao CP, et al. Ribavirin treatment of viral pneumonitis in severe combined immunodeficiency syndrome. *Lancet* 1983;2:732–733.
61. McIntosh K, Kurachek SC, Cairns LM, et al. Treatment of respiratory viral infection in an immunodeficient infant with ribavirin aerosol. *Am J Dis Child* 1984;138:305–308.
62. Wendt CH, Weisdorf DJ, Jordan C, et al. Parainfluenza virus respiratory infection after bone marrow transplantation. *N Engl J Med* 1992;326:921–926.
63. Josephs S, Kim HK, Prandt CD, et al. Parainfluenza 3 virus and other common respiratory pathogens in children with human immunodeficiency virus infection. *Pediatr Infect Dis J* 1988;7:207–209.
64. Groothius JR, Gutierrez KM, Lauer BA. Respiratory syncytial virus infection in children with bronchopulmonary dysplasia. *Pediatrics* 1988;82:199–203.
65. Chandwani S, Borkowsky W, Krasinski K, et al. Respiratory syncytial virus infection in human immunodeficiency virus–infected children. *J Pediatr* 1990;117:251–254.
66. King JC Jr, Burke AR, Clemens JD, et al. Respiratory syncytial virus illnesses in human immunodeficiency virus- and noninfected children. *Pediatr Infect Dis J* 1993;12:733–739.
67. Englund JA, Sullivan CJ, Jordan C, et al. Respiratory syncytial virus infection in immunocompromised adults. *Ann Intern Med* 1988;109:203–208.
68. Hertz MI, Englund JA, Snover D, et al. Respiratory syncytial virus–induced acute lung injury in adult patients with bone marrow transplants: a clinical approach and review of the literature. *Medicine (Baltimore)* 1989;68:269–281.
69. Harrington RD, Hooton TM, Hackman RC, et al. An outbreak of respiratory syncytial virus in a bone marrow transplant center. *J Infect Dis* 1992;165:987–993.
70. Whimbey E, Crouch RB, Englund JA, et al. Respiratory syncytial virus pneumonia in hospitalized adults with leukemia. *Clin Infect Dis* 1995;21:376–379.
71. Klemola E, Stenstrom R, von Essen R. Pneumonia as a clinical manifestation of cytomegalovirus infection in previously healthy adults. *Scand J Infect Dis* 1972;4:7–10.
72. Cohen JI, Corey GR. Cytomegalovirus infection in the normal host. *Medicine (Baltimore)* 1985;64:100–114.
73. Stagno S, Brasfield DM, Brown MB, et al. Infant pneumonitis associated with cytomegalovirus, *Chlamydia, Pneumocystis,* and *Ureaplasma:* a prospective study. *Pediatrics* 1981;68:322–329.
74. Smith CB. Cytomegalovirus pneumonia: state of the art. *Chest* 1989;95:182S–187S.
75. Smyth RL, Scott JP, Borysiewicz LK, et al. Cytomegalovirus infection in heart-lung transplant recipients: risk factors, clinical associations, and response to treatment. *J Infect Dis* 1991;164:1045–1050.
76. Millar AB, Patou G, Miller RF, et al. Cytomegalovirus in the lungs of patients with AIDS: respiratory pathogen or passenger? *Am Rev Respir Dis* 1990;141:1474–1477.
77. Jacobson MA, Mills J, Rush J, et al. Morbidity and mortality of patients with AIDS and first-episode *Pneumocystis carinii* pneumonia unaffected by concomitant pulmonary cytomegalovirus infection. *Am Rev Respir Dis* 1991;144:6–9.
78. Wallace JM, Hannah J. Cytomegalovirus pneumonitis in patients with AIDS: findings in an autopsy series. *Chest* 1987;92:198–203.
79. Squire SB, Lipman MCI, Bagdades EK, et al. Severe cytomegalovirus pneumonitis in HIV infected patients with higher than average CD4 counts. *Thorax* 1992;47:301–304.
80. Lundgren JD, Vestbo J, Junge J, et al. CMV pneumonia and response to ganciclovir treatment in an AIDS patient. *Respir Med* 1991;85:437–439.
81. Duchin JS, Koster FT, Peters CJ, et al. Hantavirus pulmonary syndrome: a clinical description of 17 patients with a newly recognized syndrome. *N Engl J Med* 1994;330:949–955.
82. Ketai LH, Williamson MR, Telepak RJ, et al. Hantavirus pulmonary syndrome: radiographic finding in 16 patients. *Radiology* 1994;191:665–668.
83. Zurlo JJ, O'Neill D, Polis MA, et al. Lack of utility of cytomegalovirus blood and urine cultures in patients with HIV infection. *Ann Intern Med* 1993;118:12–17.
84. Centers for Disease Control and Prevention. Progress in the development of *Hantavirus* diagnostic assays–United States. *MMWR* 1993;42:770–771.
85. Bartlett JG, Breiman RF, Mandell LA, et al. Community-acquired pneumonia in adults: guidelines for management. *Clin Infect Dis* 1998;26:811–838.
86. American Thoracic Society. Guidelines for the management of adults with community-acquired pneumonia: diagnosis, assessment of severity, antimicrobial therapy, and prevention. *Am J Respir Crit Care Med* 2001;163:1730–1754.
87. Skehel JJ, Hay AJ, Armstrong JA. On the mechanism of inhibition of influenza virus replication by amantadine hydrochloride. *J Gen Virol* 1977;38:97–110.
88. Dolin R, Reichman RC, Madore HP, et al. A controlled trial of amantadine and rimantadine in the prophylaxis of influenza A infection. *N Engl J Med* 1982;307:580–584.
89. Hayden FG, Gwaltney JM Jr, Van de Castle RL. Comparative toxicity of amantadine hydrochloride and rimantadine hydrochloride in healthy adults. *Antimicrob Agents Chemother* 1981;19:226–233.
90. Younkin SW, Betts RF, Roth FK, et al. Reduction in fever and symptoms in young adults with influenza A/Brazil/78 H1N1 infection after treatment with aspirin or amantadine. *Antimicrob Agents Chemother* 1983;23:577–582.
91. Hayden FG, Osterhaus AD, Treanor JJ, et al. Efficacy and safety of the neuraminidase inhibitor zanamivir in the treatment of influenzavirus infections. GG167 Influenza Study Group. *N Engl J Med* 1997;337:874–880.
92. Monto AS, Robinson DP, Herlocher ML, et al. Zanamivir in the prevention of influenza among healthy adults: a randomized controlled trial. *JAMA* 1999;282:31–35.
93. Hayden FG, Atmar RL, Schilling M, et al. Use of selective oral neuraminidase inhibitor oceltamivir to prevent influenza. *N Engl J Med* 1999;341:1336–1343.
94. Committee on Infectious Diseases. Use of ribavirin in the treatment of respiratory syncytial virus infection. *Pediatrics* 1993;92:501–504.
95. AIDS Clinical Trials Group. Mortality in patients with the acquired immunodeficiency syndrome treated with either ganciclovir or foscarnet for cytomegalovirus retinitis. *N Engl J Med* 1992;326:213–220.
96. Emanuel D, Cunningham I, Jules-Elysee K, et al. Cytomegalovirus pneumonia after bone marrow transplantation successfully treated with the combination of ganciclovir and high-dose intravenous immune globulin. *Ann Intern Med* 1988;109:777–782.
97. Huggins JW, Hsiang CM, Cosgriff TM, et al. Prospective, double-blinded, concurrent, placebo-controlled clinical trial of intravenous ribavirin therapy of hemorrhagic fever with renal syndrome. *J Infect Dis* 1991;164:1119–1127.
98. Sayer WJ, Entwhisleg, Uyeno B, et al. Cortisone therapy of early epidemic hemorrhagic fever: a preliminary report. *Ann Intern Med* 1955;42:839–851.
99. Chapman LE, Mertz GJ, Peters CJ, et al. Intravenous ribavirin for hantavirus pulmonary syndrome: safety and tolerance during 1 year of open-label experience. Ribavirin Study Group. *Antiviral Ther* 1999;4:211–219.
100. Nichol KL, Margolis KL, Wourenma J, et al. The efficacy and cost effectiveness of vaccination against influenza among elderly persons living in the community. *N Engl J Med* 1994;331:778–784.

101. Centers for Disease Control and Prevention. Prevention and control of influenza recommendations of the Advisory Committee on Immunization Practices (ACIP). *MMWR* 1995;44(RR-3):1–22.
102. Kapikian AZ, Mitchell RH, Chanock RM, et al. An epidemiologic study of altered clinical reactivity to respiratory syncytial (RS) virus infection in children previously vaccinated with an inactivated RS vaccine. *Am J Epidemiol* 1969;89:405–421.
103. Dudas RA, Karron RA. Respiratory syncytial virus vaccines. *Clin Microbiol Rev* 1998;11:430–439.
104. Pullan CR, Toms GL, Martin AJ, et al. Breast feeding and respiratory syncytial virus infection. *BMJ* 1980;281:1034–1036.
105. Groothuis JR, Simoes EAF, Levin MJ, et al. Prophylactic administration of respiratory syncytial virus immune globulin to high risk infants and young children. *N Engl J Med* 1993;329:1524–1530.
106. Leclair JM, Freeman J, Sullivan BF, et al. Prevention of nosocomial respiratory syncytial virus infections through compliance with glove and gown isolation precautions. *N Engl J Med* 1987;317:329–334.
107. Madge P, Paton JY, McColl JH, et al. Prospective controlled study of four infection-control procedures to prevent nosocomial infection with respiratory syncytial virus. *Lancet* 1992;340:1079–1083.
108. Gala CL, Hall CB, Schnabel KC, et al. The use of eye-nose goggles to control nosocomial respiratory syncytial virus infection. *JAMA* 1986;256:2706–2708.
109. Meyers JD, Reed EC, Shepp DH, et al. Acyclovir for prevention of cytomegalovirus infection and disease after allogeneic marrow transplantation. *N Engl J Med* 1988;318:70–71.
110. Singh N, Yu VL, Mieles L, et al. High-dose acyclovir compared with short-course preemptive ganciclovir therapy to prevent cytomegalovirus disease in liver transplant recipients: a randomized trial. *Ann Intern Med* 1994;120:375–381.
111. Winston DJ, Ho WG, Cheng-Hsien L, et al. Intravenous immune globulin for prevention of cytomegalovirus infection and interstitial pneumonia after bone marrow transplantation. *Ann Intern Med* 1987;106:12–18.
112. Goodrich JM, Bowden RA, Fisher L, et al. Ganciclovir prophylaxis to prevent cytomegalovirus disease after allogeneic marrow transplant. *Ann Intern Med* 1993;118:173–178.
113. Brennan DC, Garlock KA, Singer GG, et al. Prophylactic oral ganciclovir compared with deferred therapy for control of cytomegalovirus in renal transplant recipients. *Transplantation* 1997;66:1843–1846.
114. Gane EF, Saliba GJ, Valdecaas OGJ, et al. Randomised trial of efficacy and safety of oral ganciclovir in the prevention of cytomegalovirus disease in liver-transplant recipients. *Lancet* 1997;350:1729–1733.
115. Avery RK, Adal KA, Longworth DL, et al. A survey of allogeneic bone marrow transplant programs in the United States regarding cytomegalovirus prophylaxis and pre-emptive therapy. *Bone Marrow Transplant* 2000;26:763–767.
116. Spector SA, McKinley GF, Lalezari JP, et al. Oral ganciclovir for the prevention of cytomegalovirus disease in persons with AIDS. *N Engl J Med* 1996;334:1491–1497.
117. Singh N. Premptive therapy versus universal prophylaxis with ganciclovir for cytomegalovirus in solid organ transplant recipients. *Clin Infect Dis* 2001;32:742–751.
118. Peiris JSM, Lai ST, Poon LLM, et al. Coronavirus as a possible cause of severe acute respiratory syndrome. *Lancet* 2003;361:1319–1325.
119. Tsang KW, Ho PL, Ooi GC, et al. A cluster of cases of severe acute respiratory syndrome in Hong Kong. *N Engl J Med* 2003;348:1977–1985.
120. Lee N, Hyui D, Wu A, et al. A major outbreak of severe acute respiratory syndrome in Hong Kong. *N Engl J Med* 2003;348:1986–1994.
121. Poutanen SM, Low DE, Henry B, et al. Identification of severe acute respiratory syndrome in Canada. *N Engl J Med* 2003;348:1995–2005.
122. Seto WH, Tsang D, Yung RWH, et al. Effectiveness of precautions against droplets and contact in prevention of nosocomial transmission of severe acute respiratory syndrome (SARS). *Lancet* 2003;361:1519–1520.

CHAPTER 52

Mycoplasma Pneumonia

Maurice A. Mufson

HISTORY

Mycoplasma pneumoniae was isolated and recognized as the etiologic agent of Mycoplasmal pneumonia in the 1960s. Eaton first attempted to isolate a pathogen from persons with "primary atypical pneumonia" (PAP) in the 1940s. Then, PAP encompassed a diverse group of nonbacterial pneumonias of undefined causes characterized by patchy infiltrates on chest radiography, rather than lobar consolidation as in bacterial pneumonia,

and a lack of response to the few available antimicrobial drugs available. Although Eaton proved the presence of an infectious pathogen in sputum from persons with PAP because intranasal inoculation of cotton rats with such sputum caused pneumonia, he failed to isolate a pathogen (1,2). A few years later, Liu demonstrated the pathogen (designated the "Eaton agent" and later renamed *Mycoplasma pneumoniae*) in embryonated eggs experimentally infected with sputum from persons with PAP using an indirect immunofluorescence procedure (3). Subsequently, Chanock and colleagues succeeded in isolating *M. pneumoniae* on agar from the sputum of persons with serologically confirmed *M. pneumoniae* pneumonia, establishing it as the first *Mycoplasma* species pathogenic for humans (4–6).

MICROBIOLOGY

M. pneumoniae belongs to the class Mollicutes, order Mycoplasmatales, family Mycoplasmataceae, and genus *Mycoplasma* (7). The smallest organisms capable of replicating on complex cell-free medium, mycoplasmas lack a cell wall, require cholesterol for growth and divide by binary fission. *M. pneumoniae* also metabolizes glucose, exhibits hemadsorption, is motile, and produces hydrogen peroxide and superoxide anion. The GC content of *M. pneumoniae* is approximately 40 mol%, higher than for any other *Mycoplasma* species (7).

The genome of *M. pneumoniae* comprises about 816394 base pairs, with 677 putative coding sequences (open reading frames); the sequence of the complete genome is available on GenBank (www.ncbi.nlm.gov) (8). It contains one ribosomal ribonucleic acid (rRNA) operon, and its RNA gene order is 5'-16S-23S-5S-3' (9). *M. pneumoniae* contains several specific proteins of molecular masses 168/170, 130, 110, 92, 90, 45, and 35 kDa, two of which are adhesins (7). The P1 adhesin protein (168/170 kDa) and a P30 adhesin (30 kDa) mediate attachment to cells by recognition of either sulfated glycolipids or α_{2-3}-linked sialyloligosaccharides on glycoproteins (10–13). Erythrocyte binding requires only the α_{2-3}-linked-sialyloligosaccharide receptor; sialoglycolipids inhibit adhesion of *M. pneumoniae* to erythrocytes (14–16). Two distinct genomic types of *M. pneumoniae* have been classified based on variation of the gene encoding P1 adhesin protein, type 1 (prototype strain PI 1428) and type 2 (prototype strain MAC), which differ by substantial sequence variation (12,13,17,18). Restriction fragment length profile also identified five subtypes of the P1 of type 1 and three subtypes of the P1 of type 2 (12,13). The P1 adhesin resides on the tiplike configuration of *M. pneumoniae*. The gene for the P1 protein has been cloned, the amino acid sequence deduced, and a single 13-amino acid site-specific epitope synthesized that reacts with a cytadherence-blocking monoclonal antibody (8,19,20). In *M. pneumoniae*, cytadherence undergoes spontaneous reversible switching involving five high-molecular-weight proteins (9).

EPIDEMIOLOGY

M. pneumoniae occurs endemically and sometimes epidemically at 4- to 7-year intervals among all age groups (21). Pneumonia develops in 3% to 10% of persons infected with *M. pneumoniae*. It accounts for approximately 5% to 15% of all community-acquired pneumonias, although the rate may be two to three times higher in high-risk groups. The incidence of community-acquired *M. pneumoniae* pneumonia among adults is approximately 15 per 100,000 persons (22). It occurs commonly in children and young adults, causing approximately one-third to two-thirds of the pneumonias in these groups; peak incidence of *M. pneumoniae* pneumonia occurs among teenagers (21). Approximately 5% of patients with mycoplasmal pneumonia require in-hospital care (22,23).

M. pneumoniae spreads by infectious droplets. Particles less than 5 nm in diameter reach the lungs and the larger droplets deposit on the nasal and upper respiratory tract passages. It spreads slowly, especially in families and in semiclosed populations during several months. Persons in semi-closed populations not yet affected during a *M. pneumoniae* outbreak may be prevented from becoming ill by administering azithromycin prophylaxis (24). The incubation period of *M. pneumoniae* is approximately 3 weeks. School-age children introduce the organism into the household and eventually it spreads to all susceptible family members. Pneumonia may develop in as many as one-half of family members.

PATHOGENESIS

The pathogenic mechanisms of *M. pneumoniae* involve several components including the attachment of cytadhesins, the secretion of hydrogen peroxide and superoxide anion, and the formation of autoantibodies (25). *M. pneumoniae* attaches to the ciliated epithelium of the respiratory tract by two adhesins, one of which is the P1 protein, that bind to α_{2-3}-linked sialyloligosaccharides of glycoproteins and to $Gal(3SO_4)\beta 1$ residues of sulfated glycolipids. These sites are abundant in the bronchial epithelium (10,26,27). The close attachment of the organism through these cytadherence receptors probably promotes its destructive effects on ciliated cells. The P1 protein evokes a homologous antibody response (28). The formation of complexes between the receptors of host cells and the organism may be the stimulus for the formation of a number of autoantibodies in *M. pneumoniae* infection (14,29–31). *M. pneumoniae* attaches to erythrocytes also by means of the α_{2-3}-linked sialyloligosaccharides of Ii antigen, and these complexes may induce the formation of cold hemagglutinins (16,18). Circulating autoantibodies may be involved in the pulmonary and extrapulmonary manifestations of *M. pneumoniae* infection (10).

Hydrogen peroxide and superoxide anion produced by *M. pneumoniae* damage respiratory tract cells and erythrocytes (32,33). Viable organisms inhibit catalase activity of host cells, thus averting inactivation of the peroxide and superoxide anion. Circulating and cell surface antibodies may also influence recovery from *M. pneumoniae* infection (5). Cellular immunity may be implicated in recovery from infection; because *M. pneumoniae* induces release of interferon from human lymphocytes (33).

CLINICAL MANIFESTATIONS

Mycoplasmal pneumonia begins insidiously, with fever, nonproductive cough, chills, headache, and malaise. Several days elapse before the patient seeks medical care (Table 52.1). More than one-half of patients suffer all of these symptoms (34–36). Nearly all patients experience fever, usually a temperature between 100°F and 103°F, accompanied by a chilly sensation, but frank shaking chills do not occur. After a few days, cough becomes productive of small amounts of white mucoid or watery sputum. Hemoptysis rarely occurs. The paucity of physical findings at the beginning of the pneumonia contrasts with its apparent severity. Rales and rhonchi develop in more than three-fourths of patients, often appearing several days after the onset. Rhinorrhea, myal-

---

TABLE 52.1. Salient Clinical Features of Mycoplasmal Pneumonia

Onset is insidious with cough, fever, headache, chills, and malaise.
Mucoid sputum develops several days later.
Sputum is rarely blood tinged.
Rhonchi and rales appear, usually several days after first physical examination.
On radiographic examination, pneumonic infiltrates appear diffusely reticulonodular or interstitial, often leading from the hilum to the lung base.
The pneumonia is unilateral in most cases; in approximately one fourth of cases, it is bilateral.
Pleural effusion may be present in about one fifth of cases.
Leukocytosis occurs in about one fourth of cases.
Cold hemagglutinins develop in about one half of cases, usually in the more serious illnesses.
Other organ systems are infrequently involved.
Treatment with tetracycline or erythromycin effectively reduces the duration of symptoms and signs and shortens the duration of illness; however, shedding of *M. pneumoniae* continues for 1 or 2 wk after antibiotic treatment is begun.
Fatalities rarely occur.

---

gias, chest pain, sore throat, and hoarseness occur in one-fourth to one-half of patients. Tympanitis or bullous myringitis develop in only a few patients (37).

Untreated mycoplasmal pneumonia abates in 10 to 14 days; in a minority of patients, the course of illness may be protracted, lasting as long as 6 weeks (6). Some patients experience persistent cough, and about one fifth of patients manifest radiographic abnormalities for up to four months (6). Pleural effusions develop in about one-fourth of pneumonias among adults. Small pleural effusions develop in approximately one-half of the cases among children (38). Rarely, *M. pneumoniae* can be isolated from pleural fluid (39). Interleukin-18 (IL-18) levels form in pleural fluid of *M. pneumoniae* pneumonia, possibly related to fibrotic changes in the lungs, and *M. pneumoniae* deoxyribonucleic acid could be detected in the pleural fluid of these cases and other cases of pleuritis with polymerase chain reaction (40,41). In nearly all instances, mycoplasmal pneumonia heals without pulmonary sequelae. Pulmonary complications occur rarely and include residual pleural abnormalities, lung abscesses, lobar consolidation, necrotizing pneumonitis, severe respiratory failure, and adult respiratory distress syndrome (42–45). Fatal infection occurs rarely (45,46).

The differential diagnosis of mycoplasmal pneumonia includes psittacosis; Q fever; and common viral pneumonias, especially influenza virus pneumonia, *Legionella* pneumonia, and *Chlamydia pneumoniae* pneumonia. These pneumonias can cause similar clinical features and radiographic findings. Bacterial pneumonia should be considered in the differential diagnosis, because mycoplasmal pneumonia uncommonly shows a lobar pattern at radiography. Mycoplasmal pneumonia may present as an apical pneumonia mimicking pulmonary tuberculosis.

Mycoplasmal pneumonia tends to occur in one lung, more often the right lung, and in the lower lobes. The infiltrates appear diffusely reticulonodular or interstitial, segmental or non-segmental, and often appear as streaks from the hilum to the base (47). Bilateral pneumonia develops in one-fourth of patients, sometimes involving both hilar regions and producing a "butterfly-like" infiltrate. Modest pleural effusions are found at radiography in approximately one-fourth of adults with *M. pneumoniae* pneumonia, but an associated pleuritis occurs uncommonly.

The results of routine clinical laboratory tests are normal in the majority of cases of mycoplasmal pneumonia. However, leukocytosis develops in approximately one-fourth of patients, and an elevated erythrocyte sedimentation rate develops in approximately one-third of patients.

Serious extrapulmonary complications of *M. pneumoniae* infection occur at exceedingly low rates. About one per 1,000 *M. pneumoniae* infections becomes complicated by central nervous system disease (48). The leading complications involve diverse central nervous system diseases, mainly meningoencephalitis, meningitis, and encephalitis and rarely acute cerebellar ataxia, cranial nerve neuritis, Guillain-Barré syndrome, and mononeuritis multiplex with brachial plexus neuropathy (49–55). Uncommon complications include pericarditis, nephritis, Stevens-Johnson syndrome, erythema nodosum, aplastic anemia, and cold hemagglutinin–mediated hemolytic anemia (56–61). The altered immune reactivity in *M. pneumoniae* infection may contribute to the pathogenesis of extrapulmonary involvement (10,27).

DIAGNOSIS

A specific laboratory diagnosis of *M. pneumoniae* infection can be made by isolation on agar of the organism from sputum, throat swab, pleural fluid, or tissue; demonstration of a diagnostic rise in antibody to *M. pneumoniae* during convalescence by complement fixation, enzyme-linked immunosorbent assay or latex agglutination assay; detection of a high-titer immunoglobulin M- or immunoglobulin A-specific antibody to *M. pneumoniae* in an acute-phase serum specimen; or amplification of genomic sequences in sputum specimens by polymerase chain reaction using primer sets from variable regions of 16S rRNA specific for *M. pneumoniae* (62). Detection of high levels (above 1:40) of cold hemagglutinin antibody in a single serum specimen provides only presumptive evidence of *M. pneumoniae* infection. They develop in approximately one-half of cases of M. pneumoniae pneumonia, usually among the more severely ill persons (34,63). Although this antibody occurs in other clinical conditions, it serves as a rapid and easily done test upon which to base initiating antibiotic treatment of *M. pneumoniae* infection

Culture of *M. pneumoniae* from clinical specimens represents the "gold standard" for diagnosis of infection; however, *M. pneu-moniae* grows slowly and its isolation usually requires about 10 to 14 days. It grows as small colonies on mycoplasma agar plates that can be seen adequately only by low-power microscopy, but colonial morphology does not differentiate *M. pneumoniae* from other nonpathogenic mycoplasmas that inhabit the oropharynx. *M. pneumoniae* can be identified by metabolic characteristics or growth (disk) neutralization employing antibody-impregnated disks. In SP-4 diphasic medium, growth of the organism produces acid metabolites that change the indicator from blue to yellow or cause turbidity in the liquid. Isolates in SP-4 diphasic medium must be subcultured onto agar and identified either by a rapid direct plate immunofluorescence antibody test or by disk neutralization procedures (64).

Rapid identification of *M. pneumoniae* infection facilitates early appropriate antibiotic treatment. Polymerase chain reaction applied to sputum specimens holds promise as a rapid albeit complex procedure of high sensitivity and specificity (65–68). Different primer sets of the variable region of 16S rRNA successfully amplify genomic sequences specific to *M. pneumoniae* (69,70). These procedures can detect 5 to 50 fg of *M. pneumoniae* DNA or approximately 100 colony-forming units/mL (71). Polymerase chain reaction can rapidly identify *M. pneumoniae* DNA in cerebrospinal fluid of persons with central nervous system infections (49). The determination of immunoglobulin A– and immunoglobulin M–specific antibody also has the advantage of quickly identifying *M. pneumoniae* as the infecting organism. The detection of immunoglobulin A– and immunoglobulin M–specific antibody in high titers measured by enzyme-linked immunosorbent assay in an acute serum specimen collected approximately 7 to 10 days after the onset of illness provides a sensitive and specific means of serologic diagnosis (72). Immunoglobulin A-specific antibody to *M. pneumoniae* occurs in reinfection. Peak titers of these antibodies develop about 1 week later. Immunoglobulin M anti-P1 antibody detected by enzyme immunoassay (ELISA) as a rapid procedure for the diagnosis of *M. pneumoniae* infections (73).

Routine antibody tests for detection of *M. pneumoniae* infection include complement fixation, enzyme-linked immunosorbent assay, and growth inhibition. These procedures are sensitive and specific and command wide use in clinical laboratories and in epidemiologic studies. However, serologic diagnosis of infection requires the demonstration of a rise in antibody level by testing paired serum specimens obtained during the acute and convalescent phases of illness. In these cases, the convalescent-phase

TABLE 52.2. Laboratory Diagnosis of *Mycoplasma pneumoniae* Infection

Target	Procedure	Reagent	Use as routine test	Significance
Isolation	Culture on agar		Yes	Gold standard for diagnosis
Direct	Polymerase chain reaction	Primer sets	No	Rapid detection of amplification is diagnostic
Specific antibody	Complement fixation	Glycolipid	Yes	Increase is diagnostic
	Metabolic inhibition	Whole organism	Yes	Increase is diagnostic
	Enzyme immunoassay	Protein; purified P1 protein	Yes	Increase is diagnostic
	Mycoplasmacidal assay	Whole organism	No	Increase is diagnostic
	Immunofluorescence	Membrane	No	Increase is diagnostic
	Indirect hemagglutination	Whole organism	No	Increase is diagnostic
	Immunoblotting	Sonicated, solubilized organism	No	Specific peptide lines diagnostic
Nonspecific antibody	Cold hemagglutination	Anti-I agglutinins	Yes	Increase is presumptive
	Venereal Disease Research Laboratory Test	False-positive serologic test result for syphilis	No	None
	Streptococcus agglutination	Streptococcus MG	No	None
	Complement fixation	Autoantibodies	No	None
		Rheumatoid factor	No	False-positive results

serum specimen should be obtained 18 to 21 days after the acute-phase serum specimen. Other antibody assays, such as immunofluorescence and indirect hemagglutination, are less often used routinely for the diagnosis of infection (Table 52.2).

TREATMENT

The treatment of mycoplasmal pneumonia consists of the administration of appropriate antibiotics and supportive therapy to lessen the discomfort of the illness. The majority of children and adults in whom mycoplasmal pneumonia (or an atypical pneumonia) develops can be treated on ambulatory basis. Among children and adults treated in-hospital or as outpatients, the recommended antibiotics include macrolides, doxycycline and fluoroquinolones, which show excellent activity to *M. pneumoniae* isolates (74). The treatment schedules of oral antibiotics for adults are: erythromycin, 2 g daily in divided doses for 10 to 14 days; azithromycin, 500 mg on day 1 and 250 mg daily for 5 days; clarithromycin, 500 mg twice daily for 10 to 14 days; doxycycline, 100 mg twice daily for 10 to 14 days; and, levofloxacin 250 mg twice daily or moxifloxacin 400 mg daily for 10 to 14 days or another new fluoroquinolone. In children, the dosage of these antibiotics must be adjusted. Among infants and children 3 months to 5 years of age treated as outpatients, administer orally erythromycin in a dose of 10 mg/kg four times a day or clarithromycin 7.5 mg/kg twice daily for 7 to 10 days or azithromycin 10 mg/kg on the first day and 5 mg/kg daily for 5 days and for children 5 to 18 years of age administer 500 mg four times a day or clarithromycin 500 mg twice daily for 7 to 10 days or azithromycin 500 mg on the first day and 250 mg daily for 5 days or doxycycline 100 mg twice daily. Adults and children admitted to hospital with severe mycoplasmal pneumonia, which may be not differentiated from other bacterial and atypical pneumonias before the need to initiate antibiotics, will require treatment on an empiric basis with two antibiotics, one which must be a macrolide or a fluorquinolone. *In vitro* tests show that *M. pneumoniae* is sensitive to macrolide, doxycycline and fluoroquinolone antibiotics. Supportive therapy includes bed rest, ample fluids, bronchodilators, antipyretic medications (avoid aspirin in infants and children), and antitussive syrups.

PREVENTION

Recommended general preventive measures are handwashing and use of disposable paper tissues, rather than handkerchiefs, to wipe the nose and hands.

There is no commercially available vaccine for *M. pneumoniae*. During the past two decades, experimental inactivated whole-organism vaccines and live attenuated vaccines were tested in volunteers for antigenicity and efficacy (75). However, they failed to produce the levels of protection necessary for use in high-risk groups or the general population. Studies of vaccines center on the use of purified components of the organism as vaccines, principally the P1 adhesin (76). An acellular extract vaccine composed of several *M. pneumoniae* proteins including the P1 adhesin protein administered to chimpanzees protected them from serious illness during subsequent challenge (77).

REFERENCES

1. Eaton MD, Meiklejohn G, Van Herick W. Studies on the etiology of primary atypical pneumonia: I. Filterable agent transmissible to cotton rats, hamsters, and chick embryos. *J Exp Med* 1944;79:649–668.
2. Eaton MD, Meiklejohn G, Van Herick W. Studies on the etiology of primary atypical pneumonia. II. Properties of the virus isolated and propagated in chick embryos. *J Exp Med* 1945;82:317–328.
3. Liu C. Studies on primary atypical pneumonia. I. Localization, isolation, and cultivation of a virus in chick embryos. *J Exp Med* 1957;106:455–466.
4. Chanock RM, Hayflick L, Barile MF. Growth on artificial medium of an agent associated with atypical pneumonia and its definition as a PPLO. *Proc Natl Acad Sci USA* 1962;48:41–48.
5. Rifkind D, Chanock RM, Kravetz H, et al. Ear involvement (myringitis) and primary atypical pneumonia following inoculation of volunteers with Eaton agent. *Am Rev Respir Dis* 1962;85:479–489.
6. Kingston JR, Chanock RM, Mufson MA, et al. Eaton Agent pneumonia. *JAMA* 1961;176:118–123.
7. Razin S, Yogev D, Naot Y. Molecular biology and pathogenicity of mycoplasmas. *Microbiol Mol Biol Rev* 1998;62:1094–1156.
8. Himmelreich R, Hilbert H, Plagens H, et al. Complete sequence analysis of the genome of the bacterium Mycoplasma pneumoniae. *Nucleic Acids Res* 1996;24:4420–4449.
9. Bove JM. Molecular features of mollicutes. *Clin Infect Dis* 1993;17[Suppl 1]:S10–31.
10. Dallo SF, Lazzell AL, Chavoya A, et al. Biofunctional domains of the Mycoplasma pneumoniae P30 adhesin. *Infect Immun* 1996;64:2595–2601.
11. Layh-Schmitt G, Himmelreich R, Leibfried U. The adhesin related 30-kDa protein of Mycoplasma pneumoniae exhibits size and antigen variability. *FEMS Microbiol Lett* 1997;152:101–108.
12. Dorigo-Zetsma JW, Wilbrink B, Dankert J, et al. Mycoplasma pneumoniae P1 type 1- and type 2-specific sequences within the P1 cytadhesin gene of individual strains. *Infect Immun* 2001;69:5612–5618.
13. Dorigo-Zetsma JW, Dankert J, Zaat SA. Genotyping of *Mycoplasma pneumoniae* clinical isolates reveals eight P1 subtypes within two genomic groups. *J Clin Microbiol* 2000;38:965–970.
14. Krivan HC, Olson LD, Barile MF, et al. Adhesion of *Mycoplasma pneumoniae* to sulfated glycolipids and inhibition by dextran sulfate. *J Biol Chem* 1989;264:9283–9288.
15. Petrovsky T. *Mycoplasma pneumoniae* infection and post-infection asthma [letter]. *Med J Aust* 1990;152:391
16. Loomes LM, Uemura K, Feizi T. Interaction of *Mycoplasma pneumoniae* with erythrocyte glycolipids of I and i antigen types. *Infect Immun* 1985;47:15–20.
17. Dallo SF, Horton JR, Su CJ, et al. Restriction fragment length polymorphism in the cytadhesin P1 gene of human clinical isolates of *Mycoplasma pneumoniae*. *Infect Immun* 1990;58:2017–2020.
18. Su CJ, Dallo SF, Baseman JB. Molecular distinctions among clinical isolates of *Mycoplasma pneumoniae*. *J Clin Microbiol* 1990;28:1538–1540.
19. Su CJ, Chavoya A, Dallo SF, et al. Sequence divergency of the cytadhesin gene of *Mycoplasma pneumoniae*. *Infect Immun* 1990;58:2669–2674.
20. Wray W, Scully C, Rennie J, et al. Major and minor salivary gland swelling in *Mycoplasma pneumoniae* infection. *BMJ* 1980;280:1421.
21. Foy HM. Infections caused by *Mycoplasma pneumoniae* and possible carrier state in different populations of patients. *Clin Infect Dis* 1993;17[Suppl 1]:S37–S46.
22. Marston BJ, Plouffe JF, File TM Jr, et al. Incidence of community-acquired pneumonia requiring hospitalization. Results of a population-based active surveillance Study in Ohio. The community-based pneumonia incidence study group. *Arch Intern Med* 1997;157:1709–1718.
23. Mufson MA, Chang V, Gill V, et al. The role of viruses, mycoplasmas and bacteria in acute pneumonia in civilian adults. *Am J Epidemiol* 1967;86:526–544.
24. Hyde TB, Gilbert M, Schwartz SB, et al. Azithromycin prophylaxis during a hospital outbreak of *Mycoplasma pneumoniae* pneumonia. *J Infect Dis* 2001;183:907–912.
25. Baseman JB, Tully JG. Mycoplasmas: sophisticated, reemerging, and burdened by their notoriety. *Emerg Infect Dis* 1997;3:21–32.
26. Krause DC. *Mycoplasma pneumoniae* cytadherence: unravelling the tie that binds. *Mol Microbiol* 1996;20:247–253.
27. Baseman JB, Reddy SP, Dallo SF. Interplay between mycoplasma surface proteins, airway cells, and the protean manifestations of mycoplasma-mediated human infections. *Am J Respir Crit Care Med* 1996;154:S137–S44.
28. Morrison-Plummer J, Leith DK, Baseman JB. Biological effects of anti-lipid and anti-protein monoclonal antibodies on *Mycoplasma pneumoniae*. *Infect Immun* 1986;53:398–403.
29. Roberts DD, Olson LD, Barile MF, et al. Sialic acid-dependent adhesion of *Mycoplasma pneumoniae* to purified glycoproteins. *J Biol Chem* 1989;264:9289–9293.
30. Loveless RW, Feizi T. Sialo-oligosaccharide receptors for *Mycoplasma pneumoniae* and related oligosaccharides of poly-N-acetylgalactosamine series are polarized at the cilia and apical-microvillar domains of the ciliated cells in human bronchial epithelium. *Infect Immun* 1989;57:1285–1289.
31. Konig AL, Kreft H, Hengge U, et al. Coexisting anti-I and anti-F1/Gd cold agglutinins in infections by *Mycoplasma pneumoniae*. *Vox Sang* 1988;55:176–180.
32. Almagor M, Kahane I, Yatziv S. Role of superoxide anion in host cell injury induced by mycoplasma pneumoniae infection. A study in normal and trisomy 21 cells. *J Clin Invest* 1984;73:842–847.
33. Arai S, Munakata T, Kuwano K. Mycoplasma interaction with lymphocytes and phagocytes: role of hydrogen peroxide released from M. pneumoniae. *Yale J Biol Med* 1983;56:631–638.

34. Mufson MA, Manko MA, Kingston JR, et al. Eaton agent pneumonia: Clinical features. *JAMA* 1961;178:369–374.

35. Lieberman D. Atypical pathogen pneumonia. *Curr Opin Pulm Med* 1997;3:111–115.

36. Marrie TJ, Peeling RW, Fine MJ, et al. Ambulatory patients with community-acquired pneumonia: the frequency of atypical agents and clinical course. *Am J Med* 1996;101:508–515.

37. Mansel JK, Rosenow EC, 3d, Smith TF, et al. *Mycoplasma pneumoniae* pneumonia. *Chest* 1989;95:639–646.

38. Hutchison AA, Landau LI, Phelan PD. Severe mycoplasma pneumonia in previously healthy children. *Med J Aust* 1981;1:126–128.

39. Loo VG, Richardson S, Quinn P. Isolation of *Mycoplasma pneumoniae* from pleural fluid. *Diagn Microbiol Infect Dis* 1991;14:443–445.

40. Narita M, Tanaka H, Abe S, et al. Close association between pulmonary disease manifestation in *Mycoplasma pneumoniae* infection and enhanced local production of interleukin-18 in the lung, independent of gamma interferon. *Clin Diagn Lab Immunol* 2000;7:909–914.

41. Narita M, Matsuzono Y, Itakura O, et al. Analysis of mycoplasmal pleural effusion by the polymerase chain reaction. *Arch Dis Child* 1998;78:67–69.

42. Baum H, Strubel A, Nollert J, et al. Two cases of fulminant *Mycoplasma pneumoniae* pneumonia within 4 months. *Infection* 2000;28:180–183.

43. Radisic M, Torn A, Gutierrez P, et al. Severe acute lung injury caused by *Mycoplasma pneumoniae:* potential role for steroid pulses in treatment. *Clin Infect Dis* 2000;31:1507–1511.

44. Oermann C, Sockrider MM, Langston C. Severe necrotizing pneumonitis in a child with *Mycoplasma pneumoniae* infection. *Pediatr Pulmonol* 1997;24:61–65.

45. Chan ED, Welsh CH. Fulminant *Mycoplasma pneumoniae* pneumonia [clinical conference]. *West J Med* 1995;162:133–142.

46. Takiguchi Y, Shikama N, Aotsuka N, et al. Fulminant *Mycoplasma pneumoniae* pneumonia. *Intern Med* 2001;40:345–348.

47. Reittner P, Muller NL, Heyneman L, et al. *Mycoplasma pneumoniae* pneumonia: radiographic and high-resolution CT features in 28 patients. *AJR* 2000;174:37–41.

48. Smith R, Eviatar L. Neurologic manifestations of *Mycoplasma pneumoniae* infections: diverse spectrum of diseases. A report of six cases and review of the literature. *Clin Pediatr (Phila)* 2000;39:195–201.

49. Bitnun A, Ford-Jones EL, Petric M, et al. Acute childhood encephalitis and *Mycoplasma pneumoniae*. *Clin Infect Dis* 2001;32:1674–1684.

50. Goebels N, Helmchen C, Abele-Horn M, et al. Extensive myelitis associated with Mycoplasma pneumoniae infection: magnetic resonance imaging and clinical long-term follow-up. *J Neurol* 2001;248:204–208.

51. Thomas NH, Collins JE, Robb SA, et al. *Mycoplasma pneumoniae* infection and neurological disease [see comments]. *Arch Dis Child* 1993;69:573–576.

52. Rabay-Chacar H, Rizkallah E, Hakimeh NI, et al. Neurological complications associated with Mycoplasma pneumoniae infection. A case report. *J Med Liban* 2000;48:108–111.

53. Pellegrini M, O'Brien TJ, Hoy J, et al. Mycoplasma pneumoniae infection associated with an acute brainstem syndrome. *Acta Neurol Scand* 1996;93:203–206.

54. Fernandez CV, Bortolussi R, Gordon K, et al. *Mycoplasma pneumoniae* infection associated with central nervous system complications. *J Child Neurol* 1993;8:27–31.

55. Jacobs BC, Rothbarth PH, van der Meche FG, et al. The spectrum of antecedent infections in Guillain-Barre syndrome: a case-control study. *Neurology* 1998;51:1110–1115.

56. Berger RP, Wadowksy RM. Rhabdomyolysis associated with infection by *Mycoplasma pneumoniae:* a case report. *Pediatrics* 2000;105:433–436.

57. Said MH, Layani MP, Colon S, et al. *Mycoplasma pneumoniae*-associated nephritis in children [see comments]. *Pediatr Nephrol* 1999;13:39–44.

58. Stephan JL, Galambrun C, Pozzetto B, et al. Aplastic anemia after *Mycoplasma pneumoniae* infection: a report of two cases. *J Pediatr Hematol Oncol* 1999;21:299–302.

59. Sadler JP, Gibson J. *Mycoplasma pneumoniae* infection presenting as Stevens-Johnson syndrome: a case report. *Dent Update* 1997;24:367–368.

60. Tay YK, Huff JC, Weston WL. *Mycoplasma pneumoniae* infection is associated with Stevens-Johnson syndrome, not erythema multiforme (von Hebra). *J Am Acad Dermatol* 1996;35:757–760.

61. Leaute-Labreze C, Lamireau T, Chawki D, et al. Diagnosis, classification, and management of erythema multiforme and Stevens-Johnson syndrome. *Arch Dis Child* 2000;83:347–352.

62. Hindiyeh M, Carroll KC. Laboratory diagnosis of atypical pneumonia. *Semin Respir Infect* 2000;15:101–113.

63. Jacobs E. Serological diagnosis of *Mycoplasma pneumoniae* infections: a critical review of current procedures. *Clin Infect Dis* 1993;17[Suppl 1]:S79–S82.

64. Tully JG. New laboratory techniques for isolation of *Mycoplasma pneumoniae*. *Yale J Biol Med* 1983;56:511–515.

65. Dorigo-Zetsma JW, Wilbrink B, van der Nat H, et al. Results of molecular detection of *Mycoplasma pneumoniae* among patients with acute respiratory infection and in their household contacts reveals children as human reservoirs. *J Infect Dis* 2001;183:675–678.

66. Dorigo-Zetsma JW, Verkooyen RP, van Helden HP, et al. Molecular detection of *Mycoplasma pneumoniae* in adults with community-acquired pneumonia requiring hospitalization. *J Clin Microbiol* 2001;39:1184–1186.

67. Ferwerda A, Moll HA, De Groot R. Respiratory tract infections by *Mycoplasma pneumoniae* in children: a review of diagnostic and therapeutic measures. *Eur J Pediatr* 2001;160:483–491.

68. Abele-Horn M, Busch U, Nitschko H, et al. Molecular approaches to diagnosis of pulmonary diseases due to *Mycoplasma pneumoniae*. *J Clin Microbiol* 1998;36:548–551.

69. Cousin-Allery A, Charron A, de Barbeyrac B, et al. Molecular typing of *Mycoplasma pneumoniae* strains by PCR-based methods and pulsed-field gel electrophoresis. Application to French and Danish isolates. *Epidemiol Infect* 2000;124:103–111.

70. Kong F, Gordon S, Gilbert GL. Rapid-cycle PCR for detection and typing of *Mycoplasma pneumoniae* in clinical specimens. *J Clin Microbiol* 2000;38:4256–4259.

71. Kai M, Kamiya S, Yabe H, et al. Rapid detection of *Mycoplasma pneumoniae* in clinical samples by the polymerase chain reaction. *J Med Microbiol* 1993;38:166–170.

72. Waris ME, Toikka P, Saarinen T, et al. Diagnosis of *Mycoplasma pneumoniae* pneumonia in children. *J Clin Microbiol* 1998;36:3155–3159.

73. Tuuminen T, Suni J, Kleemola M, et al. Improved sensitivity and specificity of enzyme immunoassays with P1-adhesin enriched antigen to detect acute *Mycoplasma pneumoniae* infection. *J Microbiol Methods* 2001;44:27–37.

74. Plouffe JF. Importance of atypical pathogens of community-acquired pneumonia. *Clin Infect Dis* 2000;31[Suppl 2]:S35–S39.

75. Barile MF. Immunization against *Mycoplasma pneumoniae* disease: a review. *Isr J Med Sci* 1984;20:912–915.

76. Dallo SF, Su CJ, Horton JR, et al. Identification of P1 gene domain containing epitope(s) mediating *Mycoplasma pneumoniae* cytoadherence. *J Exp Med* 1988;167:718–723.

77. Barile MF, Grabowski MW, Kapatais-Zoumbois K, et al. Protection of immunized and previously infected chimpanzees challenged with *Mycoplasma pneumoniae*. *Vaccine* 1994;12:707–714.

CHAPTER 53
Pneumocystis carinii *Pneumonia*

Walter T. Hughes

Unlike the usual pneumonias caused by bacteria and viruses, that due to *Pneumocystis carinii* is unique in several ways. It occurs almost exclusively in patients whose immune systems are compromised. Even so, the organism and the disease remain localized to the lung parenchyma, whereas other infections in the immunocompromised host undergo systemic spread. This localized but complex infection requires a multidisciplinary approach by physician specialists. Because the patient almost assuredly has some underlying disease, an oncologist, organ transplanter, or clinical immunologist may be the primary physician who elicits the help of an infectious disease specialist. The diagnosis requires an invasive procedure, such as endoscopy and bronchoalveolar lavage done by the pulmonologist or thoracic surgeon, or open lung biopsy under general anesthesia. Specimens are processed and interpreted by the pathologist. Patients with *P. carinii* pneumonitis often require assisted ventilation and the services of an intensive care unit team.

HISTORY

P. carinii was first shown to be a cause of infection in humans in the early 1940s, when it was associated with epidemics of infantile interstitial plasma-cell pneumonitis in Europe. By the mid-1950s, it was recognized as a cause of diffuse alveolar disease in children and adults who had an underlying immunodeficiency disorder. As immunosuppressive therapy came to be used more extensively in cancer patients and organ transplant recipients, the prevalence of *P. carinii* pneumonitis increased. However, by far the greatest impact has been the epidemic of human immunodeficiency virus (HIV) infection (see also Chapter 115). In fact, the acquired immunodeficiency syndrome (AIDS) was first discovered because of the occurrence of *P. carinii* pneumonitis in young men with no obvious underlying disease. *P. carinii* pneumonitis occurs in about 75% of untreated patients with AIDS and 43% of patients with severe combined immuodeficiency syndrome.

EPIDEMIOLOGY

P. carinii has been found only in the lungs of humans and lower mammals. No natural habitat outside the lung has been identified. Studies in the United States and Europe show that more than 75% of normal healthy individuals have acquired antibody to *P. carinii* by 4 years of age (1, 2). Furthermore, rats, mice, ferrets, and rabbits are latently infected to the extent that when they are immunosuppressed, overt *P. carinii* pneumonia ensues. In most parts of the world, both humans and lower animals are infected, with no areas of significant predominance or clustering.

The mode of transmission of *P. carinii* to humans is not known, but experimental studies in rats have shown that the organism can be airborne from animal to animal (3). *P. carinii* DNA sequences can readily be found in air samples (4). It is believed that *P. carinii* is acquired early in life and is unassociated with discernible illness, and that the organism persists in a latent subclinical state in the immunocompetent host. However, if the immune system becomes profoundly impaired, the organisms replicate and pneumonitis becomes evident. Recent experimental studies in rats (5, 6) and genetic epidemiology of *P. carinii* in humans (7) strongly suggest that many cases of the pneumonitis result from acutely acquired organisms regardless of age (8).

PATHOGENESIS

It is likely that the trophozoite, the cyst, or both forms of *P. carinii* are inhaled and reach the alveolar lumen. From this point, the type and extent of the disease process, if any, depend on the immune response of the host and the replication of the organism. Because evidence of disease is rarely found in normal immunocompetent individuals, it is believed that the quantity of organisms is maintained at a low number. This could be explained by continuous surveillance and phagocytosis of replicating organisms at a rate sufficient to maintain a disease-free state. An alternative hypothesis is that one is exposed frequently to the organism, that immunity does not develop from asymptomatic infection, and that reinfection and pneumonitis occur in the absence of adequate host defense when the host is exposed to an infectious dose of airborne organisms. In fact, data support the latter hypothesis (5–8). With the use of molecular methods to identify specific strains of *P. carinii*, laboratory animals and humans were found to have more than one strain in the same lung, suggesting replenishment of the organism from the environment (7, 9).

The most effective component of the immune system in defense against *P. carinii* is the cell-mediated response. This has been most vividly exemplified by the results of retroviral infection and destruction of the important CD4$^+$ lymphocytes by HIV. The attack rate of *P. carinii* pneumonitis can be related directly to the quantity of CD4$^+$ cells (10). Once the CD4$^+$ cell count reaches 200/mm^3 or less, the risk for developing the pneumonitis is greatly enhanced (11). However, episodes may occur infrequently with CD4$^+$ lymphocyte counts of 200 to 500/mm^3.

The immune defect permissive to *P. carinii* pneumonitis is not limited to impaired cell-mediated response. Cases have been associated with classic X-linked agammaglobulinemia. Broad-spectrum immunodeficiency induced by corticosteroids and other immunosuppressive drugs effectively provokes the pneumonitis. Factors that enhance replication of *P. carinii* *in vivo* or *in vitro* are unknown.

Once in the alveolus, *P. carinii* attaches to the alveolar wall. As the disease evolves, an increase in trophozoites and cysts is seen, reactive alveolar macrophages appear, and organisms may be found in the cytoplasm of the phagocytes in varying stages of digestion. No intracellular phase of the life cycle has been demonstrated. The major surface glycoproteins of *P. carinii* provoke release and gene expression of interleukin-8 and tissue necrosis factor alpha (TNF-α) in monocytes (12). Eventually, the alveolar lumen becomes filled with a proteinaceous exudate and an extensive diffuse desquamative alveolopathy. The inflammatory reaction disrupts surfactant function during *P. carinii* pneumonia (13). The interstitial tissue may show mononuclear cell infiltrates. In the infantile form, an interstitial plasma cell pneumonitis predominates, but this is rarely found in the immunocompromised child and adult. Although the organism and the disease remain localized to the pulmonary parenchyma in more than 99% of cases, extrapulmonary lesions may rarely be encountered. Lesions with *P. carinii* in the bone marrow, skin, liver, heart, spleen, lymph nodes, eye, ear, thyroid, and mastoid bone have been described.

CLINICAL MANIFESTATIONS

Although the symptoms and signs of *P. carinii* pneumonia are limited to cough, shortness of breath, fever, tachypnea, dyspnea, flaring of the nasal alae, cyanosis, and occasionally chest pain, the number and extent of these manifestations vary from patient to patient. The underlying condition of the host may indicate the clinical pattern to be expected. For example, in the infantile type, seen in patients younger than 6 months, fever is usually absent and the onset is subtle; rales are usually abundant. In the immunosuppressed child or adult with cancer, the onset is usually abrupt, with fever and tachypnea in the absence of rales. In the patient with AIDS, the onset is more subtle than with the cancer patient, although fever, cough, tachypnea, and dyspnea are prominent manifestations.

The chest radiograph reveals a bilateral diffuse alveolar disease in 90% or more of cases. The infiltrates become apparent first in the perihilar area, spreading peripherally but sparing the apical areas until the disease is far advanced. The hilar nodes are not enlarged. Spontaneous pneumothorax is occasionally seen even without an invasive diagnostic procedure. Atypical forms of *P. carinii* pneumonitis, seen uncommonly, include lobar pneumonia, single-coin lesions, unilateral infiltrates, and hyperexpanded lung.

Studies of arterial blood gases are especially helpful in identifying the presence of pulmonary disease before radiographic tests can detect infiltrates, and also for assessing the extent of established pneumonitis. Although not specific for *P. carinii* pneumonitis, the presence of reduced arterial oxygen tension (Pao$_2$) and increased alveolar-arterial oxygen gradient is characteristic. These changes may be evident before abnormalities are seen radiographically but rarely before tachypnea occurs.

Serum lactate dehydrogenase activity may be increased and *P. carinii* antibody detectable, but these are not of diagnostic help.

Once the pneumonitis has become evident radiographically, few patients if any will survive without treatment.

DIAGNOSIS

A definitive diagnosis requires the demonstration of *P. carinii* in lung tissue or fluids aspirated from the lung or lower airways. Specimens may be obtained by one or more of the following procedures.

Open Lung Biopsy

This procedure provides the greatest amount of dependable information about the pulmonary disease. Adequate samples may be obtained for cultures and histologic stains. If no *P. carinii* organisms are seen in an adequate biopsy specimen, one can reliably conclude that the pneumonitis is not due to this organism. Also, concomitant infections may be detected by this method. Although this may be the most sensitive method and the "gold standard," it may not necessarily be the most appropriate for a given patient, because a general anesthetic is required and the operative procedure may jeopardize pulmonary function at a critical time in the course of the disease.

Bronchoscopy and Bronchoalveolar Lavage

This procedure is especially useful for the diagnosis of *P. carinii* pneumonitis in AIDS patients, because organisms seem generally to be more abundant in these patients than in non-AIDS patients. Organisms may be missed in about 10% of cases, and complications of pneumothorax, bleeding, and transient impairment of pulmonary functions are undesirable features.

Transbronchial Biopsy

Transbronchial biopsy may be done with bronchoscopy and bronchoalveolar lavage, adding information to that obtained from the lavage specimen. It should be done when the patient's condition will permit it without undue risk. The complications of bleeding and pneumothorax are more likely than with bronchoalveolar lavage alone.

Induced Sputum

This has been of diagnostic help when organisms are found, but the failure to find *P. carinii* in sputum samples does not exclude the diagnosis. The success of this procedure varies from institution to institution and probably depends on the development of skills in inducing the production of adequate sputum samples.

Specimens should be stained by methods that will identify the cyst and the trophozoite forms. The Gomori-Grocott methenamine-silver nitrate stain or toluidine blue 0 identifies the cyst form. Giemsa and Wright-Giemsa stains are preferred for the trophozoite forms (see Chapter 283). An immunofluorescence stain using a monoclonal antibody to *P. carinii* has been used successfully. Detection of *P. carinii* by DNA amplification with polymerase chain reaction (PCR) is a highly sensitive diagnostic test for bronchoalveolar lavage specimens, although limited problems with false-positive reactions are encountered (14). Promising results are also reported from the use of oral secretions (15). Standardized commercially available DNA tests are not available at this time.

DIFFERENTIAL DIAGNOSIS

The differential diagnosis includes infections due to *Mycobacterium avium-intracellulare,* cytomegalovirus, Epstein-Barr virus, *Toxoplasma gondii,* and *Chlamydia trachomatis;* acute bacterial pneumonia (pneumococcal, streptococcal, and so forth); pulmonary mycosis *(Cryptococcus, Histoplasma, Coccidioides);* and acute viral pneumonia (parainfluenza virus, adenovirus, respiratory syncytial virus). In infants and children with AIDS, lymphoid interstitial pneumonitis resembles *P. carinii* pneumonitis.

TREATMENT

Four drugs are approved by the U.S. Food and Drug Administration for the treatment of *P. carinii* pneumonitis. These are trimethoprim-sulfamethoxazole, pentamidine isethionate, atovaquone, and trimetrexate with leucovorin. Two other drugs in general use are dapsone plus trimethoprim and clindamycin plus primaquine. Trimethoprim-sulfamethoxazole is the drug of first choice.

Trimethoprim-Sulfamethoxazole

Trimethoprim alone has no effect on *P. carinii,* and sulfamethoxazole alone is effective; however, the combination is presumed to be synergistic, and approximately 75% of patients will recover with treatment (16, 17). The dosage for intravenous administration is trimethoprim at 15 mg/kg and sulfamethoxazole at 75 mg/kg per day in three or four equally divided doses. Orally, the dosage is based on trimethoprim at 20 mg/kg and sulfamethoxazole at 100 mg/kg per day in three or four divided doses. If treatment is initiated with the oral preparation, it is often advisable to give the first dose as half the total daily quantity as a loading dose. The subsequent total daily doses, oral or intravenous, should not exceed 640 mg of trimethoprim and 3200 mg of sulfamethoxazole. In general, doses may be modified as needed to maintain peak serum levels of trimethoprim of about 5 to 8 μg/mL, and of sulfamethoxazole, about 100 to 150 μg/mL. A course of 10 days is usually adequate in non-AIDS patients. Those with AIDS generally require 2 to 3 weeks of treatment.

Adverse reactions to trimethoprim-sulfamethoxazole include rashes, fever, leukopenia, elevated transaminase values, and gastrointestinal symptoms. AIDS patients have a unique susceptibility to react adversely to this drug. More than half of AIDS patients may have such reactions; a maculopapular erythematous rash is the most frequent effect. Less than 5% of non-AIDS patients have adverse reactions.

Pentamidine Isethionate

Pentamidine is available only for intravenous or intramuscular administration. Aerosolized pentamidine is not used for treatment. A dose of 4.0 mg/kg per day administered intravenously in a period of 1 hour is preferred.

Adverse reactions to pentamidine occur in more than 50% of both AIDS and non-AIDS patients (17). These include renal dysfunction, hypoglycemia, hypertension, neutropenia, and thrombocytopenia. The duration of treatment is the same as for trimethoprim-sulfamethoxazole. Recovery can be expected in about 75% of cases.

Atovaquone

Atovaquone is available only for oral administration. The dosage is 750 mg three times daily with meals. No significant adverse effects have been associated with atovaquone therapy. In mild and moderately severe cases of *P. carinii* pneumonitis (alveolar-arterial oxygen gradient less than 45 mm Hg), the overall therapeutic success with atovaquone was found to be equal to that of trimethoprim-sulfamethoxazole. This was due to a significantly lower rate of treatment-limiting adverse effects balanced by a lower rate of antimicrobial efficacy from atovaquone (18). Similar results were obtained when atovaquone was compared with intravenous pentamidine (19).

Trimetrexate and Leucovorin

Trimetrexate inhibits the dihydrofolate reductase of *P. carinii*. Leucovorin must be administered concomitantly to prevent antifolate toxicity in the host. In moderate to severe cases of *P. carinii* pneumonitis, this drug regimen was found effective, but it was less effective than trimethoprim-sulfamethoxazole (20). The dose is 45 mg (base)/m^2 once daily for 21 days. The drug is administered intravenously in 30 to 60 minutes. Leucovorin may be given orally or intravenously at a dose of 20 mg/m^2 every 6 hours. Treatment-limiting adverse reactions are less frequent with trimetrexate than with trimethoprim-sulfamethoxazole.

Dapsone and Trimethoprim

Although dapsone alone is effective therapy for *P. carinii* pneumonitis, the addition of trimethoprim provides a synergistic effect. The drug combination has efficacy similar to that of trimethoprim-sulfamethoxazole or pentamidine. The usual dose is dapsone at 100 mg/d and trimethoprim at 20 mg/kg per day. The adverse effects are similar to those of trimethoprim-sulfamethoxazole; however, about two-thirds of patients who have adverse reactions to trimethoprim-sulfamethoxazole are able to tolerate dapsone (21).

Clindamycin Plus Primaquine

The combination of 600 mg of clindamycin every 8 hours and 30 mg of primaquine once daily orally is effective therapy (22). The adverse effects include rash, diarrhea, and vomiting. Clinical studies have been limited at this time.

Other Therapeutic Modalities

Corticosteroid treatment has been recommended for AIDS patients with moderately severe or severe *Pneumocystis* pneumonia, as indicated by a Po$_2$ of less than 70 mm Hg. Early studies suggested that oral corticosteroids prevent early deterioration in AIDS patients with mild *P. carinii* pneumonitis (23). A recent study failed to show improved survival with corticosteroid therapy in non-HIV infected patients with *P. carinii* pneumonia (24).

PREVENTION

P. carinii pneumonitis can be prevented by chemoprophylaxis. Several drugs are available for this purpose. Trimethoprim-sulfamethoxazole is the drug of first choice. The dose of 160 mg of trimethoprim and 800 mg of sulfamethoxazole may be given orally in single or divided doses daily or only 3 days a week

(25–27). For patients who have mild to moderate adverse reactions to trimethoprim-sulfamethoxazole, it is often possible to rechallenge or attempt desensitization to the drug (28), or an alternative drug may be selected. Dapsone alone in the dose of 100 mg/d is effective. Studies have shown that 50 mg of dapsone daily plus 50 mg of pyrimethamine per week plus 25 mg of leucovorin per week, or 200 mg of dapsone plus 75 mg of pyrimethamine plus 25 mg of leucovorin once a week, provides effective prophylaxis against toxoplasmosis as well as *P. carinii* pneumonitis (29–31).

Aerosolized pentamidine, 300 mg once monthly by Respirgard II-like nebulizer, is also effective in the prevention of the pneumonitis. Atovaquone 1500 mg daily is as effective as dapsone and aerosolized pentamidine and is safe (32).

Recommendations for prophylaxis of *P. carinii* in AIDS patients have been proposed by the U.S. Public Health Service and the Infectious Diseases Society of America (11). It is recommended that prophylaxis as described above be given to patients who have had one or more episodes of *P. carinii* pneumonia and others who have a CD4$^+$ lymphocyte count of less than 200/mm^3 or a history of oropharyngeal candidiasis. *P. carinii* prophylaxis can be safely discontinued in patients responding to highly active antiretroviral therapy (HAART) with a sustained increase in CD4$^+$ lymphocyte count from <200 cells/mm^3 to >200 cells/mm^3 (33).

REFERENCES

1. Pifer LL, Hughes WT, Stagno S, et al. *Pneumocystis carinii* infection: Evidence for high prevalence in normal and immunosuppressed children. *Pediatrics* 1978;61:35–44.
2. Meuwissen JH, Tauber I, Leeuwenberg AD, et al. Parasitologic and serologic observations of infection with *Pneumocystis* in humans. *J Infect Dis* 1977;136:43–48.
3. Hughes WT. Natural mode of acquisition for de novo infection with *Pneumocystis carinii*. *J Infect Dis* 1982;145:843–848.
4. Wakefield A. Detection of DNA sequences identical to *Pneumocystis carinii* in samples of ambient air. *J Eukaryot Microbiol* 1994; 41:116S.
5. Vargas SL, Hughes WT, Wakefield AE, et al. Limited persistence in and subsequent elimination of *Pneumocystis carinii* from the lungs after *P. carinii* pneumonia. *J Infect Dis* 1995;172:506–510.
6. Cheu W, Gigliotti F, Harmsen AG. Latency is not an inevitable outcome of infection with *Pneumocystis carinii*. *Infect Immun* 1993;61:5405–5409.
7. Beard CB, Carter JL, Keely SP, et al. Genetic variation in *P. carinii* isolates from different geographic regions: implications for transmission. *Emerg Infect Dis* 2000;6:265–272.
8. Hughes WT. Current issues in the epidemiology, transmission and reactivation of *Pneumocystis carinii*. *Sem Resp Infect* 1998;13:283–288.
9. Armstrong MYH, Cushion MT. Animal models. In: Walzer PD, ed. *Pneumocystis carinii pneumonia*, 2nd ed. New York: Marcel Dekker, 1993:181–222.
10. Phair J, Munoz A, Retels R, et al. The risk of *Pneumocystis carinii* pneumonia among men infected with human immunodeficiency virus type I. *N Engl J Med* 1990;322:161–165.
11. Centers for Disease Control and Prevention. 1999 Guidelines for the prevention of opportunistic infections in persons with human immunodeficiency virus. *MMWR* 1999;48(RR-10):1–66.
12. Benefield TL, Lundgren B, Levine SJ, et al. The major surface glycoprotein of *Pneumocystis carinii* induces release and gene expression of interleukin-8 and tissue necrosis factor alpha in monocytes. *Infect Immun* 1997;65:4790–4796.
13. Wright TW, Notter RH, Wang Z, et al. Pulmonary inflammation disrupts surfactant function during *Pneumocystis carinii* pneumonia. *Infect Immun* 2001;69:758–764.
14. Torres J, Goldman M, Wheat J, et al. Diagnosis of *Pneumocystis carinii* in human immunodeficiency virus–infected patients with polymerase chain reaction: a blinded comparison to standard methods. *Clin Infect Dis* 2000;30:141–145.
15. Helweg-Larsen J, Jensen J, Bentfield T, et al. Diagnostic use of PCR for detection of *Pneumocystis carinii* in oral wash samples. *J Clin Microbial* 1998;36:2068–2072.
16. Hughes WT, Feldman S, Chaudhary SC, et al. Comparison of pentamidine isethionate and trimethoprim-sulfamethoxazole in the treatment of *Pneumocystis carinii* pneumonia. *J Pediatr* 1978;92:285–291.
17. Sattler FR, Cowan R, Nielsen DM, et al. Trimethoprim-sulfamethoxazole

compared with pentamidine for treatment of *Pneumocystis carinii* pneumonia in the acquired immunodeficiency syndrome: A prospective, noncrossover study. *Ann Intern Med* 1988;109:280–287.

18. Hughes WT, Leoung G, Kramer F, et al. Comparison of atovaquone (566C80) with trimethoprim-sulfamethoxazole to treat *Pneumocystis carinii* pneumonia in patients with AIDS. *Engl J Med* 1993;328:1521–1527.

19. Dohn MN, Weinberg WG, Torres RA, et al. Oral atovaquone compared with intravenous pentamidine for *Pneumocystis carinii* pneumonia in patients with AIDS. *Ann Intern Med* 1994;121:174–180.

20. Sattler FR, Frame P, Davis R, et al. Trimetrexate with leucovorin versus trimethoprim-sulfamethoxazole for moderate to severe episodes of *Pneumocystis carinii* pneumonia in patients with AIDS: A prospective, controlled multicenter investigation of the AIDS Clinical Trials Group Protocol 029/031. *J Infect Dis* 1994;170:165–172.

21. Hughes WT. Use of dapsone in the prevention and treatment of *Pneumocystis carinii* pneumonia: A review. *Clin Infect Dis* 1998;27:197–204.

22. Toma E, Thorne A, Singer J, et al. Clindamycin with primaquine vs. trimethroprim-sulfamethoxazole therapy for mild and moderately severe *Pneumocystis carinii* pneumonia in patients with AIDS: A multicenter, double-blind, randomized trial (CTN 004). *Clin Infect Dis* 1998;27:524–530.

23. Bozzette SA, Sattler FR, Chiu J, et al. A controlled trial of early adjunctive treatment with corticosteroids for *Pneumcystis carinii* pneumonia in acquired immunodeficiency syndrome. *N Engl J Med* 1990;323:1451–1457.

24. Delclaux C, Zahar J-R, Armstrong G, et al. Corticosteroids as adjuctive therapy for severe *Pneumocystis carinii* pneumonia in non-human immunodeficiency virus-infected patients: A retrospective study of 31 patients. *Clin Infect Dis* 1999;29:670–672.

25. Schneider MME, Hoepelman AIM, Schattenkerk JKME, et al. A controlled trial of aerosolized pentamidine or trimethoprim-sulfamethoxazole as primary prophylaxis against *Pneumocystis carinii* pneumonia in patients with human immunodeficiency virus infection. *N Engl J Med* 1992;327:1836–1841.

26. Hardy WD, Feinberg J, Finkelstein DM, et al. A controlled trial of trimethoprim-sulfamethoxazole or aerosolized pentamidine for secondary prophylaxis of *Pneumocystis carinii* pneumonia in patients with acquired immunodeficiency syndrome. *N Engl J Med* 1992; 327:1842–1848.

27. Hughes WT, Rivera GK, Schell MJ, et al. Successful intermittent chemoprophylaxis for *Pneumocystis carinii* pneumonitis. *N Engl J Med* 1987;316:1627–1632.

28. Gluckstein D, Ruskin J: Rapid oral desensitization to trimethoprim-sulfamethoxazole (TMP-SMZ) use in prophylaxis for *Pneumocystis carinii* pneumonia in patients with AIDS who were previously intolerant to TMP-SMZ. *Clin Infect Dis* 1995;20:849–853.

29. Girard PM, Landman R, Gandebout C, et al. Dapsone-pyrimethamine compared with aerosolized pentamidine as primary prophylaxis against *Pneumocystis carinii* pneumonia and toxoplasmosis in HIV infection. *N Engl J Med* 1993;328:1514–1520.

30. Mallolas J, Zamora L, Gatell JM, et al. Primary prophylaxis for *Pneumocystis carinii* pneumonia: A randomized trial comparing cotrimoxazole, aerosolized pentamidine and dapsone plus pyrimethamine. *AIDS* 1993;7:59–64.

31. Opravil M, Heald A, Lazzarin A, et al. Once-weekly administration of dapsone-pyrimethamine vs. aerosolized pentamidine for *Pneumocystis carinii* pneumonia and toxoplasmic encephalitis in human immunodeficiency virus–infected patients. *Clin Infect Dis* 1995;20:531–541.

32. El-Sadr WM, Murphy RL, Yurik TM, et al. Atovaquone compared with dapsone for the prevention of *Pneumocystis carinii* pneumonia in patients with HIV infection who cannot tolerate trimethoprim, sulfonamides, or both. *N Engl J Med* 1998;339:1889–1895.

33. Furrer H, Opravil M, Rossi, M, et al. Discontinuation of primary prophylaxis in HIV-infected patients at high risk of *Pneumocystis carinii* pneumonia: A prospective multicenter study. *AIDS* 2001;15:501–507.

CHAPTER 54
Fungal Pneumonias

Susan Hadley and Donald B. Louria

Fungal pneumonias occur in normal hosts, those with pulmonary anatomic abnormalities, and those with compromised immune status. Pathogens causing primary fungal pneumonia are the dimorphic endemic fungi and *Cryptococcus neoformans*. These community-acquired mycoses occur in normal or immunocompromised hosts. Secondary fungal pneumonias, caused by opportunistic fungal pathogens, occur primarily in patients with abnormal pulmonary architecture or compromised immunity (Table 54.1). Increased mobility of the population and larger numbers of immunocompromised patients contribute to the growing numbers of patients with fungal pneumonias.

COMMUNITY-ACQUIRED MYCOSES

Organisms causing community-acquired infections naturally occupy environmental niches, most with geographic specificity, and include the dimorphic fungi and *Cryptococcus neoformans*. Several common features of the dimorphic fungi are worth noting. In nature, the organism exists in the mycelial form. Infection occurs with inhalation of conidia. Once at body temperature, transition to a tissue invasive yeast phase occurs. In the endemic geographic areas, a large proportion of the population is asymptomatically infected at some time. Although the infection is usually asymptomatic with spontaneous resolution in normal hosts, it may reactivate at a later date. These fungi may also disseminate from the lungs to other organs particularly in the immunocompromised host. In general, the clinical patterns of disease are acute asymptomatic or symptomatic infections, chronic progressive infection and disseminated disease. The outcome of infection is determined by host defenses primarily characterized by a granulomatous response involving alveolar macrophages and T cell immunity at the local level. The geographic specificity of some of the dimorphic fungi, *Histoplasma capsulatum*, *Coccidioides immitis*, and *Blastomyces dermatiditis*, is an important epidemiologic clue to causes of undiagnosed pneumonias in persons with an appropriate environmental exposure and should be sought in the history of all patients.

Histoplasmosis

Histoplasma capsulatum was originally described in Panama by Darling and subsequently determined to be a dimorphic fungus by DeMonbreun (1). Although it is now known that this soil-residing dimorphic fungus has a worldwide distribution, the preponderance of clinical cases occur in the Ohio and Mississippi River valleys of the United States, and to lesser extents in Mexico, Puerto Rico, and other islands of the Caribbean basin. Sporulation of the organism is promoted by growth in bird guano, and epidemiologic links to non-commercial chicken coops, bird roosts, and avian feces products such as chicken manure exist. Unlike uninfected avians, bats are infected with the organism without evidence of disease (2). The organism is found in bat guano such that Histoplasmosis is a hazard to spelunkers who explore caves laden with bat and bird guano. There have been more than 40 cave-associated outbreaks; the majority of spelunkers in many areas are exposed and should expect to have a positive histoplasmin skin test result (3). Because cell-mediated immunity is the major defense against *H. capsulatum*, those with underlying diseases characterized by its defects such as Hodgkin's disease or acquired immunodeficiency syndrome (AIDS), are inordinately susceptible to *H. capsulatum* infection. Indeed, in some geographic areas, histoplasmosis is a major cause of morbidity and death in AIDS patients (4).

In soil, *H. capsulatum* is mycelial in form, possessing characteristic tuberculate chlamydospores. After the spores are inhaled, there is prompt phagocytosis by in situ lung mononuclear phagocytes and thereafter a rapid morphologic metamorphosis to the tissue invasive yeast form. Mycelia may be found within chronic lung cavities and rarely on the surface of cardiac vegetations.

TABLE 54.1. Community Acquired and Opportunistic Pathogens Causing Fungal Pneumonias

Community acquired mycoses		Opportunistic mycoses
		Mostly in compromised hosts
Mostly in normal hosts	**About equally in normal and compromised persons**	
Histoplasma capsulatum	*Cryptococcus neoformans*	*Aspergillus* sp.
Blastomyces dermatitidis	*Sporothrix schenckii*	*Zygomycetes*
Coccidioides immitis	*Penicillium marneffei*	*Fusarium* sp.
Paracoccidioides brasiliensis		*Pseudallescheria boydii*
		(Scedosporium apiospermum)
		Scedosporium prolificans
		Scopulariopsis sp.
		Curvularia lunata
		Paecilomyces varioti
		Candida sp.
		Trichosporon sp
		Geotrichum sp.

Three stages of transition to the yeast phase with associated alterations in the molecular, biochemical and physical properties of the organism have been identified (5). Recent identification of the yeast phase-specific gene (*ysp-3*) is expected to yield a greater understanding of the molecular mechanisms of thermotolerant fungi (6). Survival of yeast cells within the phagolysosome is accomplished by alkalinization of the environment, avoiding the acid proteinases of the phagolysosome while maintaining a pH suitable for iron acquisition (7). After early infection, the organism disseminates via the bloodstream in infected macrophages. The balance between intracellular germination and intracellular control is determined by the efficacy of cell-mediated immunity. Cytokine induced T-cell activation of macrophages is essential for such controls occurring via interleukin-3, macrophage colony stimulating factor and granulocyte-macrophage stimulating factors (8). Reinfection of persons with established specific cellular immunity usually produces an intense inflammatory response resulting in a shortened illness. However the intensity of the response may contribute to complications of mediastinal and/or pulmonary fibrosis (9).

The clinical syndromes associated with *H. capsulatum* infection have been extensively reviewed by Wheat (10,11). Together with the amount of inoculum, the host pulmonary and immune status influence the clinical presentation and outcome of the infection (Table 54.2). Asymptomatic disease occurs in more than 95% of persons with low exposure to *H. capsulatum* (10). When a heavy inoculum exposure occurs, the likelihood for symptomatic disease typified by a flu-like illness with signs of bronchopneu-

monia is much higher. Five to ten percent of these patients may manifest pericardial, rheumatologic, or dermatologic inflammatory complications. While dissemination of the organism typically occurs in all patients, disseminated disease manifests primarily in the immunocompromised host.

ACUTE ASYMPTOMATIC PRIMARY INFECTION

This is the most prevalent clinical form of the disease. In the majority of cases, the infection is so mild that it comes to the attention of physicians relatively infrequently. Chest radiographs may show minimal to no parenchymal infiltrates followed by either complete healing or residual calcification. Usually, no antifungal treatment is required.

ACUTE PROGRESSIVE SYMPTOMATIC PRIMARY INFECTION

Occurring 1 to 2 weeks after exposure, this syndrome is characterized by fever, chills, sweats, cough, chest pain, headache, myalgia, fatigue, and, in some cases, sputum production or dyspnea. Physical findings are variable. There may be no abnormalities or only sticky inspiratory rales or areas with dullness to percussion and altered breath sounds; occasionally, there may be evidence of frank consolidation. Pleural rubs are observed infrequently. In a small number of cases, there may be a pleural effusion; in such cases, the fluid can be serous, serosanguinous, or even frankly bloody. The predominant cell type in the effusion is usually the lymphocyte, but there can be a striking number of eosinophils (12). Chest radiographs typically show one or more areas of focal nodular infiltrates or, less commonly, consolidation. Hilar adenopathy is frequently present (13). In most cases, the nodules heal over several months (2). Calcification of the lymph nodes and pulmonary lesions may occur later.

DIFFUSE RETICULONODULAR AND MILIARY DISEASE

This syndrome may occur after heavy exposure and is characterized by severe illness that can progress to respiratory failure and disseminated disease. Diffuse reticulonodular or miliary lesions occur on chest radiograph (2). Typically, patients recover without treatment but residual pulmonary fibrosis and restrictive lung physiology may result (2).

CHRONIC DISEASE

Chronic pulmonary histoplasmosis occurs primarily in patients with underlying lung disorders. Enlarging pleural-based

TABLE 54.2. Classification of *H. capsulatum* Pulmonary Syndromes by Host Status

Normal host	Abnormal host (immunocompromised or structural pulmonary defect)
Acute primary infection	Progressive disseminated infection
Asymptomatic	Chronic pulmonary infection
Symptomatic	Excessive fibrotic response
Reinfection	Mediastinal fibrosis
	Histoplasmoma

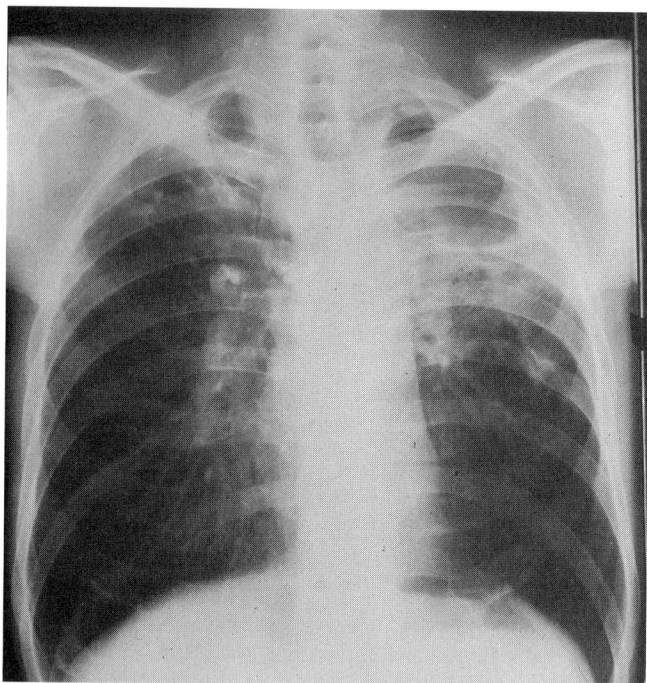

Figure 54.1. Upper lobe cavitary lesion in person with chronic pulmonary histoplasmosis. (Courtesy of Harriet Provine, Harvard Medical School, Boston, MA.)

cavitary lesions associated with productive cough, dyspnea, chest pain, hemoptysis, fevers, and sweats may be confused with active tuberculosis. The majority of patients suffering from chronic histoplasmosis have radiographic evidence of one or more cavities, usually in the upper lobes (Fig. 54.1). These may rupture into the pleural space with resultant empyema or bronchopleural fistula. Superinfection of the cavities and aspergilloma formation may lead to massive hemoptysis.

COMPLICATIONS OF ACUTE OR CHRONIC HISTOPLASMOSIS

Calcified nodes can erode into the bronchus; these broncholiths can cause either hemoptysis or recurrent pneumonia and may require surgical intervention. They can also obstruct major bronchi, with resultant localized wheeze. There has been increased interest in histoplasma-induced mediastinal fibrosis resulting from an exuberant fibrotic response to previous infection (14,15). Manifestations include dyspnea, hemoptysis, and postobstructive pneumonia resulting from tracheal or bronchial stenosis. Superior vena caval or pulmonary artery occlusion may occur. Fibrosing mediastinitis may also affect the esophagus, with the potential for traction diverticula or fistulae; symptoms include dysphagia, chest pain, and odynophagia (16). Dysphagia can also result from extrinsic lymph node pressure. The nodes on the right side of the mediastinum are involved more frequently than those on the left side.

In addition to localized complications, a systemic, noninfectious, rheumatoid inflammation may occur in 5% to 10% of patients with acute infection. Polyarticular arthritis and arthralgias occur more commonly in women and may be associated with erythema nodosum or erythema multiforme (10).

PROGRESSIVE DISSEMINATED DISEASE

Progressive histoplasmosis occurs most often in patients at the extremes of ages and in those with compromised immunity. The clinical spectrum ranges from chronic progressive pulmonary disease to disseminated disease resulting in acute fulminant sepsis syndrome and death. Three forms of chronic progressive disease exist. The chronic progressive form presents most commonly as painful oral ulcers involving the tongue, buccal mucosa, gingiva, and occasionally the larynx. Hepatosplenomegaly occurs in 30%. A subacute form is characterized by more constitutional symptoms over a prolonged period of 1 to 3 months and multiple organ involvement including the gastrointestinal tract, bone marrow, reticuloendothelial system, and central nervous system. Life-threatening adrenal insufficiency may develop in 5% to 10% of patients. If untreated, death results usually within 2 years. The acute progressive form is seen commonly in patients with the acquired immune deficiency syndrome. Pulmonary symptoms and radiographic abnormalities are common as are manifestations of disseminated disease. A hyperacute syndrome may occur in 10% to 20% of patients associated with adult respiratory distress syndrome, disseminated intravascular coagulation, and multiorgan failure despite treatment.

The diagnosis of histoplasmosis varies according to severity of infection and, in many cases, the index of suspicion for disease. Culture, tissue staining, serology, and antigen detection are diagnostic methods with high specificity for the infection and varying sensitivity depending on the extent of infection. Culture is the most sensitive method in disseminated disease. Blood (by lysis centrifugation) and bone marrow cultures yield the highest results (11,17). Diagnosis of diffuse or miliary pulmonary histoplasmosis may be made by culture of expectorated sputum or, if required, by culture of bronchoalveolar lavage fluid (18). Fungal staining of tissues samples may be positive in about 50% of cases; however, detection is largely dependent upon the experience of the pathologist in reading the results (19). In most cases the diagnosis is made serologically using precipitation, immunodiffusion, complement fixation, and latex agglutination tests. More than 90% of patients with acute symptomatic pulmonary infection will have positive serologic test results by 6 weeks (20). Detection of *Histoplasma* glycoprotein antigen in blood or urine provides rapid diagnosis in patients with disseminated or diffuse pulmonary disease (21).

No treatment is required for most cases of acute pulmonary histoplasmosis. Treatment is advisable for those with severe, persistent, or progressive disease and for those who are immunocompromised and do not improve rapidly without treatment. Amphotericin B is fungicidal for *H. capsulatum* and remains the most predictable agent in severe or life-threatening disease, especially in immunocompromised hosts. Itraconazole is the alternative agent; a dosage of 200 to 400 mg/day given for 1 to 12 months, depending on the clinical circumstances, is usually effective in pulmonary and disseminated histoplasmosis, particularly in non-immunocompromised hosts. Immunocompromised patients may require chronic maintenance therapy to prevent infection relapse. Treatment cessation in patients with AIDS with sustained immune reconstitution from highly active antiretroviral therapy is being addressed in an ongoing clinical trial. However, *in vitro* data measuring histoplasmin skin tests, lymphoproliferative responses and interferon gamma production in patients with or without human immunodeficiency virus (HIV) and infection demonstrated a poor response in patients with HIV with CD4 cells less than 500 mm^3, suggesting a need for ongoing maintenance therapy (22). Those with chronic cavitary disease should almost always be treated with either amphotericin B or itraconazole; treatment must often be prolonged (6 to 12 months). Fluconazole by mouth is less effective than itraconazole and generally not recommended for maintenance therapy or secondary prophylaxis in patients with AIDS (23). The efficacy of treatment can be evaluated in many cases by monitoring blood and urine *Histoplasma* antigen levels (24). Patients with mediastinal fibrosis, obstructing nodes, obstructing histoplasmomas, broncholith-induced bleeding, or esophageal diverticula or fistulae frequently require surgical intervention (14).

Blastomycosis

Described by Gilchrist in 1894, blastomycosis is an acute or chronic disease caused by the endemic dimorphic fungus *Blastomyces dermatitidis*. Although soil is clearly the reservoir during the infectious mycelial phase, it has been remarkably difficult to recover *B. dermatitidis* from soil samples. However, in an outbreak in Wisconsin, the fungus was isolated repeatedly from environmental samples, and the attack rate of exposed persons was a surprisingly high 51%; approximately one half were symptomatic after an incubation period ranging from 21 to 106 days (25,26). For 70 years, blastomycosis was thought to be confined geographically to the central and southeastern United States. Now the disease appears to have a more global distribution; cases have been reported from Canada, Mexico, the Middle East, Africa, and India (27). Although most of those acquiring *B. dermatitidis* infection are immunocompetent males, disease in immunocompromised patients may be severe (28).

In the United States, inhalation of spores results in pulmonary infection. Experimental data indicate that lung macrophages have some ability to ingest and kill *B. dermatitidis*, as do polymorphonuclear cells (29). Transformation from the mycelial to the yeast phase appears to result from temperature-dependent changes in oxidative phosphorylation and respiratory rates (29,30). The critical shunt pathways are sulfhydryl dependent. Subsequent dissemination of the organism via the bloodstream to the skin and other organs may occur. Once host immunity develops, a pyogranulomatous inflammatory response to the yeast forms, unique to blastomycosis, occurs.

Clinical presentations of pulmonary blastomycosis include asymptomatic infection, acute pneumonia and chronic pneumonia. The clinical features of disease were elucidated in a Wisconsin epidemic that involved enough persons to permit a better understanding of symptom and sign frequency (25,31). In decreasing frequency, the following occurred in the 26 symptomatic persons: cough, fever, night sweats, chest pain, weight loss, myalgias, and hemoptysis. The onset of illness is usually abrupt (but may be insidious) and is characterized by cough productive of mucopurulent sputum that may be confused with acute bacterial pneumonia. Myalgias and arthralgias may accompany the pulmonary manifestations, producing an influenza-like clinical picture. On occasion, the pulmonary infection may be overwhelming, mimicking severe acute bacterial pneumonia; the adult respiratory distress syndrome has also been noted (32).

Physical findings on lung examination range from none to inspiratory rales to evidence of frank consolidation. Radiographic findings are likewise variable, including consolidation of part or all of a lobe, multilobar infiltrates, perihilar infiltrates, multiple nodules, and mediastinal node involvement. Miliary infiltrates are occasionally noted. Pleural effusion occurs infrequently. In patients with HIV, the characteristic findings are diffuse or miliary infiltrates (33). Acute lung involvement may resolve spontaneously, persist, or progress. Chronic lesions are characterized by fibrosis and cavitation.

The fungus may be seen in sputum or bronchoalveolar lavage specimens as spherical 5- to 20-μm cells with a thick double-contoured refractile wall (Fig. 54.2). Characteristic broad-based budding yeast cells may be detected on potassium hydroxide (KOH) preparations of sputum. The fungus grows slowly; colonies appear 3 to 35 days after incubation. Serologic tests for diagnosis are not entirely satisfactory. Enzyme immunoassay appears to have greater sensitivity than either immunodiffusion or complement fixation, but test results of a significant percentage of those who are infected remain negative (26). The immunodiffusion and complement fixation tests have greater specificity.

Amphotericin B is clearly an effective agent in both acute and chronic pulmonary blastomycosis and should be used in overwhelming or life-threatening infection. In mild-to-moderate disease, itraconazole appears equally effective (34). Fluconazole may also be useful (35).

Coccidioidomycosis

Originally described in 1892, the disease has a variety of sobriquets—valley fever, desert rheumatism, San Joaquin Valley fever. The major endemic area is confined to the lower Sonoran life zone in the United States, where the soil is arid and alkaline and the ambient temperature is usually in the 80°F to 100°F range. Parts or all of California, Nevada, Arizona, Texas, Utah,

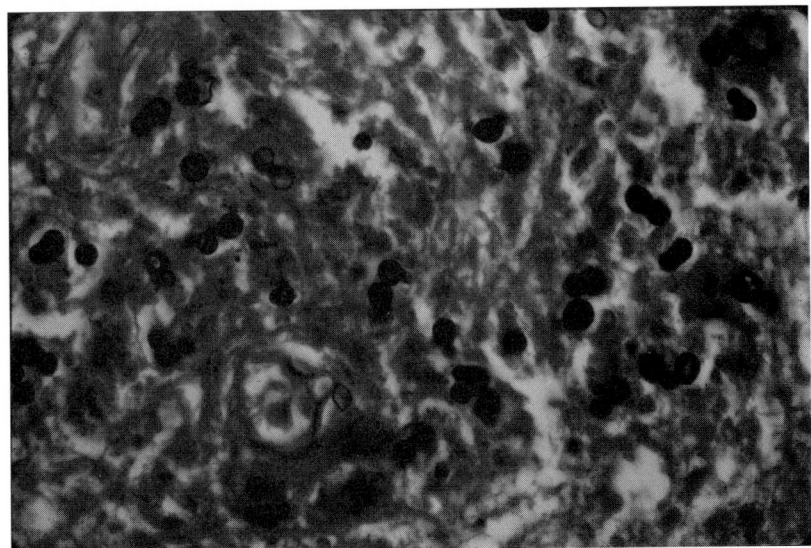

Figure 54.2. Bronchoalveolar lavage specimen revealing spherical cells of *B. dermatiditis*. (Courtesy of Harriet Provine, Harvard Medical School, Boston, MA.)

and New Mexico lie in this zone, but coccidioidal infections are not limited to this area. Some desert regions of Mexico are also endemic areas, and small numbers of cases have been reported from Central and South America.

In endemic areas, the attack rate is high. At least 15% of persons entering such an area can expect to have a positive skin test result within a year, and 30% to more than 50% will have a positive skin test result after 2 to 4 years of residence (36–38). Cell-mediated immunity is necessary for host control after *Coccidioides immitis* invasion (39). Therefore, persons at the extremes of age, with AIDS or lymphomas, receiving corticosteroids or immunosuppressive treatments, or undergoing organ transplantation show increased susceptibility to coccidioidal infection (36–38,40). Case-control studies have demonstrated an increased risk for infection in elderly persons who have recently translocated to the endemic area (41). Moreover, diabetic patients, women in the second half of pregnancy, those of Filipino, African-American, Hispanic, or Oriental race are at increased risk for disseminated infection (36,38,42).

In at least 95% and probably more than 99% of cases of acute pneumonia, coccidioidomycosis is a self-limited disease, requiring no treatment and having no sequelae. Symptoms occur in only 30% to 40% of acutely infected individuals (43). They include, in descending order of frequency, cough, fever, chest pain, headache, chills, shortness of breath, malaise, myalgias, and rash (erythema nodosum or erythema multiforme). The chest pain may be pleuritic, centrally located and severe on occasion, and may mimic acute costochondritis. The pulmonary infection can occasionally be overwhelming, can mimic bacterial septic shock, and can be accompanied by adult respiratory distress syndrome (44). Physical examination is often unrewarding. Rales, rhonchi, or wheezes may be detected; in some cases, there may be evidence of frank consolidation or pleural effusion.

Radiographs may show only hilar adenopathy (on occasion massive), or there may be a variety of soft or nodular infiltrates, most frequently found in the upper lobes. In those with persistent or progressive disease, infiltrates are most often bilateral in the upper lobes (often apical), are fibronodular and contain multiple cavities that are characteristically thin walled, and may have air-fluid levels. These cavities may close spontaneously. Chronic cavitary diseases may be complicated by bacterial or fungal superinfection, significant hemoptysis, pyopneumothorax, or bronchopleural fistulae (36–38,45). *C. immitis* infection usually develops in patients with HIV after CD4+ lymphocyte counts are less than 200/mm^3; their pulmonary disease may manifest as focal pneumonic infiltrates but is usually characterized by diffuse reticulonodular or nodular patterns (40).

In some cases, solitary nodules—coccidioidomas—may be the only manifestation of lung involvement; some of these may calcify. Miliary disease is seen in a small percentage of those with primary lung involvement, usually in patients suffering from severe underlying diseases, such as diabetes or AIDS, or in those being treated with immunosuppressive agents or corticosteroids. On rare occasions, lung lesions may be accompanied by striking tissue eosinophilia and some peripheral eosinophilia (46).

Dissemination from the lungs ordinarily occurs early during the course of the acute infection; only rarely does dissemination occur after several months of infection in those with chronic pulmonary coccidioidomycosis. The lung lesion can be complicated by fistula formation that is not necessarily restricted to the thorax; extraordinary examples have been reported of pulmonary-gluteal or pulmonary-thigh fistulae.

The diagnosis can be established by isolation of the fungus and by serologic tests. In some cases, examination of sputum treated with sodium hydroxide will demonstrate the yeast phase, the spherule, which ranges from 20 to 80 μm in diameter and may contain small (2 to 4 μm) endospores. *C. immitis* grows readily in culture, producing white cottony mycelia in 2 to 8 days; the hyphae contain characteristic rectangular arthrospores. Serologic studies include precipitation, latex agglutination, complement fixation, immunodiffusion, counter-immunodiffusion, and enzyme immunoassay. The precipitation test, reflecting immunoglobulin M early in the course of the infection, and the complement fixation test, reflecting immunoglobulin G somewhat later, are still the two most useful studies. In coccidioidomycosis limited to the lungs, the complement fixation titers usually do not exceed 1:16. Complement fixation titers are often deceptively low in patients with chronic cavitary disease and in those with coccidioidomas.

Most patients with acute pulmonary coccidioidomycosis do not require therapy. In persistent or progressive disease or in chronic cavitary disease, amphotericin B remains the agent of choice. The triazoles, fluconazole and itraconazole, given in a dosage of at least 400 mg/day appear to be reasonable alternatives for non–life-threatening disease (38,47). Surgery may be required for severe hemoptysis, cavities that rupture or enlarge despite treatment, empyema, or fistulae.

Sporotrichosis

Sporothrix schenkii is a dimorphic fungus with worldwide distribution. Decaying vegetation is the environmental niche for the mold form. Frequently manifested as a subacute to chronic cutaneous or lymphocutaneous infection caused by direct inoculation of the organism, the rarer pulmonary form is presumed to be due to inhalation of aerosolized conidia. Those at risk for pulmonary disease often have underlying lung disease or are immunosuppressed by virtue of alcoholism, diabetes, sarcoidosis or exogenous or endogenous immunodeficiency. Constitutional symptoms of fever, night sweats, weight loss, and fatigue often accompany the pulmonary symptoms of dyspnea and productive cough sometimes complicated by hemoptysis (48,49). Primary pulmonary sporotrichosis may be associated with pneumonitis and hilar or paratracheal lymphadenopathy (50,51). Upper lobe cavities occur frequently, and disease is progressive if untreated. Diagnosis is made by culture of the organism from sputum, bronchoalveolar lavage fluid or tissue; non-caseating granulomas may be seen on biopsy without evidence of organisms, however. Itraconazole is now the mainstay of therapy for mild-to-moderate disease; amphotericin B with or without surgical resection remains the drug of choice for severe infection (52).

Paracoccidioidomycosis

Paracoccidioides brasiliensis is endemic to Central and South America typically causing pulmonary disease in young adult males in rural settings. Like the other dimorphic fungi, pneumonia may be acute, chronic or lead to disseminated disease (53). Symptoms include productive cough, dyspnea, hemoptysis, chest pain, fever, weight loss, and night sweats and may be very indolent. Fibrocavitary disease is evident on chest radiography, and obstructive pulmonary function results from extensive fibrosis over time. Itraconazole is successful treatment in mild-to-moderate disease; sulfadiazine may also be used with success when cost is a consideration. Amphotericin B may be required for severe pulmonary disease. Treatment duration is long (at least 6 months) due to late relapses.

Cryptococcosis

Cryptococcius neoformans is ubiquitous in nature, residing in soil, and ordinarily infects through the respiratory route. Cryptococcal pneumonia not infrequently arises in ostensibly healthy persons; however, more often the yeast attacks those with defects in delayed immune mechanisms, those receiving corticosteroids, and those being treated simultaneously with immunosuppressive drugs and corticosteroids as therapy for malignant neoplasms or after organ or tissue transplantation. Those with hematologic malignancies are susceptible in the absence of therapy, but that susceptibility is markedly increased during treatment. Other less well-established risk factors include the presence of sarcoidosis, diabetes, and hepatic cirrhosis. Of course, AIDS has become the major risk factor; *C. neoformans* infection develops in as many as 10% of patients with AIDS (54,55).

The symptoms and signs of pulmonary cryptococcal infection are variable and lack specificity. Indeed, there may be no symptoms referable to the chest. Mild temperature elevation and nonproductive or slightly productive cough are found frequently, but there may also be chest pain, and substantial hemoptysis has been reported rarely (56). The sputum may rarely appear purulent. Although the clinical pattern is usually characterized by insidious onset and slow progression, the disease can be fulminating; this pattern is found with considerable frequency in those with AIDS. Cryptococcosis can also be a nosocomial infection, but it is unclear in such cases whether the infection arises from the hospital environment or the patient's respiratory tract (57). Rarely, endobronchial lesions have caused obstructive phenomena.

Findings on chest radiography are variable. Patterns include one or more nodular lesions that are often round and devoid of surrounding inflammation, patchy infiltrates, lobar or lobular consolidation, pneumonia with cavitation, diffuse reticulonodular or interstitial infiltrates, and miliary disease (Fig. 54.3). Pleural effusions occur infrequently. Focal lesions can mimic lung carcinoma. Mediastinal lymphadenitis due to cryptococcal infection in patients with HIV responding to highly active antiretroviral therapy has been described in patients with and without previous cryptococcal infection even while receiving fluconazole as secondary prophylaxis (58).

The diagnosis is best made by isolating the organism from cultures of sputum, bronchoalveolar lavage fluid, or blood. In some cases, lung biopsy is necessary. Serologic studies may be helpful if antigen titers exceed 1:8, but titers of less than 1:8 may represent false-positive findings. Serum antibody determinations are not useful. Dual pulmonary infection is not infrequent; pneumonias due concomitantly to *C. neoformans* and *Mycobacterium tuberculosis*, *H. capsulatum*, *Nocardia asteroides*, or *Legionella pneumophila* are well described (59).

Some advocate no treatment for isolated pulmonary cryptococcosis in an apparently healthy host (60). Others, concerned by reports of persistence of the infection or spread to the central nervous system, recommend treatment for all those suffering from pulmonary cryptococcal infection (61,62). There is no debate about immunocompromised patients—all should be treated. Amphotericin B is the most effective agent; there are no data documenting the need to add a second agent in isolated pulmonary disease. Some would treat with two agents, particularly lower doses of amphotericin B plus 5-fluorocytosine. Fluconazole is an alternative agent but the optimal dose and route of administration have not been fully established (63). Itraconazole has been effective in some cases, but data at present are meager.

OPPORTUNISTIC PULMONARY MYCOSES

Aspergillosis

There are three forms of sinopulmonary aspergillosis: the noninvasive allergic, colonizing or saprophytic, and the invasive form (Table 54.3). Persons with immunocompromise by virtue of underlying malignancy (primarily hematologic) or HIV are at highest risk for invasive pulmonary aspergillosis, although there are increasing reports of this disease in normal hosts (64). *Aspergillus* spores are inhaled into the alveoli and if not ingested and killed by the pulmonary macrophages germinate into the

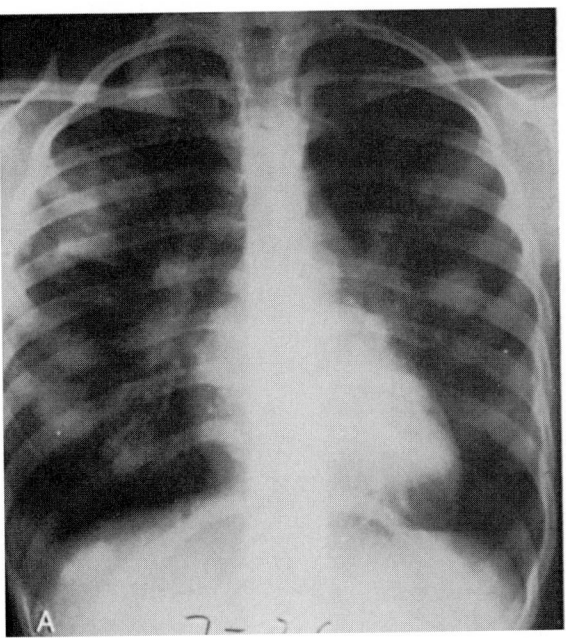
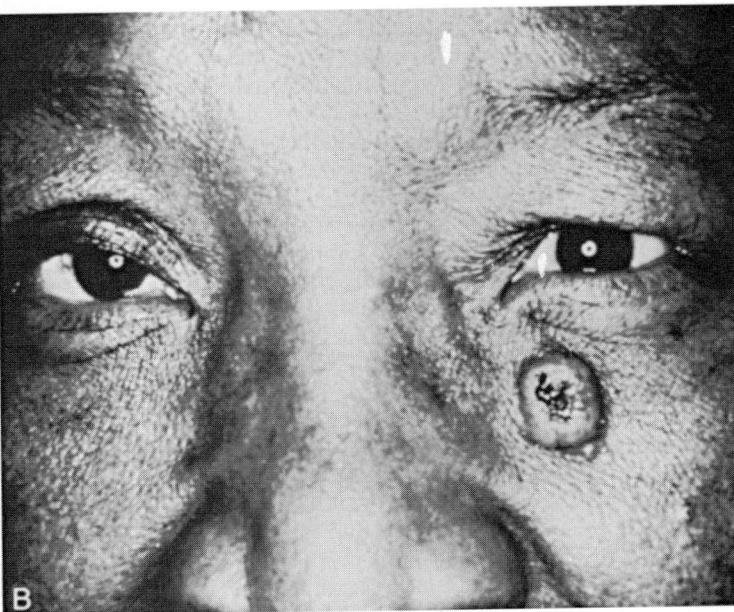

Figure 54.3. Cryptococcal nodular lung lesions (**A**) and ulcerating skin nodules (**B**) in a 72-year-old woman during steroid treatment for chronic lymphatic leukemia.

TABLE 54.3.   Types of Sino-pulmonary Aspergillosis: Host Characteristics and Treatment Recommendations

Type	Host	Treatment
Noninvasive allergic		
Extrinsic allergic alveolitis	Normal - overexposure	Remove from exposure
Extrinsic asthma	Normal - overexposure	Remove from exposure; bronchodilators
Acute bronchopulmonary aspergillosis	Normal	
Allergic sinusitis	Normal	
Colonizing		
Aspergilloma	Chronic lung disease, lung cavity	Observation; surgical resection for hemoptysis
Invasive	Immunocompromised	Amphotericin B or lipid preparations
Sinusitis		Triazoles
Tracheobronchitis	Occasionally normal host	Itraconazole, voriconazole; investigational agents
Bronchopneumonia		Echinocandins
Chronic necrotizing pneumonia		Caspofungin; investigational agents
Disseminated		Surgical resection
		Growth factors
		Granulocyte transfusions
		Cytokine immunomodulators

mycelial form. Corticosteroids inhibit the actions of pulmonary macrophages thereby permitting spore germination to the invasive mycelial form. Polymorphonuclear cells are critical in killing both the spore and mycelial forms by the actions of cationic proteins and those of the myeloperoxidase-halide system (65,66). Neutropenia is therefore a significant risk for invasion by the mycelial form.

Noninvasive Aspergillosis

Noninvasive aspergillosis primarily occurs in normal hosts. Allergic aspergillosis results from either overexposure to *Aspergillus* antigens such as occurs in farmers or from reactions of an allergic host. Symptoms of cough, fever, and myalgias associated with interstitial infiltrates on chest radiograph occur soon after overexposure and are alleviated within hours of removal from exposure. In this setting, repeated exposure may result in intractable pulmonary fibrosis. Peripheral eosinophilia, elevated total serum quantitative IgE, demonstration of precipitating antibodies against aspergillus and central bronchiectasis are characteristic of allergic bronchopulmonary aspergillosis (ABPA) (67,68). Immune complex formation and a Type III reaction are responsible for the peribronchial inflammation and evanescent pulmonary infiltrates characteristic of this disorder. A recent study investigating the role of antifungal agents in the treatment of ABPA demonstrated a role for treatment with itraconazole (69). Corticosteroids may also successfully treat this allergic condition (70). Allergic fungal sinusitis occurs in persons with atopy, nasal polyposis, and chronic sinusitis (71). Colonization by *Aspergillus* spp. of an existing pulmonary cavity may result in development of a fungus ball, or aspergilloma, within the cavity (Fig. 54.4). This asymptomatic condition may remain undetected until erosion of organisms into the cavity wall leads to hemorrhage within the cavity or erosion into a blood vessel causing massive hemoptysis. No treatment is required for an aspergilloma arising in an established neoplastic or tuberculous cavity; if severe hemoptysis or bacterial superinfection occurs, surgical excision is the treatment of choice. Chronic necrotizing pulmonary aspergillosis is a distinct entity occurring in patients with altered lung architecture by virtue of chronic lung

diseases such as chronic obstructive pulmonary disease, sarcoidosis, bronchiectasis, radiation fibrosis or prior tuberculosis with or without concomitant immunosuppression. In contrast with asymptomatic aspergillomas, patients with chronic necrotizing aspergillosis usually complain of constitutional symptoms, which may include productive cough with or without hemoptysis, pleuritic chest pain, fatigue, or weight loss (72,73). The pathologic features of the condition suggest cavity formation as a result of lung necrosis caused by the organism with possible invasion of the cavity wall and surrounding lung tissue. Antifungal therapy is warranted for treatment of chronic necrotizing aspergillosis. The *Aspergillus* active azole class of antifungal agents

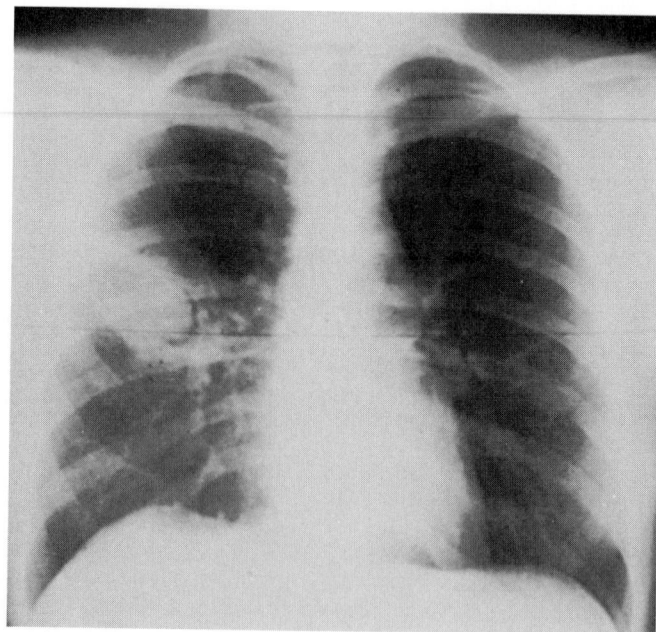

Figure 54.4. Huge aspergilloma within a lung cyst. (Courtesy of Dr. Baynard Tynes, University of Alabama School of Medicine, Birmingham, AL.)

offer the convenience of oral therapy in an otherwise ambulatory host and have demonstrated suppressive efficacy in this setting (73). Ultimately, surgical resection of the affected area may be necessary and curative.

Invasive Aspergillosis

The advances in treatment of hematologic malignancies and growing numbers of patients with HIV in the past two decades have contributed to the significant increase in invasive aspergillosis (IA) in immunocompromised hosts. Mortality due to invasive fungal infections has increased by 357% since 1980 (74,75). In hematopoietic stem cell transplant recipients, IA is the most common cause of infectious-related mortality and results in death in over 85% of cases (76). The significant host risk factors for IA include prolonged granulocytopenia, graft vs. host disease and its immunosuppressive treatment, and corticosteroid use. Thus, hematopoietic stem cell or solid organ transplant recipients, those with underlying malignancies requiring high doses of corticosteroid treatment or prolonged periods of neutropenia, and persons with advanced AIDS are at risk for IA. In addition, *Aspergillus* pneumonia may complicate viral influenza and endogenous Cushing's syndrome (77,78). Diabetic ketoacidosis also increases the risk of invasive disease in diabetic patients (Fig. 54.5).

Invasive *Aspergillus* pneumonia is primarily caused by *A. fumigatus*, but other species are well known causes including *A. flavus*, *A. niger*, and *A. terreus*. The most frequent manifestations are cough, fever, and dyspnea; pleuritic chest pain from lung infarction by the angioinvasive organism may also occur. In some cases, persistent fever despite broad-spectrum antibiotics in a neutropenic patient may be the only sign of IA. Fever and sputum production, however, are variable. Because of the tendency for blood vessel invasion by the organism, hemoptysis occurs frequently; its occurrence in the proper clinical setting should suggest the presence of *Aspergillus*. Although *Aspergillus* pneumonia is often characterized by relatively rapid onset and inexorable progression, its onset may be surprisingly indolent,

and in some cases, the pneumonia may progress slowly or may appear to improve temporarily without treatment. Infrequently, ulcerative or pseudomembranous tracheobronchial aspergillosis with or without concomitant lung infiltrates may be accompanied by prominent expiratory wheezes (79).

The high mortality associated with IA makes early diagnosis imperative, however the diagnosis of *Aspergillus* pneumonia is often difficult. Recent advances in early diagnosis of IA have included antigen detection, polymerase chain reaction detection of *Aspergillus* DNA in peripheral blood samples and early use of computed tomography scanning of the chest (80,81). Chest radiographs may reveal infarct-like nodular lesions, but this is usually a late finding (Fig. 54.6). Detection of *A. galactomannan* antigen in serum by sandwich enzyme-linked immunosorbent assay is associated with a positive predictive value of >92% and may precede clinical suspicion of IA (82). A positive test result is defined as more than one positive sample collected on 2 different days with an optical density of greater than 1.0; false-positive rates are less than 10% (81). Approval of this serologic test by the US Food and Drug Administration (FDA) is expected shortly. Mycelia can sometimes be visualized in expectorated sputum (or expectorated blood), and the fungus can be cultivated on standard media. However, sputum smears and cultures are often unrevealing. Cytologic examination of bronchoalveolar lavage fluid is more rewarding diagnostically, but can be misleadingly negative. Often, lung biopsy is required for definitive diagnosis by pathology and/or microbiology.

It is important to establish the diagnosis because vigorous therapy may be effective. Amphotericin B has long been the mainstay of treatment but is associated with significant infusion related and renal toxicities (83). Renal toxicity from amphotericin B is in itself associated with increased morbidity and mortality (84–86) Lipid formulations of amphotericin B have proven to be less nephrotoxic with similar efficacy (87). Azoles play a role in *Aspergillus* infection treatment. Itraconazole is effective in some refractory cases (88). The newly FDA-approved broad-spectrum triazole, voriconazole, has proven efficacy and superior survival rates when compared with amphotericin B followed by other licensed antifungal therapies (if required) with significantly less nephrotoxicity and is therefore expected to be utilized as a mainstay of therapy (89,90). Other extended spectrum triazoles, posaconazole and ravuconazole, are currently under clinical investigation for treatment of invasive mold infections and may have similar efficacy. The new class of antifungal agents, the echinocandins, have also shown efficacy in refractory IA cases, and much interest in combining these cell wall active agents with cell membrane active agents, such as the polyenes or triazoles, for early treatment of IA is mounting. In the presence of severe neutropenia, response to anti-*Aspergillus* agents may depend on the reversal of the neutropenia. Thus, adjuvant therapy with growth factors or immunomodulating agents to improve neutrophil counts or enhance the immune response is warranted when feasible. Surgical excision of solitary nodules or localized infection with concomitant antifungal therapy is the treatment of choice if possible.

Zygomycosis (Mucormycosis)

Pulmonary zygomycosis caused by the Zygomycetes class of fungi is a rare but frequently fatal opportunistic infection. Fungi of the order Murcorales are most commonly associated with respiratory infections. Most cases are caused by species of *Rhizopus*, *Absidia*, or *Mucor*, but a small number have been caused by other Zygomycetes, including *Cunninghamella elegans*, *Cunninghamella bertholletiae*, *Conidiobolus incongruus*, and *Saksenaea vasiformis* (91–97).

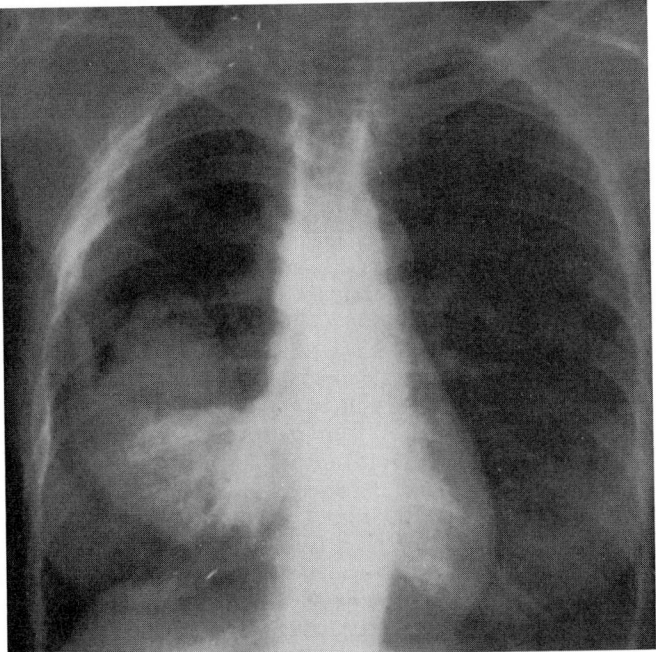

Figure 54.5. Severe aspergillosis complicating diabetic ketoacidosis in a 54-year-old woman, presenting as progressive hemoptysis.

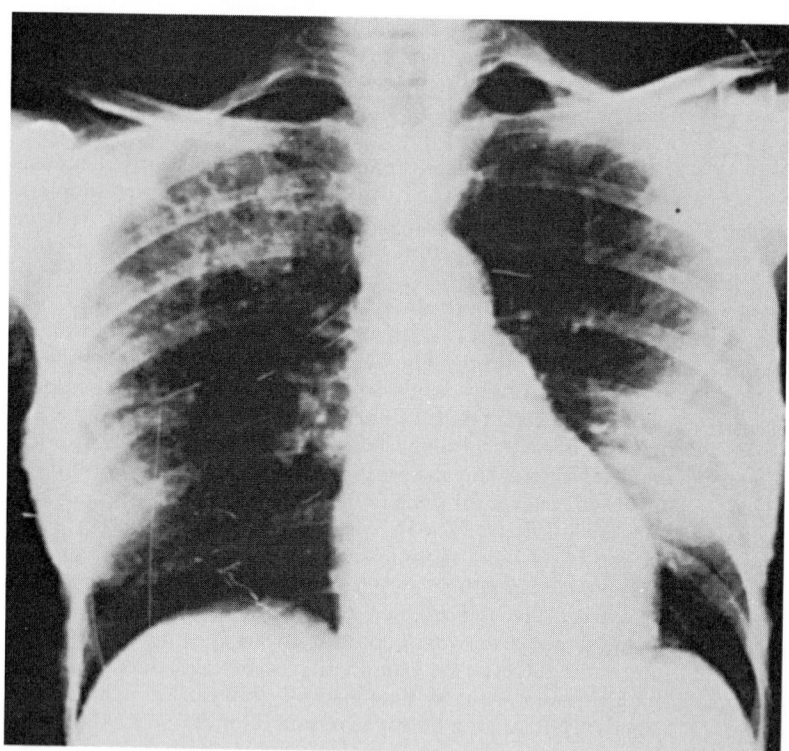

Figure 54.6. *Aspergillus* pneumonia presenting as an infarct-like lesion in a patient with subacute myelogenous leukemia after antileukemia therapy and multiple antibiotics for bacterial sepsis. (Courtesy of Dr. Donald Armstrong, Memorial Sloan-Kettering Cancer Center, New York.)

Inhalation of spores from environmental sources is the predominant mode of transmission of pulmonary disease. Both pulmonary macrophages and polymorphonuclear leukocytes appear to be important in host defenses against spores and hyphae of Zygomycetes (65,98,99). Spores are ingested by pulmonary macrophages and are killed or controlled by inhibition of germination. Hyphal elements either are ingested by neutrophils or are damaged extracellularly. Hosts with impaired pulmonary macrophage function, such as diabetics, or those with neutrophil deficiency or disorder are therefore at highest risk for invasive zygomycosis. Those suffering from hematologic malignancies ordinarily develop zygomycotic pneumonia during periods of profound treatment related neutropenia. In experimental models, diabetic mice show multiple defects in pulmonary macrophage function, including diminished capacity to attach to hyphal elements and reduced ability to prevent spore germination (99). Although ketoacidosis increases susceptibility to zygomycotic superinfection, nonketotic diabetic patients are also susceptible; indeed, zygomycosis can occur before clinical manifestations of diabetes (100). Administration of deferoxamine for iron overload is also associated with zygomycotic superinfection (101). It appears that the organisms use the iron bound to the chelators to enhance growth (102–105). Rarely, zygomycotic pneumonia occurs in those without any demonstrable underlying defect (92,100).

There is no characteristic clinical pattern; cough, fever, dyspnea, and pleuritic pain are all noted frequently (94). Zygomycetes are angioinvasive; consequently, hemoptysis (sometimes massive) may occur and infarct-like lesions may be observed on radiographic examination. In other cases, solitary nodules, cavitary lesions or patchy lobular or lobar infiltrates are found (94,106). Occasionally, despite extensive disease, standard chest films are normal but lung computed tomography scans show diffuse involvement (107). Tracheal lesions may occur and bronchopleural fistula followed by fatal hemoptysis has also been described (108).

There are no useful serologic diagnostic tests. Diagnosis can sometimes be made at bronchoscopy, but lung biopsy is often required.

Treatment is often unsuccessful. Amphotericin B is the only potentially effective agent; unfortunately, Zygomycetes are not particularly sensitive to it *in vitro*. In addition to administration of amphotericin B, successful treatment may be accomplished with control of underlying diseases such as diabetes, restoration of neutrophils via granulocyte transfusions or growth factors and discontinuation of iron chelation and immunosuppressive therapies when feasible. Surgical resection of isolated pulmonary disease offers a survival benefit over medical management (109).

Pseudallescheriasis

Pseudallescheria boydii has been described as the cause of necrotizing pneumonia in normal hosts, especially after exposure to brackish water following trauma or near drowning, but usually *Pseudallescheria* pneumonia with or without dissemination affects those with chronic lung disease during corticosteroid therapy and the immunocompromised host (110,111). The clinical signs and symptoms are indistinguishable from those of invasive aspergillosis, and like *Aspergillus* spp. and the Zygomycetes, the fungus has a proclivity for angioinvasion. This fungus, however, also invades across tissue planes and may extend beyond the lung parenchyma. The pneumonia can be acute, subacute, or chronic. Radiographic features are likewise variable and may include bronchopneumonia, lobar consolidation, cavitary lesions or multiple pulmonary nodules. Unlike *Aspergillus* spp. or the Zygomycetes, this fungus can sometimes be recovered from blood cultures. Dissemination to the central nervous system and other organs is not uncommon and is associated with high mortality (112–114). *Pseudallescheria boydii* and its asexual anamorph *Scedosporium apiospermum* are relatively resistant to most antifungal agents including amphotericin B. However, successful treatment with the newer broad-spectrum triazoles has been reported (115,116).

EMERGING FUNGAL PATHOGENS: MISCELLANEOUS FUNGI AND YEASTS

It is inevitable that as the pool of patients with severe underlying diseases—especially those undergoing treatment of hematologic malignancies and those with advanced AIDS—increases, there will be a growing number of unusual pulmonary fungal and yeast infections (Table 54.1). Two emerging pathogens are worth noting. *Scedosporium prolificans* (*inflatum*) is a dematiaceous (pigmented) mold that causes pneumonia and disseminated disease in immunocompromised hosts. Mortality is extremely high because this pathogen is usually resistant to all currently available antifungal agents (117,118). *Fusarium* spp. are hyaline molds that cause a variety of human infections, but may cause isolated pneumonia or that associated with disseminated disease. Clinically, it may be indistinguishable from aspergillosis. Recent investigations have implicated hospital water supply as a source of fusariosis in nosocomial infections (118a). Treatment with amphotericin B is not always successful; however, activity of the newer broad-spectrum triazoles against this organism is encouraging.

Three yeasts can also cause pneumonia. The most common of the three are *Candida* spp. These can be acquired via the upper respiratory tract in severely immunocompromised hosts during antibiotic, corticosteroid, or antitumor therapy and appears radiographically as unilateral or bilateral lobar or segmental infiltrates (119–121). Alternatively, diffuse lesions can arise by hematogenous spread. Diagnosis of invasive pneumonia due to *Candida* spp. is difficult especially in immunocompromised hosts. The positive predictive value of sputum or bronchoalveolar lavage cultures is low in immunocompromised patients; the yield of biopsy specimens is higher (122). *Candida* pneumonia occasionally occurs in reasonably normal hosts after aspiration, and may cause cavitary lesions (123,124). *Trichosporon beigelii* and *T. capitatum* (*Blastoschizomyces pseudotrichosporon*) are yeasts that can produce bilateral infiltrates as part of systemic infection, particularly during treatment for underlying malignant disease (125–128). For each of these yeast infections, initial treatment with amphotericin B is warranted; antifungal susceptibilities may help to guide the remainder of therapy.

REFERENCES

1. DeMonbreun WA. The cultivation and cultural characteristics of Darling's Histoplasma capsulatum. *Am J Trop Med* 1934;14:93–125.
2. Goodwin RA, Lloyd JE, Des Prez RM. Histoplasmosis in normal hosts. *Medicine* 1981;60:231–266.
3. Sacks JJ, Ajello L, Crockett LK. An outbreak and review of cave-associated histoplasmosis capsulati. *J Med Vet Mycol* 1986;24:313–325.
4. Sarosi GA, Johnson PC. Disseminated histoplasmosis in patients infected with human immunodeficiency virus. *Clin Infect Dis* 1992;14[Suppl 1]:S60–S67.
5. Medoff G, Kobayashi GS, Painter A, et al. Morphogenesis and pathogenicity of Histoplasma capsulatum. *Infect Immun* 1987;55:1355–1358.
6. Keath EJ, Abidi FE. Molecular cloning and sequence analysis of yps-3, a yeast-phase-specific gene in the dimorphic fungal pathogen Histoplasma capsulatum. *Microbiology* 1994;140[Pt 4]:759–767.
7. Eissenberg LG, Goldman WE, Schlesinger PH. Histoplasma capsulatum modulates the acidification of phagolysosomes. *J Exp Med* 1993;177:1605–1611.
8. Deepe GSJ, Bullock WE. Histoplasmosis: a granulomatous inflammatory response. In: Gallin I, Goldstein IM, Snyderman R, eds. *Inflammation: basic principles and clinical correlates*, 2nd ed. New York: Raven Press, 1992;2:943–948.
9. Goodwin RA, Nickell JA, Des Prez RM. Mediastinal fibrosis complicating healed primary histoplasmosis and tuberculosis. *Medicine* 1972;51:227.
10. Wheat LJ. Diagnosis and management of histoplasmosis. *Eur J Clin Microbiol Infect Dis* 1989;8:480–490.
11. Wheat J. Histoplasmosis: experience during outbreaks in Indianapolis and review of the literature. *Medicine* 1997;76:339–354.
12. Swinburne AJ, Fedullo AJ, Wahl GW, et al. Histoplasmoma, pleural fibrosis, and slowly enlarging pleural effusion in an asymptomatic patient. *Am Rev Respir Dis* 1987;135:502–503.
13. Wheat LJ, Slama TG, Eitzen HE, et al. A large urban outbreak of histoplasmosis: clinical features. *Ann Intern Med* 1981;94:331–337.
14. Garrett HE, Jr., Roper CL. Surgical intervention in histoplasmosis. *Ann Thorac Surg* 1986;42:711–722.
15. Mathisen DJ, Grillo HC. Clinical manifestation of mediastinal fibrosis and histoplasmosis. *Ann Thorac Surg* 1992;54:1053–1057.
16. Coss KC, Wheat LJ, Conces DJ Jr., et al. Esophageal fistula complicating mediastinal histoplasmosis. Response to amphotericin B. *Am J Med* 1987;83:343–346.
17. Paya CV, Roberts GD, Cockerill FR III. Transient fungemia in acute pulmonary histoplasmosis: detection by new blood-culturing techniques. *J Infect Dis* 1987;156:313–315.
18. Baughman RP, Kim CK, Bullock WE. Comparative diagnostic efficacy of bronchoalveolar lavage, transbronchial biopsy, and open-lung biopsy in experimental pulmonary histoplasmosis. *J Infect Dis* 1986;153:376–377.
19. Sathapatayavongs B, Batteiger BE, Wheat J, et al. Clinical and laboratory features of disseminated histoplasmosis during two large urban outbreaks. *Medicine* 1983;62:263–270.
20. Wheat LJ, French MLV, Kohler RB, et al. The diagnostic laboratory tests for histoplasmosis: analysis of experience in a large urban outbreak. *Ann Intern Med* 1982;97:680–685.
21. Wheat LJ, Kohler RB, Tewari RP. Diagnosis of disseminated histoplasmosis by detection of Histoplasma capsulatum antigen in serum and urine specimens. *N Engl J Med* 1986;314:83–88.
22. Vail GM, Mocherla S, Wheat LJ, et al. Cellular immune response in HIV-infected patients with histoplasmosis. *J Acquir Immune Defic Syndr* 2002;29:49–53.
23. McKinsey DS, Kauffman CA, Pappas PG, et al. Fluconazole therapy for histoplasmosis. *Clin Infect Dis* 1996;23:996–1001.
24. Wheat LJ, Connolly-Stringfield P, Blair R, et al. Effect of successful treatment with amphotericin B on Histoplasma capsulatum variety capsulatum polysaccharide antigen levels in patients with AIDS and histoplasmosis. *Am J Med* 1992;92:153–160.
25. Klein BS, Vergeront JM, Weeks RJ, et al. Isolation of Blastomyces dermatitidis in soil associated with a large outbreak of blastomycosis in Wisconsin. *N Engl J Med* 1986;314:529–534.
26. Klein BS, Vergeront JM, Kaufman L, et al. Serological tests for blastomycosis: assessments during a large point-source outbreak in Wisconsin. *J Infect Dis* 1987;155:262–268.
27. Berkowitz I, Diamond TH. Disseminated Blastomyces dermatitidis infection in a non-endemic area. A case report. *S Afr Med J* 1987;71:717–719.
28. Pappas PG, Threlkeld MG, Bedsole GD, et al. Blastomycosis in immunocompromised patients. *Medicine* 1993;72:311.
29. Sugar AM, Brummer E, Stevens DA. Fungicidal activity of murine bronchoalveolar macrophages against Blastomyces dermatitidis. *J Med Microbiol* 1986;21:7–11.
30. Medoff G, Painter A, Kobayashi GS. Mycelial- to yeast-phase transitions of the dimorphic fungi Blastomyces dermatitidis and Paracoccidioides brasiliensis. *J Bacteriol* 1987;169:4055–4060.
31. Baumgardner DJ, Buggy BP, Mattson BJ, et al. Epidemiology of blastomycosis in a region of high endemicity in north central Wisconsin. *Clin Infect Dis* 1992;15:629–635.
32. Meyer KC, McManus EJ, Maki DG. Overwhelming pulmonary blastomycosis associated with the adult respiratory distress syndrome. *N Engl J Med* 1993;329:1231–1236.
33. Pappas PG, Pottage JC, Powderly WG, et al. Blastomycosis in patients with the acquired immunodeficiency syndrome. *Ann Intern Med* 1992;116:847–853.
34. Dismukes WE, Bradsher RW Jr, Cloud GC, et al. Itraconazole therapy for blastomycosis and histoplasmosis. NIAID Mycoses Study Group. *Am J Med* 1992;93:489–497.
35. Pappas PG, Bradsher RW, Chapman SW, et al. Treatment of blastomycosis with fluconazole: a pilot study. The National Institute of Allergy and Infectious Diseases Mycoses Study Group. *Clin Infect Dis* 1995;20:267–271.
36. Einstein HE, Johnson RH. Coccidioidomycosis: new aspects of epidemiology and therapy. *Clin Infect Dis* 1993;16:349–354.
37. Pappagianis D. Coccidioidomycosis. *Infect Med* 1991;8:19.
38. Stevens DA. Coccidioidomycosis. *N Engl J Med* 1995;332:1077–1082.
39. Beaman LV, Pappagianis D, Benjamini E. Mechanisms of resistance to infection with Coccidioides immitis in mice. *Infect Immun* 1979;23:681–685.
40. Ampel NM, Dols CL, Galgiani JN. Coccidioidomycosis during human im-

munodeficiency virus infection: results of a prospective study in a coccidioidal endemic area. *Am J Med* 1993;94:235–240.

41. Leake JA, Mosley DG, England B, et al. Risk factors for acute symptomatic coccidioidomycosis among elderly persons in Arizona, 1996–1997. *J Infect Dis* 2000;181:1435–1440.

42. Pappagianis D. Coccidioidomycosis. *Semin Dermatol* 1993;12:301–309.

43. Snyder LS, Galgiani JN. Coccidioidomycosis: the initial pulmonary infection and beyond. *Semin Resp Crit Care Med* 1997;18:235–247.

44. Larsen RA, Jacobson JA, Morris AH, et al. Acute respiratory failure caused by primary pulmonary coccidioidomycosis. Two case reports and a review of the literature. *Am Rev Respir Dis* 1985;131:797–799.

45. Hyde L. Coccidioidal pulmonary cavitation. *Am J Med* 1958;25:890–897.

46. Lombard CM, Tazelaar HD, Krasne DL. Pulmonary eosinophilia in coccidioidal infections. *Chest* 1987;91:734–736.

47. Galgiani JN, Ampel NM, Catanzaro A, et al. Practice guideline for the treatment of coccidioidomycosis. Infectious Diseases Society of America. *Clin Infect Dis* 2000;30:658–661.

48. Kauffman CA. Sporotrichosis. *Clin Infect Dis* 1999;29:231–237.

49. Pluss JL, Opal SM. Pulmonary sporotrichosis: review of treatment and outcome. *Medicine* 1986;65:143–153.

50. Ridgeway NA, Whitcomb FC, Erickon EE, et al. Primary pulmonary sporotrichosis. *Am J Med* 1962;32:153–160.

51. Michelson E. Primary pulmonary sporotrichosis. *Ann Thorac Surg* 1977;24:83–86.

52. Kauffman CA, Hajjeh RA, Chapman SW. Practice guidelines for the management of patients with sporotrichosis. Infectious Diseases Society of America. *Clin Infect Dis* 2000;30:684–687.

53. Sugar AM. Paracoccidioidomycosis. *Infect Dis Clin North Am* 1988;2:913–924.

54. Clark RA, Greer D, Atkinson W, et al. Spectrum of *Cryptococcus neoformans* infection in 68 patients infected with human immunodeficiency virus. *Rev Infect Dis* 1990;12:768–777.

55. Rozenbaum R, Goncalves AJ. Clinical epidemiological study of 171 cases of cryptococcosis. *Clin Infect Dis* 1994;18:369–380.

56. Henson DJ, Hill AR. Cryptococcal pneumonia: a fulminant presentation. *Am J Med Sci* 1984;288:221–222.

57. Kauffman CA, Severance PJ. Nosocomial cryptococcal infection. *South Med J* 1980;73:267.

58. Lanzafame L, Trevenzoli M, Carretta G, et al. Mediastinal lymphadenitis due to cryptococcal infection in HIV-positive patients on highly active antiretroviral therapy. *Chest* 1999;116:848–849.

59. Korvick J, Yu VL. Simultaneous infection with *Cryptococcus neoformans* and *Legionella pneumophila*. In vivo expression of common defects in cell-mediated immunity. *Respiration* 1988;53:132–136.

60. Aberg JA, Mundy LM, Powderly WG. Pulmonary cryptococcosis in patients without HIV infection. *Chest* 1999;115:734–740.

61. Louria DB. Controversies in the treatment of cryptococcal infections. *Infect Med* 1985;2:187.

62. Sarosi GA. Cryptococcal lung disease in patients without HIV infection. *Chest* 1999;115:610–611.

63. Nunez M, Peacock JE Jr, Chin R Jr. Pulmonary cryptococcosis in the immunocompetent host. Therapy with oral fluconazole: a report of four cases and a review of the literature. *Chest* 2000;118:527–534.

64. Clancy CJ, Nguyen M, et al. Acute community-acquired pneumonia due to Aspergillus in presumably immunocompetent hosts: clues for recognition of a rare but fatal disease. *Chest* 1998;114:629–634.

65. Levitz SM, Selsted ME, Ganz T, et al. In vitro killing of spores and hyphae of *Aspergillus fumigatus* and *Rhizopus oryzae* by rabbit neutrophil cationic peptides and bronchoalveolar macrophages. *J Infect Dis* 1986;154:483–489.

66. Schaffner A, Douglas H, Braude A. Selective protection against conidia by mononuclear and against mycelia by polymorphonuclear phagocytes in resistance to Aspergillus. Observations on these two lines of defense in vivo and in vitro with human and mouse phagocytes. *J Clin Invest* 1982;69:617–631.

67. Murali PS, Kurup VP, Bansal NK, et al. IgE down regulation and cytokine induction by Aspergillus antigens in human allergic bronchopulmonary aspergillosis. *J Lab Clin Med* 1998;131:228–235.

68. Wang JL, Patterson R, Rosenberg M, et al. Serum IgE and IgG antibody activity against *Aspergillus fumigatus* as a diagnostic aid in allergic bronchopulmonary aspergillosis. *Am Rev Respir Dis* 1978;117:917–927.

69. Stevens DA, Schwartz HJ, Lee JY, et al. A randomized trial of itraconazole in allergic bronchopulmonary aspergillosis. *N Engl J Med* 2000;342:756–762.

70. Cockrill BA, Hales CA. Allergic bronchopulmonary aspergillosis. *Ann Rev Med* 1999;50:303–316.

71. Allphin AL, Strauss M, Abdul-Karim FW. Allergic fungal sinusitis: problems in diagnosis and treatment. *Laryngoscope* 1991;101:815–820.

72. Binder RE, Faling LJ, Pugatch RD, et al. Chronic necrotizing pulmonary aspergillosis: a discrete clinical entity. *Medicine* 1982;61:109–124.

73. Caras WE, Pluss JL. Chronic necrotizing pulmonary aspergillosis: pathologic outcome after itraconazole therapy. *Mayo Clin Proc* 1996;71:25–30.

74. McNeil MM, Nash SL, Hajjeh RA, et al. Trends in mortality due to invasive

mycotic diseases in the United States, 1980–1997. *Clin Infect Dis* 2001;33:641–647.

75. Lortholary O, Meyohas MC, Dupont B, et al. Invasive aspergillosis in patients with acquired immunodeficiency syndrome: report of 33 cases. French cooperative study group on aspergillosis in AIDS. *Am J Med* 1993;95:177–187.

76. Lin S, Schranz J, Teutsch S. Aspergillosis case-fatality rate: systematic review of the literature. *Clin Infect Dis* 2001;32:358–366.

77. Graham BS, Tucker WS Jr. Opportunistic infections in endogenous Cushing's syndrome. *Ann Intern Med* 1984;101:334–338.

78. Lewis M, Kallenbach J, Ruff P, et al. Invasive pulmonary aspergillosis complicating influenza A pneumonia in a previously healthy patient. *Chest* 1985;87:691–693.

79. Kemper CA, Hostetler JS, Follansbee SE, et al. Ulcerative and plaque-like tracheobronchitis due to infection with Aspergillus in patients with AIDS. *Clin Infect Dis* 1993;17:344–352.

80. Williamson EC, Leeming JP, Palmer HM, et al. Diagnosis of invasive aspergillosis in bone marrow transplant recipients by polymerase chain reaction. *Br J Haematol* 2000;108:132–139.

81. Denning DW. Early diagnosis of invasive aspergillosis. *Lancet* 2000;355:423–424.

82. Maertens J, Verhaegen J, Demuynck H, et al. Autopsy-controlled prospective evaluation of serial screening for circulating galactomannan by a sandwich enzyme-linked immunosorbent assay for hematological patients at risk for invasive Aspergillosis. *J Clin Microbiol* 1999;37:3223–3228.

83. Sabra R, Branch RA. Amphotericin B nephrotoxicity. *Drug Safety* 1990;5:94–108.

84. Harbarth S, Pestotnik SL, Lloyd JF, et al. The epidemiology of nephrotoxicity associated with conventional amphotericin B therapy. *Am J Med* 2001;111:528–534.

85. Bates DW, Su L, Yu DT, et al. Mortality and costs of acute renal failure associated with amphotericin B therapy. *Clin Infect Dis* 2001;32:686–693.

86. Wingard JR, Kubilis P, Lee L, et al. Clinical significance of nephrotoxicity in patients treated with amphotericin B for suspected or proven aspergillosis. *Clin Infect Dis* 1999;29:1402–1407.

87. Walsh TJ, Hiemenz JW, Seibel NL, et al. Amphotericin B lipid complex for invasive fungal infections: analysis of safety and efficacy in 556 cases. *Clin Infect Dis* 1998;26:1383–1396.

88. Stevens DA, Lee JY. Analysis of compassionate use itraconazole therapy for invasive aspergillosis by the NIAID Mycoses Study Group criteria. *Arch Intern Med* 1997;157:1857–1862.

89. Denning DW, Ribaud P, Milpied N, et al. Efficacy and safety of voriconazole in the treatment of acute invasive aspergillosis. *Clin Infect Dis* 2002;34:563–571.

90. Herbrecht R, Denning DW, Patterson TF, et al. Open, randomised comparison of voriconazole (VRC) and amphotericin B (AmB) followed by other licensed antifungal therapy (OLAT) for primary therapy of invasive aspergillosis (IA). *N Engl J Med* 2002;347:408–415.

91. Hay RJ, Campbell CK, Marshall WM, et al. Disseminated zygomycosis (mucormycosis) caused by *Saksenaea vasiformis*. *J Infect* 1983;7:162–165.

92. Ingram CW, Sennesh J, Cooper JN, et al. Disseminated zygomycosis: report of four cases and review. *Rev Infect Dis* 1989;11:741–754.

93. Kontoyianis DP, Vartivarian S, Anaissie EJ, et al. Infections due to *Cunninghamella bertholletiae* in patients with cancer: report of three cases and review. *Clin Infect Dis* 1994;18:925–928.

94. Lee FY, Mossad SB, Adal KA. Pulmonary mucormycosis: the last 30 years. *Arch Intern Med* 1999;159:1301–1309.

95. Ventura GJ, Kantarjian HM, Anaissie E, et al. Pneumonia with *Cunninghamella* species in patients with hematologic malignancies. A case report and review of the literature. *Cancer* 1986;58:1534–1536.

96. Walsh TJ, Renshaw G, Andrews J, et al. Invasive zygomycosis due to *Conidiobolus incongruus*. *Clin Infect Dis* 1994;19:423–430.

97. Ribes JA, Vanover-Sams CL, Baker DJ. Zygomycetes in human disease. *Clin Microbiol Rev* 2000;13:236–301.

98. Diamond RD, Clark RA. Damage to *Aspergillus fumigatus* and *Rhizopus oryzae* hyphae by oxidative and nonoxidative microbicidal products of human neutrophils in vitro. *Infect Immun* 1982;38:487–495.

99. Waldorf AR, Ruderman N, Diamond RD. Specific susceptibility to mucormycosis in murine diabetes and bronchoalveolar macrophage defense against *Rhizopus*. *J Clin Invest* 1984;74:150–160.

100. Blankenberg HW. Mucormycosis of the lung: a case without significant predisposing factor. *Am Rev Tuberc* 1959;79:357.

101. Rex JH, Ginsberg AM, Fries LF, et al. *Cunninghamella bertholletiae* infection associated with deferoxamine therapy. *Rev Infect Dis* 1988;10:1187–1194.

102. Verdonck AK, Boelaert JR, Gordts BZ, et al. Effect of ferrioxamine on the growth of *Rhizopus*. *Mycoses* 1993;36:9–12.

103. Van Cutsem J, Boelaert JR. Effects of deferoxamine, feroxamine and iron on experimental mucormycosis (zygomycosis). *Kidney Int* 1989;36:1061–1068.

104. Boelaert JR, de Locht M, Van Cutsem J, et al. Mucormycosis during deferoxamine therapy is a siderophore-mediated infection. In vitro and in vivo animal studies. *J Clin Invest* 1993;91:1979–1986.

105. Boelaert JR, Van Cutsem J, de Locht M, et al. Deferoxamine augments growth

and pathogenicity of *Rhizopus*, while hydroxypyridinone chelators have no effect. *Kidney Int* 1994;45:667–671.

106. Libshitz HI, Pagani JJ. Aspergillosis and mucormycosis: two types of opportunistic fungal pneumonia. *Radiology* 1981;140:301–306.

107. Aderka A, Sidi Y, Garfinkel D, et al. Roentgenologically invisible mucormycosis pneumonia. *Respiration* 1983;44:158–160.

108. Watts WJ. Bronchopleural fistula followed by massive fatal hemoptysis in a patient with pulmonary mucormycosis. A case report. *Arch Intern Med* 1983;143:1029–1030.

109. Tedder M, Spratt JA, Anstadt MP, et al. Pulmonary mucormycosis: results of medical and surgical therapy. *Ann Thorac Surg* 1994;57:1044–1050.

110. Jabado N, Casanova JL, Haddad E, et al. Invasive pulmonary infection due to *Scedosporium apiospermum* in two children with chronic granulomatous disease. *Clin Infect Dis* 1998;27:1437–1441.

111. Saadah HA, Dixon T. *Petriellidium boydii* (*Allescheria boydii*). Necrotizing pneumonia in a normal host. *JAMA* 1981;245:605–606.

112. Berenguer J, Diaz-Mediavilla J, Urra D, et al. Central nervous system infection caused by *Pseudallescheria boydii*: case report and review. *Rev Infect Dis* 1989;11:890–896.

113. Welty FK, McLeod GX, Ezratty C, et al. *Pseudallescheria boydii* endocarditis of the pulmonic valve in a liver transplant recipient. *Clin Infect Dis* 1992;15:858–860.

114. Galgiani JN, Stevens DA, Graybill JR, et al. *Pseudallescheria boydii* infections treated with ketoconazole. Clinical evaluations of seven patients and in vitro susceptibility results. *Chest* 1984;86:219–224.

115. Walsh TJ, McLelland R, Driscoll T, et al. Voriconazole in the treatment of aspergillosis, scedosporiosis and other invasive fungal infections in children. *Pediatr Infect Dis J* 2002;21:240–248.

116. Mellinghoff IK, Winston DJ, Mukwaya G, et al. Treatment of *Scedosporium apiospermum* brain abscesses with posaconazole. *Clin Infect Dis* 2002;34:1648–1650.

117. Berenguer J, Rodriguez-Tudela JL, Richard C, et al. Deep infections caused by *Scedosporium prolificans*. A report on 16 cases in Spain and a review of the literature. *Scedosporium prolificans* Spanish Study Group. *Medicine* 1997;76:256–265.

118. Idigoras P, Perez-Trallero E, Pineiro L, et al. Disseminated infection and colonization by *Scedosporium prolificans*: a review of 18 cases, 1990–1999. *Clin Infect Dis* 2001;32:e158–e165.

118a. Anaissie EJ, Kuchar RT, Rex JH, et al. Fusariosis associated with pathogenic fusarium species colonization of a hospital water system: a new paradigm for the epidemiology of opportunistic mould infections. *Clin Infect Dis* 2001;33:1871–1878.

119. Buff SJ, McLelland R, Gallis HA, et al. *Candida albicans* pneumonia: radiographic appearance. *AJR* 1982;138:645–648.

120. Haron E, Vartivarian S, Anaissie E, et al. Primary *Candida* pneumonia. Experience at a large cancer center and review of the literature. *Medicine* 1993;72:137–142.

121. Masur H, Rosen PP, Armstrong D. Pulmonary disease caused by *Candida* species. *Am J Med* 1977;63:914–925.

122. Kontoyianis DP, Rolston K, Whimbey K, et al. Pulmonary candidiasis (PC) in cancer patients (pts): an autopsy study. Abstracts of the 41st Interscience Conference on Antimicrobial Agents and Chemotherapy, Chicago, September 22–25, 2001. Abstract No J-677, 2001.

123. Sihvo EI, Vilkko PS, Salminen JT, et al. Subacute primary *Candida* lung abscess. *Scand J Infect Dis* 1999;31:592–595.

124. Worthington M. Fatal *Candida* pneumonia in a non-immunosuppressed host. *J Infect* 1983;7:159–161.

125. Hoy J, Hsu KC, Rolston K, et al. *Trichosporon beigelii* infection: a review. *Rev Infect Dis* 1986;8:959–967.

126. Martino P, Venditti M, Micozzi A, et al. *Blastoschizomyces capitatus*: an emerging cause of invasive fungal disease in leukemia patients. *Rev Infect Dis* 1990;12:570–582.

127. Saul SH, Khachatoorian T, Poorsattar A, et al. Opportunistic *Trichosporon* pneumonia. Association with invasive aspergillosis. *Arch Pathol Lab Med* 1981;105:456–459.

128. Walling DM, McGraw DJ, Merz WG, et al. Disseminated infection with *Trichosporon beigelii*. *Rev Infect Dis* 1987;9:1013–1019.

CHAPTER 55
Legionnaires' Disease (Clinical)

Robert R. Muder

INTRODUCTION

Legionnaire's disease is a bacterial pneumonia caused by organisms of the genus *Legionella*, members of which are fastidious gram-negative aerobic bacilli. The disease and the genus take their name from an outbreak occurring at the American Legion convention in Philadelphia in 1976 (1), during which over 200 people became ill and 34 died. The causative organism, *Legionella pneumophila*, was isolated from lung tissue by workers at the Centers for Disease Control (2). Although previous workers had isolated *Legionella* species in animals or embryonated eggs as early as 1943, isolation onto artificial media and phenotypic characterization did not occur until the investigation of the 1976 epidemic. Since that time, over 40 species of *Legionella* have been described; 19 have been isolated in cases of human infection (3) (Table 55.1). *Legionella* species may also cause a non-pneumonic, self-limited febrile illness known as "Pontiac Fever."

EPIDEMIOLOGY

Legionella have a widespread distribution in both natural and manmade aquatic habitats, including fresh water (4), cooling towers (5) and evaporative condensers (6), whirlpool spas (7), and potable water systems (8,9). Members of the genus grow well at and can often be found readily in warm, nutrient-rich water (10,11). Humans acquire infection from environmental sources; there is no evidence for direct person-to-person transmission. Ninety percent of human infections are caused by *L. pneumophila*, and of these, over 80% are due to a single serogroup, serogroup 1 (12).

Legionnaires' disease was initially recognized following a point-source epidemic of *L. pneumophila* infection linked to a hotel (1). Similar occurrences linked to hotels, hospitals and other structures have subsequently been reported, with several to hundreds of persons affected. Most cases of community-acquired disease are not associated with recognized outbreaks. More recent studies have demonstrated that *Legionella* species are relatively common causes of community-acquired pneumonias occurring in an endemic or sporadic fashion (Table 55.2). There is considerable difference in the frequency of legionellosis as a cause of pneumonia from study to study based at least in part upon differences in location, population, time, and use of culture in diagnosis among the various studies. Extrapolation of findings from a large population based study of pneumonia etiology estimated the annual number of community-acquired cases in the United States to be 10,800 to 18,000 annually (13). Although nosocomial legionellosis has been discovered in apparent outbreaks (5,14), when specifically sought, endemic disease has been found in a number of hospitals (15). Colonization of a hospital's potable water supply by *Legionella* may predict the occurrence of nosocomial infection (16). The precise mode of transmission from aquatic habitats is often uncertain. A number of community outbreaks of *L. pneumophila* infection have been linked to point sources; studies of several of these have

TABLE 55.1. *Legionella* spp. Isolated from Cases of Pneumonia

Legionella pneumophila
L. micdadei
L. bozemanii
L. dumoffii
L. longbeachae
L. jordanis
L. gormanii
L. feeleii
L. hackeliae
L. maceachernii
L wadsworthii
L. birminghamensis
L. cincinnatiensis
L. tucsonensis
L. anisa
L. sainthelensi
L. lansingensis
L. oakridgensis
L. parisiensis

implicated aerosol generating devices, such as cooling towers and evaporative condensors, contaminated with *Legionella* (6). Other community outbreaks have been traced to whirlpool spas (17), a grocery store mist machine (18), and a decorative fountain (19) contaminated with *L. pneumophila*. Several community outbreaks have occurred in which no potential source of *Legionella* could be identified despite extensive investigation (20,21). Potable water systems of large buildings such as hospitals and hotels are often extensively colonized by *Legionella*; these systems may be associated with human infection (8,9,22–24). Residential water systems have been implicated in community-acquired cases (25–27).

Nosocomial infection is particularly associated with colonization of hospital hot water systems by *Legionella* (8,24). In addition to *L. pneumophila*, *L. micdadei* (9), *L. dumoffii* (28), and *L. bozemanii* (29) may cause nosocomial disease in the presence of colonized water. Contamination of aerosol-generating respiratory therapy equipment by tap water has been implicated as a source (30,31). Aerosolization from showers and taps is a possible mode of transmission (32,33). Aspiration of contaminated water as a mode of transmission is supported by several epidemiologic studies (34–36). Major oncologic surgery of the head and neck, in which postoperative aspiration is nearly universal, predisposes

to *Legionella* infection (37). Introduction of contaminated water into nasogastric tubes is also associated with nosocomial pneumonia (38,39), presumably due to aspiration of gastric contents. An outbreak of postoperative wound infection was associated with washing of the wound area with *Legionella*-contaminated tap water (40).

Factors associated with an increased risk of infection include male sex, advanced age, cigarette smoking, chronic obstructive pulmonary disease, organ transplantation, use of immunosuppressive medications, malignancy, and chronic renal failure (12,41). Patients with acquired immune deficiency syndrome also have an elevated risk of *Legionella* infection compared to the general population (12). In addition, risk of nosocomial infection is further increased by general anesthesia and by endotracheal intubation (15,42,43). Infection in children is rare, but has been reported in both immunocompromised and immunocompetent children (44). There are reports of nosocomial *Legionella* infection in premature neonates requiring mechanical ventilation (45,46).

Pontiac Fever occurs after exposure to aerosols contaminated by *Legionella*. Implicated sources include air conditioning systems (47), industrial equipment (48), and whirlpool spas (49). In addition to *L. pneumophila*, *L. feeli* (48), *L. micdadei* (50), and *L. ansia* (51) may cause Pontiac fever.

PATHOGENESIS

Although capable of multiplying freely in the environment and on artificial media, *Legionella* are considered intracellular parasites. *Legionella* can multiply within fresh water amoebae and protozoa (52). Although these protozoa have been found in potable water distribution systems (53), it is unclear if this growth in protozoa is related to pathogenesis.

The organisms enter the respiratory tract via aerosolization or aspiration. *L. pneumophila* is phagocytosed by polymorphonuclear leukocytes and mononuclear cells. Data from several *in vitro* models of infection demonstrate that specific antibody, complement and neutrophils are ineffective in killing *L. pneumophila* (54).

L. pneumophila is phagocytized by monocytes and alveolar macrophages; uptake is mediated by complement fixed to the bacterial surface through the alternate pathway (55) and enhanced in the presence of specific antibody (56). A major virulence determinant of *L. pneumophila* is the Mip protein, a 24-kDal molecule that promotes infection of mononuclear phagocytes (57). Inside the phagocye, *L. pneumophila* multiplies

TABLE 55.2. Proportion of Community-Acquired Pneumonia due to *Legionella* Species

Year	Site	No. of patients	Diagnostic methods				
			Culture	Serology	Urinary antigen	*Legionella*	Reference
1991	US	2,060	yes	yes	yes	3%	(13)
1994–1996	US	145	yes	yes	yes	14%	(105)
1994–1996	US	522	yes	yes	no	8%	(124)
1994–1996	Spain	392	yes	yes	yes	12%	(125)
1994–1997	Japan	326	yes	yes	no	0.8%	(126)
1996–1997	Spain	385	yes	yes	no	8%	(127)
1996–1997	Slovenia	211	no	yes	yes	2.8%	(128)
1996–1999	US	104	yes	yes	yes	9%	(129)
1998–1999	Great Britain	267	yes	yes	yes	3%	(130)

within a ribosome-lined vacuole and inhibits phagosome-lysome fusion (58). Multiplication occurs until the phagocytic cell ruptures.

Cell-mediated immunity is the primary host defense. Lymphocyte proliferation and cutaneous delayed hypersensitivity to *L. pneumophila* occur in the first 2 weeks of infection (53,59,60). Lymphocytes from patients and experimental animals surviving *Legionella* infection demonstrate proliferation and lymphokine production in the presence of the organism (61,62). Monocytes activated by interferon gamma do not support intracellular multiplication of *Legionella* (63). Interferon gamma causes downregulation of transferrin receptors in human monocytes, limiting the availability of iron, an essential growth factor for *L. pneumophila* (64).

In addition to the Mip protein, several other potential virulence factors have been identified (54). The 60-kDa heat shock protein appears to enhance attachment and entry of *L. pneumophila* into eukaryotic cells. The Dot/ICM type IV secretion system consists of bacterial proteins that promote secretion of bacterial virulence factors postulated to play a role in inhibition of phagosome-lysosome fusion.

The pathogenesis of Pontiac fever does not involve infection of host cells by *Legionella* species. The clinical manifestations appear to be related to inhalation of endotoxin contained in aerosols from water sources colonized with *Legionella* (65).

PATHOLOGY

The characteristic pathologic presentation is a fibrinopurulent pneumonia with inflammatory cellular exudate composed of neutrophils and macrophages in the terminal airspaces. A characteristic lysis of the exudate has been described (66). Diffuse alveolar damage especially to the capillaries and hyaline membrane formation are seen. *Legionella* can be demonstrated in phagocytes and alveolar spaces by Dieterle silver staining or direct immunofluorescence. Invasion of blood vessels and lymphatics can be seen by immunofluorescent staining. *Legionella* have been seen in extrapulmonary tissues including spleen, liver, kidney, myocardium, brain, prostate gland, thyroid gland, and muscle (67,68), consistent with hematogenous spread.

CLINICAL MANIFESTATIONS

The overwhelming majority of *Legionella* infections are caused by *L. pneumophila*. Pneumonia (Legionnaires' disease) is the major clinical manifestation of *Legionella* infection, although extrapulmonary infection and non-pneumonic disease (Pontiac fever) occur.

Based on data from point-source outbreaks, the usual incubation period of *Legionella* pneumonia is estimated to be 2 to 10 days after exposure (1). There may be a prodrome of several days with the insidious onset of fever, malaise, and nonproductive cough. Nearly all patients will be febrile at presentation, and half will have a temperature of 103°F or greater (69). Cough is usually nonproductive at first, but 50% to 75% of patients will produce sputum within several days of presentation. Chest pain and dyspnea occur in approximately 50% of patients (70). Respiratory failure necessitating ventilatory support occurs in 15% to 50% of community-acquired cases (69–72). Gastrointestinal symptoms including diarrhea and abdominal pain are common. Myalgias may be a prominent presenting feature. Initial reports emphasized the multi-systemic

nature of *Legionella* pneumonia. Confusion, hematuria, renal failure, and hepatic dysfunction were symptoms reported to be typical of Legionnaires' disease. However, *Legionella* infection does not appear to be distinguishable from other pneumonias on clinical grounds alone (73). Early reports included many patients given inadequate therapy; the multiple organ dysfunction reported is probably nonspecific and can be seen in overwhelming bacterial pneumonia of any etiology. In recent reports, multiorgan system failure appears to be associated with the requirement for mechanical ventilation or pressors during treatment of pneumonia (74,75).

Syndromes such as acute tubular necrosis, pancreatitis, cerebellar ataxia, peripheral neuropathy, rhabdomyolysis, hemolytic anemia, thrombotic thrombocytopenic purpura, and various rashes have been reported with *Legionella* infection (76–79); the mechanism by which *Legionella* could cause these manifestations is unclear.

Extrapulmonary *Legionella* infection occurs infrequently. In most, but not all, cases, such infections have occurred during the course of pneumonia, presumably through hematogenous spread. Renal abscess, soft tissue infection, endocarditis, myocarditis, pericarditis, peritonitis, and hemodialysis fistula infection have been reported (80).

In highly immunocompromised hosts (e.g., transplant patients), the presentation of *Legionella* infection may not suggest bacterial pneumonia initially. The onset may be abrupt, and typical pneumonic symptoms may be absent; fever may be the only symptom (81). Localized pleuritic pain and dyspnea may suggest the diagnosis of pulmonary embolism (82).

Laboratory data are likewise nonspecific. The majority of patients will have a polymorphonuclear leukocytosis on presentation. Early reports of Legionnaires' disease suggested elevated creatinine concentration, abnormal hepatic function, hypophosphatemia, and hematuria as characteristic manifestations. Subsequent comparative studies have concluded that the laboratory manifestations of *Legionella* infection are not distinctive when compared with those of other bacterial pneumonias (83–85). Hyponatremia appears to occur more frequently in Legionnaires' disease than in pneumonia of other etiology (83).

RADIOLOGY

Most patients present with abnormal chest radiographs, and essentially all will have radiographic evidence of pneumonia by the third day of illness (86). There is a slight predominance of lower lobe involvement, but any area may be affected. The infiltrates are alveolar, and may be segmental, lobar, or diffuse on presentation. Pleural-based, rounded opacities with poorly defined margins may resemble pulmonary infarction or neoplasm (Fig. 55.1). Although the majority of cases present with single lobe involvement, there is a notable tendency for the radiographic extent of pneumonia to increase during the first several days after presentation (87), and to involve additional lobes in 25% to 50% of patients (Fig. 55.2) (88). This progression may occur in the face of appropriate antibiotic therapy and does not, of itself, predict clinical failure. The extent of radiologic involvement in *Legionella* infection bears little relationship to prognosis (89). Small to moderate pleural effusions occur in at least one-third of patients and can occasionally precede the appearance of the infiltrate; in a few patients pleural effusion is the only radiographic abnormality (86,90). Loculated effusion and empyema occur occasionally, and require drainage.

Cavitation is unusual in the immunologically intact patient, but is frequent in the patient receiving corticosteroids or immunosuppressive medications (86). In these patients, the initial

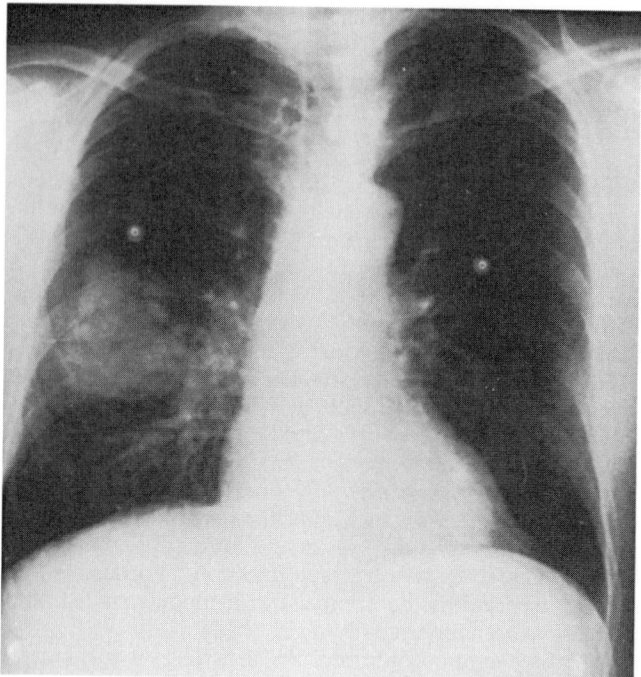

Figure 55.1. A 64-year-old smoker presented with fever and nonproductive cough. Chest radiograph showed a rounded density in the right upper lobe. Malignancy was suspected. Culture of respiratory secretions obtained at bronchoscopy yielded *L. pneumophila.* (From Muder RR, Yu VL, Fang GD. Community-acquired legionnaires' disease. *Semin Resp Infect* 1989;4:32–39.

infiltrate tends to appear as a rounded density that undergoes progressive central cavitation until a thin-walled cavity remains. The progression of cavitation may occur during the course of successful antibiotic therapy. The cavity usually closes spontaneously over time.

Radiographic clearing of infiltrates after *Legionella* infection tends to be slower than that seen in other bacterial pneumonias. Residual infiltrates are present in 30% to 40% at 3 months or beyond after illness (86,88).

OTHER LEGIONELLA SPECIES

Nineteen *Legionella* species other than *L. pneumophila* have been isolated from cases of human infection (3), Of the 10% of *Legionella* infections are due to these other species, most caused by four species: *L. micdadei, L. longbeachae, L. bozemanii,* and *L. dumoffi.* Patients with non-pneumophila infections appear to be more likely to be immunocompromised than patients infected with *L. pneumophila* (91). Otherwise, the clinical and radiologic features are similar to those described for *L. pneumophila* infection. Cases of simultaneous infection by multiple *Legionella* species have been documented (92,93).

PONTIAC FEVER

Pontiac fever is an acute febrile illness occurring after exposure to aerosolized *L. pneumophila* (47), *L. feeleii* (48), *L. micdadei* (50), or *L. anisa* (51). The attack rate may exceed 90% in exposed individuals. The illness has a superficial resemblance to influenza, with associated chills, myalgia, headache, and malaise (94). Although nonproductive cough and chest pain are present in approximately one half of the patients, radiographic evidence of pneumonia does not develop. The symptoms occur 1 to 2 days after exposure and resolve spontaneously in 2 to 5 days without specific therapy.

DIAGNOSIS

Legionella species are fastidious and cannot be recovered on the usual bacteriologic media used in the diagnosis of pneumonia.

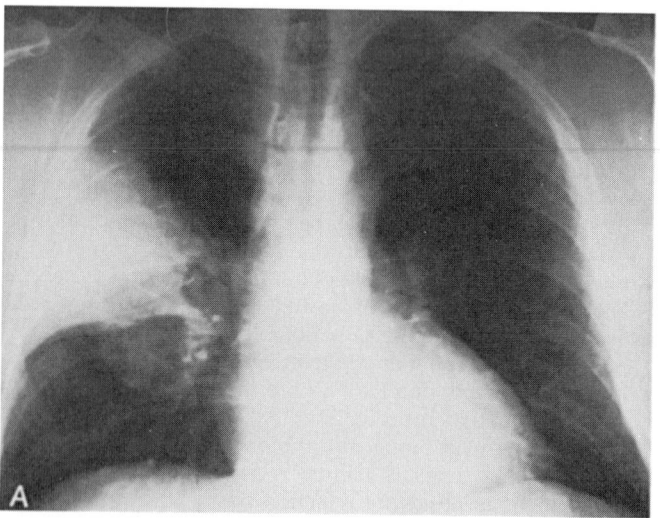
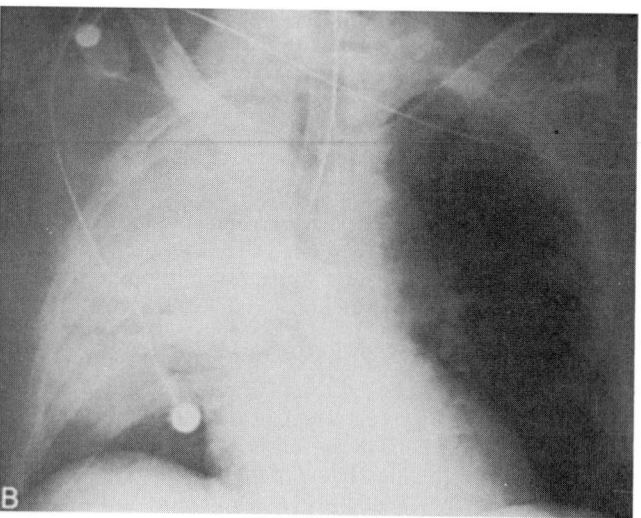

Figure 55.2. A 47-year-old man presented with chills and slightly productive cough. His history was remarkable only for cigarette smoking and essential hypertension. Chest x-ray showed a segmental infiltrate in the lower portion of the right upper lobe (**A**). Cephalosporin therapy was begun. By the third hospital day, the infiltrate had progressed to the right upper lobe and the upper portion of the right lower lobe (**B**). Sputum culture obtained on admission yielded heavy growth of *L. pneumophila*. Erythromycin and rifampin were begun followed by clinical response and ultimate recovery. (From Muder RR, Yu VL, Parry M. Radiology of *Legionella pneumonia. Semin Resp Infect* 1987;2:242–254, with permission.)

Although gram negative, they are generally not visible on Gram stain of respiratory specimens. *L. micdadei* is weakly acid fast and can be visualized in clinical specimens. Specialized microbiologic and immunologic techniques are needed for the diagnosis of *Legionella* infection.

Recovery from clinical specimens by culture is hampered by the tendency for overgrowth of commensal flora. The base media is buffered charcoal yeast extract (BCYE) agar. Antibacterial and antifungal agents are added to inhibit competing flora and dyes are added to enhance visibility. *L. pneumophila* can be isolated from expectorated sputum in 70% if multiple selective media are used (95,96). Specimens obtained via bronchoscopy probably do not give a significantly better yield than sputum. Transtracheal aspirate specimens that are free of contaminating oral flora gives the highest yield (sensitivity of 90%). Acid buffer pretreatment of sputum samples reduces competing flora and improves sensitivity (97). Characteristic " ground glass colonies" can be identified in 48 to 72 hours with a dissecting microscope. Rapid speciation of the isolate is accomplished by direct fluorescent antibody (DFA) staining or slide agglutination. Isolation of *Legionella* from the sputum of a patient with pneumonia is presumed to be diagnostic of infection, as colonization of the oropharynx has not yet been demonstrated.

Legionella can be isolated from the blood of patients by specially supplemented media or by "blind" direct subculture of nonsupplemented aerobic blood culture media onto BCYE agar (98).

Direct visualization of *Legionella* in clinical specimens can be accomplished in approximately two hours by use of DFA staining. This test has a sensitivity in detecting *L. pneumophila* in respiratory secretions of 30% to 70% (95). The test is highly specific, although false-positive results occur due to cross-reactions with other species of bacteria. The test is species and serogroup specific; conjugates containing multiple antisera are commercially available. A monoclonal antibody that reacts with multiple serogroups of *L. pneumophila* is commercially available (Bio-Rad Laboratories, Redmond, WA); sensitivity and specificity appear to be superior to the polyclonal DFA reagent. DFA reagents for other *Legionella* species are available; sensitivity and specificity have not been rigorously evaluated. Deoxyribonucleic acid amplification shows promise for detection of *Legionella* clinical specimens. A commercial kit designed for the detection of *Legionella* species in environmental samples (Enviro-Amp, Perkin-Elmer Cetus) showed a sensitivity of 90% and a specificity of 100% when compared to culture (99); however, this product is no longer commercially available.

Rapid diagnosis can be achieved by detection of *L. pneumophila* antigens in the urine. Sensitivity is 80% by day 3 of illness and specificity is 99% (100,101). The test is commercially available but limited to *L. pneumophila*, serogroup 1 (Binax, Portland, ME; Wampole Laboratories, Princeton, NJ). Antigenuria may persist for months after clinical illness.

Serologic diagnosis can be accomplished using a variety of methods, although the indirect fluorescent antibody (IFA) and enzyme-linked immunoabsorbent assay are most widely used (95,102). Eighty percent of patients infected with *L. pneumophila* will show a diagnostic rise in titer within 2 to 6 weeks. A fourfold rise to a titer of 1:128 by IFA is considered diagnostic; a single elevated titer of 1:256 accompanying a compatible clinic illness can be considered presumptive. The specificity of serology is estimated to be 95% in the diagnosis infection due to *L. pneumophila* serogroup 1. Neither sensitivity nor specificity has been established for other species, and diagnosis of a *Legionella* infection other than *L. pneumophila* based solely on serology should be made with caution.

Diagnosis of non-pneumonic legionellosis (Pontiac fever) is based on antibody seroconversion following a compatible clinical illness. *Legionella* have not been demonstrated in clinical specimens by either culture or DFA.

THERAPY

In the 1976 Philadelphia outbreak, therapy with erythromycin or tetracycline was associated with markedly improved survival compared to treatment with beta-lactam or aminoglycoside antibiotics (1). Although *Legionella* are susceptible *in vitro* to a variety of antibiotics, animal and egg model studies have demonstrated that agents that penetrate intracellularly have therapeutic efficacy. Erythromycin, rifampin, tetracycline, trimethoprim-sulfamethoxazole, and 5-fluoroquinolones all have demonstrated *in vitro* and *in vivo* activity against *Legionella*.

Erythromycin was the historical drug of choice for *Legionella* infection. However, the newer macrolides such as clarithromycin and azithromycin have excellent activity against *Legionella in vitro* and *in vivo* (103,104). These agents have the advantage of high tissue levels following oral administration, and gastrointestinal upset is much less than with oral erythromycin. Because of better in vitro activity, favorable pharmacokinetics, and better tolerability, these newer agents have largely supplanted erythromycin. A 10-day course of therapy is adequate for immunocompetent patients (105).

The 5-fluoroquinolones, including ciprofloxacin, levofloxacin and ofloxacin, are highly active against *Legionella in vitro* and *in vivo* (106,107). Quniolones have been used successfully in the treatment of *Legionella* pneumonia, including cases in which erythromycin has failed (108). Quniolones are preferable to macrolides in the treatment of transplant patients receiving cyclosporine, as the latter interferes with cyclosporine metabolism (109). Quinolones are also preferable in patients with hepatic and renal failure, who are at risk for erythromycin ototoxicity.

Tetracycline (110), trimethoprim-sulfamethoxazole (111), and imipenem-cilastin (112) have been used successfully in limited number of patients.

Mortality of patients receiving erythromycin for treatment of community-acquired illness is approximately 10% and is dependent on the severity of underlying illness and the timing of initiation of specific antibiotic therapy. Risk of mortality is increased by advanced age and the presence of underlying conditions such as immunosuppression, malignancy and end-stage renal disease. Mortality in nosocomially acquired disease approaches 40% (12), reflecting the severity of the patients' underlying illnesses.

PREVENTION AND CONTROL

Colonization of a hospital water system with *L. pneumophila* predicts the occurrence of nosocomial legionellosis (15,113,114). Surveillance of hospital water systems for *Legionella* is a reasonable precaution (115). The isolation of *Legionella* from a hospital's water system mandates, as a minimum, surveillance for cases of nosocomial infection. One potential strategy is to apply diagnostic tests for *Legionella* infection to cases of nosocomial pneumonia among patients at highest risk, including patients receiving immunosuppressive therapy, undergoing general anesthesia, or suffering from chronic pulmonary disease (116).

Various biocides have been used to decontaminate cooling towers, but microbiologic control has been inconsistent and clinical correlation has been lacking (117). Several methods have been successfully used to decontaminate potable water systems linked to nosocomial infection; a decrease in *Legionella* colonization has been followed by decrease in the incidence of disease. Elevation of hot water temperature to 70°C followed by flushing of distal sites (faucets, shower heads) (9,117) is effective at providing immediate reduction in *Legionella* concentrations; colonization tends to recur rapidly. Continuous hyperchlorination causes accelerated corrosion of pipes and may lead to release of carcinogenic chlorine byproducts (118,119). Chlorine dioxide appears to be a more effective agent than chlorine with fewer of its disadvantages (120). A system using electrodes that continuously generate copper and silver ions (Liquitech, Burr Ridge, IL) is highly effective in eliminating *Legionella* (121,122). Unlike chlorine, metal ions do not promote corrosion of pipes. Ultraviolet light treatment of water near the point of use (123) is a means of providing a locally disinfected water supply to a high-risk patient group.

REFERENCES

1. Fraser DW, Tsai T, Ornstein W, et al. Legionnaires' disease: description of an epidemic of pneumonia. *N Engl J Med* 1977;297:1189–1197.
2. McDade J, Shepard C, Fraser D, et al. Legionnaires' disease: isolation of a bacterium and demonstration of its role in other respiratory disease. *N Engl J Med* 1977;297:1197–1203.
3. Muder RR, Yu VL. Infection due to *Legionella* speies other than *L. pneumopila*. *Clin Infect Dis* 2002;35:990–998.
4. Fliermans CB, Cherry WB, Orrison LH, et al. Ecological distribution of *Legionella pneumophila*. *Appl Environ Microbiol* 1981;41:9–16.
5. Dondero TJ, Jr., Rendtorff RC, Mallison GF, et al. An outbreak of Legionnaires' disease associated with a contaminated air-conditioning cooling tower. *N Engl J Med* 1980;302:365–370.
6. Cordes L, Fraser D, Skaliy P. Legionnaires' disease outbreak at Atlanta, Georgia, country club: evidence for spread from an evaporative condenser. *Am J Epidemiol* 1980;11:425–431.
7. Groothius DG, Havelaar AH, Veenendaal HR. A note on legionellas in whirlpools. *J Appl Bacteriol* 1985;58:479–482.
8. Stout JE, Yu VL, Vickers RM, et al. Ubiquitousness of *Legionella pneumophila* in the water supply of a hospital with endemic Legionnaires' disease. *N Engl J Med* 1982;36:466–468.
9. Best M, Yu VL, Stout J, et al. *Legionellaceae* in the hospital water supply—epidemiological link with disease and evaluation of a method of control of nosocomial Legionnaires' disease and Pittsburgh pneumonia. *Lancet* 1983;2:307–310.
10. Wadowsky RM, Yee RB, Mezmar L, et al. Hot water systems as sources of *Legionella pneumophila* in hospital and nonhospital plumbing fixtures. *Appl Environ Microbiol* 1982;43:1104–1110.
11. Tison DL, Baross JA, Seidler RJ. Legionella in aquatic habitats in the Mount Saint Helens blast zone. *Curr Microbiol* 1983;9:345–348.
12. Marston BJ, Lipman HB, Breiman RF. Surveillance for Legionnaires' disease. Risk factors for morbidity and mortality. *Arch Intern Med* 1994;154:2417–2422.
13. Marston BJ, Plouffe JF, File TM, et al. Incidence of community-acquired pneumonia requiring hospitalization; results of a population based active surveillance study in Ohio. *Arch Intern Med* 1997;157:1709–1718.
14. Thacker SB, Bennet JV, Tsai T. An outbreak in 1975 of severe respiratory illness caused by Legionnaires' disease bacteriium. *J Infect Dis* 1978;238:512–519.
15. Muder RR, Yu VL, McClure J, et al. Nosocomial Legionnaires' disease uncovered in a prospective pneumonia study: implications for underdiagnosis. *JAMA* 1983;249:3184–3188.
16. Yu VL. Resolving the controversy on environmental cultures for *Legionella*. *Infect Cont Hosp Epidemiol* 1998;19:893–897.
17. Den Boor JW, Yzerman EPF, Schellekens J, et al. A large outbreak of Legionnaires' disease at a flower show, The Netherlands, 1999. *Emerg Infect Dis* 2002;184:1289–1292.
18. Mahoney FJ, Hoge CW, Farley TA, et al. Community-wide outbreak of Legionnaires' disease associated with a grocery store mist machine. *J Infect Dis* 1992;165:736–739.
19. Hlady C. Outbreak of Legionnaires' disease linked to a decorative fountain by molecular epidemiology. *Am J Epidemiol* 1993;138:555–562.
20. Mamolen M, Breiman RF, Barbaree JM. Use of multiple molecular subtyping techniques to investigate a Legionnaires' disease outbreak due to identical strains at two tourist lodges. *J Clin Microbiol* 1993;31:2584–2588.
21. Redd SC, Yeng F, Lin C, et al. A rural outbreak of Legionnaires' disease linked to visiting a retail store. *Am J Pub Health* 1990;80:431–434.
22. Nolte FS, Conlin C, Roisin A. Plasmids as epidemiological markers in nosocomial Legionnaires' disease. *J Infect Dis* 1984;149:251–256.
23. Schlech WF III, Gorman GW, Payne MD, et al. Legionnaires' disease in the caribbean: an outbreak associated with a resort hotel. *Arch Intern Med* 1985;145:2076–2079.
24. Helms CM, Massanari R, Zeiter S, et al. Legionnaires' disease associated with a hospital water system: a cluster of 24 nosocomial cases. *Ann Intern Med* 1983;99:172–178.
25. Stout JE, Yu VL, Muraca P, et al. Potable water as the cause of sporadic cases of community-acquired Legionnaires' disease. *N Engl J Med* 1992;326:151–154.
26. Castellani Pastoris M, Vigano EF, Passi C. A family cluster of *Legionella pneumophila* infections. *Scand J Infect Dis* 1988;20:489–493.
27. Chen YS, Lin WR, Liu YC, et al. Residential water supply as a likely cause of community-acquired Legionnaires' disease in an immunocompromised host. *Eur J Clin Microbiol Infect Dis* 2002;21:706–709.
28. Joly JR, Diery P, Gauvrau L, et al. Legionnaires' disease caused by *Legionella dumoffi* in distilled water. *Can Med Assoc J* 1986;135:1273–1277.
29. Parry MF, Stampleman L, Hutchinson J, et al. Waterborne *Legionella bozemanii* and nosocomial pneumonia in immunosuppressed patients. *Ann Intern Med* 1985;103:205–210.
30. Arnow P, Chou T, Weil D, et al. Nosocomial Legionnaires' disease caused by aerosolized tap water from respiratory devices. *J Infect Dis* 1982;146:460–467.
31. Mastro TD, Fields BS, Breiman RF, et al. Nosocomial Legionnaires' disease and use of medication nebulizers. *J Infect Dis* 1991;163:667–671.
32. Bollin GE, Plouffe JF, Para MF, et al. *Legionella pneumophila* generated by shower heads and hot water faucets. *Appl Environ Microbiol* 1986;50:1128–1131.
33. Woo AH, Goetz A, Yu VL. Transmission of *Legionella* by respiratory equipment aerosol generating devices. *Chest* 1992;102:1586–1590.
34. Muder RR, Yu VL, Woo A. Mode of transmission of *Legionella pneumophila*: a critical review. *Arch Intern Med* 1986;146:1607–1612.
35. Yu VL. Could aspiration be the major mode of transmission for *Legionella*? *Am J Med* 1993;95:13–15.
36. Marrie TJ, Macdonald S, Clarke K, et al. Nasogastric tubes flushed with contaminated potable water are a risk factor for nosocomial Legionnaires' disease. Interscience Conference on Antimicrobial Agents and Chemotherapy, 1988.
37. Johnson JT, Yu VL, Best M, et al. Nosocomial legionellosis uncovered in surgical patients with head and neck cancer: implications for epidemiologic reservoir and mode of transmission. *Lancet* 1985;2:298–300.
38. Blatt SP, Parkinson MD, Pace E, et al. Nosocomial Legionnaires' disease: aspiration as a primary mode of transmission. *Am J Med* 1993;95:16–22.
39. Venezia RA, Agresta MD, Hanley EM, et al. Nosocomial legionellosis associated with aspiration of nasogastric feedings diluted in tap water. *Infect Cont Hosp Epidemiol* 1994;15:529–533.
40. Lowry PW, Blankenship RJ, Gridley W, et al. A cluster of *Legionella* sternal wound infections due to postoperative topical exposure of contaminated tap water. *N Engl J Med* 1991;324:109–112.
41. England AC, Fraser DW. Sporadic and epidemic nosocomial legionellosis in the United States. *Am J Med* 1981;70:707–711.
42. Tompkins LS, Roessler BJ, Redd SC, et al. Legionella prosthetic-valve endocarditis. *N Engl J Med* 1988;318:530–535.
43. Strebel P, Ramos J, Eidelman I, et al. Legionnaires' disease in a Johannesburg teaching hospital. Investigation and control of an outbreak. *S Afr Med J* 1988;19:329–333.
44. Brady M. Nosocomial legionnaires' disease in a children's hospital. *J Pediatr* 1989;115:46–50.
45. Womack P, Liang KC, Llagan N, et al. *Legionella pneumophila* in a preterm infant - a case report. *J Perinatol* 1992;12:303–305.
46. Luck PC, Dinger D, Helbig JH, et al. Analysis of *Legionella pneumophila* strains associated with nosocomial pneumonia in a neonatal intensive care unit. *Eur J Clin Microbiol Infect Dis* 1994;13:565–571.
47. Kaufman AF, McDade J, Patton C, et al. Pontiac fever: isolation of the etiologic agent (*Legionella pneumophila*) and demonstration of its mode of transmission. *Am J Epidemiol* 1981;114:337–347.
48. Herwaldt LA, Gorman GW, McGrath T, et al. A new legionella species: *Legionella feeleii* species nova, causes pontiac fever in an automobile plant. *Ann Intern Med* 1984;100:333–338.
49. Spitalny KC, Voot RL, Orciarl LE, et al. Pontiac fever associated with a whirlpool spa. *Am J Epidemiol* 1984;120:809–817.
50. Goldberg DJ, Wrench JG, Collier PW, et al. Lochgoihead fever: outbreak of non-pneumonic legionellosis due to *Legionella micdadei*. *Lancet* 1989;1:316–318.
51. Fenstersheib M, Miller M, Diggins C, et al. Outbreak of Pontiac fever due to *Legionella anisa*. *Lancet* 1990;336:35–37.
52. Fields BS. Legionella and protozoa: interaction of a pathogen and its natural host. In: Barbaree JM, Breiman JF, Dufour AP, eds. *Legionella: current status and emerging perspectives*. Washington DC: American Society for Microbiology, 1993:129–136.
53. Breiman R, Fields B, Sanden G, et al. Association of shower use with legionnaires' disease: possible role of amoebae. *JAMA* 1990;263:2924–2926.
54. Swanson MS, Hammer BK. *Legionella pneumophila* pathogenesis: a fateful

journey from amoebae to macrophages. *Annu Rev Microbiol* 2000;54:567–613.

55. Payne NR, Horwitz MA. Phagocytosis of *Legionella pneumophila* is mediated by human monocyte complement receptors. *J Exp Med* 1987;166:1377–1389.

56. Nash TW, Libby D, Horwitz MA. Interaction between the legionnaires' disease bacterium (*L. pneumophila*) and human alveolar macrophages: influence of antibody lymphokine, and hydrocortisone. *J Clin Invest* 1984;74:771–782.

57. Cianciotto NP, Eisenstein BI, Mody CH, et al. A *Legionella pneumophila* gene encoding a species-specific surface protein potentiates initiation of intracellular infection. *Infect Immun* 1989;57:1255–1262.

58. Horwitz MA. The legionnaires' disease bacterium (*Legionella pneumophila*) inhibits phagosome-lysosome fusion in human monocytes. *J Exp Med* 1983;158:2108–2126.

59. Plouffe JF, Baird IM. Lymphocyte blastaogenic responses to *Legionella pneumophila* in acute legionellosis. *J Clin Lab Immunol* 1982;7:43–44.

60. Friedman H, Widen R, Lee I, et al. Cellular immunity to *L. pneumophila* in guinea pigs assessed by direct and indirect migration inhibition; reaction in vitro. *Infect Immun* 1983;41:1132–1137.

61. Horwitz MA, Silverstein SC. Intracellular multiplication of legionnaires' disease bacteria (*Legionella pneumophila*) in human monocytes is reversibly inhibited by erythromycin and rifampin. *J Clin Invest* 1983;71:15–26.

62. Skerrett SJ, Schmidt R, Martin TR. Impaired clearance of aerosolized *L. pneumophila* in corticosteroid treated rats: a model of legionnaires' disease in the compromised host. *J Infect Dis* 1989;160:261–268.

63. Horwitz MA, Silversteen SC. Interaction of the legionnaires' disease bacterium (*Legionella pneumophila*) with human phagocytes II. Antibody promotes binding of *L. pneumophila*. *J Exp Med* 1981;153:398–406.

64. Byrd TF, Horwitz MA. Interferon gamma-activated human monocytes downregulate transferrin receptors and inhibit the intracellular multiplication of *Legionella pneumophila* by limiting the availability of iron. *J Clin Invest* 1989;83:1457–1465.

65. Fields BS, Haupt T, Davis JP, et al. Pontiac fever due to *Legionella micdadei* from a whirlpool spa: possible role of bacterial endotoxin. *J Infect Dis* 2001;15:1289–1292.

66. Winn WC, Myerowitz RL. The pathology of the legionella pneumonias. *Hum Pathol* 1981;12:401–422.

67. Monforte R, Maro F, Estruch R, et al. Multiple organ involvement by *L. pneumophila* in a fatal case of legionnaires' disease. *J Infect Dis* 1989;159:809.

68. White H, Felton W, Sun CN. Extrapulmonary histopathologic manifestations of legionnaires' disease. *Arch Pathol Lab Med* 1980;104:287–289.

69. Fang GD, Fine M, Orloff J, et al. New and emerging etiologies for community-acquired pneumonia with implications for therapy: a prospective multicenter study of 359 cases. *Medicine* 1990;69:307–316.

70. Woodhead MA, MacFarlane JT. Legionnaires' disease; a review of 79 community acquired cases in Nottingham. *Thorax* 1986;41:635–640.

71. Falco V, Fernandez de Sevilla T, Alegre J, et al. *Legionella pneumophila*—a cause of severe community-acquired pneumonias. *Chest* 1991;100:1007–1011.

72. Tsai TF, Finn DR, Pilikaytis B, et al. Clinical features of the epidemic in Philadelphia. *Ann Intern Med* 1979;90:509–517.

73. Mulazimoglu L, Yu VL. Can legionnaires' disease be diagnosed by clinical criteria: a critical review. *Chest* 2001;120:1049–1951.

74. Hubbard RB, Mathur RM, MacFarlane JT. Severe community-acquired legionella pneumonia: treatment, complications and outcome. *Q J Med* 1993;86:327–332.

75. Kociuba KR, Buist M, Munro R, et al. Legionnaires' disease outbreak in southwestern Sydney, 1992: clinical aspects. *Med J Austr* 1994;160:274–277.

76. Posner MR, Caudill A, Brass R, et al. Legionnaires' disease associated with rhabdomyolysis and myoglobinuria. *Arch Intern Med* 1980;848.

77. Fenves AZ. Legionnaires' disease associated with acute renal failure: a report of two cases and review of the literature. *Clin Nephrol* 1985;23:96–100.

78. Johnson JT, Raff M, VanArsdall J. Neurologic manifestations of legionnaires' disease. *Medicine* 1984;63:303–310.

79. Westblom T, Hamory BH. Acute pancreatitis caused by *Legionella pneumophila*. *South Med J* 1988;81:1200–1201.

80. Lowry PW, Tompkins LS. Nosocomial legionellosis: a review of pulmonary and extrapulmonary syndromes. *Am J Infect Cont* 1993;21:21–27.

81. Fuller J, Levinson MD, Kline JR, et al. Legionnaires' disease after heart transplantation. *Ann Thoracic Surg* 1985;39:308–311.

82. Moore EH, Webb WR, Gamsu G, et al. Legionnaires' disease in the renal transplant patient: clinical presentation and radiographic progression. *Radiology* 1984;153:583–593.

83. Yu VL, Kroboth FJ, Shonnard J, et al. Legionnaires' disease: new clinical perspective from a prospective pneumonia study. *Am J Med* 1982;73:357–361.

84. Woodhead MA, MacFarlane JT. Comparative clinical and laboratory features of *Legionella* with pneumococcal and mycoplasma pneumonias. *Br J Dis Chest* 1987;81:133–139.

85. Woodhead MA, MacFarlane JT, McCracken JS, et al. Prospective study of the aetiology and outcome of pneumonia in the community. *Lancet* 1987;i:671–674.

86. Muder RR, Yu VL, Parry M. Radiology of *Legionella pneumonia*. *Semin Resp Infect* 1987;2:242–254.

87. Tan MJ, Tan JS, Hamor R, et al. The radiologic manifestations of legionnaires disease. The Ohio community-based pneumonia incidence study group. *Chest* 2000;117:398–403.

88. MacFarlane JT, Miller AC, Smith RWH. Comparative radiographic features of community acquired legionnaires' disease, pneumococcal pneumonia, mycoplasma pneumonia, and psittacosis. *Thorax* 1984;39:28–33.

89. Fairbank JT, Mamourian AC, Dietrich PA, et al. The chest radiograph in legionnaires' disease. Further observations. *Radiology* 1983;147:33–34.

90. Bornstein N, Mercatello A, Marmet D, et al. Pleural infection caused by *Legionella anisa*. *J Clin Microbiol* 1989;27:2100–2101.

91. Fang GD, Yu VL, Vickers RM. Disease due to *Legionellaceae* (other than *Legionella pneumophila*): historical, microbiological, clinical and epidemiological review. *Medicine* 1989;68:116–139.

92. Muder RR, Yu VL, Vickers R, et al. Simultaneous infection with *Legionella pneumophila* and Pittsburgh pneumonia agent—clinical features and epidemiological implications. *Am J Med* 1983;74:609–614.

93. Tompkins LS, Trout N, Wood ST, et al. Molecular epidemiology of legionella speies by restriction endonuclease and alloenzyme analysis. *J Clin Microbiol* 1987;25:1875–1880.

94. Glick TH, Gregg MB, Berman B, et al. Pontiac fever. An epidemic of unknown etiology in a health department. I. Clinical and epidemiologic aspects. *Am J Epidemiol* 1978;107:149–160.

95. Zuravleff JJ, Yu VL, Shonnard J, et al. Diagnosis of legionnaires' disease: an update of laboratory methods with new emphasis on isolation by culture. *JAMA* 1983;250:1981–1985.

96. Vickers RM, Stout JE, Yu VL, et al. Culture methodology for the isolation of *Legionella pneumophila* and other *Legionellaceae* from clinical and environmental specimens. *Semin Resp Infect* 1987;2:274–279.

97. Vickers RM, Yee YC, Rihs JD, et al. Prospective assessment of sensitivity, quantitation, and timing of urinary antigen, serology, direct immunofluorescence (DFA) for diagnosis of legionnaires' disease (LD). (C-17) Abstracts Annual Meeting of American Society for Microbiology, 1994.

98. Rihs JD, Yu VL, Zuravleff JJ, et al. Isolation of *Legionella pneumophila* from blood with the BACTEC system: a prospective study yielding positive results. *J Clin Microbiol* 1985;22:422–424.

99. Matsiota-Bernard P, Pitsouni E, Legakis N, et al. Evaluation of commercial amplification kit for detection of *Legionella pneumophila* in clinical samples. *J Clin Microbiol* 1994;32:1503–1505.

100. Kohler RB, Winn WC Jr, Wheat LJ. Onset and duration of urinary antigen excretion in Legionnaires' disease. *J Clin Microbiol* 1984;20:605–607.

101. Vickers RM, Yee YC, Rihs JD, et al. Prospective assessment of sensitivity, quantitation, and timing of urinary antigen, serology, and direct fluorescent antibody for diagnosis of legionnaires' disease. (Abstract C17.) Presented at the 93rd annual meeting of the American Society of Microbiology, 1994.

102. Wilkinson H, Cruce D, Brome C. Validation of *Legionella pneumophila* indirect immunofluorescence assay with epidemic sera. *J Clin Microbiol* 1981;13:139–146.

103. Fitzgeorge RB, Featherstone ASR, Baskerville A. Efficacy of azithromycin in the treatment of guinea pigs infected with *Legionella pneumophila* by aerosol. *J Antimicrob Chemother* 1990;25[Suppl. A]:101–108.

104. Edelstein PH, Edelstein MAC. In vitro activity of azithromycin against clinical isolates of legionella species. *Antimicrob Agents Chemother* 1991;35:180–181.

105. Vergis EN, Indorf A, File TM, et al. Azithromycin vs. cefuroxime plus erythromycin for empirical treatment of community-acquired pneumonia in hospitalized patients: a prospective, randomized, multicenter trial. *Arch Intern Med* 2000;160:1294–1300.

106. Saito A, Koga H, Shigeno H, et al. The antimicrobial activity of ciprofloxacin against *Legionella* species and the treatment of experimental legionella pneumonia in guinea pigs. *J Antimicrob Chemother* 1986;18:251–260.

107. Saito A, Sawatari K, Fukuda Y, et al. Susceptibility of *Legionella pneumophila* to ofloxacin in vitro and in experimental legionella pneumonia in guinea pigs. *Antimicrob Agents Chemother* 1985;28:15–20.

108. Unertl KE, Lenhart FP, Forst H, et al. Brief report: ciprofloxacin in the treatment of legionellosis in critically ill patients including those cases unresponsive to erythromycin. *Am J Med* 1989;87[Suppl. 5A]:128S–131S.

109. Hooper T, Gould F, Swinburn CR, et al. Ciprofloxacin: a preferred treatment for legionella infection in patients receiving cyclosporin. *J Antimicrob Chemother* 1988;6:952–953.

110. Miller AC. Erythromycin in legionnaires' disease: a reappraisal. *J Antimicrob Chemother* 1981;7:217–222.

111. Rudin JE, Evans TL, Wing EJ. Failure of erythromycin in treatment of *Legionella micdadei* pneumonia. *Am J Med* 1984;76:318–320.

112. Piagnerelli M, Jacobs O, Carlier E, et al. Successful treatment of severe legionella pneumonia with imipenem. *Intensive Care Med* 1999;25:1030.

113. Yu VL, Beam TR, Lumish RM, et al. Routine culturing for legionella in the hospital environment may be a good idea: a three-hospital prospective study. *Am J Med Sci* 1987;294:97–99.

114. Goetz AM, Stout JE, Jacobs SL, et al. Nosocomial legionnaires' disease

discovered in community hospitals following cultures of the water system: seek and ye shall find. *Am J Infect Control* 1998;26:6–11.

115. Stout JE, Yu VL. *Legionella* in the hospital water supply: a plea for decision making based on evidence-based medicine. *Infect Control Hosp Epidemiol* 2001;22:670–672.

116. Goetz A, Yu VL. Screening for nosocomial legionellosis by culture of the water supply and targeting of high-risk patients for specialized laboratory testing. *Am J Infect Cont* 1991;19:63–66.

117. Muraca P, Yu VL, Goetz A. Disinfection of water distribution systems for Legionella: a review of application procedures and methodologies. *Infect Control Hosp Epidemiol* 1990;11:79–88.

118. Grosserode M, Helms C, Pfaller M, et al. Continuous hyperchlorination for control of nosocomial legionnaires' disease: a ten year follow-up of efficacy, environmental effects, and cost. In: Barbaree JM, Breiman RF, Dufour AP, eds. *Legionella—current status and emerging perspectives.* Washington DC: American Society for Microbiology, 1993:226–229.

119. Lin YE, Stout JE, Yu VL. Disinfection of water distribution systems for Legionella. *Semin Resp Infect* 1998;13:147–159.

120. Hamilton E, Seal DV, Hay J. Comparison of chlorine and chlorine dioxide disinfection for control of legionella in a hospital water supply. *J Hosp Infect* 1996;32:156–160.

121. Stout JE, Lin YSE, Goetz AM, et al. Controlling *Legionella* in hospital water systems: experience with the superheat-and-flush method and copper-silver ionization. *Infect Contr Hosp Epidemiol* 1998;19:911–914.

122. Stout JE, Lin YE, Yu VL. Survey of hospitals using copper-silver ionization for control of legionella. Presented at the 5th International Conference on Legionella; American Society of Microbiology, Ulm, Germany, 2000.

123. Farr BM, Gratz J, Tartaglino J, et al. Evaluation of ultraviolet light for disinfection of hospital water contaminated with legionella. *Lancet* 1988;2:669–672.

124. Park DR, Sherbin VL, Goodman MS, et al. The etiology of community-acquired pneumonia at an urban public hospital: influence of human immunodeficiency virus infection and initial severity of illness. *J Infect Dis* 2001;184:268–277.

125. Sopena N, Sabria-Leal M, Pedro-Botet ML, et al. Comparative study of the clinical presentation of legionella pneumonia and other community-acquired pneumonias. *Chest* 1998;113:1195–1200.

126. Ishida T, Hashimoto T, Arita M, et al. Etiology of community-acquired pneumonia in hospitalized patients: a 3-year prospective study in Japan. *Chest* 1998;114:1588–1593.

127. Ruiz M, Ewig S, Marcos MA, et al. Etiology of community-acquired pneumonia: impact of age, comorbidity, and severity. *Am J Respir Crit Care Med* 1999;160:397–405.

128. Socan M, Marinic-Fiser N, Kraigher A, et al. Microbial aetiology of community-acquired pneumonia in hospitalised patients. *Eur J Clin Microbiol Infect Dis* 1999;18:777–782.

129. El-Solh AA, Sikka P, Ramadan F, et al. The etiology of severe pneumonia in the very elderly. *Am J Respir Crit Care Med* 2001;163:645–651.

130. Lim WS, MacFarlane JT, Boswell TC, et al. Study of community acquired pneumonia aetiology (SCAPA) in adults admitted to hospital: implications for management guidelines. *Thorax* 2001;56:296–301.

CHAPTER 56
Chlamydia *Pneumonia*

Margaret R. Hammerschlag

Chlamydiae are obligate intracellular pathogens that have established a unique niche within the host cell. Chlamydiae cause a variety of diseases in animal species at virtually all phylogenic levels. The standard classification of the order contains one genus, *Chlamydia*, with four recognized species: *C. trachomatis*, *C. psittaci*, *C. pneumoniae*, and *C. pecorum* (1). *C. trachomatis* and *C. pneumoniae* are the most significant human pathogens. *C. psittaci* is an important zoonosis. Recent taxonomic analysis using the 16S and 23S ribosomal ribonucleic acid (rRNA) genes has suggested splitting the genus *Chlamydia* into two genera, *Chlamydia* and *Chlamydophila* (1). Two new species, *Chlamydia muridarum* (formerly the agent of mouse pneumonitis-MoPn) and *C. suis* would join *C. trachomatis*. *Chlamydophila* would contain *C. pecorum*, *C. pneumoniae* and *C. psittaci* and three new species split off from *C. psittaci*: *C. abortus*, *C. caviae* (formerly *C. psittaci* Guinea pig conjunctivitis strain) and *C. felis*. There

is continuing controversy regarding this reclassification, but for the purposes of this chapter, we will continue to refer to *Chlamydia*. *C. pneumoniae*, *C. psittaci*, and *C. trachomatis* all cause pneumonia in humans, although the routes of transmission, susceptible populations, and clinical presentation differ (Table 56.1). The microbiology of *Chlamydia* is described in detail in Chapter 222.

RESPIRATORY INFECTION CAUSED BY *CHLAMYDIA PNEUMONIAE*

The first isolates of *C. pneumoniae* were serendipitously obtained during trachoma studies in the 1960s (2). On the basis of inclusion morphology and staining characteristics in cell culture, *C. pneumoniae* was initially considered to be a novel strain of *C. psittaci* (3). Subsequent analyses, however, have demonstrated that this organism is distinct from both *C. psittaci* and *C. trachomatis* (4,5). Ultrastructural studies demonstrated that the elementary bodies of *C. pneumoniae* had a pear-shaped appearance caused by a loose periplasmic membrane, whereas the elementary bodies of *C. trachomatis* and *C. psittaci* are round (6). However, ultrastructural studies of IOL-207 and other strains of *C. pneumoniae* isolated in Japan and Finland revealed round elementary bodies similar in appearance to those of the other two chlamydial species (7,8). Only one serotype has been identified so far. Studies analyzing genomic amplified fragment length polymorphism fingerprints suggest a high degree of genetic relatedness (greater than 95%) among the *C. pneumoniae* isolates tested (9).

Epidemiology

C. pneumoniae appears to be a common human respiratory pathogen; however, the organism has also been isolated from nonhuman species, including a horse, koalas, and amphibians, although the role these infections may play in human disease is unknown (10,11). The mode of transmission remains uncertain but probably occurs through infected respiratory secretions. Acquisition of infection by droplet aerosol was described during a laboratory accident (12). *C. pneumoniae* can remain viable on Formica countertops for 30 hours and can survive small-particle aerosolization (13,14). Spread within families and enclosed populations, such as military recruits, have been described (15,16).

Several serologic surveys have documented rising chlamydial antibody prevalence rates beginning in school-age children and reaching 30% to 45% by adolescence (2). Seroprevalence of antibody, as determined by the microimmunofluorescence (MIF) method, can exceed 80% in some adult populations (17,18). The proportion of community-acquired pneumonias associated with *C. pneumoniae* infection has ranged from 3% to 29%, varying with geographic location, the age group examined, and the methods used to determine infection (i.e., serology or culture) (2,19–24). Studies that have used culture have found the prevalence of infection in children to be similar to rate seen in adults; however, these studies also noted a poor correlation between culture and serology, especially in children (21,23).

Coinfections with other organisms, specifically *Streptococcus pneumoniae* and *M. pneumoniae* may occur frequently (21,23,25). Clinically, these patients cannot be differentiated from those infected with a single organism. In these cases, *C. pneumoniae* may not be the primary cause of the pneumonia but might disrupt the normal clearance mechanisms and enable other pathogens to invade. *C. pneumoniae* has been found to inhibit ciliary motion of bronchial epithelial cells (26).

TABLE 56.1. Epidemiologic and Clinical Characteristics of Respiratory Disease Caused by *Chlamydia*

Feature	*C. pneumoniae*	*C. trachomatis*	*C. psittaci*
Natural host	Humans, koalas, frogs	Humans	Birds, mammals
Population	All ages	Infants, immunocompromised adults	Veterinarians, bird fanciers, poultry workers
Mode of transmission	Person to person: by aerosol droplets	Vertical: mother to infant	Bird to person: by aerosolized fecal material
Major respiratory diseases	Pneumonia, bronchitis, reactive airway disease	Pneumonia	Pneumonia

In studies to date, acute infection with *C. pneumoniae* does not appear to vary by season. There are reports of cycles in Seattle and Scandinavia lasting several years during which the incidence of new infection with *C. pneumoniae* waxes and wanes. In contrast, the infection appears to be endemic in Brooklyn, which may be a function of the greater population density.

Prolonged culture positivity after acute infection, lasting several weeks to more than a year, has also been described (27). Asymptomatic respiratory infection may occur in 2% to 5% of adults and children (17,28). It is not known what role asymptomatic carriage plays in the epidemiology of *C. pneumoniae*.

Pathogenesis

The pathogenic mechanisms of *C. pneumoniae* infection in humans are largely unknown. Experimental infection has been produced in nonhuman primates and mice (29–31). The infection in monkeys is largely asymptomatic, and the animals may shed the organism from the respiratory tract for 12 months or longer (29). Infection in mice is also largely asymptomatic. The lung disorder is characterized by patchy interstitial pneumonitis with predominantly polymorphonuclear leukocyte infiltration in the early stage and mononuclear cell infiltration in the later stage of infection (30,31). *C. pneumoniae* can be isolated from the lungs for several weeks after inoculation as well as from other organs including the spleen. Administration of corticosteroids results in reactivation of lung infection in mice after apparent resolution (31).

Clinical Presentation

The spectrum of disease associated with *C. pneumoniae* is expanding. Most infections are probably mild or asymptomatic. Initial reports emphasized mild atypical pneumonia clinically resembling that associated with *M. pneumoniae* (2). In several subsequent studies, however, pneumonia associated with *C. pneumoniae* has been clinically indistinguishable from other pneumonias (19,21).

C. pneumoniae has been associated with severe illness and even death, although the role of preexisting chronic conditions as contributing factors in many of these patients is difficult to assess. *C. pneumoniae* can be a serious pathogen even in the absence of underlying disease. *C. pneumoniae* was isolated from the respiratory tract and the pleural fluid of a previously healthy adolescent boy with severe pneumonia complicated by respiratory failure and pleural effusions (33).

The role of host factors remains to be determined. Although *C. pneumoniae* has been detected in bronchoalveolar lavage fluid from 10% of a group of patients with acquired immunodeficiency syndrome and pneumonia, its clinical role in these patients is uncertain because most were coinfected with other well-recognized pathogens such as *Pneumocystis carinii* and *M. tuberculosis* (34). Gaydos and colleagues (35) identified *C. pneumoniae* infection by polymerase chain reaction (PCR) in 11% of a group of immunocompromised adults with human immunodeficiency virus infection, malignant neoplasms, and other immune disorders including systemic lupus erythematosus, sarcoidosis, and common variable immunodeficiency. *C. pneumoniae* appeared to be responsible for 6 of 31 (19%) episodes of acute chest syndrome in children with sickle cell disease (36). *C. pneumoniae* infection in these patients appeared to be associated with more severe hypoxia than was infection with *M. pneumoniae*.

C. pneumoniae may also act as an inflammatory trigger for asthma. Hahn and colleagues (37) reported an association between serologic evidence of acute *C. pneumoniae* infection and wheezing in adults seen for lower respiratory tract illness. However, they were able to isolate the organism from only 1 of 365 patients. Emre et al. (28) isolated *C. pneumoniae* from 13 of 118 (11%) children 5 to 15 years of age who were initially evaluated for either new or acute exacerbations of asthma. Treatment of the infection appeared to result in both clinical improvement and improvement in pulmonary function test scores. One child who was noncompliant with his antibiotic therapy had positive culture results on five occasions over a 3-month period. Specific anti-*C. pneumoniae* IgE was detected in 85.7% of children with asthma and positive culture results compared to 9% of children with *C. pneumoniae* pneumonia who were not wheezing (38). This suggests that bronchial reactivity seen with *C. pneumoniae* infection may be IgE-mediated. The potential of *C. pneumoniae* to cause prolonged, persistent infection may produce chronic inflammation and trigger bronchospasm in susceptible individuals.

Diagnosis

A specific laboratory diagnosis of *C. pneumoniae* infection can be made by isolation of the organism from nasopharyngeal swabs and pleural fluid. The nasopharynx appears to be the optimal site for isolation of the organism (21). The organism can also be isolated from throat swabs and sputum, but the relative yield from these sites is not known. The isolation of *C. pneumoniae* requires culture in tissue; the organism cannot be propagated in cell-free media. *C. pneumoniae* grows readily in a number of cell lines derived from respiratory tissue, specifically HEp-2 and HL cells (39). Culture with an initial inoculation and one passage should take 4 to 7 days. Nasopharyngeal culture specimens can be obtained with Dacron-tipped wire-shafted swabs. Specimens for culture should be placed in appropriate transport media, usually a sucrose phosphate buffer with antibiotics and fetal calf serum, and stored immediately at 4°C for no longer than 24 hours. Viability decreases if specimens are held at room temperature. If the specimen cannot be processed within 24 hours, it should be frozen at −70°C until culture can be performed. After 72 hours of incubation, culture confirmation can be performed by staining with either a *C. pneumoniae* species-specific or a *Chlamydia* genus-specific (anti-lipopolysaccharide [LPS]) fluorescein-conjugated monoclonal antibody (39). Inclusions of *C. pneumoniae* do not contain glycogen; thus, they will not stain with iodine. Unfortunately, there is limited availability of commercially produced *C. pneumoniae*-specific reagents. If a genus-specific antibody is used, *C. pneumoniae* should be confirmed by differential staining with a specific *C. trachomatis* antibody; if this is negative, then the isolate is either *C. pneumoniae* or *C. psittaci*. If there were no avian exposure, psittacosis would be highly unlikely.

Because isolation of *C. pneumoniae* was initially considered to be difficult and limited, more emphasis was placed on serologic diagnosis. However, performance of the MIF test is also limited to a small number of research laboratories. The MIF was modified from the test for *C. trachomatis* by use of elementary bodies from TW-183 or other *C. pneumoniae* strains as the antigen. With the MIF test, one can detect IgG, IgM, and IgA antibodies. Grayston and colleagues (2) proposed a set of criteria for serologic diagnosis of *C. pneumoniae* infection with the MIF test that is used by many laboratories and clinicians. For acute infection, the patient should have a fourfold rise in IgG titer, a single IgM titer of 16 or greater, or a single IgG titer of 512 or higher. Previous or preexisting infection is defined as an IgG titer of 16 or higher but less than 512. It was further proposed that the pattern of antibody response in primary infection differed from that seen in reinfection. In initial infection, the IgM response appears about 3 weeks after the onset of illness, and the IgG response appears at 6 to 8 weeks. In reinfection, the IgM response may be absent and the IgG occurs earlier, within 1 to 2 weeks. A fourfold titer rise or a titer of 64 or higher with the complement fixation (CF) test is also thought to be diagnostic. In a report of a small outbreak of *C. pneumoniae* infections among University of Washington students, all seven patients with pneumonia had CF titers of 64 or greater (40). However, the CF test is genus-specific.

Because of the relatively long period until the development of a serologic response in primary infection, the antibody response may be missed if convalescent serum samples are obtained too soon, that is, earlier than 3 weeks after the onset of illness. Use of paired serum samples also affords only a retrospective diagnosis, which is of little help in terms of deciding how to treat the patient. The criteria for use of a single serum sample have not been correlated with the results of culture and are based mainly on data from adults. The antibody response in acute infection may take longer than 3 months to develop. Acute, culture-documented infection can also occur without seroconversion, especially in children (21,26,28).

Hyman and co-workers, (17) as part of a study of asymptomatic *C. pneumoniae* infection among subjectively healthy adults in Brooklyn, New York, found 81% to have IgG or IgM titers of 16 or greater. Seventeen percent also met the criteria for acute infection using a single serum sample: IgG titer equal to or greater than 512, or IgM titer equal to or greater than 16. However, none of these individuals had positive culture or PCR results. Similar results were reported by Kern and associates (18) among healthy firefighters and police officers in Rhode Island. The specificity of the MIF IgM assay can be affected by the presence of rheumatoid factor in the study. A study from the Netherlands found that an increased probability of false-positive results was due to rheumatoid factor with increasing age (41). Sera should be routinely absorbed before MIF IgM testing. Hyman and colleagues absorbed all the IgM-positive sera; the titers did not change (17). Some IgG antibody may result from a heterotypic response to other chlamydial species because there are cross-reactions with the major outer membrane protein between the three species as well as cross-reactions due to the genus LPS antigen. Moss and colleagues (42) reported that anti-

bodies to *C. pneumoniae* and *C. psittaci* accounted for up to half of all chlamydial IgG-positive persons attending a sexually transmitted disease clinic. Other organisms that have been reported as possibly causing cross-reactions with the MIF are *Bartonella* (43) and *Bordetella pertussis* (44). The latter could be significant as adults with pertussis frequently present with a chronic cough or severe bronchitis, which is a clinical presentation often ascribed to *C. pneumoniae*. Recent studies have found significant homology between human and *C. pneumoniae* HSP60, and *Escherichia coli* GroEL (45). Picornavirus proteins have also been reported to share antigenic determinants with HSP60/65, including the HSP60s of humans and *C. pneumoniae*, which conceivably could also lead to cross reactions with the MIF assay (46).

The MIF test is not standardized, and many laboratories use assays developed in-house. As of this writing, at least two MIF assay kits are commercially available, although neither has approval or clearance by the US Food and Drug Administration (FDA) for this indication. The two best-characterized kits are from MRL (MRL Diagnostics, Cypress, CA), which uses elementary bodies of *C. pneumoniae* isolate AR-39, and Lab Systems (Helsinki, Finland), which uses Kajaani 6. The Labsystems kit also uses a higher concentration of antigen and contains *C. trachomatis* and *C. pneumoniae* antigens as negative and positive controls, respectively. Neither kit has been evaluated in comparison with culture or PCR.

Reading the result of the MIF assay is highly subjective. Recent studies by Peeling et al. (47,48) attempted to address the problem of interlaboratory variation in the performance of the MIF test. The overall agreement among all laboratories (within one twofold dilution of the "gold-standard" at the University of Washington) was 80%. The range was 50% to 100% depending on the antibody isotype. Agreement for serodiagnostic criteria was 69% for negative, 68% for "chronic," and 87% for a fourfold increase of IgG. In a subsequent study, they compared the performance of the University of Washington assay and the commercially available MRL kit. A panel of ten sera was sent to 17 laboratories in the United States and Europe (48). When the University of Washington kit was used, agreement for IgM titers of individual serum samples ranged from 53% to 100%, and agreement for IgG titers ranged from 47% to 100%. For the MRL kit, the agreement ranged from 80% to 100% for IgM and 60% to 100% for IgG.

Although enzyme immunoassays (EIAs) offer the promise of standardized performance and objective endpoints, none have been adequately evaluated compared with culture or PCR (49,50). Most have been compared only with MIF. None have FDA approval for use in the United States. One kit uses a recombinant LPS antigen, and others are based on LPS-extracted elementary bodies or synthetic peptides (50). These kits can measure IgG, IgM, and IgA antibodies, but the cutoff points vary from kit to kit, and the criteria for interpreting positive results (acute or past infection) can be very complex (49,50). One study from the United States, comparing the recombinant LPS EIA with culture, found sensitivities ranging from 13% for IgM antibody in children to 78% for either IgA or IgG antibody in adults with respiratory infection. Specificities compared to culture ranged from 21% to 91% (50).

The Centers for Disease Control and Prevention (CDC) have recently proposed some modifications of the serologic criteria for diagnosis of *C. pneumoniae* infections (39). The MIF test is still considered to be the only currently acceptable serologic test. When the MIF test is used, acute infection is defined by a fourfold rise in IgG titer or an IgM titer of greater than 16; use of a single elevated IgG titer for diagnosis is discouraged. An IgG titer of >16 was thought to indicate previous exposure, but neither elevated IgA titers nor other serologic markers were thought to be valid indicators of persistent infection.

Deoxyribonucleic acid amplification methods (e.g., PCR) appear to be the most promising technology in the development of a rapid, nonculture method for detection of *C. pneumoniae*. At least 18 in-house PCR assays for detection of *C. pneumoniae* in clinical specimens have been reported in the literature (38,51). None of these assays are standardized or have been extensively validated compared to culture for detection of *C. pneumoniae* in respiratory specimens. None are commercially available or have FDA approval. Major variations in these methods include in collecting and processing specimens, primer design, nucleic acid extraction, amplification product detection and identification, and ways to prevent possible false-positive and inhibitory reactions. The most frequently used primers have been those based on the *omp1* gene, the 16S ribosomal ribonucleic acid (rRNA) gene, the 16S and 16S-23S spacer rRNA genes, and a *C. pneumoniae*–specific cloned *Pst* I fragment (39,51). Some assays have used single amplification; some have been nested. Methods for detecting the amplification product include agarose gel electrophoresis, Southern blot, EIA, and polyacrylamide gel electrophoresis (51). Recent studies suggest significant interlaboratory variation in performance of PCR for *C. pneumoniae* (52). The CDC does not recommend any specific assay, citing the lack of comparative data (38) and suggested that more studies need to be conducted with proper controls and larger numbers of clinical specimens from patients. The CDC suggested that any new PCR assay be compared with a sensitive culture system.

Treatment

Chlamydia species are susceptible to tetracyclines, macrolides, and quinolones (53). *C. pneumoniae* and *C. psittaci* are resistant to sulfonamides To date, there have also been few published data describing the response of *C. pneumoniae* to antimicrobial therapy. Most of the treatment studies of pneumonia caused by *C. pneumoniae* published so far have relied entirely on diagnosis by serology; thus, microbiologic efficacy could not be assessed. Results of several multicenter treatment studies that utilized culture demonstrated 70% to 86% efficacy of treatment with erythromycin, clarithromycin, azithromycin, levofloxacin and moxifloxacin in eradicating *C. pneumoniae* from the nasopharynx of children and adults with community-acquired pneumonia (21,26,54–56). Most patients improved clinically despite persistence of the organism. Persistence does not appear to be secondary to the development of antibiotic resistance (54–57).

On the basis of these few data, the following regimens can be used for respiratory infection due to *C. pneumoniae* in adults, doxycycline, 100 mg orally twice daily for 14 to 21 days; tetracycline, 250 mg orally four times daily for 14 to 21 days; azithromycin, 1.5 g orally over 5 days; clarithromycin, 500 mg orally, twice a day for 10 days; levofloxacin, 500 mg, intravenously or orally, once a day for 7 to 14 days; or moxifloxacin, 400 mg orally, once a day for 10 days. For children, erythromycin suspension, 50 mg/kg per day for 10 to 14 days; clarithromycin suspension, 15 mg/kg per day for 10 days; or azithromycin suspension, 10 mg/kg once on day 1 followed by 5 mg/kg, once daily for 4 days. Some patients may require re-treatment.

RESPIRATORY INFECTION CAUSED BY *CHLAMYDIA TRACHOMATIS*

Although *C. trachomatis* is primarily a sexually transmitted pathogen, it can cause respiratory tract infection, including pneumonia in specific circumstances. Pregnant women who have cervical infection with *C. trachomatis* can transmit the infection to their infants, who may subsequently develop neonatal conjunctivitis and pneumonia. Epidemiologic evidence strongly suggests that the infant acquires chlamydial infection from the mother during vaginal delivery (58). Infection after caesarean section is rare and usually occurs after early rupture of the amniotic membrane. There is no evidence supporting postnatal acquisition from the mother or other family members. Approximately 50% to 75% of infants born to infected women become infected at one or more anatomic sites, including the conjunctiva, rectum, and vagina. The nasopharynx is by far the most frequent site of infection. Approximately 70% of infected infants have positive culture results from that site. Most of these nasopharyngeal infections are asymptomatic and may persist for 3 years or more (59).

Pneumonia develops in only approximately 30% of infants with nasopharyngeal infection; the reasons are unknown. In those in whom pneumonia develops, the presentation and clinical findings are characteristic. The children are usually seen between 4 and 12 weeks of age; a few cases have been reported as early as 2 weeks of age, but no cases have been seen beyond 4 months. The infants frequently have a history of cough and congestion with an absence of fever. On physical examination, the infant is tachypneic, and rales are heard on auscultation of the chest; wheezing is distinctly uncommon. There are no specific radiographic findings except hyperinflation (58). Significant laboratory findings include peripheral eosinophilia (greater than 300 cells per mm^3) and elevated serum immunoglobulin levels (58).

Although asymptomatic perinatally acquired nasopharyngeal infection with *C. trachomatis* may persist for at least 2 years, respiratory tract infection in older children and adults appears to be distinctly uncommon. The reasons for this are not clear. Studies of the interaction of *C. trachomatis* and alveolar macrophages from normal healthy adults have demonstrated that these cells kill both biotypes of *C. trachomatis* efficiently (60). *C. trachomatis* has been isolated from the pharynx of some adults, apparently related to certain sexual practices. These infections have been asymptomatic.

There are two specific situations in which *C. trachomatis* can cause pneumonia in older children or adults. One is in immunosuppressed individuals. There have been several well-documented cases of pneumonia due to *C. trachomatis* in individuals with leukemia, bone marrow transplant recipients, and those with acquired immunodeficiency syndrome (61–63). In all of these cases, *C. trachomatis* was isolated from biopsy specimens of lung tissue or bronchoalveolar lavage fluid. Several patients also had a serologic response that was diagnostic of acute *C. trachomatis* infection. Unfortunately, there was no characteristic clinical presentation. These adults had none of the findings that are characteristic of infantile chlamydial pneumonia. There have also been several reports of pulmonary infection after exposure to *C. trachomatis* serotypes L$_1$ and L$_2$ in the laboratory (64). The infections were probably acquired by inhalation of aerosolized organisms. These patients presented clinically with high fever, night sweats, and cough and were found to have mediastinal lymphadenopathy or pneumonitis and splenomegaly. In two cases, the diagnosis of lymphoma was considered seriously. These findings are not unexpected given the severity of lymphogranuloma venereum genital infection. Accidental exposure to aerosolized *C. trachomatis* trachoma biotype has not been associated with significant illness.

Diagnosis

The definitive diagnosis of *C. trachomatis* pneumonia in infants is made by isolation of the organism from nasopharyngeal wash or swab specimens. *C. trachomatis* culture is usually performed in cycloheximide-treated McCoy cells with culture confirmation by staining with a specific fluorescein-conjugated monoclonal antibody (65). *C. trachomatis* can also be identified in nasopharyngeal specimens by nonculture antigen detection methods including EIA and direct fluorescent antibody tests. Although preliminary data suggests that PCR (Amplicor, Roche Molecular Diagnostics, NJ) may be more sensitive than culture in respiratory specimens from infants with *C. trachomatis* pneumonia and conjunctivitis (66), none of the currently available commercial nucleic acid amplification tests have FDA approval for detection of *C. trachomatis* in respiratory specimens from children or adults.

Infants with pneumonia should have IgM titers of specific anti–*C. trachomatis* antibody equal to or greater than 1:32 as determined by the MIF method. The CF test is not sensitive enough to detect antibody in infants with *C. trachomatis* pneumonia.

Treatment

The treatment of choice for *C. trachomatis* pneumonia in infants is oral erythromycin ethylsuccinate suspension, 50 mg/kg per day in three or four divided doses, for 10 to 14 days. There are no data on the treatment of *C. trachomatis* respiratory infections in adults, but one can extrapolate and assume that erythromycin, tetracycline, doxycycline, and levofloxacin in the dosage regimens recommended for genital infection may be effective. Azithromycin and clarithromycin may also be useful, but with use of dosage regimens suggested for *C. pneumoniae* infection.

RESPIRATORY INFECTION CAUSED BY *CHLAMYDIA PSITTACI*

Human infection with *C. psittaci* was probably first described by Juergensen in 1874 or Ritter in 1876. Ritter described seven cases of an unusual pneumonia that appeared to be caused by parrots and finches that were caged in the study of his brother's home in Switzerland. After these reports, there were several outbreaks of a similar disease in Europe that established the association with an exposure to birds (67). The term psittacosis was coined by Morange in 1892 from the Greek word for parrots, *psittakos* (67).

Organism

C. psittaci is a diverse species that affects nonpsittacine birds and many mammalian species as well. The known host range includes 15 mammalian species and 130 avian species, representing 10 orders (68). There is only 5% to 10% DNA homology between *C. psittaci* and *C. trachomatis* and *C. pneumoniae* (1,8,9). *C. psittaci*, like *C. pneumoniae*, lacks glycogen in its inclusions and is resistant to sulfonamides. Strains of *C. Psittaci* have been analyzed by pathogenicity patterns, growth characteristics, inclusion morphology in cell culture, DNA restriction endonuclease analysis, monoclonal antibodies, and numerous serologic tests, which indicate that there are nine mammalian serotypes, and seven avian serotypes (68). The mammalian strains differ greatly from avian strains in their antigenic characteristics. Two of the avian serotypes, psittacine and turkey, are of major importance in the avian population of the United States. Each is associated with important host preferences and disease characteristics (69). Strains of the turkey serotype have all been associated with a serious disease in either birds or human beings, with major epizootics in turkeys often resulting in disease in humans. The psittacine serotype has also been associated with serious disease in humans; however, human involvement is usually limited to sporadic cases after exposure to pet birds or pigeons. The pathogenicity of each *C. psittaci* strain to humans is unclear.

Epidemiology

According to the most recent report from the CDC (70), 813 cases of psittacosis were reported in the United States from 1988 to 1998, which is probably underreported. Approximately 70% of the cases were the result of exposure to pet birds, usually cockatiels, parakeets, parrots, and macaws. Those at highest risk for acquiring psittacosis included bird owners or fanciers (43% of cases), pet shop employees (10% of cases), and pigeon fanciers. Since 1984, there have been several major outbreaks of psittacosis in the United States in turkey-processing plants; approximately 300 individuals contracted the infection (71,72). Workers exposed to turkey viscera were at the highest risk for infection. In Australia, outbreaks of psittacosis have been associated with duck farming (73). An outbreak in Philadelphia was associated with an aviary (74). In 1995, the CDC investigated an outbreak of avian chlamydiosis in a shipment of over 700 pet birds from a Florida bird distributor to the Atlanta area (75). Affected birds included parrots, parakeets, finches, lovebirds, cockatiels, conures, and canaries. Clinical psittacosis or serologic evidence of *C. psittaci* infection was found in 30.7% of households with birds from the infected flock. An average of 21 days (range, 1 to 47 days) elapsed between purchase of the bird and the onset of symptoms. The majority of infected individuals had mild or asymptomatic illnesses. Among persons in exposed households, illness was more frequent if the recently purchased bird had become sick or had died. Kissing or nuzzling the bird, handling the bird, feeding the bird were all significantly associated with the development of clinical psittacosis, but in contrast to earlier studies, cleaning the bird's cage was not. The risk of developing clinical psittacosis varied significantly by type of bird to which the individual was exposed. The attack rate was highest for individuals exposed to parrots.

Inhalation of infectious aerosols derived from feces, fecal dust, or secretions of *C. psittaci*–infected animals is believed to be the primary route of infection. The source birds can be infected asymptomatically or can show signs of infection, such as anorexia, ruffled feathers, depression, and watery green droppings. Psittacosis is frequently a systemic infection in birds. The turkey strains can induce severe pericarditis. The gastrointestinal tract is also infected frequently. The psittacine serotype appears to be much less virulent in both turkeys and pigeons than in psittacine birds.

Clinical Manifestations

Infection with *C. psittaci* in humans may range from clinically inapparent to severe systemic infection involving multiple organs as well as pneumonia. Overall mortality now is low compared with that in the past, usually less than 1%. The mean incubation period is 15 days after exposure, and the range is 5 to 21 days. The onset is usually abrupt, with complaints of fever, cough, and headache. The fever is high and frequently associated with rigors and sweats. The headache can be so severe that meningitis can be considered a possibility; 33% of the patients in a series of cases from Australia had lumbar punctures (76). The cough is usually nonproductive. Rales may be heard on auscultation. Chest radiographs are usually abnormal, with variable infiltrates. Pleural effusions may also be present. The white cell count is usually not elevated, but there may be a mild leukocytosis. Almost 50% of the patients in the Australian series had abnormal liver function tests, including elevated levels of aspartate aminotransferase, alkaline phosphatase, and bilirubin (76). Psittacosis can be fulminant and has been associated with acute renal failure and acute thrombocytopenic purpura (77,78). *C. psittaci* has also been implicated as a cause of endocarditis (79,80). Patients may also present with fever of unknown origin. In contrast, the majority of the individuals in the Atlanta outbreak had very mild disease characterized by fever, headache and cough (75).

Initial infection does not appear to be followed by long-term immunity. Reinfection and clinical disease can develop within 2 months of treatment. There are several well-documented cases of reinfection (81,82). The second episodes tend to be severe.

Diagnosis

Because of the varying clinical presentation, the diagnosis of psittacosis can be difficult. History of exposure to birds is important. In the Australian series, 85% of the patients had a history of recent bird contact; 71% of these described a strong history of bird contact (76). Exposure to poultry was found in only five patients. Pneumonia due to *C. pneumoniae* can also have a similar clinical presentation. Data from Sweden, Denmark, and England have suggested that many cases of "psittacosis" with no history of bird exposure are probably due to *C. pneumoniae* (83–85). Infection with *C. pneumoniae* is more likely if there has been evidence of person-to-person spread, which is extremely unusual with human psittacosis. Other infections that can produce the syndrome of pneumonia with high fever, unusually severe headache, and myalgia include *M. pneumoniae* infection, tularemia, tuberculosis, fungal infections, Legionnaires' disease, and various bacterial infections.

Diagnosis of psittacosis in the human population is primarily based on clinical presentation, epidemiology, and serology. Although many laboratories are able to isolate *C. psittaci*, it is not a service provided by most clinical microbiology laboratories on a routine basis mainly because of the potential biohazard. The diagnosis of human infection due to *C. psittaci* has not changed substantially for many years. The mainstay of diagnosis remains serology using the CF test. According to the 2000 recommendations from the CDC (70), a confirmed case of psittacosis requires a compatible clinical illness, usually with a good history of avian exposure. Laboratory confirmation can be made by one of the three following methods: (i) culture of *C. psittaci* from respiratory secretions, (ii) greater than fourfold increase in CF or MIF titer in sera collected at least 2 weeks apart, and (iii) MIF IgM titer of greater than 16. A probable case should be epidemiologically linked to a confirmed case or have a single CF or MIF antibody titer of greater than 32 in a least one serum obtained after onset of symptoms. As with use of the MIF for diagnosis of *C. pneumoniae* infections, cross-reactions with other *Chlamydia* species and bacteria can occur. Recently a cross-reaction with *Legionella longbeachae* was described in a patient with fulminant pneumonia due to *C. psittaci* (86).

Several in-house PCR assays for detection of *C. psittaci* have been reported in the literature (87–91). Use of PCR for diagnosis of psittacosis has the same limitations as use of PCR for diagnosis of *C. pneumoniae*. Most reported studies have assessed only the ability of these assays to amplify laboratory isolates; they have not been extensively evaluated for detection of *C. psittaci* in clinical specimens from humans with suspected psittacosis. Only a small number of human cases of psittacosis documented by PCR have been reported in the literature (87,88,90). In 1997,

the CDC reported one of the most extensive evaluations of the use of PCR in investigation of a psittacosis outbreak (89). The majority of specimens tested were from birds. The target sequence of the assay was the 16S rRNA gene. The first-step amplification was genus specific, and the second amplification was multiplexed and could differentiate between *C. psittaci*, *C. pneumoniae*, and *C. trachomatis* on the basis of the molecular weight of the amplicon. By use of this assay, *C. psittaci* was detected in 13 (17.3%) of 75 sick or dead birds involved in three avian psittacosis outbreaks; five of the 13 PCR-positive birds were also culture-positive. None of the throat swab specimens from four humans involved in this outbreak were positive by PCR or culture, but one individual had a *C. psittaci*–specific MIF IgG titer of 512.

The CDC (70) provides a list of laboratories that test human specimens in its current recommendations for the control of *C. psittaci* infection among humans and pet birds.

Treatment

The recommended treatment for psittacosis in humans is 500 mg of tetracycline every 6 hours, orally, for 7 to 10 days. For initial treatment of severely ill patients, doxycycline hyclate can given intravenously at a dose of 4.4 mg/kg twice daily (up to 100 mg per dose) (70). Remission of symptoms usually occurs within 48 to 72 hours. Relapses can occur and treatment should be continued for at least 10 to 14 days after the patient becomes afebrile. Erythromycin, 2 g/day for 7 to 10 days, can also be used. However, the experience of the Australian series and anecdotal reports suggest that tetracycline may be more effective than erythromycin (76,87).

REFERENCES

1. Everett KDE, Bush RM, Anderson AA. Emended description of the order *Chlamydiales*, proposal of *Parachlamydiaceae* fam. nov. and *Simkaniaceae* fam. nov., each containing one monotypic genus, revised taxonomy of the family *Chlamydiaceae*, including a new genus and five new species, and standards for identification of organisms. *Int J Syst Bacteriol* 1999;49:425–440.
2. Grayston JT, Campbell LA, Kuo C-C, et al. A new respiratory tract pathogen: *Chlamydia pneumoniae* strain TWAR. *J Infect Dis* 1990;161:618–625.
3. Grayston JT, Kuo C-C, Wang S-P, et al. A new *Chlamydia psittaci* strain, TWAR, isolated in acute respiratory tract infections. *N Engl J Med* 1986;315:161–168.
4. Kalman S, Mitchell W, Marathe R, et al. Comparative genomes of *Chlamydia pneumoniae* and *C. trachomatis*. *Nature Gen* 1999;21:385–389.
5. Grayston JT, Kuo C-C, Campbell LA, et al. *Chlamydia pneumoniae* sp. nov. for *Chlamydia* sp. strain TWAR. *Int J Syst Bacteriol* 1989;39:88–90.
6. Chi EY, Kuo C-C, Grayston JT. Unique ultrastructure in the elementary body of *Chlamydia* sp. strain TWAR. *J Bacteriol* 1987;169:3757–3763.
7. Myashita A, Kanamoto Y, Matsumoto A. The morphology of *Chlamydia pneumoniae*. *J Med Microbiol* 1993;38:418–425.
8. Carter MW, Al-Mahdawi SAH, Treharne JD, et al. Nucleotide sequence and taxonomic value of the major outer membrane protein gene of *Chlamydia pneumoniae* IOL-207. *J Gen Microbiol* 1991;137:465–475.
9. Meijer A, Morr SA, Van Den Brule AJC, et al. Genomic relatedness of *Chlamydia* isolates determined by amplified fragment length polymorphism analysis. *J Bacteriol* 1999;181:4469–4475.
10. Jackson M, White N, Giffard P, et al. Epizootiology of *Chlamydia* infections in two free-range koala populations. *Vet Microbiol* 1999;65:255–264.
11. Reed KD, Ruth GR, Meyer JA, et al. *Chlamydia pneumoniae* infection in a breeding colony of African clawed frogs (*Xenopus tropicalis*). *Emerg Infect Dis* 2000;6:196–199.
12. Hyman CL, Augenbraun MH, Roblin PM, et al. Asymptomatic respiratory tract infection with *Chlamydia pneumoniae*. *J Clin Microbiol* 1991;29:2082–2083.
13. Falsey AR, Walsh EE. Transmission of *Chlamydia pneumoniae*. *J Infect Dis* 1993;168:493–496.
14. Theunissen HJH, Lemmens-den Toom NA, Burggraaf A, et al. Influence of temperature and relative humidity on the survival of *Chlamydia pneumoniae* in aerosols. *Appl Environ Microbiol* 1993;59:2589–2593.
15. Yamazaki T, Nakada H, Sakurai N, et al. Transmission of *Chlamydia pneumoniae* in young children in a Japanese family. *J Infect Dis* 1990;162:1390–1392.

16. Kleemola M, Saikku P, Visakorpi R, et al. Epidemics of pneumonia caused by TWAR, a new *Chlamydia* organism, in military trainees in Finland. *J Infect Dis* 1988;157:230–236.

17. Hyman CL, Roblin PM, Gaydos CA, et al. Prevalence of asymptomatic nasopharyngeal carriage of *Chlamydia pneumoniae* in subjectively healthy adults: assessment by polymerase chain reaction-enzyme immunoassay and culture. *Clin Infect Dis* 1995;20:1174–1178.

18. Kern DG, Neill MA, Schachter J. A seroepidemiologic study of *Chlamydia pneumoniae* in Rhode Island. *Chest* 1993;104:208–213.

19. Marrie TJ, Grayston JT, Wang SP, et al. Pneumonia associated with the TWAR strain of *Chlamydia*. *Ann Intern Med* 1987;106:507–511.

20. Saikku P, Ruutu P, Leinonen M, et al. Acute lower-respiratory-tract infection associated with chlamydial TWAR antibody in Filipino children. *J Infect Dis* 1988;158:1095–1097.

21. Block S, Hedrick J, Hammerschlag MR, et al. *Mycoplasma pneumoniae* and *Chlamydia pneumoniae* in pediatric community-acquired pneumonia: comparative efficacy and safety of clarithromycin vs. erythromycin ethylsuccinate. *Pediatr Infect Dis* 1995;14:471–477.

22. Harris J-A, Kolokathis A, Campbell M, et al. Safety and efficacy of azithromycin in the treatment of community acquired pneumonia in children. *Pediatr Infect Dis J* 1998;17:865–871.

23. Marston BJ, Plouffe JF, File TM, et al. Incidence of community-acquired pneumonia requiring hospitalization. *Arch Intern Med* 1997;157:1709–1718.

24. Hammerschlag MR. Community-acquired pneumonia due to atypical organisms in adults: diagnosis and treatment. *Infect Dis Clin Pract* 1999;8:232–240.

25. Kauppinen MT, Herva E, Kujula P, et al. The etiology of community-acquired pneumonia among hospitalized patients during a *Chlamydia pneumoniae* epidemic in Finland. *J Infect Dis* 1995;172:1330–1335.

26. Shemer-Avni Y, Lieberman D. *Chlamydia pneumoniae*-induced ciliostasis in ciliated bronchial epithelial cells. *J Infect Dis* 1995;171:1274–1278.

27. Hammerschlag MR, Chirgwin K, Roblin PM, et al. Persistent infection with *Chlamydia pneumoniae* following acute respiratory illness. *Clin Infect Dis* 1992;14:178–182.

28. Emre U, Roblin PM, Gelling M, et al. The association of *Chlamydia pneumoniae* infection and reactive airway disease in children. *Arch Pediatr Adolesc Med* 1994;148:727–732.

29. Holland SM, Taylor HR, Gaydos CA, et al. Experimental infection with *Chlamydia pneumoniae* in nonhuman primates. *Infect Immun* 1990;58:593–597.

30. Yang ZP, Kuo CC, Grayston JT. A mouse model of *Chlamydia pneumoniae* strain TWAR pneumonia. *Infect Immun* 1993;61:2037–2040.

31. Kaukoranta-Tolvanen SS, Laurila AL, Saikku P, et al. Experimental infection of *Chlamydia pneumoniae* in mice. *Microb Pathog* 1993;15:293–302.

32. Malinvemi R, Kuo C-C, Campbell LA, et al. Reactivation of *Chlamydia pneumoniae* lung infection in mice by cortisone. *J Infect Dis* 1995;172:593–594.

33. Augenbraun MH, Roblin PM, Mandel LJ, et al. *Chlamydia pneumoniae* pneumonia, with pleural effusion: diagnosis by culture. *Am J Med* 1991;43:437–438.

34. Augenbraun MH, Roblin PM, Chirgwin K, et al. Isolation of *Chlamydia pneumoniae* from the lungs of patients infected with the human immunodeficiency virus. *J Clin Microbiol* 1991;29:401–402.

35. Gaydos CA, Fowler CL, Gill VJ, et al. Detection of *Chlamydia pneumoniae* by polymerase chain reaction-enzyme immunoassay in an immunocompromised population. *Clin Infect Dis* 1993;17:718–723.

36. Miller ST, Hammerschlag MR, Chirgwin K, et al. The role of *Chlamydia pneumoniae* in acute chest syndrome of sickle cell disease. *J Pediatr* 1991;118:30–33.

37. Hahn DL, Dodge RW, Galubjatnikov R. Association of *Chlamydia pneumoniae* (strain TWAR) infection with wheezing, asthmatic bronchitis and adult-onset asthma. *JAMA* 1991;266:225–230.

38. Emre U, Sokolovskaya N, Roblin PM, et al. Detection of anti-*Chlamydia pneumoniae* IgE in children with reactive airway disease. *J Infect Dis* 1995;172:265–267.

39. Dowell SF, Peeling RW, Boman J, et al. Standardizing *Chlamydia pneumoniae* assays: Recommendations from the Centers for Disease Control and Prevention (USA) and the Laboratory Centre for Disease Control (Canada). *Clin Infect Dis* 2001;33:492–503.

40. Grayston JT, Aldous MB, Easton A, et al. Evidence that *Chlamydia pneumoniae* causes pneumonia and bronchitis. *J Infect Dis* 1993;168:1231–1235.

41. Verkooyen RP, Hazenberg MA, Van Haaren GH, et al. Age related interference with *Chlamydia pneumoniae* microimmunofluorescence serology due to circulating, rheumatoid factor. *J Clin Microbiol* 1992;30:1287–1290.

42. Moss TR, Darougar. S, Woodland RM, et al. Antibodies to *Chlamydia* species in patients attending a genitourinary clinic and the impact of antibodies to *C. pneumoniae* and *C. psittaci* on the sensitivity and the specificity of *C. trachomatis* serology tests. *Sex Transm Dis* 1993;20:61–65.

43. Maurin M, Eb F, Etienne J, et al. Serologic cross-reactions between *Bartonella* and *Chlamydia* species: implications for diagnosis. *J Clin Microbiol* 1997;35:2283–2287.

44. Jackson LA, Cherry JD, Wang SP, et al. Frequency of serological evidence of *Bordetella* infections and mixed infections with other respiratory pathogens in university students with cough illnesses. *Clin Infect Dis* 2000;31:3–6.

45. Ochiai Y, Fukushi H, Yan C, et al. Comparative analysis of the putative amino acid sequences of chlamydial heat shock protein 60 and *Escherichia coli* GroEL. *J Vet Med Sci* 2000;62:941–945.

46. Harkonen T, Puolakkainen M, Sarvas M, et al. Picornavirus proteins share antigenic determinants with heat shock proteins 60/65. *J Med Virol* 2000;62:383–391.

47. Peeling R, Wang S, Grayston J. *Chlamydia pneumoniae* serology: interlaboratory variation in microimmunofluorescence assay results. *J Infect Dis* 2000;181[Suppl 3]:s426–s429.

48. Peeling RW, Wang SP, Grayston JT, et al. Inter-laboratory comparison of microimmuno-fluorescence results. In: Saikku P, ed. *Proceedings of the fourth meeting of the european society for chlamydia research*. Helsinki: Universitas Helsingiensis, 2000:130.

49. Tuuminen T, Palomki P, Paavonen J. The use of serologic tests for the diagnosis of chlamydial infections. *J Microbiol Methods* 2000;42:265–279.

50. Kutlin A, Tsumura N, Roblin PM, et al. Evaluation of chlamydia IgM, IgG, IgA rELISAs medac for diagnosis of *Chlamydia pneumoniae* infection. *Clin Diag Lab Immunol* 1997;4:213–216.

51. Boman J, Gaydos CA, Quinn TC. Molecular diagnosis of *Chlamydia pneumoniae* infection. *J Clin Microbiol* 1999;37:3791–3799.

52. Apfalter P, Blasi F, Boman J, et al. Multicenter comparison trial of DNA extraction methods and PCR assays for detection of *Chlamydia pneumoniae* in endarterectomy specimens. *J Clin Microbiol* 2001;39:519–524.

53. Hammerschlag MR. Activity of gemifloxacin and other new quinolones against *Chlamydia pneumoniae*: a review. *J Antimicrob Chemother* 2000;45:[Suppl S1]:35–39.

54. Roblin PM, Hammerschlag MR. Microbiologic efficacy of azithromycin and susceptibility to azithromycin of isolates of *Chlamydia pneumoniae* from adults and children with community acquired pneumonia. *Antimicrob Agents Chemother* 1998;42:194–196.

55. Hammerschlag MR, Roblin PM. Microbiologic efficacy of levofloxacin for the treatment of community-acquired pneumonia due to *Chlamydia pneumoniae*. *Antimicrob Agents Chemother* 2000;44:1409.

56. Hammerschlag MR, Roblin PM. Microbiologic efficacy of moxifloxacin for the treatment of community-acquired pneumonia due to *Chlamydia pneumoniae*. *Int J Antimicrob Agents* 2000;15:149–152.

57. Roblin PM, Montalban G, Hammerschlag MR. Susceptibility to clarithromycin and erythromycin of isolates of *Chlamydia pneumoniae* from children with pneumonia. *Antimicrob Agents Chemother* 1994;38:1588–1589.

58. Hammerschlag MR. Chlamydial infections. *J Pediatr* 1989;114:727–734.

59. Bell TA, Stamm WE, Wang SP, et al. Chronic *Chlamydia trachomatis* infections in infants. *JAMA* 1992;267:400–402.

60. Nakajo MN, Roblin PM, Hammerschlag MR, et al. Chlamydicidal activity of human alveolar macrophages. *Infect Immun* 1990;58:3640–3644.

61. Ito JI, Comess KA, Alexander ER, et al. Pneumonia due to *Chlamydia trachomatis* in an immunocompromised adult. *N Engl J Med* 1982;307:95–98.

62. Meyers JD, Hackman RC, Stamm WE. *Chlamydia trachomatis* infection as a cause of pneumonia after human marrow transplantation. *Transplantation* 1983;36:130–134.

63. Moncada JV, Schachter J, Wofsy C. Prevalence of *Chlamydia trachomatis* lung infection in patients with acquired immune deficiency syndrome. *J Clin Microbiol* 1986;23:986.

64. Bernstein DI, Hubbard T, Wenman WM, et al. Mediastinal and supraclavicular lymphadenitis and pneumonitis due to *Chlamydia trachomatis* serovars L_1 and L_2. *N Engl J Med* 1984;311:1543–1546.

65. Centers for Disease Control and Prevention. 2001 guidelines for the laboratory detection of *Chlamydia trachomatis* and *Neisseria gonorrhoeae* infections. *MMWR*, 2001 (in press).

66. Hammerschlag MR, Roblin PM, Gelling M, et al. Use of polymerase chain reaction for the detection of *Chlamydia trachomatis* in ocular and nasopharyngeal specimens from infants with conjunctivitis. *Pediatr Infect Dis J* 1997;16:293–297.

67. MacFarlane JT, MacRae AD. Psittacosis. *Br Med Bull* 1983;39:163–167.

68. van Buuren CE, Dorrestein GM, ban Dijk JE: *Chlamydia psittaci* in birds: a review on the pathogenesis and histopathological features. *Vet Q* 1994;16:38–41.

69. Andersen AA, Tappe JP. Genetic, immunologic and pathologic characterization of avian chlamydial strains. *J Am Vet Med Assoc* 1989;195:1512–1516.

70. Centers for Disease Control and Prevention. Compendium of measures to control *Chlamydia psittaci* infection among humans (psittacosis) and pet birds (avian chlamydiosis). *MMWR* 2000;49(RR-8):3–17.

71. Centers for Disease Control. Psittacosis at a turkey processing plant—North Carolina, 1989. *MMWR* 1990;39:460–461, 467–469.

72. Hedberg K, White KE, Forfang JC, et al. An outbreak of psittacosis in Minnesota turkey industry workers: implications for modes of transmission and control. *Am J Epidemiol* 1989;130:569–577.

73. Hinton DG, Shipley A, Galvin JW, et al. Chlamydiosis in workers at a duck farm and processing plant. *Aust Vet J* 1993;70:174–176.

74. Schlossberg D, Delgado J, Moore MM, et al. An epidemic of avian and human psittacosis. *Arch Intern Med* 1993;153:2594–2596.

75. Moroney JF, Guevara R, Iverson C, et al. Detection of chlamydiosis in a shipment of pet birds, leading to recognition of an outbreak of clinically mild psittacosis in humans. *Clin Infect Dis* 1998;26:1425–1429.

76. Yung AP, Grayson ML. Psittacosis—a review of 135 cases. *Med J Aust* 1988;148:228–233.

77. Mason AB, Jenkins P. Acute renal failure in fulminant psittacosis. *Respir Med* 1994;88:239–240.

78. Day CJ, Fawcett IW. Psittacosis and acute thrombocytopenia. *J R Ind Soc Med* 1992;85:360–361.

79. Shapiro DS, Kenney SC, Johnson M, et al. *Chlamydia psittaci* endocarditis diagnosed by blood culture. *N Engl J Med* 1992;325:1192–1195.
80. Laumaury I, Sotto A, Le Quellec A, et al. *Chlamydia psittaci* as a cause of lethal bacterial endocarditis. *Clin Infect Dis* 1993;17:821–822.
81. Cartwright KAV, Caul EO, Lamb RW. Symptomatic *Chlamydia psittaci* reinfection (letter). *Lancet* 1988;1:1004.
82. Gosbell IB, Ross AD, Turner IB. *Chlamydia psittaci* infection and reinfection in a veterinarian. *Aust Vet J* 1999;77:511–513.
83. Fryden A, Kihlstrom E Maller R, et al. A clinical and epidemiological study of "ornithosis" caused by *Chlamydia psittaci* and *Chlamydia pneumoniae* (strain TWAR). *Scand J Infect Dis* 1989;21:681–691.
84. Bruu AL, Haukenes G, Aasen S, et al. *Chlamydia pneumoniae* infections in Norway 1981–87 earlier diagnosed as ornithosis. *Scand J Infect Dis* 1991;23:299–304.
85. Pether JVS, Wang SP, Grayston JT. *Chlamydia pneumoniae* strain TWAR, as the cause of an outbreak in a boys' school previously called psittacosis. *Epidemiol Infect* 1989;103:395–400.
86. Soni R, Seale JP, Young IH. Fulminant psittacosis requiring mechanical ventilation and demonstrating serological cross-reactivity between *Legionella longbeachae* and *Chlamydia psittaci*. *Respirology* 1999;4:203–205.
87. Oldach DW, Gaydos CA, Mundy LM, et al. Rapid diagnosis of *Chlamydia psittaci* pneumonia. *Clin Infect Dis* 1993;17:338–343.
88. Tong CYW, Sillis M. Detection of *Chlamydia pneumoniae* and *Chlamydia psittaci* in sputum samples by PCR. *J Clin Pathol* 1993;46:313–317.
89. Messmer TO, Skelton SK, Moroney JF, et al. Application of a nested, multiplex PCR to psittacosis outbreaks. *J Clin Microbiol* 1997;35:2043–2046.
90. Tong CY, Donnelly C, Harvey G, et al. Multiplex polymerase chain reaction for simultaneous detection of *Mycoplasma pneumoniae, Chlamydia pneumoniae* and *Chlamydia psittaci* in respiratory outbreaks. *J Clin Pathol* 1999;52:257–263.
91. Madico G, Quinn TC, Boman J, et al. Touchdown enzyme time release-PCR for detection and identification of *Chlamydia trachomatis, C. pneumoniae,* and *C. psittaci* using the 16S and 16S-23S spacer rRNA genes. *J Clin Microbiol* 2000;38:1085–1093.

CHAPTER 57
Aspiration Pneumonia

John G. Bartlett

Aspiration pneumonia refers to the pulmonary consequences that follow abnormal entry of fluid, particulate exogenous substances, or endogenous secretions into the lower airways. There are usually two requirements. First, there needs to be a compromise in the usual defenses that protect the tracheobronchial tree, such as glottic closure, cough reflex, or other clearing mechanisms of the lower airways. Second, the inoculum must be deleterious to the lower airways by a direct toxic effect, a bacterial inoculum sufficient to initiate an inflammatory process, or a sufficient volume or form to cause obstruction.

PREDISPOSING CONDITIONS

Numerous studies indicate that even healthy persons aspirate, but this is usually inconsequential. For example, Amberson (1) placed contrast material in the mouths of sleeping patients and showed by chest radiographs the following day that, although the contrast material was regularly detected in the lower airways in the majority of patients, there was no apparent clinical disease. Similarly, dye markers placed in the stomachs of postoperative patients can be aspirated from the tracheobronchial tree at surgery to demonstrate aspiration of gastric contents during general anesthesia in 7% to 16% of patients (2,3). Scintigraphic methods have been used to document frequent aspiration in patients with tracheostomies, endotracheal tubes, nasogastric tubes, gastrostomy tubes, and dysphagia (4–10). In most studies, the frequency of aspiration of the marker placed in the stomach of patients with these conditions is 10% to 40%;

elimination from the airways is complete or nearly complete by 3 hours. The frequency of aspiration during endoscopy of the upper gastrointestinal tract has been reported at 25% (11–13). These observations show that aspiration is relatively common and usually resolves unrecognized without detectable sequelae. The decisive factor in the development of pulmonary complications appears to depend on the frequency, volume, and character of the material in the inoculum, and the host's ability to clear it.

Aspiration pneumonia accounts for about 5% to 15% of all community-acquired pneumonias (14–16). The rate is particularly high in patients at risk due to dysphagia or reduced consciousness (Table 57.1). Aspiration pneumonia is the most common cause of death in patients with dysphagia associated with strokes (17,18). It is especially common in elderly debilitated nursing home residents (19). Aspiration pneumonia is found in 5% to 15% of patients hospitalized with drug overdoses (20), and it accounts for 10% to 20% of anesthesia deaths (21). In many of these conditions, the major factor is suppressed consciousness, and the risk of aspiration has been directly correlated with degree of unconsciousness (22).

PREVENTION

Prevention of aspiration has been most extensively studied in patients hospitalized in intensive care units, patients with neurologic or esophageal conditions that predispose to aspiration, and patients who receive enteral feedings. The usual methods for detection of dysphagia with vocal fold motion impairment is pharyngoesophagography (23), and for stroke patients it is fiberoptic endoscopic examination of swallowing, or observed swallowing of 50 mL of water in 10-mL aliquots with or without blood gases to determine oxygen desaturation (24). The most convincing preventive measure in the intensive care unit is use of a semirecumbent or upright position. Other methods to address this issue include tracheostomy, reduction of gastric volume by suction or metoclopramide, feedings by nasogastric tube or gastrostomy, and gastric acid neutralization by antacids or H_2 blockers (25–42). The effectiveness of these maneuvers is variable and often confounded by the fact that the remedy itself predisposes to aspiration. For example, inflation of the balloon on the tracheostomy tube may occlude the esophagus to promote aspiration. Feeding tubes are associated with aspiration (40). Percutaneous gastrostomy tubes may improve nutrition, but do not consistently reduce rates of aspiration pneumonia (32–35,39). Postpyloric feeding tubes may, however, have a role in patients with large gastric residuals due to gastroparesis (41). Neutralization of gastric acid effectively reduces the risk of chemical pneumonitis due to acid aspiration (10,16,17,21), but elimination of the gastric barrier promotes bacterial growth and bacterial pneumonia after gastric aspiration (26,30,31). Surgery is the major preventive method with some esophageal lesions, such as Zenker diverticula (37); it is more controversial with gastroesophageal reflux (38).

CLASSIFICATION

Aspiration pneumonia refers to distinctive syndromes that may be distinguished on the basis of the character of the inoculum, pathogenesis of pulmonary complications, clinical presentation, and management guidelines (43) (Table 57.2). Although there may be overlap in individual cases and some patients are difficult to classify, this classification scheme provides a useful

TABLE 57.1. Conditions That Predispose to Aspiration

Altered consciousness
    Alcoholism, seizures, cerebrovascular accident, head trauma, general anesthesia, drug overdose
Dysphagia
    Esophageal disorder: stricture, neoplasm, diverticula, tracheoesophageal fistula, incompetent cardiac sphincter
Gastroesophageal reflux
Neurologic disorder
    Multiple sclerosis, Parkinson disease, myasthenia gravis, pseudobulbar palsy
Mechanical disruption of the usual defense barriers
    Nasogastric tube, endotracheal intubation, tracheostomy, upper gastrointestinal endoscopy, bronchoscopy
Protracted vomiting, gastric outlet obstruction, large-volume nasogastric tube feedings
Pharyngeal anesthesia
General debility
Recumbent position

conceptual approach to a complex topic. The three syndromes include chemical pneumonitis, bacterial infection, and airway obstruction.

INCIDENCE

Many population-based studies of pneumonia include a category of aspiration pneumonia that is variously defined, but common criteria are a predisposition to aspiration, an infiltrate involving a dependent pulmonary segment, and no competing diagnosis. These cases account for 5% to 15% of patients in most series; although the distribution of cases using the three categories of aspiration pneumonia is rarely attempted, most consider infections involving anaerobic bacteria to account for the majority (15,16), and the *Medical Letter* recommendations for empiric treatment make this assumption (44). In studies of selected populations of patients, the frequency of aspiration is probably much higher. These include the elderly, patients in nursing homes, victims of head trauma, patients with multiple sclerosis, and patients with dysphagia.

CHEMICAL PNEUMONITIS

Chemical pneumonitis refers to the aspiration of substances that are inherently toxic to the lower airways. These substances initiate an inflammatory reaction that is independent of bacterial infection and cannot be ascribed to bronchial obstruction. Examples include acid, animal fats such as milk and mineral oil, and volatile hydrocarbons such as gasoline or kerosene. The prototypic example and best studied of these is the chemical pneumonitis associated with aspiration of gastric acid, as classically described by Mendelson in 1946 (45).

Clinical Presentation

The classic study by Mendelson included 61 obstetric patients who aspirated gastric contents during ether anesthesia. When the aspiratory event was witnessed, respiratory distress became apparent within 2 hours (46) accompanied by abrupt onset of cyanosis, tachypnea, and tachycardia. Nearly all patients had bronchospasm, leading Mendelson to compare this with an acute asthmatic attack. Chest radiographs showed infiltrates that were generally located in one or both lower lobes. Despite the severity of illness, all patients recovered and most were clinically stable within 24 to 36 hours. Radiographs generally showed clearing of infiltrates within 4 to 7 days.

Extensive studies of acid pneumonitis since this original report have shown an increased frequency of fever, reduced frequency of observed bronchospasm, and a substantial mortality (47–51). Acid aspiration is now recognized as one of the three most common causes of the adult respiratory distress syndrome (52). The most striking difference compared with Mendelson's experience concerns mortality, which later reports showed to be in the range of 30% to 60%, possibly because the patients described by Mendelson were young, previously healthy obstetric patients, whereas those reviewed in the later reports were often debilitated with multiple associated conditions. Analysis of blood gases shows partial pressure of oxygen is often in the 35- to 50-mm Hg range, usually with a normal or low partial pressure of carbon dioxide and a respiratory alkalosis. If hypoxemia is severe, the partial pressure of carbon dioxide may be elevated with a metabolic acidosis. Factors contributing to the hypoxemia include pulmonary edema, reduced surfactant activity, reflex airway closure, alveolar hemorrhage, and hyaline membrane

TABLE 57.2. Classification of Aspiration Pneumonia

Inoculum	Pulmonary sequelae	Clinical features	Therapy
Acid	Chemical pneumonitis	Acute dyspnea, tachypnea, tachycardia; ± cyanosis, bronchospasm, fever Sputum: pink, frothy Radiograph: infiltrates in one or both lower lobes Hypoxemia	Positive-pressure breathing Intravenous fluids Tracheal suction
Oropharyngeal bacteria	Bacterial infection	Usually insidious onset Cough, fever, purulent sputum Radiograph: infiltrate involving dependent pulmonary segment or lobe ± cavitation	Antibiotics
Inert fluids	Mechanical obstruction Reflex airway closure	Acute dyspnea, cyanosis ± apnea Pulmonary edema	Tracheal suction Intermittent positive-pressure breathing with oxygen and isoproterenol
Particulate matter	Mechanical obstruction	Dependent on level of obstruction, ranging from acute apnea and rapid death to irritating chronic cough ± recurrent infections	Extraction of particulate matter Antibiotics for superimposed infection

formation. Pulmonary function tests show decreased compliance, abnormalities of ventilation-perfusion, and reduced diffusing capacity. Many patients have hypotension owing to an immediate reflex reaction or fluid aggregation in the lung with intravascular volume depletion. Pulmonary artery pressure is usually low or normal because of reduced cardiac output with decreased intravascular volume. Patients with severe disease often progress to the adult respiratory distress syndrome. Another potential complication is superimposed infection because the acid-injured lung appears to be predisposed to bacterial infection (46).

Clinical features that specifically suggest chemical pneumonitis include the abrupt onset of symptoms, dyspnea, cyanosis, low-grade fever, diffuse rales, hypoxemia, and infiltrates in dependent pulmonary segments (53,54). The course of the disease has been examined in a retrospective review of 50 cases by Bynum and Pierce (46), who divided patients into three categories: The first group accounted for 12% and was characterized by a fulminant course with death shortly after aspiration, presumably due to the adult respiratory distress syndrome. The second group accounted for 62% and had a rapid improvement of the chest radiograph in a fashion analogous to the course described by Mendelson (45); in these patients, the radiographic changes cleared in a mean time of 4.5 days. The third group accounted for 26% and resembled the second group in terms of rapid improvement; however, these individuals subsequently had new or extending infiltrates on the chest radiograph associated with fever, which was ascribed to pulmonary superinfection.

Pathophysiology

Acid pneumonitis has been studied extensively *in vivo* or *ex vivo* using experimental animals with intratracheal instillations of acid (55–62). There are two essential requirements in these experiments. First, challenge using graded acids indicates that the pH must be 2.5 or less to initiate an inflammatory reaction. Substances with a higher pH, including saline, saliva, buffered gastric acid, and so forth, demonstrate only a transient, self-limited period of respiratory distress, which is probably due to brief airway obstruction or reflex airway closure. The severity of the pneumonitis correlates with the pH of the inoculum at levels below 2.5. The second requirement is a relatively large inoculum, generally 0.3 mL/kg. Translation of these observations to the clinical setting indicates that aspiration of gastric contents in adult patients should involve at least 25 mL, with a pH of 2.5 or lower. Smaller volumes may produce a more subtle process that either escapes clinical detection or causes a less fulminant form of pneumonitis. In support of this contention is the observation of frequent bouts of recurrent pneumonitis or otherwise unexplained pulmonary fibrosis in patients with esophageal disease or gastric reflux (63–68).

The pathologic changes in acid pneumonitis occur with extraordinary rapidity (59). Atelectasis is apparent within seconds and becomes extensive at 3 minutes. Additional early changes include peribronchial hemorrhage, pulmonary edema, and degeneration of bronchial epithelial cells. By 4 hours, the alveolar spaces are filled with polymorphonuclear leukocytes in fibrin. Hyaline membranes can be seen at 48 hours. At this time, the lung is grossly edematous and hemorrhagic with alveolar consolidation. Resolution begins on the third day and may be complete or result in residual parenchymal scarring. Virtually all of these findings have been noted on autopsy studies of patients with fatal aspiration pneumonia. The pathophysiology of these events is ascribed to the release of proinflammatory cytokines, especially tumor necrosis factor and interleukin-8,

which are responsible for recruitment and activation of neutrophils. The neutrophil and complement appear to play a major role in lung injury associated with acid pneumonitis, but methods to exploit this information with therapy are ill-defined (69–71). Long-term follow-up studies in patients who survive this condition show either complete recovery or radiographic evidence of pulmonary fibrosis with disturbances in gas exchange (72,73).

Diagnosis

Acid pneumonitis is usually a presumed diagnosis that is based on clinical observations and supported by radiographic findings. A highly characteristic feature of the disease is its precipitous onset and its rapid evolution to complete clearing within days, progression to the adult respiratory distress syndrome, or secondary bacterial infection. Despite the drama of the classical presentation, some patients simply present with cough, wheezing with or without O_2 desaturation (74). If the aspiratory event is observed, the chest radiograph will demonstrate pulmonary infiltrates within 1 to 2 hours (46). Bronchoscopy is sometimes advocated to remove particulate matter that may be aspirated concurrently. Bronchoscopy will demonstrate erythema of the bronchi, which suggests acid injury.

Treatment

Tracheal suction is often appropriate to clear fluids and particulate matter that may cause obstruction as a compounding feature. Intravenous fluid support is necessary to expand intravascular space. Tracheal inoculation of buffering solutions and pulmonary lavage in an attempt to neutralize the acid inoculum is futile because of the rapidity with which acid is neutralized by the normal defense mechanisms. This disease has been compared with a "flash burn" of the lung in which most of the damage has occurred by the time the patient is initially treated. The major therapeutic modality is support of pulmonary function. Beyond this and tracheal suction, there are no interventions with established merit.

One of the previously controversial areas concerned the use of corticosteroids, but two well-designed therapeutic trials have failed to show benefit (75,76). These agents also appear to be contraindicated for the adult respiratory distress syndrome, which is a relatively frequent complication (77). There is no good evidence that bacteria play any important role in the acute events in animal or clinical studies. Indeed, the pH of the inoculum necessary to initiate a chemical pneumonitis is inhospitable to bacterial survival. Antimicrobial agents are commonly given because it is difficult to eliminate bacterial infection as a contributing factor. Studies in experimental animals have shown that the acid-injured lung is highly susceptible to bacterial challenge (78). Clinical studies indicated that 13% to 26% of patients acquire pulmonary superinfections during the course of recovery (46,47,79). Available evidence does not support the use of prophylactic antibiotics in aspiration-prone patients, but it is hard to dissuade use of these agents in critically-ill patients who often have no clearly established diagnosis.

BACTERIAL INFECTION

The most common form of aspiration pneumonia is bacterial infection due to aspiration of bacteria that normally reside in the upper airways or stomach. There is a potential problem here with semantics, because the majority of bacterial pneumonias probably occur as a result of aspiration, including most cases caused by *Streptococcus pneumoniae*, *Haemophilus influenzae*, gram-negative bacilli, and *Staphylococcus aureus*. These are relatively virulent in the lower airways so that only a small inoculum is required. The process might be referred to as microaspiration, which is subtle and relatively common in the patient who is not necessarily aspiration prone. By contrast, aspiration pneumonia due to bacterial pathogens usually refers to pneumonia in a patient who is predisposed to aspiration of relatively large volumes, most commonly as a result of altered consciousness or dysphagia (see Table 57.1). This diagnosis is suspected when a susceptible host develops typical findings for a pulmonary infection, including fever, purulent sputum, and a pulmonary infiltrate in a dependent pulmonary segment (43,80–82).

Clinical Features

The presenting findings are highly variable, depending to a large extent on the bacteria involved and the host's status. The predominant pathogens are anaerobic bacteria that normally reside in the gingival crevice. The tempo of the disease in this process tends to be relatively slow. The initial lesion is pneumonitis, which may be clinically similar to other forms of acute bacterial pneumonias with cough, fever, purulent sputum, and dyspnea (80–84). If the patient is less seriously ill and does not seek medical attention in this early stage, there is often progression to the late stages, which are characterized by suppuration including lung abscess, necrotizing pneumonia, or empyema associated with bronchopleural fistula (43,80–84).

Factors that specifically suggest pneumonia due to aspiration of anaerobic bacteria are the associated conditions predisposing to aspiration, lack of rigors, failure to recover likely pathogens with cultures of expectorated sputum, indolent course, and sputum that is often putrid in late stages. Many of these patients show evidence of periodontal disease, because the organisms involved generally reside in the periodontal pockets. Chest radiographs usually show infiltrates in segments that are dependent in the recumbent position: the superior segment of the lower lobes or posterior segments of the upper lobes. Abscess formation empyema and putrid sputum are late complications that usually occur after more than 7 days. Basilar segments of the lower lobes are favored in patients who aspirate in the sitting or upright position.

Bacteriology

Aspiration of oropharyngeal or gastric contents usually results in an infection involving a polymicrobial flora. The major pathogens are anaerobic bacteria, which are found in 60% to 85% of cases according to studies using appropriate diagnostic methods (43,82–89). Establishing the microbial diagnosis is hard for all and may be impossible for most. Expectorated sputum is unsuitable for anaerobic culture because of inevitable contamination by the normal flora of the upper airways. Preferred specimens are transtracheal aspirate, transthoracic needle aspirate, empyema fluid, and quantitative cultures of bronchoscopy specimens obtained with the protected brush or of bronchoalveolar lavage specimens (80–93). Most clinical studies that included uncontaminated specimens for bacteriologic analysis in aspiration pneumonia were done from 1970 to 1980, when transtracheal aspiration was common (82–85,88,89). This procedure is now rarely performed; there is increasing interest in quantitative cultures of bronchoscopic specimens, although the experience with this technique in anaerobic bacterial infections of the lung is limited (91–93).

The major bacterial isolates in patients with aspiration pneumonitis or lung abscess include anaerobic streptococci (*Peptostreptococcus* spp.), *Fusobacterium nucleatum*, and *Prevotella melaninogenica* (formerly *Bacteroides melaninogenicus*) (80–93). Most of these patients have multiple species of anaerobic bacteria in the lower airways, 15% to 25% of which are resistant to penicillin due to penicillinase production. Aerobic or microaerophilic bacteria are concurrently present in at least half of cases of pulmonary infections involving anaerobic bacteria. Gram-negative bacilli are especially common in patients with hospital-acquired aspiration pneumonia (97). These organisms are not considered to be components of the normal oral flora. However, studies indicate that the rate of colonization of the upper airways by gram-negative bacilli is directly correlated with the severity of associated conditions (98). This observation presumably accounts for the marked difference in bacteriologic patterns between community-acquired and hospital-acquired aspiration pneumonia. It also appears that gastric contents may be the source of gram-negative bacteria in aspiration pneumonia, and this especially applies to patients who have lost the acid gastric barrier from medication (antacids or H_2-blocking agents) or aging (29–31).

Treatment

The mainstay of treatment is antibiotics, and the selection of specific agents is obviously simplified if definitive bacteriologic studies have been done. As noted previously, a microbial diagnosis with anaerobic bacteria requires invasive diagnostic techniques that are generally not performed except for thoracocentesis in patients with empyema. As a consequence, antibiotics are usually selected empirically. Expectorated sputum cultures are often used to guide the selection of agents for aerobic bacteria that may be present concurrently (99). This may help with nosocomial cases; it is not likely to be helpful with community-acquired cases.

Historically, the standard drug for aspiration pneumonia or lung abscess due to anaerobic bacteria has been penicillin given intravenously or high doses given orally (100,101). Several trials performed from 1950 through 1975, primarily on patients with lung abscess, showed that the great majority of patients responded (102–104). These recommendations have been confounded in more recent years by the observation that up to 40% of *Fusobacterium* spp. and 60% of non-fragilis *Bacteroides* spp. produce penicillinase (94–96). In two comparative therapeutic trials of lung abscess, clindamycin was significantly superior to intravenous penicillin in terms of response rates and time to defervescence (105,106). Alternative regimens in which the anecdotal experience is favorable include amoxicillin-clavulanate (107) and penicillin plus metronidazole (108). Metronidazole should not be used as a single agent because extensive studies have shown that approximately 50% of patients do not respond, presumably due to the contributing role of aerobic and microaerophilic streptococci (109,110). It is not clear that the findings with trials for lung abscess can be extrapolated to aspiration pneumonia, even though the bacteriology is the same. Further, it seems likely that many antibiotics may successfully treat anaerobic pneumonitis, but recommendations are limited to the few that have been tested. Patients with nosocomial aspiration pneumonia are likely to have a polymicrobial flora that includes aerobic gram-negative bacilli or *S. aureus*, as well as anaerobic bacteria. The need to treat all components of a mixed flora in such cases is not well established. However, the high mortality for gram-negative bacillary pneumonia suggests that these organisms should clearly be treated in patients who are seriously ill and those who have hospital-acquired infection.

MECHANICAL OBSTRUCTION

Aspiration pneumonia may involve fluid or particulate matter that is not inherently toxic to the lung, but may cause airway obstruction or reflux airway closure.

Fluids

Typical fluids that may be aspirated and are not inherently toxic to the lung include saline, barium, water, most ingested fluids, and gastric contents with a pH exceeding 2.5. When these fluids are instilled intratracheally into animals in limited quantities, the result is a transient, self-limited hypoxemia. On occasion, there is pulmonary edema with more severe hypoxemia and reduced compliance (111). This reaction is reversible by vagotomy or administration of atropine or isoproterenol, suggesting intrinsic pulmonary reflex closure that is not related to the chemical composition of the inoculum (60,111,112). A possible clinical counterpart of this observation in experimental animals is apparently seen in some drowning victims (111–113). Appropriate treatment consists of intermittent positive-pressure breathing with 100% oxygen combined with isoproterenol.

The usual consequence of aspirating fluids is simple mechanical obstruction. Most patients tolerate aspiration of relatively large volumes well, as verified by tolerance of the large volumes used in pulmonary lavage with bronchoscopy. Patients at risk for mechanical obstruction are those who have profound neurologic deficit with no cough reflex, unconscious patients, or drown victims. The obvious critical therapeutic intervention is tracheal suction. If a subsequent chest radiograph fails to show any pulmonary infiltrate, no additional therapy is required except that intended to prevent further episodes of aspiration.

Solid Particles

The severity of respiratory obstruction after aspiration of particulate matter depends on the relative size of the object aspirated and the caliber of the lower airways. Foreign body aspiration usually occurs in children during the oral stage of development, at one to three years of age, and the most common objects are peanuts, other vegetable particles, inorganic materials, and teeth (114–117). Vegetable materials, including peanuts, are especially a problem because they are not apparent on a radiograph, they tend to swell because of their hydroscopic properties, and the undigested cellulose acts as a local irritant to produce the inflammation.

The clinical consequences of aspiration depend on the level of obstruction. Large objects that lodge in the larynx or trachea cause sudden respiratory distress, cyanosis, and aphonia and can lead quickly to death. This has been referred to as the cafe coronary syndrome because the symptoms may simulate those of acute myocardial infarction and often involve a piece of meat that is aspirated during restaurant dining (118). In these cases, there is little opportunity for diagnostic evaluation or even transfer to an acute care facility. The suggested maneuver is the Heimlich maneuver, consisting of firm, rapid pressure applied to the upper abdomen in an effort to force the diaphragm up and dislodge the particle.

Aspiration of smaller particles causes less severe obstruction or simply partial obstruction unless multiple small airways are involved. The usual initial symptom is an irritating cough. When major bronchi are involved, there may be cyanosis, dyspnea, wheezing, chest pain, and vomiting. Chest radiographs may show atelectasis or obstructive emphysema. When the obstruction is partial, there may be unilateral wheezing, and an expiration radiograph will often demonstrate a shift in the mediastinum. Bacterial infection is a frequent complication when obstruction or partial obstruction persists for longer than 1 week (119). The usual pathogens are anaerobic bacteria from the upper airways, as described previously. This alleged bacteriologic pattern is supported only by anecdotal cases studied with appropriate diagnostic techniques and using uncontaminated specimens and by experimental animal studies using cotton plugs to obstruct the lower airways in dogs; the subsequent pneumonia that occurred distal to the obstructing lesion involved anaerobic bacteria from the upper airways (120). Patients with this complication may respond well to antibiotics, but infections are likely to recur. An important clue is that the infections tend to involve the same anatomic site as shown by chest radiography.

The primary therapeutic modality is removal of the foreign object from the lower airways. Fiberoptic bronchoscopy has been used successfully alone, but many authorities prefer the Jackson bronchoscope because of its superior visualization and larger channel, which facilitates mechanical removal (121).

REFERENCES

1. Amberson JB. Aspiration bronchopneumonia. *Int Clin* 1937;3:126.
2. Berson W, Adiani J. "Silent" regurgitation and aspiration of gastric contents during anesthesia. *Anesthesiology* 1954;15:644.
3. Gardner AMN. Aspiration of food and vomit. *Q J Med* 1958;27:227.
4. Cameron JL, Reynolds J, Zuidema GD. Aspiration in patients with tracheostomies. *Surg Gynecol Obstet* 1973;136:68.
5. Spray SB, Zuidema GD, Cameron JL. Aspiration pneumonia: incidence of aspiration with endotracheal tubes. *Am J Surg* 1976;121:701.
6. Stewardson RH, Nyhus LM. Pulmonary aspiration. *Arch Surg* 1977;112:1192.
7. Cole MJ, Smith JT, Molnar C, et al. Aspiration after percutaneous gastrostomy: assessment by Tc-99m labeling of the enteral feed. *J Clin Gastroenterol* 1987;9:90.
8. Coben RM, Weintraub A, DiMarino AJ Jr, et al. Gastroesophageal reflux during gastrostomy feeding. *Gastroenterology* 1994;106:13.
9. Silver KH, Van Nostrand D. The use of scintigraphy in the management of patients with pulmonary aspiration. *Dysphagia* 1994;9:107.
10. Martin BJ, Corlew MM, Wood H, et al. The association of swallowing dysfunction and aspiration pneumonia. *Dysphagia* 1994;9:1.
11. Prout BJ, Metreweli C. Pulmonary aspiration after fibre-endoscopy of the upper gastrointestinal tract. *BMJ* 1972;4:269.
12. Vennes JA. Infectious complications of gastrointestinal endoscopy. *Dig Dis Sci* 1981;26:60S.
13. Lipper B, Simon D, Cerrone F. Pulmonary aspiration during emergency endoscopy in patients with upper gastrointestinal hemorrhage. *Crit Care Med* 1991;19:330.
14. Mandell LA, Marrie TJ, Grossman RF, et al. Canadian guidelines for the initial management of community-acquired pneumonia. *Clin Infect Dis* 2000;31:383.
15. Bartlett JG, Dowell S, Mandell LA, et al. Practice guidelines for the management of community-acquired pneumonia in adults. *Clin Infect Dis* 2000;31:347.
16. Fine MJ, Smith MA, Carson CA, et al. Prognosis and outcomes of patients with community-acquired pneumonia. *JAMA* 1996;275:134.
17. Holas MA, DePippo KL, Reding MJ. Aspiration and relative risk of medical complications following stroke. *Arch Neurol* 1994;51:1051.
18. Daniels SK, Brailey K, Priestly DH, et al. Aspiration in patients with acute stroke. *Arch Phys Med Rehabil* 1998;79:14.
19. Marrie TJ, Durant H, Kwan C. Nursing home-acquired pneumonia: a case-control study. *J Am Geriatr Soc* 1986;34:697.
20. Roy TM, Ossorio MA, Cipolla LM, et al. Pulmonary complications after tricyclic antidepressant overdose. *Chest* 1989;96:852.
21. Warner MA, Warner ME, Weber JG. Clinical significance of pulmonary aspiration during the perioperative period. *Anesthesiology* 1993;78:56.
22. Adnet F, Baud F. Relation between Glasgow coma scale and aspiration pneumonia. *Lancet* 1996;348:123.

23. Heitmiller RF, Tseng E, Jones B. Prevalence of aspiration and laryngeal penetration in patients with unilateral vocal fold motion impairment. *Dysphagia* 2000;15:184.

24. Lim SH, Lien PK, Phan SY, et al. Accuracy of bedside clinical methods compared with fiberoptic endoscopic examination of swallowing (FEES) in determining the risk of aspiration in acute stroke patients. *Dysphagia* 2001; 16:1.

25. Lam AM, Grace DM, Penny FJ, et al. Prophylactic intravenous cimetidine reduces the risk of acid aspiration in morbidly obese patients. *Anesthesiology* 1986;65:684.

26. Mehta S, Archer JF, Mills J. pH-dependent bactericidal barrier to gram-negative aerobes: its relevance to airway colonization and prophylaxis of acid aspiration and stress ulcer syndromes—study in vitro. *Intensive Care Med* 1986;12:134.

27. Ciocon JO, Silverstone FA, Graver LM, et al. Tube feedings in elderly patients: indications, benefits, and complications. *Arch Intern Med* 1988;148: 429.

28. Chang JH, Coln CD, Stickland AD, et al. Surgical management of gastroesophageal reflux in severely mentally retarded children. *J Merit Defic Res* 1987;31:1.

29. Kowalsky SF. Cimetidine in anesthesia: does it minimize the complications of acid aspiration? *Drug Intell Clin Pharmacol* 1984;18:382.

30. Driks MR, Craven DE, Celli BR, et al. Nosocomial pneumonia in intubated patients given sucralfate as compared with antacids or histamine type 2 blockers: the role of gastric colonization. *N Engl J Med* 1987;317:1376.

31. Toung TJ, Rosenfeld BA, Yoshiki A, et al. Sucralfate does not reduce the risk of acid aspiration pneumonitis. *Crit Care Med* 1993;21:1359.

32. Mathus-Vliegen LM, Louwerse LS, Merkus MP, et al. Percutaneous endoscopic gastrostomy in patients with amyotrophic lateral sclerosis and impaired pulmonary function. *Gastrointest Endosc* 1994;40:463.

33. Park RH, Allison MC, Lang J, et al. Randomised comparison of percutaneous endoscopic gastrostomy and nasogastric tube feeding in patients with persisting neurological dysphagia. *BMJ* 1992;304:1406.

34. Fay DE, Poplausky M, Gruber M, et al. Long-term enteral feeding: a retrospective comparison of delivery via percutaneous endoscopic gastrostomy and nasoenteric tubes. *Am J Gastroenterol* 1991;86:1604.

35. Weltz CR, Morris JB, Mullen JL. Surgical jejunostomy in aspiration risk patients. *Ann Surg* 1992;215:140.

36. MacFadyen BV Jr, Ghobrial R, Catalano M, et al. Concomitant placement of percutaneous endoscopic gastrostomy and jejunostomy. *Surg Endosc* 1992;6:289.

37. Schmit PJ, Zuckerbraun L. Zenker's diverticula by cricopharyngeus myotomy under local anesthesia. *Am Surg* 1992;58:710.

38. Kiviluoto T, Luukkonen P, Salo J. Laparoscopic gastro-oesophageal antireflux surgery. *Ann Chir Gynaecol* 1994;83:101.

39. Drakulovic MB, Torres A, Bauer TT, et al. Supine body position as a risk factor for nosocomial pneumonia in mechanically ventilated patients: a randomised trial. *Lancet* 1999;354:1851.

40. Balan KK, Vinjamuri S, Maltby P, et al. Gastroesophageal reflux in patients fed by percutaneous endoscopic gastrostomy (PEG): detection by a simple scintigraphic method. *Am J Gastroenterol* 1998;93:946.

41. Montecalvo MA, Steger KA, Farber HW, et al. Nutritional outcome and pneumonia in critical care patients randomized to gastric versus jejunal tube feedings. *Crit Care Med* 1992;20:1377.

42. Burtch GD, Shatney CH. Feeding gastrostomy: assistant or assassin? *Am Surg* 1985;51:204.

43. Bartlett JG, Gorbach SL. The triple threat of aspiration pneumonia. *Chest* 1975;68:560.

44. Med Letter Consultants. Choice of antibacterial drugs. *Med Lett* 2001;43: 69.

45. Mendelson CL. The aspiration of stomach contents into the lungs during obstetric anesthesia. *Am J Obstet Gynecol* 1946;52:191.

46. Bynum LJ, Pierce AK. Pulmonary aspiration of gastric contents. *Am Rev Respir Dis* 1976;114:1129.

47. Cameron JL, Mitchell WH, Zuidema GD. Aspiration pneumonia. *Arch Surg* 1973;106:49.

48. Awe WC, Fletcher WS, Jacob SW. The pathophysiology of aspiration pneumonitis. *Surgery* 1966;50:232.

49. Broe PJ, Toting TJ, Cameron JL. Aspiration pneumonia. *Surg Clin North Am* 1980;60:1551.

50. Hamelberg WV, Bosomworth PP. Aspiration pneumonitis. Springfield, IL: Charles C Thomas, 1968.

51. Lewis RT, Burgess JH, Hampson LG. Cardiorespiratory studies in critical illness. *Arch Surg* 1971;103:335.

52. Doyle RL, Szarflarski N, Modin GW, et al. Identification of patients with acute lung injury. *Am J Respir Crit Care Med* 1995;152:1818.

53. DePaso WJ. Aspiration pneumonia. *Clin Chest Med* 1991;12:269.

54. Marik PE. Aspiration pneumonitis and aspiration pneumonia. *N Engl J Med* 2001;344:665.

55. Toting TJ, Bordos D, Benson DW, et al. Aspiration pneumonia: experimental evaluation of albumin and steroid therapy. *Ann Surg* 1976;183:179.

56. Wolfe JE, Bone RC, Ruth WE. Effects of corticosteroids in the treatment of patients with gastric aspiration. *Am J Med* 1977;63:719.

57. Chapman RL Jr, Downs JB, Modell JH, et al. The ineffectiveness of steroid therapy in treating aspiration of hydrochloric acid. *Arch Surg* 1974;108: 858.

58. Fisk RL, Symes JF, Aldridge LL, et al. The pathophysiology and experimental therapy of acid pneumonitis in ex vivo lungs. *Chest* 1970;57:364.

59. Greenfield LJ, Singleton RP, McCaffree DR, et al. Pulmonary effects of experimental graded aspiration of hydrochloric acid. *Ann Surg* 1969;170: 74.

60. Halmagyi DJF. Lung changes and incidence of respiration arrest in rats after aspiration of sea and fresh water. *J Appl Physiol* 1961;16:41.

61. Teabeaut J II. Aspiration of gastric contents: an experimental study. *Am J Pathol* 1952;28:51.

62. Toung TJ, Cameron JL, Kimera T, et al. Aspiration pneumonia: treatment with osmotically active agents. *Surgery* 1981;89:588.

63. Hiebert CA, Belsey R. Incompetency of the gastric cardia without radiologic evidence of hiatus hernia. *J Thorac Cardiovasc Surg* 1961;42:352.

64. Mays EE, Dubois JJ, Hamilton GB. Pulmonary fibrosis with tracheobronchial aspiration. *Chest* 1976;69:512.

65. Urschel HC Jr, Paulson DL. Gastroesophageal reflux and hiatal hernia. *J Thorac Cardiovasc Surg* 1967;53:21.

66. Crausaz FM, Favez G. Aspiration of solid food particles into lungs of patients with gastroesophageal reflux and chronic bronchial disease. *Chest* 1988;93: 376.

67. Johnson LF, Rajagopal KR. Aspiration resulting from gastroesophageal reflux: a cause of chronic bronchopulmonary disease (editorial). *Chest* 1988;93: 676.

68. Wynne JW, Modell JH. Respiratory aspiration of stomach contents. *Ann Intern Med* 1977;87:466.

69. Folkesson HG, Matthay MA, Hebert CA, et al. Acid aspiration-induced lung injury in rabbits is mediated by interleukin-8-dependent mechanisms. *J Clin Invest* 1995;96:107.

70. Weiser MR, Pechet TT, Williams JP, et al. Experimental murine acid aspiration injury is mediated by neutrophils and the alternative complement pathway. *J Appl Physiol* 1997;83:1090.

71. Matthay MA, Rosen GD. Acid aspiration induced lung injury. *Am J Respir Crit Care Med* 1996;154:277.

72. Steiner J, Bachofen M, Bachofen H. Recovery from aspiration pneumonia. *Pneumologie* 1974;151:127.

73. Sladen A, Zanca P, Hadnott WH. Aspiration pneumonitis: the sequelae. *Chest* 1971;59:448.

74. Gipson SL, Stovall TG, Elkins TE, et al. Pharmacologic reduction of the risk of aspiration. *South Med J* 1986;79:1356.

75. Sukumaran M, Granada MJ, Berger HW, et al. Evaluation of corticosteroid treatment in aspiration of gastric contents: a controlled clinical trial. *Mt Sinai J Med* 1980;47:335.

76. Wolfe JE, Bone RC, Ruth WE. Effects of corticosteroids in the treatment of patients with gastric aspiration. *Am J Med* 1977;63:719.

77. Bernard GR, Luce JM, Sprung CL, et al. High-dose corticosteroids in patients with the adult respiratory distress syndrome. *N Engl J Med* 1987;317: 1565.

78. Johanson WG Jr, Jay SJ, Pierce AK. Bacterial growth in vivo: an important determinant of the pulmonary clearance of *Diplococcus pneumoniae* in rats. *J Clin Invest* 1974;53:1320.

79. Dines DE, Titus JL, Sessler AD. Aspiration pneumonitis. *Mayo Clin Proc* 1970;45:347.

80. Bartlett JG. Anaerobic bacterial infections of the lung and pleural space. *Clin Infect Dis* 1993;4:S248.

81. Finegold SM. Aspiration pneumonia. *Rev Infect Dis* 1991;9:S737.

82. Bartlett JG, Finegold SM. Anaerobic infections of the lung and pleural space. *Am Rev Respir Dis* 1974;110:56.

83. Bartlett JG. Anaerobic bacterial infections of the lung. *Chest* 1987;6:901.

84. Bartlett JG. Anaerobic bacterial pneumonitis. *Am Rev Respir Dis* 1979;119: 19.

85. Yamashita Y, Kohno S, Tanaka K, et al. Anaerobic respiratory infection-evaluation of methods of obtaining specimens. *Kansenshogaku Zasshi* 1994; 68:631.

86. Beerens H, Tahon-Castel M. *Infection humaines a bacteries anaerobies non-toxigenes.* Brussels: Presses Academiques Europeennes, 1965:91.

87. Finegold SM, George WL, Mulligan ME. Anaerobic infections. *Dis Mon* 1985;31:8.

88. Brook I, Finegold SM. Bacteriology of aspiration pneumonia in children. *Pediatrics* 1980;65:1115.

89. Lorber B, Swenson RM. Bacteriology of aspiration pneumonia. *Ann Intern Med* 1974;81:329.

90. Wimberly NW, Bass JB, Boyd BW, et al. Use of a bronchoscopic protected catheter brush for the diagnosis of pulmonary infections. *Chest* 1982;81: 556.

91. Henriquez AH, Mendoza J, Gonzalez PC. Quantitative culture of bronchoalveolar lavage from patients with anaerobic lung abscesses. *J Infect Dis* 1991;164:414.

92. Bartlett JG. Diagnostic accuracy of transtracheal aspiration bacteriologic studies. *Am Rev Respir Dis* 1977;115:777.

93. Verma P. Laboratory diagnosis of anaerobic pleuropulmonary infections. *Semin Respir Infect* 2000;15:114.

94. Appelbaum PC, Spangler SK, Jacobs MR. Beta-lactamase production and susceptibilities to amoxicillin, amoxicillin-clavulanate, ticarcillin, ticarcillin-clavulanate, cefoxitin, imipenem and metronidazole of 320 non-*Bacteroides fragilis Bacteroides* isolates and 129 fusobacteria from 28 U.S. centers. *Antimicrob Agents Chemother* 1990;34:1546.

95. Fosse T, Madinier I, Hitzig C, et al. Prevalence of beta lactamase-producing strains among 149 anaerobic gram negative rods isolated from periodontal pockets. *Oral Microbiol Immunol* 1999;14:352.
96. Kleinkauf N, Ackermann G, Schaumann R, et al. Comparative in vitro activities of gemifloxacin, other quinolones, and nonquinolone antimicrobials against obligately anaerobic bacteria. *Antimicrobial Agents Chemother* 2001;45:1896.
97. Bartlett JG, O'Keefe P, Tally FP, et al. The bacteriology of hospital-acquired pneumonia. *Arch Intern Med* 1986;146:868.
98. Johanson WG, Pierce AK, Sanford JP. Changing pharyngeal bacterial flora of hospitalized patients: emergence of gram-negative bacilli. *N Engl J Med* 1969;281:1137.
99. Mathai D, Lewis MT, Kugler KC, et al. Antimicrobial activity of 41 antimicrobials tested against 2773 bacterial isolates from hospitalized patients with pneumonia. *Diag Microbiol Infect Dis* 2001;39:105.
100. Bartlett JG. Treatment of anaerobic pleuropulmonary infections. *Ann Intern Med* 1975;83:376.
101. Bartlett JG, Gorbach SL. A comparison of penicillin and clindamycin in the treatment of aspiration pneumonia and lung abscess. *JAMA* 1975;234:935.
102. Weiss W. Oral antibiotic therapy of acute primary lung abscess: comparison of penicillin and tetracycline. *Curr Ther Res* 1970;12:154.
103. Weiss W. Delayed cavity closure in acute nonspecific primary lung abscess. *Am J Med Sci* 1968;255:313.
104. Weiss W. Cavity behavior in acute, primary nonspecific lung abscess. *Am Rev Respir Dis* 1973;108:1273.
105. Levison ME, Mangura CT, Lorber B, et al. Clindamycin compared with penicillin for the treatment of anaerobic lung abscess. *Ann Intern Med* 1983;98:466.
106. Gudiol F, Manressa F, Pallares R, et al. Clindamycin vs. penicillin for anaerobic lung infections. *Arch Intern Med* 1990;158:2525.
107. Germaud P, Poirier J, Jacqueme P, et al. Monotherapy using amoxicillin/clavulanic acid as treatment of first choice in community-acquired lung abscess. Apropos of 57 cases. *Rev Pneumol Clin* 1993;49:137.
108. Eykyn SJ. Therapeutic use of metronidazole in anaerobic infection: six years' experience in a London hospital. *Surgery* 1983;93:209.
109. Perlino CA. Metronidazole vs clindamycin treatment of anaerobic pulmonary infection. *Arch Intern Med* 1981;141:1424.
110. Sanders CV, Hanna BJ, Lewis AB. Metronidazole in the treatment of anaerobic infections. *Am Rev Respir Dis* 1979;120:337.
111. Colebatch HJH, Halmagyi DFJ. Reflex airway reaction to fluid aspiration. *J Appl Physiol* 1964;17:787.
112. Modell JH, Moya F, Newby EJ, et al. The effects of fluid volume in seawater drowning. *Ann Intern Med* 1967;67:68.
113. Modell JH, Moya F, Williams HD, et al. Changes in blood gases and A-aDO$_2$ during near drowning. *Anesthesiology* 1968;29:456.
114. Yuksel H, Coskun S, Onag A. Pumpkin seed aspiration into the middle of the trachea in a wheezy infant unresponsive to bronchodilators. *Pediatr Emerg Care* 2001;17:312.
115. Kuschner WG, Sarinas PS, Chitkara R. Foreign body aspiration diagnosed by microscopy. *Am J Med Sci* 2001;322:44.
116. Abdulmajid OA, Ebeid AM, Motaweh MM, et al. Aspirated foreign bodies in the tracheobronchial tree: report of 250 cases. *Thorax* 1976;31:635.
117. Kim IG, Brummitt WM, Humphry A, et al. Foreign body in the airway: a review of 202 cases. *Laryngoscope* 1973;83:347.
118. Haugen RK. The cafe coronary: sudden deaths in restaurants. *JAMA* 1963;186:142.
119. Hedblom CA. Foreign bodies of dental origin in a bronchus pulmonary complication. *Ann Surg* 1920;71:568.
120. Lansing AM, Jamieson WG. Mechanisms of fever in pulmonary atelectasis. *Arch Surg* 1963;87:184.
121. Zavala DC, Rhodes ML. Foreign body removal: a new role for the fiberoptic bronchoscope. *Ann Otol Rhinol Laryngol* 1975;84:650.

CHAPTER 58
Lung Abscess and Necrotizing Pneumonia

John G. Bartlett

Lung abscess is described as necrosis of the pulmonary parenchyma caused by a microbial infection. Some authorities categorize necrotizing pneumonia and lung gangrene separately in reference to multiple small pulmonary abscesses in contiguous areas of the lung. Numerous microbiologic agents can be responsible for lung abscess, but the usual agents are bacteria other than mycobacteria. Before the era of penicillin, lung abscess was a relatively common infection with considerable morbidity and mortality. Since that time, the incidence of lung abscess has been decreased by approximately tenfold, and the mortality has decreased from 30% to 40% to 5% to 10%. Despite the apparent progress, there continues to be considerable controversy regarding methods to determine microbial agents and select antimicrobial agents.

CLASSIFICATION

A number of criteria have been used to classify lung abscess. Many of these were developed decades ago when the infection was far more common. Lung abscess may be classified as acute or chronic on the basis of the duration of symptoms before the patient seeks medical care. The usual dividing line is 4 to 6 weeks. Lung abscess may also be considered primary or secondary on the basis of associated conditions. Abscesses in patients prone to aspiration or in previously healthy individuals are considered primary; secondary lesions are a complication of a primary condition in the lungs, such as a bronchogenic neoplasm or systemic disease that compromises immune defenses. Nonspecific lung abscess refers to lung abscess with no likely pathogen recovered from expectorated sputum. The presumed pathogens in most of these cases are anaerobic bacteria. Putrid lung abscess indicates the offensive odor of sputum or breath that is considered diagnostic of anaerobic infection, although 30% to 40% of patients with lung abscess due to anaerobic bacteria do not have this characteristic feature. In extensive experience with more than 1,000 reported cases of lung abscess during the antibiotic era, approximately 80% were considered primary, 60% putrid, 40% nonspecific, and 40% chronic (1–23).

CLINICAL FEATURES

The most frequent pathogens are anaerobic bacteria. Patients with this type of infection usually have indolent symptoms combined with associated conditions that predispose to aspiration (see Chapter 57). The most common associated conditions are those that compromise consciousness or cause dysphagia (5,24–26). A second characteristic-associated condition is periodontal infection with pyorrhea or gingivitis. The dominant organisms are located in the gingival crevice or gingival pockets, which represent the space separating the gum and tooth. Nevertheless, approximately 10% to 15% of patients with lung abscesses due to anaerobic bacteria have no apparent predisposition to aspiration or periodontal disease (5,24–26).

Symptoms associated with lung abscesses due to anaerobic bacteria are usually chronic with complaints dating for weeks or months. The usual symptoms are fever, fatigue, and cough with sputum production, often associated with pleuritic pain and sometimes hemoptysis. Weight loss and anemia are often present and provide testimony to the chronicity of these infections, even in patients who report an abbreviated illness. Studies using sequential radiographs in experimental animals or in patients who have a defined period of aspiration indicate that the initial lesion is pneumonitis followed by cavitation, which usually appears at least 7 to 14 days later. The sputum is usually purulent, and approximately 60% of those with lung abscesses due to anaerobic bacteria will have putrid sputum, empyema fluid, or putrid breath. Most have leukocytosis with peripheral white cell counts of 15,000 to 20,000/mm^3. Empyema develops in approximately one-third of patients.

Occasional patients have a more fulminant course characterized by high fever, high white blood cell (WBC) count, rapid spread to involve contiguous lung segments, and early involvement of the pleural space. This process is usually caused by anaerobic bacteria and is sometimes referred to as pulmonary gangrene.

EVALUATION

The diagnosis of lung abscess is generally established with a chest radiograph showing an infiltrate in the pulmonary parenchyma with a cavity indicating necrosis of tissue, often in association with an air-fluid level. The differential diagnosis for radiographs with this finding is provided in Table 58.1. The infiltrate is usually confined to a pulmonary segment or lobe, and there is no associated lymphadenopathy. Associated pleural effusions are common and may represent empyema. Other diagnostic considerations with lucent areas on the chest radiograph are cysts, blebs, bullae, and pneumatoceles; all have walls with a thickness less than 1 mm, which distinguishes them from abscesses. Computed tomography is an especially sensitive method to detect lung abscesses. With computed tomography, compared with chest radiography, the abscess is apparent earlier and anatomic definition is better. Computed tomography is regarded as more sensitive, and it clearly distinguishes air-fluid levels in the pleural space from those due to lung abscess in the pulmonary parenchyma (27–30). The usual anatomic locations of anaerobic lung abscesses are the segments that are dependent in the recumbent position, including the superior segments of the lower lobe and the posterior segments of the upper lobe.

Microbiologic studies in patients with cavitary lesions of the lung should include stains and cultures of expectorated sputum for detecting fungi, mycobacteria, and aerobic bacteria. Thoracocentesis should be performed on patients with an associated pleural effusion; the fluid is used for standard analysis, which includes WBC count, protein, pH, Gram stain, and culture for aerobic and anaerobic bacteria. Other acceptable methods of obtaining specimens for anaerobic culture include transtracheal aspiration, transthoracic aspiration, and fiberoptic bronchoscopy using the protected brush or bronchoalveolar lavage and quantitative cultures (31–37). Experience with quantitative cultures of bronchoscopy specimens using bronchoalveolar lavage or the protected brush catheter for quantitative culture for anaerobes is limited but promising (35–37). Blood cultures should be performed in patients with a "septic" clinical picture, but these are commonly positive only in infections due to pyogenic bacteria other than anaerobes. The typical presentation is a patient who is prone to aspiration with an abscess in a dependent pulmonary segment and putrid sputum. In such cases, a presumptive diagnosis of anaerobic infection can be made without the need for invasive diagnostic studies. When the etiologic agent is less apparent and other culture results (pleural fluid, blood, and expectorated sputum) are negative, invasive tests are better justified. The indications and the specific technique used are variable, depending to a large extent on the available resources and the likely pathogens according to the clinical setting. Any of these diagnostic tests for bacteria are considered unreliable after antimicrobial agents are given; this especially applies to fragile organisms such as anaerobes. The greatest mistake that is made is credibility given to an expectorated sputum culture that yields potential pathogens that are unlikely causes of lung abscess such as *Streptococcus pneumoniae*, *Pseudomonas aeruginosa*, coliforms, etc. Gram stain of sputum showing a mixed flora with morphotypes suggesting anaerobes may help, but the validity of this simple method is not well confirmed. Putrid discharge is diagnostic—helpful if present but less helpful if absent.

A common recommendation in previous years was to perform bronchoscopy in virtually all patients with lung abscess to facilitate drainage and detect underlying pulmonary lesions. However, there has been no convincing evidence that this procedure is therapeutically beneficial, and the need to detect underlying pulmonary lesions in patients with typical presentations is not cost-effective. As a consequence, bronchoscopy is now generally reserved for patients who have an atypical presentation, who fail to respond to antibiotic treatment directed against likely pathogens, or in whom there is a specific reason to suspect a localized lesion, especially bronchogenic neoplasms (38).

BACTERIOLOGY

The usual bacteria responsible for lung abscess are anaerobic bacteria that colonize the gingival crevice. The prominent role of these organisms in lung abscess was established by the pioneering work of David Smith (39–41) in the late 1920s.

My experience with bacteriologic studies of patients with lung abscess based on cultures of transtracheal aspirate specimens, empyema fluid, thoracotomy aspirate specimens, or positive blood cultures is summarized in Table 58.2. The results show that 89% of infections involved anaerobic bacteria. The major isolates were *Peptostreptococcus* spp., *Prevotella melaninogenica* (formerly *Bacteroides melaninogenicus*), and *Fusobacterium nucleatum*. Other investigators have found similar results regarding the frequency of recovery of anaerobic bacteria with uncontaminated specimens and the frequency of specific organisms (42,43).

TABLE 58.1.   Differential Diagnosis of a Cavitary Lesion on Chest Radiograph

Necrotizing infections
  Bacteria: anaerobes *Staphylococcus aureus*, enteric gram-negative bacteria, *Pseudomonas aeruginosa*, *Legionella* spp., *Haemophilus influenzae*, *Streptococcus pyogenes*, *Klebsiella pneumoniae*, *Pasteurella multocida*, *Rhodococcus*, *Actinomyces*
  Mycobacteria: *Mycobacterium tuberculosis*, *Mycobacterium kansasii*, *Mycobacterium avium-intracellulare*
  Bacteria-like: *Nocardia* spp.
  Fungi: *Coccidioides immitis*, *Histoplasma capsulatum*, *Blastomyces hominis*, *Aspergillus* spp., *Mucor* spp.
  Parasitic: *Entamoeba histolytica*, *Paragonimus westermani*, *Echinococcus*
Cavitary infarction
  Bland infarction (with or without superimposed infection)
Septic embolism
  S. aureus, anaerobes, others
Vasculitis
  Wegener granulomatosis, periarteritis
Neoplasms
  Bronchogenic carcinoma, metastatic carcinoma, lymphoma
Miscellaneous lesions
  Cysts, blebs, bullae, or pneumatocele with or without fluid collections
Sequestration
Empyema with air-fluid level
Bronchiectasis

TABLE 58.2. Bacteriology of Lung Abscess

Total cases	93
Aerobic bacteria only	10 (11%)
Anaerobic bacteria only	43 (46%)
Mixed aerobes-anaerobes	40 (43%)
Predominant isolates	
Aerobes	
Staphylococcus aureus	13 (4)[a]
Escherichia coli	9
Klebsiella pneumoniae	7 (3)
Pseudomonas aeruginosa	7 (1)
Streptococcus pneumoniae	6 (1)
Anaerobes	
Peptostreptococcus spp.	40 (12)
Fusobacterium nucleatum	34 (5)
Prevotella melaninogenica	32 (1)
Bacteroides fragilis group	14

[a]Frequency of isolation; number in parentheses is frequency of isolation in pure culture.
Adapted from Bartlett JG. Anaerobic bacterial infections of the lung. *Chest* 1987;91:901.

Common bacterial agents of lung abscess in immunocompromised patients include *Nocardia* (44,45), *Legionella pneumophila*, or *Legionella micdadei* (46–49). In immunocompetent patients, the most common pathogens other than anaerobes are microaerophilic streptococci, especially *Streptococcus milleri* (50,51). Other bacteria that occasionally cause lung abscess include *Staphylococcus aureus* (52,53), *Klebsiella pneumoniae* (54), other gram-negative bacilli (55), *Streptococcus pyogenes* (56), *Pseudomonas pseudomallei* (57), *Haemophilus influenzae* (primarily type b), *Brucella* (58), *Selenomonas* (59), *P. cepacia* (60,61), *Actinomyces* spp., *Salmonella* (62), and *Rhodococcus equi* (63–65). Embolic abscesses often involve *S. aureus* as a complication of tricuspid valve endocarditis in injection drug users. Occasional cases represent complications of septic thrombophlebitis due to jugular thrombophlebitis (Lemierre syndrome) or pelvic thrombophlebitis; the usual pathogens in these cases are anaerobes. Unique features of septic emboli are the associated conditions and the involvement of multiple noncontiguous areas of the lung.

TREATMENT

The natural history of pyogenic lung abscess was described by Allen and Blackman (66) in the pre-chemotherapeutic era. These investigators reviewed 2,114 cases reported before 1936 when there was nearly equal division between conservative management, bronchoscopic or postural drainage, and surgery. They noted a mortality of 32% to 34% with all three therapeutic approaches. Of the surviving patients, approximately one-half had persistent illness with recurrent abscesses, chronic empyema, debilitating bronchiectasis, and other sequelae. A subsequent review by Smith (41) of 1,650 cases reported from 1935 to 1945, when sulfonamides were available, showed that these agents had no effect on outcome.

Resectional surgery was developed at the time when penicillin became available so that during the early 1950s, the relative merits of surgery and penicillin became the subject of great controversy. However, by the late 1950s, there was general agreement that most patients with primary lung abscess should be treated with a trial of antibiotics. The favored agent of the time was penicillin; tetracycline was used in patients who did not respond (25,26,67–71). Important contributions were made by Weiss and Cherniack (71) at Philadelphia General Hospital, who showed that oral penicillin (750 mg of penicillin V four times daily) was as effective as high-dose intravenous penicillin G. Weiss showed that even patients with "delayed closure" (persistent cavity shown by chest radiograph after 4 to 6 weeks of treatment) would eventually respond to antibiotics, that more than 90% of patients responded to penicillin (67–72), and that the occasional penicillin failure generally responded to tetracycline (68).

In more recent years, there has been concern about penicillin as the preferred agent. *In vitro* sensitivity data show that 15% to 25% of lung abscesses involve anaerobic bacteria that are resistant to this agent, primarily by the production of penicillinase. These include *P. melaninogenica*, *Bacteroides ruminicola*, *Campylobacter* (formerly *Bacteroides*) *gracilis*, *Bacteroides ureolyticus*, and others (42,72). More recent data suggest that up to 40% of fusobacteria and 60% of non-fragilis *Bacteroides* species may produce penicillinase (73). Nevertheless, it is not clear that many or most patients with these strains will not respond to treatment with penicillins.

The only large-scale prospective studies in modern times that compared antibiotic regimens for anaerobic lung abscesses were reported by Levison and co-workers (74) in 1983 and Gudiol and colleagues (75) in 1990. Both groups compared clindamycin with high-dose intravenous penicillin and concluded that clindamycin was superior on the basis of rate of response, time to defervescence, time to resolution of putrid sputum, and rate of relapses. Another option is metronidazole combined with penicillin, which provides relatively low cost as well as excellent in vitro activity against anticipated pathogens. The published experience with metronidazole plus penicillin is favorable but limited (76); however, the experience with metronidazole alone is poor despite excellent *in vitro* activity against virtually all anaerobes (77,78). The presumed explanation is that clinically important aerobic and microaerophilic streptococci are resistant to metronidazole, and this accounts for the recommendation for concurrent use of penicillin. A prospective but uncontrolled trial of ampicillin-clavulanate (4 g/day for 7 days or longer followed by 2 g/day for 14 days or longer) showed that 52 of 57 patients responded (79).

Recommendations for the duration of therapy are variable and range from 3 weeks to several months. My practice is to continue these drugs according to serial chest radiographs (25,26). Drugs are discontinued when the radiograph is either clear or shows only a small stable residual lesion. The risk with premature discontinuation is relapse.

Drainage is commonly viewed as the most important aspect in managing abscesses at virtually all anatomic sites, but with lung abscess, the air-fluid level that is characteristically found on the chest radiograph usually indicates communication with the bronchus, meaning that spontaneous drainage has already taken place. Improved drainage may be facilitated with physical therapy or bronchoscopy. However, as noted previously, initial studies with bronchoscopy in the pre-chemotherapeutic era showed no advantage. Aggressive attempts to drain substantial collections may result in spillage to other pulmonary segments with the immediate complication of airway obstruction (80).

Surgery is reserved for a minority of patients, 10% to 12% in the cumulative literature experience for the past two decades (Table 58.3). The usual indications are failure to respond to medical management, suspected neoplasm, or hemorrhage (81–83). Failure to respond to antibiotics usually results from an obstructed bronchus, an extremely large abscess (greater than 6 cm diameter), an abscess that has been present long before

TABLE 58.3.   Mortality Rates for Lung Abscess

Date of report	No. of patients	Surgical treatment (%)	Mortality (%)
1889–1935	2,114	49	34
1936–1945	1,650	45	34
1946–1955	460	32	5
1956–1965	496	38	8
1966–1998	1,900	14	10

Adapted from Bartlett JG. Anaerobic bacterial infections of the lung. *Chest* 1987;91:901. Data from Bartlett JG. Anaerobic bacterial infections of the lung and pleural space. *Clin Infect Dis* 1993;4:5248.

treatment, or an abscess due to relatively resistant organisms such as *Pseudomonas aeruginosa*. The usual procedure in such cases is lobectomy or pneumonectomy. An alternative is percutaneous drainage, which is being used with increasing frequency, primarily in patients who fail to respond to medical therapy. This is often done under computed tomographic guidance, and the reported experience showed nearly uniform response (84–89). The aspirate specimen should be submitted for microbiologic studies (bacteria, fungi, mycobacteria) and cytologic studies.

RESPONSE TO THERAPY

Patients with lung abscess usually show clinical improvement with decreased fever within 3 to 4 days of initiation of antibiotic treatment. Defervescence is expected within 7 to 10 days (5,67–71,74,75,90). Patients with fevers persisting for 7 to 14 days should undergo bronchoscopy or other diagnostic tests to better define anatomic changes and microbiologic findings. Cultures of expectorated sputum are not likely to be helpful at this juncture, except for detecting nonbacterial pathogens such as mycobacteria and fungi. The response to therapy by serial chest radiographs is delayed. In fact, infiltrates usually show progression during the first 3 days in approximately one-half of patients, continuing for at least 1 week in approximately one-third (27). Pleural involvement is relatively common and may occur in an explosive fashion. The most frequent causes of failures with medical management include the failure to drain pleural collections, inappropriate choice of antimicrobial agents, an obstructed bronchus that prevents drainage, or refractory lesions due to an inadequate host, resistant organisms, or large cavity size.

Mortality rates for primary lung abscess are generally reported at 5% to 15% (see Table 58.3). Clinical findings suggesting a poor prognosis include large cavity size, usually greater than 6 cm in diameter; symptoms that have persisted for 8 weeks or longer before presentation; necrotizing pneumonia or lung gangrene; elderly, debilitated, or immunologically compromised patients; abscesses that complicate bronchial obstruction; abscesses due to aerobic bacteria; and nosocomial acquisition. Perlman and colleagues (14) found only a single death among 57 patients with primary lung abscess, compared with a 75% mortality rate among patients who had abscesses associated with obstructing lesions or compromised host defense mechanisms. A review of lung abscess cases in Japan showed the mortality rate to be 2% in community-acquired cases and 67% for nosocomial cases (22).

REFERENCES

1. Abernathy RS. Antibiotic therapy of lung abscesses: effectiveness of penicillin. *Dis Chest* 1968;53:592.
2. Anderson MN, McDonald KE. Prognostic factors of results of treatment in pyogenic pulmonary abscess. *J Thorac Surg* 1970;39:573.
3. Barnett TB, Herring CL. Lung abscess. *Arch Intern Med* 1971;127:217.
4. Bartlett JG. Treatment of anaerobic pleuropulmonary infections. *Ann Intern Med* 1975;83:376.
5. Bartlett JG, Gorbach SL, Tally FP, et al. Bacteriology and treatment of primary lung abscess. *Am Rev Respir Dis* 1974;109:510.
6. Block JA, Wagley PF, Fisher MA. Delayed closure in lung abscess: a re-evaluation of the indications for surgery. *Johns Hopkins Med J* 1969;126:19.
7. Collins HA, Guest JL, Daniel RA Jr. Primary lung abscess. *J Thorac Cardiovasc Surg* 1964;47:383.
8. Drake EH, Stones FM Jr. The management of lung abscess with special reference to the place of antibiotics in therapy. *Ann Intern Med* 1951;35:1218.
9. Fox JR, Hughes FA, Sutliff WD. Nonspecific lung abscess: experience with fifty-five consecutive cases. *J Thorac Surg* 1953;26:255.
10. Gopalakrishna KV, Lerner PI. Primary lung abscess. *Clev Clin Q* 1975;42:3.
11. Hagan JL, Hardy JD. Lung abscess revisited: a survey of 184 cases. *Ann Surg* 1983;197:755.
12. Harber P, Terry PB. Fatal lung abscesses: review of 11 years' experience. *South Med J* 1981;74:281.
13. Jensen H, Amdrup E. Nonspecific abscesses of the lung 129 cases. *Acta Chir Scand* 1964;127:487.
14. Perlman LV, Lerner E, D'Esopo N. Clinical classification and analysis of 97 cases of lung abscess. *Am Rev Respir Dis* 1969;99:390.
15. Pohlson EC, McNamara J, Char C, Kurata B. Lung abscess: a changing pattern of the disease. *Ann Surg* 1985;150:97.
16. Rambaugh IF, Prior JA. Lung abscess: a review of forty-one cases. *Ann Intern Med* 1961;55:223.
17. Schweppe HI, Knowles JH, Kane L. Lung abscess: an analysis of the Massachusetts General Hospital cases from 1943 through 1956. *N Engl J Med* 1961;265:1039.
18. Shafron RD, Tate CF Jr. Lung abscess: a five-year evaluation. *Dis Chest* 1968;53:12.
19. Shoemaker EH, Yow EM, Byrd WC. Antibiotic therapy of primary pulmonary abscess. *Arch Intern Med* 1955;96:683.
20. Wolcott MW, Coury OH, Baum GL. Changing concepts in the therapy of lung abscess: a twenty year survey. *Dis Chest* 1961;40:1.
21. Hirshberg B, Skair-Levi M, Nir-Paz R, et al. Factors predicting mortality of patients with lung abscess. *Chest* 1999;115:746.
22. Mori T, Eb T, Takahashi M, et al. Lung abscess: analysis of 66 cases from 1979 to 1991. *Intern Med* 1993;32:278.
23. Hammond JM, Potgieter PD, Hanslo D, et al. The etiology and antimicrobial susceptibility patterns of microorganisms in acute community-acquired lung abscess. *Chest* 1995;108:937.
24. Bartlett JG, Finegold SM. Anaerobic infections of the lung and pleural space. *Am Rev Respir Dis* 1974;110:56.
25. Bartlett JG. Lung abscess. *Johns Hopkins Med J* 1982;150:141.
26. Bartlett JG. Anaerobic bacterial infections of the lung and pleural space. *Clin Infect Dis* 1993;4:S248.
27. Landay MJ, Christensen EE, Bynum LJ, et al. Anaerobic pleural and pulmonary infections. *AJR* 1980;134:233.
28. Stark DD, Federle MP, Goodman PC, et al. Differentiating lung abscess and empyema: radiography and computed tomography. *AJR* 1983;141:163.
29. Williford ME, Godwin JD. Computed tomography of lung abscess and empyema. *Radiol Clin North Am* 1983;21:575.
30. Johnson JF, Shiels WE, White CB, et al. Concealed pulmonary abscess: diagnosis by computed tomography. *Pediatrics* 1986;78:283.
31. Bartlett JG. Diagnostic accuracy of transtracheal aspiration bacteriology. *Am Rev Respir Dis* 1977;115:777.
32. Bartlett JG. The technique of transtracheal aspiration. *J Crit Illness* 1986;1:43.
33. Bartlett JG, Rosenblatt JE, Finegold SM. Percutaneous transtracheal aspiration in the diagnosis of anaerobic pulmonary infection. *Ann Intern Med* 1973;79:535.
34. Bandt PD, Blank N, Casstellino RA. Needle diagnosis of pneumonitis: value in high-risk patients. *JAMA* 1972;220:1578.
35. Wimberley NW, Bass JB, Boyd BW, et al. Use of a bronchoscopic protected catheter brush for the diagnosis of pulmonary infections. *Chest* 1982;81:556.
36. Henriquez AH, Mendoza J, Gonzalez PC. Quantitative culture of bronchoalveolar lavage from patients with anaerobic lung abscesses. *J Infect Dis* 1991;164:414.
37. Verma P. Laboratory diagnosis of anaerobic pleuropulmonary infections. *Semin Respir Infect* 2000;15:114.
38. Sosenko A, Glassroth J. Fiberoptic bronchoscopy in the evaluation of lung abscesses. *Chest* 1985;87:489.
39. Smith DT. Experimental aspiratory abscess. *Arch Surg* 1927;14:231.
40. Smith DT. Fuso-spirochetal disease of the lungs. *Tubercle* 1928;9:420.
41. Smith DT. Medical treatment of acute and chronic pulmonary abscesses. *J Thorac Surg* 1948;17:72.

42. Finegold SM, George WL, Mulligan ME. Anaerobic infections. *Dis Mon* 1985;31:8.
43. Civen R, Jousimies-Somer H, Marina M, et al. A retrospective review of cases of anaerobic empyema and update of bacteriology. *Clin Infect Dis* 1995; 20[Suppl 2]:S224.
44. Stack WA, Richardson PD, Logan RP, et al. Nocardia asteroides lung abscess in acute ulcerative colitis treated with cyclosporine. *Am J Gastroenterol* 2001;96: 225.
45. vanBurik JA, Hackman RC, Nadeem SO, et al. Nocardiosis after bone marrow transplantation: a retrospective study. *Clin Infect Dis* 1997;24: 1154.
46. Ernst A, Gordon FD, Hayek J, et al. Lung abscess complicates *Legionella micdadei* pneumonia in a liver transplant recipient: a case report and review. *Transplantation* 1998;65:130.
47. Johnson KM, Huseby JS. Lung abscess caused by *Legionella micdadei*. *Chest* 1997;111:252.
48. Senecal JL, St-Antoine P, Beliveau C. *Legionella pneumophila* lung abscess in a patient with systemic lupus erythematosus. *Am J Med Sci* 1987;293:309.
49. Halberstam M, Isenberg HD, Hilton E. Abscess and empyema caused by *Legionella micdadei*. *J Clin Microbiol* 1992;30:512.
50. Kobayashi K. *Streptococcus milleri* as a cause of pulmonary abscess. *Acta Paediatr* 2001;90:233.
51. Jerng JS, Hsueh PR, Teng LJ, et al. Empyema thoracic and lung abscess caused by viridians streptococci. *Am J Respir Crit Care* 1997;156:1508.
52. Wollenman OJ, Finland M. Pathology of staphylococcal pneumonia complicating clinical influenza. *Am J Pathol* 1943;19:23.
53. Fisher AM, Trever RW, Curtin JA, et al. Staphylococcal pneumonia: a review of 21 cases in adults. *N Engl J Med* 1958;258:919.
54. Bullowa JGM, Chess J, Friedman NJ. Pneumonia due to *Bacillus friedlanderi*. *Arch Intern Med* 1937;60:735.
55. Williams DM, Krick JA, Remington JS. Pulmonary infections in the compromised host. *Am Rev Respir Dis* 1976;114:359.
56. Frieden TR, Biebuyck J, Hierholzer WJ Jr. Lung abscess with group: a beta-hemolytic streptococcus. Case report and review. *Arch Intern Med* 1991;151:1655.
57. Howe C, Sampath A, Spotnitz M. The pseudomallei group: a review. *J Infect Dis* 1971;124:596.
58. Papiris SA, Maniati MA, Haritou A, et al. *Brucella* haemorrhagic pleural effusion. *Eur Respir J* 1994;7:1369.
59. Bisiaux-Salauze B, Perez C, Sebald M, et al. Bacteremias caused by *Selenomonas artemidis* and *Selenomonas infelix*. *J Clin Microbiol* 1990;28:140.
60. Snell GI, de Hoyos A, Krajden M, et al. *Pseudomonas cepacia* in lung transplant recipients. *Chest* 1993;103:466.
61. Poe RH, Marcus HR, Emerson GL. Lung abscess due to *Pseudomonas cepacia*. *Am Rev Respir Dis* 1977;115:861.
62. Ankobiah WA, Salehi F. *Salmonella* lung abscess in a patient with acquired immunodeficiency syndrome (letter). *Chest* 1991;100:591.
63. Harvey RL, Sunstrum JC. *Rhodococcus equi* infection in patients with and without human immunodeficiency virus infection. *Rev Infect Dis* 1991;13: 139.
64. Verville TD, Huycke MM, Greenfield RA, et al. *Rhodococcus equi* infections of humans. 12 cases and a review of the literature. *Medicine (Baltimore)* 1994;73: 119.
65. Shapiro JM, Romney BM, Weiden MD, et al. *Rhodococcus equi* endobronchial mass with lung abscess in a patient with AIDS. *Thorax* 1992;47:62.
66. Allen CI, Blackman JF. Treatment of lung abscess with report of 100 consecutive cases. *J Thorac Surg* 1936;6:156.
67. Weiss W. Delayed cavity closure in acute nonspecific primary lung abscess. *Am J Med Sci* 1968;255:313.
68. Weiss W. Oral antibiotic therapy of acute primary lung abscess: comparison of penicillin and tetracycline. *Curr Ther Res* 1970;12:154.
69. Weiss W. Cavity behavior in acute, primary, nonspecific lung abscess. *Am Rev Respir Dis* 1973;108:1273.
70. Weiss W. Letter to the editor. *Chest* 1975;67:625.
71. Weiss W, Cherniack NS. Acute nonspecific lung abscess: a controlled study comparing orally and parenterally administered penicillin G. *Chest* 1974;66: 348.
72. Finegold SM, Rolfe RD. Susceptibility testing of anaerobic bacteria. *Diagn Microbiol Infect Dis* 1983;1:33.
73. Appelbaum PC, Spangler SK, Jacobs MR. Beta-lactamase production and susceptibilities to amoxicillin, amoxicillin-clavulanate, ticarcillin, ticarcillin-clavulanate, cefoxitin, imipenem and metronidazole of 320 non-*Bacteroides fragilis* isolates and 129 fusobacteria from 28 U.S. centers. *Antimicrob Agents Chemother* 1990;34:1546.
74. Levison ME, Mangura CT, Lorber B, et al. Clindamycin compared with penicillin for the treatment of anaerobic lung abscess. *Ann Intern Med* 1983;98: 466.
75. Gudiol F, Manressa F, Pallares R, et al. Clindamycin vs. penicillin for anaerobic lung infections. *Arch Intern Med* 1990;158:2525.
76. Eykyn SJ. The therapeutic use of metronidazole in anaerobic infection: six years' experience in a London hospital. *Surgery* 1983;93:209.
77. Perlino CA. Metronidazole vs. clindamycin treatment of anaerobic pulmonary infection. *Arch Intern Med* 1981;141:1424.
78. Sanders CV, Hanna BJ, Lewis AC. Metronidazole in the treatment of anaerobic infections. *Am Rev Respir Dis* 1979;120:337.
79. Germaud P, Poirier J, Jacqueme P, et al. Monotherapy using amoxicillin/clavulanic acid as treatment of first choice in community-acquired lung abscess. Apropos of 57 cases. *Rev Pneumol Clin* 1993;49:137.
80. Rasanen J, Bools JC, Downs JB. Endobronchial drainage of undiagnosed lung abscess during chest physical therapy: a case report. *Phys Ther* 1988;68: 371.
81. Cordice JW Jr, Chitkara RK. The role of surgery in treating pleuropulmonary suppurative disease—review of 77 cases managed at Queens Hospital Center between 1986 and 1989. *J Natl Med Assoc* 1992;84:145.
82. Pfitzner J, Peacock MJ, Tsirgiotis E, et al. Lobectomy for cavitating lung abscess with haemoptysis: strategy for protecting the contralateral lung and also the non-involved lobe of the ipsilateral lung. *Br J Anaesth* 2000;85:791.
83. Tseng YL, Wu MH, Lin MY, et al. Surgery for lung abscess in immunocompetent and immunocompromised children. *J Pediatr Surg* 2001;36:470.
84. Al-Salem, AH Ali EA. Computed tomography-guided percutaneous needle aspiration of abscesses in neonates and children. *Pediatr Surg Int* 1997;12: 417.
85. Ha HK, Kang MW, Park JM, et al. Lung abscess. percutaneous catheter therapy. *Acta Radiol* 1993;34:362.
86. VanSonnenberg E, D'Agostino HB, Casola G, et al. Lung abscess: CT-guided drainage. *Radiology* 1991;178:347.
87. Shim C, Santos GH, Zelefsky M. Percutaneous drainage of lung abscess. *Lung* 1990;168:201.
88. Aizumi K, Watanabe A, Saito A, et al. Yield of percutaneous needle lung aspiration in lung abscess. *Chest* 1990;97:69.
89. Klein JS, Schultz S, Heffner JE. Interventional radiology of the chest: image-guided percutaneous drainage of pleural effusions, lung abscess, and pneumothorax. *AJR* 1995;164:581.
90. Bartlett JG, Finegold SM. Anaerobic pleuropulmonary infections. *Medicine (Baltimore)* 1972;51:413.

CHAPTER 59
Empyema

John G. Bartlett

Most empyemas represent complications of bacterial pneumonias; less common predisposing causes are prior thoracic surgery, chest trauma, esophageal rupture, subdiaphragmatic infection, and septicemia. Approximately 40% of patients with bacterial pneumonias have pleural effusions, but only about 1% represent empyemas. The major challenge to clinicians is to determine which effusions require specific therapy, that is, which require drainage, which require chest tube drainage, and which require thoracic surgery.

DEFINITION

The classic definition is pleural pus. Subsequent definitions include pleural fluid with a leukocyte count exceeding $25,000/mm^3$ with a predominance of polymorphonuclear leukocytes, pleural fluid with microorganisms demonstrated by stain and/or culture, and pleural fluid pH levels of 7.0 or lower (1,2). Nevertheless, low pH levels may also be noted in pleural effusions associated with tuberculosis, malignancy, or rheumatoid arthritis.

PATHOPHYSIOLOGY

The most common cause of empyema is extension of bacterial infection of the lung to the pleural space. This accounts for 40% to 60% of cases in most series (2–20). Previous thoracic surgery accounts for 15% to 30% of cases, and extension from subdiaphragmatic infection accounts for 5% to 10%. Less frequent antecedent predisposing conditions are perforation of the esophagus, chest trauma (especially with hemothorax), embolic lesions (including tricuspid valve endocarditis), extension from perimandibular or neck space infection, inadvertent contamination of the pleura by drug users attempting injection into cervical veins, septicemia, and thoracentesis with inadequate sterile technique. These miscellaneous causes collectively account for 10% to 20%. Rare cases are idiopathic (2–23).

Empyema after bacterial pneumonitis or lung abscess is the most common form. The usual mechanism is direct extension of the infection to an adjacent parapneumonic effusion. In the pre-antibiotic era, the dominant agent of pneumonia and empyema was clearly *Streptococcus pneumoniae*. Empyema was noted as a complication of pneumococcal pneumonia in 11% of 3,131 cases reported by Finland in 1939 (24). A review of 3,000 cases of empyema reported between 1934 and 1939 showed that 80% were associated with pneumonia; *S. pneumoniae* accounted for 64% (25). The second mechanism of a postpneumonic empyema is by a bronchopleural fistula due to necrosis of the airways, which then provides a direct conduit to the pleural cavity. These account for 10% to 20% of empyemas and are generally ascribed to the organisms most likely to cause pulmonary necrosis, most commonly anaerobic bacterial (1,10,17,26); less common causes are microaerophilic streptococci such as *Streptococcus milleri*, *Staphylococcus aureus*, Enterobacteriaceae, and pseudomonads (27).

The host response to microorganisms in the pleural space is divided into three stages that merge indistinguishably. The time frame in this sequence largely accounts for the variations noted with analysis of pleural fluid and also dictates the appropriate methods of drainage (2,17). The initial stage is the exudated stage in which there is a collection of thin, free-flowing fluid that shows a low number of leukocytes that are predominantly neutrophils, normal blood chemistries (pH higher than 7.2; lactate dehydrogenase values lower than 1,000 IU/L), and negative microbial studies including Gram stain and culture. Adequate antibiotic treatment at this stage usually stops progression of the illness. The second stage is the fibropurulent stage in which a large number of polymorphonuclear leukocytes and fibrin accumulate. Pleural fluid analysis at this stage shows low pH, lactate dehydrogenase values higher than 1,000 IU/L, and low glucose values; bacteria are seen on a Gram stain and culture results are positive. Fibrin is deposited in both the parietal and the visceral pleurae, at the site of involvement, causing loculation and fixation of the lung. These loculi make adequate drainage with chest tubes progressively difficult. The final stage is the organizing stage in which fibroblasts produce a pleural peel of fibrous tissue. At this stage the empyema is regarded as chronic, the exudate is composed of thick pus, and the empyema may drain spontaneously through the chest wall (empyema necessitatis), or it may drain into the lung via a bronchopleural fistula. The lung at this stage is trapped and essentially nonfunctional.

INCIDENCE

Empyema was once a relatively common complication of bacterial infections of the lung. In the prepenicillin era, it complicated 10% to 20% of cases of pneumococcal pneumonia (24,28,29). Infection of the pleural space occurred relatively late in the disease course and was referred to as metapneumonic; this was in contrast to streptococcal empyema, which generally occurred early in the course of pneumonia and was referred to as synpneumonic (30,31). Since that time, the frequency of empyema has decreased to about 1% of cases of community-acquired pneumonia requiring hospitalization (32), and the frequency of *S. pneumoniae* has

decreased even more. The implication is that previous antibiotic treatment successfully prevents this relatively late complication. At present, the reported incidence of empyema is generally on the order of 0.5 to 0.8 per 1,000 admissions (4,5,7,17). The frequency of empyema as a complication of lung resection is 1% to 5% (33,34); most of these empyemas are associated with a bronchopleural fistula.

BACTERIOLOGY

Microbiologic studies of empyema may be divided into three stages: the preantibiotic era, the early postantibiotic era, and the five decades of the antibiotic era (Table 59.1).

Preantibiotic Era

Multiple studies of empyema in the preantibiotic era showed that *S. pneumoniae* consistently accounted for 60% to 70% of all cases in adults; group A β-hemolytic streptococci accounted for 10% to 15%; and *S. aureus* accounted for 5% to 8% (25,28,35–37). In a review of 5,393 cases of pneumococcal pneumonia reported from 1926 to 1933, there were 286 with empyema, for a frequency of 5.3% (29). Coliforms were so rare as to be the subject of anecdotal case reports. Anaerobic cultures were infrequently done, but 5% to 7% of cases were noted to have putrid pleural fluid.

Early Antibiotic Era

Bacteriologic studies of empyema fluid after the introduction of penicillin in the mid-1940s through the late 1960s showed that *S. pneumoniae* accounted for only 5% to 10%, *S. aureus* accounted for 20% to 60%, and coliforms accounted for 30% to 60% (3,4,38–40). Many of these infections were polymicrobial. Cultures for anaerobic bacteria were infrequently done, with the exception of the report by Beerens and Tahon-Castel (38).

More Recent Experience

During the past two decades increasing attention has been paid to the role of anaerobic bacteria, although the recovery rate of these organisms with empyema complicating community-acquired pneumonia or lung abscess is highly variable, ranging from 11% to 76% (6–13,20,41,43,44). Important clues to these organisms are the presence of putrid pleural fluid, which is diagnostic of anaerobic infection, and a Gram stain showing a polymicrobial flora or a Gram stain showing bacteria with the morphologic characteristics of anaerobes. Important factors contributing to differences in bacteriology results are the host population, the associated conditions, the adequacy of anaerobic cultures, and the use of antibiotics before pleural fluid culture. Empyemas associated with thoracic surgery or chest trauma are usually caused by *S. aureus*; gram-negative bacteria are less frequent. Most infections involving anaerobes are polymicrobial; monomicrobial infections are most likely to involve *S. pneumoniae*, *S. aureus*, or gram-negative bacteria.

CLINICAL FEATURES

The usual clinical presentation cannot be distinguished from that of pneumonitis or lung abscess. Common features include fever, cough, sputum production, and dyspnea. Approximately 60% of patients complain of pleurisy. Physical examination usually

TABLE 59.1. Bacteriology of Empyema

Literature source	Years reviewed	Patients	No. of cases	Bacteriologic findings[a]							
				Sterile	SP	β-Streptococci	SA	GNB	Anaerobes	More than one species
Ehler (25)	1934–1939	Literature review; all cases	3000	NS	1920 (64)	282 (9)	195 (7)	NS	5% putrid	NS
Novak (35)	1932–1939	All cases	500	NS	317 (63)	92 (16)	38 (5)	NS	7% putrid	NS
Hochberg and Kramer (36)	1929–1936	Children	267	NS	122 (46)	82 (31)	35 (13)	NS	NS	28 (10)
Yeh et al. (3)	1956–1963	All cases	103	42 (4)	1 (2)	1 (2)	26 (43)	36 (59)	NS	16 (26)
Beerens and Tahon-Castel (38)	1948–1965	All cases	45	0	0	1 (2)	13 (29)	13 (29)	23 (51)	21 (47)
Stiles et al. (39)	1955–1961	Children	152	84 (55)	6 (9)	NS	78 (51)	NS	NS	NS
Snider and Seleh (4)	1952–1967	Adults; VA hospital	79	15 (16)	7 (11)	6 (9)	42 (66)	36 (56)	6 (9)	25 (52)
Lutz et al. (40)	1948–1962	All cases	638	NS	35 (5)	16 (3)	255 (40)	238 (37)	86 (13)	141 (22)
Simmons et al. (6)	1957–1971	All cases	60	13 (22)	3 (6)	NS	11 (23)	23 (49)	0	29 (62)
Sullivan et al. (41)	1950–1972	All cases	482	256 (53)	32 (13)	NS	31 (12)	16 (6)	42 (19)	58 (39)
Weese et al. (5)	1967–1969	All cases	49	15 (31)	4 (12)	9 (26)	12 (35)	19 (56)	NS	6 (17)
Bartlett et al. (10)	1971–1973	Adults	83	0	5 (6)	0	17 (20)	21 (25)	63 (76)	60 (72)
Varkey et al. (7)	1969–1978	Adults	72	10 (14)	6 (10)	3 (5)	7 (11)	11 (18)	28 (39)	20 (32)
Benfield (11)	1968–1978	All cases	117	38 (32)	12 (15)	NS	20 (25)	23 (29)	9 (11)	NS
Mauroudis et al. (8)	1970–1980	Adults	100	3 (3)	17 (17)	NS	33 (34)	35 (36)	25 (26)	42 (43)
Lemmer et al. (12)	1978–1982	Adults	70	4 (6)	4 (6)	NS	27 (26)	13 (20)	20 (30)	41 (62)
Grant and Finley (9)	1970–1980	All cases	90	9 (10)	NS	NS	NS	NS	26 (32)	30 (37)
Mayo (13)	1955–1979	All cases	63	18 (29)	0	5 (11)	17 (38)	10 (22)	6 (13)	14 (31)
Caplan et al. (42)	1982–1983	Trauma	31	0	0	3 (10)	14 (45)	11 (35)	3 (10)	14 (43)
Brook (43)	1974–1978	Children	72	0	13 (18)	3 (4)	10 (14)	8 (11)	24 (33)	14 (19)
Alfageme et al. (18)	1984–1990	All cases	82	6 (7)	9 (11)	NS	11 (13)	21 (26)	32 (39)	30 (37)
Kelly and Morris (44)	1985–1993	Adults	60	13 (22)	5 (6)	NS	10 (17)	22 (27)	10 (17)	14 (17)
LeMense et al. (20)	1989–1993	All cases	43	16 (37)	1 (2)	NS	11 (26)	1 (2)	5 (12)	7 (16)

[a] Numbers of cases, with percentage in parentheses, are given.
SP, *Streptococcus pneumoniae*; SA, *Staphylococcus aureus*; GNB, gram-negative bacteria; NS, not specified.
Adapted from Bartlett JG: Bacterial infections of the pleural space. *Semin Respir Infect* 1998;3:309.

shows dullness and reduced breath sounds on the affected side, but it is usually not possible to distinguish empyema with sterile parapneumonic effusions on the basis of history or physical examination. Chest radiographs show pleural effusions, which are most readily apparent at the costophrenic angles on the posteroanterior view and the posterior gutters on the lateral view. A lateral decubitus radiograph will reveal smaller effusions. Some authorities consider the lateral decubitus radiograph to be essential in the evaluation of small pleural effusions detected by blunting of a costophrenic angle (2). If the distance from the inside chest wall to the bottom of the lung measures more than 10 mm, there should be a thoracentesis; smaller pleural effusions are considered insignificant (45). In practice, these recommendations are seldom followed. Computed tomography or ultrasonography is generally unnecessary but will distinguish pleural collections from parenchymal infiltrates (46,47). The differential diagnosis of a pleural effusion includes pulmonary embolism, mycobacterial infection, viral infection, fungal infection, postcardiotomy syndrome, collagen-vascular disease (lupus or rheumatoid effusions), malignant effusion, drug-induced pulmonary disease, congestive heart failure, and sympathetic effusion reflecting subdiaphragmatic disease such as pancreatitis or subphrenic abscess. Patients with empyema usually show concurrent evidence of pneumonitis or lung abscess.

DIAGNOSTIC STUDIES

Recommended routine tests include leukocyte count and differential, total protein, pH determination, levels of lactate dehydrogenase and glucose, Gram stain, and cultures for aerobic and anaerobic bacteria. Grossly purulent pleural fluid generally requires no diagnostic studies beyond culture. For patients without grossly purulent fluid, the findings on pleural fluid analysis often dictate management (2,17,48–52) (Table 59.2). A meta-analysis of seven studies reporting values for pH, lactate dehydrogenase, and glucose showed that pleural fluid pH had the highest diagnostic accuracy for identifying parapneumonic effusions that require drainage (51). The decision threshold in this analysis varied between 7.21 and 7.29.

The Gram stain usually provides immediate information regarding the presence or absence of bacteria as well as morphologic features of the implicated organism to guide the initial selection of antimicrobial agents. Putrid odor to the fluid is considered diagnostic of anaerobic infection, although anaerobic organisms may be difficult to recover with culture due to faulty laboratory techniques or antecedent antibiotic treatment.

THERAPY

The usual treatment for patients with empyema includes administration of antibiotics, supportive care, arbitrary use of thrombolytic agents, and drainage. The greatest controversy and most important decision concern the drainage procedure.

Antibiotic Selection

Antibiotic selection is simplified if the bacteriologic diagnosis is established with a Gram stain and/or cultures of the empyema fluid. The major concern is relatively fastidious organisms that may be difficult to recover, especially after antibiotic treatment, such as *S. pneumoniae* and anaerobic bacteria. By contrast,

TABLE 59.2. Classification and Therapy of Parapneumonic Effusions and Empyema

Class	Diagnostic criteria	Treatment
Insignificant effusion	Small (<10 mm fluid on a lateral decubitus film; see text)	Antibiotics Thoracentesis usually unnecessary
Parapneumonic effusion	>10 mm thick on lateral decubitis film	Antibiotics Thoracentesis
Borderline complicated effusion	pH 7–7.2 and/or lactate dehydrogenase value >1,000 IU/L; glucose level >40 mg/dL; negative Gram stain and culture	Antibiotics and serial thoracentesis Tube thoracostomy sometimes necessary
Simple complicated effusion	pH <7 and/or glucose value <40 mg/dL and/or positive Gram stain or culture	Antibiotics and tube thoracostomy
Complex-complicated effusion	Above plus multiple loculi	Antibiotics Tube thoracostomy and thrombolytics
Simple empyema	Pus Single loculus or free-flowing fluid	Antibiotics Tube thoracostomy ± decortication
Complex empyema	Pus Multiple loculi	Antibiotics Tube thoracostomy and thrombolytics Thoracostomy or decortication

S. aureus and aerobic gram-negative bacilli should be easily recovered. *In vitro* sensitivity tests are required as a guide to therapeutic agents. Most diffuse well into pleural fluid with or without infection so that local instillation is usually not advocated. Nevertheless, there is variation between agents in penetration, and some are relatively inactive because of the presence of pus, low pH, and β-lactamase (53,54).

Thrombolytic Agents

Streptokinase and urokinase are often advocated for patients with loculated effusions. The goal is to dissolve fibrin membranes to facilitate drainage. The usual regimen is 250,000 units of streptokinase or 100,000 units of urokinase in a volume of 100 mL, delivered through the chest tube that is clamped for 1 to 2 hours. This may be given daily for up to 14 days. The reported experience is variable (21,55–58). In experimental empyema, varidase (streptokinase and streptodornase) was superior to streptokinase or urokinase (55).

Drainage

The main principle is that empyemas must be drained and the space obliterated, a concept that has not changed since Hippocrates 2000 years ago (59). Nevertheless, the timing and method of drainage remain highly controversial. General guidelines are dictated largely by radiographic findings and analyses of pleural fluid that reflect the stage of the infection (2,9,17, 22,23,60–69). Specific guidelines are summarized in Table 59.2. An alternative approach offered by LeMense and colleagues (20) is a decision tree based on chest computed tomography. If there are no multiple loculi, the treatment is thoracentesis or thoracostomy drainage; if repeated computed tomography shows inadequate drainage at 24 hours, thrombolytics are added. If there are multiple loculi or an inadequate response to thrombolytics, the preferred treatment is thoracostomy drainage or decortication. Others have found CT scan to be useless in these management decisions (70) and also found thrombolytics to have high rates of failure (23).

During the initial exudative phase, the fluid is thin and free flowing and the lung is easily reexpanded. This may resolve with antibiotic therapy for the associated pneumonia, or repeated thoracentesis or tube thoracostomy drainage may be required (65). The necessity for thoracostomy drainage increases the lower the pH, the lower the glucose level, and the higher the lactate dehydrogenase level. Some authorities base the decision to perform thoracostomy in patients with nonpurulent effusions on the pleural fluid pH. Nearly all patients with a pH below 7.0 require tube drainage, and nearly all with a pH above 7.3 experience resolution without sequelae with appropriate antibiotics alone (2,17,52,68). Pleural fluid pH levels of 7.0 to 7.3 represent a gray zone; repeated pleural fluid analyses and careful clinical follow-up are required to evaluate the response to antibiotics. Some authorities use repeated thoracentesis, resorting to thoracostomy only if there are persistent signs of sepsis after 3 or 4 days or rapid reaccumulation of fluid regardless of pleural fluid pH levels.

During the fibropurulent phase the fluid is too thick for adequate drainage by thoracentesis, so thoracostomy is required. Large-bore needles may be required to obtain diagnostic material. Drainage may be facilitated by fluoroscopic, computed tomographic, or ultrasonic guidance for catheter placement (71–74). This type of closed drainage with suction is recommended as the initial procedure when the fluid is thick, there is evidence of a bronchopleural fistula, or the pleural fluid is putrid. The tubes are left in place until the cavity is obliterated by expansion of the lung, pleural drainage is small (less than 25 mL per day), infection is controlled with no fever (usually within 7 to 10 days), and any prior bronchopleural fistula is sealed airtight. Failure to respond with clinical improvement in 48 to 72 hours indicates inadequate drainage, occluded tube, improperly placed tube, debilitated host, inappropriate antibiotic selection, or severe pneumonia. The adequacy of tube placement may be evaluated with radiography or preferably computed tomography.

Open drainage with rib resection or decortication is required if the closed procedure fails. Indications are persistent signs of sepsis, failure to demonstrate reduction in cavity size, or inadequate removal of infected material despite reinsertion of tubes (2,17). Open drainage requires a pleural cavity with margins that are adherent to the chest wall. This usually occurs 1 to 2 weeks after thoracostomy drainage and can be demonstrated radiographically after the chest tube is opened. The procedure is performed in the operating room. Adhesions are lysed under direct vision and chest tubes are placed in appropriate sites, or a pleurocutaneous fistula is created (Eloesser procedure). Open drainage is seldom necessary when empyema is adequately treated early in its course.

During the late organizing phase, extensive fibrous material may compromise pulmonary function with a pleural peel and entrapment of the lung. This generally represents a complication of chronic empyema and requires decortication (21,23).

MORTALITY

There is considerable variation in mortalities reported for empyema in different series. This variation is perhaps best ascribed to variations in the population studied at the time of the report, studies from thoracic surgery versus medical services, the type of treatment used, and the distinction between mortality ascribed directly to empyema versus mortality with empyema as a contributing factor. However, even studies from the prepenicillin era, when 60% to 70% of cases were associated with pneumococcal pneumonia and involved patients with a relatively consistent demographic profile, mortalities ranged from 7% to 41% (25,35–38,75). During the antibiotic era, most studies have indicated mortalities ranging from 8% to 20% (3–12,76,77); these include series published in the 1990s (18,20–23) Of particular note is the report by Finland and Barnes (78) of 452 patients seen at Boston City Hospital. Approximately half were seen in the prepenicillin era and half thereafter, and there was minimal change between the results before and after the availability of penicillin. Factors that bore an ominous prognosis included the presence of a bronchopleural fistula, chronic empyema, nosocomial acquisition, cases involving aerobic gram-negative bacilli, old age (or adults versus children), and association with malignant neoplasms. By excluding patients with serious or ultimately lethal associated conditions, some investigators have reported mortality rates of only 3% to 6% (3,4,7,16,76).

REFERENCES

1. Bartlett JG. Bacterial infections of the pleural space. *Semin Respir Infect* 1988;3:309.
2. Light RW. A new classification of parapneumonic effusions and empyema. *Chest* 1995;108:299.
3. Yeh T, Hall D, Ellison R. Empyema thoracis: a review of 110 cases. *Am Rev Respir Dis* 1963;88:785.
4. Snider G, Saleh S. Empyema of the thorax in adults: review of 105 cases. *Dis Chest* 1968;54:12.
5. Weese W, Shindler E, Smith I, et al. Empyema of the thorax then and now. *Arch Intern Med* 1973;131:516.
6. Simmons E, Sauer P, Elkadi A, et al. Review of nontuberculous empyema at the University of Missouri Medical Center from 1957 to 1971. *J Thorac Cardiovasc Surg* 1972;64:578.
7. Varkey B, Rose H, Kutty K, et al. Empyema thoracis during a ten-year period. *Arch Intern Med* 1981;141:1771.
8. Mauroudis C, Symmonds J, Minagi H, et al. Improved survival in management of empyema thoracis. *J Thorac Cardiovasc Surg* 1981;82:49.
9. Grant D, Finley R. Empyema: analysis of treatment techniques. *Can J Surg* 1985;28:449.
10. Bartlett J, Thadepalli H, Gorbach S, et al. Bacteriology of empyema. *Lancet* 1974;1:338.
11. Benfield G. Recent trends in empyema thoracis. *Br J Dis Chest* 1981;75:358.
12. Lemmer J, Rotham M, Orringer M. Modern management of adult thoracic empyema. *J Thorac Cardiovasc Surg* 1985;90:849.
13. Mayo P. Early thoracotomy and decortication for nontuberculous empyema in adults with and without underlying disease: a 25-year review. *Am Surg* 1985;51:230.
14. LeBlanc K, Tucker W. Empyema of the thorax. *Surg Gynecol Obstet* 1984;158:66.
15. Meyerovitch J, Shohet I, Rubinstein E. Analysis of 37 cases of pleural empyema. *Eur J Clin Microbiol* 1985;4:337.
16. Geha A. Pleural empyema: changing etiologic, bacteriologic, and therapeutic aspects. *J Thorac Cardiovasc Surg* 1971;61:626.
17. Light RW. *Pleural diseases.* Baltimore: Williams & Wilkins, 1995.
18. Alfageme I, Munoz F, Pena N, Umbria S. Empyema of the thorax in adults: etiology, microbiologic findings, and management. *Chest* 1993;103:839.
19. Wiedemann HP, Rice TW. Lung abscess and empyema. *Semin Thorac Cardiovasc Surg* 1995;7:119.
20. LeMense GP, Strange C, Sahn SA. Empyema thoracis: therapeutic management and outcome. *Chest* 1995;107:1532.
21. deSousa A, Offner PJ, Moore EE, et al. Optimal management of complicated empyema. *Am J Surg* 2000;180:507.
22. Chen KY, Hsueh PR, Liaw YS. A 10-year experience with bacteriology of acute thoracic empyema with emphasis on *Klebsiella pneumoniae* in patients with diabetes mellitus. *Chest* 2000;117:1685.
23. Powell LL, Allen R, Brenner M, et al. Improved patient outcome after surgical treatment for loculated empyema. *Am J Surg* 2000;179:1.
24. Finland M. The significance of pneumococcal types in disease, including types IV to XXXII (Cooper). *Ann Intern Med* 1939;15:1531.
25. Ehler AA. Non-tuberculous thoracic empyema: collective review of literature from 1934 to 1939. *Int Abstr Surg* 1941;72:17.
26. Bartlett JG. Anaerobic bacterial infections of the lung and pleural space. *Clin Infect Dis* 1993;16[Suppl 4]:S248.
27. Molina JM, Leport C, Bure A, et al. Clinical and bacterial features of infections caused by *Streptococcus milleri*. *Scand J Infect Dis* 1991;23:659.
28. Finland M, Brown J, Ruegegger J. Anatomic and bacteriologic findings in infections with specific types of pneumococci, including types I to XXXII. *Arch Pathol* 1937;23:801.
29. Heffron R. Pneumonia. Cambridge, MA: Harvard University Press, 1939:566–585.
30. Keefer C, Rantz L, Rammelkamp C. Hemolytic streptococcal pneumonia and empyema: a study of 55 cases with special reference to treatment. *Ann Intern Med* 1941;14:1533.
31. Welch C, Tombridge T, Baker W, et al. Beta-hemolytic streptococcal pneumonia: report of an outbreak in a military population. *Am J Med Sci* 1961;242:157.
32. Fine MJ, Smith MA, Carson CA, et al. Prognosis and outcomes of patients with community-acquired pneumonia. *JAMA* 1996;275:134.
33. Deschamps C, Allen MS, Trastek VA, Pairolero PC. Empyema following pulmonary resection. *Chest Surg Clin North Am* 1994;4:583.
34. Bernard A, Pillet M, Goudet P, Viard H. Antibiotic prophylaxis in pulmonary surgery: a prospective randomized double-blind trial of flash cefuroxime versus forty-eight-hour cefuroxime. *J Thorac Cardiovasc Surg* 1994;107:896.
35. Novak S. Empyema thoracis: an analytical study of 500 cases with general remarks. *Med Clin North Am* 1939;23:1355.
36. Hochberg LA, Kramer B. Acute empyema of the chest in children: review of 300 cases. *Am J Dis Child* 1939;57:1310.
37. Shank P. Empyema of the lung: review of literature and analysis. *Am J Surg* 1944;66:224.
38. Beerens H, Tahon-Castel M. *Infection humaines a bacteries anarobes non-toxigenes.* Brussels: Academiques Européennes, 1965:92.
39. Stiles QR, Lindesmith GG, Tucker BL, et al. Pleural empyema in children. *Ann Thorac Surg* 1970;10:37.
40. Lutz A, Grooten O, Berger M. Considerations apropos of germs isolated in 638 cases of purulent pleurisy. *Strasbourg Med* 1963;2:119.
41. Sullivan K, O'Toole R, Fisher R, et al. Anaerobic empyema thoracis. *Arch Intern Med* 1973;131:521.
42. Caplan ES, Hoyt N, Rodrigues A, et al. Empyema occurring in the multiply traumatized patient. *J Trauma* 1984;24:785.
43. Brook I. Microbiology of empyema in children and adolescents. *Pediatrics* 1990;85:722.
44. Kelly JW, Morris MJ. Empyema thoracis: medical aspects of evaluation and treatment. *South Med J* 1994;87:1102.
45. Sokolowski JW Jr, Burgher LW, Jones FL Jr, et al. Guidelines for thoracentesis and needle biopsy of the pleura. *Am Rev Respir Dis* 1989;140:257.
46. Schabel SL. Imaging of pleural infections. *Semin Respir Infect* 1988;3:298.
47. Levin DL, Klein JS. Imaging techniques for pleural space infections. *Semin Resp Infect* 1999;14:31.
48. Storey D, Dines D, Coles D. Pleural effusion: a diagnostic dilemma. *JAMA* 1976;236:2183.
49. Sahn S, Targl DA, Good JT. Experimental empyema: time course and pathogenesis of pleural fluid acidosis and low pleural fluid glucose. *Am Rev Respir Dis* 1979;120:355.
50. Potts DE, Taryle DA, Sahn SA. The glucose-pH relationship in parapneumonic effusions. *Arch Intern Med* 1978;138:1378.
51. Heffner JE, Brown LK, Barbieri C, DeLeo JM. Pleural fluid chemical analysis in parapneumonic effusions: a meta-analysis. *Am J Respir Crit Care Med* 1995;151:1700.
52. Light RW, Rodriguez RM. Management of parapneumonic effusions. *Clin Chest Med* 1998;19:373.
53. Teixeira LR, Sasse SA, Villarino MA, et al. Antibiotic levels in empyema fluid. *Chest* 2000;117:1734.
54. Hughes CE, Van Scoy RE. Antibiotic therapy of pleural empyema. *Semin Respir Infect* 1991;6:94.
55. Light RW, Nguyen T, Mulligan ME, Sasse SA. The in vitro efficacy of varidase versus streptokinase or urokinase for liquefying purulent exudative material from locutated empyema. *Lung* 2000;178:13.
56. Henke CA, Leatherman JW. Intrapleurally administered streptokinase in the treatment of acute loculated nonpurulent parapneumonic effusions. *Am Rev Respir Dis* 1992;45:680.
57. Robinson LA, Moulton AL, Fleming WH, et al. Intrapleural fibrinolytic treatment of multiloculated thoracic empyemas. *Ann Thorac Surg* 1994;57:803.
58. Pollak JS, Passik CS. Intrapleural urokinase in the treatment of loculated pleural effusions. *Chest* 1994;105:868.

59. Miller JI Jr. The history of surgery of empyema, thoracoplasty, eloesser flap, and muscle flap transposition. *Chest Surg Clin North Am* 2000;10:45.
60. Frimodt-Moller P, Vejlsted H. Early surgical intervention in nonspecific pleural empyema. *J Thorac Cardiovasc Surg* 1985;33:41.
61. Morgan JF. Surgical management of pleural space infections. *Semin Respir Infect* 1988;3:383.
62. le Roux BT, Mohlala ML, Odell JA et al. Suppurative diseases of the lung and pleural space: empyema thoracis and lung abscess. *Curr Probl Surg* 1986;23:5.
63. Iioka S, Sawamura K, Mori T, et al. Surgical treatment of chronic empyema: a new one-stage operation. *J Thorac Cardiovasc Surg* 1985;90:179.
64. Okada M, Tsubota N, Yoshimura M, et al. Surgical treatment for chronic pleural empyema. *Surg Today* 2000;30:506.
65. Sasse S, Nguyen T, Teixeira LR, Light R. The utility of daily therapeutic thoracentesis for the treatment of early empyema. *Chest* 1999;116:1703.
66. Kaplan DK. Treatment of empyema thoracis. *Thorax* 1994;49:845.
67. Odell JA. Management of empyema thoracis. *J R Soc Med* 1994;87:466.
68. Strange C, Sahn SA. The clinician's perspective on parapneumonic effusions and empyema. *Chest* 1993;103:259.
69. Ashbaugh DG. Empyema thoracis: factors influencing morbidity and mortality. *Chest* 1991;99:1162.
70. Kearney SE, Davies CW, Davies RJ, Gleeson FV. Computed tomography and ultrasound in parapneumonic effusions and empyema. *Clin Radiol* 2000;55:542.
71. Yim AP, Ho JK, Lee TW, Chung SS. Thoracoscopic management of pleural effusions revisited. *Aust NZ J Surg* 1995;65:308.
72. Hunnam GR, Flower CD. Radiologically-guided percutaneous catheter drainage of empyemas. *Clin Radiol* 1988;39:121.
73. Stavas J, vanSonnenberg E, Casola G, Wittich GR. Percutaneous drainage of infected and noninfected thoracic fluid collections. *J Thorac Imaging* 1987;2:80.
74. O'Moore PV, Mueller PR, Simeone JF, et al. Sonographic guidance in diagnostic and therapeutic interventions in the pleural space. *AJR* 1987;149:1.
75. Maes U. Mortality of empyema analysis of 100 consecutive deaths from records of charity hospital in New Orleans. *J Thorac Surg* 1935;4:615.
76. Jess P, Brynitz, S, Friis Moller A. Mortality in thoracic empyema. *Scand J Thorac Cardiovasc Surg* 1984;18:85.
77. Cohn L, Blaisdell E. Surgical treatment of nontuberculous empyema. *Arch Surg* 1970;100:376.
78. Finland M, Barnes M. Changing ecology of acute bacterial empyema: occurrence and mortality at Boston City Hospital during 12 selected years from 1935 to 1972. *J Infect Dis* 1978;137:274.

Cardiovascular System

CHAPTER 60
Bloodstream Invasion

John G. Bartlett, John E. McGowan, Jr., and Jonas A. Shulman

Bloodstream invasion (which for the purposes of this chapter means the presence of bacteria, fungi, or mycobacteria in the bloodstream) remains a major problem for patient and physician alike. Bloodstream infections remain common, and new patterns of occurrence and cause have made it more difficult for the physician to provide appropriate treatment. Moreover, rates of bacteremia and fungemia are useful sentinel indicators for overall change in severe infections, because study of bloodstream invasion avoids some of the difficulties involved in defining infection at other sites (1).

This chapter reviews bloodstream invasion by bacteria, fungi, and mycobacteria. Endocarditis is excluded from the discussion because it is the subject of Chapter 62. Septic shock, which is often associated with bloodstream invasion, is covered separately as well (Chapter 61).

OCCURRENCE

Several investigators have defined a variety of sepsis syndromes, usually in association with trials of therapeutic agents given for a heterogeneous and broad range of severe illness. Systemic inflammatory response syndrome, sepsis, severe sepsis, and septic shock have all been defined and used in various studies (2,3). This presentation focuses on the classic and more conservative entity of bloodstream invasion as defined by demonstration of bacteremia, fungemia, or viremia. Such restriction may correlate with the definition of sepsis (a systemic inflammatory response syndrome caused by documented infection) in some studies and not in others, depending on whether a given study's authors accept documentation of the infection by culture from sources other than the bloodstream.

Approximately 300,000 to 500,000 cases of bacteremia occur annually in the United States, and between 20% and 30% of the affected patients die (4,5). The rate of discharge diagnoses reporting bloodstream invasion increased from 74 cases per 10,000 patients in 1979 to 110 to 180 per 10,000 in the 1990s (7). Table 60.1 lists incidence rates of bloodstream invasion for some hospitals reporting overall incidence rates for nosocomial or community-acquired infection or both since 1975 (8–41). Incidence rates are expressed in terms of admissions or discharges from the hospital. The hospitals represented reported markedly different characteristics and overall attack rates of nosocomial bacteremia and fungemia. The table shows that reported rates of nosocomial bacteremia have increased dramatically in the 1990s.

ETIOLOGIC FACTORS

Major changes have occurred in the cause of septicemia in the past few decades (42–46). The relative frequency of some organisms and organism groups in selected studies since 1991 is shown in Table 60.2 (16,26,46). Some of the changes are discussed in the following sections. In terms of microbial patterns, the most remarkable change has been the increasing rate of bacteremia due to gram-positive cocci, especially coagulase-negative staphylococci, *Staphylococcus aureus*, and enterococcus.

Polymicrobial Sepsis

In a longitudinal study of bloodstream invasion at Boston City Hospital from 1935 to 1972, single isolates from cases of nosocomial bloodstream invasion were the rule in the early years (47). In succeeding years, the average number of isolates per case gradually increased. This trend has continued to the present (4). Polymicrobial sepsis is as likely in community-acquired as in nosocomial bloodstream invasion (32). The likelihood of isolating multiple pathogens is particularly high for patients in intensive care, for children, for diabetic patients, for patients with burns, and for those with malignancies (48). In a study from France, 43% of patients with sepsis acquired in the intensive care unit (ICU) had polymicrobial infection, compared with 31% of those outside the ICU (2).

SEQUENTIAL EPISODES OF INFECTION IN THE SAME PATIENT AND AT MULTIPLE SITES

Not only are more organisms being found in each episode, but many patients now have more than one episode of bloodstream invasion (49).

TABLE 60.1. Occurrence of Bacteremia and Fungemia in Selected Incidence Studies Since 1975

Year	Location	Incidence (cases per 1,000 admissions or discharges)			Reference
		Overall	Community acquired	Nosocomial	
1975	Copenhagen, Denmark	7.2	3.5	3.7	8
1976	London, UK	1.3–6.6[a]			9
1977	Hackensack, NJ	5.6	3.3	2.3	10
1977	Houston, TX	3.8			11
1977	Madison, WI	3.4	2.2	1.2	12
1977	Atlanta, GA	14.7	9.9	4.8	13
1977	New York City, NY			1.5	14
1977	Charlottesville, VA			4.0	15
1974–1979	Bergen, Norway	4.3	2.1	2.4	16
1979	London, UK	6.1–8.0[b]			17
1981	Columbia, SC	2.8–15.4[c]	1.9–6.8	0.9–9.8	18
1981	Madison, WI			7.5	19
1981	Iowa City, IA			6.7	6
1982	Madison, WI	3.4			20
1983	Denver, CO	12.5	4.4	8.1	21
1984	Huddinge, Sweden	4.3	2.1	2.4	22
1985	Kuwait	10.9	6.8	4.1	23
1985	Newcastle, Australia	5.4	3.3	2.1	24
1985	Atlanta, GA			5.8	25
1970–1986	London, UK		4.3[e]	2.9[e]	26
1986	Columbia, SC	10.0[d]	4.9	5.1	27
1986	Virginia			2.6[f]	28
1984–1987	Vancouver, Canada	14.6			29
1987	Madison, WI	10.3			20
1987	Nottingham, UK	7.1			30
1987	Gainesville, FL; Iowa City, IA	2.6			31
1988	Barcelona, Spain	19.1	11.5	7.6	32
1979–1989	Berlin, Germany	8.1	3.8	4.3	33
1988–1989	Bergen, Norway	8.7	4.2	4.5	16
1981–1990	Oviedo, Spain	15.7			34
1990–1991	Hadyai, Thailand			15.5	35
1991	Iowa City, IA			21.3	6, 37
1989–1992	Newcastle, UK	11.7			36
1992	Iowa City, IA			18.4	6
1995	Denmark	9.6	6.8	2.8	38
1997	Tel Aviv		1.4		39
1998–1999	Saudi Arabia	23			40
1999–2000	Finland			2.2	41

[a]Range of annual figures for the 10-y period 1966–1975.
[b]Range of annual figures for the 5-y period 1972–1976.
[c]Range of figures for four hospitals in one city during the 3-y period 1977–1979.
[d]Mean value for four hospitals in one city during the 5-y period 1977–1981.
[e]Episodes of bacteremia from 1969 to 1989; rate was calculated by using discharges for 1988–1989.
[f]Combined data for average of 44 hospitals reporting data for 6 mo or more during the period 1978–1984.
Adapted in part from McGowan JE Jr: Septicaemia: changing patterns of causative organisms and underlying conditions. In: Shanson DC, ed. *Septicaemia and endocarditis: clinical and microbiological aspects.* London: Oxford University Press, 1989:8, by permission of Oxford University Press.

Gram-Positive Organisms

A dramatic increase has been noted in the cases of bacteremia caused by gram-positive cocci both in the United States and around the world (6). Infections with gram-positive bacilli are now becoming more frequent as well (5). In large measure this is due to increasing occurrence of antimicrobial resistance. Major organisms accounting for this change are listed below.

1. *Streptococcus pneumoniae.* This organism remains important in community-acquired infections, especially in association with pneumonia. Mortality has not changed significantly in the past few decades (50). Bacteremic pneumococcal strains resistant to penicillin and other commonly used antimicrobial including fluoroquinolones and macrolides have been associated with treatment failure (51,52). These strains are often multidrug resistant (53). This brings renewed interest in pneumococcal vaccine, which may reduce the risk of pneumococcal bacteremia in high-risk patients (54–57).

2. Group A and group B streptococci. Endemic cases of sepsis caused by group A streptococci are seen in both adults and children (58,59). Toxic shock syndrome may be part of the presentation of adults with bacteremia caused by group A streptococci (59,60). Group B streptococcal sepsis continues to occur with some frequency, especially in older persons and in those with serious underlying conditions (61,62).

3. *Enterococcus.* Enterococcal sepsis can have severe consequences; overall mortality is 30% or higher, with significantly higher mortality in burn patients and other immunocompromised patients (62). The appearance of resistance to vancomycin, added to resistance to aminoglycosides and

TABLE 60.2. Relative Frequency of Selected Organisms in Community-Acquired and Nosocomial Bloodstream Invasion from Two Studies Published Since 1991

Organism group and selected organisms	Relative frequency of organism (range) (%)	
	Community-acquired cases[a]	Nosocomial cases[b]
Gram-positive cocci		
Staphylococcus aureus	7–22	18–20
Coagulase-negative staphylococci	<2–11	8–15
Enterococcal species	<2–2	5–11
S. pneumoniae	7–13	0–2
Viridans streptococcus	2–10	0–4
β-Hemolytic streptococci	4–5	0–2
Gram-positive rods	0–3	0–3
Gram-negative aerobic bacilli and coccobacilli		
Escherichia coli	21–27	16–19
Klebsiella species	<2–4	9–12
Proteus species	3–4	5–6
Pseudomonas species	0–5	4–9
Haemophilus influenzae	4–6	<1
Neisseria meningitidis	3–6	<1
Anaerobes		
Bacteroides species	1–6	<1–5
Candida species	<2	1–8

Does not include data from the National Nosocomial Infections Surveillance (NNIS) Study of the CDC36 as the NNIS program uses a definition of "primary bloodstream invasion" that differs from that in the included studies.
[a]Range of values for cases of community-acquired bacteremia in 1969–1989 (23) and 1988–1997 (13, 43).
[b]Range of values for cases of nosocomial bacteremia in 1969–1989 (23) and 1988–1989 (13).

β-lactam drugs, has made therapy for enterococcal bacteremia much more difficult although most strains are sensitive to linezolid and most vancomycin-resistant *Enterococcus faecium* are sensitive to quinupristin-dalfopristin (63). Prior use of broad-spectrum cephalosporins has been implicated as a risk factor for nosocomial bacteremia with *Enterococcus faecalis* (64). Other risk factors include organ transplantation, hematologic malignancy, renal failure, severe underlying illness, and use of multiple antibiotics (65).

4. Nonenterococcal group D, group C, and group G streptococci. The ability of the hospital laboratory to perform routine serogrouping of streptococcal isolates has shed new light on these organisms as a source of sepsis. Group C streptococcal bacteremia affects primarily older patients with severe underlying diseases and has an underlying focus in skin or soft tissue (66,67). Group G streptococcal bacteremia is commonly a community-acquired infection, seen especially in parenteral drug abusers and older patients (67,68). Biotyping of *Streptococcus bovis* has distinguished strains closely associated with bacteremia and colonic neoplasm (biotype 1) from other bacteremic strains of the organisms (59).

5. *Streptococcus viridans*. Soft tissue, skin, and respiratory tract infections are the most prominent conditions associated with sepsis caused by this group of organisms (70). Neutropenic patients, especially those undergoing bone marrow transplantation, are at higher risk (71–73). Treatment is complicated by the presence of high-level resistance to aminoglycosides and resistance to penicillins in some strains (74).

6. *Staphylococcus aureus*. This organism has continued to be a frequent source of both community-acquired and nosocomial bloodstream invasion in the United States and in other countries (75–78). Mortality remains high in series of bacteremia, especially those associated with methicillin-resistant strains. Methicillin-resistant strains are prominent in many hospitals and are becoming more frequent in community-acquired infections as a clonally distinct group (78,79). When bacteremic episodes recur they are often associated with the presence of intravascular foreign bodies (e.g., catheters) (77). Other risks are injection drug use, advanced HIV infection, nasal colonization, and antibiotic exposure (65). The risk of endocarditis is high so echocardiograms are commonly advocated (80). Antibiotic treatment is complicated for nosocomial strains of multiple-resistant *S. aureus* because these are usually resistant to most antibiotics other than vancomycin, linezolid, and quinupristin-dalfopristin (81,82). Vancomycin resistance has been reported (83).

7. Coagulase-negative staphylococci and other components of endogenous flora. Many isolates of coagulase-negative staphylococci from blood do not represent true pathogens (84,85). Nevertheless, in the right host setting the organism must be considered virulent (86). Occurrence is often related to the presence of indwelling vascular catheters (77,87). Bacteremia related to this organism has been shown to increase mortality and duration of hospital stay (88). Treatment is complicated by resistance to common antibiotics and the frequent need to remove artificial devices including central catheters (77,81).

Other components of endogenous flora are now known to have a potential similar to that of coagulase-negative staphylococci for infecting the patient whose host defenses are sufficiently impaired. For example, antibiotic-resistant corynebacteria cause bacteremia, especially in patients with compromised host defenses (89,90). Vancomycin-resistant gram-positive bacilli such as *Lactobacillus* spp. are usually community-acquired (91). In immunosuppressed patients, *Bacillus* spp. organisms can cause septicemia, especially in association with Hickman and other long-term indwelling catheters (92).

Gram-Negative Bacilli

Bacteremia caused by these organisms remains common (5,71,93). In large measure this is due to highly vulnerable patients and extensive use of antibiotics increasing occurrence of antimicrobial resistance. Among major organisms causing bacteremia in this group are

1. Enterobacteriaceae. Organisms of this group (e.g., *Escherichia coli*, *Klebsiella* spp., *Enterobacter* spp., *Proteus mirabilis*, *Serratia marcescens*) continue to be a major cause of gram-negative aerobic bacillary bacteremia (5,77,94,95). Bloodstream invasion caused by gram-negative bacilli has increased, perhaps because the organisms translocate more efficiently from the gastrointestinal tract than do other bacteria (96). Although antimicrobial resistance has been a problem in some areas, it has been less so in others (97). *E. coli* is usually the most common blood culture isolate in community-acquired infections (26,94,98). In some settings, antimicrobial resistance is as frequent in community-acquired bacteremic strains of *E. coli* as in those of nosocomial origin (75,99). *Klebsiella pneumoniae* continues to be important in both nosocomial and community-acquired bacteremias (5,94,100). *Enterobacter* spp. have accounted for a sizable proportion (between 3% and 10%) of nosocomial

bacteremic infections since the 1970s in both the United States and Europe (5,94,101–103). The role of *Enterobacter* spp. has been enhanced by frequent resistance to multiple antimicrobial agents and by association with vascular catheters and prior antimicrobial therapy (94,102,103). *Salmonella* bacteremia remains prominent in developing nations, in children, and in patients with AIDS (104,105). The major contexts in which bacteremic Enterobacteriaceae have been noted are hospital outbreaks associated with intestinal colonization, urinary catheterization, and resistance to many antimicrobial agents.

2. *Pseudomonas* spp. For decades, *Pseudomonas aeruginosa* has been an appreciable source of both community-acquired and nosocomial bacteremias. High case-fatality rates have characterized cases associated with this organism (106). Factors especially important in fatal outcomes of *P. aeruginosa* infection are shock, granulocyte count less than $500/mm^3$, inappropriate antimicrobial therapy, development of secondary foci of infection, and presence of AIDS (106–108). Community-acquired cases of bacteremia caused by *Pseudomonas* species other than *P. aeruginosa* have been rare, but nosocomial infections with these organisms are seen with increased frequency (75,109). Nosocomial infections with these organisms tend to appear in association with contamination of a commercial product such as respiratory therapy equipment, disinfectants, blood gas analyzers, or blood products (110).

3. Gram-negative bacilli other than *Pseudomonas*. So-called nonfermenters (gram-negative aerobic bacilli that do not ferment the sugars commonly tested in clinical laboratories) include *Pseudomonas* spp., *Acinetobacter*, *Flavobacterium*, *Aeromonas*, and *Stenotrophomonas* species. Of these, *Acinetobacter* spp. are probably the most prominent. Although the organism on occasion is found in community disease, its major importance is as a nosocomial pathogen. The spectrum of illness caused by *Acinetobacter* spp. ranges from mild and possibly self-limiting to serious and life-threatening. Life-threatening infection is especially likely in those with compromised host defenses, burns, and trauma, especially after antimicrobial agents have been given (111). Nosocomial strains frequently demonstrate resistance to many antimicrobial agents. *Flavobacterium meningosepticum* has caused a variety of nosocomial infections, and bacteremia is one of the situations in which it has been found (112). Most hospital outbreaks associated with *Flavobacterium* spp. have involved environmental contamination of fluids, notably solutions, medications for respiratory therapy, or antiseptics. *Aeromonas* spp. cause infection more frequently in patients with underlying hepatic cirrhosis (113). Several pseudo-outbreaks with *Stenotrophomonas* (formerly *Xanthomonas*) *maltophilia* frequently make it difficult to assess the clinical impact of blood isolates of this organism (109).

Gram-Negative Coccobacilli

Sepsis caused by *Haemophilus influenzae* type B has nearly disappeared since the introduction of an effective vaccine (114). *Haemophilus* bacteremia in adults occurs more frequently in the elderly or patients with AIDS and is usually due to nontypable strains of *H. influenza* (115).

Meningococcemia still occurs in epidemic as well as endemic fashion (116). *Branhamella* (*Moraxella*) *catarrhalis* bacteremia is typically accompanied by pneumonia in adults but may present without an obvious focus in neutropenic patients (117).

Anaerobes

Cases of bacteremia associated with anaerobes have declined substantially in frequency in nearly all centers presumably due to the empiric use of appropriate antibiotics in settings where they are most likely to cause bacteremia, especially intra-abdominal sepsis (118–121). *Bacteroides fragilis* and *Clostridium* spp. remain the most frequently reported anaerobic organisms causing bacteremia. Virtually all obligate anaerobes are sensitive to metronidazole, imipenem or meropenem, chloramphenicol, and any beta-lactam–beta-lactamase combination; cefoxitin and clindamycin are also usually active (120). Mortality associated with organisms of the *B. fragilis* group is still appreciable (120,122).

Fungi

Rates of fungemia have increased at most hospital centers (5,6,123–126). For bloodstream invasion by *Candida* spp., attributable mortality is high and hospital stay is prolonged (106). Previous antimicrobial therapy, indwelling intravascular catheters, parenteral alimentation, urinary catheterization, central intravascular lines, burns, surgery, and neutropenia are significant risk factors for candidal bloodstream invasion (124–126). *Candida albicans* accounts for 60% to 80% of isolates; *C. glabrata*, *C. tropicalis*, *C parapsilosis*, and *C. krusei* account for most of the rest. Catheter-associated sepsis has also increased the frequency and virtually always requires catheter removal (77). Some strains, especially *C. krusei* and some *C. glabrata*, are resistant to fluconazole (127).

PATHOGENESIS

Organisms frequently enter the bloodstream, but host defenses usually clear these invaders without adverse effects on the patient. When host defenses become compromised or the organism's virulence is enhanced, illness may result (128). Host defenses may be impaired by the patient's primary disease, but bloodstream invasion today arises commonly in association with therapy (e.g., antimicrobial agents, immunosuppressives) or with instruments used for the patient's care (26). Even when no underlying disorder is present, consequences of bacteremia may be severe (128).

Infection may occur as a result of invasion by an exogenous source. Today, however, bacteremic infection is more frequently due to organisms that are usually among the endogenous flora of the patient or that have replaced or joined the usual microbial flora at one or more body sites. Changes in usual flora are especially frequent after hospitalization.

Bacteremia occurs more frequently in neonates and older persons than in persons in age groups in between (129). Septicemia in children has different implications and a different pattern than that in adults (130). In the elderly, bloodstream infection acquired in the community is often as severe as cases acquired in the hospital, in contrast to the greater hazard from nosocomial infection in most other age groups (30,75).

The relationship between sepsis and hematologic malignancy is especially prominent (16,26) as is the link between sepsis and other neoplasms (106,131). Intravenous drug abusers are at higher risk of septicemia than many other population groups and rates of endocarditis are about 1,000-fold greater in this population (132). Other frequently associated infections include soft tissue, abscess, and cellulitis (68).

Although opportunistic infections are considered more characteristic of those infected with HIV, bacteremia and fungemia still occur with considerable frequency (133). The most common causes of bacteremia are *S. aureus*, line-associated *S. epidermidis*, *P. aeruginosa*, Salmonella, *Mycoplasma avium*, and *Mycoplasma tuberculosis* (105,134,135).

Other groups at high risk of bloodstream invasion include patients with liver or splenic dysfunction (98,136), patients with burns (137), patients in ICUs, patients in long-term care facilities (138), patients with implanted foreign bodies, and patients with indwelling urinary catheters. In particular, the profusion of intravascular catheters used in providing modern medical care in both hospital and community settings has led to greater risks of sepsis than in the past (77). These features account in large part for the increased frequency of bloodstream invasion in patients in ICUs (2,16,94,124).

Previous antimicrobial therapy is associated with the presence of antimicrobial resistance in bloodstream isolates (64,65). However, the cause and effect relationship is by no means a general one and probably holds only for specific organism-drug combinations (65,97,134).

CLINICAL MANIFESTATIONS

No specific clinical findings are diagnostic of bacteremia or fungemia (138–140). Early signs of bloodstream invasion are nonspecific: malaise, lethargy, confusion, nausea, vomiting, and/or hyperventilation. Progression to a more classic history of fever, sweating, and shivering (chills) may or may not be noted (141). Hypothermia may occur and is a sign of a particularly bad prognosis. On occasion, the only subjective manifestation may be a general feeling of unease or apprehension.

Objective signs of bloodstream invasion may be few. Fever may be absent, especially in the elderly, the newborn, and patients receiving immunosuppressive drugs. In the absence of septic shock (see Chapter 61), the patient may or may not have tachycardia or tachypnea. Various rashes, evidence of embolization, or bleeding and clotting abnormalities may be present, especially in association with certain invading organisms (meningococcus, *Salmonella typhi*, *P. aeruginosa*). Skin findings accompany some cases (142), and gastrointestinal symptoms, mental confusion symptoms, and mental or other brain dysfunction may be noted in others. Acute respiratory distress syndrome (shock lung) may appear during the course. Renal manifestations become prominent as an acute or subacute process (140).

More prominent may be the signs and symptoms related to an underlying site of infection from which the organisms reach the bloodstream. Infections of the urinary tract, surgical wounds, and gastrointestinal tract (including the biliary tree) are especially likely sources for bloodstream invasion; these often have associated local manifestations. Infants and children with fever of unclear etiology may have occult bacteremia, and their evaluation often includes blood culture (130,141).

Changes in the white blood cell differential count and sustained neutrophilia often accompany sepsis. However, neither vital signs nor white blood cell count may be abnormal in bacteremic patients with AIDS (143). Leukopenia or neutropenia may be characteristic of some infections (e.g., typhoid fever); however, in cases related to other pathogens neutropenia sometimes occurs and often indicates a poor prognosis. Of course, many patients with nosocomial bacteremia have extremely low neutrophil counts because of cancer chemotherapy or immunosuppressive drugs. Isolated thrombocytopenia is more frequently observed than disseminated intravascular coagulation

(140). At times, however, clotting disturbances may produce serious sequelae.

DIAGNOSIS

Early recognition of bacteremia and its complications is the most important part of care (140,144). The physician must maintain a healthy suspicion for bloodstream invasion, by searching for the clinical clues that lead to culture of blood, ancillary diagnostic testing, and/or empirical therapy (145). Blood culture results have had a measurable positive impact on antibiotic treatment (146). However, the cost-effectiveness of blood culture in some settings remains unclear (147). Studies have led to models that predict patients at high and low risk for bacteremia (148,149) as well as algorithms developed to help determine whether or not a positive blood culture result represents contamination (150).

Microbiologic cultures must be done before antimicrobial agents are given. Blood cultures are the most important part of the process, but cultures of other potential sources of bloodstream invasion are appropriate when present (concurrent urinary tract infection, surgical wound infection, pneumonia, skin sites of sepsis). Culture of other sites is also necessary when complications of sepsis (e.g., meningitis) are suspected. Gram staining of material from local sites of infection (e.g., sputum, wound exudate, abscess drainage) may be useful. Additional nonculture tests (e.g., buffy coat smears, polymerase chain reaction, or other amplification techniques) are sometimes helpful; however, their use has not been beneficial in most situations and is, in general, reserved for carefully selected cases. Molecular typing has been used to distinguish infection versus contamination with coagulase-negative staphylococci (84). False-positive blood culture results can lead to diagnostic confusion and incorrect treatment, with grave consequences for the patients (84,151,152).

The recovery of infecting organisms is dependent on methods used for culture (145). For example, at least 20, and preferably 30 mL, should be collected with each venipuncture (153–155). Two separate venipunctures should be done as a routine practice. The blood for culture should be drawn separately from blood for other determinations, such as blood gas, blood chemistry, and hematologic studies; if this is not possible, the blood culture vials must be filled before the other containers. Failing to observe this order can lead to epidemics of pseudobacteremia (152). Blood cultures should be obtained by separate venipunctures, but there is no evidence that any particular interval between the collections is more efficient in demonstrating bacteremia (155). Culture obtained through venous catheters are equally sensitive compared to peripheral blood, but more likely to be contaminated (156). Arterial rather than venous blood for cultures has little justification. The effectiveness of adding ion-exchange resins to blood culture media to remove antimicrobials in blood is controversial, as is the use of iodine rather than iodophor antiseptics before the skin is punctured.

A major change in the past decade has been marked and rapid improvements in laboratory techniques for isolating and identifying organisms from culture of blood (151–159). These technologic advances alone may account for some of the absolute increase in frequency of septicemia seen in the past five decades. The classic way to detect organisms in blood cultures was to incubate a liquid medium; observe it for a number of days for hemolysis, gas bubbles, or other change in physical characteristics; and then subculture to solid media if evidence of the presence of microorganisms was found. Newer methods detect gas production or other metabolic activity by organisms.

This can be signaled by a variety of methods (e.g., infrared spectroscopy, color change in an indicator, pressure measurement). Instrumented approaches for detecting these signals are now widely used (157). Another approach to diagnosis is lysis-centrifugation, in which the initial blood culture is treated with chemical agents to lyse the blood cells, centrifuged to concentrate any organisms, and then plated on a variety of media specific for bacteria, fungi, mycobacteria, or other organisms. These different methods vary in their ability to detect different groups of organisms. Lysis-centrifugation is more sensitive for detection of noncandidal fungi and mycobacteria in blood and is regarded as the method of choice for recovering these organisms (159). However, for bacterial infection this method is more labor-intensive than use of automated instruments (160,161). No single method is satisfactory in identifying the presence of all bacterial organisms in blood or in recovering detected organisms in culture. Thus, in most hospitals one system is designated as the standard set for routine use to detect most common blood pathogens; supplemental methods are made available for special circumstances.

Processing of cultures depends on the system used. Most systems provide for distribution of the blood from venipuncture among at least two vials, one for aerobic incubation and one vial for anaerobic incubation. The time for which vials must be incubated before the culture is called negative varies with the processing method; with most of the newer systems, a 72-hour period of incubation detects most of the common pathogens (162). In view of the frequency with which polymicrobial cases now occur (discussed previously), the laboratory must continue to look for pathogens in a blood culture even after one organism is recovered. Further steps in the processing of the vials are crucial if the laboratory intends to obtain a good yield; these steps have been reviewed in detail.

When a patient with bloodstream invasion responds well clinically, follow-up blood cultures are rarely indicated. However, if the patient fails to improve despite what seems to be appropriate therapy, cultures must be repeated in an attempt to detect "breakthrough" bacteremia (163). This condition may indicate inadequate antimicrobial therapy, an undrained focus of infection, or an infected prosthesis. Emergence of resistance to antimicrobial drugs during therapy is perhaps more likely in patients with *Enterobacter* spp. bacteremia (101). These patients must be monitored closely for this possibility.

TREATMENT

For most cases of bloodstream invasion, prompt initiation of aggressive, appropriate therapy is vital (139,140,144). The crude mortality rate for nosocomial bacteremia is 27% and the attributable mortality rate is estimated at 15% (7). Beginning correct therapy before complications develop can reduce the mortality in bacterial sepsis (164) and probably affects mortality in cases related to other organisms as well. Treatment includes several steps other than antimicrobial therapy (3,140). Ancillary measures to manage complications such as hypovolemia, metabolic problems, and organ dysfunction (e.g., renal failure) must be started immediately. Intravenous fluids, oxygen, or β-adrenergic agents may be required.

Antimicrobial drugs are important not only for clearing the bloodstream but also for preventing secondary infection from developing as a result of bloodstream invasion, especially in *S. aureus* bacteremia. Dealing with bloodstream invasion is easiest when information is available about the site of infection, the identity of the infecting agent, or results of susceptibility testing for the causative organism. The site of infection can often

be determined and at times can help the physician plan initial antimicrobial therapy and adjunctive measures (e.g., drainage of pus, removal of a foreign body) when antibiotics are chosen. However, it is rare to have information about the exact infecting pathogen or its susceptibilities when initial therapy must be given. Thus, empirical therapy based on site of infection and results of immediate tests (e.g., Gram stain, discussed later) is the rule rather than the exception. Treatment regimens are empirically chosen to try to eradicate the most likely etiologic agents in the hope that the choice can be modified on the basis of culture results and other subsequent information. Appropriate smears and cultures must be obtained before antimicrobial therapy is begun.

No single antimicrobial regimen is adequate to deal with all episodes of bloodstream invasion (165). The choice depends on the range of organisms commonly encountered in a given institution and the susceptibility patterns prevalent in these organisms. These factors determine whether single or combination therapy is preferred (106,166). Thus, empirical therapy for infection must be tailored for the individual patient, but a variety of suitable regimens should be available at most centers.

Therapy should cover the sites of infection that seem likely from initial examination of the patient. No symptom or sign can clearly differentiate infection caused by gram-negative bacilli from those caused by gram-positive cocci or other organism groups, although appropriate Gram stains from localized sites of infection may help make this distinction. Some laboratory data may assist the clinician at this point; for example, a suspected urinary tract infection may be treated more logically after a urine specimen is examined. This can help in determining whether organisms are present and (if they are) deciding whether the infecting organism is a gram-positive coccus (suggesting *Enterococcus* as the source of sepsis), a gram-negative rod (suggesting a different group of antibacterial drug choices to deal with gram-negative aerobic bacilli), or yeast (suggesting *Candida* spp. or other fungi).

The status of the patient's host defenses is another major factor. A patient with defective defenses has less margin of error for tolerating an inappropriate drug regimen. The prescriber should err on the side of increasing the spectrum of coverage for a brief period in such patients. The possible emergence of antimicrobial resistance during the course of therapy must be considered when patients fail to respond (168).

COURSE

Bloodstream infection increases mortality (169). Nosocomial cases increase attributable mortality, lead to an alarming increase in length of acute hospital stay, and substantial extra costs for care (170). The fearsome toll of septicemia is dramatically illustrated by Table 60.3, which portrays case-fatality rates from a variety of the studies reported in Table 60.1.

Patients in intensive care experience case-fatality rates in the neighborhood of 50% (2). This holds true for both directly related mortality (24% case-fatality rate for nosocomial cases versus 13% in community-acquired sepsis) and unrelated deaths. Bacteremia associated with lower respiratory tract sites or abdominal wound infections is associated with the highest mortality rates and the highest costs. Bloodstream invasion arising from other sources can be dealt with more readily in today's medical practice.

Antibiotic resistance is thought to increase risk of death. However, neither vancomycin resistance nor gentamicin resistance has led to greater mortality in patients with bacteremic enterococcal infection in comparison with those bacteremic with

TABLE 60.3. Case Fatality Rates Associated With Bloodstream Invasion in Selected Series Published Since 1975

Year published	Location	Case-fatality rates (%)			
		Overall	Community acquired	Nosocomial	Reference
1975	Copenhagen, Denmark	25	18	33	8
1977	Hackensack, NJ	35	37	32	10
1977	Madison, WI	20	—	—	12
1977	New York City NY	—	—	17	14
1977	Charlottesville, VA	—	—	34	15
1979	London, UK	42[a]		—	17
1981	Columbia, SC	—	11–28[b]	23–58[b]	18
1981	Madison, WI	—		40	19
1981	Iowa City, IA	—		51	6
1982	Madison, WI	21		—	20
1983	Denver, CO	42	21	52	21
1984	Huddinge, Sweden	13	—	—	22
1985	Newcastle, Australia	—	—	29	23
1986	Columbia, SC	30[c]	20[c]	40[c]	27
1986	Berlin, Germany	22	—	—	33
1987	Nottingham, UK	29	23	36	30
1987	Gainesville, FL; Iowa City, IA	20	—	—	31
1988	Barcelona, Spain	—	—	18	32
1989	Berlin, Germany	21	—	—	33
1989	Bergen, Norway	19	—	—	16
1990–1991	Hadyai, Thailand	—	—	37	35
1989–1992	Newcastle, UK	7	9	5	36
1992	Iowa City, IA	—	—	32	6
1996	Denmark	16	—	—	38
2000	Saudi Arabia	34	—	—	40
2002	Tel Aviv	—	21%	—	39
2002	Finland	16	—	—	41

[a]Range of annual figures for the 5-y period 1972–1976.
[b]Range of figures for four hospitals in one city during the 3-y period 1977–1979.
[c]Mean value for four hospitals in one city during the 5-y period 1977–1981.
Adapted in part from McGowan JE. Septicaemia: changing patterns of causative organisms and underlying conditions. In: Shanson DC, ed. *Septicaemia and endocarditis: clinical and microbiological aspects.* London: Oxford University Press, 1989:9; by permission of Oxford University Press.

susceptible strains, after adjustment for factors such as underlying illness (171).

PREVENTION

Rapid and effective attention to other sites of infection can prevent the infection from reaching a level of severity at which bloodstream invasion can occur. The key to minimizing the occurrence of nosocomial bloodstream invasion is effective control of initial infection, as many hospital-acquired infections may lead to sepsis. Proper use of instruments, especially intravascular catheters, is the key to preventing their infection and resultant bloodstream invasion (172). New vaccines against common agents of bacteremia are in clinical trial, but their effectiveness and cost-efficiency have not yet been established. Use of prophylactic antimicrobial drugs to attempt to "decontaminate" the gut and other endogenous sites for nosocomial pathogens has been proposed, but carefully controlled studies have not documented a benefit for this.

REFERENCES

1. Freeman J, McGowan JE Jr. Methodologic issues in hospital epidemiology. I. Rates, case-finding, and interpretation. *Rev Infect Dis* 1981;3:658.
2. Brun-Buisson C, Doyon F, Carlet J, et al. Incidence, risk factors, and outcome of severe sepsis and septic shock in adults. A multicenter prospective study in intensive care units. *JAMA* 1995;274:968.
3. Bernard RG. Efficacy and safety of recombinant human activated protein C for severe sepsis. *N Engl J Med* 2001;344:699.
4. Wenzel RP. Anti-endotoxin monoclonal antibodies: a second look. *N Engl J Med* 1992;326:1151.
5. Edmond MB. Nosocomial bloodstream infections in U.S. hospitals: a three-year analysis. *Clin Infect Dis* 1999;29:239.
6. Pittet D, Wenzel RP. Nosocomial bloodstream infections. Secular trends in rates, mortality, and contribution to total hospital deaths. *Arch Intern Med* 1995;155:1177.
7. Wenzel RP, Edmond MB. The impact of hospital-acquired bloodstream infections. *Emerg Infect Dis* 2001;7:14.
8. Jepsen OB, Kerner B. Bacteremia in a general hospital: a prospective study of 102 consecutive cases. *Scand J Infect Dis* 1975;7:179.
9. Williams GT, Houang ET, Shaw EJ, Tabaqchali S. Bacteraemia in a London teaching hospital 1966–75. *Lancet* 1976;2:1291.
10. Setia U, Gross PA. Bacteremia in a community hospital. *Arch Intern Med* 1977;137:1698.
11. Quadri SMH, Evans LJ, Wende RD, Williams RP. Bacteremia in a metropolitan teaching hospital. *Tex Med* 1977;73:59.
12. Scheckler WE. Septicemia in a community hospital 1970 through 1973. *JAMA* 1977;237:1938.
13. McGowan JE Jr, Parrott PL, Duty VP. Nosocomial bacteremia: potential for prevention. *JAMA* 1977;237:2727.
14. Holzman RS, Florman AL, Toharsky B. The clinical usefulness of an ongoing bacteremia surveillance program. *Am J Med Sci* 1977;274:13.
15. Rose RC, Hunting KJ, Townsend TR, Wenzel RP. Morbidity/mortality and economics of hospital-acquired bloodstream infections: a controlled study. *South Med J* 1977;70:1267.
16. Haug JB, Harthug S, Kalager T, et al. Bloodstream infections at a Norwegian university hospital, 1974–1979 and 1988–1989: changing etiology, clinical features, and outcome. *Clin Infect Dis* 1994;19:246.
17. Abeysundere RL, Bradley JM, Chipping P, et al. Bacteraemia in the Royal Free Hospital 1972–1976. *J Infect* 1979;1:127.

18. Brenner ER, Bryan CS. Nosocomial bacteremia in perspective: a community-wide study. *Infect Control* 1981;2:219.

19. Maki DG. Epidemic nosocomial bacteremias. In: Wenzel RP, ed. *CRC handbook of hospital-acquired infections.* West Palm Beach, FL: CRC Press, 1981:371.

20. Scheckler WE, Scheibel W, Kresge D. Temporal trends in septicemia in a community hospital. *Am J Med* 1991;91[Suppl 3B]:90S.

21. Weinstein MP, Reller LB, Murphy JR, Lichtenstein KA. The clinical significance of positive blood cultures: a comprehensive analysis of 500 episodes of bacteremia and fungemia in adults. I. Laboratory and epidemiologic observations. *Rev Infect Dis* 1983;5:35.

22. Ljungman P, Malmborg AS, Nystrom B, Tillegard A. Bacteremia in a Swedish university hospital: A one-year prospective study in 1981 and a comparison with 1975–76. *Infection* 1984;12:243.

23. Elhag KM, Mustafa AK, Sethi SK. Septicaemia in a teaching hospital in Kuwait. I: Incidence and aetiology. *J Infect* 1985;10:17.

24. Duggan JM, Oldfield GS, Ghosh HK. Septicaemia as a hospital hazard. *J Infect* 1985;6:406.

25. McGowan JE Jr. Changing etiology of nosocomial bacteremia and fungemia and other hospital-acquired infections. *Rev Infect Dis* 1985;7[Suppl]:S357.

26. Gransden WR. Predictors for bacteraemia. *J Hosp Infect* 1991;18[Suppl A]:308.

27. Bryan CS, Reynolds KL, Brenner ER. Analysis of 1,186 episodes of gram-negative bacteremia in non-university hospitals: the effects of antimicrobial therapy. *Rev Infect Dis* 1986;5:629.

28. Morrison AJ Jr, Freer CV, Searcy MA, et al. Nosocomial bloodstream infections: Secular trends in a statewide surveillance program in Virginia. *Infect Control* 1986;7:550.

29. Roberts FJ, Geere IW, Coldman A. A three-year study of positive blood cultures, with emphasis on prognosis. *Rev Infect Dis* 1991;13:34.

30. Ispahani P, Pearson NJ, Greenwood D. An analysis of community and hospital-acquired bacteraemia in a large teaching hospital in the United Kingdom. *Q J Med* 1987;241:427.

31. Haddy RI, Klimberg S, Epting RJ. A two-center review of bacteremia in the community hospital. *J Fam Pract* 1987;24:253.

32. Gatell JM, Trilla A, Latorre X, et al. Nosocomial bacteremia in a large Spanish teaching hospital: analysis of factors influencing prognosis. *Rev Infect Dis* 1988;10:203.

33. Geerdes HF, Ziegler D, Lode H, et al. Septicemia in 980 patients at a university hospital in Berlin: prospective studies during 4 selected years between 1979 and 1989. *Clin Infect Dis* 1992;15:991.

34. Vazquez F, Mendoza MC, Villar MH, et al. Survey of bacteraemia in a Spanish hospital over a decade (1981–1990). *J Hosp Infect* 1994;26:111.

35. Jamulitrat S, Meknavin U, Thongpiyapoom S. Factors affecting mortality, outcome and risk of developing nosocomial bloodstream infection. *Infect Control Hosp Epidemiol* 1994;15:163.

36. Gray J, Pedler SJ. The changing face of bacteraemia. *J Hosp Infect* 1994;28:317.

37. Pittet D, Davis CS, Li N, Wenzel RP. Identifying the hospitalized patient at risk for nosocomial bloodstream infection: a population-based study. *Proc Assoc Am Physicians* 1997;109:58.

38. Jensen AG, Kirstein A, Jensen I, et al. A 6-month prospective study of hospital-acquired bacteremia in Copenhagen county. *Scand J Infect Dis* 1996;28:601.

39. Siegman-Igra Y, Fourer B, Orni-Wasserlauf R, et al. Reappraisal of community-acquired bacteremia: a proposal of a new classification for the spectrum of acquisition of bacteremia. *Clin Infect Dis* 2002;34:1431.

40. Akbar DH. Adult bacteremia. Comparative study between diabetic and non-diabetic patients. *Saudi Med J* 2000;21:40.

41. Lyytikainen O, Lumio J, Sarkkinen H, et al. Nosocomial bloodstream infections in Finnish hospitals during 1999–2000. *Clin Infect Dis* 2002;35:e14.

42. Weinstein MP, Towns ML, Quartey SM, et al. The clinical significance of positive blood cultures in the 1990's. *Clin Infect Dis* 1997;24:584.

43. Edmond MB, Wallace SE, McClish DK, et al. Nosocomial bloodstream infections in U.S. hospitals: a three-year analysis. *Clin Infect Dis* 1999;29:239.

44. Pittet D. Nosocomial bloodstream infections. In: Wenzel RP, et al, ed. *Prevention and control of nosocomial infection,* 3rd ed. Baltimore: Williams & Wilkins, 1997:711–769.

45. Filice GA, Van Etta LL, Darby CP, Fraser DW. Bacteremia in Charleston County, South Carolina. *Am J Epidemiol* 1986;123:128.

46. Horan TC, White JW, Jarvis WR, et al. Nosocomial infection surveillance, 1984. *MMWR CDC Surveill Summ* 1986;35:17SS.

47. McGowan JE Jr, Barnes MW, Finland M. Bacteremia at Boston City Hospital: occurrence and mortality during 12 selected years (1935–1972), with special reference to hospital-acquired cases. *J Infect Dis* 1975;132:316.

48. Reuben AG, Musher DM, Hamill RJ, Broucke I. Polymicrobial bacteremia: clinical and microbiologic patterns. *Rev Infect Dis* 1989;11:161.

49. Capdevila JA, Almirante B, Pahissa A, et al. Incidence and risk factors of recurrent episodes of bacteremia in adults. *Arch Intern Med* 1994;154:411.

50. Afessa B, Greaves WL, Frederick WR. Pneumococcal bacteremia in adults: a 14-year experience in an inner-city university hospital. *Clin Infect Dis* 1995;21:345.

51. Whitney CG. Increasing prevalence of multidrug-resistant *Streptococcus pneumoniae* in the United States. *N Engl J Med* 2000;243:1917.

52. Davidson R. Resistance to levofloxacin and failure of treatment in pneumococcal pneumonia. *N Engl J Med* 2002;346:747.

53. Hyde TB. Macrolide resistance among invasive *Streptococcus pneumoniae* isolates. *JAMA* 2001;286:1857.

54. Breiman RF. Evaluation of effectiveness of the 23-valent pneumococcal capsular polysaccharide vaccine in HIV-infected patients. *Arch Intern Med* 2000;160:2633.

55. Cristenson B. Effects of large scale intervention with influenza and 23-valent pneumococcal vaccines in adults aged 65 years or older: a prospective study. *Lancet* 2001;357:1008.

56. Watson L, Wilson BJ, Waugh N. Pneumococcal polysaccharide vaccine: a systemic review of clinical effectiveness in adults. *Vaccine* 2002;20:2166.

57. Farr BM, Johnston BL, Cobb DK, et al. Preventing pneumococcal bacteremia in patients at risk: results of a matched case-control study. *Arch Intern Med* 1995;155:1336.

58. Moses AE, Mevorach D, Rahav G, et al. Group A streptococcus bacteremia at the Hadassah Medical Center in Jerusalem. *Clin Infect Dis* 1995;20:1393.

59. Sharkawy A. Severe group A streptococcal soft tissue infections in Ontario: 1992–1996. *Clin Infect Dis* 2002;34:454.

60. Forni AL, Kaplan EL, Schlievert PM, Roberts RB. Clinical and microbiological characteristics of severe group A streptococcus infections and streptococcal toxic shock syndrome. *Clin Infect Dis* 1995;21:333.

61. Jackson LA, Hilsdon R, Farley MM, et al. Risk factors for group B streptococcal disease in adults. *Ann Intern Med* 1995;123:415.

62. Colford JM Jr, Mohle-Boetani J, Vosti KL. Group B streptococcal bacteremia in adults. Five years' experience and a review of the literature. *Medicine (Baltimore)* 1995;74:176.

63. Vergis EN. Determinants of vancomycin resistance and mortality rates in enterococcal bacteremia. *Ann Intern Med* 2001;135:484.

64. Noskin GA, Peterson LR, Warren JR. *Enterococcus faecium* and *Enterococcus faecalis* bacteremia: acquisition and outcome. *Clin Infect Dis* 1995;20:296.

65. Safdar N, Maki DG. The commonality of risk factors for nosocomial colonization and infection with antimicrobial-resistant *Staphylococcus aureus,* enterococcus, gram-negative bacilli, *Clostridium difficile* and Candida. *Ann Intern Med* 2002;136:834.

66. Carmeli Y, Schapiro JM, Neeman D, et al. Streptococcal group C bacteremia. Survey in Israel and analytic review. *Arch Intern Med* 1995;155:1170.

67. Kristensen B, Schonheyder HC. A 13-year survey of bacteraemia due to β-haemolytic streptococci in a Danish county. *J Med Microbiol* 1995;43:63.

68. O'Connor PG, Selwyn PA, Schottenfeld RS. Medical care for injection-drug users with human immunodeficiency virus infection. *N Engl J Med* 1994;331:450.

69. Ruoff KL, Miller SI, Garner CV, et al. Bacteremia with *Streptococcus bovis* and *Streptococcus salivarius:* clinical correlates of more accurate identification of isolates. *J Clin Microbiol* 1989;27:305.

70. Jacobs JA, Pietersen HG, Stobberingh EE, Soeters PB. Bacteremia involving the "*Streptococcus milleri*" group: analysis of 19 cases. *Clin Infect Dis* 1994;19:704.

71. Collin BA. Evolution, incidence and susceptibility of bacterial bloodstream isolates from 519 bone marrow transplant patients. *Clin Infect Dis* 2001;33:947.

72. Carratala J, Alcaide F, Fernandez-Sevilla A, et al. Bacteremia due to viridans streptococci that are highly resistant to penicillin: increase among neutropenic patients with cancer. *Clin Infect Dis* 1995;20:1169.

73. Rolston KVI, Elting LS, Bodey GP. Bacteremia due to viridans streptococci in neutropenic patients. *Am J Med* 1995;99:450.

74. Bochud P-Y, Calandra T, Francioli P. Bacteremia due to viridans streptococci in neutropenic patients: a review. *Am J Med* 1994;97:256.

75. Lark RL. Four year prospective evaluation of community-acquired bacteremia: epidemiology, microbiology and patient outcome. *Diagn Microbiol Infect Dis* 2001;41:15.

76. Morin CA. Population-based incidence and characteristics of community-onset *Staphylococcus aureus* infections with bacteremia in four metropolitan Connecticut areas, 1998. *J Infect Dis* 2001;184:1029.

77. Mermel LA. guidelines for management of intravascular catheter-related infection. *Clin Infect Dis* 2001;32:1249.

78. Baba T. Genome and virulence determinants of high virulence community-acquired MRSA. *Lancet* 2002;359:1819.

79. Groom AV. Community-acquired methicillin-resistant *Staphylococcus aureus* in a rural American Indian community. *JAMA* 2001;12:1201.

80. Rosen AB. Transesophageal echocardiography can be used to direct antibiotic decision for bacteremia. *Ann Intern Med* 1999;130:810.

81. Deem DJ. Survey of infections due to *Staphylococcus* species. *Clin Infect Dis* 2001;32[Suppl 2]:S114.

82. Stevens DL. Linezolid versus vancomycin for the treatment of methicillin-resistant *Staphylococcus aureus* infections. *Clin Infect Dis* 2002;34:1481.

83. Centers for Disease Control and Prevention. *Staphylococcus aureus* resistant to vancomycin—United States, 2002. *MMWR* 2002;51:565.

84. Seo SK. Molecular typing of coagulase-negative staphylococci from blood

cultures does not correlate with clinical criteria for true bacteremia. *Am J Med* 2000;109:697.

85. Viagappan M, Kelsey MC. The origin of coagulase-negative staphylococci isolated from blood cultures. *J Hosp Infect* 1995;30:217.

86. Rupp ME, Archer GL. Coagulase-negative staphylococci: pathogens associated with medical progress. *Clin Infect Dis* 1994;19:231.

87. Dahmash NS, Chowdhury MN, Fayed DF. Coagulase-negative staphylococcal bacteraemia with special reference to septic shock: experience in an intensive care unit. *J Infect* 1994;29:295.

88. Martin MA, Pfaller MA, Wenzel RJ. Coagulase-negative staphylococcal bacteremia: mortality and hospital stay. *Ann Intern Med* 1989;110:9.

89. Tumbarello M, Tacconelli E, Del Forno A, et al. *Corynebacterium striatum* bacteremia in a patient with AIDS. *Clin Infect Dis* 1994;18:1007.

90. Wood CA, Pepe R. Bacteremia in a patient with non-urinary-tract infection due to *Corynebacterium urealyticum*. *Clin Infect Dis* 1994;19:367.

91. Woodford N, Johnson AP, Morrison D, Speller DCE. Current perspectives on glycopeptide resistance. *Clin Microbiol Rev* 1995;8:585.

92. Blue SR, Singh VR, Saubolle MA. *Bacillus licheniformis* bacteremia: Five cases associated with indwelling central venous catheters. *Clin Infect Dis* 1995;20:629.

93. Uzun O, Akalin HE, Hayran M, Unal S. Factors influencing prognosis in bacteremia due to gram-negative organisms: evaluation of 448 episodes in a Turkish university hospital. *Clin Infect Dis* 1992;15:866.

94. Diekema DJ. Survey of bloodstream infections due to gram-negative bacilli. *Clin Infect Dis* 1999;29:595.

95. Chamberland S, L'Ecuyer J, Lessard C, et al. Antibiotic susceptibility profiles of 941 gram-negative bacteria isolated from septicemic patients throughout Canada. *Clin Infect Dis* 1992;15:615.

96. Steffen EK, Berg RD, Deitch EA. Comparison of translocation rates of various indigenous bacteria from the gastrointestinal tract to the mesenteric lymph node. *J Infect Dis* 1988;157:1032.

97. McGowan JE Jr. Do intensive hospital antibiotic control programs prevent the spread of antibiotic resistance? *Infect Control Hosp Epidemiol* 1994;17:478.

98. Thulstrup AM. Population-based study of the risk and short-term prognosis for bacteremia in patients with liver cirrhosis. *Clin Infect Dis* 2000;31:1357.

99. Gransden WR, Eykyn SJ, Phillips I, Rowe B. Bacteremia due to *Escherichia coli*: a study of 861 episodes. *Rev Infect Dis* 1990;12:1008.

100. Lee KH, Hui KP, Tan WC, Lim TK. *Klebsiella* bacteraemia: a report of 101 cases from National University Hospital, Singapore. *J Hosp Infect* 1994;27:299.

101. Chow JW, Fine MJ, Shlaes DM, et al. *Enterobacter* bacteremia: clinical features and emergence of antibiotic resistance during therapy. *Ann Intern Med* 1991;115:585.

102. Al Ansari N, McNamara EB, Cunney RJ, et al. Experience with *Enterobacter* bacteraemia in a Dublin teaching hospital. *J Hosp Infect* 1994;27:69.

103. Weischer M, Kolmos HJ. Retrospective 6-year study of *Enterobacter* bacteraemia in a Danish university hospital. *J Hosp Infect* 1992;20:15.

104. Ramos JM, Garcia-Corbiera P, Aguado JM, et al. Clinical significance of primary vs. secondary bacteremia due to nontyphoid *Salmonella* in patients without AIDS. *Clin Infect Dis* 1994;19:777.

105. Galofre J, Moreno A, Mensa J, et al. Analysis of factors influencing the outcome and development of septic metastasis or relapse in *Salmonella* bacteremia. *Clin Infect Dis* 1994;18:873.

106. Chatzinikolaou I. Recent experience with *Pseudomonas aeruginosa* bacteremia in patients with cancer: retrospective analysis of 245 episodes. *Arch Intern Med* 2000;160:501.

107. Fergie JE, Shema SJ, Lott L, et al. *Pseudomonas aeruginosa* bacteremia in immunocompromised children: analysis of factors associated with a poor outcome. *Clin Infect Dis* 1994;18:390.

108. Mendelson MH, Gurtman A, Szabo S, et al. *Pseudomonas aeruginosa* bacteremia in patients with AIDS. *Clin Infect Dis* 1994;18:886.

109. Gales AC. Characterization of *Pseudomonas aeruginosa* isolates: occurrence rates, antimicrobial susceptibility patterns and molecular typing in the global SENTRY antimicrobial surveillance program, 1997–1999. *Clin Infect Dis* 2001;32[Suppl 2]:S146.

110. Henderson DK, Baptiste R, Parrillo J, Gill VJ. Indolent epidemic of *Pseudomonas cepacia* bacteremia and pseudobacteremia in an intensive care unit traced to a contaminated blood gas analyzer. *Am J Med* 1988;84:75.

111. Tilley PAG, Roberts FJ. Bacteremia with *Acinetobacter* species: risk factors and prognosis in different clinical settings. *Clin Infect Dis* 1994;18:896.

112. Pokrywka M, Viazano K, Medvick J, et al. A *Flavobacterium meningosepticum* outbreak among intensive care patients. *Am J Infect Control* 1993;21:139.

113. Ko W-C, Chuang Y-C. *Aeromonas* bacteremia: review of 59 episodes. *Clin Infect Dis* 1995;20:1298.

114. Bothner. J, Lelyveld S, Losek JD, Cunningham SJ. *Haemophilus influenzae* bacteremia: a vanishing entity. *Pediatr Emerg Care* 1995;11:127.

115. Najm WI, Cesario TC, Spurgeon L. Bacteremia due to *Haemophilus* infections: a retrospective study with emphasis on the elderly. *Clin Infect Dis* 1995;21:213.

116. Powars D, Larsen R, Johnson J, et al. Epidemic meningococcemia and purpura fulminans with induced protein C deficiency. *Clin Infect Dis* 1993;17:254.

117. Ioarmidis JPA, Worthington M, Griffiths JK, Snydman DR. Spectrum and significance of bacteremia due to *Moraxella catarrhalis*. *Clin Infect Dis* 1995;21:390.

118. Dorsher CW, Rosenblatt JE, Wilson WR, Ilstrup DM. Anaerobic bacteremia: decreasing rate over a 15-year period. *Rev Infect Dis* 1991;13:633.

119. Zaidi AK, Knaut AL, Mirrett S, Reller LB. Value of routine anaerobic blood cultures for pediatric patients. *J Pediatr* 1995;127:263.

120. Nguyen MH. Antimicrobial resistance and clinical outcome of bacteroides bacteremia: findings of a multicenter prospective observational trial. *Clin Infect Dis* 2000;30:870.

121. Arzese A, Trevisan R, Menozzi MG. Anaerobe-induced bacteremia in Italy: a nationwide survey. *Clin Infect Dis* 1995;20[Suppl 2]:S230.

122. Redondo MC, Arbo MDJ, Grindlinger J, Snydman DR. Attributable mortality of bacteremia associated with the *Bacteroides fragilis* group. *Clin Infect Dis* 1995;20:1492.

123. Beck-Sague CM, Jarvis WR, National Nosocomial Infections Surveillance System. Secular trends in the epidemiology of nosocomial fungal infection in the United States, 1980–1990. *J Infect Dis* 1993;167:1247.

124. Blumberg HM. Risk factors for Candidal bloodstream infections in surgical intensive care unit patients. *Clin Infect Dis* 2001;33:177.

125. Sobel J, Rex J. Invasive candidiasis: turning risk into a practical prevention policy? *Clin Infect Dis* 2001;33:187.

126. Pfaller MA. International surveillance of bloodstream infections due to Candida species. *J Clin Microbiol* 2001;39:3254.

127. Liebowitz LD. A two year global evaluation of the susceptibility of Candida species to fluconazole by disk diffusion. *Diag Microbiol Infect Dis* 2001;4:27.

128. Amit M, Pitlik SD, Samra Z, et al. Bacteremia in patients without known underlying disorders. *Scand J Infect Dis* 1994;26:605.

129. Gransden WR, Eykyn SJ, Phillips I. Septicaemia in the newborn and elderly. *J Antimicrob Chemother* 1994;34[Suppl A]:101.

130. Baker MD, Bell LM, Avner JR. Outpatient management without antibiotics of fever in selected infants. *N Engl J Med* 1993;329:1437.

131. Beebe JL, Koneman EW. Recovery of uncommon bacteria from blood: association with neoplastic disease. *Clin Microbiol Rev* 1995;8:336.

132. Wilson LE. Prospective study of infective endocarditis among injection drug users. *J Infect Dis* 2002;185:1761.

133. Vugia DJ, Kiehlbauch JA, Yeboue K, et al. Pathogens and predictors of fatal septicemia associated with human immunodeficiency virus infection in Ivory Coast, West Africa. *J Infect Dis* 1993;168:564.

134. Jacobson MA, Gellermann H, Chambers H. *Staphylococcus aureus* bacteremia and recurrent staphylococcal infection in patients with acquired immunodeficiency syndrome and AIDS-related complex. *Am J Med* 1988;85:172.

135. Chin DP, Reingold AL, Horsburgh CR Jr, et al. Predicting *Mycobacterium avium* complex bacteremia in patients infected with human immunodeficiency virus: a prospectively validated model. *Clin Infect Dis* 1994;19:668.

136. Jong GM, Hsiue TR, Chen CR, et al. Rapidly fatal outcome of bacteremic *Klebsiella pneumoniae* pneumonia in alcoholics. *Chest* 1995;107:214.

137. McManus AT, Mason AD Jr, McManus WF, Pruitt BA Jr. A decade of reduced gram-negative infections and mortality associated with improved isolation of burned patients. *Arch Surg* 1994;129:1306.

138. Richardson JP. Bacteremia in the elderly. *J Gen Intern Med* 1993;8:89.

139. Cunha BA. Antibiotic treatment of sepsis. *Med Clin North Am* 1995;79:551.

140. Rivers E. Early goal-directed therapy in the treatment of severe sepsis and septic shock. *N Engl J Med* 2001;345:1368.

141. Finch RG. Septicaemia: clinical features. In: Shanson DC, ed. *Septicaemia and endocarditis: clinical and microbiological aspects*. London: Oxford University Press, 1989:49.

142. Kingston ME, Mackey D. Skin clues in the diagnosis of life-threatening infections. *Rev Infect Dis* 1986;8:1.

143. Saviteer SM, Samsa GP, Rutala WA. Nosocomial infections in the elderly. Increased risk per hospital day. *Am J Med* 1988;84:661.

144. Natsch S. Earlier initiation of antibiotic treatment for severe infections after interventions to improve the organization and specific guidelines in the emergency department. *Arch Intern Med* 2000;160:1317.

145. Chandrasekar PH, Brown WJ. Clinical issues of blood cultures. *Arch Intern Med* 1994;154:841.

146. Schonheyder HC, Hojbjerg T. The impact of the first notification of positive blood cultures on antibiotic therapy: a one-year survey. *APMIS* 1995;103:37.

147. Chalasani NP, Valdecanas MA, Golpal AK, et al. Clinical utility of blood cultures in adult patients with community-acquired pneumonia without defined underlying focus. *Chest* 1995;108:932.

148. Mylotte JM, Pisano MA, Ram S, et al. Validation of a bacteremia prediction model. *Infect Control Hosp Epidemiol* 1995;16:203.

149. Pfitzenmeyer P, Decrey H, Auckenthaler R, Michel JP. Predicting bacteremia in older patients. *J Am Geriatr Soc* 1995;43:230.

150. Bates DW, Lee TH. Rapid classification of positive blood cultures. Prospective validation of a multivariate algorithm. *JAMA* 1992;267:1962.

151. Emmanuel FXS, Aucken H, Watt B, et al. False-positive blood cultures from contaminated ESR tubes. *Lancet* 1993;341:111.

152. Jumaa PA, Chattopadhyay B. Pseudobacteraemia. *J Hosp Infect* 1994;27:167.

153. Mermel LA, Maki DG. Detection of bacteremia in adults: consequences of culturing an inadequate volume of blood. *Ann Intern Med* 1993;119:270.

154. Kellogg JA, Bankert DA, Manzella JP, et al. Occurrence and documentation of low-level bacteremia in a community hospital's patient population. *Am J Clin Pathol* 1995;104:524.
155. Li J Plorde JJ, Carlson LG. Effects of volume and periodicity on blood cultures. *J Clin Microbiol* 1994;32:2829.
156. Everts RJ, Vinson EN, Adholla PO, et al. Contamination of catheter drawn blood cultures. *J Clin Microbiol* 2001;39:3393.
157. Schwabe LD Thomson RB Jr, Flint KK, Koontz FP. Evaluation of BACTEC 9240 blood culture system by using high-volume aerobic resin media. *J Clin Microbiol* 1995;33:2451.
158. Wilson ML, Weinstein MP, Mirrett S, et al. Controlled evaluation of BacT/Alert standard anaerobic and FAN anaerobic blood culture bottles for the detection of bacteremia and fungemia. *J Clin Microbiol* 1995;33:2265.
159. Lyon R, Woods G. Comparison of the BacT/Alert and isolator blood culture systems for recovery of fungi. *Am J Clin Pathol* 1995;103:660.
160. Cockerill FR, Torgerson CA, Reed GS, et al. Clinical comparison of Difco ESP, Wampole Isolator, and Becton Dickinson Septi-Chek aerobic blood culturing systems. *J Clin Microbiol* 1996;34:20.
161. Pohlman JK, Kirkley BA, Easley KA, Washington JA. Controlled clinical comparison of Isolator and BACTEC 9240 Aerobic/F resin bottle for detection of bloodstream infections. *J Clin Microbiol* 1995;33:2525.
162. Masterson KC, McGowan JE Jr. Detection of positive blood cultures by the Bactec NR660. The clinical importance of five versus seven days of testing. *Am J Clin Pathol* 1988;90:91.
163. Weinstein MP, Reller LB: Clinical importance of "breakthrough" bacteremia. *Am J Med* 1984;76:175.
164. Gross PA, Barrett TL, Dellinger EP, et al. Quality standard for the treatment of bacteremia. *Clin Infect Dis* 1994;18:428.
165. Medical Letter Consultants. The choice of antibacterial drugs. *Med Lett* 2001;43:69.
166. Korvick JA, Bryan CS, Farber B, et al. Prospective observational study of *Klebsiella* bacteremia in 230 patients: outcome for antibiotic combinations versus monotherapy. *Antimicrob Agents Chemother* 1992;36:2639.
167. Wiener J, Itokazu G, Nathan C, et al. A randomized, double-blind, placebo-controlled trial of selective digestive decontamination in a medical-surgical intensive care unit. *Clin Infect Dis* 1995;20:861.
168. Siebert JD, Thomson RB Jr, Tan JS, Gerson LW. Emergence of antimicrobial resistance in gram-negative bacilli causing bacteremia during therapy. *Am J Clin Pathol* 1993;100:47.
169. Bates DW, Pruess KE, Lee TH. How bad are bacteremia and sepsis? Outcomes in a cohort with suspected bacteremia. *Arch Intern Med* 1995;155:593.
170. Pittet D, Tarara D, Wenzel RP. Nosocomial bloodstream infection in critically ill patients. Excess length of stay, extra costs, and attributable mortality. *JAMA* 1994;271:1598.
171. Shay DK, Maloney SA, Montecalvo M, et al. Epidemiology and mortality risk of vancomycin-resistant enterococcal bloodstream infection. *J Infect Dis* 1995;172:993.
172. Maki DG. Yes, Virginia, aseptic technique is very important: maximal barrier precautions during insertion reduce the risk of central venous catheter-related bacteremia. *Infect Control Hosp Epidemiol* 1994;15:227.

CHAPTER 61

Sepsis

David W. Hines, Jeffrey M. Lisowski,
Roger C. Bone, and John G. Bartlett

Sepsis, the inflammatory response to an infection, is a leading cause of death in intensive care units (1). Mortality rates range from 20% to 90% despite both our growing understanding of the pathogenesis of sepsis and advances in its therapy (1–7). Every year in the United States, there are an estimated 500,000 cases of sepsis; and only 55% to 65% of patients survive (7–10). Clearly, early recognition of sepsis and appropriate therapy before shock ensues are paramount in reducing the high mortality (11–15).

This chapter reviews some of the microbiologic and host factors related to sepsis, its pathogenesis, and its protean clinical manifestations. This chapter also provides practical recommendations on optimal therapy for this medical emergency and a brief review of potentially useful adjunctive therapies involving the various mediators of sepsis that are currently under investigation.

DEFINITIONS

As investigators delineate the pathogenesis of sepsis and the inflammatory response to it, new and confusing terms have arisen to describe disease states that defy pigeonholing into separate and discrete categories. Sepsis, septic shock, sepsis syndrome, systemic inflammatory response syndrome (SIRS), and other terms have been applied to various groups of patients whose responses to therapy may be divergent.

To better understand sepsis and therefore better treat patients, consistent definitions must be employed (16). To this end, a consensus conference met in August 1991 to provide a set of definitions that could be applied to patients with sepsis and its sequelae (17) (Fig. 62.1).

SIRS may be associated with either infectious or noninfectious injuries (e.g., pancreatitis, trauma, and burns) and can be identified by the presence of at least two of the following manifestations:

1. Body temperature greater than 38°C or less than 36°C
2. Heart rate greater than 90 beats per minute
3. Tachypnea with a respiratory rate of more than 20 breaths per minute, or arterial carbon dioxide tension ($Paco_2$) less than 32 mm Hg
4. White blood cell counts greater than 12,000/mm^3 or less than 4,000/mm^3, or more than 10% immature forms (bands)

These criteria are by no means specific in identifying septic patients, but they are quite sensitive (18).

The patient with sepsis meets all the criteria for SIRS, of which it is a subset; however, it is the result of an infection. Severe sepsis is defined as sepsis associated with organ dysfunction, perfusion abnormalities, or hypotension (Table 61.1). Septic shock is sepsis with hypotension despite adequate fluid resuscitation. Multiorgan dysfunction syndrome emphasizes the search for early signs of organ dysfunction, rather than waiting for its failure.

From one large prospective epidemiologic study, it was evident that there is a clinical progression from SIRS to sepsis to severe sepsis and septic shock (18). There was also a progressive increase in mortality rates along this continuum, from 7% to 16% to 20% and 46%, respectively. In subgroups of patients meeting two, three, and all four criteria for SIRS, mortality rates increased directly with the number of criteria present (19).

Others have suggested using severity-of-illness scales to predict outcome more accurately (16). Given the protean manifestations of sepsis and the unpredictable response in an individual patient, these scoring systems are perhaps more useful to compare groups of patients in clinical trials.

The rationale for making the new definitions broad based and standardized is twofold. Foremost is the rapid identification and treatment of potentially septic patients, and second is to improve research efforts in comparative trials of new therapies for septic patients.

MICROBIOLOGY AND HOST FACTORS

Sepsis may complicate infections with bacteria, viruses, rickettsiae, mycobacteria, fungi, and parasites. Gram-positive organisms were responsible for most cases of bacteremias in the preantibiotic era (10). Gram-negative infections emerged during the antibiotic era and eventually surpassed bacteremias with gram-positive organisms (8–11,15). The reasons for this may be related to (a) antibiotic pressure; (b) use of invasive devices in a nosocomial environment; and (c) immunosuppression. Gram-negative sepsis and septic shock became synonymous,

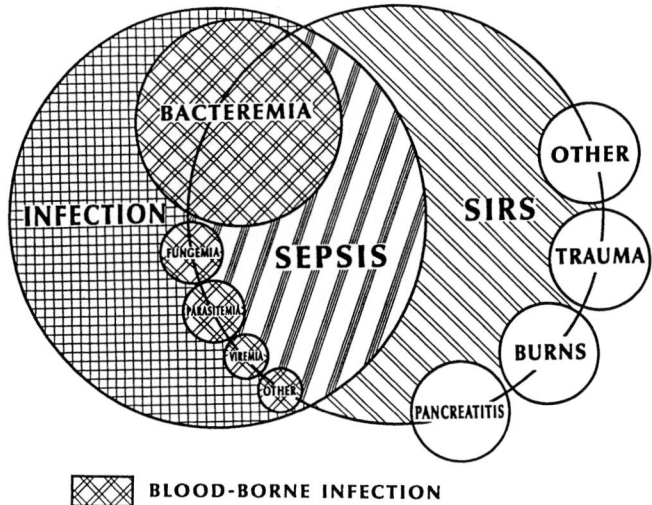

BLOOD-BORNE INFECTION

Figure 61.1. The interrelationship among systemic inflammatory response syndrome, sepsis, and infection.

which has in part contributed to the confusion surrounding sepsis.

More recently, gram-positive organisms have reemerged as important pathogens in sepsis (20–25). In a review of several studies of sepsis, gram-positive infections accounted for about one half of the cases (23–26). Factors that predispose patients to infections with gram-positive organisms include (a) the aggressive use of catheters and prosthetic devices, (b) antibi-otic pressure [methicillin-resistant *Staphylococcus aureus* (MRSA), vancomycin-resistant enterococci, etc.], and (c) immunosup-pressed states and chemotherapy (27).

Although it is impossible to clinically distinguish gram-negative or gram-positive bacterial sepsis from that caused by other pathogens, knowledge of predisposing host factors can give valuable clues to organisms of particular importance (27,28) (Table 61.2). Oncologists, well experienced with septicemia, have learned that gram-negative bacterial sepsis is rapidly fa-tal, whereas sepsis with gram-positive bacteria progresses less rapidly (27,28). Whether this experience can be generalized is unclear.

The nature of the underlying illness markedly influences the likelihood of surviving an episode of gram-negative bacteremia (2,3,5,11,12). In patients with rapidly fatal diseases, it is diffi-cult even to show that antibiotics increase survival at all (12). In patients with nonfatal or ultimately fatal conditions, however, appropriate antibiotic use seems to correlate with improved sur-vival (2,4,11,12,15). Infections with some organisms, for exam-ple, *Pseudomonas* species, may have a higher mortality (11,12). Whether this is related to properties of the bacteria or is just an association with an underlying disease remains to be proved. Other factors that seem to be associated with an increased mor-tality are listed in Table 61.3.

CLINICAL MANIFESTATIONS

Classic Signs

Fever, chills, and hypotension are classic signs of septic shock and should prompt cultures of blood and other likely sources of infection. Two and three sets of blood cultures from a bacteremic

---

TABLE 61.1. New Definitions for Sepsis and Related Disorders[a]

Infection	A microbial phenomenon characterized by an inflammatory response to the presence of microorganisms or the invasion of normally sterile host tissue by those organisms.
Bacteremia	The presence of viable bacteria in the blood (the presence of other organisms in the blood should be described in a similar manner—viremia, fungemia, and so on).
Systemic inflammatory response syndrome (SIRS)	The systemic inflammatory response to a variety of severe clinical insults, including infection, pancreatitis, ischemia, multiple trauma and tissue injury, hemorrhagic shock, immune-mediated organ injury, and exogenous administration of inflammatory mediators such as tumor necrosis factor or other cytokines. SIRS is manifested by (but not limited to) two or more of the following conditions: • Temperature: >38°C or <36°C • Heart rate: >90 beats/min • Respiratory rate: >20 breaths/min or arterial carbon dioxide tension of <32 mm Hg • White cell count: >12,000 cells/mm^3, <4,000 cells/mm^3, or >10% immature (band) forms These changes should represent an acute alteration from baseline in the absence of another known cause for the abnormalities.
Sepsis	The systemic response to infection. This response is identical to SIRS, except that it must result from infection.
Severe sepsis	Sepsis associated with organ dysfunction, perfusion abnormalities, or hypotension. Perfusion abnormalities may include (but are not limited to) lactic acidosis, oliguria, and an acute alteration in mental status. Hypotension is defined as a systolic blood pressure <90 mm Hg or a reduction of >40 mm Hg from baseline in the absence of another known cause for hypotension.
Septic shock	Sepsis with hypotension (as defined above) despite adequate fluid resuscitation, in conjunction with perfusion abnormalities (as defined above). Patients who are receiving inotropic or vasopressor agents may not be hypotensive at the time that perfusion abnormalities are measured, yet they may still be considered to have septic shock.
Multiorgan dysfunction syndrome (MODS)	Presence of altered organ function in an acutely ill patient, such that homeostasis cannot be maintained without intervention. Primary MODS is the direct result of a well-defined insult in which organ dysfunction occurs early and can be directly attributable to the insult itself. Secondary MODS develops as a consequence of a host response and is identified within the context of SIRS.

[a]These definitions were developed at a consensus conference jointly sponsored by the American College of Chest Physicians and the Society for Critical Care Medicine held in August 1991.
Source: From Bone RC. Why new definitions of sepsis and organ failure are needed. *Am J Med* 1993;95:348–350 with permission.

TABLE 61.2. Pathogens Associated with Immunodeficiency

Condition	Usual conditions	Pathogens
Neutropenia (<500/mL)	Cancer chemotherapy; adverse drug reaction; leukemia	Bacteria: Aerobic GNB (coliforms and pseudomonads); *Staphylococcus aureus*, viridans streptococcus, *Staphylococcus epidermidis* Fungi: *Aspergillus, Candida* species
Cell-mediated immunity	Organ transplantation; HIV infection; lymphoma (especially Hodgkin's disease); corticosteroid therapy	Bacteria: *Listeria, Salmonella, Nocardia,* mycobacteria (*Mycobacterium tuberculosis* and *Mycobacterium avium*), *Legionella* Viruses: CMV, herpes simplex, varicella-zoster, JC virus Parasites: *Pneumocystis carinii; Toxoplasma; Strongyloides stercoralis;* cryptosporidia Fungi: *Candida, Cryptococcus, Histoplasma, Coccidioides*
Hypogammaglobulinemia or dysgammaglobulinemia	Multiple myeloma; congenital or acquired deficiency; chronic lymphocytic leukemia	Bacteria: *Streptococcus pneumoniae, Haemophilus influenzae* (type B) Parasites: *Giardia* Viruses: Enteroviruses
Complement deficiencies C2, 3 C5 C6-8 Alternative pathway	Congenital	Bacteria: *S. pneumoniae, H. influenzae* *S. pneumoniae, S. aureus, Enterobacteriaceae* *Neisseria meningitidis* *S. pneumoniae, H. influenzae,* salmonella
Hyposplenism	Splenectomy; hemolytic anemia	*S. pneumoniae, H. influenzae, Capnocytophaga canimorsus*
Defective chemotaxis	Diabetes, alcoholism, renal failure, lazy leukocyte syndrome, trauma, SLE	*S. aureus,* streptococci, *Candida*
Defective neutrophilic killing	Chronic granulomatous disease, myeloperoxidase deficiency	Catalase-positive bacteria: *S. aureus, Echerichia coli; Candida* species

CMV, cytomegalovirus; GNB, gram-negative bacteria; HIV, human immunodeficiency virus; SLE, systemic lupus erythematosus.

patient will yield the organism 89% and 99% of the time, respectively (29). Nevertheless, only 30% of patients who have the classic features of sepsis will have positive blood culture results (6). Many patients, especially the elderly and debilitated, may not manifest the classic symptoms. Hypothermia may be seen with gram-negative sepsis and usually indicates a poorer prognosis (4,12,15). Hyperventilation may precede any other changes in vital signs and can lead to respiratory alkalosis. Diaphoresis, apprehension, and a change in mental status, none of which is specific for sepsis, may also occur early.

Skin Findings

Cutaneous manifestations of sepsis due to gram-negative bacilli are varied and include cellulitis, erythema multiforme, diffuse bullous lesions, symmetric peripheral gangrene with disseminated intravascular coagulation (DIC), and the classic lesions associated with endocarditis (Janeway lesions, Osler nodes) (30). A peculiar lesion most frequently seen in neutropenic patients with *Pseudomonas* sepsis is ecthyma gangrenosum (31–33). These are discrete rounded lesions that begin as dark red or purplish macules and progress to "bull's-eye" erythematous halos sur-

rounding a central vesicle or ulcer. They have also been described in bacteremias with other gram-negative rods and fungi (33,34). Sometimes biopsies or aspirations of a skin lesion with cultures and Gram stain may yield a diagnosis before blood cultures.

The most dramatic skin lesions occur with fulminant meningococcemia. These are diffuse petechial, purpuric, ecchymotic lesions that signal the presence of DIC. Petechiae may also be seen in infections with gram-positive organisms (e.g., in asplenic patients with pneumococcal infection) and in association with endocarditis. During the early phases of sepsis, the skin will be warm and flushed because of reduced peripheral vascular resistance. As the patient progresses to clinical shock, blood supply to the skin is reduced and the extremities become mottled, cyanotic, and cool.

Cardiovascular Manifestations

The hemodynamic picture of septic shock is complex and not static. It is often thought to begin with a hyperdynamic phase characterized by increased cardiac output and decreased systemic vascular resistance (SVR) (warm shock) (35). This is considered a classic example of distributive shock, that is, a maldistribution of blood flow to different body compartments. As the various mediators of septic shock contribute to microvascular dysregulation, cardiac output becomes inadequate to maintain normal perfusion pressures and shock ensues (6,7,13,35–39). Swan-Ganz catheter monitoring would then show decreased cardiac output and increased SVR (cold shock). As perfusion to tissues decreases, energy requirements are partially met by anaerobic metabolism, which leads to lactic acidemia. Whether the decreased perfusion and microvascular abnormalities are primary causes of organ failure in sepsis or just other associated events is unclear (1).

Despite normal to high measurements of cardiac output, there is growing evidence of significant myocardial dysfunction in septic shock (38,39). A myocardial depressant factor is

TABLE 61.3. Factors Influencing Survival with Bacteremia

Severity of the underlying disease (2, 3, 5, 11, 12)
Appropriate antibiotic use (2, 4, 11, 12, 15)
Microorganism (3, 5, 7, 11, 12, 28)
Advanced age (11, 15)
Site of infection (respiratory → abdominal → urinary) (3, 11)
Nosocomial versus community-acquired infection (2, 3, 10)
Magnitude of bacteremia (2, 3)
Polymicrobial bacteremia (2, 4, 9)
Complications of sepsis (shock, hypothermia, anuria) (12, 15)

most likely responsible, although nothing definite has been isolated as yet (1,40). Tumor necrosis factor (TNF) has properties that inhibit myocyte contractility and may be one of several cytokines responsible for myocardial dysfunction in patients with sepsis (41).

When measured serially, significant differences in cardiac indices and oxygen use were noted in survivors and nonsurvivors of septic shock 8 hours before the hypotensive crisis (42). This suggests that a patient's outcome may be determined before any evidence of shock exists. Others have demonstrated the prognostic significance of heart rate and SVR in survivors of septic shock. Survivors are more likely to have heart rates of less than 106 beats per minute initially, then progressively slower heart rates and higher SVR measurements during the first 24 hours (35).

In late shock, tissue hypoperfusion leads to progressive acidosis as cardiac output falls, accompanied by refractory hypotension and inevitable death. Efforts to increase cardiac output with fluids and inotropic agents often prove futile (38). This has led some researchers to postulate that a metabolic block triggered by sepsis prevents tissues from the normal oxidative use of available substrate (43,44).

Pulmonary Manifestations

The earliest response to sepsis is tachypnea, which may be followed by a wide array of respiratory signs. These may range from hyperventilation and respiratory alkalosis to adult respiratory distress syndrome (ARDS) and finally failure of the respiratory muscles. The exact pathophysiologic mechanism of the lung damage is unclear; it probably involves numerous mediators activated by sepsis and a resultant increased alveolar-capillary permeability. The increase in pulmonary edema is associated with a ventilation-perfusion mismatch, a widened alveolar-arterial oxygen gradient, and reduced lung compliance (45,46).

ARDS may complicate sepsis 10% to 40% of the time, increasing the mortality to 80% to 90% (7,47,48). Establishing a diagnosis is arbitrary at times but usually includes arterial oxygen tension of less than 50 mm Hg despite a fraction of inspired oxygen more than 50%, diffuse alveolar infiltrates without cardiomegaly or other signs of heart failure, and a pulmonary capillary wedge pressure less than 15 mm Hg. Host factors do not seem to predispose patients to ARDS, but infections with gram-negative organisms are more often associated with ARDS (47–49).

In the later stage of ARDS, as a preterminal event, oxygenation becomes impossible despite 100% inspired oxygen and high levels of positive end-expiratory pressure.

Hematologic Findings

Most patients with sepsis will exhibit a neutrophilic leukocytosis from both a stress-related demargination early and a release of less mature granulocytes from the marrow reserve later. Leukemoid reactions with leukocyte counts of 50,000/mm³ or more are sometimes observed. Significant neutropenia is seen in overwhelming bacteremias. A low platelet count and observance of toxic granulation, Döhle bodies, and vacuolization of the neutrophil on a complete blood cell count may be early clues to bacteremia (50). DIC is characterized by fibrin deposition and thrombosis of the microvasculature. Hemorrhage results from consumption of platelets and clotting factors (51). Elevated fibrin degradation products, prolonged prothrombin time, and decreased platelets, fibrinogen, and clotting factors are diagnos-

tic of DIC. Hemolytic anemias may complicate infections with *Clostridium* and *Mycoplasma* species and may occur in association with DIC.

Renal and Gastrointestinal Manifestations

Renal insufficiency in sepsis is multifactorial. It depends to varying degrees on the host, the microbe, and the therapeutic interventions (52). Glomerular lesions are seen with endocarditis (especially staphylococcal) and other unrelated infectious processes. Tubulointerstitial disease related to various bacteria and antibiotic therapy is well known. Most often, renal failure is attributed to acute tubular necrosis, which may be caused by hypotension, volume depletion, or any one of the numerous mediators of septic shock.

Sepsis is also associated with upper gastrointestinal tract bleeding (53) and is often seen in patients with coagulopathies and mechanical ventilation (54). Liver dysfunction usually causes a cholestatic jaundice and may result from red blood cell lysis or hepatocellular dysfunction (55). For unexplained reasons, sepsis with *Bacteroides* species is often accompanied by hyperbilirubinemia (56). Precipitous increases in transaminase levels usually indicate shock liver from a hypotensive episode and generally decrease rapidly as blood pressure is restored.

Hypoglycemia may complicate sepsis with various bacteria and should be looked for in patients who have any change in mental status or seizures (57). The pathogenesis is unclear, but patients with underlying liver disease are more likely to become hypoglycemic with sepsis (58). Inhibition of gluconeogenesis and depletion of hepatic glycogen stores have been implicated (59).

Multiorgan Dysfunction

When there is evidence of dysfunction in two or more systems (pulmonary, renal, gastrointestinal, central nervous, and hepatic), the diagnosis of multiorgan dysfunction syndrome can be made. Mortality rises in proportion to the number of organ systems involved (60,61). When four or more systems are involved, mortality is nearly 100%.

MEDIATORS OF THE INFLAMMATORY RESPONSE SYNDROME

The systemic response to insult such as overwhelming infection or trauma involves a complicated cascade of biologic events culminating in hemodynamic compromise and organ damage. Triggering substances such as bacteria-derived endotoxin induce the production of endogenous mediators, which in turn act in an interdependent fashion to stimulate the reticuloendothelial, complement, and coagulation systems. It seems reasonable that the coordinated effect of localized inflammation is an attempt to physiologically contain and overcome offenses such as bacterial invasion. However, when the inflammatory response is no longer contained and regulatory mechanisms are overwhelmed, systemic complications such as sepsis may occur (Fig. 61.2). Research in the last two decades has concentrated on characterizing and moderating these mediators of sepsis.

The events leading to sepsis typically involve the production and release of microbial toxins. In sepsis associated with gram-negative infection, the cell wall constituent known as *endotoxin* induces the release of proinflammatory mediators (7). Endotoxin, or lipopolysaccharide (LPS), consists of a three-part complex of species-specific O antigens, core polysaccharide, and

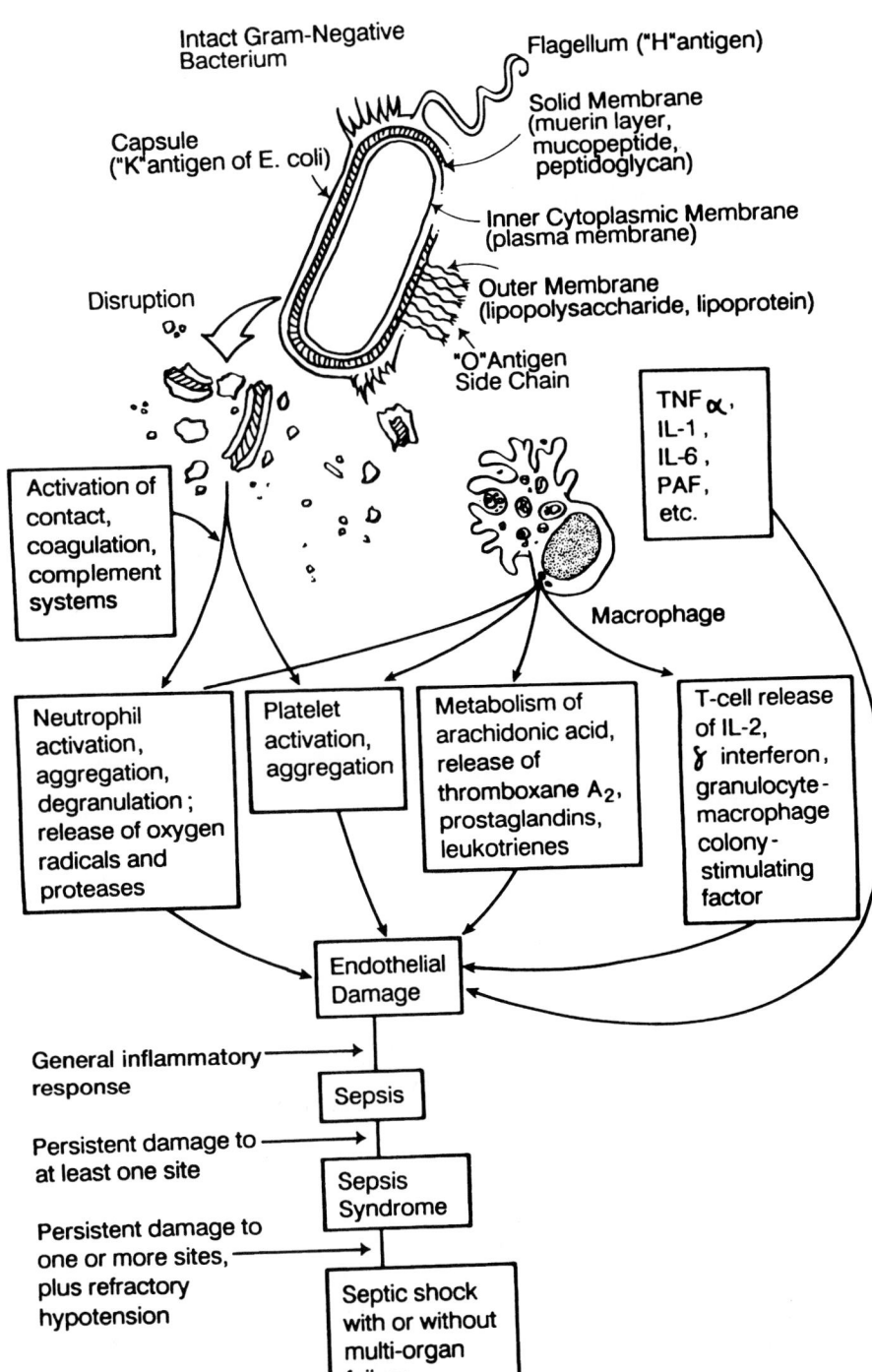

Figure 61.2. Mechanisms underlying gram-negative sepsis. This figure provides a framework for understanding how sepsis and systemic inflammatory response syndrome may occur. The pathways are not distinct, however, and effects may vary from individual to individual, depending on physiologic conditions. If general homeostasis is not restored, the systemic inflammatory response will produce clinical evidence of sepsis, and persistent endothelial damage at one site will ultimately result in organ dysfunction. GM-CSF, granulocyte-macrophage colony-stimulating factor; IFN-γ, interferon-γ; IL, interleukin; PAF, platelet-activating factor; TNF-α, tumor necrosis factor-α. (From Bone RC. The pathogenesis of sepsis. *Ann Intern Med* 1991;115:457–469, with permission.)

glucosamine-based phospholipid (lipid A). The core lipid A portion is antigenically conserved among gram-negative species and possesses most of the complex's biologic activity. Endotoxin is known to be a potent stimulus for the production of TNF-α and other cytokines and inflammatory cells. Endotoxin potency is augmented by LPS-binding protein found in human serum. In addition to facilitating bacterial opsonization, the resulting endotoxin–LPS-binding protein complexes bind readily to CD14 receptors on monocytes and macrophages (62). Complement and coagulation cascades are affected by endotoxin through the activation of Hageman factor (factor XII) (63).

Toxin production is also seen with the other microbes such as the toxic shock syndrome toxin produced by *S. aureus* in toxic

shock syndrome. Gram-positive bacterial, fungal, viral, and even parasitic organisms may elicit cell wall and other antigenic products that trigger the inflammatory response (26).

Development of SIRS in the absence of gram-negative infection suggests other principal mediators unrelated to endotoxin. Of these, TNF-α has received the most attention. TNF-α is released early in SIRS by activated monocyte/macrophages and endothelial cells and stimulates the induction of secondary proinflammatory cytokines such as interleukin (IL)-1, IL-6, and platelet-activating factors (PAFs) (64). Additional reactions include the induction of endothelial adhesion molecules, which promote neutrophil adherence to endothelium, and the enhancement of phagocytosis. Although TNF-α is considered pivotal in the production of the inflammatory cascade, the half-life of TNF-α is brief and significant levels are not necessary to maintain the inflammatory response of sepsis (65).

Cytokines may behave independently or in concert with other modulators to provoke the inflammatory cascade. IL-1 acts synergistically with TNF-α to promote fever, hypotension, and shock. Other actions include release of IL-6 and PAF, as well as endothelial cell activation and increased endothelial adhesion molecule expression (62). PAF similarly functions to amplify the release of cytokines (62). IL-6, on the other hand, while promoting neutrophil activation and accumulation also acts in an antiinflammatory fashion by down-regulating TNF-α production and release. Similar antiinflammatory cytokines include IL-8, a potent chemoattractant for neutrophils but a substance that may also function to limit neutrophil–endothelial cell adherence, and IL-10, which decreases production of IL-1, IL6, and TNF-α (66).

Sepsis mediator activation results in damage to endovascular tissue with subsequent vascular disruption, hemodynamic compromise, and end-organ tissue damage. TNF-α and IL metabolism of arachidonic acid results in the manufacture of leukotrienes, thromboxane A_2, and prostaglandins, which increase vascular permeability and vasodilation. Endotoxin-induced nitric oxide production by macrophage and endothelial cells acts as a potent vasodilator (67). TNF-α probably acts as a myocardial-depressant substance (41). Stimulated neutrophils release lysosomal enzymes and oxygen radicals, augmenting vascular and tissue compromise. Platelet aggregation and activation of the complement and coagulation cascades lead to thrombosis and hemorrhage and further impair tissue perfusion (64).

Table 61.4 provides examples of the numerous mediators of sepsis and highlights steps that have been or are currently being investigated as targets for immunomodulation therapies.

TABLE 61.4. Mediators of Sepsis

Mediator	Effect	Possible treatment modalities
Endotoxin	Induces TNF and other cytokine release	Polyclonal antisera
	Activates Hageman's factor	Monoclonal antibodies
	Activation of complement and coagulation	
TNF-α	Induces IL-1, IL-6, and PAF release	Monoclonal antibodies
	Arachidonic acid metabolism to produce leukotrienes, thromboxane A_2, and prostaglandins	Recombinant TNF receptors
	Induces endothelial adhesion molecule expression	
	Enhances neutrophil phagocytosis	
IL-1	Induces TNF, IL-6, and PAF release	IL-1 receptor antagonists
	Arachidonic acid metabolism	Soluble IL-1 receptors
	T-cell activation to produce interferon-γ, other ILs, and GM-CSF	
	Provides synergy for TNF function	
IL-6	Neutrophil chemoattractant and activator	
	Stimulates activated B cells	
	Induces acute-phase response	
	May down-regulate TNF production (antiinflammatory)	
IL-8	Neutrophil chemoattractant and activator	
	Limits adherence to IL-1–activated endothelial cells (antiinflammatory)	
IL-10	Decreases production of IL-1, IL-6, and TNF	
PAF	Amplifies cytokine release	PAF antagonists
	Arachidonic acid metabolism	
Hageman's factor	Initiates coagulation cascade and fibrinolysis (may lead to disseminated intravascular coagulation)	Monoclonal antibodies
	Activates complement	
	Induces production of bradykinin	
Leukotrienes	Increase vascular permeability and resistance	
Thromboxane A_2	Increases vascular permeability and resistance	Inhibitors or antagonists
	Induces EDRF	
Prostaglandins	Effect vasodilation and increased permeability	Inhibitors or antagonists
Interferon-γ	Induces and augments TNF, ILs, and adhesion molecules	
GM-CSF	Stimulates production and activation of PMNs and mononuclear cells	
EDRF (? nitrous oxide)	Relaxes vascular smooth muscle	
	Inhibits platelet aggregation	
Complement	PMN activation and mast cell degranulation	
PMN leukocytes	Promote mediator release	
	Free radical and lysosomal enzyme release	
Adhesion molecule	Augments PMN and monocyte adherence to endothelial cells	Monoclonal antibodies to adhesion molecules
Platelets	Induce EDRF	
	Vasoconstriction and PMN stimulation	
Bradykinin	Promotes EDRF release	
Thrombin	Induces PAF and EDRF	
	Encourages fibrinogen consumption and factor inactivation	
Myocardial depressant substance (? TNF)	Reversible myocardial depression, ventricular dilation, and decreased left ejection fraction	
Nitrous oxide	Potent vasodilator	

EDRF, endothelial derived relaxing factor; GM-CSF, granulocyte-macrophage colony-stimulating factor; IL, interleukin; PAF, platelet-activating factor; PMN, polymorphonuclear; TNF, tumor necrosis factor.
Source: From Bone RC. The pathogenesis of sepsis. *Ann Intern Med* 1991;115:457–469, with permission.

THERAPY

Patients in septic shock are probably best managed in an intensive care unit with Swan-Ganz and arterial catheters. Rapid implementation of diagnostic and therapeutic interventions correlates with favorable outcome (13,14). The implication is that treatment should start on the ward or in the emergency department (68,69). Proof that invasive monitoring improves survival is from retrospective studies only. Measurements of right-sided heart pressures, pulmonary artery wedge pressures, and cardiac outputs are useful both in diagnosing sepsis (decreased SVR, increased cardiac output) and in following the response to volume replacement (avoiding pulmonary edema) (70,71). The value of monitoring central circulation with pulmonary artery catheters is unclear but appears justified with shock, particularly if there is end-organ failure (7).

The essential therapies for septic shock include (a) antibiotics, (b) fluid replacement, (c) oxygen, and (d) vasopressors.

Antibiotic treatment: Early antibiotic administration may dampen the inflammatory cascade. Although studies have shown increased levels in serum endotoxin as a response to antimicrobial use, there is clearly a therapeutic advantage to using antibiotics that are active *in vitro* against the blood culture isolate (2,5,8,72). Antibiotics should be chosen on the basis of potential sources of infection, epidemiologic concerns (community-acquired vs. nosocomial infection), and underlying host factors (see Table 61.2). For empiric treatment, the *Medical Letter* recommendation for severe sepsis is an aminoglycoside combined with (a) an advanced-generation cephalosporin (e.g., cefotaxime, ceftazidime, cefepime, or ceftriaxone); (b) a carbapenem (imipenem or meropenem); or (c) a β-lactam–β-lactamase inhibitor (piperacillin-tazobactam or ticarcillin-clavulanate) (73). For suspected MRSA, vancomycin is added. Guidelines for empiric treatment of sepsis in patients with cancer with neutropenia include (a) dual therapy with an aminoglycoside combined with an antipseudomonal penicillin, cefepime, ceftazidime, or carbapenem or (b) monotherapy with cefepime, ceftazidime, or a carbapenem (74). The addition of vancomycin is an option to be used if there is suspected catheter-related infection resulting from colonization by MRSA, a positive blood culture result for gram-positive cocci, or hypotension.

Many cases are associated with intravenous catheters. The predominant pathogens in such cases are gram-negative bacilli, *S. aureus*, and *Staphylococcus epidermidis*; less common are enterococci and *Candida* (75). For the diagnostic evaluation, the recommendation for a nontunneled catheter is two blood cultures (at least one peripheral culture), removal of the catheter for semiquantitative or quantitative culture (roll-plate vortex or sonication), and insertion of a new catheter (76). Nontunneled central venous catheters may be managed similarly with replacement over a guidewire. For tunneled central venous catheters, it may be possible to retain the catheter and treat infections caused by coagulase-negative staphylococci; this tactic is less commonly effective with *S. aureus* and almost never works with *Candida* species and gram-negative bacilli. Antibiotic treatment should be 7 to 14 days but longer if there are complications such as septic thrombosis, endocarditis, or osteomyelitis.

Fluid replacement: Hypovolemia results from fluid losses, capillary leakage, and increased venous capacitance. Most patients require 4 to 6 L of crystalloid. Colloid has no proven benefit over crystalloid. Fluid administration is based on results of monitoring blood pressure, urinary output, clinical response, cardiac index, and oxygen saturation.

Pressors: Persistent hypotension reflects low systemic resistance sometimes combined with reduced cardiac output. Advocated interventions are α-adrenergic agonists for vasoconstriction with or without β-adrenergic stimulation to increase cardiac output. Dopamine (2–20 μg/kg per minute) is often used for its α-adrenergic effect and potential to maintain urine output. Norepinephrine (5–20 μg per minute) is often given for refractory oliguria and hypotension (77,78).

Intubation: Respiratory failure may progress rapidly and require intubation and mechanical ventilation.

Corticosteroids: Initial studies with small numbers of patients seemed to show that high-dose short-course corticosteroid therapy was beneficial, but subsequent large controlled trials and a metaanalysis refuted this conclusion (79–82). More recently, the issue has been readdressed in the context of corticosteroids therapy in replacement doses for patients who have reduced adrenal reserve (83).

Activated protein C: Drotrecogin-α has antiinflammatory, antithrombotic, and profibrinolytic properties. This activity offers the potential to modulate coagulation and inflammation associated with sepsis. A controlled trial with 1,690 participants showed a statistically significant survival benefit (31% vs. 25%) in patients with severe sepsis as indicated by an acute physiologic assessment and chronic health evaluation (APACHE) score of 25 or higher (84). The major drawbacks are bleeding and price. This current recommendation is severe sepsis with failure of at least one organ, an APACHE score of more than 25, and no preexisting bleeding diathesis.

REFERENCES

1. Parillo JE. Pathogenetic mechanisms of septic shock. *N Engl J Med* 1993;328:1471.
2. Dupont HL, Spink WW. Infections due to gram-negative organisms: an analysis of 860 patients with bacteremia at the University of Minnesota Medical Center 1959–1966. *Medicine (Baltimore)* 1969;48:307.
3. Kreger BE, Craven DE, Carling PC, et al. Gram-negative bacteremia, III: reassessment of etiology, epidemiology and ecology in 612 patients. *Am J Med* 1980;68:332.
4. Weinstein MP, Murphy JR, Reller LB, Lichtenstein KA. The clinical significance of positive blood cultures: a comprehensive analysis of 500 episodes of bacteremia and fungemia in adults, II: clinical observations, with special reference to factors influencing prognosis. *Rev Infect Dis* 1983;5:54.
5. McCabe WR, Jackson GG. Gram-negative bacteremia, II: clinical, laboratory, and therapeutic observations. *Arch Intern Med* 1962;110:856.
6. Wheeler AP, Bernard GR. Treating patients with severe sepsis. *N Engl J Med* 1999;340:207.
7. Parillo JE. Septic shock in humans: advances in the understanding of pathogenesis, cardiovascular dysfunction, and therapy. *Ann Intern Med* 1990;113:227.
8. McCabe WR, Treadwell TL, De Maria A. Pathophysiology of bacteremia. *Am J Med* 1983;75:7018.
9. McCabe WR, Jackson GG. Gram-negative bacteremia, I: etiology and ecology. *Arch Intern Med* 1962;110:847.
10. McGowen JE, Barnes MW, Finland MW. Bacteremia at Boston City Hospital: occurrence and mortality during 12 selected years (1935–1972) with special reference to hospital-acquired cases. *J Infect Dis* 1975;132:316.
11. Bryan CS, Reynolds KL, Brenner ER. Analysis of 1,186 episodes of gram-negative bacteremia in non-university hospitals: the effects of antimicrobial therapy. *Rev Infect Dis* 1983;5:629.
12. Bryant RE, Hood AF, Hood CE, et al. Factors affecting mortality of gram-negative rod bacteremia. *Arch Intern Med* 1971;127:120.
13. Rivers E, Nguyen B, Havstad S, et al. Early goat-directed therapy in the treatment of severe sepsis and septic shock. *N Engl J Med* 2001;345:1368.
14. Nguyen HB, Rivers EP, Havstad S, et al. Critical care in the emergency department. *Acad Emerg Med* 2000;7:1354.
15. Kreger BE, Craven DE, McCabe WR. Gram-negative bacteremia, IV: reevaluation of clinical features and treatment in 612 patients. *Am J Med* 1980;68:344.
16. Bone RC. Why new definitions of sepsis and organ failure are needed. *Am J Med* 1993;95:348.
17. Bone RC, Balk RA, Cerra FB, et al. Definitions of sepsis and organ failure and guidelines for the use of innovative therapies in sepsis. *Chest* 1992;101:1644.
18. Rangel-Frausto MS, Pittet D, Costigan M, et al. The natural history of the systemic inflammatory response syndrome (SIRS). *JAMA* 1995;273:117.
19. Knaus WA, Wagner DP, Draper EA, et al. The APACHE III prognostic prediction of hospital mortality for critically ill hospitalized adults. *Chest* 1991;100:1619.
20. Bannerjee SN, Emori TG, Culver DH, et al. Secular trends in nosocomial

primary bloodstream infections in the United States, 1980–1989. *Am J Med* 1991;91:865.

21. Schaberg DR, Culver DH, Gaynes RP. Major trends in the microbial etiology of nosocomial infection. *Am J Med* 1991;91:725.

22. Bamberger DM, Gurley MB. Microbial etiology and clinical characteristics of distributive shock. *Clin Infect Dis* 1994;18:726.

23. Collin BA, Leather HL, Wingard JR, et al. Evolution, incidence and susceptibility of bacterial bloodstream isolates from 519 bone marrow transplant patients. *Clin Infect Dis* 2001;33:947.

24. Lark RL, Saint S, Chenoweth C, et al. Four-year prospective evaluation of community-acquired bacteremia: epidemiology, microbiology, and patient outcome. *Diagn Microbiol Infect Dis* 2001;41:15.

25. Edmond MB, Wallace SE, McClish DK, et al. Nosocomial bloodstream infections in United States hospitals: a three-year analysis. *Clin Infect Dis* 1999;29:239.

26. Bone RC. Gram-positive organisms and sepsis. *Arch Intern Med* 1994;154:26.

27. Peacock JE Jr, Herrington DA, Wade JC, et al. Ciprofloxacin plus piperacillin compared with tobramycin plus piperacillin as empirical therapy to febrile neutropenic patients. *Ann Intern Med* 2002;137:137.

28. Baden LR, Rubin RH. Fever, neutropenia and the second law of thermodynamics. *Ann Intern Med* 2002;137:123.

29. Washington JA. Blood cultures: principles and techniques. *Mayo Clin Proc* 1975;50:91.

30. Musher DM. Cutaneous and soft tissue manifestations of sepsis due to gram-negative enteric bacilli. *Rev Infect Dis* 1980;2:854.

31. Greene SL, Su WP, Muller SA. Ecthyma gangrenosum: report of clinical, histopathologic and bacteriologic aspects of eight cases. *J Am Acad Dermatol* 1984;11:781.

32. Dorff GJ, Geimer NF, Rosenthal DR, et al. *Pseudomonas* septicemia: illustrated evolution of its skin lesion. *Arch Intern Med* 1971;128:591.

33. Bonduel M, Santos P, Turienzo CF, et al. Atypical skin lesions caused by *Curvularia* sp and *Pseudoallescheria boydii* in two patients after allogeneic bone marrow transplant. *Bone Marrow Transplant* 2001;27:1311.

34. Shackelford PG, Ratzan SA, Shearer WT. Erythema gangrenosum produced by *Aeromonas hydrophila*. *J Pediatr* 1973;83:100.

35. Parker MM, Shelhamer JH, Natanson C, et al. Serial cardiovascular variables in survivors and nonsurvivors of human septic shock: heart rate as an early predictor of prognosis. *Crit Care Med* 1987;15:923.

36. Weil MH, Nishijima H. Cardiac output in bacterial shock. *Am J Med* 1978;64:920.

37. Parrillo JE. The cardiovascular pathophysiology of sepsis. *Annu Rev Med* 1989;40:469.

38. Ognibene FP, Parker MM, Natanson C, et al. Depressed left ventricular performance: response to volume infusion in patients with sepsis and septic shock. *Chest* 1988;93:903.

39. Parker MM, Shelhamer JH, Bacharach SL, et al. Profound but reversible myocardial depression in patients with septic shock. *Ann Intern Med* 1984;100:483.

40. Parrillo JE, Burch C, Shelhamer JH, et al. A circulating myocardial depressant substance in humans with septic shock. *J Clin Invest* 1985;76:1539.

41. Cunnion RE. Myocardial depressant substance. *Ann Intern Med* 1990;113:237.

42. Abraham E, Bland RD, Cobo JC, et al. Sequential cardiorespiratory patterns associated with outcome in septic shock. *Chest* 1984;85:75.

43. Siegel JH, Cerra FB, Coleman B, et al. Physiological and metabolic correlations in human sepsis. *Surgery* 1979;86:163.

44. Mizock B. Septic shock: a metabolic perspective. *Arch Intern Med* 1984;144:579.

45. Dantzker DR, Brock CJ, De Hart P, et al. Ventilation perfusion distributions in the adult respiratory distress syndrome. *Am Rev Respir Dis* 1979;120:1039.

46. Clowes G. Pulmonary abnormalities in sepsis. *Surg Clin North Am* 1974;54:993.

47. Fein AM, Lippmann M, Holtzman H, et al. The risk factors, incidence, and prognosis of ARDS following septicemia. *Chest* 1983;83:40.

48. Fowler AA, Hamman RI, Good JT, et al. Adult respiratory distress syndrome in gram-negative sepsis. *Ann Intern Med* 1983;98:593.

49. Kaplan RL, Sahn SA, Petty TL. Incidence and outcome of the respiratory distress syndrome in gram-negative sepsis. *Arch Intern Med* 1979;139:867.

50. Malcolm ID, Fogel KM, Katz M. Vacuolization of the neutrophil in bacteremia. *Arch Intern Med* 1979;139:675.

51. Mant MJ, King EG. Severe, acute disseminated intravascular coagulation. *Am J Med* 1979;67:557.

52. Spector DA, Millan J, Zauber N, et al. Glomerulonephritis and *Staphylococcus aureus* infections. *Clin Nephrol* 1980;14:256.

53. Altemeier WA, Fullen WO, McDonough JJ. Sepsis and gastrointestinal bleeding. *Ann Surg* 1972;175:759.

54. Schuster DP, Rowley H, Feinstein S, et al. Prospective evaluation of the risk of upper gastrointestinal bleeding after admission to a medical intensive care unit. *Am J Med* 1984;76:623.

55. Zimmerman HJ, Fang M, Utili R, et al. Jaundice due to bacterial infection. *Gastroenterology* 1979;77:362.

56. Chow AW, Guze LB. Bacteroidaceae bacteremia: a clinical experience with 112 patients. *Medicine (Baltimore)* 1974;53:93.

57. Miller SR, Wallace RJ, Musher DM, et al. Hypoglycemia as a manifestation of sepsis. *Am J Med* 1980;68:649.

58. Nouel O, Bernuau J, Rueff B, et al. Hypoglycemia: a common complication of septicemia in cirrhosis. *Arch Intern Med* 1981;141:1477.

59. Filkins JP, Cornell RP. Depression of hepatic gluconeogenesis and the hypoglycemia of endotoxic shock. *Am J Physiol* 1974;227:778.

60. Fry DE, Pearlstein L, Fulton RL, et al. Multiple system organ failure. *Arch Surg* 1980;115:136.

61. Bell RC, Coalson JJ, Smith JD, et al. Multiple organ system failure and infection in adult respiratory distress syndrome. *Ann Intern Med* 1983;99:293.

62. Giroir BP. Mediators of septic shock: new approaches for interrupting the endogenous inflammatory cascade. *Crit Care Med* 1993;21:780.

63. Kalter ES, Daha MR, ten Cate SW, et al. Activation and inhibition of Hageman factor–dependent pathways and the complement system in uncomplicated bacteremia or bacterial shock. *J Infect Dis* 1985;151:1019.

64. Bone RC. The systemic inflammatory response syndrome: does the new name mean new therapies? *Clin Immunother* 1994;1:369.

65. St. John RC, Dorinsky PM. Immunologic therapy for ARDS, septic shock, and multiple-organ failure. *Chest* 1993;103:932.

66. Glauser MP, Heumann D, Baumgartner JD, et al. Pathogenesis and potential strategies for prevention and treatment of septic shock: an update. *Clin Infect Dis* 1994;18:S205.

67. Lorente JA, Landin L, Renes E, et al. Role of nitric oxide in the hemodynamic changes of sepsis. *Crit Care Med* 1993;21:759.

68. Li TCM, Phillips MC, Shaw L, et al. On site physician staffing in a community hospital intensive care unit: impact on test and procedure use and on patient outcome. *JAMA* 1984;252:2023.

69. Reynolds HN, Raupt MT, Thill-Baharozian, et al. Impact of critical care physician staffing on patients with septic shock in a university hospital medical intensive care unit. *JAMA* 1988;260:3446.

70. Ognibene FP. Management of septic shock. *Ann Intern Med* 1990;113:240.

71. Packman MI, Rackow C. Optimum left heart filling pressure during fluid resuscitation of patients with hypovolemic and septic shock. *Crit Care Med* 1983;11:165.

72. Shenap JL, Flynn PM, Barrett FF, et al. Serial quantitation of endotoxemia and bacteremia during therapy for gram-negative bacterial sepsis. *J Infect Dis* 1988;157:565.

73. Medical Letter Consultants. Choice of antibacterial drugs. *Med Lett* 2001;43:71.

74. Hughes WT, Armstrong D, Bodey GP, et al. 2002 guidelines for the use of antimicrobial agents in neutropenic patients with cancer. *Clin Infect Dis* 2002;34:730.

75. Raad II, Hanna HA. Intravascular catheter-related infections. *Arch Intern Med* 2002;162:871.

76. Mermel LA, Farr BM, Sherertz RJ, et al. Guidelines for the management of intravascular catheter-related infections. *Clin Infect Dis* 2001;32:1249.

77. Desjars P, Pinaud M, Potel G, et al. A reappraisal of norepinephrine therapy in human septic shock. *Crit Care Med* 1987;15:134.

78. Meadows D, Edwards D, Wilkins RG, et al. Reversal of intractable septic shock with norepinephrine therapy. *Crit Care Med* 1988;16:663.

79. Sprung CL, Caralis PV, Marcial E, et al. The effects of high-dose corticosteroids in patients with septic shock: a prospective, controlled study. *N Engl J Med* 1987;311:1137.

80. Bone RC, Fisher CJ Jr, Clemmer TP, et al. A controlled clinical trial of high-dose methylprednisolone in the treatment of severe sepsis and septic shock. *N Engl J Med* 1987;317:653.

81. Hinshaw L, Peduzzi P, Young E, et al. Effect of high-dose glucocorticoid therapy on mortality in patients with clinical signs of systemic sepsis. The Veterans Administration Systemic Sepsis Cooperative Study Group. *N Engl J Med* 1987;317:659.

82. Cronin L, Cook DJ, Carlet J, et al. Corticosteroid treatment for sepsis: a critical appraisal and meta-analysis of the literature. *Crit Care Med* 1995;23:1430.

83. Annane D, Sebille V, Charpentier C, et al. Effect of treatment with low doses of hydrocortisone and fludrocortisone on mortality in patients with septic shock. *JAMA* 2002;288:862.

84. Bernard GR, Vincent JL, Laterre PF, et al. Efficacy and safety of recombinant human activated protein C for severe sepsis. *N Engl J Med* 2001;344:699.

CHAPTER 62
Infective Endocarditis

Donald Kaye

Until the 1940s, infective endocarditis was a progressively debilitating, incurable, fatal disease that usually affected young people (1). The advent of antibiotics made it possible to eradicate infection in nearly all cases of infective endocarditis, provided that the diagnosis was made and treatment was begun sufficiently early. Fatalities occurred from irreversible anatomic injury, resulting in complications such as heart failure or cerebral hemorrhage (2).

In the last 50 years, the population susceptible to disease, the predisposing lesions, and the infecting agents have changed; nevertheless, the incidence of infective endocarditis in non–intravenous drug users (IVDUs) (about 20–50 cases per million population per year) has remained the same as in the preantibiotic era (3,4). However, depending on the number of IVDUs in the population, this frequency can at least double (5).

CHARACTERISTICS OF THE DISEASE

Infective endocarditis usually refers to bacterial or fungal infection within the heart. Extracardiac endothelium can also be colonized by microorganisms, and the infection (more properly called *endarteritis*) produces a clinical syndrome indistinguishable from infective endocarditis (6). Endocarditis was initially classified as acute or subacute on the basis of the clinical course as observed before availability of antimicrobial therapy and in a population at risk that consisted mainly of patients with congenital heart disease (CHD) or rheumatic heart disease (RHD) (7).

Acute endocarditis denoted infection of a normal valve by a virulent organism such as *Staphylococcus aureus* or *Streptococcus pneumoniae*, which rapidly destroyed the heart valve and frequently caused widespread metastatic foci. Death occurred in less than 6 weeks. Subacute endocarditis referred to infection of abnormal valves with relatively avirulent organisms, such as viridans streptococci. The course was indolent (up to 2 years) and metastatic foci were uncommon. Such classic presentations of infective endocarditis are now encountered less frequently. Currently, patients with prosthetic cardiac valves, IVDUs, and persons with mitral valve prolapse (MVP), instead of patients with RHD, account for most cases of endocarditis. CHD is still an important underlying lesion. The bacteriology in each population differs, and correlations between organism and course of disease are variable. Current useful classifications refer to underlying anatomy and infecting organism and serve as a basis for therapy and clinical prognosis.

Native Valve Endocarditis

Sixty percent to eighty percent of persons with native valve endocarditis who do not use parenteral drugs have an identifiable predisposing cardiac lesion (8). In recent series, MVP has been the underlying lesion in about one third of cases (9). Although the frequency of MVP is three times greater in women than in men, men with MVP and a systolic murmur are at considerably higher risk of developing infective endocarditis. Men older than 45 years and those with thickening and redundancy of the mitral leaflets are particularly at risk (10,11).

In the United States and most other industrialized nations, RHD accounts for a diminishing proportion of the heart lesions in patients with endocarditis (probably less than 20% in the United states) (12,13). Most patients with RHD and endocarditis in the United States are middle-aged or older, reflecting the decline in the occurrence of rheumatic fever and carditis. In RHD with endocarditis, the mitral valve is most commonly involved, followed by the aortic valve. Both valves are infected simultaneously in less than 5% of patients (14). A tricuspid valve may occasionally be affected by RHD (15). RHD remains a common underlying disease for endocarditis in many of the developing nations.

CHD is the underlying lesion in 10% to 20% of patients. Routine closure of a patent ductus arteriosus by medical or surgical means has considerably reduced the number of young people at risk. Other predisposing lesions include ventricular septal defects, subaortic and valvular aortic stenosis, bicuspid aortic valve, tetralogy of Fallot, coarctation of the aorta, lesions associated with Marfan syndrome, and pulmonary stenosis. Uncomplicated atrial septal defect does not predispose to endocarditis.

Degenerative heart disease, particularly calcific aortic stenosis, is important in predisposing the elderly to infective endocarditis (16). Degenerative heart disease is very likely underestimated as a predisposing lesion, because the lesion may be difficult to demonstrate (e.g., a degenerative nodule on a valve or a fleck of calcium). Syphilitic aortic valves are unusual as underlying lesions in infective endocarditis.

Infective endocarditis on a native valve in non-IVDUs remains predominantly a disease of men (observed male-to-female ratio, 1.2:1 to 3:1) and has become a disease of older people with a mean age of about 60 years (13,17).

CAUSES

Streptococci including *Streptococcus bovis* and nutritionally deficient streptococci (now classified as *Abiotrophia* species) are the cause of about 20% to 55% of cases of endocarditis on native valves in non-IVDUs; enterococci (5%–10%) and staphylococci (25%–40%) account for most of the remaining cases (13,18,19) (Table 62.1). Viridans streptococci, normal inhabitants of the oropharynx, account for more than half of all streptococcal infections. This group includes a variety of *Streptococcus* species, including *Streptococcus sanguis, Streptococcus salivarius, Streptococcus mutans*, and *Streptococcus mitior*, most of which are highly susceptible to penicillin (20). Because of the recent emergence of occasional strains resistant to penicillin, determination of penicillin susceptibility of the infecting organism is necessary (21). Infections caused by these organisms occur mainly on abnormal heart valves. Although about 15% to 20% of patients infected with these organisms report recently having undergone dental procedures, a recent case-control study indicated that no more than 5% to 10% of endocarditis cases caused by oral microflora can be attributed to procedures in the oropharynx (13).

Enterococci (formerly classified as streptococci) are members of Lancefield group D and are isolated from about 5% to 10% of patients with endocarditis. The genus *Enterococcus* contains at least 12 species including *Enterococcus faecalis, Enterococcus faecium, Enterococcus durans, Enterococcus avium*, and *Enterococcus gallinarum* (22). Most of the cases of endocarditis have been caused by *E. faecalis* (about 85%) and most of the remainder by *E. faecium*. Enterococci are α-, β-, or γ-hemolytic and normally inhabit the gastrointestinal (GI) tract and the anterior urethra. Enterococci can attack normal or damaged heart valves. Most patients with enterococcal endocarditis are men 60 years or older who may give a recent history of genitourinary manipulation

TABLE 62.1.   Approximate Frequency of Microbial Pathogens in Infective Endocarditis

Organisms	Native valve (%)		Prosthetic valve (%)	
	Non-IVDU	IVDU	Early (<2 mo)	Late (>2 mo)
Streptococci	20–55	10–20	5–10	30–40
Enterococci	5–10	2–7	5–15	10
Staphylococci				
Staphylococcus aureus	20–35	55–75	10–20	10–20
Coagulase-negative staphylococci	5	2	20–35	10–30
Gram-negative bacilli	<1–5	<1–8	10–15	<1–10
Fungi	<1–2	2–5	5–15	1–5
Diphtheroids	<1–5	<1	5–15	3–5
Miscellaneous organisms	5–10	1	2–10	5–10[a]
Culture-negative results	5–10	7	5–10	5–10

[a]The miscellaneous organisms are more frequent in areas of the world where *Coxiella burnetii* is a frequent cause of prosthetic valve endocarditis.
IVDU, intravenous drug users.

(cystoscopy, urethral catheterization, or prostatectomy), trauma, or disease; less often, women younger than 40 years who may have undergone abortion, pregnancy, or cesarean section are affected. However, case-control studies have not been able to demonstrate a relationship between these procedures and enterococcal endocarditis (probably because of lack of adequate numbers of cases in the studies). Correct biochemical identification and *in vitro* susceptibility testing are critical because of the worldwide emergence and nosocomial spread of multidrug-resistant strains (23). Enterococci are highly resistant to cephalosporins, relatively resistant to penicillins, and usually are not killed by penicillins alone. This is because of intrinsic low-level resistance to penicillins conferred by low-affinity penicillin-binding proteins. Therefore, large doses of penicillin must be used in therapy and an aminoglycoside must be added to achieve a bactericidal effect (24). *E. faecium* are generally more resistant to penicillins than *E. faecalis*, and many are so resistant that penicillins cannot be used in therapy. Enterococci, particularly *E. faecium*, are capable of acquiring new resistance determinants from other species (25). Uncommonly, resistance to β-lactams has been acquired as the result of the transfer of a β-lactamase gene from staphylococci (26). Transfer of genes encoding aminoglycoside-modifying enzymes through plasmids and transposons has resulted in increasing prevalence of strains with high-level resistance to all aminoglycosides (27). Nosocomially acquired enterococcal strains, especially *E. faecium*, may be highly resistant to vancomycin, penicillin, and aminoglycosides (28). Two new agents linezolid and quinupristin-dalfopristin have activity against *E. faecium* infection, and linezolid also has activity against *E. faecalis* infection; however, their efficacy in treatment of enterococcal endocarditis remains to be determined (28,29).

S. bovis and *Streptococcus equinus* are group D streptococci that are normal inhabitants of the bowel. They differ biochemically from enterococci and are usually highly susceptible to penicillin. *S. bovis*–related endocarditis occurs principally in persons older than 60 years and is frequently associated with the presence of colonic polyps or colonic malignant neoplasms (30). *S. bovis* infection accounts for about 10% of cases of endocarditis.

Other Lancefield group streptococci account for less than 5% of cases of endocarditis. Group A and group B streptococci can attack normal valves with rapid destruction and can produce distant metastases. Group B streptococci often produce large vegetations (31). Diabetics are particularly at risk for group B organism infection. Susceptibility of group B streptococci to penicillins varies.

Staphylococci cause about 25% to 40% of cases of native valve endocarditis (13,18,32). Most are coagulase-positive (*S. aureus*); coagulase-negative species (most often *S. epidermidis*) account for 10% to 20% of staphylococcal isolates (13,18,19,33). The great majority of staphylococci, whether acquired in the hospital or in the community, are highly resistant to penicillin G because of their ability to produce penicillinase. In the past 20 years, an increasing prevalence has been noted of methicillin-resistant isolates of *S. aureus* and *S. epidermidis* in hospitals, nursing homes, and even community settings; this has rendered β-lactam agents ineffective in some geographic locales as empiric therapy before demonstration of susceptibility (34). A recent phenomenon has been the emergence of methicillin-resistant *S. aureus* (MRSA) with intermediate susceptibility to vancomycin (i.e., inhibited by 8–16 μg of vancomycin), and even more recently, a strain was isolated that was highly resistant to vancomycin (35,36). Neither β-lactam antibiotics nor vancomycin is likely to be useful as a single agent in treatment of infections with these bacteria. These organisms are usually susceptible to linezolid and quinupristin-dalfopristin (29,37).

S. aureus–related endocarditis is usually fulminant, and there may be multiple metastatic abscesses. Normal or damaged valves can be affected and are rapidly destroyed. Coagulase-negative staphylococci usually cause an indolent infection of abnormal valves. However, *Staphylococcus lugdunensis*, a coagulase-negative staphylococcus causes marked destruction of valves (38).

The HACEK group of organisms (*Haemophilus, Actinobacillus, Cardiobacterium, Eikenella,* and *Kingella*) account for up to 5% of cases of endocarditis on native valves of non-IVDUs. These are slow-growing fastidious gram-negative bacilli that tend to cause large friable vegetations (39).

Almost all species of bacteria are occasionally identified as causes of native valve endocarditis. Some examples are *S. pneumoniae, Neisseria gonorrhoeae, Pseudomonas, Listeria, Bartonella, Tropheryma whippleii, Spirillum minus, Legionella, Chlamydia, Coxiella burnetii,* and diphtheroids (40–43). The clinical course can be fulminant or indolent. Gram-negative enteric organisms that are killed by serum and anaerobic organisms are less capable of sustaining endocardial infection (44).

Fungi rarely cause native valve endocarditis in the absence of intravenous drug use. Factors that predispose to fungemia resulting in endocarditis are intravenous catheters, severe underlying illness, corticosteroids, prolonged use of broad-spectrum antibiotics, and cytotoxic agents. *Candida* and *Aspergillus* species are usually implicated. The course is indolent but grave; large vegetations frequently embolize to major vessels in the lower extremities (45).

Endocarditis in Intravenous Drug Users

The frequency of endocarditis in IVDUs is difficult to estimate, although studies have documented that approximately 13% of febrile IVDUs presenting to urban emergency departments have infective endocarditis (46,47). In urban tertiary medical centers, patients who are IVDUs account for up to 50% of infective endocarditis cases. There appear to be differences in relative risk for infection based on the drugs used, the frequency of use, and the modes of drug preparation (48). IVDUs with endocarditis are usually men (male-to-female ratio, 3:1), and their mean age is 30 years (49). Approximately 20% have underlying cardiac disease, usually either congenital lesions or residua of previous endocarditis. Echocardiographic studies have demonstrated mild degrees of tricuspid valve insufficiency in IVDUs, which may explain the predilection for right-sided infective endocarditis among drug users. The tricuspid valve is infected in about 54% of patients, the aortic valve in 25%, and the mitral valve in 20%. Mixed right- and left-sided endocarditis occurs in 6% of patients (49,50) The skin is the most frequent source of the microorganisms responsible for endocarditis, although contamination of drugs and associated paraphernalia also contributes to bacteremia (51).

S. aureus is isolated in about 55% to 75% of patients, various species of streptococci and enterococci in about 10% to 30%, gram-negative bacilli (predominantly *Pseudomonas* and *Serratia* species) in up to 8%, and fungi (usually *Candida*) in up to 5% of patients (18,52) (see Table 62.1). More than one microorganism is isolated from the blood of about 5% of drug-addicted patients (52). Multiple organisms either can cause the primary infection or can be acquired during the course of therapy. *S. aureus* accounts for 80% of clinical isolates in tricuspid valve endocarditis (49–52). Similarly, in 70% to 80% of IVDUs with *S. aureus*–related endocarditis, only the tricuspid valve is involved.

The majority (more than 70%) of IVDUs with tricuspid valve endocarditis are noted to have pneumonia or multiple pulmonary septic emboli, but the murmur of tricuspid valve insufficiency frequently is not present or may be misinterpreted as a functional or flow murmur (52,53). Moreover, patients with a syndrome compatible with tricuspid valve endocarditis may actually have an extracardiac focus of endovascular infection (i.e., septic thrombophlebitis involving the subclavian or femoral venous system) rather than endocarditis (52).

There do not appear to be important clinical or pathophysiologic differences in endocarditis in IVDUs with concurrent human immunodeficiency virus (HIV) infection (47,52,54,55). Although infective endocarditis is usually reported in the early stages of HIV infection, the clinical stage of HIV infection does not appear to affect the outcome of treatment. Valve-replacement surgery does not seem to accelerate HIV-related disease (52,56,57).

Prosthetic Valve Endocarditis

Prosthetic valve infections account for 10% to 20% of all patients with endocarditis. The overall frequency of endocarditis in patients with prosthetic valves is 1% to 4% (58–61). By convention, prosthetic valve endocarditis (PVE) is termed early when symptoms appear within 60 days of valve insertion and late when they occur thereafter. The early and late groups differ in clinical features, microbial patterns, and mortality rates.

Early PVE generally reflects contamination during the perioperative period. Most contamination probably occurs intraoperatively through direct wound inoculation or contamination of the bypass machine. Postoperative sources include intravenous catheters (particularly central lines), arterial lines, urethral catheters, cardiac pacing wires, and endotracheal tubes. The attack rate for early PVE before 1969 was 2.5% of all patients undergoing valve replacement and has been 0.75% of all such patients subsequently. Despite use of prophylactic antibiotics, staphylococcal infection accounts for about 30% to 55% of early PVE. *S. epidermidis* is the organism most often isolated (frequency about 20%–35%); *S. aureus* causes 10% to 20% of infections (see Table 62.1). The remaining cases are caused by gram-negative aerobic bacilli (10%–15%), fungi (particularly *Candida* and *Aspergillus*, 5%–15%), streptococci and enterococci (10%–25%), and diphtheroids (5%–15%) (18,19,61,62).

The incidence of late PVE depends on the length of follow-up. It has been estimated to occur at an overall incidence of 0.3% to 0.6% per patient-year (61). The source of infection is presumed to be transient bacteremia seeding the valve. Thus, the bacteriology more closely resembles that of native valve endocarditis. Streptococci are the organisms isolated most often (about 30%–40%) (see Table 62.1); median time to onset of PVE is 24 months after valve implantation. Enterococci account for about 10%. Infections with staphylococci (coagulase-negative staphylococci usually *S. epidermidis*, about 10%–30%; *S. aureus*, about 10%–20%); gram-negative bacilli (up to 10%); fungi (1%–5%); and diphtheroids (3%–5%) account for the great majority of the remaining cases (18,19,61). Infections caused by coagulase-negative staphylococci, gram-negative bacilli, fungi, and diphtheroids occur far more frequently in the first 18 months after implantation of the valve than thereafter. These infections (i.e., other than those caused by streptococci, enterococci, and *S. aureus*) often reflect delayed clinical appearance of infections acquired perioperatively (61,63).

In contrast to native valve endocarditis, the aortic prosthetic valve is more prone to infection than the mitral prosthetic valve. There seems to be no significant difference in the frequency of infection between mechanical and heterograft valves. The frequency of PVE after replacement of an infected native valve is approximately 4%, much higher than after replacement of an uninfected valve. However, it is usually not caused by the originally infecting organism. An increased occurrence of PVE has been associated with the black race, male sex, and longer cardiopulmonary bypass time.

Early PVE is often associated with valve dysfunction or dehiscence, paravalvular abscesses, a fulminant course, and a high mortality rate. Depending on the infecting organism, late PVE is commonly indistinguishable clinically from that in patients without a prosthesis, but it may also present with a fulminant course (61).

PATHOGENESIS

Three hemodynamic cardiac factors predispose patients to the development of infective endocarditis: a high-velocity jet stream, flow from a high- to a low-pressure chamber, and a comparatively narrow orifice separating the two chambers that creates a pressure gradient (64,65). The lesions of infective endocarditis tend to form just beyond the narrowed orifice through which the high-velocity jet stream passes (i.e., on the ventricular surfaces of the incompetent aortic valve, on the atrial surface of the incompetent mitral or tricuspid valve, and on the walls of the pulmonary artery at the orifice of the patent ductus arteriosus). Satellite lesions can also grow where the jet stream strikes the endocardium (e.g., the atrial wall opposite the mitral orifice in mitral regurgitation, the papillary muscle of the left ventricle in aortic regurgitation, and the surface of the pulmonary artery opposite the patent ductus arteriosus). The force of the jet stream against these sites presumably denudes the endothelium and promotes deposition of clumps of fibrin and platelets, which form sterile vegetations called *nonbacterial thrombotic endocarditis*. Sterile vegetations can also occur in patients with wasting disease, particularly malignant neoplasia (marantic endocarditis); in areas surrounding foreign bodies, such as intracardiac catheters; and at surgical sites, particularly vascular incisions and implants (66,67).

Infective endocarditis occurs when microorganisms are deposited onto the sterile vegetation during the course of bacteremia (67–69). Organisms that adhere well to platelets, fibrin, or fibronectin by means of specific surface molecules and are resistant to host defense mechanisms such as complement and other serum factors are most likely to colonize sterile vegetations and at lower inocula (67,70,71). Subsequent deposition of platelets and fibrin over the bacteria forms a "protected site" into which phagocytic cells penetrate poorly, allowing survival and proliferation of the microorganisms. Fresh vegetations of infective endocarditis are composed of clumps of microorganisms, platelets, fibrin, occasional red blood cells, and few leukocytes attached to the surface of a valve leaflet, chorda, or ventricular endocardium (72). Underlying valve destruction may coexist. The morphologic characteristics of vegetations can vary, depending on the nature of the infecting organism and the activity of the disease, from small, flat, granular lesions to large, pedunculated, friable masses. Unimpaired bacterial growth results in extremely high colony counts (10^9 to 10^{10} bacteria per gram of tissue). As vegetations heal during the process of bacteriologic cure, infiltration by polymorphonuclear leukocytes and fibroblasts leads to fibrosis, hyalinization, and sometimes calcification. Finally, the lesion is covered by endothelium (73).

A disparity in clinical course and response to antimicrobial therapy between left-sided and right-sided infective endocarditis has long been noted in animal models of infective endocarditis and in patients. The exact mechanisms for this disparity remain largely undefined. However, some of the following factors may account for the increased severity of left-sided versus right-sided endocarditis: increases in oxygen tension resulting in increased intravegetation bacterial populations, higher rates of spontaneous emergence of antimicrobial-resistant strains, more frequent establishment of extracardiac foci of infection with resultant sustained bacteremia and valvular reseeding, reduced intralesional penetration of antibiotics, and attenuated penetration of the vegetation by phagocytic cells (74).

Organisms that possess little inherent pathogenicity, such as viridans streptococci, usually implant only on sites of preexisting nonbacterial thrombotic endocarditis; more virulent organisms, such as *S. aureus* or *S. pneumoniae,* may be able to infect apparently normal valves.

Conditions that predispose to bacteremia, particularly with the common causative organisms for infective endocarditis, have been examined extensively. Transient bacteremia occurs whenever a mucosal surface or other tissue heavily colonized with bacteria is traumatized. The degree of bacteremia is proportional to the number of organisms that inhabit the area. The number of organisms in blood usually does not exceed 10/mL, and intravascular residence is transient, lasting no more than 15 to 30 minutes (75,76). Transient bacteremias are most commonly associated with dental extraction; periodontal surgery; and invasive oropharyngeal, GI tract, urologic, or gynecologic diagnostic

or surgical procedures. Spontaneous bacteremia in the absence of trauma occurs with lung and skin infections and in patients with severe periodontal disease. Viridans streptococci are the bacteria most commonly isolated from blood, alone or mixed with other species, after trauma to tissues of the mouth (76). A wide variety of trivial events, such as chewing and tooth brushing, induce bacteremia caused by viridans streptococci and other mouth organisms. This may explain why no more than an estimated 5% to 10% of cases of endocarditis caused by mouth organisms can be related to dental procedures (13).

Enterococcal and gram-negative bacillus bacteremias occur commonly after genitourinary or GI tract surgery or instrumentation. Although about half of patients with enterococcal endocarditis have reported genitourinary tract manipulation before the onset of their disease, case-control studies have not demonstrated a relationship between enterococcal endocarditis and preceding genitourinary or GI tract procedures (77,78). Furthermore very few cases of enterococcal endocarditis possibly related to GI tract diagnostic procedures have been described (79). An antecedent staphylococcal infection has been reported in about 30% of patients with staphylococcal endocarditis.

PATHOPHYSIOLOGY

The symptoms and signs of infective endocarditis are highly variable. Clinical features result from the local intracardiac infectious process and its attendant complications, bland or septic embolization of fragments of vegetations to virtually any organ, constant bacteremia with seeding of distant foci, and development of immune complex–associated disease (65,80).

Intracardiac infection can lead to perforation of the valve leaflet or rupture of the chordae tendineae, interventricular septum, or papillary muscle (81). Infections, particularly with *S. aureus,* may result in valve ring abscesses and may extend into the myocardium to produce burrowing abscesses and purulent pericardial effusions. Conduction abnormalities, fistulas between chambers of the heart and pericardium or major vessels, and aneurysms of the sinus of Valsalva may result (81). Large vegetations such as those caused by fungi, group B streptococci, or the HACEK group of organisms can interfere with valve function and may occasionally occlude a valve orifice. Healing of the infection may cause scar formation and subsequent valvular stenosis or insufficiency. Myocarditis and myocardial infarction may be due to coronary artery emboli, myocardial abscesses, or immune complex vasculitis.

Embolic phenomena are common in infective endocarditis. Most often, the renal, splenic, coronary, and cerebral circulatory systems are involved. Pulmonary emboli occur in right-sided endocarditis, and large emboli suggest fungal infection. Infarcts or abscesses may result, depending on whether septic or bland embolization has occurred. Septic embolization to the vasa vasorum or direct bacterial invasion of the arterial wall produces mycotic aneurysms (81). The most commonly involved vessels include the cerebral arteries, aorta, sinus of Valsalva, ligated ductus arteriosus, and the superior mesenteric, splenic, coronary, and pulmonary arteries (82,83). Rupture of the weakened vessel may occur acutely or years later.

The persistent bacteremia of endocarditis stimulates both the humoral and the cellular immune systems (84,85). Specific antibodies of the immunoglobulin M (IgM), G (IgG), or A (IgA) class, having opsonic, agglutinating, and complement-fixing properties, as well as cryoglobulins and macroglobulins have been described in infective endocarditis. Nonspecific generalized hypergammaglobulinemia also develops, as in many other chronic infections. Circulating immune complexes are found in virtually all patients. Immune complex deposition along the glomerular basement membrane may result in the development of glomerulonephritis (focal, membranoproliferative, or diffuse) (81,86). Arthritis and peripheral manifestations of infective endocarditis, such as Osler nodes, have been attributed to immune complex deposition in joints and in mucocutaneous vessels. Effective treatment leads to disappearance of circulating immune complexes. Rheumatoid factor (anti-IgG/IgM antibody) develops in about 50% of patients with subacute infective endocarditis. The titer correlates with the level of hypergammaglobulinemia and decreases in response to therapy.

CLINICAL MANIFESTATIONS

Symptoms of endocarditis generally start within 2 weeks of the precipitating bacteremia (65,87–88). Nonspecific symptoms such as malaise, fatigue, night sweats, anorexia, and weight loss are common, particularly with organisms of low pathogenicity (e.g., viridans streptococci). The onset of infection with organisms of high pathogenicity (e.g., *S. aureus*) is usually explosive. Fever is present in almost all patients with endocarditis but may be absent in elderly persons, in persons with severe debility, renal failure, or congestive heart failure, or in those treated previously with antibiotics. The fever is usually low grade (temperature <39°C) except with acute disease (80).

Heart murmurs are almost always present, except in acute infections and with right-sided or mural infection. The appearance of a new regurgitant murmur or significant changes in a preexisting murmur (not changes in intensity caused by anemia or changes in heart rate or cardiac output) are uncommon but when present suggest acute disease (usually staphylococcal) and correlate with development of congestive heart failure (80).

Splenomegaly (present in up to 30% of cases), petechiae (20%–40%), and clubbing of the fingers (10%–20%) tend to occur in disease of long duration (more than 6 weeks) (80). Petechiae are most frequently found on the conjunctivae, palate, buccal mucosa, and extremities; they may be embolic or vasculitic. Splinter hemorrhages (subungual, linear, dark red streaks) are nonspecific, as they are often related to trauma. Lesions located proximally in the nail bed are more suggestive of endocarditis than are distal lesions. Osler nodes (small, tender nodules, usually on the finger or toe pads, that persist for hours to days) occur in 10% to 25% of patients but are also a feature of other diseases (80). Immune complexes have been demonstrated in dermal vessels of Osler nodes. Janeway lesions are due to septic emboli and are most commonly seen in acute endocarditis. They are nontender hemorrhagic areas on the palms and soles. Roth spots (oval retinal hemorrhages with a pale center located near the optic disk) occur in less than 5% of patients with endocarditis and are also found in patients with connective tissue disease and hematologic disorders. Musculoskeletal complaints (arthralgia or arthritis) may mimic rheumatologic disorders.

Systemic emboli may occur during or after therapy and are recognized in about one third of patients. Pulmonary emboli are common in IVDUs with tricuspid valve endocarditis (49,52) and can also be seen in left-sided endocarditis with left-to-right cardiac shunts. Neurologic manifestations are present in about one third of patients with endocarditis (89,90). Major emboli to the middle cerebral artery system occur in up to 25% of patients with endocarditis and mycotic aneurysms occur in 2% to 10%. Brain abscesses and purulent meningitis, cerebral arteritis, intracerebral bleeding, and encephalomalacia have also been documented in endocarditis. Although mycotic aneurysms are usually silent,

symptoms may be those of an expanding mass or a catastrophic hemorrhage. Congestive heart failure is the most common complication of infective endocarditis. Contributing factors include valve destruction, myocarditis, coronary artery emboli with infarction, and myocardial abscesses. Renal disease is present in most patients with endocarditis and is due to abscesses (uncommon), infarction (50%), or glomerulonephritis (up to 80%). Renal insufficiency may result.

LABORATORY FEATURES

A normochromic, normocytic anemia is present in 70% to 90% of cases of endocarditis and worsens with duration of illness. The white blood cell count is usually normal (91,92). In acute endocarditis (particularly staphylococcal), leukocytosis may be present. The erythrocyte sedimentation rate is almost always elevated (exceptions may occur in patients with heart or kidney failure). Rheumatoid factor is present in 50% of patients with endocarditis for at least 3 to 6 weeks. Circulating immune complexes are present in virtually all patients, but hypergammaglobulinemia is detected in only about 25%. High serum titers of antibodies directed against teichoic acid constituents of the cell wall of staphylococci suggest endocarditis or other deepseated infection (93). Unfortunately, false-positive reactions and cross-reactions with other gram-positive bacteria limit their usefulness in diagnosis. Large mononuclear cells can occasionally be seen in peripheral blood smears; the yield is increased to as high as 25% if the first drop of blood obtained after massage and puncture of the earlobe is examined. Intraleukocytic bacteria can be seen in buffy coat preparations of blood in about 50% of patients (94).

The urinalysis usually shows abnormalities, with proteinuria or microscopic hematuria in most patients. Reduction in serum complement parallels the occurrence of abnormal renal function, especially that caused by diffuse glomerulonephritis (95).

The blood culture is the critical diagnostic laboratory test in endocarditis, and blood cultures are positive in more than 95% of patients. The bacteremia in endocarditis is continuous, so if any culture is positive, all are likely to be positive. Because the magnitude of bacteremia is constant, timing of cultures based on temperature is not rational. In subacute disease, in the absence of previous therapy, three cultures should be obtained in 3 to 6 hours, after which time therapy is initiated. Cultures should be obtained at least 30 minutes apart to prove that the bacteremia is continuous. Results of blood cultures may be negative in as many as 25% of patients who recently received outpatient antibiotic therapy (96). Therefore, depending on clinical status, it may be necessary to judiciously delay treatment for a number of days while continuing to obtain cultures. This will increase the chances of obtaining positive blood cultures. Therapy for acute disease should not be delayed for more than 2 to 3 hours.

Only one culture should be obtained from each venipuncture using anaerobic and aerobic methods. If antibiotics have already been administered, media containing antibiotic removal or neutralization methods are available commercially. Modern commercially available automated blood culture systems will demonstrate most pathogens within 5 days of incubation (97). Subculturing onto enriched media at 5 days is a strategy to increase the yield of cultures in patients with suspected endocarditis. The yield of positive cultures may be further increased by observing them for 3 to 4 weeks and making periodic blind Gram stains and subcultures. Hypertonic media may improve recovery of cell wall–deficient bacteria from previously treated patients (98). Addition of pyridoxine hydrochloride or cysteine to media will improve chances of isolating *Abiotrophia* species (nutritionally deficient variant streptococci) on plates (99); most commercially available media now contain this supplementation (97). Arterial blood cultures or cultures of bone marrow offer no advantage over venipuncture (100).

Results of blood cultures may be negative in infections with fastidious organisms such as *Brucella* species and *Bartonella* species. Up to 17% of patients with *Candida* endocarditis and almost all with *Aspergillus, Histoplasma, C. burnetii,* or *Chlamydia psittaci* endocarditis have negative blood culture results (97,101,102). Because large peripheral emboli are common in fungal endocarditis, embolectomy with histologic examination and culture of the embolus may be diagnostic. Serologic procedures have not proved useful in the diagnosis of fungal endocarditis. Serologic tests are of particular value in endocarditis caused by *C. burnetii* and *Bartonella* species (101).

Cardiac ultrasonography has assumed an increasingly important role in the assessment and management of patients with suspected infective endocarditis (103–109). Two-dimensional echocardiography combined with Doppler echocardiography has become widely accepted as the technique for identifying underlying valvular abnormalities and their hemodynamic consequences. In selected cases, serial echocardiography findings can contribute to decisions for surgical intervention and intraoperatively guide the eventual cardiac repairs. Transesophageal echocardiography (TEE) has proven to be much more sensitive than transthoracic echocardiography (TTE) in detecting vegetations and structural cardiac complications of endocarditis such as mycotic aneurysms, intracardiac shunts, and valve ring abscesses. Limitations of TTE include relative insensitivity to small vegetations, poor visibility of periannular complications, and inability to detect abnormalities on prosthetic valves as a result of acoustic shadowing and poor acoustic windows. Compared with TTE, TEE is superior in delineating small (<5 mm) vegetations (sensitivity in multiple studies of 90%–95% vs. 70%–75% for TTE), perivalvular abscesses (sensitivity of 87% vs. 28% for TTE), and prosthetic valve abnormalities (sensitivity of 82% vs. 36% for TTE). The negative predictive value for infective endocarditis of a single TEE is greater than 90%, depending on the clinical circumstances and the absence of a prosthetic valve. Repeated TEE should be performed when suspicion of infection remains high and the initial study is not diagnostic.

DIAGNOSIS

The protean manifestations of infective endocarditis duplicate the clinical findings of atrial myxoma, acute rheumatic fever, marantic endocarditis, collagen-vascular diseases, and thrombotic thrombocytopenic purpura. Endocarditis should be suspected when a heart murmur and unexplained fever are present for at least 1 week, in febrile IVDUs, in young persons with a sudden neurologic event, and in patients with a prosthetic valve who have fever or valve dysfunction. Because overdiagnosis and underdiagnosis are common, particularly in patients with atypical presentations, clinical guidelines have been developed to aid in the accuracy of diagnosis. Currently the most frequently used guidelines are the Duke criteria proposed by Durack et al. (110), with modifications and refinements suggested by others (111–114). These criteria rely heavily on echocardiography in addition to blood culture evidence, which has always been the key to diagnosis. Table 62.2 shows a modification of the Duke criteria, as proposed by Li, Sexton, and Mick (114). In the final analysis, these criteria are guidelines; nothing can replace clinical judgment.

TABLE 62.2. Clinical Diagnosis of Infective Endocarditis

Definite infective endocarditis: two major criteria; or one major plus three minor criteria; or five minor criteria
Possible infective endocarditis: one major criterion plus one minor; or three minor criteria
A. Major criteria
 1. Evidence of sustained bacteremia: (a) at least two positive blood cultures for an organism that is typical for endocarditis (e.g., viridans streptococci; *Streptococcus bovis;* HACEK group; *Staphylococcus aureus;* community acquired-enterococcus with no primary focus) or (b) any organism that is not a typical cause of infective endocarditis but is consistent with endocarditis, isolated from all three or a majority of at least four blood cultures drawn over 1 or more hours or isolated from two blood cultures 12 or more hours apart; or (c) one blood culture positive for *Coxiella burnetii* or serological evidence of active infection with *C. burnetii.*
 2. Echocardiographic evidence of a vegetation or abscess or partial dehiscence of a prosthetic valve (if absent on transthoracic study, transesophageal echocardiogram required)
 3. New valvular regurgitation
B. Minor criteria
 1. Predisposing heart lesion or intravenous drug user
 2. Temperatures >38°C
 3. Vascular phenomena: Arterial emboli, septic pulmonary emboli, mycotic aneurysm, intracranial hemorrhage, conjunctival hemorrhages, Janeway lesions
 4. Immunologic phenomena: glomerulonephritis, Osler nodes, Roth spots, rheumatoid factor
 5. Positive blood culture not meeting (A.1.) above; or serologic evidence of active infection with an organism consistent with infective endocarditis (excludes single positive cultures for coagulase negative staphylococci or other organisms unlikely to be a cause of endocarditis)

TREATMENT

Inside the vegetation, infecting organisms exist at high densities in a state of reduced metabolic activity, protected from host defenses (115). Because cure requires eradication of all the organisms by antimicrobial agents, bactericidal rather than bacteriostatic agents must be used in high enough concentrations and for a long enough period to sterilize the vegetation (116). Parenteral therapy is preferable because it achieves higher and more predictable serum antibiotic levels than oral treatment. The antimicrobial susceptibility of the infecting organism should be determined accurately. The organism should be saved for (a) further antimicrobial susceptibility testing if a change in therapy is indicated, (b) determination of synergistic combinations of antibiotics if necessary, (c) comparison with a relapse strain, and (d) if indicated, future testing of serum bactericidal activity. A peak serum bactericidal titer (the highest dilution of the serum that kills a standard inoculum of the infecting organism *in vitro*) of 1:8 or greater generally indicates adequate therapy (117). Adequate therapeutic efficacy may be anticipated in streptococcal, enterococcal, staphylococcal, and HACEK group endocarditis with regimens containing penicillins, cephalosporins, or vancomycin, provided that the organisms are susceptible to these drugs. In these instances, routine assays of serum bactericidal titers are unnecessary. Determination of the titer is most valuable when response to therapy is suboptimal, when endocarditis is due to an unusual organism, or when an unconventional treatment regimen is used (24).

In the past several years, a trend toward outpatient management of patients with uncomplicated infective endocarditis has evolved. Parenteral regimens using intravenous catheters and antibiotics with long therapeutic half-lives have given results comparable to those achieved with treatment rendered in inpatient settings (118,119).

Blood cultures should be obtained soon after antimicrobial therapy is instituted to ensure that the bacteremia has been eradicated. Use of anticoagulants should be avoided if possible, because of an increased risk for intracranial hemorrhage.

SPECIFIC ANTIMICROBIAL REGIMENS

While awaiting the results of blood cultures, empiric antimicrobial therapy should be directed at the organism or organisms most likely to cause infection in the clinical setting. For patients with a native valve and a subacute clinical course, therapy should be directed against enterococci, which are more antibiotic resistant than streptococci; in those patients with an acute course, treatment should cover *S. aureus*. In IVDUs, therapy should be directed against *S. aureus* (including methicillin-resistant organisms in cities with high rates of this organism among IVDUs) and gram-negative bacilli (e.g., a regimen of nafcillin or vancomycin plus gentamicin). Patients with prosthetic valves should receive empiric antibiotic coverage for methicillin-resistant *S. epidermidis* and gram-negative bacilli. When the organism has been identified, the antimicrobial coverage should be adjusted according to the results of *in vitro* susceptibility testing. If cultures remain negative but endocarditis is likely and a clinical response has occurred, the empiric treatment is continued. Recommendations for the specific antimicrobial treatment of streptococcal, enterococcal, staphylococcal, and HACEK group endocarditis have been published by the American Heart Association (24).

Streptococci and Enterococci

Regimens for streptococcal endocarditis are based principally on the minimum inhibitory concentration (MIC) of the isolate to penicillin G (24).

HIGHLY PENICILLIN-SUSCEPTIBLE VIRIDANS AND OTHER STREPTOCOCCI (MIC NO MORE THAN 0.1 μg/mL)

These recommendations (Table 62.3) also apply to infection with *S. bovis*, a penicillin-susceptible nonenterococcal group D streptococcus. Penicillin G alone for 4 weeks (regimen A) gives cure rates of up to 98%. Ceftriaxone alone for 4 weeks (regimen B) gives equivalent results. Addition of gentamicin (regimen C or D) produces synergistic killing and sterilizes cardiac vegetations more rapidly. Equivalent cure rates are obtained in 2 weeks (24,120). Two-week regimens (i.e., regimens C and D) are appropriate only for uncomplicated infections. Regimen A or B is preferred for patients who are likely to have side effects with aminoglycosides (those with renal insufficiency, with eighth nerve disease, or older than 65 years). Alternative regimens for

---

TABLE 62.3. Treatment of Infective Endocarditis (See text for details)

Streptococci and enterococci
Viridans streptococci and *Streptococcus bovis*
  Penicillin G susceptible (MIC ≤ 0.1 μg/mL)
    Regimen A: Penicillin G 12–18 million units/d i.v. in divided doses q4h or ampicillin 6–12 g/d in divided doses q4h for 4 wk
    [a]Regimen B: Ceftriaxone 2 g/d i.v. or i.m. in a single dose for 4 wk
    Regimen C: Penicillin as in regimen A plus gentamicin 1 mg/kg q8h or 1.5 mg/kg q12h i.v. or i.m. both for 2 wk
    [a]Regimen D: Ceftriaxone as in regimen B plus gentamicin as in regimen C both for 2 wk
    [a]Regimen E: Vancomycin 15 mg/kg i.v. q12h for 4 wk
  Relatively penicillin G resistant (MIC > 0.1 μg/mL but <0.5 μg/mL)
    Regimen F: Penicillin G 18 million units/d i.v. for 4 wk plus gentamicin as in regimen C for the first 2 wk
    [a]Regimen G: Ceftriaxone as in regimen B plus gentamicin as in regimen C for the first 2 wk
    [a]Regimen E (see above)
  Enterococci, viridans streptococci (MIC ≥ 0.5 μg/mL) and nutritionally variant streptococci (*Abiotrophia* species)
    Regimen H: Penicillin G 18–30 million units/d or ampicillin 12 g/d i.v. in divided doses q4h plus gentamicin 1 mg/kg i.v. q8h or streptomycin 7.5 mg/kg (not to exceed 500 mg) i.m. q12h, both for 4–6 wk
    [a]Regimen I: Vancomycin 15 mg/kg i.v. q12h plus gentamicin or streptomycin as in regimen H, both for 4–6 wk
  Prosthetic valve (see text)
Staphylococci
Native valve
  Methicillin susceptible (*Staphylococcus epidermidis, Staphylococcus aureus*)
    Regimen J: Nafcillin 2 g i.v. q4h for 4–6 wk with or without gentamicin 1 mg/kg i.v. q8h for the first 3–5 d
    [a]Regimen K: Cefazolin 2 g i.v. q8h for 4–6 wk with or without gentamicin as in regimen J
    [a]Regimen L: Vancomycin 15 mg/kg i.v. q12h for 4–6 wk
  Methicillin resistant
    [a]Regimen L (see above)
Prosthetic valve
  Methicillin susceptible
    Regimen M: Nafcillin 2 g i.v. q4h or cefazolin 2 g i.v. q8h plus rifampin 300 mg p.o. q8h for 6–8 wk with gentamicin 1 mg/kg i.v. q8h for the first 2 wk
    [a]Regimen N: Vancomycin 15 mg/kg i.v. q12h plus rifampin 300 mg p.o. q8h for 6–8 wk with gentamicin as in regimen M for the first 2 wk
  Methicillin resistant
    Regimen N (see above)

i.m., intramuscularly; i.v., intravenously; MIC, minimal inhibitory concentration.
[a]Regimens for patients allergic to penicillin. Cephalosporins should not be used in individuals with immediate-type hypersensitivity (urticaria, angioedema, or anaphylaxis) to penicillins.
With gentamicin 1 mg/kg i.v. or i.m. q8h, a peak serum concentration of about 3 μg/mL is desirable 1 hr after a 20–30-min i.v. infusion or i.m. injection. The trough level should be <1 μg/mL. In obese patients, dosage on a milligram-per-kilogram basis should be based on ideal body weight.
With vancomycin, peak serum concentrations should be 30–45 μg/mL 1 hour after completion of a 1-hour infusion. Daily dosage should not exceed 2 g/24 hr unless serum levels are monitored. In obese patients, dosing should be based on ideal body weight.

penicillin-allergic patients include regimens B and D for those with a history of penicillin rash and regimen E for those who have experienced immediate-type hypersensitivity (i.e., urticaria angioedema or anaphylaxis). A 6-week regimen of penicillin with an aminoglycoside for at least the first 2 weeks is recommended for patients with PVE.

Regimens B, D, and E can be used more easily for home therapy. In fact, single daily doses of gentamicin (3 mg/kg), together with single daily doses of ceftriaxone, have used successfully in 2-week courses (120).

RELATIVELY PENICILLIN-RESISTANT STREPTOCOCCI (MIC >0.1 AND <0.5 μg/mL)

Treatment with 18 million units daily of penicillin in combination with an aminoglycoside (regimen F) is recommended for strains of viridans streptococci and strains of *S. bovis* relatively resistant to penicillin (24). When penicillin cannot be used because of development of a rash, a cephalosporin can be substituted for the penicillin (regimen G). For patients with immediate-type allergic reactions, vancomycin alone (regimen E) for 4 weeks is the substitute of choice.

ENTEROCOCCI, VIRIDANS STREPTOCOCCI (MIC OF AT LEAST 0.5 μg/mL), AND NUTRITIONALLY VARIANT STREPTOCOCCI (ABIOTROPHIA SPECIES)

Enterococci are relatively resistant to penicillin G (median MIC, 2 μg/mL) and uniformly resistant to cephalosporins. Because penicillin, ampicillin, and vancomycin alone are not bactericidal for enterococci, treatment of enterococcal endocarditis requires the addition of an aminoglycoside to achieve a synergistic bactericidal effect [regimen H routinely, or regimen I for persons allergic to penicillin or where high-level penicillin resistance is present (usually *E. faecium*)]. This has resulted in cure rates of approximately 75%. Therapy usually lasts 4 weeks but should be extended to 6 weeks when symptoms have existed for more than 3 months or the course is complicated and to 6 or more weeks when infection is present on a prosthetic valve.

The synergistic bactericidal effect of aminoglycosides on enterococci occurs only when growth *in vitro* is inhibited by 2,000 μg/mL of the aminoglycoside. The degree of resistance and the susceptibility to individual aminoglycosides is highly variable, so testing *in vitro* should be routine. Synergism is more likely with gentamicin than with streptomycin. In many locales, enterococci resistant to 2,000 μg/mL or more of gentamicin have become common (121). Although some of these gentamicin-resistant strains are inhibited by streptomycin, most are resistant to all aminoglycosides. It is unlikely with strains resistant to all aminoglycosides that the addition of an aminoglycoside would be of benefit. For these organisms, aminoglycosides probably should be excluded from the regimen, and the duration of therapy should be prolonged to 8 to 12 weeks. Relapse is more likely in infections with these organisms.

Patients infected with β-lactamase–producing enterococci should receive either ampicillin-sulbactam or vancomycin plus an aminoglycoside antibiotic if they do not demonstrate concurrent aminoglycoside resistance. Nosocomially acquired enterococcal strains (especially *E. faecium*) may be resistant to vancomycin, penicillins, and aminoglycosides, thus posing a major therapeutic dilemma (122). Antibiotic selection should be based on *in vitro* susceptibility and synergy by testing. If teicoplanin susceptibility is demonstrated in a vancomycin- and β-lactam–resistant strain, this agent should be used if it can be obtained (not available in the United States). When organisms are resistant to β-lactam antibiotics, aminoglycosides, vancomycin, and teicoplanin, the best option is probably to use linezolid (*E. faecalis* or *E. faecium*) or quinupristin-dalfopristin (*E. faecium*

only) with or without other antibiotics depending on *in vitro* testing results. Experience with these agents in treatment of enterococcal endocarditis is minimal (123). However, because they are bacteriostatic, their effectiveness is in question, and it is likely that many cases would require cardiac surgery to achieve cure. In addition, various combinations of penicillins, vancomycin, cephalosporins, and aminoglycosides have been effective in experimental models (122).

Staphylococci

Most staphylococci are resistant to penicillin G because they elaborate penicillinase. Drugs of choice for the treatment of most patients with native valve staphylococcal endocarditis are semisynthetic penicillinase-resistant penicillins such as nafcillin (regimen J) or first-generation cephalosporins (regimen K). Patients who cannot tolerate penicillins or cephalosporins should receive intravenous vancomycin (regimen L). A large percentage of coagulase-negative staphylococci (*S. epidermidis*) and an increasing percentage of coagulase-positive strains (*S. aureus*) are methicillin resistant; these strains are resistant to all penicillins and cephalosporins, and intravenous vancomycin (regimen L) is the only option. Addition of an aminoglycoside to these regimens for the first 3 to 5 days hastens clearing of bacteremia, but evidence of improved outcome is lacking, so routine administration of an aminoglycoside is not recommended (124). Treatment for 4 weeks is standard; prolonged courses of 6 weeks or longer are indicated for patients with metastatic or intracardiac abscesses or otherwise complicated courses. As vancomycin use for the treatment of *S. aureus* infective endocarditis has increased, suboptimal clinical outcomes have been documented and concerns have been raised regarding the comparative efficacy of glycopeptide antibiotics (i.e., vancomycin, teicoplanin) versus the β-lactam agents (3). Delays in *in vitro* bacterial killing, as well as prolonged fever and bacteremia in patients, have been documented with vancomycin and teicoplanin even with uncomplicated right-sided endocarditis caused by methicillin-susceptible strains (125). More disturbing have been reports of bacteriologic failures even when organisms are demonstrably vancomycin susceptible. Failures of the antibiotic have been variously attributed to high protein binding, poor penetration of drug into vegetations, inadequate killing of stationary-phase bacteria, and rapid renal clearance (32).

S. aureus tricuspid valve infections in IVDUs are much more responsive to antimicrobial therapy than aortic or mitral valve infections. Two-week courses of a penicillinase-resistant penicillin plus an aminoglycoside have been highly successful in treatment of *S. aureus* tricuspid valve disease (52,126,127). In fact one study reported a high cure rate with the penicillinase-resistant penicillin alone for 2 weeks (126). Outcome depends on careful selection of patients without large vegetations, left-sided endocarditis, or extracardiac metastatic foci of infection. Because of unacceptably high failure rates, short-course therapy with a vancomycin-aminoglycoside combination is not recommended (128,129). There has also been some advocacy for oral treatment of uncomplicated right-sided infective endocarditis. An oral regimen consisting of a fluoroquinolone and rifampin showed promise in preliminary trials; however, bacteriologic and clinical failures have been documented (130–132). The linkage of quinolone resistance with methicillin resistance further limits the widespread usefulness of these agents in IVDUs with staphylococcal-infective endocarditis.

There is scant experience with methicillin-resistant strains of *S. aureus* that are of intermediate resistance to vancomycin or completely resistant to vancomycin (35,36). If endocarditis was caused by one of these organisms, linezolid or quinupristin-dalfopristin would probably be the treatment of choice (29,37).

STAPHYLOCOCCAL ENDOCARDITIS IN THE PRESENCE OF INTRACARDIAC PROSTHETIC MATERIAL

In the absence of contradictory evidence *in vitro*, all *S. epidermidis* organisms causing PVE should be assumed to be methicillin resistant. Optimal antibiotic therapy is provided by vancomycin plus rifampin for 6 to 8 weeks, with an aminoglycoside added for the first 2 weeks of therapy (regimen N). If myocardial abscess or valve dysfunction is present, surgery is required. Similar combination therapy is also recommended for MRSA PVE. Methicillin-susceptible strains should be treated with a penicillinase-resistant penicillin, together with rifampin for 6 to 8 weeks, with gentamicin added for the first 2 weeks (regimen M) unless a penicillin can not be used because of hypersensitivity, in which case, regimen N is used.

HACEK Group

Endocarditis caused by one of the HACEK group organisms should be treated with ceftriaxone (2 g i.v. or i.m. in a single daily dose for 4 weeks with a native valve and for 6 weeks with a prosthetic valve) (24). In patients who cannot be treated with ceftriaxone, a fluoroquinolone such as ciprofloxacin is the agent of choice.

Other Organisms

Endocarditis caused by gram-negative bacilli, anaerobes, and other uncommon pathogens should be treated with the regimen of bactericidal drugs that demonstrates the best activity *in vitro* (133). If efficacy *in vitro* can be demonstrated, the best results are obtained by combining β-lactam antibiotics (e.g., penicillins, cephalosporins, imipenem, and aztreonam) or vancomycin with an aminoglycoside and administering the drugs for 4 to 6 weeks. Quinolone antibiotics, such as ciprofloxacin, have expanded treatment options for gram-negative bacillary endocarditis by allowing prolonged oral administration of these agents. Although clinical experience is limited, reports indicate successful outcomes even in *Pseudomonas* endocarditis (52,134). Serum bactericidal titers should be monitored. Valve replacement may be necessary in addition to antimicrobial therapy.

Currently available antifungal agents are unlikely to cure fungal endocarditis, so a combined medical (amphotericin B, alone or with other antifungal agents) and early surgical approach (excision of the vegetation or valve replacement) is advocated. The role of caspofungin and the new triazoles (posaconazole and voriconazole) in treatment of fungal endocarditis has not been determined. Outcome of medical therapy alone is poor at best, and relapses are common after discontinuation of therapy. The availability of oral azole agents active against *Candida* and *Aspergillus* species provides feasible agents for long-term oral antifungal treatment and suppression. A report of fungal infective endocarditis on prosthetic valves has indicated a marked improvement in outcome when postoperative antifungal suppression is maintained indefinitely (62).

SURGERY IN THE MANAGEMENT OF ENDOCARDITIS

The four principal indications for cardiac surgical intervention in infective endocarditis are as follows: (a) moderate to severe congestive heart failure resulting from valve dysfunction, (b) uncontrolled infection, (c) prosthetic valve dysfunction or dehiscence, and (d) paravalvular abscess (135–141). In patients with acute aortic regurgitation from endocarditis complicated by congestive heart failure, mortality exceeds 50% (137,138). Immediate valve replacement is essential. Valve replacement for uncontrolled infection is indicated (a) when blood cultures remain persistently positive (over 7 days) despite appropriate antimicrobial therapy, (b) when appropriate microbicidal therapy is not available (e.g., infections caused by fungi or certain gram-negative bacilli), or (c) when recurrent relapse occurs despite appropriate antimicrobial therapy. Surgery often becomes necessary for PVE caused by organisms other than streptococci. Persistence of infection with the same organism has been uncommon after valve replacement. Postoperative antimicrobial therapy should be continued long enough to eradicate metastatic foci of infection. Valvulectomy without valve implantation may suffice in right-sided endocarditis (52). Myocardial invasion extending from the valve annulus is common in PVE. Prompt surgical intervention may be life saving (136).

Surgery should be considered when large vegetations are demonstrated by echocardiography and there are recurrent (at least two) arterial emboli during appropriate antimicrobial therapy (136). However, several studies have now determined that the rate at which emboli occur during treatment is time dependent; a twofold to threefold reduction of embolic events occurs between the first week and the second to third week of effective antibiotic treatment, regardless of the size, shape, mobility, and location of the vegetations (142–144). Therefore, after 1 week of therapy, reembolization is much less likely to occur.

Headache or transient or persistent central nervous system symptoms must suggest the possibility of a leaking or enlarging mycotic aneurysm. Radiologic evaluation is required, and in the presence of symptoms and an aneurysm, intervention by either interventional radiology or neurosurgery is indicated.

PROGNOSIS

The fever of most patients subsides by 3 to 5 days after antimicrobial therapy is begun. Persistence or recurrence of fever may be due to associated myocardial or metastatic abscesses, recurrent emboli, superinfection of the vegetation, or most often febrile reactions to antimicrobial agents (145). Petechiae, Osler nodes, emboli, rupture of mycotic aneurysms, and congestive heart failure may continue or develop during or even after effective antimicrobial therapy. Blood cultures performed 2 to 4 weeks after completion of therapy will detect most relapses but are not necessary if the patient has remained well.

The factors that predispose to a poor prognosis in infective endocarditis are nonstreptococcal disease, development of heart failure, aortic valve involvement, presence of large vegetations, infection of a prosthetic valve, older age, and valve ring or myocardial abscesses (146).

With a native valve, the cure rate for streptococcal endocarditis is about 90%. Failures are due to heart failure, embolic phenomena, rupture of mycotic aneurysms, complications of cardiac surgery, or renal failure (24). For non-IVDUs, mortality from *S. aureus* endocarditis ranges from 25% to 40%, whereas cure rates in IVDUs exceed 90% (147). Death is more likely to occur during the initial 2 weeks of therapy as a consequence of congestive heart failure, rupture of mycotic aneurysms, or widespread metastatic infection. Results of medical therapy alone are poor in endocarditis caused by fungi and gram-negative bacilli.

The overall mortality rate from PVE has been reduced by earlier and more aggressive cardiac surgery, coupled with antibiotic therapy, and has been reported to be as low as 10% to 30% in selected series from centers with extensive experience with this type of surgery (61,148–153). The mortality for early disease has classically been significantly higher than that for late disease, but this is probably mainly related to the organisms involved and the higher frequency of invasion of paravalvular tissue. Early and radical cardiac surgery for early PVE may narrow the differences in prognosis between early and late PVE (154). Seemingly clear is that the prognosis of *S. aureus* infection on a prosthetic valve is poor and is significantly improved by aggressive surgical intervention (61,155). About 10% of patients with native valve endocarditis or PVE will have additional episodes of endocarditis.

PREVENTION

In an effort to prevent infective endocarditis, the American Heart Association has recommended antibiotic prophylaxis in patients with predisposing cardiac lesions who are to undergo certain traumatic procedures to the oral mucosa or genitourinary or GI tracts (156). Prophylaxis for oral procedures is directed at the oral flora, mainly viridans streptococci, and prophylaxis for genitourinary tract or below-the-diaphragm GI tract procedures is directed at enterococci. There is no direct proof that antibiotic prophylaxis reduces the risk for endocarditis, and recent studies have indicated that the large majority of cases of endocarditis occur from bacteremias produced by activities of daily living (e.g., brushing teeth and chewing), rather than from the occasional bacteremia associated with traumatic procedures (13,77,78). However, it is generally accepted that at least some cases of endocarditis are related to the bacteremias caused by traumatic procedures to mucosal surfaces with high titers of an indigenous microflora, and prophylaxis is used in an attempt to prevent these cases.

The conditions for which prophylaxis is recommended are classified as high risk or moderate risk (156). High-risk conditions are prosthetic cardiac valves (including bioprosthetic valves and homografts), previous infective endocarditis, complex cyanotic CHD, and surgically constructed systemic pulmonary shunts or conduits. Moderate-risk conditions are most other congenital heart malformations (except for uncomplicated atrial septal defects or surgically corrected cardiac lesions more than 6 months after operation), acquired valvular heart disease (e.g., rheumatic or degenerative), and hypertrophic cardiomyopathy. MVP is a common lesion, and the risk for endocarditis is only moderately increased. Therefore, prophylaxis is recommended only for patients with valvular regurgitation and/or thickened leaflets; these patients are considered to be at moderate risk.

Prophylaxis is recommended for dental and other traumatic procedures in the mouth, nose, throat, or esophagus that are likely to cause bleeding and is aimed at viridans streptococci (156). The specific dental procedures for which prophylaxis is recommended are dental extractions, periodontal procedures, dental implant placement, subgingival placement of antibiotic fibers or strips, initial placement of orthodontic bands, intraligamentary injections, and prophylactic cleaning of the teeth or implants where bleeding is expected. Prophylaxis is recommended for root canal procedures only if surgery or instrumentation is beyond the apex. The specific respiratory tract and esophageal procedures for which prophylaxis is recommended are tonsillectomy, adenoidectomy, surgery on the respiratory mucosa, and bronchoscopy only with a rigid bronchoscope. Prophylaxis aimed at viridans streptococci is recommended for sclerotherapy of esophageal varices and esophageal stricture dilation for patients with high-risk cardiac lesions and is optional for medium-risk lesions.

TABLE 62.4. Recommendations for Prophylaxis Against Endocarditis

Procedure	Risk factors	Patient-related factors determining choice of regimen	Recommended regimen
Dental, oral, respiratory tract, or esophageal procedures (aimed at viridans streptococci)	High- and moderate-risk patients	Ability to take oral antibiotic and no allergy to amoxicillin/amplicillin	Amoxicillin 2.0 g orally 1 hr before procedure
		Inability to take oral antibiotic and no allergy to amoxicillin/ampicillin	Ampicillin, i.v. or i.m. 2.0 g 30 min before procedure
		Allergy to amoxicillin/ampicillin	Clindamycin 600 mg p.o. 1 hr before procedure or cephalexin[a] or cefadroxil[a] 2.0 g p.o. 1 hr before procedure or azithromycin or clarithromycin 500 mg p.o. 1 hr before procedure
		Inability to take oral antibiotic and allergy to amoxicillin/ampicillin	Clindamycin 600 mg i.v. 30 min before procedure or cefazolin[a] 1 g i.m. or i.v. 30 min before procedure
Genitourinary or gastrointestinal tract (excluding esophageal procedures) (aimed at enterococci)	High-risk patients	No allergy to amoxicillin/ampicillin	Ampicillin 2.0 g i.v. or i.m. plus gentamicin 1.5 mg/kg[b] i.v. or i.m. within 30 min of starting procedure; 6 hr later ampicillin 1 g i.v. or i.m. or amoxicillin 1 g p.o.
		Allergy to amoxicillin/ampicillin	Vancomycin 1 g i.v. over 1–2 hr plus gentamicin 1.5 mg/kg[b] i.v. or i.m.; complete injection/infusion within 30 min of starting procedure
	Moderate-risk patients	No allergy to amoxicillin/ampicillin	Amoxicillin 2 g p.o. 1 hr before procedure, or ampicillin 2.0 g i.v. or i.m. within 30 min of starting procedure
		Allergy to amoxicillin/ampicillin	Vancomycin 1 g i.v. over 1–2 hr: complete infusion within 30 min of starting procedure

[a]Cephalosporins should not be used in individuals with immediate-type hypersensitivity reactions (urticaria, angioedema, or anaphylaxis) to penicillins.
[b]Not to exceed 120 mg.
i.m., intramuscularly; i.v., intravenously; p.o., per os.

Prophylaxis aimed against enterococci is recommended for certain procedures involving the genitourinary tract and the GI tract below the diaphragm (156). The specific genitourinary tract procedures for which prophylaxis is recommended are prostatic surgery, cystoscopy, and urethral dilation. Prophylaxis is recommended for endoscopic retrograde cholangiography with biliary obstruction, biliary tract surgery, and surgery on intestinal mucosa for patients with high-risk cardiac lesions and is optional for medium-risk lesions. Prophylaxis is optional for high-risk cardiac lesions for bronchoscopy with a flexible bronchoscope with or without biopsy, TEE, endoscopy with or without biopsy, vaginal hysterectomy, and vaginal delivery. Recommendations for prophylaxis by the American Heart Association are outlined in Table 62.4.

Prophylaxis for cardiac surgery, including implantation of prosthetic devices, patches, and sutures, is directed against staphylococci. The usual regimen is intravenous administration of cefazolin, 2 g, immediately before surgery, with additional doses to maintain levels interoperatively and no more than 24 hours postoperatively. With the emergence of methicillin-resistant *S. epidermidis* (and more recently MRSA) as important nosocomial pathogens, it has been necessary to consider the substitution of vancomycin for cefazolin, especially in institutions with postoperative cardiac valve infections with these organisms (157). Vancomycin is also used for patients who are hypersensitive to penicillin and cephalosporins. It is reasonable to consider adding gentamicin to cefazolin or vancomycin to achieve a synergistic bactericidal effect and for better coverage of gram-negative bacilli.

REFERENCES

1. Kelson SR, White PD. Notes on 250 cases of subacute bacterial streptococcal endocarditis studied and treated between 1927 and 1939. *Ann Intern Med* 1940;22:40.
2. Christie RV. Penicillin in subacute bacterial endocarditis. *Br Med J* 1948;1:4539.
3. Bayer AS. Infective endocarditis. *Clin Infect Dis* 1993;17:313.
4. Hoesley CJ, Cobbs CG. Endocarditis at the millennium. *J Infect Dis* 1999;179[Suppl 2]:S360.
5. Berlin JA, Abrutyn E, Strom BL, et al. Incidence of infective endocarditis in the Delaware Valley, 1988–1990. *Am J Cardiol* 1995;76:933.
6. Parkhurst GF, Decker JP. Bacterial aortitis and mycotic aneurysms of the aorta: a report of 12 cases. *Am J Pathol* 1955;31:821.
7. Kerr A Jr. *Subacute bacterial endocarditis.* Springfield, IL: Charles C Thomas, 1955:3–343.
8. Weinberger I, Rotenberg Z, Zacharovitch D, et al. Native valve infective endocarditis in the 1970's versus the 1980's: underlying cardiac lesions and infecting organisms. *Clin Cardiol* 1990;13:94.
9. McKinsey DS, Ratts TE, Bisno AL. Underlying cardiac lesions in adults with infective endocarditis. *Am J Med* 1987;82:681.
10. Frary CJ, Devereux RB, Kramer-Fox R, et al. Clinical and health care cost consequences of infective endocarditis in mitral valve prolapse. *Am J Cardiol* 1993;73:263.
11. Marks AR, Choong CY, Chir MBB, et al. Identification of high-risk and low-risk subgroups of patients with mitral valve prolapse. *N Engl J Med* 1989;320:1031.
12. Kaye D. Changing pattern of infective endocarditis. *Am J Med* 1985;78[Suppl 6B]:157.
13. Strom BL, Abrutyn E, Berlin JA, et al. Dental and cardiac risk factors for infective endocarditis. *Ann Intern Med* 1998;129:761.
14. DiNubile MJ, Calderwood SB, Steinhaus DM, et al. Cardiac conduction abnormalities complicating native valve active infective endocarditis. *Am J Cardiol* 1986;58:1213.
15. Pelletier LL, Petersdorf RG. Infective endocarditis: a review of 125 cases from the University of Washington Hospital, 1963–72. *Medicine (Baltimore)* 1977;56:287.
16. Stekelberg JM, Melton LJ IV, Ilstrup DM, et al. Influence of referral bias on the apparent clinical spectrum of infective endocarditis. *Am J Med* 1990;88:582.
17. Harris SL. Definitions and demographic characteristics. In: Kaye D, ed. *Infective endocarditis*, 2nd ed. New York: Raven Press, 1992:1.
18. Tunkel AR, Mandell, GL. Infecting microorganisms. In: Kaye D, ed. *Infective endocarditis*, 2nd ed. New York: Raven Press, 1992:85.
19. Castillo JC, Anguita MP, Ramirez A. Long term outcome of infective endocarditis in patients who were not drug addicts: a 10 year study. *Heart* 2000;83:525.
20. Tuazon CU, Gill V, Gill F. Streptococcal endocarditis: single vs. combination antibiotic therapy and role of various species. *Rev Infect Dis* 1986;8:54.
21. Guiot HF, Corel LJ, Vossen JM. Prevalence of penicillin-resistant viridans streptococci in healthy children and in patients with malignant hematological disorders. *Eur J Clin Microbiol Infect Dis* 1994;13:645.
22. Murray BE. The life and times of the enterococcus. *Clin Microbiol Rev* 1990;3:46.
23. Martone WJ. Spread of vancomycin-resistant enterococci: why did it happen in the United States? *Infect Control Hosp Epidemiol* 1998;19:539.
24. Wilson W, Karchmer AW, Dajani AS, et al. Antibiotic treatment of adults with infective endocarditis due to streptococci, enterococci, staphylococci, and HACEK microorganisms. *JAMA* 1995;274:1706.
25. Low DE, Willey BM, Betschel S, et al. Enterococci: pathogens of the 90's. *Eur J Surg Suppl* 1994;573:19.
26. Murray BE, Singh KV, Markowitz SM, et al. Evidence for clonal spread of a single strain of β-lactamase producing *Enterococcus (Streptococcus) faecalis* to six hospitals in five states. *J Infect Dis* 1991;163:780.
27. Eliopoulos GM. Aminoglycoside resistant enterococcal endocarditis. *Infect Dis Clin North Am* 1993;7:117.
28. Lundstrom TS, Sobel JD. Antibiotics for gram-positive bacterial infections. *Infect Dis Clin North Am* 2000;14:464.
29. Chien JW, Kucia ML, Salata RA. Use of linezolid, an oxazolidinone, in the treatment of multidrug-resistant gram-positive bacterial infections. *Clin Infect Dis* 2000;30:146.
30. Leport C, Bure A, Leport J, et al. Incidence of colonic lesions in *Streptococcus bovis* and enterococcal endocarditis. *Lancet* 1987;1:748.
31. Sambola A, Miro JM, Tornos MP. Streptococcus agalactiae infective endocarditis: analysis of 30 cases and review of the literature, 1962–1998. *Clin Infect Dis* 2002;34:1576.
32. Mortara LA, Bayer AS. *Staphylococcus aureus* bacteremia and endocarditis—new diagnostic and therapeutic concepts. *Infect Dis Clin North Am* 1993;7:53.
33. Whitener C, Caputo GM, Weitekamp MR, et al. Endocarditis due to coagulase-negative staphylococci: microbiologic, epidemiologic and clinical considerations. *Infect Dis Clin North Am* 1993;7:81.
34. Voss A, Milatovic D, Wallrauch-Schwarz C, et al. Methicillin-resistant *Staphylococcus aureus* in Europe. *Eur J Clin Microbiol Infect Dis* 1994;13:50.
35. Fridkin SK. Vancomycin-intermediate and -resistant *Staphylococcus aureus*: what the infectious disease specialist needs to know. *Clin Infect Dis* 2001;32:108.
36. *Staphylococcus aureus* resistant to vancomycin—United States. *MMWR Morb Mortal Wkly Rep* 2002;51:565.
37. Drew RH, Perfect JR, Srinath L, et al. Treatment of methicillin-resistant *Staphylococcus aureus* infections with quinupristin-dalfopristin in patients intolerant of or failing prior therapy. *J Antimicrob Chemother* 2000;46:775.
38. Burgert SJ, LaRocco MT, Wilansky S. Destructive native valve endocarditis caused by *Staphylococcus lugdunensis*. *South Med J* 1999;92:812.
39. Geraci JE, Wilson WR. Symposium on infective endocarditis, III: endocarditis due to gram-negative bacteria, report of 56 cases. *Mayo Clin Proc* 1982;57:145.
40. Bruyn GAW, Thompson J, Vandermeer JWM. Pneumococcal endocarditis in adult patients: a report of five cases and review of the literature. *Q J Med* 1990;74:33.
41. Owens JE, Kelchak JA: Gonococcal endocarditis: report of a case and review of the literature. *J S C Med Assoc* 1990;86:93.
42. Fenollar F, Lepidi H, Raoult D. Whipple's endocarditis: review of the literature and comparisons with Q fever, *Bartonella* infection and blood culture-positive endocarditis. *Clin Infect Dis* 2001;33:1309.
43. Brouqui P, Raoult D. Endocarditis due to rare and fastidious bacteria. *Clin Microbiol Rev* 2001;14:177.
44. Yersin B, Glauser MP, Guze PA, et al. Experimental *Escherichia coli* endocarditis in rats: roles of serum bactericidal activity and duration of catheter placement. *Infect Immun* 1988;56:1273.
45. Rubinstein E, Noriega ER, Simberkoff MS, et al. Fungal endocarditis: analysis of 24 cases and review of the literature. *Medicine (Baltimore)* 1975;54:331.
46. Bayer AS, Ward FL, Ginzton LE, et al. Evaluation of new clinical criteria for diagnosis of infective endocarditis. *Am J Med* 1994;96:211.
47. Weisse AB, Heller DR, Schimenti RJ, et al. The febrile parenteral drug user: a prospective study in 121 patients. *Am J Med* 1993;94:274.
48. Chambers HF, Morris DL, Tauber MG, et al. Cocaine use and the risk for endocarditis in intravenous drug users. *Ann Intern Med* 1987;106:833.
49. Reisberg BE. Infective endocarditis in the narcotic addict. *Prog Cardiovasc Dis* 1979;22:193.
50. Hecht SR, Berger M. Right-sided endocarditis in intravenous drug users. Prognostic features in 102 episodes. *Ann Intern Med* 1992;117:560.
51. Vlahov D, Sullivan M, Astemborski J. Bacterial infections and skin cleaning prior to injection among intravenous drug users. *Public Health Rep* 1992;107:595.
52. Miro JM, del Rio A, Mestres CA. Infective endocarditis in intravenous drug abusers and HIV-1 infected patients. *Infect Dis Clin North Am* 2002;16:273.
53. Chambers HF, Korzeniowski OM, Sande MA, the National Collaborative Endocarditis Study Group. *Staphylococcus aureus* endocarditis: clinical manifestations in addicts and nonaddicts. *Medicine (Baltimore)* 1983;62:170.

54. Valencia ME, Guinea J, Soriano V, et al. Study of 164 episodes of infective endocarditis in drug addicts: comparison of HIV positive and negative patients. *Rev Clin Esp* 1994;194:535.

55. Carrel T, Schaffner A, Vogt P, et al. Endocarditis in intravenous drug addicts and HIV infected patients: possibilities and limitations of surgical treatment. *J Heart Valve Dis* 1993;2:140.

56. Lemma M, Vanelli P, Beretta L, et al. Cardiac surgery in HIV positive intravenous drug addicts: influence of cardiopulmonary bypass on the progression to AIDS. *Thorac Cardiovasc Surg* 1992;40:279.

57. Brau N, Esposito RA, Simberkoff MS. Cardiac valve replacement in patients infected with the human immunodeficiency virus. *Ann Thorac Surg* 1992;54: 552.

58. Cowgill LD, Addonizio VP, Hopeman AR, et al. Prosthetic valve endocarditis. *Curr Probl Cardiol* 1986;11:617.

59. Heimburger TS, Duma RJ. Infections of prosthetic heart valves and cardiac pacemakers. *Infect Dis Clin North Am* 1989;3:221.

60. Grover FL, Cohen DJ, Oprian C, et al. Determinants of the occurrence of and survival from prosthetic valve endocarditis. Experience of the Veteran's Affair Cooperative Study on Valvular Heart Diseases. *J Thorac Cardiovasc Surg* 1994;108:207.

61. Karchmer AW, Longworth DL. Infections of intracardiac devices. *Infect Dis Clin North Am* 2002;16:477.

62. Muehrcke DD. Fungal prosthetic valve endocarditis. *Thorac Cardiovasc Surg* 1995;7:20.

63. Bayer AS, Nelson RJ, Slama TG. Current concepts in prevention of prosthetic valve endocarditis. *Chest* 1990;97:1203.

64. Rodbard S. Blood velocity and endocarditis. *Circulation* 1963;27:18.

65. Weinstein L, Schlesinger JJ. Pathoanatomic, physiologic and clinical correlates in endocarditis. *N Engl J Med* 1974;291:832, 1122.

66. Lopez JA, Ross RS, Fishbein MC, et al. Nonbacterial thrombotic endocarditis: a review. *Am Heart J* 1987;113:773.

67. Moreillon P, Que YA, Bayer AS. Pathogenesis of streptococcal and staphylococcal endocarditis. *Infect Dis Clin North Am* 2002;16:297.

68. Baddour LM, Christensen GD, Lowrance JH, et al. Production and progress of the disease in rabbits. *Br J Exp Pathol* 1973;54:142.

69. Baddour LM, Christensen GD, Lowrance JH, et al. Pathogenesis of experimental endocarditis. *Rev Infect Dis* 1989;11:452.

70. Bisno AL. Probing the pathogenesis of infective endocarditis. *J Lab Clin Med* 1988;112:1.

71. Sullam PM, Drake TA, Sande MA. Pathogenesis of endocarditis. *Am J Med* 1985;78[Suppl 6B]:110.

72. Vegetations, valves, and echocardiography [Editorial]. *Lancet* 1988;2:1118.

73. Roberts WC, Buchbinder NA. Healed left-sided infective endocarditis: a clinicopathological study of 59 patients. *Am J Cardiol* 1977;40:876.

74. Bayer AS, Norman DC. Valve site-specific pathogenic differences between right sided and left sided bacterial endocarditis. *Chest* 1990;98:200.

75. VanderMeer JTM, VanWijk W, Thompson J, et al. Efficacy of antibiotic prophylaxis for prevention of native valve endocarditis. *Lancet* 1992;339:135.

76. Hall G, Heimdahl A, Nord CE. Bacteremia after oral surgery and antibiotic prophylaxis for endocarditis. *Clin Infect Dis* 1999;29:1.

77. Lacassin F, Hoen B, Leport C, et al. Procedures associated with infective endocarditis in adults. A case control study. *Eur Heart J* 1995;16:1968.

78. Strom BL, Abrutyn E, Berlin JA, et al. Risk factors for infective endocarditis: oral hygiene and nondental exposures. *Circulation* 2000;102:2842.

79. Durack DT. Current issues in the prevention of infective endocarditis. *Am J Med* 1985;78[Suppl 6B]:149.

80. Bush LM, Johnson CC. Clinical syndrome and diagnosis. In: Kaye D, ed. *Infective endocarditis*, 2nd ed. New York: Raven Press, 1992:99–115.

81. McFarland MM. Pathology of infective endocarditis. In: Kaye D, ed. *Infective endocarditis*, 2nd ed. New York: Raven Press, 1992:57–83.

82. Mansur AJ, Grinberg M, Leao PP, et al. Extracranial mycotic aneurysms in infective endocarditis. *Clin Cardiol* 1986;9:65.

83. Brust JCM, Dickinson PCT, Hughes JEO. The diagnosis and treatment of cerebral mycotic aneurysms. *Ann Neurol* 1990;27:238.

84. Phair JP, Clarke J. Immunology of infective endocarditis. *Prog Cardiovasc Dis* 1979;22:137.

85. Bayer AS, Theofilopoulos AN. Immunopathogenetic aspects of infective endocarditis. *Chest* 1990;97:204.

86. McKinsey DS, McMurray TL, Flynn JM. Immune complex glomerulonephritis associated with *Staphylococcus aureus* bacteremia: response to corticosteroid therapy. *Rev Infect Dis* 1990;12:125.

87. Starkebaum M, Durack D, Beeson P. The "incubation period" of subacute bacterial endocarditis. *Yale J Biol Med* 1977;50:49.

88. Lemer PL, Weinstein L. Infective endocarditis in the antibiotic era. *N Engl J Med* 1966;274:388.

89. Salgado AV, Furlan AJ, Keys TF, et al. Neurologic complications of endocarditis: a 12-year experience. *Neurology* 1989;39:173.

90. Tunkel AR, Kaye D. Neurologic complications of infective endocarditis. *Neurol Clin* 1993;11:419.

91. Weinstein L, Rubin RH. Infective endocarditis—1973. *Prog Cardiovasc Dis* 1973;26:239.

92. Kaye KM, Kaye D. Laboratory findings including blood cultures. In: Kaye D, ed. *Infective endocarditis*, 2nd ed. New York: Raven Press, 1992:117–124.

93. Bayer AS, Lam K, Ginzton L, et al. *Staphylococcus aureus* bacteremia: clinical, serologic, and echocardiographic findings in patients with and without endocarditis. *Arch Intern Med* 1987;147:457.

94. Powers DL, Mandell GL. Intraleukocytic bacteria in endocarditis patients. *JAMA* 1974;227:312.

95. Gutman RA, Striker GE, Gilliland BC, et al. The immune complex glomerulonephritis of bacterial endocarditis. *Medicine (Baltimore)* 1972;51:1.

96. Pazin GJ, Saul S, Thompson ME. Blood culture positivity: suppression by outpatient antibiotic therapy in patients with bacterial endocarditis. *Arch Intern Med* 1982;142:263.

97. Towns ML, Reller LB. Diagnostic methods: current best practices and guidelines for isolation of bacteria and fungi in infective endocarditis. *Infect Dis Clin North Am* 2002;16:363.

98. Washington JA II. The role of the microbiology laboratory in the diagnosis and antimicrobial treatment of infective endocarditis. *Mayo Clin Proc* 1982;57: 22.

99. Carey RB, Gross KC, Roberts RB. Vitamin B$_6$–dependent *Streptococcus minor* (mitis) isolated from patients with systemic infections. *J Infect Dis* 1975;131:722.

100. Beeson PB, Brannon ES, Warren JV. Observations on the sites of removal of bacteria from the blood in patients with bacterial endocarditis. *J Exp Med* 1945;81:9.

101. Houpikian P, Raoult D. Diagnostic methods: current best practices and guidelines for identification of difficult-to-culture pathogens in infective endocarditis. *Infect Dis Clin North Am* 2002;16:377.

102. Tunkel AR, Kaye D. Endocarditis with negative blood cultures. *N Engl J Med* 1992;326:1215.

103. Shapiro SM, Young E, DeGuzman S, et al. Transesophageal echocardiography in the diagnosis of infective endocarditis. *Chest* 1994;105:377.

104. Grayburn PA. Southwestern Internal Medicine Conference: clinical applications of transesophageal echocardiography. *Am J Med Sci* 1994;307:151.

105. Daniel WG, Muggi A, Grote J, et al. Comparison of transthoracic and transesophageal echocardiography for detection of abnormalities of prosthetic and bioprosthetic valves in the mitral and aortic positions. *Am J Cardiol* 1993;71:210.

106. Lowry RW, Zoghbi WA, Baker WB, et al. Clinical impact of transesophageal echocardiography in the diagnosis and management of infective endocarditis. *Am J Cardiol* 1994;73:1089.

107. Ryan EW, Bolger AF. Transesophageal echocardiography (TEE) in the evaluation of infective endocarditis. *Cardiol Clin* 2000;18:773.

108. Lerakis S, Robert Taylor W, Lynch M, et al. The role of transesophageal echocardiography in the diagnosis and management of patients with aortic perivalvular abscesses. *Am J Med Sci* 2001;321:152.

109. Sachdev M, Peterson GE, Jollis JG. Imaging techniques for diagnosis of infective endocarditis. *Infect Dis Clin North Am* 2002;16:319.

110. Durack DT, Lukes AS, Bright DK, et al. New criteria for diagnosis of infective endocarditis: utilization of specific echocardiographic findings. *Am J Med* 1994;96:200.

111. Von Reyn CF, Arbier RD. Case definitions for infective endocarditis. *Am J Med* 1994;96:220.

112. Bayer AS. Diagnostic criteria for identifying cases of endocarditis: revisiting the Duke criteria two years later. *Clin Infect Dis* 1996;23:303.

113. Lamas CC, Eyken SJ. Suggested modifications to the Duke criteria for the clinical diagnosis of native valve and prosthetic valve endocarditis analysis of 118 pathologically proven cases. *Clin Infect Dis* 1997;25:713.

114. Li JS, Sexton DJ, Mick N. Proposed modifications to the Duke criteria for the diagnosis of infective endocarditis. *Clin Infect Dis* 2000;30:633.

115. Durack DT, Beeson PB. Experimental bacterial endocarditis II. Survival of bacteria in endocardial vegetations. *Br J Exp Pathol* 1972;53:50.

116. Bayer AS, Crowell D, Nast CC. Intravegetation antimicrobial distribution in aortic endocarditis analyzed by computer-generated model. *Chest* 1990;97: 611.

117. Wolfson JS, Swartz MN. Drug therapy: serum bactericidal activity as a monitor of antibiotic therapy. *N Engl J Med* 1985;312:968.

118. Francioli P, Etienne J, Hoigne R, et al. Treatment of streptococcal endocarditis with a single daily dose of ceftriaxone sodium for 4 weeks. Efficacy and outpatient treatment feasibility. *JAMA* 1992;267:264.

119. Francioli PB. Ceftriaxone and outpatient treatment of infective endocarditis. *Infect Dis Clin North Am* 1993;7:97.

120. Sexton DJ, Tenenbaum MJ, Wilson WR. Ceftriaxone once daily for four weeks compared with ceftriaxone plus gentamicin once daily for two weeks for treatment of endocarditis due to penicillin-susceptible streptococci. *Clin Infect Dis* 1998;27:1470.

121. Kaye KS, Fraimow HS, Abrutyn E. Pathogens resistant to antimicrobial agents. *Infect Dis Clin North Am* 2000;14:293.

122. Hoen B. Special issues in the management of infective endocarditis caused by gram-positive cocci. *Infect Dis Clin North Am* 2002;16:437.

123. Babcock HM, Ritchie DJ, Christiansen E, et al. Successful treatment of vancomycin-resistant enterococcus endocarditis with oral linezolid. *Clin Infect Dis* 2001;32:1373.

124. Korzeniowski O, Sande MA, the National Collaborative Endocarditis Study Group. *Staphylococcus aureus* endocarditis: clinical manifestations in patients addicted to parenteral drugs and in nonaddicts. *Ann Intern Med* 1982;97:496.

125. Levine DP, Fromm BS, Reddy BR. Slow response to vancomycin or vancomycin plus rifampin therapy among patients with methicillin-resistant *Staphylococcus aureus* endocarditis. *Ann Intern Med* 1991;115:674.

126. Ribera E, Gomez V, Cortes E, et al. Effectiveness of cloxacillin with or without gentamicin in short-term therapy for right-sided *Staphylococcus aureus* endocarditis: a randomized controlled trial. *Ann Intern Med* 1996;125:969.

127. Fortun J, Navas E, Martinez-Beltran J. Short-course therapy for right-sided endocarditis due to *Staphylococcus aureus* in drug abusers: cloxacillin versus glycopeptides in combination with gentamicin. *Clin Infect Dis* 2001;33:120.

128. Chambers HF. Short-course combination and oral therapies of *Staphylococcus aureus* endocarditis. *Infect Dis Clin North Am* 1993;7:69.

129. DiNubile MJ. Short-course antibiotic therapy for right-sided endocarditis caused by *Staphylococcus aureus* in injecting drug users. *Ann Intern Med* 1994;121:873.

130. Tebas P, Ruiz M, Roman F, et al. Early resistance to rifampin and ciprofloxacin in the treatment of right-sided *Staphylococcus aureus* endocarditis. *J Infect Dis* 1991;163:204.

131. Chambers HF. Treatment of infection and colonization caused by methicillin-resistant *Staphylococcus aureus*. *Infect Control Hosp Epidemiol* 1994;12:29.

132. Heldman AW, Hartert TV, Ray RC, et al. Oral antibiotic treatment of right-sided staphylococcal endocarditis in injection drug users: prospective randomized comparison with parenteral therapy. *Am J Med* 1996;101:68.

133. Cohen PS, Maguire JH, Weinstein L. Infective endocarditis caused by gram-negative bacteria: a review of the literature 1945–1977. *Prog Cardiovasc Dis* 1980;22:205.

134. Ugun O, Akalin HE, Unal S, et al. Long-term oral ciprofloxacin in the treatment of prosthetic valve endocarditis due to *Pseudomonas aeruginosa*. *Scand J Infect Dis* 1992;24:797.

135. Alsip SG, Blackstone EH, Kirklin JW, et al. Indications for cardiac surgery in patients with active infective endocarditis. *Am J Med* 1985;78:138.

136. Olaison L, Pettersson G. Current best practices and guidelines. Indications for surgical intervention in infective endocarditis. *Infect Dis Clin North Am* 2002;16:453.

137. Abdelnoor M, Nitter-Hauge S, Trettli S. Relative survival of patients after heart valve replacement. *Eur Heart J* 1990;11:23.

138. Jones EL, Weintraub WS, Craver JM, et al. Ten-year experience with the porcine bioprosthetic valve: interrelationship of valve survival and patient survival in 1,050 valve replacements. *Ann Thorac Surg* 1990;49:370.

139. David TE. The surgical treatment of patients with prosthetic valve endocarditis. *Semin Thorac Cardiovasc Surg* 1995;7:47.

140. Yu VL, Fand GD, Keys TF. Prosthetic valve endocarditis: superiority of surgical valve replacement versus medical therapy only. *Ann Thorac Surg* 1994;58:1073.

141. Grover FL, Cohen DJ, Oprian C, et al. Determinants of the occurrence of and survival from prosthetic valve endocarditis. *J Thorac Cardiovasc Surg* 1994;108:207.

142. Steckelberg JM, Murphy JG, Ballard D, et al. Emboli in infective endocarditis: the prognostic value of echocardiography. *Ann Intern Med* 1991;114:635.

143. Alestig K, Hogevik H, Olaison L. Infective endocarditis: a diagnostic and therapeutic challenge for the new millennium. *Scand J Infect Dis* 2000;32:343.

144. Heiro M, Nikoskelainen J, Engblom E, et al. Neurologic manifestations of infective endocarditis: a 17-year experience in a teaching hospital in Finland. *Arch Intern Med* 2000;160:2781.

145. Wilson WR, Guiliani ER, Danielson GK, et al. Management of complications of infective endocarditis. *Mayo Clin Proc* 1982;57:162.

146. Verheul HA, Van den Brink RB, Van Vreeland T, et al. Effects of changes in management of active infective endocarditis on outcome in a 25 year period. *Am J Cardiol* 1993;72:682.

147. Karchmer AW. Staphylococcal endocarditis: laboratory and clinical basis for antibiotic therapy. *Am J Med* 1985;78[Suppl 6B]:116.

148. Jault F, Gandjbakheh I, Chastre JC, et al. Prosthetic valve endocarditis with ring abscesses: surgical management and long-term results. *J Thorac Cardiovasc Surg* 1993;105:1106.

149. David TE. The surgical treatment of patients with prosthetic valve endocarditis. *Semin Thorac Cardiovasc Surg* 1995;7:47.

150. Lytle BW, Priest BP, Taylor PC, et al. Surgery for acquired heart disease: surgical treatment of prosthetic valve endocarditis. *J Thorac Cardiovasc Surg* 1996;111:198.

151. d'Udekem Y, David TE, Feindel CM, et al. Long term results of operation for paravalvular abscess. *Ann Thorac Surg* 1996;62:48.

152. Dossche KM, Defauw JJ, Ernst SM, et al. Allograft aortic root replacement in prosthetic aortic valve endocarditis: a review of 32 patients. *Ann Thorac Surg* 1997;63:1644.

153. Pansini S, di Summa M, Patane F, et al. Risk of recurrence after reoperation for prosthetic valve endocarditis. *J Heart Valve Dis* 1997;6:84.

154. Calderwood SB, Swinski LA, Karchmer AA, et al. Prosthetic valve endocarditis: analysis of factors affecting outcome of therapy. *J Thorac Cardiovasc Surg* 1986;92:776.

155. John MVD, Hibberd PL, Karchmer AW, et al. *Staphylococcus aureus* prosthetic valve endocarditis: optimal management and risk factors for death. *Clin Infect Dis* 1998;26:1302.

156. Dajani AS, Taubert KA, Wilson W, et al. Prevention of bacterial endocarditis. Recommendations by the American Heart Association. *Circulation* 1997;96:358.

157. Lark RL, VanderHyde K, Deeb GM, et al. An outbreak of coagulase-negative staphylococcal surgical-site infections following aortic valve replacement. *Infect Control Hosp Epidemiol* 2001;22:618.

CHAPTER 63
Vascular Graft Infections

Thomas F. O'Donnell, Jr., Harold J. Welch, and Richard A. Nitzberg

Vascular infections are fortunately rather rare, averaging about 2% in most series. Although improvements in surgical techniques and perioperative management have led to decreased mortality and amputation rates (Table 63.1), graft infections always present a formidable challenge to both the vascular surgeon and the infectious disease consultant. Vascular infections can be divided into (a) those that involve the native vessel primarily, without a previous vascular reconstruction, and (b) those that are associated with the insertion of a synthetic graft or with a vascular reconstructive procedure. Although the most frequent causes of primary vascular infections in the 1970s and 1980s were organisms such as salmonellae, which are hematogenously spread from an initial enteric portal of entry, this cause is now rare. Now, direct inoculation of bacteria into the vessels, associated with drug abuse, is much more common in primary arterial infection. This chapter focuses on those infections related to vascular surgery.

INCIDENCE

The incidence of graft infection varies with the site of the graft. With intraabdominal aortic level procedures, the infection rate is approximately 1%; with infrainguinal reconstructions, the rate is 2% to 4%. The primary culprit in these cases is groin dissection, as seen in the higher rates of aortofemoral grafts versus intraabdominal aortic procedures. For various reasons, the rate of graft infections is higher with emergency operations, such as those performed for ruptured aneurysms, than with elective procedures. Mortality rates also vary with the anatomic location of the graft and are highest at the aortic level. In contrast, limb loss may be higher with infrainguinal vascular infections, perhaps because alternative routes of revascularization are limited. The data in Table 63.1 underline the fact that graft infections, though rare, are a lethal problem confronting both the surgeon and the infectious disease consultant.

ETIOLOGY

Although the bacterium responsible for most graft infections is usually identified, the origin of the infection often remains unclear. Two probable mechanisms of graft infection are bacteremic seeding and direct contamination at the time of surgery (Table 63.2). Bacteremic seeding of grafts, such as has been described with *Pseudomonas* infections of autogenous vein grafts after *Pseudomonas* urinary tract infections (1), and with aortic infections after angiograms (2), supports the theory of hematogenous seeding of vascular prostheses. Reports of aortic graft sepsis from *Pasteurella multocida* after a dog bite confirm bacteremic seeding as a mechanism of late graft infection (3).

The timing of hematogenous bacterial contamination appears to be critical to infectivity. In experimental studies, all dogs challenged with an intravenous bolus infusion of *Staphylococcus aureus* immediately after graft implantation developed graft infection (4), whereas only 30% developed sepsis when the same

TABLE 63.1.   Graft Infections

Author	Number	Type of infection	Time to infection (mo)	Treatment	Mortality (%)	Amputation (%)
Aortic level						
Kuestner et al., 1995 (21)	33	AEF	73.2	IGR/EAB	27.3	9.1
Sharp et al., 1994 (55)	27	18 PGI/9 AEF	62.5	IGR/EAB ISR, PGE	3.7	0
Kieffer et al., 1993 (15)	43	34 PGI/9 AEF	63.6	ISAGR	12	0
Bacourt and Koskas, 1992 (56)	98	PGI/AEF	37	IGR/EAB	24	10
McCarthy et al., 1992 (57)	17	PGI	—	IGR/EAB	18	0
Ricotta et al., 1991 (58)	32	24 PGI/8 AEF	34	PGE ± EAB IGR ± EAB	25	13
Quiniones-Baldrich et al., 1991 (59)	45	PGI/AEF	40.3	PGE ± EAB	24	11
Reilly et al., 1984 (60)	92	59 PGI	25	IGR ± EAB	10	25
		33 AEF	33	IGR/EAB	21	24
Infrainguinal level						
Calligaro et al., 1991 (52)	35	PGI/VGI	—	IGR ± EAB, PGE, GP	2.8	7
Cherry et al., 1992 (14)	39	PGI	2	IGR + EAB; GP	7.6	28
Mertens et al., 1995 (61)	67	PGI	3	GP; IGR; PGE	18	40

AEF, aortoenteric fistula; EAB, extraanatomic bypass; GP, graft preservation; IGR, infected graft removal; ISAGR, in situ allograft replacement; ISR, in situ replacement; PGE, partial graft excision; PGI, prosthetic graft infection; VGI, vein graft infection.

bacterial challenge was given at 1 year. Obviously, the degree of graft endothelialization in such experimental models determines "infectability" because an intact luminal surface provides a barrier against infection. Studies with endothelium-seeded prosthetic graft show that these grafts are more resistant to infection than are their nonseeded counterparts (5). In humans, the lack of complete endothelialization of a prosthesis and the presence of defects in the pseudointima probably account for instances of late graft infection via a hematogenous route that occurs 4 to 5 years after implantation. Certainly, in the perioperative period, when the pseudointima consists of various proteins and cellular elements from the blood that afford only a weak barrier against bacterial invasion, numerous opportunities exist for hematogenous contamination, such as from central venous and arterial lines or urinary catheters.

Bacterial colonization of grafts by direct contamination is another mechanism for prosthetic graft infection that is probably the most common. This conclusion is supported by studies such as those of Schwartz et al. (6), who demonstrated that when cultured, more than 10% of abdominal aortic aneurysms grew bacteria—a potential source of graft contamination. The relationship between positive bacterial culturing from aortic aneurysm walls and subsequent graft infection was first emphasized by Ernst et al. (7), who cultured bacteria from the aneurysm wall in 12 of 78 patients. One patient subsequently developed graft sepsis. Ernst et al. (7) observed that those patients with ruptured

aneurysms had a fourfold higher positive culture rate (38%) than those who underwent elective surgery for aneurysms (10%). The clinical studies of Malone et al. (8) revealed that the incidence of graft infections rose with the number of "redo" vascular operations; that is, reoperative surgery for failed grafts carries with it a greater risk of vascular infections. Later studies by Durham, Malone, and Bernhard (9) showed that patients with negative arterial wall cultures failed to develop graft infections, whereas a significant number of patients with positive arterial wall cultures went on to develop graft infections. Like Malone et al. (8), Durham, Malone, and Bernhard (9) demonstrated that patients undergoing reoperative vascular surgery had a significant increase in the incidence of graft infection, especially if the arterial wall culture was positive. On the basis of these studies, these investigators recommended that intraoperative cultures be done for all patients undergoing vascular *reoperation.* If arterial wall cultures are positive, long-term antibiotics may be indicated. This recommendation is supported by the work of Bergamini (10), who found a 24% positive culture rate in patients undergoing reoperation for anastomotic aneurysms without signs of suppuration or frank sepsis. Eighteen patients with positive cultures in the studies by Bandyk et al. (11) and Schmitt et al. (12) represented reoperations, and the predominant bacterium was *Staphylococcus epidermidis.*

Direct contamination of vascular prostheses usually occurs at the time of implantation, which implies a break in surgical technique. *In vitro* models of bacterial adherence demonstrate that microorganisms readily adhere to prosthetic grafts. Knitted Dacron grafts exhibited the greatest degree of adherence (12). Direct graft contamination can occur at the time of implantation by contact with skin flora, especially in inguinal incisions. Alternatively, this contamination may occur after contact of the graft, surgeon's hands, or instruments with the patient's skin for a prolonged period.

Known or occult enteric injury also can directly contaminate grafts, whereas inadequate sterilization can rarely cause graft infection. The lymphatic system appears to play an important role in preventing graft infection, especially in patients with ischemic limbs. In a study using a canine model, femoral polytetrafluoroethylene (PTFE) interposition grafts were implanted after procedures that produced unilateral limb ischemia (13). Ipsilateral inoculation of both *Escherichia coli* and *S. aureus*

TABLE 63.2.   Causes of Graft Infection

Bacteremic seeding
  Source: urinary tract, arteriographic puncture site, or other distant inoculation site
Direct contamination
  Source: aortic wall, e.g., aneurysm, break in surgical technique
    Surgeon's hands or instruments
    Graft contact with skin
    Entertomy—planned or inadvertent
    Lymphatic disruption
    Direct extension from septic site
    Aortoenteric fistula
    Wound breakdown that exposes graft

into the ischemic limb produced graft infections in those animals that had their lymphatics transected or preserved. By contrast, there was a significant reduction in positive graft cultures in the group of animals that had either excision or ligation of the lymphatics in the ischemic limb. These findings suggest that the lymphatics may contribute to graft infection, possibly by absorbing and then transporting bacteria to the site of graft implantation. The clinical implications of this work are important and dictate that careful isolation, transection, and ligation of groin lymphatics may reduce the incidence of graft infections.

Finally, direct extension of superficial wound infections can cause graft infection. This is the most common mechanism in the groin, where either excessive moisture, poor technique, or both in wound closure, particularly in obese patients, will result in wound breakdown. This mechanism is also seen in grafts tunneled subcutaneously, such as femoropopliteal, axillofemoral, and axilloaxillary bypasses. Direct extension is also the mechanism for aortoenteric fistula formation. Adherence of bowel, most commonly the duodenum, to aortic grafts results in erosion of the bowel wall, allowing the luminal bacteria to infect the graft.

BACTERIOLOGY

The time interval from surgery to graft infection may be as short as 2 days (14) to as long as 18 years (15). Early graft infections are caused by virulent strains, particularly *S. aureus* and gram-negative bacteria such as *Pseudomonas, Klebsiella, Proteus,* and *Enterobacter. S. aureus* has been the most common organism causing graft infections, which has been isolated in one third to one half of patients (16,17). The common skin contaminant *S. epidermidis* now accounts for a greater number of infections. Although *E. coli* and other gram-negative organisms are more commonly found in classic late graft infections (Table 63.3), Bandyk et al. (18) found *S. epidermidis* to be the responsible organism in more than 50% of their cases of late graft infections. They related this increase in frequency to the unique protective mechanism of this bacterium. *S. epidermidis* can produce a biofilm of mucin "slime" that surrounds the organism as a protective barrier. The organism remains dormant and is usually associated with late infections months to years after graft implantation. The infection commonly presents as an anastomotic aneurysm that is often accompanied by a mucinous perigraft cavity. These organisms induce a complex host–organism response that causes weakening at the graft-to-host artery anastomosis.

The role of anaerobic bacteria, especially in aortofemoral graft infections, has been elucidated by Brook (19). In a 10-year review of aortofemoral graft infections, anaerobes were cultured from 13 (82%) of 16 specimens. Predisposing conditions, which included leg ulcers, gangrene, reoperation, and diabetes, existed in more than 50% of these patients.

Culture results show mixed flora in many instances. Calligaro et al. (20) grew both gram-positive and gram-negative organisms from 16 of 42 wounds, whereas many other cultures were positive for several species of gram-positive or gram-negative bacteria. Keustner et al. (21) grew multiple organisms in 44% of cultures from secondary aortoenteric fistulas.

Adhesion of bacteria to vascular grafts varies among types of grafts and bacteria. Schmitt et al. (12) examined the adherence of four strains of bacteria to three types of graft materials. All strains had a higher affinity for velour knitted Dacron than for expanded PTFE, and both *S. aureus* and *E. coli* had a higher affinity for velour knitted Dacron than for woven Dacron. When a mucin-producing strain of *S. epidermidis* was compared with a non–mucin-producing strain, the former had a much higher adherence to both expanded PTFE and knitted Dacron. The authors also showed that longer incubation allowed greater adhesion for the mucin-producing strain. In addition, the mucin-producing strain of *S. epidermidis* adhered to the graft wall in clusters, whereas the non–mucin-producing strain of *S. epidermidis, S. aureus,* and *E. coli* primarily adhered as single organisms.

Despite clinically obvious graft infections, cultures are sometimes negative, or intraoperative culture results may not agree with preoperative culture results. Perioperative antibiotics may be responsible for negative postoperative cultures. Goldstone and Effeney (22), who noted negative cultures in 40% of proven graft infections, urged that the graft material itself be submitted for culture. Padberg, Smith, and Eng (23) used the techniques of ultrasonic bath treatment, direct ultrasonic disruption, and Vortex mixing to quantitatively culture bacteria from seeded Dacron grafts. They found the 5-minute ultrasonic bath treatment to be consistently better than the other two methods.

Fungal infections of vascular prosthetics are rare and are usually associated with disseminated infection. Graft infections with *Candida, Coccidioides, Aspergillus,* and other fungi may be the presenting manifestation of more widespread involvement.

TABLE 63.3. Bacteriology of Graft Infection

Organism	Types of bacteria in culture (%)						
	Szilagy et al., 1972 (25) (n = 48)	Liekweig and Greenfield, 1977 (17) (n = 22)	Bunt, 1983 (41) (n = 205)	Bandyk et al., 1984 (11) (n = 30)	Calligaro et al., 1990 (20) (n = 30)	Quinones-Baldrich et al., 1991 (59) (n = 45)	Cherry et al., 1992 (14) (n = 39)
Staphylococcus (coagulase positive)	33	41	43	8	24	13	31
Staphylococcus (coagulase negative)	15	—	—	42	24	21	10
Sreptococcus (nonhemolytic)	5	—	—	6	51	5	18
Escherichia coli	23	9	17	11	10	18	(28% gram negative)
Proteus	6	1	8	—	20	5	
Pseudomonas	2	14	10	3	33	21	8
Mixed						39	20
Negative culture						21	10

TABLE 63.4. Prospective Evaluation of the Role of Prophylactic Antibiotics in Vascular Surgery

Author	Antibiotic	Number in trial	Incidence of infection (%)	
			Placebo	Treated
Kaiser et al., 1978 (24)	Cefazolin	462	6.8	0.9
Pitt et al., 1980 (34)	Cephradine	231	22.6	2.6

PROPHYLACTIC ANTIBIOTICS

Antibiotics are routinely given before vascular surgery for two reasons: (a) the synthetic graft acts as a foreign body and (b) there is a high risk of mortality or limb loss from graft infections. Usually, a first-generation cephalosporin such as cefazolin (Kefzol) is infused 1 to 2 hours before the skin incision is made and is continued for 24 to 48 hours after the vascular procedure. In a prospective randomized study of more than 450 patients, Kaiser et al. (24) showed that such a regimen reduced wound infections from 6.8% in a placebo-treated group to 0.9% in a cefazolin-treated group (Table 63.4). Although graft infections were also reduced in the antibiotic-treated group, this finding only *approached* statistical significance; all four graft infections occurred in the placebo group. Before this report, retrospective studies by Szilagyi et al. (25) and Fry and Lindenauer (26) noted a low incidence of graft infections in patients not treated with prophylactic antibiotics, 1.2% and 1.34%, respectively. These authors thought that a low rate of graft infections in the absence of routine prophylaxis argued against the use of prophylactic antibiotics. To the contrary, in their retrospective studies, Goldstone and Moore (27) found a threefold decrease in graft sepsis with the use of antibiotics. In a review of 2,614 arterial prosthetic graft procedures carried out for an 11-year period, Edwards et al. (16) observed that prophylactic antibiotics had been given in 22 of 24 cases of graft infection. In only 7 of the 22, however, antibiotics were given according to the usual and appropriate protocol.

What has not yet been settled is how long to administer the prophylactic antibiotics. Edwards et al. (16) noted that more than 50% of surgical wound infections had a distant site of infection, of which 30% were related to urinary tract infections and 25% to respiratory tract sepsis. Despite routine administration of antibiotics, May et al. (28) found that 14% of their patients had positive Foley catheter cultures and that 16% had positive sputum cultures. Certainly, such findings would argue for both prompt removal of Foley catheters and antibiotic protection until their removal.

PREVENTION

Recognized risk factors for graft infections include reoperation, septic complications, and inadvertent or planned entry into the gastrointestinal (GI) tract at the time of graft placement. Obviously, reoperation cannot be avoided, but avoidance of GI tract mishaps helps prevent graft infections.

Placement of autogenous grafts, when possible, as opposed to synthetic grafts, can also reduce the incidence of vascular infections. It is well known that graft infections occur more frequently when a synthetic graft is used (29). As noted earlier, careful division and ligation of groin lymphatics are helpful in preventing graft infections (13). Attention to detail in excluding the graft from contact with the bowel postoperatively is imperative. This involves covering the graft with aneurysm sac (when appropriate), carefully closing the retroperitoneum, and using omental patches where necessary. Earnshaw et al. (30) showed that although pathogenic organisms could be isolated from the skin preoperatively in 35% of patients studied, none of these organisms could be cultured from inguinal lymph nodes. Other studies have shown no benefit from the use of prophylactic closed suction drainage of inguinal wounds in patients undergoing vascular reconstruction (31). Despite the occurrence of hematomas, seromas, and lymphoceles, closed suction drainage demonstrated no advantage over primary wound closure. The benefit of topical antibiotic wound irrigation has been shown. The retrospective studies of Lord, Rossi, and Daliawa (32) showed a 0.23% incidence of wound infections in 434 patients who had topical wound irrigation, whereas Halasz (33) showed equal efficacy between topical and systemic antibiotics. In one of the few prospective trials to examine this issue, Pitt et al. (34) demonstrated a beneficial effect of wound irrigation, but the higher than usual wound infection rate in the control group weakened the impact of the study.

Further attempts to reduce graft infections have focused on either bonding or saturating prosthetic grafts with antibiotics, including rifampin, gentamicin, and ciprofloxacin. The risk of graft infection is probably greatest in the perioperative period; one study demonstrated that when antibiotics were added to the blood used for preclotting Dacron grafts, the frequency of graft sepsis was lowered (35). Greco et al. (36) and others (37,38) showed that antibiotic bonding to prosthetic grafts may be useful when a new graft must be placed in the setting of an infection. Torsello et al. (39) had no early (6-month) infections in rifampin-soaked aortic grafts placed *in situ*. Further work on the binding process is necessary because antibiotics can be leached out quickly with flowing blood (40).

General measures that surgical staff can follow, such as showering with antiseptic soap 24 to 48 hours before surgery, not shaving the operative area until the patient is in the operating room, and using iodine- and povidone-impregnated drapes, help reduce wound and graft infection when coupled with meticulous surgical technique. Prophylactic antibiotics are beneficial but probably do not need to be given beyond 48 hours.

CLASSIFICATION

Graft infection is classified in the following ways: (a) level of septic involvement, (b) distal or proximal site, (c) type of bacteria, and (d) type of graft (Table 63.5). A type 1 infection involves the skin only; and type 2, the subcutaneous tissue and skin. Type 3 is considered a true graft infection, in which the shaft with or without the anastomosis is involved. In his extensive clinical review, Bunt (41) suggested that vascular graft infection should be classified as (a) graft infection, (b) graft enteric erosion,

TABLE 63.5. Classification of Graft Infections

Level of involvement: Type 1—skin only
Type 2—skin and subcutaneous tissue
Type 3—graft involvement: shaft alone or shaft and anastomosis
Site: proximal (aortic) or distal (infrainguinal)
Type of bacteria
Type of graft: synthetic or autogenous; proximal and distal anastomotic locations
Bunt classification: Graft infection
Graft—enteric erosion
Graft—enteric fistula
Aortic stump infections

(c) graft enteric fistula, or (d) aortic stump sepsis. He observed that the incidences of graft infection and graft enteric fistula were comparable, whereas the incidences of graft enteric erosion and aortic stump sepsis were much less, approximately 10% of the former. The clinical diagnosis and subsequent management are clearly related to the type of infection; therefore, they are discussed separately.

CLINICAL PRESENTATION

The incidence of graft infection has not changed significantly over the past 20 years, although there has been a slight decline. More than three fourths of graft infections occur in the groin (25,27). Although earlier studies show that a significant portion of graft infections occurred early, most later studies show infection developing an average of 4 to 6 years after implantation. The type of graft also influences the onset of graft sepsis. Infections associated with aortofemoral grafts tend to present earlier than aortoiliac grafts, probably because of the superficial location of the femoral limb. With grafts located in the femoral region, patients usually exhibit localized signs of sepsis—an inguinal mass accompanied or unaccompanied by redness, pain, and fever (Table 63.6). The mass frequently progresses to frank drainage so that a sinus tract develops. A false aneurysm may be a sign of graft infection in approximately 10% of patients, whereas a smaller number present with evidence of hemorrhage, graft occlusion, or septic emboli. For infections involving grafts that are

TABLE 63.7. Aortoenteric Fistula: New England Medical Center and University of California, San Francisco, Experiences

	NEMC	UCSF
Number of patients	13	33
Original procedure		
Aneurysm	7	15
Occlusive	6	17
Both		1
Occurrence after implantation (yr)	5.5	6.1
Site of AEF		
Duodenum	9	23
Jejunum	4	6
Other		5
Presenting symptoms		
Gastrointestinal bleeding	8	22
Shock	0	8
Fever	7	22
Sinus tract	0	5
Septic emboli	0	9
Positive blood culture results	8	11 (n = 15)
Diagnosis (diagnostic for AEF)		
Upper gastrointestinal tract series	2/7	1/8
Arteriography	0/9	0/30
Endoscopy	4/10	2/17
Computed tomography		8/24

AEF, aortoenteric fistula; NEMC, New England Medical Center; UCSF, University of California, San Francisco.

contained entirely within the abdomen, such as a tube or an aortoiliac graft, localized signs are unusual. Generally, the patient complains of recurrent febrile episodes, malaise, and weight loss, which are typical signs of occult sepsis. Blood cultures may be positive.

Graft enteric fistulas usually present with bleeding from the GI tract (Table 63.7). The degree of bleeding depends on the site of the fistula. Massive acute bleeding is characteristic of fistulas that involve the graft-to-aorta anastomosis (Fig. 63.1), whereas fistulas involving the shaft of the graft more commonly bleed in low volume. In these situations, the bleeding is usually from the mucosa of the GI tract, which has become irritated by the prosthetic graft (42,43). Patients in these cases may be febrile, but if blood cultures are positive, the prognosis is less good (44).

TABLE 63.6. Clinical Diagnosis of Graft Infections (Average from Literature)

Type of infection	%
General	
Localized cellulitis or abscess	50
Fever	37
Systemic infection	25
Leukocytosis	26
Draining sinus	20
False aneurysm	16
Anastomotic bleeding	12
Graft occlusion	8
Septic emboli	6
Aortic level	
Herald bleeding	76
Acute gastrointestinal tract bleeding	56
Chronic gastrointestinal tract bleeding	40

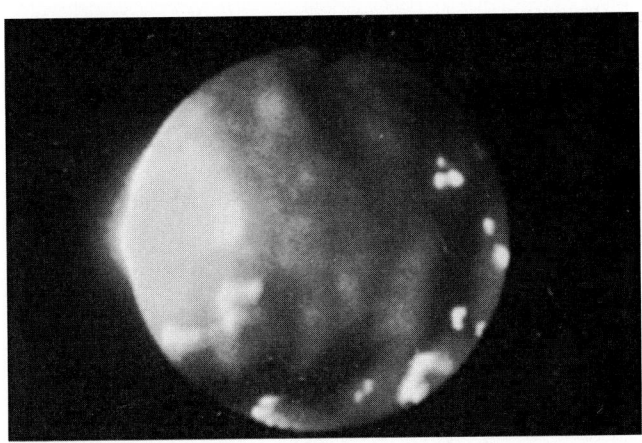

Figure 63.1. Endoscopic view of an aortoenteric fistula. Whitish, highly reflective material at the left (at 9-o'clock position) represents graft fabric; mucosa with hemorrhage is seen to fill the remainder of the circle.

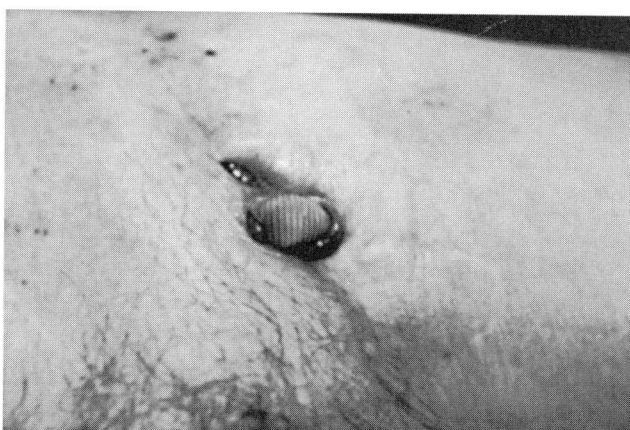

Figure 63.2. Obvious extrusion of graft through inguinal wound in a patient with a draining sinus and graft infection. This patient had an aortofemoral bypass graft several years ago and was referred for management of this infection.

DIAGNOSIS

The diagnosis of graft infection may leave the surgeon with the uneasy sense of a suspected rather than a confirmed infection at a time when a major procedure associated with potentially high mortality and morbidity rates must be undertaken. Some clues can be derived from the physical examination. A erythematous, tender, pulsatile mass in the inguinal region or elsewhere suggests graft sepsis (see Table 63.6). A draining sinus in the area of a graft is clear-cut evidence of graft infection (Fig. 63.2). Nonspecific studies include laboratory measurements of white blood cell count, erythrocyte sedimentation rate, and blood cultures. The yield of specific diagnostic studies depends on the site and the type of infection. Radiologic techniques for detailing infections can be divided into those that detect anatomic abnormalities and those that reveal sites of inflammation. In patients with suspected graft infection, we have found that anatomic definition by computed tomography (CT) is the most helpful diagnostic study because it examines both the retroperitoneum and the perigraft tissue (45). CT may reveal a collection of fluid around the main body of the graft or its limbs, blurring of the usual tissue planes in the retroperitoneum, or air collections around the graft (Fig. 63.3). False aneurysms may be detected (Fig. 63.4). With an

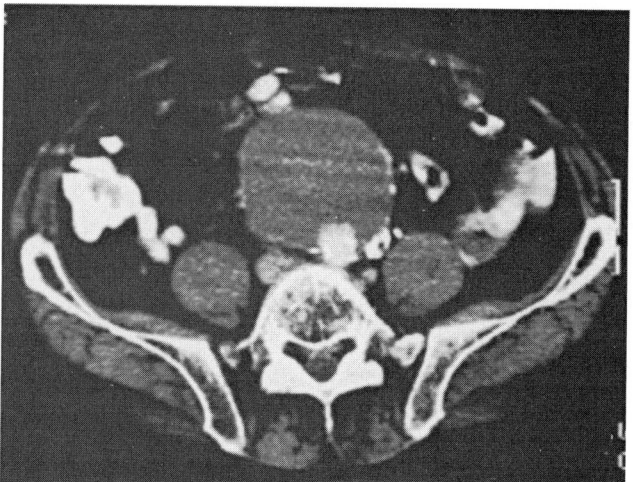

Figure 63.4. Computed tomographic scan of a false aneurysm in a patient with an aortoenteric fistula. The presence of the aortic anastomotic aneurysm was inferential evidence of a suspected aortoenteric fistula. This view is above the graft anastomosis and reveals the false aneurysm and overlying bowel.

aortoenteric fistula, oral contrast medium may sometimes be seen delineating the contour of the graft (Fig. 63.5). Another attractive feature of CT is that it may delineate other possible sites of infection unrelated to the graft.

Magnetic resonance imaging (MRI) is also useful, particularly in identifying perigraft fluid. However, fluid persists in up to 22% of patients at 12 weeks and may not be completely resolved for up to 24 weeks. Combined use of axial spin echo and short-tau inversion recovery imaging has been shown to be highly accurate for diagnosing graft infections (46).

Ultrasonography has also been used. However, other than confirming the presence of a false aneurysm, ultrasound techniques have been disappointing in the evaluation of graft sepsis.

Contrast studies (Fig. 63.6) may also be helpful not only in diagnosing the presence of infection but also in planning the operative approach and the procedure. A patient with a clearly evident draining sinus should undergo sinography to define the level of wound infection as superficial or deep, the latter with graft involvement. In addition to demonstrating

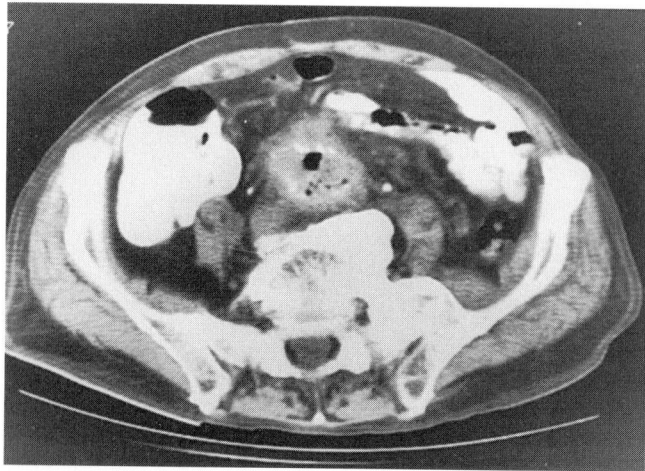

Figure 63.3. Computed tomographic scan of a patient with a graft infection. Blurring of the usual tissue planes in the retroperitoneum and air are observed around the shaft of the aortic graft.

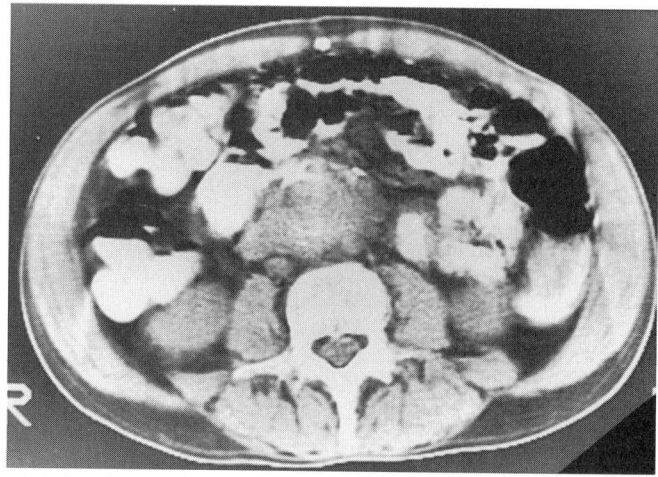

Figure 63.5. Computed tomographic scan of an aortoenteric fistula with oral contrast medium from the duodenum delineating the aortic graft (11-o'clock position of the graft).

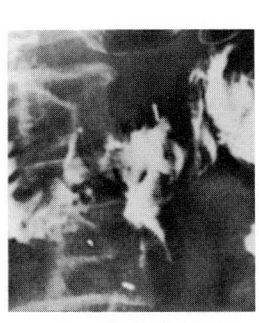
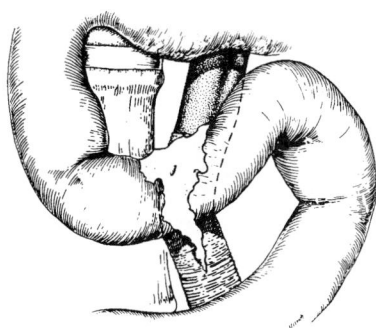

Figure 63.6. Upper gastrointestinal tract series in a patient with an aortoenteric fistula. The schematic drawing on the right illustrates the barium study on the left. The ulcer appeared in the fourth portion of the duodenum overlying the aortic anastomosis.

the runoff, arteriography may reveal an unsuspected false aneurysm, which provides suggestive evidence of graft sepsis (Fig. 63.7).

Radionuclide scans enjoyed an initial rush of enthusiasm, but this enthusiasm has been tempered by their overall lower than expected sensitivity. Because of normal postoperative inflammation, these scans are not useful in the first 3 to 5 months after graft implantation. Labeling leukocytes with indium-111 or technetium-99m–hexamethylpropyleneamine oxime has produced a diagnostic accuracy of 80% to 100% (47,48). Polyclonal human immunoglobulin G scans and gallium scans are other options, each with its own advantages and disadvantages (49). Radionuclide studies should be combined with other imaging techniques, such as CT or MRI, to increase diagnostic accuracy.

Endoscopy is extremely useful in stable patients suspected of having an aortoenteric fistula. Gastroduodenoscopy must be carried out to the fourth portion of the duodenum. Occasionally, the graft material itself will be visualized (see Fig. 63.1), but any mucosal abnormality must be viewed with suspicion. Endoscopy must exclude other sources of bleeding, such as

varices and ulcers; however, normal examination results do not necessarily exclude an aortoenteric fistula. Stable patients with lower GI tract bleeding or guaiac-positive stools and normal upper GI tract endoscopic results should undergo flexible sigmoidoscopy to evaluate a possible graft sigmoid fistula.

If the diagnosis of graft sepsis is made preoperatively, attempts to determine the extent of infection (e.g., an entire graft or just one limb of an aortobifemoral graft) should be made. This may aid in planning the scope of the graft removal surgery. Unfortunately, a diagnosis of graft infection may be suspected but not confirmed despite multiple tests, and the patient must undergo exploration in the operating room. The major finding at surgery determining graft infection is how well the graft itself is incorporated, or healed, in the perigraft tissue. Findings of perigraft mucin or slime, bile staining, and easy dissection of perigraft tissue indicate graft infection. Using culture techniques described earlier, Padberg, Smith, and Eng (50) compared graft incorporation and graft culture results. They found that graft disincorporation correlated with the presence of bacteria in 71% of cases and that graft incorporation excluded bacteria in 97%.

THERAPY

The "gold standard" for treating an infected vascular prosthetic is complete removal of the graft with revascularization through clean, noninfected tissue planes. Additional tenets include (a) complete resection and débridement of infected perigraft tissue, with special care to obtain a clean proximal arterial stump; (b) drainage or irrigation of the perigraft infection; (c) appropriate perioperative and long-term antibiotics; and (d) use of monofilament (vice-braided) sutures for arterial closure (Fig. 63.8).

Unfortunately, the gold standard of therapy carries the greatest risks of morbidity and mortality to the patient. As a result, clinicians have challenged the gold standard with a variety of treatments aimed at decreasing these risks. Even the gold

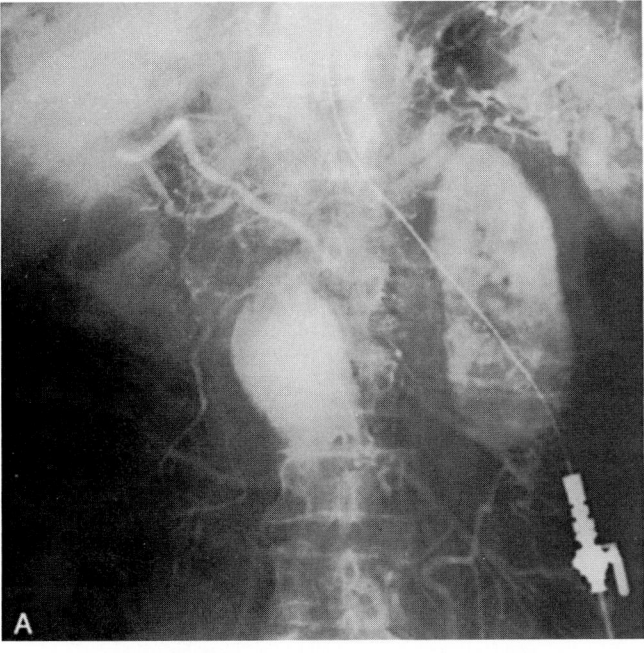
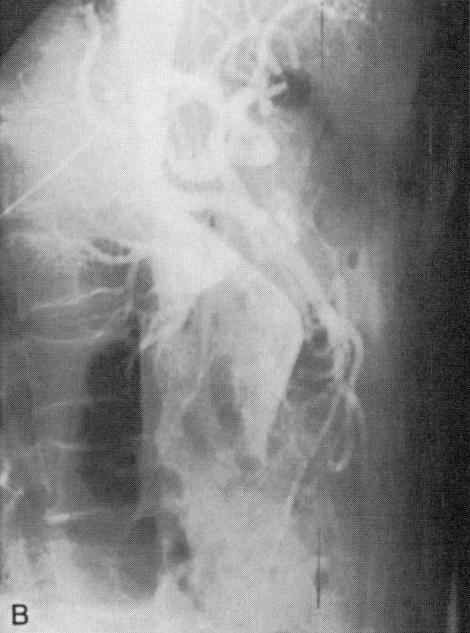

Figure 63.7. Anteroposterior **(A)** and lateral **(B)** arteriograms of a patient with an false aortic aneurysm and gastrointestinal tract bleeding. Subsequent exploration revealed an aortoenteric fistula that was treated by graft excision and extraanatomic bypass by axillofemoral bypass.

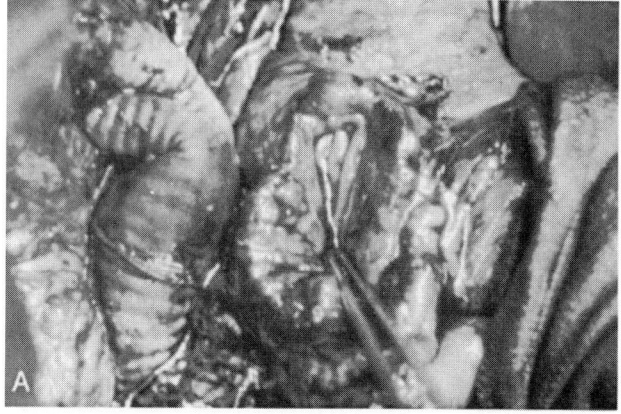
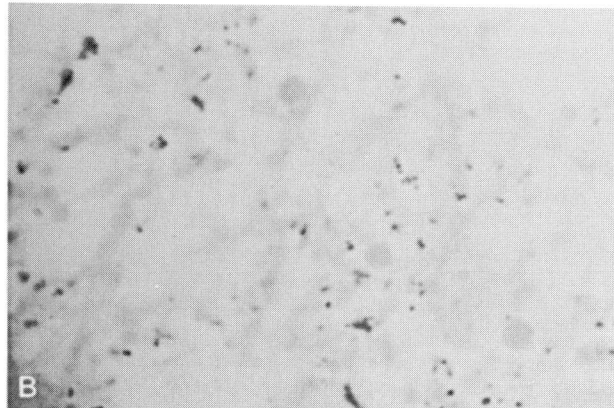
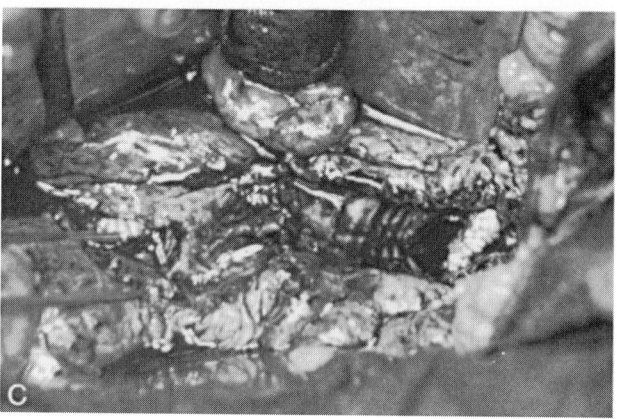

Figure 63.8. A.: Bile-stained aortofemoral graft secondary to an aortoenteric fistula. Forceps point to the duodenum, which was densely adherent to the shaft of the aortic limb. **B:** Immediate Gram stain of periaortic tissue shows multiple gram-positive organisms. **C:** Completed aortic stump closure and fistula. Forceps point to open bowel, which was subsequently closed.

standard has variations in management, particularly for infected aortic grafts (51). Removal of the infected graft and revascularization can be performed in a staged manner, in which the extraanatomic bypass is done, followed by graft removal a few days later. Although the theoretical risk for infecting the new extraanatomic bypass exists, in practice the risk is quite low. This approach allows the patient to have two shorter, less stressful procedures. Alternatively, the procedures may be done in a sequential approach, in which the lower extremities are perfused via an extraanatomic bypass, immediately followed by total aortic graft excision. Another option is the synchronous approach, which includes graft resection either before or after an in-line reconstruction. All these approaches include total resection of the infected graft.

Less extensive options include partial graft resection and nonresection of the infected graft. The former is an option for aortobifemoral grafts when only one limb is involved and for infrainguinal grafts with only a short portion infected. In patients with superficial wound infections involving exposed grafts, several authors have reported successful preservation of the graft using local wound care, irrigation, and long-term antibiotics. One dictum has been that infections involving anastomoses require graft excision. Calligaro et al. (52) examined this issue. The authors were able to preserve patent grafts with infections involving the anastomosis in 10 of 11 patients having vein or PTFE grafts. They recommended graft excision if (a) there was bleeding from the anastomosis, (b) the graft was occluded, (c) the patient was in a septic condition from the graft infection, or (d) the graft was made of Dacron (52).

Another alternative to the gold standard includes infected graft resection and regrafting *in situ* (i.e., simply replacing the graft). The new graft should be autogenous tissue (vein or endarterectomized artery), PTFE, or antibiotic-treated graft. The virulence of the primary pathogen will influence this decision. Cryopreserved aortic allografts have been used as *in situ* replacements with good success (15), as have venous allografts (53,54).

REFERENCES

1. Campbell OR, Bartlett FF. Postoperative *Pseudomonas* urinary tract infections as a source of bacterial contamination of an autogenous vein graft. *J Vasc Surg* 1987;5:492.
2. Cullen PJ, Leahy AL, McBride KD, et al. Angiographically induced infection of the aorta. *Ann Vasc Surg* 1986;1:386.
3. Sannella NA, Tavano P, McGoldrick DM, et al. Aortic graft sepsis caused by *Pasteurella* multocida. *J Vasc Surg* 1987;5:887.
4. White JV, Freda J, Kozar R, et al. Does bacteremia pose a threat to synthetic vascular graft? *Surgery* 1987;102:498.
5. Keller JD, Falk J, Bjorson HS, et al. Bacterial infectability of chemically implanted endothelial cell-seeded expanded polytetrafluoroethylene vascular grafts. *J Vasc Surg* 1988;7:524.
6. Schwartz JA, Powell TW, Burnham SJ, Johnson G Jr. Culture of abdominal aortic aneurysm contents. An additional series. *Arch Surg* 1987;122:777.
7. Ernst CB, Campbell HC Jr, Daugherty ME, et al. Incidence and significance of intraoperative bacterial cultures during abdominal aortic aneurysmectomy. *Ann Surg* 1977;185:626.
8. Malone JM, et al. Bacteremic infectibility of vascular grafts: the influence of pseudointimal integrity and duration of graft function. *Surgery* 1975;78:211.
9. Durham JR, Malone JM, Bernhard VM. The impact of multiple operations on the importance of arterial wall cultures. *J Vasc Surg* 1987;5:160.
10. Bergammi TM. Vascular prostheses: infections caused by bacterial biofilms. *Semin Vasc Surg* 1990;3:101.
11. Bandyk DF, Berni GA, Thide BL, et al. Aortofemoral graft infection due to *Staphylococcus epidermidis*. *Arch Surg* 1984;119:102.
12. Schmitt DD, Bandyk DF, Pequet AJ, et al. Bacterial adherence to vascular prostheses. A determinant of graft infectivity. *J Vasc Surg* 1986;3:732.
13. Rubin JR, Malone JM, Goldstone J. The role of the lymphatic system in acute arterial prosthetic graft infections. *J Vasc Surg* 1985;2:92.
14. Cherry KJ, Roland CF, Pairolero PC, et al. Infected femorodistal bypass: is graft removal mandatory? *J Vasc Surg* 1992;15:295.

15. Kieffer E, Bahini A, Koskas F, et al. In situ allograft replacement of infected infrarenal aortic prosthetic grafts: results in forty-three patients. *J Vasc Surg* 1993;17:349.
16. Edwards WH Jr, Martin RS 3rd, Jenkins JM, et al. Primary graft infections. *J Vasc Surg* 1987;6:235.
17. Liekwig WJ Jr, Greenfield LJ. Vascular prosthetic infections: collected experience and results of treatment. *Surgery* 1977;81:335.
18. Bandyk DF, Beramini TM, Kinney EV, et al. *In situ* replacement of vascular prostheses infected by bacterial biofilms. *J Vasc Surg* 1991;13:575.
19. Brook I. Role of anaerobic bacteria in aortofemoral graft infection. *Surgery* 1988;104:843.
20. Calligaro KD, Veith FJ, Schwartz ML, et al. Are gram-negative bacteria a contraindication to selective preservation of infected prosthetic arterial grafts? *J Vasc Surg* 1992;16:337.
21. Keustner LM, Reilly LM, Jicha DL, et al. Secondary aortoenteric fistula: contemporary outcome with use of extraanatomic bypass and infected graft excision. *J Vasc Surg* 1995;21:184.
22. Goldstone J, Effeney DJ. Prevention of arterial graft infections. In: Bernhard VM, Towne JB, eds. *Complications in vascular surgery*, 2nd ed. New York: Grune & Stratton, 1985:487–498.
23. Padberg FT, Smith SM, Eng RH. Optimal method for culturing vascular prosthetic grafts. *J Surg Res* 1992;53:384.
24. Kaiser AB, Clayson RR, Mulherin JL, et al. Antibiotic prophylaxis in vascular surgery. *Ann Surg* 1978;188:283.
25. Szilagyi DE, Smith RF, Elliott JP, et al. Infection in arterial reconstruction with synthetic grafts. *Ann Surg* 1972;176:321.
26. Fry WJ, Lindenauer SM. Infection complicating the use of plastic arterial implants. *Arch Surg* 1967;94:600.
27. Goldstone J, Moore WS. Infection in vascular prostheses: clinical manifestations and surgical management. *Am J Surg* 1974;128:225.
28. May AL, Darling RC, Brewster DC, et al. A comparison of the use of cephalothin and oxacillin in vascular surgery. *Arch Surg* 1980;115:56.
29. Keller JD, Falk J, Bjorston HS, et al. Bacterial infectability of chemically implanted endothelial cell-seeded expanded polytetrafluoroethylene vascular grafts. *J Vasc Surg* 1988;7:524.
30. Earnshaw JJ, Berridge DC, Slack RC, et al. Do preoperative chlorhexidine baths reduce the risk of infection after vascular reconstruction? *Eur J Vasc Surg* 1989;3:323.
31. Healy DA, Keyser J 3rd, Holcomb GW 3rd, et al. Prophylactic closed suction drainage of femoral wounds in patients undergoing vascular reconstruction. *J Vasc Surg* 1989;10:166.
32. Lord JM, Rossi G, Daliawa M. Intraoperative antibiotic wound lavage: an attempt to eliminate postoperative infections in arterial and clean procedures. *Ann Surg* 1977;185:634.
33. Halasz NA. Wound infection and topical antibiotics: the surgeon's dilemma. *Arch Surg* 1977;112:1240.
34. Pitt HA, Postier RG, MacGowan WA, et al. Prophylactic antibiotics in vascular surgery: topical, systemic or both? *Ann Surg* 1980;192:356.
35. White JV, Benvenisty AI, Reemtsma K, et al. Simple methods for direct antibiotic protection of synthetic vascular grafts. *J Vasc Surg* 1984;1:372.
36. Greco RS, Trooskin SZ, Donetz AP, et al. The application of antibiotic bonding to the treatment of established vascular prosthetic infection. *Arch Surg* 1985;120:71.
37. Modak SM, Sampath L, Fox CL, et al. A new method for the direct incorporation of antibiotics in prosthetic vascular grafts. *Surg Gynecol Obstet* 1987;164:143.
38. Shah PM, Modak S, Fox CL, et al. PTFE graft treated with silver norfloxacin (AGNF): drug retention and resistance to bacterial challenge. *J Surg Res* 1987;42:298.
39. Torsello G, Sandmann W, Gehrt A, et al In situ replacement of infected vascular prostheses with rifampin-soaked vascular grafts: early results. *J Vasc Surg* 1993;17:768.
40. Birinyi LK, Douville EC, Lewis SA, et al. Increased resistance to bacteremic graft infection after endothelial cell-seeding. *J Vasc Surg* 1987;5:193.
41. Bunt TJ. Synthetic vascular graft infections, I: graft infections. *Surgery* 1983;93:733.
42. Champion MC, Sullivan SN, Coles JC, et al. Aortoenteric fistula. Incidence, presentation, recognition, management. *Ann Surg* 1982;195:314.
43. Bunt TJ. Synthetic vascular graft infections, II: graft-enteric erosion and graft-enteric fistulas. *Surgery* 1983;94:1.
44. O'Donnell TF, Scott G, Shepard A, et al. Improvements in the diagnosis and management of aortoenteric fistula. *Am J Surg* 1985;149:481.
45. Qvarfordt PG, Reilly LM, Mark AS, et al. Computerized tomographic assessment of graft incorporation after aortic reconstruction. *Am J Surg* 1985;150:227.
46. Hansen ME, Yucel EK, Waltman AC. STIR imaging of synthetic vascular graft infection. *Cardiovasc Intervent Radiol* 1993;16:30.
47. LaMurglia GM, Fischman AJ, Strauss HK, et al. Utility of indium 111–labeled human immunoglobulin G scan for the detection of focal vascular graft infection. *J Vasc Surg* 1989;10:20.
48. Prats E, Banzo J, Abos MD, et al. Diagnosis of prosthetic vascular graft infection by technetium-99m-HMPAO–labeled leukocytes. *J Nucl Med* 1994;35:1303.
49. Wakefield TW. Diagnosis of aortic graft infection. In: Ernst CB, Stanley JC, eds. *Current therapy of vascular surgery*. Philadelphia: BC Decker, 1991.
50. Padberg FT, Smith SM, Eng RH. Accuracy of disincorporation for identification of vascular graft infection. *Arch Surg* 1995;130:183.
51. Reilly LM, Stoney RJ, Goldstone J, et al. Improved management of aortic graft infection: the influence of operation sequence and staging. *J Vasc Surg* 1987;5:412.
52. Calligaro KD, Westcott CJ, Buckley RM, et al. Infrainguinal anastomotic arterial graft infections treated by selective graft preservation. *Ann Surg* 1992;216:74.
53. Fujitani RM, Bassiouny HS, Gewertz BL, et al. Cryopreserved saphenous vein allogenic homografts: an alternative conduit in lower extremity arterial reconstruction in infected fields. *J Vasc Surg* 1992;15:519.
54. Snyder SO, Wheeler JR, Gregory RT, et al. Freshly harvested cadaveric venous homografts as arterial conduits in infected fields. *Surgery* 1987;101:283.
55. Sharp WJ, Hoballah JJ, Moran CR, et al. The management of the infected aortic prosthesis: a current decade of experience. *J Vasc Surg* 1994;19:844.
56. Bacourt F, Koskas F. Axillobifemoral bypass and aortic exclusion for vascular septic lesions: a multicenter retrospective study of 98 cases. *Ann Vasc Surg* 1992;6:119.
57. McCarthy WJ, McGee GS, Lin WW, et al. Axillary-popliteal bypass provides successful limb salvage after removal of infected aortofemoral grafts. *Arch Surg* 1992;127:974.
58. Ricotta JJ, Faggioli GL, Stella A, et al. Total excision and extraanatomic bypass for aortic graft infection. *Am J Surg* 1991;162:145.
59. Quinones-Baldrich WJ, Hernandez JJ, Moore WS. Long-term results following surgical management of aortic graft infection. *Arch Surg* 1991;126:507.
60. Reilly LM, Ahmay H, Lusby RJ, et al. Late results following surgical management of vascular graft infection. *J Vasc Surg* 1984;1:36.
61. Mertens RA, O'Hara PJ, Hertzer NR, et al. Surgical management of infrainguinal arterial prosthetic graft infections: review of a thirty-five year experience. *J Vasc Surg* 1995;21:782.

CHAPTER 64
Pericarditis and Myocarditis

Catherine Diamond and Jeremiah Tilles

In this chapter, we review the etiology, pathogenesis, clinical presentation, diagnosis, treatment, and prognosis of infections of the pericardium and myocardium. Because the pericardium is anatomically close to the myocardium, infections of the heart frequently involve both tissues. Because inflammation of one of the two tissues usually predominates, the clinical diagnosis becomes either pericarditis or myocarditis.

PERICARDITIS

Etiology

The causes of acute pericarditis include infectious and noninfectious etiologies (Table 64.1). Noninfectious causes include systemic diseases (e.g., collagen-vascular disease or uremia), malignancy, injuries (e.g., thoracic surgery, radiation, trauma, or myocardial infarction), or a drug reaction (e.g., against hydralazine or procainamide). In most cases of idiopathic pericarditis, the etiologic agent is likely infectious, in general, and a virus, in particular. The viruses that cause pericarditis also cause myocarditis, and concurrent myocarditis is frequently present.

The most common of the diagnosed infectious caused of pericarditis is viral infection, for example, enteroviruses such as coxsackievirus group A or B and echoviruses (1,2). Human immunodeficiency virus (HIV), influenza virus, and herpesviruses such as Epstein-Barr virus and cytomegalovirus (CMV) also may cause viral pericarditis. About one fifth of patients with acquired immunodeficiency syndrome (AIDS) have pericardial effusion, although the effusions are usually small, asymptomatic, and

TABLE 64.1. Causes of Acute Pericarditis

Infectious	Noninfectious
Viruses	Injuries
Adenovirus	Cardiac surgery
Coxsackieviruses A and B	Chest trauma
Cytomegalovirus	Chylopericardium
Epstein-Barr virus	Dissecting aortic aneurysm
Echovirus	Myocardial infarction
Hepatitis B virus	Postirradiation
Herpes simplex virus	Diseases
Human immunodeficiency	Familial Mediterranean fever
virus	Hypothyroidism
Influenza virus	Inflammatory bowel disease
Mumps virus	Metastatic tumor
Varicella-zoster virus	Mixed connective tissue disease
Fungi	Polymyositis/dermatomyositis
Aspergillus species	Rheumatoid arthritis
Blastomyces dermatitidis	Rheumatic fever
Candida species	Sarcoidosis
Coccidioides immitis	Scleroderma
Cryptococcus neoformans	Systemic lupus erythematosus
Histoplasma capsulatum	Uremia
Parasites	Wegener's granulomatosis
Entamoeba histolytica	Drugs
Schistosoma species	Heparin
Toxocara canis	Methysergide
Toxoplasma gondii	Minoxidil
Bacteria	Phenytoin
Actinomyces species	Procainamide
Bacteroides	Hydralazine
Borrelia burgdorferi	
Brucella species	
Campylobacter	
Chlamydia	
Haemophilus influenzae	
Enteric gram-negative rods	
Legionella pneumophila	
Listeria monocytogenes	
Neisseria meningitidis and	
Neisseria gonorrhoeae	
Mycoplasma	
Prevotella	
Propionibacterium acnes	
Salmonella species	
Staphylcoccus aureus	
Anaerobic streptococci	
Streptococcus pneumoniae	
Other *Streptococcus* species	
Mycobacterium tuberculosis	
Mycobacterium avium	
complex	
Nocardia asteroides	

idiopathic (3). When effusions are large and symptomatic, various nonviral causes such as bacteria (e.g., *Staphylococcus aureus* or *Streptococcus pneumoniae*), mycobacteria (e.g., *Mycobacterium tuberculosis* or *Mycobacterium avium*), or malignancy (e.g., non-Hodgkin's lymphoma or Kaposi's sarcoma) are in the differential diagnosis (4).

Before the advent of antibiotics, bacterial pericarditis was a common disease that occurred in previously healthy children and adults with pneumonia (5–7). Bacterial pericarditis has become unusual with the widespread use of antibiotics and generally afflicts chronically ill adults as a complication of another illness. Although *S. pneumoniae* was the predominant pathogen in the past, *S. aureus* has been the most common bacterial cause of pericarditis more recently (7,8). In addition, the proportion of bacterial pericarditis caused by gram-negative rods is

increasing (6,9). Pericarditis caused by gram-negative rods is usually a nosocomial infection occurring in a compromised host (6,9). Anaerobes occasionally cause pericarditis in the setting of esophageal perforation and mediastinitis, head and neck infections, or through bacteremia (10,11). *Haemophilus influenzae* was a prominent cause in children before the introduction of the conjugate vaccine (12). On the other hand, the meningococcus still causes either sterile or purulent pericarditis (13,14). Lastly, pathogens that cause atypical pneumonia, such as *Mycoplasma pneumoniae* and *Legionella pneumophila*, may also cause pericarditis (15,16).

Tuberculosis is a major cause of pericarditis in underdeveloped countries and in patients with AIDS. There is pericardial involvement in approximately 1% of cases of untreated pulmonary tuberculosis (17). Fungal pericarditis is infrequent, but *Candida* species, *Aspergillus* species, or *Cryptococcus neoformans* may cause pericarditis either as part of disseminated infection in immunocompromised hosts or as a complication following cardiothoracic surgery (18–20). Although *Coccidioides immitis* rarely causes pericarditis with disseminated disease, *Histoplasma capsulatum* may infect pericardial tissue during disseminated infection and has caused sterile reactive pericarditis in outbreak settings (21). Pericarditis caused by parasitic infections is also rare but may accompany primary infection at other sites with *Toxoplasma gondii*, *Entamoeba histolytica*, or *Schistosoma* species.

Pathogenesis

The visceral pericardium adheres to the epicardial surface of the heart, whereas the parietal pericardium attaches to the sternum, great vessels, and diaphragm. Between the two layers, there is usually about 30 mL of clear fluid that drains into the thoracic and the right lymphatic ducts. Inflammation of the pericardium may be accompanied by accumulation of pericardial fluid if the inflammatory infiltrate impairs lymphatic drainage. Viruses usually reach the pericardium hematogenously, whereas bacteria frequently infect by direct extension from local structures, such as the lungs, endocardium, or mediastinum (22). Bacterial pericarditis can also result from inoculation of organisms into the pericardium from penetrating injuries of the chest wall or thoracic surgery (23) or less commonly from seeding of the pericardium by bacteremia. In pericarditis, the pericardial fluid may be serous, fibrinous, suppurative, or hemorrhagic. Cardiac tamponade occurs when the volume of the accumulated fluid restricts ventricular filling during diastole, reducing cardiac output and increasing in systemic and pulmonary venous pressures (24). Recurrent pericarditis is thought to be autoimmune in mechanism, but routine immunologic testing is usually unrevealing and histopathologic examination usually shows only fibrosis (25). Constrictive pericarditis occurs when the pericardium becomes fibrotic; the motion of the heart is impaired and the filling pressures of the right and left ventricles equalize.

Clinical Presentation

The most common symptom of acute viral pericarditis is sharp precordial chest pain (26) (Table 64.2). The pain may radiate to the back and is often worse with movement, inspiration, or coughing. The pain is exacerbated by resting supine and alleviated by leaning forward. Patients may also have fever, cough, and constitutional symptoms such as fatigue, myalgia, and arthralgia. Patients with bacterial pericarditis are usually acutely ill with their symptoms, reflecting the underlying disease that precipitated pericarditis. In contrast, tuberculosis pericarditis is insidious in onset.

TABLE 64.2. Clinical and Laboratory Features of Acute Pericarditis

Symptoms	Signs
Chest pain	Evidence of tamponade
Cough	Hypotension
Dyspnea	Jugular venous distention
Fatigue	Muffled heart sounds
Arthralgias	Peripheral edema
Myalgias	Pulsus paradoxus
	Tachycardia
	Fever
	Pericardial friction rub

Laboratory abnormalities
  Elevated creatinine phosphokinase
  Elevated erythrocyte sedimentation rate
  Leukocytosis
Electrocardiographic changes
  ST-segment elevation in most leads
  ST-segment depression in a VR and V$_1$
  T-wave inversions
  PR-segment depression
Imaging studies
  Pericardial thickening by computed tomography
  Enlarged heart silhouette on chest radiograph (if effusion present)
  Pericardial effusion on echocardiogram

The most frequent finding of pericarditis on physical examination is a friction rub (27). Classically, it is a three-part rub, reflecting contact of the inflamed parietal pericardial tissue with the visceral pericardium during ventricular and atrial systole and rapid ventricular filling in early diastole. Although the triphasic friction rub is characteristic of acute pericarditis, lack of a rub does not preclude the diagnosis. In one study, 56% of patients with acute pericarditis had a three-component friction rub present on physical examination (28). Physical findings in the setting of tamponade include hypotension, distended neck veins, edema, muffled heart sounds, tachycardia, and paradoxic pulse.

Laboratory abnormalities consistent with acute pericarditis include elevations of the erythrocyte sedimentation rate, white blood cell count, cardiac isoenzymes, and troponin-I (29,30). Patients with acute pericarditis typically have electrocardiographic (ECG) changes (31). Diffuse ST-segment elevation is the most sensitive ECG feature, and PR-segment depression is specific but not sensitive in acute pericarditis. ST-segment depression in leads aVR and V$_1$, and widespread T-wave inversion may also occur. Decreased QRS voltage signifies a large pericardial effusion. The rhythm is usually sinus rhythm or sinus tachycardia unless there is underlying heart disease or myocarditis. The chest radiograph will show cardiac enlargement if an effusion of at least 250 mL is present. Echocardiography is the easiest method to evaluate the size of the pericardial effusion and assess for tamponade (24,32). Computed tomography (CT) or magnetic resonance imaging (MRI) may be useful to demonstrate pericardial fluid, thickening, or masses (33–35).

Diagnosis

When patients have concomitant conditions known to cause pericarditis, such as uremia, myocardial infarction, or metastatic cancer (see Table 64.1), the cause of pericarditis may be self-evident (36). Similarly, documentation of infection in the chest near the pericardium or systemic infection with bacteria, mycobacteria, or fungi allows a presumptive etiologic diagnosis. The diagnosis of viral pericarditis is usually clinical. Given the

number of potential viruses that cause pericarditis, the pursuit and confirmation of a definitive diagnosis may be frustrating. The clinician may pursue the diagnosis of a concomitant viral infection by obtaining viral culture samples from sites such as blood, throat, or rectum, although these cultures may be negative. Serologic tests showing a fourfold rise in specific antibody titers against coxsackie B viruses or other locally prevalent enteroviruses between acute and convalescent serum samples or the presence of specific immunoglobulin M antibody may support the clinical suspicion of a viral infection. Evidence of systemic viral infection would support the diagnosis of a viral etiology of the pericarditis but would not prove it. Viral culture of the pericardial fluid is usually negative, although a positive polymerase chain reaction (PCR) for the suspected viral pathogen in either the pericardial fluid or the tissue would confirm the diagnosis. HIV testing is recommended in the setting of idiopathic pericarditis.

Pericardiocentesis is not recommended in an otherwise healthy individual with suspected viral or idiopathic pericarditis. In a study of 256 patients with pericarditis, 221 (86%) had idiopathic, 12 (5%) neoplastic, 11 (4%) tuberculous, 4 (2%) collagen vascular, 3 (1%) viral, 2 (1%) toxoplasmal, and 3 (1%) purulent pericarditis (37). When the patients in the study received pericardiocentesis to relieve tamponade, the diagnostic yield was 28%, which was more than five times that found when the procedure was undertaken for diagnostic purposes only. On the other hand, when the patients received a pericardial biopsy or pericardectomy for tamponade, the diagnostic yield was 54%. In a similar study of patients with large-volume effusions without tamponade in whom purulent pericarditis was considered unlikely, only 7% of patients who underwent pericardiocentesis or pericardial biopsy emerged with a diagnosis as a result of the procedure. Of 45 patients who did not undergo these procedures, none developed tamponade or died and only 2 had persistent moderate or large effusions (38). Based on these studies, diagnostic pericardiocentesis is indicated only in cases involving patients with suspected purulent effusion (a nonviral infection), immunocompromised status, cardiac tamponade, or an unusually prolonged course (more than 3 weeks) (39) (Table 64.3). When an invasive procedure is necessary, biopsy and drainage is more likely to result in a diagnosis than pericardiocentesis alone (40).

Historically, the diagnosis of purulent pericarditis is often missed premortem. The percentage of cases diagnosed postmortem varies from approximately 30% to 80% depending on the series (6,7,9,23,41). Patients with purulent pericarditis often do not have classic symptoms such as chest pain or friction rub, resulting in a high rate of postmortem diagnosis. Also, many of these patients have underlying illnesses that cause symptoms of fever, shortness of breath, and tachycardia; this is particularly characteristic of patients postthoracotomy (23). Thus, the treating physician attributes these symptoms to the patient's underlying illness. Because purulent pericarditis can progress rapidly, we recommend an aggressive approach in patients for whom this diagnosis is suspected.

TABLE 64.3. Indications for Pericardiocentesis in Acute Pericarditis

Suspected purulent effusion
Immunocompromised patient
Cardiac tamponade
Suspected malignancy
Prolonged course without a clear diagnosis

Treatment

Pain management, bed rest, and hemodynamic monitoring are standard therapy for all patients with acute pericarditis. It is best to avoid the use of anticoagulants because of the risk of hemorrhage and tamponade. Patients with cardiac tamponade and unstable hemodynamic status require emergency pericardiocentesis. In stable patients with tamponade, surgical drainage with pericardial biopsy is preferable to pericardiocentesis (see the previous section, "Diagnosis"). Recurrent tamponade is an indication for a pericardial window or pericardectomy.

IDIOPATHIC (VIRAL) PERICARDITIS

Nonsteroidal antiinflammatory drugs (NSAIDs) such as ibuprofen or indomethacin are recommended for viral pericarditis. Patients infected with a virus sensitive to specific antiviral therapy should receive the appropriate antiviral for up to 4 weeks (e.g., intravenous acyclovir for varicella-zoster). Corticosteroids are useful only in those unusual cases of relapsing disease or cases unresponsive to NSAIDs. Surgical pericardectomy is rarely necessary and employed only in patients in whom drug therapy either fails or is not tolerated.

BACTERIAL PERICARDITIS

A prolonged course of an intravenous antibiotic must be used for a patient with bacterial pericarditis. For example, pericarditis caused by methicillin-sensitive *S. aureus* should be treated for 4 to 6 weeks with high doses of intravenous nafcillin. Because intravenous antibiotics achieve high levels in the inflamed pericardium, antibiotic irrigation is unnecessary. Most cases of bacterial pericarditis require surgical drainage of the pericardial fluid (42). There has been a single case report of the successful use of intrapericardial streptokinase for purulent pericarditis (43).

TUBERCULOUS PERICARDITIS

Antibiotic treatment for tuberculous pericarditis is the same as that for pulmonary tuberculosis. Most experts recommend corticosteroids to reduce inflammation and prevent the development of constrictive pericarditis in the setting of tuberculous pericarditis (44,45). A systemic review from the Cochrane collaboration concluded that although corticosteroids might have a large impact on survival, further placebo-controlled trials of steroids are needed because the completed trials have been too small to prove it (46). In patients with pulmonary tuberculosis, pericardial infection may be clinically inconspicuous until the hemodynamic consequences of constrictive pericarditis occur late in the disease course. Constrictive pericarditis develops in 30% to 50% of cases of tuberculous pericarditis, despite appropriate therapy, and the risk is higher in patients with a history of tamponade (47,48). Pericardectomy is required for those patients with hemodynamic compromise caused by progressive pericardial thickening or recurrent tamponade (49).

Course and Prognosis

ACUTE PERICARDITIS

Because most cases of bacterial pericarditis occur in debilitated hosts, the prognosis must be guarded. In previous reports, the mortality in patients diagnosed antemortem and treated with combined medical and surgical therapy was 16% to 45% (7,9,41). Morality is highest in older patients, debilitated patients, patients in whom the diagnosis is delayed, and in patients who do not receive appropriate therapy. Patients with pericarditis caused by gram-negative rods or with an intracardiac or postoperative source also tend to do poorly. In contrast to bacterial pericarditis, viral pericarditis is usually a self-limited illness lasting 1 to 3 weeks.

RECURRENT PERICARDITIS

Recurrent pericarditis is defined as pericarditis occurring at least 3 months after a documented resolved episode of acute pericarditis in a patient without active systemic disease (25). Among patients with idiopathic acute pericarditis, 15% to 30% of patients have one or more recurrences (50,51). Recurrences may occur as late as several years after the initial episode. The duration, frequency, and number of recurrences are variable, but recurrent episodes tend to be less severe than the original disease. Deaths are rare and the incidence of cardiac tamponade or constrictive pericarditis appears to be less than 10% (52). Most patients respond to intermittent courses of NSAIDs, although a few patients require prolonged therapy. Colchicine is useful in patients with relapsing pericarditis to prevent recurrence (53,54). Corticosteroid therapy should be considered only for patients who are unresponsive to NSAIDs and colchicine (25). Although one study showed benefit from pericardiectomy (55), most experts recommend the procedure only for patients with extremely severe or frequent episodes unresponsive to medical therapy or for patients with constrictive pericarditis.

CONSTRICTIVE PERICARDITIS

Constrictive pericarditis may follow acute pericarditis of almost any cause. Although viral infection is unlikely to result in constrictive pericarditis, untreated bacterial infections, connective tissue diseases, and tuberculosis, in particular, are the most common causes. Constrictive pericarditis involves fibrosis of the visceral and parietal pericardium with obliteration of the pericardial space, reduced expansion of the heart during filling, and decreased venous return and cardiac output. The onset is insidious, with patients eventually presenting with dyspnea, orthopnea, dry cough, malaise, and abdominal swelling. Physical examination shows signs of elevated venous pressure, such as jugular venous distention, ascites, hepatomegaly, peripheral edema, pleural effusion, and pulsus paradoxus. Although patients with restrictive cardiomyopathy may present with similar clinical findings, echocardiographic and hemodynamic criteria and the presence of pericardial thickening on CT (56,57) can distinguish them. Although sodium restriction and diuretics may be used preoperatively, the treatment for most patients is pericardiectomy. Corticosteroids are not useful in the treatment of constrictive pericarditis.

MYOCARDITIS

Etiology

There are multiple infectious and noninfectious causes of myocarditis (Table 64.4). Viruses are the most frequent cause of myocarditis, especially the group B coxsackieviruses and other enteroviruses such as coxsackie A virus and echovirus (58). Influenza causes myocarditis that is often subclinical detected by ECG changes in patients without cardiac symptoms (59). Coxsackie B viruses have the highest proportion of infections manifesting cardiac disease (34.6 per 1,000 infections), followed by influenza B (17.4 per 1,000 infections), influenza A (11.7 per 1,000 infections), coxsackie A (9.1 per 1,000 infections), and CMV (8.0 per 1,000 infections) (60). In the past, virologists viewed adenovirus as a frequent cause of myocarditis in children, but studies

TABLE 64.4. Causes of Myocarditis

Infectious	Noninfectious
Viruses	Diseases
Adenovirus	Acute necrotizing eosinophilic
Argentinian hemorrhagic	myocarditis
fever	Hyperthyroidism
Bolivian hemorrhagic fever	Hypothyroidism
Chikungunya virus	Metastatic tumor
Coxsackieviruses A and B	Peripartum
Cytomegalovirus	Pheochromocytoma
Dengue virus	Drugs
Echovirus	Alcohol
Epstein-Barr virus	Anthracyclines (daunorubicin,
Hepatitis B and C virus	doxorubicin)
Herpes simplex virus	Clozapine
Human immunodeficiency	Cocaine
virus	Cyclophosphamide
Influenza viruses A and B	Dobutamine
Lymphocytic choriomeningitis	Emetine
virus	Interferons
Measles virus	Interleukin-2
Mumps virus	Methyldopa
Parvovirus B19	Opiates
Poliomyelitis virus	Sulfonamides
Rabies virus	Tetracycline
Rubella virus	Autoimmune and rheumatic
Respiratary syncytial virus	Inflammatory myositis
Vaccinia	Kawasaki's disease
Variola	Rheumatoid arthritis
Varicella-zoster virus	Rheumatic fever
Bacteria	Scleroderma
Actinomyces species	Still's disease
Borrelia burgdorferi	Systemic lupus erythematosus
Brucella species	Toxins and poisons
Chlamydia species	Arsenic
Clostridium perfringens	Carbon monoxide
Corynebacterium diphtheriae	Lead
Ehrlichia	Radiation
Legionella pneumophilia	Stings (scorpion, wasp, spider)
Listeria monocytogenes	
Mycoplasma pneumoniae	
Neisseria species	
Salmonella species	
Staphylococcus species	
Streptococcus species	
Treponema pallidum	
Vibrio cholera	
Parasites	
Trichinella spiralis	
Entamoeba histolytica	
Toxoplasma gondii	
Trypanosoma species	
Fungi	
Aspergillus species	
Candida species	
Cryptococcus neoformans	

in the 1990s detected adenovirus deoxyribonucleic acid in myocardial tissue samples from cases of adult myocarditis (61,62). Patients with HIV infection have an elevated risk of myocarditis and dilated cardiomyopathy (63).

Myocarditis caused by nonviral infections is uncommon in the United States. Diphtheric myocarditis occurs when the toxin produced by *Corynebacterium diphtheriae* damages the myocardium and the conduction system. Lyme myocarditis caused by *Borrelia burgdorferi* also affects the conduction system. Myocarditis with bacterial pathogens may occur when infectious foci are established in the myocardium of bacteremic patients or in association with bacterial pericarditis. In addition, perivalvu-

lar abscesses may complicate some cases of bacterial endocarditis. Fungal myocarditis may occur in the setting of disseminated infection in either the normal or the immunocompromised host. Parasitic infections of the myocardium are most common in underdeveloped countries. For instance, *Trypanosoma cruzi*, acquired through the bite of the reduviid bug, is a common cause of myocarditis in South and Central America (64).

Pathogenesis

Although extracellular toxins such as those elaborated by *C. diphtheriae* may directly injure the myocardium, most cases of myocarditis are due to viruses, with the pathogenesis in humans not completely clear. There are a variety of mouse models of viral myocarditis in which young mice are injected intraperitoneally with coxsackie B3 virus and multiple mechanisms of tissue damage demonstrated. Typically, the virus is easily isolated from the heart and blood during this acute phase of viral replication. During this phase, depending on the model, cardiac histology may show inflammatory infiltrates, myocyte necrosis, and/or coronary artery microvascular spasm causing myocardial hypoperfusion. In some models, during the subsequent chronic phase, congestive heart failure (CHF) may develop, characterized by myocardial fibrosis, and results in a dilated cardiomyopathy. Although viral infection of myocytes usually occurs early, most of the tissue damage often occurs later with infiltration of T lymphocytes. Cytokines are induced at that time and contribute to the inflammatory response. In this postviral autoimmune myocarditis, heart-specific autoantibodies against heavy-chain cardiac myosin may develop. In rats with autoimmune myocarditis induced by immunization with cardiac myosin, inflammation increases expression of the common cell surface receptor, coxsackie adenoviral receptor (65,66). This may worsen the severity of viral infection and consequently amplify the inflammatory process.

Epidemiology

Although most cases of myocarditis occur in children and young adults, the disease is most severe in neonates and the immunocompromised (67,68). Coxsackie myocarditis generally occurs in the summer and autumn, and influenza myocarditis presents in the winter and spring. Because viral myocarditis is usually subclinical and thus undiagnosed, the incidence of viral myocarditis in the general population is unknown (69). The prevalence of histologic myocarditis among unselected deaths is 1% to 3% versus 7% to 24% among young people with sudden unexpected natural death (70–76). The incidence of clinically diagnosed acute myocarditis was 0.17 per 1,000 person-years among young Finnish military men (77). As many as 5% of coxsackie B infections have associated cardiac signs and symptoms but the risk of cardiac involvement may be increased in the setting of a coxsackie B outbreak (2,68,78,79). During influenza infection, up to 43% of infected individuals have ECG changes that are usually transient (80,81).

Clinical Presentation

Commonly, acute myocarditis typically is either entirely asymptomatic or causes a mild undiagnosed illness that resolves without treatment. In immunocompetent adults, viral myocarditis may occur after a nonspecific illness manifest with fever, arthralgias, malaise, or coryza. There is usually no preceding illness in infants and the immunocompromised or in patients with either nonviral infectious causes or noninfectious causes. When acutely

TABLE 64.5. Clinical and Laboratory Features of Myocarditis

Symptoms	Signs
Chest pain	Tachycardia
Palpitations	Muffled first heart sound
Shortness of breath	Third heart sound (S_3 gallop)
Cough	Mitral regurgitant murmur
Fever	Pericardial friction rub
Arthralgias	Paradoxical pulse
Coryza	Congestive heart failure
	(jugular venous distention,
	hepatomegaly, edema)
Electrocardiographic changes	Laboratory abnormalities
imaging studies	Creatine phosphokinase
Chest x-ray	elevation
Echocardiogram	Troponin elevation
Cardiac catheterization	Erythrocyte sedimentation rate
Radionucleotide scan	elevation
(indium-111–labeled	C-reactive protein elevation
monoclonal antimyosin	Leukocytosis or leukopenia
antibody or gallium scan)	
Magnetic resonance imaging	

symptomatic, myocarditis may present as myocardial infarction (chest pain, ECG changes, and elevated cardiac isoenzymes) or with cardiogenic shock, serious arrhythmia, or sudden death. Patients may also present subacutely with mild ventricular dysfunction and CHF. Although chest pain, either pleuritic or substernal, is the most common symptom, shortness of breath and palpitations are also common complaints (82) (Table 64.5). Fever, tachycardia, a muffled first heart sound, pericardial friction rub, third heart sound (S_3 gallop), mitral regurgitant murmur, tachypnea, and signs of CHF may be evident on physical examination.

Patients with myocarditis may have an elevated erythrocyte sedimentation rate or C-reactive protein and either leukocytosis or leukopenia. Creatinine kinase MB or troponin may be elevated, but neither is specific for myocarditis (83,84). ST-segment elevation and T-wave inversions may occur on serial ECG recordings but usually resolve over a few months. Supraventricular tachycardia and ventricular extrasystoles may be present, but ventricular tachycardia, complex ventricular arrhythmias, atrioventricular block, and bundle-branch blocks are infrequent (82). Echocardiography detects intracardiac thrombus, pericardial effusion, or tamponade, assesses left ventricular wall motion, and estimates ejection fraction. Chest radiography shows an enlarged heart with or without signs of heart failure in about half of patients with myocarditis (82). Nuclear imaging such as indium-111–labeled monoclonal antimyosin antibodies or gallium scanning may demonstrate myocardial injury (85–87). MRI was highly sensitive and specific in reflecting the presence of acute myocarditis present on endomyocardial biopsy in a small pediatric case series (88).

Diagnosis

The definitive diagnosis of myocarditis rests on the histologic interpretation of an endomyocardial biopsy or myocardial tissue specimens at autopsy. Because viruses are the most common cause of myocarditis and there is currently no specific therapy for viral myocarditis other than antivirals, endomyocardial biopsy is generally not recommended (89). On the other hand, in the face of progressive clinical deterioration, the risk of cardiac

perforation associated with biopsy may be justifiable. Biopsy is definitely indicated when there is a suspicion of a potentially treatable cause of myocarditis that cannot be diagnosed by noninvasive means. If a patient undergoes endomyocardial biopsy, the specimen should be sent for stains and cultures for viruses, parasites, fungi, bacteria, and mycobacteria, as well as routine histology. In immunocompetent adults, viruses are usually not isolated from endomyocardial biopsy specimens, but specimens from immunocompromised patients are frequently productive.

The prevalence of histologically proven myocarditis in patients thought to have the diagnosis ranged from less than 10% to almost 90% in various studies (89–96). Diverse histologic criteria, as well as sampling error, may account for some of this variability. A group of cardiac pathologists developed the stringent Dallas criteria to standardize microscopic criteria for the interpretation of endomyocardial biopsy. The Dallas criteria require "lymphocytic myocarditis," a lymphocytic infiltrate in the myocardium with associated myocyte necrosis, and exclude 90% of persons suspected of having myocarditis based on clinical criteria (93).

A positive immunoglobulin M titer for a specific virus, a four-fold rise in titer of specific viral antibody between acute and convalescent serum samples, or isolation of a virus from cerebrospinal fluid, throat, or stool provides evidence of recent viral infection and a presumptive cause of clinical myocarditis. In addition to the viral studies mentioned, HIV testing is indicated for patients with acute myocarditis. Because the same viruses that cause myocarditis commonly cause infection without myocarditis, serologic tests or viral culture from a noncardiac site should be interpreted cautiously. In one study, approximately one fourth of patients without myocarditis had serologic evidence of infection with agents known to cause myocarditis (97). Firm evidence of a causal role for a virus is identification of virus in cardiac tissue, either by culture, immunofluorescence or peroxidase-labeled antibody (98), or PCR.

Treatment

Because most diagnosed cases of myocarditis are either idiopathic or caused by viruses for which there is no proven specific therapy, supportive therapy is the mainstay of treatment. Based on studies that show that exercise worsens the outcome of coxsackie myocarditis in mice (99) and exacerbates wall motion abnormalities in humans (100), bed rest is recommended. Hospitalization with oxygen therapy and cardiac monitoring for arrhythmias is beneficial. Antiarrhythmics, electrophysiologic evaluation, a pacemaker, or an implantable defibrillator may be necessary to treat serious arrhythmias. Patients with CHF usually respond to diuretics, salt restriction, and afterload reduction. Afterload reduction with an angiotensin-converting enzyme inhibitor is recommended. Substitute hydralazine and isorbide dinitrate only if there is a contraindication. Captopril ameliorated cardiac inflammation, necrosis, and myocyte hypertrophy in a mouse model (101). Because digoxin increases expression of proinflammatory cytokines and mortality in a mouse model, it should be administered only at low doses (102). Aggressive support measures including intensive care, intraaortic balloon pump, extracorporeal membrane oxygenation, or a left ventricular assist device may be useful in patients with cardiogenic shock. Cardiac transplantation may ultimately be necessary in the setting of persistent heart failure.

When the clinician has diagnosed an acute infection caused by a specific virus, administration of antiviral agents such as ganciclovir or foscarnet for CMV, M2 (amantadine, rimantadine) or oral neuraminidase inhibitors (oseltamivir) for influenza, antiretrovirals for HIV, or pleconaril (investigational) for enterovirus may be beneficial. Pleconaril (VP63843), a novel oral compound that integrates into the capsid of picornaviruses, is available for compassionate use for severe picornaviral illness and decreased symptoms and shortened disease duration in enteroviral meningitis with minimal side effects (103,104). A precursor drug, WIN 54954, decreased myocardial coxsackievirus replication and improved survival in a mouse model of myocarditis, but adverse events associated with the compound prevented its development for human use (105,106). Patients with mycobacterial, bacterial, fungal, or parasitic myocarditis should receive the appropriate specific chemotherapy.

Because postviral myocarditis may be autoimmune in its pathogenesis, researchers have experimented with various immunosuppressant and immunomodulating agents to treat myocarditis. The use of NSAIDs increased coxsackievirus titers and mortality in a mouse model and thus should be avoided (107). Corticosteroids also were deleterious in a mouse model, causing extensive and disseminated myocardial necrosis (108). The only controlled human study that showed benefit with corticosteroids had serious methodologic flaws and the best designed study thus far, the Myocarditis Treatment Trial, showed no benefit (93,109). Thus, corticosteroids are not recommended for myocarditis. Although immunoglobulin treatment showed benefit in a mouse model (110), a study of intravenous immune globulin therapy in patients with recent-onset dilated cardiomyopathy did not show benefit from immunoglobulin beyond the expected improvement in left ventricular ejection fraction that was seen in both treated subjects and controls (111). Although interferon demonstrated benefit in two murine models of viral myocarditis, clinical experience in the treatment of myocarditis with this agent is still lacking (112–114).

Course and Prognosis

Because most viral myocarditis is mildly symptomatic and never diagnosed, it is likely that most patients with viral myocarditis recover within a few weeks and have a good long-term prognosis (115). In more severe cases, the left ventricular ejection fraction typically improves about 10% to 15% in 6 months (111,116). Symptomatic coxsackie B myocarditis may evolve to chronic dilated cardiomyopathy in up to 50% of diagnosed patients (117,118). In the Myocarditis Treatment Trial, a higher left ventricular ejection fraction at baseline, less intensive conventional therapy, and a shorter duration of disease predicted improvement in left ventricular ejection fraction (93). In that study, which enrolled patients with a histopathologic diagnosis of myocarditis and a left ventricular ejection fraction of less than 0.45, the mortality rate was 20% at 1 year and 56% at approximately 4 years despite an early improvement in mean left ventricular ejection fraction. Sustained recovery after mechanical support for acute myocarditis is unpredictable (119). However, fulminant myocarditis with severe hemodynamic compromise, rapid onset, and fever is a distinct clinical entity that has an excellent long-term prognosis. Thus, aggressive hemodynamic support is warranted for patients with this condition (120).

ACKNOWLEDGMENT

This work was sponsored in part by the California Collaborative Treatment Group (CC99-SD-003).

REFERENCES

1. Brodie HR, Marchessault V. Acute benign pericarditis caused by coxsackie group B. *N Engl J Med* 1960;262:1278–1280.
2. Grist NR, Bell EJ. Coxsackie viruses and the heart. *Am Heart J* 1969;77:295–300.
3. Rerkpattanapipat P, Wongpraparut N, Jacobs LE, et al. Cardiac manifestations of acquired immunodeficiency syndrome. *Arch Intern Med* 2000;160:602–608.
4. Chen Y, Brennessel D, Walters J, et al. Human immunodeficiency virus–associated pericardial effusion: report of 40 cases and review of the literature. *Am Heart J* 1999;137:516–521.
5. Boyle JD, Pearce ML, Guze LB. Purulent pericarditis: review of literature and report of eleven cases. *Medicine* 1961;40:119–144.
6. Klacsmann PG, Bulkley BH, Hutchins GM. The changed spectrum of purulent pericarditis. An 86 year autopsy experience in 200 patients. *Am J Med* 1977;63:666–673.
7. Rubin RH, Moellering RC. Clinical, microbiologic and therapeutic aspects of purulent pericarditis. *Am J Med* 1975;59:68–78.
8. Kauffman CA, Watanakumnakorn C, Phair JP. Purulent pneumococcal pericarditis. *Am J Med* 1973;54:743–750.
9. Gould K, Barnett JA, Sanford JP. Purulent pericarditis in the antibiotic era. *Arch Intern Med* 1974;134:923–927.
10. Brook I, Frazier EH. Microbiology of acute purulent pericarditis. A 12 year experience in a military hospital. *Arch Intern Med* 1996;156:1857–1860.
11. Skiest DJ, Steiner D, Werner M, et al. Anaerobic pericarditis: case report and review. *Clin Infect Dis* 1994;19:435–440.
12. Fyfe DA, Hagler DJ, Puga FJ et al. Clinical and therapeutic aspects of *Haemophilus influenzae* pericarditis in pediatric patients. *Mayo Clin Proc* 1984;59:415–422.
13. Blaser MJ, Reingold AL, Alsever RN, et al. Primary meningococcal pericarditis: a disease of adults associated with serogroup C *Neisseria meningitidis. Rev Infect Dis* 1984;6:625–632.
14. Finkelstein Y, Adler Y, Nussinovitch M, et al. A new classification for pericarditis associated with meningococcal infection. *Eur J Pediatr* 1997;156:585–588.
15. Kenney RT, Li JS, Clyde WA, et al. Mycoplasmal pericarditis: evidence of invasive disease. *Clin Infect Dis* 1993;17[Suppl I]:S58–S62.
16. Maycock R, Skale B, Kohler RB. Legionella pneumophila pericarditis proved by culture of pericardial fluid. *Am J Med* 1983;75:534–536.
17. Larrieu AJ, Tyers FO, Williams EH, et al. Recent experience with tuberculous pericarditis. *Ann Thorac Surg* 1980;29:464–468.
18. Schrank JH, Dooley DP. Purulent pericarditis caused by *Candida* species: case report and review. *Clin Infect Dis* 1995;21:182–187.
19. Walsh TJ, Bulkley BH. *Aspergillus* pericarditis: clinical and pathological features in the immunocompromised patient *Cancer* 1982;49:48–54.
20. Acierno LJ. Cardiac complications in acquired immunodeficiency syndrome (AIDS): a review. *J Am Coll Cardiol* 1989;13:1144–1154.
21. Wheat LJ, Stein L, Corya BC, et al. Pericarditis as a manifestation of histoplasmosis during two large urban outbreaks. *Medicine* 1983;62:110–119.
22. Buchbinder NA, Roberts WC. Left-sided valvular active infective endocarditis: a study of 45 necropsy patients. *Am J Med* 1972;53:20–35.
23. Bulkley BH, Klacsmann PG, Hutchins GM. A clinicopathological study of post-thoracotomy purulent pericarditis. A continuing problem of diagnosis and therapy. *J Thorac Cardiovasc Surg* 1977;73:408–412.
24. Engel PJ, Hon H, Fowler NO, et al. Echocardiographic study of right ventricular wall motion in cardiac tamponade. *Am J Cardiol* 1982;50:1018–1021.
25. Fowler NO. Recurrent pericarditis. *Cardiol Clin* 1990;8:621–626.
26. Smith WG. Coxsackie B myopericarditis in adults. *Am Heart J* 1970;80:34–46.
27. Spodick DH. Acoustic phenomena in pericardial disease. *Am Heart J* 1971;81:114–124.
28. Spodick DH. Pericardial rub: prospective multiple observer investigation of pericardial friction rub in 100 patients. *Am J Cardiol* 1975;35:357–362.
29. Shabetai R. Acute pericarditis. *Cardiol Clin* 1990;8:639–644.
30. Brandt RR, Filzmaier K, Hanrath P. Circulating cardiac troponin I in acute pericarditis. *Am J Cardiol* 2001;87:1326–1328.
31. Spodick DH. Electrocardiogram in acute pericarditis. Distributions of morphologic and axial changes by stages. *Am J Cardiol* 1974;33:470–474.
32. Horowitz MS, Schultz CS, Stinson EB, et al. Sensitivity and specificity of echocardiographic diagnosis of pericardial effusion. *Circulation* 1974;50:239–247.
33. Stark DD, Higgins CB, Lanzer P, et al. Magnetic resonance imaging of the pericardium: normal and pathologic findings. *Radiology* 1984;150:469–474.
34. Isner JM, Carter BL, Bankoff MS, et al. Computed tomography in the diagnosis of pericardial heart disease. *Ann Intern Med* 1982;97:473–479.
35. Sechtem U, Tscholakoff D, Higgins CB. MRI of the abnormal pericardium. *AJR Am J Roentgenol* 1986;147:245–252.
36. Spodick DH. Pericarditis in systemic diseases. *Cardiol Clin* 1990;8:709–716.
37. Soler-Soler J, Permanyer-Miralda G, Sagrista-Sauleda J. A systematic diagnostic approach to primary acute pericardial disease. The Barcelona experience. *Cardiol Clin* 1990;8:609–620.

38. Merce J, Sagrista-Sauleda J, Permanyer-Miralda G, et al. Should pericardial drainage be performed routinely in patients who have a large pericardial effusion without tamponade? *Am J Med* 1998;105:106–109.

39. Permanyer-Miralda G, Sagrista-Sauleda J, Soler-Soler J. Primary acute pericardial disease: a prospective series of 231 consecutive patients. *Am J Cardiol* 1985;56:623–630.

40. Corey GR, Campbell PT, Van Trigt P, et al. Etiology of large pericardial effusions. *Am J Med* 1993;95:209–213.

41. Sagrista-Sauleda J, Barrabes JA, Permanyer-Miralda G, et al. Purulent pericarditis: review of a 20-year experience in a general hospital. *J Am Coll Cardiol* 1993;22:1661–1665.

42. Morgan RJ, Stephenson LW, Woolf PK, et al. Surgical treatment of purulent pericarditis in children. *J Thorac Cardiovasc Surg* 1983;85:527–531.

43. Defouilloy C, Meyer G, Slama M, et al. Intrapericardial fibrinolysis: a useful treatment in the management of purulent pericarditis. *Intensive Care Med* 1997;23:117–118.

44. Strang JIG, Kakaza HHS, Gibson DG, et al. Controlled trial of prednisolone as adjuvant in the treatment of tuberculous constrictive pericarditis in Transkei. *Lancet* 1987;2:1418–1422.

45. Strang JIG, Kakaza HHS, Gibson DG, et al. Controlled clinical trial of complete open surgical drainage and of prednisone in treatment of tuberculous pericardial effusion in Transkei. *Lancet* 1988;2:759–764.

46. Mayosi BM, Volmink JA, Commerford PJ. Interventions for treating tuberculous pericarditis (Cochrane Review). In: *The Cochrane Library*, issue 4. Oxford: Update Software, 2001.

47. Carson TJ, Murray GF, Wilcox BR, et al. The role of surgery in tuberculous pericarditis. *Ann Thorac Surg* 1974;17:163–167.

48. Suwan PK, Potjalongsilp S. Predictors of constrictive pericarditis after tuberculous pericarditis. *Br Heart J* 1995;73:187–189.

49. Fowler NO. Tuberculous pericarditis. *JAMA* 1991;266:99–103.

50. Connolly DC, Burchell HB. Pericarditis: a ten year survey. *Am J Cardiol* 1961;7:7–14.

51. Carmichael DB, Sprague HB, Wyman SM, et al. Acute nonspecific pericarditis. *Circulation* 1951;3:321–331.

52. Fowler NO, Harbin AD. Recurrent acute pericarditis: follow-up study of 31 patients. *J Am Coll Cardiol* 1986;7:300–305.

53. Adler Y, Finkelstein Y, Guindo J, et al. Colchicine treatment for recurrent pericarditis a decade of experience. *Circulation* 1998;97:2183–2185.

54. Millaire A, de Groote P, Decoulx E, et al. Treatment of recurrent pericarditis with colchicine. *Eur Heart J* 1994;15:120–124.

55. Hatcher CR, Logue RB, Logan WD, et al. Pericardiectomy for recurrent pericarditis. *J Thorac Cardiovasc Surg* 1971;62:371–378.

56. Vaitkus PT, Kussmaul WG. Constrictive pericarditis versus restrictive cardiomyopathy: a reappraisal and update of diagnostic criteria. *Am Heart J* 1991;122:1431–1441.

57. Sutton FJ, Whitley NO, Applefield MM. The role of echocardiography and computed tomography in the evaluation of constrictive pericarditis. *Am Heart J* 1985;109:350–355.

58. Hirschman SZ, Hammer GS. Coxsackievirus myopericarditis. *Am J Cardiol* 1974;34:224–232.

59. Karjalainen J, Heikkila J, Nieminen MS, et al. Etiology of mild acute infectious myocarditis. *Acta Med Scand* 1983;213:65–73.

60. Grist NR, Reid D. Epidemiology of viral infections of the heart. In: Banatvala JE, ed. *Viral infections of the heart*. London: Hodder and Stoughton, 1993:23–31.

61. Martin AB, Webber S, Fricker FJ, et al. Acute myocarditis rapid diagnosis by PCR. *Circulation* 1994;90:330–339.

62. Pauschinger M, Bowles NE, Fuentes-Garcia FJ, et al. Detection of adenoviral genome in the myocardium of adult patients with idiopathic left ventricular dysfunction. *Circulation* 1999;99:1348–1354.

63. Cheitlin, MD. Cardiovascular complications of HIV infection. In: Sande MA, Volberding PA, eds. *The medical management of AIDS*, 6th ed. Philadelphia: WB Saunders, 1999:275–284.

64. Rosenbaum MB. Chagasic myocardiopathy. *Prog Cardiovasc Dis* 1964;7:199–225.

65. Bergelson JM, Cunningham JA, Droguett G, et al. Isolation of a common receptor for coxsackie B viruses and adenoviruses 2 and 5. *Science* 1997;275:1320–1323.

66. Ito M, Kodama M, Masuko M, et al. expression of coxsackievirus and adenovirus receptor in hearts of rats with experimental autoimmune myocarditis. *Circ Res* 2000;86:275–280.

67. Rosenberg HS, McNamara DG. Acute myocarditis in infancy and childhood. *Prog Cardiovasc Dis* 1964;7:179–197.

68. BMJ Publishing Group. Coxsackie B5 virus infections during 1965. A report to the Director of the Public Health Laboratory Service from various laboratories in the United Kingdom. *Br Med J* 1967;4:575–577.

69. Friman G, Wesslen L, Fohlman J, et al. The epidemiology of infectious myocarditis, lymphocytic myocarditis and dilated cardiomyopathy. *Eur Heart J* 1995;16[Suppl O]:36–41.

70. Blankenhorn MA, Gall EA. Myocarditis and myocardiosis: a clinicopathologic appraisal. *Circulation* 1956;12:217–223.

71. Gore I, Saphir O. Myocarditis: a classification of 1402 cases. *Am Heart J* 1947;34:827–830.

72. Molander N. Sudden natural death in later childhood and adolescence. *Arch Dis Child* 1982;57:572–576.

73. Neuspiel DR, Kuller LH. Sudden and unexpected natural death in childhood and adolescence. *JAMA* 1985;254:1321–1325.

74. Saphir O. Myocarditis: a general review, with an analysis of two hundred and forty cases. *Arch Pathol* 1941;32:1000–1051.

75. Topaz O, Edward JE. Pathologic features of sudden death in children, adolescents, and young adults. *Chest* 1985;87:476–482.

76. Wentworth P, Jentz LA, Croal AE. Analysis of sudden unexpected death in Southern Ontario with emphasis on myocarditis. *Can Med Assoc J* 1979;120:676–680.

77. Karjalainen J, Heikkila J. Incidence of three presentations of acute myocarditis in young men in military service. *Eur Heart J* 1999;20:1120–1125.

78. Helin M, Savola J, Lapinleimu K. Cardiac manifestations during a coxsackie B5 epidemic. *Br Med J* 1968;3:97–99.

79. Woodruff JF. Viral myocarditis. *Am J Pathol* 1980;101:426–84.

80. Karjalainen J, Nieminen MS, Heikkila J. Influenza A1 myocarditis in conscripts. *Acta Med Scand* 1980;207:27–30.

81. Verel D, Warrack AJN, Potter CW, et al. Observations on the A2 England influenza epidemic. *Am Heart J* 1976;92:290–296.

82. Karjalainen J. Clinical diagnosis of myocarditis and dilated cardiomyopathy. *Scand J Infect Dis* 1988;S88:33–43.

83. Lauer B, Niederau C, Kuhl U, et al. Cardiac troponin T in patients with clinically suspected myocarditis. *J Am Coll Cardiol* 1997;30:1354–1359.

84. Smith SC, Ladenson JH, Mason JW, et al. Elevations of cardiac troponin I associated with myocarditis. *Circulation* 1997;95:163–168.

85. Kuhl U, Lauer B, Souvatzoglu M, et al. Antimyosin scintigraphy and immunohistologic analysis of endomyocardial biopsy in patients with clinically suspected myocarditis-evidence of myocardial cell damage and inflammation in the absence of histologic signs of myocarditis. *J Am Coll Cardiol* 1998;32:1371–1376.

86. O'Connell JB, Henkin RE, Robinson JA, et al. Gallium-67 imaging in patients with dilated cardiomyopathy and biopsy-proven myocarditis. *Circulation* 1984;70:58–62.

87. Yasuda T, Palacios IF, Dec GW, et al. Indium 111-monoclonal antimyosin antibody imaging in the diagnosis of acute myocarditis. *Circulation* 1987;76:306–311.

88. Gagliardi MG, Bevilacqua M, Di Renzi P, et al. Usefulness of magnetic resonance imaging for diagnosis of acute myocarditis in infants and children, and comparison with endomyocardial biopsy. *Am J Cardiol* 1991;68:1089–1091.

89. Chow LC, Dittrich HC, Shabetai R. Endomyocardial biopsy in patients with unexplained congestive heart failure. *Ann Intern Med* 1988;109:535–539.

90. Dec GW, Palacios IF, Fallon JT, et al. Active myocarditis in the spectrum of acute dilated cardiomyopathies. *N Engl J Med* 1985;312:885–890.

91. Feldman AM, McNamara D. Myocarditis. *N Engl J Med* 2000;343:1388–1398.

92. Herskowitz A, Campbell S, Deckers J, et al. Demographic features and prevalence of idiopathic myocarditis in patients undergoing endomyocardial biopsy. *Am J Cardiol* 1993;71:982–986.

93. Mason JW, O'Connell JB, Herskowitz A, et al. A clinical trial of immunosuppressive therapy for myocarditis. *N Engl J Med* 1995;333:269–275.

94. Nippoldt TB, Edwards WD, Holmes DR, et al. Right ventricular endomyocardial biopsy. *Mayo Clin Proc* 1982;57:407–418.

95. Parrillo JE, Aretz HT, Palacios I, et al. The results of transvenous endomyocardial biopsy can frequently be used to diagnose myocardial diseases in patients with idiopathic heart failure. *Circulation* 1984;69:93–101.

96. Vasiljevic JD, Kanjuh V, Seferovic P, et al. The incidence of myocarditis in endomyocardial biopsy specimens from patients with congestive heart failure. *Am Heart J* 1990;120:1370–1377.

97. Vikerfors T, Stjerna A, Olcen P, et al. Acute myocarditis: serologic diagnosis, clinical findings and follow-up. *Acta Med Scand* 1988;223:45–52.

98. Lerner AM, Wilson FM, Reyes MP. Enteroviruses and the heart (with special emphasis on the probable role of coxsackieviruses group B types 1–5). II. Observations in humans. *Modern Concepts Cardiovasc Dis* 1975;44:11–15.

99. Tilles JG, Elson SH, Shaka JA, et al. Effects of exercise on Coxsackie A9 myocarditis in adult mice. *Proc Soc Exp Biol Med* 1964;117:777–782.

100. Damm S, Andersson LG, Henriksen E, et al. Wall motion abnormalities in male elite orienteers are aggravated by exercise. *Clin Physiol* 1999;19:121–126.

101. Rezkalla SH, Raikar S, Kloner RA. Treatment of viral myocarditis with focus on captopril. *Am J Cardiol* 1996;77:634–637.

102. Matsumori A, Igata H, Ono K, et al. High doses of digitalis increase the myocardial production of proinflammatory cytokines and worsen myocardial injury in viral myocarditis: a possible mechanism of digitalis toxicity. *Jpn Circ J* 1999;63:934–940.

103. Rotbart HA, O'Connell JF, McKinlay MA. Treatment of human enterovirus infection. *Antiviral Res* 1998;38:1–14.

104. Rotbart HA, Webster AD, for the Pleconaril Treatment Group. Treatment of potentially life-threatening enterovirus infections with pleconaril. *Clin Infect Dis* 2001;32:228–235.

105. Fohlman J, Pauksen K, Hyypia T, et al. Antiviral treatment with WIN 54 954 reduces mortality in murine coxsackievirus B3 myocarditis. *Circulation* 1996;94:2254–2259.

106. See DM, Tilles JG. Treatment of coxsackievirus A9 myocarditis in mice with WIN 54954. *Antimicrob Agents Chemother* 1992;36:425–428.

107. Khatib R, Reyes MP, Smith F, et al. Enhancement of coxsackievirus B4 virulence by indomethacin. *J Lab Clin Med* 1990;116:116–120.

108. Kilbourne ED, Wilson CB, Perrier D. The induction of gross myocardial lesions by a coxsackie (pleurodynia) virus and cortisone. *J Clin Invest* 1956;35:362–370.

109. Camargo PR, Snitcowsky R, da Luz PL, et al. Favorable effects of

immunosuppressive therapy in children with dilated cardiomyopathy and active myocarditis. *Pediatr Cardiol* 1995;16:61–68.

110. Takada H, Kishimoto C, Hiraoka Y. Therapy with immunoglobulin suppresses myocarditis in a murine coxsackie B3 model. *Circulation* 1995;92:1604–1611.
111. McNamara DM, Holubkov R, Starling RC, et al. Controlled trial of intravenous immune globulin in recent-onset dilated cardiomyopathy. *Circulation* 2001;103:2254–2259.
112. Miric M, Miskovic A, Vasiljevic JD, et al. Interferon and thymic hormones in the therapy of human myocarditis and idiopathic dilated cardiomyopathy. *Eur Heart J* 1995;16[Suppl O]:150–152.
113. Lutton CW, Guantt CJ. Ameliorating effects of interferon beta and anti-interferon beta on coxsackievirus B3–induced myocarditis in mice. *J Interferon Res* 1985;5:137–146.
114. Matsumori A, Tomioka N, Kawai C. Protective effect of recombinant alpha interferon on coxsackievirus B3 myocarditis in mice. *Am Heart J* 1988;115:1229–1232.
115. Remes J, Helin M, Vaino P, et al. Clinical outcome and left ventricular function 23 year after acute coxsackie virus myopericarditis. *Eur Heart J* 1990;11:182–188.
116. Garg A, Shiau J, Guyatt G. The ineffectiveness of immunosuppressive therapy in lymphocytic myocarditis: an overview. *Ann Intern Med* 1998;128:317–322.
117. Levi G, Scalvini S, Volterrani M, et al. Coxsackie virus heart disease: 15 years after. *Eur Heart J* 1988;9:1303–1307.
118. Quigley PJ, Richardson PJ, Meany BT, et al. Long-term follow-up of acute myocarditis. Correlation of ventricular function and outcome. *Eur Heart J* 1987;8[Suppl J]:39–42.
119. Houel R, Vermes E, Tixier DB, et al. Myocardial recovery after mechanical recovery for acute myocarditis: is sustained recovery predictable? *Ann Thorac Surg* 1999;68:2177–2180.
120. McCarthy RE, Boehmer JP, Hruban RH, et al. Long-term outcome of fulminant myocarditis as compared with acute (nonfulminant) myocarditis. *N Engl J Med* 2000;342:690–695.

Gastrointestinal Tract

CHAPTER 65
Approach to the Patient with Diarrhea

Alain R. Bouckenooghe and Herbert L. DuPont

Diarrhea is defined as output of more than 200 g of unformed feces per day or by decreased stool consistency (unformed or loose) and increased stool frequency (three or more bowel movements in 24 hours). On a global level, diarrhea is the second most important cause of overall death, the main cause of pediatric mortality, and generally a major cause of severe morbidity. The mean annual attack rate for children younger than 5 years is typically 1 to 2 for persons of all ages in the United States, versus 8 to 12 for children in most developing regions. The high incidence of diarrhea in the United States was illustrated in a cross-sectional telephone survey, in which diarrhea was reported to have occurred in 27% of respondents in the month before the survey was conducted (Sandler et al., 2000). Diarrhea is therefore considered also in the United States a major morbidity factor.

DEFINITIONS

Diarrhea severity is graded based on its clinical impact on the patient.

Mild diarrhea: Diarrhea is typically mild if the number of bowel movements is three or less and if the symptoms allow the patient to have normal activities.

Moderate diarrhea: The production of four or more unformed stools, often associated with intestinal and systemic symptoms (abdominal cramps, nausea, vomiting, tenesmus, fever, malaise, dehydration) which characteristically force a change in activities.

Severe diarrhea: Diarrhea leading to incapacitation.

Diarrhea is *acute* if the onset is within the last 14 days, *persistent* if it lasts longer than 14 days, and *chronic* if it lasts longer than 30 days.

Moderate and severe diarrhea requires special attention to workup and treatment.

ETIOLOGY AND PATHOPHYSIOLOGY

The etiology of diarrhea is diverse. Some of the causes of diarrhea include infections (viral, bacterial, and protozoal), inflammatory bowel disease (Crohn's disease, ulcerative colitis, diverticulitis), syndromes of malabsorption (pancreatic insufficiency, lactase insufficiency, nontropical sprue, tropical sprue and bacterial overgrowth syndrome, Whipple's disease, short bowel syndrome, postgastrectomy), irritable bowel syndrome, change in food and fluid status, and alcohol consumption, but can also be due to less common causes including endocrine abnormalities, neoplasms (gastrinoma, carcinoid syndrome, secretory adenoma), bowel ischemia, or radiation induced. As diverse as the etiology is the treatment that goes with it. A proper diagnosis is important to select an effective treatment. We further focus on infectious etiologies in this chapter. In analysis of the epidemiology of enteric infections, one must consider pathogen, host factors, and the environment just as in other infections.

There are several pathophysiologic mechanisms through which pathogens can act, resulting in diarrhea with specific clinical features (Table 65.1). In addition, diarrhea can be divided by disease pathophysiology as follows:

1. *Osmotic diarrhea:* Because of presence of nonabsorbable osmotically active products in the lumen of the gut leading to imbalance in oncotic pressure, net water is attracted to the gut lumen. Causes include use of some laxatives, pancreatic insufficiency, lactulose and sorbitol ingestion, sprue, short bowel syndrome after extensive bowel resection, or presence of intestinal fistulas and lactase deficiency (either genetically determined or secondary due to previous infectious gastroenteritis). The osmolar gap, calculated by the formula stool osmolar gap = $290 - 2$ (fecal $Na^+ + K^+$), is typically greater than 50 in osmotic diarrhea and the symptoms often abate with fasting. Osmotic diarrhea is more important in chronic diarrhea than acute diarrhea.

2. Secretory diarrhea is clinically noted as a profuse watery diarrhea and is caused by active ion secretion into the gut lumen. The classic example is toxin-mediated diarrhea caused by enterotoxigenic *Escherichia coli*; the heat-labile LT-toxin subunit A_2 activates intestinal adenylate cyclase, leading to an increase in cyclic adenosine monophosphate (cAMP), which promotes active chloride ion secretion into the lumen. Similarly the heat-stable ST toxin activates enterocytic guanylate cyclase, leading to increased levels of cyclic guanosine monophosphate (cGMP). The presence of these ions then attracts water to the gut lumen. The osmolar gap in secretory diarrhea, calculated by the formula stool osmolar gap = $290 - 2$ (fecal $Na^+ + K^+$), is typically less than 50, because of the high Na content in

TABLE 65.1. Clinical Features of Acute Diarrhea

Clinical observation	Anatomic consideration	Pathogens to consider	Fecal leukocytes, fecal lactoferrin
Passage of few, voluminous stools	Diarrhea of proximal small bowel origin	*Vibrio cholerae*, enterotoxigenic. *Escherichia coli*, *Shigella* strains early in the infection, *Giardia*	Absent
Passage of many small-volume stools	Diarrhea of large bowel origin or distal small bowel	*Shigella*, *Salmonella*, *Campylobacter*, *E. coli* O157:H7 and Shiga toxin–producing *E. coli* *Entamoeba histolytica*	Present for bacteria
Tenesmus, fecal urgency, dysentery	Colitis or proctitis	*Shigella*, *Salmonella*, *Campylobacter*, *E. coli* O157:H7 and Shiga toxin–producing *E. coli*, *E. histolytica*, sexually transmitted diseases	Present for bacteria
Vomiting as the predominant symptom	Gastroenteritis	Viral agents (rotavirus, Norwalk virus) or intoxication (*Staphylococcus aureus*, *Bacillus cereus*)	Absent
Fever as an important finding	Mucosal inflammation	*Shigella*, *Salmonella*, *Campylobacter*, viral agents (rotavirus, Norwalk), *Clostridium difficile*	Present
Fever and systemic toxicity	Mucosal inflammation	*Shigella*, *Salmonella*, *Campylobacter*	Present

the gut. Secretory alterations explain the pathophysiology of most cases of acute diarrhea.

3. Exudative diarrhea is the result of diffuse inflammation and mucosal damage to the colon. Markers of inflammation (see section "Fecal Leukocyte or Lactoferrin Examination") include the presence of fecal leukocytes, fecal lactoferrin, presence of occult or gross blood in the stool, and clinical signs of fever, tenesmus, or mucus visible in the stool. Dysenteric inflammatory diarrhea is defined as exudative diarrhea with gross blood visible in the stool and is typically caused by bacteria, for example, *Shigella*, *Campylobacter*, and occasionally *Salmonella*, or parasites such as *Entamoeba histolytica*, or is toxin mediated (e.g., *Clostridium difficile*, *E. coli* O157:H7 (and other Shiga toxin–producing *E. coli*)], whereas dysenteric or nondysenteric inflammatory diarrhea can be caused by various bacteria (e.g., *Salmonella*, *Shigella*, *Yersinia*, *Campylobacter*, diarrheagenic *E. coli*), toxins, and noninfectious causes (e.g., inflammatory bowel disease, diverticulitis, radiation enterocolitis, and ischemic bowel disease). Enteric fever is caused by invasive organisms that penetrate the mucosa and lead to fever, diarrhea, and abdominal pain (e.g., *Yersinia enterocolitica*, *Salmonella typhi*). In inflammatory diarrhea, a gut secretory component is important, often mediated by intestinal cytokine release.

4. *Diarrhea due to altered motility:* This is often the result of hormonal disorders [e.g., hyperthyroidism, diabetes mellitus, adrenal insufficiency, and gastrin and vasoactive intestinal polypeptide hypersecretion], use of antibiotics (e.g., erythromycin), use of cholinergic and other products (e.g., caffeine), neurologic disorders (e.g., Parkinson's disease), presence of intraintestinal blood [e.g., major gastrointestinal (GI) tract bleeding], or autonomic hyperresponsiveness, as seen in irritable bowel syndrome. This mechanism is particularly important in chronic diarrhea.

HOST FACTORS

It is a common observation that not everyone exposed to a virulent enteric pathogen will become ill. Most of the enteric pathogens are commonly isolated from stools of persons without symptoms, which characteristically represents asymptomatic infection, rather than colonization, because in many instances, the presence of the organisms elicits an intestinal secretory immunoglobulin A (IgA) reaction. Host factors and organism inoculum size are likely important in determining who is at highest risk of becoming ill.

Host genotype is a major yet not fully unraveled determinant, as suggested by the higher susceptibility to cholera for individuals with blood group O. The extremes of age are accompanied by relative immune deficiency, although the influence of age to susceptibility to enteric infections is more obvious in children, in whom a number of pathogens such as *rotavirus* and enteropathogenic *E. coli* (EPEC) characteristically occur. With exposure and development of a humoral immune reaction and possibly the loss of intestinal receptors, the susceptibility to a number of pathogens reduces with age.

Most of the organisms are neutralized in the stomach because of the gastric barrier. People who are low acid secretors because of the presence of atrophic gastritis, achlorhydria, history of gastric surgery, chronic gastric *Helicobacter pylori* infection, or use of antacid medication (not including sucralfate), particularly the potent proton pump inhibitors, are at increased risk of symptomatic infection after exposure.

The infectious dose of the various organisms is variable and can be remarkably low (as low as 10 to 100 organisms) in *Shigella*, *Giardia*, *Cryptosporidium*, Norwalk virus, and Shiga toxin–producing *E. coli*. As such, host hygiene is of great importance. Many organisms are food-borne or waterborne, but person-to-person transmission is seen, particularly with organisms or cysts transmittable with low infective doses in the setting of care for young children or mentally disadvantaged hosts. Host behavior can further influence exposure, for example, transmission of enteric pathogens or sexually transmitted organisms through homosexual contact. Intestinal motility helps to mechanically clear pathogenic organisms and assist the host in maintaining normal bowel flora. Conditions that cause stasis of the small bowel (short-bowel syndrome, diabetic diarrhea, scleroderma, and small-bowel diverticulosis) frequently result in diarrhea. It has therefore been postulated that changes in motility may influence intestinal defense mechanisms. Normal bacterial enteric flora is effective in resisting colonization by certain pathogenic organisms, such as *Salmonella*, on basis of competition. Loss of the normal flora during antibiotic use may lead to major increases in susceptibility, as documented with salmonellosis and *C. difficile* enterocolitis. Young infants may find protection, if breast-fed, by exclusion of contaminated food and drink and possibly through transfer from antibodies and presence of lactoferrin and perhaps other factors with bacteriostatic effect in the breast milk.

Specific Hosts

TRAVELER'S DIARRHEA

Travelers may be exposed to a wider range of pathogens depending on the geographic region they travel to, the host's country of origin, and the level of precautions taken (Table 65.2). Europeans and North Americans experience more GI tract infections as travelers, than travelers from Asia, Africa, and South America. On a global level, there are three major areas of risk based on the incidence of traveler's diarrhea (TD) among international travelers. Low-risk areas for a traveler from developed nations include the industrialized nations such as the United States and Canada, most of Europe, Japan, Australia, and New Zealand. The risk is medium (up to 7%) for southern Europe, Israel, the Middle East, China, Russia, and some Caribbean nations. The highest incidence (20%–50%) is seen in travelers to Africa, Central, and South America, and Southern Asia. The attack rates are higher in small children and younger travelers (especially 7- to 20-year-olds). The risk of TD further increases with increased dietary risk taking.

TD typically occurs within the first 2 weeks of arrival in an area of increased endemicity. Signs and symptoms are variable and depend to some extend on the infecting organism. The average duration of untreated TD is typically 3 to 5 days, although untreated infection with *Campylobacter, Shigella, Entamoeba, Giardia,*

and enteroaggregative *E. coli* (EAEC) tends to persist longer. Isolation rates of pathogens in studies of TD vary between 40% and 60% on average depending on the study, with bacterial causes representing approximately 80% of the defined pathogens and with viruses and parasites contributing approximately 10% and 5%, respectively. The large number of cases of TD without identified pathogen is suspected to be due to a bacterial pathogen, as empiric antibiotic treatment often reduces the length and severity of illness in these patients (see section "Treatment"), and includes underdiagnosed ETEC, EAEC, and other bacteria currently not identified.

Pseudomembranous enterocolitis caused by *C. difficile* is a concern in travelers with diarrhea and a history of use of antibiotics, including for prophylactic purposes, although the frequency appears to be low.

DIARRHEA AND AIDS

Hosts with acquired immunodeficiency syndrome (AIDS) are at increased risk of severe bacterial, viral, and protozoal enteric infections (see Table 65.2), contributing to a wasting syndrome that was commonly observed before the arrival of antiretroviral therapy. The human immunodeficiency virus (HIV) itself can cause an enteropathy leading to chronic diarrhea. The severity of immunosuppression correlates with the incidence and severity of diarrhea caused by the various pathogens. The most

TABLE 65.2. Pathogenic Organisms in Specific Syndromes of Infectious Diarrheal Diseases

Host	Bacteria	Parasites	Viruses

Traveler's diarrhea	*Escherichia coli*
	    Enterotoxigenic
	    Enteroaggregative
	    Enteroinvasive
	Yersinia
	Campylobacter species
	Salmonella species
	Shigella
	Aeromonas
	Plesiomonas
	Vibrio species
		Entamoeba histolytica
		Giardia lamblia
		Cyclospora
		Cryptosporidium
		Microsporidium
			Rotavirus
			Norwalk virus
			Enterovirus

AIDS and diarrhea	*Salmonella* species *Campylobacter* *Shigella* MAC EAEC *Clostridium difficile*	*Cryptosporidium* *Isospora belli* *Microsporidia* *Cyclospora*	HIV CMV HSV
Food poisoning and Food-borne disease	*Salmonella* species *Staphylococcus aureus* *Bacillus cereus* *Shigella* *Clostridium perfringens* *Vibrio* species *Campylobacter* *Yersinia* species *E. coli* O157:H7 and other Shiga toxin–producing *E. coli* *Listeria monocytogenes*	*Cryptosporidium* *Giardia lamblia* *Trichinella spiralis*	Norwalk virus Hepatitis A Astrovirus Calicivirus
Proctitis	*Neisseria gonorrhoeae* *Chlamydia trachomatis* *Treponema pallidum* *Salmonella* species *Shigella* MAC	*Cryptosporidium* *Isospora* *Entamoeba*	Herpes simplex CMV HIV

AIDS, acquired immunodeficiency syndrome; CMV, cytomegalovirus; EAEC, enterotoxigenic *E. coli;* HIV, human immunodeficiency virus; HSV, herpes simplex virus; MAC, *Mycobacterium avium* complex.

important organisms causing diarrhea in patients with AIDS include most importantly the parasites (*Cryptosporidium, Isospora, Cyclospora,* and *Microsporidia*), bacteria (*Shigella, Salmonella, Campylobacter,* EAEC, *C. difficile, Mycobacterium avium-intracellulare* [MAI]), and viruses (HIV as mentioned, herpes simplex, and cytomegalovirus).

OTHER IMMUNODEFICIENT HOSTS

Neutropenic patients are at increased risk for "typhlitis," mainly due to anaerobic organisms and gram-negative bacilli. Patients with immunoglobulin deficiencies are more susceptible to *Shigella, Salmonella, Campylobacter, Giardia,* and rotavirus.

DRUG-RELATED DIARRHEA, NOSOCOMIAL DIARRHEA

Diarrhea is a common problem after the use of an antimicrobial agent. Sometimes an alteration in the bowel flora produces limited and mild changes of the stool pattern. At other times, the cause is the proliferation of *C. difficile,* which is facilitated by the loss of inhibition usually delivered by the normal intestinal flora. Once *C. difficile* is allowed to proliferate, it produces toxins that cause characteristic mucosal damage consisting of pseudomembranous or plaquelike lesions, usually in the distal colon. Patients typically present with a watery, bloody diarrhea and occasionally systemic symptoms such as fever. The diagnosis is suggested by the history of prior ingestion of an antibiotic, recent or current hospitalization, and a positive fecal leukocyte examination, and it is confirmed by identification of *C. difficile* toxin or the organism in stool specimens or by endoscopic demonstration of the condition.

Other agents that often cause diarrhea include magnesium antacids, laxatives, and high-fiber foods. Oral contraceptives and other drugs can cause allergic vasculitis and production of bloody diarrhea caused by hemorrhagic colitis. Conventional enteric pathogens including *Shigella, Salmonella, Campylobacter,* and the parasitic pathogens should not be routinely sought in nosocomial diarrhea. They are rarely identified.

ACUTE DIARRHEA AND PROCTITIS IN MALE HOMOSEXUALS

Diarrhea and acute proctitis are common problems for homosexual men. The reasons include (a) the higher frequency of fecal-oral transmission of organisms (illness can be caused by any enteric pathogen in this setting; multiple agents often are present); (b) direct inoculation of *Neisseria gonorrhoeae,* herpes simplex virus, *Chlamydia trachomatis,* or *Treponema pallidum* into the rectum during receptive anal intercourse; and (c) the immunosuppression of patients who have AIDS (see organisms important in this infection listed in Table 65.2).

FOOD POISONING AND FOOD-BORNE DIARRHEA AND VOMITING

Often this process is caused by a bacterium or a virus, by toxic chemicals or preformed enterotoxins, or more rarely by parasites (see Tables 65.2 and 65.3) present in water or food. As a general rule, syndromes that appear within minutes after the ingestion of contaminated food or water are due to chemical poisons; onset during 2 to 7 hours implicates preformed enterotoxins, as elaborated by *Staphylococcus aureus* or *Bacillus cereus;* onset between 8 and 16 hours suggests *Clostridium perfringens* toxin or a second *B. cereus* enterotoxin; and appearance of symptoms more than 12 hours later is characteristically due to viruses (Norwalk virus) or bacterial agents (*Shigella, Salmonella, Campylobacter,* or diarrheagenic *E. coli*). In epidemic gastroenterocolitis, the history often gives important clues. By considering clinical features in a common source outbreak with an estimated incubation period, a potential etiology should be suspected. The important clinical findings include vomiting, fever, and dysentery (see Table 65.3). In the case of food-borne disease in which bloody stools are commonly passed, an important clinical finding is the presence or absence of clinically significant fever. Fever (higher than 101°F) in epidemic or sporadic dysentery is more suggestive of *Shigella, Salmonella,* and *Campylobacter,* whereas low-grade or absent fever in outbreaks of bloody diarrhea suggests the likelihood of finding *E. coli* O157:H7 or other Shiga toxin–producing *E. coli* as a responsible agent.

TABLE 65.3. Characteristics of Diarrhea Associated with Ingestion of Contaminated Food or Water

Incubation period (h)	Vomiting	Abdominal cramps and pain	Fever	Watery diarrhea	Dysentery (bloody stools)	Causative agent	Diagnostic tests
2–7	++	−	−	±	−	*Staphylococcus aureus, Bacillus cereus* enterotoxin (preformed)	Detection of toxin in food (usually clinical diagnosis)
8–16	−	+	−	+	−	*Clostridium perfringens, B. cereus* enterotoxin (produced *in vivo*)	Isolation of organisms from food or stools
12–72	± to +	+	±	++	−	*Shigella, Salmonella, Campylobacter jejuni, Vibrio* species, Enterotoxigenic *Escherichia coli,* Norwalk virus	Isolation of organisms from food or stools
12–72	± to +	+	++	+	++	*Shigella, Salmonella, Campylobacter jejuni*	Isolation of organisms from food or stools
12–72	± to +	++	− to ±	+	+ to ++	*E. coli* O157:H7 and Shiga toxin–producing *E. coli*	Detection of organism from food or stool or Shiga toxin from stool
12–72	++	+	± to +	+	−	Norwalk virus	Stool assay by reverse transcriptase polymerase chain reaction

−, absent; ±, mild; +, moderate; ++, severe.

DIARRHEAL SYNDROMES

Diarrhea must be evaluated for its severity and must be differentiated from a problem of GI tract bleeding or fecal incontinence through proper history. Recurrent diarrhea and constipation is more suggestive of irritable bowel syndrome or colonic obstruction. Although diarrheal illness may not show important specific differences according to the causative agent, a number of enteric disease syndromes when associated with common-source outbreaks suggest a cause or category of causal agents (see Table 65.3). An important distinction to be made in patients with enteric disease is whether the patient has noninflammatory watery diarrhea or inflammatory diarrhea, with or without dysentery (passage of bloody stools). Large volumes of watery diarrhea are typically caused by noninflammatory infections involving the small bowel (large volume, small number) such as ETEC, *Vibrio cholerae*, and viral agents including rotavirus, Norwalk virus, and other caliciviruses. If vomiting is a predominant symptom, enterotoxin-mediated gastroenteritis caused by *S. aureus* or *Bacillus cereus* preformed toxin, or Norwalk virus or Rotavirus infection should be considered. Passage of many small-volume stools is often a symptom of inflammatory disease located in the distal small bowel and colon. This type of process is typically accompanied by presence of occult fecal red blood cells and leukocytes but may be accompanied also by passage of gross blood and mucus; patients may or may not be febrile and they characteristically have abdominal cramps. As mentioned earlier, presence or absence of fever and sporadic versus food-borne or waterborne outbreak often provides evidence that invasive bacterial pathogens (*Shigella*, *Salmonella*, or *Campylobacter*) or *E. coli* O157:H7 or other Shiga toxin–producing *E. coli* are responsible for the illness (see Table 65.3). Tenesmus and fecal urgency are symptoms of colitis often caused by *Shigella*, *Salmonella*, *Campylobacter* or *Entamoeba*. In patients undergoing receptive anal intercourse, other pathogens must be considered (see Table 65.2). Enteric fever is caused by invasive organisms (e.g., *Salmonella*) and high fever is often a dominant symptom. Symptoms of weight loss and anorexia may help differentiate between acute and chronic processes. Loss of fluid and electrolytes may lead to fatigue, hypotension, and dehydration.

DIAGNOSIS

Many tests can help narrow the differential diagnosis of diarrhea and allow for proper therapy. The history and physical examination (including examination of the stool) are important, but certain laboratory tests should be considered in the general approach to patients with diarrhea to look for specific pathogens (see Table 65.1). Not all tests may need to be done, depending on history, severity, symptoms, and differential diagnosis.

Fecal Leukocyte or Lactoferrin Examination

An inflammatory diarrhea is clinically suspected if there are clinical signs of fever, tenesmus, and gross blood or mucus visible in the stool. Because these signs are neither sensitive nor specific, a fecal laboratory examination may be done to confirm presence of a treatable enteric pathogen. A specimen of fresh stool (mucus is preferred and often can be obtained by applicator stick) is mixed with two drops of dilute Loeffler's methylene blue and is examined under the microscope. The presence of a few white blood cells is usually considered an indeterminate result, and arbitrar-

ily, presence of five or more polymorphonuclear leukocytes per high-power field examined is considered positive. A positive test result usually indicates the presence of diffuse colonic mucosal inflammation or proctitis that is caused by either an invasive bacterium, a sexually transmitted disease, or an idiopathic inflammatory disease. A negative test result indicates preformed toxin; an infection by a virus, a parasite, a toxigenic bacterium; or a small-bowel process. Fresh stool is preferred over diaper or swab specimens. If a stool specimen cannot be examined freshly, the morphology of the white blood cells may not be preserved, leading to a "false-negative" result. Presence of fecal lactoferrin is a more sensitive neutrophil marker and is unaffected by stool storing procedures and conditions; this may be an easier and more useful "field test," although cost and very high sensitivity are often disadvantages.

Examination for Parasites

Examination of feces for parasites is indicated in patients with a history of diarrhea that persists more than 7 to 14 days or after traveling to mountainous areas, to Russia, or to Nepal, those who have been in contact with day care centers, immunocompromised patients including HIV-infected patients, and homosexual men. Sometimes this examination should include duodenal aspirate and specimens from duodenal biopsy. The most important parasitic causes of diarrhea are *Giardia lamblia*, *E. histolytica*, *Cryptosporidium*, *Cyclospora*, *Microsporidia* and *Strongyloides* (often in HIV-infected patients). Three different specimens should be examined carefully if parasites are strongly suspected because these organisms are not always detectable when present. Different techniques can be used to concentrate the specimens and improve the sensitivity of the test. Commercial enzyme immunoassays are available for *Giardia*, *Entamoeba*, and *Cryptosporidium* and are the preferred methods for detecting these pathogens in most laboratories.

Stool Culture

COMMUNITY-ACQUIRED OR TRAVELER'S DIARRHEA

Material for stool cultures should be taken from every patient with severe diarrhea requiring hospitalization, from those with high fever, those with a positive test result for fecal leukocytes, and those with persistent diarrhea. In travelers with moderate to severe diarrhea, empiric treatment without studies is recommended; stool cultures and parasite studies are recommended in those clinically failing empiric treatment, where antibiotic-resistant *Campylobacter* and parasitic agents are to be sought, whereas stool examination for parasites is recommended in all cases (travelers and nontravelers) of persistent diarrhea. Most laboratories can identify the common bacterial pathogens: *Salmonella*, *Shigella*, *Campylobacter*, and *Yersinia*, but every effort should be made to direct the laboratory to the likely pathogen when the clinical setting suggests another diagnosis. In cases in which *Vibrio parahaemolyticus* or *V. cholerae* is suspected (after ingestion of contaminated seafood or a visit to an area endemic for cholera with a dehydrating form of diarrhea), the stool specimens should be plated on thiosulfate citrate bile salts sucrose (TCBS) medium that is not used routinely. The stool culture should be screened for *E. coli* O157:H7, and Shiga toxin–producing *E. coli* in the case of food-borne diarrhea outbreaks, especially when cases of bloody diarrhea without high fever, have been reported. Screening tests for presence of toxins of *C. difficile* are indicated if antibiotics or chemotherapy was used within the last 12 weeks and the patient is currently or was recently hospitalized.

NOSOCOMIAL DIARRHEA

There is ample documentation that the yield of routine stool cultures from patients who develop diarrhea after 3 days of hospitalization is very low, with perhaps the exception of patients 65 years or older, presence of comorbidities, neutropenia, and HIV. With the exception of these groups, the stool specimens from these patients should not be submitted for culture. Stools from nosocomial cases of diarrhea should routinely be examined for the presence of toxins of *C. difficile,* the most common nosocomial enteric pathogen.

Virus Detection

Rotavirus and enteric adenoviruses can be identified in stool specimens with a commercial assay. Norwalk virus and non-Norwalk calicivirus infections currently can be diagnosed only in research centers.

Proctosigmoidoscopy

Proctoscopy may be helpful in the diagnosis of inflammatory colitis. Proctosigmoidoscopy in patients with diarrhea should also be considered in homosexual men, patients with moderate to severe diarrhea that becomes persistent or chronic, and in patients in whom the diagnosis of *E. histolytica* is suspected or the hospitalized patient on antibacterial drugs develops colitis and the diagnosis cannot be confirmed by other simpler methods. Rectal mucosa biopsy specimens may sometimes be useful in the identification of *E. histolytica,* Whipple's disease, sprue, possibly *G. lamblia,* and other conditions.

Other Studies

Steatorrhea is determined by Sudan III stain of a stool sample or a 72-hour quantitative fecal fat measurement. Measurement of fecal Na^+ and K^+ levels and the stool osmolar gap (see the section "Etiology and Pathophysiology") can help to discern the physiologic type of diarrhea. Values greater than 50 suggest an osmotic diarrhea and values less than 50 suggest presence of secretory diarrhea. Barium contrast x-ray studies may be important in the diagnosis of problems such as malabsorption, inflammatory bowel syndrome, motility disorders, and presence of fistula.

TREATMENT

Four types of interventions can be considered in all patients with diarrhea: (a) fluids and electrolytes, (b) diet, (c) nonspecific antidiarrheal therapy, and (d) antimicrobial therapy. Rehydration is always the first goal of therapy, and all patients with significant vomiting or diarrhea, particularly very young and elderly patients, should be encouraged to drink fluids and to consume salt (e.g., from saltine crackers and soups). Oral rehydration solutions (ORSs) are available in prepared forms to treat cholera-like diseases in developing countries and characteristically contain 3.5 g of sodium chloride, 1.5 g of potassium chloride, 2.5 g of sodium bicarbonate, and 20 g of glucose in a liter of previously boiled water. Homemade recipes should reflect the same mixes of ingredients. New formulations include rice powder or other starches that provide fluid, electrolytes, and calories and may actually improve diarrhea, and use of amino acids such as glutamine have the advantages stated for starches and reduced healing time of gut mucosa.

Patients should avoid dairy products for the first 2 days of illness because transient lactase deficiency resulting from small bowel mucosal inflammation often perpetuates the symptoms when dairy products are consumed. Intravenous rehydration is indicated for those with more severe dehydration or intense or protracted vomiting. Patients with diarrhea should ingest food, mainly soups, toast, bananas, and boiled and baked meats and vegetables. Food is important to take in during bouts of diarrhea to encourage enterocyte repair and intestinal recovery from the inflammatory process.

The two most successful types of nonspecific drugs are the antisecretory agents [bismuth subsalicylate (BSS)] and antimotility preparations (loperamide, diphenoxylate). BSS, 30 mL every 30 minutes for eight doses per day for 2 days in adult patients, reduces diarrhea symptoms by about 40%. No other salicylate products should be taken with BSS because of the potential for salicylate intoxication. Opiates are even more effective, reducing the number of stools passed by 60%. The customary initial dose of loperamide is 4 mg, followed by 2 mg after each loose bowel movement, not to exceed 8 to 16 mg per day. Diphenoxylate atropine is equally effective but has greater central opiate effect when taken in overdosage, and the atropine may produce objectionable symptoms without improving diarrhea. Tincture of opium is used as 0.5 to 1 mL orally every 4 to 6 hours. These drugs should not be taken by patients who have known shigellosis, diarrhea caused by *C. difficile* infection, or diarrhea caused by Shiga toxin–producing *E. coli* or by patients who have fever or are passing bloody stools because they could potentiate inflammatory/invasive bacterial disease. Antimotility drugs should not be used in pediatric patients younger than 2 years.

Antimicrobial drugs are restricted for use in a limited subset of patients; possible side effects and risk of emerging resistance are to be put in balance with potential clinical benefit. In moderate to severe traveler's diarrhea, empiric use of antibiotics is recommended, and the treatment of choice for adults is fluoroquinolones for 1 day or up to 3 days if symptoms continue, if no contraindication is known. Combinations of an antibiotic with loperamide have been found to be superior to either agent alone in this setting. Azithromycin and rifaximin, which is unlicensed in the United States, are alternatives for treatment of traveler's diarrhea. For certain travelers with a clinical picture of moderate to severe disease suggesting bacterial or parasitic infection, empiric treatment with antibiotics should be started after one or more stool samples are obtained for studies described earlier.

TABLE 65.4.   Antimicrobial Agents Suggested for Laboratory-confirmed Enteric Infections and Traveler's Diarrhea in Adults

Diagnosis	Drug	Adults
Shigellosis	Norfloxacin	400 mg b.i.d. for 3 d
	Levofloxacin	500 mg q.d. for 3 d
	Ciprofloxacin	500 mg b.i.d. for 3 d
Campylobacter jejuni enterocolitis	Erythromycin	500 mg q.d. for 5 d
	Azithromycin	500 mg q.d. for 3–5 d
	Norfloxacin	400 mg b.i.d. for 5 d
	Levofloxacin	500 mg b.i.d. for 3 d
	Ciprofloxacin	500 mg q.d. for 5 d
Traveler's diarrhea	As for shigellosis	Treat 1–3 d
	Azithromycin	500 mg q.d. for 1–3 d
	Rifaximin	200 mg t.i.d. for 3 d
Giardiasis	Metronidazole	250 mg t.i.d. for 10 d
	Furazolidone	100 mg t.i.d. for 7 d
	Tinidazole	2-g single dose
Amebiasis	Metronidazole *plus*	750 mg t.i.d. for 5 d
	Iodoquinol	650 mg t.i.d. for 21 d
Cryptosporidiosis	Nitazoxanide	(Licensed for children)

b.i.d., twice daily; t.i.d., three times a day; q.d., every day.

The empiric treatment for the specific pathogens is listed in Table 65.4.

PROPHYLAXIS AND PREVENTION

General Measures

Prevention of infectious diarrhea is usually based on rules of personal hygiene, consumption of clean water, and safe food preparation. This is particularly important when traveling to hyperendemic areas, but education is also essential in immuno-compromised patients. Only food or water heated to 60°C (a temperature that is considered too hot to touch) can be considered safe to consume. For travelers, the old adagio "Clean it, peel it, cook it, or forget it" is still valid as a guide for safe food choices. It should be remembered that just because a food has been cooked does not mean it is safe. Cooked foods should be heated just before consumption because recontamination after cooking is a common problem in tropical regions. Alcoholics and patients with chronic liver disease are at increased risk of developing *Vibrio* infections and must further avoid raw shellfish. Patients with cell-mediated immune deficiencies must be cautioned against sources of *Listeria monocytogenes* infection including soft cheeses and deli meat. All patients should avoid consuming raw dairy products. Prevention of nosocomial diarrhea includes contact isolation of known and suspected *C. difficile* carriers and cases.

Prophylaxis

A new live oral cholera vaccine and a killed whole-cell (cholera or ETEC) cholera B-subunit vaccine are available in some countries outside the United States for the prevention of cholera and possibly ETEC. Rotavirus vaccine is effective but currently not on the market because of an association with the development of infantile intussusception. Various other vaccines against a variety of enteric pathogens are currently under study.

Different regimens have been used for prophylaxis of diarrhea for travelers in endemic areas. Both antimicrobial drugs (e.g., quinolones) and to a lesser degree non-antimicrobial agents (BSS and *Lactobacillus* GG) have been proven effective for short-term travel to areas of high risk. Travelers should not be encouraged to use antimicrobial chemoprophylaxis except in special situations.

REFERENCES

1. Adachi JA, Ostrosky-Zeichner L, et al. Empirical antimicrobial therapy for traveler's diarrhea. *Clin Infect Dis* 2000;31:1079–1083.
2. DuPont HL, and the Practice Parameters Committee of the American College of Gastroenterology. Guidelines on acute diarrhea in adults. *Am J Gastroenterol* 1997;92:1962–1975.
3. Ericsson CD. Travelers' diarrhea: epidemiology, prevention, and self-treatment. *Infect Dis Clin North Am* 1998;12:285–303.
4. Guerrant RL, Van Gilder T, Steiner TS, et al. Practice guidelines for the management of infectious diarrhea. *Clin Infect Dis* 2001;32:331–350.
5. Sandler RS, Stewart WF, Liberman JN, et al. Abdominal pain, bloating and diarrhea in the United States: prevalence and impact. *Dig Dis Sci* 2000;45:1166–1171.

CHAPTER 66
Shigellosis

Gerald T. Keusch

Shigella causes acute inflammatory colitis and bloody diarrhea, which in its most characteristic clinical presentation is manifested by the dysentery syndrome, a clinical triad consisting of cramps, painful straining to pass stools (tenesmus), and a frequent small-volume, bloody mucoid discharge (1) (Fig. 66.1). In the United States and other highly industrialized societies, *Shigella sonnei* is the most common isolate, whereas *Shigella flexneri* predominates in developing countries (2,3). Since the late 1960s, after an absence of half a century, epidemics caused by *Shigella dysenteriae* type 1 have occurred in Latin America, Africa, and Asia and have been associated with high morbidity and, in infants and young children and elderly patients, high mortality rates (4).

EPIDEMIOLOGY

Transmission of *Shigella* infection is primarily from person to person, facilitated by the ability of as few as a few hundred organisms to cause infection and illness (5). Thus, it is relatively easy to transfer an infectious inoculum by the fingers, by food or water (which may lead to common-source epidemics), and even by contaminated fomites. The genus is highly adapted to the human host, and only a few higher primates appear to become naturally infected (4).

Shigellosis is primarily a pediatric disease, presumably because of the lack of preexisting immunity and the greater likelihood that children will transfer the organism by the fecal-oral route (1–4). In the United States, most cases of *S. sonnei* occur in patients younger than 10 years, with most infections occurring in children younger than 5 years (2–4). In contrast, the average age of patients in the United States with *S. flexneri* infection has steadily risen, particularly among young adult men (6). It is presumed that this is the consequence of sexually transmitted infection among young male homosexuals. Shigellosis remains a problem among developmentally delayed and mentally retarded individuals (7), and it has become a particular problem in day care settings (8). The rates of bacteriologically documented infections, as reported to the Centers for Disease Control and Prevention, have averaged approximately 6 per 100,000 population, increasing in some years to more than 9 per 100,000, primarily as the result of large outbreaks of *S. sonnei* (9). Infections in young children accounted for most of these cases. The incidence in children younger than 4 years was 27 per 100,000, compared with approximately 2 per 100,000 in adults older than 20 years. Infections were also most commonly reported from urban regions with large populations of low-income minority groups and from Native American reservations. However, because most cases in the United States are not bacteriologically documented and, indeed, may be so mild that medical attention is not sought or obtained, these data represent gross underestimates.

The aforementioned rates should be compared with those documented in prospective cohort studies in a typical rural village in Guatemala, where the isolation rate for *Shigella* was 9,800 per 100,000 children younger than 4 years with diarrheal illness (10). More than 50% of the children had more than one documented *Shigella* infection, yielding an overall incidence rate of approximately 125,000 per 100,000 children per year. Similar

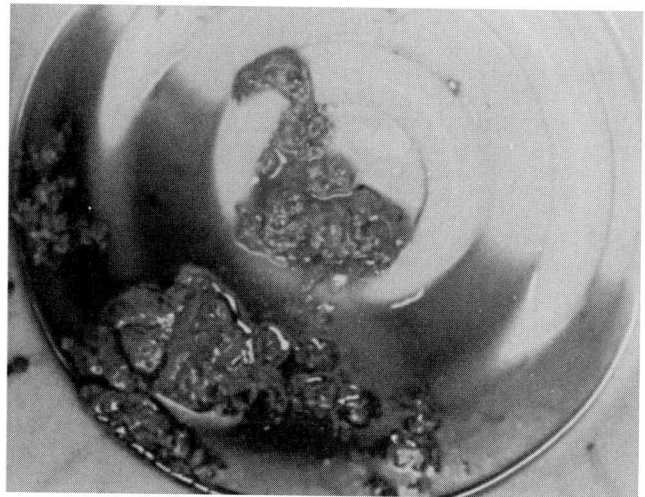

Figure 66.1. A characteristic stool of shigellosis, with mucoid stool mixed with a small amount of bloody fluid. The typical dysenteric stool, consisting of a small amount of grossly bloody mucus, is actually uncommon. (From Keusch GT, Formal SB, Bennish ML. Shigellosis. In: Warren KS, Mahmoud AAF, eds. *Tropical and geographical medicine,* vol 2. New York, McGraw-Hill, 1990:762–776, with permission.)

isolation rates of 9,700 per 100,000 children with diarrhea have been reported from Bangladesh (3).

Because of the small inoculum needed, the infection is readily transmitted in families (11). The index case is usually a preschool child; secondary attack rates average approximately 20% and may be as high as 40%, with young children generally developing symptomatic infection and adults having asymptomatic disease. Mild infection is self-limited, with a typical duration of 5 to 7 days. Prolonged carriage beyond 2 months in convalescence is uncommon unless there is evidence of protein-energy malnutrition.

CLINICAL MANIFESTATIONS

Although commonly described as *bacillary dysentery,* implying a bloody dysenteric presentation, most clinical shigellosis caused by S. sonnei in the United States is a watery diarrhea quite indistinguishable from other bacterial and viral causes of mild to moderate diarrhea. More severe inflammatory manifestations occur when S. flexneri is isolated and are especially common when S. dysenteriae type 1 is the causative agent (1). The initial symptom is usually fever, followed by the onset of watery diarrhea that contains numerous leukocytes that are detectable by light microscopy. In a few hours to a few days, depending on the species of the infecting organism and perhaps on host resistance, the diarrhea may turn bloody (see Fig. 66.1), with or without the other signs and symptoms of dysentery (12). The initial symptoms of clinical illness in children may be respiratory or central nervous system findings, but cultures of airway secretions and cerebrospinal fluid in these patients are negative, and the true diagnosis becomes apparent when the diarrhea begins and the stools are cultured. However, such extraintestinal presentations are quite rare, although the initial manifestation of infection in young children may be a seizure associated with rapidly rising fever (13). The episode is generally a single seizure, and except for affecting somewhat older children, it is otherwise clinically similar to a febrile seizure. Neurologic findings, such as altered consciousness, may be due to either electrolyte abnormalities or hypoglycemia (discussed in the section "Therapy"). Occasionally, patients present with encephalopathic manifestations, most

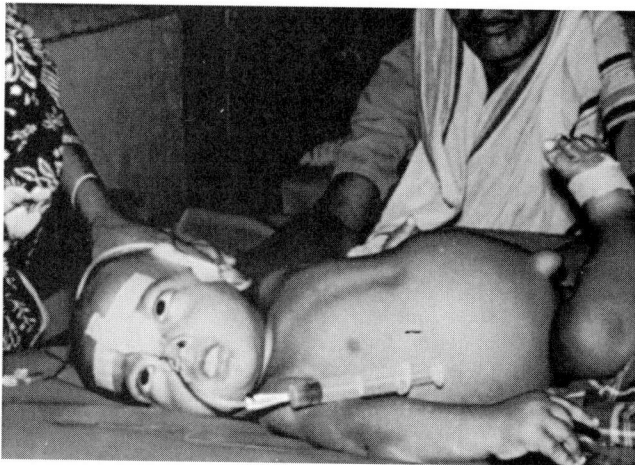

Figure 66.2. Encephalopathic manifestations of *Shigella flexneri* infection. Posturing, staring, and unresponsiveness can be appreciated in this Bangladeshi child. (Courtesy Dr. Michael L. Bennish, New England Medical Center, Boston, Massachusetts.)

commonly in S. flexneri infection, with bizarre posturing and unresponsiveness (14) (Fig. 66.2).

Either local or systemic manifestations may complicate the illness. The most severe colonic complication, toxic megacolon (Fig. 66.3), occurs primarily during S. dysenteriae type 1 infection and is related to the severity of the colitis (15). Perforation of the colon can also occur, with a significant increase in the

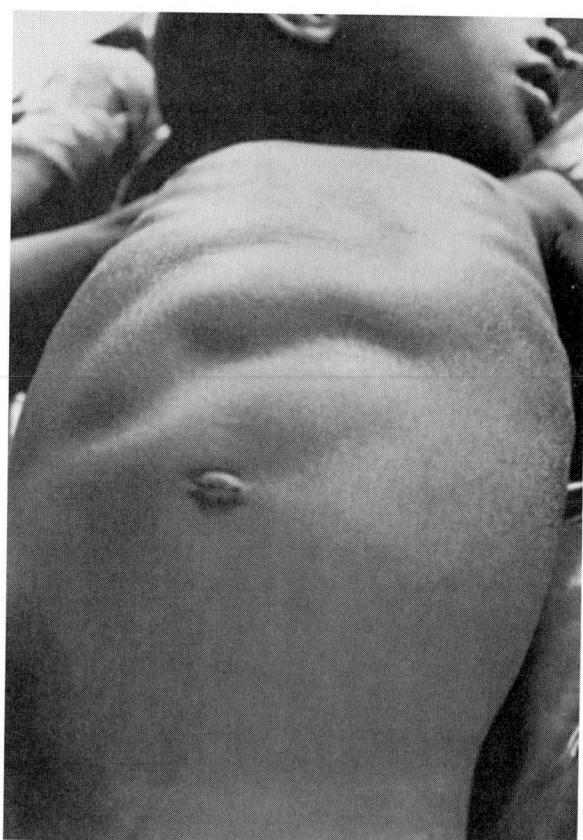

Figure 66.3. Toxic megacolon caused by shigellosis in a Bangladeshi infant. The dilated bowel is easily seen. (From Keusch GT, Formal SB, Bennish ML. Shigellosis. In: Warren KS, Mahmoud AAF, eds. *Tropical and geographical medicine,* vol 2. New York: McGraw-Hill, 1990:762–776, with permission.)

case-fatality rate. In some young children, continued straining at stool and poorly developed ligamentous support of the terminal colon and the rectum results in rectal prolapse. The prolapse usually reduces spontaneously and does not require intervention except to keep the mucosa moist. Protein-losing enteropathy of varying severity occurs in most patients with colonic inflammation, but in children in developing countries, it is a major factor in the later development of protein-energy malnutrition (16).

Systemic complications include bacteremia with the infecting strain or other Enterobacteriaceae originating from the stool, occurring especially in young, malnourished, weaned infants and occasionally resulting in disseminated intravascular coagulopathy (17), leukemoid reactions, and the hemolytic-uremic syndrome, with the last two complications seen almost exclusively in *S. dysenteriae* type 1 infection (18). In addition, reactive arthritis and even full-blown Reiter's syndrome, both of which are strongly associated with *S. flexneri* infection, particularly in patients with human leukocyte antigen B27 (19), and profound metabolic abnormalities such as hyponatremias (20) and hypoglycemia (21) can be significant problems.

PATHOGENESIS

In humans, the major pathologic findings are in the colon, where *Shigella* invades the mucosa and results in an inflammatory colitis of varying severity (22). Lesions are more common and profound in the distal colon and become progressively less severe in the transverse colon and ascending colon (23). Histologic findings include mucosal edema and hemorrhage, crypt hyperplasia, goblet cell discharge, a marked inflammatory infiltrate in the lamina propria, epithelial cell damage and death, superficial ulcerations, and an inflammatory exudate in the lumen and the stool (Fig. 66.4). The invasive process is quite complex, requires the contribution of multiple genetic loci in the organism, both

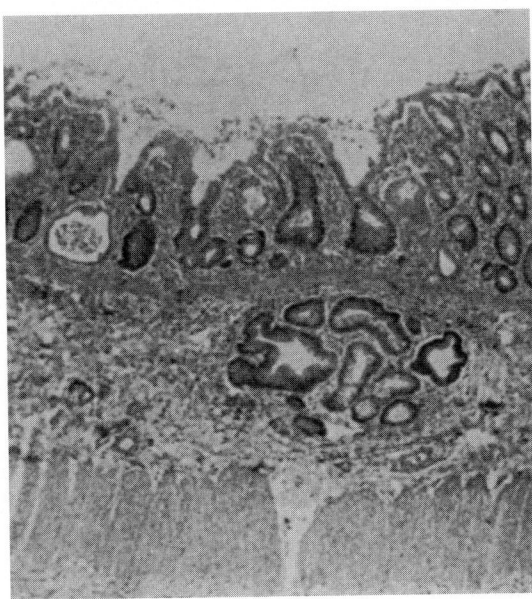

Figure 66.4. Section of colon from a fatal *Shigella flexneri* infection in a 1-year-old Bangladeshi infant with a 1-month history of dysentery, presenting with rectal prolapse and acute kwashiorkor. There are disruption and sloughing of the epithelial cell layer, an inflammatory exudate in the lamina propria, a crypt abscess on the left, and an extension of glands into the submucosa on the right. (From Butler T, Dunn D, Dahms B, et al. Causes of death and the histopathologic findings in fatal shigellosis. *Pediatr Infect Dis J* 1989;8:767–772, with permission.)

chromosomal and plasmid, and is essential for virulence (24). The nature of the initial contact between the nonmotile organism and the target host cell is not understood; however, contact of the pathogen with the surface of the colonic cell triggers ingestion within membrane-bounded vesicles as the organism induces the polymerization of actin fibrils in a process analogous to that of phagocytosis (25). This process is followed by rapid lysis of the phagocytic vacuole with release of the invading organism into the cytoplasm, where it is able to multiply. Actin polymerization then occurs at one pole of the organism, resulting in a propulsive force dubbed the "actin motor," which drives the bacteria to the plasma membrane of the host cell, using energy derived from hydrolysis of adenosine triphosphate resulting from a bacterial adenosine triphosphatase (26). This force is enough to propel the bacterium, still within the host cell and bounded by the host cell membrane, to protrude into adjacent cells (27). Subsequent fusion of the host cell membranes results in transfer of *Shigella* organisms from one cell to the next without ever exiting the intracellular milieu (28). In this manner, foci of infection develop, leading to local cell injury, death, and sloughing, as well as the production of the characteristic ulcerations of the intestinal mucosa associated with dysentery.

Various data suggest the importance of the induced inflammatory response early in the course of mucosal infection to pathogenesis. In *in vitro* studies in cultured human intestinal cell monolayers, addition of bacteria to the apical surface of the cells and of human neutrophils to the basal surface results in considerably increased transfer of bacteria across the monolayer, occurring primarily at intracellular tight junctions (29). Invasion of *Shigella in vivo* in the ligated rabbit ileal loop model also supports this role of the host cell neutrophilic response because the number of invading bacteria increases dramatically when neutrophilic infiltration occurs. Introduction of antibody to the neutrophil surface antigen, CD18, can reduce the extent of the neutrophilic response (30). Perfusion of animals with the cytokine antagonist interleukin-1 receptor antagonist before infection of ileal loops with *S. flexneri* significantly reduces bacterial invasion, the extent of mucosal inflammation, and tissue destruction (31).

The cellular inflammatory response is accompanied by the production of inflammatory cytokines, which are detectable in both serum and stool (32). An increase in all cytokine-producing cells in the rectal mucosa has been demonstrated in humans with dysentery (33). This increase persists for several weeks, perhaps explaining why anorexia and the metabolic consequences of shigellosis are so severe in these cases (34) and why malnutrition is a major associated factor in morbidity (18).

In addition to effecting invasion, *S. dysenteriae* type 1 produces the cytotoxin protein Shiga toxin. In an experimental primate model of shigellosis, an isogenic toxin-negative *S. dysenteriae* type 1 strain caused much milder illness, with much less inflammation and bleeding, compared with that caused by the parental wild-type toxin-positive strain (35). Shiga toxin binds to host cells expressing the blood group–active glycolipid Gb3 (globotriaosylceramide), specifically to its terminal galactose-α1→4-galactose disaccharide (36). Tissue culture and rabbit intestinal cells that express this determinant are able to bind toxin. When toxin is translocated to the cytoplasm by a receptor-mediated endocytosis, the ribonucleic acid (RNA) glycohydrolase enzymatic activity of the α subunit cleaves a specific residue in the 28S ribosomal RNA of the 60S ribosomal subunit, irreversibly inhibiting protein synthesis and leading to cell death (1). Biologic effects are determined in large part by selectivity in toxin binding. In the rabbit small bowel, for example, only villous cells express the principal glycolipid toxin receptor (Gb3), bind toxin, and are inhibited in protein synthesis (37). These findings are associated with depressed sodium absorption, which is a major function of the villus cell. Because the crypt cell is not affected, basal fluid secretion continues. The combination of diminished absorption and normal secretion results in the net accumulation of fluid within the lumen. Although no studies have documented a small bowel phase in human shigellosis, this mechanism could explain the observed "net secretory" state described in monkey jejunum in the course of experimental *S. flexneri* type 2a infection, (38) and the early watery diarrhea phase in human shigellosis (1).

Because the genes for Shiga toxin are restricted to *S. dysenteriae* type 1 strains, this mechanism would not account for watery diarrhea caused by other *Shigella* species. Two new enterotoxins, designated ShET1 and ShET2, have been described in *Shigella* (39,40). Both alter electrolyte transport in rabbit small bowel mucosa *in vitro* and result in fluid accumulation in ligated ileal loops *in vivo*. ShET1 is encoded by a chromosomal gene in *S. flexneri* type 2 but not other serotypes or *Shigella* species (41). ShET2 is plasmid encoded and is significantly homologous to a previously described enterotoxin of enteroinvasive *Escherichia coli* (42). Humans develop neutralizing antibody to the ShET toxins, indicating that these substances are produced during infection. Their role, however, remains speculative, intriguing, and unproven.

It is likely that Shiga toxin directly contributes to the pathogenesis of hemolytic-uremic syndrome associated with *S. dysenteriae* type 1 infection, because the same complication occurs after infection with Shiga toxin–producing serotypes of *E. coli*, such as O157:H7, but not with non–toxin-producing serotypes (43). Although the mechanism is not known with certainty, it is postulated to be related to the ability of Shiga toxin to bind to and damage endothelial cells, initiating the microangiopathic hemolysis and glomerular lesions of hemolytic-uremic syndrome.

Hyponatremia in shigellosis is common in children in developing countries and is likely a consequence of inappropriate antidiuretic hormone secretion (18,20). If this is true, the mechanism by which excess antidiuretic hormone is released remains to be determined. Hypoglycemia also occurs frequently and appears to be due in large part to inadequate gluconeogenic responses (21). Other metabolic responses generally associated with inflammatory bowel diseases, such as muscle catabolism and protein-losing enteropathy, may be manifestations of the release of metabolically active cytokines such as interleukin-6 and tumor necrosis factor or other similar mediator peptides in the inflamed bowel so characteristic of the infection (44).

THERAPY

Because the fluid losses in shigellosis are not great, dehydration is not typically an important problem, even when the insensible losses secondary to fever and rapid respiration are included. If dehydration occurs, it is readily managed in most patients by oral rehydration therapy (45).

The keystone to specific management is the use of effective antimicrobial agents, which lower mortality and reduce the duration of illness (1). The major problem is to select antimicrobial drugs to which the organism remains sensitive (46). It should be remembered that the phenomenon of transferable multidrug resistance was described for the first time among patients with *Shigella* infections in Japan in the mid-1950s, and multidrug resistance remains a problem (47). In addition to their common resistance to the penicillins and to the extended-spectrum, second-generation penicillins—streptomycin, tetracycline, and chloramphenicol—many strains are now also resistant to trimethoprim-sulfamethoxazole, especially those originating in developing countries. In the United States, documented drug resistance can be overcome by use of a third-generation cephalosporin or in adults a 4-fluoroquinolone (47). The quinolones are not currently approved for use in patients younger than 17 years because of the possibility of associated cartilage damage similar to that reported in young rodents receiving long-term high doses of these drugs. Although the risk to humans appears remote, only when there are sufficient clinical data on the safety of quinolones in young children from controlled clinical trials will we be able to determine when and in whom they can be safely used.

In developing countries, the high frequency of multidrug resistance now often necessitates the use of nalidixic acid (although it is not licensed in the United States for this indication) because other effective drugs either are not available or are too expensive. Five days of therapy with an effective drug is the usual regimen, but it is likely that shorter and less expensive courses will also be effective, an idea that is currently being evaluated (48). It is not certain that early and appropriate treatment will reduce the prevalence of complications such as hemolytic-uremic syndrome, and indeed some authors have suggested that antibiotic therapy increases the risk of some of these complications (49).

Severe shigellosis in children in Bangladesh is frequently accompanied by clinically significant hyponatremia, with serum sodium levels lower than 120 mmol/L (20). Infusion of 3% saline has been advocated by some (12 mL/kg in 2 hours, which is sufficient to produce an increase in serum sodium levels of approximately 10 mmol/L), and rapid reversal of the associated central nervous system depression has been observed (18). Once there is a response, free access to water should be restricted because hyponatremia recurs if patients are allowed to drink as much as they want. Because severe hyponatremia occurs primarily with infection caused by *S. dysenteriae* type 1 and *S. flexneri*, particularly in young, poorly nourished infants and children, it is only rarely observed in the United States.

Hypoglycemia in shigellosis is most frequently associated with *S. flexneri* and may be seen in both developed and developing countries, especially in young children (21). Pathogenesis appears to be an inadequate gluconeogenic response, and a blood glucose level lower than 1 mmol/L requires rapid infusion of glucose—for example, 5.6 mmol (1 g) of dextrose per kilogram of body weight in 5 to 10 minutes—followed by intravenous fluids containing 278 mmol (50 g) of dextrose per liter at a rate determined by the patient's fluid needs. Ultimately, management depends on control of infection per se, which restores glucose metabolism to normal.

In poorly nourished infants and children, special attention should be given to continuing nutritional rehabilitation because the catabolic stress of shigellosis is known to continue well into the convalescent period. Malnourished patients may require months of special nutritional therapy to replete body stores of protein, energy, and minerals (50).

The typical febrile seizure of shigellosis usually does not require more than appropriate measures to reduce body temperature, including use of antipyretics (13). Only uncommonly is it necessary to administer barbiturates or other anticonvulsive medication.

REFERENCES

1. Acheson DWK, Keusch GT. *Shigella* and enteroinvasive *Escherichia coli*. In: Blaser MJ, Smith PD, Ravdin JI, et al., eds. *Infections of the gastrointestinal tract*. New York: Raven Press, 1995:763–784.

2. *Laboratory confirmed* Shigella *surveillance annual summary, 1991–1992.* Atlanta: Centers for Disease Control and Prevention, Foodborne and Diarrheal Diseases Branch, 1995.

3. Zaman K, Yunus M, Baqui AH, et al. Surveillance of shigellosis in rural Bangladesh: a 10 year review. *J Pakistan Med Assoc* 1991;41:75–78.

4. Keusch GT, Bennish ML. Shigellosis. In: Evans AS, Brachman P, eds. *Bacterial infections of humans,* 3rd ed. New York: Plenum Publishing, 1998.

5. DuPont HL, Levine MM, Hornick RB, et al. Inoculum size in shigellosis and implications for expected mode of transmission. *J Infect Dis* 1989;159:1126–1128.

6. Tauxe RV. The persistence of *Shigella flexneri* in the United States: the increased role of the adult male. *Am J Public Health* 1988;78:1432–1435.

7. Coles FB, Kondracki SF, Gallo RJ, et al. Shigellosis outbreaks at summer camps for the mentally retarded in New York State. *Am J Epidemiol* 1989;130:966–975.

8. Bartlett AV, Moore M, Gary GW, et al. Diarrheal illness among infants and toddlers in day care centers, I: epidemiology and pathogens. *J Pediatr* 1985;107:495–502.

9. Lee LA, Shapiro CN, Hargrett-Bean N, et al. Hyperendemic shigellosis in the United States: a review of surveillance data for 1967–1988. *J Infect Dis* 1991;164:894–900.

10. Cruz JR, Cano F, Bartlett AV, et al. Infection, diarrhea and dysentery caused by *Shigella* species and *Campylobacter jejuni* among Guatemalan rural children. *Pediatr Infect Dis J* 1994;13:216–223.

11. Wilson R, Feldman RA, Davis J, et al. Family illness associated with *Shigella* infection: the interrelationship of age of the index patient and the age of the household members in acquisition of illness. *J Infect Dis* 1981;143:130–132.

12. DuPont HL, Hornick RB, Dawkins A, et al. The response of man to virulent *Shigella flexneri* 2a. *J Infect Dis* 1969;119:296–299.

13. Askenazi S, Dinari G, Zenulunov A, et al. Convulsions in shigellosis: evaluation of possible risk factors. *Am J Dis Child* 1987;141:208–210.

14. Goren A, Freier S, Passwell JH. Lethal toxic encephalopathy due to childhood shigellosis in a developed country. *Pediatrics* 1992;89:1189–1193.

15. Bermish ML, Azad KA, Yousefzadeh D. Intestinal obstruction during shigellosis: incidence, clinical features, risk factors, and outcome. *Gastroenterology* 1991;101:626–634.

16. Bennish ML, Salam MA, Wahed MA. Enteric protein loss during shigellosis. *Am J Gastroenterol* 1993;88:53–57.

17. Struelens MJ, Patte D, Kabir I, et al. *Shigella* septicemia: prevalence, presentation, risk factors and outcome. *J Infect Dis* 1985;152:784–790.

18. Bennish ML, Harris JR, Wojtyniak BJ, et al. Death in shigellosis: incidence and risk factors in hospitalized patients. *J Infect Dis* 1990;161:500–506.

19. Stieglitz H, Lipsky P. Association between reactive arthritis and antecedent infection with *Shigella flexneri* carrying a 2-Md plasmid and encoding an HLA-B27 mimetic epitope. *Arthritis Rheum* 1993;36:1387–1391.

20. Samadi AR, Wahed MA, Islam MR, et al. Consequences of hyponatraemia and hypernatraemia in children with acute diarrhoea in Bangladesh. *Br Med J* 1983;286:671–673.

21. Bennish ML, Azad AK, Rahman O, et al. Hypoglycemia during diarrhea in childhood. Prevalence, pathophysiology, and outcome. *N Engl J Med* 1990;3222:1357–1363.

22. Islam MM, Azad K, Bardhan PK, et al. Pathology of shigellosis and its complications. *Histopathology* 1994;24:65–71.

23. Speelman P, Kabir I, Islam M. Distribution and spread of colonic lesions in shigellosis: a colonoscopic study. *J Infect Dis* 1984;150:899–903.

24. Parsot C. *Shigella flexneri:* Genetics of entry and intercellular dissemination in epithelial cells. *Curr Top Microbiol Immunol* 1994;192:217–241.

25. Goldberg MB, Sansonetti PJ. *Shigella* subversion of the cellular cytoskeleton: a strategy for epithelial colonization. *Infect Immun* 1993;61:4941–4946.

26. Zychlinsky A, Perdomo JJ, Sansonetti PJ. Molecular and cellular mechanisms of tissue invasion by *Shigella flexneri. Ann N Y Acad Sci* 1994;730:197–208.

27. Bernardini ML, Mounier J, d'Hauteville H, et al. Identification of icsA, a plasmid locus of *Shigella flexneri* that governs bacterial intra- and intercellular spread through interactions with F-actin. *Proc Natl Acad Sci USA* 1989;86:3867–3871.

28. Allaoui A, Mounier J, Prevost MC, et al. icsB: a *Shigella flexneri* virulence gene necessary for the lysis of protrusions during intercellular spread. *Mol Microbiol* 1992;6:1605–1616.

29. Perdomo JJ, Gounon P, Sansonetti PJ. Polymorphonuclear leukocyte transmigration promotes invasion of colonic epithelial monolayer by *Shigella flexneri. J Clin Invest* 1994;93:633–643.

30. Perdomo OJ, Cavaillon JM, Huerre M, et al. Acute inflammation causes epithelial invasion and mucosal destruction in experimental shigellosis. *J Exp Med* 1994;180:1307–1319.

31. Sansonetti PJ, Arondel J, Cavaillon J-M, et al. Role of interleukin-1 in the pathogenesis of experimental shigellosis. *J Clin Invest* 1995;96:884–892.

32. Raqib R, Wretlind B Andersson J, et al. Cytokine secretion in acute shigellosis is correlated to disease activity and directed more to stool than to plasma. *J Infect Dis* 1995;171:376–384.

33. Raqib R, Lindberg AA, Wretlind B, et al. Persistence of local cytokine production in shigellosis in acute and convalescent stages. *Infect Immun* 1995;63:289–296.

34. Rahman MM, Kabir I, Mahalanabis D, et al. Decreased food intake in children with severe dysentery due to *Shigella dysenteriae* 1 infection. *Eur J Clin Nutr* 1992;46:833–838.

35. Fontaine A, Arondel J, Sansonetti PJ. Role of Shiga toxin in the pathogenesis of bacillary dysentery, studied by using a Tox⁻ mutant of *Shigella dysenteriae* 1. *Infect Immun* 1988;56:3099–3109.

36. Jacewicz M, Clausen H, Nudelman E, et al. Pathogenesis of shigella diarrhea, XI: isolation of a shigella toxin–binding glycolipid from rabbit jejunum and HeLa cells and its identification as globotriaosylceramide. *J Exp Med* 1986;163:1391–1404.

37. Kandel G, Donohue-Rolfe A, Donowitz A, et al. Pathogenesis of *Shigella* diarrhea, XVI: selective targeting of Shiga toxin to villus cells of rabbit jejunum explains the effect of the toxin on intestinal electrolyte transport. *J Clin Invest* 1989;84:1509–1517.

38. Rout WR, Formal SB, Giannella RA, et al. Pathophysiology of *Shigella* diarrhea in the rhesus monkey: Intestinal transport, morphological, and bacteriological studies. *Gastroenterology* 1975;68:270–278.

39. Fasano A, Noriega FR, Maneval DR Jr, et al. *Shigella* enterotoxin 1: an enterotoxin of *Shigella flexneri* 2a active in rabbit small intestine *in vivo* and *in vitro. J Clin Invest* 1995;95:2853–2861.

40. Nataro JP, Seriwatana J, Fasano A, et al. Cloning and sequencing of a new plasmid-encoded enterotoxin in enteroinvasive *E. coli* and *Shigella.* Presented at the 29th Joint Conference on Cholera and Related Diseases. Bethesda, MD: National Institutes of Health, 1993:144–147.

41. Noriega FR, Liao FM, Formal SB, et al. Prevalence of *Shigella* enterotoxin 1 (ShET1) among *Shigella* clinical isolates of diverse serotypes. *J Infect Dis* 1995;172:1408–1411.

42. Fasano A, Kay BA, Russell RG, et al. Enterotoxin and cytotoxin production by enteroinvasive *Escherichia coli. Infect Immun* 1990;58:3717–3723.

43. Hofmann SL. Southwestern Internal Medicine Conference: Shiga-like toxins in hemolytic-uremic syndrome and thrombotic thrombocytopenic purpura. *Am J Med Sci* 1993;306:398–406.

44. de Silva DG, Mendis LN, Sheron N, et al. Concentrations of interleukin 6 and tumour necrosis factor in serum and stools of children with *Shigella dysenteriae* 1 infection. *Gut* 1993;34:194–198.

45. Varavithya W, Sunthornkachit R, Eampokalap B. Oral rehydration therapy for invasive diarrhea. *Rev Infect Dis* 1991;13[Suppl 4]:325–331.

46. Bennish ML, Salam MA. Rethinking options for the treatment of shigellosis. *J Antimicrob Chemother* 1992;30:243–247.

47. Bermish ML, Levy SB. Antimicrobial resistance of enteric pathogens. In: Blaser MJ, Smith PD, Ravdin JI, et al., eds. *Infections of the gastrointestinal tract.* New York: Raven Press, 1995:1499–1523.

48. Bermish ML, Salam MA, Khan WA, et al. Treatment of shigellosis, III: comparison of one- or two-dose ciprofloxacin with standard 5-day therapy. *Ann Intern Med* 1992;117:727–734.

49. Butler T, Islam MR, Azad MAK, et al. Risk factors for development of hemolytic-uremic syndrome during shigellosis. *J Pediatr* 1987;110:894–897.

50. Keusch GT, Scrimshaw NS. Selective primary health care: strategies for control of disease in the developing world: XXIII: control of infection to reduce the prevalence of infantile and childhood malnutrition. *Rev Infect Dis* 1986;8:273–287.

CHAPTER 67
Food Safety

David W. K. Acheson

Food safety is a broad topic that encompasses a multitude of disciplines involving physicians, other health care professionals, manufacturers, regulators, and consumers. However, for the purposes of this text, the focus is on current trends in food-borne disease, with the goal of providing the reader with an update on topical issues in relation to food safety. This encompasses recent trends in the epidemiology of food-borne pathogens and the mechanisms used to track such changes. The text also addresses various food-borne pathogens from the perspective of the types of symptoms they cause and what can be undertaken to diagnose and prevent the important food-borne diseases.

It is only recently, in the past 10 or 20 years, that the importance of food safety has gained wide recognition among health care professionals, manufacturers, federal regulators and consumers. Part of the reason for this is the emergence of new food-borne pathogens such as *Escherichia coli* O157:H7, and the recognition of old pathogens such as *Listeria monocytogenes* as causes of significant food-borne morbidity and mortality. One of the seminal events in this change was the infamous *E. coli* O157:H7 outbreak on the West Coast in late 1992 (1). This outbreak was the first large *E. coli* O157:H7 outbreak reported in the United States that was linked with the consumption of undercooked ground beef. The report by Bell (1) indicates that more than 500 individuals in Washington State became infected, of whom 45 developed hemolytic-uremic syndrome (HUS) and 3 died. The outbreak actually involved several other states, resulting in close to 750 cases. After this outbreak, for the first time large sections of the general public became aware of the dangers lurking in certain types of food if not either cooked or handled properly. This outbreak served to emphasize a number of facts that had not been well recognized in the past. First, the fact that previously healthy individuals, especially children, can develop life-threatening food-borne illness after normal daily activities such as eating at a fast-food restaurant. Second, food-borne illness can be much more than just a few uncomfortable days of gastroenteritis. Third, there was a critical need to educate consumers, improve the microbiologic quality of certain types of food, and strengthen the public health infrastructure to recognize, control, and prevent outbreaks.

During the 1990s, the Presidential Food Safety Initiative was instrumental in moving the food safety arena forward. This has been accomplished in a variety of ways but especially in relation to surveillance and the recognition of outbreaks. Consumer awareness has improved through intensive education campaigns, and manufacturers pay a great deal more attention to producing safer products. The following sections first describe the tools used to follow the epidemiology of food-borne disease and then discuss the important food-borne pathogens from a symptomatic perspective and how they may result in a wide range of clinical presentations. It is not the aim of this chapter to provide exhaustive detail on the myriad food-borne pathogens because many of these are covered in other parts of this volume.

EPIDEMIOLOGY OF FOOD-BORNE DISEASE

Several hundred different agents that have been associated with human disease may be transmitted via food or water (2). Exposure to such agents may have both short- and long-term consequences, resulting in either acute disease or longer term sequelae such as the effects from exposure to carcinogenic agents. The list of potentially harmful agents is long and includes chemicals, metals, toxins, and the more classic infectious agents such as bacteria, parasites, and viruses. New threats have also emerged recently such as prions. As already stated, the list of microbes that are linked with food-borne disease either directly or indirectly through the production of toxins is long; Table 67.1 summarizes many of them.

There have been at least two major developments in recent years in relation to getting a better understanding of the epidemiology of food-borne diseases; these are the implementation of FoodNet and PulseNet. In 1996 the Foodborne Diseases Active Surveillance Network (FoodNet) was established and is a cooperative venture between the Centers for Disease Control and Prevention (CDC), state health departments, the Food Safety and Inspection Service of the U.S. Department of Agriculture (USDA), and the Food and Drug Administration (FDA). FoodNet is a sentinel network that is designed to produce national estimates of the burden and sources of specific food-borne illnesses. FoodNet currently focuses on obtaining information on nine important and emerging food-borne infections agents (Table 67.2).

FoodNet operates by conducting population-based active surveillance for confirmed cases of the various pathogens shown

TABLE 67.1. Various Bacterial, Viral, Protozoal, Helminthic, and Toxic Agents that Are Associated with Food-borne Illness in Humans

1. Bacterial food-borne pathogens[a]
   Bacteria causing disease primarily mediated by a preformed toxin
   Clostridum botulinum
   Staphylococcus aureus
   Bacillus cereus
   Bacteria causing disease by production of toxins within the intestine
   Vibrio species
   Clostridum perfringens
   Shiga toxin–producing *Escherichid coli*
   Enterotoxigenic *E. coli*
   Bacteria causing disease primarily by invading the intestinal epithelial cells
   Salmonella species
   Camplylobacter species
   Yersinia species
   Listeria monocytogenes
   Shigella species
   Enteroinvasive *E. coli*
   Other bacterial causes of food-borne illness
   Aeromonas species
   Plesiomonas shigelloids
   Enteropathogenic *E. coli*
   Enteroaggregative *E. coli*
2. Viral food-borne pathogens
   Hepatitis A virus
   Hepatitis E virus
   Rotavirus
   Small round structured virus
   Enteric adenovirus
   Sapporo-like viruses
   Coronaviruses
   Toroviruses
   Reoviruses
   Caliciviruses
   Astroviruses
   Parvoviruses
   Picobirnaviruses
3. Protozoal food-borne pathogens
   Toxoplasma gondii
   Cryptosporidium parvum
   Giardia lamblia
   Entamoeba histolytica
   Cyclospora cayetanensis
   Microsporidium (Enterocytozon bieneusi, Septata intestinalis)
   Isospora belli
   Dientamoeba fragilis
   Blastocystis hominis
4. Cestodes and worms
   Taenia saginata
   Taenia solium
   Diphyllobothrium latum
   Hymenolepis nana
   Ascariasis
   Trichuriasis
   Trichinella spiralis
5. Natural toxins
   Ciguatera
   Scombroid
   Shellfish poisoning (neurotoxic, diarrheic, and toxic encephalopathic)
   Tetrodotoxin
   Mushroom toxins
   α toxins

[a]Several of the bacterial foodborne pathogens have been broken down into three basic pathogenetic mechanisms: preformed toxins, production of toxins *in vivo*, and invasive organisms.

TABLE 67.2. Food-borne Pathogens Routinely Under Surveillance As Part of FoodNet

Bacteria
   Campylobacter species
   Escherichia coli O157:H7
   Listeria monocytogenes
   Salmonella spp
   Shigella spp
   Vibrio species
   Yersinia
Protozoa
   Cryptosporidium
   Cyclospora

in Table 67.2. Since the initiation of FoodNet in 1996 the population under surveillance has grown from five sites and a population of 14.2 million to nine sites and 37.8 million in 2001. This now represents 13% of the U.S. population. The nine sites that are part of FoodNet include Minnesota, Oregon, California, Connecticut, Georgia, Maryland, New York, Colorado, and Tennessee.

The objectives of FoodNet are to determine the frequency and severity of food-borne diseases. This includes examining the association of common food-borne diseases with eating specific foods. To achieve these goals, FoodNet uses active surveillance and conducts epidemiologic studies. To identify cases of food-borne disease, FoodNet contacts more than 450 clinical laboratories serving the catchment areas either weekly or monthly

depending on the size of the laboratory. (More specific information about FoodNet can be found at *www.cdc.gov/foodnet.*) The most recent complete FoodNet report is from the year 2000 in which only eight sites were involved (Colorado was added in 2001) (3), with preliminary data available on the 2001 survey (4). During 2000 a total of 12,930 laboratory-confirmed cases caused by the various pathogens under surveillance were identified. Figure 67.1 shows the clear seasonal effects seen with *Campylobacter, Salmonella, Shigella,* and *E. coli* O157 where the number of cases for all three pathogens rises markedly in the warmer summer months. Interestingly, there is a spike in *Yersinia* during the colder months, with 47% of cases reported in January, February, or December (see Fig. 67.1). Another striking difference seen is the variation in the incidence rates by site. For example, the incidence rates for *Campylobacter* varied from 6.4 per 100,000 in Tennessee to 37.4 per 100,000 in California; and for *Shigella* infections from 1.04 per 100,000 in New York to 18.4 per 100,000 in Minnesota (3). Some of these variations may be due to differences in laboratory practices, but this is unlikely to be the sole explanation. Age is also an important factor, with the incidence rates for *Salmonella* and *Campylobacter* infection being markedly higher in children younger than 1 year (Fig. 67.2).

Obviously not all food-borne diseases have the same degree of morbidity and mortality. This is well illustrated by the hospitalization and death rates seen in the FoodNet sites from the nine pathogens that are tracked. Overall, 14.9% of patients with culture-confirmed infection were hospitalized. As shown in Table 67.3, this varies markedly between pathogens, with *Listeria* being well ahead with approximately 90% of infected patients requiring hospitalization. Similarly, the fatality rates vary

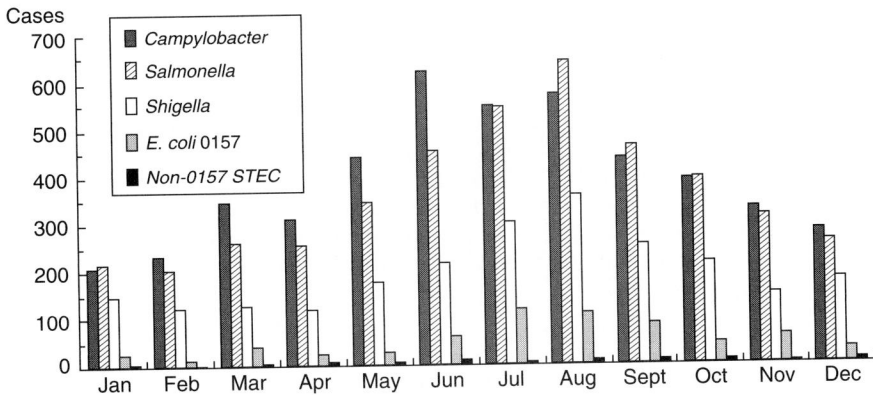

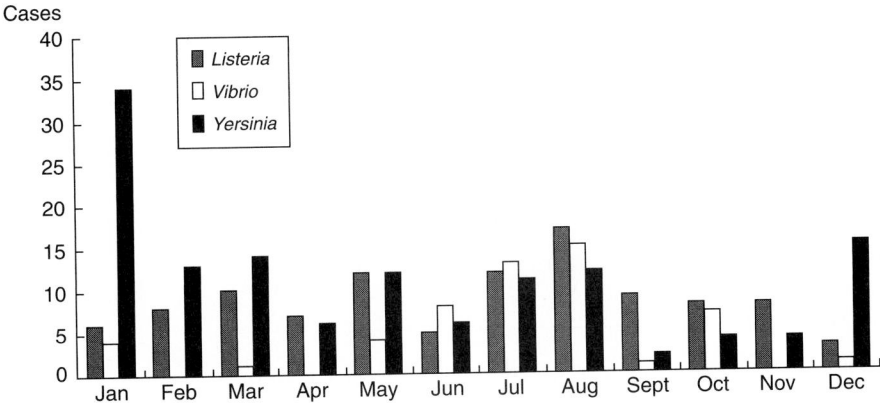

Figure 67.1. Cases of food-borne disease caused by specific pathogens, by month, FoodNet sites, 2000. (From Centers for Disease Control and Prevention. FoodNet surveillance report for 2000. Available at: *www.cdc.gov/foodnet/annuals.htm,* with permission.)

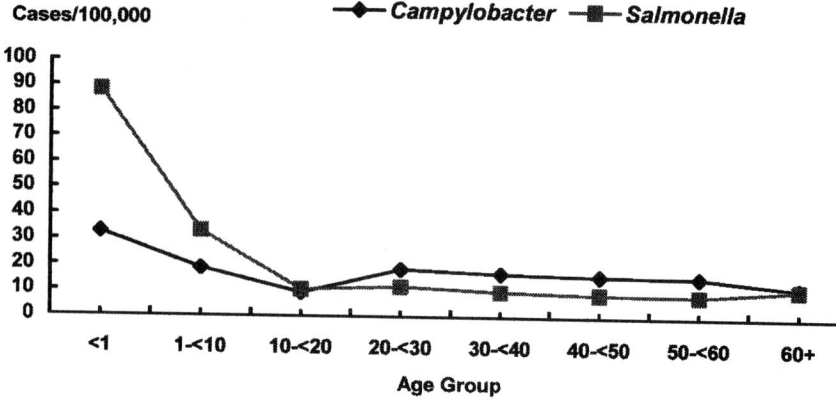

Cases/100,000

◆—*Campylobacter*   ■—*Salmonella*

Age Group

Figure 67.2. Incidence of *Campylobacter* and *Salmonella* infections by age-group, FoodNet sites, 2000. (From Centers for Disease Control and Prevention. FoodNet surveillance report for 2000. Available at: *www.cdc.gov/foodnet/annuals.htm,* with permission.)

markedly between pathogens. During 2000 there were 58 deaths in those with culture-confirmed food-borne diseases in FoodNet sites; of these 58 deaths, 20% were associated with *Listeria.* The fatality rates of the more common infections (such as *Campylobacter* or *Salmonella*) were among the lowest.

When food safety is lax, one of the outcomes may be an outbreak of disease. It is often the outbreaks that cause the most attention, especially from the media. However, outbreaks account for only a relatively small number of infections overall. A recently published summary of documented outbreaks, which occurred between 1993 and 1997, illustrates the important pathogens and food-borne agents that are most often linked to outbreaks (5). During that period, 2,751 outbreaks were investigated by the CDC, averaging about 500 outbreaks per year. A total of 86,058 people were sick in connection with the outbreaks, and although only 32% had a known cause, they accounted for 59% of the 86,058 infections. Table 67.4 summarizes some of these outbreak data, illustrates the importance of *Salmonella* and *E. coli* as causes of outbreaks and outbreak-related death, and demonstrates the importance of two preformed toxins, scombroid toxin and ciguatoxin, as causes of outbreaks. FoodNet data in 2000 also looked at outbreaks during that year. It is interesting to note that of those outbreaks in which a pathogen was found, outbreaks caused by Norwalk-like virus (NLV) far outnumbered any other pathogens (Table 67.5).

The most recent data from FoodNet is the 2001 preliminary data, which show some interesting trends in food-borne disease and suggests that some aspects of food safety may be working (Table 67.6). Again there were variations in the incidence of specific pathogens, with California having the highest rates for *Campylobacter* and young children (younger than 1 year) having the highest incidence of most food-borne infections. For the first time, the CDC used a log-linear Poisson regression model to estimate the effect of time on the incidence of various pathogens using 1996 as the reference year, because it was the first year for FoodNet surveillance. By doing this, the data show that the incidence of most pathogens decreased from 1996 to 2001. *Salmonella* is an interesting case in point however. Although there was an overall decrease in the incidence of *Salmonella* infection, there was considerable variation among the different serotypes. From 1996 to 2001, *Salmonella typhimurium* infection decreased 24% [95% confidence interval (CI), 13%–34% decrease], *Salmonella enteritidis* infection decreased 22% (95% CI, 41% decrease to 3% increase), but *Salmonella* Newport increased 32% (95% CI, 24% decrease to 128% increase), *Salmonella* Heidelberg increased 34% (95% CI, 7%–66% increase), and *Salmonella* Javiana increased 228% (95% CI, 75%–513% increase) (5).

These overall downward trends are very encouraging and are likely due to a number of factors, including the implementation by the U.S. Department of Agriculture's Food Safety

TABLE 67.3.   Comparison of Infections, Hospitalizations and Deaths (as a Percentage) for Each of the Pathogens Tracked by FoodNet.

Pathogen	Percent of total infections	Percent of those infected who were hospitalized	Case-fatality rate (actual numbers of deaths)
Campylobacter	36.5	9.8	0.1 (4)
Escherichia coli O157:H7	4.8	41.8	1.1 (7)
Non-O157 Shiga toxin–producing, *E. coli*	0.4	5.3	0 (0)
Listeria	0.8	90.5	20.6 (22)
Salmonella	33.5	16.7	0.3 (13)
Shigella	18.2	10	0.1 (2)
Vibrio	0.4	24.1	1.9 (1)
Yersinia	1.0	27.1	0 (0)
Cryptosporidium	4.1	18.9	1.7 (9)
Cyclospora	0.2	0	0 (0)

Source: From Preliminary FoodNet data on the incidence of foodborne illnesses—selected sites, United States, 2001. *MMWR* 2002;51:325–329.

TABLE 67.4. Major Causes of Food-borne Disease Outbreaks in the United States Between 1993 and 1997

Etiology	No. of outbreaks (%)	No. of cases (%)	No. of deaths (%)
Salmonella	357 (13.0)	32,610 (37.6)	13 (44.8)
Escherichia coli	84 (3.1)	3,260 (3.8)	8 (27.6)
Scrombroid toxin	69 (2.5)	297 (0.3)	0
Ciguatoxin	60 (2.2)	205 (0.2)	0
Clostridium perfringens	57 (2.1)	2,772 (3.2)	0
Shigella	43 (1.6)	1,555 (1.8)	0
Staphylococcus aureus	42 (1.5)	1,413 (1.6)	1 (3.4)
Campylobacter	25 (0.9)	539 (0.6)	1 (3.4)
Hepatitis A	23 (0.8)	729 (0.8)	0
Bacillus cereus	14 (0.5)	691 (0.8)	0
Clostridium botulinum	13 (0.5)	56 (0.1)	1 (3.4)
Norwalk virus	9 (0.3)	1,233 (1.4)	0
Listerid monocytogenes	3 (0.1)	100 (0.1)	2 (6.9)

Source: Modified from Surveillance for food-borne disease outbreaks—United States, 1993–1997. *MMWR Morb Mortal Wkly Rep* 2000;49:1–51, with permission.

Inspection Service the Pathogen Reduction/Hazard Analysis Critical Control Point (HACCP) systems regulating meat and poultry slaughter and processing plants. Significant efforts toward consumer education and safe food-handling practices have also likely contributed to these downward trends. Other important innovations that have taken effect since 1996 include the egg quality-assurance programs for *S. enteritidis*, increased attention to the safety of fresh produce, introduction of HACCP in the seafood industry, regulation of fresh fruit and vegetable juice, and increased regulation of imported foods. Overall these trends are very encouraging, but we must not lose sight of emerging pathogens such as *Salmonella* Newport, antibiotic-resistant food-borne pathogens, and new food safety entities such as the transmissible spongiform encephalopathies.

One of the recently developed most useful tools in relation to food safety is the ability to undertake molecular epidemi-

ologic investigations. This has provided public health officials with the tools necessary to identify outbreaks that would have previously gone unrecognized. Although many tools are available for molecular epidemiology including techniques such as randomly amplified polymeric deoxyribonucleic acid typing (RAPD), pulsed field gel electrophoresis (PFGE), ribotyping (6), or even microarrays (7), the CDC has made great use of PFGE in conjunction with a national molecular subtyping network named *PulseNet* (8). PulseNet, which began in 1996, is an early warning system for outbreaks of food-borne disease. It is a national network of public health laboratories that performs deoxyribonucleic acid (DNA) "fingerprinting" on bacteria that may be food borne. The network identifies and labels each "fingerprint" pattern and permits rapid comparison of these patterns through an electronic database at the CDC to identify related strains. By 2001 the network included 46 state and 2 local laboratories, as well as the USDA and FDA laboratories. PulseNet is used to type *E. coli* O157:H7, nontyphoidal *Salmonella*, *L. monocytogenes*, and *Shigella*, and other pathogens will come on line in the future (8). The use of PulseNet in combination with local epidemiology has allowed links to be made between human disease and specific food products that have resulted in recalls of contaminated products, thus limiting consumer exposure to contaminated food (9). However, it is important to remember that obtaining a match between a bacterial isolate from a patient and an isolate from food does not give a 100% guarantee that the two are linked. Ensuring that there is an epidemiologic link is all part of an appropriate investigation.

TABLE 67.5. Reported Outbreaks with Ten or More Persons Ill, by Pathogen, FoodNet Sites, 2000

Etiology	No. of outbreaks	Median no. ill
Bacillus cereus	1	10
Campylobacter	1	13
Clostridium perfringens	2	53
Cyclospora	1	29
Escherichia coli O157	4	40
Hepatitis A virus	1	38
Norwalk-like virus	34	26
Salmonella	8	14
Scrombroid toxin	1	11
Shigella	1	24
Staphylococcus	4	95
Unknown, viral profile[a]	7	18
Unknown, other	35	24
Total	100	25

Note: Outbreaks reported as of January 22, 2002. Does not include multistate or multicounty outbreaks as all involved sites were not in FoodNet catchment area. FoodNet sites were involved in seven multistate outbreaks and six multicounty outbreaks.
[a]Unconfirmed viral etiology largely based on symptoms.
Source: From FoodNet surveillance report for 2000. Available at: www.cda.gov/foodnet/annuals.htm, with permission.

CLINICAL SPECTRUM OF FOOD-BORNE DISEASE

With the large number of agents that may cause food-borne disease, that a wide range of clinical presentations exist is not surprising. Typically, one expects food-borne illness to present with various gastrointestinal (GI) tract symptoms such as nausea, vomiting, abdominal pain, diarrhea, and fever. However, food-borne illness can present in very different ways, with neurologic symptoms, such as headaches, paralysis, or tingling, hepatitis, or renal failure. Some food-borne agents may act very quickly, within a matter of minutes (in the case of chemical poisons) to hours (in the case of preformed toxins), whereas others may not cause disease until several weeks after exposure (e.g., hepatitis

TABLE 67.6.   Changes in Incidence of the Various Pathogens Surveyed by FoodNet between 1996 and 2001

Pathogen	Percent change (95% confidence intervals)	Notes
Yersinia	49% decrease (35%–60% decrease)	—
Listeria	35% decrease (9%–53% decrease)	—
Campylobacter	27% decrease (19%–35% decrease)	—
Salmonella	15% decrease (7%–22% decrease)	There was marked variation between serotypes (see text)
Escherichia coli O157:H7	21% decrease (41% decrease to 5% increase)	This decline reflects a decrease in 2001 only
Shigella	35% decrease (57% decrease to 3% increase)	There was considerable variation by year and by site
Vibrio	83% increase (3%–224% increase	This is largely due to the emergence of *Vibrio parahemolyticus* O3:K6.
Cryptosporidium	33% decrease (4%–53% decrease)	Surveillance did not begin until 1997
Cyclospora	Too few cases to calculate	Surveillance did not begin until 1997

Source: From Preliminary FoodNet data on the incidence of food-borne illnesses—selected sites, United States, 2001. *MMWR Morb Mortal Wkly Rep* 2002;51:325–329, with permission.

A or *L. monocytogenes*). With this range of clinical presentations, one has to ask what can be done to narrow down the diagnosis clinically? One also has to determine whether all patients should have stool cultures, which patients should be prescribed antimicrobial therapy, and what are the public health implications of a patient with a food-borne disease? Physicians treating such patients have a responsibility not only to the patient, but also to the community as a whole in terms of alerting public health officials to minimize spread within the general community, and educating the patient on how to reduce the chance of spreading the infection to other members of their household or close contacts.

As already stated, the spectrum of food-borne disease is wide (10), with the majority having some type of GI tract component. However, it is important to remember that some food-borne diseases may manifest in a way that is not focused on the GI tract, for example, in the form of paralysis (e.g., botulism or some types of shellfish poisoning), as headaches and tingling (e.g., ciguatera fish poisoning or scombroid), with amnesia (e.g., amnesic shellfish poisoning), with hepatitis (e.g., hepatitis A and E), or with meningitis or spontaneous abortion (e.g., *L. monocytogenes*). The physician should consider a number of important factors when trying to determine the differential diagnosis of food-borne diseases: first, the presenting symptoms; second, exposure to a particular type of food associated with food-borne disease; and third, the time interval between exposure to the suspect food and the onset of symptoms.

PRESENTING SYMPTOMS

As stated, there are many different ways in which food-borne pathogens may result in clinical illness and each one may have a different type of clinical presentation. It is beyond the scope of this chapter to discuss the myriad pathogens and symptoms they may invoke. However, it is possible to give some broad-based examples of how to approach the problems and how one can use this to determine the more likely causes of the illness. This overall approach is summarized in Table 67.7. One way to categorize the differences between bacterial food-borne pathogens is to think about them in the context of their mechanism of action, such as whether they exert their effects from the pro-

duction of a preformed toxin (e.g., *Staphylococcus aureus* enterotoxin, *Bacillus cereus* toxin, *Clostridium botulinum* neurotoxins); whether a toxin is produced once the organism has been ingested [e.g., *Clostridium perfringens*, enterotoxigenic *E. coli* (ETEC) Shiga toxin–producing *E. coli* (STEC), *Vibrio cholerae*]; or whether the organism is invasive (*Shigella, Campylobacter, Salmonella*, enteroinvasive *E. coli, Yersinia enterocolitica*). In an attempt to simplify the situation, the key food-borne pathogens have been classified based on the predominant symptom they produce, whether it be GI (vomiting and diarrhea) or non-GI (see Table 67.7). At the outset, it is important to recognize that there are literally dozens of chemicals that could be added to food either accidentally or deliberately with significant consequences. It is not the goal of this chapter to discuss these, but health professionals always need to keep that in the back of their minds when dealing with food-borne disease or a patient who appears to have a food-borne disease.

Vomiting as the Major Presenting Symptom

A sudden onset of nausea and vomiting is likely due to the ingestion of a preformed toxin such as *S. aureus* enterotoxin or *B. cereus* toxin or a chemical irritant. Both microbial toxins will lead to vomiting as the primary symptom. In the case of *S. aureus* toxin, symptoms usually begin within 1 to 6 hours of ingestion, with nausea, vomiting, and abdominal cramps. Fever and/or diarrhea may occur in a minority of patients. *S. aureus* toxin is heat stable and is often associated with the consumption of prepared food such as dairy produce, meats, eggs, and salads that have been prepared by a food handler (11). There are a variety of different staphylococcal enterotoxins designated A through F, although type F, associated with toxic shock syndrome, has not been linked with food-borne disease (12,13). It is usually the food handler who contaminates the product, which when held at room temperature allows multiplication of the organisms and subsequent toxin production. Vomitus and/or food can be tested for the enterotoxin, but the diagnosis is usually clinical.

B. cereus is capable of producing at least two types of food-borne disease (14). The most dramatic is due to the heat-stable enterotoxin, which is typically found in starchy foods such as rice (15). The preformed *B. cereus* enterotoxin causes a rapid (within 1–6 hours) onset of nausea and profuse vomiting. The disease is

TABLE 67.7. Some of the Principle Presenting Symptoms Linked with the Major Food-borne Microbes that May Be Responsible for that Symptom

Major presenting symptom	Likely microbes	Incubation period	Likely food sources
Gastrointestinal			
Vomiting	*Staphylococcus aureus*	1–6 hr	Prepared food, for example, salads, dairy, meat
	Bacillys cereus	1–6 hr	Rice, meat
	Norwalk-like viruses	24–48 hr	Shellfish, prepared foods, salads, sandwiches, fruit
Watery diarrhea	*Clostridium perfringens*	8–16 hr	Meat, poultry, gravy
	Enterotoxigenic *Escherichia coli*	1–3 d	Fecally contaminated food or water
	Enteric viruses	10–72 hr	Fecally contaminated food or water
	Cryptosporidium parvum	2–28 d	Vegetables, fruit, unpasturized milk, water
	Cyclospora cayetanensis	1–11 d	Imported berries, basil
Inflammatory diarrhea	*Campylobacter* species	2–5 d	Poultry, unpasteurized milk, water
	Non-typhoidal *Salmonella*	1–3 d	Eggs, poultry, meat, unpasteurized milk or juice, fresh produce
	Shiga toxin–producing *E. coli*	1–8 d	Ground beef, unpasteurized milk and juice, raw vegetables, water
	Shigella species	1–3 d	Fecal contamination of food and water
	Vibrio parahaemolyticus	2–48 hr	Raw shellfish
Nongastrointestinal			
Neurologic	Botulism (*Clostridium botulinum*)	12–72 hr	Home canned foods, fermented fish, herb-infused oils, bottled garlic, foods held warm for long periods
	Ciguatera toxin	2–6 hr	Large reef fish: grouper, red snapper, Amberjack, barracuda
	Scrombroid	1 min to 3 hr	Fish: bluefin, tuna, skipjack, mackerel, marlin, mahi mahi
Systemic	*Listeria monocytogenes* (listeriosis)	2–6 wk	Ready to eat deli meats, hot dogs, unpasturized soft cheese and milk
	Vibrio vulnificus	1–7 d	Shellfish
Hepatitis	Hepatitis A	15–50 d	Shellfish, prepared foods infected by a food handler

Source: Modified from Centers for Disease control and Prevention. Diagnosis and management of food borne illness, a primer for physicians. *MMWR Murb Mortal Wkly Rep* 2001;50(RR-2), with permission.

usually self-limiting, although it has been very rarely associated with acute hepatic necrosis (16). Diagnosis is usually clinical, but reference laboratories will have the capability of testing food or vomitus for the toxin. Because these are preformed toxins, there is no risk of spread to others; however, they may be responsible for outbreaks (17). The other syndrome associated with *B. cereus* is more likely to cause diarrhea, has a longer incubation period (8–16 hours), and is due to a different toxin (18).

Another group of food-borne diseases that typically cause vomiting as the predominant symptom are viral infections such as NLVs. NLVs (also known as *small round structured virus*) are now considered one of the most common food-borne diseases and typically cause nausea, vomiting, and watery diarrhea (2). NLVs have been associated with large outbreaks on cruise ships, are readily transmitted from vomitus of an infected person, and may be transmitted in aerosol form (19). A recent outbreak of NLV associated with salad is another example of how infectious agents may be transmitted from food handlers to food (20). Infection with NLV is usually self-limiting, and there are no routine diagnostic assays available for it. Reverse transcriptase polymerase chain reaction (RT-PCR)–based assays and electron microscopy can be used in reference settings. Shellfish are known to harbor NLVs, but otherwise they are usually transmitted from a food handler via food. Therefore, exposure to prepared food such as salads, sandwiches, and fruit is a risk factor.

Exposure to certain metals such as copper, zinc, and cadmium can also lead to a rapid onset of vomiting (within 5–15 minutes) and has been linked with outbreaks through consumption of contaminated food (21–23).

Diarrhea as the Major Symptom

When trying to categorize diarrhea in the context of food-borne pathogens, one has to think in the context of the type of diarrhea (e.g., watery or bloody), the extent of the diarrhea (numbers of times per day, volume each time), the timing of the diarrhea in relation to the putative exposure, and other associated symptoms (e.g., nausea, vomiting, abdominal pain, and fever).

WATERY DIARRHEA

Many food-borne microbes cause watery diarrhea and the presence of watery diarrhea alone is of little help in the differential diagnosis. The degree of diarrhea may be some help because some food-borne microbes such as *V. cholerae* may cause massive watery diarrhea, but this is unlikely to be seen in the United States. *C. perfringens* is a much more likely cause of watery diarrhea in patients in the United States (24). Of the five types of *C. perfringens* enterotoxin described, type A is the one predominantly associated with food-borne disease. Type A results in a noninflammatory diarrhea that is usually linked to the consumption of meat or poultry (typically foods that are high in protein) that has been prepared and allowed to remain between 15°C and 60°C for more than 2 hours. During this period, clostridial spores germinate and begin vegetative growth. When around 10^5 vegetative cells are ingested, they are present in large enough numbers to transiently colonize portions of the intestine and produce enough toxin to cause disease. Ingestion of preformed toxin or nongerminated spores will not usually result in disease.

Vibrio parahaemolyticus has recently become an increasingly common cause of watery diarrhea. Consumption of raw or undercooked seafood is the most common route for acquiring infection with *V. parahaemolyticus,* and clinically the presentation is usually one of watery diarrhea and abdominal pain. Occasionally, the stool is bloody and there may be a low-grade fever. The upsurge in worldwide incidence of *V. parahaemolyticus* infection in the last 5 years has been attributed to the recent appearance of three serotypes with pandemic potential: O3:K6, O4:K68, and O1:K untypeable (25).

Other microbial causes of watery diarrhea include ETEC, *B. cereus,* and many of the enteric viruses such as rotavirus, astroviruses, enteric adenoviruses, and NLV. ETEC have been the cause of outbreaks in the United States (2), including a recent one in Illinois linked to potato salad, and are a frequent cause of traveler's diarrhea. Both ETEC and enteric viruses are transmitted via fecal contamination of food or water from an infected person. Prepared food is therefore at the top of the list of likely sources. There are no specific tests for ETEC in routine use. ETEC look like any other *E. coli* on standard laboratory media, and if they are suspected, a special request should be made to the testing laboratory.

As already discussed, the role of viruses as a cause of food-borne disease is gaining increasing recognition (2,26). However, the lack of diagnostic methods and the absence of specific treatment have dampened physician's enthusiasm for diagnosing viral food-borne disease. The vast majority of viral food-borne disease seems to be due to NLVs. NLVs are small, single-stranded ribonucleic acid (RNA) viruses that were previously called *small round structured* viruses because of their appearance under an electron microscope. They constitute a genus in the family Caliciviridae and are divided into three distinct genogroups (GI, GII, and GIII) (26). Other common viruses that may cause watery diarrhea include rotavirus, enteric adenovirus, astrovirus, and Sapporo-like viruses. Although these other viruses have occasionally been linked to spread in food and the cause of food-borne outbreaks, food-borne transmission is not considered a major component in their spread (26). As with certain other food-borne pathogens such as *Shigella* and hepatitis A, the aforementioned viruses do have a tendency to be transmitted from food handlers. Thus, in outbreak situations, this route of transmission must be considered.

Two other food-borne pathogens worth discussing that may cause predominantly watery diarrhea are *Cryptosporidium parvum* and *Cyclospora cayetanensis* (27). *C. parvum* causes a lot of disease (2), but only 10% of it is considered to be food borne, in contrast *C. cayetanensis* causes a lot less disease, but 90% of it is considered to be food borne (2). *C. parvum,* for which proven effective therapy does not exist, has gained notoriety for causing persistent chronic diarrhea in immunocompromised patients (28). *C. parvum* is endemic in cattle and is usually acquired in humans from contaminated water, fresh produce, unpasteurized milk, or person-to-person spread. The incubation period is typically about a week but can be as long as 28 days. *C. parvum* is known to cause large outbreaks, the largest of which was waterborne in Milwaukee, in which around 400,000 individuals became sick (29). As with some of the other pathogens discussed already, *C. parvum* outbreaks have also been linked to infected food handlers (30). *Cyclospora* is considered an emerging pathogen because of its recent association with food-borne disease (31). Susceptible humans are infected by ingesting sporulated oocysts. Though unknown, the infectious dose is presumed to be low. Symptoms of infection may include watery diarrhea, mild to severe nausea, anorexia, abdominal cramping, fatigue, and weight loss. Diarrhea can be intermittent and protracted (32–34). Outbreaks of cyclosporiasis in the United States have been associated with consumption of fresh raspberries, mesclun lettuce, and basil (35,36). An important feature of the biology of *Cyclospora* is that oocysts excreted in feces require days to weeks outside the host to sporulate and thus to become infectious. This makes person-to-person transmission very unlikely. It can be diagnosed by direct acid-fast microscopy of stool, but it is important to note that most microbiology laboratories will not routinely look for *C. parvum* and/or *C. cayetanensis,* so they must be asked for specifically. Diagnosis of *C. cayetanensis* is important because it is readily treatable with trimethoprim-sulfamethoxazole.

INFLAMMATORY DIARRHEA

As already mentioned, the presence of inflammatory cells in the stool indicates that the illness may be due to a different spectrum of agents to those discussed. Making the diagnosis of inflammatory diarrhea requires, by definition, the presence of inflammatory cells or a marker of inflammatory cells such as lactoferrin (37). However, there are clinical clues based on the patient's history that should increase suspicion that one is dealing with a food-borne microbe that is causing inflammatory diarrhea. Such symptoms and signs include the following (a) passage of diarrhea with blood or mucus; (b) the presence of severe abdominal pain; and/or (c) fever. Statistically in the context of food-borne disease, a patient with inflammatory diarrhea in the United States is far more likely to be infected with *Salmonella* or *Campylobacter* than any of the other causes of inflammatory diarrhea. The typhoidal salmonellae, such as *Salmonella typhi* or *Salmonella paratyphi,* primarily colonize humans, are transmitted via the consumption of fecally contaminated food or water, and cause a systemic illness usually with little or no diarrhea. The much broader group of nontyphoidal salmonellae are found in the intestines of other animals and are therefore acquired from the consumption of products that have become contaminated with animal feces (38). Thus, much of the salmonellosis is due to either cross-contamination or undercooking of raw meat or poultry products or contamination of fresh produce. The major exception to this is *S. enteritidis,* which may be present in the ovaries of chickens, resulting in transovarian contamination of eggs as they are being formed in the chicken.

As discussed in section "Epidemiology of Food-borne Disease," the epidemiologic trends of salmonellosis are changing. One of the more recent trends has been the emergence of multidrug-resistant *Salmonella* Newport (39). Investigation of a recent outbreak that involved 47 patients in five states revealed that isolates were resistant to amoxicillin-clavulanate, ampicillin, cefoxitin, ceftiofur, cephalothin, chloramphenicol, streptomycin, sulfamethoxazole, and tetracycline. In addition, two of three isolates tested were resistant to kanamycin, and two had decreased susceptibility or resistance to ceftriaxone (39). This was thought to have been transmitted via ground beef and raises the important question of the need to control the development of antibiotic resistance in food-borne pathogens (40).

Food-borne disease caused by *Campylobacter* species was not recognized until the mid-1970s. *Campylobacter jejuni* accounts for the vast majority of food-borne campylobacteriosis and *Campylobacter coli* accounts for most of the remainder. The incubation period is usually about 2 to 5 days, and poultry is a common source of the organism. Studies from various locations including the United States indicate that 70% to 80% of retail poultry is contaminated with *Campylobacter* (41), thus making cross-contamination during food preparation an important hazard. Although *Campylobacter* are fastidious and slow growing, they can be diagnosed using routine microbiologic techniques on selective plates.

Of the other food-borne pathogens that may cause inflammatory diarrhea, STEC, *Shigella,* and *Y. enterocolitica* are the most important ones. STEC are now the most frequent cause of acute renal failure in the United States (42,43). Although *E. coli* O157:H7 is the serotype most often associated with human disease, it is now clear there are more than 50 other STEC serotypes that have been associated with diarrheal disease and HUS. STEC typically have been found in ground beef, unpasteurized juice, raw fruits, and vegetables including alfalfa sprouts. The incubation period ranges from about 1 day to 1 week. The presentation usually begins with watery diarrhea that may become bloody. Recent data from the United States indicate that close to 50% of STEC clinical isolates are non-O157:H7 STEC (44). As more data are generated on the importance of non-O157 STEC, it is becoming clear that several serotypes are predominant, including O111, O26, O121, and O103. An O111 STEC was responsible for a large outbreak of disease in the United States in 1999, with at least two cases of HUS (45). STEC can be diagnosed using Shiga toxin–based assays, which have advantages over the more conventional sorbitol-MacConkey agar test. Most clinical microbiology laboratories will test only for O157:H7 STEC using sorbitol-MacConkey plates (O157:H7 ferments sorbitol only slowly compared with other *E. coli*). Use of sorbitol-MacConkey plates will fail to detect non-O157:H7 strains and appear to have diminished sensitivity compared with Shiga toxin–based tests (46). Determining whether a patient is positive for STEC has important implications in relation to antibiotic therapy. In the past, a number of small studies have indicated that antibiotic therapy may increase the risk of serious complications following STEC infection (47). However, a recent metaanalysis indicted that these risks may have been exaggerated (48). It is likely that there is some middle ground in this argument. *In vitro* and *in vivo* studies in animals have shown that certain antibiotics, such as quinolones, can increase Shiga toxin production from STEC through their ability to induce the Shiga toxin–encoding bacteriophage (49). Currently, it is still unclear what the degree of danger is in treating STEC infection with antibiotics, but current data suggest that certain antibiotics are best avoided (50).

Shigella will only colonize humans and some nonhuman primates; therefore, transmission of *Shigella* in food or water is most likely from either fecal contamination or direct contamination from a food handler. *Shigella sonnei* and *Shigella flexneri* are the two species most likely to be seen in the United States. A variety of foods have been implicated in the spread of *Shigella,* including salads (potato, tuna, shrimp, macaroni, and chicken), raw vegetables, milk and dairy products, and poultry, as well as common-source water supplies. Diagnosis is routine in clinical microbiology laboratories. Another important cause of food-borne disease that will cause an inflammatory diarrhea is *Y. enterocolitica,* which is typically associated with consumption of undercooked pork, unpasteurized milk, and fecally contaminated water.

Nongastrointestinal Presentations

There are a wide range of food-borne agents whose ingestions may cause significant effects on systems other than the GI tract. Such agents or illnesses may be bacterial (*L. monocytogenes, Vibrio vulnificus,* tuberculosis, anthrax, Q fever), viral (hepatitis A), caused by toxins (*C. botulinum,* ciguatera, scombroid toxin, mushroom toxins, tetrodotoxin, aflatoxins), parasitic (*Toxoplasma gondii,* trichinosis), or helminthic (tapeworms). Plus there is a wide range of chemicals, such as nitrites or rat poison (51), that may get into food either deliberately or in error that can cause major systemic illness and death. It is beyond the scope of this chapter to review all of these agents, but some of the more important ones do warrant further comment.

L. monocytogenes is the cause of listeriosis, which is a rare but deadly food-borne disease with a mortality rate of approximately 20%. It is most likely to occur in the immunocompromised, elderly, or pregnant women. Exposure to deli meat, raw hot dogs, and unpasteurized soft cheese are risk factors that need to be considered, but the incubation period may be as long as 6 weeks. The diagnosis is usually made by culturing *L. monocytogenes* from blood or cerebrospinal fluid (CSF). Five percent to ten percent of the population have *L. monocytogenes* in their stool, so stool culture is unhelpful. *L. monocytogenes* has occasionally been known to cause GI tract symptoms and fever with a short (10–48-hour) incubation period in normal adults. The most renowned time this happened was following contamination of chocolate milk in which 45 individuals became sick(52).

V. vulnificus is another unusual but deadly microbe that affects the immunocompromised, and especially those with chronic liver disease. It is a frequent contaminant of oysters in the U.S., especially in the summer (53). It is associated with exposure to raw shellfish and has an incubation period of 1 to 7 days. It may present with GI symptoms or skin infection that rapidly develop into bacteremia and systemic disease. Because of its ability to invade the blood stream without causing gastroenteritis there may be no GI symptoms, even though the organisms is acquired via food. Culture for Vibrios requires special media and is not done routinely, therefore a special request should be made to the laboratory if *V. vulnificus* is suspected.

Of the toxins, botulism (due to *C. botulinum* toxin) is one of the most important because of its life-threatening consequences. In the context of visual disturbance and/or descending paralysis, a food history may be critical because botulism is associated with the consumption of foods in which *C. botulinum* spores have germinated and the resulting vegetative cells have produced toxin. Typical foods associated with botulism are those canned at home, fermented fish, herb-infused oils, and foods held warm for extended periods. Stool, serum, and stool can be tested for toxin by reference laboratories. Although the worldwide incidence of infant botulism is rare, most cases are diagnosed in the United States. An infant can acquire botulism by ingesting *C. botulinum* spores, which are found in soil or honey products. The spores germinate into bacteria that colonize the bowel and synthesize toxin. As the toxin is absorbed, it irreversibly binds to acetylcholine receptors on motor nerve terminals at neuromuscular junctions. The infant with botulism becomes progressively weak, hypotonic, and hyporeflexic, showing bulbar and spinal nerve abnormalities. Presenting symptoms include constipation, lethargy, a weak cry, poor feeding, and dehydration. A high index of suspicion for the diagnosis of botulism and prompt treatment of infant botulism are important, because this disease can quickly progress to respiratory failure (54).

Ciguatera toxin may initially (2–6 hours) cause nausea, vomiting, diarrhea, and abdominal pain, followed by the onset of paresthesia, weakness, and/or reversal of hot or cold among other neurologic symptoms that can progress to cardiovascular abnormalities in 2 to 5 days. Occasionally long-term complications may develop (55). Ciguatera toxin disease is associated with consumption of large reef fish such as grouper, red snapper, Amber jack, and barracuda contaminated by their consumption of algal blooms containing dinoflagellates, which produce the heat-stable ciguatoxin that becomes concentrated as it moves up the food chain (56).

Scombroid occurs within minutes to hours of consumption of certain fish, or occasionally cheese, in which there has been a buildup of biogenic amines, especially histamine (57). Patients

TABLE 67.8.   Items that Patients Should Be Specifically Questioned about in the Context of a Potential Exposure that May Link to Specific Food-borne Pathogens

Item	Commonly associated microbes[a]
Raw seafood	Norwalk-like virus, *Vibrio* species, hepatitis A
Raw eggs	*Salmonella*
Undercooked meat or poultry	*Salmonella, Campylobacter,* STEC, *Clostridium perfringens*
Unpasteurized milk or juice	*Salmonella, Campylobacter,* STEC, *Yersinia*
Unpasteurized soft cheeses	*Salmonella, Campylobacter,* STEC, *Yersinia, Listeria*
Home made canned goods	Botulism *(Clostridium botulinum)*
Raw hot dogs, deli meat	*Listeria*
Sprouts	*Salmonella,* STEC

[a]This association lists the commonly associated organisms and is not fully comprehensive.
STEC, Shiga toxin–producing *Escherichia coli.*

complain of flushing, burning sensation, urticaria, dizziness, and paresthesia after consumption of certain types of fish that typically are either blue fish, tuna, mackerel, marlin, or mahi mahi.

Shellfish may also contain toxins that fall into three groups (diarrheic, neurotoxic, and amnesic) that cause various symptoms as their names imply. Symptoms usually occur within 30 minutes to several hours after exposure. A variety of mushroom toxins result in a mixture of GI tract and neurologic disturbances including hallucinations and confusion. Tetrodotoxin from puffer fish causes a rapid onset (less than 30 minutes) of neurologic, respiratory tract, and cardiac complications that are usually fatal. Taking a food history is key if tetrodotoxin is in the differential diagnosis.

Of the parasites, *T. gondii* is responsible for a significant number of deaths in the United States (2). It is usually ingested from the accidental contamination of food with the parasite oocytes from cat litter boxes, the garden, or undercooked hamburger (steak tartar). It is often asymptomatic in normal hosts but may be deadly in the immunocompromised patient with pneumonitis, myocarditis, and neurologic symptoms. It is on occasion transferred vertically from mother to child during pregnancy, leading to congenital toxoplasmosis.

LINKING THE DIAGNOSIS WITH A POSSIBLE EXPOSURE

Patients who have acute gastroenteritis with nausea, vomiting, diarrhea, and abdominal pain will often arrive at the physician having decided they have a food-borne disease and with a clear idea of what they think is the cause. Often a patient will consider their malady to be due to the last thing they ate before the onset of symptoms. Clearly, however, there is a need to go further back in the food history. Overall, a number of valuable pieces of information can be gleaned from taking a food history from the patient. Although it is generally not practical to go back more than 72 hours, it is helpful to ask about specific exposures. Not only can this help the physician narrow down the cause of the patient's symptoms (e.g., did they eat raw oysters in the last few days?), but it may also yield useful epidemiologic information that public health departments can use to identify the causes of outbreaks and thus issue warnings or work with federal agencies to initiate recalls. In the previous sections of this chapter, a number of specific foods have been alluded to in relation to specific pathogens. Clearly, it is possible to contaminate almost any type of food with almost any type of microbe. Yet there are a number of well-established links between certain types of food and certain microbes. Several of the major ones are summarized

in Table 67.8, which can be used as a quick reference to cover the principle food-borne exposures.

PREVENTION

The watchword for food safety is *prevention,* because essentially all food-borne disease may be considered preventable, although in practice there will always be situations in which the unexpected happens, such as a failure in processing that goes undetected. Despite these unexpected situations, there is a great deal that manufacturers and consumers can do to safeguard themselves against food-borne disease. There is a large volume of information available on the Internet from various federal agencies including the CDC, the USDA, and the FDA relating to food safety and how to best protect one's self from illness. It is therefore not necessary here to go into this in great detail, save to focus on a few important points.

It is now very clear that certain groups are especially susceptible to food-borne disease. Generally these groups are those with compromised immune responses, whether this be because of age (very young or elderly), underlying chronic disease (e.g., diabetes), other infections (e.g., human immunodeficiency virus), as a consequence of therapy (e.g., immunosuppressives posttransplantation), physiologic (pregnancy), genetic, or some other cause is immaterial. The basic message is the same. It is important to prevent cross-contamination between raw potentially contaminated products and ready-to-eat products that will not be further thermally processed. It is important to cook food adequately. It is important to keep appropriate products in the refrigerator to prevent bacterial growth, although there are some classic exceptions to this, such as with *L. monocytogenes* that will continue to grow at refrigeration temperatures. Thus, in the case of *L. monocytogenes,* there are a number of separate and important preventive strategies one should adopt if one falls into a high-risk group: (a) not eating hot dogs and luncheon meats, unless they are reheated until steaming hot; (b) not eating soft cheeses such as Feta, brie, and camembert cheeses, blue-veined cheeses, and Mexican-style cheeses such as "queso blanco fresco;" (c) not eating refrigerated pates or meat spreads, although canned or shelf-stable pates and meat spreads may be eaten; (d) not eating refrigerated smoked seafood, unless it is contained in a cooked dish, such as a casserole; (e) not drinking unpasteurized milk or eating foods that contain unpasteurized milk.

Preventing spread of food-borne pathogens to others through education and informing public health authorities is also an important function of the health care professional treating a patient with a food-borne disease. There are numerous examples of person-to-person spread of food-borne pathogens within families, nursing homes, and schools. Education of infected patients is an important part of preventing this type of spread.

CONCLUSION

This chapter has reviewed some of the latest trends in food-borne disease and attempted to group the myriad agents that may cause food-borne disease into symptom-related groups. Many food-borne diseases are transient, self-limiting, and of little consequence other than social inconvenience. Yet some food-borne diseases are clearly life threatening and may have significant long-term consequences. In many cases, all that is required is supportive care and rehydration. It is important to pay close attention to both the clinical status and the causative agent before prescribing antibiotics for what is perceived to be "infectious gastroenteritis;" sometimes antibiotic therapy may do more harm than good. Though unusual, infection with some food-borne agents such as botulism, *L. monocytogenes*, or *V. vulnificus* can be rapidly life threatening, and speedy therapy may be life saving. Maintaining an open mind in relation to the plethora of presentations of food-borne disease and remembering to ask about food exposures are both key elements in the diagnosis and treatment of food-borne disease. The field of food safety is constantly changing as old pathogens are better controlled and new threats such as antibiotic resistance, transmissible spongiform encephalopathies, and an increasingly susceptible population emerge. Finally, prevention is a critical part of food safety. This involves education on how to prepare, handle, and maybe even avoid certain types of food. Health care professionals have a duty to inform their high-risk patients of what types of food to avoid, for example, avoiding foods likely to be contaminated with *L. monocytogenes* in pregnant women. Keeping an open mind about the variety of clinical presentations and remembering that all food-borne disease is essentially preventable is key in ensuring food safety.

REFERENCES

1. Bell BP, Goldoft M, Griffin PM, et al. A multistate outbreak of *Escherichia coli* O157:H7–associated bloody diarrhea and hemolytic uremic syndrome from hamburgers. The Washington experience. *JAMA* 1994;272:1349–1354.
2. Mead PS, Slutsker L, Dietz V, et al. Food-related illness and death in the United States. *Emerg Infect Dis* 1999;5:607–625.
3. Centers for Disease Control and Prevention. FoodNet surveillance report for 2000. Available at: *www.cdc.gov/foodnet/annuals.htm.*
4. Preliminary FoodNet data on the incidence of foodborne illnesses—selected sites, United States, 2001. *MMWR Morb Mortal Wkly Rep* 2002;51:325–329.
5. Surveillance for foodborne disease outbreaks—United States, 1993–1997. *MMWR Morb Mortal Wkly Rep* 2000;49:1–51.
6. Avery SM, Liebana E, Reid CA, et al. Combined use of two genetic fingerprinting methods, pulsed-field gel electrophoresis and ribotyping, for characterization of *Escherichia coli* O157 isolates from food animals, retail meats, and cases of human disease. *J Clin Microbiol* 2002;40:2806–2812.
7. Liang P. A decade of differential display. *Biotechniques* 2002;33:338–344.
8. Swaminathan B, Barrett TJ, Hunter SB, et al, and the CDC PulseNet Task Force. PulseNet: the molecular subtyping network for foodborne bacterial disease surveillance, United States. *Emerg Infect Dis* 2001;7:382–389.
9. Multistate outbreak of *Escherichia coli* O157:H7 infections associated with eating ground beef—United States, June–July 2002. *MMWR Morb Mortal Wkly Rep* 2002;51:637–639.
10. Centers for Disease Control and Prevention. Diagnosis and management of food borne illness, a primer for physicians. *MMWR Morb Mortal Wkly Rep* 2001;50:RR-2.
11. Balaban N, Rasooly A. Staphylococcal enterotoxins. *Int J Food Microbiol* 2000;61:1–10.
12. Bergdol MS, Crass BA, Reiser RF, et al. A new staphylococcal enterotoxin, enterotoxin F, associated with toxic shock syndrome *Staphylococcus aureus* isolates. *Lancet* 1981;1:1017.
13. Bergdol MS. The enterotoxins. In: Cohen JO, ed. *The staphylococci.* New York: Wiley, 1972:301–321.
14. Granum PE. *Bacillus cereus* and its toxins. *J Appl Bacteriol* 1994;23[Suppl]:61S–66S.
15. Drobniewski FA. *Bacillus cereus* and related species. *Clin Microbiol Rev* 1993;6:324–338.
16. Mahler H, Pasi A, Kramer JM, et al. Fulminant liver failure in association with the emetic toxin of *Bacillus cereus. N Engl J Med* 1997;336:1142–1148.
17. Ghelardi E, Celandroni F, Salvetti S, et al. Identification and characterization of toxigenic *Bacillus cereus* isolates responsible for two food-poisoning outbreaks. *FEMS Microbiol Lett* 2002;208(1):129–134.
18. Terranova W, Blake PA. *Bacillus cereus* food poisoning. *N Engl J Med* 1978;298:143–144.
19. Becker KM, Moe CL, Southwick KL, et al. Transmission of Norwalk virus during football game. *N Engl J Med* 2000;26:1223–1227.
20. Holtby I, Tebbutt GM, Green J, et al. Outbreak of Norwalk-like virus infection associated with salad provided in a restaurant. *Commun Dis Public Health* 2001;4(4):305–310.
21. Semple AB, Parry WH, Phillips DE. Acute copper poisoning: an outbreak traced to contaminated water from a corroded geyser. *Lancet* 1960;2:700.
22. Brown MA, Thom JV, Orth GL, et al. Food poisoning involving zinc contamination. *Arch Environ Health* 1964;8:657.
23. Baker TD, Hafner WG. Cadmium poisoning from a refrigerator shelf used as an improvised barbecue grill. *Public Health Rep* 1961;76:543.
24. Shandera WX, Tacket CO, Blake PA. Food poisoning due to *Clostridium perfringens* in the United States. *J Infect Dis* 1983;147:167–170.
25. Chowdhury NR, Chakraborty S, Ramamurthy T, et al. Molecular evidence of clonal *Vibrio parahaemolyticus* pandemic strains. *Emerg Infect Dis* 2000;6:631–636.
26. Bresee JS, Widdowson MA, Monroe SS, et al. Foodborne viral gastroenteritis: challenges and opportunities. *Clin Infect Dis* 2002;35(6):748–753.
27. Slifko TR, Smith HV, Rose JB. Emerging parasite zoonoses associated with water and food. *Int J Parasitol* 2000;30:1379–1393.
28. Mosier DA, Oberst RD. Cryptosporidiosis. A global challenge. *Ann N Y Acad Sci* 2000;916:102–111.
29. MacKenzie WR, Schell WL, Blair KA, et al. A massive outbreak in Milwaukee of *Cryptosporidium* infection transmitted through the public water supply. *N Engl J Med* 1994;331:161–167.
30. Quiroz ES, Bern C, MacArthur JR, et al. An outbreak of cryptosporidiosis linked to a food handler. *J Infect Dis* 2000;181(2):695–700.
31. Sterling CR, Ortega YR. Unraveling *Cyclospora:* an enigma worth. *Emerg Infect Dis* 1999;5:48–53.
32. Ortega YR, Nagle R, Gilman RH, et al. Pathologic and clinical findings in patients with cyclosporiasis and a description of intracellular parasite life-cycle stages. *J Infect Dis* 1997;176:1584–1589.
33. Ortega YR, Sterling CR, Gilman RH, et al. *Cyclospora* species—a new protozoan pathogen of humans. *N Engl J Med* 1993;328:1308–1312.
34. Ortega YR, Sterling CR, Gilman RH. A new coccidian parasite (Apicomplexa:Eimeriidae) from humans. *J Parasitol* 1994;80:625–629.
35. Ho AY, Lopez AS, Eberhart MG, et al. Outbreak of cyclosporiasis associated with imported raspberries, Philadelphia, Pennsylvania, 2000. *Emerg Infect Dis* 2002;8(8):783–788.
36. Lopez AS, Dodson DR, Arrowood MJ, et al. Outbreak of cyclosporiasis associated with basil in Missouri in 1999. *Clin Infect Dis* 2001;32:1010–1017.
37. Guerrant RL, Van Gilder T, Steiner TS, et al. Practice and guidelines for the management of infectious diarrhea. *Clin Infect Dis* 2001;32:331–350.
38. Hohmann EL. Nontyphoidal salmonellosis. *Clin Infect Dis.* 2001;32:263–269.
39. Zansky S, Wallace B, Schoonmaker-Bopp D, et al, and the Centers for Disease Control and Prevention. Outbreak of multi-drug resistant *Salmonella* Newport—United States, January–April 2002. *JAMA* 2002;288(8):951–953.
40. Barza M, Gorbach SB eds. The need to improve antimicrobial use in agriculture. *Clin Infect Dis,* 2002 34 supp 3 S71–S144.
41. Kramer JM, Frost JA, Bolton FJ, Wareing DR. Campylobacter contamination of raw meat and poultry at retail sale: identification of multiple types and comparison with isolates from human infection. *J Food Protect* 2000;63:1654–1659.
42. Nataro JP, Kaper JB. Diarrheagenic *Escherichia coli. Clin. Microbiol. Rev.* 1998;11:142–201.
43. Paton JC, Paton AW. Pathogenesis and diagnosis of Shiga toxin–producing *Escherichia coli* infections. *Clin Microbiol Rev* 1998;11:450–479.
44. Fey PD, Wicket RS, Rupp ME, et al. Prevalence of non-O157:H7 Shiga toxin–producing *Escherichia coli* in diarrheal stool samples in Nebraska. *Emerg Infect Dis* 2000;6:530–533.
45. *Escherichia coli* O111:H8 outbreak among teenage campers—Texas, 1999. *MMWR Morb Mortal Wkly Rep* 2000;49:321–324.
46. Kehl KS, Havens P, Behnke CE, et al. Evaluation of the premier EHEC assay for detection of Shiga toxin–producing *Escherichia coli. J Clin Microbiol* 1997;35:2051–2054.
47. Wong CS, Jelacic S, Habeeb RL, et al. The risk of the hemolytic-uremic syndrome after antibiotic treatment of *Escherichia coli* O157:H7 infections. *N Engl J Med* 2000;342(26):1930–1936.
48. Safdar N, Said A, Gangnon RE, et al. Risk of hemolytic uremic syndrome after antibiotic treatment of *Escherichia coli* O157:H7 enteritis: a meta-analysis. *JAMA* 2002;288(8):996–1001.

49. Zhang X, McDaniel AD, Wolf LE, et al. Quinolone antibiotic induces Shiga toxin–encoding bacteriophages, toxin production and death in mice. *J Infect Dis* 2000;181:664–670.
50. Molbak K, Mead PS, Griffin PM. Antimicrobial therapy in patients with *Escherichia coli* O157:H7 infection. *JAMA* 2002;288(8):1014–1016.
51. Food poisoning, fatal-China (Nanjing). A ProMED-mail post; September 18, 2002; no. 20020918.5347. Available at: *www.promedmail.org.*
52. Dalton CB, Austin CC, Sobel J, et al. An outbreak of gastroenteritis and fever due to *Listeria monocytogenes* in milk. *N Engl J Med* 1997;336(2):100–105.
53. Neill MA, Carpenter CCJ. Other pathogenic vibrios. In: Mandell GL, Bennett JE, Dolin R, eds. *Principles and practice of infectious diseases.* Philadelphia: Churchill Livingstone, 2000:2272–2276.
54. Cox N, Hinkle R. Infant botulism. *Am Fam Physician* 2002;65(7):1388–1392.
55. Farstad DJ, Chow T. A brief case report and review of ciguatera poisoning. *Wilderness Environ Med* 2001;12:263–269.
56. Lewis RJ. The changing face of ciguatera. *Toxicon* 2001;39(1):97–106.
57. Lehane L, Olley J. Histamine fish poisoning revisited. *Int J Food Microbiol* 2000;58(1-2):1–37.

CHAPTER 68
Salmonella *Infections*

Arthur Y. Kim, Marcia B. Goldberg, and Robert H. Rubin

The genus *Salmonella* includes approximately 2,500 serovars, which are capable of infecting a wide array of hosts, ranging from humans and domestic animals to reptiles, birds, and insects. With the important exception of *Salmonella typhi* and *Salmonella paratyphi*, for which there are no zoonotic reservoirs, the various salmonellae are almost ubiquitous as both commensals and pathogens in the animal kingdom. Those that are pathogens cause various clinical syndromes in both animals and humans (1).

Salmonellae are facultative anaerobic gram-negative bacilli that generally express peritrichous flagella, which make them motile (2). The genus *Salmonella*, which is classified within the family Enterobacteriaceae, was named in honor of D. E. Salmon, an American veterinarian who first isolated *Salmonella choleraesuis* from pigs with hog cholera in 1884 (3). *S. typhi*, the causative agent of typhoid fever, was discovered in the mesenteric nodes and spleens of persons dying of typhoid fever in 1880 by Eberth and was first cultured in 1884 by Gaffky (4).

The nomenclature and classification of salmonellae have been changed and restructured over the years. Traditionally, *Salmonella* species were named in accordance with the Kaufmann-White typing system, defined by surface antigens, resulting in more than 2,000 different species names. Recently, all salmonellae have been reclassified into two species, *Salmonella enterica* and *Salmonella bongori*, with the serologically defined names appended as serovars or serotypes. For instance, the current nomenclature of *S. typhi* is *S. enterica* serovar *typhi*. *S. enterica* is preferred over the confusing name *S. choleraesuis*, which is also the name of a commonly isolated serotype (5). *S. bongori* consists of approximately 17 serotypes that are rarely isolated from people or animals; it is believed to be a progenitor of *S. enterica*. (6). This chapter refers to the various *Salmonella* serovars by the conventional, albeit less stringent, system used in the literature. For a more detailed discussion of the taxonomy, microbiology, and molecular pathogenesis of this important group of organisms, the reader is directed to Chapter 196. The scope of this chapter includes the epidemiology, clinical syndromes, diagnosis, and management of both typhoidal and nontyphoidal *Salmonella* infection.

EPIDEMIOLOGY

Typhoid Fever

Improvements in sanitation, quality of water supplies, and food hygiene since the 1920s have dramatically decreased the prevalence of typhoid fever in the United States (Fig. 68.1). In 1920, there were 35,994 cases of typhoid fever reported. Since 1965, the number of cases per year has seldom exceeded 500 (7). Between 1990 and 1999, a mean of 420 cases and a mean of less than one death per year have been attributed to typhoid fever (8). This trend holds in other industrialized countries as well. It was originally hoped that as carriers slowly died from natural causes and fewer individuals became carriers because of the low prevalence, the incidence of typhoid fever would continue to decrease, leading to eventual eradication of the illness. However, since 1965, the number of reported cases has remained fairly constant, largely because of the importation of the disease by returning tourists, immigrants, and migrant laborers (7).

Because there is no zoonotic reservoir of *S. typhi*, the two principal sources of transmission are patients with acute disease and more commonly chronic carriers. Both patients with acute disease and chronic carriers excrete large numbers of organisms, approximately 1 to 10 billion organisms per gram of stool (1). Carriers are defined as persons who have recovered from the acute illness and continue to shed *S. typhi* for longer than 1 year. In endemic areas, contaminated water is the most common source, whereas in nonendemic areas, food contaminated by a carrier is the most common source.

In endemic areas, the highest attack rates occur in children. In contrast, in the United States, typhoid fever is most prevalent in age-groups most likely to travel to endemic areas. Large-scale outbreaks related to contamination of food or water with *S. typhi* have become rare in the United States; a large proportion of cases are imported. A review of 2,666 cases of acute typhoid fever between 1975 and 1984 revealed that 62% (70% between 1983 and 1984) were acquired through foreign travel. From 1982 to 1984, the countries that contributed the most travel-associated cases were Peru, India, Pakistan, Chile, and Haiti (7). A review of typhoid fever in New York City from 1980 through 1990 revealed a similar trend, with 66% of cases related to foreign travel

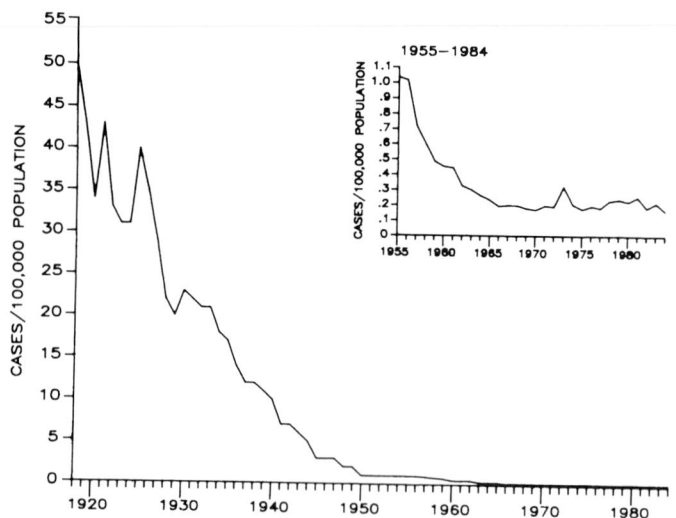

Figure 68.1. Incidence of typhoid fever in the United States, by year, 1918 to 1984. (From Ryan CA, Hargrett-Bean NT, Blake PA. *Salmonella typhi* infections in the United States, 1975–1984: increasing role of foreign travel. *Rev Infect Dis* 1989;11:1–8, with permission.)

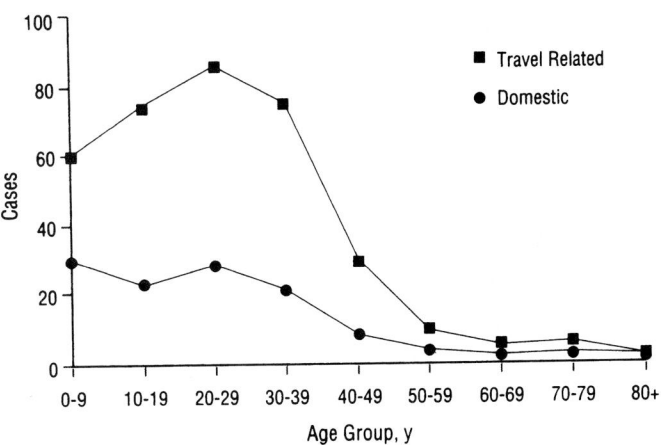

Figure 68.2. Typhoid fever in New York City. Distribution is given by age-group, 1980 through 1990. (From Mathieu JJ, Henning KJ, Bell E, et al. Typhoid fever in New York City, 1980 through 1990. *Arch Intern Med* 1994;154:1713–1718, with permission.)

(9) (Fig. 68.2). Infrequently, microbiology technicians, nurses, nurse's aides, and physicians acquire *S. typhi* through occupational exposure, presumably related to lack of attention to both barrier isolation techniques and proper hand washing. Direct person-to-person transmission is rare, but anal-oral transmission has been described in homosexual men (10). Because of the relatively low incidence of typhoid fever in the United States, there is a paucity of information on the incidence of typhoid fever among

patients with acquired immunodeficiency syndrome (AIDS). In Lima, Peru, where typhoid fever is endemic, the reported rate of *S. typhi* and *S. paratyphi* for individuals infected with human immunodeficiency virus (HIV) is estimated to be approximately 60 times that of the general population (11).

Nontyphoidal Salmonellosis

The incidence of human nontyphoidal salmonellosis in the United States steadily increased from 1955 to 1985. Since then, with the exception of 1985, when the largest food-borne outbreak ever reported to the Centers for Disease Control and Prevention (CDC) occurred, the reported incidence of nontyphoidal salmonellosis has remained fairly constant, with an average of 45,566 cases per year (8) (Fig. 68.3). Reported cases, which are tabulated primarily in outbreak investigations, are thought to represent only 1% of the actual number of nontyphoidal *Salmonella* infections; the total number is estimated to be between 1 and 4 million per year (12). The average number of deaths attributed to nontyphoidal salmonellosis annually from 1989 to 1998 was 54.8. In the United States, *Salmonella* infections account for approximately 30% of deaths resulting from food-borne illness (13).

There is a marked seasonal variation in the occurrence of nontyphoidal *Salmonella* infections; peak incidence occurs in summer and fall, due to many small outbreaks of contaminated food, often associated with picnics and other outdoor eating. The highest rates of nontyphoidal *Salmonella* infections are in children younger than 5 years, particularly infants; rates in

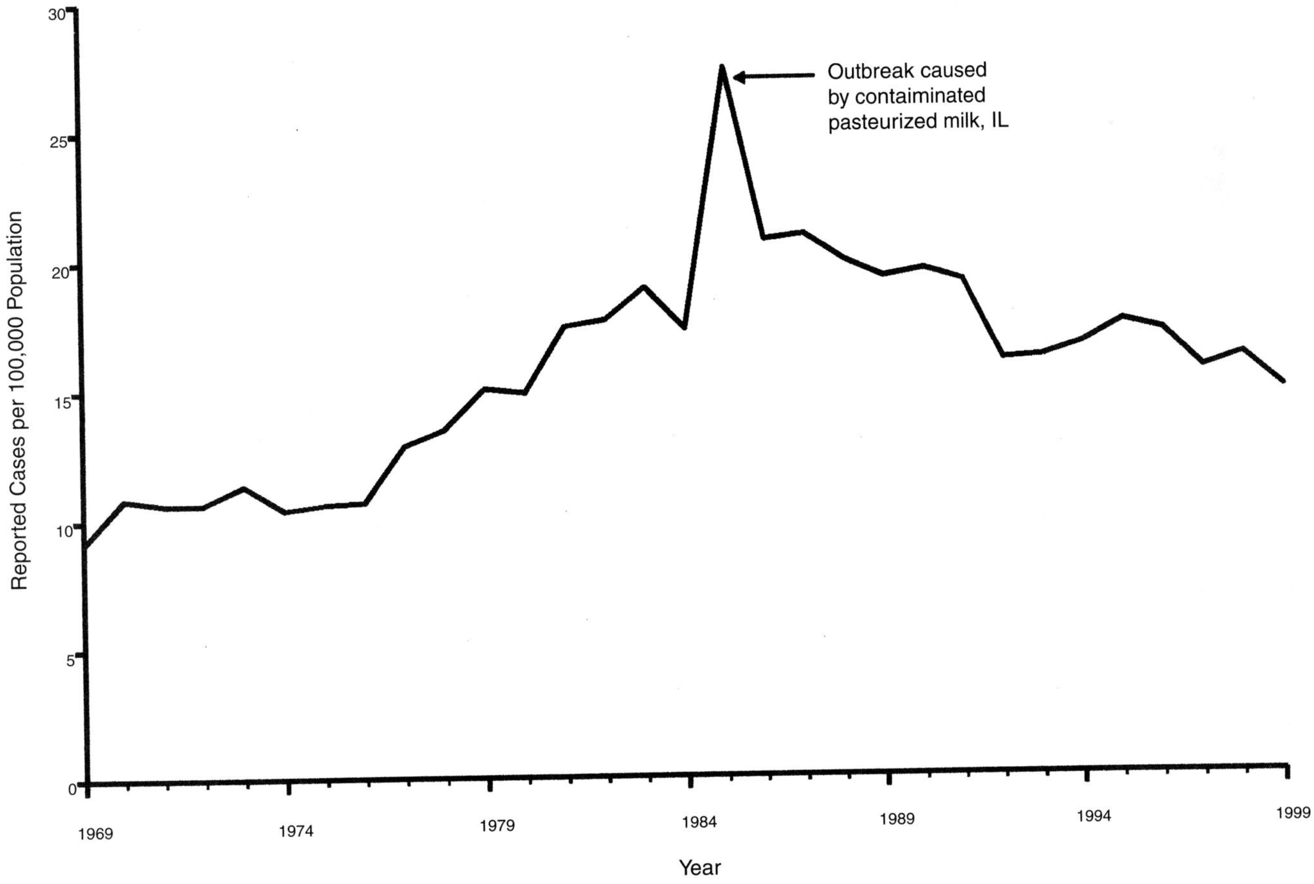

Figure 68.3. Nontyphoidal salmonellosis in the United States, by year, 1969 to 1999. (From Centers for Disease Control and Prevention. Summary of notifiable diseases, United States—1999. *MMWR Morb Mortal Wkly Rep* 2001;48:1, with permission.)

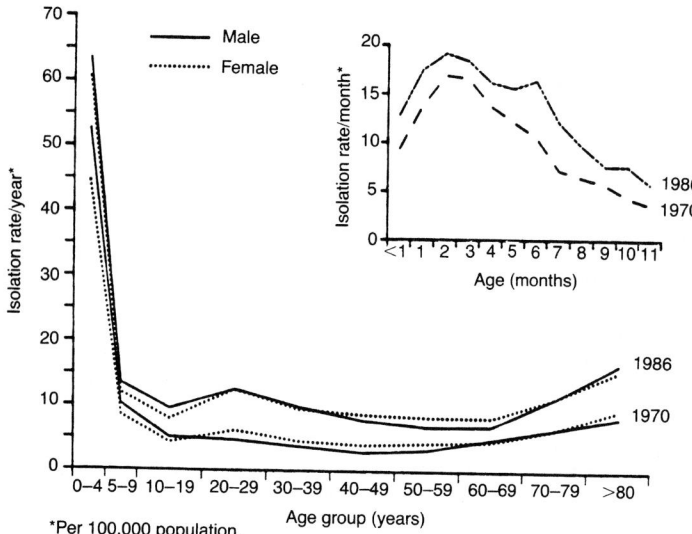

Figure 68.4. *Salmonella* isolation rates in the United States, by age and gender of patient and by year, 1970 and 1986. (From Hargrett-Bean NT, Pavia AT, Tauxe RV. *Salmonella* isolates from humans in the United States, 1984–1986. *MMWR CDC Surveill Summ* 1988;2:25–31, with permission.)

persons 20 to 40 years old and in persons older than 70 years are also slightly higher than those in the general population (14) (Fig. 68.4).

In contrast to the limited species tropism of *S. typhi*, which only causes disease in humans, nontyphoidal *Salmonella* infections are widely distributed among different animal species. A wide variety of agricultural products, processed foods, and domestic animals have been vectors in *Salmonella* outbreaks. Chicken, egg products, beef, turkey, and pork are responsible for the largest proportion of *Salmonella* cases that have an identified origin (15). The most common isolates in human infections (Table 68.1) closely resemble those isolated from these animal sources (16). In addition to consumption of eggs, poultry, and dairy products, consumption of items such as chocolate, fruit,

TABLE 68.1. *Salmonella* **Isolates from Human Infections, United States, 1997**

Serotype	Isolates	
	No.	% of total
Salmonella typhimurium	9,116	26.3
Salmonella enteritidis	7,924	22.9
Salmonella heidelberg	2,104	6.1
Salmonella newport	1,584	4.6
Salmonella agona	739	2.1
Salmonella montevideo	718	2.1
Salmonella thompson	695	2.0
Salmonella javiana	675	1.9
Salmonella infantis	651	1.9
Salmonella hadar	643	1.9
Salmonella oranienberg	623	1.8
Other	9,136	26.4
Total	34,608	100.0

Source: From Olsen SJ, Bishop R, Brenner FW, et al. The changing epidemiology of *Salmonella:* trends in serotypes isolated from humans in the United States, 1987–1997. *J Infect Dis* 2001;183:753, with permission.

TABLE 68.2. **Recommendations for Preventing Transmission of *Salmonella* from Reptiles to Humans**

- Pet-store owners, veterinarians, and pediatricians should provide information to owners and potential purchasers of reptiles about the risk for acquiring salmonellosis from reptiles.
- Persons should always wash their hands thoroughly with soap and water after handling reptiles or reptile cages.
- Persons at increased risk of infection or serious complications of salmonellosis (e.g., children aged <5 years and immunocompromised persons) should avoid contact with reptiles.
- Pet reptiles should be kept out of households where children aged <5 years or immunocompromised persons live. Families expecting a new child should remove the pet reptile from the home before the infant arrives.
- Pet reptiles should not be kept in child care centers.
- Pet reptiles should not be allowed to roam freely throughout the home or living area.
- Pet reptiles should be kept out of kitchens and other food-preparation areas to prevent contamination. Kitchen sinks should not be used to bathe reptiles or to wash dishes, cages, or aquariums used by reptiles. If bathtubs are used for these purposes, they should be cleaned thoroughly and disinfected with bleach before use by humans.

Source: From Centers for Disease Control and Prevention. Reptile-associated salmonellosis—selected states, 1996–1998. *MMWR Morb Mortal Wkly Rep* 1999;48:1009, with permission.

rattlesnake meat, kangaroo meat, alfalfa sprouts, and marijuana have been implicated in *Salmonella* outbreaks (17–22). Outbreaks related to ice cream (23) and orange juice (24) have been linked to failure or lack of pasteurization during preparation. Contact with infected pets, such as turtles, iguanas, lizards, snakes, and ducklings, has resulted in *Salmonella* infection, particularly in children and immunocompromised hosts (25–29). Cases associated with reptiles have recently increased in frequency; thus, public health recommendations for children younger than 5 years and immunocompromised hosts currently include avoidance of contact with reptiles (30,31) (Table 68.2).

Following *Campylobacter jejuni, Salmonella* is the second most common pathogenic bacterium isolated from fecal specimens from individuals with diarrhea (32). Yet, *Salmonella* accounts for the vast majority of food-borne outbreaks caused by bacteria that are investigated. Of the 2,751 outbreaks of food-borne illness reported to the CDC from 1993 to 1997, *Salmonella* accounted for 55% of those attributed to bacteria and was the most frequently reported bacterial pathogen in each year. The most commonly reported food preparation practice that contributed to food-borne disease was improper storage or holding temperature. The second most commonly reported practice was inadequate cooking. Delicatessens, cafeterias, and restaurants were the most frequent establishments in which contaminated food was eaten (33).

Since the mid-1980s, egg-borne *Salmonella* infections, largely due to *Salmonella enteritidis*, have become a major health problem in the United States. The annual rate of isolation of *S. enteritidis* reported to the CDC increased sixfold between 1976 and 1996 (34). *S. enteritidis* outbreaks were initially reported in the New England states but have since spread to the remainder of the country (34) (Fig. 68.5). Of the 380 outbreaks of *S. enteritidis* infection occurring in the United States from 1985 to 1991, grade A shell eggs were implicated in 82% (35). In the past, egg-borne salmonellosis was caused by cracked or dirty eggs, but more recent outbreaks have involved intact eggs. Approximately 1 per 10,000 shell eggs contains *S. enteritidis* (36). The organism is known to infect and localize in the ovaries of laying hens;

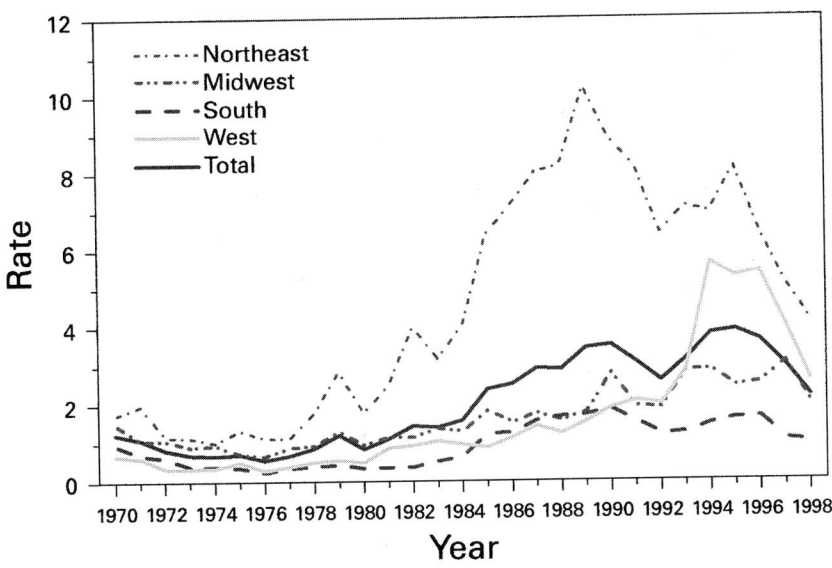

Figure 68.5. Rate of isolation of *Salmonella* serotype *enteritidis*, by region and year, United States, 1970–1988. Rates are per 100,000 population. *Northeast* = Connecticut, Main, Massachusetts, New Hampshire, New Jersey, New York, Pennsylvania, Rhode Island, and Vermont; *Midwest* = Illinois, Indiana, Iowa, Kansas, Michigan, Minnesota, Missouri, Nebraska, North Dakota, Ohio, South Dakota, and Wisconsin; *South* = Alabama, Arkansas, Delaware, District of Columbia, Florida, Georgia, Kentucky, Louisiana, Maryland, Mississippi, North Carolina, Oklahoma, South Carolina, Tennessee, Texas, Virginia, and West Virginia; *West* = Alaska, Arizona, California, Colorado, Hawaii, Idaho, Montana, Nevada, New Mexico, Oregon, Utah, Washington, and Wyoming. (From Centers for Disease Control and Prevention. Outbreaks of *Salmonella* serotype *enteritidis* infection associated with eating raw or undercooked shell eggs—United States, 1996–1998. *MMWR Morb Mortal Wkly Rep* 2000;49:73, with permission.)

transovarian transmission may be one mode of egg contamination. *Salmonella* species can penetrate and enter an egg through an intact as well as a cracked shell. Similarly, both transovarian and horizontal transmissions can sustain infection in flocks being raised for meat. *Salmonella* are present on a small number of broiler chickens at the time of slaughter, and unsanitary conditions in slaughterhouses allow spread of the bacteria among carcasses (15,37). Strategies that are being explored to combat contamination of chicken include the addition of additives such as propionic acid and lactose to feeds, γ-ray irradiation, quarantine of contaminated birds, development of vaccines for chickens, and introduction of nonpathogenic bacteria to make chickens more resistant to colonization with *Salmonella* (15,38–40). Reported multistate outbreaks of food contaminated with *S. enteritidis* illustrate the persistence of this problem (41).

Mass production and wide geographic distribution of foodstuffs can greatly increase the scope and extent of a *Salmonella* outbreak. In particular, contamination of processing equipment, conveyor belts, and other machinery associated with mass processing of foodstuffs can markedly amplify the outbreak (1). A prime example of this is a 1985 *Salmonella typhimurium* epidemic that affected more than 16,000 persons in a six-state area of the midwestern United States. In this epidemic, contamination of valves through which huge volumes of raw milk passed resulted in secondary infection of previously sterile milk with the epidemic strain. Because the dairy supplied the contaminated milk to large population centers throughout the Midwest, a major epidemic ensued (42).

Since the source of most nontyphoidal *Salmonella* infection in humans is animals raised for food, animal husbandry practices have a significant impact on human disease. For example, feeding domestic animals *Salmonella*-contaminated fishmeal or other contaminated feeds has resulted in widespread infection both in domestic animals and in the humans who consume these animals (43,44). In addition, the use of subtherapeutic concentrations of antibiotics as nonspecific growth factors added to the feed has been shown to foster development of antibiotic-resistant strains of *Salmonella* that can ultimately cause human disease (45).

When such agricultural practices are combined with the selective pressures of antibiotic use in humans and the propensity of salmonellae to acquire plasmids that carry genes that mediate antibiotic resistance, it is not surprising that antibiotic resistance is common among these bacteria. Since the mid-1980s, there has

been a significant increase in the frequency of infection caused by antimicrobial-resistant *Salmonella* in the United States (Fig. 68.6). Moreover, organisms isolated from patients have been resistant to a wide range of antimicrobial agents (46) (Table 68.3).

Of primary concern is the worldwide emergence of plasmid-mediated resistance in strains that exhibit drug resistance to multiple major antibiotics. The isolate of *S. typhimurium* known as definitive type 104 (DT104) has emerged during the past decade and is resistant to ampicillin, chloramphenicol, streptomycin, tetracycline, and sulfonamides. In the western United States, this resistance pattern is found in more than 40% of *S. typhimurium* isolates (47) (Fig. 68.7). Ominously, the DT104 strain also can demonstrate resistance to nalidixic acid and reduced susceptibility to fluoroquinolones (48). Patients with resistant isolates are more likely to have a history of travel to the developing world and to have severe manifestations of *Salmonella* infection, such as bacteremia, and thus require hospitalization (46,49–51).

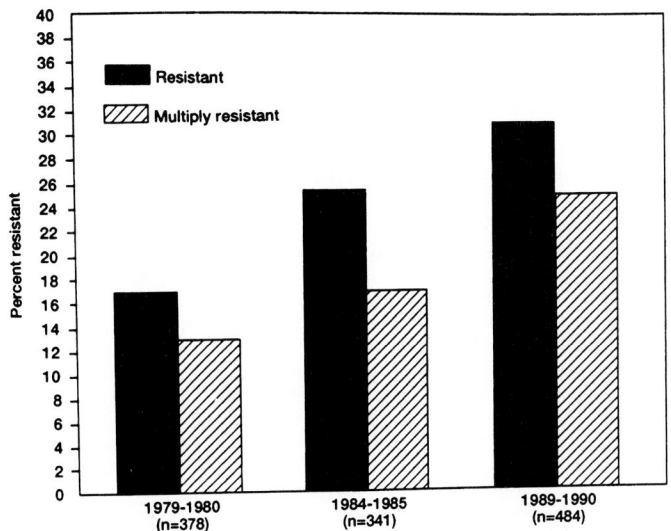

Figure 68.6. Percentage of patients in the United States with resistant *Salmonella* infections from 1979 to 1980, from 1984 to 1985, and from 1989 to 1990. (From Lee LA, Puhr ND, Maloney EK, et al. Increase in antimicrobial-resistant *Salmonella* infections in the United States, 1989–1990. *J Infect Dis* 1994;170:128–134, with permission.)

TABLE 68.3.   Number (Percentage) of Antibiotic Resistant *Salmonella* Organisms Isolated During Three Periods of Study

Antimicrobial agent	1979–1980 (n = 378)	1984–1985 (n = 341)	1989–1990 (n = 484)
Streptomycin	47 (12)	45 (13)	112 (23)
Tetracycline	33 (9)	52 (15)	114 (24)
Ampicillin	36 (10)	35 (10)	70 (14)
Sulfisoxazole	31 (8)	25 (7)	68 (14)
Kanamycin	15 (4)	17 (5)	38 (8)
Gentamicin	0	3 (1)	20 (4)
Chloramphenicol	4 (1)	9 (3)	14 (3)
Nitrofurantoin	5 (1)	13 (4)	7 (1)
Trimethoprim-sulfamethoxazole	0	2 (1)	2
Cephalothin	6 (2)	4 (1)	1
Nalidixic acid	0	5 (1)	1
Colistin	0	2 (1)	0

Source: From Lee LA, Puhr ND, Maloney EK, et al. Increase in antimicrobial-resistant *Salmonella* infections in the United States, 1989–1990. *J Infect Dis* 1994;170:128, with permission.

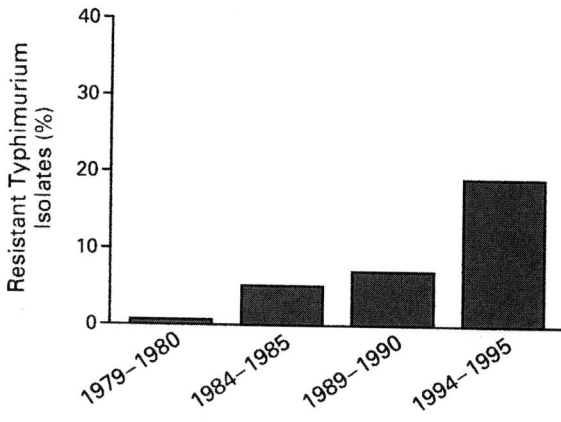

Figure 68.7. Prevalence of resistance to ampicillin, chloramphenicol, streptomycin, sulfonamides, and tetracycline among *S. typhimurium* isolates identified by surveys of antimicrobial drug resistance in sentinel counties. (From Glynn MK, Bopp C, Dewitt W, et al. Emergence of multidrug-resistant *Salmonella enterica* serotype *typhimurium* DT104 infections in the United States. *N Engl J Med* 1998;338:1333, with permission.)

Resistance to fluoroquinolones and third-generation cephalosporins remains rare among *Salmonella* isolates from the United States; however, the rapid increase in use of these agents in both humans and livestock has translated into a rise in infections caused by isolates resistant to these agents (52–54). A case-control analysis of an outbreak of nosocomial quinolone-resistant *S. schwartzgrund* revealed that patients were much more likely to have received fluoroquinolones during the 6 months before developing disease (55). A ceftriaxone-resistant isolate from a 12-year-old boy was found to be indistinguishable from an isolate found in the source cattle herd (56). Prevention of resistance in *Salmonella* species will require both a reduction in unnecessary use of these classes of antibiotics in people and a ban of their subtherapeutic use in livestock feed (57).

Because of the frequent presence of salmonellae in our food sources, it is important to emphasize that despite at times heroic public health measures, the major defense against human infection is appropriate food-handling and cooking practices. Cooking food to temperatures higher than 70°C for longer than 12 minutes decreases the risk of salmonellosis. Because salmonellae have been shown to survive in boiled, fried, and scrambled eggs, particularly if some of the yolk remains liquid, the use of pasteurized eggs has been advocated for individuals in nursing homes and hospitals and for patients with immunodeficiencies (34,58–60). Food safety measures for eggs and egg-containing foods, as outlined by the World Health Organization and the CDC, are listed in Table 68.4 (34,61).

Outbreaks of salmonellosis in nursing homes and hospitals pose a particular threat because the case-fatality rate is much higher in these settings. Of all food-borne disease outbreaks in nursing homes from 1975 to 1987, *Salmonella* was the most frequently reported pathogen, accounting for 52% of outbreaks and 81% of deaths (58). Of the 380 outbreaks of *S. enteritidis* from 1985 to 1991, 59 of those that occurred in nursing homes or hospitals accounted for 90% of all reported deaths. The case-fatality rate

TABLE 68.4.   Food Safety Measures for Eggs and Foods Containing Eggs

- Shell eggs should be refrigerated at ≤45°F (≤7.2°C) during storage.
- Eating raw or undercooked eggs should be avoided, especially by young children, the elderly, and immunocompromised persons.
- If available, eggs already processed for safety (i.e., pasteurized eggs) should be used, particularly in hospitals, nursing homes, food-service establishments, day care centers, elementary schools, and commercial kitchens. Dried egg powder presents a lesser risk of contamination, provided that it is handled properly during storage and after reconstitution.
- Eggs that have not been processed for safety should be cooked until all parts reach a minimum temperature of 70°C (158°F), at which point both the yolk and the white have become firm. Scrambled eggs need to be cooked in small batches until they are firm (not runny) throughout. Boiled eggs, depending on their initial size and temperature, may require a minimum boiling period of 7–9 min so that the yolk becomes firm. Similarly, dishes made with raw eggs should be well cooked.
- Leftovers and foods prepared in advance should be refrigerated at ≤45°F (≤7.2°C). Stored food must be reheated thoroughly before eating so that all parts of the food again reach a minimal temperature of 70°C (158°F).
- Hands, cooking utensils, and food-preparation surfaces should be washed with hot water and soap after contact with raw eggs or foods containing raw eggs.
- Food handlers should wash their hands thoroughly before preparing food, after handling foods likely to be contaminated, including shell eggs, and after every interruption in food preparation, particularly after using the toilet.
- Shell eggs should not be washed. If they are soiled with fecal matter, blood, or some other substance, they may be washed and should be used without delay.
- Cracked eggs are more likely to be contaminated and present a higher health risk.

Source: From Centers for Disease Control and Prevention. Outbreaks of *Salmonella* serotype *enteritidis* infection associated with eating raw or undercooked shell eggs—United States, 1996–8. *MMWR Morb Mortal Wkly Rep* 2000;49:73, and World Health Organization. Food safety measures for eggs and foods containing eggs. *World Health Forum* 1993;14:437, with permission.

in these settings was estimated to be 70 times greater than that in other settings (35).

Several case series have demonstrated that nontyphoidal salmonellosis tends to be more prolonged, severe, and recurrent in patients with immunosuppression such as AIDS (62–65). One review reported a 20-fold increase in the annual incidence of *Salmonella* infections in men with AIDS compared to men without AIDS (66). The proportion of *Salmonella* blood isolates among 25- to 49-year old men in states with a high incidence of AIDS increased by about fourfold from 1978 to 1987 (67). The increased incidence and severity of salmonellosis in patients with AIDS underline the importance of safe food-handling procedures and food counseling in this population (68). Moreover, in patients with prolonged or invasive *Salmonella* infection, clinicians should consider the presence of underlying immunosuppression (69).

From both clinical and public health perspectives, a great deal of emphasis is placed on the full identification of a particular *Salmonella* isolate. Because different *Salmonella* serotypes are more or less likely to produce a particular syndrome, this information is useful in predicting what clinical events are apt to occur. From the public health standpoint, identification of the organism is the primary tool for delineating and tracing epidemics. Such identification includes serotyping and when an outbreak is suspected, the use of molecular epidemiologic techniques, such as plasmid profiles, restriction endonuclease digestion of plasmid and chromosomal DNA, nucleic acid hybridization, and phage typing (70–71). Outbreak detection depends on the complete identification of isolates because major clues to the presence of an outbreak include clustering of cases due to a rare serotype, an unusually large number of isolations of a particular serotype from a defined area, and changes in the normal geographic distribution of a particular serotype. Molecular techniques can then be applied to prove that different isolates of the same serotype are indeed identical and thus likely to emanate from the same source (72). Routine subtyping of isolates using pulsed field gel electrophoresis can rapidly identify outbreaks of a common serotype such as *S. typhimurium* and facilitate timely public health interventions (73)

PATHOGENESIS AND HOST DEFENSES

The likelihood that an organism will cause infection in humans depends on a variety of factors, including the infective dose, the pathogenicity of the organism for humans, and the level of host defenses. After salmonellae are ingested, if they survive the low acidity of the stomach, they progress to the distal small bowel, where they penetrate the epithelial barrier. Ileal M cells are a type of specialized intestinal epithelial cell found overlying Peyer's patches. These cells normally function in antigen sampling by internalizing organisms and small particles from the intestinal lumen and transferring them to underlying macrophages and leukocytes. They may be the primary site of *Salmonella* entry. In enteric fever, salmonellae are transported across M cells in vacuoles and are released by exocytosis at the cellular basal membrane into the lamina propria and lymphatic system, where they gain access to the bloodstream, spleen, liver, and other components of the reticuloendothelial system. Some organisms may reach the liver through the portal circulation. *Salmonella* species that cause gastroenteritis remain localized in the intestinal mucosa (1,74,75). The molecular basis for *Salmonella* virulence is detailed in Chapter 196.

The minimum infective dose of *Salmonella* for humans is imprecisely characterized. Volunteer studies suggested that a large inoculum of salmonellae was necessary to produce infection.

However, in one human volunteer, as few as 25 organisms caused disease. In one review of 12 outbreaks of typhoid fever, the estimated number ingested ranged from 17 organisms to 100 billion organisms, and in more than 50% of the outbreaks, the estimated number ingested was fewer than 1,000 organisms. In addition to the dose, the serotype of the organism is relevant. For example, *Salmonella pullorum*, which is adapted to chickens, produces infection in humans rarely and only when a large number of organisms (more than 1 billion) are ingested. In contrast, *S. typhimurium* and *S. enteritidis* may cause infection in humans with a relatively small number of organisms (76).

Human host resistance to infection from salmonellae can be divided into two general categories: nonspecific host defenses, which are well delineated, and specific host defenses, which are poorly understood. Three nonspecific host defense mechanisms have been identified as protective against *Salmonella* infection: gastric acidity, normal gastrointestinal (GI) tract motility, and normal intestinal flora. Abnormalities in one or more of these mechanisms will result in an increased incidence and severity of clinical disease due to *Salmonella* infections (77,78) (Table 68.5). Salmonellae will generally be killed instantly at a pH level of less than 2 and more slowly at a pH level between 2 and 3 (79). Thus, impairment of gastric acid secretion due to achlorhydria, gastric resection, vagotomy, or administration of antacids, histamine H_2 blockers, or proton pump inhibitors allows salmonellae to escape the bactericidal environment of the stomach. Age has been shown to be an important factor in *Salmonella* infections. Because infants produce little hydrochloric acid and the incidence of achlorhydria is increased in persons older than 60 years, these factors likely contribute to the higher risk of infection within these age groups (79). Rapid gastric emptying may allow bacteria to escape from the stomach into the duodenum. Medication-dependent diabetics have been shown to be at increased risk of *Salmonella* infection, possibly because of reduced gastric acid secretion and motility (80). Finally, abrogation of resistance conferred by normal GI tract flora as a result of treatment with broad-spectrum antibiotics or purgatives or bowel surgery predisposes patients to infection (77). Prior exposure to antimicrobial agents increases the risk of infection with either antimicrobial-sensitive or resistant salmonellae, presumably by changing the GI tract flora (81). In experimental infections with *S. typhi*, treatment with streptomycin before exposure to bacteria reduces the number of organisms necessary to cause disease in both mice and humans (82,83). In this last category, a not uncommon clinical scenario is the transformation of the asymptomatic *Salmonella* carrier state into symptomatic disease after either administration of antibiotics or abdominal surgery.

TABLE 68.5. Conditions that Predispose to *Salmonella* Infection

Decreased gastric acidity (e.g., secondary to antacids, H_2 blockers, H^+,K^+-ATPase inhibitors, or gastric resection)
Decreased gastrointestinal motility (e.g., secondary to opiates)
Alterations of normal intestinal flora (e.g., secondary to broad-spectrum antibiotics, purgatives, or bowel surgery)
Acquired immunodeficiency syndrome
Lymphoproliferative disease
Conditions associated with macrophage dysfunction (hemolysis, bartonellosis, malaria, histoplasmosis)
Inflammatory bowel disease (possible predisposing condition)
Schistosomiasis
Diabetes mellitus

Specific host defenses against salmonellae are incompletely understood. Clinical observations suggest that intracellular killing of these organisms by activated macrophages is of critical importance. Thus, patients with defects of macrophage function, such as those with AIDS or chronic granulomatous disease, are less able to eradicate *Salmonella*. Moreover, illnesses in which macrophage function is disrupted, including sickle cell anemia, other hemoglobinopathies, malaria, bartonellosis, louse-borne relapsing fever, disseminated histoplasmosis, and certain forms of malignancy, are associated with an increased incidence and severity of *Salmonella* infection (84–86). Less information is available about the impact of T-lymphocyte deficiencies and antibody deficiencies on the course of salmonellosis, although severe infections have been reported in transplant recipients and in patients with antibody-deficiency syndromes. In normal hosts, the correlation between protection against *S. typhi* and the levels of specific antibodies to different *Salmonella* antigens is poor. Protection from reinfection after the occurrence of natural infection has been shown to be partial at best (1,87).

CLINICAL MANIFESTATIONS

The clinical manifestations of *Salmonella* infection can be divided into four distinct syndromes, each of which requires a specific diagnostic and therapeutic approach: (a) gastroenteritis, (b) enteric fever, (c) bacteremia with or without metastatic infection, and (d) the asymptomatic carrier state. In addition, there are specific populations, particularly immunocompromised hosts, for which the effects of *Salmonella* infection require special attention. Theoretically, any *Salmonella* serotype can cause any of the clinical syndromes. In fact, certain serotypes are particularly associated with certain constellations of clinical manifestations. For example, *S. newport* and *S. anatum* commonly cause gastroenteritis; *S. typhi*, *S. paratyphi* A, *S. schottmülleri*, and *S. hirschfeldii* (the last three are the paratyphoid strains and were formerly known as *S. paratyphi* A, B, and C, respectively) are the principal causes of enteric fever; and *S. choleraesuis*, although it enters the host through a GI tract portal, rarely causes GI tract manifestations but commonly causes bacteremia or metastatic infection. One organism, *S. typhimurium*, stands out for its propensity to cause the full array of clinical syndromes. In the United States, *S. typhimurium* is the most common cause of gastroenteritis, bacteremia, and the asymptomatic carrier state (87,88) (Table 68.6).

Gastroenteritis

The most commonly recognized clinical syndrome caused by *Salmonella* is gastroenteritis, which can be caused by any serotype. Typically, symptoms of nausea and vomiting begin 8 to 48 hours after exposure to the organism and subside a few hours later. Very soon thereafter, diarrhea and colicky abdominal pain develop, primarily in the periumbilical area and the right lower quadrant. The extent of diarrhea is quite variable, ranging from a few loose stools, to cholera-like profuse watery diarrhea, to dysentery like with bloody slimy stools and associated symptoms of rectal urgency and tenesmus. Similarly, abdominal findings on physical examination can range from very mild to an extreme that suggests acute appendicitis, cholecystitis, or a ruptured viscus. In particular, *Salmonella* gastroenteritis (like bacterial gastroenteritis caused by *Campylobacter jejuni* and *Yersinia enterocolitica*) is an important cause of "pseudoappendicitis," a clinical syndrome that usually occurs in the first two decades of life and closely mimics typical appendicitis. A moderate elevation in temperature (less than 39°C) is present in 50% of patients and usually returns to normal within 1 or 2 days. Patients may complain of chills. Transient bacteremia probably occurs in 1% to 4% of patients. In most situations, it is trivial, but in patients with certain underlying conditions, it is a major concern because of the possibility of metastatic seeding (1,87,89).

Underlying conditions that are associated with more severe gastroenteritis syndromes include advanced age, malnutrition, AIDS, achlorhydria, and inflammatory bowel disease. Each is associated with more severe and prolonged diarrhea and a higher rate of bloodstream invasion with its potential consequences (87).

The diagnosis of *Salmonella* gastroenteritis is based on the history and the stool culture. The diagnosis should be suspected in any patient who presents with a febrile gastroenteritis syndrome, particularly if there is an epidemiologic history that includes eating at a fast-food establishment, the possibility of having ingested inadequately cooked chicken or eggs, or a history of contact with persons with a similar clinical syndrome. Stools of patients with *Salmonella* gastroenteritis are usually not bloody, but they may contain occult blood and a moderate number of polymorphonuclear leukocytes. Mild leukocytosis may be present, but the white blood cell count is most often normal (87). Stool cultures are preferable to rectal swabs, and enrichment broth and media are important for isolation of the organisms (90,91). After resolution of the illness, repeating fecal cultures is generally not recommended because results may be intermittently positive and are of unclear utility (69).

TABLE 68.6.   Summary of Clinical Syndromes of *Salmonella* Infection

Syndrome	Most common causative serotypes	Symptoms and findings
Gastroenteritis	*Salmonella typhimurium* *Salmonella enteritidis* *Salmonella newport* *Salmonella anatum*	Moderate fever, nausea, vomiting, diarrhea, variable abdominal discomfort
Enteric fever	*Salmonella typhi* *Salmonella paratyphi A* *Salmonella schottmuelleri* *Salmonella hirschfeldii*	Prolonged fever, headache, myalgias, nausea, constipation or diarrhea, hypertrophy of reticuloendothelial system, possible metastatic infection, possible immune complex deposition
Bacteremia, with or without metastatic disease	*Salmonella typhimurium* *Salmonella choleraesuis* *Salmonella heidelberg*	Fever, possible nausea, vomiting, possible diarrhea, abdominal discomfort, possible cardiovascular infection, possible metastatic infection
Chronic carrier state	*Salmonella typhimurium*	Asymptomatic

Enteric Fever

Enteric fever is a *Salmonella* infection with multiorgan involvement that is characterized by (a) prolonged fever; (b) sustained bloodstream infection without endothelial or endocardial seeding; (c) profound hypertrophy and activation of the reticuloendothelial system, particularly the intestinal and the mesenteric lymphoid tissue, the liver, and the spleen; and (d) metastatic infection and immunologic complications such as immune complex deposition, leading to multiorgan dysfunction (1,87).

In theory, any *Salmonella* serotype is capable of producing an enteric fever syndrome. In fact, most cases of enteric fever are caused by *S. typhi* and the paratyphoid strains (*S. paratyphi* A, *S. schottmülleri*, and *S. hirschfeldii*). Regardless of the serotype involved, the clinical manifestations of enteric fever are qualitatively identical. However, the disease's severity, mortality rate, relapse rate, duration, and associated incidence of complications are greater in patients infected with *S. typhi* (1,87).

The incubation period of enteric fever depends on the size of the inoculum. It may be as short as 3 days or as long as 60 days, but it is typically 1 to 2 weeks. Approximately 10% of patients experience diarrhea during the first week after exposure. Many individuals who are asymptomatic during this period have transiently positive stool cultures. Fever is usually the earliest indication of disease; it rises in a stepwise fashion over 2 to 3 days up to 39°C to 40°C. Appropriate antibiotic therapy eliminates fever within 3 to 5 days (92). Signs and symptoms associated with enteric fever include fever, chills, myalgias, abdominal pain, headache, rose spots, cough, and sore throat. A comparison of signs and symptoms noted in three large outbreaks of typhoid fever shows that although fever is almost always present, the other findings are quite variable (Table 68.7). Interestingly, symptoms such as sore throat, weakness, myalgias, constipation, and anorexia were apparently more common in patients with typhoid fever during the preantibiotic era (93). Physical examination of the abdomen may reveal some tenderness, distention, hepatomegaly, or splenomegaly. Although relative bradycardia and rose spots are classically associated with enteric fever, they are absent in most patients (94,95).

The clinical syndrome caused by *S. typhi* in infants and young children is often different from that seen in adults. In its severe form, it may present as sepsis, especially in children younger than 2 years. One large 1983 study of 197 infants in Chile during the peak season for typhoid (January to March) revealed that *S. typhi* and *S. paratyphi* can cause a mild self-limited bacteremic illness that was previously often misdiagnosed as a respiratory tract illness or a viral syndrome (96). In addition, in young children, diarrhea is more common than constipation (96,97).

The major complications of enteric fever are perforation of the terminal ileum or proximal colon and hemorrhage from ulcerations in the same area. These complications occur in patients whose disease has progressed for 2 weeks or more. They remain the leading causes of death in patients with typhoid fever. Other complications include psychosis, hepatitis, cholecystitis, pneumonitis, pericarditis, and meningitis. With prompt specific therapy, complications are rare. Relapses occur in up to 10% to 15% of patients treated with ampicillin, chloramphenicol, or trimethoprim-sulfamethoxazole, usually 2 weeks after cessation of therapy. Frequently, the relapse is a self-limited febrile illness, but a few patients may require an additional short course of an antibiotic (83).

Many signs and symptoms can be related to the known toxic and pyrogenic effects of endotoxin (83). It has been postulated that endotoxin in localized sites is responsible for cytotoxic and ischemic damage, which may result in intestinal hemorrhage and perforation. Circulating endotoxin has been demonstrated only in patients infected with *S. typhi* who present with septic shock.

Laboratory test results in patients with enteric fever may reveal leukopenia or leukocytosis, but the leukocyte count is usually normal. Elevations in liver function test results, specifically of aspartate transaminase, alanine transaminase, alkaline phosphatase, and lactate dehydrogenase, may be seen. Examination of the stool often reveals a moderate number of polymorphonuclear leukocytes (1,87).

Definitive diagnosis depends on the isolation of the organism from the patient. Sites commonly cultured include bone marrow aspirate, blood, urine, feces, bile, and rose spots. The yield of culture varies, depending on the site (Table 68.8). Cultures of bone marrow aspirates are the most sensitive, being positive in 90% of cases. They are usually positive more quickly than cultures of other specimens, and unlike with blood cultures, the prior use of antibiotics does not diminish their yield. Blood cultures are positive in approximately 50% to 70% of patients. Stool cultures yield the organism in approximately 90% of patients if numerous samples are cultured. The duodenal string test yields the organism in about 70% of patients but is probably no more reliable than blood cultures. The most sensitive diagnostic approach is a combination of two or more cultures from different sites (98–100).

Several serologic methods have been developed for the detection of *S. typhi* antigens and antibodies. The classic Widal test, a serum agglutination test for *Salmonella* O and H antigens, is still widely used in developing countries. Limitations of the test include poor standardization of the antigens and difficult interpretation in areas endemic for *S. typhi* infection, where baseline antibody titers of the population are unknown (101,102). In addition, vaccine administration, other systemic inflammatory processes, and infection with nontyphoidal strains of *Salmonella* can cause elevations in these antibody levels (1). Other serologic tests include enzyme-linked immunosorbent assay for

TABLE 68.7. Symptoms in Typhoid Fever during Three Periods of Study (Percentage)

Symptoms	1939–1944[a] (n = 360)	1964[b] (n = 507)	1973 (n = 105)
Fever	100	75	93
Headache	90	78	59
Diarrhea	43	37	57
Anorexia	91	NA	39
Abdominal pain	19	35	39
Chills	37	16	37
Vomiting	54	24	35
Cough	86	37	28
Nausea	54	NA	23
Muscle pains	91	25	12
Constipation	79	38	10
Weakness	87	NA	10
Dysuria	3	NA	7
Sore throat	84	NA	6
Dizziness	25	NA	3
Seizures	0	0	1

[a] See reference 93.
[b] See reference 179.
NA, not available.
Source: From Hoffman TA, Ruiz CJ, Counts GW, et al. Waterborne typhoid fever in Dade County, Florida. Clinical and therapeutic evaluation of 105 bacteremic patients. *Am J Med* 1975;59:481–487, with permission.

TABLE 68.8. Yield of Cultures from Various Sites during the Course of Untreated Typhoid Fever

Time course	Incubation period Ingestion ↓	Stage of active invasion Wk 1	Wk 2	Established disease Wk 3	Convalescent period Wk 4 — Wk 5	Period of late focal complications Indefinite
Blood cultures	Negative	←——— 80%–90% ———→			Negative unless continued disease or relapse occurs	
Stool cultures	Transiently positive	Negative	←——— 80% Positive ———→		←— 50% Positive —→	Decreasing incidence of positive cultures with time: 20% at 2 mo 10% at 3 mo 3% at 1 yr
Urine cultures	Negative	Negative	←——— 25% Positive ———→		←— 10% Positive —→	Decreasing incidence of positive cultures
Ancillary cultures	Negative	Negative		Decreasing incidence of positive cultures		
Bone marrow			←— 80%–90% Positive —→			
Rose spot			←— 60% Positive —→			
Wadal test	Negative	←— 20% Positive —→	←— 50% Positive —→		←— 80% Positive ———————→	

immunoglobulins M and G antibodies against *S. typhi* lipopolysaccharide, the coagglutination test, counterimmunoelectrophoresis, and radioimmunoassay (103,104). None of these tests is widely used because of cost or lack of sensitivity, specificity, or rapidity.

Bacteremia and Metastatic Infection

Invasion of the bloodstream by *Salmonella* organisms, whether during transient bacteremia that can occur in the setting of the gastroenteritis syndrome or during the more sustained bacteremia of enteric fever, carries the potential for metastatic infection. Salmonellae have a unique capacity to metastasize, particularly to sites of preexisting structural abnormality. Major sites of concern are cardiovascular lesions, skeletal lesions, malignancies, and the meninges (spread to the meninges is particularly common in infants); however, almost any organ in the body may be affected (105). The serotype that is most predisposed to both sustained bacteremia and metastatic infection is *S. choleraesuis* (106). Because of major improvements in the pork industry, however, human infection with this particular serotype has become much less common, and *S. typhimurium*, *S. enteritidis*, and *S. heidelberg* are now the serotypes most likely to cause this array of clinical problems (1,87,107).

The consequences of *Salmonella* bacteremia depend on several host factors including age and immune status. Children older than 1 year with *Salmonella* bacteremia have a much lower rate of metastatic complication than adults (108–110), whereas neonates and infants younger than 1 year remain more susceptible (111). Immunosuppressed patients with bacteremia secondary to *Salmonella* species infection have a significantly higher rate of relapse and higher mortality (112–113).

CARDIOVASCULAR INFECTIONS

Most critical in a case of *Salmonella* bacteremia is the degree of bacteremia. High-grade bacteremia (defined as more than 50% of three or more cultures of blood drawn over several hours grow the organism) is suggestive of focal intracardiac or intravascular infection. Salmonellae have a unique propensity to localize on abnormal cardiovascular surfaces, particularly atherosclerotic aneurysms, plaques of the aorta and ileofemoral vessels, and abnormal surfaces of the endocardium (89,114). *Salmonella* vascular infections have been reported in the thoracic and abdominal portions of the aorta, the coronary arteries, the peripheral arteries, arteriovenous fistulas, and a Dacron bypass graft. Most

common are abdominal aortic infections, followed by infections of the femoral arteries, the thoracic aorta, and the iliac arteries. Most commonly isolated in *Salmonella* infections of abdominal aortic aneurysms is *S. typhimurium*, followed by *S. choleraesuis* and *S. enteritidis*. Complications include psoas abscess, lumbar vertebral osteomyelitis, aortoduodenal fistula, and rupture (115,116). Because the presentation is usually subacute and may be subtle, Rubin and Weinstein (1) identified five presentations suggestive of cardiovascular infection: (a) a prolonged fever after an episode of gastroenteritis; (b) pain in the back, abdomen, or chest accompanied by *Salmonella* bacteremia; (c) recurrence of *Salmonella* bacteremia during or after adequate therapy; (d) vertebral osteomyelitis or paravertebral masses associated with *Salmonella* bacteremia; and (e) *Salmonella* bacteremia in patients with prosthetic vascular grafts.

The mortality rate of *Salmonella* vascular infection is high; both early surgical intervention and early medical therapy are important. Surgical excision of the infected sites and reconstruction along clean tissue planes, under the coverage of antibiotic therapy, should be performed. Surgery should not be delayed in an attempt to eradicate the infection with antibiotics alone because the mortality rate associated with medical therapy alone is as high as 100%. Even with appropriate surgery, most patients require 6 weeks of antibiotic therapy; patients who are immunosuppressed or at high risk for reinfection or recrudescence may require longer courses of therapy or lifelong suppression. (114,117–119).

Endocarditis caused by salmonellae is rare. Most patients with *Salmonella* endocarditis have preexisting heart disease. Most cases involve the mitral or the aortic valve. However, the incidence of isolated mural endocarditis caused by *Salmonella* infection is relatively high, which underscores the organism's propensity for seeding abnormal surfaces of the endocardium. The most frequent serotypes to cause *Salmonella* endocarditis are *S. choleraesuis*, *S. typhimurium*, and *S. enteritidis*. Complications include valve perforation, valve ring abscess, atrial septal abscess, atrioventricular wall perforation, and rupture of the cusps. In addition, *Salmonella* infection has been reported to cause myocarditis, pericarditis, coronary arteritis, and pacemaker infections (117).

Because of the high incidence of underlying cardiovascular disease in persons older than 50 years, endothelial and endocardial infection with *Salmonella* is predominantly a disease of the elderly: As many as 25% of patients older than 50 years who have documented *Salmonella* bacteremia develop cardiovascular infection (120). These data suggest that although antibiotics may prolong fecal excretion of salmonellae, they may be justified for *Salmonella* gastroenteritis in the subset of patients with underlying cardiovascular disease.

BONE AND JOINT INFECTIONS

Although any skeletal site can become infected, *Salmonella* infections of bone typically involve the long bones, the chondrosternal junctions, and the spine. Skeletal infection is particularly common at sites of skeletal injury or abnormality, at sites of trauma, in areas that have been injured in the setting of sickle cell disease, and on skeletal prostheses. Most patients have involvement of one bone, but many patients with sickle cell disease may have two or more sites affected. Predisposing conditions include diabetes mellitus, corticosteroid therapy, systemic lupus erythematosus, sickle cell anemia, and age younger than 5 years. With 2 to 4 weeks of antibiotic therapy, the overall prognosis is good (1,87,117).

Suppurative arthritis may occur as an extension from a contiguous site of osteomyelitis or as a distinct site of metastatic infection. Predisposing conditions include young age, immunosuppression, corticosteroid administration, and sickle cell anemia. Most commonly involved are the knee, the shoulder, the hip, and the sacroiliac joints. The most common causative serotype is *S. typhimurium*. Blood cultures are frequently positive. The high incidence of positive blood cultures in both *Salmonella* osteomyelitis and septic arthritis suggests that most cases are hematogenous in origin. Antibiotic therapy for 4 weeks with repeated arthrocentesis generally produces favorable results (1,87,117).

Salmonella gastroenteritis may be complicated by reactive arthritis, which is usually a migratory polyarthritis occurring an average of 10 days after the gastroenteritis. Most frequently affected are knees, ankles, and wrist joints. In one review, human leukocyte antigen B27 was present in 90% of patients with *Salmonella* reactive arthritis and was associated with a more severe course (121). Approximately 25% of patients have the triad of arthritis, conjunctivitis, and urethritis that constitute Reiter's syndrome. Conjunctivitis and urethritis usually occur before or at the onset of arthritis. The average duration of symptoms of postinfectious reactive arthritis is 5.5 months. Cultures of blood, urine, urethral secretions, and joint fluid are negative. The pathogenesis is unclear, but *Salmonella*-specific antibodies (particularly immunoglobulin A) have been identified in the serum and synovial fluid. In addition, there is direct evidence that *Salmonella* antigens and lipopolysaccharide are present in the joint space. Antiinflammatory agents are the mainstay of therapy (122,123).

CENTRAL NERVOUS SYSTEM INFECTIONS

Meningitis caused by *Salmonella* infection is primarily a disease of young children: More than 50% of cases occur in newborns, and in these infants, it tends to have a fulminant course. In those patients who survive, there is a high rate of neurologic sequelae, including residual seizures, hydrocephalus, ventriculitis, abscess formation, subdural empyema, and permanent disability. Four weeks of intravenous antibiotic therapy is usually necessary. Because of the long-term sequelae associated with *Salmonella* meningitis, even with optimal therapy, it is recommended that physicians attempt to prevent this condition by administering antibiotics to all children younger than 1 year with *Salmonella* gastroenteritis (124,125).

Focal intracranial *Salmonella* infections, such as brain abscesses, subdural empyemas, and epidural abscesses, are rare. Unlike meningitis, focal intracranial infections occur in adults and in children. Brain abscesses occur more often in adults, and

subdural empyemas more often in children. Predisposing factors include meningitis, trauma, and intracranial hematoma. Surgical drainage with antibiotic therapy is generally associated with a good prognosis (126).

ABDOMINAL INFECTIONS

Intraabdominal *Salmonella* infection usually involves the hepatobiliary system and the spleen. The most frequent intraabdominal infection is cholecystitis. Liver abscesses most often occur in patients with preexisting liver disease, and splenic abscesses most often occur in patients with sickle cell disease. Other reported intraabdominal infections include pancreatic abscesses, subphrenic abscesses, adrenal abscesses, and peritonitis (117).

PULMONARY INFECTIONS

Pleuropulmonary infection caused by *Salmonella* is rare and generally occurs in patients with abnormalities of either the pulmonary parenchyma or the pleura. Typically, these patients present with an acute onset of symptoms and a lobar infiltrate. Blood and stool cultures are positive in 50%. Complications develop often and include abscesses, empyemas, hemoptysis, pleural effusions, and bronchopleural fistulas. Most patients with uncomplicated pneumonia do well with a 2-week course of antibiotic therapy. Complicated pneumonias often require surgical intervention and prolonged antibiotic therapy (127).

GENITOURINARY TRACT INFECTIONS

Salmonella urinary tract infections generally occur in patients with preexisting genitourinary structural abnormalities (e.g., obstruction, reflux, calculous disease, or abnormalities secondary to tuberculosis or schistosomiasis), malignancy, or immunosuppression. In addition to antibiotic therapy, correction of the structural abnormality is often necessary for cure. Because of the high rate of relapse, performance of surveillance urine cultures during follow-up is recommended (128,129).

Genital infections caused by *Salmonella* are rare but have been reported in testicular and ovarian abscesses, epididymitis, prostatitis, and septic abortion (117).

SOFT TISSUE INFECTIONS

Burns, trauma, sickle cell disease, diabetes mellitus, and immunosuppression predispose patients to soft tissue infections with *Salmonella*. Mastitis, endophthalmitis, parotid abscess, thyroiditis, and thyroid abscess caused by *Salmonella* infection have been reported. However, the most frequent site of *Salmonella* soft tissue infection is the skin. Skin infections caused by *Salmonella dublin* may be seen in veterinarians and farmers exposed to birthing cattle (117).

Chronic Carrier State

The *chronic carrier state* refers to the persistence of salmonellae in stool or urine for periods of a year or longer. It develops in less than 1% of persons who have had nontyphoidal salmonellosis and in approximately 2% to 3% of patients who have had typhoid fever. The principal site in the GI tract where these organisms are harbored is the biliary tree; difficulty in eradicating the carrier state is highly correlated with the presence of gallstones or biliary scarring.

The urinary carrier state has been reported in 0.2% to 3.3% of patients with typhoid fever. The urinary carrier state is strongly associated with obstructive uropathy from stones, strictures, tumors, tuberculosis, or schistosomiasis. Chronic urinary carriage is uncommon, except in areas of endemic schistosomiasis, where it may reach 5% (1,87,128,129).

A transient, asymptomatic carrier state that persists for less than 1 year is probably the most common outcome of ingesting salmonellae. In one review of 32 studies of nontyphoidal salmonellae excretion, patients younger than 5 years were found to have a median duration of excretion of 7 weeks, and 40% were culture positive at 20 weeks. In older children and adults, the median duration of excretion was 3 to 4 weeks, and 90% were culture negative at 9 weeks (130). After *S. typhi* infection, organisms can be recovered in 50% of cases after 1 month, in 20% after 2 months, and in 10% after 3 months. Although children are more likely to have relatively prolonged convalescent carriage, they usually do not carry the organism long enough to meet the criteria for the carrier state, which is carriage for longer than 2 years. Women are three times as likely as men to develop the carrier state after infection with *S. typhi* (1,87). In addition to stool cultures, a simple passive hemagglutination test based on highly purified Vi antigen can be used to identify chronic *S. typhi* carriers (100).

Importantly, the chronic carrier state has been associated with an increased incidence of carcinoma of the gallbladder (131). Case-control studies from India have demonstrated a strong epidemiologic link, particularly in patients with concomitant gallstones and culture-positive carriers (132,133). Thus, eradication of the chronic carrier state on a population level may result in a decrease in the incidence of this malignancy (134). The mechanisms of carcinogenesis remain unknown.

Infection in Special Clinical Settings

SALMONELLA AND HUMAN IMMUNODEFICIENCY VIRUS INFECTIONS

Since the first reports of *Salmonella* infection in patients with AIDS in 1983, it has become clear that patients with HIV infection are more susceptible than the normal host to infection with *Salmonella*. These individuals are more prone to bacteremic events, prolonged infections, complications, and relapses after adequate antimicrobial therapy, particularly at lower CD4 counts (135). The incidence of bacteremia caused by *Salmonella* infection in HIV-infected individuals has been calculated to be 20 to 100 times that of the general population (66,136). Recurrence of bacteremia caused by *Salmonella* infection is a criterion for the CDC classification of AIDS. Infections caused by *Salmonella* may occur before any other manifestations of HIV infection, such that *Salmonella* bacteremia in a patient at risk of HIV infection may suggest the diagnosis of AIDS. Often, in the presence of bacteremia, characteristic GI tract symptoms are absent. Metastatic complications include meningitis, peritonitis, septic arthritis, mycotic aortic aneurysm, necrotizing pneumonia, empyema, subcutaneous abscess, brain abscess, and splenic abscess (136–140).

Because the relapse rate is high, treatment of *Salmonella* infection in HIV-infected patients poses a particular problem (141). Although there is no consensus on the duration of antibiotic therapy in these patients, appropriate intravenous therapy followed by one to several months of suppressive therapy seems reasonable; however, some patients may require lifelong suppression (62–65). Some authors have reported success with 1 to 8 months of ciprofloxacin therapy (142). Because the antiviral zidovudine has a direct bactericidal effect against *Salmonella*, it should be considered as part of the antiviral regimen for HIV-infected individuals with recurrent *Salmonella* (143).

SALMONELLA AND MALIGNANCY

In patients with neoplastic disease, bacteremia occurs in 35% to 49% of *Salmonella* infections. Focal infections are seen frequently, particularly pleuropulmonary disease. Patients with hematologic malignancies are at particular risk of disseminated salmonellosis. Predisposing factors in patients with neoplasia include chemotherapy and other antineoplastic therapy, antacid use, corticosteroids, granulocytopenia, and surgery. The use of rattlesnake capsules, an alternative therapy for cancer, has resulted in infections with *S. arizonae* (144). Despite appropriate and prolonged therapy, the rates of mortality and relapse are relatively high (145,146).

SALMONELLA AND TRANSPLANT RECIPIENTS

Like other patients with immunosuppression, transplant recipients have extremely high rates of bacteremia (about 60%) and extraintestinal complications (about 35%) when infected with *Salmonella*. Most cases reported in the literature are in renal transplant recipients, who are particularly susceptible at the point of maximal immunosuppression (147). In renal transplant recipients, unusual sites of focal infections include the maxillary sinus, axillary vein thrombosis, hemodialysis fistula, and testes. Asymptomatic bacteriuria is often present and may be prolonged (longer than 3 months). Many transplant recipients present with a gastroenteritis prodrome, followed by bacteremia and metastatic infection. Antimicrobial therapy of febrile gastroenteritis syndromes in this group of patients is warranted, with direction of such therapy against nontyphoidal *Salmonella* and *Listeria* (148,149).

SALMONELLA AND INFLAMMATORY BOWEL DISEASE

The relationship between *Salmonella* infection and idiopathic inflammatory bowel disease, particularly ulcerative colitis, is complex and at present incompletely understood. At least three different clinical scenarios have been noted. (a) Acute *Salmonella* gastroenteritis can mimic acute idiopathic disease in its clinical, radiographic, endoscopic, and pathologic presentation; yet, the process resolves completely with recovery from the infection. (b) Patients with a history of inflammatory bowel disease who acquire *Salmonella* infection have a much more severe clinical syndrome than other individuals with *Salmonella* gastroenteritis. In these patients, the disease involves a high rate of bowel invasion with bacteremia, toxic megacolon, systemic toxicity, and even death. (c) Uncommonly, a patient with no previous history of inflammatory bowel disease who presents with *Salmonella* gastroenteritis develops chronic inflammatory bowel disease, suggesting that the infection triggered the disease diathesis (150,151).

SALMONELLA AND SCHISTOSOMIASIS

Patients with schistosomiasis are at risk of the development of a chronic, systemic *Salmonella* syndrome. The bacteria infect the schistosomes and appear to be sequestered therein, protected from the effects of antimicrobial therapy. The clinical syndrome that ensues is characterized by chronic *Salmonella* bacteremia that can persist for years, marked hypertrophy of the reticuloendothelial system (most profoundly demonstrated by massive hepatosplenomegaly), wasting, and hyperglobulinemia. The clinical presentation may mimic kala azar or lymphoma. Eradication requires effective treatment of both the schistosomiasis and the salmonellosis (152–155).

CLINICAL MANAGEMENT

Although each of the clinical syndromes caused by *Salmonella* requires a different series of management decisions (Table 68.9), three general principles underlie antimicrobial management of all forms of salmonellosis: (a) *Salmonella* exhibits a high rate of

TABLE 68.9.   Management of *Salmonella* Infections

Clinical syndrome	Treatment	Antibiotics of choice

Gastroenteritis
  Normal host
  Newborn infants
  Persons older than 50 yr
  Lymphoproliferative disease
  Anatomic cardiovascular disease
  Bone or joint disease, especially in
    patients with prostheses
  Sickle cell disease or other chronic
    hemolysis
  Transplant recipients
  HIV infection
	No antibiotics
	Antibiotic prophylaxis until patient
	  is afebrile for 24 hr
		Ciprofloxacin p.o., trimethoprim-sulfamethoxazole p.o.,
		  amoxicillin p.o., cefriaxone i.v., cefoperazone i.v.,
		  ciprofloxacin i.v., trimethoprim-sulfamethoxazole i.v.,
		  ampicillin i.v.

Enteric fever	Antibiotic therapy for 10–14 d	Ciprofloxacin p.o./i.v., ceftriaxone i.v., cefoperazone
		  i.v., chloramphenicol p.o./i.v., ampicillin i.v.,
		  trimethroprim-sulfamethoxazole i.v.

Bacteremia
  Without metastatic infection
  With extraintestinal nonvascular
    metastatic infection
 	
  Vascular metastatic infection
	Antibiotic therapy for 7–14 d
	Antibiotic therapy for 2–4 wk and
	  drainage of focal infection,
	  where appropriate
	Antibiotic therapy for 4–6 wk and
	  excision of infected sites where
	  possible
		Chloramphenicol i.v., ampicillin i.v., trimethoprim-
		  sulfamethoxazole i.v./p.o., ciprofloxacin i.v./p.o.,
		  cefriaxone i.v., cefoperazone i.v.

Chronic carrier state
  Normal biliary tract
 	
  Biliary tract disease
	Antibiotic therapy for 4–6 wk
	
	Parenteral antibiotics for 10–14 d
	  and cholecystectomy
		Ampicillin p.o., amoxicillin p.o., trimethoprim-
		  sulfamethoxazole p.o., ciprofloxacin p.o.
		Chloramphenicol i.v., ampicillin i.v., trimethoprim-
		  sulfamethoxazole i.v./p.o., ciprofloxacin i.v./p.o.,
		  ceftriaxone i.v., cefoperazone

HIV, human immunodeficiency virus; i.v., intravenously; p.o., orally.

plasmid-mediated antibiotic resistance, particularly to traditionally used drugs such as ampicillin; (b) there is incomplete correlation between results of antimicrobial susceptibility testing *in vitro* and the possible clinical efficacy of a particular antibiotic; (c) although *in vitro* resistance correlates with clinical failure, *in vitro* sensitivity does not necessarily correlate with clinical benefit. At present, effective anti-*Salmonella* drugs (if *in vitro* testing reveals sensitivity) include the traditional drugs chloramphenicol, ampicillin, amoxicillin, and trimethoprim-sulfamethoxazole, as well as third-generation cephalosporins, such as ceftriaxone and cefoperazone, and the fluoroquinolones (87).

Gastroenteritis

The primary approach to *Salmonella* gastroenteritis includes fluid and electrolyte replacement, control of nausea and vomiting, and, under certain circumstances, antibiotic prophylaxis. The use of agents that alter bowel motility is discouraged, as such therapy can increase the incidence and the extent of bacteremia. Antibiotic treatment of gastroenteritis per se does not alter the course of this infection in normal hosts. In addition, antibiotic therapy has been associated with an increased duration and frequency of the intestinal carrier state. Although the quinolones have a favorable pharmacokinetic profile against *Salmonella,* ciprofloxacin was shown in one randomized, placebo-controlled, double-blind trial to have a high bacteriologic relapse rate in patients with salmonellosis and to be associated with prolonged fecal carriage (156). Finally, antibiotic treatment of enterohemorrhagic *Escherichia coli* infection may increase the risk of developing hemolytic-uremic syndrome (157); therefore, empiric institution of antibiotics for a diarrheal syndrome that might be consistent with either *Salmonella* or enterohemorrhagic *E. coli,*

before having a laboratory diagnosis, may increase the risk of this complication.

At present, therapy with antibiotics for patients with *Salmonella* gastroenteritis should be viewed principally as a prophylactic effort aimed at persons for whom even transient bacteremia could have catastrophic consequences. In the setting of possible or demonstrated *Salmonella* gastroenteritis, the following groups of patients should be considered for such prophylaxis: (a) newborn infants, because of the high risk of meningitis; (b) patients older than 50 years, because of the high risk of infecting atherosclerotic plaques or an aneurysm; (c) those who have lymphoproliferative disorders; (d) those who have suspected or known anatomic cardiovascular disease; (e) those who have significant bone or joint disease, including the presence of prostheses or other foreign bodies; (f) those with sickle cell disease or other forms of chronic hemolysis; (g) those with transplants; and (h) those with HIV infection (87).

The best antimicrobial regimen for prophylaxis of bacteremia is unknown. When oral therapy is feasible, our preference is ciprofloxacin, 500 mg two times per day; trimethoprim-sulfamethoxazole, two double-strength tablets two times per day; or amoxicillin, 500 mg three times per day. If parenteral therapy is necessary, intravenous ceftriaxone, ciprofloxacin, trimethoprim-sulfamethoxazole, or ampicillin in full doses is prescribed. Therapy is continued until the patient has been afebrile for more than 24 hours.

Enteric Fever

Unlike the situation with *Salmonella* gastroenteritis, antimicrobial therapy is clearly efficacious in the treatment of enteric fever. Chloramphenicol was first used to treat *S. typhi* infections in

1948. It became the drug of choice because there was a uniform response pattern: The temperature returned to normal in 3½ to 5 days, patients felt better within 24 to 48 hours, and recovery was complete in 10 to 14 days. Mortality rates were reduced from 15% to 20% to 1.0% to 1.5%. Chloramphenicol, ampicillin, and trimethoprim-sulfamethoxazole have been the mainstays of therapy. The emergence of chloramphenicol-resistant strains and fear of the infrequent, but severe bone marrow toxicity of chloramphenicol have curtailed use of this drug in some countries. However, because of its low cost and excellent oral bioavailability, chloramphenicol is still widely used in developing countries (158,159).

The fluoroquinolones (e.g., ciprofloxacin, 500 mg two times per day for 10 to 14 days) have been shown to be effective in the treatment of enteric fever. For several reasons, they have emerged as the drugs of choice in the treatment of enteric fever. Multidrug-resistant organisms have been reported in areas such as Latin America, the Indian subcontinent, and the Middle East. Currently, the incidence of antimicrobial resistance to the fluoroquinolones is lower than that to the traditional agents used against typhoid fever. The fluoroquinolones achieve high concentrations in the bile, the bowel, and the urinary tract. In addition, they reach high concentrations within macrophages, where they are bactericidal (160–162).

The third-generation cephalosporins cefotaxime, ceftriaxone, and cefoperazone are effective against *S. typhi,* with overall cure rates of approximately 90% and relapse rates of approximately 5%. Second-generation cephalosporins, despite *in vitro* susceptibility, have an unacceptably low cure rate and are not recommended. Similarly, aminoglycoside antibiotics and aztreonam are effective *in vitro* but do not effect clinical cure (163,164). An alternative to third-generation cephalosporins is azithromycin, which, as with fluoroquinolones, achieves high intracellular levels (165–167).

Although fluoroquinolones and third-generation cephalosporins remain the primary effective treatment choices against *S. typhi,* the clinician should remain vigilant for the possibility of resistance to these agents, particularly in travelers from developing countries (168,169). Reduced susceptibility to nalidixic acid or ciprofloxacin has been correlated with treatment failure (170,171). In a survey of 293 cases of symptomatic typhoid fever with positive *S. typhi* isolates in the United States from 1996 to 1997, 20 (7%) patients, each with a history of foreign travel, yielded strains that were resistant to nalidixic acid (172). Formal minimum inhibitory concentration testing should be considered for isolates from areas known to be endemic for this strain, particularly the Indian subcontinent.

High-dose dexamethasone therapy in conjunction with chloramphenicol therapy was shown to reduce the case-fatality rate of severe enteric fever from 55.6% to 10.0% in one study involving 38 patients (173). Patients included in the study had severe disease with either abnormal state of consciousness (delirium, obtundation, stupor, or coma) or shock. There was no significant difference in the incidence of complications among the survivors of the two groups. Thus, the use of high-dose glucocorticoid therapy seems justified in the small subset of patients with severe enteric fever (173,174).

Bacteremia with or without Metastatic Infection

Bacteremic *Salmonella* infection merits antimicrobial therapy once sufficient blood cultures have been drawn to delineate the level of bacteremia. When sustained bacteremia is present, an effort should be made to rule out a cardiovascular site of infection. Transient bacteremia with extraintestinal nonvascular infection

requires 2 to 4 weeks of antibiotic therapy and when appropriate surgical drainage of the focal infection. Transient bacteremia without metastatic infection should be treated for 7 to 14 days, preferably with a bactericidal drug. If relapse occurs, an aggressive search for a metastatic focus, particularly within the cardiovascular system, should be undertaken, as well as a 4- to 6-week course of treatment initiated, coupled with surgical intervention (1,87).

Chronic Carrier State

Success of antimicrobial treatment of the chronic carrier state depends on whether anatomic abnormalities of the biliary tract are present. In the absence of biliary tract disease, a 4- to 6-week course of ampicillin or amoxicillin at doses of 2 to 4 g per day or trimethoprim-sulfamethoxazole at doses of one to two double-strength tablets two times per day is effective in more than 80% of patients. For chronic carriers with gallbladder disease, the rate of failure with ampicillin treatment is approximately 75%. Because of the high achievable concentrations in bile, ceftriaxone and fluoroquinolones are considered preferred agents. In some small studies, fluoroquinolones have been shown to be successful in eradicating the carrier state (175–178).

When biliary tract disease is present, medical therapy fails in most patients. Cholecystectomy without concomitant antibacterial therapy results in a 70% to 80% cure rate, but with significant morbidity and mortality, because of dissemination of *Salmonella* at the time of surgery. The best results are obtained with the combination of cholecystectomy and a 10- to 14-day course of parenteral antibiotics that is initiated before surgery. The level of serum antibodies to the Vi antigen serves as a useful marker of the success of the treatment of chronic carriers because carriers will usually revert to seronegative after successful treatment (9,87).

PREVENTION

Recommendations for typhoid vaccination are discussed in Chapter 196.

REFERENCES

1. Rubin RH, Weinstein L. *Salmonellosis: microbiologic, pathologic, and clinical features.* New York: Stratton International, 1977.
2. Holt JG, Kreig NR, Sneath PHA, et al, eds. *Bergey's manual of determinative bacteriology,* 9th ed. Baltimore: Williams & Wilkins, 1994.
3. Foster WD. *A history of medical bacteriology and immunology.* London: Cox and Wyman, 1970.
4. Burrows W. *Textbook of microbiology.* Philadelphia: WB Saunders, 1985.
5. Brenner FW, Villar RG, Angulo FJ, et al. *Salmonella* nomenclature. *J Clin Microbiol* 2000;38:2465.
6. Fierer J, Swancutt M. Non-typhoid *Salmonella:* a review. *Curr Clin Top Infect Dis* 2000;20:134.
7. Ryan CA, Hargrett-Bean NT, Blake PA. *Salmonella typhi* infections in the United States, 1975–1984: increasing role of foreign travel. *Rev Infect Dis* 1989; 11:1.
8. Centers for Disease Control and Prevention. Summary of notifiable diseases, United States, 1999. *MMWR Morb Mortal Wkly Rep* 2001;48:1.
9. Mathieu JJ, Henning KJ, Bell E, et al. Typhoid fever in New York City, 1980 through 1990. *Arch Intern Med* 1994;154:1713.
10. Dritz SK, Braff EH. Sexually transmitted typhoid fever. *N Engl J Med* 1977;296:1359.
11. Gotuzzo E, Frisancho O, Sanchez J, et al. Association between the acquired immunodeficiency syndrome and infection with *Salmonella typhi* or *Salmonella paratyphi* in an endemic typhoid area. *Arch Intern Med* 1991;151:381.
12. Chalker RB, Blaser MJ. A review of human salmonellosis, III: magnitude of *Salmonella* infection in the United States. *Rev Infect Dis* 1988;10:111.
13. Mead P, Slutsker L, Dietz V, et al. Food-related illness and death in the United States. *Emerg Infect Dis* 1999;5:607.

14. Hargrett-Bean NT, Pavia AT, et al. *Salmonella* isolates from humans in the United States, 1984–1986. *MMWR CDC Surveill Summ* 1988;2:25.
15. Hui YH, Gorham JR, Murrell KD, et al, eds. *Foodborne disease handbook, diseases caused by bacteria,* vol 1. New York: Marcel Dekker, 1994.
16. Olsen SJ, Bishop R, Brenner FW, et al. The changing epidemiology of *Salmonella:* trends in serotypes isolated from humans in the United States, 1987–1997. *J Infect Dis* 2001;183:753.
17. Gill ON, Sockett PN, Bartlett CL, et al. Outbreak of *Salmonella napoli* infection caused by contaminated chocolate bars. *Lancet* 1983;1:547.
18. Centers for Disease Control and Prevention. Multistate outbreak of *Salmonella poona* infections—United States and Canada, 1991. *MMWR Morb Mortal Wkly Rep* 1991;40:549.
19. Babu K, Sonnenberg M, Kathpalia S, et al. Isolation of salmonellae from dried rattlesnake preparations. *J Clin Microbiol* 1990;28:361.
20. Bensink JC, Ekaputra L, Taliotis C. The isolation of *Salmonella* from kangaroos and feral pigs processed for human consumption. *Aust Vet J* 1991;68:106.
21. Van Beneden CA, Keene WE, Strang RA, et al. Multinational outbreak of *Salmonella enterica* serotype Newport infections due to contaminated alfalfa sprouts. *JAMA* 1999;281:158.
22. Taylor DN, Wachsmuth IK, Shangkuan Y, et al. Salmonellosis associated with marijuana. *N Engl J Med* 1982;306:1249.
23. Hennessy TW, Hedberg CW, Slutsker L, et al. A national outbreak of *Salmonella enteritidis* infections from ice cream. *N Engl J Med* 1996;334:1281.
24. Cook KA, Dobbs, TE, Hlady WG, et al. Outbreak of *Salmonella* serotype Hartford infections associated with unpasteurized orange juice. *JAMA* 1998;280:1504.
25. Cohen ML, Potter M, Pollard R, et al. Turtle-associated salmonellosis in the United States. *JAMA* 1980;243:1247.
26. Centers for Disease Control and Prevention. Iguana-associated salmonellosis—Indiana. *MMWR Morb Mortal Wkly Rep* 1992;41:38.
27. Centers for Disease Control and Prevention. Lizard-associated salmonellosis—Utah. *MMWR Morb Mortal Wkly Rep* 1992;41:610.
28. Fonseca RJ, Dubey LM. *Salmonella montevideo* sepsis from a pet snake. *Pediatr Infect Dis J* 1994;13:550.
29. Centers for Disease Control and Prevention. *Salmonella hadar* associated with pet ducklings—Connecticut, Maryland, and Pennsylvania 1991. *MMWR Morb Mortal Wkly Rep* 1992;41:185.
30. Mermin J, Hoar B, Angulo FJ. Iguanas and *Salmonella* Marina infection in children: a reflection of the increasing incidence of reptile-associated salmonellosis in the United States. *Pediatrics* 1997;99:399.
31. Centers for Disease Control and Prevention. Reptile-associated salmonellosis—selected states, 1996–1998. *MMWR Morb Mortal Wkly Rep* 1999;48:1009.
32. Centers for Disease Control and Prevention. Preliminary FoodNet data on the incidence of foodborne illnesses—selected sites, United States, 2000. *MMWR Morb Mortal Wkly Rep* 2001;50:241.
33. Olsen SJ, MacKinnon LC, Goulding JS, et al. Surveillance for foodborne disease outbreaks, 1993–1997. *MMWR CDC Surveill Summ* 2000;49:SS-1.
34. Centers for Disease Control and Prevention. Outbreaks of *Salmonella* serotype enteritidis infection associated with eating raw or undercooked shell eggs—United States, 1996–8. *MMWR Morb Mortal Wkly Rep* 2000;49:73.
35. Mishu B, Koehler J, Lee L, et al. Outbreaks of *Salmonella enteritidis* infections in the United States, 1985–1991. *J Infect Dis* 1994;169:547.
36. Centers for Disease Control and Prevention. Update: *Salmonella enteritidis* infections and shell eggs—United States, 1990. *MMWR Morb Mortal Wkly Rep* 1990;39:909.
37. Cox NA, Bailey JS, Mauldin JM, et al. Extent of salmonellae contamination in breeder hatcheries. *Poult Sci* 1991;70:416.
38. Clavero MR, Monk JD, Beuchat LR. Inactivation of *Escherichia coli* O157:H7, salmonellae, and *Campylobacter jejuni* in raw ground beef by gamma irradiation. *Appl Environ Microbiol* 1994;60:2069.
39. Cooper GI, Venables LM, Woodbard MJ, et al. Vaccination of chickens with strain CVL30, a genetically defined *Salmonella enteritidis* aroA live oral vaccine candidate. *Infect Immun* 1994;62:4747.
40. Stephensen J. Fighting flora with flora: FDA approves an anti-*Salmonella* spray for chickens. *JAMA* 1998;279:1152.
41. Centers for Disease Control and Prevention. Outbreak of *Salmonella enteritidis* associated with nationally distributed ice cream products—Minnesota, South Dakota, and Wisconsin, 1994. *MMWR Morb Mortal Wkly Rep* 1994;43:740.
42. Ryan CA, Nickels MK, Hargrett-Bean NT, et al. Massive outbreak of antimicrobial resistant salmonellosis traced to pasteurized milk. *JAMA* 1987;258:3269.
43. Clark GM, Kaufmann AF, Gangarosa EJ, et al. Epidemiology of an international outbreak of *Salmonella agona*. *Lancet* 1973;2:490.
44. Gangarosa EJ, Barker WH, Barne WB, et al. Man vs. animal feeds as the source of human salmonellosis. *Lancet* 1973;1:878.
45. Holmberg SD, Osterholm MT, Senger KA, et al. Drug-resistant *Salmonella* from animals fed antimicrobials. *N Engl J Med* 1984;311:617.
46. Lee LA, Puhr ND, Maloney EK, et al. Increase in antimicrobial-resistant *Salmonella* infections in the United States, 1989–1990. *J Infect Dis* 1994;170:128.
47. Glynn MK, Bopp C, Dewitt W, et al. Emergence of multidrug-resistant *Salmonella enterica* serotype *typhimurium* DT104 infections in the United States. *N Engl J Med* 1998;338:1333.
48. Mølbak K, Baggesen DL, Aarestrup FM, et al. An outbreak of multidrug-resistant, quinolone-resistant *Salmonella enterica* serotype *typhimurium* DT104. *N Engl J Med* 1999;341:1420.
49. Frost JA, Kelleher A, Rowe B. Increasing ciprofloxacin resistance in salmonellas in England and Wales 1991–1994. *J Antimicrob Chemother* 1996;37:85.
50. Hakanen A, Siitonen A, Kotilainen P, et al. Increasing fluoroquinolone resistance in salmonella serotypes in Finland during 1995–1997. *J Antimicrob Chemother* 1999;43:145.
51. Yang YJ, Liu CC, Wang SM. High rates of antimicrobial resistance among clinical isolates of nontyphoidal *Salmonella* in Taiwan. *Eur J Clin Microbiol Infect Dis* 1998;17:880.
52. Herikstad H, Hayes P, Mokhtar M, et al. Emerging quinolone-resistant *Salmonella* in the United States. *Emerg Infect Dis* 1997;3:371.
53. Mølbak K, Baggesen DL, Aarestrup FM, et al. An outbreak of multidrug-resistant, quinolone-resistant *Salmonella enterica* serotype *typhimurium* DT104. *N Engl J Med* 1999;341:1420.
54. Dunne EF, Fey PD, Kludt P, et al. Emergence of domestically acquired ceftriaxone-resistant *Salmonella* infections associated with AmpC beta-lactamase. *JAMA* 2000;284:3151.
55. Olsen SJ, DeBess EE, McGivern TE, et al. A nosocomial outbreak of fluoroquinolone-resistant *Salmonella* infection. *N Engl J Med* 2001;344:1572.
56. Fey PD, Safranek TJ, Rupp ME, et al. Ceftriaxone-resistant *Salmonella* infection acquired by a child from cattle. *N Engl J Med* 2000;342:1242.
57. Gorbach SL. Antimicrobial use in animal feed—time to stop. *N Engl J Med* 2001;345:1202.
58. Levine WC, Smart JF, Archer DL, et al. Foodborne disease outbreaks in nursing homes, 1975 through 1987. *JAMA* 1991;266:2105.
59. Humphrey TJ, Greenwood M, Gilbert RJ, et al. The survival of salmonellas in shell eggs cooked under simulated domestic conditions. *Epidemiol Infect* 1989;103:35.
60. Altekruse S, Hyman F, Klontz K, et al. Foodborne bacterial infections in individuals with the human immunodeficiency virus. *South Med J* 1994;87:170.
61. World Health Organization. Food safety measures for eggs and foods containing eggs. *World Health Forum* 1993;14:437.
62. Nadelman RB, Mathur-Wagh U, Yancovitz, Mildvan D. *Salmonella* bacteremia associated with the acquired immunodeficiency syndrome (AIDS). *Arch Intern Med* 1985;145:1968.
63. Smith PD, Macher AM, Bookman MA, et al. *Salmonella typhimurium* enteritis and bacteremia in the acquired immunodeficiency syndrome. *Ann Intern Med* 1985;102:207.
64. Jacobs JL, Gold JW, Murray HW, et al. *Salmonella* infections in patients with the acquired immunodeficiency syndrome. *Ann Intern Med* 1985;102:186.
65. Glaser JB, Morton-Kute L, Berger SR. Recurrent *Salmonella typhimurium* bacteremia associated with the acquired immunodeficiency syndrome. *Ann Intern Med* 1985;102:189.
66. Cecum CL, Chaisson RE, Rutherford GW, et al. Incidence of salmonellosis in patients with AIDS. *J Infect Dis* 1987;156:998.
67. Levine WC, Buehler JW, Bean NH, et al. Epidemiology of nontyphoidal *Salmonella* bacteremia during the human immunodeficiency virus epidemic. *J Infect Dis* 1991;164:81.
68. USPHS/IDSA Prevention of Opportunistic Infections Working Group. 2001 USPHS/IDSA guidelines for the prevention of opportunistic infections in persons infected with human immunodeficiency virus. Available at: *www.hivatis.org*.
69. Hohmann EL. Nontyphoidal salmonellosis. *Clin Infect Dis* 2001;32:263.
70. Gershman M. Single phage-typing set for differentiating salmonellae. *J Clin Microbiol* 1977;5:302.
71. Wachsmuth IK, Kiehlbauch JA, Bopp DN, et al. The use of plasmid profiles and nucleic acid probes in epidemiologic investigations of foodborne, diarrheal diseases. *Int J Food Microbiol* 1991;12:77.
72. O'Brien TF, Hopkins JD, Gilleece ES, et al. Molecular epidemiology of antibiotic resistance in *Salmonella* from animals and human beings in the United States. *N Engl J Med* 1982;307:1.
73. Bender JB, Hedberg CW, Boxrud DJ, et al. Use of molecular subtyping in surveillance for *Salmonella enterica* serotype *typhimurium*. *N Engl J Med* 2001;344:189.
74. Formal SB, Hale TL, Sansonetti PJ. Invasive enteric pathogens. *Rev Infect Dis* 1983;5:702.
75. Finlay BB, Falkow S. Common themes in microbial pathogenicity. *Microbiol Rev* 1989;53:210.
76. Blaser MJ, Newman LS. A review of human salmonellosis, I: infective dose. *Rev Infect Dis* 1982;4:1096.
77. Hook EW. Salmonellosis: certain factors influencing the interaction of *Salmonella* and the human host. *Bull N Y Acad Med* 1961;37:499.
78. Giannella RA, Broitman SA, Zamcheck N. *Salmonella* enteritis, I: role of reduced gastric secretion in pathogenesis. *Am J Dig Dis* 1971;16:1000.
79. Gorden J, Small PLC. Acid resistance in enteric bacteria. *Infect Immun* 1993;61:364.
80. Telzak EE, Greenberg MS, Budnick LD. Diabetes mellitus—a new described risk factor for infection from *Salmonella enteritidis*. *J Infect Dis* 1991;164:538.
81. Pavia AT, Shipman LD, Wells JG. Epidemiologic evidence that prior antimicrobial exposure decreases resistance to infection by antimicrobial-sensitive *Salmonella*. *J Infect Dis* 1990;161:255.

82. Miller CP, Bohnhoff M. Changes in the mouse's enteric microflora associated with enhanced susceptibility to *Salmonella* infection following streptomycin treatment. *J Infect Dis* 1963;113:59.

83. Hornick RB, Greisman SE, Woodward TE, et al. Typhoid fever: pathogenesis and immunologic control. *N Engl J Med* 1970;283:686.

84. Kaye D, Gill FA, Hook EW. Factors influencing host resistance to *Salmonella* infections: the effects of hemolysis and erythrophagocytosis. *Am J Med Sci* 1967;254:205.

85. Gill FA, Kaye D, Hook EW. The influence of erythrophagocytosis on the interaction of macrophages and *Salmonella in vitro*. *J Exp Med* 1966;124:173.

86. Wheat LJ, Rubin RH, Harris NL, et al. Systemic salmonellosis in patients with disseminated histoplasmosis. *Arch Intern Med* 1987;147:561.

87. Goldberg MB, Rubin RH. The spectrum of *Salmonella* infection. *Infect Dis Clin North Am* 1988;2:571.

88. Olsen SJ, Bishop R, Brenner FW, et al. The changing epidemiology of *Salmonella*: trends in serotypes isolated from humans in the United States, 1987–1997. *J Infect Dis* 2001;183:753, 2001.

89. Saphra I, Winter JW. Clinical manifestations of salmonellosis in man: an evaluation of 7779 human infections identified at the New York *Salmonella* Center. *N Engl J Med* 1957;256:1128.

90. McCall CE, Martin WT, Boring JR. Efficiency of cultures of rectal swabs and faecal specimens in detecting *Salmonella* carriers: correlation with numbers of salmonellae excreted. *J Hyg (Lond)* 1966;64:261.

91. Chattopadhyay B, Pilfold JN. The effect of prolonged incubation of selenite F broth on the rate of isolation of *Salmonella* from faeces. *Med Lab Sci* 1976;33: 191.

92. Hornick RB, Greisman SE, Woodward TE, et al. Typhoid fever: pathogenesis and immunologic control. *N Engl J Med* 1970;283:686.

93. Stuart BM, Pullen RL. Typhoid fever: clinical analysis of 360 cases. *Arch Intern Med* 1946;78:629.

94. Hoffman TA, Ruiz CJ, Counts GW. Waterborne typhoid fever in Dade County, Florida: clinical and therapeutic evaluation of 105 bacteremic patients. *Am J Med* 1975;59:481.

95. Davis TM, Makepeace AE, Dallimore EA, et al. Relative bradycardia is not a feature of enteric fever in children. *Clin Infect Dis* 1999;28:582.

96. Ferreccio C, Levine MM, Manterola A, et al. Benign bacteremia caused by *Salmonella typhi* and *paratyphi* in children younger than two years. *J Pediatr* 1984;104:899.

97. Mahle WT, Levine MM. *Salmonella typhi* infection in children younger than five years of age. *Pediatr Infect Dis* 1993;12:627.

98. Gilman RH, Terminel M, Levine MM, et al. Relative efficacy of blood, urine, rectal swab, bone marrow, and rose-spot cultures for recovery of *Salmonella typhi* in typhoid fever. *Lancet* 1975;1:1211.

99. Hoffman SL, Punjabi NH, Rockhill RC. Duodenal string-capsule culture compared with bone-marrow, blood and rectal-swab cultures for diagnosing typhoid and paratyphoid fever. *J Infect Dis* 1984;149:157.

100. Edelman R, Levine MM. Summary of an international workshop on typhoid fever. *Rev Infect Dis* 1986;8:329.

101. Schroeder SA. Interpretation of serologic test for typhoid fever. *JAMA* 1968;206:839.

102. Pang V, Puthucheary SD. Significance and value of the Widal test in the diagnosis of typhoid fever in an endemic area. *J Clin Pathol* 1983;36:471.

103. Nardiello S, Pizzella T, Russo M, et al. Serodiagnosis of typhoid fever by enzyme-linked immunosorbent assay determination of anti–*Salmonella typhi* lipopolysaccharide antibodies. *J Clin Microbiol* 1984;20:718.

104. Shetty NP, Srinivasa H, Bhat P. Coagglutination and counter immunoelectrophoresis in the rapid diagnosis of typhoid fever. *Am J Clin Pathol* 1985;84: 80.

105. Black PH, Kunz LJ, Swartz MN. Salmonellosis—a review of some unusual aspects. *N Engl J Med* 1960;262:864.

106. Saphra I, Wasserman M. *Salmonella choleraesuis*: a clinical and epidemiologic evaluation of 329 infections identified between 1940 and 1954 in the New York *Salmonella* Center. *Am J Med Sci* 1954;228:525.

107. Cherubin CE, Neu HC, Imperato PJ, et al. Septicemia with non-typhoid salmonella. *Medicine (Baltimore)* 1974;53:365.

108. Zaidi E, Bachur R, Harper M. Non-typhi *Salmonella* bacteremia in children. *Pediatr Infect Dis J* 1999;18:1073.

109. Shimoni Z, Pitlik S, Leibovici L, et al. Nontyphoidal salmonella bacteremia: age-related differences in clinical presentation, bacteriology, and outcome. *Clin Infect Dis* 1999;28:822.

110. Lee SC, Yang PH, Shieh WB, et al. Bacteremia due to non-typhi Salmonella: analysis of 64 cases and review. *Clin Infect Dis* 1994;19:693.

111. Sirinavin S, Jayanetra P, Thakkinstian A. Clinical and prognostic categorization of extraintestinal nontyphoidal *Salmonella* infections in infants and children. *Clin Infect Dis* 1999;29:1151.

112. Galofre J, Moreno A, Mensa J, et al. Analysis of factors influencing the outcome and development of septic metastasis or relapse in *Salmonella* bacteremia. *Clin Infect Dis* 1994;18:873.

113. Lester A, Eriksen NH, Nielsen H, et al. Non-typhoid *Salmonella* bacteraemia in Greater Copenhagen 1984 to 1988. *Eur J Clin Microbiol Infect Dis* 1991;10: 486.

114. Oskoui R, Davis WA, Gomes MN. *Salmonella* aortitis: a report of a successfully treated case with a comprehensive review of the literature. *Arch Intern Med* 1993;153:517.

115. Brooks DJ, Cant AJ, Lambert HP, et al. Recurrent salmonella septicaemia with aortitis, osteomyelitis and psoas abscess. *J Infect* 1983;7:156.

116. Morrow C, Safi H, Beall AC Jr. Primary aortoduodenal fistula caused by *Salmonella* aortitis. *J Vasc Surg* 1987;6:415.

117. Cohen JI, Bartlett JA, Corey GR. Extra-intestinal manifestations of *Salmonella* infections. *Medicine (Baltimore)* 1987;66:349.

118. Donabedian H. Long-term suppression of *Salmonella* aortitis with an oral antibiotic. *Arch Intern Med* 1989;149:1452.

119. Soravia-Dunand VA, Loo VG, Salit IE. Aortitis due to *Salmonella*: report of 10 cases and comprehensive review of the literature. *Clin Infect Dis* 1999;29: 862.

120. Cohen PS, O'Brien TF, Schoenbaum S, et al. The risk of endothelial infection in adults with *Salmonella* bacteremia. *Ann Intern Med* 1978;89:931.

121. Leirisalo-Repo M, Helenius P, Hannu T, et al. Long-term prognosis of reactive salmonella arthritis. *Ann Rheum Dis* 1997;56:516.

122. Granfors K, Jalkanen S, Lindberg A. *Salmonella* lipopolysaccharide in synovial cells from patients with reactive arthritis. *Lancet* 1990;335:685.

123. Maki-Ikola O, Yli-Kerttula U, Saario R, et al. *Salmonella* specific antibodies in serum and synovial fluid in patients with reactive arthritis. *Br J Rheumatol* 1992;31:25.

124. Rabinowitz SG, MacLeod NR. *Salmonella* meningitis. A report of three cases and a review of the literature. *Am J Dis Child* 1972;123:259.

125. Rodriguez RE, Valero V, Watanakunakorn C. *Salmonella* focal intracranial infections: review of the world literature (1894–1984) and report of an unusual case. *Rev Infect Dis* 1986;8:31.

126. Rodriguez RE, Valero V, Watanakunakorn C. *Salmonella* focal intracranial infections: review of the world literature (1894–1984) and report of an unusual case. *Rev Infect Dis* 1986;8:31.

127. Aguado JM, Obeso G, Cabanillas JJ, et al. Pleuropulmonary infections due to nontyphoidal strains of *Salmonella*. *Arch Intern Med* 1990;150:54.

128. Scott MB, Cosgrove MD. *Salmonella* infection and the genitourinary system. *J Urol* 1977;118:64.

129. Melzer M, Altmann G, Rakowszcyk M, et al. *Salmonella* infections of the kidney. *J Urol* 1965;94:23.

130. Buchwald DS, Blaser MJ. A review of human salmonellosis, II: duration of excretion following infection with nontyphi *Salmonella*. *Rev Infect Dis* 1984;6: 345.

131. Welton JC, Marr JS, Friedman SM. Association between hepatobiliary cancer and typhoid carrier state. *Lancet* 1979;1:791.

132. Shukla VK, Singh H, Pandey M, et al. Carcinoma of the gallbladder—is it a sequel of typhoid?. *Dig Dis Sci* 2000;45:900.

133. Dutta U, Garg PK, Kumar R, et al. Typhoid carriers among patients with gallstones are at increased risk for carcinoma of the gallbladder. *Am J Gastroenterol* 2000;95:784.

134. Nath G, Singh H, Shukla VK. Chronic typhoid carriage and carcinoma of the gallbladder. *Eur J Cancer Prev* 1997;6:557–559.

135. Nelson MR, Shanson DC, Hawkins DA, et al. *Salmonella, Campylobacter,* and *Shigella* in HIV-seropositive patients. *AIDS* 1992;6:1495.

136. Sperber SJ, Schleupner CJ. Salmonellosis during infection with human immunodeficiency virus. *Rev Infect Dis* 1987;9:925.

137. Gouny P, Valverde A, Vincent D, et al. Human immunodeficiency virus and infected aneurysm of the abdominal aorta: report of three cases. *Ann Vasc Surg* 1992;6:239.

138. Satue JA, Aguado JM, Ramon Costa J, et al. Pulmonary abscess due to non-*typhi Salmonella* in a patient with AIDS [Letter]. *Clin Infect Dis* 1994;19:555.

139. Olive AT, Tena X. *Salmonella* septic arthritis in patients with human immunodeficiency virus. *J Rheumatol* 1994;21:1172.

140. Torres JR, Rodriguez Casas J, Balda E, et al. Multifocal *Salmonella* splenic abscess in a HIV-infected patient. *Trop Geogr Med* 1992;44:66.

141. Fischl MA, Dickinson GM, Sinave C, et al. *Salmonella* bacteremia as manifestation of acquired immunodeficiency syndrome. *Arch Intern Med* 1986;146: 113.

142. Jacobson MA, Hahn SM, Gerberding JL, et al. Ciprofloxacin for *Salmonella* bacteremia in the acquired immunodeficiency syndrome. *Ann Intern Med* 1989;110:1027.

143. Casado JL, Valdezate S, Calderon C, et al. Zidovudine therapy protects against Salmonella bacteremia recurrence in human immunodeficiency virus–infected patients. *J Infect Dis* 1999;179:1553.

144. Sharma J, Von Hoff DD, Weiss GR. *Salmonella arizonae* peritonitis secondary to ingestion of rattlesnake capsules for gastric cancer. *J Clin Oncol* 1993;11:2288.

145. Wolfe MS, Louria DB, Armstrong D, et al. Salmonellosis in patients with neoplastic disease. A review of 100 episodes at Memorial Cancer Center over a 13-year period. *Arch Intern Med* 1971;128:546.

146. Noriega LM, Van der Auwera P, Daneau D, et al. *Salmonella* infections in a cancer center. *Support Care Cancer* 1994;2:116.

147. Dhar JM, al-Khader AA, al-Sulaiman M, et al. Non-typhoid *Salmonella* in renal transplant recipients: a report of twenty cases and review of the literature. *Q J Med* 1991;78:235.

148. Samra Y, Shaked Y, Maier MK. Nontyphoid salmonellosis in renal transplant recipients: report of five cases and review of the literature. *Rev Infect Dis* 1986;8:431.

149. Rubin RH, Young LS. *Clinical approach to infection in the compromised host*, 3rd ed. New York: Plenum Publishing, 1994.

150. Szilagyi A, Gerson M, Mendelson J, et al. *Salmonella* infections complicating inflammatory bowel disease. *J Clin Gastroenterol* 1985;7:251.

151. Martinez Aviles P, Moreno Carazo A, Bellkessam N, et al. Salmonellosis and ulcerative colitis. A case report and review of the literature. *Rev Clin Esp* 1993;192:116.

152. Neves J, Raso P, Marinko PP. Prolonged septicemic salmonellosis intercurrent with *Schistosoma mansoni* infection. *J Trop Med Hyg* 1971;74:9.
153. Rocha H, Kirk JW, Hearey CD Jr. Prolonged *Salmonella* bacteremia in patients with *Schistosoma mansoni* infection. *Arch Intern Med* 1971;128:254.
154. Young SW, Higashi G, Kamel R, et al. Interactions of salmonellae and schistosomes in host-parasite relations. *Trans R Soc Trop Med Hyg* 1973;67:797.
155. Gendrel D, Richard-Lenoble D, Kombila M, et al. *Schistosoma intercalatum* and relapses of *Salmonella* infection in children. *Am J Trop Med Hyg* 1984;33:1166.
156. Neill MA, Opal SM, Heelan J, et al. Failure of ciprofloxacin to eradicate convalescent fecal excretion after acute salmonellosis: experience during an outbreak in health care workers. *Ann Intern Med* 1991;114:195.
157. Wong C, Jelacic S, Habeeb R, et al. The risk of the hemolytic-uremic syndrome after antibiotic treatment of *Escherichia coli* O157:H7 infections. *N Engl J Med* 2000;342:1930.
158. Vazquez V, Calderon E, Rodriquez R. Chloramphenicol-resistant strains of *Salmonella* typhosa. *N Engl J Med* 1972;286:1220.
159. Gilman RH, Terminel M, Levine MM, et al. Comparison of trimethoprim-sulfamethoxazole and amoxicillin in therapy chloramphenicol-resistant and chloramphenicol-sensitive typhoid fever. *J Infect Dis* 1975;132:630.
160. Asperilla MO, Smego RA Jr, Scott LK. Quinolone antibiotics in the treatment of *Salmonella* infections. *Rev Infect Dis* 1990;12:873.
161. Lewin CS. Treatment of multiresistant *Salmonella* infection. *Lancet* 1991;337:47.
162. Reid TMS. The treatment of non-typhic salmonellosis. *J Antimicrob Chemother* 1992;29:4.
163. Soe GB, Overturf GD. Treatment of typhoid fever and other systemic salmonelloses with cefotaxime, ceftriaxone, cefoperazone, and other newer cephalosporins. *Rev Infect Dis* 1987;9:719.
164. Choo KE, Ariffin WA, Ong KH, et al. Aztreonam failure in typhoid fever. *Lancet* 1991;337:498.
165. Girgis NI, Butler T, Frenck RW. Azithromycin versus ciprofloxacin for treatment of uncomplicated typhoid fever in a randomized trial in Egypt that included patients with multidrug resistance. *Antimicrob Agents Chemother* 1999;43:1441.
166. Butler T, Sridhar CB, Daga MK. Treatment of typhoid fever with azithromycin versus chloramphenicol in a randomized multicenter trial in India. *J Antimicrob Chemother* 1999;44:243.
167. Frenck RW, et al. Azithromycin versus ceftriaxone for the treatment of uncomplicated typhoid fever in children. *Clin Infect Dis* 2000;31:1134.
168. Saha SK, Tulukder S, Islam M, et al. A highly ceftriaxone-resistant *Salmonella typhi* in Bangladesh. *Pediatr Infect Dis J* 1999;18:387.
169. Murdoch DA, Banatvala NA, Bone A, et al. Epidemic ciprofloxacin-resistant *Salmonella typhi* in Tajikistan. *Lancet* 1998;351:339.
170. Wain J, Hoa NT, Chinh NT, et al. Quinolone-resistant *Salmonella typhi* in Viet Nam: molecular basis of resistance and clinical response to treatment. *Clin Infect Dis* 1997;25:1404.
171. Threlfall EJ, Ward LR, Skinner JA, et al. Ciprofloxacin-resistant *Salmonella typhi* and treatment failure. *Lancet* 1999;353:1590.
172. Ackers ML, Puhr ND, Tauxe RV, et al. Laboratory-based surveillance of *Salmonella* serotype *typhi* infections in the United States. *JAMA* 2000;283:2668.
173. Hoffman SL, Punjabi NH, Kumala S, et al. Reduction of mortality in chloramphenicol-treated severe typhoid fever by high-dose dexamethasone. *N Engl J Med* 1984;310:82.
174. Kamath PS, Jalihal A, Chakraborty A. Differentiation of typhoid fever from fulminant hepatic failure in patients presenting with jaundice and encephalopathy. *Mayo Clin Proc* 2000;75:462.
175. Dinbar A, Altman G, Tulcinsky DB. The treatment of chronic biliary *Salmonella* carriers. *Am J Med* 1969;47:236.
176. Diridl G, Pichler H, Wolf D. Treatment of chronic *Salmonella* carriers with ciprofloxacin. *Eur J Clin Microbiol* 1986;5:260.
177. Cherubin CE, Kowalski J. Nontyphoidal *Salmonella* carrier state treated with norfloxacin. *Ann Intern Med* 1990;85:100.
178. Raymond J, Moulin F, Badoual J, et al. Eradication of convalescent-phase *Salmonella* carriage in children with two oral doses of pefloxacin. *Eur J Clin Microbiol Infect Dis* 1994;13:307.
179. Walker W. The Aberdeen typhoid outbreak of 1964. *Scottish Med J* 1965;10:466.

CHAPTER 69
Infections Due to Escherichia coli

Michael S. Donnenberg

Escherichia coli is a pluripotential pathogen. Although this organism is the most abundant facultative anaerobe in the human intestine and most strains are poorly suited to cause disease in normal hosts, an impressive array of specialized pathogenic *E. coli* strains exists that can cause a variety of illnesses. These strains can be grouped into "pathotypes" on the basis of common genetic determinants that specify the ability to carry out common pathogenetic mechanisms, which result in more or less distinct pathophysiologic and clinical syndromes (1). The *E. coli* strains that cause urinary tract infections are discussed separately in Chapter 99. Those that cause other extraintestinal infections including neonatal meningitis share many virulence attributes with the uropathogenic strains and are not discussed here (2). Instead, this chapter focuses on the pathotypes of *E. coli* that cause gastrointestinal (GI) tract infections (Table 69.1).

Pathogenic strains share with nonpathogenic *E. coli* certain basic attributes that are important to their biology. Most ferment lactose (and other sugars) and are indole positive. They have a highly reactive lipopolysaccharide, many produce capsule, and most are motile because of the production of peritrichous flagellae. The various *E. coli* pathotypes are able to cause disease because they possess virulence genes that encode factors that allow them to navigate pathogenic pathways. These virulence genes are packaged in bacteriophages, exchanged on plasmids, or presented in sets on discrete chromosomal domains known as *pathogenicity islands*. The complete genomic sequences of two *E. coli* strains, one a harmless laboratory workhorse K-12 strain, the other a highly pathogenic serotype O157:H7 strain, have lent tremendous insight into the composition of a pathogen (3,4). These strains diverged from a common ancestor an estimated 4.5 million years ago and have therefore had ample opportunity to acquire and dispose of nonessential genetic information. The two strains share 3,573 genes, which are for the most part colinear. In addition, the pathogenic strain has 1,387 genes absent from the K-12 strain, whereas 528 genes are unique to the latter. These genes are distributed within the genomes among hundreds of islands of various sizes. In addition to previously described virulence factors, the genome of the pathogenic strain reveals many additional sequences that suggest a role in pathogenesis, as well as a large number of genes of unknown function. Investigators studying the molecular pathogenesis of *E. coli* infections thus have a large number of new factors to investigate. It is anticipated that this number will multiply as the genomes of additional pathogenic *E. coli* strains are published.

ENTEROTOXIGENIC *E. COLI*

Definition

Enterotoxigenic *E. coli* (ETEC) strains were first recognized on the basis of their ability to cause diarrhea in animal models and later in volunteers (5,6). These strains are defined by production of either or both a heat-labile enterotoxin (LT) and a heat-stable enterotoxin (ST).

TABLE 69.1.   Features of Infections Caused by Pathotypes of *Escherichia coli* that Cause Diarrhea

Pathotype	Epidemiology	Clinical manifestations	Virulence factors	Diagnosis	Treatment
ETEC	Contaminated food and water. Children in developing countries, travelers.	Watery diarrhea	Colonization factor antigens; heat-labile and heat-stable enterotoxins	PCR or probes for toxin genes	Rehydration; fluoroquinolones + loperimide
EPEC	Person-to-person. Infants in developing countries.	Watery diarrhea and vomiting	Bundle-forming pili (localized adherence), type III secretion system, intimin-Tir	PCR for intimin and bundle forming pilin genes and to exclude Shiga toxin genes	Rehydration; antibiotics if susceptible
STEC including EHEC	Contaminated food and water, person-to-person. Developed countries.	Watery diarrhea, hemorrhagic colitis, hemolyticuremic syndrome	Shiga toxins. In EHEC type III secretion system, intimin-Tir	Sorbitol MacConkey agar (O157:H7 only), PCR for Shiga toxin genes	Rehydration; supportive care. Avoid antimotility agents and antibiotics
EAEC	Children in developing countries, outbreaks in developed countries, HIV-infected patients.	Mucoid diarrhea, chronic diarrhea	Fimbria that mediate aggregative adherence, toxins.	Tissue culture adherence assay	Rehydration; fluoroquinolones may be of benefit if HIV positive
DAEC	Older children in developing countries.	Not well described	Fimbria and afimbrial adhesins that mediate diffuse adherence	Tissue culture adherence assay	Rehydration
EIEC	Outbreaks from contaminated food, endemic in developing countries.	Watery diarrhea, dysentery	Plasmid mediated invasion, cell–cell spread, macrophage apoptosis	PCR or probes for invasion genes	Rehydration; antibiotics may be of benefit if susceptible.

ETEC, enterotoxigenic *E. coli;* EPEC, enteropathogenic *E. coli;* STEC, Shiga toxin–producing *E. coli;* EHEC, enterohemorrhagic *E. coli;* EAEC, enteroaggregative *E. coli;* DAEC, diffuse adhering *E. coli;* EIEC, enteroinvasive *E. coli;* HIV, human immunodeficiency virus; PCR, polymerase chain reaction.

Epidemiology

Because ETEC infections are transmitted via contaminated food and water, infections are common where sanitation is inadequate. Thus, ETEC strains are a leading cause of watery diarrhea in children throughout the nations of the developing world where they make a major contribution to the burden of diarrheal disease and are the most common recognized cause of diarrhea among travelers to such countries (7). ETEC are also pathogens of major importance to armed forces because of their potential to disrupt military operations overseas (8). Endemic ETEC infections predominate among children who have recently been weaned. Because of the antigenic diversity of ETEC strains, children can suffer multiple ETEC infections.

Pathogenesis

The pathogenesis of ETEC infections has been recognized for years to be the result of two types of plasmid-encoded factors: colonization factors and toxins. Recently, the description of additional potential virulence determinants encoded on pathogenicity islands on the chromosome has led to the appreciation that ETEC pathogenesis may be more complex than hitherto thought.

Experiments with ETEC strains that cause disease in animals established the concept that the ability to produce adhesins is a requirement for illness. A large number of adhesins, often referred to as *colonization factors antigens* (CFAs), have been described for ETEC strains that infect humans. Many of these CFAs are fimbriae, but some are thinner less rigid surface appendages called *fibrillae.* CFAs are encoded on plasmids. Individual strains may produce several CFAs, but no particular CFA is found in most strains. CFAs are antigenically distinct and play an important role in strain specific protective immunity.

The LT produced by many ETEC strains shares with cholera toxin a limited degree of its amino acid sequence, a virtually identical three-dimensional (3D) structure, and a common mechanism of action. Both toxins are composed of a single, catalytic A subunit that has its α-helical carboxyl terminus inserted into the

hollow center of a ring-shaped pentamer of identical receptor-binding B subunits (Fig. 69.1). The A and B subunits are encoded by adjacent genes on plasmids. After the B subunits bind to the glycolipid GM$_1$ ganglioside, LT is taken up by enterocytes into endosomes and is transported retrograde into the Golgi apparatus. The A subunit enters the cytoplasm where it acts as a nicotinamide adenine dinucleotide (NAD) ribosyl transferase, covalently modifying the A subunit of the stimulatory

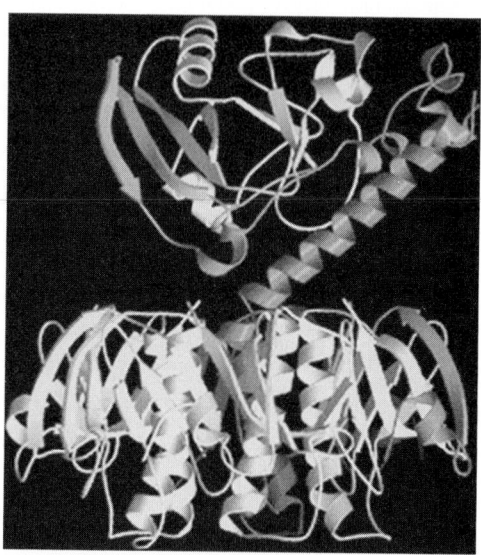

Figure 69.1. The structure of enterotoxigenic *Escherichia coli* heat-labile toxin (LT). LT is depicted in a ribbons diagram. The catalytic A subunit is perched atop the receptor-binding B-subunit pentamer with its α-helical amino terminus projecting through a pore surrounded by the B pentamer. [This figure was downloaded from the Protein Data Bank (PDB ID: 1LTS, *www.rcsb.org/pdb/*); Berman HM, Westbrook J, Feng Z, et al. The Protein Data Bank. *Nucleic Acids Res* 2000;28:235–242. Available at: *www.rcsb.or/pdb/*] and is based on published crystallographic data from reference 128.]

heterotrimeric G protein on the basolateral cytoplasmic membrane. This modification locks the signaling protein in the guanosine triphosphate (GTP)–bound "on" position, which causes it to persistently activate adenylate cyclase. The elevated levels of cyclic adenosine monophosphate (cAMP) that result lead to activation of protein kinase A, which in turn leads to phosphorylation of the cystic fibrosis transmembrane conductance regulator (CFTR) and the active secretion of chloride by intestinal crypt cells. To maintain charge and solute equilibrium, sodium and water follow passively and fluid accumulates in the intestinal lumen. ETEC strains may produce in addition or instead of LT an ST, a small peptide that has six cysteine residues involved in three intramolecular disulfide bonds. ST resembles the endogenous peptide guanilyn and like its mammalian homolog binds to guanylyl cyclase C in the enterocyte apical membrane (9). Binding of ST results in activation of the receptor and production of cyclic guanosine monophosphate (cGMP), which also leads to activation of protein kinase A and opening of CFTR.

Recently several loci present in chromosomal pathogenicity islands have been identified that may encode factors that play a role in ETEC pathogenesis. Two of these factors, Tia and TibA encode outer membrane proteins that may play a role in ETEC adherence and perhaps in cellular invasion (10,11). Another gene, *leoA*, located near *tia* appears to be involved in LT secretion (12). Thus, it seems that pathogenicity islands as well as plasmids contribute to the ability of ETEC to cause disease.

Clinical Manifestations

After ingestion of heavily contaminated food or water and an incubation period of hours to 2 days, ETEC infections induce watery diarrhea sometimes accompanied by cramps. Vomiting, fever, and mucus or blood in the stools are not common. The illness is self-limited, usually lasting less than 5 days. Occasionally, severe diarrhea resulting in serious dehydration can occur. The diagnosis is suspected in travelers, outbreaks, or in endemic areas on the basis of these symptoms. Confirmation requires assays for the enterotoxins or the genes that produce them and therefore is not routinely available in clinical microbiology laboratories.

Therapy and Prevention

The cornerstone of therapy of diarrheal disease, to maintain adequate hydration, usually with oral rehydration solution, applies to ETEC infections. The addition of antibiotics to which the organism is susceptible can reduce the duration of symptoms, as can antimotility agents. A commonly used and successful approach for the treatment of traveler's diarrhea is to provide the traveler with a fluoroquinolone antibiotic, along with loperamide for immediate use should diarrhea develop during a trip to a developing country. Those with fever, bloody stools, or symptoms of dysentery should not take loperamide. A single dose of the fluoroquinolone is effective (13).

Many studies have been conducted on the prevention and treatment of traveler's diarrhea, which is often caused by ETEC. Meticulous avoidance of beverages that are not bottled, ice, cooked food that is not served steaming hot, raw vegetables, and fruit that is not peeled can reduce the incidence of traveler's diarrhea, as can prophylactic ingestion of bismuth subsalicylate (7,14). However, many vacationers find it difficult to comply with these measures. The use of prophylactic antibiotics should be strongly discouraged because of the mild nature of the illness in travelers, the potential for adverse effects of the medication,

and the potential for the emergence of resistant strains. The possibility of a multivalent ETEC vaccine is the subject of extensive investigation.

ENTEROPATHOGENIC *E. COLI*

Definition

Enteropathogenic *E. coli* (EPEC) strains were the first *E. coli* recognized to cause disease when it was appreciated that strains isolated from infants during devastating outbreaks of neonatal diarrhea differed serologically from those isolated from control infants (15). For many years, these strains were identified antigenically, defined as belonging to particular serotypes associated with outbreaks. More recently, as an understanding of the pathogenesis of these infections has emerged, they have been identified by the virulence attributes that make them unique (16). Thus, EPEC strains do not produce Shiga toxins (see the section "Enterohemorrhagic and Other Shiga Toxin–producing *E. coli*," later in this chapter) and are able to modify the apical cytoskeleton of enterocytes and attach intimately to the surface of these cells in a process known as the attaching and effacing effect (Fig. 69.2). In addition, "typical" EPEC strains are able to auto-aggregate and to adhere in 3D microcolonies to host cells by virtue of their ability to express bundle-forming pili (Fig. 69.3), whereas "atypical" strains lack these features.

Epidemiology

EPEC strains cause disease almost exclusively in infants; most cases occur in those younger than 6 months (17). EPEC infections are common in impoverished urban settings in developing countries all over the world (18–26). In developed countries, a few outbreaks associated with attendance in child day care centers have been reported (27,28). Although occasional nosocomial outbreaks similar to those described in the middle part of the last century still occur (29,30), most cases appear to be sporadic. Person-to-person spread appears to be the main mode of transmission (29), whereas outbreaks resulting from contaminated food are rare (31). Lack of breast-feeding has emerged in several studies as an important risk factor for infection, and in one study, recent prior hospitalization was also more common in cases than controls (32).

Pathogenesis

Two critical virulence attributes have been proven in volunteer studies to be required for full virulence in typical EPEC strains: the ability to produce functional bundle-forming pili and the ability to induce the attaching and effacing effect.

The bundle-forming pilus is encoded by the *bfp* operon, a locus containing 14 genes present on a large plasmid common to typical EPEC strains. The first gene in the operon, *bfpA*, encodes bundlin, the major structural subunit of the pilus. Recent studies have shown that different strains of EPEC have *bfpA* alleles that specify variable bundlin proteins and that most of the *bfpA* sequence variation is confined to regions of the protein predicted to be exposed on the surface of the pilus fibers (33). The rest of the genes of the operon specify the pilus biogenesis machinery, which is poorly understood. The bundle-forming pilus is a member of a family of type IV pili that are widely distributed among gram-negative bacteria and are critical for the virulence of diverse human and animal pathogens. Production of the pili is required for two phenotypes characteristic of EPEC strains: the ability to form 3D microcolonies on the surface of tissue culture

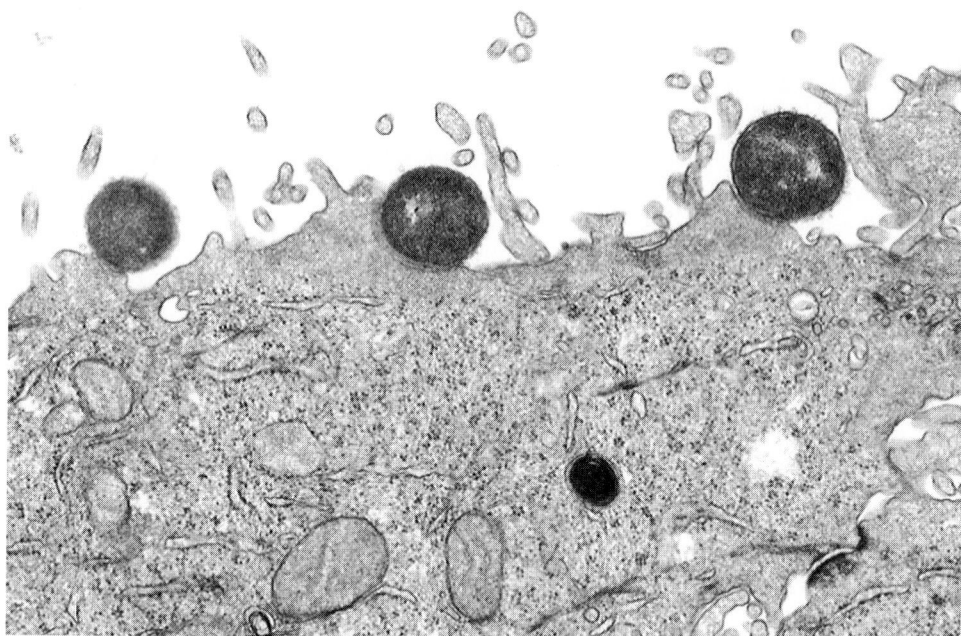

Figure 69.2. Attaching and effacing activity of enteropathogenic *Escherichia coli* (EPEC). EPEC bacteria can be seen attaching intimately to the surface of a tissue culture cell. The cell responds by losing its microvilli and embracing the bacteria on adherence pedestals composed of actin and other cytoskeletal proteins. Attaching and effacing activity is exhibited by EPEC in biopsies from infected infants, in animal models and *in vitro*. Attaching and effacing activity has also been demonstrated in animal models and *in vitro* for enterohemorrhagic *E. coli*.

cells, a pattern known as *localized adherence* (see Fig. 69.3), and the ability to form reversible aggregates in liquid media. Mutations at the *bfpF* locus result in bacteria that are hyperpiliated and form larger microcolonies than do wild-type bacteria, but the microcolonies and aggregates of these bacteria fail to disperse (34–36). Proteins similar to BfpF from other bacteria that make type IV fimbria are required for the generation of mechanical force that results in pilus retraction (37). Curiously, the *bfpF* mutant bacteria are as attenuated in the ability to cause diarrhea in volunteers, as are *bfpA* mutants that are unable to synthesize pili at all (34).

The ability to induce the attaching and effacing effect (see Fig. 69.2) is specified by a pathogenicity island containing 41 genes that is located on the EPEC chromosome (38). This locus of enterocyte effacement (LEE) encodes a type III secretion system, proteins secreted via this system, an outer membrane adhesin protein known as *intimin* and proteins of unknown function. The type III secretion system delivers several proteins directly to the host cell cytoplasm or membrane. One of these proteins, the translocated intimin receptor (Tir), is inserted into the host cell membrane by the bacteria where it serves as the receptor for intimin (39). Actin is recruited to this site and assembled

into filaments by host cell machinery (40). The crystal structure of the complex formed by the extracellular domains of both intimin and Tir has been solved and reveals that two molecules of intimin contact a Tir dimer in a plane roughly parallel to the membranes of both bacteria and host cells, which explains the intimate attachment of the bacteria to the enterocyte (41). Both intimin and EspB, one of several secreted proteins required for the translocation of Tir to the host cell membrane, have been proven in volunteer studies to be essential for full EPEC virulence (42,43).

Despite advances in our understanding of the molecular pathogenesis of EPEC infection, the mechanisms by which EPEC causes diarrhea remain incompletely understood. The EspF protein, encoded within the LEE and translocated by EPEC into host cells via the type III secretion system, induces an increase in permeability across intestinal epithelial cell monolayers by loosening tight junctions (44). This compromise of intestinal barrier function could lead to loss of fluid and solute into the lumen and contribute to diarrhea. An LEE-dependent transient membrane depolarization and ion flux has been detected and may be indicative of an active solute secretion mechanism that contributes to fluid loss (45,46). Finally, loss of absorptive surface

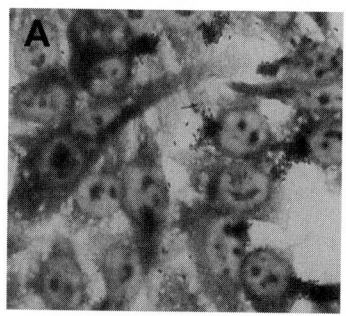 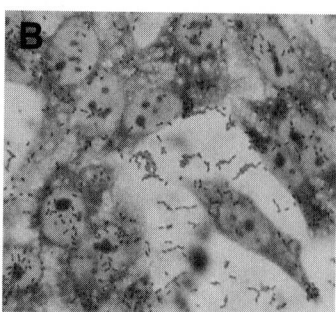 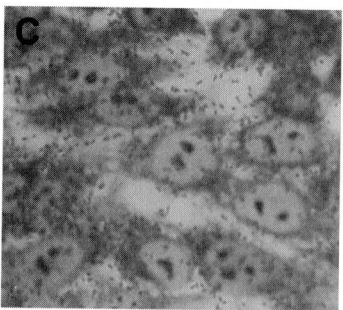

Figure 69.3. Adherence patterns of *Escherichia coli* that cause diarrhea. **A:** Typical enteropathogenic *E. coli* strains produce the bundle-forming pilus and adhere to epithelial cells in three-dimensional microcolonies in a pattern termed *localized adherence*. **B:** Enteroaggregative *E. coli* strains adhere to epithelial cells and often to the substrata in two-dimensional aggregates. **C:** Diffuse-adhering *E. coli* stains blanket the surface of epithelial cells.

due to extensive attaching and effacing effects could explain the resolution of diarrhea in some patients upon institution of total parenteral nutrition (47). It is interesting to note that although mutant strains unable to produce the bundle-forming pilus or unable to induce the attaching and effacing effect are highly attenuated, they remain able to cause diarrhea in a minority of volunteers (34,42,43).

Clinical Manifestations

Infection with EPEC may induce a broad range of illness severity, including asymptomatic colonization, transient watery diarrhea, profuse watery diarrhea with vomiting, and persistent diarrhea (17,18,47–49). Thus, EPEC infection is clinically indistinguishable from other causes of diarrhea. Blood and mucus are rarely present in the stool, however, and fever is usually low grade or absent. However, in contrast to other bacterial causes of diarrhea, vomiting may be prominent in EPEC infection and may render oral rehydration therapy problematic. Many laboratories lack the capabilities to make the diagnosis of EPEC infection. Traditionally, a presumptive diagnosis was made with the use of typing sera that recognize O (lipopolysaccharide) antigens that are common among EPEC strains, but this method is neither sensitive nor specific. A positive polymerase chain reaction (PCR) assay using primers specific for the *eae* gene, which encodes intimin, in conjunction with a negative result using primers specific for *stx* genes, which encode Shiga toxins found in enterohemorrhagic *E. coli* (EHEC), may be used for the diagnosis of EPEC infection (50). The addition of primers specific for the *bfpA* gene encoding the bundle-forming pilus pilin protein allows one to differentiate between typical and atypical EPEC strains.

Therapy and Prevention

As with other types of diarrhea, rehydration with oral or if necessary parenteral solutions is of paramount importance in the therapy of EPEC infections. A single randomized double-blind placebo-controlled trial has suggested that antibiotics can reduce the duration of symptoms caused by EPEC infection (51). Unfortunately, many strains of EPEC possess plasmids that render them resistant to multiple antibiotics (52,53). In a double-blind placebo-controlled trial of hospitalized children aged 3 to 35 months with acute diarrhea in Peru, racecadotril, an enkephalinase inhibitor, in addition to oral rehydration therapy significantly reduced stool output, duration of diarrhea, and use of oral rehydration therapy (54). Most of these children had rotavirus infection, but racecadotril was equally efficacious in the group of children with bacterial infections, among which EPEC was the most commonly isolated pathogen. These results suggest that racecadotril may be useful in the treatment of diarrhea caused by EPEC. Racecadotril is presumed to act by increasing the concentrations of GI tract enkephalins, which lower cAMP levels in enterocytes and counteract hypersecretion.

The risk of EPEC infection is higher in infants who are bottle-fed (32); thus, breast-feeding seems to be a practical and inexpensive means of preventing EPEC disease. Indeed, human milk inhibits EPEC adherence and contains antibodies against several EPEC virulence factors (32,55–57). Person-to-person spread of EPEC infection can be interrupted by attention to hand washing (29). Enthusiasm for an EPEC vaccine based on intimin, the bundle-forming pilus, or secreted proteins is tempered by the sequence variability of these antigens (33,58) and the daunting task of delivering any potential vaccine to the population at risk.

ENTEROHEMORRHAGIC AND OTHER SHIGA TOXIN–PRODUCING *E. COLI*

Definition

By definition, Shiga toxin–producing *E. coli* (STEC) strains produce Shiga toxins. EHEC strains are a subgroup of STEC that in addition share with EPEC the ability to induce the attaching and effacing effect in host cells (Fig. 69.4). Like EPEC, these EHEC strains have the LEE pathogenicity island encoding the type III secretion system, intimin, Tir, and EspF (59). They also have a large plasmid, but unlike typical EPEC strains, they lack the genes for and do not produce the bundle-forming pilus. Among the EHEC, strains of serotype O157:H7 reign supreme as lethal human pathogens.

Epidemiology

EHEC strains cause sporadic episodes and common-source outbreaks of disease. EHEC strains of serotype O157:H7 have caused the vast majority of outbreaks as well as those that have involved the greatest numbers of patients (60,61). Other EHEC serotypes including the closely related O157:NM strains, O26:H11 strains, and O111 strains have also been involved in outbreaks (62,63). In contrast, non-EHEC STEC strains have only rarely been involved in outbreaks. EHEC infections are contracted by consumption of contaminated food, water, or other beverages, by swimming in contaminated water, by contact with animals, or by close contact with infected people (60,61,64–75). The reservoir for EHEC is infected ruminants, particularly cattle. Many outbreaks can be traced directly or indirectly to contamination with bovine excrement. Undercooked ground beef is the vehicle most commonly implicated in EHEC outbreaks and in sporadic cases (76), but a wide variety of other foods and beverages have been to blame. EHEC infections are more common in the summer and appear to be more prevalent in the northern than the southern parts of the United States and Great Britain.

Pathogenesis

One of the remarkable features of EHEC infections is the extremely low infectious dose, 100 or fewer organisms, required

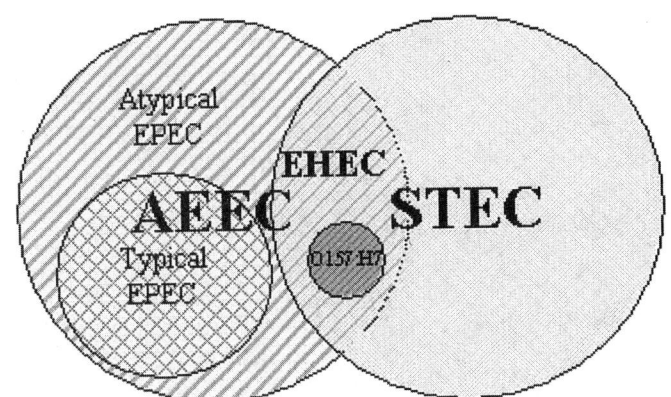

Figure 69.4. The relationships among Shiga toxin–producing *Escherichia coli* (STEC), enterohemorrhagic *E. coli* (EHEC), and enteropathogenic *E. coli* (EPEC) strains. EPEC and EHEC strains are both capable of inducing the attaching and effacing effect and can therefore be grouped together as attaching and effacing *E. coli* (AEEC). EHEC are also a subset of STEC. Among the EHEC, strains of serotype O157:H7 stand out as particularly important pathogens. Among the EPEC, typical strains produce the bundle-forming pilus, whereas atypical strains do not.

for infection (69). This feature of EHEC accounts for its propensity to cause disease in patients who consume ground meat that is less than well done and its potential to spread person to person. An enhanced ability of EHEC in comparison to other *E. coli* strains to survive low pH levels and hence to transit the stomach intact may be relevant to this low infectious dose and its survival in certain acidic foods and beverages (77,78).

Once resident in the lower GI tract, it is assumed that EHEC adhere to epithelial cells via the intimin–Tir interaction and induce the attaching and effacing effect, as do EPEC. However, attaching and effacing lesions have been reported only for EHEC *in vitro* and in animal models of infection, rather than in patients. Unlike EPEC, which predominantly infect the small intestine but may colonize the GI tract from the duodenum to the rectum, EHEC colonization is restricted to the colon. This different tissue tropism is difficult to account for on the basis of the Tir–intimin interaction, because the Tir receptor can be translocated into many types of epithelial cells. Recently nucleolin has been identified as an additional, host cell receptor for EHEC intimin (79). It has been proposed that differences in the EPEC and EHEC intimin sequences may account for different tissue tropism, but the potential contribution of other adhesins has not been excluded (80). The mechanisms by which non-EHEC STEC colonize the gut remain to be described.

The principal virulence factor of STEC is Shiga toxin. Shiga toxins are encoded by bacteriophages that resemble the classic *E. coli* phage lambda (81). Production of the toxin is linked to that of the proteins produced when the bacteriophage exits the lysogenic state and lyses the bacteria. Conditions that induce the bacterial SOS response, including antibiotics such as fluoroquinolones and trimethoprim, lead to induction of toxin production (82). Shiga toxins, which come in several varieties and are produced by *Shigella dysenteriae,* have a quaternary structure that is very similar to that of cholera toxin and LT with a single enzymatic A subunit inserted into a pentamer of identical receptor-binding B subunits (83). However, the enzymatic activity and pathologic effects of Shiga toxin are vastly different than those of LT. The B subunits of Shiga toxin bind to globotriaosylceramide (84). The toxin is taken up into endosomes and transported retrograde into the endoplasmic reticulum (85). The target of the A subunit is the 28S ribosomal ribonucleic acid (RNA), which it depurinates at a specific adenine residue. The result is a cessation of protein synthesis and death of the intoxicated cell. Endothelial cells, particularly those of the renal microvasculature, are particularly relevant targets (86). How the toxin is translocated across the intestinal epithelium and into the bloodstream to reach these cells is incompletely understood. Experiments *in vitro* indicate that the toxin can pass through polarized intestinal epithelial cells (87). Circulating neutrophils may disseminate the toxin (88).

Clinical Manifestations

The severity of illness that may be caused by STEC varies widely from asymptomatic infection to severe manifestations with lethal complications. EHEC illness often begins as watery diarrhea, which may progress to hemorrhagic colitis (89–91). The resulting hematochezia may be severe enough to resemble GI tract hemorrhage. Diarrhea is often accompanied by severe abdominal pain and cramps. Nausea, vomiting, and fever are not prominent features of EHEC infection. Fecal leukocytes are often present. The dreaded complication of STEC infections is the hemolytic-uremic syndrome (HUS), which may resemble thrombotic thrombocytopenic purpura in adults. HUS occurs in approximately 5% to 10% of patients who acquire *E. coli* O157:H7 in common-source outbreaks and is more common in young children and the elderly. Risk factors for HUS include prior consumption of antibiotics, leukocytosis, and according to some studies the use of antimotility agents (92–95). HUS is a microangiopathic illness, presumed to result from intoxication of endothelial cells by Shiga toxin, resulting in activation of coagulation in the microvasculature with platelet and thrombin deposition and distal ischemic necrosis. Anemia (resulting from intravascular hemolysis) and thrombocytopenia result and schistocytes are noted on peripheral smear. The kidney is particularly susceptible and uremia ensues. However, any organ may be affected and complications include strokes, toxic megacolon, blindness, and digital autoamputation.

The diagnosis of STEC infection should be suspected in anyone with bloody diarrhea or with watery diarrhea accompanied by severe cramps. Infection with *E. coli* O157:H7 strains can be diagnosed by culture on sorbitol-MacConkey agar, a differential medium that takes advantage of the inability of these strains to ferment sorbitol (90). Hence, these colonies are white in contrast to the pink colonies formed by most *E. coli* strains. The microbiology laboratory should be alerted when this infection is suspected, to ensure that the proper medium is used. The diagnosis of STEC infection is extremely important both for care of the patient and for the public health. Recognition of a single case of *E. coli* O157:H7 infection is cause for a full epidemiologic investigation to identify the source of the infection and prevent additional cases. Unfortunately non-O157:H7 STEC usually ferment sorbitol. Therefore, diagnosis of infection caused by other STEC strains and confirmation of *E. coli* O157:H7 infection requires assays, either immunologic such as enzyme-linked immunosorbent assay (ELISA) or deoxyribonucleic acid (DNA) based such as PCR, that detect Shiga toxins or the genes that encode them. These assays are available in many reference laboratories, state health laboratories, and at the Centers for Disease Control and Prevention.

Therapy and Prevention

Therapy of STEC infections is entirely supportive, consisting of fluid resuscitation, monitoring for complications, and when required support for organ failure. Antibiotics are contraindicated because they induce the bacteriophages that encode the Shiga toxins, increase production, and release of toxin and increase the risk of HUS (82,95). The risk of acquiring STEC infections can be reduced by thorough cooking of ground beef, by avoidance of unpasteurized beverages, and by standard practices to prevent cross-contamination of potentially infected and ready-to-serve foods. In addition, infants and toddlers should be restricted from swimming areas if they have recently had diarrhea, and people should wash their hands after contact with animals in farms and petting zoos. Several approaches to additional preventive measures including vaccines, receptor-binding analogs, and alteration of cattle flora are under active investigation.

ENTEROAGGREGATIVE AND DIFFUSE-ADHERING *E. COLI*

Definition

Enteroaggregative *E. coli* (EAEC) and diffuse-adhering *E. coli* (DAEC) are two distinct pathotypes of diarrheagenic *E. coli* that are both defined by the patterns of adherence to tissue culture cells that they exhibit (see Fig. 69.3). It is widely accepted, however, that strains that exhibit either of these tissue culture adherence patterns are highly heterogeneous and that information gained from studying a prototype strain may not have generalized relevance (5,96,97). Nonetheless, epidemiologic studies have established an association between strains identified on the basis of these adherence patterns and diarrhea (see the next section, "Epidemiology"). In the case of EAEC, volunteer studies have confirmed that at least one such strain is capable of causing diarrhea in humans under experimental conditions (98). The same cannot be said of DAEC strains (99).

Epidemiology

Studies from several developing countries have identified an association between diarrhea and the isolation of EAEC strains from children (100–102). Intriguingly, there is an association between EAEC and persistent diarrhea, which carries with it a great burden of morbidity and mortality. In addition, EAEC have been implicated as a cause of diarrhea and crampy abdominal pain in Europe (103) and have been isolated from patients with acquired immunodeficiency syndrome (104,105). There have also been outbreaks of EAEC infections in children and adults (106,107). DAEC have also been associated with diarrhea in developing countries (108), particularly when the analysis is limited to older infants and children (109,110).

Pathogenesis

The pathogenesis of EAEC infection is poorly understood. Two related plasmid-encoded pili have been shown to mediate the characteristic aggregative pattern of adherence, but many EAEC strains produce neither of these fimbriae (97,111). Several toxins have been described in EAEC strains including Pet and Pic, both members of the serine protease auto-transporter of the Enterobacteriaceae (SPATE) family (112), and EAST, which resembles ST from ETEC (113). An understanding of the roles of these toxins in pathogenesis requires further investigation. It has recently been appreciated that the feces of children colonized by EAEC contains elevated levels of interleukin-8 (IL-8), a neutrophil-attractant chemokine (114). Further study has revealed that the flagellin of a prototype EAEC strain is a potent inducer of IL-8 expression by epithelial cells (115).

Although a number of fimbrial (116) and afimbrial (117) adhesins and a novel form of envelopment within surface appendages of epithelial cells (118) have been described for certain DAEC strains, our understanding of the pathogenesis of infection caused by these organisms remains rudimentary.

Clinical Manifestations

The striking clinical feature of EAEC infection is its tendency to cause persistent diarrhea (100). Diarrhea caused by EAEC is often mucoid and may have gross blood. Fever and vomiting are each found in a minority of patients with EAEC infection (119). The clinical features of DAEC infection have not been well defined. The diagnosis of either infection is based on characteristic adherence patterns in assays using tissue culture cells and is thus not available in most clinical laboratories. The use of molecular techniques for diagnosis has been problematic because of strain heterogeneity with regard to the prevalence of various putative virulence genes.

Therapy and Prevention

The mainstay of therapy for all diarrheal diseases is oral rehydration. In a double-blind crossover trial of ciprofloxacin versus placebo in the treatment of human immunodeficiency

virus–infected patients with chronic diarrhea and EAEC infection, the organism was eradicated and symptoms improved during the treatment phase (120). Whether these results are applicable to other patient populations is unknown. There are no data on which to base treatment recommendations for DAEC infections. Strategies for the prevention of these infections have yet to be developed.

ENTEROINVASIVE *E. COLI*

Definition

The enteroinvasive *E. coli* (EIEC) are capable of efficiently invading a variety of epithelial cells, induce inflammatory responses in the conjunctivae of laboratory animals (Sereny's test) and resemble in all other important features members of the genus *Shigella*. They share with these organisms biochemical properties, virulence genes, pathogenetic mechanisms, and molecular phylogeny. In fact *Shigella* organisms are so closely related to other *E. coli* that they fall well within the latter genus by all molecular criteria but retain their former designation for historical reasons (121). Because infections caused by *Shigella* are presented in detail Chapter 66, EIEC strains will receive only brief discourse here.

Epidemiology

EIEC infections occur as occasional outbreaks in developed countries and endemic infections in developing countries (5,122,123). Many outbreaks are associated with contaminated food or water, and the potential for person-to-person spread appears to be lower than that of *Shigella*, as is the infectious dose in volunteer experiments (6).

Pathogenesis

Based on the presence of similar virulence determinants, the pathogenesis of EIEC infection is presumed to be similar to that of infections caused by *Shigella* species, which depend on the presence of a large plasmid that confers upon these organisms the ability to invade epithelial cells, exit the phagocytic vacuole, and commandeer the host cell actin machinery to spread in the cytoplasm, spread directly from cell to cell, and induce apoptosis in and release of proinflammatory cytokines by macrophages (124). Chromosomal factors, including an enterotoxin, may also play a role in infection (125).

Clinical Manifestations

EIEC commonly cause watery diarrhea that is indistinguishable from that due to other pathogens. In a minority of cases, EIEC infection causes the clinical syndrome known as *bacterial dysentery*, manifested as the passage of frequent low-volume mucoid or bloody stools accompanied by fever, abdominal pain, and tenesmus (5). The diagnosis of EIEC infection is difficult. Like *Shigella*, many EIEC strains are lactose and lysine decarboxylase negative. A variety of molecular probes and PCR assays have been developed for the identification of factors common to EIEC and *Shigella*, but these are not available in most clinical laboratories.

Therapy and Prevention

Like patients with diarrhea caused by other organisms, patients with EIEC infection must be evaluated for dehydration and if necessary treated with rehydration solutions. There are no data regarding the role of antimicrobial therapy in the treatment of patients with EIEC infection, but antibiotics such as fluoroquinolones are effective in the treatment of diarrhea caused by *Shigella* (126). However, one must be careful not to administer antibiotics to patients in whom the diagnosis of EHEC infection has not been excluded.

REFERENCES

1. Donnenberg MS, Whittam TS. Pathogenesis and evolution of virulence in enteropathogenic and enterohemorrhagic *Escherichia coli*. *J Clin Invest* 2001;107:539–548.
2. Russo TA, Johnson JR. Proposal for a new inclusive designation for extraintestinal pathogenic isolates of *Escherichia coli*: ExPEC. *J Infect Dis* 2000;181:1753–1754.
3. Blattner FR, Plunkett G III, Bloch CA, et al. The complete genome sequence of *Escherichia coli* K-12. *Science* 1997;277:1453–1462.
4. Perna NT, Plunkett G III, Burland V, et al. Genome sequence of enterohaemorrhagic *Escherichia coli* O157:H7. *Nature* 2001;409:529–533.
5. Nataro JP, Kaper JB. Diarrheagenic *Escherichia coli*. *Clin Microbiol Rev* 1998;11:142–201.
6. DuPont HL, Formal SB, Hornick RB, et al. Pathogenesis of *Escherichia coli* diarrhea. *N Engl J Med* 1971;285:1–9.
7. DuPont HL, Ericsson CD. Drug therapy: prevention and treatment of traveler's diarrhea. *N Engl J Med* 1993;328:1821–1827.
8. Hyams KC, Bourfeois AL, Merrell BR, et al. Diarrheal disease during operation desert shield. *N Engl J Med* 1991;325:1423–1428.
9. Schulz S, Lopez MJ, Kuhn M, et al. Disruption of the guanylyl cyclase-C gene leads to a paradoxical phenotype of viable but heat-stable enterotoxin-resistant mice. *J Clin Invest* 1997;100:1590–1595.
10. Fleckenstein JM, Kopecko DJ, Warren RL, et al. Molecular characterization of the *tia* invasion locus from enterotoxigenic *Escherichia coli*. *Infect Immun* 1996;64:2256–2265.
11. Elsinghorst EA, Weitz JA. Epithelial cell invasion and adherence directed by the enterotoxigenic *Escherichia coli tib* locus is associated with a 104-kilodalton outer membrane protein. *Infect Immun* 1994;62:3463–3471.
12. Fleckenstein JM, Lindler LE, Elsinghorst EA, et al. Identification of a gene within a pathogenicity island of enterotoxigenic *Escherichia coli* H10407 required for maximal secretion of the heat-labile enterotoxin. *Infect Immun* 2000;68:2766–2774.
13. Adachi JA, Ostrosky-Zeichner L, DuPont HL, et al. Empirical antimicrobial therapy for traveler's diarrhea. *Clin Infect Dis* 2000;31:1079–1083.
14. Ericsson CD, DuPont HL. Travelers' diarrhea: approaches to prevention and treatment. *Clin Infect Dis* 1993;16:616–626.
15. Bray J. Isolation of antigenically homogeneous strains of *Bact. coli neapolitanum* from summer diarrhoea of infants. *J Pathol Bacteriol* 1945;57:239–247.
16. Kaper JB. Defining EPEC. *Rev Microbiol Sao Paulo* 1996;27[Suppl 1]:130–133.
17. Gomes TAT, Rassi V, Macdonald KL, et al. Enteropathogens associated with acute diarrheal disease in urban infants in São Paulo, Brazil. *J Infect Dis* 1991;164:331–337.
18. Robins-Browne R, Still CS, Miliotis MD, et al. Summer diarrhoea in African infants and children. *Arch Dis Child* 1980;55:923–928.
19. Thorén A, Stintzing G, Tufvesson B, et al. Aetiology and clinical features of severe infantile diarrhoea in Addis Ababa, Ethiopia. *J Trop Pediatr* 1982;28:127–131.
20. Cravioto A, Reyes R, Ortega R, et al. Prospective study of diarrhoeal disease in a cohort of rural Mexican children: incidence and isolated pathogens during the first two years of life. *Epidemiol Infect* 1988;101:123–134.
21. Cobeljic M, Mel D, Arsic B, et al. The association of enterotoxigenic and enteropathogenic *Escherichia coli* and other enteric pathogens with childhood diarrhoea in Yugoslavia. *Epidemiol Infect* 1989;103:53–62.
22. Kain KC, Barteluk RL, Kelly MT, et al. Etiology of childhood diarrhea in Beijing, China. *J Clin Microbiol* 1991;29:90–95.
23. Gunzburg ST, Chang BJ, Burke V, et al. Virulence factors of enteric *Escherichia coli* in young Aboriginal children in north-west Australia. *Epidemiol Infect* 1992;109:283–289.
24. Begaud E, Jourand P, Morillon M, et al. Detection of diarrheogenic *Escherichia coli* in children less than ten years old with and without diarrhea in New Caledonia using seven acetylaminofluorene-labeled DNA probes. *Am J Trop Med Hyg* 1993;48:26–34.
25. Molbak K, Wested N, Hojlyng N, et al. The etiology of early childhood diarrhea: A community study from Guinea-Bissau. *J Infect Dis* 1994;169:581–587.
26. Echeverria P, Taylor DN, Bettelheim KA, et al. HeLa cell-adherent enteropathogenic *Escherichia coli* in children under 1 year of age in Thailand. *J Clin Microbiol* 1987;25:1472–1475.
27. Bower JR, Congeni BL, Cleary TG, et al. *Escherichia coli* O114:nonmotile as a pathogen in an outbreak of severe diarrhea associated with a day care center. *J Infect Dis* 1989;160:243–247.

28. Paulozzi LJ, Johnson KE, Kamahele LM, et al. Diarrhea associated with adherent enteropathogenic *Escherichia coli* in an infant and toddler center, Seattle, Washington. *Pediatrics* 1986;77:296–300.
29. Wu S-X, Peng R-Q. Studies on an outbreak of neonatal diarrhea caused by EPEC O127:H6 with plasmid analysis restriction analysis and outer membrane protein determination. *Acta Paediatr Scand* 1992;81:217–221.
30. Senerwa D, Olsvik O, Mutanda LN, et al. Enteropathogenic *Escherichia coli* serotype O111:HNT isolated from preterm neonates in Nairobi, Kenya. *J Clin Microbiol* 1989;27:1307–1311.
31. Makino S, Asakura H, Shirahata T, et al. Molecular epidemiological study of a mass outbreak caused by enteropathogenic *Escherichia coli* O157:H45. *Microbiol Immunol* 1999;43:381–384.
32. Blake PA, Ramos S, Macdonald KL, et al. Pathogen-specific risk factors and protective factors for acute diarrheal disease in urban Brazilian infants. *J Infect Dis* 1993;167:627–632.
33. Blank TE, Zhong H, Bell AL, et al. Molecular variation among type IV pilin (*bfpA*) genes from diverse enteropathogenic *Escherichia coli* strains. *Infect Immun* 2000;68:7028–7038.
34. Bieber D, Ramer SW, Wu CY, et al. Type IV pili, transient bacterial aggregates, and virulence of enteropathogenic *Escherichia coli*. *Science* 1998;280:2114–2118.
35. Anantha RP, Stone KD, Donnenberg MS. The role of BfpF, a member of the PilT family of putative nucleotide-binding proteins, in type IV pilus biogenesis and in interactions between enteropathogenic *Escherichia coli* and host cells. *Infect Immun* 1998;66:122–131.
36. Knutton S, Shaw RK, Anantha RP, et al. The type IV bundle-forming pilus of enteropathogenic *Escherichia coli* undergoes dramatic alterations in structure associated with bacterial adherence, aggregation and dispersal. *Mol Microbiol* 1999;33:499–509.
37. Merz AJ, So M, Sheetz MP. Pilus retraction powers bacterial twitching motility. *Nature* 2000;407:98–102.
38. McDaniel TK, Jarvis KG, Donnenberg MS, et al. A genetic locus of enterocyte effacement conserved among diverse enterobacterial pathogens. *Proc Natl Acad Sci USA* 1995;92:1664–1668.
39. Kenny B, DeVinney R, Stein M, et al. Enteropathogenic *E. coli* (EPEC) transfers its receptor for intimate adherence into mammalian cells. *Cell* 1997;91:511–520.
40. Kalman D, Weiner OD, Goosney DL, et al. Enteropathogenic *E. coli* acts through WASP and Arp2/3 complex to form actin pedestals. *Nat Cell Biol* 1999;1:389–391.
41. Luo Y, Frey EA, Pfuetzner RA, et al. Crystal structure of enteropathogenic *Escherichia coli* intimin-receptor complex. *Nature* 2000;405:1073–1077.
42. Donnenberg MS, Tacket CO, James SP, et al. The role of the *eaeA* gene in experimental enteropathogenic *Escherichia coli* infection. *J Clin Invest* 1993;92:1412–1417.
43. Tacket CO, Sztein MB, Losonsky G, et al. Role of EspB in experimental human enteropathogenic *Escherichia coli* infection. *Infect Immun* 2000;68:3689–3695.
44. McNamara BP, Koutsouris A, O'Connell CB, et al. Translocated EspF protein from enteropathogenic *Escherichia coli* disrupts host intestinal barrier function. *J Clin Invest* 2001;107:621–629.
45. Stein MA, Mathers DA, Yan H, et al. Enteropathogenic *Escherichia coli* (EPEC) markedly decreases the resting membrane potential of Caco-2 and HeLa human epithelial cells. *Infect Immun* 1996;64:4820–4825.
46. Collington GK, Booth IW, Donnenberg MS, et al. Enteropathogenic *Escherichia coli* virulence genes encoding secreted signaling proteins are essential for modulation of Caco-2 cell electrolyte transport. *Infect Immun* 1998;66:6049–6053.
47. Rothbaum R, McAdams AJ, Giannella R, et al. A clinicopathological study of enterocyte-adherent *Escherichia coli*: a cause of protracted diarrhea in infants. *Gastroenterology* 1982;83:441–454.
48. Clausen CR, Christie DL. Chronic diarrhea in infants caused by adherent enteropathogenic *Escherichia coli*. *J Pediatr* 1982;100:358–361.
49. Taylor J, Powell BW, Wright J. Infantile diarrhea and vomiting: a clinical and bacteriological investigation. *Br Med J* 1949;2:117–141.
50. Tornieporth NG, John J, Salgado K, et al. Differentiation of pathogenic *Escherichia coli* strains in Brazilian children by PCR. *J Clin Microbiol* 1995;33:1371–1374.
51. Thorén A, Wolde-Mariam T, Stintzing G, et al. Antibiotics in the treatment of gastroenteritis caused by enteropathogenic *Escherichia coli*. *J Infect Dis* 1980;141:27–31.
52. Antai SP, Anozie SO. Incidence of infantile diarrhoea due to enteropathogenic *Escherichia coli* in Port Harcourt metropolis. *J Appl Bacteriol* 1987;62:227–229.
53. Lim YS, Ngan CCL, Tay L. Enteropathogenic *Escherichia coli* as a cause of diarrhoea among children in Singapore. *J Trop Med Hyg* 1992;95:339–342.
54. Salazar-Lindo E, Santisteban-Ponce J, Chea-Woo E, et al. Racecadotril in the treatment of acute watery diarrhea in children. *N Engl J Med* 2000;343:463–467.
55. Loureiro I, Frankel G, Adu-Bobie J, et al. Human colostrum contains IgA antibodies reactive to enteropathogenic *Escherichia coli* virulence–associated proteins: intimin, BfpA, EspA, and EspB. *J Pediatr Gastroenterol Nutr* 1998;27:166–171.
56. Parissi-Crivelli A, Parissi-Crivelli JM, Girón JA. Recognition of enteropathogenic *Escherichia coli* virulence determinants by human colostrum and serum antibodies. *J Clin Microbiol* 2000;38:2696–2700.

57. Silva MLM, Giampaglia CMS. Colostrum and human milk inhibit localized adherence of enteropathogenic *Escherichia coli* to HeLa cells. *Acta Paediatr Scand* 1992;81:266–267.

58. McGraw EA, Li J, Selander RK, et al. Molecular evolution and mosaic structure of α, β, and γ intimins of pathogenic *Escherichia coli*. *Mol Biol Evol* 1999;16:12–22.

59. Perna NT, Mayhew GF, Pósfai G, et al. Molecular evolution of a pathogenicity island from enterohemorrhagic *Escherichia coli* O157:H7. *Infect Immun* 1998;66:3810–3817.

60. Michino H, Araki K, Minami S, et al. Massive outbreak of *Escherichia coli* O157:H7 infection in schoolchildren in Sakai City, Japan, associated with consumption of white radish sprouts. *Am J Epidemiol* 1999;150:787–796.

61. Bell BP, Goldoft M, Griffin PM, et al. A multistate outbreak of *Escherichia coli* O157:H7-associated bloody diarrhea and hemolytic uremic syndrome from hamburgers: the Washington experience. *JAMA* 1994;272:1349–1353.

62. Lerman Y, Cohen D, Gluck A, et al. A cluster of cases of *Escherichia coli* O157 infection in a day-care center in a communal settlement (kibbutz) in Israel. *J Clin Microbiol* 1992;30:520–521.

63. Caprioli A, Luzzi I, Rosmini F, et al. Communitywide outbreak of hemolytic-uremic syndrome associated with non-O157 verocytotoxin-producing *Escherichia coli*. *J Infect Dis* 1994;169:208–211.

64. Banatvala N, Magnano AR, Cartter ML, et al. Meat grinders and molecular epidemiology: two supermarket outbreaks of *Escherichia coli* O157:H7 infection. *J Infect Dis* 1996;173:480–483.

65. Besser RE, Lett SM, Weber JT, et al. An outbreak of diarrhea and hemolytic uremic syndrome from *Escherichia coli* O157:H7 in fresh-pressed apple cider. *JAMA* 1993;269:2217–2220.

66. Breuer T, Benkel DH, Shapiro RL, et al. A Multistate Outbreak of *Escherichia coli* O157:H7 infections linked to alfalfa sprouts grown from contaminated seeds. *Emerg Infect Dis* 2001;7:977–982.

67. Cieslak PR, Noble SJ, Maxson DJ, et al. Hamburger-associated *Escherichia coli* O157:H7 infection in Las Vegas: a hidden epidemic. *Am J Public Health* 1997;87:176–180.

68. Hilborn ED, Mermin JH, Mshar PA, et al. A multistate outbreak of *Escherichia coli* O157:H7 infections associated with consumption of mesclun lettuce. *Arch Intern Med* 1999;159:1758–1764.

69. Tilden J Jr, Young W, McNamara AM, et al. A new route of transmission for *Escherichia coli*: infection from dry fermented salami. *Am J Public Health* 1996;86:1142–1145.

70. CDC. Lake-associated outbreak of *Escherichia coli* O157:H7—Illinois, 1995. *MMWR Morb Mortal Wkly Rep* 1996;45:437–439.

71. Keene WE, McAnulty JM, Hoesly FC, et al. A swimming-associated outbreak of hemorrhagic colitis caused by *Escherichia coli* O157:H7 and *Shigella sonnei*. *N Engl J Med* 1994;331:579–584.

72. Swerdlow DL, Woodruff BA, Brady RC, et al. A waterborne outbreak in Missouri of *Escherichia coli* O157:H7 associated with bloody diarrhea and death. *Ann Intern Med* 1992;117:812–819.

73. Banatvala N, Debeukelaer MM, Griffin PM, et al. Shiga-like toxin–producing *Escherichia coli* O111 and associated hemolytic-uremic syndrome: a family outbreak. *Pediatr Infect Dis J* 1996;15:1008–1011.

74. Belongia EA, Osterholm MT, Soler JT, et al. Transmission of *Escherichia coli* O157:H7 infection in Minnesota child day-care facilities. *JAMA* 1993;269:883–888.

75. Centers for Disease Control and Prevention. Outbreaks of *Escherichia coli* O157:H7 infections among children associated with farm visits—Pennsylvania and Washington, 2000. *MMWR Morb Mortal Wkly Rep* 2001;50:293–297.

76. Slutsker L, Ries AA, Maloney K, et al. A nationwide case-control study of *Escherichia coli* O157:H7 infection in the United States. *J Infect Dis* 1998;177:962–966.

77. Benjamin MM, Datta AR. Acid tolerance of enterohemorrhagic *Escherichia coli*. *Appl Environ Microbiol* 1995;61:1669–1672.

78. Waterman SR, Small PLC. Characterization of the acid resistance phenotype and *rpoS* alleles of Shiga-like toxin–producing *Escherichia coli*. *Infect Immun* 1996;64:2808–2811.

79. Sinclair JF, O'Brien AD. Cell-surface localized nucleolin is a eucaryotic receptor for the adhesin intimin-γ of enterohemorrhagic *Escherichia coli* O157: H7. *J Biol Chem* 2001;277:2876–2885.

80. Tzipori S, Gunzer F, Donnenberg MS, et al. The role of the *eaeA* gene in diarrhea and neurological complications in a gnotobiotic piglet model of enterohemorrhagic *Escherichia coli* infection. *Infect Immun* 1995;63:3621–3627.

81. O'Brien AD, Newland JW, Miller SF, et al. Shiga-like toxin–converting phages from *Escherichia coli* strains that cause hemorrhagic colitis or infantile diarrhea. *Science* 1984;226:694–696.

82. Zhang XP, McDaniel AD, Wolf LE, et al. Quinolone antibiotics induce Shiga toxin–encoding bacteriophages, toxin production, and death in mice. *J Infect Dis* 2000;181:664–670.

83. Fraser ME, Chernaia MM, Kozlov YV, et al. Crystal structure of the holotoxin from *Shigella dysenteriae* at 2.5 A resolution. *Nat Struct Biol* 1994;1:59–64.

84. Keusch GT, Jacewicz M, Mobassaleh M, et al. Shiga toxin: intestinal cell receptors and pathophysiology of enterotoxic effects. *Rev Infect Dis* 1991;13[Suppl 4]:S304–S310.

85. Sandvig K, Garred O, Prydz K, et al. Retrograde transport of endocytosed Shiga toxin to the endoplasmic reticulum. *Nature* 1992;358:510–512.

86. Louise CB, Obrig TG. Specific interaction of *Escherichia coli* O157:H7-derived Shiga-like toxin II with human renal endothelial cells. *J Infect Dis* 1995;172:1397–1401.

87. Acheson DWK, Moore R, De Breucker S, et al. Translocation of Shiga toxin across polarized intestinal cells in tissue culture. *Infect Immun* 1996;64:3294–3300.

88. Te Loo DM, van Hinsbergh VW, van den Heuvel LP, et al. Detection of verocytotoxin bound to circulating polymorphonuclear leukocytes of patients with hemolytic uremic syndrome. *J Am Soc Nephrol* 2001;12:800–806.

89. Griffin PM, Ostroff SM, Tauxe RV, et al. Illnesses associated with *Escherichia coli* O157:H7 infections: a broad clinical spectrum. *Ann Intern Med* 1988;109:705–712.

90. Tarr PI. *Escherichia coli* O157:H7: clinical, diagnostic, and epidemiological aspects of human infection. *Clin Infect Dis* 1995;20:1–10.

91. Boyce TG, Swerdlow DL, Griffin PM. Current concepts: *Escherichia coli* O157:H7 and the hemolytic-uremic syndrome. *N Engl J Med* 1995;333:364–368.

92. Bell BP, Griffin PM, Lozano P, et al. Predictors of hemolytic uremic syndrome in children during a large outbreak of *Escherichia coli* O157:H7 infections. *Pediatrics* 1997;100:E121–E126.

93. Ostroff SM, Tarr PI, Neill MA, et al. Toxin genotypes and plasmid profiles as determinants of systemic sequelae in *Escherichia coli* O157:H7 infections. *J Infect Dis* 1989;160:994–998.

94. Siegler RL, Pavia AT, Christofferson RD, et al. A 20-year population-based study of postdiarrheal hemolytic uremic syndrome in Utah. *Pediatrics* 1994;94:35–40.

95. Wong CS, Jelacic S, Habeeb RL, et al. The risk of the hemolytic-uremic syndrome after antibiotic treatment of *Escherichia coli* O157:H7 infections. *N Engl J Med* 2000;342:1930–1936.

96. Okeke IN, Lamikanra A, Czeczulin J, et al. Heterogeneous virulence of enteroaggregative *Escherichia coli* strains isolated from children in southwest Nigeria. *J Infect Dis* 2000;181:252–260.

97. Czeczulin JR, Whittam TS, Henderson IR, et al. Phylogenetic analysis of enteroaggregative and diffusely adherent *Escherichia coli*. *Infect Immun* 1999;67:2692–2699.

98. Nataro JP, Yikang D, Cookson S, et al. Heterogeneity of enteroaggregative *Escherichia coli* virulence demonstrated in volunteers. *J Infect Dis* 1995;171:465–468.

99. Tacket CO, Moseley SL, Kay B, et al. Challenge studies in volunteers using *Escherichia coli* strains with diffuse adherence to HEp-2 cells. *J Infect Dis* 1990;162:550–552.

100. Bhan MK, Raj P, Levine MM, et al. Enteroaggregative *Escherichia coli* associated with persistent diarrhea in a cohort of rural children in India. *J Infect Dis* 1989;159:1061–1064.

101. Bhatnagar S, Bhan MK, Sommerfelt H, et al. Enteroaggregative *Escherichia coli* may be a new pathogen causing acute and persistent diarrhea. *Scand J Infect Dis* 1993;25:579–583.

102. Wanke CA, Schorling JB, Barrett LJ, et al. Potential role of adherence traits of *Escherichia coli* in persistent diarrhea in an urban Brazilian slum. *Pediatr Infect Dis J* 1991;10:746–751.

103. Huppertz HI, Rutkowski S, Aleksic S, et al. Acute and chronic diarrhoea and abdominal colic associated with enteroaggregative *Escherichia coli* in young children living in western Europe. *Lancet* 1997;349:1660–1662.

104. Polotsky Y, Nataro JP, Kotler D, et al. HEp-2 cell adherence patterns, serotyping, and DNA analysis of *Escherichia coli* isolates from eight patients with AIDS and chronic diarrhea. *J Clin Microbiol* 1997;35:1952–1958.

105. Wanke CA, Mayer H, Weber R, et al. Enteroaggregative *Escherichia coli* as a potential cause of diarrheal disease in adults infected with human immunodeficiency virus. *J Infect Dis* 1998;178:185–190.

106. Itoh Y, Nagano I, Kunishima M, et al. Laboratory investigation of enteroaggregative *Escherichia coli* O untypeable:H10 associated with a massive outbreak of gastrointestinal illness. *J Clin Microbiol* 1997;35:2546–2550.

107. Smith HR, Cheasty T, Rowe B. Enteroaggregative *Escherichia coli* and outbreaks of gastroenteritis in UK. *Lancet* 1997;350:814–815.

108. Girón JA, Jones T, Millán-Velasco F, et al. Diffuse-adhering *Escherichia coli* (DAEC) as a putative cause of diarrhea in Mayan children in Mexico. *J Infect Dis* 1991;163:507–513.

109. Gunzburg ST, Chang BJ, Elliott SJ, et al. Diffuse and enteroaggregative patterns of adherence of enteric *Escherichia coli* isolated from aboriginal children from the Kimberley region of Western Australia. *J Infect Dis* 1993;167:755–758.

110. Levine MM, Ferreccio C, Prado V, et al. Epidemiologic studies of *Escherichia coli* diarrheal infections in a low socioeconomic level peri-urban community in Santiago, Chile. *Am J Epidemiol* 1993;138:849–869.

111. Nataro JP, Deng Y, Maneval DR, et al. Aggregative adherence fimbriae I of enteroaggregative *Escherichia coli* mediate adherence to HEp-2 cells and hemagglutination of human erythrocytes. *Infect Immun* 1992;60:2297–2304.

112. Henderson IR, Nataro JP. Virulence functions of autotransporter proteins. *Infect Immun* 2001;69:1231–1243.

113. Savarino SJ, Fasano A, Watson J, et al. Enteroaggregative *Escherichia coli* heat-stable enterotoxin 1 represents another subfamily of *E. coli* heat-stable toxin. *Proc Natl Acad Sci USA* 1993;90:3093–3097.

114. Steiner TS, Lima AAM, Nataro JP, et al. Enteroaggregative *Escherichia coli* produce intestinal inflammation and growth impairment and cause interleukin-8 release from intestinal epithelial cells. *J Infect Dis* 1998;177:88–96.

115. Steiner TS, Nataro JP, Poteet-Smith CE, et al. Enteroaggregative *Escherichia coli* expresses a novel flagellin that causes IL-8 release from intestinal epithelial cells. *J Clin Invest* 2000;105:1769–1777.

116. Bilge SS, Clausen CR, Lau W, et al. Molecular characterization of a fimbrial adhesin, F1845, mediating diffuse adherence of diarrhea-associated *Escherichia coli* to HEp-2 cells. *J Bacteriol* 1989;171:4281–4289.

117. Benz I, Schmidt MA. Isolation and serologic characterization of AIDA-I, the adhesin mediating the diffuse adherence phenotype of the diarrhea-associated *Escherichia coli* strain 2787 (O126: H27). *Infect Immun* 1992;60:13–18.

118. Cookson ST, Nataro JP. Characterization of HEp-2 cell projection formation induced by diffusely adherent *Escherichia coli*. *Microb Pathog* 1996;21:421–434.

119. Nataro JP, Steiner T, Guerrant RL. Enteroaggregative *Escherichia coli*. *Emerg Infect Dis* 1998;4:251–261.

120. Wanke CA, Gerrior J, Blais V, et al. Successful treatment of diarrheal disease associated with enteroaggregative *Escherichia coli* in adults infected with human immunodeficiency virus. *J Infect Dis* 1998;178:1369–1372.

121. Pupo GM, Karaolis DKR, Lan RT, et al. Evolutionary relationships among pathogenic and nonpathogenic *Escherichia coli* strains inferred from multilocus enzyme electrophoresis and *mdh* sequence studies. *Infect Immun* 1997;65:2685–2692.

122. Gordillo ME, Reeve GR, Pappas J, et al. Molecular characterization of strains of enteroinvasive *Escherichia coli* O143, including isolates from a large outbreak in Houston, Texas. *J Clin Microbiol* 1992;30:889–893.

123. Echeverria P, Sethabutr O, Serichantalergs O, et al. *Shigella* and enteroinvasive *Escherichia coli* infections in households of children with dysentery in Bangkok. *J Infect Dis* 1992;165:144–147.

124. Sansonetti PJ, Tran VN, Egile C. Rupture of the intestinal epithelial barrier and mucosal invasion by *Shigella flexneri*. *Clin Infect Dis* 1999;28:466–475.

125. Maurelli AT, Fernandez RE, Bloch CA, et al. "Black holes" and bacterial pathogenicity: a large genomic deletion that enhances the virulence of *Shigella* spp. and enteroinvasive *Escherichia coli*. *Proc Natl Acad Sci USA* 1998;95:3943–3948.

126. Bennish ML, Salam MA, Khan WA, et al. Treatment of shigellosis, III: comparison of one- or two-dose ciprofloxacin with standard 5-day therapy: a randomized, blinded trial. *Ann Intern Med* 1992;117:727–734.

127. Berman HM, Westbrook J, Feng Z, et al. The Protein Data Bank. *Nucleic Acids Res* 2000;28:235–242. Available at: *www.rcsb.or/pdb/*.

128. Sixma TK, Kalk KH, van Zanten BA, et al. Refined structure of *Escherichia coli* heat-labile enterotoxin, a close relative of cholera toxin. *J Mol Biol* 1993;230:890–918.

CHAPTER 70
Escherichia coli O157:H7 and Other Shiga Toxin–producing E. coli

Megan E. Reller and Patricia M. Griffin

[1]*Escherichia coli* O157:H7 is the most important of the Shiga toxin–producing *E. coli* (STEC). Named for its somatic (O) and flagellar (H) antigens, *E. coli* O157:H7 was first recognized as a human pathogen in 1982, when it was isolated from persons with diarrhea and hemorrhagic colitis (HC) in two outbreaks traced to the same chain of fast-food restaurants in the United States and one outbreak in a nursing home in Canada (1,2). Around the same time, Canadian investigators isolated Shiga toxin–producing strains of *E. coli* from the feces of children with hemolytic-uremic syndrome (HUS) (3). Since its discovery, *E. coli* O157:H7 has emerged as a major cause of both outbreak-

associated and sporadic diarrhea in North America and is now known to be the most frequent cause of HUS, the leading etiology of acute renal failure in children. Many *E. coli* serotypes produce Shiga toxins, but only a few commonly cause human illness. The term enterohemorrhagic *E. coli* (EHEC) was first used to describe those serotypes that mimic *E. coli* O157:H7 clinically, possess a 60-megadalton virulence plasmid, produce one or more phage-encoded Shiga toxins, and provoke attaching-effacing lesions in an animal model (4,5). The term *EHEC* is now generally used to refer to those STEC that cause human illness.

ESCHERICHIA COLI O157:H7

Epidemiology

E. coli O157:H7 has been found in most areas of the world in which it has been sought, including Europe, Asia, Australia, Africa, and South America. Cases are reported most frequently in Canada, the United Kingdom, the United States, and Japan. Within North America, cases are reported more frequently in western than in eastern Canada, in Canada than in the United States, and in northern states than in southern states within the United States (6,7). Recent data from the Foodborne Diseases Active Surveillance Network (FoodNet) and a large multicenter study confirm that these regional differences do not merely reflect differential testing and reporting (7,8).

Improved screening for *E. coli* O157:H7 infection and reporting of outbreaks likely explain the sharp increase in infections reported to the Centers for Disease Control and Prevention (CDC) between 1992 and 2000. Although the number of states that mandate the reporting of *E. coli* O157:H7 infections increased from 2 in 1987 to 49 by 2000 (unpublished data) (Fig. 70.1), sporadic cases and outbreaks still go undetected, even in states where it is a reportable disease, because many clinical laboratories do not routinely screen for the organism. Based on data compiled from active and passive surveillance systems with adjustment for regional variation and underreporting, the CDC has estimated that *E. coli* O157:H7 causes approximately 73,000 illnesses that lead to more than 2,000 hospitalizations and 60 deaths in the United States each year (9). The incidence of *E. coli* O157:H7 infection also varies by season. The summer peak in human *E. coli* O157:H7 infections mirrors that of bovine shedding of *E. coli* O157:H7 (9). Whether the seasonal difference reflects direct contact with cattle or their feces or other human behaviors, such as ground beef consumption, cooking practices, cross-contamination of foods, or swimming in pools, is unknown.

Much epidemiologic evidence ties human *E. coli* O157:H7 infection to cattle, and the observation that 10% of healthy beef cattle excrete *E. coli* O157:H7 (10) makes the link biologically plausible. Two Canadian studies suggested that consumption of undercooked ground beef was associated with sporadic cases of *E. coli* O157:H7 infection (11,12), and a subsequent nationwide case-control study in the United States found that among a number of possible exposures, only consumption of undercooked beef was independently associated with *E. coli* O157:H7 infection in multivariate analysis (13). More than 250 outbreaks were reported in the United States between 1982 and 2001, and more than half of the foods implicated were of bovine origin (CDC, unpublished data, 2001). Although undercooked ground beef, in which the combination of meat from multiple animals increases the probability of contamination, has been the most common vehicle, other incriminated bovine products have included roast beef (14), dry cured salami (15), dry fermented sausage (16), venison jerky (17), unpasteurized milk (18), and cheese curds (19). When nonbovine vehicles have been implicated in outbreaks,

---

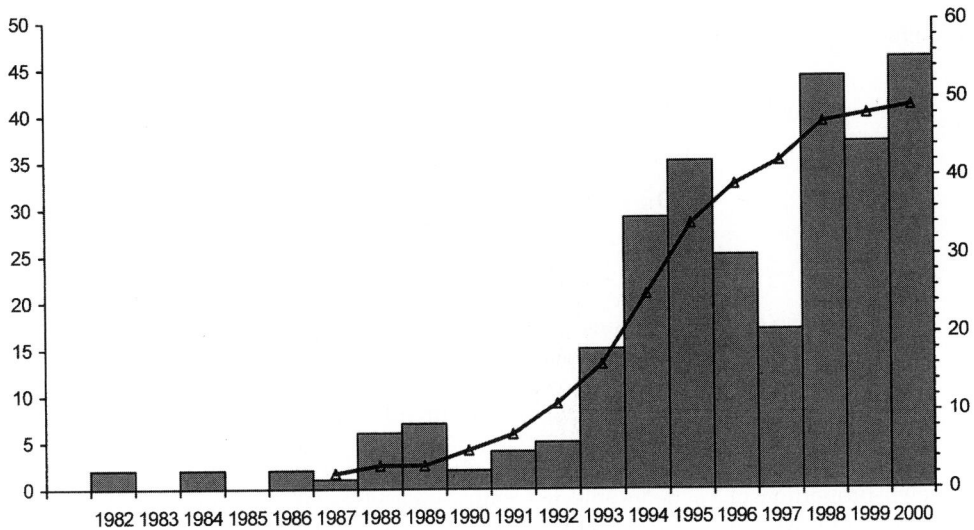

Figure 70.1. Number of reported outbreaks of *Escherichia coli* O157:H7 infection in the United States and number of states requiring reporting of *E. coli* O157:H7 infections, from 1982 to 2000.

cross-contamination by beef products or manure often has been deemed likely, as in one by an outbreak traced to vegetables contaminated by cow manure (20) and another caused by unpasteurized cider made from apples collected from the ground (21).

Other modes of transmission of *E. coli* O157:H7 include drinking water from unchlorinated municipal drinking water supplies (22), swallowing water while swimming in a lake (23), direct animal contact (24), and person-to-person transmission in child care centers and long-term care settings (25–27). Nosocomial spread and laboratory-acquired infections have also have been reported (28).

The efficiency of person-to-person transmission suggests that the infectious dose is low; three outbreaks, in which contaminated ground beef, dry fermented salami, and dry fermented sausage were implicated, suggest that the requisite inoculum is likely between 2 and 700 organisms (16,29,30).

Young children excrete *E. coli* O157:H7 longer than older children and adults. Shedding of *E. coli* O157:H7 may be intermittent (31) and may last longer in patients with HUS (32). In a study of sporadic cases, 53% of children 4 years or younger shed *E. coli* O157:H7 for more than 3 weeks after onset of diarrhea compared with 8% of older children and adults (33). In a day care center outbreak, the median duration of shedding was 17 days, and 38% shed *E. coli* O157:H7 for more than 20 days (25). Carriage rates of up to 124 days have been reported (32).

Pathogenesis

Although the pathogenesis of *E. coli* O157:H7–induced diarrhea and HUS is not fully understood, the production of Shiga toxin appears to be an important part of the process; indeed, the histologic pattern of colonic injury seen in *E. coli* O157:H7 infection is similar to that of *Clostridium difficile* colitis (34), which is also toxin mediated. Shiga toxin-1 is identical to that of *Shigella dysenteriae* type 1, the only pathogen other than STEC that is known to cause HUS. Shiga toxin-2 has 60% nucleotide homology to Shiga toxin-1 (35). *E. coli* O157:H7 and other STEC can produce one or both of these toxins. Targeted delivery of the toxin is facilitated by the organism's ability to dissolve the brush border at the site of its attachment to the mucosal surface of the large intestine (36). Animal models suggest that circulating toxin also contributes to colonic injury (37–39).

HUS may occur when the denuded colonic mucosa allows Shiga toxin, lipopolysaccharide, and other inflammatory medi-

ators, such as interleukin-1 and tumor necrosis factor, to reach the systemic circulation and to bind to Gb3 on renal endothelial cells (40–42). Although Shiga toxin has not been isolated from human sera, Shiga toxin-2 has been found in circulating polymorphonuclear leukocytes of patients with HUS (43).

Young children and the elderly are more susceptible not only to *E. coli* O157:H7 infection (6,44) but also to its complications, which suggests that immunity may contribute to protection. However, children without known immune deficiencies have been infected twice (45,46).

Clinical Manifestations

The clinical spectrum of *E. coli* O157:H7 infection includes asymptomatic carriage, nonbloody diarrhea, bloody diarrhea (hemorrhagic colitis), HUS, thrombotic thrombocytopenic purpura (TTP), and death (47). The average incubation period is 3 days (within a range of 1–8 days) (48); many of those with apparent incubation periods longer than 8 days are likely secondary cases (49,50).

Illness usually begins with severe abdominal cramps and nonbloody diarrhea. Although diarrhea may remain nonbloody (50,51), most people who seek care have developed bloody diarrhea, ranging from streaks to gross hemorrhage, usually by the second or third day of illness (7). One third have nausea and vomiting (7). Fever may be low grade or absent.

Although patients with *E. coli* O157:H7 infection are less likely to have fever than those with other bacterial enteric infections (7), the symptoms and signs of O157 diarrhea are not distinctive enough to distinguish it definitively from other infections. Because few clinical laboratories routinely screen for *E. coli* O157:H7, other diagnoses, such as inflammatory bowel disease, ischemic colitis, pseudomembranous colitis in adults or intussusception in children, are often considered (Table 70.1). Severe abdominal pain may lead to exploratory laparotomy (47,48). The presence of similar illness in others or patchy right-sided colonic inflammation should suggest *E. coli* O157:H7 infection (47). At colonoscopy, the mucosa often appears edematous and hyperemic with superficial ulcerations (47); a thumb-printing pattern, resulting from edema and submucosal hemorrhage in the ascending and transverse colon, is seen with barium enema (47). Rarely, extraintestinal sites are involved; *E. coli* O157:H7 has been isolated from the glans penis (52), urine (52), and blood (53).

**TABLE 70.1.   Differential Diagnosis of Colitis Caused by
Escherichia coli O157:H7**

Infectious causes	Noninfectious causes
Shigella	Ulcerative colitis
Salmonella	Crohn disease
Campylobacter	Intussusception
Yersinia enterocolitica	Ischemic colitis
Clostridium difficile	Diverticulosis
Entamoeba histolytica	Appendicitis

Source: From Boyce TG, Swerdlow DL, Griffin PM. *Escherichia coli* O157:H7 and the hemolytic-uremic syndrome. *N Engl J Med* 1995;333:364–368, with permission.

Symptoms of infection with *E. coli* O157:H7 usually subside within 1 week without sequelae. An unknown proportion of adults and approximately 8% of children with culture-proven *E. coli* O157:H7 develop HUS; among children younger than 5 years, the rate was 13% in one study (54). HUS is the most common cause of acute renal failure in children and is characterized by microangiopathic hemolytic anemia, thrombocytopenia, renal failure, and often central nervous system manifestations (55). Host predictors of HUS include extremes of age (56–58), leukocytosis (26,58,59), treatment with antimotility agents or antidiarrheal agents (56,59), fever (26,59), short enteric prodrome (58), and in some studies bloody diarrhea (27). The toxin genotype of the infecting strain also may influence development of HUS (60).

Population-based studies suggest that about 90% of cases of HUS are preceded by diarrhea (61). Most patients with postdiarrheal HUS in Europe and North America can be linked to *E. coli* O157:H7; antibody responses to O157 lipopolysaccharide were identified in 73% of patients with HUS in the United Kingdom (62), 91% in Germany (63), 73% in central Europe (64), and 80% in the United States (65). Many fewer patients have positive fecal cultures because HUS is usually diagnosed about 6 days (within a range of 2–14 days) after the onset of diarrhea (3), when the number of pathogens in the stool is decreasing (66). However, when fecal specimens were obtained promptly in two studies in the United States and Canada, 87% to 96% (66,67) yielded *E. coli* O157:H7. Outside the United States, non-O157 STEC serogroups, especially O111 and O26 (68), are commonly isolated from patients with HUS.

TTP, which is usually diagnosed in adults, includes all the clinical features of HUS, except the renal injury is typically less severe and the neurologic involvement is more prominent (69). Few cases are preceded by a diarrheal prodrome (47); however, postdiarrheal TTP is probably the same disorder as HUS (47,69,70). We prefer to use the term *HUS* for this severe complication of *E. coli* O157:H7 infection, whatever the age of the patient.

Predictors of severe HUS include an elevated white blood cell count (61,71,72), a shorter (72) and more severe diarrheal prodrome (71), early onset of anuria (61), seizures (71), age younger than 2 years (61,71), and female sex (71). Overall, one fourth of patients develop neurologic impairment, including focal or generalized seizures in 18% and other signs (e.g., coma or hemiparesis) in 18% (61); children and those exposed to antimotility agents appear particularly susceptible (73). Approximately one half of patients with HUS require dialysis, and three fourths require red blood cell transfusions (61). The mortality rate of HUS is 3% to 5% (61,72), and 5% of surviving patients have severe sequelae, such as permanent neurologic injury and renal disease (61).

Although HUS is the most common severe complication of *E. coli* O157:H7, others occur, and not all *E. coli* O157:H7–related

deaths are related to HUS (74). Intussusception (75), appendicitis (76), and rectal prolapse (76,77) have been reported in patients with *E. coli* O157:H7 infection without HUS, as has inflammation of the small bowel, predominantly the terminal ileum (78).

Diagnosis

E. coli O157:H7 infection should be suspected in any patient with bloody stools, a history of bloody stools, or HUS. The diagnosis should also be considered for persons with nonbloody diarrhea who have a history of exposure to a risky vehicle, such as undercooked ground beef or unpasteurized milk. During an outbreak, clinical suspicion should be raised to detect milder cases; if only bloody stools are cultured for *E. coli* O157:H7, some infections will be missed.

Although one study reported that fecal specimens of patients infected with *E. coli* O157:H7 more often contained fecal leukocytes than those of patients infected with *Salmonella*, *Shigella*, or *Campylobacter* (7), the leukocytes usually were not abundant; only 24% of specimens had more than 10 leukocytes per high-power field (7). A national consensus conference recommended that all stool samples submitted for culture of bacterial enteric pathogens also be examined for *E. coli* O157:H7 (79), a precautionary measure that the Infectious Disease Society of America (IDSA) reiterated more recently in its practice guidelines (80). Still, not all clinical laboratories routinely culture even bloody stools for *E. coli* O157:H7; thus, clinicians should specifically request testing for *E. coli* O157:H7 when clinically or epidemiologically warranted, to ensure proper processing of stool specimens.

Although routine stool cultures will not detect *E. coli* O157:H7, screening for the organism is neither difficult nor expensive. Unlike 80% to 90% of human fecal flora, almost no *E. coli* O157:H7 ferments sorbitol rapidly (81), which enables laboratories to screen for it using sorbitol-MacConkey (SMAC) agar (82). However, sorbitol-positive strains of *E. coli* O157 have been reported in Europe (83). The colorless sorbitol-negative colonies are selected and tested for the O157 antigen using commercially available reagents. *E. coli* that are both sorbitol negative and agglutinate in O157 antisera may be presumptively identified as *E. coli* O157:H7; confirmation requires either identification of the flagellar H7 antigen or determination that the strain produces Shiga toxin (35). If the flagellar H7 antigen is not detected, toxin testing should be performed because only the toxin-producing strains of nonmotile *E. coli* O157 have been linked to human illness.

Because non-O157 STEC cannot be distinguished from nonpathogenic *E. coli* on SMAC media (84) and no media selects for non-O157 STEC serogroups, testing for these organisms is more difficult. Culture for non-O157 STEC is indicated for patients with HUS, bloody diarrhea, or a history of bloody diarrhea (80,85). Testing stool samples after broth enrichment with an enzyme-linked immunoassay (EIA) kit is a sensitive method of detecting Shiga toxin. However, false-positive results may occur (86); therefore, a positive EIA test result should be followed by stool culture. If the organism is not identified as *E. coli* O157, the isolate should be sent to the state public health laboratory for serotyping. Presumptive isolates of *E. coli* O157 also should be sent so that molecular subtyping (e.g., by pulsed field gel electrophoresis) can be performed to detect outbreaks (35). These typing techniques aid investigation of outbreaks and assessment of interventions, and as such are important tools in protecting the public's health.

Immunomagnetic separation increases the proportion of specimens that yield *E. coli* O157:H7, especially when *E. coli*

O157:H7 are not abundant in the stool, such as late in the course of a patient's illness (35). Research laboratories use DNA probes and polymerase chain reaction (PCR) to demonstrate the presence of genes encoding Shiga toxins. PCR assays can detect potential virulence-associated genes such as *eae*, the enterohemolysin gene EHEC-*hlyA*, and *katP*, a gene on the large plasmid of *E. coli* O157:H7 that encodes a novel catalase peroxidase (35). These assays have contributed to the identification of different pathogenic groups of STEC.

Treatment

No specific therapy for patients with *E. coli* O157:H7 or other STEC infections has been proven effective. The challenge is to identify patients at increased risk for HUS and to rapidly provide appropriate supportive care. Adequate fluid replacement and vigilance for the development of pallor and oliguria are appropriate for all patients; patients at high risk for HUS also merit monitoring of peripheral blood cell counts, blood smears, and urinalyses. Those who develop HUS require meticulous attention to fluid and electrolyte balance, and often dialysis (50). Antimotility agents, which should not be used in any patient with bloody diarrhea, are especially dangerous with *E. coli* O157:H7 infection, because they have been associated with an increased risk of HUS (56,59). The use of antimicrobial agents to treat STEC infections has long been debated. Although most *E. coli* O157:H7 strains are susceptible to antibiotics, in retrospective analyses, antimicrobial treatment has not decreased the duration of diarrhea (59) and may even prolong bloody diarrhea (87). Moreover, antimicrobial treatment may increase the risk of HUS. *In vitro*, subinhibitory doses of some antimicrobial agents can increase toxin production through induction of a Shiga toxin–encoding bacteriophage (88–90). In a mouse model, treatment with subtherapeutic doses of ciprofloxacin increased fecal levels of Shiga toxin (91).

Whether therapeutic doses of antibiotics are helpful or harmful in humans is not clear. To date, most studies have not been randomized and so potentially have been confounded by the greater likelihood of sicker patients to seek treatment and receive antibiotics. In small, nonrandomized, retrospective studies, a higher proportion of patients treated with an antimicrobial agent developed HUS (13,59,92); however, one study found antibiotics to be protective (76) and in none of the studies was the difference between groups statistically significant. Four prospective studies, only one of which was randomized, do not resolve the issue. Pavia et al. (26) found that those treated with sulfonamides tended to be more likely to develop HUS, but only 17 patients were followed and the difference was not significant. Wong et al. (93) reported a positive association between antimicrobial treatment and HUS, which was significant; however, Ikeda et al. (94) found that early treatment with fosfomycin reduced the risk of HUS. In the only randomized trial, in which patients were randomized late in illness, trimethoprim-sulfamethoxazole neither predicted nor protected against progression to HUS (95). Finally, because antimicrobial agents are of uncertain efficacy in preventing HUS, agents that bind Shiga toxin in the gut have been developed (96,97) but remain investigational.

Prevention

Control of *E. coli* O157:H7 is hindered by several factors: It commonly colonizes healthy cattle, can survive in food and water, is tolerant of acidic conditions, and has a low infectious dose. Prevention measures aimed at all steps from farm to table are needed.

E. coli O157:H7 is common in cattle and ubiquitous in beef feedlots (98). Though definitive, on-farm control measures are elusive and efforts to improve sanitation of animal feeds, minimize animal crowding, and improve disposal and composting of manure may be important control measures on the farm. Cattle arrive at slaughter with O157 in their gastrointestinal tracts and caked in dung on their hides. Critical points during processing include limiting cross-contamination of carcasses and equipment, ensuring that meat patties sold as "ready to eat" are either cooked to temperatures high enough to kill STEC (160°F) or irradiated, and pasteurizing juice and milk. In the home, people should use a meat thermometer when cooking ground beef to verify that meat at the center reaches 160°F and should prevent contamination of other foodstuffs with raw meat.

Persons visiting county fairs, farms, and petting zoos should wash their hands after contact with animals and before eating. Secondary spread is common in day care centers and can result in HUS (25); one study suggested that person-to-person spread may account for more illness than direct exposure to ground beef (99). Supervised hand washing and exclusion of infected children from day care until two consecutive stool cultures are negative has been shown to prevent ongoing transmission (25). Because STEC are highly sensitive to chlorine, chlorination of public water supplies can prevent infections resulting from ingesting contaminated water while at agricultural fairs or in swimming pools.

After a presumptive *E. coli* O157:H7 is isolated, the local health department must be notified immediately. Once a case is detected in a nursing home or day care center, enhanced surveillance and control measures may avert an outbreak. Cases of HUS and clusters of bloody diarrhea should be reported promptly also. In a large outbreak in the western United States in 1993, early detection and reporting of *E. coli* O157:H7 infections and HUS enabled a rapid recall of contaminated ground beef and prevented an estimated 800 infections (51).

OTHER SHIGA TOXIN–PRODUCING *ESCHERICHIA COLI*

More than 400 Shiga toxin–producing serogroups of *E. coli* have been isolated from humans. However, a small number of serogroups cause most illnesses, and some serotypes appear not to be human pathogens. Like *E. coli* O157:H7, non-O157 STEC can cause nonbloody or bloody diarrhea and HUS. In the United States, non-O157 STEC are isolated at a similar frequency as *E. coli* O157 from persons with diarrhea (100–102); in parts of continental Europe, non-O157 STEC are isolated up to five times as frequently as *E. coli* O157 (103). In contrast, *E. coli* O157 is associated with most cases of HUS in both areas (65). In the 1983 to 2000 CDC database of non-O157 STEC isolates from patients with diarrhea or HUS, the most common serogroups were O26 (22%), O111 (18%), O103 (10%), O121 (8%), O45 (5%), O145 (5%), O165 (2%), and O113 (1%) (104). In continental Europe, the top non-O157 serogroups from the pooled results of eight studies of diarrhea conducted between 1988 and 1997 are similar: O26 (16%), O103 (15%), O111 (6%), O91 (4%), O113 (3%), O145 (3%), and O128 (2%) (103). Stool specimens from clusters of patients with bloody diarrhea or HUS should be tested for Shiga toxin and for *E. coli* O157 and the causative agent serotyped.

Outbreaks caused by non-O157 STEC are less common and more difficult to detect than those caused by *E. coli* O157. Noteworthy examples include an outbreak in Montana in 1994 of

E. coli 104:H21 infections caused by contaminated milk (105), an outbreak in South Australia of *E. coli* O111:NM infections caused by sausage (106), and an outbreak of *E. coli* O111:H8 infections among teenage campers in Texas in 1999 in which consuming ice and salad were associated with illness (107).

CONCLUSION

Among STEC, *E. coli* O157:H7 is the most important serotype for clinicians and public health agencies alike. In addition to bloody and nonbloody diarrhea, it causes most cases of HUS in North America and Europe. Clinicians need to communicate with their colleagues in the laboratory when STEC infection is suspected. Prompt diagnosis may help the individual avoid unnecessary complications, including surgical procedures, and may help the community avert an outbreak. Other STEC, especially O111 and O26 serotypes, are becoming increasingly recognized as important pathogens as laboratories develop the capability to detect them.

REFERENCES

1. Riley LW, et al. Hemorrhagic colitis associated with a rare *Escherichia coli* serotype. *N Engl J Med* 1983;308(12):681–685.
2. Johnson WM, Lior H, Bezanson GS. Cytotoxic *Escherichia coli* O157:H7 associated with haemorrhagic colitis in Canada. *Lancet* 1983;1(8314-5):76.
3. Karmali MA, et al. The association between idiopathic hemolytic uremic syndrome and infection by verotoxin-producing *Escherichia coli*. *J Infect Dis* 1985;151(5):775–782.
4. Levine MM, Edelman R. Enteropathogenic *Escherichia coli* of classic serotypes associated with infant diarrhea: epidemiology and pathogenesis. *Epidemiol Rev* 1984;6:31–51.
5. Levine MM, et al. A DNA probe to identify enterohemorrhagic *Escherichia coli* of O157:H7 and other serotypes that cause hemorrhagic colitis and hemolytic uremic syndrome. *J Infect Dis* 1987;156(1):175–182.
6. Griffin PM, Tauxe RV. The epidemiology of infections caused by *Escherichia coli* O157:H7, other enterohemorrhagic *E. coli*, and the associated hemolytic uremic syndrome. *Epidemiol Rev* 1991;13:60–98.
7. Slutsker L, et al. *Escherichia coli* O157:H7 diarrhea in the United States: clinical and epidemiologic features. *Ann Intern Med* 1997;126(7):505–513.
8. Centers for Disease Control and Prevention. FoodNet surveillance report for 1999 [Final Report]. Atlanta, GA: Centers for Disease Control and Prevention, 2000.
9. Mead PS, Griffin PM. *Escherichia coli* O157:H7. *Lancet* 1998;352(9135):1207–1212.
10. Synge B, Paiba G. Verocytotoxin-producing *E coli* O157. *Vet Rec* 2000;147(1):27.
11. Bryant HE, Athar MA, Pai CH. Risk factors for *Escherichia coli* O157:H7 infection in an urban community. *J Infect Dis* 1989;160(5):858–864.
12. Le Saux N, et al. Ground beef consumption in noncommercial settings is a risk factor for sporadic *Escherichia coli* O157:H7 infection in Canada. *J Infect Dis* 1993;167:500–502.
13. Slutsker L, et al. A nationwide case-control study of *Escherichia coli* O157:H7 infection in the United States. *J Infect Dis* 1998;177(4):962–966.
14. Rodrigue DC, et al. A university outbreak of *Escherichia coli* O157:H7 infections associated with roast beef and an unusually benign clinical course. *J Infect Dis* 1995;172(4):1122–1125.
15. *Escherichia coli* O157:H7 outbreak linked to commercially distributed dry-cured salami–Washington and California, 1994. *MMWR Morb Mortal Wkly Rep* 1995;44(9):157–160.
16. Paton AW, et al. Molecular microbiological investigation of an outbreak of hemolytic-uremic syndrome caused by dry fermented sausage contaminated with Shiga-like toxin-producing *Escherichia coli*. *J Clin Microbiol* 1996;34(7):1622–1627.
17. Keene WE, et al. An outbreak of *Escherichia coli* O157:H7 infections traced to jerky made from deer meat. *JAMA* 1997;277(15):1229–1231.
18. Keene WE, et al. A prolonged outbreak of *Escherichia coli* O157:H7 infections caused by commercially distributed raw milk. *J Infect Dis* 1997;176(3):815–818.
19. Outbreak of *Escherichia coli* O157:H7 infection associated with eating fresh cheese curds—Wisconsin, June 1998. *MMWR Morb Mortal Wkly Rep* 2000;49(40):911–913.
20. Cieslak PR, et al. *Escherichia coli* O157:H7 infection from a manured garden. *Lancet* 1993;342(8867):367.
21. Besser RE, et al. An outbreak of diarrhea and hemolytic uremic syndrome from *Escherichia coli* O157:H7 in fresh-pressed apple cider. *JAMA* 1993;269:2217–2220.
22. Swerdlow DL, et al. A waterborne outbreak in Missouri of *Escherichia coli* O157:H7 associated with bloody diarrhea and death [see Comments]. *Ann Intern Med* 1992;117(10):812–919.
23. Keene WE, et al. A swimming-associated outbreak of hemorrhagic colitis caused by *Escherichia coli* O157:H7 and *Shigella sonnei*. *N Engl J Med* 1994;331(9):579–584.
24. Crump JA, et al. An outbreak of *Escherichia coli* O157:H7 infections among visitors to a dairy farm. *N Engl J Med* 2002;347:555–560.
25. Belongia EA, et al. Transmission of *Escherichia coli* O157:H7 infection in Minnesota child day-care facilities. *JAMA* 1993;269(7):883–888.
26. Pavia AT, et al. Hemolytic-uremic syndrome during an outbreak of *Escherichia coli* O157:H7 infections in institutions for mentally retarded persons: clinical and epidemiologic observations. *J Pediatr* 1990;116(4):544–551.
27. Carter AO, et al. A severe outbreak of *Escherichia coli* O157:H7–associated hemorrhagic colitis in a nursing home. *N Engl J Med* 1987;317(24):1496–1500.
28. Coia JE, Nosocomial and laboratory-acquired infection with *Escherichia coli* O157. *J Hosp Infect* 1998;40(2):107–113.
29. Tuttle J, et al. Lessons from a large outbreak of *Escherichia coli* O157:H7 infections: insights into the infectious dose and method of widespread contamination of hamburger patties. *Epidemiol Infect* 1999;122(2):185–192.
30. Tilden J, et al. A new route of transmission for *Escherichia coli*: infection from dry fermented salami. *Am J Public Health* 1996;86(8)(pt 1):1142–1145.
31. Swerdlow DL, Griffin PM. Duration of faecal shedding of *Escherichia coli* O157:H7 among children in day-care centres. *Lancet* 1997;349(9054):745–746.
32. Karch H, et al. Long-term shedding and clonal turnover of enterohemorrhagic *Escherichia coli* O157 in diarrheal diseases. *J Clin Microbiol* 1995;33(6):1602–1605.
33. Pai CH, et al. Epidemiology of sporadic diarrhea due to verocytotoxin-producing *Escherichia coli*: a two-year prospective study. *J Infect Dis* 1988;157(5):1054–1057.
34. Griffin PM, Olmstead LC, Petras RE. *Escherichia coli* O157:H7–associated colitis. A clinical and histologic study of 11 cases. *Gastroenterology* 1990;99(1):142–149.
35. Strockbine NA, et al. Overview of detection and subtyping methods. In: Kaper JB, O'Brien AD, eds. Escherichia coli *O157:H7 and other Shiga toxin–producing* E. coli *strains*. Washington, DC: ASM Press, 1998:331–356.
36. Moon HW. Comparative histopathology of intestinal infections. *Adv Exp Med Biol* 1997;412:1–19.
37. Barrett TJ, Potter ME, Wachsmuth IK. Continuous peritoneal infusion of Shiga-like toxin II (SLT II) as a model for SLT II–induced diseases. *J Infect Dis* 1989;159(4):774–777.
38. Richardson SE, et al. Experimental verocytotoxemia in rabbits. *Infect Immun* 1992;60(10):4154–4167.
39. Padhye VV, et al. Colonic hemorrhage produced in mice by a unique vero cell cytotoxin from an *Escherichia coli* strain that causes hemorrhagic colitis. *J Infect Dis* 1987;155(6):1249–1253.
40. van de Kar NC, et al. Tumor necrosis factor and interleukin-1 induce expression of the verocytotoxin receptor globotriaosylceramide on human endothelial cells: implications for the pathogenesis of the hemolytic uremic syndrome. *Blood* 1992;80(11):2755–2764.
41. Kaye SA, Obrig TG. Effect of TNF-alpha, Shiga toxin and calcium ionophore on Weibel-Palade body content of endothelial cells: possible implications for the hemolytic uremic syndrome. *Thromb Res* 1995;79(4):415–421.
42. Louise CB, Obrig TG. Shiga toxin–associated hemolytic-uremic syndrome: combined cytotoxic effects of Shiga toxin, interleukin-1 beta, and tumor necrosis factor alpha on human vascular endothelial cells in vitro. *Infect Immun* 1991;59(11):4173–4179.
43. Te Loo DM, et al. Detection of verocytotoxin bound to circulating polymorphonuclear leukocytes of patients with hemolytic uremic syndrome. *J Am Soc Nephrol* 2001;12(4):800–806.
44. Olsen SJ, et al. A waterborne outbreak of *Escherichia coli* O157:H7 infections and hemolytic uremic syndrome: implications for rural water systems. *Emerg Infect Dis* 2002;8(4):370–375.
45. Siegler RL, et al. Recurrent hemolytic uremic syndrome secondary to *Escherichia coli* O157:H7 infection. *Pediatrics* 1993;91(3):666–668.
46. Robson WL, Leung AK, Miller-Hughes DJ. Recurrent hemorrhagic colitis caused by *Escherichia coli* O157:H7. *Pediatr Infect Dis J* 1993;12(8):699–701.
47. Griffin PM, et al. Illnesses associated with *Escherichia coli* 0157:H7 infections. A broad clinical spectrum [Review]. *Ann Intern Med* 1988;109(9):705–712.
48. Ostroff SM, et al. A statewide outbreak of *Escherichia coli* O157:H7 infections in Washington State. *Am J Epidemiol* 1990;132(2):239–247.
49. Salmon RL, et al. A christening party outbreak of haemorrhagic colitis and haemolytic uraemic syndrome associated with *Escherichia coli* O157:H7. *Epidemiol Infect* 1989;103(2):249–254.
50. Tarr PI. *Escherichia coli* O157:H7: clinical, diagnostic, and epidemiological aspects of human infection. *Clin Infect Dis* 1995;20(1):1–8; quiz 9–10.
51. Bell BP, et al. A multistate outbreak of *Escherichia coli* O157:H7–associated bloody diarrhea and hemolytic uremic syndrome from hamburgers. The Washington experience. *JAMA* 1994;272(17):1349–1353.
52. Grandsen WR, et al. Haemorrhagic cystitis and balanitis associated with verotoxin-producing *Escherichia coli* O157:H7 [letter]. *Lancet* 1985;2(8447):150.
53. Krishnan C, et al. Laboratory investigation of outbreak of hemorrhagic colitis caused by *Escherichia coli* O157:H7. *J Clin Microbiol* 1987;25(6):1043–1047.

54. Rowe PC, et al. Risk of hemolytic uremic syndrome after sporadic *Escherichia coli* O157:H7 infection: results of a Canadian collaborative study [see Comments]. *J Pediatr* 1998;132(5):777–782.

55. Neild GH, Hemolytic uremic syndrome/thrombotic thrombocytopenic purpura: pathophysiology and treatment. *Kidney Int Suppl* 1998;64:S45–S49.

56. Cimolai N, et al. A continuing assessment of risk factors for the development of *Escherichia coli* O157:H7–associated hemolytic uremic syndrome. *Clin Nephrol* 1994;42(2):85–89.

57. Tarr PI, Hickman RO. Hemolytic uremic syndrome epidemiology: a population-based study in King county, Washington, 1971–1980. *Pediatrics* 1987;80(1):41–45.

58. Buteau C, et al. Leukocytosis in children with *Escherichia coli* O157:H7 enteritis developing the hemolytic-uremic syndrome. *J Pediatr Infect Dis* 2000;19(7):642–647.

59. Bell BP, et al. Predictors of hemoytic urmeic syndrome in children during a large outbreak of *Escherichia coli* O157:H7 infections. *Pediatrics* 1997;100:e12.

60. Ostroff SM, et al. Toxin genotypes and plasmid profiles as determinants of systemic sequelae in *Escherichia coli* O157:H7 infections. *J Infect Dis* 1989;160(6):994–998.

61. Siegler RL, et al. A 20-year population-based study of postdiarrheal hemolytic uremic syndrome in Utah. *Pediatrics* 1994;94(1):35–40.

62. Chart H, et al. Serological identification of *Escherichia coli* O157:H7 infection in haemolytic uraemic syndrome. *Lancet* 1991;337(8734):138–140.

63. Bitzan M, et al. High incidence of serum antibodies to *Escherichia coli* O157 lipopolysaccharide in children with hemolytic-uremic syndrome. *J Pediatr* 1991;119(3):380–385.

64. Bitzan M, et al. The role of *Escherichia coli* O157 infections in the classical (enteropathic) haemolytic uraemic syndrome: results of a Central European, multicentre study. *Epidemiol Infect* 1993;110(2):183–196.

65. Banatvala N, et al. The United States national prospective hemolytic uremic syndrome study: microbiologic, serologic, clinical, and epidemiologic findings. *J Infect Dis* 2001;183(7):1063–1070.

66. Tarr PI, et al. *Escherichia coli* O157:H7 and the hemolytic uremic syndrome: importance of early cultures in establishing the etiology. *J Infect Dis* 1990;162(2):553–556.

67. Rowe PC, et al. A prospective study of exposure to verotoxin-producing *Escherichia coli* among Canadian children with haemolytic uraemic syndrome. *Epidemiol Infect* 1993;110(1):1–7.

68. Scheutz F, Beutin L, Smith HR. Characterisation of non-O157 verocytotoxigenic *E. coli* (VTEC) isolated from patients with haemolytic uraemic syndrome (HUS) world-wide from 1982 to 2000. In Fourth International Symposium and Workshop on Shiga toxin (verocytotoxin)–producing *Escherichia coli* Infections. Kyoto, Japan: VTEC 2000 Organizing Committees, 2000.

69. Ruggenenti P, Remuzzi G. Pathophysiology and management of thrombotic microangiopathies. *J Nephrol* 1998;11(6):300–310.

70. Ashkenazi S. Role of bacterial cytotoxins in hemolytic uremic syndrome and thrombotic thrombocytopenic purpura. *Annu Rev Med* 1993;44:11–18.

71. Rowe PC, et al. Epidemiology of hemolytic-uremic syndrome in Canadian children from 1986 to 1988. The Canadian Pediatric Kidney Disease Reference Centre. *J Pediatr* 1991;119(2):218–224.

72. Martin DL, et al. The epidemiology and clinical aspects of the hemolytic uremic syndrome in Minnesota. *N Engl J Med* 1990;323(17):1161–1167.

73. Cimolai N, Morrison BJ, Carter JE. Risk factors for the central nervous system manifestations of gastroenteritis-associated hemolytic-uremic syndrome. *Pediatrics* 1992;90(4):616–621.

74. Boyce TG, Swerdlow DL, Griffin PM. *Escherichia coli* O157:H7 and the hemolytic-uremic syndrome. *N Engl J Med* 1995;333(6):364–368.

75. Lopez EL, et al. Intussusception associated with *Escherichia coli* O157:H7. *Pediatr Infect Dis J* 1989;8(7):471–473.

76. Cimolai N, et al. *Escherichia coli* O157:H7 infections associated with perforated appendicitis and chronic diarrhoea. *Eur J Pediatr* 1990;149(4):259–260.

77. Bhimma R, et al. Post-dysenteric hemolytic uremic syndrome in children during an epidemic of *Shigella* dysentery in Kwazulu/Natal. *Pediatr Nephrol* 1997;11(5):560–564.

78. Tarr PI, et al. Bacterial ileocecitis caused by *Escherichia coli* O157:H7. *J Pediatr Gastroenterol Nutr* 1992;14(3):261–263.

79. Consensus conference statement. *Escherichia coli* O157:H7 infections—an emerging national health crisis, July 11–13, 1994. *Gastroenterology* 1995;108(6):1923–1934.

80. Guerrant RL, et al. Practice guidelines for the management of infectious diarrhea. *Clin Infect Dis* 2001;32(3):331–351.

81. Ratnam S, et al. Characterization of *Escherichia coli* serotype O157:H7. *J Clin Microbiol* 1988;26(10):2006–2012.

82. March SB, Ratnam S. Sorbitol-MacConkey medium for detection of *Escherichia coli* O157:H7 associated with hemorrhagic colitis. *J Clin Microbiol* 1986;23(5):869–872.

83. Bielaszewska M, et al. Isolation and characterization of sorbitol-fermenting Shiga toxin (Vero cytotoxin)–producing *Escherichia coli* O157:H strains in the Czech Republic. *J Clin Microbiol* 1998;36(7):2135–2137.

84. Stapp JR, et al. Comparison of *Escherichia coli* O157:H7 antigen detection in stool and broth cultures to that in sorbitol-MacConkey agar stool cultures. *J Clin Microbiol* 2000;38(9):3404–3406.

85. Guidelines for the control of infection with Vero cytotoxin producing *Escherichia coli* (VTEC). Subcommittee of the PHLS Advisory Committee on Gastrointestinal Infections. *Commun Dis Public Health* 2000;3(1):14–23.

86. University outbreak of calicivirus infection mistakenly attributed to Shiga toxin–producing *Escherichia coli* O157:H7—Virginia, 2000. *MMWR Morb Mortal Wkly Rep* 2001;50(23):489–491.

87. Cimolai N, Anderson JD, Morrison BJ. Antibiotics for *Escherichia coli* O157:H7 enteritis? *J Antimicrob Chemother* 1989;23(5):807–808.

88. Grif K, et al. Strain-specific differences in the amount of Shiga toxin released from enterohemorrhagic *Escherichia coli* O157 following exposure to subinhibitory concentrations of antimicrobial agents. *Eur J Clin Microbiol Infect Dis* 1998;17(11):761–766.

89. Walterspiel JN, et al. Effect of subinhibitory concentrations of antibiotics on extracellular Shiga-like toxin I. *Infection* 1992;20(1):25–29.

90. Murakami J, et al. Macrolides and clindamycin suppress the release of Shiga-like toxins from *Escherichia coli* O157:H7 *in vitro*. *Int J Antimicrob Agents* 2000;15(2):103–109.

91. Zhang X, et al. Quinolone antibiotics induce Shiga toxin–encoding bacteriophages, toxin production, and death in mice. *J Infect Dis* 2000;181(2):664–670.

92. Gilbert L, et al. Antimicrobial use is not a risk factor for hemolytic uremic syndrome after *E. coli* O157 infection: results of a 1996–1997 FoodNet study [Abstract]. In: Programs and abstracts of the International Conference on Emerging Infectious Diseases; 2000; Atlanta, Georgia.

93. Wong CS, et al. The risk of the hemolytic-uremic syndrome after antibiotic treatment of *Escherichia coli* O157:H7 infections [see Comments]. *N Engl J Med* 2000;342(26):1930–1936.

94. Ikeda K, et al. Effect of early fosfomycin treatment on prevention of hemolytic uremic syndrome accompanying *Escherichia coli* O157:H7 infection. *Clin Nephrol* 1999;52(6):357–362.

95. Proulx F, Seidman E. Is antibiotic therapy of mice and humans useful in *Escherichia coli* O157:H7 enteritis [Editorial, Comment]. *Eur J Clin Microbiol Infect Dis* 1999;18(8):533–534.

96. Armstrong GD, McLaine PN, Rowe PC. Clinical trials of Synsorb-Pk in preventing hemolytic-uremic syndrome. In: Kaper JB, O'Brien AD, ed. *Escherichia coli O157:H7 and other Shiga toxin–producing* E. coli *strains*. Washington, DC: ASM Press, 1998:374–384.

97. Takeda T, et al. *In vitro* assessment of a chemically synthesized Shiga toxin receptor analog attached to chromosorb P (Synsorb Pk) as a specific absorbing agent of Shiga toxin 1 and 2. *Microbiol Immunol* 1999;43(4):331–337.

98. Hancock DD, et al. Multiple sources of *Escherichia coli* O157 in feedlots and dairy farms in the northwestern USA. *Prev Vet Med* 1998;35(1):11–19.

99. Rowe PC, et al. Diarrhoea in close contacts as a risk factor for childhood haemolytic uraemic syndrome. *Epidemiol Infect* 1993;110(1):9–16.

100. Fiorentino T, et al. *Emergence of nonculture methods for detecting Shiga toxin–producing* E. coli *(STEC) in Connecticut (CT) laboratories, 2000 [Abstract C-166]; Proceedings of the American Society for Microbiology 101st General Meeting*. Orlando, FL: American Society for Microbiology, 2001:187.

101. Nims L, et al. *Isolation of Shiga toxin–producing* Escherichia coli *in New Mexico [Abstract C-165]; Proceedings of the American Society for Microbiology 101st General Meeting*. Orlando, FL: American Society for Microbiology, 2001:187.

102. Acheson DW. How does *Escherichia coli* O157:H7 testing in meat compare with what we are seeing clinically? *J Food Protection* 2000;63(6):819–821.

103. Caprioli A, Tozzi AE. Epidemiology of Shiga toxin–producing *Escherichia coli* infections in continental Europe. In: Kaper JB, O'Brien AD, eds. Escherichia coli *O157:H7 and other Shiga toxin–producing* E. coli *strains*. Washington, DC: ASM Press, 1998:38–48.

104. Brooks JT, et al. Non-O157 Shiga toxin–producing *Escherichia coli* reported to CDC, 1983–2000. In: Program and abstracts of the 39th annual Meeting of the Infectious Diseases Society of America. San Francisco: IDSA, 2001:185. Abstract no. 856.

105. Outbreak of acute gastroenteritis attributable to *Escherichia coli* serotype O104:H21—Helena, Montana, 1994. *MMWR Morb Mortal Wkly Rep* 1995; 44(27):501–503.

106. Community outbreak of hemolytic uremic syndrome attributable to *Escherichia coli* O111:NM—South Australia 1995. *MMWR Morb Mortal Wkly Rep* 1995;44(29):550–551, 557–558.

107. Centers for Disease Control and Prevention. *Escherichia coli* O111:H8 outbreak among teenage campers—Texas, 1999. *MMWR Morb Mortal Wkly Rep* 2000;49(15):321–324.

CHAPTER 71
Campylobacter *Infections*

Ban Mishu Allos

Campylobacter species are an important cause of gastrointestinal (GI) tract infections in both the developing and the developed world. These previously underrecognized microorganisms now are known to be one of the most common causes of bacterial diarrhea worldwide. In the United States, more than 99% of reported *Campylobacter* isolates are *Campylobacter jejuni* (1). A description of the clinical features of this organism as well as its microbiology and epidemiology are contained in Chapter 198.

Because the selective media commonly used to detect *C. jejuni* may not permit growth of other campylobacters, these "atypical" isolates may not be detected despite their presence in stools. In parts of the world where *Campylobacter* isolation procedures are used, which permit growth of atypical campylobacters (other than *C. jejuni* or *C. coli*) only one third of strains are *C. jejuni* (2). Indeed, worldwide, only 80% of identified campylobacters are *C. jejuni* (3). This chapter highlights the microbiology, epidemiology, and clinical characteristics of campylobacters and *Campylobacter*-like organisms (CLOs) other than *C. jejuni* and *C. coli*.

CAMPYLOBACTER FETUS

Campylobacter (formerly *Vibrio* and *C. fetus* subspecies *fetus*) *fetus* was first recognized as a cause of abortion in sheep and cattle in the early twentieth century (4). Later the organism was recognized as a human pathogen causing bacteremia and other extraintestinal illness in immunocompromised persons.

Prolonged incubation of blood cultures is required for detection of *C. fetus* bacteremia, because 3 to 25 days may be required for primary isolation from blood. The organisms grow better in aerobic bottles. Isolation of *C. fetus* from stools presents additional difficulties. Because most *C. fetus* strains are susceptible to cephalothin, use of cephalothin-containing media (commonly used to isolate *C. jejuni* from stools) will not permit the growth of *C. fetus* or other atypical campylobacters. Therefore, an alternative detection method is needed. Because campylobacters are quite small (0.3–0.6 μm in diameter), stools may be filtered through a 0.45- to 0.65-μm filter onto an antibiotic-free medium. This filtration technique is now considered the optimal method for isolation of *Campylobacter* species from stools.

Like other campylobacters, *C. fetus* is microaerophilic, requiring 3% to 5% oxygen for growth. The organism does not ferment carbohydrates; most strains are nitrate, catalase, and oxidase positive. *C. fetus* grows well at 25°C and 37°C, but unlike most *C. jejuni* strains, it does not grow at 42°C. [However, exceptional *C. fetus* strains are able to grow at this higher temperature (5).] *C. fetus* is resistant to nalidixic acid, susceptible to cephalothin, and lacks pyrazinamidase activity—features that help distinguish it from *C. jejuni* (Table 71.1).

C. fetus infections remain quite rare; only 265 isolates were reported to the Centers for Disease Control and Prevention (CDC) *Campylobacter* Surveillance System between 1982 and 1989 (6). Most *C. fetus* infections are extraintestinal and occur in immunocompromised persons (Table 71.2); 75% of infected persons have underlying malignancy, diabetes, alcoholism, cirrhosis or other liver disease, or acquired immunodeficiency syndrome (AIDS), or they are receiving immunosuppressive therapy (7,8). Among adults with *C. fetus* infection, men outnumber women by a ratio of 3:1 (7).

Because *C. fetus* has a tropism for vascular tissue, any patient with *C. fetus* infection should be carefully evaluated for septic thrombophlebitis. Infections also may be associated with endocarditis or mycotic aneurysms (9–11). In pregnant animals, intestinal infection with *C. fetus* may lead to hematogenous spread, followed by placental and fetal infection and death (12). Similarly, in pregnant women, GI tract *C. fetus* infection (with or without symptoms) may be followed by placental infection or chorioamnionitis (13,14); 80% of fetuses and neonates die even when maternal infection is mild and appropriate antibiotics are given (15,16). *C. fetus* infections also may cause salpingitis, septic arthritis, cellulitis, abscesses, meningitis, peritonitis, osteomyelitis, urinary tract infections, cholecystitis, or hypersplenism (17–27). Occasionally, *C. fetus* infection may produce uncomplicated enteritis in healthy persons (5,7,28).

The most likely route of human infection with *C. fetus* is via the GI tract. The organism is rarely isolated from stools, however, 40% of patients with *C. fetus* bacteremia report diarrhea (29). Perhaps normal hosts are able to contain infection within the gut, whereas compromised hosts cannot. Although only one third of patients with *C. fetus* bacteremia report contact with farm animals, it is likely that humans acquire infection from animals. *C. fetus* is isolated from sheep, cattle, poultry, reptiles, and swine (30) (Table 71.3). Human consumption of food or water contaminated with intestinal contents of infected animals probably results in transmission of infection (31). Outbreaks of *C. fetus* infection have resulted from consumption of unpasteurized milk (5,32) and raw liver (33,34). One outbreak of *C. fetus* occurred via nosocomial spread in a neonatal intensive care unit (35).

The resistance of *C. fetus* to the bactericidal activity of normal human serum could account for the high proportion of *C. fetus* infections that results in bacteremia (36,37). Human *C. fetus* isolates are covered by a surface (S)-layer protein forming a paracrystalline surface array that functions as capsule and strongly inhibits binding of C3b (38). Disruption of C3b binding explains both the serum and the phagocytosis resistance that has been observed; S-positive strains are not recognized by the alternative pathway of complement.

Serious *C. fetus* infections may be treated with ampicillin or third-generation cephalosporins (21). Imipenem and meropenem also may be effective (39). An aminoglycoside may be added to the regimen when treating endocarditis; the duration of therapy should last at least 4 weeks. Two to three weeks of therapy is needed to treat *C. fetus* infections of the central nervous system. Tetracycline and erythromycin are usually not effective for the treatment of *C. fetus* infections. Some strains of *C. fetus* may be resistant to quinolones (40,41).

The prognosis of patients with *C. fetus* infections depends largely on their general state of health. Immunocompetent patients with uncomplicated enteritis do quite well without antibiotic therapy. Immunocompromised persons with systemic infections require parenteral antibiotics but may still have a poor outcome. The overall mortality associated with *C. fetus* infections is 20% (42,43).

CAMPYLOBACTER UPSALIENSIS

Campylobacter upsaliensis is a thermotolerant *Campylobacter* that can cause gastroenteritis and bacteremia in humans. It was first identified in the stools of dogs (44) but in 1985 was recognized

TABLE 71.1. Biochemical Characteristics of *Campylobacter* and Related Species

Organism	CAT	NIT RED	IND ACE	ARYLSULF	PYRAZIN	HIPP	NAL	CEPH	H2S Rapid[a]	H2S Lead Ace	H2S TSI	Growth 25°C	Growth 37°C	Growth 42°C	H2 required
Campylobacter jejuni bio. 1[b]	+	+	+	-	+	+	S	R	-	++	-	-	+	+	-
Campylobacter jejuni bio. 2[b]	+	+	+	+	+	+	S	R	+	++	-	-	+	+	-
Campylobacter coli	+	+	+	-	+	-	S	R	-	++	-	-	+	+	-
Campylobacter fetus	+	+	-	-	-	-	R	S	-	+	-	+	+	(+)	d
Campylobacter upsaliensis	(+)	+	+	-	+	-	S	S	-	(+)	-	-	+	+	-
Campylobacter lari	+	+	-	-	+	-	R	R	+	+	-	(+)	+	+	d
Campylobacter hyointestinalis	+	+	-	+	+	-	R	S	+	5+	3+	-	+	-	-
Helicobacter fennelliae[c,d]	+	-	+	+	-	-	S	(S)	-	+	-	-	+	(+)	d
Helicobacter cinaedi[b]	(+)	+	+	-	-	(+)	S	(S)	-	(+)	-	-	+	(+)	-
Campylobacter jejuni subspecies *doylei*	(+)	-	+	-	+	-	S	(S)	-	-	-	-	+	(+)	-
Arcobacter cryaerophilus[e]	+	+	+	-	-	-	S	(R)	-	-	-	+	+	-	-
Arcobacter butzleri[e]	(+)	+	-	+	+	-	R	(R)	+	5+	3+	-	+	+	-
Campylobacter sputorum bio. *sputorum*	-	+	-	+	-	-	R	S	+	5+	3+	-	+	(+)	-
Campylobacter sputorum bio. *bubulus*	-	+	-	+	+	-	R	S	+	5+	3+	-	+	+	-
Campylobacter sputorum bio. *faecalis*	+	+	-	+	+	-	S	S	-	3+	(+)	-	+	(-)	+
Campylobacter concisus	-	+	-	+	+	-	(R)	S	-	3+	(+)	(-)	+	(-)	+
Campylobacter mucosalis	-	+	-	-	-	-	R	S	-	5+	+	-	+	(-)	+
Campylobacter curvus	-	+	+	+	+	-	R	S	-	5+	+	-	+	+	+
Campylobacter rectus	-	+	+	+	+	-	S	R	-	3+	+	-	+	+	+

[a]Rapid H₂S method of Skirrow and Benjamin (Skirrow MB, Benjamin J: Differentiation of enteropathogenic *Campylobacter* [Letter]. *J Clin Pathol* 33:1122, 1980).

[b]*Campylobacter jejuni* subsp. *jejuni* biotypes 1 and 2 refer to Skirrow's scheme. Susceptibilities are based on 30-μg disks.

[c]Spreading, noncolonial growth.

[d]Hypochlorite odor.

[e]Aerobic growth occurs at 30°C.

CAT, catalase; NIT RED, nitrate reduction; IND ACE, indole acetate; ARYLSULF, arylsulfatase; PYRAZIN, pyrazinamidase; HIPP, hippurate hydrolysis; NAL, nalidixic acid resistance; CEPH, cephalothin resistance; Lead Ace, lead acetate; TSI, triple sugar iron; +, positive; (+), most strains positive; −, negative; (−), most strains negative; R, resistant; (R), most strains resistant; S, susceptible; (S), most strains susceptible; d, some isolates grow much better in hydrogen-enhanced growth conditions.

TABLE 71.2.   Clinical Features Associated with *Campylobacter* and Related Species Implicated us Causes of Human Illness

Species	Commonly encountered clinical features	Less commonly encountered clinical features
Campylobacter jejuni	Fever, diarrhea, abdominal pain	Bacteremia
Campylobacter coli	Fever, diarrhea, abdominal pain	Bacteremia
Campylobacter fetus	Bacteremia, sepsis, meningitis, vascular infections	Diarrhea, relapsing fevers
Campylobacter upsaliensis	Watery diarrhea, low-grade fever, abdominal pain	Bacteremia, abscesses
Campylobacter lari	Gastroenteritis, abdominal pain, diarrhea	Colitis, appendicitis
Campylobacter hyointestinalis	Watery or bloody diarrhea, vomiting, abdominal pain	Bacteremia
Helicobacter fennelliae	Chronic, mild diarrhea; abdominal cramps; proctitis	Bacteremia in persons infected with human immuno-deficiency virus and in children
Helicobacter cinaedi	Chronic, mild diarrhea; abdominal cramps; proctitis	Bacteremia in persons infected with human immuno-deficiency virus and in children
Campylobacter jejuni subspecies *doylei*	Gastroenteritis	Chronic gastritis, bacteremia in children
Arcobacter cryaerophilus	Gastroenteritis	
Arcobacter butzleri	Fever, diarrhea, abdominal pain, nausea	Bacteremia
Campylobacter sputorum	Lung, perianal, groin, axillary abscesses	Bacteremia, appendicitis
Hydrogen-requiring *Campylobacter* species[a]	Periodontitis	Diarrhea, osteomyelitis, bacteremia in children

[a]Includes *Campylobacter rectus, Campylobacter curvus,* and *Campylobacter concisus.*

as a human pathogen (45). The name *C. upsaliensis* was validated in 1991 (46).

C. upsaliensis is distinguished from other campylobacters by its susceptibility to nalidixic acid and cephalothin (47) (see Table 71.1). As with *C. fetus, C. upsaliensis* cannot grow on commonly used *Campylobacter* selective media–containing antibiotics; stools suspected of harboring this organism must be filtered onto an antibiotic-free medium (48). Other microbiologic characteristics of most *C. upsaliensis* strains include a negative hippurate hydrolysis test result, positive nitrate reductase and indoxyl acetate test results, and a negative or weakly positive catalase test result (49).

Like many other campylobacters, *C. upsaliensis* is principally a GI tract pathogen; typical illness is characterized by watery diarrhea, abdominal cramps, and low-grade fever (see Table 71.2). Symptoms are usually milder than those associated with *C. jejuni* infection (50). Onset of symptoms usually is abrupt and illness usually is self-limited; occasionally, prolonged or relapsing illness occurs (51–53). Prolonged diarrhea appears to occur more frequently in *C. upsaliensis* infections in human immunodeficiency virus (HIV)–positive persons (54). Few patients have bloody stools or fecal leukocytes. *C. upsaliensis* may cause bacteremia, usually in persons with other chronic underlying illness (47,52,55). The GI tract is likely the source of these systemic

infections. Both Guillain-Barré syndrome (GBS) and hemolytic-uremic syndrome (HUS) have been reported following enteric infection with *C. upsaliensis* (56–58).

Humans acquire *C. upsaliensis* infections via contact with dogs and cats (see Table 71.3) (44,52,59,60). When polymerase chain reaction (PCR) methods are used, as many as 7% of dogs and cats with acute or chronic diarrhea have *C. upsaliensis* detected in their stools (61). The incidence appears to increase during the fall (53). At least one outbreak of diarrhea caused by *C. upsaliensis* has been described among children attending a day care center in Brussels (62). Although the incidence of *C. upsaliensis* infections is not known with certainty, when filtration methods (i.e., antibiotic-free media) are used to culture stools, 12% to 22% of isolated campylobacters are *C. upsaliensis* (63–65). When other methods are used for culture, less than 1% of isolated campylobacters are identified as *C. upsaliensis* (66–67). Currently, the rate of recognized infection, even in persons with GI tract illness is quite low (50,68), but this may be due to inadequate isolation methods rather than the rarity of infection (69). Newer PCR assays provide highly specific and rapid identification of *C. upsaliensis* but are not yet in widespread clinical use (70). Fluoroquinolones are the drug of choice for treatment of *C. upsaliensis* infections (71). Erythromycin resistance is encountered in 4% to 18% of *C. upsaliensis* isolates (52,64,72).

TABLE 71.3.   Animal Reservoirs for Atypical *Campylobacter* Species

Campylobacter fetus	Cattle, sheep
Campylobacter hyointestinalis	Pigs, cattle, hamsters
Campylobacter lari	Seagulls, crows, kittiwakes, poultry, monkeys, seals
Helicobacter cinaedi and *Helicobacter fennelliae*	Hamsters, dogs
Arcobacter cryaerophila and *Arcobacter butzleri*	Pigs, primates, ostrich, cattle
Campylobacter jejuni subspecies *doyleii*	None known
Hydrogen-requiring campylobacters	Lambs, pigs
Campylobacter sputorum and subspecies	Cattle, sheep

CAMPYLOBACTER HYOINTESTINALIS

Campylobacter hyointestinalis is principally known as a cause of enteritis in swine (see Table 71.3), but this organism also may cause diarrhea in immunocompromised persons and homosexual men. The organism is catalase and nitrate reductase positive, which helps distinguish it from other campylobacters (see Table 71.1). *C. hyointestinalis* is thermotolerant in that it survives at 42°C but grows most abundantly at 37°C (73). Some *C. hyointestinalis* strains require a hydrogen-enhanced atmosphere for growth (74).

Several published studies report the isolation of *C. hyointestinalis* from stools of patients with watery diarrhea; however, the organism has also been isolated from stools of asymptomatic persons (74–76). Symptomatic *C. hyointestinalis* infections usually occur in homosexual men and immunocompromised or elderly persons (3) (see Table 71.2). The organism is also found in the stools of very young or malnourished children with diarrhea (48). *C. hyointestinalis* has been cultured from the blood of one patient following bone marrow transplantation (3). All clinical *C. hyointestinalis* isolates tested have been susceptible to erythromycin.

CAMPYLOBACTER LARI

Campylobacter lari, formerly *Campylobacter laridis*, is a nalidixic acid–resistant *Campylobacter* that may cause acute diarrheal illness in normal hosts and bacteremia in immunocompromised persons. Few microbiologic features distinguish *C. lari* from other campylobacters. Most *C. lari* strains are oxidase and catalase negative; the hippurate hydrolysis test is negative for the organism (77) (see Table 71.1). Unlike *C. jejuni*, *C. lari* strains do not hydrolyze indoxyl acetate (78).

C. lari is isolated with high frequency from seagulls, kittiwakes, and crows (77,79–81) (see Table 71.3), which may be a source of transmission to humans; the organism is infrequently found in poultry (82). Rivers and other surface waters also may be a source of *C. lari* infection (29,83). A waterborne outbreak of gastroenteritis caused by *C. lari* infection occurred in Ontario after drinking water became contaminated by surface waters frequented by seagulls (84).

Several reports document the presence of *C. lari* in stools of immunocompetent and compromised persons with diarrhea (84–86). *C. lari* bacteremia occurs in immunocompromised persons (67,88–91) (see Table 71.2). It has been reported as a cause of pleurisy (92) as well as an infected pacemaker (93). Patients with uncomplicated diarrheal disease caused by *C. lari* may not require treatment with antibiotics. For patients with more severe disease, antibiotics are indicated; the organism is susceptible to erythromycin, clindamycin, chloramphenicol, aminoglycosides, and imipenem (85,87,88). In addition to nalidixic acid resistance, most *C. lari* isolates are resistant to penicillin, vancomycin, all cephalosporins, and trimethoprim (85,87). Quinolone-resistant strains have been reported in HIV-infected persons (85).

HELICOBACTER CINAEDI AND HELICOBACTER FENNELLIAE

Helicobacter cinaedi and *Helicobacter fennelliae* were first called campylobacter-like organisms (CLOs), and later *Campylobacter cinaedi* and *Campylobacter fennelliae*; in 1991, they were recognized as members of the *Helicobacter* genus (94). These microorganisms cause enteritis and proctocolitis in homosexual men; they also may cause bacteremia.

H. cinaedi and *H. fennelliae* grow best at 37°C and not at all at 42°C or 25°C (30,95) (see Table 71.1). *H. fennelliae* colonies have an odor similar to household chlorine bleach. *H. cinaedi* and *H. fennelliae* may be distinguished by serologic tests (96), sodium dodecyl sulfate polyacrylamide gel electrophoresis (97), and arylsulfatase activity (28).

CLOs were first identified in the stools of homosexual men with GI tract symptoms (98,99). Up to 8% of homosexual men's stools contained CLOs (100), whereas stools from women and heterosexual men did not (99). The source of human infection with *H. cinaedi* and *H. fennelliae* is not known; however, the organisms have been isolated from dogs and hamsters (101,102) (see Table 71.3), suggesting possible animal-to-human transmission.

Infections with *H. cinaedi* and *H. fennelliae* may produce illness that is quite mild and consists only of a few loose stools per day (103). However, they may produce illness similar to *C. jejuni* gastroenteritis with fever, diarrhea, and abdominal cramps. These infections also may be associated with anal discharge and pain, tenesmus, and hematochezia (99) (see Table 71.2). Blood and leukocytes may be found in stools. Sigmoidoscopic examination may show ulceration and mucosal bleeding; histopathologically, crypt abscesses and polymorphonuclear leukocytes are found scattered through the lamina propria (99).

Numerous reports document *H. cinaedi* bacteremia in patients with HIV infection or AIDS (104–108); there are fewer reports of *H. fennelliae* bacteremia (105,109). Bacteremia caused by these organisms may present only with low-grade fevers, malaise, and lethargy, but some patients report a preceding GI tract illness. Hypotension and other signs of sepsis are usually not present, although *H. fennelliae* bacteremia was reported to have caused septic shock in a heterosexual man with cirrhosis and diabetes mellitus (110). *H. fennelliae* may also cause cellulitis and arthritis (108,110–112). No fatal outcomes resulting from *H. cinaedi* and *H. fennelliae* infection have been described.

Recent reports from South Africa suggest *H. cinaedi* and *H. fennelliae* infections also may cause gastroenteritis in heterosexual men and in women and children (48,101,103,113,114). *H. cinaedi* has caused septic arthritis in a heterosexual, immunocompetent man (110). One report documents the presence of *H. cinaedi* in the cerebrospinal fluid of a neonate whose mother reported a third-trimester diarrheal illness (115).

All *H. cinaedi* and *H. fennelliae* isolates are resistant to trimethoprim; most are also resistant to metronidazole. Thirteen percent of pediatric isolates are resistant to erythromycin (48), and twenty-eight percent of isolates from adult men are erythromycin and clindamycin resistant (116). Oral fluoroquinolones (ciprofloxacin, 500 mg orally every 12 hours, or ofloxacin, 200–400 mg orally every 12 hours) are the treatment of choice for persistent *H. cinaedi* and *H. fennelliae* infections (117,118). Other antimicrobial agents that have documented *in vitro* activity against these organisms include ampicillin, gentamicin, tetracycline, doxycycline, ceftriaxone, rifampin, streptomycin, nalidixic acid, and chloramphenicol (116). Infections have been successfully treated with ceftazidime, ampicillin, sulbactam, ciprofloxacin, clarithromycin, and rifampin (106,107,110,119).

ARCOBACTER CRYAEROPHILUS AND ARCOBACTER BUTZLERI

Arcobacter (formerly *Campylobacter*) *cryaerophilus* and *Arcobacter* (formerly *Campylobacter*) *butzleri* are aerobic organisms that may cause bacteremia and gastroenteritis. The organisms were removed from the genus *Campylobacter* to *Arcobacter* in 1991 (94). *Arcobacter* species may be detected in healthy dairy cattle (120). *A. butzleri* is frequently isolated from nonhuman primates (121–122) (see Table 71.3). *A. cryaerophilus* is frequently isolated from urban sewage, especially near swine slaughter houses (123) and from pig fetuses (124–125). The route of transmission of these organisms to humans is not known. Only four *A. cryaerophilus* human isolates have been confirmed: three from blood and one from stool (126–127). Human *A. butzleri* infection occurs more commonly. Among 631 Thai children with diarrhea, *A. butzleri* was the most common atypical *Campylobacter* isolated from stools (66). Of 43 patients with *A. butzleri* isolated from their stools, more than 50% had abdominal pain and nausea, and many also had fever, chills, vomiting, and malaise (126). Abdominal cramps may be the predominant symptom associated with *A. butzleri* infection. In an outbreak of *A. butzleri* infection at an Italian elementary school, all 10 affected children had recurrent attacks of abdominal cramps, two to three times per day for about 10 days; none had diarrhea (128). *A. butzleri* has been isolated from the blood of a man with hepatic cirrhosis and from a preterm neonate (129,130).

CAMPYLOBACTER JEJUNI SUBSPECIES DOYLEI

C. jejuni subspecies *doylei* is only recently being recognized for its pathogenic potential in humans. During a 30-month study in South Africa, *C. jejuni* subspecies *doylei* made up more than 10% of campylobacters isolated from children with gastroenteritis. Of the 142 *C. jejuni* subspecies *doylei*–infected children, 81% had diarrhea, 14% had bloody stools, and 20% has fecal leukocytes (48). Eleven patients were bacteremic (see Table 71.2). Studies in other parts of the world have not shown as high a frequency of *C. jejuni* subspecies *doylei;* however, even in these studies, infection with the organism was associated with diarrhea in children (48,63,64,66,131–133). *C. jejuni* subspecies *doylei* may be distinguished from other campylobacters by its ability to reduce nitrate to nitrite (134) (see Table 71.1). The organism is susceptible to both cephalothin and nalidixic acid (135).

HYDROGEN-REQUIRING CAMPYLOBACTER ORGANISMS

Four species of *Campylobacter*—*Campylobacter concisus, Campylobacter mucosalis, Campylobacter rectus,* and *Campylobacter curvus*—are known to require hydrogen for growth. A strong association exists between *C. concisus* and human periodontal disease (136–138). At one point, *C. concisus* was associated with GI tract illness because studies in South Africa (48,139) and Belgium (140,141) detected *C. concisus* in 2.4% to 12.3% of adults and children with gastroenteritis. However, later studies showed that although *C. concisus* was detected in 13% of patients with diarrhea, the rate of isolation was not significantly different (9%) in healthy controls (142). Similarly, in another Danish study, *C. concisus* was found in the stools of many patients with diarrhea but was also detected in healthy persons (143). Currently, no good evidence suggests *C. concisus* is a cause of human GI tract illness. *C. rectus* is also associated with periodontal disease and is isolated in 80% of adults and children with this condition (144). *C. rectus* has not been associated with GI tract illness. The role of *C. curvus* in causing human disease is not yet known, but this organism also may be associated with periodontal disease (145) and gastroenteritis (123,141). *C. mucosalis* is an important veterinary pathogen causing proliferative enteritis in lambs and pigs (146,147). Only three human isolates (two from stool, one from blood) have been reported (89,148).

CAMPYLOBACTER SPUTORUM

Campylobacter sputorum and its subspecies have occasionally been associated with human disease (149–152), but a causal role has not been established. A close phylogenetic neighbor *Campylobacter hominis* (species nova) is a newly discovered species that is found in the feces of healthy people and has not been associated with disease (153).

CONCLUSION

As detection methods for *Campylobacter* and related organisms improve, other new species may be identified as human pathogens and the isolation rate of atypical species may rise. Increasing understanding of the source of infection and pathogenesis of these infections will enhance the ability to both prevent and treat these illnesses.

REFERENCES

1. Tauxe RV, Hargrett-Bean N, Patton CM, et al. *Campylobacter* isolates in the United States, 1982–1986. *MMWR Morb Mortal Wkly Rep* 1988;37: 1–13.
2. Lastovica AJ. Efficient isolation of *Campylobacter* from stools. *J Clin Microbiol* 2000;38:2798–2799.
3. Allos BM, Lastovica A, Blaser MJ. Atypical campylobacters and related organisms. In: Blaser MJ, Smith PD, Ravdin JI, et al, eds. *Infections of the gastrointestinal tract.* New York: Raven Press, 1995:849–866.
4. McFadyean J, Stockman S. *Report of the department of committee appointed by the Board of Agriculture and Fisheries to inquire into epizootic abortions. Appendix to Part III abortion in sheep.* London: His Majesty's Stationery Office, 1913:1–29.
5. Klein BS, Vergeront JM, Blaser MJ, et al. *Campylobacter* infection associated with raw milk: an outbreak of gastroenteritis due to *Campylobacter jejuni* and thermotolerant *Campylobacter fetus* subsp. *fetus. JAMA* 1986;255:361–364.
6. Mishu B, Patton C, Tauxe RV. Clinical and epidemiologic features of non–*jejuni campylobacters.* In: Nachamkin I, Blaser MJ, Tompkins LS, eds. Campylobacter jejuni: *current status and future trends.* Washington, DC: American Society of Microbiology, 1992:31–41.
7. Guerrant RL, Lahita RG, Winn EC Jr, et al. Campylobacteriosis in man: pathogenic mechanisms and review of 91 bloodstream infections. *Am J Med* 1978;65:484–592.
8. Francioli P, Herztein J, Grob JP, et al. *Campylobacter fetus* subspecies *fetus* bacteremia. *Arch Intern Med* 1985;145:289–292.
9. Montero A, Corbella X, Lopez JA, et al. *Campylobacter fetus*–associated aneurysms: report of a case involving the popliteal artery and review of the literature. *Clin Infect Dis* 1997;24:1019–1021.
10. Peetermans WE, De Man F, Moerman P, et al. Fatal prosthetic valve endocarditis due to *Campylobacter fetus. J Infect* 2000;41:180–182.
11. Mii S, Tanaka K, Furugaki K, et al. Infected abdominal aortic aneurysm caused by *Campylobacter fetus* subspecies *fetus*: report of a case. *Sung Today* 1998;28:661–664.
12. Miller VA, Jenson R, Gilroy JJ. Bacteremia in pregnant sheep following oral administration of *Vibrio fetus. Am J Vet Res* 1959;20:677–679.
13. Lowrie DB, Pearce JH. The placental localisation of *Vibrio fetus. J Med Microbiol* 1970;3:607–614.
14. Viejo G, Gomez B, De Miguel D, et al. *Campylobacter fetus* subspecies *fetus* bacteremia associated with chorioamnionitis and intact fetal membranes. *Scand J Infect Dis* 2001;33:1 26–27.
15. Eden AH. Perinatal mortality caused by *Vibrio fetus.* Review and analysis. *J Pediatr* 1966;68:297–304.
16. Simor AE, Karmali MA, Jadavji T, et al. Abortion and perinatal sepsis associated with *Campylobacter* infection. *Rev Infect Dis* 1986;8:397–402.
17. Franklin B, Ulmer DD. Human infection with *Vibrio fetus. West J Med* 1974;120:200–204.
18. Kilo C, Hagemann PO, Maryi J. Septic arthritis and bacteremia due to *Vibrio fetus. Am J Med* 1965;38:962.
19. Brown WJ, Sautter R. *Campylobacter fetus* septicemia with concurrent salpingitis. *J Clin Microbiol* 1977;6:72–75.
20. Wens R, Dratwa M, Potvliege C, et al. *Campylobacter fetus* peritonitis followed by septicemia in a patient on continuous ambulatory peritoneal dialysis. *J Infect* 1985;10:249–251.
21. Neuzil K, Wang E, Haas D, et al. Persistence of *Campylobacter fetus* bacteremia associated with absence of opsonizing antibodies. *J Clin Microbiol* 1994;32:1 718–720.
22. Yao JDC, Ng HMC, Campbell I. Prosthetic hip joint infection due to *Campylobacter fetus. J Clin Microbiol* 1993;31:3323–3324.
23. Takatsu M, Ichiyama S, Nada T, et al. *Campylobacter fetus* subsp. *fetus* cholecystitis in a patient with advanced hepatocellular carcinoma. *Scand J Infect Dis* 1997;29:197–198.
24. Yamashita K, Aoki Y, Hiroshima K. Pyogenic vertebral osteomyelitis caused by *Campylobacter fetus* subspecies *fetus.* A case report. *Spine* 1999;24:582–584.
25. Anstead G, Jorgensen J, Craig F, et al. Thermophilic multidrug-resistant *Campylobacter fetus* infection with hypersplenism and histiocytic phagocytosis in a patient with acquired immunodeficiency syndrome. *Clin Infect Dis* 2001;32:295–296.
26. Dronda F, Garcia-Arata I, Navas E, et al. Meningitis in adults due to *Campylobacter fetus* subspecies *fetus. Clin Infect Dis* 1998;27:906–907.
27. Ichiyama S, Hirai S, Minami T, et al. *Campylobacter fetus* subspecies *fetus* cellulitis associated with bacteremia in debilitated hosts. *Clin Infect Dis* 1998;27:256–258.
28. Burnens AP, Nicolet J. Three supplementary diagnostic tests for *Campylobacter* species and related organisms. *J Clin Microbiol* 1993;31:708–710.

29. Brennhound O, Kapperud G, Langeland G. Survey of thermotolerant *Campylobacter* spp and *Yersinia* spp. in three surface water sources in Norway. *Int J Food Microbiol* 1992;15:327–338.

30. Smibert RM. Genus *Campylobacter*. Sebald and Veron 1963, 907[AL]. In: Krieg NR, HG Holt, eds. *Bergey's manual of systematic bacteriology*, vol 1. Baltimore: Williams & Wilkins, 1984:111–118.

31. Blaser MJ, Taylor DN, Feldman RA. Epidemiology of *Campylobacter jejuni* infections. *Epidemiol Rev* 1983;5:157–176.

32. Taylor PR, Weinstein WM, Bryner JH. *Campylobacter fetus* infection in human subjects: association with raw milk. *Am J Med* 1979;66:779–783.

33. Centers for Disease Control and Prevention. *Campylobacter* sepsis associated with "nutritional therapy"—California. *MMWR Morb Mortal Wkly Rep* 1981;30:294–295.

34. Centers for Disease Control and Prevention. Premature labor and neonatal sepsis caused by *Campylobacter fetus* subsp. Fetus—Ontario. *MMWR Morb Mortal Wkly Rep* 1984;33:483–489.

35. Morooka T, Umeda A, Fujita M, et al. Epidemiologic application of pulsed-field gel electrophoresis to an outbreak of *Campylobacter fetus* meningitis in a neonatal intensive care unit. *Scand J Infect Dis* 1996;28:269–270.

36. Blaser MJ, Smith PF, Kohler PA. Susceptibility of *Campylobacter* isolates to the bactericidal activity in human serum. *J Infect Dis* 1985;151:227–235.

37. Blaser MJ, Smith PF, Hopkins JA, et al. Pathogenesis of *Campylobacter fetus* infections. Serum-resistance associated with high molecular weight surface proteins. *J Infect Dis* 1987;155:696–706.

38. Blaser MJ, Smith PF, Repine JE, et al. Pathogenesis of *Campylobacter fetus* infections. Failure of C3b to bind explains serum and phagocytosis resistance. *J Clin Invest* 1988;81:1434–1444.

39. Tremblay C, Gaudreau C. Antimicrobial susceptibility testing of 59 strains of *Campylobacter fetus* subsp. *fetus*. *Antimicrob Agents Chemother* 1998;42:1847–1849.

40. Meier PA, Dooley DP, Jorgensen JH, et al. Development of quinolone-resistant *Campylobacter fetus* bacteremia in human immunodeficiency virus–infected patients. *J Infect Dis* 1998;177:951–954.

41. Font C, Cruceta A, Moreno A, et al. A study of 30 patients with bacteremia due to *Campylobacter* spp. [in Spanish]. *Med Clin* 1997;108:336–340.

42. Dickgiesser N, Kasper G, Kihm W. *Campylobacter fetus* ssp. *fetus* bacteremia. A patient with liver cirrhosis. *Infection* 1983;11:288.

43. Rao GG, Karim QN, Maddocks A, et al. *Campylobacter fetus* infections in two patients with AIDS. *J Infect* 1990;20:170–172.

44. Sandstedt K, Ursing J, Walder M. Thermotolerant *Campylobacter* with no or weak catalase activity isolated from dogs. *Curr Microbiol* 1983;8:209–213.

45. Steele TW, Sangster N, Lanser JA. DNA relatedness and biochemical features of *Campylobacter* spp. isolated in Central and South Australia. *J Clin Microbiol* 1985;72:71–74.

46. International Union of Microbiological Societies. Validation of the publication of new names and new combinations previously effectively published outside the IJSB. *Int J Syst Bacteriol* 1991;41:580–581.

47. Lastovica AJ, Le Roux E, Penner JL. *Campylobacter upsaliensis* isolated from blood cultures of pediatric patients. *J Clin Microbiol* 1989;27:657–659.

48. Lastovica AJ, Le Roux E. Prevalence and distribution of *Campylobacter* spp. in the diarrheic stools and blood cultures of pediatric patients. *Acta Gastroenterol Belg* 1993;56[Suppl]:34.

49. Sandstedt K, Ursing J. Description of *Campylobacter upsaliensis* sp. nov. previously known as the CNW group. *Syst Appl Microbiol* 1991;14:39–48.

50. Jimenez SG, Heine RG, Ward PB, et al. *Campylobacter upsaliensis* gastroenteritis in childhood. *Pediatr Infect Dis J* 1999;18:988–992.

51. Megraud F, Bonnet F. Unusual campylobacters in human feces. *J Infect* 1986;12:275–276.

52. Patton CM, Shaffer N, Edmonds P, et al. Human disease associated with *Campylobacter upsaliensis* (catalase-negative or weakly positive *Campylobacter* species) in the United States. *J Clin Microbiol* 1989;27:66–73.

53. Walmsley SL, Karmali MA. Direct isolation of thermophilic *Campylobacter* species from human feces on selective agar medium. *J Clin Microbiol* 1989;27:668–670.

54. Jenkin GA, Tee W. *Campylobacter upsaliensis*–associated diarrhea in human immunodeficiency virus–infected patients. *Clin Infect Dis* 1998;27:816–821.

55. Chusid MJ, Wortmann DW, Dunne WM. *Campylobacter upsaliensis* sepsis in a boy with acquired hypogammaglobulinemia. *Diagn Microbiol Infect Dis* 1990;13:367–369.

56. Koga M, Yuki N, Takahashi M, et al. Are *Campylobacter curvus* and *Campylobacter upsaliensis* antecedent infectious agents in Guillain Barré and Fisher's syndromes? *J Neurol Sci* 1999;163:53–57.

57. Ho TW, Hsieh ST, Nachamkin I, et al. Motor nerve terminal degeneration provides a potential mechanism for rapid recovery in acute motor axonal neuropathy after *Campylobacter* infection. *Neurology* 1997;48:695–700.

58. Carter JE, Cimolai N. Hemolytic-uremic syndrome associated with acute *Campylobacter upsaliensis* gastroenteritis. *Nephron* 1996;74:489.

59. Owen RJ, Hernandez J. Occurrence of plasmids in *Campylobacter upsaliensis* (catalase negative or weak group) from geographically diverse patients with gastroenteritis or bacteremia. *Eur J Epidemiol* 1990;6:111–117.

60. Hald B, Madsen M. Healthy puppies and kittens as carriers of *Campylobacter* spp., with special reference to *Campylobacter upsaliensis*. *J Clin Microbiol* 1997;35:3351–3352.

61. Steinhauserova I, Fojtikova K, Klimes J. The incidence and PCR detection of *Campylobacter upsaliensis* in dogs and cats. *Lett Applied Microbiol* 2000;31:209–212.

62. Goossens H, Giesendorf BA, Vandamme P, et al. Investigation of an outbreak of *Campylobacter upsaliensis* in day care centers in Brussels: analysis of relationships among isolates by phenotypic and genotypic typing methods. *J Infect Dis* 1995;172:1298–1305.

63. Albert MJ, Tee W, Leach A, et al. Comparison of a blood-free medium and a filtration technique for the isolation of *Campylobacter* spp. from diarrhoeal stools of hospitalized patients in central Australia. *J Med Microbiol* 1997;37:176–179.

64. Goossens H, Vlaes L, De Boeck M, et al. Is *Campylobacter upsaliensis* an unrecognised cause of human diarrhoea? *Lancet* 1990;336:584–586.

65. Goossens H, Pot B, Vlaes L, et al. Characterization and description of *Campylobacter upsaliensis* isolated from human feces. *J Clin Microbiol* 1990;28:1039–1046.

66. Taylor DN, Diehlbauch JA, Tee W, et al. Isolation of group 2 aerotolerant *Campylobacter* species from Thai children with diarrhea. *J Infect Dis* 1991;163:1062–1067.

67. Skirrow MB, Jones DM, Sutcliffe E, et al. *Campylobacter* bacteremia in England and Wales, 1981–91. *Epidemiol Infect* 1993;110:567–573.

68. Lopez L, Castillo FJ, Clavel A, et al. Use of a selective medium and a membrane filter method for isolation of *Campylobacter* species from Spanish paediatric patients. *Eur J Clin Microbiol Infect Dis* 1998;17:489–492.

69. Bourke B, Chan VL, Sherman P. *Campylobacter upsaliensis:* waiting in the wings. *Clin Microbiol Rev* 1998;11:440–449.

70. Van Doorn U, Vershuuren-van Haperen A, Burnens A, et al. Rapid identification of thermotolerant *Campylobacter jejuni, Campylobacter coil, Campylobacter lari,* and *Campylobacter upsaliensis* from various geographic locations by a GTPase-based PCR-reverse hybridization assay. *J Clin Microbiol* 1999;37:1790–1796.

71. Preston MA, Simor AE, Walmsley SL, et al. *In vitro* susceptibility of *Campylobacter upsaliensis* to twenty-four antimicrobial agents. *Eur J Clin Microbiol Infect Dis* 1990;9:822–824.

72. da Silva-Tatley FM, Lastovica AJ, Steyn LM. Plasmid profiles of *Campylobacter upsaliensis* isolated from blood cultures and stools of pediatric patients. *J Med Microbiol* 1992;37:8–14.

73. Edmonds P, Patton CM, Griffin PM, et al. *Campylobacter hyointestinalis* associated with human gastrointestinal disease in the United States. *J Clin Microbiol* 1987;25:685–691.

74. Vandamme P, De Ley J. Proposal for a new family, Campylobacteraceae. *Int J Syst Bacteriol* 1991;41:451–455.

75. Salana SM, Tabor H, Richter M, et al. Pulsed-field gel electrophoresis for epidemiologic studies of *Campylobacter hyointestinalis* isolates. *J Clin Microbiol* 1992;30:1982–1984.

76. Minet J, Growbois B, Megraud F. *Campylobacter hyointestinalis*: an opportunistic enteropathogen? *J Clin Microbiol* 1988;26:2659–2660.

77. Von Graevgenitz A. A revised nomenclature of *Campylobacter landis, Enterobacter intermedium,* and "*Flavobacterium branchiophilum*. *Int J Syst Bacteriol* 1990;40:211.

78. Popovic-Uroic T, Patton CM, Nicholson MA, et al. Evaluation of indoxylacetate hydrolysis test for rapid differentiation of *Campylobacter, Helicobacter,* and *Wolinella* species. *J Clin Microbiol* 1990;28:2335–2339.

79. Glunder G, Petermann S. The occurrence and characterization of *Campylobacter* spp. in silver gulls (*Larus argentatus*), three-toed gulls (*Rissa tridactyla*), and house sparrows (*Passer domesticus*). *Zentralbl Veterinarmed B* 1989;36:123–130.

80. Kakkar M, Dogra SC. Prevalence of *Campylobacter* infections in animals and children in Haryana, India. *J Diarrhoeal Dis Res* 1990;8:34–36.

81. Maruyama S, Tanaka T, Katube Y, et al. Prevalence of thermophilic campylobacters in crows (*Corvus lavaillantii, Corvus corne*) and serogroups of the isolates. *Jpn J Vet Sci* 1990;52:1237–1244.

82. Kazawala RR, Jiwa SF, Nkya AE. The role of management systems in the epidemiology of thermophilic campylobacters among poultry in eastern zone Tanzania. *Epidemiol Infect* 1993;110:273–278.

83. Bolton FJ, Coates D, Hutchinson DN, et al. A study of thermophilic *Campylobacter* in a river system. *J Appl Bacteriol* 1987;62:167–176.

84. Borczyk A, Thompson S, Smith D, et al. Water-borne outbreak of *Campylobacter landis*–associated gastroenteritis. *Lancet* 1987;1:164–165.

85. Evans TG, Riley D. *Campylobacter landis* colitis in a human immunodeficiency virus–positive patient treated with a quinolone. *Clin Infect Dis* 1992;15:172–173.

86. Tauxe RV, Patton CM, Edmonds P, et al. Illness associated with *Campylobacter landis*, a newly recognized *Campylobacter* species. *J Clin Microbiol* 1985;21:222–225.

87. Simor AE, Wilcox L. Enteritis associated with *Campylobacter landis*. *J Clin Microbiol* 1987;25:10–12.

88. Nachamkin I, Stowell C, Skalina D, et al. *Campylobacter landis* causing bacteremia in an immunosuppressed patient. *Ann Intern Med* 1984;101:55–57.

89. Soderstrom C, Schalen C, Walder M. Septicaemia caused by unusual *Campylobacter* species (*C. landis* and *C. mucosalis*). *Scand J Infect Dis* 1991;23:369–371.

90. Vargas J, Carzo JE, Perez MJ, et al. Enfermedades infecciosas. *Microbiol Clin* 1992;10:155–157.

91. Chiu CH, Kuo CY, Ou JT. Chronic diarrhea and bacteremia caused by *Campylobacter lari* in a neonate. *Clin Infect Dis* 1995;21:700–701.

92. Bruneau B, Burc L, Bizet C, et al. Purulent pleurisy caused by *Campylobacter ian. Eur J Clin Microbiol Infect Dis* 1998;17:185–188.

93. Morris CN, Scully B, Garvey GJ. *Campylobacter lari* associated with permanent pacemaker infection and bacteremia. *Clin Infect Dis* 1998;27:220–221.

94. Vandamme P, Falsen E, Rossau R, et al. Revision of *Campylobacter, Helicobacter,* and *Wolinella* taxonomy: emendation of generic descriptions and proposal of *Arcobacter* gen. nov. *Int J Syst Bacteriol* 1991;41:88–103.

95. Griffiths PL, Moreno GS, Park RW. Differentiation between thermophilic *Campylobacter* species by species-specific antibodies. *J Appl Bacteriol* 1992; 72:467–472.

96. Flores BM, Fennell CL, Stamm WE. Characterization of *Campylobacter cinaedi* and *C. fennelliae* antigens and analysis of human immune response. *J Infect Dis* 1989;159:635–660.

97. On SLW, Owen RJ, Lastovica A, et al. Taxonomic study of *Helicobacter (Campylobacter) fennelliae* from clinical material by numerical analysis of one-dimensional electrophoretic protein patterns. *Microb Ecol Health Dis* 1991;4:S103.

98. Quinn TC, Stamm WE, Goodell SE, et al. The polymicrobial origin of intestinal infections in homosexual man. *N Engl J Med* 1983;309:76–82.

99. Quinn TC, Goodell SE, Fennell CL, et al. Infections with *Campylobacter jejuni* and *Campylobacter*-like organisms in homosexual men. *Ann Intern Med* 1984;101:187–192.

100. Laughon BE, Vernon AA, Druckman DA, et al. Recovery of *Campylobacter* species from homosexual men. *J Infect Dis* 1988;158:464–467.

101. Burnens AP, Angeloy-Wick B, Nicolet J. Comparison of *Campylobacter* carriage rates in diarrheic and healthy pet animals. *J Vet Med Ser B* 1992;39:175–180.

102. Gebhart CJ, Fennell CL, Murtaugh MP, et al. *Campylobacter cinaedi* is the normal intestinal flora in hamsters. *J Clin Microbiol* 1989;27:1692–1694.

103. Grayson ML, Tee W, Dwyer B. Gastroenteritis associated with *Campylobacter cinaedi. Med J Aust* 1989;150:214–215.

104. Burman WJ, Cohn DL, Reves RR, et al. Multifocal cellulitis and monoarticular arthritis as manifestations of *Helicobacter cinaedi* bacteremia. *Clin Infect Dis* 1995;20:564–571.

105. Ng VL, Hadley WK, Fennell CL, et al. Successive bacteremias with *Campylobacter cinaedi* and *Campylobacter fennelliae* in a bisexual male. *J Clin Microbiol* 1987;25:2008–2009.

106. Mammen MP Jr, Aronson NE, Edenfield WJ, et al. Recurrent *Helicobacter cinaedi* bacteremia in a patient infected with human immunodeficiency virus: case report. *Clin Infect Dis* 1995;21:1055.

107. Hung CC, Hsueh PR, Chen MY, et al. Bacteremia caused by *Helicobacter cinaedi* in an AIDS patient. *J Formosan Med Assoc* 1997;96:558–560.

108. Tee W, Street AC, Spelman D, et al. *Helicobacter cinaedi* bacteraemia: varied clinical manifestations in three homosexual males. *Scand J Infect Dis* 1996;28:199–203.

109. Kemper CA, Mickelson P, Morton A, et al. *Helicobacter (Campylobacter) fennelliae*–like organisms as an important but occult cause of bacteremia in a patient with AIDS. *J Infect Dis* 1993;26:97–101.

110. Hsueh PR, Teng U, Hung CC, et al. Septic shock due to *Helicobacter fennelliae* in a non-human immunodeficiency virus–infected heterosexual patient. *J Clin Microbiol* 1999;37:2084–2086.

111. Burman WJ, Cohn DL, Reves RR, et al. Multifocal cellulitis and monoarticular arthritis as manifestations of *Helicobacter cinaedi* bacteremia. *Clin Infect Dis* 1995;20:564–570.

112. van der Ven AJ, Kullberg BJ, Vandamme P, et al. *Helicobacter cinaedi* bacteremia associated with localized pain but not with cellulitis. *Clin Infect Dis* 1996;22:710–711.

113. Wilcox CM, Byford BA, Forsmark CE, et al. *Campylobacter*-like organisms are uncommon pathogens in patients infected with the human immunodeficiency virus. *J Clin Microbiol* 1990;28:2370–2371.

114. Burnens AP, Stanley J, Schaad VB, et al. Novel *Campylobacter*-like organism resembling *Helicobacter fennelliae* isolated from a boy with gastroenteritis and from dogs. *J Clin Microbiol* 1993;31:1916–1917.

115. Orlicek SL, Welch DF, Kuhls TL. Septicemia and meningitis caused by *Helicobacter cinaedi* in neonate. *J Clin Microbiol* 1993;31:569–571.

116. Flores BM, Fennell CL, Holmes KK, et al. *In vitro* susceptibility of *Campylobacter*-like organisms to twenty antimicrobial agents. *Antimicrob Agents Chemother* 1985;28:188–191.

117. Sacks LV, Labriola AM, Gill VJ, et al. Use of ciprofloxacin for successful eradication of bacteremia due to *Campylobacter cinaedi* in a human immunodeficiency virus–infected patient. *Rev Infect Dis* 1993;13:1066–1068.

118. Decker CF, Martin GJ, Barham WB, et al. Bacteremia due to *Campylobacter cinaedi* in a patient infected with human immunodeficiency virus. *Clin Infect Dis* 1992;15:178–179.

119. Lasry S, Simon J, Marais A, et al. *Helicobacter cinaedi* septic arthritis and bacteremia in an immunocompetent patient. *Clin Infect Dis* 2000;31:201–202.

120. Wesley IV, Wells SJ, Harmon KM, et al. Fecal shedding of *Campylobacter* and *Arcobacter* spp. in dairy cattle. *Appl Environ Microbiol* 2000;66:1994–2000.

121. Anderson KF, Kiehlbauch JA, Anderson DC, et al. *Arcobacter (Campylobacter) butzleri*–associated diarrheal illness in a nonhuman primate population. *Infect Immun* 1993;61:2220–2223.

122. Russell RG, Kiehlbauch JA, Gebhart CJ, et al. Uncommon *Campylobacter* species in infant *Macaca nemestrina* monkeys housed in a nursery. *J Clin Microbiol* 1992;30:3024–3027.

123. Stamp S, Varoli O, Zanetti F, et al. *Arcobacter cryaerophilus* and thermophilic campylobacters in a sewage treatment plant in Italy: two secondary treatments compared. *Epidemiol Infect* 1993;110:633–639.

124. Neill SD, Ellis WA, Obrien JJ. The biochemical characteristics of *Campylobacter*-like organisms from cattle and pigs. *Res Vet Sci* 1978;25:368–372.

125. Boudreau M, Higgins R, Mittal KR. Biochemical and serological characterization of *Campylobacter cryaerophilus. J Clin Microbiol* 1991;29:54–58.

126. Kiehlbauch JA, Brenner DJ, Nicholson MA, et al. *Campylobacter butzleri* sp. nov. isolated from humans and animals with diarrheal illness. *J Clin Microbiol* 1991;29:376–385.

127. Hsueh PR, Teng U, Yang PC, et al. Bacteremia caused by *Arcobacter cryaerophilus* 1B. *J Clin Microbiol* 1997;35:489–491.

128. Vandamme P, Pigina P, Benzi G, et al. Outbreak of recurrent abdominal cramps associated with *Arcobacter butzleri* in Italian school. *J Clin Microbiol* 1992;30:23356–23337.

129. Yan JJ, Ko WC, Huang AH, et al. *Arcobacter butzleri* bacteremia in a patient with liver cirrhosis. *J Formosan Med Assoc* 2000;99:166–169.

130. On SL, Stacey A, Smyth J. Isolation of *Arcobacter butzleri* from a neonate with bacteraemia. *J Infect* 1995;31:225–227.

131. Lastovica AJ, Kirby R, Ambrosio RE. Clinical isolates of thermophilic *Campylobacter* spp. with no or weak catalase activity [Abstract]. In: Pearson AD, Skirrow MB, Lior H, et al., eds. *Campylobacter* III. London: Public Health Laboratory Service, 1985:201.

132. Musmanno RA, Russi M, Figura N, et al. Unusual species of campylobacters isolated in the Siena Tuscany area, Italy. *New Microbiol* 1998;21:15–22.

133. Fernandez H, Fagundes Neto U, Ogatha S. Acute diarrhea associated with *Campylobacter jejuni* subsp. *doylei* in Sao Paulo, Brazil. *Pediatr Infect Dis J* 1997;16:1098–1099.

134. Steele TW, Owen RJ. *Campylobacter jejuni* subspecies *doylei* (subsp. nov.), a subspecies of nitrate-negative campylobacters isolated from human clinical specimens. *Int J Syst Bacteriol* 1988;38:316–318.

135. Firehammer BD. The isolation of vibrios from ovine feces. *Cornell Vet* 1965;55:482–494.

136. Tanner ACR, Badger S, Lai CH, et al. *Wolinella* gen. nov., *Wolinella succinogenes* (*Vibrio succinogenes* Wolin et al.) comb. nov., and description of *Bacteroides gracilis* sp. nov., *Wolinella recta* sp. nov., *Campylobacter concisus* sp. nov., and *Eikenella corrodens* from humans with periodontal disease. *Int J Syst Bacteriol* 1981;31:432–435.

137. Tanner ACR, Dzink JL, Ebersole JL, et al. *Wolinella recta, Campylobacter concisus, Bacteroides gracilis,* and *Eikenella corrodens* from periodontal lesions. *J Periodont Res* 1987;22:327–330.

138. Badger SJ, Tanner ACR. Serological studies of *Bacteroides gracilis, Campylobacter concisus, Wolinella recta,* and *Eikenella corrodens,* all from humans with periodontal disease. *Int J Syst Bacteriol* 1981;31:446–451.

139. Lastovica AJ, Le Roux E, Warren R, et al. Clinical isolates of *Campylobacter mucosalis. J Clin Microbiol* 1993;31:2835–2836.

140. Vandamme P, Falsen E, Pot B, et al. Identification of EF group 22 campylobacters from gastroenteritis cases as *Campylobacter concisus. J Clin Microbiol* 1989;27:1775–1781.

141. Lauwers S, Kevreker T, Van Etterijck R, et al. Isolation of *Campylobacter concisus* from human feces. *Microbiol Ecol Health Dis* 1991;4:591.

142. Van Etterijck R, Breynaert J, Revets H, et al. Isolation of *Campylobacter concisus* from feces of children with and without diarrhea. *J Clin Microbiol* 1996;34:2304–2306.

143. Engberg J, On SL, Harrington CS, et al. Prevalence of *Campylobacter, Arcobacter, Helicobacter,* and *Sutterella* spp. In human fecal samples as estimated by a reevaluation of isolation methods for campylobacters. *J Clin Microbiol* 2000;38:2798–2799.

144. Rams TE, Feik D, Slots J. *Campylobacter rectus* in human periodontitis. *Oral Microbiol Immunol* 1993;8:230–235.

145. Tanner ACR, Listgarten MA, Ebersole JL. *Wolinella curva* sp. nov.: *Vibrio succinogenes* of human origin. *Int J Syst Bacteriol* 1984;34:275–282.

146. Lawson GHK, Rowland AC. *Campylobacter sputorum* subsp. *mucosalis*. In: Butzler JP, ed. Campylobacter *infection in man and animals*. Boca Raton, FL: CRC Press, 1984:207–225.

147. Megraud F, Elharrif Z. Isolation of *Campylobacter* species by filtration. *Eur J Clin Microbiol* 1985;4:437–438.

148. Figura N, Guglielmetti P, Zanchi A, et al. Two cases of *Campylobacter mucosalis* enteritis in children. *J Clin Microbiol* 1993;31:727–728.

149. Raffi F, Derriennic M, Michault A, et al. Infections humaines a *Campylobacter sputorum*: A propos de deux observations. *Med Mal Infect* 1985:65–68.

150. Borczyk A, Lior H, McKeown A, et al. Isolations of *Campylobacter sputorum* associated with human infection [Abstract 211]. In: Kaijser B, Falsen E, eds. *Campylobacter* IV. Götenborg, Sweden: University of Götenborg, 1987:166.

151. On SL, Ridgewell F, Cryan B, et al. Isolation of *Campylobacter sputorum* biovar *sputorum* from an axillary abscess. *J Infect* 1992:175–179.

152. Josebe Unzaga M, Rojo P, Melero P, et al. Isolation of *Campylobacter sputorum* bio van sputorum from a bed sore [in Spanish]. *Enfermedades Infecciosas Microbiol Clin* 1997;15:43.

153. Lawson AJ, On SL, Logan JM, et al. *Campylobacter hominis* sp. nov., from the human gastrointestinal tract. *Int J Syst Evolution Microbiol* 2001;51:651–660.

CHAPTER 72
Yersinia enterocolitica *Infections*

Douglas A. Finch and Edward J. Bottone

Yersinia enterocolitica, a gram-negative coccobacillus, was first isolated in the United States in 1934 by McIver and Pike (1) from a 53-year-old farm dweller with two facial abscesses. Retrospective examination of the previously unidentified isolate on deposit at the New York State Department of Health by Schleifstein and Coleman (2), along with three additional isolates from enteric contents, led these investigators to propose the name *Bacterium enterocoliticum* for these microorganisms (3). Interestingly, while the major emphasis in studying the basic microbiology and clinical manifestations of *Y. enterocolitica* and *Yersinia* pseudotuberculosis was taking place in European countries (4), heightened awareness of *Y. enterocolitica* in the United States was propelled in 1976 by the food-borne outbreak of *Y. enterocolitica* gastrointestinal infection involving 222 subjects in upstate (Holland Patent) New York (5).

The genus *Yersinia* is composed of ten species, of which three, *Yersinia pestis* (plague bacillus), *Y. enterocolitica*, and *Y. pseudotuberculosis*, are well recognized human pathogens. Whereas isolates of *Y. pestis* and *Y. pseudotuberculosis* are inherently pathogenic, virulence among *Y. enterocolitica* isolates differs by biogroup and serogroup.

MICROBIOLOGY

Many of the basic microbiologic attributes of *Y. enterocolitica* are influenced by growth temperature. For instance, *Y. enterocolitica* is nonmotile at 37°C but motile at 25°C; acetylmethylcarbinol (Voges-Proskauer test) is produced at 25°C but not at 37°C; plasmid-encoded virulence factors are expressed at 37°C and lost at 25°C. Therefore, full characterization of an isolate as *Y. enterocolitica* should include tests determined at two incubation temperatures (4).

Y. enterocolitica grows on a variety of bacteriologic media, including media used for the isolation of other enteric bacterial species. On these media, however, *Y. enterocolitica* produces pinpoint colonies after 24 hours of incubation and may be overlooked in clinical specimens (e.g., feces) containing a multiplicity of bacterial species (Fig. 72.1). Thus, awareness of growth patterns on widely used enteric isolation media will aid recognition and recovery (Table 72.1). Although routine enteric media such as MacConkey agar support the growth of *Y. enterocolitica*, the use of cefsulodin-irgasan-novobiocin agar greatly aids recovery when *Y. enterocolitica* is strongly suspected (Table 72.1). A modification of this medium by the addition of esculin can distinguish pathogenic non–esculin-hydrolyzing *Y. enterocolitica* (biogroup 1B) from nonpathogenic esculin-hydrolyzing environmental isolates (6). Pathogenic isolates will produce red colonies, and nonpathogenic isolates will produce dark colonies with a dark peripheral zone.

The stools of patients with acute gastroenteritis due to commonly occurring pathogenic *Y. enterocolitica* serogroups (O3, O5,27, O8, O9) are productive of numerous colonies on routine isolation media (7). However, in those instances when *Y. enterocolitica* is sought during convalescence from acute enteritis, or for surveillance during an "outbreak," cold (4°C) enrichment of

stool specimens in phosphate-buffered saline for up to 4 weeks with periodic subculture may enhance recovery (8). *Y. enterocolitica* isolates recovered after prolonged cold enrichment should be biogrouped and serogrouped before clinical significance is ascribed to the isolate. In many instances, such isolates are of an environmental origin (biogroup 1A) and lack virulence attributes (7,8).

Compared with *Y. pestis* and *Y. pseudotuberculosis*, *Y. enterocolitica* strains are biochemically heterogeneous, a characteristic that is linked to ecologic distribution, virulence potential, and serogroup designation. Biochemical characteristics distinguishing *Y. enterocolitica* from *Y. pseudotuberculosis* and *Y. pestis* and from closely related species are noted in Table 72.2. *Y. enterocolitica* biogrouping schemas based on 12 biochemical reactions have been revised by Wauters and colleagues (9) (Table 72.3). On the basis of these 12 reactions, six biogroups have been established that also correlate with human pathogenic potential (Table 72.4). In the United States, biogroup 4, serogroup O3 has emerged as the most frequently isolated serogroup, exceeding serogroup O8 (10). This trend was first noted in New York in the 1980s (10–12). Wauters and co-workers (9) proposed six biogroups of *Y. enterocolitica*, with biogroup 6 being composed of strains designated biogroups 3A and 3B by Bercovier and colleagues (13). Characterization of strains in biogroups 3A and 3B has led to species ascription as *Yersinia bercovieri* and *Yersinia mollaretii* (14) (Table 72.2). API 20 is the semi-automated system of choice for identifying pathogenic and nonpathogenic species (15).

Y. enterocolitica isolates may be serologically grouped by slide agglutination with rabbit antisomatic O antisera into approximately 60 serogroups (16), which, as noted before, correlate with human pathogenic strains and their ecologic distribution. Because cross-reactions may occur with other *Yersinia* species, and because some *Yersinia* isolates showing specific antigens were later reclassified as separate species, serogrouping is useful in conjunction with biogrouping as an index of the clinical significance of a *Y. enterocolitica* isolate (17). Further assessment of the pathogenicity and epidemiology of a given *Y. enterocolitica* isolate may be achieved through bacteriophage typing, which also relates biogroups and serogroups to secondary autoimmune sequelae and epidemiologic distribution (Table 72.5).

EPIDEMIOLOGY

Y. enterocolitica is widely distributed in terrestrial and freshwater ecosystems, and it has been recovered from the intestinal tract of numerous mammalian species and from birds, insects, frogs, crabs, and oysters. In many instances, yersinial isolates recovered from these reservoirs are nonpathogenic members of biogroup 1A.

In the late 1970s, most reports of *Y. enterocolitica* infections originated from Europe, with incipient reports appearing from South Africa (20), Japan (21), and the United States (6). Today, however, as a consequence of heightened awareness by clinicians and microbiologists, *Y. enterocolitica* infections have been documented almost globally (22). Whereas a cooler seasonal prevalence has long been recognized in European countries, such a correlation with cases has not been found in the United States or other countries (22). It has been speculated that the frequency of infection is correlated with the porcine reservoir of pathogenic serogroups (O3, O5,27, O8, O9) (23) and consumption of undercooked or raw pork products (24) or even their preparation (25,26).

In terms of pathogenic serogroups, the pig is the only animal source clearly associated with serogroups O3, O5,27, O8, and

TABLE 72.1. Colony Characteristics of *Yersinia enterocolitica* on Commonly Used Isolation Media

Medium	Growth pattern
MacConkey agar	Pinpoint, colorless (pink), 24 h; 0.5–1.0 mm, 48 h
Hektoen enteric agar	Pinpoint, salmon colored due to sucrose fermentation; mimics "coliform" colonies
Xylose-lysine-deoxycholate agar	Pinpoint, yellow colonies due to xylose fermentation; mimics coliform colonies
Eosin-methylene blue agar	Pinpoint, lavender colonies with metallic sheen (48 h) due to sucrose fermentation; mimics colonies of *Escherichia coli*
Cefsulodin-irgasan-novobiocin agar	Red colonies with a transparent border 0.5–1.0 mm after 24 h at 25°C

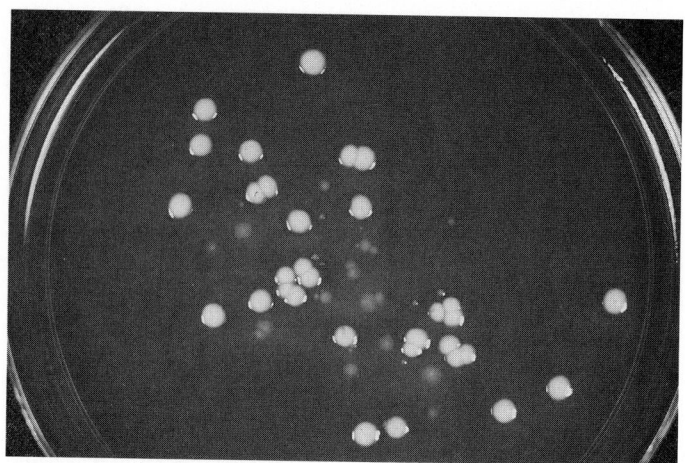

Figure 72.1. Stool cultured on MacConkey agar with pinpoint *Yersinia enterocolitica* colonies scattered between large colonies of *Salmonella* and large, lactose-fermenting colonies of *Escherichia coli*.

O9, especially in regions where the frequency of *Y. enterocolitica* infection is particularly elevated (26).

Although most sporadic infections with *Y. enterocolitica* cannot be traced to a specific exposure, ingestion of contaminated milk (27) or other dairy foods, contact with sick animals or perhaps, index cases, and transfusion of contaminated blood seem to be the main reported routes of transmission and acquisition of this bacterial pathogen. At present, in the United States, most sporadic cases have been associated with serogroup O3 isolates (10,12,22). Five of eight common-source food outbreaks have been caused by serogroup O8; and one each by serogroup O13a,13b and O3. (4,22–26) Two outbreaks of O3 infection in children have been associated with the household preparation of chitterlings from pig intestines (25). Reasons accounting for serogroup O8 involvement in the majority of food-borne outbreaks in the United States may center on its innate virulence, which is analogous to that of *Salmonella typhi* among salmonellae.

PATHOGENESIS

Gastrointestinal disease, the most common clinical manifestation of *Y. enterocolitica* infection, ensues subsequent to ingestion of a pathogenic strain of the bacterium. To gain access to the lamina propria, *Y. enterocolitica* traverse the host lumen through M cells (28), which are especially abundant over Peyer's patches in the terminal ileum. *Y. enterocolitica* motility is necessary for migration to host cells and for establishing contact prior to invasion (29). Studies in animal models with *Y. enterocolitica* serogroups O3 and O8 have established that the initial site of involvement is Peyer's patches of the distal ileum, which results in the formation of microabscesses, ulceration of the overlying epithelium, and an inflammatory reaction (30,31). Infection subsequently spreads to the mesenteric lymph nodes, which may lead to abscesses in the medullary region and pain in the lower quadrant mimicking appendicitis. Acute enteritis with inflammatory cells

TABLE 72.2. Select Biochemical Tests Differentiating *Yersinia enterocolitica* from Closely Related Species

Test	Yersinia							
	Enterocolitica[a]	Pseudotuberculosis	Pestis	Frederiksenii	Intermedia	Kristensenii	Mollaretii	Bercovieri
Fermentation								
Glucose	+	+	+	+	+	+	+	+
Sucrose	+	0	0	+	+	0	+	+
Rhamnose	0	+	0	+	+	0	+	+
Raffinose	0	0	0	0	+	0	0	0
Melibiose	0	+	v	0	+	0	0	0
Cellobiose	+	0	0	+	+	+	+	+
Sorbose	v	0	0	+	+	+	+	+
Ornithine decarboxylase	+	0	0	+	+	+	+	+
Voges-Proskauer	+ (25°C)	0	0	+	+	0	0	0
Indole	v	0	0	+	+	v	0	0
Urease production	+	+	0	+	+	+	+	+
Motility (25°C)	+	+	0	+	+	+	+	+

[a]Biotype 5 strains may vary in some reactions. See Table 72.3.
+, positive; 0, negative; v, variable.

TABLE 72.3. Biochemical Characteristics Used to Determine Biogroups of *Yersinia enterocolitica*

	Biogroup					
Characteristic	1A	1B[a]	2	3	4	5
Lipase activity	+	+	0	0	0	0
Salicin (acid 24 h)	+	0	0	0	0	0
Esculin hydrolysis (24 h)	+/0	0	0	0	0	0
Xylose (acid production)	+	+	+	+	0	v
Trehalose (acid production)	+	+	+	+	+	0
Indole production	+	+	0	0	0	0
Ornithine decarboxylase	+	+	+	+	+	+(+)
Voges-Proskauer test	+	+	+	+	+	+(+)
Pyrazinamidase activity	+	0	0	0	0	0
Sorbose (acid production)	+	+	+	+	+	0
Inositol (acid production)	+	+	+	+	+	+
Nitrate reduction	+	+	+	+	+	0

[a]Biogroup 1B is composed mainly of strains isolated in the United States.
+, positive; 0, negative; (+), delayed positive; v, variable.
Modified from Wauters G, Kandolo K, Janssens M Revised biogrouping scheme of *Yersinia enterocolitica. Contrib Microbiol Immunol* 1987;9:14–21, with permission.

TABLE 72.4. Correlation of Pathogenic Potential of *Yersinia enterocolitica* with Biogroup, Serogroup, and Ecologic Distribution

Associated with human infections	Biogroup	Serogroups	Ecologic distribution
Yes	1B	O8; O4; O13a, 13b; O18; O20; O21	Environment? Pig (O8); mainly in the United States
	2	O9; O5,27	Pigs
	3	O1,2,3; O5,27	Chinchilla
	4	O3	Pigs
	5	O2,3	Hare
No[a]	1A	O5; O6, 30; O7,8; numerous	Environment, food, water, animal and human feces

[a]*Y. enterocolitica* isolates comprising biogroup 1A may be recovered from asymptomatic humans as commensals. These strains, however, may be opportunistic pathogens in patients with underlying disorders.

TABLE 72.5. Correlation Between Serogroup, Biogroup, and Phage Type of Pathogenic *Yersinia enterocolitica* with Geographic Distribution and Secondary Sequelae of Infection[a]

Geographic distribution	Serogroup	Biogroup	Phage type	Secondary sequelae
United States	O8	1B	10[b]	No
	O3	4	9B	No
Canada	O3	4	9B	No
Europe	O3	4	8	Yes
	O9	2	10	Yes
Japan	O3	4	8	Rare (21)
South Africa	O3	4	9A	?[c]

[a]Secondary sequelae are arthritis and erythema nodosum.
[b]New bacteriophage typing system developed (18).
[c]Probable but not definitive (19).

TABLE 72.6. Spectrum of *Yersinia enterocolitica* Infections

Gastrointestinal infections
  Enterocolitis, especially in young children; concomitant bacteremia may also be present
  Pseudoappendicitis syndrome (children older than 5 yr, adults)
    Acute mesenteric lymphadenitis
    Terminal iletis
  Peritonitis
Septicemia
  Especially in immunosuppressed individuals and those with iron overload or being treated with iron-chelating agents
  Transfusion related
Metastatic infections after septicemia
  Focal abscesses: liver, kidney, spleen, lung
  Cutaneous manifestations: cellulitis, pyomyositis, pustules, and bullous lesions
  Pneumonia, cavitary pneumonia
  Meningitis
  Panophthalmitis
  Endocarditis, infected mycotic aneurysm
  Osteomyelitis
Postinfection sequelae; associated with human leukocyte antigen B27
  Arthritis
  Myocarditis
  Glomerulonephritis
  Uveitis
  Erythema nodosum
Pharyngitis

and occasionally bloody, watery stools characterize infection in children. Furthermore, concomitant *Y. enterocolitica* bacteremia may be present in infants with enteritis (12). In young adults, acute terminal ileitis and mesenteric adenitis are the more common presentations (32) (Table 72.6). Extensive ulceration of the intestinal tract and death have occurred in the course of *Y. enterocolitica* serogroup O8 infection (33,34). The role of heat-stable enterotoxin in this process is unclear (35).

Although *Y. enterocolitica* is primarily a gastrointestinal tract pathogen, extraintestinal disease depends on the host immune status and the pathogenic potential of the infecting strain. For instance, primary *Y. enterocolitica* serogroup O8 septicemia mimicking typhoid fever has been reported in a previously healthy 75-year-old individual from upstate New York (36). Also, primary septicemia with pulmonary embolization was reported in a 47-year-old Japanese man without gastrointestinal symptoms and without usual predisposing factors (37).

Secondary manifestations of bacteremia may involve every organ of the body, including the endovasculature and the central nervous system, and may even lead to cutaneous lesions (38–41) (Table 72.6).

A striking characteristic of *Y. enterocolitica* is the increased incidence of invasive infection in people with iron overload diseases or in those being administered iron-chelating agents (42,43). *Y. enterocolitica* serogroups O3, O5,27, and O9 require iron overload to cause septicemia or show animal lethality, and are typically regarded as low virulence species in healthy people (42). By way of contrast, the highly virulent serogroup O8 *Y. enterocolitica* does not require exogenous iron to cause septicemia or lethality in animals (44,45).

Bacteremia with *Y. enterocolitica* may also occur by transfusion of contaminated blood (46). Since the first report in 1975 (47), 26 cases of *Y. enterocolitica* transfusion-associated bacteremia had been documented up to 1994 (48). Of these, 11 occurred in the United States from 1985 through 1992. An additional 10 cases were reported to the Centers for Disease Control and Prevention through 1996 (46). These cases were predominantly associated with transfusion of packed red blood cells (including autologous transfusion). Shock, with and without disseminated intravascular coagulation, occurred in all 36 recipients, and death occurred in 19 patients. The source of *Y. enterocolitica* contamination was asymptomatic bacteremia in the donor.

Secondary nonsuppurative sequelae of *Y. enterocolitica* infection include polyarticular arthritis and erythema nodosum reported mainly among northern Europeans (49–52). Polyarthritis onset is acute and is preceded by a history of fever and gastrointestinal disturbance. Symptoms of polyarthritis are manifested predominantly in weight-bearing joints (e.g., knees, ankles, and fingers). Joint involvement with pain and swelling occurs in rapid succession during a 2-week course. Synovial fluid may show a polymorphonuclear response, but although cultures are sterile, yersinial antigen may be present. Symptoms may persist for up to 4 months with a tendency toward chronicity in the absence of rheumatoid factor (51). Predisposing factors for reactive arthropathy, but not erythema nodosum, include the presence of human leukocyte antigen B27 (in 80% of individuals) (53). In these patients, joint symptoms were more severe. Reiter's syndrome (53), uveitis (54), myocarditis (55), and glomerulonephritis (56) have also been reported as late sequelae associated with *Y. enterocolitica* infection. In glomerulonephritis, patients presented with proteinuria and hematuria, and *Yersinia* antigen complexed with immunoglobulin G and complement could be demonstrated in basement membranes by immunofluorescence (57).

A case-control study of patients with chronic fatigue syndrome (CFS) did not find a significant difference in the presence of antibodies to *Yersinia* outer membrane proteins in patients with and without CFS. It was concluded that *Y. enterocolitica* was unlikely to cause CFS (58).

In Europe and northern European (Scandinavian) countries, *Y. enterocolitica* serogroup O3, phage type 8, and serogroup O9 are the common causes of yersiniosis. Phage type 8 isolates of serogroup O3 are unique to Europe, where the majority, if not all, secondary postinfectious sequelae occur, in contrast to Canada and South Africa, for example, where *Y. enterocolitica* serogroup O3, phage types 9B and 9A, respectively, predominate but cases of reactive arthritis or other secondary sequelae have not been definitively documented (4,19).

Through serologic studies, *Y. enterocolitica* has also been associated with various thyroid disorders, including Graves' disease, nontoxic goiter, and Hashimoto's thyroiditis (59). Antibody titers to serogroup O3 *Y. enterocolitica* have been detected in up to 52% of patients with thyroid disorders in the United States (60) and Israel (61). At the time of these studies, however, serogroup O3 *Y. enterocolitica* had not yet emerged as a significant pathogen in the United States and was rarely encountered in Israel. These data suggest nonspecific serologic cross-reactions between *Y. enterocolitica* O3 or cross-reactivity with human thyrotropin receptor rather than a causal role for *Y. enterocolitica* in thyroid disorders (62).

VIRULENCE FACTORS

In concert with the plague bacillus, *Y. pestis*, and *Y. pseudotuberculosis*, human pathogenic strains of *Y. enterocolitica* possess a variety of plasmid- and chromosome-encoded virulence determinants that promote human infection and disease. Those specified

by a 70- to 75-kb plasmid are under exquisite temperature control, being expressed mainly at 37°C and in reduced copy number at 25°C (63). Thus, with acquisition of the bacterium from an inanimate reservoir (e.g., food or water), adaptation to host temperature (37°C) results in synthesis of several virulence determinants that confer resistance to phagocytosis by polymorphonuclear leukocytes (64), intracellular killing by macrophages (65), and resistance to serum bactericidal activity (66). Also shared with *Y. pestis* and *Y. pseudotuberculosis* is plasmid-encoded V and W surface antigens, which may also provide antiphagocytic activity (67).

Chromosomally encoded determinants include production of an outer membrane protein named invasin. When the gene (*inv*) encoding this surface component is introduced into a noninvasive *Escherichia coli*, invasiveness for several cultured epithelial cell lines is conferred on the recipient (68). The binding sites for invasin on host cells are a group of β_1 integrins (69). Binding of *Y. enterocolitica* to these integrins results in cytoskeletal alteration of the host cell and, subsequently, internalization of the bacterium via parasite-mediated endocytosis (69). Nonmotile strains have been noted to be less invasive than motile strains, despite having adequate invasin levels (70). Therefore, flagella-dependent motility may ensure that the pathogenic bacterium contacts the host cell. Interestingly, functional invasin is absent from *Y. pestis*, which gains access to host tissue by direct inoculation through a flea bite or by inhalation.

Of significance is that invasin is maximally produced at 25°C, which may aid initial colonization of host tissues when the bacterium is obtained from an environmental source. Subsequent adaptation to 37°C triggers the plasmid-encoded virulence attributes, and another chromosomally encoded outer membrane protein is necessary to establish an infectious nidus in the human host. The latter surface component, which also confers invasiveness on *Y. enterocolitica* (71), is coded by a specified chromosomal locus termed *ail* for the attachment/invasion locus. Presence of the *ail* gene also allows *Yersiniae* to resist serum bactericidal activity (72).

In contrast to *inv*, *ail* is expressed at 37°C and may therefore augment the initial invasive attribute contributed by *inv*, while the bacterium undergoes a thermal transition from ambient or refrigerated temperatures to host (37°C) temperature. The *ail* locus is commonly found among *Y. enterocolitica* serogroups associated with human infections and is absent from environmental isolates (73).

Y. enterocolitica also produces a heat-stable enterotoxin, but its role in diarrheal disease is disputed because it is maximally produced below 30°C in late log-phase broth cultures (35).

The difference in virulence between 08 and the O3, O5,27, and O9 serogroups resides in the production under conditions of iron starvation of an iron-complexing siderophore and an outer membrane receptor for chelated iron by the highly pathogenic O8 serogroup (44). The gene coding for the iron-regulated synthesis of the outer membrane protein is absent in low pathogenicity strains (e.g., O3) (44), necessitating their need for exogenous free or chelated iron (42). Although it is not conclusive, the nonanimal lethal group of *Y. enterocolitica* has been shown to express an outer membrane protein of 82,000 daltons that cross-reacts serologically with the O8 siderophore and may serve a similar function in iron transport (45).

TREATMENT

Older surveys had shown that isolates of *Y. enterocolitica* are susceptible *in vitro* to trimethoprim-sulfamethoxazole (TMP-SMX), third-generation cephalosporins, aminoglycosides, imipenem, aztreonam, and quinolones (74,75). More recently, there is a trend of increasing resistance to TMP-SMX and chloramphenicol in Spain (76).

Y. enterocolitica isolates produce two distinct chromosomally encoded β-lactamases (A and B) (77) that inactivate a wide variety of penicillins and first-generation cephalosporins. Differences in β-lactamase susceptibility in biogroup 2 (serogroup O9, O5,27), biogroup 4 (serogroup O3) and biogroup 5 (serogroup O2,3) have been attributed to variable expression of β-lactamases A and B due to antibiotic induction (78). Biogroups 1A, 1B, 3 also have β-lactamases A and B and variable susceptibility has again been attributed to induction (79).

Despite antibiotic susceptibility to common agents (e.g., TMP-SMX), there is still controversy over the need to treat uncomplicated *Y. enterocolitica* enteritis (22,32,74). The mean duration of symptoms in untreated enteritis in children is 14 days (80). In a placebo-controlled, double-blind study of TMP-SMX in *Y. enterocolitica* enteritis in children, Pai and co-workers (81) not only failed to show earlier resolution of symptoms but also showed prolongation (relapse) of bacteriologic cure as well. These investigators, however, began therapy late (eleventh or twelfth day) in the course of enteritis of the 19 children studied. As they noted, treatment begun at the outset of symptoms might have had a different outcome. A retrospective chart review of children with stool cultures positive for *Y. enterocolitica* in Michigan found no difference in resolution or improvement of diarrhea in ambulatory patients treated and not treated with TMP-SMX (82). No isolates were resistant to TMP-SMX.

Extraintestinal infection, such as bacteremia in infants with enteritis (12,83), in immunocompromised hosts, or in people with iron overload disease, merits antiyersinial therapy. Bacteremia complicated by focal disease of liver, bones, joints, and central nervous system may require prolonged (3 weeks or more) therapy. A retrospective analysis of 43 cases of bacteremia in the French national registry showed that third-generation cephalosporins in combination with other antibiotics resulted in a successful outcome in 85% of cases (84). In this series, fluoroquinolones alone, or in combination with an aminoglycoside, or a third-generation cephalosporin, were shown to be highly effective in 15 of 43 patients treated. Resolution of symptoms, and of bacteremia, ensued within 1 to 4 days. Monotherapy with earlier generation β-lactams failed in 18 cases, and amoxicillin-clavulanate failed in all except six cases. These authors concluded that antibiotic regimens including fluoroquinolones constitute the best treatment of *Y. enterocolitica* septicemia.

PREVENTION

Prevention of food-borne outbreaks requires adherence to known preventive measures (e.g., pasteurization, and maintenance of sanitation policies for food-processing equipment, establishment of programs for minimizing contamination of finished products) as have been instituted for another food-borne pathogen, *Listeria monocytogenes* (85–88). A public education campaign in Belgium emphasizing the importance of good hygiene in the handling and preparation of food and avoiding eating raw or undercooked pork was associated with a significant decrease in the number of *Y. enterocolitica* infections between 1987 and 1996 (26).

Numerous efforts have been proposed to reduce the incidence of transfusion-associated yersiniosis, including screening donors for a history of gastrointestinal illness within 4 weeks of donation (89). Recently, a polymerase chain reaction assay was developed

for the screening and rapid identification of *Y. enterocolitica* in blood (90).

REFERENCES

1. McIver MA, Pike RM. Chronic glanders-like infection of face caused by an organism resembling *Flavobacterium pseudomallei*. In: Clinical miscellany. Cooperstown, NY: Mary Imogene Bassett Hospital, 1934:16–20.
2. Schleifstein J, Coleman MB. An unidentified microorganism resembling *A. lignieri* and *Past. pseudotuberculosis* and pathogenic for man. *N Y State J Med* 1939;39:1749–1753.
3. Schleifstein J, Coleman MB. *Bacterium enterocoliticum*. In: *Annual report of Division of Laboratories and Research*. Albany, NY: New York State Department of Health, 1943:56.
4. Bottone EJ. *Yersinia enterocolitica*: a panoramic view of a charismatic microorganism. *Crit Rev Microbiol* 1977;5:211–241.
5. Black RE, Jackson RJ, Tsai T, et al. Epidemic *Yersinia enterocolitica* infection due to contaminated chocolate milk. *N Engl J Med* 1978;298:76–79.
6. Fukushima H. New selective agar medium for isolation of virulent *Yersinia enterocolitica*. *J Clin Microbiol* 1987;25:1068–1073.
7. Van Noyen R, Vandepitte J, Wauters G. Nonvalue of cold enrichment of stools for isolation of *Yersinia enterocolitica* serotype 3 and 9 from patients. *J Clin Microbiol* 1980;11:127–131.
8. Pai CH, Sorger S, Lafleur L, et al. Efficacy of cold enrichment techniques for recovery of *Yersinia enterocolitica* from human stools. *J Clin Microbiol* 1979;9:712–715.
9. Wauters G, Kandolo K, Janssens M. Revised biogrouping scheme of *Yersinia enterocolitica*. *Contrib Microbiol Immunol* 1987;9:14–21.
10. Bottone EJ. Current trends of *Yersinia enterocolitica* isolates in the New York City area. *J Clin Microbiol* 1983;17:63–67.
11. Shayegani M, DeForge I, McGlynn DM, et al. Characteristics of *Yersinia enterocolitica* and related species isolated from human, animal and environmental sources. *J Clin Microbiol* 1981;14:304–312.
12. Bottone EJ, Gullans CR, Sierra MF. Disease spectrum of *Yersinia enterocolitica* serogroup 0:3, the predominant cause of human infection in New York City. *Contrib Microbiol Immunol* 1987;9:56–60.
13. Bercovier H, Brault J, Barre N, et al. Biochemical, serological and phage types characteristics of 459 *Yersinia* strains isolated from a terrestrial ecosystem. *Curr Microbiol* 1978;1:353–357.
14. Wauters GM, Janssens M, Steigerwalt AG, et al. *Yersinia mollaretii* sp. nov. and *Yersinia bercovieri* sp. nov., formerly called *Yersinia enterocolitica* biogroups 3A and 3B. *Int J Syst Bacteriol* 1988;38:424.
15. Neubauer H, Sauer T, Becker H, et al. Comparison of systems for identification and differentiation of species within the genus *Yersinia*. *J Clin Microbiol* 1998;36:3366–3368.
16. Wauters G. Antigens of *Yersinia enterocolitica*. In: Bottone EJ, ed. *Yersinia enterocolitica*. Boca Raton, FL: CRC Press, 1981:41–53.
17. Chiesa C, Pacifico L, Ravagnan G. Identification of pathogenic serotypes of *Yersinia enterocolitica*. *J Clin Microbiol* 1993;31:2248–2249.
18. Baker PM, Farmer JJ III. New bacteriophage typing system for *Yersinia enterocolitica*, *Yersinia kristensenii*, *Yersinia frederiksenii*, and *Yersinia intermedia*: correlation with serotyping, biotyping and antibiotic susceptibility. *J Clin Microbiol* 1982;15:491–502.
19. Robins-Browne RM, Rabson AR, Koornhoff HJ. *Yersinia enterocolitica* in South Africa. In: Bottone EJ, ed. *Yersinia enterocolitica*. Boca Raton, FL: CRC Press, 1981:193–203.
20. Rabson AR, Hallett AF, Koornhoff HJ. Generalized *Yersinia enterocolitica* infection. *J Infect Dis* 1975;131:447–451.
21. Zen-Yoji H. Epidemiologic aspects of yersiniosis in Japan. In: Bottone EJ, ed. *Yersinia enterocolitica*. Boca Raton, FL: CRC Press, 1981:206–216.
22. Cover TL, Aber RC. *Yersinia enterocolitica*. *N Engl J Med* 1989;321:16–24.
23. Doyle MP, Hugdahl MB, Taylor SL. Isolation of virulent *Yersinia enterocolitica* from porcine tongues. *Appl Environ Microbiol* 1981;42:661–666.
24. Tauxe RV, Vandepitte J, Wauters G, et al. *Yersinia enterocolitica* infections and pork: the missing link. *Lancet* 1987;1:1129–1132.
25. Lee LA, Gerber AR, Lonsway DR, et al. *Yersinia enterocolitica* infections in infants and children associated with the household preparation of chitterlings. *N Engl J Med* 1990;322:984–987.
26. Verhagen J, Charlier J, Lemmens P, et al. Surveillance of human *Yersinia enterocolitica* infections in Belgium: 1967–1996. *Clin Infect Dis* 1998;27:59–64.
27. Ackers ML, Schoenfeld S, Markman J, et al. An outbreak of *Yersinia enterocolitica* O:8 infections associated with pasteurized milk. *J Infect Dis* 2000;181:1834–1837.
28. Grützkau A, Hanski C, Naumann M. Comparative study of histopathological alterations during intestinal infection of mice with pathogenic and non-pathogenic strains of *Yersinia enterocolitica* serotype O:8. *Virchows Arch [A]* 1993;423:97–103.
29. Young GM, Badger JL, Miller VL. Motility is required to initiate host cell invasion by *Yersinia enterocolitica*. *Infect Immun* 2000;68:4323–4326.
30. Carter PB. Human *Yersinia enterocolitica* infection: laboratory models. In: Bottone EJ, ed. *Yersinia enterocolitica*. Boca Raton, FL: CRC Press, 1981:74–81.
31. Robins-Browne RM, Tzopori S, Gonis G, et al. The pathogenesis of *Yersinia*

enterocolitica infection in gnotobiotic piglets. *J Med Microbiol* 1985;19:297–308.

32. Ehara A, Egawa K, Kuroki F, et al. Age-dependent expression of abdominal symptoms in patients with *Yersinia enterocolitica* infection. *Pediatr Int* 2000;42:364–366.

33. Gutman LT, Ottesen EA, Quan TJ, et al. An interfamilial outbreak of *Yersinia enterocolitica* enteritis. *N Engl J Med* 1973;288:1372–1376.

34. Bradford WD, Noce PS, Gutman LT. Pathologic features of enteric infection with *Yersinia enterocolitica*. *Arch Pathol* 1974;98:17–22.

35. Boyce JM, Evans EJ Jr, Evans DG, et al. Production of heat-stable, methanol-soluble enterotoxin by *Yersinia enterocolitica*. *Infect Immun* 1979;25:532–537.

36. Keet EE. *Yersinia enterocolitica* septicemia. Source of infection and incubation period identified. *N Y State J Med* 1974;74:2226–2230.

37. Hosaka S. Uchiyama M, Ishikawa M, et al. *Yersinia enterocolitica* serotype O:8 septicemia in an otherwise healthy adult: analysis of chromosome DNA pattern by pulse-field gel electrophoresis. *J Clin Microbiol* 1997;35:3346–3347.

38. Sonnenwirth AC. Bacteremia with and without meningitis due to *Yersinia enterocolitica, Edwardsiella tarda, Commamonas terrigena,* and *Pseudomonas maltophilia. Ann N Y Acad Sci* 1970;174:L488–L502.

39. Reed RP, Robins-Browne RM, Williams ML. *Yersinia enterocolitica* peritonitis. *Clin Infect Dis* 1997;25:1468–1469.

40. Olbrych TG, Zarconi J, File TM Jr, et al. Bullous skin lesions associated with *Yersinia enterocolitica* septicemia. *Am J Med Sci* 1094;287:38–39.

41. Bonnet E, Archambaud M, Sommabera A, et al. Endocarditis due to *Yersinia enterocolitica. Infection* 1998;26:320–321.

42. Robins-Browne RM, Prpic JK. Effects of iron and desferrioxamine on infections with *Yersinia enterocolitica. Infect Immun* 1985;43:774–779.

43. Adamkiewicz TV, Berkovitch M, Krishnan C, et al. Infection due to *Yersinia enterocolitica* in a series of patients with beta-thalassemia: incidence and predisposing factors. *Clin Infect Dis* 1998;27:1362–1366.

44. Carniel E, Mercereau-Puijalon O, Bonnefoy S. The gene coding for the 190,000 dalton iron-regulated protein of *Yersinia* species is present only in highly pathogenic strains. *Infect Immun* 1989;57:1211–1217.

45. Heesemann J, Hantke K, Vocke T, et al. Virulence of *Yersinia enterocolitica* is closely associated with siderophore production expression of an iron-repressible outer membrane polypeptide of 65,000 Da and pesticin sensitivity. *Mol Microbiol* 1993;8:397–408.

46. Anonymous. Red blood cell transfusions contaminated with *Yersinia enterocolitica*—United States, 1991–1996, and initiation of a national study to detect bacteria-associated transfusion reactions. *MMWR* 1997;46:553–555.

47. Bruining A, DeWilde-Beekhuizen CCM. A case of contamination of donor blood by *Yersinia enterocolitica* type 9. *Medilon* 1975;4:30–31.

48. Haditsch M, Binder C, Gabriel C, et al. *Yersinia enterocolitica* septicemia in autologous blood transfusion. *Transfusion* 1994;34:907–909.

49. Ahvonen P, Sievers K, Aho K. Arthritis associated with *Yersinia enterocolitica* infection. *Acta Rheumatol Scand* 1969;15:232–253.

50. Laitenen O, Tuuhea J, Ahvonen P. Polyarthritis associated with *Yersinia enterocolitica* infection. Clinical features and laboratory findings in nine cases with severe joint symptoms. *Ann Rheum Dis* 1972;31:34–39.

51. Winblad S. Arthritis associated with *Yersinia enterocolitica* infections. *Scand J Infect Dis* 1975;7:191–193.

52. van-der-Heijden IM, Res PC, Wilbrink B, et al. *Yersinia enterocolitica:* a cause of chronic polyarthritis. *Clin Infect Dis* 1997;25:831–837.

53. Laitinen O, Leirisalo M, Skylv G. Relation between HLA-B27 and clinical features in patients with *yersinia* arthritis. *Arthritis Rheum* 1977;20:1121–1124.

54. Careless DJ, Chiu B, Rabinovitch T, et al. Immunogenetic and microbial factors in acute anterior uveitis. *J Rheumatol* 1997;24:102–108.

55. Agner E, Larsen JH, Leth A. *Yersinia enterocolitica* carditis as a differential diagnosis—and the prognosis of this disease. *Scand J Rheumatol* 1978;7:26–28.

56. Denneberg T, Friedberg M, Samuelsson T, et al. Glomerulonephritis in infections with *Yersinia enterocolitica* O-serotype 3. I. Evidence for glomerular involvement in acute cases of yersiniosis. *Acta Med Scand* 1981;209:97–101.

57. Denneberg T, Friedberg M, Brun C, et al. Glomerulonephritis in infections with *Yersinia enterocolitica* O-serotype 3. II. The incidence and immunological features of *Yersinia* infection in a consecutive glomerulonephritis population. *Acta Med Scand* 1981;209:103–110.

58. Swanink CM, Stolk-Engelaar VM, van-der-Meer JW, et al. *Yersinia enterocolitica* and the chronic fatigue syndrome. *J Infect* 1998;36:269–272.

59. Bech K, Nerup J, Larsen JH. *Yersinia enterocolitica* infection and thyroid diseases. *Acta Endocrinol* 1977;84:87–92.

60. Shenkman L, Bottone EJ. Antibodies to *Yersinia enterocolitica* in thyroid disease. *Ann Intern Med* 1976;85:735–739.

61. Weiss M, Rubinstein E, Bottone EJ, et al. *Yersinia enterocolitica* antibodies in thyroid disorders. *Isr J Med Sci* 1979;15:553–555.

62. Toivanen P, Toivanen A. Does *Yersinia* induce autoimmunity? *Int Arch Allergy Immunol* 1994;104:107–111.

63. Straley SC, Skrzypek E, Plano GV, Bliska JB. Yops of *Yersinia* spp. pathogenic for humans. *Infect Immun* 1993;61:3103–3110.

64. Lian C, Hwang WS, Pai CH. Plasmid-mediated resistance to phagocytosis in *Yersinia enterocolitica. Infect Immun* 1987;55:1176–1183.

65. Une T. Studies on the pathogenicity of *Yersinia enterocolitica*. II. Interaction with cultured cells *in vitro. Microbiol Immunol* 1977;21:365–367.

66. Pai CH, DeStephano L. Serum resistance associated with virulence in *Yersinia enterocolitica. Infect Immun* 1982;35:605–611.

67. Perry RD, Brubaker RR. Vwa+ phenotype of *Yersinia enterocolitica. Infect Immun* 1983;40:166–177.

68. Isberg RR, Falkow S. A single genetic locus encoded by *Yersinia pseudotuberculosis* permits invasion of cultured animal cells by *Escherichia coli* K-12. *Nature* 1985;317:262–264.

69. Isberg RR, Leong JM. Multiple β_1 chain integrins and receptors for invasin, a protein that promotes bacterial penetration into mammalian cells. *Cell* 1990;60:861–871.

70. Young GM, Badger JL, Miller VL. Motility is required to initiate host cell invasion by *Yersinia enterocolitica. Infect Immun* 2000;68:4323–4326.

71. Miller VL, Falkow S. Evidence for two genetic loci from *Yersinia enterocolitica* that can promote invasion of epithelial cells. *Infect Immun* 1988;56:1242–1248.

72. Bliska JB, Falkow S. Bacterial resistance to complement killing mediated by the Ail protein of *Yersinia enterocolitica. Proc Natl Acad Sci USA* 1992;89:3561–3565.

73. Miller VL, Farmer JJ III, Hill WE, et al. The *ail* locus is found uniquely in *Yersinia enterocolitica* serotypes commonly associated with disease. *Infect Immun* 1989;57:121–131.

74. Hoogkamp-Korstanje JA. Antibiotics in *Yersinia enterocolitica* infections. *J Antimicrob Chemother* 1987;20:123–131.

75. Hornstein MJ, Jupeau AM, Scavizzi MR, et al. *In vitro* susceptibilities of 126 clinical isolates of *Yersinia enterocolitica* to 21 beta-lactam antibiotics. *Antimicrob Agents Chemother* 1985;27:806–811.

76. Prats G, Mirelis B, Llovet T, et al. Antibiotic resistance trends in enteropthogenic bacteria isolated in 1985–1987 and 1995–1998 in Barcelona. *Antimicrob Agents Chemother* 2000;44:1140–1145.

77. Cornelis G. Distribution of beta-lactamases A and B in some groups of *Yersinia enterocolitica* and their role in resistance. *J Gen Microbiol* 1975;91:391–402.

78. Stock I, Heisig P, Wiedemann B. Expression of β-lactamases in *Yersinia enterocolitica* strains of biovars 2, 4, and 5. *J Med Microbiol* 1999;48:1023–1026.

79. Stock I, Heisig P, Wiedemann B. β-lactamase expression in *Yersinia enterocolitica* biovars 1A, 1B and 3. *J Med Microbiol* 2000;49:403–408.

80. Marks MI, Pai CH, Lafleur L, et al. *Yersinia enterocolitica* gastroenteritis: a prospective study of clinical, bacteriologic, and epidemiologic features. *J Pediatr* 1980;96:26–31.

81. Pai CH, Gillis F, Tuomanen E, et al. Placebo-controlled double-blind evaluation of trimethoprim-sulfamethoxazole treatment of *Yersinia enterocolitica* gastroenteritis. *J Pediatr* 1984;104:308–311.

82. Abdel-Haq NM, Asmar BI, Abuhammour WM, et al. *Yersinia* enterocolitica infection in children. *Pediatr Infect Dis J* 2000;19:954–958.

83. Shapiro ED. *Yersinia enterocolitica* septicemia in normal infants. *Am J Dis Child* 1981;135:477–478.

84. Gayraud M, Scavizzi MR, Mollaret HH, et al. Antibiotic treatment of *Yersinia enterocolitica* septicemia: a retrospective review of 43 cases. *Clin Infect Dis* 1993;17:405–410.

85. Tappero JW, Schuchat A, Deaver RA, et al. Reduction in the incidence of human listeriosis in the United States. Effectiveness of prevention efforts? *JAMA* 1995;273:1118–1122.

86. Shayegani M, Morse D, DeForge T. Microbiology of a food-borne outbreak of gastroenteritis caused by *Yersinia enterocolitica* serogroup O:8. *J Clin Microbiol* 1983;17:35–40.

87. Tackett CO, Ballard J, Harris N. An outbreak of *Yersinia enterocolitica* infection caused by contamination of tofu (soybean curd). *Am J Epidemiol* 1985;121:705–711.

88. Aber RC, McCarthy MA, Berman R, et al. An outbreak of *Yersinia enterocolitica* gastrointestinal illness among members of a Brownie group in Centre County, Pennsylvania. In: *Program and abstracts of the 72nd Interscience Conference on Antimicrobial Agents and Chemotherapy.* Washington, DC: American Society for Microbiology, 1982.

89. Bottone EJ, *Yersinia enterocolitica:* the charisma continues. *Clin Microbiol Rev* 1997;10:257–276.

90. Sen, K. Rapid identification of *Yersinia enterocolitica* in the blood by the 5′ nuclease PCR assay. *J Clin Microbiol* 2000;38:1953–1958.

CHAPTER 73

Cholera and Related Illnesses Caused by Vibrio, Aeromonas, and Plesiomonas Species*

David A. Sack

Cholera is an acute diarrheal disease that, in severe cases, can lead to such massive fluid loss that normal, healthy people die of dehydration and shock within a few hours. In developing countries, epidemics can occur in massive outbreaks, leading to thousands of cases and deaths in a few days or weeks. Thus, cholera has earned respect as one of the great epidemic diseases. Cholera is caused by enterotoxigenic strains of *Vibrio cholerae* belonging to serogroup O1 or O139. These strains are members of the Vibrionaceae family, along with other serogroups of *V. cholerae* and other species of *Vibrio*. The pathogenic species of *Vibrio* include *V. mimicus*, *V. vulnificus*, *V. fluvialis*, *V. parahaemolyticus*, *V. hollisae*, *V. furnissii*, *V. alginolyticus*, *V. metschnikovii*, *V. damsela*, and *V. cincinnatiensis*. Formerly, the vibrios were simply classified as either *V. cholerae* O1, with epidemic potential, or nonagglutinating vibrios, which were unlikely to spark an epidemic. Now it is clear that many of the *Vibrio* strains have characteristic pathogenic patterns and need to be speciated beyond simply carrying out agglutination tests with the O1 antiserum.

The vibrios share several common features. They are all motile, gram-negative, rod-shaped organisms with a single polar flagellum. Their natural habitat is environmental waters, and their spread and epidemic patterns are highly linked to the ecologic changes of the water in which they persist. Thus, in temperate climates they are more common during the warmer summer months, when they can be isolated from water, plankton, and shellfish. Most infections in humans occur during this time. In tropical areas, their seasonality is more complex, because transmission may occur throughout the year. Halophilic (salt-loving) species require salt for growth and are generally isolated from saltwater sources. As with the illness caused by *V. cholerae* O1, most of the illnesses caused by the vibrios are diarrheal; however, certain species, especially *V. vulnificus*, may cause bacteremia and wound infections. The pathogenicity of *Aeromonas* species and *P. shigelloides* is less certain, but these bacteria probably cause diarrheal illness in some cases and rarely also lead to systemic infections.

VIBRIOS GENERALLY ASSOCIATED WITH DIARRHEA

Vibrio cholerae O1 and O139

HISTORY

Cholera has been endemic to the Indian subcontinent and other parts of the world for centuries. It was inadvertently introduced into Europe in 1817 during the age of colonial expansion.

Subsequently, it spread around the world in successive pandemics and reached U.S. port cities in the mid-1800s. Cholera even followed pioneers across the American West, contaminating the drinking water of the wagon trains. The current seventh pandemic, involving *V. cholerae* biotype El Tor, serogroup O1, began in Indonesia in 1961 and is continuing in Asia and Africa. A focus of infection continues on the Gulf Coast of the United States even without environmental contamination with sewage (1). In most years, a few persons who eat undercooked seafood from the Gulf Coast in August develop cholera (2).

There have been two more recent landmarks in the history of cholera. First, Latin America had remained free of cholera for 100 years until 1991, when cholera appeared in Peru and subsequently spread to nearly all other Latin American countries (3). After initial epidemics, the number of Latin American cases has dropped. By 2002, cholera had not spread to any of the Caribbean islands.

Second, in 1992, a new serogroup of epidemic cholera, *V. cholerae* O139, appeared in Bangladesh and India along the Bay of Bengal (4). Previously, all epidemic strains of cholera belonged to serogroup O1, but this new strain caused epidemics like previous epidemics with serogroup O1. Because of its association with the Bay of Bengal, it was given the name *V. cholerae* O139 (synonym Bengal). Scientists are monitoring this new strain to determine whether it will continue its expansion outside Asia, invade other regions, and become the eighth pandemic strain (5,6).

Because of its high case-fatality rates, physicians throughout history desperately attempted to develop effective treatments. Unfortunately, these treatments had more to do with the popular medical philosophy of the day than with a reasonable approach to the disease. In the nineteenth century, cholera was treated with bleeding, laxatives, enemas, and a variety of herbs, and the therapy undoubtedly contributed to high case-fatality rates. Even Osler's textbook advocated injections of morphine, ice by mouth, brandy, and tannic acid enemas. A few physicians, however, realized that the key event of cholera was loss of fluids and attempted to replace them with intravenous fluids. For example, Latta used intravenous saline as early as 1831 (7,8), and a few of his patients survived, but sterile fluids and supplies were not available then, and case-fatality rates remained high, with many deaths caused by sepsis.

By the early 1900s, Rogers (9), working in Calcutta, began using improved intravenous fluids to treat cholera, and gradually the case-fatality rates began to decrease. Still, the case-fatality rates did not reach their current low level of less than 1% until the 1960s, when physicians learned to use isotonic intravenous fluids that approximated the electrolyte composition of the diarrhea stool being lost. The development of rational intravenous fluids saved patients who were able to get this treatment (10,11), but the important public health breakthrough came with the development of oral rehydration fluids in the late 1960s in Calcutta and Dhaka (12–14).

In terms of etiology, Snow (15) in 1855 first described the relationship between risk of cholera and the use of contaminated water and hypothesized the presence of a toxin that was being spread by way of water. Koch is generally credited with discovering the bacterium in 1884, although Pacini may have found the *Vibrio* organism as early as 1854. Regardless of this earlier claim, Koch's discovery quickly led to an appreciation of the infectious nature of the disease. Within a year, scientists developed a killed, whole-cell injectable vaccine, variations of which were widely used for many decades and which is still available, even though its use is discouraged.

EPIDEMIOLOGY

Cholera is spread by eating or drinking contaminated food or water. In common-source outbreaks, a specific food (16) or water

---

*Although they share many characteristics, these species are now classified into different families. Vibrios are included under the Vibrionaceae, under the Order *Vibrionales*, whereas *Aeromonas* belongs to a new family, *Aeromonadaceae*, under the Order *Aeromonadales*. *Plesiomonas* now belongs to the Order *Enterobacteriales*, Family *Enterobacteriaceae*.

supply (17) can often be identified; however, the two sources usually overlap, because market food is often washed with contaminated water or leftover food is mixed with water. Because the environmental reservoir for *Vibrio* is water and shellfish, seafood has often been implicated, especially in the United States, where other vehicles are not present (18). In endemic areas, many foods and water sources can spread the bacterium.

The risk of cholera in the United States and other industrialized countries is small. A few cases have resulted from contaminated seafood from the Gulf Coast and a few cases have resulted from imported food (19). Thus, cholera is primarily a disease of developing countries in areas where water and hygiene are substandard. Internationally, cholera is a reportable disease; however, the true global disease burden from cholera remains uncertain. On the basis of sample reporting, there are an estimated 6 million cases of cholera per year, associated with about 600,000 hospitalizations and about 120,000 deaths in the world (20). Unfortunately, the national stigma associated with cholera and the fear of economic reprisals led many countries in Asia and Africa to avoid reporting cases, so it has not been possible to detect trends in cholera epidemiology outside the Americas.

Cholera can be divided, somewhat arbitrarily, into endemic cholera and epidemic cholera. In areas with endemic cholera, such as the Ganges Delta, cholera occurs regularly, with most cases appearing during cholera seasons. In some areas, two seasons are seen before and after the rainy season, whereas in other regions a single peak season is observed. In Asia, the highest rate of cholera occurs in childhood, naturally acquired immunity apparently protecting older individuals from the high illness rates seen in childhood (21). Still, most cases are seen in older children and adults because they represent a much larger segment of the population (22,23). In Latin America, case rates have remained highest in adult men, perhaps because of increased exposure, even though cholera has become endemic. Interestingly, rates of serotype O139 remain higher in adults than in children in Asia where this strain has become endemic (unpublished data, D.A. Sack).

Epidemic cholera occurs among populations that have had no previous exposure to cholera but become exposed suddenly. The explosive outbreaks of cholera in Africa caused by contaminated water sources, especially in refugee camps, are examples of epidemic cholera (24,25). Incidence rates and fatality rates in these epidemics are generally high because the population has little immunity and facilities for case management are not developed.

Certain factors have been identified that increase the risk of cholera infection and, in those who become infected, increase the disease's severity. Because vibrios are acid sensitive, hypochlorhydria, antacids, and gastric resection increase the risk for developing cholera (26–29). For reasons that are not understood, persons with blood group O are at higher risk for El Tor cholera (but not classic cholera) than persons with other blood groups (30,31). Breast-feeding has a strong protective effect, and cholera is rare in infants who are nursing. Although nursing infants have less exposure to pathogens, the breast milk itself is protective (32).

PATHOGENESIS

Cholera occurs when the bacterium is ingested in sufficient numbers to pass through the gastric acid barrier and enter the small intestine, where they colonize the upper small intestine. Colonization is facilitated by colonization pili, the best known being the toxin-coregulated pilus (33,34) and mannose-sensitive hemagglutinin pilus (35,36). An electron micrograph of *V. cholerae* is shown in Fig. 73.1.

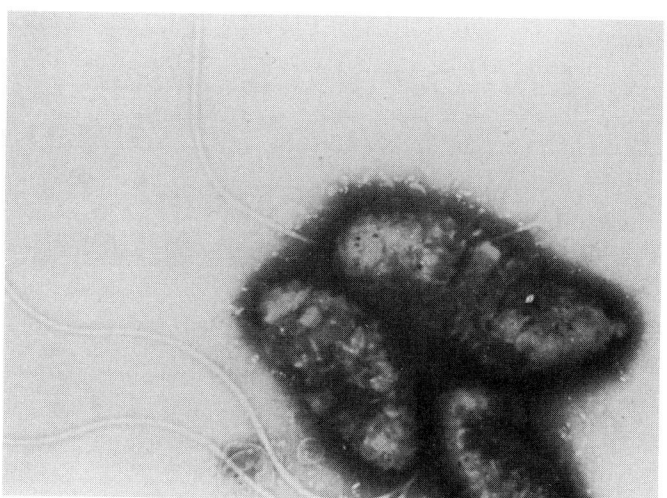

Figure 73.1. Electron photomicrograph of *Vibrio cholerae*.

When they have colonized the intestine, the bacteria secrete cholera toxin, a protein (molecular weight 84,000) with a central active (A) subunit surrounded by five binding (B) subunits. The B subunit attaches irreversibly to its mucosal cell receptor, GM1 ganglioside, which makes up part of all mammalian cell membranes. The A subunit is injected into the cell, and in a process involving stimulation of adenylate cyclase, it leads to the secretion of chloride and water (37–39). The rate of fluid secretion overwhelms the reabsorptive capacity of the small and large intestines, and the net secretions pass out as watery diarrhea. Although the functions of the mucosal cells are disturbed by the biochemical changes, the mucosa is not inflamed and there is no cytotoxic effect. Cholera toxin is similar in structure and function to a toxin of *Escherichia coli* called heat-labile toxin, and antibodies to cholera toxin also neutralize heat-labile toxin.

The volume and biochemical characteristics of the diarrhea fluid are important to the pathogenesis of cholera and its complications, because all of the signs and symptoms of cholera are explained by the loss of this fluid. The diarrhea fluid is an isotonic filtrate of serum that is modified only by exchange mechanisms that can take place before the fluid is excreted; in severe cases the transit time is so short that there is little time for exchange of electrolytes. Thus, the cholera stool contains a high concentration of sodium and bicarbonate and a low concentration of potassium, similar to serum (40). Because the mucosa is not inflamed, the stool contains little protein. Thus, the effect of the toxin is to induce the rapid loss of an isotonic, alkaline fluid, and because the loss occurs rapidly, the fluid comes from the circulating and extracellular spaces. This results in dehydration, hypovolemia, hemoconcentration, potassium deficiency, and metabolic acidosis. Models of the pathogenesis of cholera and the cholera toxin molecule are shown in Figs. 73.2 and 73.3.

CLINICAL MANIFESTATIONS

The spectrum of severity in cholera varies tremendously. Some individuals infected with this bacterium may experience no symptoms and some have mild diarrhea, whereas others develop severe, dehydrating watery diarrhea and excrete large volumes of nonbloody rice-water stool (Fig. 73.4; see also Color Fig. 73.4). The latter syndrome, often called cholera gravis, is a life-threatening condition in which perfectly healthy persons can become moribund and die within a few hours (24). These severely affected patients generally have associated symptoms of nausea, vomiting, and muscle cramps and signs of shock. Volumes of stools may exceed 1 L per hour in adults or more

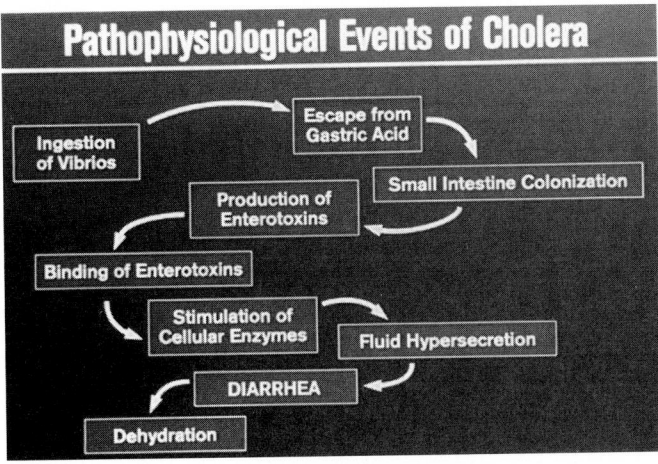

Figure 73.2. Model of the pathogenesis of cholera.

than 10 mL/kg per hour in children. As the fluid loss continues, dehydration progresses, the radial pulse becomes weak, the blood pressure drops to undetectable levels, the mental status becomes depressed, and coma ensues. Gasping hyperventilation frequently occurs because of metabolic acidosis. If cholera gravis is left untreated, at least 50% of patients with it die, yet almost all of these patients survive if given effective rehydration therapy.

DIAGNOSIS

Cholera should be suspected in persons with severe watery diarrhea, especially if they live in a cholera-endemic area, have just returned from a cholera-endemic area, or have eaten high-risk foods during the warm months. Except for travelers returning from cholera-endemic areas and a few exceptional cases resulting from imported contaminated foods, all U.S. cases occur in the summer (usually August) after consumption of shellfish from the Gulf of Mexico. In the United States, fecal specimens from all suspected cases should be cultured for vibrios, generally using thiosulfate citrate bile salts sucrose (TCBS) agar. Positive isolates should be reported immediately to the state health department, and the isolate should be sent for confirmation.

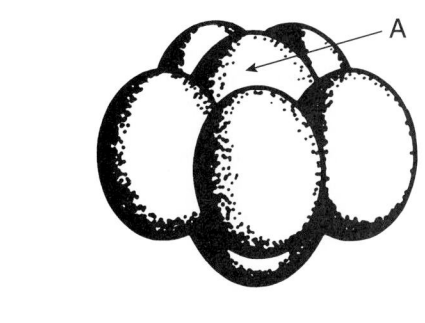

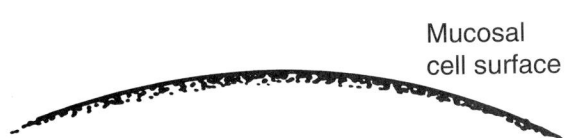

Figure 73.3. Model of cholera toxin showing the five binding subunits surrounding a single active (*A*) subunit.

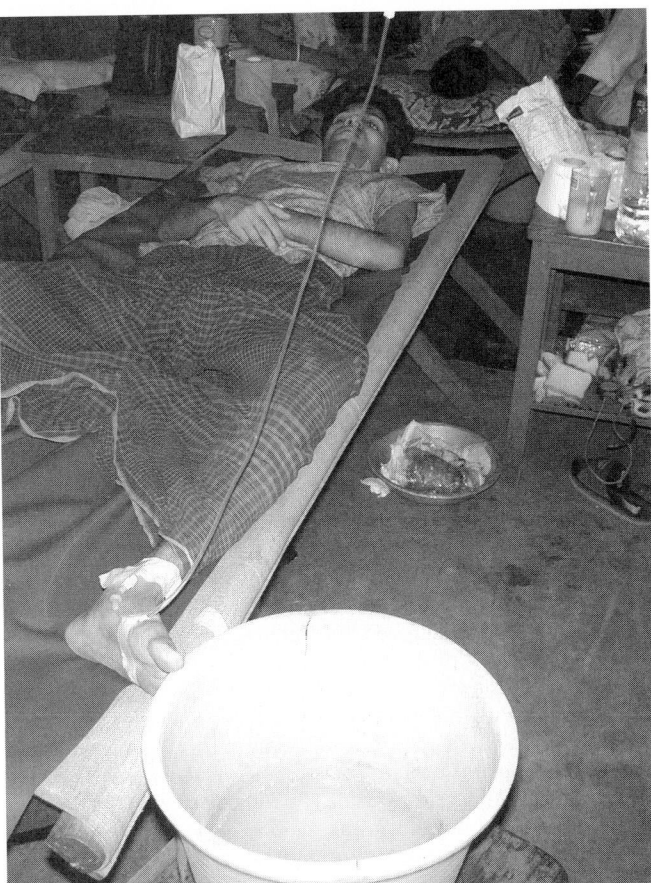

Figure 73.4. (See also Color Fig. 73.4.) Patient excreting large volumes of nonbloody rice-water stool.

In cholera-endemic areas, the diagnosis of new cases in the region should be confirmed with stool cultures, and a sample surveillance system is advisable to confirm a proportion of cases. During epidemics, most patients who have cholera symptoms do in fact have cholera, and culture confirmation of every case is not necessary. Cultures from a systematic sample of cases are useful for monitoring antibiotic sensitivity patterns, which can change during an epidemic season.

Patients with cholera develop a serologic response. If confirmation of the diagnosis is needed, acute serum and convalescent serum samples show a fourfold increase in vibriocidal antibodies (41).

TREATMENT

Treatment of cholera consists of rehydration therapy and antibiotics. Of these, rehydration is by far the more important because even severely affected patients survive without antibiotics but not without rehydration. To rehydrate appropriately, the hydration status of the patient is first assessed and a determination of the degree of dehydration is made. The stage of dehydration is generally categorized as not dehydrated, some dehydration, or severely dehydrated. For severely dehydrated patients, intravenous fluids with Ringer's lactate (or another suitable polyelectrolyte solution) are given to rapidly (e.g., in 2–4 hours) correct the fluid deficit. This requires a large-bore needle and may require more than one infusion at a time. Severely dehydrated patients are assumed to have lost 10% of their body weight, and this volume needs to be replaced. Thus, a 50-kg patient needs 5 L of Ringer's lactate. Moderately dehydrated patients can generally be rehydrated with oral rehydration solution (ORS) and

TABLE 73.1. Assessment of the Diarrhea Patient for Dehydration

	No dehydration	Some dehydration (two or more of these signs, including one in bold)	Severe dehydration[a] (two or more of these signs, including one in bold)
General appearance	Well, alert	**Restless, irritable**	**Lethargic or unconscious; floppy**
Eyes	Normal	Sunken	Very sunken and dry
Tears	Present	Absent	Absent
Mouth and tongue	Moist	Dry	Very dry
Thirst	Drinks normally, not thirsty	**Thirsty, drinks eagerly**	**Drinks poorly or not able to drink**
Skin pinch	Goes back quickly	**Goes back slowly**	**Goes back very slowly**

[a]In adults and in children over 5 years of age, other signs of severe dehydration are **absent radial pulse** and **low blood pressure**. The skin pinch may be less useful in patients with marasmus (severe wasting) or kwashiorkor (severe malnutrition with edema), or obese patients. Tears are a relevant sign only for infants and young children.

are assumed to have lost 7.5% of their body weight. Those without signs of dehydration are not critically ill, but signs of dehydration do not appear until more than 5% of the body weight has been lost. Thus, those who have watery stools and are suspected of having cholera should be rehydrated with ORS, with volumes to approximate 5% of the body weight.

Clinical criteria are used to determine the state of dehydration and are shown in Table 73.1, but laboratory tests can be used to confirm the patient's condition. The laboratory changes include an elevated plasma protein level and elevated hematocrit (resulting from hemoconcentration) and a decreased serum bicarbonate value (resulting from the metabolic acidosis). The potassium concentration generally remains in the normal range, but it decreases as acidosis is corrected during rehydration unless potassium is included in the rehydration fluids.

While the patient is being rehydrated, continuing stool losses are noted, and equivalent volumes of ORS are provided to replace these ongoing losses. If possible, a cholera cot (a camping cot with a hole cut beneath the buttock area to allow stool to pass into a bucket underneath) is used to facilitate the measuring of these ongoing losses. The patient's hydration status must be monitored especially carefully during the critical first 24 hours, and occasional passing of urine is a helpful sign of hydration.

ORS is generally prepared from packets, although some workers prepare it from locally available ingredients. The recommended concentration of the sodium and glucose in the standard formula of World Health Organization (WHO) ORS has recently been lowered to 75 mmoles of each, and this new formula results in a solution that has a lower osmolarity than previously. Although the new solution is not superior to the previous formula for cholera (with a sodium concentration of 90 mmoles), it does appear superior for noncholera diarrhea and is safe for cholera patients (42). Thus, both solutions (e.g., with sodium of either 75 or 90 mEq) are acceptable for cholera.

ORS that contains 40 to 80 g of rice in place of 20 g of glucose per liter is superior for cholera patients, in that the purging rate and duration of diarrhea are lessened by about 30% to 40% (43). Commercial preparations of rice ORS are now available, and its use has been validated in cholera (44). Rehydration solutions used to treat cholera patients are shown in Table 73.2.

Oral antibiotics are given to kill the *Vibrio* and thus to decrease the duration of the illness (45–47). They should be given as early in the illness as possible, although a few hours' delay may be needed to rehydrate and to allow vomiting to cease. A single dose of doxycycline, 300 mg, is effective against sensitive strains. Resistant strains also frequently cause epidemics, and alternative antibiotics (e.g., ciprofloxacin as a 1-g single dose) may be used (48–52). Antibiotics used to treat cholera patients are shown in Table 73.3.

TABLE 73.2. Composition of Cholera Stools and the Electrolyte Rehydration Solutions Used to Replace Stool Losses

Fluid	Na+ (mM)	Cl− (mM)	K+ (mM)	HCO3 (mM)	Carbohydrate (g/L)	Osmolality (mM)
Cholera stool						
Adults	130	100	20	44		
Children	100	90	33	30		
Oral rehydration						
Glucose ORS (WHO)	75	65	20	10[a]	13.5[b]	245
Rice ORS	75	65	20	10[a]	30 to 50[c]	About 180
Intravenous fluids						
Lactated Ringer's	130	109	4	28[d]		271
Dhaka solution	133	154	13	48[e]		292
Normal saline	154	154	0	0		308

[a]Base is given as trisodium citrate having 30 mEq (10 mM).
[b]Glucose (13.5 g) containing 75 mM.
[c]30 to 50 g of rice contains about 30 mM depending on degree of hydrolysis.
[d]Base in Ringer's is lactate.
[e]Base in Dhaka solution is acetate.

TABLE 73.3. Antimicrobial Agents Used in the Treatment of Cholera

Antibiotic	Adult dose	Pediatric dose
Doxycycline	300 mg single dose[a] or 100 mg b.i.d. for 3 days	
Tetracycline	500 mg q.i.d. for 3 days	12.5 mg/kg q.i.d. for 3 days[b]
Furazolidone	100 mg q.i.d. for 3 days[c]	1.25 mg/kg q.i.d. for 3 days
TMP-SMX	TMP at 160 mg + SMX at 800 mg b.i.d. for 3 days	TMP at 5 mg/kg + SMX at 25 mg/kg b.i.d. for 3 days[d]
Ciprofloxacin[e]	250 mg b.i.d. for 3 days	Not approved for children

[a]The drug of choice for most situations because a single dose can be used.
[b]Be aware of policies against using tetracycline for children in whom teeth staining can occur.
[c]Furazolidone is the drug of choice for pregnant women.
[d]TMP-SMX is the preferred drug for children.
[e]Reserve for strains resistant to all other antibiotics.
b.i.d., twice daily; q.i.d., four times daily; TMP-SMX, trimethoprim-sulfamethoxazole.

COMPLICATIONS

Oral Rehydration Solution Failure

After initial rehydration, a few patients with severe cholera again become dehydrated even while being given ORS. This is generally due to severe vomiting and severe purging in excess of oral intake. For example, if the purging rate exceeds 10 mL/kg per hour, it is difficult to administer sufficient ORS to maintain hydration (53). Likewise, vomiting in some patients prevents efficient oral replacement. In these cases, the patients should be rehydrated again with intravenous fluids.

Renal Failure

Acute tubular necrosis can occur if rehydration is insufficient (e.g., if fluid replacement prevents death but does not correct the shock). These patients need to be rehydrated to reestablish the circulating volume, but their potassium levels need to be monitored to avoid hyperkalemia. Occasionally, dialysis may be needed, but usually the renal failure is reversible.

Cholera Sicca

Signs of dehydration and shock can occur in the absence of severe purging when fluid collects in the intestine without being expelled. The abdominal swelling and shock can be mistaken for an acute surgical emergency. Treatment is the same as with other severe cases: replacement of fluids.

Hypokalemia

Hypokalemia may occur if potassium is not adequately replaced. Symptoms include abdominal distention and ileus, urinary retention, and cardiac arrhythmias. Generally, potassium concentrations are normal or high prior to the start of treatment, but they decrease quickly as the acidosis is corrected. Thus, potassium replacement is a standard part of the rehydration solutions.

Pulmonary Edema

This may result from overhydration with intravenous fluids. It is more likely if saline rather than Ringer's lactate is used, because the acidosis is not corrected.

Hypoglycemia

Hypoglycemia, manifested by seizures, is a rare complication in children with cholera. If seizures should occur, a bolus of intravenous glucose should be given while the blood glucose level is being measured. Most cholera patients experience decreasing levels of blood glucose during treatment, but only rarely do they develop profound hypoglycemia.

Abortion and Premature Delivery

Pregnant women with cholera frequently abort or deliver prematurely, apparently because of placental circulatory insufficiency (54). Rapid rehydration decreases the likelihood of this complication. Centers that see many cases of cholera need to make provisions for delivering premature infants.

Fever and Chills

These are not a part of the cholera syndrome, but if they occur, pyrogens in the intravenous fluid or an intravenous line infection is the most likely cause. Chills without fever can occur from rapid infusion of cool intravenous fluids.

PREVENTION

Improvements in water quality and sanitation are the long-term strategies for prevention. Because these goals cannot be realized quickly, persons traveling in cholera areas should use boiled or bottled water and avoid high-risk foods and drinks (e.g., raw seafood, foods from street vendors, and drinks with ice).

Oral vaccines are becoming available in Europe and may be available soon in other parts of the world, and they will be recommended for persons traveling to cholera-endemic areas. Two types of vaccines have been developed: a killed oral vaccine (23,55) and a live attenuated vaccine (56). The killed vaccine provides about 60% protection for 3 years and is recommended in high-risk situations like refugee camps. Its use for routine use in endemic areas is not yet established. The live vaccine was very effective in North American volunteers and therefore is likely to protect travelers, but it failed to induce significant protection in an endemic area (57), so additional data are needed from such endemic areas before its use as a public health tool is known. The currently available killed injectable vaccine is not recommended because of local inflammatory reactions, short duration of protection (6 months), and low level of protection (50%) (58).

Prophylactic antibiotics are sometimes used during cholera outbreaks when the strain is tetracycline sensitive. If used, a single dose of doxycycline, 300 mg, can be given to members of the immediate household but not to others in the neighborhood or community. Wide-scale use of prophylactic antibiotics quickly leads to the development of resistant strains (59,60).

Non-O1 *Vibrio cholerae*

Strains of *V. cholerae* that do not agglutinate with antiserum O1 or O139 are termed non-O1 *V. cholerae*. They may still induce severe diarrhea, even though they do not cause epidemics, and thus they do not present the same public health risk as serotypes O1 and O139.

EPIDEMIOLOGY

The ecologic niche of the non-O1 *V. cholerae* is similar to that of cholera. These strains are associated with contaminated water or with shellfish, especially raw oysters and crabs. However, non-O1 *V. cholerae* strains are more widely distributed than O1 *V. cholerae* and are frequently isolated in the estuaries and bays of the United States, as well as in developing countries (61–63). In developing countries, these organisms are usually not distinguished from the many bacterial pathogens causing diarrhea; hence, less is known about their transmission. In the United States or Mexico, however, patients with non-O1 *V. cholerae* infection have generally eaten raw or undercooked shellfish. In temperate climates, nearly all cases occur during the summer months.

PATHOGENESIS

Many of the non-O1 *V. cholerae* strains have been found to produce an enterotoxin nearly identical to cholera toxin, and a few other strains produce a heat-stable toxin closely related to the heat-stable enterotoxin of *E. coli* (64,65). However, the presence of these toxins has not altogether explained the mechanism of illness, because some strains have been associated with diarrhea yet produced neither of these two toxins (66). Also, some episodes have been associated with significant fevers, a feature not seen in O1 cholera. Thus, multiple virulence factors are likely responsible for illnesses.

Non-O1 *V. cholerae* strains occasionally cause wound infection and sepsis, especially in patients with predisposing illnesses, such as liver cirrhosis or immunosuppression (67).

CLINICAL MANIFESTATIONS

Diarrhea is the most common presentation for non-O1 *V. cholerae* infections, and these illnesses cannot be distinguished clinically from watery diarrhea caused by other organisms. Although individual patients can have a severe cholera-like illness with severe dehydration, diarrhea caused by non-O1 *V. cholerae* tends to be less severe than that in cholera. Fever and severe abdominal cramps may be seen, and occasionally blood is present in the stool. The illness is self-limited, with diarrhea lasting a few days. Wound infections and sepsis present in a manner similar to those seen with *V. vulnificus*.

DIAGNOSIS

Persons with acute diarrhea should have a stool culture for vibrios with TCBS medium, especially if there is a recent history of eating shellfish. Suspected colonies should be confirmed, and if there is doubt about their identity they should be referred to the state health department.

TREATMENT

Treatment for diarrhea caused by non-O1 *V. cholerae* is the same as the treatment in cholera, following principles of rehydration therapy according to the degree of dehydration using intravenous and/or oral rehydration fluids. The benefit of antibiotics has not been shown, but in severe cholera-like cases, doxycycline, a 300-mg single dose, or ciprofloxacin, 250 to 500 mg twice a day for 3 days, can be used. (Note: There have been no clinical trials for non-O1 *V. cholerae* infections; hence, these doses are based on treatment of O1 *V. cholerae*.) Those with milder cases need no antibiotics. Systemic infections require antibiotics according to sensitivity patterns. Tetracycline is generally used, but others may also be effective, according to sensitivity patterns.

PREVENTION

There are no vaccines for non-O1 *V. cholerae* and the illness is sufficiently rare that one is not needed. Persons traveling to areas where there is a risk of ingesting vibrios should use boiled or bottled water and should avoid high-risk seafood, especially during the warmer months. Persons with predisposing factors (liver cirrhosis or immunosuppression) should especially avoid high-risk foods.

Vibrio mimicus

Diarrhea caused by *V. mimicus* is similar to that caused by *V. cholerae* except that it does not occur in epidemics. The pathogenesis involving the cholera toxin is the same, although additional toxins may also play a role (68,69). Like other vibrios, *V. mimicus* is associated with seafood consumption. Treatment according to the degree of dehydration is the same as that for cholera (70,71). Rarely, *V. mimicus* may cause systemic infections (72,73).

Vibrio parahaemolyticus

V. parahaemolyticus is a halophilic vibrio that generally causes diarrhea but may rarely cause wound and systemic infections as well (74,75). Like the other vibrios, *V. parahaemolyticus* is associated with saltwater and seafood, and many of the U.S. cases result from eating raw oysters. Cases are reported from all continents, but this infection is especially common in Japan, where it accounts for a majority of bacterial gastroenteritis cases (76). The popularity of raw fish in Japan probably accounts for the high number of cases there.

Most cases of diarrhea associated with *V. parahaemolyticus* cannot be distinguished from watery diarrhea caused by other agents, but in some cases the stool becomes bloody and patients may have fever. The stool is described as a "washed meat" stool that is watery but bloody (Fig. 73.5; see also Color Fig. 73.5). Virulence of *V. parahaemolyticus* is thought to be related to a hemolysin that is found in most clinical isolates and can be detected using Wagatsuma agar or molecular methods. Treatment follows the same guidelines for rehydration as described for cholera. Antibiotics have not been shown to be helpful.

Although *V. parahaemolyticus* usually infects persons with normal immune systems, studies have shown increased risk for persons immunosuppressed because of human immunodeficiency virus infection or immunosuppressive drugs. Persons with these conditions should avoid raw seafood, especially during the warmer months.

Recently, a strain of *Vibrio parahaemolyticus* emerged as a pandemic strain. Initially the marker for this pandemic strain was the serotype O3 (77–80). Now genetic markers for this strain have been identified, and it appears that the virulence properties are not limited to the O3 serotype. This strain appears to have spread from South Asia to other parts of Asia and is now found in North America as well.

Vibrio fluvialis

V. fluvialis (formerly called group EF-6 and group F *Vibrio*) is closely related biochemically to *Aeromonas*. It is ubiquitous in brackish waters and, like other vibrios, can infect persons by way of seafood. Patients infected with *V. fluvialis* have had diarrhea symptoms often with vomiting, abdominal pain, and fever. The fluid loss can lead to severe dehydration, similar to that in cholera. Treatment is similar to that for cholera with regard to

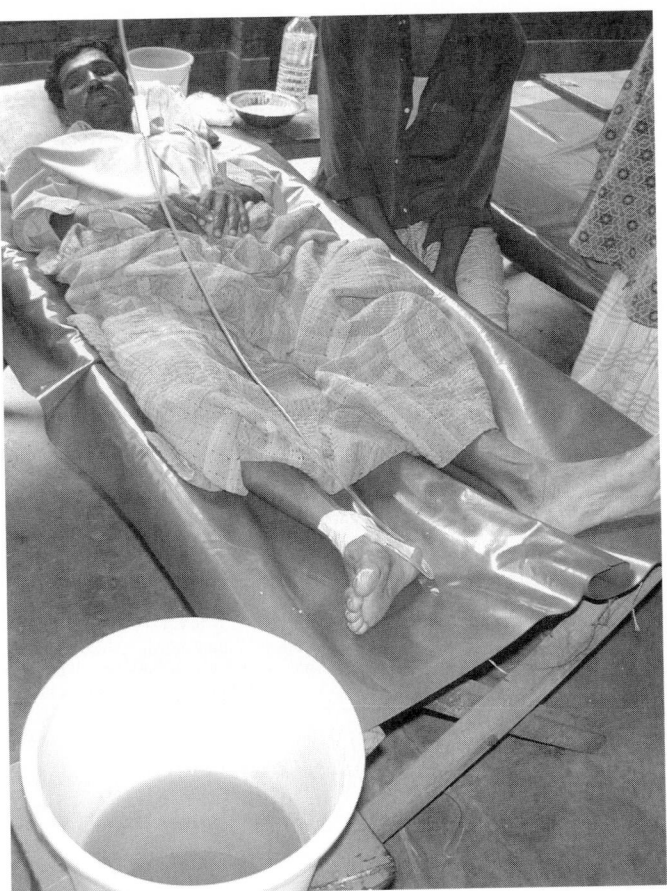

Figure 73.5. (See also Color Fig. 73.5.) Patient excreting "washed meat" stool that is watery but bloody.

fluid replacement, depending on the degree of dehydration. A major outbreak of *V. fluvialis* infection occurred in Bangladesh in 1977, but similar large-scale outbreaks have not been reported since then (81).

Vibrio furnissii

As with other vibrios, transmission of *V. furnissii* is associated with seafood and has been linked to diarrhea (82–84). Rehydration therapy for this illness uses the strategy described for cholera.

Vibrio hollisae

V. hollisae has been associated with diarrhea caused by eating seafood. Few cases have been reported, but the bacterium grows poorly on TCBS agar; hence, little is known of its true incidence. Rehydration, using guidelines as for cholera, is needed for patients with severe dehydration (85–88). It also may rarely cause septicemia in a manner similar to *V. vulnificus.*

Vibrios Generally Associated with Wound and Systemic Infections

All of the vibrios described above may cause wound or systemic infections, but their predominant syndrome is diarrhea. The ones that are described in the section below rarely cause diarrhea, and are more often found as pathogens causing severe wound infections and septicemia. The systemic infections frequently occur in

patients with predisposing risk factors, including chronic liver disease, iron overload syndromes, immunosuppression (e.g., transplant patients or HIV-AIDS), and, less commonly, diabetes. The species include *V. vulnificus, V. alginolyticus, V. damsela,* and possibly *V. cincinnatiensis.*

Vibrio vulnificus

V. vulnificus is primarily an extraintestinal pathogen, causing severe illness characterized by sepsis and wound infections, especially in persons with certain underlying diseases, including cirrhosis (related to alcohol, hepatitis B, hepatitis C, or other causes), hemochromatosis (or other conditions with an excess of iron), thalassemia, acquired immunodeficiency syndrome, and diabetes (75,89–92). Although this is a rare infection for normal hosts in the United States, it is a major risk for persons with these conditions who become exposed, and because of its high case-fatality rate, it is the leading cause of death among the *Vibrio*-caused illnesses in the United States and in many other countries. Risk of exposure is highly related to seawater temperature, because the organism prospers in warmer waters (more than 15°C). Oysters are an especially high-risk food during warm months because the bacteria can multiply in mollusks. They also are found in high concentrations in intestines of certain fishes; hence, cleaning fish can also be risky.

Vibrio sepsis, which generally occurs within a day or two after eating undercooked seafood, is a nonspecific acute fever that progresses rapidly to hypotension and septic shock. Case-fatality rates for this syndrome have exceeded 50% (75), and patients require immediate supportive care and antibiotics, especially tetracycline or ciprofloxacin.

Wound infections occur after trauma with contamination by seawater, especially during the warmer months. Typical injuries have been cuts sustained while cleaning fish or shelling crabs. During the next 1 to 2 days, the wound becomes inflamed and may be associated with bullous skin lesions. The case-fatality rate for this infection is also substantial, about 25%, and aggressive treatment is needed with antibiotics and possibly wound débridement (92,93).

Rarely *V. vulnificus* can infect other organs, causing peritonitis, corneal ulcer, epiglottitis, meningitis, endometritis, and osteomyelitis.

Virulence of *V. vulnificus* is thought to be due to a bacterial capsular polysaccharide that makes the organism resistant to serum. A high proportion of the isolates from infections produce this capsule, but most environmental isolates do not; thus, the presence of the capsule appears to be a marker of pathogenicity (94–97). This species is also able to utilize iron from the host tissue and from heme to promote growth and production of toxins (98–100). Several toxins and extracellular enzymes have been identified that contribute to its pathogenicity (101–103).

Because case-fatality rates are so high, persons at high risk must be warned of the dangers of exposure to undercooked seafood and of wounds sustained while in saltwater, especially during summer months.

Vibrio alginolyticus

V. alginolyticus is rarely isolated from humans but, like other vibrios, is associated with marine environments. Most infections have been associated with wounds sustained while in saltwater, and some of these infections have been severe. It has also been associated with ear infections. As with other *Vibrio* wound infections, immunocompromised persons are at higher risk.

Other Vibrios

V. metschnikovii, a common bacterium in marine environments, is an extremely rare pathogen in people. *V. damsela*, previously known as EF-5, a pathogen for damselfish, has infected wounds of persons exposed to seawater and caused severe necrotizing infections (104,105). The species may be confused with *Aeromonas* in the laboratory, so additional studies may be needed to differentiate these two (106). *V. cincinnatiensis* was reported to cause meningitis and sepsis in a case report of a patient with no marine exposure (107).

AEROMONAS SPECIES

Aeromonas species are gram-negative, oxidase-positive, motile rods that are part of the normal flora of surface waters. On the basis of biochemical characteristics, three species have been designated: *A. hydrophila*, *A. sobria*, and *A. caviae*. Initially it was thought that speciation would help identify clinically relevant features, but this has not yet become clear. They are considered to be causes of diarrhea by some, but their etiologic role in diarrhea is not yet clear because case-control studies have found similar rates of isolation in cases and control subjects, depending on the method of isolation (108), although one did find an association with diarrhea (109). In most cases, their isolation is probably a marker for surface water consumption because the species is a common naturally occurring water bacteria. If *Aeromonas* species are enteropathogens, probably only some strains are pathogens. Markers of pathogenicity have been proposed, such as exotoxin production, but the correlation of these with virulence is not yet clear. Recently it was suggested that a combination of virulence factors are needed to cause diarrhea, but that a single factor by itself may not render the organism pathogenic (110). Syndromes of diarrhea that have been seen in patients from whom *Aeromonas* species were isolated have included acute watery diarrhea, bloody diarrhea, and persistent diarrhea; hence, a typical clinical syndrome has not emerged (111). Some patients with *Aeromonas*-associated diarrhea have responded to trimethoprim-sulfamethoxazole or tetracycline, but *Aeromonas* is generally resistant to ampicillin.

Two unique features of *Aeromonas* species are their ability to multiply in cold conditions and relative resistance to chlorine. Thus, refrigerated foods are more likely to become contaminated, and water from municipal systems with lower levels of chlorine is more likely to contain *Aeromonas* species.

Although their etiologic role in diarrhea remains undefined, they are the occasional causes of systemic infection, including wound infection, bacteremia, and meningitis.

PLESIOMONAS SHIGELLOIDES

P. shigelloides is a motile gram-negative, oxidase-positive rod that also lives in surface waters. It is also considered a potential enteropathogen, but its true relationship to diarrhea is not clear. A few cases of diarrhea have been ascribed to this agent, but clinical studies have shown little difference between the rates of isolation in case and control subjects (109), and volunteers who were challenged with *P. shigelloides* have not developed illness (112), nor have travelers with this infection developed serologic responses. Cases that have been described were related to oysters or other seafood or were related to travel to developing countries (113). Tests for specific virulence factors, such as invasiveness or enterotoxins, have generally been negative.

Among the 43 serogroups of *P. shigelloides*, the most common serotype, type 17, has a cell wall identical to that of *Shigella sonnei*. It is speculated that repeated exposure to this serotype by drinking surface water may stimulate a local intestinal immune response and protect people in developing countries from infection with *S. sonnei* (114).

P. shigelloides is a rare cause of systemic infection and sepsis, usually in immunocompromised hosts.

REFERENCES

1. Blake PA, Allegra DT, Snyder JD, et al. Cholera—a possible endemic focus in the United States. *N Engl J Med* 1980;302(6):305–309.
2. Blake PA. Epidemiology of cholera in the Americas. *Gastroenterol Clin North Am* 1993;22(3):639–660.
3. Glass RI, Claeson M, Blake PA, et al. Cholera in Africa: lessons on transmission and control for Latin America. *Lancet* 1991;338(8770):791–795.
4. Cholera Working Group. Large epidemic of cholera-like disease in Bangladesh caused by Vibrio cholerae O139 synonym Bengal. *Lancet* 1993;342(8868):387–390.
5. Bodhidatta L, Echeverria P, Hoge CW, et al. Vibrio cholerae O139 in Thailand in 1994. *Epidemiol Infect* 1995;114(1):71–73.
6. Siddique AK, Akram K, Zaman K, et al. Vibrio cholerae O139: how great is the threat of a pandemic? *Trop Med Int Health* 1996;1(3):393–398.
7. Latta T. Letter from Dr. Latta to the Secretary of the Central Board of Health, London, affording a view of the rationale and results of his practice in the treatment of cholera by aqueous and saline solutions. *Lancet* 1831;2:274–277.
8. O'Shaughnessy WB. Proposal of a new method of treating blue epidemic cholera by the injection of highly oxygenated salts into the venous system. *Lancet* 1831(1):366–371.
9. Rogers LE. *Bowel diseases in the tropics*. London: Froude, Hodder, & Stoughton, 1921.
10. Carpenter CCJ, Mondal A, Sack RB, et al. Clinical studies in Asiatic cholera. *Bull Johns Hopkins Hospital* 1966;118:174–196.
11. Cash RA, Toha KMM, Nalin DR. Acetate in the correction of acidosis secondary to diarrhoea. *Lancet* 1969;2:302–303.
12. Pierce NF, Banwell JG, Mitra RC, et al. Oral maintenance of water-electrolyte and acid-base balance in cholera: a preliminary report. *Ind J Med Res* 1968;56(5):640–645.
13. Hirschhorn N, Kinzie JL, Sachar DB, et al. Decrease in net stool output in cholera during intestinal perfusion with glucose-containing solutions. *N Engl J Med* 1968;279:176–181.
14. Nalin DR, Cash RA, Islam R, et al. Oral maintenance therapy for cholera in adults. *Lancet* 1968;2(7564):370–373.
15. Snow J. *Cholera and the water supply in the south districts of London in 1854*. London: T. Richards, 1856.
16. St Louis ME, Porter JD, Helal A, et al. Epidemic cholera in West Africa: the role of food handling and high-risk foods. *Am J Epidemiol* 1990;131(4):719–728.
17. Khan MU, Shahidullah M. Role of water and sanitation in the incidence of cholera in refugee camps. *Trans R Soc Trop Med Hyg* 1982;76(3):373–377.
18. Weber JT, Levine WC, Hopkins DP, et al. Cholera in the United States, 1965–1991. Risks at home and abroad. *Arch Intern Med* 1994;154(5):551–556.
19. Taylor JL, Tuttle J, Pramukul T, et al. An outbreak of cholera in Maryland associated with imported commercial frozen fresh coconut milk. *J Infect Dis* 1993;167(6):1330–1335.
20. Institute of Medicine. *New vaccine development, establishing priorities*. Vol. II. Diseases of importance in developing countries. Washington, DC: Institute of Medicine, 1986.
21. Glass RI, Becker S, Huq MI, et al. Endemic cholera in rural Bangladesh, 1966–1980. *Am J Epidemiol* 1982;116(6):959–970.
22. Siddique AK, Zaman K, Baqui AH, et al. Cholera epidemics in Bangladesh: 1985–1991. *J Diarrhoeal Dis Res* 1992;10(2):79–86.
23. Clemens JD, Sack DA, Harris JR, et al. Field trial of oral cholera vaccines in Bangladesh: results from three-year follow-up. *Lancet* 1990;335(8684):270–273.
24. Siddique AK, Salam A, Islam MS, et al. Why treatment centres failed to prevent cholera deaths among Rwandan refugees in Goma, Zaire. *Lancet* 1995;345(8946):359–361.
25. Goma Epidemiology Group. Public health impact of Rwandan refugee crisis: what happened in Goma, Zaire, in July, 1994? *Lancet* 1995;345(8946):339–344.
26. van Loon FP, Clemens JD, Shahrier M, et al. Low gastric acid as a risk factor for cholera transmission: application of a new non-invasive gastric acid field test. *J Clin Epidemiol* 1990;43(12):1361–1367.
27. Nalin DR, Levine RJ, Levine MM, et al. Cholera, non-vibrio cholera, and stomach acid. *Lancet* 1978;2(8095):856–859.
28. Cash RA, Alam J, Toaha KM. Gastric acid secretion in cholera patients. *Lancet* 1970;2(7684):1192.
29. Sack GH Jr, Pierce NF, Hennessey KN, et al. Gastric acidity in cholera and noncholera diarrhoea. *Bull World Health Organ* 1972;47(1):31–36.

30. Barua D, Paguio AS. ABO blood groups and cholera. *Ann Hum Biol* 1977;4(5):489–492.

31. Clemens JD, Sack DA, Harris JR, et al. ABO blood groups and cholera: new observations on specificity of risk and modification of vaccine efficacy. *J Infect Dis* 1989;159(4):770–773.

32. Glass RI, Svennerholm AM, Stoll BJ, et al. Protection against cholera in breast-fed children by antibodies in breast milk. *N Engl J Med* 1983;308(23):1389–1392.

33. Taylor RK, Miller VL, Furlong DB, et al. Identification of a pilus colonization factor that is coordinately regulated with cholera toxin. *Ann Sclavo Collana Monogr* 1986;3(1-2):51–61.

34. Herrington DA, Hall RH, Losonsky G, et al. Toxin, toxin-coregulated pili, and the toxR regulon are essential for *Vibrio cholerae* pathogenesis in humans. *J Exp Med* 1988;168(4):1487–1492.

35. Osek J, Svennerholm AM, Holmgren J. Protection against *Vibrio cholerae* El Tor infection by specific antibodies against mannose-binding hemagglutinin pili. *Infect Immun* 1992;60(11):4961–4964.

36. Osek J, Jonson G, Svennerholm AM, et al. Role of antibodies against biotype-specific *Vibrio cholerae* pili in protection against experimental classical and El Tor cholera. *Infect Immun* 1994;62(7):2901–2907.

37. Field M. Modes of action of enterotoxins from *Vibrio cholerae* and *Escherichia coli. Rev Infect Dis* 1979;1(6):918–926.

38. Holmgren J. Actions of cholera toxin and the prevention and treatment of cholera. *Nature* 1981;292(5822):413–417.

39. Holmgren J, Lonnroth I, Mansson J, et al. Interaction of cholera toxin and membrane GM1 ganglioside of small intestine. *Proc Natl Acad Sci USA* 1975;72(7):2520–2524.

40. Molla AM, Rahman M, Sarker SA, et al. Stool electrolyte content and purging rates in diarrhea caused by rotavirus, enterotoxigenic *E. coli,* and *V. cholerae* in children. *J Pediatr* 1981;98(5):835–838.

41. Benenson AS, Saad A, Mosley WH. Serological studies in cholera. 2. The vibriocidal antibody response of cholera patients determined by a microtechnique. *Bull WHO* 1968;38(2):277–285.

42. Alam NH, Majumder RN, Fuchs GJ. Efficacy and safety of oral rehydration solution with reduced osmolarity in adults with cholera: a randomised double-blind clinical trial. CHOICE study group. *Lancet* 1999;354(9175):296–299.

43. Gore SM, Fontaine O, Pierce NF. Efficacy of rice-based oral rehydration. *Lancet* 1996;348(9021):193–194.

44. Zaman K, Yunus M, Rahman A, et al. Efficacy of a packaged rice oral rehydration solution among children with cholera and cholera-like illness. *Acta Paediatr* 2001;90(5):505–510.

45. Alam AN, Alam NH, Ahmed T, et al. Randomised double blind trial of single dose doxycycline for treating cholera in adults. *BMJ* 1990;300(6740):1619–1621.

46. Sack DA, Islam S, Rabbani H, et al. Single-dose doxycycline for cholera. *Antimicrob Agents Chemother* 1978;14(3):462–464.

47. De S, Chaudhuri A, Dutta P, et al. Doxycycline in the treatment of cholera. *Bull WHO* 1976;54(2):177–179.

48. Khan WA, Bennish ML, Seas C, et al. Randomised controlled comparison of single-dose ciprofloxacin and doxycycline for cholera caused by *Vibrio cholerae* 01 or 0139. *Lancet* 1996;348(9023):296–300.

49. Pastore G, Rizzo G, Fera G, et al. Trimethoprim-sulphamethoxazole in the treatment of cholera. Comparison with tetracycline and chloramphenicol. *Chemotherapy* 1977;23(2):121–128.

50. Uylangco C, Santiago L, Pescante M, et al. Pivmecillinam, co-trimoxazole and oral mecillinam in gastroenteritis due to *Vibrio* spp. *J Antimicrob Chemother* 1984;13(2):171–175.

51. Khan WA, Begum M, Salam MA, et al. Comparative trial of five antimicrobial compounds in the treatment of cholera in adults. *Trans R Soc Trop Med Hyg* 1995;89(1):103–106.

52. Burans JP, Podgore J, Mansour MM, et al. Comparative trial of erythromycin and sulphatrimethoprim in the treatment of tetracycline-resistant *Vibrio cholerae* O1. *Trans R Soc Trop Med Hyg* 1989;83(6):836–838.

53. Sack DA, Huda S, Neogi PK, et al. Microtiter ganglioside enzyme-linked immunosorbent assay for *Vibrio* and *Escherichia coli* heat-labile enterotoxins and antitoxin. *J Clin Microbiol* 1980;11(1):35–40.

54. Ayangade O. The significance of cholera outbreak in the prognosis of pregnancy. *Int J Gynaecol Obstet* 1981;19(5):403–407.

55. Sanchez JL, Vasquez B, Begue RE, et al. Protective efficacy of oral whole-cell/recombinant-B-subunit cholera vaccine in Peruvian military recruits. *Lancet* 1994;344(8932):1273–1276.

56. Tacket CO, Cohen MB, Wasserman SS, et al. Randomized, double-blind, placebo-controlled, multicentered trial of the efficacy of a single dose of live oral cholera vaccine CVD 103-HgR in preventing cholera following challenge with *Vibrio cholerae* O1 El tor inaba three months after vaccination. *Infect Immun* 1999;67(12):6341–6345.

57. Richie EE, Punjabi NH, Sidharta YY, et al. Efficacy trial of single-dose live oral cholera vaccine CVD 103-HgR in North Jakarta, Indonesia, a cholera-endemic area. *Vaccine* 2000;18(22):2399–2410.

58. Mosley WH, Aziz KM, Rahman AS, et al. Field trials of monovalent Ogawa and Inaba cholera vaccines in rural Bangladesh—three years of observation. *Bull WHO* 1973;49(4):381–387.

59. Khan MU. Efficacy of short course antibiotic prophylaxis in controlling cholera in contacts during epidemic. *J Trop Med Hyg* 1982;85(1):27–29.

60. Sack RB. Prophylactic antibiotics? The individual versus the community. *N Engl J Med* 1979;300(19):1107–1108.

61. Morris JG Jr, Black RE. Cholera and other vibrioses in the United States. *N Engl J Med* 1985;312(6):343–350.

62. Finch MJ, Valdespino JL, Wells JG, et al. Non-O1 *Vibrio cholerae* infections in Cancun, Mexico. *Am J Trop Med Hyg* 1987;36(2):393–397.

63. Ko WC, Chuang YC, Huang GC, et al. Infections due to non-O1 *Vibrio cholerae* in southern Taiwan: predominance in cirrhotic patients. *Clin Infect Dis* 1998;27:774–780.

64. Yamamoto K, Takeda Y, Miwatani T, et al. Evidence that a non-O1 *Vibrio cholerae* produces enterotoxin that is similar but not identical to cholera enterotoxin. *Infect Immun* 1983;41(3):896–901.

65. Arita M, Honda T, Miwatani T, et al. Purification and characterization of a new heat-stable enterotoxin produced by *Vibrio cholerae* non-O1 serogroup Hakata. *Infect Immun* 1991;59(6):2186–2188.

66. Morris JG Jr, Picardi JL, Lieb S, et al. Isolation of nontoxigenic *Vibrio cholerae* O group 1 from a patient with severe gastrointestinal disease. *J Clin Microbiol* 1984;19(2):296–297.

67. Pitrak DL, Gindorf JD. Bacteremic cellulitis caused by non-serogroup O1 *Vibrio cholerae* acquired in a freshwater inland lake. *J Clin Microbiol* 1989;27(12):2874–2876.

68. Bi K, Miyoshi SI, Tomochika KI, et al. Detection of virulence associated genes in clinical strains of *Vibrio mimicus. Microbiol Immunol* 2001;45(8):613–616.

69. Shi L, Miyoshi S, Hiura M, et al. Detection of genes encoding cholera toxin (CT), zonula occludens toxin (ZOT), accessory cholera enterotoxin (ACE) and heat-stable enterotoxin (ST) in *Vibrio mimicus* clinical strains. *Microbiol Immunol* 1998;42(12):823–828.

70. Davis BR, Fanning GR, Madden JM, et al. Characterization of biochemically atypical *Vibrio cholerae* strains and designation of a new pathogenic species, *Vibrio mimicus. J Clin Microbiol* 1981;14(6):631–639.

71. Kaper JB, Nataro JP, Roberts NC, et al. Molecular epidemiology of non-O1 *Vibrio cholerae* and *Vibrio mimicus* in the U.S. Gulf Coast region. *J Clin Microbiol* 1986;23(3):652–654.

72. Albert MJ, Kabir I, Neogi PK, et al. *Vibrio mimicus* bacteraemia in a child. *J Diarrhoeal Dis Res* 1992;10(1):39–40.

73. Klontz KC, Cover DE, Hyman FN, et al. Fatal gastroenteritis due to *Vibrio fluvialis* and nonfatal bacteremia due to *Vibrio mimicus*: unusual *Vibrio* infections in two patients. *Clin Infect Dis* 1994;19(3):541–542.

74. Daniels NA, MacKinnon L, Bishop R, et al. *Vibrio parahaemolyticus* infections in the United States, 1973–1998. *J Infect Dis* 2000;181(5):1661–1666.

75. Hlady WG, Klontz KC. The epidemiology of *Vibrio* infections in Florida, 1981–1993. *J Infect Dis* 1996;173(5):1176–1183.

76. Obata H, Kai A, Morozumi S. [The trends of *Vibrio parahaemolyticus* foodborne outbreaks in Tokyo: 1989–2000]. *Kansenshogaku Zasshi* 2001;75(6):485–489.

77. Okuda J, Ishibashi M, Hayakawa E, et al. Emergence of a unique O3:K6 clone of *Vibrio parahaemolyticus* in Calcutta, India, and isolation of strains from the same clonal group from Southeast Asian travelers arriving in Japan. *J Clin Microbiol* 1997;35(12):3150–3155.

78. Bag PK, Nandi S, Bhadra RK, et al. Clonal diversity among recently emerged strains of *Vibrio parahaemolyticus* O3:K6 associated with pandemic spread. *J Clin Microbiol* 1999;37(7):2354–2357.

79. Matsumoto C, Okuda J, Ishibashi M, et al. Pandemic spread of an O3:K6 clone of *Vibrio parahaemolyticus* and emergence of related strains evidenced by arbitrarily primed PCR and toxRS sequence analyses. *J Clin Microbiol* 2000;38(2):578–585.

80. Chiou CS, Hsu SY, Chiu SI, et al. *Vibrio parahaemolyticus* serovar O3:K6 as cause of unusually high incidence of food-borne disease outbreaks in Taiwan from 1996 to 1999. *J Clin Microbiol* 2000;38(12):4621–4625.

81. Klontz KC, Desenclos JC. Clinical and epidemiological features of sporadic infections with *Vibrio fluvialis* in Florida, USA. *J Diarrhoeal Dis Res* 1990;8(1-2):24–26.

82. Shimada T, Arakawa E, Okitsu T, et al. Additional O antigens of *Vibrio fluvialis* and *Vibrio furnissii. Jpn J Infect Dis* 1999;52(3):124–126.

83. Hickman-Brenner FW, Brenner DJ, Steigerwalt AG, et al. *Vibrio fluvialis* and *Vibrio furnissii* isolated from a stool sample of one patient. *J Clin Microbiol* 1984;20(1):125–127.

84. Brenner DJ, Hickman-Brenner FW, Lee JV, et al. *Vibrio furnissii* (formerly aerogenic biogroup of *Vibrio fluvialis*), a new species isolated from human feces and the environment. *J Clin Microbiol* 1983;18(4):816–824.

85. Hickman FW, Farmer JJ III, Hollis DG, et al. Identification of Vibrio hollisae sp. nov. from patients with diarrhea. *J Clin Microbiol* 1982;15(3):395–401.

86. Nishibuchi M, Doke S, Toizumi S, et al. Isolation from a coastal fish of *Vibrio hollisae* capable of producing a hemolysin similar to the thermostable direct hemolysin of *Vibrio parahaemolyticus. Appl Environ Microbiol* 1988;54(8):2144–2146.

87. Yamasaki S, Shirai H, Takeda Y, et al. Analysis of the gene of *Vibrio hollisae* encoding the hemolysin similar to the thermostable direct hemolysin of *Vibrio parahaemolyticus. FEMS Microbiol Lett* 1991;64(2–3):259–263.

88. Vuddhakul V, Nakai T, Matsumoto C, Oh T, et al. Analysis of *gyrB* and *toxR* gene sequences of *Vibrio hollisae* and development of *gyrB-* and *toxR*-targeted PCR methods for isolation of *V. hollisae* from the environment and its identification. *Appl Environ Microbiol* 2000;66(8):3506–3514.

89. Armstrong CW, Lake JL, Miller GB Jr. Extraintestinal infections due to halophilic vibrios. *South Med J* 1983;76(5):571–574.

90. Bonner JR, Coker AS, Berryman CR, et al. Spectrum of *Vibrio* infections in a Gulf Coast community. *Ann Intern Med* 1983;99(4):464–469.

91. Hoge CW, Watsky D, Peeler RN, et al. Epidemiology and spectrum of *Vibrio* infections in a Chesapeake Bay community. *J Infect Dis* 1989;160(6):985–993.

92. Said R, Volpin G, Grimberg B, et al. Hand infections due to non-cholera *Vibrio* after injuries from St Peter's fish (*Tilapia zillii*). *J Hand Surg [Br]* 1998;23(6):808–810.

93. Reed KC, Crowell MC, Castro MD, et al. Skin and soft-tissue infections after injury in the ocean: culture methods and antibiotic therapy for marine bacteria. *Milit Med* 1999;164(3):198–201.

94. Zuppardo AB, Siebeling RJ. An epimerase gene essential for capsule synthesis in *Vibrio vulnificus*. *Infect Immun* 1998;66(6):2601–2606.

95. Reddy GP, Hayat U, Bush CA, et al. Capsular polysaccharide structure of a clinical isolate of *Vibrio vulnificus* strain B062316 determined by heteronuclear NMR spectroscopy and high-performance anion exchange chromatography. *Anal Biochem* 1993;214:106–115.

96. Hayat U, Reddy GP, Bush CA. Capsular types of *Vibrio vulnificus*: an analysis of strains from clinical and environmental sources. *J Infect Dis* 1993;168:758–762.

97. Amako K, Okada E, Miake S. Evidence for the presence of a capsule in *Vibrio vulnificus*. *J Gen Microbiol* 1984;130:2741–2743.

98. Amaro C, Biosca EG, Fouz B. Role of iron, capsule, and toxins in the pathogenicity of *Vibrio vulnificus* biotype 2 for mice. *Infect Immun* 1994;62:759–763.

99. Zakaria-Meechan Z, Massad G, Simpson LM. Ability of *Vibrio vulnificus* to obtain iron from hemoglobin–haptoglobin complexes. *Infect Immun* 1988;56:275–277.

100. Simpson LM, Oliver JD. Siderophore production by *Vibrio vulnificus*. *Infect Immun* 1983;41:644–649.

101. Miyoshi S, Hirata Y, Tomochika K, et al. *Vibrio vulnificus* may produce a metalloprotease causing an edematous skin lesion *in vivo*. *FEMS Microbiol Lett* 1994;121:321–325.

102. Wright AC, Morris JG Jr. The extracellular cytolysin of *Vibrio vulnificus*: inactivation and relationship to virulence in mice. *Infect Immun* 1991;59:192–197.

103. Nishina Y, Miyoshi S, Nagase A, et al. Significant role of an exocellular protease in utilization of heme by *Vibrio vulnificus*. *Infect Immun* 1992;60:2128–2132.

104. Kreger AS. Cytolytic activity and virulence of *Vibrio damsela*. *Infect Immun* 1984;44(2):326–331.

105. Perez-Tirse J, Levine JF, Mecca M. *Vibrio damsela*. A cause of fulminant septicemia. *Arch Intern Med* 1993;153:1838–1840.

106. Abbott SL, Seli LS, Catino M Jr, et al. Misidentification of unusual *Aeromonas* species as members of the genus *Vibrio*: a continuing problem. *J Clin Microbiol* 1998;36(4):1103–1104.

107. Bode RB, Brayton PR, Colwell RR. A new *Vibrio* species, *Vibrio cincinnatiensis*, causing meningitis: successful treatment in an adult. *Ann Intern Med* 1986;104:55–56.

108. Sack DA, Chowdhury KA, Huq A, et al. Epidemiology of *Aeromonas* and *Plesiomonas* diarrhoea. *J Diarrhoeal Dis Res* 1988;6(2):107–112.

109. Albert MJ, Faruque AS, Faruque SM, et al. Case-control study of enteropathogens associated with childhood diarrhea in Dhaka, Bangladesh. *J Clin Microbiol* 1999;37(11):3458–3464.

110. Albert MJ, Ansaruzzaman M, Talukder KA, et al. Prevalence of enterotoxin genes in *Aeromonas* spp. isolated from children with diarrhea, healthy controls, and the environment. *J Clin Microbiol* 2000;38(10):3785–3790.

111. Agger WA, McCormick JD, Gurwith MJ. Clinical and microbiological features of *Aeromonas hydrophila* associated diarrhea. *J Clin Microbiol* 1985;21:909–913.

112. Herrington DA, Tzipori S, Robins-Browne RM. *In vitro* and *in vivo* pathogenicity of *Plesiomonas shigelloides*. *Infect Immun* 1987;55:979–985.

113. Holmberg SD, Farmer JJ III. *Aeromonas hydrophila* and *Plesiomonas shigelloides* as causes of intestinal infections. *Rev Infect Dis* 1984;6:633–639.

114. Sack DA, Hoque AT, Huq A, et al. Is protection against shigellosis induced by natural infection with *Plesiomonas shigelloides*? *Lancet* 1994;343(8910):1413–1415.

Clostridium difficile–Associated Diarrhea and Colitis

John G. Bartlett

Clostridium difficile, the major recognized agent of antibiotic-associated diarrhea and colitis, was originally reported as an agent of enteric disease in 1977 (1). This organism produces a spectrum of disease, ranging from simple and self-limited diarrhea to its most advanced and characteristic form, pseudomembranous colitis (PMC). *C. difficile* produces at least two toxins, toxin A and toxin B, which are responsible for clinical expression and pathologic changes (2). An unusual feature of *C. difficile* is that it causes disease almost exclusively in the presence of antibiotic exposure.

HISTORICAL PERSPECTIVE

A retrospective review of *C. difficile*-induced enteric disease shows three quite different lines of investigation: studies of the anatomy of PMC, studies of *C. difficile*, and studies of antibiotic-associated cecitis in rodent models (2).

The anatomic studies began with the initial report of pseudomembranous lesions of the intestinal tract by Finney in 1893 (3). The case involved a 22-year-old patient of William Osler who underwent gastric surgery and postoperatively developed severe diarrhea that proved to be a lethal complication. Autopsy showed lesions that appeared as "diphtheritic membranes" in the small bowel. Pseudomembranous enterocolitis remained a relatively rare condition until the introduction of antibiotics. In the early 1950s, pseudomembranous enterocolitis became a relatively common complication of antibiotic therapy, especially with tetracycline and chloramphenicol. *Staphylococcus aureus* was the major nosocomial pathogen at the time, and it was implicated as the agent of this disease by virtue of recovery from stool (4). A retrospective review of the data did not provide persuasive evidence for a causal role for *S. aureus* because the majority of the patients receiving antimicrobial agents harbored the organism; however, the role of *S. aureus* as the agent of antibiotic-associated colitis was not seriously challenged until there was renewed interest in the disease during the 1970s. The most important study was of a condition that became known as clindamycin colitis, conducted by Tedesco and co-workers (5) at Barnes Hospital in 1974. This was a prospective evaluation of 200 patients treated with clindamycin; 42 (21%) developed diarrhea and 20 (10%) had PMC at endoscopy. Stool cultures from these patients failed to grow *S. aureus* despite the relative ease of detecting this organism with selective media. A retrospective review of the Barnes Hospital experience indicates that the extraordinary frequency of this complication presumably reflects an epidemic of *C. difficile*, an impression supported by analysis of stored stool specimens from that epidemic, which revealed *C. difficile* toxin after the tissue culture assay was described 5 years later (2).

The second series of relevant experiments in the history of *C. difficile* concerns the rodent model of antibiotic-associated colitis. Hambra and co-workers (6) reported in 1943 that attempts to determine the potential utility of penicillin for the treatment of gas gangrene in a guinea pig model were complicated by lethality that was ascribed to penicillin. Necropsy examinations showed large ceca filled with hemorrhagic fluid, and subsequent work showed that nearly all antibiotics may be lethal to guinea pigs and that hamsters are equally susceptible. A particularly important contribution was reported by Green (7). In 1974, he noted that stools and tissues of affected animals showed cytotoxic changes in cultured cells. No virus could be propagated, but he concluded that a latent virus was responsible. A similar observation was made in 1977 by Larson and colleagues (8), who used stool specimens from patients with PMC.

Studies of *C. difficile* itself began with the demonstration of *C. difficile* as a component of the normal intestinal flora of newborn infants by Hall and O'Toole (9) in 1935. These investigators noted that this organism produced a "neurotoxin"; they observed that the cell-free supernatant of broth cultures was lethal when injected into experimental animals. In spite of this finding, the clinical significance of *C. difficile* remained enigmatic. The most comprehensive report on the organism before that time was the doctoral thesis of Hafiz (10) at the University of Leeds under the supervision of Professor Oakley, a noted authority on *Clostridium* organisms. Hafiz noted that the organism was widespread and could be recovered from stools of various animals. He also observed that most strains produced the lethal toxin, although in varying quantities, *in vitro*.

The three landmark studies were all reported in 1974 (3,7,10). Nevertheless, there was no way at that time to know that the organism described in detail by Hafiz produced the cytotoxin noted by Green that caused the lesions described by Tedesco.

What subsequently brought these three lines of investigation together were studies using the hamster model of antibiotic-associated colitis. This work showed that cecal contents contained a filterable protein toxin that was cytopathic in cell culture and would reproduce typical lesions when injected intracecally into healthy recipient animals (1). Both the organism and its cytopathic toxin could be detected in all hamsters with antibiotic-induced disease and in nearly all patients with antibiotic-associated PMC (11).

PATHOPHYSIOLOGY

Factors contributing to the pathogenesis of *C. difficile*–associated diarrhea and colitis include (a) a source of the organism, presumably the host's normal flora or an environmental source (the latter is especially important in epidemics); (b) an altered intestinal flora that results from antibiotic exposure; (c) toxin production, reflecting rapid growth of toxigenic strains at the time the competing flora is suppressed; (d) a poorly understood, age-related susceptibility; and (e) immunologic susceptibility.

Colonization Rates

C. difficile may be detected in stool with the use of selective media, such as the media containing cycloserine and cefoxitin (12). The recovery rate for healthy adults is usually 2% to 3% (12–14) (Table 74.1); for patients who recently received antimicrobial agents and do not have diarrhea, it is 5% to 15% (14); and for hospitalized patients the range is 20% to 30% whether or not they were exposed to an antibiotic (15). The isolation rate in healthy infants is highly variable, ranging from 5% to 70% (9,14,16,17). Variable but often high carrier rates persist during the first 8 months of life, until the "normal adult flora" becomes established and the isolation rate subsequently approximates the 2% to 3% rate noted in healthy adults (14,16,17).

TABLE 74.1. Clinical Experience with Tissue Culture Assay for *Clostridium difficile* Toxin and Culture for *C. difficile*

Patient's category	Isolation of *C. difficile* (%)	*C. difficile* toxin assay (%)
Antibiotic-associated diarrhea/colitis		
Antibiotic-associated diarrhea without colitis	15–30	15–25
Pseudomembranous colitis	90–100	90–100
Antibiotic exposure without diarrhea	10–20	2–8
Gastrointestinal diseases unrelated to antibiotics	2–3	0–1
Healthy adults	2–3	0–0.5
Healthy neonates	30–70	5–60

Antibiotic Exposure

A striking feature of *C. difficile* is that it appears to cause enteric disease almost exclusively in the presence of antibiotic exposure. Virtually all drugs with an antibacterial spectrum of activity have been implicated, most frequently those that have a pronounced impact on the colon flora, primarily cephalosporins, ampicillin or amoxicillin, and clindamycin (18–20). The most frequent inducing agents in more recent years have been cephalosporins, especially in nosocomial cases (21–25). Less frequently implicated are penicillins other than ampicillin, erythromycin, quinolones, and trimethoprim-sulfamethoxazole. Rare inducing agents include fluoroquinolones, rifampin, parenteral aminoglycosides, sulfonamides, metronidazole, and tetracycline. For most drugs, the dose, the route of administration, and the duration of treatment seem to have little effect on the frequency or the severity of this complication. In addition, activity *in vitro* against *C. difficile* bears little apparent relevance. For example, the minimal inhibitory concentrations (MICs) of vancomycin and ampicillin are nearly identical, despite the fact that the former is highly effective therapy, and the latter is one of the most common offending agents (26).

Toxins

There are two toxins, designated A and B; both are produced by *C. difficile* during log-phase growth of vegetative forms (27–29). Most strains are toxigenic, and virtually all toxigenic strains produce both toxins under identical culture conditions, although there are strain variations in the amount of toxin produced, and there are differences between the toxins in biologic activity (27–32). Toxin B is a 270- to 279-kd protein that is a potent cytotoxin causing nonlethal disruption of actin microfilaments of the cytoskeleton (27,28,33,34). Toxin A is a 308-kd protein that causes similar cytotoxic changes but is about 1,000 times less potent in tissue culture assays. Toxin A induces neutrophilic infiltration, increased myoelectric activity, and severe mucosal damage in loop assays of small bowel or colon of guinea pigs, hamsters, rats, mice, and rabbits (27–29,35). Toxin B has no activity in these loop assays using rodent models, suggesting that toxin B is responsible for tissue culture changes and toxin A is responsible for enteric disease. Studies with human intestinal cells (T84) in Ussing chambers showed that toxin B was about 10 times more potent in permeability and morphologic changes (36). Furthermore, there are now several case reports of typical cases involving toxin A–negative, toxin B–positive strains of *C. difficile* (37,38). The implication is that both toxins may be important in clinical expression in patients.

Age-Related Risk

Numerous studies have shown high carriage rates of both *C. difficile* and its toxin among healthy neonates (14,16,17). This is the only population in which the toxin is found in the stool at high frequency in the absence of clinical expression. One suggested explanation is that the infant gut simply is not susceptible (39). In addition, population-based studies in Sweden have shown that the incidence of *C. difficile* toxin–positive stools is 20 to 100 times greater for persons over 60 years than for those 10 to 20 years of age (13). Serologic assays indicate that most healthy persons over 5 to 10 years of age have circulating antibody to toxin A, toxin B, or both, but this apparently does not confer protection (40). These data suggest that the aging process is associated with increasing susceptibility to colonization, toxin production, and disease caused by *C. difficile*, although the mechanism is not known.

HUMORAL IMMUNITY

The potential role of humoral immunity in clinical expression of *C. difficile* toxin was reported by Kyne et al. (41,42). The initial report showed that clinical expression with diarrhea in hospitalized patients with *C. difficile* colonization correlated with the absence of serum antibody to toxin A (41). A subsequent report showed a similar observation for relapses of *C. difficile* enteric disease (42).

CLINICAL FEATURES

Signs and Symptoms

The single symptom that is found in nearly all patients with PMC is diarrhea. Only 10% to 25% of all patients with antibiotic-associated diarrhea have positive toxin assays for *C. difficile* (2,20). The majority of the toxin-negative cases are enigmatic. Clinical features that specifically suggest *C. difficile*–associated enteric disease in the patient with antibiotic-associated diarrhea are: exposure to common inducing agents (clindamycin, broad-spectrum penicillins, and cephalosporins), evidence of colitis (fecal white blood cells, cramps, fever, leukocytosis, and tenesmus), hypoalbuminemia, and toxic megacolon. Most patients with *C. difficile*–negative, antibiotic-associated diarrhea (43) have modest diarrhea without evidence of colitis that is most commonly due to reduced fecal flora with disruptive carbohydrate or bile acid metabolism (44).

  C. difficile most often causes mild or moderate diarrhea that resolves when the implicated agent is simply discontinued. Other features in more seriously ill patients (24,45–51) include fever, which is usually low grade but the temperature may reach 105°F; leukocytosis that averages 15,000 cells per mm^3 but may reach leukemoid levels of 50,000 cells per mm^3 or higher (52); and loose stools that may be as frequent as 15 to 30 per day. Because this is a protein-losing enteropathy, hypoalbuminemia is common, and pedal edema or anasarca is a late complication in advanced cases (53). Stool examinations for fecal leukocytes are positive by direct methylene blue stain in 40% to 50% of cases and by stool lactoferrin in 60% to 80% (22,54,55).

  Serious complications in patients with *C. difficile*–induced diarrhea or colitis include severe dehydration, electrolyte imbalance, hypotension, hypoalbuminemia with anasarca, toxic megacolon, and colonic perforation. Extraintestinal symptoms are infrequent, except for the complications noted, which are ascribed largely to severe colitis and diarrhea, although occasional

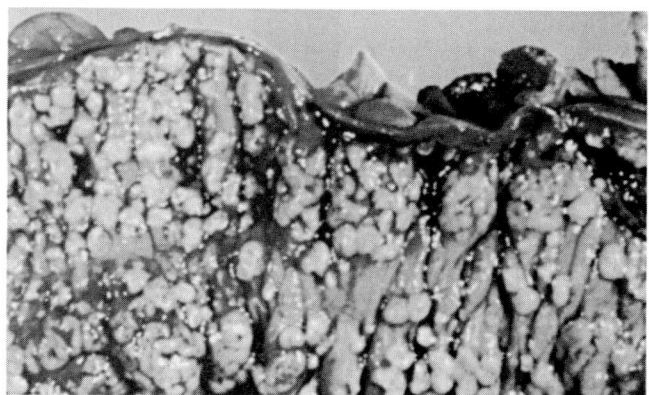

Figure 74.1. Resected colon showing pseudomembranous colitis.

patients have polyarthritis (56–58). Three findings that appear to be somewhat unique to *C. difficile* diarrhea (compared with that caused by other bacterial agents) include its propensity to chronicity, the characteristic anatomic feature of PMC, hypoalbuminemia, and the nearly uniform lack of small bowel involvement.

Pathologic Changes

Endoscopy in patients with antibiotic-associated diarrhea shows a spectrum of changes on gross inspection, including an entirely normal mucosa, erythema, edema, severe inflammation, or, the most characteristic feature, pseudomembranous lesions. With PMC, gross inspection shows multiple, elevated, yellowish white plaques that vary in size from a few millimeters to 5 to 10 mm (5,59,60) (Fig. 74.1). Early lesions are punctate, but with advanced disease the pseudomembranes may coalesce and eventually slough to leave large denuded areas.

  Histologic studies indicate that the pseudomembrane typically arises from a point of superficial ulceration and is accompanied by acute or chronic inflammatory changes in the lamina propria (47,48). The pseudomembrane is composed of fibrin mucin inflammatory cells and sloughed mucosal epithelial cells (Fig. 74.2). There is no evidence of bacterial invasion of the bowel mucosa, and no typical organisms are found within the pseudomembrane.

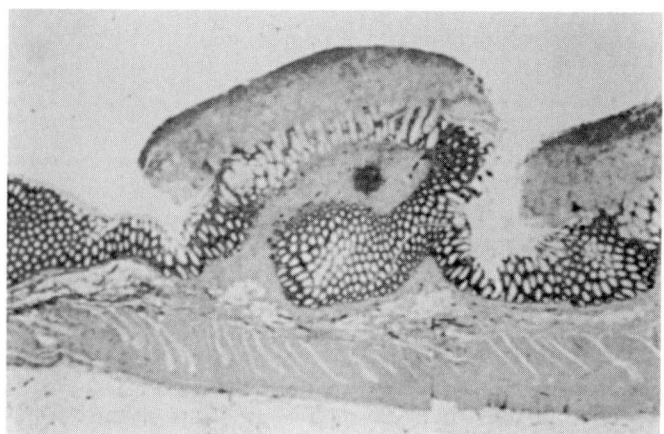

Figure 74.2. Histopathology of the lesion seen in Fig. 74.1 showing the pseudomembrane.

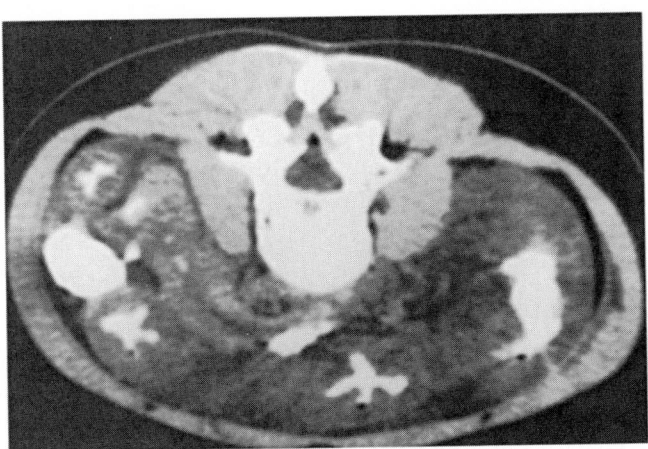

Figure 74.3. Computed tomographic scan of abdomen showing colitis due to *Clostridium difficile*, with thickened colonic mucosa.

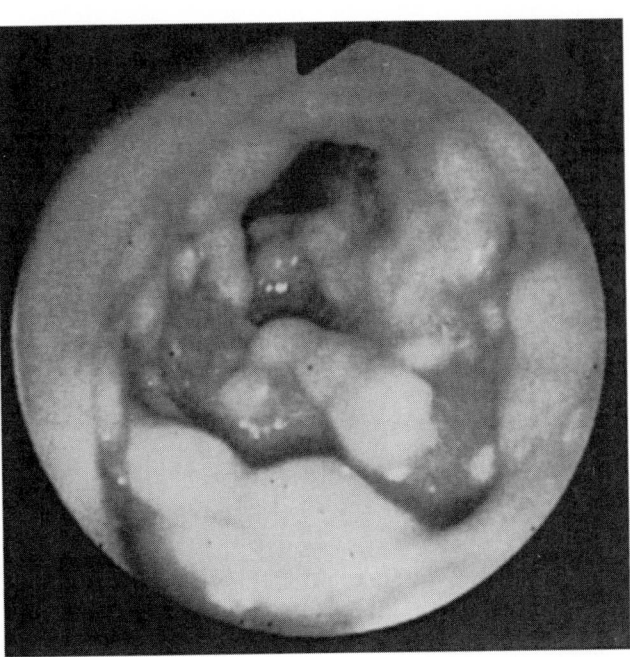

Figure 74.4. Pseudomembranous plaques seen with colonoscopy in a patient with *Clostridium difficile*–associated pseudomembranous colitis.

DIAGNOSTIC STUDIES

Diagnostic studies in patients with antibiotic-associated diarrhea or colitis are separated into those used to define anatomic changes and those used to detect the agent of disease. For anatomic studies, radiographs are usually nonspecific, although plain films of the abdomen in patients with colitis may show a markedly edematous colon with distention and distorted haustral markings (61,62). Characteristic findings with computed tomography are changes restricted to the colon without small bowel involvement, colonic thickening that averages 10 to 15 mm, and ascites fluid (63–65) (Fig. 74.3). Changes in the colon may be focal or pancolonic. Only approximately 50% of patients with positive toxin assays show changes on the computed tomography scan.

The preferred method for determining anatomic changes is endoscopy. In most patients the distal colon is involved, so sigmoidoscopy is often adequate; however, as many as one third of the patients have lesions restricted to the right colon, necessitating colonoscopy (66). The typical changes are those noted previously: punctate lesions that stud the colonic mucosa with an intervening mucosa that is normal or erythematous (Fig. 74.4). The role of endoscopy in these patients is often controversial. Because the procedure is unpleasant, because it is expensive, and because therapeutic decisions are usually based on the severity of clinical symptoms, the *C. difficile* toxin assay is the preferred diagnostic test.

Most authorities consider the tissue culture assay to be the gold standard (48–52). This requires the demonstration of a cytopathic toxin that is neutralized by *C. difficile* or *Clostridium sordellii* antitoxin (67–68). Results with this assay in various populations are summarized in Table 74.1. The major disadvantages of the test are that many laboratories do not offer tissue culture technology, and there is a 24- to 48-hour delay for results. The toxin titer may be evaluated using serial dilutions of stool, but there appears to be little correlation between the severity of disease and toxin titers. False-negative results are unusual, provided the specimen is processed by a competent laboratory using a sufficiently low dilution of the specimen.

The preferred test in most laboratories in the current era is the enzyme immunoassay. Reagents are now available from multiple suppliers for detection of toxin A or toxins A and B. Major advantages of these assays compared with tissue culture assays are the ease of technical performance and the speed with which results are completed, usually 2 to 3 hours. Sensitivity is 10% to 15% less compared with the tissue culture assay, but specificity is good (51,69–72) if enzyme immunoassays are done; the preferred method is technology to recognize toxin A and B due to cases involving toxin A–negative, B–positive strains (37,38). Other techniques being developed are a polymerase chain reaction to amplify gene fragments that encode for toxin A or B (73,74). Some authorities advocate stool cultures to supplement toxin assays (75,76). Advantages are that sensitivity is good when experienced technicians perform the assay, and this permits strain identity in epidemics. Disadvantages are the technical expertise required, the 48- to 72-hour delay for results, and the relative nonspecificity of results due to high rates of carriage in the population of greatest interest: hospitalized patients and patients receiving antibiotics (Table 74.1). Recommendations of the Society for Hospital Epidemiology of America (SHEA) (51) are to test only diarrheal stools, test only specimens from persons over 1 year of age, and do not use this assay for a "test-of-cure." Sending multiple specimens increases sensitivity and cost (22).

EPIDEMIOLOGY

C. difficile is a sporulating organism that survives well in nature and appears to be widely distributed in the environment (10). It is also a transferable pathogen that poses a threat to patients in hospitals and in chronic care facilities where there is nosocomial exposure and a large population of susceptible hosts, owing to the frequency of antibiotic use (5,15,47–51,77–87). Within such institutions, *C. difficile* may be endemic or epidemic in selected areas. Several investigators have found environmental sources of *C. difficile*, primarily in case-associated areas (82,83). For example, Kim and associates (82) isolated the organism in environmental samplings from 37 of 114 (32%) case-associated areas but in only 6 of 445 (1.3%) controlled sites. The primary sources for positive cultures in such studies have been toilets, bed pans, floors, and the hands of personnel. The hospital environment may pose considerable risk for acquisition of *C. difficile*, even in the absence of an epidemic of clinically apparent disease. McFarland and co-workers (15) sampled rectal swab material sequentially from 428 hospitalized patients and found that 112 (26%) harbored *C. difficile* at some time during their hospital course; of these 112, 6 (6%) were apparently colonized before hospitalization, 23 (21%) had been in a nursing home before their hospitalization, and 83 (74%) acquired the organism during hospitalization. Most of the patients had no symptoms. Risks identified for both increased rates of carriage and increased rates of diarrhea include advanced age, severe underlying disease, and exposure to selected antibiotics, especially clindamycin and cephalosporins (5,22,23,48–51,88–90).

Epidemiologic studies often include methods to type strains to monitor epidemiology and to correlate strain types with virulence according to clinical correlations and *in vivo* toxin production. Strain-typing methods include plasmid fingerprinting, protein analysis, immunoblotting, polyacrylamide gel electrophoresis, serotyping, restriction endonuclease analysis, polymerase chain reaction, ribotyping, bacteriocin typing, and restriction fragment length polymorphism (80,91–93). Although strain typing facilitates hospital epidemiologic investigation, most laboratories do not culture stool for *C. difficile*, most do not do strain typing, and management decisions based on these results are unclear.

TREATMENT

Treatment of *C. difficile*–associated diarrhea or colitis includes discontinuation of the implicated agent, implementation of supportive measures, and, in selected cases, oral administration of metronidazole or vancomycin. Antiperistaltic agents should be avoided (94,95). Some patients require continued antibiotic treatment of the underlying condition; in these cases, it is advised to give oral metronidazole or vancomycin and change the suspected inducing agent to an alternative agent that infrequently causes this complication, such as fluoroquinolone, doxycycline, parenteral aminoglycoside, trimethoprim-sulfamethoxazole, sulfonamide, parenteral vancomycin, or metronidazole.

Antimicrobial Treatment

Many patients respond when the implicated agent is simply discontinued and do not require antibiotic treatment of the antibiotic-induced complication (96). The major advantage is avoidance of the risk of relapsing *C. difficile*–associated diarrhea or colitis. Indications for antibiotic treatment are arbitrary and include severe diarrhea, diarrhea accompanied by systemic signs or evidence of colitis, ileus, and persistent symptoms after antibiotics have been discontinued. The drug usually administered in these cases is oral metronidazole, which is preferred to oral vancomycin treatment based on cost, demonstrated efficacy that is comparable with vancomycin (97,98), and the opportunity to avoid vancomycin, which may promote vancomycin-resistant *Enterococcus faecium* in nosocomial cases. Thus, oral metronidazole (250 mg four times daily or 500 mg three times daily for 10 days) is viewed as the preferred antimicrobial by the Centers for Disease Control and Prevention, (98) SHEA (51), and the Infectious Diseases Society of America (95). A theoretical disadvantage of metronidazole is nearly complete absorption so that levels in the colonic lumen are nil. This is a toxin-mediated disease, with *C. difficile* retained entirely in the colonic lumen without invasion, meaning that drug in the colonic lumen is the

assumed goal of therapy. Additionally, a small number of strains of *C. difficile* are resistant to metronidazole, but vancomycin resistance has never been reported. With either drug, the usual response is impressive; fever usually resolves within 1 day, and diarrhea resolves in 4 to 5 days (2,24,49,96–98). Patients who do not improve promptly usually have toxic megacolon or ileus, or they have an alternative or concurrent condition that accounts for symptoms.

Treatment Failure

Patients who fail to respond should be evaluated for ileus and alternative diagnoses with various studies, including stool culture, computed tomography, and/or endoscopy. Oral vancomycin is the preferred agent for patients who are pregnant or intolerant of metronidazole, and some consider it preferred in patients who are seriously ill or unresponsive to metronidazole. Options in patients with ileus are parenteral administration of metronidazole, which usually does not work (99), and enteric administration of vancomycin by tube from above or below. Approximately 0.4% of patients fail to respond and are candidates for surgery (100). The usual indications for surgery are persistent or progressive signs of systemic toxicity, persistent diarrhea, signs of peritonitis (although perforation is rare), and progressive colonic disease as seen on sequential computed tomography scans. In these cases, the procedure of choice is a total colectomy.

Relapse

The major complication with either oral metronidazole or vancomycin is relapse. This occurs only with antimicrobial treatment; it is found with equal frequency after treatment with vancomycin, bacitracin, and metronidazole, and the frequency is reported at 5% to 50% (96–98), with a rate of 24% in the largest series. Most patients respond well to a second course of antibiotics, but approximately 2% to 5% have multiple relapses, defined as four or more relapses after antimicrobial treatment. The clinical features of relapses are quite stereotyped: the patient responds to standard treatment, but 2 to 28 days (usually 3–7 days) after antimicrobial treatment is discontinued, he or she reports that the same symptoms have recurred. Stool assays for toxin at that time will be positive, and cultures yield *C. difficile* that may be the same strain as the original isolate or may represent infection with a newly acquired strain (101).

There are several methods that can be used to treat the patients with multiple relapses; all work some of the time and none work all of the time (Table 74.2). The method we prefer is a 10- to 14-day course of vancomycin or metronidazole, followed by a second stage of treatment consisting of pulse dose vancomycin, 125 mg given orally every second day for 6 weeks (9). An alternative method for the second phase of treatment is administration of cholestyramine, 4-g packet three times per day, plus *Lactobacillus* (e.g., Lactinex; Hynson, Westcott & Dunning, Baltimore, Maryland), 1 g four times per day or *Lactobacillus* GG ("culturelle") or *Saccharomyces boulardii*, all for 4 to 6 weeks (102–104). The theory used to justify these tactics is that the first phase is given to gain control of the disease, and the second phase is an attempt to inhibit *C. difficile* until the normal flora becomes reestablished. Other methods used to manage relapses include intravenous immunoglobulin (105,106), based on studies showing relapses reflect failure to mount a humoral response to toxin A (41,42); rectal instillations of stool from healthy donors (107); and rectal instillations of broth cultures of stool isolates (108).

TABLE 74.2. Treatment of *Clostridium difficile*-Induced Diarrhea and Colitis

I. Nonspecific treatment
  A. Discontinuation of implicated antimicrobial agent (i.e., discontinuation of treatment or change to an alternative regimen unlikely to cause this complication)
  B. Implementation of supportive measures: correction of fluid losses and electrolyte imbalances essential; parenteral hyperalimentation rarely indicated; role of corticosteroids in seriously ill patients not established
  C. Avoidance of antiperistaltic agents
  D. Observance of enteric isolation precautions for hospitalized patients
II. Specific treatment and dosages
  A. Antimicrobial agents (advocated only if symptoms are severe or persist)
    1. Oral agent (preferred)
      (a) Vancomycin: 125 mg p.o. q.i.d. for 7–14 days (efficacy is established)
      (b) Metronidazole: 250 mg p.o. t.i.d. for 7–14 days (efficacy is established)
      (c) Alternative: bacitracin, 25,000 units p.o. q.i.d. for 7–14 days (efficacy is established)
    2. Oral treatment precluded by NPO status, ileus, intolerance of medicines
      (a) Parenteral agents: metronidazole—500 mg i.v. every 6 h (experience is anecdotal and variable; oral treatment should be given whenever feasible)
      (b) Vancomycin (0.5–2 g/d) via long tube in small bowel or via endoscopy or rectal tube in colon
III. Multiple relapses
  A. Vancomycin or metronidazole p.o. for 10 days, followed by
    1. Cholestyramine 4-g packet p.o. t.i.d. plus *Lactobacillus* l g p.o. q.i.d., or *Lactobacillus* GG (see below) for 6 wk
    2. Vancomycin, 125 mg PO qod × 6 wks
  B. Experimental agents
    1. *Saccharomyces boulardii:* vancomycin 500 mg p.o. q.i.d. for 10 days, add on day 6 *S. boulardii* as two 250-mg capsules b.i.d. for 4 wk (103)
    2. *Lactobacillus* GG: 1 tab (10^{10} organisms) b.i.d. for 4 wk after course of vancomycin or metronidazole (104)
    3. Intravenous immunoglobulin: 400 mg/kg every 3 wk (reported primarily in pediatric patients and in an adult with immunoglobulin A deficiency) (105,106)
    4. Rectal instillation of feces: 50 g fresh stool from healthy donor in 500 mL saline delivered by enema (107)
    5. Rectal instillation of broth cultures of bacterial isolates from healthy donors: strains selected based on *in vitro* inhibition of *C. difficile,* cultured to 10^9/mL, 2 mL of each mixed in anaerobic glovebox with 180 mL, saline and given by enema (108)

p.o., by mouth; q.i.d., four times daily; t.i.d., three times daily; b.i.d., twice daily; tab, tablet; NPO, nothing by mouth; i.v., intravenously.

Infection Control

C. difficile–induced enteric disease may be endemic or epidemic in acute care hospitals, chronic care facilities, and day care centers, all settings where there is clustering of people rendered vulnerable by high rates of antibiotic use (47–49,51,77–99). Patients in acute and chronic care facilities should be in private rooms with bathroom facilities until diarrhea resolves. There should be enteric precautions, with careful attention to hand washing, use of vinyl gloves (109), avoidance of rectal thermometers, and terminal room cleansing with a sporicidal agent (51). In epidemics it may be necessary to institute controls on use of major inducing agents, primarily clindamycin and cephalosporins (89,90).

REFERENCES

1. Bartlett JG, Onderdonk AB, Cisneros AB, et al. Clindamycin-associated colitis due to toxin-producing species of *Clostridium* in hamsters. *J Infect Dis* 1977;136:701.
2. Bartlett JG. *Clostridium difficile:* clinical considerations. *Rev Infect Dis* 1990;12(suppl):243.
3. Finney JMT. Gastroenterostomy for cicatrizing ulcer of pylorus. *Bull Johns Hopkins Hosp* 1893;4:53.
4. Hummel RO, Altemeier WA, Hill EO. Iatrogenic staphylococcal enterocolitis. *Ann Surg* 1964;160:551.
5. Tedesco FJ, Barton RW, Alpers DH. Clindamycin-associated colitis: a prospective study. *Ann Intern Med* 1974;81:429.
6. Hambra DM, Rake G, McKeet CM, et al. The toxicity of penicillin as prepared for clinical use. *Am J Med Sci* 1943;206:642.
7. Green RH. The association of viral activation with penicillin toxicity in guinea pigs and hamsters. *Yale J Biol Med* 1974;47:166.
8. Larson HE, Parry JV, Price AB, et al. Undescribed toxin in pseudomembranous colitis. *BMJ* 1977;1:1246.
9. Hall IC, O'Toole E. Intestinal flora in newborn infants with a description of a new pathogenic anaerobe, *Bacillus difficiles. Am J Dis Child* 1935;49:380.
10. Hafiz S. *Clostridium difficile* and its toxins [PhD dissertation]. Leeds, England: University of Leeds, 1974.
11. Bartlett JG, Chang TW, Gurwit M, et al. Antibiotic-associated pseudomembranous colitis due to toxin-producing clostridia. *N Engl J Med* 1978;298:531.
12. George WL, Sutter VL, Citron D, et al. Selective and differential medium for isolation of *Clostridium difficile. J Clin Microbiol* 1979;9:214.
13. Karlstrom O, Fryklund B, Tullus K, et al. A prospective nationwide study of *Clostridium difficile*–associated diarrhea in Sweden. *Clin Infect Dis* 1998;26:141.
14. Viscidi R, Willey S, Bartlett JG. Isolation rates and toxigenic potential for *Clostridium difficile* isolates from various patient populations. *Gastroenterology* 1981;81:5.
15. McFarland LV, Mulligan ME, Kwok RYY, et al. Nosocomial acquisition of *Clostridium difficile* infection. *N Engl J Med* 1989;320:204.
16. Larson HE, Barclay FE, Honour P, et al. Epidemiology of *Clostridium difficile* in infants. *J Infect Dis* 1982;146:727.
17. Holst E, Helin I, Mardh P. A recovery of *Clostridium difficile* in children. *Scand J Infect Dis* 1981;13:41.
18. Bartlett JG. Antimicrobial agents implicated in *Clostridium difficile* toxin-associated diarrhea or colitis. *Johns Hopkins Med J* 1981;149:6.
19. George WL, Rolfe RD, Finegold SM. *Clostridium difficile* and its cytotoxin in feces of patients with antimicrobial agent-associated diarrhea and miscellaneous conditions. *J Clin Microbiol* 1982;15:1049.
20. Wilcox MH. Cleaning up *Clostridium difficile* infection. *Lancet* 1996;348:767.
21. Golledge CL, McKenzie T, Riley TV. Extended spectrum cephalosporins and *Clostridium difficile. J Antimicrob Chemother* 1989;23:929.
22. Manabe YC, Vinetz JM, Moore RD et al. *Clostridium difficile* colitis: an efficient clinical approach to diagnosis. *Ann Intern Med* 1995;123:835.
23. Anand A, Bashey B, Mir T, et al. Epidemiology, clinical manifestation, and outcome of *Clostridium difficile*-associated diarrhea. *Am J Gastroenterol* 1994;89:519.
24. Mylonakis M, Ryan ET, Calderwood SB. *Clostridium difficile*–associated diarrhea. *Arch Intern Med* 2000;161:525.
25. Fekety R. Guidelines for the diagnosis and management of *Clostridium difficile*–associated diarrhea and colitis. *Am J Gastroenterol* 1997;92:739.
26. Dzink JA, Bartlett JG. *In vitro* susceptibility of *Clostridium difficile* isolates from patients with antibiotic-associated diarrhea or colitis. *Antimicrob Agents Chemother* 1980;17:695.
27. Taylor NS, Thome G, Bartlett JG. Comparison of two toxins produced by *Clostridium difficile. Infect Immun* 1981;34:1036.
28. Sullivan NM, Pettett S, Wilkins TD. Purification and characterization of toxins A and B of *Clostridium difficile. Infect Immun* 1982;35:1032.
29. Lima AM, Lyerly DM, Wilkins TD, et al. Effects of *Clostridium difficile* toxins A and B in rabbit small and large intestine *in vivo* and cultured cells *in vitro. Infect Immun* 1988;56:582.
30. Fluit AC, Wolfhagen MJHM, Verdonk GPHT, et al. Nontoxigenic strains of *Clostridium difficile* lack the genes for both toxin A and toxin B. *J Clin Microbiol* 1991;29:2666.

31. Borriello SP, Wren BW, Hyde S, et al. Molecular, immunological, and biological characterization of a toxin A-negative, toxin B-positive strain of *Clostridium difficile*. *Infect Immun* 1992;60:4192.

32. Johnson S, Sypura WD, Gerding DN, et al. Selective neutralization of a bacterial enterotoxin by serum immunoglobulin A in response to mucosal disease. *Infect Immun* 1995;63:3166.

33. Fiorentini C, Malorni W, Paradisi S, et al. Interaction of *Clostridium difficile* toxin A with cultured cells: cytoskeletal changes and nuclear polarization. *Infect Immun* 1990;58:2329.

34. Just I, Selzer J, Wilm M, et al. Glucosylation of Rho proteins by *Clostridium difficile* toxin B. *Nature* 1995;375:500.

35. Burakoff R, Zhao L, Celifarco AJ, et al. Effects of purified *Clostridium difficile* toxin A on rabbit distal colon. *Gastroenterology* 1995;190:348.

36. Riegler M, Sedivy R, Pothoulakis C, et al. *Clostridium difficile* toxin B is more potent than toxin A in damaging human colonic epithelium *in vitro*. *J Clin Invest* 1995;95:2004.

37. Limaye AP, Turgeon DK, Cookson BT, et al. Pseudomembranous colitis caused by a toxin A- B+ strain of *Clostridium difficile*. *J Clin Microbiol* 2000;38:1696.

38. Kato H, Kato N, Watanabe K, et al. Identification of a toxin-negative toxin B positive *Clostridium difficile* by PCR. *J Clin Microbiol* 1998;26:2178.

39. Eglow R, Pothoulakis C, Itzkowitz S, et al. Diminished *Clostridium difficile* toxin A sensitivity in newborn rabbit ileum is associated with decreased toxin A receptor. *J Clin Invest* 1992;90:822.

40. Viscidi R, Laughon BE, Yolken R, et al. Serum antibody response to toxins A and B of *Clostridium difficile*. *J Infect Dis* 1983;148:93.

41. Aronsson B, Mollby R, Nord CE. Antimicrobial agents and *Clostridium difficile* in acute disease: epidemiological data from Sweden, 1980–1982. *J Infect Dis* 1985;151:476.

42. Kyne L, Warny M, Oamar A, et al Asymptomatic carriage of *Clostridium difficile* and serum levels of IgG antibody against toxin A. *N Engl J Med* 2000;342:390.

43. Gilbert DN. Aspects of the safety profile of oral antimicrobial agents. *Infect Dis Clin Pract* 1995;4(suppl 2):103.

44. Hogenauer C, Hammer HF, Krejis GJ, et al. Mechanisms and management of antibiotic-associated diarrhea. *Clin Infect Dis* 1998;27:702.

45. George WL, Rolfe RD, Finegold SM. *Clostridium difficile* and its cytotoxin in feces of patients with antimicrobial agent–associated diarrhea and miscellaneous conditions. *J Clin Microbiol* 1982;15:1049.

46. Bartlett JG, Taylor NW, Chang TW, et al. Clinical and laboratory observations in *Clostridium difficile* colitis. *Am J Clin Nutr* 1981;33:2521.

47. Mogg GM, Keighley M, Burdon D, et al. Antibiotic-associated colitis: a review of 66 cases. *Br J Surg* 1979;66:738.

48. Bartlett JG. Antibiotic-associated diarrhea. *Clin Infect Dis* 1992;15:573.

49. Fekety R, Shah AB. Diagnosis and treatment of *Clostridium difficile* colitis. *JAMA* 1993;269:71.

50. Kelly C, Pothoulakis C, LaMont JT. *Clostridium difficile* colitis. *N Engl J Med* 1994;330:257.

51. Gerding DN, Johnson S, Peterson LR, et al. *Clostridium difficile*–associated diarrhea and colitis: the SHEA position paper. *Infect Control Hosp Epidemiol* 1995;16:459.

52. Bulusu M, Narayan S, Shetler K, et al. Leukocytosis as a harbinger and surrogate marker of *Clostridium difficile* infection in hospitalized patients with diarrhea. *Am J Gastroenterol* 2000;95:3137.

53. Rybolt AH, Laughon BE, Greenough WB, et al. Protein-losing enteropathy associated with *Clostridium difficile* infection. *Lancet* 1989;1:1353.

54. Yong WH, Mattia AR, Ferraro MJ. Comparison of fecal lactoferrin latex agglutination assay and methylene blue microscopy for detection of fecal leukocytes in *Clostridium difficile*–associated disease. *J Clin Microbiol* 1994;32:1360.

55. Schleupner MA, Garner DC, Sosnowski KM, et al. Concurrence of *Clostridium difficile* toxin A enzyme-linked immunosorbent assay, fecal lactoferrin assay, and clinical criteria with *C. difficile* cytotoxin titer in two patient cohorts. *J Clin Microbiol* 1995;33:1755.

56. Putterman C, Rubinow A. Reactive arthritis associated with *Clostridium difficile* pseudomembranous colitis. *Semin Arthritis Rheum* 1993;22:420.

57. Jacobs A, Barnard K, Fishel R, et al. Extracolonic manifestations of *Clostridium difficile*: presentation of two cases and review of the literature. *Medicine* 2001;80:88.

58. Rollins DE, Moeller D. Polyarthritis associated with clindamycin-induced colitis. *JAMA* 1975;231:1228.

59. Price AB, Davies DR. Pseudomembranous colitis. *J Clin Pathol* 1977;30:1.

60. Summer HW, Tedesco FJ. Rectal biopsy in clindamycin-associated colitis. *Arch Pathol* 1975;99:237.

61. Stanley RJ, Melson GL, Tedesco FJ. The spectrum of radiographic findings in antibiotic-related pseudomembranous colitis. *Radiology* 1974;111:519.

62. Stanley RJ, Melson GL, Tedesco FJ, et al. Plain-film findings in severe pseudomembranous colitis. *Radiology* 1976;118:7.

63. Fishman E, Kavuru M, Kulzlman JE, et al. CT of pseudomembranous colitis: radiologic, clinical and pathologic correlation. *Radiology* 1991;180:57.

64. Boland GW, Lee MJ, Cats AM, et al. Antibiotic-induced diarrhea: specificity of abdominal CT for the diagnosis of *Clostridium difficile* disease. *Radiology* 1994;191:103.

65. Kirkpatrick ID, Greenberg HM. Evaluating the CT diagnosis of *Clostridium difficile* colitis: should CT guide therapy? *AJR* 2001;176:635.

66. Tedesco FJ, Corless JK, Brownstein RE. Rectal sparing in antibiotic-associated pseudomembranous colitis: a prospective study. *Gastroenterology* 1982;83:1259.

67. Chang TW, Lauermann M, Bartlett JG: Cytotoxicity assay in antibiotic-associated colitis. *J Infect Dis* 1979;140:765.

68. Bartlett JG. Laboratory diagnosis of antibiotic-associated colitis. *Lab Med* 1981;12:347.

69. Laughon BE, Viscidi RP, Gdovin SL, et al: Enzyme immunoassays for detection of *Clostridium difficile* toxins A and B in fecal specimens. *J Infect Dis* 1984;149:781.

70. Merz CS, Kramer C, Forman M, et al. Comparison of four commercially available rapid enzyme immunoassays with cytotoxin assay for detection of *Clostridium difficile* toxins(s) from stool specimens. *J Clin Microbiol* 1994;32:1142.

71. Lozniewski A, Rabaud C, Dotto E, et al. Laboratory diagnosis of *Clostridium difficile*–associated diarrhea and colitis: usefulness of premier cytoclone A+B enzyme immunoassay for combined detection of stool toxins and toxigenic *C. difficile* strains. *J Clin Microbiol* 2001;39:1996.

72. Landry ML, Topal J, Ferguson D, et al. Evaluation of biosite triage *Clostridium difficile* panel for rapid dete4ction of *Clostridium difficile* in stool samples. *J Clin Microbiol* 2001;39:1855.

73. Kato N, Ou C-Y, Kato H, et al. Detection of toxigenic *Clostridium difficile* in stool specimens by the polymerase chain reaction. *J Infect Dis* 1993;167:455.

74. Kuhl SJ, Tang YJ, Navarro L, et al. Diagnosis and monitoring of *Clostridium difficile* infections with the polymerase chain reaction. *Clin Infect Dis* 1993;16(suppl 4):234.

75. Peterson LR, Kelly PJ, Nordbrock HA. Role of culture and toxin detection in laboratory testing for diagnosis of *Clostridium difficile*–associated diarrhea. *Eur J Clin Microbiol Infect Dis* 1996;15:330.

76. Bond F, Payne G, Borriello SP, et al. Usefulness of culture in the diagnosis of *Clostridium difficile* infection. *Eur J Clin Microbiol Infect Dis* 1995;14:223.

77. Gerding DN, Johnson S, Peterson LIZ, et al. *Clostridium difficile*–associated diarrhea and colitis. *Infect Control Hosp Epidemiol* 1995;16:459.

78. McFarland LV, Surawicz CM, Stamm EW. Risk factors for *Clostridium difficile* carriage and *C. difficile*-associated diarrhea in a cohort of hospitalized patients. *J Infect Dis* 1990;162:678.

79. Samore MH, DeGirolami PC, Tlucko A, et al. *Clostridium difficile* colonization and diarrhea at a tertiary care hospital. *Clin Infect Dis* 1994;18:181.

80. Samore MH, Venkataraman L, DeGirolami PC, et al. Clinical and molecular epidemiology of sporadic and clustered cases of nosocomial *Clostridium difficile* diarrhea. *Am J Med* 1996;100:32.

81. Simor AE, Yake SL, Tsimidis K. Infection due to *Clostridium difficile* among elderly residents of a long-term care facility. *Clin Infect Dis* 1993;17:672.

82. Kim KH, Fekety R, Botts DH, et al. Isolation of *Clostridium difficile* from the environment and contacts of patients with antibiotic-associated colitis. *J Infect Dis* 1981;143:42.

83. Mulligan ME, George WL, Rolfe RD, et al. Epidemiological aspects of *Clostridium difficile*–induced diarrhea and colitis. *Am J Clin Nutr* 1981;33:2533.

84. Mody LR, Smith SM, Dever LL. *Clostridium difficile*–associated diarrhea in a VA medical center: clustering of cases, association with antibiotic usage, and impact on HIV-infected patients. *Infect Control Hosp Epidemiol* 2001;22:42.

85. Johnson S, Samore MH, Farrow KA, et al. Epidemics of diarrhea caused by a clindamycin-resistant strain of *Clostridium difficile* in four hospitals. *N Engl J Med* 1999;341:1645.

86. Chang VT, Nelson K. The role of physical proximity in nosocomial pneumonia diarrhea. *Clin Infect Dis* 2000;31:717.

87. Samore MH, Venkataraman L, De Girolami PC, et al. Clinical and molecular epidemiology of sporadic and clustered cases of nosocomial *Clostridium difficile* diarrhea. *Am J Med* 1996;100:32.

88. Pear SM, Williamson TH, Bettin KM, et al. Decrease in nosocomial *Clostridium difficile*–associated diarrhea by restricting clindamycin use. *Ann Intern Med* 1994;120:272.

89. McNulty C, Logan M, Donald IP, et al. Successful control of *Clostridium difficile* infection in an elderly care unit through use of a restrictive antibiotic policy. *J Antimicrob Chemother* 1997;40:707.

90. Climo MN, Israel DS, Wong ES, et al. Hospital-wide restriction of clindamycin: effect on the incidence of *Clostridium difficile*–associated diarrhea and cost. *Ann Intern Med* 1998;128:989.

91. Brazier JS. An international study on the unification of nomenclature for typing *Clostridium difficile*. *Clin Infect Dis* 1995;20(suppl 2):325.

92. Gerding DN, Olson M, Peterson R, et al. *Clostridium difficile*–associated diarrhea and colitis in adults. A prospective case controlled epidemiologic study. *Arch Intern Med* 1986;146:95.

93. Brazier JS. An international study on the unification of nomenclature for typing *Clostridium difficile*. *Clin Infect Dis* 1995;20(suppl 2):325.

94. Novak E, Lee JE, Seckman CE, et al. Unfavorable effect of atropine-diphenoxylate (Lomotil) therapy in lincomycin-caused diarrhea. *JAMA* 1976;235:1451.

95. Guerrant RL. Practice guidelines for the management of infectious diarrhea. *Clin Infect Dis* 2001;32:331.

96. Bartlett JG. Treatment of *Clostridium difficile* colitis. *Gastroenterology* 1985; 89:1192.
97. Wenisch C, Parschalk B, Hasenhundl M, et al. Comparison of vancomycin, metronidazole, and fusidic acid for the treatment of *Clostridium difficile*–associated diarrhea. *Clin Infect Dis* 1996;22:813.
98. Centers for Disease Control and Prevention. Recommendation for preventing the spread of vancomycin resistance. *MMWR* 1995;44(RR-12):1.
99. Guzman R, Kirkpatrick J, Forward K, et al. Failure of parenteral metronidazole in the treatment of pseudomembranous colitis [Letter]. *J Infect Dis* 1988;158:1146.
100. Lipsett PA, Samantaray DK, Tam ML, et al. Pseudomembranous colitis: a surgical disease? *Surgery* 1994;116:491.
101. Walters BA, Roberts R, Stafford R, et al. Relapse of antibiotic-associated colitis: endogenous persistence of *Clostridium difficile* during vancomycin therapy. *Gut* 1983;24:206.
102. McFarland LV, Surawicz CM, Greenberg RN, et al. A randomized, placebo-controlled trial of *Saccharomyces boulardii* in combination with standard antibiotics for *Clostridium difficile* disease. *JAMA* 1994;271:1913.
103. McFarland LV, Surawicz CM, Greenberg RN, et al. A randomized placebo-controlled trial of *Saccharomyces boulardii* in combination with standard antibiotics for *Clostridium difficile* disease. *JAMA* 1994;271:1913.
104. Gorbach S, Chang T-W Goldin B. Successful treatment of relapsing *C. difficile* colitis with *Lactobacillus* GG. *Lancet* 1987;2:1519.
105. Leung DY, Kelly CP, Boguniewicz M, et al. Treatment with intravenously administered gamma globulin of chronic relapsing colitis induced by *Clostridium difficile* toxin. *J Pediatr* 1991;118:633.
106. Hassett J, Meyers S, McFarland L, et al. Recurrent *Clostridium difficile* infection in a patients with selective IgG1 deficiency treated with intravenous immune globulin and *Saccharomyces boulardii*. *Clin Infect Dis* 1885;20(suppl 2):266.
107. Schwan A, Sjolin S, Trottestam U, et al. Relapsing *Clostridium difficile* enterocolitis cured by rectal infusion of normal feces. *Scand J Infect Dis* 1984;16:211.
108. Tvede M, Rask-Madsen J: Bacteriotherapy for chronic relapsing *Clostridium difficile* diarrhoea in six patients. *Lancet* 1989;6:1156.
109. Johnson S, Gerding DS, Olson MM, et al. Prospective controlled study of vinyl glove use to interrupt *Clostridium difficile* nosocomial transmission. *Am J Med* 1990;88:137.

CHAPTER 75
Viral Gastroenteritis

Neil R. Blacklow

Viral gastroenteritis is an extremely common illness that affects all age groups worldwide. Both epidemic and endemic patterns of infection occur. In a comprehensive 10-year study of illnesses among American families, viral gastroenteritis was found to be second in frequency only to the common cold (1). It is responsible for a considerable loss of time from work and school (2), aside from the distress it produces in those afflicted. In the United States, viral gastroenteritis is a relatively benign and self-limited illness, although it can be severe, and even lethal, in infants and in elderly or debilitated patients (3).

HISTORY

The agents responsible for this common illness were not defined until the 1970s and 1980s. This is in marked contrast to the viruses of acute respiratory tract disease and common childhood febrile and exanthematous illnesses, which were defined in the 1950s and 1960s. The reason for the delay was the inability to cultivate the responsible organisms from diarrheal stools in cell cultures and laboratory animals. Controlled epidemiologic studies in the 1950s and 1960s had shown that known cultivatable enteric viruses such as echovirus and coxsackievirus were not important causes of gastroenteritis (4). Studies performed during the 1940s and 1950s established that the disease syndrome could be induced and serially propagated in volunteers

by oral administration of bacteria-free filtrates of diarrheal stool, but these infectious materials failed to yield cultivatable agents (5). The causative viruses were discovered only when electron microscopy and advanced laboratory techniques that could identify agents without *in vitro* cultivation were available. The result was the discovery in the 1970s of two major medically important causes of viral gastroenteritis, rotavirus and Norwalk virus (6,7). It is interesting that the various viral gastroenteritis agents known today still are not cultivatable or replicate inefficiently *in vitro*. Thus, antigen and nucleic acid detection techniques and electron microscopy are the mainstays for detecting viral gastroenteritis agents.

ETIOLOGIC AGENTS

There are four viruses that are medically important causes of gastroenteritis (Table 75.1). Detailed discussion of the characteristics of each of these viruses is provided in Part VII of this text. The four agents for which an important role in diarrhea is well established are rotavirus (group A), calicivirus (for which Norwalk virus is the prototype), astrovirus, and enteric adenovirus types 40 and 41 (8–11). Several other viruses may cause gastroenteritis, but their medical importance is uncertain. These include non–group A rotavirus, coronavirus/torovirus, Aichi virus, picobirnavirus, and pestivirus. Non–group A rotavirus (particularly groups B and C) definitely causes gastroenteritis, but the extent to which and frequency with which this occurs are unclear (12–16). Coronavirus-like particles, including torovirus, have been detected in feces in some studies, but clearcut and confirmed disease associations have been difficult to establish (17–19). A novel picornavirus, Aichi virus, has been identified in gastroenteritis outbreaks in Japan and in travelers to Southeast Asia, but worldwide epidemiologic studies of its medical importance are lacking (20,21). Picobirnavirus, an agent containing bisegmented double-stranded RNA, has been detected in stools of children with diarrhea, but no epidemiologic studies have been reported (22,23). Pestivirus antigens have been found in preliminary studies of the stools of some infants with gastroenteritis (24); however, viral particles have yet to be detected, and the medical significance of these findings is unclear.

The four medically important agents of viral gastroenteritis belong to diverse virologic groupings (Table 75.1). Two are larger agents (rotavirus and enteric adenovirus) and the other two are small round viral particles (calicivirus and astrovirus, which are discussed together in Chapter 263). All of the viral gastroenteritis agents (except enteric adenovirus) contain RNA. Only rotavirus, enteric adenovirus, and astrovirus have replicated in and been adapted to cell culture, and for each of these viruses, the efficiency of viral isolation from human stools is low. Thus, cell culture is not used for clinical diagnosis of viral gastroenteritis.

The individual viral gastroenteritis agents have unique characteristics. Rotavirus possesses 11 segments of double-stranded RNA, and four types (defined by glycoprotein and protease-sensitive protein analysis) are medically important causes of diarrhea; Norwalk virus is the prototype 27-nm virus for the calicivirus family which contains multiple strains classified in two genuses called Norwalk-like viruses and Sapporo-like viruses; enteric adenovirus types 40 and 41 are specific serotypes that are quite fastidious in their requirements for cultivation *in vitro*, in contrast to the other conventional adenoviruses; and astrovirus has a star shape contained within a sphere.

Despite our knowledge of viral gastroenteritis agents, a specific agent has not been identified for approximately one third

TABLE 75.1. Medically Important Agents of Viral Gastroenteritis

Virus	Virion diameter (nm)	Nucleic acid type	Replication in cell culture	Laboratory diagnostic tests
Rotavirus	70–75	dsRNA	Yes	ELISA, EM, NAA
Calicivirus (e.g., Norwalk virus[a])	27–40	ssRNA	No	ELISA, NAA, IEM in research laboratories
Enteric adenovirus	70–80	dsDNA	Yes	ELISA, EM, NAA
Astrovirus	27–32	ssRNA	Yes	EM, ELISA, NAA

ss, single-stranded; ds, double-stranded; ELISA, enzyme-linked immunosorbent assay; EM, electron microscopy; IEM, immunoelectron microscopy; NAA, viral nucleic acid analysis.
[a]Also called Norovirus.

of all suspected cases of viral gastroenteritis when all available research diagnostic techniques are employed. Presumably, additional agents remain to be discovered.

EPIDEMIOLOGY

Viral gastroenteritis occurs primarily in two epidemiologically distinct clinical forms (25). One entity develops predominantly in infants and young children and is usually sporadic and occasionally epidemic. This form of illness is typified by rotavirus, a major human pathogen that produces severe diarrhea that lasts for 3 to 9 days and is usually accompanied by vomiting and fever (26). Disease typically occurs during the winter months in temperate climates (27). The incubation period is short (1–3 days) and spread is by the fecal-oral route. Infants and children 4 to 24 months old, who are affected most often (27), are usually symptomatic and may develop severe diarrhea and dehydration requiring oral, or even parenteral, fluid replacement. Adult contacts of ill infants usually develop asymptomatic infections, and only rarely severe clinical disease (28,29). Nosocomial rotaviral outbreaks are well described. Rotavirus accounts for 30% to 50% of pediatric cases of gastroenteritis that necessitate hospitalization and probably a similar proportion of outpatient diarrhea in this age group. It is estimated that 50,000 children are hospitalized with rotaviral diarrhea in the United States each year and about 20 die (30). Enteric adenovirus types 40 and 41 are agents of pediatric diarrhea in temperate climates; they are reported to produce 3% to 10% of cases (10,31). Some calicivirus strains also cause this syndrome (32) and in one study were responsible for 3% of diarrhea cases in day care settings (33). Astrovirus causes about 2% to 10% of endemic pediatric diarrhea worldwide, and is an important pathogen in day care center diarrhea (11,34,35).

The second clinical entity is characteristically epidemic and consists of family and community-wide outbreaks of gastroenteritis among school-aged children, family contacts, and adults. This form of illness is typified by the prototype calicivirus strain, Norwalk virus. In contrast to the first clinical entity, infants and young children are typically spared. Outbreaks occur throughout the year without a seasonal predilection (9). The incubation period is quite short (12–48 hours), and spread is by the fecal-oral route (36). Because of the short incubation period and explosive disease onset, a respiratory route of spread is hypothesized, and some limited epidemiologic evidence exists to back this theory (37,38). Vomiting, diarrhea, or both develop rapidly and typically last only 1 to 2 days (36). A variety of descriptive labels have been applied to this clinical entity, such as winter vomiting disease, epidemic collapse, epidemic diarrhea and vomiting, and acute infectious nonbacterial gastroenteritis (5). Approximately 96% of viral gastroenteritis outbreaks in the United States are associated with Norwalk virus (39). Epidemiologic settings often involve fecally contaminated foods (most common), contaminated drinking or swimming water, ingestion of raw or inadequately cooked shellfish, recreational camps, military populations, cruise ships, nursing homes, schools, and community or family locations. Calicivirus strains other than Norwalk virus (e.g., Snow Mountain, Hawaii, Mexico, Southampton, and Toronto) are all derived from epidemic outbreaks, similar to Norwalk virus itself, and their epidemiologic settings appear to be similar to those of Norwalk virus (40–42).

Non–group A rotavirus (group B) has been described as producing medically important disease primarily in China, where severe outbreaks of diarrheal disease with a waterborne route of spread have affected many adults as well as children (13,14). Enteric coronavirus, also called torovirus, remains a controversial potential pathogen; some reports associate it with severe necrotizing diarrhea in newborns (43) and with infection, sometimes including bloody diarrhea, in immunocompromised hospitalized children (19). Its pathogenic potential is obscured by its presence in the stools of both ill and well persons, particularly in developing countries (17).

PATHOGENESIS

The pathogenesis of viral gastroenteritis is similar for each agent. The most comprehensive data available are derived from studies of human volunteers infected experimentally by oral administration of Norwalk virus. At the time of disease onset, a mucosal lesion develops in the proximal small intestine, which has been examined in biopsy specimens taken at the duodenojejunal junction (44). This lesion (Fig. 75.1) has also been found in volunteers infected with another calicivirus, Hawaii virus (45). Villi are blunted, and there is an intense inflammation of the lamina propria with ingress of mononuclear cells and polymorphonuclear leukocytes. The crypts of the villi are hypertrophic, and although the intestinal mucosal surface epithelial cells are grossly intact, they are clearly damaged, as evidenced by their vacuolization. Electron microscopic examination of these epithelial cells reveals damage to their microvillous architectural substructure. The virus and its antigens have not been detected within involved mucosal cells by electron microscopy or immunofluorescence, probably because of the virus's small size and patchy distribution. These histopathologic changes seen with the Norwalk or Hawaii strain of calicivirus persist for up to 2 weeks, long after clinical recovery has taken place.

Accompanying this small intestinal lesion is bowel dysfunction manifested by malabsorption of fat and xylose (4,5,44). Malabsorption has been found for at least 1 week after disease onset. Decreased levels of intestinal brush border enzymes occur during disease, whereas adenylate cyclase levels remain normal within epithelial cells of the small intestine.

In contrast to the small intestine, the gastric mucosa remains histologically normal during Norwalk virus illness, as does its

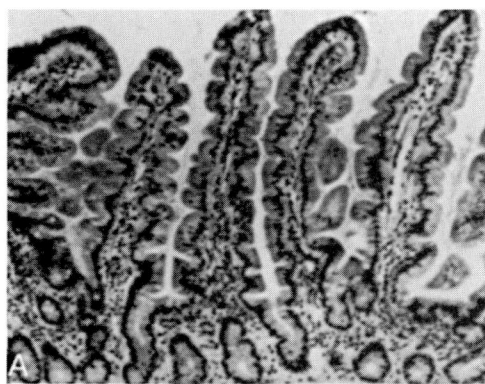
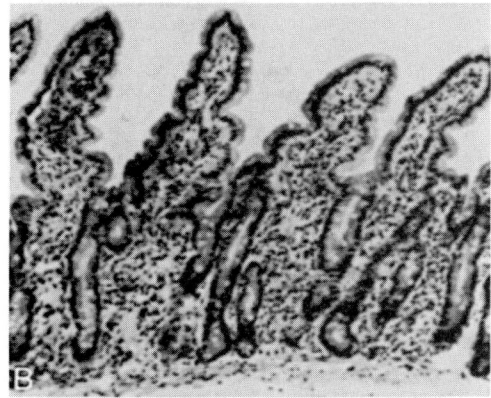
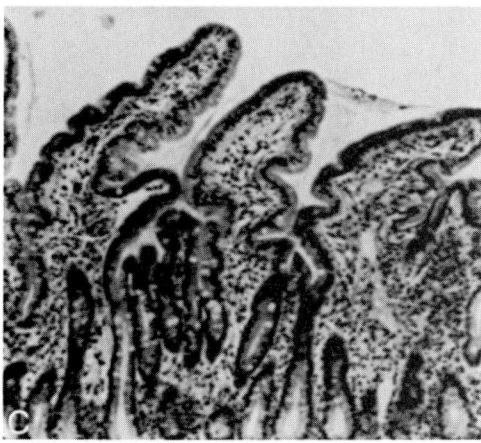

Figure 75.1. Biopsy specimens of the small intestine before and after oral ingestion of Norwalk agent (hematoxylin and eosin, original magnification ×100). **A:** Before ingestion, villi are tall, and the cellularity of the lamina propria is normal. **B:** Two days after ingestion, the villi are shortened, the crypts are hypertrophied and contain increased numbers of mitoses, and the cellularity of the lamina propria is increased. **C:** Six days after ingestion, shortened villi, hypertrophied crypts, and increased mitoses persist. (From Schreiber DS, Blacklow NR, Trier JS. The mucosal lesion of the proximal small intestine in acute infectious non-bacterial gastroenteritis. *N Engl J Med* 1973;288:1319, with permission.)

secretions of acid, pepsin, and intrinsic factor (46); however, gastric emptying is markedly delayed, as evidenced by physiologic studies that indicate altered gastric motor function (47). This may explain the frequency of nausea and vomiting seen with Norwalk virus illness. Thus, use of the term *gastroenteritis,* rather than just *enteritis,* seems justified for this infection. The colonic mucosa remains normal, a finding that is consistent with the usual absence of fecal leukocytes in this syndrome.

The pathogenesis of human rotavirus infection has been studied in naturally infected children, and the findings resemble those seen with Norwalk virus–infected volunteers (48). In contrast to Norwalk virus, however, rotavirus and its antigens have been detected within the mucosal epithelial cells of the small intestine (49), and in rare fatal cases the involvement of the virus may extend from its usual duodenal and jejunal location to the large bowel (50). The major pathophysiologic mechanism for rotaviral diarrhea seems to be decreased absorption of salt and water because of selective infection of the absorptive intestinal villus cells, resulting in net fluid secretion, isotonic dehydration, and compensated metabolic acidosis (51). In this regard, the rotavirus nonstructural glycoprotein NSP4 causes a toxin-like effect, inducing diarrhea in a murine model (52), and the virus also activates the murine enteric nervous system that regulates intestinal fluid absorption and secretion (53). Dehydration occurs frequently but is normally less than 5%, except in severe cases, the most extreme of which require hospitalization.

CLINICAL MANIFESTATIONS

Viral gastroenteritis can vary widely in its clinical features, ranging from asymptomatic or mild illness to complete prostration, dehydration, and circulatory collapse. Diarrhea is typical for a noninflammatory form of gastroenteritis, with watery stools lacking fecal leukocytes and blood. The clinical characteristics of rotavirus and calicivirus (e.g., Norwalk virus) illnesses are often indistinguishable, but there can be differences.

Rotavirus illness usually has a sudden onset of fever and vomiting in infants and young children, and watery diarrhea often develops later (26). Although fever is typically low grade, it can be high in some dehydrated patients. Diarrhea normally lasts from 3 to 9 days and is self-limited, although relapses occasionally occur. Chronic or prolonged diarrhea can occur in patients who are immunosuppressed (e.g., for bone marrow transplantation) or have primary immunodeficiency diseases. Findings referable to the respiratory tract may occur, such as pharyngeal or tympanic membrane erythema (54), but the virus has not been detected in the respiratory tract of patients with gastroenteritis. Severe dehydration is more common with rotavirus disease than with other enteric viral, bacterial, or parasitic pathogens. There are numerous reports of rotavirus in association with a variety of syndromes such as intussusception, Kawasaki syndrome, Reye's syndrome, and inflammatory bowel disease; however, the relationships are probably not causal. A disease association seems strongest for some cases of neonatal necrotizing enterocolitis (43).

Calicivirus (e.g., Norwalk virus) illness develops abruptly. Some patients experience primarily vomiting, others diarrhea, and still others both (36). Affected persons often also have abdominal cramps, myalgia, low-grade fever, headache, or malaise. The illness typically renders the patient prostrate and unable to work; however, it is short-lived, usually resolving spontaneously 24 to 48 hours after the onset of symptoms. Some patients have developed a transient leukocytosis, but the white cell count remains normal in most. Fatalities are extremely rare and are limited to elderly and debilitated persons (3).

DIAGNOSIS

Clinical and epidemiologic features of an acute diarrheal illness may suggest viral gastroenteritis, but usually the findings are not distinctive enough to confirm the diagnosis. Some nonviral pathogens commonly produce a noninflammatory diarrhea with watery stools lacking fecal leukocytes—a clinical picture that is indistinguishable from viral gastroenteritis. Thus, to diagnose viral diarrhea with certainty, the specific causal agent must be detected. The primary diagnostic tests are immunoassays, principally enzyme-linked immunosorbent assay (ELISA), and electron microscopy, which can detect the presence of the virus or its antigens in stool specimens. Nucleic acid hybridization and reverse transcription polymerase chain reaction (RT-PCR) assays are also available in research laboratory settings (Table 75.1).

Rotavirus infection can be diagnosed in stool specimens rapidly in many hospital diagnostic laboratories with the use of commercially available ELISA test kits. More sensitive than rotavirus latex agglutination tests, ELISAs permit a specific diagnosis within 4 hours. Tests that use monoclonal antibodies against rotavirus seem to be more specific and sensitive than those that use polyclonal sera (55). Rotavirus in feces usually correlates with acute diarrhea caused by this pathogen.

Infection with enteric adenovirus types 40 and 41 can be diagnosed rapidly in stool specimens using commercially available ELISA test kits (56) as can diagnosis of astrovirus gastroenteritis (57).

Specific diagnosis of calicivirus infection is limited to specialized research centers. Electron microscopy, specifically immuno-electron microscopy, is available as a diagnostic tool in only a few medical centers, and considerable technical experience is necessary with the use of an electron microscope specifically for the diagnosis of calicivirus gastroenteritis. Nucleic acid hybridization and RT-PCR assays are developed to diagnose calicivirus infection in research centers, and while very sensitive, are still too strain specific for widespread diagnostic use (58–61).

TREATMENT

Specific antiviral therapy is not available for any of the agents of viral gastroenteritis, so therapy is directed at fluid replacement. Most patients can be managed with oral rehydration solutions that are commercially available and contain glucose or sucrose plus electrolytes (62,63) (see Chapter 78). Severely dehydrated patients, usually those who are elderly, debilitated, or infant, may require parenteral fluid and electrolyte replacement (62). Immunodeficient children with chronic rotavirus infection have responded to therapy with human milk containing rotavirus antibody. Normal children with rotavirus diarrhea have received treatment with oral immunoglobulins with varying results, perhaps related to the small amounts of antibodies used in some studies (64). Chicken egg yolk immunoglobulin, hyperimmunized with human rotavirus, when used as therapy in infected children, has produced modest improvement in the severity of diarrhea (65). In experimentally infected volunteers, bismuth subsalicylate reduced the severity and duration of abdominal cramping caused by Norwalk virus.

PREVENTION

Considerable effort has been directed at the development of a live attenuated oral vaccine to prevent rotavirus infection by the four medically important types. A rhesus rotavirus-based tetravalent vaccine was licensed for use in the United States in August 1998 based on several vaccine trials demonstrating 49% to 68% efficacy in preventing rotavirus diarrheal episodes and 69% to 91% in preventing severe rotavirus disease (30,66,67). Fourteen months later the vaccine was withdrawn from use because of an

apparent association with an increased rate of intussusception in vaccine recipients during the first 2 weeks postvaccination (68), representing an additional risk of 1 in 10,000 for intussusception. Subsequent analyses have challenged the risk of this association, particularly in the context that up to 1 in 200 children die of rotavirus disease in some developing regions (69–71). Considerable discussion is ongoing about risk/benefit calculations for this vaccine; meanwhile, other candidate vaccines are being evaluated. A candidate Norwalk virus vaccine, composed of viral capsid protein, is under evaluation for potential use in prevention of illness in the short term, as for travelers (72).

Standard infection control measures for enteric infections, emphasizing hand washing, are required for prevention of nosocomial viral gastroenteritis in hospital and nursing home units as well as in homes and day care centers. Cohorting of infected patients and staff can control disease transmission in hospitals, nursing homes, and day care centers. Use of proper food preparation and water purification practices can prevent Norwalk virus and other calicivirus disease outbreaks.

Controversy exists over whether some infants may derive protection against severe rotavirus diarrhea from breast-feeding (73), but if this protection exists, it clearly is not complete, nor is it seen in all infants. Oral administration of human serum globulin possessing rotaviral antibodies provides significant protection against illness for low-birth-weight infants (74).

REFERENCES

1. Dingle JH, Badger GF, Feller AE, et al. A study of illness in a group of Cleveland families. I. Plan of study and certain general observations. *Am J Hyg* 1953; 58:16.
2. National Center for Health Statistics. *Current estimates from the Health Interview Survey, United States.* Rockville, MD: National Center of Health Statistics, 1973. U.S. Dept. of Health, Education, and Welfare publication (HRA) 74-1512.
3. Gangarosa RE, Glass RI, Lew JF, et al. Hospitalizations involving gastroenteritis in the United States, 1985: the special burden of the disease among the elderly. *Am J Epidemiol* 1992;135:281.
4. Schreiber DS, Trier JS, Blacklow NR. Recent advances in viral gastroenteritis. *Gastroenterology* 1977;73:174.
5. Blacklow NR, Dolin R, Fedson DS, et al. Acute infectious nonbacterial gastroenteritis: etiology and pathogenesis. *Ann Intern Med* 1972;76:993.
6. Kapikian AZ, Wyatt RG, Dolin R, et al. Visualization by immune electron microscopy of a 27-nm particle associated with acute infectious nonbacterial gastroenteritis. *J Virol* 1972;10:1075.
7. Bishop RF, Davidson GP, Holmes IH, et al. Detection of a new virus by electron microscopy of faecal extracts from children with acute gastroenteritis. *Lancet* 1974;1:149.
8. Brandt CD, Kim HW, Yolken RH, et al. Comparative epidemiology of two rotavirus serotypes and other viral agents associated with pediatric gastroenteritis. *Am J Epidemiol* 1979;110:243.
9. Kaplan JE, Gary GW, Baron RC, et al. Epidemiology of Norwalk gastroenteritis and the role of Norwalk virus in outbreaks of acute nonbacterial gastroenteritis. *Ann Intern Med* 1982;96:756.
10. Kotloff KL, Losonsky GA, Morris JG, et al. Enteric adenovirus infection and childhood diarrhea: an epidemiological study in three clinical settings. *Pediatrics* 1989;84:219.
11. Herrmann JE, Taylor DN, Echeverria P, et al. Astroviruses as a cause of gastroenteritis in children. *N Engl J Med* 1991;324:1757.
12. Dolin R, Treanor JJ, Madore HP. Novel agents of viral enteritis in humans. *J Infect Dis* 1987;155:365.
13. Hung T, Chen G, Wang C, et al. Waterborne outbreak of rotavirus diarrhoea in adults in China caused by a novel rotavirus. *Lancet* 1984;2:1139.
14. Sen A, Kobayashi N, Das S, et al. The evolution of human group B rotaviruses. *Lancet* 2001;357:198.
15. Nilsson M, Svenungsson B, Hedlund KO, et al. Incidence and genetic diversity of group C rotavirus among adults. *J Infect Dis* 2000;182:678.
16. Kuzuya M, Fujii R, Hamano M, et al. Seroepidemiology of human group C rotavirus in Japan based on a blocking enzyme-linked immunosorbent assay. *Clin Diag Lab Immunol* 2001;8:161.
17. Ashley C, Caul EO. Human enteric coronavirus. In: Farthing MJG, ed. *Viruses and the gut.* London: Swan Press, 1989:91–95.
18. Krishnan T, Naik TN. Electronmicroscopic evidence of torovirus like particles in children with diarrhoea. *Ind J Med Res* 1997;105:108.
19. Jamieson FB, Wang EEL, Bain C, et al. Human torovirus: a new nosocomial gastrointestinal pathogen. *J Infect Dis* 1998;178:1263.

20. Yamashita T, Sugiyama M, Tsuzuki K, et al. Application of a reverse transcription-PCR for identification and differentiation of Aichi virus, a new member of the picornavirus family associated with gastroenteritis in humans. *J Clin Microbiol* 2000;38:2955.

21. Yamashita T, Ito M, Tsuzuki H, et al. Identification of Aichi virus infection by measurement of immunoglobulin responses in an enzyme-linked immunosorbent assay. *J Clin Microbiol* 2001;39:4178.

22. Cascio A, Bosco M, Vizzi E, et al. Identification of picobirnavirus from faeces of Italian children suffering from acute diarrhea. *Eur J Epidemiol* 1996;12:545.

23. Chandra R. Picobirnavirus, a novel group of undescribed viruses of mammals and birds: a minireview. *Acta Virol* 1997;41:59.

24. Yolken R, Leister F, Almeido-Hill J, et al. Infantile gastroenteritis associated with excretion of pestivirus antigens. *Lancet* 1989;1:517.

25. Blacklow NR, Greenberg HB. Viral gastroenteritis. *N Engl J Med* 1991;325:252.

26. Rodriguez WJ, Kim HW, Arrobio JO, et al. Clinical features of acute gastroenteritis associated with human reovirus-like agent in infants and young children. *J Pediatr* 1977;91:188.

27. Kapikian AZ, Kim HW, Wyatt RG, et al. Human reovirus-like agent as the major pathogen associated with winter gastroenteritis in hospitalized infants and young children. *N Engl J Med* 1976;294:965.

28. Wenman WM, Hinde D, Feltham S, et al. Rotavirus infection in adults: results of a prospective family study. *N Engl J Med* 1979;301:303.

29. Echeverria P, Blacklow NR, Cukor G, et al. Rotavirus as a cause of severe gastroenteritis in adults. *J Clin Microbiol* 1983;18:663.

30. Centers for Disease Control and Prevention. Rotavirus vaccine for the prevention of rotavirus gastroenteritis among children. *MMWR* 1999;48(suppl):1–19.

31. Uhnoo I, Goran W, Lennart S, et al. Importance of enteric adenoviruses 40 and 41 in acute gastroenteritis in infants and young children. *J Clin Microbiol* 1984;20:365.

32. Pang XL, Joensuu J, Vesikari T. Human calicivirus-associated sporadic gastroenteritis in Finnish children less than two years of age followed prospectively during a rotavirus vaccine trial. *Pediatr Infect Dis* 1999;18:420.

33. Matson DO, Estes MK, Glass RI, et al. Human calicivirus-associated diarrhea in children attending day care centers. *J Infect Dis* 1989;159:71.

34. Lew JF, Moe CL, Monroe SS, et al. Astrovirus and adenovirus associated with diarrhea in children in day care settings. *J Infect Dis* 1991;164:673.

35. Blacklow NR, Herrmann JE. Astrovirus gastroenteritis. *Trans Am Clin Climatol Assoc* 1994;106:58.

36. Dolin R, Blacklow NR, DuPont H, et al. Transmission of acute infectious nonbacterial gastroenteritis to volunteers by oral administration of stool filtrates. *J Infect Dis* 1971;123:307.

37. Sawyer LA, Murphy JJ, Kaplan JE, et al. 25- to 30-nm virus particle associated with a hospital outbreak of acute gastroenteritis with evidence for airborne transmission. *Am J Epidemiol* 1988;127:1261.

38. Marks PJ, Vipond IB, Carlisle D, et al. Evidence for airborne transmission of Norwalk-like virus (NLV) in a hotel restaurant. *Epidemiol Infect* 2000;124:481.

39. Fankhauser RL, Noel JS, Monroe SS, et al. Molecular epidemiology of "Norwalk-like viruses" in outbreaks of gastroenteritis in the United States. *J Infect Dis* 1998;178:1571.

40. Ando T, Monroe SS, Gentsch JR, et al. Detection and differentiation of antigenically distinct small round-structured viruses (Norwalk-like viruses) by reverse transcription-PCR and Southern hybridization. *J Clin Microbiol* 1995;33:64.

41. Lew JF, Kapikian AZ, Valdesuso J, et al. Molecular characterization of Hawaii virus and other Norwalk-like viruses: evidence for genetic polymorphism among human caliciviruses. *J Infect Dis* 1994;170:535.

42. Wang J, Jiang X, Madore HP, et al. Sequence diversity of small, round-structured viruses in the Norwalk virus group. *J Virol* 1994;68:5982.

43. Vaucher YE, Ray CG, Minnich LL, et al. Pleomorphic, enveloped, virus-like particles associated with gastrointestinal illness in neonates. *J Infect Dis* 1982;145:27.

44. Schreiber DS, Blacklow NR, Trier JS. The mucosal lesion of the proximal small intestine in acute infectious non-bacterial gastroenteritis. *N Engl J Med* 1973;288:1318.

45. Schreiber DS, Blacklow NR, Trier JS. The small intestinal lesion induced by Hawaii agent acute infectious nonbacterial gastroenteritis. *J Infect Dis* 1974;129:705.

46. Widerlite L, Trier JS, Blacklow NR, et al. Structure of the gastric mucosa in acute infectious nonbacterial gastroenteritis. *Gastroenterology* 1975;68:425.

47. Meeroff JC, Schreiber DS, Trier JS, et al. Abnormal gastric motor function in viral gastroenteritis. *Ann Intern Med* 1980;92:370.

48. Davidson GP, Barnes GL. Structural and functional abnormalities of the small intestine in infants and young children with rotavirus enteritis. *Acta Paediatr Scand* 1979;68:181.

49. Bishop RF, Davidson GP, Holmes IH, et al. Virus particles in epithelial cells of duodenal mucosa from children with acute nonbacterial gastroenteritis. *Lancet* 1973;2:1281.

50. Carolson JAK, Middleton PJ, Szymanski MT, et al. Fatal rotavirus gastroenteritis: an analysis of 21 cases. *Am J Dis Child* 1978;132:477.

51. Tallett S, MacKenzie C, Middleton P, et al. Clinical laboratory and epidemiological features of viral gastroenteritis in infants and children. *Pediatrics* 1977;60:217.

52. Ball JM, Tian P, Zeng CQY, et al. Age-dependent diarrhea induced by a rotaviral nonstructural glycoprotein. *Science* 1996;272:101.

53. Lundgren O, Peregrin AT, Persson K, et al. Role of the enteric nervous system in the fluid and electrolyte secretion of rotavirus diarrhea. *Science* 2000;287:491.

54. Lewis HM, Parry JV, Davies HA, et al. A year's experience of the rotavirus syndrome and its association with respiratory illness. *Arch Dis Child* 1979;54:339.

55. Dennehy PH, Gauntlet DR, Tente WE. Comparison of nine commercial immunoassays for the detection of rotavirus in fecal specimens. *J Clin Microbiol* 1988;26:1630.

56. Vizzi E, Ferraro D, Cascio A, et al. Detection of enteric adenoviruses 40 and 41 in stool specimens by monoclonal antibody-based enzyme immunoassays. *Res Virol* 1996;147:333.

57. Glass RI, Noel J, Mitchell DK, et al. The changing epidemiology of astrovirus-associated gastroenteritis: a review. *Arch Virol* 1996;12(suppl):287.

58. Jiang X, Wang J, Graham DY, et al. Detection of Norwalk virus in stool by polymerase chain reaction. *J Clin Microbiol* 1992;30:2529.

59. DeLeon R, Matsui SM, Baric RS, et al. Detection of Norwalk virus in stool specimens by reverse transcriptase-polymerase chain reaction and nonradioactive oligoprobes. *J Clin Microbiol* 1992;30:3151.

60. Altmar RL, Estes MK. Diagnosis of noncultivatable gastroenteritis viruses, the human caliciviruses. *Clin Microbiol Rev* 2001;14:15.

61. Centers for Disease Control and Prevention. "Norwalk-like viruses." Public health consequences and outbreak management. *MMWR* 2001;50(suppl):1–17.

62. Santosham M, Daun RS, Dillman L, et al. Oral rehydration therapy of infantile diarrhea. A controlled study of well-nourished children hospitalized in the United States and Panama. *N Engl J Med* 1985;306:159.

63. Santosham M, Burns B, Nadkarni V, et al. Oral rehydration therapy for acute diarrhea in ambulatory children in the United States: a double-blind comparison of four different solutions. *Pediatrics* 1985;76:159.

64. Hammarstrom L. Passive immunity against rotavirus in infants. *Acta Paediatr Suppl* 1999;430:127.

65. Sarker SA, Casswall TH, Juneja LR, et al. Randomized, placebo-controlled, clinical trial of hyperimmunized chicken egg yolk immunoglobulin in children with rotavirus diarrhea. *J Pediatr Gastroenterol Nutr* 2001;32:19.

66. Rennels MB, Glass RI, Dennehy PH, et al. Safety and efficacy of high-dose rhesus-human reassortant rotavirus vaccines—report of the national multicenter trial. *Pediatrics* 1996;97:7.

67. Perez-Schael I, Guntinas MJ, Perez M, et al. Efficacy of the rhesus rotavirus-based quadrivalent vaccine in infants and young children in Venezuela. *N Eng J Med* 1997;337:1181.

68. Murphy TV, Gargiullo PM, Massoudi MS, et al. Intussusception among infants given an oral rotavirus vaccine. *N Engl J Med* 2001;344:564.

69. Weijer C. The future of research into rotavirus vaccine. *BMJ* 2000;321:525.

70. Chang HGH, Smith PF, Ackelsberg J, et al. Intussusception, rotavirus diarrhea, and rotavirus vaccine use among children in New York state. *Pediatrics* 2001;108:54.

71. Simonsen L, Morens DM, Elixhauser A, et al. Effect of rotavirus vaccination programme on trends in admission of infants to hospital for intussusception. *Lancet* 2001;358:1224.

72. Tackett CO, Mason MS, Losonsky G, et al. Human immune responses to a novel Norwalk virus vaccine in transgenic potatoes. *J Infect Dis* 2000;182:302.

73. Cushing AH, Anderson L. Diarrhea in breast-fed and non-breast-fed infants. *Pediatrics* 1982;70:921.

74. Barnes GL, Doyle IW, Hewson PH, et al. A randomised trial of oral gamma-globulin in low-birth-weight infants infected with rotavirus. *Lancet* 1982;1:1371.

CHAPTER 76
Traveler's Diarrhea

Sherwood L. Gorbach

On the scale of life's tribulations, traveler's diarrhea (TD) is neither the most perilous nor the most debilitating illness, but an episode of intestinal agonies during a trip abroad can certainly rank among the more memorable events of a lifetime. Diarrheal disease has plagued travelers for centuries. Whether the trip is for business or pleasure, military conquest or amusement, TD has infiltrated all ranks, given rise to numerous theories of causation, and achieved worldwide fame by its various euphemisms, some of which are lilting, others scatologic. Among the approximately 300 million travelers who cross their national borders each year, about 16 million travel from industrialized countries to developing countries. In view of an incidence of diarrhea in the range of 30% to 50%, it can be said, at least for these hapless travelers, that travel broadens their minds as it loosens their bowels.

Diarrheal disorders have been noted in hippocratic writings and in the Bible. Travelers throughout the ages have referred discreetly in their journals to episodes of intestinal indisposition. But the credit for scientific study of TD belongs to Kean, who undertook a classic series of investigations in the 1950s of students traveling to Europe and Mexico (1,2). Besides describing the clinical and epidemiologic features, he made the seminal observation, in a well-designed, placebo-controlled trial, that antimicrobial drugs can provide protection against the illness, thereby implicating bacterial pathogens as the cause (3). In his final contribution to this subject, Kean participated in the team effort that led to the discovery of enterotoxigenic *Escherichia coli* (ETEC) as the major culprit in this illness (4).

CHARACTERISTICS OF THE PATHOGENS

Traditional folklore of TD has spawned such etiologic theories as change in the water, too much noonday sun, spicy foods, and the general vicissitudes of travel. As improved laboratory methods became available, particularly testing for ETEC (4,5), it became apparent that TD is caused in the main by infectious microorganisms that are acquired in food and drink (6–9). Several studies have isolated specific microbial pathogens from the feces of sick tourists. The causal link between infection and clinical disease has been solidified by field trials that have demonstrated the efficacy of antibacterial drugs in preventing and treating TD (8,10–13); indeed, prevention rates of 80% or more, achieved with a variety of antimicrobial drugs, strongly implicate bacterial pathogens, and probably gram-negative enteric organisms, as the cause of most TD cases.

Etiologic studies of TD have been carried out in many parts of the world. Travelers to Mexico have undergone the most intensive scrutiny: 21 reports have been published since 1974 (4,5,14–32). There have also been 9 investigations of TD in other parts of Latin America (6,32–39) and the Caribbean (31,32) as well as 11 investigations of travelers to Asia (31,32,40–48), 5 studies of travelers to Africa (32,39,49–51), and other studies of around-the-world journeys (52) and cruise ships (53). An array of pathogens have been found, but it is apparent that the leading culprits are various forms of *E. coli*, particularly ETEC and enteroaggregative *E. coli* (EAEC) (Table 76.1). Some geographic differences have become apparent in the isolation rates of ETEC in travelers. In Latin America, for example, the median isolation rate of ETEC in TD cases has been 42% (range 26%–72%), compared with a median

of 16% in Asia (range 0%–37%) (9,51,52,54–56). EAEC has been recognized as a major cause of TD. These strains were isolated in 26% of travelers to Mexico, Jamaica, and Goa (57). EAEC was second only to ETEC, and decreased the prevalence of cases with unexplained cause from 51% to 37% (31). Enteroinvasive strains of *E. coli* similar to *Shigella* account for 5% of TD cases in Mexico, according to one study (58).

Shigella species have been encountered in approximately 10% of TD cases, although the rate of isolation varies from 0% to more than 20% (15,22,24,25). The disease caused by *Shigella* tends to be more severe than the usual form of TD. In a report from Cancun, Mexico, *Shigella dysenteriae* type 1 was isolated from tourists (59). This is the most virulent strain of *Shigella*, and in some of these cases the disease was associated with the hemolytic-uremic syndrome. In addition, many of these strains were resistant to trimethoprim-sulfamethoxazole (TMP-SMX).

Salmonella organisms are found in less than 5% of TD cases, although the incidence is higher among travelers to Asia, particularly in the more developed areas of Asia, than in travelers to Latin America or Africa (6,7,9). There is also a geographic difference in isolation rates of *Campylobacter jejuni*, which accounts for 15% to 20% of TD cases in Thailand and Bangladesh (47,60), compared with less than 5% in Mexico (27) and elsewhere. Vibrios, particularly *Vibrio parahaemolyticus*, and *Aeromonas* species have also been isolated more often in travelers to Asia and North Africa than to Latin America or Africa (6,7,9,42,43,45–47, 61,62).

Intestinal protozoa are found in 0% to 12% of travelers with acute diarrhea (1). *Giardia lamblia* is a hazard to travelers in Leningrad (63), and was also common in persons who stayed in Nepal for more than 2 weeks (64), but not necessarily in Latin America and other parts of Asia (4,13,14,47,60). Amebiasis, which has been characterized by Elsdon Dew as the "refuge of the diagnostically destitute," is relatively uncommon in Mexico (4,14) and Asia (42,47,60). *Cryptosporidium* has been isolated only sporadically in travelers (65–67). Microsporidium has been found in a few travelers, especially when polymerase chain reaction on stool is used, and it seems to be a particular hazard in travelers infected with with human immunodeficiency virus (68,69). *Cyclospora* has been identified in the stools of travelers with chronic diarrhea in Nepal and South America (70).

Viral diarrhea is generally thought to be more common in children than in adults, but rotavirus has been isolated from adult travelers in Mexico (14,18,20,25,71) and Honduras (34,35), as well as Asia (32,40,41,47). In a study of viral pathogens in the stools of U.S. military personnel with diarrhea who were deployed in South America and West Africa, rotavirus was found in 11% and Norwalk virus in 10% (39). Rotaviruses and enteric adenoviruses were found in 9% of travelers to East Africa, Jamaica, and Goa (72).

Several studies have reported more than one pathogen in TD cases, up to 15% in Mexico (14,29) and 33% in Thailand (47) and in multiple destinations (52). To confuse the issue further, no pathogens have been identified, despite careful laboratory study, in more than 40% of cases, from all parts of the world (4,5,12–15,19,21,22,25–27,33,41,47,49,52,73). The high incidence of mixed infections, along with the inability to isolate pathogens in many cases, casts some doubt on the veracity of etiologic studies altogether. Nevertheless, the striking efficacy of prophylaxis and treatment directed against bacterial pathogens suggests that TD is indeed a bacterial infection in most cases.

EPIDEMIOLOGY

TD is a syndrome consisting of a twofold or greater increase in the frequency of bowel movements, usually unformed, and commonly associated with other symptoms such as abdominal

TABLE 76.1.   Microbial Pathogens in Traveler's Diarrhea

Pathogen	Frequency Average (%)	Frequency Range (%)
Enterotoxigenic *Escherichia coli*	40–60	0–72
Enteroadherent *E. coli*	15	—
Invasive *E. coli*	<5	0–5
Shigella	10	0–30
Salmonella	<5	0–15
Campylobacter	<5	0–15
Vibrio	<5	0–30
Aeromonas	<5	0–30
Rotavirus	5	0–36
Giardia lamblia	<5	0–6
Entamoeba histolytica	<5	0–6
Cryptosporidium	<5	—
No pathogen identified	40	22–83

cramps, nausea, bloating, and urgency (74). Travelers at risk are defined as persons from industrialized countries visiting for a period of up to 1 month a region or country where there is increased risk for contracting the disease.

The major determinant of risk is the destination. According to studies of nearly 20,000 European tourists to various locations, it has been possible to define three zones of risk. High-risk destinations, where the incidence of TD ranges from 20% to 65%, include Latin America, Africa, the Middle East, and Asia. Intermediate-risk destinations, with a 10% to 20% incidence of TD, include southern European countries, Israel, and a few Caribbean islands. Low-risk areas, where the incidence is less than 8%, include Canada, the United States, Northern Europe, Australia, New Zealand, and a number of the Caribbean islands (75). These estimates, however, are based on questionnaires filled out by returning travelers. In summarizing the experience from 34 prospective studies, a somewhat greater TD risk emerges: median TD rates of 53% (21%–100%) in Latin America, 54% (21%–57%) in Asia, and 54% (36%–62%) in Africa (9,32).

The national origin of the traveler is another important factor in TD liability. At an international conference in Teheran held in 1968, participants from the United States and Northern Europe had a 36% attack rate, compared with only 8% for colleagues from developing countries and 2% for local Iranians (76). Similar findings were noted in an international congress in Mexico (77). Longer residence in the tropical country also leads to increased resistance to TD (16), but previous short-term travel to areas of high risk does not necessarily confer protection (4,42).

The purpose of travel and eating style both play significant roles in risk of developing this illness. The greatest frequency of diarrhea occurs in people traveling as students or itinerant tourists, the lowest risk in those visiting relatives, and intermediate risk in business travelers (66,78). Most diarrhea occurs in people who eat in restaurants and school cafeterias, and the risk is particularly high, as might be imagined, for those who succumb to the wares of street vendors. The safest place to eat is in a private home (75,78). Younger travelers, particularly those 20 to 29 years of age, have the highest risk, and the lowest TD rates are noted in those over 55 years of age (2,78). In accordance with the general susceptibility of younger travelers, it appears that small children are even more vulnerable. In a retrospective Swiss survey of children and adolescents, most with a destination of Latin America or Africa, TD occurred within 2 weeks in 40%, 9%, 22%, and 36% in the age groups 0 to 2 years, 3 to 6 years, 7 to 14 years, and 15 to 20 years, respectively. Thereafter, the incidence declined to 23% at the age of 70 years or more (79). Whether this apparent respect for advancing age is due to immunity gained after frequent attacks or to less adventuresome eating habits is a source of speculation.

TD is acquired through ingestion of fecally contaminated food or beverages (19,75,78,80,81). In one study, foods in Mexico were more likely to contain fecal coliforms and enteric pathogens than similar foods from Houston, Texas (81). Especially risky foods include uncooked vegetables, meat, and seafood. Tap water, ice, unpasteurized milk and dairy products, and unpeeled fruits are also associated with increased risk. High-level contamination with enteric bacteria is found in food from school cafeterias, restaurants, and street vendors; the highest counts are found in dairy products, although some contamination is found even in cooked foods (19,80,82). Tabletop sauces in Mexican restaurants are heavily contaminated with ETEC and EAEC (83). Bottled carbonated beverages (especially flavored beverages), beer, wine, hot coffee or tea, and water boiled or appropriately treated with chlorine are relatively safe. Some studies, however, show that drinking bottled uncarbonated mineral water increased the risk of waterborne infection (84–86). Enteropathogens can be killed in water hotter than 65°C, which is too hot to touch when it comes from a faucet; in one study only 1 of 14 hotels in Mexico had hot tap water that was hotter than 65°C (87). Dietary indiscretion is penalized by an increased risk of TD. Yet, even the most conscientious travelers were unable to resist such temptations, and 98% of Swiss travelers consumed unsafe food and beverages during the first 3 days of an overseas journey: 71% consumed salads or uncooked vegetables, and 53% accepted ice cubes in drinks (88). Hence, dietary advice, although universally recognized as important and of proven efficacy, is rarely heeded by even the most informed, responsible travelers.

CLINICAL FEATURES

The definition of TD has varied according to investigator (4,11,14,42,75). Most studies define TD as the passage of three or more loose stools in a 24-hour period in association with at least one of the following symptoms or signs of enteric disease: nausea, vomiting, abdominal cramps, fever, fecal urgency, tenesmus, or the passage of bloody or mucoid stools (89). This definition has been modified to require either four or more loose stools in a 24-hour period or three or more loose stools in an 8-hour period with at least one of these additional symptoms or signs (90,91). As a working definition, however, any bowel movement that fits the shape of the container is considered diarrhea. The disease does not begin immediately after the traveler's arrival but generally 2 to 3 days later (75,78). Although most people have three to five loose stools per day, about 20% can have 6 to 15 watery motions (4,14). The average duration of illness in untreated subjects is 3 to 5 days, but a few unfortunate ones have persistent diarrhea throughout their stay (4,75,78).

Watery, loose stools are the most common complaint, along with an array of associated symptoms (Table 76.2). Approximately 2% to 10% have fever, bloody stools, or both, and they are more likely to have shigellosis (92). In general, persons with a milder clinical presentation, regardless of the pathogen, experience more rapid resolution of disease than those with more severe symptoms, but even mild disease can produce an illness that lasts 4 to 5 days. Travelers with identifiable pathogens in their stools had a longer duration of diarrhea and more symptoms than those with culture-negative stools; invasive bacteria, especially *Campylobacter*, produced the most severe disease (93). Despite the impressive list of symptoms, less than

TABLE 76.2. Associated Symptoms in Traveler's Diarrhea

Symptom	% of subjects
Gas	79
Fatigue	74
Cramps	68
Nausea	61
Fever	56
Abdominal pain	53
Anorexia	53
Headache	39
Chills	38
Back pain	35
Dizziness	34
Vomiting	29
Malaise	24
Arthralgia	23

1% of travelers are admitted to a local hospital, and no reports of death caused by diarrhea have been recorded among several hundred thousand insured travelers from Switzerland (75,78).

TREATMENT

Treatment of all forms of diarrhea entails two modalities: fluid replacement and appropriate drugs (94,95). In TD cases, severe dehydration is encountered rarely, so fluid losses can be repaired generally with soft drinks, fruit juices, and some clear fluids. Drug treatment is directed at suppressing the pathogen, as with antibiotics, or at reducing fluid and electrolyte losses with antisecretory agents. Not all patients require drug treatment, however, as shown by an analysis of U.S. adult travelers to Guadalajara, Mexico (89). If diarrhea was mild, defined as one or two loose stools per 24 hours with only one symptom of enteric disease, 60% of affected persons did well by the second day and only 22% continued to have mild diarrhea. Because the cause was essentially the same in patients with mild or severe TD, the results suggest that travelers with mild TD be advised to wait before instituting antimicrobial therapy until at least three unformed stools are passed during 24 hours.

Several antibiotics have been used successfully in treatment of TD (Table 76.3). TMP-SMX or TMP alone reduced duration of diarrhea from 93 hours to approximately 30 hours (21). Ciprofloxacin was as effective as TMP-SMX (29). Fleroxacin (96), norfloxacin (97), and aztreonam (98) have also been used successfully for treatment of TD. Studies have shown that a single dose of ciprofloxacin (99) or fleroxacin (96) is effective, although one study found that a 3-day regimen of ciprofloxacin was more effective than a single dose (100). Ciprofloxacin was also effective in treating TD caused by EAEC (57). On the other hand, furazolidone and ampicillin were disappointing as therapeutic measures (101).

Antimotility drugs have enjoyed considerable support among tourists for providing relief from the intestinal indignities of travel, and their approbation is supported by good scientific studies (38,102,103). Loperamide induces rapid improvement demonstrable even on the first day of therapy, when the results were significantly better than those obtained with either placebo or bismuth subsalicylate (BSS) (38). The concern about potentially exacerbating a case of dysentery with an antimotility drug (104) has largely been dispelled by clinical experience; patients with shigellosis, even infection with *S. dysenteriae* type 1, have been treated inadvertently with loperamide as the only drug, and they had a normal resolution without evidence of prolonged illness or delayed expulsion of the pathogen (38, 102,103).

The most effective relief from symptoms of TD has been provided by a combination of an antimicrobial drug and an antimotility drug. In a study of travelers to Mexico, the combined use of loperamide and TMP-SMX curtailed diarrhea in 1 hour, compared with 30 hours with either drug alone or 59 hours with placebo (105). Even in the severest forms of TD, those with fecal leukocytes or blood-tinged stool, the median duration of illness was 4.5 hours, a remarkable result in this setting. Other investigators, however, have not seen any benefit in adding loperamide to an effective antibiotic such as ciprofloxacin in treating TD (100).

BSS has been effective in treating mild to moderate TD. BSS is an insoluble complex of trivalent bismuth and salicylate. The drug possesses antimicrobial activity on the basis of the bismuth

TABLE 76.3. Antimicrobial Treatments for Traveler's Diarrhea

Treatment regimen		Duration of diarrhea (h)	Reference
TMP-SMX	1 DS tablet b.i.d. for 5 days	29[a]	22
TMP	200 mg b.i.d. for 5 days	31[a]	
Placebo		93	
Furazolidone	100 mg q.i.d. for 5 days	57	90
Ampicillin	500 mg q.i.d. for 5 days	72	
Bicozamycin	500 mg q.i.d. for 3 days	28[a]	25
Placebo		64	
Ciprofloxacin	500 mg b.i.d. for 5 days	29[a]	29
TMP-SMX	1 DS tablet b.i.d. for 5 days	20[a]	
Placebo		81	
TMP-SMX	2 DS tablets for 1 dose	28[a]	94
Loperamide	4 mg; then 2 mg for 3 days	33	
TMP-SMX + loperamide		1[a]	
Placebo		59	
Ciprofloxacin	500 mg for 1 dose	25[a]	88
Placebo		54	
Ciprofloxacin	750 mg for 1 dose	36	89
Ciprofloxacin + loperamide	750 mg for 1 dose 4 mg; then 2 mg q.i.d.	34	
Ciprofloxacin + loperamide	750 mg b.i.d. for 3 days 4 mg; then 2 mg q.i.d.	44	
Aztreonam	100 mg p.o. t.i.d. for 5 days	33[a]	87
Placebo		68	
Rifaximin	200, 400 or 600 mg t.i.d. for 5 days	43[a]	Add 24
TMP-SMX	1 DS b.i.d. for 5 days	68[a]	
Placebo (historical)		82	

[a]Significantly shorter than with placebo.
DS, double-strength; b.i.d., twice daily; q.i.d., four times daily; p.o., orally; TMP-SMX, trimethoprim-sulfamethoxazole.

and antisecretory properties related to the salicylate moiety (106). In the four therapeutic trials conducted in Mexico or West Africa, BSS reduced frequency of diarrhea significantly over placebo, but results were generally better when the higher dose (4.2 g per day) was used (38,107–110). These studies demonstrate that BSS has modest efficacy in ameliorating symptoms and reducing fluid losses in TD when higher doses are used and a low incidence of side effects (107).

The current recommendations for treating TD are somewhat different from those made by the National Institutes of Health Consensus Conference (111,112). For mild to moderate diarrhea, generally less than four bowel movements per day, without blood or fever, either loperamide or BSS can be used effectively. For more severe forms of diarrhea, the optimal therapy at present seems to be a combination of an antimotility drug and an effective antimicrobial drug (13,105).

PREVENTION

It is certainly beneficial to prevent an attack of diarrhea, especially one that can interfere with an overseas journey. Having stated the obvious, such prevention is not easy to accomplish, unless one travels with sterile, hermetically sealed containers of food and drink. Four approaches to preventing TD can be conceived: avoiding unsafe foods and beverages, use of antiinfective drugs, use of other medications, and immunization.

Certain precautions about eating habits should be observed to prevent not only diarrhea but other food- and waterborne diseases as well. An association between consumption of salads with raw vegetables and TD risk has been found (14), but not in all studies (77). High risk of TD has also been associated with eating raw meat and fish and dairy products (80–82,113,114). Although there is a direct relationship between dietary indiscretions and the incidence of TD (92), other studies have failed to show any benefit from dietary restriction, probably because this advice is followed more in theory than in practice (78,80,115–117). Bottled beverages are generally safe, although some reported epidemics have been associated with contaminated bottled drinks (84–86,118). Carbonated beverages are safer than noncarbonated ones, owing to the low pH, generally 4.0 to 5.0, which has antibacterial properties (82,119). Tea or coffee prepared with boiling water is generally safe when consumed while it is still hot. Because the venue of food consumption determines the risk of TD, travelers are advised not to eat food from street vendors. Despite these recommendations it is apparent that most travelers are unable to maintain perfect vigilance during a pleasure trip; so this approach, although universally recommended, does not in reality provide complete protection (88).

Antimicrobial drugs have been used extensively for prevention of TD. Since the classic study by Kean and colleagues in 1962 (3,16), placebo-controlled trials have been conducted (3,10,21,24,26,28,35,36,46,30,120–124) (Table 76.4). Significant protection compared with placebo was noted in all but three studies, two of which involved neomycin (3,120) and the third doxycycline in twice-weekly doses rather than the usual daily doses (35). Protection rates have varied from 28% to 100%; the lower rates have been seen with what would now be recognized as poorly effective antimicrobial drugs, such as sulfonamides and streptomycin (3,120), or when a high level of resistance to the drug is found in ETEC isolated in the area (36,46). In studies using TMP-SMX, protection rates have ranged from 71% to 95% (21,24); with norfloxacin or ciprofloxacin the protection rates are 68% to 94% (26,122–124).

The incidence of side effects has also varied considerably, depending in part on how carefully the subjects are followed. The lowest rates are recorded in studies in which retrospective questionnaires are used to tabulate side effects. On the other hand, when the research team is on site, making frequent data collections, a higher incidence of untoward effects is observed (11). With TMP-SMX, 14% of subjects reported a rash with the higher dose (21) and 2% to 3% with the lower dose (24). In the doxycycline trials, nausea and vomiting were the most common complaints (4%–12% of subjects) (10). In one of the studies involving norfloxacin (25), 2% of subjects developed a rash related to the study drug.

Antimicrobial resistance can develop in the intestinal flora of subjects taking antibiotic prophylaxis (46,50,125,126). In addition, travelers tend to acquire the microflora of their new environment (126), and in developing countries the general enteric flora has many resistant organisms (36,46,51,127). For this reason travel to Mexico, even without taking antibiotics, can lead to acquisition of an antibiotic-resistant enteric flora (128).

Resistance to antimicrobial drugs is a universal occurrence, and the bacteria causing TD are involved in this trend. The enteric pathogens, especially *Shigella* (48,127,129) and ETEC (36,46,50,127,130), have a high degree of resistance to several antimicrobial agents in many developing countries. Resistance has been increasing to TMP-SMX (39,129) and tetracycline (129), which are widely used for TD, yet resistance to quinolones was not observed in strains isolated from TD in two studies (39,129). Fluoroquinolones have the most reliable activity against the pathogens of TD, although resistance may be increasing in Southeast Asia and needs to be monitored (130).

When considering the use of antimicrobial prophylaxis, it is necessary to balance the benefits of widespread prophylactic use in several million travelers each year with the potential drawbacks (131). The known risks include allergy and adverse effects such as rashes, photosensitivity of the skin, blood disorders, Stevens-Johnson syndrome, staining of children's teeth, and induction of other infections by the antimicrobial drug, for example, antibiotic-associated colitis, *Candida* vaginitis, and possibly salmonellosis. In addition, excessive use of these agents would apply pressure to select for bacterial resistance to antimicrobial drugs in general, which is a problem that exists already in many developing countries (127,130).

Antimicrobial agents are not recommended for universal use by travelers (13,111,112,132,133). This position is justified by the excellent results of early and aggressive treatment of TD, which, as outlined earlier, can reduce the duration of diarrhea to an average of 1 hour if a combination of antimicrobial and antimotility drugs is used (105). By avoiding prophylactic antimicrobial agents, only people traveling to high-risk areas who actually develop moderate to severe TD (less than 30% of travelers at risk) are exposed to the side effects of antimicrobial agents, and this exposure is restricted to a period of 1 to 3 days.

BSS has been used for prevention of TD because of its antimicrobial and antisecretory activities (106). The bismuth moiety has been shown to suppress several bacterial pathogens *in vitro* (134,135) at concentrations that can be achieved in the intestinal tract. Indeed, the isolation of bacterial pathogens from the stools of patients with infectious diarrhea is markedly reduced in BSS-treated patients compared with placebo-treated control subjects (108,136,137). In clinical prevention trials, the larger dose of 4.2 g per day (60 mL four times a day) in the liquid form, or 2.1 g per day (two tablets four times a day) in the tablet form, produced protection rates of 62% and 65%, respectively (20,30); the lower dose of 1.05 g per day (one tablet four times a day) gave protection of only 35% to 40% (30,137). A severe form of TD was studied in a laboratory setting in which ETEC was administered to volunteers, and the efficacy of BSS as a prophylactic agent was convincingly established (136). It appears that BSS provides

TABLE 76.4. Antimicrobial Prophylaxis of Traveler's Diarrhea

Year (ref.)	Country	Antimicrobial agent	Dosage	TD (%)	Protection
1962 (3)	Mexico	Neomycin	500 mg b.i.d.	16	24
		Phthalylsulfathiazole	1,000 mg b.i.d.	12	51[a]
		Placebo		24	—
1967 (109)	Various	Streptotriad	1 tablet b.i.d.	13	28[a]
		Neomycin-sulfa	1 tablet b.i.d.	17	0
		Placebo		17	—
1976 (48)	Kenya	Doxycycline	100 mg q.i.d.	6	86[a]
		Placebo		43	—
1977 (49)	Morocco	Doxycycline	100 mg q.i.d.	8	83[a]
		Placebo		46	—
1978 (33)	Honduras	Doxycycline	100 mg twice weekly	33	27
		Placebo		45	—
1980 (34)	Honduras	Doxycycline	100 mg q.i.d.	32	68[b]
		Placebo		100	—
1980 (44)	Thailand	Doxycycline	100 mg q.i.d.	10	59[b]
		Placebo		24	—
1981 (110)	Mexico	Doxycycline	100 mg q.i.d.	4	81[a]
		Placebo		21	—
1983 (40)	Egypt and Far East	Mecillinam	200 mg q.i.d.	13	75[a]
		Placebo		53	—
1982 (21)	Mexico	TMP-SMX	1 DS tablet b.i.d.	16	71[a]
		Placebo		55	—
1983 (24)	Mexico	TMP-SMX	1 DS tablet q.i.d.	2	95[a]
		TMP	200 mg q.i.d.	14	59[a]
		Placebo		33	—
1985 (28)	Mexico	Bicozamycin	500 mg q.i.d.	0	100[a]
		Placebo		53	—
1986 (26)	Mexico	Norfloxacin	400 mg q.i.d.	7	88[a]
		Placebo		60	—
1987 (111)	Various	Norfloxacin	200 mg b.i.d.	11	68[a]
		Placebo		34	—
1990 (112)	Egypt	Norfloxacin	400 mg q.i.d.	2	92[a]
		Placebo		26	—
1989 (113)	Tunisia	Ciprofloxacin	500 mg q.i.d.	4	94[a]
		Placebo		64	—

[a]Significantly different from placebo.
[b]High incidence (~50%) of doxycycline-resistant enterotoxigenic *Escherichia coli*.
b.i.d., twice daily; q.i.d., four times daily; DS, double-strength; TMP-SMX, trimethoprim-sulfamethoxazole.

modest protection against TD but only when the traveler is conscientious about taking the higher dose.

Among drugs other than antimicrobials, halogenated hydroxyquinolines have enjoyed popular use. In a review of field trials, some studies have shown benefit and others have failed to find any salutary effect (138). Notwithstanding its questionable efficacy for prophylaxis of TD, this class of drug should not be used by travelers, or in other situations, because of the reported association with subacute myelooptic neuropathy (139,140).

Various commercial preparations of *Lactobacillus* and *Streptococcus faecium* (68) have been used prophylactically for TD, and the effects have generally been negative (17,107,141). A study in animals has shown that lactobacilli that have the ability to adhere to the intestinal mucosa can prevent colonization with *E. coli* (142). This concept was incorporated in a preparation known as *Lactobacillus* GG, which was shown to reduce TD by 40% in one of two hotels studied in Turkey (143).

Various starches, talcs, chalks, and absorbent compounds have been prescribed for diarrheal diseases for as long as recorded history. Kaolin and pectin, for example, are included in several proprietary formulations, yet there is no substantive evidence that these products can alter the volume or electrolyte content of diarrhea stool (144–146), and they are not recommended for use in TD (147).

Although several avenues appear promising, there is no current vaccine or immunologic intervention that can be recommended for preventing TD. Most work is focused on controlling ETEC, because it is the major pathogen (39,148,149). Another approach employs cholera vaccine or the toxin B subunit, which induces protection against ETEC (150). These various approaches are being pursued vigorously in several laboratories, and active vaccine or passive antibodies may become available in the future for use in TD as well as the important problem of diarrhea in developing countries.

REFERENCES

1. Kean BH, Waters SR. The diarrhea of travelers. *N Engl J Med* 1959;216:71.
2. Kean BH. The diarrhea of travelers to Mexico: summary of five-year study. *Ann Intern Med* 1963;59:605.
3. Kean BH, Schaffner W, Brennan RW, et al. The diarrhea of travelers. V. Prophylaxis with phthalylsulfathiazole and neomycin sulphate. *JAMA* 1962;180:367.
4. Gorbach SL, Kean BH, Evans DG, et al. Travelers' diarrhea and toxigenic *Escherichia coli*. *N Engl J Med* 1975;292:933.
5. Shore EG, Dean AG, Holik KJ, et al. Enterotoxin-producing *Escherichia coli* and diarrheal disease in adult travelers: a prospective study. *J Infect Dis* 1974;129:577.
6. Black RE. Pathogens that cause travelers' diarrhea in Latin America and Africa. *Rev Infect Dis* 1990;12(suppl 1):131.

7. Taylor DN, Echeverria P. Etiology and epidemiology of travelers' diarrhea in Asia. *Rev Infect Dis* 1990;12(suppl 1):5136.
8. Sack RB. Travelers' diarrhea: microbiologic bases for prevention and treatment. *Rev Infect Dis* 1990;12(suppl 1):559.
9. Black RE, Epidemiology of traveler's diarrhea and relative importance of various pathogens. *Rev Infect Dis* 1990;12(suppl 1):573.
10. Sack RB. Antimicrobial prophylaxis of travelers' diarrhea: a selected summary. *Rev Infect Dis* 1986;8(suppl 2):5160.
11. DuPont HL, Ericsson CD, Johnson PC, et al. Antimicrobial agents in the prevention of travelers' diarrhea. *Rev Infect Dis* 1986;8(suppl 2):5167.
12. DuPont HL, Ericcson CD, Reves RR, et al. Antimicrobial therapy for travelers' diarrhea. *Rev Infect Dis* 1986;8(suppl 2):217.
13. DuPont HL. Travellers' diarrhoea. Which antimicrobial? *Drugs* 1993;45:910.
14. Merson MH, Morris GK, Sack DA, et al. Travelers' diarrhea in Mexico: a prospective study of physicians and family members attending a congress. *N Engl J Med* 1976;294:1299.
15. DuPont HL, Olarte J, Evans DG, et al. Comparative susceptibility of Latin America and United States students to enteric pathogens. *N Engl J Med* 1976;295:1520.
16. DuPont HL, Haynes GA, Pickering LK, et al. Diarrhea of travelers to Mexico: relative susceptibility of United States and Latin American students attending a Mexican university. *Am J Epidemiol* 1977;105:37.
17. Pozo-Olano J de D, Warram JH Jr, Gómez RG, et al. Effect of a lactobacilli preparation on travelers' diarrhea: a randomized double-blind clinical trial. *Gastroenterology* 1978;74:829.
18. Vollett JJ, Ericsson CD, Gibson G, et al. Human rotavirus in an adult population with travelers' diarrhea and its relationship to the location of food consumption. *J Med Virol* 1979;4:81.
19. Ericsson CD, Pickering LK, Sullivan P, et al. The role of location of food consumption in the prevention of travelers' diarrhea in Mexico. *Gastroenterology* 1980;79:812.
20. DuPont HL, Sullivan P, Evans DG, et al. Prevention of travelers' diarrhea (emporiatric enteritis): prophylactic administration of subsalicylate bismuth. *JAMA* 1980;243:237.
21. DuPont HL, Evans DG, Rios N, et al. Prevention of travelers' diarrhea with trimethoprim-sulfamethoxazole. *Rev Infect Dis* 1982;4:533.
22. DuPont HL, Reves RR, Galindo E, et al. Treatment of travelers' diarrhea with trimethoprim-sulfamethoxazole alone. *N Engl J Med* 1982;307:841.
23. Freeman LD, Hooper DR, Lathen DF, et al. Brief prophylaxis with doxycycline for the prevention of travelers' diarrhea. *Gastroenterology* 1983;84:276.
24. DuPont HL, Galindo E, Evans DG, et al. Prevention of travelers' diarrhea with trimethoprim-sulfamethoxazole and trimethoprim alone. *Gastroenterology* 1983;84:75.
25. Ericsson CD, DuPont HL, Sullivan P, et al. Bicozamycin, a poorly absorbable antibiotic, effectively treats travelers' diarrhea. *Ann Intern Med* 1983;98:20.
26. Johnson PC, Ericsson CD, Morgan DR, et al. Prophylactic norfloxacin for acute travelers' diarrhea. *Clin Res* 1984;32:870A.
27. Mathewson JJ, Johnson PC, DuPont HL, et al. A newly recognized cause of travelers' diarrhea: enteroadherent *Escherichia coli*. *J Infect Dis* 1985;151:471.
28. Ericsson CD, DuPont HL, Galindo E, et al. Efficacy of bicozamycin in preventing travelers' diarrhea. *Gastroenterology* 1985;88:473.
29. Ericsson CD, Johnson PC, DuPont HL, et al. Ciprofloxacin or trimethoprim-sulfamethoxazole as initial therapy for travelers' diarrhea. *Ann Intern Med* 1987;106:216.
30. DuPont HL, Ericsson CD, Johnson PC, et al. Prevention of travelers' diarrhea by the tablet formulation of bismuth subsalicylate. *JAMA* 1987;257:1347.
31. Adachi JA, Jiang Z-H, Mathewson JJ, et al. Enteroaggregative *Escherichia coli* as a major etiologic agent in traveler's diarrhea in 3 regions of the world. *Clin Infect Dis*. 2001;32:1706–1709.
32. von Sonnenburg F, Tornieporth N, Waiyaki P, et al. Risk and aetiology of diarrhoea at various tourist destinations. *Lancet* 2000;356:133–134.
33. Guerrant RL, Rouse JD, Hughes JM, et al. Turista among members of the Yale Glee Club in Latin America. *Am J Trop Med Hyg* 1980;29:895.
34. Sheridan JF, Aurelian L, Barbour G, et al. Travelers' diarrhea associated with rotavirus infection: analysis of virus-specific immunoglobulin classes. *Infect Immun* 1981;31:419.
35. Santosham M, Sack RB, Froehlich J, et al. Biweekly prophylactic doxycycline for travelers' diarrhea. *J Infect Dis* 1981;143:598.
36. Sack RB, Santosham M, Froehlich JL, et al. Doxycycline prophylaxis of travelers' diarrhea in Honduras, an area where resistance to doxycycline is common among enterotoxigenic *Escherichia coli*. *Am J Trop Med Hyg* 1984;33:460.
37. Sack RB, Froehlich JL, Orskov F, et al. Doxycycline is an effective treatment for travellers' diarrhoea. *J Diarrhoeal Dis Res* 1986;3:144.
38. Johnson PC, Ericsson CD, DuPont HL, et al. Comparison of loperamide with bismuth subsalicylate for the treatment of acute travelers' diarrhea. *JAMA* 1986;255:757.
39. Bourgeois AL, Gardiner CH, Thornton SA, et al. Etiology of acute diarrhea among United States military personnel deployed to South America and West Africa. *Am J Trop Med Hyg* 1993;48:243.
40. Escheverria P, Hodge FA, Blacklow NR, et al. Travelers' diarrhea among United States Marines in South Korea. *Am J Epidemiol* 1978;108:68.
41. Escheverria P, Ramirez G, Blacklow NR, et al. Travelers' diarrhea among US Army troops in South Korea. *J Infect Dis* 1979;139:215.
42. Escheverria P, Blacklow NR, Sanford LB, et al. Travelers' diarrhea among American Peace Corps volunteers in rural Thailand. *J Infect Dis* 1981;143:767.
43. Black FR, Gaarslev K, Orskov F, et al. Mecillinam, a new prophylactic for travellers' diarrhoea: a prospective double-blind study in tourists travelling to Egypt and the Far East. *Scand J Infect Dis* 1983;15:189.
44. Kudoh Y. Imported bacterial diarrheal disease in Tokyo (in Japanese). *Medico* 1984;15:6392.
45. Abe H, Ichiki S, Hashimoto S, et al. Isolation and characterization of enterotoxigenic *Escherichia coli* from patients with travellers' diarrhoea in Osaka. *J Diarrhoeal Dis Res* 1984;2:83.
46. Echeverria P, Sack RB Blacklow NR, et al. Prophylactic doxycycline for travelers' diarrhea in Thailand. Further supportive evidence of *Aeromonas hydrophila* as an enteric pathogen. *Am J Epidemiol* 1984;120:912.
47. Taylor DN, Echeverria P, Blaser MK, et al. Polymicrobial aetiology of travellers' diarrhoea. *Lancet* 1985;1:381.
48. Taylor DN, Houston R, Shum DR, et al. Etiology of diarrhea among travelers and foreign residents in Nepal. *JAMA* 1988;260:1245.
49. Sack DA, Kaminsky DC, Sack RB, et al. Enterotoxigenic *Escherichia coli* diarrhea of travelers: a prospective study of American Peace Corps volunteers. *Johns Hopkins Med J* 1977;141:63.
50. Sack DA, Kaminsky DC, Sack RB, et al. Prophylactic doxycycline for travelers' diarrhea: results of a prospective double-blind study of Peace Corps volunteers in Kenya. *N Engl J Med* 1978;298:758.
51. Sack RB, Froehlich JL, Zulich AW, et al. Prophylactic doxycycline for travelers' diarrhea: results of a prospective double-blind study of Peace Corps volunteers in Morocco. *Gastroenterology* 1979;76:1368.
52. Keskimaki M, Mattila L, Peltola H, et al. Prevalence of diarrheagenic *Escherichia coli* in Finns with or without diarrhea during a round-the-world trip. *J Clin Microbiol* 2000;38:4425–4429.
53. Daniels NA, Neimann J, Karpati A, et al. Traveler's diarrhea at sea: three outbreaks of waterborne enterotoxigenic Escherichia coli on cruise ships. *J Infect Dis* 2000;181:1491–1495.
54. Tacket CO, Moseley SL, Kay B, et al. Challenge studies in volunteers using *Escherichia coli* strains with diffuse adherence to HEp-2 cells. *J Infect Dis* 1990;162:550.
55. Cohen MB, Hawkins JA, Weckbach LS, et al. Colonization by enteroaggregative *Escherichia coli* in travelers with and without diarrhea. *J Clin Microbiol* 1993;31:351.
56. Wanger AR, Murray BE, Echeverria P, et al. Enteroinvasive *Escherichia coli* in travelers with diarrhea. *J Infect Dis* 1988;158:640.
57. Glandt M, Adachi JA, Mathewson JJ, et al. Enteroaggregative *Escherichia coli* as a cause of traveler's diarrhea: clinical response to ciprofloxacin. *Clin Infect Dis* 1999;29:335–338.
58. Orskov I, Orskov F. Significance of surface antigens in relation to enterotoxigenicity of *E. coli*. In: Ouchterlony O, Holmgren J, eds. *Cholera and related diarrheas*. New York: S Karger, 1980:134–141.
59. Parsonnet J, Greene KD, Gerber AR, et al. *Shigella dysenteriae* type I infections in US travelers to Mexico 1988. *Lancet* 1989;2:543.
60. Speelman P, Struelens MJ, Sanyal SC, et al. Detection of *Campylobacter jejuni* and other potential pathogens in travelers' diarrhoea in Bangladesh. *Scand J Gastroenterol* 1983;84(suppl):19.
61. Spiratanaban A, Reinprayoon S. *Vibrio parahaemolyticus*: a major cause of travelers' diarrhea in Bangkok. *Am J Trop Med Hyg* 1982;31:128.
62. Hanninen ML, Salmi S, Mattila L, et al. Association of *Aeromonas* spp. with travellers' diarrhoea in Finland. *J Med Microbiol* 1995;42:26.
63. Jokipii L, Jokipii AMM. Giardiasis in travelers: a prospective study. *J Infect Dis* 1974;130:295.
64. Shlim DR, Hoge CW, Rajah R, et al. Persistent high risk of diarrhea among foreigners in Nepal during the first 2 years of residence. *Clin Infect Dis* 1999;29:613–616.
65. Jokipii L, Pohjola S, Jokipii AMM. *Cryptosporidium*: a frequent finding in patients with gastrointestinal symptoms. *Lancet* 1983;2:358.
66. Sterling CR, Seegar K, Sinclair NA. *Cryptosporidium* as a causative agent of travelers' diarrhea [Letter]. *J Infect Dis* 1986;153:380.
67. Soave R, Ma P. Cryptosporidiosis: travelers' diarrhea in two families. *Arch Intern Med* 1985;145:70.
68. Muller A, Bialek R, Kamper A, et al. Detection of microsporidia in travelers with diarrhea. *J Clin Microbiol* 2001;39:1630–1632.
69. Lopez-Velez R, Turrientes MC, Garron C, et al. Microsporidiosis in travelers with diarrhea from the tropics. *J Travel Med* 1999;6(4):223–227.
70. Hoge CW, Shlim DR, Rajah R, et al. Epidemiology of diarrhoeal illness associated with coccidian-like organism among travellers and foreign residents in Nepal. *Lancet* 1993;341:1175.
71. Bolivar R, Conklin RH, Vollett JJ, et al. Rotavirus in travelers' diarrhea: study of an adult student population in Mexico. *J Infect Dis* 1978;137:324.
72. Jiang ZD, Lowe B, Verenkar MP, et al. Prevalence of enteric pathogens among international travelers with diarrhea acquired in Kenya (Mombasa), India (Goa), or Jamaica (Montego Bay). *J Infect Dis* 2002;185:497–502.
73. Luscher D, Altwegg M. Detection of shigellae, enteroinvasive and enterotoxigenic *Escherichia coli* using the polymerase chain reaction (PCR) in patients returning from tropical countries. *Mol Cell Probes* 1994;8:285.
74. Peltola H, Gorbach SL. Traveler's diarrhea. In: DuPont HL, Steffen R, eds. *Travel medicine*, 2nd ed. London: Decker, 2001:151–159.

75. Steffen R. Epidemiologic studies of travelers' diarrhea, severe gastrointestinal infections, and cholera. *Rev Infect Dis* 1986;8(suppl 2):122.

76. Kean BH. Turista in Teheran: travelers' diarrhoea at the Eighth International Congress of Tropical Medicine and Malaria. *Lancet* 1969;2:583.

77. Lowenstein MS, Balows A, Gangarosa EJ. Turista at an international congress in Mexico. *Lancet* 1973;1:529.

78. Steffen R, van der Linde F, Gyr K, et al. Epidemiology of diarrhea in travelers. *JAMA* 1983;249:1176.

79. Pitzinger B, Steffen R, Tschopp A. Incidence and clinical features of traveler's diarrhea in infants and children. *Pediatr Infect Dis J* 1991;10:719.

80. Tjoa WS, DuPont HL, Sullivan P, et al. Location of food consumption and travelers' diarrhea. *Am J Epidemiol* 1977;106:61.

81. Wood LV, Ferguson LE, Hogan P, et al. Incidence of bacterial enteropathogens in foods from Mexico. *Appl Environ Microbiol* 1983;46:328.

82. Blaser MJ. Environmental interventions for the prevention of travelers' diarrhea. *Rev Infect Dis* 1986;8(suppl 2):5142.

83. Adachi JA, Mathewson JJ, Jiang ZD, et al. Enteric pathogens in Mexican sauces of popular restaurants in Guadalajara, Mexico, and Houston, Texas. *Ann Intern Med* 2002;136:884–887.

84. Blake PA, Rosenberg ML, Florencia J, et al. Cholera in Portugal, 1974. II. Transmission by bottled mineral water. *Am J Epidemiol* 1977;105:344.

85. Harris JR. Are bottled beverages safe for travelers? [Editorial]. *Am J Public Health* 1982;72:787.

86. Communicable Diseases (Scotland) Unit. Outbreak of illness associated with holiday in Soviet central Asia. *Commun Dis Scotl Wkly Rep* 1984;19:7.

87. Bandres JC, Mathewson JJ, DuPont HL. Heat susceptibility of bacterial enteropathogens. Implications for the prevention of travelers' diarrhea. *Arch Intern Med* 1988;148:2261.

88. Kozicki M, Steffen R, Schar M. "Boil it, cook it, peel it, or forget it": Does this rule prevent travelers' diarrhoea? *Int J Epidemiol* 1985;14:169.

89. Ericsson CD, DuPont HL. Travelers' diarrhea: approaches to prevention and treatment. *Clin Infect Dis* 1993;16:616.

90. Hyams KC, Bourgeois AL, Merrell BR, et al. Diarrheal disease during Operation Desert Shield. *N Engl J Med* 1991;325:1423.

91. Turner AC. Travellers diarrhoea. *Ann Soc Belg Med Trop* 1979;59:109.

92. Ericsson CD, Patterson TF, DuPont HL. Clinical presentation as a guide to therapy for travelers' diarrhea. *Am J Med Sci* 1987;294:91.

93. Mattila L. Clinical features and duration of traveler's diarrhea in relation to its etiology. *Clin Infect Dis* 1994;19:728.

94. De Bruyn G. Hahn S. Borwick A. Antibiotic treatment for travellers' diarrhoea [Review] [49 refs]. *Cochrane Database Syst Rev* 2000;(3):CD002242.

95. DuPont HL, Ericsson CD, Mathewson JJ, et al. Rifaximin: a nonabsorbed antimicrobial in the therapy of travelers' diarrhea. *Clin Infect Dis* 2001;33:1807–1815.

96. Steffen R, Jori R, DuPont HL, et al. Efficacy and toxicity of fleroxacin in the treatment of travelers' diarrhea. *Am J Med* 1993;94:1825.

97. Mattila L, Peltola H, Siitonen A, et al. Short-term treatment of traveler's diarrhea with norfloxacin: a double-blind, placebo-controlled study during two seasons. *Clin Infect Dis* 1993;17:779.

98. DuPont HL, Ericsson CD, Mathewson JJ, et al. Oral aztreonam, a poorly absorbed yet effective therapy for bacterial diarrhea in US travelers to Mexico. *JAMA* 1992;267:1932.

99. Salam I, Katelaris P, Leigh-Smith S et al. Randomised trial of single-dose ciprofloxacin for travellers' diarrhoea. *Lancet* 1994;344:1537.

100. Petruccelli BP, Murphy GS, Sanchez JL, et al. Treatment of traveler's diarrhea with ciprofloxacin and loperamide. *J Infect Dis* 1992;165:557.

101. DuPont HL, Ericsson CD, Galindo E, et al. Furazolidone versus ampicillin in the treatment of travelers' diarrhea. *Antimicrob Agents Chemother* 1984;26:160.

102. Schiller LIZ, Santa Ana CA Morawksi SG, et al. Mechanism of the antidiarrheal effect of loperamide. *Gastroenterology* 1984;86:1475.

103. Van Loon FPL, Bennish ML, Speelman P, et al. Double-blind trial of loperamide for treating acute watery diarrhoea in expatriates in Bangladesh. *Gut* 1989;30:492.

104. DuPont HL, Hornick RB. Adverse effect of Lomotil therapy in shigellosis. *JAMA* 1973;226:1525.

105. Ericsson CD, DuPont HL, Mathewson JJ, et al. Treatment of traveler's diarrhea with sulfamethoxazole and trimethoprim and loperamide. *JAMA* 1990;263:257.

106. Gorbach SL. Bismuth therapy in gastrointestinal diseases. *Gastroenterology* 1990;99:863.

107. Steffen R. Worldwide efficacy of bismuth subsalicylate in the treatment of travelers' diarrhea. *Rev Infect Dis* 1990;12(suppl 1):80.

108. DuPont HL, Sullivan P, Pickering LK, et al. Symptomatic treatment of diarrhea with bismuth subsalicylate among students attending a Mexican university. *Gastroenterology* 1977;73:715.

109. Steffen R, Mathewson JJ, Ericsson CD, et al. Travelers' diarrhea in West Africa and in Mexico: Fecal transport systems and liquid bismuth subsalicylate for self-therapy. *J Infect Dis* 1988;57:1008.

110. Steffen R, Heusser R, Tschopp A, et al. Efficacy and side effects of six agents in the self-treatment of travelers' diarrhea. *Travel Med Int* 1988;6:153.

111. Gorbach SL, Edelman R, eds. Travelers' diarrhea: National Institutes of Health Consensus Development Conference. *Rev Infect Dis* 1986;8:109.

112. Consensus Conference. Travelers' diarrhea. *JAMA* 1985;253:2700.

113. Kendrick MA. Summary of study on illness among Americans visiting Europe, March 31, 1969–March 30, 1970. *J Infect Dis* 1972;126:685.

114. Gangarosa EJ, Kendrick MA, Loewenstein MS, et al. Global travel and travelers' health. *Aviat Space Environ Med* 1980;51:265.

115. Turner AC. Travellers diarrhoea. *Trans Med Soc Lond* 1975–1977;92–93:64.

116. Chang T-W. Traveler's diarrhea [Letter]. *Ann Intern Med* 1978;89:428.

117. Ryder RW, Oquist CA, Greenberg H, et al. Travelers' diarrhea in Panamanian tourists in Mexico. *J Infect Dis* 1981;144:442.

118. Gonzales-Cortes A, Gangarosa EJ, Parrilla C, et al. Bottled beverages and typhoid fever: the Mexican epidemic of 1972–73. *Am J Public Health* 1982;72:844.

119. Koser SA, Skinner WW. Viability of the colon typhoid group in carbonated water and carbonated beverages. *J Bacteriol* 1922;7:111.

120. Turner AC. Traveler's diarrhoea: a survey of symptoms, occurrence, and possible prophylaxis. *BMJ* 1967;4:453.

121. Freeman LD, Hooper DR, Lathen DF, et al. Brief prophylaxis with doxycycline for the prevention of travelers' diarrhea. *Gastroenterology* 1983;84:276.

122. Wistrom J, Norrby SR, Burman LG, et al. Norfloxacin versus placebo for prophylaxis against travellers' diarrhoea. *J Antimicrob Chemother* 1987;20:563.

123. Scott DA, Haberberger RL, Thornton SA, et al. Norfloxacin for the prophylaxis of travelers' diarrhea in US military personnel. *Am J Trop Med Hyg* 1990;42:160.

124. Rademaker CM, Hoepelman IM, Wolfhagen MJ, et al. Results of a double-blind placebo-controlled study using ciprofloxacin for prevention of travelers' diarrhea. *Eur J Clin Microbiol Infect Dis* 1989;8:690.

125. Murray BE, Rensimer ER, DuPont HL. Emergence of high-level trimethoprim resistance in fecal *Escherichia coli* during oral administration of trimethoprim or trimethoprim-sulfamethoxazole. *N Engl J Med* 1982;306:130.

126. Stenderup J, Orskov I, Orskov F. Changes in serotype and resistance pattern of the intestinal *Escherichia coli* flora during travel. Results from a trial of mecillinam as a prophylactic against travellers' diarrhea. *Scand J Infect Dis* 1983;15:367.

127. Murray BE. Resistance of *Shigella, Salmonella,* and other selected enteric pathogens to antimicrobial agents. *Rev Infect Dis* 1986;8(suppl 2):172.

128. Murray BE, Mathewson JJ, DuPont HL, et al. Emergence of resistant fecal *Escherichia coli* in travelers not taking prophylactic antimicrobial agents. *Antimicrob Agents Chemother* 1990;34:515.

129. Vila J, Gascon J, Abdalla S, et al. Antimicrobial resistance of *Shigella* isolates causing traveler's diarrhea. *Antimicrob Agents Chemother* 1994;38:2668.

130. Gomi H. Jiang ZD, Adachi JA, et al. *In vitro* antimicrobial susceptibility testing of bacterial enteropathogens causing traveler's diarrhea in four geographic regions. *Antimicrob Agents Chemother* 2001;45:212–216.

131. Rendi-Wagner P. Kollaritsch H. Drug prophylaxis for travelers' diarrhea. *Clin Infect Dis* 2002;34:628–633.

132. Preventing travellers' diarrhoea [Editorial]. *Lancet* 1988;2:144.

133. Steffen R, Boppart I. Travellers' diarrhoea. *Baillieres Clin Gastroenterol* 1987;1:361.

134. Cornick NA, Silva M, Gorbach SL. *In vitro* antibacterial activity of bismuth subsalicylate. *Rev Infect Dis* 1990;12(suppl 1):9.

135. Manhart MD. *In vitro* antimicrobial activity of bismuth subsalicylate and other bismuth salts. *Rev Infect Dis* 1990;12(suppl 1):11.

136. Graham DY, Estes MK, Gentry LO. Double-blind comparison of bismuth subsalicylate and placebo in the prevention and treatment of enterotoxigenic *Escherichia coli*-induced diarrhea in volunteers. *Gastroenterology* 1983;85:1017.

137. Steffen R, DuPont HL, Heusser R, et al. Prevention of travelers' diarrhea by the tablet form of bismuth subsalicylate. *Antimicrob Agents Chemother* 1986;29:625.

138. Steffen R, Heusser R, DuPont HL. Prevention of travelers' diarrhea by nonantibiotic drugs. *Rev Infect Dis* 1986;8(suppl 2):151.

139. Tsubaki T, Honma Y, Hoshi M. Neurologic syndrome associated with clioquinol. *Lancet* 1971;1:696.

140. Baumgartner G, Gawel MJ, Kaeser HE, et al. Neurotoxicity of halogenated hydroxyquinolines: clinical analysis of cases reported outside Japan. *J Neurol Neurosurg Psychiatry* 1979;42:1073.

141. Clemens ML, Levine MM, Black RE, et al. *Lactobacillus* prophylaxis for diarrhea due to enterotoxigenic *Escherichia coli. Antimicrob Agents Chemother* 1981;20:104.

142. Itoh K, Freter R. Control of *Escherichia coli* populations by a combination of indigenous clostridia and lactobacilli in gnotobiotic mice and continuous-flow cultures. *Infect Immun* 1989;57:559.

143. Oksanen PJ, Salminen S, Saxelin M, et al. Prevention of travellers' diarrhoea by *Lactobacillus* GG. *Ann Med* 1990;22:53.

144. Durrington PN, Manning AP, Bolton CH, et al. Effect of pectin on serum lipids and lipoproteins, whole-gut transit time, and stool weight. *Lancet* 1976;2:394.

145. Cummings JH, Southgate DAT, Branch WJ, et al. The digestion of pectin in the human gut and its effect on calcium absorption and large bowel function. *Br J Nutr* 1979;41:477.

146. Portnoy BL, DuPont HL, Pruitt D, et al. Antidiarrheal agents in the treatment of acute diarrhea in children. *JAMA* 1976;236:844.

147. Donowitz M, Wicks J, Sharp GWG. Drug therapy for diarrheal diseases: a look ahead. *Rev Infect Dis* 1986;8(suppl 2):188.

148. Sack RB, Mine RL, Spira WM. Oral immunization of rabbits with enterotoxigenic *Escherichia coli* protects against intraintestinal challenge. *Infect Immun* 1988;56:387.

149. Svennerholm A-M, Vidal YL, Holmgren J, et al. Role of PCF8775 antigen and its *coli* surface subcomponents for colonization, disease, and protective immunogenicity of enterotoxigenic *Escherichia coli* in rabbits. *Infect Immun* 1988;56:523.

150. Clemens JD, Sack DA, Harris JR, et al. Cross-protection by B subunit-whole cell cholera vaccine against diarrhea associated with heat-labile toxin-producing enterotoxigenic *Escherichia coli*: results of a large-scale field trial. *J Infect Dis* 1988;158:372.

CHAPTER 77
Food Poisoning

Davidson H. Hamer and David R. Snydman

Food-borne illness is a significant public health problem. It is a major cause of morbidity and an infrequent cause of mortality in the United States (1). From 1993 to 1997, 2,751 outbreaks of food-borne disease were reported to the Centers for Disease Control and Prevention (CDC) from virtually all 50 states. The number of ill individuals in these outbreaks exceeded 80,000 and there were 29 deaths. Surveillance suggests that these outbreaks are grossly underreported; the true scope of disease related to food is probably 10 to 100 times more frequent. Estimates of 6 million to 99 million cases at a cost of $5 billion to $23 billion have been made (2).

For most public health authorities, a food-borne disease outbreak is defined by two criteria: (a) two or more persons experiencing a similar illness, usually gastrointestinal, after ingestion of a common food, and (a) epidemiologic analysis implicating food as the source of the illness. There are certain exceptions to this definition. For example, one case of botulism or chemical poisoning constitutes an outbreak for epidemiologic investigation and control purposes.

Reported food-borne outbreaks are generally divided into two categories: (a) laboratory confirmed, that is, outbreaks in which evidence of a specific etiologic agent is obtained and specific laboratory criteria are met, and (b) undetermined, that is, outbreaks in which epidemiologic evidence implicates a food source but adequate laboratory confirmation is not obtained.

Food poisoning is defined as an illness caused by the consumption of food contaminated with pathogenic microorganisms, their toxins, or chemicals (3). Food poisoning can be related to bacteria, bacterial toxins, parasites (e.g., trichinosis), viruses (e.g., hepatitis A or E), and chemicals (e.g., in mushrooms). Food poisoning caused by bacteria constitutes approximately two thirds of the recognized food-borne outbreaks in the United States for which an etiology can be determined. However, it should be noted that only 32% of outbreaks fulfill the criteria for a confirmed etiology (1) (Table 77.1).

The major recognized causes of bacterial food poisoning are generally limited to about a dozen bacteria, namely *Salmonella*, *Staphylococcus aureus*, *Clostridium perfringens*, *Shigella*, toxigenic or enterohemorrhagic *Escherichia coli*, *Bacillus cereus*, *Clostridium botulinum*, vibrios including *Vibrio cholerae*, *Campylobacter*, *Yersinia*, *Aeromonas*, and *Listeria*. Other agents such as streptococci and *Arizona* species have also infrequently been implicated as agents in food-borne illness in the United States.

Salmonella outbreaks predominate among the confirmed outbreaks and constitute almost a third of all reported cases of food-borne illness. This may be due in part to ease of recognition and to the awareness of physicians and the public. Among other bacterial causes of food-borne outbreaks, *E. coli*, followed by *C. perfringens*, *Shigella*, and *S. aureus*, have been among the most commonly recognized. However, two chemical causes, ciguatoxin and scombrotoxin, have increasingly been recognized as among the more common causes of food-borne outbreak (1).

Etiologic patterns vary throughout the world. These patterns are dependent on many factors, such as food preferences, physician and public awareness, and laboratory capabilities. For example, in the United States *Salmonella* and *E. coli* are among the agents most commonly involved in food-borne outbreaks, being present in more than 50% of bacterial food-borne outbreaks (1). In contrast, *Salmonella* is implicated in more than 90% of the recognized food-borne illness in England and Wales (4). Japan, on the other hand, has different etiologic patterns, probably related to many of the aforementioned factors. *Vibrio parahaemolyticus* gastroenteritis was first described in that country; *V. parahaemolyticus* is the dominant pathogen in food-borne outbreaks and is present in more than 50% of the reported outbreaks (5).

In the past decade in the United States, there has been a marked change in the epidemiology of food-borne disease (6). The decline in food-borne outbreaks caused by *S. aureus* and *C. perfringens* has been accompanied by increasing rates of salmonellosis and the recognition of major new food-borne pathogens, such as *E. coli* O157:H7, *Cyclospora cayetanensis*, and *Listeria monocytogenes* (7–10). Furthermore, a greater appreciation for *Campylobacter jejuni* and Norwalk virus, described in the 1970s as agents of food-borne disease, has emerged (10,11).

Some of these changes may be due to a shift in dietary habits with a marked increase in per capita consumption of fresh vegetables, fresh fruit, cheese, and poultry (6). Furthermore, importation of exotic fruits and vegetables, especially from Mexico and South America, has grown. There has also been a trend toward increased consumption of food from commercial service establishments, leading to the potential for outbreaks caused by infected food handlers.

In addition to exotic foods and changing practices, unusual outbreaks such as thyrotoxicosis related to consumption of bovine thyroid glands in ground beef (12) and eosinophilic myalgia syndrome related to contaminated L-tryptophan (13) point not only to the impact widespread food distribution may have in multistate outbreaks but also to unusual clinical manifestations that may occur as a result of food poisoning.

This chapter focuses primarily on the major toxin-mediated, short-incubation food poisoning syndromes. For a complete discussion of individual pathogens, the reader is referred to the respective chapters.

BACTERIAL CAUSES OF FOOD-BORNE ILLNESS

Many microorganisms are associated with food-borne disease. Table 77.2 lists the major bacterial causes, some epidemiologic and clinical features, and diagnostic media. For a more complete discussion of each bacterial pathogen, the reader is referred to individual chapters in the text.

Staphylococcus aureus

Dack and co-workers (14) were the first to prove that staphylococcal food poisoning was due to toxin production by *S. aureus*. They performed classic experiments with human volunteers, demonstrating that culture filtrates of staphylococci isolated from a cream-filled sponge cake, which had been the implicated vehicle in a food-borne outbreak, could cause gastroenteritis (15). After these reports appeared, staphylococcal food poisoning became widely appreciated, and today staphylococci are among the most common agents implicated in food-borne disease.

PATHOPHYSIOLOGY

The microbiologic distinguishing characteristics of *S. aureus* are outlined in Chapter 182. Six immunologically distinct *S. aureus* enterotoxins have been described, termed A, B, C, D, E, and F (15,16). These enterotoxins are heat-resistant, single-polypeptide

TABLE 77.1.   Confirmed Food-Borne Disease Outbreaks, Cases, and Deaths, 1993 to 1997, United States, as reported to the Centers for Disease Control and Prevention

Etiology	Outbreaks		Cases		Deaths	
	No.	%	No.	%	No.	%
Bacterial						
Bacillus cereus	14	0.5	691	0.8	0	0.0
Brucella	1	0.0	19	0.0	0	0.0
Campylobacter	25	0.9	539	0.6	1	3.4
Clostridium botulinum	13	0.5	56	0.1	1	3.4
Clostridium perfringens	57	2.1	2,772	3.2	0	0.0
Escherichia coli	84	3.1	3,260	3.8	8	27.6
Listeria monocytogenes	3	0.1	100	0.1	2	6.9
Salmonella	357	13.0	32,610	37.9	13	44.8
Shigella	43	1.6	1,555	1.8	0	0.0
Staphylococcus aureus	42	1.5	1,413	1.6	1	3.4
Streptococcus, group A	1	0.0	122	0.1	0	0.0
Streptococcus, other	1	0.0	6	0.0	0	0.0
Vibrio cholerae	1	0.0	2	0.0	0	0.0
Vibrio parahaemolyticus	5	0.2	40	0.0	0	0.0
Yersinia enterocolitica	2	0.1	27	0.0	1	3.4
Other bacterial	6	0.2	609	0.7	1	3.4
Total bacterial	**655**	**23.8**	**43,821**	**50.9**	**28**	**96.6**
Chemical						
Ciguatoxin	60	2.2	205	0.2	0	0.0
Heavy metals	4	0.1	17	0.0	0	0.0
Monosodium glutamate	1	0.0	2	0.0	0	0.0
Mushroom poisoning	7	0.3	21	0.0	0	0.0
Scombrotoxin	69	2.5	297	0.3	0	0.0
Shellfish	1	0.0	3	0.0	0	0.0
Other chemical	6	0.2	31	0.0	0	0.0
Total chemical	**148**	**5.4**	**576**	**0.7**	**0**	**0.0**
Parasitic						
Giardia lamblia	4	0.1	45	0.1	0	0.0
Trichinella spiralis	2	0.1	19	0.0	0	0.0
Other parasitic	13	0.5	2,261	2.6	0	0.0
Total parasitic	**19**	**0.7**	**2,325**	**2.7**	**0**	**0.0**
Viral						
Hepatitis A	23	0.8	729	0.8	0	0.0
Norwalk	9	0.3	1,233	1.4	0	0.0
Other viral	24	0.9	2,104	2.4	0	0.0
Total viral	**56**	**2.0**	**4,066**	**4.7**	**0**	**0.0**
Confirmed etiology	878	31.9	50,788	59.0	28	96.6
Unknown etiology	1,873	68.1	35,270	41.0	1	3.4
Total 1993–1997	**2,751**	**100.0**	**86,058**	**100.0**	**29**	**100.0**

From Olsen SJ, MacKinnon LC, Goulding JS, et al. Surveillance for foodborne disease outbreaks—United States. *MMWR* 2000;49(SS-1):1–62, with permission.

chains that contain large quantities of lysine, aspartic and glutamic acids, and tyrosine. They range in molecular weight from 28,366 to 34,700. The precise mechanism of action is not yet known; however, when they were tested in a rat intestinal loop model, net transport of water and solute occurred (17). These toxins were emetic when administered to monkeys and cats (18). The toxic shock–producing toxin, enterotoxin F, has not been associated with food-borne disease (19).

Enterotoxins A, B, C, D, and E have all been implicated in outbreaks of staphylococcal food poisoning in the United States and United Kingdom. Most implicated strains produce A or both A and D. Surprisingly, from 1979 to 1981 all the reported staphylococcal food-borne outbreaks were due to enterotoxin A (20).

There are three requisites for staphylococcal food poisoning to occur: (a) contamination of a food with enterotoxin-producing staphylococci, (b) a food that has suitable growth requirements for the organisms, and (c) a permissive temperature and amount of time at which the organism can multiply.

EPIDEMIOLOGY

S. aureus was the fifth most common bacterial agent implicated in bacterial food poisoning from 1993 to 1997 (1). Outbreaks are characterized by explosive onset between 1 and 6 hours after consumption of a contaminated vehicle (median 3 hours). Attack rates are usually quite high because small quantities of enterotoxin can cause illness. Secondary cases are not of concern in this type of food poisoning.

Outbreaks related to staphylococci can occur at all times of the year, but most outbreaks are reported during the warm weather months.

Many different foods have been implicated in staphylococcal food poisoning. However, certain foods are frequently implicated: ham, canned beef, pork, or any salted meat and cream-filled cakes or pastries such as cream puffs. Potato and macaroni salads are occasionally involved. Foods that have a high salt content (ham) or sugar content (custard) selectively favor the growth of staphylococci, which generally occurs when there is inadequate refrigeration of the implicated foods.

TABLE 77.2. Characteristics of Bacterial Food Poisoning

Organism	Common vehicles	Median incubation period (h)[a]	Toxin, primary in pathogenesis	Clinical features	Median duration (days)[a]	Secondary attack rates (%)	Sources of diagnostic material	Laboratory diagnosis
Bacillus cereus	Fried rice, vanilla sauce, cream	2 (1–6)	Heat stable	N, V, C, D (33%)	0.4 (0.2–0.5)	—	Vomitus, stool, or food	>10^5 colonies on peptone-beef extract egg yolk agar; need controls for stool analysis (may be normal flora), serotyping
	Vanilla sauce, meatballs, boiled beef, barbecued chicken	9 (6–14)	Heat labile	D, C, N, V	1 (1–2)	—		
Bacillus anthracis	Beef, other livestock?	48? (24–188)	Lethal and edema factors	N, V, B, C, F	?? (2–7)	0	Blood, food	
Campylobacter jejuni	Milk, chicken, pets, beef	48 (24–240)	?	D, F, C, B, H, M, N, V	7 (2–30)	25	Stool or rectal swab	Brucella agar base with vancomycin, polymyxin, and trimethoprim grown in reduced oxygen
Clostridium perfringens	Beef, turkey, chicken	12 (8–22)	Heat labile	D, C (N, V, F rare)	1 (0.3–3)	—	Stool or rectal swab; food, food contact surfaces	Egg yolk-free tryptose-sulfite-cycloserine agar; Hobbs or bacteriocin typing
Escherichia coli	Salads, beef, salami, sprouts, unpasteurized milk, apple cider	24 (8–14)	Heat labile (ETEC)	D, C, N, H, F, M	3 (1–4)	0	Stool or rectal swab	MacConkey medium; E. coli must be tested for toxin production (see Chapter 73)
		72 (24–112)	Heat stable Verotoxin (EHEC)	F, M, D, C B, C, F hemolytic-uremic syndrome	5 (?)	20	Stool or rectal swab, serum	Sorbital MacConkey medium, serotyping, ELISA, PCR, antibody
Listeria monocytogenes	Milk, raw vegetables, coleslaw, dairy products, poultry, beef, soft cheese	? (9–48)	?	D, F, C, M, N, V	?	10	Stool or rectal swab, blood, CSF	Cold enrichment, nutrient broth potassium thiocyanate and nalidixic acid
Staphylococcus aureus	Ham, pork, canned beef, cream-filled pastry	3 (1–6)	Heat stable	V, N, C, D, F (rare)	1 (0.3–2)	—	Stool, vomitus; food or food contact surfaces; nasal, hand, purulent lesion from food preparer	Egg yolk-tellurite-glycine-pyruvate agar or mannitol salt; phage type isolates; enterotoxin testing
Salmonella	Eggs, meat, poultry, tomatoes, cantaloupe	24 (5–72)	—	D, C, N, V, F, H, B (rare); enteric fever	3 (0.5–14)	30–50	Stool or rectal swab from patients and food preparation workers; raw food	Salmonella-Shigella, deoxycholate-citrate, Hektoen enteric, or xylose-lysine-deoxycholate; phage typing for Salmonella typhimurium
Shigella	Milk, salads (potato, tuna, turkey)	24 (7–168)	—	C, F, D, B, H, N, V	3 (0.5–14)	40–60	Stool or rectal swab from patients or food preparation workers; food	Same media as above; colicin typing
Vibrio parahaemolyticus	Seafood, rarely salt water or salted vegetables	12 (2–18)	?	D, C, N, V, H, F (25%), B (rare)	3 (2–10)	—	Stool or rectal swab; food, food contact surfaces; seawater	Thiosulfate citrate bile salts agar; test for Kanagawa phenomenon (see text); serotyping
Yersinia enterocolitica	Chocolate or raw milk, pork	?72 (2–144)	Heat stable (see text)	F, C, D, V, pharyngitis, arthritis, mesenteric adenitis, rashes	7 (2–30)	20	Stool from food preparer	Cold enrichment; serotyping, serology

[a]Ranges are given in parentheses.

B, Bloody diarrhea; C, crampy abdominal pain; D, diarrhea; F, fever; H, headache; M, myalgias; N, nausea; V, vomiting; ELISA, enzyme-linked immunosorbent assay; PCR, polymerase chain reaction. ETEC, enterotoxigenic Escherichia coli; EHEC, enterohemorrhagic E. coli.

CLINICAL FEATURES

The symptoms of staphylococcal food poisoning are primarily profuse vomiting, nausea, and abdominal cramps, often followed by diarrhea. In severe cases, blood may be observed in the vomitus or stool. Rarely, hypotension and marked prostration occur. Fatalities are unusual and recovery is complete in 24 to 48 hours. Fever is not a common accompaniment but may be present if dehydration is severe.

DIAGNOSIS

Staphylococcal food poisoning should be considered in anyone who presents with severe vomiting, nausea, cramps, and some diarrhea. A history of ingesting meats of high salt or protein content may be helpful. Usually, the best epidemiologic clue is the short incubation period (1–7 hours). Of the agents of bacterial food-borne diseases, only B. cereus has a similar incubation period with a marked vomiting syndrome (21). Because the B. cereus vomiting syndrome is often closely associated with fried rice, an easy epidemiologic distinction can usually be made (22).

The diagnosis can be confirmed by culturing the epidemiologically incriminated food, the skin or nose of the food handler, or occasionally the vomitus or stools of affected individuals. Any S. aureus recovered can be typed using phage or molecular methods such as pulsed-field gel electrophoresis to prove that the isolated strains are identical.

Several methods have been developed for detection of staphylococcal enterotoxin, including immunofluorescence, hemagglutination, radioimmunoassay, and enzyme-linked immunoassay, which can detect nanogram quantities of enterotoxin (23). These should be considered research tools.

TREATMENT

Most people with staphylococcal food poisoning do not report their symptoms to a physician and recover without the need for any treatment. More severe cases may require supportive care, particularly rehydration and correction of alkalosis. As is the case for all the toxin-producing bacteria responsible for food poisoning except C. botulinum, no specific therapy is available.

Bacillus cereus

The classic description of the illness caused by B. cereus was that of Hauge (24), who described four Norwegian outbreaks involving 600 people in 1955. Interestingly, the vehicle in all four outbreaks appeared to be a vanilla sauce. Samples of sauce in each instance contained B. cereus in concentrations greater than 10^6/mL. After an incubation of about 10 hours, the patients developed profuse, watery diarrhea that was associated with abdominal pain and nausea but rarely with vomiting. Fever was distinctly uncommon, and all symptoms usually abated within 12 hours.

Hauge demonstrated in himself that vanilla sauce inoculated with a strain of B. cereus isolated from an outbreak of gastrointestinal illness and allowed to incubate for 24 hours caused severe abdominal pain and diarrhea 13 hours after consumption. He was able to culture B. cereus from his stool as well.

The first well-documented outbreak of gastrointestinal disease in the United States was reported in 1970 (25). In 1974 a vomiting syndrome caused by B. cereus that involved fried rice was recognized (26). This report heralded the realization that this organism may be responsible for two distinct food-borne syndromes.

MICROBIOLOGY AND PATHOPHYSIOLOGY

B. cereus is a gram-positive, catalase-positive, aerobic spore–forming rod. Most strains are β-hemolytic. Several extracellular toxins are produced by strains of B. cereus and may contribute to their virulence (27). An enterotoxin has been described that produces fluid accumulation in rabbit ileal loops, alters vascular permeability in the skin of rabbits, kills mice when injected intravenously, and stimulates the adenylate cyclase–cyclic AMP system in intestinal epithelial cells (28).

A second heat-stable toxin with a molecular weight of 5,000 kd has been isolated from a strain of B. cereus implicated in an outbreak of vomiting-type illness that produced vomiting when fed to rhesus monkeys (29).

EPIDEMIOLOGY

Fourteen outbreaks of B. cereus gastroenteritis affecting 691 persons were reported to the CDC from 1993 to 1997 (1). Most reported outbreaks have attack rates of 50% to 75%. In the reported vomiting-type outbreaks, virtually all individuals who consumed contaminated fried rice became ill. There is no risk for secondary cases.

The median incubation period for the diarrheal outbreaks reported in the United States was 9 hours (range 6–14 hours). The median incubation period for the outbreaks of emetic illness has been 2 hours (range 1–6 hours).

The reports of most outbreaks of the vomiting syndrome in the United States and of outbreaks in Great Britain implicated fried rice as the vehicle, whereas inadequately refrigerated meats have been less commonly involved. The diarrheal illness, however, has been related to a variety of vehicles, including boiled beef, sausage, chicken soup, vanilla sauce, dried milk, spaghetti sauces, spices, cream sauces, and puddings.

Illness characterized by vomiting as the major finding can be attributed to the common practice in Chinese restaurants of allowing large portions of boiled rice to drain unrefrigerated to avoid clumping. The flash frying in the final preparation of the fried rice does not produce enough heat to destroy the preformed heat-stable toxin (29).

CLINICAL FEATURES

The diarrheal, long-incubation illness is characterized by diarrhea (96%), abdominal cramps (75%), and vomiting (23%) (20). Fever is uncommon. The duration of illness has ranged from 20 to 36 hours, with a median of 24 hours.

The emetic form of the illness has the predominant symptoms of vomiting (100%) and abdominal cramps (100%). Diarrhea is present in only one third of affected individuals. The duration of this illness has ranged from 8 to 10 hours (median 9 hours). In both types of illness the disease is usually mild and self-limited.

DIAGNOSIS

The diagnosis of B. cereus food poisoning should be considered in any individual who has diarrhea without fever in association with lower abdominal cramps. The disease caused by C. perfringens is so similar to that of B. cereus that they cannot be differentiated clinically or epidemiologically; culture methods are required.

The vomiting syndrome must be differentiated from S. aureus food poisoning. The association with fried rice is useful in differentiating the two organisms.

The diagnosis can be made by the isolation of 10^5 or more B. cereus organisms per gram from the incriminated food item. B. cereus can sometimes be found in the stools of healthy persons; therefore, isolation of the organism from feces may not be suitable confirmation unless negative stool cultures are obtained from an appropriate control group.

Bacillus anthracis

Although most anthrax infections are the result of cutaneous exposure to or inhalation of infected spores, the ingestion of infected animal tissue can lead to gastrointestinal disease. This organism is a rare cause of food-borne disease.

The consumption of endospore-contaminated meat from infected animals is the primary mode of transmission of gastrointestinal anthrax. Point source outbreaks within households are common. This form of anthrax has never been conclusively documented in the United States, presumably because livestock are vaccinated for anthrax in endemic areas and because animals are routinely inspected by federal and state meat inspectors. A recent outbreak of gastrointestinal illness characterized by diarrhea, abdominal pain, and fever was identified in two family members who had consumed meat from a carcass that was found to be contaminated with *B. anthracis* (30).

Approximately 1 to 7 days after the ingestion of raw or undercooked meat from infected animals, patients experience initial symptoms including nausea, vomiting, abdominal pain, and fever. These are often followed by the development of bloody diarrhea, diffuse abdominal pain with rebound tenderness, and, occasionally, hematemesis. Ascites, which may be purulent, develops 2 to 4 days later. More than 50% of episodes are fatal, with death developing as a consequence of toxemia, intestinal perforation, or shock from hemorrhage and fluid losses.

Oropharyngeal anthrax is a less common form of infection that develops when spores are deposited in the oropharynx. Symptoms include fever, a severely sore throat, and dysphagia, which may progress to respiratory distress. Examination often reveals swelling of the neck, lymphadenitis, and pharyngeal ulcers covered by a pseudomembrane. Despite the relatively severe symptoms, this form of infection tends to be milder than gastrointestinal disease and is rarely fatal.

Details on the diagnosis, treatment, and prevention of gastrointestinal anthrax can be found in Chapters 164 and 188.

Clostridium perfringens

C. perfringens was first recognized and confirmed in the United States as a food-borne pathogen in 1945 by McClung (31), who studied four outbreaks of diarrhea related to the consumption of chickens steamed 24 hours before consumption. *C. perfringens* was isolated from the cooked chickens.

Shortly after McClung's discovery, filtrates from strains of *C. perfringens* were administered by mouth to human subjects (31). Cramps and diarrhea occurred in some individuals, but the incubation period was short, 45 to 80 minutes. Living cultures induced cramps and bloating in 4 hours and diarrhea several hours thereafter. Hobbs and colleagues (32) elegantly confirmed these results and outlined the epidemiologic features of the disease in Great Britain in 1953.

Another discovery in the late 1940s was the outbreak of a severe and often lethal intestinal condition termed enteritis necroticans or Darmbrand that affected more than 400 people in Germany (33). This outbreak was similar to others described later in New Guinea and termed pigbel (34). Both conditions were due to *C. perfringens*. The diarrheal form of disease is caused by an enterotoxin elaborated by strains of *C. perfringens* type A, whereas enteritis necroticans and pigbel are caused by type C.

MICROBIOLOGY

Clostridia are gram-positive, spore-forming obligate anaerobes. The microbiologic features are outlined in Chapter 213. Although all species grow better under anaerobic conditions, *C. perfringens* is remarkably aerotolerant and may survive exposure to oxygen for as long as 72 hours.

PATHOPHYSIOLOGY

C. perfringens is known to produce 12 toxins that are active in tissues, as well as several enterotoxins. Diarrheal disease is caused by a heat-labile, protein enterotoxin with a molecular weight of approximately 34,000 daltons (35). This toxin is nondialyzable, precipitated by ammonium sulfate, antigenic, and inactivated by pronase but not by trypsin, lipase, or amylase (36). Duncan and colleagues (35–39) have shown that the toxin is a structural component of the spore coat and is formed during sporulation. The toxin can be shown to cause fluid accumulation in the rabbit ileal loop model (36,38) (the toxin is described in greater detail in Chapter 213).

An enterotoxin has been isolated from strains of *C. perfringens* type C implicated in the pigbel syndrome in New Guinea in the 1950s. This enterotoxin seems to be quite similar if not identical to the one described for type A strains (39).

EPIDEMIOLOGY

C. perfringens food poisoning is the third most common food-borne disease in the United States (1). Epidemics of *C. perfringens* illness are usually characterized by high attack rates with a large number of affected individuals; the average number of affected individuals per outbreak was nearly 50 from 1993 to 1997. There is no risk for secondary transmission. The incubation period in most outbreaks varies between 8 and 14 hours (median 12 hours) but can be as long as 72 hours.

Virtually every outbreak has roasted, boiled, stewed, or steamed meats or poultry as the vehicle of infection. The organism is ubiquitous, usually found in the gastrointestinal tract or in soil. The implicated food invariably undergoes a period of inadequate cooling during which the redox potential of the food is in a reduced state that allows the spores to germinate. This usually happens below 50°C. More cases of *C. perfringens* food poisoning are reported in the fall and winter months, presumably because stews and turkey are more likely to be consumed in winter.

CLINICAL FEATURES

C. perfringens food poisoning is characterized by watery diarrhea, nausea, and severe, crampy abdominal pain, usually without vomiting, beginning 8 to 24 hours after the incriminated meal. Fever, chills, headache, or other signs of infection are usually not present. The illness is of short duration, usually 24 hours or less. Rare fatalities have been recorded in debilitated or hospitalized patients.

Enteritis necroticans or pigbel is a much more severe, necrotizing disease of the small intestine with high mortality. After a 24-hour incubation period, illness ensues with intense abdominal pain, bloody diarrhea, vomiting, and shock. The mortality rate in this illness is about 40%, and death is usually due to intestinal perforation. Outbreaks of pigbel in New Guinea have been clearly related to orgiastic consumption of pig in large native feasts. The pig is improperly cooked, and large quantities are usually consumed. This syndrome has also been encountered in the United States after the consumption of pig intestines (chitterlings) (40).

DIAGNOSIS

The diagnosis of *C. perfringens* food poisoning should be considered in any diarrheal illness characterized by abdominal pain and moderate to severe diarrhea, unaccompanied by fever or chills. Many other individuals are usually involved in the outbreak, and the suspect food is beef or chicken that has been stewed, roasted, or boiled earlier and then allowed to sit without proper refrigeration.

The major laboratory criterion for diagnosis is the isolation of the same organism from epidemiologically incriminated food and from the stools of ill individuals. If no food specimens are available, the isolation of organisms with the same serotype in stools of most ill individuals, and not in the stools of suitable control subjects, would suffice for the diagnosis. In the absence of either of these findings, a culture of the incriminated food containing 10^5 organisms per gram or more is suggestive. Studies have demonstrated *C. perfringens* toxin in the stools of affected individuals (41). Serologic diagnosis is difficult because a high proportion of healthy individuals have antibody to *C. perfringens*.

Clostridium botulinum

The growth of *C. botulinum* in food is associated with the production of a potent neurotoxin. Ingestion of this toxin causes botulism, a neuroparalytic disease that may be fatal (42). Outbreaks and sporadic cases have been associated with meat, fish, and vegetables that are contaminated and improperly processed. Between 1993 and 1997 there were a total of 13 outbreaks of botulism in the United States, which were responsible for 56 cases and 1 death (1).

Toxin production occurs after germination of *C. botulinum* spores in inadequately processed foods, most commonly in the presence of anaerobic, low-solute, and low-acid conditions. The toxins can result in the development of an acute gastrointestinal illness, usually within 18 to 24 hours after ingestion of the toxin. When neurologic disease occurs, constipation is most common, but nausea, vomiting, and even diarrhea may occur before the onset of paralysis. This disease is caused by one of three distinct heat-labile neurotoxins designated A, B, and E (43). Neurotoxin-producing strains of *C. butyricum* and *C. baratii* are less commonly encountered causes of human botulism. The syndrome of infant botulism is thought to result from ingestion of spores with toxin production *in vivo* (44). A more complete discussion of this illness may be found in Chapter 212.

Botulism outbreaks have been generally associated with ingestion of low-acidity home-canned vegetables, fruits, or fish (43). Outbreaks have been associated with ingestion of sauteed onions, chopped garlic, and baked potatoes (45,46). A disproportionate number of cases in recent years have occurred in the Pacific Northwest and Alaska. These cases have been associated with native American foods such as seal or whale that have been fermented or preserved using traditional methods. Botulism may be confirmed by the demonstration of toxin in the serum or stool of ill people and in the incriminated food or by the isolation of *C. botulinum* from feces of ill people. Therapy is discussed in Chapter 212.

Escherichia coli

In the past 10 years, the emergence of verotoxin-producing *E. coli* of serotype O157:H7 (along with other serotypes) as a major food-borne pathogen has been remarkable (7,47). Furthermore, these verotoxin-producing strains have been associated with the development of the hemolytic-uremic syndrome (48).

The significance of this pathogen as a cause of food-borne disease was not evident in CDC surveillance data from 1988 to 1992 (49). However, in the period 1993 to 1997, the number of outbreaks reported to the CDC increased to 84, making *E. coli* the second most common cause of food-borne outbreaks after *Salmonella* (1). Some of this increase can be attributed to increased screening for the organism and reporting to public health authorities. In the past decade, multistate outbreaks with hundreds of cases and a number of deaths, especially among children, have been linked to contaminated, undercooked beef (50). Furthermore, these outbreaks have resulted in clusters of cases of hemolytic-uremic syndrome. Additional vehicles of transmission such as cold-pressed apple cider (51), dry-cured salami (52), unpasteurized milk (53), and mesclun lettuce have been recognized (54).

E. coli O157:H7 is present in the intestines of approximately 1% of healthy cattle. The process of slaughter and grinding presumably leads to contamination of beef, which, if the beef is undercooked, may lead to subsequent transmission. It should be noted that there are many other verotoxin-producing *E. coli* serotypes that may cause diarrheal illness (55); therefore, screening for the O157:H7 serotype clearly underrepresents the frequency of such infections.

The spectrum of disease may vary from nonbloody to bloody diarrhea, even frank hemorrhagic colitis, the hemolytic-uremic syndrome, thrombocytopenic purpura, and death. In *E. coli* O157:H7 outbreaks, about 25% of the patients have required hospitalization, about 5% developed hemolytic-uremic syndrome, and about 1% died (56).

The secondary attack rate in outbreaks in nursing homes and day care centers has been reported to be as high as 20%, perhaps reflecting a low inoculum necessary for transmissions (57). For a more complete discussion of this pathogen the reader is referred to Chapter 70.

Listeria monocytogenes

This organism is also becoming increasingly recognized as a food-borne pathogen (58). *Listeria* is a gram-positive, motile rod that is relatively heat-resistant. *Listeria* is widely distributed in nature, found in the intestinal tracts of various animals and humans and in sewage, soil, and water.

There is now sufficient evidence that *Listeria* is causally related to food-borne illness from investigations of a number of epidemics. Contaminated cole slaw, raw vegetables, raw and pasteurized milk, and Mexican-style soft cheeses have been implicated as vehicles for epidemic listeriosis (58). The sources of sporadic *Listeria* infection are less well understood, although one can culture the organism from raw poultry, beef, or pork, prepackaged meat products, cheeses, and raw vegetables (59).

The syndromes usually associated with *Listeria* include meningitis, bacteremia, and focal metastatic disease. It has frequently been noted that gastrointestinal symptoms, such as diarrhea, precede the recognized onset of bacteremic disease. The organism has a propensity to affect adults who are either immunosuppressed or pregnant. As a reflection of this host susceptibility, the most common cause of mortality associated with food-borne illness from 1983 to 1987 was epidemic listeriosis, which accounted for 70 deaths (60).

Immunocompetent hosts occasionally suffer from gastroenteritis characterized by fever, headache, abdominal pain, nausea, and diarrhea—this form of listeriosis is usually not complicated by bacteremia (9). The exact rate of food-borne transmission in sporadic cases of listeriosis is not known. Because the incubation period to disease onset may be more than a week, it may be difficult to pinpoint the food exposures that occurred before case recognition. However, a commercial food monitoring program initiated by the U.S. Food and Drug Administration detected *L. monocytogenes* in 2% to 3% of all processed dairy products that were tested, reflecting the widespread distribution of this organism in nature (61). There has been a reduction in the incidence of human listeriosis in the United States, perhaps as a result of industry, regulatory, and educational efforts (62). Surveillance estimates suggest about a 45% reduction in illness and death related to *L. monocytogenes*.

This organism is discussed in greater detail in Chapter 190.

Salmonella

Salmonella is the most commonly documented cause of food poisoning in the United States. Between 1993 and 1997, this organism was responsible for 357 recorded outbreaks and 32,610 cases, resulting in 13 fatalities (1). Given estimates that as few as 10% of cases are actually reported, infections caused by this pathogen are probably even more common. The marked increase in salmonellosis has in part been attributed to increasing contamination of poultry and grade A eggs (63,64). Certain serotypes have been epidemiologically linked to particular animal species, for example, *Salmonella enteriditis* with chicken eggs (65), *Salmonella hadar* with turkey products (66), and *Salmonella dublin* with raw cow's milk (67). Details regarding *Salmonella* pathogenesis and therapy are provided in Chapters 68 and 196.

Vibrio parahaemolyticus

V. parahaemolyticus was first recognized as a potential food-borne pathogen by Fujino and co-workers (68,69) when it was isolated from autopsy materials collected in relation to a food-poisoning outbreak. During the next decade, many other outbreaks in Japan were associated with a pleomorphic, halophilic, hemolytic gram-negative organism similar to the one described by Fujino and co-workers and variously named *Pasteurella parahaemolytica*, *Pseudomonas enteritis*, and *Oceanomonas parahaemolytica* (69). The vehicles in these outbreaks were usually raw fish, shellfish, and cucumbers in brine. Extensive taxonomic studies by Sakazaki and colleagues (70) and Fujino (69) revealed that the organisms in question belonged to the genus *Vibrio*, and the new species designation *V. parahaemolyticus* was officially adopted.

Volunteer feeding experiments in Japan in the 1960s supplied further evidence of the pathogenicity of this organism. Kato and co-workers (71) made the next major advance when they observed that strains isolated from ill humans caused hemolysis on Wagatsuma blood agar, whereas strains obtained from routine food samples lacked this characteristic. It was suggested that this trait correlated with pathogenicity. Indeed, this was borne out in volunteer studies, because only hemolytic strains were pathogenic in humans. This has been termed the Kanagawa phenomenon.

Japanese workers, using various culture media with a high salt content, showed that *V. parahaemolyticus* accounts for 50% to 70% of reported food-borne disease in Japan during the summer months (5). This organism has also been implicated in outbreaks in the United States (72).

MICROBIOLOGY AND PATHOPHYSIOLOGY

V. parahaemolyticus is a gram-negative, straight or curved rod that is pleomorphic, halophilic, and facultatively anaerobic. This organism is part of the genus *Vibrio*, which includes *V. cholerae*, *V. alginolyticus*, *V. vulnificus*, and other species (see Chapter 199).

Pathogenic strains produce a number of toxins, including a lethal toxin, which is also hemolytic. In some studies, these organisms have been shown to produce an enterotoxin that causes fluid accumulation in the rabbit ileal loop model and a cytotoxic

toxin that causes damage to HeLa cells. Some strains have the ability to invade the intestinal mucosa and cause bacteremia in experimental animals (73).

EPIDEMIOLOGY

Although most outbreaks of *V. parahaemolyticus* gastroenteritis have been recorded in Japan, many other countries in Southeast Asia, as well as Australia, Great Britain, and the United States, have documented this infection. The organism itself is ubiquitous in marine waters and can be found on the U.S. coastline, in Canada, Great Britain, the Netherlands, and virtually all of Southeast Asia. In the United States, outbreaks have been related to crabs (both steamed and processed), shrimp (both cooked and uncooked), and raw oysters.

There has been a striking association of *V. parahaemolyticus* infection in the United States with coastal states. Maryland, Massachusetts, Louisiana, New Jersey, Texas, and Washington have all reported outbreaks. In addition, there have been several epidemics on cruise ships. The majority of reported cases have occurred during the warm months (June to October).

It is difficult to assess the real incidence of food poisoning caused by *V. parahaemolyticus* in the United States. Between 1973 and 1998, 40 outbreaks caused by this organism were reported (72). The attack rates in epidemics reported in the United States have varied from as low as 3% to as high as 100% of exposed individuals, and the number of affected individuals from 2 to nearly 300. No secondary cases have been reported in either the United States or Japan, although two individuals with long incubation periods (96 hours) may have been secondary cases in one outbreak. The median incubation period for most outbreaks has been 13 to 23 hours; the range has been quite variable, from 4 to 48 hours.

CLINICAL FEATURES

Explosive watery diarrhea is the cardinal manifestation of more than 90% of cases. Abdominal cramps, nausea, vomiting, and headache are common. Fever and chills occurred in approximately 25% of cases. Clinically, this illness resembles that produced by nontyphoidal salmonellosis. However, in one epidemic case in the United States, a bloody dysenteric syndrome was observed with fecal leukocytes and superficial ulcerations on sigmoidoscopic examination; a small percentage of cases in a cruise ship outbreak also reported bloody diarrhea.

The illness has generally been mild, with a median duration of 3 days (range 2 hours to 10 days). There have been few deaths in the more than 1,000 cases reported in the United States. This has generally been the experience in Japan, although in the first outbreak reported by Fujino (68), 20 of 272 ill individuals died. The diarrhea is usually not as profuse as that of *V. cholerae*. Yet, in one outbreak in Great Britain, hypotension and shock occurred in three of five cases. The spectrum of disease is thus quite varied.

V. parahaemolyticus can occasionally cause wound infections and primary septicemia. Most cases in the United States have been related to trauma associated with a marine environment.

DIAGNOSIS

V. parahaemolyticus should be considered in any outbreak of diarrheal illness related to seafood occurring in the warm months. The occurrence of mild but explosive watery diarrhea with or without dysentery (bloody, mucoid stools) in association with abdominal cramps, nausea, vomiting, and headache is most characteristic.

Rectal swabs or stool specimens should be streaked onto thiosulfate citrate bile salts agar or bromothymol blue-Teepol agar plates and incubated at 35° to 37°C for 18 to 24 hours. Studies have shown mannitol salt agar to be an acceptable alternative medium.

Other Organisms

A number of other bacteria have been implicated in food-borne diarrheal illness. Many reports are unconvincing or unconfirmed.

ARIZONA

The organism *Arizona* is a motile gram-negative rod now classified as a subspecies of *Salmonella* (74). It has been implicated in outbreaks of gastroenteritis and enteric fever. Various vehicles have included eggs or poultry as the contaminated product (75). Because of the similarities to *Salmonella,* contaminated animal products should be considered the usual vehicle.

The syndromes caused by *Arizona* are also similar to salmonellosis. Gastroenteritis, enteric fever, bacteremia, and localized infection have been described. The incubation period is similar to that of *Salmonella.* Usually 24 to 48 hours after ingestion of contaminated food, symptoms develop, including fever, headache, nausea, vomiting, abdominal pain, and watery diarrhea. Marked prostration may occur. Symptoms may persist for several days. Therapy and prevention are also similar to the methods used for salmonellosis.

AEROMONAS AND PLESIOMONAS

The role of *Aeromonas* species as food-borne pathogens is unclear (76,77). The organisms can be isolated from a number of environmental sources, including fresh water, brackish water, and sewage (78). *Aeromonas* species have also been isolated from raw meats and unpasteurized milk. Gastroenteritis caused by this organism is more prevalent during warmer months.

Case-control studies in some series have implicated *Aeromonas* species as a cause of diarrhea (79). However, there have been few reports of outbreaks caused by this organism. Symptomatic infections are usually characterized by watery diarrhea with nausea and vomiting. Rarely, bloody, mucoid diarrhea may also occur. Most infections are self-limited, so antimicrobial therapy is generally not necessary.

Plesiomonas shigelloides is a gram-negative rod from the family Vibrionaceae, which also has been associated with diarrheal illness (80). At least two outbreaks have been reported, including one related to ingestion of raw oysters (81). Individuals who became ill did so 48 hours after consuming raw oysters. It is thought that the organism is enteroinvasive on the basis of lack of discernible toxins and the presence of blood and fecal polymorphonuclear leukocytes in stools of individuals with diarrhea (81).

PROVIDENCIA

Although the enteropathogenicity of *Providencia alcalifaciens* has not been well established, this organism was implicated as the cause of gastroenteritis in a large food-borne outbreak in Japan in 1996 (82). Presenting symptoms included diarrhea and abdominal pain; fever was present in about a quarter of patients. A clonal isolate of *P. alcalifaciens* was isolated from several symptomatic patients, whereas no other potential pathogens were isolated. The role of this organism as a cause of food-borne disease needs to be prospectively evaluated.

CHRONIC DIARRHEA

A chronic diarrheal syndrome has been described in individuals drinking raw milk. It was described originally in Brainerd, Min-

nesota, where individuals developed acute watery diarrhea that persisted for an average of 2 years (83). The etiologic agent has not been identified. Diarrhea began approximately 2 weeks after ingestion of the product. In addition, there has been a second outbreak of a similar illness associated with a restaurant, suggesting that a food vehicle other than raw milk may be involved (84).

VIRUSES

The two most common viral causes of food poisoning are the hepatitis A and Norwalk viruses (1). Humans are the only known reservoir for both viruses.

Hepatitis A infections have been linked to raw shellfish, but efficient transmission from infected food handlers can also occur (85). High secondary attack rates are common, especially in household contacts.

Outbreaks of Norwalk virus have been associated with raw shellfish, frosting, and contaminated salads (86,87). Waterborne outbreaks have also been described (88). Norwalk virus food poisoning is marked by high attack rates, presumably because of the low inoculum necessary to transmit infection (89,90). For a complete discussion of hepatitis A and Norwalk virus, the reader is referred to Chapters 251 and 263, respectively.

PARASITIC DISEASE

A number of parasites have been implicated in food-borne disease, including *Trichinella spiralis, Entamoeba histolytica, Giardia lamblia, Cryptosporidium parvum, Cyclospora cayetanensis, Ascaris lumbricoides, Taenia saginata, Taenia solium, Anisakis,* and *Diphyllobothrium latum.* From 1993 to 1997, four outbreaks caused by *G. lamblia* and two by *T. spirallis* were reported to the CDC (1). In addition, 13 other outbreaks due to parasites were reported. Outbreaks associated with these parasites are much less common than those due to bacteria.

Water-borne outbreaks caused by *Cryptosporidium* have reached national prominence (91). In addition, one reported outbreak was related to fresh-pressed apple cider (92) and a recent outbreak at a university was linked to an infected food handler (93). Food-borne outbreaks of *C. cayetanensis* have also been increasingly described during recent years, with imported raspberries implicated as the probable vehicle of transmission (8,94). The life cycles, modes of transmission, and discussions of these parasites can be found in Chapter 284.

SYNDROMES RELATED TO CHEMICALS

In addition to bacterial food poisoning, which primarily causes diarrheal syndromes with abdominal cramps and fever, a number of food-borne diseases are related to chemicals, many of which are not due to microbial pathogens. Individuals who develop nausea and vomiting with or without abdominal cramps within an hour of food consumption usually have disease primarily related to heavy metal poisoning. Copper, zinc, tin, and cadmium have generally caused such outbreaks (95,96). The time from consumption to onset of disease is generally 5 to 15 minutes. Nausea, vomiting, and cramps usually occur and resolve several hours after removal of the offending agent by vomiting.

Several syndromes are characterized by paresthesias occurring within 1 to several hours after ingestion of the toxin. The major ones include fish poisoning, Chinese restaurant syndrome, and niacin poisoning (97–100). The Chinese restaurant syndrome is characterized by a burning sensation in the neck, abdomen, and arms along with chest tightness. Headache, flushing, weakness, nausea, and abdominal cramps have also been described. Symptoms are thought to be caused primarily by excessive amounts of monosodium L-glutamate, although not all the substances that cause this syndrome have been well defined (98). This illness is treated symptomatically and usually resolves within hours. Another syndrome that is associated with burning or facial flushing is niacin poisoning, which can occur within less than an hour of ingestion and generally resolves rapidly (99).

The fish and shellfish poisoning syndromes are outlined in Table 77.3. Several different syndromes have been described, namely scombroid, ciguatera, paralytic shellfish, diarrhetic shellfish, amnestic shellfish, and neurotoxic shellfish poisoning (100–102). Most of these syndromes occur within hours of ingestion, although symptoms of illness can last for months in some cases.

SCOMBROID

Scombroid poisoning is characterized by symptoms that are typical of a histamine reaction (103). Burning of the mouth and throat, flushing, and headache frequently occur. In many cases urticaria and bronchospasm can also be present. Symptoms are the result of histamine that is produced by enzymatic decarboxylation of histidine by marine-associated bacteria. Elevated plasma histamine levels may be present in patients at the time of initial evaluation (104) but more commonly are not increased (102). Histamine, cadaverine, and putrescine were detected in samples from one outbreak that was associated with a nonscombroid fish, a bluefish (105). Treatment with oral antihistamines and/or parenteral histamine-2 blockers have been shown to help relieve symptoms of scombroid poisoning (106).

SHELLFISH POISONING SYNDROMES

There are several types of shellfish poisoning, including paralytic, diarrhetic, amnesic, and neurotoxic (101). Each syndrome is associated with a different toxin. These syndromes are generally confined to coastal areas of the world. Symptoms in paralytic shellfish poisoning are due to saxitoxins produced by marine microalgae (*Gonyaulax catenella, Gonyaulax tamarensis*); these typically include paresthesias, shortness of breath, muscle weakness or paralysis, and respiratory insufficiency (97,107,108). Saxitoxin is heat stable and blocks nerve and muscle action potential by interfering with sodium permeability. Brevetoxins produced by the dinoflagellates responsible for red tide (*Gymnodinium breve*) are responsible for neurotoxic shellfish poisoning. This form of seafood poisoning tends to be milder, and respiratory paralysis has not been reported.

Diarrhetic shellfish poisoning is characterized by a predominance of gastrointestinal symptoms. Dinophysisoxins, lipophilic polyether compounds, produced by dinoflagellates of the genera *Dinophysis* and *Prorocentrum*, are responsible for this syndrome. Although the acute illness may be relatively severe, it is self-limited, with most patients recovering within a few days.

Amnestic shellfish poisoning was first described in an outbreak in Canada associated with the consumption of mussels that had been harvested from Prince Edward Island. A diatomous red seaweed, Pseudo-nitzschia multiseries, was eventually found to be the source of the toxin, domoic acid. This toxin is a water-soluble, heat-stable amino acid that is a potent glutamate agonist (101). Subsequently, several other outbreaks have occurred in the United States, Spain, and United Kingdom. One U.S. outbreak was found to be due to toxic Californian anchovies.

CIGUATERA

Ciguatera is one of the most commonly reported illnesses that is attributable to seafood. Most cases in the United States have been reported from Hawaii, Florida, and the territories of Puerto Rico and the Virgin Islands (102). The toxin is produced by the dinoflagellate *Gambierdiscus toxicus*. The ciguatoxin is heat stable, lipid soluble, and acid resistant, and is found in carnivorous reef-dwelling fish species, including barracuda, snapper, and grouper.

Ciguatera fish poisoning can be distinguished from paralytic shellfish poisoning by symptoms characterized by a more abdominal component, including abdominal cramps, nausea, vomiting, and diarrhea (108–110). Although patients may have numbness and paresthesias of the lips and tongue, dry mouth, myalgias, blurred vision, photophobia, transient blindness, and a sharp shooting pain in the legs have also been reported. In addition, there may be a sensation of looseness and pain in the teeth and a reversal of cold and hot sensation. Respiratory paralysis may occur. Ciguatoxin has been demonstrated to be similar to the toxins described in paralytic shellfish poisoning (111). The duration of ciguatoxin poisoning tends to be longer than that seen with the neurotoxic or paralytic shellfish poisonings (112). Acute illness may range for days to months, and pain has been reported to occur for years after an episode. Treatment is supportive; rehydration is often necessary early in the acute illness.

TETRODOTOXIN

Intoxication from the tetrodotoxin has been primarily reported from Japan (101), where it has been associated with consumption of the flesh of puffer fish (Fugu). This expensive delicacy can result in a range of symptoms depending on individual response and the amount of residual tetrodotoxin in the fish flesh. Symptoms usually develop within a few hours and include lethargy, peripheral and facial paresthesias, hyperemesis, salivation, weakness, and ataxia. More severe cases proceed to ascending paralysis, autonomic irregularities, respiratory failure, and death (102).

MUSHROOM POISONING SYNDROMES

A number of clinical syndromes associated with the ingestion of toxic mushrooms have been described (Table 77.4). A syndrome with a short incubation period in which patients develop confusion, restlessness, visual disturbances, and lethargy has been described (113). Several *Amanita* species of mushrooms that contain ibotenic acid or muscimol are responsible for this syndrome. Another species of mushroom causes an illness in which parasympathetic hyperactivity is pronounced with salivation, blurred vision, sweating, and diarrhea. In addition, patients may develop bradycardia or bronchospasm. Symptoms usually resolve in 24 hours. This syndrome is caused by the chemical muscarine found in *Inocybe* and *Clitocybe* species (114). An acute psychotic reaction caused by toxins found in several species of mushrooms

TABLE 77.3. Fish and Shellfish Poisoning Syndromes

Syndrome	Fish	Incubation period	Symptoms	Duration	Geographic location	Toxin
Scombroid	Tuna, mackeral, bonito, skipjack, mahi-mahi	5 min–3 h	Histamine reaction, burning, flushing, urticaria, nausea, vomiting, bronchospasm	Hours	Coast (Hawaii, California)	Histamine and saurine
Ciguatera	Barracuda, snapper, grouper, amberjack	1–6 h	Nausea, vomiting, diarrhea, blurred vision, photophobia, shooting pains, hot-cold temperature reversal, bradycardia hypotension, respiratory paralysis	Days–months	35 degrees north 35 degrees south latitude (Hawaii, Florida)	Ciguatoxin
Paralytic shellfish	Shellfish	5 min–4 h	Perioral paresthesias, peripheral paresthesia, dizziness, nausea, vomiting, dysphagia, respiratory paralysis	Hours–days	>30 degrees north and <30 degrees south New England, West Coast	Saxitoxin
Neurotoxic shellfish	Shellfish	5 min–4 h	Paresthesias, myalgias, dizziness, hot-cold temperature reversal, vomiting, diarrhea	Hours–days	Gulf Coast, Atlantic Coast (Florida)	Saxitoxin
Amnestic shellfish	Shellfish, anchovies	Gastrointestinal <24 h; neurologic <48 h	Nausea, vomiting, cramps, diarrhea, headache, dizziness, weakness, confusion, ataxia, memory loss, seizures, coma	Days–months	Coastal Canada, USA, and Europe	
Diarrhetic shellfish	Shellfish	30 min–12 h	Acute diarrhea, nausea, vomiting, abdominal pain, chills	Hours–days	Coastal Europe, Japan	
Puffer fish poisoning	Puffer fish (Fugu)	10 min–3 h	Lethargy, paraesthesias, salivation, hyperemesis, weakness, ataxia, dysphagia, respiratory failure, hypotension, bradycardia	Hours–days	Japan, Mexico	

Data from Whittle et al. (101), Eastaough (102), Gilbert et al. (103), Bagnis et al. (110), and Morris et al. (113).

TABLE 77.4. Mushroom Poisoning Syndromes

Syndrome	Incubation period (h)	Species	Toxin
Confusion, restlessness, visual disturbances, lethargy	2	*Amanita muscaria* *Amanita pantherina*	Ibotenic acid, muscimol
Parasympathetic activity	2	*Inocybe* species *Clitocybe* species	Muscarine
Hallucinations	2	*Psilocybe* species *Panaeolus* species	Psilocybin Psilocin
Disulfiram	2	*Coprinus atramentarius*	Disulfiram-like substances
Gastroenteritis	2	Many	Unknown
Hepatorenal failure	6–24	*Amanita phalloides* *Amanita virosa* *Amanita verna* *Galerina autumnalis* *Galerina marginata* *Galerina venenata*	Amatoxins Phallotoxins
Hepatic failure	6–24	*Gyromitra* species	Gyromitrin

has been described. Mushroom intoxication can also cause a disulfiram-like reaction if alcohol is consumed. A number of mushrooms can cause gastroenteritis. The toxins responsible for this syndrome have not been well characterized.

By far the most lethal mushroom poisoning syndromes are due to the amatoxins and phallotoxins found in the species *Amanita phalloides, Amanita virosa, Amanita verna, Galerina autumnalis, Galerina marginata,* and *Galerina venenata.* After ingestion the syndrome is heralded by abdominal cramps and diarrhea; however, after apparent improvement in symptoms, patients develop both liver and renal failure (115). A mortality rate of at least 50% has been reported. A similar syndrome without renal failure has been described after ingestion of *Gyromitra.* The toxin associated with this species does not appear to cause acute renal failure; however, significant hepatic failure has been described.

WATERBORNE DISEASE

Occasionally clusters of waterborne disease that may mimic a food-borne epidemic are reported. The most common causes of waterborne disease have been *G. lamblia* (see Chapter 278), which has been responsible for several large outbreaks associated with municipal water supplies, and *Cryptosporidium* (see Chapter 284), which has caused large, community-wide outbreaks (91). Other waterborne outbreaks have been caused by *Shigella,* hepatitis A virus, nontyphoid *Salmonella, Salmonella typhi,* enterotoxigenic *E. coli, C. jejuni,* and viral agents, including Norwalk virus and others.

TREATMENT

For each of the pathogens enumerated here, treatment is beyond the scope of this chapter. In general, for the illnesses that are self-limited and mediated by toxins, antibiotics play little role in either therapy or prophylaxis. Invasive disease caused by *Salmonella* or *Campylobacter* may require antibiotic therapy. Disease caused by *Shigella* or *Listeria* requires antibiotic treatment, a discussion of which can be found in their respective chapters. Fluid replacement and supportive therapy are the major considerations in all of these illnesses.

CONTROL AND PREVENTION

The common theme that ties all food-borne illnesses together is the presence of an improper food-handling procedure before food consumption. In a review of the factors responsible for food-borne outbreaks in the United States during a 15-year period, inadequate refrigeration was the single factor most frequently implicated in food-borne outbreaks (1,116) (Table 77.5). Usually more than one factor is associated with an outbreak, and inadequate refrigeration, advance preparation of food without adequate storage, and improper reheating or cooling are usually present to one degree or another. To a lesser degree, contaminated equipment, cross-contamination, and food preparation personnel with poor personal hygiene may contribute to outbreaks. Contaminated raw ingredients are frequently part of the process as well. The ubiquity of *B. cereus* and *C. perfringens* makes it mandatory that food be cooked properly and, when stored, cooled properly. The failure to refrigerate food properly is the major problem in staphylococcal disease, the only difference being the contamination of the food by a carrier at some point before service. It becomes obvious that control must be based

TABLE 77.5. Factors Contributing to Food-Borne Disease Outbreak in the United States from 1961 to 1976

Factor	% Implicated[a]
Inadequate refrigeration	47
Food prepared too far in advance of service	21
Infected person with poor personal hygiene	21
Inadequate cooking	16
Inadequate holding temperature	16
Inadequate reheating	12
Contaminated raw ingredients	11
Cross-contamination	7
Dirty equipment	7

[a]Values total more than 100% because more than one factor may contribute to foodborne outbreaks.
From Bryan FL. Epidemiology of foodborne diseases. In: Reimann H, Bryan FL eds. *Foodborne infections and intoxications,* ed 2. New York: Academic, 1979;3–69, with permission.

on inhibiting bacterial growth, preventing contamination after preparation, and killing potential pathogens with cooking. In general, foods should be heated to an internal temperature of 165°F, but lower temperatures for longer periods may be equally effective. Once cooked or processed, foods must be held at a temperature of 40°F or below.

Although these control measures are standard, many places where food preparation takes place do not abide by these guidelines. It is through diligent efforts by public health officials that reported outbreaks are investigated and food preparation techniques corrected. Therefore, recognition and reporting of food-borne illness are instrumental in the control of the problem. Education of the public, nurses, physicians, and eating establishments is crucial to the control of food-borne illness. Carriage of most of the organisms considered in this chapter is not a problem, with the exception of staphylococci and Salmonella. Because staphylococcal carriage is a necessary step in the development of staphylococcal food-borne illness, education of food handlers to watch for boils and pustules should be emphasized. Except for *S. typhi*, carriage of *Salmonella* is not the usual means of transmission of these organisms.

IMMUNIZATION

In general, immunization has not been attempted in these diseases. The immunogenicity of many of the toxins described has not been totally defined, and the populations at risk are so vast that immunization may not be practical. An interesting report on using a clostridial toxoid prepared from type C cultures in New Guinea suggests the prevention of pigbel in children (117). However, for viral diseases, the use of hepatitis A vaccine is very effective in prevention of food-borne hepatitis A, even in an outbreak situation (118).

REFERENCES

1. Olsen SJ, MacKinnon LC, Goulding JS, et al. Surveillance for foodborne disease outbreaks—United States. *MMWR* 2000;49(SS-1):1–62.
2. Todd E. Epidemiology of foodborne illness: North America. *Lancet* 1990;336:788–790.
3. Centers for Disease Control and Prevention. Diagnosis and management of foodborne illnesses. A primer for physicians. *MMWR* 2001;50(RR-2):1–48.
4. Bryan FL, Fanelli MJ, Reimann H. Salmonella infections. In: Reimann H, Bryan FL, eds. *Foodborne infections and intoxications*, 2nd ed. New York: Academic, 1979:73–130.
5. Sakazaki R. Halophilic *Vibrio* infections. In: Reimann H, ed. *Foodborne infections and intoxications*. New York: Academic, 1969:115–119.
6. Hedberg CW, MacDonald KL, Osterholm MT. Changing epidemiology of foodborne disease: a Minnesota perspective. *Clin Infect Dis* 1994;18:671–682.
7. Slutzker LA, Ries AA, Green JG, et al. Escherichia coli O157:H7 diarrhea in the United States: clinical and epidemiological features. *Ann Intern Med* 1997;126:505–513.
8. Herwaldt BL, Ackers ML. An outbreak in 1996 of cyclosporiasis associated with imported raspberries. The Cyclospora Working Group. *N Engl J Med* 1997;336:1548–1556.
9. Aureli P, Fiorucci GC, Caroli D, et al. An outbreak of febrile gastroenteritis associated with corn contaminated by *Listeria monocytogenes*. *N Engl J Med* 2000;342:1236.
10. Skirrow MB. *Campylobacter* perspectives. Public Health Laboratory Service. *Microbiol Diagn* 1989;6:113–117.
11. Morse DL, Guzewich JJ, Hanrahan JP, et al. Widespread outbreaks of clam- and oyster-associated gastroenteritis: role of Norwalk virus. *N Engl J Med* 1986;314:678–681.
12. Hedberg CW, Fishbein DB, Janssen RS, et al. An outbreak of thyrotoxicosis caused by consumption of bovine thyroid gland in ground beef. *N Engl J Med* 1987;316:993–998.
13. Belongia EA, Hedberg CW, Gleich GJ, et al. An investigation of the cause of the eosinophilia-myalgia syndrome associated with tryptophan use. *N Engl J Med* 1990;323:357–365.
14. Dack GM, Cary WE, Woolpert O, et al. An outbreak of food poisoning proved to be due to a yellow hemolytic *Staphylococcus*. *J Prev Med* 1930;4:167–175.
15. Dack GM, Jordan EO, Woolpert O. Attempts to immunize human volunteers with *Staphylococcus* filtrates that are toxic to man when swallowed. *J Prev Med* 1931;5:151–159.
16. Dack GM. *Staphylococcus* food poisoning. In: Dack GM, ed. *Food poisoning*. Chicago: University of Chicago Press, 1956:109–158.
17. Sullivan R, Asano T. Effects of staphylococcal enterotoxin B on intestinal transport in the rat. *Am J Physiol* 1971;222:1793–1799.
18. Minor TE, March EH. *Staphylococcus aureus* and staphylococcal food poisoning. *J Milk Food Technol* 1972;34:21–29, 77–83, 227–241; 1973;35:447–476.
19. Bergdoll MS, Crass BA, Reiser RF, et al. A new staphylococcal enterotoxin, enterotoxin F, associated with toxic-shock-syndrome *Staphylococcus aureus* isolates. *Lancet* 1981;1:1017–1021.
20. Holmberg SD, Blake PA. Staphylococcal food poisoning in the United States. New facts and old misconceptions. *JAMA* 1984;25:487–489.
21. Terranova W, Blake PA. Bacillus cereus food poisoning. *N Engl J Med* 1978;298:143–144.
22. Mortimer PR, McCann G. Food-poisoning episodes associated with *Bacillus cereus* in fried rice. *Lancet* 1974;1:1043–1045.
23. Saunders GC, Bartlett ML. Double-antibody solid-phase enzyme immunoassay for the detection of staphylococcal enterotoxin A. *Appl Environ Microbiol* 1977;34:518–522.
24. Hauge S. Food poisoning caused by aerobic spore forming bacilli. *J Appl Bacteriol* 1955;18:591–595.
25. Midura T, Gerber M, Wood R, et al. Outbreak of food poisoning cause by *Bacillus cereus*. *Public Health Rep* 1970;85:45–48.
26. Portnoy BL, Goepfert JM, Harmon SM. An outbreak of *Bacillus cereus* food poisoning resulting from contaminated vegetable sprouts. *Am J Epidemiol* 1976;103:589–594.
27. Turnbull PCB, Nottingham JF, Ghosh AC. A severe necrotic enterotoxin produced by certain food, food poisoning and other clinical isolates of *Bacillus cereus*. *Br J Exp Pathol* 1977;58:273–280.
28. Turnbull PCB. Studies on the production of enterotoxins by *Bacillus cereus*. *J Clin Pathol* 1976;29:941–948.
29. Lund BM. Foodborne disease due to *Bacillus* and *Clostridium* species. *Lancet* 1990;336:982–986.
30. Morbidity and Mortality Weekly Report. Human ingestion of *Bacillus anthracis*–contaminated meat—Minnesota, August 2000. *MMWR* 200049:813–816.
31. McClung LS. Human food poisoning due to growth of *Clostridium perfringens* (*C. welchii*) in freshly cooked chicken: a preliminary note. *J Bacteriol* 1945;50:229–233.
32. Hobbs BC, Smith ME, Oakley CL, et al. *Clostridium welchii* food poisoning. *J Hyg* 1953;51:75–101.
33. Zeissler J, Rassfeld-Stemberg L. Enteritis necroticans due to *Clostridium welchii* type F. *BMJ* 1949;1:267–270.
34. Murrell TGC, Egerton JR, Rampling A, et al. The ecology and epidemiology of the pig-bel syndrome in man in New Guinea. *J Hyg* 1966;64:375–396.
35. Stark RL, Duncan CL. Biological characteristics of *Clostridium perfringens* type A enterotoxin. *Infect Immun* 1971;4:89–96.
36. Duncan CL, Strong DH. *Clostridium perfringens* type A food poisoning. I. Response of the rabbit ileum as an indication of enteropathogenicity of strains of *Clostridium perfringens* in monkeys. *Infect Immun* 1971;3:167–170.
37. Duncan CL. Time of enterotoxin formation and release during sporulation of *Clostridium perfringens* type A. *J Bacteriol* 1973;113:932–936.
38. Skjelkvale R, Duncan CL. Enterotoxin formation by different toxigenic types of *Clostridium perfringens*. *Infect Immun* 1975;11:563–575.
39. Skjelkvale R, Duncan CL. Characterization of enterotoxin purified from *Clostridium perfringens* type C. *Infect Immun* 1975;11:1061–1068.
40. Petrillo TM, Beck-Sagué CM, Songer JG, et al. Enteritis necroticans (pigbel) in a diabetic child. *N Engl J Med* 2000;342:1250–1253.
41. Bartholomew BA, Stringer MF, Watson GN, et al. Development and application of an enzyme linked immunosorbent assay for *Clostridium perfringens* type A enterotoxin. *J Clin Pathol* 1985;38:222–228.
42. Arnon SS, Midura TF, Clay SA, et al. Infant botulism: epidemiological, clinical and laboratory aspects. *JAMA* 1977;237:1946–1952.
43. Shapiro RL, Hatheway C, Swerdlow DL. Botulism in the United States: a clinical and epidemiologic review. *Ann Intern Med* 1998;129:221–228.
44. Horwitz MH, Hughes JM, Merson MH, et al. Foodborne botulism in the United States, 1970–75. *J Infect Dis* 1977;136:153–157.
45. MacDonald KL, Spengler RF, Hathaway CL, et al. Type A botulism from sauteed onions. *JAMA* 1985;253:1275–1278.
46. St. Louis ME, Peck SHS, Bowering D, et al. Botulism from chopped garlic: delayed recognition of a major outbreak. *Ann Intern Med* 1988;108:363–368.
47. Mead PS, Griffin PM. *Escherichia coli* O157:H7. *Lancet* 1998;352:1207–1212.
48. Boyce TG, Swerdlow DL, Griffin PM. *Escherichia coli* O157:H7 and the hemolytic-uremic syndrome. *N Engl J Med* 1995;333:364–368.
49. Centers for Disease Control and Prevention. Surveillance for foodborne-disease outbreaks—United States, 1988–1992. *MMWR* 1996;45(SS-5):1–66.
50. Bell BP, Goldoft M, Griffin PM, et al. A multistate outbreak of *Escherichia coli* O157:H7–associated bloody diarrhea and hemolytic uremic syndrome from hamburgers. The Washington experience. *JAMA* 1994;272:1349–1353.

51. Besser RE, Lett SM, Weber TJ, et al. An outbreak of diarrhea and hemolytic uremic syndrome from *Escherichia coli* O157:H7 in fresh-pressed apple cider. *JAMA* 1993;269:2217–2220.

52. Centers for Disease Control and Prevention. *Escherichia coli* O157:H7 outbreak linked to commercially distributed dry-cured salami—Washington and California, 1994. *MMWR* 1995;44:157–160.

53. Keene WE, Hedberg K, Herriott DE, et al. A prolonged outbreak of *Escherichia coli* O157:H7 infections caused by commercially distributed raw milk. *J Infect Dis* 1997;176:815–818.

54. Hilborn ED, Mermin JH, Mshar PA, et al. A multistate outbreak of *Escherichia coli* O157:H7 infections associated with consumption of mesclun lettuce. *Arch Intern Med* 1999;159:1758–1764.

55. Su C, Brandt LJ. *Escherichia coli* 0157:H7 infection in humans. *Ann Intern Med* 1995;123:698–714.

56. Griffin PM, Ostroff SM, Tauxe RV, et al. Illnesses associated with *Escherichia coli* O157:H7 infections. A broad clinical spectrum. *Ann Intern Med* 1988;109:705–712.

57. Belongia EA, Osterholm MT, Soler JJ, et al. Transmission of *Escherichia coli* O157:H7 infection in Minnesota child day-care facilities. *JAMA* 1993;269:883–888.

58. Schlech WF. Foodborne listeriosis. *Clin Infect Dis* 2000;31:770–775.

59. Pinner RW, Schuchat A, Swaminathan B, et al. Role of foods in sporadic listeriosis. II. Microbiologic and epidemiologic investigation. *JAMA* 1992;267:2046–2050.

60. Centers for Disease Control and Prevention. *Foodborne and waterborne disease outbreaks. Five year summary, 1983–1987.* Atlanta: Centers for Disease Control and Prevention, 1990.

61. *Listeria* contamination seen controlled by normal sanitation procedures. Washington, DC: National Association of Federal Veterinarians, 1987:2.

62. Tappero JW, Schucart A, Deaver KA, et al. Reduction in the incidence of human listeriosis in the United States. Effectiveness of prevention efforts? *JAMA* 1995;273:1118–1122.

63. Hohmann EL. Nontyphoidal salmonellosis. *Clin Infect Dis* 2001;32:263–269.

64. St. Louis ME, Morse DL, Potter ME, et al. The emergence of grade A eggs as a major source of *Salmonella enteriditis* infections. New implications for the control of salmonellosis. *JAMA* 1988;259:2103–2107.

65. Mishu B, Griffin PM, Tauxe RV, et al. *Salmonella enteritidis* gastroenteritis transmitted by intact chicken eggs. *Ann Intern Med* 1991;115:190–194.

66. Fowler NG, Mead GC. Salmonella in poultry [Letter]. *Lancet* 1991;337:118–119.

67. Maguire H, Cowden J, Jacob M, et al. An outbreak of *Salmonella dublin* infection in England and Wales associated with soft unpasteurized cows' milk cheese. *Epidemiol Infect* 1992;109:389–396.

68. Fujino T, Okuno Y, Nahada D, et al. On the bacteriological examination of shirasu-food poisoning. *Med J Osaka Univ* 1953;4:299–304.

69. Fujino T, Sakazaki R, Tamura K. Designation of the type of strain of *Vibrio parahaemolyticus* and description of 200 strains of the species. *Int J Syst Bacteriol* 1974;24:447–499.

70. Sakazaki R Tamura K, Kato T, et al. Studies on the enteropathogenic facultatively halophilic bacteria, *Vibrio parahaemolyticus*. III. Enteropathogenicity. *Jpn J Med Sci Biol* 1968;21:325–331.

71. Kato T, Obara Y, Ichinose H, et al. Hemolytic activity and toxicity of *Vibrio parahaemolyticus*. *Jpn J Bacteriol* 1966;21:442–443.

72. Daniels, NA, MacKinnon L, Bishop R, et al. *Vibrio parahaemolyticus* infections in the United States, 1973–1998. *J Infect Dis* 2000;181:1661–1666.

73. Calia FM, Johnson DE. Bacteremia in suckling rabbits after oral challenge with *Vibrio parahaemolyticus*. *Infect Immun* 1975;11:1222–1225.

74. Johnson RH, Lutwick LI, Huntley GA, et al. *Arizona hinshawii* infections. New cases, antimicrobial sensitivities, and literature review. *Ann Intern Med* 1976;85:587–592.

75. Kumar MC, Nivas SC, Bahl AK, et al. Studies on natural infection and egg transmission of *Arizona hinshawii* 7:1, 7, 8 in turkeys. *Avian Dis* 1974;18:416–426.

76. Holmberg SD, Farmer JJ III. *Aeromonas hydrophila* and *Plesiomonas shigelloides* as causes of intestinal infections. *Rev Infect Dis* 1982;6:633–639.

77. Singh DV, Sanyal SC. Enterotoxicity of clinical and environmental isolates of *Aeromonas* spp. *J Med Microbiol* 1992;36:269–272.

78. Jones BL, Wilcox MH. *Aeromonas* infections and their treatment. *J Antimicrobial Chemother* 1995;35:453–461.

79. Namdari H, Bottone EJ. Microbiologic and clinical evidence supporting the role of *Aeromonas caviae* as a pediatric enteric pathogen. *J Clin Microbiol* 1990;28:837–840.

80. Holmberg SD, Wachsmuth IK, Hickman-Brenner FW, et al. *Plesiomonas* enteric infections in the United States. *Ann Intern Med* 1986;105:690–694.

81. Rutala WA Sarubi FA Jr, Finch CS, et al. Oyster-associated outbreak of diarrhoeal disease possibly caused by *Plesiomonas shigelloides* [Letter]. *Lancet* 1982;1:739.

82. Murata T, Iida T, Shiomi Y, et al. A large outbreak of foodborne infection attributed to *Providencia alcalifaciens*. *J Infect Dis* 2001;184:1050–1055.

83. Osterholm MT, MacDonald KL, White KE, et al. An outbreak of a newly recognized chronic diarrhea syndrome associated with raw milk consumption. *JAMA* 1986;256:484–490.

84. Martin DL, Hoberman LJ. A point source outbreak of chronic diarrhea in Texas. No known exposure to raw milk [Letter]. *JAMA* 1986;256:469.

85. Snydman DR, Dienstag JL, Stedt BL, et al. Use of IgM-hepatitis A antibody testing to investigate a common-source, foodborne outbreak. *JAMA* 1981;245:827–830.

86. Kuritsky JN, Osterholm MT, Greenberg HB, et al. Norwalk gastroenteritis: a community outbreak associated with bakery product consumption. *Ann Intern Med* 1984;100:519–521.

87. Kohn MA, Farley TA, Ando T, et al. An outbreak of Norwalk virus gastroenteritis associated with eating raw oysters. Implications for maintaining safe oyster beds. *JAMA* 1995;273:466–471.

88. Kukkula M, Maunula L, Silvennoinen E, et al. Outbreak of viral gastroenteritis due to drinking water contaminated by Norwalk-like viruses. *J Infect Dis* 1999;180:1771–1776.

89. Blacklow NR, Greenberg HB. Viral gastroenteritis. *N Engl J Med* 1991;325:252–264.

90. Morse DL, Guzewich JJ, Hanrahan JP, et al. Widespread outbreaks of clam- and oyster-associated gastroenteritis. Role of Norwalk virus. *N Engl J Med* 1986;314:678–681.

91. MacKenzie WR, Hoxie NJ, Proctor ME, et al. A massive outbreak in Milwaukee of cryptosporidium infection transmitted through the public water supply. *N Engl J Med* 1994;331:161–167.

92. Millard PS, Gensheimer KF, Addiss DG, et al. An outbreak of cryptosporidiosis from fresh pressed apple cider. *JAMA* 1994;272:1592–1596.

93. Quiroz ES, Bern C, MacArthur JR, et al. An outbreak of cryptosporidiosis linked to a foodhandler. *J Infect Dis* 2000;181:695–700.

94. Fleming CA, Caron D, Gunn JE, et al. A foodborne outbreak of *Cyclospora cayetanensis* at a wedding. Clinical features and risk factors for illness. *Arch Intern Med* 1998;158:1121–1125.

95. Semple AB Parry WH, Phillips DE. Acute copper poisoning: an outbreak traced to contaminated water from a corroded geyser. *Lancet* 1960;2:700.

96. Brown MA, Thom JV, Orth GL, et al. Food poisoning involving zinc contamination. *Arch Environ Health* 1964;8:657–661.

97. Mills AR, Passmore R. Pelagic paralysis. *Lancet* 1988;1:161–163.

98. Schaumburg HH, Byck B, Gerstl R, et al. Monosodium L-glutamate: its pharmacology and role in the Chinese restaurant syndrome. *Science* 1969;163:826–828.

99. Hudson PJ, Vogt RL. A foodborne outbreak traced to niacin overenrichment. *J Food Prot* 1985;48:249–251.

100. Hughes JM, Merson MH. Current concepts fish and shellfish poisoning. *N Engl J Med* 1976;295(20):1117–1120.

101. Whittle K, Gallacher S. Marine toxins. *Br Med Bull* 2000;56:236–253.

102. Eastaough J, Sheperd S. Infections and toxic syndromes from fish and shellfish consumption. *Arch Intern Med* 1989;149:1735–1739.

103. Gilbert RJ, Hobbs G, Murray CK, et al. Scombrotoxic fish poisoning: features of the first 50 incidents to be reported in Britain (1976–1979). *BMJ* 1980;28:71–72.

104. Bédry R, Gabinski C, Paty MC. Diagnosis of scombroid poisoning by measurement of plasma histamine. *N Engl J Med* 2000;342:520–521.

105. Etkind P, Wilson ME, Gallagher K, et al. Bluefish-associated scombroid poisoning. An example of the expanding spectrum of food poisoning from seafood. *JAMA* 1987;258:3409–3410.

106. Blakesley ML. Scombroid poisoning: prompt resolution of symptoms with cimetidine. *Ann Emerg Med* 1983;12:104–106.

107. Lehane L. Paralytic shellfish poisoning: a potential public health problem. *Med J Aust* 2001;175:29–31.

108. Porkiss MEE, Horstman DA, Harpur D. Paralytic shellfish poisoning. A report of 17 cases in Cape Town. *S Afr Med J* 1979;55:1017–1021.

109. Engleberg NC, Morris JG Jr, Lewis J, et al. Ciguatera fish poisoning: a major common-source outbreak in the U.S. Virgin Islands. *Ann Intern Med* 1983;98:336–337.

110. Bagnis R, Kuberski T, Laugier S. Clinical observations on 3,009 cases of ciguatera fish poisoning in the south pacific. *Am J Trop Med Hyg* 1979;28:1067–1073.

111. Farstad DJ, Chow T. A brief case report and review of ciguatera poisoning. *Wilderness Environ Med* 2001;12:263–269.

112. Bidard JN Vijverberg HPM, Frelin C, et al. Ciguatoxin is a novel type of Na$^+$ channel toxin. *J Biol Chem* 1984;259:8353–8357.

113. Morris JG Jr, Lewin P, Hargrett NT, et al. Clinical features of ciguatera fish poisoning. A study of disease in the US Virgin Islands. *Arch Intern Med* 1982;142:1090–1092.

114. Lampe KF. Toxic fungi. *Annu Rev Pharmacol Toxicol* 1979;19:85–102.

115. Paaso B, Harrison DL. A new look at an old problem. Mushroom poisoning. *Am J Med* 1975;58:505–507.

116. Bryan FL. Epidemiology of foodborne diseases. In: Reimann H, Bryan FL, eds. *Foodborne infections and intoxications*, 2nd ed. New York: Academic, 1979:3–69.

117. Lawrence G, Shann F, Freestone DS, et al. Prevention of necrotising enteritis in Papua New Guinea by active immunisation. *Lancet* 1979;1:227–230.

118. Sagliocca L, Amoroso P, Stroffolini T, et al. Efficacy of hepatitis A vaccine in prevention of secondary hepatitis A infection: a randomised trial. *Lancet* 1999;353:1136–1139.

CHAPTER 78
Specific and Nonspecific Treatment of Diarrhea

James D. Campbell, Karen L. Kotloff, and Myron M. Levine

The worldwide burden of diarrheal diseases remains high, particularly in settings where drinking water is not potable, sanitation is poor, and personal hygiene practices are suboptimal. Research on the treatment of diarrheal diseases continues to expand and lead to identification of new diarrheal agents. Development of new antibiotics used to treat enteric infections continues to outpace development of resistance. In this chapter, we describe the various specific and nonspecific interventions in an effort to foster a rational approach to treatment of the patient with acute infectious diarrhea.

The most important principles to guide clinicians treating patients with acute infectious diarrhea are as follows: (a) rehydration, preferably with oral rehydration therapy (ORT), is the most crucial and often the sole necessary therapeutic intervention; (b) ORT is best practiced using low-osmolarity solutions containing salts and either simple or complex carbohydrates; (c) rehydration should most often be completed rapidly, and refeeding should be instituted as soon as rehydration is completed; (d) infants should be breast-fed before, during, and after episodes of diarrhea; and (e) antibiotics, antimotility agents, and antiemetics are unnecessary in most cases of diarrhea.

FLUID THERAPY

Diarrheal illnesses lead to excessive water losses, and the resulting dehydration can cause hypovolemia, acidosis, shock, and death. Although all diarrheal agents, including those classically associated with dysentery, can cause dehydration, cholera at any age and diarrhea caused by enterotoxigenic *Escherichia coli* (ETEC) or rotavirus in infants commonly result in frequent, voluminous stools. In fact, persons with cholera gravis may purge 10 to 20 mL/kg per hour, resulting in the rapid onset of hypovolemic shock. The cornerstone of therapy for all diarrheal diseases is rehydration designed to correct fluid and electrolyte deficits and to replace ongoing losses.

Hydration instituted after the onset of diarrhea but before dehydration is evident can prevent dehydration. Once a patient suffers from dehydration, rehydration must be instituted promptly. Intravenous fluid therapy is necessary for only a small proportion of patients, including those with severe dehydration and shock (for whom intravenous fluid therapy may be lifesaving), diminished mental status, symptomatic electrolyte disturbances, paralytic ileus, excessively high purging rate, or intractable vomiting. Rapid infusion of an appropriate solution, such as Ringer's lactate, to expand vigorously the intravascular volume, is followed by the administration of additional rehydration fluids, preferably by the oral route. This strategy is meant to replace the remaining deficit and to provide for ongoing losses and maintenance requirements. Those with hypertonic dehydration should be closely monitored, especially following acute rehydration, when replacement of fluids is done more slowly than following hypotonic or isotonic dehydration. Intravenous fluid therapy may be overused in industrialized countries, where it is often a route of convenience rather than the superior method.

Most patients with diarrhea in all settings can be effectively treated with oral rehydration. This therapy is simple to administer, inexpensive, and highly efficacious (1,2). It has led, over the past 20 years, to an estimated 67% reduction in diarrhea-associated deaths in children under 5 years of age (3). Glucose-based ORT rests on the observation that active transport of glucose is coupled with sodium transport in the small intestine (4), a process that is preserved during diarrheal illness. Other solutes, such as amino acids and dipeptides, are also actively and independently cotransported with sodium. Solutions containing multiple actively transported substrates have been studied in an attempt to optimize absorption and minimize stool output and duration (5–7).

Throughout the developing world, the World Health Organization (WHO) recommends the use of a single oral rehydration solution (WHO-ORS) with a sodium concentration of 90 mEq/L and osmolarity of 311 mmol/L for diarrheal illness of all causes in all ages (8). By concurrently offering appropriate amounts of low-solute fluids, WHO-ORS can be used to prevent dehydration as well as to replace deficits of body water and electrolytes (9–12). The reader is referred to a review article for a more detailed discussion of its use (13). WHO-ORS ORT is as efficacious as intravenous fluid therapy in treating hyponatremic and isotonic dehydration, and its use in hypernatremic dehydration results in a lower frequency of seizures (14,15). ORS with a reduced osmolarity (134 to 224 mmol/L) has been found to be equivalent or superior to traditional WHO-ORS (16–22). In the developed world, numerous commercial ORS products are available and recommended for use in children with acute gastroenteritis (23).

Although glucose-based ORT effectively replaces diarrheal losses, it does not abate stool output. Rice powder and electrolyte solutions, which deliver higher densities of glucose to the small intestine in the form of complex starches along with amino acids and small peptides, offer some theoretical advantages over glucose-electrolyte solutions. Potentially, they may lead to increased nutrient and caloric intake and to a decrease in the duration or volume of loose stools. Compared with WHO-ORS in a number of studies, rice powder and cereal-based ORS have been found to be equivalent or superior with regard to clinical outcomes such as ORS requirements, weight gain, and duration and volume of stools, but may lead to more mixing errors and poorer compliance (24–28).

Although in the past it was common practice to restrict or modify the diet of patients with acute diarrheal illnesses, studies in children support the resumption of a normal diet immediately after rehydration on the first day of care (29–31). In a multicenter European trial, children randomized to receive early feeding after ORS (4 hours after treatment had begun) had better weight gain, no worsening of diarrhea or vomiting, and no lactose intolerance (29).

ANTIMICROBIAL THERAPY

In general, antimicrobial agents are prescribed too liberally for treatment of diarrheal diseases. In fact, most illness is mild and self-limited and can be treated with fluid therapy alone. The widespread use of antibiotics in some areas has provided selective pressures leading to antibiotic resistance among enteropathogens, complicating the treatment of patients who warrant antibiotics. For many bacterial diarrheas, controlled studies to establish the efficacy of specific antibiotics either have not been done or have shown no benefits; viral diarrheas obviously do not respond to such treatment. Nevertheless, antibiotics have proven efficacy in the treatment of certain bacterial and protozoan enteric infections and may be warranted

TABLE 78.1. Relative Indications for Use of Antimicrobial Agents in Diarrheal Disease Caused by Specific Etiologic Agents in Immunocompetent Hosts

Clearly indicated	Sometimes indicated	Not indicated
Shigellosis	Nontyphoidal salmonellosis[b]	Rotavirus
Cholera	Enteropathogenic *E. coli* (nursery	Other viral agents
Enterotoxigenic *Escherichia coli*	outbreaks or persistent infection)	Cryptosporidiosis
traveler's diarrhea[a]	Enteroinvasive *E. coli*	Enterohemorrhagic
Amebiasis	*Campylobacter* (early treatment of	*E. coli*
Giardiasis	dysentery)	
Clostridium difficile colitis	Non–*Vibrio cholerae* vibrios	
	Enteroaggregative *E. coli* (persistent	
	diarrhea)	

[a]Enterotoxigenic *E. coli* is the most common cause of acute traveler's diarrhea, and certain antibiotics are highly effective.
[b]For high-risk patients, such as infants younger than 12 weeks of age and patients with sickle cell disease or immunodeficiencies.

for treating others when the illness is complicated or severe (Table 78.1).

Shigellosis

Shigella species infection is the most common cause of dysentery (32). One serotype, *Shigella dysenteriae* type 1, causes particularly fulminant illness and is associated with a high case-fatality rate. In controlled clinical trials, several antibiotics have been shown to shorten the duration of clinical disease and excretion of *Shigella*; therefore, antibiotics are recommended for the treatment of shigellosis. Information from clinical trials is critical because *in vitro* susceptibility does not necessarily correlate with efficacy *in vivo*. Several antibiotics, including cephalexin (33) and cefaclor (34), are of little value clinically despite favorable activity *in vitro*. In addition, as effective antibiotics have achieved broad use, widespread resistance has developed. From the 1940s through the mid-1970s, sulfa drugs, tetracycline, and ampicillin were successively the drugs of choice for treating shigellosis, until resistant strains became highly prevalent. The utility of trimethoprim-sulfamethoxazole (TMP-SMX), the drug

of choice in many areas in the 1980s, has been eroded worldwide by increasing levels of resistance (35–41), often associated with multiple other antibiotic resistances. The proportion of isolates of *Shigella* in the United States that are resistant to antibiotics is also high. From 1995 to 1998, among 430 *Shigella* isolates in the state of Oregon, 63% were resistant to ampicillin and 59% to TMP-SMX. Among *Shigella sonnei* alone, 81% were TMP-SMX resistant, and 68% were ampicillin resistant (42).

Nalidixic acid and the fluoroquinolones are useful to treat infections caused by *Shigella* strains that are resistant to other antibiotics. However, in areas of South and Southeast Asia, *S. dysenteriae* has become resistant to nalidixic acid, limiting the utility of this agent (39,43).

For sensitive strains, a 5-day course of tetracycline, ampicillin, or TMP-SMX to treat shigellosis has been shown to shorten the illness and the duration of pathogen excretion (Table 78.2). A single large dose (stosstherapy) of tetracycline has efficacy comparable to a 5-day regimen (44,45) but is not widely used. Tetracycline is contraindicated in pregnancy and in children younger than 7 years of age because of its associated tooth discoloration; the safety of stosstherapy has not been evaluated in these groups.

TABLE 78.2. Recommended Antibiotic Dosage Regimens for the Treatment of Shigellosis

Antibiotic	Dose and duration	
	Infants and children	Adults and adolescents
Oral		
TMP-SMX	10 mg/kg/d of TMP and 50 mg/kg/d of SMX in two divided doses for 5 d	160 mg of TMP and 800 mg of SMX q12h for 5 d
Ampicillin	100 mg/kg/d in four divided doses for 5 d	500 mg q6h for 5 d
Norfloxacin		400 mg q12h for 5 d
		500 mg q6h for 5 d
Tetracycline		Stosstherapy: 2.5 g in 1 dose
		500 mg q12h for 5 d (*Shigella dysenteriae*)
Ciprofloxacin		500 mg q12h for 3 d (*Shigella flexneri* and *sonnei*)
		500 mg (d 1), 250 mg (d 2–5)
Azithromycin	10–12 mg/kg/d (d 1), 5 mg/kg/d (d 2–5)	1 g q6h for 5–7 d
Nalidixic acid	55 mg/kg/d in four divided doses for 5–7 d	
Parenteral		
Ceftriaxone	50 mg/kg single daily dose for 5 d	

TMP-SMX, trimethoprim-sulfamethoxazole.

Although shorter courses of ampicillin (46) and cefixime (47) compare favorably with 5-day regimens, they are associated with significantly higher rates of bacteriologic failure. Amoxicillin is ineffective in the treatment of shigellosis for reasons that are ill understood (48). In areas where *Shigella* strains are commonly resistant to other antibiotics (38,39,41–43,49), the fluoroquinolones have become the drugs of choice for the empiric treatment of shigellosis, while awaiting sensitivities (35).

Several clinical trials have demonstrated the effectiveness of ciprofloxacin and norfloxacin in the treatment of shigellosis (49–52). Limited experience has shown that single-dose therapy with ciprofloxacin is effective treatment against disease caused by all *Shigella* species except *S. dysenteriae* type 1, for which a 5-day course of therapy is superior (53). Several of the quinolones have been associated with arthropathies in young animals (54), and case reports of ciprofloxacin-associated arthropathy in children have appeared (55). For this reason, the quinolones, except nalidixic acid, have not been approved for use in children and pregnant or nursing women. (Nalidixic acid was approved before these studies.) However, there is support for cautious use of the fluoroquinolones for treatment of severe, multidrug-resistant *Shigella* infections in children when effective alternatives are unavailable (56–58). In these situations, the risk for arthropathy must be weighed against the risk of leaving the shigellosis untreated.

Ceftriaxone, administered parenterally once daily for 2 to 5 days (59), or oral cefixime (47,60) are effective alternatives in children, but cefixime performs poorly in adults with shigellosis (61). In addition, resistance to third-generation cephalosporins, by means of an extended-spectrum β-lactamase, has been reported (62). Another alternative is azithromycin, which has been shown to have a clinical and bacteriologic success rate equivalent to ciprofloxacin for the treatment of shigellosis (63).

Salmonella Species Gastroenteritis

The effect of antibiotic treatment on uncomplicated nontyphoidal *Salmonella* gastroenteritis has been studied in several randomized placebo-controlled trials. Variously employing chloramphenicol (64), neomycin (65), TMP-SMX (66), and ampicillin and amoxicillin (67,68), these studies failed to show any benefit over placebo in terms of diminishing duration or severity of diarrheal illness or duration of pathogen excretion. Children treated with either oral amoxicillin or ampicillin have a significantly higher frequency of bacteriologic relapse, not infrequently associated with recurrence of diarrhea (68). Although the fluoroquinolones show excellent *in vitro* activity against salmonellae, a randomized, placebo-controlled, double-blind trial found that no significant clinical or bacteriologic benefit is conferred by treatment with ciprofloxacin (69). On the basis of these studies, antibiotics are not recommended for treatment of uncomplicated *Salmonella* gastroenteritis in adults, children, or infants 12 weeks of age or older.

Infants younger than 12 weeks of age, patients with hemoglobinopathies, and individuals with acquired immunodeficiency syndrome who develop *Salmonella* gastroenteritis are at increased risk for bacteremia and metastatic complications such as meningitis, septic arthritis, and osteomyelitis (70). It is recommended that these high-risk groups be treated with antibiotics. Some authorities extend this recommendation to include patients with malignant neoplasms and other immunosuppressive conditions (71), although data are lacking. Usually, ampicillin, amoxicillin, or TMP-SMX for 7 to 10 days is appropriate, although susceptibility patterns *in vitro* should guide the choice. Fluoroquinolones, ceftriaxone, or cefotaxime are alternate choices for treatment of severe or invasive nontyphoidal

Salmonella infections when isolates are resistant to other antibiotics (72,73). Spread of isolates resistant to multiple antimicrobials, including fluoroquinolones, has increased (74), reinforcing the need for susceptibility tests to guide antibiotic therapy.

Campylobacter jejuni Enteritis

Campylobacter enteritis is a common diarrheal disease worldwide, with a spectrum of illness ranging from watery diarrhea to frank dysentery. Several placebo-controlled trials of erythromycin in children and adults have demonstrated significant curtailment of pathogen excretion in treated groups (75,76). However, only one study, in which children with dysentery were treated with erythromycin within 5 days of disease onset (mean of 3 days), has demonstrated significant amelioration of diarrheal illness (77). Studies from Thailand note an increasing proportion of erythromycin-resistant *Campylobacter* isolates (39,78).

Several studies have been conducted using fluoroquinolones for treatment of campylobacteriosis in adults. In three randomized double-blind trials in which a 3- to 5-day course of either norfloxacin or ciprofloxacin was compared with placebo, a modest reduction in the duration of diarrhea was observed (79–81). Emergence of fluoroquinolone-resistant *Campylobacter* isolates in several areas has been documented, which may limit the utility of these agents in this disease (39,80,82,83). Azithromycin attains high tissue concentrations and shows good *in vitro* activity against *Campylobacter* species (84). In one trial, azithromycin was shown to be as efficacious as ciprofloxacin in treating adults with *Campylobacter* enteritis (83).

Patients presenting early with moderate to severe *Campylobacter* enteritis may be treated with a macrolide or a fluoroquinolone. Because resistance to both antibiotics may be seen (85), choice of antibiotics is best done using susceptibility profiles.

Enterotoxigenic *Escherichia coli* Infections

ETEC, which produces a toxin-mediated secretory diarrhea, is a frequent cause of diarrhea in travelers to developing areas and is also endemic among infants in such areas. In a placebo-controlled trial among Bangladeshi adults with ETEC-induced diarrhea, tetracycline significantly shortened pathogen excretion, although only limited clinical benefits were noted (86). TMP-SMX treatment has demonstrated clinical and bacteriologic efficacy compared with placebo in ETEC-induced diarrhea in three separate studies involving American volunteers (87), adult travelers in Mexico (88), and young Mexican children (89). As high rates of resistance to tetracycline, ampicillin, TMP-SMX, and other antibiotics have emerged in many areas (90–92), the fluoroquinolones, which are highly active against ETEC *in vitro* (93), have been shown to be useful. A short course of ciprofloxacin, norfloxacin, or ofloxacin shortens the duration of ETEC-associated diarrhea compared with placebo (81,94,95).

In areas where ETEC is prevalent, it is recommended that adult traveler's diarrhea be treated with ciprofloxacin or norfloxacin for 3 to 5 days. Although definitive data are not available, pediatric travelers may be treated with cefixime or azithromycin. TMP-SMX has become less valuable given widespread resistance. Antibiotics are not routinely recommended for suspected ETEC-induced diarrhea in persons who live in areas where ETEC is endemic. A vast amount of clinical experience from oral rehydration studies in which the causative agents were identified supports this contention. In persons from endemic areas, degrees of background immunity tend to make ETEC infections self-limited and amenable to ORT alone.

Enteropathogenic *Escherichia coli* Infections

Enteropathogenic *Escherichia coli* (EPEC) is an important cause of diarrhea in infants younger than 6 months of age in many developing areas of the world; occasional nursery and community outbreaks still occur in industrialized countries. In the 1960s, oral neomycin was sometimes used to treat EPEC-induced diarrhea (96), but its use is now discouraged because neomycin commonly causes intestinal malabsorption and diarrhea as adverse effects. In an Ethiopian trial, EPEC-infected infants receiving either mecillinam or TMP-SMX for 5 days had significantly better clinical and bacteriologic cure rates compared with an untreated control group (97). Two studies of EPEC-infected infants and children employing ampicillin had different outcomes: one showed a favorable clinical and bacteriologic response (98), and the other showed no difference (67) compared with placebo. Given the paucity of data, a reasonable approach is to employ an antibiotic such as TMP-SMX when EPEC is implicated as the cause of severe or persistent diarrhea in a young infant or in a nursery outbreak situation.

Enteroinvasive and Enterohemorrhagic *Escherichia coli* Infections

Enteroinvasive *Escherichia coli* (EIEC) has many similarities to *Shigella* in its virulence properties and pathogenesis. Like *Shigella*, EIEC can cause dysentery. EIEC infections are thought to be responsive to the same agents that are used to treat shigellosis, although there have been no controlled trials to support this claim, and few published antibiotic susceptibility data are available.

Enterohemorrhagic *Escherichia coli* (EHEC) causes hemorrhagic colitis and is also associated with hemolytic-uremic syndrome (HUS) and thrombotic thrombocytopenic purpura. In a 1992 study, no benefit was afforded to patients with O157:H7 EHEC-associated enteritis who received TMP-SMX (99), and retrospective analyses suggested that the use of antibiotics in EHEC diarrhea constitutes a risk factor for progression to HUS (100,101). Quinolones induce production of the Shiga toxin made in these organisms (102). In a prospective trial, antibiotic use in children with EHEC colitis increased the risk for HUS (103). Routine antibiotic therapy for EHEC-associated diarrhea or colitis is not recommended.

Yersinia enterocolitica Enteritis

Y. enterocolitica causes enteritis and dysentery in young children, particularly in certain cooler regions such as northern Europe. Older children and adolescents may instead present with mesenteric lymphadenitis, mimicking appendicitis. Extraintestinal infections, including septicemia, have been infrequently reported in patients with certain underlying conditions, most notably in iron overload states (104) and in infants (105). In general, isolates are susceptible *in vitro* to aminoglycosides, tetracycline, chloramphenicol, TMP-SMX, third-generation cephalosporins, and quinolones (106), but data are lacking to support their use in uncomplicated diarrhea. A retrospective review of 142 hospitalized children found all isolates of *Y. enterocolitica* susceptible to TMP-SMX, gentamicin, and tobramycin (107). However, in a placebo-controlled trial, in which children with *Yersinia* species enteritis were treated on average 12 days into their illness, TMP-SMX offered no beneficial clinical or bacteriologic effect (108). On the basis of available information, it is recommended that antibiotic therapy be limited to patients with particularly severe or chronic *Y. enterocolitica* enteritis, those with focal extraintestinal or systemic infections, and im-munocompromised patients. The choice of antibiotics should be guided by susceptibility testing *in vitro*, but empiric therapy with TMP-SMX or a third-generation cephalosporin and an aminoglycoside is prudent in these cases, while awaiting susceptibilities.

Cholera

Vibrio cholerae O1 and O139 strains cause a secretory diarrhea characterized by voluminous purging. As an adjunct to fluid therapy, antibiotics are of proven benefit. Tetracycline, the drug of choice for sensitive strains, markedly diminishes the volume and duration of diarrhea and fluid replacement requirements and curtails the excretion of the pathogen (109,110). Adults may be given 500 mg four times daily or 2 g once daily for 2 days, with equivalent results. Because duration of therapy is short, it is considered safe for use in children (125 mg four times daily for 2 to 4 days). Although they are inferior to tetracycline, other antibiotics, such as doxycycline (111), chloramphenicol (109), furazolidone (112), erythromycin (113), and ampicillin (113), have proven efficacy in treating cholera. In one small study, norfloxacin (400 mg twice daily for 5 days) was shown to be effective in treatment of severe cholera in adults (114), but an outbreak of norfloxacin-resistant cholera has been reported (115). Furazolidone may be used as an alternative treatment for children and pregnant women. Outbreaks associated with tetracycline-resistant strains (116) and multidrug-resistant strains (117,118) underscore the importance of antibiotic alternatives. Preliminary data suggest that antibiotics used to treat *V. cholerae* O1, including tetracycline, are also effective therapy for *V. cholerae* O139 (Bengal) (119). Both serogroups may be resistant to TMP-SMX (119,120).

Clostridium difficile Diarrhea and Colitis

C. difficile is the most common agent of antibiotic-associated pseudomembranous colitis and is less frequently implicated in antibiotic-associated diarrhea without colitis. Antimicrobial therapy is warranted for patients with *C. difficile*–induced colitis or diarrhea that does not respond to discontinuation of the offending antibiotic (121). Although multiple studies have documented the efficacy and safety of oral vancomycin (122), it is costly and has a high frequency of clinical relapse (6% to 39%). Both oral metronidazole (123) and bacitracin (124) are comparable clinically to vancomycin. Metronidazole has become the first-line agent because it is considerably less expensive than vancomycin and because of the emergence of vancomycin-resistant nosocomial pathogens. Its use is contraindicated in pregnant and nursing women because of the theoretical potential for human teratogenesis, and concurrent alcohol consumption is proscribed because of its disulfiram-like effect.

Cases of multiple relapses and relapse associated with adynamic ileus are especially problematic. For multiple relapses, uncontrolled studies have shown a favorable response to an extended course of cholestyramine in tandem with oral vancomycin as well as to bacteriotherapy (see later), although optimal therapy has not been established. In patients who are unable to tolerate oral therapy, limited anecdotal experience using parenteral metronidazole and vancomycin has met with both success and failure with each agent (125). Demonstrable achievement of therapeutic intracolonic metronidazole levels after parenteral dosing (126) favors its use, although more controlled studies with these agents and a search for other therapies need to be pursued. Others advocate vancomycin and rifampin for these recalcitrant cases (127,128).

Decisions on the use of antibiotics for the treatment of children younger than 2 years of age who are found to have *C. difficile* in the stool are complicated by their high rates of colonization: 34% to 71% (129–132).

Amebiasis, Giardiasis, Cryptosporidiosis, Microsporidiosis, Cyclosporiasis, and Isosporiasis

Amebiasis, giardiasis, cryptosporidiosis, cyclosporiasis, and isosporiasis are discussed elsewhere in this text.

CLINICAL APPROACH TO TREATMENT OF INFECTIOUS DIARRHEA

The clinician faces a series of therapeutic decisions when a patient presents with infectious diarrhea. The foremost concern should be the patient's state of hydration. After this is assessed and appropriate fluid therapy instituted, the indication for antimicrobial therapy must be determined. This decision hinges on whether the likely offending pathogen is amenable to such therapy. It is helpful to categorize the patient's disease into one of six clinical types (Table 78.3). Depending on the geographic setting, which pathogen most frequently causes each type of diarrhea varies somewhat.

Most patients present with simple diarrhea, characterized by watery stools without blood, low-grade fever, abdominal cramps, malaise, and occasional vomiting. Viral pathogens, mainly rotavirus, are the most frequent etiologic agents of pediatric diarrhea in many settings and clearly do not warrant antibiotic therapy. In developing areas, bacterial pathogens, including ETEC and EPEC, are more frequent offenders; hence, adult travelers to such areas who have moderate to severe watery diarrhea may respond to early institution of antibiotics active against ETEC.

In any setting, when the patient presents with dysentery, the physician must consider the invasive bacterial pathogens, such as *Shigella, Campylobacter,* and *Yersinia* species and EIEC, as well as amebic colitis. Empiric antibiotic therapy should not be given in settings in which EHEC is likely, given the increased risk for progression to HUS. In many areas outside the United States, *Shigella* is the most common agent, and empiric therapy may be indicated. In the United States, *Campylobacter* is the most common bacterial cause of diarrhea (133). Because the fluoroquinolones are active against both *Shigella* and *Campylobacter,* they may be used as monotherapy for dysentery in adults, although the emergence of resistance to the quinolones has disturbed this approach. Quinolones are also effective against enteroaggregative *E. coli* in travelers (134). In developing areas where *Entamoeba histolytica* is endemic, stool examination for amoebae must be performed to determine whether antiprotozoal therapy is warranted. In the appropriate setting, such as the hospitalized patient receiving antibiotics, *C. difficile* must be considered another potentially treatable cause of bloody diarrhea.

Tetracycline therapy is warranted for patients in endemic cholera areas who present with voluminous rice-water purging. Patients with persistent diarrhea may suffer profound nutritional losses, and detailed evaluation for an infectious agent may uncover a treatable cause, such as giardiasis.

NONSPECIFIC THERAPIES

A plethora of nonantibiotic antidiarrheal agents are used in the hope of achieving symptomatic relief of diarrheal illness. Few are both innocuous and effective. Kaolin-pectin preparations are innocuous but essentially ineffective. They serve to increase the consistency of the diarrheal stool, but the water and electrolyte content of the stools remains unchanged (135).

Bacteriotherapy, the oral administration of nonpathogenic microorganisms to inhibit growth of enteropathogens, has been studied as well. *Lactobacillus acidophilus* is commonly prescribed for treatment of acute diarrhea, although there is little evidence from controlled studies that such preparations can prevent or ameliorate infectious diarrheas (136,137). *Lactobacillus* GG has shown more promise. In three randomized placebo-controlled studies in children, oral administration of 10^{9-11} colony-forming units twice daily for 2 to 5 days was well tolerated and hastened recovery from acute watery diarrhea by about 1 day (138–140). When given with ORS from the outset of therapy for children with diarrhea caused by rotavirus and other pathogens, it reduces the time with diarrhea and the length of stay in the hospital (141,142). An uncontrolled study described the successful use of rectal instillation of a mixture

TABLE 78.3.   Clinical Presentations and Likely Agents of Acute Diarrheal Disease

Clinical type	Patients (approximate %)	Likely agent	
		Industrialized countries	Developing countries
Simple diarrhea	90	Rotavirus, other viruses, *Salmonella, Campylobacter jejuni*	Rotavirus, ETEC, *C. jejuni*
Dysentery	5–10	*Shigella, C. jejuni, Yersinia, Salmonella*	*Shigella, C. jejuni, Entamoeba histolytica,* EIEC
Persistent diarrhea (>14 d)	3–4	*Giardia, Salmonella, Yersinia*	EPEC, *Giardia,* EAggEC
Severe purging of rice-water stools	1[a]	Rotavirus, *Salmonella*	*Vibrio cholerae,* ETEC
Hemorrhagic colitis	<1	EHEC	EHEC, *Shigella dysenteriae* type 1
Repeated vomiting without diarrhea	1–2		
Acute	1	Norwalk virus, other viruses	Viruses, *Giardia*
Persistent	<0.5	*Giardia*	*Giardia, Strongyloides*

[a]More common in cholera endemic areas.
[b]ETEC, Enterotoxigenic *E. coli;* EIEC, enteroinvasive *E. coli;* EPEC, enteropathogenic *E. coli;* EHEC, enterohemorrhagic *E. coli;* EAggEC, enteroaggregative *E. coli.*

of 10 different bacteria in the treatment of chronic relapsing *C. difficile*–associated diarrhea. Administration of this preparation led to recolonization with *Bacteroides* species (absent in all patients before treatment) and elimination of *C. difficile*, associated with cessation of diarrhea (143).

Chlorpromazine inhibits the secretory effect of cholera toxin and *E. coli* heat-labile toxin *in vitro* (144). Clinical trials in cholera patients have shown that chlorpromazine can significantly diminish the voluminous diarrhea (145), but the doses required to achieve a therapeutic effect may induce somnolence and thereby interfere with a patient's ability to imbibe ORT. For this reason, chlorpromazine has not been approved for this use.

Opioids, including paregoric and codeine, have long been employed to relieve diarrhea. Synthetic opioids, such as diphenoxylate and loperamide, are also used; and loperamide is now available over the counter. One of their most prominent effects is to decrease intestinal motility. The synthetic opioids may also have antisecretory effects. The advisability of using antimotility agents is the subject of considerable debate among physicians experienced in the treatment of diarrheal diseases. Evidence from animal models and clinical studies speaks against the use of antimotility agents in patients with invasive bacterial infections such as shigellosis. Guinea pigs are normally resistant to *Shigella*, but if they are pretreated with paregoric, fatal enteritis follows oral inoculation with *Shigella* (146). Human volunteers experimentally challenged with *Shigella* and subsequently treated with diphenoxylate after developing clinical illness exhibited higher fever and prolonged excretion of *Shigella* compared with untreated infected volunteers (147). Case series have pointed to the dangers of antimotility agents in children (147–149). In contrast, a study of Thai adults found that treatment of shigellosis with ciprofloxacin and loperamide hastened the resolution of diarrhea in comparison to antibiotic alone, and no deleterious effects were observed (150).

We advocate a reasoned, conservative approach to the use of opioids in patients with infectious diarrheas. These drugs should not be used in the treatment of diarrheal disease in children or adults living in developing countries because invasive bacterial diarrheas are common in such areas; therapy must be as economical as possible; and any diversion from an emphasis on oral rehydration is considered ill advised. Loperamide, apparently the safest of the opioids, may be used as an adjunct to therapy in adults or older children with nonbloody diarrhea in industrialized countries, as long as appropriate precautions are taken (e.g., examination for fecal leukocytes) to ascertain that it is unlikely that the diarrhea is due to an invasive bacterial enteropathogen such as *Shigella*. Some physicians prescribe loperamide for adult travelers with mild to moderate watery diarrhea, particularly when abdominal cramps are prominent (151). We advocate a conservative approach that limits use of such agents to a single dose at the outset of antibiotic therapy (152,153).

Bismuth subsalicylate (BSS) has been widely studied as an antidiarrheal agent. Its effects are probably mediated by the salicylate component, although studies with ETEC-induced diarrhea suggest that the bismuth compound may act to inhibit intraluminal attachment or growth (154). Field studies in adults with traveler's diarrhea have shown the liquid suspension of BSS to provide moderate relief of symptoms (155), although this formulation has not been shown to diminish the water content or total weight of stools more than placebo does (156). Because of the inconvenient dosing regimen with the liquid formulation, BSS in tablet form has been studied. BSS tablets reduce the occurrence of traveler's diarrhea for up to 3 weeks when used prophylactically but have not been efficacious in relieving established diarrhea (154–157). The salicylate component of BSS is readily absorbed,

and mean serum levels of 40 μg/mL are expected after multiple doses (158,159). Patients taking aspirin, those with aspirin hypersensitivity or bleeding diathesis, and young children should avoid its use.

In two of three small inpatient studies using moderate (25 mg/kg per day) doses of aspirin to treat acute diarrhea in infants and children in developing countries, it was shown to diminish intestinal fluid losses (160,161). In the one study in which no beneficial effect was demonstrated, EPEC was the most commonly identified pathogen (162). Despite promising animal data (163), the few studies of indomethacin as an antidiarrheal agent either were poorly controlled (164) or demonstrated no efficacy (165). Until more safety and efficacy data are available, the use of aspirin or indomethacin in the symptomatic treatment of diarrhea cannot be advocated.

Cholestyramine, a nonabsorbable exchange resin, has been studied in a number of settings. It significantly shortens the duration of acute diarrhea in infants, among whom rotavirus is the most common pathogen (166). A few small uncontrolled studies suggest that cholestyramine may have a beneficial effect in treating persistent diarrhea in infants in developing countries and antibiotic-associated diarrhea and colitis, particularly in those patients who suffer multiple relapses after oral vancomycin therapy (167,168). Potential adverse effects include development of hyperchloremic acidosis in young children and in persons with renal insufficiency and interference with absorption of other drugs.

Octreotide is a somatostatin analog that has been approved for use in treating diarrhea that results from certain hormone-secreting tumors. Several case reports provide anecdotal evidence of a dramatic antidiarrheal effect when it is used in patients with acquired immunodeficiency syndrome who have severe secretory diarrhea associated with *Cryptosporidium* (169,170).

Another antidiarrheal, the enkephalinase racecadotril, is well tolerated and reduces stool output, duration of diarrhea, and required amount of rehydration fluid in the treatment of diarrhea (171,172). If future studies confirm these findings, it may prove to be helpful in ameliorating the severity of acute watery diarrhea.

Additional agents under study include immunoglobulin from bovine colostrum (173,174) and micronutrients such as zinc (175), among others. In a randomized, double-blind, placebo-controlled trial of treatment with bovine immunoglobulin concentrate against ETEC and EPEC performed in Bangladesh, the intervention group had no decrease in ORS requirements, no decrement in total stool losses or length of time with diarrhea, and no improvement in time to clearance of the organism compared with the placebo group (174). In contrast, use of a similar preparation directed against rotavirus has been shown to decrease stool output and frequency, diminish ORS volume ingested, and shorten the time of rotavirus shedding in children (173). In a randomized, double-blind, placebo-controlled trial of children receiving zinc, vitamin A, zinc and vitamin A, or neither, those receiving zinc or zinc and vitamin A had lower stool output, improved weight gain, and improved rates of early clinical recovery when compared with children receiving vitamin A alone or placebo (176).

REFERENCES

1. Santosham M, Daum RS, Dillman L, et al. Oral rehydration therapy of infantile diarrhea: a controlled study of well-nourished children hospitalized in the United States and Panama. *N Engl J Med* 1982;306:1070–1076.
2. Tamer AM, Friedman LB, Maxwell SR, et al. Oral rehydration of infants in a large urban U.S. medical center. *J Pediatr* 1985;107:14–19.

3. Victora CG, Bryce J, Fontaine O, et al. Reducing deaths from diarrhoea through oral rehydration therapy. *Bull W H O* 2000;78:1246–1255.

4. Schedl HP, Clifton JA. Solute and water absorption by human small intestine. *Nature* 1963;199:1264.

5. Nalin DR, Cash RA. Oral or nasogastric maintenance therapy for diarrhoea of unknown aetiology resembling cholera. *Trans R Soc Trop Med Hyg* 1970;64:769–771.

6. Santosham M, Burns BA, Reid R, et al. Glycine-based oral rehydration solution: reassessment of safety and efficacy. *J Pediatr* 1986;109:795–801.

7. Patra FC, Sack DA, Islam A, et al. Oral rehydration formula containing alanine and glucose for treatment of diarrhoea: a controlled trial. *BMJ* 1989;298:1353–1356.

8. World Health Organization. *The treatment and prevention of acute diarrhoea: practical guidelines.* Geneva: World Health Organization, 1989:39.

9. Ahmed SM, Islam MR, Butler T. Effective treatment of diarrhoeal dehydration with an oral rehydration solution containing citrate. *Scand J Infect Dis* 1986;18:65–70.

10. Sack DA, Islam S, Brown KH, et al. Oral therapy in children with cholera: a comparison of sucrose and glucose electrolyte solutions. *J Pediatr* 1980;96:20–25.

11. Nalin DR, Levine MM, Mata L, et al. Oral rehydration and maintenance of children with rotavirus and bacterial diarrhoeas. *Bull W H O* 1979;57:453–459.

12. Cutting WA, Belton NR, Gray JA, et al. Safety and efficacy of three oral rehydration solutions for children with diarrhoea (Edinburgh 1984–85). *Acta Paediatr Scand* 1989;78:253–258.

13. Levine MM, Pizarro D. Advances in therapy of diarrheal dehydration: oral rehydration. *Adv Pediatr* 1984;31:207–234.

14. Pizarro D, Posada G, Villavicencio N, et al. Oral rehydration in hypernatremic and hyponatremic diarrheal dehydration. *Am J Dis Child* 1983;137:730–734.

15. Pizarro D, Posada G, Levine MM. Hypernatremic diarrheal dehydration treated with "slow" (12-hour) oral rehydration therapy: a preliminary report. *J Pediatr* 1984;104:316–319.

16. Valentiner-Branth P, Steinsland H, Gjessing HK, et al. Community-based randomized controlled trial of reduced osmolarity oral rehydration solution in acute childhood diarrhea. *Pediatr Infect Dis J* 1999;18:789–795.

17. Sarker SA, Mahalanabis D, Alam NH, et al. Reduced osmolarity oral rehydration solution for persistent diarrhea in infants: a randomized controlled clinical trial. *J Pediatr* 2001;138:532–538.

18. Hahn S, Kim Y, Garner P. Reduced osmolarity oral rehydration solution for treating dehydration due to diarrhoea in children: systematic review. *BMJ* 2001;323:81–85.

19. Fuchs GJ. A better oral rehydration solution? An important step, but not a leap forward. *BMJ* 2001;323:59–60.

20. CHOICE Study Group. Multicenter, randomized, double-blind clinical trial to evaluate the efficacy and safety of a reduced osmolarity oral rehydration salts solution in children with acute watery diarrhea. *Pediatrics* 2001;107:613–618.

21. Dutta P, Mitra U, Dutta S, et al. Hypo-osmolar oral rehydration salts solution in dehydrating persistent diarrhoea in children: double-blind, randomized, controlled clinical trial. *Acta Paediatr* 2000;89:411–416.

22. Guarino A. Oral rehydration for infantile diarrhoea: toward a modified solution for the children of the world. *Acta Paediatr* 2000;89:764–767.

23. Practice parameter: the management of acute gastroenteritis in young children. American Academy of Pediatrics, Provisional Committee on Quality Improvement, Subcommittee on Acute Gastroenteritis. *Pediatrics* 1996;97:424–435.

24. Gore SM, Fontaine O, Pierce NF. Impact of rice based oral rehydration solution on stool output and duration of diarrhoea: meta-analysis of 13 clinical trials. *BMJ* 1992;304:287–291.

25. Lebenthal E, Khin MU, Rolston DD, et al. Thermophilic amylase-digested rice-electrolyte solution in the treatment of acute diarrhea in children. *Pediatrics* 1995;95:198–202.

26. Molina S, Vettorazzi C, Peerson JM, et al. Clinical trial of glucose-oral rehydration solution (ORS), rice dextrin–ORS, and rice flour–ORS for the management of children with acute diarrhea and mild or moderate dehydration. *Pediatrics* 1995;95:191–197.

27. Meyers A, Sampson A, Saladino R, et al. Safety and effectiveness of homemade and reconstituted packet cereal-based oral rehydration solutions: a randomized clinical trial. *Pediatrics* 1997;100:E3.

28. Faruque AS, Hoque SS, Fuchs GJ, et al. Randomized, controlled, clinical trial of rice versus glucose oral rehydration solutions in infants and young children with acute watery diarrhoea. *Acta Paediatr* 1997;86:1308–1311.

29. Sandhu BK, Isolauri E, Walker-Smith JA, et al. A multicentre study on behalf of the European Society of Paediatric Gastroenterology and Nutrition Working Group on Acute Diarrhoea. Early feeding in childhood gastroenteritis. *J Pediatr Gastroenterol Nutr* 1997;24:522–527.

30. Duggan C, Nurko S. "Feeding the gut": the scientific basis for continued enteral nutrition during acute diarrhea. *J Pediatr* 1997;131:801–808.

31. Szajewska H, Hoekstra JH, Sandhu B. Management of acute gastroenteritis in Europe and the impact of the new recommendations: a multicenter study. The Working Group on acute Diarrhoea of the European Society for Paediatric Gastroenterology, Hepatology, and Nutrition. *J Pediatr Gastroenterol Nutr* 2000;30:522–527.

32. Kotloff KL, Winickoff JP, Ivanoff B, et al. Global burden of Shigella infections: implications for vaccine development and implementation of control strategies. *Bull W H O* 1999;77:651–666.

33. Nelson JD, Haltalin KC. Comparative efficacy of cephalexin and ampicillin for shigellosis and other types of acute diarrhea in infants and children. *Antimicrob Agents Chemother* 1975;7:415–420.

34. Ostrower VG. Comparison of cefaclor and ampicillin in the treatment of shigellosis. *Postgrad Med J* 1979;55[Suppl 4]:82–84.

35. Salam MA, Bennish ML. Therapy for shigellosis. I. Randomized, double-blind trial of nalidixic acid in childhood shigellosis. *J Pediatr* 1988;113:901–907.

36. Griffin PM, Tauxe RV, Redd SC, et al. Emergence of highly trimethoprim-sulfamethoxazole-resistant Shigella in a native American population: an epidemiologic study. *Am J Epidemiol* 1989;129:1042–1051.

37. Tiemens KM, Shipley PL, Correia RA, et al. Sulfamethoxazole-trimethoprim-resistant *Shigella flexneri* in northeastern Brazil. *Antimicrob Agents Chemother* 1984;25:653–654.

38. Tuttle J, Ries AA, Chimba RM, et al. Antimicrobial-resistant epidemic *Shigella dysenteriae* type 1 in Zambia: modes of transmission. *J Infect Dis* 1995;171:371–375.

39. Hoge CW, Gambel JM, Srijan A, et al. Trends in antibiotic resistance among diarrheal pathogens isolated in Thailand over 15 years. *Clin Infect Dis* 1998;26:341–345.

40. Yurdakok K, Sahin N, Ozmert E, et al. Shigella gastroenteritis: clinical and epidemiological aspects, and antibiotic susceptibility. *Acta Paediatr Jpn* 1997;39:681–684.

41. Legros D, Ochola D, Lwanga N, et al. Antibiotic sensitivity of endemic Shigella in Mbarara, Uganda. *East Afr Med J* 1998;75:160–161.

42. Replogle ML, Fleming DW, Cieslak PR. Emergence of antimicrobial-resistant shigellosis in Oregon. *Clin Infect Dis* 2000;30:515–519.

43. Bennish ML, Salam MA, Hossain MA, et al. Antimicrobial resistance of Shigella isolates in Bangladesh, 1983–1990: increasing frequency of strains multiply resistant to ampicillin, trimethoprim-sulfamethoxazole, and nalidixic acid. *Clin Infect Dis* 1992;14:1055–1060.

44. Lionel ND, Abeyasekera FJ, Samarasinghe HG, et al. A comparison of a single dose and a five-day course of tetracycline therapy in bacillary dysentery. *J Trop Med Hyg* 1969;72:170–172.

45. Pickering LK, DuPont HL, Olarte J. Single-dose tetracycline therapy for shigellosis in adults. *JAMA* 1978;239:853–854.

46. Gilman RH, Spira W, Rabbani H, et al. Single-dose ampicillin therapy for severe shigellosis in Bangladesh. *J Infect Dis* 1981;143:164–169.

47. Martin JM, Pitetti R, Maffei F, et al. Treatment of shigellosis with cefixime: two days vs. five days. *Pediatr Infect Dis J* 2000;19:522–526.

48. Nelson JA, Haltalin KC. Amoxicillin less effective than ampicillin against Shigella in vitro and in vivo: relationship of efficacy to activity in serum. *J Infect Dis* 1974;129[Suppl]:7.

49. Lolekha S, Vibulbandhitkit S, Poonyarit P. Response to antimicrobial therapy for shigellosis in Thailand. *Rev Infect Dis* 1991;13[Suppl 4]:S342–S346.

50. Bennish ML, Salam MA, Haider R, et al. Therapy for shigellosis. II. Randomized, double-blind comparison of ciprofloxacin and ampicillin. *J Infect Dis* 1990;162:711–716.

51. Gotuzzo E, Oberhelman RA, Maguina C, et al. Comparison of single-dose treatment with norfloxacin and standard 5-day treatment with trimethoprim-sulfamethoxazole for acute shigellosis in adults. *Antimicrob Agents Chemother* 1989;33:1101–1104.

52. Bhattacharya SK, Bhattacharya MK, Dutta P, et al. Randomized clinical trial of norfloxacin for shigellosis. *Am J Trop Med Hyg* 1991;45:683–687.

53. Bennish ML, Salam MA, Khan WA, et al. Treatment of shigellosis. III. Comparison of one- or two-dose ciprofloxacin with standard 5-day therapy: a randomized, blinded trial. *Ann Intern Med* 1992;117:727–734.

54. Schluter G. Ciprofloxacin: toxicologic evaluation of additional safety data. *Am J Med* 1989;87:37S–39S.

55. Alfaham M, Holt ME, Goodchild MC. Arthropathy in a patient with cystic fibrosis taking ciprofloxacin. *BMJ (Clin Res Ed)* 1987;295:699.

56. Fontaine O. Antibiotics in the management of shigellosis in children: what role for the quinolones? *Rev Infect Dis* 1989;11[Suppl 5]:S1145–S1150.

57. Schaad UB, Abdus SM, Aujard Y, et al. Use of fluoroquinolones in pediatrics: consensus report of an International Society of Chemotherapy commission. *Pediatr Infect Dis J* 1995;14:1–9.

58. Salam MA, Dhar U, Khan WA, et al. Randomised comparison of ciprofloxacin suspension and pivmecillinam for childhood shigellosis. *Lancet* 1998;352:522–527.

59. Eidlitz-Marcus T, Cohen YH, Nussinovitch M, et al. Comparative efficacy of two- and five-day courses of ceftriaxone for treatment of severe shigellosis in children. *J Pediatr* 1993;123:822–824.

60. Helvaci M, Bektaslar D, Ozkaya B, et al. Comparative efficacy of cefixime and ampicillin-sulbactam in shigellosis in children. *Acta Paediatr Jpn* 1998;40:131–134.

61. Salam MA, Seas C, Khan WA, et al. Treatment of shigellosis. IV. Cefixime is ineffective in shigellosis in adults. *Ann Intern Med* 1995;123:505–508.

62. Radice M, Gonzealez C, Power P, et al. Third-generation cephalosporin resistance in Shigella sonnei, Argentina. *Emerg Infect Dis* 2001;7:442–443.

63. Khan WA, Seas C, Dhar U, et al. Treatment of shigellosis. V. Comparison of azithromycin and ciprofloxacin: a double-blind, randomized, controlled trial. *Ann Intern Med* 1997;126:697–703.

64. MacDonald WB, Friday F, McEacharn M, et al. The effect of chloramphenicol in *Salmonella* enteritis of infancy. *Arch Dis Child* 1954;29:238.

65. Effect of neomycin in non-invasive salmonella infections of the gastrointestinal tract. Joint Project by Members of the Association for the Study of Infectious Disease. *Lancet* 1970;2:1159–1161.

66. Kazemi M, Gumpert TG, Marks MI. A controlled trial comparing sulfamethoxazole-trimethoprim, ampicillin, and no therapy in the treatment of salmonella gastroenteritis in children. *J Pediatr* 1973;83:646–650.

67. Garcia DO, Trujillo H, Agudelo N, et al. Treatment of diarrhea in malnourished infants and children: a double-blind study comparing ampicillin and placebo. *Am J Dis Child* 1974;127:379–388.

68. Nelson JD, Kusmiesz H, Jackson LH, et al. Treatment of *Salmonella* gastroenteritis with ampicillin, amoxicillin, or placebo. *Pediatrics* 1980;65:1125–1130.

69. Sanchez C, Garcia-Restoy E, Garau J, et al. Ciprofloxacin and trimethoprim-sulfamethoxazole versus placebo in acute uncomplicated Salmonella enteritis: a double-blind trial. *J Infect Dis* 1993;168:1304–1307.

70. Torrey S, Fleisher G, Jaffe D. Incidence of *Salmonella* bacteremia in infants with Salmonella gastroenteritis. *J Pediatr* 1986;108:718–721.

71. Salmonella infections. In: Committee on Infectious Diseases, American Academy of Pediatrics, eds. *2000 Red book: report of the Committee on Infectious Diseases*, 25th ed. Elk Grove Village, IL: American Academy of Pediatrics; 2000:501–506.

72. Wessalowski R, Thomas L, Kivit J, et al. Multiple brain abscesses caused by *Salmonella* enteritidis in a neonate: successful treatment with ciprofloxacin. *Pediatr Infect Dis J* 1993;12:683–688.

73. Gendrel D, Raymond J, Legall MA, et al. Use of pefloxacin after failure of initial antibiotic treatment in children with severe salmonellosis. *Eur J Clin Microbiol Infect Dis* 1993;12:209–211.

74. Molbak K, Baggesen DL, Aarestrup FM, et al. An outbreak of multidrug-resistant, quinolone-resistant *Salmonella enterica* serotype *typhimurium* DT104. *N Engl J Med* 1999;341:1420–1425.

75. Anders BJ, Lauer BA, Paisley JW, et al. Double-blind placebo controlled trial of erythromycin for treatment of *Campylobacter* enteritis. *Lancet* 1982;1:131–132.

76. Pitkanen T, Pettersson T, Pomka A, et al. Effect of erythromycin on the fecal excretion of *Campylobacter fetus* subspecies *jejuni*. *J Infect Dis* 1982;145:128.

77. Salazar-Lindo E, Sack RB, Chea-Woo E, et al. Early treatment with erythromycin of *Campylobacter jejuni*-associated dysentery in children. *J Pediatr* 1986;109:355–360.

78. Taylor DN, Blaser MJ, Echeverria P, et al. Erythromycin-resistant *Campylobacter* infections in Thailand. *Antimicrob Agents Chemother* 1987;31:438–442.

79. Pichler HE, Diridl G, Stickler K, et al. Clinical efficacy of ciprofloxacin compared with placebo in bacterial diarrhea. *Am J Med* 1987;82:329–332.

80. Wistrom J, Jertborn M, Ekwall E, et al. Empiric treatment of acute diarrheal disease with norfloxacin: a randomized, placebo-controlled study. Swedish Study Group. *Ann Intern Med* 1992;117:202–208.

81. Mattila L, Peltola H, Siitonen A, et al. Short-term treatment of traveler's diarrhea with norfloxacin: a double- blind, placebo-controlled study during two seasons. *Clin Infect Dis* 1993;17:779–782.

82. Endtz HP, Ruijs GJ, van Klingeren B, et al. Quinolone resistance in *Campylobacter* isolated from man and poultry following the introduction of fluoroquinolones in veterinary medicine. *J Antimicrob Chemother* 1991;27:199–208.

83. Kuschner RA, Trofa AF, Thomas RJ, et al. Use of azithromycin for the treatment of *Campylobacter* enteritis in travelers to Thailand, an area where ciprofloxacin resistance is prevalent. *Clin Infect Dis* 1995;21:536–541.

84. Gordillo ME, Singh KV, Murray BE. In vitro activity of azithromycin against bacterial enteric pathogens. *Antimicrob Agents Chemother* 1993;37:1203–1205.

85. Murphy GS Jr, Echeverria P, Jackson LR, et al. Ciprofloxacin- and azithromycin-resistant *Campylobacter* causing traveler's diarrhea in U.S. troops deployed to Thailand in 1994. *Clin Infect Dis* 1996;22:868–869.

86. Merson MH, Sack RB, Islam S, et al. Disease due to enterotoxigenic *Escherichia coli* in Bangladeshi adults: clinical aspects and a controlled trial of tetracycline. *J Infect Dis* 1980;141:702–711.

87. Black RE, Levine MM, Clements ML, et al. Treatment of experimentally induced enterotoxigenic *Escherichia coli* diarrhea with trimethoprim, trimethoprim-sulfamethoxazole, or placebo. *Rev Infect Dis* 1982;4:540–545.

88. DuPont HL, Reves RR, Galindo E, et al. Treatment of travelers' diarrhea with trimethoprim/sulfamethoxazole and with trimethoprim alone. *N Engl J Med* 1982;307:841–844.

89. Oberhelman RA, Javier DLC, Vasquez GE, et al. Efficacy of trimethoprim-sulfamethoxazole in treatment of acute diarrhea in a Mexican pediatric population. *J Pediatr* 1987;110:960–965.

90. Echeverria P, Verhaert L, Ulyangco CV, et al. Antimicrobial resistance and enterotoxin production among isolates of Escherichia coli in the Far East. *Lancet* 1978;2:589–592.

91. Sack RB, Santosham M, Froehlich JL, et al. Doxycycline prophylaxis of travelers' diarrhea in Honduras, an area where resistance to doxycycline is common among enterotoxigenic Escherichia coli. *Am J Trop Med Hyg* 1984;33:460–466.

92. Jiang ZD, Mathewson JJ, Ericsson CD, et al. Characterization of enterotoxigenic *Escherichia coli* strains in patients with travelers' diarrhea acquired in Guadalajara, Mexico, 1992–1997. *J Infect Dis* 2000;181:779–782.

93. Goossens H, De Mol P, Coignau H, et al. Comparative in vitro activities of aztreonam, ciprofloxacin, norfloxacin, ofloxacin, HR 810 (a new cephalosporin), RU28965 (a new macrolide), and other agents against enteropathogens. *Antimicrob Agents Chemother* 1985;27:388–392.

94. Ericsson CD, Johnson PC, DuPont HL, et al. Ciprofloxacin or trimethoprim-sulfamethoxazole as initial therapy for travelers' diarrhea: a placebo-controlled, randomized trial. *Ann Intern Med* 1987;106:216–220.

95. DuPont HL, Ericsson CD, Mathewson JJ, et al. Five versus three days of ofloxacin therapy for traveler's diarrhea: a placebo-controlled study. *Antimicrob Agents Chemother* 1992;36:87–91.

96. Nelson JD. Duration of neomycin for enteropathogenic *Escherichia coli* diarrheal disease: a comparative study of 113 cases. *Pediatrics* 1971;48:248–258.

97. Thoren A, Wolde-Mariam T, Stintzing G, et al. Antibiotics in the treatment of gastroenteritis caused by enteropathogenic Escherichia coli. *J Infect Dis* 1980;141:27–31.

98. Haltalin KC, Kusmiesz HT, Hinton LV, et al. Treatment of acute diarrhea in outpatients: double-blind study comparing ampicillin and placebo. *Am J Dis Child* 1972;124:554–561.

99. Proulx F, Turgeon JP, Delage G, et al. Randomized, controlled trial of antibiotic therapy for Escherichia coli O157:H7 enteritis. *J Pediatr* 1992;121:299–303.

100. Ostroff SM, Kobayashi JM, Lewis JH. Infections with Escherichia coli O157:H7 in Washington State: the first year of statewide disease surveillance. *JAMA* 1989;262:355–359.

101. Martin DL, MacDonald KL, White KE, et al. The epidemiology and clinical aspects of the hemolytic uremic syndrome in Minnesota. *N Engl J Med* 1990;323:1161–1167.

102. Zhang X, McDaniel AD, Wolf LE, et al. Quinolone antibiotics induce Shiga toxin-encoding bacteriophages, toxin production, and death in mice. *J Infect Dis* 2000;181:664–670.

103. Wong CS, Jelacic S, Habeeb RL, et al. The risk of the hemolytic-uremic syndrome after antibiotic treatment of Escherichia coli O157:H7 infections. *N Engl J Med* 2000;342:1930–1936.

104. Adamkiewicz TV, Berkovitch M, Krishnan C, et al. Infection due to Yersinia enterocolitica in a series of patients with beta-thalassemia: incidence and predisposing factors. *Clin Infect Dis* 1998;27:1362–1366.

105. alMohsen I, Luedtke G, English BK. Invasive infections caused by Yersinia enterocolitica in infants. *Pediatr Infect Dis J* 1997;16:253–255.

106. Hoogkamp-Korstanje JA. Antibiotics in Yersinia enterocolitica infections. *J Antimicrob Chemother* 1987;20:123–131.

107. Abdel-Haq NM, Asmar BI, Abuhammour WM, et al. *Yersinia enterocolitica* infection in children. *Pediatr Infect Dis J* 2000;19:954–958.

108. Pai CH, Gillis F, Tuomanen E, et al. Placebo-controlled double-blind evaluation of trimethoprim-sulfamethoxazole treatment of Yersinia enterocolitica gastroenteritis. *J Pediatr* 1984;104:308–311.

109. Lindenbaum J, Greenough WB, Islam MR. Antibiotic therapy of cholera in children. *Bull W H O* 1967;37:529–538.

110. Wallace CK, Anderson PN, Brown TC, et al. Optimal antibiotic therapy in cholera. *Bull W H O* 1968;39:239–245.

111. Rahaman MM, Majid MA, Alam AKMJ, et al. Effects of doxycycline in actively purging cholera patients: a double-blind clinical trial. *Antimicrob Agents Chemother* 1976;10:610–612.

112. Pierce NF, Banwell JG, Mitra RC, et al. Controlled comparison of tetracycline and furazolidone in cholera. *BMJ* 1968;3:277–280.

113. Roy SK, Islam A, Ali R, et al. A randomized clinical trial to compare the efficacy of erythromycin, ampicillin and tetracycline for the treatment of cholera in children. *Trans R Soc Trop Med Hyg* 1998;92:460–462.

114. Bhattacharya SK, Bhattacharya MK, Dutta P, et al. Double-blind, randomized, controlled clinical trial of norfloxacin for cholera. *Antimicrob Agents Chemother* 1990;34:939–940.

115. Bhattacharya MK, Ghosh S, Mukhopadhyay AK, et al. Outbreak of cholera caused by Vibrio cholerae 01 intermediately resistant to norfloxacin at Malda, West Bengal. *J Indian Med Assoc* 2000;98:389–390.

116. Maimone F, Coppo A, Pazzani C, et al. Clonal spread of multiply resistant strains of Vibrio cholerae O1 in Somalia. *J Infect Dis* 1986;153:802–803.

117. Dubon JM, Palmer CJ, Ager AL, et al. Emergence of multiple drug-resistant Vibrio cholerae O1 in San Pedro Sula, Honduras. *Lancet* 1997;349:924.

118. Garg P, Chakraborty S, Basu I, et al. Expanding multiple antibiotic resistance among clinical strains of Vibrio cholerae isolated from 1992–7 in Calcutta, India. *Epidemiol Infect* 2000;124:393–399.

119. Dhar U, Bennish ML, Khan WA, et al. Clinical features, antimicrobial susceptibility and toxin production in *Vibrio cholerae* O139 infection: comparison with *V. cholerae* O1 infection. *Trans R Soc Trop Med Hyg* 1996;90:402–405.

120. Swerdlow DL, Ries AA. Vibrio cholerae non-O1—the eighth pandemic? *Lancet* 1993;342:382–383.

121. Gerding DN. Epidemiology and management of *Clostridium difficile* infection. *Contemp Intern Med* 1990;2:55.

122. Bartlett JG. Treatment of antibiotic-associated pseudomembranous colitis. *Rev Infect Dis* 1984;6[Suppl 1]:S235–S241.

123. Teasley DG, Gerding DN, Olson MM, et al. Prospective randomised trial of metronidazole versus vancomycin for Clostridium-difficile-associated diarrhoea and colitis. *Lancet* 1983;2:1043–1046.

124. Young GP, Ward PB, Bayley N, et al. Antibiotic-associated colitis due to *Clostridium difficile*: double-blind comparison of vancomycin with bacitracin. *Gastroenterology* 1985;89:1038–1045.

125. Oliva SL, Guglielmo BJ, Jacobs R, et al. Failure of intravenous vancomycin and intravenous metronidazole to prevent or treat antibiotic-associated pseudomembranous colitis. *J Infect Dis* 1989;159:1154–1155.

126. Bolton RP, Culshaw MA. Faecal metronidazole concentrations during oral and intravenous therapy for antibiotic associated colitis due to Clostridium difficile. *Gut* 1986;27:1169–1172.

127. Buggy BP, Fekety R, Silva J Jr. Therapy of relapsing *Clostridium difficile*-associated diarrhea and colitis with the combination of vancomycin and rifampin. *J Clin Gastroenterol* 1987;9:155–159.

128. Johnson S, Gerding DN. *Clostridium difficile*—associated diarrhea. *Clin Infect Dis* 1998;26:1027–1034.

129. Tina LG, Proto N, Sciacca A. Asymptomatic intestinal colonization by *Clostridium difficile* in preterm neonates. *Pediatr Infect Dis J* 1994;13:1158–1159.

130. Bolton RP, Tait SK, Dear PR, et al. Asymptomatic neonatal colonisation by *Clostridium difficile*. *Arch Dis Child* 1984;59:466–472.

131. Al Jumaili IJ, Shibley M, Lishman AH, et al. Incidence and origin of *Clostridium difficile* in neonates. *J Clin Microbiol* 1984;19:77–78.

132. Blakey JL, Lubitz L, Campbell NT, et al. Enteric colonization in sporadic neonatal necrotizing enterocolitis. *J Pediatr Gastroenterol Nutr* 1985;4:591–595.

133. Allos BM, Blaser MJ. *Campylobacter jejuni* and the expanding spectrum of related infections. *Clin Infect Dis* 1995;20:1092–1099.

134. Glandt M, Adachi JA, Mathewson JJ, et al. Enteroaggregative *Escherichia coli* as a cause of traveler's diarrhea: clinical response to ciprofloxacin. *Clin Infect Dis* 1999;29:335–338.

135. Portnoy BL, DuPont HL, Pruitt D, et al. Antidiarrheal agents in the treatment of acute diarrhea in children. *JAMA* 1976;236:844–846.

136. dios Pozo-Olano J, Warram JH Jr, Gomez RG, et al. Effect of a lactobacilli preparation on traveler's diarrhea: a randomized, double blind clinical trial. *Gastroenterology* 1978;74:829–830.

137. Zoppi G, Balsamo V, Deganello A, et al. Oral bacteriotherapy in clinical practice. II. The use of different preparations in the treatment of acute diarrhoea. *Eur J Pediatr* 1982;139:22–24.

138. Isolauri E, Juntunen M, Rautanen T, et al. A human Lactobacillus strain (*Lactobacillus casei* sp strain GG) promotes recovery from acute diarrhea in children. *Pediatrics* 1991;88:90–97.

139. Raza S, Graham SM, Allen SJ, et al. Lactobacillus GG promotes recovery from acute nonbloody diarrhea in Pakistan. *Pediatr Infect Dis J* 1995;14:107–111.

140. Shornikova AV, Isolauri E, Burkanova L, et al. A trial in the Karelian Republic of oral rehydration and *Lactobacillus* GG for treatment of acute diarrhea. *Acta Paediatr* 1997;86:460–465.

141. Rautanen T, Isolauri E, Salo E, et al. Management of acute diarrhoea with low osmolarity oral rehydration solutions and Lactobacillus strain GG. *Arch Dis Child* 1998;79:157–160.

142. Guandalini S, Pensabene L, Zikri MA, et al. *Lactobacillus* GG administered in oral rehydration solution to children with acute diarrhea: a multicenter European trial. *J Pediatr Gastroenterol Nutr* 2000;30:54–60.

143. Tvede M, Rask-Madsen J. Bacteriotherapy for chronic relapsing *Clostridium difficile* diarrhoea in six patients. *Lancet* 1989;1:1156–1160.

144. Holmgren J, Lange S, Lonnroth I. Reversal of cyclic AMP-mediated intestinal secretion in mice by chlorpromazine. *Gastroenterology* 1978;75:1103–1108.

145. Rabbani GH, Greenough WB III, Holmgren J, et al. Chlorpromazine reduces fluid-loss in cholera. *Lancet* 1979;1:410–412.

146. Formal SB, Abrams GD, Schneider H, et al. Experimental *Shigella* infections. VI. Role of the small intestine in an experimental infection in guinea pigs. *J Bacteriol* 1963;85:119.

147. DuPont HL, Hornick RB. Adverse effect of Lomotil therapy in shigellosis. *JAMA* 1973;226:1525–1528.

148. Chow CB, Li SH, Leung NK. Loperamide associated necrotising enterocolitis. *Acta Paediatr Scand* 1986;75:1034–1036.

149. Minton NA, Smith PG. Loperamide toxicity in a child after a single dose. *BMJ* (Clin Res Ed) 1987;294:1383.

150. Murphy GS, Bodhidatta L, Echeverria P, et al. Ciprofloxacin and loperamide in the treatment of bacillary dysentery. *Ann Intern Med* 1993;118:582–586.

151. Caeiro JP, DuPont HL, Albrecht H, et al. Oral rehydration therapy plus loperamide versus loperamide alone in the treatment of traveler's diarrhea. *Clin Infect Dis* 1999;28:1286–1289.

152. van Loon FP, Bennish ML, Speelman P, et al. Double blind trial of loperamide for treating acute watery diarrhoea in expatriates in Bangladesh. *Gut* 1989;30:492–495.

153. Ericsson CD, DuPont HL, Mathewson JJ, et al. Treatment of traveler's diarrhea with sulfamethoxazole and trimethoprim and loperamide. *JAMA* 1990;263:257–261.

154. Graham DY, Estes MK, Gentry LO. Double-blind comparison of bismuth subsalicylate and placebo in the prevention and treatment of enterotoxigenic *Escherichia coli*-induced diarrhea in volunteers. *Gastroenterology* 1983;85:1017–1022.

155. Steffen R, Mathewson JJ, Ericsson CD, et al. Travelers' diarrhea in West Africa and Mexico: fecal transport systems and liquid bismuth subsalicylate for self-therapy. *J Infect Dis* 1988;157:1008–1013.

156. DuPont HL, Sullivan P, Pickering LK, et al. Symptomatic treatment of diarrhea with bismuth subsalicylate among students attending a Mexican university. *Gastroenterology* 1977;73:715–718.

157. DuPont HL, Ericsson CD, Johnson PC, et al. Prevention of travelers' diarrhea by the tablet formulation of bismuth subsalicylate. *JAMA* 1987;257:1347–1350.

158. Pickering LK, Feldman S, Ericsson CD, et al. Absorption of salicylate and bismuth from a bismuth subsalicylate—containing compound (Pepto-Bismol). *J Pediatr* 1981;99:654–656.

159. Feldman S, Chen SL, Pickering LK, et al. Salicylate absorption from a bismuth subsalicylate preparation. *Clin Pharmacol Ther* 1981;29:788–792.

160. Burke V, Gracey M, Suharyono S. Reduction by aspirin of intestinal fluid-loss in acute childhood gastroenteritis. *Lancet* 1980;1:1329–1330.

161. Gracey M, Phadke MA, Burke V, et al. Aspirin in acute gastroenteritis: a clinical and microbiological study. *J Pediatr Gastroenterol Nutr* 1984;3:692–695.

162. Mohan M, Daral TS, Singh HP, et al. Aspirin in childhood gastroenteritis. *J Diarrhoeal Dis Res* 1985;3:215–218.

163. Wald A, Gotterer GS, Rajendra GR, et al. Effect of indomethacin on cholera-induced fluid movement, unidirectional sodium fluxes, and intestinal cAMP. *Gastroenterology* 1977;72:106–110.

164. Neumann SZ. Childhood diarrhoea and its treatment with indomethacin in Libya. *Trop Doct* 1980;10:24–28.

165. Rabbani GH, Butler T. Indomethacin and chloroquine fail to inhibit fluid loss in cholera. *Gastroenterology* 1985;89:1035–1037.

166. Isolauri E, Vesikari T. Oral rehydration, rapid feeding, and cholestyramine for treatment of acute diarrhea. *J Pediatr Gastroenterol Nutr* 1985;4:366–374.

167. Kreutzer EW, Milligan FD. Treatment of antibiotic-associated pseudomembranous colitis with cholestyramine resin. *Johns Hopkins Med J* 1978;143:67–72.

168. Pruksananonda P, Powell KR. Multiple relapses of Clostridium difficile-associated diarrhea responding to an extended course of cholestyramine. *Pediatr Infect Dis J* 1989;8:175–178.

169. Cook DJ, Kelton JG, Stanisz AM, et al. Somatostatin treatment for cryptosporidial diarrhea in a patient with the acquired immunodeficiency syndrome (AIDS). *Ann Intern Med* 1988;108:708–709.

170. Katz MD, Erstad BL, Rose C. Treatment of severe *Cryptosporidium*-related diarrhea with octreotide in a patient with AIDS. *Drug Intell Clin Pharm* 1988;22:134–136.

171. Salazar-Lindo E, Santisteban-Ponce J, Chea-Woo E, et al. Racecadotril in the treatment of acute watery diarrhea in children. *N Engl J Med* 2000;343:463–467.

172. Cezard JP, Duhamel JF, Meyer M, et al. Efficacy and tolerability of racecadotril in acute diarrhea in children. *Gastroenterology* 2001;120:799–805.

173. Sarker SA, Casswall TH, Mahalanabis D, et al. Successful treatment of rotavirus diarrhea in children with immunoglobulin from immunized bovine colostrum. *Pediatr Infect Dis J* 1998;17:1149–1154.

174. Casswall TH, Sarker SA, Faruque SM, et al. Treatment of enterotoxigenic and enteropathogenic *Escherichia coli*-induced diarrhea in children with bovine immunoglobulin milk concentrate from hyperimmunized cows: a double-blind, placebo-controlled, clinical trial. *Scand J Gastroenterol* 2000;35:711–718.

175. Black RE, Sazawal S. Zinc and childhood infectious disease morbidity and mortality. *Br J Nutr* 2001;85[Suppl 2]:S125–S129.

176. Khatun UH, Malek MA, Black RE, et al. A randomized controlled clinical trial of zinc, vitamin A or both in undernourished children with persistent diarrhea in Bangladesh. *Acta Paediatr* 2001;90:376–380.

CHAPTER 79
Whipple's Disease

Steven F. Solga and Theodore M. Bayless

Whipple's disease is a rare multisystem disorder caused by an actinobacterium known as *Tropheryma whippleii* (1). The periodic acid–Schiff (PAS)-positive microorganism, and the characteristic macrophage response can be identified in almost all organ systems. Small intestinal involvement is characteristic but not essential for the diagnosis. Several studies have implicated an impaired cellular immune response in patients with Whipple's disease (2,3). This host susceptibility may be inherited because Whipple's disease primarily affects white males in Europe and North America (4).

In the early phase of the disease, the clinical features are multisystemic, with relapsing arthralgias, polyserositis, and lymphadenopathy. Diarrhea with or without malabsorption, weight loss, hyperpigmentation, endocarditis, and central nervous system (CNS) abnormalities is a prominent finding in the later stages of the disease.

Before the use of antibiotics to treat this disease, its course was unrelenting and ultimately fatal. After 1960, intestinal biopsy provided a method of diagnosis, and treatment with antibiotics has greatly improved outcome. The response to antibiotics is usually rapid and sometimes complete. Cardiac and CNS involvement may make treatment difficult, and relapses can occur.

CLINICAL MANIFESTATIONS

The hallmark findings of Whipple's disease include diarrhea, weight loss, arthralgia or arthritis, and abdominal pain. A multitude of CNS and cardiovascular symptoms may also develop, and presentations can be protean and multisystemic. A common theme, however, seems to be the initial onset of joint complaints. Two thirds of 52 patients in a recent review by Durand and colleagues (5) experienced articular manifestations before the diagnosis. Indeed, rheumatological concerns were far more common than other signs or symptoms in the earliest stages of Whipple's disease. All patients reported by Durand had involvement of peripheral joints, although axial joint involvement was not uncommon. Symptoms and signs may be expressed as arthralgia or arthritis. Attacks of pain or inflammation are often sporadic and last for days to weeks. The joints are typically symmetrically involved, lack significant tissue destruction, and are seronegative.

Intestinal symptoms, in contrast, frequently manifest most often at the time of diagnosis. They are typified by diarrhea and weight loss, which occur in most patients (85% in the Durand review). Other symptoms include crampy abdominal pain, anorexia, and occult blood loss. The jejunum and ileum are most often involved, followed by the duodenum. Although gastrointestinal tract symptoms are characteristic, 15% to 25% of patients will have no gastrointestinal symptoms, and these patients could easily be overlooked.

Although joint and bowel manifestations are common, obvious CNS symptoms can be lacking. Nevertheless, in his review, Dobbins (4) asserted that all patients have some element of CNS disease even if only a minority demonstrate symptoms. Further, a small number of patients manifest dramatic CNS symptoms but lack symptoms elsewhere. For example, Knox and associates (6) reported a diagnosis of Whipple's disease based on analysis of brain and eye tissue 62 years after a patient's death. The patient had experienced dementia, supranuclear ophthalmoplegia, and monoclonic ocular or facial jerks. These symptoms typify CNS involvement in Whipple's disease, although among many possibilities are headache, seizure, ataxia, muscle weakness, and auditory changes. Notably, Knox's patient did not have symptoms outside of the CNS, and biopsies of many other tissues (including intestine) were negative. CNS Whipple's disease often includes ocular symptoms such as blurry vision, loss of vision, uveitis, and iritis.

Cardiovascular and pulmonary presentations are less common. Some amount of cardiovascular involvement is often present at autopsy, but overt symptoms are unusual. Possibilities include pericarditis, myocarditis, endocarditis, and heart failure. Pulmonary symptoms can include cough, pleural effusion, and pleuritic chest pain associated with serositis. Cough can be present in up to 50% of cases but is rarely a presenting symptom.

Presentations involving other organ systems are rare. Examples include hypothyroidism, adrenal gland involvement, and prosthetic joint infection. Skin involvement is very unusual, even though an unexplained hyperpigmentation rash occurs in about one third of patients.

Physical examination is variable, and findings vary according to disease severity, duration, and area of involvement. General features can include intermittent low-grade fever at any time during the illness and relative hypotension late in the course of disease. Lymphadenopathy, abdominal tenderness, splenomegaly, and edema are also possible.

TROPHERYMA WHIPPLEII

In 1907, George Hoyt Whipple, who later became the 1934 Nobel laureate in physiology, provided a thorough account of a 36-year-old physician's chronic illness (7). Diarrhea, weight loss, arthritis, and cough were prominent features. Whipple gave an extremely detailed and accurate description of the histologic findings in the small bowel and mesenteric lymph nodes. Whipple named the illness "intestinal lipodystrophy" despite the fact that he clearly recognized bacteria in one lymph node. The bacterial origins of Whipple's disease were later confirmed (8) by electron microscopy in 1961. During the same period, a number of groups were reporting dramatic responses of patients with Whipple's disease after treatment with various antibiotics, and an invariably fatal illness became readily curable.

Still, identification and characterization of the organism remained elusive until the application of modern molecular techniques. Wilson and colleagues (9) and, later, Relman and colleagues (1) used polymerase chain reaction (PCR) based on highly conserved sequences that are shared by all bacterial organisms on the 16s ribosomal RNA. These sequences are interspersed with variable regions that are distinct for different bacteria. The 16s bacterial ribosomal RNA was amplified by PCR with a sequential combination of broad and then specific primers. The PCR first uses broad primers that bind to the highly conserved sequence. The nucleotide sequence is then analyzed, and specific primers for the variable regions are used for a second-stage PCR. The nucleotide sequence of the amplicon provides a specific diagnostic PCR product.

With this strategy, Relman and colleagues (1) identified a specific PCR product in a patient with Whipple's disease and then used the specific primers on five other patients who all had positive tests. Ten control patients had no false-positive results. The phylogenetic position of this bacterium is believed to be related to actinomycetes. The etiologic agent of Whipple's disease was thus positively identified and named: *Tropheryma whippleii*. Of note, "trophe" translates from Greek to "nourishment," and acknowledges the symptom of malabsorption.

Most recently, Schoeden and colleagues (10) reported successful isolation and growth of *T. whippleii* using a strategy involving deactivation of macrophages with interleukin-4 (IL-4). Further landmark progress was reported by Raoult and associates (11) with the first successful cultivation of *T. whippleii*. These investigators used a human fibroblast cell line to propagate *T. whippleii* through multiple passages with an estimated doubling time of 18 days.

T. whippleii is a gram-positive, non–acid-fast, non–spore-forming rod. It measures about 0.2×1.5 to 2.5 μm. The cell wall is remarkable for a low electron density layer with an inner electron dense layer. The cystoplasmic membrane has two electron dense layers. It is the glyoprotein-containing cell wall that stains with PAS; fragments of this diastase-resistant layer accumulate in the macrophages after lysis and are responsible for the characteristic appearance on histology. The phylogenic position of *T. whippleii* suggests that it may inhabit soil or water; the bacterium has been found in sewage.

EPIDEMIOLOGY

Demography

Dobbins (4) provided an excellent analysis of demographic data in a study of 664 patients, including 574 males and 90 females. In male patients, the median age at diagnosis was 49.1 years; that for female patients was 51 years. The age at diagnosis was maximal in the fifth decade for men but in the seventh decade for women. Only 9 of the 664 patients were younger than 31 years at diagnosis. The racial distribution of the disease was almost exclusively white. Only 10 of the patients were black, of whom 8 were male and 2 were female. Of the patients analyzed by Dobbins, only 15 were nonwhite. Durand and colleagues' review (5) of 52 patients provided similar data: 73% of patients were male, and the mean age at diagnosis was 50 years for males and 58 years for females.

Occupations

There have been suggestions that Whipple's disease occurs more commonly in rural situations. Dobbins was able to confirm this in his review of the occupations of 191 patients. Farmers accounted for 23% of the total. The frequency in farm workers is three times that expected from the total number of farmers in the U.S. workforce. Combining those who work in farming and construction and those who work as machinists and those who might therefore be expected to have major contact with soil or animals, one can account for two thirds of the total known occupations of affected persons. These observations fit with the soil origin of the actinobacteria species. There are some suggestions that Whipple's disease might be a food-borne illness.

Clustering

There are three reports of siblings with the illness, including one family with possible multigenerational involvement. There have been some reports of clustering, including three patients from a French village and four patients from an Italian village. In a U.S. report, 7 of 19 patients from the state of North Carolina lived within a 20-mile radius of Fayetteville.

Prevalence

Whipple's disease is rare. Recent literature suggests a rise in the diagnosis, but it is unclear whether the true incidence is changing. PCR techniques have afforded the opportunity to apply a sensitive diagnostic test to many contexts. Some reports have suggested that *T. whippleii* is more common than previously thought and is perhaps even commensal of the human gut flora (12). Other investigators, however, have not found this to be true (13). Given that basic understanding of the natural reservoir and the mode of transmission of *T. whippleii* is lacking, controversy on this subject is likely to persist until further techniques are applied.

IMMUNOLOGY AND PATHOLOGY

Patients with Whipple's disease clearly manifest an inadequate immune response to the causative organism. They are unable to clear the organism from intracellular residues. Several small studies have suggested a defect of cellular immunity. Demonstrable abnormalities include decreased lymphocyte mitogenicity to concavalin A and phytohemagglutinin. Skin testing for recall antigens is also abnormal (14). In one study, the serum of patients with Whipple's disease manifested inhibitory properties during active disease (3). Proliferation assays showed higher proliferation rates of peripheral blood mononuclear cells among all groups of patients when cells were mixed with control serum; more important, there was decreased proliferation of control mononuclear cells when they were mixed with patients' serums. In the same study, patients with the disease manifested a persistent reduction in peripheral blood mononuclear cell CD11b expression (complement receptor 3α chain). Abnormalities of CD11b have been implicated previously in congenital leukocyte adhesion deficiency. Complement receptor 3α activity has been implicated in macrophage accumulation and cellular adhesion (15). Thus, defective CD11b expression in patients with Whipple's disease may be one of the major contributory factors in the inadequate immune response to the causative organism and may play a role in determining susceptibility to the disease. Further study has demonstrated reduced production of IL-12 and interferon-γ in patients with Whipple's disease (16).

There are also demonstrable abnormalities of mucosal immunity in Whipple's disease. Ectors and colleagues (17) found decreased phagocytic potential, decreased CD4-to-CD8 ratio, and increased numbers of intraepithelial lymphocytes in a study of small bowel mucosa from 16 Belgian patients with Whipple's disease.

The immune deficiency may be genetically determined. In the review by Dobbins (4), 14 of 53 patients (26%) were positive for human leukocyte antigen (HLA)-B27. This is considerably higher than the expected ranges of 0.3% to 6.9% in this patient population. It has been hypothesized that this genetic association may play a role in determining the presence of cellular immune deficiency. Other authors have reported similar results, although a recent small Italian study did not find any HLA-B27 association (18).

In terms of immunopathology, a granulomatous inflammatory reaction may occur in Whipple's disease. The polyvisceral granulomata resemble those in sarcoidosis. Nine percent of the cases reviewed by Dobbins (4) contained evidence of granulomatous changes, especially in the liver, mesentery, and peripheral lymph nodes as well as intestine, brain, and lung. Other sites of granulomata reported in the literature include synovium and kidneys (19,20). PAS staining of lymph nodes containing granulomata has sometimes led to a conclusive diagnosis of Whipple's disease in patients with an otherwise elusive diagnosis.

DIAGNOSIS

Given the rarity of the disease, clinical suspicion is critical to successful diagnosis. Physical exam findings are nonspecific but may include intermittent fever, abdominal tenderness, lymphadenopathy, splenomegaly, and hyperpigmentation on sun-exposed areas. Laboratory and radiologic testing tends to be nonspecific. Many patients will have a mildly elevated erythrocyte sedimentation rate. Computed tomography examination may be notable only for abdominal lymphadenopathy, whereas small bowel series may identify small bowel inflammation through thickened or edematous folds, or may be normal.

Histology remains the most useful test. A classic diagnosis involves the finding of PAS positive, diastase-resistant, acid-fast negative bodies in the cytoplasm of foamy macrophages located in the lamina propria of the small intestine in a patient with an appropriate clinical syndrome. Upper endoscopy is the easiest route to acquiring such tissue. Endoscopic findings range from normal to mild inflammatory changes and edema. Dilated lipid laden lacteals can give a "tuffed rug" appearance. Multiple biopsies should be obtained from the distal duodenum and jejunum to maximize diagnostic yield. Although PAS-positive macrophages can occur in other intestinal syndromes (e.g., *Mycobacterium avium*), additional testing (e.g., acid-fast staining) and clinical context rarely cause confusion with Whipple's disease.

Even in patients with primarily extraintestinal manifestations of Whipple's disease, biopsy of the small intestine is often the most useful single test given its high sensitivity. Nevertheless, the characteristic macrophages have been located in many types of extraintestinal tissue. In these instances, however, confirmatory electron microscopy or PCR is useful because PAS-positive macrophages are more likely to be confused with other disease processes (e.g., sarcoidosis) compared with intestinal biopsy. Intestinal biopsies have, at times, been negative late in the course when neurologic manifestations were predominant or after antibiotic administration.

The utility of PCR in the diagnosis of Whipple's disease is unclear. Lowsky and coworkers (21) described two patients for whom the diagnosis was made by molecular analysis of peripheral blood. With whole-blood DNA, PCR yielded an amplicon, and subsequent sequence analysis demonstrated 100% homology of an examined variable portion to *T. whippleii*. Rickman and colleagues (22) reported a patient with chronic uveitis and little clinical evidence of Whipple's disease in whom the diagnosis of ocular Whipple's disease was made by PCR of vitreous fluid. The described patient also had molecular evidence of duodenal infection without clinical symptoms. These reports suggest that PCR may yet be the most sensitive and accurate method of diagnosing Whipple's disease.

Finally, Raoult and associates (11), in their report on the cultivation of *T. whippleii*, described the development of an indirect immunofluorescence serologic assay. Their description included a small number of patients tested for immunoglobulin G and M antibodies at various titer cutoff values. Although such serologic tests may prove valuable in the future, their use is presently investigational.

TREATMENT AND PROGNOSIS

Before the observation of the effectiveness of antibiotics in 1952, Whipple's disease was invariably fatal; it continued to be so until the early 1960s. The immediate response to antibiotics is often described as spectacular. Responses have occurred to a variety of antibiotics, including tetracycline, trimethoprim-sulfamethoxazole (TMP-SMX), chloramphenicol, erythromycin, penicillin G alone and with streptomycin, and third-generation cephalosporins. The optimal regimen and length of treatment are not defined. A combination of theory and practice, however, has yielded some guidelines.

Given that many patients have neurologic involvement, antibiotic regimens ensuring CNS penetration seem requisite. Such regimens might include, for example, TMP-SMX with or without a third-generation cephalosporin. Although many treatment successes have occurred without a CNS penetrant drug, many relapses have also been documented. This is particularly true of tetracycline (5,23). When the CNS has not been involved, treatment successes occur more readily. Antibiotic treatment should be given for a long period, probably at least 1 year, although there is some evidence that 3 months of therapy may be sufficient for some patients.

There are several different initial treatment regimens advocated in the literature. The current recommendations by Dobbins (4), based on extensive review of the literature in 1986, include parenteral penicillin plus streptomycin for 10 to 14 days, followed by one double-strength tablet of sulfamethoxazole given twice daily for 1 year. Although treatment failures are rare, Durand and associates (5) have questioned the need for induction with penicillin and streptomycin given their poor CNS penetration. Instead, in 1997, these authors proposed therapy with TMP-SMX alone. Given the length of treatment under consideration, supplemental treatment with folinic acid to prevent folic acid deficiency has been suggested.

An alternative treatment regimen features third-generation cephalosporins. Schnider (24) reported success by substituting ceftriaxone for the penicillin in combination with streptomycin and also recommend its use in CNS relapse, particularly after the use of TMP-SMX. A novel approach introduced by Schneider and colleagues (25) involves the inclusion of interferon-γ to the regimen.

Relapses are more common than had been appreciated originally. In the largest review, by Keinath and colleagues (26), there were 31 relapses among 88 treated patients. The relapses may be manifested by recurrence of the patient's original symptoms or may be characterized by development of new symptoms, particularly in the CNS. Only 1 of 11 patients who suffered CNS manifestations and relapse of symptoms responded to new courses of antibiotics, whereas 19 of 20 patients with intestinal symptoms responded to reinstitution of therapy (26). Knox and coworkers (27) had emphasized the phenomenon of CNS relapses after inadequate antibiotic therapy. In the review by Keinath's group, 13 of the 31 patients who suffered a relapse had a CNS relapse (26). Regimens ensuring CNS penetration, as described earlier, may be less prone to relapse.

The histologic correlation with successful treatment (or relapse) remains unclear. Certainly, in many treatment successes, the condition of the surface epithelium in the intestine improves within 1 week, whereas free bacteria may exist in the lamina propria for up to 9 weeks during therapy. The PAS-positive macrophages, however, clear at a much lower rate, so that 6 months or even 12 months after beginning therapy, prominent macrophages may still be present. The membranous materials of the macrophages, which presumably represent bacterial cell walls, are eventually replaced by granular material. We had previously used disappearance of the membranous material within the PAS-positive macrophages as a sign that therapy had been adequate, but we have no data to support this view. If all symptoms disappear and there is a complete remission, there is probably no need for routine follow-up with intestinal biopsy; however, intestinal biopsy should be done at the time of any symptomatic relapse regardless of the system involved. Recovery of free bacilli by electron microscopy or persistently positive PCR results can also aid in the assessment of relapse from extraintestinal sites (e.g., from cerebrospinal fluid).

A Jarisch-Herxheimer reaction has been reported on four occasions during initial treatment with oral or intravenous penicillin. A systemic reaction developed within 12 to 24 hours, including temperature elevations, chills, headache, hypertension, and, in two patients, severe abdominal pain and chest pain (28).

Adrenocorticosteroids were given for 1 week to one patient to control a presumed Jarisch-Herxheimer reaction. This reaction is similar to that seen 42 hours after the initial treatment of syphilis with penicillin. Presumably, endotoxin or some other product released from the bacteria causes this reaction. Other possible explanations are depletion of endogenous opioids and activation of the complement system.

SUMMARY

Whipple's disease is a rare infectious disease that seems to occur in a specific population of middle-aged white men who have significant exposure to soil or to a rural environment. There is evidence that there are subtle immune defects in these patients; the predominance of HLA-B27 suggests a genetic predisposition.

The etiologic agent is *T. whippleii*, a gram-positive actinomycete that stains positively with PAS. The organism multiplies in the lamina propria of the intestinal mucosa and in other organs without exciting a vigorous immune response. The bacterium is sensitive to a variety of antibiotics; however, eradication and cure usually require prolonged antibiotic therapy. CNS involvement requires specific attention. Current recommendations include combinations of either penicillin or a third-generation cephalosporin with streptomycin for 2 weeks, followed by 1 year of TMP-SMX therapy versus TMP-SMX monotherapy.

Relapses, especially in the CNS, can be extremely resistant to therapy. Deaths from Whipple's disease continue to occur, largely because of late recognition of the illness or because of CNS and cardiac involvement.

The ability to recognize and treat this disease should continue to improve with the identification of the causative organism and the description of newer molecular techniques of detection in tissues and body fluids.

REFERENCES

1. Relman DA, Schmidt TM, MacDermott RP, et al. Identification of the uncultured bacillus of Whipple's disease. *N Engl J Med* 1992;327:293–301.
2. Martin F, Vilseck J, Dobbins WO, et al. Immunological alterations in patients with treated Whipple's disease. *Gastroenterology* 1972;63:6–18.
3. Marth T, Roux M, von Herbay AV, et al. Persistent reduction of complement receptor 3 alpha-chain expressing mononuclear blood cells and transient inhibitory serum factors in Whipple's disease. *Clin Immunol Immunopathol* 1994;72:217–226.
4. Dobbins WO III. *Whipple's disease.* Springfield, IL: Charles C Thomas, 1987.
5. Durand D, et al. Whipple's disease: clinical review of 52 cases. *Medicine* 1997;76(3):170–184.
6. Knox DL, et al. Cerebral ocular Whipple's disease: a 62 year odyssey from death to diagnosis. *Neurology* 1995;45(4):617–625.
7. Whipple GH. A hitherto undescribed disease characterized anatomically by deposits of fat and fatty acids in the intestinal and mesenteric lymphatic tissue. *Bull Johns Hopkins Hosp* 1907;18:381–391.
8. Yardley JH, Hendrix TR. Combined electron and light microscopy in Whipple's disease. *Bull Johns Hopkins Hosp* 1961;109:80–87.
9. Wilson KH, et al. Phylogeny of the Whipple's disease-associated bacterium. *Lancet* 1991;338:474–475.
10. Schoedon G, et al. Deactivation of macrophages with interleukin-4 is the key to the isolation of *T. whippleii. J Infect Disease* 1997;176:672–677.
11. Raoult D, et al. Cultivation of the bacillus of Whipple's disease. *N Engl J Med* 2000;342(9):62–625.
12. Ehrbar HU, et al. PCR-positive test for *T. whippleii* in patients without Whipple's disease. *Lancet* 1999;354:1178–1179.
13. Maiwald M, et al. *Tropheryma whippleii* DNA is rare in the intestinal mucosa of patients without other evidence of Whipple disease. *Ann Intern Med* 2001;134(2):115–119.
14. Feurle GE, Dorken B, Schopf E, et al. HLA B27 and defects in the T-cell system in Whipple's disease. *Eur J Clin Invest* 1979;9:385–389.
15. Ding A, Wright SD, Nathan C. Activation of mouse peritoneal macrophages by monoclonal antibody to Mac-1 (complement receptor type 3). *J Exp Med* 1987;165:733–749.
16. Marth T, et al. Defects of monocyte interleukin 12 production and humoral immunity in Whipple's disease. *Gastroenterology* 1997;113:442–448.
17. Ectors N, Geboes K, De Vos R, et al. Whipple's disease: a histological, immunocytochemical and electron microscopic study of the immune response in the small intestinal mucosa. *Histopathology* 1992;21:1–12.
18. Olivieri I, et al. Lack of association with spondyloarthritis and HLA-B27 in Italian patients with Whipple's disease. *J Rheumatol* 2001;28(6):1294–1297.
19. Dhib M, Heron F, Francois A, et al. Kidney granuloma in Whipple's disease. *BMJ* 1993;307:1067–1068.
20. Rouillon A, Menkes CJ, Gerster JC, et al. Sarcoid-like forms of Whipple's disease: report of 2 cases. *J Rheumatol* 1993;20:1070–1072.
21. Lowsky R, Archer GL, Fyles G, et al. Diagnosis of Whipple's disease by molecular analysis of peripheral blood. *N Engl J Med* 1994;331:1343–1346.
22. Rickman LS, Freeman W, Green R, et al. Brief report: uveitis caused by *Tropheryma whippleii* (Whipple's bacillus). *N Engl J Med* 1995;332:363–366.
23. Feurle GE, Marth T. An evaluation of antimicrobial treatment for Whipple's disease: tetracycline versus trimethoprim-sulfamethoxazole. *Dig Dis Sci* 1994;39:1642–1648.
24. Schnider PJ. Long-term follow-up in cerebral Whipple's disease. *Eur J Gastroenterol Hepatol* 1996;8(9):899–903.
25. Schneider T, et al. Treatment of refractory Whipple disease with interferon gamma. *Ann Intern Med* 1998;129(11):875–877.
26. Keinath RD, Merrell DE, Vlietstra R, et al. Antibiotic treatment and relapse in Whipple's disease: long-term follow-up of 88 patients. *Gastroenterology* 1985;88:1867–1873.
27. Knox DL, Bayless TM, Pittman FE. Neurologic disease in patients with treated Whipple's disease. *Medicine* (Baltimore) 1976;55:467–476.
28. Reed JI, Sipe JD, Wohlgethan JR, et al. Response of the acute-phase reactants, C-reactive protein and serum amyloid A protein, to antibiotic treatment of Whipple's disease. *Arthritis Rheum* 1985;28:352–355.

CHAPTER 80

Approach to the Patient with Intraabdominal Infections

Dietmar H. Wittmann and Robert E. Condon

The approach to patients suffering from intraabdominal infections is governed by the limited time to establish proper treatment. An exact diagnosis, although the ultimate goal, may not be possible before treatment must be initiated. Some authors discuss this entity under the term *acute abdomen*, meaning the presence of abnormal abdominal signs and symptoms that require an immediate workup to initiate appropriate treatment. Early treatment of potentially life-threatening peritonitis may result in a better outcome. Any delay may correlate with exponentially increasing mortality.

The most valuable information is obtained from the patient's presentation and description of the circumstances of the presenting symptoms. The specific time of onset and the duration of complaints are important guides to the correct diagnosis, which is purely clinical. Sophisticated technology such as an abdominal computed tomography scan or time-consuming laboratory tests and similar nonessential diagnostic procedures may delay appropriate therapy and increase mortality.

The accepted classification of intraabdominal infection is a division into primary, secondary, and tertiary peritonitis (Table 80.1). Although in primary peritonitis, hematogenous bacterial spread to the peritoneum prevails, secondary peritonitis follows a spontaneous or traumatic perforation of a hollow viscus or cystic structure, and tertiary peritonitis denotes ongoing inflammation without a bacterial trigger (1–3).

TABLE 80.1. Classification of Intraabdominal Infection

Primary peritonitis
  Spontaneous peritonitis of childhood
  Spontaneous peritonitis of adulthood
  Peritonitis in patients with continuous ambulatory peritoneal
    dialysis
  Tuberculosis peritonitis
Secondary peritonitis
  Spontaneous peritonitis (spontaneous acute)
    Gastrointestinal tract perforation
    Bowel wall necrosis
    Pelvic peritonitis
    Peritonitis after translocation of bacteria
  Postoperative peritonitis
    Leak of an anastomosis
    Leak of a suture line
    Stump insufficiency (leak of a blind bowel end)
    Other iatrogenic leaks
  Posttraumatic peritonitis
    Peritonitis after blunt abdominal trauma
    Peritonitis after penetrating abdominal trauma
Tertiary peritonitis
  Peritonitis without pathogens
  Peritonitis with fungi
  Peritonitis with low-grade pathogenic bacteria
Intraabdominal abscess
  Intraabdominal abscess with primary peritonitis
  Intraabdominal abscess with secondary peritonitis

DEFINITION

Intraabdominal infection and peritonitis are not synonymous, although both terms are used clinically to describe a suppurative intraabdominal process. *Peritonitis* simply means inflammation of the peritoneum or of a part of it with or without bacteria being involved. The peritoneum is formed by a single layer of mesothelial cells together with underlying loose connective tissue (4) and composes a total area of about 1.8 m². It covers all of the intestinal organs and the abdominal wall, the diaphragm, the retroperitoneum, and the pelvis. In older textbooks, the area of the peritoneum is described as about equal to the area of the skin, drawing an analogy of the systemic responses in intraabdominal infection with those of burn injuries to the skin.

Intraabdominal infection implies the presence of a bacterial source from which identifiable microorganisms gain access into the peritoneal cavity. The host response to the bacterial challenge is localized peritoneal inflammation, progressing if infection is unchecked to a systemic inflammatory response. Peritonitis can be regarded as a general class of peritoneal inflammation, of which a specific entity is intraabdominal infection.

The leviathan inflammatory response of the peritoneum to any injuring challenge influences all of the varieties of clinical presentation of intraabdominal infection. Inflammatory edema resulting in thickening of the peritoneum by only 1 mm would require shifting over 8 L of fluid into the peritoneum from the extracellular space, leading to abdominal hypertension (5), hypovolemia, and deleterious effects on systemic tissue perfusion. Bacteria may flow quickly from the peritoneal cavity into systemic circulation through the diaphragmatic lymphatic and other lymph channels. Consequently, intraabdominal infections are not solely a local disease but affect the entire body, resulting in early signs of organ dysfunction that may be detected at the initial workup (5,6).

HOST RESPONSE

The inflammatory reaction of secondary peritonitis that occurs in intraabdominal infection is triggered by the influx into the abdominal cavity of bacteria-laden gastrointestinal contents or chemical irritants. In primary peritonitis, with a lower initial bacterial inoculum, this reaction is not as fulminant. Bacteria and their toxins ultimately play a key role in all forms of intraabdominal infection. Immediately after the initial influx of bacteria into the free peritoneal cavity, the bacteria multiply at a rate that depends on their adaptability to the new environment (6,7). The damage caused by these events takes the following course.

Histamine and other vasoactive substances are released, owing to mast cell degranulation after cell damage to the peritoneum (Fig. 80.1). The complement system is activated, and chemotaxis is induced. Vasoactive substances increase the permeability of vessels. In combination with chemotaxis, this promotes an influx of polymorphonuclear granulocytes. Both inmigrating and local macrophages phagocytose bacteria as well as detritus and foreign bodies. This process is supported by the activated complement system, which promotes opsonization. Finally, phagocytosed bacteria are destroyed, and the dead bacteria and phagocytic cells are carried away, primarily through the lymphatic stomata and channels in the diaphragm.

Owing to increased vascular permeability, plasma exudes into the free peritoneal cavity, leading to fibrin formation. Necrotic, bacteria-containing detritus is delimited, leading to abscess formation (Fig. 80.2). In the developing abscess, bacteria continue to divide, producing toxins and enzymes that, together with the proteolytic enzymes of macrophages, liquefy the abscess content, creating high osmotic pressure. Because oxygen and nutrients cannot easily cross the abscess membrane, anaerobic glycolysis is promoted within the abscess, which finally results in an anaerobic environment of high pressure in which growth of obligate anaerobic bacteria is promoted. Rupture of such an

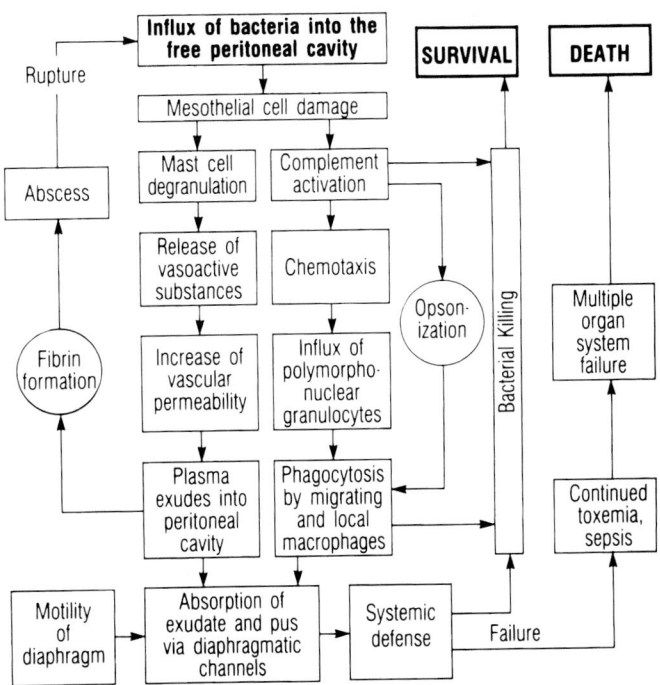

Figure 80.1. The evolution of intraabdominal infection. Bacterial contamination of the peritoneal cavity initiates a sequence of local and systemic responses that culminate in the survival or death of the patient.

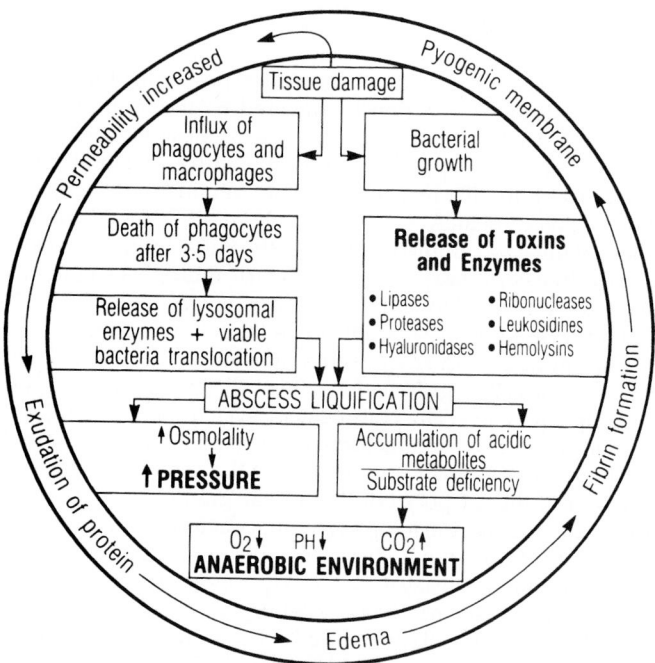

Figure 80.2. Pathophysiologic processes during formation of an abscess.

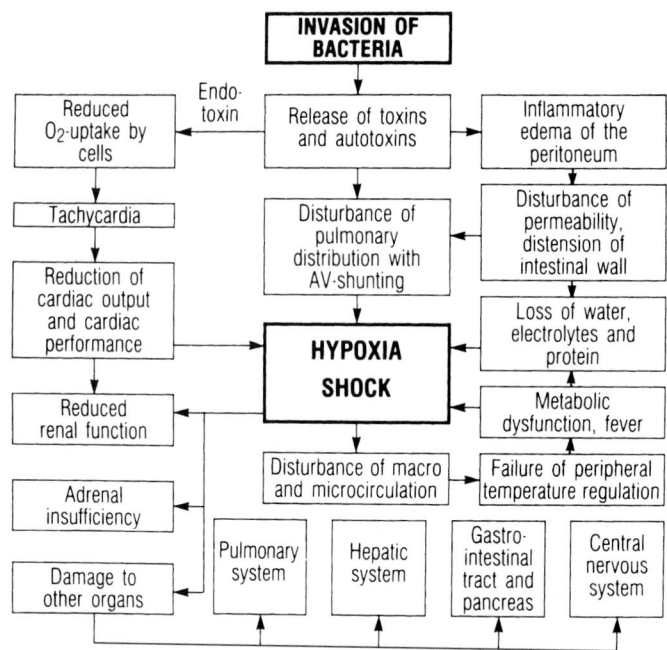

Figure 80.3. The systemic pathophysiologic responses in intraabdominal infection are largely mediated through disturbed oxygen-dependent processes.

abscess into the peritoneal cavity may reinitiate the process of diffuse bacterial peritonitis, but with a different primary causative microorganism.

Absorption of exudate and pus through diaphragmatic lymphatic channels represents an important defense mechanism of the peritoneal cavity. This defense reaction is enhanced by respiratory motion in connection with the diaphragmatic lymphatic "valves." Eight tenths of the exudate and toxins generated in most intraabdominal infections is eventually absorbed through the diaphragmatic-thoracic lymphatic channels into the central venous circulation. Intraabdominal infection thus affects the entire organism at an early stage. Rapid intraabdominal clearance of considerable amounts of bacteria and noxious material can lead to damage in all organ systems (8–12). In effect, a local-regional infection turns into a severe systemic infection mediated by cytokines, autacoids, eicosanoids, nitric oxide, and other inflammatory mediators (13).

The inflammatory reaction of the peritoneum produces significant sequestration of fluid in the peritoneal cavity. The inflammatory edema expanding the peritoneum may result in a relatively acute fluid loss of 5 to 8 L from the circulation. This leads initially to hypovolemic shock, followed by dehydration and, finally, death in connection with toxin-induced shock. The signs and symptoms of sepsis are mainly due to the products of bacterial breakdown. Hypoxia forms the turnstile of all the involved pathophysiologic mechanisms (Fig. 80.3). Hypoxia results from the inability of cells to utilize oxygen for energy-generating processes.

A hyperdynamic cardiovascular response occurs that attempts to compensate for what is perceived by the body as a cellular oxygen deficit. Clinically, high cardiac output and low systemic vascular resistance are seen, coupled with deficient cellular oxygen use, so that highly oxygenated blood returns to the venous system. Compounding factors may be toxic respiratory insufficiency with reduced pulmonary oxygen transport, thus further reducing oxygen delivery to the tissues. This process contributes to cell death and aggravates the endotoxin–macrophage–nitric oxide inhibition of adenosine triphosphate

synthesis in the mitochondria. Gradual cell death of organs leads to sequential organ system failure (13).

PATHOPHYSIOLOGIC CHANGES THAT LEAD TO VITAL ORGAN DAMAGE

Heart: dehydration, tachycardia, hypotension, reduction of cardiac output and venous return with decreased peripheral resistance (blood pooling), hypoxia, and shock. Progressive peripheral cell death eventually leads to a hypodynamic circulation and the low cardiac output of the failing or dying heart.

Lung: decreased ventilatory space due to inflammatory edema and increased abdominal pressure, disturbance of pulmonary ventilation-perfusion with atrial venous shunting, increased pulmonary resistance, nitric oxide–induced alveolar cell destruction, increased oxygen transfer distance, pulmonary insufficiency (acute respiratory distress syndrome), hypoxia

Kidney: reduced perfusion secondary to hypovolemia and increased intraabdominal pressure, retention of toxic metabolites, hypoxic and toxic damage to renal epithelia, increase in urea nitrogen and creatinine, renal insufficiency

Intestine: local hypoxia, increased sympathetic activity, disproportionate bacterial growth, bowel distention, increased intraabdominal pressure, abdominal compartment syndrome

Liver: hypoxic cell damage, reduced protein synthesis, impaired Kupffer's cell function, reduced metabolic detoxification, reduced perfusion due to increased intraabdominal pressure

BACTERIOLOGY

Normal Bowel Flora

Bacterial counts in the gastrointestinal tract vary greatly, from nearly sterile in the fasting, normal, low-pH stomach to high concentrations of bacteria approaching 10^{12} per milliliter of feces in the distal colon. Of the more than 400 different species of intestinal bacteria, most are symbiotic saprophytes, and only a few are capable of survival outside the bowel (6,14–17).

ESOPHAGUS AND STOMACH

Normally, there are fewer than 1,000 organisms per milliliter of fluid in the esophagus and stomach. There are no obligate anaerobes; the flora is composed chiefly of α-hemolytic streptococci, lactobacilli, yeasts, and some swallowed oral bacteria. There is a direct correlation between the pH of the stomach (normally between 2 and 3) and the bacterial concentration. In achlorhydria, the count ranges from 100,000 to 10 million per milliliter. Anesthesia reduces gastric acid secretion and thus permits an increase in the microbial count. Higher bacterial concentrations in the stomach are also associated with the administration of histamine-2 (H_2)-receptor antagonist and proton pump inhibitor drugs; this needs to be considered when upper gastrointestinal tract perforation occurs in patients receiving such drugs, especially patients who are being treated in the intensive care unit for other reasons. Studies of stomach bacteria after resection or vagotomy consistently show an increased bacterial count (18).

DUODENUM AND JEJUNUM

In the duodenum and jejunum, there are 100 to 10,000 bacteria per milliliter, primarily hemolytic streptococci, lactobacilli, transitory oral flora, and in rare cases, *Enterobacter* species and some *Bacteroides* species. Duodenal diverticula and biliary calculous disease contribute to higher bacterial counts, as does previous gastrectomy with a blind duodenal stump or ileus of any cause.

ILEUM

With decreasing distance from the ileocecal valve, the bacterial count increases, reaching values of 1 to 10 million per milliliter in the distal ileum (15). Lactobacilli and streptococci are most frequent; *Bacteroides* and *Enterobacter* species are found in equal concentrations in the terminal ileum. High counts are found in any pathologic bowel state, such as ileus, obstruction, or chronic inflammatory disease.

COLON

Two thirds of dry fecal matter consists of bacteria. Less than 0.3% of these bacteria are Enterobacteriaceae. Moore and Holdeman (7) identified 400 to 500 different bacterial species in the large bowel. The ratio of anaerobic to aerobic organisms is 3,000:1 to 10,000:1. The total bacterial count is 3.8×10^{12} per milligram dry stool (Table 80.2).

TABLE 80.2. Mean Concentration^a of Selected Intraluminal Bacteria

Bacteria	Concentration
Streptococci	$10^{6.5}$
Bacillus species	$10^{7.0}$
Enterococci	$10^{7.5}$
Escherichia coli	$10^{8.0}$
Bifidobacteria	$10^{8.3}$
Anaerobic cocci	10^{10}
Eubacteria	$10^{10.5}$
Clostridia	$10^{10.5}$
Bacteroides species	10^{11}

^{a}Per milligram of dried feces.

Pathogen Virulence Selection

The pathogens that cause intraabdominal infections come primarily from the intestine and associated hollow organs. Knowledge of the types and frequency of pathogenic bacteria usually resident in various segments of the bowel provides the basis for a presumptive diagnosis of the most likely pathogens before culture and sensitivity findings are available. The intestinal flora, however, is dependent on other factors: age, race, diet, previous operations, malnutrition, gastric acidity, bile salt excretion, gut motility, immune mechanisms, and prior administration of antibiotics (7,18). These factors alter the spectrum of possible target bacteria for therapy. In addition, the qualitative distribution of bacteria within their normal environment may be altered by various virulence factors outside the gastrointestinal tract (19–23).

Once outside the intestines, most of the intestinal bacteria die in the new hostile extraluminal environment, and only those few bacteria that can withstand the host defense system survive (19). The consequence is a selection of virulent species after viscus perforation and other forms of intraabdominal infection (Fig. 80.4). Information about the pathogenicity of individual bacterial species is particularly important in the mixed infections usually seen with intraabdominal infection because there are multiple possibilities of synergistic interactions, and there may also be antagonistic ones.

Current microbiologic identification and sensitivity testing methods available in hospitals do not meet the optimal requirements for management of antibacterial chemotherapy (24). Results need to be available within a short time (minutes) after the cultures are taken if the physician is to be able to institute selective antibiotic therapy without risking increased mortality and morbidity due to delay in starting that therapy. The desired time frame is in the range of minutes and will probably never be achieved. Therefore, presumptive antimicrobial therapy should be started as soon as an intraabdominal infection is diagnosed (25).

The initial therapy may be modified when specific sensitivity data are available, but changing antibiotics is not indicated unless the initial regimen is failing. Often, results of the initial bacteriologic assessment may be impaired because of inadequate specimen sampling or inappropriate transport time, especially in patients who have their laparotomy outside of the regular working hours of the laboratory. Antibiotic choice should not be based on such potentially flawed bacteriologic reports, which usually show predominance of transport-resistant bacteria such as enterococci that are of little pathogenic importance. The duration of antibiotic therapy should be short. Only when the source of infection cannot be controlled operatively as, for example, in infected pancreatic necrosis may an antibiotic regimen of more than 5 days' duration be justified (26).

Isolation of Pathogens

The isolation of pathogens poses many problems for the usual hospital clinical laboratory. Almost any bacterium known to be pathogenic for humans (Fig. 80.4) may be seen on a Gram stain obtained from the infected peritoneum. Except to confirm that a mixed bacterial flora is present, the Gram stain is of little help and even routine culture is of questionable help. Many pathogens die off rapidly after the initial sampling and cannot be cultured easily by the hospital bacteriologist. Subsequent antibiotic therapy may fail if it is based on bacteriologic test results gained under suboptimal conditions. It is surprising, however, how similar are the results concerning distribution and frequency of pathogens

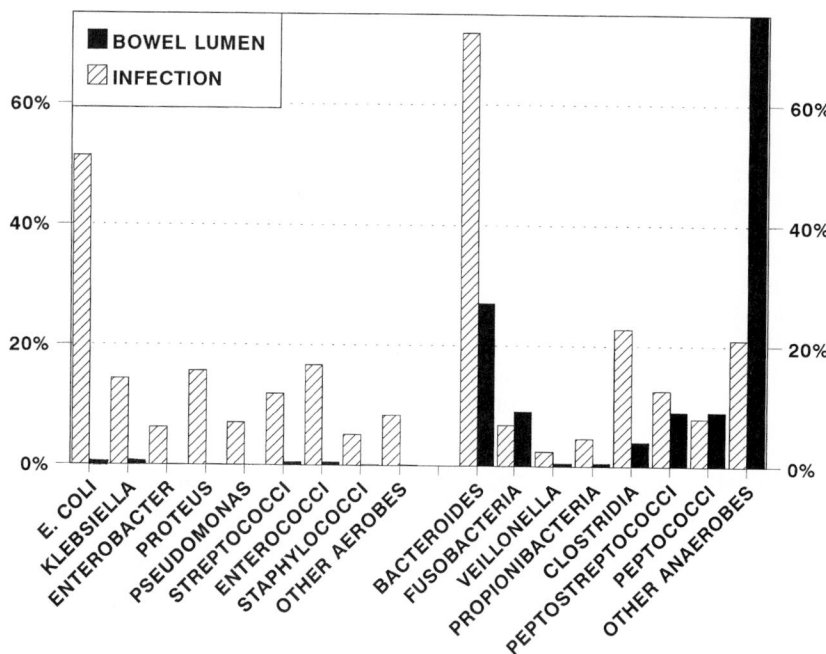

Figure 80.4. There is a disparity between the proportions of bacteria found in the lumen of the bowel in a normal person and bacteria recovered in intraabdominal infections. Aerobic organisms are relatively rare in the normal bowel but grow preferentially in infections. *Escherichia coli*, normally present in low concentration, becomes the dominant aerobe and the second most frequently recovered bacterium in infection. Anaerobic organisms that predominate in the bacterial population of the normal bowel are, with the exception of *Bacteroides* species, relatively less predominant. (Adapted from Wittmann DH. Die Bedeutung der Infektionserreger fur die Therapie der eitrigen Peritonitis. *Chirurgie* 1985;56:363–370, 1985, with permission.)

from different studies using the best available technique (25,27) (Table 80.3).

The data of Table 80.3 record the important pathogens that should be considered target bacteria for therapy. *Escherichia coli* is the most commonly isolated pathogen. Its relative frequency

in abdominal infections exceeds its intraluminal frequency by about 300 times, indicating that *E. coli* has a better chance of survival outside its natural environment, thus confirming its pathogenicity. The second most commonly isolated bacteria in intraabdominal infections are gram-negative obligate anaerobes, particularly *Bacteroides fragilis*. These organisms, in combination with other nonobligate anaerobes, are responsible for abscess formation (21–23). Other important organisms to be covered by initial chemotherapy are clostridia and gram-positive anaerobic cocci. Staphylococci and pseudomonads are unimportant as initial pathogens in peritonitis. Enterococci are frequently isolated, but their pathogenic role is not yet defined; these organisms may act as a cofactor in the development of abscesses induced by obligate anaerobes. Even the recent emergence of resistant gram-positive bacteria does not play a major role as initial pathogens. They typically are seen in tertiary peritonitis as contaminants of the peritoneal cavity.

TABLE 80.3.   Pathogens of 900 Intraabdominal Infections Isolated in Six Independent Studies

	Isolates	
Pathogen	No.	%
Aerobes		
Escherichia coli	462	38
Klebsiella species	129	10
Enterobacter species	56	5
Proteus species	141	11
Pseudomonas aeruginosa	63	5
Staphylococcus aureus	46	4
Enterococcus faecalis	150	12
Other streptococci	107	9
Other aerobes	75	6
Total	1,229	48
Anaerobes		
Bacteroides fragilis	329	24
Other *Bacteroides* species	318	24
Fusobacteria	61	5
Veillonella	22	2
Peptococci	71	5
	113	8
Clostridia	205	15
Propionibacteria	41	3
Other	189	14
Total	1,349	52
Grand total	2,578	

Data from Wittmann DH. Treatment of peritonitis: antibiotic concentration dynamics at the site of infection as criterion of antimicrobial chemotherapy [Thesis]. Habilitation. Hamburg: Medizinische Fakultät der Universität, 1985, with permission.

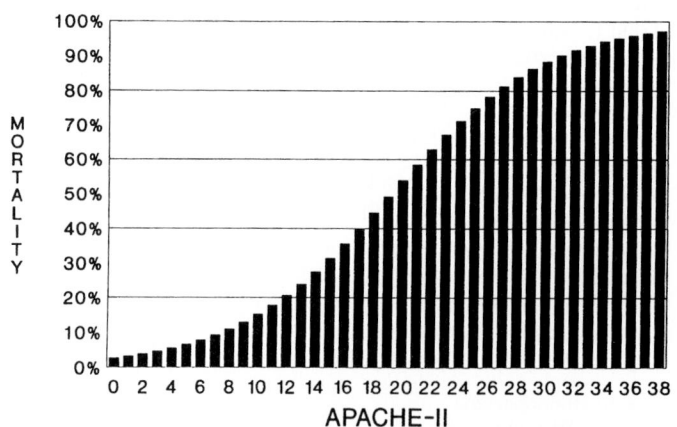

Figure 80.5. Relation between the Acute Physiology and Chronic Health Evaluation (APACHE) II score and predicted mortality for patients with intraabdominal infection. (From Wittmann DH, Condon RE, Walker AP. Peritonitis and intraabdominal infection. In: Schwartz S, ed. Principles of surgery, 6th ed. New York: McGraw-Hill, 1993:1449–1483, with permission of The McGraw-Hill Companies.)

Sepsis

Patients with intraabdominal infections die of the deleterious effects of their own immune response to infection, a process defined as sepsis and septic shock, and best measured by the Acute Physiology and Chronic Health Evaluation II (APACHE II) score (3,13) (Fig. 80.5). Sepsis is most commonly induced by endotoxin released from dying facultative bacteria such as E. coli (28). The term *sepsis* has been used to denote the systemic response to infection and its pathophysiologic changes. Sepsis is the most common cause of death in the intensive care unit and is the thirteenth most common cause of death in the United States; 400,000 patients develop sepsis annually, in 200,000, it progresses to septic shock, and 100,000 patients die annually (24). Microorganisms (such as E. coli) therefore constitute the major target for antibiotic therapy if the threat of mortality and organ failure is to be reduced (13,25,27).

CLINICAL FEATURES OF INTRAABDOMINAL INFECTION

Every case of intraabdominal infection, of whatever cause, initiates a sequence of responses involving the peritoneum, the bowel, and the body fluid compartments, which then produces secondary endocrine, cardiac, respiratory, renal, and metabolic responses (Figs. 80.1 and 80.3). In certain forms of peritonitis, notably acute suppurative peritonitis, additional responses due to the presence of infection also occur. These pathophysiologic responses form the basis of schemes to stratify mortality risk among patients with peritonitis (2,3,10,13).

Abdominal pain is almost always the predominant symptom, unless its perception is masked by the administration of analgesics or the presence of a fresh surgical wound. The pain may have been sudden in onset, associated with rupture of a viscus, or more insidious. When fully developed, pain is steady, unrelenting, burning, and aggravated by any motion. Pain is usually most intense in the region of most advanced peritoneal inflammation. Decreasing intensity and extent of pain with time suggest localization of the inflammatory process, whereas increasing intensity and extent imply the presence of spreading peritonitis.

Anorexia is almost always present. Nausea is frequent and may be accompanied by vomiting. The patient usually complains of thirst and of feeling feverish, often with intermittent chills. Temperature usually ranges between 38°C and 40°C; the fever is more spiking in character in younger and healthier patients, whereas older or debilitated patients may exhibit only a modest febrile response. Tachycardia and a diminished palpable peripheral pulse volume are indicative of hypovolemia. As hypovolemia progresses, compensatory initial vasoconstrictive responses may be overwhelmed with the rapid appearance of hypovolemic shock. Respirations are typically rapid and shallow: rapid because of greater tissue demands for oxygen and the need to correct developing acidosis, and shallow because deep respiration intensifies the perception of abdominal pain.

The abdomen is distended and may be stiff from increased intraabdominal pressure and decreased abdominal wall compliance (5). The abdomen is quiet to auscultation and tender to palpation. Tenderness is present over the entire extent of the peritoneum involved in the inflammatory process and is maximal usually in the region of the organ in which the process originated. In some cases, maximal tenderness is found over the advancing edge of peritoneal inflammation. Direct, percussive, and referred rebound tenderness confirms the presence of peritoneal irritation. Percussion tenderness sometimes is more accurate than direct palpation in locating the point of maximal tenderness and in delineating the extent of peritoneal irritation.

Rigidity of the abdominal muscles is produced—initially by voluntary guarding—after involvement of the parietal peritoneum by inflammation but also by reflex muscle spasm. Reflex spasm may become so severe that boardlike abdominal rigidity is produced. Hyperresonance due to accumulating gas in the paralyzed, distended intestines usually can be demonstrated easily by percussion.

Some bowel sounds may be audible on auscultation early in intraabdominal infection, but as inflammation spreads, the nearly silent abdomen of adynamic ileus ("atonia") supervenes. Rectal and vaginal examinations are essential steps to locate the extent of tenderness and the possible presence of a pelvic mass. Vaginal examination of the cervix may provide clues to the origin of the inflammatory process.

Leukocytosis is common in acute intraabdominal infection, but the total white cell count, taken alone without a differential count, can be misleading. Massive peritoneal inflammation may mobilize sufficient numbers of leukocytes into the diseased area to produce peripheral leukopenia. Leukocytosis of more than 25,000 and leukopenia of less than 4,000 white cells/mm^3 are both associated with higher mortality. The differential count provides the essential evidence of the presence of acute inflammation by showing a moderate to marked leftward shift even if the total white cell count is normal.

The radiologic picture in an acute intraabdominal infection is of paralytic ileus. Inflammatory exudate and edema of the intestinal wall may produce widening of the spaces between adjacent bowel loops noted on a flat film of the abdomen. Peritoneal flank fat lines and the retroperitoneal psoas shadows may be obliterated. Free air may be visible on an upright abdominal or lateral decubitus film if a ruptured hollow viscus is the cause of peritonitis or if peritonitis is well established and due to gas-forming bacteria such as E. coli. Air beneath the diaphragm also may be noted on radiographs of the chest, especially if the patient remains in an upright position for 5 minutes before the film is made.

THERAPY

The therapeutic goal is reduction of mortality. The mortality of intraabdominal infection was about 90% at the turn of the nineteenth century, when management was mainly nonoperative and supportive. Through the application of the following surgical principles of early, definitive treatment, mortality in the worst cases has been reduced by more than 50% (29,30):

- Closure, resection, or exteriorization to control the source of infection
- Elimination or reduction of the concentration of bacteria, toxins, and necrotic material in the peritoneal cavity
- Treatment of residual bacteria with antimicrobial drugs
- Decompression of abdominal compartment syndrome
- Restoration of organ function

After its initial introduction into medical practice, antibiotic therapy did not reduce the mortality of intraabdominal infection, although it was successful in treating many other surgical infections. Poor isolation techniques that obscured the participation of anaerobes in peritonitis, and the limited activity of the antimicrobials initially available against endotoxin-producing Enterobacteriaceae, were major factors responsible for the initial failure of antibiotic therapy in peritonitis.

TABLE 80.4.   Causes of Peritonitis

Causes of peritonitis	All patients		Patients who died	
	No.	%	No.	%
Perforation	331	58	58	18
Bowel wall necrosis	116	20	42	36
Trauma	10	2	2	20
Postoperative leak	80	14	23	29
Abscess	26	5	5	19
Not specified	4	1	2	
Total	567	100	132	23

During the past two decades, however, the mortality risk of peritonitis has diminished. Reliable studies of advanced peritonitis reporting mortality rates of 30% and less (13,30–34) have been published. The improvement can be attributed to a better understanding of the true pathogens of intraabdominal infections and to antimicrobial therapy targeted at these microorganisms. Improved surgical technique is another important factor (1). Some authors have reported better survival rates in a subset of high-risk patients with intraabdominal infection treated more aggressively by leaving the abdomen open or planned repeated laparotomies. These advanced procedures introduce two new operative principles that supplement the classic two principles of (a) source control and (b) cleaning the abdominal cavity of bacteria, toxins, and adjuvants. The newly introduced principles include (c) decompression of an abdominal compartment syndrome by leaving the abdomen open, and (d) quality control by reopening the abdomen and checking out suture lines and completeness of removal of bacteria, toxins, and adjuvants (13,30–32,35) (Table 80.4).

The staged abdominal repair (STAR) program combines the benefits of the classic operation with both new procedures of the open abdomen technique and planned relaparotomy (Fig. 80.6) (30,35). Concomitant mandatory antibiotic therapy should start as early as possible after diagnosis but not before the operative

reduction of the bacterial inoculum, which helps to reduce the threat of endotoxemia (25,35–37).

Antibiotic therapy should be started as early as possible after confirming diagnosis intraoperatively. Specific, directed treatment is not possible, however, because the infecting microorganisms and their sensitivities are not precisely known. Consequently, the choice of antimicrobial must be based on other criteria (32,38). Antimicrobial therapy should be directed against the most frequently expected pathogens and should achieve an antimicrobially active concentration of drug at the site of infection. The potential for adverse interaction of antibiotics with host defenses, and possible toxic effects such as the ototoxicity of aminoglycosides, must also be considered. Controlled clinical trial reports of antimicrobial efficacy are often of little help; the most severely diseased patients have been excluded from most trials (39,40). Sampling of pus for bacteriologic studies is done as an early step in operative treatment.

Perforation Peritonitis

Perforation peritonitis is the most common form of acute intraabdominal infection. In major hospitals, about 80% of cases are due to a variety of primary necrotic lesions of the gastrointestinal tract or of other intraabdominal organs; 10% to 20% of perforations are seen in patients after abdominal operations (postoperative peritonitis). In 58% of patients, frank perforation of the gastrointestinal tract due to peptic ulcer disease, diverticulitis, appendicitis, or a malignant lesion leads to the infection (Table 80.5). Bowel wall necrosis, either after strangulation caused by incarcerated hernia or due directly to impaired vascular flow, is the cause of infection in 20% of cases.

Infection after Perforation of Stomach and Duodenum

Infection after peptic ulcer perforation presents acutely; the patient is usually able to identify the exact time at which the perforation occurred. This form of peritonitis is initially chemical in

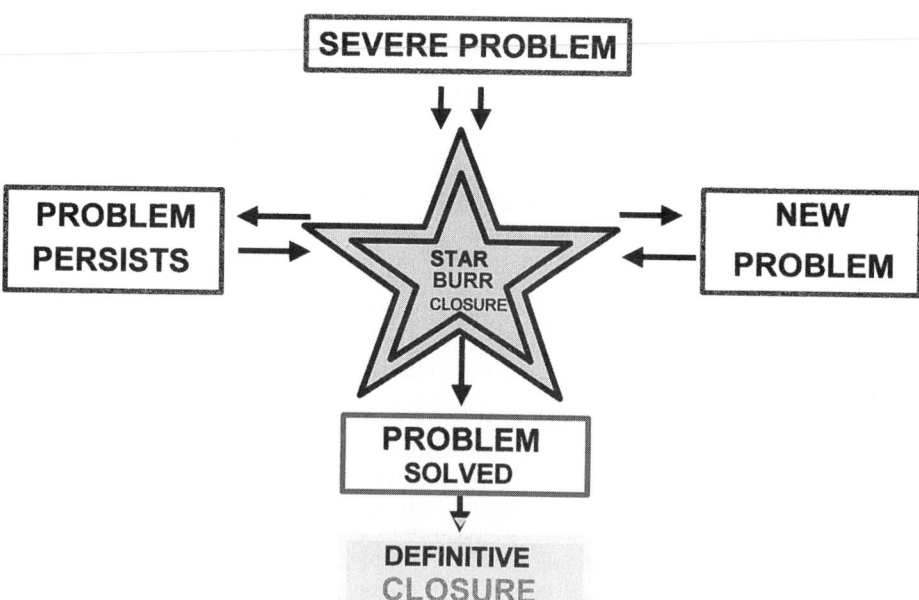

STAR STRATEGY

Figure 80.6. Staged abdominal repair (STAR) procedure.

TABLE 80.5. Organ Source of Origin of Peritonitis

Origin of peritonitis	All patients		Those who died	
	No.	%	No.	%
Stomach and duodenum	175	31	38	22
Biliary tract	50	9	8	16
Pancreas	11	2	4	36
Small bowel	71	13	27	38
Appendix	125	22	16	13
Colon	117	21	43	37
Genitourinary system	14	2	3	21
Other	4	1	1	25
Total	567	100	140	25

nature but with the passage of a short time becomes infected through bacterial translocation. The patient most often seeks help early owing to severe pain, and operative repair is often possible before systemic dissemination of infection and organ failure occur. The proper management is simple closure. Antibiotic therapy either is not required (chemical peritonitis) or may be given over a very short period in the range of 1 to 3 days because bacterial numbers are generally small and the source can be closed safely (26).

The high mortality rate of anastomotic leakage or suture line breakdown after gastroduodenal operations is explained by the fact that the duodenum is retroperitoneally fixed and cannot be exteriorized, and the source of infection often cannot be adequately controlled or closed. Consequently, infective material and proteolytic enzymes are delivered continuously into the peritoneal cavity, sustaining the infection.

Infection after Pancreatitis

Translocation of bacteria is probably the mechanism of progression from initial chemical inflammation to later intraabdominal infection. The combination of tissue necrosis due to proteolytic and lipolytic pancreatic juice and the presence of intestinal bacteria is the reason for the high mortality rate of infected pancreatic necrosis. The diagnosis of pancreatitis is not difficult; a history of midepigastric pain radiating to the back, in combination with elevated levels of amylase and lipase in serum and urine, suggests the correct diagnosis. The transition from pancreatitis to infected pancreatic necrosis and diffuse peritonitis is more difficult to diagnose, and thus antimicrobial therapy is often started late, when deterioration and multiorgan system failure have already occurred. In this type of advanced disease, multiple planned reoperations may be necessary (38,41).

Infection after Small Bowel Perforation

Symptoms of intraabdominal infection after small bowel perforation fall into two major categories:

1. Ileus precedes peritonitis. Colic and other features of bowel obstruction are the leading signs and symptoms initially, gradually changing to those of localized or diffuse peritonitis with fever and leukocytosis.
2. Bowel wall necrosis due to inadequate vascular supply or inflammation leads to perforation. Peritonitis may be diagnosed at a late stage, owing to a lack of initial symptoms. Often, these patients are operated on late in the evolution of their peritonitis, and the mortality rate is more than 50%. This contributes to the mortality figure of 38% in patients who had peritonitis after bowel wall necrosis (Table 80.5).

Infection and Appendicitis

In formal usage, appendicitis meets the criteria of a local peritonitis, but this disease is not usually included under secondary suppurative peritonitis because of the strictly localized inflammation and the extremely low mortality in typical cases. If the appendix has perforated, however, the disease may become life threatening, especially when the omentum is not able to contain the infection, diffuse suppurative peritonitis then results. The symptoms of appendicitis are outlined in Chapter 83. When peritonitis develops, usually there is a sudden deterioration in the clinical status. Treatment is more likely to be successful once the appendix is removed and the source of infection is thus controlled. This explains the lower mortality rate of 13% in the series recorded in Table 80.6.

Disseminated intraabdominal infection from appendicitis is not seen as often today as in the first decades of the twentieth century, when vital statistics showed that appendicitis was the major cause of peritonitis seen in hospitals (29). Because the human life span has increased, other organ origins of peritonitis are now seen more often, and diseases of aged persons, cancer and diverticulitis for example, are more frequently the cause of intraabdominal infections.

Infection after Colon Perforation

Colon perforation due to diverticulitis or cancer is a common cause of diffuse, suppurative peritonitis. Postoperative peritonitis due to a disrupted anastomosis is seen most frequently after a colon operation. A myriad of bacteria gain access to the peritoneal cavity through the perforated colon. This factor, together with the many associated diseases in the population of elderly patients with colon disease, contributes to the high mortality rate of 37% (Table 80.6). This group of patients particularly

TABLE 80.6. Principles of Operative Management of Advanced Peritonitis

		Indication: When to do
Principle 1	Source control: close or eliminate all bacterial leaks	Simple IAI Advanced IAI
Principle 2	Abdominal toilet: purge (cleanse) the abdominal cavity from bacteria, toxins, and adjuvants	Simple IAI Advanced IAI
Principle 3	Decompression of increased intraabdominal pressure to improve organ perfusion and function	Only advanced IAI
Principle 4	Quality control of principle 1 and 2 by daily abdominal reentries	Only advanced IAI

benefits from STAR, for which the overall mortality rate is less than 20% (30,31,35). The basis for successful treatment is elimination of the infectious source. With the STAR procedure, anastomotic healing following resection of the diseased colon can be directly observed, thus diminishing the need for colostomy. Because additional complications are associated with the formation and takedown of colostomies, and because STAR rarely requires more than two abdominal reentries for assurance of proper anastomotic healing, colostomies are less often performed in modern surgery. Antibiotic therapy needs to cover both facultative and obligate anaerobic bacteria and can be discontinued after 5 days (13,34,40,42).

Infection after Perforation of the Genitourinary Tract

A variety of conditions may cause peritonitis originating from the genitourinary tract. Ruptured perinephric abscess and ruptured chronic cystitis after radiation therapy for female reproductive tract cancer are examples. Pelvic peritonitis due to sexually transmitted infection is seen in young women; usually, there is acute, severe abdominal pain. The condition is easily diagnosed by Gram stain if it is suspected. Treatment is only with antimicrobials in nearly all cases.

Postoperative Peritonitis

Postoperative peritonitis is usually due to a leak from a suture line and was discovered only after some delay, as a rule between the fifth and seventh postoperative days. Delay contributed to the high mortality rate. A suture line leak is easier to repair if it is observed in the colon, small bowel, or stomach, compared with leaks of the duodenum or esophagus. Upper gastrointestinal tract disease after an operation allows only a limited therapeutic correction to control the source because these organs are fixed or closely attached to the retroperitoneum, and the infectious source cannot be totally excluded under most circumstances. Resection of the anastomosis or of the diseased bowel segment is better than repair. STAR using a temporary abdominal closure device may be of particular benefit to this subset of patients with intraabdominal infections; we were able to reduce the mortality rate to 24% (30,31,35).

Posttraumatic Peritonitis

Peritonitis may develop in patients with injuries after blunt trauma who have unrecognized intraabdominal conditions, such as ruptured mesentery with obliteration of the vascular supply to the small or large bowel or a frank bowel perforation. This type of intraabdominal infection is usually severe because it is masked by other injuries. Treatment does not differ from that of intraabdominal infection generally.

Contamination of the abdominal cavity seen after penetrating abdominal trauma is usually not considered an intraabdominal infection. Only one third of patients with penetrating trauma to the colon actually sustain documented contamination of the peritoneal cavity, although many trials testing the efficacy of antimicrobials erroneously use this subset of patients as representative of peritonitis (40).

Tertiary Peritonitis

Patients who are unable to contain an infection, whether because of inadequate host defense mechanisms or overwhelm-

ing infection, may go on to develop persistent inflammation and diffuse peritonitis, which Rotstein and Meakins (43) have called *tertiary peritonitis*. The clinical picture is one of occult sepsis manifested by hyperdynamic cardiovascular findings, low-grade fever, and a general hypermetabolic state. These patients have the clinical picture of sepsis without the presence of a well-defined focus of infection and are often subjected to laparotomies in the hope of improving drainage of recurrent or residual collections of infected fluid. These infected fluid collections are different from true abscesses because they are not delimited by an inflammatory membrane or capsule. These patients frequently die with multiorgan system failure as the result of cellular asphyxia. Bacteria of low pathogenic potential, usually selected by antimicrobial therapy, are isolated from these patients. The bacterial isolates may include multiresistant, coagulase-negative staphylococci, enterococci, and species of pseudomonads and fungi. These microorganisms do not seem to be readily affected by antimicrobial treatment, which suggests an underlying problem of generalized failure of host defenses.

REFERENCES

1. Wittmann DH. Symposium of intra-abdominal infections: Introduction. *World J Surg* 1990;14:145.
2. Dellinger EP, Wertz MJ, Meakins JL, et al. Surgical infection stratification system for intra-abdominal infection. *Arch Surg* 1985;120:21.
3. Nyström PO, Bax R, Dellinger EP, et al. Proposed definitions for diagnosis, severity scoring, stratification, and outcome for trials on intraabdominal infection. *World J Surg* 1990;14:148.
4. Lierse W. Das Peritoneum. Anatomische Grundlagen. *Chirurgie* 1985;56:357.
5. Wittmann DH, Iskander GA. The abdominal compartment syndrome: state-of-the-art review. *J Intens Care Med* 2000;15:201–220.
6. Hau T, Ahrenholz DH, Simmons RL. Secondary bacterial peritonitis: the biologic basis of treatment. In: Ravitch MM, Steinchen FM, eds. *Current problems in surgery*. Chicago: Year Book Medical Publishers, 1979.
7. Moore WEC, Holdeman LV. Human fecal flora: the normal fecal flora of 20 Japanese-Hawaiians. *Appl Microbiol* 1974;27:961.
8. Baue AE. Multiple, progressive, or sequential systems failure: a syndrome of the 1970's. *Arch Surg* 1975;110:779.
9. Fry DE, Pearlstein L, Fulton RL, et al. Multiple system organ failure: the role of uncontrolled infection. *Arch Surg* 1981;115:136.
10. Stahl TJ, Cerra FB. Hemodynamic and metabolic response to infection. In: Simmons RL, Howard RJ, eds. *Surgical infectious disease*. Norwalk, CT: Appleton & Lange, 1988:209–232.
11. Goris RJA. Pathophysiology of multiple organ failure with "sepsis." *Med Link* 1987;82:546.
12. Tighe D, Moss R, Boghossian S, et al. Multi-organ damage resulting from experimental faecal peritonitis. *Clin Sci* 1989;76:269.
13. Wittmann DH, Schein M, Condon RE. Management of secondary peritonitis. *Ann Surg* 1996;224:10–18.
14. Drasar BS, Hill MJ. *Human intestinal flora*. London: Academic Press, 1974.
15. Finegold SM. Microflora of the gastrointestinal tract. In: Wilson SE, Finegold SM, Williams RA, eds. *Intra-abdominal infection*. New York: McGraw-Hill, 1982:1–22.
16. Bentley DW, Nichols RL, Condon RE, et al. The microflora of the human ileum and intra-abdominal colon: Results of direct needle aspiration at surgery and evaluation of technique. *J Lab Clin Med* 1972;79:421.
17. Clark JS, Bartlett JG, Finegold SM. Bacteriology of the gut and its clinical implications. *West J Med* 1976;121:359.
18. Greenlee HB, Gelbart SM, DeOrio AJ. The influence of gastric surgery on intestinal flora. *Am J Clin Nutr* 1977;30:1826.
19. Collee JG. Factors contributing to loss of anaerobic bacteria in transit from the patient to laboratory. *Infection* 1980;8:145.
20. Meleney FL, Ollp J, Harvey HD, et al. Peritonitis. II. Synergism of bacteria commonly found in peritoneal exudates. *Arch Surg* 1932;25:709.
21. Bartlett JG, Onderdonk AB, Louie TJ, et al. A review: lesson from an animal model of intra-abdominal sepsis. *Arch Surg* 1978;113:853.
22. Onderdonk AB, Weinstein W, Sullivan NM, et al. Experimental intraabdominal abscesses in rats: quantitative bacteriology of infected animals. *Infect Immun* 1974;10:1256.
23. Hagen CJ, Wood WS, Hashimoto T. In vitro stimulation of *Bacteroides fragilis* growth by *Escherichia coli*. *Eur J Clin Microbiol* 1982;1:338.
24. Parrillo JE: Pathogenic mechanisms of septic shock. *N Engl J Med* 1993;328:1471.
25. Wittmann DH, Syrrakos B, Wittmann MM. Advances in the diagnosis and treatment of intra-abdominal infection. In: Nyhus L, Nichols RL, eds. *Problems*

in general surgery: surgical sepsis, 1992 and beyond. Philadelphia: JB Lippincott, 1993:604–627.

26. Wittmann, DH, Schein, M. Let us shorten antibiotic prophylaxis and therapy in surgery. *Am J Surg* 1996;172(6A):26S–32S.

27. Wittmann DH. *Treatment of peritonitis: antibiotic concentration dynamics at the site of infection as criterion of antimicrobial chemotherapy.* Habilitation. Hamburg: Medizinische Fakultät der Universität, 1984.

28. Prins JM, van Deventer SJH, Kuijper EJ, et al. Clinical relevance of antibiotic-induced endotoxin release. *Antimicrob Agents Chemother* 1995;38:121.

29. Kirschner M. Die Behandlung der akuten eitrigen freien Bauchfellentzündung. *Langenbecks Arch Chir* 1926;142:53.

30. Wittmann DH, Bansal N, Bergstein JM, et al. Staged abdominal repair compares favorably when adjusting for prognostic factors with a logistic model. *Theor Surg* 1994;9:201.

31. Aprahamian C, Wittmann DH. Operative management of intraabdominal infection. *Infection* 1991;19:453.

32. Schein M, Hirshberg A, Hashmonai M. The surgical management of severe intra-abdominal infection. *Surgery* 1992;112:489.

33. Ohmann C, Wittmann DH, Wacha H. Prospective evaluation of prognostic scoring systems in peritonitis. *Eur J Surg* 1994;159:167.

34. Wittmann DH, Bergstein JM, Frantzides CT. Calculated empiric antimicrobial therapy for mixed surgical infections. *Infection* 1991;19(Suppl 6): 345.

35. Wittmann DH. Staged abdominal repair: development and current practice of an advanced operative technique for diffuse suppurative peritonitis. *Eur Surg* 2000;32:171–178.

36. Hurley JC. Antibiotic-induced release of endotoxin: a reappraisal. *Clin Infect Dis* 1992;15:840.

37. Shenep JL. Antibiotic-induced bacterial cell lysis: a therapeutic dilemma. *Eur J Clin Microbiol* 1986;5:11.

38. Bradley EL. The necessity for a clinical classification of acute pancreatitis. The Atlanta System. In: Bradley EL, ed. *Acute pancreatitis, diagnosis and therapy.* New York: Raven Press, 1994:27–35.

39. Solomkin JS, Meakins JL Jr, Allo MD, et al. Antibiotic trials in intra-abdominal infections: a critical evaluation of study design and outcome reporting. *Ann Surg* 1984;200:29.

40. Wittmann DH. Standard cephalosporin for surgical infections. *Diagn Microbiol Infect Dis* 1995;22:173.

41. Stone HH, Strom PR, Mullins RJ. Pancreatic abscess management by subtotal resection and packing. *World J Surg* 1984;8:340.

42. Bohnen JMA, Solomkin JS, Dellinger EP, et al. Guidelines for clinical care: anti-infective agents for intra-abdominal infection. A Surgical Infection Society policy statement. *Arch Surg* 1992;127:83.

43. Rotstein OD, Meakins JL. Diagnostic and therapeutic challenges of intra-abdominal infections. *World J Surg* 1990;14:159.

CHAPTER 81
Peritonitis

Ronald Lee Nichols

Although many types of intraabdominal infections are reported in the surgical literature, peritonitis, which follows the interruption of the continuity of the gastrointestinal tract by trauma, intrinsic disease, or surgery, is most common. The degree of dissemination of the infection within the peritoneal cavity depends primarily on five factors: (a) the location and size of the primary leak, (b) the nature of the underlying injury or disease, (c) the presence of peritoneal adhesions from previous disease states or operations, (d) the duration of the present illness, and (e) the efficiency of the local and systemic host defense mechanisms.

THE PERITONEAL MEMBRANE

The adult peritoneal membrane, made up of a single layer of mesothelial cells, measures about 1.7 m^2, which closely approximates the total cutaneous surface area. This membrane lines the peritoneal cavity and viscera within this space, forming the largest preformed extravascular space in the body. The space is normally lubricated with about 20 to 50 mL of clear yellow fluid transudate, which has been reported to possess some intrinsic an-

tibacterial activity (1,2). This peritoneal fluid normally contains less than 300 cells per mm^3, mostly macrophages and lymphocytes; however, when inflammation or infection is present, rapid increases of the total fluid volume and cell counts occur, with a shift in cell type to neutrophils predominantly.

The ability of the peritoneal membrane to participate in fluid exchange and absorption is well documented. The hyperosmolar nature of the peritoneal fluid in bacterial peritonitis can result in a rapid inflow of 300 to 500 mL of fluid per hour into the peritoneal space, which can lead to a hypovolemic condition unless therapy is initiated promptly. Some have likened the hemodynamic effect of acute generalized peritonitis to that of burns covering 50% or more of the body surface (1).

Although the entire peritoneal membrane participates in fluid and solute exchange, the diaphragmatic lymphatics specifically absorb particulate matter (3). It is only in this region that lymphatic collecting vessels (lacunae) form small pores (stomata) that penetrate the mesothelial basement membrane and open directly into the peritoneal cavity. Peritoneal fluid flows through the stomata into the lacunae during relaxation of the diaphragm while contraction empties the lymphatics into efferent ducts. Flow is aided by one-way valves in the thoracic lymphatics that prevent reversal of these dynamics. Because each stoma ranges from 8 to 12 μm in size and most bacteria are 0.5 to 2 μm in diameter, the bacteria are cleared rapidly from the peritoneal cavity by this mechanism. This clearance is delayed when the patient is in the upright position and increased by the bent-down position. During peritonitis, it has been observed that intraabdominal fibrin formation is enhanced, whereas fibrinolytic activity is reduced. The fibrin clots within the peritoneum can trap bacteria and reduce clearance, increase abscess formation, and protect bacteria caught in the fibrin from antimicrobial agents and immunologic defense mechanisms. Fibrin alone is readily lysed by the fibrinolytic enzymes present in the healthy peritoneal cavity (4). The use of heparin has been shown to be of benefit in experimental peritonitis by preventing the additional apposition of fibrin and therefore improving the clearing mechanisms (5).

The effect of recombinant tissue plasminogen activator was studied in a rat model of generalized *Escherichia coli* and *Bacteroides fragilis* peritonitis by van Goor and co-workers (6). The tissue plasminogen activator was shown to reduce abscess formation but also resulted in early bacteremia and increased mortality. Abscesses that formed consisted of *E. coli* and other species of intestinal origination, thus showing bacterial translocation. It is apparent that further studies should be performed to ascertain whether this treatment modality would be of clinical benefit.

Experimental investigations have shown that the peritoneal mesothelium sloughs readily even after only brief exposure to air or saline solution; rapid regeneration begins within hours of these exposures and is completed within a week of the injury (7). Whether this healing occurs from differentiation of local macrophages into mesothelium or from the mesothelial cells from the opposing peritoneal surfaces is unclear.

EXPERIMENTAL INTRAPERITONEAL INFECTIONS

Experimental studies of intraperitoneal sepsis have contributed much to our understanding of the pathophysiologic and microbiologic events as well as the therapeutic considerations significant in clinical infection. Weinstein and co-workers (8) studied antimicrobial agents in the treatment of experimentally induced intraperitoneal sepsis in rats. In their experimental model, pooled colonic contents from the rats were placed into gelatin capsules and then surgically positioned within the peritoneal cavity (9). They used a constant inoculum and observed that a two-stage disease developed in untreated rats. Initially, death caused by acute peritonitis was observed in 37% of the rats, whereas all of the survivors developed late intraabdominal abscesses. In the antibiotic-treated rats, gentamicin alone (aerobic coverage) reduced the acute mortality rate to 4%, but 98% of the survivors later developed abscesses. Clindamycin therapy alone (anaerobic coverage) was associated with an acute mortality rate of 35%, but the frequency of late intraabdominal abscesses in survivors was only 5%. A combination of gentamicin and clindamycin produced the salutary effects of each agent—an acute mortality rate of 7% and a frequency of late abscess formation of 6% in the survivors. These studies, which were done with appropriate microbiologic manipulations, suggested that coliform organisms caused the early deaths due to peritonitis and that anaerobes were principally responsible for the late complications of intraabdominal abscess formation.

Subsequent experimental studies by Onderdonk and colleagues (10) stressed the importance of *E. coli* in acute mortality in experimental peritonitis. Their results also suggested that intraabdominal abscesses are formed by a synergistic relationship between anaerobic and facultative bacteria. They were unable to cause early septicemic death or late abscess formation when only *B. fragilis* was used as the inoculum. They also found that implanting 5×10^7 enterococci alone in the capsule placed in the peritoneal cavity caused neither early septicemic mortality nor late abscess formation, whereas the placement of a mixed inoculum of *E. coli plus* enterococci failed to result in abscess formation. However, when combinations of *B. fragilis* or *Fusobacterium* organisms with enterococci were used, a high rate of intraperitoneal abscess was observed. These investigators thought that the pathogenicity of the enterococcus rested in its ability to act synergistically with the anaerobes in the formation of abscesses.

Further experimental studies (11,12), however, identified a polysaccharide capsule external to the outer membrane in some strains of the *B. fragilis* group. On the basis of slight differences in biochemical reactions, it has been determined that of the many different subspecies of *B. fragilis*, only *B. fragilis* subspecies *fragilis* has this capsule. This subspecies is more frequently isolated from clinical infections, despite its relatively low numbers in human stool, than are the other subspecies (13).

Our laboratory (14,15) modified these techniques and thereby widened the spectrum of experimental intraabdominal sepsis so that a disease more similar to that observed in humans could be induced. We found that in the rats studied, the mortality rate due to acute peritonitis increased with increasing doses of human stool inoculum (14). The results of this study revealed that only the broad-spectrum antibiotic agents with aerobic and anaerobic coverage significantly decreased the early mortality rate due to peritonitis in the large-inoculum group compared with the control group, whereas all the tested agents singly or in combination significantly decreased the mortality rate in the middle-inoculum group compared with the control group.

Other experimental studies have disclosed the adjuvant action that hemoglobin plays in peritonitis (16). Although the exact mechanism of this action is unproved, most authors agree that it is based on the ability of hemoglobin to delay the clearance of the bacteria from the peritoneal cavity (17). Hall and associates (18) have presented evidence that this mechanism may rest on the ability of hemoglobin to inhibit the chemotactic response of the polymorphonuclear neutrophils by interfering with the effective interaction of the cytotoxin to the receptor on the cell wall.

The value of intraperitoneal irrigation with both antibiotic solutions and povidone-iodine has also been studied in experimental fecal peritonitis (19). In this study, lethal fecal peritonitis was prevented in 5 of 17 (29%) animals after 0.1% kanamycin peritoneal irrigation; all other groups treated by irrigation with saline solution or varying concentrations of povidone-iodine (and no parenteral antibiotics) had no survivors. When appropriate systemic antibiotics were administered before peritoneal irrigation to animals with fecal peritonitis, the results indicated no better survival or less abscess formation after lavage with aminoglycoside than with saline alone (20). Intraperitoneal lavage with a dilute solution of hydrogen peroxide appeared to have a significantly greater toxic effect than benefit compared with a control group treated with saline solution (21).

Despite aggressive surgical intervention and antibiotic therapy, morbidity and mortality can remain high in patients with diffuse peritonitis. A possible explanation is that the immune system is adversely affected by the infectious process causing an immunosuppression. This suppression may be mediated by the increased release of cytokines such as interleukin-1 or tumor necrosis factor (TNF) or by a decreased ability of immune system cells to identify and destroy infecting bacteria (22,23).

Brown and co-investigators (24) have shown an improved survival rate when the immunomodulator muramyl dipeptide is given 24 hours before the onset of experimental peritonitis, whereas no protection has been observed when this or another immunostimulant is given at the time of bacteria inoculation (25,26). Dunn and co-workers (26) showed a clearly defined additive effect of muramyl dipeptide pretreatment given with a prophylactic dose of cefoxitin in a human fecal peritonitis rat model.

Sawyer and associates (27) studied the effects of pretreatment with cefoxitin and anti-TNF antibody on mortality and serum TNF levels in a murine model of mixed *E. coli* and *B. fragilis* peritonitis. At low- and intermediate-inoculum levels, only the cefoxitin prevented death, and all groups demonstrated low serum TNF levels. At the high-inoculum level, mortality was uniform in all groups except the cefoxitin and anti-TNF antibody group. This group and the anti-TNF antibody group both showed significantly reduced levels of serum TNF at 6 hours. The authors concluded that the cytokine response was dependent on both the nature of the insult (inoculum level) and the therapeutic intervention.

McMasters and Cheadle (28) pretreated experimental peritonitis in mice with the immunomodulator compounds muramyl dipeptide or monophosphoryl lipid A. Neither agent altered the expression of TNF-α during peritonitis. They concluded that peritonitis is associated with an early increase in peritoneal macrophage TNF-α. Tissues remote from the infection demonstrated less marked changes, indicating that the immunosuppression is related to the proximity to the infectious process.

SECONDARY BACTERIAL PERITONITIS

Secondary bacterial peritonitis is a frequently encountered clinical condition that usually arises after gastrointestinal tract leakage within the peritoneal cavity. This leakage may follow perforation of diseased viscera or blunt or penetrating trauma to the abdomen.

Characteristics of the Pathogen

Altemeier (29), in 1938, was the first to stress the polymicrobial aerobic and anaerobic nature of the bacterial flora of peritonitis resulting from acute appendiceal perforation. In 1942, he reported on the pathogenicity of the aerobic and anaerobic bacteria isolated from the peritoneal exudate of these 100 cases of acute perforated appendicitis in experimental animals (30). The primary conclusions of this study were as follows: (a) the great majority of the bacteria did not produce fatal peritonitis when injected in pure culture; (b) many avirulent strains of bacteria, particularly *E. coli*, became highly virulent in the presence of dead sterile tissue within the peritoneal cavity; (c) in mixed culture, these bacteria show a synergistic action producing a high degree of pathogenicity; and (d) acute perforated appendicitis peritonitis appears to be an infection resulting from the synergistic activities of the various bacterial symbionts present in a given case. These important studies were not elaborated on for nearly three decades, until modern techniques for the isolation and growth of anaerobic bacteria allowed better classification in both normal flora and postoperative infection studies (31–33).

INTESTINAL MICROFLORA

The numbers and types of microorganisms increase progressively down the gastrointestinal tract. In normal humans, the stomach and proximal small intestine support a sparse bacterial flora of both aerobes and anaerobes [less than 10^4 colony-forming units (CFU)/mL] (34). Acidity and motility appear to be the major factors that inhibit the growth of bacteria in the stomach. Diseases of the stomach and duodenum may compromise these factors. Thus, in cases of bleeding or obstructing duodenal ulcer, gastric ulcer, or carcinoma, the microflora of the stomach usually increases, being composed principally of anaerobes from the oral cavity and aerobic coliforms.

The microflora of the distal small bowel represents a transitional zone between the microfloras of the upper and lower gastrointestinal tract; modest numbers of aerobic and anaerobic microorganisms (up to 10^8 CFU/mL) are usually present (35,36). The largest concentrations of anaerobes are in the colon, where up to 10^{11} CFU per gram of stool or milliliter of intestinal aspirate can be identified (37). Coliforms are also present in the colon in concentrations of 10^8 CFU/g.

This anatomic location of microorganisms within the gastrointestinal tract in part accounts for the differences in septic complications associated with injuries to the upper and lower tract. Sepsis that occurs after upper intestinal leaks is generally less severe and associated with less morbidity and mortality than is sepsis due to leaks that follow colon injuries.

Microbiology of Intraperitoneal Infection

The numbers of aerobic and anaerobic bacteria isolated from sites of intraabdominal sepsis depend on the nature of the microflora of the diseased or traumatized organ. A complex polymicrobial flora results from contamination from the gastrointestinal tract. The polymicrobial nature of the pathogens in patients with intraabdominal infection is evident from several reports (38–41), which, when combined, showed that the average number of strains of bacteria isolated from the infected sites ranged from 2.5 to 5.0. These figures included an average of 1.4 to 2.0 aerobes and 2.4 to 3.0 anaerobes per infection. One or more anaerobic species were isolated from 65% to 94% of the patients (Table 81.1).

The commonly isolated aerobes in all of the studies included *E. coli* and *Klebsiella, Streptococcus, Proteus,* and *Enter-*

obacter species; the anaerobes isolated most frequently were *Bacteroides, Peptostreptococcus,* and *Clostridium* species. *B. fragilis* was the anaerobe most often isolated. Along with other species of *Bacteroides, B. fragilis* accounted for 30% to 60% of all the anaerobic isolates in these studies. Purely anaerobic intraabdominal sepsis was usually reported in less than 15% of the cases, whereas purely aerobic infections were noted in about 10%. Both aerobes and anaerobes were involved in more than 75% of the cases of intraabdominal infections.

In addition, highly antibiotic-resistant strains, such as *Pseudomonas aeruginosa, Serratia marcescens,* and *Acinetobacter* and *Providencia* species, are frequently isolated from patients who have an intraabdominal septic event within the hospital setting (42). The microbiology of persistent peritonitis in patients with long hospitalizations, repeated courses of antibiotics, multiple operations, or admissions to the intensive care unit favors the growth of breakthrough microorganisms such as *Staphylococcus epidermidis* or *Enterococcus* and *Candida* species (43,44). Other more rare organisms have infrequently been recovered from patients with peritonitis, especially after continuous ambulatory peritoneal dialysis (CAPD). These include *Nocardia, Lactobacillus, Listeria, Aeromonas, Campylobacter, Mycobacterium,* and *Brevibacterium* species and *Streptococcus pneumoniae* (45–52). The origin of these organisms has been shown to include both internal and external sources.

Clinical Features

Secondary bacterial peritonitis occurs after the leakage of endogenous microorganisms from a diseased or traumatized intraperitoneal hollow viscus. The extent of dissemination of the infections within the peritoneal cavity depends primarily on many local factors, including the presence of adhesions from previous operations, the presence of a well-functioning omentum, and the size and location of the primary site of leakage. Localization of the spread usually results in the formation of intraperitoneal, retroperitoneal, or visceral abscesses, whereas generalized peritonitis is most commonly seen after penetrating or blunt abdominal trauma and rarely after organ perforation when the spread of infection is not localized.

Abdominal pain is present in all cases of peritonitis; when it is localized to one region of the abdomen, it is associated with rebound tenderness and muscle guarding in the area of organ perforation. In generalized peritonitis, the pain and tenderness are found over the entire abdomen and are aggravated by any movement, including coughing or jarring the hospital bed. Associated muscle rigidity is present, which in extreme cases may result in the so-called boardlike abdomen. Patients with peritonitis also have fever and a progressive tachycardia that occurs secondary to the third-space loss within the peritoneal cavity. If treatment is delayed, hypovolemia develops rapidly, and shock follows. Early shock is usually due to hypovolemia alone, whereas later it is due to both hypovolemia and sepsis. Abdominal distention is due to the accumulation of fluid and debris

| | | | Average number | Average number | Average number | Number of cases with |
Reference	Number of cases studied	Average number of microorganisms per infection	of aerobes per infection	of anaerobes per infection	anaerobes/number studied (%)
Altemeier et al. (1973)[38]	501	2.5	Not available	Not available	Not available (65)
Gorbach et al. (1974)[40]	46	5.0	2.0	3.0	40/60 (87)
Swenson et al. (1974)[39]	64	3.8	1.4	2.4	52/64 (81)
Gorbach et al. (1975)[41]	67	4.8	1.9	2.9	63/67 (94)

TABLE 81.1. Microorganisms Isolated from Patients with Intraabdominal Infections

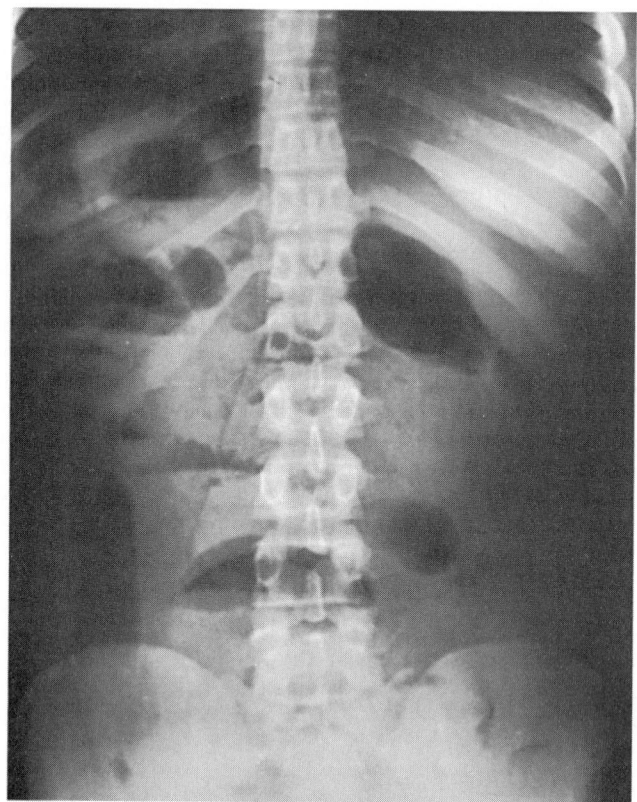

Figure 81.1. Upright radiograph of the abdomen demonstrates the presence of small intestinal air-fluid levels in addition to the free peritoneal fluid.

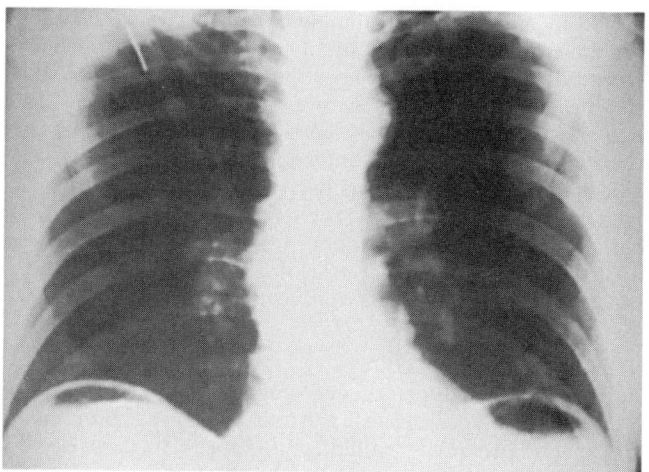

Figure 81.2. Preoperative chest radiograph demonstrates the presence of free air, obvious under both hemidiaphragms.

in the peritoneal cavity as well as to increases in the intraluminal bowel gas and liquid due to the associated paralytic ileus (Fig. 81.1). Bowel sounds are usually diminished early in the course of disease and become absent as time passes.

Diagnosis

The diagnosis of diffuse peritonitis is usually based on the clinical history and typical physical findings. Associated increases of the peripheral leukocyte counts are frequently observed, most often exceeding 15,000/mm^3 with a shift to the left. Basic radiographic examination may be helpful in showing evidence of free air below the diaphragm on chest films (Fig. 81.2) or the finding of mild distention of the small and large intestine associated with an intraperitoneal fluid collection between the bowel loops. Specialized radiographic procedures are most helpful in searching for localized intraabdominal collections and are rarely necessary to make the diagnosis. Paracentesis may be required to confirm the diagnosis. If gross pus, intestinal contents, or feces is aspirated, the diagnosis is confirmed. A Gram stain of the aspirated fluid offers immediate insights concerning the cause of the peritonitis. Aerobic and anaerobic bacterial cultures should always be performed so that further therapy can be based on knowledge of the pathogens and their antibiotic susceptibility patterns.

Attempts have been made to evaluate the severity of peritonitis by use of a variety of scoring systems. These include the acute physiologic assessment and chronic health evaluation (APACHE) II scores, the Mannheim Peritonitis Index, and the Peritonitis Index Altona II. Although they have limited value in clinical trials to define risk, compare treatments, and define inclusion criteria, they have not been shown to be of diagnostic value in individual patients to predict outcomes (53).

Treatment

The most critical aspect of the treatment of secondary bacterial peritonitis is early diagnosis and prompt surgical intervention. Preoperative care requires rapid monitoring of arterial and venous pressures as well as of urinary output. Frequent monitoring allows better fluid resuscitation during the perioperative course. Optimal preoperative care includes oxygenation of the tissues aided by the use of nasal cannula, administration of blood products in anemic patients, and use of vasoactive or inotropic agents as indicated. Intubation and respiratory assistance initiated at the time of operation are continued for varying periods during the postoperative period to prevent hypoxia. Preoperative placement of a nasogastric tube helps to decompress the accumulated gastrointestinal gas and fluid contents, which reduces pressure on the diaphragm and improves pulmonary ventilation. It appears that early bowel decompression also facilitates early return of intestinal motility during the postoperative course. The use of sedatives, analgesics, and antibiotics should be initiated only after the diagnosis of peritonitis has been made and the surgical procedure planned.

The nutritional requirements of these septic patients can be enormous, depending on the severity of the infection and the patient's prior health. Parenteral alimentation or enteral feedings delivered by a jejunostomy tube placed at the time of surgery are routinely recommended in severely septic patients and those with preoperative malnutrition.

Despite advances in the understanding of the pathophysiologic events that occur in patients with intraabdominal infection, the mortality and morbidity remain significant. Some investigators believe that improvement in these rates may be possible if study design and outcome reporting become standardized. This will allow better comparison of different treatment regimens in equivalent populations of patients, steps that may help to detect small differences (54,55). In addition to the general aspects of perioperative care just addressed, the true mainstays of treatment for peritonitis remain antibiotic selection and operative therapy.

ANTIBIOTIC SELECTION

Unlike superficial wound abscesses, for which surgical drainage alone usually suffices, intraabdominal sepsis is best managed by a combination of surgical repair, diversion, or drainage plus appropriate parenterally administered antibiotic agents. The antibiotic therapy should be initiated a soon as the diagnosis is made during the preoperative course and continued during the operative procedure and into the postoperative period. The choice of the ideal agent or agents and the necessary length of the therapeutic course remain controversial and unproven; however, the spectrum of activity of the chosen antibiotics based on early experimental (8,15) and clinical (43,56) studies must have activity against both the colonic aerobes and anaerobes including *B. fragilis*.

Instead of a list of the countless antibiotic studies that report equal efficacy in intraabdominal sepsis, a list of agents commonly used singly or in combination is offered (Table 81.2).

The importance of using antibiotic agents that are effective against both aerobic and anaerobic gastrointestinal bacteria was demonstrated in a prospective study of 100 abdominal trauma patients reported in 1973 (56). This study revealed a significantly increased rate of anaerobic septicemia and intraabdominal infections in the group of patients treated with cephalothin-kanamycin (aerobic coverage) compared with those treated with clindamycin-kanamycin (aerobic and anaerobic coverage). The authors appropriately stated on the basis of these results that anaerobic bacteria appear to be a significant cause of infection in abdominal trauma.

Hofstetter and co-investigators (57) in 1984 reported on their prospective study of 119 abdominal trauma patients. Results of this heterogeneous group appeared to indicate that a short-term course with a single drug, cefoxitin, was as safe and effective as the use of a triple-drug regimen of aminoglycoside, ampicillin, and clindamycin. The authors also suggested that it might be prudent to consider leaving the skin and subcutaneous tissues open in patients who had hollow viscus injury because of the high rate of localized wound infection in this clinical setting. Prospective randomized studies of purely penetrating abdominal trauma carried out during the same period reached similar conclusions in regard to the efficacy of antibiotic therapy (58–60). Results of cefoxitin alone were found to be equal to those of combination therapy (58–60). The antibiotic agents used

in these studies generally lacked efficacy against the enterococci, which were frequently isolated from infected sites in mixed culture. Despite their isolation, rarely was it necessary to alter the original antibiotic therapy to have a successful outcome; however, a similar study has stressed the ability of certain broad-spectrum cephalosporins to result in enterococcal overgrowth in this clinical setting (61).

A trend has developed during the past decade to reduce the duration of antibiotic therapy to less than 48 hours in patients with penetrating abdominal trauma with gastrointestinal contamination (62–64). A study by Nichols and colleagues (65) allocated patients who had sustained penetrating abdominal trauma to either 2 or 5 days of antibiotics on the basis of the severity of their injuries and predicted infection risk. The patients predicted to have a low probability of infection who received 2 days of treatment showed the same rates of infection (10% major, 12% minor) as historical control patients who had received 5 days of treatment (9% major, 14% minor). Results of this study indicate that risk factors can be used to identify low-risk patients who require only short-term antibiotic therapy. Other patients are at greater risk for infection despite prolonged antibiotics and delayed wound closure. The use of the initial peritoneal culture in penetrating abdominal trauma and in other clinical settings in which there is no established intraabdominal infection has been reported to have no predictive value for the development of postoperative infection or for the pathogen identified from such infections when they occurred (59,66).

The Surgical Infection Society in 1992 issued guidelines for the use of antiinfective agents in intraabdominal infections (67). The guidelines were restricted to infections derived from the gastrointestinal tract and took into account various factors, including results from experimental and clinical studies and the pharmacokinetics, mechanisms of action, resistance, and safety of antibiotics. They stressed that antimicrobial coverage must provide a sufficient spectrum of activity against both facultative (aerobic) gram-negative bacilli and obligate anaerobic gram-negative bacilli. Regimens with little or no activity against these organisms are not acceptable. Their recommendations include the following: single-agent therapy with cefoxitin, cefotetan, cefmetazole, or ticarcillin-clavulanate for community-acquired infections of mild to moderate severity; single-agent therapy with imipenem-cilastatin or combination therapy with either a third-generation cephalosporin, aztreonam, or an aminoglycoside plus clindamycin or metronidazole for more severe infections.

Finally, the choice of individual antibiotic agents or combinations must be influenced by many factors, including efficacy, toxicity, local hospital microbial sensitivity patterns, and price.

SURGICAL TECHNIQUES

The type of surgical procedure to be performed depends on what intraperitoneal disease is identified. The goals of the procedure should be to arrest peritoneal contamination and to débride necrotic tissue, remove debris and foreign bodies, and drain all localized purulent collections. Many mechanical techniques designed to reduce the bacterial burden within the peritoneal cavity have been advocated in addition to the primary surgical procedure (Table 81.3) (68).

The first of these techniques, intraoperative peritoneal irrigation, is used almost universally to treat secondary bacterial peritonitis. The irrigation is carried out at the end of the operative procedure either with a pour-in technique or with a jet lavage device using 2 or 3 L of irrigant. The evidence indicates that this technique does reduce the number of bacteria present, especially when it is done before fibrin has been deposited within the peritoneal cavity (69).

TABLE 81.2. Parenteral Antibiotic Agents Used for Coverage of Aerobic and Anaerobic Components of the Human Colonic Microflora

Combination Therapy
Aerobic coverage—to be combined with a drug having anaerobic activity
  Amikacin
  Aztreonam
  Ceftriaxone
  Ciprofloxacin
  Gentamicin
  Levofloxacin
  Tobramycin
Anaerobic coverage—to be combined with a drug having aerobic activity
  Clindamycin
  Metronidazole
Single-drug therapy
Aerobic-anaerobic coverage—single agent
  Ertapenem
  Cefoxitin
  Imipenem-cilastatin[a]
  Meropenem[a]
  Piperacillin-tazobactam
  Ticarcillin-clavulanate

[a]If selected, should be used for the treatment of hospital-acquired infection.

TABLE 81.3.   Intraoperative Mechanical Techniques Used in Intraabdominal Sepsis

Irrigation of the peritoneal cavity (pour-in or jet lavage)
   Saline solution
   Antibiotic solutions
   Povidone-iodine
Closed peritoneal catheter lavage
Radical surgical débridement
Leaving the peritoneal cavity open
Reoperation
   Use of surgical zipper or other temporary closure techniques
   Classic techniques

The use of antibiotic irrigation of the peritoneal cavity in the face of peritonitis became popular in the mid-1960s (70,71). A review of 29 investigators' descriptions of the use of various antibiotic solutions in intraperitoneal irrigations for peritonitis has failed to prove the efficacy of the technique (72). Until definite evidence of clinical efficacy is available, physicians must exercise caution before routinely using this technique, which may result in significant toxic effects because of peritoneal absorption (73), increased expense, and increased deposition of peritoneal adhesions (74). The use of varying concentrations of povidone-iodine irrigations in the bacterially contaminated abdomen was first recommended by Sindelar and Mason (75) in 1979. In their study, which did not completely standardize the use of systemic antimicrobial administration, they reported the frequency of postoperative intraabdominal abscesses was reduced from 9 of 88 patients (10.2%) with saline irrigation alone to 1 of 80 patients (1.3%) by irrigation with 0.1% iodine. Despite initial clinical enthusiasm, experimental studies of peritonitis have demonstrated that this technique can actually increase the mortality rate in peritonitis, presumably by damaging host defense mechanisms (19,76). In contrast, wound irrigation alone with local antibiotics or antiseptics continues to be a safe, commonly used technique, especially when primary wound closure is done.

In 1987, Leiboff and Soroff (77) published their critical review of 39 studies concerning the use of closed postoperative catheter peritoneal lavage in generalized peritonitis. Three of four prospective randomized studies showed unfavorable results with this technique, whereas 25 of 27 noncomparative studies showed favorable results. The authors concluded that the therapeutic value of this procedure remains unknown and that there remains a need for a large-scale, prospective, randomized study to evaluate the efficacy of closed postoperative catheter peritoneal lavage in the treatment of generalized peritonitis. As yet, this has not been done.

Radical surgical débridement was advocated by Hudspeth (78) in 1975. To date, no clinical study has confirmed the remarkable results of this study, and one prospective randomized study has shown no advantages of the radical over the conservative approach (79).

Reoperation for intraabdominal sepsis, based on clinical judgment, has been recommended on the basis of a retrospective study of 50 patients (80). The authors found that laboratory tests were not helpful in predicting the presence of infections on reexploration, but if reoperation was performed before the development of organ failure, the authors believed that the risk associated with a negative exploration is worth taking.

Teichmann and colleagues (81) were among the first to report a prospective study of a new concept of scheduled multiple laparotomies with abdominal lavage in 61 patients for the treatment of diffuse peritonitis. This process, which they named *Etappenlavage*, consists of scheduled reoperations of the abdominal cavity to ensure exclusion of the infected source, promote maximal elimination of necrotic material, and allow prompt recognition of complications to effect immediate repair. They modified the technique for the last 31 patients in that reoperation was facilitated by closing the abdomen with a zipper. This technique was revised and further studied by Wittmann and co-workers (82) in a series of 117 patients with severe advanced suppurative peritonitis. They compared the technique using retention sutures, simple zippers, slide fasteners, and a Velcro analog (artificial bur). The patients required an average of 6.1 reoperations and showed a reduction of 34% to 93% predicted mortality (APACHE II or Surgical Infection Society Modified APACHE II scoring) to 24%. More complications were seen with retention sutures, and decompression of the abdomen was not allowed by retention sutures or the simple zipper. The Velcro analog was seen to be the most practical method of temporary abdominal closure. An additional study by this group further showed the usefulness and safety of this artificial bur (83). There is some thought among surgeons that operations after multiple scheduled reoperations and lavage might prove difficult because of increased amounts of adhesions and a generally "hostile" abdomen. This, however, was not seen in a series of 12 patients requiring later operations to restore bowel continuity or for abdominal wall reconstruction (84).

I favor the technique of scheduled reoperations for high-risk patients with diffuse peritonitis and think that daily unzipping should be accomplished in the operating room until evidence of continued peritoneal sepsis is absent. Other investigators have recommended reoperation only when clinical findings or laboratory tests indicate continued intraabdominal infection (85,86).

In summary, the treatment of secondary bacterial peritonitis requires prompt initial diagnosis followed by adequate surgery and efficacious parenteral antibiotics. For high-risk patients, I recommend that the abdomen be closed with a surgical zipper to allow daily reoperation until the evidence of continued sepsis is absent.

PRIMARY PERITONITIS

Less than 1% of the cases of bacterial peritonitis occur spontaneously, without evidence of intraabdominal organ perforation, and are referred to as *primary peritonitis*. Presumably, in most cases, the bacterial offenders reach the peritoneal cavity by hematogenous spread. Although this syndrome is seen more frequently in infants and children, it appears to be decreasing. Primary peritonitis has been diagnosed most frequently in the following groups: normal infants and children, patients with cirrhosis, and children with nephrotic syndrome. Even more rarely, it has been diagnosed in patients with systemic lupus erythematosus or Fitz-Hugh-Curtis syndrome.

The occurrence of primary peritonitis in normal infants and children accounts for more than 10% of cases of diffuse peritonitis (87). In infants, the peak occurrence is before 2 months of age, predominantly in girls; in children, it usually occurs between 5 and 9 years of age with equal frequency in boys and girls. In children with the nephrotic syndrome, boys predominate, and the mean age of presentation of the primary peritonitis is about 4 years (88). In this group, the most important pathogens are streptococci, particularly pneumococci, followed by coliforms such as *E. coli*.

The first cases of this disease in patients with cirrhosis were observed about 40 years ago. The frequency of primary peritonitis in cirrhosis patients appears to be about 6% (89).

The causative bacterial flora in primary peritonitis associated with cirrhosis is a single microorganism in more than 90% of cases (89). Although pneumococci were the most frequently isolated pathogen earlier in this century, the rate has decreased in more recent times. Today, the coliforms, especially *E. coli*, are most commonly implicated, followed by streptococci. Anaerobic bacteria are rarely found in primary peritonitis and if isolated would suggest secondary bacterial peritonitis. With the perihepatitis of the Fitz-Hugh-Curtis syndrome, the organisms isolated would generally be a gonococcus or *Chlamydia* species (90).

The four most frequently implicated routes of bacterial contamination in primary peritonitis are hematogenous, direct from the female genital tract, contagious spread of infection from the retroperitoneal or supradiaphragmatic region, and migration of endogenous intestinal bacteria.

In a patient with cirrhosis or nephrosis, the presence of ascites is of great importance in the pathogenesis of primary peritonitis because it provides a nutritious and protective environment for the invading bacteria.

The symptoms and finding of primary peritonitis are generally less acute and develop slowly compared with those of secondary bacterial peritonitis. Nevertheless, they can mimic both early appendicitis and a catastrophic abdominal illness (91). Fever associated with abdominal pain and tenderness and muscle guarding or rigidity with rebound are common. Leukocytosis is characteristic, and abdominal radiographs rarely provide any clues to the presence of intraabdominal disease, including masses or free air.

If primary peritonitis is suspected, it can be diagnosed by paracentesis, with or without peritoneal lavage. Infected fluid contains at least 300 white cells per mm^3, and usually more than 500 (92). Gram stain of the peritoneal fluid usually provides insights to the offending microorganism, and culture provides definitive identification. The finding on Gram stain of mixed flora of gram-positive and gram-negative microorganisms is highly suggestive of secondary bacterial peritonitis.

The mortality rate associated with primary peritonitis in children early in this century approached 100%, with or without operation. Since the advent of effective antibiotics and vaccines, the rate has fallen below 10% for children and below 50% for neonates (87). The development of primary peritonitis in cirrhosis is associated with a high mortality rate, approaching 90% to 95%, owing principally to the complications of cirrhosis, including hepatic decompensation.

The treatment of primary peritonitis most frequently includes an exploratory laparotomy to rule out surgically correctable lesions that cause secondary bacterial peritonitis. In high-risk patients who have suggestive findings clinically and on peritoneal tap, appropriate empiric antibiotic therapy may be successful. This treatment regimen can be modified when culture and sensitivity results are available for organisms in the peritoneal fluid.

OTHER ATYPICAL FORMS OF INFECTIVE PERITONITIS

Barium Peritonitis

Perforation of the gastrointestinal tract during the course of a radiographic procedure that uses barium sulfate is a dreaded complication. Experimental models have indicated that the combination of barium and intestinal contents produces a more virulent peritonitis than either does alone (13,14). It is thought that the water-insoluble barium tenaciously binds to intestinal bacteria. This lethal mixture, which is difficult if not impossible to remove surgically, results in multiple foci of intraabdominal infection. The best chance for survival occurs when the disease is localized. The best treatment is prevention! Several recommendations have been offered to decrease the risk for this occurrence (93). Once the diagnosis is made, successful therapy depends largely on the general health of the patient before this event; on

appropriate choice of parenteral antibiotics aimed at the intestinal flora; and on multiple surgical procedures designed to divert, débride, and drain the affected areas.

Peritonitis Associated with Intraperitoneal Prosthesis

Peritonitis may occur in patients who have indwelling synthetic catheters for peritoneal dialysis or peritoneal venous or ventriculoperitoneal shunts. This complication is most common in CAPD patients owing to the relatively large numbers of these procedures; however, the frequency has decreased with general improvements in catheter design (94). The repeated connecting and disconnecting of the administration sets to the indwelling catheter and any breakdown of aseptic technique are the major causes of CAPD peritonitis. The average rate of peritonitis is reported to be 1.3 to 1.4 episodes per patient-year (95). The most frequently isolated organisms, usually originating from the skin flora, are coagulase-negative staphylococci (30% to 45%) (96,97). A lesser number of cases are due to *Staphylococcus aureus* (10% to 20%), streptococci (10% to 15%), and gram-negative organisms (20% to 35%). Peritonitis in CAPD patients may result from decreased host phagocytic efficiency with depressed phagocytosis and bactericidal capacity of peritoneal macrophages. Diagnosis is usually made when a cloudy effluent is seen, with or without clinical signs or symptoms such as abdominal pain or tenderness, fever, nausea, vomiting, chills, or increased dialysate white cell count. The intraperitoneal route for antibiotic administration allows most patients with uncomplicated peritonitis to be treated as outpatients. A large number of antibiotics, including cephalosporins, aminoglycosides, and penicillins, have been used to treat CAPD peritonitis (95). Vancomycin (intravenously or intraperitoneally) is the most commonly used antibiotic for gram-positive bacteria; aminoglycosides (intravenously or intraperitoneally) are commonly used for gram-negative infections. Although there have been several reports of successful therapy with oral quinolones such as ciprofloxacin and ofloxacin, their efficacy has not been proved conclusively (98,99).

Successful treatment mandates large doses of specific systemic antimicrobials, and frequently it is necessary to remove and subsequently replace the affected foreign body; however, peritoneal dialysis catheters rarely need to be removed unless

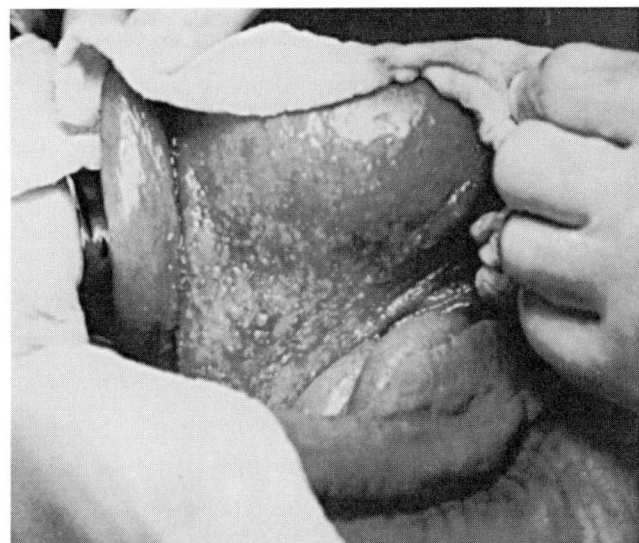

Figure 81.3. Operative picture of a patient with tuberculous peritonitis. The multiple tubercles can be seen on the intestinal serosa and on the root of the mesentery.

there is associated infection of the subcutaneous tunnel. In this setting, continuous dialysis is instituted to prevent fluid loculation and adhesion formation until the patient is asymptomatic.

Tuberculous Peritonitis

Tuberculous peritonitis is today a rare disease (100). In most cases, a primary pulmonary focus is present, which allows the spread of *Mycobacterium tuberculosis* hematogenously to the peritoneal cavity. Abdominal pain, progressively increasing abdominal girth, fever, weight loss, night sweats, and ascites are common. Paracentesis rarely is helpful, but laparoscopy or exploratory surgery discloses multiple tubercles scattered throughout the peritoneal cavity (Fig. 81.3). Treatment with triple antituberculosis drugs is most often successful.

REFERENCES

1. Ahrenholz DH, Simmons RL. Peritonitis and other intraabdominal infections. In: Howard RJ, Simmons RL, eds. *Surgical infectious diseases*, 2nd ed. Norwalk, CT: Appleton & Lange, 1988:605–646.
2. Bercovici B, Michel J, Miller J, et al. Antimicrobial activity of human peritoneal fluid. *Surg Gynecol Obstet* 1975;141:885.
3. Tsilibary EC, Wissig SL. Absorption from the peritoneal cavity: SEM study of the mesothelium covering the peritoneal surface of the muscular portion of the diaphragm. *Am J Anat* 1977;149:127.
4. Dunn DL, Rotstein OD, Simmons RL. Fibrin in peritonitis. *Arch Surg* 1984;119:139.
5. Hau T, Simmons RL. Heparin in the treatment of experimental peritonitis. *Ann Surg* 1978;187:294.
6. van Goor H, de Graaf JS, Kooi K, et al. Effect of recombinant tissue plasminogen activator on infra-abdominal abscess formation in rats with generalized peritonitis. *J Am Coll Surg* 1994;179:407.
7. Watters WB, Buck RC. Scanning election microscopy of mesothelial regeneration in the rat. *Lab Invest* 1972;26:604.
8. Weinstein WM, Onderdonk AB, Bartlett JG, et al. Antimicrobial therapy of experimental intraabdominal sepsis. *J Infect Dis* 1975;132:282.
9. Weinstein WM, Onderdonk AB, Bartlett JG, et al. Experimental intraabdominal abscesses in rats: development of an experimental model. *Infect Immun* 1974;10:1250.
10. Onderdonk AB, Bartlett JG, Louie T, et al. Microbial synergy in experimental intraabdominal abscess. *Infect Immun* 1976;13:22.
11. Kasper DL. The polysaccharide capsule of *Bacteroides fragilis* subspecies *fragilis*: immunochemical and morphologic definition. *J Infect Dis* 1976;133:79.
12. Onderdonk AB, Kasper DL, Cisneros RL, et al. The capsular polysaccharide of *Bacteroides fragilis* as a virulence factor; comparison of the pathogenic potential of encapsulated and unencapsulated strains. *J Infect Dis* 1977;136:82.
13. Bartlett JG, Onderdonk AB, Louie T, et al. A review: lessons from an animal model of intraabdominal sepsis. *Arch Surg* 1978;113:853.
14. Nichols RL, Smith JW Balthazar ER. Peritonitis and intraabdominal abscess: an experimental model for the evaluation of human disease. *J Surg Res* 1978;25:129.
15. Nichols RL, Smith JW, Fossedal EN, et al. Efficacy of parenteral antibiotics in the treatment of experimentally induced intraabdominal sepsis. *Rev Infect Dis* 1979;1:302.
16. Davis JH, Hull AB. A possible toxic factor in abdominal injury. *J Trauma* 1962;2:291.
17. Filler RM, Sleeman HK. Pathogenesis of peritonitis. I. The effect of *Escherichia coli* and hemoglobin on peritoneal absorption. *Surgery* 1967;61:385.
18. Hall T, Nelson RD, Fiegel VD, et al. Mechanisms of the adjuvant action of hemoglobin in experimental peritonitis.2. Influence of hemoglobin on human leukocyte chemotaxis in vitro. *J Surg Res* 1977;22:194.
19. Lally KP, Nichols RL. Various intraperitoneal irrigation solutions in treating experimental fecal peritonitis. *South Med J* 1981;74:789.
20. Lally KP, Shorr LD, Nichols RL. Adjunctive aminoglycoside lavage: lack of efficacy in experimental fecal peritonitis. *J Pediatr Surg* 1985;20:541.
21. Lawson KJ, Lavery I. Hydrogen peroxide vs normal saline lavage in experimental fecal peritonitis. *Cleve Clin J Med* 1987;54:279.
22. Brown JM, Grosso MA, Harken AH. Cytokines, sepsis and the surgeon. *Surg Gynecol Obstet* 1988;169:568.
23. Ertel W, Morrison MH, Wang P, et al. The complex pattern of cytokines in sepsis. *Ann Surg* 1991;214:141.
24. Brown GL, Foshee H, Pietsch J, et al. Muramyl dipeptide enhances survival from experimental peritonitis. *Arch Surg* 1986;121:47.
25. Browder W, Williams D, Sherwood E, et al. Synergistic effect of nonspecific immunostimulation and antibiotics in experimental peritonitis. *Surgery* 1987;102:206.
26. Dunn CW Horton JW, Walker PB. Additive effect of an immunomodulator and broad-spectrum antibiotic in fecal peritonitis. *Am J Surg* 1989;157:548.
27. Sawyer RG, Adams RB, May AK, et al. Anti-tumor necrosis factor antibody reduces mortality in the presence of antibiotic-induced tumor necrosis factor release. *Arch Surg* 1993;128:73.
28. McMasters KM, Cheadle WG. Regulation of macrophage TNFα, IL-1β, and Ia (I-Au) mRNA expression during peritonitis is site dependent. *J Surg Res* 1993;54:426.
29. Altemeier WA. The bacterial flora of acute perforated appendicitis with peritonitis: a bacteriologic study based upon one hundred cases. *Ann Surg* 1938;107:517.
30. Altemeier WA. The pathogenicity of the bacteria of appendicitis peritonitis: an experimental study. *Surgery* 1942;11:374.
31. Nichols RL, Smith JW. Modern approach to the diagnosis of anaerobic sepsis. *Surg Clin North Am* 1975;55:21.
32. Bentley DN, Nichols RL, Condon RE, et al. The microflora of the human ileum and intraabdominal colon: results of direct needle aspiration at surgery and evaluation of the techniques. *J Lab Clin Med* 1972;79:421.
33. Nichols RL. Intraabdominal sepsis: characterization and treatment. *J Infect Dis* 1977;135[Suppl]:S54.
34. Nichols RL, Smith JW. Intragastric microbial colonization in common disease states of the stomach and duodenum. *Ann Surg* 1975;182:557.
35. Gorbach SL, Bartlett JG. Anaerobic infections. *N Engl J Med* 1974;290:1177.
36. Nichols RL, Condon RE, Bentley DW, et al. Real microflora in surgical patients. *J Urol* 1971;105:351.
37. Nichols RL, Condon RE, Gorbach SL, et al. Efficacy of preoperative antimicrobial preparation of the bowel. *Ann Surg* 1972;176:227.
38. Altemeier WA, Culbertson WR, Fullen WD, et al. Intraabdominal abscesses. *Am J Surg* 1973;125:701.
39. Swenson RM, Lorber B, Michaelson TC, et al. The bacteriology of intraabdominal infections. *Arch Surg* 1974;109:398.
40. Gorbach SL, Thadepalli H, Norsen J. Anaerobic microorganisms in intraabdominal infections. In: Balows A, DeHaan RM, Dowell VR Jr, et al., eds. *Anaerobic bacteria: role in disease.* Springfield, IL: Charles C Thomas, 1974:399–407.
41. Gorbach SL. Anaerobic infections: treatment of intraabdominal sepsis. *Ann Intern Med* 1975;83:377.
42. Tally FP, McGowan K, Kellum JM, et al. A randomized comparison of cefoxitin with or without amikacin and clindamycin plus amikacin in surgical sepsis. *Ann Surg* 1981;193:318.
43. Rotstein DD, Pruett TL, Simmons RL. Microbiologic features and treatment of persistent peritonitis in patients in the intensive care unit. *Can J Surg* 1986;29:247.
44. Nichols RL, Musik AC. Enterococcal infections in surgery: the mystery continues! *Clin Infect Dis* 1992;15:72.
45. Lopes JO, Alves SH, Benevenga JP, et al. *Nocardia asteroides* peritonitis during continuous ambulatory peritoneal dialysis. *Rev Inst Med Trop Sao Paulo* 1993;35:377.
46. Sanyal D, Bhandari S. CAPD peritonitis caused by *Lactobacillus rhamnosus*. *J Hosp Infect* 1992;22:325.
47. Kent SJ, Van Scoy MS, Skerrett S. *Listeria monocytogenes* peritonitis with review of the literature. *Aust N Z J Med* 1994;24:405.
48. Schoenmakers EAJM, Brummer RM, van Tiel FH. Spontaneous bacterial peritonitis due to *Streptococcus pneumoniae* in a male who did not have another concurrent infection. *Clin Infect Dis* 1994;19:551.
49. Muñoz P, Femández-Baca V, Peláez T, et al. *Aeromonas* peritonitis. *Clin Infect Dis* 1994;18:32.
50. Perkins DJ, Newstead GL. *Campylobacter jejuni* enterocolitis causing peritonitis, ileitis and intestinal obstruction. *Aust N Z J Surg* 1994;64:55.
51. Gruner E, Pfyffer GE, von Graevenitz A. Characterization of *Brevibacterium* ssp. from clinical specimens. *J Clin Microbiol* 1993;31:1408.
52. Giladi M, Lee BE, Berlin OG, et al. Peritonitis caused by *Mycobacterium kansasii* in a patient undergoing continuous ambulatory peritoneal dialysis. *Am J Kidney Dis* 1992;19:597.
53. Ohmann C, Wittmann DH, Wacha H, and the Peritonitis Study Group. Prospective evaluation of prognostic scoring systems in peritonitis. *Eur J Surg* 1993;159:267.
54. Dellinger EP, Wertz MJ, Meakins JL, et al. Surgical infection stratification system for intraabdominal infection. *Arch Surg* 1985;120:21.
55. Solomkin JS, Meakins JL, Allo MD, et al. Antibiotic trials in intraabdominal infections: a critical evaluation of study design and outcome reporting. *Ann Surg* 1984;200:29.
56. Thadepalli H, Gorbach SL, Broido PW, et al. Abdominal trauma, anaerobes and antibiotics. *Surg Gynecol Obstet* 1973;173:270.
57. Hofstetter SR Pachter HL, Bailey AA, et al. A prospective comparison of two regimens of prophylactic antibiotics in abdominal trauma: cefoxitin versus triple drug. *J Trauma* 1984;24:307.
58. Gentry LO, Feliciano DV, Lea AS, et al. Perioperative antibiotic therapy for penetrating injuries of the abdomen. *Ann Surg* 1984;200:561.
59. Nichols RL, Smith JW, Klein DB, et al. Risk of infection after penetrating abdominal trauma. *N Engl J Med* 1984;311:1065.
60. Jones RC, Thal ER, Johnson NA, et al. Evaluation of antibiotic therapy following penetrating abdominal trauma. *Ann Surg* 1985;201:576.
61. Feliciano DV, Gentry LO, Bitondo CG, et al. Single agent cephalosporin prophylaxis for penetrating abdominal trauma: results and comment on the emergence of the enterococcus. *Am J Surg* 1986;152:674.

62. Dellinger EP, Wertz MJ, Lennard ES, et al. Efficacy of short-course antibiotic prophylaxis after penetrating abdominal injury: a prospective randomized trial. *Arch Surg* 1986;121:23.
63. Fabian TC, Croce MA, Payne LW, et al. Duration of antibiotic therapy for penetrating abdominal trauma: a prospective trial. *Surgery* 1992;112:788.
64. Bozorgzadeh A, Pizzi WF, Barie PS, et al. The duration of antibiotic administration in penetrating abdominal trauma. *Am J Surg* 1999;177:125.
65. Nichols RL, Smith JW, Robertson GD, et al. Prospective alterations in therapy for penetrating abdominal trauma. *Arch Surg* 1993;128:55.
66. Browder W, Smith JW, Vivoda LM, et al. Nonperforative appendicitis: a continuing surgical dilemma. *J Infect Dis* 1989;159:1088.
67. Bohnen JMA, Solomkin JS, Dellinger AP, et al. Guidelines for clinical care: anti-infective agents for intra-abdominal infection: a Surgical Infection Society policy statement. *Arch Surg* 1992;127:83.
68. Nichols RL. The treatment of intraabdominal infections in surgery. *Diagn Microbiol Infect Dis* 1989;12:195(S).
69. Schumer W, Lee DK, Jones B. Peritoneal lavage in postoperative therapy of late peritoneal sepsis: preliminary report. *Surgery* 1964;55:841.
70. DiVincenti FC, Cohn I Jr. Intraperitoneal kanamycin in advanced peritonitis: a preliminary report. *Am J Surg* 1966;3:147.
71. Noon GP, Beall AC Jr, Jordan GL Jr, et al. Clinical evaluation of peritoneal irrigation with antibiotic solution. *Surgery* 1967;62:73.
72. Roth RM, Gleckman RA, Gantz NM, et al. Antibiotic irrigations: a plea for controlled clinical trials. *Pharmacotherapy* 1985;5:222.
73. Pissiotis CA, Nichols RL, Condon RE. Absorption and excretion of intraperitoneally administered kanamycin sulfate. *Surg Gynecol Obstet* 1972;134:995.
74. Rappaport WD, Holcomb M, Valente J, et al. Antibiotic irrigation and the formation of intraabdominal adhesions. *Am J Surg* 1989;158:435.
75. Sindelar WF, Mason GR. Intraperitoneal irrigation with povidone-iodine solution for the prevention of intraabdominal abscesses in the bacterially contaminated abdomen. *Surg Gynecol Obstet* 1979;148:409.
76. Ahrenholz DH, Simmons RL. Povidone-iodine in peritonitis. I. Adverse effects of local instillation in experimental *E. coli* peritonitis. *J Surg Res* 1979;26:458.
77. Leiboff AR, Soroff HS. The treatment of generalized peritonitis by closed postoperative peritoneal lavage. *Arch Surg* 1987;122:1005.
78. Hudspeth AS. Radical surgical debridement in the treatment of advanced generalized bacterial peritonitis. *Arch Surg* 1975;110:1233.
79. Polk HC, Fry DE. Radical peritoneal débridement for established peritonitis: the results of a prospective randomized clinical trial. *Ann Surg* 1980;192:350.
80. Machiedo GW, Tikellis J, Suval W, et al. Reoperation for sepsis. *Am Surg* 1985;51:149.
81. Teichmann W, Wittmann DH, Andreone PA. Scheduled reoperations (*Etappenlavage*) for diffuse peritonitis. *Arch Surg* 1986;121:147.
82. Wittmann DH, Aprahamian C, Bergstein JM. Etappenlavage: advanced diffuse peritonitis managed by planned multiple laparotomies utilizing zippers, slide fastener, and Velcro analogue for temporary abdominal closure. *World J Surg* 1990;14:218.
83. Wittmann DH, Aprahamian C, Bergstein JM, et al. A burr-like device to facilitate temporary abdominal closure in planned multiple laparotomies. *Eur J Surg* 1993;159:75.
84. Sleeman D, Sosa JL, Gonzalez A, et al. Reclosure of the open abdomen. *J Am Coll Surg* 1995;180:200.
85. Andrus C, Doering M, Herrmann VM, et al. Planned reoperation for generalized intraabdominal infection. *Am J Surg* 1986;152:682.
86. Butler JA, Huang J, Wilson SE. Repeated laparotomy for postoperative intraabdominal sepsis. *Arch Surg* 1987;122:702.
87. McDougal WS, Izant RJ Jr, Zollinger RM Jr. Primary peritonitis in infancy and childhood. *Ann Surg* 1975;181:310.
88. Speck WT, Dresdale SS, McMillan RW. Primary peritonitis and the nephrotic syndrome. *Am J Surg* 1974;127:267.
89. Correra JP, Conn HO. Spontaneous bacterial peritonitis in cirrhosis: endemic or epidemic? *Med Clin North Am* 1975;59:963.
90. Wilner-Hanssen P, Westrom L, Mardh PA. Chlamydial perihepatitis. *Scand J Infect Dis* 1982;32(Suppl):77.
91. Golden GT, Shaw A. Primary peritonitis. *Surg Gynecol Obstet* 1972;135:513.
92. Conn HO. Spontaneous bacterial peritonitis: multiple revisitations. *Gastroenterology* 1976;70:455.
93. Grobmyer AJ III, Kerlan RA, Peterson CM, et al. Barium peritonitis. *Am Surg* 1984;2:116.
94. Rubin J, Ray R, Barnes T, et al. Peritonitis in continuous ambulatory peritoneal dialysis patients. *Am J Kidney Dis* 1983;2:602.
95. Balaie GR, Eisele G. Continuous ambulatory peritoneal dialysis: a review of its mechanics, advantages, complications, and areas of controversy. *Ann Pharmacother* 1992;26:1409.
96. von Graevenitz A, Amsterdam D. Microbiological aspects of peritonitis associated with continuous ambulatory peritoneal dialysis. *Clin Microbiol Rev* 1992;5:36.
97. Saklayen MG. CAPD peritonitis: incidence, pathogens, diagnosis and management. *Med Clin North Am* 1990;74:997.
98. Smith JA. Treatment of intra-abdominal infections with quinolones. *Eur J Clin Microbiol Infect Dis* 1991;10:330.
99. Janknegt R. CAPD peritonitis and fluoroquinolones: a review. *Perit Dial Int* 1991;11:53.
100. Dineen P, Homan WP, Grafe WR. Tuberculous peritonitis: 43 years' experience in diagnosis and treatment. *Ann Surg* 1976;184:717.

CHAPTER 82
Intraabdominal Abscesses

Rachel G. Khadaroo, Avery B. Nathens, and Ori D. Rotstein

Intraabdominal abscesses are localized collections of purulent material that are walled off from the rest of the peritoneal cavity by inflammatory adhesions, loops of intestine and their mesentery, the greater omentum, and other viscera. The development of an abscess reflects the successful prevention of disseminated infection by local host defense mechanisms in the peritoneal cavity. However, complete resolution of infection is thwarted by the inability of immune cells to function within the microenvironment of the abscess cavity.

Abscesses may occur in the peritoneal cavity, either within or outside the abdominal viscera, or in the retroperitoneum. Nonvisceral abscesses within the peritoneal cavity represent a consequence of the disruption of the gastrointestinal tract, whether occurring spontaneously or posttraumatically. Visceral abscesses most commonly occur from hematogenous or lymphatic spread of bacteria to the particular organ. Retroperitoneal abscesses originate through one of several mechanisms, including perforation of the gastrointestinal tract into the retroperitoneal space or hematogenous or lymphatic spread of bacteria to the retroperitoneal organs, particularly into the inflamed pancreas.

In the peritoneal cavity, visceral abscesses refer primarily to abscesses present in the liver or spleen. These, as well as retroperitoneal abscesses related to the pancreas and kidney, are discussed in Chapters 89, 91, 92, and 101. The present discussion focuses on the etiology, pathogenesis, diagnosis, and management of nonvisceral abscesses of the peritoneal cavity.

ETIOLOGY

Intraabdominal abscesses arise in three general settings: (a) following perforation of the gastrointestinal tract with resolution of diffuse peritonitis in which a loculated area of infection persists and evolves into an abscess, (b) following a spontaneous or traumatic perforation of the gastrointestinal tract, and (c) in the postoperative period following anastomotic disruption or through contamination of a perianastomotic hematoma or fluid collection.

Reports in the literature regarding the etiology and location of abscesses have described a change over time, an effect that is likely due to the maturation of our understanding of antibiotic therapy as well as improvements in surgical technique. Altemeier and colleagues (1) reviewed a series of 540 abscesses in 501 patients over an 11-year period spanning 1961 to 1972. Nonvisceral intraperitoneal abscesses constituted about 36% of all cases reviewed. Most of these were located in the right lower quadrant (44%), and appendicitis was deemed to be the underlying pathology in 50%. More recent series have documented that more than 80% of intraabdominal abscesses occur in the postoperative period, with most following pancreaticobiliary or colorectal surgery (2,3) (Table 82.1). More than 30% of abscesses are associated with clear evidence of an anastomotic leak (3,4). By contrast, intraabdominal abscesses unassociated with prior operation are most commonly due to inflammatory processes with a small, localized perforation as in appendicitis, diverticulitis, and Crohn's disease (3,5).

TABLE 82.1.   Incidence of Postoperative Abscess Formation in Relation to Site of Initial Operation

Site of initial operation	Incidence of postoperative abscess (%)
Pancreas and biliary tract	20
Colon	15
Stomach	9
Retroperitoneum	9
Trauma	9
Duodenum	8
Appendix	6
Kidney and adrenal gland	5
Small intestine	4
Spleen	4
Liver	4
Vascular	2
Uterus and ovary	1
Others	11

From Levison MA, Zeigler D. Correlation of APACHE II score, drainage technique and outcome in postoperative intra-abdominal abscess. *Surg Gynecol Obstet* 1991;172:89–94, with permission.

The spectrum of organisms inoculating the peritoneum following perforation of the gastrointestinal tract is diverse. The distal small bowel and colon contain more than 500 species of bacteria at a concentration of 10^{12} bacteria per gram of luminal contents with an anaerobe-to-aerobe ratio of 1000:1 (6,7). Although large numbers of bacteria may contaminate the peritoneal cavity, early events involved in abscess formation result in both a marked simplification and change in the rank order of their prevalence from that found in the gastrointestinal tract (Table 82.2). Cultures obtained from abscesses under optimal conditions usually reveal mixed aerobic and anaerobic species, with *Escherichia coli*, *Enterococcus* species, *Bacteroides fragilis* predominating. A recent bacteriologic study of patients in Japan with intraabdominal infection revealed a total of 125 bacterial strains, which consisted of 52.8% anaerobes, 43.2% aerobes, and 4% fungi. In this study, the major aerobic pathogen was Enterobacteriaceae, and the major anaerobes were *Bacteroides* species (8). A recent study has shown that the microbiology of postoperative peritonitis differs greatly from community-acquired peritonitis (9). This report showed that there was a significantly greater proportion of enterococci, *Enterobacter* species and *Staphylococcus aureus*, and decreased isolates of *E. coli* and streptococci (Table 82.3). Antibiotic treatment before reintervention correlated with the increase in the number of resistant organisms. There was also an increase in opportunistic fungal infections, *Candida* species being the most common fungi isolated in abscesses (Table 82.2). In the postoperative patient, this may be due to the use of immunosuppressive therapy, chemotherapy, radiation therapy, and broad-spectrum antimicrobial therapy. The alterations in the normal flora by antimicrobial therapy can promote the colonization and overgrowth of *Candida* species. Additional risk factors for developing candidal infections include diabetes, malnutrition, hyperalimentation, neoplasia, and multiple surgeries (10). Experimental studies have also shown that *Candida* can work synergistically with *E. coli*, leading to higher mortality rates in experimental peritonitis (11). Clinically, it has also been shown that surgical patients who remained untreated with fungemia had an increased rate of mortality. Autopsies performed on many of these patients revealed *Candida* intraabdominal abscesses as the most common sources of the fungi (12).

The central role of *B. fragilis* in abscess formation has been delineated in a series of experiments. Early studies focused on the role of polymicrobial infections in the pathogenesis on intraabdominal abscess formation. In these reports, known quantities of *E. coli*, *B. fragilis*, *Fusobacterium varium*, or enterococcus within gelatin capsules were inoculated into the peritoneal cavity. Neither *E. coli* nor enterococci produced intraabdominal abscesses, nor did combinations of the two aerobes or the two anaerobes. By contrast, a mixed anaerobe-aerobe inoculum consistently produced intraperitoneal abscesses. More recent work has delineated the important role of the capsular polysaccharide complex

TABLE 82.2.   Comparison of Common Bacterial Isolates from Normal Colonic Flora and from Intraabdominal Abscesses

Colonic isolates[a]		Abscess isolates[b]	
Rank	Organism	Rank	Organism
1	*Bacteroides vulgatus*	1	*Escherichia coli*
2	*Fusobacterium prausnitzii*	2	*Enterococcus* species
3	*Bifidobacterium adolescentis*	3	*Klebsiella* species
4	*Eubacterium aerofaciens*	4	*Bacteroides fragilis*
5	*Peptostreptococcus productus II*	5	*Pseudomonas* species
6	*Bacteroides thetaiotaomicron*	6	*Staphylococcus* species
7	*Eubacterium eligens*	7	*Candida* species
8	*Peptostreptococcus productus I*	8	*Enterobacter* species
9	*Eubacterium biforme*	9	*Clostridium* species
10	*Eubacterium aerofaciens III*	10	*Proteus* species
11	*Bacteroides distasonis*	11	*Serratia* species
28	*Bacteroides ovatus*		
29	*Bacteroides fragilis*		
59–75	*Enterococcus* species		
76–113	*Escherichia coli*, *Klebsiella* species		

[a]From Moore WEC, Holdeman LV. Human fecal flora: the normal flora of 20 Japanese-Hawaiians. *Appl Microbiol* 1974;27:961–979, with permission.
[b] From Olson MM, Allen MO. Nosocomial abscess: results of an eight-year prospective study of 32,284 operations. *Arch Surg* 1989;124:356–361, with permission; and Olak J, Christou NV, Stein LA, et al. Operative vs percutaneous drainage of intraabdominal abscesses: comparison of morbidity and mortality. *Arch Surg* 1986;121:141–146.

TABLE 82.3.	Bacteriology of Postoperative Versus Community-acquired Peritonitis		
	No. (%) of isolates of		
Strain	Postoperative peritonitis (n = 111)	Community-acquired peritonitis (n = 118)	*p*
Enterococci	23 (21)	6 (5)	0.001
Escherichia coli	21 (19)	42 (36)	0.005
Enterobacter species	13 (12)	4 (3)	<0.05
Bacteroides species	8 (7)	12 (10)	
Klebsiella species	8 (7)	8 (7)	
Staphylococcus aureus	7 (6)	1 (1)	<0.05
Coagulase-negative staphylococci	6 (5)	1 (1)	0.05
Candida species	4 (4)	8 (7)	
Pseudomonas species	7 (6)	2 (2)	
Streptococci	4 (4)	17 (14)	0.005
Hemolyzing streptococci		4 (3)	
Other	10 (9)	13 (11)	
Total	111	118	

From Roehrborn A, Thomas L, Potreck O, et al. The microbiology of postoperative peritonitis. *Clin Infect Dis* 2001; 33:1513–1519, with permission.

derived from *B. fragilis* or *S. aureus* as a primary virulence determinant necessary for abscess formation (13–15). Intraperitoneal administration of this complex without live organisms resulted in sterile abscesses, which were histologically identical to those formed in response to viable bacteria.

PATHOGENESIS OF ABSCESS FORMATION

Bacterial contamination of the peritoneal cavity initiates a complex series of events that ultimately result in abscess formation. Following peritoneal soiling, massive bacterial contamination is limited by mechanical clearance through the diaphragmatic lymphatics such that more than 60% of organisms are cleared within the first 60 minutes of contamination (16). Locally, peritoneal macrophages and mesothelial cells elaborate proinflammatory mediators in response to the inflammatory stimuli, leading to hyperemia, exudation of protein-rich fluid containing fibrinogen, and a massive influx of phagocytic cells (17,18). The regulation of early peritoneal neutrophils migration in response to infection was also shown to be dependent on macrophage inflammatory protein-2 and mast cells (19). This phagocytic phase lasts about 48 to 72 hours, during which time most organisms are ingested either by neutrophils during the early inflammatory response or by peritoneal macrophages at later time points.

Experimentally, bacterial adherence to mesothelial cells seems to be one of the most important steps in the pathogenesis of intraabdominal abscesses. This process has been shown to be enhanced in encapsulated bacteria, which have a polysaccharide capsule. This capsule aids both in the prevention of engulfment by phagocytes and in attachment. The capsular polysaccharide from *B. fragilis* has been shown to elicit the release of tumor necrosis facto-α (TNF-α), interleukin-1α (IL-1α), IL-8, and IL-10 from phagocytic cells (20). These cytokines may play a role in recruitment of immune cells to the peritoneal cavity following contamination. In addition to the role of chemokines in attracting cells, TNF-α production can stimulate intercellular adhesion molecule-1 (ICAM-1) production by mesothelial cells. The enhanced ICAM-1 expression can aid in increased polymorphonuclear leukocyte binding to the mesothelium (21).

The early events set the stage for the localization phase in which residual bacteria and inflammatory cells are localized within fibrinous exudates, loops of bowel, and omentum. Fibrin deposition is mediated by the procoagulant effect of activated macrophages and damaged peritoneal mesothelial cells through the cellular expression of tissue factor, which initiates the coagulation cascade (22–24). Further, fibrin deposition is facilitated through a reduction in peritoneal fibrinolytic activity mediated by a marked increase in peritoneal fluid plasminogen activator inhibitor (25). The initiation of coagulation in response to bacterial infection is recognized as a mechanism that is both protective and potentially harmful. During the early phases of peritonitis, fibrin matrices serve to sequester bacteria within the peritoneal cavity and further localize the contamination by causing loops of intestine to adhere both to each other and to the omentum, thereby preventing disseminated infection and bacteremia. The protective role of fibrin is demonstrated by studies in which fibrin deposition is prevented through the administration of tissue plasminogen activator (26) or systemic fibrinogen depletion (27). Both interventions significantly increased bacteremia and mortality in a rodent model of intraabdominal infection.

By virtue of its ability to wall off and contain infection locally, peritoneal fibrin deposition plays an important role in abscess formation. The ability of fibrin to enmesh microorganisms appears to protect the bacteria from normal host clearance mechanisms, thereby permitting unopposed proliferation and ultimately the establishment of an abscess (28,29). That fibrin deposition is a necessary component of abscess formation has been outlined in a series of experiments in which aerosolized fibrinogen administered into the contaminated peritoneum augments abscess formation (30), whereas fibrinolytic agents almost completely abrogate their development (26).

The contribution of the specific and the nonspecific cellular immune responses to the localization phase of abscess formation remains poorly defined. Classically, phagocytic cells have been considered to constitute the major cellular defense against intraabdominal infection. As described earlier, peritoneal macrophages appear to be important in abscess development through induction of procoagulant activity upon exposure to bacterial lipopolysaccharide (22,31). However, evidence suggests that the ability of the capsular polysaccharide complex of *B. fragilis* to induce the formation of abscesses is dependent on the presence of nonimmune CD4$^+$ and CD8$^+$ T cells (32). Another study showed that CD4$^+$ T lymphocytes played a central role

TABLE 82.4. Local Factors in Abscesses that Favor Microbial Persistence

Factor	Effect	References
Microenvironmental		
Hypoxia	Impairs neutrophil migration and killing	125–127
Low pH	Impairs neutrophil migration, phagocytosis, and killing	125, 128–130
Hyperosmolarity	Impairs neutrophil phagocytosis, cell degranulation, and killing	131, 132
Hypercarbia	Reduced phagocytic cell cytoplasmic pH leads to cell dysfunction	133
Microbiologic		
Bacterial synergy	Optimizes microenvironment for bacterial growth, provision of nutrients between bacterial partners	134, 135
High concentrations of bacterial by-products, cell wall components, proteases	Impaired phagocytic function, local tissue damage, complement depletion	136
Adjuvant materials		
Necrotic debris	Complement depletion, neutrophil deactivation	137, 138
Blood, hemoglobin, fibrin	Impaired phagocytic cell function, reduced access of cell to bacteria	29, 139
Barium sulfate	Reduced access of cells to bacteria	140
Bile salts	Toxic to neutrophils	141
Hemostatic agents	Impaired neutrophil function	142
Foreign body	Premature activation of neutrophils	143, 144
Unknown	Impaired macrophage antigen presenting capacity	145

in the pathophysiology of abscess formation in murine model of transient bacterial infection (33). In these studies, treating animals with the most potent polysaccharide from *B. fragilis*, termed *polysaccharide A*, shortly before or after bacterial challenge, has also been shown to protect animals from abscess formation. This protective immune response seems to be dependent on CD4+ T-cell–dependent response, which is mediated through IL-2 production (34). Furthermore, rodent studies have demonstrated that abscess formation can be prevented by preimmunization with capsular polysaccharide complex, an effect dependent on specific CD8+ T lymphocytes (32,35). Adoptive transfer with these cells prevented abscess formation in naive mice, as did the passive transfer of a soluble cell lysate derived from these immune T cells (36). These findings, while demonstrating seemingly contradictory effects of T cells in abscess formation, represent novel concepts implicating specific cell-mediated immunity in the pathogenesis of intraabdominal abscesses.

Having defined the importance of the localization phase in the initiation of abscesses, it is important to consider the subsequent processes involved in abscess formation and persistence. A mature abscess consists of a central core containing necrotic debris, dead cells, and bacteria; a surrounding ring of neutrophils and macrophages; and a peripheral ring consisting of smooth muscle cells and fibroblasts within a collagen capsule (37). The evolution from an infected phlegmonous mass to a well-defined abscess suggests a process by which bacteria are able to sequester themselves within a milieu where they are protected from the host's attempts to effect ultimate resolution of the infection. The chemical, bacterial, and physical microenvironments of an abscess lead to microbial persistence. Table 82.4 summarizes the potential mechanisms whereby bacterial clearance is frustrated, leading to persistent localized infection.

CLINICAL MANIFESTATIONS

In contrast to diffuse generalized peritonitis, in which the symptoms and physical findings are obvious, patients with intraabdominal abscesses frequently have less profound findings. The

local symptoms and signs of an intraabdominal abscess may vary with the source and location of the abscess and with the underlying status of the patient, whereas low-grade fever, anorexia, general malaise, and weakness are frequent systemic symptoms. Enteroparietal abscesses may produce pain, tenderness, and a palpable, diffuse abdominal mass. The latter may be interpreted as "fullness" due to the surrounding omentum and adherent intestinal loops. Interloop, intramesenteric, and subphrenic abscesses are usually less obvious clinically because the visceral peritoneum is innervated by splanchnic rather than somatic pain fibers, and no mass can be palpated. Additionally, patients with subphrenic abscesses may have hiccoughs, cough, tachypnea, or jaundice (38). Nonspecific thoracic manifestations include pleural effusions, elevation of the diaphragm, and decreased basilar breath sounds (39,40). Retroperitoneal abscesses may only produce lumbar or ileopsoas muscle spasm or referred pain to the hip, groin, or knee (41). Chronic psoas abscesses may present with leg and back pain with a flexion deformity of the hip and wasting of the quadriceps femoris (42). Pelvic abscesses may occasionally be palpated on rectal examination but usually give few symptoms. Intractable diarrhea may occur as the presenting feature in as many as 20% of patients owing to irritability of the sigmoid colon as a result of the adjacent inflammatory process (43). Systemic evidence of inflammation is often reflected in peripheral leukocyte count, as noted by a leukocytosis or a left shift toward immature forms. Additional laboratory investigation adds little to confirm the diagnosis.

In the postoperative patient, the abdominal symptoms may be masked by incisional pain and postoperative analgesics. Physical examination is notoriously unreliable in this period; most patients are distended and tender. Additionally, the clinical findings associated with an intraabdominal abscess may be abrogated by the administration of antibiotics to the patient. The median time from initial operation to clinical presentation in a series of 114 abscesses was 8 days (4). In this series, the median time from presentation of abscess symptoms to drainage was 4 days. The systemic response to antibiotic therapy in the postoperative period following surgery for peritonitis may also provide a clue to the presence of residual intraabdominal infection. In two commonly cited papers, it has been suggested that antibiotics could be discontinued when defined clinical end points were reached with a low probability of subsequent infection (less than 1%). These were an afebrile patient, a normal leukocyte count, and a band count less than 3% (44,45). This normalization usually occurred within 5 to 10 days. Extension beyond this period suggests persistent infection and should direct the physician to more intensive radiologic investigation (44,45). At times, the first sign of postoperative abscess formation may be progressive organ dysfunction leading to multiple organ failure (46). Immunocompromised patients may present with shock as the only indication of ongoing intraabdominal infection. Occasionally, the reporting of an unexpected positive blood culture, particularly if it is polymicrobial or contains an anaerobe, will provide the first evidence of an intraabdominal abscess (47,48).

DIAGNOSIS

Definitive diagnosis of an intraabdominal abscess is most commonly made by abdominal imaging. Conventional plain film radiographs of the abdomen may reveal loculated extraluminal gas collections or mottled soft tissue masses, either of which is indicative of abscess formation. More subtle signs include the presence of a localized ileus or obliteration of the psoas muscle margins. Chest radiographs may document the presence of a pleural effusion or atelectasis, features that may indicate the presence of a subphrenic collection (49). A limited contrast examination may be useful to investigate the integrity of an anastomosis in the postoperative period or to evaluate localized spontaneous perforations of the gastrointestinal tract such as a walled-off perforated duodenal ulcer. At best, conventional radiographic techniques offer indirect evidence of an abscess. Clinical suspicion of an abscess should direct the physician to the use of more advanced imaging techniques to confirm the diagnosis and anatomically define its extent.

Ultrasonography and computed tomography (CT) have largely replaced conventional radiography and nuclear scintigraphy, whereas new techniques such as magnetic resonance imaging have yet to achieve a significant role. Ultrasonography is a sensitive tool for the detection and localization of fluid collections in the abdomen and pelvis. It is rapid and noninvasive and does not expose the patient to additional radiation. It has real-time capabilities that can visualize bowel peristalsis, thereby enhancing differentiation between fluid-filled bowel and abscesses. The availability of mobile machines permits bedside examination, allowing for safe examination of critically ill patients in the intensive care unit (ICU) without the added risk of transporting them to the radiology department. Sensitivity and specificity of ultrasonography in the detection of abscesses are in the range of 80% to 90%, depending on the site of the abscess and skill of the operator (50,51). The right upper quadrant, pelvis, and left upper quadrants (when the spleen is present) are best visualized using ultrasound, owing to the lack of intestinal loops. Interloop abscesses are not well visualized (52). Additionally, the use of endoluminal probes allows transvaginal or transrectal visualization and drainage of deep pelvic abscesses, an advantage not offered by other techniques (53,54). The principal disadvantages of ultrasound are related to its technical limitations and lack of specificity in the postoperative setting. Intestinal gas reflects transmitted sound waves and prevents imaging of large areas of the abdomen, pelvis, and retroperitoneum. This may be a particular problem in the postoperative setting in patients with an ileus in whom multiple distended air-filled bowel loops make examination difficult. Patients with open wounds, extensive dressings drains, or stomas are poorly suited for ultrasound examination because of the lack of acoustic windows.

CT has several advantages over ultrasound and appears to be the most accurate technique available for the diagnosis of intraabdominal abscesses (50,55). Sensitivity and specificity are in the range of 97.5% and 85%, respectively (50). Its advantages include higher resolution, operator independence, and an ability to see deep to bone and gas-filled structures without the need for an intact abdominal wall. It has proved excellent in visualizing the retroperitoneum, with a sensitivity approaching 100%, in contrast to 67% using ultrasonography (41). Optimal detection by CT depends on the administration of intravenous contrast material and gastrointestinal contrast to opacify bowel. The combination of rectal plus oral contrast, in addition to intravenous contrast, improves the diagnosis of abscesses by enhancing differentiation of fluid-filled bowel from extraluminal collections. Criteria for the identification of an abscess by CT include identification of an area of low attenuation in an extraluminal location (0 to 40 Hounsfield units), the presence of intracavitary gas or heterogeneous internal debris, contrast enhancement of the wall, and displacement of surrounding viscera or edema of the adjacent tissue planes (52). A long air-fluid level within an abscess suggests a fistulous connection to the bowel (56).

The major disadvantages of CT scanning are the requirement for a cooperative patient who will remain immobile and the lack of portability of the unit. Several settings exist in which accuracy of CT scans may be compromised. The accuracy of the scan is reduced in patients in whom the gastrointestinal tract is not opacified with contrast. In this setting, the scans are limited in their ability to distinguish fluid-filled bowel loops from an abscess. Interloop abscesses, which represent 4% of all abscesses, are also poorly visualized with CT scanning (57). Further, artifacts related to the presence of surgical clips or residual barium in the gastrointestinal tract may limit the accuracy of this technique. Finally, although both ultrasound and CT scanning demonstrate a high degree of accuracy with respect to anatomic localization of fluid collections, both are somewhat limited in their ability to discern the origin of the collection. Fluid-filled collections simulating abscesses include hematomas, bilomas, lymphoceles, seromas, and urinomas.

Early postoperative fluid collections may be difficult to identify definitively as abscesses. In two prospective studies, 19% to 23% of asymptomatic patients had evidence of fluid collections on the fourth or fifth postoperative day (58,59). Most of these were crescent shaped and conformed to the peritoneal recesses. Only 6% of patients still demonstrated fluid on the eighth postoperative day, suggesting that most were sterile collections relating to the surgical procedure, rather than early abscesses (59). In those patients in whom diagnosis is in doubt, ultrasound or CT-guided diagnostic aspiration can help to provide an accurate diagnosis by providing fluid for Gram stain and culture. Percutaneous needle aspiration of intraabdominal collections for the purpose of diagnosis therefore represents an important adjuvant technique to scanning (60). In one study, the authors used the analysis of intraabdominal fluid for pH and Po_2 measurements to determine bacterial infection and concluded that pH was a sensitive indicator of infection. A pH less than or equal to 7.04 was a good indicator of infection and suggested drainage of the collection. By contrast, it was suggested that drainage could be delayed pending culture results if the above pH criteria were not met (61). Further evaluation of this general approach appears warranted. For example, rapid microbiologic diagnostics might be applied to such specimens to discern need for drainage and adjustments of antibiotic therapy.

CT scanning has proved particularly effective in the analysis of patients in the ICU setting where clinical examination is difficult because of altered level of consciousness, immunosuppression, or comorbidities. Barkhausen and colleagues evaluated the use of CT in 63 ICU patients with sepsis of unknown origin.

TABLE 82.5. Role of Computed Tomography and Ultrasonography in the Diagnosis of Intraabdominal Abscesses

	Ultrasound	Computed tomography
Advantages	Rapid	Higher resolution
	Portable	Superior imaging of the retroperitoneum
	No ionizing radiation	Operator independent
	Visualize bowel peristalsis—may allow differentiation of bowel from abscess	
	Greatest sensitivity in right upper quadrant, pelvis	
Disadvantages	Limited sensitivity in obese patients due to signal attenuation	Requires patient transport—difficult in the critically ill patient
	Limited sensitivity in patients with gaseous abdominal distention (e.g., ileus)	Barium sulfate, metallic clips may cause image distortion
	Operator dependent	Not available in all centers
	Technically difficult in presence of open abdominal wounds, stomas, or bulky abdominal dressings	Expensive

They identified the source of sepsis in the chest or abdomen in 19% of patients, most commonly owing to the presence of a localized abscess (62). In another study, CT scan identified a septic focus in the abdomen in more than half of a group of critically ill major trauma patients with sepsis of unknown origin. Importantly, in this sick group of patients, significant adverse events such as hypotension and oxygen desaturation did not occur during transport from the ICU to the radiology suite (63).

Studies comparing ultrasonography with CT imaging generally demonstrate the latter to be the superior modality with respect to accuracy (64,65). However, the advantages and disadvantages of each technique (summarized in Table 82.5) must be considered in the particular clinical setting and with consideration of the resources and expertise available.

Nuclear scintigraphy using either gallium-67 citrate or indium-111 has a limited role in the diagnosis of intraabdominal abscesses. Gallium has an affinity for iron-binding proteins present on leukocytes and on bacterial surfaces and thus is concentrated at sites of infection (66). The detection of an abscess is based on increased uptake outside of expected sites. However, gallium is excreted in the colon and accumulates in the stool. An enema is necessary to clear radiolabeled stool and allow for interpretation of the study. Other disadvantages of this technique include the false-positive imaging of neoplasms and the 24- to 72-hour delay required between injection of the radionuclide and the scanning procedure. Recent experimental work has evaluated the use of technetium-99m–labeled polyethylene glycol–coated liposomes in scintigraphic identification of abscesses. This agent proved to be promising in terms of its ability to image abscesses *in vivo* without the prolonged time delay (67). Further studies are required.

For white blood cell scanning, indium-111 in the form of the chelate indium-111 oxyquinoline is used to label leukocytes drawn from the patient (50,68). After labeling, the cells are reinjected into the patient, and the patient is scanned with a gamma camera. Although conceptually attractive, this technique has several shortcomings. Labeling of granulocytes with indium-111 requires a highly skilled technician. In addition, because this technique depends on delivery of neutrophils to a site of acute inflammation, it may be associated with a significant number of false-negative test results in patients with chronic infection (50). Neither indium-111 nor gallium scans are effective in the early postoperative period. Peritoneal inflammation at this time will attract the isotopes, and all sites at which dissection has occurred will show isotope localization. There may be some benefit

from these scanning techniques in the later postoperative period (greater than 2 weeks), once inflammation has quiesced (69). Finally, these tests do not provide sufficiently accurate localization of the collection to permit diagnostic needle aspiration or insertion of a percutaneous drainage catheter. In general, these two techniques do not add much to the diagnostic armamentarium of intraabdominal infection. They may be useful as an initial screening examination in patients who are not critically ill and do not have a localizing site of infection. If uptake is noted in the abdomen, subsequent CT or ultrasound scanning may be used to better define the lesion.

The role of magnetic resonance imaging in the diagnosis of intraabdominal abscesses requires further evaluation. Initial studies have suggested potential advantages (70). Surgical clips do not interfere with imaging, and intravenous contrast is not necessary to outline the abscess or distinguish it from adjacent structures. In addition, sagittal section may be useful in the pelvis to provide improved anatomic definition. However, although gadolinium-enhanced magnetic resonance imaging demonstrates excellent accuracy in the diagnosis of abdominal abscesses, it is not clearly superior to the excellent sensitivity and specificity of CT and ultrasound (71). The use of spectroscopy to evaluate parameters such as tissue pH may ultimately be helpful in differentiating between various fluid collections, an ability presently lacking with ultrasound and CT.

MANAGEMENT

Three basic principles guide the management of intraabdominal abscesses: (a) supportive care of the patient, (b) antibiotic administration, and (c) drainage of the abscess–either percutaneous or operative.

Supportive Management

Patients with intraabdominal abscess exhibit a spectrum of clinical presentations, ranging from a low-grade fever to septic shock. In general, these patients have intravascular volume depletion that calls for fluid resuscitation and monitoring. The intensity of resuscitation and monitoring depends on the status of the patient. Hourly monitoring of vital signs, urine output, and mental status may be necessary. In the critically ill individual, Swan-Ganz catheterization and invasive arterial monitoring are essential to direct initial resuscitation, particularly if administration of inotropic agents is necessary. Hypoxemia may be present for several reasons. Atelectasis, basilar pneumonia, and pleural effusions may exist secondary to abdominal distention and elevation of the diaphragm or a subdiaphragmatic inflammatory process. Intraabdominal infection is intimately associated with the development of a host-derived systemic inflammatory response mediated by several proinflammatory mediators, perhaps the most important of which are TNF, IL-1, and IL-6 (72,73). If the process is advanced, early signs of organ dysfunction may develop, resulting in hemodynamic instability, acute respiratory distress syndrome, and renal dysfunction. At present, the role of mediator-directed therapy as an adjuvant in the management of intraabdominal abscess remains to be defined, and its use should be limited to carefully controlled clinical trials.

Nutritional support is important to minimize debilitation. Patients in whom abscesses develop in the postoperative period are usually already at a nutritional disadvantage because they have usually spent 7 to 10 days without adequate caloric intake. The marked catabolic response associated with sepsis further aggravates this problem. Total parenteral nutrition has been preferred in patients with intraabdominal infection particularly in patients with an abscess related to an anastomotic leak. Enteral feeding, even in the early postoperative period, appears to be well tolerated in most patients. In addition, patients with enterocutaneous fistulas may be managed using this approach as long as adequate drainage prevents further contamination of the peritoneal cavity (74). One recent metaanalysis supports the concept that enteral feeding should be started early after surgery, compared with maintaining nothing by mouth. In this analysis, early feeding (either oral or enteral) reduced the risk for infection and length of hospital stay. The risk for vomiting was slightly increased. This result has clear relevance to the nutritional support of patients during management of abscesses (75).

Antimicrobial Therapy

Empiric antibiotic therapy should be initiated once the diagnosis of intraabdominal abscess is suspected. Antimicrobial therapy should include an agent or agents with activity against both aerobic and anaerobic organisms. Virtually all studies performed that compare different regimens have shown equivalence between treatment arms when these general principles are applied (76). Table 82.6 lists several antibiotic regimens that have been shown to be effective in the management of intraabdominal infection. It is noteworthy that most trials are performed using patients with the spectrum of intraabdominal infection, including both peritonitis and abscesses. The numbers of patients in the subgroup analysis of abscesses are too small to make conclusions specifically regarding abscesses, but it is reasonable to conclude, based on microbiology, that comparable principles should apply to antibiotic selection for abscesses as those for intraabdominal infection in general. Most experts recommend regimens with a somewhat more extended spectrum of coverage to treat complex abscesses such as those postoperatively following treatment of peritonitis, those that are recurrent, or those occurring in immunocompromised patients or patients receiving prolonged antibiotics. The potential for resistant microbes in those patient groups is augmented; therefore, altered antimicrobial therapy is warranted as noted in Table 82.3. These patients have altered microbiology characterized by reduced isolates of E. coli and increased isolates of enterococci and Enterobacter species. Accordingly, recent guidelines published by the Surgical Infection Society recommend that advanced spectrum therapies—such as imipenem-cilastatin; piperacillin-tazobactam; meropenem; ertapenem; or a second-generation cephalosporin with anaerobic coverage; as well as combination regimens—such as cefuroxime (or a third- or fourth-generation cephalosporin or an aminoglycoside) plus an antianaerobe; aztreonam plus clindamycin;

TABLE 82.6. Antibiotic Therapy for Intraabdominal Infections

Monotherapy	References
Imipenem-cilastatin	77
Piperacillin-tazobactam	146, 147
Ertapenem	148
Meropenem	149, 150
Cephalosporins (e.g., cefotetan, ceftizoxime, cefoxitin)	151–153
Ampicillin-sulbactam	151
Cefmetazole	154, 155

Combination therapy	
Antianaerobe plus quinolone (e.g., ciprofloxacin plus metronidazole)	77, 156
Antianaerobe plus third-generation cephalosporin (e.g., cefotaxime plus metronidazole, cefepime plus metronidazole)	149, 157
Antianaerobe plus aminoglycoside (e.g., gentamicin plus clindamycin, tobramycin plus clindamycin)	147, 158, 159
Antianaerobe plus monobactam (e.g., clindamycin plus aztreonam)	160

or ciprofloxacin plus metronidazole may be more appropriate (76a). Antibiotic usage before repeat laparotomy in the patients was shown to influence the development of resistant strains (9).

Several recent studies of antimicrobial agents in intraabdominal infection have reported the efficacy of an intravenous-to-oral switchover regimen as an alternative to an entire course consisting of intravenous therapy. One documented the ability to switch from intravenous ciprofloxacin-metronidazole to oral preparations of the same drugs at day 3 to 5 of treatment as being equivalent to intravenous imipenem-cilastatin. This intravenous-to-oral switchover regimen is particularly attractive for patients with abscesses because they frequently are able to take oral medications soon after abscess drainage (77). This would potentially reduce costs and morbidity of antimicrobial administration without compromising efficacy.

Drainage

Supportive care and antimicrobial therapy serve primarily as adjuncts to drainage of the abscess cavity. Antibiotics alone are unlikely to be effective for numerous reasons. These include poor penetration of antibiotics into the abscess center, inactivation of antibiotics in the low pH, hypoxic suppurative environment, and inactivity of the drug against a large bacterial inoculum (78,79). Drainage of an abscess reverses these adverse conditions and increases the efficacy of the antibiotics.

Percutaneous abscess drainage (PAD) has become the interventional procedure of choice for the management of intraabdominal abscesses, having superseded operative drainage as the first line of therapy. In early studies, attempts at PAD were limited to simple abscesses–well-defined, unilocular collections without evidence of enteric communication and no significant tissue necrosis. Multiple or multiloculated abscesses, those that form a fistula to adjacent organs or bowel, and abscesses containing viscous fluid, debris, or necrotic material were defined as complex and were formerly considered contraindications to PAD. However, extensive experience during the past decade has demonstrated that percutaneous management of complex abscesses is feasible and represents a reasonable initial approach in almost all cases.

The care of patients undergoing PAD is similar to that of those undergoing operative drainage. Intravenous antibiotic therapy should be administered before the procedure. Either ultrasonography or CT is used to image the abscess and provide guidance for abscess drainage. The choice of technique depends largely on the size and location of the abscess, operator preference, and the status of the patient. For example, portable ultrasound and PAD may be performed at the bedside in critically ill, unstable patients—a distinct advantage over CT. Once visualized, percutaneous drainage is achieved using a modified Seldinger technique. A fine needle (20 or 22 gauge) is guided into the collection both for localization and aspiration of a sample of fluid. A guidewire is placed through the needle into the cavity and then an 8.3 to 14 French catheter is placed into the cavity over the guidewire, followed by removal of the guidewire. Larger-bore tubes do not necessarily lead to more effective drainage. Complex abscesses, including those with multiple septa, hematoma, or thick purulent fluid within the abscess, pose particularly difficult management problems because of catheter occlusion and ineffective drainage. Recent reports have suggested the possibility that laparoscopic drainage of abscesses might be appropriate under selected circumstances in which either the abscess is not located in a site amenable to PAD or the abscess contents are too thick to be evacuated by a drain alone and require some débridement (80,81).

Close monitoring of both the patient and percutaneous drain is as vital to patient outcome as postoperative care following operative drainage. Catheters are placed to gravity drainage or low suction. Daily irrigation with 10 to 15 mL of saline should be performed to maintain catheter patency. Repeated CT or ultrasound and sinograms are necessary to ensure a progressive reduction in cavity size and to discern whether any enteral communication exists. Criteria for removal of the percutaneous catheter include (a) clinical resolution of septic parameters as judged by patient well-being, normal temperature, and normal leukocyte count; (b) minimal drainage from the catheter; and (c) radiologic evidence of abscess resolution as judged by sinogram or abdominal imaging. Some authors have recommended gradual removal of the catheter over 1 to 2 days (82), although this is not the authors' preference. The overall duration of drainage varies widely, ranging from 7 to 47 days (83). In general, the prolonged drainage periods are due to the presence of an enteric communication because drains are left in place until the fistula heals, thereby reducing the risk for recurrence. Major complications of percutaneous drainage occur in 0% to 5% of patients and include hemorrhage, intestinal perforation and enteric fistulas, and empyemas resulting from inadvertent transpleural passage of the catheter (84–86).

A clinical response to drainage should be observed within 48 to 72 hours of drainage. The development or persistence of fever and leukocytosis within 72 hours of drainage is worrisome and suggests a definite need for reevaluation (87). Possible reasons for failure include ineffective drainage due to inadequate catheter size or position, an undrained area of contiguous abscess, a large enteric communication, or the presence of a second unrecognized abscess. A repeat CT scan with or without a sinogram will elucidate the cause of persistent infection. Residual abscesses can then be percutaneously drained or the catheter repositioned if necessary (Fig. 82.1). If residual infections exist that cannot be adequately drained, or if no residual collections are seen, then a formal laparotomy should be performed.

Outcome following percutaneous drainage is stratified as curative success, palliative success, or failure (88,89). A curative success provides complete cure without the need for additional percutaneous or operative intervention. Palliative success implies the use of percutaneous drainage where cure is impossible.

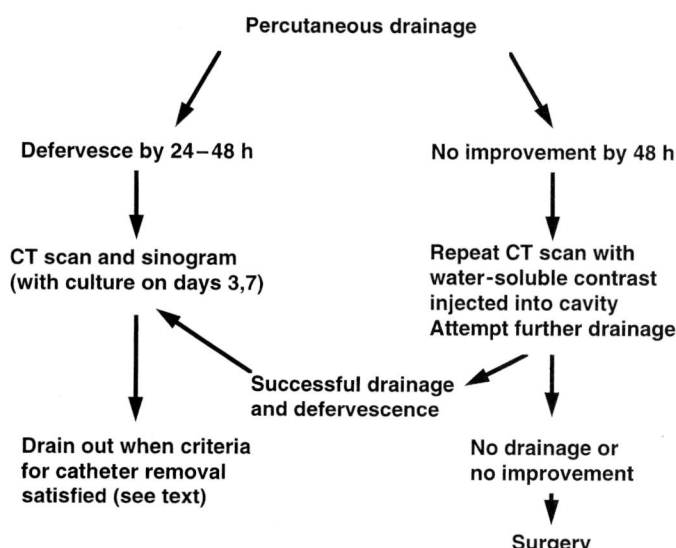

Figure 82.1. Algorithm for the management of patients with intraabdominal abscesses using percutaneous drainage. (Adapted from Rotstein OD, Nathens AB. Peritonitis and intra-abdominal abscesses. In: Wilmore DW, Cheung LY, Harken AH, et al., eds. *ACS surgery: principles and practice,* 2nd ed. New York: WebMD Professional Publishing, 2003.)

Most frequently, palliative success refers to the ability of percutaneous drainage to act as a temporizing measure, providing for patient stabilization before definitive operative management. This is particularly important in the management of diverticular abscesses. Before the use of PAD, patients presenting with a diverticular abscess required a two- or three-stage procedure including abscess drainage, proximal diverting colostomy, sigmoid colectomy and anastomosis, and reversal of colostomy. However, in more than two thirds of patients, local control of the abscess with PAD allows for single-stage sigmoid colectomy and primary anastomosis in an elective setting (90). Similarly, patients presenting with spontaneous abscesses as a result of a perforated viscus may be treated with initial percutaneous drainage. Operative intervention may then be postponed or deemed unnecessary, depending on nature of the underlying disease (91). Most spontaneous and postoperative abscesses occur as a result of perforation of a viscus or anastomotic leak. The enteral communication often presents as a sudden increase in drainage of gastrointestinal contents from the catheter. Many of these fistulas may be managed conservatively providing that the intraabdominal infection is controlled. Various factors, including local conditions and site of origin of the fistula, influence the likelihood of spontaneous closure (Table 82.7). These warrant consideration in the clinical decision-making process. Occasionally, an unresectable, infected tumor mass may be successfully decompressed, thereby minimizing systemic signs of sepsis. However, this is clearly palliative in nature.

An overall success rate exceeding 80% has been reported for PAD (92–96). The type, location, and etiology of the abscess have a significant influence on outcome. Simple abscesses are successfully drained in 82% to 95% of cases, whereas complex collections are associated with a 45% to 69% success rate. Equivalent rates of success have been documented using PAD or operative drainage for simple abscesses, whereas complex abscesses may be treated successfully more often by operation (97), although it is probably reasonable to attempt PAD as a first-line approach. In certain situations, operative management should be undertaken without primary PAD. Clearly, when the abscess in inaccessible or ill-defined, or when CT demonstrates multiple small abscesses or an infected phlegmon, an operative approach is necessary to

TABLE 82.7. Probability of Fistula Closure in Relation to Underlying Disease and Location

I	Local factor	Spontaneous closure rate (%)
	Local infection and abscess	Virtually 0
	Complete anastomotic dehiscence	Virtually 0
	Retained foreign body	Virtually 0
	Epithelialization of tract	Virtually 0
	Distal obstruction	Virtually 0
	Crohn's disease	8
	Irradiation of small bowel	14
	Tract <2 cm	17
	Malignancy	26
	Closure rate with none of these factors	32
II	**Origin of fistula**	
	Esophagus	82
	Stomach	43
	Duodenum (end)	50
	Duodenum (lateral)	27
	Jejunum	21
	Ileum	19
	Pancreas	67
	External biliary tree	60
	Cecum and appendix	44
	Colon	30
	Rectum	30

Adapted from Reber H, Roberts C, Way LW, et al. Management of external gastrointestinal fistulas. *Ann Surg* 1978;188:460, with permission.

ensure adequate drainage. With accurate CT localization, a direct (often extraserous) approach to abscesses in the subphrenic, subhepatic, or pelvic regions or retroperitoneum can be performed. A general laparotomy under these circumstances is unnecessary and may be detrimental, leading to complications such as enteric fistulas and bleeding. On the other hand, laparotomy is usually necessary when abscesses are in the lesser sac or when multiple abscesses are present. Additionally, one should consider PAD of fluid collections developing in the early postoperative period (less than 72 hours) with some caution because the collections are rarely localized and may result from an anastomotic dehiscence. A laparotomy to deal with both the dehisced anastomosis and the diffuse peritoneal contamination may be a preferable approach.

In most patients, normal host defense mechanisms localize the infectious process as an abscess, allowing for relatively straightforward management using either percutaneous or operative drainage. There is a subset of critically ill patients at risk for intraabdominal abscesses who manifest a systemic inflammatory response yet demonstrate no evidence of intraabdominal abscesses on imaging studies. At laparotomy, only poorly defined, serosanguinous collections are found, rather than discrete purulent abscesses (98,99). Peritoneal cultures yield organisms that are traditionally considered to be of low virulence, including *Enterococcus* and *Candida* species, coagulase-negative staphylococci, and *Pseudomonas aeruginosa* (98–100). Associated organ dysfunction is common. This triad of organ dysfunction, poorly localized intraabdominal infection, and atypical pathogens constitutes a syndrome coined *tertiary peritonitis* (98). It is believed that the impaired host defense mechanisms of critical illness render the localization process and subsequent abscess formation ineffective. The significance of these organisms is unclear. Their presence may relate to selection by antibiotic pressures or an indication of impaired systemic immunity. Management is complex and usually involves multiple laparotomies and intensive supportive therapy. Despite this, the mortality rate is as high as 64% (99).

PREVENTION

Intraabdominal abscesses most frequently occur following surgery on the gastrointestinal tract as a result of anastomotic leak. In this setting, prevention of postoperative sepsis is dependent on meticulous surgical technique. Anastomoses should be performed between ends of bowel that are free from tension and are well vascularized. Meticulous hemostasis should be achieved and foreign bodies avoided.

Abscesses following surgery for secondary peritonitis usually represent foci of residual infection. Prevention of recurrent infection involves (a) elimination of the source of contamination, (b) reduction of bacterial contamination, and (c) prevention of recurrent infection. The source of contamination is controlled by closing, excluding, or resecting the perforated viscus. Primary anastomoses are at increased risk for dehiscence when performed in the setting of acute inflammation or in the immunocompromised patient (101). Bowel exteriorization should be performed to circumvent the potential dangers of anastomotic breakdown, although in selected circumstances, primary anastomosis may be feasible (102).

Following secondary peritonitis, normal host defense mechanisms are overwhelmed by massive bacterial contamination. Techniques aimed at controlling bacterial contamination are geared toward reducing the bacterial inoculum to a level at which normal host defense mechanisms can eliminate the few remaining organisms. At operation, gross purulent exudates are aspirated, and loculations are gently opened and débrided. Particulate debris, such as fecal matter or other gross intestinal contents, is removed to optimize bacterial clearance. Intraoperative peritoneal lavage using saline or saline-antibiotic combinations have been attempted with variable success. A recent prospective study by Schein and colleagues did not demonstrate any improvement in mortality or postoperative abscess formation in patients receiving saline lavage or saline lavage with chloramphenicol (103). Peritoneal lavage may have deleterious effects on endogenous clearance mechanisms. Saline lavage may impair phagocytosis and leukocyte migration (104). Antibiotics or antiseptics in the lavage fluid may impair neutrophil chemotaxis (105) and microbicidal killing (106) and may potentiate adhesion formation (107). These data suggest a limited or potential deleterious impact of intraoperative lavage. As a result, reduction of bacterial contamination should be limited to thorough cleansing with suction and moist swabs (108).

In the setting of diffuse peritonitis, a variety of adjuvant surgical techniques have been advocated to prevent residual infection and abscess formation. Based on the theoretical arguments that fibrin deposited within the peritoneal cavity in response to bacterial contamination served as a nidus for abscess formation, Hudspeth advocated the use of radical peritoneal débridement in patients with fibrinopurulent peritonitis (109). This technique involved the meticulous débridement of fibrinous exudates off the peritoneal surface. The sole randomized study in which this technique was compared with standard techniques demonstrated no advantage to its use and, in fact, suggested a potentially deleterious effect due to the induction of hemorrhage (110).

Postoperative peritoneal lavage represents another measure designed to limit recurrent infection. At the time of operation for secondary peritonitis, drains are left *in situ*, and lavage using saline with or without antibiotics is started in the immediate postoperative period. Numerous studies have evaluated the role of postoperative peritoneal lavage in the treatment of general peritonitis (111). However, most are limited by severe flaws in study design. Nonrandomized comparative studies have generally shown improved outcome with postoperative peritoneal lavage. However, those using a prospective randomized study design were unable to confirm these encouraging results (103). The technique is extremely labor intensive, requires ICU monitoring, and is potentially complicated by the development of enteric fistulas due to catheter erosion. As a result, there appears to be no strong justification for its use at the present time. Randomized prospective studies using well-defined high risk patient population are necessary to further define its role.

In critically ill patients with significant peritoneal contamination, two additional operative approaches designed to limit recurrent intraabdominal infection have been suggested. *Scheduled* or *planned relaparotomy* is the practice of performing repeat operations at fixed intervals (24 to 72 hours) regardless of the patients clinical condition. Difficulties encountered with this approach center around the need for repeated, forceful closure of the abdominal wall in the presence of significant visceral edema. Abdominal closures under tension are at risk for dehiscence and may compromise perfusion of the abdominal wall, viscera, and kidneys as well as limit ventilation (112,113). Further, the development of abdominal compartment syndrome may compromise cardiac output and consequently tissue perfusion (114). As a result, an *open abdomen* approach has been proposed to obviate the need for abdominal closure—in effect treating the entire abdominal cavity as an abscess. Complications of this technique include evisceration, massive fluid losses, spontaneous fistulas, and contamination of the open wound. Additionally, patient sedation and mechanical ventilation are required and necessitate management in an intensive care setting.

As a result of difficulties encountered with scheduled relaparotomy and the open abdomen approach, a compromise has been reached by using various means of temporary abdominal closure. Various absorbable and nonabsorbable mesh products as well as synthetic barriers such as a sterile intravenous bag, the so-called Bogota bag, have been used. Closure with these barriers reduces the requirement for mechanical ventilation, prevents evisceration, and may lower the rate of iatrogenic fistulas. During relaparotomy, the entire abdomen should be explored manually, breaking down adhesions between loops and débriding fibrinous exudates, fluid, and necrotic debris. Additionally, frequent explorations allow for early recognition of enteric fistula, a problem that may significantly complicate management in these patients. Repeated explorations are continued until clinical sepsis has subsided, and the abdominal cavity appears clean as judged by the presence of healthy granulation tissue and adhesion formation. Nonabsorbable barriers may be removed after 7 to 9 days, once adhesions eliminate the possibility of evisceration. One major technical problem with this technique relates to an inability to explore the entire abdomen once the peritoneal surface starts to granulate and loops of bowel become adherent to each other and the abdominal wall. This problem has been circumvented by performing sequential CT scans in these patients. Inaccessible collections (usually in the subphrenic spaces) may be managed by percutaneous drainage.

A major difficulty in interpreting the efficacy of these approaches is the heterogeneous nature of intraabdominal infection. This is compounded by the lack of adequate prospective studies comparing these treatment modalities. Despite these concerns, early reports evaluating the outcome of this approach

---

TABLE 82.8. Components of the APACHE II Severity of Illness Scoring System

I—Acute physiology parameters (0; normal to 4 points; markedly abnormal)
Temperature
Mean blood pressure
Heart rate
Respiratory rate
Oxygenation
Arterial pH
Serum sodium
Serum potassium
Hematocrit
Glasgow coma scale
White blood cell count
Serum creatinine value

II—Age points

Age (yr)	Points
<44	0
45–54	2
55–64	3
65–74	5
>75	6

III—Chronic health points
If the patient has a history of severe organ system insufficiency or is immunocompromised, points are assigned as follows:
Nonoperative or emergency postoperative patients—5
Elective postoperative patients—2

APACHE II score = I + II + III

APACHE, acute physiologic assessment and chronic health evaluation.
Data from Knaus WA, Draper EA, Wagner DP, et al. APACHE II: a severity of disease classification system. *Crit Care Med* 1985;13:818–829, with permission.

---

were quite optimistic. A report by Walsh and colleagues (115) examined the use of the Marlex mesh technique in the treatment of diffuse nonlocalizing peritonitis in patients stratified using the acute physiologic assessment and chronic health evaluation (APACHE) II severity of illness scoring system (116) (Table 82.8). In patients with postoperative peritonitis, the mortality rate in patients receiving a mesh at the time of reoperation had a mortality rate that was one third that expected based on APACHE II scoring. The greatest benefit occurred in those patients with mid-range APACHE II scores, a finding confirmed in studies by Garcia-Sabrido and associates (117). More recently, in a prospective evaluation of 239 patients with severe peritonitis, there was no difference in mortality rate among patients who were treated with conventional abdominal closure, a mesh zipper, or open gauze packing (118). Based on a compilation of 642 patients from 22 series, Schein and colleagues concluded that there was insufficient evidence to recommend either open management or scheduled relaparotomy in patients with severe peritonitis (108). Additionally, the use of mesh is not without complications. In excess of 10% of patients develop fistulas as a result of small bowel perforations directly attributable to the presence of the mesh (119). One recent study suggested that scheduled repeat laparotomy may actually be detrimental to patients insofar as it was shown to induce systemic mediator response and increased organ dysfunction, ICU stay, and mortality (120). Patients were assigned prospectively in a nonrandomized fashion to be treated with either primary closure or scheduled repeat laparotomy. Both groups had comparable APACHE II scores, although the relaparotomy group tended to be sicker based on the Multiple Organ Failure Score and the Sepsis-related Organ Failure Assessment. Interestingly, even the anticipated benefit in oxygenation related to the open abdomen was not realized in this study.

PROGNOSIS

Intraabdominal abscesses are associated with rates of mortality in the range of 7% to 29% (2,92,117,121,122). This broad range reflects the heterogeneity of the patient populations described in the literature. The principal determinant of outcome relates to the severity of illness at abscess presentation—a measure easily quantitated using APACHE II scores described earlier. The risk for mortality correlates with the APACHE II score at abscess presentation (2,92,122) (Fig. 82.2). In 1980, Fry and colleagues reported a mortality rate of 32% in patients with intraabdominal abscesses (123). Organ failure, bacteremia, recurrent or multiple abscesses, and subphrenic or lesser sac abscesses were predictive of mortality. In most cases, deaths were attributed to inadequate drainage. Olson and Allen demonstrated persistent abscesses in 41% of patients at autopsy, again implicating inadequate drainage as a factor contributing to mortality (4).

Several unrandomized, retrospective studies have compared the outcomes of percutaneous and operative drainage in patients stratified by severity of illness. All demonstrate equivalent mortality rates (2,92,122). There may be a slight benefit to operative drainage in patients with APACHE II scores greater than 15, although the small number of patients in this particular study precludes any definitive conclusion (2). Deveney compared the mortality rates of patients with intraabdominal abscesses treated between 1973 and 1978 before the use of CT, ultrasound, and percutaneous drainage to patients treated between 1981 and 1986, when these modalities were available. The mortality rate dropped from 39% to 21% over this period. This reduction in mortality was accompanied by a greater proportion of patients with predrainage localization, successful initial drainage, and a decreased incidence of predrainage organ failure. There was no difference in mortality in patients in the later group treated with PAD or operation, suggesting that the reduction in mortality was due to earlier and more precise localization, rather than the particular drainage technique used (124). Duration of drainage appears to be longer in patients treated percutaneously (2,122), but this does not appear to affect the length of hospital stay (92). Most patients may be discharged from the hospital with the drainage tube in place, once evidence of systemic sepsis has abated.

SUMMARY

Intraabdominal abscesses may occur following diffuse peritonitis, after spontaneous or traumatic perforation of the gastrointestinal tract, or in the postoperative period as a result of anastomotic disruption. Abscess formation occurs as a result of the unique suppurative environment leading to bacterial proliferation and frustration of local host defenses. Diagnosis is made by abdominal imaging with either CT or ultrasonography. Drainage remains the most important intervention in facilitating abscess resolution. Percutaneous drainage is highly successful and may be carried out with either curative or palliative intent. Antimicrobial therapy is an important adjunct to drainage and should be directed against aerobic and anaerobic organisms. Intraabdominal abscesses are associated with a mortality rate of 7% to 29%, with the most important outcome predictor being the severity of illness at the time of abscess drainage.

REFERENCES

1. Altemeier WA, Culbertson WR, Fullen WD, et al. Intra-abdominal abscesses. *Am J Surg* 1973;125:70–79.
2. Levison MA, Zeigler D. Correlation of APACHE II score, drainage technique and outcome in postoperative intra-abdominal abscess. *Surg Gynecol Obstet* 1991;172:89–94.
3. Lambiase RE, Deyoe L, Cronan JJ, et al. Percutaneous drainage of 335 consecutive abscesses: results of primary drainage with 1-year follow-up. *Radiology* 1992;184:167–179.
4. Olson MM, Allen MO. Nosocomial abscess: results of an eight-year prospective study of 32,284 operations. *Arch Surg* 1989;124:356–361.
5. Field TC, Pickleman J. Intra-abdominal abscess unassociated with prior operation. *Arch Surg* 1985;120:821–824.
6. Stone HH, Kolb LD, Geheber CE. Incidence and significance of intraperitoneal anaerobic bacteria. *Ann Surg* 1975;181:705–715.
7. Moore WE, Holdeman LV. Human fecal flora: the normal flora of 20 Japanese-Hawaiians. *Appl Microbiol* 1974;27:961–979.
8. Ito Y, Kato N, Kato H, Watanabe K. Bacteriological study of 28 patients with intraabdominal infection in Japan. *J Infect Chemother* 2000;6:168–172.
9. Roehrborn A, Thomas L, Potreck O, et al. The microbiology of postoperative peritonitis. *Clin Infect Dis* 2001;33:1513–1519.
10. Gaines JD, Remington JS. Disseminated candidiasis in the surgical patient. *Surgery* 1972;72:730–736.
11. Klaerner HG, Uknis ME, Acton RD, et al. *Candida albicans* and *Escherichia coli* are synergistic pathogens during experimental microbial peritonitis. *J Surg Res* 1997;70:161–165.
12. Solomkin JS, Flohr AM, Simmons RL. Indications for therapy for fungemia in postoperative patients. *Arch Surg* 1982;117:1272–1275.
13. Tzianabos AO, Wang JY, Lee JC. Structural rationale for the modulation of abscess formation by Staphylococcus aureus capsular polysaccharides. *Proc Natl Acad Sci U S A* 2001;98:9365–9370.
14. Tzianabos AO, Onderdonk AB, Zaleznik DF, et al. Structural characteristics of polysaccharides that induce protection against intra-abdominal abscess formation. *Infect Immun* 1994;62:4881–4886.
15. Tzianabos AO, Onderdonk AB, Rosner B, et al. Structural features of polysaccharides that induce intra-abdominal abscesses. *Science* 1993;262:416–419.
16. Steinberg B. *Infections of the peritoneum*. New York: Hoeber, 1944.
17. Lanfrancone L, Boraschi D, Ghiara P, et al. Human peritoneal mesothelial cells produce many cytokines (granulocyte colony-stimulating factor [CSF], granulocyte-monocyte-CSF, macrophage-CSF, interleukin-1 [IL-1], and IL-6) and are activated and stimulated to grow by IL-1. *Blood* 1992;80:2835–2842.
18. Dunn DL, Barke RA, Ewald DC, et al. Macrophages and translymphatic absorption represent the first line of host defense of the peritoneal cavity. *Arch Surg* 1987;122:105–110.
19. Mercer-Jones MA, Shrotri MS, Heinzelmann M, et al. Regulation of early peritoneal neutrophil migration by macrophage inflammatory protein-2 and mast cells in experimental peritonitis. *J Leukoc Biol* 1999;65:249–255.
20. Gibson FC, Tzianabos AO, Onderdonk AB. The capsular polysaccharide complex of *Bacteroides fragilis* induces cytokine production from human and murine phagocytic cells. *Infect Immun* 1996;64:1065–1069.
21. Gibson FC 3rd, Onderdonk AB, Kasper DL, et al. Cellular mechanism of intraabdominal abscess formation by *Bacteroides fragilis*. *J Immunol* 1998;160:5000–5006.

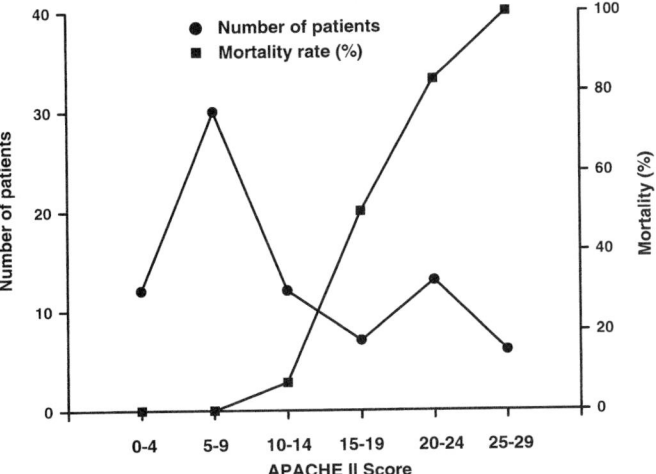

Figure 82.2. Distribution of patients and mortality with respect to acute physiologic assessment and chronic health evaluation (APACHE) II scores. Although most patients with intraabdominal abscesses have relatively low APACHE II scores, the mortality rate arises from the 10% to 20% of patients with APACHE II scores higher than 15. (Adapted from Levison MA, Zeigler D. Correlation of APACHE II score, drainage technique and outcome in postoperative intra-abdominal abscess. *Surg Gynecol Obstet* 1991;172:89, with permission.)

22. Sawyer RG, Pruett TL. Cellular mechanisms of abscess formation: macrophage procoagulant activity and major histocompatibility complex recognition. *Surgery* 1996;120:488–495.

23. Hau T, Ahrenholz DH, Simmons RL. Secondary bacterial peritonitis: the biologic basis of treatment. *Curr Probl Surg* 1979;16:1–65.

24. Rosenthal GA, Levy G, Rotstein OD. Induction of macrophage procoagulant activity by *Bacteroides fragilis*. *Infect Immun* 1989;57:338–343.

25. van Goor H, de Graaf JS, Grond J, et al. Fibrinolytic activity in the abdominal cavity of rats with faecal peritonitis. *Br J Surg* 1994;81:1046–1049.

26. van Goor H, de Graaf JS, Kooi K, et al. Effect of recombinant tissue plasminogen activator on intra-abdominal abscess formation in rats with generalized peritonitis. *J Am Coll Surg* 1994;179:407–411.

27. McRitchie DI, Girotti MJ, Glynn ME, et al. Effect of systemic fibrinogen depletion on intraabdominal abscess formation. *J Lab Clin Med* 1991;118:48–55.

28. Ciano PS, Colvin RB, Dvorak AM, et al. Macrophage migration in fibrin gel matrices. *Lab Invest* 1986;54:62–70.

29. Rotstein OD, Pruett TL, Simmons RL. Fibrin in peritonitis. V. Fibrin inhibits phagocytic killing of *Escherichia coli* by human polymorphonuclear leukocytes. *Ann Surg* 1986;203:413–419.

30. Dubrow T, Schwartz RJ, McKissock J, et al. Effect of aerosolized fibrin solution on intraperitoneal contamination. *Arch Surg* 1991;126:80–83.

31. Chapman HA Jr, Vavrin Z, Hibbs JB Jr. Coordinate expression of macrophage procoagulant and fibrinolytic activity in vitro and in vivo. *J Immunol* 1983;130:261–266.

32. Shapiro ME, Kasper DL, Zaleznik DF, et al. Cellular control of abscess formation: role of T cells in the regulation of abscesses formed in response to Bacteroides fragilis. *J Immunol* 1986;137:341–346.

33. Sawyer RG, Adams RB, May AK, et al. CD4+ T cells mediate preexposure-induced increases in murine intraabdominal abscess formation. *Clin Immunol Immunopathol* 1995;77:82–88.

34. Tzianabos AO, Russell PR, Onderdonk AB, et al. IL-2 mediates protection against abscess formation in an experimental model of sepsis. *J Immunol* 1999;163:893–897.

35. Shapiro ME, Onderdonk AB, Kasper DL, et al. Cellular immunity to *Bacteroides fragilis* capsular polysaccharide. *J Exp Med* 1982;155:1188–1197.

36. Zaleznik DF, Finberg RW, Shapiro ME, et al. A soluble suppressor T cell factor protects against experimental intraabdominal abscesses. *J Clin Invest* 1985;75:1023–1027.

37. Joiner KA, Onderdonk AB, Gelfand JA, et al. A quantitative model for subcutaneous abscess formation in mice. *Br J Exp Pathol* 1980;61:97–107.

38. Sherman NJ, Davis JR, Jesseph JE. Subphrenic abscess: a continuing hazard. *Am J Surg* 1969;117:117–123.

39. Carter R, Brewer LA. Subphrenic abscess: a thoracoabdominal clinical complex. *Am J Surg* 1964;108:165.

40. Boyd DP. The intrathoracic complications of subphrenic abscess. *J Thorac Cardiovasc Surg* 1959;38:771.

41. Crepps JT, Welch JP, Orlando R 3rd. Management and outcome of retroperitoneal abscesses. *Ann Surg* 1987;205:276–281.

42. Durning P, Schofield PF. Diagnosis and management of psoas abscess in Crohn's disease. *J R Soc Med* 1984;77:33–34.

43. Longo WE, Milsom JW, Lavery IC, et al. Pelvic abscess after colon and rectal surgery—what is optimal management? *Dis Colon Rectum* 1993;36:936–941.

44. Stone HH, Bourneuf AA, Stinson LD. Reliability of criteria for predicting persistent or recurrent sepsis. *Arch Surg* 1985;120:17–20.

45. Lennard ES, Dellinger EP, Wertz MJ, et al. Implications of leukocytosis and fever at conclusion of antibiotic therapy for intra-abdominal sepsis. *Ann Surg* 1982;195:19–24.

46. Polk HC Jr, Shields CL. Remote organ failure: a valid sign of occult intra-abdominal infection. *Surgery* 1977;81:310–313.

47. Ing AF, McLean AP, Meakins JL. Multiple-organism bacteremia in the surgical intensive care unit: a sign of intraperitoneal sepsis. *Surgery* 1981;90:779–786.

48. Fry DE, Garrison RN, Polk HC Jr. Clinical implications in *Bacteroides* bacteremia. *Surg Gynecol Obstet* 1979;149:189–192.

49. DeCrosse JJ, Poulin TL, Fox PS, et al. Subphrenic abscess. *Surg Gynecol Obstet* 1974;138:841–846.

50. Knochel JQ, Koehler PR, Lee TG, et al. Diagnosis of abdominal abscesses with computed tomography, ultrasound, and 111In leukocyte scans. *Radiology* 1980;137:425–432.

51. Taylor KJ, Wasson JF, De Graaff C, et al. Accuracy of grey-scale ultrasound diagnosis of abdominal and pelvic abscesses in 220 patients. *Lancet* 1978;1:83–84.

52. Gazelle GS, Goldberg MA, Wittenberg J, et al. Efficacy of CT in distinguishing small-bowel obstruction from other causes of small-bowel dilatation. *AJR Am J Roentgenol* 1994;162:43–47.

53. vanSonnenberg E, D'Agostino HB, Casola G, et al. US-guided transvaginal drainage of pelvic abscesses and fluid collections. *Radiology* 1991;181:53–56.

54. Bennett JD, Kozak RI, Taylor BM, et al. Deep pelvic abscesses: transrectal drainage with radiologic guidance. *Radiology* 1992;185:825–828.

55. Dobrin PB, Gully PH, Greenlee HB, et al. Radiologic diagnosis of an intra-abdominal abscess. Do multiple tests help? *Arch Surg* 1986;121:41–46.

56. Jaques P, Mauro M, Safrit H, et al. CT features of intraabdominal abscesses: prediction of successful percutaneous drainage. *AJR Am J Roentgenol* 1986;146:1041–1045.

57. Baker ME, Blinder RA, Rice RP. Diagnostic imaging of abdominal fluid collections and abscesses. *Crit Rev Diagn Imaging* 1986;25:233–278.

58. Aveline B, Guimaraes R, Bely N, et al. Intraabdominal serous fluid collections after appendectomy: a normal sonographic finding. *AJR Am J Roentgenol* 1993;161:71–73.

59. Neff CC, Simeone JF, Ferrucci JT Jr, et al. The occurrence of fluid collections following routine abdominal surgical procedures: sonographic survey in asymptomatic postoperative patients. *Radiology* 1983;146:463–466.

60. Haaga JR, Weinstein AJ. CT-guided percutaneous aspiration and drainage of abscesses. *AJR Am J Roentgenol* 1980;135:1187–1194.

61. Wong JK, Mustard R, Gray RR, et al. Predicting infection in localized intraabdominal fluid collections: value of pH and pO$_2$ measurements. *J Vasc Interv Radiol* 1999;10:421–427.

62. Barkhausen J, Stoblen F, Dominguez-Fernandez E, et al. Impact of CT in patients with sepsis of unknown origin. *Acta Radiol* 1999;40:552–555.

63. Velmahos GC, Kamel E, Berne TV, et al. Abdominal computed tomography for the diagnosis of intra-abdominal sepsis in critically injured patients: fishing in murky waters. *Arch Surg* 1999;134:831–836; discussion 836–838.

64. Korobkin M, Callen PW, Filly RA, et al. Comparison of computed tomography, ultrasonography, and gallium-67 scanning in the evaluation of suspected abdominal abscess. *Radiology* 1978;129:89–93.

65. Moir C, Robins RE. Role of ultrasonography, gallium scanning, and computed tomography in the diagnosis of intraabdominal abscess. *Am J Surg* 1982;143:582–585.

66. Hoffer P. Gallium: mechanisms. *J Nucl Med* 1980;21:282–285.

67. Dams ET, Reijnen MM, Oyen WJ, et al. Imaging experimental intraabdominal abscesses with 99mTc-PEG liposomes and 99mTc-HYNIC IgG. *Ann Surg* 1999;229:551–557.

68. Dutcher JP, Schiffer CA, Johnston GS. Rapid migration of 111indium-labeled granulocytes to sites of infection. *N Engl J Med* 1981;304:586–589.

69. Fry DE, Clevenger FW. Reoperation for intra-abdominal abscess. *Surg Clin North Am* 1991;71:159–174.

70. Wall SD, Fisher MR, Amparo EG, et al. Magnetic resonance imaging in the evaluation of abscesses. *AJR Am J Roentgenol* 1985;144:1217–1221.

71. Noone TC, Semelka RC, Worawattanakul S, et al. Intraperitoneal abscesses: diagnostic accuracy of and appearances at MR imaging. *Radiology* 1998;208:525–528.

72. Casey LC, Balk RA, Bone RC. Plasma cytokine and endotoxin levels correlate with survival in patients with the sepsis syndrome. *Ann Intern Med* 1993;119:771–778.

73. Bellomo R. The cytokine network in the critically ill. *Anaesth Intens Care* 1992;20:288–302.

74. Levy E, Frileux P, Cugnenc PH, et al. High-output external fistulae of the small bowel: management with continuous enteral nutrition. *Br J Surg* 1989;76:676–679.

75. Lewis SJ, Egger M, Sylvester PA, et al. Early enteral feeding versus "nil by mouth" after gastrointestinal surgery: systematic review and meta-analysis of controlled trials. *BMJ* 2001;323:773–776.

76. Holzheimer RG, Dralle H. Antibiotic therapy in intra-abdominal infections—a review on randomised clinical trials. *Eur J Med Res* 2001;6:277–291.

76a. Mazuski JE, Sawyer RG, Nathens AB, et al. The Surgical Infection Society guidelines on antimicrobial therapy for intra-abdominal infections: an executive summary. *Surg Infect* 2002;3:161–173.

77. Solomkin JS, Reinhart HH, Dellinger EP, et al. Results of a randomized trial comparing sequential intravenous/oral treatment with ciprofloxacin plus metronidazole to imipenem/cilastatin for intra-abdominal infections. The Intra-Abdominal Infection Study Group. *Ann Surg* 1996;223:303–315.

78. Galandiuk S, Lamos J, Montgomery W, et al. Antibiotic penetration of experimental intra-abdominal abscesses. *Am J Surg* 1995;61:521–525.

79. Bryant RE. *New dimensions in antimicrobial therapy.* New York: Churchill Livingstone, 1984.

80. Balint A, Batorfi J, Mate M, et al. Intraabdominal abscess managed successfully via the laparoscopic approach. *Surg Endosc* 2000;14:593–594.

81. Horvath KD, Kao LS, Wherry KL, et al. A technique for laparoscopic-assisted percutaneous drainage of infected pancreatic necrosis and pancreatic abscess. *Surg Endosc* 2001;15:1221–1225.

82. vanSonnenberg E, Ferrucci JT Jr, Mueller PR, et al. Percutaneous drainage of abscesses and fluid collections: technique, results, and applications. *Radiology* 1982;142:1–10.

83. Stabile BE, Puccio E, vanSonnenberg E, et al. Preoperative percutaneous drainage of diverticular abscesses. *Am J Surg* 1990;159:99–104; discussion.

84. Samelson SL, Ferguson MK. Empyema following percutaneous catheter drainage of upper abdominal abscess. *Chest* 1992;102:1612–1614.

85. Stylianos S, Martin EC, Starker PM, et al. Percutaneous drainage of intra-abdominal abscesses following abdominal trauma. *J Trauma* 1989;29:584–588.

86. Schechter S, Eisenstat TE, Oliver GC, et al. Computerized tomographic scan-guided drainage of intra-abdominal abscesses: preoperative and postoperative modalities in colon and rectal surgery. *Dis Colon Rectum* 1994;37:984–988.

87. Brolin RE, Flancbaum L, Ercoli FR, et al. Limitations of percutaneous catheter drainage of abdominal abscesses. *Surg Gynecol Obstet* 1991;173:203–210.

88. Rotstein OD. *Peritonitis and intra-abdominal abscesses.* New York: Scientific American, 1992.

89. Pruett TL, Rotstein OD, Crass J, et al. Percutaneous aspiration and drainage for suspected abdominal infection. *Surgery* 1984;96:731–737.

90. Montgomery RS, Wilson SE. Intraabdominal abscesses: image-guided diagnosis and therapy. *Clin Infect Dis* 1996;23:28–36.

91. Flancbaum L, Nosher JL, Brolin RE. Percutaneous catheter drainage of abdominal abscesses associated with perforated viscus. *Am Surg* 1990;56:52–56.

92. Hemming A, Davis NL, Robins RE. Surgical versus percutaneous drainage of intra-abdominal abscesses. *Am J Surg* 1991;161:593–595.

93. Haaga JR. Imaging intraabdominal abscesses and nonoperative drainage procedures. *World J Surg* 1990;14:204–209.

94. Gerzof SG, Johnson WC, Robbins AH, et al. Expanded criteria for percutaneous abscess drainage. *Arch Surg* 1985;120:227–232.

95. Brolin RE, Nosher JL, Leiman S, et al. Percutaneous catheter versus open surgical drainage in the treatment of abdominal abscesses. *Am Surg* 1984;50:102–108.

96. Goletti O, Lippolis PV, Chiarugi M, et al. Percutaneous ultrasound-guided drainage of intra-abdominal abscesses. *Br J Surg* 1993;80:336–339.

97. Malangoni MA, Shumate CR, Thomas HA, et al. Factors influencing the treatment of intra-abdominal abscesses. *Am J Surg* 1990;159:167–171.

98. Rotstein OD, Pruett TL, Simmons RL. Microbiologic features and treatment of persistent peritonitis in patients in the intensive care unit. *Can J Surg* 1986;29:247–250.

99. Nathens AB, Rotstein OD, Marshall JC. Tertiary peritonitis: clinical features of a complex nosocomial infection. *World J Surg* 1998;22:158–163.

100. Sawyer RG, Rosenlof LK, Adams RB, et al. Peritonitis into the 1990s: changing pathogens and changing strategies in the critically ill. *Am Surg* 1992;58:82–87.

101. Schrock TR, Deveney CW, Dunphy JE. Factor contributing to leakage of colonic anastomoses. *Ann Surg* 1973;177:513–518.

102. Jimenez MF, Marshall JC. Source control in the management of sepsis. *Intensive Care Med* 2001;27[Suppl 1]:S49–62.

103. Schein M, Gecelter G, Freinkel W, et al. Peritoneal lavage in abdominal sepsis: a controlled clinical study. *Arch Surg* 1990;125:1132–1135.

104. Dunn DL, Simmons RL. The role of anaerobic bacteria in intraabdominal infections. *Rev Infect Dis* 1984;6[Suppl 1]:S139–S146.

105. Majeski JA, McClellan MA, Alexander JW. Evaluation of leukocyte chemotactic response in the presence of antibiotics. *Surg Forum* 1975;26:83–85.

106. Hansbrough JF, Zapata-Sirvent RL, Cooper ML. Effects of topical antimicrobial agents on the human neutrophil respiratory burst. *Arch Surg* 1991;126:603–608.

107. Rappaport WD, Holcomb M, Valente J, et al. Antibiotic irrigation and the formation of intraabdominal adhesions. *Am J Surg* 1989;158:435–437.

108. Schein M, Hirshberg A, Hashmonai M. Current surgical management of severe intraabdominal infection. *Surgery* 1992;112:489–496.

109. Hudspeth AS. Radical surgical debridement in the treatment of advanced generalized bacterial peritonitis. *Arch Surg* 1975;110:1233–1236.

110. Polk HC Jr, Fry DE. Radical peritoneal debridement for established peritonitis: the results of a prospective randomized clinical trial. *Ann Surg* 1980;192:350–355.

111. Leiboff AR, Soroff HS. The treatment of generalized peritonitis by closed postoperative peritoneal lavage: a critical review of the literature. *Arch Surg* 1987;122:1005–1010.

112. Richards WO, Scovill W, Shin B, et al. Acute renal failure associated with increased intra-abdominal pressure. *Ann Surg* 1983;197:183–187.

113. Richardson JD, Trinkle JK. Hemodynamic and respiratory alterations with increased intra-abdominal pressure. *J Surg Res* 1976;20:401–404.

114. Nathens AB, Brenneman FD, Boulanger BR. The abdominal compartment syndrome. *Can J Surg* 1997;40:254–258.

115. Walsh GL, Chiasson P, Hedderich G, et al. The open abdomen: the Marlex mesh and zipper technique: a method of managing intraperitoneal infection. *Surg Clin North Am* 1988;68:25–40.

116. Knaus WA, Draper EA, Wagner DP, et al. APACHE II: a severity of disease classification system. *Crit Care Med* 1985;13:818–829.

117. Garcia-Sabrido JL, Tallado JM, Christou NV, et al. Treatment of severe intra-abdominal sepsis and/or necrotic foci by an 'open-abdomen' approach: zipper and zipper-mesh techniques. *Arch Surg* 1988;123:152–156.

118. Christou NV, Barie PS, Dellinger EP, et al. Surgical Infection Society intra-abdominal infection study: prospective evaluation of management techniques and outcome. *Arch Surg* 1993;128:193–198.

119. Mastboom WJ, Kuypers HH, Schoots FJ, et al. Small-bowel perforation complicating the open treatment of generalized peritonitis. *Arch Surg* 1989;124:689–692.

120. Zugel N, Siebeck M, Geissler B, et al. Circulating mediators and organ function in patients undergoing planned relaparotomy vs conventional surgical therapy in severe secondary peritonitis. *Arch Surg* 2002;137:590–599.

121. Mughal MM, Bancewicz J, Irving MH. 'Laparostomy': a technique for the management of intractable intra-abdominal sepsis. *Br J Surg* 1986;73:253–259.

122. Olak J, Christou NV, Stein LA, et al. Operative vs percutaneous drainage of intra-abdominal abscesses. Comparison of morbidity and mortality. *Arch Surg* 1986;121:141–146.

123. Fry DE, Garrison RN, Heitsch RC, et al. Determinants of death in patients with intraabdominal abscess. *Surgery* 1980;88:517–523.

124. Deveney CW, Lurie K, Deveney KE. Improved treatment of intra-abdominal abscess: a result of improved localization, drainage, and patient care, not technique. *Arch Surg* 1988;123:1126–1130.

125. Rotstein OD, Fiegel VD, Simmons RL, et al. The deleterious effect of reduced pH and hypoxia on neutrophil migration in vitro. *J Surg Res* 1988;45:298–303.

126. Mandell GL. Bactericidal activity of aerobic and anaerobic polymorphonuclear neutrophils. *Infect Immun* 1974;9:337–341.

127. Knighton DR, Halliday B, Hunt TK. Oxygen as an antibiotic: the effect of inspired oxygen on infection. *Arch Surg* 1984;119:199–204.

128. Simchowitz L. Intracellular pH modulates the generation of superoxide radicals by human neutrophils. *J Clin Invest* 1985;76:1079–1089.

129. Liberek T, Topley N, Jorres A, et al. Peritoneal dialysis fluid inhibition of phagocyte function: effects of osmolality and glucose concentration. *J Am Soc Nephrol* 1993;3:1508–1515.

130. Tonetti M, Cavallero A, Botta GA, et al. Intracellular pH regulates the production of different oxygen metabolites in neutrophils: effects of organic acids produced by anaerobic bacteria. *J Leukoc Biol* 1991;49:180–188.

131. Hampton MB, Chambers ST, Vissers MC, et al. Bacterial killing by neutrophils in hypertonic environments. *J Infect Dis* 1994;169:839–846.

132. Kazilek CJ, Merkle CJ, Chandler DE. Hyperosmotic inhibition of calcium signals and exocytosis in rabbit neutrophils. *Am J Physiol* 1988;254:C709–C718.

133. Simchowitz L, Cragoe EJ Jr. Regulation of human neutrophil chemotaxis by intracellular pH. *J Biol Chem* 1986;261:6492–6500.

134. Rotstein OD, Pruett TL, Simmons RL. Mechanisms of microbial synergy in polymicrobial surgical infections. *Rev Infect Dis* 1985;7:151–170.

135. Sawyer RG, Spengler MD, Adams RB, et al. The peritoneal environment during infection: the effect of monomicrobial and polymicrobial bacteria on pO2 and pH. *Ann Surg* 1991;213:253–260.

136. Howard RJ. *Surgical infectious disease,* 2nd ed. Norwalk, CT: Appleton & Lange, 1988.

137. Finlay-Jones JJ, Kenny PA, Nulsen MF, et al. Pathogenesis of intra-abdominal abscess formation: abscess-potentiating agents and inhibition of complement-dependent opsonization of abscess-inducing bacteria. *J Infect Dis* 1991;164:1173–1179.

138. Yamada Y, Hefter K, Burke JF, et al. An in vitro model of the wound microenvironment: local phagocytic cell abnormalities associated with in situ complement activation. *J Infect Dis* 1987;155:998–1004.

139. Pruett TL, Rotstein OD, Fiegel VD, et al. Mechanism of the adjuvant effect of hemoglobin in experimental peritonitis. VIII. A leukotoxin is produced by *Escherichia coli* metabolism in hemoglobin. *Surgery* 1984;96:375–383.

140. Yamamura M, Nishi M, Furubayashi H, et al. Barium peritonitis: report of a case and review of the literature. *Dis Colon Rectum* 1985;28:347–352.

141. Cho J, Rotstein OD, Pruett TL. The adjuvant effect of bile salts in experimental peritonitis. *Surg Forum* 1984;35:231.

142. Hill GB. Enhancement of experimental anaerobic infections by blood, hemoglobin, and hemostatic agents. *Infect Immun* 1978;19:443–449.

143. Zimmerli W, Waldvogel FA, Vaudaux P, et al. Pathogenesis of foreign body infection: description and characteristics of an animal model. *J Infect Dis* 1982;146:487–497.

144. Zimmerli W, Lew PD, Waldvogel FA. Pathogenesis of foreign body infection. Evidence for a local granulocyte defect. *J Clin Invest* 1984;73:1191–1200.

145. Gallinaro RN, Naziri W, McMasters KM, et al. Alteration of mononuclear cell immune-associated antigen expression, interleukin-1 expression, and antigen presentation during intra-abdominal infection. *Shock* 1994;1:130–134.

146. Vestweber KH, Grundel E. Efficacy and safety of piperacillin/tazobactam in intra-abdominal infections. *Eur J Surg Suppl* 1994;57–60.

147. Results of the North American trial of piperacillin/tazobactam compared with clindamycin and gentamicin in the treatment of severe intra-abdominal infections. Investigators of the Piperacillin/Tazobactam Intra-abdominal Infection Study Group. *Eur J Surg Suppl* 1994:61–66.

148. Yellin AE, Hassett JM, Fernandez A, et al. Ertapenem monotherapy versus combination therapy with ceftriaxone plus metronidazole for treatment of complicated intra-abdominal infections in adults. *Int J Antimicrob Agents* 2002;20:165–173.

149. Sitges-Serra A, Guirao X, Diaz J, et al. [Prospective randomized trial of meropenem versus cefotaxime and metronidazole in the treatment of intraabdominal infections]. *Med Clin (Barc)* 1998;111:88–91.

150. Lowe MN, Lamb HM. Meropenem: an updated review of its use in the management of intra-abdominal infections. *Drugs* 2000;60:619–646.

151. Walker AP, Nichols RL, Wilson RF, et al. Efficacy of a beta-lactamase inhibitor combination for serious intraabdominal infections. *Ann Surg* 1993;217:115–121.

152. Bumgardner GL, Simmons RL. Newer cephalosporins: lessons to be learned from clinical trials in intraabdominal infections. *Am J Surg* 1988;155:5–10.

153. Wilson SE, Boswick JA Jr, Duma RJ, et al. Cephalosporin therapy in intraabdominal infections: a multicenter randomized, comparative study of cefotetan, moxalactam, and cefoxitin. *Am J Surg* 1988;155:61–66.

154. Schentag JJ. Cefmetazole sodium: pharmacology, pharmacokinetics, and clinical trials. *Pharmacotherapy* 1991;11:2–19.

155. Bohnen JM, Solomkin JS, Dellinger EP, et al. Guidelines for clinical care: anti-infective agents for intra-abdominal infection: a Surgical Infection Society policy statement. *Arch Surg* 1992;127:83–89.

156. Cohn SM, Lipsett PA, Buchman TG, et al. Comparison of intravenous/oral ciprofloxacin plus metronidazole versus piperacillin/tazobactam in the treatment of complicated intraabdominal infections. *Ann Surg* 2000;232:254–262.

157. Barie PS, Vogel SB, Dellinger EP, et al. A randomized, double-blind clinical trial comparing cefepime plus metronidazole with imipenem-cilastatin in the treatment of complicated intra-abdominal infections. Cefepime Intra-abdominal Infection Study Group. *Arch Surg* 1997;132:1294–1302.

158. Shyr YM, Lui WY, Su CH, et al. Piperacillin/tazobactam in comparison with clindamycin plus gentamicin in the treatment of intra-abdominal infections. *Zhonghua Yi Xue Za Zhi (Taipei)* 1995;56:102–108.

159. Condon RE, Walker AP, Sirinek KR, et al. Meropenem versus tobramycin plus clindamycin for treatment of intraabdominal infections: results of a prospective, randomized, double-blind clinical trial. *Clin Infect Dis* 1995;21:544–550.

160. Ballow CH, Wels PB, Welage LS, et al. A double-blind, randomized comparison of aztreonam plus clindamycin with tobramycin plus clindamycin in abdominal infections. *Am J Ther* 1995;2:373–377.

CHAPTER 83
Appendicitis

Gordon L. Telford, John A. Weigelt, and
Robert E. Condon

Appendicitis can occur at any age; it accounts for about 1% of all surgical operations (1). Although rare in infants, appendicitis becomes increasingly common throughout childhood, reaching its maximal frequency between the ages of 10 and 30 years.

PATHOPHYSIOLOGY

Obstruction followed by infection is the most likely pathogenesis of appendicitis (2,3). The appendiceal lumen first becomes obstructed by hyperplasia of submucosal lymphoid follicles, fecalith, foreign body, stricture, tumor, pinworms (*Enterobius vermicularis*), or other pathologic state. Once it is obstructed, mucus accumulates within the lumen of the appendix, and intraluminal pressure increases. The accumulated mucus is converted into pus by luminal bacteria; continued secretion, combined with the relative inelasticity of the serosa, leads to a further increase in pressure in the lumen. Lymphatic obstruction ensues, leading to edema, diapedesis of bacteria, and mucosal ulceration. Continued secretion results in a further rise in intraluminal pressure, leading to venous obstruction, increasing edema, and ischemia of the appendix, and acute suppurative appendicitis ensues.

Progression of this pathologic process results in venous and arterial thromboses in the wall of the appendix and gangrenous appendicitis. The final stage in the progression of acute appendicitis is perforation through a gangrenous infarct and spilling of accumulated pus.

MICROBIOLOGY

The flora of the lumen of the appendix is that of the lumen of the colon, a mixture of aerobic and anaerobic organisms (4). The flora cultured from infections resulting from acute appendicitis is representative of the flora of the lumen of the appendix (Table 83.1). More than 90% of wound infections resulting from an episode of acute appendicitis are polymicrobial; most commonly, five different species of bacteria are cultured. In order of prevalence, bacterial isolates include *Bacteroides* species, *Escherichia coli*, other gram-negative aerobes, and anaerobic and aerobic streptococci.

SYMPTOMS

Although the symptom history varies, the cardinal symptoms of acute appendicitis are usually present (1,5). The symptoms usually begin with epigastric or periumbilical abdominal pain, followed by anorexia and nausea. Vomiting, if it occurs, appears next. After a variable time, usually about 8 hours, the pain becomes localized to the right side and usually into the right lower quadrant.

Pain

Acute appendicitis typically begins with diffuse, central, minimally severe visceral pain. This is followed in 8 hours by somatic pain that is more severe and usually well localized to the right lower quadrant. Atypical pain that does not follow the classic visceral-somatic sequence is common in acute appendicitis, however, occurring in up to 45% of patients. Atypical pain, while it is localized to the right lower quadrant, may remain visceral. Conversely, the pain may never become localized. Atypical pain is found more frequently in older patients.

Patients with high retrocecal appendicitis may present with only diffuse pain in the right flank. Similarly, patients whose entire appendix is within the true pelvis may never develop somatic pain and, instead, may have tenesmus and vague discomfort in the suprapubic area.

Anorexia, Nausea, and Vomiting

Anorexia and nausea are present in almost all cases of acute appendicitis. The presence or absence of vomiting should not be a criterion for the diagnosis of appendicitis. When vomiting does occur, it is not persistent and begins after the onset of pain with such regularity that if it antedates pain, the diagnosis of appendicitis should be questioned. If vomiting is persistent, the diagnosis should also be questioned.

Constipation and Diarrhea

A history of constipation or diarrhea of recent onset is not exceptionally helpful in the diagnosis of appendicitis.

PHYSICAL EXAMINATION

Typical physical signs of acute appendicitis include localized tenderness, muscle guarding, and rebound tenderness. Cutaneous hyperesthesia, right-sided pelvic tenderness on rectal examination, and the presence of a psoas or obturator sign are less common and tend to be dependent on the examiner. Although a normal temperature is often present, temperature up to 38°C occurs, but in the typical case of appendicitis, high fever is uncommon.

If the appendix ruptures, the physical findings change. If the infection is contained, the patient often develops a soft, tender mass in the right lower quadrant, and the area of tenderness now encompasses the entire right lower quadrant. Involuntary guarding becomes evident and rebound tenderness more marked. The patient's temperature is more like that seen with abscess formation and may rise to 39°C and be associated with tachycardia.

If appendiceal rupture fails to localize, the patient develops the signs and symptoms of diffuse peritonitis. Tenderness and guarding become generalized, the temperature remains above 38°C and spikes to 40°C, and the pulse rises above 100 beats per minute.

Tenderness and Muscle Guarding

On routine abdominal examination, an area of maximal tenderness is often elicited in the area of the McBurney point. In high retrocecal appendicitis, tenderness may occur over a large area, and there may be no signs of muscle spasm. In pelvic appendicitis, neither sign may be present. Both signs are often absent or minimal in aged persons.

Signs of peritoneal inflammation or irritation in the right lower quadrant are also helpful in the diagnosis. Coughing or bouncing on the heels produces this type of pain. Rebound tenderness and muscle guarding can usually be elicited. Rovsing's sign, pain elicited in the right lower quadrant by palpation

TABLE 83.1. Relative Prevalence of Bacterial Flora of the Appendix

Aerobes	Percentage	Anaerobes	Percentage
Escherichia coli	80	*Bacteroides fragilis* group	89
Klebsiella-Enterobacter species	57	Other *Bacteroides* species	25
Enterococcus faecalis group	26	Streptococci	64
Other gram-positive cocci	8	Clostridia	13
Other aerobes	43	Other anaerobes	41
No growth	1	No growth	4

Data from the Surgical Microbiology Research Laboratory, Medical College of Wisconsin, Milwaukee, Wisconsin, 1990.

pressure in the left lower quadrant, is another type of rebound tenderness and can be present in acute appendicitis.

Abdominal Mass

As the disease process progresses, it may be possible to palpate a tender mass in the right lower quadrant. Although the mass may be due to an abscess, it can also result from adherence of the omentum and loops of intestine to an inflamed appendix.

Rectal Examination

Rectal examination, although essential for all patients in whom appendicitis is suspected, is helpful only in those few whose appendix lies almost wholly within the pelvis. In these patients, a thorough rectal examination may be the only way to elicit tenderness.

LABORATORY TESTS

Laboratory tests have little value in the early diagnosis of acute appendicitis. Up to one third of patients, particularly older ones (6), have a normal total leukocyte count with acute appendicitis (1,7). The differential white cell count often reveals a shift to the left with an increase in the percentage of polymorphonuclear neutrophils (7). In considering the diagnosis of appendicitis, clinical findings take precedence over the white cell count or other laboratory observations when they are at variance.

The urinalysis is helpful in the differential diagnosis of patients with lower abdominal pain only when it reveals that a urinary tract lesion is causing the symptoms. Patients with advanced appendicitis and abscess formation or generalized peritonitis may have abnormal results of liver function tests.

RADIOLOGIC EXAMINATION

Abdominal radiographs are seldom helpful in the diagnosis of acute appendicitis, except when they demonstrate a fecalith or exclude other diagnoses such as acute cholecystitis, perforated duodenal ulcer, perforated colon cancer, and acute diverticulitis. Cecal distention or a sentinel loop of distended small intestine in the right lower quadrant is frequently present in appendicitis.

A mass can often be demonstrated extrinsic to the cecum late in the course of appendicitis. There may be scoliosis to the right, absence of the right psoas shadow, and signs of edema of the abdominal wall. With late appendicitis and generalized peritonitis, there will be an ileus pattern with generalized gas throughout the small and large intestines.

Barium enema examination, although not indicated in cases in which the diagnosis of acute appendicitis is evident on clinical grounds, can be helpful in some situations (8,9). It can be helpful in young women, in whom the diagnosis is still in question after observation and in whom the negative laparotomy rate is high. It can also be helpful in patients with a debilitating systemic disease such as leukemia, for whom the operative risk is markedly increased. Findings of significance on barium enema examination are nonfilling or partial filling of the appendix and an extrinsic defect on the cecum (the reversed-three sign) (9,10).

An experienced radiologist is able to diagnose acute appendicitis using ultrasonography with an accuracy greater than 90% (11–13). Appendicitis is diagnosed if the maximal cross-sectional diameter of the appendix exceeds 6 mm, if the appendix is noncompressible, if an appendicolith is present, or if a complex mass is demonstrated. Other criteria that are not universally agreed on include rigidity and nonmobility. Nonvisualization of the appendix is not a criterion for appendicitis. More prospective studies are necessary to identify the most appropriate criteria for the ultrasound diagnosis of acute appendicitis. Ultrasonography is also useful in the diagnosis of perforated appendicitis with abscess formation.

Although more expensive, computed tomography (CT) has been demonstrated to be effective in the diagnosis of acute appendicitis with an accuracy greater than 90% (14,15). The cost can be reduced by performing a limited, unenhanced CT scan with no significant loss in diagnostic accuracy (14). Appendicitis is diagnosed when the appendix is thickened with a diameter greater than 6 mm and there are inflammatory changes in the periappendiceal fat (streaking and poorly defined increased attenuation) (14–16). Both the presence of pericecal inflammation without an inflamed appendix and an appendicolith without the presence of periappendiceal inflammation are insufficient to diagnose acute appendicitis.

ACUTE APPENDICITIS IN INFANTS AND YOUNG CHILDREN

The diagnosis of acute appendicitis can be difficult in this age group. The patient is usually unable to give an accurate history. Appendicitis is uncommon, and acute nonspecific abdominal pain is common in infants and children. Because of such factors, diagnosis and treatment are delayed, and complications develop (17). The suspicion of appendicitis is often not aroused until the appendix has ruptured and the child is obviously ill (18). Two thirds of young children with appendicitis have symptoms for more than 3 days before appendectomy (17). Vomiting, fever, irritability, flexing of the thighs, and diarrhea are likely early signs. Abdominal distention is the most consistent physical finding. As in adults, the total leukocyte count is not a reliable test.

The frequency of perforation in infants younger than 1 year of age is almost 100%, and although it decreases with age, it is still 50% at age 5 years. The mortality rate in this age group remains as high as 5% because of the aforementioned factors.

APPENDICITIS IN YOUNG WOMEN

Whereas the overall frequency of "negative laparotomy" in patients suspected of having appendicitis is as high as 20%, the frequency in women younger than 30 years of age is as high as 45%. Most the misdiagnoses are accounted for by pain associated with ovulation; diseases of the ovaries, tubes, and uterus; and urinary tract infections (cystitis). If a young woman has atypical pain, muscle guarding in the right lower quadrant is absent, and there is no fever, leukocytosis, or leftward shift in the differential white cell count, then it is best to observe the patient and to perform frequent reexaminations. If the patient's signs and symptoms remain stable after several hours, it is appropriate to perform a barium enema examination or a CT scan.

APPENDICITIS DURING PREGNANCY

The risk for appendicitis during pregnancy is the same as in nonpregnant women of the same age; the frequency is 1 in every 2,000 pregnancies. Appendicitis occurs more often during the first two trimesters, during which period the symptoms are similar to those seen in nonpregnant women (13). Surgery should be performed during pregnancy when appendicitis is suspected just as it would be in a nonpregnant woman. As in nonpregnant patients, the effects of a negative laparotomy are minor, whereas the effects of ruptured appendicitis can be catastrophic. If peritonitis and sepsis ensue, the infant mortality rate, due both to prematurity and to the effects of sepsis, increases.

The mortality rate for appendicitis during pregnancy is due mainly to delay in diagnosis. In the final analysis, early appendectomy is the appropriate therapy in suspected appendicitis during all stages of pregnancy (19).

APPENDICITIS IN ELDERLY PERSONS

Appendicitis has a much greater mortality rate among elderly people than among young adults. The increased risk appears to be due both to delay in seeking medical care and to delay in making the diagnosis (20,21). Elderly persons have the classic symptoms, but they are often less pronounced. Right lower quadrant pain localizes later and may be milder. On initial physical examination, the findings are often minimal, although right lower quadrant tenderness eventually develops (22). Distention of the abdomen and a clinical picture suggestive of small bowel obstruction are commonly seen. More than 30% of elderly patients have a ruptured appendix at the time of operation (22).

DIFFERENTIAL DIAGNOSIS

When the classic symptoms of appendicitis are present, the diagnosis is usually made easily and is seldom missed. It is most im-portant to rule out diseases that do not require operative therapy and can be made worse by operation, for example, pancreatitis, myocardial infarction, and basilar pneumonia.

The diseases in young children that are most frequently mistaken for acute appendicitis are gastroenteritis, *Yersinia enterocolitica* enterocolitis and associated mesenteric lymphadenitis, Meckel's diverticulitis, pyelitis, small intestinal intussusception, enteric duplication, and basilar pneumonia.

In teenagers and young adults, the differential diagnosis is different for men and women. In young women, it includes diseases of the ovaries and tubes, such as ruptured ectopic pregnancy, mittelschmerz, endometriosis, and salpingitis (23); chronic constipation also needs to be considered. In young men, the differential diagnosis is smaller and includes the acute onset of regional enteritis, right-sided renal or ureteral calculus, torsion of the testes, and acute epididymitis. In both young men and young women, *Y. enterocolitica* enterocolitis and associated mesenteric lymphadenitis should be considered.

In older persons, the differential diagnosis of acute appendicitis includes diverticulitis, perforated peptic ulcer, acute cholecystitis, acute pancreatitis, intestinal obstruction, perforated cecal carcinoma, mesenteric vascular occlusion, rupturing aortic aneurysm, and the disease entities mentioned before for young adults. Although rare, amebic infection of the cecum with cecal dilation can mimic appendicitis. Because it can cause leukocytosis, fever, nausea, vomiting, and abdominal cramps, *Salmonella* species infection can also mimic appendicitis and must be considered in patients with diarrhea who report that other family members or friends have gastroenteritis.

TREATMENT

Preoperative Preparation

It is not necessary to rush a patient with a presumed diagnosis of acute appendicitis directly to the operating room. All patients, especially those with a presumed diagnosis of peritonitis, should be adequately prepared and then taken to the operating room. Patients with a palpable right lower quadrant mass may be managed initially without operation (24).

Intravenous fluid replacement should be initiated and the patient resuscitated. Once urine output reaches acceptable levels (more than 30 mL per hour), it can be assumed that resuscitation is complete. Nasogastric suction is helpful for patients with peritonitis and a profound ileus. If the patient's body temperature is greater than 39°C, measures should be taken to reduce fever before beginning an operation.

Antibiotic Therapy

Before antibiotics were available, the mortality rate for acute appendicitis was in the range of 8% to 15%. Today, it is less than 1%. Although other factors are involved, antibiotic therapy is a major factor in improving the mortality rate.

The risk for an infectious complication becomes greater as the state of the appendix worsens. The frequency of wound infection after removal of a normal appendix or an appendix in the early stages of appendicitis is in the range of 5% to 10%. The risk increases by threefold or fourfold with gangrene and to one of every two patients with perforation.

More than 100 clinical trials have now been conducted at a number of institutions to measure the efficacy of antibiotics in appendicitis. The results of these studies clearly indicate that antibiotics decrease infectious complications for all stages of appendicitis so that a preoperative "single shot" of an efficacious antibiotic regimen is indicated in every patient having an operation for suspected appendicitis. The same cannot be said for the use of antimicrobial and antiseptic solutions to irrigate the abdominal cavity and the wound. Few studies in which irrigants were used have demonstrated reduction of the infection rate.

Infections resulting from acute appendicitis are polymicrobial, and aerobe–anaerobe synergy plays a pathogenic role. An antibiotic that is active against both aerobes and anaerobes is needed. A large number of antibiotics and antibiotic combinations have been demonstrated to be effective. These include second-generation cephalosporins (cefoxitin, cefotetan), third-generation cephalosporins (ceftazidime, ceftizoxime) combined with an antianaerobe agent (metronidazole, clindamycin), the expanded-spectrum penicillins combined with β-lactamase inhibitors (ampicillin-sulbactam, ticarcillin clavulanate), aztreonam plus clindamycin, and doxycycline as well as the traditional but now outmoded aminoglycoside-antianaerobe and "triple-antibiotic" combinations. Although all of these antibiotic regimens are effective, current recommendations emphasize single-agent coverage for uncomplicated infections. For mild to moderate infections, ampicillin-sulbactam (3 g every 6 hours) or cefoxitin (2 g every 8 hours) is recommended. The risk for enterococcal infection makes a penicillin more desirable then a broad-spectrum cephamycin. In severe infections, single-agent coverage is still feasible with the carbapenems. Imipenem-cilastatin is one option (750 mg every 12 hours). The use of double and triple antimicrobial coverage for infections with appendicitis is not recommended.

All patients suspected of having acute appendicitis should receive antibiotics once a decision is made to proceed with operative therapy. If the appendicitis is uncomplicated or if the diagnosis is incorrect, antibiotics are discontinued.

Antibiotics should be continued postoperatively as the clinical condition indicates in patients who have a gangrenous or ruptured appendix and localized or generalized peritonitis. This often entails treatment for a week or so. More important is the selection of an end point for therapy; we stop giving antibiotics when the white cell count is normal with a normal differential count, the temperature has not been elevated for 24 hours, and the patient is taking food without problems. If these conditions have not been achieved by the tenth postoperative day, CT for an abdominal or pelvic abscess may be appropriate. Antibiotic therapy should be changed or stopped, depending on the clinical circumstances.

Examination under Anesthesia

After the induction of anesthesia, the patient's abdomen should be palpated systematically. Such an examination may, on occasion, demonstrate other disease to be the cause of the patient's symptoms, such as acute cholecystitis. It may also be possible to palpate an appendiceal mass that will confirm the suspected diagnosis.

Uncomplicated Appendicitis without a Palpable Mass

When the diagnosis of uncomplicated acute appendicitis has been made, appendectomy should be performed as an emergency procedure. The earlier the diagnosis is made and the sooner the appendectomy is performed, the better is the prognosis. Uncomplicated appendectomy should have a surgical mor-

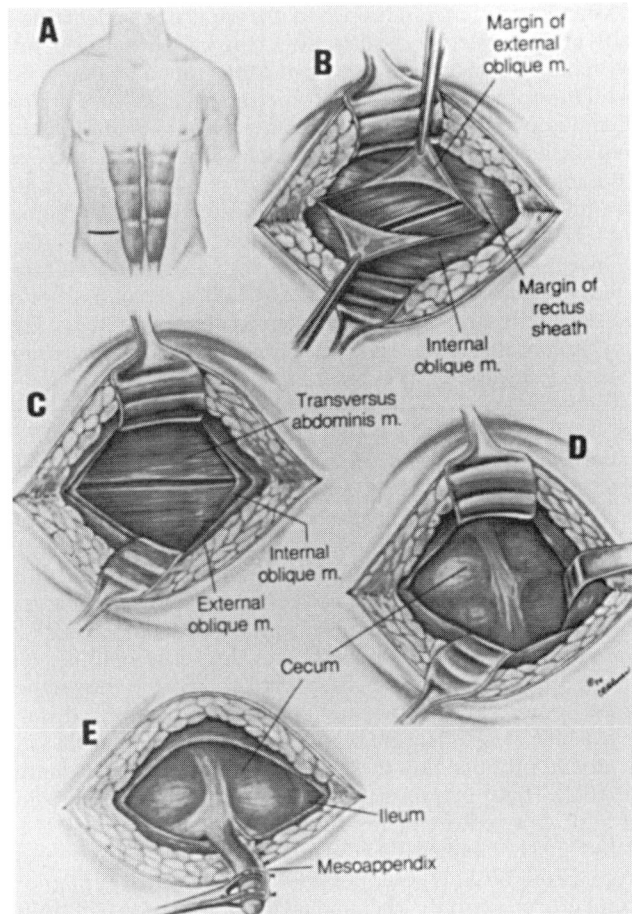

Figure 83.1. Steps in performing an appendectomy through a transverse incision. **A:** Placement of the skin incision. **B, C:** External and internal oblique and transversus abdominis muscles are divided in the direction of their fibers. **D:** After incision of the peritoneum, the cecum is exposed, and the appendix is located by following the anterior cecal taenia inferiorly. **E:** The cecum is mobilized into the wound by incising its lateral peritoneal reflections. (From Condon RE. Appendicitis. In: Moody FG, Carey LC, Jones RS, et al., eds. *Surgical treatment of digestive diseases.* Chicago: Year Book Medical Publishers, 1986, with permission.)

tality rate of less than 0.1%. In contrast, the mortality rate for ruptured appendicitis can be as high as 10%.

The recommended incision for a routine appendectomy is a transverse incision (Rockey-Davis, Fowler-Weir-Mitchell; Fig. 83.1). Exposure of the appendix through this incision is much better than that obtained through the classic McBurney incision, particularly in patients who have a retrocecal appendix or are obese.

The gridiron, or muscle-splitting, incision (McBurney incision) is the one most widely used for uncomplicated appendicitis, largely because of surgical tradition rather than its particular utility. The exposure through a McBurney incision can be awkward, especially for a retrocecal appendix, unless the appendix lies immediately below the incision. If necessary, the incision can be extended medially, partially transecting the rectus sheath, but this maneuver is usually helpful only for a pelvic appendix.

If the diagnosis of acute appendicitis is in doubt and exploratory laparotomy is indicated, a vertical midline incision is appropriate. If an appendiceal mass is encountered, the midline incision can be closed and a more direct approach to the lesion made through a right lower quadrant incision.

After the peritoneum is opened, the appendix is identified by following the anterior cecal taenia to the base of the appendix. The inflamed appendix is coaxed into the wound by gentle traction. If the appendix is retrocecal or retroperitoneal, or if the local inflammation and edema are intense, exposure is improved by dividing the lateral peritoneal reflection of the cecum. At the end of the maneuver, the cecum should lie within the wound, and the appendix should be at the level of the anterior abdominal wall (Fig. 83.1).

Once the appendix has been freed, the mesoappendix is transected, beginning at its free border by taking small bites of the mesoappendix between pairs of hemostats placed about 1 cm from and parallel to the appendix. This process is repeated until the base of the appendix is reached.

There are three ways to handle the appendiceal stump: simple ligation, inversion, and a combination of the two. Either simple ligation or inversion is acceptable, and both have comparable rates of complications. The combination of ligation and inversion is not recommended because it does not reduce the risk for septic complications (25) but does create conditions conducive to development of an intramural abscess or a mucocele. Also, the ligated and inverted appendiceal stump can appear later as a cecal "tumor," a source of diagnostic difficulties in the future (26).

Simple ligature of the appendiceal stump is accomplished by crushing the appendix at its base with a hemostat, then removing the hemostat and replacing it on the appendix just distal to the crushed line. A ligature of monofilament suture is placed in the groove produced by the crushing clamp and is tied tightly (Fig. 83.2). The appendix is transected just proximal to the hemostat and removed. Inversion of an unligated stump using a Z stitch (Fig. 83.3), rather than the more conventional purse-string suture, is preferred. The upper level of the Z stitch is placed as a Lembert suture in the cecum, just distal to the base of the appendix. The suture is brought around the base of the appendix and continued as a second Lembert suture beneath the base of the appendix.

The appendix is transected between clamps; the stump is inverted into the cecum; the proximal clamp is removed; and the ends of the Z stitch are tied over the stump of the appendix, which is not ligated. If the appendiceal stump is unsuitable for inversion because of edema, it should be simply ligated and not inverted.

Laparoscopy has gained acceptance in the diagnosis and treatment of acute appendicitis (27). If uncomplicated appendicitis is encountered at the time of laparoscopy, an appendectomy can be

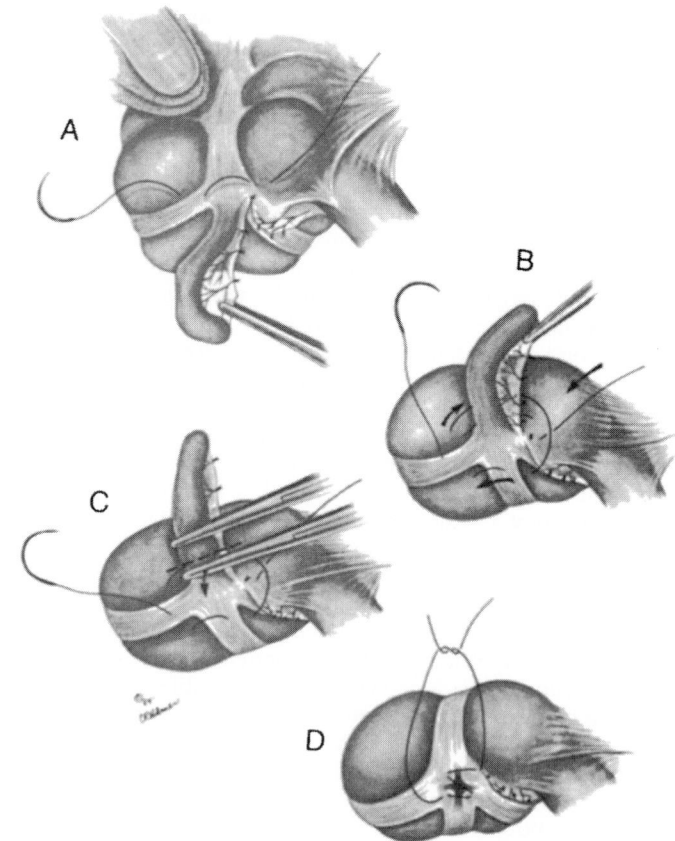

Figure 83.3. Use of a Z stitch to invert the unligated appendiceal stump. **A:** Two bites of the suture are placed in the cecum 1 cm distal to the base of the appendix. **B:** The suture is then brought around the appendix medially, and two additional bites are placed beneath the base of the appendix. **C:** The appendix is then transected. **D:** The stump of the appendix is inverted into the cecum, and the clamp is removed as the suture is tightened. (From Adams JT. Z stitch suture for inversion of the appendiceal stump. *Surg Gynecol Obstet* 1968;127:1321, with permission of *Surgery, Gynecology & Obstetrics*, now known as the journal of the *American College of Surgeons*.)

performed with relative ease. If a normal appendix is encountered, the abdomen can be examined with the laparoscope, thus avoiding a large abdominal incision.

Perforated or Gangrenous Appendicitis with a Periappendiceal Mass

When a mass is detected by examination under anesthesia that was not appreciated preoperatively, a transverse incision is made over the most prominent portion of the mass. The muscles and aponeuroses are split along their lines of cleavage in gridiron fashion. If the peritoneal cavity is entered, the wound should be packed immediately to prevent contamination of the abdominal cavity. Any fluid or pus is aspirated, and a specimen is sent for culture and sensitivity studies. A finger should be used to break up any loculations. As mentioned earlier, the mass may be made up of omentum and loops of small intestine that are adherent to the inflamed appendix, and an abscess may not be present. If feasible, appendectomy is then performed; it is usually not possible to invert the stump; hence, simple ligation is preferred.

In a patient with a gangrenous appendix and little or no periappendiceal pus, it is not necessary to place a subfascial drain. If there is a periappendiceal abscess and the tissues are so fixed as to create a dead space, the cavity should be drained with one or

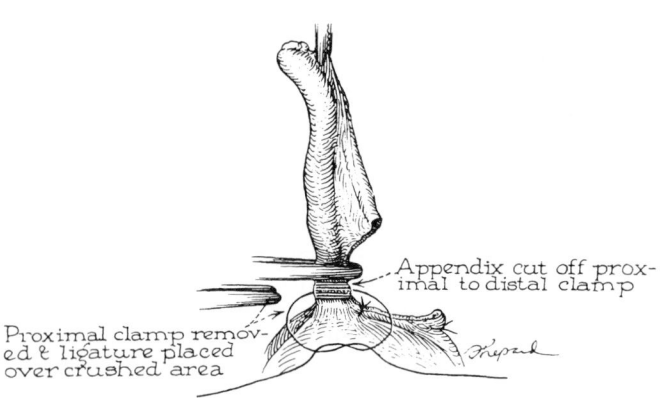

Figure 83.2. Ligation of the stump of the appendix in the groove formed by a crushing clamp. (From Partipilo AV. *Surgical technique and principles of operative surgery*, 6th ed. Philadelphia: Lea & Febiger, 1957, with permission.)

more closed suction drains brought out through a separate stab incision.

Before fascial closure, the right iliac fossa and the wound should be liberally irrigated. Muscles and aponeuroses should be closed with interrupted sutures. Whether the skin should be closed is a matter of controversy. Studies in children indicate that primary closure is a safe practice (28,29). The practice of primary wound closure in adults remains controversial. Delayed primary closure is acceptable and will result in a low wound infection rate. However, open wounds create clinical problems for the patient and surgeon. Primary wound closure is associated with a low incidence of wound infection. The morbidity is not excessive after wound closure even in patients with perforated or gangrenous appendicitis (30). Using a decision analysis model, patients preferred primary wound closure to delayed closure. Parenteral antibiotics should be given for 5 days after operation or until clinical signs indicate absence of infection and the white cell count and differential count are normal. Rectal examination for a pelvic abscess is performed daily. The patient should be discharged from the hospital only after discontinuing antibiotics for 24 hours without developing a fever.

Perforated Appendicitis with Localized Abscess Formation

If, at the time of initial physical examination, a well-localized periappendiceal mass is found and the patient's symptoms are improving, it is acceptable in healthy adults to initiate parenteral antibiotic treatment and to observe the patient expectantly. This form of therapy is not appropriate for children, pregnant women, or elderly patients. For two thirds of cases, expectant treatment of an appendix mass succeeds, and interval appendectomy can be performed later. If the patient's symptoms do not subside, an emergency operation should be performed with the diagnosis of localized abscess.

The skin incision for drainage of a periappendiceal abscess is made just medial to the crest of the ileum at the level of the abscess. With use of a muscle-splitting technique, the lateral edge of the peritoneum is exposed and pushed medially so that the abscess is approached from its lateral aspect. Once it is entered, a finger should be used to break up the loculations. Any fluid or pus is sent for culture and sensitivity study. If the appendix can be freed without breaking down adhesions, appendectomy should be performed. If an appendectomy is not performed, an interval appendectomy should be done 3 to 6 months after the abscess has ceased to drain and the wound is completely healed.

After the wound has been thoroughly irrigated with normal saline, a closed suction drain should be inserted into the abscess cavity and brought out through a separate stab wound in the flank. The muscles and aponeuroses are closed with interrupted nonabsorbable sutures, and the skin and subcutaneous tissues are packed open with saline-soaked gauze. The drain should be left in place until it is draining less than 50 mL per day; then it is advanced progressively until it is removed.

Systemic antibiotics should be continued for 5 days postoperatively or until signs of sepsis have cleared and the white cell count and differential count are normal. A daily rectal examination should be done to detect pelvic abscess. The patient should be discharged from the hospital only after having discontinued antibiotics for 48 hours without developing a fever.

Perforated Appendicitis with Diffuse Peritonitis

The major cause of mortality from appendicitis is generalized peritonitis; thus, for a patient with a diagnosis of acute appendicitis whose physical signs are consistent with diffuse peritonitis, immediate exploration is indicated. If a perforated appendix and diffuse peritonitis are documented at operation, an appendectomy should be performed and the abdomen thoroughly irrigated. The use of drains in diffuse peritonitis is not recommended unless there are localized abscesses that require drainage (31). The wound and postoperative care should be handled as described in a patient with a periappendiceal abscess.

Normal Appendix when Appendicitis Is Suspected

Whenever a patient undergoes exploratory laparotomy, especially through a right lower quadrant incision, for the diagnosis of acute appendicitis, and a normal appendix is found, a careful search for other disease should be made, and an appendectomy should be performed. The cause of the symptoms should be identified and treated, or the surgeon should be sure that no lesion requiring treatment is present. The normal appendix is removed to avoid diagnostic confusion in the future.

If the history and physical examination findings are appropriate for the diagnosis of acute appendicitis, it is not an error to perform an exploratory laparotomy and remove what appears to be a normal appendix. A policy of early surgical intervention on the basis of clinical suspicion has been demonstrated overall to reduce both the morbidity and mortality of acute appendicitis.

Complications

Postoperative complications occur in 5% of patients with an unperforated appendix but in more than 30% of those with a gangrenous or perforated appendix. The most frequent complications after appendectomy are wound infection, intraabdominal abscess, fecal fistula, pylephlebitis, and intestinal obstruction.

Subcutaneous tissue infection is the most common complication after appendectomy. The organisms most frequently cultured are anaerobic *Bacteroides* species and the aerobes *Klebsiella* and *Enterobacter* species and *E. coli* (32). When early signs of wound infection (undue pain and edema) are present, the skin and subcutaneous tissue should be opened. The wound should be packed with saline-soaked gauze and reclosed with Steri-Strips in 4 to 5 days.

Pelvic, subphrenic, or other intraabdominal abscesses occur in up to 20% of patients with a gangrenous or perforated appendix. Such abscesses are accompanied by recurrent fever, malaise, and anorexia. CT is a great help in making the diagnosis of intraabdominal abscess. When abscesses are diagnosed, they should be drained either operatively or percutaneously under CT or ultrasound guidance.

Some fecal fistulas close spontaneously, provided that there is no anatomic reason for the fistula to remain open. Obviously, those that do not close spontaneously require operation. Pylephlebitis, or portal pyemia, is characterized by jaundice, chills, and high fever. It is a serious illness that frequently leads to multiple liver abscesses. The infecting organism is usually *E. coli*. This complication has become rare with the routine use of antibiotics in complicated appendicitis. Although not frequent, true mechanical bowel obstruction may occur as a complication of acute appendicitis. As for any other mechanical small bowel obstruction, operative therapy is indicated.

REFERENCES

1. Lewis FR, Holcroft JW, Boey J, et al. Appendicitis: a critical review of diagnosis and treatment in 1,000 cases. *Arch Surg* 1975;110:677.

2. Wangensteen OH, Dennis C. Experimental proof of obstructive origin of appendicitis in man. *Ann Surg* 1939;110:629.
3. Dennis C. Physiologic behavior of the human appendix and the problem of appendicitis: reaction of the appendix to drugs. *Arch Surg* 1941;43:1021.
4. Altemeier WA. The bacterial flora of acute perforated appendicitis with peritonitis: a bacteriologic study based upon one hundred cases. *Ann Surg* 1938;107:517.
5. Pieper R, Kager L, Nasman P. Acute appendicitis: a clinical study of 1018 cases of emergency appendectomy. *Acta Chir Scand* 1982;148:51.
6. Hubbell DS, Barton WK, Soloman OD. Leukocytosis in appendicitis in older patients. *JAMA* 1961;175:139.
7. Bolton JP, Craven ER, Croft RJ, et al. An assessment of the value of the white cell count in the management of suspected acute appendicitis. *Br J Surg* 1975;62:906.
8. Rajagopalan AE, Mason JH, Kennedy M, et al. The value of the barium enema in the diagnosis of acute appendicitis. *Arch Surg* 1977;112:531.
9. Jona JZ, Belin RP, Selke AC. Barium enema as a diagnostic aid in children with abdominal pain. *Surg Gynecol Obstet* 1977;44:351.
10. Smith DE, Kirchmer NA, Stewart DR. Use of the barium enema in the diagnosis of acute appendicitis and its complications. *Am J Surg* 1979;138:829.
11. Hayden CK, Kuchelmeister J, Lipscomb TS. Sonography of acute appendicitis in childhood: perforation versus nonperforation. *J Ultrasound Med* 1992;11:209.
12. Sivit CJ, Newman KD, Boenning DA, et al. Appendicitis: usefulness of US in diagnosis in a pediatric population. *Radiology* 1992;185:549.
13. Rioux M. Sonographic detection of the normal and abnormal appendix. *AJR Am J Roentgenol* 1992;158:773.
14. Malone AJ, Wolf CR, Malmed AS, et al. Diagnosis of acute appendicitis: value of unenhanced CT. *AJR Am J Roentgenol* 1993;160:763.
15. Balthazar EJ, Megiban AJ, Siegel SE, et al. Appendicitis: prospective evaluation with high-resolution CT. *Radiology* 1991;180:21.
16. Shapiro MP, Gale ME, Gerzof SG. CT of appendicitis: diagnosis and treatment. *Radiol Clin North Am* 1989;27:753.
17. Stone HH, Sanders SL, Martin JD. Perforated appendicitis in children. *Surgery* 1971;69:673.
18. Graham JM, Pokorny WJ, Harberg FJ. Acute appendicitis in preschool age children. *Am J Surg* 1980;139:247.
19. Gomez A, Wood M. Acute appendicitis during pregnancy. *Am J Surg* 1979;137:180.
20. Owens BJ III, Hamit HE. Appendicitis in the elderly. *Ann Surg* 1978;187:392.
21. Thorbjarnarson B, Loehr WJ. Acute appendicitis in patients over the age of sixty. *Surg Gynecol Obstet* 1967;125:1277.
22. Burns RP, Cochran JL, Russell WL, et al. Appendicitis in mature patients. *Ann Surg* 1985;201:695.
23. Bongard F, Landers DV, Lewis F. Differential diagnosis of appendicitis and pelvic inflammatory disease: a prospective analysis. *Am J Surg* 1985;150:90.
24. Hoffman J, Lindhard A, Jensen H-E. Appendix mass: conservative management without interval appendectomy. *Am J Surg* 1984;1248:379.
25. Kingsley DPE. Some observations on appendectomy with particular reference to technique. *Br J Surg* 1969;56:491.
26. Myllariemi H, Perttala Y, Peltokallio P. Tumor-like lesions of the cecum following inversion of the appendix. *Dig Dis* 1974;19:547.
27. Gotz F, Pier A, Badier C. Modified laparoscopic appendectomy in surgery: a report of 388 operations. *Surg Endosc* 1990;4:6.
28. Neilson IR, Laberge JM, Nguyen LT, et al. Appendicitis in children: current therapeutic recommendations. *J Pediatr Surg* 1990;25:1113.
29. Burnweit C, Bilik R, Shandling B. Primary closure of contaminated wounds in perforated appendicitis. *J Pediatr Surg* 1991;26:1362.
30. Brasel KJ, Borgstrom DC, Weigelt JA. Cost-utility analysis of contaminated appendectomy wounds. *J Am Coll Surg* 1997;184:23.
31. Haller JA, Shaker IJ, Donahoo JS, et al. Peritoneal drainage versus nondrainage for generalized peritonitis from ruptured appendicitis in children. *Ann Surg* 1973;177:595.
32. Leigh DA, Simmons K, Normal E. Bacteria flora of the appendix fossa in appendicitis and postoperative wound infection. *J Clin Pathol* 1974;27:997.

CHAPTER 84
Diverticulitis

Dietmar H. Wittmann

Acute diverticulitis is the inflammation of congenital or acquired colonic diverticula. The terms *diverticulosis* and *diverticulitis* must not be confused. Diverticulosis indicates the presence of symptomatic or silent diverticular disease. Diverticulitis signifies an infectious process developing in the former. The incidence of the disease increases with age. Most often it occurs as a complication of acquired diverticulosis of the sigmoid colon (1,2). In the Western world, the sigmoid colon is the segment affected in 90% of the cases of diverticulitis (3), whereas in Asian countries, such as Japan, right-sided disease is more common (4,5). It is estimated that the annual risk for acute diverticulitis in the population with diverticulosis of the colon is 1% to 3% (6). Diverticulosis affects 30 million Americans annually, bringing 200,000 to the hospital and incurring health care costs that may exceed a third of a billion dollars (6). Several studies strongly suggest that symptomatic diverticulosis in younger patients (i.e., younger than 40 to 50 years) is prone to severe complications and would usually require, at some stage, surgical treatment (7,8).

PATHOGENESIS

The pathophysiologic mechanism of colonic diverticulum formation is complex. It must, however, involve spaces of high intracolonic pressure and areas of relative weakness in the colon wall. In manometric and cinematographic studies, high-pressure waves coincide with bandlike contractions that occlude short segments, thus leading to herniation of the mucosa (9). This mechanism is not uniformly accepted, and other theories have been proposed. The tensile strength and elasticity of the colon decline with age and are more marked in the left colon, which is the narrowest and thickest part, suggesting that the mechanical properties of the bowel wall are the main etiologic factors. Because tensile strength is a probable factor in the firmness of the colon wall and the process of aging is associated with an increase in type I collagen and a decrease in type III collagen (10) in some tissues, this could explain the increased incidence of diverticulosis with age.

The striking differences in the incidence of diverticulosis, so common in the Western world and almost nonexistent in African populations, must be emphasized. Disparities in nutritional habits probably are responsible: high-residue diets of Africans produce bulkier feces and as a result a thinner and more elastic colon wall. Conversely, the end result of the low-residue Western dietary habits is the narrow, contracted, diverticulum-prone colon (11). Acute diverticulitis usually originates in a narrow-necked diverticulum with impacted fecal material. A reactive inflammatory edema obstructs the neck and prevents intraluminal drainage of the fecal material, which can contain about 400 different species of bacteria in large numbers (12). This leads to the development of diverticular microempyema, an accumulation of pus in the preformed diverticulum. Increased pressure in the diverticulum leads to microperforation of the mucosa, promoting leakage of intraluminal feces, including lots of bacteria into adjacent sterile tissues or the free abdominal cavity. The patient's host defense mechanisms respond with the formation of a peridiverticular infiltrate, consisting of omentum and adjacent structures, to prevent fecal contamination of the peritoneal cavity.

A wide variety of disease processes may follow, ranging in severity from acute inflammation without pus formation to simple acute fecal peritonitis, or abscess formation representing the middle of the spectrum (Table 84.1 and Fig. 84.1). The end result of the initial insult depends on the size of the perforation and the magnitude of the bacterial challenge versus the local host response. Intact host defense mechanisms will foster abscess formation rather than free bacterial peritonitis. Omentum may adhere to the perforating diverticular area to confine the initial infectious process. The abscess develops when, in the inflammatory mass, bacterial toxins and the host's proteolytic enzymes liquefy the central oxygen- and nutrient-depleted necrotic areas,

TABLE 84.1. The Spectrum of Perforative Diverticular Disease

Acute simple diverticulitis (acute inflammation without pus formation)
Localized purulent process
   Local peritonitis (peridiverticular infiltrate)
   Abscess
   Fistula (vagina, bladder, bowel, skin)
Diffuse fecal peritonitis
   After perforation of a diverticulum
   After perforation of a peridiverticular abscess

creating an ideal condition for further growth of obligate and facultative anaerobic bacteria. The abscess might perforate into the free peritoneal cavity, releasing a selection of more pathogenic bacteria that have been shown to survive or even thrive in the extracolonic environment. Free perforation now overloads the peritoneal cavity and quickly reaches entire organism via thoracic lymphatics and the bloodstream, evoking a systemic inflammatory response and septic shock.

On the other hand, the abscess may become a fistula by perforating into adjacent organs, most commonly the urinary bladder. Occasionally, it spreads along retroperitoneal tissue planes into the skin, especially in the left groin. The prevalence of fistula formation among patients with colonic diverticular disease is reported to be 12% (13,14).

The free perforation via the bowel wall (Fig. 84.2) occurs early. Perforation of a peridiverticular abscess wall comes about late. A fresh perforation releases high inocula of nonselected bowel flora. A late perforation discharges more proliferating and selected bacteria into the peritoneal cavity, resulting in a more serious generalized peritonitis that may be associated with a higher rate of mortality. It is well recognized that nonsteroidal antiinflammatory drugs interfere with local "walling off" mechanisms. Hence, free perforation and associated complications of acute diverticulitis are significantly more common in patients who ingest these drugs (15).

CLINICAL MANIFESTATIONS

A careful history may lead to the diagnosis because diverticulitis often is recurrent. The most prominent symptom is steady,

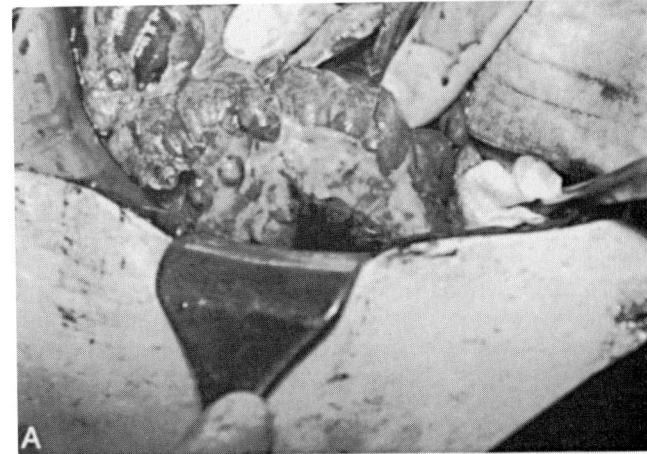
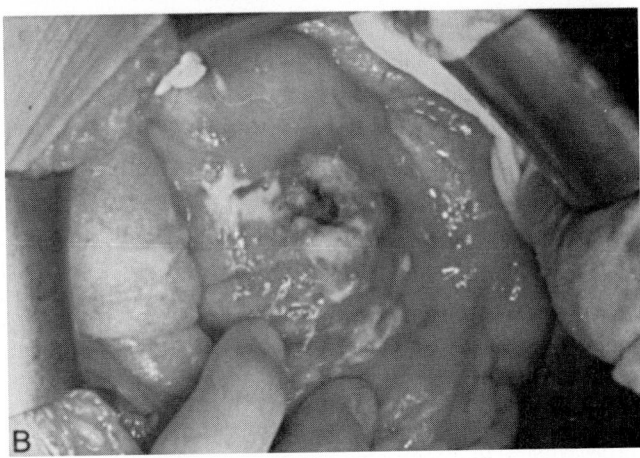

Figure 84.1. Peritonitis caused by perforated diverticulum. **A:** Peritonitis with fibrinous exudate and diverticula of the sigmoid colon. **B:** Inflammation of the peritoneum caused by a perforated diverticulum of the sigmoid colon.

deep-seated, left lower quadrant pain, which may at times be crampy and intermittent. Because the sigmoid colon is mobile, the symptoms and signs may present in other quadrants of the abdomen. Changes in bowel function may occur: usually constipation but sometimes diarrhea or alternating diarrhea and constipation. Low-grade or spiking fever with chills is usually

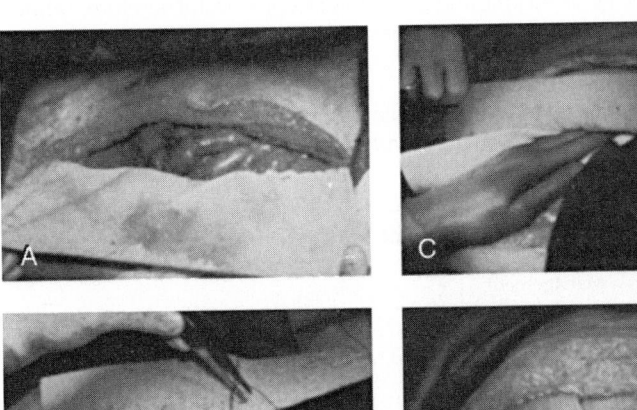

Figure 84.2. Abdominal wound with artificial bur fascial expander (Wittmann Patch) sutured to the abdominal fascias to ease temporary abdominal closure between planned abdominal reentries every 24 to 36 hours (staged abdominal repair). **A:** The looped sheet of the artificial bur is sutured to the abdominal fascia on one side of the abdominal wound. **B:** The hooked sheet of the artificial bur is sutured to the opposite abdominal fascia. **C:** The looped sheet is pushed underneath the hooked sheet covering the intestines. **D:** The hooked sheet adheres to the looped sheet and the abdominal wound is closed, leaving a gap between the fascias to decompress the abdominal compartment syndrome that is often seen in diffuse peritonitis after diverticular perforation.

present if the disease is severe. Nausea and vomiting are not common unless there is perforation, peritonitis, or bowel obstruction. Urinary symptoms such as frequency, urgency, and dysuria may be present when the inflammation extends to the bladder. Dysuria and urinary frequency associated with pneumaturia and fecaluria are pathognomonic for colovesical fistulas.

The physical examination usually reveals left lower quadrant abdominal tenderness with or without muscle guarding. Occasionally on deep palpation a tender, fixed mass may be felt, which is indicative of suppurative pericolitis. When severe inflammation is present, abdominal muscle guarding makes the palpation of such a mass impossible. On rectal digital examination, however, the mass can be felt occasionally. Blood and mucus may be seen on the examining finger, but profuse hemorrhage is uncommon. In cases with free perforation into the peritoneal cavity, the symptoms and signs of generalized peritonitis prevail.

DIAGNOSIS

Chest and abdominal radiographs should be obtained at the time of admission to the hospital to rule out free perforation or bowel obstruction. If indicated, contrast-enhanced studies should always be performed with low-pressure and water-soluble contrast media. Sigmoidoscopy should never be performed with insufflation of air. There is little, if any, indication for these diagnostic procedures during the acute phase of the disease, although they may be of great value when performed after the symptoms have subsided, to exclude inflammatory bowel disease or neoplasia. Colonoscopy in patients with symptomatic sigmoid diverticular disease has revealed an associated carcinoma in 7 of 105 (6.6%) patients and adenomatous polyps in 29 (27.6%). Barium enema examination has been inaccurate (16). Studies suggest that computed tomography might be helpful not only in the diagnosis of diverticulitis and its complications (17), but also in selecting the therapeutic regimen. (18–20).

The triad of a diverticulum, a segmentally thickened colon, and extraluminal fluid collection, with or without associated gas, correctly identifies an abscess. The combination of diverticulum, thickened colon, and an adjacent, gas-containing edematous bladder points to a colovesical fistula (21). Computed tomography combined with diatrizoate meglumine (Gastrografin) enema has been used prospectively to assess the severity of the acute attack. Mild diverticulitis has been defined as localized colon wall thickening of less than 5 mm with inflammation of pericolic fat. The same findings associated with an abscess, extraluminal air, or extraluminal Gastrografin suggest a severe attack of diverticulitis. Most patients classified as having a mild disease responded to conservative treatment, whereas those considered to have a severe attack required an urgent operation or an interval procedure after nonoperative treatment (8). Because a pericolic phlegmon should be managed differently than a pericolic abscess, the differentiation of these conditions may obviate undue delay or undue rush for management. Although laboratory and radiologic findings can at times be valuable in the evaluation of acute diverticulitis, we believe that the diagnosis should be based principally on the clinical evaluation. Computed tomography is helpful in patients in whom abscess or fistulization is suspected after they fail to improve rapidly with conservative therapy.

TREATMENT

General Considerations

Treatment of acute sigmoid diverticulitis is best considered under the following headings: (a) medical (nonoperative) management, (b) operative management of infectious complications, and (c) medical and surgical prevention of recurrent episodes.

Generally, our practical therapeutic approach (Table 84.2) is based on the extent of the process (Table 84.1). Acute inflammation without pus formation is managed conservatively, localized suppuration requires an immediate or delayed operation, and the diffuse process is treated with an emergency laparotomy. About 80% of patients admitted to the hospital for diverticulitis are managed medically with antibiotics and a low-residue diet. Only 10% to 20% require an emergency operation, and at operation generalized or fecal peritonitis is found in 20% to 60% of these patients (22).

Medical (Nonoperative) Treatment

An attack of mild, noncomplicated, acute phlegmonous diverticulitis usually responds to conservative therapy. The colon is "rested" with a low-residue diet. If ileus develops, the patient is given nothing by mouth. If analgesics are required, the agent of choice appears to be pentazocine, which has been shown to reduce the motility of the sigmoid in patients with diverticulitis (23), although hydromorphone may be preferred because it is less likely to produce disorientation.

Antibiotic therapy is initiated based on the assumption that pathogenic bacteria within the stool flora are responsible for the acute infectious process. Antimicrobials should suppress growth of both endotoxin-producing facultative aerobes and obligate anaerobes, even if blood cultures grow only a single species. The microbial pathogenicity of the disease process favors the development of synergistic infection by organisms that include *Escherichia coli*, *Bacteroides fragilis* and other *Bacteroides* species, clostridia, and anaerobic streptococci. Therefore, "blind" or even empiric antimicrobial chemotherapy is antiquated and should be discarded in favor of calculated antibiotic therapy (24) (Table 84.3).

Because it is impossible to investigate pathogens directly in infected diverticula, pathogens isolated in peritonitis after

---

TABLE 84.2. Management of Acute Diverticulitis (Authors' Recommendations)

Disease process	Management
Acute simple diverticulitis	Nonoperative treatment
Diverticular abscess	Percutaneous drainage plus delayed elective sigmoid resection
Diverticular fistula	Resection of fistula and sigmoid colon
	Colocutaneous fistula may heal spontaneously
Diffuse peritonitis	Sigmoid resection and primary anastomosis plus staged abdominal repair (STAR) using the Wittmann Patch for temporary fascial closure (see Chapter 80)
	Hartmann procedure in desperate situations (no longer recommended)

TABLE 84.3.   Essentials of Calculated Antimicrobial Therapy

Consideration of typical spectrum of infecting bacteria
Consideration of pathogenicity of different bacteria and synergistic or
  antagonistic interactions
Consideration of the antibiotic concentration sustained at the
  infectious site after a given dose
Consideration of toxicity of antibiotics under the specific
  circumstances
Consideration of antibiotic interaction with host defense
Consideration of results of controlled clinical trials

perforation of the colon most closely delineate the target bacteria (24,25) (Table 84.4). The antibiotic concentration at the site of infection should surpass the minimum inhibitory concentration (MIC) for the targeted bacteria. Antimicrobial concentrations measured in peritoneal fluid (26) have been shown to be more representative of drug levels at the infectious site than the serum concentration. After a dose of 500 mg of metronidazole, a concentration of 2 to 4 mg/L is present in peritoneal fluid for about 12 hours, a concentration sufficient for most anaerobic bacteria. *B. fragilis* generally cannot survive at this concentration of metronidazole. A dose interval of 12 hours is sufficient. Because its bioavailability is greater than 90% after oral or rectal administration, the route of administration does not significantly influence the concentration at the infectious site (27).

With all the previous information in mind, the antimicrobial choice should include activity against *E. coli* and other less common gram-negative enteric organisms. In 104 studies, 10,413 strains of *E. coli* were tested using standardized techniques (test inoculum 6.0 $\log_{10}$ colony-forming units per milliliter) against cefotaxime, ceftazidime, and moxalactam and other β-lactam antibiotics. No strain had an MIC higher than the concentrations achieved in peritoneal fluid for 2 g of cefotaxime, ceftazidime, or moxalactam. Of the *E. coli* strains, 26%, 19%, and 13% had MICs higher than the antibiotic concentrations achieved at the infec-

tious site for 2 g of cefoxitin, 1.5 g of cefuroxime, and 2 g of cefoperazone, respectively. More than 35% of the *E. coli* strains had MICs that were greater than the peritoneal fluid concentrations for 5 g of mezlocillin and piperacillin at 50 mg/kg given intravenously (26,28). No properly conducted prospective randomized antibiotic trial has dealt with diverticulitis only. Other trials of antibiotics for so-called intraabdominal infections provided insufficient information to help in choosing the right antibiotic because they excluded the most seriously ill patients from being enrolled in the studies (29,30). Furthermore, many patients in these studies were described as having intraabdominal infections and had just simple abdominal contamination resulting from penetrating bowel injury. Therefore, the choice of antibiotic is better based on the pharmacodynamics mentioned earlier.

The antibiotic of choice should include cefotaxime, ceftizoxime, or similar third-generation cephalosporins in combination with 500 mg of metronidazole (Table 84.5) or clindamycin for coverage of the pathogenic anaerobes. Clindamycin, 1,200 mg every 12 hours intravenously (31) (or the traditional but not so good 600 mg every 6 hours), may be combined with 2,000 mg of aztreonam for effective treatment. Ceftazidime should not be used for diverticulitis (it should be reserved for *Pseudomonas aeruginosa* infections). Monotherapy with an intravenous drug such as moxalactam, 2 g every 12 hours; or cefotetan, 2 g every 12 hours, may have the same effect as combinations owing to their excellent activity against *E. coli* and obligate anaerobes. Fixed combinations such as imipenem-cilastatin, 1,000 mg every 8 hours, and the newly approved penicillin-β-lactamase inhibitor combinations are alternative choices. Combinations with metronidazole and quinolones seem attractive because both drugs can be given orally.

Today the value of aminoglycosides seems to be limited to certain classes of patients who may be infected by bacteria that are resistant to the third-generation cephalosporins, monobactams or quinolones. In such patients who have in previous weeks been exposed to antibiotics or to a hospital environment, the additive effect or synergy of amino glycosides plus β-lactams on certain strains of multidrug-resistant bacteria may be utilized.

The classic combination of an aminoglycoside plus clindamycin has been widely used. At present, this regimen may be used under specific circumstances when potentially less toxic alternatives cannot be administered. When diverticulitis progresses to peritonitis, renal function may be impaired as a result of the systemic repercussions of the infectious process. The nephrotoxic potential of aminoglycosides may become clinically relevant even if serum levels are monitored.

Because there have been few randomized controlled clinical studies of diverticulitis, one may be tempted to base patients' management on the results of numerous antibiotic trials for intraabdominal infection of gut origin, but the value of these trials is limited by the excessively restrictive criteria for selection of patients (29,30).

Patients with milder symptoms of acute diverticulitis, such as low-grade fever and minimal signs of peritoneal irritation, might be given oral antibiotics to avoid hospitalization. Among the drugs suggested have been oral ciprofloxacin in combination with clindamycin or metronidazole. Another possibility is amoxicillin-clavulanate potassium (Augmentin), which gives good aerobic and anaerobic coverage.

TABLE 84.4.   Bacteria Isolated in Intraabdominal Infections After Perforation of the Large Bowel in 48 Patients

Organism	Isolates	
	n	%
Aerobes (facultative anaerobes)		
Escherichia coli	39	81
Klebsiella species	10	21
Enterobacter cloacae	1	2
Proteus mirabilis	7	15
Proteus vulgaris	1	2
Streptococci group A	3	6
Streptococci groups C and D	2	4
Enterococcus faecalis	16	33
Pseudomonas aeruginosa	2	4
Other aerobes	7	15
Total aerobes	88	
Anaerobes (obligate anaerobes)		
Bacteroides fragilis	25	52
Other *Bacteroides* species	22	46
Fusobacterium	1	2
Peptostreptococci	7	15
Clostridium perfringens	9	19
Other clostridia	4	8
Other anaerobes	6	13
Total anaerobes	74	

Surgical Treatment

OPERATIVE TREATMENT OF INFECTIOUS COMPLICATIONS
The perforation of a diverticulum allows a direct communication between the lumen of the colon and adjacent sterile tissues

TABLE 84.5.   Recommendations for Antimicrobial Therapy for Diverticulitis

Agent	Dose (mg)	Administration
Fixed combinations		
Imipenem-cilastatin	1,000	every 8 h i.v.
Ampicillin-sulbactam	3,000	every 6 h i.v.
Ticarcillin-clavulanate	3,100	every 8 h i.v.
Piperacillin-tazobactam	4,500	every 8 h i.v.
Amoxicillin-clavulanate	500/125	every 8 h p.o.
Combinations of antianaerobic drugs with cephalosporins and monobactams		
Metronidazole	500	every 12 h i.v., or p.o. or rectally
	or	
Clindamycin	1,200	every 12 h i.v. or 600 mg every 8 h p.o.
	in combination with	
Cefotaxime	2,000	every 8–12 h i.v.
	or	
Ceftizoxime	2,000	every 12 h i.v.
	or	
Ceftriaxone	2,000	every 12 h i.v.
Alternative combinations		
Clindamycin	1,200	every 12 h i.v.
	in combination with	
Aztreonam	2,000	every 8 h i.v.

i.v., Intravenously; p.o., orally.

or the free abdominal cavity, resulting in a spectrum of conditions (Table 84.1) that require selective therapy. The choice of the specific surgical technique has been controversial for many decades (22). Previously, the surgical management of complicated diverticulitis has been based on guidelines suggested by Mayo (32), Lockhart-Mummary (33), and Smithwick (34). During the past 50 years, surgeons have relied on a diverting colostomy or multiple-stage repair that involves high risk for mortality and morbidity. There is currently a trend that favors a single-stage repair with resection of the sigmoid colon without protective colostomy (35–40). The existence of several published studies that report unfavorable results for staged repair, the availability of potent antibiotics, and better surgical intensive care are probably reasons for this rapid change. Some investigators believe that primary anastomosis can be performed even in the presence of obstruction or perforation (41–46). This can be accomplished without an intraoperative colonic preparation (45).

A collective review of the literature (22) outlined the superiority of the one-stage resection over all other more "conservative" procedures. ["Secure suture of a perforation has never really been possible" (47).] Poor outcome seen with suture closure and drainage plus colostomy confirms this statement. Nevertheless, one might reason that multiple-stage procedures are usually performed on the most severely ill patients and represent a negative selection. In 1981, Sakai and colleagues (44) published a report of multiple-stage series, an operative strategy similar to staged abdominal repair, with no associated mortality in this high-risk group of patients (48). In it, primary resection was performed and the abdomen was temporarily closed to allow repeated débridement and control of the healing of the anastomosis.

Staged abdominal repair (e.g., multiple planned abdominal reentries) (Fig. 84.2) may be the best treatment option for a high-risk group (49): If the patient's physiologic derangement predicts a high risk for death on the basis of the Acute Physiology and Chronic Health Evaluation II (APACHE II) score (50) and if débridement cannot be accomplished in a single procedure, staged abdominal repair should be considered. In this proce-

dure the infected abdominal cavity is treated like an open wound that is closed temporarily. This allows daily reexploration and débridement until the septic focus is under control and anastomotic healing is ensured. Temporary abdominal closure can be accomplished by using various meshes, or the artificial bur (Wittmann Patch) (49). In one series, planned, abdominal reexplorations were performed in 10 consecutive patients suffering from diffuse fecal peritonitis. There was no mortality, attesting to the importance of aggressive, repeated peritoneal "toilet" when fecal contamination is massive (48).

Occasionally the invading bacteria and adjuvants of infection are confined in a localized abscess, which may be demonstrable at the time of diagnosis. Computed tomography–guided percutaneous drainage may be a good treatment option (51,52). The bacterial inoculum is reduced considerably, optimizing the effectiveness of antimicrobials. The resection of the diseased colon could be delayed and subsequently performed electively. If clinical resolution is not seen within 48 hours, an urgent operation should be performed. It is hoped that in the future there will be more controlled trials to determine the best treatment options. Our current therapeutic recommendations are summarized in Table 84.2.

Laparoscopic Surgery. Many surgeons now recommend laparoscopic colon resections for elective operations, and some investigators have assessed the value of laparoscopic colon resections for emergency operations (53–58). The current consensus is that laparoscopic procedures are safe 2 to 6 months after an acute episode for simple cases excluding advanced stages with adhesions (59,60). There is no final word concerning laparoscopic techniques for diffuse peritonitis following a perforated diverticulitis or perforated diverticular abscess.

MEDICAL AND SURGICAL PREVENTION OF RECURRENT EPISODES

After the successful conservative management of the acute episode, a high-fiber diet to relieve pain and bowel dysfunction is recommended. The role of the high-fiber diet, which reduces the pressure in the diseased colon segment, is generally accepted for uncomplicated diverticular disease. Clinical evidence demonstrating a reduction in the recurrence rate has been found in a prospective analysis of almost 50,000 men in the United States (61). Men who consumed a high-fiber diet, consisting of primarily fruit and vegetables, had a 3.32% reduced relative risk compared with those who consumed a diet low in fiber and high in red meet and fat diet. Five slices (150 g) of whole wheat bread or varying amounts of widely marketed cereals may furnish adequate fiber intake (62).

Prevention of recurrences by primary resection of the diseased colon segment has been advocated for recurrent disease, which is seen in 50% of the cases. The risk for life-threatening complications is the basis for indicating interval sigmoid resection after conclusion of acute inflammatory symptoms (63). Currently, the interval sigmoid colon resection is advocated by most surgeons (63), although it is not uniformly agreed upon whether it should follow the first or the second acute episode (64). Common indications for delayed elective sigmoidectomy after the first attack include the following:

1. Young patients (40 to 50 years old) who are prone to complicated recurrences
2. Suspicion of an underlying carcinoma
3. Demonstrable complications such as fistulas, residual abscess, or colonic stenosis

A recurrent episode of acute diverticulitis is certainly an indication for a sigmoidectomy. If appropriate, elective surgical resection should be performed 8 to 10 weeks after the acute episode. This time interval permits resolution of the inflammatory reaction. The operation of choice is primary resection of the sigmoid colon without colostomy. The entire distal sigmoid colon needs to be resected and anastomosed to the upper rectum to avoid recurrent diverticulitis (65). More proximal diverticula-bearing colon segments should be left alone, because the risk for symptomatic disease originating proximal to the resected sigmoid is minimal (66). It is difficult to assess the overall benefit of this management. In one study, 7% of patients who had resection for diverticular disease suffered recurrent disease (66). In a separate series, long-term follow-up (3 to 15 years) demonstrated that half of the patients had only one repeated episode of acute diverticulitis (63).

ACUTE DIVERTICULITIS IN A SOLITARY CECAL DIVERTICULUM

This rare condition is encountered during 1 of 500 emergency laparotomy procedures. When compared with acute appendicitis, it is encountered at a ratio of 1:220. Thus, even busy surgeons would not treat more than a few such cases during their lifetime. The condition usually develops in an age group intermediate to those of patients with acute appendicitis and sigmoid diverticulitis. The clinical presentation mimics that of acute appendicitis but is perhaps less dramatic. In the majority of patients, a diagnosis of acute appendicitis is made, leading to an operation. Occasionally, a correct initial diagnosis is established, with the help of a contrast study or computed tomographic examination, ordered because of atypical symptoms or the history of a previous appendectomy.

When a definitive diagnosis of cecal diverticulitis is established, nonoperative treatment, along lines similar to those described for sigmoid diverticulitis, should be attempted and in most cases is successful. Most patients, however, undergo laparotomy, during which the typical finding consists of a cecal mass (phlegmon). Differentiation from carcinoma or Crohn's disease may be extremely difficult. When the possibility of cecal diverticulitis is entertained, a correct intraoperative diagnosis can be made by palpation (a fecalith within the diverticulum) or through a colotomy. In such a situation the procedure should consist of local excision of the diverticulum followed by primary closure of the colonic defect. When accurate diagnosis is in doubt, most researchers agree that an immediate right hemicolectomy with an ileocolic anastomosis is the safest option (67).

REFERENCES

1. Boles RS Jr, Jordan SM. The clinical significance of diverticulosis. *Gastroenterology* 1958;35:579.
2. Homer JL. Natural history of diverticulosis of the colon. *Am J Dig Dis* 1958;3:343.
3. Rodkey GV, Welch CE. Changing patterns in the surgical treatment of diverticular disease. *Ann Surg* 1984;200:466.
4. Kovalcik PJ, Surstarsic DL. Cecal diverticulitis. *Ann Surg* 1981;47:72.
5. Schuler JG, Bayley J. Diverticulitis of the cecum. *Surg Gynecol Obstet* 1983;156:743.
6. Griffin HE, Mendeloff AL. *Epidemiology of digestive disease.* National Institutes of Health, U.S. Department of Health, Education, and Welfare Publication No. 79-1887. Washington, DC: U.S. Government Printing Office, 1978:11–33.
7. Quriel K, Schwartz SI. Diverticular disease in the young patient. *Surg Gynecol Obstet* 1983;156:1.
8. Ambrosetti P, Robert J, Witzig JA, et al. Prognostic factors from computed tomography in acute left colonic diverticulitis. *Br J Surg* 1992;79:117.
9. Painter NS, Truelove SC, Ardran GM, et al. Segmentation and the localization of intraluminal pressures in the human colon, with special reference to the pathogenesis of colonic diverticula. *Gastroenterology* 1965;49:169.
10. Bornstein P. Disorders of connective tissue function and the aging process: a synthesis and review of current concepts and findings. *Mech Ageing Dev* 1976;5:305.
11. Watters DAK, Smith AN. Strength of the colon wall in diverticular disease. *Br J Surg* 1990;77:257.
12. Bentley DW Nichols RL, Condon RE, et al. The microflora of the human ileum and intra-abdominal colon: results of direct needle aspiration at surgery and evaluation of technique. *J Lab Clin Med* 1972;79:421.
13. Fazio WV, Church MJ, Jagelman GD, et al. Colocutaneous fistulas complicating diverticulitis. *Dis Colon Rectum* 1987;30:89.
14. Woods JR, Lavery CI, Fazio WV, et al. Internal fistulas in diverticular disease. *Dis Colon Rectum* 1988;31:591.
15. Campbell K, Steele RJ. Non-steroidal anti-inflammatory drug and complicated diverticular disease: a case-control study. *Br J Surg* 1991;78:190.
16. Boulos PB, Cowen AP, Karamanolis DG, et al. Diverticula, neoplasia, or both? Early detection of carcinoma in sigmoid diverticular disease. *Ann Surg* 1985;202:607.
17. Morris J, Stellato TA, Lieberman J, et al. The utility of computed tomography in colonic diverticulitis. *Ann Surg* 1986;104:128.
18. Lieberman JM, Haagar JR. Computed tomography of diverticulitis. *J Comput Assist Tomogr* 1983;7:431.
19. Goldman SM, Fishman EK, Gatewood OMB, et al. Demonstration of colovesical fistulae secondary to diverticulitis. *J Comput Assist Tomogr* 1984;8:462.
20. Raval B, Lamki N, St. Ville E. Role of computed tomography in diverticulitis. *J Comput Assist Tomogr* 1987;11:144.
21. Labs JD, Sarr MG, Fishman EK, et al. Complications of acute diverticulitis of the colon: improved diagnosis with computerized tomography. *Am J Surg* 1988;155:331.
22. Krukowski ZH, Matheson NA. Emergency surgery for diverticular disease complicated by generalized and faecal peritonitis: a review. *Br J Surg* 1984;71:921.
23. Stanciu C, Bennett JR. Colonic response to pentazocine. *BJM* 1974;1:312.
24. Wittmann DH, Bergstein JM, Frantizdes C. Calculated empiric antimicrobial therapy for mixed surgical infections. *Infection* 1991;19(suppl):345.
25. Onderdonk AB, Kaspar DL, Mansheim BJ, et al. Experimental animal models for anaerobic infections. *Rev Infect Dis* 1979;1:291.
26. Wittmann DH, Schassan H-H. Penetration of eight beta-lactam antibiotics into peritoneal fluid. *Arch Surg* 1983;118:205–212.
27. Wittmann DH, Frommelt V. Metronidazole in intra-abdominal infections [in German]. *Fortschr Antimicrob Antineoplast Chemother* 1983;2:703–706.
28. Wittmann DH: Treatment of peritonitis: antibiotic concentration dynamics at the site of infection as criterion of antimicrobial chemotherapy [Habilitation]. Hamburg University Medical School, Hamburg, Germany, 1984.
29. Solomkin JS, Meakins JL Jr. Antibiotic trials in intra-abdominal infections: a critical evaluation of study design and outcome reporting. *Ann Surg* 1984;201:29.
30. Schein M, Wittmann DH, Lorenz W. Forum Statement: a plea for selective and controlled postoperative antibiotic administration Europ. *J Surg* 1996;162(suppl 576):66–75.
31. Plaisance KI, Drusano GL, Forrest A, et al. Pharmacokinetic evaluation of two dosage regimens of clindamycin phosphate. *Antimicrob Agents Chemother* 1989;33:618.

32. Mayo WJ. Acquired diverticulitis of the large intestine. *Surg Gynecol Obstet* 1907;5;8.
33. Lockhart-Mummary JP. Late results in diverticulitis. *Lancet* 1938;2;1041.
34. Smithwick RH. Experiences with the surgical management of diverticulitis of the sigmoid. *Ann Surg* 1942;115;969.
35. Eng K, Ranson JHC, Locaslio SA. Resection of the perforated segment: a significant advance in treatment of diverticulitis with free perforation or abscess. *Am J Surg* 1977;133;67.
36. Grief JM, Fried G, McSherry CK. Surgical treatment of perforated diverticulitis of the sigmoid colon. *Dis Colon Rectum* 1980;23;483.
37. Eisenstat TE, Rubin RJ, Salrari EP. Surgical management of diverticulitis: the role of the Hartmann procedure. *Dis Colon Rectum* 1983;26;429.
38. Auguste L, Borrero E, Wise L. Surgical management of perforated colonic diverticulitis. *Arch Surg* 1985;120;450.
39. Lambert ME, Knox RA, Schofield RF, et al. Management of the septic complications of diverticular disease. *Br J Surg* 1986;73;576.
40. Silvis R, Keeman JN. Complicated diverticulitis in acute surgery. *Neth J Surg* 1988;40;117.
41. Dandekar NV, McCann WJ. Primary resection and anastomosis in the management of perforation of diverticulitis of the sigmoid flexure and diffuse peritonitis. *Dis Colon Rectum* 1969;12;172.
42. Farkouh E, Hellon G, Allard M, et al. Resection and primary anastomosis for diverticulitis with perforation and peritonitis. *Can J Surg* 1982;25;314.
43. Madden JL. Primary resection in the treatment of acute perforations of the colon with abscess or diffuse peritonitis. In Delaney JP, Varco RL, eds. *Controversies in surgery II.* Philadelphia: WB Saunders, 1983;349.
44. Wittmann DH, Kellinghusen C, Frommelt L. Peritonitis after perforations of sigma diverticula. In: Wittmann DH, ed. *Intra-abdominal infections.* Munich: Futuramed Verlag, 1983;535–542.
45. Saadia R, Schein M. Intra-operative colonic lavage. *Dis Colon Rectum* 1988;32;78.
46. Mealy K, Salman A, Arthur G. Definitive one-stage emergency large bowel surgery. *Br J Surg* 1988;75;1216.
47. Condon RE. Management of the acute complications of diverticular disease: peritonitis and septicemia. *Dis Colon Rectum* 1976;19;296.
48. Sakai L, Daake J, Kaminski DL. Acute perforation of sigmoid diverticuli. *Am J Surg* 1981;142;12.
49. Wittmann DH, Aprahamian C, Bergstein J. Etappenlavage: advanced diffuse peritonitis managed by planned multiple laparotomies utilizing zippers, slide fastener, and Velcro for temporary abdominal closure. *World J Surg* 1990;14;218.
50. Wittmann DH, Nyström PO. Multicenter validation of APACHE II score for intraabdominal infection. *Surg Res Commun* 1990;8(suppl);27.
51. Neff CC, van Sonnenberg E, Casola G, et al. Diverticular abscesses: percutaneous drainage. *Radiology* 1987;163;15.
52. Saini S, Mueller PR, Wittenberg J, et al. Percutaneous drainage of diverticular abscess. *Arch Surg* 1986;121;475.
53. Carbajo MA, Caballero Martin del Olmo JC, Blanco Alvarez JI, et al. Acute diverticulitis and diverticular disease of the colon: a safe indication for laparoscopic surgery, *Rev Esp Enferm Dig* 2000;92;718.
54. Hildebrandt U, Kreissler-Haag D, Lindemann W. Laparoscopy-assisted colorectal resections: morbidity, conversions, outcomes of a decade, *Zentralbl Chir* 2001;126;323.
55. Schlachta CM, Mamazza J, Seshadri PA, et al. Defining a learning curve for laparoscopic colorectal resections, *Dis Colon Rectum* 2001;44;217.
56. Cox JA, Rogers MA, Cox SD. Treating benign colon disorders using laparoscopic colectomy, *AORN J* 2001;73;377.
57. Vargas HD, Ramirez RT, Hoffman GC, et al. Defining the role of laparoscopic-assisted sigmoid colectomy for diverticulitis. *Dis Colon Rectum* 2000;43;1726.
58. Tuech JJ, Pessaux P, Rouge C, et al. Laparoscopic vs open colectomy for sigmoid diverticulitis: a prospective comparative study in the elderly. *Surg Endosc* 14:1031 (2000).
59. Nyström PO, Kald A. Laparoscopic sigmoid resection in diverticulitis. *Zentralbl Chir* 1999;124;1147.
60. Kockerling F, Schneider C, Reymond MA, et al. Laparoscopic resection of sigmoid diverticulitis. Results of a multicenter study. Laparoscopic Colorectal Surgery Study Group. *Surg Endosc* 1999;13;567.
61. Aldoori WH, Giovannucci EL, Rockett HR, et al. A prospective study of dietary fiber types and symptomatic diverticular disease in men. *J Nutr* 1998;128;714.
62. The high-fiber diet: its effect on the bowel. *Med Lett* 1975;17;93.
63. Chappuis CW, Cohn I Jr. Acute colonic diverticulitis. *Surg Clin North Am* 1988;68;301.
64. Manousos ON. Diverticular disease of the colon. *Dig Dis* 1989;7;86.
65. Bern PL, Wolff BG, Ilstrup DM. Level of anastomosis and recurrent colonic diverticulitis. *Am J Surg* 1986;151;269.
66. Wolff BG, Ready RL, MacCarty RL, et al. Influence of sigmoid resection on progression of diverticular disease of the colon. *Dis Colon Rectum* 1984;27;645.
67. Schmit PJ, Bennion RS, Thompson JE. Cecal diverticulitis: a continuing diagnostic dilemma. *World J Surg* 1991;15;367.

Liver and Biliary Tract

CHAPTER 85
Type A Viral Hepatitis

Stanley M. Lemon

Type A viral hepatitis occurs as a result of infection with a hepatotropic picornavirus, hepatitis A virus (HAV) (1–3). The virus is transmitted between persons via the fecal-oral route, and appears to undergo primary replication within epithelial cells of the small intestine (4). This is associated with a low-level viremia that leads to subsequent spread of the virus to the liver where, following an incubation period of approximately 4 weeks, it causes an acute necroinflammatory hepatitis. The signs and symptoms of the acute illness reflect infection of the hepatocyte with HAV and its subsequent clearance by several different immune mechanisms. The disease itself is probably largely immunopathologic in nature. During the acute phase of the illness, copious amounts of virus are shed from the infected liver into the gastrointestinal track via the hepatobiliary system, completing the infectious cycle (5). Chronic viral hepatitis is not associated with HAV infection, and, unlike the viruses responsible for hepatitis B, hepatitis delta, and hepatitis C, there is no strong evidence for long-term persistence of HAV in infected persons. HAV also differs from these other viruses in its strong potential for epidemic spread, since its transmission (like that of hepatitis E virus) is predominantly enteric and can occur through fecally contaminated ground waters or food. It is a frequent cause of common source outbreaks of hepatitis (6,7).

VIROLOGY

The biology of HAV is considered in greater detail in Chapter 251; only selected aspects relevant to the clinical features of hepatitis A are considered here. HAV is currently classified within the genus *Hepatovirus* of the family *Picornaviridae* (8). The HAV particle is 27 nm in diameter, nonenveloped, and consists of a 7.5-kb, positive-sense, single-stranded RNA molecule (the HAV genome) tightly encapsidated within a protein shell composed of 60 copies each of three (perhaps four) different structural proteins (3,9). HAV is distantly related to enteroviruses and the human rhinoviruses, causative agents of the common cold, but has very little nucleotide sequence relatedness with these viruses. There is no antigenic cross-relatedness evident between HAV and other picornaviruses, nor any antigenic relatedness with other viruses that cause acute hepatitis in humans (10). HAV replication occurs in the cytoplasm of hepatocytes, and appears to follow a general scheme resembling that of poliovirus, the best studied member of the picornavirus family (9) (see Chapter 248).

The HAV particle demonstrates exceptional physical stability (11–14). Like the enteroviruses, HAV is stable at very low pH, consistent with its ability to survive gastric acidity. The thermal stability of the HAV virion is also significantly greater than that of poliovirus and other human picornaviruses. In suspension, the infectivity of HAV is not appreciably affected by incubation for brief periods at temperatures up to 60°C. It is likely that the stability of the virus under adverse conditions of temperature and pH promotes its spread in the environment and its propensity for causing epidemics. Because of the absence of a lipid envelope, the virus is resistant to lipid solvents and is not inactivated by the solvent-detergent inactivation procedures that are commonly used to ensure the virus safety of blood products (15).

The nucleotide sequences of human HAV isolates generally differ from each other by less than 20%; even greater conservation (>95%) is evident in the amino acid sequences of the capsid proteins (16). Thus, HAV displays significantly less genetic variability than that observed among different types of poliovirus. Nonetheless, the analysis of a large number of HAV strains has indicated the existence of at least seven distinct HAV genotypes that differ from each other at greater than 15% of nucleotide positions within regions of the genome encoding the structural proteins (17). HAV strains recovered from humans comprise four of these genotypes (genotypes I, II, III, and VII), while viruses in the remaining three genotypes (IV, V, and VI) are simian strains that display subtle antigenic differences and have thus far only been recovered from naturally infected nonhuman primates (cynomolgus monkeys and African green monkeys). The high level of antigenic conservation that is evident at the molecular level is associated with an absence of significant antigenic variability among human HAV strains worldwide (10,18), and even the simian viruses can be considered members of the same single HAV serotype. Infection with any one of these viruses is likely to elicit neutralizing antibodies that are protective against all strains of HAV.

The simian viruses (genotypes IV, V, VI) are considered to have low pathogenicity for humans. Evidence suggests that they constitute a biologically distinct group of viruses that are capable of causing disease in experimentally infected cynomolgus and African green monkeys, but not chimpanzees, which (like New World owl monkeys and certain tamarin species) develop acute liver disease following challenge with human strains of HAV (19–21). In contrast, human strains of HAV generally do not cause disease in the former primate species. These differences in virus host range could be due, at least in part, to differences in the cellular receptors utilized by these HAV strains since there appear to be associated differences in the surface features of the virus particle. Strain-specific differences in virulence have not been described among human HAV strains.

It is notable that HAV is the only human hepatitis virus that has been reliably propagated in conventional cell culture systems (22–24). The virus replicates in several types of primate cell cultures, but it does so slowly and less efficiently than poliovirus. HAV infection does not induce a shut-down of host cell macromolecular synthesis, and replication in vitro usually is not associated with a cytopathic effect (25). It is not known for certain whether replication in vivo might differ from what is generally observed in cultured cells with respect to the prolonged replication cycle and absence of cytopathic effect. However, it seems likely that these features of the HAV replication cycle may contribute to the lengthy incubation period of hepatitis A.

The virus can be adapted to more efficient growth in cell culture by continued passage, and such virus has often been shown to be attenuated when used to challenge otherwise susceptible nonhuman primates (chimpanzees, owl monkeys, tamarins) (26,27). Several strains of virus that are highly adapted to growth in cell culture are cytopathic in cell culture and have the capacity to form plaques when inoculated onto cells that are then cultured under an agar overlay (28,29). Although the pathogenicity of such viruses has not been tested in animal models, these viruses are also likely to be highly attenuated in vivo. Cell culture–adapted viruses were evaluated as candidate attenuated vaccine

strains in humans, but the development of these vaccines was dropped when they demonstrated an unacceptably low level of immunogenicity (30,31) (see Chapter 251). On the other hand, virus recovered from infected cell cultures remains highly immunogenic following formalin inactivation, and such material serves as a very effective vaccine when alum is used as an adjuvant (32–35).

Infection of permissive cell cultures almost always results in the establishment of a persistent HAV infection in vitro (22–24). Nevertheless, there are no strong clinical or virologic data supporting long-term persistence of HAV infection in humans. A possible exception may be infected premature infants, in which epidemiologic evidence supports the occasional persistence of virus for periods of months, presumably secondary to the immaturity of the immune system (36). Despite the absence of evidence for persistence of the virus in vivo, relapses have been reported up to 4 months after the acute illness in adults. Although some studies have described the presence of virus in clinical samples during such relapses (37,38), such patients have provided no conclusive evidence of long-term persistence of virus. The failure of the virus to establish persistent infection in infected humans suggests that immune responses to the virus are usually very effective, even in severely immunocompromised individuals such as those with advanced human immunodeficiency virus (HIV) infection and the acquired immunodeficiency syndrome (AIDS). Relevant immune clearance mechanisms include the development of antibodies capable of neutralizing HAV (39), the proliferation of virus-specific, HLA-restricted cytotoxic T cells (40), and the induction of interferons with antiviral activity (41).

EPIDEMIOLOGY

Transmission

Transmission of HAV almost always occurs by the fecal-oral route (2,6,7,42,43). Spread of the virus is facilitated by the exceptional stability of the virus capsid as described above, which may promote the spread of HAV through contaminated ground water or via contaminated food (44,45). Common source outbreaks may also be related to infected food handlers who are involved in the preparation of uncooked foods (46). A large number of different food vehicles have been incriminated in transmission of the virus. Remarkably, in several outbreaks it seems likely that lettuce or other produce may have been contaminated at its source or in the wholesale distribution chain, leading to widely distributed infections (45,47). However, despite the impressive nature of common source outbreaks, the vast majority of hepatitis A occurs in a sporadic and endemic fashion.

While rare, the occasional transmission of HAV by blood or blood products is well documented (36,48). Viremia occurs only during the early and acute stages of the infection, and is greatly reduced once symptoms become apparent. Thus, for transmission to occur through blood transfusion, a potential donor must give blood during the early stages of the infection when viremic, but not yet ill (since any illness would result in exclusion of the donor). The transmission of HAV to hemophilic patients by some high purity, solvent-detergent inactivated factor VIII preparations can be attributed to use of commercially procured plasma in very large donor plasma pools, the high purity of the material with resultant removal of potentially protective immunoglobulins, and the absence of a virus inactivation process with efficacy against HAV (49,50).

In some settings, transmission of HAV among users of illicit injectable drugs dominates the local epidemiology of hepatitis A (51–53). It has been controversial as to whether such transmission

TABLE 85.1.   Commonly Reported Risk Factors for Acquisition of Hepatitis A in the United States

Risk factor	Patients with hepatitis A (%)[a]
Household or other close contact with person with hepatitis A	12%–26%
Associated with day care center	11%–16%
Foreign travel	4%–6%
Associated with food or waterborne outbreak	2%–3%
Male homosexual activity	<10%[b]
Illicit injection drug use	<10%[b]
Transfusion of blood or blood product	Uncommon
Unknown	~50%

[a]Adapted from Prevention of hepatitis A through active or passive immunization: recommendations of the Advisory Committee on Immunization Practices (ACIP). *MMWR* 1999;48, with permission.
[b]Higher in years with outbreaks.

is due to the parenteral spread of virus via contaminated drug injection paraphernalia, or the enteric spread of virus due to poor hygiene among drug users, but the fact that the incidence of hepatitis A among drug users in the United States has closely paralleled that of other parenterally transmitted forms of hepatitis over the past two decades suggests the former. This hypothesis is also supported by the stability of the virus particle and its resistance to drying and heat. All forms of blood-borne transmission of HAV reflect the fact that viremia persists for several weeks during acute infection.

Incidence and Prevalence

Serologic surveys have shown that the prevalence of previous infection (ascertained by the presence of antibody to the virus, anti-HAV) is directly related to age, socioeconomic status, and the general level of public health sanitation (6,43,54). Thus, the prevalence of HAV varies widely among different geographic regions, largely reflecting previous and existing sanitation conditions. Infection is common early in life in many developing countries, and generally rare among the well-developed economies of northern Europe. The United States can be considered to have an intermediate level of endemicity (6,43). Hepatitis A is most prevalent in the southwestern part of the country, and generally less common in the northeast. Many cases of hepatitis A appear to be acquired as part of extended, community-based outbreaks that do not have readily apparent sources.

Although 30,021 clinical cases of hepatitis A were reported to the Centers for Disease Control and Prevention in the United States during 1997 (7), a much greater number of cases probably go unreported each year. In studies carried out in the 1970s, approximately one half of Americans over the age of 50 had serologic evidence of prior infection, most likely reflecting a higher national incidence of HAV infection earlier in this century (55). Current surveys indicate that the majority of young adults from North America and Northern Europe are susceptible to infection with this virus, explaining why foreign travel (particularly to developing regions or regions with poor sanitation) remains an important risk factor for acquisition of hepatitis A for persons from these regions.

Long-term fluctuations in the rates of infectious hepatitis (presumed to be largely hepatitis A) have been reported over periods spanning decades in European countries and the United States (6,7,43). However, within the United States, this cyclical variation in incidence seems to have flattened out in recent years. There are no apparent differences in the virulence of HAV strains circulating in different regions of the world, although the typical age at which infection occurs varies widely and influences the incidence of accompanying disease (55–58). Overt liver injury is uncommon in infected children, particularly those under the age of 2, and is much more likely to be severe in older adults.

Risk Factors for Acquisition

Risk factors that have been associated with hepatitis A within the United States are shown in Table 85.1. With the exception of illicit drug use and the use of high-purity clotting factor concentrates (as discussed above), all of these risk factors are easily related to an increased probability of fecal-oral transmission. The risk of infection associated with the administration of high-purity clotting factors appears to have been relatively low and has been further reduced by the implementation of additional virus inactivation procedures such as heat treatment (14). Day care centers caring for preschool children are worth noting as frequent sites of transmission of HAV, as they are for many other enteric pathogens (57,59,60). In such settings, the risk for secondary transmission is greatest from children under the age of 2 years who are not yet toilet trained. This risk may be increased by the fact that the infection in these young children is often clinically silent. In contrast, the risk for disease is substantially greater in older siblings and caregivers (57).

PATHOGENESIS

Virologic Events

An understanding of the pathogenesis of hepatitis A has been gained from studies of experimentally infected humans and nonhuman primates (chimpanzees, tamarins, and owl monkeys) (5,20,61–64). Such studies suggest that there is replication of HAV within gastrointestinal epithelial cells in orally infected animals. HAV antigen has been described in the intestinal cells of infected tamarins (65), a finding confirmed in orally challenged owl monkeys in which viral antigen was identified in epithelial cells within the crypts of the small intestine (4). In addition, small amounts of virus have been found in the saliva during acute hepatitis A, suggesting that replication might occur in the oropharynx (66).

It is not clear how the virus reaches the liver from the gastrointestinal track following its ingestion by the host, but this seems likely to occur as a result of a primary viremia stemming from replication of virus within the gut. One suggestion has been that the virus may be transported to the hepatocyte in the form of an infectious complex with nonneutralizing IgA antibodies (67). According to this model, it is subsequently taken up by the hepatocyte via the asialoglycoprotein receptor. Whatever the mechanism, virus is present in the liver within a week of oral inoculation of nonhuman primates (4).

The dominant site of virus replication *in vivo* is the hepatocyte, although small amounts of viral antigen have been found in lymph nodes, spleen, and along the glomerular basement membrane in infected primates (68). Virus replicated within hepatocytes is shed into the bile via the biliary canaliculi (5), and from the large bile ducts reaches the intestines and is shed into the environment with feces. A high level of replication and shedding of virus may occur in completely asymptomatic individuals during the incubation phase of the disease (Fig. 85.1). This suggests that virus replication is by itself noncytopathic. The clinical findings thus correlate well with the characteristically slow, noncytopathic replication of wild-type HAV in cell culture (described in detail in Chapter 251). Studies carried out in experimentally infected primates indicate that infectious virus first appears in the stool within a week of oral or intravenous inoculation (4,63). The amount of virus shed in feces increases over the subsequent 2 to 3 weeks, generally reaching a maximum just prior to the onset of biochemical evidence of liver injury and clinical symptoms.

Lesser amounts of virus are found in the blood. At any point in time, the titer of virus in serum is approximately 1,000-fold less than the titer of virus in feces (69). However, the temporal course of the viremia follows fecal shedding closely, suggesting that it also derives primarily from the liver. Viremia typically persists for up to 3 weeks and occasionally longer (66,69). It usually decreases markedly in magnitude with the occurrence of symptoms and the first appearance of antibodies to the virus in serum.

Nonetheless, small quantities of infectious virus may continue to be present in the serum for a week or more after such antibodies are present, and virus may be detected for a considerably longer period of time using sensitive reverse transcription polymerase chain reaction (RT-PCR)–based methods. During experimental HAV infections in primates, up to 10^4 to 10^5 infectious virus particles have been found per milliliter of serum (62,69). Maximum viremia titers may be even higher in humans. This brief window of viremia during the asymptomatic, prodromal phase of the infection explains why the parenteral transmission of virus is possible with donation of blood, or sharing of injection paraphernalia among drug users. During this period, still higher titers of virus are generally found in liver tissue (69).

The symptoms of hepatitis A usually have their onset about 4 weeks after exposure, but this interval may range from 2 to 6 weeks (2). In experimentally infected primates, higher dose inocula tend to lead to shorter incubation periods. Acute liver cell injury is marked chemically by elevations of serum alanine aminotransferase (ALT) and aspartate aminotransferase (AST), and is followed somewhat later by increases in serum bilirubin levels reflective of impaired biliary transport. The onset of disease is usually coincident with the appearance of virus-specific antibody (Fig. 85.1). Histopathologically, hepatitis A is marked by hepatocellular necrosis, centrilobular cholestasis, and periportal infiltration of the liver with mononuclear inflammatory cells (70–73) (Fig. 85.2). The cellular infiltrates that characterize the histopathology of hepatitis A and the fact that the disease develops concurrent with the first evidence of an immune response to the virus suggests that the liver injury is to a large extent an immunopathologic condition. Curiously, however, unlike the case with hepatitis B, there is no clinical evidence to

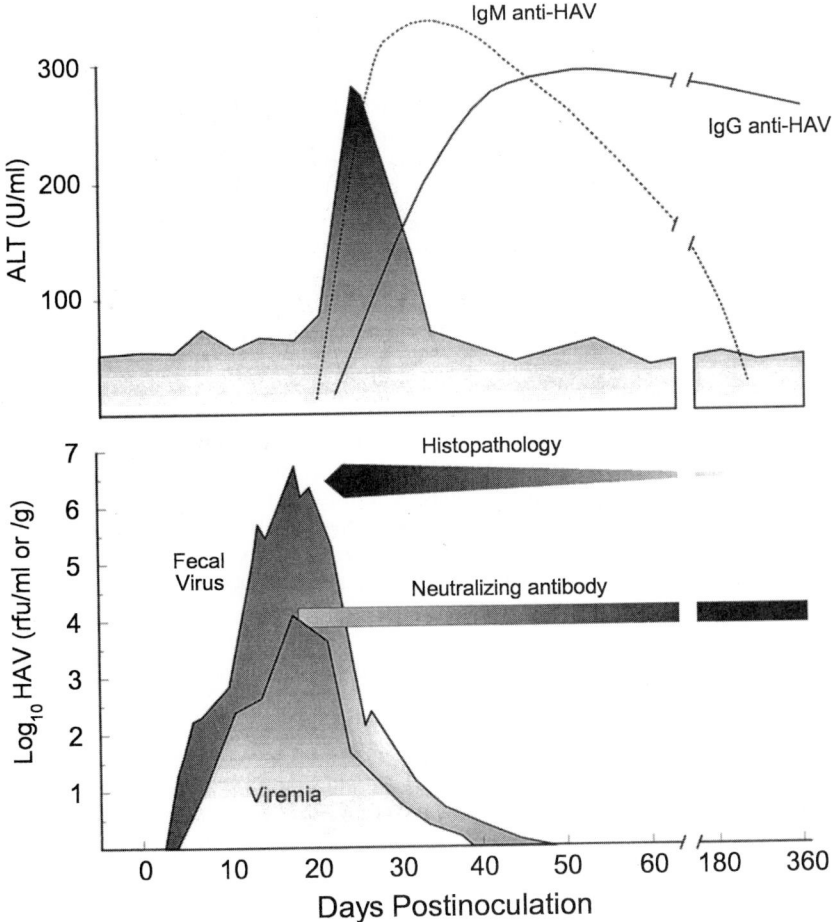

Figure 85.1. Virologic events accompanying hepatitis A virus infection in an experimentally inoculated owl monkey. The events mimic hepatitis A in humans. The top panel depicts serum alanine aminotransferase activity (*thick line*), and the antibody response as determined by an immunoglobulin isotype-nonspecific competitive inhibition assay (*solid line*) and an immunoglobulin M–specific immunoassay (*dashed line*). The bottom panel depicts the recovery of infectious virus from feces (radioimmunofocus-forming units [rfu]/g) and serum (rfu/mL). The shaded box represents the presence of detectable neutralizing antibody to the virus, while the intensity of the histopathologic findings are depicted at the top of the panel.

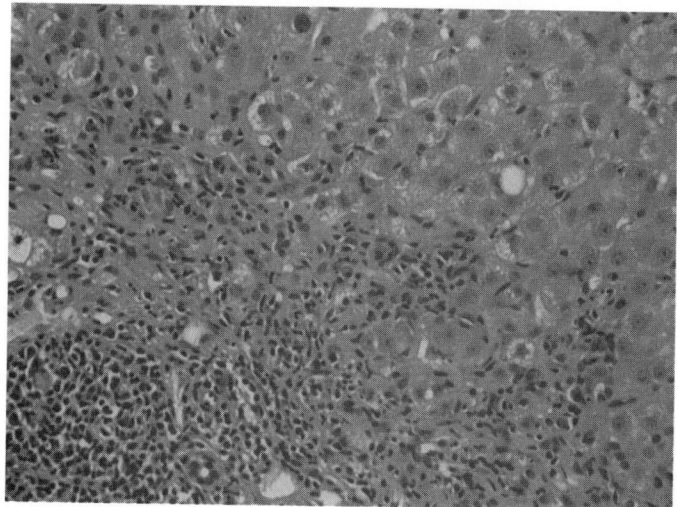

Figure 85.2. Histopathologic features of acute hepatitis A include inflammation of the portal and periportal zones of the liver with infiltration of mononuclear cells (lower left field), and disarray of the normal lobular architecture of the liver (upper right field). There is also prominent hepatocellular ballooning degeneration (cytoplasmic vacuolization). (Courtesy of Dr. Shu-Yuan Xiao, hematoxylin and eosin stain, original magnification ×40.)

suggest that immunologically impaired persons are less likely to develop symptomatic hepatitis A following infection with the virus.

Immune Response to HAV Infection

Total serum immunoglobulins are often nonspecifically elevated during hepatitis A, and rheumatoid factor (IgM antibodies to IgG) is often present. Virus-specific antibodies of all three major isotypes—IgM, IgG, and IgA—appear early in the course of the illness (2,74,75). Immunoglobulin M (IgM) antibody is the most useful diagnostic marker for acute hepatitis A, because the duration of the IgM response is generally limited to less than 6 months following infection. On the other hand, IgG antibody to HAV persists for many years, and perhaps for life in most patients. Both IgG and IgM antibodies have been shown to have virus-neutralizing activity.

Liver injury is mediated by virus-specific, cytotoxic CD8+ T cells and less specific natural killer cells, both of which have been described in acute hepatitis A infections (40,76,77). As proposed for hepatitis B, the elaboration of interferon-γ by virus-specific CD8+ cells (41) probably results in the recruitment of nonspecific inflammatory cells to the site of virus replication. These inflammatory cells likely play an important role in the production of the disease as well as in the control of the infection. Virus replication is sensitive to interferon (78), and interferons and other cytokines probably contribute substantially to the ultimate elimination of the virus in acutely infected persons. Recent studies in experimentally infected nonhuman primates indicate that inducible nitric oxide synthetase is expressed within the infected liver prior to the appearance of necroinflammatory lesions (79). Thus, the production of nitric oxide also may contribute to the liver injury as well as the clearance of virus.

Lifelong immunity is afforded by persisting levels of serum-neutralizing antibody, although there is limited, indirect evidence that asymptomatic reinfection may occur in older individuals living in areas of high HAV endemicity (80). In such cases, primary infection presumably occurred at an early age and was followed by a loss of detectable serum antibody later in life. Rein-

fection then occurs in the setting of household exposure to HAV and is marked by reappearance of serum antibody (IgG, without an IgM response) in the absence of clinically evident disease.

Surprisingly, secretory immunity appears not to play a major role in defense against hepatitis A. While virus-specific IgA has been detected in fecal extracts by immunoassays, viral-neutralizing activity has not been found to be reproducibly present in saliva or fecal extracts (81,82). The lack of a significant neutralizing secretory IgA response may reflect low levels of virus replication in intestinal tissues, but it remains somewhat perplexing. It has important implications for vaccine-induced immunity, and is consistent with the high level of protection afforded by passive immunization with parenterally administered immunoglobulins. Because the presence of circulating neutralizing antibodies prevents infection of the liver, such antibodies also limit the amount of virus that can be shed in the feces. Thus, serum antibodies will limit the extent to which an exposed person can transmit the virus to others. This is important, because it makes for a situation quite different from that seen with poliovirus, in which serum antibodies elicited by inactivated poliovirus vaccine do not prevent transmission of poliovirus among immunized individuals (83). In contrast, serum-neutralizing antibodies produced by inactivated HAV vaccines are very effective in preventing transmission of HAV within immunized populations (7,84). As mentioned above, nonneutralizing IgA antibodies have been suggested to play a role in the uptake of the virus by the hepatocyte (67).

CLINICAL MANIFESTATIONS

Acute Hepatitis A

The clinical manifestations accompanying infection with HAV are listed in Table 85.2. These differ between adults and young children, as most children under the age of two experience asymptomatic infection or an infection marked with symptoms other than those suggestive of hepatic inflammation (2,57). On the other hand, the majority of adults over the age of 18 years develop clinical evidence of hepatitis in association with HAV infection, with up to two thirds becoming clinically icteric (58). The most common symptoms are nausea, dark urine, and light stools. Fever may be impressive by history, but is most often not present by the time the patient seeks medical attention. Diarrhea is reported more often by children (or their parents) than by adults, although the reason for this difference remains uncertain.

The acute illness associated with HAV infection lasts from 1 to 3 weeks, but it is often followed by a period of prolonged convalescence. Serum ALT and AST elevations may persist for a number of weeks, although they are always normal on long-term follow-up (1 year). There is no evidence for progression to chronic viral hepatitis. However, it has been suggested that acute hepatitis A may trigger the onset of chronic autoimmune hepatitis in certain genetically predisposed individuals (85). If so, this must be a rare event.

Cholestatic Hepatitis A

Some patients may experience a prolonged period of jaundice (at times greater than 12 weeks in length) following an episode of acute hepatitis A and the subsidence of serum ALT and AST levels toward normal (86,87). In addition to pruritis associated with cholestasis, patients with this condition (which has been termed cholestatic hepatitis A) may complain of diarrhea and weight loss. Eventually, the serum bilirubin returns to normal

TABLE 85.2.   Symptoms Associated with Hepatitis A, B, and non-A, non-B in Adults

Finding	Prevalence of symptoms (%)		
	Hepatitis A (18 patients)	Hepatitis B (214 patients)	Hepatitis non-A, non-B (68 patients)
Jaundice	88%	83%	82%
Dark urine	68	79	89
Fatigue	63	74	77
Light-colored stools	58	48	37
Loss of appetite	42	56	62
Distaste for cigarettes (smokers only)	45	57	63
Nausea or vomiting	26	46	56
Abdominal pain	37	51	51
Fever or chills	32	25	25
Headache	26	26	25
Muscle pain	26	21	17
Diarrhea	16	30	15
Constipation	16	17	19
Joint pain	11	30	21
Sore throat	0	12	14

Findings in U.S. Army personnel admitted to hospital with a serologically proven hepatitis virus infection (2,105). Most cases of "hepatitis non-A, non-B" were probably due to hepatitis C virus infection.

over a period of weeks, with complete resolution of the illness. Most often, the challenge to the clinician is to avoid inappropriate clinical maneuvers in such patients. The pathogenic basis for this condition is not known. In rare cases, cholestatic disease may be associated with renal failure.

Relapsing Hepatitis A

Relapsing hepatitis A occurs following an episode of otherwise typical acute hepatitis A (37,38,88). Persons with this syndrome develop recrudescent clinical signs and symptoms and worsening biochemical indices of liver inflammation following a period of apparent convalescence from a bout of acute hepatitis 1 to 4 months previously. Some affected individuals may demonstrate an associated increase in the titer of total serum antibodies against HAV, and in most cases there is persistence of IgM anti-HAV. It is not clear, however, whether IgM anti-HAV persists in such patients for longer periods of time than in most uncomplicated cases of acute hepatitis A. HAV has been putatively identified in feces collected during such clinical relapses, and viral RNA was reportedly found in serum using an RT-PCR assay (37,38).

Although supervening infections with other hepatitis agents have not been excluded in all cases, reports of relapsing hepatitis A have occurred with sufficient frequency to suggest that the phenomenon is real. Such relapses are not well explained by existing concepts of the pathogenesis of hepatitis A, but suggest the selection of a persisting virus variant that has the potential to partially escape cellular or humoral immune responses late in the course of infection. Even in cases of relapsing hepatitis A, however, complete recovery is the rule. Occasional patients may complain of persisting fatigue beyond 12 months, but it is difficult to relate these symptoms specifically to previous infection with HAV.

Fulminant Hepatitis A

Fulminant hepatitis is marked by the clinical failure of hepatic synthetic functions with associated bleeding diathesis and coma.

This complication of hepatitis A has been described in approximately 0.14% of hospitalized cases, making this complication of HAV infection relatively rare. HAV accounts for approximately 10% to 20% of all cases of fulminant viral hepatitis (89). Risk factors for development of fulminant disease include age above 50 years and preexisting chronic liver disease due to other viral or nonviral causes (6). There is no evidence that a fulminant course of disease is due to greater than usual virulence on the part the infecting strain of virus (90). Interestingly, however, this rare outcome of HAV infection was reported recently in a group of three previously healthy siblings, suggesting a possible host genetic determinant (91). Fulminant hepatitis A may be fatal, although survival rates are higher than with fulminant hepatitis B or non-A, non-B, non-C disease. Liver transplantation may be lifesaving in this setting.

DIAGNOSIS

Importantly, the clinical signs and symptoms of hepatitis A do not allow its differentiation from hepatitis B or other forms of acute viral hepatitis in individual cases (Table 85.2). A specific diagnosis may be suggested by the epidemiologic setting, such as involvement in a common-source epidemic, or recent travel to a region where the prevalence of the infection is high. However, serologic confirmation is always required.

The diagnosis of acute hepatitis A rests on the specific detection of IgM anti-HAV (74,75,92) (see Chapter 251). The presence of this serum marker is usually indicative of HAV infection having occurred within the preceding 6 months, although detectable IgM antibody may persist for up to 12 months after acute infection in some patients. Total serum antibody to HAV may also be measured as an index of immunity to the virus. Non–isotype-specific tests for anti-HAV antibodies are relatively insensitive, having a detection threshold of about 100 mIU/mL based on use of a World Health Organization reference reagent. Thus, such tests often do not detect protective levels of antibody present after administration of immune globulin (IG) or following a single dose of inactivated hepatitis A vaccine.

TREATMENT

Although interferon inhibits HAV replication in cell cultures (78), it has never been evaluated as a therapeutic agent in acute hepatitis A. It would seem unlikely that it would have any significant impact on the course of the disease given present understanding of the respective roles of viral replication versus the immune response to the virus in liver injury. Similarly, there are no clinically useful antiviral drugs with activity against HAV. The management of patients with acute hepatitis A is thus directed at alleviating symptoms and has at best a limited impact on the clinical course of the infection.

Hospitalization is usually not recommended for the typical patient with acute hepatitis A. However, it is indicated for patients who are severely ill, who have evidence of liver failure, or in elderly patients who are more likely to develop complications (93). In particular, evidence of confusion or prolongation of the prothrombin time should prompt early hospitalization. Bed rest has never been shown to have any effect other than improving the patient's comfort, and patients may be returned to full activity as soon as symptoms subside. A brief course of corticosteroid therapy has been advocated for those patients with persistent jaundice and high serum bilirubin levels (cholestatic hepatitis) (86), but this should be used with caution even in this very special circumstance. No specific therapy has been shown to be of benefit in patients with fulminant hepatitis A. General medical support, including vitamin K for bleeding diathesis and measures to reduce cerebral edema, should be aggressively pursued. Orthotopic liver transplantation may be life-saving (94).

PREVENTION

Immune Globulin

The administration of pooled human IG by intramuscular injection has been used for prevention of symptomatic hepatitis A in exposed individuals for over 50 years. It was shown to be approximately 80% effective in preventing infectious hepatitis among American soldiers overseas (95). When given as an intramuscular preparation for postexposure prophylaxis, IG probably limits viremia and secondary intrahepatic spread of the virus. This most likely results in a reduction in the number of hepatocytes that are ultimately infected, thereby explaining the ability of IG to limit symptoms while allowing development of normal immunity (so-called passive-active immunization) (96,97).

Generally speaking, IG (0.02 mL/kg) is considered effective only if it is administered within 2 weeks after exposure (7), although it may have some beneficial effects even later in the course of the infection. Administration of IG at this dosage will lead to serum antibody levels of about 40 mIU/mL that do not interfere with diagnostic antibody tests for hepatitis A (98). Higher doses of IG given prior to exposure (0.02–0.06 mL/kg) are capable of preventing infection for periods of 1 to 6 months. IG administration generally has few side effects, but does carry a risk for anaphylaxis in individuals with IgA deficiency, especially with repeated administration.

Postexposure prophylaxis with intramuscular IG is indicated following close, personal exposure to a person with hepatitis A, or in persons with other well-defined exposures that are considered likely to result in transmission (Table 85.3). This includes sexual contacts of persons with hepatitis A, and those who are known to have recently shared illicit drugs or injection paraphernalia with a person developing hepatitis A.

The administration of IG is a useful control measure when HAV transmission is documented within a preschool day care setting (7). Its use should be considered for nonimmunized staff and attendees, and possibly also for members of the households of children attending the center. The administration of IG is generally not recommended in a common-source outbreak setting, however, due to the delay that is inherent in recognition of an outbreak and the fact that most exposures will have occurred more than 2 weeks prior to when prophylaxis is first considered (7). In all of these postexposure settings, IG is not required for persons who have received at least one dose of inactivated hepatitis A vaccine more than 2 weeks previously.

TABLE 85.3. Prevention of Hepatitis A

Candidates for immunization with inactivated hepatitis A vaccine
    Children living in areas in which the incidence of hepatitis A is ≥20 cases/100,000 population per year (approximately twice the U.S. national average).
    Persons traveling to or working in countries with intermediate or high endemicity of hepatitis A; intramuscular immune globulin (IG) should be administered simultaneously at a separate anatomic site if travel is to occur within 2–4 weeks, and is an alternative to vaccine for short-term protection.
    Men engaging in sexual acts with other men.
    Users of illicit injectable or noninjectable drugs.
    Occupational exposure to HAV-infected primates or to HAV in a laboratory setting.
    Anti-HAV negative individuals receiving clotting factor concentrates.
    Susceptible individuals with underlying chronic liver disease.
    Preschool and school-aged children and/or certain groups of adults in communities experiencing outbreaks of hepatitis A, subject to specific epidemiologic circumstances and possibly in conjunction with IG.
Candidates for postexposure prophylaxis with IG
    Close personal and/or sexual contact within the previous 2 weeks with a person developing hepatitis A.
    Nonimmunized staff, attendees, or family of attendees of a preschool day care center within which transmission of HAV has occurred.

HAV, hepatitis A virus.
[a]Adapted from Prevention of hepatitis A through active or passive immunization: recommendations of the Advisory Committee on Immunization Practices (ACIP). *MMWR* 1999;48.

Preexposure prophylaxis with intramuscular IG is used less frequently now than in previous decades, having been replaced largely by active immunization with inactivated hepatitis A vaccine. Its use is generally confined to travelers going to endemic regions for whom immediate protection is desired (Table 85.3). Detailed recommendations on the use of IG that have been developed by the U.S. Public Health Service may be found elsewhere (7).

Hepatitis A Vaccines

Inactivated hepatitis A vaccines have been developed by several vaccine manufacturers. Two different but quite similar hepatitis A vaccines (Havrix, Glaxo-SmithKline, Research Triangle Park, NC, U.S.A.; and Vaqta, Merck, West Point, PA, U.S.A.) have been approved for sale in the United States, while a third vaccine (TwinRix, Glaxo-SmithKline) is a combined hepatitis A and hepatitis B vaccine containing the Havrix antigen (7,99). These vaccines contain formaldehyde-inactivated HAV particles produced in infected diploid human cells, with the inactivated viral antigen subsequently adsorbed to aluminum hydroxide for its adjuvant effect. The purity of the inactivated viral particles varies considerably between manufacturers, but this has not been shown to correlate with differences in safety, immunogenicity, or efficacy, and in almost all respects these hepatitis A vaccines appear to be quite comparable (7,99,100). The vaccines are very safe, with minor local and systemic side effects similar in frequency and severity to those seen with the recombinant hepatitis B vaccine (7,99). More serious adverse events have been described (anaphylaxis, Guillain-Barré syndrome), but these occur only at low frequencies. Anaphylaxis is likely related to the vaccine or its vehicle, while infrequently reported neurologic events such as Guillain-Barré syndrome have an uncertain association with vaccine administration because they do not appear to occur with a frequency greater than the background frequency expected in nonimmunized persons (7).

Generally speaking, a single dose of inactivated hepatitis A vaccine is sufficient to induce levels of antibodies to HAV that, while much lower than those following natural infection, are significantly greater than those present following a single 0.02 mL/kg dose of IG (7,98,100,101). This level of antibody is protective against clinical hepatitis A. Although evidence supports the presence of protective antibody levels within 2 weeks of administration of a single dose of vaccine, it is preferable to immunize travelers at least 4 weeks prior to departure. IG can be given simultaneously with the vaccine (at alternate anatomic sites), allowing travelers immediate protection with little effect on vaccine immunogenicity (7). Booster doses of the vaccine generally lead to marked increases in antibody titer, and are recommended because they extend the duration of protection.

Two prospective clinical trials have confirmed that inactivated hepatitis A vaccines are extremely efficacious in preventing hepatitis A in immunized children (33,34). In one study, protection against clinical disease was 100% within 3 weeks following administration of a single dose of inactivated vaccine (Vaqta) (33). One month after this immunization, the median level of anti-HAV antibody was approximately 40 mIU/mL. In a second study using a different vaccine (Havrix), an equivalent level of clinical protection was observed among Thai school children who had received multiple doses of the vaccine (34). Although comparable controlled clinical studies are lacking in adults, the vaccine is almost certainly equivalently protective based on a comparison of the levels of antibody that are induced with active immunization, and those that are present following administration of IG.

General recommendations for the use of these vaccines are shown in Table 85.3 (7). Because the doses and schedules vary for vaccines provided by different manufacturers, this information should be obtained from the package insert. While IG remains the measure of choice for postexposure prophylaxis for persons who have had close personal contact with an infected individual, vaccine is generally preferable for most preexposure indications. Due to costs, immunization with inactivated hepatitis A vaccines is generally targeted to high-risk populations, including either those at significantly increased risks for acquiring the infection, or those with chronic underlying liver disease in whom there is an increased risk for more serious disease should infection occur. Although immunization is recommended for persons with chronic hepatitis C because of an increased risk for fulminant hepatitis A, the cost effectiveness of this practice has engendered some controversy (102,103).

Hepatitis A vaccines remain relatively costly, and this has had a continuing negative impact on the extent to which they have been used. Cost-effectiveness studies generally do not support the universal immunization of children, although this has been recommended recently within the United States in regions where the annual incidence of hepatitis A exceeds twice the national average (7,104). It has yet to be shown whether these vaccines will receive wide enough use to cause a reduction in the overall incidence of hepatitis A in the United States, or in other countries with even higher rates of hepatitis A. Effective control of hepatitis A is likely to require universal immunization of children, but this will require the development of vaccines that are less expensive to manufacture and administer. Candidate attenuated vaccines have been tested in limited clinical trials, but have not proven sufficiently immunogenic to warrant further development (see Chapter 251).

REFERENCES

1. Cuthbert JA. Hepatitis A: old and new. *Clin Microbiol Rev* 2001;14:38–58.
2. Lemon SM. Type A viral hepatitis: new developments in an old disease. *N Engl J Med* 1985;313:1059–1067.
3. Lemon SM, Robertson BH. Current perspectives in the virology and molecular biology of hepatitis A virus. *Semin Virol* 1993;4:285–295.
4. Asher LVS, Binn LN, Mensing TL, et al. Pathogenesis of hepatitis A in orally inoculated owl monkeys (*Aotus trivirgatus*). *J Med Virol* 1995;47:260–268.
5. Schulman AN, Dienstag JL, Jackson DR, et al. Hepatitis A antigen particles in liver, bile, and stool of chimpanzees. *J Infect Dis* 1976;134:80–84.
6. Lemon SM, Shapiro CN. The value of immunization against hepatitis A. *Infect Agents Dis* 1994;3:38–49.
7. Prevention of hepatitis A through active or passive immunization: recommendations of the Advisory Committee on Immunization Practices (ACIP). *MMWR* 1999;48.
8. Regenmortel MHV, Fauquet CM, Bishop DL, et al. Virus *taxonomy: the classification and nomenclature of viruses*. The Seventh Report of the International Committee on Taxonomy of Viruses. San Diego: Academic, 2000.
9. Martin A, Lemon SM. The molecular biology of hepatitis A virus. In: Ou J-H, ed. Hepatitis viruses. Norwell, MA: Kluwer Academic, 2002:23–50.
10. Lemon SM, Jansen RW, Brown EA. Genetic, antigenic, and biologic differences between strains of hepatitis A virus. *Vaccine* 1992;10(suppl):40–44.
11. Scholz E, Heinricy U, Flehmig B. Acid stability of hepatitis A virus. *J Gen Virol* 1989;70:2481–2485.
12. Siegl G, Weitz M, Kronauer G. Stability of hepatitis A virus. *Intervirology* 1984;22:218–226.
13. Lemon SM, Amphlett E, Sangar D. Protease digestion of hepatitis A virus: disparate effects on capsid proteins, antigenicity, and infectivity. *J Virol* 1991;65:5636–5640.
14. Murphy P, Nowak T, Lemon SM, Hilfenhaus J. Inactivation of hepatitis A virus by heat treatment in aqueous solution. *J Med Virol* 1993;41:61–64.
15. Lemon SM, Murphy PC, Smith A, et al. Removal/neutralization of hepatitis A virus during manufacture of high purity, solvent/detergent factor VIII concentrate. *J Med Virol* 1994;43:44–49.
16. Ticehurst JR, Cohen JI, Feinstone SM, et al. Replication of hepatitis A virus: new ideas from studies with cloned cDNA. In: Ehrenfeld E, Semler BL, eds.

Molecular aspects of picornavirus infection and detection. Washington, DC: ASM Press, 1989:27–50.

17. Robertson BH, Jansen RW, Khanna B, et al. Genetic relatedness of hepatitis A virus strains recovered from different geographic regions. *J Gen Virol* 1992;73:1365–1377.

18. Lemon SM, Binn LN. Antigenic relatedness of two strains of hepatitis A virus determined by cross-neutralization. *Infect Immun* 1983;42:418–420.

19. Tsarev SA, Emerson SU, Balayan MS, et al. Simian hepatitis A virus (HAV) strain AGM-27: comparison of genome structure and growth in cell culture with other HAV strains. *J Gen Virol* 1991;72:1677–1683.

20. Dienstag JL, Feinstone SM, Purcell RH, et al. Experimental infection of chimpanzees with hepatitis A virus. *J Infect Dis* 1975;132:532–545.

21. Emerson SU, Tsarev SA, Govindarajan S, et al. A simian strain of hepatitis a virus, AGM-27, functions as an attenuated vaccine for chimpanzees. *J Infect Dis* 1996;173:592–597.

22. Provost PJ, Giesa PA, McAleer WJ, et al. Isolation of hepatitis A virus *in vitro* in cell culture directly from human specimens. *Proc Soc Exp Biol Med* 1981;167:201–206.

23. Binn LN, Lemon SM, Marchwicki RH, et al. Primary isolation and serial passage of hepatitis A virus strains in primate cell cultures. *J Clin Microbiol* 1984;20:28–33.

24. Daemer RJ, Feinstone SM, Gust ID, et al. Propagation of human hepatitis A virus in African Green Monkey kidney cell culture: primary isolation and serial passage. *Infect Immun* 1981;32:388–393.

25. Gauss-Muller V, Deinhardt F. Effect of hepatitis A virus infection on cell metabolism *in vitro*. *Proc Soc Exp Biol Med* 1984;175:10–15.

26. Provost PJ, Conti PA, Giesa PA, et al. Studies in chimpanzees of live, attenuated hepatitis A vaccine candidates. *Proc Soc Exp Biol Med* 1983;172:357–363.

27. Cohen JI, Rosenblum B, Ticehurst JR, et al. Complete nucleotide sequence of an attenuated hepatitis A virus: comparison with wild-type virus. *Proc Natl Acad Sci U S A* 1987;84:2497–2501.

28. Lemon SM, Murphy PC, Shields PA, et al. Antigenic and genetic variation in cytopathic hepatitis A virus variants arising during persistent infection: evidence for genetic recombination. *J Virol* 1991;65:2056–2065.

29. Cromeans T, Fields HA, Sobsey MD. Kinetic studies of a rapidly replicating, cytopathic hepatitis A virus. In: Zuckerman AJ, ed. *Viral hepatitis and liver disease.* New York: Alan R. Liss, 1988:24–26.

30. Sjogren MH, Purcell RH, McKee K, et al. Clinical and laboratory observations following oral or intramuscular administration of a live, attenuated hepatitis A vaccine candidate. *Vaccine* 1992;10(suppl 1):135–137.

31. Midthun K, Ellerbeck E, Gershman K, et al. Safety and immunogenicity of a live attenuated hepatitis A virus vaccine in seronegative volunteers. *J Infect Dis* 1991;163:735–739.

32. Armstrong ME, Giesa PA, Davide JP, et al. Development of the formalin-inactivated hepatitis A vaccine, VAQTA, from the live attenuated virus strain CR326F. *J Hepatol* 1993;18(suppl 2):20–26.

33. Werzberger A, Mensch B, Kuter B, et al. A controlled trial of a formalin-inactivated hepatitis A vaccine in healthy children. *N Engl J Med* 1992;327:453–457.

34. Innis BL, Snitbhan R, Kunasol P, et al. Protection against hepatitis A by an inactivated vaccine. *JAMA* 1994;271:1328–1334.

35. Andre FE, Hepburn A, D'Hondt E. Inactivated candidate vaccines for hepatitis A. *Prog Med Virol* 1990;37:72–95.

36. Rosenblum LS, Villarino ME, Nainan OV, et al. Hepatitis A outbreak in a neonatal intensive care unit: risk factors for transmission and evidence of prolonged viral excretion among preterm infants. *J Infect Dis* 1991;164:476–482.

37. Sjogren MH, Tanno H, Fay O, et al. Hepatitis A virus in stool during clinical relapse. *Ann Intern Med* 1987;106:221–226.

38. Glikson M, Galun E, Oren R, et al. Relapsing hepatitis A. Review of 14 cases and literature survey. *Medicine (Baltimore)* 1992;71:14–23.

39. Lemon SM, Binn LN. Serum neutralizing antibody response to hepatitis A virus. *J Infect Dis* 1983;148:1033–1039.

40. Vallbracht A, Gabriel P, Maier K, et al. Cell-mediated cytotoxicity in hepatitis A virus infection. *Hepatology* 1986;6:1308–1314.

41. Maier K, Gabriel P, Koscielniak E, et al. Human gamma interferon production by cytotoxic T lymphocytes sensitized during hepatitis A virus infection. *J Virol* 1988;62:3756–3763.

42. Shapiro CN, Shaw FE, Mandel EJ, et al. Epidemiology of hepatitis A in the United States. In: Hollinger FB, Lemon SM, Margolis HS, eds. Viral hepatitis and liver disease. Baltimore: Williams & Wilkins, 1991:71–76.

43. Bell BP, Shapiro CN, Alter MJ, et al. The diverse patterns of hepatitis A epidemiology in the United States—implications for vaccination strategies. *J Infect Dis* 1998;178:1579–1584.

44. Friedman LS, O'Brien TF, Morse LJ, et al. Revisiting the Holy Cross football team hepatitis outbreak (1969) by serological analysis. *JAMA* 1985;254:774–776.

45. Hutin YJ, Pool V, Cramer EH, et al. A multistate, foodborne outbreak of hepatitis A. National Hepatitis A Investigation Team. *N Engl J Med* 1999;340:595–602.

46. Hooper RR, Juels CW, Routenberg JA, et al. Outbreak of type A viral hepatitis at the naval training center, San Diego: epidemiologic evaluation. *Am J Epidemiol* 1977;105:148–155.

47. Rosenblum LS, Mirkin IR, Allen DT, et al. A multifocal outbreak of hepatitis A traced to commercially distributed lettuce. *Am J Public Health* 1990;80:1075–1079.

48. Sherertz RJ, Russell BA, Reuman PD. Transmission of hepatitis A by tranfusion of blood products. *Arch Intern Med* 1984;144:1579–1580.

49. Lemon SM. The natural history of hepatitis A: the potential for transmission by transfusion of blood or blood products. *Vox Sang* 1994;67(suppl 4):19–23.

50. Mannucci PM, Gdovin S, Gringeri A, et al. Transmission of hepatitis A to patients with hemophilia by factor VIII concentrates treated with organic solvent and detergent to inactivate viruses. *Ann Intern Med* 1994;120:1–7.

51. Shaw DD, Whiteman DC, Merritt AD, et al. Hepatitis A outbreaks among illicit drug users and their contacts in Queensland, 1997. *Med J Aust* 1999;170:584–587.

52. Centers for Disease Control and Prevention. Hepatitis A among drug abusers. *MMWR* 1988;37:297–305.

53. Widell A, Hansson BG, Moestrup T, et al. Increased occurrence of hepatitis A with cyclic outbreaks among drug addicts in a Swedish community. *Infection* 1983;11:198–200.

54. Dienstag JL, Szmuness W, Stevens CE, et al. Hepatitis A virus infection: new insights from seroepidemiologic studies. *J Infect Dis* 1978;137:328–340.

55. Szmuness W, Dienstag JL, Purcell RH, Stevens et al. The prevalence of antibody to hepatitis A antigen in various parts of the world: a pilot study. *Am J Epidemiol* 1977;106:392–398.

56. Burke DS, Snitbhan R, Johnson DE, et al. Age-specific prevalence of hepatitis A virus antibody in Thailand. *Am J Epidemiol* 1981;113:245–249.

57. Hadler SC, Webster HM, Erben JJ, et al. Hepatitis A in day-care centers: a community-wide assessment. *N Engl J Med* 1980;302:1222–1227.

58. Lednar WM, Lemon SM, Kirkpatrick JW, et al. Frequency of illness associated with epidemic hepatitis A virus infections in adults. *Am J Epidemiol* 1985;122:226–233.

59. Hadler SC, Erben JJ, Matthews R, et al. Effect of immunoglobulin on hepatitis A in day-care centers. *JAMA* 1983;249:48–53.

60. Benenson MW, Takafuji ET, Bancroft WH, et al. A military community outbreak of hepatitis type A related to transmission in a child care facility. *Am J Epidemiol* 1980;112:471–481.

61. Purcell RH, Emerson SU. Animal models of hepatitis A and E. *ILAR J* 2001;42(2):161–177.

62. Provost PJ, Villarejos VM, Hilleman MR. Suitability of the rufiventer marmoset as a host animal for human hepatitis A virus. *Proc Soc Exp Biol Med* 1977;155:283–286.

63. LeDuc JW, Lemon SM, Keenan CM, et al. Experimental infection of the New World owl monkey (*Aotus trivirgatus*) with hepatitis A virus. *Infect Immun* 1983;40:766–772.

64. Krawczynski KK, Bradley DW, Murphy BL, et al. Pathogenetic aspects of hepatitis A virus infection in enterally inoculated marmosets. *Am J Clin Pathol* 1981;76:698–706.

65. Karayiannis P, Jowett T, Enticott M, et al. Hepatitis A virus replication in tamarins and host immune response in relation to pathogenesis of liver cell damage. *J Med Virol* 1986;18:261–276.

66. Cohen JI, Feinstone S, Purcell RH. Hepatitis A virus infection in a chimpanzee: duration of viremia and detection of virus in saliva and throat swabs. *J Infect Dis* 1989;160:887–890.

67. Dotzauer A, Gebhardt U, Bieback K, et al. Hepatitis A virus-specific immunoglobulin A mediates infection of hepatocytes with hepatitis A virus via the asialoglycoprotein receptor. *J Virol* 2000;74:10950–10957.

68. Mathiesen LR, Drucker J, Lorenz D, et al. Localization of hepatitis A antigen in marmoset organs during acute infection with hepatitis A virus. *J Infect Dis* 1978;138:369–377.

69. Lemon SM, Binn LN, Marchwicki R, et al. *In vivo* replication and reversion to wild-type of a neutralization-resistant variant of hepatitis A virus. *J Infect Dis* 1990;161:7–13.

70. Teixera MR J., Weller IVD, Murray A, et al. The pathology of hepatitis A in man. *Liver* 1982;2:53–60.

71. Dienstag JL, Popper H, Purcell RH. The pathology of viral hepatitis types A and B in chimpanzees. *Am J Pathol* 1976;85:131–144.

72. Keenan CM, Lemon SM, LeDuc JW, et al. Pathology of hepatitis A infection in the owl monkey (*Aotus trivirgatus*). *Am J Pathol* 1984;115:1–8.

73. Abe H, Beninger PR, Ikejiri N, et al. Light microscopic findings of liver biopsy specimens from patients with hepatitis type A and comparison with type B. *Gastroenterology* 1982;82:938–947.

74. Lemon SM, Brown CD, Brooks DS, et al. Specific immunoglobulin M response to hepatitis A virus determined by solid-phase radioimmunoassay. *Infect Immun* 1980;28:927–936.

75. Decker RH, Kosakowski SM, Vanderbilt AS, et al. Diagnosis of acute hepatitis A by HAVAB(R)-M, a direct radioimmunoassay for IgM anti-HAV. *Am J Clin Pathol* 1981;76:140–147.

76. Vallbracht A, Maier K, Stierhof Y-D, et al. Liver-derived cytotoxic T cells in hepatitis A virus infection. *J Infect Dis* 1989;160:209–217.

77. Kurane I, Binn LN, Bancroft WH, et al. Human lymphocyte responses to hepatitis A virus–infected cells: interferon production and lysis of infected cells. *J Immunol* 1985;135:2140–2144.

78. Vallbracht A, Hofmann L, Wurster KG, et al. Persistent infection of human fibroblasts by hepatitis A virus. *J Gen Virol* 1984;65:609–615.

79. Pinto MA, Marchevsky RS, Pelajo-Machado M, et al. Inducible nitric oxide synthase (iNOS) expression in liver and splenic T lymphocyte rise are associated with liver histological damage during experimental hepatitis A virus (HAV) infection in Callithrix jacchus. *Exp Toxicol Pathol* 2000;52(1):3–10.

80. Villarejos VM, Serra CJ, Anderson-Visona K, et al. Hepatitis A virus infection in households. *Am J Epidemiol* 1982;115:577–586.
81. Locarnini SA, Coulepis AG, Stratton AM, et al. Solid-phase enzyme-linked immunosorbent assay for detection of hepatitis A–specific immunoglobulin M. *J Clin Microbiol* 1979;9:459–465.
82. Stapleton JT, Lange DK, LeDuc JW, et al. The role of secretory immunity in hepatitis A virus infection. *J Infect Dis* 1991;163:7–11.
83. Ogra PL, Karzon DT. Formation and function of poliovirus antibody in different tissues. *Prog Med Virol* 1971;13:156–193.
84. Werzberger A, Kuter B, Nalin D. Six years' follow-up after hepatitis A vaccination. *N Engl J Med* 1998;338:1160.
85. Vento S, Garofano T, di Perri G, et al. Identification of hepatitis A virus as a trigger for autoimmune chronic hepatitis type 1 in susceptible individuals. *Lancet* 1991;337:1183–1187.
86. Gordon SC, Reddy KR, Schiff L, et al. Prolonged intrahepatic cholestasis secondary to acute hepatitis A. *Ann Intern Med* 1984;101:635–637.
87. Corpechot C, Cadranel JF, Hoang C, et al. [Cholestatic viral hepatitis A in adults. Clinical, biological and histopathological study of 9 cases]. *Gastroenterol Clin Biol* 1994;18:743–750.
88. Bornstein JD, Byrd DE, Trotter JF. Relapsing hepatitis A: a case report and review of the literature. *J Clin Gastroenterol* 1999;28:355–356.
89. Mathiesen LR, Skinoj P, Nielsen JO, et al. Hepatitis type A, B, and non-A non-B in fulminant hepatitis. *Gut* 1980;21:72-77.
90. Fujiwara K, Yokosuka O, Fukai K, et al. Analysis of full-length hepatitis A virus genome in sera from patients with fulminant and self-limited acute type A hepatitis. *J Hepatol* 2001;35:112–119.
91. Durst RY, Goldsmidt N, Namestnick J, et al. Familial cluster of fulminant hepatitis A infection. *J Clin Gastroenterol* 2001;32:453–454.
92. Duermeyer W, van der Veen J. Specific detection of IgM-antibodies by ELISA, applied in hepatitis-A. *Lancet* 1978;2:684–685.
93. Willner IR, Uhl MD, Howard SC, et al. Serious hepatitis A: an analysis of patients hospitalized during an urban epidemic in the United States [see comments]. *Ann Intern Med* 1998;128:111–114.
94. Debray D, Cullufi P, Devictor D, et al. Liver failure in children with hepatitis A. *Hepatology* 1997;26:1018–1022.
95. Gellis SS, Stokes J Jr, Brother GM, et al. The use of human immune serum globulin (gamma globulin) in infectious (epidemic) hepatitis in the Mediterranean theater of operations. I. Studies on prophylaxis in two epidemics of infectious hepatitis. *JAMA* 1945;128:1062–1063.
96. Winokur PL, Stapleton JT. Immunoglobulin prophylaxis for hepatitis A. *Clin Infect Dis* 1992;14:580–586.
97. Krugman S, Ward R, Giles JP, et al. Infectious hepatitis: studies on the effect of gamma globulin and on the incidence of inapparent infection. *JAMA* 1960;174:323–330.
98. Lemon SM, Murphy PC, Provost PJ, et al. Immunoprecipitation and virus neutralization assays demonstrate qualitative differences between protective antibody responses to inactivated hepatitis A vaccine and passive immunization with immune globulin. *J Infect Dis* 1997;176:9–19.
99. Lemon SM, Thomas DL. Vaccines to prevent viral hepatitis. *N Engl J Med* 1997;336:196–204.
100. Ashur Y, Adler R, Rowe M, et al. Comparison of immunogenicity of two hepatitis A vaccines—VAQTA and HAVRIX—in young adults. *Vaccine* 1999;17:2290–2296.
101. Ambrosch F, Widermann G, Andre FE, et al. Comparison of HAV antibodies induced by vaccination, passive immunization, and natural infection. In: Hollinger FB, Lemon SM, Margolis HS, eds. Viral hepatitis and liver disease. Baltimore: Williams & Wilkins, 1991:98–100.
102. Myers RP, Gregor JC, Marotta PJ. The cost-effectiveness of hepatitis A vaccination in patients with chronic hepatitis C. *Hepatology* 2000;31:834–839.
103. Arguedas MR, Heudebert GR, Fallon MB, et al. The cost-effectiveness of hepatitis A vaccination in patients with chronic hepatitis C viral infection in the United States. *Am J Gastroenterol* 2002;97:721–728.
104. Beutels P, Edmunds WJ, Antonanzas F, et al. Economic evaluation of vaccination programmes: a consensus statement focusing on viral hepatitis. *Pharmacoeconomics* 2002;20:1–7.
105. Lemon SM, Lednar WM, Bancroft WH, et al. Etiology of viral hepatitis in American soldiers. *Am J Epidemiol* 1982;116:438–450.

CHAPTER 86
Hepatitis B and Hepatitis D

Raymond S. Koff

HEPATITIS B

Epidemiology

INCUBATION PERIOD
The incubation period of hepatitis B, defined as the interval between exposure to hepatitis B virus (HBV) and elevation of the serum aminotransferase levels, has a broad peak of between 60 and 90 days, with a range of 30 to 180 days. The incubation period, if taken as the period between exposure to HBV and the initial appearance of the hepatitis B surface antigen (HBsAg) in serum, the earliest marker of infection routinely detected, may be as short as 1 to 2 weeks. Biochemical evidence of hepatitis is usually present within a month or two after HBsAg is identified.

EPIDEMIOLOGIC PATTERNS
HBV infection occurs throughout the world: more than 2 billion people have been infected, and HBV-related deaths occur at a rate of over 1 million per year. HBV transmission is not dependent on serial propagation from acutely infected to susceptible individuals; a human reservoir, currently estimated to be approximately 350 million persistently infected individuals, is present in nearly all communities of the world (Fig. 86.1). Without treatment, as many as 25% to 40% of those with chronic hepatitis B will succumb from cirrhosis or hepatocellular carcinoma. HBV infection has been identified in highly endemic zones in geographically remote and culturally isolated populations (e.g., South Pacific Islanders and Alaskan Natives) as well as in large, densely populated regions (e.g., sub-Saharan Africa and Asia). In the United States, infections due to HBV have declined to less than 80,000 cases annually (1). This decline has been seen among both sexes, all racial groups, and in those age groups with the highest infection rates, namely young adults (2). The decline began after the introduction of HBV vaccines but before widespread implementation of a national vaccination program. Therefore, in large part, changes in high-risk behaviors may be responsible. Despite the decline in new infections in the United States, approximately 0.4% (1.25 million individuals) are chronically infected and 5,000 deaths are annually attributed to sequelae of chronic HBV infection.

HBV infection occurs early in life in most high-prevalence areas. As a consequence of maternal-neonatal transmission and horizontal spread between young children, markers of prior HBV infection may be found in most children by 10 to 15 years of age in these endemic regions.

In contrast, in lower-prevalence populations, the rate of infection peaks later; a substantial proportion of the population may have markers of HBV infection by age 25 years. Sexual activity plays an important role in this pattern. In the United States, as in many low-prevalence areas, markers of HBV infection are found in less than 5% of the general population (2). They are found more frequently in Alaskan Eskimos, Pacific Islanders, immigrants from countries where hepatitis B is endemic, Asian Americans, and blacks and Hispanics than in white persons. In general, in low-prevalence populations, such as in the United States sexual activity, injection drug use, occupationally-acquired

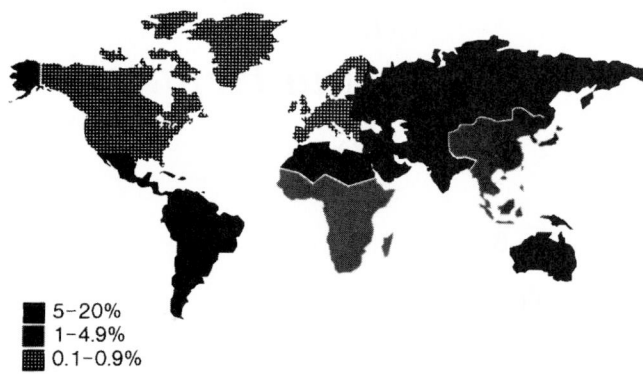

Figure 86.1. The global prevalence of the hepatitis B virus carrier state. High-endemicity zones, in which the hepatitis B surface antigen carrier rate approaches or occasionally exceeds 20%, are found in Southeast Asia and in sub-Saharan Africa. (Courtesy of the Clinical Teaching Project, American Gastroenterological Association.)

infection, nonsexual household or intrafamilial spread, hemodialysis, and use of multiple blood products have been the principal identified mechanisms of HBV transmission (Fig. 86.2). Imported cases in immigrants and travelers returning from high-prevalence countries are of minor importance. In about 25% to 30% of cases, no risk factor can be identified; unrecognized or inapparent permucosal or percutaneous spread (e.g., via tattooing, body-piercing, shared razor blades, etc.) is likely to be responsible for some of these infections. Transfusion-associated hepatitis B has become a rare event in the United States since the introduction of an all-volunteer donor system and serologic screening. The introduction of nucleic acid testing of donor blood in minipools should reduce the risk even further. Recipients of certain pooled blood products, such as patients with hemophilia, who have had a substantial risk for HBV infection in the past, are also less likely to be infected since virus inactivation procedures to treat these products and recombinant clotting factors were introduced.

In the United States, the risk for HBV transmission among young children appears to be low (2). Peak attack rates of HBV are seen in the 15- to 39-year-old age group and have represented nearly 75% of all reported cases, thereby supporting the concept of HBV infection as a sexually transmitted disease in this country.

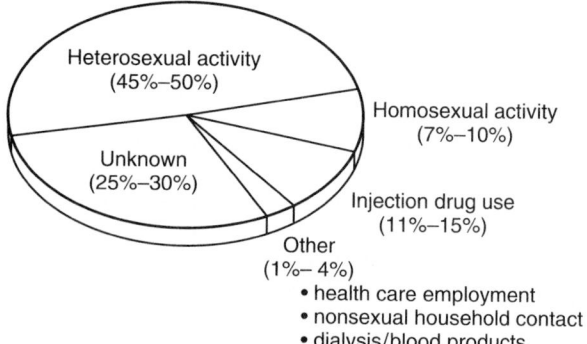

Figure 86.2. Major risk factors for the acquisition of hepatitis B virus infection in the United States. (Adapted from McQuillan G, Alter MJ, Everhart JE. Viral hepatitis. In: Everhart JE, ed. *Digestive diseases in the United States.* National Institutes of Health Publication No. 94-1447. Washington, DC: U.S. Government Printing Office, 1994:127–156.)

MODES OF TRANSMISSION

Contact Transmission

Although blood contains the highest HBV concentrations of all body fluids, horizontal transfer of HBV-contaminated body secretions, including semen, cervicovaginal secretions, and saliva, is involved in contact transmission between sexual partners and between some household members not engaging in sexual activity. Transfer of contaminated body fluids to nonsexual household and family contacts is most likely to occur by child-to-child spread and may involve such diverse mechanisms as shared eating utensils, teething rings, toys, and toothbrushes. Efficient transmission may be especially common when the infected individual is mentally retarded and institutionalized. Exposure to open wounds in contact sports such as sumo wrestling and football may result in horizontal transmission (3). The infectivity of body fluids and the contagiousness of persistently infected individuals may decrease with increasing age, concomitantly with a reduction in levels of viral replication. In fact, small amounts of plasma positive for HBV DNA by polymerase chain reaction (PCR) testing but negative for HBsAg is not invariably infectious (4).

Maternal-Neonatal Transmission

No more than 5% to 10% of neonatal HBV infections appear to result from *in utero* infection prior to delivery (5). The presumed mechanism of most neonatal infections is transplacental leakage of HBV-contaminated maternal blood resulting from uterine contractions and disruption of placental barriers during labor and delivery. Some neonatal HBV infections may occur in the early postpartum period by mechanisms that are less well-defined. HBV DNA has been identified by PCR amplification in colostral specimens, but breast-feeding does not increase the risk for transmission to infants provided that they are immunized shortly after birth with hepatitis B immune globulin (HBIG) and hepatitis B vaccine. Data on the efficacy of delivery by cesarean section in reducing the risk for infection are conflicting.

Maternal-neonatal HBV transmission occurs most frequently when the mother is an HBV carrier who is also hepatitis B e antigen (HBeAg)-positive or when she develops HBV infection during the third trimester or early postpartum period. Nearly 90% of the infants of HBeAg-positive carrier women will be infected; about 10% to 15% of the infants of HBeAg-negative women will be infected (6) (Fig. 86.3). In contrast to infections in adults, most neonatal infections will be persistent (i.e., the infant becomes an HBV carrier). The strongest independent predictor of the risk for persistent infection in the infant is the maternal HBV DNA level (6). The risk increases with increasing maternal HBV load.

Percutaneous Transmission

Percutaneous inoculation appears to be a highly efficient mode of HBV transfer. HBV infection is common in injecting drug users who share needles and other inoculation equipment, in those who inject frequently, and in those who attend "shooting galleries" (7). Within the first year of injection drug use, 50% acquire HBV infection (8). It was also common among health care workers exposed through accidental needlesticks with contaminated equipment in the era before widespread use of HBV vaccines in this occupational group.

Tissue penetrations with any form of contaminated instruments (e.g., acupuncture needles, tattoo needles, and ear-piercing equipment) may be responsible for sporadic cases as well as for mini-outbreaks of infection. Communal use of water for bathing has been implicated in the development of outbreaks of HBV among track-finders with multiple cuts and scratches. An extreme example of percutaneous transmission, HBV infection

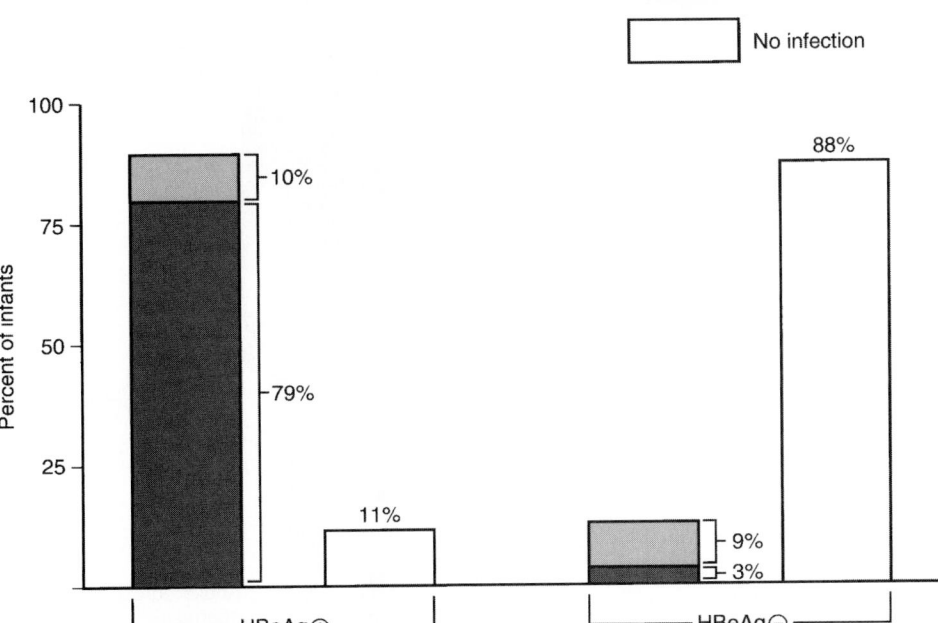

Figure 86.3. Infant hepatitis B virus infection rates and the hepatitis B e antigen (HBeAg) status of the hepatitis B surface antigen–positive carrier mother. As shown here, most infections in the infants of HBeAg-positive mothers are persistent. (Adapted from Burk RD, Hwang L-Y, Ho GYF, et al. Outcome of perinatal hepatitis B virus exposure is dependent on maternal virus load. *J Infect Dis* 1994;170:1418–1423, with permission.)

after transplantation of HBV-contaminated organs, has become uncommon since appropriate donor screening for HBsAg has been implemented. However, livers from donors who are HBsAg negative but positive for antibody to hepatitis B core antigen (anti-HBc) can transmit HBV to transplant recipients (9).

In the medical office, in the hospital laboratory, or at the bedside, permucosal transfer may result from splashing accidents when mucosal surfaces are exposed to contaminated biomaterials, such as blood or other body fluids. Percutaneous, iatrogenic transmission of hepatitis B remains a concern in many countries due to reuse of inoculation equipment with inadequate sterilization or inappropriate multidose syringe techniques (10). The use of human plasma to stabilize vaccines is no longer acceptable, but when it did occur during World War II, over 300,000 U.S. soldiers acquired hepatitis B from HBV-contaminated yellow fever vaccine (11).

Unestablished Routes of Spread

Respiratory or airborne transmission and food- and water-borne spread are not accepted epidemiologic entities. The role of biting insects (e.g., bedbugs) remains speculative (12).

Pathogenesis and Pathology

The principal histologic lesions of acute HBV infection are foci of hepatocyte necrosis, with loss of cells (dropout), ballooning degeneration, and acidophilic (Councilman-like) bodies, which are mummified hepatocytes that have undergone apoptosis. Necrosis and inflammation may be most prominent in the centrilobular zones; an endophlebitis may be present. Whereas the lobular architecture is intact, a diffuse mononuclear cell infiltrate may be prominent within the lobule and within expanded portal tracts, which may demonstrate segmental erosion of the limiting plate. The CD8+ cytotoxic lymphocyte appears to be the predominant mononuclear cell in the liver of the patient with HBV infection; it is closely associated with infected hepatocytes. Natural killer lymphocytes are also prominent. The mononuclear macrophages of the liver, the Kupffer cells, appear enlarged and hyperplastic.

Hepatocyte injury in HBV infection does not appear to be due to a direct cytopathic effect of the virus or its gene products because liver histology and function may be entirely normal in HBV carriers. Nonetheless, in some instances (e.g., after liver transplantation for end-stage chronic hepatitis B with active viral replication), the rapid onset of HBV reinfection of the graft and the development of severe hepatitis in the immunosuppressed recipient suggest a direct cytotoxic role for the virus in these settings.

Cell-mediated immune mechanisms are thought to be key in the pathogenesis of liver injury in hepatitis B. The precise mechanisms are still poorly understood. Major histocompatibility complex–restricted cytotoxic T-lymphocyte activity, antibody-dependent cell-mediated cytotoxicity, and natural killer cell activity have been postulated to be involved, but it is the polyclonal and multispecific cytotoxic T-lymphocyte response to HBV that appears to be predominantly responsible for liver injury. After recovery, this response persists indefinitely and is thought to be maintained by continued antigenic stimulation resulting from residual and largely innocuous virus in the liver. Activation of cytotoxic T-lymphocytes directed against specific target viral antigens (e.g., HBcAg) expressed on the hepatocyte membrane are thought to be important for controlling HBV replication (13). Viral antigen-independent activation of cytotoxic T lymphocytes may also play a role.

In acutely infected chimpanzees, noncytopathic mechanisms mediated by intrahepatic induction of inflammatory cytokines (interferon-γ, tumor necrosis factor-α, and interferon-α and -β) contribute to HBV clearance from the hepatocyte well before maximal T-cell infiltration of the liver and before immune-mediated destruction of infected hepatocytes (14). These observations indicate that cell necrosis is not essential for purging HBV from infected hepatocytes.

The mechanisms responsible for the development of chronic HBV infection also remain incompletely understood. The high frequency of chronic infection in those infected early in life and in the immunocompromised suggests that immunologic tolerance may play a key role. In general, the cytotoxic T-lymphocyte response to HBV is relatively weak in chronic hepatitis B patients. However, during acute exacerbations or during treatment with interferon, the cytotoxic T-lymphocyte response becomes prominent. Genetically determined host factors also appear to play a role in HBV persistence (15). In the presence of a quantitatively weak or delayed T-lymphocyte response to HBV or inadequate generation of antiviral cytokines, low-level hepatocyte necrosis and continuing HBV replication in hepatocytes result in the development of chronic hepatitis B.

Clinical Manifestations of Acute Hepatitis B

CLINICAL FEATURES

Acute hepatitis B occurs in two major forms: asymptomatic and symptomatic hepatitis.

Asymptomatic Hepatitis

Asymptomatic HBV infection can be either subclinical or inapparent. In subclinical infection, abnormal blood test results reflecting hepatic injury (i.e., elevated serum aminotransferase levels) are present, but jaundice and symptoms are absent. In inapparent infection, neither symptoms nor biochemical abnormalities are detected; inapparent infections are identified by serologic studies. In neonates and young children with HBV infection, asymptomatic infection is typical. The ratio of subclinical and inapparent infection remains ill defined. In contrast to experience in children, symptomatic disease is more frequently encountered in adolescents and adults.

Symptomatic Hepatitis

In adults with symptomatic disease, about one in four patients will have jaundice. Symptomatic hepatitis without jaundice is termed anicteric hepatitis. The clinical features of anicteric hepatitis are identical, save for the absence of jaundice, to those of icteric hepatitis, but they are milder and often abbreviated. Gastrointestinal symptoms, either alone or in combination with influenza-like symptoms, including mild fever, may be the predominant clinical features of anicteric hepatitis. Malaise, fatigue, weakness, and anorexia may or may not be present.

Preicteric (Prodromal) Features

The onset of symptoms in hepatitis B is usually insidious, and in a few patients no symptoms occur before the onset of jaundice. However, more typically, a set of constitutional, gastrointestinal, and to a lesser extent respiratory symptoms may be seen during a preicteric prodromal phase that may last for several weeks. In about 25% of patients, the preicteric phase may be less than 1 week long. Lassitude, fatigue, myalgias and arthralgias, anorexia, and nausea and vomiting may be the most prominent complaints. In less than 10% of patients, an immune complex–mediated (HBsAg–anti-HBs or HBeAg–anti-HBe) extrahepatic serum sickness–like syndrome may be the initial or major preicteric feature. In affected patients, combinations of polyarthritis, angioedema, urticaria, maculopapular eruptions, and more rarely hematuria and proteinuria reflecting glomerular involvement or cutaneous or systemic vasculitis are observed (Fig. 86.4). The polyarthritis is typically symmetric, involves chiefly the distal joints (e.g., the proximal interphalangeal joints and, to a lesser extent, the larger axial and appendicular joints), and usually subsides with the development of jaundice.

Icteric and Recovery Phases

Darkening of the urine to a brownish color and lightening of stool color are often observed for a few days before the appearance of jaundice. Anorexia, malaise, nausea, and vomiting transiently worsen with the development of jaundice, and pruritus may be

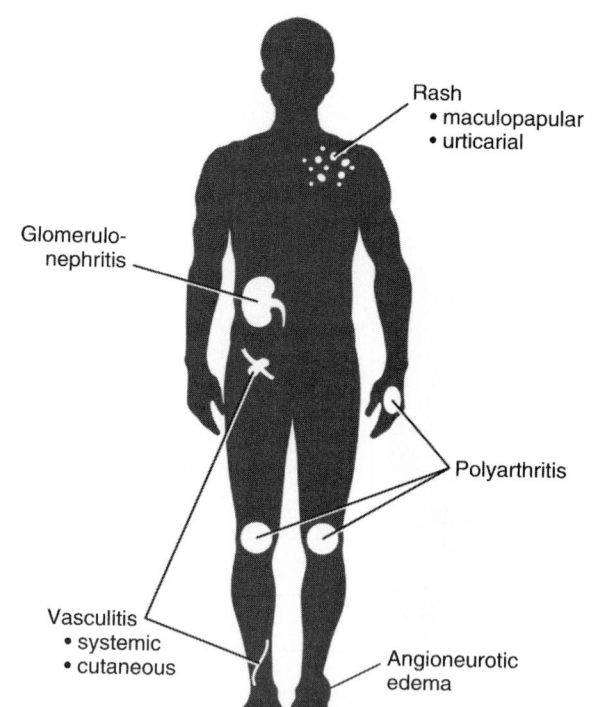

Figure 86.4. Extrahepatic manifestations of the hepatitis B virus–associated, immune complex–mediated, serum sickness–like syndrome seen in the prodrome of acute hepatitis B. (Courtesy of the Clinical Teaching Project, American Gastroenterological Association.)

noted. Mild weight loss may occur. Within a few days, as jaundice deepens, the constitutional symptoms become less severe, and gustatory and olfactory acuity return with an improvement in appetite. Jaundice peaks and then disappears gradually, usually within a month or two after its onset.

PHYSICAL FINDINGS

In the prodrome, the physical examination may be entirely normal or may reveal slight hepatomegaly or signs of joint or skin involvement. In the jaundiced patient, the liver may be moderately tender as well as mildly enlarged. The liver edge is usually rounded, and the spleen tip may be palpated in as many as 20% of patients. Posterior cervical lymphadenopathy is detected in a similar proportion. Small spider angiomas may be recognized. These findings disappear during the recovery phase.

LABORATORY STUDIES

Blood Chemistries

Serum alanine aminotransferase and aspartate aminotransferase elevations are found in the late prodromal phase and reach peak levels, usually 10 to 100 times the upper limits of normal, during the early icteric phase. Serum bilirubin levels peak 1 to 8 days after peak aminotransferase levels. In most icteric patients, maximal serum bilirubin levels are below 10 mg/dL. Higher levels suggest severe disease or a cholestatic element to the hepatitis. In the convalescent phase, serum aminotransferase and bilirubin levels decline toward normal; minor elevations of the aminotransferases may persist for a few months even after serum bilirubin levels are normal. Typically, serum alkaline phosphatase levels are normal or only mildly elevated, and only minimal alterations in hepatic synthetic function (prothrombin time and serum albumin levels) are found.

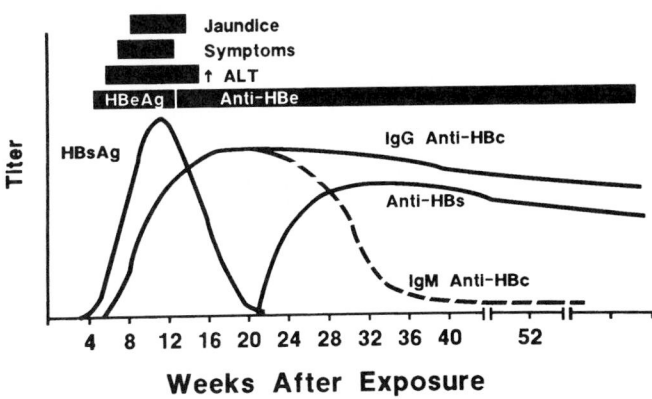

Figure 86.5. The sequential appearance of the major antigen-antibody systems in acute hepatitis B and their relative titers. *ALT,* alanine aminotransferase. (From Koff RS. Acute and chronic hepatitis B. In: Seeff LB, Lewis JH, eds. *Current perspectives in hepatology.* New York: Plenum, 1989:23–33, with permission.)

Serologic Tests

Hepatitis B Surface Antigen. The first readily identifiable and widely available serologic marker of acute HBV infection is the HBsAg (Fig. 86.5). It appears before the development of elevated levels of serum alanine or aspartate aminotransferase. In patients in whom the HBV-associated prodromal serum sickness–like syndrome is recognized, HBsAg may be the only marker present in serum samples. In most HBV-infected patients, HBsAg becomes serologically undetectable, by conventional radioimmunoassay or enzyme-linked immunosorbent assay, within a few weeks to a few months after its appearance. In about 10% of patients, HBsAg has disappeared by the time symptoms develop. In contrast, persistence of HBsAg beyond 6 months indicates the development of chronic HBV infection. Pre-S proteins (pre-S1 and pre-S2), a component of HBsAg, and their corresponding antibodies are transiently present in the sera of HBV-infected patients but are not routinely measured.

Hepatitis B e Antigen. This derivative of the HBcAg is usually detected within a few days to a few weeks after the appearance of HBsAg in acute HBV infection. The HBcAg is not generally detected in serum. HBeAg is a marker of active HBV replication because its presence is correlated, imperfectly, with the presence of HBV particles and HBV DNA in serum in both acute and chronic hepatitis B. However, mutations in the precore (pre-C) region of HBV DNA result in HBV infections in which HBeAg is not produced but active viral replication may be present. In uncomplicated acute HBV infection, HBeAg disappears before HBsAg disappears. Shortly after the disappearance of HBeAg, its corresponding antibody, anti-HBe, becomes detectable. This marker may persist for prolonged periods. Detection of HBeAg in serum has served as an index of viral replication, infectivity, and response to treatment.

Hepatitis B Virus DNA. Tests for HBV DNA are sensitive but vary in sensitivity; a World Health Organization international standard of a titer of 10^6 IU/mL has been established (16). Circulating HBV DNA can be detected during the early phase of acute HBV infection, well before the appearance of HBsAg; during this period, it is the single best marker of active HBV replication. Several weeks later in the acute infection, it, as well as HBeAg, is generally undetectable when measured by hybridization techniques. In most patients, HBeAg clearance occurs before clearance of HBV DNA (17). However, in self-limited acute hepatitis B, HBV DNA may be detected by the more sensitive technique

of PCR amplification in serum, peripheral blood mononuclear cells, and liver, years after clinical, biochemical, and apparent serologic remission (18).

In contrast, the prolonged presence of HBV DNA detected by the less sensitive hybridization techniques usually indicates persistent infection with continuing viral replication and continued infectivity. Whereas HBV DNA has been identified in an extrachromosomal site in the hepatocytes of patients with active HBV replication, it seems likely that integration of HBV DNA into the DNA of the hepatocyte may occur randomly throughout the infectious process.

Antibody to the Hepatitis B Core Antigen. Freely circulating HBcAg is not detectable in HBV infection, and testing for this antigen is not available in clinical laboratories. Testing for its corresponding antibody, anti-HBc, is widely available. Anti-HBc is detected shortly after HBsAg is detected and before the appearance of anti-HBs. Initially, the predominant immunoglobulin class of anti-HBc is IgM. Peak levels of IgM anti-HBc are reached within several weeks of the onset of infection; IgM anti-HBc persists considerably longer than HBsAg. A positive test response for IgM anti-HBc is the most sensitive test for the identification of acute HBV infection. IgM anti-HBc will be detected in the 10% of patients who have lost HBsAg by the time of first testing. After reaching peak levels, IgM anti-HBc diminishes in titer and disappears in most patients with acute HBV infection by 4 to 8 months after its appearance. Test results for total anti-HBc remain positive: the predominant form of anti-HBc found during late convalescence and thereafter for years to decades after acute HBV infection is IgG anti-HBc. Levels of IgG anti-HBc decline slowly during a prolonged period.

Antibody to the Hepatitis B Surface Antigen. As the titer of HBsAg declines with time in acute, self-limited HBV infection, its corresponding antibody (anti-HBs) becomes detectable and reaches peak levels within a few months. This antibody is believed to be the neutralizing, protective antibody. During the late convalescent phase of acute HBV infection, anti-HBs titers begin to decrease but the rate of decline is slow; anti-HBs remains detectable for many years to decades. In some patients, a distinct minority, anti-HBs may eventually become undetectable but may reappear if reexposure to HBV occurs. In a small proportion of patients, anti-HBs is lost early or never becomes detectable.

Diagnosis

The diagnosis of HBV infection is a serologic one. Through use of serologic markers, it is possible to identify acute HBV infection, the replicative and nonreplicative phases of chronic HBV infection, and the recovery phase (Table 86.1).

SPECIFIC SEROLOGIC DIAGNOSIS OF ACUTE HEPATITIS B
The serologic diagnosis of acute HBV infection is based on the presence of HBsAg and IgM anti-HBc. Although nearly all patients with acute infection are HBsAg positive for some time, HBsAg will have disappeared by the time illness is recognized and serologic testing is undertaken in about 10%. Testing for IgM anti-HBc identifies all acutely infected patients, regardless of whether HBsAg is still present. HBeAg and HBV DNA are typically present during the acute phase of illness, but because their identification adds little clinically useful information, they are not routinely measured.

DIFFERENTIAL DIAGNOSIS
Acute hepatitis, as defined by symptoms and signs and the presence of typical laboratory abnormalities indicating hepatocellular injury, in an HBsAg-positive individual, is not necessarily

TABLE 86.1. Serologic Markers of Hepatitis B Virus Infection

Phase	HBsAg/anti-HBs	HBeAg/anti-HBe	Anti-HBc	HBV DNA
Acute infection	HBsAg	HBeAg	IgM	Present
Chronic infection				
Replicative phase	HBsAg	HBeAg	IgG	Present
Nonreplicative phase	HBsAg	Anti-HBe	IgG	Absent
Recovery	Anti-HBs	Anti-HBe	IgG	Absent

HBsAg, hepatitis B surface antigen; anti-HBs, antibody to HBsAg; HBeAg, hepatitis B e antigen; anti-HBe, antibody to HBeAg; anti-HBc, antibody to hepatitis B core antigen; HBV, hepatitis B virus; IgM, immunoglobulin M; IgG, Immunoglobulin G.

pathognomonic of acute HBV infection. Differential diagnosis in this setting includes reactivation of chronic HBV infection, a seroconversion flare in chronic hepatitis B in which elevated aminotransferase levels may occur during the transition from HBeAg-positive to anti-HBe-positive, superinfection by other hepatitis viruses in an individual who is a carrier of HBsAg (IgM anti-HBc is usually not detectable), and liver injury due to other causes such as alcohol or drugs. Precise serologic diagnosis may require assessment of multiple markers and sequential serologic studies.

Clinical Variants

ACUTE LIVER FAILURE

In less than 1% of adult patients, hepatic encephalopathy and striking prolongation of the prothrombin time, the clinical hallmarks of acute liver failure (fulminant hepatitis), develop within a few days to 8 weeks after the onset of HBV infection. Precore and core HBV mutants are commonly found (19) and transmission of precore HBV mutants from HBV infected, HBeAg-negative mothers to their newborns may also result in acute liver failure in the newborn (20). Examination of liver tissue, obtained at necropsy or liver transplantation, reveals massive destruction and dropout of hepatocytes, and HBV DNA may be detected. The few surviving hepatocytes may form thickened plates and pseudoglandular structures. Small round cells, plasma cells, and polymorphonuclear leukocytes may be present.

The major complication of acute liver failure is cerebral edema (21) which often signals the development of brain death or brainstem involvement, which in turn may lead to cardiopulmonary arrest and central hypotension. Severe coagulopathy is usually present and may be manifested by gastrointestinal bleeding. Sepsis may be prominent; in some patients, severe, life-threatening hypoglycemia or insulin-resistant nonketotic hyperglycemia may dominate the clinical findings. In addition to hepatic failure, other organ systems eventually fail, reducing the likelihood of recovery. Fatality rates in patients with severe disease often exceed 75%. Emergency liver replacement for patients near death from fulminant hepatitis, by means of orthotopic liver transplantation, is associated with a survival rate of about 60% to 75%.

Chronic Hepatitis B Virus Infection

Chronic HBV infection is defined operationally as the persistence of HBsAg for at least 6 months. In rare instances, in the absence of detectable HBsAg and even more rarely in the absence of anti-HBc, HBV may be responsible for chronic hepatitis; in this circumstance HBV DNA may be detected in both serum and liver (22). The highest risk for HBV persistence is found in neonates born to HBV carrier women who are HBeAg positive and have high levels of HBV DNA (6). Of these infected neonates, as many as 90% progress to chronic infection (23). In

contrast, approximately 30% of children infected before 6 years of age develop chronicity. Among adults infected by HBV, more than 98% recover completely. In the remainder, persistent infection may be associated with chronic hepatitis or an asymptomatic carrier state. In general, persistent infection occurs with a higher frequency in males than in females and among individuals with impaired immunity.

NATURAL HISTORY

Asymptomatic Carriers

In the absence of symptoms related to liver disease, persistently HBsAg-positive individuals with normal serum aminotransferase levels, as well as other normal liver chemistries, are termed asymptomatic or healthy carriers. Most of these individuals are HBeAg negative, HBV DNA negative by hybridization, and most have normal or minimally abnormal results of liver biopsy on initial evaluation. Short-term (10 years) follow-up studies indicate that reactivation of HBV replication and hepatic histologic progression are infrequent, although some patients develop mild or transient serum aminotransferase elevations on sequential study (24). Carriers who develop sustained serum aminotransferase elevations may experience HBV reactivation and histologic progression to chronic hepatitis. Spontaneous HBsAg clearance in asymptomatic HBsAg carriers appears to occur at an annual rate of about 0.8%. In contrast, HBsAg clearance in patients with chronic hepatitis B is slightly lower at a rate of about 0.5% annually (25).

Chronic Hepatitis B

The natural history of chronic hepatitis B also is variable. A large body of data indicates that continuing viral replication and cellular immune responses to infected hepatocytes are highly correlated with progression of disease and reduced life expectancy. In typical patients with chronic hepatitis B, a large proportion of hepatocytes are infected. It is estimated that approximately 10% of patients with chronic hepatitis B spontaneously cease to have detectable viral replication, as reflected in loss of HBeAg or HBV DNA, during the first year after identification and each year thereafter. Unless these patients experience relapse, hepatic inflammation and hepatocyte necrosis are diminished, and the likelihood of developing cirrhosis, liver failure, and premature death are reduced. Relapses, often called reactivation, are recognized by the reappearance of HBeAg or HBV DNA and occur in about 7% of those who have lost HBeAg in the first year and in about 3% per year thereafter. Among patients with chronic hepatitis B in whom viral replication continues, the annual probability of developing cirrhosis has been estimated to be 12%, and the annual probability that liver failure will ensue in those with cirrhosis is estimated to be close to 6% (26). Limited studies suggest that concomitant alcohol consumption may enhance the risk for cirrhosis and liver failure in patients with chronic hepatitis B.

Hepatocellular carcinoma, an extraordinarily prevalent malignant neoplasm in many parts of the world, has been etiologically linked with chronic HBV infection and may be seen in both asymptomatic carriers and those with chronic hepatitis B with or without cirrhosis. Most hepatocellular carcinomas arise in the setting of HBV-associated cirrhosis. Patients with chronic hepatitis B associated with cirrhosis have an annual incidence of hepatocellular carcinoma estimated to be close to 2.5% (26). The risk for hepatocellular carcinoma therefore increases over time, and in regions in which HBV infection rates are high, hepatocellular carcinoma is a leading cause of cancer-related death. Although the precise oncogenic mechanisms remain ill-defined, immune-mediated hepatocyte injury may be responsible for the initiation of hepatocarcinogenesis (27).

The natural history of chronic hepatitis B associated with the pre-C HBV mutant remains incompletely understood. In individuals with chronic HBV infection in whom the pre-C mutant has emerged, either an asymptomatic carrier state with normal serum aminotransferase levels or a more severe and progressive liver disease may be predominant (28). The natural history of individuals with chronic hepatitis B in whom no serologic markers of infection other than HBV DNA can be found in serum or liver remains to be determined.

PATHOLOGY

Portal and periportal inflammation with small round cells, hepatocyte degeneration, apoptotic changes, and necrosis that may be confluent (bridging necrosis), and the formation of fibrous septa are the characteristic histologic features. The predominant inflammatory cell is the cytotoxic T-lymphocyte; plasma cells are also present. The inflammatory infiltrate may spill over and erode the limiting plate of the portal triad, producing the lesion termed interface hepatitis (previously called piecemeal necrosis). During active phases of disease and during relapses, lobular inflammation may be similar to that seen in acute hepatitis B, with scattered acidophilic (apoptotic) bodies. In most patients with chronic hepatitis B, HBsAg may be demonstrated in hepatocyte cytoplasm with immunostaining or routine orcein staining. Hepatocytes rich in HBsAg may have a ground-glass appearance.

CLINICAL MANIFESTATIONS

Patients with chronic hepatitis B may be asymptomatic, may experience fatigue, or may have symptoms of end-stage liver disease due to cirrhosis. During active phases of the disease, malaise and weakness may be striking. Elevated serum aminotransferase levels are usually found; levels may be increased from 2- to 20-fold. In patients with elevated serum bilirubin levels, prolonged prothrombin times, and reduced serum albumin levels, severe disease should be anticipated. The development of edema, ascites, splenomegaly and hypersplenism, or esophageal varices strongly suggests the presence of cirrhosis and portal hypertension. In no more than 1% to 3% of patients with chronic hepatitis B, extrahepatic manifestations resembling the immune complex–mediated serum sickness–like syndrome seen in the prodrome of acute hepatitis B may be striking. These include cryoglobulinemia, arthritis, membranous or membranoproliferative glomerulonephritis, and generalized vasculitis.

Episodes of acute flares with striking elevations of serum aminotransferase levels in chronic hepatitis B are common and in as many as 20% of cases may be due to superinfection by other hepatitis viruses. In the remainder, spontaneous exacerbations may occur as a consequence of an enhanced immune-mediated response to the virus as a result of increased HBV replication, the emergence of HBV mutants, or the restoration of immune competence after treatment with cytotoxic or immunosuppressive therapy (29). The role of alcohol in the pathogenesis of spontaneous exacerbations is uncertain.

SPECIFIC SEROLOGIC DIAGNOSIS OF CHRONIC HEPATITIS B

HBsAg and anti-HBc (IgG) are present in nearly all patients with chronic hepatitis B (Fig. 86.6); the exceptions are those few patients in whom HBV DNA in serum or liver is the sole indicator of chronic infection. In the more typical and most common form of chronic hepatitis B, HBeAg and HBV DNA are detected in those HBsAg-positive patients with active viral replication (Table 86.1), with the notable exception that HBeAg may be absent in patients with the pre-C HBV variant. Surprisingly, a small proportion of patients may have low-titer, low-affinity heterotypic anti-HBs nonreactive with their circulating HBsAg. In this circumstance, the presence of anti-HBs has no clinical importance. In patients in whom HBV reactivation occurs, HBV DNA, HBeAg, and even IgM anti-HBc may reappear in serum concurrently with elevation of serum aminotransferases.

Treatment

ACUTE HEPATITIS B

Effective and safe antiviral treatment of acute HBV infection, were it available, might be targeted to infected infants and young children in whom the risk of chronic infection is high without treatment, to patients with severe disease in whom acute liver failure is a major concern, and to patients with acute HBV infection after liver transplantation. Studies of the efficacy of antiviral treatment of acute hepatitis B with interferon-α or lamivudine, drugs used in the treatment of chronic hepatitis B, are extremely limited (30,31). Because interferon may induce a flare in disease activity, its use in patients with severe acute hepatitis B may be dangerous. Only supportive and symptomatic measures are currently available. Physical activity restrictions are best determined by the patient and should be based on the patient's sense of well-being. Dietary restrictions are usually unnecessary as long as a well-balanced diet can be consumed. Corticosteroids should not be used.

ASYMPTOMATIC CARRIERS

No effective treatment of asymptomatic, healthy HBsAg carriers is currently available. Treatment with interferon-α or lamivudine is not recommended. Repeated administration of HBV vaccine with concurrent administration of lamivudine, a nucleoside analog capable of suppressing HBV replication, is under study in this setting as well as in chronic hepatitis B.

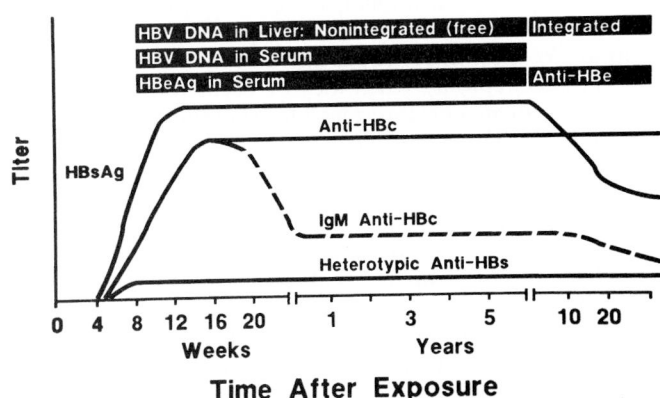

Figure 86.6. The sequential serologic appearance of the major antigen-antibody systems and hepatitis B virus DNA (in serum and liver) in chronic hepatitis B. (From Koff RS. Acute and chronic hepatitis B. In: Seeff LB, Lewis JH, eds. *Current perspectives in hepatology*. New York: Plenum, 1989:23–33, with permission.)

CHRONIC HEPATITIS B

Currently, two therapeutic agents have been approved by the U.S. Food and Drug Administration for the treatment of chronic hepatitis B: interferon-α and lamivudine. Interferon was the first approved therapy. A large number of prospective, controlled studies have shown that treatment with interferon-α of patients with chronic hepatitis B in whom HBV replication is active will induce a long-term response in about 35% to 40% (26). Response is defined by serum HBV clearance by non-PCR assays, loss of HBeAg, development of anti-HBe, biochemical resolution, and histologic improvement. Loss of circulating HBsAg and appearance of anti-HBs may occur in as many as one third of responding patients but is often delayed for years. Relapse after ending therapy may occur in about 10% of patients. Among patients with or without compensated cirrhosis, virologic remission is associated with improved survival (32–34). Recommended regimens are 10 million units of interferon-α2b three times a week for 16 to 24 weeks by subcutaneous injection or 5 million units daily for the same period. A flare-up in the hepatitis, with a mild to moderate increase in serum aminotransferase levels beginning at about week 4 to 8 of interferon treatment, is typical in responding patients but may also occur in some nonresponders. Interferon-associated adverse events—including depression, fatigue, granulocytopenia, and thrombocytopenia, to name only a few—require dose reductions in about 35% of treated patients and premature cessation of treatment in about 5% of patients (26). Interferon-α treatment has been reported to be cost saving, increasing life expectancy by more than 3 years and decreasing lifetime health care costs (26). Seroconversion from HBeAg to anti-HBe usually occurs during the last month of interferon treatment or within 3 months after ending treatment, while HBV DNA clearance usually occurs earlier. Interferon treatment may also induce remissions in patients with extrahepatic disorders (e.g., glomerulonephritis) associated with chronic HBV infection.

The second therapeutic agent available for treatment of chronic hepatitis B is lamivudine, given in an oral dose of 100 mg daily. This nucleoside analog, which inhibits HBV DNA synthesis by chain termination, is effective in inhibiting HBV replication in as many as 60% of patients after 1 year of therapy, but sustained viral clearance occurs in less than 20%. Lamivudine has been administered for periods of 1 year or longer; the optimal length of treatment remains uncertain (35). The drug is exceedingly well tolerated. Drug discontinuation is usually attempted after 1 year of treatment if the patient is HBeAg negative, anti-HBe positive, and has cleared HBV DNA (36). Although liver biopsy results improve in just over half of treated patients, viral resistance emerges in 15% to 20% of patients treated for 1 year and in nearly 60% when therapy is extended to 3 years. However, treatment for 3 years resulted in HBeAg seroconversion in up to 65% (37). Lamivudine infrequently induces biochemical flare-ups; typically when they do occur it is after discontinuation of treatment. Resistance to lamivudine is associated with mutations in the tyrosine, methionine, aspartate, aspartate (YMDD) motif of the HBV polymerase gene, leading to steric hindrance between the mutant amino acid side chain and the nucleoside (38). The HBV mutants associated with lamivudine resistance are not responsive to treatment with famciclovir or emtricitabine (other drugs currently being studied as therapy for chronic hepatitis B) but may be responsive to other nucleotide analogs such as adefovir. Despite this resistance, which may lead to the reappearance of HBV DNA in the circulation, the mutant viruses appear to be replication defective and less pathogenic than the wild-type virus (39).

Pharmacoeconomic studies suggest that therapy with lamivudine may be more cost effective than therapy with interferon (40).

Combining lamivudine with interferon-α does not seem to confer any added benefit compared to treatment with either agent alone. New approaches to treatment include the use of long-acting pegylated interferons alone, the combination of pegylated interferon with lamivudine, other combinations of antiviral nucleoside or nucleotide analogs (adefovir, entecavir, emtricitabine), therapeutic vaccines incorporating a cytotoxic T-lymphocyte epitope derived from the hepatitis B core protein, thymosin, antisense oligonucleotides, and ribozymes. Limited studies have suggested that repeated inoculations of the recombinant HBV vaccines used in immunoprophylaxis may decrease HBV replication in patients with chronic hepatitis B (41). Whether the combination of immunotherapy with vaccine and antiviral drugs will enhance the likelihood of sustained viral clearance is unknown.

END-STAGE CHRONIC HEPATITIS B WITH CIRRHOSIS

In patients with HBV-associated cirrhosis, in whom clinical evidence of decompensation is present (e.g., jaundice, ascites, encephalopathy, or previous esophageal variceal bleeding), treatment with interferon-α, even in low doses, is unlikely to be beneficial and may lead to sepsis and severe acute flare-ups of hepatic inflammation and injury, both of which are life threatening (42). For the patient with cirrhosis and decompensation, lamivudine is therefore the agent of choice. In well-compensated cirrhosis, interferon may be used but very close monitoring is required. Liver transplantation has had considerable success since the administration of HBIG during the operative procedure and routinely thereafter has been adopted. Posttransplantation treatment with lamivudine and other antiviral drugs is also under study.

HEPATOCELLULAR CARCINOMA

Although screening of patients with chronic hepatitis B for hepatocellular carcinoma by serial measurement of serum α-fetoprotein and ultrasound examination of the liver has been advocated, the benefits of screening remain controversial; the costs are high, many of the lesions detected have been unresectable, prolonged survival has been infrequently reported, and lead-time and length biases may have confounded some of the studies suggesting a benefit. In patients without cirrhosis and well-preserved hepatic function, resection of single small tumors, less than 2 cm in diameter is more effective than chemotherapy or radiotherapy, but new lesions may appear on follow-up. In patients with cirrhosis, orthotopic liver transplantation for pretransplantation-identified solitary tumors under 5 cm in diameter or less than 3 tumors each less than 3 cm in diameter or those small tumors discovered incidentally at the time of surgery appears to prolong life expectancy (43). The role of percutaneous ethanol injection, radiofrequency thermoablation, and chemoembolization in the treatment of unresectable disease before transplantation or in the noncandidate for transplantation remains under study.

Prevention

GENERAL MEASURES

Although changing high-risk behaviors reduces the risk for HBV infection, modification of such behaviors if often exceedingly difficult. Furthermore, in as many as 25% to 30% of patients with acute HBV infection, the specific route of infection and likely source remain uncertain. Hence, the key to control of HBV infection is immunoprophylaxis.

IMMUNIZATION

Anti-HBs is the protective, neutralizing antibody responsible for immunity to HBV infection. Passive immunization, the administration of exogenous, preformed anti-HBs in the form of HBIG prepared from donors who have recovered from HBV infection, is rarely used alone. Active immunization with HBV vaccine and combined active-passive immunization (HBV vaccine and HBIG) are the preferred approaches. Anti-HBs is induced by HBsAg, the active immunogenic material in the yeast-recombinant HBV vaccines (Recombivax HB [Merck & Co, Inc., Warehouse Station, New Jersey] and Engerix-B [GlaxoSmithKline Biologicals, Rixensart, Belgium]) commercially available in the United States (Table 86.2). These vaccines contain HBsAg particles but lack HBV DNA, HBcAg, HBeAg, or pre-S sequences. Transiently positive serum test results for HBsAg have been obtained within 24 hours following vaccine administration and rarely may remain detectable for days to weeks after vaccine administration before disappearance. The recombinant vaccines are safe, immunogenic, and close to 95% effective in preventing HBV infection or clinical hepatitis B. Although the vaccines are rendered impotent by freezing, heating for 1 week at 45°C or for 1 month at 37°C has not affected immunogenicity. The immune response to active immunization by vaccination is limited to anti-HBs alone; the response to natural infection with HBV involves induction of both anti-HBc and anti-HBs 48 (Fig. 86.7). Titers of anti-HBs after vaccination are usually lower than those found after natural infection. Breakthrough infections in vaccinated individuals can be attributed to hyporesponsiveness or nonresponsiveness to HBV vaccine or, very rarely, to infection by the HBV escape mutant in which the "a" determinant of HBsAg cannot be neutralized by vaccine-induced anti-HBs (44). This HBV vaccine-induced escape mutant has been identified in Italy, Singapore, Japan, Africa, and less frequently in the United States.

Postvaccination anti-HBs levels peak at 1 to 3 months after the third dose and then titers diminish with time. Whereas anti-HBs levels also decrease after natural infection, the duration of protection is lifelong in nearly all instances of natural infection. The duration of protection after vaccine-induced immunity remains uncertain but may also be lifelong. A specific, critical threshold value of anti-HBs above which immunity is solid and below which immunity is uncertain has yet to be unequivocally established. Nonetheless, a threshold level of greater than 10 mIU/mL has been considered indicative of seroprotection. The duration of anti-HBs persistence is highly correlated with the peak titer after the third or fourth dose (45).

Although the available recombinant, yeast-derived vaccines contain different amounts of HBsAg protein, postvaccination anti-HBs levels in young, healthy recipients are probably similar, and it is assumed that they offer similar early protective efficacy. Whether long-term protection will differ remains to be estab-

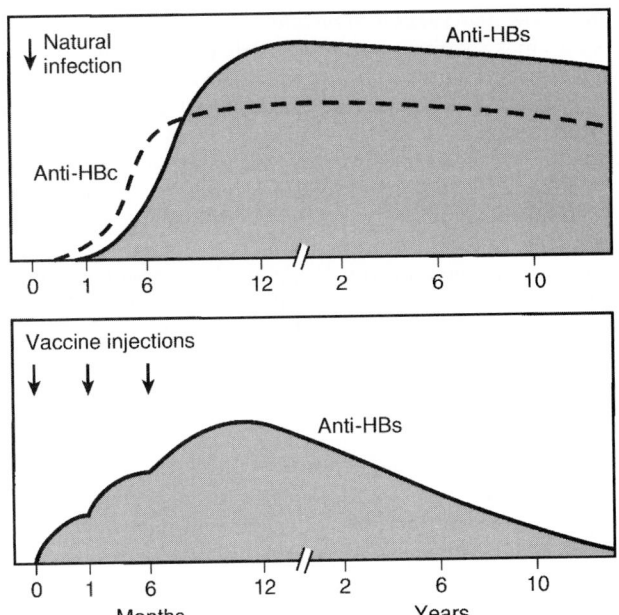

Figure 86.7. The immune response to natural infection with hepatitis B virus (HBV) **(top)** involves induction of both the antibody to hepatitis B core antigen and the antibody to hepatitis B surface antigen (high-titer anti-HBs). In contrast, the response to HBV vaccine **(bottom)** is limited to anti-HBs.

lished, but it may well be that the higher dose vaccine provides longer protection. At 10 years after initial vaccination, when the titer of anti-HBs may have fallen below 10 mIU/mL in as many as 40% or is undetectable, continued protection against clinical hepatitis and persistent HBV infection has been demonstrated and has been attributed to immunologic memory. Recent evidence indicates that since immunologic memory persists for at least 15 years and probably considerably longer (46), booster doses are not needed through the first 15 years after successful vaccination. However, boosters are recommended in immunosuppressed populations such as patients undergoing maintenance hemodialysis if, on annual testing, anti-HBs levels fall below 10 mIU/mL.

The major host factors affecting vaccine immunogenicity are age and immunocompetency. HIV infection, obesity, smoking, chronic cardiopulmonary and renal disease, maintenance hemodialysis, and receipt of an organ transplant are each linked to a diminished responsiveness. In these groups and in older individuals there may be some advantage in using the recombinant vaccine with higher concentrations of HBsAg protein.

TABLE 86.2.   Monovalent, Recombinant, Yeast-Derived Hepatitis B Virus Vaccines Approved by the U.S. Food and Drug Administration

	Engerix-B	Recombivax HB
Manufacturer	GlaxoSmithKline	Merck and Co.
Yeast source	*Saccharomyces cerevisae*	*Saccharomyces cerevisiae*
Chemical treatment	None	Formaldehyde
HBsAg subtype	adw	adw
HBsAg protein content		
Adult dose	>19 yr: 20 μg	>19 yr: 10 μg
Pediatric dose	≤19 yr: 10 μg	≤19 yr: 5 μg
Approved schedules	0, 1, and 6 mo	0, 1, and 6 months
	0, 1, 2, and 12 mo	0, 4–6 mo: 10 μg for
	0, 12, and 24 mo: 10 μg	ages 11–15 yr
	for ages 5–16 yr	

Route, Dose, and Vaccine Schedule

HBV vaccines are given intramuscularly into the deltoid muscle in children and adults and into the anterolateral muscle of the thigh in infants in a three-dose schedule (0, 1–2, and 4–6 months for adults, adolescents or older children; 0, 1–4, and 6–18 months for infants of HBsAg-negative mothers; and within 12 hours of birth, 1–2, and 6 months of age for infants of HBsAg-positive mothers) (Table 86.2). A two-dose schedule has been approved for Recombivax-HB for adolescents, age 11 to 15 years, and a four-dose schedule (at birth, 1, 2, and 12 months) has been approved for Engerix-B. Other schedules (e.g., first dose at 2 months of age, second at 4 months, and third at 12 months) may also be used in infants. Regardless of the schedule selected, the second and third doses should be separated by an interval of at least 2 months.

Adverse Effects of Immunization

The vaccines are very well-tolerated. The major side effect of both HBIG and HBV vaccine is transient pain at the injection site. Thimerosol is no longer used as a preservative in either vaccine. No causal association with autism, autoimmune disorders, or neurologic disorders has been established (47).

CANDIDATES FOR IMMUNOPROPHYLAXIS

Preexposure Prophylaxis

Shortly after the introduction of HBV vaccines, only high-risk groups were targeted for vaccination, a policy with limited impact on the overall infection rate. The current strategy for HBV control in the United States is screening of pregnant women for HBsAg and administration of HBIG and HBV vaccine to their neonates, combined with universal vaccination of all other infants, "catch-up" vaccination of unimmunized adolescents through 18 years of age, and continuing vaccination of high-risk populations. Currently, over 130 countries have adopted HBV vaccination into their immunization programs. Proof of effectiveness has become available (48,49).

Preexposure HBV vaccination is recommended for individuals in high-risk categories: household contacts of HBsAg-positive individuals; homosexual or bisexual men; individuals with a history of episodes of sexually transmitted diseases; health care workers regularly exposed to blood or blood-contaminated secretions (such as surgeons and pathologists; medical technicians and blood bank technologists; dialysis staff; operating room, intensive care, and emergency room nurses; and dentists and dental professionals); first responders (e.g., police, firefighters); parenteral drug users; workers and residents in institutions for the mentally retarded; recurrent recipients of high-risk blood products; and inmates of prisons in which parenteral drug use or homosexual behavior may continue. Immunization at an early age, for example, for health care students and other trainees, is more likely to be effective than later immunization.

Travelers to HBV-endemic regions who are likely to require medical assistance or in whom intimate contact with the local population is anticipated are also candidates for preexposure vaccination. Other high-risk groups appropriately considered for universal immunization include Alaskan Natives and Pacific Islanders. Refugees or adopted children from countries at high risk for HBV infection (Southeast Asia, sub-Saharan Africa, eastern Europe, and the former Soviet Union) should probably be screened for HBV infection; if the carrier state or chronic hepatitis B is identified, susceptible household contacts should be vaccinated.

Postexposure Prophylaxis

For susceptible health care workers who have not been vaccinated but are inadvertently exposed to HBV through needlesticks, lacerations, or splashing accidents, combined passive-active immunization with HBIG and HBV vaccine has been recommended. HBIG is given intramuscularly in a dose of 0.06 mL/kg body weight as early as possible after exposure, and the first of three doses of HBV vaccine is given at another site in the deltoid muscle at the same time or within several days. The second and third vaccine doses are given 1 and 6 months later. The efficacy of earlier administration of the second and third vaccine doses, in an accelerated schedule, with or without prior HBIG is uncertain.

Sexual contacts of patients with acute HBV infection should receive a single dose of HBIG (0.06 mL/kg body weight) within 14 days of exposure; there is no current evidence that vaccination of contacts of acutely infected individuals is necessary, although failure to vaccinate individuals who will be at future risk may be considered a missed opportunity. For the very high risk individual (e.g., susceptible male homosexuals or promiscuous heterosexuals), HBV vaccine should be initiated at the same time.

HBV vaccine alone has been recommended for susceptible intimate and household contacts of index cases with chronic HBV infection. Immunoprophylaxis is not recommended for the casual contacts of HBsAg-positive persons, whether they are acutely or chronically infected.

Prevention of maternal-neonatal transmission of HBV requires screening of all pregnant women to determine HBsAg status. For neonates of HBsAg-positive women, a dose of 0.5 mL of HBIG should be given within 12 hours of birth into the anterolateral muscle of the thigh of the neonate; HBV vaccine is given in the contralateral thigh at the same time and repeated at 1 and 6 months. The protective efficacy of the combined program approaches 90% to 95% (50). Immunized infants should be tested for HBV markers at about 12 months of age. The presence of HBsAg indicates treatment failure; the presence of both anti-HBs and anti-HBc suggests that infection occurred but was modified by immunoprophylaxis; the presence of anti-HBs alone suggests vaccine-induced immunity.

Remaining Issues

New HBV vaccines are on the drawing boards. These include microencapsulated synthetic HBsAg peptide vaccines (51), vaccines composed of the HBV DNA encoding HBsAg (naked DNA vaccines) (52), conjugation of nuclear localization signal peptides to HBV DNA to enhance the immune response (53), as well as others. Combination vaccines incorporating HBV with hemophilus influenza B and HBV with HAV are now available in the United States as well as elsewhere. The HAV/HBV bivalent vaccine (Twinrix [GlaxoSmithKline Biologicals, Rixensart, Belgium]) contains 750 ELISA units (EL.U.) of inactivated HAV and 20 μg of HBsAg protein in each dose, is highly immunogenic, and is well tolerated when given in three doses (0, 1, and 6 months) (54). In the United States it is approved for use in individuals over 18 years of age. Vaccine-induced antibodies are long-lasting: 100% of the vaccinees were anti-HAV positive and more than 95% had seroprotective levels of anti-HBs 4 years after the first dose (55). The vaccine has been targeted to groups at risk for both hepatitis A and B and should improve ease of administration and reduce costs.

A small number of otherwise healthy, immunocompetent individuals may be nonresponsive or hyporesponsive (anti-HBs levels of less than 10 mIU/mL) after three doses of the current HBV vaccines. An additional three doses may produce a more vigorous response in about half. Nonresponsiveness after a total of six doses appears to be genetically determined and related to the presence of a specific extended HLA haplotype (56). Attempts to overcome such nonresponsiveness by vaccination with preparations that contain both HBsAg and the pre-S proteins are under study. Whether nonresponsiveness may be circumvented by immunization with HBV vaccine in conjunction with a helper T-cell peptide recognized by the major histocompatibility complex class II molecules remains to be determined.

HEPATITIS D

Epidemiology

Although hepatitis D virus (HDV) infection has been identified in nearly all parts of the world, the epidemiology of HDV infection remains incompletely understood. It shares many epidemiologic features with HBV infection, and as in the case of HBV, large geographic variations in HDV infection rates have been identified. Somewhat surprisingly, given the close biologic interrelationship of HDV with HBV, the prevalence of HDV infection among HBV-infected patients with chronic liver disease is highly variable. In some areas, such as Southeast Asia, HDV infections are uncommon; in others, such as the Amazon region of South America, HDV infection appears to be hyperendemic with periodic outbreaks. Among the 350 million worldwide HBsAg carriers, it is estimated that as many as 15 million (5%) are infected by HDV (57). Although available data are limited, currently the prevalence of HDV infection appears to be rapidly declining in developed countries (58).

INCUBATION PERIOD

The incubation period of HDV infection may range from a few weeks to several weeks or months, based on limited observations in transfusion-associated cases and experimental transmission studies in chimpanzees (59). The incubation period, when measured from HDV exposure to the development of serum alanine aminotransferase elevations, was related to the size of the HDV inoculum in infected chimpanzees; it varied from 24 days when an undiluted inoculum was given to 51 days in the animal given the highest dilution inoculum.

EPIDEMIOLOGIC PATTERNS

Modes of transmission are similar to those associated with HBV infection. Although HDV infections can be either acute or persistent, it is the latter that are believed to facilitate the spread of HDV among individuals infected by HBV. HDV may spread rapidly in susceptible populations and may spill over into other populations within communities. Two different epidemiologic patterns are recognized: one that appears to be endemic, and the other nonendemic. The endemic pattern has been seen in the countries of the Mediterranean littoral, in the Balkans, in European regions of the former Soviet Union, in parts of Africa and the Middle East, and in the Amazon basin of South America. Outbreaks in these areas may result from the introduction of HDV-infected individuals into susceptible (HBV carrier) populations; horizontal transmission among children may contribute to the rapid spread of infection (60). HDV is spread in endemic regions chiefly by person-to-person direct contact between HDV infected individuals and HBV carriers; intrafamilial and sexual routes of spread are common.

HDV infection is infrequent in the general population of nonendemic regions such as North America and northern Europe. In these areas, HDV infections occur with moderate frequency in HBsAg-positive persons at risk for percutaneous exposure (i.e., injecting drug users and hemophiliacs). Outbreaks of HDV infection have been noted in such individuals and in their intimate contacts. A high prevalence of HDV infections has been identified in prisoners. In this case, HDV infection is assumed to result from the increased frequency of injecting drug use among those incarcerated. These data suggest that in nonendemic regions, HDV infection is largely confined to that narrow segment of the population that is exposed by direct percutaneous inoculation.

MODES OF TRANSMISSION

HDV is a blood-borne pathogen, and concentrations of HDV in blood may be as high as 10^{10} to 10^{12}/mL. Few studies have evaluated the presence of HDV in body fluids other than blood. Percutaneous spread, as among injecting drug users, is clearly a major mode of transmission. Posttransfusion acquisition of HDV infection also has been recognized, particularly among hemophiliac patients who have received large quantities of clotting factors. Other modes of transmission include person-to-person contact spread through intimate or inapparent transmission through open skin lesions or spread through household contamination. These observations suggest that HDV and HBV may be present in the same body fluids. Contact transmission of HDV is believed to involve the same mechanisms as in contact transmission of HBV but is likely to be far less efficient. High-risk sexual behavior (i.e., with multiple sex partners) has been associated with acquisition of HDV among HBV carriers. For example, among HBsAg-positive prostitutes, HDV infection rates are considerably higher than those seen in the general population of HBsAg-positive individuals. HDV infection rates in homosexual or bisexual men have been independently associated with injecting drug use, the number of sexual partners, and rectal trauma. Maternal-neonatal spread may also occur, but its epidemiologic importance seems minor. Persistence of active HDV and HBV infections provides a reservoir of HDV and HBV carriers who may serve as sources of infection in some populations.

Pathogenesis and Pathology

The pathogenesis of HDV infection is poorly understood. Although the presence of microvesicular steatosis, vacuolization, and focal hepatocyte necrosis, with a paucity of parenchymal mononuclear inflammatory cells, is suggestive of a direct cytopathic effect on the hepatocyte, studies in transgenic mice in which both HDV antigen isoforms are expressed revealed no evidence of hepatocyte injury (61). No relationship between the severity of the initial lesions of acute hepatitis D and the development of HDV associated chronic hepatitis has been recognized. In contrast, a significant positive relationship was observed between the expression of HDV antigens and the presence of inflammation in the liver in chronic hepatitis D, suggesting the importance of immune mechanisms in perpetuating injury. Furthermore, in the patient with HDV and HBV infection in whom liver transplantation is undertaken, HDV can be demonstrated immunohistochemically within 1 week in the transplanted graft, but hepatocellular injury is delayed until HBV reinfection ensues, usually more than 3 months after transplantation (62). These observations support the notion that HDV requires HBV for its pathogenicity and that immune-mediated mechanisms are responsible for hepatic injury. T-lymphocyte cytotoxic responses are probably involved in both the induction of injury and the control of viral spread in chronic infection.

Serologic Diagnosis

Serologic diagnosis of HDV infection should be sought only in patients shown to be HBsAg-positive or in those in whom HBsAg-negative acute hepatitis B is recognized by demonstration of IgM anti-HBc and in whom coinfection with HDV is considered possible. In all other settings, HDV infection in persons who are HBsAg negative must be exceedingly rare. Whereas

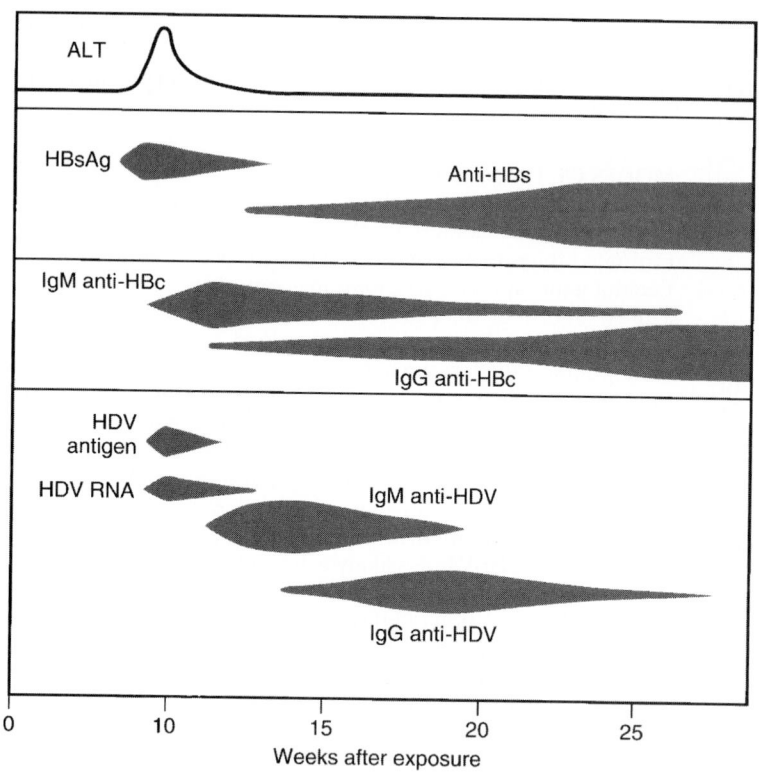

Figure 86.8. Schematic illustration of the sequence of biochemical and serologic events seen in self-limited hepatitis D virus and hepatitis B virus coinfection. *ALT*, alanine aminotransferase.

immunohistochemical demonstration of intrahepatic HDV antigen appears to be a sensitive marker of active HDV infection, this approach is impractical because it requires liver biopsy. Detection of HDV RNA in serum by PCR also appears to be highly sensitive and specific for ongoing viral replication in chronic hepatitis D (63), but approved assays are not yet available.

COINFECTION
A variety of serologic responses indicative of HDV infection have been identified in patients with acute, self-limited HDV coinfection with HBV (Fig. 86.8). Circulating HDV antigen and serum HDV RNA (detected by dot blot analysis or PCR) appear during the late incubation period and early acute phase of illness concurrently with the detection of HBsAg but are present transiently (64). Research assays indicate that HDV antigen disappears early from serum, before or concurrently with the clearance of HBsAg and coincident with the development of the corresponding antibodies to HDV (anti-HDV). Although viremia is usually short-lived, HDV RNA may persist in some instances for prolonged periods even when HDV antigen and anti-HDV are undetectable. Assays for serum HDV antigen and HDV RNA are research tools. As a consequence, detection of antibodies to HDV is the principal widely available tool used for serologic diagnosis.

Seroconversion to IgM anti-HDV, as determined by either radioimmunoassay or enzyme-linked immunosorbent assay, usually occurs within several days to a few weeks after the onset of illness. IgM anti-HDV is seldom detectable for longer than 2 to 8 weeks. It is usually followed by IgG anti-HDV, which may also disappear in a number of weeks, or it may persist for as long as 6 months in low titers or occasionally for as long as 1 to 2 years (65,66). One or more of these markers may be absent in a typical case of acute HDV infection or, curiously, may appear during the convalescent phase.

SUPERINFECTION
In HDV superinfection of HBsAg-positive individuals, HDV antigen and HDV RNA are detectable in serum, and HDV anti-

gen is identifiable in the liver. Simultaneously, a reduction in HBV replication and a consequent decrease in the titer of circulating HBsAg may ensue. Rarely, this HDV inhibition of HBV replication results in the termination of the HBsAg carrier state. As shown in Fig. 86.9, IgM anti-HDV appears during the superinfection and may be followed or accompanied by the brisk and sustained production of IgG anti-HDV in high titers. In a large proportion of superinfected patients, HDV infection becomes persistent, and HDV antigen and HDV RNA may remain detectable in serum; large quantities of HDV antigen can also be detected in hepatocytes by immunofluorescent techniques. High titers of IgG anti-HDV, variable titers of IgM anti-HDV, and serum HDV RNA positivity by PCR are maintained in persistent HDV infection.

Clinical Spectrum

COINFECTION
In HDV and HBV coinfections, the acute illness resembles uncomplicated hepatitis B in the majority of instances (Fig. 86.10). In a small proportion, probably less than 15%, the disease may be severe, as reflected by the development of a prolonged prothrombin time or hepatic encephalopathy, and fatalities may occur in a few cases as a consequence of acute liver failure with extensive hepatic necrosis. In some outbreaks, case fatality rates have been high. For example, in a major outbreak of virulent HDV infection among injecting drug users in the city of Worcester, Massachusetts, in which serologic analysis revealed that most cases resulted from coinfection, a case-fatality rate of 8% was observed (67). Because most HBV infections in adults are short lived, and because HDV infection cannot persist after recovery from HBV, the majority of coinfections are self-limited and chronic HDV infection is distinctly uncommon.

SUPERINFECTION
In HDV superinfection of HBV carriers (Fig. 86.10), the acute disease is more likely to be severe, and chronic, progressive hepatitis

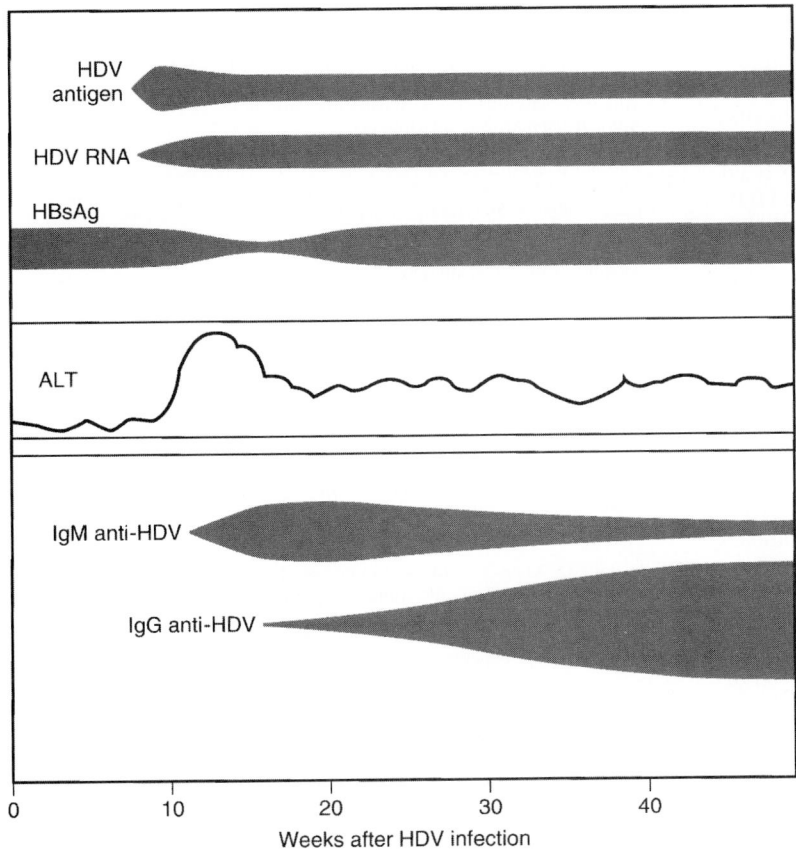

Figure 86.9. Schematic illustration of the sequence of serologic and biochemical events in hepatitis D virus superinfection of hepatitis B virus carriers. *ALT,* alanine aminotransferase.

is far more frequent than in coinfection. Furthermore, in some but probably not all populations with chronic hepatitis D, cirrhosis or hepatic failure has appeared to be a common sequela of persistent HDV infection. In a prospective study of HBV carriers among the Yucpa Indians of Venezuela in whom the consequences of HDV superinfection were evaluated, more than half of HDV-superinfected persons had moderate to severe chronic liver disease compared with none of the non–HDV-infected individuals (68). Mortality rates in HDV-infected individuals varied from 7% to 9% per year; most deaths were due to rapidly progressive chronic liver disease or the development of acute liver failure. The risk for progression from chronic hepatitis D to cirrhosis appears to be greater than for patients with chronic hepatitis B alone, and the rate of progression may be striking. In one study, progression to cirrhosis was observed in more than 50% of patients with chronic hepatitis D after a little more than 2 years of follow-up (69). The role of HDV superinfection in the development of hepatocellular carcinoma in HBsAg-positive patients remains ill defined.

The preceding facts notwithstanding, the morbidity and mortality associated with HDV infection may have been overestimated in early studies of the natural history of HDV infection. Increasingly, as more data are collected, evidence of less severe infections has accumulated, indicating that the spectrum of disease severity associated with HDV is considerably broader than initially believed and that HDV infections may not invariably be highly pathogenic. Furthermore, HBsAg clearance rates may be higher in HDV-infected patients when compared with HBsAg carriers without HDV infection, a potentially beneficial effect (70).

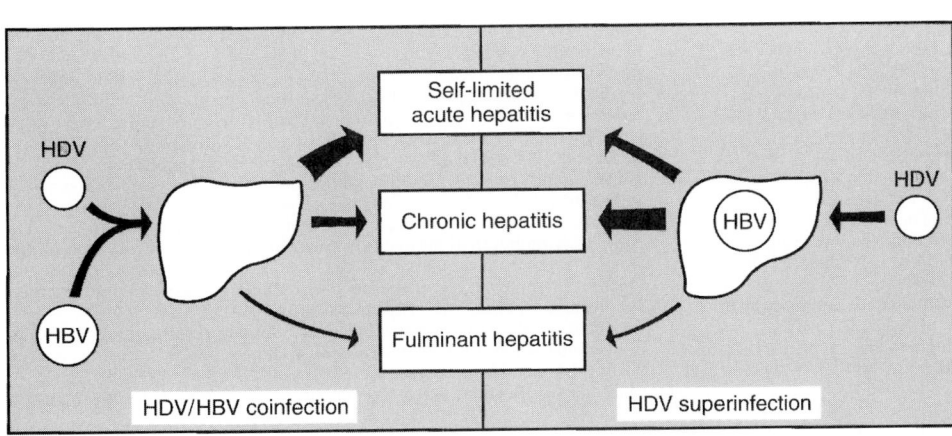

Figure 86.10. Schematic illustration of the sequelae of hepatitis D virus (HDV) and hepatitis B virus (HBV) coinfection **(left)** and HDV superinfection of HBV carriers **(right).**

Treatment

No specific therapy has yet been shown to alter the natural history of acute HDV infection. Treatment of chronic hepatitis D with high doses of interferon-α for 12 years has induced a sustained response in a single reported case (71); lamivudine alone (72) or the addition of lamivudine to interferon has not been beneficial (73). Drugs that inhibit prenylation of the large HDV antigen and interfere with the life cycle of HDV are under development (74).

Liver transplantation in patients with HDV-associated cirrhosis, when combined with long-term passive administration of anti-HBs, has been associated with a 5-year actuarial survival of 88%, a figure comparable to that found after liver transplantation for other diseases (75).

Prevention

Because HDV infection requires the helper functions of HBV, HBV vaccination of susceptible individuals will prevent coinfection. In HBsAg-positive individuals, neither passive immunoprophylaxis with conventional or an HDV-specific immune globulin nor active immunization with an HDV vaccine are available for the prevention of HDV superinfection. Experimental DNA vaccines composed of plasmids encoding the large hepatitis D antigen or coexpressing this antigen and HBsAg have induced both humoral and cellular immune responses in mice (76), but clinical studies in humans are not yet available. Potential candidates for vaccination would be HBsAg-positive hemodialysis patients, injecting drug users, recipients of multiple blood products, and individuals with multiple sexual contacts. Until a safe and effective HDV vaccine becomes a reality, for HBsAg-positive injection drug abusers, needle exchange programs and education about cleaning needles might reduce the risk of infection. For HDV infected individuals, safe sex practices should reduce the risk for transmitting infection to sexual contacts.

REFERENCES

1. Coleman PJ, McQuillan GM, Moyer LA, et al. Incidence of hepatitis B virus infection in the United States, 1976–1994: estimates from the National Health and Nutrition Examination Surveys. *J Infect Dis* 1998;178:954–959.
2. McQuillan GM, Coleman PJ, Kruszon-Moran D, et al. Prevalence of hepatitis B virus infection in the United States: the National Health and Nutrition Examination Surveys 1976 through 1994. *Am J Public Health* 1999;89:14–18.
3. Tobe K, Matsuura K, Ogura T, et al. Horizontal transmission of hepatitis B virus among players of an American football team. *Arch Intern Med* 2000;160:2541–2545.
4. Prince AM, Lee D-H, Brotman B. Infectivity of blood from PCR-positive, HBsAg-negative, anti-HBs-positive cases of resolved hepatitis B infection. *Transfusion* 2001;41:329–332.
5. Stevens CE, Toy PT, Tong MJ, et al. Perinatal hepatitis B virus transmission in the United States. Prevention by passive-active immunization. *JAMA* 1985;253:1740–1745.
6. Burk RD, Hwang L-Y, Ho GYF, et al. Outcome of perinatal hepatitis B virus exposure is dependent on maternal virus load. *J Infect Dis* 1994;170:1418–1423.
7. Levine OS, Vlahov D, Nelson KE. Epidemiology of hepatitis B virus infections among injecting drug users: seroprevalence, risk factors, and viral interactions. *Epidemiol Rev* 1994;16:418–436.
8. Garfein RS, Vlahov D, Galai N, et al. Viral infections in short-term injection drug users: the prevalence of the hepatitis C, hepatitis B, human immunodeficiency, and human T-lymphotropic viruses. *Am J Public Health* 1996;86:655–661.
9. Dickson RC, Everhart JE, Lake JR, et al. Transmission of hepatitis B by transplantation of livers from donors positive for antibody to hepatitis B core antigen. The National Institute of Diabetes and Digestive and Kidney Diseases Liver Transplantation Database. *Gastroenterology* 1997;113:1668–1674.
10. Mast EE, Alter MJ, Margolis HS. Strategies to prevent and control hepatitis B and C virus infections: a global perspective. *Vaccine* 1999;17:1730–1733.
11. Seeff LB, Beebe GW, Hoofnagle JH, et al. A serologic follow-up of the 1942 epidemic of post-vaccination hepatitis in the United States Army. *N Engl J Med* 1987;316:965–970.
12. Silverman AL, Qu LH, Blow J, et al. Assessment of hepatitis B virus DNA and hepatitis C RNA in the common bedbug (*Cimex lectularius* L.)and kissing bug (*Rodnius prolixus*). *Am J Gastroenterology* 2001;96:2194–2198.
13. Matsumura S, Yamamoto K, Shimada N, et al. High frequency of circulating HBcAg-specific CD8 T cells in hepatitis B infection: a flow cytometric analysis. *Clin Exp Immunol* 2001;124:435–444.
14. Guidotti LG, Rochford R, Chung J, et al. Viral clearance without destruction of infected cells during acute HBV infection. *Science* 1999;284:825–829.
15. Thursz MR, Kwiatkowski D, Allsopp CEM, et al. Association between an MHC class II allele and clearance of hepatitis B virus in the Gambia. *N Engl J Med* 1995;332:1065–1069.
16. Saldanha J, Gerlich W, Lelie N, et al. An international collaborative study to establish a World Health Organization international standard for hepatitis B viral DNA nucleic acid amplification techniques. *Vox Sang* 2001;80:63–71.
17. Tassopoulos NC, Kuhns MC, Koutelou MG, et al. Quantitative detection of hepatitis B virus DNA in sera from patients with acute hepatitis B. *Dig Dis Sci* 1993;38:2156–2162.
18. Marasuwa H, Uemoto S, Hijikata M, et al. Latent hepatitis B virus infection in healthy individuals with antibodies to hepatitis B core antigen. *Hepatology* 2000;31:488–495.
19. Teo E-K, Ostapowicz G, Hussain M, et al. Hepatitis B infection in patients with acute liver failure in the United States. *Hepatology* 2001;33:972–976.
20. Hawkins AE, Gilson RJC, Beath SV, et al. Novel application of a point mutation assay: evidence for transmission of hepatitis B viruses with precore mutations and their detection in infants with fulminant hepatitis B. *J Med Virol* 1994;44:13–21.
21. Shakil AO, Kramer D, Mazariego GV, et al. Acute liver failure: clinical features, outcome analysis and applicability of prognostic criteria. *Liver Transplant* 2000;6:163–169.
22. Chemin I, Zoulim F, Merle P, et al. High incidence of hepatitis B infections among chronic hepatitis cases of unknown etiology. *J Hepatol* 2001;34:447–454.
23. Hyams KC. Risks of chronicity following acute hepatitis B virus infection: a review. *Clin Infect Dis* 1995;20:992–1000.
24. de Franchis R, Meucci G, Vecchi M, et al. The natural history of asymptomatic hepatitis B surface antigen carriers. *Ann Intern Med* 1993;118:191–194.
25. Liaw Y -F, Sheen I-S, Chen T-J, et al. Incidence, determinants and significance of delayed clearance of serum HBsAg in chronic hepatitis B virus infection: a prospective study. *Hepatology* 1991;13:627–631.
26. Wong JB, Koff RS, Tine F, et al. Cost-effectiveness of interferon-alfa 2b treatment for hepatitis B e antigen-positive chronic hepatitis B. *Ann Intern Med* 1995;122:664–675.
27. Nakamoto Y, Guidotti LG, Kuhlen C, et al. Immune pathogenesis of hepatocellular carcinoma. *J Exp Med* 1998;188:341–350.
28. Lai ME, Solinas A, Mazzoleni AP, et al. The role of the pre-core hepatitis B virus mutants on the long-term outcome of chronic hepatitis B virus hepatitis. A longitudinal study. *J Hepatol* 1994;20:773–781.
29. Perrillo RP. Acute flares in chronic hepatitis B: the natural and unnatural history of an immunologically mediated liver disease. *Gastroenterology* 2001;120:1009–1022.
30. Andreone P, Caraceni P, Grazi GL, et al. Lamivudine treatment for acute hepatitis B after liver transplantation. *J Hepatol* 1998;29:985–989.
31. Reshef R, Sbeit W, Kaspa RT. Lamivudine in the treatment of acute hepatitis B. *N Engl J Med* 2000;343:1123–1124.
32. Fattovich G, Giustina G, Realdi G, et al. Long-term outcome of hepatitis B e antigen-positive patients with compensated cirrhosis treated with interferon alfa. *Hepatology* 1997;26:1338–1342.
33. Niederau C, Heintges T, Lange S, et al. Long-term follow-up of HBeAg-positive patients treated with interferon alfa for chronic hepatitis B. *N Engl J Med* 1996;334:1422–1427.
34. Lin SM, Sheen IS, Chien RN, et al. Long-term beneficial effect of interferon therapy in patients with chronic hepatitis B virus infection. *Hepatology* 1999;29:971–975.
35. Dienstag JL, Schiff ER, Wright TL, et al. Lamivudine as initial treatment for chronic hepatitis B in the United States. *N Engl J Med* 1999;341:1256–1263.
36. Dienstag JL, Schiff ER, Mitchell M, et al. Extended lamivudine retreatment for chronic hepatitis B: maintenance of viral suppression after discontinuation of therapy. *Hepatology* 1999;30:1082–1087.
37. Leung NWY, Lai C-L, Chang T-T, et al. Extended lamivudine treatment in patients with chronic hepatitis B enhances hepatitis B e antigen seroconversion rates: results after 3 years of therapy. *Hepatology* 2001;33:1527–1532.
38. Das K, Xiong X, Yang H, et al. Molecular modeling and biochemical characterization reveal the mechanism of hepatitis B virus polymerase resistance to lamivudine (3TC) and emtricitabine (FTC). *J Virol* 2001;75:4771–4779.
39. Melegari M, Scaglioni PP, Wands JR. Hepatitis B virus mutants associated with 3TC and famciclovir administration are replication defective. *Hepatology* 1998;27:628–633.
40. Brooks EA, Lacey LF, Payne SL, et al. Economic evaluation of lamivudine compared with interferon-alpha in the treatment of chronic hepatitis B in the United States. *Am J Manag Care* 2001;7:677–682.
41. Pol S, Nalpas N, Driss F, et al. Efficacy and limitations of a specific immunotherapy in chronic hepatitis B. *J Hepatol* 2001;34:917–921.
42. Perrillo R, Tamburro C, Regenstein F, et al. Low-dose, titratable interferon alfa in decompensated liver disease caused by chronic infection with hepatitis B virus. *Gastroenterology* 1995;109:908–916.
43. Mazzaferro V, Regalia E, Doci R, et al. Liver transplantation for the treatment

of small hepatocellular carcinomas in patients with cirrhosis. *N Engl J Med* 1996;334:693–699.

44. Fortuin M, Karthigesu V, Allison L, et al. Breakthrough infections and identification of a viral variant in Gambian children immunized with hepatitis B vaccine. *J Infect Dis* 1994;169:1374–1376.

45. Gesemann M, Scheiermann N. Quantification of hepatitis B vaccine–induced antibodies as a predictor of anti-HBs persistence. *Vaccine* 1995;13:443–447.

46. Watson N, West DJ, Chilkatowsky A, et al. Persistence of immunologic memory for 13 years in recipients of a recombinant hepatitis B vaccine. *Vaccine* 2001;19:3164–3168.

47. Monteyne P, Andre FE. Is there a causal link between hepatitis B vaccination and multiple sclerosis? *Vaccine* 2000;18:1994–2001.

48. Chen H-L, Chang M-H, Ni Y-H, et al. Seroepidemiology of hepatitis B virus infection in children. Ten years of mass vaccination in Taiwan. *JAMA* 1996;276:906–908.

49. Harpaz R, McMahon BJ, Margolis HS, et al. Elimination of new chronic hepatitis B virus infections: results of the Alaska immunization program. *J Infect Dis* 2000;181:413–418.

50. Andre FE, Zuckerman AJ. Review: protective efficacy of hepatitis B vaccines in neonates. *J Med Virol* 1994;44:144–151.

51. Moynhan JS, Jones DH, Farrar GH, et al. A novel microencapsulated peptide vaccine against hepatitis B. *Vaccine* 2001;19:3292–3300.

52. Prince AM, Whalen R, Brotman B. Successful nucleic acid based immunization of newborn chimpanzees against hepatitis B virus. *Vaccine* 1997;15:916–919.

53. Schirmbeck R, Konig-Merediz SA, Riedl P, et al. Priming of immune response to hepatitis B surface antigen with minimal DNA expression constructs modified with a nuclear localization signal peptide. *J Mol Med* 2001;79:343–350.

54. Knoll A, Hottentrager B, Kainz J, et al. Immunogenicity of a combined hepatitis A and B vaccine in healthy young adults. *Vaccine* 2000;18:2029–2032.

55. Thoelen S, Van Damme P, Leentvaar-Kuypers A, et al. The first combined vaccine against hepatitis A and B: an overview. *Vaccine* 1999;17:1657–1662.

56. Alper CA, Kruskall MS, Marcus-Bagley BS, et al. Genetic prediction of nonresponse to hepatitis B vaccine. *N Engl J Med* 1989;321:708–712.

57. Rizzetto M, Ponzetto A, Forzani I. Epidemiology of hepatitis delta virus: Overview. *Prog Clin Biol Res* 1991;364:1–20.

58. Gaeta GB, Stroffolini T, Charamonte M, et al. Chronic hepatitis D: a vanishing disease? An Italian multicenter study. *Hepatology* 2000;32:824–827.

59. Ponzetto A, Hoyer BH, Popper H, et al. Titration of the infectivity of hepatitis D virus in chimpanzees. *J Infect Dis* 1987;155:72–78.

60. Manock SR, Kelley PM, Hyams KC, et al. An outbreak of fulminant hepatitis delta in the Waorani, an indigenous people of the Amazon basin of Ecuador. *Am J Trop Med Hyg* 2000;63:209–213.

61. Guilhot S, Huang S-N, Xia YP, et al. Expression of the hepatitis delta virus large and small antigens in transgenic mice. *J Virol* 1994;68:1052–1058.

62. Davies S, Lau JY, O'Grady JG, et al. Evidence that hepatitis D virus needs hepatitis B virus to cause hepatocellular damage. *Am J Clin Pathol* 1992;98:554–558.

63. Simpson LH, Battegay M, Hoofnagle JH, et al. Hepatitis delta virus RNA in serum of patients with chronic delta hepatitis. *Dig Dis Sci* 1994;39:2650–2655.

64. Gupta S, Govindarajan S, Cassidy WM, et al. Acute delta hepatitis: serological diagnosis with particular reference to hepatitis delta virus RNA. *Am J Gastroenterol* 1991;86:1227–1231.

65. Hoofnagle JH. Type D (delta) hepatitis. *JAMA* 1989;261:1321–1325.

66. Shattock AG, Morris M, Kinane K, et al. The serology of delta hepatitis and the detection of IgM anti-HD by EIA using serum derived delta antigen. *J Virol Methods* 1989;23:233–240.

67. Lettau LA, McCarthy JG, Smith MH, et al. Outbreak of severe hepatitis due to delta and hepatitis B viruses in parenteral drug abusers and their contacts. *N Engl J Med* 1987;317:1256–1262.

68. Hadler SC, de Monzon MA, Rivero D, et al. Epidemiology and long-term consequences of hepatitis delta virus infection in the Yucpa Indians of Venezuela. *Am J Epidemiol* 1992;136:1507–1516.

69. Buti M, Mas A, Sanchez-Tapias JM, et al. Chronic hepatitis D in intravenous drug addicts and non-addicts. A comparative clinico-pathological study. *J Hepatol* 1988;7:169–174.

70. Niro GA, Gravinese E, Martini E, et al. Clearance of hepatitis B surface antigen in chronic carriers of hepatitis delta antibodies. *Liver* 2001;21:254–259.

71. Lau DT, Kleiner DE, Park Y, et al. Resolution of chronic delta hepatitis after 12 years of interferon alfa therapy. *Gastroenterology* 1999;117:1229–1233.

72. Lau DT, Doo E, Park Y, et al. Lamivudine for chronic delta hepatitis. *Hepatology* 1999;30:546–549.

73. Wolters LM, van Nunen AB, Honkoop P, et al. Lamivudine-high dose interferon combination therapy for chronic hepatitis B patients co-infected with the hepatitis D virus. *J Viral Hepatol* 2000;7:428–434.

74. Glenn JS, Marsters JC Jr, Greenberg HB. Use of a prenylation inhibitor as a novel antiviral agent. *J Virol* 1998;72:9303–9306.

75. Samuel D, Zignego A-L, Reynes M, et al. Long-term clinical and virological outcome after liver transplantation for cirrhosis caused by chronic delta hepatitis. *Hepatology* 1995;21:333–339.

76. Huang YH, Wu JC, Tao MH, et al. DNA-based immunization produces Th1 immune responses to hepatitis delta virus in a mouse model. *Hepatology* 2000;32:104–110.

CHAPTER 87
Hepatitis C

Raymond S. Koff

EPIDEMIOLOGY

Incubation Period

The incubation period of hepatitis C virus (HCV) varies widely between 2 and 20 weeks, with a mean of about 6 to 9 weeks from exposure to elevation of serum aminotransferase levels or onset of symptoms (1). Viremia, as determined by the detection of circulating HCV RNA, generally can be detected within 10 to 20 days after exposure during the early incubation period, although low-level viremia may occur even earlier.

Epidemiologic Patterns

HCV infections are widely distributed throughout the world; in the United States, HCV infection is the most common chronic blood-borne viral infection (2). In fact, no more than 15% to 45% of acutely infected patients recover completely (i.e., losing HCV RNA and normalizing serum alanine aminotransferase [ALT] levels, and probably eventually losing antibody to HCV [anti-HCV] after many years) (3). As shown in Table 87.1, high seroprevalence rates of HCV infection have been reported from geographically diverse regions; infection rates exceed 20% in some areas, whereas infection rates in neighboring areas are no higher than 1% to 2%. Although not completely understood, high rates may be a consequence of iatrogenic transmission through the reuse of contaminated needles, syringes, or other instruments (4). Genotype patterns vary widely, as shown in Fig. 87.1. Phylogenic analyses based on genomic sequencing suggest that genotypes 1a and 1b, the predominant HCV infections in the United States, may have originated about 100 years ago and spread rapidly, while type 6 (reported from Asia) may have arisen about 700 years ago and has a slower and more localized rate of spread (5).

Hepatitis C accounted for about 10% to 15% of the acute viral hepatitis reported in the United States during the past decade; in recent years a dramatic decline in incidence was reported, presumably due to a reduction in transfusion and illicit injection drug-associated cases. Most acute HCV infections occur in young adults, although all age groups are affected. Currently about 1.8% of the population, or roughly 4 to 5 million individuals, have evidence of past or present HCV infection, and nearly 3 million are viremic (6). Seroprevalence rates are higher in black than in white persons and peak in the 30- to 39-year-old age group. It is estimated that as many as 10,000 deaths annually can be attributed to the sequelae of chronic hepatitis C.

Modes of Transmission

PERCUTANEOUS TRANSMISSION

Direct percutaneous exposure to infectious blood is the most efficient mode of HCV spread, and individuals with chronic infection are the major source of infection for others. Prior to the serologic identification of HCV in 1989, hepatitis C was the major complication related to transfusion of blood and blood products. By the mid-1990s, as a consequence of changes in blood banking resulting from exclusion of individuals with risk factors for human immunodeficiency virus (HIV) infection, from

TABLE 87.1.   Global Hepatitis C Virus Antibody Seroprevalence: the General Population Endemicity Rates of Hepatitis C Virus Based on Data (First- or Second-Generation Assays) from the General Population or Blood Donors in Selected Countries

Endemicity pattern	Country	Seroprevalence (%)
Low endemicity (0%–2.5%)	United Kingdom	0.1
	Hong Kong	0.5
	Sweden	0.7
	Australia	0.8
	South Africa	0.9
	United States	1.8
	Ethiopia	2.0
	Taiwan	2.5
Moderate endemicity (>2.5%–5%)	Yemen	2.6
	South Sudan	3
	Peru	3
	China	3.9
	Malawi	3.9
	Japan	4
	Kiribati	5
	Philippines	5
High endemicity (>5%)	Zaire	6
	Gabon	6.5
	Italy	7
	Libya	8
	Cameroon	15
	Egypt	22

TABLE 87.2.   Risk Factors Associated with Hepatitis C Virus Infection in the Centers for Disease Control and Prevention's Four-Sentinel County Study (1992)

Risk factor	%
Injection drug use	29
Heterosexual activity	8
Household contact	4
Transfusion	4
Health care employment	2
Low socioeconomic status or high-risk behavior or contacts[a]	45
Unknown	8

[a]Behavior or contacts more than 6 months before onset of illness.

Injection drug use with shared needles or equipment has been the principal mode of HCV transmission in the United States, and 50% to 95% of injection drug users have been infected. In the Centers for Disease Control and Prevention's four-sentinel (now six) county study (Table 87.2) of acute hepatitis C, just under 30% were associated with injection drug use. A limited number of studies indicate that the infection rate after accidental needlesticks with HCV-contaminated equipment among health care workers varies between 0% and 10%.

As many as 10% to 45% of hemodialysis patients are HCV infected, and outbreaks continue to occur in this setting. Blood transfusions are not the probable source: nosocomial spread via dialysis machines and intraunit spread due to failure to follow appropriate infection control practices is more likely.

Acupuncture performed without sterilization between patients and the use of nonsterilized, contaminated needles, syringes, and knives by practitioners of folk medicine may be responsible for some episodes of community-acquired HCV infection. Furthermore, in developing countries, nosocomial transmission due to reuse of syringes, needles, or endoscopes without adequate sterilization may contribute to the spread of infection. In developed countries, occasional outbreaks in pediatric oncology, hematology, and other hospital-related sites usually have been related to breaks in infection control, but the mode of transmission sometimes remains elusive (8).

the introduction of surrogate testing of blood donors (serum ALT and anti-hepatitis B core antigen), and from markedly improved anti-HCV screening techniques (second-generation and then third-generation assays), the risk for HCV infection was reduced to 1 per 100,000 transfused units (7). With the introduction of nucleic acid testing of donors in minipools, the estimated risk, as of 2001, is less than 1 per 1 million transfused units, and ALT testing is of no longer of any value. Clotting factor concentrates, derived from plasma, also were a source of HCV for recipients until the introduction of viral inactivation procedures in 1987. All immune globulin preparations made in the United States also undergo viral inactivation.

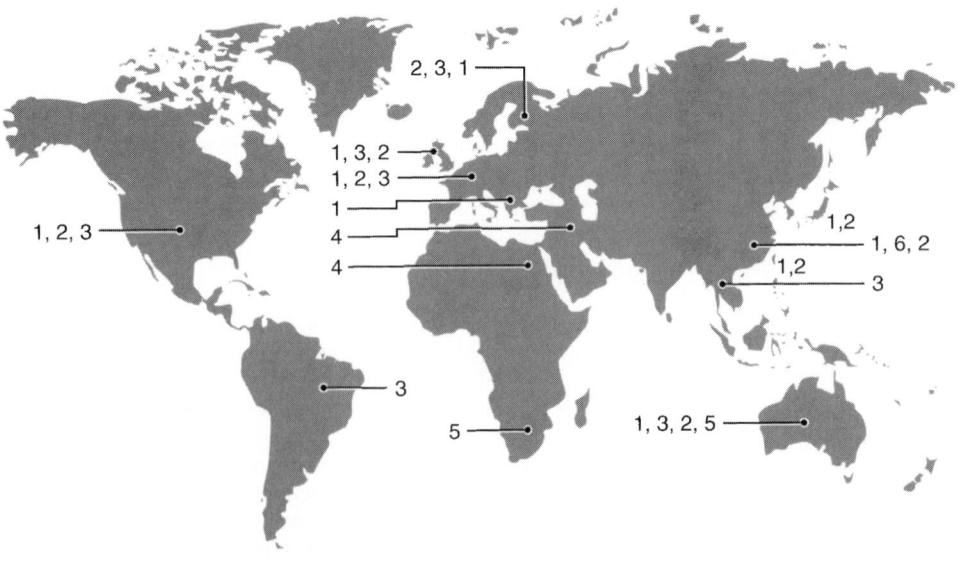

Figure 87.1. Global distribution of hepatitis C virus genotypes in blood donors. Order reflects decreasing prevalence of genotype. (Adapted from van der Poel CL, Cuypers HT, Reesink HW. Hepatitis C virus six years on. *Lancet* 1994;344(89351):1475–1479, with permission.)

Organ transplantation from anti-HCV–positive donors has been another recognized mode of transmission, but screening of donors has reduced the risk. Nonetheless, transplantation of HCV-positive organs into HCV-positive recipients is undertaken in some transplantation centers. Other percutaneous routes of spread include tattooing (9) and cosmetic tissue penetrations (body piercing).

CONTACT TRANSMISSION

Person-to-person spread from acutely or chronically infected individuals to their intimate, sexual contacts has been reported and supported by nucleotide sequencing studies (10). The risk for sexual transmission is generally low and probably correlated with the frequency, duration, and nature of sexual exposure. As might be anticipated, anti-HCV prevalence rates in female prostitutes and in sexually active homosexual men are increased, although injection drug use may confound the association with HCV infection. However, even after controlling for percutaneous exposures, the number of lifetime sexual partners and the number of oral- or anal-receptive partners were weakly associated with HCV seroprevalence (11). As shown in Table 87.2, about 12% of identified cases in the sentinel county study could be linked with either heterosexual activity or household contact, which included exposure to a sexual partner or a household member with hepatitis or exposure to multiple sexual partners. HCV transmission from men to women seems to be more efficient than transmission from women to men. Intrafamilial clustering of HCV infection among nonsexual household members also occurs, but the frequency of such clustering is uncertain. Whether saliva or crevicular fluid plays a role is also unknown, and the responsible modes of transmission remain uncertain.

MATERNAL-NEONATAL TRANSMISSION

About 1% to 5% of newborns of anti-HCV–positive women are found to be HCV RNA positive when studied during the first year after birth (12). Increased rates of transmission are seen with concomitant HIV infection and high levels of maternal viremia. Neither breast-feeding nor cesarian section have been implicated in transmission.

UNESTABLISHED ROUTES OF SPREAD

Although about 10% of HCV-infected patients do not admit to a specific risk factor associated with transmission, some high-risk behaviors may have been forgotten or so emotionally charged that they cannot be discussed. Other patients, often from low socioconomic strata, do admit to high-risk behaviors but not in the 6 months preceding the onset of illness (Table 87.2). Respiratory or airborne transmission and food-borne or waterborne spread are unlikely. A role for arthropod vectors in transmission is unknown.

PATHOGENESIS

HCV is not directly cytopathic except perhaps in unusual circumstances (e.g., in the immunosuppressed liver transplant recipient in whom levels of viral replication are high and gene products are overexpressed). Hence, in most HCV infections the pathogenesis of acute and chronic liver injury is believed to be a consequence of the host immune response, which comprises both a nonspecific immune response, including interferon and other cytokines, natural killer cell activity, and a cell-mediated and (less importantly) humoral HCV-specific immune response. The occurrence of severe chronic hepatitis C in some patients with primary antibody deficiencies indicates that humoral immune responses are unlikely to be responsible for hepatic injury or rapid progression of the liver disease (13). The precise mechanisms responsible for liver injury remain to be defined. In self-limited HCV infection, liver-produced cytokines and chemokines may contribute to hepatocyte injury, and a polyclonal, multispecific CD8+ T-lymphocyte response (14) along with a coordinated CD4+ T-lymphocyte response appears to be associated with eradication of HCV infection, and the latter response may be maintained indefinitely (15). Similarly, in a study of chimpanzees who had recovered from an initial HCV infection and rapidly cleared viremia, a strong T-cell proliferative response was identified when the animals were rechallenged with homologous or heterologous HCV genotypes (16).

In general, when HCV is cleared from serum in acute infection or as a consequence of effective therapy in chronic infection, hepatocyte clearance also occurs and hepatic inflammation disappears. In patients who develop chronic infection, the immune and cytokine response appears inadequate to eliminate HCV from infected hepatocytes, but contributes to ongoing liver injury. An effect of HCV gene products on cytokine- or oncogene-mediated apoptosis also may contribute to either liver injury or HCV persistence, but (17) further studies will be needed to elucidate the importance of this mechanism. The role of immune-mediated selection of resistant HCV and quasispecies in persistent infection remains uncertain because these are not essential for the development of chronic infection (18). More research will be needed to better understand why the immune response is blunted, permitting the persistence of HCV infection.

PATHOLOGY

In patients with acute HCV infection, liver biopsy reveals, in general, a mild form of hepatitis with portal lymphocytic inflammation, parenchymal inflammation, focal hepatocyte necrosis in the form of ballooning degeneration, and apoptosis with scattered acidophilic bodies.

Histopathologic analysis of liver specimens from patients with chronic hepatitis C reveals typical changes of chronic inflammation with a variable amount of fibrosis. Four histologic lesions useful in distinguishing hepatitis C from B are bile duct damage; lymphoid follicles or aggregates, occasionally with germinal centers; large-droplet steatosis; and periportal Mallory body–like material (19). The steatosis may be related to HCV-induced alterations in apolipoprotein B metabolism and may be associated with an increased risk for hepatic fibrosis (20).

Multiple granulomata and multinucleated giant cells may be found in about 10% of patients with chronic hepatitis C and cirrhosis. HCV RNA replicative intermediates may be demonstrated in as few as 5% to as many as 30% of hepatocytes in chronic infection.

CLINICAL MANIFESTATIONS

Clinical Features

Symptomatic hepatitis with jaundice is seen in no more than 20% of acute hepatitis C cases. Fever is uncommon, and hepatomegaly is present in less than one third of patients.

Patients with chronic hepatitis C may experience fatigue, although many are asymptomatic at time of diagnosis.

Blood Chemistries

Peak serum levels of the aminotransferases and bilirubin tend to be lower than in acute hepatitis A or B. Fluctuations in the aminotransferase levels are frequently seen in both acute and chronic hepatitis C. Hematologic studies are usually unremarkable during the course of uncomplicated acute hepatitis C. However, autoimmune markers (e.g., rheumatoid factor, and low-level antinuclear and anti–smooth muscle antibodies) are common in chronic hepatitis C.

EXTRAHEPATIC DISEASES

Cryoglobulinemia may be present in one third to one half of patients with chronic hepatitis C (21), and HCV RNA is present both in serum and in the isolated cryoglobulins of affected patients. However, only 1% to 2% of patients with HCV-associated cryoglobulinemia have symptomatic disease manifested as purpura, vasculitis, or peripheral neuropathy. Membranoproliferative glomerulonephritis, usually linked with HCV-associated cryoglobulinemia, is also unusual; glomerular deposition of immune complexes of HCV and anti-HCV appears responsible. In addition to HCV-associated mixed cryoglobulinemia, other disorders putatively linked with chronic HCV infection include autoimmune thyroiditis; diabetes mellitus; porphyria cutanea tarda; sialadenitis, resembling Sjögren's syndrome; membranous glomerulonephritis; B-cell non-Hodgkin's lymphoma; lichen planus; and Mooren's corneal ulcer, an extremely rare form of chronic ulcerative keratitis (22).

SEROLOGIC STUDIES AND DIAGNOSIS

Acute Hepatitis C

The first identifiable marker of acute HCV infection is the appearance in serum of HCV RNA (which may be detected by polymerase chain reaction amplification tests approved by the U.S. Food and Drug administration) within 10 to 20 days after exposure and 3 to 5 weeks before elevation of serum aminotransferase levels and 6 to 9 weeks before the development of anti-HCV (Fig. 87.2). Low-level viremia undetectable by current tests or intermittently undetectable viremia may precede the period of detection of HCV (23). Serologic diagnosis of acute HCV infection rests on the detection of both HCV RNA and antibodies to recombinant HCV antigens, associated with

elevations of serum aminotransferases, and the absence of evidence of preexisting hepatitis. Second- and third-generation enzyme immunoassays and recombinant immunoblot assays that use multiple antigens from both structural and nonstructural regions of the HCV genome have increased sensitivity and specificity. As shown in Fig. 87.2, antibodies to C22-3 and C33c may be the first anti-HCV antibodies to appear in HCV infection. Anti-NS5 appears somewhat later; anti–C100-3 appears to be the last antibody to be detected in acute, self-limited infection.

Antibodies to HCV antigens may be detected in more than 60% of patients during the acute phase of illness; seroconversion occurs weeks to months later in another 35%. In perhaps 5% of infected patients, current assays for anti-HCV may remain persistently negative, although the presence of circulating HCV RNA indicates the presence of infection.

Anti-HCV titers generally decline over time following recovery from acute infection and may eventually become undetectable (24) although cellular immune responses persist.

Chronic Hepatitis C

In chronic hepatitis C, anti-HCV is almost invariably present, and circulating HCV RNA is detected consistently throughout the course of infection, but viral levels may vary by 0.5 log from determination to determination. Nonetheless, the viral load appears to generally increase over time (25), and viremia is probably lifelong. Transient clearance and then reappearance of HCV RNA has been well documented but may reflect errors in assay because spontaneous prolonged HCV clearance must be extremely rare once the infection has become chronic. Serum aminotransferase levels are persistently or intermittently elevated in about 60% to 70% of patients; in the remainder the levels are within the normal range.

NATURAL HISTORY

The majority of patients infected by HCV develop persistent infection with histologic and biochemical evidence of chronic hepatitis. Most patients are relatively asymptomatic, and their infections remain clinically silent for decades after onset of infection. Progression of chronic hepatitis C to cirrhosis may be seen in as few as 2% to as many as 20% of patients after 20 years of infection. Despite studies supporting the lower risk figure (26,27), by the middle of the 1990s, end-stage liver disease due to chronic hepatitis C with cirrhosis had become the single most common form of liver disease for which liver transplantation was undertaken in the United States. Furthermore, the risk for HCV-related hepatocellular carcinoma has been estimated to be about 2.5% annually in patients with cirrhosis, and in the United States the incidence of HCV-related hepatocellular carcinoma has been increasing (28). Predictors of disease progression to cirrhosis include concomitant alcohol consumption, male gender, early or late age at onset of infection, immunodeficiency, and coinfections with HIV or HBV (29).

CLINICAL VARIANTS

Acute Liver Failure

In the United States, HCV is a rare cause of acute liver failure. It may be more common in some countries, for example, Taiwan, where HCV infection has been identified in nearly one half of patients with fulminant non-A, non-B hepatitis (30). Because of the

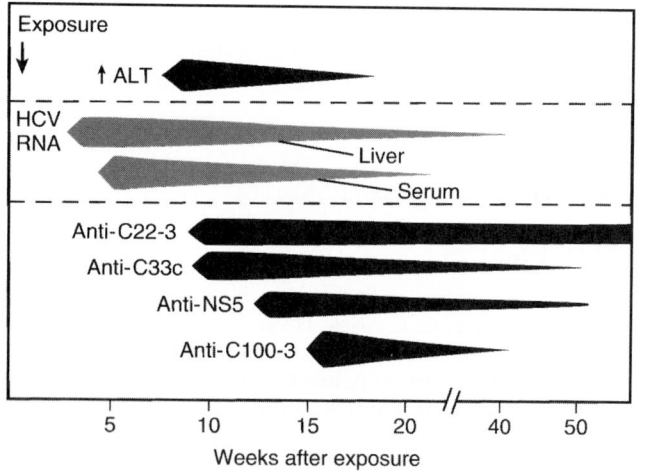

Figure 87.2. Sequence of serum alanine aminotransferase (*ALT*) elevation and appearance and clearance of serologic markers of hepatitis C virus infection in self-limited acute hepatitis C.

delayed appearance of anti-HCV in acute hepatitis C, detection of HCV RNA may be necessary for diagnosis.

TREATMENT

Acute Hepatitis C

The benefit of treatment for individuals who become HCV RNA positive following accidental exposure to HCV is uncertain. Randomized, controlled trials of interferon-α monotherapy in patients with acute hepatitis C indicate that a 3-month course significantly increased the likelihood of a sustained loss of HCV RNA (31). However, treatment of acute hepatitis C with interferon is not approved in the United States and should be considered experimental. The efficacy of high-dose interferon, interferon plus ribavirin (a guanosine analog), or pegylated interferon plus ribavirin in the setting of acute hepatitis C remains to be determined.

Chronic Hepatitis C

The goals of treatment of chronic hepatitis C have been to relieve symptoms, when present; to eradicate HCV, thereby eliminating infectivity and hepatic inflammation and decreasing ongoing HCV-induced liver injury; and to prevent histologic and clinical progression to cirrhosis and end-stage liver disease and hepatocellular carcinoma. Administration of the monovalent HAV and HBV vaccines, or the combined HAV/HBV vaccine, is appropriate to prevent superinfection by these viruses in susceptible patients with chronic hepatitis C. At present, the therapy of choice is the combination of recombinant interferon-α conjugated to polyethylene glycol (pegylated interferon) given once per week subcutaneously in a dose of 1 μg/kg or 180 μg, depending on the product selected, and the daily oral administration of ribavirin in a dose of 800 to 1,200 mg for 1 year (32,33). Interferon treatment results in a very rapid and dose-dependent decline in viral load, presumably due to inhibition of HCV replication, followed by a slower and more variable decline thought to be related to the death rate of infected hepatocytes (34). Depending on the genotype of the treated patient, sustained virologic response rates, defined as the absence of detectable HCV RNA 6 months after ending therapy, are about 50% for genotype 1 to 90% for genotypes 2 and 3 (32,33). Pegylated interferons alone are less beneficial and avoid the hemolysis induced by ribavirin (35,36) but may be nearly equivalent in efficacy to the combination of nonpegylated interferon thrice weekly plus ribavirin. Among patients achieving a sustained virologic response, 95% maintain that response indefinitely, with normal serum aminotransferases and improvement or complete recovery of liver injury (37). Relapses later than 2 years after discontinuation of therapy are rare.

The major adverse events associated with pegylated interferon therapy and ribavirin include a flu-like illness, fatigue, depression, irritability, insomnia, granulocytopenia, thrombocytopenia, hair thinning, and thyroid dysfunction, all attributable to the interferon component, and hemolytic anemia and bronchospasm, consequences of ribavirin. Drug reductions may be necessary in about 25% of treated patients and discontinuation in about 5% in controlled trials.

Although data are still limited, chronic hepatitis C patients with persistently normal serum aminotransferase levels (who in general have milder liver disease and slower progression to cirrhosis than those with elevated aminotransferase levels) respond similarly to interferon therapy as those with elevated levels (38).

Sustained virologic response rates are higher in whites than blacks, in genotypes 2 and 3 compared to genotype 1, in women, in younger patients, in those with lower viral loads, in noncirrhotic patients, in the immunocompetent, and in nondrinkers of alcohol.

Resistance to antiviral therapy in HCV remains poorly understood, but the HCV NS5A protein has been implicated. For patients who do not respond to pegylated interferon plus ribavirin, no clearly effective treatment is currently available. Long-term therapy with pegylated interferon alone in an attempt to halt progression of liver disease in the absence of viral clearance is under study in patients with histologically advanced disease, as are combinations of interferon, ribavirin, amantidine, and other drugs. Limited available data suggest that interferon therapy may have a beneficial long-term effect even if HCV remains detectable (29,39).

Patients with end-stage cirrhosis due to HCV are candidates for liver transplantation, but recurrence of infection is invariable. The disease is generally mild and often clinically silent; progressive disease leading to hepatic failure is uncommon in the first 5 years of follow-up. Treatment of HCV-related hepatocellular carcinoma remains problematic, but liver transplantation offers the best results in these cirrhotic patients.

Interferon treatment of patients with cryoglobulinemia may result in symptomatic improvement, and a reduction of cryoglobulin levels. Among patients with HCV-associated glomerulonephritis, proteinuria may decrease during treatment with interferon, but renal function appears unlikely to improve, and proteinuria may recur after cessation of treatment. Experiences with treatment of the other extrahepatic disorders is limited.

PREVENTION

General Measures

Needle exchange programs have the potential for reducing HCV infection among injection drug users but only if sharing of needles and other injection equipment is discontinued. Continued screening of blood donors for anti-HCV and HCV RNA, screening of blood products such as immune globulin products for HCV RNA and viral inactivation procedures, and implementation of universal precautions in health care settings may further reduce the frequency of blood-borne HCV infection, but the risk is already relatively low in these settings. Safe sex practices may reduce the risk for transmission among sexual partners, but compliance with this approach is far from assured, and measurement of effectiveness will be difficult.

Passive Immunization

Although HCV can elicit a neutralizing antibody, it appears to be a restricted, isolate-specific response (40). Conventional immune globulin provides no clear protection, but an experimental high titer anti-HCV–containing immune globulin is under study.

Active Immunization

Among the known obstacles to vaccine development, the heterogeneity of HCV looms large: HCV reinfections and superinfections by other HCV genotypes have been reported in both chimpanzees and humans (41,42). If cross-protection between the recognized genotypes is limited or nonexistent, a broadly effective HCV vaccine would need to incorporate antigenic domains from the most common genotypes. The limited availability and high cost of the only other susceptible primate—the chimpanzee—is another obstacle. The absence of a tissue culture system supporting high-level HCV replication may be less of an obstacle given recent reports of the cultivation of RNA replicons permitting high-level RNA replication (43,44). Nonetheless, HCV vaccine development is being pursued through the use of purified recombinant HCV antigens (45), recombinant viruses incorporating HCV antigenic material (46), synthesis of HCV-like particles in insect cells (47), and the use of genetic, DNA-based immunization (48).

Although a safe and effective HCV vaccine that provided sterilizing immunity would be highly desirable, one that prevented persistent HCV infection would be very acceptable because it is chronic HCV infection that leads to important morbidity and mortality. Despite the declining incidence of acute hepatitis C in the United States, no major reductions have been reported for nations of the less affluent, developing world, where HCV infection continues to occur at high rates. For these countries, HCV vaccines, once available, should be incorporated into childhood immunization programs. In developed nations, such as the United States, HCV vaccine would be initially targeted to high-risk groups and only later recommended for childhood immunization.

REFERENCES

1. Centers for Disease Control and Prevention. Recommendations for prevention and control of hepatitis C virus (HCV) infection and HCV-related chronic disease. *MMWR* 1998;47(RR-19):1–39.
2. Alter MJ, Margolis HS, Krawczynski K, et al. The natural history of community-acquired hepatitis C in the United States. *N Engl J Med* 1992;327:1899–1905.
3. Vogt M, Lang T, Frosner G, et al. Prevalence and clinical outcome of hepatitis C infection in children who underwent cardiac surgery before the implementation of blood-donor screening. *N Engl J Med* 1999;341:866–870.
4. Hayashi J, Kishihara Y, Yamaji K, et al. Transmission of hepatitis C virus by health care workers in a rural area of Japan. *Am J Gastroenterol* 1995;90:794–799.
5. Pybus OG, Charleston MA, Gupta S, et al. The epidemic behavior of the hepatitis C virus. *Science* 2001;292:2323–2325.
6. Alter MJ, Kruszon-Moran D, Nainan OV, et al. The prevalence of hepatitis C virus infection in the United States, 1988 through 1994. *N Engl J Med* 1999;341:556–562.
7. Schreiber GB, Busch MP, Kleinman SH, et al. The risk of transfusion-transmitted viral infections. *N Engl J Med* 1996;334:1685–1690.
8. Knoll A, Helmig M, Peters O, et al. Hepatitis C virus transmission in a pediatric oncology ward: an analysis of an outbreak and review of the literature. *Lab Invest* 2001;81:251–262.
9. Haley RW, Fischer RP. Commercial tattooing as a potentially important source of hepatitis C infection. *Medicine* 2001;80:134–151.
10. Halfon P, Riflet H, Renou C, et al. Molecular evidence of male-to-female sexual transmission of hepatitis C virus after vaginal and anal intercourse. *J Clin Microbiol* 2001;39:1204–1206.
11. Osmond DH, Charlebois E, Sheppard HW, et al. Comparison of risk factors for hepatitis C and hepatitis B virus infection in homosexual men. *J Infect Dis* 1993;167:66–71.
12. Yeung LTF, King SM, Roberts EA. Maternal-to-infant transmission of hepatitis C virus. *Hepatology* 2001;34:223–229.
13. Chapel HM, Christie JML, Peach V, et al. Five-year follow-up of patients with primary antibody deficiencies following an outbreak of acute hepatitis C. *Clin Immunol* 2001;99:320–324.
14. Gruner NH, Gerlach TJ, Jung M-C, et al. Association of hepatitis C virus–specific CD8+ T cells with viral clearance in acute hepatitis C. *J Infect Dis* 2000;181:1528–1536.
15. Chang K-M, Thimme R, Melpolder JJ, et al. Differential CD4+ and CD8+ T-cell responsiveness in hepatitis C virus infection. *Hepatology* 2001;33:267–276.
16. Bassett SE, Guerra B, Brasky K, et al. Protective immune response to hepatitis C virus in chimpanzees rechallenged following clearance of primary infection. *Hepatology* 2001;33:1479–1487.
17. Machida K, Tsukiyama-Kohara K, Seike E, et al. Inhibition of cytochrome c reductase in Fas-mediated signaling pathway in transgenic mice induced to express hepatitis C viral proteins. *J Biol Chem* 2001;276:12140–12146.
18. Forns X, Thimme R, Govindarajan S, et al. Hepatitis C virus lacking the hypervariable region 1 of the second envelope protein is infectious and causes acute resolving or persistent infection in chimpanzees. *Proc Natl Acad Sci U S A* 2000;97:13318–13323.
19. Lefkowitch JH, Schiff ER, Davis GL, et al. Pathological diagnosis of chronic hepatitis C: a multicenter comparative study with chronic hepatitis B. *Gastroenterology* 1993;104:595–603.
20. Serfaty L, Andreani T, Giral P, et al. Hepatitis C virus induced hypobetalipoproteinemia: a possible mechanism for steatosis in chronic hepatitis C. *J Hepatol* 2001;34:428–434.
21. Pawlotsky J-M, Roudot-Thoraval F, Simmonds P, et al. Extrahepatic immunologic manifestations in chronic hepatitis C and hepatitis C virus serotypes. *Ann Intern Med* 1995;122:169–173.
22. Koff RS, Dienstag JL. Extrahepatic manifestations of hepatitis C and the association with alcoholic liver disease. *Semin Liver Dis* 1995;15:101–109.
23. Schuttler CG, Caspan G, Jursch CA, et al. Hepatitis C virus transmission by a blood donation negative in nucleic acid amplification tests for viral RNA. *Lancet* 2000;355:41–42.
24. Takaki A, Wiese M, Maertens G, et al. Cellular immune responses persist and humoral responses decrease two decades after recovery from a single-source outbreak of hepatitis C. *Nat Med* 2000;6:578–582, 2000.
25. Fanning L, Kenny-Walsh E, Levis J, et al. Natural fluctuations of hepatitis C viral load in a homogeneous patient population: a prospective study. *Hepatology* 2000;31:225–229.
26. Kenny-Walsh E for the Irish Hepatology Research Group. Clinical outcomes after hepatitis C infection from contaminated anti-D immune globulin. *N Engl J Med* 1999;340:1228–1233.
27. Seeff LB, Miller RN, Rabkin CS, et al. 45-Year follow-up of hepatitis C virus infection in healthy young adults. *Ann Intern Med* 2000;132:105–111.
28. El-Serag HB, Mason AC. Rising incidence of hepatocellular carcinoma in the United States. *N Engl J Med* 1999;340:745–750.
29. Niederau C, Lange S, Heintges T, et al. Prognosis of chronic hepatitis C: results of a large, prospective cohort study. *Hepatology* 1998;28:1687–1695.
30. Chu C-M, Sheen I-S, Liaw Y-F. The role of hepatitis C virus in fulminant viral hepatitis in an area with endemic hepatitis A or B. *Gastroenterology* 1994;107:189–195.
31. Thevenot T, Regimbeau C, Ratziu V, et al. Meta-analysis of interferon randomized trials in the treatment of viral hepatitis C in naïve patients: 1999 update. *J Viral Hepatitis* 2001;8:48–62.
32. Manns MP, McHutchison JG, Gordon SC, et al. Peginterferon alfa-2b plus ribavirin compared with interferon alfa-2b plus ribavirin for initial treatment of chronic hepatitis C: a randomised trial. *Lancet* 2001;358:958–965.
33. Fried M, Shiffman ML, Reddy RK, et al. Pegylated (40 kDa) interferon alfa-2a (Pegasys) in combination with ribavirin: efficacy and safety results from a phase III, randomized, actively-controlled, multicenter trial. *Gastroenterology* 2001;120:A-55.
34. Zeuzem S, Herrmann E, Lee J-L, et al. Viral kinetics in patients with chronic hepatitis C treated with standard or peginterferon alfa2a. *Gastroenterology* 2001;120:1438–1447.
35. Zeuzem S, Feinman SV, Rasenack J, et al. Peginterferon alfa-2a in patients with chronic hepatitis C. *N Engl J Med* 2000;343:1666–1672.
36. Lindsay KL, Trepo C, Heintges T, et al. A randomized, double-blind trial comparing pegylated interferon alfa-2b as initial treatment for chronic hepatitis C. *Hepatology* 2001;34:395–403.
37. Marcellin P, Boyer N, Gervais A, et al. Long-term histologic improvement and loss of detectable intrahepatic HCV RNA in patients with chronic hepatitis C and sustained response to interferon-alpha therapy. *Ann Intern Med* 1997;127:875–881.
38. Shiffman ML, Stewart CA, Hofmann CM, et al. Chronic infection with hepatitis C virus in patients with elevated or persistently normal serum alanine aminotransferase levels: comparison of hepatic histology and response to interferon therapy. *J Infect Dis* 2000;182:1595–1601.
39. Shiffman ML, Hofmann CM, Contos MJ, et al. A randomized, controlled trial of maintenance interferon for treatment of chronic hepatitis C non-responders. *Gastroenterology* 1999;117:1164–1172.
40. Farci P, Alter HJ, Wong DC, et al. Prevention of hepatitis C virus infection in chimpanzees after antibody-mediated *in vitro* neutralization. *Proc Natl Acad Sci U S A* 1994;91:7792–7796.
41. Farci P, Alter HJ, Govindarajan S, et al: Lack of protective immunity against reinfection with hepatitis C virus. *Science* 1992;258:135–140.
42. Kao J-H, Chen P-J, Lai M-Y, et al. Superinfection of heterologous hepatitis C virus in a patient with chronic type C hepatitis. *Gastroenterology* 1993;105:583–587.
43. Lohmann V, Korner F, Dobierzewska A, et al. Mutations in hepatitis C virus RNAs conferring cell culture adaptation. *J Virol* 2001;75:1437–1449.
44. Blight KJ, Kolykhalov AA, Rice CM. Efficient initiation of HCV RNA replication in cell culture. *Science* 2000;290:1972–1975.
45. Choo QL, Kuo G, Ralston R, et al. Vaccination of chimpanzees against infection by the hepatitis C virus. *Proc Natl Acad Sci U S A* 1994;91:1294–1298.
46. Pancholi P, Liu Q, Tricoche N, et al. DNA prime-canarypox boost with polycistronic hepatitis C virus (HCV) genes generates potent immune responses to HCV structural and nonstructural proteins. *J Infect Dis* 2000;182:18–27.
47. Lechmann M, Murata K, Satoi J, et al. Hepatitis C virus-like particles induce virus-specific humoral and cellular immune responses in mice. *Hepatology* 2001;34:417–423.
48. Forns X, Payette PJ, Satterfield W, et al. Vaccination of chimpanzees with plasmid DNA encoding the hepatitis C virus (HCV) envelope E2 protein modified the infection after challenge with homologous monoclonal HCV. *Hepatology* 2000;32:618–625.

CHAPTER 88

Hepatitis E

Raymond S. Koff

EPIDEMIOLOGY

Incubation Period, Virus Shedding, and Viremia

The incubation period of hepatitis E has a reported range of 15 to 65 days and a mean of about 40 days. Elevation of serum aminotransferase levels may persist for 3 to 13 weeks. The hepatitis E virus (HEV) is shed in the stools after transport from the liver into bile and then into the intestinal contents. Shedding may occur during the second half of the incubation period, through the onset of illness, and continue for 2 to 3 weeks in most cases (1). The maximal duration of fecal shedding is probably no more than 1 to 2 months. Whether replication occurs in the intestine remains uncertain; the presence of replicative intermediates of HEV in extrahepatic tissues and other body fluids has yet to be reported. The duration of viremia is generally believed to be short-lived (Fig. 88.1) but viremia has been identified as late as 4 months after the onset of jaundice. Protracted viremia may be present in 15% of patients (2). Neither an intestinal carrier state nor persistent viremia have been established.

Epidemiologic Patterns

HEV has been linked with epidemic and endemic disease in developing countries, particularly in the Indian subcontinent, Asia, and Africa. Limited seroprevalence data suggest that less than 3% of the population of developed countries have detectable antibody to HEV (Table 88.1); in contrast, higher seroprevalence rates have been identified in developing countries, but rates may vary widely depending on the population studied and sources of drinking water. The specificity of anti-HEV detection in developed nations, in the absence of known epidemic or endemic disease, remains to be established. There is evidence that HEV is endemic, at relatively low levels, in some developing countries

of the New World (e.g., Mexico, Venezuela, Brazil, and Cuba). It may be present in others. Outbreaks of HEV infection have been recognized in Mexico (3). Acute hepatitis E is seen in developed nations throughout the world in very low frequencies, but in most cases the infection is imported by travelers and immigrants from the developing world; rare instances of sporadic infection have been reported in the United States in the absence of a travel history or exposure to a traveler. Because a virus closely related to human HEV has been found in swine and possibly other animals, exposure to feces from infected animals may be responsible for transmission in these otherwise unexplained cases (4). In endemic regions of the developing world, sporadic human cases of HEV infection or HEV infection in swine or other animals may serve as a reservoir of infection.

Although the epidemiology of HEV infection resembles that of hepatitis A and immunity to reinfection is probably lifelong for each, there are distinct differences. HEV infection is thought to be the most common form of clinically apparent sporadic hepatitis in the young adult population of developing countries; hepatitis A may be the most common form of subclinical or inapparent infection in children in these same areas, with seroprevalence rates of nearly 100% in the first years of life. However, in some of the same regions, the seroprevalence of HEV infection has exceeded 60% at the end of the first decade and 75% by the second (5). Whereas hepatitis A is generally mild, even during pregnancy, hepatitis E is often a severe disorder in pregnancy with high case-fatality rates.

Modes of Transmission

Outbreaks of hepatitis E have been repeatedly linked to fecal contamination of drinking water. Both human and animal sewage may be responsible. Some endemic infections also appear to result from fecal-oral transmission due to continuing contamination of water and breakdown in purification techniques. Intrafamilial person-to-person transmission may occur but is unusual (6). Maternal-neonatal transmission has been documented; intrauterine infection may be responsible (7). A high frequency of abortions and intrauterine deaths results from such infections. Affected surviving infants may have clinical and biochemical evidence of HEV infection.

In endemic regions, transfusion-associated transmission of HEV from asymptomatic viremic blood donors has led to hepatitis E in recipients (8). The importance of percutaneous, blood-borne transmission in the spread of HEV requires further study, as does the frequency and mechanisms responsible for nosocomial spread of HEV in health care facilities (9).

PATHOGENESIS AND PATHOLOGY

The pathogenesis of HEV infection remains poorly understood. A direct HEV-induced cytopathic effect is possible, but an immunologically mediated mechanism of hepatocyte injury seems more likely. Infiltration of both lymphocytes and monocytes in areas of hepatocyte loss and direct contact between lymphocytes and hepatocytes are prominent features in experimentally infected nonhuman primates and in human cases. The possibility of two phases of HEV infection was raised in one study in cynomolgus macaques (10). In the first, HEV might replicate in the liver, and a mild hepatitis may be seen as a consequence of a viral or immune-mediated effect. The second phase might begin with the development of a humoral immune response that results in clearing of HEV but worsening of the hepatic histologic changes. Further studies will be needed to confirm this notion of

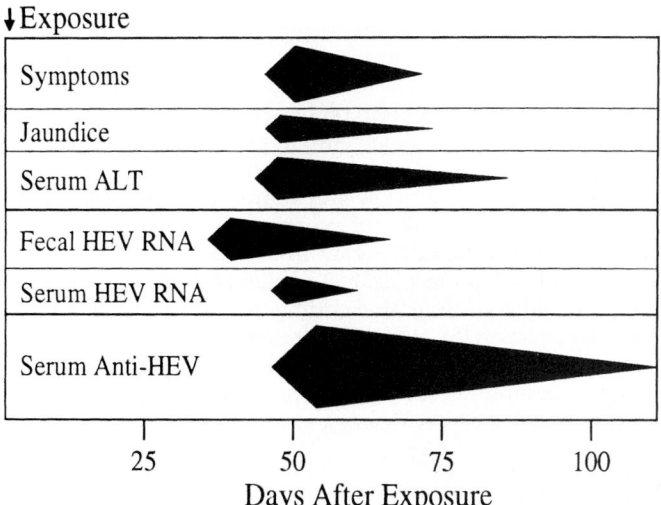

Figure 88.1. Proposed scheme of clinical, biochemical, virologic, and serologic events in acute hepatitis E infection. *ALT,* alanine aminotransferase.

TABLE 88.1. Seroprevalence of Antibodies to Hepatitis E Virus (Anti-HEV) in Selected Countries and Regions

Country or region	Anti-HEV prevalence (%)
Taiwan	0–11 (healthy subjects)
United States	0.5–2 (blood donors)
Ukraine	0.5
South Africa	<2
Europe	<2–3
Italy	0.74 (healthy subjects)
	0.9 (blood donors)
Thailand	2
Spain	2.8 (blood donors)
	6.3 (hemodialysis patients)
Venezuela	1.6 (pregnant women, Caracas)
	4 (rural population)
	5 (rural Amerindians)
Tajikistan	8.5
Saudi Arabia	9.5 (blood donors)
Egypt	25–75 (blood donors and rural villagers)
Malaysia	45–50 (aboriginal communities)
	2 (blood donors)

biphasic infection because patterns of HEV infection in nonhuman primates vary widely. In some instances, for example in the chimpanzee model, infection following intravenous inoculation of HEV may occur without evidence of liver injury (11).

In general, liver biopsy specimens of patients with acute hepatitis E resemble those seen in other forms of acute viral hepatitis, and cholestatic features may be prominent with canalicular bile plugs. Although the presence of regenerating liver cells arranged in a duct-like pattern known as pseudoglandular transformation may be more common in hepatitis E than other forms of hepatitis, it is nonspecific.

CLINICAL MANIFESTATIONS

In typical outbreaks, highest attack rates of clinically apparent disease are usually found in individuals between 15 and 40 years of age. In children, most infections are anicteric. In most adult patients with hepatitis E, the disease is clinically indistinguishable from other forms of viral hepatitis (12). Serum enzyme elevations are usually monophasic. Jaundice may last for 2 to 3 weeks; serum bilirubin and serum alanine aminotransferase levels return to normal within 3 months (Fig. 88.1). Cholestasis may be prominent. In one study of hepatitis E in a predominantly adult population (13), cholestasis was evident, as identified by the presence of pruritus and clay-colored stools, in 25%. About 5% of patients may develop generalized lymphadenopathy during the course of the illness. Overall case-fatality rates due to acute liver failure in hepatitis E are usually in the range of 0.5% to 3%.

SEROLOGIC STUDIES AND DIAGNOSIS

Immunoglobulin M (IgM) antibodies to HEV (IgM anti-HEV), IgA antibodies to HEV (IgA anti-HEV), and IgG antibodies to HEV (IgG anti-HEV) appear following HEV infection. The IgM anti-HEV is detectable in most acute specimens, early in hepatitis E and may persist for at least 6 weeks after the peak of the illness (14). IgG anti-HEV is also present early, peaks about 2 weeks or more after the onset of clinical disease, and remains detectable at declining levels for at least 20 months (14). Relative to testing for HEV RNA (a research assay) in acute hepatitis E, IgM and IgG anti-HEV had sensitivities of 53% and 87%, respectively, while the specificities were 99% and 92%, respectively (15). Enzyme immunoassays for IgM and IgG anti-HEV are commercially available: none have been approved by the U.S. Food and Drug Administration. The presence of IgG anti-HEV in low-prevalence populations without evidence of endemic or epidemic disease may reflect false-positive test results because of cross-reactivity with another closely related agent or nonspecificity of these assays.

CLINICAL VARIANTS AND SEQUELAE

The acute hepatitis associated with HEV infection has been shown to be self-limiting, except in the few patients in whom acute liver failure ensues. Coinfection with HAV may result in a more severe course (16). In pregnant women, particularly in the third trimester, a surprisingly high proportion (10% to 20%) of HEV infections result in acute liver failure with a high risk for maternal and intrauterine fetal or neonatal mortality. The mechanism underlying the enhanced virulence of HEV in the third trimester of pregnancy remains to be determined.

TREATMENT

No specific treatment of hepatitis E is available, and management is largely symptomatic and supportive. Early delivery of pregnant women with acute liver failure due to hepatitis E may be beneficial, as is referral for liver transplantation; in developing countries where the disease is most prevalent, neither may be feasible.

PREVENTION

In developing countries, assuring clean water supplies is likely to reduce the risk of HEV infection. Effective immunoprophylaxis is not yet available but is under study.

Passive Immunization

Conventional immune globulin manufactured in the United States is unlikely to contain anti-HEV and is not likely to be useful for immunoprophylaxis of travelers to endemic regions. Unfortunately, immune globulin prepared in developing countries where the disease is endemic also appears to have insufficient anti-HEV levels to prevent infection, although in one study the incidence of infection was lower in immunized pregnant women (17). Passive immunization of cynomolgus monkeys with anti-HEV–titered convalescent serum from experimentally infected animals did not protect against challenge with live HEV, although it did reduce fecal shedding of the virus and ameliorated the disease (18). Whether administration of HEV-specific monoclonal antibodies to the ORF-2 capsid protein (19) or high-titered, hyperimmune globulin can provide pre- or postexposure protection remains to be determined.

Active Immunization

The ORF-2 capsid protein of HEV has been the most promising immunogen used in vaccine development. Immunization of cynomolgus monkeys with a 55-kd recombinant HEV fusion protein from ORF-2 protected against challenge with live HEV (18), and administration of a plasmid construct expressing the ORF-2 protein protected monkeys from challenge with a heterologous strain (20). In rhesus monkeys, a recombinant ORF-2 protein vaccine did not provide sterilizing immunity but did reduce the duration and extent of viremia and fecal shedding (21). A candidate, two-dose recombinant ORF-2 protein–containing vaccine is now in clinical trials.

REFERENCES

1. Aggarwal R, Kini D, Sofat S, et al. Duration of viraemia and faecal viral excretion in acute hepatitis E. *Lancet* 2000;356:1081–1082.
2. Nanda SK, Ansan IH, Acharya SK, et al. Protracted viremia during acute sporadic hepatitis E virus infection. *Gastroenterology* 1995;108:225–230.
3. Yelazquez O, Stetler HC, Avila C, et al. Epidemic transmission of enterically transmitted non-A, non-B hepatitis in Mexico, 1986–1987. *JAMA* 1990;263:3281–3285.
4. Halbur PG, Kasorndorkbua C, Gilber C, et al. Comparative pathogenesis of infection of pigs with hepatitis E virus recovered from a pig and human. *J Clin Microbiol* 2001;39:918–923.
5. Fix AD, Abdel-Hamid M, Purcell RH, et al. Prevalence of antibodies to hepatitis E in two rural Egyptian communities. *Am J Trop Med Hyg* 2000;62:519–523.
6. Arankalle YA, Chadha MS, Mehendale SM, et al. Epidemic hepatitis E: serological evidence for lack of intrafamilial spread. *Ind J Gastroenterol* 2000;19:24–28.
7. Khuroo MS, Kamili S, Jameel S. Vertical transmission of hepatitis E virus. *Lancet* 1995;345:1025–1026.
8. Arankalle YA, Chobe LP. Hepatitis E virus: can it be transmitted parenterally? *J Viral Hepatitis* 1999;6:161–164.
9. Robson SC, Adams S, Brink N, et al. Hospital outbreak of hepatitis E. *Lancet* 1992;339:1424–1425.
10. Longer CF, Denny SL, Caudill JD, et al. Experimental hepatitis E: pathogenesis in cynomolgus macaques (*Macaca fascicularis*). *J Infect Dis* 1993;168:602–609.
11. McCaustland KA, Krawczynski K, Ebert JW, et al. Hepatitis E virus infection in chimpanzees: a retrospective analysis. *Arch Virol* 2000;145:1909–1918.
12. Aggarwal R, Krawczynski K. Hepatitis E: an overview and recent advances in clinical and laboratory research. *J Gastroenterol Hepatol* 2000;15:9–20.
13. Khuroo MS, Rustgi VK, Dawson GJ, et al. Spectrum of hepatitis E virus infection in India. *J Med Virol* 1994;42:281–286.
14. Bryan JP, Tsarev SA, Iqbal M, et al. Epidemic hepatitis E in Pakistan: patterns of serologic response and evidence that antibody to hepatitis E virus protects against disease. *J Infect Dis* 1994;170:517–521.
15. Lin CC, Wu JC, Chang TT, et al. Diagnostic value of immunoglobulin G (IgG) and IgM anti-hepatitis E virus (HEV) tests based on HEV RNA in an area where hepatitis E is not endemic. *J Clin Microbiol* 2000;38:3915–3918.
16. Zanetti AR, Schlauder GG, Romano L, et al. Identification of a novel variant of hepatitis E virus in Italy. *J Med Virol* 1999;57:356–360.
17. Arankalle YA, Chadha MS, Dama BM, et al. Role of immune serum globulin in pregnant women during an epidemic of hepatitis E. *J Viral Hepatitis* 1998;5:199–214.
18. Tsarev SA, Tsareva TS, Emerson SU, et al. Successful passive and active immunization of cynomolgus monkeys against hepatitis E. *Proc Natl Acad Sci U S A* 1994;91:10198–10202.
19. Schofield DJ, Glamann J, Emerson SU, et al. Identification by phage display and characterization of two neutralizing chimpanzee monoclonal antibodies to the hepatitis E virus capsid protein. *J Virology* 2000;74:5548–5555.
20. Kamili 5, Spelbring J, Krawczynski K. DNA vaccination protects non-human primates against hepatitis E virus. *Hepatology* 2000;32:380a.
21. Tsarev SA, Tsareva TS, Emerson SU, et al. Recombinant vaccine against hepatitis E: dose response and protection against heterologous challenge. *Vaccine* 1997;15:1834–1838.

CHAPTER 89
Pyogenic Liver Abscess

John G. Bartlett

Because the liver is exposed to bacteria in both the systemic and the portal circulations, it would seem relatively vulnerable to bacterial infections. Nevertheless, the extensive network of reticuloendothelial cells that lines the sinusoids seems highly protective, and this appears to be one of the most effective sites of bacterial clearance (1). The most common bacterial infection is pyogenic abscess. Even this is relatively rare, but when it occurs it often represents a life-threatening infection that may be difficult to detect and controversial with respect to management strategies.

HISTORY

Hepatic abscesses were originally described in 1836 by John Bright (2). Ochsner (3) published his classic review in 1938, which included 575 cases culled from the literature: 35% were amebic and 34% occurred in association with appendicitis. The mortality rate at that time was 80%, and it remained in the 65% to 80% range until the mid-1960s. During the past 30 years, there have been three important changes in our understanding and management of pyogenic liver abscesses: (a) imaging techniques were developed that remarkably facilitated detection; (b) refinements in the microbiology showed that anaerobic bacteria were major pathogens; and (c) percutaneous drainage methods were introduced as an alternative to surgery. Pyogenic liver abscess continues to be a somewhat elusive clinical condition, but the aforementioned developments have driven mortality rates down to the 10% to 20% range.

INCIDENCE

Hepatic abscesses accounted for 0.007% to 0.04% of all hospitalizations in the preantibiotic era (4,5). A review of 18,300 autopsies in 1932 by Collins (5) showed 111 cases, for an autopsy incidence of 0.6%. Since that time the incidence has declined, possibly owing to the availability of antibiotic therapy. A review of nine cases from the Henry Ford Hospital from 1950 to 1960 indicated that these accounted for 0.005% of all hospital admissions, and another review published in 1973 indicated an incidence of 0.007% (6,7). A review at Duke showed 58 patients with this diagnosis during the period 1968 to 1982, representing 15 cases per 100,000 admissions (8).

PATHOPHYSIOLOGY

Pyogenic abscesses usually are secondary to another condition, although 15% to 30% are considered "cryptogenic." The most common associated conditions are biliary tract disease, hepatic neoplasms, infections of the portal system, infections at distant anatomic sites, and trauma (8–36). The distribution of associated conditions is reviewed in Table 89.1, which presents data from a review of 885 cases reported in the literature from 1954 to 1979 by McDonald and Howard (9) and a review of 55 cases at Duke from 1968 to 1982 by McDonald and co-workers (8).

The most common associated condition at present is ascending cholangitis secondary to biliary obstruction or manipulation secondary to calculus, stricture, or malignancy. This accounted for only 14% of hepatic abscesses in the prechemotherapy era, according to the review of 575 cases by Ochsner (3), but it now accounts for approximately 30% (8,13–19,22,24–40).

Hematogenous infection of the liver may occur via the hepatic artery or, more frequently, the portal vein. In the report by Ochsner and colleagues (3), 34% were associated with appendicitis, but these now account for less than 1%. Other associated infections that may reach the liver via the portal circulation include inflammatory diseases of the small and large bowel, diverticulitis, pancreatic infections, splenic infections, peritonitis, intraabdominal abscesses, and omphalitis The most common of these at present are infections involving the colon. There has

TABLE 89.1. Associated Conditions in Liver Abscess

	McDonald and Howard (Literature review)	McDonald et al. (Duke University Hospital)
Cases	885	55
Period	1954–1979	1968–1982
Associated conditions (%)		
Biliary tract disease	33	36
Neoplastic disease	10	22
Portal system infection	12	12
Other infection	13	15
Trauma	3	4
Unknown	21	15

Data from McDonald AP, Howard RJ. Pyogenic liver abscess. *World J Surg* 1980;4:369; and McDonald MI, Corey GA, Gallis HA, et al. Single and multiple pyogenic liver abscesses: natural history, diagnosis and treatment, with emphasis on percutaneous damage. *Medicine (Baltimore)* 1984;63:291.

been increasing recognition of hepatic abscesses in patients with Crohn's disease, an incidence reported at 0.5% to 3% (41–43). Hematogenous infection of the liver may occur from primary foci at extraabdominal sites through the hepatic artery. These include diverse conditions, may occur in association with hepatic trauma, and often involve a relatively unusual bacterium, such as *Staphylococcus aureus*. A distinctive variant of this pattern is jugular septic thrombophlebitis, with bacteremia almost invariably due to *Fusobacterium necrophorum* and multiple hepatic abscesses as described by Lemierre and popularly referred to as Lemierre's syndrome (44).

Infections that may reach the liver parenchyma by direct extension include penetrating tumors of the gastrointestinal tract, cholecystitis, pancreatitis, perihepatic abscess, and penetrating duodenal or gastric ulcer.

Miscellaneous conditions of the liver that may be complicated by pyogenic abscesses include trauma, tumors (hepatomas or metastatic cancer), infected cysts, and foreign bodies. Malignancies were second only to biliary tract disease in the Duke series (8), but most were extrahepatic tumors involving the biliary tract or pancreas accompanied by biliary tract obstruction. Nevertheless, Robertson and colleagues (10) reported that 16% of all hepatic abscesses reported during a 25-year interval represented secondary infections of neoplastic lesions of the liver.

Hepatic abscess is being recognized more often in immunosuppressed hosts, including those with defective B-cell function (45,46), chronic granulomatous disease (47), diabetes (48,49), sickle cell disease (50), or defective cell-mediated immunity (51–53), including recipients of liver transplants (54) and patients with acquired immunodeficiency syndrome (55–57). As expected, those associated with defective cell-mediated immunity usually involve opportunistic fungi.

Cirrhosis is another important predisposing condition based on a survey of the National Registry of Patients in Denmark (58). This showed that the frequency of pyogenic liver abscesses was 15-fold higher in patients with versus those without cirrhosis.

Approximately 20% of pyogenic liver abscesses have no associated underlying condition and are referred to as cryptogenic. Cryptogenic liver abscesses are usually solitary (8,14,25).

MICROBIOLOGY

The review of 575 reported cases of hepatic abscess by Ochsner (3) in 1938 indicated that approximately one third were due to amebiasis and the balance were "pyogenic." Since that time, the relative incidence of amebic liver abscesses in industrialized countries has declined. In the United States, they now account for only about 10% of all liver abscesses, although there may be great interhospital differences according to the population served. In U.S. hospitals serving a large population of Hispanic immigrants, amebic abscesses may account for the majority of cases (58,58a), and in developing countries these clearly constitute the majority (58–62).

Microbiologic studies of pyogenic abscesses in the preantibiotic era implicated *Escherichia coli* in 30%, *Streptococcus* in 27%, and *Staphylococcus* in 26%; cultures for the remaining 30% were sterile (3). The literature review by McDonald and Howard (9) showed that the major isolates in 604 patients reported from 1954 to 1979 included *E. coli* (37%), *S. aureus* (23%), *Proteus* (13%), *Klebsiella* or *Enterobacter* species (12%), and *Streptococcus* (17%). Anaerobic bacteria accounted for 6% in this review, and 7% of patients had sterile lesions. A major revision of the bacteriology of pyogenic liver abscess followed the 1972 report by Sabbaj and associates (11), which showed anaerobes in 25 of 47 cases (45%; Table 89.2). A subsequent review by Finegold (12) summarized the anaerobic bacteriology in 310 reported patients with liver abscesses ascribed to anaerobic bacteria reported before 1976. The most common of the 379 strains reported were microaerophilic

TABLE 89.2. Bacteriology of Liver Abscess: 25 Cases Involving Anaerobic Bacteria

Bacteria	No. of liver isolates	No. of blood isolates
Anaerobes	30	14
Peptostreptococci	6	2
Microaerophilic streptococci	7	7
Fusobacteria	5	1
Bacteroides fragilis	5	2
Other *Bacteroides* species	5	2
Aerobes	7	6
Streptococci	4	3
Escherichia coli	2	2
Proteus	1	0

From Sabbaj J, Sutter VL, Finegold SM. Anaerobic pyogenic liver abscess. *Ann Intern Med* 1972;77:629, with permission.

and anaerobic streptococci (96 isolates), *F. necrophorum* (47), *Bacteroides fragilis* (33), *Clostridium* (38), *Actinomyces* (32), and unspeciated strains of *Bacteroides* (39) and of *Fusobacterium* (34). The reports by Finegold (12) and Sabbaj (11) both include a substantial number of "microaerophilic streptococci." Many of these are now properly classified as *Streptococcus milleri*, which appear to be especially common in cryptogenic liver abscesses and hepatic abscess associated with Crohn's disease (63,64).

Most studies show that 30% to 50% of blood cultures of patients with pyogenic abscesses are positive and that cultures of liver aspirates usually show a polymicrobial flora.

Many of these infections are due to mixtures of aerobic and anaerobic bacteria. The most common isolates from blood or aspirates are coliforms, various streptococci (aerobic, microaerophilic, and anaerobic), and anaerobic gram-negative bacilli, principally *Fusobacterium* and *Bacteroides* species.

Less common causes of pyogenic liver abscess include *Listeria monocytogenes* (65,66), *Yersinia enterocolitica* (especially in patients who have hemachromatosis or who receive iron therapy) (67–70), *Pasteurella multocida* (with animal exposure) (71), *Actinomyces* (usually cryptogenic) (72–74), *Pseudomonas pseudomallei* (which causes the majority of pyogenic abscesses in countries where melioidosis is endemic) (75), and tuberculosis (76). In children, the major pathogen is *S. aureus* (77–81), although some have found that the mixed flora with anaerobes predominate (82). A distinctive syndrome of hepatic candidiasis with multiple microabscesses is recognized with increasing frequency in immunocompromised hosts, especially patients with acute granulocytic leukemia (83–85).

CLINICAL FEATURES

Age

In the preantibiotic era the predominant age group consisted of 30- to 40-year-old individuals, but the reduction in cases associated with appendicitis has been accompanied by a shift in age prevalence, so that most more recent series show a predominance of patients in the sixth and seventh decades of life. Nevertheless, there appears to be little difference in presentation or response to therapy that is age related (40).

Symptoms

The usual systemic signs of infection include fever, chills, malaise, and anorexia. Most patients appear severely ill and have spiking fever, although the fever pattern is quite varied and may be continuous or intermittent. Most patients also complain of right side upper quadrant pain that may radiate to the right shoulder. In some instances, the infection persists for long periods and is associated with signs of chronic infection, such as weight loss and anemia. This was noted in 30% to 50% of cases in the extensive literature review by McDonald and Howard (9).

Physical Examination

Approximately two thirds of patients with pyogenic liver abscesses have a large, tender liver. Perhaps the most useful specific finding is a localized point of tenderness, which must be carefully sought by a fingertip march over the intercostal spaces of the right upper quadrant. Before scanning technology was available, this technique was used to identify the site for needle aspiration in an effort to confirm the diagnosis, and the relatively

TABLE 89.3. Laboratory Findings in Liver Abscess

Parameter	No. abnormal/no. tested (%)
Leukocytosis	
White cells >10,000/mm³	316/445 (71)
Anemia	
Hemoglobin <12 g/dL	165/349 (47)
Elevated bilirubin level	
>2 mg/dL	117/299 (39)
Hypoalbuminemia	
<2 g/dL	130/238 (55)
Elevated alkaline phosphatase level	139/300 (46)
Abnormal chest radiograph	181/344 (53)

Adapted from McDonald AP, Howard RJ. Pyogenic liver abscess. *World J Surg* 1980;4:369, with permission.

low yield may be one of the reasons that these lesions were often detected only at autopsy. Jaundice is unusual and often reflects extrahepatic biliary disease rather than involvement of the liver itself. Breath sounds may be reduced or absent at the right base, owing to an overlying pleural effusion or splinting.

Laboratory Tests

The typical findings are those of systemic infection and impaired hepatic function (Table 89.3). Most patients have leukocytosis with a leftward shift and anemia. Indicators of hepatic dysfunction commonly include slight elevation in the bilirubin value, elevated alkaline phosphatase and hepatic aminotransferase levels, and hypoalbuminemia. Especially characteristic are elevated alkaline phosphatase and low serum albumin values. Chest radiographs show abnormalities in at least half the cases, but the findings are nonspecific. Typical features include an elevation of the right diaphragm, a right side pleural effusion, and atelectasis of the right lower lobe. Gas in the liver parenchyma on plain films of the abdomen is considered virtually diagnostic, but it is present infrequently (86). Also, it may be difficult to distinguish gas collections in the biliary tract, the portal vein, or the bowel. A right side lateral view or contrast studies may be helpful in making this distinction.

Hepatic Scans

The availability of scanning techniques is probably the most important development in management guidelines for suspected liver abscesses and is largely credited with the substantial reduction in mortality rate in more recent series (87–95). There are now numerous scanning techniques from which to choose, and the selection depends on the clinical setting and availability (Fig. 89.1).

Ultrasonography demonstrates areas of echogenicity that may be quite variable. Most lesions are round with irregular walls; they may be cystic, multiloculated, or septate, or they may show internal echoes indicating debris. The sensitivity of the test is somewhat technician dependent, but most report that it is 70% to 90% sensitive (92,95). False-negative results are ascribed to suboptimal technique, failure to detect small abscesses, difficult interpretation confounded by overlying bowel gas, and misinterpretation of subcapsular collections as ascites. An advantage of ultrasonography is the ability to perform the test at the bedside, which is a notable advantage for seriously ill patients. Sonograms complement the technetium scan in distinguishing

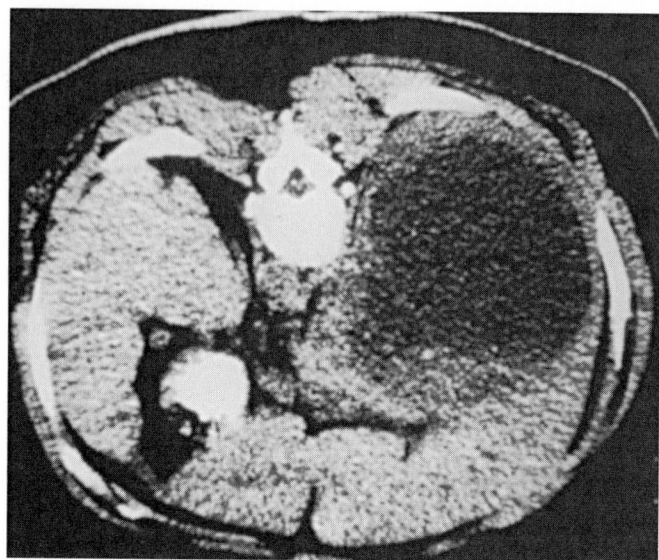

Figure 89.1. Magnetic resonance image showing a large hepatic abscess.

solid from cystic lesions, and they may also be used to guide drainage.

Computed tomography is generally regarded as the most sensitive and specific method of detecting pyogenic abscesses of the liver. Typical lesions are sharply demarcated low-density masses of 20 to 30 Hounsfield units. Gas is detected within the abscess in 20% to 30% of patients, presumably produced by gas-forming organisms, primarily anaerobic bacteria, or occasionally coliforms such as *E. coli* or *Klebsiella*. The use of intravenous contrast medium increases the sensitivity of the test, which is usually reported to be 90% to 100% (87,88,93–97). Advantages of computed tomography include the potential for guided aspiration, the ability to detect smaller lesions (resolution limit 0.5 cm), the utility of the test in defining other sites of intraabdominal pathology, and the ability to distinguish tumors, cysts, and hematomas as causes of the focal defects. Nevertheless, such distinctions are not always easy, and occasional false-negative readings have been reported. Relative merits of magnetic resonance imaging compared with computed tomography are unclear (98).

It should be noted that all scanning techniques are considered unreliable early in the course of hepatic candidiasis in the neutropenic host (83–85). With resolution of neutropenia, ultrasonography or computed tomography will usually demonstrate typical lesions (84).

ETIOLOGIC DIAGNOSIS

The major diagnostic challenge in many cases is the differentiation of pyogenic and amebic abscesses because this distinction dictates therapeutic decisions. The distinction is important because amebic abscesses usually respond to medical management, and pyogenic abscesses require drainage. With pyogenic abscesses, blood culture results are often positive, and there are the common associated diseases (e.g., biliary tract disease, inflammation involving the bed of portal circulation, hemochromatosis, cirrhosis or Crohn's disease). Amebic abscesses are most common in immigrants from or travelers to endemic areas, and these persons are usually young, previously healthy adults. Most do not have concurrent amebic colitis, although a stool examination will sometimes yield the parasite. The most reliable diagnostic test is serology using enzyme-linked immunosorbent

assays, which are almost invariably positive with invasive disease (99,100). Aspirates from patients who have needle aspiration should have stains and culture for acid-fast bacteria, aerobic and anaerobic bacteria, and fungi; the sniff test indicating putrid discharge is considered diagnostic of anaerobic infection. Hepatic candidiasis in the neutropenic host may be extremely elusive because scans are often negative, as are cultures of blood and liver.

TREATMENT

The treatment of amebic liver abscess is antibiotic therapy, usually using metronidazole followed by diloxanide furoate, iodoquinol, or paromomycin. About 10% of patients require surgery owing to extrahepatic complications, rupture, or failure to respond (59–62). Some patients undergo a diagnostic aspiration, which appears to hasten the initial response but provides no clear advantage with long-term follow-up in uncomplicated amebic abscesses (100). Some authorities think that there is an advantage with routine percutaneous aspiration for amebic abscesses, especially those that exceed 6 cm in diameter (100–102).

Pyogenic abscesses sometimes respond to antimicrobial treatment alone (103), but most authorities advocate drainage. The major issue is the method of drainage, with three options: surgery, percutaneous drainage with insertion of a drain, or percutaneous aspiration. Each approach is accompanied by antibiotic treatment.

Surgical Drainage

Operative approaches are extraserous drainage and transperitoneal drainage (104,105). Extraserous drainage was previously preferred because it avoids contamination of the peritoneal cavity. The extraserous approach involves a subcostal incision for anterior abscesses or a transpleural approach for a more posterior abscess. The problems are the limited ability to explore the liver (which increases the likelihood that adjacent or accessory abscesses will be overlooked) and the inability to identify sites of intraabdominal disease that may represent underlying lesions. With progress in surgical sepsis control, most surgeons now favor the transperitoneal approach using appropriate antibiotic coverage and peritoneal toilet. This affords the surgeon the opportunity to palpate the liver, aspirate suspicious lesions, and detect associated conditions in the abdominal cavity. The postoperative complication rate is generally reported at 30% to 40%, and the principal problems are recurrence of abscesses, intraabdominal abscesses, and wound infections.

Percutaneous Drainage

Percutaneous drainage offers the advantages of reduced cost, no need for general anesthesia, avoidance of postoperative complications, and apparently shorter recovery period (106–111). Potential disadvantages are that the liver cannot be explored and that sites of intraabdominal pathology may go undetected. Multiple drains may be placed for patients with multiple hepatic abscesses, and as many as eight discrete abscesses have been drained in this fashion in a single patient (S. Gerzof, personal communication). The published experience shows morbidity and mortality rates that are as low or lower than those achieved with surgery (32,37–39,93,95,106–111). Most authorities now conclude that surgery should be reserved for patients who fail to respond to percutaneous drainage.

Antibiotic Treatment

McFadzean and colleagues (104) reported the successful treatment of 14 patients with solitary liver abscesses using both parenteral and percutaneous instillation of antibiotics in 1953. At that time prompt surgical drainage was considered the mainstay of therapy. Although researchers occasionally reported successful antibiotic management of anecdotal cases, this impression that surgery was required prevailed until the late 1970s. In 1979, Maher and colleagues (103) from the Los Angeles County–University of Southern California Medical Center reported successful medical treatment of six patients. Since then, other reports have supported the impression that antibiotic treatment alone is satisfactory (112–114). In many of these cases, percutaneous aspiration was used to determine the microbiology to facilitate antibiotic selection, and this assisted drainage as well. Others have been less successful with this approach (115). In some instances, patients have been treated empirically with metronidazole for suspected amebic abscess; subsequent serology excluded this diagnosis, although the prompt clinical response implicated anaerobic infection and the possibility of avoiding a drainage procedure.

Antibiotic Selection

Most hepatic abscesses contain pathogens similar to those in intraabdominal sepsis-coliforms and anaerobic bacteria. Common regimens include ampicillin, gentamicin plus metronidazole, or cefotaxime/ceftriaxone plus metronidazole. This decision is obviously simplified if the bacterial population of the lesion is defined, as by aspiration of the abscess, although the clinical experience has taught that bacteriologic patterns are largely predictable. Problematic organisms that may not be addressed with commonly used regimens include *Pseudomonas aeruginosa*, enterococci, and *S. aureus*. Metronidazole is often included in the initial regimen owing to the possibility of amebiasis as well as optimal activity versus anaerobes.

PROGNOSIS

The mortality rate reported by Ochsner for his series in the preantibiotic era was 80% (3). During the early antibiotic era, numerous reports indicated a persistently high mortality rate in the range of 65% to 80%. More recent reports have shown decreased mortality rates of 10% to 25%, presumably owing to more accurate and earlier diagnosis. The major factor that now influences outcome is the number of abscesses (8). Most studies show that, regardless of the type of therapy or the period of review, substantially higher mortality rates are associated with multiple abscesses than with single abscesses (116). In the series by Ochsner (3), the difference was 37% versus 90%; in the Duke series representing the modern experience, the difference was 15% versus 41% (8). Mortality also seems to correlate directly with age and with associated diseases (116,117), including cirrhosis (58).

REFERENCES

1. Beeson PB, Brannon ES, Warren JV. Observations on the sites of removal of bacteria from the blood in patients with bacterial endocarditis. *J Exp Med* 1945;81:9.
2. Bright J. Observations on jaundice: more particularly on that form of the disease which accompanies diffused inflammation of the liver. *Guys Hosp Rep* 1836;1:630.
3. Ochsner A, Debakey M, Murray S. Pyogenic abscesses of the liver. II. An analysis of forty-seven cases with review of the literature. *Am J Surg* 1938;40:292.
4. Norris GW, Farley DC. Abscess of the liver. *Med Clin North Am* 1926;10:17.
5. Collins AN. Abscess of the liver. *Minn Med* 1932;15:756.
6. Knowles R, Rinaldo JA. Pyogenic hepatic abscess secondary to sigmoid diverticulitis. *Gastroenterology* 1960;38:262.
7. Ribaudo JM, Ochsner A. Intrahepatic abscesses: amebic and pyogenic. *Am J Surg* 1973;125:570.
8. McDonald MI, Corey GR, Gallis HA, et al. Single and multiple pyogenic liver abscesses: natural history, diagnosis and treatment, with emphasis on percutaneous drainage. *Medicine (Baltimore)* 1984;63:291.
9. McDonald AP, Howard RJ. Pyogenic liver abscess. *World J Surg* 1980;4:369.
10. Robertson RD, Foster JH, Peterson CG. Pyogenic liver abscess studies by cholangiography: case report and 25 year review. *Ann Surg* 1966;32:521.
11. Sabbaj J, Sutter VL, Finegold SM. Anaerobic pyogenic liver abscess. *Ann Intern Med* 1972;77:629.
12. Finegold SM. *Anaerobic bacteria in human disease.* New York: Harcourt, 1977.
13. de la Maza LM, Naeim F, Berman L. The changing etiology of liver abscess. *JAMA* 1974;227:161.
14. Heymann AD. Clinical aspects of grave pyogenic abscess of the liver. *Surg Gynecol Obstet* 1979;149:209.
15. McFadzean AJS, Chang KPS, Wong CC. Solitary pyogenic abscess of the liver treated by closed aspiration and antibiotics. *Br J Surg* 1953;41:141.
16. Pitt HA, Zuideman GD. Factors influencing mortality in the treatment of pyogenic hepatic abscess. *Surg Gynecol Obstet* 1975;140:228.
17. Pyrtek LJ, Bartus SA. Hepatic pyemia. *N Engl J Med* 1965;272:551.
18. Rubin RH, Swartz MN, Malt R. Hepatic abscess: changes in clinical, bacteriologic and therapeutic aspects. *Am J Med* 1974;57:601.
19. Warren KW, Hardy KJ. Pyogenic hepatic abscess. *Arch Surg* 1968;97:40.
20. Altemeier WA. Pyogenic liver abscess. In: Schiff L, Schiff ER, eds. *Diseases of the liver.* Philadelphia: JB Lippincott, 1983.
21. Balasegaram M. Management of hepatic abscess. *Curr Probl Surg* 1981;18:285.
22. Chattopadhyay B. Pyogenic liver abscess. *J Infect* 1983;6:5.
23. DeBakey ME, Jordan GL. Hepatic abscesses, both intra- and extra-hepatic. *Surg Clin North Am* 1977;57:325.
24. Pyogenic liver abscess [Editorial]. *BMJ* 1980;280:1155.
25. Lee JF, Block GE. The changing clinical pattern of hepatic abscesses. *Arch Surg* 1972;104:465.
26. Brodine WN, Schwartz SI. Pyogenic liver abscess. *Br J Hosp Med* 1981;26:47.
27. Neoptolemos JP, Macpherson DS. Pyogenic liver abscess. *Br J Hosp Med* 1981;26:47.
28. Dietrich RB. Experience with liver abscess. *Am J Surg* 1984;147:288.
29. Perera MR, Kirk A, Noone P. Presentation, diagnosis and management of liver abscess. *Lancet* 1980;2:629.
30. Price JE, Joseph WL, Mulder DG. Diagnosis and treatment of intra-hepatic abscess. *Am Surg* 1967;33:820.
31. Wintch RW, Reines HD, Rambo WM. Liver abscess: a changing entity. *Am Surg* 1982;48:11.
32. Yinnon AM, Hadas-Halpern I, Shapiro M, et al. The changing clinical spectrum of liver abscess: the Jerusalem experience. *Postgrad Med J* 1994;70:436.
33. Georges RN, Deitch EA. Pyogenic hepatic abscess. *South Med J* 1993;86:1233.
34. Teh LB, Ng HS, Kwok KC, et al. Liver abscess—a clinical study. *Ann Acad Med Singapore* 1986;15:176.
35. Mehta RB, Parija SC, Chetty DV, et al. Management of 240 cases of liver abscess. *Int Surg* 1986;71:91.
36. Levitt MD, Quinlan MF, Sheiner HJ. Liver abscess in Western Australia (1974–1983). *Aust N Z J Surg* 1986;56:341.
37. Perez JA, Gonzalez JJ, Baldonedo RF, et al. Clinical course, treatment, and multivariate analysis of risk factors for pyogenic liver abscess. *Am J Surg* 2001;181:177.
38. Barrio J, Cosme A, Ojeda E, et al. Pyogenic liver abscesses of bacterial origin: a study of 45 cases. *Rev Esp Enferm Dig* 2000;92:232.
39. Barakate MS, Stephen MS, Waugh RC, et al. Pyogenic liver abscess: a review of 10 years' experience in man. *Aust N Z Surg* 1999;69:205.
40. Smoger SH, Mitchell CK, McClave SA. Pyogenic liver abscesses: a comparison of older and younger patients. *Age Ageing* 1998;27:443.
41. Mir-Madjlessi SH, McHenry MC, Farmer RG. Liver abscess in Crohn's disease. Report of four cases and review of the literature. *Gastroenterology* 1986;91:987.
42. Vakil N, Hayne G, Sharma A, et al. Liver abscess in Crohn's disease. *Am J Gastroenterol* 1994;89:1090.
43. Greenstein AJ, Sachar DB, Lowenthal D, et al. Pyogenic liver abscess in Crohn's disease. *Q J Med* 1985;56:505.
44. Hagelskjaer KL, Prag J. Human necrobacilliosis with emphasis on Lemierre's syndrome. *Clin Infect Dis* 2000;31:524.
45. Tweedy CR, White WB. Multiple *Fusobacterium nucleatum* liver abscesses. Association with a persistent abnormality in humoral immune function. *J Clin Gastroenterol* 1987;9:194.
46. Francis IR, Glazer GM, Amendola MA, et al. Hepatic abscesses in the immunocompromised patient: role of CT in detection, diagnosis, management, and follow-up. *Gastrointest Radiol* 1986;11:257.
47. Skibber JM, Lotze MT, Garra B, et al. Successful management of hepatic abscesses by percutaneous catheter drainage in chronic granulomatous disease. *Surgery* 1986;99:626.
48. Chew SK, Lim HS, Mah PK, et al. Pyogenic hepatic abscess and diabetes mellitus–a probable association. *Ann Acad Med Singapore* 1985;14:261.
49. Saccente M. *Klebsiella pneumoniae* liver abscess, endophthalmitis, and meningitis in a man with newly recognized diabetes mellitus. *Clin Infect Dis* 1999;29:1570.

50. Shulman ST, Beem MO. A unique presentation of sickle cell disease. Pyogenic hepatic abscess. *Pediatrics* 1971;47:1019.

51. Shirkhoda A, Lopez-Berestein G, Holbert JM, et al. Hepatosplenic fungal infection: CT and pathologic evaluation after treatment with liposomal amphotericin B. *Radiology* 1986;159:349.

52. Shenep JL, Kalwinsky DK, Feldman S, et al. Mycotic cervical lymphadenitis following oral mucositis in children with leukemia. *J Pediatr* 1985;106:243.

53. DeVoe PW, Buckley RH, Shirley LIZ, et al. Successful immune reconstitution in severe combined immunodeficiency despite Epstein-Barr virus and cytomegalovirus infections. *Clin Immunol Immunopathol* 1985;34:48.

54. Kusne S, Dummer JS, Singh N, et al. Infections after liver transplantation. An analysis of 101 consecutive cases. *Medicine (Baltimore)* 1988;57:132.

55. Pottipati AR, Dave PB, Gumaste V, et al. Tuberculosis abscess of the liver in acquired immunodeficiency syndrome. *J Clin Gastroenterol* 1991;13:549.

56. Liu CJ, Hung CC, Chen MY, et al. Amebic liver abscess and human immunodeficiency virus infection: a report of three cases. *J Clin Gastroenterol* 2001;33:64.

57. Filice C, Brunett E, Bruno R, et al. Clinical management of hepatic abscesses in HIV patients. *Am J Gastroenterol* 2000;95:1092.

58. Nordestgaard AG, Stapleford L, Worthen N, et al. Contemporary management of amebic liver abscess. *Am Surg* 1992;58:315.

58a. Molle I, Thulstrup AM, Vilstrup H, et al. Increased risk and case fatality rate of pyogenic liver abscess in patients with liver cirrhosis: a nationwide study in Denmark. *Gut* 2001;48:260.

59. Hoffner RJ, Kilaghbian T, Esekogwu VI, et al. Common presentations of amebic liver abscess. *Ann Emerg Med* 1999;34:351.

60. Chuah SK, Chang-Chien CS, Sheen IS, et al. The prognostic factors of severe amebic liver abscess: a retrospective study of 125 cases. *Am J Trop Med Hyg* 1992;46:398.

61. Meng XY, Wu JX. Perforated amebic liver abscess: clinical analysis of 110 cases. *South Med J* 1994;87:985.

62. Hai AA, Singh A, Mittal VL, et al. Amoebic liver abscess. Review of 220 cases. *Int Surg* 1991;76:81.

63. Moore-Gillon JC, Eykyn SJ, Phillips I. Microbiology of pyogenic liver abscess. *BMJ* 1981;283:819.

64. Chua D, Reihart HH, Sobel JD. Liver abscess caused by *Streptococcus milleri*. *Rev Infect Dis* 1989;11:197.

65. Braun TI, Travis D, Dee RR, et al. Liver abscess due to *Listeria monocytogenes*: case report and review. *Clin Infect Dis* 1993;17:267.

66. Lopez-Prieto MD, Garciia AI, Garciia A, et al. Liver abscess due to *Listeria monocytogenes*. *Clin Microbiol Infect* 2000;6:226.

67. Vadillo M, Corbella X, Pac V, et al. Multiple liver abscesses due to *Yersinia enterocolitica* discloses primary hemochromatosis: three case reports and review. *Clin Infect Dis* 1994;18:938.

68. Leighton PM, MacSween HM. *Yersinia* hepatic abscesses subsequent to long-term iron therapy. *JAMA* 1987;257:964.

69. Hopewood AH, Riddle BW. *Yersinia enterocolitica* hepatic abscesses. *J Ky Med Assoc* 1986;84:13.

70. Hopfner M, Nitsche R, Rohr A, et al. *Yersinia enterocolitica* infection with multiple liver abscesses uncovering primary hemochromatosis. *Scand J Gastroenterol* 2001;36:220.

71. Cortez JC, Shapiro M, Awe RJ. *Pasteurella multocida* liver abscess. *Am J Med Sci* 1986;292:107.

72. Mongiardo N, De Rienzo B, Zanchetta G, et al. Primary hepatic actinomycosis. *J Infect* 1986;12:65.

73. Roesler PJ Jr, Willis JS. Hepatic actinomycosis: CT features. *J Comput Assist Tomogr* 1986;10:335.

74. Miyamoto MI, Fang FC. Pyogenic liver abscess involving *Actinomyces*: case report and review. *Clin Infect Dis* 1993;16:303.

75. Vatcharapreechasakul T, Suputtamongkol Y, Dance DA, et al. *Pseudomonas pseudomallei* liver abscesses: a clinical, laboratory, and ultrasonographic study. *Clin Infect Dis* 1992;14:412.

76. Kubota H, Ageta M, Kubo H, et al. Tuberculous liver abscess treated by percutaneous infusion of antituberculous agents. *Intern Med* 1994;33:351.

77. Moore SW, Millar AJ, Cywes S. Conservative initial treatment of liver abscesses in children. *Br J Surg* 1994;81:872.

78. Vachon L, Diament MJ, Stanley P. Percutaneous drainage of hepatic abscesses in children. *J Pediatr Surg* 1986;21:366.

79. Bilfinger TV, Hayden CK, Oldham KT, et al. Pyogenic liver abscesses in non-immunocompromised children. *South Med J* 1986;79:37.

80. Diament MJ, Stanley P, Kangarloo H, et al. Percutaneous aspiration and catheter drainage of abscesses. *J Pediatr* 1986;108:204.

81. Karrar ZA, Abdullah MA. Pyogenic liver abscess in children: a report of three patients and review of the literature. *Ann Trop Paediatr* 1985;5:97.

82. Brook I, Fraizer EH. Role of anaerobic bacteria in liver abscesses in children. *Pediatr Infect Dis J* 1993;12:743.

83. Gorg C, Weide R, Schwerk WB, et al. Ultrasound evaluation of hepatic and splenic microabscesses in the immunocompromised patient: sonographic patterns, differential diagnosis, and follow-up. *J Clin Ultrasound* 1994;22:525.

84. Thaler M, Pastakia B, Shawker T, et al. Hepatic candidiasis in cancer patients: the evolving picture of the syndrome. *Ann Intern Med* 1988;108:88.

85. Flannery MT, Simmons DB, Saba H, et al. Fluconazole in the treatment of hepatosplenic candidiasis. *Arch Intern Med* 1992;152:406.

86. Lee TY, Wan TY, Tsai CC. Gas-containing liver abscess: radiological findings and clinical significance. *Abdom Imaging* 1994;19:47.

87. Owaga T, Shimizu S, Morisaki T, et al. The role of percutaneous transhepatic abscess drainage for liver abscess. *J Hepatobil Pancreat Surg* 1999;6:263.

88. Gabata T, Kadoya M, Matsui O, et al. Dynamic CT of hepatic abscesses. *AJR* 2001;176:675.

89. Conter RL, Pitt HA, Tompkins RK, et al. Differentiation of pyogenic from amebic hepatic abscesses. *Surg Gynecol Obstet* 1986;162:114.

90. Kandel G, Marcon NE. Pyogenic liver abscess: new concepts of an old disease. *Am J Gastroenterol* 1984;79:65.

91. Kuligowska E, Noble J. Sonography of hepatic abscesses. *Semin Ultrasound* 1983;4:102.

92. Newlin N, Silver TM, Stuck KJ, et al. Ultrasonic features of pyogenic liver abscess. *Radiology* 1981;139:155.

93. Donovan AJ, Yellin AE, Ralls PW. Hepatic abscess. *World J Surg* 1991;15:162.

94. Barreda R, Ros PR. Diagnostic imaging of liver abscess. *Crit Rev Diagn Imaging* 1992;33:29.

95. Philips RL. Computed tomography and ultrasound in the diagnosis and treatment of liver abscesses. *Aust Radiol* 1994;38:165.

96. Buchman TG, Zuideman GD. The role of computerized tomographic scanning in the surgical management of pyogenic hepatic abscess. *Surg Gynecol Obstet* 1981;153:1.

97. Callen PW. Computed tomographic evaluation of abdominal and pelvic abscesses. *Radiology* 1979;131:171.

98. Balci NC, Semelka RC, Noone TC, et al. Pyogenic hepatic abscesses: MRI findings on T1-T2 weighted serial gadolinium-enhanced gradient-echo images. *J Magn Reson Imaging* 1999;9:285.

99. Abd-Alla MD, Jackson TF, Gathiram V, et al. Differentiation of pathogenic *Entamoeba histolytica* infections from nonpathogenic infections by detection of galactose-inhibitable adherence protein antigen in sera and feces. *J Clin Microbiol* 1993;31:2845.

100. Flores BM, Reed SL, Ravdin JI, et al. Serologic reactivity to purified recombinant and native 29-kilodalton peripheral membrane protein of pathogenic *Entamoeba histolytica*. *J Clin Microbiol* 1993;31:1403.

101. Ramini A, Ramani R, Kumar MS, et al. Ultrasound-guided needle aspiration of amoebic liver abscess. *Postgrad Med J* 1993;69:38.

102. Adams EB, MacLeod IN. Invasive amebiasis. II. Amebic liver abscess and its complications. *Medicine* 1977;56:325.

103. Maher JA, Reynolds TB, Yellin AE. Successful medical treatment of pyogenic liver abscess. *Gastroenterology* 1979;77:618.

104. Hansen N, Vargish T. Pyogenic hepatic abscess: a case for open drainage. *Am Surg* 1993;59:219.

105. Nosher JL, Giudici M, Needell GS, et al. Elective one-stage abdominal operations after percutaneous catheter drainage of pyogenic liver abscess. *Am Surg* 1993;59:658.

106. McFadzean AJR, Chang KPS, Wong CC. Solitary abscess of the liver treated by closed aspiration and antibiotics: fourteen cases with recovery. *Br J Surg* 1953;41:141.

107. Kraulis JE, Bird BL, Colapinto ND. Percutaneous catheter drainage of liver abscess: an alternative to open drainage. *Br J Surg* 1980;67:400.

108. Gerzof SG, Robbins AH, Johnson WC, et al. Percutaneous catheter drainage of abdominal abscesses: a five-year experience. *N Engl J Med* 1981;305:653.

109. Porter JA Loughry CW, Cook AJ. Use of the computerized tomographic scan in the diagnosis and treatment of abscesses. *Am J Surg* 1985;150:257.

110. Gerzof SG, Johnson WC, Robbins AH, et al. Intrahepatic pyogenic abscesses: treatment by percutaneous drainage. *Am J Surg* 1985;149:487.

111. Moulds-Merritt C, Frazee RC. Therapeutic approach to hepatic abscesses. *South Med J* 1994;87:884.

112. Berger LA, Osborne DR. Treatment of pyogenic liver abscesses by percutaneous needle aspiration. *Lancet* 1982;1:132.

113. Herbert DA, Rothman J, Fogel DA, et al. Pyogenic liver abscess: successful non-surgical therapy. *Lancet* 1982;1:134.

114. Reynolds TB. Medical treatment of pyogenic liver abscess. *Ann Intern Med* 1982;96:373.

115. McCorkell SJ, Niles NL. Pyogenic liver abscesses: another look at medical management. *Lancet* 1985;1:803.

116. Chou FF, Sheen-Chen SM, Chen YS. Prognostic factors for pyogenic abscess of the liver. *J Am Coll Surg* 1994;179:727.

117. Land MA, Moinuddin M, Bisno AL. Pyogenic liver abscess: changing epidemiology and prognosis. *South Med J* 1985;78:1426.

CHAPTER 90
Cholecystitis and Cholangitis

Juan Carlos Jimenez, Yale Podnos, Russell A. Williams, and Samuel Eric Wilson

ACUTE CALCULOUS CHOLECYSTITIS

Gallstones and their complications are among the most common acquired diseases of the population of developed countries, and operations on the biliary tree are the most frequently performed abdominal procedures. Up to 500,000 cases are reported annually in the United States. Acute cholecystitis is associated with gallstones in 95% of cases, and only 5% are acalculous.

Epidemiology

PREVALENCE AND INCIDENCE
The prevalence of gallstones is difficult to estimate accurately. A British study, based on a stratified random sample of 1,896 adults screened using real-time ultrasonography, demonstrated that at 60 to 69 years, 11.5% of men and 22.4% of women either had gallstones or previously underwent cholecystectomy (1). In another study performed in Denmark, individuals were screened with abdominal ultrasonography at 5-year intervals, which demonstrated that incidence increased with age. In men 30, 40, and 50 years of age, the incidence of gallstone disease was 0.3%, 2.9%, and 2.5%, respectively. At 60 years of age, the 5-year incidence of gallstones increased to 3.3% (2) (Table 90.1).

NATURAL HISTORY

Pathogenesis
In the majority of symptomatic patients, pain is caused by gallstone obstruction of the cystic duct, resulting in a marked elevation in the hydrostatic pressure within the gallbladder lumen. Pain is usually localized to the right upper quadrant or the epigastric region for 30 minutes or more (3). Bile salts and phospholipases (which transform phospholipids to cytotoxic lyso compounds) cause an initial chemical cholecystitis. Prostaglandin production increases in the inflamed gallbladder and stimulates secretion of fluid by the epithelium and contraction of the gallbladder wall. The fluid secretion results in increased hydrostatic pressure, which impairs the microcirculation and decreases both the viability of the gallbladder wall and the clearance rate of noxious intraluminal agents.

Bacteriology
Infection of the gallbladder is a secondary phenomenon, with up to 60% of patients' gallbladder bile cultures being positive and the percentage increasing with the duration of cholecystitis (4). Aerobic gram-negative rods predominate (55%), followed by streptococci (30%) and anaerobes (15%) (Table 90.2). Single species are found in 30% of patients, but the majority have multiple organisms (5). In most patients, cultures from the gallbladder wall and gallbladder bile grow the same organisms.

The incidence of infection with anaerobes is increased in older patients and in patients with current choledocholithiasis (6). Invasion of an ischemic or necrotic gallbladder wall by gas-forming bacteria (especially *Clostridium* species) is most common in elderly, male, diabetic patients; the result is emphysematous cholecystitis.

The biliary tract of healthy persons usually does not harbor bacteria (7). Contamination from the duodenum may occur via the bile ducts. Supportive evidence for this is that the incidence of infected bile is lower when tumors completely obstruct the biliary tree than when partially obstructing stones or iatrogenic strictures retain communication with the duodenum. Bile may also be contaminated by portal venous bacteremia or via the lymphatics.

Pathology
The gallbladder becomes tense and edematous, and the surface is a lusterless gray-red color. As the serosal inflammation progresses, adhesions form to adjacent structures (gastrohepatic omentum, duodenum, porta hepatis, colon). If the obstruction is not relieved, the tension causes ischemia and gangrene, particularly in the fundus, where the blood supply is poorest. Most cases do not progress beyond the initial chemical phase, with resolution leading to changes of chronic cholecystitis. In 15% of cases, complications may occur, with gangrene and perforation.

Histologic examination of gallbladder tissue shows hemorrhage and edema with an inflammatory infiltrate consisting mostly of monocytes, with relatively few neutrophils and bacteria (Fig. 90.1).

Clinical Manifestations
Acute cholecystitis usually follows an attack of biliary colic that persists longer than 6 hours. Initially the pain may be epigastric, but later it becomes localized to the right upper quadrant and radiates to the angle of the right subscapular region. Severe and constant, it is often associated with nausea and vomiting. Fever develops in most patients, but rigors are unusual unless there are associated bile duct stones and cholangitis. Mild jaundice occurs in some patients, but deeper jaundice usually indicates choledocholithiasis.

The main findings on physical examination are tenderness and guarding in the right upper quadrant; in some patients a mass may be palpable. Generalized peritoneal tenderness is found in patients with free perforation, but clinical signs do not always correlate with severity of the disease, especially in older patients.

TABLE 90.1.   Factors Associated with Incidence of Gallstones

Factor	Effect on incidence
Ethnicity	Marked increase in Pima Indians, Mexicans, and Swedes
Geography	High incidence in United States, Great Britain, and Australia
Age	Increases with age
Sex	More common in females than in males
Pregnancy	Increases with parity
Obesity	
Cirrhosis	Increases two- to threefold (40,41)
Total parenteral nutrition	Increases with prolonged therapy (42)
Hemolysis	

TABLE 90.2.   Microorganisms in Bile in Acute Cholecystitis: Classification of 199 Organisms

Aerobes (n = 174; 87%)				
Gram-negative (n = 132; 66%)		Gram-positive (n = 42; 21%)		
Escherichia coli	77	*Enterococcus faecalis*	30	
Klebsiella	22	*β*-hemolytic streptococci	4	
Proteus	13	*Staphylococcus epidermidis*	4	
Enterobacter	8	*Streptococcus viridans*	1	
Pseudomonas	4			
Anaerobes (n = 25; 13%)				
Gram-negative (1%)		Gram-positive (n = 23; 12%)		
Bacteroides species	2	*Clostridium perfringens*	16	
		Peptostreptococcus	7	

From Keighley MRB. Micro-organisms in the bile. A preventable cause of sepsis after biliary surgery. *Ann R Col Surg Engl* 1977;59:328, with permission.

Acute Cholecystitis During Pregnancy

The incidence of acute cholecystitis in pregnant women has been reported as 0.5 to 0.8 cases per 1,000 births (8). Several studies support a strong association between pregnancy and gallstone formation, but acute cholecystitis in pregnancy remains rare (9). Landers et al. studied 30 cases of acute cholecystitis over a 12-year period. Twenty-one patients were managed with medical therapy alone, while nine underwent cholecystectomy following failure of conservative treatment. One patient underwent surgery in the first trimester and subsequently aborted. The remaining patients underwent cholecystectomy in the second trimester without serious complication. It has therefore been recommended that conservative management, consisting of antibiotics and bowel rest, can be successfully used as the primary treatment for acute cholecystitis in pregnancy. Surgical intervention should be reserved for patients failing medical management (10).

Cholecystitis in Elderly Persons

Acute cholecystitis in patients over 65 years of age is a serious condition associated with a high incidence of complications and a significantly greater mortality rate. Often the diagnosis is made late because of minimal or masked signs (11), and early surgery is recommended unless there are serious medical contraindica-

tions. The increased incidence of complications (gangrene, perforation, and empyema) and the frequently associated cardiovascular and pulmonary disorders in these patients account for a 9% mortality rate, as opposed to 1.6% in younger persons.

Diagnosis

There is usually mild leukocytosis with minor biochemical abnormalities (elevated transaminase and alkaline phosphatase values). Slightly elevated serum amylase values are common, but marked elevation is associated with biliary pancreatitis. At Harbor-UCLA Medical Center, the mean serum amylase level in patients with biliary pancreatitis was 2,465 mU/mL (normal 20 to 110 mU/mL).

The plain radiograph of the abdomen is only occasionally helpful in establishing the diagnosis (calcified stones in 10% of patients and gas in the gallbladder with emphysematous cholecystitis), but it is valuable for excluding other disease.

Ultrasonography with real-time scanning has become the most widely used test for acute cholecystitis. At the same examination, other intraabdominal sites (pancreas, liver, and appendix) can be screened. Its accuracy in detecting gallstones is 90% to 95% (12), but the interpretation of the criteria for diagnosing acute cholecystitis—which include stone impaction, focal gallbladder tenderness, pericholecystic fluid collections, and changes in the gallbladder wall—in many cases depends on the experience of the technician (Fig. 90.2).

Radionuclide imaging with technetium 99m–labeled agents [lidofenin (hepatoiminodiacetic acid), iminodiacetic acid, or iprofenin (*p*-isopropyliminodiacetic acid)] has enabled clinicians to diagnose or exclude acute cholecystitis with great accuracy. It is noninvasive, easy to read, and applicable even in jaundiced patients, and it provides good images of the intra- and extrahepatic ducts. It is sensitive for determining patency of the cystic duct, and visualization of the gallbladder effectively excludes the diagnosis of acute cholecystitis (Figs. 90.3 and 90.4). False-positive results (failure to visualize a gallbladder not involved by acute cholecystitis) are encountered in patients who are receiving parenteral nutrition, have severe intercurrent illness, are alcoholic, or have gallstone pancreatitis.

Initially ultrasonography should be used to screen for gallstones and signs of acute cholecystitis. If no stones are present on ultrasonography, the physician then performs radionuclide studies in search of acute acalculous cholecystitis. The conditions that simulate acute cholecystitis include acute pancreatitis, perforated peptic ulcer, retrocecal appendicitis, liver abscess,

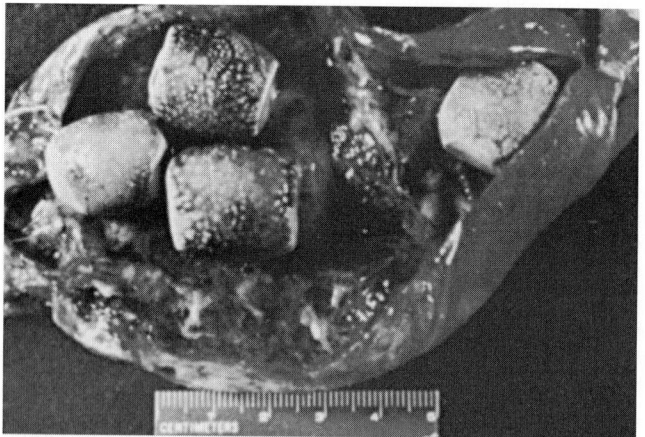

Figure 90.1. Acute cholecystitis with an obstructing stone at the neck of the gallbladder, which is thick walled and edematous, with serosal inflammation.

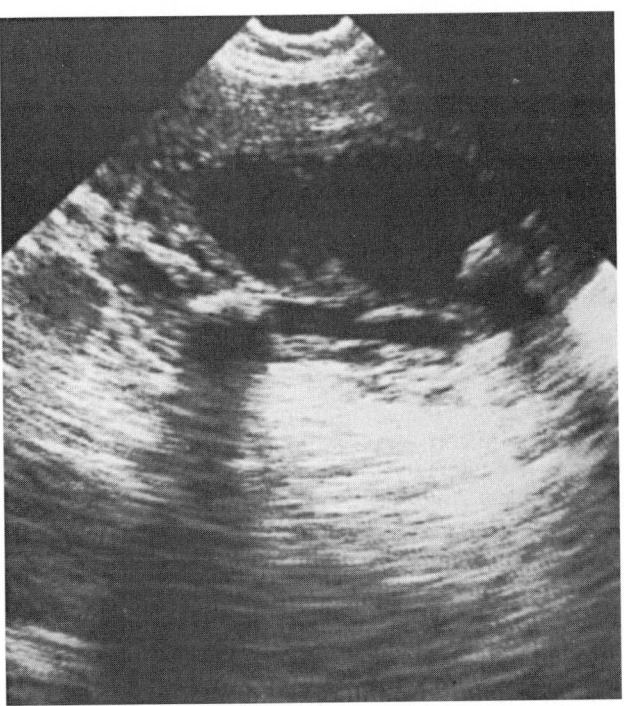

Figure 90.2. Ultrasonographic examination shows a distended gallbladder with a calculus causing acoustic shadowing.

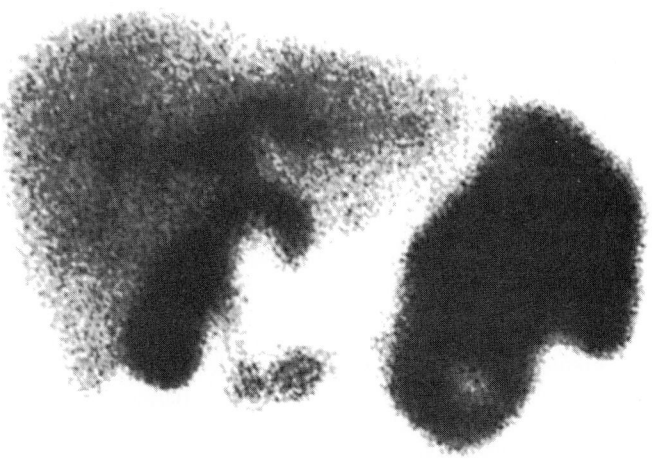

Figure 90.4. Lidofenin scan shows normal filling of the gallbladder and biliary tree with free flow into the duodenum and proximal bowel.

hepatitis, pyelonephritis, myocardial infarction, and right side lower lobe pneumonia.

Gangrene and Perforation

Patchy gangrene affecting the fundus of the gallbladder is found in 8% of patients, and perforation affects a like number. Perforation of the gallbladder may be acute (with generalized peritonitis), subacute (with a pericholecystic abscess), or chronic (with fistulous communication involving another viscus).

Perforation is more common in older patients and in those who have diabetes or acalculous or emphysematous cholecysti-

tis. The reported incidence varies widely between series, ranging from 1% to 15% (13). An incidence of approximately 5.4% to 6% is close to the experience of most surgeons who perform operations in the acute phase of the disease (14–16).

The mechanism of perforation is probably related to vascular congestion and subsequent ischemia and necrosis. The signs and symptoms are not distinctive; many cases are diagnosed late or are missed, which accounts for the 30% to 50% mortality rate for patients with free perforation.

Empyema

The reported frequency of empyema varies from 1% to 9%, but the higher figures may overestimate the incidence because milky contents of the acutely inflamed gallbladder may represent precipitate of calcium carbonate and cholesterol rather than true pus (Fig. 90.5). It usually affects older patients, and fever, leukocytosis, and a tender mass are typical, but as with perforation, minimal disturbance with few signs is not uncommon in debilitated, elderly patients. As many as 15% of older patients may have liver abscess or subphrenic abscess (11).

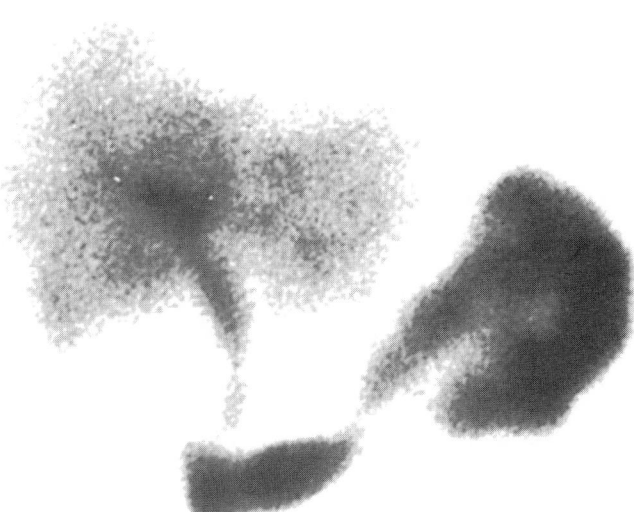

Figure 90.3. Lidofenin scan in acute cholecystitis shows absence of gallbladder filling and normal free-draining bile duct.

Figure 90.5. Lidofenin scan shows free flow of tracer in the bile duct and proximal bowel but absence of gallbladder filling and a large defect in the inferior aspect of the liver due to a gallbladder empyema.

Emphysematous Cholecystitis

Emphysematous cholecystitis, an uncommon variant of acute cholecystitis, is associated with gallbladder infection by gas-forming organisms (most commonly *Clostridium perfringens*, often with *Escherichia coli* and anaerobic streptococci as co-pathogens). It is associated with gallstones in 72% of cases and has a predilection for older male diabetic patients.

The presentation varies from a mild illness simulating the more usual form of acute cholecystitis to a serious fulminant disease associated with rapid clinical deterioration. The diagnosis may be confirmed by use of a radiograph that shows gas in the gallbladder lumen or wall. Gangrene and perforation occur with greater frequency than in ordinary forms of cholecystitis and may be related to obliterative vascular changes in the cystic artery, particularly in diabetic patients. The treatment recommended is immediate cholecystectomy and aggressive antibiotic therapy with anaerobic coverage (penicillin and metronidazole). The mortality rate in reported series averages 15%.

Pancreatitis

The incidence of pancreatitis associated with acute cholecystitis varies widely, depending on whether the diagnosis is established with serum amylase value, imaging technique, or operative findings. It is interesting to note how infrequently acute pancreatitis is reported in patients who undergo surgery for acute cholecystitis immediately or early in the disease. For patients who undergo surgery during their hospitalization for gallstone pancreatitis, the incidence of acute cholecystitis ranges from 13% to 14% (17,18). In our series of 46 patients who had early surgery for gallstone pancreatitis at Harbor-UCLA Medical Center, only 6 (13%) had acute cholecystitis by histologic criteria. The pancreatitis is usually the edematous interstitial type. Other rare complications include hemobilia and hemoperitoneum. Cholangitis is unusual unless there are also stones in the bile duct, a condition that occurs in about 15% of patients (17). Cholangitis and jaundice may occasionally be caused by obstruction of the common hepatic duct by a large cystic duct stone (18). Rarely, biliary peritonitis may occur without perforation of the gallbladder.

Treatment

Treatment options for acute cholecystitis include medical therapy and surgery (19–22). The two approaches are compared in Table 90.3.

MEDICAL THERAPY

Initial management for all patients is medical: intravenous fluids, analgesia, nasogastric suction if vomiting occurs, and antibiotics. Antibiotics probably do not influence the progression of the disease and have not been shown to decrease the incidence of local complications such as empyema and pericholecystic collections. When used preoperatively, however, they do decrease the incidence of septicemia and wound infection.

Antibiotics effective against gram-negative rods should be used. Second- and third-generation cephalosporins (e.g., cefotetan, cefoxitin, defotaxime), β-lactam / β-lactamase inhibitors (e.g., piperacillin-tazobactam), and aminoglycosides have been shown to be effective against the usual forms of acute cholecystitis. The antibiotic regimen may need to be refined for patients who are found at operation to have extensive sepsis, for patients with emphysematous cholecystitis or cholangitis, and for those whose clinical status deteriorates in response to the aforementioned regimens. Additional coverage for gram-positive aerobes and anaerobes may be required in such situations.

LAPAROSCOPIC CHOLECYSTECTOMY AND ACUTE CHOLECYSTITIS

Laparoscopic cholecystectomy was introduced by French surgeons who performed the first operation in 1989. Since then, general surgeons and the public alike have strongly embraced minimally invasive gallbladder surgery. More than 85% of all cholecystectomies in the United States were estimated to have been performed laparoscopically in 1993. Shea et al. found that the number of nonincidental cholecystectomies increased 26% from 1989 to 1993 at five Pennsylvania community hospitals (20). Several studies have confirmed its safety and efficacy in the setting of acute cholecystitis and gallstone disease. Chahin conducted a retrospective analysis of 557 patients with either acute or chronic cholecystitis over a 3-year period (1994 to 1996) (21). He found that patients who underwent laparoscopic cholecystectomy had shorter operating time and shorter length of stay than patients undergoing open cholecystectomy. An overall lower complication rate was also noted. Similar results were published by Willsher (22) on the treatment of 152 patients who underwent laparoscopic cholecystectomy. Conversion to open cholecystectomy was performed in only 9% of cases. However, conversion was less likely in patients undergoing surgery within 2 days of admission rather than patients undergoing surgery beyond 2 days when adhesions are more dense and the inflamed tissues bleed easily. Early laparoscopic cholecystectomy is therefore the preferred treatment in the setting of acute cholecystitis in conjunction with bowel rest and antibiotics.

TABLE 90.3. Mortality in Acute Cholecystitis: Comparison of Medical Therapy and Surgical Treatment

| | Medical therapy | | Surgical therapy | | | | | |
| | | | Delayed | | Early | | Urgent | |
Author	Patients	Deaths	Patients	Deaths	Patients	Deaths	Patients	Deaths
Payne (28)	265	0	265	7	133	0		
Essenhigh (29)	312	20	137	a	22	1	95	12
Kune and Birks (30)			73	0	162	1	27	5
Reiss et al. (37)					182	1		
Van der Linden and Edlund (38)	185	4	141	7			10	3
Rosi and Midel (39)	107	5	173	9	234	5	31	6

a Deaths were not reported.

URGENT SURGICAL TREATMENT

Most patients can improve clinically with the medical regimen followed by early cholecystectomy, and only a few require urgent intervention, for reasons such as the following: (a) failure of medical therapy with clinical deterioration, (b) generalized peritonitis, (c) emphysematous or acalculous cholecystitis, (d) empyema, and (e) diagnostic uncertainty, when other intraabdominal conditions cannot be excluded. Many patients who require urgent intervention are old and infirm, and for those who are a high operative risk, cholecystostomy may be performed under local anesthesia, provided extensive gangrene, perforation, or associated bile duct stones and cholangitis are not present. Percutaneous cholecystostomy has been performed successfully in unfit patients (23).

Cholecystostomy is rarely performed today, which may reflect improvements in anesthesia and resuscitation and the broader training of residents in elective biliary surgery. Nevertheless, cholecystostomy is indicated in cases in which the anatomy is obscured by inflammation and persistent prolonged attempts to perform cholecystectomy are not in the patient's best interest.

Planned cholecystectomy is usually performed after cholecystostomy, and the procedure has not been associated with greater morbidity or mortality than elective cholecystectomy, but in many elderly patients no further treatment or stone dissolution therapy may be appropriate.

ACUTE ACALCULOUS CHOLECYSTITIS

Acute acalculous cholecystitis, a variant of acute cholecystitis, accounts for 5% of cases of acute cholecystitis and has been described in a variety of settings. Half of all cases of acute cholecystitis in children are acalculous disease. Clinical cholecystitis is a well-known complication of infusion chemotherapy and of primary systemic diseases such as typhoid fever, brucellosis, and miliary tuberculosis and *Campylobacter*, cytomegalovirus, *Cryptosporidium*, and *Candida albicans* infections.

The more usual settings in which acalculous cholecystitis occurs are in association with critical illness, parenteral nutrition, trauma, and thermal injury. It may develop after intra- or extraabdominal procedures.

Pathophysiology

Numerous factors have been implicated in the pathogenesis of acalculous cholecystitis, including (a) bile stasis after massive transfusions, prolonged fasting, or dehydration, leading to cystic duct obstruction; (b) functional obstruction of the ampulla of Vater by opiates; and (c) ischemic mucosal injury in low-flow states and multisystem failure. Anatomic variants that cause cystic duct obstruction (adhesions, enlarged cystic duct node, and tortuous cystic artery) rarely cause cholecystitis. Cullen studied the effects of endotoxin on the gallbladder wall of adult opossums (24). He found that ischemic changes (coagulation necrosis, hemorrhage, fibrin deposition, and extensive mucosal loss) to the gallbladder wall similar to that seen in acalculous cholecystitis could be induced following administration of intravenous endotoxin. A decreased contractile response was also seen in response to hormonal and neural stimuli.

Clinical Aspects

Acute acalculous cholecystitis demonstrates a male predominance, higher incidences of gangrene and perforation, and a higher mortality rate than ordinary acute cholecystitis. The clinical settings in which it occurs account for the fact that the disease is often unsuspected and the diagnosis delayed. The symptoms and signs are often subtle and not characteristic, particularly in patients who are recovering from an abdominal procedure or are critically ill.

A mass may be palpable in up to 40% of patients, but the most useful investigation is ultrasonography, which may show a large gallbladder with a thickened wall and a pericholecystic collection. Computed tomography has proved to be a valuable alternative, but radionuclide studies are unreliable because in many of the clinical settings associated with acalculous cholecystitis these studies yield false-positive results.

Treatment

Cholecystectomy should be performed as soon as possible because progression to gangrene (52%) or perforation (11%) is likely to be fatal if diagnosis and treatment are delayed until cholecystostomy is no longer possible.

ASCENDING AND SUPPURATIVE CHOLANGITIS

Jaundice, chills and fever, and abdominal pain are the sentinel findings of cholangitis. Charcot first appreciated the significance of this triad in 1877. Pathologically, Charcot's triad is the result of biliary tract obstruction and infection.

Captain Leonard Rogers suggested the necessity for surgical drainage of the obstructed infected bile duct in 1803, and he was inspired to operate on a patient with cholangitis and to insert a glass tube to drain the bile duct. Before this, all patients died of suppurative cholangitis.

Charcot's triad was expanded in 1959, when Reynolds and Dargan (25) added two more signs of severe cholangitis: shock and central nervous system depression. These signs indicate not only infection in the biliary tree, but also the presence of pus under pressure, which needs urgent intervention (26–30).

Bacteriology

Organisms are grown from the bile duct of up to 90% of patients with cholangitis. The flora typically is composed of multiple organisms, the majority of which are aerobic, predominantly *E. coli* and *Klebsiella* and *Streptococcus* species. These same organisms are isolated from the gallbladder of patients with cholecystitis; however, in cholangitis, particularly in patients who had previous bile duct surgery that has been complicated by stricture formation, anaerobic organisms are more common. The anaerobic organisms are *Bacteroides fragilis* and *C. perfringens*.

Animal experiments have shown that particles of a size comparable with gram-negative bacteria translocate rapidly from within the hepatic duct to the bloodstream in response to only modest pressure gradients across the biliary system wall (31). Similarly, infection itself generates elevated pressure, leading to unremitting bacteremia and septic shock if the bile duct is not decompressed by drainage (32).

Epidemiology

Most often, cholangitis develops as a complication of stones in the biliary tree. Although stone disease of the biliary tract is among the most common surgical diseases in the United States and choledocholithiasis is common, cholangitis is a rare complication of gallstones. It accounted for 2 of every 1,000 hospital admissions and 17 of 955 patients with biliary disease in one series seen by a gastroenterologist.

In surgical series, approximately 10% of patients with a prior diagnosis of biliary disease develop suppurative cholangitis, and one third of all patients who have a common duct operation have had cholangitis. About half the patients who develop cholangitis are over 70 years of age.

Pathogenesis

The clinical presentations of the two forms of cholangitis, ascending and suppurative, have overlapping features. The difference between the two is in the degree of biliary obstruction: with partial obstruction and bacterial multiplication in the bile ducts, pressure does not increase dramatically. Bacteria are showered intermittently into the bloodstream, producing the characteristic remitting and relapsing clinical course of ascending cholangitis.

Suppurative cholangitis develops in a completely obstructed biliary system. Pressure increases rapidly as the infection evolves into frank purulence within the biliary system, and there is unremitting translocation of bacteria into the bloodstream. The clinical course in suppurative cholangitis is toward rapidly progressive septic shock and death.

Ascending cholangitis can evolve into suppurative cholangitis, as complete bile duct occlusion develops secondary to inflammatory thickening of the duct wall and production of tenacious mucopurulent material and "biliary mud" within the bile ducts.

Multiple abscesses often develop in the liver, which may be the source of persistent sepsis even though bile duct obstruction is relieved. The bile ducts dilate and become thick walled; at times they may even resemble the small bowel. With continued unrelenting obstruction, biliary cirrhosis may supervene.

Bactibilia, the presence of bacteria in the bile, occurs with varying frequency, depending on the patient's age and other conditions in the biliary tract. It is more likely to be found in elderly persons who have stones in the duct and obstructive jaundice, particularly if they have previously had surgery in the biliary area. Asymptomatic bactibilia evolves to symptomatic, clinical disease with increasing biliary obstruction.

Stones most often obstruct the ducts. In some cases there are stones in the gallbladder as well. In other cases they were missed during a previous operation, particularly cholecystectomy, or they have formed since that time. Cholangitis may be the first indication of the presence of a stone in the patient's bile duct.

Clinical Manifestations

The majority of patients have Charcot's triad. The fever develops suddenly and can be associated with paroxysmal shaking; mild jaundice often follows; and pain develops in the right upper quadrant that radiates to the back and is associated with deep tenderness.

Many patients experience this triad of signs and symptoms intermittently over a protracted period, even years, but some patients present with the triad plus shock and nervous system depression, indicating severe suppuration in the biliary tree.

Diagnosis

Charcot's triad is not exclusively a manifestation of cholangitis; it occurs also in other inflammatory diseases of the gallbladder and pancreas and with hepatitis. The constellation may not always be complete, and at times a patient with cholangitis may present with septicemia or fever of undetermined origin. A pos-

itive blood culture, particularly one that grows one or more of the organisms that are characteristic of the biliary flora, should prompt the physician to consider cholangitis.

The most common biochemical abnormality among liver function tests is a modest elevation in bilirubin level. Accompanying this, the serum alkaline phosphatase value is often elevated, indicating bile duct obstruction.

Plain radiographs of the abdomen rarely show gas in the bile ducts (produced by gas-forming pathogens such as *Clostridium*). Radiopaque stones in the gallbladder or along the course of the bile duct are rare findings and serve as sentinels to direct attention to the biliary system.

If cholangitis is suspected, imaging of the biliary system is done expeditiously. If cholangitis is present, this demonstrates a dilated thick-walled duct, typically containing stones, and often indicates the level of obstruction, usually in the larger, more distal bile duct, but sometimes in the more proximal ducts, including either the right or left hepatic duct system. The most likely cause of obstruction is gallstones, but if no stones are found, other causes, such as previous bile duct injury leading to stricture or carcinoma in the biliary system, must be considered.

As part of the ultrasonographic investigation of suspected cholangitis, the liver is examined for the presence of abscesses and the gallbladder for accompanying disease, particularly gallstones. Usually ultrasonographic examination of the biliary system is sufficient to confirm the diagnosis of cholangitis. Computed tomography is less efficient for showing stones in the biliary system but does show duct lesions and abscesses in the liver.

Studies performed to outline the biliary tract, such as transhepatic cholangiography and endoscopic retrograde cholangiopancreatography, are invasive and demand special equipment and personnel. Each elevates the pressure in the biliary tree and produces bacteremia and an exacerbation of the patient's clinical condition, so at times, in the examination study room or after returning to the ward from the examination suite, the patient develops florid septic shock. This should be anticipated, and patients undergoing these examinations need pretreatment with intravenous fluids and antibiotics well before the study is performed. These studies not only outline the biliary tree but also define the specific obstructive lesion.

Such invasive studies are not obtained routinely but are considered if the cause of the biliary obstruction is unusual (e.g., traumatic stricture, which needs good definition to plan for surgery) or if the patient is unfit for surgery and it is thought that endoscopic sphincterotomy or transhepatic biliary drainage is the safest means of decompression and, at times, particularly with choledocholithiasis, of curing the obstruction.

Treatment

Most patients with cholangitis respond well to antimicrobial therapy against the biliary flora and fluid administration to expand intravascular volume. Some patients respond well initially to this regimen then relapse into shock soon thereafter. Rarely, the treatment is ineffective because the septic shock is profound. Both situations are life threatening and require urgent decompression of the biliary system. This may be accomplished by endoscopic sphincterotomy and insertion of a drainage tube into the bile duct via the endoscope, or, less satisfactory, drainage can be achieved percutaneously. The latter technique often aggravates sepsis and leads to biliary cutaneous fistulas.

Endoscopic biliary drainage has become the treatment of choice for patients with severe acute cholangitis due to choledocholithiasis. Lai et al. studied 82 patients over a 43-month period with severe acute cholangitis due to retained gallstones

(33). Patients were either randomly assigned to endoscopic biliary decompression or surgical decompression. The complication rate was significantly lower in the group treated with endoscopic sphincterotomy. Mortality was significantly lower in this group as well (4 vs. 13 deaths) (32). Boender et al. studied 95 patients undergoing endoscopic sphincterotomy for retained stones (34). They found that for patients with good response to antibiotics prior to stone extraction, delay in biliary drainage did not influence the risk of complications. However, in patients with persistent fever for several days prior to arrival and poor response to antibiotics, delay in biliary drainage led to increased risk for septic complications (34).

Surgery should be reserved for cases where endoscopic drainage has failed (35,36). At operation it is usually possible to effect permanent relief of the obstruction, either by removing refractory stones from the bile duct or by draining a bile duct obstructed by fibrous stricture or malignant disease into adjacent bowel. The simplest means for draining the bile duct operatively is to insert a large T tube.

REFERENCES

1. Heaton KW, Braddon FE, Mountford RA, et al. Symptomatic and silent gallstones in the community. *Gut* 1991;32:316–320.
2. Jensen KH, Jorgensen T. Incidence of gallstones in a Danish population. *Gastroenterology* 1991;100:790–794.
3. Diehl AK, Sugarek NJ, Todd KH. Clinical evaluation for gallstone disease; usefulness of symptoms and signs in diagnosis. *Am J Med* 1990;89(1):29–33.
4. Claesson BEB, Holmlund DEW, Matzsch TW. Microflora of the gallbladder related to duration of acute cholecystitis. *Surg Obstet Gynecol* 1986;162:531.
5. Keighley MRB. Microorganisms in the bile. A preventable cause of sepsis after biliary surgery. *Ann R Coll Surg Engl* 1977;59:329.
6. Shimada K, Inamatsu T, Yamashiro M. Anaerobic bacteria in biliary disease in elderly patients. *J Infect Dis* 1977;135:850.
7. Csendes A, Fernandez M, Uribe P. Bacteriology of the gallbladder bile in normal subjects. *Am J Surg* 1975;129:629.
8. Ramin KD, Ramsey PS. Disease of the gallbladder and pancreas in pregnancy. *Obstet Gynecol Clin* 2001;28(3).
9. Landers D, Carmona R, Crombleholme W, et al. Acute cholecystitis in pregnancy. *Obstet Gynecol* 1987;69(1):131–133.
10. Hiatt JR, Hiatt JCG, Williams RA. Biliary disease in pregnancy: strategy for surgical management. *Am J Surg* 1986;150:263.
11. Morrow DJ, Thompson J, Wilson SE. Acute cholecystitis in the elderly: a surgical emergency. *Arch Surg* 1978;118:1149.
12. Cooperberg PL, Burhenne HJ. Real-time ultrasonography diagnostic technique of choice in calculous gallbladder disease. *N Engl J Med* 1980;302:1277.
13. Diffenbaugh WG, Sarver FE, Strohl EL. Gangrenous perforation of the gallbladder. *Arch Surg* 1949;59:742.
14. Lee AE. The management of acute cholecystitis. *Br J Surg* 1958;45:523.
15. Essenhigh DM. Perforation of the gall-bladder. *Br J Surg* 1968;55:175.
16. Pines B, Rabinovitch J. Perforation of the gallbladder in acute cholecystitis. *Ann Surg* 1954;140:170.
17. Stone HH, Fabian TS, Dunlop WE. Gallstone pancreatitis. Biliary tract pathology in relation to timing of operation. *Ann Surg* 1981;194:305.
18. Frei GJ, Frei VT, Thirlby RC, et al. Biliary pancreatitis: clinical presentation and surgical management. *Am J Surg* 1986;151:170.
19. Soper NJ, Brunt LM, Kerbl K. Laparoscopic general surgery. *N Engl J Med* 1994;330(6):409–419.
20. Shea JA, et al. Indications for and outcomes of cholecystectomy: a comparison of the pre and postlaparoscopic eras. *Ann Surg* 1998;227(3).
21. Chahin F, Elias N, Paramesh A, et al. The efficacy of laparoscopy in acute cholecystitis. *JSLS* 1999;3(2):121–125.
22. Willsher PC. Early laparoscopic cholecystectomy for acute cholecystitis: a safe procedure. *J Gastrointest Surg* 1999;3(1):50–53.
23. Klimberg S, Hawkins I, Vogel SB. Percutaneous cholecystostomy for acute cholecystitis in high-risk patients. *Am J Surg* 1987;153:125.
24. Cullen JJ. Effect of endotoxin on opossum gallbladder motility: a model of acalculous cholecystitis. *Ann Surg* 2000;232(2):202–207.
25. Reynolds BM, Dargan EL. Acute obstructive cholangitis. *Ann Surg* 1959;150:299.
26. Coelho JC, Buffara M, Pozzoban CE, et al. Incidence of common bile duct stones in patients with acute and chronic cholecystitis. *Surg Obstet Gynecol* 1984;158:76.
27. Koehler RE, Melson GL, Lee JKT, et al. Common hepatic duct obstruction by cystic duct stone: Mirizzi syndrome. *AJR* 1977;132:1007.
28. Payne RA. Evaluation of the management of acute cholecystitis. *Br J Surg* 1969;56:200.
29. Essenhigh DM. Management of acute cholecystitis. *Br J Surg* 1966;53:1032.
30. Kune GA, Birks D. Acute cholecystitis. An appraisal of current methods of treatment. *Med J Aust* 1970;2:218.
31. Huang T, Bass JA, Williams RD. The significance of biliary pressure in cholangitis. *Arch Surg* 1969;98:629.
32. Andrew DJ, Johnson SE. Acute suppurative cholangitis, a medical and surgical emergency: a review of ten years' experience emphasizing early recognition. *Am J Gastroenterol* 1970;54:141.
33. Lai EC, et al. Endoscopic biliary drainage for severe acute cholangitis. *N Eng J Med* 1992;326(24):1582–1586.
34. Boender J, et al. Endoscopic sphincterotomy and biliary drainage in patients with cholangitis due to common bile duct stones. *Am J Gastroenterol* 1995;90(2).
35. Duensing RA, Williams RA, Collins JC, et al. Managing choledocholithiasis in the laparoscopic era. *Am J Surg* 1995;170(6):619–623.
36. Duensing RA, Williams RA, Collins JC, et al. Common bile duct stone characteristics: correlation with treatment choice during laparoscopic cholecystectomy. *J Gastrointest Surg* 2000;4(1):6–12.
37. Reiss R, Pikelnie S, Engelberg M. The value of early surgery and routine operative cholangiography in the management of acute cholecystitis. *World J Surg* 1979;3:107.
38. Van der Linden W, Edlund G. Early versus delayed cholecystectomy: the effect of a change in management. *Br J Surg* 1981;68:753.
39. Rosi PA, Midell AI. Acute cholecystitis. An analysis of current treatment. *Surg Clin North Am* 1967;47(1):147–156.
40. Cohen S, Kaplan M, Gottlieb L, et al. Liver disease and gallstones in regional enteritis. *Gastroenterology* 1971;60:237.
41. Bouchier IAD. Postmortem study of the frequency of gallstones in patients with cirrhosis of the liver. *Gut* 1969;10:705.
42. Roslyn JJ, Pitt HA, Mann L, et al. Parenteral nutrition-induced gallbladder disease: a reason for early cholecystectomy. *Am J Surg* 1984;148:58.

Pancreas and Spleen

CHAPTER 91
Infection after Acute Pancreatitis

Thomas Foitzik, Ernst Klar, and Andrew L. Warshaw

Acute pancreatitis is an inflammatory process originating in the pancreas. In 80% to 85% of the cases inflammation remains localized in the pancreas and subsides uneventfully without specific treatment. These cases are termed mild or edematous pancreatitis and involve (almost) no mortality. In 15% to 20% of the cases, however, the inflammatory process exacerbates and is accompanied by the development of pancreatic and peripancreatic tissue (fat) necrosis and by a systemic inflammatory response syndrome (SIRS), which also affects remote organ systems and may lead to multiple organ dysfunction syndrome (MODS). Mortality is biphasic in this group of patients with severe necrotizing pancreatitis. In the first week or two, it is caused by the overwhelming sequelae of SIRS to pancreatic injury and is not related to infection or sepsis. Today, few patients die from these early disease sequelae, largely as a result of improved intensive care medicine. In contrast, late mortality occurring after several (more than 3) weeks is usually caused by septic MODS and still exceeds 10%.

Although infection may occur in various circumstances after acute pancreatitis, sepsis mainly develops in patients in whom necrotic pancreatic and peripancreatic tissue becomes infected. The devitalized tissue provides an ideal culture medium for bacterial replication and the septic focus that fuels SIRS and MODS in the later course of the disease.

DEFINITION

Infected Peripancreatic Fluid Collections and Infected Pancreatic Necrosis

Peripancreatic fluid collections arising from a combination of escaped enzyme-rich pancreatic secretions and exudate are a hallmark of acute pancreatitis. In severe cases, they can extend from the bursa omentalis to the retroperitoneal spaces (e.g., perirenal, retrocolic) and the abdominal cavity. They are poorly confined by the tissue spaces and lack a granulation or fibrous wall. Probably as a consequence of the pancreatic enzymes, focal or confluent necrosis evolves in the pancreas and surrounding peripancreatic (fatty) tissue. There are no reliable morphologic criteria to determine whether bacteria are present in the pancreatic tissue or surrounding collections unless there is gas in the tissue. Once bacteria have been detected by percutaneous fine-needle aspiration (see later section on Percutaneous Needle Aspiration of Pancreatic Tissue), we generally speak of infected pancreatic (or peripancreatic) necrosis. Today, this term is used when the content of the infected material includes tissue debris (1).

Pancreatic Phlegmon

The term *pancreatic phlegmon* was suggested by Kune and King (2) and Warshaw (3) to describe the ligneous pancreatic and peripancreatic tissue swelling and inflammation that may persist for weeks or even months after the attack. This process can resolve spontaneously or evolve into frank necrosis in either small (even microscopic) patches or large, confluent areas. The latter are particularly at risk for becoming infected, but infection is not obligatory and may even occur in the absence of grossly apparent necrosis (4,5). Although the use of the term *pancreatic phlegmon* has been discouraged (1), we find it important because it reflects a state of uncertainty, evolution of change, and the need for continuous surveillance.

Infected Acute Pseudocyst

An acute pseudocyst has developed when glandular destruction creates a collection of escaped secretion, blood, and necrotic tissue that becomes walled off by adjacent structures and eventually encapsulated by granulation tissue (which may mature with fibrosis into a chronic pseudocyst). Bacterial infection of this debris, although relatively uncommon, converts the collection into an infected (acute) pseudocyst (6,7). The feature that distinguishes this entity from a peripancreatic fluid collection containing bacteria is its mural definition. When pus is present, the lesion is more correctly termed a pancreatic abscess (1,7,8).

Pancreatic Abscess

A pancreatic abscess is a circumscribed collection of pus and thus the easiest of the pancreatic infections to recognize. It is probably the end result of tissue destruction, liquefaction, and infection. In the late stage, it may be morphologically similar to other intraabdominal abscesses. Earlier in its evolution (as with the infected pseudocyst), there are usually considerable semisolid chunks of necrotic tissue debris in the cavity.

The term *pancreatic abscess* has in the past been (improperly) used for all forms of pancreatic infections. Beger et al. (9,10) suggested distinguishing between pancreatic abscesses and infected pancreatic necrosis because the mortality rate associated with infected pancreatic necrosis developing early in the course of the disease is considerably higher than that of a pancreatic abscess that evolves later in the aftermath of the attack. Therapy for these two conditions may differ depending on the amount of residual solid components of necrotic tissue (see later sections on Indication and Timing, and on Aim and Approach).

Although there are several variations of pancreatic infections with overlapping symptoms, it is likely that most of the morphologic differences do not characterize uniquely different entities but reflect the same process modified by time and endogenous defense processes, which determine the point at which infection becomes evident (11).

PATHOGENESIS

Pancreatic infection is rare in mild/edematous pancreatitis but a common complication in the severe/necrotizing form of the disease. Ten percent to 20% of patients with acute pancreatitis develop necrosis, and that necrotic pancreatic tissue becomes infected in approximately 40% to 50%; pancreatic infection occurs in 5% to 10% of all cases of acute pancreatitis. Although it has been suggested that patients with alcohol-associated pancreatitis may have a lower risk for developing infection than others, a strong relationship between pancreatic infection and the antecedent cause of the disease has not been convincingly demonstrated (12–20).

The microorganisms most commonly found in infected pancreatic tissue are coliforms and other gram-negative enteric species, as well as anaerobes like *Clostridium* and *Bacteroides* species (5,9,21–24) (Table 91.1). Infection is multimicrobial in approximately 30%. Fungi are initially rare but recovered more frequently (in 24% of patients in a recent report [24]) once patients have been treated with antibiotics. Although the majority of fungal pancreatic infections have been with *Candida* species, reports of haploid yeasts like *Torulopsis glabrata* are appearing (25). In recent years, there has also been a shift toward nonenteric gram-positive organisms, which now represent up to 40% of all isolates (23,24). These changes may be related to the widespread use of antibiotics given prophylactically or for nosocomial infections in patients with severe pancreatitis.

Whether the type of bacteria identified in infected pancreatic necrosis influences the course of the disease is not known. Luiten et al. (26) found no significant difference in the morbidity and mortality of patients with gram-negative vs. gram-positive infection of pancreatic necrosis. However, gram-negative intestinal colonization was associated with an increased risk for developing pancreatic infection and complications (27). Grewe et al. (28) reported that patients with fungal infection of pancreatic necrosis tend to have more systemic complications and poorer outcome, while Gloor et al. (24) found no such evidence. Fungal infection may be a marker of late premortem colonization rather than the cause of the deterioration.

Primary fungal or tuberculous abscesses of the pancreas (29–32) or opportunistic pancreatic infections in patients with AIDS (33,34) are not the subject of this chapter.

The Relationship Between the Severity of Pancreatitis and Pancreatic Infection

The healthy pancreas is highly resistant to infection, even if challenged by the injection of bacteria into the pancreatic duct (35–37). Using percutaneous needle aspiration of pancreatic tissue in patients with acute pancreatitis, Gerzof et al. (5) found extremely low rates of bacterial infection in peripancreatic fluid collections, moderate rates in phlegmons, and high rates in necrotic tissues. Furthermore, experimental and clinical evidence suggests that the extent of pancreatic necrosis influences the likelihood of

TABLE 91.1. Microorganisms Found in Pancreatic Infections

Organism	Period 1974–1983 (N = 45 patients)		Period 1990–1996 (N = 36 patients)	
	No. of isolates	(%)[a]	No. of isolates	(%)[a]
Gram-negative bacteria				
Escherichia coli	22	(27)	9	(13)
Klebsiella species	6	(7)	7	(10)
Enterobacter species	n.d.		4	(6)
Pseudomonas species	3	(4)	2	(3)
Proteus species	4	(5)	1	
Others	n.d.		1	
Gram-positive cocci				
Enterococcus species	17	(21)	12	(18)
Staphylococcus species	16	(19)	12	(18)
Nonenteric streptococci	2	(2)	7	(10)
Anaerobic bacteria	n.d.			
Clostridium species			2	(3)
Other			1	
Candida species	3	(4)	4	(6)
Other	9	(11)	5	(7)
Total	82		67	
Polimicrobial	20/45 (44%)		16/36 (44%)	

[a]Percentage of total isolates.
n.d., not determined.

pancreatic infection (5,9,36). The relationship found between the number of Ranson's prognostic signs and subsequent infection (13,16) also reflects this relationship between the extent of tissue injury and the prevalence of infection.

Bacterial Translocation

The finding that the bacteria identified in necrotic pancreatic tissue resemble the typical spectrum of intestinal flora has fostered the hypothesis that infection in acute pancreatitis is gut derived. Experimental evidence for gut-derived infection in acute pancreatitis has been provided by Widdison et al. (38), who placed a specific strain of *Escherichia coli* in the colon of cats given pancreatitis. After 24 hours they retrieved the same strain from the pancreas, but enclosing the colon in an impermeable bag prevented the passage. In another experiment, Medich et al. (39) fed fluorescent microbeads to rats: the beads were found in the pancreas of 90% of animals with acute pancreatitis but in none of the healthy controls. Other investigators confirmed these findings and also recovered intestinal bacteria in the blood and extrapancreatic tissue after induction of pancreatitis (40–44). These studies suggest that bacteria migrate from the gut lumen through the gut wall to mesenteric lymph nodes, blood, and transperitoneally to necrotic pancreatic and other tissues. This phenomenon, known as bacterial translocation, is believed to be promoted by three factors: (a) gut mucosal barrier dysfunction, (b) bacterial overgrowth, and (c) impaired host defense (45). Two additional factors may explain why infection of extraintestinal sites is facilitated in acute pancreatitis: (d) necrotic tissues providing ideal culture conditions for bacterial replication, and (e) the use of total parenteral nutrition leading to deficiency of immune defenses and the gut barrier. Clearly, these risk factors for infection are much more likely to accumulate in severe pancreatitis than in a mild attack.

GUT BARRIER DYSFUNCTION

Electrophysiologic measurements demonstrate decreased gut wall resistance and increased flux of molecules like mannitol through the grossly and microscopically intact gut wall in acute pancreatitis (46,47). The degree of barrier loss correlates with disease severity (48). In patients with acute pancreatitis, Ammori et al. (49) found evidence for gut barrier dysfunction by demonstrating increased intestinal permeability for macromolecules. Increased gut wall permeability is thought to develop as a consequence of the systemic inflammatory reaction to pancreatic injury. Like renal and respiratory failure, gut barrier failure can be regarded as part of pancreatitis-associated multiple organ dysfunction syndrome. Factors contributing to gut barrier dysfunction in acute pancreatitis are listed in Table 91.2. Like any other organ, the gut remains intact only if it is supplied with sufficient oxygen and nutrients. Measurements in animals and patients indicate that splanchnic oxygen consumption is increased in acute pancreatitis, while perfusion, microcirculation, and nutrient flow are compromised (50–52). In the face of this abnormal stress, which may be further aggravated by exogenous factors such as catecholamines, which further impair mucosal perfusion, the

TABLE 91.2. Extrapancreatic Factors Contributing to Gut Barrier Dysfunction, Bacterial Translocation, and Pancreatic Infection in Acute Pancreatitis

Decreased gut oxygenation
  Increased oxygen consumption/reduced splanchnic perfusion
  Microcirculatory disorders
Insufficient supply of (essential) nutrients
  Increased demand under stress (SIRS)/decreased endogenous synthesis
  Decreased exogenous supply (e.g., of glutamine)
  Decreased delivery via disturbed (micro)circulation
Overgrowth of pathogenic bacteria
  Decreased gut motility, pH changes, MALT dysfunction
Exogenous adverse factors
  Catecholamines, morphines, total parenteral nutrition

MALT, mucosa-associated lymphoid tissue.

mucosa becomes leaky to endotoxins, bacteria, and other macro-molecules.

BACTERIAL OVERGROWTH

Experimental and clinical findings suggest an overgrowth of fac-ultative pathogenic bacteria in acute pancreatitis, which has been explained by decreased gut motility and paralysis, pH alterations due to bile and pancreatic juice flow changes, and immunologic disturbances (53–56).

IMPAIRED HOST DEFENSE

Bacterial overgrowth is a challenge even for an intact gut bar-rier. Gut barrier and mucosa-associated lymphoid tissue (MALT) function are, however, impaired in severe pancreatitis, thereby facilitating bacterial migration through the gut wall. Once hav-ing breached the mucosal barrier, bacteria and endotoxin may reach the free abdominal cavity or pass through the interstitium to the lymph or venous system. Mesenteric lymph nodes and hepatic Kupffer's cells are the first immune defense stations, but experimental and clinical evidence suggests that both regional and systemic immune defenses are also impaired in acute pan-creatitis (56–58).

EXTRAINTESTINAL (PANCREATIC) NECROSIS

Viable, well-perfused tissues are resistant to infection. However, poorly perfused and necrotic pancreatic and peripancreatic tis-sues are fertile soil for bacterial beachheads and replication. These necrotic areas are probably the *conditio sine qua non* for postpancreatitis infection. This requirement also explains why infection is rarely if ever seen in mild/edematous pancreatitis (see earlier section on The Relationship Between the Severity of Pancreatitis and Pancreatic Infection).

Time Course of Pancreatic Infection

Beger et al. (9) reported a 24% prevalence of pancreatic infection in patients who underwent surgery in the first week after the on-set of acute pancreatitis, 36% in the second week, and 71% in the third. A similar time course was found with computed tomogra-phy (CT)-guided fine-needle aspirates from pancreatic tissue (5). Experimental findings and increased endotoxin plasma levels in patients (36,50) also support the assertion that bacterial translo-cation and infection occur early during the first disease week. Infection may be present for an indeterminate time before caus-ing clinical signs. Later in the course of the disease, probably after the population of bacteria in the damaged tissue reaches critical levels (perhaps after 2 or 3 weeks), this septic focus begins to fuel SIRS and triggers MODS (Fig. 91.1).

Other Sources and Routes of Infection

The route or routes by which microorganisms reach the pan-creas has not yet been fully established and may comprise direct transmural spread of bacteria from the colon across the peri-toneal cavity as well as lymphatic and hematogenous seeding (38,42,59). Insight into the pathogenesis of pancreatic infections and sepsis in acute pancreatitis was gained by applying differ-ent antibiotic regimens in a rodent model of severe necrotizing pancreatitis (42). Because early pancreatic infection could be re-duced by either gut decontamination (see later section on Selec-tive Gut Decontamination) or a systemic antibiotic concentrated in the pancreas, there appears to be an interplay between di-rect bacterial spread from the gut and hematogenous seeding from necrotic tissues. Infection in other sites such as the kidney could only be prevented by systemic antibiotic therapy, a finding suggesting that intact tissues are less susceptible to transmural contamination than necrotic tissues.

Although the colon is thought to be the predominant source of bacteria infecting the pancreas, some experimental data suggest that infections may also spread from the gallbladder (60–64). The biliary tree may be a likely source of infection in patients with common duct stones and associated cholangitis. Infection of pancreatic necrosis by bacteria originating in the urinary or respiratory tract is possible, but unproven.

Pancreatic infections frequently spread out from the pancreas, usually following retroperitoneal tissue planes down the para-colic gutters or between the mesenteric leaves of the large and small intestines. It is thought that these extensions are facili-tated by the activated pancreatic proteolytic enzymes, which are admixed in the debris contents and potentiate the erosion of tissue along the advancing front. Pancreatic abscesses have been known to reach the groin and scrotum or travel up the me-diastinum to the neck. Along the way, they can perforate the

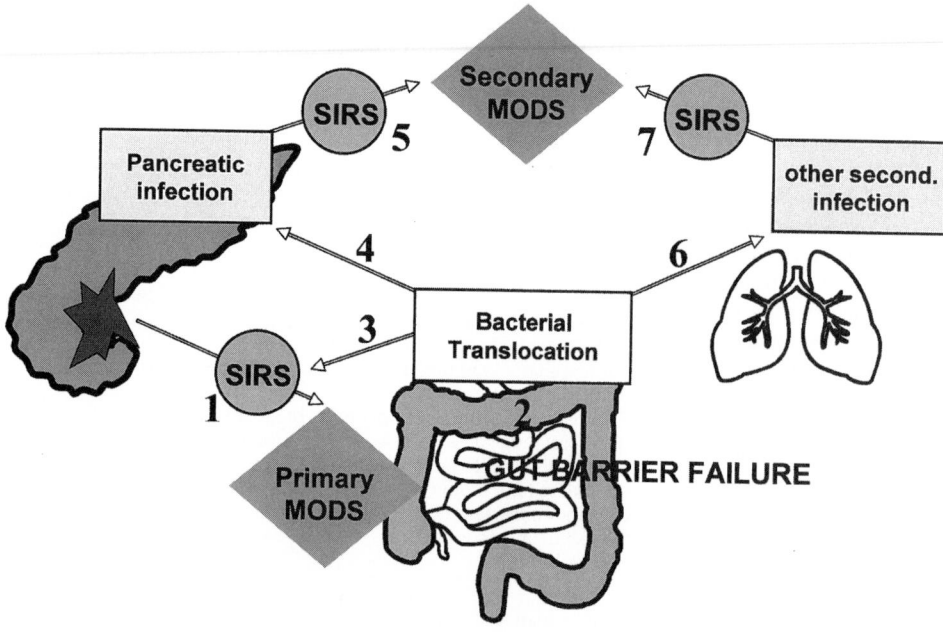

Figure 91.1. The enteral factor in pancreatic infection. (*1*) The gut is a target organ of the systemic inflammatory response syndrome (*SIRS*) to pancreatic injury and involved in the pancreatitis-associated multiple organ dys-function syndrome (*MODS*). (*2*) The gut bar-rier becomes insufficient, thereby allowing bacteria and (endo)toxin to translocate. (*3*) Translocated bacteria and endotoxins may directly aggravate SIRS, thereby promoting primary/early MODS. (*4*) Translocated bacte-ria find ideal conditions to replicate in pan-creatic necrosis. (*5*) The secondary infectious focus in the pancreas promotes SIRS and trig-gers secondary/late (septic) MODS (after the gut barrier has stabilized again). (*6*) Translo-cated bacteria may also infect other tissue, thereby (*7*) promoting secondary MODS.

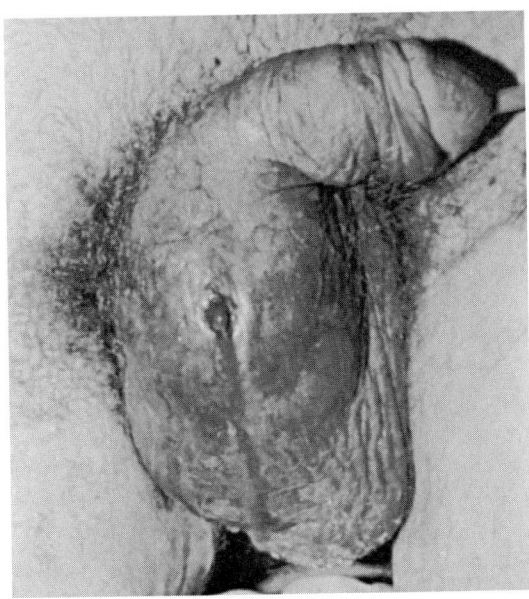

Figure 91.2. Retroperitoneal extension of a pancreatic abscess with necessitation out through the scrotum.

peritoneal cavity, an intraabdominal hollow viscus, the pleural space, or even a bronchus (65–67) (Fig. 91.2). Their aggressive migrating behavior is not matched by any other form of intraabdominal abscess.

CLINICAL MANIFESTATIONS

The symptoms of pancreatic infection are nonspecific (16,18,67). Patients with severe pancreatitis almost always fulfill SIRS criteria. Theoretically, infection makes these patients septic (SIRS + infection = sepsis) (68), but there is no sign specific for sepsis. Even fever, the typical and most common sign of infection, may be absent, as illustrated in Table 91.3, which shows our experience with pancreatic abscesses. On the contrary, sterile necrosis can also produce fever and leukocytosis.

The spectrum of clinical severity of pancreatic infections ranges from silent to fulminant, but two relatively distinct patterns are archetypal (10,16,18,67,69,70). In the first, the patient seems to recover from the acute attack, appears to be well for 1 to 5 weeks (latent period), and then develops fever, leukocytosis, and perhaps other signs of intraabdominal infection. These patients usually have distinct, well-demarcated pancreatic ab-

scesses, which are the final product of infected necrosis that has liquefied. In the second, the patient never recovers from the presenting inflammatory episode but continues to be acutely ill with clinical signs of fluid sequestration, hyperdynamic cardiac function, circulatory instability, fever, and leukocytosis. These patients appear to be more sick than those in the first group. Their illness usually accelerates earlier, and the threshold for intervention is reached an average of 2 weeks earlier than in patients with pancreatic abscesses (18,70). CT or surgical exploration will show that the infected necrotic tissue has not yet fully liquefied and cannot be distinguished from sterile necrosis in most cases (4,5,71). We suggest that these two processes do not represent different pathologic entities but different points in the evolution of pancreatic infection after acute pancreatitis. In the first group, the acute phase of SIRS subsides, the infection remains subclinical, and the infected necrosis advances to liquefaction. In the second, the combination of continuing pancreatitis, progressive pancreatic necrosis, and infection produces significantly greater toxicity and multiple organ failure, and is more likely to compel intervention before liquefaction leads to an abscess.

DIAGNOSIS

Clinical Signs and Laboratory Tests

Because the local or systemic effects of pancreatic necrosis may exactly mimic those of an infected process (including the hyperdynamic, high-output cardiocirculatory dysfunction (72), the clinical picture cannot be relied on to make the diagnosis of pancreatic infection. Consequently, infection in acute pancreatitis must be considered in any patient with the severe necrotizing form of the disease (as best indicated by CT; see later section on Imaging) or unremitting SIRS. Patients at particular risk are those who have had a fulminant presentation with multiple clinical and laboratory signs of severity (12,16,73), those in whom necrosis exceeds 50% of the gland, and those with elevated serum levels of C-reactive protein (greater than 100 mg/L at the end of the first disease week) and phospholipase A (74–77). Patients who remain febrile after the first several days or who become febrile after a period of quiescence are suspects for pancreatic infection. High-spiking fevers are suggestive but not specific. Routine laboratory parameters (white blood cell count, C-reactive protein) indicate inflammation but are not specific for pancreatic infection. Other sources of infection, such as the lungs, urinary tract, and intravenous lines, must be evaluated. Conversely, pancreatic infection may be present even in the absence of fever, leukocytosis, abdominal signs, or palpable masses. Table 91.4 shows

TABLE 91.3. Presenting Symptoms and Signs of Pancreatic Infections in 45 Patients

Sign or symptom	n	%
Fever	39	87
Abdominal pain	37	82
Abdominal tenderness	28	62
Palpable mass	22	50
Nausea or vomiting	21	47
Distention	12	27
Jaundice	7	16
Systemic sepsis	3	7
Pulmonary failure	2	4
Gastrointestinal bleeding	1	2

TABLE 91.4. Routine Laboratory Findings in 45 Pancreatic Infections

Parameter		n
White blood cell count (/mm³)	>20,000	6
	15,000–20,000	7
	10,000–15,000	26
	<10,000	6
Serum amylase	<25 Russell	19
Alkaline phosphatase	>40 IU	18
Serum aspartate aminotransferase	>40 units	23
Bilirubin	>1.2 mg/dL	17
Calcium	<8.5 mg/dL	25
Albumin	<3 g/dL	20

data from 45 patients with a confirmed pancreatic abscess. The findings are not striking in many of these cases and even normal in some. The white blood cell count usually did not exceed 15,000/mm³, and 13% of the patients had results in the normal range. These findings have been confirmed in several studies and emphasize the difficulties of separating patients with infected necrosis from those with a sterile process by routine tests (10,12,18,67,69).

Elevated serum levels of cytokines such as interleukin-6 indicate the severity of the inflammatory response but do not distinguish between sterile and infected necrosis, but serum procalcitonin levels have recently been reported to identify patients with infected pancreatic necrosis with high accuracy. Mandi et al. (78) found high concentrations (8.5 ± 4.8 ng/mL) only in patients with infected necrosis, whereas none of the serum samples of those with sterile necrosis was higher than 1.2 ng/mL. Further prospective studies are needed to verify these promising data.

Imaging

Radiographic abnormalities are common in severe pancreatitis, but most are also insensitive and nonspecific with regard to infection. The classic soap bubble sign (mottled lucencies that are a combination of necrotic tissue and gas bubbles in retroperitoneal tissues; Fig. 91.3) occurs infrequently (4 of 45 patients in one series [18]). Contrast studies of the upper gastrointestinal tract yielded only indirect evidence of visceral displacement, stenosis, or obstruction, albeit commonly (40 of 45). Seventy-one percent of our patients had an abnormal chest radiograph that showed pleural effusion, atelectasis, or pneumonitis, the presence of which may indicate severe pancreatitis but do not provide information on the presence of infection.

Ultrasonographic examination is technically unsatisfactory in 30% of patients with pancreatitis because of excess bowel gas. CT is superior in this respect, and for detecting areas of liquefaction within and around pancreatic inflammatory masses (18,70,79). At least 75% of abscesses can be demonstrated with CT, and many more can be suspected (12,18,70,80). Although gas in the fluid collection (Fig. 91.4) is widely accepted as proof of infection, it is absent in the majority of patients with confirmed infection and can sometimes occur in association with an enteric fistula (81–85).

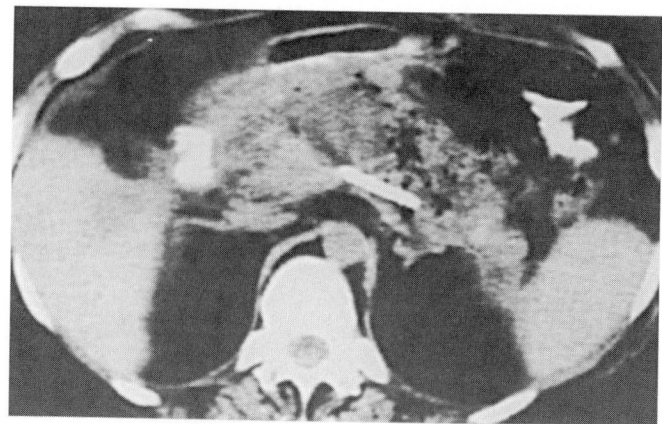

Figure 91.4. Computed tomography scan of a pancreatic abscess showing gas bubbles in a large volume of regional necrosis.

Because pancreatic necrosis is the major risk factor for developing pancreatic infection, there has been a concerted effort to use CT for identifying those patients at risk and to correlate the CT finding with the prevalence of infection. Clavien et al. (85) found that the majority of patients with extensive phlegmonous extrapancreatic inflammation within 36 hours of admission developed a pancreatic abscess. Balthazar, Ranson, and co-workers (86,87) established a grading system that uses the extent of the inflammatory process and the number of collections in and around the pancreas to estimate the probability of subsequent infection. The incidence of infection in patients graded as having the most severe disease was as high as 60% to 80%. Ascites and pleural effusions appear to have less prognostic importance (88).

Dynamic angio- or contrast-enhanced CT performed during rapid injection of a large volume of intravenous contrast medium has become established as the best method for detecting poorly perfused or nonperfused tissue, which is either necrotic or at risk for becoming necrotic and thus infected (89–91). The principle of this technique is that well-perfused pancreatic parenchyma will be contrast enhanced in the CT image and will be easily distinguishable from nonperfused areas (91–93) (Fig. 91.5). Studies in experimental pancreatitis have suggested that nonperfused or poorly perfused areas are likely to be or become nonviable (94). Clinical studies have tended to confirm that defects visualized by contrast-enhanced CT reflect microcirculatory failure as confirmed by corresponding microangiographic findings in resected human specimens (95).

There is experimental evidence that both ionic and nonionic intravenous contrast medium aggravates the microcirculatory perfusion defect, impairs pancreatic tissue oxygenation, and increases the degree of pancreatic tissue injury and mortality when given early after the onset of pancreatitis (96–99). Clinical studies (100,101) do not dispel this concern. Since the findings of contrast-enhanced CT are rarely needed to detect or map necrosis in the first few days, and are unlikely to have any impact on clinical decisions at this early stage, it may be safer to defer the use of intravenous contrast media for at least several days after the attack. A CT without intravenous contrast medium may be equally helpful if the diagnosis of acute pancreatitis is unclear. Contrast-enhanced CT can be reserved to identify necrotic areas in patients whose attack does not resolve, to follow the evolution of the necrosis, and to plan débridement if necessary.

Magnetic resonance imaging (MRI) has not proven to be superior to CT in demonstrating the presence and extent of pancreatic fluid collections and necrosis and also cannot distinguish between infected and sterile necrosis (102,103). Unlike the contrast

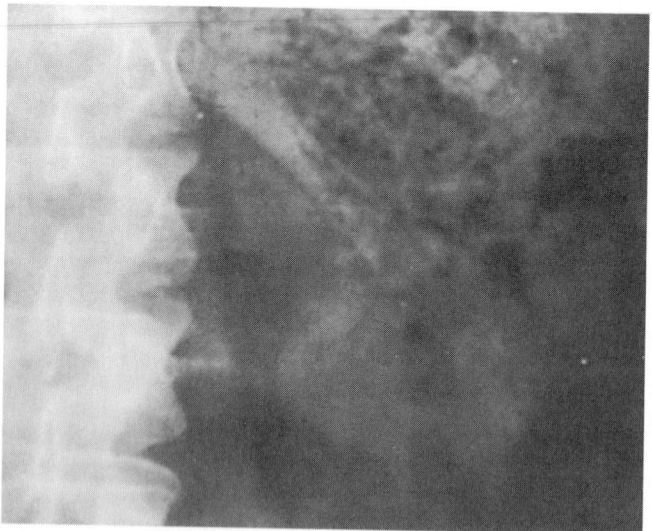

Figure 91.3. Abdominal radiograph showing the classic soap bubble sign of a pancreatic abscess.

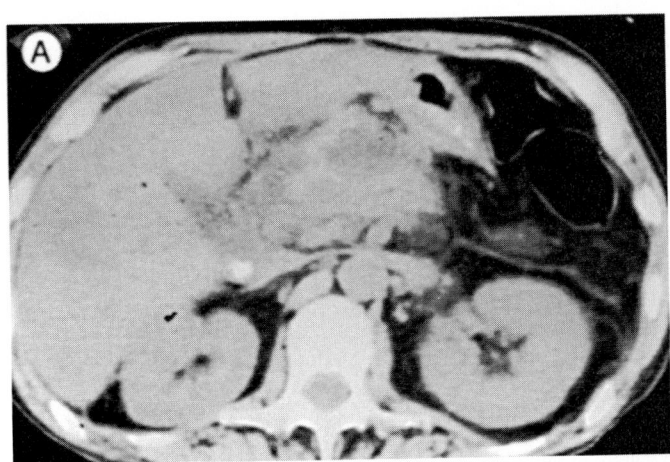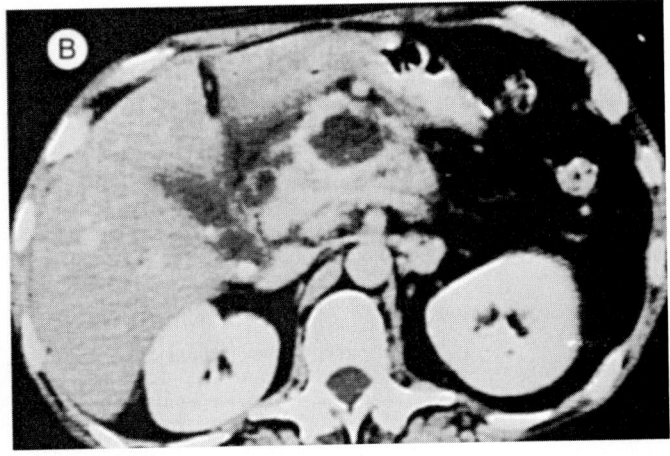

Figure 91.5. Contrast-enhanced computed tomography scan in pancreatic necrosis. **A:** Without contrast. **B:** With use of intravenous contrast medium. Note the enhancement of the viable pancreas and improved delineation of the nonenhanced necrotic area.

medium used for CT, the use of gadolinium for contrast enhancement in MRI had no negative effects on pancreatic microcirculation or disease severity in the animal model (104). However, even the indication for MRI early in the course of the disease should be considered carefully, since a first case of gadolinium-induced acute pancreatitis has recently been reported (105).

Percutaneous Needle Aspiration of Pancreatic Tissue

The only diagnostic test that reliably identifies infection of pancreatic tissue (and has a high probability of excluding it) is a sampling of those tissues for microscopic and bacteriologic examination. Blood cultures are of lesser value, although positive results may indicate patients at increased risk to die (70).

Studies have proven that it is safe to sample peripancreatic fluid collections, inflammatory masses, and parenchyma by percutaneous fine-needle aspiration under CT or ultrasound guidance (5,106–108). They have shown a remarkable 90% to 95% accuracy in both proving and disproving infection. Gerzof et al. (5) showed that about 60% of patients suspected of harboring infection were infected. Peripancreatic fluid collections were not commonly infected (15%), whereas phlegmons or acute pseudocysts and necrotic areas frequently were (more than 50%). They had no false-positive cultures, no false-negatives, and no contamination caused by needle aspiration (testimony to the excellence of their technique). In their patients, 22% of the infections were found within 7 days after the onset of the attack and 55% within 14 days, confirming the observations of Beger et al. (9), who obtained cultures during surgical débridement for necrotizing pancreatitis. Percutaneous needle aspiration under CT guidance is the undisputed technique of choice for confirming pancreatic infection after acute pancreatitis and is almost as good for confirming contemporaneous sterility of the process. It must be kept in mind, however, that sampling at a single point in time cannot assure continuing sterility.

MEDICAL TREATMENT

There is no firm evidence that pancreatic necrosis can be prevented by any known therapy. Recent studies, however, suggest that antibiotics reduce the prevalence of pancreatic infection and subsequent complications, provided that therapy is started early and that the agents cover the spectrum of bacteria usually found

in pancreatic infection and penetrate into necrotic pancreatic tissue.

Limiting Pancreatic Necrosis

Because there is a general proportional relationship between the extent of pancreatic necrosis and the development of pancreatic infection (see earlier section on The Relationship Between the Severity of Pancreatitis and Pancreatic Infection), limiting necrosis in the early stage of the disease should be an important objective toward reducing pancreatic infection after acute pancreatitis. Because pancreatic ischemia plays a key role in the evolution of pancreatic necrosis (109–112), stabilization and improvement of pancreatic perfusion and microcirculation may be of crucial value. Besides avoiding factors like catecholamines, which impair pancreatic capillary blood flow (113), enhancement of pancreatic microcirculation by vasoactive mediator blockade or hemodilution therapy using plasma expanders like dextran or hemodilution therapy using plasma expanders like dextran has been shown to reduce pancreatic necrosis in animals if therapy was started early enough (114–116). In the clinical situation, however, patients appear for treatment 1 or 2 days after the onset of symptoms. At this point, necrosis has already occurred (117) and it may no longer be possible to prevent it by any therapeutic means. A number of drugs successful in animal experiments have failed to reduce pancreatic necrosis or secondary complications in human pancreatitis (for a review see references 118 and 119). However, recent animal studies have suggested that therapy aimed at improving microcirculation may be beneficial in other ways, even if pancreatic necrosis can no longer be influenced (120). Enhancement of hepatic and colonic microcirculation, for example, was associated with improved reticuloendothelial system and gut barrier function, reduced bacterial translocation, and reduced pancreatic infection (121,122). This fits with the recognition of microcirculatory disorders as a systemic phenomenon in acute pancreatitis which contribute to pancreatitis-associated MODS (123–125).

Limiting Bacterial Translocation

Provided that the gut is the principal source of bacteria infecting pancreatic necrosis, then the incidence of pancreatic infection could be reduced by the following three strategies: (a) eliminating pathogenic bacteria in the gut lumen; (bi) avoiding bacterial migration through the gut wall; or (cii) killing bacteria outside

TABLE 91.5.   Therapeutic Strategies Aimed at Reducing Bacterial Translocation and Pancreatic Infection in Acute Pancreatitis

	Evidence[a]
Eliminating bacteria in the gut lumen/decreasing bacterial overgrowth	
Selective decontamination of the digestive tract	C
Gut irrigation	
Avoiding bacterial migration through the gut wall/strengthening the gut barrier	
Optimizing gut oxygenation	
Stabilizing cardiorespiratory function (intensive care therapy)	
Enhancing microcirculation (e.g., hemodilution)	
Optimizing nutrition	
Early enteral (tube) feeding	C
Supplementation of (conditionally essential) substrates (e.g., glutamine)	
Reducing bacteria in the gut lumen (gut decontamination, irrigation, see above)	
Avoiding exogenous adverse factors	
Enhancing local (MALT) immune defense (enteral feeding, immunonutrition?)	
Eliminating bacteria behind the gut barrier	
Adequate i.v. antibiotics	B
Enhancing regional and systemic immune defense	

[a]Levels of evidence [modified according to Sackett 1989 (215,216)]:

Grade
A: supported by more than one level I investigation
B: supported by one level I investigation
C: supported by level II investigations

Level
I: large randomized controlled trial (RCT) with clear-cut results
II: small RCT

MALT, mucosa-associated lymphoid tissue; i.v., intravenous.

the gut. Measures to achieve these goals are summarized in Table 91.5 and discussed as follows.

SELECTIVE GUT DECONTAMINATION (FOR ELIMINATING PATHOGENIC BACTERIA IN THE GUT)

Selective decontamination of the digestive tract (SDD) by orally administered nonabsorbable antibiotics is a clinically established tool for eliminating the particularly dangerous gram-negative bacteria from the gut and reducing extraintestinal infections by organisms originating in the intestine. In a randomized controlled multicenter trial on the effect of SDD in 102 patients with severe acute pancreatitis, Luiten et al. (126) showed that patients who underwent SDD had significantly fewer pancreas infections (30%) and lower late mortality (6% after 2 weeks) than did those without SDD (75% and 19%). This study was criticized because patients in the SDD group also received an intravenous antibiotic. Experimental and clinical data, however, show that the parenteral antibiotics not only provide systemic prophylaxis but are also necessary for gut decontamination, perhaps because the drug is also secreted into the gut lumen or concentrates in the mucosa, where it eliminates bacteria (127–129).

Enteric bacteria may also be reduced by gut irrigation, performed most effectively via loop ileostomy or split colonostomy. Experimental data (130,131) and positive experience in a small series of patients (132) support this principle, but the approach is too extreme to be acceptable.

AVOIDING BACTERIAL TRANSLOCATION BY STABILIZING THE GUT BARRIER

If gut barrier failure is a consequence of the systemic inflammatory response to pancreatic injury, then attenuating pancreatic injury and the concomitant SIRS should reduce the prevalence of gut failure, bacterial translocation, and secondary infections. Experimental data suggest that limiting SIRS may be possible by early immunomodulation using certain anticytokines (133,134),

but as previously noted, the events triggering the systemic inflammatory response are already in progress long before the patient arrives at the hospital.

Optimizing Oxygenation. The prerequisites for optimal gut oxygenation are stable cardiocirculatory and respiratory function. Adequate volume resuscitation is essential. A hematocrit of 30% to 35% guarantees optimal blood flow at the capillary level (135). Due to capillary leakage with massive fluid loss from the intra- into the extravascular space, patients with severe acute pancreatitis usually present with extreme hemoconcentration. Isovolemic hemodilution with plasma expanders like dextran or hydroxyethyl starch, which rapidly decreases hematocrit and improves microcirculation, has been successfully tested in animals and in a pilot study of patients with severe acute pancreatitis (113,136). Experimental studies have demonstrated that hemodilution improves capillary blood flow in the colon to the same extent as in the pancreas and is associated with reduced bacterial translocation, secondary pancreatic infection, and mortality (137).

Optimizing Nutrition. Experimental and clinical evidence suggests that enteral nutrition is a prerequisite for normal gut motility, bacterial growth in the gut, and the functional and morphologic integrity of the mucosa. Controlled randomized clinical trials have shown that enteral nutrition significantly reduced bacterial translocation and nosocomial infections in certain patients, including those with acute pancreatitis (138–141). These studies indicate that early enteral feeding is superior to parenteral nutrition (142–145). However, patients with severe acute pancreatitis may have an ileus, making them intolerant of adequate feeding. These patients will require supplemental parenteral nutrition if enteral feeding cannot be resumed after a week. It is now recognized as well that glutamine is a conditionally essential amino acid for the gut in stress and that glutamine is significantly depleted in patients with severe acute pancreatitis

(146,147) because the increased demand under stress cannot be compensated for by endogenous synthesis. Experimental studies in a rodent model of severe acute pancreatitis have demonstrated that glutamine supplementation, now available as a stable dipeptide for intravenous application, decreases gut wall permeability and is associated with reduced pancreatic infections (46).

Systemic Antibiotic Therapy (for Eliminating Bacteria Beyond the Gut Barrier)

The role of antibiotic treatment for preventing pancreatic infection in acute pancreatitis continues to be debated. Two controlled clinical trials conducted in the 1970s reached the conclusion that prophylactic antibiotic therapy was useless (148,149). These studies, however, enrolled a population of patients with mild pancreatitis not at risk for developing infection (see earlier section on The Relationship Between the Severity of Pancreatitis and Pancreatic Infection) and tested an antibiotic (ampicillin) that did not concentrate in the pancreas. In the 1990s Bassi et al. (150) and Büchler et al. (151) further characterized the pathogens commonly responsible for pancreatic infection and investigated the pharmacokinetics of antibiotics in the pancreas. They demonstrated that the penetration of antibiotics into pancreatic tissue was not reduced during pancreatitis. Quinolones and imipenem appeared to be most suitable for treating pancreatic infection because they not only penetrate the pancreas at sufficient concentrations but have a spectrum of effectiveness against the flora usually found in infected pancreatic necrosis. In rats with severe pancreatitis, we found that early treatment with imipenem and ciprofloxacin during the first disease week significantly reduced pancreatic infection, late septic complications, and mortality (42,152). Clinically, the effect of prophylactic therapy with imipenem (0.5 g given intravenously three times daily for 14 days) was studied in a controlled multicenter trial (153) in 74 patients with necrotizing pancreatitis documented by contrast-enhanced CT. Pancreatic infection, assessed microbiologically in specimens obtained by fine-needle aspiration, occurred significantly less frequently in the treated group (12%) than in the controls (30%; $p < 0.01$). However, the need for surgical intervention and mortality (7% vs. 12%) was not lessened. In another randomized controlled study (154) of 60 patients with severe ethanol-induced pancreatitis confirmed by contrast-enhanced CT, cefuroxime (4.5 g per day intravenously) was shown to reduce infectious complications and mortality (even though cefuroxime does not reach high tissue concentrations in the pancreas and does not cover all the microorganisms usually found in infected pancreatic tissue). Similar results were reported in other studies (155,156). A metaanalysis by Sharma and Howden (157) finds a nonsignificant trend toward a decrease in pancreatic infections and a significant reduction in sepsis (by 21%) and mortality (12%) in patients with severe pancreatitis with appropriate antibiotic therapy. We suggest imipenem or a quinolone in combination with metronidazole to be given in all patients with necrotizing pancreatitis.

OPERATIVE TREATMENT

Indication and Timing

Once necrosis is infected or an abscess is present, medical treatment is unlikely to cure it. There may be exceptions to this rule, but it is not currently possible to predict which patients with infected pancreatic necrosis have a better chance to re-

TABLE 91.6. Indications for Surgical Débridement of Pancreatic Necrosis in Acute Pancreatitis

Indication	Early (<6 weeks) (n = 37 patients)	Late (>6 weeks) (n = 27 patients)
Infected necrosis	30%	18%
Pancreatic abscess	11%	11%
Sepsis syndrome	35%	11%
Persistent pancreatitis	24%	59%
APACHE II score (no. of patients)	11.4 ± 6	5.7 ± 4

cover without débridement. The standard of treatment for infected pancreatic necrosis and abscesses is still débridement and drainage for local control of infection. Prophylactic débridement of sterile necrosis remains a focus of controversy. Early surgical débridement or packing of pancreatic necrosis is not known to curtail further necrosis or prevent infection. Patients subjected to early operation (extensive débridement or pancreatic resections) demonstrated unacceptably high mortality rates of up to 60% (158–161).

If the necrosis is infected (as documented by culture-positive fine-needle aspirates), débridement is probably mandatory (162–165). Immediate surgical débridement of infected pancreatic necrosis to prevent septic organ complications (166), however, is probably unnecessary. Recent studies have shown that most patients with infected necrosis can be treated with antibiotics and profit from delaying surgery until they have stabilized (23,167). The indication for and timing of surgery are now better determined by the severity of systemic reactions than by local findings (23) (Table 91.6). Following surgery, we and others found no difference in mortality or other outcome parameters between patients with infected or sterile necrosis (23,168) (Table 91.7). This should not, however, obscure the fact that infection of pancreatic necrosis is a major risk factor for late mortality: perceived need for surgical intervention, whether for proven infection or for severe SIRS or MODS, defines the population of pancreatitis patients at greatest risk, and infection is present in at least two thirds of this population.

The fact that patients profit from delaying operative intervention has been most impressively confirmed by Mier et al. (169). Their prospective randomized study had to be terminated prematurely because the patients undergoing surgery in the first 3 days after disease onset had a considerably higher mortality rate (59%) than those whose surgery was delayed at least until the second week (27%). Other centers (170–174) have also been moving toward later intervention, especially to take advantage of more clear demarcation and definition of the areas to be débrided.

In our experience (23), the most favorable time point for surgery was in the fourth week of the disease. When the necrosectomy was performed in this period, outcome scores were optimized, and no additional advantage accrued with further delay (but costs increased).

It is still unclear how often and which patients with infected necrosis may be treated with antibiotics but no invasive intervention, as has been advocated for sterile necrosis (175–178). In a prospective clinical study, Ruenzi et al. (179) reported that 7 of 13 patients (54%) with infected pancreatic necrosis recovered without surgery, while surgical removal of collections in six patients could be delayed until after the fourth week of disease by using intermittent percutaneous drainage; one patient died. In another series of 42 patients with culture-positive pancreatic

TABLE 91.7. Comparison of Outcome Parameters in Patients after Surgical Débridement for Infected versus Sterile Necrosis

Complication	Early		Late	
	Infected (n = 23 patients)	Sterile (n = 14 patients)	Infected (n = 13 patients)	Sterile (n = 14 patients)
APACHE II (no. of patients)	13 ± 6	9 ± 5	7 ± 4	5 ± 3
Organ failure (%)	39	50	31	0
Reoperations (%)	35	7	8	0
Postoperative percutaneous drain (%)	22	21	38	14
Enteric fistula (%)	30	7	8	14
Pancreatic fistula (%)	52	64	38	57
Postoperative hospital stay (days)	54 ± 37	40 ± 24	32 ± 23	28 ± 22
Mortality (%)	9	7	8	0

necrosis, Baril et al. (180) reported that six patients (14%) recovered without débridement, 25 (60%) had percutaneous catheter drainage as the primary therapy, and 11 (26%) had surgery as the primary treatment.

Although surgery for infected pancreatic necrosis may be delayed or occasionally obviated, there is no apparent advantage to avoid drainage of a fully formed pancreatic abscess (see later sections on Aim and Approach, and Minimally Invasive Methods). There is no precedent that abscesses can resolve with antibiotics alone.

Aim and Approach

In general, surgical débridement (necrosectomy), lavage, and drainage are considered the definitive therapy (12,16,18,23,162–165,181,182). There are two general techniques: "closed" procedures in which a relaparotomy is not planned unless complications occur, and "open" procedures with planned reexploration and necrosectomies every day or two until no further necrotic areas are found. The choice between the two depends in part on the timing of surgery (how well demarcated the necrosis is found to be) and the experience (or bias) of the center. A new less invasive approach uses an operating nephroscope with a 4-mm working channel inserted under CT guidance and catheter dilatation under general anesthesia to perform the necrosectomy (183). There was resolution of symptoms in 7 of 10 patients after a median of three percutaneous explorations and drainage, but two patients (20%) died. The risk for uncontrollable hemorrhage or enteric injury, as well as the success rate, will need to be addressed if this technique is pursued. The aim of any strategy for removal of pancreatic necrosis should be the complete elimination of the dead tissue that comprises the culture medium for bacteria. Failure is most often a consequence of inadequate clearance requiring reoperation.

Minimally Invasive Methods

Although percutaneous CT-guided catheter drainage has been highly successful (up to 90%) in other kinds of intra-abdominal abscesses, the results have been less encouraging for pancreatic collections (between 30% in infected necrosis and 90% in abscesses), mainly because of the incomplete separation of necrotic tissue and the size of the sequestered debris, which cannot readily pass through the drainage catheters (184–189). Use of multiple large-bore double-lumen catheters for continuous irrigation and suction may improve results in the future. Placing an average of three catheters in 41 patients with infected necrosis or abscesses,

Gouzi et al. (190) reported a 70% success rate. However, the 15% mortality rate and the 59% complication rate in survivors is unacceptably high. Nevertheless, percutaneous catheterization may have a valid place in selected cases: (a) as a preliminary means of decompressing and stabilizing a critically ill septic patient; (b) when surgical access to the abscess is particularly difficult or dangerous; and (c) for drainage of small recurrent or satellite abscesses, especially after multiple surgical drainage procedures (23,191,192). Endoscopic transpapillary drainage as recently described by Venu et al. (193) may be an option for the rare patient whose pancreatic abscess communicates with the main pancreatic duct.

Conventional Surgical Procedures

CLOSED PACKING

In our opinion, an upper midline incision provides the best access, allowing wide exposure to thoroughly explore the entire abdomen in search of multiple locations, present in up to 30% of the patients (8,70). Others favor upper abdominal transverse incisions (9,181). The transmesocolic approach to the pancreas (Fig. 91.6) is often the most expeditious and safest for avoiding

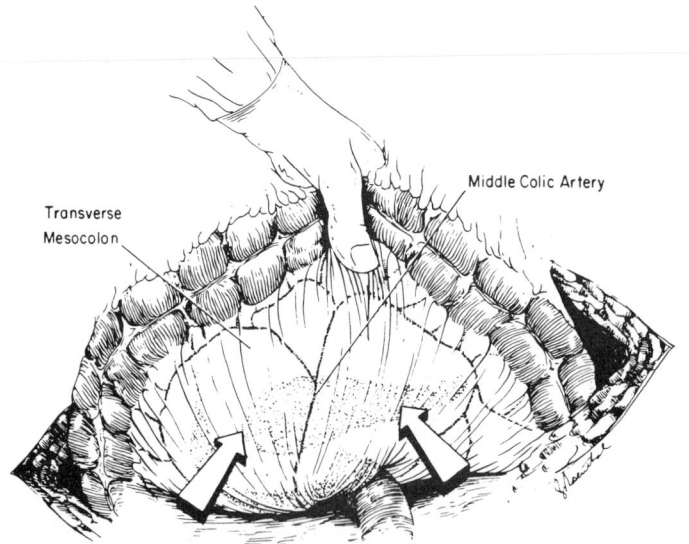

Transverse Mesocolon

Middle Colic Artery

Figure 91.6. Transmesocolic approach to drainage and débridement of the pancreas.

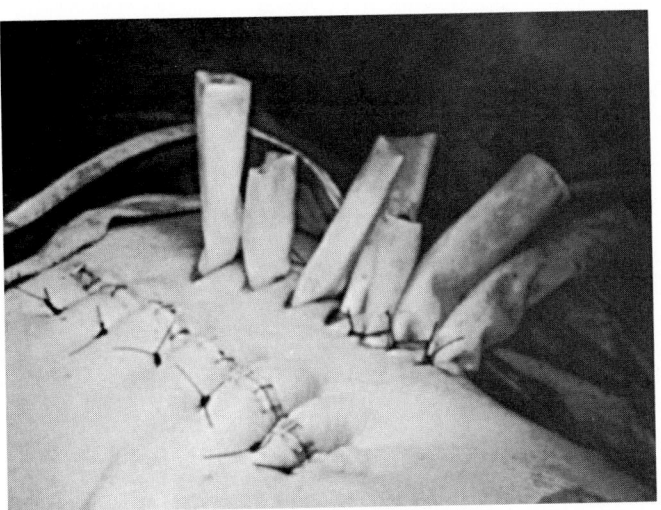

Figure 91.7. Multiple closed-system suction and stuffed drains placed in the cavity left after drainage and débridement of pancreatic abscess.

damage to the transverse colon and the stomach when they are closely adjacent to the pancreas. After the bursa is emptied of pus and debris, special attention must be directed toward the evacuation of necrotic tissue. Blunt digital dissection is most discriminating between debris and viable tissue, including major vascular structures, which often line the walls or traverse abscess cavities. External drainage should be carefully implemented in all extensions of the cavity and is best accomplished with multiple soft suction drains and stuffed rubber drains brought out through several separate stab wounds (Fig. 91.7). This technique has the advantage of providing both packing and large paths for slough and drainage of devitalized tissue and yet minimizes the risk for incisional hernia. The stuffed drains should be left in place for at least 1 week and subsequently be removed one at a time to allow the cavity to contract around the remaining drains. The suction drains should remain in place until the drainage volume is minimal and any fistulas have closed. Using this technique, we have observed a striking decrease in mortality rates for pancreatic abscesses and infected necrosis, from 38% to 6% between 1973 and today (18,23).

In our latest series, a single surgical procedure sufficed in more than two thirds of the 64 consecutive patients with necrotizing pancreatitis (56% of whom had infected necrosis) who underwent surgery using this technique between 1990 and 1996. A second surgical procedure was required in only 17% of patients, and additional percutaneous drainage of residual or recurrent collections in 20% (23). This positive experience parallels a trend seen with comparable techniques elsewhere (194–196) and may be attributed not only to the improvement in intensive care medicine and imaging techniques but also to this thoughtful approach regarding timing, adequate débridement, and drainage.

An extended period of irrigation or programmed relaparotomies with open lavage may be indicated for those patients who have to undergo surgery early and in whom sufficient débridement cannot be achieved at the first operation.

CLOSED LAVAGE
The concept behind this technique advocated by Beger et al. (194) is that (local) lavage is more effective than drains alone in facilitating the egress of sloughed material. Thus, the cavity is continuously irrigated with saline for up to several weeks (me-

dian 25 days), usually until the return no longer contains debris or increased quantities of pancreatic enzymes. Results with this technique are comparable with those of our series (194–196).

OPEN PACKING
The concept of the open packing of pancreatic necrosis (168, 181,197–199) is based on the tendency of the necrotizing process to continue and spread, involving and destroying more tissue, and on the inability to define the extent of the damage and to safely débride at the primary operation. The packs are changed every day or two, which requires repeated surgery under general anesthesia. Wound management may be eased by using a zipper sewn to the abdominal wall (168,198). Later, as the wound defines and granulates, the packing may be changed with the patient under sedation in the intensive care unit. A few groups have reported better salvage in the difficult subset of pancreatic infections with early fulminant presentation. Current mortality rates for these patients are down to 9% to 22% (168,181,200). Open packing with repeated changes has the disadvantage of multiple procedures and perhaps a higher incidence of postoperative enteric fistulas and abdominal wall hernias (181).

Postinterventional Complications and Their Management

Débridement of pancreatic necrosis (whether infected or not) is associated with significant postsurgical complications (Table 91.8) and mortality rates of up to 50% (168,169,181,201). Death from infected pancreatic necrosis and abscesses is principally caused by a combination of the ongoing necrotizing process, uncontrolled sepsis, hemorrhage, and multiple organ failure (18,23,70,168). A recent series did not confirm previous reports that patients who underwent surgery for infected necrosis develop more complications and have a higher mortality than those with sterile necrosis (23,168). Differences in outcome appear to be mainly due to presurgical disease severity requiring more frequent and earlier surgery in patients with infected necrosis compared to those with sterile necrosis (see earlier section on Indication and Timing)

RECURRENT ABSCESSES
Recurrent abscesses, which in some cases may be additional abscesses missed in the first procedure, have been described in 30% to 40% in earlier series (8,202,203). We and others have found that a technique of thorough abdominal exploration and débridement reduces the rate of this complication to 13% to 16% (18,23,168). Although the principal strategy should still consist of surgical drainage, percutaneous catheter drainage can be beneficial here as an adjunct therapeutic tool, if directed toward small additional abscesses, in which surgical access is hazardous due to previous operations (18,187,189–192).

BLEEDING
Intraoperative bleeding most likely results from decompression of necrotic vessels or vascular trauma caused by the débridement and is best controlled by packing if direct ligation is difficult. Serious problems can arise from hemorrhage at later stages due to difficulties in surgical access and localization of the bleeding source. Transcatheter arterial embolization or balloon occlusion has proved to be beneficial with regard to the temporary control of bleeding and allows reexploration, débridement, and repacking under more favorable conditions (18,23,168,204,205). In our latest series, we experienced massive intraoperative hemorrhage in 6% of patients and postoperative bleeding in 3% (23). Other series have reported incidences of 18% to 26% (168,199,201,206).

TABLE 91.8. Complications after Surgical Débridement of Pancreatic Necrosis

Complications	Period 1974–1983 (n = 45 patients)		Period 1990–1996 (n = 64 patients)	
	No.	%	No.	%
Hemorrhage	10	22	2	3
GI bleeding	0	0	3	5
Pancreatic fistula	14	31	34	53
Enteric fistulas	5	11	10	16
Biliary fistula	0	0	1	
Splenic vein thrombosis	1	2	0	
Wound infection	6	13	9	14
Wound deshiscence/hernia	1	2	1	
Systemic sepsis	8	18		
Renal failure	4	9	2	3
Respiratory failure, ARDS	3	7	3	5
Pulmonary emboli	1	2	1	
Pneumonia	9	20	1	
Endocarditis	0	0	1	
Diabetes mellitus	3	7	6	9
Exocrine insufficiency	n.d.		16	25
Total no. of deaths	11	24	4	6

GI, gastrointestinal; ARDS, adult respiratory distress syndrome; n.d., not determined.

PANCREATIC FISTULAS

The prevalence of fistulas occurring after débriding pancreatic necrosis and abscesses is as high as 50% even in recent series (12,18,168,181,207–210) (Table 91.8). They develop presumably because of a combined effect of enzymatic digestion and local ischemia due to small vessel thrombosis (210). Direct injury by the surgeon or the drains is also a possibility. More than 50% of these fistulas are reported to close spontaneously within weeks or months (18,23,168,210), but persistence may indicate an isolated pancreatic segment, usually the tail, which later requires resection or closure with a jejunal Roux-en-Y loop (210). In our recent series, all patients with pancreatic fistulas went home with drains in the surgical site and were treated conservatively (sometimes with adjunctive octreotide) with gradual drain advancement. Only 9% required surgical closure (23).

ENTERIC FISTULAS AND COLON INJURY

The incidence of enteric fistulas varies from 4% to 35% (23, 168,181,201,206,207,211–214). Although some may heal spontaneously if they are small and well channeled, colocutaneous fistulas usually require a proximal colostomy to help control sepsis, a subsequent segmental resection of the damaged colon, and later reanastomosis. Healing of lesser colon injuries may lead to a symptomatic stenosis that requires resection. Duodenal fistulas often do not heal spontaneously and may require internal drainage into a Roux-en-Y jejunal loop or even pancreatoduodenectomy. Gastric fistulas have additional potential for major hemorrhage, possibly due to digestion by high-volume acid output. Some gastric fistulas close, but it has been recommended that gastric resection and reconstruction be undertaken after 4 weeks of unsuccessful waiting (211–214).

REFERENCES

1. Bradley EL. A clinically based classification system for acute pancreatitis. *Arch Surg* 1993;128:586–590.
2. Kune GA, King R. The late complications of acute pancreatitis: pancreatic swelling, cyst and abscess. *Med J Aust* 1973;1:1241–1246.
3. Warshaw AL. Inflammatory masses following acute pancreatitis. Phlegmon, pseudocyst, and abscess. *Surg Clin North Am* 1974;54:621–634.
4. Sostre CF, Flournoy JG, Bova JG, et al. Pancreatic phlegmon. Clinical features and course. *Dig Dis Sci* 1985;30:918–927.
5. Gerzof SG, Banks PA, Robbins AH, et al. Early diagnosis of pancreatic infection by computed tomography-guided aspiration. *Gastroenterology* 1987;93:1315–1320.
6. Colhoun E, Murphy JJ, MacEarlean DP. Percutaneous drainage of pancreatic pseudocysts. *Br J Surg* 1984;71:131–132.
7. Glazer G, Dudley HAP. Pancreatic abscess: an incomplete descriptive phrase. *Br J Surg* 1984;71:401.
8. Warshaw AL. Pancreatic abscesses. *N Engl J Med* 1972;287:1234–1236.
9. Beger HG, Bittner R, Block S, et al. Bacterial contamination of pancreatic necrosis. A prospective clinical study. *Gastroenterology* 1986;91:433–438.
10. Bittner R, Block S, Buechler M, et al. Pancreatic abscess and infected pancreatic necrosis. Different local septic complications in acute pancreatitis. *Dig Dis Sci* 1987;32:1082–1087.
11. Warshaw AL. Lowering the level of uncertainty in late pancreatitis. *Gastroenterology* 1987;93:1434–1437.
12. Renner IG, Savage WT III, Pantoja JL, et al. Death due to acute pancreatitis. A retrospective analysis of 405 autopsy cases. *Dig Dis Sci* 1985;30:1005–1018.
13. Becker JM, Pemberton JH, DiMagno EP, et al. Prognostic factors in pancreatic abscess. *Surgery* 1984;96:455–461.
14. Allardyce DB. Incidence of necrotizing pancreatitis and factors related to mortality. *Am J Surg* 1987;154:295–299.
15. Donahue PE, Nyhus LM, Baker RJ. Pancreatic abscess after alcoholic pancreatitis. *Arch Surg* 1980;115:905–909.
16. Ranson JHC, Spencer FC. Prevention, diagnosis, and treatment of pancreatic abscess. *Surgery* 1977;82:99–106.
17. Appelros S, Lindgren S, Borgstrom A. Short and long term outcome of severe acute pancreatitis. *Eur J Surg* 2001;167:281–286
18. Warshaw AL, Jin G. Improved survival in 45 patients with pancreatic abscess. *Ann Surg* 1985;202:408–417.
19. Ranson JHC. Acute pancreatitis. *Curr Probl Surg* 1997;16:1–84.
20. Widdison AL, Karanjia ND. Pancreatic infection complicating acute pancreatitis. *Br J Surg* 1993;80:148–154.
21. Banks PA, Gerzof SG, Chong FK, et al. Bacteriologic status of necrotic tissue in necrotizing pancreatitis. *Pancreas* 1990;5:330–333.
22. Bassi C, Falconi M, Girelli R, et al. Microbiological findings in severe pancreatitis. *Surg Res Commun* 1989;5:1–4.
23. Fernandez-del Castillo C, Rattner DW, Makary MA, et al. Debridement and closed packing for the treatment of necrotizing pancreatitis. *Ann Surg* 1998;228:676–684.
24. Gloor B, Muller CA, Worni M, et al. Pancreatic infection in severe pancreatitis: the role of fungus and multiresistant organisms. *Arch Surg* 2001;136:592–596.

25. Robbins EG, Sollman NH, Bierman P, et al. Pancreatic fungal infections: a case report and review of the literature. *Pancreas* 1996;12:308–312.

26. Luiten EJ, Hop WC, Lange JF, et al. Differential prognosis of gram-negative versus gram-positive infected and sterile pancreatic necrosis: results of a randomized trial in patients with severe acute pancreatitis treated with adjuvant selective decontamination. *Clin Infect Dis* 1997;25:811–816.

27. Luiten EJ, Hop WC, Endtz HP, et al. Prognostic importance of gram-negative intestinal colonization preceding pancreatic infection in severe acute pancreatitis. Results of a controlled clinical trial of selective decontamination. *Intens Care Med* 1998;24:438–445.

28. Gewe M, Tsiotos GG, Luque de-Leon E, et al. Fungal infection in acute necrotizing pancreatitis. *J Am Coll Surg* 1999;188:408–414.

29. Richter JM, Jacoby GA, Schapiro RH, et al. Pancreatic abscess due to *Candida albicans. Ann Intern Med* 1982;97:221–222.

30. Howard JM, Bieluch VB. Pancreatic abscess secondary to *Candida albicans. Pancreas* 1989;4:120–122.

31. Stambler JB, Kilbaner MI, Bliss CM, et al. Tuberculous abscess of the pancreas. *Gastroenterology* 1982;83:922–925.

32. Khuroo MS. Hepatobiliary and pancreatic ascariasis. *Ind J Gastroenterol* 2001;20(suppl 1):C28–C32.

33. Keaveny AP, Karasik MS. Hepatobiliary and pancreatic infections in AIDS: Part I. *AIDS Patient Care STDS* 1998;12:347–357.

34. Keaveny AP, Karasik MS. Hepatobiliary and pancreatic infections in AIDS: Part II. *AIDS Patient Care STDS* 1998;12:451–456.

35. Senninger N, Moody FG, Coelho JC, et al. The role of biliary obstruction in the pathogenesis of acute pancreatitis in the opossum. *Surgery* 1986;99:688–693.

36. Foitzik T, Mithöfer K, Ferraro MJ, et al. Time course of bacterial infection of the pancreas and its relation to disease severity in a rodent model of acute necrotizing pancreatitis. *Ann Surg* 1994;220:193–198.

37. Hansson K. Experimental and clinical studies in aetiologic role of bile reflux in acute pancreatitis. *Arch Chir Scand Suppl* 1967;375:102.

38. Widdison AL, Karanjia ND, Reber HA. Routes of spread of pathogens into the pancreas in a feline model of acute pancreatitis. *Gut* 1994;35:1306–1310.

39. Medich DS, Lee TK, Melhem MF. Pathogenesis of pancreatic sepsis. *Am J Surg* 1993;165:46–52.

40. Cicalese L, Sahai A, Sileri P, et al. Acute pancreatitis and bacterial translocation. *Dig Dis Sci* 2001;46:1127–1132.

41. Kazantsev GB, Hecht DW, Rao R, et al. Plasmid labeling confirms bacterial translocation in pancreatitis. *Am J Surg* 1994;167:201–207.

42. Foitzik T, Fernández-del Castillo C, Ferraro MJ, et al. Pathogenesis and prevention of early pancreatic infection in experimental acute necrotizing pancreas. *Ann Surg* 1995;222:179–185.

43. Runkel NS, Rodriguez LF, Moody FG. Mechanisms of sepsis in acute pancreatitis in opossums. *Am J Surg* 1995;169:227–232.

44. Runkel NS, Moody FG, Smith GS, et al. The role of the gut in the development of sepsis in acute pancreatitis. *J Surg Res* 1991;51:18–23.

45. Deitch EA. The role of intestinal barrier failure and bacterial translocation in the development of systemic infection and multiple organ failure. *Arch Surg* 1990;125:403–404.

46. Foitzik T, Stufler M, Hotz HG, et al. Glutamine stabilizes intestinal permeability and reduces pancreatic infection in acute experimental pancreatitis. *J Gastrointest Surg* 1997;1:40–47.

47. Hotz HG, Foitzik T, Rohweder J, et al. Intestinal microcirculation and gut permeability in acute pancreatitis: early changes and therapeutic implications. *J Gastrointest Surg* 1998;2:518–525.

48. Ryan CM, Schmidt J, Lewandrowski K, et al. Gut macromolecular permeability in pancreatitis correlates with severity of disease in rats. *Gastroenterology* 1993;104:890–895.

49. Ammori BJ, Leeder PC, King RF, et al. Early increase in intestinal permeability in patients with severe acute pancreatitis: correlation with endotoxemia, organ failure, and mortality. *J Gastrointest Surg* 1999;3:252–262.

50. Ruokonen E, Uusaro A, Alhava E, et al. The effect of dobutamine infusion on splanchnic blood flow and oxygen transport in patients with acute pancreatitis. *Intens Care Med* 1997;23:732–737.

51. Krzewicki J. Disturbances of blood flow in the large bowel during acute pancreatitis. *Wiad Lek* 1989;42:330–333.

52. Foitzik T, Eibl G, Hotz HG, et al. Endothelin receptor blockade in severe acute pancreatitis leads to systemic enhancement of microcirculation, stabilization of capillary permeability, and improved survival rates. *Surgery* 2000;128:399–407.

53. Runkel NS, Moody FG, Smith GS, et al. Alterations in rat intestinal transit by morphine promote bacterial translocation. *Dig Dis Sci* 1993;38:1530–1536.

54. Leveau P, Wang X, Soltesz V, et al. Alterations in intestinal motility and microflora in experimental acute pancreatitis. *Int J Pancreatol* 1996;20:119–125.

55. Gianotti L, Solomkin JS, Munda R, et al. Failure of local and systemic bacterial clearance in rats with acute pancreatitis. *Pancreas* 1995;10:78–84.

56. Curley PJ. Endotoxin, cellular immune dysfunction and acute pancreatitis. *Ann R Coll Surg Engl* 1996;78:531–535.

57. Buttenschoen K, Berger D, Hiki N, et al. Endotoxin and antiendotoxin antibodies in patients with acute pancreatitis. *Eur J Surg* 2000;166:459–466.

58. Forgacs B, Wudel E, Franke J, et al. Impairment of RES-function early in acute pancreatitis [Abstract]. *Pancreas* 1998;17:433.

59. Beger HG, Block S, Bittner R. The significance of bacterial infection in acute pancreatitis. In: Beger HG, Büchler M, eds. *Acute pancreatitis*. Berlin: Springer, 1987:79–86.

60. Webster MW, Pasculle AW, Myerowitz RL, et al. Postinduction bacteremia in experimental acute pancreatitis. *Am J Surg* 1979;138:418–420.

61. Hanke E, Marklien G. Bacterial contamination of the pancreas with intestinal germs: A cause of acute suppurative pancreatitis? In: Beger HG, Büchler M, eds. *Acute pancreatitis*. Berlin: Springer, 1987:87–89.

62. Semsch B, Heitz G, Berger G, et al. Influence of *E. coli* on the course of acute pancreatitis in mini pigs. In: Beger HG, Büchler M, eds. *Acute pancreatitis*. Berlin: Springer, 1987:90–99.

63. Tarpila E, Nystrom PO, Franzen L, et al. Bacterial translocation during acute pancreatitis in rats. *Eur J Surg* 1993;159:109–115.

64. Arendt T, Nizze H, Stuber E, et al. Infected bile-induced acute pancreatitis in rabbits. The role of bacteria. *Int J Pancreatol* 1998;24:111–116.

65. Iglehart JD, Mansback C, Postlethewait R, et al. Pancreaticobronchial fistula: case report and review of the literature. *Gastroenterology* 1986;90:759–763.

66. Balazs A, Lukovich P, Flautner L. A case of retroperitoneal pancreatic abscess spreading to the femoral region. *Orv Hetil* 2000;141:241–244.

67. Fink AS, Hiatt JR, Pitt HA, et al. Indolent presentation of pancreatic abscess. Experience with 100 cases. *Arch Surg* 1988;123:1067–1072.

68. American College of Chest Physicians/Society of Critical Care Medicine Consensus Conference. Definitions for sepsis and organ failure guidelines for the use of innovative therapies in sepsis. *Crit Care Med* 1992;20:864–874.

69. Block S, Buchler M, Bittner R, et al. Sepsis indicators in acute pancreatitis. *Pancreas* 1987;2:499–505.

70. Malangoni MA, Richardson JD, Shallcross JC, et al. Factors contributing to fatal outcome after treatment of pancreatic abscess. *Ann Surg* 1986;203:605–613.

71. White EM, Wittenberg J, Mueller PR, et al. Pancreatic necrosis: CT manifestations. *Radiology* 1986;158:343–346.

72. Beger HG, Bittner R, Buchler M, et al. Hemodynamic data pattern in patients with acute pancreatitis. *Gastroenterology* 1986;90:74–79.

73. Ranson JHC, Rifkind KM, Turner JW. Prognostic signs and nonoperative peritoneal lavage in acute pancreatitis. *Surg Gynecol Obstet* 1976;143:209–219.

74. Wilson C, Heads A, Shenkin A, et al. C-reactive protein, antiproteases and complement factors as objective markers of severity in acute pancreatitis. *Br J Surg* 1989;76:177–181.

75. Büchler M, Malfertheiner P, Schoetensack C, et al. Sensitivity of antiproteases, complement factors and C-reactive protein in detecting pancreatic necrosis. Results of a prospective clinical study. *Int J Pancreatol* 1986;1:227–235.

76. Mayer AD, McMahon MJ, Bowen M, et al. C-reactive protein: an aid to assessment and monitoring of acute pancreatitis. *J Clin Pathol* 1984;37:207–211.

77. Puolakkainen P, Valtonen V, Paananen A, et al. C-reactive protein (CRP) and serum phospholipase A2 in the assessment of the severity of acute pancreatitis. *Gut* 1987;28:764–771.

78. Mandi Y, Farkas G, Takacs T, et al. Diagnostic relevance of procalcitonin, IL-6, and sICAM-1 in the prediction of infected necrosis in acute pancreatitis. *Int J Pancreatol* 2000;28:41–49.

79. Block S, Maier W, Bittner R, et al. Identification of pancreas necrosis in severe acute pancreatitis: Imaging procedures versus clinical staging. *Gut* 1986;27:1035–1045.

80. Saxon A, Reynolds JT, Doolas A. Management of pancreatic abscesses. *Ann Surg* 1981;194:545–552.

81. Jeffrey RB, Federle MP, Cello JP, et al. Early computed tomography in severe acute pancreatitis. *Surg Gynecol Obstet* 1982;154:170–174.

82. Siegelman SS, Copeland BE, Saba GP, et al. CT of fluid collections associated with pancreatitis. *AJR* 1980;134:1121–1132.

83. Federle MP, Jeffrey RB, Crass RA, et al. Computed tomography of pancreatic abscesses. *AJR* 1981;136:879–882.

84. White M, Simeone JF, Wittenberg J. Air within a pancreatic inflammatory mass: not necessarily a sign of abscess. *J Clin Gastroenterol* 1983;5:173–175.

85. Clavien PA, Hauser H, Meyer P, et al. Value of contrast-enhanced computerized tomography in the early diagnosis and prognosis of acute pancreatitis. A prospective study of 202 patients. *Am J Surg* 1988;155:457–466.

86. Balthazar EJ, Ranson JHC, Naidich DP, et al. Acute pancreatitis: prognostic value of CT. *Radiology* 1985;156:767–772.

87. Ranson JHC, Balthazar E, Caccavale R, et al. Computed tomography and the prediction of pancreatic abscess in acute pancreatitis. *Ann Surg* 1985;201:656–665.

88. Vernacchia FS, Jeffrey RB Jr, Federle MP, et al. Pancreatic abscess: predictive value of early abdominal CT. *Radiology* 1987;162:435–438.

89. London NJM, Neoptolemos JP, Lavelle J, et al. Contrast-enhanced abdominal computed tomography scanning and prediction of severity of acute pancreatitis: a prospective study. *Br J Surg* 1989;76:268–272.

90. Bradley EL, Murphy F, Ferguson C. Prediction of pancreatic necrosis by dynamic pancreatography. *Ann Surg* 1989;210:495–504.

91. Nuutinen P. Contrast-enhanced computed tomography in acute oedematous pancreatitis. *Surg Res Commun* 1987;1:251.

92. Schroder T, Kivisaari L, Standertskjold-Nordenstam CG, et al. The clinical significance of contrast-enhanced computed tomography in acute pancreatitis. *Ann Chir Gynaecol* 1984;73:268–272.

93. Kivisaari L, Somer K, Standertskjold-Nordenstam CG, et al. A new method for the diagnosis of acute hemorrhagic-necrotizing pancreatitis using contrast-enhanced CT. *Gastrointest Radiol* 1984;9:27–30.

94. Nuutinen P, Kivisaari L, Standertskjold-Nordenstam CG, et al. Microangiography of the pancreas in experimental hemorrhagic pancreatitis. *Eur J Radiol* 1986;6:187–190.

95. Nuutinen P, Kivisaari L, Schroder T. Contrast-enhanced computed tomography and microangiography of the pancreas in acute human hemorrhagic/necrotizing pancreatitis. *Pancreas* 1988;3:53–60.

96. Lund G, Einzig S, Rysavy J, et al. Role of ischemia in contrast-induced renal damage. *Circulation* 1984;69:783–789.

97. Schmidt J, Hotz HG, Foitzik TH, et al. Intravenous contrast medium aggravates the impairment of pancreatic microcirculation in necrotizing pancreatitis in the rat. *Ann Surg* 1995;221:257–264.

98. Foitzik TH, Bassi DG, Schmidt J, et al. Intravenous contrast medium accentuates the severity of acute necrotizing pancreatitis in the rat. *Gastroenterology* 1994;106:207–214.

99. Foitzik TH, Bassi DG, Fernández-del Castillo C, et al. Intravenous contrast medium impairs oxygenation of the pancreas in acute necrotizing pancreatitis in the rat. *Arch Surg* 1994;129:706–711.

100. McMenamin DA, Gates LK Jr. A retrospective analysis of the effect of contrast-enhanced CT on the outcome of acute pancreatitis. *Am J Gastroenterol* 1996;91:1384–1387.

101. Carmona-Sanchez R, Uscanda L, Bezaury-Rivas P, et al. Potential harmful effect of iodinated intravenous contrast medium on the clinical course of mild acute pancreatitis. *Arch Surg* 2000;135:1280–1284.

102. Robinson PJ, Sheridan MB. Pancreatitis: computed tomography and magnetic resonance imaging. *Eur Radiol* 2000;10:401–408.

103. Piironen A, Kivisaari R, Kemppainen E, et al. Detection of severe acute pancreatitis by contrast-enhanced magnetic resonance imaging. *Eur Radiol* 2000;10:354–361.

104. Werner J, Schmidt J, Warshaw AL, et al. The relative safety of MRI contrast agent in acute necrotizing pancreatitis. *Ann Surg* 1998;227:105–111.

105. Terzi C, Sokmen S. Acute pancreatitis induced by magnetic-resonance-imaging contrast agent. *Lancet* 1999;354:1789–1790.

106. Hiatt JR, Fink AS, King W III, et al. Percutaneous aspiration of peripancreatic fluid collections: a safe method to detect infection. *Surgery* 1987;101:523–530.

107. Rau B, Pralle U, Mayer JM, et al. Role of ultrasonographically guide fine-needle aspiration cytology in the diagnosis of infected pancreatic necrosis. *Br J Surg* 1998;85:179–184.

108. Malecka-Panas E, Juszynski A, Chrzastek J, et al. Pancreatic fluid collections: diagnostic and therapeutic implications of percutaneous drainage guide by ultrasound. *Hepatogastroenterology* 1998;45:873–878.

109. Popper HL, Necheles H, Russel KC: Transition of pancreatic edema into pancreatic necrosis. *Surg Gynecol Obstet* 1948;87:79.

110. Pfeffer RB, Lazzarini-Robertson A, Safadi D, et al. Gradations of pancreatitis edematous through hemorrhagic, experimentally produced by controlled injection of microspheres into blood vessels in dogs. *Surgery* 1992;51:764–769.

111. Warshaw AL, O'Hara PJ. Susceptibility of the pancreas to ischemic injury in shock. *Ann Surg*, 1978;188:197–201.

112. Klar E, Messmer K, Warshaw AL, et al. Pancreatic ischaemia in experimental acute pancreatitis: mechanism, significance and therapy. *Br J Surg* 1990;77:1205–1210.

113. Klar E, Rattner DW, Compton C, et al. Adverse effect of therapeutic vasoconstrictors in experimental acute pancreatitis. *Ann Surg* 1991;214:168–174.

114. Klar E, Herfarth CH, Messmer K. Therapeutic effect of isovolemic hemodilution with dextran 60 on the impairment of pancreatic microcirculation in acute biliary pancreatitis. *Ann Surg* 1990;211:346–353.

115. Foitzik T, Faulhaber J, Hotz HG, et al. Endothelin receptor blockade improves fluid sequestration, pancreatic capillary blood flow, and survival in severe experimental pancreatitis. *Ann Surg* 1998;22:670–675.

116. Schmidt J, Fernandez-del Casillon C, Rattner DW, et al. Hyperoncotic ultra-high molecular weight dextran solutions reduce trypsinogen activation, prevent acinar necrosis, and lower mortality in rodent pancreatitis. *Am J Surg* 1993;165:40–45.

117. Isenmann R, Büchler B, Uhl W, et al. Pancreatic necrosis: an early finding in severe acute pancreatitis. *Pancreas* 1993;8:358–361.

118. Steinberg WM, Schlesselman SE. Treatment of acute pancreatitis. Comparison of animal and human studies. *Gastroenterology* 1987;93:1420–1427.

119. Niederau C. Experimentelle Therapieansätze bei akuter Pankreatitis. In: Mössner J, Adler G, Fölsch UR, et al., eds. *Erkrankungen des exkretorischen Pankreas*. Jena: G. Fischer, 1995:293–302.

120. Foitzik T, Eibl G, Buhr HJ. Therapy for microcirculatory disorders in severe acute pancreatitis: comparison of delayed therapy with ICAM-1 antibodies and a specific endothelin A receptor antagonist. *J Gastrointestinal Surg* 2000;4:240–246.

121. Eibl G, Foitzik T, Forgacs B, et al. Reduktion sekundärer Pankreasinfektionen bei akuter Pankreatitis durch Verbesserung der intestinalen Mikrozirkulation. *Langenbecks Arch Chir* 1999;(suppl 1):33–36.

122. Forgacs B, Eibl G, Wudel E, et al. RES function and liver microcirculation in the early stage of acute experimental pancreatitis. *Hepatogastroenterology* 2001 (in press).

123. Foitzik T, Eibl G, Hotz B, et al. Persistent multiple organ microcirculatory disorders in severe acute pancreatitis. *Dig Dis Sci* 2001 (in press).

124. Kirckpatrick CJ, Bittinger F, Klein CL, et al. The role of the microcirculation in multiple organ dysfunction syndrome (MODS): a review and perspective. *Virchows Arch* 1996;427:461–476.

125. Gullo A, Berlot G. Ingredients of organ dysfunction or failure. *World J Surg* 1996;20:430–436.

126. Luiten EJ, Hop WC, Lange JF, et al. Controlled clinical trial of selective decontamination for the treatment of severe acute pancreatitis. *Ann Surg* 1995;222:57–65.

127. Van der Waaij D, Manson WL, Arends JP, et al. Clinical use of selective decontamination: the concept. *Intens Care Med* 1990;16(suppl 3):212–216.

128. Stoutenbeek CP. The role of systemic antibiotic prophylaxis in infection prevention in intensive care by selective decontamination of the digestive tract (SDD). *Infection* 1989;17:418–421.

129. Jackson RJ, Smith SD, Rowe MI. Selective bowel decontamination results in gram-positive translocation. *J Surg Res* 1990;48:444–447.

130. Sahin M, Yol S, Ciftci E, et al. Does large bowel enema reduce septic complications in acute pancreatitis. *Am J Surg* 1998;176:331–334.

131. Yol S, Ozer S, Aksoy F, et al. Whole gut washout ameliorates the progression of acute experimental pancreatitis. *Am J Surg* 2000;180:121–125.

132. Horn J. Ileostoma as part of a surgical therapy concept in acute pancreatitis. *Chirurgie* 1983;54:320–322.

133. Denham W, Norman J. The potential role of therapeutic cytokine manipulation in acute pancreatitis. *Surg Clin North Am* 1999;79:767–781.

134. Denham W, Fink G, Yang J, et al. Small molecule inhibition of tumor necrosis factor gene processing during acute pancreatitis prevents cytokine cascade progression and attenuates pancreatitis severity. *Am Surg* 1997;63:1045–1050.

135. Messmer K. Hemodilution—possibilities and safety aspects. *Acta Anaesthesiol Scand* 1988;89(suppl):49–53.

136. Klar E, Foitzik T, Buhr HJ, et al. Isovolemic hemodilution with dextran 60 as treatment of pancreatic ischemia in acute pancreatitis. *Ann Surg* 1993;217:369–374.

137. Foitzik T, Eibl G, Kahrau S, et al. Nachweis persistierender systemischer Mikrozirkulationsstörungen bei der akuten Pankreatitis—Ansatz für neue Therapiekonzepte. *Langenbecks Arch Chir* 2000;29(suppl 1):595–599.

138. Kalfarentzos F, Kehagias J, Mead N, et al. Enteral nutrition is superior to parenteral nutrition in severe acute pancreatitis. Results of a randomized pospective trial. *Br J Surg* 1997;84:1665–1669.

139. Powell JJ, Murchison JT, Fearon KC, et al. Randomized clinical trial: randomized controlled trial of the effect of early enteral nutrition on markers of the inflammatory response in predicted severe acute pancreatitis. *Br J Surg* 2000;87:1385–1381.

140. Olah A, Pardavi G, Belagyi T. Early jejunal feeding in acute pancreatitis: prevention of septic complications and multiorgan failure. *Magy Seb* 2000;53:7–12.

141. Lehocky P, Sarr MG. Early enteral feeding in severe acute pancreatitis: can it prevent secondary pancreatic (super) infection? *Dig Surg* 2000;17:571–577.

142. Alexander JW. Bacterial translocation during enteral and parenteral nutrition [Review]. *Proc Nutr Soc* 1998;57:389–393.

143. Deitch EA, Xu D, Naruhn MB, et al. Elemental diet and i.v. TPN-induced bacterial transocation is associated with loss of intestinal mucosal barrier function against bacteria. *Ann Surg* 1995;221:299–307.

144. Kueppers PM, Miller TA, Chen CY, et al. Effect of total parenteral nutrition plus morphine on bacterial translocation. *Ann Surg* 1993;217:286–292.

145. Gianotti L, Alexander JW, Gennari R, et al. Oral glutamine decreases bacterial translocation and improves survival in experimental gut origin sepsis. *JPEN* 1995;19:69–74.

146. Wernermann J, Hammarqvist F. Glutamine: a necessary nutrient for the intensive care patient. *Int J Colorectal Dis* 1999;14:137–142.

147. Roth E. Die Bedeutung des Glutamins in der Intensivmedizin. *Intensivmed* 1997;34:91–100.

148. Finch WT, Sawyers JL, Schenker SA. A prospective study to determine the efficacy of antibiotics in acute pancreatitis. *Ann Surg* 1976;183:667–671.

149. Craig RM, Dordal E, Myles L. The use of ampicillin in acute pancreatitis. *Ann Intern Med* 1975;83:831–832.

150. Bassi C, Pederzoli P, Vesentini S. Behavior of antibiotics during human necrotizing pancreatitis. *Antimicrob Agents Chemother* 1994;38:830–836.

151. Büchler M, Malfertheiner P, Friess H. Human pancreatic tissue concentration of bactericidal antibiotics. *Gastroenterology* 1992;103:1902–1908.

152. Mithöfer K, Fernández-del Castillo C, Ferraro MJ, et al. Antibiotic treatment improves survival in experimental acute necrotizing pancreatitis. *Gastroenterology* 1996;110:232–240.

153. Pederzoli P, Bassi C, Vesentini S, et al. A randomized multicenter clinical trial of antibiotic prophylaxis of septic complications in acute necrotizing pancreatitis with imipenem. *Surg Gynecol Obstet* 1993;176:480–483.

154. Sainio V, Kemppainen E, Puolakkainen P, et al. Early antibiotic treatment in acute necrotising pancreatitis. *Lancet* 1995;346:663–667.

155. Schwarz M, Isenmann R, Meyer H, et al. Antibiotic use in necrotizing pancreatitis. Results of a control study. *Dtsch Med Wochenschr* 1997;122:356–361.

156. Nordback I, Sand J, Saaristo R, et al. Early treatment with antibiotics reduces the need for surgery in acute necrotizing pancreatitis—a single-center randomized study. *J Gastrointest Surg* 2001;5:113–120.

157. Sharma VK, Howden CW. Prophylactic antibiotic administration reduces sepsis and mortality in acute necrotizing pancreatitis: a meta-analysis. *Pancreas* 2001;17:571–577.

158. Aldidge MC, Ornstein M, Glazar G, et al. Pancreatic resection for severe acute pancreatitis. *Br J Surg* 1985;72:796–800.

159. Alexandre JH, Guerrieri MT. Role of total pancreatectomy in the treatment of necrotizing pancreatitis. *World J Surg* 1981;5:369–377.

160. Kivilaakso E, Fraki O, Nikki P, et al. Resection of the pancreas for acute fulminant pancreatitis. *Surg Gynecol Obstet* 1981;151:493–498.

161. Norton L, Eisemann B. Near-total pancreatectomy for hemorrhagic pancreatitis. *Am J Surg* 1974;127:191–195.

162. McFadden DW, Reber HA. Indications for surgery in severe acute pancreatitis. *Int J Pancreatol* 1994;15:83–90.

163. Bradley EL III. Indications for debridement of necrotizing pancreatitis. *Pancreas* 1996;13:219–223.

164. Fernández-del Castillo, Warshaw AL. Parenchymal necrosis: infection and other indications for debridement and drainage. *Chirurgie* 2000;71:269–273.

165. Büchler P, Reber A. Surgical approach in patients with acute pancreatitis. Is infected or sterile necrosis an indication-in whom should this be done, when, and why? *Gastroenterol Clin North Am* 1999;28:661–671.

166. Schoenberg MH, Rau B, Beger HG. New approaches in surgical management of severe acute pancreatitis. *Digestion* 1999;60(suppl 1):22–26.

167. Tenner S, Sica G, Hughes M, et al. Relationship of necrosis to organ failure in severe acute pancreatitis. *Gastroenterology* 1997;113:899–903.

168. Tsiotos GG, Lugue-de León E, Söreide JA, et al. Management of necrotizing pancreatitis by repeated operative necrosectomy using a zipper technique. *Am J Surg* 1998;175:91–97.

169. Mier J, Lugue-de León E, Castillo A, et al. Early versus late necrosectomy in severe necrotizing pancreatitis. *Am J Surg* 1997;173:71–75.

170. Rattner DW, Legermate DA, Lee MJ, et al. Early surgical debridement of symptomatic pancreatic necrosis is beneficial irrespective of infection. *Am J Surg* 1992;163:105–110.

171. Foitzik T, Klar E, Runkel N, et al. Stellenwert der Klassifikation für die Therapie und Prognose der akuten Pankreatitis. Analyse des Krankengutes der Chirurgischen Klinik Heidelberg 1986–1989. *Chirurgie* 1991;62:486–492.

172. Foitzik T, Klar E, Buhr HJ, et al. Improved survival in acute necrotizing pancreatitis despite limiting the indications for surgical debridement. *Eur J Surg* 1995;161:187–192.

173. Gebhardt Ch, Bödeker H, Blinzler D, et al. Wandel in der Therapie der schweren akuten Pankreatitis. *Chirurgie* 1994;65:33–41.

174. Pederzoli P, Bassi C, Vesentini S, et al. Necrosectomy by lavage in the surgical treatment of severe necrotizing pancreatitis. *Acta Chir Scand* 1990;156:775–780.

175. Rau B, Pralle U, Uhl W, et al. Management of sterile necrosis in instances of severe acute pancreatitis. *J Am Coll Surg* 1995;181:279–288.

176. Rau B, Pralle U, Schoenberg MH, et al. Nonsurgical treatment of necrotizing pancreatitis. Is there a rationale in patients with infected necrosis? [Abstract]. *Pancreas* 1997;15:452.

177. Uomo G, Visconti M, Manes G, et al. Nonsurgical treatment of acute necrotizing pancreatitis. *Pancreas* 1996;12:142–148.

178. Büchler MW, Gloor B, Müller CA, et al. Acute necrotizing pancreatitis: treatment strategy according to the status of infection. *Ann Surg* 2000;232:619–626.

179. Rünzi M, Layer P. Nonsurgical management of acute pancreatitis. Use of antibiotics. *Surg Clin North Am* 1999;79:759–765.

180. Baril NB, Ralls PW, Wren SM, et al. Does an infected peripancreatic fluid collection or abscess mandate operation? *Ann Surg* 2000;231:361–367.

181. Bradley EL. Management of infected pancreatic necrosis by open drainage. *Ann Surg* 1987;206:542–550.

182. Foitzik T. Die Indikaion zur Operation der akuten Pankreatitis—ein Streitthema. *Chir Gastroenterol* 1999;15:342–348.

183. Carter CR, McKay CJ, Imrie CW. Percutaneous necrosectomy and sinus tract endoscopy in the management of infected pancreatic necrosis: an initial experience. *Ann Surg* 2000;232:175–180.

184. Gerzof SG, Robbins AH, Johnson WC, et al. Percutaneous catheter drainage of abdominal abscesses: a five-year experience. *N Engl J Med* 1981;305:653–657.

185. Gerzof SG, Johnson WC, Robbins AH, et al. Expanded criteria for percutaneous abscess drainage. *Arch Surg* 1985;120:227–232.

186. Gerzof SG, Johnson WC, Robbins AH, et al. Percutaneous drainage of infected pancreatic pseudocysts. *Arch Surg* 1984;119:888–893.

187. Pickleman J, Moncada R. The role of percutaneous drainage of pancreatic abscess. *Am Surg* 1987;8:451–455.

188. Steiner E, Mueller PR, Hahn PF, et al. Complicated pancreatic abscesses: problems in interventional management. *Radiology* 1988;167:443–446.

189. Lee MJ, Wittich GR, Mueller PR. Percutaneous intervention in acute pancreatitis. *Radiographics* 1998;18:711–724.

190. Gouzi JL, Bloom E, Julio C, et al. Percutaneous drainage of infected pancreatic necrosis: an alternative to surgery. *Chirurgie* 1999;124:31–37.

191. Mithöfer K, Mueller PR, Warshaw AL. Interventional and surgical treatment of pancreatic abscess. *World J Surg* 1997;21:162–168.

192. Walters R, Herman CM, Neff R, et al. Percutaneous drainage of abscesses in the postoperative abdomen that is difficult to explore. *Am J Surg* 1985;149:623–626.

193. Venu RP, Brown RD, Marrero JA, et al. Endoscopic transpapillary drainage of pancreatic abscess: technique and results. *Gastrointest Endosc* 2000;51:391–395.

194. Beger HG, Buchler M, Bittner R, et al. Necrosectomy and postoperative local lavage in necrotizing pancreatitis. *Br J Surg* 1988;75:207–212.

195. Beger HG, Rau B, Isenmann R, Mayer J. Surgical treatment of acute pancreatitis. *Ann Chir Gynecol* 1998;87:183–189.

196. Gloor B, Muller CA, Worni M, et al. Late mortality in patients with severe acute pancreatitis. *Br J Surg* 2001;88:975–979.

197. Bradley EL III. Operative management of acute pancreatitis: ventral open packing. *Hepatogastroenterology* 1991;38:134–138.

198. Garcia-Sabrido JL, Tallado JM, Christou NV, et al. Treatment of severe intraabdominal sepsis and/or necrotic foci by an "open-abdomen" approach. Zipper and zipper-mesh techniques. *Arch Surg* 1988;123:152–156.

199. Sarr MG, Nagorney DM, Mucha P Jr, et al. Acute necrotizing pancreatitis: management by planned, staged pancreatic necrosectomy/debridement and delayed primary wound closure over drains. *Br J Surg* 1991;78:576–581.

200. Branum G, Galloway J, Hirchowitz W, et al. Pancreatic necrosis. Results of necrosectomy, packing, and ultimate closure over drains. *Ann Surg* 1998;227:870–877.

201. Doglietto GB, Gui D, Pacelli F, et al. Open vs. closed treatment of secondary pancreatic infections: a review of 42 cases. *Arch Surg* 1994;129:689–693.

202. Aranha GV, Prinz RA, Greenlee HB. Pancreatic abscess: an unresolved surgical problem. *Am J Surg* 1982;144:534–538.

203. Holden JL, Berne TV, Rossoff L. Pancreatic abscess following acute pancreatitis. *Arch Surg* 1976;111:858–861.

204. Waltman AC, Luers PR, Athanasoulis CA, et al. Massive arterial hemorrhage in patients with pancreatitis. Complementary role of surgery and transcatheter occlusive techniques. *Arch Surg* 1986;121:439–443.

205. Stanten R, Frey CF. Comprehensive management of acute necrotizing pancreatitis and pancreatic abscess. *Arch Surg* 1990;125:1269–1275.

206. Fagniez PL, Rotman N, Kracht M. Direct retroperitoneal approach to necrosis in severe acute pancreatitis. *Br J Surg* 1989;76:264–267.

207. Pemberton JH, Nagomey DM, Becker JM, et al. Controlled lesser sack drainage for pancreatic abscess. *Ann Surg* 1986;203:600–604.

208. Stone HH, Strom PR, Mullins RJ. Pancreatic abscess management by subtotal resection and packing. *World J Surg* 1984;8:340.

209. Fielding GA, McLatchie GR, Wilson C, et al. Acute pancreatitis and pancreatic fistula formation. *Br J Surg* 1989;76:1126–1128.

210. Schmidt J, Warshaw AL. Surgical treatment of pancreatic fistulas: rationale, timing and technique. In: Bassi C, Vesentini S, eds. *Topics on pancreatic fistulas.* Berlin: Springer-Verlag, 1993:176–194.

211. Warshaw AL, Moncure AC, Rattner DW. Gastrocutaneous fistulas associated with pancreatic abscesses. An aggressive entity. *Ann Surg* 1989;210:603–607.

212. Russell JC, Welch JP, Clark DG. Colonic complications of acute pancreatitis and pancreatic abscess. *Am J Surg* 1983;146:558–564.

213. Bouillot JL, Alexandre JH, Vuong NP. Colonic involvement in acute necrotizing pancreatitis. Results of surgical treatment. *World J Surg* 1967;13:84.

214. Bradley EL. Enteropathies. In: Bradley EL, eds. *Complications of pancreatitis.* Philadelphia: WB Saunders, 1982:265–292.

215. Sackett DL. Resules of evidence and clinical recommendations on the use of antithrombotic agents. *Chest* 1989;95(2)(suppl):2–4.

216. Pulmonary artery catheter consensus conference participants. Consensus statement. *Crit Care Med* 1997;25:910–925.

CHAPTER 92
Splenic Abscess

Basam Helou and Thomas R. Gadacz

Splenic abscess is an unusual source of intraabdominal sepsis. However, the incidence of splenic abscess has been increasing (1–4). Autopsy studies report an incidence of 0.14% to 0.7% (5,6). In this chapter, the classification, etiology, diagnosis, and treatment of splenic abscess are discussed.

CLASSIFICATION AND ETIOLOGY

Splenic abscesses can be classified in several ways. The most common classification is based on the organism cultured from the abscess. Table 92.1 shows the incidence of various organisms based on several reviews (1,5,6). Aerobic organisms make up the vast majority of organisms isolated and include *Staphylococcus, Streptococcus,* and *Salmonella* species. Anaerobes account for 10%, mycobacteria 4%, and fungi 11%. Almost unheard of before 1977, mycobacteria and fungi have increased in incidence (5). The increase in incidence of these organisms has been attributed to the increasing incidence of immunosuppressed states such as human immunodeficiency virus (HIV) infection and intravenous drug abuse. *Candida* is the most frequent fungal pathogen, but *Aspergillus, Blastomyces,* and *Cryptococcus* have also been cultured. In 16% of splenic abscess, no organism is isolated.

TABLE 92.1. Organisms Found in Splenic Abscesses

Bacterial findings	Cases	%
Aerobic bacteria		
Streptococcus	65	12
Staphylococcus	95	17
Salmonella	72	13
Pseudomonas	18	3
Escherichia coli[a]	49	12
Proteus[a]	10	2
Klebsiella[a]	8	2
Enterococcus[a]	20	5
Others[a]	43	10
Anaerobes	53	10
Mycobacteria	21	4
Fungi	60	11
Sterile cultures	85	16

Based on cumulative data from reviews by Ooi and Leong, Nelken et al., and Chun et al. (N = 543).
[a]Data only available from Ooi and Leong and Nelken (N = 414).

TABLE 92.2. Predisposing Conditions in 281 Patients with Splenic Abscess

Risk factor	%
Infectious etiology	
Systemic infection	36.7
Intraabdominal infection	13.9
Unidentified infection	7.8
Contiguous spread	6.8
Embolic	
Endocarditis	17.4
Hemoglobinopathy	4.9
Trauma	7.2
Immunosuppression	
Intravenous drug abuse	12.1
Disease states	9.3
Human immunodeficiency virus	8.9
Steroids	2.1
Chemotherapy	1.8

Splenic abscesses can also be classified as solitary or multiple (7) (Fig. 92.1). Solitary splenic abscesses are usually detected at an early stage. These abscesses have a better prognosis and are usually not associated with multiorgan sepsis. Multiple splenic abscesses are clinically covert, have a high mortality rate, and are part of multiorgan sepsis. In several reports, multiple splenic abscesses have accounted for increasing numbers of cases. They appear to be associated with immunosuppressed states.

There are several predisposing factors for splenic abscess (Table 92.2). The most common cause is metastatic infection (1). Endocarditis and intraabdominal infection are the most common sources. Metastatic infection is present in 62% of cases. Less commonly, splenic abscess may develop as a result of contiguous spread such as from a perinephric abscess or perforated colon carcinoma. Hemoglobinopathies, including sickle cell disease and thalassemia, can lead to splenic infarction. Five percent of

all splenic abscesses in Leong's review occurred in patients with splenic infarction (1). Splenic trauma is also associated with an increased risk for abscess. In this case, the abscess usually presents weeks to several months after the trauma, but has been reported up to 10 years posttrauma (8). A third and steadily increasing predisposing factor is immunosuppression. Nearly 35% of patients have some form of immunocompromise. The most common are HIV infection, various disease states (e.g., systemic lupus erythematosus, myeloma, etc.), and intravenous drug abuse. Other conditions included cancer chemotherapy and long-term steroid use.

DIAGNOSIS

History and Physical Examination

The signs and symptoms of splenic abscess are nonspecific. They are often related to the underlying disease process (i.e.,

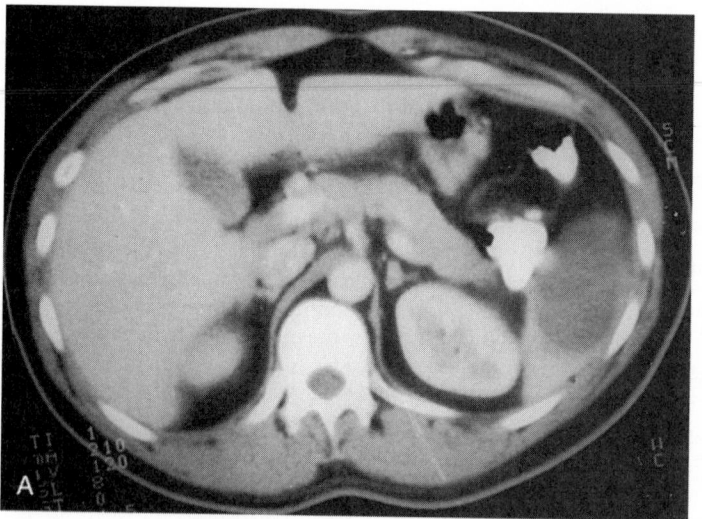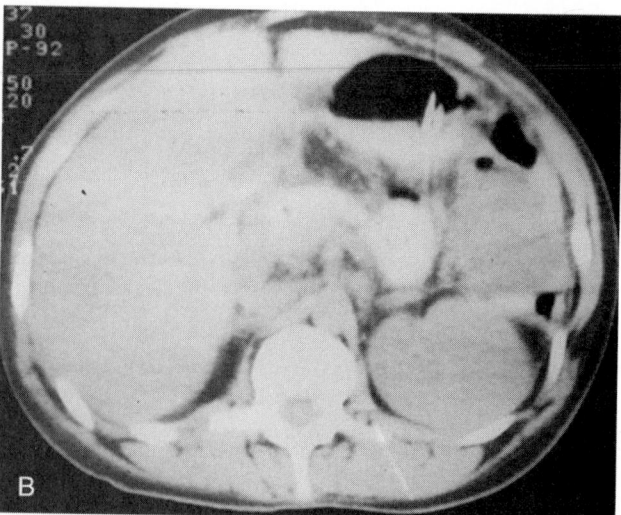

Figure 92.1. A: Unilocular hypodense splenic abscess secondary to endocarditis. The infecting organism was *Staphylococcus.* The patient was treated successfully with a splenectomy. **B:** A hypodense spleen with an air bubble seen on a computed tomographic scan. The contiguous colonic and pancreatic process mandated a splenectomy. Multiple enteric organisms were cultured.

endocarditis). In Leong's review of 287 cases, fever is the most common finding, present in 91% of cases (1). Left upper quadrant pain and splenomegaly are present in 50% and 30% of cases, respectively. Pain may also be noted in the left shoulder. This is due to referred pain from irritation of the left hemidiaphragm. Despite these signs and symptoms, many patients with splenic abscess are critically ill and show little more than an unexplained fever. Due to the lack of specific findings on history and physical examination, as well as the wide availability of accurate imaging studies, the diagnosis of splenic abscess is a radiographic one.

Laboratory Findings

Leukocytosis is present in 70% to 88% of patients but is a variable finding. In one large series, the white blood cell count varied between 2,400 and 41,000/mm^3 (5). In general, other serum laboratory studies are not helpful.

Radiographic Findings

Multiple imaging modalities can be used to aid in the diagnosis with varying levels of sensitivity and specificity. Plain films of the abdomen reveal a left pleural effusion in 20% of cases (1,9). Other findings on plain film include a left upper quadrant mass, elevation of the left hemidiaphragm, and an air-fluid level in the left upper quadrant. Barium studies may show a medial displacement of the stomach. Although these studies may be suggestive, definitive studies such as ultrasonography or computed tomography (CT) are needed to establish the diagnosis.

Radioisotope scanning with technetium or gallium has a reported accuracy of 80% to 90%. Abscesses larger than 2 cm are frequently demonstrated, but 80% to 90% of the smaller abscesses are not well seen. This type of study is not as widely available as ultrasonography or CT scan. In addition, the latter two modalities are equal or superior to nuclear medicine imaging in terms of accuracy. Consequently, radioisotope scanning is not recommended in the diagnosis of splenic abscess (10).

Ultrasonography

Ultrasonography is an accurate means of diagnosing splenic abscess, with sensitivity approaching 90% (11). Furthermore, ultrasonography has the advantage of being widely available, relatively inexpensive, and portable. Splenic abscesses are usually anechoic or hypoechoic. Often multiple septa and variable internal echo patterns are seen. However, when compared with CT scan, ultrasound investigations of the spleen are slightly less effective in establishing a diagnosis of a splenic abscess.

Computed Tomography

CT scan to diagnose splenic abscess is quite accurate, with sensitivity up to 96% (1). When a scan is enhanced with intravenous contrast material, the spleen is homogenous. Abscesses are typically low-density lesions with a center of fluid or necrotic tissue. If a capsule has developed, mild enhancement may be seen (12). Air within an intrasplenic collection is diagnostic of an abscess, although most do not contain air. In patients with fungal etiology, fluid collections are typically less then 2 cm in diameter, multiple, and hypodense. Occasionally, a central focus of higher attenuation or wheel-within-a-wheel pattern may be seen (13). Granulomatous infections of the spleen are often seen as multiple irregular hypodense lesions in patients with mild splenomegaly. This population of patients may also have abdominal lymphadenopathy, high-attenuation ascites, nodular peritoneal thickening, and hepatomegaly (14).

TREATMENT

Untreated splenic abscess is uniformly fatal (1). The gold standard treatment of a splenic abscess is splenectomy and intravenous antibiotics (1,2,6). A second option is percutaneous drainage. This option should be considered if the patient has a unilocular abscess, is too unstable to undergo a splenectomy, has had multiple previous operations, or has significant risks for standard surgical drainage (15,16). A third option, splenotomy, was once the procedure of choice, but now is largely of historical interest (2).

Percutaneous Drainage

Percutaneous abscess drainage of the spleen can be safely employed only when a drainage window that avoids adjacent thoracic, gastrointestinal, and vascular structures is present (17). In general, anterior approaches on the abdominal wall should be avoided. The posterior abdominal wall offers dependent drainage and increased safety. The catheter should be placed at the most dependent portion of the cavity, and a Gram stain and culture for aerobes, anaerobes, fungi, and mycobacteria should be done routinely. At the time of catheter placement, the catheter should be irrigated copiously when the cavity has been evacuated so as to remove necrotic debris.

While the catheter remains in place, irrigation with 10 to 25 mL of saline should be done routinely. The catheter can be removed when the drainage is scant and the cavity has decreased in size as evidenced by ultrasonography or CT scan. Failure of the cavity to resolve or lack of clinical improvement mandates splenectomy. Percutaneous drainage is most likely to succeed when the abscess collection is unilocular and has a discrete wall and no internal septation. Abscesses containing thick, necrotic debris are less likely to be successfully drained percutaneously, as are phlegmons, poorly defined cavities, microabscesses, multiple abscesses, and abscesses originating from a contiguous process. Percutaneous drainage of a multiloculated abscess is almost uniformly unsuccessful; however, for a single loculation, percutaneous drainage has been reported to be effective 75% to 90% of the time (1,2,10). It should be noted that for patients who undergo nonoperative treatment, multiple percutaneous drainages may be required (2). In cases of failure of percutaneous drainage, splenectomy is the remaining option.

Splenectomy

For most patients undergoing surgical treatment, a midline operative approach allows examination of the entire abdomen if other areas of sepsis are suspected; otherwise, a subcostal incision is acceptable. In the presence of previous trauma or an enlarged spleen, vascular control of the splenic artery is obtained at the celiac axis. The splenic attachments are incised, and short gastric vessels are ligated and divided. The hilar vessels are identified and ligated, and the spleen is removed. After copious irrigation, the splenic bed is drained.

Laparoscopic splenectomy has many advantages over the open procedure. However, laparoscopic splenectomy for splenic abscess is controversial. Several researchers have expressed concern that the infectious process may potentially be spread

TABLE 92.3. Outcome of Treatment

Treatment	n	Initial resolution (%)	Salvage required (%)	Mortality (%)
Splenectomy	148	100	0	16.9
Salvage splenectomy	21	100	0	14.3
Partial splenectomy	2	100	0	0
Open drainage	3	100	0	0
Percutaneous aspiration	31	64.5	38.7	3.2
Percutaneous catheter drainage	45	51.1	31.1	0
Antibiotics only	49	59.2	22.5	24.5
No treatment	9	0	—	100

further and consider splenic abscess a relative contraindication to laparoscopic splenectomy (18).

Broad-spectrum antibiotics should be initiated when a splenic abscess is diagnosed. This therapy should include agents effective against staphylococcal, streptococcal, and gram-negative bacteria. If a contiguous abdominal process is suspected, an anaerobic agent should be added. Once culture data are known, treatment may be tailored appropriately. In immunosuppressed patients, antifungal coverage should be initiated early in the disease process.

OUTCOME

In Ooi and Leong's review, the mortality rate associated with splenic abscess was 12.4% (1). All untreated patients had a fatal outcome (Table 92.3). With antibiotics alone there is a 24.5% mortality rate. Percutaneous drainage and open drainage involved no mortality, and splenectomy carried a 16.9% mortality rate. Immunosuppressed patients accounted for a significant amount of the mortality associated with splenectomy, with the mortality rate in this group exceeding 25%. Except for splenectomy, the number of cases in each treatment group is too small to make definitive comparisons. The lack of mortality in the percutaneous group may be due to patient selection.

The best treatment of an established fungal abscess is unclear because individual experiences are small in number. Most patients are cured by a combination of antifungal agents and splenectomy. One report has confirmed that 12 of 16 patients with a fungal abscess were cured with antifungal agents alone, and the mortality rate did not differ from that of an immediate splenectomy. These data suggest that confirmed fungal abscesses in the spleen may be treated with prolonged antifungal agents alone provided that CT confirms complete resolution. Exceptions include patients with a large fungal abscess, which should be treated by percutaneous abscess drainage or by splenectomy. Splenectomy is also the treatment for patients who do not respond to antifungal therapy.

CONCLUSION

Splenic abscess remains an uncommon clinical entity. However, with the increasing population of immunosuppressed patients,

its incidence is increasing. Definitive diagnosis is established with ultrasonography or CT scan. Once diagnosis is established, treatment with broad-spectrum antibiotics should be initiated, and consideration of splenectomy or percutaneous drainage should be made. Splenectomy is the usual treatment. As the role of the spleen in immune function has become better understood and as percutaneous drainage techniques have become more refined, percutaneous drainage is becoming a more attractive option as first-line treatment. The success rates of this technique would suggest that in patients with small solitary lesions, percutaneous drainage with salvage splenectomy (if needed) is appropriate treatment.

REFERENCES

1. Ooi LL, Leong SS. Splenic abscesses from 1987 to 1995. *Am J Surg* 1997;174:87–93.
2. Green BT. Splenic abscess: report of six cases and review of the literature. *Am Surg* 2001;67:80–85.
3. Alsono-Cohen MA, Galera MJ, Ruiz M, et al. Splenic abscess. *World J Surg* 1990;14:513–517.
4. Tikkakoski T, Siniluoto T, Paivasalo M, et al. Splenic abscess: imaging and intervention. *Acta Radiol* 1992;33:561–565.
5. Chun CH, Raff MJ, Conteras L. Splenic abscess. *Medicine (Baltimore)* 1980;59:50–65.
6. Nelken N, Ignatius J, Skinner M, et al. Changing clinical spectrum of splenic abscess. A multicenter study and review of the literature. *Am J Surg* 1987;154:27–34.
7. Gadacz TR. Splenic abscess. *World J Surg* 1985;9:410–415.
8. Toevs CC, Beilman GJ. Splenic abscess ten years after splenic trauma: a case report. *Am Surg* 2000;66:204–205.
9. Van Der Laan RT, Verbeeten B Jr, Smits NJ, et al. Computed tomography in the diagnosis and treatment of solitary splenic abscess. *J Comput Assist Tomogr* 1989;13:71–74.
10. Chou YH, Hsu CC, Tiu CM, et al. Splenic abscess: sonographic diagnosis and percutaneous drainage. *Gastrointest Radiol* 1992;17:262–266.
11. Rabushka LS, Kawashima A, Fishman ER. Imaging of the spleen with supplemental MR examination. *Radiographics* 1994;14:307–332.
12. Coslowitz PL, Labs JD, Fishman EK, et al. The changing spectrum of splenic abscess. *Clin Imag* 1989;13:201–207.
13. Choi BI, Im JC, Han MC, et al. Hepatosplenic tuberculosis with hypersplenism: CT evaluation. *Gastrointest Radiol* 1989;14:265–267.
14. Gleich S, Wolin DA, Herbsman H. A review of percutaneous drainage in splenic abscess. *Surg Gynecol Obstet* 1988;167:211–216.
15. Quinn SF, van Sonnenberg E, Casola G, et al. Interventional radiology in the spleen. *Radiology* 1986;161:289–291.
16. Sarr MG, Zuidema GD. Splenic abscess: prevention, diagnosis and treatment. *Surgery* 1982;92:480–485.
17. Faught WE, Gilbertson JJ, Nelson EW. Splenic abscess: presentation, treatment options and results. *Am J Surg* 1989;158:612–614.
18. Flowers JL, Lefor AT, Steers JS. Laparoscopic splenectomy in patients with hematologic disease. *Ann Surg* 1996;224:19–26.

Other Surgical Infections

CHAPTER 93
Approach to the Patient with Postoperative Fever

E. Patchen Dellinger

Postoperative fever is common and is a source of concern to physician and patient. Most doctors and patients associate fever with infection, and the empiric prescription of antibiotics is a common response. To put these concerns into perspective and to analyze the best approach to this common phenomenon, I will consider the definition of fever, the correlation between postoperative fever and postoperative infection, and other possible causes of postoperative fever.

DEFINITIONS AND INCIDENCE

Fever can be defined as any temperature above 37°C, but the normal variability of temperature among individuals and the even greater variability of temperature in the postoperative period render this definition too nonspecific to be useful clinically. Dykes found that 82% of 162 nonobstetric postoperative patients had a recorded temperature above 37°C in the first postoperative week (1). Figure 93.1 illustrates the range of unexplained fevers observed after four different representative surgical procedures. Other definitions of postoperative fever use 37.8° to 38.9°C, accept one reading above the limit or require more, and follow

the patient for 2 to 10 days with or without including the first 1 or 2 days following the operation (2–23). These papers report the incidence of postoperative fever as 14% to 91%. In the same reports, the prevalence of infection varied from 0% to 13% for all patients and from 0% to 62% for febrile patients, but not all infected patients meet the definition of fever. The proportion of febrile patients who are infected appears to increase as the definition of fever becomes more rigorous (Table 93.1). However, as the definition of postoperative fever becomes more rigorous, a greater proportion of infected patients no longer meet the definition of fever. The result is that the overall accuracy of fever as an index of infection changes little, if at all (6,24–26). Triulzi reported 109 patients having spinal fusion procedures with an infection rate of 7%. The average duration of fever in infected patients was 4 days compared with 3 days in patients without infection (27). The mean day for diagnosis of infection was 8 with a median of 14. Clearly, the great majority of febrile postoperative patients are not infected, and indeed, as many as 50% of infected patients may not be febrile (7,13,17,19), depending on the definition of postoperative fever.

Because fever is common in the absence of infection, it is important to consider causes other than infection. Atelectasis without infection is commonly cited as a cause of postoperative fever, although the mechanism is not known. Atelectasis may be responsible for some postoperative fevers, but many patients with postoperative fever show no physical or radiographic signs of atelectasis, and many patients with radiographic evidence of atelectasis are not febrile (11,26). Roberts found that 37 of 109 febrile patients did not have radiographic evidence of atelectasis, whereas 82 of 154 patients with atelectasis did not have fever (26). Similarly, in patients who had no preexisting cardiac or pulmonary disease Ejlertsen found a large group with atelectasis but no fever following upper abdominal operations (28). In reports where a careful effort is made to identify the causes of postoperative fever, the proportion of fevers that are unexplained or noninfectious varies from 11% to 100% (1,2,6,9,25,26). Any condition that can cause the release of interleukin-1, interleukin-6, or tumor necrosis factor—hematoma formation and direct tissue trauma, pulmonary embolism, or atelectasis—could theoretically cause fever. These explanations are, however, poorly documented as causes of fever, and many individual examples of each exist without significant fever. Frank and colleagues followed 271 patients having noncardiac thoracic or vascular operations and recorded frequent core temperatures and serum interleukin-6 levels. Average preoperative temperature was 36.6° ± 0.6°C and the mean maximum temperature during the next 24 hours was 38.0° ± 1.0°C. Twenty-five percent of the patients had a postoperative temperature of at least 38.5°C and 10% at least 38.8°C. Only one patient had evidence of infection. Elevated temperatures correlated with measured interleukin-6 levels and longer operating times but not with intraoperative temperatures or efforts for intraoperative warming (29). In another study of 205 patients having a cardiac operation with cardiopulmonary bypass, patients were randomized to receive dexamethasone 0.6 mg/kg or placebo after anesthesia induction. Shivering, a key mechanism of fever, occurred in only 13% of patients in the treatment arm compared with 33% in the placebo arm (30).

Whatever the noninfectious causes of postoperative fever, they are nearly all self-limited and do not require specific therapy. Most experienced clinical surgeons have noted that some temperature elevation is a common part of the complex metabolic response to surgical injury. In many patients one can observe a series of changes beginning 3 to 6 days after the operation. Within a 24-hour period, temperature normalizes, the pulse rate decreases to preoperative levels, bowel function returns, fluid balance sheets show diuresis of the interstitial (third space) fluid

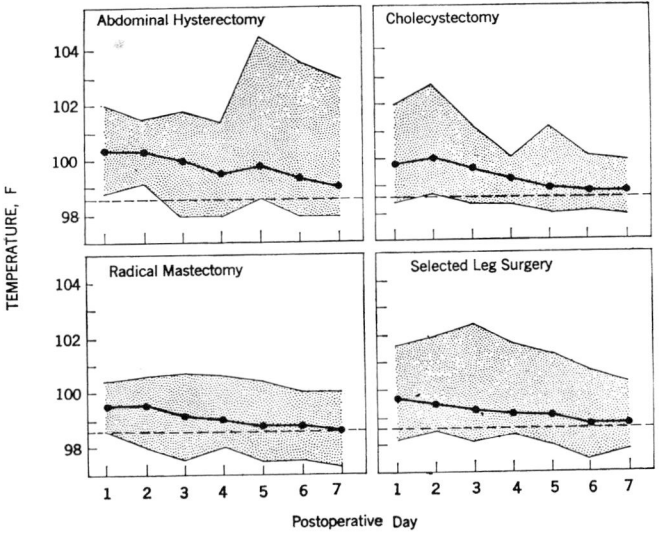

Figure 93.1. Mean, maximal, and minimal daily temperatures in four groups of 20 consecutive patients with unexplained fevers. (From Dykes MHM. Unexplained postoperative fever. Its value as a sign of halothane sensitization. *JAMA* 1971;216:641–644, with permission.)

TABLE 93.1. Postoperative Fever Definitions, Incidence of Fever, and Infection

Investigator	Patients/Operation	Fever criterion (°C)	Duration	No. of patients	Patients		Febrile patients infected (%)
					No. febrile (% of total)	No. infected (% of total)	
Dykes (1)	Nonobstetric	>37	Any, days 1–7	133	104 (78)	31[a] (23)	30[a]
Yeung et al. (3)	Pediatric	≥38	Any, days 1–3	256	73 (29)	4 (2)	5
Miholic et al. (4)	Open heart	>38	Any	115	102 (89)	7 (6)	7
Pien et al. (5)	Coronary bypass	>38	Any, days 1–9	263	174[b] (66)	24 (9)	14
Mellors et al. (6)	Abdominal operations	≥38.1	Any, days 1–7	434	163 (38)	26 (6)	16
Garibaldi et al. (2)	General surgical	>38	2 consecutive days	871	194 (22)	113 (13)	58
Galicier and Richet (7)	General surgical	≥38	Persists 48 h in hospital	570	78 (14)	48 (8)	62
Freischlag and Busuttil (8)	Abdominal operations	≥38.5	Twice in 8 h, days 1–6	464	71 (15)	19 (4)	27
Le Gall et al. (9)	ICU patients/abdominal operations	≥39	Any, days 3–10	Only febrile patients	100 (100)	89 (89)	89
Engoren (11)	Open heart	>38	Days 0–2	100	37 (37)	0	0
Petrelli et al. (12)	Colorectal operations	>38.5	Days 0–2	100	14 (14)	0	0
Rantala et al. (10)	Abdominal operations	>38.5	Any, days 1–7 >24 h post surgery	77	37 (48) 107 (107)	0 48 (45)	0 45
Giangobbe et al. (13)	Cholecystectomy	>38.4 or >38	Any time in hospital twice, 4 h apart	176	28 (16)	10 (6)	7
Lyon et al. (23)	Benign gynecologic operations	>38	Any time in hospital	257	147 (57)	6 (2)	4
Circiumaru et al. (22)	Postoperative ICU patients	≥38.4	Any time in ICU	64	45 (70)	11 (17)	24
Kennedy et al. (21)	Total knee replacement	≥37.8	Any	90	82 (91)	0[c]	0
Guinn et al. (20)	Total knee replacement	>38.3	Any	90	46 (51)	0[c]	0
McNally et al. (19)	Vaginal or abdominal hysterectomy	>38 >38	Any Any during first 72 h	117 112	80 (68) 51 (46)	10[d] (9) 7[e] (6)	13 8
Schwandt et al. (18)	Major gynecologic operation	≥38.5	Twice ≥4 h apart	105	28 (27)	4 (4)	14
Shackelford et al. (17)	Vaginal operations	>38	Twice ≥4 h apart after the first 24 h	431	54 (13)	35[f] (8)	24
Angel et al. (16)	Pediatric orthopaedic operations	>38	Any	174	127 (73)	2 (1)	2
Merjanian et al. (15)	Pediatric orthopaedic operations	39 ≥38	Any	174 177	17 (10) 103 (58)	1 (1) 5 (3)	1 5
Velazquez et al. (14)	Endovascular aortic aneurysm repair	>38.5	Any	12	8 (67)	0	0

[a] Includes both infected patients and patients with diagnosed, noninfectious causes of fever (atelectasis and hematoma).
[b] Number projected from incidence in subset of uninfected patients.
[c] No joint infections.
[d] Reporting on joint infections only.
[e] Three not febrile.
[f] Twenty-two not febrile.

accumulated during the procedure, and the patient begins to smile spontaneously and take an interest in personal appearance again (positive lipstick sign). Two exceptions to this self-limited course include major pulmonary collapse, which should be treated by physical measures for reexpansion, and pulmonary embolism, which is treated with anticoagulation or other specific measures. The clinician's primary approach to a postoperative fever, therefore, is appropriately focused on the possibility of infection, although in most cases none is found. While the surgical incision is the natural area of concern, it is not the location of the majority of postoperative infections, and in fact, often is not even the most common (3,6–8,31,32). The two most common sites of infection are wounds and the urinary tract. Following these are respiratory tract infections and then a number of less common ones, including intravenous catheter–associated infections, other bloodstream infections, sinusitis, and infections entirely unrelated to the operative procedure.

THE IMPORTANCE OF TIMING

The approach to a patient with postoperative fever must account for the relative likelihood that different causes will produce fever at different times after operation and the importance or urgency of diagnosis of the different causes. Garibaldi found that 38% of all postoperative fevers occurred within 48 hours after an operation, but the great majority (73%) of these early fevers were noninfectious in origin (2) (Fig. 93.2). Eighty percent of fevers originating on the first day were noninfectious, whereas most of the remaining 20% were respiratory in origin. On the second and third days, new fevers were still 55% to 65% noninfectious. Only on the fifth postoperative day was a new fever as likely to represent a surgical site infection as to be noninfectious (2). Of all fevers that began 5 days or longer after operation, 42% were due to wound infections, 29% to urinary tract infections, 12% to respiratory tract infections, and only 10% were noninfectious. Galicier found that the majority of fevers due to infection began on the third postoperative day or later, whereas almost 95% of fevers without an infectious origin began within 4 days of the operation (7). Pien and co-workers found that less than 10%

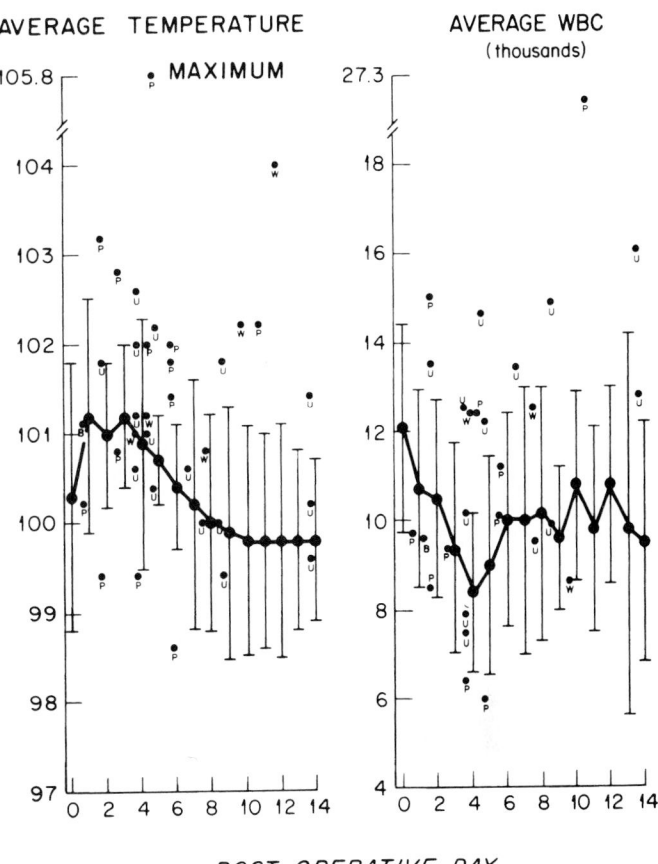

POST OPERATIVE DAY

Figure 93.3. Curves represent mean values ± 1 SD for daily maximal temperature and white blood cell count for 154 patients without infection. Individual points represent values for the 35 patients with infection on the day infection was documented. *P,* pneumonia; *W,* wound infection; *U,* urinary tract infection; *B,* bacteremia. (From Bell DM, Goldmann DA, Hopkins CC, et al. Unreliability of fever and leukocytosis in the diagnosis of infection after cardiac valve surgery. *J Thorac Cardiovasc Surg* 1978;75:87–90, with permission.)

of patients with noninfectious fevers after coronary artery bypass operations were febrile after the fourth postoperative day, whereas 25% of fevers that were still present or began after the fourth day were due to infections (5). Data also do not support the commonly held belief that the intensity of the fever (above 39° or 40°C) during the first 5 to 7 postoperative days is more likely to distinguish infected from uninfected patients or severe from minor infections (2,6,24,25) (Figs. 93.3 and 93.4).

URGENT CAUSES OF EARLY FEVER

These data influence the approach to early (within 48 hours) postoperative fever. The great majority of early fevers are noninfectious and self-limited. This does not mean that such fevers can be ignored, but it does mean that an extensive laboratory or radiographic workup is not indicated. Two rare but lethal infections should be considered when high fever presents in the first 24 to 48 hours after an operation. Both should be detected by physical examination, and each febrile postoperative patient should be examined to rule them out. After an abdominal operation, an unnoticed injury to the bowel or a leaking anastomosis that causes peritoneal soiling with intestinal contents can result in an early, high fever. It also causes striking cardiovascular

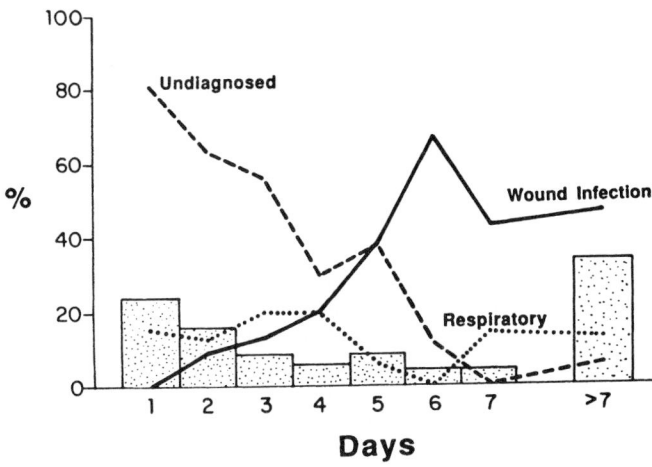

Figure 93.2. Vertical bars indicate the percentage of all fevers that appear each respective day. Lines indicate the percentage of new fevers on each day that are due to wound infection (*solid line*) or respiratory infection (*dotted line*), or are unexplained (*dashed line*). (Data from Garibaldi RA, Brodine S, Matsumiya S, et al. Evidence for the non-infectious etiology of early postoperative fever. *Infect Control* 1985;6:273–277, with permission.)

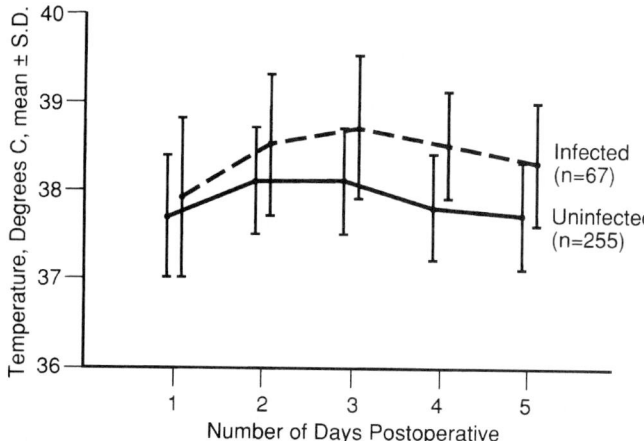

Figure 93.4. Mean daily maximal temperature ± 1 SD for 67 patients with (*dashed line*) and 255 patients without (*solid line*) postoperative infection after celiotomy for penetrating abdominal injury.

disturbances, marked fluid sequestration, and specific physical findings. Abdominal examination and review of the clinical setting should suffice to discover this problem, although the abdominal examination is made more difficult by the proximity of a recent incision. This potential complication is best evaluated by the operating surgeon, who is aware of the details of the operative procedure, including any unusual or untoward intraoperative events.

Most wound infections are not evident on physical examination before the fourth postoperative day; in fact, most are discovered considerably later. However, an invasive soft tissue infection due to either β-hemolytic streptococci or a histotoxic *Clostridium* species may become symptomatic within 24 hours of the operation. Infections caused by these organisms are discussed in detail in other chapters. Diagnosis is made by inspection of the wound and Gram smear of any wound fluid.

An even rarer cause of fever in the first 48 hours after operation is toxic shock syndrome associated with a *Staphylococcus aureus* wound infection. During an 18-month period in 1980 and 1981, the Centers for Disease Control (CDC) confirmed 13 such cases among 16 suspected (33). This represented less than 1% of all cases of toxic shock reported to the CDC during that interval. Seven of the 13 cases had their onset within 48 hours after operation. Fever, diarrhea, and vomiting were the earliest signs. The most characteristic presentation was fever, profuse watery diarrhea, erythroderma, and hypotension. Local signs of wound infection were often absent initially. The best treatment is not known, but drainage and irrigation of the wound in combination with a systemic antistaphylococcal antibiotic seems reasonable (34). Raab and colleagues examined the records related to 390,000 surgical procedures in two community hospitals between 1981 and 1993. They found 12 (0.003%) cases of associated toxic shock occurring 2 to 8 days following operation with an average of 4 days to onset. The cases followed hysterectomy, cholecystectomy, orthopedic procedures, breast biopsy, pilonidal cyst excision, rhinoplasty, and chest tube insertion (35). Signs and symptoms were as previously described, and the surgical site often had minimal findings.

Antibiotic-associated enterocolitis due to *Clostridium difficile* is another potential cause of postoperative fever. It can occur within 1 or 2 days after operation and antibiotic administration but is often delayed and can occur several weeks later. It should be considered in any hospitalized patient who has received antibiotics and who has diarrhea. Cases have been reported after

a single short course of prophylactic antibiotics (36,37). In one report, 55% of all cases of *C. difficile* colitis over a 10-year period occurred on the surgical service. Perioperative prophylaxis was the most common indication for preceding antibiotics, and accounted for 25% of all cases (36). Many, but not all, patients will have fever, and abdominal cramps and leukocytosis are also common (38,39). Full details of diagnosis and treatment are covered in Chapter 74.

USE OF ANTIBIOTICS

There is no place for empiric antibiotic administration to a postoperative patient with fever without a specific diagnosis, and usually adjunctive surgical therapy. Both intraabdominal emergencies and invasive soft tissue infections fail to resolve if treated with antibiotics but without operation. Other wound infections, with or without toxic shock, require wound drainage, and enterocolitis is best treated by stopping the original antibiotic and withholding new parenteral antibiotics while initiating treatment with oral metronidazole or, in certain cases, vancomycin. Other infectious causes of early fever, such as urinary tract infection and pneumonia, are amenable to diagnosis by directed examination before treatment is instituted. Existing evidence suggests that prolonging the duration of administration of perioperative prophylactic antibiotics does not reduce the incidence of wound infection (40–44), although this is often done (45–47).

THE ROLES OF TESTING AND EXAMINATION

After the third or fourth postoperative day, the likelihood that a new or persistent fever is infectious in origin is greater and begins to exceed the probability that a noninfectious cause is responsible (Fig. 93.2). A variety of diagnoses should be considered in decreasing order of likelihood: surgical site infection (in either the incision or a deeper operative site), urinary tract infection, respiratory tract infection, intravascular catheter-associated infection, and others unrelated to the operation. Here the clinician may be tempted to order a series of standardized tests to begin the workup, such as white blood cell count and differential count, chest film, and blood, urine, sputum, and wound cultures. In one report, an average of 3.8 such tests were ordered for febrile postoperative patients (8). Unfortunately, such testing is neither efficient nor economical. Only 7% of such tests ordered routinely gave information useful in the care of the patient. Mellors found that only 1 in 73 radiographs and cultures ordered for patients who had fever but no other specific findings was positive (6). Of 60 patients with fever following hysterectomy but without physical findings suggestive of infection, 102 blood cultures (1.7 per patient) were all negative (48).

In the postoperative setting, an elevated white blood cell count is common in both infected and uninfected patients (8,24,25,49). Freischlag found that leukocytosis had only 74% sensitivity and 45% specificity (8). Other routine tests were even less helpful. Mellors, however, found that greater specificity was obtained by considering a white blood cell count that was either greater than 10×10^9 cells per liter or less than 5×10^9 cells per liter, as compared with a count simply greater than a specific level (6). Physical examination by a physician with knowledge of the recent history and details of the operative procedure is most helpful for diagnosing postoperative infections. Tests suggested by this examination are likely to confirm a clinical diagnosis. A wound infection is diagnosed by inspecting the wound. Urinary tract infections are rare in postoperative patients who have not been catheterized and have no history of prior urinary tract infections or acute symptoms. Urinalysis and Gram smear of an unspun drop of urine give valuable information about the likelihood of a urinary tract infection a day before culture results are available. Ordering a sputum culture for a patient who does not have a productive cough and thoracic findings on physical examination is unrewarding and merely produces information regarding the bacterial content of the oropharynx.

Blood cultures should be part of the evaluation of any fever that occurs after the fourth postoperative day in a patient with a permanent intravascular device such as a cardiac valve or vascular graft. Blood cultures obtained from postoperative patients with fever whose course is otherwise routine rarely grow organisms. They are indicated for patients who are clinically septic, but only as an adjunct, and even then they are most often negative in postoperative patients, even among those with documented bacterial infection (9). In a study of the utility of blood cultures for diagnosis in febrile postoperative patients, Theuer reported on 364 cultures obtained during 108 febrile events in 72 patients. All patients had temperatures above 38.6°C, and the average temperature was 38.9°C in patients both with and without positive blood cultures. Among the 364 cultures obtained, there were 5 positive cultures, 4 contaminants, and 355 cultures without growth. None of the 85 cultures obtained on the first 3 days after operation were positive. Eight percent of cultures obtained on days 4 through 10 were positive (50).

A postoperative patient with signs of systemic sepsis must be assumed to have a life-threatening infection at the operative site unless it is proven otherwise, and this nearly always demands direct diagnostic procedures and finally operative intervention. In none of these settings does a patient benefit from empiric administration of antibiotics before a presumptive clinical diagnosis is made and appropriate operative intervention is instituted. Antibiotic administration without diagnosis and indicated operative intervention may temporarily suppress clinical evidence of infection, such as fever, cause a delay in diagnosis, and increase the risk for secondary complications such as the multiple organ failure syndrome.

INTRAABDOMINAL INFECTIONS

A deep intraabdominal infection is a less common but more serious complication of abdominal surgery than wound infection, urinary tract infection, respiratory tract infection, or infection of intravascular devices. Approximately 4% of all abdominal operations are followed by an urgent reoperation within the next month, and about half of these are required for a deep infectious complication (51–54) (Table 93.2). However, a patient with high fever and systemic sepsis who qualifies for intensive care unit admission after an abdominal operation is much more likely to have an intraabdominal infection (9). Intraabdominal infection

is associated with a mortality rate in the range of 15% to 50%, depending on the patient population and other risk factors (55–58). Delay in diagnosis is common and increases mortality, especially in the immediate postoperative period (58).

The seriousness of a postoperative intraabdominal infection is the stimulus for much testing in patients with postoperative fever. As discussed above for other potential postoperative infections, blind reliance on blood tests and radiographs is not an effective strategy. Only about 11% to 29% of patients with documented intraabdominal infection have positive blood cultures (9,56,57). Specialized radiographic tests are needed for diagnosis in the minority of cases (59). In the specific circumstance of septic intensive care unit patients, computed tomography used as the primary study often fails to yield information that is helpful in determining the management of the patient (60). The most sensitive instrument for suspecting infection and determining its most likely location continues to be a conscientious physician using the time-honored skills of history and physical examination. Computed tomography can be extremely useful, however, for confirming a suspicion and planning the best therapeutic approach (61).

LESS COMMON CAUSES OF FEVER

If the workup outlined here does not produce a diagnosis, less common causes of postoperative fever must be considered. Drug fever must be considered in any febrile patient, but it is a diagnosis of exclusion. A patient who has in place devices such as a nasogastric or nasotracheal tube may develop purulent sinusitis due to nosocomial organisms (62). Purulent nasal drainage implies the diagnosis, but drainage may not be present. In one recent study of trauma patients, serous or purulent otitis media was a sensitive and specific indicator of paranasal sinusitis (63). Sinus mucosal thickening or fluid, with or without an air-fluid level, may be detected by plain films or computed tomography, but tomography is more sensitive, especially in the presence of tubes, bandages, and fractures. Sinus puncture for Gram smear and culture, the definitive diagnostic test, also provides information about pathogens and sensitivity.

Postoperative deep venous thrombosis (DVT) is often included in the differential diagnosis of postoperative fever. Kazmers and colleagues examined the records of 1,847 postoperative patients who had duplex venous examinations to rule out DVT. Two hundred twenty-eight patients had evidence of acute DVT with an average temperature of 98.7°F, while 1,619 had no evidence of DVT with an average temperature of 98.5°F (64).

Gout can be triggered by surgical stress, which may unmask previously undiagnosed disease. In a 10-year experience at the Jackson Veterans Affairs Hospital, 295 patients with the preoperative diagnosis of gout had surgical procedures, and 45 (15%) developed postoperative gout. Another 7 patients had their first

TABLE 93.2. Repeated Laparotomy for Infection

Investigator	Primary laparotomies (n)	Repeated laparotomy		Repeated laparotomy for infection	
		n	%	n	%
Hinsdale and Jaffe (41)	5,532	119	2	77	65
Harbrecht et al. (40)	1,633	133	7	60	53
Zer et al. (39)	3,679	95	3	33	35
Bunt (38)	2,657	192	7	93	48
Total	13,501	519	3.8	263	51

diagnosed gout attack during the postoperative period during this same 10 year interval. The average temperature of these 52 patients was 38.2°C, and the attacks occurred 1 to 17 days postoperatively with a mean of 4 days. Eighty-five percent occurred in the lower extremity, while 87% were monoarticular, but only 15% had classic podagra (65).

Any patient can develop parotitis, but elderly and dehydrated patients and those with poor oral hygiene are at higher risk. It is marked by local pain and swelling, and sometimes by edema overlying the gland. In some cases pus can be expressed from the duct. It is treated with antistaphylococcal antibiotics and sometimes incision of the gland.

SUMMARY

Postoperative fever is common, both with and without postoperative infectious complications. In the first 2 to 4 days after operation most fevers are noninfectious in origin and resolve without specific therapy. It is important, however, to rule out peritoneal leak of enteric contents and invasive soft tissue infection with directed physical examination. The clinician should also be aware of the remote possibility of toxic shock syndrome associated with staphylococcal wound infection. After the fourth postoperative day, a new or persistent fever is more likely to represent an infectious complication, although many self-limited, noninfectious fevers still can occur. The most effective diagnostic approach is review of the operative and preoperative history and physical examination. Laboratory tests and radiographic examinations are best directed by the results of the physical examination rather than being ordered routinely in response to fever. Neither prolongation of perioperative prophylactic antibiotics nor initiation of empiric therapeutic antibiotics is indicated without a presumptive clinical diagnosis and a plan for operative intervention when indicated.

REFERENCES

1. Dykes M. Unexplained postoperative fever. Its value as a sign of halothane sensitization. *JAMA* 1971;216:641–644.
2. Garibaldi RA, Brodine S, Matsumiya S, et al. Evidence for the noninfectious etiology of early postoperative fever. *Infect Control* 1985;6:273–277.
3. Yeung RS, Buck JR, Filler RM. The significance of fever following operations in children. *J Pediatr Surg* 1982;17:347–349.
4. Miholic J, Hiertz H, Hudec M, et al. Fever, leucocytosis and infection after open heart surgery. A log-linear regression analysis of 115 cases. *Thorac Cardiovasc Surg* 1984;32:45–48.
5. Pien FD, Ho PWL, Fergusson DJG. Fever and infection after cardiac operation. *Ann Thorac Surg* 1982;33:382–384.
6. Mellors JW, Kelly JJ, Gusberg RJ, et al. A simple index to estimate the likelihood of bacterial infection in patients developing fever after abdominal surgery. *Am Surg* 1988;54:558–564.
7. Galicier C, Richet H. A prospective study of postoperative fever in a general surgery department. *Infect Control* 1985;6:487–490.
8. Freischlag J, Busuttil RW. The value of postoperative fever evaluation. *Surgery* 1983;94:358–363.
9. Le Gall JR, Fagniez PL, Meakins J, et al. Diagnostic features of early high post-laparotomy fever: a prospective study of 100 patients. *Br J Surg* 1982;69:452.
10. Rantala A, Niinikoski J, Lehtonen O-P. Early *Candida* isolations in febrile patients after abdominal surgery. *Scand J Infect Dis* 1993;25:479–485.
11. Engoren M. Lack of association between atelectasis and fever. *Chest* 1995;107:81–84.
12. Petrelli NJ, Stulc JP, Rodriguez-Bigas M, et al. Nasogastric decompression following elective colorectal surgery: a prospective randomized study. *Am Surg* 1993;59:632–635.
13. Giangobbe MJ, Rappaport WD, Stein B. The significance of fever following cholecystectomy. *J Fam Pract* 1992;34:437–440.
14. Velazquez OC, Carpenter JP, Baum RA, et al. Perigraft air, fever, and leukocytosis after endovascular repair of abdominal aortic aneurysms. *Am J Surg* 1999;178:185–189.
15. Merjanian RB, Kiriakos CR, Dorey FJ, et al. Normal postoperative febrile response in the pediatric orthopaedic population. *J Pediatr Orthop* 1998;18:497–501.
16. Angel JD, Blasier RD, Allison R. Postoperative fever in pediatric orthopaedic patients. *J Pediatr Orthop* 1994;14:799–801.
17. Shackelford DP, Hoffman MK, Davies MF, et al. Predictive value for infection of febrile morbidity after vaginal surgery. *Obstet Gynecol* 1999;93:928–931.
18. Schwandt A, Andrews SJ, Fanning J. Prospective analysis of a fever evaluation algorithm after major gynecologic surgery. *Am J Obstet Gynecol* 2001;184:1066–1067.
19. McNally CG, Krivak TC, Alagoz T. Conservative management of isolated posthysterectomy fever. *J Reprod Med* 2000;45:572–576.
20. Guinn S, Castro FP, Garcia R, et al. Fever following total knee arthroplasty. *Am J Knee Surg* 1999;12:161–164.
21. Kennedy JG, Rodgers WB, Zurakowski D, et al. Pyrexia after total knee replacement. A cause for concern? *Am J Orthop* 1997;26:549–552, 554.
22. Circiumaru B, Baldock G, Cohen J. A prospective study of fever in the intensive care unit. *Intens Care Med* 1999;25:668–673.
23. Lyon DS, Jones JL, Sanchez A. Postoperative febrile morbidity in the benign gynecologic patient. Identification and management. *J Reprod Med* 2000;45:305–309.
24. Bell DM, Goldmann DA, Hopkins CC, et al. Unreliability of fever and leukocytosis in the diagnosis of infection after cardiac valve surgery. *J Thorac Cardiovasc Surg* 1978;75:87.
25. Dellinger EP, Wertz MJ, Oreskovich MR, et al. Specificity of fever and leukocytosis after laparotomy for penetrating abdominal trauma. *J Trauma* 1983;23:633.
26. Roberts J, Barnes W, Pennock M, et al: Diagnostic accuracy of fever as a measure of postoperative pulmonary complications. *Heart Lung* 1988;17:166.
27. Triulzi DJ, Vanek K, Ryan DH, et al. A clinical and immunologic study of blood transfusion and postoperative bacterial infection in spinal surgery. *Transfusion* 1992;32:517–524.
28. Ejlertsen T, Nielsen PH, Jepsen S, et al. Early diagnosis of postoperative pneumonia following upper abdominal surgery; a study in patients without cardiopulmonary disorder at operation. *Acta Chir Scand* 1989;155:93.
29. Frank SM, Kluger MJ, Kunkel SL. Elevated thermostatic setpoint in postoperative patients. *Anesthesiology* 2000;93:1426–1431.
30. Yared JP, Starr NJ, Hoffmann-Hogg L, et al. Dexamethasone decreases the incidence of shivering after cardiac surgery: a randomized, double-blind, placebo-controlled study. *Anesth Analg* 1998;87:795–799.
31. Horan TC, White JW, Jarvis WR, et al. Nosocomical infection surveillance, 1984. CDC Surveillance Summaries. *MMWR* 1986;35.
32. Dellinger E, Oreskovich M, Wertz M, et al. Risk of infection following laparotomy for penetrating abdominal injury. *Arch Surg* 1984;119:20–27.
33. Bartlett P, Reingold AL, Graham DR, et al. Toxic shock syndrome associated with surgical wound infections. *JAMA* 1982;247:1448.
34. Goodpasture HC, Voth DW. Toxic shock syndrome—additional perspectives. *JAMA* 1982;247:1464.
35. Raab MG, O'Brien M, Hayes JM, et al. Postoperative toxic shock syndrome. *Am J Orthop* 1995;24:130–136.
36. Jobe BA, Grasley A, Deveney KE, et al. *Clostridium difficile* colitis: an increasing hospital-acquired illness. *Am J Surg* 1995;169:480–483.
37. Yee J, Dixon CM, McLean AP, et al. *Clostridium difficile* disease in a department of surgery. The significance of prophylactic antibiotics. *Arch Surg* 1991;126:241–246.
38. George WL. Antimicrobial agent-associated colitis and diarrhea: historical background and clinical aspects. *Rev Infect Dis* 1984;6(suppl):208.
39. Bartlett JG. Antibiotic-associated colitis. *Dis Mon* 1984;30:6.
40. Dellinger EP, Wertz MJ, Lennard ES, et al. Efficacy of short-course antibiotic prophylaxis after penetrating intestinal injury. A prospective randomized trial. *Arch Surg* 1986;121:23–30.
41. Dellinger E, Caplan E, Weaver L, et al. Duration of preventive antibiotic administration for open extremity fractures. *Arch Surg* 1988;123:333–339.
42. Dellinger E, Miller S, Wertz M, et al. Risk of infection after open fracture of the arm or leg. *Arch Surg* 1988;123:1320–1327.
43. Strachan C, Black J, Powis S, et al. Prophylactic use of cephazolin against wound sepsis after cholecystectomy. *BMJ* 1977;1:1254–1256.
44. Mendelson J, Portnoy J, deSaint Victor J, et al. Effect of single and multidose cephradine prophylaxis on infectious morbidity of vaginal hysterectomy. *Obstet Gynecol* 1979;53:31–35.
45. Shapiro M, Townsend TR, Rosner B, et al. Use of antimicrobial drugs in general hospitals: patterns of prophylaxis. *N Engl J Med* 1979;301:351–355.
46. Classen DC, Evans RS, Pestotnik SL, et al. The timing of prophylactic administration of antibiotics and the risk of surgical-wound infection [see comments]. *N Engl J Med* 1992;326:281–286.
47. Currier JS, Campbell H, Platt R, et al. Perioperative antimicrobial prophylaxis in middle Tennessee, 1989–90. *Rev Infect Dis* 1991;12(suppl):874–878.
48. Swisher ED, Kahleifeh B, Pohl JF. Blood cultures in febrile patients after hysterectomy. Cost-effectiveness. *J Reprod Med* 1997;42:547–550.
49. Goodman JS, Shaffner W, Collins HA, et al. Infection after cardiovscular surgery: clinical study including examination of antimicrobial prophylaxis. *N Engl J Med* 1968;278:117.
50. Theuer CP, Bongard FS, Klein SR. Are blood cultures effective in the evaluation of fever in perioperative patients? *Am J Surg* 1991;162:615–619.
51. Bunt TJ. Urgent relaparotomy: the high-risk, no-choice operation. *Surgery* 1985;98:555–560.
52. Zer M, Dix S, Dintsman M. The timing of relaparotomy and its influence on prognosis. *Am J Surg* 1980;139:338–343.

53. Harbrecht PJ, Garrison RN, Fry DE. Early urgent relaparotomy. *Arch Surg* 1984;119:369–374.
54. Hinsdale JG, Jaffe BM. Re-operation for intraabdominal sepsis: indications and results in modern critical care setting. *Ann Surg* 1984;199:31–36.
55. Hau T, Ahrenholz DH, Simmons RL. Secondary bacterial peritonitis: the biologic basis of treatment. *Curr Probl Surg* 1979;16:1–65.
56. Lennard ES, Minshew BH, Dellinger EP, et al. Stratified outcome comparison of clindamycin-gentamicin vs chloramphenicol-gentamicin for treatment of intra-abdominal sepsis. *Arch Surg* 1985;120:889–898.
57. Dellinger EP, Wertz MJ, Meakins JL, et al. Surgical infection stratification system for intra-abdominal infection. Multicenter trial. *Arch Surg* 1985;120:21–29.
58. Bohnen J, Boulanger M, Meakins JL, et al. Prognosis in generalized peritonitis: relation to cause and risk factors. *Arch Surg* 1983;118:285–290.
59. Wright HK, Dunn E, MacArthur JD, et al. Specific but limited role of new imaging techniques in decision making about intraabdominal abscesses. *Am J Surg* 1982;143:456.
60. Norwood SH, Civetta JM. Abdominal CT scanning in critically ill surgical patients. *Ann Surg* 1985;202:166–175.
61. Hoogewoud H-M, Rubli E, Terrier F, et al. The role of computerized tomography in fever, septicemia and multiple system organ failure after laparotomy. *Surg Gynecol Obstet* 1986;162:539.
62. Deutschman C, Wilton P, Sinow J, et al. Paranasal sinusitis associated with nasotracheal intubation: a frequently unrecognized and treatable source of sepsis. *Crit Care Med* 1986;14:111–114.
63. Christensen L, Schaffer S, Ross SE. Otitis media in adult trauma patients: incidence and clinical significance. *J Trauma* 1991;31:1543–1545.
64. Kazmers A, Groehn H, Meeker C. Do patients with acute deep vein thrombosis have fever? *Am Surg* 2000;66:598–601.
65. Craig MH, Poole GV, Hauser CJ. Postsurgical gout. *Am Surg* 1995;61:56–59.

CHAPTER 94
Surgical Site Infection

Ronald Lee Nichols

Wound infections remain a major source of postoperative morbidity, accounting for about a quarter of the total number of nosocomial infections (1,2). Today many of these infections are first recognized in the outpatient clinic or in the patient's home because of the large number of operations done in the outpatient setting (2). This leads to errors in establishing the true frequency of their occurrence but undoubtedly decreases the overall real cost and prolongation of hospital stay. The pathogens implicated in the development of wound infections remain largely the microorganisms from the exogenous environment and the endogenous organ microflora. Many perioperative factors have been identified that increase the frequency of the development of postoperative wound infection. Avoidance of these factors as well as the appropriate use of perioperative antibiotic prophylaxis has decreased the incidence of wound infection.

The rate of wound infection varies from surgeon to surgeon, from hospital to hospital, and from one surgical procedure to another, and most important from one patient to another (Table 94.1). One of the earliest comprehensive reviews showed that the overall postoperative infection rate was approximately 7.4% (3). In 1976, wound infections accounted for approximately 24% of the total number of nosocomial infections (4). This figure represented more than 500,000 wound infections, or about 2.8 per 100 operations performed. Previous published data have shown that the average hospital stay was noted to double and the cost of hospitalization was correspondingly increased when postoperative wound infection developed after six commonly performed operations during the mid-1970s (5). These figures of real cost and length of hospital stay are undoubtedly lower today for most surgical procedures that are performed as outpatient procedures or those that require only a short postoperative stay. In these cases, most of the wound infections are diagnosed and treated in the outpatient clinic or in the patient's home. However, major complications such as deep sternal wound infections continue to a have grave impact, increasing the duration of hospitalization as much as 20-fold and the cost of hospitalization fivefold (6). The development of any surgical wound infection after open heart surgery has also been shown to result in a significant net loss of reimbursement to the hospital compared with uninfected cases, a factor that should serve as a potent incentive to hospitals to minimize the occurrence of postoperative wound infections (7).

During the 1980s, many significant observations were reported from data collected by the ongoing Study on the Efficacy of Nosocomial Infection Control (SENIC) project (8). In addition to the benefits from well-organized infection surveillance and control program improvements, significant advances have occurred in the appropriate use of prophylactic antibiotics in the surgical patient and in the accurate identification of those patients who are at greatest risk for the development of surgical wound sepsis in the various surgical procedures. The identification of high-risk patients in each specific surgical procedure will allow prospective alteration in therapy studies, which will be conducted and reported during the next decade (2).

DESCRIPTION OF CLINICAL WOUND INFECTIONS

To carry out surveillance, prevention, and control of surgical wound infections, it is necessary to use a commonly employed set of definitions. The Hospital Infections Program, Center for Infectious Diseases of the Centers for Disease Control and Prevention (CDC), previously developed a set of definitions to be used for the surveillance of nosocomial infections in the hospitals participating in the National Nosocomial Infections Surveillance System (9). These definitions were modified in 1992 to include specific sites of deep organ or space surgical site infections and to replace the term *wound infections* with *surgical site infections* (10). The wound site infections are divided into superficial and deep incisional and organ/space and are considered to be nosocomial (hospital acquired) only if there is no evidence that the infection was present or incubating at the time of hospital admission. The definitions for superficial and deep incisional and organ/space surgical site infections are presented in Table 94.2.

Most superficial surgical site infections are diagnosed sometime between the fourth and eighth postoperative day (late). When infection occurs during the first 48 hours after surgery (early), it is characteristically a rapidly moving gangrenous infection caused by a single type of microorganism, either a *Clostridium* species or β-hemolytic *Streptococcus*. In these rare cases, the dramatic clinical presentation may include profound systemic toxic effects and rapid local advance of the infection, often involving all layers of the body wall.

TRADITIONAL WOUND CLASSIFICATION: A TIME FOR REASSESSMENT

Classification of the surgical wound in the operating room by surgeons and nurses is a time-honored routine that has been practiced for at least 40 years, since the study by the National Academy of Sciences National Research Council on the influence of ultraviolet irradiation on surgical wound infection (3). This traditional method uses four classes of wounds based on the risk level and type of contamination expected or observed at operation. Clean surgical wounds (class I) are those in which only exogenous (airborne) contamination is expected or observed; the predicted rate of wound infection, largely due to gram-positive microorganisms such as *Staphylococcus aureus*,

TABLE 94.1. Overall Rate of Wound Infections after Surgical Procedures

Reference	Reported rate (%)	Comments
National Academy of Sciences, 1964 (3)	7.4	5-hospital 2.5-yr survey (15,613 operations)
Cruse, 1981 (43)	4.7	10-yr single-hospital study, standardized definitions, 28-day follow-up (62,939 operations)
Haley et al., 1985 (4)	2.8	1-yr (1975–1976) nationwide survey (18,271,858 operations)
Olson and Lee, 1990 (44)	2.5	10-yr review at a single medical center (40,915 operations)

was approximately 2%. Clean-contaminated (class II) wounds are those in which generally both exogenous and endogenous (aerobic-anaerobic) bacterial contamination occurs during elective operations; the infection rate in this category was estimated at 5% to 15% and is usually due to the polymicrobial endogenous flora. Contaminated wounds (class III) are those with early endogenous leakage or delayed exogenous contamination in the absence of established clinical infection; they carried a greater than 15% infection rate. In dirty-infected wounds (class IV), in which active infection was encountered during operation, a postoperative infection rate of greater than 30% was anticipated.

During the last decade, problems have been identified with the use of this traditional wound classification system and the accuracy of the predicted infection rates in each category. The major limitation lies in the lack of attention to the varying risk for infection among subjects in each class of wound. Haley and co-workers (11) at the CDC were among the first to describe the importance of identifying the varying individual risks for infection among patients in each of the traditional four categories of wounds. This and other timely studies on risk factors for surgical wound infection are discussed in Chapter 39. From this analysis,

TABLE 94.2. Criteria for Defining a Surgical Site Infection (SSI)

Superficial incisional SSI

Infection occurs within 30 days after the operation

and infection involves only skin or subcutaneous tissue of the incision

and at least one of the following:

1. Purulent drainage, with or without laboratory confirmation, from the superficial incision.
2. Organisms isolated from an aseptically obtained culture of fluid or tissue from the superficial incision.
3. At least one of the following signs or symptoms of infection: pain or tenderness, localized swelling, redness, or heat and superficial incision is deliberately opened by surgeon, unless incision is culture-negative.
4. Diagnosis of superficial incisional SSI by the surgeon or attending physician.

Do not report the following conditions as SSIs:

1. Stitch abscess (minimal inflammation and discharge confined to the points of suture penetration).
2. Infection of an episiotomy or newborn circumcision site.
3. Infected burn wound.
4. Incisional SSI that extends into the fascial and muscle layers (see deep incisional SSI).

Note: Specific criteria are used for identifying infected episiotomy and circumcision sites and burn wounds.

Deep incisional SSI

Infection occurs within 30 days after the operation if no implant[a] is left in place or within 1 year if implant is in place and the infection appears to be related to the operation

and infection involves deep soft tissues (e.g., fascial and muscle layers) of the incision

and at least one of the following:

1. Purulent drainage from the deep incision but not from the organ/space component of the surgical site.
2. A deep incision spontaneously dehisces or is deliberately opened by a surgeon when the patient has at least one of the following signs or symptoms: fever (>38°C), localized pain, or tenderness, unless site is culture-negative.
3. An abscess or other evidence of infection involving the deep incision is found on direct examination, during operation, or by histopathologic or radiologic examination.
4. Diagnosis of a deep incisional SSI by a surgeon or attending physician.

Notes:

1. Report infection that involves both superficial and deep incision sites as deep incisional SSI.
2. Report an organ/space SSI that drains through the incision as a deep incisional SSI.

Organ/space SSI

Infection occurs within 30 days after the operation in no implant[a] is left in place or within 1 year if implant is in place and the infection appears to be related to the operation

and infection involves any part of the anatomy (e.g., organs or spaces), other than the incision, which was opened or manipulated during an operation

and at least one of the following:

1. Purulent drainage from a drain that is placed through a stab wound[b] into the organ/space.
2. Organisms isolated from an aseptically obtained culture of fluid or tissue in the organ/space.
3. An abscess or other evidence of infection involving the organ/space that is found on direct examination, during reoperation, or by histopathologic or radiologic examination.
4. Diagnosis of an organ/space SSI by a surgeon or attending physician.

[a]National Nosocomial Infection Surveillance definition: a nonhuman-derived implantable foreign body (e.g., prosthetic heart valve, nonhuman vascular graft, mechanical heart, or hip prosthesis) that is permanently placed in a patient during surgery.
[b]If the area around a stab wound becomes infected, it is not an SSI. It is considered a skin or soft tissue infection, depending on its depth.
From Horan TC, Gaynes RP, Martone WJ, et al. CDC definitions of nosocomial surgical site infections, 1992: a modification of CDC definitions of surgical wound infections. *Am J Infect Control* 1992;20:271, with permission.

TABLE 94.3. Comparison of Rates of Surgical Wound Infections Using Either the Traditional Classification System or the Simplified Risk Index for 58,498 Patients Undergoing Surgical Procedures at 338 SENIC Hospitals in 1970

Traditional wound class	Infection rate (%) for a simplified risk index[a] of					
	0	1	2	3	4	All
Class I: Clean	1.1	3.9	8.4	15.8	—	2.9
Class II: Clean-contaminated	0.6	2.8	8.4	17.7	—	3.9
Class III: Contaminated	—	4.5	8.3	11.0	23.9	8.5
Class IV: Dirty-infected	—	6.7	10.9	18.8	27.4	12.6
All	1.0	3.6	8.9	17.2	27.0	4.1

[a]Total number of the following risk factors: abdominal operation; operation longer than 2 hours; contaminated or dirty-infected operation; three or more diagnoses.
SENIC, Study on the Efficacy of Nosocomial Infection Control.
Data from Haley RW, Culver DH, Morgan WM, et al. Identifying patients at high risk of surgical wound infection. *Am J Epidemiol* 1985; 121:206.

we understand today that the risk for infection in each traditional category of surgical procedures varies greatly, depending on the individual patient's risk factors. The infection rate in clean surgical procedures cannot be assumed to be low (12). Haley and colleagues (11) created a simplified index of the risk for infection that consists of the total number of the following risk factors: abdominal operation, operation longer than 2 hours, contaminated (class III) or dirty-infected operation (class IV), and three or more diagnoses. They compared this risk index with the traditional wound classifications (Table 94.3) and found a great range of infection rates among each of the traditional classes, from 1% to 16% for clean surgery to 7% to 27% in dirty-contaminated cases. Realization of the presence of the patient's risk factors in each surgical procedure will result in more accurate assessment of the initial risk for wound infection and will allow prophylactic or therapeutic interventions, which may ideally lead to an overall decrease in the occurrence of wound infection.

Most recently, the National Nosocomial Infection Surveillance (NNIS) risk index has been developed, which is operation specific and applies to all prospectively collected surveillance data (13). The index values range from 0 to 3 points and are defined by these independent and equally weighted variables. One point is scored for each of the following when present: (a) American Society of Anesthesiologists (ASA) Physical Status Classification of greater than 2; (b) either contaminated or dirty infected wound classification (class III or IV) and; (c) length of operation greater than T hours, where T is the approximate 75th percentile of the duration of specific operations being performed.

In conclusion, the traditional four-class system of estimating risk for postoperative wound infection is largely dependent on the nature and extent of perioperative contamination, reflecting little focus on the individual patient's risk factors (14). In addition, the classification levels overlap. Although this system has served well, the data presented indicate that newer developed systems are more effective. The risk for postoperative wound infection depends largely on the combined effects of the nature and extent of perioperative contamination as well as the individual patient's risk factors. More attention should now be focused on delineating the general risk factors, including specific disease or operative factors, for infection in the surgical patient.

PATHOGENS IMPLICATED IN SURGICAL WOUND INFECTIONS

The pathogens that are isolated from surgical wound infections vary, primarily on the basis of the type of surgical procedure

undertaken (Table 94.4). In clean surgical procedures in which the gastrointestinal, gynecologic, and respiratory tracts have not been entered, *Staphylococcus aureus* from the exogenous environment or the patient's skin flora is the usual cause of infection. In the other categories of surgical procedures, including clean-contaminated, contaminated, and dirty-infected, the polymicrobial aerobic-anaerobic flora closely resembling the normal endogenous microflora of the surgically resected organ constitutes the most frequently isolated pathogens (15).

The importance of thoughtfully carried out epidemiologic and microbiologic investigations of the changing patterns of nosocomial pathogens both in outbreak investigations and in national surveillance data has been stressed since the early 1960s (16). Evidence reported from the SENIC project and the

TABLE 94.4. Common Potential Pathogens Causing Surgical Wound Infections

Type of surgical procedure	Potential pathogens
Clean	
Cardiac, vascular, orthopedic	*Staphylococcus aureus*, *Staphylococcus epidermidis*, enteric gram-negative bacilli
Clean-contaminated or contaminated	
Gastroduodenal	Aerobic and anaerobic streptococci, enteric gram-negative bacilli, *Bacteroides species* (not *fragilis*)
Biliary	Enteric gram-negative bacilli, enterococci, clostridia
Colorectal (elective)	Enteric gram-negative bacilli, *B. fragilis*, peptostreptococci, clostridia
Small intestine	Enteric gram-negative bacilli, *B. fragilis*, peptostreptococci
Appendectomy	Enteric gram-negative bacilli, *B. fragilis*, peptostreptococci, enterococci
Vaginal or abdominal hysterectomy; cesarean section; abortion	Enteric gram-negative bacilli, *B. fragilis*, enterococci, clostridia, group B streptococci
Dirty-infected	
Penetrating abdominal trauma	Enteric gram-negative bacilli, *B. fragilis*, peptostreptococci, clostridia, enterococci
Other traumatic wounds	*S. aureus*, clostridia, group A streptococci

NNIS system has shown that the rate of nosocomial infections caused by different pathogens continues to change (17). The number of nosocomial infections caused by gram-positive cocci, which had been declining, is again increasing, with the emergence of coagulase-negative staphylococci as important nosocomial pathogens (18,19). Edmiston and colleagues (19) have observed that the majority of prosthetic vascular graft infections are now caused by mucin-producing strains of *Staphylococcus epidermidis,*which express varying degrees of adherence to the synthetic substrates.

Antibiotic-resistant strains of both gram-positive and gram-negative microorganisms are being increasingly isolated from infections in postoperative patients and from the hospital environment (20,21). Rapidly growing mycobacteria, *Rhodococcus bronchialis,* and *Candida tropicalis* have been implicated in outbreaks of both deep and superficial wound infections after open heart surgery (22–24). In the case of the mycobacterial infections, about 80% of the cardiac isolates were from the southern coastal states, and the heterogeneity of the isolates suggests that most are unrelated but are derived from local environmental sources rather than from contaminated commercial surgical materials or devices (22). This finding of heterogeneity among the isolates of rapidly growing mycobacteria has also been reported in wound infections after augmentation mammaplasty despite case clustering in Texas and other southern coastal states (25). The outbreaks of wound infection due to both *R. bronchialis* and *C. tropicalis* were identified to be common-source cluster epidemics; the removal of the sources from the cardiac team terminated the outbreaks (23,24).

The importance of the strict enforcement of infection control policies within the operating room has been the subject of two reports (26,27). An outbreak of infection due to *Serratia marcescens* was reported in eight patients who had undergone cardiovascular surgery in one hospital (26). Two of the patients became bacteremic, and one died. The epidemiologic investigation identified the cause of the outbreak to be contaminated skin cream used by a scrub nurse. This nurse also wore artificial nails, which are known to increase the carriage rate of gram-negative bacteria. The outbreak stopped after the use of the cream was discontinued. In the other study, a relatively new intravenous anesthetic, propofol, was implicated in a large number of postoperative wound and other infections (27). This drug has a unique lipid base that can support microbial growth if it is contaminated. Sixty-two patients at seven hospitals developed infections after administration of propofol. These infections, at first, were attributed to the surgeon or procedure performed. Subsequently, it was found that extrinsic contamination of the drug had resulted from numerous breaks in infection control technique by the anesthesia personnel (27,28). Contaminated drug was then administered to the patients, resulting in the infections.

FACTORS THAT RELATE TO SURGICAL WOUND INFECTION AND THE PATIENT'S RISK FACTORS

Many factors, including length of preoperative hospital stay, use of antibiotic prophylaxis, preoperative cleansing and shaving techniques, use of prophylactic drains, and elective operation done in the presence of an active remote infection, have been proved to influence the development of postoperative wound infections (29). Many other factors have been considered, without convincing evidence, to influence postoperative wound infection, including preoperative scrub technique, surgical glove damage, barrier materials, and laminar flow air-handling systems in the operating room. Anecdotal experience and commercial interests rather than scientific studies usually account for these associations. A thoughtful review by Sebben (30) offered recommendations that are thought to be essential elements of infection control for office-based surgical practice, including modern concepts of instrument sterilization, skin cleansing, and insights into the use of prophylactic antibiotics.

These factors as well as general risk factors related to the patient are described in Chapter 39 and therefore are not reviewed again here.

RISK FACTORS FOR INFECTION IN SPECIFIC OPERATIVE PROCEDURES

Many clinical studies of risk factors for infection in specific operative procedures were published during the 1980s. Knowledge of the presence or absence of these risk factors in the perioperative period may allow alterations of infection control techniques in the studies conducted in the future (Table 94.5).

Shapiro and coinvestigators (31) in 1982 were the first to use logistic regression analysis to identify the risk factors for operative site infections in abdominal or vaginal hysterectomy. They observed that an increasing duration of operative time was associated with a decreasing effect of antibiotic prophylaxis in preventing operative site infection. The statistically significant benefit of antibiotic prophylaxis in procedures lasting 1 hour or less was lost in operations lasting more than 3.3 hours. Using a similar logistic regression analysis of the risks for infection after penetrating abdominal trauma, we showed that a statistically higher risk for infection was associated with the increasing age of the patient, an injury to the left colon necessitating colostomy, a large number of transfusions at surgery, and a large number of injured organs identified at operation (32). The presence of shock on arrival to the hospital, which was found to increase the risk for infection when this factor was analyzed individually, did not add predictive power. We then conducted a double-blind, randomized study of 170 patients with traumatic perforation of the gastrointestinal tract who were administered an advanced-generation cephalosporin (33). At surgical closure, patients were divided into infection risk groups (below 40%, low; 40% to 70%, middle; and above 70%, high) by use of the logistic regression formula based on four proven risk factors: age, blood replacement, ostomy, and number of organs injured. Patients in the low-risk group received 2 days of antibiotic therapy; those in the middle- and high-risk groups received 5 days of antibiotic therapy. Those patients in the low- and middle-risk groups had primary wound closure; those in the high-risk group had their wounds packed open and closed later. Most of the patients (n = 144, or 85%) were in the low-risk group. Their major and minor infection rates (10% and 12%, respectively) were not significantly different from 145 historical control subjects receiving 5 days of antibiotic therapy (9% major, 14% minor). Patients in the middle- and high-risk groups showed a greater rate of major infections (46%) but a similar rate of minor infections (12%). The results indicated that risk factors can be used to identify low-risk patients who require only short-term antibiotic therapy and primary wound closure. The remaining patients were shown to be at greater risk for infection despite prolonged antibiotic therapy and delayed wound closure.

In a published large single-hospital study of wound infections after cesarean section, significantly higher rates of infections were observed in clinic patients (15.8%) compared with private patients (6.0%) (34). All significant individual risk factors for infection, including emergency versus elective operation, number of vaginal examinations before operation, duration of

TABLE 94.5.   Risk Factors Implicated[a] in Increased Surgical Wound Infection Rates after Specific Operative Procedures

Procedure	Risk factors
Penetrating abdominal trauma	Increased age
	Left colon injury requiring colostomy
	Increased transfusions at surgery
	Increased number of injured organs or associated injuries
	Increased colon injury score
	Significant intraperitoneal contamination
Elective colonic resection	Duration of operation
	Location of resection
Nonperforative appendicitis	Nonuse of perioperative antibiotics
	Surgeon's determination of gangrenous appendix
Abdominal or vaginal hysterectomy	Increased operative time
Cardiac surgery	Obesity
	Diabetes
	Prolonged hospitalization
	Prolonged stay in intensive care unit
	Prolonged mechanical ventilation
	Preexisting chronic pulmonary disease or postoperative pneumonia
	Increased age
	Prolonged use of Foley catheter
	Reexploration
	Postoperative weight gain
	Placement of intraaortic balloon pump
	Postoperative blood products
	Male sex
Vascular surgery for lower limb arterial ischemia	Rest pain
	Skin necrosis
	Increased age
Gastroduodenal surgery	Low gastric acidity
	Reduced gastrointestinal motility
Biliary surgery	Age >70 yr
	Previous biliary tract surgery
	Jaundice, acute cholecystitis, or common duct stones

[a]One or more controlled clinical studies.

operation, vertical skin incision, and category of surgeon, were overrepresented in the group of clinic patients. There was no difference in the wound infection rate among potentially infected patients whether or not prophylactic antibiotics were used.

A prospective study of nonperforated appendicitis, using a logistic regression analysis of risk factors, has shown that the risk for postoperative wound infection related only to the failure to use perioperative antibiotics and the surgeon's determination of the appendix as gangrenous (35). The highest infection probability (77%) was predicted in those patients receiving placebo and having a gangrenous appendix, the lowest (2%) in those receiving an antibiotic perioperatively and not having a gangrenous appendix at surgery. Perioperative antibiotic prophylaxis had a beneficial effect in decreasing hospital stay.

Kaiser and associates (36), studying elective colon resection and different approaches to preoperative antibiotic prophylaxis, have shown a direct correlation between the duration of operation and the postoperative infection rate. In operations lasting less than 3 hours, no infections were identified when the antibiotic prophylaxis was with a parenteral agent alone or a combination of oral and parenteral agents. However, in operations lasting more than 4 hours, a significant reduction of infection was observed in those patients receiving the combination prophylactic regimen. Coppa and Eng (37), in a similar study of elective colon resection, have stressed that postoperative wound infections are associated with the length of operation and location of the colonic resection (intraperitoneal colon resection vs. rectal resection). These researchers showed that the wound infec-

tion rate in high-risk patients with long operations (longer than 215 minutes) and rectal resection could be reduced significantly by the use of a combination of oral and parenteral prophylactic antibiotics. Whether to repair the injured colon primarily or to do a colostomy has been the subject of a prospective study of colonic injuries after penetrating abdominal trauma (38). Using logistic regression analysis, the researchers identified that transfusion of four or more units, more than two associated injuries, significant intraperitoneal contamination, and increasing colon injury severity scores significantly correlate with increased frequencies of postoperative wound and intraabdominal infections. They concluded that nearly all penetrating colon wounds can be repaired primarily regardless of risk factors.

Many current studies have been published concerning the risk factors for wound and deep sternal infections after median sternotomy for cardiac surgical procedures. Knowledge of these risk factors is required to aid surgeons and patients in making judgments about the relative benefits of surgery and to alert nursing personnel to be particularly aware of early signs of infection in patients at high risk (39). This may also be helpful in planning additional prophylactic measures for high-risk patients. Numerous individual risk factors have been identified in this population of patients (2) (Table 94.5). The use of bilateral internal mammary arterial grafting in coronary revascularization procedures has been shown to be a risk factor for infection in some studies.

The risk factors for wound infection after vascular surgery have been reported after a study of 100 consecutive patients with lower limb arterial ischemia (40). The researchers found a significant number of patients harboring pathogenic organisms on their skin preoperatively in those with rest pain and skin necrosis. Another risk factor was increasing age of the patient, whereas claudication or the presence of an aneurysm was not.

Undoubtedly, risk factor studies accomplished in the next decade, for other operative procedures, will aid in our discovery of the high-risk patient, which will allow prospective alterations in preventive techniques in this group.

SURVEILLANCE OF THE SURGICAL WOUND

Traditional surveillance of the surgical wound, which was practiced widely into the 1970s, depended primarily on infection control personnel's searching for positive cultures from the microbiology laboratory. The finding of a positive culture of wound drainage or exudate triggered a review of the patient's chart and of the patient if he or she was still hospitalized. Errors in this approach were due to inadequate and widely varying definitions of surgical wound infection in addition to the missing of clinical infection when cultures were not done for infected patients or when the culture result was negative in infected patients.

With use of a representative sample of U.S. general hospitals (SENIC project), the efficacy of infection surveillance and control on the prevention of nosocomial infections was established by the CDC in 1985 (41). A 32% reduction in nosocomial infections was noted from 1970 to the period from 1975 to 1976 in the participating hospitals where the essential components of the intensive infection surveillance and control programs were practiced. These effective programs included conducting organized concurrent surveillance and control activities and having a trained effectual infection control physician, an infection control nurse per 250 beds, and a system for reporting infection rates to practicing surgeons. It was estimated that because only a few hospitals had these programs, only 6% of the nation's approximately 2 million nosocomial infections were actually being prevented by the mid-1970s, leaving another 26% to be prevented by universal adoption of these programs. Among hospitals without effective programs, the overall infection rate increased by 18% from 1970 to 1976. In an update of the SENIC project (42) using information collected in 1983 from a random sample of hospitals, it was found that the intensity of infection surveillance and control activities had greatly increased from 1976. The number of hospitals with an infection control nurse per 250 beds increased from 22% to 57%, although the number with a physician trained in infection control remained low (15%). There was an increase in the number of hospitals having effective programs to prevent urinary tract infections, bacteremias, and pneumonias, but this was not the case for surgical wound infection. Also noted was that the percentage of hospitals doing surgical wound infection surveillance had decreased (from 90% to 79%), and those reporting surgeon-specific infection rates to surgeons had decreased (from 19% to 13%). At this point, it is estimated that 9% of the nosocomial infections were being prevented, whereas 32% could be prevented if all hospitals adopted the most effective programs. The NNIS program has resulted in additional benefits during the past decade and will continue to in the decade ahead (13).

The first comprehensive, single-hospital, 10-year prospective study of wound infection surveillance was reported in 1981 (43) (Table 94.1). In this study, all wounds were inspected by a single surgical nurse. Definitions of wound infections were standardized, and surveillance was continued by telephone for up to 28 days, when a final report on each wound was made. An overall infection rate of 4.7% was identified. Each surgeon received an annual report showing the surgeon's individual rate of infection in clean wounds as well as the average clean wound infection rate of the patients of the other surgeons in corresponding surgical divisions. A monthly computer report of the infection rates, especially stressing the clean wound, was discussed at the division of surgery and the infection control committee meetings. The bottom line of this report was a reduction of almost 50% in the overall wound infection rate as well as of the clean infection rate within 6 months after institution of this surveillance program.

In a later 10-year wound infection surveillance program, procedure-specific rates rather than surgeon-specific rates were calculated annually (44). The results of this study (Table 94.1) showed a significant reduction in wound infection rates in the past 9 years of surveillance in every class of surgical wound compared with the index year rates. Estimated savings in hospital room costs alone reached $3 million during the 10 years.

The improvement in wound infection rates in all of these studies was the direct result of periodic clinical interventions based on the surveillance data, which have already been described in the section on the factors that prevent surgical wound infections. The use of computer surveillance to improve the use of antibiotic administration in both the prevention and treatment of nosocomial infections, including wound infections, has also been stressed (45,46). Many different computer-based programs have been developed for the monitoring of surgical wound infections and the identification of risk factors for the development of infection (47,48).

Shorter lengths of hospitalization and the increasing numbers of outpatient operations have heightened our awareness of the importance of posthospital surveillance to accurately document the presence of surgical wound infection. Follow-up of patients for at least 30 days after surgery is generally required to rule out the presence of a superficial wound infection. Large studies have shown that at present, about 50% of all infections can be identified after hospital discharge if adequate surveillance is performed (49,50). In addition to the data obtained from clinic visits, questionnaires for the physician and patient sent out approximately 30 days after discharge from the hospital have appeared to offer the best efficacy in determining the true rate of surgical wound infection (49).

Most studies concerning the collection and confidential distribution of surgeon-specific wound infection rates, especially in clean surgical procedures, have shown a reduction of surgical wound infection after the use of this approach (51,52). However, an editorial has stressed that to prove the validity of surgeon-specific wound infection rates, one must adjust for surgical procedure as well as for the severity of the patient's illness (53).

A standardized effective surveillance program to detect and control surgical wound infection has proved to be of benefit in reducing the frequency of these infections. It is urged that all hospitals implement these programs (54).

IMPLICATIONS FOR THE FUTURE

The number of patients admitted to hospitals for inpatient surgery will continue to decrease while the numbers of outpatient surgical procedures will continue to increase. The severity of the patient's illness and the risk for postoperative wound infection and other septic events in hospitalized patients will increase. These trends will require effective infection surveillance in both the hospital and the outpatient setting for collection of meaningful data (29). Continued advances in computer technology will improve the collection and integration of pertinent clinical, laboratory, and surgical information and will greatly facilitate surveillance, analysis, and control of infections in the surgical wound.

Specific patient-related risk factors for each operative procedure will be reported, and these risk factors will be used to plan prospective alterations in therapy studies with the intention of doing less for the low-risk patient and increasing the preventive and therapeutic modalities in the high-risk patient.

Further progress in the area of chemotherapeutic development will occur, with the emphasis being placed on the use of oral or local regimens. The use of antibiotic prophylaxis before operative procedures will continue to be streamlined, largely on the basis of further pharmacokinetic data that will influence administration techniques and limit the total dosage. Operative procedures that use foreign body implants may be performed with implants that have been commercially bonded or prepared with antibiotics or antiseptics. Immunomodulators will be used to help prevent infectious complications in the immunosuppressed host. Infection control committees will ideally direct more attention to proper surveillance of the surgical wound than to the discussion of the relative merits of sacred cows.

REFERENCES

1. Nichols RL. Postoperative wound infection. *N Engl J Med* 1982;307:1701.
2. Nichols RL. Preventing surgical site infections: a surgeon's perspective. *Emerg Infect Dis* 2001;7(2)220.
3. National Academy of Sciences, National Research Council. Postoperative wound infections: the influence of ultraviolet irradiation of the operating room and of various other factors. *Ann Surg* 1964;160(suppl 2):1.
4. Haley RW, Culver DH, White JW, et al. The nationwide nosocomial infection rate: a new need for vital statistics. *Am J Epidemiol* 1985;121:159.
5. Green JW, Wenzel RP. Postoperative wound infection: a controlled study of the increased duration of hospital stay and direct cost of hospitalization. *Ann Surg* 1977;185:264.
6. Taylor GJ, Mikell FL, Moses HW, et al. Determinants of hospital charges for coronary artery bypass surgery: the economic consequences of postoperative complications. *Am J Cardiol* 1990;65:309.
7. Boyce JM, Potter-Bynoe G, Dziobek L. Hospital reimbursement patterns among patients with surgical wound infections following open heart surgery. *Infect Control Hosp Epidemiol* 1990;11:89.
8. Haley RW, Quade D, Freeman HE, et al. The SENIC Project. Study on the efficacy of nosocomial infection control (SENIC Project). Summary of study design. *Am J Epidemiol* 1980;111:472.
9. Garner JS, Jarvis WR, Emori TG, et al. CDC definitions for nosocomial infections, 1988. *Am J Infect Control* 1988;16:128.
10. Horan TC, Gaynes RP, Martone WJ, et al. CDC definitions of nosocomial surgical site infections, 1992: a modification of CDC definitions of surgical wound infections. *Am J Infect Control* 1992;20:271.
11. Haley RW, Culver DH, Morgan WM, et al. Identifying patients at high risk of surgical wound infection. *Am J Epidemiol* 1985;121:206.
12. Nichols RL. Wound infection rates following clean operative procedures: can we assume them to be low? *Infect Control Hosp Epidemiol* 1992;13:455.
13. Culver DH, Horan TC, Gaynes RP, et al. Surgical wound infection rates by wound class, operative procedure, and patient risk index. National Nosocomial Infection Surveillance System. *Am J Med* 1991;91:152.
14. Nichols RL. Classification of the surgical wound: a time for reassessment and simplification. *Infect Control Hosp Epidemiol* 1993;14:253.
15. Nichols RL. Prevention of infection in high risk gastrointestinal surgery. *Am J Med* 1984;76:111.
16. Kundsin RB, Walter CW, Morin P. *Staphylococcus aureus* UC-18: agent of nosocomial infections. *Science* 1964;145:1322.
17. Hughes JM. Study on the efficacy of nosocomial infection control (SENIC Project): results and implications for the future. *Chemotherapy* 1988;34:553.
18. Large M, Stubbs E, Berm R, et al. A study of coagulase-negative staphylococci isolated from clinically significant infections at an Australian teaching hospital. *Pathology* 1989;21:19.
19. Edmiston CE Jr, Schmitt DD, Seabrook GR. Coagulase-negative staphylococcal infections in vascular surgery: epidemiology and pathogenesis. *Infect Control Hosp Epidemiol* 1989;10:111.
20. Andersen BM, Sorlie D, Hotvedt R, et al. Multiply beta-lactam resistant *Enterobacter cloacae* infections linked to the environmental flora in a unit for cardiothoracic and vascular surgery. *Scand J Infect Dis* 1989;21:181.
21. The Hospital Infection Control Practices Advisory Committee (HICPAC). Recommendations for preventing the spread of vancomycin resistance—special communication. *Am J Infect Control* 1995;23:87.
22. Wallace RJ Jr, Musser JM, Hull SI, et al. Diversity and sources of rapidly growing mycobacteria associated with infections following cardiac surgery. *J Infect Dis* 1989;159:708.
23. Isenberg HD, Tucci V, Cintron F, et al. Single-source outbreak of *Candida tropicalis* complicating coronary bypass surgery. *J Clin Microbiol* 1989;27:2426.
24. Richet HM, Craven PC, Brown JM, et al. *Rhodococcus bronchialis* sternal wound infections following coronary artery bypass graft surgery. *N Engl J Med* 1991;324:104.
25. Wallace RJ Jr, Steele LC, Labidi A, et al. Heterogeneity among isolates of rapidly growing mycobacteria responsible for infections following augmentation mammoplasty despite case clustering in Texas and other southern coastal states. *J Infect Dis* 1989;160:281.
26. Centers for Disease Control and Prevention. Sleuths track nosocomial outbreak to skin cream. *Hosp Infect Control* 1995;22:65.
27. Bennett SN, McNeil MM, Bland LA, et al. Postoperative infections traced to contamination of an intravenous anesthetic, propofol. *N Engl J Med* 1995;333:147.
28. Nichols RL, Smith JW. Bacterial contamination of an anesthetic agent. *N Engl J Med* 1995;333:184.
29. Mangram AJ, Horan TC, Pearson ML, et al. Guideline for Prevention of Surgical Site Infection, 1999. *Infect Control Hosp Epidemiol* 1999;20:247.
30. Sebben JE. Sterile technique and the prevention of wound infection in office surgery—part II. *J Dermatol Surg Oncol* 1989;15:38.
31. Shapiro M, Munoz A, Tager IB, et al. Risk factors for infection at the operative site after abdominal or vaginal hysterectomy. *N Engl J Med* 1982;307:1661.
32. Nichols RL, Smith JW, Klein DB, et al. Risk of infection after penetrating abdominal trauma. *N Engl J Med* 1984;311:1065.
33. Nichols RL, Smith JW, Robertson GD, et al. Prospective alterations in therapy for penetrating abdominal trauma. *Arch Surg* 1993;128:55.
34. Webster J. Post-caesarean wound infection: a review of the risk factors. *Aust N Z J Obstet Gynaecol* 1988;28:201.
35. Browder W, Smith JW, Vivoda LM, et al. Nonperforative appendicitis: a continuing surgical dilemma. *J Infect Dis* 1989;159:1088.
36. Kaiser AB, Herrington JL Jr, Jacobs JK, et al. Cefoxitin versus erythromycin, neomycin, and cefazolin in colorectal operations. *Ann Surg* 198:525, 1983.
37. Coppa GF, Eng K: Factors involved in antibiotic selection in elective colon and rectal surgery. *Surgery* 1988;104:853.
38. George SM Jr, Fabian TC, Voeller GR, et al. Primary repair of colon wounds: a prospective trial in nonselected patients. *Ann Surg* 1989;209:728.
39. Lillienfeld DE, Vlahov D, Tenney JH, et al. Obesity and diabetes as risk factors for postoperative wound infections after cardiac surgery. *Am J Infect Control* 1988;16:3.
40. Earnshaw JJ, Slack RCB, Hopkinson BR, et al. Risk factors in vascular surgical sepsis. *Ann R Coll Surg Engl* 1988;70:139.
41. Haley RW, Culver DH, White JW, et al. The efficacy of infection surveillance and control programs in preventing nosocomial infections in US hospitals. *Am J Epidemiol* 1985;121:182.
42. Haley RW, Morgan WM, Culver DH, et al. Update from the SENIC project. Hospital infection control: recent progress and opportunities under prospective payment. *Am J Infect Control* 1985;13:97.
43. Cruse P. Wound infection surveillance. *Rev Infect Dis* 1981;3:734.
44. Olson MM, Lee JT Jr. Continuous, 10-year wound infection surveillance: results, advantages, and unanswered questions. *Arch Surg* 1990;125:794.
45. Evans RS, Larsen RA, Burke JP, et al. Computer surveillance of hospital-acquired infections and antibiotic use. *JAMA* 1986;256:1007.
46. Larsen RA, Evans RS, Burke JP, et al. Improved perioperative antibiotic use and reduced surgical wound infection through use of computer decision analysis. *Infect Control Hosp Epidemiol* 1989;10:316.
47. Bremmelgaard A, Raahave D, Beier-Holgersen R, et al. Computer-aided surveillance of surgical infections and identification of risk factors. *J Hosp Infect* 1989;13:1.
48. Kjaeldgaard P, Cordtz T, Sejberg D, et al. The DANOP-DATA system: a low cost personal computer based program for monitoring of wound infections in surgical ward. *J Hosp Infect* 1989;13:273.
49. Brown RB, Bradley S, Opitz E, et al. Surgical wound infections documented after hospital discharge. *Am J Infect Control* 1987;15:54.
50. Krukowski ZH, Matheson NA. Ten-year computerized audit of infection after abdominal surgery. *Br J Surg* 1988;75:857.
51. Condon RE, Schulte WJ, Malangoni MA, et al. Effectiveness of a surgical wound surveillance program. *Arch Surg* 1983;118:303.
52. Mead PB, Pories SE, Hall P. Decreasing the incidence of surgical wound infection. *Arch Surg* 1986;121:458.
53. Scheckler WE. Surgeon-specific wound infection rates—a potentially dangerous and misleading strategy. *Infect Control Hosp Epidemiol* 1988;9:145.
54. Nichols RL. Surveillance of the surgical wound. *Infect Control Hosp Epidemiol* 1990;11:513.

CHAPTER 95

Gas Gangrene and Other Clostridial Skin and Soft Tissue Infections

Sherwood L. Gorbach

Clostridial species are associated with a variety of skin and soft tissue infections. The clinical presentation may be acute and dramatic, with tissue destruction and gangrene that progresses over a few hours to an inexorably lethal outcome, or these organisms can coexist in apparent symbiosis with other bacteria in a chronic, suppurative infection, such as diabetic foot ulcer, which can persist for months and even years. The most important distinction in classifying clostridial infections is clinical evidence of toxin production, which causes local effects on muscle, with destruction and gangrene, and systemic effects such as hypotension, renal failure, and hemolysis. In a classic paper, MacLennan (1) described what he termed "the histotoxic clostridial infections," a classification based mostly on his experiences with clostridial infections in wartime. This simple approach has become somewhat outdated since other forms of toxigenic clostridial infections have been described in civilian practice. Besides the typical traumatic injuries described by MacLennan, whether associated with war wounds, civilian violence, or major trauma, serious, nontraumatic cases have been recognized, some of which occur with classic myonecrosis and others with spreading cellulitis and overwhelming toxinosis but without direct involvement of muscle (Table 95.1).

Gas gangrene is a necrotizing, gas-forming process of muscle associated with systemic signs of toxemia (1–10). The appearance of affected muscle is distinctive, and the diagnosis of gas gangrene can be made on direct inspection of the open wound. Histologically, there is gelatinous necrosis of muscle cells, with early loss of striations and nuclei, in the absence of acute inflammation or infiltration of polymorphonuclear leukocytes.

MICROBIOLOGY

Clostridium perfringens type A is the leading cause of gas gangrene, reported in about 80% of such cases (ranging from 50% to 100%) (4,8,10). *Clostridium novyi* or *Clostridium septicum* is the pathogen in most of the remaining cases. Some reports have implicated *Clostridium histolyticum, Clostridium bifermantans, Clostridium sporogenes,* and *Clostridium fallax,* although the evidence for their role is rather tenuous (4,10–12). *Clostridium difficile* was implicated in a case of necrotizing fasciitis and gas gangrene (13). The incriminated pathogen is isolated in pure culture in about half of cases, and in the remainder an assortment of aerobic and anaerobic organisms coexist in the contaminated wound (10).

PATHOPHYSIOLOGY

Among the 12 toxins elaborated by *C. perfringens,* the α toxin, which has phospholipase C (PLC; lecithinase) and sphingomyelinase activities, is the major toxin responsible for the clinical manifestations of gas gangrene (see Chapter 213) (14). Minute amounts of α toxin are lethal to mice; in rabbits, it causes

bradycardia, hypotension, and a dose-dependent reduction in myocardial function (15). PLC directly suppresses myocardial contractility and is associated with reductions in cardiac output and hypotension (16). Guinea pigs immunized with α toxin are protected against challenge by the organism itself or the purified toxin. The availability of purified α toxin and knowledge of the genetics of the toxin have brought additional data confirming the central role of this toxin in the clinical presentation of gas gangrene. By using *Escherichia coli* protein comprising the C-terminal domain of α toxin, it was possible to provide protection in a mouse model against lethal effects of a challenge of *C. perfringens* type A organisms (17). The role of α toxin was also examined by a genetic approach that used "knockout" mutants of *C. perfringens* type A. The mutant strain that failed to produce α toxin could not cause gas gangrene in a mouse myonecrosis model, whereas the parent strain with intact α toxin production had full virulence in this model (18). A hemolysin, θ toxin (perfingolysin O, PFO) is also lethal to mice, and it causes a decrease in peripheral vascular resistance, resulting in "warm shock" (16,19). PLC and PLO appear to act synergistically to produce hypotension, hypoxia, and reduced cardiac output, which are the systemic hallmarks of gas gangrene.

The physiologic state of the wound site is critical to allowing the organism to germinate and produce its toxins. The proper conditions are a low oxidation-reduction potential, anoxia, and the availability of various peptides and amino acids (7). Calcium

TABLE 95.1. Classification of Clostridial Skin and Soft Tissue Infections

Toxigenic infections
  Traumatic gas gangrene
    Wounds of violence: gunshot, projectile missiles, stabbings, anal impalement
    War wounds
    Civilian violence
    Major traumatic injuries
      Motor vehicle and motorcycle accidents
      Industrial accidents
      Open fractures
    Minor trauma
      Puncture wounds
      Insect bites
      Intramuscular injections
      Subcutaneous injections, especially epinephrine
  Postoperative gas gangrene
    Gastrointestinal operations
    Gallbladder operations
  Uterine gas gangrene
    Post partum
    Septic abortion
    Nonpregnant women
  Spontaneous (nontraumatic) myonecrosis
    Local (contiguous spread from a focus)
      Colon cancer
      Intraabdominal abscess
    Distant (metastatic) spread
      Colon cancer, various other types
      Neutropenia (leukemia, cyclic neutropenia)
    Crepitant cellulitis or fasciitis, with systemic toxinosis
Nontoxigenic infections
  Crepitant cellulitis or fasciitis, localized
  Suppurative skin and soft tissue infections
    Diabetic foot ulcer and stump infections
    Decubitus ulcers
  Suppurative myositis
    Intravenous drug abuse
    Intramuscular injection

ion is also needed because α toxin requires this ion for interaction with substrate (20). Because α toxin has a high affinity for lipids, it is bound locally to tissue, and circulating toxin is not generally found (21–23). In animal experiments, the minimal infecting dose of the organism is 1,000 times greater for normal muscle tissue than for devitalized muscle. The infecting dose can be reduced by 10^6 when devitalized tissue is contaminated with sterile dirt (24). Many of these promoting factors are found in traumatic wounds.

EPIDEMIOLOGY

Estimates of the annual number of cases of gas gangrene in the United States range from 1,000 to 3,000 (6,10). In Great Britain, a case of gas gangrene was seen in a general hospital every 2 years (25), a figure not unlike that reported in Cincinnati, Ohio (4). Referral centers admit approximately 10 cases per year (10). Throughout history, gas gangrene has been tied intimately to the battlefield (1–7). Because of improved treatment in combat zones, there has been a gratifying reduction in the incidence of gas gangrene associated with war wounds: 5% in World War I, 0.7% in World War II, 0.2% in the Korean War, and 0.02% in the Vietnam War (1–3,26,27). *C. perfringens* is often present in war wounds: MacLennan (1) reported that 20% to 30% of wounds were contaminated by the organism, but only 0.32% of them developed gas gangrene. A review of 187,936 open traumatic wounds showed a contamination rate with clostridia of 3.8% to 39%, but less than 2% of patients actually developed gas gangrene (3,4).

In peacetime practice, traumatic injuries account for half of the cases of gas gangrene, the remainder being divided between postoperative complications (30%) and spontaneous (nontraumatic) gas gangrene (20%) (6,8–10,28–30). Among the trauma cases, major trauma is responsible for more than 70%; the most common causes are motor vehicle accidents, particularly those involving motorcycles, followed by crush injuries, industrial accidents, gunshot wounds, and burns. Minor injury is noted in 30% of the trauma category: puncture wounds, insect bites, simple lacerations, intramuscular injections, and subcutaneous injections, especially with epinephrine (31). Postoperative gas gangrene, which accounts for 30% of cases, is related to the following operative sites, in order of frequency: appendix, biliary tract, colon, small intestine, and upper gastrointestinal tract (32). Those in the spontaneous gas gangrene group have diverse underlying diagnoses, including colon cancer, diabetes, vascular disease, neutropenia, and intraabdominal infection.

Gas gangrene is two to three times more common in males than females. The average age is 35 to 40 years, but children and elders are also affected. The location of gas gangrene is important in terms of management and overall survival. In 80% of traumatic cases the disease originates in an extremity, and in the head or trunk area in 20%, whereas in postoperative cases the figures are reversed. In spontaneous cases, the head and trunk are the favored sites (10).

Because clostridia are distributed so widely in nature—they can be cultured from virtually all soil samples (7) as well as from multiple environmental sites in a hospital, including air and dust (even in the operating room)—it is difficult to know where the infecting strain originated (33,34). Nevertheless, it is believed that most infections, particularly those involving trauma or surgery, are associated with endogenous strains from the patient's own flora, although outbreaks within a hospital have been recognized (33,34). In battlefield conditions, a soldier's uniform is covered with a patina of excrement that harbors large numbers of clostridial spores; a penetrating wound is liable to be contaminated with pieces of this soiled clothing, as well as dirt and other particulate matter. Not all clostridial strains are equally capable of causing gas gangrene. In animal challenge experiments, those strains isolated from feces or from infected wounds are considerably more virulent than are strains obtained from soil samples (7,24).

CLINICAL FEATURES

Gas Gangrene

Although gas gangrene is relatively rare, its dramatic presentation and often devastating outcome make each case a memorable event in the personal experience of a physician. Local destruction of muscle and soft tissues and systemic signs of toxemia and hypotension dominate the clinical picture. The onset generally comes 1 to 4 days after the initiating event, although it can start as early as 8 hours or as late as 3 weeks. The initial symptom is gnawing pain in the wound that persists after surgical repair, increasing in severity and extending somewhat beyond the original borders over the next few hours. The skin becomes intensely edematous. It changes from an initial pallor to a magenta hue, often accompanied by large, hemorrhagic bullae. A thin, watery discharge appears early in the course. The discharge has an unpleasant, foul-sweet odor. Microscopic examination reveals abundant gram-positive rods and a remarkable paucity of inflammatory cells. Tachycardia, which cannot be explained by the degree of fever or circulatory changes, is an early finding. Profuse sweating is a constant feature. The temperature can be elevated or even normal. Later, hypotension that is unresponsive to fluid administration and renal failure ensue.

In gas gangrene, the appearance of the involved muscles is characteristic and quite unlike that of any other surgical infection. It must be viewed by direct operative exposure, because many of the changes are not apparent on inspection through the edges of a traumatic wound. Initially, the muscle is pale and edematous, looking like a piece of steak that has been seared over a charcoal fire. The muscle does not contract when stimulated. Further dissection reveals beefy, red, nonviable muscle tissue. A brownish, watery discharge with bubbles of gas seeps through the wound. As the disease progresses, the muscle becomes frankly gangrenous, black, and extremely friable, but by this time the patient is near death. It is important to establish the diagnosis of myonecrosis as early as possible, so that all devitalized, necrotic muscle can be resected. Gas production is often a late finding, and although highly suggestive of gas gangrene, it should not be used as a pathognomonic sign, nor should its absence be allowed to disparage the diagnosis (see Chapter 213 for additional discussion of gas production) (35,36).

The mental status of a patient with gas gangrene is an extraordinary feature of the disease process. Despite profound hypotension, renal failure, and advancing crepitation, these patients may be remarkably alert and extremely sensitive to their surroundings. They are aware of their impending doom, and a sense of terror can be read in their furtive gaze. This intense mental awareness is mercifully suspended just before death, when the patient lapses into toxic delirium and eventually into a coma.

Minor trauma may precipitate a severe, even lethal, case of gas gangrene. Insect bites, puncture wounds, and superficial lacerations have been incriminated (10). Intramuscular injections have been the predisposing cause in a number of patients, particularly those with diabetes (31,37,38). Epinephrine and other vasoconstrictors are most dangerous in this regard (39); other drugs have included insulin, barbiturate, potassium chloride, and pentazocine (37). Diabetes patients appear to be at increased risk for developing gas gangrene, not only from injections but also from injuries in the lower extremity (40,41).

Gas gangrene of the eye and orbit usually follows traumatic panophthalmitis (42–46). A penetrating wound of the globe is the portal of entry. The ensuing infection destroys vision, and it is usually necessary to enucleate the eye or eviscerate the orbit. Surprisingly, the postoperative course is uneventful, and these patients are not at as high a risk for death as are those with other forms of gas gangrene. There are also mild cases of clostridial conjunctivitis (43,47). A laboratory report of the organism in a conjunctival discharge is greeted with considerable skepticism owing to the benign clinical course.

Uterine Gas Gangrene

Clostridial invasion of the myometrium can produce an overwhelming infection that starts 2 to 3 days after the inciting event (48–52). Before abortion was legalized in the United States and in many European countries, septic abortion was the major cause of uterine gas gangrene. This complication occurred in 0.5% to 10% of septic abortions. In the United States, gas gangrene was a leading cause of maternal death, a situation that still prevails in countries where unsanitary abortions are performed (48,53). Although rare, uterine gas gangrene can complicate normal delivery (53,54), cesarean section (53,55,56), and amniocentesis (57). Both mother and newborn are endangered by the infection. Nonpregnant women can develop uterine gas gangrene in association with uterine cancer, leiomyoma, and curettage for choriocarcinoma (58,59).

Uterine gas gangrene is heralded by the dramatic onset of fever, rapid pulse, and severe toxemia. Hypotension is a regular feature of the syndrome, and for some patients unexplained hypotension is the initiating event. Renal output is invariably reduced, accompanied in the early stages by "port wine" urine secondary to hemoglobinuria; it usually progresses to anuria and acute cortical necrosis, which necessitates renal dialysis. Jaundice may progress with extraordinary rapidity, owing to massive intravascular hemolysis caused by α toxin (lecithinase) (60). As a result, the patient's skin and sclerae assume a deep, mahogany discoloration in a matter of hours. Peripheral blood smears show crinkled and shaggy erythrocytes. Pelvic findings may be minimal even at this point, although an radiography can demonstrate the presence of gas in the midline, related to the uterine wall but distinct from the intestine, as well as in surrounding pelvic structures. Computed tomography can demonstrate gas bubbles in the uterine wall even when the standard radiograph and ultrasonogram do not.

Two forms of pathologic process are recognized. A milder form consists of a superficial decidual infection limited to the uterine contents. This infection can liberate large amounts of toxin so that the clinical features are fully expressed with only minimal local disease. Simple curettage is usually sufficient to remove the necrotic tissue at the site of infection. The second-and more serious form of gas gangrene involves invasion of uterine muscle and gelatinous necrosis of tissue. As in the disease associated with skeletal muscle, remarkably few inflammatory cells are associated with this process. The infection can spread beyond the uterus itself into the structures of the pelvis. Mortality rates of up to 70% have been reported for uterine gas gangrene, but total hysterectomy, when performed early for the more severe form of invasive disease, can reduce the mortality rate to less than 10% (49).

Clostridium sordellii has been associated with fatal postpartum infection (61,62). In each of the reported cases, the postpartum infection occurred in a rather limited, inconspicuous site, such as a retained vaginal sponge or cesarean section operative site, or

associated with endometritis. A galloping, downhill course with hypotension and shock was observed in each of these women. Cases of soft tissue infections and bacteremia have also been reported with *C. sordellii* with a better outcome than in the postpartum cases (63). Neither uterine myonecrosis nor gas formation was present. *C. sordellii* elaborates a factor known as β toxin, which when injected in animals causes necrosis, edema, hemorrhage, and death (64,65). This lethal toxin may actually consist of two toxins, which seem to be similar to toxin A and toxin B of *Clostridium difficile* (66,67). The gene of the cytotoxin of *C. sordellii*, known as L, shares homologies with the C-terminal of the *C. difficile* cytotoxin gene, although there are clear structural differences (68). There are also immunologic and cytotoxic effects that are different among the two toxins of *C. difficile* and toxin L of *C. sordellii* (69).

Spontaneous (Nontraumatic) Myonecrosis

A variant of the classic picture of gas gangrene is one that arises spontaneously, without an apparent source, at least at onset. Three clinical forms are recognized (Table 95.1). The local form is associated with an intraabdominal or pelvic focus of infection from which clostridia spread into surrounding muscle. The usual setting is "silent" colon cancer or occasionally a diverticular abscess. The disease is characterized by the presence of gas in the flank or thigh muscles, along with hypotension and renal failure (10,37,70). The initiating event may also be perforation of a viscus during bladder catheterization or barium enema (71,72).

The second form of spontaneous gas gangrene is distant "metastatic" spread of the infection, which originates in a colon cancer or in neutropenic enterocolitis, and rarely in non-Hodgkin's lymphoma, but presents as a gas-forming, necrotizing infection of an extremity or, less commonly, the abdominal wall (37,70,73–77). The unique features of this form of gas gangrene are the absence of trauma, the isolation of *Clostridium* as the sole pathogen, and an abbreviated course, with spreading crepitation and rapid clinical deterioration. The crepitation advances relentlessly during a period of hours, until the entire limb, and even the trunk, is involved. Unlike classic gas gangrene, which tends to be a more localized process, the organism spreads rapidly in these cases through tissue planes, producing massive volumes of gas and advancing far beyond the border of necrotic muscle. Renal failure, hemolytic anemia, and hypotension are usually present, and the patient succumbs 1 to 3 days after onset (73,74). More than 90% of these cases are associated with colon cancer, which is occult in nearly half the patients (73).

The third form of spontaneous gas gangrene is a related, and perhaps earlier, stage of this metastatic process: crepitant cellulitis and fasciitis with overwhelming toxinosis in the absence of direct muscle invasion (70,73,78,79). The disease manifests with dramatic abruptness, spreading through fascial planes with widespread gas formation, moving in a virtually visual fashion. Physical examination reveals diffuse crepitation but relatively little pain over the muscles. The process usually begins in an extremity and spreads rapidly to the trunk. Systemic signs of overwhelming clostridial toxemia are present, often leading rapidly to death less than 24 hours from onset (74,78).

It can be said of this infection, as it was said of cholera in the past, that it is a disease that begins where other diseases end—with death. Pathologic examination fails to show the muscle necrosis characteristic of gas gangrene, although an inflammatory reaction can be seen in the muscle groups adjacent to the affected fascial planes. (A condition analogous to crepitant cellulitis caused by *C. sordellii* occurs in the uterus as noted earlier.)

In spontaneous gas gangrene, the pathogen has been *C. perfringens* in two thirds of cases and *C. septicum* in the remainder (70,73,74), although *C. septicum* may be the more common pathogen in the variety associated with crepitant cellulitis and fasciitis (74). Colon cancer (80), leukemia, and various forms of neutropenia, including cyclic neutropenia and neutropenic enterocolitis (81), have been the underlying cause. Overall mortality in the cases associated with malignancy is 70%, and the highest mortality rates are noted in patients with *C. septicum* infection, who have a short incubation period and a rapid course. (See Chapter 213 for a discussion of *C. septicum* bacteremia.)

Nontoxigenic Clostridial Infections

Clostridial cellulitis, without signs of systemic toxinosis, is a localized suppurative process that tracks along fascial planes with abundant gas formation yet lacks the systemic signs of clostridia toxin activity. It has a rather leisurely progression: an incubation period of 3 to 5 days and a slower course than that of gas gangrene (1,4). Clostridial cellulitis, along with anaerobic streptococcal cellulitis, was reported frequently during World War II, but both conditions are rare in more recent times, probably because of more aggressive treatment of traumatic wounds and large-dose antibiotic therapy.

Suppurative skin and soft tissue infections may involve clostridia, usually along with other organisms. About one third of foot ulcers in diabetic patients harbor clostridia (82,83); careful bacteriologic studies reveal several different species, most commonly *C. perfringens* (84,85). Gas formation is a frequent finding in diabetic foot ulcer, but most cases are caused by gram-negative enteric bacilli and streptococci rather than by clostridia (35). Gas gangrene is rare in diabetic foot ulcers, although crepitant cellulitis has been described arising from the ulcer or an infected stump amputation. Decubitus ulcer is another site of infection with clostridia, which can even invade the bloodstream (86–88).

Clostridia cause a form of suppurative myositis. This condition differs from gas gangrene because it lacks systemic findings, has a relatively benign course, and produces less muscle destruction. The infection is localized in a single muscle, and it can be managed with simple drainage, leaving a functional muscle group (89). In intravenous drug abusers, clostridial suppurative myositis manifests with local pain and tenderness, eventually developing into a discrete area of fluctuance that requires surgical drainage. The main sites are the thigh and the forearm. The pathologic findings include subcutaneous abscess in the muscle with an intense inflammatory response that may involve adjacent soft tissues and fascia. A similar condition has been associated with injections of various therapeutic drugs, particularly in diabetic patients (38). These clinical forms resemble tropical myositis, although the tropical disease is usually caused by *Staphylococcus aureus*. Cases of severe systemic sepsis and soft-tissue inflammation related to clostridial infections have been reported among injection drug users in the United Kingdom, Ireland, and Canada (90).

DIAGNOSIS

In its severe forms, gas gangrene produces an unmistakable clinical picture: myonecrosis, shock, and renal failure. By the time gas gangrene is clinically evident, however, the patient is usually doomed. Thus, it is important to make the diagnosis at the earliest moment to halt the progression of the disease and avoid dire complications that might require mutilating surgery. Initial suspicion should be aroused when the patient complains of unrelenting pain in a wound site even after it has been surgically repaired. Tight, bulging retention sutures or a tight cast over a compound fracture should be warning signs. A rapid pulse in an afebrile patient who has sustained trauma is another ominous sign. The diagnosis of myonecrosis is established by direct examination of the incriminated muscle. The typical appearance, along with failure of the muscle to respond to stimuli and poor blood supply, indicates its nonviable nature. The watery, brownish, foul-smelling discharge shows under the microscope an abundance of gram-positive rods and no inflammatory cells. Culture, which usually propagates the organism within 24 hours, shows *C. perfringens* in most cases. Gas, when present, is useful in diagnosis, but it also can be misleading. Crepitation can be found in nontoxigenic clostridial infections as well as in streptococcal infections. It can also be seen with infections caused by coliforms. These conditions can be excluded by careful examination of the muscle and Gram stain examination of the discharge. Patients with spontaneous gas gangrene present with crepitant cellulitis and severe systemic signs, often before direct muscle invasion occurs. Material from the fascial plane is obtained by needle aspiration, and a Gram stain examination can establish the diagnosis. Radiography, ultrasonography, and computed tomography may be useful to indicate the presence of incipient gas and to delineate the margins of infection. Such examinations are particularly valuable when the muscle is relatively inaccessible, as in the flank or pelvis.

TREATMENT

The most important therapeutic modality in gas gangrene is adequate surgical débridement. All necrotic muscle must be removed because it provides a nidus for proliferation of the organism and toxin production. This may involve amputation of an involved limb, wide resection of limb muscles, removal of abdominal musculature, or hysterectomy. In the absence of adequate resection, antibiotics do not quell this infection (4,10–12,32,91–93).

Antibiotic therapy is an important adjunct to surgical management. It is generally agreed that penicillin is the drug of choice (4,10,93–95). For experimental clostridial infections, several drugs, including penicillin, chloramphenicol, and tetracycline, are effective as prophylaxis or therapy (3,96–100). Antibiotics that inhibit protein synthesis, such as clindamycin, tetracycline, and chloramphenicol, are superior to cell wall–active agents such as penicillin, probably owing to suppression of toxin production by the former group of drugs (101,102). The combination of penicillin and clindamycin produces better results than either drug alone in some animal experiments (103). Because resistance to penicillin among clostridia is still rather uncommon (see Chapter 213) and the clinical experience with this drug remains favorable, the drug regimen for treatment of gas gangrene should include penicillin. At least 50% of these wounds are contaminated by other aerobic and anaerobic bacteria (10), and additional drugs are often needed. Clindamycin would be a reasonable choice for anaerobic bacteria and to add synergistic activity to penicillin against clostridia (103); another drug, such as an aminoglycoside or a third-generation cephalosporin, should be used for gram-negative organisms. Because there has never been a controlled trial of antibiotic therapy for gas gangrene, such recommendations are based on clinical experience, supported by data from *in vitro* studies and from animal experiments.

Antitoxin was recommended in earlier times, based primarily on the excellent results published from the wartime experiences (1,8,9). The antiserum was raised in horses against five clostridial species. Severe allergic reactions were reported, and several authorities (28,93,104) including Altemeier, (3,4) who had not used the antitoxin since 1943, recommended against using it. This view was endorsed by the National Research Council and the U.S. Department of Defense (4), and the production of antitoxin has been discontinued; all current supplies are outdated.

Hyperbaric oxygen (HBO) therapy, a procedure used for treating gas gangrene during the past 35 years (105), is still highly controversial, mostly because its adherents are so convinced of its efficacy that they have not conducted a randomized clinical trial. *In vitro*, oxygen at 3.0 atmospheres is bactericidal to many strains of clostridia (106) and inhibits production of α toxin (107). In a dog model of clostridial infection, neither surgery nor HBO therapy produced survivors; antibiotic treatment alone was associated with a 50% rate of survival, the addition of surgery resulted in 70% survival, and the use of HBO along with surgery and antibiotics produced 95% survival (108). HBO also reduced morbidity and mortality in a mouse model of clostridial infection (29,109). Clearly, animals treated with surgery alone fare worse than those treated with surgery and HBO (110). When antibiotics are added to the equation, which simulates the clinical situation, the results are less convincing for HBO. In one study, either clindamycin or metronidazole improved survival in challenge experiments, but HBO did not have an additive effect (111); in the other study, the best results were seen with clindamycin compared with metronidazole, penicillin, or HBO, and its superior efficacy was not further enhanced by HBO (112). Several groups have reported good experiences with HBO in clinical cases of gas gangrene (10,41,79,93,113–116), the overall mortality rate being 25% (10). It is difficult to judge its value from reading the literature, but this author can aver from limited personal experience that the effect of HBO therapy for gas gangrene can be quite dramatic. Having stated this, there are certain problems with such a therapeutic modality, not the least of which is the logistic challenge of moving desperately ill patients to appropriately equipped centers. In addition, HBO has certain untoward effects, including oxygen toxicity, barotrauma, decompression sickness, lung damage, and fire hazard (10,117,118), but these complications are infrequently encountered (10,119–122). During the acute period, HBO is administered at 2.0 to 2.5 atmospheres, three times a day, and this regimen has not caused a chamber-related death in more than 20,000 compressions (10). It would be reasonable to conclude that patients with gas gangrene should be treated with HBO when a facility is readily available. To be sure, some centers without an HBO chamber have reported excellent results; for example, Altemeier and Fullen (4) had a 15% mortality rate in their cases, one of the best records in the literature.

PROGNOSIS

Survival from gas gangrene is related to several factors (Table 95.2). The best results (90% survival or better) are seen in younger patients with traumatic myonecrosis involving a single extremity (10). At the other extreme, only 20% of patients with spontaneous gas gangrene, particularly those with leukemia or *C. septicum* infection, survive (4,37,73,79,104). Treatment also influences survival. During the world wars, before antibiotic and HBO treatments, mortality rates of 30% were common (2). When the full range of treatment options—surgery, antibiotics, and HBO—is applied in experienced centers, cases of traumatic gas gangrene are associated with mortality rates of less than 10%, and the overall mortality rate for all cases is 25% (10,123). Amputations are required in 15% to 20% of patients with gas gangrene, most often in those patients with traumatic or spontaneous myonecrosis in

TABLE 95.2. Features of Gas Gangrene Associated with Poor Outcome

Shock
Long incubation period (>30 h)
Spontaneous or postoperative cause
Location in trunk
Older age
Male sex
Underlying disease (cancer, diabetes)
Leukopenia
Renal failure
Hemolysis

Adapted from Hart GB, Lamb RC, Strauss MB. Gas gangrene. *J Trauma* 1983;23: 991–1000, with permission.

an extremity (10). Risk factors associated with a poor outcome are evidence of shock on admission, incubation period longer than 30 hours, and cancer or leukemia as an underlying disease (10,73).

PREVENTION

The best prevention of gas gangrene in trauma cases is good surgical management at the earliest moment, because antibiotics by themselves cannot prevent the disease. The basic principles were articulated more than 70 years ago by Wilensky: "The opening up completely of the entire wound including all pockets; the removal of all dirt and the mechanical cleansing of the wound; the removal of all foreign bodies; the eradication of all hematomata, small and large; the removal of all muscle tissue which is in any way compromised; complete hemostasis. It is imperative to institute wide and abundant drainage" (10,124).

REFERENCES

1. MacLennan JD. The histotoxic clostridial infections of man. *Bacteriol Rev* 1962;26:177.
2. MacLennan JD. Anaerobic infections of war wounds in the Middle East. *Lancet* 1943;2:94.
3. Finegold SM. *Anaerobic bacteria in human disease.* New York: Academic, 1977:418–428.
4. Altemeier, WA Fullen WD. Prevention and treatment of gas gangrene. *JAMA* 1971;217:806.
5. Weinstein L, Barza M. Gas gangrene. *N Engl J Med* 1973;289:1129.
6. Hitchcock CR, Demello FJ, Haglin JJ. Gangrene infection: new approaches to an old disease. *Surg Clin North Am* 1975;55:1403.
7. Smith LDS. The pathogenic anaerobic bacteria, 2nd ed. Springfield, IL: Charles C Thomas, 1975:115–324.
8. Caplan ES, Kluge RM. Gas gangrene: review of 34 cases. *Arch Intern Med* 1976;136:788.
9. Cameron HU, Ford M. Gas gangrene—need it occur? *Can Med Assoc J* 1978;119:1207.
10. Hart GB, Lamb RC, Strauss MB. Gas gangrene. *J Trauma* 1983;23:991.
11. DeHaven KE, Evarts CM. The continuing problem of gas gangrene: a review and report of illustrative cases. *J Trauma* 1971;11:983.
12. Hitchcock CR, Haglin JJ, Arnar O. Treatment of clostridial infection with hyperbaric oxygen. *Surgery* 1967;62:759.
13. Bhargava A, Sen P, Swaminathan A, et al. Rapidly progressive necrotizing fasciitis and gangrene due to *Clostridium difficile*: case report. *Clin Infect Dis* 2000;30:954–955.
14. Rood JI. Virulence genes of *Clostridium perfringens. Annu Rev Microbiol* 1998;52:333–360.
15. Alouf JE, Jolivet-Reynaud C. Purification and characterization of *Clostridium perfringens* S toxin. *Infect Immun* 1981;31:536.
16. Stevens DL, Bryant AE. The role of clostridial toxins in the pathogenesis of gas gangrene. *Clin Infect Dis* 2002;35(suppl):93–100.
17. Williamson ED, Titball RW. A genetically engineered vaccine against the alpha-toxin of *Clostridium perfringens* protects mice against experimental gas gangrene. *Vaccine* 1993;11:1253.

18. Awad MM, Bryant AE, Stevens DL, et al. Virulence studies on chromosomal alpha-toxin and theta-toxin mutants constructed by allelic exchange provide genetic evidence for the essential role of alpha-toxin in *Clostridium perfringens*–mediated gas gangrene. *Mol Microbiol* 1995;15:191.

19. Awad MM, Ellemor DM, Boyd RL, et al. Synergistic effects of alpha-toxin and perfringolysin O in *Clostridium perfringens*–mediated gas gangrene. *Infect Immun* 2001;69(12):7904–7910.

20. Jolivet-Reynaud C, Moreau H, Alouf JE. Purification of a toxin from *Clostridium perfringens. Methods Enzymol* 1988;165:91.

21. Stevens DL, Troyer BE, Merrick DT, et al. Lethal effects and cardiovascular effects of purified a and 6 toxins from *Clostridium perfringens. Infect Dis* 1988;157:272.

22. Ellner PD. Fate of partially purified ^{14}C-labeled toxin of *Clostridium perfringens. J Bacteriol* 1961;82:275.

23. Bullen JJ. Role of toxins in host-parasite relationships. In: Montie TC, Kadis S, Aji SJ, eds. *Microbial toxins.* Vol. 2. London: Academic, 1972:109–158.

24. Altemeier WA, Furste WL. Studies in virulence of *Clostridium welchii. Surgery* 1949;25:12.

25. Parker MT. Postoperative clostridial infections in Britain. *BMJ* 1969;3:671.

26. Simeone F. Clostridial myositis. In: Symposium on Military Medicine in the Far East Command. *Surg Circ Lett Med* 1951;September(Suppl).

27. Brown PW, Kinman PB. Gas gangrene in a metropolitan community. *J Bone Joint Surg Am* 1974;56:1445.

28. Eraklis AJ, Filler RM, Pappas AM, et al. Evaluation of hyperbaric oxygen as an adjunct in the treatment of anaerobic infections. *Am J Surg* 1969;117:485.

29. Holland JA, Hill GB, Wolfe WG, et al. Experimental and clinical experience with hyperbaric oxygen in the treatment of clostridial myonecrosis. *Surgery* 1975;77:75.

30. Skiles MS, Covert GK, Fletcher HS. Gas-producing clostridial and non-clostridial infections. *Surg Gynecol Obstet* 1978;147:65.

31. Hallagan LF, Scott JL, Horowitz BC, et al. Clostridial myonecrosis resulting from subcutaneous epinephrine suspension injection. *Ann Emerg Med* 1992;21:434.

32. Fromm D, Siles W. Postoperative clostridial sepsis of the abdominal wall. *Am J Surg* 1969;118:517.

33. Lowbury EJL, Lilly HA. The sources of hospital infection of wound with *Clostridium welchii. J Hyg* 1958;56:169.

34. Eickhoff TC. An outbreak of surgical wound infections due to *Clostridium perfringens. Surg Gynecol Obstet* 1962;114:102.

35. Bessman AN, Wagner W. Nonclostridial gas gangrene: report of 48 cases and review of the literature. *JAMA* 1975;233:958.

36. Nichols RL, Smith JW. Gas in the wound: What does it mean? *Surg Clin North Am* 1975;55:1289.

37. Nordkild P, Crone P. Spontaneous clostridial myonecrosis: a collective review and report of a case. *Ann Chir Gynaecol* 1986;75:274.

38. Kershaw CJ, Bulstrode CJK. Gas gangrene in a diabetic after intramuscular injection. *Postgrad Med J* 1988;64:812.

39. Harvey PW, Purnell GV. Fatal case of gas gangrene associated with intramuscular injection. *BMJ* 1968;1:744.

40. Kahn O. The incidence and significance of gas gangrene in a diabetic population. *Angiology* 1974;25:462.

41. Kofoed H, Riegels-Nielsen P. Myonecrotic gas gangrene of the extremities. *Acta Orthop Scand* 1983;54:220.

42. Walker S. Prognosis of *Bacillus welchii* panophthalmitis. *Arch Ophthalmol* 1938;19:406.

43. Henkind P, Fedukowicz H. *Clostridium welchii* conjunctivitis. *Arch Ophthalmol* 1963;70:791.

44. Leavitt JM, Stam J. *Clostridium perfringens* panophthalmitis. *Arch Ophthalmol* 1970;84:227.

45. Duke-Elder S. *System of ophthalmology.* London: Kimpton, 1872:405–410.

46. Crock GW, Heriot WJ, Janakiraman P, et al. Gas gangrene infection of the eyes and orbits. *Br J Ophthalmol* 1985;69:143.

47. Walsh T. Clostridial ocular infection. Case report of gas gangrene panophthalmitis. *Br J Ophthalmol* 1965;49:472.

48. Ragan WD. Gas gangrene complicating term pregnancy. *Obstet Gynecol* 1960;15:332.

49. Decker WH, Hall W. Treatment of abortions infected with *Clostridium welchii. Am J Obstet Gynecol* 1966;19:545.

50. Pritchard JA, Whaley PJ. Abortion complicated by *Clostridium perfringens* infection. *Am J Obstet Gynecol* 1971;111:484.

51. Smith LP, McLean AP, Maughan GB. *Clostridium welchii* septicotoxemia: a review and report of 3 cases. *Am J Obstet Gynecol* 1971;110:135.

52. Patchell RD. Gas gangrene complicating term pregnancy. *Obstet Gynecol* 1966;28:64.

53. Dylewski J, Wisenfeld H, Latour A. Postpartum uterine infection with *Clostridium perfringens. Rev Infect Dis* 1989;2:470.

54. Kirkpatrick CJ, Werdehausen K, Jaeger J, et al. Fatal *Clostridium perfringens* infection after normal term pregnancy. *Arch Gynecol* 1982;231:167.

55. Browne JT, Van Derhor AH, McConnell TS, et al. *Clostridium perfringens* myometritis complicating cesarean section: report of 2 cases. *Obstet Gynecol* 1966;28:64.

56. Halpin TF, Molinari JA. Diagnosis and management of *Clostridium perfringens* sepsis and uterine gas gangrene. *Obstet Gynecol Surv* 2002;57:53–57.

57. Fray RE, Davis TP, Brown EA. *Clostridium welchii* infection after amniocentesis. *BMJ* 1984;288:901.

58. Lacey CG, Futoran R, Murrow CP. *Clostridium perfringens* infection complicating chemotherapy for choriocarcinoma. *Obstet Gynecol* 1976;47:337.

59. Braverman J, Adachi A, Lev-Gur M, et al. Spontaneous clostridia gas gangrene of uterus associated with endometrial malignancy. *Am J Obstet Gynecol* 1987;156:1205.

60. Becker RC, Giuliani M, Savage RA, et al. Massive hemolysis in *Clostridium perfringens* infections. *J Surg Oncol* 1987;35:13.

61. Soper DD. Clostridial myonecrosis arising from an episiotomy. *Obstet Gynecol* 1986;68:265.

62. McGregor JA, Soper DE, Lovell G, et al. Maternal deaths associated with *Clostridium sordellii* infection. *Am J Obstet Gynecol* 1989;161:987.

63. Spera RV Jr, Kaplan MH, Allen SL. *Clostridium sordellii* bacteremia: case report and review. *Clin Infect Dis* 1992;15:950.

64. Willis AT. *Clostridia of wound infection.* London: Butterworth, 1969.

65. Nakamura SN, Tanabe K, Yamakawa K, et al. Cytotoxin production by *Clostridium sordellii* strains. *Microbiol Immunol* 1983;27:495.

66. Popoff MR. Purification and characterization of *Clostridium sordellii* lethal toxin and cross-reactivity with *Clostridium difficile* cytotoxin. *Infect Immun* 1987;55:35.

67. Martinez RD, Wilkins TD. Purification and characterization of *Clostridium sordellii* hemorrhagic toxin and cross-reactivity with *Clostridium difficile* toxin A (enterotoxin). *Infect Immun* 1988;56:1215.

68. Green GA, Schue V, Monteil H. Cloning and characterization of the cytotoxin L-encoding gene of *Clostridium sordellii*: homology with *Clostridium difficile* cytotoxin B. *Gene* 1995;161:57.

69. Baldacini O, Girardot R, Green GA, et al. Comparative study of immunological properties and cytotoxic effects of *Clostridium difficile* toxin B and *Clostridium sordellii* toxin L. *Toxicon* 1992;30:129.

70. Jendrzejewski JW Jones S, Newcombe R, et al. Nontraumatic clostridial myonecrosis. *Am J Med* 1978;65:542.

71. Amar AD, Ratiff RK. Gas gangrene of the urinary bladder and abdominal wall following catheterization. *J Urol* 1958;80:130.

72. Reckman LS, Short WF, Cooper WM. Barium enema septicemia—occurrence in a patient with leukemia. *JAMA* 1973;226:62.

73. Kornbluth AA, Danzig JB, Bernstein LH. *Clostridium septicum* infection and associated malignancy: report of 2 cases and review of the literature. *Medicine (Baltimore)* 1989;68:30.

74. Stevens DL, Musher DM, Watson DA, et al. Spontaneous, nontraumatic gangrene due to *Clostridium septicum. Rev Infect Dis* 1990;12:286.

75. Buckley D, Kudsk K. Occult gastrointestinal carcinoma causing metastatic clostridial soft-tissue infection: report of two cases. *Dis Colon Rectum* 1988;31:306.

76. Bretzke ML, Bubrick MP, Hitchcock CR. Diffuse spreading *Clostridium septicum* infection, malignant disease and immune suppression. *Surg Gynecol Obstet* 1988;166:197.

77. Garcia-Suarez J, de Miguel D, Krsnik I, et al. Spontaneous gas gangrene in malignant lymphoma: an underreported complication? *Am J Hematol* 2002;70(2):145–148.

78. Gorbach SL. Case records of the Massachusetts General Hospital, case 49-1979. *N Engl J Med* 1979;301:1276.

79. Hitchcock CF, Bubrick MP. Gas gangrene infections of the small intestine, colon and rectum. *Dis Colon Rectum* 1976;19:112.

80. Lorimer JW, Eidus LB. Invasive *Clostridium septicum* infection in association with colorectal carcinoma. *Can J Surg* 1994;37:245.

81. Lev R, Sweeney KG. Neutropenic enterocolitis: two unusual cases with review of the literature. *Arch Pathol Lab Med* 1993;117:524.

82. Manson MH. Pathogenic gas-producing anaerobic bacilli in chronic ulcers. *Arch Surg* 1932;24:752.

83. Louie TJ, Bartlett JG, Tally FP, et al. Aerobic and anaerobic bacteria in diabetic foot ulcers. *Ann Intern Med* 1976;85:461.

84. Sapico FL, Canawati HN, Witte JL, et al. Quantitative aerobic and anaerobic bacteriology of infected diabetic feet. *J Clin Microbiol* 1980;12:413.

85. Sapico FL, Witte JL, Canawati HN, et al. The infected foot of the diabetic patient: quantitative microbiology and analysis of clinical features. *Rev Infect Dis* 1984;6:5171.

86. Wilson WR, Martin WJ, Wilkowske CJ, et al. Anaerobic bacteremia. *Mayo Clin Proc* 1972;47:639.

87. Rissing JP, Crowder JG, Dunfee T, et al. *Bacteroides* bacteremia from decubitus ulcers. *South Med J* 1974;67:1179.

88. Chow AW, Galpin JE, Guze LB. Clindamycin for treatment of sepsis caused by decubitus ulcers. *J Infect Dis* 1977;135(suppl):65.

89. Gorbach SL, Thadepalli H. Isolation of *Clostridium* in human infections: evaluation of 114 cases. *J Infect Dis* 1975;131:581.

90. Williamson N, Archibald C, Van Vliet JS. Unexplained deaths among injection drug users: a case of probable *Clostridium myonecrosis. CMAJ* 2001;165(5):609–611.

91. Duff JH, McLean APH, MacLean LD. Treatment of severe anaerobic infections. *Arch Surg* 1970;101:314.

92. Klein RS, Berger SA, Yekutiel P. Wound infection during the Yom Kippur war: observations concerning antibiotic prophylaxis and therapy. *Ann Surg* 1975;182:15.

93. Darke SG, King AM, Slack WK. Gas gangrene and related infection: classification, clinical features and aetiology, management and mortality: a report of 88 cases. *Br J Surg* 1977;64:104.

94. Knight RJ. Reception and resuscitation of casualties in South Vietnam. Experience at the First Australian Field Hospital. *Lancet* 1972;2:29.

95. Finegold SM, George WL, Mulligan ME. Anaerobic infections. Part II. *Dis Mon* 1985;31:1.
96. Hac LR. Experimental *Clostridium welchii* infection. IV Penicillin therapy. *J Infect Dis* 1944;71:164.
97. Altemeier WA, McMurrin JA, Alt LP. Chloromycetin and aureomycin in experimental gas gangrene. *Surgery* 1950;28:621.
98. Freeman WA, McFadzean JA, Whelan JPF. Activity of metronidazole against experimental tetanus and gas gangrene. *J Appl Bacteriol* 1968;31:443.
99. Irvin TT, Moir ERS, Smith G. Treatment of *Clostridium welchii* infection with hyperbaric oxygen. *Surg Gynecol Obstet* 1968;127:1058.
100. Owen-Smith MS, Matheson JM. Successful prophylaxis of gas gangrene of the high-velocity missile wound in sheep. *Br J Surg* 1968;55:36.
101. Stevens DL, Maier KA, Laine BM, et al. Comparison of clindamycin, rifampin, tetracycline, metronidazole, and penicillin for efficacy in prevention of experimental gas gangrene due to *Clostridium perfringens*. *J Infect Dis* 1987;155:220.
102. Stevens DL, Maier KA, Mitten JE. Effect of antibiotics on toxin production and viability of *Clostridium perfringens*. *Antimicrob Agents Chemother* 1987;31:213.
103. Stevens DL, Laine BM, Mitten JE. Comparison of single and combination antimicrobial agents for prevention of experimental gas gangrene caused by *Clostridium perfringens*. *Antimicrob Agents Chemother* 1987;31:312.
104. Roding B, Groeneveld PHA, Boerema I. Ten years of experience in the treatment of gas gangrene with hyperbaric oxygen. *Surg Gynecol Obstet* 1972;134:579.
105. Brummelkamp WH, Hogendjik J, Boerema I. Treatment of anaerobic infections (clostridial myositis) by drenching the tissues with oxygen under high atmospheric pressure. *Surgery* 1961;49:299.
106. Hill GB, Osterhout S. Experimental effects of hyperbaric oxygen on selected clostridial species. I. In-vivo studies. *J Infect Dis* 1972;125:17.
107. Van Unnik AJM. Inhibition of toxin production in *Clostridium perfringens in vitro* by hyperbaric oxygen. *Antonie Van Leeuwenhoek* 1965;31:181.
108. Demello FJ, Haglin JJ, Hitchcock CR. Comparative study of experimental *Clostridium perfringens* infection in dogs treated with antibiotics, surgery, and hyperbaric oxygen. *Surgery* 1973;73:936.
109. Hill GB, Osterhout S. Experimental effects of hyperbaric oxygen on selected clostridial species. II. *In vivo* studies in mice. *J Infect Dis* 1972;125:26.
110. Him M. Hyperbaric oxygen in the treatment of gas gangrene and perineal necrotizing fasciitis: a clinical and experimental study. *Eur J Surg Suppl* 1993;570:1.
111. Muhvich KH, Anderson LH, Mehm WJ. Evaluation of antimicrobials combined with hyperbaric oxygen in a mouse model of clostridial myonecrosis. *J Trauma* 1994;36:7.
112. Stevens DL, Bryant AE, Adams K, et al. Evaluation of therapy with hyperbaric oxygen for experimental infection with *Clostridium perfringens* [see comments]. *Clin Infect Dis* 1993;17:231.
113. Unsworth IF, Sharo PA. Gas gangrene. An 11-year review of 73 cases managed with hyperbaric oxygen. *Med J Aust* 1984;140:256.
114. Gibson A, Davis FM. Hyperbaric oxygen therapy in the management of *Clostridium perfringens* infections. *N Z Med J* 1986;99:617.
115. Him M, Niinikoski J. Hyperbaric oxygen in the treatment of clostridial gas gangrene. *Ann Chir Gynaecol* 1988;77:37.
116. Grim PS, Gottlieb LJ, Boddie A, et al. Hyperbaric oxygen therapy. *JAMA* 1990;263:2216.
117. Brummelkamp WH, Boerema I, Hogendjik L. Treatment of clostridial infections with hyperbaric oxygen drenching. A report on 26 cases. *Lancet* 1963;1:235.
118. Slack WK, Hanson GC, Chew HER. Hyperbaric oxygen in the treatment of gas gangrene and clostridial infections. A report of 40 patients treated in a single-person hyperbaric oxygen chamber. *Br J Surg* 1969;56:505.
119. Bernhard WF, Filler RM. Hyperbaric oxygenation: current concepts. *Am J Surg* 1968;115:661.
120. DeHaven KE, Evarts CM. The continuing problem of gas gangrene: a review and report of illustrative cases. *J Trauma* 1971;11:983.
121. Davis JC, Dunn JM, Hagood CO, et al. Hyperbaric medicine in the US Air Force. *JAMA* 1973;224:205.
122. Johnson JT, Gillespie TE, Cole JR, et al. Hyperbaric oxygen therapy for gas gangrene in war wounds. *Am J Surg* 1969;118:839.
123. Heimbach RD. Gas gangrene: review and update. *HBO Rev* 1980;1:41.
124. Wilensky AO. Gas gangrene. *Surg Gynecol Obstet* 1918;27:187.

CHAPTER 96
Skin and Soft Tissue Infections

Sherwood L. Gorbach

SUPERFICIAL SKIN AND SOFT TISSUE INFECTIONS

Superficial skin and soft tissue infections are among the most common infections seen in clinical practice (1). These infections occur in three sites within the skin structures: (a) just below the stratum corneum (impetigo); (b) in the hair follicles (furuncles) or apocrine glands (hidradenitis suppurativa); and (c) below the epidermis, penetrating the dermis to subcutaneous tissues (cellulitis). They do not involve the fascia (as in necrotizing fasciitis) or muscle.

It is necessary to make the diagnosis of these superficial skin lesions by direct inspection (a) in order to initiate appropriate antimicrobial drugs immediately, if indicated; (b) because many lesions will not yield a positive culture (cellulitis) or it is unnecessary to order a culture since the result is predictable (furunculosis); and (c) to avoid surgery (erysipelas) or recommend surgery (carbuncle).

Pyodermas

STAPHYLOCOCCUS AUREUS INFECTIONS

This organism is present in the anterior nares in 10% to 40% of people, depending on their underlying health, association with hospitals, and age; less commonly, it also colonizes the skin. *S. aureus* skin infections are more common in diabetics and immunocompromised hosts.

Clinical Manifestations

Folliculitis involves the ostium of a hair follicle, usually on the face or extensor surface of an extremity; it has an uncomplicated evolution from a vesicle that points to the outside, to drainage, encrustment, and finally spontaneous healing. (*Pseudomonas aeruginosa* can cause extensive folliculitis 2 days following exposure to a contaminated swimming pool or whirlpool. Pruritic papulourticarial lesions that progress to vesicle formation are seen in various stages at multiple sites, sparing the palms and soles.

Furuncles (boils) develop from folliculitis, spreading to the subcutaneous layers of the skin. There is a firm, discrete nodule with purulent drainage. Systemic manifestations are not seen.

Carbuncles, more extensive, multiloculated lesions involving subcutaneous fat, occur in skin that is thick and inelastic, such as that found on the back of the neck, the back, or thighs. Abundant pus drains along hair follicles from deep, septated pockets. They are painful, indurated, and often associated with systemic signs of fever, headache, and malaise.

Recurrent furunculosis occurs most often in otherwise healthy individuals. The strain of *S. aureus* is usually identical on each recurrence and does not display antibiotic resistance or special virulence factors. The organism is usually carried in the anterior nares or on the skin.

Differential Diagnosis

It is important to distinguish these staphylococcal infections from acne vulgaris, which involves the sebaceous follicles and is infected with *Propionibacterium acnes* and *S. epidermitis*, but rarely *S. aureus*; and from hidradenitis suppurativa, which is an inflammation of the apocrine glands of the axilla or perineal and inguinal areas.

Management

Folliculitis and milder furuncles are treated with warm, moist packs to encourage localization and drainage. No medical or surgical therapy is necessary. More severe furuncles and localized carbuncles require judicious incision and drainage.

Extensive, multiloculated carbuncles should be drained with a small wick inserted to encourage drainage and to prevent closure of the incision. Drainage, while often necessary, also carries some risk for spreading infection to distant sites since the incision destroys the demarcation by pyogenic membranes, which can lead to dissemination and septicemia.

Antibiotics are indicated for furuncles when drainage is performed and for carbuncles. Oral drugs are usually sufficient. The preferred treatment is an antistaphylococcal penicillin (cloxacillin, by mouth, or oxacillin or nafcillin, by parenteral route) or a cephalosporin. For methicillin-resistant *S. aureus* (MRSA), vancomycin or linezolid is preferred.

Recurrent furunculosis is difficult to manage. An attempt should be made to eliminate nasal carriage by intranasal application of 2% mupirocin for 5 days. Prolonged antistaphylococcal treatment (for 2 months) is sometimes helpful. A mostly successful, although admittedly difficult, treatment is use of low-dose (150 mg per day) oral clindamycin for 3 months.

STREPTOCOCCUS PYOGENES INFECTIONS

Group A *Streptococcus pyogenes* is the most common strain, although some cases are caused by organisms in group C or G, and in newborns, in group B (2). Rarely, *S. aureus* can produce erysipelas. The incriminated *Streptococcus* is carried in the nasopharynx or on the skin. It is acquired from the host or by person-to-person transmission from a carrier.

Erysipelas

CLINICAL MANIFESTATIONS

Occurring more commonly in children, especially infants, and in the elderly, erysipelas presents as a hyperacute cellulitis with involvement of underlying lymphatics (3). It is a painful condition that starts as a raised, bright red, indurated lesion that spreads circumferentially over a period of minutes to hours, with an advancing red border that sometimes shows small streaks from the edge. Because of underlying lymphatic obstruction, the lesion is edematous, with a peau d'orange appearance. The extremities are the most common sites of involvement, followed by the face, especially over the bridge of the nose ("butterfly") or the cheeks. Some cases occur spontaneously, but most cases are associated with traumatic wounds, skin ulcers, psoriatic lesions, or the umbilical stump of newborns. Facial erysipelas is often preceded by a respiratory infection. Patients at risk are those with diabetes, venous stasis, underlying skin ulcers, alcohol abuse, and nephrotic syndrome. Systemic findings are prominent, with high fever and shaking chills and altered mental status. This condition, before the antibiotic era, was associated with a high mortality rate.

DIAGNOSIS

The diagnosis is based on clinical findings since it is uncommon for a positive culture to be obtained. An open skin lesion is usually absent; needle aspiration from the advancing edge is a fruitless exercise, being positive in less than 10%. Blood cultures are rarely positive. Serology for streptococcal infection is usually positive, but this is retrospective.

Differential diagnosis includes cellulitis and necrotizing fasciitis, which have a more leisurely course and are not associated with such systemic toxicity at the onset, and streptococcal gangrene, which is a more localized condition. Contact dermatitis and giant urticaria deserve consideration, but they are pruritic and do not have the systemic manifestations. Erythema chronicum migrans (ECM) of Lyme disease is another consideration, but it generally has the central zone of clearing, it moves more slowly, and has only low-grade fever.

TREATMENT

Penicillin is the preferred treatment, orally (as penicillin V-K) or by intramuscular injection (as procaine penicillin). Most cases are severe enough to require hospitalization, where intravenous penicillin can be given in high doses (2 to 4 million units every 4 to 6 hours). Erythromycin can be used but is often unsatisfactory in terms of therapeutic response. Treatment should be continued for 2 to 3 weeks, usually with oral penicillin to complete the course. There is risk for relapse, so the patient should be warned of this possibility and followed at least by phone. Surgery is not a consideration in erysipelas.

Recurrent Erysipelas

This condition is associated with chronic edema due to lymphatic or venous obstruction in a limb: axillary dissection secondary to breast cancer surgery, or any lymph node resection for cancer or trauma, Milroy's disease, or chronic venous stasis. In individuals with an initial attack, the recurrence rate is about 10% per year, but in some persons it can recur several times a year.

Each event is rather stereotypic for that individual; it usually begins with some pain or discomfort in the limb at a specific site, where within hours, a red, tender lesion appears, which rapidly advances up the limb, often with lymphatic streaking. The patient experiences pain and fever with shaking chills. Blood cultures are, as a rule, negative. Aspiration of the lesion does not yield a microbiologic diagnosis. In the rare cases where positive cultures have been obtained, they are invariably *Streptococcus*, but not necessarily group A. Added weight to the association with *Streptococcus* is the rapid and universal response to penicillin.

Penicillin G, administered in high doses intravenously, is the treatment of choice. The treatment should be extended to 2 to 4 weeks depending on the rapidity of initial response. Oral penicillin can be given in the final phase. Cephalosporins are also effective, and erythromycin or clindamycin can be used in allergic individuals.

Preventive measures are sometimes effective. Pressure devices are available to "milk" the affected limb during the night in order to reduce edema. Physiotherapy to improve muscle tone can also be effective in selected cases. Suppression by antibiotics can be tried in cases with multiple relapses. Low-dose, oral penicillin (penicillin V-K, 250 mg per day) is given for 3 to 6 months, and then stopped. If recurrences continue after stopping, continuous oral penicillin should be given.

Streptococcal Gangrene

Caused in the main by group A *Streptococcus*, although rarely by group C or G, this condition starts at the site of previous skin damage, either trauma, which may be minor, puncture wound, or surgical incision. The initial lesion is painful and erythematous and may have surrounding edema and an advancing edge.

Within 1 to 2 days the center of the lesion becomes dark red, then blue-black, with frank necrosis. Bullae that contain dark red fluid are sometimes present. Deeper fascia and muscle may also be involved, and if untreated, septicemia and shock can ensue.

Surgical management involves débridement of the gangrenous skin and incision and drainage of the surrounding tissues and fascial planes. Because it is important to release the pressure on the skin and subcutaneous tissues, the incisions should be extended beyond the areas of gangrene and far enough into the superficial fascia to establish good drainage. The limb should be elevated in order to promote drainage, and dressed with moist packs for superficial débridement. High-dose, intravenous penicillin G is administered in doses of 2 to 4 million units every 4 to 6 hours.

Impetigo

Either together or separately, group A *Streptococcus* and *S. aureus* cause this most superficial of the skin infections. While the streptococcal and mixed forms predominated in the past, recent studies suggest that the pure staphylococcal form is becoming the most common.

CLINICAL MANIFESTATIONS

Bullous impetigo is composed of superficial flaccid bullae containing neutrophils and gram-positive cocci; upon rupture, the fluid dries on the skin surface to form a brown lacquered patina. In nonbullous impetigo, thin-walled vesicles and pustules form on an erythematous base.

The lesions appear on the face or on extremities (at the site of minor trauma or insect bites or eczema). Impetigo is most common during the hot, humid summer season, related to skin colonization by the microorganisms. They can also be spread from nasopharyngeal colonization during any season. The condition is highly contagious, and is spread by direct person-to-person contact, often in school or day care facilities. Poor hygiene and crowded living conditions can facilitate spread. Because the lesions are pruritic, scratching can spread the infection to uninvolved sites or to other persons.

TREATMENT

Antimicrobial therapy is the preferred approach to impetigo. Oral drugs active against *S. aureus* should be used. Either dicloxacillin, amoxicillin-clavulanate, or a cephalosporin is preferred, although erythromycin can also be used in allergic children. Penicillin or ampicillin treatment was used in the past, but may be associated with failures due to the presence of resistant staphylococcal strains. Treatment should be given for 1 week.

A topical antimicrobial is an alternative in some patients. Mupirocin is the preferred agent, given three times per day for 7 days. Disadvantages of the topical regimen are the inconvenience of application when lesions are widespread on the skin, less effectiveness in bullous impetigo, and the inability to eradicate the site of colonization in the respiratory tract.

Mechanical débridement with soaps or antibacterial soaks may produce a satisfactory cosmetic effect, but there is little evidence that it hastens healing.

Cellulitis

Cellulitis is a spreading inflammatory process involving the deep dermis and subcutaneous fat (4). It can occur acutely and then proceed to a chronic phase. The infection is caused mainly by *Streptococcus pyogenes* or *Staphylococcus aureus* in normal hosts.

Several other bacteria can cause cellulitis, often with distinguishing physical findings and in special clinical settings.

CLINICAL MANIFESTATIONS

The infection often develops in association with an initial portal of entry, either local (a traumatic injury, puncture wound, insect bite, or surgical incision) or distant (a foot lesion, such as interdigital tinea pedis or skin fissures, or a hand wound, which spreads to cause cellulitis of the limb).

Intense erythema, pain, and advancing edema develop within a few days after the inciting event. The process moves more slowly than erysipelas, whose progression is measured in hours, compared with cellulitis, which moves over days. The appearance of cellulitis is also different from that of erysipelas, which has a discrete, expanding red margin. The advancing edge of cellulitis is elevated but is not well demarcated. Systemic complaints (chills, fever, and malaise) are common. Bacteremia is seen in a minority of patients, usually those with more aggressive infection. A more indolent form of cellulitis can develop in the lower leg in association with chronic edema and venous insufficiency.

STREPTOCOCCAL CELLULITIS

Group A *S. pyogenes* (GAS) is a major cause of cellulitis. It occurs acutely, often associated with a previous injury. The appearance is a diffuse, intense erythema with pain, tenderness, and swelling of the entire area of skin. Patients with dependent edema due to venous insufficiency or lymphatic obstruction are at high risk for streptococcal cellulitis.

Postoperative wound infection with GAS is a life-threatening occurrence. The incubation period is shorter than with most such wounds, ranging from 6 to 48 hours, often in the first postoperative day. In most cases there is no drainage, at best only a minimal amount of serous discharge that contains polymorphonuclear leukocytes (PMNs) and abundant gram-positive cocci in chains. Profound systemic manifestations are present, such as high fever, tachycardia, and hypotension. Bacteremia, which may be accompanied by hemolysis, is common in this setting, and the associated hypotension may be the heralding event. The route of spread is direct inoculation into the wound from a carrier of the organism, usually someone in direct contact during or just after the operation. Streptococcal cellulitis can be the presenting condition in a more ominous form, necrotizing fasciitis with septic shock.

Non–group A streptococci, such as those belonging to groups B, C, and G, can cause cellulitis, particularly when there is a chronic condition present, such as lymphatic obstruction or fissures between the toes. Such organisms have been associated with postoperative cellulitis at the saphenous vein donor site in patients who have undergone cardiac bypass surgery.

STAPHYLOCOCCAL CELLULITIS

Staphylococcus aureus is the main pathogen. Other staphylococci, such as *S. epidermitis,* can cause cellulitis in immunocompromised hosts. Most strains of community-acquired *S. aureus* are sensitive to methicillin (MSSA), although an increasing number of methicillin-resistant strains (MRSA) are causing infections in otherwise healthy individuals. Staphylococci tend to spread through the subcutaneous tissues of the skin in a circumferential, slowly progressive fashion over a period of days. The usual appearance is different from that of streptococcal cellulitis, although there is enough overlap that the etiology cannot be distinguished with certainty even when a "classic" lesion is present. This organism is still the major cause of postoperative wound infection, which is usually transferred by person-to-person contact either on the hands of medical personnel or from a carrier who harbors the organism in the nares. Clinically, a staphylococcal wound infection becomes obvious 3 to 4 days after the procedure. The suture line becomes reddened, tender, and somewhat tense. A slow ooze of odorless, yellow pus can be discerned at the edges and on the dressing. MRSAs are common in many U.S. hospitals, accounting for 40% to 80% of all staphylococcal infections.

OTHER GRAM-POSITIVE ORGANISMS THAT CAUSE CELLULITIS

Erysipelothrix rhusiopathiae, a gram-positive bacillus, causes a distinctive form of cellulitis known as erysipeloid. It occurs mostly on the fingers and hands, presenting as purplish red, indurated, painful or burning lesions with a sharp margin that spreads peripherally with some central clearing. The surrounding area of skin is rather swollen. The organism is ubiquitous in nature, found in fish, mammals, birds, insects, organic matter, and contaminated water, and the patient invariably has a history of contact with a known source.

Streptococcal pneumoniae is a rare cause of cellulitis as a result of bacteremia from a primary site, usually in the lung.

GRAM-NEGATIVE ORGANISMS CAUSING CELLULITIS

Pseudomonas aeruginosa can cause several types of cellulitis in normal, as well as immunocompromised, hosts. Its usual habitat is water, so the infection is often associated with exposure to water sources or moist sites. Besides its intrinsic virulence, invading small arterioles leading to avascular necrosis of skin and soft tissues, *Pseudomonas* is difficult to treat because of its resistance to many antibiotics.

Swimmer's ear, paronychia, and aggressive interdigital infections are caused by *Pseudomonas* in persons who have prolonged contact with a contaminated water source. Exposure to hot tubs, spas, or whirlpools can lead to a diffuse, pruritic maculopapular or vesiculopustular eruption caused by *Pseudomonas*. The bathing suit area is often spared. Outbreaks of such infections are common due to contamination of the water and poor environmental control. The condition is self-limited, without need for medical intervention.

A severe form of cellulitis, known as malignant external otitis, involves the ear pinna in diabetics, usually preceded by a chronic otitis externa or trauma from a hearing aid or irrigation of the ear canal to remove cerumen. The condition advances rapidly, causing local destruction of cartilage and bone and invasion of the central nervous system. Puncture wounds of persons wearing sneakers or old shoes, which harbor *Pseudomonas* in their moist, warm crevices, can lead to cellulitis of the sole of the foot with underlying osteomyelitis. In immunocompromised hosts, *Pseudomonas* bacteremia can produce cellulitis, as well as discrete, necrotic ulcers (ecthyma gangrenosum).

Aeromonas is found in fresh or brackish waters. It causes cellulitis in persons with previous lacerations or traumatic injuries who are exposed to such conditions.

Vibrios, which are found in sea water, can cause cellulitis and ear infections. The following species have been incriminated: *Vibrio cholerae* non-0:1, *V. parahaemolyticus*, *V. vulnificus*, and *V. mimicus* (the first three also cause septicemia).

V. vulnificus is particularly virulent. It can cause severe cellulitis in persons who develop skin injuries while swimming in sea water or have prior lacerations. A life-threatening form of cellulitis develops from bacteremia associated with eating raw oysters in persons with underlying liver disease.

Haemophilus influenzae type b can cause cellulitis of the face, neck, or arms in young children with bacteremia from a primary site in the middle ear or upper respiratory tract. This infection can also occur in adults with epiglottis or lower respiratory tract infections. The classic form has a purple or blue hue, but most cases have an erythematous appearance that is indistinguishable from other forms of cellulitis.

DIAGNOSIS

When cellulitis is associated with an open wound, there is usually an exudate that can be used for gram stain and culture. In the setting of cellulitis with unbroken skin, a needle aspiration from the advancing edge can sometimes (10%) yield a positive diagnosis. A positive blood culture is diagnostic. Bacteremia is uncommon in staphylococcal cellulitis but is frequent in cellulitis caused by *Streptococcus* or gram-negative bacteria. Clues can be gleaned from the patient's underlying disease (diabetes, cirrhosis, malignancy), recent exposures (swimming in fresh or salt water), or occupation (fisherman).

MANAGEMENT

As a rule cellulitis is not treated by surgical intervention. Antimicrobial therapy is required, often administered on an empirical basis, awaiting laboratory confirmation:

Streptococcal infection: large doses of intravenous penicillin or ampicillin.

Staphylococcal infection: oxacillin or nafcillin, or a first-generation cephalosporin (e.g., cefazolin).

When the diagnosis of streptococcal versus staphylococcal infection is unclear, a combination of ampicillin and oxacillin or a first-generation cephalosporin should be used.

Pseudomonas infection: a quinolone with an aminoglycoside (for more serious infections such as malignant external otitis). Swimmer's ear and hot-tub folliculitis do not require antibiotics. Aeromonas and *Vibrio* infections are treated with a quinolone or a tetracycline. The life-threatening forms should treated with an intravenous quinolone with an aminoglycoside.

Streptococcal Necrotizing Fasciitis with Toxic Shock

In the past decade there has been a dramatic increase in the number of severe, life-threatening cases of GAS infections associated with necrotizing fasciitis and toxic shock syndrome (5). In 1995, it was estimated that 10,000 to 15,000 cases of severe GAS infections occur annually in the United States, of which 5% to 10% are cases of necrotizing fasciitis with toxic shock.

DEFINITIONS

Confirmed cases involve necrosis of subcutaneous tissue together with severe systemic illness (including one or more of the following: sudden death; shock with a systolic blood pressure of less than 90 mm Hg; disseminated intravascular coagulation; system failure such as respiratory, hepatic, or renal failure) and with GAS isolated from the affected site or a normally sterile site.

Probable cases involve the clinical criteria above, along with serologic or histologic evidence of streptococcal infection but without a culture of GAS from the affected site or a normally sterile site.

CLINICAL MANIFESTATIONS

The age range is 20 to 50 years. There is usually no underlying disease. The portal of entry is found in 50% of cases, often the local skin site. A mucus membrane (throat, vagina) site of GAS infection is uncommon. The initial symptom is pain (in 85%), which is abrupt and severe.

Signs and Symptoms

	Percentage
Fever greater than 38°C	70
Confusion	55
Heart rate greater than 100 beats/min	80
Hypotension	100
Skin changes	80
Swelling	10
Swelling and erythema	65
Bullae	5
Desquamation (late)	20

Laboratory Findings

	Mean Values on Admission/at 48 Hours
Leukocytes	11,765/…
Immature granulocytes	43%/…
Platelets	216,000/129,000
Creatinine	2.5/3.4
Calcium	8.1/6.6
Albumin	3.3/2.3
Creatine phosphokinase (CPK)	3,000/100,000

MICROBIOLOGY

Bacteremia is present in 60% of cases. When available, culture from the skin site is positive for GAS. GAS M types are 1, 3, 28, and 12. Mucoid colonies are rare. The strains contain pyogenic serotoxin A or B.

Complications

	Percentage
Shock	95
Adult respiratory distress syndrome	55
Renal impairment	80
Irreversible	10
Reversible	70
Death	30

MANAGEMENT

Penicillin G is the treatment of choice; however, failures are noted in humans and experimental animals. In experimental animals with GAS infections results are as follows: clindamycin better than erythromycin better than penicillin. Results may be related to inhibition of M protein and toxin production. Ceftriaxone has a greater affinity for streptococcal penicillin-binding proteins. Based on experimental results, clindamycin should be used either with penicillin or ceftriaxone. Treatment with intravenous immunoglobulin G is recommended for severe cases. Surgical treatment includes drainage, débridement, fasciotomy, or amputation, according to the clinical situation.

NECROTIZING SKIN AND SOFT TISSUE INFECTIONS

The severe skin and soft tissue infections differ from the milder, superficial infections by clinical presentation, coexisting systemic manifestations, and treatment strategies (6,7) (Table 96.1). They are often deep and devastating: deep because they involve the fascial or muscle compartments; devastating because they cause major destruction of tissue and can lead to a fatal outcome. These conditions are usually "secondary" infections in that they develop from an initial break in the skin related to

trauma or surgery. They can be monomicrobial, usually streptococci or staphylococci, or polymicrobial, involving a mixed aerobe-anaerobe bacterial flora.

Five clinical features suggest the presence of a deep and severe infection of the skin and its deeper structures:

1. Severe pain, which is constantly present.
2. Bullous lesions, related to occlusion of deep blood vessels that traverse the fascia or muscle compartments. Bullae are not diagnostic of deep infections because they can also be found in association with superficial infections (erysipelas, cellulitis, toxic shock syndrome, disseminated intravascular coagulation, purpura fulminans), some toxins (e.g., brown recluse spider bites), and primary dermatologic conditions (e.g., pyoderma gangrenosum).
3. Gas in the soft tissues, which is detected by palpation, radiography, or scanning. Gas is produced by metabolic activity of the aerobic or anaerobic bacteria. When anaerobes are present, there is also a distinctive odor of putrefaction.
4. Systemic toxicity, manifested by fever, leukocytosis, delirium and renal failure.
5. Rapid spread centrally along fascial planes.

Another distinction from the milder skin infections is that necrotizing deep infections usually require surgical intervention along with antimicrobial drugs for cure. While attempting to preserve as much viable tissue as possible, it is necessary to perform bold resection of all necrotic material and incise the fascial planes until the full extent of purulence is realized.

The choice of antimicrobial drugs is based on the specific organisms present (Table 96.2).

Necrotizing Fasciitis

Necrotizing fasciitis is a relatively rare infection involving subcutaneous tissues with extensive undermining and tracking along fascial planes (8,9).

CLINICAL FEATURES

Extension from a skin lesion is seen in 80% of cases. The initial lesion often is trivial, such as a minor abrasion, insect bite, injection site (in the case of heroin addicts), or boil. Rare cases have arisen in Bartholin's gland abscesses or perianal abscesses, from which the infection spreads to fascial planes of the perineum, thigh, groin, and abdomen. The remaining 20% of patients have no visible skin lesion. The initial presentation is that of cellulitis, which advances rather slowly. Over the next 2 to 4 days, however, there is systemic toxicity with high temperatures. The patient is disoriented and lethargic. The local site shows the following features: cellulitis (90%); edema (80%); skin discoloration or gangrene (70%); and anesthesia of involved skin (frequent, but true incidence is unknown).

The most distinguishing clinical feature is the wooden-hard feel of the subcutaneous tissues. In cellulitis or erysipelas, the subcutaneous tissues can be palpated and are yielding. But in fasciitis the underlying tissues are firm, and the fascial planes and muscle groups cannot be discerned by palpation. It is often possible to observe a broad erythematous tract in the skin, along the route of the fascial plane, as the infection advances cephalad in an extremity. If there is an open wound, probing the edges with a blunt instrument permits ready dissection of the superficial fascial planes well beyond the wound margins. There is remarkably little pain associated with this procedure.

BACTERIOLOGY

In the monomicrobial form, pathogens are group A β-hemolytic *S. pyogenes*, *S. aureus*, and anaerobic streptococci (*Peptostreptococcus*). Staphylococci and hemolytic streptococci occur with

TABLE 96.1. Necrotizing Soft Tissue Infections

Parameter	Gas-forming cellulitis	Synergistic necrotizing cellulitis	Gas gangrene	Streptococcal myonecrosis	Necrotizing fasciitis	Infected vascular gangrene	Streptococcal infection
Predisposing conditions	Traumatic	Diabetes, prior local lesions, perirectal lesions	Traumatic or surgical wound	Trauma, surgery	Diabetes, trauma, surgery, perineal infection	Arterial insufficiency	Traumatic or surgical wound
Incubation period	>3 days	3–14 days	1–4 days	3–4 days	1–4 days	>5 days	6 h to 2 days
Etiologic organisms	Clostridia, others	Mixed aerobic-anaerobic flora	Clostridia, especially *Clostridium perfringens*	Anaerobic streptococci	Mixed aerobic-anaerobic flora	Mixed aerobic-anaerobic flora	*Streptococcus pyogenes*
Systemic toxicity	Minimal	Moderate to severe	Severe	Minimal until late in course	Moderate to severe	Minimal	Severe
Course	Gradual	Acute	Acute	Subacute	Acute to subacute	Subacute	Acute
Wound findings							
Local pain	Minimal	Moderate to severe	Severe	Minimal until late in course	Minimal to moderate	Variable	Severe
Skin appearance	Swollen, minimal discoloration	Erythematous or gangrene	Tense and blanched, yellow-bronze, necrosis with hemorrhagic bullae	Erythema or yellow-bronze	Blanched, erythema, necrosis with hemorrhagic bullae	Erythema or necrosis	Erythema, necrosis
Gas	Abundant	Variable	Usually present	Variable	Variable	Variable	No
Muscle Involvement	No	Variable	Myonecrosis	Myonecrosis	No	Myonecrosis limited to area of vascular insufficiency	No
Discharge	Thin, dark, sweetish or foul odor	Dark pus or "dishwater," putrid	Serosanguineous, sweet or foul odor	Seropurulent	Seropurulent or dishwater, putrid	Minimal	None or sero sanguineous
Gram stain	PMNs, gram-positive bacilli	PMNs, mixed flora	Sparse PMNs, gram-positive bacilli	PMNs, gram-positive cocci	PMNs, mixed flora	PMNs, mixed flora	PMNs, gram-positive cocci in chains
Surgical therapy	Débridement	Wide filleting incisions	Extensive excision, amputation	Excision of necrotic muscle	Wide filleting incisions	Amputation	Débridement of necrotic tissue

PMNs, polymorphonuclear leukocytes.
From Bartlett JG. Clostridial myonecrosis and other clostridial diseases. In: Wyngaarden JB, Smith LH Jr, Bennett JC, eds. *Cecil textbook of medicine,* 19th ed. Philadelphia; WB Saunders, 1992:1679, with permission.

TABLE 96.2.   Treatment of Necrotizing Infections of the Skin, Fascia, and Muscle

First-line	Second-line/penicillin allergic
Mixed infections	
Imipenen/cilastatin	Cefoxitin, clindamycin,
Ticarcillin/clavulanate	or metronidazole and
Ampicillin/sulbactam	an aminoglycoside
Piperacillin/tazobactam	
Streptococcus	Cefazolin
Penicillin (and Clindamycin, for toxic shock or necrotizing fasciitis)	Vancomycin
Staphylococcus aureus	
Nafcillin	Cefazolin
Cloxacillin	Vancomycin
Vancomycin (for resistant strains)	Linezolid
Linezolid (for resistant strains)	

about equal frequency, and approximately one third of patients will have both pathogens simultaneously. Most patients acquire their infection outside the hospital. The majority of these infections present in the extremities, approximately two thirds in the lower extremity. There is often an underlying cause, such as diabetes, arteriosclerotic vascular disease, or venous insufficiency with edema. In some instances a chronic vascular ulcer changes into a more acute process. The mortality rate in this group is high, approaching 50% in patients with severe vascular disease.

In the polymicrobial form, an array of anaerobic and aerobic organisms can be cultured from the involved fascial plane: from 1 to 15 bacteria, with an average of 5 pathogens in each wound. Most of the organisms originate from the bowel flora (e.g., coliforms and anaerobic bacteria).

The polymicrobial infection is associated with four clinical settings:

1. Surgical procedures, especially bowel resections and penetrating trauma, can be complicated by cellulitis, leading to a superficial fascial dissection.
2. An infection proceeding from a decubitus ulcer, minor trauma, or a perianal abscess can involve the buttocks and perineum. Due to the proximity of the anus, contamination by fecal bacteria is universally present.
3. In intravenous drug users, the upper extremities are frequently involved at the site of injection. Because the needles and "works" are contaminated, unusual organisms such as *Pseudomonas* and *Citrobacter* can be isolated, sometimes in association with anaerobes.
4. The lesion can spread from a Bartholin's abscess or a minor vulvovaginal infection. Some cases have been associated with pudendal block anesthesia during delivery. While mixed infections are usually noted in this setting, some cases are caused by a single pathogen, particularly anaerobic *Streptococcus.*

DIAGNOSIS

It may not be possible to diagnose fasciitis upon first seeing the patient. Overlying cellulitis is a frequent accompaniment. That the process involves the deeper fascial planes is suggested by the following features:

- Failure to respond to initial antibiotic therapy.
- Cellulitis usually improves, with lowering of fever and reduction in local signs, within 24 to 48 hours.

- Fasciitis is a more stubborn infection and shows little improvement in the initial few days.
- The hard, wooden feel of the subcutaneous tissue, extending beyond the area of apparent skin involvement.
- Systemic toxicity, often with altered mental status.

DIAGNOSIS

Computed tomography (CT) or magnetic resonance imaging may show exudate extending along the fascial plane. The most important diagnostic feature of necrotizing fasciitis is the appearance of the fascial planes at surgery. Upon direct inspection, the fascia is swollen and dull gray in appearance, with stringy areas of necrosis. A thin, brownish exudate emerges from the wound. Even upon deep dissection, there is no true pus. Extensive undermining of surrounding tissues is present, and the fascial planes can be dissected with a gloved finger or a blunt instrument. Gram staining of the exudate demonstrates the pathogens and provides an early clue to therapy. Gram-positive cocci in chains suggest *Streptococcus* (either group A or anaerobic). Large gram-positive cocci in clumps suggest *S. aureus*. A mixed flora suggests polymicrobial infection. Cultures are best obtained from the deep tissues. If the infection has emanated from a contaminated skin wound, such as a vascular ulcer, the bacteriology of the superficial wound is not necessarily indicative of the deep tissue infection. An array of coliforms, staphylococci, and various streptococci can be isolated from the ulcer, but the fascia may have a pure culture or single organism, such as anaerobic streptococci of *S. aureus*. Direct needle aspiration of the advancing edge has been advocated as a means of obtaining material for culture, but this technique is nearly always unproductive. A definitive bacteriologic diagnosis can be established only by culture of the fascia at operation or by positive blood culture.

TREATMENT

Surgical intervention is the major therapeutic modality in cases of necrotizing fasciitis. It should be emphasized, however, that some patients can be treated with large doses of appropriate antibiotics, thereby avoiding potentially mutilating surgery. The decision to undertake aggressive surgery should be based on the following:

1. Failure to respond to antibiotics after a reasonable trial is the most common index. A response to antibiotics should be judged by reduction in fever and toxicity and lack of advancement.
2. Profound toxicity, fever, hypotension, or advancement of the skin and soft tissue infection during antibiotic therapy is an indication for surgical intervention.
3. When the local wound shows extensive necrosis with easy dissection along the fascia by a blunt instrument, more complete incision and drainage are required.

Under general anesthesia, the skin is incised or the wound is widened down to the fascial plane for complete inspection. Finger dissection along the fascial plane determines the extent of the linear incision. Usually, multiple incisions or "filets" are required to delineate adequately the extent of involvement. Loose gauze dressings are packed into the wound and changed every 6 hours or as required. Wet-to-dry dressings are used in order to facilitate mechanical débridement. As the dressings are removed, the depth of the wound should be inspected by a gloved finger to determine any extension that requires further incision. The first procedure is almost never sufficient to determine the extent of involvement. As further tracts are discovered, the patient is returned to the operating room for additional incision and débridement. Although no discrete pus is encountered, these wounds can discharge copious amounts of tissue fluid; aggressive fluid and colloid therapy is a necessary adjunct.

Antimicrobial therapy can minimize the extent of, and even avert, surgical intervention, especially in those cases in which the distinction between cellulitis and fasciitis is difficult. The therapy must be directed at the pathogens and used in high doses for a prolonged period of time, usually 2 to 3 weeks (Table 96.2).

OUTCOME

The overall mortality rate associated with necrotizing fasciitis is 20% to 30%. Adverse risk factor include diabetes, advanced arteriosclerotic vascular disease, and lesions that involve an extremity and progress into the buttocks or back muscles or onto the chest wall.

Anaerobic Streptococcal Myositis

Anaerobic streptococci cause a more indolent process than other streptococcal infections. Involvement of the muscle and fascial planes by anaerobic streptococci usually is associated with trauma or a surgical procedure.

CLINICAL FEATURES

There may be severe local pain. The overlying skin appears as a gangrenous wound that emits a foul, watery, brown discharge. Bleb formation is common. Crepitus may be apparent in the surrounding tissue. The gas formation can be extensive, with tracking into the adjacent healthy tissues. Inspection of the muscle reveals redness and edema with some local destruction. There is no myonecrosis, however, and the muscle contracts under the scalpel. Although there is generalized toxicity and fever and even organ failure, the patient is not as ill as someone with gas gangrene.

DIAGNOSIS

The initial approach to a crepitant skin infection is to obtain a sample of exudate for Gram's stain and open the wound for inspection of muscle and soft tissue. The major distinctions between the disease caused by anaerobic streptococci and clostridia are as follows:

1. Systemic effects are less prominent with the streptococcal form. This infection does not cause hypotension and renal failure, as does clostridial disease.
2. The involved muscle remains viable in streptococcal disease, although there may be inflammatory reaction and edema. True myonecrosis is not found.
3. Considerable gas is produced, occurring early in the course, whereas clostridial infections tend to have less gas and usually as a late development.
4. The discharge from the wound is thin, brown ooze that shows gram-positive cocci and multiple PMNs in the Gram's stain slide. By contrast, the discharge in gas gangrene shows gram-positive rods but few PMNs.

TREATMENT

Incision and drainage are critical. Necrotic tissue and debris are resected, but the inflamed muscle should not be removed since it can heal and become functionally useful. The incision should be packed with moist dressings. Antibiotic treatment is highly effective. These organisms are all sensitive to penicillin or ampicillin, which should be administered in high doses.

Streptococcal Gangrene (Meleney's Streptococcal Gangrene, β-Hemolytic Streptococcal Gangrene)

A superficial streptococcal infection can progress to cause severe destruction of the superficial layers of skin. This condition occurs most frequently in the extremities, associated with minor trauma, puncture wound, or surgical incision, but can occur in postoperative abdominal incisions. The initial event is erysipelas, with the typical findings of pain, erythema, edema, and advancing border. Within 1 to 2 days the center of the lesion becomes dark red, then blue-black, with formation of bullae and gangrene of the skin and subcutaneous tissues. The surrounding tissue is fiery red, raided, and edematous. Deeper fascia and muscle may also be involved.

Surgical management involves débridement of the gangrenous skin and incision and drainage of the surrounding tissues and fascial planes. It is important to release the pressure on the skin and subcutaneous tissues, so incisions should be extended beyond the areas of gangrene and far enough into the superficial fascia to establish good drainage. The limb should be elevated in order to promote drainage, and dressed with moist packs for superficial débridement. Although no discrete pockets of pus are found, there is significant oozing of tissue fluid, which must be made up by appropriate intravenous administration of fluid and colloids. High-dose penicillin or ampicillin is also given.

Progressive Bacterial Synergistic Gangrene (Meleney's Gangrene)

This indolent process is characterized by poor wound healing with elevation and erythema of the surrounding skin. This is a postoperative infection that typically occurs in the vicinity of retention suture or in a drain site following an abdominal operation or an incision of the chest wall. In recent years this infection is rare because postoperative antibiotics are administered at the earliest sign of infection in the wound. In the classic presentation the diagnosis is recognized 1 to 2 weeks after surgery, when the lesion has extended circumferentially with three zones of involvement: a central area of necrosis; a middle zone of violaceous, tender, edematous tissue; and an outer zone of bright erythema. Local pain and tenderness are nearly always present; however, fever and systemic toxicity usually are absent.

The condition is caused by synergistic (cooperative) association between *S. aureus* and a microaerophilic or anaerobic *Streptococcus*. These organisms can be isolated from the outer zone of infection; sampling the central zone of necrosis, however, yields a mixed flora of coliforms that does not reflect the essential pathologic process. In experimental studies synergy has been demonstrated in mixed infections of *S. aureus* and *S. pyogenes* and of various aerobes and anaerobes.

In the preantibiotic era, Meleney advocated extensive resection of all nonviable tissue, as well as extension of the incision beyond the area of induration and necrosis to include some healthy tissue. The availability of antibiotics has eliminated the requirement for such radical excisions. It is now recommended that all necrotic tissue be removed, with inspection of subcutaneous structures for burrowing tracks. Wet-to-dry dressings should then be used. Daily inspection should reveal any extension of the process that requires additional débridement. A heterograft or homograft may be necessary to cover the wound. Antimicrobial therapy should be directed at the two major pathogens, *S. aureus* and the anaerobic *Streptococcus*. A semisynthetic penicillin (nafcillin or oxacillin) or a cephalosporin can be used.

Pyomyositis

Pyomyositis is a discrete abscess within an individual muscle group caused in the main by *S. aureus*. Occasionally *S. pneumoniae* or a gram-negative enteric rod is the responsible pathogen. Blood cultures are positive in 5% to 30% of cases. Because of its geographic distribution, this condition is often referred to as "tropical pyomyositis," but cases are increasingly recognized in temperate climates, especially in patients with human immunodeficiency virus infection or diabetes (10). Presenting findings are localized pain in a single muscle group, muscle spasm, and fever. The disease occurs most often in an extremity, but any muscle group can be involved, including the psoas or muscles of the trunk. Initially it may not be possible to palpate a discrete abscess because the infection is localized deep within the muscle, but the area has a firm, woody feel on palpation, along with pain and tenderness. In the early stages, ultrasonography or CT is needed to make the diagnosis, which can be confused with deep vein thrombosis, but in more advanced cases, a bulging abscess is apparent. Surgical incision and drainage are required, along with appropriate antibiotics.

Synergistic Necrotizing Cellulitis

This is a highly lethal polymicrobial infection that produces extensive necrosis of skin and soft tissues with progressive undermining along fascial planes (11–13). The process may be rather indolent at first, presenting after 7 to 10 days of mild symptoms. Patients are often afebrile or have only low-grade fever, lacking systemic toxicity in the early stages. The initial lesion in the skin is a small area of necrotic or reddish brown bleb with extreme local tenderness; however, the superficial appearance belies the widespread destruction of the deeper tissues. By direct inspection through skin incisions, there is extensive gangrene of the superficial tissues and fat, with gelatinous necrosis of fascia and muscle. Gas can be palpated in the tissues in 25% of patients. The most common site of involvement is the perineum, seen in one half of patients.

The major predisposing causes are perirectal abscess and ischiorectal abscess; these conditions track to the deeper structures of the pelvis, leading to a severe form of the disease. A more superficial form involves the buttocks without extension to deeper muscles. Approximately 40% of patients have involvement of the thigh and leg. Some infections arise in the adductor compartment of the thigh, often extending from an infected amputation stump or diabetic gangrene. Lesions in the lower leg usually are associated with vascular disease or diabetic foot ulcers. The remaining 10% of cases occur in the upper extremities or in the neck, most frequently in patients with vascular disease or diabetes. Seventy-five percent of patients have diabetes mellitus, which may be relatively mild and only discovered at the time of admission. Some patients present with ketoacidosis. Cardiovascular and renal disease are seen in 50% of patients. Obesity is common, found in over 50% of patients.

BACTERIOLOGY

The discharge is brown, rather thin and watery, with a foul odor: such exudate has been labeled "dishwater pus." This is a mixed aerobic-anaerobic infection, consisting of organisms that have their origin in the intestinal tract. Gram's stain reveals a mixed flora with abundant PMNs. Among the aerobes, coliforms are most common, such as *Escherichia coli*, *Klebsiella*, and *Proteus*. Anaerobes are usually abundant, including *Bacteroides*, *Peptostreptococcus*, *Clostridium*, and *Fusobacterium*. Approximately one third of patients have positive blood cultures, usually a coliform, *Bacteroides* or *Peptostreptococcus*.

TREATMENT

Surgical management of synergistic necrotizing cellulitis involves radical débridement of involved tissues, followed by wet-to-dry dressing and mechanical débridement. When the lower extremity is involved, as in diabetes, an amputation usually is required. In the perineum, infection that is confined to the buttocks can be managed with complete surgical excision; however, deeper infection in the pelvis, extending from perirectal disease, is difficult to approach by complete resection, and may require repeated sessions of débridement in the operating room to achieve adequate drainage. Antibiotic therapy involves a spectrum broad enough to cover both aerobes and anaerobes.

OUTCOME

A mortality rate of 50% is associated with this disease. The patient usually succumbs to septic shock and circulatory collapse. Adverse risk factors include diabetes, especially ketoacidosis, severe renal disease, and involvement of deep tissues of the pelvis and perineum.

Nonclostridial Crepitant Cellulitis

This condition is caused by gas-forming bacteria that involve the skin, either primarily or as an extension from deeper structures. The origin of infection is an abdominal wound, perianal disease, or operative incisions that have become secondarily infected. Tracking of gas-forming organisms from deeper sites of infection may also present as crepitant cellulitis without a break in the skin. Infection of the perineal area is associated with ischiorectal abscess, while those in the flank generally communicate with a perinephric abscess. Diabetics are more likely to acquire such infections, especially in the lower extremities. These emphysematous infections generally are not as serious as those associated with clostridia, since the nonclostridial pathogens do not liberate systemic toxins. Among the bacteria isolated are anaerobic organisms such as *Bacteroides* or anaerobic streptococci (*Peptostreptococcus*), or coliform bacteria, especially *E. coli* and *Klebsiella*.

TREATMENT

The surgical approach should be aggressive, but tailored specifically to the underlying cause of infection. Extensive resection usually is not required, since the gas is not an index of underlying necrosis, but rather reflects tracking of the infection along the fascial or lymphatic planes. Antibiotic therapy is directed at a mixed aerobic-anaerobic flora, until culture reports are available.

DIFFERENTIAL DIAGNOSIS

Noninfectious processes can be associated with gas in subcutaneous tissues. On the chest wall, at the site of thoracentesis, chest tube insertion, or a thoracic procedure, there may be subcutaneous emphysema that tracks extensively along subcutaneous tissues. A tracheotomy provides a portal for air to track along the tissues of the neck, even to the anterior chest wall. Transtracheal aspiration by a needle produces local emphysema in approximately 10% of cases. On rare occasion, a thin column of gas is palpated or seen by radiography along the course of an intravenous catheter in the arm. This is most likely caused by a central venous pressure line or a Swan-Ganz catheter. This is a benign condition, not associated with infection in the lines or the surrounding veins

Fournier's Gangrene

This is a variant of synergistic gangrene that involves the scrotum and penis and has an explosive onset (14,15). The average age of onset is 50 to 60 years. Most have significant underlying disease, particularly diabetes. Twenty percent of patients have no preceding cause. The remaining individuals have one of the following conditions: ischiorectal abscess; perianal fistula; erysipelas of the perineum; bowel disease (rectal carcinoma, diverticulitis); scrotal trauma; prior urogenital surgery, especially involving the periurethral glands; rarely in alcoholics who develop pressure sores of the scrotum and perineum by sitting in the same position in a drunken stupor; or dissection of pancreatic juice through the retroperitoneum and into the scrotum.

The infection can begin insidiously with a discrete area of necrosis on the scrotum, which can then move with advancing skin necrosis rapidly over 1 to 2 days. The route of infection is via Buck's fascia, spreading along the planes of the Dartos fascia of the scrotum and penis. The infection may then extend to Colles' fascia of the perineum and even to Scarpa's fascia of the abdominal wall. At the outset, it tends to be superficial gangrene, limited to skin and subcutaneous tissue, extending to the base of the scrotum. The testes, glans penis, and spermatic cord usually are spared, since they have a separate blood supply. There may be extension to the perineum and the anterior abdominal wall through the fascial planes.

BACTERIOLOGY

Most cases are caused by a mixed flora of aerobic and anaerobic bacteria, similar to those noted in synergistic necrotizing cellulitis. Staphylococci are frequently present, usually in mixed culture but occasionally as a single pathogen. *Pseudomonas* is another common organism in the mixed culture.

TREATMENT

Prompt and aggressive surgical débridement should be instituted with removal of all necrotic tissue, sparing the deeper structures when possible. It is often necessary to return to the operating room on several occasions for the necessary resection of necrotic tissue. Diversion of the fecal or urinary stream is necessary in some, but not all, cases. Antibiotic therapy should cover the range of organisms in the mixed culture. Special attention is directed to *Staphylococcus* and *Pseudomonas*.

OUTCOME

Even with optimal surgical and medical therapy, the mortality rate ranges from 10% to 40%.

REFERENCES

1. File TM Jr, Tan JS. Treatment of skin and soft-tissue infections. *Am J Surg* 1995;169(suppl):27–33.
2. Bisno AL, Stevens DL. Streptococcal infections of skin and soft tissues. *N Engl J Med* 1996;334(4):240–245.
3. Chartier C, Grosshans E. Erysipelas: an update. *Int J Dermatol* 1996;35(11):779–781.
4. Brook I, Frazier EH. Clinical features and aerobic and anaerobic microbiological characteristics of cellulitis. *Arch Surg* 1995;130:786–792.
5. Stevens DL. Streptococcal toxic shock syndrome associated with necrotizing fasciitis. *Annu Rev Med* 2000;51:271–288.
6. Ahrenholz DH. Necrotizing soft-tissue infections. *Surg Clin North Am* 1988;68:199–214.
7. Lewis RT. Necrotizing soft-tissue infections. *Infect Dis Clin North Am* 1992;6:693–703.
8. Rea WJ, Wyrick WJ Jr. Necrotizing fasciitis. *Ann Surg* 1970;172:957–964.
9. Giuliano A, Lewis F Jr, Hadley K, et al. Bacteriology of necrotizing fasciitis. *Am J Surg* 1977;134:52–57.
10. Sissolak D, Weir WR. Tropical pyomyositis. *J Infect* 1994;29:121–127.
11. Salvino C, Harford FJ, Dobrin PB. Necrotizing infections of the perineum. *South Med J* 1993;86:908–911.
12. Stone HH, Martin JD Jr. Synergistic necrotizing cellulitis. *Ann Surg* 1972;175:702–711.
13. Kingston D, Seal DV. Current hypotheses on synergistic microbial gangrene. *Br J Surg* 1990;77:260–264.
14. Laucks SS 2nd. Fournier's gangrene. *Surg Clin North Am* 1994;74:1339–1352.
15. Eke N. Fournier's gangrene: a review of 1726 cases. *Br J Surg* 2000;87(6):718–728.

CHAPTER 97
Infections in Trauma

Ronald C. Jones

Trauma is the leading cause of death before 65 years of age (1). Infection remains the most serious threat to patients who survive the initial insult. Septic complications occur in 10% to 15% of those patients (2). After hemorrhage and a closed head injury, sepsis is the next most common cause of death in patients who sustain abdominal trauma, and it is the leading cause of postoperative morbidity (3,4). A review of over 1,200 trauma patient admissions to a surgical intensive care unit noted an infection rate of 12%. The most frequently occurring infection was pneumonia, which accounted for almost half of the patients, and approximately one fourth were due to urinary tract infections and 20% to bacteremia. The most common organism in pneumonia and urinary tract infections was *Enterobacter* species, followed by *Escherichia coli* in the urinary tract group (5).

The source of a nosocomial infection is either exogenous or endogenous. Infection after penetrating abdominal trauma usually results in endogenous organisms introduced by perforation of the gastrointestinal tract. The bacterial population of the large bowel is 10^{11} to 10^{12} bacteria per gram of stool, and anaerobes outnumber aerobes by 1,000 to 10,000 (6). The large intestine provides an ideal anaerobic environment and a low oxidation-reduction potential. A less common cause of infection is exogenous bacteria, which may be carried into the wound on pieces of clothing, dirt, or foreign bodies by a knife or bullet. Gram positive infections due to staphylococcal, streptococcal, or clostridial infections may result. During the immediate resuscitation, contamination may result from a breach in sterile technique while intravenous and urinary catheters or arterial lines are inserted, or during arteriography.

LOCAL OR SYSTEMIC FACTORS

Many factors are responsible for infection following trauma, such as the number and virulence of organisms, blood supply or viability of tissue, host resistance, shock, adequacy of surgical débridement, tissue tension, dead space, hemostasis, age, and associated diseases (7).

The duration of shock correlates with the development of infections. In one series of penetrating and blunt trauma to the abdomen, the infection rate in normotensive patients was 14% versus 30% in hypotensive patients (8). It has also been noted that hypotensive patients who do not correct their lactic acidosis within 12 hours have a much higher infection rate (13% vs. approximately 50%) when the lactic acidosis is not corrected for 12 to 24 hours (9). The length of stay was also increased from 17 days to 31 days. In another study of 3,254 patients, the majority of whom were under 65 years of age compared with those patients over 65 years of age, had an infection rate of 17% in the younger population versus 39% in patients over 65. There was also an increased length of stay and mortality rate. Older patients were found to have a 2.2 times greater relative risk for infection compared with younger patients matched for injury severity score (ISS). Elderly patients had a greater percentage in relative risk for respiratory and genitourinary infections, suggesting age as a predisposing factor (10). Normal tissue has remarkable resistance to microorganisms, whereas devitalized tissue has a limited capacity for resistance (11,12). Clinical experience has long shown that there is an inverse relationship between the vascularity of an area and its susceptibility to infection. Débridement remains the most important adjunct in the prevention of infection.

HOST DEFENSE MECHANISMS

As the severity of injury increases, there are progressively more abnormalities in host defense mechanisms (13,14). Host defense mechanisms include humoral (antibody) responses, compliment, phagocytic cells, the cell-mediated system, and barrier defense of the gastrointestinal tract. There are numerous humoral mediators of acute-phase responses, including interleukin-1 and prostaglandins. Within 2 hours of sustaining severe injuries, patients have alterations in host defense mechanisms that activate the complement cascade. Chemotaxis and phagocytosis are impaired (15,16). Treatment of the patient with impaired host defense mechanisms is by parenteral nutrition, restoration of blood volume, adequate oxygenation, débridement, good hemostasis, and evaluation for a possible source of infection (17).

In another large study of almost 5,000 patients admitted to a trauma center, it was noted that the systemic inflammatory response syndrome (SIRS) predicted mortality and length of stay. Over 80% of these patients have sustained blunt trauma. The mortality rate in patients with SIRS was 7% versus 1% in patients without SIRS. A significantly increased mortality rate was also noted in older patients with an ISS of greater than or equal to 30 (61% vs. 27%). Patients with a SIRS score of 2 at admission were 11 times more likely to die as patients without manifestation of SIRS. These data suggest that the SIRS score is a more accurate predictor of mortality in blunt trauma patients compared with penetrating patients (18). This center subsequently reported that an admission SIRS score of greater than or equal to 2 is a significant independent predictor of infection and outcome in blunt trauma patients. SIRS is present when two or more of the following criteria are met: temperature greater than 38°C or less that 36°C, heart rate greater than 90 beats/min, respiratory rate greater than 20 breaths/min, or $Paco_2$ less than 32 mm Hg, and white blood cell count greater than 12,000/mm³ or less than 4,000/mm³ or the presence of 10% bands (19).

The inflammatory response to injury involves an interplay among hormones [e.g., catecholamines, adrenocorticotropic hormone, cortisol, and glucagon); cytokines [e.g., tumor necrosis factor-α, interleukin-6 (IL-6), IL-8, IL-10, IL-1B]; and other cellular products such as proteases, free radicals, eicosanoids, acutephase reactants, and growth factors. The interplay among these mediators is complex; although much is known about the activities and regulation of these mediators *in vitro* and in animal studies, these effects and regulation in human stress states are less well characterized (20).

Moore described the penetrating abdominal trauma index (PATI) in 1981. In calculating the PATI, each abdominal organ is given a risk factor of 1 to 5, and the severity of each organ injury also is graded on a scale of 1 to 5. Thus, the PATI for each abdominal organ injury may range from 1 to 25, but if multiple organs are injured, the PATI may be much higher. A PATI of 26 or more is a strong predictor of infection (21).

PROPHYLACTIC ANTIBIOTICS

Sepsis is related to the length of the interval between bacterial contamination of the traumatic wound and the initiation of treatment designed to prevent sepsis. The effectiveness of preventive antibiotics in surgical wounds has been shown to be no more that 3 hours (22). Antibiotics should be started as soon as possible after injury for which such drugs are indicated.

It has been known for over 35 years that patients in shock had a higher incidence of septic complications than normotensive patients. In 1965, more than 400 patients who sustained penetrating abdominal trauma were retrospectively reviewed to determine the preventive benefit of penicillin and tetracycline. Approximately half of the patients received antibiotics before or during their operation, and the other half in the recovery room or when infection developed or never (i.e., therapeutic group) (23). Patients sustaining gunshot wounds were four times more likely to develop sepsis than those sustaining stab wounds (Table 97.1). Patients in shock had twice as many septic complications as did normotensive patients (24% vs. 11%). The overall infection rate was reduced from 9% to 4.5% with the early use of antibiotics.

Based on the biphasic animal model experiments, a second study was initiated, which included 122 patients prospectively randomized who sustained penetrating abdominal trauma to receive clindamycin plus tobramycin, no antibiotics (as a control group), or cefoxitin (24). The infection rate for combination therapy was 16%, for no antibiotics 44%, and for the single-agent 10%. Antibiotic therapy prevented sepsis in a clinical setting, but there was no difference between single-agent and combination therapy. Thus, routine use of an aminoglycoside was shown to be unnecessary for abdominal trauma.

These findings have been documented in subsequent studies. Jones and colleagues evaluated 257 patients to determine whether single-agent therapy was comparable with combination therapy and whether anaerobes played a role in infection after trauma (25). Patients were randomized to receive combination therapy (clindamycin-tobramycin); cefamandole, which is

TABLE 97.1. Effects of Preventive Antibiotics in Penetrating Abdominal Trauma

	Preoperative or intraoperative treatment			Postoperative therapeutic			Totals		
	Patients treated	Patients with infection		Patients treated	Patients with infection		Patients treated	Patients with infection	
Type of trauma	n	n	%	n	n	%	n	n	%
Stab wounds	77	0	0	111	5	4.5	188	5	2.6
Gunshot wounds	113	8	7	102	15	15	215	23	10.7

TABLE 97.2. Penetrating Abdominal Trauma: Colon and/or Small Bowel Injuries
(N = 147)

Patient group	Antibiotic	No. of patients	No. of infections (%)	Bacteremia, abdominal abscess, operative soft tissue
I	Cleocin/tobramycin	51	15 (29)	7 (14%)
II	Mandol	44	20 (45)	11 (25%)
III	Cefoxitin	52	8 (15)	5 (10%)
I vs. III			$p = 0.086$	$p = 0.515$
II vs. I and III			$p = 0.006$	$p = 0.048$

not active against *Bacteroides fragilis*; or cefoxitin, which is active against aerobes and anaerobes. The overall infection rate with clindamycin-tobramycin was 20%; with cefamandole 29%; and with cefoxitin 13%. Among patients who sustained colon or small bowel injuries, the infection rate increased to 29%, 45%, and 15%, respectively (Table 97.2). This study demonstrated that single-agent antimicrobial therapy was as effective as combination therapy and that antibiotics active against *B. fragilis* and other anaerobes are necessary in the preoperative treatment of the trauma patient. However, in the absence of colon injury, there was no difference in infection rate, regardless of what antibiotic was given.

Several studies have confirmed that results of single-agent therapy are comparable with those of combination therapy. Fabian demonstrated that single-agent therapy with ticarcillin-clavulanate (Timentin; GlaxoSmithKline, Research Triangle Park, NC) was comparable to combination therapy with clindamycin-gentamicin for treating penetrating abdominal trauma (26). A metaanalysis of 17 trials with 1,956 patients found no difference in outcomes between single β-lactam antimicrobials versus aminoglycoside combinations in treating penetrating trauma (27).

Nichols and associates demonstrated an overall infection rate of 20% using cefoxitin, versus 23% with clindamycin-gentamicin (28). He determined risk factors for development of infection after trauma, including older age, injury to the left side of the colon, massive transfusions (probable shock), and multiple injured organs. It is known that patients with massive blood loss are at increased risk for development of postoperative infection, and these patients may require a second dose of antibiotic during the operative procedure (29). Gentry and colleagues evaluated cefamandole, cefoxitin, and ticarcillin-tobramycin for penetrating abdominal trauma, noting that the intraabdominal abscess rates were identical (6%) for cefoxitin and combination therapy and half that for cefamandole (12%) (25,28,29) (Table 97.3). Others

TABLE 97.3. Single-Agent Therapy for Penetrating Abdominal Trauma

Investigator	Patients (n)		Infections (%)		Abdominal abscess (%)	
	Cef	CT	Cef	CT	Cef	CT
Jones (25)	94	85	13	20	5	4
	Cef	TT	Cef	TT	Cef	TT
Gentry et al. (29)	50	51	6	10	6	6
	Cef	CG	Cef	CG	Cef	CG
Nichols et al. (28)	70	75	20	23	4	7

Cef, cefoxitin; TT, ticarcillin-tobramycin; CG, clindamycin-gentamicin; CT, clindamycin-tobramycin.

have demonstrated comparable outcomes comparing cefoxitin to clindamycin-gentamicin (30). Thus, preventative antibiotics, either a single agent or a combination, are beneficial when given before operation to patients having sustained abdominal trauma.

The appropriate duration of preventive antibiotic therapy appears to be no more than 24 hours, with or without gastrointestinal injury. Fabian evaluated over 500 patients sustaining penetrating abdominal trauma, prospectively and double-blinded. Patients were randomized to receive antibiotic therapy for 24 hours versus 5 days. Those patients who had no hollow viscus injury did not receive additional antibiotic therapy beyond the perioperative dose. Patients receiving antibiotic therapy for 1 day had a 17% incidence of wound infection versus 18% with a 5-day course. Thus, 24 hours of antibiotic therapy appears to be equal to 5 days of therapy (31). Subsequently, Kirton demonstrated that high-risk patients with colon or other hollow viscus injuries from penetrating abdominal trauma are at no greater risk for surgical infection when treated with only a 24-hour course of broad-spectrum antibiotics than those treated for 5 days. Ampicillin/sulbactam (Unasyn, Pfizer, New York, NY) was the antibiotic studied in a total of 317 patients from four level I trauma centers. Those receiving antibiotics for 24 hours had a surgical site infection rate of 8% versus 10% for those receiving antibiotics for 5 days. The dosage was 3 g every 6 hours. ISSs, trauma scores, and PATI scores were calculated for each patient and used to stratify patients by degree of injury (32). Even with gastrointestinal injury, antibiotics are not indicated after 24 hours, and those without gastrointestinal tract injuries can have antibiotics discontinued at the termination of surgery.

In another study by Bozorgzadeh and Barie, 300 patients were evaluated and randomized to 24 hours of 1 g of cefoxitin every 6 hours versus 5 days of therapy. The rate of infection was higher in patients having associated shock on admission or a greater number of intraabdominal organs injured, specifically colon injuries. In each group the wound infection rate was approximately 10% and the intraabdominal abscess rate was approximately 6%. There was no difference in infection between those patients receiving 24 hours versus 5 days of therapy (33).

BACTEREMIA IN TRAUMA

Bacteremia often follows gunshot wounds to the colon, and gram-negative organisms account for 70% of the isolates. Anaerobes are isolated from 20% of patients (34). The overall mortality rate for patients with bacteremia after trauma is approximately 40%. Of a group of patients with bacteremia, two thirds had sustained colon injuries and 75% were gunshot wounds. This is similar to the report of Gibson, who noted that 75% of patients who developed intraabdominal abscesses had sustained gunshot wounds (35). The most common gram-negative aerobes

TABLE 97.4. Antibiotics for Penetrating Abdominal Trauma

Antibiotic	Dose
Cefoxitin	2 g every 6 h (28)
Timentin	3 g every 4 h (26)
Unasyn	3 g every 6 h (32)
Cefotetan	2 g every 12 h (31)

isolated were *Klebsiella pneumoniae* and *Escherichia coli* followed by *Enterobacter*, *Pseudomonas*, and *Serratia* species. It was unusual to isolate anaerobes following blunt trauma, but the rate was 28% after penetrating trauma. Resistant organisms, such as *Pseudomonas aeruginosa*, *Serratia marcescens*, and *Enterobacter cloacae*, were uncommon isolates in patients who had not previously undergone surgery or had received other antibiotic therapy.

Enterococcus may be the only organism isolated from blood cultures and appears to be a significant pathogen when isolated from blood. Isolation of an *Enterococcus* species is rare immediately after trauma; more often these organisms also are present following multiple complications and having been previously treated with antibiotics.

Antibiotic coverage may not have to be as broad for patients sustaining penetrating or blunt abdominal trauma; nevertheless, several antibiotic choices are available (Table 97.4). In another group of patients who sustained pancreatic trauma, 15% developed bacteremia and half of them had an associated colon injury. Combination therapy is indicated, especially for *Pseudomonas* organisms.

In a multicenter study evaluating *Bacteroides* bacteremia, the mortality rate among patients who received an antibiotic not active against *Bacteroides* organisms was 45% compared with 16% mortality if the organism was sensitive to the antibiotic administered. In that study, 45% of the *Bacteroides* isolates were resistant to cefotan, 37% to piperacillin, 16% to clindamycin, and 8% to cefoxitin. In contrast, no *in vitro* resistance to metronidazole and imipenem was demonstrated, and there was less than 1% resistance to ampicillin/sulbactam (Unasyn) and ticarcillin/clavulanate (Timentin) to *Bacteroides* species (36).

INTRAOPERATIVE MANAGEMENT OF FECAL CONTAMINATION

Most colon injuries are managed by primary repair. Asensio and Bern have cautioned about using primary repair in patients who have greater than 6 units of blood transfused and more than 6 hours has elapsed from injury to surgery and those patients with a penetrating abdominal trauma index of 25 or more. However, the majority of patients sustaining colon trauma undergo primary repair (37–41). There appears to be no difference in right-versus left-sided colon injuries as to the incidence of infection (42,43).

PERITONITIS

Peritonitis is usually accompanied by sequestration of extracellular fluid, which requires liberal administration of a balanced salt solution. Once peritonitis is diagnosed, antibiotic therapy is initiated, the choice of drug being based on the

site of infection and the suspected pathogens. Anaerobic organisms such as *B. fragilis*, *Clostridium*, and *Peptostreptococcus* species are common in both generalized peritonitis and postoperative intraabdominal abscess. An agent active against both aerobes and anaerobes should be started. Imipenem/cilastatin 500 mg every 6 hours intravenously has been the antibiotic used to compare other antibiotics for the management of intraabdominal infections (44). Agents such as meropenem as well as ciprofloxacin plus metronidazole have yielded results comparable with imipenem/cilastatin for the management of intraabdominal infections (47). Cefotaxime (2 g) plus metronidazole 500 mg every 8 hours has been shown to be comparable with imipenem/cilastatin (45,46). Imipenem (Primaxin, Merck & Co., Inc., West Point, PA), a carbapenem, is a useful antibiotic for empirical treatment of moderate to severe intraabdominal infections, for resistant organisms, and for severe pulmonary infections in patients in a step-down intensive care unit (46). For established *Pseudomonas* sepsis, imipenem/cilastatin is combined with an aminoglycoside. Ampicillin/sulbactam and Timentin/clavulanate also have been utilized.

INTRAABDOMINAL ABSCESS AFTER SURGERY FOR TRAUMA

The majority of intraabdominal abscesses follow gunshot wounds to the abdomen and are usually associated with a gastrointestinal injury, particularly a colon injury (34). Although *Enterococcus* is often isolated from the abscess, it is almost always in association with other organisms. Most frequent organisms isolated include *Staphylococcus* species, *E. coli*, and *Enterobacter* species. *B. fragilis* was isolated from approximately 25% of patients, and *Clostridium perfringens* or other clostridia were isolated from 22%. As in bacteremia, *Pseudomonas* is not often associated with a first intraabdominal complication of trauma (34).

Of the patients with intraabdominal abscess, more than one third had associated bacteremia. Clinical findings before drainage of the abscess frequently include temperature elevations to 102°F and white blood cell counts in excess of 20,000/mm³. The mortality rate for intraabdominal abscess approaches 20% (48).

Diagnosis of intraabdominal abscess is best made by computed tomography (CT). Sonography is of little value because of overlying gas from ileus (49). It is usually possible to predict on which side a subphrenic abscess will develop, depending on whether there has been an associated liver or spleen injury (50,51). At the time of surgical or percutaneous drainage, a needle is inserted in the abscess and material is withdrawn in a syringe and sent to the laboratory for aerobic and anaerobic culture. Percutaneous drainage of an intraabdominal abscess is successful in approximately 80% of patients (52).

Closed suction drainage has decreased the incidence of intraabdominal abscess formation, formally more common following use of Penrose and older sump drains (50). Early diagnosis and drainage of an intraabdominal abscess is the most important aspect of management, along with adjuvant antibiotic therapy. Abdominal CT scans have been shown to be useful in diagnosing the cause of sepsis following major trauma. Over half the patients admitted to an intensive care unit with sepsis of unknown origin were proven on abdominal CT scan to have a focus of infection (53). Intravenous contrast and oral contrast solution are administered when possible through a nasogastric tube to patients to determine the presence of abscesses, bowel perforation, anastomotic leaks, or a necrotic bowel, particularly when air is noted within the bowel wall or mesenteric or portal veins. With a negative CT scan, exploratory laparotomy may be avoided. Early surgical drainage or percutaneous drainage of an intraabdominal abscess reduces the risk for death. Antibiotic therapy is directed to both aerobes and anaerobes. Single antibiotic therapy is usually adequate.

SEPSIS IN THE SURGICAL INTENSIVE CARE UNIT

Sepsis continues to be the leading cause of death in intensive care units, where up to 400,000 patients die annually in the United States. In one large center, 183 patients were empirically treated for sepsis using imipenem/gentamicin. This review covering slightly less than 2 years did not reveal any indication that using this combination caused antibiotic resistance. Neither did it lead to an increased incidence of fungemia. The usual duration of therapy was 72 hours, but it ranged from 1 to 71 days (54). The most common organisms isolated were *Klebsiella* and *Enterobacter* species and *pseudomonas aeruginosa*.

CLOSED CHEST DRAINAGE

The use of prophylactic antibiotics in the management of trauma patients with chest tubes remains controversial, but the majority of patients who require closed chest drainage have associated injuries and therefore other indications for antibiotic prophylaxis. A metaanalysis has demonstrated that antibiotics are effective (55).

PULMONARY INFECTION IN THE INTENSIVE CARE UNIT

It is difficult to determine whether to treat an intubated patient with antibiotics since most of these patients have abnormal chest radiographs, are semiconscious, and tend to aspirate. They may develop gram-negative pneumonia, because gram-negative organisms colonize the trachea within 3 or 4 days of admission to the intensive care unit. It is not productive to culture sputum because of the colonization of the pharynx. Transtracheal aspiration may be performed or cultures may be obtained via bronchoscopy to identify the suspected pathogen. Pneumonia may be treated by single-agent therapy, but if *Pseudomonas aeruginosa* is suspected, combination therapy with aminoglycoside is often required (56). For suspected staphylococcal infection, vancomycin is administered. The treatment for established empyema is rib resection (57).

POSTSPLENECTOMY INFECTION

Since the recognition of postsplenectomy sepsis, commonly due to the *Pneumococcus*, attempts have been made to repair the spleen or perform partial splenectomy or observe patients with minor splenic injury. In addition to pneumococcal organisms, overwhelming infection may also be due to *E. coli, Haemophilus influenzae, Meningococcus, Staphylococcus,* or *Streptococcus* species (58). Pneumovax (Merck & Co., Inc., West Point, PA) and prophylactic penicillin are frequently recommended to treat children who had undergone splenectomy. Splenectomy in childhood followed by overwhelming infection has given rise to the desire to salvage a part or all of the spleen, particularly in children and adolescents (59). *Pneumococcus* and *Haemophilus influenzae*

are encapsulated bacteria that probably gain access to the blood through the respiratory tract. The spleen usually clears the bacteria that are poorly or inadequately opsonized from the bloodstream. Splenectomy in children and adolescents is followed by a small number of patients susceptible to overwhelming sepsis. Although long-term antibiotic administration has been advocated, it has poor compliance. Polyvalent pneumococcal vaccine has been used in an attempt to prevent postsplenectomy sepsis (60). It does not provide protection against *H. influenzae*. A vaccine against *H. influenzae* is available (61). In the postsplenectomy patient, immunizations should be administered to patients during the hospitalization in which their splenectomy occurred rather than waiting until they return for a follow-up visit. Clinical studies have demonstrated adequate antibody response to immediate immunization (62). Simultaneous immunization with *H. influenzae* type B, meningococcal serogroup C, and polyvalent pneumococcal vaccine is both immunogenic and well tolerated. Some clinicians have advocated supplying patients with oral antibiotics such as amoxicillin with instructions to begin the medication if fever develops until the patients can see their physician (63). Diamond has defined late overwhelming postsplenectomy infection (OPSI) as a fulminate bacteria that usually progresses to death within 24 hours of recognition. Following splenectomy, young children are at particularly high risk for developing fulminant infections due to *Streptococcus pneumoniae*, *H. influenza*, and *Neisseria meningitidis*. Ninety percent of cases of postsplenectomy in adults are due to *S. pneumoniae* and occur within the first few years following operation. The vaccines may not be completely protective but are effective. Vaccines are not recommended for children under 2 years of age since these children rarely achieve protective antibody titers. They should received prophylactic penicillin until 2 years of age, when they can receive the vaccines (64).

A 23 valent pneumococcal vaccine (Pneumovax) should be administered to these patients. The approximate lifetime risk for an asplenic patient developing OPSI is estimated to be 1 to 3 in every 5,000. The risk in children is 2- to 10-fold higher than that of adults.

MULTIPLE-SYSTEM ORGAN FAILURE

Death results from multiple-organ failure in approximately 25% of patients in whom major infections develop (31). In multisystem organ failure, there is sequential instead of simultaneous organ failure, usually starting with the lungs and followed by liver, gastrointestinal tract, and kidneys. Fry noted pulmonary failure as the first of the failed systems. Hepatic failure and stress bleeding followed, and renal failure then became most predictive of a fatal outcome for the patient (65). Pulmonary failure is first manifested by acute respiratory distress syndrome (66). Sepsis and organ failure can be produced by activating the inflammatory response: bacteria, endotoxin, and ischemic tissue all activate this response. More than half of the patients with acute respiratory distress syndrome develop the sepsis syndrome, which is followed by multisystem organ failure. To prevent multisystem organ failure, it is important that the source of infection be identified and treated with appropriate antibiotics or surgical drainage.

ORTHOPEDIC TRAUMA

A first-generation cephalosporin such as cephalothin, nafcillin, or oxacillin can produce a significant reduction in infections that follow open fractures and hip fractures (67–69). Ampicillin/sulbactam is an alternate antibiotic for use in injuries that may be contaminated with Enterobacteriaceae (70–72). Success or failure in preventing infection after open fracture depends on the adequacy of débridement, blood supply, and presence of foreign bodies, and whether primary skin closure can be accomplished. One series reviewed antibiotic prophylaxis for open fractures and suggested that when fracture wounds were less than 1 cm long and not associated with extensive soft tissue damage, antibiotics can be administered for only 24 hours. For patients with extensive soft tissue damage and arterial injury that requires repair, a minimal of 48 hours of antibiotic prophylaxis is recommended (73).

NEUROSURGICAL TRAUMA

Sanford reported meningitis following basilar skull fractures (74). Common organisms resulting in meningitis include *Pneumococcus* and *H. influenzae*. Cerebrospinal fluid rhinorrhea is a sequela of only 2% or 3% of acute head injuries (75,76). Experts disagree whether prophylactic antibiotics should be administered to patients with cerebrospinal fluid rhinorrhea. For antibiotics to be effective, they must cross the blood-brain barrier. Those that do so most effectively are the penicillins and chloramphenicol. Klastersky and associates (77) found that penicillin reduced the incidence of bacterial meningitis in patients with rhinorrhea or otorrhea. Brawley and Kelly (75) noted only 1 case of meningitis during a 15 year period among patients treated with prophylactic antibiotics. However, MacGee (78) was unable to demonstrate a statistically significant difference in the incidence of meningitis in patients who received prophylactic antibiotics after cerebrospinal fluid rhinorrhea. Gilbert (79) reported a successful treatment of six patients noting cessation of cerebrospinal fluid leaks and conversion to sterile cerebrospinal fluid within 72 hours. The danger of administering prophylactic antibiotics over a prolonged period of time is the possible development of antibiotic-resistant organisms. Thus, it is difficult to demonstrate the beneficial effects of prophylactic antibiotics following neurosurgical trauma.

Knowledge of the hospital's antibiotic sensitivity pattern is important for appropriate antibiotic selection for an established infection.

REFERENCES

1. Update. Years of potential life lost before age 65: United States 1988 and 1999. *MMWR* 1991;40:60–62.
2. Dellinger EP. Antibiotic prophylaxis in trauma: penetrating abdominal injuries and open fractures. *Rev Infect Dis* 1991;13(suppl 10):847–857.
3. Caplan ES, Hoyt N. Infection surveillance and control in the severely traumatized patient. *Am J Med* 1981;70:638.
4. Jones RC. Management of pancreatic trauma. *Ann Surg* 1978;187:555.
5. Wallace WC. Nosocomial infection in the surgical intensive care unit: a difference between trauma and surgical patients. *Am Surg* 1999;65:990.
6. Bartlett JG. The normal flora. In: Condon RE, Gorbach SL, eds. *Surgical infections, selective antibiotic therapy.* Baltimore: Williams & Wilkins, 1981:4–5.
7. Hunt PK, Jawetz E, Hutchinson JGP, et al. A new model for the study of wound infection. *J Trauma* 1967;7:298.
8. Jones RC, Thal ER, Johnson NA, et al. Evaluation of antibiotic therapy following penetrating abdominal trauma. *Ann Surg* 1985;201:576–585.
9. Claridge JA. Persistent occult hypoperfusion is associated with a significant increase in infection rate and mortality in major trauma patients. *J Trauma* 2000;48:8–15.
10. Bochicchio GV. Impact of nosocomial infections in trauma: does age make a difference? *J Trauma* 2001;50:612–619.
11. Elek FD, Conen PE. The virulence of staphylococcal pryogenes for man. A study of the problems of wound infection. *Br J Exp Pathol* 1957;38:573.
12. Evans BG. The enhancement of bacterial infections by Adrenalin. *Br J Exp Pathol* 1948;19:20.
13. Meakins JL, MacLean APH, Kelly R, et al. Delayed hypersensitivity and neutrophil chemotaxis. Effect of trauma. *J Trauma* 1978;8:240.
14. Schneider RP, Christou NV, Meakins JL, et al. Humoral immunity in surgical patients with and without trauma. *Arch Surg* 1991;126:143.
15. MacLean LD. Host resistance in surgical patients. *J Trauma* 1979;19:297.
16. MacLean LD, Meakins JL, Taguchi K, et al. Host resistance in sepsis and trauma. *Ann Surg* 1975;182:207.
17. Pruett TL, Rothstein OD, et al. Mechanisms of the adjunct effect of hemoglobin in experimental peritonitis. *Surgery* 1984;96:375.
18. Lena M. Napolitano: systemic inflammatory response syndrome score at admission independently predicts mortality and length of stay in trauma patients. *J Trauma* 2000;49:647–653.
19. Bochicchio GV. Systemic inflammatory response syndrome score at admission independently predicts infection in blunt trauma patients: *J Trauma* 2001;50:817–820.
20. Kim PK, Deutschman CS. Inflammatory responses and mediators. *Surg Clin North Am* 2000;80:885–894.
21. Moore EE. Penetrating abdominal trauma index. *J Trauma* 1981;21:439–445.
22. Burke JF. The effective period of preventive antibiotic action in experimental incisions and dermal lesions. *Surgery* 1961;50:161.
23. Jones RC. Antibiotics in trauma. In: Condon RE, Gorbach SL eds. *Surgical infections.* Baltimore: Williams & Wilkins, 1981.
24. Jones RC. Personal communication, 1980.
25. Jones RC, Thal ER, Johnson NA. Evaluation of antibiotic therapy following penetrating abdominal trauma. *Ann Surg* 1985;201:576.
26. Fabian TC, Boldreghini SJ. Antibiotics in penetrating abdominal trauma: comparison of ticarcillin plus clavulanic acid with gentamicin plus clindamycin. *Am J Med* 1985;79(suppl 5B):157.
27. Hooker KD. Aminoglycoside combinations vs. beta lactams alone for penetrating abdominal trauma: a meta-analysis. *J Trauma* 1991;31:1155.
28. Nichols RL, Smith JW, Klein DB, et al. Risk of infection after penetrating abdominal trauma. *N Engl J Med* 1984;311:1065.
29. Gentry LO, Feliciano DV, Scott L, et al. Perioperative antibiotic therapy for penetrating injuries of the abdomen. *Ann Surg* 1984;200:561.
30. Heseltine PNR, Berne RV, Yellin AE, et al. The efficacy of cefoxitin versus clindamycin-gentamicin in surgically treated stab wounds of the bowel. *J Trauma* 1986;26:241.
31. Fabian TC. Duration of antibiotic therapy for penetrating abdominal trauma: a prospective trial surgery. *Surgery* 1992;112:788.
32. Kirton OC. Perioperative antibiotic use in high-risk penetrating hollow viscus injury: a prospective randomized, double-blind, placebo-control trial of 24 hours versus 5 days. *J Trauma* 2000;49:822–832.
33. Bozorgzadeh A. The duration of antibiotic administration in penetrating abdominal trauma. *Am J Surg* 1999;177:125–131.
34. Jones RC. New directions in antimicrobial therapy, infections in trauma. A symposium, St. James, Barbados. Stuart Pharmaceuticals, 1983:17.
35. Gibson DM, Feliciano DV, Mattox KL. Intra-abdominal abscess after penetrating abdominal trauma. *Am J Surg.* 1981;142:699.
36. Nguyen MH. Antimicrobial resistance in clinical outcome of bacteroides bacteremia: findings of a multicenter prospective observational trial. *Clin Infect Dis* 2000;30:870.
37. Cornwell EE 3rd, Velmahos GC, Berne TV, et al. The fate of colonic suture lines in high-risk trauma patients: a prospective analysis. *J Am Coll Surg* 1998;187:58.
38. Stone HH, Fabian TC. Management of perforating colon trauma: randomization between primary closure and exteriorization. *Ann Surg* 1979;190:430–435.
39. Sasaki LS, Allaben RD, Golwala R, et al. Primary repair of colon injuries: a prospective randomized study. *J Trauma* 1995;39:895–901.
40. George SM Jr, Fabian TC, Voeller GR, et al. Primary repair of colon wounds: a prospective trial in nonselected patients. *Ann Surg* 1989;209:728–734.
41. Shannon FL, Moore EE. Primary repair of the colon: when is it a safe alternative? *Surgery* 1985;98:851–859.
42. Thompson JS, Moore EE. Comparison of penetrating injuries of the right and left colon. *Ann Surg* 1981;193:414.
43. Schrock TR, Christiansen N. Management of penetrating injuries of the colon. *Surg Gynecol Obstet* 1972;135:65.
44. Solomkin JS, Wilson SE, Christou NV, et al. Results of a clinical trial of clinafloxacin versus imipenem/cilastatin for intra-abdominal infections. *Ann Surg* 2001;233:79.
45. Solomkin JS, Reinhart HH, Dellinger EP, et al. Results of a randomized trial comparing sequential intravenous/oral treatment with ciprofloxacin plus metronidazole to imipenem/cilastatin for intra-abdominal infections. *Ann Surg* 1996;223:303.
46. Wilson SE. Carbapenems: monotherapy in intra-abdominal sepsis. *Scand J Infect Dis* 1995;96(suppl):28–33.
47. Solomkin JS, Dellinger EP, Christou NV, et al. Results of a multicenter trial comparing imipenem/cilastatin to tobramycin/clindamycin for intra-abdominal infection. *Ann Surg* 1990;212:581.
48. Goins WA, Rodriguez A, Joshi M, et al. Intra-abdominal abscess after blunt abdominal trauma. *Ann Surg* 1990;212:60.
49. Saini S, Kellum JM, O'Leary MP, et al. Improved localization and survival in patients with intra-abdominal abscesses. *Am J Surg* 1983;145:136.

50. Jones RC. Management of pancreatic trauma. *Am J Surg* 1985;160:698.
51. Norwood SH, Civetta JM. Abdominal CT scanning in critically ill surgical patients. *Am Surg* 1985;202:166.
52. Gerzof S, Robbins AH, Johnson WC, et al. Percutaneous catheter drainage of abdominal abscesses: a five year experience. *N Engl J Med* 1981;305:653.
53. Velmahos GC, Kamel E, Berne TV, et al. Abdominal computed tomography for the diagnosis of intra-abdominal sepsis in critically injured patients. *Arch Surg* 1999;134:831.
54. Namias N. Empiric therapy of sepsis in the surgical intensive care unit with broad-spectrum antibiotic for 72 hours does not lead to the emergence of resistant bacteria. *J Trauma* 1998;45:887.
55. Fallon WF Jr. Prophylactic antibiotics for the prevention of infectious complications including empyema following tube thoracostomy for trauma: results of meta-analysis. *J Trauma* 1992;33:110.
56. Hoyt NJ, Kaplan ES. Identification and prevention of infections in the critically ill population. *Crit Care Q* 1983;6:17.
57. Lemmer JH, Botham MJ, Oringer MB. Modern management of adult thoracic empyema. *J Thorac Cardiovasc Surg* 1985;90:849.
58. Francke EL, Neu HC. Postsplenectomy infection. *Surg Clin North Am* 1981;61:135.
59. Eimond LK. Splenectomy in childhood and the hazards of overwhelming infection. *Pediatrics* 1969;43:886–889.
60. Broome CV. Efficacy of pneumococcal polysaccharide vaccines. *Rev Infect Dis* 1981;3(suppl):582–596.
61. Peltola H. Prevention of haemophilus influenza type b bacteraemic infections with a capsular polysaccharide vaccine. *N Engl J Med* 1984;310:1561–1566.
62. Rutherford EJ. Efficacy and safety of pneumococcal revaccination after splenectomy for trauma. *J Trauma* 1995;39:448–452.
63. Styrt B. Infection associated with asplenia: risk mechanisms and prevention. *Am J Med* 1990;85:5–33n.
64. Malangoni MA. Splenic salvage: current expectations and results. In: Maull KI, ed. *Advances in trauma.* Vol. 5. St Louis: Mosby Yearbook, 1990.
65. Fry BE. Multiple system organ failure: the role of uncontrolled infection. *Arch Surg* 1980;115:136.
66. Baue AE. Multiple, progressive or sequential systems failure: a syndrome of the 1970s. *Arch Surg* 1975;110:779.
67. Boyd JJ, Burke JF, Colton T. A double-blind clinical trial of prophylactic antibiotics in hip fractures. *J Bone Joint Surg Am* 1973;55:6.
68. Burnett JW, Gustilo RB, Williams DN, et al. Prophylactic antibiotics in hip fractures, a double-blind prospective study. *J Bone Joint Surg Am* 1980;62:457.
69. Tengve B, Kjellander J. Antibiotic prophylaxis in operations on trochanteric femoral fractures. *J Bone Joint Surg Am* 1978;60:97.
70. Gustilo RV. Prevention of infection in the treatment of 1,025 open fractures of long bones. *J Bone Joint Surg Am* 1976;58:453.
71. Patzakis MJ. The role of antibiotics and the management of open fractures. *J Bone Joint Surg Am* 1974;56:532.
72. Braun R. A double-blind clinical trial of prophylactic cloxacillin in open fractures. *J Orthop Trauma* 1987;1:12.
73. Antrum RM, Solomkin JS. A review of antibiotic prophylaxis for open fractures. *Orthop Rev* 1987;16:246.
74. Hand WL, Sanford JP. Post-traumatic bacterial meningitis. *Ann Intern Med* 1970;72:869.
75. Brawley BW, Kelly WA. Treatment of basal skull fractures with and without cerebrospinal fluid fistulae. *J Neurosurg* 1967;26:57.
76. Raaf J. Post-traumatic cerebrospinal fluid leaks. *Arch Surg* 1967;95:648.
77. Klastersky J, Sadeghi M, Brihaye J. Antimicrobial prophylaxis in patients with rhinorrhea or otorrhea: a double-blind study. *Surg Neurol* 1976;6:111.
78. MacGee EE, et al. Meningitis following an acute traumatic cerebrospinal fluid fistula. *J Neurosurg* 1970;33:312.
79. Gilbert VE, Beals JD Jr, Natelson SE, et al. Treatment of cerebrospinal fluid leaks and gram-negative bacillary meningitis with large doses of intrathecal amikacin and systemic antibiotics. *Neurosurgery* 1986;18:402.

CHAPTER 98
Burns

Basil A. Pruitt, Jr., Albert T. McManus, and Seung H. Kim

Burn injury results in damage or loss of the cutaneous microbiologic barrier. Such damage and associated microvascular injury limit the host's ability to establish and deliver both specific and non-specific immunological defenses. In addition, the residual nonviable tissue and denatured proteinaceous material in the wound adds the potential that this undefended, rich growth medium will be overgrown with residual or contaminating organisms. In the past, local wound infections frequently developed that often expanded, invaded underlying unburned tissue, and spread to remote organs and tissues by hematogenous and/or lymphatic routes in patients with extensive burn wounds. That process, termed invasive burn wound sepsis, was associated with a virtually universal mortality. With the introduction of effective topical antimicrobial chemotherapy in 1964 and the subsequent widespread use of preemptive surgical excision of colonized burn wounds, the incidence of burn wound sepsis has dramatically decreased and the survival of even massively burned patients has increased.

BURN WOUND CARE

Topical antimicrobial chemotherapy is initiated as soon as the patient is hemodynamically stable and the burn wounds have been cleansed and débrided. Such therapy limits proliferation and invasion by the bacteria that initially colonize the surface of the burn wound. There are four antimicrobial agents of documented effectiveness in controlling the microbial density in the burn wound: mafenide acetate burn cream, 0.5% silver nitrate soaks, silver sulfadiazine burn cream, and Acticoat silver-coated dressing (Table 98.1) (2,3). The physical characteristics of the latter three agents are such that they act principally on the surface of the wound and are most effective when application is begun within the first 24 to 48 hours following injury, before microbial penetration of the eschar has occurred. Mafenide acetate burn cream has similar antimicrobial activity on the wound surface, but the solubility of mafenide acetate permits it to penetrate into the burned tissue where it exerts its antimicrobial action and controls proliferation of microorganisms both within the eschar and at the viable-nonviable tissue interface.

Excision of the burn wound is commonly begun as soon as possible after resuscitation is complete (usually the third to fifth postburn day). Early excision with immediate grafting in patients with available donor sites effects wound closure and reduces the length of time that the wound is at risk for infection. There are other patients with associated injuries or other complicating conditions, who are not able to undergo excision, usually because of respiratory failure, cardiac failure, or sepsis related coagulopathy (4). In those patients and patients in whom the extent of burn prevents excision of all burn wounds at a single sitting, topical chemotherapy must be continued until resolution of organ failure occurs or excision of the burn wound can be completed. Since the protection provided by topical antimicrobial agents is imperfect, some burn patients, most commonly

TABLE 98.1.   Effective Topical Burn Wound Antimicrobial Agents

Characteristic	Mafenide acetate burn cream	0.5% Silver nitrate soaks	Silver sulfadiazine burn cream	Acticoat silver-coated dressing
Spectrum of antimicrobial activity	Gram-negative bacteria—Selectively good activity Gram-positive bacteria—Good activity Yeasts—minimal activity	Gram-negative bacteria—Good activity Gram-positive bacteria—Good activity Yeasts—good activity	Gram-negative bacteria—Selectively good activity Gram-positive bacteria—Good activity Yeasts—good activity	Gram-negative bacteria—Good activity Gram-positive bacteria—Good activity Yeasts—good activity
Method of wound care	Exposure: Applied following Daily cleansing and renewed 12 hours later	Occlusive dressings changed 2 or 3 times per day	Exposure or light dressing Impregnated with agent: Applied following daily cleansing and renewed 12 hours later if exposure method used	Applied in dressing sheets
Advantages	Easily applied Penetrates eschar Wound appearance readily monitored No resistance of Pseudomonas Joint motion unrestricted	Painless No hypersensitivity reactions Dressings reduce evaporative heat loss No gram-negative resistance Effective against yeasts	Easily applied Painless Wound appearance readily monitored when exposure method used Effective against yeasts	Painless and easily applied
Disadvantages	Painful on partial-thickness burns Inhibition of carbonic anhydrase results in self-limited acidosis Cutaneous hypersensitivity reactions in 7% of patients	Deficits of sodium, potassium, calcium, and chloride No eschar penetration Limitation of joint motion by Dressings Methemoglobinemia—rare Argyria—rare Staining of environment and equipment	Limited eschar penetration Neutropenia—usually transient Hypersensitivity—infrequent Resistance of clostridia and certain gram-negative bacteria Rapid appearance of plasmid mediated resistance to sulfonamides and multiple other antibiotics	Limited wound penetration

those with burns of more than 30% of the total body surface, may develop invasive burn wound infection (5).

BURN WOUND INFECTION

The diagnosis of infection in burn patients is confounded by the fact that most of the systemic and many of the laboratory signs of infection are mimicked by the physiologic response to severe injury (6). Because clinical and laboratory signs are not reliable in making the diagnosis of infection in severely burned patients, reliance must be placed upon daily examination of the entire burn wound to identify changes indicative of infection before systemic spread has occurred. The examination of the wound is best carried out at the time of daily cleansing when all dressings and topical applications have been removed. Focal dark red, brown, or black discoloration of the burn wound is the most common tinctorial change associated with burn wound infection, but the reliability of this sign may be compromised by hemorrhage into the burn wound due to local trauma which can produce similar changes (7). Conversion of an area of partial-thickness injury to full-thickness necrosis is the most reliable sign of burn wound infection (8). As noted in Table 98.2, there are other clinical signs typically associated with infections caused by specific organisms, for example, ecthyma gangrenosa and green discoloration of the subcutaneous fat are characteristic of *Pseudomonas* infections, while saponification of the subcutaneous fat, unexpectedly rapid spontaneous separation of the eschar, and rapidly expanding ischemic necrosis are typical of fungal infection. The appearance of vesicular lesions in the nasolabial area of healing burn wounds is typical of herpes simplex virus

TABLE 98.2.   Clinical Signs of Burn Wound Infection

I. Systemic:
  a. Temperature change[a]
     Hyperthermia: early sign
     Hypothermia: late sign of severe infection
  b. Tachycardia[a]
  c. Hyperventilation[a]
  d. Pain: may be obscured by burn wound sensitivity
  e. Ileus[a]
  f. Disorientation and obtundation[a]
  g. Glucose intolerance[a]
II. Local
  a. Conversion of partial-thickness injury to full-thickness necrosis
  b. Color change of wound: focal dark red, brown or black eschar discoloration
  c. Hemorrhagic discoloration of subeschar tissues
  d. Degeneration of granulation tissue and formation of neoeschar
  e. Edema of unburned skin at margins of wound
  f. Erythematous or violaceous discoloration of unburned skin at margins of wound
  g. Green pigment visible in subcutaneous fat[b]
     (1) Pale gray or yellow cheesy–appearing fat necrosis (soap formation)[c]
  h. Nodular necrotic lesions (ecthyma gangrenosum) in unburned skin[b]
  i. Unexpectedly rapid separation of eschar[c]
  j. Rapid centrifugal expansion of ischemic necrotic lesion with surrounding edema[c]
  k. Vesicular lesions in healed or healing partial-thickness burns[d]
  l. Crusted serrated margins of partial-thickness facial burn[d]

[a]Produced by extensive burn injury per se.
[b]Characteristic of *Pseudomonas* infections.
[c]Characteristic of fungal infections.
[d]Characteristic of herpes simplex virus I infections.

infections. The identification of any of these local signs necessitates more precise assessment of the microbial status of the burn wound.

Cultures of the burn wound surface are useful in only an epidemiologic sense and even quantitative cultures merely identify the density of colonizing organisms on or in nonviable tissue. Quantitative cultures are only helpful in a negative sense, for example, low counts in tissue obtained from a burn wound biopsy sample correlate well with the absence of invasive infection but high counts are unreliable as an indication of the presence of infection (9). The histologic examination of a burn wound biopsy is the most reliable and rapid way of making the critical differentiation between the colonization of nonviable tissue and the invasion of viable tissue.

Whenever any of the clinical signs of burn wound infection are identified, a burn wound biopsy should be obtained from that area of the wound showing the most pronounced changes. A 500 mg lenticular tissue sample (the specimen must include viable subcutaneous tissue underlying the burn eschar) is obtained using a scalpel (Fig. 98.1). Punch biopsy is usually unsatisfactory. One half of the bisected specimen is cultured to identify the organisms present and their antibiotic sensitivities. The other half of the specimen is processed for histologic examination by the pathologist using either a rapid-section technique requiring 4 hours for section preparation or a frozen-section technique requiring approximately 30 minutes for section preparation (10,11). Because the frozen-section technique is associated with a 4% false-negative diagnosis rate, a specimen initially processed by that technique should be subsequently processed by regular-section technique. The histologic identification of microorganisms in unburned viable tissue confirms the diagnosis of invasive burn wound infection. The other histologic findings listed in Table 98.3 are not diagnostic of invasive burn wound infection but should heighten the pathologist's index of suspicion and prompt a meticulous search for microorganisms in the unburned tissue included in the specimen.

The microbial status of a biopsy sample can be staged according to the scheme detailed in Table 98.4. If the histologic examination reveals only colonization, no change in wound care is required. If serial biopsy examinations reveal progression from

TABLE 98.3. Histologic Signs of Burn Wound Infection
1. Microorganisms present in unburned tissue
2. Exaggerated inflammatory reaction in unburned tissue
3. Hemorrhage into viable subeschar tissue
4. Small vessel thrombosis and ischemic necrosis of unburned tissue

5. Intracellular viral inclusions
  a. Type A Cowdry bodies—light microscopy
  b. Virions: electron microscopy

6. Dense microbial growth[a]
  a. Surrounding hair follicles and sweat glands
  b. Marked proliferation in subeschar space

7. Dense mononuclear cell infiltration with multinucleated giant cells containing fungal spores.
8. Epithelioid granuloma formation with fungal hyphae in viable soft tissue

[a]Typical of deep colonization.

stage IA to IC, such evidence of microbial proliferation and eschar penetration justifies alteration of wound care. A histologic diagnosis of stage II necessitates alteration of wound care including urgent burn wound excision as well as systemic antimicrobial therapy. A biopsy diagnosis of stage IIC, indicating involvement of the microvasculature and lymphatics portends hematogenous spread to remote tissues and organs and mandates close monitoring of the lungs and heart-common sites of metastatic spread (Fig. 98.2).

The burn wound biopsy histologic findings must always be evaluated with respect to the patient's clinical condition. A stage I histologic diagnosis, or negative biopsy report in a septic burn patient in whom no other source of infection exists, necessitates immediate biopsy of another area of the burn wound that shows changes typical of infection. If histologic examination of that biopsy specimen also fails to confirm invasive infection, wound monitoring is continued and biopsy specimens of new or expanding areas of wound changes are obtained as they appear.

A diagnosis of invasive burn wound infection should prompt immediate therapeutic intervention. If a nonabsorbable topical agent is being used, it should be discontinued and twice-daily application of mafenide acetate burn cream instituted. Supportive measures should be employed to correct and maintain organ function and to prevent initiation of the cascade of multiple

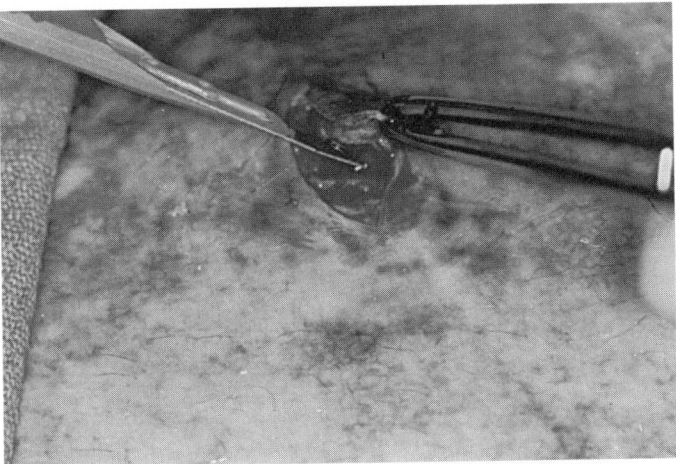

Figure 98.1. A scalpel is used to obtain a burn wound biopsy specimen from an area of the burn wound showing focal dark red and black discoloration typical of invasive infection. Elevation of the biopsy specimen demonstrates that unburned subcutaneous tissue is included in the sample. Note that bleeding into the biopsy wound also confirms viability of the tissue at the line of excision.

TABLE 98.4. Classification of Microbial Status of Burn Wounds

Stage I. Colonization of non-viable tissue
  A. Superficial colonization: microorganisms present on burn wound surface
  B. Microbial penetration: microorganisms present in variable thickness of eschar
  C. Subeschar proliferation: multiplication of microorganisms in the subeschar space or neo-colonization in which microorganisms are present on desiccated tissue exposed by prior escharectomy

Stage II. Invasion of viable tissue
  A. Microinvasion: microscopic foci of microorganisms in unburned viable tissue immediately beneath eschar
  B. Generalized invasion: Multifocal or diffuse penetration of microorganisms into viable subcutaneous tissue
  C. Microvascular invasion: microorganisms present in unburned small blood vessels and lymphatics

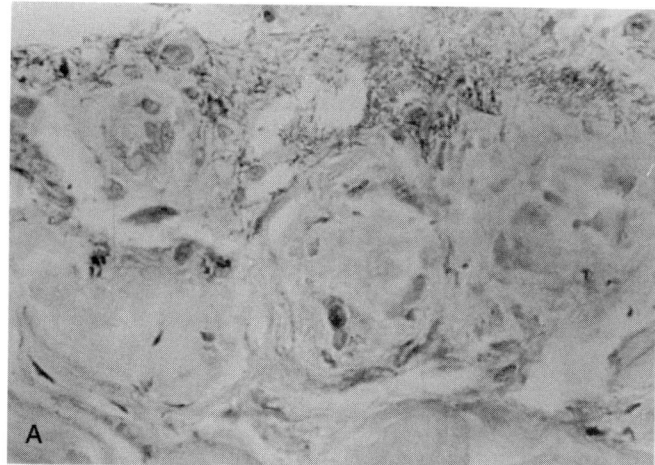

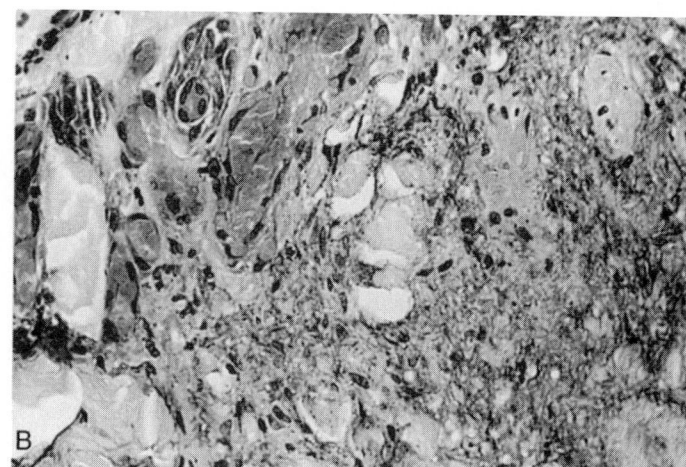

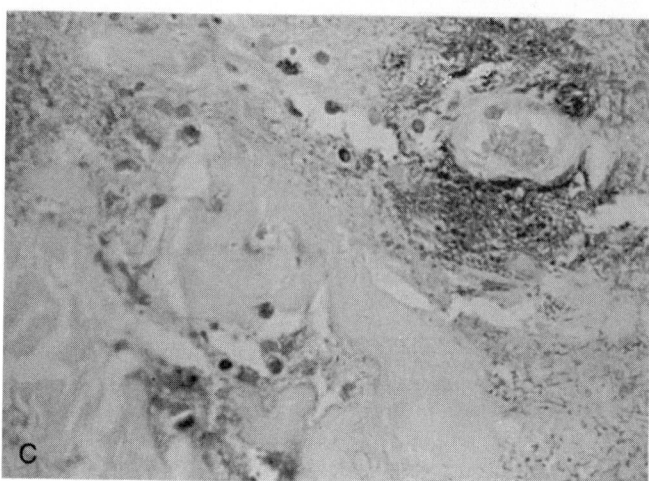

Figure 98.2. Photomicrographs of three burn wound biopsies illustrating the stages of invasive burn wound infection. **(A)** Stage IIA: Microinvasion. Note the dark staining bacilli invading the viable tissue immediately beneath the coagulated eschar visible at the upper right margin of the field. **(B)** Stage IIB: Generalized invasion. Dark staining bacilli are present throughout this section of viable subcutaneous tissue. The presence of inflammatory cells confirms that the infected tissue has an intact blood supply and is unburned. **(C)** Stage IIC: Microvascular invasion. Extensive invasion of viable tissue with palisading of dark-staining bacilli around the small blood vessel at 2 o'clock is characteristic of *Pseudomonas* vasculitis.

sequential organ failure. Systemic administration of an antibiotic active against the infecting organism should be started. If no cultures have been taken from the burn wound, the selection of antibacterial agents should be based upon the gram stain characteristics of the organisms identified in the biopsy sections. Ideally, previous microbial surveillance data from the patient's wounds or from a prior biopsy can be used to guide antibiotic selection. If such information is not available, the results of the unit's microbial surveillance program should be used to determine the antibiotics most likely to be effective (12).

The hypermetabolism and hyperdynamic circulation of the burn patient alter both the metabolism and excretion rate of antibiotic agents necessitating careful monitoring of peak and trough levels to ensure adequacy of therapy. The increased effective renal blood flow characteristic of burn patients can markedly decrease the effective half-life of antibiotics that are excreted primarily by the renal route (13,14).

Even though the overall incidence of invasive burn wound infection has decreased markedly, *Pseudomonas aeruginosa* remains the most common causative bacterium, and it is typically sensitive to high concentrations of broad-spectrum penicillins. Accordingly, one half of the daily dose of a broad-spectrum penicillin, such as piperacillin, suspended in 1,000 mL of normal saline should be immediately infused into the subeschar tissues beneath all infected areas of the wound using a no. 20 spinal needle to minimize the number of injection sites. The patient should then be scheduled for excision of the infected tissue within the next 12 hours and a second subeschar antibiotic

infusion performed immediately prior to that procedure to minimize hematogenous dissemination of viable bacteria during the excision.

The development of generalized invasive burn wound infection can be forestalled and the high mortality associated with it reduced by scheduled wound surveillance and the use of wound biopsies to identify infection at an early stage. In one study of histologically documented invasive Pseudomonas burn wound infection, subeschar antibiotic infusion and, when the patient's condition permitted, surgical excision of the infected tissue controlled the infection in ten of 19 patients (15). The importance of early diagnosis and control of the infection prior to bacterial spread through the microvasculature to the general circulation is emphasized by the finding that the five patients who survived both the episode of invasive infection and their burn injury had no positive blood culture results before excision.

Burn wound infections caused by gram-positive cocci, chief among which are the staphylococci, tend to be localized, although the initially present micro abscesses may slowly expand with time. Removal of the burned tissue overlying a solitary staphylococcal abscess may be sufficient treatment but the presence of multiple micro-abscesses may necessitate excision of extensive areas of the eschar utilizing a variant of tangential excision. A disproportionate systemic response in a patient with a staphylococcal infection should alert one to the possibility that the infecting strain is causing systemic toxicity by production of exotoxins such as TSST-l. Such patients should be treated by systemic administration of vancomycin.

The rarity of beta hemolytic streptococcal cellulitis has led most surgeons to abandon the use of prophylactic penicillin in the immediate postburn period (16). However, if cellulitic changes characterized by bright red, rapidly spreading erythema with or without lymphangiitis develop, a presumptive diagnosis of beta hemolytic streptococcal cellulitis should be made, culture specimens are obtained and penicillin therapy initiated.

Staphylococcal pustular eruptions with patchy epidermal sloughing in areas of healed partial-thickness wounds (Fig. 98.3) or healed grafts (burn wound impetigo) may be treated with topical application of mupirocin. This agent, which is derived from *Pseudomonas fluorescens*, has rapid action against most strains of staphylococci and clinical use of this agent at the authors' burn center has not been associated with the development of resistance or opportunistic overgrowth (17).

Candidal Infections

The overall incidence of bacterial burn wound infection has significantly decreased and that due to *Pseudomonas aeruginosa* has precipitously receded over the past 25 years during which time the incidence of non-bacterial burn wound infections has increased (12). *Candida* species are the most common non-bacterial colonizers of burn wounds. An example of such colonization by *Candida albicans* of nonviable eschar (biopsy stage 1A) is presented in Fig. 98.4A. This situation typically remains confined to burned tissue without invasion and thus requires no specific treatment (18). Candidal colonization of a previously excised burn wound exposed in the interstices of a mesh graft or an excised burn wound exposed by loss of skin grafts (Fig. 98.4B) requires treatment by twice-daily application of a topical antifungal agent such as clotrimazole cream or ciclopiroxolamine cream. Excision of the infected tissue may be necessary if such treatment is ineffective in preventing extension of the disease process. In patients requiring excision of foci of candidal infection, systemic administration of amphotericin B should be instituted.

During the period 1985 to 2000, 219 candidal infections were documented in 3,898 burn patients treated at the US Army Institute of Surgical Research's Burn Center (Table 98.5).

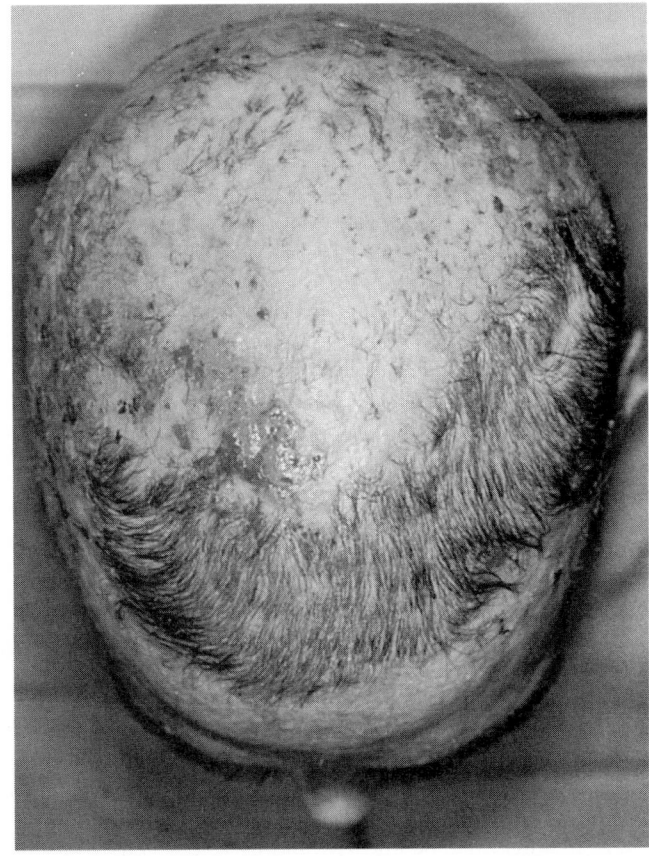

Figure 98.3. Superficial staphylococcal infection with patchy epidermal loss surrounding hair follicles in a previously healed partial-thickness scalp burn (45th postburn day).

Those infections included 141 of the urinary tract, 50 of the blood, and only eight of the burn wound. Infection with this non-bacterial opportunist commonly occurred in patients with extensive burns, many of whom had received broad-spectrum antibiotics perioperatively at the time of burn wound excisions and for the treatment of other infections. The average time of

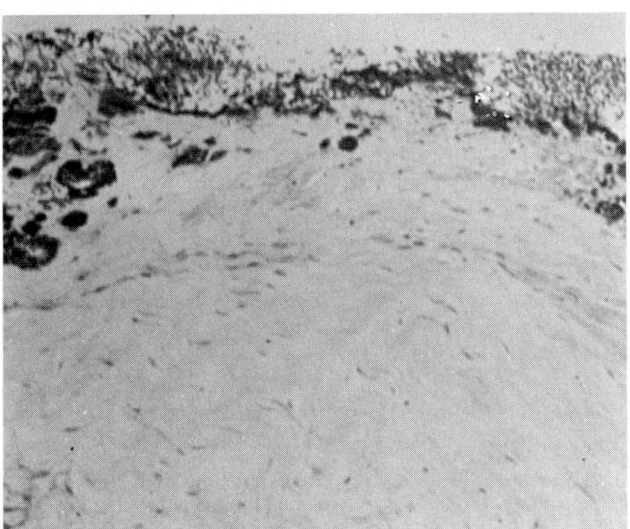

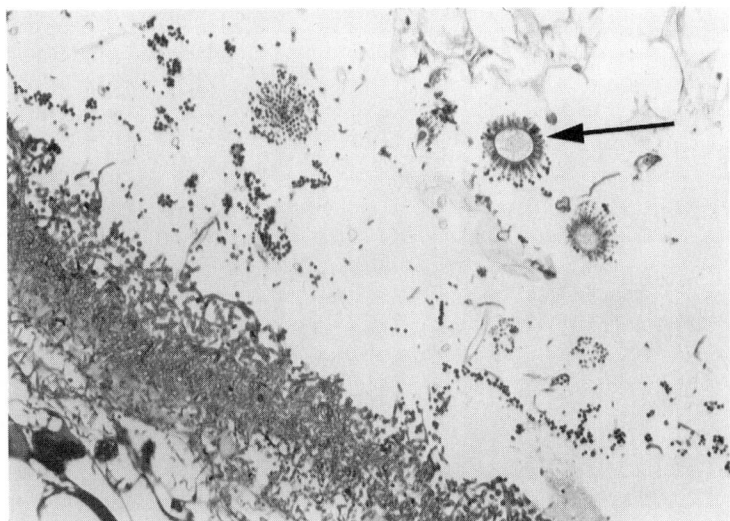

A   B

Figure 98.4. **(A)** Colonization of non-viable eschar with *Candida albicans* (stage IA). **(B)** Neocolonization of previously excised burn wound by *Aspergillus* sp. with several sunflower-head shaped conidiospores (fruiting bodies) *(arrow)*, which show numerous branchings of fungal hyphae.

TABLE 98.5. *Candida* Infection in Burn Patients, 1985–2000

Site of infection	Number of infections
Urinary tract	141
Blood	50
Burn wound	8
Respiratory tract	9
Pneumonia	8
Tracheitis	1
Eye	4
Vagina	3
Vein	2

candidal colonization of the burn wound (27th PBD), of candidal urinary tract infection (44th PBD), and of other candidal infections (37th PBD) are all consistent with that possibility. Irrigation of the bladder with amphotericin B solution (50 mg/L sterile water per day for 5 days) is recommended for the treatment of *Candida* cystitis, but the urine may not clear until the urethral catheter is removed. Candidemia requires a full course of systemic amphotericin B therapy (0.5 to 0.7 mg/kg per day for 7 to 10 days).

Fungal Infections

Filamentous fungi are much more apt to cause invasive burn wound infection than are candidal organisms. Between 1985 and 2000 at this institute, 80 burn wound invasions caused by filamentous (true) fungi were observed. These infections occurred at an average of 22 days after burn in a group of severely burned patients who had burns involving an average of 61% of the total body surface. The infections occurred earlier than the candidal wound infections noted above. *Aspergillus* species, the most common filamentous fungi that caused burn wound infections, typically remained confined to the subcutaneous tissue and rarely traversed tissue planes (19). As with invasive bacterial burn wound infection, the diagnosis of invasive fungal infection is best made by the histologic examination of a burn wound biopsy specimen (Fig. 98.5). Treatment of such infections consists of twice-daily topical application of an antifungal

agent such as clotrimazole cream or ciclopiroxolamine cream, institution of systemic amphotericin B therapy, and prompt excision of the infected tissue.

Members of the genera *Phycomycetes*, particularly *mucor* species, are the most aggressive of the filamentous fungi (20). Infections caused by these organisms spread rapidly along tissue planes and readily cross fascial barriers. The predilection of phycomycotic hyphae to invade vessels accounts for the rapidly expanding ischemic necrosis and the frequency of distant metastases characteristic of infections caused by these organisms (Fig. 98.6). The diagnosis is best made by the identification of broad non-septate hyphae in unburned tissue. All forms of topical therapy appear to be ineffective in controlling phycomycotic infections and immediate surgical intervention is required. The extent of surgical excision required is often defined by a rim of edema at the outermost limit of the disease process. What has been termed radical debridement is carried out to ensure removal of all infected tissue and reduce the risk of further local extension and hematogenous dissemination to remote tissues. If a phycomycotic infection in a limb has traversed the investing fascia and involves significant amounts of underlying muscle, amputation may be necessary to control the infectious process as was the case in 26 (35%) of 75 patients with phycomycotic burn wound infections treated between 1954 and 1983 (21). A full course of parenteral amphotericin B should be administered to all patients with invasive phycomycotic wound infections.

Viral Infections

Viral infections in burn patients are relatively uncommon as indicated by the occurrence of only 13 herpes simplex virus I infections in the 3,898 patients treated at this institution from 1985 to 2000. Herpetic infections occur most commonly in healing or recently healed partial-thickness burns, particularly those in the nasolabial area (Fig. 98.7A). The diagnosis of herpetic burn wound infection is most reliably made by the histologic examination of a biopsy or scrapings from the cutaneous lesions. Because the vesicles are easily ruptured and readily colonized by bacteria from the surrounding skin, the light microscopic characteristics

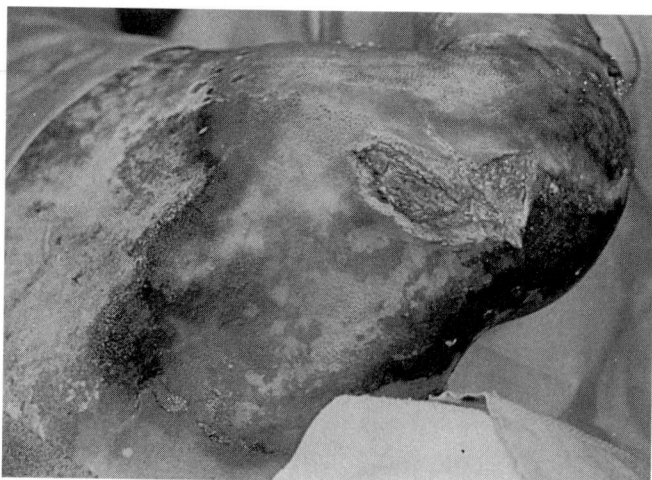

Figure 98.6. Invasive mucormycosis of the burn wound of the left shoulder of this patient necessitated a forequarter amputation. Note the black ischemic discoloration over the top of the shoulder and at the margin of the expanding infection near the midline of the upper back and at the lower margin of the scapula inferiorly. Involvement of the unburned underlying muscles was confirmed by biopsy of the ischemic muscle exposed at the upper margin of the scapula.

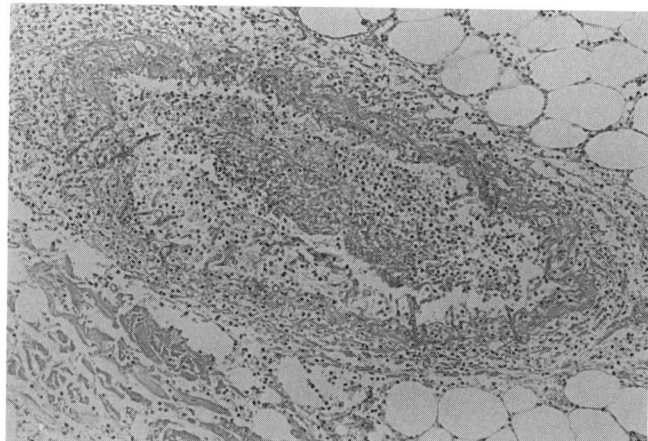

Figure 98.5. Invasive fungal (*Aspergillus* sp.) burn wound infection. Stage IIC. Note hyphal penetration into the lumen of the small vessel in the center of the field. Such microvascular involvement increases the likelihood of hematogenous spread of the infection to remote tissues and organs.

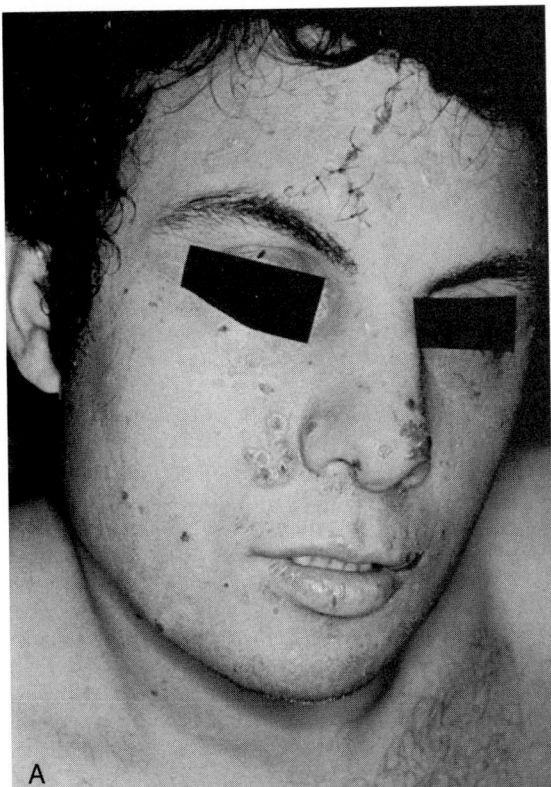

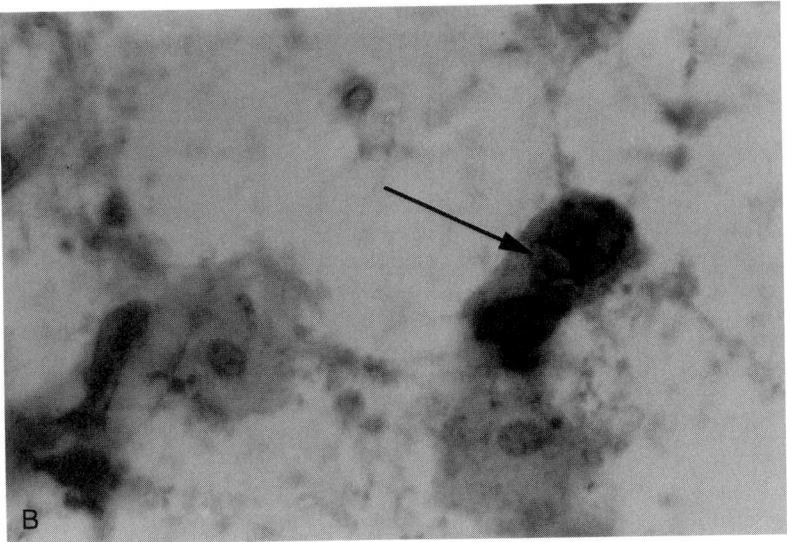

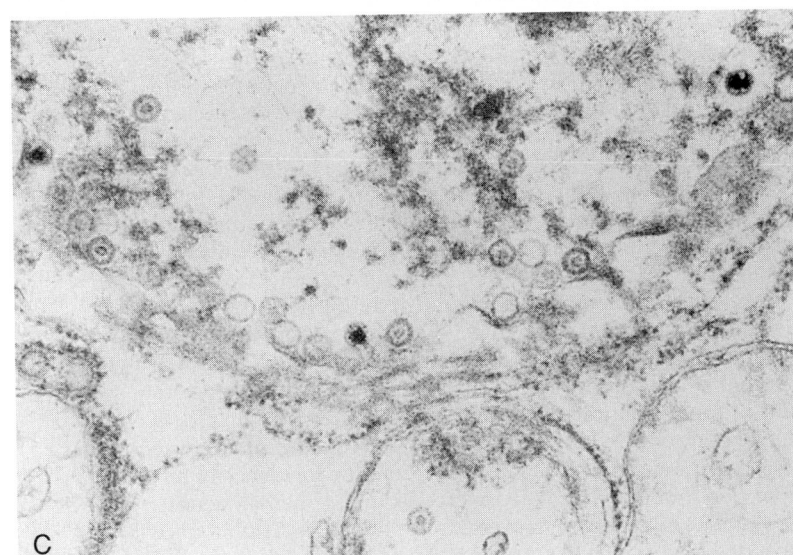

Figure 98.7. (A) The circular lesions with a narrow rim of thickened epithelium are characteristic of herpes simplex virus infection. Crusts have formed on the base of the lesions following rupture of the vesicles that developed in the healing partial-thickness facial burns of this patient. **(B)** Demonstration of Herpes simplex virus intranuclear inclusion body (Cowdry type A) *(arrow)* in multinucleated giant cell in skin scraping. **(C)** Mature Herpes simplex virus demonstrated by electron microscopic examination of skin scraping.

of herpes simplex virus I infections, that is, type A Cowdry bodies (Fig. 98.7B; *arrow*), may be obscured. In this case, electron microscopy can be used to identify intracellular virions (Fig. 98.7C) (22). Topical application of acyclovir (Zovirax®) which may inactivate the virus and prevent further development of cutaneous lesions is most effective when done early in the course of lesion development.

Although herpetic infections occur most commonly in healing partial-thickness burns and remain localized, such infections may occur in other tissues as documented by autopsy evidence of herpetic involvement of the airway in three patients from 1985 and 1994. No cases have been recognized since then. Occasionally, systemic herpes virus infections involving multiple organs such as the liver, lung, spleen, adrenal, and bone marrow occur (22). Unexplained hypotension or other signs of systemic sepsis in a burn patient with no other source of infection and rapidly spreading cutaneous herpetic lesions, should alert one to the possibility of a systemic herpes simplex virus infection. If the patient has an intact coagulation system, a percutaneous hepatic biopsy may confirm hepatic involvement and justify the institution of systemic anti-viral therapy using either acyclovir (10 mg/kg three times a day for 10 days) or adenine arabinoside, Vidarabine®, (15 mg/kg per day for 10 days) (23).

Cytomegalovirus (CMV) is the other virus most commonly recovered from burn patients (24,25). The majority of CMV infections have involved the aerodigestive tract as documented by autopsy findings in four patients with airway involvement from 1985 to 1994. Systemic CMV infection may produce varying degrees of jaundice associated with the clinical signs of low-grade infection. In such patients, documentation of rising CMV titers in successive serum samples will enable one to avoid the potentially deleterious effects of inappropriate broad-spectrum antibiotic administration. Ganciclovir is the antiviral agent of choice for the treatment of CMV infection (7.5 to 10 mg/kg per day for up to 20 days).

Other Infections

That infection remains the most frequent cause of morbidity and mortality in burn patients indicates the pervasive effect of the global immunosuppression, which is induced in direct proportion to the extent of burn injury. From 1985 to 1999, infection was considered the primary cause of death in 117 (36%) of 323 fatal burns (Table 98.6). The effectiveness of topical chemotherapy and current wound care techniques is attested to by the fact that invasive burn wound infection was considered to be the primary

TABLE 98.6.   Infections as Cause of Death in Fatal Burns: 1985–1999

Number of fatal burns	323
Pneumonia	85
Invasive burn wound infection	14
Sepsis	6
Abscess	3
Bacterial endocarditis	2
Enterocolitis	2
Staphylococcal scalded skin syndrome	1
Viral infection	2
Herpes simplex virus	1
Cytomegalovirus infection	1
Peritonitis	1
Gastrointestinal infection	1
Total	117 (36.2%)

cause of death in 13 patients whereas pneumonia was present in 85 (26%) of the 323 fatal burns. Over the past two decades, the predominant organisms causing infections in burn patients have also changed dramatically (7,26,27). Gram-negative opportunistic organisms, initially predominant, receded in importance and *Staphylococcus aureus* became the most frequent infecting organism, recovered from 27% of all infections in patients treated at the US Army Institute of Surgical Research Burn Center (Fig. 98.8). In the past 6 years, there has been a resurgence of gram-negative bacteria, which now represent a slight majority of causative organisms.

Control of the microbial population of the burn wound has altered the predominant site of infection in burn patients, the types of organisms causing pneumonia, and the predominant form of pneumonia that occurs in those patients. Before the development of topical antimicrobial burn wound therapy, hematogenous pneumonia occurred with twice the frequency of airborne or bronchopneumonia, but since that time the incidence of airborne pneumonia has greatly exceeded that of hematogenous pneumonia and at present represents less than 10% of pulmonary infections. The frequency of pneumonia necessitates close clinical and radiologic monitoring to make a timely diagnosis of pneumonia and differentiate between the two forms of pulmonary infection.

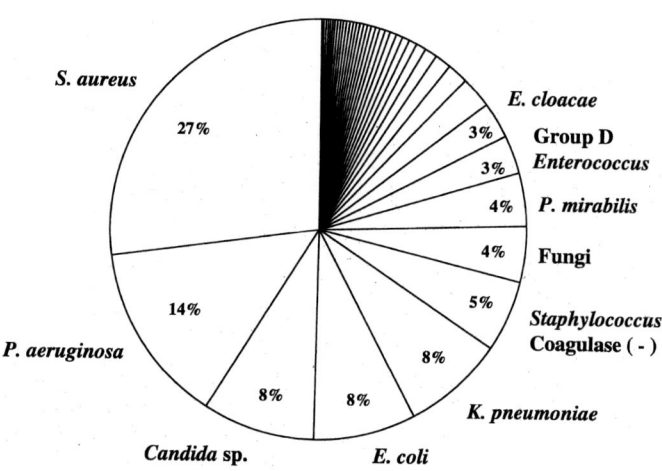

Figure 98.8. Frequency of recovery of microorganisms from infections in burn patients treated at the US Army Burn Center from 1985 to 2000. Unlabeled segments represent organisms causing less than 3% of infections.

BRONCHOPNEUMONIA

Airborne, or bronchopneumonia, usually begins as a tracheobronchitis that causes necrosis of the airway mucosa, and subsequently extends distally to involve the alveoli (28). The infectious process then spreads to involve a variable volume of pulmonary parenchyma. This disease process is nonrandom in distribution, involves mainly dependent areas of the lung, and is a frequent complication in patients with inhalation injury (29). The incidence of bronchopneumonia in burn patients with moderate or severe inhalation injury is 38.4% as compared to 9.1% for patients without inhalation injury (30). This form of pneumonia is fatal in only approximately one third of patients, but is the primary cause of death in 80% of burn patients who die of the disease (28).

The pathogenesis, clinical presentation, diagnosis, and treatment of bronchopneumonia in burn patients are the same as in other critically ill patients. With improvements in burn wound management and in patient isolation, *S. aureus* has replaced *P. aeruginosa* and other gram-negative opportunists as the most common causative organism of bronchopneumonia in burn patients (12,31,32). Consequently, the initial selection of antibiotics should be based on the results of the microscopic examination of bronchial secretions and the current results of the patient's surveillance cultures. The presence of resistance to the penicillinase resistant penicillins such as methicillin proscribes the use of all beta lactam antibiotics. To avoid the selection of cross-resistant strains by such agents and insure effectiveness of treatment, vancomycin is always used for the treatment of staphylococcal infections at the US Army Burn Center. Even with such common use of vancomycin, we have recovered only three resistant enterococcal isolates, two resistant *Corynebacterium* species, one resistant *Lactobacillus* species, and no resistant staphylococci since 1986 (33). The initial antibiotic therapy may subsequently be altered, if necessary, on the basis of the patient's endobronchial culture and sensitivity results.

In a patient with clinical signs of infection but no roentgenographically evident infiltrates or other source of infection, an endobronchial aspirate indicative of respiratory tract infection is consistent with the diagnosis of tracheobronchitis. That process should be treated with antibiotics selected on the basis of the microscopic examination of the aspirate and the predominant nosocomial flora.

HEMATOGENOUS PNEUMONIA

Hematogenous pneumonia begins as a necrotizing capillaritis caused by blood-borne bacteria. The infection then spreads to adjacent alveoli forming a nodular lesion that may ultimately erode into bronchi. This form of pneumonia, which occurs in a random distribution depending upon the location of the vessels in which bacteria lodge, presents relatively late in the postburn course with the average time of diagnosis being the 17th postburn day (28). The sudden appearance of a dense rounded infiltrate on the chest roentgenogram is consistent with a diagnosis of hematogenous pneumonia and should prompt a search for the primary site of infection and the initiation of systemic antibiotic therapy based on surveillance cultures from the patient (Fig. 98.9). If patient culture data are not available, the institution's current surveillance information should be used. Endobronchial cultures should be obtained but may be of little assistance in identifying the causative organisms since these organisms erode into the bronchi only late in the disease process.

Although occult visceral perforation and inapparent soft tissue infections may serve as primary sources of hematogenous pneumonia, an invasive burn wound infection or a focus of suppurative thrombophlebitis is the primary source in 98% of cases. The primary infection must be controlled either by excision of

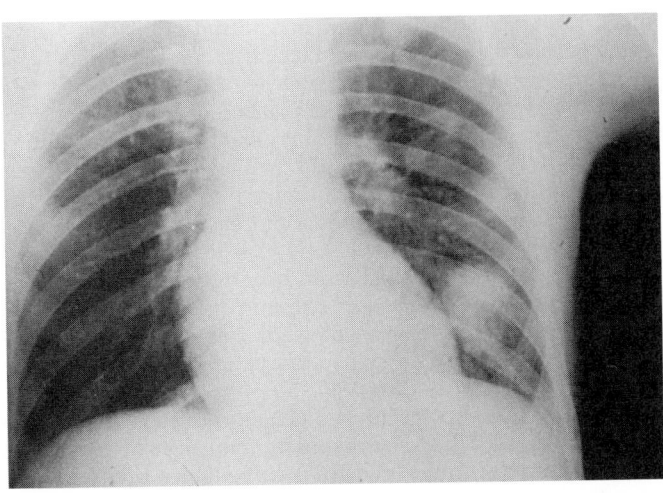

Figure 98.9. The dense, solitary, rounded infiltrate that appeared in the left lower lung field of this burn patient with open infected wounds on the 60th postburn day is characteristic of hematogenous pneumonia.

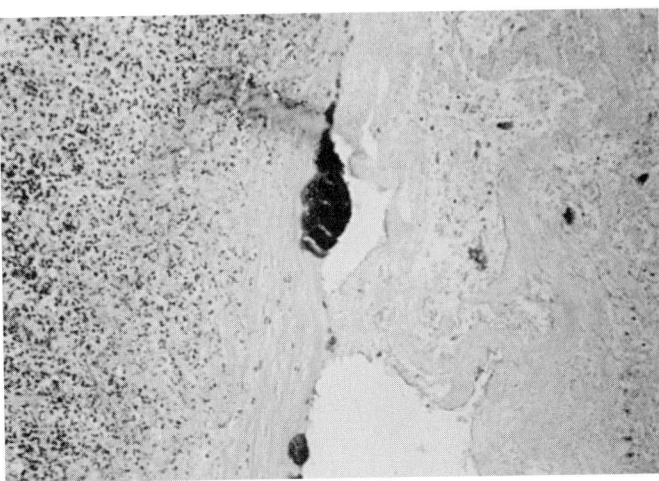

Figure 98.10. Histologic section of vein wall and infected thrombus in specimen obtained from a site of suppurative thrombophlebitis. Note focal collections of dark staining bacteria on endothelial surface of inflamed vein and foci of dark staining bacteria within organizing intraluminal thrombus.

an infected burn wound (as described previously) or excision of an infected vein (as described below) to prevent continued pulmonary and systemic seeding. The mortality associated with hematogenous pneumonia exceeds 90%, but as a reflection of its being secondary to a remote infection, it is infrequently the primary cause of death (28).

SUPPURATIVE THROMBOPHLEBITIS

Intraluminal suppuration can occur in any previously cannulated vein. Cannula composition, the characteristics of the infused fluids, the duration of cannulation, microbial seeding of the infusion system, and lodgment of blood-borne bacteria on the fibrin sleeve that forms around the cannula can all serve as contributory factors in the development of suppurative thrombophlebitis (34). The risk of microbial seeding of the fibrin sleeve on the intravascular cannula is particularly high in burn patients, in whom bacteremia may occur in association with wound debridement procedures, with the incidence of positive blood culture results related directly to the extent of the burn, and the magnitude of wound manipulation (35). Since 1979, strict limitation of venous cannulation duration to no more than 72 hours has reduced the incidence of this infection. From 1982 to 1990, the incidence was 0.71% compared to 6.9% before the initiation of that policy (7).

Suppurative thrombophlebitis typically begins at the site of cannula tip placement and can extend for surprisingly long distances both proximally and distally from the site. The diagnosis of suppurative thrombophlebitis should be considered in any burn patient with a pulmonary infiltrate characteristic of hematogenous pneumonia and no other apparent source of infection. Local signs of infection are present in less than 30% of the burn patients in whom this disease develops (36). Consequently, all previously cannulated veins, beginning with the most recently cannulated vessel and progressing to the most remotely cannulated vessel, may have to be explored to locate the infection. The site of cannula tip residence should be surgically exposed and the vein incised. The diagnosis of suppurative thrombophlebitis is confirmed if intraluminal pus is identified. If a nonsuppurative intraluminal clot is present, however, that section of vein should be excised and both the vein and the clot cultured and subjected to histologic examination. A positive culture or the presence of microorganisms in the clot or the vein wall confirms the diagnosis of suppurative thrombophlebitis (Fig. 98.10).

Suppurative thrombophlebitis is treated by excision of the infected vein and the systemic administration of antibiotics active against the infecting organism. Since multiple areas of intraluminal infection may be present proximal to the relatively normal-appearing "skip areas," the excision should continue to the point at which the vein becomes a tributary of the next higher order of veins or to that point at which the vein wall is unequivocally normal and brisk retrograde flow of unaltered blood is noted. Following excision of the infected vein and any grossly involved tributaries, the venectomy wounds should be loosely packed and covered with an occlusive dressing.

Skin grafting or secondary closure is carried out following resolution of the infection and the local inflammatory changes.

Suppuration may occur even in high-flow central veins that cannot be readily excised. Central vein suppuration should be treated by a full maximum-dose course of antibiotic therapy with addition of heparin anticoagulation if pulmonary emboli develop. Balloon catheter extraction of an infected thrombus from a central vein has been reported, but re-thrombosis at the site of vein wall inflammation limits the effectiveness of such intervention (37).

Persistence of the septic state following excision of a focus of suppurative thrombophlebitis may be due to residual infection proximal to the level of excision, requiring proximal extension of the previous level of excision. Alternatively, it may be due to suppuration within another vein, requiring identification and excision of the other infected vein. Hematogenous pneumonia or acute bacterial endocarditis secondary to dissemination of the infection before excision of the involved vein also may cause persistence of the septic state, necessitating specific therapy as described for those processes.

ACUTE ENDOCARDITIS

The prolonged need for intravenous infusions, the high incidence of suppurative thrombophlebitis, and the previously noted frequency of bacteremia related to burn wound manipulation have all been incriminated in the relatively high incidence of acute endocarditis in burn patients. From 1969 to 1974, acute bacterial endocarditis developed in 1.3% (22 of 1,699) of patients treated at this burn center; in the past two decades, however, only seven cases have occurred. The incidence has decreased in concert with the declining incidence of invasive burn wound infections (38). In burn patients, acute endocarditis is slightly more common on the right side of the heart, although either or both sides may be involved. The identification of murmurs characteristic of this disease is difficult in the presence of the markedly hyperdynamic circulation of the burn patient.

The diagnosis of acute bacterial endocarditis should be entertained if the same organism, particularly coagulase-positive *S. aureus*, is recovered from two or more blood cultures in a burn patient with sepsis and no other apparent infection. Two-dimensional echocardiographic examination can be used to identify valvular lesions, but small foci of infection may go undetected. If no other source of infection is identified, systemic antibiotic therapy should be initiated and treatment continued for at least 3 weeks or until the blood cultures clear. Cardiac catheterization should be performed if antibiotic therapy fails to clear the septicemia or if valvular insufficiency occurs along with other signs of infection. Treatment can be delayed and repeat blood cultures obtained when a positive blood culture result is obtained from a patient whose general condition is inconsistent with sepsis. If exogenous contamination can be excluded, systemic antibiotic therapy should be initiated if the same organism is recovered from two successive blood cultures, even if the patient is not clinically septic. False-negative culture results can be minimized if the blood cultures are drawn as the patient's temperature is rising or, in a patient already receiving antibiotic therapy, immediately prior to a scheduled antibiotic dose, when circulating levels of the antibiotic will be lowest.

Bacteremia

Recovery of multiple organisms from a single blood culture or different organisms from successive blood cultures in critically ill burn patients with life-threatening complications is indicative of loss of effective host resistance and should not be discounted as a consequence of technical error. Maximum doses of an antibiotic or antibiotics active against all of the recovered organisms should be administered to such patients, and the septic focus from which the microorganisms arose should be identified and controlled.

The organism recovered from the blood determines the impact of septicemia on the burn patient. A review spanning 24 years has demonstrated that gram-negative septicemia and candidemia significantly increased mortality above that predicted on the basis of the extent of burn, while gram-positive septicemia had no demonstrable effect upon expected mortality (39). In recent years improvements in wound care and general care have resulted in a reduction of the comorbid effect of gram-negative septicemia.

INFECTION CONTROL

The types of organisms causing infection in burn patients can be influenced by manipulating the patient environment (40,41). During a recent 10-year period at this institution, improvement in patient isolation was associated with significant reductions in both the frequency and comorbid effect of infection. The changes observed were related to the use of single bed isolation of seriously burned patients and reduction in between-patient contact. Assignment of nursing personnel to specific patients, regulating other staff traffic to flow from new patients to convalescent patients and prevention of contact with convalescent patients who serve as a reservoir for multiply resistant organisms were effective in reducing inter-patient transfer of organisms and pre-

vented the establishment of endemic burn center strains. Environmental control measures included strict enforcement of hand washing, gowning, and gloving policies.

The quality assurance of patient isolation and infection control were based on a microbial surveillance program. Culture specimens were obtained from the wound surface, upper respiratory system (sputum) and urinary tract at admission and then three times per week throughout each patient's hospital course. Antibiotic sensitivity testing was done on *S. aureus* and *P. aeruginosa* or the principal gram-negative species isolated at each site. Patients with multiply resistant organisms acquired in other hospitals before burn center admission or detected during hospitalization were assigned to a patient-specific care team (41).

The high incidence of infectious complications in burn patients mandates that every burn center establish its own infection control committee and a microbial surveillance program. The surveillance database can document the organism types and antimicrobial sensitivity patterns for the individual patient's flora from time of admission throughout the hospital course. This permits temporal documentation of colonization and the early identification of specific microorganisms when clinical signs of infection develop. The availability of antibiotic sensitivity data also permits selection of pathogen-specific agents, which reduces the high costs associated with empirical use of newer broad-spectrum agents.

Each burn center should establish an infection control committee that can use clinically relevant and appropriate definitions of infections that occur in burn patients to monitor the results of the microbial surveillance program in order to identify temporal changes in the endemic flora, clusters of infection, changes in the types of infections that occur, and the predominant causative organisms (7). The committee should also assess the appropriateness of antibiotic use. Lastly, outcome analyses must be conducted to identify organism-related effects on morbidity and mortality in order to modify patient care and environmental control procedures as needed.

REFERENCES

1. Pruitt BA Jr, Mason AD Jr. Epidemiological, demographic and outcome characteristic of burn injury. In: Herndon DN, ed. *Total burn care*. London: WB Saunders, 1996:5–15.
2. Pruitt BA Jr. The burn patient: II. Later care and complications of thermal injury. *Curr Probl Surg* 1979;XVI(5):6–10.
3. Tredget EE, Shankowsky HA, Groeneveid A, Burrell R. A matched-pair, randomized study evaluating the efficacy and safety of Acticoat silver-coated dressing for the treatment of burn wounds. *J Burn Care Rehabil* 1998;19:531–537.
4. McManus WF, Mason AD Jr, Pruitt BA Jr. Excision of the burn wound in patients with large burns. *Arch Surg* 1989;124:718–720.
5. Goodwin CW, Pruitt BA Jr. Management of surgical infections: pathogenesis, diagnosis, and treatment. In: Davis JH, Sheldon OF, eds. *Clinical surgery*. St. Louis: Mosby, 1995:355–412.
6. Pruitt BA Jr. Infection: cause or effect of pathophysiologic change in burn and trauma patients. In: Paubert-Braquet M, ed. *Lipid mediators in the immunology of shock*. New York: Plenum Press, 1987:31–42.
7. Pruitt BA Jr, McManus AT. The changing epidemiology of infection in burn patients. *World J Surg* 1992;16:57–67.
8. Pruitt BA Jr, McManus AT, Kim SH, et al. Use of burn wound biopsy in the diagnosis and treatment of burn wound infection. In: Lorenz S, Zellner PR, eds. *Die Infektion beim Brandverletzten*. Darmstadt, Germany: Steinkopf Verlag, 1993:55–63.
9. McManus AT, Kim SH, McManus WF, et al. Comparison of quantitative microbiology and histopathology in divided burn wound biopsy specimens. *Arch Surg* 1987;122:74–76.
10. Kim SH, Hubbard GB, Worley BL, et al. A rapid section technique for burn wound biopsy. *J Burn Care Rehabil* 1985;6:433–435.
11. Kim SH, Hubbard GB, McManus WF, et al. Frozen section technique to evaluate early burn wound biopsy: a comparison with the rapid section technique. *J Trauma* 1985;25:1134–1137.

12. McManus AT, Mason AD Jr, McManus WF, et al. Control of *Pseudomonas aeruginosa* infection in burned patients. *Surg Res Commun* 1992;12:61–67.
13. Aulick LH, Goodwin CW Jr, Becker BA, et al. Visceral blood flow following thermal injury. *Ann Surg* 1981;193:112–116.
14. Zaske DE, Sawchuk RJ, Gerding DN, et al. Increased dosage requirements of gentamicin in burn patients. *J Trauma* 1976;16:824–828.
15. McManus WF, Goodwin CW Jr, Pruitt BA Jr. Subeschar treatment of burn wound infection. *Arch Surg* 1983;118:291–294.
16. McManus AT, McManus WF, Mason AD Jr, et al. Beta-hemolytic streptococcal burn wound infections are too infrequent to justify penicillin prophylaxis (letter). *Plast Reconstr Surg* 1994;93:650.
17. Pruitt BA Jr, McManus AT, Kim SH, Goodwin CW. Burn wound infection: current status. *World J Surg* 1998;22:135–144.
18. Bruck HM, Nash G, Stein JM, et al. Studies on the occurrence and significance of yeast and fungi in the burn wound. *Ann Surg* 1972;176:108–110.
19. Becker WK, Cioffi WG, McManus AT, et al. Fungal burn wound infection: a 10 year experience. *Arch Surg* 1991;126:44–48.
20. Majeski JA, MacMillan BG. Fatal systemic mycotic infections in the burned child. *J Trauma* 1977;17:320–322.
21. Pruitt BA Jr. Phycomycotic infections. In: Alexander JW, ed. *Problems in general surgery.* Vol. I, no. 4. Philadelphia: J.B. Lippincott, 1984, pp 664–678.
22. Foley FD, Greenawald KA, Nash G, et al. Herpesvirus infection in burned patients. *N Engl J Med* 1970;282:652–656.
23. Brandt SJ, Tribble CG, Lakeman AD, et al. Herpes simplex burn wound infections: epidemiology of a case cluster and responses to acyclovir therapy. *Surgery* 1985;98:338–343.
24. Deepe GS Jr, MacMillan BG, Linnemann CC Jr. Unexplained fever in burn patients due to cytomegalovirus infection. *JAMA* 1982;248:2299–2301.
25. Bale JF Jr, Kealey GP, Massanari PM, et al. The epidemiology of cytomegalovirus infection among patients with burns. *Infect Control Hosp Epidemiol* 1990;11:17–22.
26. Pruitt BA Jr. Cadaverous particles and infections in injured man-clinical review based on the Semmelweis lecture. *Eur J Surg* 1993;159:515–520.
27. McManus AT, Mason AD Jr, McManus WE, et al. A decade of reduced gram-negative infections and mortality associated with improved isolation of burned patients. *Arch Surg* 1994;129:1306–1309.
28. Pruitt BA Jr, DiVincenti FC, Mason AD Jr, et al. The occurrence and significance of pneumonia and other pulmonary complications in burned patients: comparison of conventional and topical treatments. *J Trauma* 1970;10:519–531.
29. Shirani KZ, Pruitt BA Jr, Mason AD Jr. The influence of inhalation injury and pneumonia on burn mortality. *Ann Surg* 1987;205:82–87.
30. Rue LW, Cioffi WG, Mason AD, et al. Improved survival of burned patients with inhalation injury. *Arch Surg* 1993;128:772–780.
31. Taylor GD, Kibsey P, Kirkland T, et al. Predominance of staphylococcal organisms in infections occurring in a burns intensive care unit. *Burns* 1992;18:332–335.
32. Frame JD, Kangesu L, Malik WM. Changing flora in burn and trauma units: experience in the United Kingdom. *J Burn Care Rehabil* 1992;13:281–286.
33. McManus AT, Goodwin CW, Pruitt BA Jr. Observations on the risk of resistance with the extended use of Vancomycin. *Arch Surg* 1998;133:1207–1210.
34. Pruitt BA Jr, McManus WF, Kim SH, et al. Diagnosis and treatment of cannula related intravenous sepsis in burn patients. *Arch Surg* 1980;191:546–554.
35. Mozingo DW, McManus AT, Kim SH, Pruitt BA Jr. Incidence of bacteremia after wound manipulation in the early postburn period. *J Trauma* 1997;42:1006–1011.
36. Pruitt BA Jr, Stein JM, Foley FD, et al. Intravenous therapy in burn patients: suppurative thrombophlebitis and other life threatening complications. *Arch Surg* 1970;100:399–404.
37. Stein JM. In discussion: Pruitt BA Jr, Stein JM, Foley FD, et al. Intravenous therapy in burn patients: suppurative thrombophlebitis and other life threatening complications. *Arch Surg* 1970;100:399–404.
38. Baskin TW, Rosenthal A, Pruitt BA Jr. Acute bacterial endocarditis: a silent source of sepsis in the burn patient. *Ann Surg* 1976;184:618–621.
39. Mason AD Jr, McManus AT, Pruitt BA Jr. Association of burn mortality and bacteremia: a twenty-five year review. *Arch Surg* 1986;121:1027–1031.
40. McManus AT, McManus WF, Mason AD Jr, et al. Microbial colonization in a new intensive care burn unit: a prospective cohort study. *Arch Surg* 1985;120:217–223.
41. Shirani KZ, McManus AT, Vaughan GM, et al. Effects of environment on infection in burn patients. *Arch Surg* 1986;121:31–36.

Urinary Tract

CHAPTER 99

Approach to the Patient with Urinary Tract Infection

Walter E. Stamm and Ann E. Stapleton

The term urinary tract infection (UTI) is applied to a variety of clinical conditions, ranging from asymptomatic bacteriuria to acute pyelonephritis with gram-negative septicemia. Many designations have been used to subdivide UTIs: symptomatic and asymptomatic, complicated and uncomplicated, upper tract and lower tract infection, among others. These schemes frequently overlap and do not correspond well to epidemiologically related groups of patients recognized by clinicians. In this chapter, symptomatic UTI in adults is subdivided into three groups: acute uncomplicated cystitis in women; acute uncomplicated pyelonephritis in women; and complicated UTIs in men or women. Most acute symptomatic UTIs in adults fall into one of these categories. Asymptomatic bacteriuria is discussed separately; it may be associated with any of the three groups. Being able to place a patient's complaint in one of the groups allows the physician to predict the likely infecting organisms and to choose an agent for empirical therapy.

CAUSATIVE PATHOGENS

More than 95% of UTIs are caused by a single bacterial species. *Escherichia coli* is the agent in more than 80% of cases of uncomplicated cystitis and pyelonephritis (Table 99.1). Interestingly, relatively few O serogroups produce the majority of these uncomplicated infections (02, 04, 08, O18ab, 075, 0150); they are known collectively as uropathogenic *E. coli* clones (1). In recurrent UTIs, the proportion of cases due to other organisms (usually *Klebsiella*, *Proteus*, or *Enterobacter* species or enterococci) is greater, as is the likelihood of isolating an organism with increased antibiotic resistance. From hospital-acquired UTIs a much wider range of organisms other than *E. coli* are isolated (see Table 99.1). Antibiotic-resistant isolates are common in nosocomial UTIs, particularly if the patient received previous courses of antimicrobial treatment.

Coagulase-negative staphylococci are often considered urinary contaminants, but studies have clearly demonstrated a pathogenic role for *Staphylococcus saprophyticus* (2, 3). In urine specimens, this species can be reliably identified as a coagulase-negative staphylococcus that is resistant to novobiocin (4). The vast majority of *S. saprophyticus* infections occur in young women, most commonly in the spring and summer. In northern Europe (5,6), *S. saprophyticus* has accounted for up to one third of acute uncomplicated UTIs in young women, whereas in the United States *S. saprophyticus* has usually accounted for 5% to 15% of acute cystitis episodes (7). Anaerobic bacteria, lactobacilli, corynebacteria, streptococci (other than enterococci),

TABLE 99.1. Microbial Species Most Often Associated with Specific Types of Urinary Tract Infections

Microbe	Acute uncomplicated cystitis (%)	Acute uncomplicated pyelonephritis (%)	Complicated UTI (%)	Catheter-associated UTI (%)
Escherichia coli	79	89	32	24
Staphylococcus saprophyticus	11	0	1	0
Proteus	2	4	4	6
Klebsiella	3	4	5	8
Enterococci	2	0	22	7
Pseudomonas	0	0	20	9
Mixed	3	5	10	11
Other	0	2	5	10
Yeast	0	0	1	28
S. epidermidis	0	0	15	8

Data in columns one and two are from 607 episodes of cystitis and 84 episodes of pyelonephritis in Seattle; data from columns 3 and 4 from Platt R, Polk BF, Murdock B, Rosner B. Risk factors for nosocomial urinary tract infection. *Am J Epidemiol* 1986;124:977, and Gasser TC, et al. Treatment of complicated UTIs with ciprofloxacin. *Am J Med* 1987;82 [Suppl 4]:278.

and *Staphylococcus epidermidis* are the predominant organisms isolated from the normal flora of the perineum and distal urethra, but they seldom cause UTI (8). These organisms are among the most common contaminants in urine cultures.

Staphylococcus aureus bacteriuria often indicates metastatic infection of the kidney following bacteremia; ascending cystitis or pyelonephritis due to *S. aureus* is extremely unusual in patients who have not undergone instrumentation (9). Adenoviruses (especially type 11) cause epidemic hemorrhagic cystitis in children, particularly boys (10), and may be underestimated as an endemic cause of cystitis.

The role of other organisms in urinary infection remains unclear. Using special media, Maskell and colleagues (11) have isolated fastidious microaerophilic organisms from many women with the acute dysuria-frequency syndrome, but the causal role of these organisms is disputed by others (12). *Gardnerella vaginalis* can be isolated from the urine of women with and without urinary tract symptoms, but its pathogenic role is likewise often uncertain (13). *Ureaplasma urealyticum* and *Mycoplasma hominis* probably account for some cases of acute pyelonephritis, and perhaps some cases of cystourethritis (14,15). *Haemophilus influenzae* may, on occasion, cause community-acquired UTI.

EPIDEMIOLOGY

Table 99.2 summarizes the prevalence of UTI, the male/female ratio, and major risk factors for patients by age group. Prevalence of bacteriuria in the neonatal period is approximately 1% (16), and infections during this period are often associated with bacteremia. Many are associated with functional or anatomic abnormalities of the urinary tract. In the first year of life, the frequency of UTI is higher in males than in females (17). Between ages 1 and 5 years, the prevalence of bacteriuria in girls rises to 4.5%, whereas in boys it decreases to 0.5% (18). Infections in young boys are often associated with congenital anomalies of the urinary tract. More recently, an intact foreskin has been identified as an important risk factor for UTIs in this group (19). Between one third and one half of UTIs in girls in the first 5 years of life are associated with vesicoureteral reflux, and this appears to be a critical period in determining whether renal scarring will occur (20,21).

The prevalence of bacteriuria in schoolgirls in the United States is approximately 1%; 5% of girls experience bacteriuria at some time. Most such episodes are not associated with renal abnormalities (22,23). Bacteriuria is rare in elementary school-age boys.

TABLE 99.2. Overview of the Epidemiology of Urinary Tract Infections by Age Group

Age group (y)	Females Prevalence (%)	Females Risk factors	Males Prevalence (%)	Males Risk factors
<1	1	Anatomic or functional urologic abnormalities	1	Anatomic or functional urologic abnormalities
1–5	4–5	Congenital abnormalities, vesicoureteral reflux	0.5	Congenital abnormalities, uncircumcised penis
6–15	4–5	Vesicoureteral reflux	0.5	None
16–35	20	Sexual intercourse, spermicide use, diaphragm use	0.5	Homosexuality, uncircumcised, human immunodeficiency virus infection
36–65	35	Gynecologic surgery, bladder prolapse, postmenopausal estrogen deficiency	20	Prostatic hypertrophy, obstruction, catheterization, surgery
>65	40	As for those age 36–65, plus incontinence, chronic catheterization	35	As for those age 36–65, plus incontinence, long-term catheterization

During late adolescence, the occurrence of UTI increases strikingly in young women. Approximately 20% of young women have at least one episode of acute dysuria each year, most due to bacterial infections (24). An estimated 7 million cases of acute cystitis occur in young women each year, making these among the most frequent infections in this age group (25). This figure probably understates the true incidence of these infections, because at least half of all UTIs resolve without coming to medical attention. During this period of life, UTIs are 50 times more common in women than in men. Major risk factors in women of this age group appear to be sexual intercourse and diaphragm and spermicide use (see later). Among young men in whom an uncomplicated UTI develops, homosexuality (perhaps due to exposure of the urethra to E. coli during rectal intercourse), lack of circumcision, and human immunodeficiency virus infection appear to be important risk factors (26,27).

In the later years of life, the incidence of UTI increases in both sexes and the female/male ratio declines. Many of these infections occur in the setting of catheterization, instrumentation, and bladder outlet obstruction due to prostatic hypertrophy (28).

PATHOGENESIS

Community-acquired UTIs usually result from entry into the bladder of bacteria that colonize the anterior urethra or the vaginal introitus (28,29). Bloodborne or lymphatic spread of pathogens from distant sites of infection occurs occasionally. Relapsing infection from unresolved foci in the prostate, kidney, or calculi may seed other parts of the urinary tract. Rarely, bacteria spread from the bowel to the bladder via a fistulous communication, as in Crohn's disease or malignancy. Characteristically, polymicrobial infection and pneumaturia result in such cases.

The pathogenesis of community-acquired UTI has been studied most carefully in young women, because they have the most infections (30). The short female urethra allows bacteria colonizing the distal urethra to enter the bladder after urethral massage, which in part explains the association of UTIs and bacteriuria with sexual activity (31). In addition, the proximity of the urethral meatus to the rectum in women facilitates colonization of the periurethral area with coliform bacteria.

In prospective studies, it has been repeatedly observed that the organisms that eventually cause UTIs usually colonize the vagina and the periurethral area beforehand (32). Factors that promote colonization of the vaginal introitus are poorly understood. Both colonization of the vaginal introitus and bacteriuria due to E. coli have been strongly associated with diaphragm and spermicide use (33), which may account for the apparently increased risk of UTI associated with sexual activity (34). Although the mechanism of this association is not yet clear, it is probably at least partly a perturbation of the vaginal flora caused by spermicides. Certain antibiotics, especially β-lactam, also promote introital colonization with E. coli (35).

Bacterial adherence to vaginal and uroepithelial cells represents the initial step in colonization of the lower urinary tract (36). An important unresolved question is the extent to which epithelial cells vary in their susceptibility to bacterial attachment, either from person to person or in one person at different times. Several studies have demonstrated that uroepithelial cells from women prone to recurrent UTI bind larger numbers of bacteria than do cells from women with no history of UTI (37,38). This observation suggests that some women may be genetically predisposed to UTI, a hypothesis that is further supported by the fact that nonsecretors of blood group antigens have an increased risk of recurrent UTI and their uroepithelial cells bind E. coli in greater numbers than do cells from secretors (39,40). The biochemical basis for these observations may lie in the fact that vaginal epithelial cells from nonsecretors contain unique uropathogenic E. coli–binding glycosphingolipids that are not present in cells from secretors (41). Alternatively, other factors such as estrogenic hormones appear to influence bacterial binding to epithelial cells and may alter the risk of UTI (42). Spermicide use could also influence the likelihood of bacterial attachment to uroepithelial cells, either by directly altering the epithelial cell surface or by eliminating the normal vaginal flora.

BACTERIAL VIRULENCE FACTORS

In comparison with "nonuropathogeneic" E. coli from the normal fecal flora, uropathogenic E. coli strains appear to belong to distinct clonal groups that exhibit specific virulence factors, including increased adherence to vaginal (43) and uroepithelial cells (44), resistance to the bactericidal activity of human serum (45), production of hemolysin (46) and of cytotoxic necrotizing factor-1 (47), carboxylesterase B electrophoretic pattern (48), presence of chromosomal aerobactin (49), and increased amounts of K capsular antigen (50). These organisms belong to a limited number of O, K, and H serogroups. Their adhesive properties are important determinants not only of infectivity but also in some cases of a propensity to develop upper tract infections. Adhesion is mediated by specific bacterial ligands, usually small proteins located at the tips of bacterial fimbriae which act as lectins to host cell membrane glycoconjugate moieties (51,52). Most E. coli strains (and many other Enterobacteriaciae) possess type 1 fimbriae, which bind mannoside residues on mannose-containing glycoproteins, such as uroplakins Ia and Ib on uroepithelial cells (53). Binding can be competitively inhibited by α-methyl mannoside and is thus mannose sensitive. Type 1 pili appear to be important in animal models of UTI and likely play a pathogenic role in mediating attachment to the bladder epithelium in humans as well (54). E. coli strains that cause upper UTIs usually express other adhesins that cannot be inhibited by an α-methyl mannoside and were thus originally called mannose-resistant adhesins. Eighty percent to 90% of uropathogenic E. coli strains that express mannose-resistant adhesins recognize a specific glycolipid receptor found on human erythrocytes and uroepithelial cells (55). The minimal recognition structure for this adhesin is a disaccharide moiety, α-D-galactopyranosyl-(1→4)-β-galactopyranoside, which is present on the globoseries glycosphingolipid on epithelial and erythrocyte membranes (56). For this reason, these fimbriae have been called gal-gal fimbriae by some workers. Because this structure also constitutes a major part of the P blood group antigen on erythrocytes (57), it has been named the P fimbria. Other mannose-resistant adhesins that do not recognize this disaccharide moiety are termed X adhesins (58); the specific recognition sites for several X adhesins have been determined (58).

Considerable evidence supports the importance of specific bacterial virulence factors in the pathogenesis of UTI. The importance of adhesion in uropathogenicity, for example, is demonstrated in experiments in which E. coli colonization of the mouse bladder can be prevented by mannose (i.e., *competitive blockade* of the mannose-sensitive adhesin) (59). Antibodies directed against P fimbriae block adherence to epithelial cells in vitro and prevent upper tract infection in a mouse model of pyelonephritis (60). An E. coli vaccine using gal-gal pili as the immunogen prevents pyelonephritis in the same model (61). Similarly, an immunogen using a portion of the FimH receptor binding protein for the type 1 pilus prevents UTIs in mice (62). Adhesion, often fimbria mediated, probably also plays a central role in the uropathogenicity of other bacterial species, such as *S. saprophyticus* and *Klebsiella*, but has been less studied.

Once attachment to uroepithelial cells occurs, bacterial virulence factors other than adhesins become important. These virulence determinants are often closely linked genes on the bacterial chromosome referred to as virulence or pathogenicity islands. These genes appear to have been acquired horizontally from other organisms (63). Most uropathogenic strains produce hemolysin, which may be important in initiating tissue invasion and cell damage or in making iron available to invading *E. coli*. Siderophores, such as aerobactin, are iron-scavenging proteins that are found with increased frequency in uropathogenic strains. The presence of K antigen protects bacteria from phagocytosis by leukocytes. Endotoxin derived from the *E. coli* cell wall is an important initiator of the inflammatory process in the kidney. Other virulence determinants are present in pathogenicity islands but their function has not been defined. Many or all of these virulence factors characteristically are found in *E. coli* strains isolated from infections, especially those involving the kidney, in urologically normal patients. Thus, these factors appear necessary for such strains to infect the intact host; however, they are less important in patients with structural or functional abnormalities of the urinary tract. *E. coli* strains infecting the upper tracts of children with vesicoureteral reflux or adults with urologic abnormalities, for example, do not exhibit the typical virulence factors found in the uropathogenic *E. coli* strains infecting nonimpaired hosts.

HOST DEFENSE MECHANISMS IN THE URINARY TRACT

Small numbers of bacteria presumably enter the female bladder frequently, but established infection rarely ensues. A variety of host factors act in concert to protect against infection (64). The flushing and diluting effects of urine accumulation and voiding help to clear infection. The acidity, high urea concentration, and extremes of osmolality in urine make it a poor culture medium for many anaerobic and fastidious bacteria and inhibit growth of many other organisms. Bacteria grow less avidly in urine collected from men than from women, probably because of the inhibitory activity of prostatic secretions (65). Tamm-Horsfall protein may act as a barrier to infection with Enterobacteriaceae, because it contains large numbers of mannose residues, which bind the mannose-sensitive adhesins on these bacteria and competitively inhibit attachment to epithelial cells and to uroplakins Ia and Ib (66). Taken together, these factors often successfully defend the bladder against small bacterial inocula, but they may be overcome by larger inocula or by more virulent bacteria. Foreign bodies such as stones and structural abnormalities provide such good refuge for bacteria that they may be extremely difficult or impossible to eradicate with antimicrobial agents.

Bacterial binding to glycolipid and glycoprotein receptors on urinary epithelial cells activates signaling pathways that eventuate in the secretion from these cells of IL-6, IL-8, and other cytokines and chemokines (67). IL-8 binds to the neutrophil chemokine receptors CXCR1 and CXCR2, inducing neutrophils to migrate from capillaries to the bladder where pyuria results and the neutrophils ingest and destroy bacteria (68,69). Urine inhibits phagocytic functions of polymorphonuclear leukocytes, including migration, aggregation, and killing. The inflammatory response itself is in part responsible for the symptoms of cystitis. In contrast to pyelonephritis (70), cystitis is seldom associated with a marked systemic or local antibody response to the infecting organism (71), and reinfection with the same strain may occur.

OVERVIEW OF CLINICAL MANIFESTATIONS

The symptoms of UTI in young children are notoriously nonspecific; often the major manifestations are fever, poor feeding, and vomiting. Abdominal discomfort may be present. UTI must always be excluded when a child has unexplained fever. After early childhood, the classic symptoms of dysuria, urgency, and frequency are more common. Adult women with cystitis generally void frequently and urgently, usually in small volumes (73), and often experience a sensation of lower abdominal heaviness or lower back pain. The urine may be turbid, and it is frankly bloody in one third of cases. Onset of symptoms is usually abrupt. Most cases respond rapidly to antimicrobial treatment, and many resolve even without therapy. If untreated, some patients progress over several days to develop signs and symptoms of upper tract involvement: fever, rigors, vomiting, and flank pain. Studies that compared clinical signs and symptoms with the localization of bacteria to the upper or lower urinary tract by laboratory techniques have demonstrated a poor correlation between clinical manifestations and site of infection (74,75).

In elderly persons, UTIs often produce no symptoms, and, as in childhood, when symptoms and signs are present they are frequently nonspecific. In addition, frequency, urgency, nocturia, and incontinence may have multiple causes in this age group. Physicians should not hesitate to collect urine for culture when an elderly patient has unexplained fever, mental status changes, increased urinary frequency, incontinence, or lower abdominal discomfort. Patients with neurogenic bladders or an indwelling catheter usually have few or no symptoms referable to the bladder when a UTI develops; signs and symptoms of pyelonephritis and unexplained fever or septicemia are more common.

Acute Uncomplicated Cystitis

Acute uncomplicated cystitis generally occurs in young women, but it may also be seen in older men and women and in children. Typical symptoms include dysuria, urinary frequency, urgency, voiding of small volumes, incontinence, and suprapubic or pelvic pain. Suprapubic tenderness is present in about 20% of patients with cystitis, and gross hematuria in approximately 30%, but both are relatively specific findings for cystitis in this group of patients (76).

Acute cystitis must be differentiated from other conditions in which dysuria may be a prominent symptom, especially vaginitis and urethral infections caused by sexually transmitted pathogens. Table 99.3 summarizes the characteristic features that are useful in assigning a patient with dysuria to one of these diagnostic categories (77).

Approximately 10% to 35% of patients with characteristic symptoms of acute uncomplicated cystitis may also have unrecognized infection of the upper urinary tract (occult renal infection) when localization studies such as the bladder washout test, selective ureteral catheterization, or antibody-coated bacteria tests are performed (78–80). The likelihood of occult renal infection in a patient presumed to have acute cystitis appears to be greater for women whose symptoms have persisted at least 7 days or who have a history of recent UTI and for those in lower socioeconomic groups.

Acute Pyelonephritis

Patients with acute pyelonephritis characteristically present with the symptoms of localized flank, low back, or abdominal pain and systemic symptoms such as fever, rigors, sweats, headache, nausea, vomiting, malaise, and prostration (81). Antecedent or

TABLE 99.3.   Factors That Distinguish Acute Cystitis from Vaginitis and Urethritis

Factor	Acute cystitis	Acute urethritis	Vulvovaginitis
Pathogen	*Escherichia coli, Staphylococcus saprophyticus*	*Chlamydia trachomatis, Neisseria gonorrhoeae*, herpes simplex virus	*Candida, Trichomonas*
Symptoms	Internal dysuria, frequency, urgency, hematuria	Internal dysuria, frequency, urgency, vaginal discharge	External dysuria, vaginal discharge, vaginal odor
Onset	Abrupt; symptoms severe	Gradual; symptoms mild	Gradual; symptoms mild
History	Prior UTI, diaphragm use	New sexual partner	Dyspareunia
Physical findings	Suprapubic tenderness	Cervicitis; vulvar lesions (HSV)	Vulvovaginitis

HSV, herpes simply virus; UTI, urinary tract infection.

concomitant symptoms of cystitis may or may not be present. Fever and flank pain are relatively specific indicators of acute renal infection.

A wide spectrum of illness is encountered among patients with acute pyelonephritis, ranging from mild disease to full-blown gram-negative sepsis. Volume contraction from recurrent vomiting may necessitate intravenous administration of fluids and antimicrobial agents. Complications, such as necrotizing intrarenal and perinephric abscesses (82) or gram-negative sepsis (83), develop in a minority of patients with acute pyelonephritis. These severe manifestations occur primarily in patients with associated urinary tract obstruction, diabetes, or other immunosuppressive conditions (84,85) and often necessitate aggressive diagnostic and therapeutic efforts, including emergency ultrasonography or computed tomography, and in some cases, hemodynamic monitoring, pressors, assisted ventilation, or urologic surgical procedures.

COMPLICATED URINARY TRACT INFECTIONS

In addition to being classified by the presumed anatomic site of infection, UTIs are often categorized as complicated or uncomplicated, depending on the presence or absence of host conditions known to promote infection, account for persistence of infection, or lead to a recurrence (85,86) (Table 99.4). Generally, uncomplicated cystitis and uncomplicated pyelonephritis occur in young women who lack evidence of structural or functional urologic abnormalities; thus, among females, complicated infections primarily affect premenarchal girls and postmenopausal women. All UTIs in males should be considered complicated until proved otherwise. As indicated earlier, the clinical manifestations that accompany complicated UTI are more often atypical and nonspecific. When complicating host factors or antimicrobial resistance is present, response to therapy is often disappointing (even with agents active against the patient's pathogen) (85), and severe complications of infection are more frequent. Antimicrobial and

TABLE 99.4.   Complicating Factors in Urinary Tract Infection

Male sex
Pregnancy
Diabetes
Immunosuppression
Hospital-acquired urinary tract infection
Recent antibiotic use
Catheterization or instrumentation of the urinary tract
Stone or urinary tract structural abnormality

adjunctive therapies may require modification in the presence of complicating factors (see later).

DIAGNOSIS

Confirmation of a UTI requires documentation of bacteriuria by culture. Suprapubic aspiration avoids potential contamination of the urine during collection but is rarely used in practice, except in children and certain other patients. Urethral catheterization can also be used to collect a specimen for urine culture; contamination of specimens collected by in-and-out catheterization is infrequent compared with that of voided specimens, but the procedure is uncomfortable for the patient, time-consuming, and thus rarely used. If a patient has an indwelling catheter, specimens for culture should be obtained from the specimen collection port on the catheter.

Urine Culture

In clinical practice, urine for culture is usually voided unless a catheter is in place, so specimens are often contaminated with perineal bacteria. Quantitative cultures and specific identification of the organisms in urine are used to distinguish culture contaminants (usually in small numbers and usually nonpathogenic species, often several of them) from true infective agents (usually larger numbers of typical uropathogens only) (87). The urine bacterial concentration is usually determined by inoculating a culture dish with a known volume of urine (10^{-2} or 10^{-3} mL), or it can be estimated using a dip-culture method (88). The finding of more than 10^5 bacteria per milliliter of voided urine was shown by Kass, Sanford, and others to differentiate infected from contaminated urine of women with asymptomatic bacteriuria or acute pyelonephritis (87–89). Since these studies were published, many physicians have considered at least 10^5 colony-forming units (CFU) per milliliter to be a necessary criterion for the diagnosis of any urinary infection; however, approximately one third of women with acute cystitis caused by *E. coli, S. saprophyticus*, and *Proteus* species have colony counts in midstream urine between 10^2 and 10^4 CFU/mL (90,91). Similarly, acute pyelonephritis has been reported in association with low bacterial counts in voided urine (92). Thus, in acutely symptomatic women, a more appropriate threshold value for defining "significant bacteriuria" is more than 10^2 CFU/mL of a known uropathogen (90,91). Failure to use this criterion for such patients seriously compromises the sensitivity of the urine culture. Many microbiology laboratories use culture techniques that accurately detect 10^3 but not 10^2 CFU/mL, so a 10^3 CFU/mL criterion may be more practical for many clinicians and laboratorians. Clinicians should encourage their clinical laboratory to use techniques that detect 10^3 CFU/mL and to report the results of cultures that grow 10^3 to 10^5 CFU/mL of a uropathogen.

As alternatives to standard culture methods, several rapid methods for the detection of bacteriuria have been developed and are reviewed in detail elsewhere (93). These methods detect bacterial growth by using photometry or bioluminescence and can provide results in as little as 2 hours. In general, these methods achieve a sensitivity of 95% to 98% and better than 99% negative predictive value compared with conventional cultures when bacteriuria is defined as at least 10^5 CFU/mL. Thus, they are excellent for screening out negative culture results by this definition of bacteriuria. Unfortunately, the sensitivity of these tests falls to unsatisfactory levels when they are asked to detect bacteriuria between 10^2 and 10^4 CFU/mL, which is necessary in patients with symptoms of acute disease.

Rapid Noncultural Diagnostic Tests

Rapid tests for detecting urinary leukocytes, erythrocytes, and bacteria permit presumptive confirmation of UTI at the time of initial evaluation without the expense and delays associated with urine culture. Among women with acute uncomplicated infection, when pyuria in voided urine specimens is carefully assessed using the hemocytometer method and when UTI is defined as more than 10^2 CFU/mL of a uropathogen plus acute urinary tract symptoms, pyuria is a highly sensitive indicator of UTI (93). In fact, its absence should call into question the diagnosis of UTI in this group of patients. Unfortunately, assessment of pyuria using the centrifuged urine sediment method that is employed in many laboratories is far less accurate and reproducible than counting leukocytes in uncentrifuged urine using a chamber method. The former method should be discouraged. The leukocyte esterase dipstick method is somewhat less sensitive in identifying pyuria than the hemocytometer method (94), but it can serve as an alternative approach when microscopy is not available. Pyuria is a less sensitive and specific indicator of complicated or catheter-associated UTI than of uncomplicated infection, but assessment of pyuria should be undertaken in such patients suspected of having a UTI.

Microscopic hematuria is found in 40% to 60% of cases of acute cystitis and is uncommon in other dysuric syndromes of young women; therefore, for this group, hematuria is a highly specific indicator of cystitis. In elderly persons, urinary calculi or tumors must be considered when hematuria is observed. Microscopic bacteriuria, which is most conveniently assessed using Gram-stained, uncentrifuged urine, is found in more than 90% of UTIs in which colony counts are at least 10^5 CFU/mL and is a highly specific finding (95). Bacteria are not readily detected microscopically with infections of lower colony counts (10^2 to 10^4 CFU/mL). Thus, microscopic hematuria and bacteriuria lack sensitivity but are reasonably specific for UTI in most groups of patients. Failure to detect them in a patient whose symptoms are consistent with UTI should not be interpreted as evidence against the diagnosis. At the same time, the presence of bacteriuria or hematuria in a patient with acute dysuria is strong evidence of bacterial UTI.

Selection of Laboratory Tests

Many authorities recommend that urine culture and antimicrobial susceptibility testing be performed whenever a UTI is suspected. However, the spectrum of infecting bacterial species and their antimicrobial susceptibility profiles are reasonably predictable in patients with acute cystitis. Further, treatment decisions are usually made, and therapy is often completed, before culture and susceptibility tests results are known in such patients. Thus, it may be more cost-effective to manage patients who have symptoms and urinalysis findings characteristic of acute, uncomplicated cystitis without an initial urine culture. In a study of women with uncomplicated infection, pretreatment urine cultures were not predictive of the therapeutic outcome and were considered unnecessary (96). Another study (97) estimated that the routine use of pretherapy urine cultures in acute cystitis increased costs by 40% but decreased the overall duration of symptoms by only 10%.

In view of these data, when patients have symptoms and signs suggestive of acute cystitis but no complicating factors, one approach that is increasingly used is to provide empirical antimicrobial therapy and do no laboratory testing unless the patient fails to improve. Alternatively, a urinalysis or a leukocyte esterase dipstick test can be performed (98). If results indicate pyuria or bacteriuria, these tests provide sufficient documentation of UTI, and urine culture and susceptibility testing can be omitted. Urine culture should be performed, however, when symptoms and urine examination findings leave the diagnosis of cystitis in question. Pretreatment culture and susceptibility tests are also essential to the management of patients with suspected upper tract infections and those who have complicating factors, because in these situations a variety of pathogens may be present and antibiotic therapy is best tailored to the individual organism (99).

TREATMENT

General Principles

All symptomatic UTIs should be treated with antimicrobial drugs. Ideally, the most effective, least toxic, least expensive drug should be prescribed for a period long enough to eradicate the infection. The antibacterial spectrum of the drug should cover the likely infecting organisms but should minimally disrupt the normal gut and perineal flora. Successful treatment of uncomplicated lower UTIs correlates with the inhibitory concentration of antimicrobial agent achieved in the urine, not in plasma or tissue (79) Some antimicrobial agents that are used successfully to treat cystitis (e.g., nitrofurantoin [79]) do not achieve microbicidal blood or tissue levels but are excreted in high concentrations in the urine. Urinary concentrations of many antibiotics are much higher than corresponding levels in other body fluids and may even exceed the minimal inhibitory concentration of some resistant organisms. This probably accounts for the clinical observation that some patients with cystitis are cured by antibiotics to which the infecting organism was apparently resistant. Urinary pH is an important determinant of the in vitro antibacterial activity of some antimicrobials, such as erythromycin and the aminoglycosides, but it is rarely important clinically.

A variety of nonspecific adjunctive measures is recommended to supplement antimicrobial treatment of UTIs (100). Patients with UTIs are usually advised to drink as much water as they can. The diluting and flushing out of nonadherent bacteria from the bladder may rapidly reduce the bacteria count in the urine and provide temporary symptomatic relief. In some cases, a large fluid load may be sufficient to clear the infection, but often as urine flow diminishes, bacterial counts rise again and symptoms appear. Other effects of "forcing fluids" may not be beneficial: urinary acidification is reduced, antibacterial substances in the urine are diluted, and obstruction or reflux may be exacerbated. Nonspecific treatment to reduce bladder discomfort and dysuria such as potassium citrate and phenazopyridine have little place in the management of bacterial cystitis. Phenazopyridine is occasionally helpful in women with recurrent dysuria, who have no documented infection.

Acute Cystitis

The traditional approach to treating acute cystitis was 7 to 10 days' therapy with an oral antibiotic; however, single-dose therapy (SDT) is effective in treating most women with acute cystitis, is less costly, and is associated with significantly fewer side effects than longer therapy (101,102). However, in controlled trials in which the sample size was adequate to allow detection of 15% to 20% differences in efficacy, SDT has been less effective than 7- to 10-day therapy (103,104). In addition, high-risk patients such as pregnant women; those with diabetes, immunosuppressive conditions, or urinary tract anomalies; and those who experienced symptoms for at least 7 days before therapy started are more likely to have occult upper tract infection and to not be cured by SDT or to develop complications if the infection is not eradicated (103,104).

Cure rates with SDT are in part related to the drug used. Higher cure rates have generally been observed with trimethoprim, trimethoprim-sulfamethoxazole, and fluoroquinolones, whereas lower cure rates have been observed with ampicillin, amoxicillin, and other β-lactam agents. This probably results mainly from the rapid urinary excretion of the latter compounds and the prolonged urinary excretion of the former. In addition, trimethoprim is concentrated in renal tissues to a greater extent than is ampicillin (105). The high incidence of resistance to ampicillin among pathogens from community-acquired UTIs (Table 99.5) also contributes substantially to the decreased efficacy of ampicillin and amoxicillin in antibody-coated bacteria-positive infections. SDT may also be less effective because it does not eradicate E. coli from the vaginal reservoir as effectively as 10-day therapy. The majority of "relapses" after SDT probably represent failure of such therapy to eliminate E. coli from the vaginal reservoir, followed rapidly by ascending reinfection.

More recently, many studies have evaluated the use of a 3-day course of therapy for treatment of cystitis. On theoretical grounds, 3-day therapy can be expected to be more effective than SDT, especially in patients with unrecognized complicating factors, and may be more effective than SDT in eradicating E. coli from the vaginal reservoir. In controlled trials, 3-day regimens of trimethoprim, trimethoprim-sulfamethoxazole, or fluoroquinolones have been associated with an incidence of adverse effects as low as that seen with SDT, and with cure rates that appear comparable to those achieved with longer courses of therapy (106). Thus, 3-day therapy is currently the preferred short course regimen for treating acute uncomplicated lower UTI with trimethoprim-sulfamethoxazole, trimethoprim, ciprofloxacin and levofloxacin being the most commonly used

drugs. Over the last 5-10 years, however, the prevalence of resistance to TMP-SMX among strains causing acute uncomplicated cystitis has increased to 20% in many parts of the United States (107). Most of these strains that are TMP-SMX resistant are also multidrug resistant, often demonstrating resistance to TMP, TMP-SMX, amoxicillin, tetracycline, and oral cephalosporins. Because these TMP-SMX resistant strains are associated with high rates of clinical failure if TMP-SMX is used for therapy, alternative agents should be given (108). Most of these strains remain susceptible to fluoroquinolones and to nitrofurantoin, which are alternative agents for use in areas with a high (greater than 20%) prevalence of TMP-SMX resistance. Short-course therapy (Table 99.6; see Table 99.5) should be reserved for patients presumed to have acute cystitis and no known complicating factors. When complicating factors are present in such patients, therapy should be continued for at least 7 days.

Acute Pyelonephritis

Patients with acute pyelonephritis can be subdivided into three groups: (a) those with mild acute pyelonephritis that can be managed in an outpatient setting; (b) those with acute uncomplicated pyelonephritis who are sufficiently ill to require hospitalization for initial parenteral therapy; and (c) those with complicated infection occurring in the setting of prior catheterization, hospitalization, urologic surgery, or known urologic abnormalities. The first group can be treated successfully as outpatients with 7 to 14 days of oral antibiotics, provided adequate compliance and follow-up can be ensured (108). Some physicians also provide a single loading dose of parenteral antibiotic given in the office or emergency department for such patients. A cost analysis showed that outpatient therapy for acute pyelonephritis was considerably less expensive than inpatient therapy (109).

Therapy for the second group of patients with acute pyelonephritis, who generally have severe abdominal and/or flank pain, nausea, vomiting and hypotension, necessitates hospital admission, intravenous fluids, and parenteral antibiotics because of the patient's degree of debility and inability to take oral medications. The majority of these cases of community-acquired pyelonephritis are caused by E. coli or other gram-negative bacilli. If enterococcal infection can be excluded using the urine Gram stain, we recommend initiation of therapy for acute uncomplicated pyelonephritis due to gram-negative bacilli with a single intravenous agent, generally a fluoroquinolone, an aminoglycoside or a third generation cephalosporin while awaiting culture results. The choice of which of these drugs to

---

TABLE 99.5. Susceptibility of Urinary Tract Infection Pathogens to Commonly Used Antibiotics in Selected Situations[a]

Antibiotic	Cystitis (%)	Acute pyelonephritis (%)	Complicated UTI (%)
Ampicillin	62	57	30
First-generation cephalosporin	72	60	51
Third-generation cephalosporin	N/A	95	95
Gentamicin	99	95	81
Nitrofurantoin	94	N/A	N/A
Trimethoprim-sulfamethoxazole	81	70	63
Fluoroquinolone	99	98	95

[a]Author's unpublished data. N/A indicates not available.
UTI, urinary tract infection.
Modified from Johnson JR, Stamm WE. Diagnosis and treatment of acute urinary tract infections. *Infect Dis Clin North Am* 1987;1:773–791.

TABLE 99.6.   Empirical Treatment Regimens for Selected Clinical Situations

Clinical situation	Expected pathogens	Antibiotic therapy[a]	Expected outcome	Comments
Acute uncomplicated cystitis	Escherichia coli (>90%) Staphylococcus saprophyticus	Therapy for 3 d with TMP-SMX,[b] TMP,[b] norfloxacin, ofloxacin, ciprofloxacin, or nitrofurantoin for 7 d	Cure >95%, relapse rare; subsequent reinfection possible	Therapy is extended to 7 d for following situations: unreliable patient, recent infection, ≥7 d of symptoms, diabetes, pregnancy, age <12 or >65 y
Acute pyelonephritis, no clinical evidence of stones or urologic disease, no evidence of sepsis, mild illness	E. coli (>90%)	7–14-d course of ofloxacin, ciprofloxacin, or TMP-SMX[c] given orally to outpatient[d]	Cure >90%; ~10% reinfection; relapse rare	With relapse, calculi or urologic disease is ruled out; then 2–6 wk with appropriate drug treatment eradicates focus
Acute pyelonephritis with suspected gram-negative sepsis or severe illness	E. coli (>90%), Klebsiella, Proteus	14-d course of therapy; start with initial IV. Gentamicin, fluoroquinolone or third-generation for 3d followed by PO therapy	Cure >80%; may relapse as described above	Hospitalization, parenteral antibiotics, other measures to manage shock; obstruction relieved if present
Complicated infection with calculi or urologic abnormality	E. coli, Proteus, Klebsiella, Pseudomonas, occasionally Staphylococcus or Enterococcus	At least 14-d course directed by culture results and sensitivities; begin with ampicillin plus gentamicin or other alternatives include piperacillin-tazobactam, ticarcilliin-clavulanate, imipenem, fluoroquinolone	Dependent on relief of underlying condition	Therapy before culture results are known depends on degree of illness and local sensitivity patterns (see text)
Nosocomial infection in catheterized patient; no clinical evidence of pyelonephritis or sepsis	E. coli, Proteus, Klebsiella, Pseudomonas, Serratia, Enterococcus	Often none if catheter can be withdrawn and patient is asymptomatic; if catheter cannot be withdrawn, treat symptomatic patients and selected asymptomatic patients such as immunosuppressed patients (especially renal transplant recipients), and those at high risk of sepsis. (old age, severe underlying disease)	Usually eradicated if catheter is withdrawn; treatment usually fails otherwise	Therapy based on culture results and sensitivities
Asymptomatic bacteriuria	E. coli (>90%) in young women; diverse spectrum in elderly	Treatment not always needed (see text); pregnant women and men about to undergo urologic surgery are treated as for acute uncomplicated cystitis	Cure 70%	Two culture results should be positive before treatment is undertaken

[a]TMP-SMX, Trimethoprim-sulfamethoxazole; IV, intravenous; PO, oral.
[b]Where resistance prevalence ≥20%, use alternative agent for empiric therapy.
[c]Do not use TMP-SMX unless organism is known to be susceptible.
[d]Can give first dose of these regimens IV in office or emergency room, followed by oral therapy.

use depends on cost considerations and on local antimicrobial sensitivity patterns. TMP-SMX should not be used for empiric therapy since resistance to this drug among acute pyelonephritis strains now exceeds 30% in many parts of the United States (108). Therapy can be modified after 24 to 48 hours, when susceptibility testing results are available. Parenteral therapy should be used until symptoms improve, fever disappears, and the patient is able to take fluids by mouth.

The duration of therapy for acute uncomplicated pyelonephritis in women need not be longer than 14 days (110). Shorter courses of therapy are curative for some cases of acute pyelonephritis, as reflected in reports of success with as little as 5 days' therapy (111). However, in one controlled trial, 1 week of therapy using the combination of pivampicillin and pivmecillinam resulted in significantly more bacteriologic recurrences than 3 weeks of therapy (112). On the other hand, 7 days of oral ciprofloxacin provided highly effective therapy (113). Thus, 7 to 14 days of therapy is supported by the currently available comparative clinical trials.

The presence of complicating factors in patients with upper UTI argues for more aggressive management, closer follow-up,

and a longer course of therapy. Reference to recent urine culture reports or to the Gram stain examination of the initial urine specimen may be used to better define the spectrum of empirical antimicrobial coverage. Consideration should be given to making urologic consultation part of the initial management of such patients. Similarly, patients with suspected pyelonephritis who have symptoms of renal colic or a stone on their admission abdominal radiograph or who fail to improve after 3 days appropriate antibiotic therapy should be suspected of harboring a stone or of having an underlying anatomic abnormality, urinary tract obstruction, or an acquired complication of infection such as intrarenal abscess. In such cases, ultrasonography, computed tomography, or excretory urography should be performed and urologic consultation obtained if indicated. Empiric treatment of complicated pyelonephritis should generally provide coverage for enterococci and pseudomonas (see Table 99.6).

Asymptomatic Bacteriuria

Generally, children with asymptomatic bacteriuria should be treated. Bacteriuria in pregnancy is associated with a high risk of developing acute pyelonephritis and may jeopardize the pregnancy (114). Women should thus be screened for bacteriuria during pregnancy and treated promptly (see later). For adults who are not pregnant, there is little convincing evidence that treating asymptomatic bacteriuria is beneficial (115,116). Exceptions may include selected high-risk patients such as those with neutropenia or a renal transplant. At present, there is no reason to treat asymptomatic bacteriuria in elderly patients. Although the mortality rate for hospitalized patients with bacteriuria has been higher than that for patients without bacteriuria (117), this probably relates to the frequency with which seriously ill patients are catheterized and the mortality associated with bacteremic catheter-associated UTI. Therefore, asymptomatic bacteriuria should not be treated in most cases of catheter-associated UTI.

Prophylaxis of Recurrent Infection in Women

Many women have occasional episodes of cystitis, but in a minority, recurrent episodes occur with such frequency (three or more per year) that antimicrobial prophylaxis is justified. These patients can be divided into two groups: (a) those with structural or functional abnormalities of the urinary tract (and an associated tendency to develop pyelonephritis or relapsing infection), and (b) the great majority, those who have a normal urinary tract infection confined to the lower urinary tract, and repeated reinfections. In some of these women, infections can be temporally related to sexual intercourse or diaphragm use, but in the majority no predisposing factor is apparent. The recurrent infections tend to cluster in time (118); that is, the likelihood of a subsequent infection is greatest at the end of the treatment course and then diminishes progressively the longer that the woman is infection free.

Simple measures such as voiding immediately after sexual intercourse or substituting an alternative form of contraception for a diaphragm may be effective for women for whom these factors are related to recurrent infection. Three antimicrobial strategies can be used: (a) continuous low-dose prophylaxis (119); (b) self-administered single-dose treatment (120), and (c) postcoital single-dose prophylaxis (121).

For continuous low-dose prophylaxis, trimethoprim (with or without sulfamethoxazole), nitrofurantoin, and norfloxacin have been evaluated extensively and are highly effective (119). Most experience has been gained with trimethoprim-sulfamethoxazole; it is tolerated well and produces an excellent therapeutic index when used long term. Side effects are rare but usually develop in the first few weeks of therapy. While emergence of resistant strains on prophylaxis has been unusual in the past with these drugs, this may be expected to occur more often with increased TMP-SMX resistance in UTI strains. Other drugs such as nitrofurantoin and fluoroquinolones may thus be better alternatives for long-term prophylaxis.

The choice of management strategy depends on the factors that predispose to recurrent infection, the numbers of infections per year, and the preference of the patient (122). In general, continuous prophylaxis is preferred for women who experience three infections or more per year. Patient-administered 3-day therapy should be reserved for women who have two infections per year, and postcoital prophylaxis for women who relate their infections to sexual activity. The costs of prophylaxis and patient-administered SDT with trimethoprim-sulfamethoxazole are approximately the same (120). There are no clear guidelines as to when to stop prophylaxis, but most often, it is given for at least 6 months. Most women's infections return at the pre-prophylaxis rate when the drug is withdrawn (123).

Among postmenopausal women, estrogen deficiency is associated with an increased risk of recurrent UTI (124) and with alterations of the vaginal flora favoring colonization with uropathogens (125). In a double-blind, placebo-controlled trial, treatment with topical intravaginal estradiol cream was shown to ameliorate these derangements of the vaginal flora and to dramatically reduce the risk of recurrent UTI among these women (126).

Urinary Tract Infection in Pregnancy

Asymptomatic bacteriuria occurs in 4% to 7% of pregnancies (127), the risk increasing with parity, lower socioeconomic status, and age. Several physiologic changes account for this predisposition to infection in pregnancy, including estrogen-induced and progesterone-induced dilation of the uterus, bladder, and renal pelvis; increased bladder capacity; hydroureter and decreased ureteral peristalsis; and vesicoureteral reflux. Approximately one third of untreated pregnant women with bacteriuria develop upper tract infections, usually in the third trimester, in contrast with a rate of less than 1% in patients without bacteriuria in early pregnancy (128). The incidence of pyelonephritis in bacteriuric women can be reduced to less than 5% by appropriate therapy. Thus, more than 75% of cases of acute pyelonephritis in pregnancy can be prevented by screening for and treating asymptomatic bacteriuria early in pregnancy. Prevention of pyelonephritis in pregnancy also prevents associated fetal morbidity (principally prematurity).

Women should be screened for bacteriuria at their first antenatal clinical visit. Sulfonamides, nitrofurantoin, ampicillin, cephalexin, and nalidixic acid are all considered safe to use early in pregnancy. Sulfonamides should not be used near term, owing to the theoretical risk that kernicterus may be induced in the newborn by sulfonamide displacement of bilirubin from plasma albumin binding sites. Trimethoprim, a dihydrofolate reductase inhibitor, is not generally recommended in pregnancy because there is some evidence of fetal toxicity with high doses in experimental animals; however, in pregnant humans there is no evidence of teratogenicity or other adverse effects. Tetracyclines and fluoroquinolones are contraindicated in pregnancy.

At present, a 7-day course of antimicrobial agent would *seem a* reasonable treatment of choice for asymptomatic bacteriuria or uncomplicated lower UTI during pregnancy if careful follow-up is possible (129). Patients should be followed up 2 weeks after completing therapy and then at monthly intervals. The aim of follow-up is to detect and treat asymptomatic bacteriuria as promptly as possible and therefore to prevent the development of acute pyelonephritis.

CATHETER-ASSOCIATED INFECTIONS

Catheter-associated UTIs constitute 35% to 40% of all hospital-acquired infections (130). The majority of these infections are asymptomatic, but some produce the clinical manifestations of cystitis described earlier. More important, catheter-associated bacteriuria is a common source of gram-negative bacteremia in hospitalized patients (131) and has been associated with a three-fold increase in mortality (132), prolonged hospital stay, and increased hospital costs.

Bacteria gain entry to the catheterized bladder in three ways: they may be introduced during catheterization, they may enter on the external surface of the catheter in the urethral mucus sheath (periurethral route) (133), or they may enter the drainage system by contamination of the collecting bag or disconnection of the junction between the catheter and collecting tube and ascend through the lumen of the catheter (intraluminal route) (133). The importance of the intraluminal route is illustrated by the marked reduction in the incidence of catheter-associated UTI because of the introduction of sterile, closed drainage systems. Presently, in hospitals where closed, sterile drainage is used, the periurethral route of infection appears to be the most frequent route of bacterial entry, especially in women. Antecedent rectal and periurethral colonization plays an important role in the subsequent development of catheter-associated bacteriuria, as it does in women with cystitis (133). In one study, urethral colonization preceded the development of catheter-associated UTI in 67% of women and 29% of men (133).

The overall risk of infection increases with the time that the catheter is in place. Bacteriuria develops in approximately 50% of men and women catheterized for 2 weeks, and all patients with permanent indwelling catheters eventually become infected. Risk of catheter-associated UTI is greater in women, in patients whose sterile, closed drainage system is disconnected, and in patients who are not receiving systemic antibiotics.

Prevention of Infection

Closed, sterile drainage systems significantly reduce the incidence of catheter-associated infection. Provided that the system is not breached, bacteriuria can be prevented in the majority of patients for up to 10 days with modern collecting systems and catheters. In general, antibiotic ointments and creams applied to the urethral meatus have not been protective; however, one study showed that twice-daily application of a polyantimicrobial cream to the urethral meatus significantly reduced infection in women with periurethral colonization at the time of catheterization (134). Silver-impregnated catheters may prevent bacteriuria, especially in patients catheterized long term (135,136). Systemic antibiotic treatment has a definite short-term effect in reducing the prevalence of UTIs in catheterized patients, but in the long term it predisposes to infection by resistant strains. This approach may be appropriate for short-term coverage of high-risk patients, but it is unwise for periods of catheterization longer than 1 week.

Treatment

In general, catheter-associated bacteriuria should be treated only in patients with symptomatic infection. When treatment is to be started, it is preferable to remove the catheter, start appropriate therapy, and then reintroduce a new catheter and drainage system if indwelling catheterization is still necessary. Concretions on the internal surface of the catheter often serve as a reservoir for bacteria, where they may be protected from antimicrobial drugs much as they are in urinary calculi. If such "infected" catheters are left in place, relapsing infection will occur when antimicrobial therapy is stopped. If fever and flank pain are present, parenteral treatment should be started immediately. Evidence is insufficient to cite an optimal duration of treatment for catheter-associated UTI; 7 days' therapy is usual. Resistant bacteria and fungi (usually *Candida*) are often isolated in catheterized patients receiving multiple courses of broad-spectrum antimicrobials. Symptomatic bacterial infections should be treated based on antimicrobial sensitivities. Yeast isolation does not necessarily require treatment, because many episodes clear without treatment, but repeated isolations or symptomatic infections should be treated with oral fluconazole or amphotericin B irrigations (137,138).

REFERENCES

1. Orskov F, Orskov I. Summary of a workshop on the clone concept in the epidemiology, taxonomy and evolution of the enterobacteriaceae and other bacteria. *J Infect Dis* 1983;148:346.
2. Latham RH, Running K, Stamm WE. Urinary tract infections in young women caused by *Staphylococcus saprophyticus*. *JAMA* 1983;250:3063.
3. Mabeck CD. Significance of coagulase-negative staphylococcal bacteriuria. *Lancet* 1969;2:1150.
4. Pereira AT. Coagulase-negative strains of staphylococcus possessing antigen 51 as agents of urinary infection. *J Clin Pathol* 1962;15:252.
5. Hovelius B, Mardh P-A. *Staphylococcus saprophyticus* as a common cause of urinary tract infections. *Rev Infect Dis* 1984;6:328.
6. Wallmark G, Arremark I, Telander B. *Staphylococcus saprophyticus*: A frequent cause of urinary tract infection among female outpatients. *J Infect Dis* 1978;138:791.
7. Jordan PA, Irvani A, Richard GA, et al. Urinary tract infection caused by *Staphylococcus saprophyticus*. *J Infect Dis* 1980;142:510.
8. Marrie TJ, Swantee CA, Hartlen M. Aerobic and anaerobic urethral flora of healthy females in various physiological age groups and females with urinary tract infections. *J Clin Microbiol* 1980;11:654.
9. Demuth PJ, Gerding DN, Crossley K. *Staphylococcus aureus* bacteriuria. *Arch Intern Med* 1979;139:78.
10. Manalo D, Mufson MA, Zollar IM, Mandad VN. Adenovirus infection in acute hemorrhagic cystitis: a study in 25 children. *Am J Dis Child* 1971;121:281.
11. Maskell R, Pead L, Sanderson RA. Fastidious bacteria and the urethral syndrome. *Lancet* 1983;2:1277.
12. Gargan RA, Brumfitt W, Hamilton-Miller JMT. Do anaerobes cause urinary infection? *Lancet* 1980;1:37.
13. Fairley KF, Birch DF. Unconventional bacteria in urinary tract disease: *Gardnerella vaginalis*. *Kidney Int* 1983;23:862.
14. Stamm WE, Running K, Hale J, Holmes KK. Etiologic role of *M. hominis* and *U. urealyticum* in women with the acute urethral syndrome. *Sex Transm Dis* 1983;10:3185.
15. Thomsen AC. Mycoplasmas in human pyelonephritis: demonstration of antibodies in serum and urine. *J Clin Microbiol* 1978;8:197.
16. Bran JL, Levison ME, Kaye D. Entrance of bacteria into the female urinary bladder. *N Engl J Med* 1972;259:626.
17. Abbott GD. Neonatal bacteriuria: a prospective study in 1460 infants. *BMJ* 1972;1:267.
18. Randolph MF, Greenfield M. The incidence of asymptomatic bacteriuria and pyuria in infancy. A study of 400 infants in private practice. *J Pediatr* 1964;65:57.
19. Herzog LW. Urinary tract infections and circumcision. *Am J Dis Child* 1989;143:348.
20. Smellie JM, Normand ICS. Bacteriuria, reflux and renal scarring. *Arch Dis Child* 1975;50:581.
21. Editorial: Bacteriuria-When does it matter? *Lancet* 1979;2:1155.
22. Kunin CM. The natural history of recurrent bacteriuria in school girls. *N Engl J Med* 1970;282:1443.
23. Gillenwater JY, Harrison RB, Kunin CM. Natural history of bacteriuria in schoolgirls: a long-term case-control study. *N Engl J Med* 1979;301:369.
24. Sanford JP. Urinary tract symptoms and infections. *Annu Rev Med* 1975;26:485.
25. National Center for Health Statistics. Ambulatory medical care rendered in physicians' offices-United States-1975. *Adv Data* 1977;12:1.
26. Barnes RC, Daifuku R, Roddy RE, Stamm WE. Urinary tract infection in sexually active homosexual men. *Lancet* 1986;2:171.
27. Spach DH, Stapleton AE, Stamm WE. Lack of circumcision increases the risk of urinary tract infection in young men. *JAMA* 1992;267:679.
28. Lipsky BA. Urinary tract infections in men. Epidemiology, pathophysiology, diagnosis, and treatment. *Ann Intern Med* 1989;110:138.
29. Stamey TA, Timothy M, Millar M, Mikhara G. Recurrent urinary tract infections in adult women. The role of introital enterobacteria. *Calif Med* 1971;115:1.
30. Svanborg-Eden C, Hausson S, Jodal U, et al. Host-parasite interaction in the urinary tract. *J Infect Dis* 1988;157:421.
31. Nicolle LE, Harding GKM, Preiksaitis J, Ronald AR. The association of urinary tract infections with sexual intercourse. *J Infect Dis* 1982;146:579.
32. Stamey TA. *Pathogenesis and treatment of urinary tract infections*. Baltimore: Williams & Wilkins, 1972.
33. Hooton TM, Hillier S, Johnson C, et al. *Escherichia coli* bacteriuria and contraceptive method. *JAMA* 1991;265:64.
34. Strom BL, Collins M, West SL, et al. Sexual activity, contraceptive use, and other risk factors for symptomatic and asymptomatic bacteriuria: a case-control study. *Ann Intern Med* 1987;107:816.
35. Herthelius BM, Hedstrom KG, Mollby R, et al. Pathogenesis of urinary tract infections-amoxicillin induces genital *E. coli* colonization. *Infection* 1988;5:263.
36. Reid G, Sobel JD. Bacterial adherence in the pathogenesis of urinary tract infection: a review. *Rev Infect Dis* 1987;9:470.
37. Svanborg-Eden C, Jodal U. Attachment of *E. coli* to urinary sediment epithelial cells from urinary tract infection-prone and healthy children. *Infect Immun* 1979;26:837.
38. Schaeffer AJ, Jones JM, Dunn JK. Association of in vitro *E. coli* adherence to

vaginal and buccal epithelial cells with susceptibility of women to recurrent urinary tract infections. *N Engl J Med* 1981;304:1062.

39. Kinane DF, Blackwell CC, Brettle RP, et al. ABO blood group, secretor state, and susceptibility to recurrent urinary tract infection in women. *BMJ* 1982;285:7.
40. Lomberg H, Cedergren B, Leffler H, et al. Influence of blood group on the availability of receptors for attachment of uropathogenic *E. coli*. *Infect Immun* 1986;51:919.
41. Stapleton A, Nudelman E, Clausen H, et al. Binding of uropathogenic *Escherichia coli* R45 to glycolipids extracted from vaginal epithelial cells is dependent on the histo-blood group secretor status. *J Clin Invest* 1992;90:965.
42. Reid G, Brooks HJK, Bacon DF. In vitro attachment of *E. coli* to human epithelial cells: variation in receptivity during the menstrual cycle and pregnancy. *J Infect Dis* 1983;148:412.
43. Schaefer AJ, Jones JM, Falkowski WS, et al. Variable adherence of uropathogenic *Escherichia coli* to epithelial cells from women with recurrent urinary tract infection. *J Urol* 1982;128:1227.
44. Svanborg-Eden C, Hanson LA, Jodal U, et al. Variable adherence to normal urinary tract epithelial cells of *Escherichia coli* strains associated with various forms of urinary tract infections. *Lancet* 1976;2:490.
45. Bjorksten B, Kaijser B. Interaction of human serum and neutrophils with *Escherichia coli* strains: difference between strains isolated from urine of patients with pyelonephritis or asymptomatic bacteriuria. *Infect Immun* 1978;22:308.
46. Hughs C, Hacker J, Roberts A, Boegel A. Hemolysin production as a virulence marker in symptomatic and asymptomatic urinary tract infections caused by *Escherichia coli*. *Infect Immun* 1983;39:546.
47. Blanco J, Blanco M, Alonso MP, et al. Characteristics of haemolytic *Escherichia coli* with particular reference to production of cytotoxic necrotizing factor type 1 (CNF1). *Res Microbiol* 1992;143:869.
48. Johnson JR, Goullet P, Picard B, et al. Association of carboxylesterase B electrophoretic pattern with expression of urovirulence factor determinants and antimicrobial resistance among strains of *Escherichia coli* that cause urosepsis. *Infect Immun* 1991;59:2311.
49. Johnson JR, Moseley SL, Roberts PL, Stamm WE. Aerobactin and other virulence genes among strains of *E. coli* causing urosepsis: association with patient characteristics. *Infect Immun* 1988;56:405.
50. Roberts AP, Phillips R. Bacteria causing symptomatic urinary tract infection or bacteriuria. *J Clin Pathol* 1979;32:492.
51. Reid G, Sobel JD. Bacterial adherence in the pathogenesis of urinary tract infection - a review. *Rev Infect Dis* 1987;9:470.
52. Korhonen TK, Leffler H, Svanborg-Eden C. Binding specificity of piliated strains of *Escherichia coli* and *Salmonella typhimurium* to epithelial cells, *Saccharomyces cerevisiae* cells and erythrocytes. *Infect Immun* 1981;32:796.
53. Wu X-R, Sun T-T, Medina JJ. In vitro binding of type 1-fimbriated *Escherichia coli* to uroplakins I1 and Ib: relation to urinary tract infection. *Proc Natl Acad Sci* 1996;93:9630–9635.
54. Mulvey MA, Lopez-Boado YS, Wilson CL, et al. Induction and evasion of host defenses by type 1-piliated uropathogenic *E. coli*. *Science* 1998;282:1494–1497.
55. Donnenberg MS, Welch RA. *Virulence determinants of uropathogenic E. coli in urinary tract infections: molecular pathogenesis and clinical management*. Washington DC: ASM Press, 1996:135–174.
56. Källenius G, Mollby R, Svenson SB, et al. Identification of a carbohydrate receptor recognized by uropathogenic *Escherichia coli*. *Infection* 1980;8(Suppl 3):S288.
57. Källenius G, Svenson SB, Hultberg H, et al. Occurrence of P-fimbriated *Escherichia coli* in urinary tract infections. *Lancet* 1981;2:1369.
58. Nowicki B, Moulds J, Hull R, Hull S. A hemagglutinin of uropathogenic *E. coli* recognizes the Dr blood group antigen. *Infect Immun* 1988;56:1057.
59. Aronson M, Medalia O, Schori L, et al. Prevention of colonization of the urinary tract of mice with *Escherichia coli* by blocking of bacterial adherence with methyl-α-D-mannopryanoside. *J Infect Dis* 1979;139:329.
60. O'Hanley PD, Lark D, Falkow S, Schoolnik G. A globoside binding *E. coli* pilus vaccine prevents pyelonephritis (abstract). *Clin Res* 1983;31:372.
61. O'Hanley P, Lark D, Falkow S, Schoolnik G. Molecular basis of *Escherichia coli* colonization of the upper urinary tract in BALB/c mice: Gal-Gal pili immunization prevents *Escherichia coli* pyelonephritis in the BALB/c mouse model of human pyelonephritis. *J Clin Invest* 1985;75:347.
62. Langermann S, Palaszynski S, Barnhart M, et al. Prevention of mucosal *E. coli* infection by FimH-adhesin based systemic vaccination. *Science* 1997;276:607–611.
63. Johnson J. Virulence factors in *E. coli* urinary tract infections. *Clin Micro Rev* 1991;4:80–128.
64. Agace W, Connell H, Svanborg C. Host resistance to urinary tract infection. In: *Urinary tract infections, molecular pathogenesis and clinical management*. Washington DC: AMS Press, 1996:176–221.
65. Stamey TA, Fair WR, Timothy MM. Antibacterial nature of prostatic fluid. *Nature* 1968;218:444.
66. Pak J, Pu Y, Zhang ZT, Hasty DL, Wu XR. Tamm-Horsfall protein binds to type 1 fimbriated *Escherichia coli* and prevents *E. coli* from binding to uroplakin Ia and Ib receptors. *J Biol Chem* 2001;276(13):9924–9930.
67. Hedlund M, Duan RD, Nilsson A, et al. Fimbriae, transmembrane signalling and cell activation. *J Infect Dis* 2001;183:S47–S50.
68. Svanborg C, Frendeus B, Godaly G. Toll-like receptor signalling and chemokine receptor expression influence the severity of urinary tract infection. *J Infect Dis* 2001;183:S61–S65.

69. Schaeffer AJ: What do we know about the UTI-prone individual? *J Infect Dis* 2001;183:S66–S70.
70. Rene P, Silverblatt FJ. Serological response to *Escherichia coli* pili in pyelonephritis. *Infect Immun* 1982;37:749.
71. Rene P, Dinolfo M, Silverblatt FJ. Serum and urogenital antibody response to *Escherichia coli* pili in cystitis. *Infect Immun* 1982;38:542.
72. Stamm WE, Norrby SR. Urinary tract infections: disease panorama and challenges. *J Infect Dis* 2000;183:S1–S4.
73. Komaroff AL. Acute dysuria in women. *N Engl J Med* 1984;310:368.
74. Jones SR, Smith JW, Sanford JP. Localization of urinary tract infection by detection of antibody-coated bacteria in urine sediment. *N Engl J Med* 1974;290:591.
75. Latham RH, Stamm WE. Role of fimbriated *Escherichia coli* in urinary tract infection in adult women: correlation with localization studies. *J Infect Dis* 1984;49:835.
76. Wong ES, Fennell CL, Stamm WE. Urinary tract infection among women attending a clinic for sexually transmitted diseases. *Sex Transm Dis* 1984;11:18.
77. Johnson JR, Stamm WE. Diagnosis and treatment of acute urinary tract infections. *Infect Dis Clin North Am* 1987;1:773.
78. Fairley KF, Carson NE, Gutch RC, et al. Site of infection in acute urinary tract infection in general practice. *Lancet* 1971;2:615.
79. Stamey TA, Govan DE, Palmer JM. The localization and treatment of urinary tract infections: the role of bactericidal urine levels as opposed to serum levels. *Medicine (Baltimore)* 1965;44:1.
80. Thomas V, Shelokov A, Forland M. Antibody-coated bacteria in the urine and the site of urinary tract infection. *N Engl J Med* 1974;290:588.
81. Johnson JR, Lyons MF 2d, Pearce W, et al. Therapy for women hospitalized with acute pyelonephritis: a randomized trial of ampicillin versus trimethoprim-sulfamethoxazole for 14 days. *J Infect Dis* 1991;103:325.
82. Ahlering TE, Boyd SD, Hamilton CL, et al. Emphysematous pyelonephritis: a 5-year experience with 13 patients. *J Urol* 1985;134:1086.
83. Bahnson RR. Urosepsis. *Urol Clin North Am* 1986;13:627.
84. Cattell WR. Urinary tract infections in adults-1985. *Postgrad Med J* 1985;61:907.
85. Nicolle LE. Urinary tract pathogens in complicated infection and in elderly individuals. *J Infect Dis* 2001;183:S5–S8.
86. Preheim LC. Complicated urinary tract infections. *Am J Med* 1985;79:62.
87. Sobel JD, Kaye D. Urinary tract infections. In Mandell GL, Douglas RG Jr, Bennett JE, eds: *Principles and practice of infectious diseases*, 2nd ed. New York: John Wiley & Sons, 1985.
88. Cohen SN, Kass EH. A simple method for quantitative urine culture. *N Engl J Med* 1967;277:176.
89. Stamm WE. Recent developments in the diagnosis and treatment of urinary tract infections. *West J Med* 1982;137:213.
90. Stamm WE, Counts GW, Running KR, et al. Diagnosis of coliform infection in acutely dysuric women. *N Engl J Med* 1982;307:463.
91. Stamm WE. Quantitative urine cultures revisited (editorial). *Eur J Clin Microbiol* 1984;3:279.
92. Bollgren I, Engstrom CF, Hammarlind M, et al. Low urinary counts of P-fimbriated *Escherichia coli* in presumed acute pyelonephritis. *Arch Dis Child* 1984;59:102.
93. Pappas PG. Laboratory in the diagnosis and management of urinary tract infections. *J Gen Intern Med* 1991;75:313.
94. Carroll KC, Hale DC, Von Boerum DH, et al. Laboratory evaluation of urinary tract infections in an ambulatory clinic. *Am J Clin Pathol* 1994;101:100.
95. Jenkins RD, Fenn JP, Matsen JM. Review of urine microscopy for bacteriuria. *JAMA* 1986;255:3397.
96. Schultz HJ, McCaffrey LA, Keys TF, Nobrega FT. Acute cystitis: a prospective study of laboratory tests and duration of therapy. *Mayo Clin Proc* 1984;59:391.
97. Carlson KJ, Mulley AG. Management of acute dysuria: a decision-analysis model of alternative strategies. *Ann Intern Med* 1985;102:244.
98. Stamm WE, Hooton TM. Management of urinary tract infections in adults. *N Engl J Med* 1993;329:1328.
99. Stamm WE. When should we use urine cultures? *Infect Control* 1986;7:431.
100. Kunin CM. *Detection, prevention and management of urinary tract infections*, 4th ed. Philadelphia: Lea & Febiger, 1987.
101. Bailey RR. Single-dose therapy for uncomplicated urinary tract infections. *NZ Med J* 1985;98:327.
102. Sheehan G, Harding GKM, Ronald AR. Advances in the treatment of urinary tract infection. *Am J Med* 1984;76:141.
103. Finn SD. Single-dose antimicrobial therapy for urinary tract infections: "Less is more"? or "Reductio ad absurdum"? (editorial). *J Gen Intern Med* 1986;1:62.
104. Philbrick JT, Bracikowski JP. Single-dose antibiotic treatment for uncomplicated urinary tract infections. *Arch Intern Med* 1985;145:1672.
105. Glauser MP, Lyons JM, Braude AI. Prevention of pyelonephritis due to *Escherichia coli* in rats with gentamicin stored in kidney tissue. *J Infect Dis* 1979;139:172.
106. Warren JW, Abrutyn E, Hebel JR, Johnson JR, Schaeffer AJ, Stamm WE. Guidelines for antimicrobial treatment of uncomplicated acute bacterial cystitis and acute pyelonephritis in women. *Clin Infect Dis* 1999;29:745–758.
107. Gupta K, Scholes D, Stamm WE. Increasing prevalence of antimicrobial resistance among uropathogens causing acute uncomplicated cystitis in women. *JAMA* 1999;218:736–738.
108. Gupta K, Hooton TM, Stamm WE. Increasing antimicrobial resistance and the management of uncomplicated community-acquired urinary tract infections. *Ann Intern Med* 2001;135:41–50.

109. Patton JP, Nash DB Abrutyn E. Urinary tract infections: cost considerations. *Med Clin North Am* 1991;75:495.
110. Ronald AR. Optimal duration of treatment for kidney infection (editorial). *Ann Intern Med* 1987;106:467.
111. Bailey RR, Peddie BA. Treatment of acute urinary tract infection in women (letter). *Ann Intern Med* 1987;107:430.
112. Jernelius H, Zbomik J, Bauer C. One or three week treatment of acute pyelonephritis. A double-blind comparison using a fixed combination of pivampicillin plus pivmecillinam. *Acta Med Scand* 1988;223:469.
113. Talan DA, Stamm WE, Hooton TM, et al. Comparison of ciprofloxacin (7 days) and trimethoprim-sulfamethoxazole (14 days) for acute uncomplicated pyelonephritis in women—a randomized trial. *JAMA* 2000;283:1583–1590.
114. Kaitz AL, Hodder EW. Bacteriuria and pyelonephritis of pregnancy: a prospective study of 616 women. *N Engl J Med* 1961;265:667.
115. Nicolle LE, Mayhew WJ, Bryan C. Prospective randomized comparison of therapy and no therapy for asymptomatic bacteriuria in elderly institutionalized women. *Am J Med* 1987;83:27.
116. Wong EW, Stamm WE. Urethral infections in men and women. *Annu Rev Med* 1983;34:337.
117. Dontas AS, Kasviki-Charvati P, Papanayiotou PC. Bacteriuria and survival in old age. *N Engl J Med* 1981;304:939.
118. Kraft JK, Stamey TA. The natural history of symptomatic recurrent bacteriuria in women. *Medicine (Baltimore)* 1947;56:55.
119. Stamm WE, Counts GW, Wagner KF, et al. Antimicrobial prophylaxis of recurrent urinary tract infection. *Ann Intern Med* 1980;92:770.
120. Gupta K, Hooton TM, Roberts PL, Stamm WE. Patient-initiated treatment of uncomplicated recurrent urinary tract infection in young women. *Ann Intern Med* 2001;135:9–16.
121. Stapleton A, Latham R, Johnson C, Stamm WE. Post-coital antimicrobial prophylaxis for recurrent urinary tract infection: a randomized, double-blind, placebo-controlled trial. *JAMA* 1990;264:703.
122. Stamm WE. Prevention of urinary tract infections. *Am J Med* 1984;76[Suppl 5A]:148.
123. Stamm WE, Counts GW, McKevitt M, et al. Urinary prophylaxis with trimethoprim and trimethoprim-sulfamethoxazole—efficacy, influence on the natural history of recurrent bacteriuria, and cost control. *Rev Infect Dis* 1982;4:450.
124. Romano JM, Kaye D. UTI in the elderly: common yet atypical. *Geriatrics* 1981;36:113.
125. Stamey TA, Sexton CC. The role of vaginal colonization with enterobacteriaceae in recurrent urinary tract infections. *J Urol* 1975;113:214.
126. Raz R, Stamm WE. A controlled trial of intravaginal estrogen in postmenopausal women with recurrent urinary tract infection. *N Engl J Med* 1993;329:753.
127. Norden CW, Kass EH. Bacteriuria of pregnancy: a critical appraisal. *Annu Rev Med* 1968;19:431.
128. Kincaid-Smith P. Bacteriuria in pregnancy. *Lancet* 1965;1:395.
129. Vercaigne LM, Zhanel GG. Recommended treatment for urinary tract infection in pregnancy. *Ann Pharmacother* 1994;28:248.
130. Stamm WE, Martin SM, Bennett JV. Epidemiology of nosocomial infections due to gram-negative bacilli: aspects relevant to the use of vaccines. *J Infect Dis* 1977;136[Suppl]:S151.
131. Kreger BE, Craven DE, Carling PC, McCabe WR. Gram-negative bacteriuria. III: Reassessment of aetiology, epidemiology, and ecology in 612 patients. *Am J Med* 1980;68:332.
132. Platt R, Polk BF, Murdock B, Rosner B. Mortality associated with nosocomial urinary tract infection. *N Engl J Med* 1982;307:637.
133. Stamm WE. Catheter-associated urinary tract infections: epidemiology, pathogenesis, and prevention. *Am J Med* 1991;91[Suppl 3B]:3B–65S.
134. Butler HK, Kunin CM. Evaluation of polymyxin catheter lubricant and impregnated catheter. *J Urol* 1968;100:560.
135. Schaeffer AJ, Story KO, Johnson SM. Effect of silver oxide/trichlorolsoganuric acid antimicrobial drainage system on catheter-associated bacteriuria. *J Urol* 1988;139:69.
136. Johnson JR, Roberts PR, Olsen RJ, et al. Prevention of catheter-associated urinary tract infection with a silver oxide-coated urinary catheter: clinical and microbiological correlates. *J Infect Dis* 1990;162:1145.
137. Wong-Beringer A, Jacobs RA, Guglielmo BJ. Treatment of funguria. *JAMA* 1992;267:2780.
138. Sanford JP. The enigma of candiduria: evolution of bladder irrigation with amphotericin B for management-from anecdote to dogma and a lesson from Machiavelli. *Clin Infect Dis* 1993;16:145.

CHAPTER 100
Urethritis, Prostatitis, Epididymitis, and Orchitis

Clayton S. Lau and Grannum R. Sant

URETHRITIS

Inflammations and infections of the urethra are exceedingly common in male and female patients and arise from a wide range of inciting causes. In male patients, urethritis most commonly is caused by sexually transmitted organisms: *Neisseria gonorrhoeae*, *Chlamydia trachomatis*, and *Ureaplasma urealyticum* (1,2). In female patients, urethritis most often presents as the acute urethral syndrome or urethrocystitis, caused by infections with coliforms and *Staphylococcus saprophyticus*, and less often with *C. trachomatis* and *N. gonorrhoeae* (3).

Gonococcal Urethritis in Men

Urethritis, the most common clinical manifestation of gonorrhea in men, typically occurs after an incubation period of 2 to 7 days. It accounts for approximately 35% of urethritis in males. Most patients present with dysuria, frequency, and a purulent yellow urethral discharge, singly or in combination. Approximately 20% to 30% of heterosexual men with symptomatic gonococcal urethritis are also infected with *C. trachomatis* (1). Unless therapy is given concurrently for this organism, these men develop postgonococcal urethritis after single-dose, gonococcus-specific therapy. An estimated 1% to 5% of men with gonococcal urethritis are asymptomatic, do not seek medical attention, and serve as a reservoir, transmitting disease to uninfected sexual partners (1). Furthermore, 40% to 60% of the contacts of partners with known gonorrhea are asymptomatic. Acute epididymitis and urethral strictures are the most common genitourinary tract complications of gonococcal urethritis.

The diagnosis of gonococcal urethritis in symptomatic men is confirmed with about 95% sensitivity and specificity when Gram-stained smears of urethral discharge or a urethral smear disclose gram-negative diplococci within polymorphonuclear leukocytes (1). Absolute confirmation is made by culture of urethral specimens on selective media (e.g., Thayer-Martin medium), incubation in a moist environment in 5% carbon dioxide atmosphere at 34°C to 36°C, and identification of *N. gonorrhoeae* organisms. Antimicrobial susceptibility tests are desirable if available.

THERAPY

The following guidelines for therapy comply with the recommendations of the Center for Disease Control and Prevention (CDC) (4). The following antimicrobials are recommended for the treatment of gonorrhea: cefixime, 400 mg orally as a single dose; ceftriaxone, 250 mg intramuscularly (with local anesthetic) as a single dose; ciprofloxacin, 500 mg orally as single dose; and ofloxacin, 400 mg orally as a single dose.

Because gonorrhea is frequently accompanied by chlamydial infection, an anti-chlamydial therapy should also be added. The following treatments have been successfully applied in *C. trachomatis* infections (5). First choice treatment is usually azithromycin, 1 g orally as a single dose or doxycycline, 100 mg orally twice daily for 7 days. Second-line choices are erythromycin, 500 mg orally four times daily for 7 days; or ofloxacin 200 mg orally twice daily for 7 days.

Doxycycline and azithromycin are considered equally effective in the treatment of chlamydial infections. Erythromycin is less effective and causes more side effects. If therapy fails, one should consider treating infections by *Trichomonas vaginalis* and/or *Mycoplasma* with a combination of metronidazole (2 g orally as single dose) and erythromycin (500 mg four times daily orally for 7 days). As in other STDs, the treatment of sexual partners is necessary.

Non-Gonococcal Urethritis in Men

Non-gonococcal urethritis (NGU), caused mainly by *C. trachomatis* and occasionally by *U. urealyticum*, is the most common form of male urethritis in the United States (1,2). Its incidence is 2.5 times that of gonococcal urethritis. The incubation period is typically 7 to 21 days. The clinical manifestation is dysuria or urethral discharge, or both. The dysuria is variable, often absent, and sometimes associated with urethral itching; the discharge is typically mucoid to watery, white, and is less pronounced and purulent than that of gonorrhea. An estimated 10% of men with NGU are asymptomatic (2).

The diagnosis of NGU is usually established by failure to demonstrate gonococci on Gram stain examination and on culture in a male patient who has four or more polymorphonuclear leukocytes per high-power field at microscopy of a urethral smear or sediment from a 10-mL sample of first-voided urine. Infection caused by *C. trachomatis* can be confirmed by direct immunofluorescence with monoclonal antibodies when this test is available; otherwise, infection caused by *C. trachomatis* or *U. urealyticum* is confirmed only by means of special tissue culture techniques. Potential genitourinary tract complications of NGU include epididymitis and urethral strictures; however, the most serious consequence is the potential transmission of *C. trachomatis* to a female sexual partner, who may develop ascending infection and serious sequelae.

The recommended treatment of NGU is doxycycline, 100 mg by mouth twice daily for 7 days; azithromycin, 1 g orally once; or ofloxacin, 400 mg orally twice daily for 7 days. Whenever possible, sexual partners should be treated simultaneously.

PROSTATITIS

Prostatitis is the most common urologic diagnosis in men younger than 50 years of age, and also the third most common diagnosis in men older than 50. Men with prostatitis represent 8% of urology office visits (6).

For two decades, the traditional classification system of acute and chronic bacterial prostatitis, nonbacterial prostatitis, and prostatodynia has been misleading. Many urologists mistakenly ascribed symptoms to prostate gland disease in patients without any prostatic anomaly, thus many patients were wrongly treating a prostatic infection or inflammation that did not exist. In most cases, the etiology, pathogenesis, and pathophysiology of prostatitis are unknown. However, a few general comments can be made. First, acute bacterial prostatitis, a well-defined infectious disease of the lower urinary tract disease, represents an entirely different disease process from the chronic prostatitis syndromes. The chronic form of the syndrome is caused by possible infectious and noninfectious prostatic inflammation, with the various syndromes poorly demarcated.

In December 1995, The National Institutes of Health (NIH) convened in a consensus conference on prostatitis in Bethesda,

---

TABLE 100.1. National Institutes of Health Classification and Definition of Categories of Prostatitis (1995)

Category I: Acute Bacterial Prostatitis
- Acute infection of the prostate gland

Category II: Chronic Bacterial Prostatitis
- Recurrent urinary tract infection
- Chronic infection of prostate gland

Category III: Chronic Abacterial Prostatitis/Chronic Pelvic Pain Syndrome
- Discomfort or pain in the pelvic region (for at least 3 months) with variable voiding and sexual symptoms
- No demonstrable infection

Category IIIA: Inflammatory Chronic Pelvic Pain Syndrome
- White blood cells in semen/expressed prostatic secretion/VB3

Category IIIB: Noninflammatory Chronic Pelvic Pain Syndrome
- No white blood cells in semen/expressed prostatic secretion/VB3

Category IV: Asymptomatic Inflammatory Prostatitis
- Evidence of inflammation in biopsy, semen/expressed prostatic secretion/VB3
- No symptoms

Data from National Institutes of Health summary statement. Presented at the NIH/NIDDK workshop on chronic prostatitis. National Institutes of Health, Bethesda, MD, December 1995.

Maryland, and created a newer classification system. (Table 100.1) (7,8). Acute bacterial prostatitis (ABP) is associated with UTI, positive cultures localizing the pathogen to the prostatic secretions, and excessive inflammatory cells (leukocytes and macrophages containing fat particles) in the expressed prostatic secretions (EPS). ABP is an abrupt, febrile illness with marked constitutional and genitourinary tract signs and symptoms. Chronic bacterial prostatitis is a less dramatic disorder featuring relapsing recurrent UTI caused by persistence of the pathogen in the prostatic secretory system despite courses of antibacterial therapy. Patients with inflammatory CPPS, in contrast, have excessive numbers of inflammatory cells in their EPS despite a typically negative history of documented UTI and negative results of urinary and prostatic fluid cultures. Here no infectious organism can be localized. Patients with noninflammatory CPPS have symptoms that suggest prostatitis but have no history of UTI and normal EPS by microscopy and culture.

Etiology and Pathogenesis

The pathogens in bacterial prostatitis are similar in type and distribution to those that cause UTIs: strains of *Escherichia coli* predominate; however, infections caused by other Enterobacteriaceae and *Pseudomonas* species also occur (8).

Among the patients who have documented CBP, about 82% are infected with a single pathogen and the remainder by two or more pathogens (7,8). The role of gram-positive bacteria as agents of prostatitis is controversial. Enterococci do cause bacterial prostatitis and associated recurrent enterococcal bacteriuria. The causative role in prostatitis of other gram-positive bacteria (e.g., coagulase-negative staphylococci, micrococci, non-group D streptococci, diphtheroids) is doubtful. These organisms are not reproducibly localized to the prostate and do not cause relapsing recurrent UTI as do gram-negative pathogens and enterococci (7). These non-enterococcal gram-positive bacteria may represent colonization of the prostate gland rather than infection (8).

Possible routes of bacterial infection of the prostate include (a) ascending urethral infection, (b) reflux of infected urine into prostatic ducts that empty into the posterior urethra, (c) invasion by rectal bacteria by direct extension or lymphatic spread, and (d) hematogenous infection. Some men probably develop bacterial prostatitis because of ascending urethral infection resulting from urethral inoculation during sexual relations (9).

Urine commonly refluxes into prostatic ducts and intraprostatic urinary reflux probably is an important route for introducing bacteria into the prostate gland (9,10). Moreover, high-grade intraprostatic urinary reflux with sterile urine may be the cause of nonbacterial, "chemical" forms of prostatitis (11).

Diagnosis

GENERAL LABORATORY FINDINGS

Prostatic massage for microscopy and culture of the EPS aids in the diagnosis of prostatitis syndromes; however, accurate interpretation is impossible unless the first-voided 10 mL of urine (urethral specimen) and a midstream urine sample (bladder specimen) obtained immediately before prostatic massage are also evaluated. Inflammatory cells and bacteria of non-prostatic origin can easily contaminate the EPS and lead to erroneous conclusions (12). The same concerns apply to isolated microscopy and culture of semen. When urethral and midstream urine specimens show insignificant pyuria, the finding of at least 15 white blood cells per high power field denotes prostatic inflammation (8,12). Another important sign of prostatitis is large numbers of macrophages containing fat droplets in the prostatic secretions (12). Whereas an excessive number of inflammatory cells in the prostatic secretions denotes prostatic inflammation, it does not distinguish bacterial prostatitis from nonbacterial forms.

Bacterial prostatitis is associated with secretory dysfunction of the prostate gland (12). Although most of the physical and chemical characteristics of the prostatic secretions are altered, the most important changes are increased alkalinity of the secretions and depressed levels of zinc. This secretory dysfunction, especially increased alkalinity of the secretions, affects pharmacokinetics, and the depressed zinc level may increase the susceptibility of the prostate to bacterial infection (13). Zinc serves as a potent antibacterial factor against bacterial prostatitis and ascending UTI in men (14). The specificity of these markers in the differential diagnosis of prostatitis syndromes, however, remains undefined.

Bacterial prostatitis quickly leads to the elaboration of pathogen-specific antibody in the serum and especially in the prostatic fluid of patients (15). In patients with ABP cured by antimicrobial therapy, antigen-specific immunoglobulin (Ig) G in both serum and prostatic fluid is elevated at the onset of the infection but declines slowly in the ensuing 6 to 12 months (16). On the other hand, the level of antigen-specific IgA in prostatic fluid rises significantly at the onset of infection and begins to decline only after 12 months, whereas an initial elevation of IgA in the serum disappears after only 1 month.

In patients with CBP that is cured by antimicrobial therapy, levels of antigen-specific IgA and IgG in prostatic fluid are elevated at the onset of treatment but begin to decline slowly to normal levels-IgG after about 6 months and IgA not until about 24 months. Patients with CBP that is not cured by antimicrobial therapy have persistently elevated levels of antigen-specific IgG and IgA in prostatic fluid.

BACTERIOLOGIC LOCALIZATION CULTURES

The clinician can easily and accurately confirm the diagnosis of bacterial prostatitis, especially CBP, by performing bacterial localization cultures. This method, first introduced in 1968 by Meares and Stamey (17) is reliable when carried out properly. Culture specimen of prostatic fluid from a man with CBP often grows small numbers of bacteria. Because CBP is usually a focal tissue infection, no absolute count of bacterial colonies on culture is diagnostic. Instead, the bacterial counts in specimens of

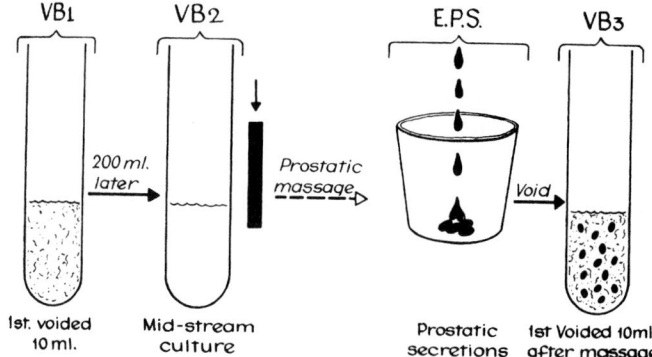

Figure 100.1. Segmented cultures of the lower urinary tract in the male. (From Meares EM, Stamey TA. Bacteriologic localization patterns in bacterial prostatitis and urethritis. *Invest Urol* 1968;5:492–518, with permission.)

urethral and midstream bladder urine and of EPS—all obtained at the same time—must be compared. Both careful collection of segmented specimens and immediate culturing after collection (Fig. 100.1, Table 100.2) and the application of microbiologic techniques capable of quantifying small numbers of bacteria are essential for proper diagnosis.

If the bladder urine is sterile or nearly so, urethral colonization or infection is indicated by a much higher count in the first 10 mL of urine that is passed (VB₁) than in either the EPS or the first 10 mL of urine voided after prostatic massage (VB₃). With bacterial prostatitis, the reverse is true. If culture of bladder urine (VB₂) shows heavy bacteriuria, 2 or 3 days' treatment with an antimicrobial agent that is active in urine but not in prostatic tissue (e.g., 500 mg penicillin G by mouth every 6 hours or 100 mg nitrofurantoin by mouth every 8 hours) should be given before segmented specimens are collected. The diagnosis of CBP is best confirmed when the numbers of pathogenic bacteria in the prostatic specimens exceed by at least 10-fold those in the VB₁ and VB₂ specimens. Recently a post massage urine culture has been advocated as a more practical method of obtaining a localization culture (7,8).

Acute Bacterial Prostatitis

ABP is an acute infection of the prostate typically caused by enteric bacteria, mainly coliforms (especially *E. coli*) and *Pseudomonas aeruginosa* (7,8,16). Because the clinical presentation of ABP is well defined, the clinician usually makes the diagnosis without difficulty, although the non-urologist may mistakenly think the patient has acute pyelonephritis. The typical clinical picture is sudden onset of chills; fever; perineal, suprapubic, and low back pain; and symptoms of both irritative and obstructive voiding dysfunction. On examination, the prostate gland is tender, swollen, indurated, and warm. These findings alone are usually sufficient for a presumptive diagnosis of ABP. Acute bacterial epididymitis develops in some patients; some experience transient bacteremia. Other findings are generalized malaise and prostration, arthralgia, myalgia, and acute urinary retention.

Prostatic massage is not recommended, however, because it is painful for the patient and may lead to bacteremia. Because bacteriuria usually accompanies ABP, the causative agent can usually be identified by culture of voided urine. Patients with ABP usually respond promptly to pathogen specific therapy, even with antimicrobial agents that normally diffuse poorly into prostatic secretions. The intense inflammation of ABP appears to allow drugs that are normally excluded to accumulate at

TABLE 100.2. Segmented Cultures of 15 Men with Chronic Bacterial Prostatitis

Patient	Antibiotic	Colonies per milliliter				Organism
		VB$_1$[a]	VB$_2$[a]	EPS[a]	VB$_3$[a]	
1	Yes	90	0	800	20	*Escherichia coli*
	No	10	0	1,000	20	*E. coli*
2	Yes	0	0	1,000	0	*Enterococcus*
3	Yes	20	0	4,000	10	*Enterococcus*
	Yes	50	0	165	150	*E. coli*
		0	0	50	20	*Enterobacter aerogenes*
		0	0	560	50	*Proteus mirabilis*
		0	0	140	0	*Proteus morganii*
	Yes	0	0	660	190	*E. coli*
		10	0	400	40	*E. aerogenes*
		0	0	500	20	*P. mirabilis*
4		0	0	200	0	*P. morganii*
	Yes	20	0	5,000	50	*Klebsiella*
	Yes	50	0	100,000	1,000	*Klebsiella*
5	No	60	0	1,000	20	*E. coli*
	No	640	40	100,000	220	*E. coli*
6	Yes	0	0	5,000	100	*E. coli*
	Yes	50	10	10,000	1,500	*E. coli*
7	Yes	120	0	3,600	370	*E. coli*
	No	2,000	200	100,000	4,000	*E. coli*
8	Yes	250	20	5,000	330	*Klebsiella*
	No	0	0	50	0	*Klebsiella*
	No	20	0	10,000	2,000	*Klebsiella*
9	Yes	10,000	150	100,000	10,000	*E. coli*
	Yes	110	0	1,500	810	*E. coli*
10	No	2,000	60	4,000	250	*Enterococcus*
	No	600	60	4,000	2,000	*Enterococcus*
	No	260	20	7,200	90	*Enterococcus*
	Yes	20	20	500	30	*Enterococcus*
11	Yes	30	0	10,000	—	*E. coli*
	Yes	0	0	3,600	—	*E. coli*
12	Yes	800	20	—	5,000	*E. coli*
	Yes	10,000	800	100,000	10,000	*E. coli*
13	No	0	0	10,000	600	*E. coli*
	Yes	0	0	7,000	10	*E. coli*
	Yes	0	0	4,000	120	*E. coli*
14	Yes	0	0	700	200	*P. mirabilis*
	Yes	30	0	1,000	10	*P. mirabilis*
15	Yes	2,500	300	20,000	10,000	*Pseudomonas*
	Yes	110	70	30,000	750	*Pseudomonas*

[a]VB$_1$, First 10 mL of urine voided (urethral culture); VB$_2$, midstream aliquot (bladder culture); EPS expressed prostatic secretions from prostatic (prostatic culture), VB$_3$, first 10 mL of urine voided immediately after prostatic massage (prostatic culture).
From Meares EM Jr. Prostatitis and related disorders. In Walsh PC, Retik AB, Stamey TA, Vaughan ED Jr, eds: *Campbell's urology,* 6th ed. Philadelphia: WB Saunders, 1986:807–822; with permission.

therapeutic levels in the prostatic secretory system, interstitium, and stroma. Hospitalization may be necessary for patients who develop acute urinary retention or who need parenteral antimicrobial therapy.

Pathogen-specific antimicrobial therapy should be administered when the infecting organism can be identified by culture and sensitivity tests. While these results are pending, empirical therapy is indicated. APB can be a serious infection with fever, intense local pain and general symptoms. Parenteral administration of high doses of bactericidal antibiotics, such as aminoglycosides, a broad-spectrum penicillin derivative or a third-generation cephalosporin, are required until defeverescence and the normalization of infection parameters. In less severe cases, a fluoroquinolone may be given orally for 10 days. For parenteral therapy, excellent choices are Ciprofloxacin 400 mg every 12 hours, TMP-SMX, 8 to 10 mg/kg body weight (based on the TMP component) in two to four divided doses every 6, 8, or 12 hours intravenously, or gentamicin plus ampicillin (1 mg/kg gentamicin intravenously every 8 hours; 2 g ampicillin intra-

venously every 6 hours). If the clinical response and results of susceptibility tests are favorable, therapy should be continued at full dosage for a minimum of 30 days to prevent the development of CBP. Patients receiving parenteral therapy can usually be switched to a suitable oral agent within 1 week or as early as 48 hours after the fever subsides. Adjunctive therapy includes adequate hydration, analgesics, antipyretics, and stool softeners. Acute urinary retention is best managed by placing a punch suprapubic catheter under local anesthesia. Transurethral catheterization or instrumentation should be avoided.

With proper management, most patients with ABP are cured. Careful follow-up is indicated, however, because persistent infection of the prostate may develop. Another potential complication of ABP is prostatic abscess. Because prostatic abscess is seldom cured by antimicrobial therapy alone, a suspected abscess should be confirmed by means of transrectal ultrasonography or pelvic computed tomography. In addition to antimicrobial therapy, surgical or percutaneous drainage of the abscess is usually necessary (18).

Chronic Bacterial Prostatitis

CBP has variable clinical features, many patients having no history of a preceding bout of ABP. Some men are asymptomatic and are found to have CBP only when bacteriuria is discovered incidentally. Most patients, however, complain of mild to moderate symptoms of irritative voiding dysfunction: urinary urgency, frequency, nocturia, and dysuria. Many patients complain of pain and discomfort in the low back and in the perineal, suprapubic, penile, scrotal, or groin areas. Some patients have hemospermia and postejaculatory discomfort, but chills and fever are unusual unless ABP evolves. Single or recurrent bouts of bacterial epididymitis occasionally develop. Rectal palpation of the prostate reveals nothing specific: the prostate may feel normal, variably indurated, tender, or boggy. The most characteristic feature of CBP is its unique role in causing relapsing, recurrent UTIs (8,12,16). Because in patients with CBP most antimicrobial agents accumulate poorly in the prostatic secretory system (where the bacteria reside), these bacteria persist unaltered within the prostate gland during treatment. Therapy may sterilize the urine and resolve the symptoms, but after the patient stops the medication, the prostatic pathogen typically reinfects the urine and the symptoms of CBP recur (8,12).

Prostatic calculi develop in post pubertal men with astonishing frequency. Transrectal ultrasonography indicates that prostatic stones are detected in about 75% of middle-aged men and in about 100% of elderly men (19). Furthermore, ultrasonography demonstrates prostatic stones in about 70% of men who have no other radiographic signs of prostatic stones. Calculi within the prostate typically are not infected and cause no symptoms or harm, provided they remain confined to the prostate. In certain men with prostatic stones and relapsing, recurrent UTIs, however, the stones have proved to be infected and are the source of the relapsing UTIs (20,21).

In chronic bacterial prostatitis (CBP) and CPPS, a fluoroquinolone or TMP-SMX should be given orally for 2 weeks after the initial diagnosis (7,8). The patient should then be re-assessed and antibiotics continued only if pre-treatment cultures were positive or if the patient reports a positive effect of the treatment in terms of pain relief. A total treatment period of 4 to 6 weeks is then recommended.

Several antimicrobial agents are effective in the treatment of CBP, but the fluoroquinolones have demonstrated the best cure rates (7). The fluoroquinolones have favorable pharmacokinetics, excellent prostatic penetration, good bioavailability and good activity against the common causes of bacterial prostatitis (8,22,23). Most studies with trimethoprim-sulfamethoxazole show efficacy rates between 30% and 50% (13). Despite this, the most commonly used antimicrobial agent used for CP is trimethoprim-sulfamethoxazole (40). Other agents with reported efficacy in selected cases of CBP are carbenicillin indanyl sodium, erythromycin, minocycline, doxycycline, and cephalexin (13). The recommended dosage in CBP is ciprofloxacin 500 mg or ofloxacin, 300 or 400 mg orally twice daily for a minimum of 30 days. Trimethoprim-sulfamethoxazole has no activity against *Pseudomonas*, certain *Enterococci* and some *Enterobacteriaceae* (8).

Patients who are not cured by medical therapy generally can be managed satisfactorily with long-term suppressive therapy using low-dose medication (8,12,13). Three preferred regimens are ciprofloxacin 500 mg by mouth daily, TMP-SMX, one single-strength tablet (80 mg TMP, 400 mg SMX) by mouth daily; or nitrofurantoin, 100 mg once or twice daily by mouth. Patients who cannot be treated satisfactorily by medical therapy should be further evaluated by transrectal ultrasound to rule out infected prostatic calculi or prostatic abscess, and potentially receive endoscopic management (24).

Chronic Prostatitis/Chronic Pelvic Pain Syndrome

This subgroup of syndromes constitutes the majority (90%–95%) of patients with prostatitis seen in clinical practice (7,8). Furthermore, they are the most difficult to manage. The presenting symptoms between the two are indistinguishable, with the predominant symptom being pain localized to the perineum, suprapubic area, penis, testis, or groin. In addition, they may have variable irritative and obstructive voiding symptoms, including urgency, frequency, hesitancy, and intermittency (25).

A lower urinary tract evaluation should be done to rule out uropathogens, and microscopy of post prostatic massage urine sediment to differentiate inflammatory form noninflammatory CPPS. Because large multicenter randomized placebo-controlled trials are not available, best-evidence medicine would suggest antibiotic therapy in those with inflammatory CPPS, α-adrenergic blocking agent for those with voiding symptoms, and anti-inflammatory agents (7,8). In addition, prostatic massage, myofascial trigger point release, and biofeedback should be considered (8).

Those with significant voiding symptoms should be evaluated for interstitial cystitis, because they may be misdiagnosed with CPPS. These two conditions may be the same syndrome (26).

EPIDIDYMITIS

Etiology and Pathogenesis

Inflammation of the epididymis is sometimes the result of trauma or chemical irritation associated with reflux of sterile urine from the urethra through the vas deferens. Most cases of acute epididymitis, however, are infections that can be divided into (a) a sexually transmitted type associated with urethritis and usually caused by *C. trachomatis*, *N. gonorrhoeae*, or both; and (b) an essentially non-sexually transmitted type associated with UTI and prostatitis caused mainly by *Enterobacteriaceae* or *Pseudomonas* species (27,28).

Ascending infection from the urethra, prostate, or bladder urine appears to cause most cases of infectious epididymitis. Infected urine or secretions are thought to enter the ejaculatory ducts by reflux or direct extension and ascend the vas deferens to colonize and infect the epididymis (27). A congenital abnormality, especially an ectopic ureter draining into the ipsilateral seminal vesicle, should be suspected in cases of recurrent epididymitis in a young boy. Bacteriuric males who undergo genitourinary tract instrumentation, catheterization, or surgery are at high risk for epididymitis.

Clinical Manifestations

Painful swelling of the affected side of the scrotum is the basic manifestation. At the onset, an enlarged, indurated, and tender epididymis can usually be distinguished from the testis; however, within a few hours, the epididymis and testis may seem to become one tender mass. Acute epididymitis is typically a unilateral, febrile illness that is variably associated with a urethral discharge or signs and symptoms of prostatitis or UTI. Rectal examination may suggest an underlying acute bacterial prostatitis. Scrotal ultrasonography helps distinguish acute epididymitis from other conditions such as torsion or neoplasia, especially when an acute reactive hydrocele evolves. Urethral swabs and voided urethral (VB$_1$) and midstream (VB$_2$) specimens should be subjected to a Gram stain and culture for proper diagnosis before treatment is initiated. When sexually transmitted acute epididymitis is suspected, stain and culture for *N. gonorrhoeae* should always be performed. Likewise, attempts should be made to test for *Chlamydia* as the pathogen.

Non–Sexually Transmitted Acute Epididymitis

Non-venereal acute epididymitis occurs mainly in middle-aged and older men and is usually caused by coliform bacteria or *Pseudomonas* organisms (27,28). When the infecting organism can be identified, prompt initiation of pathogen-specific antimicrobial therapy is indicated. Severe cases may require hospitalization and the administration of parenteral antibiotics (e.g., an aminoglycoside plus ampicillin, cephalosporin, fluoroquinolone, or piperacillin/tazobactam); less severe cases may be treated at home with oral antimicrobial agents. Especially when an underlying bacterial prostatitis is suspected, our preference is to prescribe ciprofloxacin, 500 mg twice by mouth for 4 weeks, or TMP SMX, one double-strength tablet (160 mg TMP, 800 mg SMX) twice daily for 4 weeks, or ofloxacin, 400 mg twice daily by mouth for 4 weeks. When parenteral therapy is used initially, after about 1 week, a suitable oral agent should be given instead and continued for 3 weeks. Some clinicians recommend short courses of therapy (about 10 days); however, like bacterial prostatitis, acute epididymitis is a tissue infection that is likely to relapse if the duration of therapy is insufficient.

Sexually Transmitted Acute Epididymitis

Sexually transmitted acute epididymitis usually occurs before age 35 years, in association with urethritis in men who have no underlying genitourinary tract abnormalities (27,28). Absence of gram-negative rods or intracellular diplococci or positive cultures are diagnostic for infection by *N. gonorrhoeae*. When available, urethral cultures or immunologic tests should be used to identify *C. trachomatis*; otherwise, chlamydial infection is assumed by exclusion.

Preferred therapy consists of ceftriaxone 250 mg IM once and doxycycline 100 mg by mouth twice daily for 10 days. Alternatively, ofloxacin, 400 mg by mouth once, followed by a 10-day regimen of 300 mg by mouth twice daily for 10 days may be given.

ORCHITIS

Orchitis, a relatively uncommon inflammation of the testicle, is usually the result of a bloodborne viral infection. The leading cause of viral orchitis is mumps, which rarely causes orchitis in prepubertal males but involves one or both testes in 20% to 30% of post-pubertal males (29). Orchitis, unilateral in about two thirds of cases, usually follows the onset of the parotitis by a 4 to 6 days. The clinical course varies considerably. Some patients have only slight testicular swelling and tenderness and minimal constitutional signs; others experience severe testicular swelling and pain with high fever and marked constitutional signs. The illness may last only 4 to 5 days in mild cases but up to 4 weeks in severe cases. Post infectious atrophy occurs in about 50% of involved testes; patients with marked bilateral atrophy may become infertile. Because no antiviral agent is currently available to treat the mumps virus specifically, only supportive therapy can be given. This includes bedrest, scrotal elevation, and analgesics.

Pyogenic orchitis is usually a result of contiguous spread of a bacterial infection originating in the ipsilateral epididymis, but it may also result from rickettsial or parasitic infections (27). The responsible pathogens are usually coliforms or *Pseudomonas*, al-

though strains of staphylococci or streptococci are occasionally involved. Affected patients usually have fever and marked pain and swelling of the affected testes. Parenteral antimicrobial therapy, specific for the pathogen when possible, should be administered. Orchiectomy may be needed if an abscess or testicular infarction develops.

Granulomatous orchitis is rare but is sometimes seen in patients who have actinomycosis or a systemic fungal disease, such as blastomycosis, histoplasmosis, and coccidioidomycosis. Tuberculous orchitis and syphilitic orchitis are seldom seen today. Anti-infective agents that are appropriate for the underlying disease are indicated in therapy.

Testicular trauma or torsion of the spermatic cord may lead to marked swelling and progressive ischemia of the testis with resultant noninfectious orchitis. Scrotal ultrasonography and Doppler blood flow studies may assist in diagnosis, but surgical exploration is often necessary.

REFERENCES

1. Dallabetta G, Hook EW III. Gonococcal infections. *Infect Dis Clin North Am* 1987;1:25.
2. Hooton TM, Barnes RC. Urethritis in men. *Infect Dis Clin North Am* 1987;1:165.
3. Stamm WE, Counts GW, Running KR, et al. Diagnosis of coliform infection in acutely dysuric women. *N Engl J Med* 1982;307:463.
4. Center for Disease Control and Prevention. 1998 Guidelines for treatment of sexually transmitted diseases. *MMWR* 1998;47:1–111.
5. Weber JT, Johnson RE. New treatments for *Chlamydia trachomatis* genital infection. *Clin Infect Dis* 1995;20[Suppl 1]:S66.
6. McNaughton-Collins M, Stafford RS, O' Leary MP, Barry MJ. How common is prostatitis? A national survey of physician visits. *J Urol* 1998;159:1224–1228.
7. Schaeffer AJ. Prostatitis: U.S. perspective. *Int J Antimicrob Agents* 1999;11:205.
8. Nickel JC. Prostatitis: evolving management strategies. *Urol Clin North Am* 1999b;26:743–751.
9. Blacklock NJ. Anatomical factors in prostatitis. *Br J Urol* 1974;46:47.
10. Meares EM Jr, Barbalias GA. Prostatitis: bacterial, nonbacterial and prostatodynia. *Semin Urol* 1983;1:146.
11. Kirby RS, Lowe D, Bultitude MI, et al. Intraprostatic urinary reflux: an aetiological factor in abacterial prostatitis. *Br J Urol* 1982;54:729.
12. Meares EM Jr. Prostatitis syndromes: new perspectives about woes. *J Urol* 1980;123:141.
13. Meares EM Jr. Prostatitis: review of pharmacokinetics and therapy. *Rev Infect Dis* 1982;4:475.
14. Fair WR, Couch J, Wehner N. Prostatic antibacterial factor: identity and significance. *Urology* 1976;7:169.
15. Shortliffe LMD, Wehner N, Stamey TA. The defection of a local prostatic immunologic response to bacterial prostatitis. *J Urol* 1981;125:509.
16. Meares EM Jr. Prostatitis and related disorders. In Walsh PC, Gittes RF, Perlmutter AD, Stamey TA, eds: *Campbell's urology*, 5th ed. Philadelphia: WB Saunders, 1986:868–887.
17. Meares EM, Stamey TA. Bacteriologic localization patterns in bacterial prostatitis and urethritis. *Invest Urol* 1968;5:492.
18. Meares EM Jr. Prostatic abscess (editorial). *J Urol* 1986;136:1281.
19. Peeling WB, Griffiths GJ. Imaging of the prostate by ultrasound. *J Urol* 1984;132:217.
20. Meares EM Jr. Infection stones of the prostate gland. Laboratory diagnosis and clinical management. *Urology* 1974;4:560.
21. Eykyn S, Bultitude MI, Mayo ME, et al. Prostatic calculi as a source of recurrent bacteriuria in the male. *Br J Urol* 1974;46:527.
22. Larsen EH, Gasser TC, Dorflinger T, et al. The concentration of various quinolone derivatives in the human prostate. In Weidner W, Brunner H, Krause W, Rothauge CF, eds: *Therapy of prostatitis*. Munich: W Zuckschwerdt Verlag, 1986:35–39.
23. Naber KG. Use of quinolones in urinary tract infection and prostatitis. *Rev Infect Dis* 1989;11[Suppl 5]:S1321.
24. Meares EM Jr. Chronic bacterial prostatitis: role of transurethral prostatectomy (TURP) in therapy. In Weidner W, Brunner H, Krause W, Rothauge CF, eds: *Therapy of prostatitis*. Munich: W Zuckschwerdt Verlag, 1986:193–197.
25. Barbalias GA, Meares EM Jr, Sant GR. Prostatodynia: clinical and urodynamic characteristics. *J Urol* 1983;130:514.
26. Sant GR, Nickel JC. Interstitial cystitis and chronic prostatitis: the same syndrome? In Nickel JC, ed: *Textbook of prostatitis*. Oxford, UK: ISIS Medical Media, 1999:169–176.
27. Krieger JN. Epididymitis, orchitis, and related conditions. *Sex Transm Dis* 1984;11:173.
28. Berger RE. Urethritis and epididymitis. *Semin Urol* 1983;1:138.
29. Beard CM, Benson RC, Kelalis PP, et al. The incidence and outcome of mumps orchitis in Rochester, Minnesota, 1935 to 1974. *Mayo Clin Proc* 1977;52:3.

CHAPTER 101
Renal Abscess

Clayton S. Lau and Grannum R. Sant

INTRARENAL ABSCESS

Renal Cortical Abscess

ETIOLOGY AND PATHOGENESIS

Most renal cortical abscesses, or renal carbuncles, develop from hematogenous spread of *Staphylococcus aureus* (90% of cases) infection at distant sites, most often skin lesions (1). Intravenous (IV) drug abuse, diabetes mellitus, immunosuppression, and hemodialysis are predisposing factors (2,3). In contrast to other intrarenal abscesses, renal cortical abscesses rarely result from ascending infection (2,3). Initially microabscesses develop and then enlarge and coalesce to form a fluid-filled mass with a thick wall. This cortical abscess can eventually rupture through the renal capsule to form a perinephric abscess. Most renal carbuncles are unilateral (97%), solitary lesions (77%); 63% affect the right kidney (2,3).

CLINICAL FEATURES

Renal carbuncles most often develop in patients who are 20 to 50 years old, with men affected three times more often than women (2,3). Chills, fever, and localized costovertebral angle tenderness are typical clinical features. Early in the course of this condition when the abscess does not communicate with the collecting system, there are no urinary symptoms. Physical examination may disclose a flank mass or loin bulge with loss of lumbar lordosis.

Blood count typically reveals a moderate-to-marked leukocytosis, mainly neutrophils with many bands. When there is no communication between the cortical abscess and the collecting system, urinalysis is usually normal and urine culture negative. Blood culture results are often negative.

DIAGNOSIS

Imaging studies are essential for identifying the renal cortical abscess and for a differential diagnosis. Results of excretory urography are nonspecific and seldom contribute to diagnosis. Radionuclide scanning using gallium citrate (Ga 67) and indium 111–labeled white blood cells may assist in diagnosis, but certain conditions, such as renal cell carcinoma, ureteral obstruction, and severe nonsuppurative pyelonephritis, can produce false-positive findings (2,5). Ultrasonography (US) can readily confirm a renal abscess, especially after the microabscesses coalesce to form a fluid-filled, thick-walled mass. Unfortunately, the US appearance of a renal abscess in its early stages may be mistaken for a renal neoplasm (5,6). Renal arteriography often fails to differentiate a renal abscess from a hypovascular or cystic renal neoplasm. Computed tomography (CT), with or without use of contrast agents, is the most accurate diagnostic imaging modality for identifying renal abscess (5–7) (Fig. 101.1). Aspiration of the abscess under US or CT guidance not only assists in diagnosis and identification of the causative agent but also establishes a site for therapeutic drainage.

TREATMENT

The traditional mainstays of therapy have been the administration of appropriate antimicrobial agents and percutaneous or surgical drainage (1–3). However, renal cortical abscesses, partic-

ularly those caused by *S. aureus*, have been treated successfully with antimicrobial agents alone (2,3). Recommended antistaphylococcal agents are oxacillin and nafcillin; either drug is given in IV doses of 100 to 200 mg/kg per day every 4 hours. Alternative therapy might be ampicillin/sulbactam, 1.5 to 3 g IV every 4 hours or vancomycin 500 mg to 2 g daily divided in three doses IV. Parenteral therapy is continued for 10 to 14 days and followed by oral antistaphylococcal therapy for another 14 to 28 days.

If no favorable clinical response (relief of pain, reduction of fever) is evident after 48 hours' therapy, the clinician should suspect a resistant pathogen or complicating factors, such as a perinephric abscess. In such cases, an attempt at aspiration and drainage by placing an appropriate percutaneous catheter with use of US or CT guidance is indicated (3,5,6,8). If this proves unsuccessful, open surgical drainage is necessary. Nephrectomy is rarely needed.

Renal Corticomedullary Abscess

ETIOLOGY AND PATHOGENESIS

Renal corticomedullary abscesses generally evolve from an underlying urinary tract abnormality, such as an obstruction or a vesicoureteral reflux (2,3,9). Whereas staphylococcal infections most often are responsible for renal carbuncles, coliform bacteria, especially strains of *Escherichia coli, Klebsiella, Proteus,* and *Pseudomonas* are the common causative pathogens for corticomedullary abscesses (1,2).

Several types of severe acute and chronic infectious processes are related to or associated with corticomedullary abscesses. Acute focal bacterial nephritis, also called acute lobar nephronia or focal pyelonephritis, is a severe acute parenchymal infection without liquefaction (3,5,10). The infection is thought to be limited to the lobes affected by intrarenal reflux. That this solid inflammatory mass, if untreated, may eventually liquefy and become a corticomedullary abscess is an interesting postulate.

Xanthogranulomatous pyelonephritis (XPG) is a rare but important severe chronic renal inflammatory disease, which

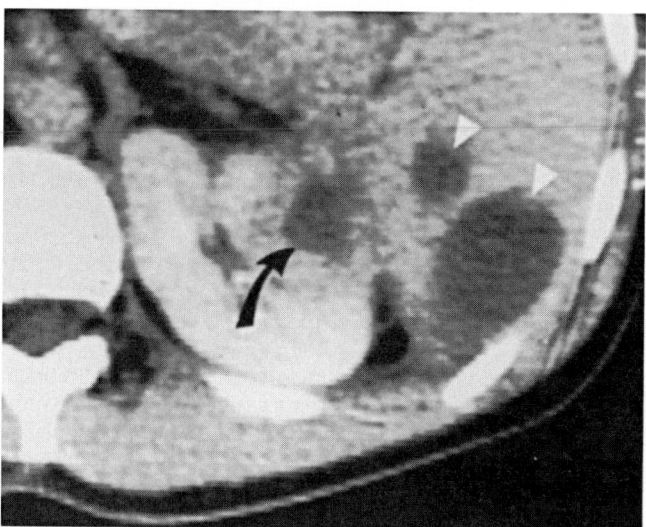

Figure 101.1. Renal cortical abscess and splenic abscesses in a 35-year-old woman with hematogenous spread of a *Staphylococcus aureus* skin infection. Computed tomography after intravenous injection of contrast material shows a cystic lesion in the left kidney with a low-density center and enhancing thick wall (*curved arrow*) and two similar lesions in the spleen (*arrowheads*).

typically results in diffuse renal destruction. Most cases are unilateral, and result in a nonfunctioning, enlarged kidney associated with obstructive uropathy secondary to nephrolithiasis. *Proteus* is the most common organism cultured (17). The typical histologic changes of xanthogranulomatous pyelonephritis include severe acute and chronic inflammation plus characteristic xanthoma cells, which are macrophages containing phagocytosed cholesterol and lipid materials (1,2,11). By radiographic studies, it is often misdiagnosed as a renal tumor. If a malignant tumor can't be excluded, nephrectomy should be performed. If incision and drainage is performed rather than nephrectomy, the patient may continue to experience symptoms and a renal cutaneous fistula may develop.

In adults, most corticomedullary abscesses are associated with renal calculi, obstructive uropathy, and damaged kidneys whereas in children, they are generally associated with vesicoureteral reflux (2,9). Another important predisposing condition, especially in adults, is diabetes mellitus (1,2). Aerobic, gram-negative bacilli are the usual pathogens in all age groups (1–3). An initial infection of the renal medulla, subsequent liquefaction, and eventual involvement of the renal cortex apparently constitute the pathogenic process of a corticomedullary abscess. Inadequately treated intrarenal abscesses may eventually perforate the renal capsule to form a perinephric abscess.

Most renal corticomedullary abscesses occur as a result of ascending urinary tract infection in patients who have a predisposing condition, which explains the differences in bacterial pathogens and anatomic location between corticomedullary abscesses and staphylococcal cortical abscesses.

CLINICAL FEATURES

The incidence of corticomedullary abscesses is similar in men and women but rises with advancing age (2,3). Chills, fever, and loin or abdominal pain are prominent features. Dysuria and other urinary tract symptoms are variably present. Nausea and vomiting affect about 65% of patients, often causing the clinician to suspect gastrointestinal disease (2,3). Constitutional symptoms (malaise, fatigue, weight loss) occur in patients with chronic disease, especially xanthogranulomatous pyelonephritis and associated abscesses. Physical findings are often nonspecific. Costovertebral angle tenderness and loin or abdominal tenderness are the rule; however, a palpable flank or abdominal mass is an inconsistent finding (2,3).

Because corticomedullary abscesses usually communicate with the collecting system, the findings of urinalysis typically are abnormal and the infecting pathogens (mainly coliforms, less often *Pseudomonas* species, *S. aureus*, and others) generally grow readily in urine culture (1–3). Compared with patients who have renal cortical abscesses, patients with corticomedullary abscesses more often have positive blood culture results. Other laboratory abnormalities include anemia (75%), hypoalbuminemia (60%), and hypergammaglobulinemia (α_1- and α_2-globulin, 79%) (2,3).

DIAGNOSIS

Because the medical history, physical findings, and results of routine laboratory tests are nonspecific, imaging studies, especially CT and US, are imperative for making the diagnosis of corticomedullary abscess. In acute focal bacterial nephritis, the renal US image may appear normal or show a solid hypoechoic mass that is poorly demarcated from adjacent normal parenchyma but deforms the renal contour and obliterates corticomedullary definition (5). Non–contrast-enhanced CT usually fails to demonstrate the lesion. Contrast-enhanced CT, however, usually demonstrates a poorly defined, wedge-

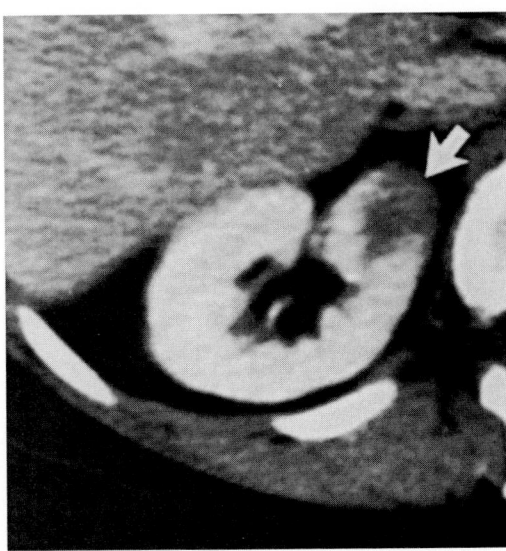

Figure 101.2. CT of acute focal bacterial nephritis (acute lobar nephronia). After injection of contrast agent, the scan demonstrates a poorly marginated, wedge-shaped, hypodense area of renal parenchyma without liquefaction (*arrow*).

shaped, hypodense area without liquefaction (5) (Fig. 101.2). The inflammatory mass may involve one or several renal lobes. The varied radiographic characteristics of xanthogranulomatous pyelonephritis were reviewed in detail by Piccirillo and coworkers (5). An obstructed, poorly functioning or nonfunctioning kidney containing calculi is a characteristic finding (Fig. 101.3).

The sonographic appearance of intrarenal abscesses, whether cortical or corticomedullary, is variable: they may lack internal echoes (mimicking cysts or calyceal diverticula), appear highly reflective (simulating neoplasms), or may contain sparse, low-density echoes (5,6). CT, with or without the use of IV contrast material, is the most definitive imaging technique for diagnosing intrarenal abscesses. CT shows a low-attenuation (0 to 20 HU), distinctly marginated parenchymal lesion that fails to enhance after IV administration of contrast medium (5,6).

TREATMENT

Experience shows that, like cortical abscesses caused by staphylococci, corticomedullary abscesses caused by coliform bacteria can sometimes be treated with antimicrobial agents alone without drainage (2,3). This is especially true for acute focal bacterial nephritis and often for small lesions with minimal liquefaction that are confined to the renal parenchyma. In addition to intensive antimicrobial therapy, moderate to large unilocular abscesses must usually be drained, preferably by insertion of a percutaneous catheter (6). Multilocular abscesses frequently must be drained by open surgical incision. Patients with xanthogranulomatous pyelonephritis and poorly functioning kidneys usually require nephrectomy.

Initial antibacterial therapy should include a combination of ampicillin, 1 g every 4 to 6 hours, or cefazolin, 1 g every 8 hours, IV, plus an aminoglycoside-gentamicin or tobramycin, 1 mg/kg every 8 hours, IV, adjusting the dose appropriately for decreased renal function. A fluoroquinolone, such as ciprofloxacin or ofloxacin, is a good choice for infection caused by gram-negative bacteria; the drug can be given IV at first, followed by the oral form (12,16). Alternatively, ampicillin/sulbactam and

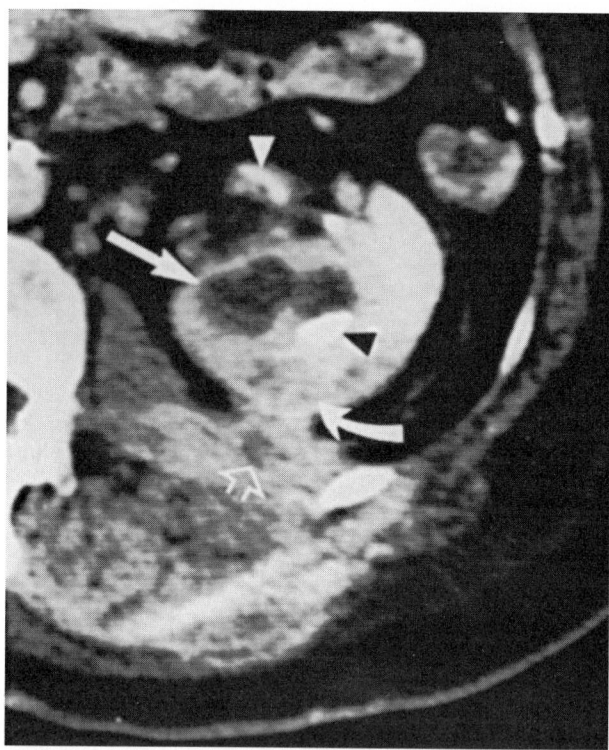

Figure 101.3. Xanthogranulomatous pyelonephritis with suppurative process extending into the perinephric space in a 51-year-old woman. CT of the left kidney after IV injection of contrast material shows calculi (*arrowheads*), hydronephrosis (*straight white arrow*), parenchymal suppuration with liquefaction (*curved white arrow*), and extension of the process through the renal capsule into the perinephric space (perinephric abscess, *short open arrow*).

piperacillin/tazobactam are each appropriate initial antibiotics. Depending on the clinical response and results of culture and sensitivity tests, combination therapy is continued or adjusted appropriately. Parenteral therapy is continued until symptoms abate, fever has resolved for at least 48 hours, and repeated imaging demonstrates a favorable response. A suitable oral antimicrobial agent is eventually given for 2 to 4 weeks, until clinical and radiologic examinations demonstrate complete resolution of the process. Early diagnosis and proper therapy usually ensure a favorable outcome. Isoniazid plus rifampin is indicated for *Mycobacterium tuberculosis* infection, while amphotericin B is necessary for abscesses caused by fungi.

PERINEPHRIC ABSCESS

A perinephric abscess is a collection of suppurative material in the perinephric space and it frequently poses a significant diagnostic challenge even to experienced physicians. Delay in diagnosis may lead to significant mortality and morbidity.

Etiology and Pathogenesis

Perinephric abscesses form mainly as a result of rupture of an intrarenal abscess into the perinephric space, so the agents are the same as those of intrarenal abscesses: *S. aureus* (cortical abscess) and aerobic, gram-negative bacteria, mainly strains of *E. coli*, *Proteus*, and *Klebsiella* (corticomedullary abscess). Other coliforms, *Pseudomonas* species, gram-positive bacteria, and obligate anaerobic bacteria are occasionally involved (1,2,4,14,15). Fungi, especially *Candida* species, and *Mycobacterium tuberculosis* are occasionally responsible. Cultures reveal multiple microbes in about 25% of cases (2). The abscess is usually confined by Gerota's fascia to the perinephric space but may extend throughout the retroperitoneum to affect surrounding structures. Predisposing factors are the same as those involved with intrarenal abscesses.

The most common mechanism for gram-negative bacterial abscess to develop is rupture of a corticomedullary abscess, while staphylococcal infection is due to rupture of a cortical abscess.

Clinical Features

The often insidious nature and confusing clinical presentation of a perinephric abscess make early recognition difficult. Data from reported series indicate that most patients with a perinephric abscess have symptoms for 2 to 3 weeks before they consult a physician (2,4). Depending on the clinical acumen of the physician, the diagnosis of perinephric abscess may be delayed several days longer. Presenting symptoms are nonspecific. The most common symptoms are fever (80%), flank or abdominal pain (40% to 50%), chills (40%), dysuria (40%), weight loss, lethargy, and gastrointestinal symptoms (25%). Pleuritic pain may occur as a result of diaphragmatic irritation. If the abscess in pressing on adjacent nerves, referred pain may be felt in the groin, thighs, or knees.

Fever, the only universal sign, may early on be considered of unknown origin. Pain in the affected flank eventually develops in most patients. Costovertebral angle tenderness and flank tenderness, with or without a palpable loin or abdominal mass, are the most prominent findings at physical examination. The diaphragm on the affected side may be elevated and fixed, with or without an associated ipsilateral pleural effusion. Scoliosis (concavity to the affected side) commonly develops from spasm of the psoas muscle, which may also cause pain on bending away from the affected side, active flexion of the ipsilateral thigh against resistance, or extension of the thigh during ambulation. Likewise, irritation of the psoas muscle or iliohypogastric, ilioinguinal, genitofemoral, or femorocutaneous nerves may refer pain to the ipsilateral hip area. Abdominal tenderness and guarding, suggestive of intraperitoneal disease, sometimes confound the diagnosis. A painful bulge in the loin with overlying erythema and edema of the tissues is a late sign but is suggestive of perinephric abscess.

Routine laboratory test results are variably altered. Blood tests usually show only mild leukocytosis with neutrophilia, an elevated erythrocyte sedimentation rate, and variable anemia. Azotemia is uncommon unless bilateral renal disease is present. Pyuria and proteinuria are often found, but hematuria is not. Approximately 30% of patients have a normal urinalysis result, and about 40% have sterile urine cultures (1,2,4). Blood culture results are positive in only 40% of cases (2).

Diagnosis

A perinephric abscess has an insidious onset and clinical course with highly variable features, often making early recognition difficult. Although uncommon, the classic patient has a cutaneous infection or urinary tract infection that is followed by 1 to 2 weeks by fever and unilateral flank pain. The most important aspect of early diagnosis is a high index of suspicion on the part of the clinician, coupled with the performance of appropriate radiographic imaging studies.

CHEST AND ABDOMINAL RADIOGRAPHY

Chest radiographs are helpful if they show an elevated or fixed hemidiaphragm, pleural effusion, empyema, lung abscess, lower lobe infiltrate or atelectasis, or apical scarring, especially in patients with tuberculous abscesses. Abdominal radiography may demonstrate thoracolumbar scoliosis (concavity toward the affected side), mass effect, renal calculi, poorly visualized or effaced renal outline, poorly visualized or effaced psoas shadows, gas in the renal or perirenal area, and Mathe sign of renal fixation (4). It must be emphasized, however, that none of these findings are specifically diagnostic of a perinephric abscess.

EXCRETORY UROGRAPHY

Excretory urography with tomography demonstrates an abnormality on the affected side in 80% to 85% of cases (4). Findings include variable abnormalities: poor or no visualization of the affected kidney; mass effect; displacement of the kidney, renal pelvis, or ureter; calculi; calicectasis; and obstruction (with or without a calculus). None of these findings is specifically diagnostic of a perinephric abscess.

ULTRASONOGRAPHY AND COMPUTED TOMOGRAPHY

Both CT and US are useful in the diagnosis of perinephric abscess, but CT best demonstrates the full extent of involvement (6,7). Piccirillo and coworkers provided an excellent detailed review of specific US and CT findings in perinephric abscess (5). CT abnormalities include a soft tissue mass of low central attenuation (0 to 20 HU), an inflammatory wall with slightly higher attenuation on noncontrast views, the rind sign (a rim of increased density in the abscess wall after IV injection of contrast medium), obliteration of surrounding tissue planes, ipsilateral enlargement of the kidney or psoas muscle, thickening of Gerota's fascia, and gas or air-fluid level in the lesion (4–6) (see Fig. 101.3). Absolute confirmation and identification of the causative agent or agents are made by percutaneous aspiration of the abscess with use of US or CT guidance.

CT scanning is the diagnostic modality of choice because it is more sensitive and accurate in diagnosis of intra-abdominal abscess (90%) than ultrasonography. It is also more effective in defining the precise location, size, degree, and extent of the abscess. The typical appearance is that of a soft-tissue mass (approximately 20 HU) with a thick wall that may enhance after contrast material administration ("rind" sign).

Ultrasonography is used as a screening tool to exclude obstructive uropathy, urolithiasis and other intraabdominal or retroperitoneal processes. US findings include hypoechoic or nearly anechoic masses, fluid-debris levels, thick irregular abscess wall, and gas. The advantages of US include noninvasiveness, lack of radiation exposure, portability, and accessibility.

Treatment

Although antimicrobial agents are useful to control sepsis and prevent spread of infection, the primary treatment in percutaneous drainage. If the former fails, traditional open surgical drainage, including copious irrigation, débridement, and placement of drains exiting the retroperitoneum is necessary. Nephrectomy is reserved for those renal units that are severely infected or nonfunctional.

Parenteral antimicrobial therapy is initially directed against staphylococci and coliforms, the most likely pathogens, until culture and sensitivity test results are available. The same agents and dosage outlined for treatment of intrarenal abscesses are recommended. Depending on the clinical response and culture and sensitivity results, appropriate changes can be made as indicated. Parenteral, and ultimately oral, antimicrobial therapy is given until clinical and repeated imaging findings indicate resolution of the infectious process.

In the past, owing to errors and delays in diagnosis, the mortality rates for patients with perinephric abscess have ranged from 20% to 57%; up to 34% were diagnosed only at autopsy (2,4,14,15). It is encouraging that Sheinfeld and coworkers reported a series of 15 patients with perinephric abscess, treated at their institution between 1979 and 1983, who had excellent outcomes and no deaths (4). Fowler and Perkins cured all 57 patients who were diagnosed and underwent drainage; in four patients, the abscess escaped detection, contributing to their deaths (7). This emphasizes what can be accomplished by early recognition by means of modern imaging techniques and prompt drainage combined with proper antimicrobial therapy.

Percutaneous drainage of perinephric abscess has a high success rate approaching 80% to 90%. Poor results may occur in fungal abscesses, thick purulent content, multiloculated cavities, and the presence of underlying disease such as diabetes and urinary calculi. Nephrectomy is reserved usually in cases of emphysematous pyelonephritis, diffusely damaged renal parenchyma and in elderly septic patients.

Appropriate antibiotics are give throughout the drainage or perisurgical period and for 1 to 3 weeks thereafter. Follow-up examination with urine culture, CT, or US is done at 1 and 3 months to rule out recurrent infection or abscess formation.

REFERENCES

1. Dembry LM, Andriole VT. Renal and perirenal abscess. *Infect Dis Clin North Am* 1997;11:663.
2. Patterson JE, Andriole VT. Renal and perirenal abscesses. *Infect Dis Clin North Am* 1987;1:907.
3. Andriole VT. Renal and perirenal abscess. In Schrier RW, Gottschalk CW, eds: *Diseases of the kidney,* 4th ed. Boston: Little, Brown, 1987:1049–1064.
4. Sheinfeld J, Erturk E, Spataro RD, et al. Perinephric abscess: current concepts. *J Urol* 1987;137:191.
5. Piccirillo M, Rigsby C, Rosenfield AT. Contemporary imaging of renal inflammatory disease. *Infect Dis Clin North Am* 1987;1:927.
6. Gerzof SG, Gale ME. Computed tomography and ultrasonography for diagnosis and treatment of renal and retroperitoneal abscesses. *Urol Clin North Am* 1982;9:185.
7. Fowler JE Jr, Perkins T. Presentation, diagnosis and treatment of renal abscesses: 1972–1988. *J Urol* 1994;151:847.
8. Gerzof SC, Robbins AH, Johnson WC, et al. Percutaneous catheter drainage of abdominal abscesses. A five-year experience. *N Engl J Med* 1981;305:653.
9. Timmons JW, Perlmutter AD: Renal abscess: a changing concept. *J Urol* 1976;115:229.
10. Nosher JL, Tamminen JL, Amorosa JK, et al. Acute focal bacterial nephritis. *Am J Kidney Dis* 1988;11:36.
11. Malek RS, Elder JS. Xanthogranulomatous pyelonephritis. A critical analysis of 26 cases and of the literature. *J Urol* 1978;119:589.
12. Andriole VT. Use of quinolones in treatment of prostatitis and lower urinary tract infections. *Eur J Clin Microbiol Infect Dis* 1991;10:342.
13. Rubenstein E, Keller N. Fluoroquinolones: present uses. *Infect Dis Clin Pract* 1994;3[Suppl 3]:5195.
14. Salvatierra O Jr, Bucklew WB, Morrow JW. Perinephric abscess: a report of 71 cases. *J Urol* 1967;98:296.
15. Thorley JD, Jones SR, Sanford JP. Perinephric abscess. *Medicine (Baltimore)* 1974;53:41.
16. Siegel JF, Smith A, Moldwin R. Minimally invasive treatment of renal abscess. *J Urol* 1996;155:52.
17. Tolia BM, Newman HR, Fruchtmann B, et al. Xanthogranulomatous pyelonephritis: segmental or generalized disease? *J Urol* 1980;124:122.

Sexually Transmitted Diseases

CHAPTER 102
Approach to the Patient with Sexually Transmitted Disease

Matthew R. Golden and H. Hunter Handsfield

Sexually transmitted diseases (STDs) are among the most common causes of infectious morbidity in the world. Excluding human immunodeficiency virus (HIV), an estimated 12 million new cases of STD occur in the United States annually at a cost of $10 billion (1). In many developing nations, STD excluding HIV is the second greatest cause of disability-adjusted years of life lost (2). Over the past decade, scientific developments, including the discovery of new sexually transmitted pathogens (e.g. human herpes virus-8), the continued emergence of antimicrobial resistance (gonorrhea, chancroid), recognition of the importance of bacterial and viral STD in facilitating HIV transmission (3), and increasing understanding of the incidence and morbidity resulting from viral STD other than HIV have elevated the importance of STD as a public health concern. Social and demographic trends, including increased global travel and trade, urbanization, war and its associated social dislocations, and the declining median age of persons in the developing world ensure that STDs will remain a major health problems in the decades to come.

The recognized spectrum of STDs includes at least 50 distinct clinical syndromes caused by more than 25 pathogenic organisms and viruses. Table 102.1 lists the predominant syndromes and complications of STDs, in the approximate order of their importance to human health, and the pathogens associated with them. In each instance, sexual contact is an important mode of transmission if not the only one. This chapter presents some general principles for clinicians who care for patients who have or are at risk for STDs.

GENERAL PRINCIPLES AND EMERGING TRENDS

STDs exact their greatest health toll on women and their newborn children. Many STDs, including gonorrhea, HIV, chlamydial infection, and genital herpes are transmitted more efficiently from men to women than the reverse, probably because of a greater surface area of exposed skin and mucous membranes and because the vagina serves as a reservoir that prolongs exposure to infectious secretions. Women are more likely than men to have asymptomatic or minimally symptomatic infections early in the clinical course, fostering delays in seeking health care. Diagnosis of STDs is often more difficult in women because the clinical findings are less specific. Finally, with the exception of HIV, infected women are at greater risk than are men for severe or permanent sequelae, such as infertility, ectopic pregnancy, chronic pelvic pain, cancer, and serious consequences for the fetus and

newborn. Thus, the prevention, treatment, and control of most STDs are important primarily to protect and preserve the health of women and their children.

STDs are often asymptomatic. Most gonococcal and chlamydial infections in women are probably either asymptomatic or are associated with mild or nonspecific symptoms that do not prompt women to seek care. While gonorrhea and chlamydial infections in men more frequently cause symptoms, significant reservoirs of asymptomatic infections exist (4). Similarly, the majority of infections with HSV are subclinical, and viral STDs such as HIV, HPV, and HBV typically remain asymptomatic for years following primary infection. Thus, screening tests and partner notification are often the only practical means to identify those who are infected.

The increasing recognition of chronic viral STDs in the past three decades requires fundamental changes in historical clinical and public health approaches to STD. Rising rates of infection with HIV, herpes simplex virus-2 (HSV-2), human herpes virus 8 (HHV8), hepatitis B virus (HBV), the human papillomaviruses (HPV), and cytomegalovirus (CMV) probably reflect both enhanced recognition and true increases in incidence and prevalence (5). Because most viral STDs persist for months or years, these infections achieve high prevalences in virtually all populations, including those in which low partner change rates limit the sustained transmission of the traditional bacterial STDs. Primary care clinicians increasingly require expertise in the management of chronic STD, addressing issues related to the psychosocial impact of disease and the affect of infections on childbearing and future relationships. From a public health perspective, in the absence of new vaccines or curative therapy, primary prevention relies primarily on inducing and sustaining behavior change in the population, although noncurative, suppressive anti-viral therapy may ultimately prove to have a prevention impact for infections such as HSV and HIV (6–8).

Most STDs, including but not limited to those that cause overt genital ulceration, enhance the efficiency of HIV transmission (3). This 'epidemiologic synergy' is thought to reflect enhanced HIV transmissibility among infected persons due to increased HIV replication by inflammatory cells that accumulate at sites of genital infection, and enhanced susceptibility in persons with STD due to breaches in epithelial integrity and the increased presence of immune cells susceptible to HIV infection. For example, recent data suggest that HSV-2 seropositivity in a person sexually exposed to HIV infection may be a more potent determinant of HIV acquisition than plasma viral load in the HIV-infected partner (9).

Two community level randomized trials have assessed the potential impact of interventions to control STD as a means of preventing HIV. The first of these, conducted in Tanzania (10), found that institution of STD clinical services, without specific HIV prevention efforts, resulted in a reduced rate of HIV seroconversion compared with control communities where STD services were not offered. However, a second community level randomized trial in which several villages in rural Uganda were randomly assigned to receive mass STD treatment or vitamins and antihelminthic therapy did not show an impact of STD therapy on HIV incidence (11). The disparity in these findings emphasizes the difficulty in attempting to establish the principle that treating STD can reduce HIV transmission; the impact of interventions focusing on STD will likely vary depending on the prevalence of different STDs and HIV in the populations affected as well as the strength of the intervention itself (12). However, despite uncertainties regarding the impact of STD control as an HIV prevention STD strategy, the preponderance of evidence supports the role of STDs as cofactors enhancing HIV transmission, and in many settings preventing the traditional STDs may be one of

TABLE 102.1.   Sexually Transmitted Pathogens, Copathogens, and Clinical Syndromes[a]

Syndrome	Primary pathogen	Secondary pathogens and copathogens
Acquired immunodeficiency syndrome and related disorders	HIV (types 1 and 2)	Numerous opportunistic pathogens
Neoplasia (squamous cell cancer of cervix, anus, vulva, penis: Kaposi's sarcoma; lymphoma; hepatocellular carcinoma)	Human papillomavirus (types 16, 18, 34, 45, others), HIV, hepatitis B virus, HHV-8	
Acute pelvic inflammatory disease and its primary complications, female infertility, ectopic pregnancy, chronic pelvic pain	*Neisseria gonorrhoeae, Chlamydia trachomatis*	*Mycoplasma hominis, Prevotella* sp., *Peptococcus* sp., *Bacteroides* sp., coliform bacteria, other vaginal flora
Neonatal or perinatal complications (premature delivery, chorioamnionitis, TORCHES syndrome, pneumonia, conjunctivitis, cognitive impairment, immunodeficiency)	*N. gonorrhoeae, C. trachomatis,* CMV, HSV (types 1 and 2), *Treponema pallidum,* group B streptococcus, HIV	*Ureaplasma urealyticum, M. hominis,* vaginal anaerobes
Lower genital tract infections in women		
Mucopurulent cervicitis and urethritis	*C. trachomatis, N. gonorrhoeae,* HSV	*Trichomonas vaginalis*
Vaginitis	*Trichomonas vaginalis, Candida* sp.	Anaerobic vaginal flora, other yeasts
Bacterial vaginosis	Primary pathogen(s) unknown	*Gardnerella vaginalis, M. hominis, Mobiluncus* sp., anaerobic vaginal flora
Anogenital warts	Human papillomaviruses (especially types 6 and 11)	
Viral hepatitis	Hepatitis viruses (A, B, C, D)	
Male urethritis	*N. gonorrhoeae, C. trachomatis, Mycoplasma genitalium, U. urealyticum* (?)	*T. vaginalis,* HSV-1 and HSV-2
Genital ulcer-lymphadenopathy syndromes	*T. pallidum,* HSV-1, HSV-2, *Haemophilus ducreyi, C. trachomatis* (LGV strains), *Calymmatobacterium granulomatis*	Pyogenic bacteria, *Candida* sp., *other fungi*
Arthritis	*N. gonorrhoeae, C. trachomatis,* hepatitis B virus, HIV (?)	*U. urealyticum, M. hominis*
Epididymitis	*C. trachomatis, N. gonorrhoeae*	Genitourinary pathogens
Tertiary syphilis	*T. pallidum*	
Proctitis, proctocolitis	Same as for urethritis, cervicitis	
Enteric infections, enterocolitis	*Shigella* sp., *Giardia lamblia, Entamoeba histolytica, Salmonella, Campylobacter* sp., HIV (?)	
Mononucleosis	CMV, human herpesvirus type 6 (?), Epstein-Barr virus, HIV	
Ectoparasite infestation	*Sarcoptes scabiei* (scabies mite), *Phthirus pubis* (crab louse)	Pyogenic bacteria
Molluscum contagiosum	Molluscum contagiosum virus	

[a] Listed in approximate order of importance to human health.
TORCHES, Toxoplasmosis, rubella, cytomegalovirus, herpes, syphilis; HIV, human immunodeficiency virus; CMV, cytomegalovirus; HSV, herpes simplex virus, LGV, lymphogranuloma venereum.

the most cost-effective approaches to preventing HIV infection (13).

TRANSMISSION DYNAMICS OF SEXUALLY TRANSMITTED DISEASES AND ASSOCIATED EPIDEMIOLOGIC PRINCIPLES

The transmission of an STD through a population can be conceptualized mathematically according to the formula $R_0 = \beta cD$, in which R_0 is the reproductive number of an infection, the average number of secondary cases generated by each primary infection in a population (14). When each case generates an average of one additional case, R_0 is 1.0 and the prevalence remains stable; values below 1.0 and above 1.0 are associated with declining or rising prevalences, respectively. As shown by the formula, the reproductive number is the product of three factors: β, the average probability of transmission per partnership; c the average number of sexual partnerships formed per unit of time; and D the mean duration of infection.

While each of the terms in this equation is complex, this simplification can explain a great deal about the distribution of different STDs in the population and provides a framework for conceptualizing STD epidemiology and prevention. For example, gonorrhea is thought to be efficiently transmitted ($\beta = .5$), but has a relatively short duration of infection, especially in setting where medical care and therapy is readily available (14). Consequently, to maintain $R_0 \geq 1$, c must be relatively high and infection tends to concentrate in a population of highly sexually active persons. In contrast, HSV-2 has a very long duration of infection, $R_0 > 1.0$ even in populations with very low rates of partner change, and genital herpes is widely disseminated throughout the population.

Each term in the equation is affected by different prevention strategies. The efficiency of transmission (β) can be altered by the use of condoms and by altering sexual repertoire to encourage behaviors that are less likely to transmit disease (e.g., oral sex instead of anal or vaginal sex). Immunization can also lower B by reducing the uninfected partner's susceptibility to infection. Encouraging persons at risk to have fewer partners directly targets the partner change rate (*c*), while screening, education efforts designed to improve patients' recognition of symptoms, and partner notification all seek to diminish the mean duration of infection in the population (*D*).

Core Populations

Simple models of transmission dynamics, like those presented previously, focus on average individual behavior and the host-parasite relationship to explain transmission dynamics. However, the distribution of sexual behavior within a population is probably more important. A potentially small minority of persons with STD, the 'core group,' disproportionately contributes to the transmission of infection and is essential to maintaining an infection in a population (14). The extent to which that group mixes with persons with lower levels of sexual activity largely determines both the susceptibility of a population to the introduction of a new STD epidemic and the extent to which that epidemic can become widespread. The concept of the core group was originally developed to explain the persistence of gonorrhea endemicity in the United States (15–17) and studies have provided empirical support for the central role of core transmission in the epidemiology of this infection (18–20). While useful conceptually, defining 'core groups' in actual practice has been difficult, with investigators variously defining core groups geographically, by the occurrence of repeated infections, by their number of infected sexual contacts, and by their participation in commercial sex (21).

Sexual Networks

When assessing a patient's risk of STD, clinicians often focus on behavioral risk. However, the risk of acquiring an STD reflects not only that person's own behavior, but also the behavior of his or her sex partners, as well as broader patterns of sexual mixing, STD prevalence, and health care seeking and access in their sexual network. For example, virtually all studies of selective screening for chlamydial infection have found that self-reported behavior is insensitive in predicting infection (22,23), whereas demographic factors such as age, race, socioeconomic status, source of clinical care, and geography are closely associated with infection (24–27). These factors, which organize human society and dictate sexual mixing patterns, play a critical role in defining an individual's risk of STD (28). STDs exist within a social context and clinicians and public health professionals must alter their assessment of risk depending on the practice setting and the patients' social milieu. Moreover, stigmatizing stereotypes related to sexual behavior and STD should be tempered by the realization that persons with low levels of risky behavior can be at relatively high risk of STD simply by virtue of their sexual network, a population that is often socially proscribed by factors such as race and economic status.

CLINICAL AND PUBLIC HEALTH CONSIDERATIONS

Several unique aspects of STDs and the populations at risk affect clinical management. The Centers for Disease Control and Prevention (CDC) periodically issues guidelines for management of patients with STDs, including recommendations for clinical assessment, prevention, and control (29) as well as guidelines for HIV testing and counseling (30).

Clinical Evaluation and Risk Assessment

In addition to routine clinical care, the management of patients with STDs entails efforts to assess risk, reduce the likelihood of future infections and complications, and protect the health of the patients' sexual partners and the public at large.

Assessment of risk requires an accurate social and sexual history, including appraisal of factors that influence sexuality, such as substance abuse. Although taking such a history is daunting to some clinicians, a forthright and sensitive approach often results in candid acknowledgment of high-risk behaviors and need not be time-consuming. Typically, a sexual history should include questions related to sexual orientation, numbers of sex partners, sexual practices (i.e., sexual repertoire), condom use, history of STD, and, among persons at significant risk of HIV, knowledge of partners' HIV serostatus. This sets the stage for counseling and education that can maximize compliance with treatment and follow-up and reduce the risk of future STD episodes.

Education and Counseling

Counseling and education are important not only for patients who currently have an STD or are at risk, but also for all young people in primary health care settings for primary prevention. When practical, such counseling should begin before the patient becomes sexually active. Clinicians should strive to provide 'client-centered' counseling. This approach involves encouraging patients to identify the behaviors and circumstances that place him or her at risk for STD and to commit to specific steps to reduce that risk (Table 102.2). This approach is outlined in depth in the CDC's HIV Counseling and Testing Guidelines (30) and has been shown to reduce the rate of STD acquisition in heterosexual STD clinic patients (31).

Diagnostic Testing

Optimally, clinicians who provide STD care should have immediate access to tests for HIV infection; syphilis serology; specific tests for *Neisseria gonorrhoeae* and *C. trachomatis*, and virologic and type-specific tests for HSV; microscopy for examination of Gram-stained smears and wet mounts of vaginal secretions; and Papanicolaou smears, which should be routinely obtained for women at risk for STDs. Those few providers who serve populations with high prevalences of syphilis should also have access to darkfield microscopy for detection of *Treponema pallidum*.

TABLE 102.2.   Elements of Prevention Counseling

1) Keep the discussion focused on STD risk reduction
2) Include an in-depth, personalized risk assessment—discuss past efforts to reduce risk. Avoid global risk reduction steps, instead concentrating on specific actions (e.g. carry a condom next time you go out, not always use condoms).
3) Acknowledge and provide support for positive steps already made
4) Clarify critical rather than general misconceptions
5) Negotiate a concrete, achievable behavior-change step that will reduce risk
6) Seek flexibility in the prevention approach and counseling process
7) Provide skill-building opportunities

STD, sexually transmitted disease.

Commonly available tests for *Chlamydia trachomatis* vary in sensitivity from as low as 40% for some enzyme immunoassays and unamplified genetic probes, to 95% or more for nucleic acid amplification tests (NAAT) (32–34). Clinicians should know what testing technology their laboratory routinely uses and should request NAAT whenever possible. New type-specific serologic tests for HSV antibody and HSV western blots, both based on HSV glycoprotein G, are the only assays that accurately distinguish HSV-1 from HSV-2 antibody. These tests are clearly useful for diagnostic testing of persons with histories of genital ulcer but no lesion for immediate culture, and for the evaluation of the sexual partners of persons with genital herpes. The role of these tests in routine screening remains controversial.

Screening

In the context of STD care, screening refers to laboratory testing for STDs for which the patient is at risk in the absence of symptoms or other clinical indications, and thus is distinct from diagnostic testing. The occurrence of an STD is a "sentinel event" that reflects unprotected sexual activity and exposure to partner(s) at risk for STD, and diagnosis of any STD usually should trigger screening for additional ones. However, most STD screening is done in persons without known infection on the basis of regional STD prevalence, individual risks, and social context. For example, in most settings, all sexually active women age 25 and under should be screened annually for *C. trachomatis*. Screening also has a central role in the control of gonorrhea, syphilis, and HIV infection, though specific recommendations are less well defined. Establishing practical screening criteria depends on the epidemiology of STDs in the local population and a balance among cost, test performance, anticipated yield, potential impact of case detection on public health, and frequency of complications. Recently, the importance of screening men who have sex with men for bacterial STD, including rectal infections, and perhaps HSV-2 has been reemphasized (35). Screening has been proposed in various settings for HSV infection, human papillomavirus infection, and other STDs, but its value in preventing these infections has not been determined.

A difficult dilemma is that screening yields that are high on a population basis may not be sufficient to sustain a clinician's resolve to continue testing his or her patients at risk. For example, a 5% prevalence of chlamydial infection in sexually active young women demands routine testing, but a yield of only one infection in 20 persons screened may tempt a clinician to restrict testing to patients who seem to be at particular risk, a strategy that almost always fails to detect most infections in the population. The development of urine-based testing for *C. trachomatis* and *N. gonorrhoeae* has simplified screening decisions and procedures for these infections.

Whenever possible, patients should be rescreened for bacterial STD 3 to 5 months after treatment. Rescreening is distinct from test-of-cure, which is advocated only in a few instances, such as for patients with syphilis and for pregnant women with other bacterial STDs. Several studies have documented 10% to 15% prevalences of *C. trachomatis* in women diagnosed with chlamydial infections when retested 3 to 5 months after treatment (36,37). The rationale for rescreening is reinforced by the well-documented observation that PID, tubal infertility, and ectopic pregnancy occur with increased frequency following recurrent as compared with initial infections (38). Although data are not available regarding re-screening in men and for persons diagnosed with gonorrhea or syphilis, clinicians should strongly consider routinely reevaluating such patients given the fact that these infections tend to be more concentrated than chlamydial infection in highly sexually active core groups (39).

Principles of Treatment

Ideally, a specific diagnosis should be made and treatment and counseling guided accordingly. In some instances, an etiologic diagnosis is known before treatment is given, such as when a positive result is received for a screening test for *C. trachomatis* or a Gram-stained smear is diagnostic of gonorrhea. More often, however, a management decision must be made before the etiologic diagnosis is known, as when a patient presents with mucopurulent cervicitis, pelvic inflammatory disease, a genital ulcer or as the partner of a person with STD. Acute symptoms usually require immediate therapy, and some patients may not defer sexual activity while awaiting test results. Accordingly, clinicians must be cognizant of the usual causes of the common STD syndromes in the populations they serve, recognizing that the causes vary geographically and fluctuate over time. However, even when initial care must be based on clinical grounds ("syndromic management"), it is good practice to obtain specific diagnostic tests whenever practical, even when the results will not be known until after treatment is started (29).

Historically, STD patients have been considered unlikely to comply with prolonged treatment, resulting in an emphasis on single-dose therapy. In fact, persons with STDs may be no less adherent than other patients, but an STD carries implications for continued transmission that magnify the importance of therapeutic compliance. Directly observed, single-dose treatment should therefore be used whenever practical; it is indicated for most cases of uncomplicated gonorrhea, chlamydial infection, primary or secondary syphilis, and many cases of nongonococcal urethritis and chancroid. If multiple-dose treatment must be given, the clinician should make a special effort to counsel the patient about the necessity of compliance. When practical, even multiple-dose drugs should be given directly to the patient in the office and the first dose should be observed, rather than giving a prescription to be filled, especially when the patient must pay for therapy. In a study of women with acute pelvic inflammatory disease diagnosed in an urban emergency department, 30% failed to fill their prescriptions for doxycycline (40).

Partner Management

Management of patients' sex partners is an integral part of treating patients with STDs. In areas where public health departments routinely provide partner notification services to all or most patients, clinicians should actively assist those efforts and should routinely advise patients with selected STD to anticipate being contacted regarding partner treatment. However, most health departments in the U.S. do not routinely provide partner notification services to patients for STDs other than syphilis, or, to a lesser extent, HIV infection. As a result, diagnosing clinicians are usually responsible for ensuring that partners are treated. Nonspecific advice to "make sure your partner gets checked" is often not heeded, and recent studies have found that between 20% and 50% of all patients with gonorrhea or chlamydial infection do not notify all of their partners (41–43). Failure to ensure treatment of the partner is often tantamount to not treating the index case, because reinfection is exceedingly common.

The traditional recommendation is that all partners of infected patients should be examined and that it is inappropriate to provide "blind" treatment without examination or referral. Indeed, referral and examination of partners remains the ideal standard. Direct assessment of partners allows for diagnosis of co-infections and opportunities to bring other partners to treatment. Compliance with treatment may be poor among partners who are not directly counseled, and education and counseling opportunities are lost. Nevertheless, for the bacterial STD the overriding goal is to assure that patients' partners are treated. Two observational studies of women with *C. trachomatis* reported lower rates of infection at follow-up among women given antibiotics to treat their partners than in women whose partners were referred for therapy (44,45). This practice appears to be common (42) and has been instituted by at least one health department as part of routine partner management (43). Although the clinician should always attempt to arrange for examination and diagnostic testing of the partner, blind treatment may be appropriate if the traditional approach is unsuccessful or impractical.

Reporting

Documentation of STD morbidity locally and nationally is integral to control. Prevention programs can be rationally designed only when such data are available, and resources can be targeted to the core populations only if their occurrence, location, and demographic characteristics are known. Thus, even when health departments do not provide partner notification services, health care providers should report all cases of designated STDs to health authorities according to local regulations; failure to do so contributes to the continued spread of STDs.

REFERENCES

1. Institute of Medicine (U.S.). Committee on Prevention and Control of Sexually Transmitted Diseases. Eng TR, Butler WT. *The hidden epidemic: confronting sexually transmitted diseases.* Washington DC: National Academy Press, 1997.
2. Gerbase AC, Rowley JT, Heymann DH, Berkley SF, Piot P. Global prevalence and incidence estimates of selected curable STDs. *Sex Transm Infect.* 1998;74[Suppl 1]:S12–S16.
3. Fleming DT, Wasserheit JN. From epidemiological synergy to public health policy and practice: the contribution of other sexually transmitted diseases to sexual transmission of HIV infection. *Sex Transm Infect* 1999;75:3–17.
4. Handsfield HH, Lipman TO, Harnisch JP, Tronca E, Holmes KK. Asymptomatic gonorrhea in men. Diagnosis, natural course, prevalence and significance. *N Engl J Med* 1974;290:117–123.
5. Fleming DT, McQuillan GM, Johnson RE, et al. Herpes simplex virus type 2 in the United States, 1976 to 1994. *N Engl J Med* 1997;337:1105–1111.
6. Blower SM, Porco TC, Darby G. Predicting and preventing the emergence of antiviral drug resistance in HSV-2. *Nat Med* 1998;4:673–678.
7. White PJ, Garnett GP. Use of antiviral treatment and prophylaxis is unlikely to have a major impact on the prevalence of herpes simplex virus type 2. *Sex Transm Infect* 1999;75:49–54.
8. Wood E, Braitstein P, Montaner JS, et al. Extent to which low-level use of antiretroviral treatment could curb the AIDS epidemic in sub-Saharan Africa. *Lancet* 2000;355:2095–2100.
9. Gray RH, Brookmeyer R, Wawer MJ. The probability of HIV-1 transmission per coital act in monogamous HIV-discordant couples, Rakai, Uganda. Presented at the 8th conference on retroviruses and opportunistic infections, sponsored by the Foundation for Retrovirology and Human Health. Chicago, 2001;121.
10. Grosskurth H, Mosha F, Todd J, et al. Impact of improved treatment of sexually transmitted diseases on HIV infection in rural Tanzania: randomised controlled trial. *Lancet* 1995;346:530–536.
11. Wawer MJ, Sewankambo NK, Serwadda D, et al. Control of sexually transmitted diseases for AIDS prevention in Uganda: a randomised community trial. Rakai Project Study Group. *Lancet* 1999;353:525–535.
12. Grosskurth H, Gray R, Hayes R, Mabey D, Wawer M. Control of sexually transmitted diseases for HIV-1 prevention: understanding the implications of the Mwanza and Rakai trials. *Lancet* 2000;355:1981–1987.
13. Roseberry W. (The World Bank). AIDS prevention and mitigation in sub-Saharan Africa: an updated world bank strategy. Report no. 15569-AFR, 1996.
14. Anderson RM. Transmission dynamics of sexually transmitted infections. In KK H, ed: *Sexually transmitted diseases,* 3rd ed. New York: McGraw-Hill, 1999:25–38.
15. Yorke JA, Hethcote HW, Nold A. Dynamics and control of the transmission of gonorrhea. *Sex Transm Dis* 1978;5:51–56.
16. Hethcote H, Yorke J, Nold A. Gonorrhea modeling. *Math Biosci* 1982;58:93–109.
17. Hethcote H, York J. Gonorrhea transmission dynamics and control. *Lecture Notes Biomath* 1984;56:1–105.
18. Rice RJ, Roberts PL, Handsfield HH, Holmes KK. Sociodemographic distribution of gonorrhea incidence: implications for prevention and behavioral research. *Am J Public Health* 1991;81:1252–1258.
19. Rothenberg RB, Potterat JJ. Temporal and social aspects of gonorrhea transmission: the force of infectivity. *Sex Transm Dis* 1988;15:88–92.
20. Rothenberg RB. The geography of gonorrhea. Empirical demonstration of core group transmission. *Am J Epidemiol* 1983;117:688–694.
21. Thomas JC, Tucker MJ. The development and use of the concept of a sexually transmitted disease core. *J Infect Dis* 1996;174[Suppl 2]:S134–S143.
22. Marrazzo JM, Fine D, Celum CL, DeLisle S, Handsfield HH. Selective screening for chlamydial infection in women: a comparison of three sets of criteria. *Fam Plann Perspect* 1997;29:158–162.
23. Handsfield HH, Jasman LL, Roberts PL, Hanson VW, Kothenbeutel RL, Stamm WE. Criteria for selective screening for *Chlamydia trachomatis* infection in women attending family planning clinics. *JAMA* 1986;255:1730–1734.
24. Marrazzo JM, White CL, Krekeler B, et al. Community-based urine screening for *Chlamydia trachomatis* with a ligase chain reaction assay. *Ann Intern Med* 1997;127:796–803.
25. Morris M. Concurrent partnerships and syphilis persistence: new thoughts on an old puzzle. *Sex Transm Dis* 2001;28:504–507.
26. Laumann EO, Youm Y. Racial/ethnic group differences in the prevalence of sexually transmitted diseases in the United States: a network explanation. *Sex Transm Dis* 1999;26:250–261.
27. Sucato G, Celum C, Dithmer D, Ashley R, Wald A. Demographic rather than behavioral risk factors predict herpes simplex virus type 2 infection in sexually active adolescents. *Pediatr Infect Dis J* 2001;20:422–426.
28. Laumann E, Gagnon J, Michaels S. *The social organization of sexuality: sexual practices in the United States.* Chicago: University of Chicago Press, 1994.
29. Centers for Disease Control and Prevention. 1998 guidelines for treatment of sexually transmitted diseases. *MMWR* 1998;47:1–111.
30. Centers for Disease Control and Prevention. Revised guidelines for HIV counseling, testing and referral and revised recommendations for HIV screening of pregnant women. *MMWR* 2001;50.
31. Kamb ML, Fishbein M, Douglas JM Jr, et al. Efficacy of risk-reduction counseling to prevent human immunodeficiency virus and sexually transmitted diseases: a randomized controlled trial. Project RESPECT Study Group. *JAMA* 1998;280:1161–1167.
32. Marrazzo JM, Stamm WE. New approaches to the diagnosis, treatment, and prevention of chlamydial infection. *Curr Clin Top Infect Dis* 1998;18:37–59.
33. Black CM. Current methods of laboratory diagnosis of *Chlamydia trachomatis* infections. *Clin Microbiol Rev* 1997;10:160–184.
34. Johnson RE, Green TA, Schachter J, et al. Evaluation of nucleic acid amplification tests as reference tests for *Chlamydia trachomatis* infections in asymptomatic men. *J Clin Microbiol* 2000;38:4382–4386.
35. Sexually transmitted disease and hiv screening guidelines for men who have sex with men (comment). *Sex Transm Dis* 2001;28:457–459.
36. Whittington WL, Kent C, Kissinger P, et al. Determinants of persistent and recurrent *Chlamydia trachomatis* infection in young women: results of a multicenter cohort study. *Sex Transm Dis* 2001;28:117–123.
37. Burstein GR, Gaydos CA, Diener-West M, Howell MR, Zenilman JM, Quinn TC. Incident *Chlamydia trachomatis* infections among inner-city adolescent females. *JAMA* 1998;280:521–526.
38. Westrom L, Joesoef R, Reynolds G, Hagdu A, Thompson SE. Pelvic inflammatory disease and fertility. A cohort study of 1,844 women with laparoscopically verified disease and 657 control women with normal laparoscopic results. *Sex Transm Dis* 1992;19:185–192.
39. Hook EW 3rd, Reichart CA, Upchurch DM, Ray P, Celentano D, Quinn TC. Comparative behavioral epidemiology of gonococcal and chlamydial infections among patients attending a Baltimore, Maryland, sexually transmitted disease clinic. *Am J Epidemiol* 1992;136:662–672.
40. Brookoff D. Compliance with doxycycline therapy for outpatient treatment of pelvic inflammatory disease. *South Med J* 1994;87:1088–1091.
41. Oh MK, Boker JR, Genuardi FJ, Cloud GA, Reynolds J, Hodgens JB. Sexual contact tracing outcome in adolescent chlamydial and gonococcal cervicitis cases. *J Adolesc Health* 1996;18:4–9.
42. Golden MR, Whittington WL, Gorbach PM, Coronado N, Boyd MA, Holmes KK. Partner notification for chlamydial infections among private sector clinicians in Seattle-King County: a clinician and patient survey. *Sex Transm Dis* 1999;26:543–547.
43. Golden MR, Whittington WHL, Handsfield HH, et al. Partner management for gonococcal and chlamydial infection: expansion of public health services to the private sector and expedited sex partner treatment through a partnership with commercial pharmacies. *Sex Transm Dis* 2001;28:658–665.
44. Kissinger P, Brown R, Reed K, et al. Effectiveness of patient delivered partner medication for preventing recurrent *Chlamydia trachomatis*. *Sex Transm Infect* 1998;74:331–333.
45. Ramstedt K, Forssman L, Johannisson G. Contact tracing in the control of genital *Chlamydia trachomatis* infection. *Int J STD AIDS* 1991;2:116–118.

CHAPTER 103
Gonorrhea

Khalil G. Ghanem, Edward W. Hook,
and Jonathan M. Zenilman

Gonorrhea is the result of infection by *Neisseria gonorrhoeae*, a gram-negative diplococcus that only infects humans, and causes a wide spectrum of clinical syndromes (Table 103.1). The failure of clinicians to appreciate all possible manifestations of the disease, including the sub clinical ones, can result in missed diagnostic and therapeutic opportunities. A better understanding of the molecular biology of the disease, coupled with recent advances in diagnostic techniques, have lead to modifications in our approach to the proper diagnosis and management of this infection. Proper diagnosis and successful management of this disease requires an understanding of its epidemiology, an awareness of the entire spectrum of possible clinical presentations, and an appreciation for the appropriate therapeutic choices geared toward the sensitivity patterns of the strains that are prevalent in the geographical area of interest.

EPIDEMIOLOGY

In 2001, 361,705 cases of gonorrhea were reported to the Centers for Disease Control and Prevention (CDC). This is certainly an underestimate of the true number of cases. It has been estimated that as many as half of all gonorrhea cases are not reported owing to either poor compliance with reporting requirements, or symptomatic treatment of patients without culture confirmation. In one study, the estimated annual number of undiagnosed gonococcal infections approached or exceeded the numbers that were diagnosed and treated (1). Between 1975 and 1997, there was a 73.8% reduction in the reported rate of gonorrhea in the United States. However, by 1998, this trend had reversed and there was a 7.8% rate increase not accounted for by changes in sensitivity of diagnostic tests or improved reporting practices (2).

TABLE 103.1. Clinical Presentations of Gonorrhea

Neonates
  Asymptomatic mucosal infection
  Conjunctivitis
  Disseminated gonococcal infection
Men
  Asymptomatic mucosal infection
  Urethritis
  Proctitis
  Pharyngitis
  Epididymitis
  Disseminated gonococcal infection
Women
  Asymptomatic mucosal infection
  Cervicitis
  Urethritis
  Proctitis
  Pharyngitis
  Skene or Bartholin gland infection
  Pelvic inflammatory disease (endometritis, salpingitis, peritonitis)
  Disseminated gonococcal infection

There is geographic variation for gonorrhea infections: The rates were highest in the southern parts of the United States (177.5 per 100,000 population). There is also a racial predilection: Blacks have the highest reported rates, even after controlling for potential confounders such as socio-economic status and access to health care (3,4). Although the rate of gonorrhea in African Americans in the United States has continued to decline since 1998 (782.3 per 100,000 in 2001), it is still 27 times higher than for non-Hispanic whites (29.4 per 100,000). On the other hand, the rates in Hispanics (74.2 per 100,000) and non-Hispanic whites have increased by 6.9% and 6.1%, respectively, from the corresponding rates in 2000. The rate in men (128.4 per 100,000 men) is similar to that in women (128.2 per 100,000 women); however, rates in the former are decreasing whereas those in the latter have remained unchanged over the past several years (2). Gonorrhea is primarily a disease of adolescents and young adults (1,2). Fifteen- to 19-year-old women had the highest rates of gonorrhea infection in 2001 (703.2 per 100,000), as did 20- to 24-year-old men (563.6 per 100,000). Except in neonates, gonococcal infections are nearly always the consequence of sexual transmission, and risk for gonorrhea acquisition is influenced by a number of covariates related to individual susceptibility, sexual partners, and practices. The high gonorrhea rates for young women probably reflect not only relatively rapid accrual of sexual partners soon after young persons become sexually active, but possibly also a biologically based increase in susceptibility among young women compared with older women. This increased susceptibility appears to be related to the presence of larger areas of cervical ectropion (columnar epithelial cells on the surface of the ectocervix) in younger women, which affords a larger area of susceptible target cells for inoculation of gonococcal infection (5,6). Persons who have multiple sexual partners and prostitutes and their clients have long been considered to be at increased risk for gonorrhea (7,8). Sexual activity associated with illicit drug use (parenteral or nonparenteral) and sex with casual partners are also risk factors (7). Thus, epidemiologic considerations are sometimes useful as a guide in making decisions regarding whom to screen for gonorrhea. In a given population, for instance, the yield of routine gonorrhea screening is usually highest among younger persons, those who have recently had sex with new partners, and those who use illicit drugs. Demographic variation in gonorrhea rates also affects the yield of routine gonorrhea screening; rates are higher among lower socioeconomic class, minority, and inner-city populations than in nearby suburban middle- or upper-class populations.

Diagnostic Considerations

The exceptional performance characteristics and widespread availability of nucleic acid amplification tests (NAAT) have revolutionized testing for *N. gonorrhoeae*. Tests based on methods such as polymerase chain reaction (PCR), transcription-mediated amplification (TMA), and strand displacement amplification testing on both urogenital specimens and urine are now available. In addition, nucleic acid hybridization tests are also available. However, it is important to state that gram stain evaluation and culture isolation (especially in men) still remain sensitive, specific, practical, and inexpensive for making the diagnosis. Nevertheless, even in situations when Gram stain and culture were expected to have high yield, nucleic acid amplification tests have been proven to be superior (9,10). The frequent absence or nonspecificity of symptoms, the potential complications of untreated infection, and the proven benefit of routine screening of populations at risk, make the time and cost for gonorrhea detection important considerations in choosing methods for diagnosis.

Specimen Collection

Proper specimen collection is important to ensure optimal yield of most gonorrhea tests. In men with detectable urethral discharge, non-amplified expressed urethral exudate may be used for Gram staining or culture (11,12). Proper specimen collection from asymptomatic men or men with symptoms who lack expressible discharge involves insertion 1.5 to 2 cm into the urethra of a wire-shafted swab tipped with calcium alginate or synthetic fibers by a rotatory motion. For diagnosis of urogenital tract gonorrhea in women, specimens should always be collected from the uterine endocervix. If the endocervical specimen is to be evaluated by Gram stain, adherent cervicovaginal secretions should be removed from the cervical os with use of large cotton-tipped swabs before the specimen is obtained. Specimens obtained for Gram stain should be rolled, rather than rubbed, onto a glass microscope slide, lest the morphologic features of inflammatory cells be distorted. Specimens collected for culture from any site should always use calcium alginate or synthetic fiber-tipped swabs. Substances contained in wooden-shafted, cotton-tipped swabs may be toxic to *N. gonorrhoeae*, particularly if the swab is to be placed in transport medium for transfer to the laboratory rather than plated directly onto culture media (11). As for the nucleic acid–based tests, swabs and transport media for the amplification tests are supplied by the manufacturer. Probe swabs for the hybridization tests can be held at 2°C to 25°C for up to 7 days whereas amplification swabs can be held at 2°C to 25°C for up to 5 days or 2°C to 8°C for up to 7 days. Urine for amplification testing can be held at room temperature for up to 24 hours or up to 5 days at 2°C to 8°C (13).

Gram Stain

For detection of gonococcal urethritis or cervicitis in persons who have symptoms or are at high risk, Gram stain examination rapidly provides accurate diagnostic information. The examination can be performed in minutes; the reagents cost pennies per test; and, if positive, the results are highly specific (12). The result of a Gram stain preparation is considered positive if gram-negative diplococci are seen within polymorphonuclear leukocytes. If gram-negative diplococci are seen extracellularly in the presence of polymorphonuclear leukocytes, the Gram stain is termed equivocal for gonorrhea, and in most instances this is sufficient indication to warrant initiation of treatment. The presence of gram-negative diplococci without associated polymorphonuclear leukocytes is difficult to interpret and does not necessarily indicate the presence of gonococcal infection.

For symptomatic men with gonococcal urethritis, the sensitivity of Gram stain is approximately 95% to 98%, and the specificity is in excess of 95%. For women with gonococcal cervicitis, sensitivity is somewhat less (40% to 60%); however, specificity again exceeds 95%. For asymptomatic men, Gram stain of urethral specimens has a sensitivity similar to that for cervical specimens (e.g., 40% to 60%), and although specificity is slightly lower than that for other sites, it still exceeds 90%. Gram stain of rectal specimens is sometimes complicated by the presence of nongonococcal, gram-negative diplococci, which may be mistaken for *N. gonorrhoeae*; nonetheless, it is sometimes useful for evaluation of symptomatic proctitis in persons who practice receptive rectal intercourse. In contrast, owing to the high prevalence of nongonococcal *Neisseria* species and other gram-negative cocci in the pharynx, Gram stain examination is not a recommended means for diagnosis of pharyngeal gonorrhea.

Culture Diagnosis

For optimal recovery of *N. gonorrhoeae*, mucosal specimens obtained for culture should be inoculated directly onto selective media and placed into a 35°C to 37°C incubator containing a 5% to 7% carbon dioxide atmosphere. Many effective transport media are available that sustain the viability of *N. gonorrhoeae* for several hours, permitting specimens to be transported to the laboratory from areas where it is not possible to stock culture media. In general, these transport media sustain gonococcal viability for periods in excess of 6 to 12 hours.

Selective media for isolation of *N. gonorrhoeae* from mucosal specimens usually contain antimicrobial substances to suppress growth of other microorganisms (bacteria and fungi) that might overgrow and obscure the presence of the relatively small colonies characteristic of *N. gonorrhoeae* (14).

Comparative studies have shown that although antimicrobial agents contained in selective media may inhibit growth of a small proportion of gonococcal isolates, that proportion is no larger than the proportion that goes undetected as the result of overgrowth in specimens plated on nonselective media (14–16). The gonococcal strains that are most likely to cause disseminated gonococcal infection (DGI) are more fastidious. As a result, specimens from patients with possible DGI should routinely be cultured onto nonselective chocolate agar to optimize culture isolation rates. The selective media most widely used for *N. gonorrhoeae* culture from mucosal sites include modified Thayer-Martin, Martin-Lewis, and New York City medium. Any of these provides suitably efficient isolation of *N. gonorrhoeae*, and all are, by and large, comparable with regard to their potential usefulness. With the implementation of good quality control measures for specimen collection, transportation, and processing, the sensitivity of culture ranges from 85% to 95% with 100% specificity (17).

Nucleic Acid Hybridization and Amplification Tests

Nucleic acid hybridization tests use a probe to detect a specific nucleotide sequence on *N. gonorrhoeae* ribonucleic acid. These tests are approved by the U.S. Food and Drug Administration (FDA) for testing endocervical and urethral specimens. Compared to culture, the range of sensitivity and specificity for these tests is 85.4% to 100% and 82% to 99.7%, respectively, depending on the study, the site being tested, and whether methods to minimize bias such as discrepant analysis were used (18). The sensitivities of NAAT generally exceed those of other tests, including culture. Sensitivity for these tests range from 90% to 98.8% and specificity from 92% to 100% again depending on the size of the study, the type of sample being evaluated, and whether discrepant analysis was used. Table 103.2 compares the sensitivity and specificity of the different diagnostic modalities. NAAT are attractive alternatives to culture-based methods especially if time and specimen handling are significant issues. They can also improve diagnostic yields in certain situations such as in low-prevalence screening protocols. Testing can be performed on self-administered swabs or collected urine specimens thereby allowing more flexibility in testing certain populations such as adolescents (19) and patients living in rural communities (20). Finally, it has also been possible to test for multiple STDs by obtaining a single intra-vaginal swab, generating more sensitive results than with individual non-NAAT testing (21). However, one disadvantage of using these methods is the inability to isolate an organism for antimicrobial sensitivity testing, subtyping, or for medico-legal purposes. This is most important in trying to better define the epidemiology of emerging antimicrobial resistance to *N. gonorrhoeae*. Cost may be another limiting factor in the use of these modalities. Suffice it to say that culture remains an attractive option in most situations where the diagnosis of gonorrhoeae in sought, especially when performed by a high-proficiency laboratory.

TABLE 103.2.   Sensitivity and Specificity of Select Diagnostic Tests for *Neisseria gonorrhoeae*

Method	% Sensitivity	% Specificity
Gram stain		
Males asymptomatic	50–70	95–100
Males symptomatic	90–95	95–100
Females	50–70	95–100
Culture	80–95	100
Hybridization		
Cervical	85.4–100	96.7–100
Urethral (male)	91.5–100	98.6–100
PCR		
Cervical	92.4	99.5
Female urine	64.8	99.8
LCR		
Cervical	90.9–100	99.6–100
Urethral (Male)	98.4–100	99.8–100
Urine men	98–100	98.6–100
Urine women	94.3–100	98.2–100
Strand displacement		
Cervical	96.6	98–100
Urethral (Male)	98.5	91.9–100
Female urine	84.9	99.3–100
Male urine	97.9	92.5–100

LCR, ligase chain reaction; PCR, polymerase chain reaction.
Adapted from references 11, 13, 14, 16, 46–48.

CLINICAL PRESENTATION

Asymptomatic Mucosal Infection

Asymptomatic infections may occur at any mucosal site of gonococcal contact (urethra, cervix, rectum, pharynx, conjunctiva) and are usually detected by screening or culture evaluation of patients who report recent exposure to sexual partners with gonorrhea. Asymptomatic urethral and cervical infections are present in approximately 10% and 40% to 50%, respectively, of men and women who report exposure to sexual partners with gonorrhea. The prevalence of asymptomatic urethral gonorrhea in military recruits and other otherwise unselected populations of sexually active men has been 0.5% to 2%. More often than not, pharyngeal and rectal gonococcal infections are asymptomatic (22,23). Asymptomatic mucosal infections are also disproportionately common among patients with DGI (24,25). It is not known whether this represents a risk factor for dissemination in patients with asymptomatic (and therefore untreated) mucosal gonorrhea, or is a reflection of the propensity of the distinctive strains that most often cause disseminated infection to also cause asymptomatic mucosal infection. Detection of asymptomatic infection through screening of populations identified as high risk based on sociodemographic characteristics, age, or history is an important facet of efforts to control gonorrhea. Because persons with asymptomatic infection are less likely to abstain from sexual activity than those in whom symptoms develop, they probably contribute disproportionately to gonococcal infection rates within communities.

Local Gonococcal Infections in Men

Symptomatic urethritis is the most common presentation of gonorrhea in men. Urethral discharge and dysuria usually develop 2 to 5 days after exposure to an infected sexual partner. The majority of men with symptomatic gonococcal urethritis have a purulent urethral discharge, which may become copious if it is untreated. Dysuria may be the sole symptom

of gonococcal infection and tends to be mild to moderate in severity.

The most common local complication of gonococcal infection in men is acute epididymitis, which usually presents as gradually increasing unilateral scrotal pain. Examination of patients with epididymitis may yield an unnoticed urethral discharge as well as tenderness or swelling of the epididymis. Acute epididymitis must be expeditiously differentiated from testicular torsion, which tends to be more acute in onset and is not usually associated with urethral discharge. In cases in which clinical differentiation is difficult, an urologist should be consulted immediately to preserve testicular viability in the event of torsion. For patients younger than 40 years, treatment of epididymitis targets *N. gonorrhoeae* and *Chlamydia trachomatis* as well, because coinfection is common. In men older than 40 years, as structural abnormalities of the urinary tract become more common, epididymitis may be caused by gram-negative rods and other urinary tract pathogens as well as STD pathogens.

Rarely, men with gonococcal urethritis present with other complications of infection, such as gonococcal cellulitis, penile lymphangitis, or periurethral abscess. In such patients, routine treatment for gonorrhea usually results in rapid resolution of these findings.

Local Gonococcal Infections in Women

The uterine cervix is the primary site of infection in women with acute uncomplicated gonorrhea. Whereas gonococcal cervicitis in women is often asymptomatic, women with local gonococcal infections may complain of increased vaginal discharge, genital itch, or dysuria. Because the same symptoms may also result from urinary tract infections, vaginal infections, or cervicitis due to other causes, evaluation of such complaints in sexually active women should include urinalysis (and culture when indicated); evaluation of vaginal secretions for candidiasis, trichomoniasis, and bacterial vaginosis; and tests for *N. gonorrhoeae* and *C. trachomatis*. Urethral cultures propagate the pathogen in 40% to 60% of women with gonococcal cervicitis, and the presence of urethral infection may help to explain dysuria as a common symptom of gonorrhea in women. In hysterectomized women, the primary site of infection is the urethra, because vaginal epithelium is relatively resistant to gonococcal infection. Women with local gonococcal infection may also present with local complications resulting from infection of Skene or Bartholin glands. In either case, these complications present with local pain and swelling.

Pelvic inflammatory disease (PID) is the most important complication of gonococcal infections (26–28). PID is a generic designation that may refer to endometritis, salpingitis, peritonitis, or a combination of these findings. Gonococcal PID usually results from ascension of *N. gonorrhoeae* from the site of primary infection (the cervix) into the upper genital tract. Symptoms of PID may include unilateral or bilateral lower abdominal cramps, dyspareunia, and intramenstrual bleeding. These symptoms may be severe or so mild that women with PID do not mention them; in such cases, the signs of PID are detected at the time of physical examination. Clinical signs associated with PID on bimanual pelvic examination include fundal or adnexal (usually bilateral) tenderness, signs of peritonitis, and occasionally adnexal masses or fullness. On speculum examination, as in gonococcal cervicitis, a grossly purulent cervical discharge may be present (Fig. 103.1), although frequently it is not. PID is most often a polymicrobial illness, and women with gonococcal PID are likely to have concurrent infection with *C. trachomatis* or an array of vaginal flora, including gram-negative rods, gram-positive cocci, and anaerobic bacteria (26,27). The tubal

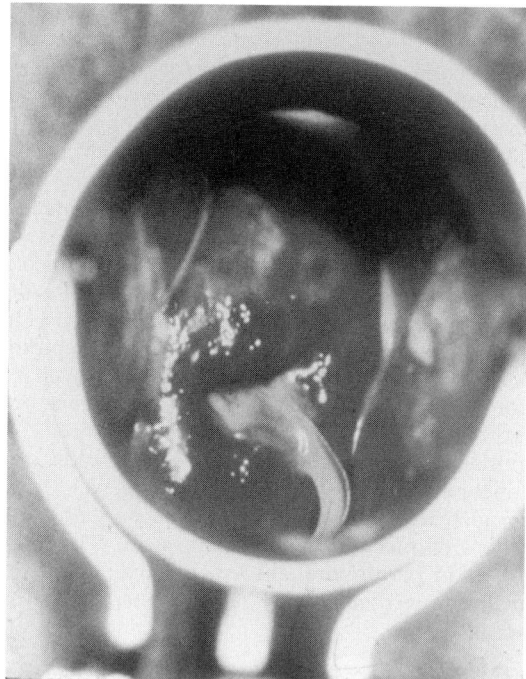

Figure 103.1. Cervical discharge in a patient with gonorrhea.

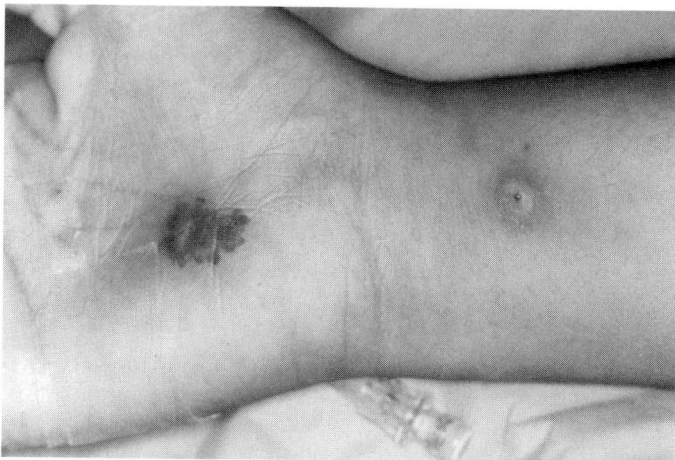

Figure 103.2. Skin lesions in a patient with disseminated gonococcal infection.

abnormalities and scarring that may result from PID or associated tuboovarian abscess are major causes of infertility, and ectopic pregnancy represents the major source of PID-associated morbidity. After a single episode of symptomatic PID, approximately 10% of women have bilateral tubal occlusion and resultant infertility, and women who do not have tubal obstruction have an approximately tenfold greater risk for ectopic pregnancy.

Anorectal Gonorrhea

Anorectal gonorrhea is unusual in heterosexual men. Asymptomatic anorectal gonococcal infection occurs in approximately 30% to 50% of women with cervical gonorrhea and is thought most often to arise from local contamination by cervicovaginal secretions. However, women and men who participate in receptive anal intercourse with infected sexual partners are also at risk for developing anorectal gonorrhea. Although most men with anorectal gonorrhea are asymptomatic, some develop signs of acute proctitis (rectal discharge, pain, tenesmus). Among homosexual men with symptomatic proctitis, coinfection with a variety of pathogens is common (23). As a result, these men who present for evaluation of symptomatic proctitis should also be thoroughly evaluated for a wide variety of other potential pathogens. The pathogens, differential diagnosis, and diagnostic approach to men with proctitis are reviewed in Chapter 113.

Disseminated Gonococcal Infections

Approximately 1% to 2% of patients with untreated gonorrhea progress to DGI, a bacteremic illness that most often presents with myalgia, arthralgia, asymmetric polyarthritis, or a characteristic dermatitis (Fig. 103.2) (24,25). Although DGI is a bacteremic illness, patients with this syndrome are often not clinically toxic. Not infrequently, the illness is characterized as influenza-like; the mean temperature of patients with

DGI is 37.9°C at time of presentation, and the mean peripheral leukocyte count is 10,550/mm³ (25). Whereas *N. gonorrhoeae* mucosal infection is present in most cases of DGI, it is frequently asymptomatic. Therefore, all potential mucosal sites of infection (urethra or cervix, pharynx, rectum) should be sampled for *N. gonorrhoeae* when the differential diagnosis includes DGI.

The two most common presentations of DGI are acute asymmetric polyarthritis and dermatitis, which sometimes may be present with painful tenosynovitis of the extremities (24,25). The arthritis of DGI tends to be asymmetric, most often involving joints of the hands, wrists, ankles, or knees, although nearly any joint may be affected. In patients with arthritis, the joint fluid polymorphonuclear leukocyte concentration may range from a few hundred cells to more than 20,000/mm³. The likelihood of isolating *N. gonorrhoeae* appears to correlate relatively well with the magnitude of synovial fluid leukocyte concentration; higher isolation rates occur in patients with higher cell counts (24). Overall, 20% to 30% of DGI patients' synovial fluid culture specimens propagate the pathogen.

The dermatitis of DGI is characteristically composed of a small number of skin lesions (usually fewer than 30) that are located predominantly on the extremities. Extremities are more often involved distally than proximally. The lesions begin as tender papules, which then progress to necrotic pustules and finally ulcerate. Many patients with such lesions characterize them as insect bites. The classic skin lesion of DGI is a necrotic pustule on an erythematous base, and lesions in different stages of evolution are often present concurrently. The lesions are often somewhat tender to the touch. Attempts at culture isolation of DGI skin lesions is rarely productive. On occasion, DGI may be complicated when seeding of heart valves or the meninges results in gonococcal endocarditis or meningitis (29–31). Either complication is potentially life threatening and should be treated aggressively and vigorously.

THERAPEUTIC CONSIDERATIONS

Drug Resistance

In the year 2003, therapy for infections due to *N. gonorrhoeae* has become complicated by an appreciation of the increasing repertoire of gonococcal antimicrobial resistance. For nearly 50 years, a penicillin was the choice for gonorrhea therapy worldwide;

however, by 1989, penicillin resistance had become widespread, severely compromising its usefulness as treatment of choice for gonorrhea (32,33). In 2001, based on data from the Gonococcal Isolate Surveillance Project (GISP), 20.9% of *N. gonorrhoeae* isolates were resistant to penicillin, tetracycline, or both (2). In the 1990s as well, resistance of *N. gonorrhoeae* to fluoroquinolones became an important public health issue. First described in the Far East (34–37), and subsequently reported in Europe (38), Africa (39), and the Middle East (40), the number of isolates in the United States has been progressively increasing. Although the number of fluoroquinolone resistant strains has remained relatively low (albeit increasing) in most of the GISP clinics (0.4% of isolates in 1999 vs. 0.7% in 2001), the number of fluoroquinolone-resistant GISP isolates in Hawaii has continued to increase dramatically (from 14.3% in 2000 to 20.3% in 2001) (2,41). A similar trend in California has also been seen, where approximately 3% of the isolates were fluoroquinolone resistant in 2001. This has lead to the recommendation that fluoroquinolones not be used as therapy in either California or Hawaii (2). The authors anticipate that this trend will be more widespread in the United States in the future.

Antimicrobial resistance of *N. gonorrhoeae* may be due to plasmid-mediated β-lactamase production; to plasmid-mediated resistance to tetracycline; or to chromosomally mediated resistance to a wide variety of antibiotics, including penicillin, tetracycline, and spectinomycin (32,42–47). Despite progressive increases in the variety and prevalence of antimicrobial resistance in *N. gonorrhoeae*, third-generation cephalosporins remain highly effective for gonorrhea therapy.

Uncomplicated Gonococcal Infections

In addition to antimicrobial resistance, other important considerations in choosing therapeutic agents for gonococcal infections include their utility against co-infecting pathogens (principally *C. trachomatis*), their ease of administration (single-dose therapy enhances compliance), and their cost (given the fact that many patients with gonorrhea have limited financial resources and so are dependent on the services of publicly funded STD clinics for therapy).

Persons at risk for one STD are often at increased risk for others as well. For patients with gonorrhea, the two most common co-infecting pathogens are *C. trachomatis* and, in women, *Trichomonas vaginalis*. It is estimated that at least 10% to 20% of men and 30% to 40% of women with uncomplicated gonorrhea have concurrent *Chlamydia* infections. No inexpensive single-dose therapy currently recommended for gonorrhea reliably eradicates *Chlamydia* organisms, and the currently recommended anti-*Chlamydia* treatment regimens are not reliable for gonorrhea. Therefore, it is recommended that patients treated for gonorrhea also be treated routinely for possible *Chlamydia* infection at the time of gonorrhea therapy. Because *Chlamydia* testing is relatively costly and usually requires several days for results, the co-treatment approach is still thought to be more cost-effective and efficient (40). However, in settings where *C. trachomatis* infection has low prevalence, if rapid methods are available to test for it, and the patient is reliable, directed therapy solely against the gonococcus may be appropriate.

In women, coexisting infection with *T. vaginalis* can often be detected by microscopic examination of saline preparations of vaginal fluid. In some women, however, the presence of trichomoniasis may become apparent only after treatment of gonorrhea. Thus, for women with persistent or new complaints of vaginal discharge or discomfort, repeated exami-

nation is necessary to differentiate failure of gonorrhea treatment from trichomoniasis or vaginal candidiasis complicating therapy.

In the past, it was recommended that repeated attempts at culture isolation be performed 4 to 7 days after completion of therapy for patients with uncomplicated gonorrhea to ensure that they had been cured (test-of-cure cultures). Since the 1989 revision of the CDC STD treatment guidelines, this recommendation was dropped for patients treated with recommended regimens. However, in the setting of persistent symptoms after therapy, it is recommended that cultures and antimicrobial susceptibility testing be performed to rule out resistant organisms. It is worth mentioning, however, that re-infection is still the predominant reason for presumed treatment failure. In many instances, this is due to the lack of treatment of the infected partners. Table 103.3 lists the approved regimens for treating uncomplicated gonococcal infections. Of note, the treatment recommendations for HIV-infected individuals are similar. For pharyngeal infections that tend to be more difficult to treat, ciprofloxacin 500 mg orally or ceftriaxone 125 mg IM in single doses are recommended (40). For gonococcal conjunctivitis, ceftriaxone 1 g IM can be used (48). Pregnant women should be treated with a cephalosporin. If penicillin allergic, then spectinomycin 2 g IM can be substituted (40).

Complicated Gonococcal Infections

In the 1970s and early 1980s, isolates from patients with DGI were found to be more sensitive to penicillin than were isolates from patients with uncomplicated gonorrhea; however as the prevalence of gonococcal antimicrobial resistance has increased, β-lactamase–producing *N. gonorrhoeae* and gonococci with clinically significant penicillin resistance have been routinely isolated from patients with disseminated infection (30,49). Therefore, penicillin is no longer recommended as initial therapy for patients with suspected DGI. Because the differential diagnosis of DGI also includes other serious infections such as endocarditis or meningococcemia, initial hospitalization is recommended to confirm the diagnosis and to ensure that patients are responding to therapy. After therapeutic response, patients with DGI may be discharged to complete therapy as outpatients with oral medications such as ciprofloxacin or even an appropriate cephalosporin depending on the organism's susceptibility.

Although the gonococcus is one of the pathogens most frequently isolated from patients with PID, the syndrome is often polymicrobial and clinical findings are not useful for determining likely pathogens. As a result, therapeutic regimens for PID should be effective not only for *N. gonorrhoeae* but also for chlamydiae, gram-negative vaginal organisms, group B streptococci, and anaerobes (see Table 103.3). In the currently recommended regimens for PID therapy, the agents with acceptable utility against the gonococcus include cefoxitin, cefotetan, ciprofloxacin and gentamicin. It is important to note that the male partners of women who have PID are often asymptomatic and should be treated (40).

In men younger than 35, epididymitis is most often caused by either *N. gonorrhoeae* or *C. trachomatis*. In those older than 35, gram-negative organisms tend to be more common, especially if they have undergone recent genitourinary surgery or instrumentation. Once testicular torsion is eliminated as the cause for the symptoms, patients can often be treated in the outpatient setting with ceftriaxone 250 mg IM and 10 days of oral doxycycline. For patients with suspected gram-negative epididymitis, a fluoroquinolone can be used for 10 days (40).

TABLE 103.3. Therapy for Gonococcal Infections

Uncomplicated gonorrhea	Pelvic inflammatory disease

Preferred regimen
Ceftriaxone, 125 mg intramuscularly (IM)
or
Ciprofloxacin, 500 mg PO[a]
or
Ofloxacin, 400 mg PO[a]
or
Levofloxacin, 250 mg PO[a]
plus
A regimen effective against *Chlamydia trachomatis*
such as
Doxycycline[b], 100 mg PO twice daily (bid) × 7 d
or
Azithromycin, 1.0 g PO as a single dose
 	
Alternative regimens
Spectinomycin, 2 g IM
or
Ceftizoxime, 500 mg IM
or
Cefotaxime, 500 mg IM
or
Cefoxitin, 2 g IM *with* probenecid, 1 g PO
or
Gatifloxacin, 400 mg PO[a]
or
Norfloxacin, 800 mg PO[a]
 	
Epididymitis
Ceftriaxone, 250 mg IM
plus
Doxycycline[b], 100 mg PO bid × 10 d
  Tetracycline, 500 mg PO four times daily, or
  erythromycin, 500 mg PO four times daily,
  may be substituted for the preferred
  doxycycline, as needed.
	Inpatient management
	Cefoxitin, 2 g intravenously (IV) q 6 h
	or
	Cefotetan, 2 g IV q 12 h
	plus
	Doxycycline, 100 mg PO[b] or IV q 12 h until improved,
	then
	Doxycycline, 100 mg PO bid[b] to complete 10–14 d course
	or
	Clindamycin, 900 mg IV q 8 h
	plus
	Gentamicin, 2 mg/kg loading dose then 1.5 mg/kg (maintenance dose) IM or
	IV q 8 h (single daily dose may be substituted) until improved,
	then
	Doxycycline, 100 mg PO bid to complete 10- to 14-d course
	
	Outpatient management
	Ofloxacin, 400 mg PO bid for 14 d[a]
	or
	Levofloxacin, 500 mg PO qd for 14 d[a]
	with or without
	Metronidazole, 500 mg PO bid for 14 d
	or
	Cefoxitin, 2 g IM
	plus
	Probenecid, 1.0 g PO
	or
	Ceftriaxone, 250 mg IM
	or
	Equivalent cephalosporin
	plus
	Doxycycline[b], 100 mg PO bid for 14 d
	with or without
	Metronidazole, 500 mg PO bid for 14 d
	
	Disseminated gonococcal infection
	(unless *C. trachomatis* coinfection is ruled out, therapy should be
	  given with doxycycline[b], 100 mg PO bid × 7 d)
	Ceftriaxone, 1 g IM or IV q 24 hr
	or
	Ceftrizoxime, 1 g IV q 8 h
	or
	Ciprofloxacin, 400 mg IV q 12 h[a]
	or
	Ofloxacin, 400 mg IV q 12 h[a]
	or
	Levofloxacin, 250 mg IV q 24 h[a]
	or
	Spectinomycin, 2 g IM q 12 h
	or
	Cefotaxime, 1 g IV q 8 h
	until 24–48 h after symptoms begin to improve,
	then
	complete 7-d course with
	Ciprofloxacin[a], 500 mg PO bid
	or
	Ofloxacin[a], 400 mg PO bid
	or
	Levofloxacin[a], 500 mg PO q 24 h

Adapted from the CDC recommendations.

[a]Quinolones should not be used for infections acquired in Asia, the Pacific, California, and other areas with known increased prevalence of quinolones resistance.

[b]Quinolone and tetracycline antibiotics are contraindicated in pregnancy.

Evaluation of Sexual Partners

The most common cause of treatment failure in patients treated for gonorrhea is repeated exposure to untreated sexual partners. Because asymptomatic partners of persons with uncomplicated or complicated gonococcal infections are at substantially increased risk for asymptomatic infection, treatment of all partners within the preceding 60 days (40) is recommended, regardless of the presence or absence of signs or symptoms of infection. This accomplishes the dual purpose of providing therapy for asymptomatically infected persons who may have infected the initial patient (source contacts) and treating partners who may have acquired infection as the result of exposure to the initial patient after his or her acquisition of infection (spread contacts), who may be asymptomatic or still incubating the infection.

REFERENCES

1. Turner CF, Rogers SM, Miller HG, et al. Untreated gonococcal and chlamydial infection in a probability sample of adults. *JAMA* 2002;287:726.
2. Division of STD Prevention. *Sexually transmitted disease surveillance 2001.* US Department of Health and Human Services, Public Health Service. Atlanta, Centers for Disease Control and Prevention, 2002.
3. Low N, Daker-White G, Barlow D, Pozniak AL. Gonorrhea in inner London: results of a cross sectional study. *BMJ* 1997;314:1719.
4. Lacey CJ, Merrick DW, Bensley DC, Fairley I. Analysis of the sociodemography of gonorrhoea in Leeds, 1989–93. *BMJ* 1997;314:1715
5. Louv WC, Austin H, Perlman J, Alexander WJ. Oral contraceptive use and the risk of chlamydial and gonococcal infections. *Am J Obstet Gynecol* 1989;160:396.
6. Critchlow CW, Wolner-Hanssen P, Eschenbach DA, et al. Determinants of cervical ectopia and cervicitis: age, oral contraception, specific cervical infection, smoking and douching. *Am J Obstet Gynecol* 1995;173:534.
7. Upchurch DM, Brady WE, Reichart CA, Hook EW III. Behavioral contributions to acquisition of gonorrhea in patients attending an inner city sexually transmitted disease clinic. *J Infect Dis* 1990;161:938.
8. Hook EW, Brady WE, Reichart CA, et al. Determinants of emergence of antibiotic-resistant *Neisseria gonorrhoeae. J Infect Dis* 1989;159:900.
9. Page-Shafer K, Graves A, Kent C, Balls JE, Zapitz VM, Klausner JD. Increased sensitivity of DNA amplification testing for the detection of pharyngeal gonorrhea in men who have sex with men. *Clin Infect Dis* 2002;34:173.
10. Stary A, Ching SF, Teodorowicz L, Lee H. Comparison of ligase chain reaction and culture for detection of *Neisseria gonorrhoeae* in genital and extragenital specimens. *J Clin Microbiol* 1997;35:239.
11. Goodhart ME, Ogden J, Zaidi AA, Kraus S. Factors affecting the performance of smear and culture tests for the detection of *Neisseria gonorrhoeae. Sex Transm Dis* 1982;9:63.
12. Lossick JG, Smeltzer MP, Curran JW. The value of the cervical gram stain in the diagnosis and treatment of gonorrhea in women in a veneral disease clinic. *Sex Transm Dis* 1982;9:124.
13. Centers for Disease Control and Prevention. Screening tests to detect *Chlamydia trachomatis* and *Neisseria gonorrhoeae* infections. *MMWR* 2002;51:RR–15.
14. Mirrett S, Reller LB, Knapp JS. *Neisseria gonorrhoeae* strains inhibited by vancomycin in selective media and correlation with auxotype. *J Clin Microbiol* 1981;14:94.
15. Bonin P, Tanino TT, Handsfield HH. Isolation of *Neisseria gonorrhoeae* on selective and nonselective media in a sexually transmitted disease clinic. *J Clin Microbiol* 1984;19:218.
16. Reichart CA, Rupkey LM, Brady WE, Hook EW III. Comparison of GC-lect and modified Thayer-Martin media for isolation of *Neisseria gonorrhoeae. J Clin Microbiol* 1989;27:808.
17. Schmale JD, Martin JE, Domescik G. Observations in the culture diagnosis of gonorrhea in women. *Am J Obstet Gynecol* 1971;109:463.
18. Koumans EH, Johnson RE, Knapp JS, St. Louis ME. Laboratory testing for *Neisseria gonorrhoeae* by recently introduced nonculture tests: a performance review with clinical and public health considerations. *Clin Infect Dis* 1998;27:1171.
19. Smith K, Harrington K, Wingood G, Oh MK, Hook EW 3rd, DiClemente RJ. Self-obtained vaginal swabs for diagnosis of treatable sexually transmitted diseases in adolescent girls. *Arch Pediatr Adolesc Med* 2001;155:676.
20. Tabrizi SN, Paterson B, Fairley CK, Bowden FJ, Garland SM. A self-administered technique for the detection of sexually transmitted diseases in remote communities. *J Infect Dis* 1997;176:289.
21. Rompalo AM, Gaydos CA, Shah N, et al. Evaluation of use of a single intravaginal swab to detect multiple sexually transmitted infections in active-duty military women. *Clin Infect Dis* 2001;33:1455.
22. Wiesner PJ, Tronca E, Bonin P, et al. Clinical spectrum of pharyngeal gonococcal infection. *N Engl J Med* 1973;288:181.
23. Quinn TC, Stamm WE, Goodell SE, et al. The polymicrobial origin of intestinal infections in homosexual men. *N Engl J Med* 1983;309:576.
24. Holmes KK, Counts GW, Beaty HN. Disseminated gonococcal infection. *Ann Intern Med* 1971;74:979.
25. Handsfield HH, Wiesner PJ, Holmes KK. Treatment of the gonococcal arthritis-dermatitis syndrome. *Ann Intern Med* 1976;84:661.
26. Eschenbach DA, Buchanan TM, Pollock HM, et al. Polymicrobial etiology of acute pelvic inflammatory disease. *N Engl J Med* 1975;293:166.
27. Wasserheit JN, Bell TA, Kiviat NB, et al. Microbial causes of proven pelvic inflammatory disease and efficacy of clindamycin and tobramycin. *Ann Intern Med* 1986;104:187.
28. Wolner-Hanssen P, Paavonen J, Kiviat N, et al. Outpatient treatment of pelvic inflammatory disease with cefoxitin and doxycycline. *Obstet Gynecol* 1988;71:595.
29. Disseminated gonorrhea caused by penicillinase-producing *Neisseria gonorrhoeae* - Wisconsin, Pennsylvania. *MMWR* 1987;36:161.
30. Black JR, Brint M, Reichart CA. Successful treatment of gonococcal endocarditis with ceftriaxone. *J Infect Dis* 1988;157:1281.
31. Centers for Disease Control and Prevention. Disseminated gonococcal infections and meningitis - Pennsylvania. *MMWR* 1984;33:158.
32. Centers for Disease Control and Prevention. 1993 Sexually transmitted diseases guidelines. *MMWR* 1993;42:57.
33. Centers for Disease Control and Prevention. Plasmid-mediated antimicrobial resistance in *Neisseria gonorrhoeae* - United States, 1988 and 1989. *MMWR* 1990;284:293.
34. Knapp JS, Mesola VP, Neal SW. Molecular epidemiology, in 1994, of *Neisseria gonorrhoeae* in Manila and Cebu City, Republic of the Phillipines. *Sex Transm Dis* 1994;24:2.
35. Tanaka M, Kumazawa J, Matsumoto T, Kobayashi I. High prevalence of *Neisseria gonorrhoeae* strains with reduced susceptibility to fluoroquinolones in Japan. *Genitourin Med* 1994;70:90.
36. Knapp JS, Wongba C, Limpakarnjanarat K. Antimicrobial susceptibilities of strains of *Neisseria gonorrhoeae* in Bangkok, Thailand: 1994–1995. *Sex Transm Dis* 1997;24:142.
37. Turner A, Gough KR, Jephcott AE, McClean AN. Importation into the UK of a strain of *Neisseria gonorrhoeae* resistant to penicillin, ciprofloxacin and tetracycline. *Genitourin Med* 1995;71:331.
38. Bogaerts J, Tello WM, Akingeneye J, Mukantabana V, VanDyck E, Piot P. Effectiveness of norfloxacin and ofloxacin for treatment of gonorrhea and decrease of in vitro susceptibility to quinolones over time in Rwanda. *Genitourin Med* 1993;69:196.
39. Dan M, Poch F, Shpitz D, Sheinberg B. High level ciprofloxacin resistance in *Neisseria gonorrhoeae:* first report from Israel. *Emerg Infect Dis* 2001;7:158.
40. Centers for Disease Control and Prevention. 2002 Sexually transmitted diseases guidelines. *MMWR* 2002;51.
41. Trees DL, Sandul AL, Neal SW, Higa H, Knapp JS. Molecular epidemiology of *Neisseria gonorrhoeae* exhibiting decreased susceptibility and resistance to ciprofloxacin in Hawaii, 1991–1999. *Sex Transm Dis* 2001;28:309.
42. Knapp JS, Biddle JW, DeWitt WE, Johnson SR. Frequency and distribution in the United States of strains of *Neisseria gonorrhoeae* with plasmid-mediated, high-level resistance to tetracycline. *J Infect Dis* 1987;155:819.
43. Morse SA, Johnson SR, Biddle JW, Roberts MC. High-level tetracycline resistance in *Neisseria gonorrhoeae* is result of acquisition of streptococcal tetM determinant. *Antimicrob Agents Chemother* 1986;30:664.
44. Handsfield HH, Sandstrom EG, Knapp JS, et al. Epidemiology of penicillinase-producing *Neisseria gonorrhoeae* infections. *N Engl J Med* 1982;306:950.
45. Boslego JW, Tramont EC, Takafuji ET, et al. Effect of spectinomycin use on the prevalence of spectinomycin-resistant and of penicillinase-producing *Neisseria gonorrhoeae. N Engl J Med* 1987;317:272.
46. Faruki H, Kohmescher RN, McKinney WP, Sparling PF. A community-based outbreak of infection with penicillin-resistant *Neisseria gonorrhoeae* not producing penicillinase (chromosomally mediated resistance). *N Engl J Med* 1985;313:607.
47. Washington AE, Browner WS, Korenbrot CC. Cost-effectiveness of combined treatment for endocervical gonorrhea. *JAMA* 1987;257:2056.
48. Haimovici R, Roussel TJ. Treatment of gonococcal conjunctivitis with single dose intramuscular ceftriaxone. *Am J Ophthalmol* 1989;107:511.
49. Buch LM, Boscia JA. Disseminated multiple antibiotic-resistant gonococcal infection: needed changes in antimicrobial therapy. *Ann Intern Med* 1987;107:692.

CHAPTER 104
Chlamydial Infections of the Genital Tract

Julius Schachter

HISTORY

Lymphogranuloma venereum (LGV), described by John Hunter in the 18th century, was the first genital tract disease caused by *Chlamydia trachomatis* to be recognized as a discrete clinical entity. Others, such as nongonococcal urethritis (NGU) and neonatal ophthalmia, were only recognized after the identification of the gonococcus (1). The introduction of Credé prophylaxis to prevent ophthalmia neonatorum, and methods to diagnose gonococcal infections, made it apparent that conjunctivitis in infants and urethritis in adult men had nongonococcal forms. Chlamydial inclusions were seen in specimens from such cases in the early 1900s, although the organism was not isolated until the late 1950s. A breakthrough was the introduction of a cell culture isolation method. Using this test, it was found that 30% to 50% of men with NGU had chlamydial infections (1,2). Since then, the clinical syndromes associated with these infections have rapidly expanded (2,3).

CHARACTERISTICS OF THE PATHOGEN

C. trachomatis is an obligate intracellular bacterium. It is one of four species within the genus *Chlamydia*. Two others, *C. psittaci* and *C. pneumoniae*, are also human pathogens. *C. trachomatis* is differentiated from the other species by sulfonamide sensitivity and having inclusions that contain glycogen. Chlamydiae are separated from other bacteria on the basis of a unique developmental cycle, which involves alternation between two morphologic forms. The infectious elementary body (EB) is a small (approximately 350 nm) rigid form that is not metabolically active, but is responsible for transmission between cells and hosts. The larger (approximately 1000 nm) intracellular form, called the reticulate body (RB), is metabolically active and divides by binary fission. It is not stable in the extracellular environment. A more detailed description of the organism's biologic properties can be found in Chapter 222.

EPIDEMIOLOGY

C. trachomatis is considered the most common sexually transmitted bacterial pathogen (4). It is estimated that greater than 3 million infections occur annually in the United States, with more than 80 million worldwide (5). With the introduction of urine-based screening using nucleic acid amplification tests (NAATs), screening studies were done on populations that could not have been readily tested using previous technology. Groups tested included high school students, and members of the job corps and the military (6–8). The results confirmed the high prevalence, and broad distribution of asymptomatic chlamydial infection in the United States.

At least 60% to 70% of perinatally exposed infants acquire the infection when they pass through the infected birth canal and pneumonia develops in approximately 18%, and conjunctivitis in 35% (9). Sporadic cases of adult conjunctivitis occur when infective genital discharges are inoculated into the eye.

Incubation periods of chlamydial infections are relatively long, typically 1 to 3 weeks, reflecting the bacterium's long (48 to 72 hours) growth cycle. The efficiency of sexual transmission of chlamydiae is not known. Contact tracing studies reveal infection rates of 85% for female source contacts of men with chlamydial urethritis (10). Inapparent infections are common. In screening settings, up to 70% of women with chlamydial infection have neither signs nor symptoms of infection (11). If untreated, chlamydial infections can persist for years.

Individuals with lower genital tract infection are at risk for upper genital tract disease (3). Clinically evident pelvic inflammatory disease will develop in approximately 10% of young women with cervical chlamydial infection. However, perhaps an even larger proportion may develop asymptomatic upper genital tract infections that can also lead to tubal factor infertility and ectopic pregnancy (12).

Several risk factors for chlamydial infection can be identified. Age is the most important one. The highest infection rates are found in sexually active adolescents where approximately 15% of girls and 5% to 10% of boys may be infected (2,7,8,11,13). Other risk factors include previous chlamydial infection, recent change in partner, a symptomatic partner, failure to use barrier contraceptives, low socioeconomic status, and use of oral contraceptives (2,8,11,13,14). One important risk factor is the diagnosis of gonorrhea (2,3). Approximately 20% of men and 40% of women with gonorrhea have concomitant chlamydial infection.

The proportions cited reflect data from studies performed before the introduction of *Chlamydia* control programs. *C. trachomatis* prevalence can drop dramatically with the introduction of broad-based screening and treatment programs. In cities where *Chlamydia* prevalence is dropping, the chlamydial contribution to various disease states changes as well.

PATHOGENESIS

Pathogenic mechanisms for chlamydial diseases are not clear. Chlamydial infection can induce local lymphoproliferation in the form of lymphoid follicles (1). The trachoma biovar of *C. trachomatis*, the common sexually transmitted pathogen, grows only in squamocolumnar cells. There is suggestive evidence that much of the pathologic process is mediated by immune responses and that second infections are more damaging. Sensitizing antigens have been identified from animal studies. The leading candidate for a sensitizing antigen has been characterized as a member of the 60-kDa heat shock protein (HSP 60) family (15). This antigen induces inflammation in previously sensitized animals. The soluble antigen is loosely bound to the EB, is excreted by infected cells, and may be produced when productive infection has been suppressed by lymphokines (16). Women suffering from tubal factor infertility or ectopic pregnancy may have high levels of antibodies to HSP 60 (17,18).

CLINICAL MANIFESTATIONS

Genital Tract Disease

The most common manifestation is NGU in men (3,4) (Table 104.1). This syndrome is defined by the failure to find *Neisseria gonorrhoeae* organisms in urethral specimens from a man with urethritis. NGU is more common than gonococcal urethritis. The age distribution is similar for NGU and gonococcal urethritis. Most cases occur in the 15- to 25-year-old group. NGU is characterized by pyuria. There is usually a mucoid to mucopurulent discharge, less purulent than the typical discharge in gonorrhea.

TABLE 104.1. Proportion of Common Genital Tract Disease Attributed to *Chlamydia trachomatis*

Condition	Percentage due to *Chlamydia*
Nongonococcal urethritis	35–50
Postgonococcal urethritis	>70
Epididymitis, young men	>60
Mucopurulent endocervicitis	30–50
Acute salpingitis	25–50

TABLE 104.2. Clinical Conditions Calling for Presumptive Therapy for *Chlamydia trachomatis* Infection

Population	Conditions
Men	Nongonococcal urethritis
	Postgonococcal urethritis
	Epididymitis
	Gonorrhea
	Female partner with conditions listed below
Women	Mucopurulent endocervicitis
	Acute salpingitis
	Gonorrhea
	Male partner with conditions listed above

However, the clinical findings in NGU and gonococcal urethritis overlap enough to render diagnosis on clinical grounds inaccurate. Men without discharge can have NGU. A common method of diagnosing NGU is to demonstrate a "significant" number of polymorphonuclear leukocytes (PMNs) in first-catch urine or a smear prepared from a urethral swab. If a Gram stain of discharge shows many PMNs but no intracellular diplococci, a presumptive diagnosis of NGU is made. There is no unanimity as to the significant number of PMNs. For resuspension of the centrifuged sediment of a 10- to 15-ml sample of first-catch urine, the usual criterion is 15 or more PMNs per 400 × high-power field; for a smear obtained by urethral swabbing, the cutoff is 5 or more PMNs per 1,000 × field (3).

Postgonococcal urethritis, a special subset of NGU, is seen in men who have been successfully treated for gonococcal infection and either develop symptoms shortly after therapy or remain symptomatic (19). *C. trachomatis* is responsible for 70% to 90% of cases. β-Lactam drugs in dosages used to treat gonorrhea are largely ineffective against chlamydiae. Because of the high (greater than 20%) double infection rate, CDC recommends that all cases of gonorrhea be treated presumptively for chlamydial infection (4).

Although NGU was long considered to be trivial, it is now recognized that serious complications can result (3). Ascending infections can result in epididymitis. *C. trachomatis* is the leading cause of epididymitis in sexually active young men. Rectal infections are not uncommon. Screening studies in gay men attending venereal disease clinics found 6% of asymptomatic men yielded *Chlamydia* from rectal swabs, compared with a 12% recovery rate from men with proctitis. *C. trachomatis* has been recovered from the pharynx of sexually active adults at risk for genital tract infection.

In the woman, the most commonly affected site is the cervix, where the organism can cause a mucopurulent endocervicitis (3). This condition is characterized by a mucopurulent endocervical discharge, with easily induced bleeding and edema within a zone of ectopy. Women with gonorrhea often have chlamydial infection. Double infection rates may be twice as high (at 35% to 45%) as those observed in men. It is even more important to treat women with gonorrhea for chlamydial infection as it reduces subsequent development of salpingitis (4,20).

Efforts have been made to establish clinical criteria for diagnosing chlamydial cervicitis. Swab tests can be used to demonstrate a purulent discharge (a white swab inserted in the endocervical canal will be colored yellow in the presence of a purulent discharge) or easily induced bleeding (a swab rubbed against the endocervical wall will be reddened by bleeding caused by pressure if the cervix is edematous and inflamed). These tests have a predictive value of 30% to 50% for *C. trachomatis* infection in different populations and have been used as a guideline for presumptive therapy (Table 104.2).

C. trachomatis is a parasite of columnar epithelium; not squamous cells. Thus, the organism does not cause vaginitis. The ma-

jor susceptible sites within the lower genital tract are in the endocervix, within the squamocolumnar junction, and in the urethra. Chlamydial infection has been associated with sterile pyuria in college-age women (3). The association of chlamydiae with the urethral syndrome should not be generalized to other female populations.

Ascending genital infection is common. Acute salpingitis is the most important complication of sexually transmitted chlamydial infection (3,4,12). *C. trachomatis* is commonly found in the endometrium or fallopian tubes of women with acute salpingitis (21–23). As expected, younger women are at higher risk (12). Chlamydial salpingitis tends to be clinically milder than salpingitis associated with gonococcal or mixed anaerobic infections. *Chlamydia*-infected women usually have a longer prodrome before being admitted to the hospital. *C. trachomatis* is also associated with the Fitz-Hugh-Curtis syndrome (perihepatitis)—a complication of salpingitis.

Chlamydiae are important causes of tubal factor infertility and ectopic pregnancy as a result of tubal damage after salpingitis (12). Unfortunately, because chlamydial salpingitis can be clinically mild, or even inapparent, evidence of chlamydial infection is often first obtained retrospectively by serologic tests performed during evaluation for infertility.

The endometrium may be involved in women with generalized pelvic inflammation (24). Endometrial infection occurs as part of a pathway involving spread from cervix to oviduct (as is likely to be the case for women with salpingitis) but there may be a discrete self-limited chlamydial endometritis. Chlamydiae have been recovered from the endometrium of asymptomatic nonpregnant women (25).

Women who test positive for *Chlamydia* in the first trimester of pregnancy may develop postpartum endometritis after vaginal delivery (26). The role of *C. trachomatis* in other pregnancy complications is controversial. Some studies found an association with fetal wastage and prematurity (27,28). Other have not confirmed these findings, or have found only a small subset of women with chlamydial infection (those with IgM antibody) had an excess prematurity rate (29). The issue is unresolved (30).

Neonatal Disease

Approximately 5 to 21 days after birth, the infant develops a mucopurulent conjunctivitis (1,2). Hyperemia and discharge are the most prominent findings. Follicles are not seen unless the condition persists for longer than 1 month. Conjunctivitis is usually self-limiting and resolves in a few months without treatment. It is not a sight-threatening condition. Corneal damage is minimal, although some keratitis and micropannus can develop. Conjunctival scarring is relatively uncommon, although sheet scarring may follow the disease in infants in whom pseudomembranes develop. These scars do not result in lid deformity. Occasional cases persist, and severe disease, which may threaten vision, can rarely develop.

The incubation period for chlamydial pneumonia of infants is usually between 2 and 12 weeks (31,32). The infants will often have had rhinitis and conjunctivitis. Affected infants are usually afebrile, are markedly tachypneic and occasionally apneic, and have a staccato cough. They are hypergammaglobulinemic, particularly in IgM. A relative eosinophilia occurs in approximately one third of affected infants. Radiographs usually show hyperinflation.

The spectrum of chlamydial respiratory involvement in infants is broad. Nasopharyngeal infections are common (31). Some infants develop a severe rhinitis, without lower respiratory tract involvement, that can occasionally interfere with respiration. The pathogenesis of chlamydial pneumonia probably reflects descending infection. Bronchiolitis can occur. Infants with chlamydial pneumonia typically fall into the category of infants with failure to thrive and often have only mild respiratory distress, with tachypnea being the prominent finding. The infants occasionally have severe respiratory problems and may become apneic and require respiratory assistance, but more often they can be managed on an outpatient basis. Most infants with chlamydial pneumonia later develop asthma or obstructive airway disease (33), even after successful treatment of the acute disease.

Conjunctivitis in Adults

Inclusion conjunctivitis in adults is an acute follicular conjunctivitis that must be differentiated from adenoviral keratoconjunctivitis by microbiologic tests. It is typically seen in sexually active young adults and results from exposure to infected genital discharges. It is similar in presentation to early trachoma but it is not considered to be sight-threatening. It can become chronic, although most cases clear spontaneously after several months if they are not treated.

DIAGNOSIS

It was long thought that isolation in a cell culture system was the most efficient way of diagnosing *C. trachomatis* infection (34). Although this procedure was only 80% to 90% sensitive in expert laboratories, it was still more sensitive than the antigen detection methods. The major variable in diagnosis has been adequate specimen collection because appropriate samples of involved epithelial cells must be collected, and it is important that specimens be processed relatively quickly and that a cold chain be maintained. Cycloheximide-treated McCoy cells are the most commonly used system. The nonculture methods that were more widely available include direct fluorescent antibody test, enzyme immunoassay, and direct DNA probes (34).

Amplified DNA probe technology is much more sensitive (34,35). There are four different technologies commercially available, polymerase chain reaction (PCR), ligase chain reaction (LCR), transcription-mediated amplification (TMA), and strand displacement assay (SDA). They have similar performance profiles and all are far more sensitive than culture. A major breakthrough was when LCR was found to be efficient in detecting chlamydial infection using urine samples from both men and women (36,37). This allows noninvasive specimen collection and opens many possibilities for screening studies. Vaginal swabs are also useful, and again the different tests are similar in performance.

Infant conjunctivitis may be diagnosed readily by any of the cytologic tests. Giemsa stain is adequate in diagnosing severe cases of conjunctivitis, whereas the antigen detection techniques are sensitive. The agent may be easily isolated. A specific diagnosis for pneumonia may be more difficult because of sampling problems, but the organism can often be isolated from the nasopharynx or tracheobronchial aspirate specimens (31). Serologic testing may be the method of choice for diagnosing chlamydial pneumonia because of the sampling problems. Infants with chlamydial pneumonia almost always develop high IgM antibody levels, and because of their defined exposure (at birth), the diagnosis may be readily established by a single high titer (greater than 1:32) of specific antichlamydial IgM antibodies in the microimmunofluorescence test (38).

Serologic tests do not play a role in diagnosing uncomplicated lower genital tract infections (39). A major problem is a high prevalence of antibodies to *C. trachomatis* in high-risk populations. The complement fixation test is relatively insensitive for diagnosing infections with the trachoma biotype. The microimmunofluorescence test is the serologic test of choice (40). Because of the high titers seen in upper genital tract disease, serology can play a supportive role in establishing a diagnosis of chlamydial salpingitis or epididymitis.

TABLE 104.3. **Treatment of Chlamydial Infections**

Organism and condition	First choice		Second choice	
	Drug	Dose	Drug	Dose
C. psittaci				
Psittacosis[a]	Tetracycline	250 mg qid × 3 wk	Erythromycin	250 mg qid × 3 wk
C. trachomatis				
Genital tract infections (e.g., urethritis, cervicitis)	Azithromycin	1 g orally, single dose[b]	Doxycycline	100 mg bid × 1 wk[b]
Pregnant women	Erythromycin	500 mg qid × 1 wk[b]	Amoxicillin	500 mg tid × 1 wk[b]
Infant pneumonia	Erythromycin	50 mg/kg/day divided into 4 doses daily × 2 wk[b]	Sulfisoxazole	37.5 mg/kg qid × 2 wk
Inclusion conjunctivitis (infants)	Erythromycin	50 mg/kg/day divided into 4 doses daily × 2 wk[b]	Sulfisoxazole	37.5 mg/kg qid × 2 wk
Inclusion conjunctivitis (adults)	Tetracycline	250 mg qid × 3 wk	Erythromycin	250 mg qid × 3 wk

[a]Similar regimens are probably effective for *C. pneumoniae* (TWAR) infection.
[b]1998 Guidelines for the Treatment of Sexually Transmitted Disease, Centers for Disease Control and Prevention.

TREATMENT

One gram of oral azithromycin given in a single dose is now considered the treatment of choice for uncomplicated lower genital tract infections with *C. trachomatis* (4). This is as effective as a week-long course of oral doxycycline (41). The currently recommended guidelines for treating these infections are shown in Table 104.3. Chlamydial infection in the infant calls for oral therapy with erythromycin. Conjunctivitis usually responds to 7 to 10 days of therapy; pneumonia should be treated for 14 to 21 days (4). Topical therapy is not recommended for conjunctivitis because of relatively high failure rates and because systemic therapy will prevent subsequent development of pneumonia. Treatment of pelvic inflammatory disease should always include antimicrobials effective against *C. trachomatis* (see Chapter 222).

PREVENTION

No vaccines are available. Guidelines for a *Chlamydia* control program have been developed, but no such control program is currently in effect because of economic constraints (42). Recommendations include screening of high-risk populations and examination and treatment of contacts. Such programs have been shown to be effective in reducing prevalence of infection among clinic attendees, and may reduce development of salpingitis (43). It is now accepted that good medical care for sexually active young women includes, as a routine, an annual test for chlamydial infection. The introduction of NAATs has allowed for non invasive specimen collection and screening of asymptomatic populations. Thus community and high-school based programs to screen for *C. trachomatis* infection of the genital tract have begun to screen both males and females (44,45).

Perinatal chlamydial infections can be prevented by a program of screening pregnant women and treating those found to be infected with erythromycin (46). Because attack rates have been fairly consistent in most studies, the prevalence of chlamydial infection in pregnant women will determine the cost-benefit relationship of this stratagem. A number of studies have found that more than 20% of pregnant women have chlamydial infection. Such prenatal clinics would clearly be appropriate sites for screening and treatment.

REFERENCES

1. Schachter J, Dawson CR. *Human chlamydial infections.* Littleton, MA: Publishing Sciences Group, 1978.
2. Schachter J. Chlamydial infections (in three parts). *N Engl J Med* 1978;298:428–435, 490–495, 540–549.
3. Stamm WE. *Chlamydia trachomatis* infections of the adult. In Holmes KK, Sparling PF, March P-A, et al, eds: *Sexually transmitted diseases,* 3rd ed. New York: McGraw Hill, 1999:407–422.
4. Centers for Disease Control and Prevention. 1998 Guidelines for treatment of sexually transmitted diseases. *MMWR* 1998;47:1–111.
5. Gerbase AC, Rowley JT, Mertens TE. Global epidemiology of sexually transmitted diseases. *Lancet* 1998;351[Suppl 3]:2–4.
6. Gaydos CA, Howell MR, Pare B, Clark KL, Ellis DA, Hendrix RM, et al. *Chlamydia trachomatis* infections in female military recruits. *N Engl J Med* 1998;339:739–744.
7. Gaydos CA, Crotchfelt KA, Howell MR, Kralian S, Hauptman P, Quinn TC. Molecular amplification assays to detect chlamydial infections in urine specimens from high school female students and to monitor the persistence of chlamydial DNA after therapy. *J Infect Dis* 1998;177:417–424.
8. Burstein GR, Gaydos CA, Diener-West M, Howell MR, Zenilman JM, Quinn TC. Incident *Chlamdyia trachomatis* infections among inner-city adolescent females. *JAMA* 1998;280:521–526.
9. Schachter J, Grossman M, Sweet RL, Holt J, Jordan C, Bishop E. Prospective study of perinatal transmission of *Chlamydia trachomatis. JAMA* 1986;255:3374–3377.
10. Oriel JD, Ridgway GL. Studies of the epidemiology of chlamydial infection of the human genital tract. In Mardh PA, Holmes KK, Oriel JD, Piot P, Schachter J, eds: *Chlamydial infections: proceedings of the 5th international symposium on human chlamydial infections, Lund, Sweden.* Amsterdam: Elsevier, 1982:425–428.
11. Schachter J, Stoner E, Moncada J. Screening for chlamydial infections in women attending family planning clinics. *West J Med* 1983;138:375–379.
12. Westrom L, Joesoef R, Reynolds G, Hagdu A, Thompson SE. Pelvic inflammatory disease and fertility. A cohort study of 1,844 women with laparoscopically verified disease and 657 control women with normal laparoscopic results. *Sex Transm Dis* 1992;19:185–192.
13. Shafer MA, Prager V, Shalwitz J, et al. Prevalence of urethral *Chlamydia trachomatis* and *Neisseria gonorrhoeae* among asymptomatic, sexually active adolescent boys. *J Infect Dis* 1987;156:223–224.
14. Handsfield HH, Jasman LL, Roberts PL, Hanson VW, Kothenbeutel RL, Stamm WE. Criteria for selective screening for *Chlamydia trachomatis* infection in women attending family planning clinics. *JAMA* 1986;255:1730–1734.
15. Morrison RP, Belland RJ, Lyng K, Caldwell HD. Chlamydial disease pathogenesis. The 57-kD chlamydial hypersensitivity antigen is a stress response protein. *J Exp Med* 1989;170:1271–1283.
16. Beatty WL, Byrne GI, Morrison RP. Morphologic and antigenic charcterization of interferon gamma-mediated persistent *Chlamydia trachomatis* infection in vitro. *Proc Natl Acad Sci USA* 1993;90:3998–4002.
17. Wagar EA, Schachter J, Bavoil P, Stephens RS. Differential human serologic response to two 60,000 molecular weight *Chlamydia trachomatis* antigens. *J Infect Dis* 1990;162:922–927.
18. Toye B, Laferriere C, Claman P, Jessamine P, Peeling R. Association between antibody to the chlamydial heat-shock protein and tubal infertility. *J Infect Dis* 1993;168:1236–1240.
19. Oriel JD, Ridgway GL, Reeve P, Beckingham DC, Owen J. The lack of effect of ampicillin plus probenecid given for genital infections with Neisseria gonorrhoeae on associated infections with *Chlamydia trachomatis. J Infect Dis* 1976;133:568–571.
20. Stamm WE, Guinan ME, Johnson C, Starcher T, Holmes KK, McCormack WM. Effect of treatment regimens for *Neisseria gonorrhoeae* on simultaneous infection with *Chlamydia trachomatis. N Engl J Med* 1984;310:545–549.
21. Mardh PA, Ripa T, Svensson L, Westrom L. *Chlamydia trachomatis* infection in patients with acute salpingitis. *N Engl J Med* 1977;296:1377–1379.
22. Wasserheit JN, Bell TA, Kiviat NB, et al. Microbial causes of proven pelvic inflammatory disease and efficacy of clindamycin and tobramycin. *Ann Intern Med* 1986;104:187–193.
23. Sweet RL, Schachter J, Robbie MO. Failure of beta-lactam antibiotics to eradicate *Chlamydia trachomatis* in the endometrium despite apparent clinical cure of acute salpingitis. *Jama* 1983;250:2641–2645.
24. Kiviat NB, Wolner-Hanssen P, Peterson M, et al. Localization of *Chlamydia trachomatis* infection by direct immunofluorescence and culture in pelvic inflammatory disease. *Am J Obstet Gynecol* 1986;154:865–873.
25. Cleary RE, Jones RB. Recovery of *Chlamydia trachomatis* from the endometrium of infertile women with serum antichlamydial antibodies. *Fertil Steril* 1985;44:233.
26. Wager GP, Martin DH, Koutsky L, et al. Puerperal infectious morbidity: relationship to route of delivery and to antepartum *Chlamydia trachomatis* infection. *Am J Obstet Gynecol* 1980;138[7 Pt 2]:1028–1033.
27. Martin DH, Koutsky L, Eschenbach DA, et al. Prematurity and perinatal mortality in pregnancies complicated by maternal *Chlamydia trachomatis* infections. *JAMA* 1982;247:1585–1588.
28. Gravett MG, Nelson HP, DeRouen T, Critchlow C, Eschenbach DA, Holmes KK. Independent associations of bacterial vaginosis and *Chlamydia trachomatis* infection with adverse pregnancy outcome. *JAMA* 1986;256:1899–1903.
29. Sweet RL, Landers DV, Walker C, Schachter J. *Chlamydia trachomatis* infection and pregnancy outcome. *Am J Obstet Gynecol* 1987;156:824–833.
30. Martin DH, Eschenbach DA, Cotch MF, et al. Double-blind placebo-controlled treatment trial of *Chlamydia trachomatis* endocervical infections in pregnant women. *Infect Dis Obstet Gynecol* 1997;5:10–17.
31. Beem MO, Saxon EM. Respiratory-tract colonization and a distinctive pneumonia syndrome in infants infected with *Chlamydia trachomatis. N Engl J Med* 1977;296:306–310.
32. Harrison HR, English MG, Lee CK, Alexander ER. *Chlamydia trachomatis* infant pneumonitis: comparison with matched controls and other infant pneumonitis. *N Engl J Med* 1978;298:702–708.
33. Weiss SG, Newcomb RW, Beem MO. Pulmonary assessment of children after chlamydial pneumonia of infancy. *J Pediatr* 1986;108[5 Pt 1]:659–664.
34. Schachter J, Stamm WE. *Chlamydia.* In Murray PR, Baron EJ, Pfaller MA, Tenover FC, Yolken RH, eds: *Manual of clinical microbiology,* 7th ed. Washington DC: American Society for Microbiology, 1999:795–806.
35. Schachter J. NAATs to diagnose *Chlamydia trachomatis* genital infection: A promise still unfulfilled. *Exp Rev Mol Diag* 2001;1:137–144.
36. Chernesky MA, Lee H, Schachter J, et al. Diagnosis of *Chlamydia trachomatis* urethral infection in symptomatic and asymptomatic men by testing first-void urine in a ligase chain reaction assay. *J Infect Dis* 1994;170:1308–1311.
37. Lee HH, Chernesky MA, Schachter J, et al. Diagnosis of *Chlamydia trachomatis* genitourinary infection in women by ligase chain reaction assay of urine. *Lancet* 1995;345:213–216.
38. Schachter J, Grossman M, Azimi PH. Serology of *Chlamydia trachomatis* in infants. *J Infect Dis* 1982;146:530–535.
39. Schachter J. Chlamydiae. In: Rose NR, Conway de Macario E, Folds JD, Lane

CH, Nakamura RM, eds. *Manual of clinical laboratory immunology*, 5th ed. Washington DC: ASM Press, 1997:552–557.

40. Wang SP, Grayston JT, Alexander ER, Holmes KK. Simplified microimmunofluorescence test with trachoma-lymphogranuloma venereum (*Chlamydia trachomatis*) antigens for use as a screening test for antibody. *J Clin Microbiol* 1975;1:250–255.

41. Martin DH, Mroczkowski TF, Dalu ZA, et al. A controlled trial of a single dose of azithromycin for the treatment of chlamydial urethritis and cervicitis. The Azithromycin for Chlamydial Infections Study Group. *N Engl J Med* 1992;327:921–925.

42. Centers for Disease Control and Prevention. Recommendations for the prevention and management of *Chlamydia trachomatis* infections, 1993. *MMWR* 1993;42:1–39.

43. Scholes D, Stergachis A, Heidrich FE, Andrilla H, Holmes KK, Stamm WE. Prevention of pelvic inflammatory disease by screening for cervical chlamydial infection. *N Engl J Med* 1996;334:1362–1366.

44. Cohen DA, Nsuami M, Etame RB, et al. A school-based *Chlamydia* control program using DNA amplification technology. *Pediatrics* 1998;101:E1.

45. Marrazzo JM, White CL, Krekeler B, et al. Community-based urine screening for *Chlamydia trachomatis* with a ligase chain reaction assay. *Ann Intern Med* 1997;127:796–803.

46. Schachter J, Sweet RL, Grossman M, Landers D, Robbie M, Bishop E. Experience with the routine use of erythromycin for chlamydial infections in pregnancy. *N Engl J Med* 1986;314:276–279.

CHAPTER 105
Syphilis

Daniel M. Musher and Robert E. Baughn

Treponema pallidum is a natural pathogen only for humans. Infection is spread from infected to uninfected individuals by sexual contact; by transplacental passage, leading to congenital syphilis; or rarely by laboratory accident or blood transfusion. The infecting organism enters the body through inapparent breaks in abraded areas of the skin. Within the tissues, local replication and dissemination via lymphatics occur simultaneously, thus setting the stage for secondary (disseminated) syphilis. Secondary syphilis resolves spontaneously, leading to a latent stage. Primary and secondary syphilis together with the first year of latency constitute early syphilis; in the absence of treatment, relapse to secondary syphilis may occur during that first year, which is called early latency. After that year of early latency, relapse to secondary syphilis does not occur, and this stage of syphilis is called late latent. Once this stage is reached, reappearance of disease is called tertiary syphilis. Human immunodeficiency virus (HIV) infection has had a major impact on the natural evolution of this disease; neurologic disease that appears after a much shorter delay is called neurosyphilis but is not designated as tertiary infection. The clinical manifestations of each stage of syphilis are listed in Table 105.1.

PATHOGENESIS AND CLINICAL MANIFESTATIONS

Primary Syphilis

Fourteen to 21 days after inoculation of *T. pallidum* into a dermal site, a red, painless papule 0.5 to 2 cm in diameter appears at the site of inoculation. Within a few days the papule ulcerates, producing the typical chancre of primary syphilis, an ulcerated area sometimes covered by a slight yellowish or grayish exudate and surrounded by a slightly indurated margin (Fig. 105.1). Remarkably, considering their location, syphilitic chancres are painless. They are generally round, although they may be elongated, following tissue lines. Modest enlargement of inguinal lymph nodes, frequently bilaterally, is observed in the majority

of patients who have genital lesions. Although solitary lesions were once said to be characteristic, multiple lesions frequently occur (1).

Because of their venereal origin, primary syphilitic chancres most frequently occur in the genital, perineal, anal, or oral area; however, any part of the body may be affected. Most chancres are found on the penis of men and on the labia, fourchette, or cervix of women. Chancres in the anus or rectum are particularly common in homosexual men. When these lesions cause pain on defecation or rectal bleeding, they can be confused with hemorrhoids or even a neoplasm (2), but they often go unnoticed, as do those on the labia and cervix. In most instances, active syphilis in women and in homosexual men is usually not diagnosed until the secondary stage. If untreated, syphilitic chancres heal spontaneously within 3 to 8 weeks. A local immune reaction, rather than a generalized one, accounts for the healing, because secondary lesions regularly appear during or after the regression of the primary one(s). Differentiating a syphilitic chancre from chancroid, the soft chancre caused by infection with *Haemophilus ducreyi*, may be impossible on clinical grounds, although a great degree of tenderness, a yellow exudate over the lesion, or striking inguinal lymphadenopathy with thin and shiny overlying skin is suggestive of chancroid. Simple trauma, especially to the penis, or a fixed drug eruption may cause lesions resembling chancre. Lesions of herpes simplex virus infection usually are not difficult to differentiate from syphilitic chancres, but coinfection by both organisms may occur.

Secondary (Disseminated) Syphilis

Lesions of secondary syphilis result from the hematogenous dissemination of treponemes from syphilitic chancres, and the term disseminated syphilis might be more appropriate (3). More than 3 weeks elapse between the deposition of *T. pallidum* in the dermis and emergence of these lesions; this delay in development compared to the primary lesions and the failure of the involved sites to develop into lesions that resemble chancres reflect a degree of humoral and/or cellular immunity that modifies the evolution of infection. Thus, secondary syphilis appears 4 to 10 weeks after the initial appearance of primary lesions. In some patients who present with disseminated lesions there is an overlap such that careful examination discloses a primary chancre. Cases of "malignant" syphilis (lues maligna), in which disseminated lesions resemble primary chancres, are rare; host factors that permit this unusual manifestation of syphilis have

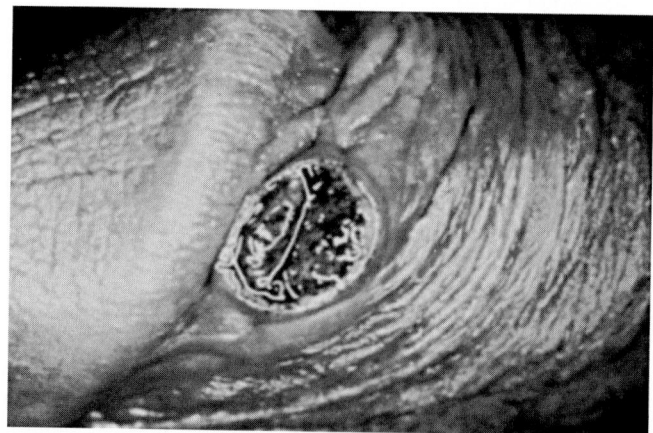

Figure 105.1. Typical syphilitic chancre with clearly demarcated, slightly indurated margin and nonpurulent base.

TABLE 105.1.   Clinical Manifestations of Syphilis by Stages[a]

Primary	Secondary	Tertiary
Chancre on penis, labia, vagina, cervix, anus, rectum, lips, mouth, nipple, navel, finger Inguinal lymphadenopathy Condyloma latum[b]	Rash Condyloma latum Lymphadenopathy Hepatitis (subclinical) Systemic: fever, malaise, weight loss Neurologic: headache, meningismus, meningitis, cranial nerve disorders (optic neuritis, deafness, otitis), cerebrovascular accident Periostitis Uveitis, iritis Glomerulonephritis Arthritis	Benign late syphilis (gummata) of skin, subcutaneous tissues, bones, testis, liver Aortitis, aortic aneurysm Neurosyphilis: tabes dorsalis, paresis, psychosis, dementia, meningitis, cerebrovascular accident, spinal cord disease

[a]Early neurosyphilis, as seen in HIV-infected persons, is specifically not included in this table (see text).
[b]Most commonly extension from a primary lesion, this condition may precede the onset of secondary (disseminated) syphilis, in which case it represents a stage intermediate between primary and secondary disease. Less frequently, condyloma latum appears in intertriginous areas during secondary (disseminated) infection.

not been identified. The clinical picture of lues maligna resembles that seen after intravenous injection of a large inoculum of *T. pallidum* into rabbits, in which multiple skin chancres appear all over the body because there has been no immune response to modify the infection.

The principal finding in disseminated syphilis is a symmetric papular eruption involving the entire trunk and the extremities, including palms of the hands and soles of the feet. The papules are red or reddish brown, discrete, and usually 0.5 to 2 cm in diameter (Fig. 105.2). They are generally scaly, although they may be smooth, follicular, or, rarely, pustular. Except for the involvement of palms and soles, syphilis may be difficult to distinguish from pityriasis rosea or psoriasis. Vesicles are said not to occur, although vesiculopustular lesions are seen on rare occasions and are common on the palms or soles. Pruritus may be present. On occasion, circular (annular) lesions may occur on the face of dark-skinned persons (4). Hypopigmentation or hyperpigmentation may be seen. Alopecia (Fig. 105.3) occurs in some cases. Mucosal lesions, either small, superficial, ulcerated areas with grayish borders that resemble painless aphthous ulcers or larger gray plaques, also occur; these are highly infectious. Erosive gastritis has been documented in rare instances.

Condyloma latum refers to one or more large, raised, whitish or gray lesions found in warm, moist areas. These lesions were originally described as a manifestation of secondary syphilis, reflecting local breakdown of secondary lesions with extension of infection in areas of tissue trauma; most frequently, the axilla and groin were involved (5). Today, it is far more common to observe condylomata in an area adjacent to a primary chancre, generally in the perineum or around the anus, resulting from extension from the primary lesion. These lesions appear before or soon after the generalized lesions. In this situation the local spread of treponemes from a primary lesion in a favorable environment is responsible; the condyloma represents an intermediate stage of infection, because, strictly speaking, it does not reflect dissemination.

Because of the widespread dissemination of treponemes and the immune response to them, secondary syphilis is a systemic disease, and symptoms other than a rash may include malaise, sore throat, headache, weight loss, low-grade fever, or muscle aches. Lymph node enlargement is present in the great majority of patients. In one prospective study, 75% of infected persons had palpable inguinal nodes, and 38% had palpable axillary, 28% posterior cervical, 18% femoral, and 17% epitrochlear nodes (6). In the preantibiotic era, periosteal inflammation

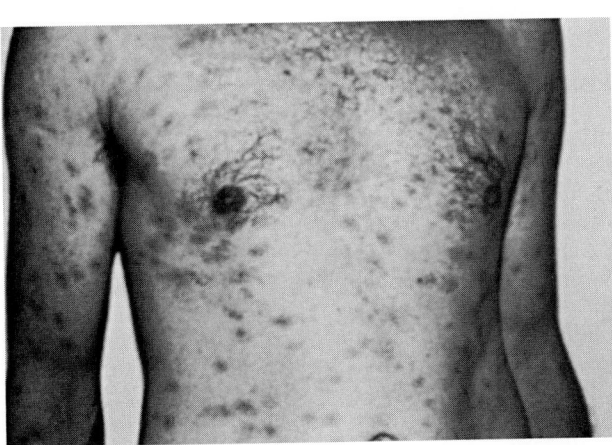

Figure 105.2. Typical generalized rash of secondary syphilis.

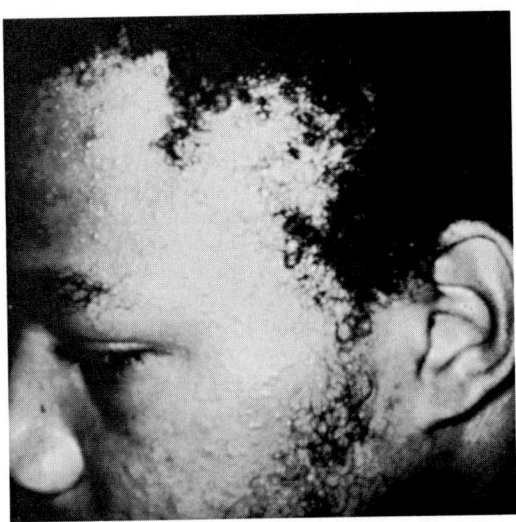

Figure 105.3. Alopecia associated with secondary syphilis. (Slide provided by the late Dr. John Knox.)

was said to be clinically apparent in one fourth of cases with skull, tibia, sternum, and ribs being involved most often; at present, symptomatic involvement occurs only rarely. Subclinical hepatitis can be detected by laboratory studies in 10% of cases and is supported by histologic findings (7). Occasionally, symptomatic hepatitis is seen, but one can not be certain that previously reported cases did not reflect concurrent viral hepatitis.

Neurologic manifestations that appear in early syphilis have received increased attention, especially because of the relation with concurrent HIV infection, which is discussed in detail later in this chapter. Before the occurrence of HIV infection, abnormalities in the cerebrospinal fluid (CSF)—increased white blood cells, elevated protein level, a positive Veneral Disease Research Laboratory (VDRL) test result, or the presence of viable *T. pallidum* organisms—were detected in up to 40% of cases of secondary syphilis in the absence of neurologic abnormalities (8,9). However, no more than 1% to 2% of patients with secondary syphilis were found to have symptoms or signs of central nervous system involvement, including meningismus, meningitis, headaches, and mental changes; cranial nerve abnormalities such as ocular palsy, deafness, or nystagmus, and internuclear ophthalmoplegia; cerebrovascular accidents; or signs of spinal cord or nerve root involvement such as tingling, weakness, and hyporeflexia. These findings are sometimes called early neurosyphilis. Before the penicillin era, they were included under the term neurorecurrence because they nearly always occurred in subjects who had received inadequate therapy for syphilis (10). There may be some degree of overlap between these neurologic manifestations of early, secondary syphilis and some of the classic manifestations of late or tertiary neurosyphilis. It is important to note, however, that at this stage the symptoms are reversible with treatment. Progression to late neurosyphilis was uncommon, even in the pre-penicillin era, if treatment was continued until the CSF returned to normal. As discussed later and reviewed elsewhere (10), both the frequency and the severity of neurologic involvement in secondary syphilis are greatly increased in persons with HIV infection.

Iritis, anterior uveitis, arthritis, and glomerulonephritis or nephrotic syndrome also occur in secondary syphilis. Circulating immune complexes that contain treponemal antigen and human fibronectin together with antibody and complement are present in this stage of infection (11), and their deposition in relevant organs is thought to play a role in the pathogenesis of these syndromes.

Latent Syphilis

The natural history of untreated secondary syphilis (Fig. 105.4) is marked by spontaneous resolution after a period of 3 to 12 weeks, leaving the patient free of lesions and symptoms. If treatment has not been given, this naturally attained asymptomatic state is called latency. In the pretreatment era, 25% of patients whose infection had become latent had a recrudescence of active, secondary syphilis (12). Because these relapses usually occurred within 1 year of the onset of latency, this period was called early latency. Relapses after this time were rare, so after 1 year without recurrence of disease and before the onset of tertiary syphilis untreated persons were said to have entered the late latent period. Patients with late latent syphilis are immune to reinfection with *T. pallidum* (13).

At present, patients are diagnosed as having latent syphilis if: (a) they have no apparent symptoms or signs of syphilis; (b) a serologic test for syphilis (STS) that measures antibody to cardiolipin (see the later section on laboratory diagnosis) is reactive; (c) a test result for specific antitreponemal antibody (*T. pallidum* hemagglutination assay) is positive; and (d) there is not a recent

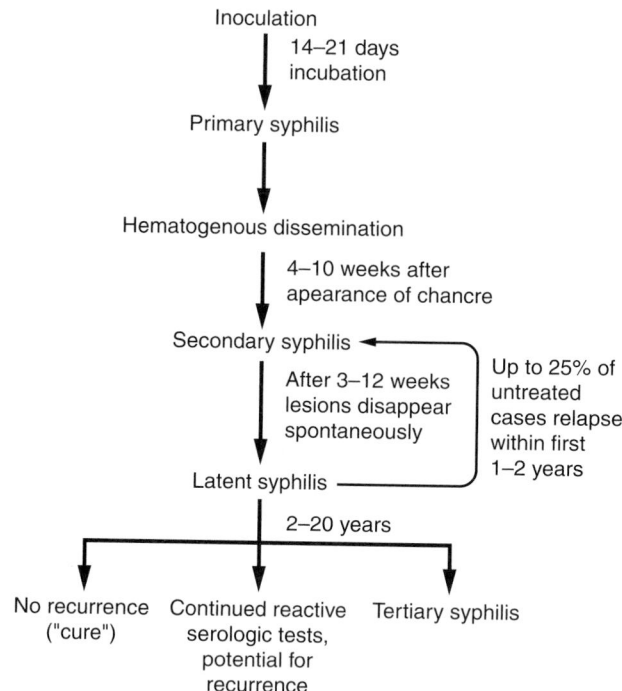

Figure 105.4. Time course of untreated syphilis. Treatment at any stage with accepted doses of penicillin nearly always eliminates disease (exceptions are late manifestations of tertiary syphilis and immunologic compromise caused by HIV infection).

and well-documented history of treatment for syphilis. Strictly speaking, the diagnosis of latent syphilis is proved only if an entirely normal CSF excludes the possibility of neurosyphilis. Patients in whom the diagnosis of latent syphilis is made persons probably represent a heterogeneous group. Some may have an unrecognized chancre. Others may have had an unrecognized chancre that healed and have not yet developed disseminated disease. Some subjects may still have a reactive test after having been given antibiotic treatment for some unrelated condition, syphilis not having been thought to be present. Others may retain reactive STS despite being cured of the infection (a "serofast" state). The majority of patients with positive STS and *T. pallidum* hemagglutination assay results but without signs of active syphilitic infection probably do not have true latent infection, although from a public health point of view they are generally regarded as if they do.

Tertiary Syphilis

Clinical manifestations of tertiary syphilis (14) develop after a highly variable latent period, usually longer than 2 years. The incidence varies greatly, depending on how careful a search is made for the manifestations. Among a large group of untreated patients who were observed for many years, benign late syphilis became clinically apparent in 15%, cardiovascular syphilis in 10%, and neurosyphilis in 7% (12). However, some authorities have stated that the longer patients are observed without treatment, the greater the percentage who develop cardiovascular syphilis (15), and, in one study, some cardiovascular abnormalities attributable to syphilis were said to be present at autopsy in up to 80% of untreated subjects (16). At present, in the United States, benign late syphilis and cardiovascular syphilis are extremely rare.

Benign late syphilis is characterized by the presence of gummata—true granulomas with epithelioid and giant cells and central necrosis that appear in nonvital structures such as skin, soft tissue, bones, cartilage, and parenchymal organs such as liver or testes. The pathogenesis of these lesions is obscure. Early reports that claimed to identify treponemes in tertiary lesions were based on examination of silver-stained tissue sections, which tended to produce false-positive results. One study used fluorescent staining to demonstrate treponemes (17), but the lesion itself was not so clearly a tertiary one. Rather than a response to the presence of large numbers of treponemes, some other kind of poorly defined immune reaction is thought to be responsible. The nature of the immune reaction is further obscured by the fact that there is no relation between the location of primary or disseminated lesions and the eventual site of gummata.

Benign late syphilis causes isolated lesions of the skin and subcutaneous tissues over the face and neck and at sites on the extremities that are exposed to minor trauma such as the elbows (18). Indurated, nodular, or ulcerated lesions that describe an arc or an irregular full circle are characteristic. Tissue destruction and scarring may result. Peripheral hyperpigmentation is seen, with central scarring. Untreated, these lesions may persist for several years. Late syphilis of bone affects the tibia, fibula, clavicle, and skull, although any bone (or bones) may be involved (14). Pain and swelling are consistent with the periosteal location of the granulomatous reaction. Destruction of cartilage also plays an important part in determining the clinical appearance of lesions. Large visceral gummata may be asymptomatic or may cause symptoms referable to the involved organ.

Syphilitic aortitis results from involvement of the vasa vasorum of the aorta and resulting medial necrosis. The majority of patients are asymptomatic. Clinical syndromes that used to be observed relatively frequently include aneurysm of the ascending aorta, sometimes with erosion into the bony thorax, aortic insufficiency, left ventricular hypertrophy, and congestive heart failure (19). Involvement of the ostia of the coronary arteries may cause symptoms of ischemic heart disease. Syphilis of the aorta is recognized radiographically by calcifications or aneurysm in the ascending aorta. This complication may become manifest years after active disease of the aorta has subsided, probably resulting from continued mechanical stress in an already damaged vital area. The VDRL reaction is negative in one third of patients at the time syphilitic disease of the aorta is diagnosed.

Late neurosyphilis may cause any of a number of syndromes, including tabes dorsalis, manic-depressive behavior, psychosis, dementia, paresis, and death. Syndromes that overlap those of early neurosyphilis include meningitis, cerebrovascular accident, and myelitis. A mixed picture may result (20). Although typical examples of "classic" cases are reported (21), the usual picture appears to be more varied (22–25). Posterior uveitis may be the sole manifestation, and is not uncommon (26). Proving a diagnosis of neurosyphilis, or, for that matter, being certain that the existing literature on the subject includes only proven cases, may be exceedingly difficult. The clinical picture is nonspecific, STS in the CSF may be negative in up to 25% of cases, and the CSF may be entirely normal in 10% to 15% of patients who are thought to have the disease (22–24). Testing CSF for anti-treponemal antibody yields false-positive reactions in an appreciable percentage of syphilitic patients who are not thought to have neurosyphilis and should not be done.

RELATION BETWEEN SYPHILIS AND HUMAN IMMUNODEFICIENCY VIRUS INFECTION

Somewhat surprisingly, there is little to suggest that the dermatologic manifestations of syphilis are more striking in HIV-infected persons, nor has an increase in syphilitic hepatitis, arthritis, or osteitis been specifically documented. This may be due, in part, to the fact that the lesions of secondary syphilis may be immunologically mediated, owing to deposition of circulating immune complexes (27). In contrast, concurrent HIV infection appears to have a profound impact on neurologic involvement in syphilis (10, 28–30). In the era of acquired immunodeficiency syndrome (AIDS), neurosyphilis has been seen often and in relatively young persons. Many cases have been described in the context of therapeutic failure with conventional doses of penicillin (see the later treatment section); their importance in terms of our understanding the pathogenesis of syphilis in these subjects is just as great. Numerous individual case reports have documented the rapid progression of early syphilis to neurosyphilis, manifested in meningitis, optic neuritis, deafness, or the symptoms of nervous system disorders (10,30–36). Cranial nerve defects appear with or without meningitis, and vasculitis with appropriate radiographic documentation has also been described, causing cerebrovascular accidents.

The term quaternary neurosyphilis has been revived to describe necrotizing encephalitis in an HIV-infected patient (35). Most important, cases of early neurosyphilis, which were nearly unheard of between 1960 and 1980, have become commonplace (10). Patients with this kind of disease may have AIDS or be at an earlier stage of infection with HIV. In many cases, the concurrent HIV infection has been documented for the first time when neurologic complications of syphilis were recognized.

LABORATORY DIAGNOSIS

The most specific and sensitive method for verifying the diagnosis of primary syphilis is the finding of treponemes by dark-field microscopic examination of fluid obtained from the chancre. This test result is nearly always positive if a good specimen can be obtained. If no exudate is present, abrading the chancre and adding a drop or two of saline yields an adequate specimen. Treponemes may also be seen if secondary lesions are examined in this fashion, but not as many organisms are present, and greater technical facility is required.

The darkfield examination is actually the only test that is required specifically to establish the diagnosis of primary syphilis. Anticardiolipin antibody, as measured by an STS such as the VDRL or the rapid plasma reagin (RPR), is present, generally at a relatively low level (less than 1:8), in about 80% of patients at the time they come to medical attention for primary syphilis. Tests that measure antibody to surface proteins of *T. pallidum* by a hemagglutination assay (*T. pallidum* hemagglutination assay or microhemagglutination assay-*T. pallidum* [MHA-TP]) are positive in approximately 90% of such cases. Thus, a negative result does not exclude the diagnosis, nor does a positive MHA-TP establish it, because antibody may be present as a result of some earlier infection. Nevertheless, STSs are generally requested to provide a baseline for follow-up after therapy. Once antibody tests for treponemal surface proteins become positive, a detectable level of antibody is likely to persist for life, a feature that greatly limits the usefulness of this test for any purpose other than excluding a diagnosis of syphilis, if results are negative.

In secondary syphilis, STS results are always positive, with the RPR nearly always reactive at a high dilution (greater than 1:32). Thus a truly negative RPR result in a patient with a disseminated rash that is thought to be syphilitic actually excludes the diagnosis. Most laboratories do not perform serum dilutions unless the physician indicates that the diagnosis of syphilis is suspected clinically and/or requests that dilution be done; in this situation, the prozone phenomenon, in which a high concentration of antibody is present but is not detected in undiluted serum, may rarely obscure a positive reading. HIV-infected subjects tend to have a positive STS result with unusually high titers.

Isolated case reports of secondary syphilis with a negative RPR result in an HIV-infected patient (37) may well be the exceptions that prove the rule.

In latent syphilis the RPR result may be positive, but the level generally subsides with time. Gummatous tertiary syphilis also has high-level RPR reactivity, presumably reflecting a continuing immune response, as the histologic picture suggests. In the case of aortitis, the decline of the VDRL titer may reflect subsidence of active inflammation, although progressive damage of the aorta results from continued mechanical stress.

The diagnosis of late neurosyphilis can be exceedingly problematic. The clinical picture is nonspecific, being consistent with a wide range of neurologic or neuropsychiatric syndromes. The serum RPR is reactive, usually at a low dilution (e.g., less than 1:4), but it may be weakly reactive or even nonreactive. A negative MHA-TP test excludes the diagnosis of late syphilis, but a positive one clearly does not establish a diagnosis. The CSF may show a modest pleocytosis with a predominance of lymphocytes, an elevated protein value, and a positive VDRL result; a positive CSF VDRL result is the one finding that establishes the diagnosis without question. The CSF MHA-TP result is often false positive and cannot be used unless immunoglobulin M reactive with *T. pallidum* antigens is measured specifically or immunoglobulin G is titrated for comparison of CSF and serum levels (38), procedures that are not generally available in the United States. CSF is said by some authorities to be entirely normal in up to 25% of cases of neurosyphilis (22–24), although others (39) do not necessarily agree. Thus, because neurosyphilis may cause any of a variety of neurologic or psychiatric findings and all laboratory studies may be normal except the serum MHA-TP, it is not possible to fully exclude this diagnosis in any older person who has ever had syphilis and who has symptoms or signs of neuropsychiatric disease. This becomes a major, unsolved, and seemingly unsolvable problem for physicians who have a hospital-based practice with elderly patients who have not been under their personal care for many years.

To summarize, even though the MHA-TP test is highly sensitive and specific for *T. pallidum* infection, clinically, it is not useful for establishing a diagnosis of syphilis in most situations because a positive result may always reflect an earlier infection. The principal usefulness of the MHA-TP test is to obtain a negative result, which excludes any diagnosis of syphilis other than early primary disease. STSs, on the other hand, are neither specific nor highly sensitive, although positivity in high titer (greater than 1:16) generally signifies active infection with *T. pallidum*. Detecting treponemes by darkfield examination remains the surest way that the laboratory can support a clinical diagnosis of syphilis. As a good general principle, consideration of one veneral disease should lead to consideration of another; for example, any person with syphilis should be studied for antibody to HIV, hepatitis B virus, and others, and vice versa.

TREATMENT

Treatment schedules for syphilis are given in standard textbooks as well as in brochures available from the Centers for Disease Control and Prevention and from state and city departments of public health.

Early Syphilis, No Human Immunodeficiency Virus Infection

After treatment with 2.4 million units of benzathine penicillin, more than 95% of all patients with primary syphilis are apparently cured of their disease. The RPR test returns to a nonre-

active state in nearly all cases within 1 to 2 years. Treatment of secondary syphilis with 2.4 million units of benzathine penicillin also seems to cure the vast majority of patients, but some authorities have recorded a serologic failure rate as high as 25% (40). Fiumara (41) has claimed that two such treatments 7 days apart cause the VDRL result to return to negative in every instance, but he tended to exclude patients whose test remained positive, regarding them as having been reinfected. It seems quite clear that a small proportion of patients who are cured of their secondary syphilis retain low-grade VDRL reactivity throughout life (the so-called serofast state) (42). These treatments probably do not produce a biologic cure; treponemes persist in lymph nodes and the central nervous system of treated patients and experimental animals (43,44), a fact that becomes important in considering treatment of HIV-infected subjects.

In the late 1970s, before AIDS was recognized, isolated case reports showed that 2.4 million units of benzathine penicillin arrested all but the neurologic manifestations of secondary syphilis (45). This finding was attributed to the miniscule levels of penicillin that are present in the central nervous system after benzathine penicillin therapy (46). The rarity of neurosyphilis before 1980 argues that, in practice, recommended doses of penicillin were remarkably successful in curing syphilis and it seems highly likely, in retrospect, that the relapses occurred in persons who had unrecognized HIV infection.

Latent and Late Syphilis, No Human Immunodeficiency Virus Infection

Latent syphilis presents a problem. As noted earlier, the diagnosis is based on a reactive RPR test in an asymptomatic subject. In the majority of instances in the United States today, this serologic result probably reflects previously treated rather than active infection. Nevertheless, the official recommendation—that two treatments of 2.4 million units benzathine penicillin be given at weekly intervals unless neurosyphilis is also present—is reasonable. Although many of these subjects may not require treatment, it is not possible to identify them, so, as a public health measure, all are treated. A problem arises from the guidelines of the Centers for Disease Control and Prevention, which consider it "desirable" to perform lumbar puncture in every patient with latent syphilis, to exclude asymptomatic neurosyphilis. Some factors help to attenuate this recommendation: (a) The character of the CSF may be within normal limits in neurosyphilis, so the lumbar puncture does not rule out the diagnosis. (b) The vast majority of latent infections are arrested or cured (i.e., no later appearance of tertiary syphilis) by two or three doses, each of 2.4 million units benzathine penicillin. (c) For all the concern about treating proven neurosyphilis with benzathine penicillin, there are few well-documented case reports of therapeutic failure. Some authorities (47) have concluded that the likelihood of serious complications resulting from lumbar puncture, as uncommon as they might be, still outweighs the potential benefits. It may be reasonable and certainly more practical to treat with three doses of benzathine penicillin at weekly intervals and do no spinal tap unless symptoms of neurologic disease are present.

Although benzathine penicillin yields barely detectable or undetectable CSF levels of penicillin, three doses of 2.4 million units at weekly intervals appear to have arrested neurosyphilis in the vast majority of cases. Nevertheless, the World Health Organization (48) has recommended against its use. It is probably preferable to treat late neurosyphilis with 2 weeks of daily procaine penicillin, 1.2 million units per day. The United States Public Health Service Centers for Disease Control and Prevention recommends larger doses of penicillin (e.g., 10 to 24 million units per day intravenously for 10 days) in the absence of any data showing that this dosage will lead to a better outcome. Syphilologists generally talk of arrest of neurosyphilis rather than cure, because in most cases return to a normal state is not expected. Those who advocate routine use of higher doses of penicillin have not advanced any data to support higher rates of cure, and enormous doses of penicillin may not eradicate *T. pallidum* from experimental animals or humans (44), especially those with AIDS (36).

Treatment of Syphilis in Patients with Human Immunodeficiency Virus

All of the foregoing considerations set the stage for discussion of this difficult subject (10). If *T. pallidum* travels to seemingly privileged areas, such as the lymph nodes and central nervous system, where it escapes the normally lethal effects of penicillin, what might be expected in the presence of severe immunosuppression? Although one early report (49) suggested that HIV-infected patients with early syphilis respond slowly to 2.4 million units of benzathine penicillin, two subsequent studies (50,51) have shown that the clinical response of early syphilis to therapy is not altered by HIV infection, although serologic responses may be delayed (52). What is impressive is the number of cases in which treatment with benzathine penicillin is followed by rapid progression to neurosyphilis (10,53–55), a clinical finding that has been supported by documentation of persisting treponemes in the CSF of HIV-infected patients (56). It is not clear, however, that larger doses or repeated injections eliminate the problem of relapse to early neurosyphilis. Treatment of primary or secondary infection without neurologic involvement in HIV-infected patients should be with 2.4 million units of benzathine penicillin. There is no benefit to adding oral amoxicillin and probenecid for 10 days (57). If a macrolide (erythromycin or azithromycin) or tetracycline is used because of history of penicillin allergy, both physician and patient should be fully aware of the need for close monitoring and the concern over failure to cure neurologic disease, since penetration of the blood brain barrier is poor and efficacy in preventing neurosyphilis is not established even in non-HIV infected persons. For syphilis with neurologic (including ophthalmologic or otologic) involvement, 10 days of intravenous penicillin, 24 million units per day, is recommended. Alternative therapy, including ceftriaxone, 1 g per day, is probably equally effective and can be administered far more easily. Both of these regimens are associated with rates of failure plus relapse that approach 30% (36,58). It is entirely possible that daily procaine penicillin for 10 to 14 days would be as effective. Clearly, with any treatment regimen, careful attention needs to be given both to clinical response and to the subsequent serum VDRL reaction.

REFERENCES

1. Chapel TA. The variability of syphilitic chancres. *Sex Transm Dis* 1978;5:68.
2. Drusin LM, Singer C, Valenti AJ, Armstrong D. Infectious syphilis mimicking neoplastic disease. *Arch Intern Med* 1977;137:156.
3. Musher DM, Knox JM. Syphilis and yaws. In Schell RF, Musher DM, eds: *Pathogenesis and immunology of treponemal infections*. New York: Marcel Dekker, 1983:101–120.
4. Friedman PS, Wright DJ. Observations on syphilis in Addis Ababa. 2. Prevalence and natural history. *Br J Vener Dis* 1977;53:276.
5. Shrivastava SN, Singh G. Extensive condyloma lata. *Br J Vener Dis* 1977;53:23.
6. Chapel TA. The signs and symptoms of secondary syphilis. *Sex Transm Dis* 1980;7:161.
7. Jozsa L, Timmer M, Somogyi T, Feher J. Hepatitis syphilitica: a clinico-pathological study of 25 cases. *Acta Hepatogastroenterol* 1977;24:344.
8. Mills CH. Routine examination of cerebrospinal fluid in syphilis: its value in regard to more accurate knowledge, prognosis and treatment. *BMJ* 1936;2:527.
9. Bauer TJ, Price EV, Cutler JC. Spinal fluid examinations among patients with primary or secondary syphilis. *Am J Syph* 1952;36:309.
10. Musher DM, Hamill RJ, Baughn RE. Effect of human immunodeficiency virus (HIV) infection on the course of syphilis and on the response to treatment. *Ann Intern Med* 1990;113:872.
11. Baughn RE, McNeely MC, Jorizzo JL, Musher DM. Characterization of the antigenic determinants and host components in immune complexes from patients with secondary syphilis. *J Immunol* 1986;136:1406.
12. Clark EG, Danbolt N. The Oslo study of the natural course of untreated syphilis: an epidemiologic investigation based on a re-study of the Boeck-Bruusgaard material. *Med Clin North Am* 1964;48:613.
13. Magnuson HJ, Thomas EW, Olansky S, et al. Inoculation syphilis in human volunteers. *Medicine (Baltimore)* 1956;35:33.
14. Kampmeier RH. The late manifestations of syphilis: skeletal, visceral and cardiovascular. *Med Clin North Am* 1964;48:667.
15. Kemp JE, Cochems KD. Studies in cardiovascular syphilis: Influence of treatment of early syphilis upon incidence of cardiovascular syphilis. *Am J Syph Gonorrhea Vener Dis* 1937;21:625.
16. Heggtveit HA. Syphilitic aortitis: a clinicopathologic autopsy study of 100 cases, 1950 to 1960. *Circulation* 1964;29:346.
17. Handsfield HH, Lukehart SA, Sell S, et al. Demonstration of *Treponema pallidum* in a cutaneous gumma by indirect immunofluorescence. *Arch Dermatol* 1983;719:677.
18. Olansky S. Late benign syphilis (gumma). *Med Clin North Am* 1964;48:653.
19. Grabau W, Emanuel R, Ross D, et al. Syphilitic aortic regurgitation: an appraisal of surgical treatment. *Br J Vener Dis* 1976;52:366.
20. Perdrup A, Jorgensen BB, Pedersen NS. The profile of neurosyphilis in Denmark: a clinical and serological study of all patients in Denmark with neurosyphilis disclosed in the years 1971–1979 incl. by Wassermann reaction (CWRM) in the cerebrospinal fluid. *Acta Derm Venereol Suppl (Stockh)* 1981;96:1.
21. Talbot MD, Morton RS. Neurosyphilis: the most common things are most common. *Genitourin Med* 1985;61:95.
22. Hooshmand H, Escobar MR, Kopf SW. Neurosyphilis: a study of 241 patients. *JAMA* 1972;219:726.
23. Catterall RD. Neurosyphilis. *Br J Hosp Med* 1977;17:585.
24. Luxon L, Greenwood RJ, Lees AJ. Neurosyphilis today. *Lancet* 1979;1:90.
25. Binder RL, Dickman WA. Psychiatric manifestations of neurosyphilis in middle-aged patients. *Am J Psychiatry* 1980;137:6.
26. Villanueva AV, Sahouri MJ, Ormerod LD, et al. Posterior uveitis in patients with positive serology for syphilis. *Clin Infect Dis* 2000;30:479.
27. Jorizzo JL, McNeely MC, Baughn RE, et al. Role of circulating immune complexes in human secondary syphilis. *J Infect Dis* 1986;153:1014.
28. Holtom PD, Larsen RA, Leal ME, Leedom JM. Prevalence of neurosyphilis in human immunodeficiency virus-infected patients with latent syphilis. *Am J Med* 1992;93:9.
29. Katz DA, Berger JA, Duncan RC. Neurosyphilis: a comparative study of the effects of infection with human immunodeficiency virus. *Arch Neurol* 1993;50:243.
30. Flood JM, Weinstock HS, Guroy ME, et al. Neurosyphilis during the AIDS epidemic, San Francisco, 1985–1992. *J Infect Dis* 1998;177:931.
31. Harris RL, Rutecki PA, Donovan DT, et al. Fever, headache and hearing loss in a young homosexual man. *Hosp Pract* 1985;20:167, 170.
32. Zaidman GW. Neurosyphilis and retrobulbar neuritis in a patient with AIDS. *Ann Ophthalmol* 1986;18:260.
33. Zambrano W, Perez GM, Smith JL. Acute syphilitic blindness in AIDS. *J Clin Neurol Ophthalmol* 1987;7:1.
34. Johns DR, Tierney M, Felsenstein D. Alteration in the natural history of neurosyphilis by concurrent infection with the human immunodeficiency virus. *N Engl J Med* 1987;316:1569.
35. Morgello S, Laufer H. Quaternary neurosyphilis. *N Engl J Med* 1989;319:1549.
36. Gordon SM, Eaton ME, George R, et al. The response of symptomatic neurosyphilis to high-dose intravenous penicillin G in patients with human immunodeficiency virus infection. *N Engl J Med* 1994;331:1469.
37. Hicks CB, Benson PM, Lupton GP, Tramont EC. Seronegative secondary syphilis in a patient infected with the human immunodeficiency virus (HIV) with Kaposi sarcoma. *Ann Intern Med* 1987;107:492.
38. Prange HW, Moskophidis M, Schipper HI, Muller F. Relationship between neurological features and intrathecal synthesis of IgG antibodies to *Treponema pallidum* in untreated and treated human neurosyphilis. *J Neurol* 1983;230:241.
39. Swartz M. Neurosyphilis. In Holmes KK, Mardh P-A, Sparling PF, Wiesner PJ, eds: *Sexually transmitted diseases*. New York: McGraw-Hill, 1984:313–334.
40. Leslie N. Treatment of early infectious syphilis with benzathine penicillin G. In *Proceedings of world forum on syphilis and other treponematoses*, September 4–8, 1962, Washington, DC. Washington DC: US Public Health Service, 1964; USPHS publication 997.
41. Fiumara NJ. Treatment of primary and secondary syphilis. Serological response. *JAMA* 1980;243:2500.
42. Schroeter AL, Lucas JB, Price EV, Falcon VH. Treatment of early syphilis and reactivity of serological tests. *JAMA* 1972;221:471.
43. Collart P, Borel L-J, Durel P. Significance of spiral organisms found, after treatment, in late human and experimental syphilis. *Br J Vener Dis* 1964;40:81.
44. Yobs AR, Clark JW Jr, Mothershed SE, et al. Further observations on the persistence of *Treponema pallidum* after treatment in rabbits and humans. *Br J Vener Dis* 1968;44:116.
45. Tramont EC. Persistence of *Treponema pallidum* following penicillin G therapy. A report of two cases. *JAMA* 1976;236:2206.
46. Goh BT, Smith GW, Samarasinghe L, et al. Penicillin concentrations in serum

and cerebrospinal fluid after intramuscular injection of aqueous procaine penicillin 0.6 MU with and without probenecid. *Br J Vener Dis* 1984;60:371.

47. Wiesel J, Rose DN, Silver AL, et al. Lumbar puncture in asymptomatic neurosyphilis. *Arch Intern Med* 1985;145:465.

48. Treponemal infections. *WHO Tech Rep Ser* 1982;674:1.

49. Frederick WR, Delapenha R, Barnes S, et al. Secondary syphilis and HIV infection (abstract 1175). Abstracts of the 28th interscience conference. *Antimicrob Agents Chemother* 1988;320.

50. Gourevitch MN, Selwyn PA, Davenny K, et al. Effect of HIV infection on the serologic manifestations and response to treatment of syphilis in intravenous drug users. *Ann Intern Med* 1993;118:350.

51. Hutchinson CM, Hook EW III, Shepherd M. Altered clinical presentation of early syphilis in patients with human immunodeficiency virus infection. *Ann Intern Med* 1994;121:94.

52. Rolfs RT, Joesoef R, Hendershot EF, et al. A randomized trial of enhanced therapy for early syphilis in patients with and without human immunodeficiency virus infection. *N Engl J Med* 1997;337:307.

53. Bayne LL, Schmidley JW, Goodin DS. Acute syphilitic meningitis. Its occurrence after clinical and serologic cure of secondary syphilis with penicillin G. *Arch Neurol* 1986;43:137.

54. Jorgensen J, Tikjob G, Weisman K. Neurosyphilis after treatment of latent syphilis with benzathine penicillin. *Genitourin Med* 1986;62:129.

55. Berry CD, Hooton TM, Collier AC, Lukehart SA. Neurologic relapse after benzathine penicillin therapy for secondary syphilis in a patient with HIV infection. *N Engl J Med* 1987;316:1587.

56. Lukehart SA, Hood EW III, Baker-Zander SA, et al. Invasion of the central nervous system by *Treponema pallidum*: implications for diagnosis and treatment. *Ann Intern Med* 1988;109:855.

57. Marra CM, Boutin P, McArthur JC, et al. A pilot study evaluating ceftriaxone and penicillin G as treatment agents for neurosyphilis in human immunodeficiency virus-infected individuals. *Clin Infect Dis* 2000;30:540.

58. Dowell ME, Ross PG, Musher DM, et al. Response of latent syphilis or neurosyphilis to ceftriaxone in persons infected with human immunodeficiency virus. *Am J Med* 1992;93:481.

CHAPTER 106
Genital Herpes

Anthony Simmons, Michael N. Oxman,
and Lawrence R. Stanberry

Genital herpes is a recurrent sexually transmitted disease caused by either herpes simplex virus type 1 (HSV-1) or HSV type 2 (HSV-2). Throughout the last decade of the twentieth century, there were great advances in the understanding of the global epidemiology of genital HSV infections (1).

Primary infection is almost always self-limited but on termination of the acute infection virus is not eliminated from the host but rather, viral genomes remain in a latent (dormant) state in sacral sensory neurons innervating initially infected skin and mucous membranes. The significance of latency is that it is a reservoir of infection that can periodically reactivate, causing virus to travel down nerve fibers to skin or mucous membranes in the dermatome of primary infection. This may be manifest clinically as recurrent genital herpes or more frequently, causes unrecognized shedding of infectious HSV (1–4) which despite being unrecognized is responsible for the majority of new HSV-2 genital infections (4). The epidemiology is further complicated by the fact that many primary infections are asymptomatic or unrecognized, which has the important implication that the first clinical presentation of genital herpes, referred to as the initial episode, may be caused by a recurrence of a prior asymptomatic primary infection.

EPIDEMIOLOGY

Transmission is by close personal contact and there is no documented transmission from inanimate objects such as toilet seats.

Further, there is no evidence of transmission by aerosols or arthropod vectors. As with many other sexually transmitted infections, transmission is more efficient from men to women than vice versa. Humans are the only natural reservoir of HSV. The latency-reactivation cycle of HSV ensures its survival in populations too small and isolated to support the continuous circulation of viruses causing epidemic diseases like measles or influenza. Clinical surveys greatly underestimate the incidence and prevalence of HSV infections. Most persons who shed HSV do so asymptomatically and many are unaware of ever having been infected. The immune responses to HSV-1 and HSV-2 are cross-reactive (5–13), which has necessitated the development of specialized type specific antibody tests to determine whether persons have been infected with one of both viruses. Besides western blot analysis (14), a new generation of type specific serologic assays exploit differences between HSV-1 and HSV-2 in a component of the viral envelope, glycoprotein G (14–19).

Type specific antibody tests have proven to be the best way to measure the prevalence of HSV-1 and HSV-2 infections. From a public health perspective, this is important because most or all HSV-2 seropositive individuals shed virus from the genital region intermittently and asymptomatically, constituting the source of virus responsible for most new infections (4). Recent research suggests that infection rates may be underestimated by this approach as HSV-2 specific lymphoproliferative responses have been reported in some HSV seronegative persons (20). Whether the responses result from infection with other herpesviruses that contain epitopes that cross react with HSV antigens or are due to HSV infection in individuals who fail to engender a humoral immune response is unknown. To date, the significance of this observation in relation to HSV latency and virus shedding is also unknown.

There are compelling data that immunity resulting from previous HSV-1 infection affords significant protection against the development of symptomatic genital HSV-2 infection, but the role of previous HSV-1 immunity in protecting against HSV-2 infection is more controversial (21–24). An increasing proportion of Americans are now reaching puberty without having been infected with HSV-1, which may be an important factor underlying the current epidemic of symptomatic genital herpes and helps explain the increasing frequency with which HSV-1 is being isolated from patients with initial episodes of genital herpes.

HSV-2 infection is rare before puberty because it is transmitted almost exclusively by sexual contact. Population-based sero-epidemiologic studies in the United States found that the prevalence of HSV-2 infection increased dramatically in the last quarter of the twentieth century (25,26). Data from the Centers for Disease Control and Prevention indicated that between 1988 and 1994 the seroprevalence of HSV-2 in Americans 12 years of age or older was 21.9%, which corresponded to 45 million infected people (26). HSV-2 seroprevalence was higher among women (25.6%) than men (17.8%) and higher among African Americans (45.9%) than whites (17.6%). Fewer than 10% of those who were seropositive reported a history of genital herpes. There have been numerous studies of selected populations including adolescents (27–29), college students (30), women attending family planning clinics (31,32), patients in family practice clinics (33), STD clinic patients (34,35), and homosexual populations (36). HSV-2 seroprevalence rates vary widely with the different populations but certain factors are frequently associated with increased risk of HSV-2 seropositivity. These include female gender, early age of first intercourse, years of sexual activity, history of other sexually transmitted infections, African-American race or Mexican-American ethnic background, less education, low family income, drug use, and a greater lifetime number of sexual partners. In heterosexual women in the United States, the probability of being infected with HSV-2 increases markedly with the number of sexual partners. It is less than 10% in women with one lifetime sexual partner and increases to 40% with two to ten, 60% with 11 to 50, and more than 80% with more than 50 lifetime sexual partners. The corresponding probabilities of HSV-2 infection in heterosexual men are less than 1%, 20%, 35%, and 70%, respectively.

Sero-epidemiologic studies using type-specific tests have demonstrated that HSV-2 infections are not just a problem in the United States but occur globally and that the prevalence of HSV-2 infections in some areas is substantially greater than in the United States (1,11,37–39). The reason for the successful spread of genital herpes probably relates to its capacity to cause unrecognized recurrent infections that are associated with shedding of virus in genital secretions or from asymptomatic lesions. All HSV-2 seropositive individuals are latently infected and probably experience reactivation at least occasionally. HSV shedding, as detected by virus culture, occurs on about 3% of days for healthy men and women, and more for persons with HIV infection. Shedding rates are also higher if shedding is detected by polymerase chain reaction as compared to virus culture (40–45).

HSV-1 is now causing disease in anatomic territory formerly inhabited almost exclusively by HSV-2 (i.e., below the waist) and vice versa. Up to 50% of initial episodes of genital herpes are now caused by HSV-1 (46–50). Although primary genital herpes caused by HSV-1 is clinically indistinguishable from primary genital herpes caused by HSV-2, the rate of subsequent recurrences, both symptomatic and asymptomatic, is five- to ten-fold lower when disease is caused by HSV-1 than by HSV-2 (51–53).

PATHOGENESIS AND IMMUNITY

The pathologic changes of herpes simplex are described in Chapter 230. In brief they are the result of cytopathic effects induced by HSV in infected cells plus local inflammatory responses. The pathogenesis of genital herpes begins with the transmission of HSV-1 or HSV-2 to anogenital sites, generally mucosal surfaces or abraded keratinized epithelium. Virus replicates locally but also quickly enters the sensory nerve fibers that innervate the skin. Virus moves from the portal of entry within nerve fibers via axoplasmic transport mechanisms to the sacral dorsal root ganglia. Within the ganglion, HSV replicates in some neurons and in others establishes a latent infection. Progeny virus produced in the ganglion neurons move back to the periphery via antero-grade axoplasmic transport process and virus is released from nerve endings at the dermal-epidermal junction where further replication in epithelial cells produce the characteristic lesions of genital HSV infection (54). Unlike other herpesvirus infections, hematogenous spread of virus does not play a role in the pathogenesis of genital HSV infection in the immunocompetent host.

In the normal host, an array of local and systemic defense mechanisms limit HSV replication and spread and destroy HSV infected cells. The host defenses fall into two categories, innate and adaptive (HSV-specific), which are most clearly differentiated during primary HSV infections (55). Only innate defenses are operative during the first several days of primary infection, that is, until specific immune responses develop, yet these are sufficient to prevent the development of clinically manifest disease in the majority of infected individuals. Clinical observations indicate that patients with deficient humoral immunity are able to limit HSV infection while those with deficient cellular immunity have difficulty controlling infection (56–58). While no defect in host immunity has been identified that accounts for recurrent HSV infections, studies suggest that interferon gamma responses may play a role in controlling recurrent infections (59,60).

CLINICAL MANIFESTATIONS AND COUNSELING

Counseling Patients

Having HSV-1 antibodies before genital exposure to HSV generally ameliorates the severity of genital HSV-2 disease (20–24). Many people experiencing their first recognized episode of symptomatic genital herpes are not, as they believe, experiencing an initial episode of exogenous infection. Instead, they are suffering their first symptomatic recurrence caused by reactivation of a latent infection established in the course of an earlier asymptomatic or unrecognized primary infection (61–63). An understanding of the fact that the initial symptomatic episode does not necessarily equate with recently acquired infection is critically important in counseling the patient with newly recognized genital herpes. The diagnosis of genital herpes frequently results in confusion and anxiety, especially when they occur in one member of a monogamous couple, neither of whom has any history of recognized genital herpes. Besides discussing the diagnosis at the time of the initial physician/healthcare provider visit, it is recommended that the patient be seen for a second visit within 1 to 2 weeks to more fully discuss issues and questions that might have been missed or not fully understood at the initial visit (64–66). The patient with genital herpes can suffer psychological morbidity that is of greater consequence to the patient than their physiological morbidity. If the patient is having difficulty adjusting to the chronic illness it is recommended that they be referred to an appropriate behavioral therapist for further counseling (66).

Primary Genital Herpes

The incubation period after sexual contact is usually 3 to 7 days, with a range of 1 day to more than 2 weeks (61,67–71). Symptomatic primary genital herpes tends to be more severe in women than in men, with a larger total area of lesions, more intense and prolonged local symptoms, more frequent constitutional symptoms, and more extragenital lesions. Complications are also more frequent in women than men, including dysuria, urethritis, meningitis, and pharyngitis (61,68–71). Classical primary herpetic vulvovaginitis may be preceded by a short period of local burning, tenderness, and erythema of the labia minora and vaginal introitus. Herpetic vesicles first appear on the external genitalia and new lesions continue to appear bilaterally, with the eruption often extending to the mons pubis, clitoris, urethral orifice, perianal skin, buttocks, and thighs. On most mucous membranes vesicles quickly rupture, leaving shallow, tender ulcers covered with a yellowish gray exudate and surrounded by a red areola. In drier areas, such as the outer surface of the labia majora and the adjacent skin, vesicles may remain intact, evolve into pustules, and then crust in several days (Fig. 106.1).

New lesions may continue to appear for a week or more and patients may develop bilateral painful inguinal and pelvic lymphadenopathy. The vaginal mucosa and vulva are inflamed and edematous. The cervix is almost always involved, and there is often a profuse watery vaginal discharge. Patients may have severe vulvar pain, exquisite tenderness of the affected tissues, and

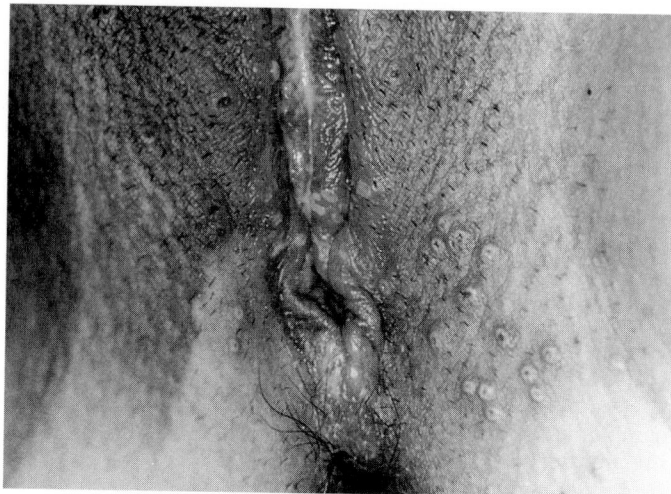

Figure 106.1. Primary genital herpes simplex virus type 2 infection in a female. (Photo courtesy of Dr. Stephen Trying, The University of Texas Medical Branch, Galveston, Texas.)

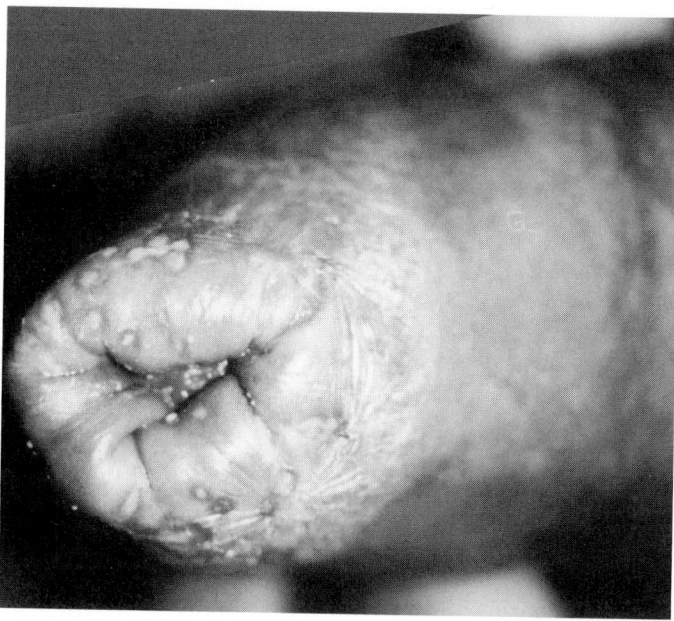

Figure 106.2. Primary genital herpes simplex virus infection in an uncircumcised male. (Photo courtesy of Dr. Stephen Trying, The University of Texas Medical Branch, Galveston, Texas.)

dysuria may be severe enough to cause urinary retention. Urethritis and detection of HSV in urine often accompany dysuria.

The majority of women with symptomatic primary genital herpes have constitutional symptoms, including fever, headache, malaise, and myalgias, which usually peaks during the first 3 to 4 days and disappears by the end of the first week. The local symptoms generally worsen during the first week, reach a peak between days 8 and 10, and then gradually subside. Even when severe, primary genital herpes is normally self-limited. Virus replication is maximal during the first 3 to 4 days and declines thereafter with a mean duration of virus shedding of 11 to 12 days. Pain usually remits in 10 to 14 days, and healing occurs without scarring in 2 to 4 weeks. Mucosal lesions heal without crusting. The cervix, which is often involved in symptomatic primary genital herpes, is a source of virus that may be shed for weeks after visible lesions have healed and symptoms have disappeared (69,72–77).

In men, the lesions of primary genital herpes usually appear bilaterally on the glans penis, the prepuce, and the shaft of the penis and less often on the scrotum, thighs, and buttocks. Their evolution is similar to that in women. In dry skin (e.g., on the shaft of the penis), they progress from papule to vesicle to pustule to crust and then heal, usually by the middle of the third week (Fig. 106.2). In moist areas (e.g., under the prepuce), the vesicles are quickly macerated and evolve into ulcers identical to those described in women. New lesions continue to appear for a week or more, and there is local pain, tenderness, inflammation, and edema. Dysuria, usually associated with herpetic urethritis and accompanied by a small amount of clear mucoid urethral discharge, occurs in 30% to 40% of men with primary genital herpes. It is generally more painful than the dysuria of gonococcal or nongonococcal urethritis, and HSV can usually be isolated from urethral swabs. There is bilateral tender inguinal and pelvic lymphadenopathy, but this is less severe and of shorter duration than in women. Less than half of men with primary genital herpes have significant constitutional symptoms. Virus is present in large amounts during the first 3 to 5 days, and the mean duration of virus shedding is 10 to 11 days. Pain usually resolves during the second week, and healing occurs without scarring in 2 to 3 weeks (61,78–81).

The clinical manifestations and course of primary genital herpes caused by HSV-1 and HSV-2 are indistinguishable. However,

the frequency of subsequent recurrences is lower after primary genital herpes caused by HSV-1 (52).

The clinical manifestations of nonprimary first-episode genital herpes are similar to those of true primary genital herpes, but the disease is less severe and of shorter duration. There is a marked reduction in the frequency of constitutional symptoms, extragenital lesions, and complications, and a smaller proportion of women shed HSV from the cervix (61,80,82–86).

Recurrent Genital Herpes

Following an initial episode of genital herpes, most people will experience one or more recurrent episodes during the subsequent year. The recurrence rate is lower for HSV-1 than for HSV-2, with a mean monthly rate of recurrence for genital herpes caused by HSV-1 of 0.02, compared with 0.33 for genital herpes caused by HSV-2 (53). Recurrent genital herpes is usually less severe and of shorter duration than the initial episode. Many patients have a prodrome of tenderness, pain, burning, tingling, or itching at the site of the impending eruption, beginning from a few hours to 1 or 2 days before the appearance of lesions. Some have a prodrome of ipsilateral sacral neuralgia, with severe burning, aching, or lancinating pain in the leg, buttock, or genital area. The lesions of recurrent genital herpes are usually fewer than seen with primary infection and are unilateral, beginning as clusters of tiny erythematous papules, which quickly develop into clusters of tiny vesicles on an erythematous base (Fig. 106.3) (61,89,90). They sometimes coalesce, and they evolve in the same manner as in primary genital herpes but more rapidly. There is also less pain, fewer days of new lesion formation, and a much smaller total area of lesions.

The clinical manifestations of recurrent genital herpes are more severe in women than in men (70,82,83,88–91). In women, the lesions are frequently painful. They are most often located on the labia minora, labia majora, or perineum but may also occur on the mons pubis, perianal skin, or buttocks. Some women have linear ulcerations in the fourchette, which resemble inflamed

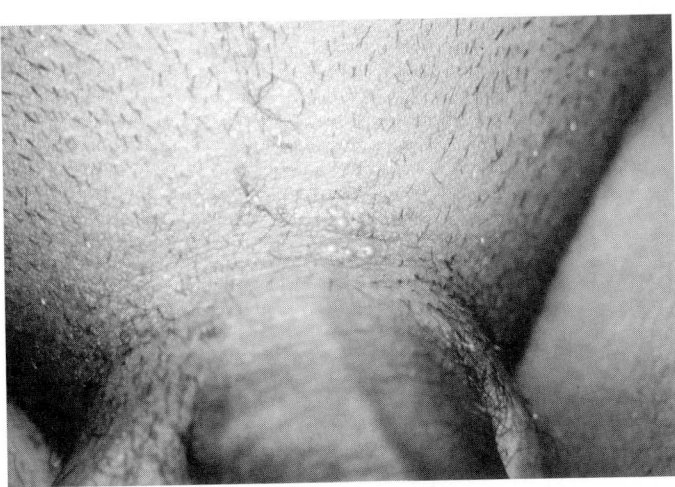

Figure 106.3. Recurrent genital herpes simplex virus infection at the base of the penile shaft. (Photo courtesy of Dr. Stephen Trying, The University of Texas Medical Branch, Galveston, Texas.)

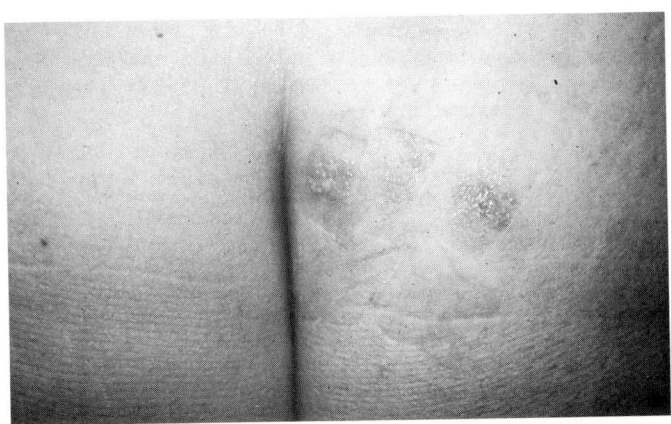

Figure 106.4. Recurrent genital herpes simplex virus infection on the buttocks. (Photo courtesy of Dr. Stephen Trying, The University of Texas Medical Branch, Galveston, Texas.)

excoriations and often are not recognized as herpetic by patients or their physicians (61,70,92). Lymphadenopathy may be present, but fever and constitutional symptoms are uncommon. Virus is present in much smaller amounts in recurrent than in primary herpetic lesions. Virus is shed for an average of 5 days, and its recovery after the seventh day is uncommon. Pain also disappears during the first week, and the lesions generally heal within 8 to 10 days. The frequency of positive cervical cultures (5% to 10%) is much lower during recurrent than during primary genital herpes. In men, recurrent genital herpes most often presents with one or more patches of grouped vesicles on the shaft of the penis, prepuce, or glans. Lesions, which are usually unilateral, begin as papules and, on dry skin, evolve into vesicles, pustules, and crusts in the same manner as the lesions of herpes labialis. Under the prepuce vesicles quickly form shallow painful ulcers. There may be mild inguinal lymphadenopathy, but constitutional symptoms and urethritis are rare. Urethral cultures are positive for HSV in less than 5% of men with recurrent genital herpes. Four or 5 days after their appearance, HSV can rarely be recovered from recrudescent lesions. Pain is present in about 60% of men with recurrent genital herpes. It is usually mild and disappears with the virus. Lesions heal in 7 to 10 days.

Symptomatic genital HSV infections are only the tip of an iceberg (3,22,40,92–101). The majority of primary genital HSV infections are asymptomatic or unrecognized, and 70% to 80% of people with antibodies to HSV-2 have no history of symptomatic genital herpes. Nevertheless, these seropositive individuals are latently infected and experience periodic virus reactivation, as evidenced by virus shedding. However, the majority of these reactivations are also asymptomatic or unrecognized. Consequently, episodes of asymptomatic virus shedding are far more frequent than episodes of symptomatic recurrent genital herpes. The rate of asymptomatic virus shedding is generally 1% to 2% in immunocompetent persons with antibody to HSV-2, but it is substantially higher (e.g., 6% or more) in the first few months after initial HSV-2 infection, in the days immediately before and after a symptomatic recurrence, and in individuals with a high rate of symptomatic recurrence (40,45,92,100–102). HSV deoxyribonucleic acid (DNA) can be detected by polymerase chain reaction (PCR) at a rate approximately eight times higher than that reported for infectious virus (101,102), but the biologic signifi-

cance of low levels of HSV DNA in the absence of infectious virus remains to be determined. Asymptomatic shedding appears to be at least as common from the usual lesion site on the vulva as from the cervix, and anal shedding is also frequently documented (3,40,93,94,102–104). The epidemiologic importance of asymptomatic genital HSV infection is underlined by the observation that the majority of the mothers of infants with neonatal herpes have had no signs or symptoms of genital herpes during pregnancy and no history of prior symptomatic genital herpes (97,105,106–111).

Genital herpes often has manifestations outside the genital region, primarily as a result of neural spread of virus to regions sharing common sensory innervation with the genitalia. Often, lesions in non-genital areas below the waist are the only symptom of HSV infection, leading potentially to difficulty in diagnosis unless the attending physician is aware of the possibility. All skin and mucous membranes below the waist are targets for HSV infections acquired genitally; the commonest sites involved are the buttocks (Fig. 106.4), perianal skin, and thighs (Fig. 106.5). No

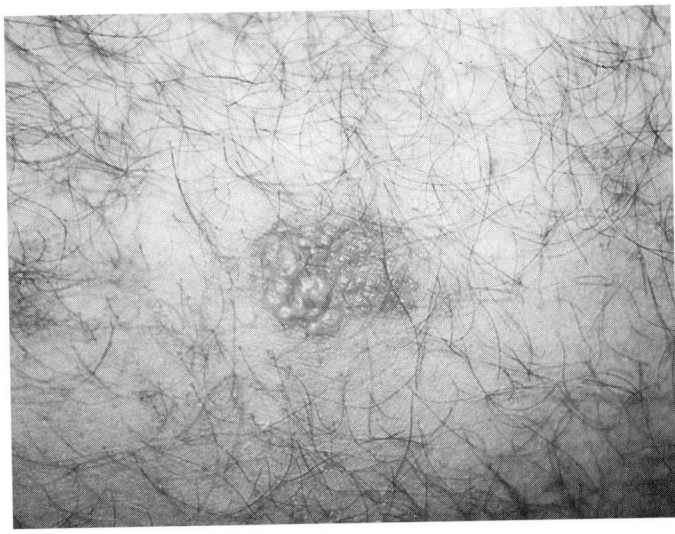

Figure 106.5. Recurrent genital herpes simplex virus infection on the thigh. (Photo courtesy of Dr. Stephen Trying, The University of Texas Medical Branch, Galveston, Texas.)

site below the waist is exempt however and it is not uncommon for recurrent blisters on the lower limbs to be misdiagnosed as recurring episodes of shingles. The latter is, in reality, an extreme rarity in the immunocompetent host (112).

Complications of Genital Herpes

Although often physically and emotionally distressing, genital herpes in the normal host is almost always self-limited and usually resolves spontaneously without major complications or sequelae. Previous infection with HSV-2 does however increase the risk for acquiring human immunodeficiency virus infection, possibly because of the capacity of HSV-2 to produce genital ulcers and/or by increasing the number of activated T-cells present in genital mucosa (113–116).

Superinfection with candida albicans may occur in males and females with either primary or recurrent genital herpes. A diagnosis of recurrent candida vaginitis should alert attention to the possibility that recurrent HSV infection is the true underlying cause. In such cases it is always prudent to take send a swab to the virology laboratory for detection of HSV. While the condition would always appear to respond to topical antifungal agents within a few days, a more appropriate and effective therapy in this scenario would be suppression of the underlying HSV infection with an anti-viral compound.

Other recognized complications are necrotizing balanitis (117), pharyngotonsillitis (118,119), sacral neuralgia (120,121), acute and recurrent meningitis (122–126), encephalitis (127), urine retention secondary to sacral radiculopathy or autonomic dysfunction (123), herpetic cystitis (128), and recurrent episodes of erythema multiforme or Stevens-Johnson syndrome (129,130). Dissemination is a rare but serious complication of either HSV-1 or HSV-2 infection that may present as acute hepatitis or rarely may resemble varicella in appearance (131–138). Disseminated HSV infection is a recognized complication of pregnancy but does respond to prompt treatment with appropriate antiviral therapy (139–141).

Genital Herpes in the Immunocompromised Host

Persons with compromised host defenses are at increased risk for severe, even fatal, HSV infections. Those at greatest risk appear to have abnormal cellular immunity, eczema, or burns (57,142–145). Most episodes of genital herpes in these patients are recurrent. Recurrent infections usually evolve normally and resolve without complications. Sometimes, however, the local lesions slowly progress to form a deep, gradually enlarging ulcer with a sharp erythematous border and a necrotic base covered with purulent exudate; there are often satellite lesions in adjacent areas of skin. These chronic progressive herpetic ulcers contain large amounts of HSV and may persist for months. They occur most frequently in patients with severely compromised cell-mediated immunity, and they often heal spontaneously with improvement of cellular immunity, as a result of remission of lymphoreticular malignant neoplasms or reduction in iatrogenic immunosuppression in organ allograft recipients.

Receptive male homosexuals with AIDS often have chronic progressive perianal herpetic ulcers (146,147). In spite of their severity, these lesions are rarely associated with constitutional symptoms or hematogenous dissemination of HSV. Asymptomatic shedding of HSV-2 is markedly increased in immunocompromised patients (148,149). In one study, the prevalence of asymptomatic shedding by HSV-2-seropositive women was found to be four times greater in human immunodeficiency virus-infected women than in uninfected control subjects, and it was greatest in those with the lowest CD4+ cell counts (148).

Neonatal Herpes Simplex Virus Infection

One of the most serious complications of genital herpes occurs when infection in a pregnant woman is transmitted to her newborn infant (105–110,150). The incidence of neonatal HSV infection in the United States is estimated to be between one in 3,000 and one in 5,000 live births, and it may be on the rise because of the increasing incidence of genital herpes. Two thirds of neonatal HSV infections are caused by HSV-2 and infection is usually acquired during passage through the infected birth canal of a mother with asymptomatic genital herpes. Intrauterine (congenital) infection is well described but uncommon (151–153). The risk for infection is much higher in infants born to mothers with initial rather than recurrent genital HSV infections (greater than 30% vs. less than 2%) (111,154,155). In some cases, ascending infection occurs shortly before birth, usually in a woman with prolonged rupture of membranes. Ascending infection can also be iatrogenic, introduced by a fetal monitor (156). In addition, asymptomatic shedding of HSV at the onset of labor due to recently acquired primary infection is associated with preterm delivery, whereas shedding due to an asymptomatic recurrence of genital herpes acquired before pregnancy is not (151). Infection may also be acquired postnatally from the mother or another adult with non-genital HSV infection or by nosocomial transmission in the nursery (157–160).

In contrast with other forms of HSV infection, infection of the newborn is virtually never asymptomatic. Its clinical presentation reflects the site and extent of virus replication. The initial clinical manifestations of neonatal herpes usually appear during the first or second week of life, but they may be present at birth or delayed until the infant is 1 month of age. Congenital (intrauterine) infection presents at birth with a triad of skin vesicles or scarring; eye disease, including chorioretinitis and often herpetic keratoconjunctivitis; and microcephaly or hydranencephaly. Mortality is high, and survivors have severe sequelae. Prepartum intrauterine (ascending) infection results in the appearance of skin lesions at birth or within 24 hours thereafter but no evidence of prepartum infection of other organs. These infants respond well to antiviral therapy. Infants infected during delivery or postnatally present with one of three patterns of disease: (a) disease localized to the portal of entry, that is, the skin, eyes, or mouth; (b) encephalitis with or without skin, eye, or mouth disease; or (c) disseminated infection involving multiple organs, including the brain, lungs, liver, heart, adrenals, and skin (107–110,150).

Infants in whom infection appears to remain localized to the skin, eyes, or mouth generally present at 10 to 11 days of life. Herpetic skin vesicles are present in about 90%, often on the presenting part, but they may be few in number. Most of these infants survive without treatment, but some develop disseminated disease or encephalitis, and 30% to 40% develop significant neurologic or ocular sequelae. Treatment has reduced the frequency of sequelae to about 10%, but even treated newborns suffer repeated recurrences during infancy (162).

Infants with encephalitis present later, at about 16 to 17 days of life, with a clinical picture resembling bacterial meningitis. Only about 60% have skin vesicles to aid diagnosis. Mortality without treatment is approximately 50%, and most survivors have severe neurologic and ocular sequelae.

Infants with disseminated neonatal HSV infections develop initial manifestations late in the first week of life. These are relatively nonspecific, consisting of lethargy, fever or hypothermia, vomiting, and poor feeding. Jaundice, purpuric rash, apneic spells, respiratory distress, and cyanosis may also appear. The clinical picture often resembles bacterial sepsis. Many of these infants have clinical evidence of central nervous system involvement, and seizures are common. The disease progresses rapidly, with the frequent development of pneumonia, shock, and disseminated intravascular coagulation. About 90% of these infants die, usually in the second week of life, and most survivors have severe neurologic sequelae. Herpetic skin lesions fail to develop in nearly one quarter of these infants. Antiviral therapy has reduced the mortality to 55% in infants with disseminated infection and to 15% in infants with encephalitis, and it has increased the proportion of survivors who function normally at 1 year of age (108).

Moreover, the availability of experimental treatment protocols has led to earlier diagnosis, increasing the proportion of infants recognized with localized infection of the skin, eyes, or mouth, many of whom would develop disseminated or central nervous system infection if untreated (163).

DIAGNOSIS

Classical genital herpes is clinically apparent, with grouped vesicles and a history of recurrent episodes. However, lesions caused by HSV are often atypical and laboratory diagnosis is recommended for all recurrent lesions below the waist, regardless of their appearance or severity. The availability of specific antiviral agents now places a high premium on early and reliable diagnosis. Virus detection using cell culture offers high sensitivity and specificity when specimens are obtained at the vesicular stage of an eruption and handled properly to avoid loss of infectivity. However, even with culture enhancement techniques (164–167) results are not available for at least 24 hours and often longer. Because many therapeutic decisions require diagnostic information in minutes to hours, much effort has been devoted to developing methods for rapid diagnosis (167–175).

Rapid direct detection of HSV antigens in clinical specimens is now a reality. These techniques are specific and sensitive when applied to herpetic lesions and can even detect viral proteins late in the course of infection, when infectious virus can no longer be recovered. However, they lack the sensitivity required to detect the small amounts of virus shed during asymptomatic recurrences of genital herpes (171,172). The application of PCR to detection of HSV DNA sequences in clinical specimens provides a solution to this problem. PCR has been useful for detection of symptomatic and asymptomatic virus shedding in patients with genital herpes (44,173–175) and recent advances in real-time PCR have increased the utility of the technique for the rapid turnaround of diagnostic samples (176).

The use of serologic tests for HSV has generated controversy in recent years. To be useful, they must be HSV type specific and it is now acknowledged that such tests are useful in defined situations. Type-specific enzyme immunoassays are simple to perform on large numbers of serum samples and have sufficient specificity for use in situations where prevalence is high (e.g. sexually transmitted disease clinics) and they have also been used in serologic surveys. In other situations, the more labor-intensive Western blot assay has greater utility. Type-specific assays (reviewed in 177) have led to a clear delineation of the epidemiology of HSV-1 and HSV-2 infections. They can assist in diagnosis and counseling of patients in certain situations, for example by confirming a diagnosis of primary HSV infection, when HSV antibodies are absent in acute-phase serum and subsequently develop during convalescence. Serologic tests can also be used to identify persons not infected with either HSV serotype, who

are therefore at risk of acquisition of infection from potential sexual partners. The use of enzyme assays for screening pregnant women for HSV-2 antibodies and identifying serologically discordant couples has been proposed as a means of reducing the incidence of neonatal herpes (178). Despite FDA approval of a test that could be used for this purpose, a recent study concluded that this approach would not be cost-effective in the USA (179) and its applicability to low prevalence populations remains a controversial issue, owing to issues of specificity.

TREATMENT

Treatment of the Normal Host

Three antiviral compounds, acyclovir, valacyclovir and famciclovir, are available in the United States for the management of first-episode and recurrent genital HSV infections in immunocompetent and immunocompromised patients. Treatment can significantly reduce the severity of genital herpes episodes and continuous administration of an anti-herpetic compound (suppressive therapy) can markedly reduce the frequency and severity of symptomatic recurrences and asymptomatic virus shedding (44,68,78–81,86,88,102,180–194). Suppressive therapy also improves the health related quality of life of patients with recurrent genital herpes (64). No treatment is presently available that can eradicate latent HSV infections or prevent the establishment of HSV latency (180). For many years, acyclovir was the mainstay of anti-herpes therapy (181–184). It is a highly effective and nontoxic inhibitor of HSV replication. The two licensed prodrugs, famciclovir and valacyclovir, provide much greater oral bioavailability than does acyclovir (195,196). This permits less frequent dosing and results in blood levels of antiviral drug previously achievable only with intravenous acyclovir. In contrast with orally and intravenously administered acyclovir or orally administered famciclovir or valacyclovir, topical acyclovir is only marginally effective and is not recommended for the treatment of genital herpes (66). Treatment options for first episode and recurrent genital herpes in immunocompetent adolescents and adults are presented in Table 106.1. Most experts recommend that the first episode of genital herpes be treated with an oral anti-herpes drug (197). The decision of whether or not to treat beyond the first episode, and of what treatment regimen to use should be guided by several factors including the severity of

---

TABLE 106.1. Antiviral Therapy of Genital Herpes Infections in the Immunocompetent Patient

First episode genital herpes
  Acyclovir 400 mg orally tid × 7–10 days
  Acyclovir 200 mg orally 5×/day × 7–10 days
  Famciclovir 250 mg orally tid × 7–10 days
  Valaciclovir 1,000 mg orally bid × 7–10 days
Recurrent genital herpes: episodic therapy
  Acyclovir 400 mg orally tid × 5 days
  Acyclovir 200 mg orally 5×/day × 5 days
  Acyclovir 800 mg orally bid × 5 days
  Acyclovir 800 mg orally tid × 2 days
  Famciclovir 125 mg orally bid × 5 days
  Valaciclovir 500 mg orally bid × 3 days
Recurrent genital herpes: suppressive therapy
  Acyclovir 400 mg orally bid
  Famciclovir 250 mg orally bid
  Valaciclovir 500 mg orally qd
  Valaciclovir 1,000 mg orally qd

the disease, the frequency of the recurrences, the psychological burden the patient feels regarding the illness, concerns regarding transmission to a susceptible sexual partner, and age of the patient (66,197).

Treatment of the Immunocompromised Host

Studies have demonstrated that oral and intravenous acyclovir is effective for the treatment (and prophylaxis) of severe mucocutaneous HSV infections in immunocompromised patients (198–204). Excellent results have been obtained with oral acyclovir dosages of 200 mg or 400 mg four or five times daily and intravenous dosages or 5 mg/kg or 250 mg/m² every 8 to 12 hours. The availability of the prodrugs valacyclovir and famciclovir has simplified dosing schedules and where investigated these drugs have been shown to be effective in the management of localized genital HSV infection of the immunocompromised host (205–207). When infection is disseminated or involves internal organs such as the liver, early initiation of systemic treatment with acyclovir (e.g., before the diagnosis has been confirmed) may be lifesaving (204). Immunosuppressive therapy should be reduced, if possible, in immunocompromised patients with HSV infection.

Acyclovir Resistance

Acyclovir resistance associated with therapeutic failure was first reported in 1982 (208). Drug resistance occurs more commonly in HIV-infected subjects than among patients with an intact immune system. The prevalence of acyclovir resistant HSV among HIV-infected patients is estimated at 7% (209). Resistance may be caused by mutations in viral genes encoding either thymidine kinase (TK) or DNA polymerase (210). Mutations in the TK gene can render the virus resistant to other nucleoside analogues that require initial phosphorylation activation, e.g., ganciclovir and penciclovir (the active form of famciclovir). Treatment of the immunocompromised patient with infection caused by acyclovir resistant HSV is difficult. Limited success has been reported with foscarnet (211), cidofovir gel (212), and topical trifluorothymidine alone (213) or combined with interferon-alpha (214).

Treatment of Genital Herpes During Pregnancy

The treatment of the pregnant women with genital herpes deserves special comment. Treatment should be considered for the pregnant woman who develops first episode genital HSV infection during pregnancy. Chronic suppressive therapy for recurrent genital herpes is generally discontinued during gestation. Daily treatment with acyclovir, famciclovir, or valacyclovir for the last four weeks of gestation has been suggested for the pregnant woman with a history of recurrent genital herpes (215). This approach is intended to prevent recurrent genital HSV infection at delivery. Although this approach has been demonstrated to be effective in reducing recurrent infections near the time of delivery (216–220), it has not been proven to reduce risk of transmission to the offspring and the safety of this therapy for the fetus or neonate has not yet been established.

Treatment of Neonatal Herpes

Intravenous acyclovir has significantly reduced mortality and increased the proportion of infants who appear to function normally at 1 year of age (108,150,183). However, considerable morbidity and mortality still exist among treated infants, and there is evidence of relapse and of progressive neurologic deterioration after cessation of therapy. In this regard, long-term suppressive therapy with oral acyclovir has been shown to markedly reduce cutaneous recurrences in infants with virologically confirmed neonatal herpes with disease confined to the skin, eyes, and mouth (162). However, the effect on neurologic outcome remains to be determined. High dose intravenous acyclovir, 60 mg/kg per day in three divided doses, is currently recommended for 14 days for neonatal herpes limited to skin, eyes, and mouth or for 21 days if disease is disseminated or involves the central nervous system (221). High dose therapy is associated with improved neurological outcome but is complicated by neutropenia (222). Infants receiving high-dose acyclovir should have assessment of their absolute neutrophils count at least twice weekly during therapy (222).

STRATEGIES FOR CONTROL OF GENITAL HERPES

Prophylaxis (Suppression) of Frequently Recurring Genital Herpes

Recurrent genital herpes is associated with substantial physical and psychological morbidity that can be reduced by treatment with antiviral drugs. Long-term prophylaxis with oral acyclovir, famciclovir, or valacyclovir has been shown to markedly reduce the rate and severity of recurrent genital herpes. However, whereas the rate of recurrence is reduced by 75% to more than 90%, many patients still experience one or more recurrences per year. Moreover, acyclovir treatment does not abolish latency or completely prevent asymptomatic HSV shedding and recurrences resume when suppressive therapy is stopped. Both dose and frequency of dosing affect the efficacy of suppression. Acyclovir, the least expensive and most widely used drug has been tested at doses ranging from 200 to 800 mg acyclovir administered as often as four times daily. Although recurrence rates were reported to be somewhat lower with 200 mg four times daily than with 400 mg twice daily, greatly increased convenience favors 400 mg acyclovir twice daily, the most extensively tested and widely recommended regimen. Patients who respond poorly to a given regimen often show improved response to higher or more frequent dosing. Thus, dosage schedules must be individualized. It seems reasonable to begin with 400 mg twice daily. Apparently compliant patients who continue to report frequent recurrences despite continuous therapy at a dose of 400 mg of acyclovir two or three times daily should be examined and cultured during one or two recurrences. It is far more common to mistake other genital signs and symptoms for recurrent genital herpes than to fail suppressive therapy. A trial of suppressive therapy with famciclovir or valacyclovir should be considered because these prodrugs have much greater oral bioavailability than acyclovir (see Table 106.1). Virus isolates should also be tested for acyclovir sensitivity. Because of the tendency of recurrences to decrease in frequency in time (measured in years) in the absence of therapy, patients receiving prophylactic acyclovir should have treatment stopped periodically (e.g., after 12 to 18 months of suppression) to reevaluate the need for its continuation. Suppression with prophylactic oral acyclovir also appears to be beneficial for patients with recurrences that are associated with severe complications, such as recurrent meningitis, herpetic whitlow, erythema multiforme, and severe neuralgia.

Prevention Against Acquiring Genital Herpes Simplex Virus Infection

Prevention of exposure is, at present, the only proven means of preventing genital HSV infection. For those with symptomatic genital herpes and a seronegative partner, abstinence is an obvious but unpopular option. Abstinence would have to be total for this strategy to work because the majority of initial genital HSV infections are acquired from a sexual partner with no history of genital herpes who is shedding virus without recognizing any signs or symptoms of infection (4,97). Further, oral-genital contact can transmit infection in either direction. Infected individuals can be educated to recognize symptoms and signs of mild recurrences (223) so that they can avoid exposing partners to some episodes of shedding but even so, some episodes remain truly asymptomatic, hence the risk of exposure to virus is unpredictable (224). Condom use offers significant but incomplete protection against HSV-2 infection in susceptible women (225) and may also afford some protection to susceptible men. Strategies to reduce the risk of transmitting genital HSV infection include avoiding intercourse during recurrences and use of condoms between recurrences.

Suppressive antiviral therapy with acyclovir, famciclovir, or valacyclovir has been proven to reduce symptomatic recurrences and asymptomatic shedding but such treatment does not completely eliminate the risk of transmission of genital HSV infection. Nevertheless, in view of the 94% reduction in asymptomatic shedding reported when recently infected women were given 400 mg of acyclovir twice daily, suppressive therapy with acyclovir (or the other prodrugs) may reduce the risk of transmission of genital HSV infection. The results of an ongoing study examining the effects of suppressive valacyclovir therapy in reducing risk of transmission are expected by 2003.

Prevention of Neonatal Herpes

Because infants born by vaginal delivery to mothers with active genital herpes at term are at significant risk for developing neonatal herpes, it is generally advised that women with active genital herpes at term be delivered by cesarean section. However, this is an ineffective strategy for significantly reducing the overall incidence of neonatal herpes because the majority of infected infants are born to mothers with no signs or symptoms of genital herpes, no history of previous episodes of genital herpes, and no history of genital herpes in their sexual partners (226). Also, prepartum ascending infections occur, and a number of infants born by cesarean section to mothers with intact membranes have developed neonatal HSV infection. The low frequency of neonatal infection and the low risk for transmission from women with asymptomatic recurrences make any strategy involving the screening of pregnant women at term by PCR for asymptomatic virus shedding very expensive. Type-specific serologic testing of pregnant women and their sexual partners could be used to identify susceptible pregnant women at risk for genital or orogenital exposure from seropositive partners (227,228), but whether effective interventions aimed at the sero-discordant couple could prevent maternal primary genital HSV infection remains to be demonstrated.

The possibility that antiviral agents might reduce asymptomatic virus shedding enough to interrupt transmission of HSV from mother-to-neonate has been an object of controversy in recent years. Neither the safety nor efficacy of this strategy has been proven beyond doubt, but it remains an option for individual mothers who are prepared to take responsibility for this approach to discuss with their obstetricians.

The Quest for a Vaccine

The most effective method for the prevention of infection by a ubiquitous virus, especially when most exposures are unrec-

ognized, is immunization (229). Despite many failed attempts to prove efficacy of vaccines against herpes simplex, there are some reasons for optimism. These include the significant reduction in the rate and severity of HSV-2 infections in persons with prior HSV-1 infections, the rarity of superinfection with different strains of the same HSV serotype in immunocompetent persons, and the antigenic stability both of HSV-1 and HSV-2. This optimism has been reinforced by a number of studies in animal models, which demonstrated significant protection from exogenous HSV-1 and HSV-2 infections by immunization with inactivated, attenuated, and replication-incompetent whole-virus vaccines, by purified and recombinant envelope glycoprotein vaccines, and by viral DNA vaccines (230–233). While two glycoprotein vaccines have failed to protect against genital herpes in clinical trials (35,234), in recent studies a subunit vaccine containing HSV-2 glycoprotein D combined with a potent adjuvant, 3-O-deacylated monophosphoryl lipid A (3dMPL), has demonstrated effectiveness in HSV seronegative women (23). The vaccine showed no effectiveness in men or HSV-1 seropositive women. It is speculated that protection was due to enhanced Th1 type cellular immunity not engendered by the previous glycoprotein vaccines. The explanation for the gender-specific protection is unknown. Further studies of this vaccine are planned.

Novel Strategies

Two new approaches to the control of genital herpes warrant mention. The first is immunomodulation as a treatment strategy (235). A pilot study has shown that resiquimod (R-848), a topically active immune response modifier, appeared to reduce the frequency of recurrences in subjects with a history of frequently recurring genital herpes (236). Further studies with this immune response modifier are planned. The second approach is the development of topical microbicides, products designed for intravaginal and/or intrarectal use for the purpose of preventing the transmission or acquisition of sexually transmitted diseases including genital herpes (237–239). Preclinical studies have shown that several candidate microbicides are effective at preventing experimental genital HSV-2 infection (240–244). Promising compounds are entering clinical trials and may afford a convenient approach to reducing the risk of genital herpes (245,246).

REFERENCES

1. Corey L, Handsfield HH. Genital herpes and public health: addressing a global problem. *JAMA* 2000;283:791–794.
2. Liu V, Bigby M. Reactivation of genital herpes simplex virus 2 infection in asymptomatic seropositive persons is frequent. *Arch Dermatol* 2000;1141.
3. Wald A, Zeh J, Selke S, et al. Reactivation of genital herpes simplex virus type 2 infection in asymptomatic seropositive persons. *N Engl J Med* 2000;342:844–850.
4. Koelle DM, Wald A. Herpes simplex virus: the importance of asymptomatic shedding. *J Antimicrob Chemother* 2000;45[Suppl T3]:1–8.
5. Schneweis KE. Serologische Untersuchungen zur Typendifferenzierung des Herpesvirus hominis. *Z Immunitaetsforsch Exp Ther* 1962;124:24.
6. Plummer G. Serological comparison of the herpesviruses. *Br J Exp Pathol* 1964;45:135.
7. Nahmias AJ, Dowdle WR. Antigenic and biologic differences in herpesvirus hominis. *Prog Med Virol* 1968;10:110.
8. Corey L Spear PG. Infections with herpes simplex viruses. *N Engl J Med* 1986;314:686, 749.
9. Spear PG. Glycoproteins specified by herpes simplex viruses. In Roizman B, ed: *The herpesviruses,* vol 3. New York: Plenum Publishing, 1985:309–373.
10. Rawls WE. Herpes simplex virus types 1 and 2 and *Herpesvirus simiae.* In Lennette EH, Schmidt NJ, eds: *Diagnostic procedures for viral, rickettsial and chlamydial infections.* Washington DC: American Public Health Association, 1979:309–373.

11. Stanberry LR, Jorgensen DM, Nahmias AJ. Herpes simplex viruses 1 and 2. In Evans AS, Kaslow RA, eds: *Viral infections of humans: epidemiology and control,* 4th ed. New York: Plenum; 1997:419–454.

12. Pereira L, Dondero DV, Gallo D, et al. Serological analysis of herpes simplex virus types 1 and 2 with monoclonal antibodies. *Infect Immun* 1982;35: 363.

13. Carmack MA, Yasukawa LL, Chang SY, et al. T cell recognition and cytokine production elicited by common and type-specific glycoproteins of herpes simplex virus type 1 and type 2. *J Infect Dis* 1996;174:899.

14. Bernstein DI, Bryson YJ, Lovett MA: Antibody response to type-common and type-unique epitopes of herpes simplex virus polypeptides. *J Med Virol* 1985;15:251–263.

15. Lee FK, Coleman RM, Pereira L, et al. Detection of herpes simplex virus type-2 specific antibody with glycoprotein G. *J Clin Microbiol* 1985;22: 641.

16. Sanchez-Martinez D, Schmid DS, Whittington W, et al. Evaluation of a test based on baculovirus-expressed glycoprotein G for detection of herpes simplex virus type-specific antibodies. *J Infect Dis* 1991;164:1196–1199.

17. Cowan FM, Johnson AM, Ashley R, et al. Antibody to herpes simplex virus type 2 as serological marker of sexual lifestyle in populations. *BMJ* 1994;309:1325.

18. Safrin S, Arvin A, Mills J, et al. Comparison of the Western immunoblot assay and a glycoprotein G enzyme immunoassay for detection of serum antibodies to herpes simplex virus type 2 in patients with AIDS. *J Clin Microbiol* 1992;30:1312.

19. Ashley RL. Sorting out the new HSV type specific antibody tests. *Sex Transm Infect* 2001;77:232–237.

20. Posavad CM. T cell immunity to HSV in seronegative persons: silent infection or acquired immunity? Abstract 25th International Herpesvirus Workshop, Portland, 2000.

21. Langenberg AG, Corey L, Ashley RL, Leong WP, Straus SE. A prospective study of new infections with herpes simplex virus type 1 and type 2. Chiron HSV Vaccine Study Group. *N Engl J Med* 1999;341:1432–1438.

22. Cowan FM, Johnson AM, Ashley R, Corey L, Mindel A. Relationship between antibodies to herpes simplex virus (HSV) and symptoms of HSV infection. *J Infect Dis* 1996;174:470–475.

23. Stanberry LR, Spruance SL, Cunningham AL, et al. (GlaxoSmithKline Herpes Vaccine Efficacy Study Group) Glycoprotein-D-adjuvant vaccine to prevent genital herpes. *N Engl J Med* 2002;347(21):1652–1661.

24. Stanberry LR, Mills L, Bernstein DI, et al. Longitudinal assessment of the acquisition of herpes simplex virus (HSV) type 2 infection by adolescent girls: effect of pre-existing HSV type 1 immunity. Submitted.

25. Johnson RE Nahmias AJ, Magder LS, et al. A seroepidemiologic survey of the prevalence of herpes simplex virus type 2 infection in the United States. *N Engl J Med* 1989;321:7.

26. Fleming DT, McQuillan GM, Johnson RE, et al. Herpes simplex virus type 2 in the United States, 1976 to 1994. *N Engl J Med* 1997;337:1105–1111.

27. Rosenthal SL, Stanberry LR, Biro FM, et al. Seroprevalence of herpes simplex virus types 1 and 2 and cytomegalovirus in adolescents. *Clin Infect Dis* 1997;24:135–139.

28. Huerta K, Berkelhamer S, Klein J, Ammerman S, Chang J, Prober CG. Epidemiology of herpes simplex virus type 2 infections in a high-risk adolescent population. *J Adolesc Health* 1996;18:384–386.

29. Sucato G, Celum C, Dithmer D, Ashley R, Wald A. Demographic rather than behavioral risk factors predict herpes simplex virus type 2 infection in sexually active adolescents. *Pediatr Infect Dis J* 2001;20:422–426.

30. Lewis LM, Bernstein DI, Rosenthal SL, Stanberry LR. Seroprevalence of herpes simplex virus-type 2 in African-American college women. *J Natl Med Assoc* 1999;91:210–212.

31. Breinig MK, Kingsley LA, Armstrong JA, Freeman DJ, Ho M. Epidemiology of genital herpes in Pittsburgh: serologic, sexual, and racial correlates of apparent and inapparent herpes simplex infections. *J Infect Dis* 1990;162:299–306.

32. Becker TM, Lee F, Daling JR, Nahmias AJ. Seroprevalence of and risk factors for antibodies to herpes simplex viruses, hepatitis B, and hepatitis C among southwestern hispanic and non-hispanic white women. *Sex Transm Dis* 1996;23:138–144.

33. Oliver L, Wald A, Kim M, Zeh J, Selke S, Ashley R, Corey L. Seroprevalence of herpes simplex virus infections in a family medicine clinic. *Arch Fam Med* 1995;4:228–232.

34. Austin H, Macaluso M, Nahmias A, et al. Correlates of herpes simplex virus seroprevalence among women attending a sexually transmitted disease clinic. *Sex Transm Dis* 1999;26:329–334.

35. Corey L, Langenberg AG, Ashley R, et al. Recombinant glycoprotein vaccine for the prevention of genital HSV-2 infection: two randomized controlled trials. Chiron HSV Vaccine Study Group. *JAMA* 1999;282:331–340.

36. Siegel D, Golden E, Washington AE, et al. Prevalence and correlates of herpes simplex infections. The population-based AIDS in Multiethnic Neighborhoods Study. *JAMA* 1992;268:1702–1708.

37. Schomogyi M, Wald A, Corey L. Herpes simplex virus-2 infection. An emerging disease? *Infect Dis Clin North Am* 1998;12:47–61.

38. Stanberry LR, Rosenthal SL. Epidemiology of herpes simplex virus infections in adolescents. *Herpes* 1999;6:12–15.

39. O'Farrell N. Increasing prevalence of genital herpes in developing countries: implications for heterosexual HIV transmission and STI control programmes. *Sex Transm Infect* 1999;75:377–384.

40. Koelle DM, Bendetti J, Langenberg A, Corey L. Asymptomatic reactivation of herpes simplex virus in women after the first episode of genital herpes. *Ann Intern Med* 1992;116:433.

41. Wald A, Zeh J, Selke S, et al. Reactivation of genital herpes simplex virus type 2 infection in asymptomatic seropositive persons. *N Engl J Med* 2000;342: 844–850.

42. Krone MR, Wald A, Tabet SR, Paradise M, Corey L, Celum CL. Herpes simplex virus type 2 shedding in human immunodeficiency virus-negative men who have sex with men: frequency, patterns, and risk factors. *Clin Infect Dis* 2000;30:261–267.

43. Krone MR, Tabet SR, Paradise M, Wald A, Corey L, Celum CL. Herpes simplex virus shedding among human immunodeficiency virus-negative men who have sex with men: site and frequency of shedding. *J Infect Dis* 1998;178:978–982.

44. Wald A, Corey L, Cone R, Hobson A, Davis G, Zeh J. Frequent genital herpes simplex virus 2 shedding in immunocompetent women. Effect of acyclovir treatment. *J Clin Invest* 1997;99:1092–1097.

45. Wald A, Zeh J, Selke S, Ashley RL, Corey L. Virologic characteristics of subclinical and symptomatic genital herpes infections. *N Engl J Med* 1995;333:770–775.

46. Lafferty WE, Downey L, Celum C, Wald A. Herpes simplex virus type 1 as a cause of genital herpes: impact on surveillance and prevention. *J Infect Dis* 2000;181:1454–1457.

47. Lowhagen GB, Tunback P, Anderson K, et al. First episodes of genital herpes in a Swedish STD population: a study of epidemiology and transmission by the use of herpes simplex virus (HSV) typing and specific serology. *Sex Transm Infect* 2000;76:179.

48. Nilsen A, Myrmel H. Changing trends in genital herpes simplex virus infection in Bergen, Norway. *Acta Obstet Gynecol Scand* 2000;79:693–696.

49. Tayal SC, Pattman RS. High prevalence of herpes simplex virus type 1 in female anogenital herpes simplex in Newcastle upon Tyne 1983–92. *Int J STD AIDS* 1994;5:359–361.

50. Lavery HA, Connolly JH, Russell JD. Incidence of herpes genitalis in Northern Ireland in 1973–83 and herpes simplex types 1 and 2 isolated in 1982–4. *Genitourin Med* 1986;62:24.

51. Benedetti JK, Corey L, Ashley R. Recurrence rates in genital herpes after symptomatic first-episode infection. *Ann Intern Med* 1994;121:847.

52. Reeves WC, Corey L, Adams HG, et al. Risk of recurrence after first episodes of genital herpes: relation to HSV type and antibody response. *N Engl J Med* 1981;304:315.

53. Lafferty WE, Coombs RW, Benedetti J, Critchlow C, Corey L. Recurrences after oral and genital herpes simplex virus infection. Influence of site of infection and viral type. *N Engl J Med* 1987;316:1444–1449.

54. Stanberry LR. The pathogenesis of herpes simplex virus infections. In Stanberry LR, ed: *Genital and neonatal herpes.* London: John Wiley and Sons, 1996:31–48.

55. Cunningham AL, Mikloska Z. The holy grail: immune control of human herpes simplex virus infection and disease. *Herpes* 2001;8[Suppl 1]:6A–10A.

56. Simmons A. Virus infections in immunocompromised patients. In Collier L, ed: *Topley and wilson microbiology and microbial infections,* vol 5. London: Edward Arnold, 1997.

57. Bustamante CI, Wade JC. Herpes simplex virus infection in the immunocompromised cancer patient. *J Clin Oncol* 1991;9:1903–1915.

58. Schmid DS, Rouse BT. The role of T cell immunity in control of herpes simplex virus. *Curr Top Microbiol Immunol* 1992;179:57–74.

59. Cunningham AL, Merigan TC. Gamma Interferon production appears to predict time of recurrence of herpes labialis. *J Immunol* 1983;130:2397–2400.

60. Posavad CM, Koelle DM, Corey L. Tipping the scales of herpes simplex virus reactivation: the important responses are local. *Nat Med* 1998;4:381–382.

61. Corey LHG, Brown ZA, Holmes KK. Genital herpes simplex virus infections: clinical manifestations, course, and complications. *Ann Intern Med* 1983;98:958–972.

62. Bernstein DI, Lovett MA, Bryson YJ. Serologic analysis of first-episode nonprimary genital herpes simplex virus infection. Presence of type 2 antibody in acute serum samples. *Am J Med* 1984;77:1055–1060.

63. Hensleigh PA, Andrews WW, Brown Z, Greenspoon J, Yasukawa L, Prober CG. Genital herpes during pregnancy: inability to distinguish primary and recurrent infections clinically. *Obstet Gynecol* 1997;89:891–895.

64. Patel R, Tyring S, Strand A, Price MJ, Grant DM. Impact of suppressive antiviral therapy on the health related quality of life of patients with recurrent genital herpes infection. *Sex Transm Infect* 1999;75:398–402.

65. Mindel A. Psychological and psychosexual implications of herpes simplex virus infections. *Scand J Infect Dis Suppl* 1996;100:27–32.

66. Stanberry L, Cunningham A, Mertz G, et al. New developments in the epidemiology, natural history and management of genital herpes. *Antiviral Res* 1999;42:1–14.

67. Breinig MK, Kingsley LA, Armstrong JA, et al. Epidemiology of genital herpes in Pittsburgh: serologic, sexual, and racial correlates of apparent and inapparent herpes simplex infections. *J Infect Dis* 1990;162:299.

68. Mindel A, Adler MW, Sutherland S, Fiddian AP. Intravenous acyclovir treatment for primary genital herpes. *Lancet* 1982;1:697.

69. Chang TW, Fiumara NJ, Weinstein L. Genital herpes: some clinical and laboratory observations. *JAMA* 1974;229:544.

70. Brown ZA, Kern ER, Spruance SL, Overall JC Jr. Clinical and virologic course of herpes simplex genitalis. *West J Med* 1979;130:414–421.

71. Vontver LA, Reeves WC, Rattray M, et al. Clinical course and diagnosis of genital herpes simplex virus infection and evaluation of topical surfactant therapy. *Am J Obstet Gynecol* 1979;133:548–554.

72. Ekwo E, Wong YW, Myers M. Asymptomatic cervicovaginal shedding of herpes simplex virus. *Am J Obstet Gynecol* 1979;134:102–103.

73. Adam E, Kaufman RH, Mirkovic RR, Melnick JL. Persistence of virus shedding in asymptomatic women after recovery from herpes genitalis. *Obstet Gynecol* 1979;54:171–173.

74. Mostad SB, Kreiss JK, Ryncarz AJ, et al. Cervical shedding of herpes simplex virus in human immunodeficiency virus-infected women: effects of hormonal contraception, pregnancy, and vitamin A deficiency. *J Infect Dis* 2000;181:58–63.

75. Wilcox RR. Necrotic cervicitis due to primary infection with virus of herpes simplex. *BMJ* 1968;1:610.

76. Peutherer JF, Smith IW, Hunter JM. Herpes simplex virus infection of the cervix. *Lancet* 1981;2:1285.

77. Koelle DM, Schomogyi M, Corey L. Antigen-specific T cells localize to the uterine cervix in women with genital herpes simplex virus type 2 infection. *J Infect Dis* 2000;182:662–670.

78. Mindel A, Adler MW, Sutherland S, Fiddian AP. Intravenous acyclovir treatment for primary genital herpes. *Lancet* 1982;1:697–700.

79. Nilsen AE, Aasen T, Halsos AM, et al. Efficacy of oral acyclovir in the treatment of initial and recurrent genital herpes. *Lancet* 1982;2:571–573.

80. Peacock JE Jr, Kaplowitz LG, Sparling PF, et al. Intravenous acyclovir therapy of first episodes of genital herpes: a multicenter double-blind, placebo-controlled trial. *Am J Med* 1988;85:301–306.

81. Bryson YJ, Dillon M, Lovett M, et al. Treatment of first episodes of genital herpes simplex virus infection with oral acyclovir. A randomized double-blind controlled trial in normal subjects. *N Engl J Med* 1983;308:916–921.

82. Guinan ME, Wolinsky SN, Reichman RC. Epidemiology of genital herpes simplex virus infection. *Epidemiol Rev* 1985;7:127–146.

83. Benedetti JK, Corey L, Ashley R. Recurrence rates in genital herpes after symptomatic first-episode infection. *Ann Intern Med* 1994;121:847.

84. Bryson Y, Dillon M, Bernstein DI, Radolf J, Zakowski P, Garratty E. Risk of acquisition of genital herpes simplex virus type 2 in sex partners of persons with genital herpes: a prospective couple study. *J Infect Dis* 1993;167:942–946.

85. Koelle DM, Bendetti J, Langenberg A, Corey L. Asymptomatic reactivation of herpes simplex virus in women after the first episode of genital herpes. *Ann Intern Med* 1992;116:433–437.

86. Mertz GJ, Critchlow CW, Benedetti J, et al. Double-blind placebo-controlled trial of oral acyclovir in first-episode genital herpes simplex virus infection. *JAMA* 1984;252:1147–1151.

87. Guinan ME, MacCalman J, Kern ER, Overall JC Jr, Spruance SL. The course of untreated recurrent genital herpes simplex infection in 27 women. *N Engl J Med* 1981;304:759–763.

88. Reichman RC, Badger GJ, Mertz GJ, et al. Treatment of recurrent genital herpes simplex infections with oral acyclovir: a controlled trial. *JAMA* 1984;251:2103–2107.

89. Reichman RC, Badger GJ, Guinan ME, et al. Topically administered acyclovir in the treatment of recurrent herpes simplex genitalis: a controlled trial. *J Infect Dis* 1983;147:336–340.

90. Adams HG, Benson EA, Alexander ER, Vontver LA, Remington MA, Holmes KK. Genital herpetic infection in men and women: clinical course and effect of topical application of adenine arabinoside. *J Infect Dis* 1976;133[Suppl]:A151–A159.

91. Guinan ME, MacCalman J, Kern ER, Overall JC Jr, Spruance SL. The course of untreated recurrent genital herpes simplex infection in 27 women. *N Engl J Med* 1981;304:759–763.

92. Koutsky LA, Stevens CE, Holmes KK, et al. Underdiagnosis of genital herpes by current clinical and viral-isolation procedures. *N Engl J Med* 1992;326:1533–1539.

93. Brock BV, Selke S, Benedetti J, Douglas JM Jr, Corey L. Frequency of asymptomatic shedding of herpes simplex virus in women with genital herpes. *JAMA* 1990;263:418–420.

94. Hankins GDV, Cunningham FG, Luby P, et al. Asymptomatic excretion of herpes simplex virus during early labor. *Am J Obstet Gynecol* 1984;150:100.

95. Arvin AM, Hensleigh PA, Prober CG, et al. Failure of antipartum maternal cultures to predict the infants risk of exposure to herpes simplex virus at delivery. *N Engl J Med* 1986;315:796.

96. Simkovich JW, Soper DE. Asymptomatic shedding of herpes virus during labor. *Am J Obstet Gynecol* 1988;158:588.

97. Mertz GJ, Schmidt O, Jourden JL, et al. Frequency of acquisition of first-episode genital infection with herpes simplex virus from symptomatic and asymptomatic source contacts. *Sex Transm Dis* 1985;12:33.

98. Brown ZA, Benedetti JK, Watts DH, et al. A comparison between detailed and simple histories in the diagnosis of genital herpes complicating pregnancy. *Am J Obstet Gynecol* 1995;172:1299.

99. Brown ZA, Benedetti J, Ashley R, et al. Neonatal herpes simplex virus infection in relation to asymptomatic maternal infection at the time of labor. *N Engl J Med* 1991;324:1247.

100. Cone RW, Hobson AC, Brown Z, et al. Frequent detection of genital herpes simplex virus DNA by polymerase chain reaction among pregnant women. *JAMA* 1994;272:792.

101. Wald A, Corey L, Cone R, et al. Frequent genital herpes simplex virus 2 shedding in immunocompetent women. *J Clin Invest* 1997;99:1092.

102. Wald A, Zeh J, Barnum G, et al. Suppression of subclinical shedding of herpes simplex virus type 2 with acyclovir. *Ann Intern Med* 1996;124:8.

103. Scher J, Bottone E, Desmond E, Simons W. The incidence and outcome of asymptomatic herpes simplex genitalis in an obstetric population. *Am J Obstet Gynecol* 1982;144:906.

104. Wittek AE, Yeager AS, Au DS, Hensleigh PA. Asymptomatic shedding of herpes simplex virus from the cervix and lesion site during pregnancy. *Am J Dis Child* 1984;138:439.

105. Prober CG, Arvin AM. Genital herpes and the pregnant woman. *Curr Clin Top Infect Dis* 1989;10:1.

106. Yeager AS, Arvin AM. Reasons for the absence of a history of recurrent genital herpes infections in mothers of neonates infected with herpes simplex virus. *Pediatrics* 1984;73:188.

107. Whitley RJ, Nahmias AJ, Soong S-J, et al. Vidarabine therapy of neonatal herpes simplex virus infection. *Pediatrics* 1980;60:495.

108. Whitley R, Arvin A, Prober C, et al. A controlled trial comparing vidarabine with acyclovir in neonatal herpes simplex virus infection. *N Engl J Med* 1991;324:444.

109. Whitley R, Arvin A, Prober C, et al. Predictors of morbidity and mortality in neonates with herpes simplex virus infections. *N Engl J Med* 1991;324:450.

110. Whitley RJ, Corey L, Arvin A, et al. Changing presentation of herpes simplex virus infection in neonates. *J Infect Dis* 1988;158:109.

111. Prober CG, Corey L, Brown ZA, et al. The management of pregnancies complicated by genital infections with herpes simplex virus. *Clin Infect Dis* 1992;15:1031.

112. Slavin HB, Ferguson JJ. Zoster-like eruptions caused by the virus herpes simplex. *Am J Med* 1950;8:456.

113. Greenblatt RM, Lukehart SA, Plummer FA, et al. Genital ulceration as a risk factor for human immunodeficiency virus infection. *AIDS* 1988;2:47.

114. Schacker T. The role of HSV in the transmission and progression of HIV. *Herpes* 2001;8:46–49.

115. del Mar Pujades Rodriguez M, Obasi A, Mosha F, et al. Herpes simplex virus type 2 infection increases HIV incidence: a prospective study in rural Tanzania. *AIDS* 2002;16:451–462.

116. Auvert B, Ballard R, Campbell C, et al. HIV infection among youth in a South African mining town is associated with herpes simplex virus-2 seropositivity and sexual behaviour. *AIDS* 2001;15:885–898.

117. Powers RD, Rein MF, Hayden FG. Necrotizing balanitis due to herpes simplex type 1. *JAMA* 1982;248:215.

118. Young EJ, Vainrub B, Musher DM, et al. Acute pharyngotonsillitis caused by herpesvirus type 2. *JAMA* 1978;239:1885–1886.

119. Tustin AW, Kaiser AB. Life-threatening pharyngitis caused by herpes simplex virus, type 2. *Sex Transm Dis* 1979;6:23.

120. Goodell SE, Quinn RC, Mkrtichian E, et al. Herpes simplex virus proctitis in homosexual men. Clinical, sigmodoscopic, and histopathological features. *N Engl J Med* 1983;308:868.

121. Oates JK, Greenhouse PRDH. Retention of urine in anogenital herpetic infection. *Lancet* 1979;1:691.

122. Stalder H, Oxman MN, Dawson DM, Levin MJ. Herpes simplex meningitis: isolation of herpes simplex virus type 2 from cerebrospinal fluid. *N Engl J Med* 1973;289:1296–1298.

123. Mertz G, Corey L. Genital herpes simplex virus infections in adults. *Urol Clin North Am* 1984;11:103–119.

124. Chambers ST, Powell KF, Croxson MC, Krishnan S, Weir RP. Demonstration of herpes simplex type 2 in the cerebrospinal fluid of two patients with recurrent lymphocytic meningitis. *NZ Med J* 1994;107[986 Pt 1]:367–369.

125. Tedder DG, Ashley R, Tyler KL, Levin MJ. Herpes simplex virus infection as a cause of benign recurrent lymphocytic meningitis. *Ann Intern Med* 1994;121:334–338.

126. Jensenius M, Myrvang B, Storvold G, Bucher A, Hellum KB, Bruu AL. Herpes simplex virus type 2 DNA detected in cerebrospinal fluid of 9 patients with Mollaret's meningitis. *Acta Neurol Scand* 1998;98:209–212.

127. Chu K, Kang DW, Lee JJ, Yoon BW. Atypical brainstem encephalitis caused by herpes simplex virus 2. *Arch Neurol* 2002;59:460–463.

128. Person DA, Kaufman RH, Gardner HL, Rawls WE. Herpesvirus type 2 genitourinary tract infections. *Am J Obstet Gynecol* 1973;116:993.

129. Huff JC. Erythema multiforme and latent herpes simplex infection. *Semin Dermatol* 1992;11:207–210.

130. Cheriyan S, Patterson R. Recurrent Stevens-Johnson syndrome secondary to herpes simplex: a follow up on a successful management program. *Allergy Asthma Proc* 1996;17:71–73.

131. Connor RW, Lorts G, Gilbert DN. Lethal herpes simplex virus type 1 hepatitis in a normal adult. *Gastroenterology* 1979;76:590.

132. Flewett TH, Parker RGF, Philip WM. Acute hepatitis due to herpes simplex virus in an adult. *J Clin Pathol* 1969;22:60.

133. Eron L, Kosinski K, Hirsch MS. Hepatitis in an adult caused by herpes simplex virus type 1. *Gastroenterology* 1976;71:500.

134. Joseph TJ, Vogt PJ. Disseminated herpes with hepatoadrenal necrosis in an adult. *Am J Med* 1974;56:735.

135. Whorton CM, Thomas DM, Denham SW. Fatal systemic herpes simplex virus type 2 infection in a healthy young woman. *South Med J* 1983;76:81.

136. Francis TJ, Osuntokum BO, Kemp GE. Fulminant hepatitis due to herpes hominis in an adult human. *Am J Gastroenterol* 1972;57:329.

137. Goyette RE, Donowho EM, Hieger LIZ, Plunkett G. Fulminant herpesvirus hominis hepatitis during pregnancy. *Obstet Gynecol* 1974;43:191.

138. Long JC, Wheeler CE, Briggaman RA. Varicella-like infection due to herpes simplex. *Arch Dermatol* 1978;114:406.

139. Gelven PL, Gruber KK, Swiger FK, Cina SJ, Harley RA. Fatal disseminated herpes simplex in pregnancy with maternal and neonatal death. *South Med J* 1996;89:732–734.

140. Young EJ, Chafizadeh E, Oliveira VL, Genta RM. Disseminated herpesvirus infection during pregnancy. *Clin Infect Dis* 1996;22:51–58.

141. Lagrew DC, Furlow TG, Hager D, Yarrish YL. Disseminated herpes simplex virus infection in pregnancy. Successful treatment with acyclovir. *JAMA* 1984;252:2058.

142. Tang IT, Shepp DH. Herpes simplex virus infection in cancer patients: prevention and treatment. *Oncology* 1992;6:101–106.

143. Vestey JP, Howie SE, Norval M, Maingay JP, Neill WA. Severe eczema herpeticum is associated with prolonged depression of cell-mediated immunity to herpes simplex virus. *Curr Prob Dermatol* 1989;18:158–161.

144. Whitley RJ, Levin M, Barton N, et al. Infections caused by herpes simplex virus in the immunocompromised host: natural history and topical acyclovir therapy. *J Infect Dis* 1984;150:323–329.

145. Bourdarias B, Perro G, Cutillas M, Castede JC, Lafon ME, Sanchez R. Herpes simplex virus infection in burned patients: epidemiology of 11 cases. *Burns* 1996;22:287–290.

146. Siegal FP, Lopez C, Hammer GS, et al. Severe acquired immunodeficiency in male homosexuals, manifested by chronic perianal ulcerative herpes simplex lesions. *N Engl J Med* 1981;305:1039.

147. Safrin S, Ashley R, Houlihan C, Cusick PS, Mills J. Clinical and serologic features of herpes simplex virus infection in patients with AIDS. *AIDS* 1991;5:1107–1110.

148. Augenbraun M, Feldman J, Chirgwin K, et al. Increased genital shedding of herpes simplex virus type 2 in HIV-seropositive women. *Ann Intern Med* 1995;123:845–847.

149. Krone MR, Wald A, Tabet SR, Paradise M, Corey L, Celum CL. Herpes simplex virus type 2 shedding in human immunodeficiency virus-negative men who have sex with men: frequency, patterns, and risk factors. *Clin Infect Dis* 2000;30:261–267.

150. Kimberlin DW, Lin CY, Jacobs RF, et al, for the National Institute of Allergy and Infectious Diseases Collaborative Antiviral Study Group. Natural history of neonatal herpes simplex virus infections in the acyclovir era. *Pediatrics* 2001;108:223–229.

151. Prober CG, Hensleigh PA, Boucher FD, et al. Use if routine viral cultures at delivery to identify neonates exposed to herpes simplex virus. *N Engl J Med* 1988;318:887.

152. Florman AL, Gershon AA, Blackett RP, Nahmias AJ. Intrauterine infection with herpes simplex virus: resultant congenital malformation. *JAMA* 1973;225:129.

153. Hutto C, Arvin A, Jacobs R, et al. Intrauterine herpes simplex virus infections. *J Pediatr* 1987;110:97.

154. Prober CG, Sullender WM, Yasukawa LL, et al. Low risk of herpes simplex virus infections in neonates exposed to the virus at the time of vaginal delivery to mothers with recurrent genital herpes simplex virus infections. *N Engl J Med* 1987;316:240.

155. Brown ZA, Benedetti J, Ashley R, et al. Neonatal herpes simplex virus infection in relation to asymptomatic maternal infection at the time of labor. *N Engl J Med* 1991;324:1247.

156. Kaye EM, Dooling EC. Neonatal herpes simplex meningoencephalitis associated with fetal monitor scalp electrodes. *Neurology* 1981;31:1045.

157. Light IJ. Postnatal acquisition of herpes simplex virus by the newborn infant. A review of the literature. *Pediatrics* 1979;63:480.

158. Adams G, Stover BH, Keenlyside RA, et al. Nosocomial herpetic infections in a pediatric intensive care unit. *Am J Epidemiol* 1981;113:126.

159. Linnemann CC Jr, Buchman TG, Light IJ, et al. Transmission of herpes simplex virus type-1 in a nursery for the newborn: identification of viral species isolated by DNA fingerprinting. *Lancet* 1978;1:964.

160. Sullivan-Bolyai JZ, Fife KH, Jacobs RF, et al. Disseminated neonatal herpes simplex virus Prober type 1 from a maternal breast lesion. *Pediatrics* 1983;71:455.

161. Baldwin S, Whitely RJ. Intrauterine herpes simplex virus infection. *Teratology* 1989;39:1.

162. Kimberlin D, Powell D, Gruber W, et al. Administration of oral acyclovir suppressive therapy after neonatal herpes simplex virus disease limited to the skin, eyes and mouth: results of a phase I/II trial. *Pediatr Infect Dis J* 1996;15:247–254.

163. Whitley RJ, Nahmias AJ, Visintine AM, Fleming CL, Alford CA. The natural history of herpes simplex virus infection of mother and newborn. *Pediatrics* 1980;66:489–494.

164. Cleaves CA, Wilson DJ, Wold AD, Smith TF. Detection and serotyping of herpes simplex virus in MRC-5 cells by use of centrifugation and monoclonal antibodies 16 h post inoculation. *J Clin Microbiol* 1985;21:29.

165. Michalski FJ, Shaikh M, Sahraie F, et al. Enzyme-linked immunosorbent assay spin amplification technique for herpes simplex virus. *J Clin Microbiol* 1986;19:548.

166. Warford AL, Chung JW, Drill AE, Steinberg E. Amplification techniques for

167. Ashley R. Laboratory techniques in the diagnosis of herpes simplex infection. *Genitourin Med* 1993;69:174.

168. Goldstein LC, Corey L, McDougall JK, et al. Monoclonal antibodies to *herpes simplex* viruses: use in antigenic typing and rapid diagnosis. *J Infect Dis* 1983;147:829.

169. Richman DD, Cleveland PH, Redfield DC, et al. Rapid viral diagnosis. *J Infect Dis* 1984;149:298.

170. Corey L. Laboratory diagnosis of herpes simplex virus infections. Principles guiding the development of rapid diagnostic tests. *Diagn Microbiol Infect Dis* 1986;4:1115.

171. Verano L, Michalski FJ. Herpes simplex virus antigen direct detection in standard transport medium by DuPont Herpchek enzyme-linked immunosorbent assay. *J Clin Microbiol* 1990;28:2555.

172. Ashley R. Current concepts in laboratory diagnosis of herpes simplex infections. In Sacks SL, Strauss SE, Whitley RJ, Griffiths PD, eds: *Clinical management of herpes viruses*. New York: IOS Press, 1995:137–174.

173. Hardy DA, Arvin AM, Yasukawa LL, et al. Use of polymerase chain reaction for successful identification of asymptomatic genital infections with herpes simplex virus in pregnant women at delivery. *J Infect Dis* 1990;162:1031.

174. Coyle PV, Desai A, Wyatt D, McCaughey C, O'Neill HJ. A comparison of virus isolation, indirect immunofluorescence and nested multiplex polymerase chain reaction for the diagnosis of primary and recurrent herpes simplex type 1 and type 2 infections. *J Virol Methods* 1999;83:75–82.

175. Cone RW, Hobson AC, Palmer J, et al. Extended duration of herpes simplex virus DNA in genital lesions detected by the polymerase chain reaction. *J Infect Dis* 1991;164:757.

176. Nichol S, Brass A, Cubie HA. Detection of herpes viruses in clinical samples using real-time PCR. *J Virol Methods* 2001;96:25.

177. Ashley RL. Sorting out the new HSV type specific antibody tests. *Sex Transm Infect* 2001;77:232–237.

178. Brown ZA. HSV-2 specific serology should be offered routinely to antenatal patients. *Rev Med Virol* 2000;10:141–144.

179. Rouse CJ, Stringer JS. An appraisal of screening for maternal type-specific herpes simplex virus antibodies to prevent neonatal herpes *Am J Obstet Gynecol* 2000;183:400.

180. Efstathiou S, Field HJ, Griffiths PD, et al. Herpes simplex virus latency and nucleoside analogues. *Antiviral Res* 1999;41:85–100.

181. Guinan ME. Oral acyclovir for treatment and suppression of genital herpes simplex virus infection: a review. *JAMA* 1986;255:1747.

182. Stone KM, Whittington WL. Treatment of genital herpes. *Rev Infect Dis* 1990;12[Suppl 6]:610.

183. Whitley RJ, Gnann JW Jr. Acyclovir: a decade later. *N Engl J Med* 1992;327:782.

184. Mertz GJ. Management of genital herpes. *Adv Exp Med Biol* 1996;394:1.

185. Centers for Diseases Control and Prevention. 2002 Sexually transmitted diseases treatment guidelines. *MMWR* 2002;51:14–15.

186. Sacks SL, Aoki FY, Diaz-Mitoma F, et al. Patient-initiated, twice-daily oral famciclovir for early recurrent genital herpes: a randomized, double-blind multicenter trial. *JAMA* 1996;276:44.

187. Saiag P, Praindhui D, Chastang C. A double-blind, randomized study assessing the equivalence of valacyclovir 1000 mg once daily versus 500 mg twice daily in the episodic treatment of recurrent genital herpes. Genival Study Group. *J Antimicrob Chemother* 1999;44:525–531.

188. Reitano M, Tyring S, Lang W, et al. Valacyclovir for the suppression of recurrent genital herpes simplex virus infection: a large-scale dose range-finding study. International Valacyclovir HSV Study Group. *J Infect Dis* 1998;178:603–610.

189. Diaz-Mitoma F, Sibbald RG, Shafran SD, Boon R, Saltzman RL. Oral famciclovir for the suppression of recurrent genital herpes: a randomized controlled trial. Collaborative Famciclovir Genital Herpes Research Group. *JAMA* 1998;280:887–892.

190. Fife KH, Barbarash RA, Rudolph T, Degregorio B, Roth R. Valacyclovir versus acyclovir in the treatment of first-episode genital herpes infection. Results of an international, multicenter, double-blind, randomized clinical trial. The Valacyclovir International Herpes Simplex Virus Study Group. *Sex Transm Dis* 1997;24:481–486.

191. Mertz GJ, Loveless MO, Levin MJ, Kraus SJ, Fowler SL, Goade D, Tyring SK. Oral famciclovir for suppression of recurrent genital herpes simplex virus infection in women. A multicenter, double-blind, placebo-controlled trial. Collaborative Famciclovir Genital Herpes Research Group. *Arch Intern Med* 1997;157:343–349.

192. Sacks SL, Aoki FY, Diaz-Mitoma F, Sellors J, Shafran SD. Patient-initiated, twice-daily oral famciclovir for early recurrent genital herpes. A randomized, double-blind multicenter trial. Canadian Famciclovir Study Group. *JAMA* 1996;276:44–49.

193. Spruance SL, Tyring SK, DeGregorio B, et al. A large-scale placebo-controlled dose-ranging trial of peroral valaciclovir for episodic treatment of recurrent genital herpes. *Arch Intern Med* 1996;156:1729–1736.

194. Wald A, Carrell D, Remington M, Kexel E, Zeh J, Corey L. Two-day regimen of acyclovir for treatment of recurrent genital herpes simplex virus type 2 infection. *Clin Infect Dis* 2002;34:944–948.

195. Vere Hodge RA. Famciclovir and penciclovir. The mode of action of

famciclovir including its conversion to penciclovir. *Antiviral Chem Chemother* 1993;4:67.

196. Weller S, Blum MR, Doucette M, et al. Pharmacokinetics of the acyclovir pro-drug valacyclovir after escalating single- and multiple-dose administration to normal volunteers. *Clin Pharmacol Ther* 1993;54:595.

197. Stanberry LR, Rosenthal SL. Genital herpes simplex virus infection in the adolescent: special considerations for management. *Paediatric Drugs* 2002;4: 291.

198. Wade JC, Newton B, McLaren C, et al. Intravenous acyclovir to treat mucocutaneous herpes simplex virus infection after marrow, transplantation: double-blind trial. *Ann Intern Med* 1982;96:265.

199. Meyers JD, Wade JC, Mitchell CD, et al. Multicenter collaborative trial of intravenous acyclovir for treatment of mucocutaneous herpes simplex virus infection in immunocompromised host. *Am J Med* 1982;73:229.

200. Shepp DH, Newton BA, Dandliker PS, et al. Oral acyclovir therapy for mucocutaneous *herpes simplex* virus infections in immunocompromised marrow transplant recipients. *Ann Intern Med* 1985;102:783.

201. Saral R, Burns WH, Laskin OL, et al. Acyclovir prophylaxis of herpes simplex virus infections: a randomized, double-blind, controlled trial in bone-marrow-transplant recipients. *N Engl J Med* 1981;305:63.

202. Wade JC, Newton B, Flournoy N. Acyclovir for prevention of herpes simplex virus reactivation after marrow transplantation. *Ann Intern Med* 1984;100:823.

203. Shepp DH, Dandliker PS, Flournoy N, Meyers JD. Sequential intravenous and twice-daily oral acyclovir for extended prophylaxis of herpes simplex virus infection in marrow transplant patients. *Transplantation* 1987;43:654.

204. Kusne S, Schwartz M, Breinig MK, et al. Herpes simplex virus hepatitis after solid organ transplantation in adults. *J Infect Dis* 1991;163:1001.

205. Conant MA, Schacker TW, Murphy RL, Gold J, Crutchfield LT, Crooks RJ, for the International Valaciclovir HSV Study Group. Valacyclovir versus acyclovir for herpes simplex virus infection in HIV-infected individuals: two randomized trials. *Int J STD AIDS* 2002;13:12–21.

206. Romanowski B, Aoki FY, Martel AY, Lavender EA, Parsons JE, Saltzman RL. Efficacy and safety of famciclovir for treating mucocutaneous herpes simplex infection in HIV-infected individuals. Collaborative Famciclovir HIV Study Group. *AIDS* 2000;14:1211–1217.

207. Schacker T, Hu HL, Koelle DM, et al. Famciclovir for the suppression of symptomatic and asymptomatic herpes simplex virus reactivation in HIV-infected persons. A double-blind, placebo-controlled trial. *Ann Intern Med* 1998;128:21–28.

208. Parris D, Harrington JE. Herpes simplex virus variants resistant to high concentrations exist in clinical isolates. *Antimicrob Agents Chemother* 1982;22:71–77.

209. Englund JA, Zimmerman ME, Swierkosz EM, Goodman JL, Scholl DR, Balfour HH Jr. Herpes simplex virus resistant to acyclovir. A study in a tertiary care center. *Ann Intern Med* 1990;112:416–422.

210. Hill EL, Hunter GA, Ellis MN. In vitro and in vivo characterization of herpes simplex virus clinical isolates recovered from patients infected with human immunodeficiency virus. *Antimicrob Agents Chemother* 1991;35:2322–2328.

211. Javaly K, Wohlfeiler M, Kalayjian R, et al. Treatment of mucocutaneous herpes simplex virus infections unresponsive to acyclovir with topical foscarnet cream in AIDS patients: a phase I/II study. *J Acquir Immune Defic Syndr* 1999;21:301–306.

212. Lalezari J, Schacker T, Feinberg J, et al. A randomized, double-blind, placebo-controlled trial of cidofovir gel for the treatment of acyclovir-unresponsive mucocutaneous herpes simplex virus infection in patients with AIDS. *J Infect Dis* 1997;176:892–898.

213. Kessler HA, Hurwitz S, Farthing C, et al. Pilot study of topical trifluridine for the treatment of acyclovir-resistant mucocutaneous herpes simplex disease in patients with AIDS (ACTG 172). *J Acquir Immune Defic Syndr* 1996;12:147–152.

214. Birch CJ, Tyssen DP, Tachedjian G, et al. Clinical effects and in vitro studies of trifluorothymidine combined with interferon-α for treatment of drug-resistant and -sensitive herpes simplex virus infections. *J Infect Dis* 1992;166:108–112.

215. ACOG Practice Bulletin No. 8. Management of herpes in pregnancy. 1999. *Int J Gynaecol Obstet* 2000;68:165–173.

216. Stray-Pedersen B. Acyclovir in late pregnancy to prevent neonatal herpes simplex. *Lancet* 1990;336:756.

217. Scott LL, Sanchez PJ, Jackson GL, Zeray F, Wendel GD. Acyclovir suppression to prevent cesarean delivery after first episode genital herpes. *Obstet Gynecol* 1996;87:69–73.

218. Brockelhurst P, Kinghorn G, Carney O, et al. A randomized placebo controlled trial of suppressive acyclovir in late pregnancy in women with recurrent genital herpes infection. *Br J Obstet Gynaecol* 1998;105:275–280.

219. Scott LL, Hollier LM, McIntire D, Sanchez PJ, Jackson GL, Wendel GD Jr. Acyclovir suppression to prevent clinical recurrences at delivery after first

episode genital herpes in pregnancy: an open-label trial. *Infect Dis Obstet Gynecol* 2001;9:75–80.

220. Braig S, Luton D, Sibony O, Edlinger C, Boissinot C, Blot P, Oury JF. Acyclovir prophylaxis in late pregnancy prevents recurrent genital herpes and viral shedding. *Eur J Obstet Gynecol Reprod Biol* 2001;96:55–58.

221. American Academy of Pediatrics. Herpes simplex. In Pickering LK, ed: *2000 Red book of the committee on infectious diseases*, 25th ed. Elk Grove Village, IL: American Academy of Pediatrics, 2000:313.

222. Kimberlin DW, Lin CY, Jacobs RF, et al, for the National Institute of Allergy and Infectious Diseases Collaborative Antiviral Study Group. Safety and efficacy of high-dose intravenous acyclovir in the management of neonatal herpes simplex virus infections. *Pediatrics* 2001;108:230–238.

223. Langenberg A, Benedetti J, Jenkins J, Ashley R, Winter C, Corey L. Development of clinically recognizable genital lesions among women previously identified as having "asymptomatic" herpes simplex virus type 2 infection. *Ann Intern Med* 1989;110:882–887.

224. Stanberry LR. Asymptomatic herpes simplex virus shedding and Russian roulette. *Clin Infect Dis* 2000;30:268–269.

225. Wald A, Langenberg AG, Link K, et al. Effect of condoms on reducing the transmission of herpes simplex virus type 2 from men to women. *JAMA* 2001;285:3100–3106.

226. Stone KM, Brooks CA, Guinan ME, Alexander ER. National surveillance for neonatal herpes simplex virus infections. *Sex Transm Dis* 1989;16:152–156.

227. Brown ZA. HSV-2 specific serology should be offered routinely to antenatal patients. *Rev Med Virol* 2000;10:141–144.

228. Qutub M, Klapper P, Vallely P, Cleator G. Genital herpes in pregnancy: is screening cost-effective? *Int J STD AIDS* 2001;12:14–16.

229. Stanberry LR, Cunningham AL, Mindel A, et al. Prospects for control of herpes simplex virus disease through immunization. *Clin Infect Dis* 2000;30:549–566.

230. Whitley RJ. Herpes simplex vaccines. In Levine MM, Woodrow GC, Kaper JB, Cobon GS, eds: *New generation vaccines*, 2nd ed. New York: Marcel Dekker, 1997:727–748.

231. Bernstein DI, Stanberry LR. Herpes simplex virus vaccines. *Vaccine* 1999;17: 1681–1689.

232. Krause PR, Straus SE. Herpesvirus vaccines. Development, controversies, and applications. *Infect Dis Clin North Am* 1999;13:61–81.

233. Stanberry LR. Genital and perinatal herpes simplex virus infections: prophylactic vaccines. In Stanberry LR, Bernstein DI, eds: *Sexually transmitted diseases: vaccines, prevention, and control*. London: Academic Press, 2000:187–216.

234. Mertz GJ, Ashley R, Burke RL, et al. Double-blind, placebo-controlled trial of a herpes simplex virus type 2 glycoprotein vaccine in persons at high risk for genital herpes infection. *J Infect Dis* 1990;161:653–660.

235. Miller RL, Tomai MA, Harrison CJ, Bernstein DI. Immunomodulation as a treatment strategy for genital herpes: review of the evidence. *Int Immunopharmacol* 2002;2:443–451.

236. Spruance SL, Tyring SK, Smith MH, Meng TC. Application of a topical immune response modifier, resiquimod gel, to modify the recurrence rate of recurrent genital herpes: a pilot study. *J Infect Dis* 2001;184:196–200.

237. Rosenthal SL, Cohen SS, Stanberry LR. Topical microbicides. Current status and research considerations for adolescent girls. *Sex Transm Dis* 1998;25:368–377.

238. Zeitlin L, Whaley KJ. Microbicides for preventing transmission of genital herpes. *Herpes* 2002;9:4–9.

239. Phillips DM, Maguire RA. The development of microbicides for clinical use to prevent sexually transmitted diseases. *Curr Infect Dis Rep* 2002;4:135–140.

240. Zacharopoulos VR, Phillips DM. Vaginal formulations of carrageenan protect mice from herpes simplex virus infection. *Clin Diagn Lab Immunol* 1997;4:465–468.

241. Zeitlin L, Whaley KJ, Hegarty TA, Moench TR, Cone RA. Tests of vaginal microbicides in the mouse genital herpes model. *Contraception* 1997;56:329–335.

242. Bourne N, Bernstein DI, Ireland J, Sonderfan AJ, Profy AT, Stanberry LR. The topical microbicide PRO 2000 protects against genital herpes infection in a mouse model. *J Infect Dis* 1999;180:203–205.

243. Bourne N, Stanberry LR, Kern ER, Holan G, Matthews B, Bernstein DI. Dendrimers, a new class of candidate topical microbicides with activity against herpes simplex virus infection. *Antimicrob Agents Chemother* 2000;44:2471–2474.

244. Maguire RA, Bergman N, Phillips DM. Comparison of microbicides for efficacy in protecting mice against vaginal challenge with herpes simplex virus type 2, cytotoxicity, antibacterial properties, and sperm immobilization. *Sex Transm Dis* 2001;28:259–265.

245. Elias CJ, Coggins C, Alvarez F, et al. Colposcopic evaluation of a vaginal gel formulation of iota-carrageenan. *Contraception* 1997;56:387–389.

246. Van Damme L, Wright A, Depraetere K, et al. A phase I study of a novel potential intravaginal microbicide, PRO 2000, in healthy sexually inactive women. *Sex Transm Infect* 2000;76:126–130.

CHAPTER 107
Chancroid, Lymphogranuloma Venereum, and Granuloma Inguinale

Allan Ronald and Michelle J. Alfa

Genital ulceration is a common presentation to health care providers who treat patients with sexually transmitted infections. In the United States, England, and Sweden, approximately 3% of patients present with ulcers. In clinics for sexually transmitted diseases in East Africa, Southeast Asia, and India, the prevalence of genital ulceration ranges from 10% to 50%. Genital herpes and primary syphilis are the first and second most common cause of genital ulcers in Western societies; chancroid accounts for a large proportion of ulcers in the developing world. Regardless of the etiology, genital ulcers are often associated with regional lymphadenopathy. Etiologic identification requires laboratory investigation owing to the nonspecificity of clinical features.

Granuloma inguinale (GI) is rare in Western countries but is endemic in Papua New Guinea, Southern Africa and in parts of India. Lymphogranuloma venereum (LGV) occurs only occasionally in the industrialized countries but is common in some developing countries including the Caribbean.

Genital ulcers have assumed increasing importance owing to their epidemiologic association with the human immunodeficiency virus type 1 (HIV-1) (1). The association between "crack" cocaine use and chancroid raises concern about outbreaks among drug users (2). The role of the genital ulcerating agents other than *Haemophilus ducreyi* as cofactors for retrovirus dissemination requires further study.

CHANCROID AND *HAEMOPHILUS DUCREYI* INFECTION

History

In 1889 at the University of Naples, Ducrey "identified" the cause of soft chancre (3,4). He inoculated three patients with pus from their own genital ulcers and at weekly intervals reinoculated a new site with material from the most recent ulcer. In each, he found a single microorganism in the ulcer exudate that he described as "short, compact streptobacillary rods with rounded ends" that were observed both within and outside of neutrophils.

Earlier investigators, including Ricord in France, differentiated the primary hard chancre of syphilis from the soft chancre, or ulcus mole, of chancroid (4). Bassereau further differentiated venereal ulcers by demonstrating that only patients with soft chancre could be reinfected at another skin site by autoinoculation of ulcer exudate (4). During the first two decades after Ducrey's discovery, several investigators studied the organism and the disease. *H. ducreyi* was cultured and its growth requirements characterized (4).

For the following six decades, there was a dearth of interest in chancroid and only rarely was *H. ducreyi* cultured from patients with genital ulcers. In 1938, Hanschell (5) described the efficacy of sulfonamides for the treatment of chancroid. The incidence declined dramatically until in 1977 only 455 cases were reported in the United States (6).

During the past 25 years, outbreaks of chancroid in Canada and the United States provided opportunities to study *H. ducreyi* and to control outbreaks (6,7). In addition, the association between genital ulcer disease and HIV transmission has identified the need to improve diagnostic procedures because of the inaccuracy of clinical diagnosis of genital ulcer disease (8). Research interest has grown and at least a dozen groups are actively investigating *H. ducreyi* and chancroid. These studies were critically reviewed by Trees and Morse (9).

Biology of *H. ducreyi*

H. ducreyi is a small, gram-negative, bipolar-staining organism. In tissue sections, the characteristic spatial features were initially described as a "school of fish" arrangement or as streptobacillary, with long parallel chains or "railway tracks." *H. ducreyi* stains poorly with both safranin and crystal violet and can readily be overlooked in the Gram stain. The non-mucoid colonies of *H. ducreyi* are yellow-grey, 0.5 to 1.0 mm in diameter (Fig. 107.1) and can be pushed intact across the surface of solid media when nudged by an inoculating loop. The organism requires hemin, serum, glutamine and cysteine for growth. Growth is enhanced in a water-saturated, 5% CO_2 environment. It grows well both aerobically and anaerobically with an optimal growth temperature of 33°C. This temperature sensitivity is thought to explain the inability of *H. ducreyi* to spread systemically in human infection (10). *H. ducreyi* is now classified in the Actinobacillus cluster of Pasteurellaceae (11). The genome is a single 1.7 MB chromosome with little diversity between isolates. *H. ducreyi* reduces nitrate and produces an alkaline phosphatase. It is cytochrome oxidase-positive when tested using tetraethyl-p-phenylenediamine. Probable virulence factors include the hemoglobin receptor, hemolysin and a cyto-lethal distending toxin (9,12). Experimental human volunteer studies have been used to study pathogenesis and identify bacterial host interactions (13,14). Following intradermal injection, *H. ducreyi* evades phagocytosis and intraepidermal pustules rapidly occur with an increase in tissue levels of the cytokines IL-6 and IL-8. *H ducreyi* infection causes both a delayed type sensitivity response and antibodies to several surface antigens (9). Despite this, volunteers and patients with chancroid are susceptible to new infections with no evidence of a protective immune response (15).

Epidemiology

H. ducreyi is confined to humans. Almost all individuals infected with *H. ducreyi* have genital ulceration (16). Women who are either source contacts or secondary contacts of men with chancroid are commonly found to have genital ulcers (16). Epidemics of chancroid have been readily controlled on numerous occasions in Western countries through intensive follow-up of female contacts, particularly prostitutes, and treatment of persons who have ulcers (7). Due to the role of prostitutes in most outbreaks, small numbers of women infect many men and the male/female ratio in most studies is about 8:1. Men with foreskins have about three times the risk of circumcised men of acquiring *H. ducreyi* infection after similar exposure (17).

Steen has argued that *H. ducreyi* can be eliminated from regions of the world in which it is endemic (18). Survival in populations requires that many men are having unprotected sex with a few infected women, most men are uncircumcised, and STD control programs are inadequate (17). The presence of chancroid in any population identifies the need for targeted interventions and enhanced STD control activities (18).

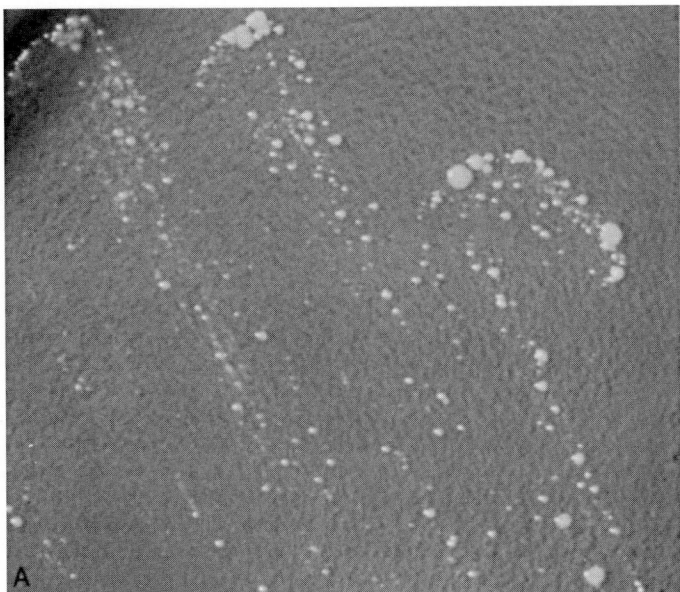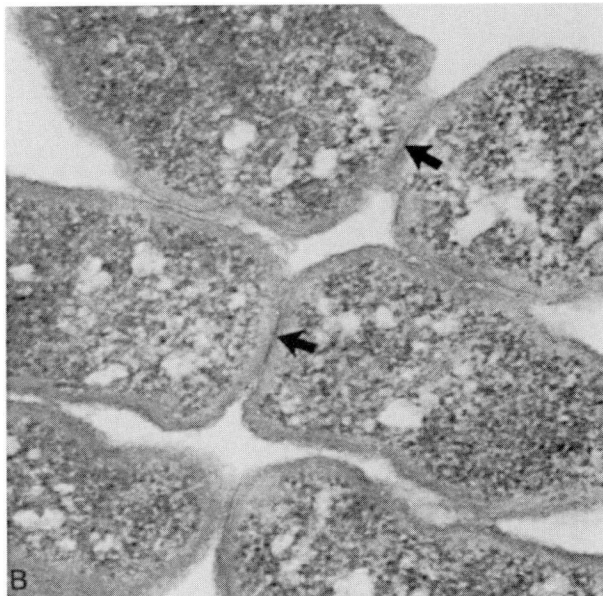

Figure 107.1. Characteristics of *H. ducreyi*. **(A)** The colonies are tan-gray and approximately 0.5 to 1 mm in diameter. The colonies can be nudged intact across the agar surface. **(B)** The intracellular adhesion shown may account for the tenacious characteristics of the colony.

H. ducreyi and Human Immunodeficiency Virus

Over 30 epidemiologic studies in resource limited societies have consistently shown that men infected with HIV-1 are three times more likely than seronegative men to have a history of genital ulcers (1,17–19). In a prospective study, HIV seronegative men who presented with chancroid had a fivefold greater risk of seroconversion during a mean follow-up period of 14 weeks compared to men who presented with urethritis (17). The risk of HIV seroconversion among men who acquired chancroid was further increased threefold in men if they were uncircumcised (17). As a result, uncircumcised men who presented with chancroid had a 48% risk of acquiring HIV presumably from the sexual liaison that transmitted *H. ducreyi* (17).

Both cross-sectional and prospective studies have demonstrated that female sex workers with genital ulcers are at greater risk of acquiring HIV-1 than similarly exposed women with no episodes of genital ulcer disease (20). Overall, among prostitutes in Nairobi, genital ulcers increase the risk of acquiring HIV-1 more than fivefold (21).

From these studies it is apparent that genital ulcers are portals of HIV-1 entry and exit. The immune response to *H. ducreyi* recruits and activates macrophages and T helper lymphocytes, which increases the susceptibility of women to HIV-1 infection (22). Viral excretion into the genital tract is increased in women with latent HIV-1 infection who develop *H. ducreyi* ulcers (23).

HIV-1 and *H. ducreyi* each interact to increase heterosexual transmission of the other pathogen and fuel the amplification cycle for each pathogen (Fig. 107.2). Control of chancroid is a critical strategy for slowing the epidemic of heterosexual HIV infection (18,24).

Histologic Features

Freinkel has described three zones in the fully developed chancroid ulcer: a narrow superficial zone of necrotic tissue, red blood cells, fibrin, and degenerate neutrophils; a broad middle zone of edematous inflammatory tissue with small dilated vessels in-

filtrated with neutrophils; and a deep zone characterized by a dense infiltrate of plasma cells, lymphocytes, and macrophages (Fig. 107.3) (25). *H. ducreyi* organisms are seen in the superficial zone. In experimental human studies, the keratinocytes and T cells expressed human leukocyte antigen DR consistent with a delayed-type hypersensitivity response (14). The histopathology of chancroid biopsy specimens demonstrates psoriasiform hyperplasia and spongiosis in the epidermis and a perivascular and interstitial mononuclear cell infiltrate are seen in the dermis (22,26). Immunoperoxidase identifies the predominant mononuclear cell types to be histiocytes and CD4-positive T lymphocytes (26). The histiocytes are mainly of Langerhans cell lineage (UCHL1-positive, S100-positive, lysozyme-negative) (22,26).

Laboratory Diagnosis

Culture of *H. ducreyi* on agar medium has supplanted older methods of culture in blood. Gonococcal fetal calf serum agar, Mueller-Hinton horse blood agar, and rabbit heart infusion blood

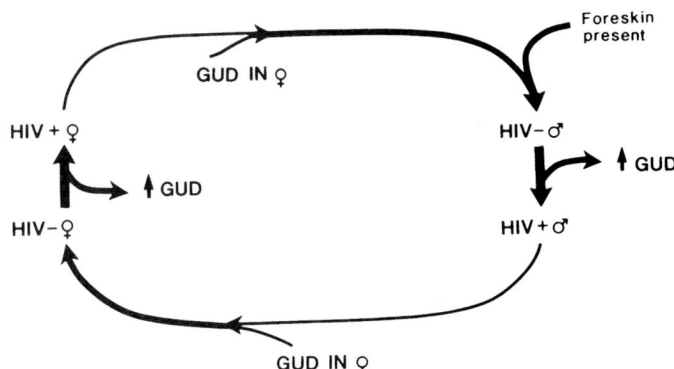

Figure 107.2. Cycle of amplification. Genital ulcer disease (GUD) augments the transmission of HIV-1 by increasing the infectiousness of women for their sexual partners and making them more susceptible to the virus.

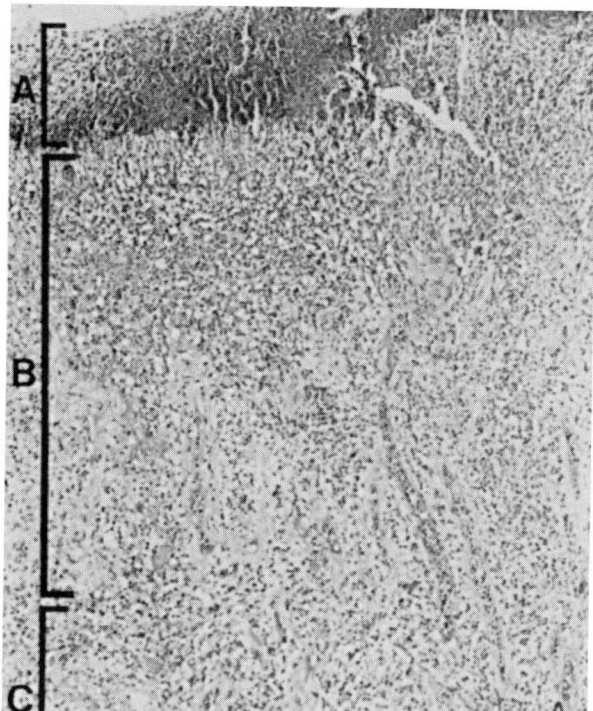
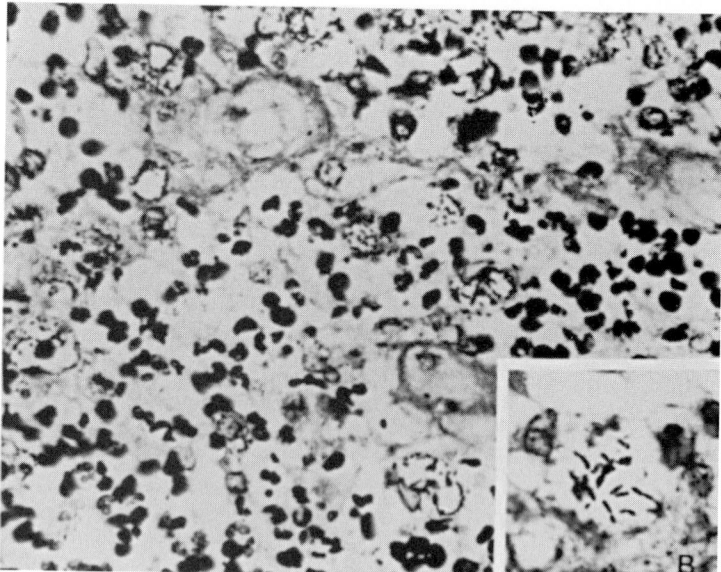

Figure 107.3. Histology of genital ulcers. **(A)** The ulcer of chancroid has three distinct zones: narrow superficial zone (*A*); broad, middle zone with vascular chancre (*B*); and deep zone (*C*). *H. ducreyi* organisms are usually seen in the superficial zone (H&E, 130×). **(B)** Granuloma inguinale shows Donovan bodies (*inset*), intracellular bipolar-staining, rod-shaped organisms (Warthin-Starry stain, 796×). (From Freinkel AL. Histological aspects of sexually transmitted genital lesions. *Histopathology* 1987;11:819–831, with permission.)

agar, each with added vancomycin (3 mg/L) to inhibit overgrowth of gram-positive bacteria, are optimal culture media with isolation rates 50% to 80% (9). Charcoal can replace fetal calf serum (27). Cotton or Dacron swabs are suitable to obtain pus for culture from the purulent ulcer base without extensive cleaning. Swabs should be plated directly or within an hour of obtaining the specimen or transported in a thioglycollate-hemin-based media. This can facilitate survival of *H. ducreyi* at 4°C for up to 4 days (28).

Cultures should be incubated at 33°C in an environment with 5% carbon dioxide and maximal humidity. A candle extinction jar with a moist paper towel is adequate if a more controlled environment is not available. Growth is usually apparent by 48 hours.

The positive predictive value of a culture that grows *H. ducreyi* is 100% (i.e., a positive culture result defines an abnormal state). The sensitivity of culture for chancroid is about 80% in males who have "clinical chancroid." All genital ulcers require dark-field microscopy and serology for syphilis, to exclude concomitant infection with *Treponema pallidum*.

Clinical Presentation

H. ducreyi gains access through a break in the epithelium of the genital mucosa or skin. In volunteer studies, the inoculum necessary for infection is one or two colony-forming units (14). After an incubation period of 3 to 10 days, an inflammatory papule appears and rapidly ulcerates. Classically, chancroid ulcers bleed readily from an irregular granulomatous base of variable depth which is often covered with a grayish, necrotic purulent exudate (Fig. 107.4). The ulcers are usually very painful, although the skin surrounding the ulcer is not inflamed. About one-half of chan-

croid ulcers are "classical" but these features can be mimicked by other pathogens.

Gaisin and Heaton (29) described several presentations, including giant ulcers formed when several smaller ones merge; a follicular type limited to hairy regions that resembles a pyogenic infection; dwarf chancroid with tiny shallow, round ulcers that resemble herpes; transient chancroid that is associated with acute regional lymphadenitis and resembles LGV; and painless single ulcers that resemble primary syphilis. About 10% of patients present with lesions that would be classified clinically as primary syphilis.

The sensitivity and specificity of the clinical diagnosis are dependent on the relative proportion of genital ulcers that are due to *H. ducreyi*. In a study from Atlanta, over 80% of typical chancroid lesions were due to herpes simplex virus (30). In Kenya, the majority of ulcers that clinically resembled herpes, were due to chancroid (8).

Certain sites on the genitalia are favored by *H. ducreyi*. In uncircumcised men, half the lesions occur on the prepuce and are about equally divided between the external and internal surface. About 10% of presentations occur as a "septic sore," usually in the prepuce but occasionally on the shaft of the penis. Several milliliters of pus can be trapped in the skin without an obvious ulcer. Lesions occur on the glans, in the urethra, on the penile shaft, and on the scrotum and skin of the perineum. "Kissing" lesions are common on adjacent cutaneous surfaces. Circumferential ulcers on the coronal sulcus are common. In women, lesions occur, in order of decreasing frequency, on the fourchette, labia, perianal area, and medial aspect of the thighs. Cervical ulcers are uncommon, and vaginal wall ulcers are rare.

Painful inguinal adenitis occurs in about 40% and is unilateral in about half of these patients. Adenitis progresses to

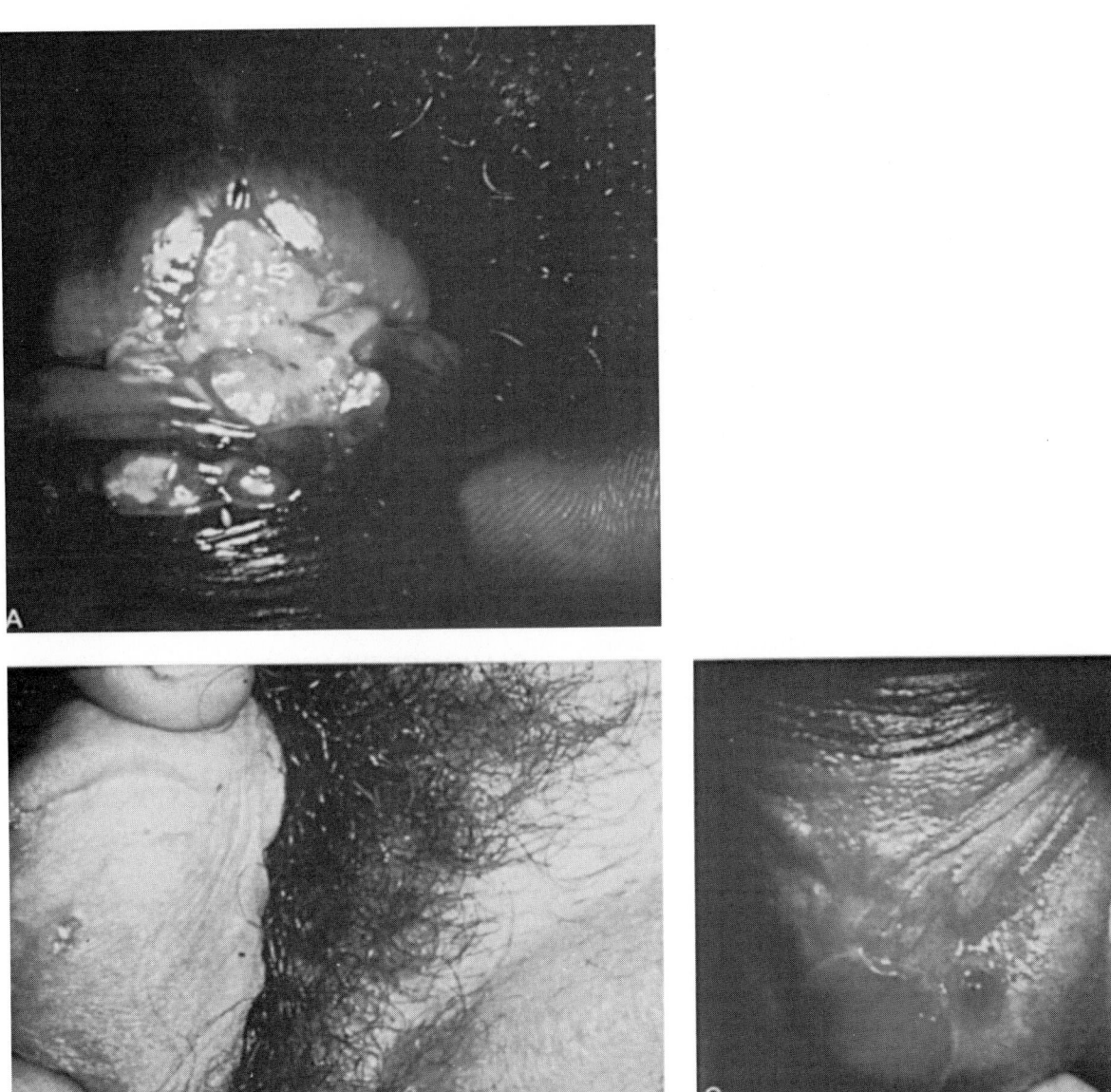

Figure 107.4. Genital ulcers. **(A)** The eroded purulent ulcer of chancroid is painful and may be associated with painful inguinal adenitis. **(B)** Lymphogranuloma venereum has a small, transient genital ulcer with swollen, extremely painful inguinal lymph nodes. **(C)** The genital lesions of GI are painless, beefy red, raised lesions. (Part C from Al-Harmozi SA, el-Tonsy MH. Granulmoa inguinale. Report of the first case in Qatar. *Sex Transm Dis* 1986;13:102, with permission.)

suppuration in untreated patients and a painful inguinal abscess or bubo develops. The overlying skin is stretched and erythematous and aspiration or incision is necessary to prevent rupture. Purulent urethritis and mucopurulent cervicitis are occasional presentations of *H. ducreyi*. Patients with concomitant HIV-1 infection appear to have more extensive ulcers.

Dual infections of *H. ducreyi* with either *T. pallidum* or herpes simplex virus occur in 5 to 20% of patients (31). In these cases, clinical features can be confusing and can only be sorted out with careful diagnostic investigation.

Antimicrobial Susceptibility and Treatment Regimens

Antimicrobial susceptibility tests should be performed with the agar dilution technique. Susceptibility varies markedly from one geographic area to another, and periodic surveys are necessary to make specific recommendations on optimal therapeutic regimens. Antimicrobial resistance has been reported to sulfonamides, tetracyclines, ampicillin and other penicillins, trimethoprim, chloramphenicol, streptomycin, and kanamycin (32).

Plasmid-mediated resistance is responsible for most antibacterial resistance. Brunton and coworkers described a 5.7 MDa β-lactamase-encoding plasmid which carried the entire sequence of the 3.2 MDa gonococcal plasmid (33). Subsequently three additional β-lactamase-encoding plasmids have been described in *H. ducreyi* (32).

Optimal chancroid treatment regimens should cure all patients with genital ulcers and inguinal buboes, rapidly eradicate *H. ducreyi* from the lesions and prevent clinical recurrence. Erythromycin, 500 mg four times a day for 7 days is predictably effective. Regimens have been prescribed successfully as a single dose (34,35). Chancroid is cured if the antibacterial activity in the serum exceeds the minimal inhibitory concentration of *H. ducreyi* for at least 48 hours (34,35). A single intramuscular dose of 250 mg of ceftriaxone can predictably cure chancroid but HIV-infected individuals have a higher failure rate (36,37). Trimethoprim, alone or together with sulfonamides, is no longer effective in most areas of the world (38). Amoxicillin combined with clavulanic acid prescribed thrice daily for 7 days is an effective regimen (39). Of the fluoroquinolones, ciprofloxacin has the greatest *in vitro* efficacy and a single dose of 500 mg in one study cured over 95% of patients (35). Thiamphenicol, kanamycin, spectinomycin, and trimethoprim combined with rifampin have all been effective treatment regimens but many studies have had small numbers of patients.

Fluctuant buboes should be aspirated or incised. Local ulcer treatment may relieve symptoms and facilitate removal of necrotic debris.

Prevention and Control

Chancroid control and eradication are an urgent priority with the increasing evidence linking it to the explosive heterosexual spread of HIV-1 (18). Studies in industrialized societies have shown that the disease can be eradicated with conventional sexually transmitted disease control strategies (7). This includes identification and treatment of contacts, examination and treatment of sex workers, and effective treatment programs. In developing countries, education linking genital ulcer disease to acquired immunodeficiency syndrome and HIV together with effective programs to provide condoms to persons who continue to take risks, may be effective to markedly reduce epidemics of chancroid (18). Targeted programs that focus on prostitutes and their clients may be particularly effective. Demonstration programs are urgently needed.

LYMPHOGRANULOMA VENEREUM

History

LGV was initially described by Wallace in 1833 and definitively characterized by Durand et al. in 1913 (40). Rake et al. grew *C. trachomatis* from patients with LGV in 1940. LGV has been known as lymphopathia venerea, tropical bubo, and lymphogranuloma inguinale (40).

Biology of Lymphogranuloma Venereum Serovars of *Chlamydia trachomatis*

C. trachomatis serovars L1, L2, and L3 are the agents of LGV. Details of *C. trachomatis* biology are presented in Chapter 222. The serovars L1, L2, and L3 differ from other chlamydial serovars in that they are more invasive in the mouse model and have a tropism for lymphatic tissue (41). Although *Chlamydia trachomatis* has been the subject of intense investigation for the past three decades, characterization of the LGV strains and the pathogenesis of this unique presentation have not kept pace, presumably owing to the infrequency of LGV infections in the industrialized world.

Epidemiology

LGV is a rare disease in Europe and North America: fewer than 600 cases are reported annually in the United States. Clinically evident infection is about ten times more common in men than in women. LGV chlamydiae are transmitted by sexual contact,

but the incidence after exposure is not known. Men are probably infectious until the primary ulcerative lesion heals, whereas women may have asymptomatic cervical infection that persists for months and serves as a reservoir for this pathogen. The incubation period varies from 5 to 21 days (42).

Laboratory Diagnosis

HISTOLOGIC FEATURES

Necrosis with invasion of neutrophils is seen in the regional lymph nodes. Vaculated macrophages with intravascular organisms, that include both elementary and reticular bodies, are also visualized in tissue specimens.

DIRECT EXAMINATION

The earliest diagnostic test for LGV was a Giemsa Stain to identify intracellular inclusions of *Chlamydia* (43). This test is specific but insensitive and it is usually positive in 50% of patients or less. Newer techniques that use antigen capture with methods incorporating immunofluorescence or enzyme-linked immunoassays have been used to detect *C. trachomatis*, but these tests are not specific for LGV serovars.

ISOLATION OF THE AGENT

Culture of *C. trachomatis* from an appropriate specimen and identification of the unique serovar is the definitive diagnostic test. Specimens for isolation of *C. trachomatis* should be collected as described in Chapter 222. To reduce cytotoxicity, bubo exudates should be diluted 1:10 before inoculating the cell culture (43). Typically, LGV strains can be inoculated directly onto eukaryotic cell lines (HeLa 229 or McCoy). The LGV serovars have a shorter growth cycle and the cell culture should be fixed and stained within 48 hours. Culture technology is substantially less sensitive in patients with more chronic disease.

SEROLOGIC TESTS

Since the description of the complement fixation test, serology has been the mainstay for the diagnosis of LGV (43). The antigen is an acid polysaccharide common to all *Chlamydia* organisms, and cross-reactions occur with antibodies to non-trachomatis *Chlamydia* species. Although 20% to 30% of a general population of a sexually transmitted disease clinic have low titers of complement fixation antibody, patients with LGV usually have a titer of 1:64 or greater. The sensitivity of this test for the diagnosis of LGV is 80% (43). A fourfold rise or fall in titer further supports this diagnosis. In the context of the appropriate syndrome, a positive results of the complement fixation test is strongly predictive of LGV, whereas a low titer of 1:16 or less tends to exclude the diagnosis.

Microimmunofluorescence tests for the detection of *C. trachomatis* serovars L1, L2, and L3 now make possible serologic diagnosis of a specific serovar. The test utilizes as antigen, yolk sac-grown serovar-specific elementary bodies (44). The antibody titer is usually in excess of 1:512.

The Frei test is an intradermal test of delayed hypersensitivity to bubo pus or egg yolk derived *C. trachomatis* antigens. It is neither sensitive nor specific for LGV and is no longer recommended.

Clinical Features

LGV is a chronic disease with three stages, not unlike syphilis. The primary lesion is an inconspicuous, usually painless transient ulcer, that heals without scarring and is recalled by no more than 20% of patients (see Fig. 107.4). Cervicitis is the common primary lesion in women. LGV chlamydiae are carried by the macrophages to the regional nodes which become exquisitely tender masses accompanied by fever, chills, malaise, headache, and weight loss. Meningoencephalitis, pneumonia, polyarthritis, and erythema nodosum can occur. Lymphadenopathy is bilateral in about 30% of patients and may be so extensive that the inguinal mass of nodes is cleaved by the inguinal ligament, the pathognomonic "groove sign." Over a course of 2 to 8 weeks, in the absence of treatment, the overlying skin becomes brawny and wrinkled with a characteristic violaceous hue, and the abscesses within the nodes coalesce and drain from one or more sinus tracts. In women, the sacral lymphatics as well as the iliac lymphatics are often involved with ongoing obstruction of lymph drainage from the rectum and uterus. Fibrosis of lymph nodes leads to lymphedema of the vulva and perineum with chronic pelvic pain.

An anorectal syndrome may be the presenting feature in women and homosexual men. A hemorrhagic proctitis can progress to perirectal abscesses, rectal strictures, and fistulae. Rectal stricture associated with LGV is etiologically linked to rectal cancer (45).

Antimicrobial Susceptibility and Treatment Regimens

The antimicrobial susceptibility of LGV strains is similar to that of other serovars of *C. trachomatis*. The organisms are susceptible to tetracyclines, erythromycin, and rifampicin (46). The prognosis of LGV is extremely variable and unpredictable. Many LGV patients have other sexually transmitted diseases, and the contribution of LGV to the overall disease process may be indeterminate. About 5% of patients who develop the inguinal lymph node syndrome develop either fistular lesions or a rectal stricture. Few controlled trials of antimicrobial therapy have been published. Although treatment has not been proved to influence the healing of the primary ulcer or the secondary lymphadenitis, most experts recommend a 3-week course of treatment with either tetracycline or erythromycin, 500 mg four times daily.

Control and Prevention

Sexual partners without apparent disease should be treated with a 2-week course of either tetracycline or erythromycin.

GRANULOMA INGUINALE

History

Granuloma tropicalis was first described in southern India in 1882 by McLeod (47). In 1905, Donovan described the intracellular "protozoan-like" inclusions (47). The bacterial nature of the Donovan body was established in 1943, when organisms were cultured in the yolk sac of embryonated eggs (47).

Biology of *Calymmatobacterium granulomatis*

Calymmatobacterium granulomatis is a gram-negative rod with a prominent capsule. In tissue smears, the bacteria are found in large histiocytic cells. They appear to reproduce in multiple foci in the cytoplasm until each vacuole contains hundreds of organisms, which are liberated on cell rupture. *C. granulomatis* has antigenic features that resemble those of the genus *Klebsiella* (48). It has only been grown recently on artificial media (48). A colormetric PCR technique for rapid diagnosis is now available (49,50).

The organism is currently classified as an "unassigned" genus associated with the family *Enterobacteriaceae*.

Epidemiology

GI is endemic in southern India, in Kwa Zulu-Natal, South Africa, Papua New Guinea, among the aboriginal community in Australia, and in the Caribbean (51,52). In the United States, fewer than 100 cases are reported annually. The disease is only moderately contagious, and repeated exposure may be necessary for transmission. Although transmission is presumed to be sexual, other modes of infection are possible. For example, GI is seen in children in regions of the world in which the disease is epidemic (52). The male/female ratio varies from 2:1 to 10:1 and studies of sexual partners report infection in about 20% of individuals (53). The incubation period is unknown but seems to vary from days to months. Rectal lesions have been described in men who have sex with men.

Laboratory Diagnosis

The ulcerative lesion is scraped and the granulation tissue is spread on the slide, air dried, and stained with a Wright or Giemsa stain (43). The classic findings are intracellular bacterial organisms, which appear as bipolar, black clusters of bacteria in the cytoplasm of large histiocytes. Performed correctly, this test is sensitive and specific for the diagnosis of GI (43). Donovan bodies can also be seen in tissue sections. Cultural and molecular techniques are under-development (49,50). No serologic test is available for the diagnosis of GI.

Clinical Features

The primary lesion is an indurated papule, generally at the portal of entry. These ulcerate but remain "clean, with a red cobblestone base", without purulence, the so-called exuberant beefy appearance (see Fig. 107.4). The lesions enlarge slowly over months, and even years, and may reach a diameter of 5 to 20 cm. The lesions are surprisingly painless. Secondary infection may result in necrosis and increased purulence. Local extension, healing, and fibrosis all occur simultaneously. Although systemic manifestations are uncommon, metastatic hematogenous spread to bones, joints, and the liver has been described. Regional lymphadenitis is rare, but the ulcerating lesion often extends onto the inguinal skin and produces pseudobuboes (52,53).

Lesions occur commonly on the prepuce of males and on the labia and cervix of females. The cervical lesions mimic cervical dysplasia and can be more aggressive during pregnancy. About 5% of patients have cutaneous sites remote from the genitalia. Anal lesions are often verrucous. Scarring may lead to phimosis. A suspected epidemiologic association with genital neoplasms has not been confirmed. Spontaneous healing is rare, and recurrences are frequent after a course of therapy. Concurrent HIV infection seems to result in delayed healing (51). GI is frequently misdiagnosed as carcinoma, and tissue biopsy should be carried out early.

Antimicrobial Susceptibility and Therapeutic Regimens

No susceptibility tests have been carried out *in vitro* so treatment regimens are empirical. Trimethoprim-sulfamethoxazole, one double-strength tablet (160 mg/800 mg) twice daily is effective (52). Ciprofloxacin, 500 mg twice daily, tetracycline and erythromycin, 500 mg four times daily, and azithromycin,

250 mg once daily are all effective (52,53). Ampicillin is ineffective. Pregnant patients should be treated with trimethoprim/sulfamethoxazole or erythromycin. After initiation of antibacterial treatment, a clinical response is usually evident within 7 to 10 days. Therapy should be continued for at least 3 weeks. Relapse occurs in 10% to 20% of patients and requires more prolonged treatment. Treatment regimens should be altered after 2 weeks if significant improvement is noted.

Prevention and Control

No information is available on primary prevention. Early diagnosis and treatment are effective in preventing the serious sequelae that can occur if treatment is delayed. Presumably, effective treatment of patients with lesions would reduce prevalence (53). GI probably increases the opportunity for HIV to be transmitted between partners analogous to chancroid.

REFERENCES

1. Simonsen JN, Cameron DW, Gakinya MN, et al. Human immunodeficiency virus infection in men with sexually transmitted diseases. *N Engl J Med* 1988;319:274.
2. Martin DH, DiCarlo RP. Recent changes in the epidemiology of genital ulcer disease in the United States. The crack cocaine connection. *Sex Trans Dis* 1994;21[Suppl]:S76.
3. Ducrey A. Experimental Untersuchungen uber den Ansteckungsstoff des weichen Schankers und uber die Bubonen. *Monatsh Prakt Dermatol* 1989;9: 387.
4. Kampmeier RH. The recognition of *Haemophilus ducreyi* as the cause of soft chancre. *Sex Transm Dis* 1982;9:212.
5. Hanschell HM. Sulfonamide in the treatment of chancroid. *Lancet* 1938;1:886.
6. Schmid GP, Sanders LL Jr, Blount JH, Alexander ER. Chancroid in the United States. Reestablishment of an old disease. *JAMA* 1987;258:3265.
7. Hammond GW, Slutchuk M, Scatliff J, Sherman E, Wilt JC, Ronald AR. Epidemiologic, clinical, laboratory and therapeutic fetures of an urban outbreak of chancroid in North America. *Rev Infect Dis* 1980;2:867–879.
8. Ndinya-Achola JO, Kihara AN, Fisher LD, et al. Presumptive specific clinical diagnosis of genital ulcer disease (GUD) in a primary health care setting in Nairobi. *Int J STD AIDS* 1996;7:201.
9. Trees DL, Morse SA. Chancroid and *Haemophilus ducreyi*: an update. *Clin Microbiol Rev* 1995;8:357.
10. Makakole SC, Sturm AW. The effect of temperature on the interaction of *Haemophilus ducreyi* with human epithelial cells. *J Med Microbiol* 2001;50:449–455.
11. Dewhirst FE, et al. Phylogeny of 54 representative strains of species in the family pasteurellaceae as determined by comparison of 16S rRNA sequences. *J Bacteriol* 1992;174:2002–2013.
12. Alfa MJ, et al. *Haemophilus ducreyi* hemolysin acts as a contact cytotoxin and damages human foreskin fibroblasts in cell culture. *Infect Immun* 1996;64:2349–2352.
13. Gelfanova V, Humphreys TL, Spinola SM. Characterization of *Haemophilus ducreyi*-specific T-cell lines from lesions of experimentally infected human subjects. *Infect Immun* 2001;69:4224–4231.
14. Al-Tawfiq JA, Harezlak J, Katz BP, Spinola SM. Cumulative experience with *Haemophilus ducreyi* 35000 in the human model of experimental infection. *Sex Transm Dis* 2000;27:111–114.
15. Al-Tawfiq JA, Palmer KL, Chen CY, et al. Experimental infection of human volunteers with *Haemophilus ducreyi* does not confer protection against subsequent challenge. *J Infect Dis* 1999;179:1283–1287.
16. Plummer FA, D'Costa LJ, Nsanze H, et al. Epidemiology of chancroid and *Haemophilus ducreyi* in Nairobi, Kenya. *Lancet* 1983;2:1293.
17. Cameron DW, Simonsen JN, D'Costa LJ, et al. Female to male transmission of human immunodeficiency virus type 1: Risk factors for seroconversion in men. *Lancet* 1989;2:403.
18. Steen R. Eradicating chancroid. *Bull WHO* 2001;79:818–826.
19. Tyndall MW, Ronald AR, Agoki E, et al. Increased risk for infection with the human immunodeficiency virus type-1 among uncircumcised men in Kenya. *Clin Infect Dis* 1996;23:449–453.
20. Plummer FA, Simonsen JN, Cameron DW, et al. Co-factors in male-female sexual transmission of HIV. *J Infect Dis* 1991;163:233.
21. Cameron WD, Nugugi EN, Ronald AR, et al. Condom use prevents genital ulcers in women working as prostitutes. Influence of human immunodeficiency virus infection. *Sex Trans Dis* 1991;18:188–191.
22. Magro CM, Crowson AN, Alfa M, et al. A morphological study of penile chancroid lesions in human immunodeficiency virus (HIV)-positive and -negative african men with a hypothesis concerning the role of chancroid in HIV transmission. *Hum Pathol* 1996;27:1066–1070.
23. Kreiss JK, Coombs R, Plummer F, et al. Isolation of human immunodeficiency virus from genital ulcers in Nairobi prostitutes. *J Infect Dis* 1989;160: 380.
24. O'Farrell N. Targeted interventions required against genital ulcers in African countries worst affected by HIV infection. *Bull WHO* 2001;79:569–577.
25. Freinkel AL. Histological aspects of sexually transmitted genital lesions. *Histopathol* 1987;11:819.
26. King R, Gough J, Ronald A, et al. An immunohistochemical analysis of naturally occurring chancroid. *J Infect Dis* 1996;174:427–430.
27. Lockett AE, Dance DAB, Mabey DCW, Drasar BS. Serum-free media for isolation of *Haemophilus ducreyi*. *Lancet* 1991;338:326.
28. Dangor Y, Radebe F, Ballard RC. Transport media for *Haemophilus ducreyi*. *Sex Transm Dis* 1993;20:5.
29. Gaisin A, Heaton CL. Chancroid: alias the soft chancre. *Int J Dermatol* 1975;3:188.
30. Salzman RS, Kraus SJ, Miller RG, et al. Chancroidal ulcers that are not chancroid. Cause and epidemiology. *Arch Dermatol* 1984;120:636.
31. Totten PA, Kuypers JM, Chen CY, et al. Etiology of genital ulcer disease in Pakar, Senegal, and comparison of PCR and serologic assays for detection of *Haemophilus ducreyi*. *J Clin Microbiol* 2000;38:268–273.
32. McNicol PJ, Ronald AR. The plasmids of *Haemophilus ducreyi*. *Antimicrob Chemother* 1984;14:561.
33. Brunton J, Neier M, Erhman N, et al. Origin of small β-lactamase-specifying plasmids in *Haemophilus* species and *Neisseria gonorrhoeae*. *J Bacteriol* 1986;168:374.
34. Plummer FA, Nsanze H, D'Costa LJ, et al. Single-dose therapy of chancroid with trimethoprim-sulfametrole. *N Engl J Med* 1983;309:67.
35. Malonza IM, Tyndall MW, Ndinya-Achola JO, et al. A randomized, double-blind, placebo-controlled trial of single-dose ciprofloxacin versus erythromycin for the treatment of chancroid in Nairobi, Kenya. *J Infect Dis* 1999;180:1886–1893.
36. Bowmer MI, Nsanze N, D'Costa LJ, et al. Single-dose ceftriaxone for chancroid. *Antimicrob Agents Chemother* 1987;31:67.
37. Tyndall M, Malisa M, Plummer FA, et al. Ceftriaxone no longer predictably cures chancroid in Kenya. *J Infect Dis* 1993;167:469–471.
38. Bogaerts J, Kestens L, Tello WM, et al. Failure of treatment for chancroid in Rwanda not related to human immunodeficiency virus infection: in vitro resistance of *Haemophilus ducreyi* to trimethoprim-sulfamethoxazole. *Clin Infect Dis* 1995;20:924–930.
39. Fast MV, Nsanze H, D'Costa LJ, et al. Treatment of chancroid by clavulanic acid with amoxicillin patients with β-lactamase-positive *Haemophilus ducreyi* infection. *Lancet* 1982;2:509.
40. Perine PL, Stamm WE. Lymphogranuloma venereum. In Holmes KK, et al, eds: *Sexually transmitted diseases*. New York: McGraw-Hill, 1999:423–432.
41. Brunham RC, Kuo C-C, Chen WJ. Systemic *Chlamydia trachomatis* infection in the mouse: a comparison of lymphogranuloma venereum and trachoma biovars. *Infect Immun* 1985;48:78.
42. Behets FM, Andriamiadana J, Rand Riamanga R, et al. Chancroid, syphilis, genital herpes, and lymphogranuloma venereum in Antananarivo, Magascar. *J Infect Dis* 1999;180:1382–1385.
43. Joseph AK, Rosen T. Laboratory techniques used in the diagnosis of chancroid, granuloma inguinale, and lymphogranuloma venereum. *Dermatol Clin* 1994;12:1.
44. Wang SP, et al. A simplified method for immunological typing of trachoma-inclusion conjunctivitis-lymphogranuloma venereum organisms. *Infect Immun* 1973;7:356.
45. Chopda NM, Desai DC, Sawant PD, et al. Rectal lymphogranuloma venereum in association with rectal adenocarcinoma. *Ind J Gastroenterol* 1994;13:103.
46. Menke HE, et al. Treatment of lymphogranuloma venereum with rifampicin. *Br J Vener Dis* 1979;55:379–383.
47. Kuberski T. Granuloma inguinale (donovanosis). *Sex Transm Dis* 1980;1:29.
48. Kharsany AB, Hoosen AA, Kiepiela P, Naicker T, Sturm AW. Culture of *Calymmatobacterium granulomatis*. *Clin Dis* 1996;22:391–392.
49. Carter J, Bowden FJ, Sriprakash KS, Bastian I, Kemp DJ. Diagnostic polymerase chain reaction for donovanosis. *Clin Infect Dis* 1999;29:1168–1169.
50. Carter J, Kemp DJ. A colorimetric detection system for *Calymmatobacterium granulomatis*. *Sex Trans Infect* 2000;76:134–136.
51. Jamkhedkar PD, Hira SK, Shroff HJ, Lanjewar DN. Clinico-epidemiologic features of GI in the era of acquired immunodeficiency syndrome. *Sex Transm Dis* 1998;25:196–200.
52. O'Farrell N. Donovanosis: an update. *Int J STD AIDS* 2001;12:423–427.
53. Hart G. Donovanosis. *Clin Infect Dis* 1997;25:24–30.

CHAPTER 108

Human Papillomaviruses and Anogenital Disease

Lawrence J. Eron

Infection by human papillomaviruses (HPVs) may be the most prevalent infectious disease, estimated to be about 100 million people in North America (1). Yet it is a hidden epidemic as less than 1% show clinical signs. While certain types of HPV may cause benign common warts of the fingers or plantar warts of the feet, other types may infect the genital area and result in severe dysplasia of the cervix and even invasive carcinomas.

CHARACTERISTICS OF PAPILLOMAVIRUSES

Taxonomy

Classified as a papovavirus along with polyomavirus and simian virus 40, HPVs form a distinct group of viruses with their own biologic and genetic characteristics. They contain an 8,000 base-pair, double-stranded, circular deoxyribonucleic acid (DNA) genome with a capsid diameter of 55 nm. Unlike the other papovaviruses, they are not easily propagated in tissue culture. It has not been possible to distinguish between HPVs with serologic methods. Rather, they are classified by DNA hybridization into more than 100 different types, 40 of which infect the genital tract (2). They are classified according to their DNA sequence, using the L-1 open reading frame as a test probe. If an HPV strain is between 90% to 98% homologous with the test probe, then it is classified as a "subtype." If the homology is greater than 98%, it is classified as a "variant" (3). Some HPV types and their clinical syndromes are listed in Table 108.1.

Virulence Factors

HPV-6, HPV-11, and other types have been associated with benign, exophytic condylomata acuminata of the anogenital region as well as dysplasias of the cervix, called "squamous intraepithelial lesions" (SILs), previously referred to as cervical intraepithelial neoplasia (CIN). SILs are further subdivided into low-grade, (corresponding to CIN I) and high-grade (corresponding to CIN II and III) lesions. HPV-6 and HPV-11 cause 90% of low-grade SILs, two thirds of which are caused by HPV-6 and one third by HPV-11 (4). HPV-16, along with other types, is most frequently found in high-grade SILs of the cervix and squamous cell carcinomas of the cervix, while HPV-18 along with other types, is most commonly associated with nonsquamous cervical neoplasms. Together, HPV-16 and HPV-18 are found in 93% of cervical carcinomas (5).

Epidemiology

HPVs that infect the anogenital area are transmitted sexually. Because they are relatively easily transmitted during intercourse, up to 40% of sexually active adults show evidence of HPV infection (6) and fully 73% of sexual partners of HPV-infected individuals show evidence of HPV infection at their initial examination (7). The prevalence is highest for females in their third decade (4). In one study, 70% of college women were infected with HPV, but the mean duration of infection was only 8 months. After 2 years, only 9% showed persistence of the same HPV type (2), indicating that in the large majority, infection is self-limited. When infection persists, it is associated with an oncogenic type such as HPV-16 or HPV-18. In general, low-grade SILs have the highest prevalence in women in their early twenties, high-grade SILs in their late twenties and early thirties, and invasive cancer of the cervix at age 40 to 50 (4).

PATHOGENESIS

At the Molecular Level

The HPV genome is organized into three distinct regions (Fig. 108.1): an "early" region that encodes viral proteins necessary for DNA replication, transcription, and cell transformation; a "late" region that encodes the viral capsid proteins; and a control region known as the upstream regulatory region (URR). The genes of the early region are designated E1 to E7 and those of the late region, L1 and L2 (Table 108.2).

In productive infection, messenger ribonucleic acid (mRNA) transcription from the early and late regions of the viral genome directs viral DNA replication and viral capsid synthesis, respectively. Mature daughter viruses assemble and infectious virions are produced. In nonproductive infection, transcription of messenger RNA is from the early region only. Viral capsid synthesis and viral assembly do not occur, and the early functions may result in transformation of the cell.

In benign condylomata caused by HPV-6 or HPV-11, productive infection produces many copies of HPV DNA per cell as extrachromosomal plasmids. In carcinomas of the genital tract from which HPV-16 and HPV-18 DNA has been isolated, the HPV DNA genome has been found to be integrated into the host chromosome, a late event in the course of infection by HPV, usually as the carcinoma becomes invasive. Integration of the virus into the host cell occurs with disruption of the circular HPV genome at the E2 gene (8). This results in the loss of the E1 and E2 genes' control of E6 and E7 function. E6 and E7 gene proteins inactivate host proteins, called "anti-oncogenes," that normally control cell growth and differentiation. The p53 protein and the pRB (retinoblastoma tumor suppressor protein) are two such examples of anti-oncogenes that are targets of HPV-induced cell transformation. These anti-oncogenes arrest host cell division in the G1 phase, to either (a) allow the cell time to repair damaged DNA before progressing to the S (DNA replication) phase, or (b) doom the damaged cell to apoptosis (9). This checkpoint is

---

TABLE 108.1.   Types of Human Papillomaviruses

Type	Source
HPV-1	Plantar warts
HPV-2, -4, -29	Verruca vulgaris
HPV-3, -10, -28, -49	Flat warts
HPV-5, -8, -9, -12, -14, -15, -17, -19 to -25	Epidermodysplasia verruciformis
HPV-6, -11	Genital warts and laryngeal papillomas
HPV-7	Butcher's warts
HPV-13, -32	Oral focal epithelial hyperplasia
HPV-16, -18, -26, -27, -30, -31, -33, -35, -39, -40, -42 to -45, -51 to -59, -61, -62, -64, -66 to -69, -71 to -74	Cervical dysplasia and carcinoma, bowenoid papulosis
HPV-30, -40	Laryngeal carcinoma

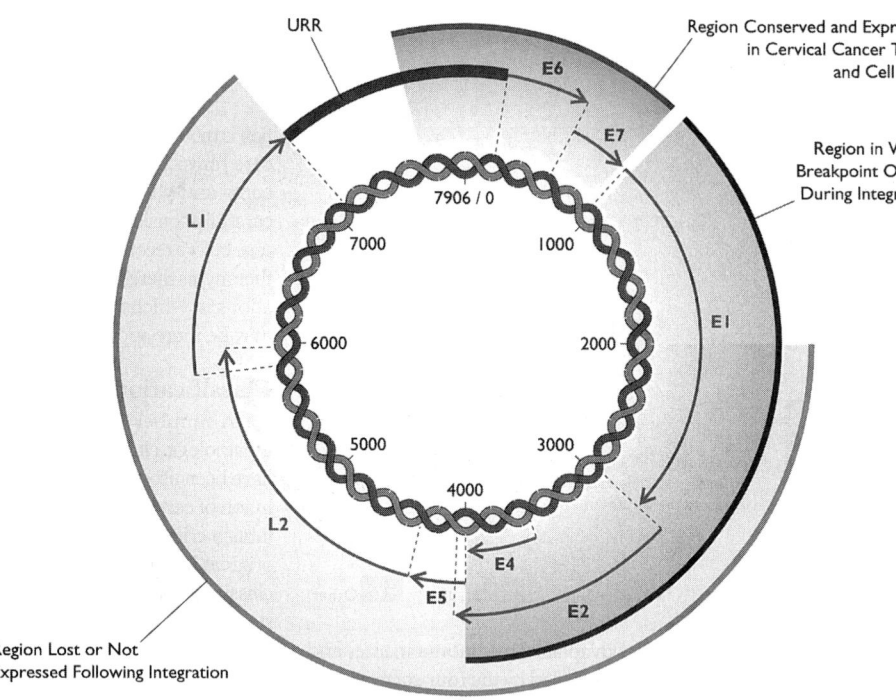

Figure 108.1. The HPV-16 genome is composed of three regions: an upstream regulatory region containing the *cis*-acting transcription and replication controls, early open reading frames for proteins E1, E2, E5, E6, and E7 that control viral replication and cell transformation, and late open reading frames L1, L2, and E4 involved in capsid formation and viral maturation. (From Burk RD. Human papillomavirus and the risk of cervical cancer. *Hosp Pract* 1999;44:103, with permission. Copyright 1999, The McGraw-Hill Companies, Inc. Illustration by Seward Hung.)

a safeguard of the integrity of the cellular genome, and loss of this repair mechanism renders the host genome genetically unstable and much more susceptible to other carcinogens such as cigarette smoke, for example (10). The pRB gene is either completely absent or has significant deletions in tumors from patients with retinoblastoma, breast cancer, and squamous cell cancers of the head and neck (4). E2 disruption caused by integration into the cellular genome induces overexpression of E6 and of E7 and consequent loss of the host cell growth and differentiation control functions via an ubiquitin-dependent degradation of p53 and degradation of pRB, respectively (11). This HPV-induced disruption of the cell cycle is mediated in a complicated way through inactivation of inhibitors of cyclins and cyclin-dependent kinases (cdks), important regulators of cell cycle progression (12).

At the Cellular and Tissue Levels

To cause an infection, HPV must penetrate through gaps in the epithelium to gain access to the basal layer of the epidermis.

Expression of the viral DNA in the basal layer induces the proliferation of keratinocytes and blood vessels resulting in a wart. The clinical features, histologic appearance, and natural history of HPV infections are determined largely by the HPV type (Table 108.3). After an incubation period of 1 to 9 months, HPV infection of the cervix, vagina, vulva, and penis may become clinically evident. HPV may also infect the perianal and intra-anal regions, occasionally above the dentate line of the distal rectum. The presence of perianal condylomata, in either males or females, need not imply a history of anal intercourse, because spread may occur merely by local extension. HPV-6 and HPV-11 may cause oral lesions and laryngeal papillomatosis in adults, transmitted by oral sex. Laryngeal papillomatosis in infants is transmitted by intrapartum contact of the neonate within an infected birth canal. Cesarean section as a measure to prevent intrapartum spread is not thought to be indicated, however.

Whereas HPV-6 and HPV-11 cause exophytic condylomata on the external genitalia, HPV-16 and HPV-18 show a predilection for the cervix and frequently progress to higher grades of SIL than HPV-6 or HPV-11. However, they do not necessarily evolve from low-grade precursors. In fact, most high-grade SILs are

---

TABLE 108.2. Papillomavirus Gene Functions

Gene	Function
E1	Extrachromosomal DNA replication down- and upregulation
E2	Transcription regulator against cell transformation
E3	Unknown
E4	Viral maturation
E5	Cellular transformation in bovine papillomavirus, control of plasmid numbers
E6	Cellular transformation, control of plasmid numbers
E7	Cellular immortalization, transcriptional transactivation
E8	DNA replication in bovine papillomavirus
L1	Major capsid protein (54,000 daltons)
L2	Minor capsid protein (76,000 daltons)

TABLE 108.3. Anogenital Lesions and Human Papillomavirus Infection

Lesion	HPV type
Condylomata acuminata	6, 11
Cervical squamous intraepithelial lesions	16, 18, 26, 27, 31, 33, 35, 39, 42–45, 51–59, 61, 62, 64, 66–69, 71–74
Bowenoid papulosis	16, 18, 33, 39
Buschke-Löwenstein tumors	6, 11
Invasive cervical carcinomas	16, 18, 31, 33, 35, 39, 45, 51, 52, 56
Vulvar carcinomas	16 (rarely 6, 11)
Penile carcinomas	16, 18

not usually preceded by low-grade SILs, and conversely most low-grade SILs do not evolve into high-grade SILs(13). In high-grade SILs, nuclear atypia and abnormal mitotic figures are observed, but koilocytosis (cytoplasmic vacuolation), seen in condylomata acuminata, is frequently absent.

Because of the long lag time between initial infection and eventual malignant conversion, estimated to be as long as 20 years, and because not all HPV-16–infected women develop cervical cancer, other cofactors are undoubtedly responsible for malignant conversion. These may include tobacco use, infection by other agents, including herpes simplex virus and *Chlamydia trachomatis*, perhaps by amplifying oncogenes and inducing mutations, and steroid hormones that may bind to the URR to initiate transcription of the E6 and E7 genes. Indeed estrogen responsiveness promoting HPV infection may be one of the explanations as to why women at menarche are so prone to HPV infection (1) and several decades later carcinoma of the cervix (13). Finally, the immune status of the host may also prevent or lead to tumor development, as described below.

Classification of cervical dysplasia by CIN grades I to III has been replaced by the Bethesda system (14), which assigns all cytologic abnormalities to either low-grade or high-grade SILs or to "atypical squamous cells of uncertain significance (ASCUS)." Most low-grade SILs regress spontaneously and consequently do not need to be treated. High-grade SILs on the other hand may have greater malignant potential and it has been proposed that HPV typing may assist in determining which high-grade SILs need to be aggressively treated and which need only be watched (15). This may also be useful for ASCUS where 5% to 40% of women with ASCUS results on Papanicolaou smears may proceed to high-grade SIL (16). On the other hand, because dysplasia associated with highly oncogenic HPV types may remit, treatment decisions must be based on the degree of dysplasia and not the HPV type (17).

Immune Responses

Because persons who are immunoincompetent often develop more numerous warts that are refractory to therapy, it is clear that the immune response is important in controlling HPV infection. Regression of warts after therapy is frequently accompanied by enhanced cell-mediated immunity responses to viral antigens. Antigen recognition is clearly type specific, as patients with regressing genital warts may have persistent plantar and common warts. Patients infected with HPV produce IgG antibodies to L1, L2, E6, and E7 gene products. Antibodies to the latter two are found more frequently in those who clear their infection. This may not indicate a causal relationship because defects of humoral immunity do not influence the natural history of HPV infection.

Patients with refractory genital warts should be screened for antibody to human immunodeficiency virus (HIV), because this condition may be a marker for HIV infection. HPV infection is closely associated with infection by HIV with a prevalence of greater than 85% among HIV-positive men who have sex with men (18). HIV-positive women have a somewhat lower prevalence of HPV infection, which ranges from 57% to 70%. In HIV-positive men, HPV is acquired through anal intercourse and manifests itself most frequently as subclinical, high-grade anal intraepithelial neoplasia (AIN). The lower the CD4 count, the greater the risk of high-grade AIN and of high-risk oncogenic HPV types. As the CD4 count rises during treatment with highly active antiretroviral therapy, cervical dysplasia may regress in some HIV-positive women, demonstrating that strengthening immunity is an effective treatment modality in and of itself.

Immunocompetent persons may also have warts that are unresponsive to therapy because of a deficiency of host response associated with HPV infection itself. While most patients with low-risk HPV types such as HPV-6 and HPV-11 clear their infection without developing SIL, the majority of patients infected with high-risk, oncogenic types also do not develop high-grade SIL presumably on the basis of an intact immune response.

Those who do not clear their infection however appear to be infected with higher risk variants of oncogenic HPV types (a variant has greater than 98% homology with the typing test probe). Higher risk HPV variants may differ by only a few amino acids from lower risk variants (19,20). A single higher risk HPV-16 variant was found in 408 of 411 cancer specimens (21). Variants of HPV-16, cluster geographically into European (E) variants, Asian (As) variants, and African variants (Af1 and Af2). Variants of HPV-16 interact with the host immune system to subvert host immunity and encourage viral persistence. They do this by altering the keratinocytes' ability to produce inflammatory cytokines.

The net result is that the Langerhans cells, which process HPV antigens and present them in the context of major histocompatibility proteins, are deficient, which leads to an ineffective immune response, persistent viral infection, and unregulated growth of cells. Variants of HPV-16 differ in their abilities to alter keratinocyte differentiation and to degrade p53 control of cell growth, in part by the avidity with which their E6 proteins bind to p53. Certain MHC haplotypes are associated with a higher risk of invasive cancer, indicating a genetic component, as well, to the hosts' immune response (22,23).

CLINICAL MANIFESTATIONS

HPV infection may become clinically apparent as one of four morphologic types—exophytic condylomata acuminata on moist surfaces, with a cauliflower-like surface (Figs. 108.2, 108.3);

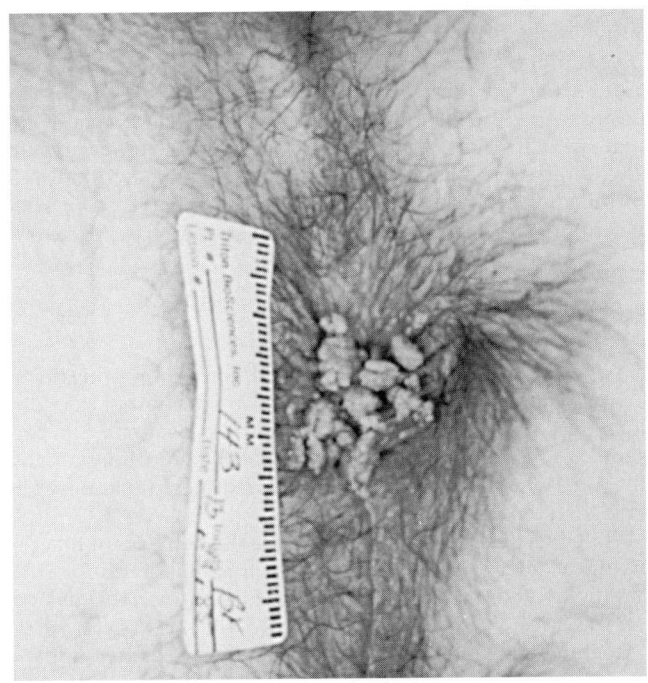

Figure 108.2. Genital warts involving the perianal region.

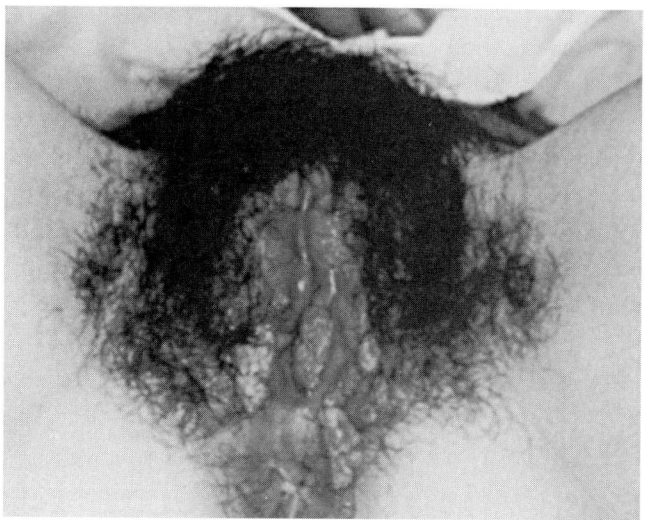

Figure 108.3. Genital warts involving the labia.

keratotic warts on keratinized skin, that may resemble seborrheic keratoses; smooth papular warts; or flat warts that can occur anywhere on the genitalia, but especially on the cervix. The latter may be visible only with the application of acetic acid and by using colposcopy. In women, exophytic warts are located most frequently in the posterior introitus, followed by the labia, clitoris, vaginal vestibule, and perianal region. They may also occur on the cervix. In uncircumcised men, the prepuce is most frequently involved, followed by the penile shaft, scrotum, and perianal area. The urethral meatus may be affected, and less frequently, the proximal urethra. While clinically apparent infection is usually asymptomatic, it may occasionally cause pruritus and burning.

DIAGNOSIS

Condylomata acuminata must be differentiated from other growths in the genital area, including molluscum contagiosum, condylomata lata, keratoses, moles, and skin tags, which may be especially difficult to distinguish in the vaginal area. If the diagnosis is in doubt, it should be confirmed with biopsy results and examination for the typical changes of koilocytosis. DNA hybridization tests are useful for identifying the type of HPV but cannot yet be advocated for routine screening purposes.

TREATMENT

Genital warts often represent chronic HPV infection, and clinical cure may merely represent reversion to latency rather than disappearance of the viral DNA. Insofar as removal of warts represents a cosmetically desirable end, their eradication appears to be a reasonable goal. However, the treatment must never be worse than the disease itself.

While it is desirable from a public health standpoint that debulking of a wart might decrease the transmissibility of HPV from the treated individual to their sexual partner, this has not been the case.

Treatment of genital warts can be classified as patient-applied or provider-administered (6). Patient-applied topical treatments include podophyllotoxin (Condylox), imiquimod (Aldara), 5-fluorouracil (Efudex), and cidofovir. Podophyllotoxin, applied

twice daily for 3 days per week, is variably effective. Imiquimod applied thrice weekly is less effective in males than other therapies. 5-fluorouracil cream is intensely irritating and patients may tolerate only one or two applications a week. It has been used after laser therapy in an attempt to prevent relapse. None of these treatments is 100% effective and each is plagued by relapse. They have however proven cost-effective in reliable patients.

Provider-administered treatments include 50% to 80% trichloroacetic acid and bichloroacetic acid, which can be used in pregnant women unlike the other topical treatments. They produce a white slough that peels in a few days. Like other topical treatments, they are essentially ineffective when applied to warts on keratinized epithelium.

A variety of provider-administered ablative procedures have been tested. Cryotherapy—two 1-minute freeze-thaw cycles induced by liquid nitrogen—is the least painful and does not require local anesthesia. However, weekly treatments are usually necessary and recurrences are common. Electrocoagulation using a battery-powered instrument may yield a somewhat higher clearance rate than cryosurgery but again there are recurrences, and a painful injection of lidocaine is required for anesthesia. Loop electrosurgical excision procedures and cold-knife cone biopsies are often used for cervical disease. These two procedures offer the advantage of providing tissue to examine for evidence of carcinoma, which is found in 2% to 3% of specimens. In contrast, laser ablation, although it does offer precise control of the depth of tissue destruction, vaporizes all treated tissue, requires local anesthesia, and is expensive to administer.

Interferons offer the potential advantage of eradicating the HPV reservoir, due to their antiviral and immune stimulating properties in addition to their antiproliferative effects. Interferon-alpha is effective when injected into the base of the wart twice or thrice weekly, but not when systemically administered. All the interferons have influenza-like side effects and relapses occur, nonetheless. The benefit of combining them with ablative therapies is still unproved. Pegylated interferon-alpha may offer additional benefits beyond its once-weekly administration, but this has yet to be demonstrated in a trial. Interferon inducers, such as imiquimod and the newer and more potent derivative resiquimod, are topically applied to warts and have none of these side effects. They do induce inflammation in and around the wart, which can be irritating.

PREVENTION

Because HPV infection develops in approximately 70% of sexual partners of those with genital warts, prevention is important, but elusive. The use of condoms and nonoxynol-9 have never been shown to be effective. Hence the need for a vaccine.

In animal models, vaccination using the capsid proteins L1 and L2 induces type-specific neutralizing antibodies and is protective against infection (5). Immunization of 60,000 beagles over a 3-year period resulted in complete protection against naturally acquired canine oral papillomavirus–induced warts (4). Prophylactic vaccines have been developed using virus-like particles (VLPs), which are morphologically quite similar to authentic virions, except they lack the DNA. They consist of the major capsid protein L1, with or without L2, produced by recombinant DNA technology, and then self-assembled into VLPs. VLP vaccines containing L2 in addition to L1 have the advantage of inducing cross-neutralizing antibodies to different HPV types and are easier to produce. Because HPV-6 and HPV-11 account for 90% of cases of condylomata acuminata (5), a bivalent vaccine would be desirable. In animals if the VLPs are administered intranasally, or with a live vaccinia virus vector, increased IgA production in the cervix can be demonstrated.

Vaccination using the early proteins E1, E2, E6, or E7 are not protective against infection but tend to induce regression of warts and dysplasia in animals. Chimeric vaccines fusing the capsid proteins L1 or L2 to the oncoproteins E6 or E7 of HPV-16 and HPV-18 are being tested to treat dysplasia and carcinomas of the cervix. Trials of an L2/E7 chimeric HPV-6 vaccine, while immunogenic, have not yet shown that the level of the immune response correlates with the frequency of wart recurrence (24).

Other vaccine trials showed some evidence of a cytotoxic response to E6 and E7 oncoproteins that correlated in a few cases with a remission (25,26). These initial studies have been done in late stage disease where a good immune response is not likely to be obtained due to downregulation of the expression of MHC molecules, required for correct processing of antigens (27). If trials are conducted in earlier disease, such as those with pre-invasive, high-grade SILs or in those patients at high risk of recurrence after primary therapy, it is possible that a better immune response to vaccination will be elicited. It will be important to develop a prophylactic vaccine for low-risk HPV types to provide an incentive for men to be vaccinated, because they are much less likely than women to develop malignancy from high-risk HPV types.

The problem of cross-neutralization can be overcome by combining HPV-16, HPV-18, HPV-31, and HPV-45, which together account for 80% of cases of cervical cancer, into one vaccine (27,28). If types HPV-33, HPV-52, and HPV-58 are added, it would account for more than 90% of cervical carcinomas (5). The development of a therapeutic and especially a prophylactic vaccine for HPVs could be an effective alternative to more expensive screening and treatment of cervical dysplasia and carcinomas and could potentially decrease the worldwide morbidity of this disease.

REFERENCES

1. McGlennen RC. Human papillomavirus oncogenesis. *Clin Lab Med* 2000; 20:383–400.
2. Burk RD. Human papillomavirus and the risk of cervical cancer. *Hosp Pract* 1999;34:103–111.
3. Kaufman RH, Adam E, Vonka V. Human papillomavirus infection and cervical carcinoma. *Clin Obstet Gynecol* 2000;43:363–380.
4. Stoler MH. Human papillomaviruses and cervical neoplasia: a model for carcinogenesis. *Int J Gynecol Pathol* 2000;19:16–28.
5. Breitburd F, Coursaget P. Human papillomavirus vaccines. *Cancer Biol* 1999;9:431–445.
6. Beutner KR, Wiley DJ, Douglas JM. Genital warts and their treatment. *Clin Infect Dis* 1999;28[suppl 1]:S37–S56.
7. Rosemberg SK, Greenberg MD, Reid R. Sexually transmitted papillomaviral infection in men. *Obstet Gynecol Clin North Am* 1987;14:495–512.
8. Tyring SK. Human papillomavirus infections: epidemiology, pathogenesis, and host immune response. *J Am Acad Dermatol* 2000;43:S18–S26.
9. Mantovani F, Banks L. The interaction between p53 and papillomaviruses. *Cancer Biol* 1999;9:387–395.
10. Zur Hausen H. Papillomaviruses causing cancer: evasion from host-cell control in early events of carcinogenesis. *J Natl Cancer Inst* 2000;92:690–698.
11. Ishiji T. Molecular mechanisms of carcinogenesis by human paillomavirus-16. *J Dermatol* 2000;27:73–86.
12. Syrjanen SM, Syrjanen KJ. New concepts on the role of human papillomavirus in cell cycle regulation. *Ann Med* 1999;31:175–187.
13. McLachlin CM. Human papillomavirus in cervical neoplasia. *Clin Lab Med* 2000;20:257–270.
14. National Cancer Institute. The 1988 Bethesda system for reporting cervical/vaginal cytological diagnoses. *JAMA* 1989;262:931–934.
15. Manos MM, Kinney WK, Hurley LB. Identifying women with cervical neoplasia. *JAMA* 1999;281:1605–1610.
16. Cox JT. Evaluating the role of HPB testing for women with equivocal papanicolaou test findings. *JAMA* 1999;281:1645–1647.
17. Kaufman RH, Adam E. Is human papillomavirus testing of value in clinical practice? *Am J Obstet Gynecol* 2000;182:479–480.
18. Collis TK, Celum CL. The clinical manifestations and treatment of sexually transmitted diseases in human immunodeficiency virus-positive men. *Clin Infect Dis* 2001;32:611–622.
19. Sedlacek TV. Advances in the diagnosis and treatment of human papillomavirus infections. *Clin Obstet Gynecol* 1999;42:206–220.
20. Conrad-Stoppler M, Ching K, Stoppler H, et al. Natural variants of the human papillomavirus type 16 E6 protein differ in their abilities to alter keratinocyte differentiation and to induce p53 degradation. *J Virol* 1996;70:6987–6993.
21. Yamada T, Manos M, Peto J, et al. Human papillomavirus type 16 sequence variation in cervical cancers: a worldwide perspective. *J Virol* 1997;71:2463–2472.
22. Apple RJ, Becker TM, Wheeler CM, et al. Comparison of human leukocyte antigen DR-DQ disease associations found with cervical dysplasia and invasive cervical carcinoma. *J Natl Cancer Inst* 1995;87:427–436.
23. Silva B, Vargas-Alarcon G, Zuniga-Ramos J, et al. Genetic features of mexican women predisposing to cancer of the uterine cervix. *Hum Pathol* 1999;30:626–628.
24. Lacy CJN, Thompson HSG, Monteiro EF, et al. Phase IIA safety and immunogenicity of a therapeutic vaccine, TA-GW, in persons with genital warts. *J Infect Dis* 1999;179:612–618.
25. Borysiewicz LK, Flander A, Nimako M, et al. A recombinant vaccinia virus encoding human papillomavirus types 6 and 18 E6 and E7 proteins as immunotherapy for cervical cancer. *Lancet* 1996;347:1523–1527.
26. Fraser IH, Tindle RW, Fernando GJP, et al. Safety and immunogenicity of HPV16 E7/algammulin. In Tindle RW, ed: *Vaccines for human papillomavirus infection and anogenital disease*, Austin, TX: RG Lands, 1999:91–104.
27. Murakami M, Gurski KJ, Stoller MA. Human papillomavirus vaccines for cervical cancer. *J Immunother* 1999;22:212–218.
28. Lowy DR, Schiller JT. Papillomavirus prophylactic vaccine prospects. *Biochim Biophys Acta* 1998;1423:M1–M8.

Gynecology and Obstetrics

CHAPTER 109
Approach to the Patient with Infection of the Pelvis

William J. Ledger

INTRODUCTION

Since the last edition of this textbook, there have been continuing changes in the practice of medicine that influence physician/patient interaction. Hospitalization is very expensive; all medical care funding agencies have intensified their focus on cost control. Fewer patients are admitted, and for those admitted, hospital stays are shorter. In gynecology, the majority of operations are now done in an ambulatory setting, with hospital admission reserved for the patient with an intra-operative complication or the rare patient with serious underlying medical problems. Patients scheduled to have more extensive operations requiring post-operative inpatient care are first admitted the day of the operation. In obstetrics, postpartum stays have been shortened. All of these patient care changes accentuate the trend of the first postoperative or postpartum indication of infection occurring when the patient is at home and not in the hospital.

There are other insidious changes in physician outpatient practice patterns. Most health maintenance organizations (HMOs) have either reduced physician payments or have granted increases that have not kept up with inflation. Over time, a trend I see is the physician booking a larger number of patients in allotted hours; an attempt to meet past levels of physician income by increasing patient visit numbers. The outcome is obvious. These new self-imposed time restraints mean less time for physician history-taking and an increasing physician reluctance to perform any office-based diagnostic testing. In one study of 150 office visits in patients with vaginitis, a microscopic examination of vaginal fluid was not done in 37% of the visits and the whiff amine test and measurement of vaginal pH were performed in only 3% of the visits (1). There are other stresses. For physicians involved in capitated care with a fixed yearly payment for each patient in their panel, there are fiscal constraints on laboratory testing, particularly the microbiology laboratory. This obviously impacts upon the evaluation of a patient with a suspected pelvic infection.

IS OUR CURRENT EMPHASIS ON PHYSICIAN DIAGNOSIS APPROPRIATE?

The current basis for physician dispensation of care may not be correct. Doctors have been inculcated with a belief in the signs and symptoms of infection that are confirmed by laboratory findings. The problem is that in many syndromes, pelvic inflammatory disease for example, these textbook findings apply to a minority of patients with infection. This makes the task of making a diagnosis difficult, because most of these women have vague signs and symptoms and the cause is usually not obvious. For example, less than half of women whose acute salpingitis was confirmed by laparoscopy were febrile (2) (Table 109.1). The traditional logic that equated fever with bacterial infection does not apply to most women with pelvic inflammatory disease. In addition, the problems of diagnosis do not end with physical signs and symptoms. Table 109.1 shows the lack of specificity of the sedimentation rate. More than half (52.7%) of the patients with no laparoscopic evidence of infection had an elevated sedimentation rate (2). Another recent study (3) evaluated the CDC minimal criteria for the diagnosis of pelvic inflammatory disease (PID), that is, lower abdominal tenderness, adnexal tenderness, and cervical motion tenderness (4). These criteria had a sensitivity of 83.3% in predicting the diagnosis of Endometritis as determined by biopsy, but these criteria had a specificity of only 21.8% (3). David Eschenbach in the discussion of this paper cogently noted that "many other diseases are known to occur independently of clinical signs and symptoms" (3). The classical hierarchy of clinical signs and laboratory findings is too inexact for this important infection in non-pregnant women. Another study by Cates et al. suggested that atypical pelvic inflammatory disease is more common than its symptomatic counterpart (5). One attempt to add more order to this diversified complex of infections now called (PID) is to categorize subgroups based on clinical and laboratory findings (6). These suggestions will need clinical testing to evaluate their effectiveness.

There is another major flaw in our emphasis upon physicians as the initiators of patient care. This implies two occurrences that guarantee patient-physician contact. In the first, the patient has sufficient symptoms to seek medical care. With this model of care, what do we do with asymptomatic patients, or those with minimal symptomatology who have *Chlamydia trachomatis*, pelvic inflammatory disease (7), or symptom-free women with *Candida* vaginitis (8), bacterial vaginosis (9), or *Trichomonas vaginalis* vaginitis (10)? A second assumption is that a mildly symptomatic patient will be seen by a physician. Private patients with minimal symptoms will have a difficult time getting past the gatekeeper who is controlling the number of patients visiting a doctor on a given day. The retrospective analyses showing symptoms in patients with *Chlamydia trachomatis*, pelvic inflammatory disease (11), and *Candida vaginitis* (12) may simply reflect the reality of patients' awareness that their symptoms were not severe enough to warrant a visit to a doctor's office, a clinic, or the emergency department. For the poor in the United States, preventive care is extremely limited, and medical care is often only sought in an Emergency Room when the patient is seriously ill and has been sick for many days. All of the Center for Disease Control's emphasis on early recognition of patient's with minimal symptoms who have an infection (4) will go for naught if the patients do not present themselves for medical care. Improvement of medical care in the future requires a refocusing of priorities. It must emphasize patient education about the risks and signs of early pelvic infection combined with over the counter test kits that are sensitive and specific enough to confirm infection.

Another troubling development in care of patients is the documented shortcomings of primary care physicians in making the diagnosis of common pelvic infections. Recently trained physicians have become less skilled in office microscopy. One study of obstetric-gynecologic residents in training at an academic medical center found only one half of the patients thought to have *Candida* vaginitis on microscopic examination of NaCl and KOH wet mounts of vaginal secretions had a positive culture result or a positive polymerase chain reaction (PCR) test result for *Candida* (13). This confirmed the findings in a previous study of primary care physicians. Only 42% of the patients with a microscopic diagnosis of a yeast infection had a positive culture result for *Candida* (14). The current emphasis upon the Gram stain of vaginal secretions evaluated in a central laboratory to make the diagnosis of bacterial vaginosis largely reflects the concern about practicing physician's competence or willingness to use a microscope (15). These doctors on the front line are anxious for a test kit that is both sensitive and specific. One recent study evaluated this technology, in which swabs obtained separately by the patient and physician were used for polymerase chain reaction testing for *Neisseria gonorrhea*, *Chlamydia trachomatis*, *Trichomonas vaginalis*,

TABLE 109.1. Classic Signs and Laboratory Findings of Salpingitis Observed in Women with a Laparoscopic Diagnosis of Salpingitis Compared with Women with Normal Pelvic Findings

Clinical and laboratory findings	% with salpingitis	% with normal findings	Statistically significant
Acute pelvic pain	94	94	No
Fever (temperature higher than 38°C)	32.9	14.1	Yes
Tender adnexal swelling or mass	49.5	24.5	Yes
Elevated erythrocyte sedimentation rate	75.9	52.7	Yes

From Jacobson L, Westrom L. Objectivized diagnosis of acute pelvic inflammatory disease. Diagnostic and prognostic value of routine laparoscopy. *Am J Obstet Gynecol* 1969;105:1088–1098; with permission.

TABLE 109.2. Key Discussion Points in the Initial Patient Interview

Why are you here?
When did the problem begin?
How does it bother you?
Are you involved with anyone?

and human papillomavirus (16). This approach detected more *N. gonorrhea*, *C. trachomatis*, and *T. vaginalis* infections than were found with standard diagnostic testing done by an examining physician.

With this as a background, I plan to highlight the workup of a patient with a pelvic infection seen by an infectious disease specialist. All too often, these patients will have had exposure to incorrect antibacterial and antifungal agents, with no diagnostic evaluation.

HISTORY

To obtain a relevant history from a patient suspected of having a pelvic infection, the physician's attitude must be open and friendly. A woman, whose symptoms cause her to seek medical care, will be alert to the physician's body language or to a dismissive tone of voice. These women deserve the same consideration and attention to the detail of care as the male with chest pain.

The patient should be allowed to describe her problem in her own words. Questioning should progress at the patient's own pace and without interruption (Table 109.2). The physician can begin the interview by asking, "Why are you here?" Subsequently, questions can be used to expand the patient's response in a nonjudgmental manner, for example, "When did the problem begin? How does it bother you?" Sometimes the patient will recall a specific event helpful to the diagnosis. The patient can be prompted to expand her description, if necessary to clarify the problem. If the patient's problem is a discharge, is she aware of an odor? Is this what is bothering her? If so, what has she done about it? If symptoms are related to her menstrual cycle, it can be a hint to the physician of some forms of vaginitis or salpingitis.

Most pelvic infections occur in sexually active women. Information about sexual activity must be sought without implying that any type of sexual activity is bad or that infection is a just punishment for the patient's transgressions. For a woman to be ill is not a sin. The questioning should be matter-of-fact and open, for example, "Are you involved with anyone?" An affirmative reply allows the physician to explore male symptoms and methods of contraception, which can help delineate some types of infection.

The initial interview ends when the physician is clear about the reasons for the patient's visit. The interview process should be the patient's unrestricted expose of problems and not the physician's checklist to fit the patient into a preordained diagnostic category.

PHYSICAL EXAMINATION

All women should receive a complete examination. Assessment of vital signs is important. In most women who have a pelvic infection, vital signs are normal, although some who have salp-

ingitis have fever, and low blood pressure could indicate a seriously ill patient with septic shock. The remainder of the general examination is important because other pathologic processes can be present not related to the symptoms that prompted the visit to the physician. Doctors can find breast lumps, a thyroid nodule, or a heart murmur that may be asymptomatic but will require future evaluation.

The focus of any physician's evaluation for pelvic infection is the pelvic examination. Anything less than this in an initial workup is inadequate care. This examination requires a table with stirrups, proper lighting, working equipment, and an assistant to aid the physician in the examination. The array of equipment needed is neither extensive nor expensive. It should include some form of magnification to evaluate lesions; slides and a microscope; saline solution; 10% potassium hydroxide; a strip of pH paper; and appropriate laboratory kits to identify herpesvirus, *Chlamydia trachomatis*, *Neisseria gonorrhoeae*, *Candida albicans*, and *Trichomonas vaginalis*. Every hospital and every office caring for women needs this as a basic requisite for care.

The pelvic examination should be unhurried and directed in part by the patient's history. The goal should be a complete evaluation without causing the patient discomfort. One aid is to inform the patient of every step of the examination. The sheets should drape the patient in such a way that she can see the physician, if this is desired.

Examination of the vulva is the first step. Too often physicians insert a speculum and omit this part of the examination. If the patient has a "sore," the location should be pinpointed. If there is a painful lesion, material is obtained for culture for herpes virus. Blood antibody studies for the herpes virus are sometimes not immediately helpful in the evaluation of a patient with a lesion; results can be negative in a patient with primary genital herpes or positive in a patient who does not have genital herpes, but has had cold sores in her mouth in the past. A positive culture for herpes virus confirms the diagnosis. However, one study showed that antibody testing is more sensitive than the culture in diagnosing genital herpes (17). There are other diagnostic problems. Some women have what appear to be *Condylomata acuminata*; biopsy can be performed to confirm the diagnosis as well as digene testing for the presence of the human papillomavirus. If a woman complains of point tenderness at the introitus with sexual penetration or the insertion of a tampon, the site of discomfort can be determined with a cotton swab. Vulvar vestibulitis is manifested by severe pain at vestibular gland sites touched with a swab.

The examination of the vagina begins with an unlubricated speculum; this prevents possible confusion when pH evaluation is performed or a culture specimen is obtained. Tap water can be alkaline, and lubricants have antibacterial substances present. If the patient's complaint is vaginal discharge, the extent and the quality of the discharge can be noted. Most gynecologic textbooks characterize the vaginal discharges associated with *Candida vulvovaginitis* and *Trichomonas vaginitis*. These clinical entities are infrequently that specific, and first impressions can be incorrect. To avoid error, the clinician must perform a number of quick diagnostic tests, the results of which will point to the diagnosis.

The test for vaginal pH is important; the sample should be from the side walls of the vagina, and not from the endocervix, which is usually alkaline. The vaginal pH is normally less than 4.5 with *Candida* vaginitis, whereas it is usually higher in *Trichomonas vaginitis* and *Bacterial vaginosis*. The physician should smell the slide when vaginal secretions are added to dilute potassium hydroxide. An unpleasant fishy amine odor is usual with bacterial vaginosis, but it can also be found in *Trichomonas vaginitis*. The hanging drop preparation of saline and 10% potassium hydroxide should be examined microscopically. Trichomonads can often be identified in the saline preparation; they are motile, and the beating flagella can be seen under high-power magnification. Clue cells have a characteristic appearance, with a speckled cytoplasm of the squamous epithelial cells and serrated cell surface. To confirm the diagnosis of bacterial vaginosis, clue cells should be present in large numbers and white blood cells should be virtually absent from the field.

The microscopic examination to confirm the diagnosis of Candida vaginitis can be difficult, because the yeast elements are often not seen. This common infectious disorder of the vagina requires a culture. Culture will propagate Candida organisms far more often than they can be detected by scanning hanging drop preparations for hyphae and mycelia (12). The culture is especially important in patients with a chronic vaginal problem. Patients should not be subjected to long-term treatment for Candida infection unless the organisms are grown in culture. Treatment does not meet their therapeutic needs, and too often a vaginal reaction will develop that is caused by local sensitivity to the propylene glycol present in most vaginal creams and suppositories (18).

A number of diagnostic tests can be helpful in some patients with vaginitis. Because the presenting sign for salpingitis can be an abnormal vaginal discharge, cervical culture for C. trachomatis and N. gonorrhoeae is appropriate when the physician suspects this possibility; however, all vaginal cultures should propagate bacteria, because the vagina has a diverse bacterial flora, similar in variety to that of the lower bowel, with much smaller numbers (19). A positive bacterial culture result should not be equated with disease. The most harmful therapeutic interventions that I have seen over the years involve antibiotic treatment of patients because vaginal cultures isolated an organism, for example, Escherichia coli. Treating a non-existent entity, E. coli vaginitis, can result in either antibiotic induced Candida vaginitis or an allergic reaction to the antibiotics. Vaginitis should not be treated with antibiotics if the cause is in doubt. The patient will not get better, and the physician can cause harm.

Finally, if the patient complains of persistent vaginal burning with no definitive findings on pH, microscopic, or culture studies, consideration should be given to the possibility of allergic vaginitis (18). Allergic vaginitis can be suspected if the patient can relate her vaginal symptoms to specific exposures, such as vaginal antifungal cream, vaginal spermicidal agents, or male ejaculate. Witkin and colleagues demonstrated the presence of immunoglobulin E and an increased number of eosinophils in the vaginal fluid of such women.

For patients with a chronic vaginal problem, a Gram stain examination of vaginal secretions can be useful. For physicians without a microscope, it can be used to diagnose bacterial vaginosis (15). It provides a permanent record of the initial cytologic findings and a standard for later comparison. In addition, culture or PCR test for T. vaginalis is in order when there is persistent vaginal discharge and microscopic findings show no trichomonads. Small numbers of trichomonads may not be seen on microscopic examination but can be detected by culture or PCR (20).

The cervix is the next site of evaluation. The gross visual evaluation of the cervix can be subject to misinterpretation. A large area of columnar epithelium on the surface can look inflamed and can bleed easily when a Papanicolaou smear is obtained. Many physicians equate this with cervicitis. One immediate diagnostic aid is a cotton-tipped applicator gently rotated in the endocervical canal and then examined against a white background. Mucopus will be evident, which confirms the diagnosis (21). It is especially important to perform this examination of the cervix when many white blood cells are seen in the vaginal hanging

drop examination. Large numbers of white blood cells should not be present on the microscopic examination of a patient with bacterial vaginosis. When they are, the physician should remember that it is possible for a patient to have concurrent conditions, bacterial vaginosis and cervicitis, due to Neisseria gonorrhea or Chlamydia trachomatis. In patients with cervicitis, tests for N. gonorrhoeae and C. trachomatis should be done. There is a deoxyribonucleic acid probe for gonorrhea and to confirm Chlamydia; the PCR test is the most sensitive for it can detect the presence of a small number of organisms not detected with culture (22).

The pelvic examination is too often not done in a postoperative patient, because the first fever occurs at night or after the patient has been discharged. The examination can be very helpful even though there is a great deal of pelvic induration after pelvic surgery and usually no purulent discharge. If the uterus is present after delivery or an abortion, the cervical os should be evaluated for the presence of purulent discharge or tissue. Forceps can be placed in the endocervical canal to remove visible retained placental tissue or membranes, and aerobic cultures are obtained. If no tissue is visible in the os, vaginal ultrasound can determine the presence of retained tissue in the uterus. In the posthysterectomy patient, the vaginal cuff should be probed for purulent material. Pelvic thrombophlebitis is the diagnosis of exclusion in a patient who remains febrile after antibiotic treatment and has no evidence of a pelvic abscess by imaging evaluation. Vaginal ultrasound examination is an excellent screening method but better delineation of pelvic disease can be achieved with magnetic resonance imaging or computed tomography if the diagnosis remains in doubt.

When salpingitis is suspected, the evaluation can be extremely important in making the diagnosis. The key to any evaluation is gentleness. Forceful pressure at the time of pelvic examination can cause pain when the pelvic viscera are inflamed. The physician's focus should be to determine whether there is adnexal tenderness or a mass. If pain is elicited and there is no pelvic mass, more forceful pressure to palpate the ovaries simply causes more discomfort without gaining any additional diagnostic information. Other important diagnostic studies should be obtained for these women. The least invasive and probably the most helpful is microscopic evaluation of a vaginal smear. Westrom has stated that he has never found salpingitis confirmed by laparoscopy when there were not a large number of white blood cells on the vaginal smear (23) and one subsequent study found this the most sensitive test for diagnosis (24). White blood cells can be present in a patient with cervicitis alone, but this simple noninvasive test is especially helpful for confirming the diagnosis. If white blood cells are absent, causes other than infection are responsible. Material should be obtained from the endocervix for detection of N. gonorrhoeae and C. trachomatis. PCR should be used as the screen for C. trachomatis. Either a simple culture, a DNA probe, or PCR can be used for N. gonorrhoeae. Imaging techniques can be helpful in some patients. For patients that have a great deal of pain, a screening vaginal ultrasound examination can demonstrate a fluid-filled mass that was not detected by pelvic examination. In some patients with pelvic pain, an adnexal pregnancy sac can be detected. Obviously, an ectopic pregnancy should not be treated with antibiotics. If the physician elicits a history of intravenous drug use by this patient or her sexual partner, blood should be drawn to screen for the antibodies to hepatitis B virus, hepatitis C, and the human immunodeficiency virus.

This is an outline of the general approach to the patient with a pelvic infection. It emphasizes a hands-on evaluation because this skill yields the most important immediate diagnostic hints.

REFERENCES

1. Wiesenfeld HC, Macio I. The infrequent use of office based diagnostic tests for vaginitis. *Am J Obstet Gynecol* 1999;181:39–41.
2. Jacobson L, Westrom L. Objectivized diagnosis of acute pelvic inflammatory disease: diagnostic and prognostic value of routine laparoscopy. *Am J Obstet Gynecol* 1969;105:1088–1098.
3. Peipert JF, Ness RB, Blume J, et al. Clinical predictors of endometritis in patients with symptoms and signs of pelvic inflammatory disease. *Am J Obstet Gynecol* 2001;184:856–864.
4. Centers for Disease Control and Prevention. 1998 Guidelines for treatment of sexually transmitted diseases. *MMWR* 1998;47:1–80.
5. Cates W Jr, Joesoef MR, Goldman MB. Atypical pelvic inflammatory disease: can we identify clinical predictors? *Am J Obstet Gynecol* 1993;169:341–346.
6. Hemsel DL, Ledger WJ, Martens M, et al. Concerns regarding the centers for disease control's published guidelines for pelvic inflammatory disease. *Clin Infect Dis* 2001;32:103–107.
7. Cates W, Wasserheit JN. Genital chlamydia infections: epidemiology and reproductive sequelae. *Am J Obstet Gynecol* 1991;164:1771–1781.
8. Sobel JD, Faro S, Force RW, et al. Vulvovaginal candidiasis: epidemiologic, diagnostic, and therapeutic considerations. *Am J Obstet Gynecol* 1988;178:203–211.
9. Eschenbach DA, Hillier S, Critchlow C, et al. Diagnosis and clinical manifestations of bacterial vaginosis. *Am J Obstet Gynecol* 1988;158:819–828.
10. Klebanoff MA, Carey C, Hauth JC, et al. Failure of metronidazole to prevent pre-term delivery among pregnant women with asymptomatic trichomonas vaginalis infection. *N Engl J Med* 2001;345:487–493.
11. Wolner-Hanssen P. Silent pelvic inflammatory disease: is it overstated? *Obstet Gynecol* 1995;86:321–325.
12. McCormack WM, Starko KM, Zinner SH. Symptoms associated with vaginal colonization with yeast. *Am J Obstet Gynecol* 1988;158:31–33.
13. Ledger WJ, Polaneczky MM, Yih MC, et al. Difficulties in the diagnosis of candida vaginitis. *Infect Dis Clin Pract* 2000;9:66–69.
14. Abbott J. Clinical and microscopic diagnosis of vaginal yeast infection: a prospective analysis. *Am Emerg Med* 1995;25:587–591.
15. Schwebke JR, Hillier SL, Sobel JD, et al. Validity of the vaginal gram stain for the diagnosis of bacterial vaginosis. *Obstet Gynecol* 1996;88:573–576.
16. Rompalo AM, Gaydos CA, Shah N, et al. Evaluation of use of a single intravaginal swab to detect multiple sexually transmitted infections in active-duty military women. *Clin Infect Dis* 2001;33:1455–1461.
17. Koutsky LA, Stevens CE, Holmes KK, et al. Underdiagnosis of genital herpes by current clinical and viral-isolation procedures. *N Engl J Med* 1992;326:1533–1539.
18. Witkin SS, Jeremias J, Ledger WJ. Vaginal eosinophils and IgE antibodies to candida albicans in women with recurrent vaginitis. *J Med Vet Mycol* 1989;27:57–58.
19. Bartlett JG, Onderdonk AB, Drude E, et al. Quantitative bacteriology of the vaginal flora. *J Infect Dis* 1977;136:271–277.
20. Jeremias J, Draper D, Zeigert M, et al. Detection of *Trichomonas vaginalis* using the polymerase chain reaction in pregnant and non-pregnant women. *Infect Dis Obstet Gynecol* 1994;2:16–19.
21. Branham RC, Paavonen J, Stevens CE, et al. Mucopurulent cervicitis: the ignored counterpart in women of urethritis in men. *N Engl J Med* 1984;311:1–6.
22. Witkin SS, Jeremias J, Toth M, Ledger WJ. Detection of *Chlamydia trachomatis* by the polymerase chain reaction in the cervices of women with acute salpingitis. *Am J Obstet Gynecol* 1993;168:1438–1442.
23. Westrom L. Clinical manifestation and diagnosis of pelvic inflammatory disease. *J Reprod Med* 1983;28:703–708.
24. Peipert JF, Boardman L, Hogan JW. Laboratory evaluation of acute upper genital tract infection. *Obstet Gynecol* 1996;87:730–736.

CHAPTER 110

Pelvic Inflammatory Disease and Tuboovarian Abscess

Richard L. Sweet

PELVIC INFLAMMATORY DISEASE

Pelvic inflammatory disease (PID) is a spectrum of upper genital tract inflammatory disorders, which includes any combination of endometritis, salpingitis, tubo-ovarian abscess, and pelvic peritonitis (1). It is one of the most frequent and important infections among non-pregnant women of reproductive age. PID is associated with major clinical, public health, and economic concerns, including diagnosis, treatment, prevention, long term sequelae, health care costs and morbidity and mortality (2). An estimated 780,000 to 1.2 million women are diagnosed with PID annually in the United States (3,4), some 10% to 25% of whom are hospitalized (3,5). The economic costs of PID and its sequelae in the United States are estimated to be more than $10.2 billion annually (4). Rein et al, taking into account a decrease in cases of PID and the change to less expensive ambulatory treatment estimated the direct medical costs of PID and its sequelae to be nearly $2 billion (3). Recently, it has been estimated that one half to two thirds of cases of PID go unrecognized (6). Thus these estimates of the medical and economic costs of PID may be understated.

Of more concern than the infection itself is that at least one of every four women who develop PID suffers serious long-term sequelae—infertility, ectopic pregnancy, tuboovarian abscess (TOA), pyosalpinx, chronic pelvic pain, or pelvic adhesive disease (7). In the most recent analysis of the Swedish laparoscopy cohort, infertility was demonstrated in 16% of PID patients compared to 3% of controls (8). Similar increases in ectopic pregnancy rates were reported. Both risks increase with recurrences. TOA, the major early complication of acute PID, is diagnosed in 10% to 15% of patients hospitalized for treatment of acute PID (9). Symptoms of chronic pelvic adhesive disease develop in nearly 20% of affected women.

Risk Factors

The importance of risk assessment in both the management and prevention of PID has been emphasized (10,11). Women who have a history of previous PID are at increased risk for recurrences. Westrom noted that nearly one in four women with PID suffers a subsequent episode (12).

A strong association exists between sexually transmitted pathogens, especially *N. gonorrhoeae* and *C. trachomatis,* and acute PID; women with a history of these sexually transmitted diseases are at increased risk for PID (13–18).

Bacterial vaginosis, a perturbation in which the lactobacilli-predominant normal vaginal microflora is replaced by high concentrations of *Gardnerella vaginalis*, anaerobic bacteria, and *Mycoplasma hominis*, has been shown to be a risk factor for acute PID (19–25). The anaerobic organisms associated with bacterial vaginosis include *Prevotella* species, *Mobiluncus* and peptostreptococci.

Women with multiple sexual partners were found to be nearly five times more likely to develop PID than were monogamous women (26). Jossens and colleagues (11) reported that women with two or more sexual partners in the previous 30 to 60 days were at significantly increased risk for PID (27). In contradistinction, these authors noted that having multiple lifetime partners was not a risk factor for acute PID.

Young age has also been associated with an increased frequency of PID. Westrom reported that nearly 70% of women with acute salpingitis were 25 years of age or younger and that 33% had their first infection before age 19 years (12). Sexually active adolescents are three times more likely to develop PID than are 25- to 29-year-old women (28). Indeed, among the group aged 13 to 15 years, this risk is increased tenfold. It is thought that this dramatic increased risk is due to the high prevalence of sexually transmitted diseases among adolescents; to multiple sexual partners; and to failure to use contraceptives, several of which (condom, diaphragm, oral contraceptives) protect against PID. The intrauterine device (IUD) is an additional risk factor in the development of acute salpingitis. Initially, it was estimated that IUD users have a threefold to fivefold greater risk for developing PID (28–32). Later studies have lowered this risk to a twofold to threefold increase compared with women who use no contraception. A syndrome of progressive endometritis has been associated with IUD use; menorrhagia, metrorrhagia, and leukorrhea were noted and were followed by progressive endometritis, parametritis, peritonitis, and pelvic abscess formation (33). Additional implicated risk factors for PID include cigarette smoking (34,35), substance abuse (36,37), menses (38), and douching (11,39–43).

Etiology

Although research in the last 20 years has provided many insights into the causation of acute PID, the exact involvement and spread of organisms and the interaction between different organisms remain unknown. PID is caused by microorganisms ascending from the lower genital tract (cervix and vagina) into the upper genital tract (endometrial cavity and fallopian tubes). As a result the etiology of PID is polymicrobic in nature with a wide variety of microorganisms recovered from the upper genital tract of women with acute PID (1,13,14,15,44–52). These putative microorganisms include *Neisseria gonorrhoeae*, *Chlamydia trachomatis*, anaerobic and aerobic bacteria from the endogenous vaginal flora such as *Prevotella* species, *Peptostreptococci* sp., *Gardnerella vaginalis*, *Escherichia coli*, *Haemophilus influenzae* and aerobic streptococci. The majority of proven cases of PID are associated with sexually transmitted pathogens, most importantly *N. gonorrhoeae* and *C. trachomatis* (2,17,53). Many of the non-STD microorganisms associated with acute PID are those involved with bacterial vaginosis (54,55).

Recently, attention has focused on "unrecognized" (subclinical) PID, a term applied to the situation where women with documented tubal factor infertility have no history of being diagnosed or treated for PID despite confirmation of chronic inflammatory residua obstructing the fallopian tubes (56). Whether the same microorganisms that cause acute symptomatic PID are similar to those associated with "unrecognized" PID remains to be elucidated. Preliminary studies by our group suggest that the STD organisms *N. gonorrhoeae* and *C. trachomatis* and the BV-associated microorganisms are also responsible for unrecognized PID (57).

Two theories emerged to explain the pathogenesis of PID. The first proposed that either *N. gonorrhoeae* or *C. trachomatis* organisms initiate the process by producing tissue damage and changing the normal environment, allowing superinfection by aerobes and anaerobes from the cervix and vagina (58–60). The second hypothesis is that PID must be a polymicrobial infection from the outset (26,46). Support for this hypothesis comes from studies that demonstrate the presence of aerobes and anaerobes in the fallopian tubes of women with salpingitis despite the absence of *N. gonorrhoeae* and *C. trachomatis*, even in the endocervix (61).

Neisseria gonorrhoeae Infection

Salpingitis was traditionally categorized as gonococcal or nongonococcal, but this distinction has become outdated. Initial work that employed cervical cultures to identify the pathogen revealed *N. gonorrhoeae* in 33% to 81% of women with PID (26,45,62–64). Except for the presence of *N. gonorrhoeae* or *C. trachomatis* cervical flora of women with acute salpingitis is not appreciably different from that of normal women (59). Comparisons of organisms obtained by culdocentesis or laparoscopy with endocervical canal specimens have shown poor correlation. This suggests that cervical flora is not representative of the tubal flora of PID (Table 110.1) (45,46,58–61,63,64).

The most widely held theory for the pathogenesis of *N. gonorrhoeae* in PID is that the pathogen gains access to the upper genital tract at or near the end of menses through the breakdown of local host defense mechanisms at the level of the cervix and can then spread directly to the adnexae. Symptoms develop in 66% to 75% of women with PID at the end of or just after menstruation (62). Similarly, Sweet and coworkers demonstrated that PID associated with *C. trachomatis* occurs at the end of or shortly after the menstrual period, with no cases of chlamydial PID noted after day 14 of the menstrual cycle (63).

Chlamydia trachomatis Infection

C. trachomatis infection is the most common bacterial sexually transmitted disease in the United States (44). Initially, it appeared

TABLE 110.1. Isolation of *Neisseria gonorrhoeae* and Anaerobic and Facultative Bacteria from Patients with Acute Salpingitis

Study	Number of patients	Endocervical *N. gonorrhoeae* (%)	Culdocentesis		
			N. gonorrhoeae only (%)	*N. gonorrhoeae* plus anaerobes/ facultatives (%)	Anaerobes/facultatives only (%)
Sweet et al.[46]	26	50	31	31	31
Eschenbach et al.[45]	54	39	28	5	24
Thompson et al.[64a]	30	80	21	21	58
Cunningham et al.[58]	104	54	22	32	46
Chow et al.[59]	20	65	0	5	90
Monif et al.[60]	17	94	31	31	38

to be more common in Scandinavia, where the organism was recovered from cervical cultures in 20% to 50% of patients with acute salpingitis (64–67) and from fallopian tube cultures in 30% (64,65,67). Initial studies in the United States failed to identify *C. trachomatis* as a major putative agent in acute PID (45,46,62,64). However, serologic studies in Seattle and San Francisco demonstrated a fourfold rise in serum antibody titer in 20% to 23% of PID patients (45,46), suggesting that the organism was important in the United States as well. One possible reason for this discrepancy is that patients in the Scandinavian studies included many with milder forms of infection who might have been treated as outpatients in the United States, whereas the US studies included only hospitalized patients. Patients with chlamydial salpingitis often have a milder clinical presentation, despite a higher erythrocyte sedimentation rate and more inflammation, resulting in more tubal damage (68). More recently U.S. investigations have clearly demonstrated that *C. trachomatis* is a principal agent in acute PID and can be recovered from the upper genital tract of roughly 20% to 40% of patients with acute disease (14,15). Moreover, our group demonstrated failure to provide antimicrobial coverage for chlamydiae results in persistent chlamydial infection in the upper genital tract despite supposed clinical cure (14).

Additional evidence that *C. trachomatis* plays a role in acute salpingitis is indirect. Epidemiologic studies have suggested that *C. trachomatis* plays a role in infertility secondary to salpingitis and tubal obstruction (69–79). These investigations demonstrated in a wide variety of populations and geographic areas that women with tubal factor infertility were significantly more likely to have had prior systemic chlamydial infection as documented serologically than pregnant controls or non tubal factor infertility patients. Similarly an association of prior chlamydial infection with ectopic pregnancy has been reported (73,80–83). Thus, the two major sequelae of acute PID, tubal infertility and ectopic pregnancy, have been associated with previous chlamydial infection.

Recent research has elucidated a model for the pathogenesis of chlamydial PID and its sequelae (84–90). It has been suggested that chlamydial PID is an immune-mediated disease resulting from host immune responses to a chlamydial heat shock protein Chsp 60 (84–90). Thus, *C. trachomatis* elicits an inflammatory response similar to a delayed hypersensitivity reaction. The fallopian tube mucosa shares a high degree of homology with Chsp and thus the immune response results in damage to the fallopian tube (84–90).

Genital Tract Mycoplasmas

M. hominis has been postulated to be a potential pathogen in PID, although the data are soft. Whereas a large percentage of women with acute salpingitis have antibodies against *M. hominis*, the organism is infrequently recovered from tubal and peritoneal fluid cultures from these women with PID (91). Experimentation using tubal organ cultures has recorded decreased ciliary activity after infection with this agent, but no cytopathic effect has yet been demonstrated (92). *M. hominis* is present in association with bacterial vaginosis (93) and thus, any role that *M. hominis* might have in the etiology of acute PID is probably related to its presence in the microflora of bacterial vaginosis.

Ureaplasma urealyticum has been frequently recovered from the lower genital tract of women with acute PID (range, 24% to 81%) but it has rarely been isolated from the fallopian tube (45,62,64,91). In general, if there is any role for *U. urealyticum* in the etiology of PID, it is minimal (8).

More recently a third genital tract *Mycoplasma, Mycoplasma genitalium* has been proposed as a putative agent for PID.

TABLE 110.2. Bacteria Frequently Recovered from the Upper Genital Tract of Women With Acute Salpingitis

Anaerobes	Aerobes
Prevotella bivia	Gardnerella vaginalis
Prevotella species	Escherichia coli
Peptostreptococcus species	Nonhemolytic streptococci
	Group B streptococci

M. genitalium has been demonstrated in the cervix with use of polymerase chain reaction technology (94) and has produced salpingitis in animal models including non-human primates (95,96). However, no investigations have demonstrated *M. genitalium* in the fallopian tubes of women with acute PID and thus its role in acute PID remains undetermined (6).

Infection with Anaerobic and Facultative Bacteria

Facultative and anaerobic bacteria are often isolated from fallopian tube and cul-de-sac cultures of women with PID (14,15,60,62). Those most often recovered are *Peptostreptococcus, Prevotella* (formerly *Bacteroides*) spp., *Escherichia coli, G. vaginalis*, and facultative streptococci (Table 110.2). These organisms are commonly found in the lower genital tract. Whether they function initially as direct pathogens or whether they require the presence of an initiating organism such as *N. gonorrhoeae* or *C. trachomatis* remains controversial. Studies reporting the results of cultures obtained from the upper genital tract of patients with acute PID are summarized in Table 110.3. In these studies, mixed anaerobic and aerobic bacteria were the most commonly recovered group of organisms (15,47–50,97). In a report, Jossens and colleagues noted that in nearly one third of acute PID cases, only anaerobic and/or aerobic bacteria were recovered from the upper genital tract (17). In addition, among the 65% of acute PID patients with *N. gonorrhoeae* or *C. trachomatis* present, half also had anaerobic or aerobic bacteria recovered.

It is apparent that many of these nongonococcal, nonchlamydial microorganisms have been implicated in bacterial vaginosis, a complex synergistic vaginal infection associated with *G. vaginalis*, members of the *Prevotella* (*Bacterioides*) spp. (especially *P. bivius, P. disiens*, and *P. capillosus*), *Peptostreptococcus* spp., the mobile curved anaerobic rod *Mobiluncus* spp., alphahemolytic streptococci, and *M. hominis* (98–102). Eschenbach initially postulated that bacterial vaginosis (BV) might be an antecedent precursor in the lower genital tract for the development of nongonococcal nonchlamydial PID (103). Several investigations have demonstrated an association between bacterial vaginosis and PID (23–25,47,50,51,55,104). Paavonen and co-workers reported that nine (29%) of 31 women with laparoscopic confirmed acute PID had BV compared with zero of 14 controls (47). All nine of these women had histologic endometritis present on endometrial biopsy. Subsequently, Eschenbach et al. noted that women with BV were significantly more likely to have adnexal tenderness (4% vs. 0.3%), uterine tenderness (4% vs. 1%), cervical motion tenderness (3% vs. 0.6%), and a diagnosis of PID (3% vs. 0%) than control women without BV (104). Hillier and colleagues reported that the BV-associated microorganisms (*Prevotella, Peptostreptococcus* and *M. hominis*) were associated with histologic endometritis in confirmed cases of PID (55). Even after controlling for chlamydial and gonococcal infection the recovery of BV associated bacteria from the endometrial cavity was independently associated with histologic endometritis (55). Recently,

TABLE 110.3.   Recovery of Microorganisms from the Upper Genital Tract of Women with Acute Pelvic Inflammatory Disease

Investigation	Number (%) of positive culture results		
	Chlamydia trachomatis	*Neisseria gonorrhoeae*	Anaerobes and facultatives
Brunham et al.[49]	21 (40%)	8 (16%)	10 (20%)
Heinonen et al.[48]	7 (19%)	15 (42%)	28 (78%)
Paavonen et al.[47]	12 (34%)	4 (11%)	24 (69%)
Sweet[97]	45 (24%)	54 (39%)	129 (68%)
Wasserheit et al.[15]	11 (44%)	8 (35%)	11 (44%)
Soper et al.[50]	1 (1.2%)[a]	32 (38%)[a]	12 (13%)[a]
	6 (7.4%)[b]	49 (98%)[b]	16 (32%)[b]
Hillier[51]	3 (4%)[a]	16 (19%)[a]	43 (50%)[a]
	23 (13%)[b]	44 (25%)[b]	168 (94%)[b]

[a]Fallopian tube/cul de sac.
[b]Endometrium.

Soper et al. noted in women with laparoscopy confirmed PID that BV was present in 61.8% (50). In addition, all the anaerobes recovered from the upper genital tract in their study were the BV associated microorganisms (50). Korn et al. noted that 10 (45%) of 22 women with BV had plasma cell endometritis compared to 1 (5%) of 19 controls (23). Peipert and co-workers reported that objective evidence (histologic, microbiologic or laparoscopic) of upper genital tract infection was present in 14 (56%) of 25 women with a clinical diagnosis of BV compared with 27 (30%) of 91 without BV ($P = .015$) (24). Using logistic regression, the presence of BV associated with a threefold increased risk of upper genital tract infection (O.R. 3.0; 95% C.I. 1.2 to 7.6). Korn et al. more recently demonstrated that plasma cell endometritis was present in 42% of women with BV versus 13% of controls (O.R. 6.5; 95%; C.I. 1.7 to 3.5) (25).

Diagnosis

Acute PID presents with a broad spectrum of manifestations that include both overt clinically apparent and unrecognized infection (2,6). As a result the specificity of any single clinical or laboratory finding is low and no symptom or sign is pathognomonic for acute PID (6). Two thirds (range, 30% to 75%) of

infertile women with post infection tubal factor infertility have no history of being diagnosed or treated for PID (72,77,105–107). Thus, unrecognized (subclinical) infection appears to be responsible for the majority of PID and tubal factor infertility post PID. At the opposite end of the spectrum, up to one-third of women presenting with abdominal/pelvic pain presumed to be acute PID are found at laparoscopy to have either other diagnosis or no disease at all (6,108–114).

Traditionally, acute PID was believed to present with lower abdominal/pelvic pain, purulent cervical discharge, cervical motion tenderness, adnexal tenderness, fever and leukocytosis (2). However, laparoscopy has shown that the diagnosis of acute PID based on these clinical criteria was often inaccurate and unsatisfactory (109). Among 814 women laparoscoped for a presumed diagnosis of acute PID by Jacobsen and Westrom, 65% had visual confirmation of the diagnosis (109).

The most common symptoms and physical findings in patients with laparoscopically confirmed acute salpingitis are listed in Table 110.4 (109). Among the presenting symptoms, only a history of fever or chills was significantly more common in the group with verified PID than in the control group whose pelvic findings at laparoscopy were normal. Whereas a documented fever, adnexal tenderness, elevated erythrocyte sedimentation

TABLE 110.4.   Frequency of Symptoms and Findings in Women with Surgically Documented Acute Pelvic Inflammatory Disease

Symptom or finding	Acute pelvic inflammatory disease ($n = 622$) No. %	Normal pelvis ($n = 184$) No. %	P
Lower abdominal pain	585 (94)	173 (94)	NS
Increased vaginal discharge	340 (55)	104 (56.5)	NS
Fever or chills	257 (41)	36 (19.6)	.001
Irregular bleeding	221 (36)	79 (42.9)	NS
Urinary symptoms	116 (19)	37 (20.1)	NS
Gastrointestinal symptoms	64 (10)	17 (9.2)	NS
Fever on admission	205 (33)	26 (14)	.001
Adnexal tenderness	573 (92)	160 (87)	.05
Increased erythrocyte sedimentation rate	473 (76)	97 (53)	.001
Abnormal vaginal discharge	394 (63)	26 (14)	.001

Adapted from Jacobsen, Westrom L. Objectivized diagnosis of acute pelvic inflammatory disease. *Am J Obstet Gynecol* 1969;105:1088.

TABLE 110.5.   Criteria for Diagnosis of Pelvic Inflammatory Disease

All three must be present:
  History of low abdominal pain and presence of low abdominal tenderness, with or without evidence of rebound
  Cervical motion tenderness
  Adnexal tenderness
  plus
One of these must be present:
  Temperature of at least 38°C
  Leukocytosis with white blood cell count above 10,000/mm³
  A culdocentesis that yields peritoneal fluid containing white blood cells and bacteria
  Presence of an inflammatory mass noted on pelvic examination or Sonography
  Elevated erythrocyte sedimentation rate
  Evidence of *N. gonorrhoeae* or *C. trachomatis* in the endocervix
    A Gram stain from the endocervix revealing gram-negative intracellular diplococci suggestive of *N. gonorrhoeae*
    A monoclonal antibody-directed smear from endocervical secretions revealing *C. trachomatis*
    Mucopurulent endocervicitis
  Presence of >10 white blood cells per oil-immersion field on Gram stain of endocervical discharge

TABLE 110.6.   Criteria for Clinical Diagnosis of PID[a]

Minimum Criteria
  • Lower abdominal tenderness
  • Adnexal tenderness
  • Cervical motion tenderness
Additional Criteria
  • Oral temperature ≥38.3°C (101°F)
  • Abnormal cervical or vaginal discharge
  • Elevated ESR or CRP
  • Laboratory documentation of cervical infection with *N. gonorrhoeae* or *C. trachomatis*
Definite criteria
  • Histopathologic endometritis on endometrial biopsy
  • Transvaginal ultrasonography or other imaging techniques showing thickened fluid-filled tubes or tubo-ovarian complex
  • Laparoscopic confirmation of PID

[a]Based on references 1, 10, 117.
CRP, C-reactive protein; ESR, erythrocyte sedimentation rate; PID, pelvic inflammatory disease.

rate, and abnormal vaginal discharge were statistically significantly more frequent among verified cases of acute PID, the differences were indistinct clinically. Most importantly, only 20% of the patients with visually confirmed acute PID had the entire constellation of the classically described signs and symptoms described above.

While laparoscopy is the "gold standard" for the diagnosis of acute PID, it is logistically and economically impractical for all patients with presumed PID. To improve the accuracy of clinical diagnosis, Hager and co-workers (115) studied clinical and laboratory information from women found to have PID by laparoscopy and formulated standardized criteria for clinical diagnosis and for grading the severity of laparoscopically confirmed salpingitis. The criteria have since been revised and are listed in Table 110.5. Kahn and co-workers (112) reviewed studies addressing the diagnosis of acute PID in which laparoscopy was considered the diagnostic "gold standard." These authors noted that the history and physical findings were reasonably sensitive but nonspecific. The only factors that had both high sensitivity and specificity were elevated erythrocyte sedimentation rate or C-reactive protein and findings on endometrial biopsy positive for plasma cell endometritis. Endometrial biopsy demonstrating acute endometrial inflammation has good sensitivity and specificity and thus has been suggested as a less invasive alternative to laparoscopy for confirming a clinical diagnosis of acute PID (15,47,106,116). However, biopsy results are not available on a rapid basis; thus limiting the clinical applicability of endometrial biopsy.

To enhance the sensitivity for diagnosing acute PID, the CDC recommends a "low threshold for diagnosis" and that in mild cases treatment for PID should be initiated utilizing the minimum criteria listed in Table 110.6 (1,10). When patients have more severe clinical findings, the CDC suggests a more elaborate diagnostic evaluation as noted in Table 110.6.

Treatment of Uncomplicated Pelvic Inflammatory Disease

The goals in the management of acute PID are to preserve fertility, prevent ectopic pregnancy, and reduce long-term inflammatory

sequelae. Optimal treatment of acute PID requires early diagnosis and prompt institution of antimicrobial therapy effective against the major pathogens known to be involved in the disease process. Studies using hysterosalpingographic and laparoscopic evaluation of tubal status have demonstrated that women treated early in the course of infection have a better chance of retaining tubal patency (118,119). Hillis and colleagues reported that women treated after 3 days or more of symptoms had a significantly greater infertility rate (19.7%) compared with those treated with less than 3 days of symptoms (8.3%) (119). Although the advent of antibiotics has reportedly decreased sequelae of salpingitis such as abscess formation, infertility, and the need for operative intervention, major complications and sequelae still occur in a large portion of treated women (7,12,120,121).

In May 2002, the Centers for Disease Control and Prevention published new recommendations for the treatment of acute PID (44). The guidelines for oral treatment of acute PID are provided in Table 110.7 and those for parenteral treatment in Table 110.8.

Lack of anaerobic coverage with ofloxacin is a concern and thus metronidazole is added to this oral treatment regimen (44).

TABLE 110.7.   Centers for Disease Control and Prevention Recommended Treatment Schedules for Oral Treatment of Acute Pelvic Inflammatory Disease, 2002

Regimen A
Ofloxacin 400 mg orally twice a day for 14 d
OR
Levofloxacin 500 mg orally once daily for 14 d
WITH OR WITHOUT
Metronidazole 500 mg orally twice a day for 14 d
Regimen B
Ceftriaxone 250 mg IM in a single dose
OR
Cefoxitin 2 g IM in a single dose and probenecid 1 g orally administered Concurrently in a single dose
OR
Other parenteral third-generation cephalosporins (e.g., ceftizoxime or cefotaxime)
PLUS
Doxycycline 100 mg orally twice a day for 14 d
WITH OR WITHOUT
Metronidazole 500 mg orally twice a day for 14 d

TABLE 110.8. Centers for Disease Control and Prevention Recommended Treatment Schedules for Parenteral Treatment of Acute Pelvic Inflammatory Disease, 2002

Regimen A
Cefotetan 2 g IV every 12 h
OR
Cefoxitin 2 g IV every 6 h
PLUS
Doxycycline 100 mg orally or IV every 12 h
Regimen B
Clindamycin 900 mg IV every 8 h
PLUS
Gentamicin loading dose IV or IM (2 mg/kg) followed by a maintenance dose every 8 h
Single-daily dosing may be substituted

TABLE 110.9. Criteria for Hospitalization of Women with Acute Pelvic Inflammatory Disease, 2002

- Surgical emergencies (e.g., appendicitis) cannot be excluded
- The patient is pregnant
- The patient does not respond clinically to oral antimicrobial therapy
- The patient is unable to follow or tolerate an outpatient oral regimen
- The patient has severe illness, nausea and vomiting, or high fever
- The patient has a tubo-ovarian abscess

Similarly, metronidazole may be added to the oral regimen with cephalosporin plus doxycycline (44,122). Because of pain associated with IV infusion, doxycycline should be administered orally, even when parenteral therapy or hospitalization is chosen (44). Parenteral therapy may be discontinued 24 hours following clinical improvement. For parenteral regimen A, oral therapy with doxycycline should continue to complete 14 days of therapy (44). With tubo-ovarian abscess clindamycin or metronidazole should also be given orally to provide more effective anaerobic coverage (44). With parenteral regimen B, parenteral therapy may also be discontinued 24 hours following clinical improvement and oral clindamycin 450 mg orally four times a day be given to complete a 14-day course of treatment (44). The CDC criteria for hospitalization are listed in Table 110.9.

Many randomized clinical trials have demonstrated the efficacy of both parenteral and oral regimens for treating PID (Table 110.10 and 110.11) (122). However, these clinical trials do not provide information regarding intermediate and long-term outcomes (eg. infertility, ectopic pregnancy, and recurrent infection). Recently, the results from the much anticipated Pelvic Inflammatory Disease Evaluation and Clinical Health (PEACH) randomized trial of the effectiveness of inpatient and outpatient strategies for treating women with acute PID was reported (123). PEACH enrolled 831 women with clinical signs and symptoms of mild-to-moderate PID into a multicenter randomized clinical trial of inpatient treatment initiated by IV cefoxitin and doxycy-

cline versus outpatient treatment with a single IM injection of cefoxitin and oral doxycycline. Short-term clinical and microbiologic improvements were similar in both groups (123). After a mean follow-up of 35 months, pregnancy rates were nearly equal (42.0% for outpatients and 41.7% for inpatients) (123). These data should help to resolve the age-old dilemma of outpatient (oral) versus inpatient (parenteral) therapy for acute PID.

TUBOOVARIAN ABSCESS

Tuboovarian abscess (TOA) is one of the major complications and early sequela of PID (2). Although most studies note a prevalence of 10% to 15% (range 3% to 16%), TOA has been reported to occur in up to one third of patients hospitalized with PID (9,124–132). Despite the clinical availability of many potent broad-spectrum antimicrobial agents for treatment of pelvic infections, pelvic abscess remains a major cause of morbidity and a diagnostic and therapeutic challenge for gynecologists.

Diagnosis

The most frequent presenting complaint (more than 90% of cases) of patients with TOA is abdominal or pelvic pain (9,125,130,133,134). Most have fever and leukocytosis, but many patients who harbor a TOA have normal temperature and white cell count (9). Temperature of at least 37.8°C has been reported in 60% to 80% of patients, and leukocytosis was reported in 66% to 80% (9,124,125,134–136). The findings of vaginal discharge, abnormal uterine bleeding, nausea, vomiting, diarrhea, dysuria, and frequency are inconsistent. Because the presenting signs and symptoms of uncomplicated PID and TOA are similar, diagnosis

TABLE 110.10. Pooled Cure Rates in the Treatment of Acute Pelvic Inflammatory Disease for Antibiotic Regimens with More Than One Study

Drug regimen	Number of studies	Number of patients	Clinical cure rate (%)	Microbiologic cure rate (%)[a]
Inpatient				
Clindamycin plus aminoglycoside	10	372	92	97
Cefoxitin plus doxycycline	7	338	93	98
Cefotetan plus doxycycline	2	86	94	100
Ciprofloxacin	4	90	94	96[b]
Metronidazole plus doxycycline	2	36	75	71
Outpatient				
Cefoxitin plus doxycycline	2	59	95	91

[a]Based on eradication of *N. gonorrhoeae* and *C. trachomatis*.
[b]High rate of persistent anaerobic bacteria.
Data from Walker CK, Kahn JG, Washington AE, et al. Pelvic inflammatory disease: meta-analysis of antimicrobial regimen efficacy. *J Infect Dis* 1993;168:969–978.

TABLE 110.11.   Reported Cure Rates in the Treatment of Acute Pelvic Inflammatory Disease for Antibiotic Regimens with Only a Single Study

Drug regimen	Number of patients	Clinical cure rate (%)	Microbiologic cure rate (%)[a]
Inpatient			
Ceftizoxime plus tetracycline	18	88	100
Cefotaxime plus tetracycline	19	94	100
Sulbactam-ampicillin plus doxycycline	37	95	100
Outpatient			
Amoxicillin-clavulanate	35	100	100
Ofloxacin	37	95	100

[a]Based on eradication of *N. gonorrhoeae* and *C. trachomatis*.
Data from Walker CK, Kahn JG, Washington AE, et al. Pelvic inflammatory disease: meta-analysis of antimicrobial regimen efficacy. *J Infect Dis* 1993;168:969–978.

relies on identification of an inflammatory adnexal mass. Patients whose severe pain and tenderness preclude an adequate pelvic examination require further evaluation for a pelvic mass. Suspicion that an inflammatory mass is present should be confirmed with appropriate imaging studies.

Various noninvasive imaging techniques facilitate the diagnosis of adnexal masses (137–148): radionucleotide scanning, ultrasonography (US), computed tomography (CT), and magnetic resonance imaging.

Ultrasound (US) has become the most frequently used technique to confirm the diagnosis of TOA. Real-time US can be used to confirm the diagnosis of TOA and to measure response to therapy. The accuracy of US in the diagnosis of pelvic abscesses has been assessed in several retrospective studies (137,143–145,149). Taylor and co-workers (143) described 220 patients with surgically proven abdominal or pelvic abscesses with the following results: 36 of 40 abdominal abscesses and 32 of 33 pelvic abscesses were correctly identified; 112 of 113 suspected abdominal abscesses and 33 of 34 suspected pelvic abscesses were correctly ruled out. Landers and Sweet (9) reported that 29 of 31 surgically confirmed TOAs were correctly diagnosed with US. TOAs were reported as complex adnexal masses or cyst-type masses with multiple internal echoes consistent with an abscess. A mass was correctly identified in all surgically confirmed TOAs and in 90% of the 67 patients with clinically diagnosed TOAs (9). In a later report, Jasinsky and co-workers (149) compared the sensitivity of US and CT in the diagnosis of intraabdominal abscess. In this study, the sensitivity of US for pelvic abscesses was 42 of 56 (75%), and the sensitivity of CT was 14 of 15 (93%). The difference was attributed to the difficulty of imaging postoperative abscesses by US in oncology patients. Thus TOAs are visualized with a high degree of accuracy by use of standard US techniques, including vaginal probe studies. In summary, transabdominal ultrasound has a sensitivity of 90% or more for detecting a pelvic abscess (150). Endovaginal ultrasonography has further enhanced the sensitivity and specificity for ultrasound confirmation of pelvic abscess (148).

CT has also been used extensively in both diagnosis and treatment of abdominal abscesses (139–142). Despite its known sensitivity in the detection of abdominal abscesses, there is less information on the accuracy of these scans for the diagnosis of TOA and other pelvic abscesses. One study on the accuracy of US, ^{67}Ga-enhanced scan, and CT in the diagnosis of abdominal abscesses reported the sensitivities as 82%, 96%, and 100%, respectively, and the specificities as 91%, 65%, and 100%, respectively (146). Thus, CT appears to be accurate in detecting the presence of an abscess, at least in the abdomen. Because CT is

significantly more expensive, the slightly higher degree of accuracy does not justify its use as a primary diagnostic tool. In general, our initial approach is to use US for the diagnosis of TOAs and to use CT as a backup. There are limited data available on the sensitivity and specificity of magnetic resonance imaging in evaluating pelvic abscess, but the technique is appealing because it discriminates between different tissue densities and fluid consistencies and does not employ ionizing radiation. Its expense precludes its use in the diagnosis of TOAs, except in unusual circumstances.

Etiology and Pathogenesis

The microorganisms isolated from TOAs are predominantly a mixed flora of anaerobes and facultative or aerobic organisms (2,9,151). When good anaerobic microbiologic methods are used, anaerobic bacteria are the most prevalent organisms isolated from TOAs. Anaerobic bacteria have been isolated from 63% to 100% of adnexal abscesses (9,152–157). The predominant organisms isolated from TOA aspirates are *E. coli, B. fragilis*, a variety of *Prevotella* species, aerobic streptococci, and *Peptostreptococcus* species (2,9,152).

It is rare to recover the gonococcus from a TOA. Landers and Sweet recovered *N. gonorrhoeae* from only 3.8% of 53 TOA aspirates despite an overall recovery rate of *N. gonorrhoeae* from the endocervix of 31% in their TOA population (9). It has been proposed that initial infection with the gonococcus leads to anaerobic invasion of the fallopian tubes (59,60). Subsequently, the facultative and anaerobic organisms may suppress the growth of *N. gonorrhoeae*, preventing its recovery (158). Similarly, *C. trachomatis* has not been recovered from the abscess content or the wall of TOAs. Whether it plays a role similar to that of *N. gonorrhoeae* in initiating the development of anaerobic overgrowth remains to be determined.

Actinomycetes, most commonly *Actinomyces israelii*, a gram-positive anaerobe, has occasionally been found in association with PID and, more specifically, TOA. This organism has been reported in association with IUD use (159–161). Burkman and co-workers reported that seven of eight (88%) PID patients with actinomycetic infection had a TOA compared with 11 of 38 (29%) without (126). In other studies of TOA, actinomycetes have not been recovered. The exact role of these organisms in the pathogenesis of TOA is unclear. Their major role may be related to an association with IUD use and subsequent abscess formation.

A variety of factors that play a role in the pathogenesis of abscess formation have been identified: exotoxins with tissue-necrotizing potential; enzymes such as collagenase and

TABLE 110.12. Comparison of Regimens with and Without Clindamycin for Treatment of Tuboovarian Abscess

Antibiotic regimen	Reduction of size at hospital discharge		Further reduction of size at 2–4 wk after discharge	
	No. responded	%	No. treated	%
Antimicrobial regimens that included clindamycin	43/63	68.3	43/50	86.0
Antimicrobial regimens that excluded clindamycin	38/104	36.5	39/84	46.4

Adapted from Landers DV, Sweet RL. Tubo-ovarian abscess: contemporary approach to management. *Rev Infect Dis* 1983;5:876–884.

heparinase; and virulence factors associated with the bacterial cell surface. The inflammatory response to antigenic stimuli has also been shown to play a role in this process. The exact mechanism of TOA formation has been difficult to establish.

Inflammatory damage to the endosalpinx results in a purulent exudate, which may spill from the fimbriated end of the fallopian tubes. In an attempt to localize and wall off the infection, the ovaries or other pelvic structures become involved in the inflammatory process. Organisms enter the ovary, presumably at an ovulation site, and subsequently invade tissue. Tissue planes are eventually lost, and the separation of tube and ovary is obscured as the abscess forms. It may remain localized, involving the tube and ovary alone, or it may involve other contiguous pelvic structures such as bowel, bladder, or the opposite adnexa. At any point in the progression, rupture may occur, exposing the peritoneal surface and other intraabdominal organs to a large amount of purulent material. This process can lead to overwhelming sepsis and further abscess formation. Fortunately, less than 1% or 2% of TOAs reach the stage when they rupture spontaneously, but a ruptured TOA is a true acute surgical emergency.

Medical Therapy of Tuboovarian Abscesses

Although it was long a clinical dictum that abscesses require surgical drainage or extirpation for cure, primary medical management with antibiotic therapy has become the initial approach to TOA as newer data have supported a conservative medical approach. Still, many patients continue to be managed primarily with surgery. Although highly effective, this approach is overzealous, because TOAs can be treated safely and effectively by conservative means. It has been suggested that even when a surgical approach is necessary, unilateral TOA can be treated with unilateral adnexectomy rather than total abdominal hysterectomy and bilateral salpingo-oophorectomy (TAH-BSO).

Numerous investigators have reported success with a conservative medical approach to the treatment of TOA (9,127,129,132,135,136,159–164). A favorable result can be expected in one half to two thirds of cases. A number of antimicrobial regimens were used in these studies.

Because these abscesses contain significant concentrations of the resistant gram-negative anaerobes, such as *B. fragilis, Prevotella bivia*, and *Prevotella disiens*, better results should accrue from aggressive treatment with antibiotics that are effective against these organisms, such as clindamycin, metronidazole, the extended-spectrum penicillins, and the newer broad-spectrum second- and third-generation cephalosporins. In addition, broad-spectrum agents combined with β-lactamase inhibitors and the penems should be efficacious as well, but further clinical trials are needed.

Landers and Sweet in a series of 232 TOAs where response to therapy was determined on the basis of improvement in symptoms, absence of fever, reduction of pelvic tenderness, and shrinking of the mass demonstrated the importance of providing antimicrobial therapy for TOAs that is effective against anaerobic bacteria, including beta-lactamase producers (9) (Table 110.12). Of 167 patients treated with antibiotics alone before discharge, reduction in mass size was observed in 25% of those who received penicillin alone, 49% who received penicillin and an aminoglycoside, and 68% who received regimens that included clindamycin (*P* < .01). Follow-up was available for 104 patients treated with antibiotic regimens that did not include clindamycin. Initial response was seen in 36.5%, compared with 68% of the 63 patients treated with regimens that included clindamycin. Surgical intervention was required for 42 patients during the initial hospitalization because of failure to respond to antimicrobial therapy alone. Of these, 64% had received drugs other than clindamycin and 36% received a regimen containing clindamycin. At follow-up 2 to 4 weeks after discharge, 46.4% of the former group and 86% of clindamycin-treated patients had further reduction or absence of adnexal masses (9).

Reed and colleagues in a study comparing cefoxitin plus doxycycline with clindamycin plus gentamicin for treatment of TOA, reported that nearly 75% of TOAs responded to medical management alone with equivalent cure rates seen in both regimens (164). Recently, McNeeley et al. assessed the efficacy of cefotetan-doxycycline, clindamycin-gentamicin, and ampicillin-clindamycin-gentamicin in the treatment of TOAs (132). They reported that overall 52 (70%) of 74 TOAs responded to antibiotic therapy alone. However, unlike Reed et al. (164), McNeeley et al. (132) noted that triple therapy (ampicillin-clindamycin-gentamicin) was significantly more effective (87.5%) than cefotetan-doxycycline (34%) or clindamycin-gentamicin (47%) (p = 0.001). These studies clearly demonstrated the importance of antimicrobial therapy with an agent effective against *B. fragilis* and *Prevotella* species and the excellent results with such therapy in the management of TOA (9,132,164).

The factor most predictive of response to antimicrobial therapy alone is TOA size. Ginsberg and co-workers (135) reported that TOAs larger than 8 cm or that were bilateral were predictive of failure to respond to antimicrobial therapy alone. Similarly Reed and co-workers (164) demonstrated that response to antimicrobial therapy was inversely proportional to abscess size.

Experience with cefoxitin, third-generation cephalosporins, or extended-spectrum penicillins in the management of TOAs is limited. In a clinical trial of 41 patients with TOA, 39 (95%) responded favorably to cefotaxime, a third-generation cephalosporin (161). No patient required surgery at initial hospitalization, and two patients needed the addition of another antibiotic. Only six patients required further surgery for persistent mass. Six patients (15%) later became pregnant, and all had had abscesses larger than 7 cm, four of them bilateral.

Treatment Rationale for Unruptured Tuboovarian Abscess

As described before, investigators have encouraged conservative management with antibiotics alone when possible (9,129,135). I treat patients with TOAs conservatively, using the following guidelines. If a ruptured TOA is suspected, the patient's condition is stabilized, antibiotic therapy is instituted, and immediate surgical intervention is undertaken. If the diagnosis is in question or there is a reasonable likelihood of an alternative surgical condition, operative intervention is undertaken, with laparoscopy or laparotomy if necessary. Otherwise, the patient is given intravenous antibiotic therapy, usually clindamycin or metronidazole plus an aminoglycoside or cefoxitin, with broad-spectrum coverage that includes the resistant gram-negative anaerobes. The initial approach of antibiotics alone is appropriate for pyosalpinx, ovarian abscess, tuboovarian complex, and TOA. Because it is often difficult to distinguish which of these entities is present, a conservative initial approach eliminates the need to resolve the question.

If the patient does not respond to appropriate antibiotic therapy within 72 hours, surgical intervention should be considered. Patients are frequently slow to respond; it can take a full 3 days' treatment before clinical improvement becomes evident. Clinical judgment is crucial, and each case must be assessed according to the patient's needs and situation. The clinician must also be aware that the abscess may rupture and become a surgical emergency. If the patient's status suddenly deteriorates, surgery should be undertaken immediately.

Several factors have been identified that are predictive of antibiotic failure. Adnexal masses larger than 8 cm or bilateral adnexal involvement has been shown to be predictive of failure (135,164). Surprisingly, the presence of fever, degree of leukocytosis, and history of PID have no predictive value (9), but persistence of fever and rising white cell count in the face of ongoing antibiotic therapy strongly suggest that surgical intervention will be necessary.

Intraabdominal rupture is one of the most serious complications of TOA. It is a surgical emergency, and the mortality rate may be increased by unnecessary delay. With expectant conservative management, Pedowitz and Bloomfield (124) noted that all of the patients who had rupture of a TOA before 1947 died. After 1947, 127 cases were treated with a more aggressive surgical approach (TAH-BSO) combined with available medical adjuvants. The mortality rate dropped to 3.1%. (124). The physician's delay in establishing the diagnosis was cited as the most common preventable cause of death. Subsequent investigators have continued to show improved survival rates with aggressive surgical management of ruptured TOA (133,165). In 1977, Rivlin and Hunt described 113 patients with ruptured TOA (166). The mortality rate was 7.1% in their series, but only 3% of the patients underwent hysterectomy. Unilateral adnexectomy, with preservation of hormonal and menstrual function, was accomplished in 73.5% of cases. Rivlin reported that only 17.5% of patients required further surgery later during the 1- to 5-year follow-up period. Landers and Sweet described four patients with ruptured TOA who underwent unilateral adnexectomy; none required further surgery in the 2- to 10-year follow-up period, and one subsequently carried an intrauterine pregnancy to term (9).

With modern antimicrobial agents and aggressive surgical intervention, ruptured unilateral TOA can be safely managed without removing the uterus and contralateral fallopian tube and ovary.

Surgical Approach to Unruptured Tuboovarian Abscess

A wide variety of surgical approaches to unruptured TOA have been employed through the years: extraperitoneal drainage, posterior colpotomy drainage, unilateral adnexectomy and TAH-BSO, and more recently, percutaneous and laparoscopic drainage. Abdominal extraperitoneal drainage of TOAs has been virtually replaced by other approaches. Posterior colpotomy, still used frequently by many clinicians, can be an effective mode of treatment when it is combined with antimicrobial therapy and restricted to patients with fluctuant abscesses in the midline that dissect the rectovaginal septum and are firmly attached to parietal peritoneum. These conditions severely limit the number of TOAs that can be safely drained by this procedure. The morbidity of this procedure can also be significant if these requirements are not met. Rubenstein and co-workers reported in 1976 that of 65 patients with pelvic abscesses drained by colpotomy or rectal incision, nearly one third subsequently required a major operation because of residual pain or infection (167). In a 1982 combined series of 348 cases of colpotomy drainage reported by Rivlin and coworkers, there were 23 cases of diffuse peritoneal sepsis (6.5%), resulting in six (26%) deaths (168). Rivlin and coworkers also described their experience with colpotomy drainage in 59 patients, of whom 24 required further surgical intervention (169). Of greatest concern, 13 (54%) of these surgeries were performed as emergency procedures. Vaginal colpotomy drainage is seldom used on our service, for the following reasons: (a) there is a high rate of complications, and more definitive surgery is frequently required after colpotomy drainage (167–169); (b) most TOAs do not meet the requirements for the vaginal approach (i.e., midline mass that adheres to pelvic peritoneum and dissects upper third of rectovaginal septum); and (c) with a conservative approach, many of these unilateral abscesses can be removed by the abdominal approach, offering a better chance for preservation of future fertility and hormone production. Whether colpotomy drainage with direct ultrasound guidance will enhance adequate drainage, prevent complications and improve results remains to be determined.

Alternative Treatment Approaches

PERCUTANEOUS DRAINAGE
Percutaneous drainage guided by CT or real-time ultrasound is commonly employed in the treatment of intraabdominal abscesses and pelvic abscess (2). US- or CT-guided drainage of intraabdominal abscesses has been reported to be successful in 75% to 89% of cases, obviating major surgery and minimizing the patient's discomfort, morbidity, and cost (170–177). In addition, patients recover more rapidly and avoid the risk of general anesthesia and surgery. CT and US are also used to observe the response of these abscesses to the drainage technique. Repeated scans are generally performed within 48 hours after drainage to evaluate response. The drainage catheters can also be used to irrigate the abscess cavities and to inject contrast material to ensure reduction of cavity size on repeated scans. Due to the excellent results with intraabdominal abscess, these interventional radiological techniques were applied to the management of pelvic abscesses. Several series have shown that percutaneous catheter drainage can be successfully used in treating pelvic abscesses.

Van Sonnenberg and co-workers (171) reported a 78% success rate for 50 abscesses. Worthen and Gunning (172) used two methods of drainage for 35 patients with TOA: small abscesses were aspirated and large abscesses were drained with a catheter. Seven patients (20%) could not be treated by drainage or aspiration for technical reasons; for the remaining patients, the success rate was 94% (18 of 19) for aspiration drainage and 77% (seven of nine) for catheter drainage. Complications included a bowel laceration and an abscess rupture that required early intervention. Tyrrel et al. (178) using CT-guided drainage reported success in seven of eight (87.5%) patients with TOAs. However, Nelson et al. (148) noted that there were technical difficulties accessing retrouterine abscesses which were approached by a transgluteal approach, thus limiting the usefulness of CT-directed drainage of TOAs and pelvic abscess.

To address this issue, endovaginal ultrasound guidance and transvaginal drainage of pelvic abscesses has been utilized resulting in success rates of approximately 85% (148,179–186). More recently, transrectal ultrasound guided drainage of pelvic abscess has been shown to have similar excellent results (187–194).

LAPAROSCOPIC DRAINAGE

Laparoscopy has been suggested as a possible approach to the management of TOA (195–198). It affords direct visualization of the abscess and confirms the diagnosis. The TOA is diagnosed under direct vision, adhesions are lysed, and purulent material is removed by suction; the peritoneal cavity can also be irrigated to remove necrotic tissue. In 1984, Henry-Suchet and coworkers (195) reported a series of 50 patients whose TOAs were managed laparoscopically. The reported overall clinical recovery rate was 90%, with almost complete disappearance of the adnexal mass and minimal adhesion formation after resolution of the acute infection. Reich and McGlynn (196) evaluated 25 women treated with this procedure. There was only one failure in the series; that woman required TAH-BSO 1 month after laparoscopic treatment. Minimal adhesions were found in five women who underwent second-look laparoscopy. Adducci (197) obtained similar results in seven cases and reported colpotomy drainage under laparoscopic control in nine patients with PID-associated pelvic abscesses. All nine responded well. More

recently, excellent results were demonstrated with laparoscopy directed drainage by Raiga et al. (199), who reported immediate clinical response in all 39 patients whose adnexal abscesses were drained via laparoscopy. Thirty-five of these patients underwent a second-look laparoscopy at 3 to 6 months; lysis of adhesions was required in all 35 and a distal tuboplasty was performed in 17 (199). Among those women not using contraception, 12 of 19 (63%) achieved a spontaneous intrauterine pregnancy. Prospective studies are needed to compare the efficacy of antimicrobial therapy alone and antimicrobial therapy with drainage in resolving the abscess and preventing long-term sequelae.

CONSERVATIVE SURGERY VERSUS TOTAL HYSTERECTOMY WITH BILATERAL ADNEXECTOMY

The extent of surgery necessary to effect a cure when antibiotic therapy alone fails remains controversial. The approaches have ranged from simple drainage to complete removal of all reproductive organs by TAH-BSO (9,124,125,164). An alternative approach is a unilateral salpingo-oophorectomy for unilateral TOAs or a bilateral salpingo-oophorectomy for bilateral disease. Whereas a TAH-BSO is curative, the more conservative unilateral adnexectomy offers the potential for future fertility, maintenance of hormonal and menstrual function, and avoidance of the physiologic and psychologic effects of hysterectomy and gonadectomy.

Several investigators have reported results of conservative surgical management of patients with unilateral TOAs (9,124,125,133,135,151,159,166). These data indicate that approximately 17% of patients treated with unilateral adnexectomy later require additional surgery. Rivlin and Hunt (166) combined conservative surgery with intraoperative and postoperative antibiotic peritoneal lavage for the treatment of 113 patients with ruptured TOA. They found that only four patients (3%) required hysterectomy during the initial hospitalization. Of the 83 patients treated with adnexal procedures (unilateral or bilateral) without removal of the uterus, 16 (19%) required further surgical intervention. An additional 19 patients reported by Landers and Sweet (9) were treated with unilateral adnexectomy; only two required subsequent surgery, and 3 subsequently became pregnant. Thus, it appears that although there is a risk that further surgery will be required, the conservative surgical approach

TABLE 110.13. Investigations of Treatment of Tuboovarian Abscess with Conservative Medical Therapy

Study	Number of cases treated	Initial response No.	Initial response %	Subsequent pregnancy in patients with follow-up No.	Subsequent pregnancy in patients with follow-up %
Landers and Sweet[9]	217	175	81	8/58	13.8
Franklin et al.[129]	120	110	90[a]	10/108	9.3
Ginsberg et al.[135]	110	76	69	9/95	9.5
Edelman and Berger[136]	318	175	55	NS	NS
Scott[160]	33	24	73	NS	NS
Manara[159]	26	11	42	1/26	3.8
Hager[127]	32	5	16	4/8	50
Hemsell et al.[161]	41	39	95	6/41	14.6
Mercer et al.[162]	20	12	60	NS	NS
Hemsell et al.[163]	24	22	92	NS	NS
Reed et al.[164]	119	90	70	NS	NS
McNeeley et al.[132]	74	52	70	NS	NS
Total	1134	791	69.8	38/336	11.3

[a]Includes some patients treated with colpotomy drainage.
NS, Not stated.

does offer the TOA patient in whom initial antibiotic therapy fails another alternative to permanent sterilization and castration.

Another potential application of unilateral adnexectomy is in patients whose disease responds to initial antimicrobial therapy but whose mass persists. These patients may benefit from unilateral adnexectomy in terms of future fertility and recurrent disease. This approach needs to be evaluated in controlled trials. With the success of in vitro fertilization techniques and as donor embryo transplantation programs improve, the demand for a conservative surgical approach will increase.

Fertility After Tuboovarian Abscess

Fertility potential after a TOA has received little attention in the medical literature. Although several investigators have reported the frequency of subsequent pregnancy following treatment of TOA, the follow-up data are limited, leaving it impossible to assess the number of patients attempting to conceive and their success rate (Table 110.13). The pregnancy rate has been reported to range from 9.5% to 13.8% after conservative medical management (9,129,135,161), 3.7% to 16% after unilateral adnexal procedures with preoperative antibiotics (9,135,151) and 10% to 15% after antibiotics plus colpotomy drainage (166,168). Hager published a series on 50 patients treated for TOA (127). A total of 11 of these patients had reproductive potential after treatment, but only eight attempted to conceive. Four of the eight (50%) conceived a total of five intrauterine pregnancies. There were no ectopic pregnancies. In addition, he described five patients who underwent unilateral salpingo-oophorectomy and attempted to conceive; four were successful (80%). Although these rates of fertility are low, we may be dramatically underestimating reproduction potential after TOA unless we consider only the number of patients who attempt to conceive. Furthermore, few data have been published about vigorous treatment with antibiotics, such as clindamycin and metronidazole, that can penetrate abscesses. More investigation is also needed to determine the effects on fertility of newer antibiotics, laparoscopic drainage, and unilateral adnexectomy for unilateral TOA.

REFERENCES

1. Centers for Disease Control. Pelvic inflammatory disease. In: *1993 Sexually transmitted diseases treatment guidelines. MMWR* 1993;42:75.
2. Sweet RL, Gibbs RS. Pelvic inflammatory disease. In: *Infectious diseases of the female genital tract.* Philadelphia: Lippincott, Williams and Wilkins, 2002.
3. Rein DB, Kassler WJ, Irwin KL, Rabiee L. Direct medical cost of pelvic inflammatory disease and its sequelae; decreasing but still substantial. *Obstet Gynecol* 2000;95:397–402.
4. Washington AE, Katz P. Cost of and payment source for pelvic inflammatory disease: trends and projections, 1983 through 2000. *JAMA* 1991;266:2565–2569.
5. Washington AE, Cates W, Zaidi AA. Hospitalizations for pelvic inflammatory disease: epidemiology and trends in the United States, 1975 to 1982. *JAMA* 1984;251:2529.
6. Westrom L, Eschenbach DA. Pelvic inflammatory disease. In Holmes KK, Sparling PF, Mardh P-A, et al, eds: *Sexually transmitted diseases.* New York: McGraw-Hill, 1999:783–809.
7. Westrom L. Incidence, prevalence and trends of acute pelvic inflammatory disease and its consequences in industrialized countries. *Am J Obstet Gynecol* 1980;38:880.
8. Westrom LV, Joesoef R, Reynolds G, et al. Pelvic inflammatory disease and fertility. A cohort study of 1,844 women with laparoscopically verified disease and 657 control women with normal laparoscopic results. *Sex Trans Dis* 1992;19:185–192.
9. Landers DV, Sweet RL. Tubo-ovarian abscess: contemporary approach to management. *Rev Infec Dis* 1983;5:876.
10. Centers for Disease Control. Pelvic inflammatory disease: guidelines for prevention and management. *MMWR* 1991;40:1–25.
11. Washington AE, Aral SO, Wolner-Hanssen P, Grimes DA, Holmes KK. Assessing risk for pelvic inflammatory disease and its sequelae. *JAMA* 1991;266:2581–2586.
12. Westrom L. Effect of acute pelvic inflammatory disease on fertility. *Am J Obstet Gynecol* 1975;122:707.
13. Mardh P-A, Lind I, Svensson L, et al. Antibodies to *Chlamydia trachomatis, Mycoplasma hominis* and *Neisseria gonorrhoeae* in serum from patients with acute salpingitis. *Br J Vener Dis* 1981;57:125–129.
14. Sweet RL, Schachter J, Robbie MO. Failure of beta-lactam antibiotics to eradicate *Chlamydia trachomatis* in the endometrium despite apparent clinical cure of acute salpingitis. *JAMA* 1983;250:2641–2645.
15. Wasserheit JN, Bell TA, Kiviat NB, et al. Microbial causes of proven pelvic inflammatory disease and efficacy of clindamycin and tobramycin. *Ann Intern Med* 1986;104:187–193.
16. Sweet RL, Schachter J, Landers DV, et al. Treatment of hospitalized patients with acute pelvic inflammatory disease: comparison of cefotetan plus doxycycline and cefoxitin plus doxycycline. *Am J Obstet Gynecol* 1988;158:736–743.
17. Jossens MOR, Schachter J, Sweet RL. Risk factors associated with pelvic inflammatory disease of differing microbial etiologies. *Obstet Gynecol* 1994;83:989–997.
18. Wolner-Hanssen P, Eschenbach DA, Paavonen J, et al. Decreased risk of symptomatic chlamydial pelvic inflammatory disease associated with oral contraceptive use. *JAMA* 1990;263:54–59.
19. Paavonen J, Teisala K, Heinonen PK, et al. Microbiological and histopathological findings in acute pelvic inflammatory disease. *Br J Obstet Gynecol* 1987;94:454.
20. Eschenbach DA, Hillier S, Critchlow C, et al. Diagnosis and clinical manifestations of bacterial vaginosis. *Am J Obstet Gynecol* 1988;158:819.
21. Hillier SL, Kiviat NB, Critchlow C, et al. Bacterial vaginosis associated bacteria as etiologic agents of pelvic inflammatory disease (abstract). In Proceedings of the Annual Meeting of the Infectious Diseases Society of Obstetrics and Gynecology, August 6–8, 1992; San Diego, CA, p 12.
22. Soper D, Brockwell NJ, Dalton HP, Johnson D. Observations concerning the microbial etiology of acute salpingitis. *Am J Obstet Gynecol* 1994;170:1008.
23. Korn AP, Bolan G, Padian N, et al. Plasma cell endometritis in women with symptomatic bacterial vaginosis. *Obstet Gynecol* 1995;85:387–390.
24. Peipert JF, Montagno AB, Cooper AS, Sung CJ. Bacterial vaginosis as a risk factor for upper genital tract infection. *Am J Obstet Gynecol* 1997;177:1184–1187.
25. Korn AP, Hessol NA, Padian NS, et al. Risk factors for plasma cell endometritis among women with cervical *Neisseria gonorrhoeae*, cervical *Chlamydia trachomatis*, or bacterial vaginosis. *Am J Obstet Gynecol* 1998;178:987–990.
26. Eschenbach DA. Epidemiology and diagnosis of acute pelvic inflammatory disease. *Obstet Gynecol* 1980;55:142S.
27. Jossens MOR, Schachter J, Sweet RL. Risk factors associated with pelvic inflammatory disease of differing microbial etiologies. *Obstet Gynecol* 1994;83:989.
28. Bell TA, Holmes KK. Age-specific risks of syphilis, gonorrhea and hospitalized pelvic inflammatory disease in sexually experienced U.S. women. *Sex Transm Dis* 1984;11:291.
29. Eschenbach DA, Harnisch JP, Holmes KK. Pathogenesis of acute pelvic inflammatory disease: role of contraception and other risk factors. *Am J Obstet Gynecol* 1977;128:838.
30. Ory HW. A review of the association between intrauterine devices and pelvic inflammatory disease. *J Reprod Med* 1978;20:200.
31. Kaufman DW, Shapiro S, Rosenberg L, et al. Intrauterine contraceptive device use and pelvic inflammatory disease. *Am J Obstet Gynecol* 1980;136:159.
32. Lee NC, Rubin GL, Ory HW, et al. Type of intrauterine device and the risk of pelvic inflammatory disease. *Obstet Gynecol* 1983;62:1.
33. Burnhill MS. Syndrome of progressive endometritis associated with intrauterine contraceptive devices. *Adv Planned Parenthood* 1973;8:144.
34. Marchbanks PA, Lee NC, Peterson HB. Cigarette smoking as a risk factor for pelvic inflammatory disease. *Am J Obstet Gynecol* 1990;162:639–644.
35. Scholes D, Daling JR, Stergachis AS. Cigarette smoking and risk of pelvic inflammatory disease. *Am J Epidemiol* 1990;132:759.
36. Wolner-Hanssen P, Eschenbach DA, Paavonen J, et al. Decreased risk of symptomatic chlamydial pelvic inflammatory disease associated with oral contraceptive use. *JAMA* 1990;263:54–59.
37. Fullilove RE, Fullilove MT, Bower BP, Gross SA. Risk of sexually transmitted diseases among black adolescent crack users in Oakland and San Francisco, CA. *JAMA* 1990;263:851–855.
38. Sweet RL, Blankfort-Doyle M, Robbie MO, Schachter J. The occurrence of chlamydial and gonococcal salpingitis during the menstrual cycle. *JAMA* 1986;255:2062–2064.
39. Forrest KA, Washington AE, Daling JR, Sweet RL. Vaginal douching as a possible risk factor for pelvic inflammatory disease. *J Natl Med Assoc* 1989;81:159–165.
40. Wolner-Hanssen P, Eschenbach DA, Paavonen J, et al. Association between vaginal douching and acute pelvic inflammatory disease. *JAMA* 1990;263:1936–1941.
41. McGregor JA, Spencer NE, French JI, et al. Psychosocial and behavioral risk factors for acute salpingitis. In: Abstracts of the Sixth International Meeting of the International Society for STD Research, July 3–August 2, 1985. Brighton, UK.
42. Scholes D, Daling JR, Stergachis A, et al. Vaginal douching as a risk factor for acute pelvic inflammatory disease. *Obstet Gynecol* 1993;81:601–606.
43. Aral SO, Mosher WD, Cates W Jr. Self-reported pelvic inflammatory disease in the United States, 1988. *JAMA* 1991;266:2570–2573.
44. Centers for Disease Control and Prevention. Pelvic inflammatory disease.

In: *2002 Sexually transmitted diseases treatment guidelines. MMWR* 2002;51:48–51.

45. Eschenbach DA, Buchanan T, Pollock HM, et al. Polymicrobial etiology of acute pelvic inflammatory disease. *N Engl J Med* 1975;293:166.

46. Sweet RL, Draper DL, Schachter J, et al. Microbiology and pathogenesis of acute salpingitis as determined by laparoscopy: what is the approach site to sample? *Am J Obstet Gynecol* 1980;138:985.

47. Paavonen J, Teisala K, Heinonen PK, et al. Microbiological and histopathological findings in acute pelvic inflammatory disease. *Br J Obstet Gynecol* 1987;94;454–460.

48. Heinonnen PK, Teisala K, Punnonen R, et al. Anatomic sites of upper genital tract infection. *Obstet Gynecol* 1985;66:384–390.

49. Brunham RC, Binns B, Gujon F, et al. Etiology and outcome of pelvic inflammatory disease. *J Infect Dis* 1988;158:510–517.

50. Soper DE, Brockwell NJ, Dalton HP, Johnston D. Observations concerning the microbial etiology of acute salpingitis. *Am J Obstet Gynecol* 1994;170:1008–1017.

51. Hillier SL, Kiviat NB, Critchlow C, et al. Bacterial vaginosis-associated bacteria as etiologic agents of pelvic inflammatory disease (abstract). In: Proceedings of the annual meeting Infectious Disease Society of Obstetrics and Gynecology, San Diego, CA, August 6, 1992.

52. Bukusi EA, Cohen CR, Stevens CE, et al. Effects of human immunodeficiency virus 1 infection in microbial origins of pelvic inflammatory disease and on efficacy of ambulatory oral therapy. *Am J Obstet Gynecol* 1999;181:1374–1381.

53. Rice PA, Schachter J. Pathogenesis of pelvic inflammatory disease. *JAMA* 1991;266:2587–2593.

54. Sweet RL. Role of bacterial vaginosis in pelvic inflammatory disease. *Clin Infect Dis* 1995;20[Suppl 2];S276–285.

55. Hillier SL, Kiviat NB, Hawes SB, et al. Role of bacterial vaginosis-associated microorganisms in endometritis. *Am J Obstet Gynecol* 1996;175:435–441.

56. Wolner-Hanssen P, Kiviat NB, Holmes KK. Atypical pelvic inflammatory disease: subacute, chronic or subclinical upper genital tract infection in women. In Holmes KK, Mardh P-A, Sparling PF, et al, eds: *Sexually transmitted diseases.* New York: McGraw-Hill, 1990:615–620.

57. Wiesenfeld HC, Hillier SL, Krohn MA, et al. Lower genital tract infection and endometritis: insight on subclinical pelvic inflammatory disease. *Obstet Gynecol* 2002;100:456–463.

58. Cunningham FG, Hauth JC, Gilstrap LC, et al. The bacterial pathogenesis of acute pelvic inflammatory disease. *Obstet Gynecol* 1978;52:161.

59. Chow AW, Malkasian KL, Marshall JR, et al. The bacteriology of acute pelvic inflammatory disease. *Am J Obstet Gynecol* 1975;122:876.

60. Monif GRG, Welkos SL, Baer H, et al. Cul-de-sac isolates from patients with endometritis-salpingitis-peritonitis and gonococcal endocervicitis. *Am J Obstet Gynecol* 1976;126:158.

61. Sweet RL, Draper D, Hadley WK. Etiology of acute salpingitis: influence of episode number and duration of symptoms. *Obstet Gynecol* 1981;58:62.

62. Eschenbach DA, Holmes KK. Acute pelvic inflammatory disease. Current concepts of pathogenesis, etiology and management. *Clin Obstet Gynecol* 1975;18;35.

63. Sweet RL, Blankfort-Doyle M, Robbie MD, Schachter J. The occurrence of chlamydial and gonococcal salpingitis during the menstrual cycle. *JAMA* 1986;255:2062.

64. Mardh -P-A, Ripa T, Swensson L, Westrom L. *Chlamydia trachomatis* infection in patients with acute salpingitis. *N Engl J Med* 1977;298:1377.

64a. Thompson SE, Hager WD, Wong KH, et al. The microbiology and therapy of acute pelvic inflammatory disease in hospitalized patients. *Am J Obstet Gynecol* 1980;136:179.

65. Osser S, Persson K. Epidemiology and serodiagnostic aspects of chlamydia salpingitis. *Obstet Gynecol* 1982;59;206.

66. Moller BR, Mardh P-A, Ahrons S, et al. Infections with *Chlamydia trachomatis, Mycoplasma hominis* and *Neisseria gonorrhoeae* in patients with acute pelvic inflammatory disease. *Sex Transm Dis* 1981;8:198.

67. Gjonnaess H, Dalaker K, Anestad G, et al. Pelvic inflammatory disease: etiologic studies with emphasis on chlamydial infection. *Obstet Gynecol* 1982;59:550.

68. Swensson L, Westrom L, Ripa KT, et al. Differences in some clinical and laboratory parameters in acute salpingitis related to culture and serologic findings. *Am J Obstet Gynecol* 1980;138;1017.

69. Henry-Suchet J, Loffredo V, Sarfaty D. Chlamydia trachomatis and mycoplasma research by laparoscopy in cases of pelvic inflammatory disease and in cases of tubal obstruction. *Am J Obstet Gynecol* 1980;138:1022.

70. Punnonen R, Terho P, Nikkanen V, et al. Chlamydial serology in infertile women by immunofluorescence. *Fertil Steril* 1979;31:656.

71. Jones RB, Ardery Br, Hui SL, Cleary RE. Correlation between serum antichlamydial antibodies and tubal factor as a cause of infertility. *Fertil Steril* 1982;38:553.

72. Moore De, Foy HM, Dalin JR, et al. Increased frequency of serum antibodies to *Chlamydia trachomatis* in infertility due to tubal disease. *Lancet* 1982;2:574.

73. Gump DW, Gibson M, Ashikaga T. Evidence of prior pelvic inflammatory disease and its relationship to *C. trachomatis* antibody and intrauterine contraceptive device use in infertile women. *Am J Obstet Gynecol* 1983;146:153.

74. Cevanini R, Possati G, LaPlaca M. *Chlamydia trachomatis* infection in infertile women. In Mardh P-A, Holmes KK, Oriel JD, Piot P, Schachter J, eds: *Chlamydial infections.* Amsterdam: Elsevier, 1982:182–192.

75. Gibson M, Gump D, Ashikaga T, Hall B. Patterns of adnexal inflammatory damage: chlamydia, the intrauterine device, and history of pelvic inflammatory disease. *Fertil Steril* 1984;41:47–51.

76. Conway D, Caul EO, Hall MR. Chlamydial serology in fertile and infertile women. *Lancet* 1984;1:191.

77. Kane JL, Woodland RM, Forsey T, et al. Evidence of chlamydial infection in infertile women with and without fallopian tube obstruction. *Fertil Steril* 1984;42:6.

78. Sellors JW, Mahoney J, Chernesky M, et al. *Chlamydia trachomatis* in fertile and infertile Canadian women. In: *Chlamydia infections,* Sixth International Symposium Proceedings June 1986. England: Cambridge University Press, 1986:233.

79. Brunham RS, MacLean IW, Binns B, et al. *Chlamydia trachomatis:* its role in tubal infertility. *J Infect Dis* 1985;152:1275.

80. Chow JM, Yonekura L, Richard GA, et al. The association between *Chlamydia trachomatis* and ectopic pregnancy: a matched-pair, case-control study. *JAMA* 1990;263;3164–3167.

81. Brunham RS, Binns B, McDowell J, et al. *Chlamydia trachomatis* infection in women with ectopic pregnancy. *Obstet Gynecol* 1986;67:722.

82. Svensson L, Mardh P-A, Ahlgren M, et al. Ectopic pregnancy and antibodies to *Chlamydia trachomatis. Fertil Steril* 1985;44:313.

83. Hartford SL, Silva PD, diZerega GS, et al. Serologic evidence of prior chlamydial infection in patients with tubal ectopic pregnancy and contralateral tubal disease. *Fertil Steril* 1987;47:118.

84. Morrison RP, Belland RJ, Lyngk, Caldwell HD. Chlamydial disease pathogenesis. The 57-KD hypersensitivity antigen in a stress response protein. *J Exp Med* 1989;170:1271–1283.

85. Witkin SS, Jeremias J, Toth M, Ledger WL. Cell-mediated immune response to the recombinant 57-KD heat-shock protein of *Chlamydia trachomatis* in women with salpingitis. *J Infect Dis* 1993;167;1379–1383.

86. Morrison RP, Manning DS, Caldwell HD. Immunology of *Chlamydia trachomatis* infections: Immunoprotective and immunopathogenic responses. In Gallin JI, Fauci AS, Quinn TC, eds: *Advances in host defense mechanisms,* vol 8: *Sexually transmitted diseases.* New York: Raven Press, 1992:57–84.

87. Patton DL, Cosgrove Sweeney YT, Kuo C-C. Demonstration of delayed hypersensitivity in *Chlamydia trachomatis* salpingitis in monkeys. A pathogenic mechanism of tubal damage. *J Infect Dis* 1994;169:680–683.

88. Brunham RC, Peeling RW. *Chlamydia trachomatis* antigens: role in immunity and pathogenesis. *Infect Agents Dis* 1994;3:218–233.

89. Peeling RW, Kimani J, Plummer F, et al. Antibody to chlamydial hsp 60 predicts an increased risk for chlamydial pelvic inflammatory disease. *J Infect Dis* 1997;175:1153–1156.

90. Eckert LO, Hawes SE, Wolner-Hanssen P, et al. Prevalence and correlates of antibody to chlamydial heat shock protein in women attending sexually transmitted diseases clinic and women with confirmed pelvic inflammatory disease. *J Infect Dis* 1997;175:1453–1458.

91. Mardh P-A, Westrom L. Tubal and cervical cultures in acute salpingitis with special reference to *Mycoplasma hominis* and T-strain mycoplasma. *Br J Vener Dis* 1970;46:179.

92. Mardh P-A, Westrom L, Ripa KT, et al. Pelvic inflammatory disease: clinical, etiologic and pathophysiologic studies. In Holmes KK, Mardh P-A, eds: *International perspectives on neglected sexually transmitted diseases.* New York: Hemisphere Publishing, 1983.

93. Amsel R, Totten, PA, Speigel CA, et al. Nonspecific vaginitis: diagnostic criteria and microbiologic and epidemiologic associations. *Am J Med* 1983;74:14.

94. Palmer HM. Detection of Mycoplasma genitalium in the genitourinary tract of women by the polymerase chain reaction. *Int J STD AIDS* 1991;2:261.

95. Taylor-Robison D. The history of *Mycoplasma genitalium* in sexually transmitted diseases. *Genitourin Med* 1995;71:1.

96. Taylor-Robinson D. Animal models of *Mycoplasma genitalium* urogenital infections. *Isr J Med Sci* 1987;23:561.

97. Sweet RL. Pelvic inflammatory disease and infertility in women. *Infect Dis Clin North Am* 1987;1:199.

98. Phiefer TA, Forsyth PS, Durfee MA, et al. Nonspecific vaginitis: role of *Haemophilus vaginalis* and treatment with metronidazole. *N Engl J Med* 1978;298:1429.

99. Holmes KK, Speigel C, Amsel R, et al. Nonspecific vaginosis. *Scand J Infect Dis* 1981;26(S):110.

100. Spiegel CA, Amsel R, Eschenbach DA, et al. Anaerobic bacteria in nonspecific vaginitis. *N Engl J Med* 1980;303:601.

101. Taylor E, Barlow D, Blackwell AL, Phillips I. *Gardnerella vaginalis,* anaerobes and vaginal discharge. *Lancet* 1982;1:1376–1379.

102. Spiegal CA, Eschenbach DA, Amsel R, Holmes KK. Curved anaerobic bacteria in bacterial (nonspecific) vaginosis and their response to therapy. *J Infect Dis* 1983;148:817.

103. Eschenbach DA. Epidemiology and diagnosis of acute pelvic inflammatory disease. *Obstet Gynecol* 1980;55:142(S).

104. Eschenbach DA, Hillier S, Critchlow C, et al. Diagnosis and clinical manifestations of bacterial vaginosis. *Am J Obstet Gynecol* 1988;158:819–828.

105. Westrom LV, Berger GS. Consequences of pelvic inflammatory disease. In *Pelvic Inflammatory Disease,* Berger GS, Westrom LV, eds. New York: Raven Press, 1992:101–114.

106. Sellors JW. Tubal factor infertility: an association with prior chlamydial infection and asymptomatic salpingitis. *Fertil Steril* 1988;49:451.

107. Smith MR. Endosalpingitis is a frequent response to intrauterine contraception. *J Reprod Med* 1976;126:159.

108. Falk V. Treatment of acute nontuberculosis salpingitis with antibiotics alone and in combination with glucocorticoids. *Acta Obstet Gynecol* 1965;44[S-16]:65.

109. Jacobsen L, Westrom L. Objectivized diagnosis of acute pelvic inflammatory disease. *Am J Obstet Gynecol* 1969;105:1088.

110. Sellors JW, Mahoney JB, Goldsmith C, et al. The diagnosis of pelvic inflammatory disease: the accuracy of clinical and laparoscopic findings. *Am J Obstet Gynecol* 1991;164:113–120.

111. Paavonen J, Westrom LV. Diagnosis of acute pelvic inflammatory disease. In Berger GS, Westrom LV, eds: *Pelvic inflammatory disease.* New York: Raven Press, 1992:49–78.

112. Kahn JG, Walker CK, Washington AE, Landers DV, Sweet RL. Diagnosing pelvic inflammatory disease. A comprehensive analysis and considerations for developing a new model. *JAMA* 1991;266:2594–2604.

113. Hadgu A. Predicting acute PID: a multivariate analysis. *Am J Obstet Gynecol* 1986;155:934.

114. Wolner-Hanssen P. Laparoscopy in women with chlamydial infection and pelvic pain: a comparison of patents with and without salpingitis. *Obstet Gynecol* 1983;61:299.

115. Hager WD, Eschenbach DA, Spence MR, Sweet RL. Criteria for diagnosis and grading of salpingitis. *Obstet Gynecol* 1983;61:113.

116. Kiviat NB, Wolner-Hanssen P, Peterson M, et al. Localization of *Chlamydia trachomatis* infection by direct immunofluorescence and culture in pelvic inflammatory disease. *Am J Obstet Gynecol* 1986;154:865–873.

117. Centers for Disease Control and Prevention. 1998 Guidelines for treatment of sexually transmitted diseases. *MMWR* 1998;47:79–86.

118. Viberg L. Acute inflammatory conditions of the uterine adnexa. *Acta Obstet Gynecol Scand* 1964;43[Suppl 4]:1.

119. Hillis SD, Joesoef R, Marchbanks PA, et al. Delayed care of pelvic inflammatory disease as a risk factor for impaired fertility. *Am J Obstet Gynecol* 1993;168:1503.

120. Washington AE, Sweet RL, Shafter M-A. Pelvic inflammatory disease and its sequelae in adolescents. *J Adolesc Health Care* 1985;6:298.

121. Sherris JD, Fox G. Infertility and sexually transmitted disease: a public health challenge. *Popul Rep L* 1983;11:113.

122. Walker CK, Kahn JG, Washington AE, et al. Pelvic inflammatory disease: meta-analysis of antimicrobial regimen efficacy. *J Infect Dis* 1993;168:969.

123. Ness RB, Soper DE, Holley RL, et al. Effectiveness of inpatient and outpatient treatment strategies for women with pelvic inflammatory disease: results from the Pelvic Inflammatory Disease Evaluation and Clinical Health (PEACH) randomized trial. *Am J Obstet Gynecol* 2002;196:929–937.

124. Pedowitz P, Bloomfield RD. Ruptured adnexal abscess with generalized peritonitis. *Am J Obstet Gynecol* 1964;88:721.

125. Nebel WA, Lucas WE. Management of tuboovarian abscess. *Obstet Gynecol* 1968;32:381.

126. Burkman R, Schlesselman S, McCaffrey L, et al. The relationship of genital tract actinomycetes and the development of pelvic inflammatory disease. *Am J Obstet Gynecol* 1982;143:585.

127. Hager WD. Follow-up of patients with tuboovarian abscess(es) in association with salpingitis. *Obstet Gynecol* 1983;61:680.

128. Benigno BB. Medical and surgical management of the pelvic abscess. *Clin Obstet Gynecol* 1981;224:1187.

129. Franklin EW, Hevron JE, Thompson JD. Management of the pelvic abscess. *Clin Obstet Gynecol* 1973;16:66.

130. Brunham RC, Binns B, Guijon F, et al. Etiology and outcome of acute pelvic inflammatory disease. *J Infect Dis* 1988;158:510.

131. Clark JFJ, Moore-Hines S. A study of tubo-ovarian abscess at Howard. *J Natl Med Assoc* 1979;71:1109–1111.

132. McNeeley SG, Hendrix SL, Mazzoni MM, et al. Medically sound, cost-effective treatment for pelvic inflammatory disease and tuboovarian abscess. *Am J Obstet Gynecol* 1998;178:1272–1278.

133. Mickal A, Sellmann AH. Management of tuboovarian abscess. *Clin Obstet Gynecol* 1969;12:252.

134. Clark JR, Moore-Hines S. A study of tubo-ovarian abscess at Howard University Hospital (1965 through 1975). *J Natl Med Assoc* 1979;71:1109.

135. Ginsberg DS, Stern JL, Hamod KA, et al. Tubo-ovarian abscess: a retrospective review. *Am J Obstet Gynecol* 1980;138:1055.

136. Edelman DA, Berger GS. Contraceptive practice and tubo-ovarian abscess. *Am J Obstet Gynecol* 1980;138:541.

137. Filly RA. Detection of abdominal abscesses: a combined approach employing ultrasonography, computed tomography and gallium-67 scanning. *J Assoc Can Radiol* 1979;30:202.

138. Norton L, Eule J, Burdick D. Accuracy of techniques to detect intraperitoneal abscess. *Surgery* 1978;84:370.

139. Hopkins GB, Kan M, Mende CW. Gallium-67 scintigraphy and intraabdominal sepsis: clinical experience in 140 patients with suspected intraabdominal abscess. *West J Med* 1976;125:425.

140. Carroll B, Silverman PM, Goodwin DA, McDougall R. Ultrasonography and indium-111 white blood cell scanning for the detection of intraabdominal abscesses. *Radiology* 1981;140:155.

141. Coleman RE, Black RE, Welch DM, et al. Indium-111-labeled leukocytes in the evaluation of suspected abdominal abscesses. *Am J Surg* 1980;139:99.

142. Bicknell TA, Kohatsu S, Goodwin DA. Use of indium-111-labeled autologous leukocytes in differentiating pancreatic abscess from pseudocyst. *Am J Surg* 1981;142:312.

143. Taylor KJK, DeGraaft MCI, Wasson JF, et al. Accuracy of grey-scale ultrasound diagnosis of abdominal and pelvic abscesses in 220 patients. *Lancet* 1978;1:83.

144. Spirtos NJ, Bernstine RL, Crawford WL, Rayle J. Sonography in acute pelvic inflammatory disease. *J Reprod Med* 1982;27:312.

145. Uhrich PC, Sanders RC. Ultrasonic characteristics of pelvic inflammatory masses. *J Clin Ultrasound* 1976;4:199.

146. Moir C, Robins RE. Role of ultrasound, gallium scanning and computed tomography in the diagnosis of intraabdominal abscess. *Am J Surg* 1982;143:582.

147. Mitchell DG, Mintz MC, Spritzer CE, et al. Adnexal masses: MR imaging observations at 15T, with US and CT correlation. *Radiology* 1987;162:319.

148. Nelson AL, Sinow RM, Renslo R, et al. Endovaginal ultrasonography guided transvaginal drainage for treatment of pelvic abscesses. *Am J Obstet Gynecol* 1995;172:1926–1935.

149. Jasinsky RW, Glazer GM, Francis IR, Harkness RL. CT and ultrasound in abscess detection at specific anatomic sites: a study of 198 patients. *Comput Radiol* 1987;11:41.

150. Ferruci TJ Jr, van Sonnenberg E. Intraabdominal abscess: radiological diagnosis and treatment. *JAMA* 1981;246:2728–2733.

151. Golde SH, Israel R, Ledger WJ. Unilateral tubo-ovarian abscess: a distinct entity. *Am J Obstet Gynecol* 1977;127:807.

152. Landers DV, Sweet RL. Current trends in the diagnosis and treatment of tubo-ovarian abscess. *Am J Obstet Gynecol* 1985;151:1098–1110.

153. Svenson RM, Michaelson TC, Daly MJ, et al. Anaerobic bacterial infections of the female genital tract. *Obstet Gynecol* 1973;42:538.

154. Thadepalli H, Gorbach SL, Keith L. Anaerobic infections of the female genital tract: bacteriologic and therapeutic aspects. *Am J Obstet Gynecol* 1973;117:1034.

155. Altemeier WA. The anaerobic streptococci in tubo-ovarian abscess. *Am J Obstet Gynecol* 1940;39:1038.

156. Ledger WJ, Campbell C, Willson JR. Postoperative adnexal infections. *Obstet Gynecol* 1968;31:83.

157. Pearson HE, Anderson GV. Genital bacteroidal abscesses in women. *Am J Obstet Gynecol* 1970;107:1264.

158. Holmes KK, Eschenbach DA, Knapp JS. Salpingitis: overview of etiology and epidemiology. *Am J Obstet Gynecol* 1980;138:893.

159. Manara LR. Management of tubo-ovarian abscess. *Am J Osteopath Assoc* 1982;81:476.

160. Scott WC. Pelvic abscess in association with intrauterine contraceptive devices. *Am J Obstet Gynecol* 1978;131:149.

161. Hemsell DL, Santos-Ramos R, Cunningham FG, et al. Cefotaxime treatment for women with community acquired pelvic abscess. *Am J Obstet Gynecol* 1985;151:771.

162. Mercer LJ, Hajj SN, Ismail MA, Block BS. Use of C-reactive protein to predict the outcome of medical management of tuboovarian abscess. *J Reprod Med* 1988;33:164.

163. Hemsell DL, Hemsell PG, Heard MC, Nobles BJ. Piperacillin and a combination of clindamycin and gentamicin for the treatment of hospital- and community-acquired acute pelvic infections including pelvic abscess. *Surg Gynecol Obstet* 1987;165:223.

164. Reed SD, Landers DV, Sweet RL. Antibiotic treatment of tuboovarian abscess: comparison or broad spectrum beta lactam agents versus clindamycin containing regimens. *Am J Obstet Gynecol* 1991;164:1556.

165. Collins CA, Jansen FW. Treatment of pelvic abscess. *Clin Obstet Gynecol* 1959;2:512.

166. Rivlin ME, Hunt JA. Ruptured tubo-ovarian abscess: is hysterectomy necessary? *Obstet Gynecol* 1977;50:518.

167. Rubenstein PR, Mishell DR, Ledger WJ. Colpotomy drainage of pelvic abscess. *Obstet Gynecol* 1976;48:142.

168. Rivlin ME, Golan A, Darling MR. Diffuse peritoneal sepsis associated with colpotomy drainage of pelvic abscess. *J Reprod Med* 1982;27:406.

169. Rivlin ME. Clinical outcome following vaginal drainage of pelvic abscess. *Obstet Gynecol* 1983;61:169.

170. Mandel SR, Body D, Jaques PF, et al. Drainage of hepatic, intraabdominal and mediastinal abscesses guided by computerized axial tomography. *Am J Surg* 1983;145:120.

171. Van Sonnenberg E, Ferrucci JT, Mueller PR, et al. Percutaneous radiographically guided catheter drainage of abdominal abscesses. *JAMA* 1982;247:190.

172. Worthen NJ, Gunning JE. Percutaneous drainage of pelvic abscess: management of tuboovarian abscess. *J Ultrasound Med* 1986;5:551.

173. Gerzof SG, Robbins AH, Johnson WC, et al. Percutaneous catheter drainage of abdominal abscesses. *N Engl J Med* 1981;305:653.

174. Gronvall S, Gammelgaard J, Haubek A, Holm HH. Drainage of abdominal abscesses guided by sonography. *Am J Radiol* 1982;138:527.

175. Van Sonnenberg E, Ferrucci JT, Mueller PR, et al. Percutaneous drainage of abscess and fluid collections. Techniques, results and applications. *Radiology* 1982;142:1.

176. Kuligowska E, Conners SK, Shapiro JH. Liver abscess: sonography in diagnosis and treatment. *AJR* 1982;138:253.

177. Jeffrey RB Jr, Federle MP, Laing FC. Computed tomography of silent abdominal abscesses. *J Comput Assist Tomogr* 1984;8:67.

178. Tyrrel RT, Murphy FB, Bernardino ME. Tuboovarian abscesses: CT-guided percutaneous drainage. *Radiology* 1990;175:87–89.

179. Abbitt PL, Goldwag S, Urbanski S. Endovaginal sonography for guidance in draining pelvic fluid collections. *AJR* 1990;154:849–850.

180. Van Der Kolk HL. Small, deep pelvic abscesses: definition and drainage guided with an endovaginal probe. *Radiology* 1991;181:283–284.

181. Van Sonnenberg E, D'Agostino HB, Casola G, Goodacre BW, Sanchez RB, Taylor B. US-guided transvaginal drainage of pelvic abscesses and fluid collections. *Radiology* 1991;181:53–56.

182. Teisala K, Heinonen PK, Punnonen R. Transvaginal ultrasound in the diagnosis and treatment of tuboovarian abscess. *Br J Obstet Gynecol* 1990;97:178–179.

183. Loy RA, Galup DG, Hill JA, et al. Pelvic abscess: examination and transvaginal drainage guided by real-time ultrasonography. *South Med J* 1989;82:788–790.

184. Nosher JL, Winchman HK, Needell CS. Transvaginal pelvic abscess drainage with US guidance. *Radiology* 1987;165:872–873.

185. Sinow R, Nelson A, Renslo R, Renslo M. Atamdede F. Ultrasound guided transvaginal aspiration of pelvic abscesses. *Surg Forum* 1992;43:520–522.

186. Abolulghar MA, Mansur RT, Serour GI. Ultrasonographically guided transvaginal aspiration of tuboovarian abscesses and pyosalpinges: an optional treatment for acute pelvic inflammatory disease. *Am J Obstet Gynecol* 1995;172:1501–1503.

187. Nelson AL, Sinow RM, Oliak D. Transrectal ultrasonographically guided drainage of gynecologic pelvic abscesses. *Am J Obstet Gynecol* 2000;182:1283–1288.

188. Kuligowska E, Keller E, Ferrucci JT. Treatment of pelvic abscesses: value of one-step sonographically guided transrectal needle aspiration and lavage. *AJR* 1995;164:201–206.

189. Bennett JD, Kozak RI, Taylor BM, Jory TA. Deep pelvic abscesses: transrectal drainage with radiologic guidance. *Radiology* 1992;185:825–828.

190. Feld R, Eschelman DJ, Sagerman JE, Segal S, Hovsepian DM, Sullivan KL. Treatment of pelvic abscesses and other fluid collections: efficacy of transvaginal sonographically guided aspiration and drainage. *AJR* 1994;163:1141–1145.

191. Chung T, Hoffer FA, Lund DP. Transrectal drainage of deep pelvic abscesses in children using a combined transrectal sonographic and fluoroscopic guidance. *Pediatr Radiol* 1996;26:874–878.

192. Kastan DJ, Nelson KM, Shetty PC, Burke MW, Sharma RP. Combined transrectal sonographic and fluoroscopic for deep pelvic abscess drainage. *J Ultrasound Med* 1996;15:235–239.

193. Hovsepian DM. Transrectal and transvaginal abscess drainage. *Radiology* 1997;8:501–515.

194. Hovsepian DM, Steele JR, Skinner CS. Transrectal versus transvaginal abscess drainage: survey of patient tolerance and effect on activities of daily living. *Radiology* 1999;212:159–163.

195. Henry-Suchet J, Soler A, Loffredo V. Laparoscopic treatment of tuboovarian abscess. *J Reprod Med* 1984;29:579.

196. Reich H, McGlynn F. Laparoscopic treatment of tuboovarian abscess and pelvic abscess. *J Reprod Med* 1987;32:747.

197. Adducci JE. Laparoscopy in the diagnosis and treatment of pelvic inflammatory disease with abscess formation. *Int Surg* 1981;66:359.

198. Kaplan AL, Jacobs WM, Ehresman JB. Aggressive management of pelvic abscess. *Am J Obstet Gynecol* 1967;98:482.

199. Raiga J, Canis M, LeBouedec G, et al. Laparoscopic management of adnexal abscesses: consequences for fertility. *Fertil Steril* 1996;66:712–717.

CHAPTER 111
Vaginitis, Cervicitis, and Endometritis

David A. Eschenbach

VAGINITIS

Complaint of an abnormal vaginal discharge is one of the most common reasons women visit primary care and specialist physicians. The discharge can be from a physiologic increase in fluid or from a vaginal or cervical infection. Vaginal infection results either from overgrowth of normal flora as in candidiasis and bacterial vaginosis (BV) or from sexual transmission as in trichomoniasis and cervicitis.

The Normal State of the Vagina

The vagina of reproductive-aged women is lined by a rather static layer of stratified squamous epithelium about 25 cells thick, containing antigen-presenting cells and T lymphocytes (1). Vaginal discharge fluid is a complex mixture of material in transudate from blood vessels just beneath the epithelial surface. Transudate egresses through intracellular channels between vaginal epithelial cells (2). Fluid is also derived from the cervix and endometrium. The remainder of vaginal discharge consists of sloughed epithelial cells, microorganisms, urea, protein (including enzymes), carbohydrates, fatty acids, and chemical by-products of microorganisms and the local cellular metabolism (3). Vaginal fluid also contain T cells, immunoglobulins, cytokines, and a multitude of other components (4).

Before puberty or at menopause, the vaginal epithelium is cuboid, and the pH of vaginal discharge is 6.0 to 8.0. Under the influence of estrogen, glycogen collects in the vaginal epithelial cells, and the epithelium markedly thickens. The glycogen is metabolized by bacteria, particularly lactobacilli. The metabolism of both lactobacilli and vaginal epithelium produces high levels of lactic acid, which results in the low pH of vaginal fluid in menstruating women of 3.5 to 4.7 (5). The normal vaginal flora in women who are producing or taking estrogen is dominated by lactobacilli, which make up about 95% of the bacterial count (6). Lactobacilli maintain their dominance over other vaginal microorganisms by producing lactic acid (and, thus, the low pH that inhibits most bacteria), hydrogen peroxide (which inhibits catalase-negative bacteria) (7), and bactericidins. Other microorganisms in vaginal flora include *Staphylococcus epidermidis*, diphtheroids, *Gardnerella vaginalis*, both aerobic and anaerobic streptococci, anaerobic *Prevotella* and *Bacteroides* species, and *Ureaplasma urealyticum* (8,9). About 15% of women carry *Escherichia coli*, group B streptococci, and *Candida* species. Lactobacilli concentration increases before menses, then decreases during menses (1). The variation of other bacteria during the menstrual cycle is relatively small. Premenarchal and postmenopausal patients have an increase number of anaerobic lactobacilli and other anaerobes.

Examination of Cervical and Vaginal Discharges

A systematic examination of the discharge is required to diagnose infection accurately in symptomatic women (10). Inspection is needed of the vulva and vagina for erythema and of the cervix for mucopus (yellow mucus on a cotton-tipped swab). Abnormal cervical discharge should be Gram stained to identify an excess of polymorphonuclear leukocytes (PMNs) of more than 30 per high-power field and tested for *Neisseria gonorrhoeae* and *Chlamydia trachomatis*. A pH of the vaginal discharge is essential to place patients in two general categories of vaginitis (Fig. 111.1). One drop of vaginal discharge is mixed with normal saline and covered with a coverslip, and another drop is mixed with 10% potassium hydroxide and smelled for the presence of amines before a coverslip is placed. In some cases, a smear for Gram stain or material for culture is collected. Therapy for vaginitis becomes relatively easy if the diagnosis is correct, and except for occasional recurrent infection, most therapeutic failures result from an incorrect diagnosis. Microscopy is essential for an accurate diagnosis of vaginitis (10). Several specific elements should be actively sought by microscopy: long *Lactobacillus* species morphotypes, small coccobacillary morphotypes, white blood cells, trichomonads, and clue cells in the saline slide and hyphae in the potassium hydroxide part of the slide (Fig. 111.1).

Candidiasis

Candida species are present as commensals in about 15% of reproductive-aged women (1,9). Several predisposing factors for candidiases have been identified in the general population, including previous vaginal candidiases, frequency of coitus, oral and vaginal contraceptive use, and more than two episodes a week of passive oral-genital contact. Special factors that

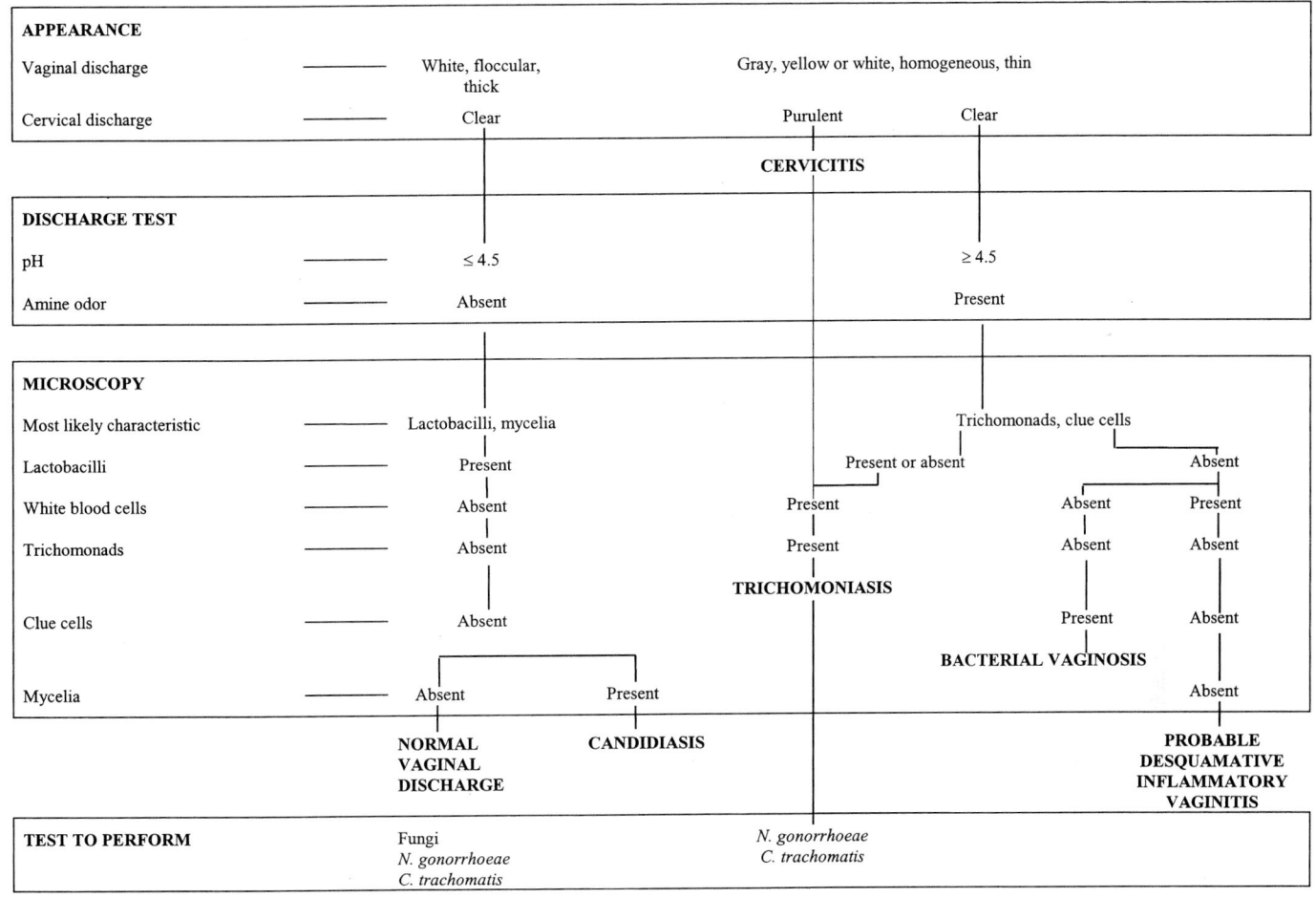

Figure 111.1. Systematic outline to ensure an accurate diagnosis of vaginitis and cervicitis.

contribute to vaginal candidiases include antibiotic and corticosteroid use, diabetes, pregnancy, and acquired immunodeficiency syndrome (AIDS) (11). In menstruating women, symptoms most commonly develop just before menses. Excessive warmth and moisture are related to vulvovaginal candidiases. Rarely, men with genital candidiases will sexually transmit *Candida* species. Tight clothing, tampon use, and douching are not related to vaginal candidiases.

Candida albicans is responsible for 85% to 90% of vaginal candidiases (12). Other *Candida* species, such as *Candida glabrata, Candida krusei, Candida tropicalis,* and *Candida pseudotropicalis,* also can cause symptomatic infection. Non-*albicans* species are particularly common in women with recurrent candidiases, and they are more resistant to azoles than *C. albicans* (13). All species of *Candida* except *C. glabrata* exist in two forms: a blastospore and a germinated form with hyphae. The blastospore attaches to the epithelial cell and colonizes the surface. The germinated form is present during infection in which *Candida* invades the superficial epithelium (11).

Typical symptoms include vulvar pruritus, a burning sensation, superficial dysuria, and a white discharge. Vulvar erythema and, at times, a geographic rash are present. The vagina is often erythematous; in about 25% of patients, a pathognomonic thick, dry, curdy vaginal discharge occurs. The vaginal pH is 4.7 or less, and hyphae usually are identified on wet mount or Gram-stained material at the low microscopic power. Among women with pruritus or other genital findings that could represent *Candida* infection, it is important to perform a culture for *Candida* when the microscopic examination result is negative. A culture identifies an increased number of symptomatic women with candidiasis compared with microscopy alone, and it also can help exclude candidiasis in symptomatic women with an unclear diagnosis (14).

Vaginal candidiasis is usually treated with one of the azoles, most commonly an intravaginal preparation. Intravaginal medication given for 3 to 7 days has better long-term efficacy than 1-day regimens. Miconazole, clotrimazole, butoconazole, and terconazole are all available for intravaginal use (15) (Table 111.1). In the unusual situation in which resistance occurs to one azole, resistance is present to all of the azoles. Oral fluconazole and itraconazole can be used to treat vaginal candidiases, but oral azole therapy is no more efficacious than local azole treatment. Particularly symptomatic women require a second oral fluconazole dose (16). Nystatin is no longer a first-line drug, but it can be useful when resistance develops to azoles. Boric acid (boric acid powder in gelatin capsules) is fungistatic, and intravaginal use helps treat strains resistant to azoles (17). Flucytosine is advocated for *C. glabrata* (18). Most patients rapidly become symptom free with any of the anti-*Candida* therapies. Allergy to the base in the vaginal preparation or other reasons for symptoms should be considered when women taking azoles have persistent or increasing symptoms. Persistent symptoms from *Candida* resistant to azoles are unusual.

Recurrent Vaginal Candidiases

Candidiasis occurs in up to 75% of women at some time in their life, usually only one to three times. However, a small number

TABLE 111.1. Treatment Regimens for Vaginal Candidiases

Imidazoles	
Clotrimazole	200-mg vaginal tablet nightly for 3 d
	or
	100-mg vaginal tablet or 1% cream, 5 g intravaginally nightly for 7 d
Miconazole nitrate	200-mg vaginal suppository nightly for 3 d
	or
	100-mg vaginal suppository or 2% cream, 5 g intravaginally nightly for 7 d
Butoconazole	2% cream, 5 g intravaginally nightly for 3 d
Terconazole	80-mg vaginal suppository nightly for 3 d
	or
	0.4% cream, 5 g intravaginally nightly for 7 d
Fluconazole	150 mg orally in a single dose
Polyenes	
Nystatin	100,000-unit vaginal tablet, 1 per vagina twice daily for 14 d
Boric acid	600 mg powder in gelatin capsules, 1 per vagina twice daily for 14 d
Treatment during pregnancy: Clotrimazole, miconazole, and terconazole may be used intravaginally for the treatment of symptomatic patients during pregnancy. It is suggested that their use be deferred until the second trimester.	

of women have frequent recurrences; those with four or more recurrences a year are considered to have frequent recurrent candidiasis (11). Such patients should be examined and culture performed for *Candida* to ensure that recurrent symptoms are actually due to *Candida* and to rule out potentially resistant species. It is not clear whether these relapses occur with the same strain or are due to rapid recolonization from the skin or gastrointestinal tract (19). Attempts to reduce *Candida* in the gastrointestinal tract only slightly influence recurrent infection (20), although continued gastrointestinal tract suppression by ingesting 4 ounces of yogurt containing lactobacilli twice daily reduces recurrence (21). Sexual partner therapy is not useful, except for men with symptomatic genital candidiasis (22).

Women with frequently recurrent candidiasis need to be scrutinized for risk factors, although few women have risk factors. Women with AIDS have an increased risk for vaginal candidiasis but AIDS is unusual even with recurrent candidiasis. Women with frequent recurrences should receive 3 weeks of standard anti-*Candida* therapy with local or oral azoles followed by 6 to 12 months of suppressive therapy. Effective suppressive therapy includes intravaginal azoles or boric acid given every third night and weekly fluconazole. Ketoconazole should no longer be used for candidiases because of hepatotoxic effects.

Trichomoniasis

Trichomonas vaginalis is a sexually transmitted protozoan. *T. vaginalis* can be recovered from the prostate gland of up to 70% of male sexual partners of women with trichomoniasis (23). Symptoms of an uncomfortable or yellow vaginal discharge occur in about 40% to 50% of patients with *T. vaginalis* infection (24,25). Symptomatic women may have vulvar erythema and edema; about 60% have a purulent vaginal discharge, and 10% have a frothy vaginal discharge (25). Pathognomonic punctate areas of red epithelium (strawberry lesions or colpitis macularis) are unusual to see with the naked eye but were observed by colposcopy in 44% of such patients (25). The vaginal pH is usually 4.7 or higher, and on saline wet mount, an elevated number of PMNs and the herky-jerky motion of the mobile trichomonad can be observed. Fortunately, most symptomatic patients have trichomonads recognized by wet mount, but only about 50% of women with *T. vaginalis* recovered from the vagina have a high enough concentration of trichomonads to be found on wet

mount. Modified Diamond media should be used for culture, although culture is usually necessary only to test for suspected metronidazole resistance.

T. vaginalis infection is treated with a 2-g single dose of metronidazole (26). Seven-day metronidazole regimens can also be used (Table 111.2). Simultaneous male partner treatment should be used to reduce failure rates from about 20% to 3% (27,28). Patients with recurrent infection should receive metronidazole for 7 days. Patients with severe symptoms in pregnancy should be treated with a 2-g single dose after the first trimester (26). *T. vaginalis* infection has not reduced preterm birth, and treatment in pregnancy is limited to symptomatic women (29).

Rarely, patients have strains of *T. vaginalis* that are relatively resistant to metronidazole, with levels of 100 μg or more of metronidazole needed for inhibition (30). These patients fail to respond to 2 g of metronidazole daily for 2 to 10 days. They often require a 1-g oral dose of metronidazole twice daily plus an intravaginal dose of 500 mg of metronidazole twice daily (tablets crushed in a base at a concentration of 500 mg per 5 mL, the volume of a vaginal applicator). This regimen causes considerable anorexia, nausea, and vomiting. Doses exceeding 3 g per day of metronidazole should be avoided because of possible irreversible peripheral neuropathy. It is possible to obtain tinidazole from the U.S. Food and Drug Administration (FDA) for metronidazole-resistant cases (31).

TABLE 111.2. Treatment Regimens for Trichomoniasis

For initial infection
Metronidazole, 2 g orally as a single dose
Metronidazole, 500 mg orally twice daily for 7 d
For treatment failures
Re-treat with metronidazole, 500 mg twice daily for 7 d
For repeated treatment failures
Re-treat with metronidazole, 1 g orally twice daily, plus 500 mg of intravaginal metronidazole twice daily for 7–10 d
Treatment during pregnancy
After the first trimester, metronidazole, 2 g orally as a single dose, for women with severe symptoms

The patient's sexual partner should be treated simultaneously.

Bacterial Vaginosis

BV is a syndrome in which the vaginal flora is no longer dominated by lactobacilli and there is an overgrowth of *G. vaginalis*, certain anaerobic bacteria, and *Mycoplasma hominis* (6). Facultative lactobacilli are found in only 20% to 25% of patients with BV, and most of these strains do not produce hydrogen peroxide. Concomitant with the drop in the concentration of facultative lactobacilli is an increase in the concentration of the other microorganisms.

In a population-based study containing a cohort of both asymptomatic and symptomatic pregnant women, those with BV have a 10-fold increase in the concentration of *G. vaginalis*, certain anaerobes, and *M. hominis* compared with those without vaginitis (6). However, symptomatic women with BV have a 100 to 1,000 times increase in the concentration of *G. vaginalis* and certain anaerobes compared to those without vaginitis. The anaerobes associated with BV include *Prevotella* species, *Prevotella bivia*, *Bacteroides ureolyticus*, *Peptostreptococcus* species, and *Mobiluncus* species (6,32). It is not clear which microorganisms are primary and which secondarily overgrow in BV. The amine trimethylamine is a metabolic product of this bacterial overgrowth that cause the fishy odor (33). These amines are bound to protein at a low pH, but alkalinization of vaginal fluid by semen during intercourse or by potassium hydroxide volatilizes the amines and produces the fishy odor characteristic of BV. A variety of inorganic acids are also produced by the microorganisms in BV, including succinate, which inhibits PMN migration (34).

Factors associated with BV include sexual activity, a new male or a female sexual partner, antibiotic use, *T. vaginalis*, and use of intrauterine device (35). However, BV is not a classic sexually transmitted disease (STD) because no specific agents in the male partner have been found, and treatment of men with metronidazole does not prevent recurrent BV (36).

About half of women with BV are asymptomatic. Women with BV complain of a fishy vaginal odor and increased vaginal discharge (37). BV is present in about 15% to 20% of a general sexually active population, but the prevalence varies widely from 5% of asymptomatic college students to 30% to 45% of women attending STD clinics and African women (38–40).

The clinical diagnosis of BV is based on the presence of three of the four following characteristics of vaginal discharge: (a) a pH above 4.5, (b) a thin (skim milk) appearance, (c) a fishy amine odor when 10% potassium hydroxide is placed on the discharge, and (d) clue cells (38). Clue cells are vaginal epithelial cells that contain so many bacteria on their surface that the cell border is obscured. On wet mount, long *Lactobacillus* morphotypes are absent, and numerous small coccobacillary forms are present. Gram stain criteria exist for BV. Gram stain diagnosis closely correlates with the diagnosis made by clinical criteria (41,42). Gram stain criteria rely on a paucity of long gram-positive lactobacilli morphotypes and numerous small gram-negative and gram-positive *Gardnerella* and *Prevotella* rod morphotypes, gram-positive cocci, and gram-variable curved-rod *Mobiluncus* morphotypes. Culture should not be used to diagnose BV because *G. vaginalis* cultures are misleading and proper anaerobic cultures are too expensive. *G. vaginalis* is isolated from virtually all women with BV but also from half of the women without vaginitis (43), and the recovery of *G. vaginalis* is too nonspecific to diagnose BV.

All symptomatic nonpregnant women and nonpregnant women undergoing selected pelvic operations with BV should be treated. Asymptomatic women should not be treated. The reason for an expansion of the treatment group relates to data associating BV with upper genital tract infection. Pregnant patients with BV have a 50% to 100% increased rate of preterm low-birth-

TABLE 111.3. Treatment Regimens for Bacterial Vaginosis

For initial infection in symptomatic patients
Nonpregnant patients
 Metronidazole, 500 mg orally twice daily for 7 d
 Metronidazole, 0.75% gel intravaginally once daily for 5 d
 Clindamycin 2% cream, intravaginally nightly for 7 d
Pregnant patients
 Metronidazole, 250 mg 3 times daily for 7 day, *after the first trimester*
 Clindamycin, 300 mg orally 3 times daily for 7 d
For recurrent infection in symptomatic patients
 Repeat treatment with vaginal metronidazole or clindamycin and consider suppressive twice weekly dosing.
For asymptomatic patients
 Antibiotic treatment should be given if the patient is at risk for upper genital tract infection from a surgical procedure.

weight delivery (44), amniotic fluid infection (45), and chorioamnion infection (46). Treatment of BV reduces the preterm low-birth-weight rate to baseline levels, in some (47,48) but not all (49) studies. Thus, BV is not routinely diagnosed and treated in pregnancy (49).

The high concentration of potentially virulent bacteria in the vagina is related to other upper genital tract infections. Patients with BV who have a cesarean section have a sixfold increased rate of postpartum endometritis (50). Patients with BV undergoing therapeutic abortion have a threefold increased rate of pelvic inflammatory disease, and metronidazole therapy reduces this rate to baseline levels (51,52). Patients with BV undergoing abdominal hysterectomy have a threefold to fourfold increased rate of vaginal cuff cellulitis (53,54).

Two antimicrobials with high activity against anaerobic bacteria provide first-line therapy (Table 111.3). Both oral and intravaginal metronidazole and clindamycin regimens produce cure rates of 80% to 90% (26,55,56). Single-dose metronidazole and 7-day amoxicillin-clavulanate regimens are also effective. Regimens with little or no activity against BV include oral ampicillin, cephalosporins, quinolones, tetracycline, and erythromycin and intravaginal triple sulfa cream and povidone-iodine (Betadine) gel. *Lactobacillus* given orally or intravaginally may help to prevent recurrence, but no proof exists. Recurrent BV has been managed with biweekly suppressive dosing following a standard 5- to 7-day regimen (57). As mentioned, metronidazole given to men has no effect on the recurrence of BV in their sexual partners (36).

CERVICITIS

Background

Terms such as *cervical erosion*, *cervical ectopy*, and *cervical hypertrophy* represent variances of the normal cervical anatomy rather than examples of cervical infection. Columnar epithelium lines the endocervical canal and secretes the mucus found in the endocervical canal. If columnar epithelium is located entirely inside the endocervical canal, it is not visible, and the cervix has a normal appearance. However, columnar epithelium can often be present on the cervical portio, where it has a red appearance because columnar epithelium is only a few cells thick and the red color is from light reflecting off superficial blood vessels. The extension of columnar epithelium onto the cervical portio is termed *ectopy* (58). Ectopy is normal variation, and the amount of ectopic tissue visible on the cervical portio varies considerably between patients. Most ectopy is unrelated to infectious agents; rather, it appears to be related to age and estrogen. Ectopy commonly appears after menarche, and patients with a high level of estrogen, such as oral contraceptive users, have increased prevalence and areas of cervical ectopy (58).

Mucopurulent cervicitis is the preferred and specific term for inflammation of cervical columnar epithelium. The presence of yellowish cervical mucus in the cervical canal or an abnormal increase in PMNs on Gram-stained material from the endocervical canal is evidence of mucopurulent cervicitis (59). A standard definition of cervicitis allows researchers to compare diseases irrespective of the microorganism recovered from the cervix. To date, microorganisms commonly correlated with the presence of mucopurulent cervicitis include *C. trachomatis, N. gonorrhoeae*, herpes simplex virus (HSV) (59,60), and most recently, *Mycoplasma genitalium* (61). Follicular cervicitis and hypertrophic cervicitis are descriptive terms used for *C. trachomatis* cervical infection. The histologic appearance of *C. trachomatis* infection in the cervix is relatively well described, but less is known about histologic changes associated with other infections. Inflammatory cells are commonly found in the cervical epithelium and in the cervical stoma of patients without mucopurulent cervicitis who undergo biopsy to diagnose cervical dysplasia. The significance of inflammatory cells with acute and chronic histologic cervicitis and their correlation with the microorganisms associated with mucopurulent cervicitis have not been determined; therefore, the remainder of this chapter focuses on mucopurulent cervicitis.

Prevalence

The true prevalence of mucopurulent cervicitis has been underestimated in most clinical settings. The frequent failure to recognize mucopurulent cervicitis has been related to nonstandard definitions, to confusion and normal anatomy, and to inattention to physical signs. The prevalence of mucopus depends on the prevalence of these microorganisms in the population under study. In an STD clinic, the prevalence of mucopurulent cervicitis in women appears to be similar to the prevalence of both nongonococcal and gonococcal urethritis in men. Mucopurulent cervicitis is reported in 24% to 40% of randomly selected female patients attending STD clinics and in 34% of consecutive women undergoing routine annual examination at a university student health clinic (60,62). Among patients with *C. trachomatis*, mucopurulent cervicitis was present in 64% to 95% of randomly sampled STD patients and in about one third of randomly sampled college students (62).

Mucopurulent cervicitis was found in only 15% of STD patients with *N. gonorrhoeae*, and the frequency of mucopus among patients with *N. gonorrhoeae* and no *C. trachomatis* is surprisingly low (62). Thus, *C. trachomatis* is more often associated with mucopus than *N. gonorrhoeae*.

Importance

Uterine cervical infections are of considerable importance because they represent an important reservoir for the spread of sexually transmitted microorganisms. Cervicitis also provides a source of intraluminal ascent of pathogenic organisms to the endometrium and endosalpinx. Cervical infections lead to the development of pelvic inflammatory disease. From 10% to 20% of women with cervical *N. gonorrhoeae* and at least 10% of patients with cervical *C. trachomatis* develop clinical manifestations of pelvic inflammatory disease. In 50% to 70% of patients with salpingitis, the infection is not recognized by the patient or her physician (63,64). Even when salpingitis is promptly recognized

and treated, most of the acute tubal damage that later caused tubal infertility appears before antibiotic therapy was instituted. Thus, the identification and treatment of cervicitis are keys to reduce rates of infertility and ectopic pregnancy secondary to salpingitis.

The second important consequence of cervicitis is the possible ascent during pregnancy of infectious agents that produce chorioamnionitis, premature rupture of membranes, amniotic fluid infection, premature delivery, and puerperal and neonatal infections. Both *C. trachomatis* and *N. gonorrhoeae* have been related to these adverse perinatal outcomes (65,66).

Microorganisms

Organisms related to mucopurulent cervicitis include *C. trachomatis, N. gonorrhoeae*, HSV, and *M. genitalium* (62). *C. trachomatis* is more closely associated with the presence of mucopus than the other agents. As mentioned earlier, a substantial proportion of patients with *C. trachomatis* have mucopus, and conversely, among patients with mucopus, 30% to 60% have *C. trachomatis* (62). Overall, *C. trachomatis* is isolated from about 40% to 50% of patients with mucopus or an increased number of PMNs on Gram stain of cervical mucus. Many patients with *C. trachomatis* also have *N. gonorrhoeae*. The strong association between *C. trachomatis* and mucopus and the weak association between *N. gonorrhoeae* and mucopus are curious. Perhaps *C. trachomatis* infection is a more chronic process, with either no symptoms or chronic symptoms and signs, whereas *N. gonorrhoeae* infection requires early treatment because of acute symptoms. Acute primary HSV infection causes ulcerative lesions and an exudate covering the cervix, but neither mucopus nor ulcers are present with recurrent HSV infections (67).

T. vaginalis and *M. hominis* and BV are not related to mucopurulent cervicitis when the presence of *C. trachomatis* is controlled. However, in one study, *U. urealyticum* remained associated with mucopurulent cervicitis after adjustment for the presence of *C. trachomatis* (62). *U. urealyticum* has also been associated with nongonococcal urethritis in men, independently of *C. trachomatis*.

Clinical Diagnosis

Manifestations of mucopurulent cervicitis are difficult to recognize for both the patient and the physician. Organisms such as *C. trachomatis* can simultaneously infect the urethra, cervix, and rectum and produce variable symptoms. Symptoms from cervical infection are often poorly localized and frequently mistaken for vaginitis. Symptoms can include an increase in yellow vaginal discharge and, less commonly, postcoital spotting, vague lower abdominal pain, and mild discomfort with intercourse. However, cervical infections usually produce no symptoms. In addition, tests for *C. trachomatis* and *N. gonorrhoeae* do not provide completely ideal information because results are positive in only about half of patients with mucopurulent cervicitis, and a large number of patients with mucopurulent cervicitis would not be detected by these tests. Further, in the past, physicians have not usually appreciated the clinical signs of cervical infection. Thus, compared with the recognition of nongonococcal urethritis in men, the recognition of cervicitis in women is more problematic.

Cervical mucus is normally clean and translucent. Yellow discharge observed on a white cotton swab best identifies cervical mucopus. However, vaginal discharge must be wiped from the face of the cervix so that it does not confuse this clinical test. Yellow mucopus is highly correlated with an increased number of PMNs on a Gram stain of cervical mucus from nonpregnant patients (60). Opaque cervical mucus is common in pregnancy, and mucopus may be more difficult to distinguish from the normal secretion in pregnant patients (68).

Easily produced bleeding of the columnar epithelium from the inflammation is the second most common manifestation of mucopurulent cervicitis (60). Bleeding occurs when the cervix is swabbed for Papanicolaou (Pap) smears or other cervical tests.

Laboratory Diagnosis

Endocervical mucus should be obtained on a swab to confirm the presence of mucopurulent cervicitis. Vaginal material must be wiped off the face of the cervix with a large cotton-tipped swab before cervical mucus is collected; otherwise, the Gram stain is likely to be uninterpretable because of vaginal bacteria or PMNs. A standard approach includes the reading of five representative fields under the high-power ($\times$1,000) microscope objective (58). An increased number of PMNs on the Gram stain is highly correlated with the presence of cervical pathogens. The exact number of PMNs needed to establish an abnormal number is population dependent. In some studies, a mean of 10 or more PMNs per high-power ($\times$1,000) field was used to define cervicitis (69). A more liberal definition of a mean of 20 to 30 PMNs increases the specificity but lowers the sensitivity to detect a cervical pathogen (59). Further evaluation of the mean number of PMNs to distinguish cervicitis is needed for pregnancy. Pap smears can also be used to detect the presence of an increased number of PMNs, and they aid in the diagnosis of cervicitis (67). DNA polymerase or ligase chain reaction tests are more sensitive than other methods used to detect *C. trachomatis* and *N. gonorrhoeae* (70).

Therapy

Therapy for mucopurulent cervicitis should cover *C. trachomatis* and *N. gonorrhoeae*. In a randomized comparison of oral tetracycline with oral amoxicillin, both agents unexpectedly treated *C. trachomatis* and cervicitis, and both equally eliminated mucopus and other cervical manifestations of cervicitis, including the PMN count in patients without *C. trachomatis* infection (71). Only about half of the patients in this study had either *C. trachomatis* or *N. gonorrhoeae*, and the disappearance of mucopus among patients without these two bacteria suggests a bacterial infection even in the culture-negative patients with cervicitis. Despite these findings, doxycycline or azithromycin is preferred to treat mucopurulent cervicitis, especially in patients with known *C. trachomatis* infection (26,72). Patients with penicillinase-producing *N. gonorrhoeae* do not usually respond to tetracyclines; thus, ceftriaxone together with azithromycin would be preferable in these cases. The regimen includes doxycycline in a dose of 100 mg twice a day for a total of 10 days, or azithromycin in a single 1-g dose.

ENDOMETRITIS

Background

Endometritis is an infection of the endometrial cavity, which is anatomically interposed between the cervix and fallopian tubes. Endometritis has only recently been described in terms of pathologic and clinical manifestations. The endometrium of patients with endometritis may contain a large variety of inflammatory cells during menstrual sloughing, but the presence of plasma cells in the endometrium is necessary to diagnose endometritis (73). Leukocytes and lymphocytes are often present in large numbers in the endometrium of patients with plasma cells, but they are also normally present just before and during menses.

However, a more acute form of endometritis may be indicated by leukocytes at other times of the menstrual cycle (73,74).

A high prevalence of plasma cell endometritis has been found among patients with mucopurulent cervicitis. Fourteen (40%) of 35 women with cervical mucopus had plasma cell endometritis (75). Endometritis is present in 80% to 90% of patients with salpingitis (73). Plasma cell endometritis appears to be infrequent among asymptomatic patients without mucopurulent cervicitis who underwent endometrial biopsy to evaluate infertility (75).

Microorganisms

Both *C. trachomatis* and, to a lesser extent, *N. gonorrhoeae* are associated with endometritis (73–75). BV also is independently associated with plasma cell endometritis (76,77). *Chlamydia* inclusions can be identified in the endometrium by use of monoclonal antibodies. In fact, *C. trachomatis* was identified more frequently in endometrial tissue by monoclonal antibody than by cultures. In unusual circumstances, HSV has also been found in endometrium (78). Recently, *M. genitalium* was related to endometritis (79).

Clinical Diagnosis

Endometritis has been associated with a history of intermenstrual vaginal bleeding and increased bleeding with menses. Up to half of the women of reproductive age who have an endometrial biopsy for abnormal uterine bleeding have had plasma cell endometritis (unpublished data). The diagnosis of endometritis was not made clinically or by usual pathologic study in most of these women. Uterine and adnexal tenderness has been recognized more frequently among patients with endometritis than among those without (74). In addition, cervical motion tenderness and elevations of the erythrocyte sedimentation rate and the peripheral white cell count can be present with endometritis.

Careful bimanual examination may reveal mild uterine tenderness (74,75); however, it is difficult to make the distinction between endometritis alone and endometritis with salpingitis on a clinical basis. Thus, in studies in which the diagnosis of salpingitis was not confirmed by laparoscopy, some patients with a clinical diagnosis of salpingitis in fact have endometritis without salpingitis. This emphasizes the difficulties inherent in the clinical diagnosis of upper genital tract infection and the overlapping clinical findings between endometritis and salpingitis.

Laboratory Diagnosis

An endometrial biopsy appears to be the only reliable means to establish a diagnosis of endometritis. Endometrial biopsy is useful to establish a diagnosis of endometritis or upper genital tract infection (75). Patients with vague complaints for whom infection is not strongly suspected benefit from endometrial biopsy if the biopsy shows endometritis; however, an absence of plasma cells in the biopsy specimen does not rule out salpingitis because about 20% of patients with laparoscopically proven salpingitis have no evidence of plasma cells on endometrial biopsy (73).

Therapy

Treatment of endometritis with ceftriaxone and azithromycin appears to eliminate plasma cells from the endometrium (unpublished data). It also appears reasonable to use the outpatient treatment of salpingitis to treat endometritis. A loading dose of antibiotic to treat gonorrhea should be followed by 14 days of antibiotics to inhibit *C. trachomatis* (26). Treating endometritis is particularly important because of risk for infertility in untreated or undertreated patients who develop salpingitis.

Two special circumstances for endometritis exist. In at least one reported case, endometritis seemed related to reversible infertility (80). The second circumstance of endometritis exists after pregnancy. This has been most closely studied among patients who have had therapeutic abortion; about 20% of patients with *C. trachomatis* before the abortion develop laparoscopically confirmed salpingitis after the procedure (81). Recently, endometritis is a possible explanation for very early loss of pregnancy in women with BV undergoing *in vitro* fertilization (82) and for mid-trimester spontaneous abortion in pregnancy (83). The rate of postabortion salpingitis is five times greater among women with *C. trachomatis* than among those without. Manifestations often begin as a low-grade abdominal pain and mild uterine tenderness indicative of endometritis. Symptoms and signs of endometritis have also been noted after term vaginal delivery, when women usually develop mild lower abdominal pain about 2 weeks after delivery. These women are usually afebrile, and half have *C. trachomatis* (84).

Endometritis may be particularly important to identify and treat before tubal damage occurs. About 50% to 70% of patients who are infertile because of occluded fallopian tubes have never had a recognized episode of salpingitis (64). Presumably, most of these patients had mild symptoms or atypical manifestations of upper genital tract infection. It is important that physicians identify and treat patients who present with mild manifestations of pelvic infection.

REFERENCES

1. Patton DL, Thwin SS, Meier A, et al. Epithelial cell layer thickness and immune cell populations in the normal human vagina at different stages of the menstrual cycle. *Am J Obstet Gynecol* 2000;183:967–973.
2. Roig de Vargas-Linares CE. Vagina as a source of immunoglobulins. In: Hafez ESE, Evans TN, eds. *The human vagina*. Amsterdam: Elsevier North Holland, 1978:42.
3. Huggins GR, Preti G. Vaginal odors and secretions. *Clin Obstet Gynecol* 1981;24:355.
4. Moghissi KS. Vaginal fluid constituents. In: Beller FK, Chumacher GFB, eds. *The biology of fluids of the female genital tract*. Amsterdam: Elsevier North Holland, 1979.
5. Cohn L. Influence of pH on vaginal discharges. *Br J Vener Dis* 1969;45:241.
6. Hillier SL, Krohn MA, Rabe LK, et al. The normal vaginal flora, H₂O₂-producing lactobacilli, and bacterial vaginosis in pregnant women. *Clin Infect Dis* 1993;16[Suppl 4]:S273.
7. Eschenbach DA, Davick PR, Williams BL, et al. Prevalence of hydrogen peroxide-producing *Lactobacillus* species in normal women and women with bacterial vaginosis. *J Clin Microbiol* 1989;27:251.
8. Bartlett JG, Moon NE, Goldstein PR, et al. Cervical and vaginal bacterial flora: ecologic niches in the female lower genital tract. *Am J Obstet Gynecol* 1978;130:658.
9. Hill GB, Eschenbach DA, Holmes KK. Bacteriology of the vagina. *Scand J Urol Nephrol Suppl* 1984;86:23.
10. Ryan Ca, Courtois BN, Hawes SE, et al. Risk assessment, symptoms, and signs as predictors of vulvovaginal and cervical infections in an urban US STD clinic: implications for use of STD algorithms. *Sex Trans Infect* 1998;74[Suppl 1]:S59–76.
11. Sobel JD, Faro S, Force RW, et al. Vulvovaginal candidiasis: epidemiologic, diagnostic and therapeutic considerations. *Am J Obstet Gynecol* 1998;179:557–558.
12. Morton RS, Raskid S. Candidal vaginitis: natural history, predisposing factors and prevention. *Proc R Soc Med* 1977;70[Suppl 4]:3.
13. Spinillo A, Pizzoli G, Colonna L, et al. Epidemiologic characteristics of women with idiopathic recurrent vulvovaginal candidiasis. *Obstet Gynecol* 1993;51:721.
14. Eckert LO, Hawes SE, Stevens CE, et al. Vulvovaginal candidiasis: clinical manifestations, risk factors, management algorithm. *Obstet Gynecol* 1998;92:757–765.
15. Sobel JD. Vaginitis. *N Engl J Med* 1997;337:1896–1903.
16. Sobel JD, Kapernick PS, Zervox M, et al. Treatment of complicated Candida vaginitis: comparison of single and sequential doses of fluconazole. *Am J Obstet Gynecol* 2001;185:363–369.
17. Van Slyke KK, Michel VP, Rein MF. Treatment of vulvovaginal candidiasis with boric acid powder. *Am J Obstet Gynecol* 1981;141:145.
18. Horowitz BJ. Topical flucytosine therapy for chronic recurrent *Candida tropicalis* infection. *J Reprod Med* 1986;31:821–824.
19. O'Connor MI, Sobel JD. Epidemiology of recurrent vulvovaginal candidiasis: identification and strain differentiation of *Candida albicans*. *J Infect Dis* 1986;154:358.
20. Nystatin Multicenter Study Group. Therapy of candidal vaginitis: the effect of eliminating intestinal *Candida*. *Am J Obstet Gynecol* 1986;155:651.
21. Hilton E, Isenberg HD Alperstein P, et al. Ingestion of yogurt containing *Lactobacillus acidophilus* as prophylaxis for candidal vaginitis. *Ann Intern Med* 1992;116:418.
22. Buck A, Christenson ES. Treatment of vaginal candidosis with natamycin and effect of treating the partner at the same time. *Acta Obstet Gynecol Scand* 1982;61:393.
23. Block E. Occurrence of trichomoniasis in sexual partners of women with trichomoniasis. *Acta Obstet Gynecol Scand* 1959;35:398.
24. Krieger JN, Tam MR, Stevens CE, et al. Diagnosis of trichomoniasis: comparison of conventional wet-mount examination with cytologic studies, cultures, and monoclonal antibody staining of direct specimens. *JAMA* 1988;259:1223.
25. Wölner-Hanssen P, Krieger JN, Stevens CE, et al. Clinical manifestations of vaginal trichomoniasis. *JAMA* 1989;261:571.
26. Centers for Disease Control and Prevention. Sexually transmitted diseases treatment guidelines 2002. *MMWR Morb Mortal Wkly Rep* 2002;51:1.
27. Pereyra AJ, Lansing JD. Urogenital trichomoniasis: treatment with metronidazole in 2002 incarcerated women. *Obstet Gynecol* 1964;499.
28. Lossick JG. Single-dose metronidazole treatment for vaginal trichomoniasis. *Obstet Gynecol* 1980;56:508.
29. Klebanoff MA, Carey JC, Hauth JC, et al. National Institute of Child Health and Human Development Network of Maternal-Fetal Medicine Units. *N Engl J Med* 2001;345:487–493.
30. Lossick JG, Muller M, Gorrell TE. In vitro drug susceptibility and doses of metronidazole required for cure in cases of refractory vaginal trichomoniasis. *J Infect Dis* 1986;153:948.
31. Sobel JD, Nyirjesy P, Brown W. Tinidazole therapy for metronidazole-resistant vaginal trichomoniasis. *Clin Infect Dis* 2001;33:1341–1346.
32. Martius J, Krohn MA, Hillier SL, et al. Relationship of vaginal *Lactobacillus* species, cervical *Chlamydia trachomatis*, and bacterial vaginosis to preterm birth. *Obstet Gynecol* 1988;71:89.
33. Brand JM, Galask RP. Trimethylamine: the substance mainly responsible for the fishy odor often associated with bacterial vaginosis. *Obstet Gynecol* 1986;63:682–685.
34. Spiegel CA, Amsel R, Eschenbach DA, et al. Anaerobic bacteria in nonspecific vaginitis. *N Engl J Med* 1980;303:601.
35. Hawes SE, Hillier SL, Benedetti J, et al. Hydrogen peroxide-producing lactobacilli and acquisition of vaginal infections. *J Infect Dis* 1996;174:1058–1063.
36. Vejtorp M, Bollerup AC, Vejtorp L, et al. Bacterial vaginosis: a double-blind randomized trial of the effect of treatment of the sexual partner. *Br J Obstet Gynaecol* 1988;95:920.
37. Pheifer TA, Forsyth PA, Durfee MA, et al. Nonspecific vaginitis: role of *Haemophilus vaginalis* and treatment with metronidazole. *N Engl J Med* 1978;198:1429.
38. Amsel R, Totten PA, Spiegel CA, et al. Nonspecific vaginitis: diagnostic criteria and microbial and epidemiologic associations. *Am J Med* 1983;74:14.
39. Eschenbach DA, Hillier SL, Critchlow CW, et al. Diagnosis and clinical features associated with bacterial vaginosis. *Am J Obstet Gynecol* 1988;158:819.
40. Martin HL, Richardson BA, Nyange PM, et al. Vaginal lactobacilli, microbial flora, and risk of human immunodeficiency virus type 1 and sexually transmitted disease acquisition. *J Infect Dis* 1999;180:1863–1868.
41. Spiegel CA, Amsel R, Holmes KK. Diagnosis of bacterial vaginosis by direct Gram stain of vaginal fluid. *J Clin Microbiol* 1983;18:170.
42. Nugent RP, Krohn MA, Hillier SL. Reliability of diagnosing bacterial vaginosis is improved by a standardized method of Gram stain interpretation. *J Clin Microbiol* 1991;29:297.
43. Totten PA, Amsel R, Hale J, et al. Selective differential human blood bilayer media for isolation of *Gardnerella (Haemophilus) vaginalis*. *J Clin Microbiol* 1982;15:141.
44. Hillier SL, Nugent RP, Eschenbach DA, et al. The association of bacterial vaginosis *Bacteroides*, and *Mycoplasma hominis* with preterm low birth weight delivery. *N Engl J Med* 1995;333:1737.
45. Gravett MG, Hummel D, Eschenbach DA, et al. Preterm labor associated with subclinical amniotic fluid infection and with bacterial vaginosis. *Obstet Gynecol* 1986;67:229.
46. Hillier SL, Martius J, Krohn MA, et al. A case-control study of chorioamniotic infection and chorioamnionitis in prematurity. *N Engl J Med* 1988;319:972.
47. Morales WJ, Schorr S, Albritton J. Effect of metronidazole in patients with preterm birth in preceding pregnancy and bacterial vaginosis: a placebo controlled double-blind study. *Am J Obstet Gynecol* 1994;171:345.
48. Hauth JC, Goldenberg RL, Andrews WW, et al. Reduced incidence of preterm delivery with metronidazole and erythromycin in women with bacterial vaginosis. *N Engl J Med* 1995;333:1732–1736.
49. Carey JC, Klebanoff MA, Hauth JC, et al. Metronidazole to prevent preterm delivery in pregnant women with asymptomatic bacterial vaginosis. National Institute of Child Health and Human Development Network of Maternal-Fetal Medicine Units. *N Engl J Med* 2000;342:534–540.
50. Watts DH, Krohn MA, Hillier SL, et al. Bacterial vaginosis as a risk factor for postcesarean endometritis. *Obstet Gynecol* 1990;75:52.
51. Larsson P, Bergman B, Forsum U, et al. *Mobiluncus* and clue cells as predictors

of PID after first-trimester abortion. *Acta Obstet Gynecol Scand* 1989;68:217.

52. Larsson P, Platz-Christensen J, Thejls H, et al. Incidence of pelvic inflammatory disease after first-trimester legal abortion in women with bacterial vaginosis after treatment with metronidazole: a double-blind, randomized study. *Am J Obstet Gynecol* 1992;166:100.

53. Soper DE, Bump RC, Hurt WG. Bacterial vaginosis and trichomoniasis vaginitis are risk factors for cuff cellulitis after abdominal hysterectomy. *Am J Obstet Gynecol* 1990;163:1016.

54. Larsson P, Platz-Christensen J, Forsum U, et al. Clue cells in predicting infections after abdominal hysterectomy. *Obstet Gynecol* 1991;77:450.

55. Hillier SL, Lipinski CM, Briselden AM, et al. Efficacy of intravaginal 0.75% metronidazole gel for the treatment of bacterial vaginosis. *Obstet Gynecol* 1993;81:963.

56. Fischbach F, Petersen EE, Weissenbacher ER, et al. Efficacy of clindamycin vaginal cream versus oral metronidazole in the treatment of bacterial vaginosis. *Obstet Gynecol* 1993;82:405.

57. Sobel JD. Bacterial vaginosis. *Annu Rev Med* 2000;51:349–356.

58. Critchlow CW, Wölner-Hanssen P, Eschenbach DA, et al. Determinants of cervical ectopia and of cervicitis: age, oral contraception, specific cervical infection, smoking and drinking. *Am J Obstet Gynecol* 1995;173:534.

59. Brunham RC, Paavonen JA, Stevens CE, et al. Mucopurulent cervicitis: the ignored counterpart in women of urethritis in men. *N Engl J Med* 1984;311:1.

60. Paavonen JA, Stevens CE, Wölner-Hanssen P, et al. Colposcopic manifestations of cervical and vaginal infection. *Obstet Gynecol Surv* 1988;43:373.

61. Manhart LE, Dutro SM, Holmes KK, et al. Mycoplasma genitalium *is associated with mucopurulent cervicitis.* Presented at the International Congress of Sexually Transmitted Infections Joint Meeting of ISSTDR/IUSTI Europe/IUSTI/DSTDG, Berlin, Germany, June 24–27, 2001, Abstract #235.

62. Paavonen JA, Critchlow CW, DeRouen T, et al. Etiology of cervical inflammation. *Am J Obstet Gynecol* 1986;154:556.

63. Eschenbach DA, Holmes KK. Acute pelvic inflammatory disease: current concepts of pathogenesis, etiology and management. *Clin Obstet Gynecol* 1975;18:35.

64. Moore DE, Spadoni LR, Foy HM, et al. Increased frequency of serum antibodies to *Chlamydia trachomatis* in women with distal tubal disease. *Lancet* 1982;2:574.

65. Elliott B, Brunham RC, Laga M, et al. Maternal gonorrheal infection as a preventable risk for low birthweight. *J Infect Dis* 1990;161:531.

66. Martin DH, Eschenbach DA, Cotch MF, et al. Double-blind placebo-controlled treatment trial of *Chlamydia trachomatis* endocervical infections in pregnant women. *Infect Dis Obstet Gynecol* 1997;5:10–17.

67. Eckert LO, Koutsky LA, Kiviat NB, et al. The inflammatory Pap smear: what does it mean? *Obstet Gynecol* 1995;86:360.

68. Rapke JT, Berlin, Spence M, et al. Reproducibility of the diagnosis of cervicitis in pregnancy. *Am J Perinatol* 1988;5:242.

69. Sellors J, Howard M, Pickard L, et al. Chlamydial cervicitis: testing the practice guidelines for presumptive diagnosis. *CMAJ* 1998;158:41–46.

70. Asbill KK, Higgins RV, Bahranii-Mostafavi Z, et al. Detection of *Neisseria gonorrhoeae* and *Chlamydia trachomatis* colonization of the gravid cervix. *Am J Obstet Gynecol* 2000;183:340–344.

71. Paavonen JA, Roberts PC, Stevens CE, et al. Treatment of mucopurulent cervicitis with doxycycline and amoxicillin. *Am J Obstet Gynecol* 1989;161:128.

72. Sendag F, Terek C, Tuncay G, et al. Single dose oral azithromycin versus seven day doxycycline in the treatment of non-gonococcal mucopurulent endocervicitis. *Aust N Z J Obstet Gynaecol* 2000;40:44–47.

73. Kiviat NB, Wölner-Hanssen P, Eschenbach DA, et al. Endometrial histopathology in patients with culture-proved upper genital tract infections and laparoscopically diagnosed acute salpingitis. *Am J Surg Pathol* 1990;14:167.

74. Piepert JF, Ness RB, Blume J, et al. Pelvic Inflammatory Disease Evaluation and Clinical Health Study Investigators. *Am J Obstet Gynecol* 2001;184:856–863.

75. Paavonen JA, Kiviat NB, Brunham RC, et al. Prevalence and manifestation of endometritis among women with cervicitis. *Am J Obstet Gynecol* 1985;152:280.

76. Korn AP, Bolang, Padian N, et al. Plasma cell endometritis in women with symptomatic bacterial vaginosis. *Obstet Gynecol* 1995;85:387–390.

77. Peipert JF, Montagno AB, Cooper AS, et al. Bacterial vaginosis as a risk factor for upper genital tract infection. *Am J Obstet Gynecol* 1997;177:1184–1187.

78. Sneider V, Behm FG, Mumaw VR. Ascending herpes endometritis. *Obstet Gynecol* 1982;59:259.

79. Cohen CR, Manhart LE, Bukusi EA, et al. Association of *Mycoplasma genitalium* with acute endometritis. *Lancet* 2002;359:765–766.

80. Gump DW, Dickstein S, Gibson N. Endometritis related to *Chlamydia trachomatis* infection. *Ann Intern Med* 1981;95:61.

81. Moller BR, Ahrons S, Laurin J, et al. Pelvic infection after elective abortion associated with *Chlamydia trachomatis.* *Obstet Gynecol* 1982;59:210.

82. Ralph SG, Rutherford AJ, Wilson JD. Influence of bacterial vaginosis in conception and miscarriage in the first trimester: cohort study. *BMJ* 1999;319:220–223.

83. Hay PE, Lament RF, Taylor-Robinson D, et al. Abnormal bacterial colonization of the genital tract and subsequent preterm delivery and late miscarriage. *BMJ* 1994;308:295–298.

84. Hoyme UB, Kiviat NB, Eschenbach DA. Microbiology and treatment of late postpartum endometritis. *Obstet Gynecol* 1986;68:226.

CHAPTER 112
Bacterial Infections Associated with Pregnancy, Delivery, and Abortion

William J. Ledger

Since the last edition of this book, continuing changes in the practice of obstetrics and gynecology have had an influence on both the presentation and the types of bacterial infections associated with pregnancy. Economic attempts to curtail medical costs have focused on the high expenses of inpatient hospital care. There have been unrelenting pressures by the payers for medical care to shorten postpartum stays, and the resulting early patient discharges mean that more postpartum infections will be discovered in the outpatient arena. This has an impact on both the diagnostic workup and the choice of antibiotics and makes it ever more difficult to gather accurate statistics on the incidence of postdelivery infections. In addition, most pregnancy terminations are now done in an outpatient setting, and this influences the selection of prophylactic antibiotics. Since the publication of Centers for Disease Control and Prevention (CDC) guidelines for the prevention of group B streptococcus neonatal sepsis in 1996 (1), there has been a huge increase in the number of pregnant women in labor receiving antibiotics, either penicillin G or ampicillin, or if penicillin allergic, clindamycin or erythromycin (2). One analysis of obstetrician applications of the guidelines indicated that many physicians have combined the risk factor strategy with the lower genital tract culture at 35 to 37 weeks' gestation strategy, treating patients in labor with risk factors who had no group B streptococcus recovered at the 35 to 37 weeks' gestation culture (3). This further increases the number of intrapartum women receiving antibiotics. This widespread use of antibiotics may influence the time of presentation and type of maternal postpartum infection. There is preliminary evidence that the strategy of ampicillin administration to prevent newborn group B streptococcal infection resulted in an increase in the number of newborn *Escherichia coli* infections (4).

Any analysis of large groups of pregnant women who develop a bacterial infection identifies risk factors. For the pregnant woman, a postpartum infection is more likely if she requires a cesarean section after being in labor and if she is from a lower socioeconomic population (5). For a patient undergoing a pregnancy termination, the earlier in the pregnancy the operation is performed, the lower are infection rate and the rate of sepsis resulting in death (6). The risk for newborn sepsis due to the group B streptococcus is increased in black women younger than 20 years of age (7) and in women with a preterm delivery (1), group B streptococcus asymptomatic bacteriuria earlier in pregnancy (1), a history of the previous delivery of an infant with group B streptococcal sepsis (1), membranes ruptured more than 18 hours after the time of delivery (1), a maternal fever during labor (1), and the use of a scalp electrode during labor (7,8). All of these risk factors have been used as markers to pinpoint patients who should receive prophylactic antibiotics.

There are individual risk factors that are just now being recognized that will influence future physician management decisions. One example is the exposition by Witkin and associates that genetic variances can modify the susceptibility to disease (9). For example, human immunodeficiency virus (HIV) patients with the 2,2 allele polymorphism who produce markedly decreased amounts of the blocker interleukin-1 receptor antagonist (IL-1-RA) have lower HIV counts than women without this gene polymorphism (10). Finally, variances in the virulence of microorganisms in the lower genital tract can influence infection presentation and severity. The best example of this is the acute onset of a serious postpartum infection due to the group A streptococcus (11).

With this as a background, I intend to evaluate postabortion infections, infections associated with preterm labor and delivery, chorioamnionitis, postpartum endomyometritis, and the role of prophylactic antibiotics.

POSTABORTION INFECTIONS

Sepsis following an abortion initiated in the community by nonmedical caregivers is fortunately a rare event in the United States in the twenty-first century. There are a number of reasons for this. The most important was the Roe v. Wade Supreme Court decision in 1973. This permitted medical care teams, led by physicians, to terminate unwanted pregnancies. In addition, increased availability of safe and effective low-dosage oral contraceptives has decreased the pregnancy risk of intercourse when no barrier contraception has been used (12).

Today, most patients with a postabortion infection have had an elective termination of their pregnancy. There are a number of situations that will increase the risk for infection in women who have had a pregnancy termination.

Asymptomatic patients whose lower genital tract is colonized by potentially serious pathogens can become infected after a termination. This can occur despite an easy and uncomplicated operative procedure. The three pathogens of most concern are *Neisseria gonorrhoeae*, *Chlamydia trachomatis*, and the group A streptococcus. The presence of *N. gonorrhoeae* increases the risk for postabortion pelvic infection (13). On services in which the incidence of *N. gonorrhoeae* infections is high, two strategies have been employed to lower the risk for infection. An endocervical test for the presence of *N. gonorrhoeae* is done, and patients with positive results can be treated with ceftriaxone, 150 mg given intramuscularly (14), before the procedure is scheduled and done. If a delay in scheduling the procedure is not possible, the ceftriaxone can be given just before the operation is to be performed.

C. trachomatis, present in the lower genital tract without symptoms, can cause postinstrumentation upper genital tract infection, which results in tubal damage and can cause subsequent infertility (15). Avoiding this outcome requires pretermination screening and treatment (15); a single dose of doxycycline may not be sufficient prophylaxis. The presence of group A streptococcus at the time of pretermination instrumentation can result in serious life-threatening infections (11). These patients present shortly after the procedure with a high temperature and few localizing signs on pelvic examination. The Eagle phenomenon is a decrease in penicillin-binding protein on the wall of these bacteria when the bacterial load is heavy (16). The antibiotic of choice in this uncommon clinical situation is clindamycin because its effectiveness is not dependent on bacterial load (17).

Some patients become infected after a pregnancy termination because not all products of conception are removed at the time of the procedure (18). This is an event that more commonly occurs in women with late pregnancy terminations, particularly those resulting from the discovery of an abnormal chromosome number in the analysis of amniotic fluid obtained by amniocentesis. Better imaging techniques, particularly transvaginal ultrasound, aid in the posttermination diagnosis. Treatment strategy requires two lines of attack: both operative removal of the retained products of conception and systemic antibiotics. Fortunately, if there

has been no uterine damage, these patients respond quickly to single or combination antibiotic therapy, which should include coverage of gram-negative anaerobes (19,20). I favor the combination of clindamycin and gentamicin or single antibiotic coverage with cefoxitin or cefotetan.

Some of the most serious infections following pregnancy termination are seen when there is soft tissue damage to the uterus. Internal bleeding can follow a uterine perforation. The subsequent hematoma can become infected. Fortunately, newer imaging techniques can delineate the problem, and directed needle aspiration with systematic antibiotic coverage usually results in recovery. The most serious posttermination pelvic infections occur when there has been bowel damage, particularly large bowel, with instrumentation. These events should be suspected when a patient becomes seriously ill after a late pregnancy termination and a collection and matted bowel are seen on imaging studies. Broad-spectrum antibiotic coverage, especially for gram-negative anaerobes, and operative intervention to repair bowel damage will be necessary for a cure (18). Combination antibiotic coverage should include metronidazole.

UTERINE INFECTION BEFORE DELIVERY

Physicians have long had an interest in the possibility of uterine infections causing premature labor and delivery. Obstetricians focus on this because preterm deliveries, which account for less than 10% of all deliveries, cause the majority of newborn cases with morbidity and mortality. Infectious disease experts are also interested in this topic because if infection caused preterm labor, there is the legitimate assumption that directed therapeutic interventions would reduce the frequency of premature labor and delivery.

Early searches for infectious causes of preterm labor and delivery sought relationships between specific bacterial agents or well-recognized and defined types of infection. Most of these relationships were determined by microbiologic screening, either by culture or Gram stain. A host of etiologic possibilities have been published in the literature. Some of these included the clinical entities of asymptomatic bacteriuria (21), bacterial vaginosis (22), untreated maternal syphilis (23), periodontal disease (24), and vaginal colonization with a variety of organisms, including genital mycoplasmas (25), *N. gonorrhoeae* (26), *C. trachomatis* (27), group B streptococcus (28), *Trichomonas vaginalis* (29,30), and gram-negative anaerobes (31). Having determined these associations, the next obvious step in the evaluation of etiologies is to analyze the impact of directed treatments on the rate of prematurity. I have always had doubts about the eventual impact of these associations on clinical efforts to lower the prematurity rate in the United States. The single most powerful determinant in the risk for a preterm delivery is the patient's history of a prior preterm delivery (22,32). This odds ratio exceeds all of the prior noted relationships in this paragraph (21–31). That suggests to me the primary importance of individual host response in seeking the cause of a preterm labor.

Studies of therapeutic trials to prevent preterm labor have been disappointing in most cases. Detection and successful antibiotic treatment of asymptomatic bacteriuria is a standard of current obstetrical care. There is uniform belief that this lowers the incidence of pyelonephritis in any obstetrical population (21,33). A favorable impact on the prematurity rate has not been found in most studies. Although reductions were noted in some studies, most have shown no benefit (33–35). Despite some early enthusiasm for the treatment of bacterial vaginosis to prevent preterm labor and delivery (36), there is increasing evidence that only selected populations will benefit from intervention.

The most successful U.S. intervention study showed benefit for women with a prior history of preterm labor who had bacterial vaginosis and were treated with metronidazole and erythromycin (37). In the largest study reported to date, the treatment of asymptomatic bacterial vaginosis in pregnant women did not reduce the rate of preterm delivery (38). Unfortunately, this was a poorly designed study in which the treatment was delayed, in many cases for weeks after the diagnosis was made. In contrast, a much smaller study in Germany showed benefit when treatment was instituted as soon as the diagnosis was made (39). More studies would be necessary to clarify this point. Treatment of pregnant women with syphilis should be approached with caution. In one evaluation of 33 pregnant women with syphilis, 15 (45%) had a Jarisch-Herxheimer reaction (40). These reactors all had either primary or secondary syphilis. The most common symptoms were fever (73%), uterine contractions (67%), and decreased fetal movement (67%). Two infants of this group did not survive (40). These patients should be admitted for observation, bed rest, hydration, and the use of antipyretics. The role for tocolysis in this clinical situation is not clear. The relationship between periodontal disease and preterm labor and delivery is an intriguing one that will be subjected to scrutiny in future antibiotic intervention studies. There is no current enthusiasm for screening and treatment of vaginal colonization with genital mycoplasmas during pregnancy. Initially, there was promise; one study reported higher infant birth weights for infants of women treated with erythromycin in the third trimester (41). There are many reasons that this has not become a standard of care. Many more pregnant women are colonized with mycoplasmas than the subsequent number who deliver prematurely (25). Tetracycline, an effective drug against many mycoplasma strains, is contraindicated in pregnancy, and a large National Institutes of Health–sponsored study showed no benefit of erythromycin therapy beyond an increase in mean birth weight (42). Our minds should not be completely closed to erythromycin intervention because one successful intervention study of pregnant women with bacterial vaginosis used a regimen of metronidazole and erythromycin (37), which is an interesting antibiotic combination because erythromycin is not a drug of choice in nonpregnant women with bacterial vaginosis. Most obstetrical units will screen for *N. gonorrhoeae* and will treat those women who are culture positive. The most popular choice for treatment is ceftriaxone, 150 mg given intramuscularly (14). Although this protects the newborn from neonatal eye infections, the impact on the prematurity rate has not been established by a controlled study (43). *C. trachomatis* has a host of adverse impacts on the newborn, including eye infection and pneumonia in the premature baby (44). Because of this, all polymerase chain reaction–positive women are treated with either 7 days of erythromycin or a single 1-g dose of azithromycin. There is also the observation that a *C. trachomatis* infection at the twenty-fourth week of pregnancy was associated with an increased prematurity rate (45). The impact of screening and treatment of *C. trachomatis*–positive patients on the prematurity rate and neonatal morbidity and mortality rates will be determined by future prospective studies. Although concerns remain about newborn infection with the group B streptococcus from colonized mothers, one large study showed no effect in attempts to prolong pregnancy or reduce the number of low-birth-weight infants (46). Although *T. vaginalis* vaginal infection has been associated with a higher-than-expected preterm delivery rate, treatment with metronidazole has not improved the outcome. In one study, treatment with metronidazole for 7 or 10 days did not improve the preterm delivery rate (47). A more adverse effect was noted in a recent study, in which metronidazole treatment resulted in an increase in preterm delivery as a result of spontaneous preterm labor (48). This study had a

bizarre protocol in which all male sexual partners were given 2 g of metronidazole orally, whereas the culture-positive pregnant women were to receive either placebo or three separate 2-g oral doses of metronidazole, at onset of treatment, 48 hours later, and then at a follow-up visit of between 24 weeks and 29 weeks, 6 days (48). Only 7.4% of the metronidazole-treated women had a positive culture at the time of the follow-up visit. This protocol used three times the recommended dose for women with vaginal trichomonas (14). The reason for this dosage selection is not made clear in this article. Bacterial vaginosis, a condition in which there is a marked increase in the number of bacteroides in the vagina, has been associated with an increased incidence of preterm labor (22,32). Despite this, therapeutic interventions with antibiotics effective against anaerobes have had mixed results. Some have reported success (36,39), some success in a small subgroup (37), and some no response (38). There is obviously more to the initiation of preterm labor than vaginal colonization with anaerobes.

The failure of these antibiotic intervention strategies to lower the prematurity rate in the United States has been a stimulus to more detailed studies on preterm labor infectious etiologies. In general, there have been two approaches. The first involves evaluation of the mechanisms in which bacterial infections initiate preterm labor and subsequent delivery. The second has been an analysis of individual variances in response to bacterial colonization and infection.

There is less mystery about the mechanisms by which infection initiates preterm labor. Bacterial infection initiates a cascade of events that increases uterine activity. This can be due to intraamniotic bacterial infection even though the membranes are still intact, an event first reported in 1977 (49). One mechanism by which intraamniotic infection causes labor was reported in the rhesus monkey in 1994 (50). The injection of a large dose of group B streptococcus into the amniotic sac was sequentially followed by an increase in the number of intraamniotic bacteria, followed by IL-1β-induced stimulation of tumor necrosis factor-α (TNF-α) production and IL-6 and led to increased production of prostaglandin E$_2$ and F$_{2\alpha}$, all of which preceded the onset of uterine contractions by several hours. Bacterial infection leading to this response does not have to be in an intraamniotic location. Women with positive chorioamniotic membrane cultures and negative amniotic fluid cultures have an active inflammatory response with high concentrations of IL-6, a proinflammatory cytokine (51). Clearly, women with no growth of bacteria in the amniotic fluid can have a bacterial infection cause for their premature labor. Injecting the proinflammatory cytokine IL-1β into the amniotic sac of rhesus monkeys induces TNF-α, prostaglandin production, and preterm contractions in pregnant rhesus monkeys (52). In this model, uterine activity diminished as the proinflammatory cytokine level returned to preinfusion levels, even though prostaglandin levels remain high. This suggests that a bacterial infection stimulating preinflammatory cytokine production is necessary for the onset of preterm labor to persist and result in preterm delivery.

These new observations could modify detection and treatment strategies in the future. Instead of using cultures as a screen for the presence of infection, measurement of elevated proinflammatory cytokines in the lower genital tract (53), amniotic fluid (54), or the blood (55) could pinpoint patients for treatment. Treatments other than antibiotics may be added to the therapeutic strategies, using proinflammatory cytokine blockers such as IL-1-RA.

Differences in patients' immune response to infection will be a major focus in the investigation of causes in premature labor in the coming decade. There are already some suggested clinical observations of such a link. The greatest risk factor for premature labor is a patient's history of prior premature labor (22,32). The most successful antibiotic treatment regimen in lowering the risk for premature delivery in patients with bacterial vaginosis was in women with a history of a prior premature birth (37). To date, much of the focus has been on women with IL-1-RA gene polymorphism. These women produce markedly diminished levels of the blocker (IL-1-RA) to the proinflammatory cytokine IL-1. This is an important observation. IL-1β is an important instigator of infection-related preterm labor (50), and in mice, IL-1-RA injection before IL-1β injection prevents preterm labor (56). The nonhuman primate studies showed that the IL-1-RA levels increased in response to either intrauterine infection or intraamniotic IL-1β infusion (57). Of interest, the source of the IL-1-RA seemed to be fetal. This is interesting to me because the two babies that I have delivered of mothers with this gene polymorphism were tested and did not have the particular allele. To date, Witkin and associates have demonstrated that the presence of this gene polymorphism in the fetus was associated with an increased prevalence of preterm birth (58). This exciting observation will be subjected to future intense studies, as will other gene polymorphisms that can influence the magnitude of the proinflammatory cytokine response in pregnant women.

CHORIOAMNIONITIS

Old concepts have impeded physician understanding of pregnancy intrauterine infection or chorioamnionitis. Because of the biologic emphasis in our premedical training, attempts to formulate scientific approaches to clinical problems have often depended on classification schemes. In obstetrics, there was a focus on the protection against bacterial infection given the pregnant woman by intact membranes and a constant emphasis on the time that membranes were ruptured with the risk for infection. These rigid guidelines need to be modified.

There are a host of examples of intrauterine infection in women with intact fetal membranes. It has been reported in women with premature (49) and term (59) labor and in women who deliver with intact membranes whose infants subsequently develop group B streptococcus sepsis (60). Maternal bacteremia can also result in chorioamnionitis with intact membranes. This has been reported with the virulent pathogen, the group A β-hemolytic streptococcus (61), which can also cause serious infectious problems in nonpregnant women (16).

The diminishment of cell-mediated immunity in pregnancy seems to account for the infrequent, but virulent, intrauterine infections due to *Listeria monocytogenes* (62). Soft cheeses and delicatessen products can be contaminated by this organism (63), and pregnant women should be advised to avoid these products. If chorioamnionitis is diagnosed in a woman with intact membranes and a listerial infection is suspected, a combination of ampicillin and gentamicin seems more effective than ampicillin alone (63).

All invasive therapeutic procedures in obstetrics have a risk for intrauterine infection. This can occur after chorionic villus sampling (64), amniocentesis, percutaneous umbilical blood sampling, and intrauterine fetal transfusion. There is also a risk after the placement of a cervical cerclage, particularly when it is done after the twentieth week of gestation (65).

In all febrile patients with intact membranes and a tender uterus, the diagnosis should be suspected when no other site of infection can be found. In this situation, amniocentesis can be performed to confirm the diagnosis (66), with microscopic examination of the amniotic fluid, a culture performed, or studies done for proinflammatory cytokines.

Most patients with chorioamnionitis will have ruptured membranes, and most care formulations equate the length of time of membrane rupture with both the risk for and severity of infection. The longer the time interval, the greater the risk (67). However, many subsequent studies have found different results. One microbiology evaluation of patients with bacteremia and postpartum endomyometritis found severity of infection related to the types of the bacterial isolates. Those with *Bacteroides fragilis* isolated in blood cultures had the most severe infections (68). Similarly, a study of all patients with postpartum endomyometritis showed no correlation with the length of time of membrane rupture and the severity of infection (69). For the clinician, this means that each patient has to be evaluated and managed as an individual and not as a member of a high-risk or a low-risk group.

The care of chorioamnionitis, presenting in the dual patient complex of mother and intrauterine fetus, is complicated. Risk for infection in the mother will influence the physician's choice of antibiotics and the route of delivery. These must be weighed against possible counter-concerns about fetal morbidity and mortality that at times require a different emphasis on antibiotic selection and delivery management.

A focus on maternal welfare in the patient with chorioamnionitis requires that attention be paid to a number of interrelated risks. The patient with chorioamnionitis is more likely to have a serious postpartum infection if a cesarean section is required (70). This is logical because it is an intraabdominal operation in an infected operative field in which a lot of foreign material suture is used to obtain homeostasis in a muscle, the uterus. In the preantibiotic era, death from sepsis was the norm, not the exception (71). To avoid postoperative intraperitoneal contamination and sepsis, the extraperitoneal cesarean section was devised and championed as a preventive measure (72). The introduction of effective antibiotics into clinical practice and the realization that gram-negative anaerobes were particularly important in the evolution of serious, life-threatening postoperative infections (69) have eliminated the need for the complicated extraperitoneal approach. Cesarean section remains a risk, and the care of these women should always include the use of antibiotics, such as metronidazole, clindamycin, cefoxitin, cefotetan, and ticarcillin, which have demonstrated effectiveness against gram-negative anaerobes. There are other factors that influence patient care. At times, logic can be dangerous for a clinician. On the face of it, it would seem that an infected pregnant uterus would be even more efficient than a noninfected uterus in emptying itself of the infected products of conception. Not so. A number of studies have demonstrated protracted labor in patients with chorioamnionitis (73,74), and this population has a much higher-than-expected cesarean section rate because of poor uterine activity (75). Despite the physician desire for a vaginal delivery to decrease the risk for infection, many of these women will require a cesarean section, which increases their risk for postpartum infectious morbidity.

Physician concern about the fetus has a number of different priorities. The first is microbiologic. For the mother, the most serious infections are caused by gram-negative anaerobes. For the fetus, the most frequent and serious pathogens are the group B streptococci (1–3,7,60) *E. coli* (76), *Haemophilus influenzae* (77), and *L. monocytogenes* (62,63). For the mother in labor with chorioamnionitis, the drugs of choice are those effective against gram-negative anaerobes. Obviously, metronidazole will not be effective against these aerobic pathogens. Clindamycin, a great selection for the mother (69), is not a good choice to protect the fetus from these bacteria. There is increasing resistance of group B streptococcus to this antibiotic (78), and it is not indicated for the other three named organisms. Cefoxitin and cefotetan have similar shortcomings. This presents a therapeutic dilemma for the physician. Although penicillin G and ampicillin alone are effective against group B streptococcus, and ampicillin in combination with gentamicin adds coverage for *E. coli, H. influenzae,* and *L. monocytogenes,* this combination does not provide the best results for high-risk mothers, those in labor who require a cesarean section (69). One strategy to combat this dilemma has been to add clindamycin to the penicillin-aminoglycoside combination after delivery (79). The fetus presents other therapeutic dilemmas for the physician caring for the mother with chorioamnionitis. There has been a dramatic shift in physician concerns because of new data. Earlier studies of chorioamnionitis (75,80–82) looked at short-term fetal results in patients with chorioamnionitis. Although the fetal survival rate was lower in women who delivered preterm infants (81,82), most newborns survived, and the newborn rate of sepsis was low (81,82). The available data indicated that antibiotics were effective and there was no reason to rush to a cesarean section, because of the stress of the chorioamnionitis, unless the fetal heart tracing indicated fetal distress. This strategy is now open to question for serious long-term fetal morbidity has been reported. Maternal infection manifested by chorioamnionitis increases the risk for cerebral palsy in preterm (83,84) and in term infants (85). Studies of fetal blood obtained by cordocentesis in women with preterm labor and preterm premature rupture of membranes found elevated levels of IL-6, a proinflammatory cytokine (86). Additional studies suggest this fetal response may contribute to the subsequent development of cerebral palsy. *Periventricular leukomalacia* is a major risk factor for the subsequent manifestation of cerebral palsy. In a study of newborn brains, expression of TNF-α and IL-6 was observed more frequently in brain lesions with *periventricular leukomalacia* (87). If these observations are borne out by subsequent studies, it will put a number of currently employed strategies in the patient with premature rupture of the membranes in question. Most services observe patients with preterm premature rupture of the membranes trying to gain more time for the fetus to mature *in utero* (88). Many services follow the same strategy in women at term (89). Would immediate induction lower the subsequent rate of chorioamnionitis? This question needs to be addressed by a prospective study with a long-term follow-up of the mental status of the newborn. For women with chorioamnionitis, the current standard is antibiotic treatment, with cesarean section reserved for those with fetal distress, failure to progress, or an abnormal fetal presentation. Are these women best treated with immediate cesarean section or adrenal cortical steroids in addition to the antibiotic treatment? These alternatives need to be evaluated by prospective study with long-term neurologic follow-up of the fetus.

POSTPARTUM ENDOMYOMETRITIS

Infection of the uterus can occur after delivery. It more commonly occurs after cesarean section and is more common in patients from a lower socioeconomic class (5). Other factors that may contribute to the development of postpartum endomyometritis include preterm delivery (90) and the maternal vaginal infection bacterial vaginosis (91).

The diagnosis of postpartum uterine infection is usually made empirically in the febrile patient. Most patients have their first temperature elevation in the evening hours (92), and many obstetricians order antibiotics to avoid the delay in therapy associated with waiting until morning rounds or until the office is open for the patient already discharged home. This is unfortunate. The pelvic examination can give valuable information about the extent of the uterine infection, and a dramatic drop in the patients'

temperature can be seen when a block to normal lochial flow, such as retained membranes, is removed. There are no effective commercial products to secure an endometrial sample for culture that is free of cervical and endocervical contamination. Despite this, I think there is value in obtaining an endocervical culture for aerobes. Occasionally, this will identify such pathogens as coagulase-positive staphylococcus, group A or B streptococcus, *S. pneumoniae,* and *N. gonorrhoeae,* all of which can be targeted by specific antibiotics. Concerns have been raised about the cost-effectiveness of blood cultures in febrile obstetrical patients (93), and the fact that bacteremia in these postpartum patients does not identify a population more likely to fail standard antibiotic regimens (94). Despite this, I still favor blood cultures in this population of infected postpartum patients. For me, the blood culture identifies the organism of most concern when I select antibiotics.

Once the diagnosis is established, the treatment is straightforward because the evidence is strong that the early use of antibiotics effective against gram-negative anaerobe achieves the best results (69). For the hospitalized patient, this is an easy therapeutic exercise. Intravenous combinations of clindamycin-gentamicin or metronidazole-gentamicin, or single agents such as imipenem, cefoxitin, cefotetan, piperacillin, ampicillin-sulbactam, mezlocillin, and ticarcillin-clavulanic acid can be employed. A major problem for the clinician today is that most of the infections will be suspected when the first temperature elevation occurs when the patient has already been discharged home. What happens most frequently is that a prescription is given to the patient for an oral antibiotic, either metronidazole, which was shown to be effective as a single agent in 80% of women who developed endomyometritis after a vaginal delivery (95), or a penicillin such as amoxicillin. The patient is usually examined the next day, with a decision made to continue the same oral antibiotic regimen or to receive intravenous antibiotics as an outpatient, depending on the clinical findings.

Despite these antibiotic interventions, some patients remain febrile and require further physician evaluation and treatment. This small subgroup should be the most interesting for readers of this text because these are the patients for whom the obstetrician-gynecologist will seek consultation from the internal medicine specialist in infectious disease. Directions to the primary care physician require an ordered approach by the consultant.

The history is important because it may define parameters of risk. This is important with an intact immune system and should be expected to respond to treatment. Systemic diseases, including human immunodeficiency virus (HIV), diabetes, and cardiovascular or connective tissue disease, increase the patient's risk for infection and the likelihood of a failure of response to care. Intrapartum care, delivery, and postpartum care specifics need to be elicited. Antibiotics administered before or at the time of delivery should be noted because the subsequent development of infection is an indication that these same agents should not be employed for treatment (96). The type of anesthesia and mode of delivery should be ascertained. Infections are more frequent and more serious after cesarean section (97), but serious infections can follow a difficult vaginal delivery, particularly when operative techniques were employed to extract the baby (98). All culture results should be reviewed, especially blood cultures and any microbiologic assessment if an abscess has been encountered and aspirated or drained. A group A streptococcus isolate should trigger the use of clindamycin and require patient isolation. Finally, any imaging studies should be reviewed to assess the extent of the infection.

The next step is the physical examination of the patient. Obesity, measured by the thickness of the subcutaneous tissue, is associated with an increased risk for a postpartum abdominal wound infection (99). There can be extrauterine sites of infection, including aspiration pneumonia, particularly if general anesthesia was used for delivery, a breast infection if the nursing postpartum woman is first evaluated many days or weeks after delivery, and pyelonephritis, which is an occasional cause of postpartum sepsis. If the uterus is deemed the primary site of infection in a patient who has undergone a cesarean section, the abdominal wound should be evaluated closely because abdominal wound infection is one source of persistent fever in the patient who has failed to respond to antibiotics (100). I have always felt that a physician other than the surgeon has the least emotionality and is best able to detect an infected abdominal wound that needs drainage.

The treatment of these women requires several considerations before a successful strategy can be formulated. Postpartum uterine infections are microbiologically mixed; that is, more than one species of bacteria is usually involved. Gram-negative anaerobic bacteria are important in the genesis of these infections and, if not successfully treated, can result in abscess formation. I believe that one arm of any antibiotic treatment has to be metronidazole. Gram-negative anaerobes, particularly *B. fragilis*, are less likely to be resistant to this antibiotic than they are to clindamycin, cefoxitin, cefotetan, or ticarcillin (101). In addition, metronidazole is more bactericidal and was the most efficient in reducing the bacterial count in the animal model abscess studies (102). The choice of other antibiotics for combination therapy will depend in part on knowledge of what antibiotics were used for prophylaxis and what aerobic organisms have been isolated in prior culture. I usually use an aminoglycoside, and in these young seriously ill women with good renal function, I believe peak and trough levels should be done to be sure that therapeutic levels have been achieved (103). Imaging studies can determine the site of a pelvic abscess collection, and these can usually be aspirated by interventional radiology. Occasionally, retained products of conception are noted, and these should be removed by curettage. Despite all of these efforts, there are some women with extensive infection who fail to respond to medical intervention and may need operative removal of the uterus for cure (104). Fortunately, these cases are much less common because of the increased physician awareness of the importance of gram-negative anaerobes in these serious infections and the prescription of effective antibiotics against these pathogens. In the past, febrile patients were seen who had spiking fevers, no evidence of abscess formation, and a dramatic temperature response when heparin was added to the antibiotic regimen (105). These cases, called *septic pelvic thrombophlebitis*, are much less common now, I believe, because of the early use of antibiotics effective against anaerobes.

PROPHYLACTIC ANTIBIOTICS

A major advance in obstetrical care came with realization that prophylactic antibiotics, used before any clinical evidence of infection, could lower subsequent infection rates. This was a remarkable development because the established medical teaching was that prophylactic antibiotics should not be used because they did not work and in fact increased the risk for infection. Documentation was published in the *New England Journal of Medicine* to support this. A study of general surgical patients undergoing laparotomy for a variety of interventions showed no benefit (106). An internal medicine report on the use of antibiotics in comatose patients to prevent pneumonia also showed no benefit, and in fact, the infections that resulted in the treated group were more likely to be caused by resistant organisms (107). The pro-

hibition against the use of prophylactic antibiotics was broken when Polk and Lopes-Mayor showed a reduction in postoperative infection rates when prophylactic antibiotics were given on the day of operation, beginning just before the procedure (108). This timing was based on the animal model research by Burke, which demonstrated the effectiveness of systemic antibiotics in reducing the extent of soft tissue infection after local contamination by the injection of bacteria (109).

As a result of this advance in care, prophylactic antibiotics are now widely used and, on some services, universally used for patients undergoing cesarean section. The evidence is convincing that prophylactic antibiotics are effective in reducing the rate of postpartum endomyometritis and abdominal wound infections (110). They are given intravenously, just after the cord is clamped, to avoid exposure of the fetus to systematic antibiotics (111). The sometimes awkward attempts to use intraperitoneal lavage instead of systemic antibiotics showed no benefit (112), and this maneuver has been dropped as an option. There is also evidence that systemic antibiotic prophylaxis in low-risk patients, that is, those undergoing elective repeat cesarean section, has benefit (113). Despite this, because of the low postoperative infection rate, I do not use prophylactic antibiotics in these patients. To achieve hospital cost savings, most services use a first-generation cephalosporin for prophylaxis, often citing studies that support this strategy (110,114). They depend on a single dose of antibiotics for prophylaxis because no benefit was seen with multiple doses (115). I support the single dose but favor either cefoxitin or cefotetan instead, because of their better coverage against gram-negative anaerobes. This reduces the chances of a late-developing pelvic abscess, but this is a very uncommon event.

The use of penicillin G, ampicillin, clindamycin, and erythromycin in laboring mothers before delivery has some long-term implications for obstetrical care. Since the publication of the 1996 CDC guidelines, I estimate that more than 1 million additional women each year receive these antibiotics in labor than occurred before (116). Studies of the effect of ampicillin prophylaxis for cesarean section showed a significant posttreatment increase of *Mycoplasma* species, *Klebsiella pneumoniae*, and *E. coli* and any gram-negative rod (117). These data must be considered if these women develop a postpartum infection and therapeutic choices about antibiotics need to be made. Clearly, a successful scheme of prevention against group B streptococcus sepsis in the newborn that does not involve this widespread use of antibiotics would be preferred. Studies are underway involving the development of a vaccine (118), and there have been trials employing a vaginal antiseptic douche in labor (119). These need further analysis.

REFERENCES

1. Centers for Disease Control and Prevention (CDC). Prevention of perinatal group B streptococcal disease: a public health perspective. *MMWR Morb Mortal Wkly Rep* 1996;45:1–24.
2. Centers for Disease Control and Prevention (CDC). Adoption of hospital policies for the prevention of perinatal group B streptococcal disease: US, 1997. *MMWR Morb Mortal Wkly Rep* 1998;47:665–670.
3. Hager WD, Schuchat A, Gibbs R, et al. Prevention of perinatal group B streptococcal infection: current controversies. *Obstet Gynecol* 2000;96:141–145.
4. Towers CV, Carr MH, Padilla G, et al. Potential consequences of widespread antepartal use of ampicillin. *Am J Obstet Gynecol* 1998;179:879–883.
5. Sweet RH, Ledger WJ. Puerperal infections morbidity. *Am J Obstet Gynecol* 1973;117:1093–1100.
6. Grimes DA, Cates W Jr, Selik RM. Fatal septic abortions in the United States, 1975–1977. *Obstet Gynecol* 1981;57:739–744.
7. Bobitt JR, Ledger WJ. Obstetric observation in eleven cases of neonatal sepsis due to the group B beta hemolytic streptococcus. *Obstet Gynecol* 1978;47:439–442.

8. Gill P, Sobeck J, Jarjourn D, et al. Mortality from early onset neonatal group B streptococcal sepsis: influence of obstetric factors. *J Matern Fetal Med* 1997;6:35–39.

9. Witkin SS, Gerber S, Ledger WJ. Influence of interleukin-1 receptor antagonist gene polymorphism on disease. *Clin Infect Dis* 2002;34(2):204–209.

10. Witkin SS, Linhares IM, Gerber S, et al. Interleukin-1 receptor antagonist gene polymorphism and circulating levels of HIV-1 RNA in Brazilian women. *J Virol* 2001;75(13):6242–6244.

11. Ledger WJ, Headington JT. Group A B-hemolytic streptococcus: an important cause of serious infections in obstetrics and gynecology. *Obstet Gynecol* 1972;39:474–482.

12. Council on Scientific Affairs, American Medical Association. Induced termination of pregnancy before and after Roe v. Wade: trends in the mortality and morbidity of women. *JAMA* 1992;268:3231–3239.

13. Burkman RT, Tonascia JA, Atienza MF, et al. Untreated endocervical gonorrhea and endometritis following elective abortion. *Am J Obstet Gynecol* 1976;126:648–651.

14. Centers for Disease Control and Prevention (CDC). 2002 Guidelines for treatment of sexually transmitted diseases. *MMWR Morb Mortal Wkly Rep* 2002;51(RR-6):1–80.

15. Moller BR, Ahrons S, Laurin J, et al. Pelvic infection after elective abortion associated with *Chlamydia trachomatis*. *Obstet Gynecol* 1982;59:210–213.

16. Garvey P, Ledger WJ. Group A streptococcus in the gynecologic patient. *Infect Dis Obstet Gynecol* 1997;5:391–394.

17. Stevens D. The toxic shock syndromes. *Infect Dis Clin North Am* 1996;10:727–747.

18. Stubblefield PG, Grimes DA. Septic abortion. *N Engl J Med* 1994;331:310–314.

19. Rotheram EB Jr, Schick SF. Nonclostridial anaerobic bacteria in septic abortion. *Am J Med* 1969;46:80–89.

20. Ledger WJ, Kriewall TJ, Gee C. The fever index: a technic for evaluating the clinical response to bacteremia. *Obstet Gynecol* 1975;45:603–608.

21. Mittendorf R, Williams MA, Kass EH. Prevention of pre-term delivery and low birth associated with asymptomatic bacteriuria. *Clin Infect Dis* 1992;14:927–932.

22. Hillier SL, Nugent RP, Eschenbach DA, et al. Association between bacterial vaginosis and pre-term delivery of a low birth weight infant. *N Engl J Med* 1995;333:1737–1742.

23. Ricci JM, Fojaco RM, O'Sullivan MJ. Congenital syphilis: the University of Miami/Jackson Memorial Medical Center experience, 1986–1988. *Obstet Gynecol* 1989;74:687–693.

24. Offenbacher S, Katz V, Fertik G, et al. Periodontal infections as a possible risk factor for pre-term low birth weight. *J Periodontal* 1996;67[Suppl]:1103–1113.

25. Braun P, Lee Y-H, Klein JO, et al. Birth weight and genital mycoplasmas in pregnancy. *N Engl J Med* 1971;284:167–171.

26. Elliot B, Brunham RC, Laga M, et al. Maternal gonococcal infection as a preventable risk factor for low birth weight. *J Infect Dis* 1990;161:513–516.

27. Gravett MG, Nelson HP, DeRouen T, et al. Independent associations of bacterial vaginosis and *Chlamydia trachomatis* infection with adverse pregnancy outcome. *JAMA* 1986;256:1899–1903.

28. Regan JA, Chao S, James LS. Premature rupture of membranes, pre-term delivery, and group B streptococcal colonization of mothers. *Am J Obstet Gynecol* 1981;141:184–186.

29. Pastorek JG, Cotch MF, Martin DH, et al. Clinical and microbiological correlates of vaginal trichomonas during pregnancy. *Clin Infect Dis* 1996;23:1075–1080.

30. Jeremias J, Draper D, Ziegert M, et al. Detection of trichomonas vaginalis using the polymerase chain reaction in pregnant and non-pregnant women. *Infect Dis Obstet Gynecol* 1994;2:16–19.

31. Krohn MA, Hillier SL, Lee ML, et al. Vaginal *Bacteroides* species are associated with an increased rate of pre-term delivery among women in pre-term delivery. *J Infect Dis* 1991;164:88–93.

32. Wang X, Zuckerman B, Coffman GA, et al. Familial aggregation of low birth weight among whites and blacks in the United States. *N Engl J Med* 1995;333:1744–1749.

33. Harris RE. The significance of eradication of bacteriuria during pregnancy. *Obstet Gynecol* 1979;53:71–73.

34. Whalley PJ, Cunningham FG. Short term vs. continuous antimicrobial therapy of asymptomatic bacteriuria in pregnancy. *Obstet Gynecol* 1977;49:262–265.

35. Romero R, Oyarzum E, Mazor M, et al. Meta-analysis of the relationship between asymptomatic bacteriuria and pre-term labor, delivery/low birth weight. *Obstet Gynecol* 1989;73:576–582.

36. McGregor JA, French JI, Seo K. Adjunctive clindamycin therapy for pre-term labor: results of a double-blind, placebo-controlled trial. *Am J Obstet Gynecol* 1991;165:867–875.

37. Hauth JC, Goldenberg RL, Andrews WW, et al. Reduced incidence of pre-term delivery with metronidazole and erythromycin in women with bacterial vaginosis. *N Engl J Med* 1995;333:1732–1736.

38. Carey JC, Klebanoff MA, Hauth JC, et al. Metronidazole to prevent pre-term delivery in pregnant women with asymptomatic bacterial vaginosis. *N Engl J Med* 2000;342:534–540.

39. Hoyme UB, Grosch A, Roemer VM, et al. Erste Resultate der Erfurter Frühgeburten-Vermeidungs-Aktion. *Z Geburtsh Neonatal* 1998;202:247–250.

40. Klein VR, Cox SM, Mitchell MD, et al. The Jarisch-Herxheimer reaction complicating syphilo therapy in pregnancy. *Obstet Gynecol* 1990;73:375–380.

41. McCormack WM, Rosner B, Lee Y-H, et al. Effect on birth weight of erythromycin treatment of pregnant women. *Obstet Gynecol* 1987;69:202–207.

42. Eschenbach DA, Nugent RP, Rao AV, et al. A randomized placebo-controlled trial of erythromycin for the treatment of *Ureaplasma urealyticum* to prevent premature delivery. *Am J Obstet Gynecol* 1991;164:734–742.

43. Donders GGG, Desmyter J, DeWet DH, et al. The association of gonorrhea and syphilis with premature birth and low birth weight. *Genitourin Med* 1993;69:98–101.

44. Alexander ER, Harrison HR. Role of *Chlamydia trachomatis* in perinatal infection. *Rev Infect Dis* 1983;5:713–719.

45. Andrews WW, Goldenberg RL, Mercer B, et al. The Pre-term Prediction Study: association of second-trimester genitourinary infection with subsequent spontaneous pre-term birth. *Am J Obstet Gynecol* 2000;183:662–668.

46. Klebanoff MA, Regan JA, Rao AV, et al. Outcome of the vaginal infections and prematurity study: results of a clinical trial of erythromycin among pregnant women colonized with group B streptococci. *Am J Obstet Gynecol* 1995;172:1540–1545.

47. Morgan I. Metronidazole treatment in pregnancy. *Int J Gynecol Obstet* 1978; 15:501–502.

48. Klebanoff MA, Carey JC, Hauth JC, et al. Failure of metronidazole to prevent pre-term delivery among pregnant women with asymptomatic *Trichomonas vaginalis* infection. *N Engl J Med* 2001;345:487–493.

49. Bobitt JR, Ledger WJ. Unrecognized amnionitis and prematurity: a preliminary report. *J Reprod Med* 1977;19:8–12.

50. Gravett MG, Witkin SS, Haluska GJ, et al. An experimental model for intra-amniotic infection and pre-term labor in rhesus monkeys. *Am J Obstet Gynecol* 1994;171:1660–1667.

51. Andrews WW, Hauth JC, Goldenberg RL, et al. Amniotic fluid interleukin-6 correlation with upper genital tract microbial colonization and gestational age in women delivered after spontaneous labor versus indicated delivery. *Am J Obstet Gynecol* 1995;173:606–612.

52. Baggia S, Gravett MG, Witkin SS, et al. Interleukin-1B intra-amniotic infusion induces tumor necrosis factor-alpha, prostaglandin production, and pre-term contractions in pregnant rhesus monkeys. *J Soc Gynecol Invest* 1996;3:121–126.

53. Inglis SR, Jeremias J, Kuno K, et al. Detection of tumor necrosis factor-alpha, interleukin-6, and fetal fibrinectin in the lower genital tract during pregnancy: relation to outcome. *Am J Obstet Gynecol* 1994;171:5–10.

54. Hillier SL, Witkin SS, Krohn MA, et al. The relationship of amniotic fluid cytokines and pre-term delivery, amniotic fluid infection, histologic chorioamnionitis, and chorioamnion infection. *Obstet Gynecol* 1993;81:941–948.

55. Murtha AP, Greig PC, Jimmerson CE, et al. Maternal serum interleukin-6 concentration as a marker for impending pre-term delivery. *Obstet Gynecol* 1998;91:161–164.

56. Romero R, Tartakousky B. The natural interleukin-1 receptor antagonist prevents interleukin-1 induced pre-term delivery in mice. *Am J Obstet Gynecol* 1992;167:1041–1045.

57. Witkin SS, Gravett MG, Haluska GJ, et al. Induction of interleukin-1 receptor antagonist in rhesus monkeys after intra-amniotic infection with group B streptococcus or interleukin-1 infusion. *Am J Obstet Gynecol* 1994;171:1688–1672.

58. Genc M, Gerber S, Nesim M, et al. Polymorphism in the interleukin-1 gene complex and pre-term labor in Hispanic women [Abstract]. In: *Program and Abstracts of the Sixth Annual Meeting of the International Diseases Society for Obstetrics and Gynecology—USA*. Chicago: April 27–29, 2001:16.

59. Romero R, Nores J, Mazor M, et al. Microbial invasion of the amniotic cavity during term labor: prevalence and significance. *J Reprod Med* 1993;38:543–548.

60. Eickhoff TC, Klein JO, Daly AK, et al. Neonatal sepsis and other infections due to group B beta-hemolytic streptococci. *N Engl J Med* 1964;271:1221–1228.

61. Monif GRG. Antenatal group A streptococcal infection. *Am J Obstet Gynecol* 1975;123:213–214.

62. Linnam MJ, Mascola L, Lou XD, et al. Epidemic listeriosis associated with Mexican style cheese. *N Engl J Med* 1988;319:823–828.

63. Lorber B. Listeriosis. *Clin Infect Dis* 1997;24:1–11.

64. Wilson RD, Hogge WA, Golbus MS. Analysis of chromosomally normal spontaneous abortions after chorionic villus sampling. *J Reprod Med* 1987;32:25–27.

65. Charles D, Edwards WR. Infectious complications of cervical cerclage. *Am J Obstet Gynecol* 1981;141:1065–1070.

66. Petrilli ES, D'Ablaing G, Ledger WJ. *Listeria monocytogenes* chorioamnionitis: diagnosis by transabdominal amniocentesis. *Obstet Gynecol* 1980;55:5S–8S.

67. Gunn GC, Mishell DR, Morton DG. Premature rupture of membranes. *Am J Obstet Gynecol* 1970;106:469–482.

68. Di Zerega GS, Yonekura ML, Keegan K, et al. Bacteremia in post-cesarean section endomyometritis: differential response to therapy. *Obstet Gynecol* 1980;55:587–590.

69. Di Zerega GS, Yonekura ML, Roy S, et al. A comparison of clindamycin-gentamicin and penicillin-gentamicin in the treatment of post-cesarean endomyometritis. *Am J Obstet Gynecol* 1979;134:238–242.

70. Tran TS, Jamulitrat S, Chongsuvivatwong V, et al. Risk factors for post cesarean surgical site infection. *Obstet Gynecol* 2000;95:367–371.

71. Ledger WJ. Evidence based medicine and outcomes research in infectious diseases. *Infect Dis Clin Pract* 1998;7:148–151.

72. Imig JR, Perkins RP. Extraperitoneal cesarean section: a new need for old skills. A preliminary report. *Am J Obstet Gynecol* 1976;125:51–54.

73. Duff F, Sanders R, Gibbs RS. The course of labor in term patients with chorioamnionitis. *Am J Obstet Gynecol* 1983;147:391–395.

74. Silver RK, Gibbs RS, Castillo M. Effect of amniotic fluid bacteria on the course of labor in nulliparous women at term. *Obstet Gynecol* 1986;65:587–592.
75. Koh KS, Chan FH, Monfared AH, et al. The changing perinatal and maternal outcome in chorioamnionitis. *Obstet Gynecol* 1979;53:730–734.
76. Gladstone IM, Ehrenkranz RA, Edberg SC, et al. A ten year review of neonatal sepsis and comparison with previous fifty year experience. *Pediatr Infect Dis J* 1990;9:819–825.
77. Rusin P, Adam RD, Petersen EA, et al. *Hemophilus influenzae*: an important cause of maternal and neonatal infections. *Obstet Gynecol* 1991;77:92–96.
78. Pearlman MD, Pierson CL, Faix RG. Frequent resistance of clinical group B streptococcal isolates to clindamycin and erythromycin. *Obstet Gynecol* 1998;92:258–261.
79. Gibbs RS, Dinsmoor MJ, Newton ER, et al. A randomized trial of intra partum versus immediate post partum treatment of women with intra-amniotic infection. *Obstet Gynecol* 1988;72:823–828.
80. Gibbs RS, Castillo MS, Rodgers PJ. Management of acute chorioamnionitis. *Am J Obstet Gynecol* 1980;136:709–713.
81. Garite TJ, Freeman R. Chorioamnionitis in the pre term gestation. *Obstet Gynecol* 1982;59:539–545.
82. Gilstrap LC III, Leveno KJ, Cox SM, et al. Intrapartum treatment of acute chorioamnionitis: impact on neonatal sepsis. *Am J Obstet Gynecol* 1988;159: 579–583.
83. Cooke RWI. Cerebral palsy in very low birth weight infants. *Arch Dis Child* 1990;65:201–206.
84. Murphy DJ, Sellers S, MacKenzie IZ, et al. Case control study of antenatal and intra partum risk factors for cerebral palsy in very pre-term singleton babies. *Lancet* 1995;346:1449–1454.
85. Grether JK, Nelson KB. Maternal infection and cerebral palsy in infants of normal birth weight. *JAMA* 1997;278:207–211.
86. Gomez R, Romero R, Ghezzi F, et al. The fetal inflammatory response syndrome. *Am J Obstet Gynecol* 1998;179:194–202.
87. Yoon BH, Romero R, Kim CJ, et al. High expression of tumor neurosis factor alpha and interleukin 6 in periventricular leukomalacia. *Am J Obstet Gynecol* 1997;177:406–411.
88. Druzin ML, Toth M, Ledger WJ. Non-intervention in premature rupture of the amniotic membranes. *Surg Gynecol Obstet* 1986;163:5–10.
89. Kappy KA, Cetrulo CL, Knuppel RA. Premature rupture of the membranes: a conservative approach. *Am J Obstet Gynecol* 1979;134:655–661.
90. Chaim W, Bashiri A, Bar-David J, et al. Prevalence and clinical significance of post partum endometritis and wound infection. *Infect Dis Obstet Gynecol* 2000;8:77–82.
91. Watts DH, Krohn MA, Hillier SL, et al. Bacterial vaginosis as a risk factor in post cesarean endometritis. *Obstet Gynecol* 1990;75:52–58.
92. Ledger WJ, Reite AM, Headington JT. A system for infectious disease surveillance on an obstetric service. *Obstet Gynecol* 1971;37:769–778.
93. Locksmith GJ, Duff P. Assessment of the value of routine blood cultures in the evaluation and treatment of patients with choriamnionitis. *Infect Dis Obstet Gynecol* 1994;2:111–114.
94. Blanco JD, Gibbs RS, Casteneda YS. Bacteremia in obstetrics: clinical course. *Obstet Gynecol* 1981;58:621–625.
95. Platt LD, Yonekura ML, Ledger WJ. The role of anaerobic bacteria in post partum endomyometritis. *Am J Obstet Gynecol* 1979;135:814–817.
96. Hillier S, Watts DH, Lee MF, et al. Etiology and treatment of post-cesarean section endometritis after cephalosporin prophylaxis. *J Reprod Med* 1990;35:322–327.
97. Ledger WJ, Kriewall TJ, Gee C. The fever index: a technique for evaluating the clinical response to bacteremia. *Obstet Gynecol* 1975;45:603.
98. Hibbard LT, Snyder EN, McVann RM. Subgluteal and retropsoal infection in obstetric practice. *Obstet Gynecol* 1972;39:137–149.
99. Vermillion ST, Lamoutte C, Soper DE, et al. Wound infection after cesarean: effect of subcutaneous tissue thickness. *Obstet Gynecol* 2000;95:923–926.
100. Martens MG, Kolrud BL, Faro S, et al. Development of wound infection or separation after cesarean delivery: prospective evaluation of 2,431 cases. *J Reprod Med* 1995;40:171–175.
101. Cuchural GJ, Snydman PR, McDermott L, et al. Antimicrobial susceptibility patterns of the *Bacteroides fragilis* group in the United States. *Clin Ther* 1992;14:122–136.
102. Bartlett JG. Recent developments in the management of anaerobic infection. *Rev Infect Dis* 1983;23:536–540.
103. Zaske DE, Cipolle RJ, Strate RG, et al. Rapid gentamicin elimination in obstetric patients. *Obstet Gynecol* 1980;56:559–564.
104. Ledger WJ, Gassner CB, Gee CL. Operative care of infections in obstetrics-gynecology. *J Reprod Med* 1974;13:128.
105. Ledger WJ, Peterson EP. The use of heparin in the management of pelvic thrombophlebitis. *Surg Gynecol Obstet* 1970;131:1115–1121.
106. Karl RC, Mertz JJ, Veith FJ, et al. Prophylactic antimicrobial drugs in surgery. *N Engl J Med* 1966;275:305–308.
107. Petersdorf RG, Curtin JA, Hoeprick PD, et al. A study of antibiotic prophylaxis in unconscious patients. *N Engl J Med* 1957;257:1001–1009.
108. Polk HC, Lopes-Mayor JF. Postoperative wound infections: a prospective study of determinant factors and prevention. *Surgery* 1969;66:97–103.
109. Burke JF. The effective period of preventive antibiotic action in experimental incisions and dermal lesions. *Surgery* 1961;50:161–168.
110. Spinnato JA, Youkilis C, Cook VD, et al. Antibiotic prophylaxis at cesarean delivery. *J Matern Fetal Med* 2000;9:348–350.
111. Wong R, Gee C, Ledger WJ. Prophylactic use of cefazolin in monitored high risk obstetrical patients undergoing cesarean section. *Obstet Gynecol* 1978;51:407–411.
112. Berkeley AS, Hirsch JC, Freedman KS, et al. Cefotaxime for cesarean section prophylaxis in labor: intravenous administration vs. lavage. *J Reprod Med* 1990;35:214–218.
113. Jakobi P, Weissman A, Sigler E, et al. Post-cesarean section febrile morbidity: antibiotic prophylaxis in low risk patients. *J Reprod Med* 1994;39:707–710.
114. Faro S, Martens MG, Hammill HA, et al. Antibiotic prophylaxis: is there a difference? *Am J Obstet Gynecol* 1990;162:900–909.
115. Gall SA, Hill GB. Single-dose vs. multiple dose piperacillin prophylaxis in primary cesarean section. *Am J Obstet Gynecol* 1987;157:502–506.
116. Ledger WJ. CDC Guidelines for the prevention of perinatal group B streptococcal disease: are they appropriate? *Infect Dis Clin Pract* 1998;7:188–193.
117. Newton ER, Wallace PA. Effects of prophylactic antibiotic on bacterial flora in women with post cesarean endometritis. *Obstet Gynecol* 1998;92:262–268.
118. Coleman RT, Sherer DM, Maniscalco WM. Prevention of neonatal group B streptococcal infections: advances in maternal vaccine development. *Obstet Gynecol* 1992;80:301–309.
119. Burman LG, Christensen P, Christensen R, et al. Prevention of excess neonatal morbidity associated with group B streptococci by vaginal chlorhexidine disinfection during labour. *Lancet* 1992;340:65–69.

AIDS and Related Infections

CHAPTER 113

Approach to the Patient with Human Immunodeficiency Virus Infection: Clinical Features

Henry Masur

In the United States, about 800,000 to 900,000 people are infected with human immunodeficiency virus type 1 (HIV-1) (1,2,3). Worldwide, more than 40 million people are infected, including males and females of all major ethnic groups and all age ranges from neonates to elders (1). Health care providers in all disciplines can expect to deal with HIV-infected patients who need health care for problems unrelated to HIV or who need diagnostic, therapeutic, or prophylactic services related to manifestations of HIV infection. Health care providers can also anticipate continued concern and awareness on the part of uninfected people who want information about the likelihood that they or their families will come into contact with or acquire HIV, either in the community or in health care facilities where they are receiving attention. Some people become concerned that a wide variety of nonspecific symptoms and signs could indicate HIV disease even if they are not engaged in any high-risk behavior. Thus, every health care provider needs to be familiar with HIV. However, health care providers need to recognize that HIV management has become sufficiently complex, and new information emerges so rapidly, that optimal care is given by practitioners who have time to focus considerable attention on HIV and who have experience with a sizable patient population (4,5). To an increasing degree, infectious disease practitioners are expected to be information resources in their medical facilities and to provide both consultations and primary care for infected persons. They are also expected to be information resources and leaders for their communities outside the hospital.

HIV produces a broad range of manifestations in humans. The range of manifestations includes an acute retroviral syndrome (6–14), an asymptomatic period, and myriad clinical syndromes that can be mild (15–20) or severe and life threatening (21–30). It is important to view untreated HIV infection as a chronic, ultimately fatal process that is punctuated by manifestations that vary dramatically in type and severity from person to person. HIV disease progresses at an unpredictable rate (19–50). The variations in rate of disease progression and specific manifestations are probably influenced by numerous factors, which may include route of HIV infection, size of HIV inoculum, specific strain of infecting HIV, gender, host genetic background, recent and past environmental exposures (including microorganisms), and medical interventions. The variation in clinical course of HIV disease, much like the variation in clinical course of most infectious and noninfectious diseases, must be recognized by health practitioners so that an appropriate respect for the unpredictability of the disease can temper the real progress that is being made in understanding the course and treatment of this retroviral process.

The clinical approach to a patient with HIV infection is predicated on the assumption that the patient is truly infected. It is essential to ascertain that the diagnosis of HIV infection has been unequivocally established (see Chapter 118). If the diagnosis is certain, the health care provider must initiate a series of assessments designed to evaluate where HIV disease is in its evolution, what processes currently present need to be diagnosed and treated, and what processes can be anticipated and either prevented or delayed. The health care provider must also initiate a process of education of the patient so that he or she can take an active role in the management of the retroviral infection, plan realistically for the future, and have the information necessary to minimize the likelihood of transmitting the virus to anyone else.

NATURAL HISTORY

Acute Retroviral Syndrome

One to 6 weeks after acquiring HIV infection, many patients experience a nonspecific febrile illness that is transient and self-limiting over several weeks (6–14). The clinical features of this illness are variable but may include fever, malaise, fatigue, rash (maculopapular, urticarial, or roseola like), arthralgias, myalgias, generalized adenopathy, pharyngitis, headache, photophobia, meningismus, diarrhea, peripheral neuropathy, and encephalitis. These manifestations are usually self-limiting during a few days to several weeks. There is nothing specific and diagnostic in the history and physical examination except a temporal relationship to a possible exposure. Because the symptoms and signs are nonspecific and most patients do not necessarily undergo a laboratory evaluation focused on HIV, it has been difficult to estimate what fraction of patients do develop this type of syndrome. One study reported an acute clinical syndrome in 41 of 46 (89%) individuals (9). Another prospective study reported an acute syndrome in 55% of 22 seropositive patients; however, 21% of 44 HIV-uninfected persons reported similar symptoms, emphasizing the nonspecific nature of the manifestation (8). Many health care workers who have acquired HIV occupationally have reported a symptomatic acute illness.

The relationship of an acute syndrome to HIV infection can be established by laboratory tests. The erythrocyte sedimentation rate and transaminase levels may be elevated. Granulocytope-

nia, lymphopenia, and thrombocytopenia may be seen. Counts of total lymphocytes (including both CD4+ and CD8+ cells) characteristically fall, followed by transient increases in CD8+ lymphocytes (6,8,9,44). CD4+ lymphocytes have been reported in one series to be 244 to 1,055 cells/mm^3 within the first 4 weeks after acquisition of HIV (9). CD4+ lymphocytes may recover to preinfection numbers, but most patients demonstrate a decrease of 100 to 200 cells in the first 6 months after seroconversion and a decline of an additional 100 cells in the next 6 months. In one review of 318 seroconverters, mean CD4+ cell counts in the initial 12 months after seroconversion fell from 999 to 673 cells/mm^3 (46). If a spinal tap is performed, cerebrospinal fluid (CSF) pleocytosis with normal protein and glucose levels is often seen (50). The CSF will have HIV detectable by polymerase chain reaction (PCR) in many patients.

HIV serologic studies often show p24 antigen in the serum or CSF within 2 weeks of exposure (6,49,50). This p24 antigen often appears concurrently with acute symptoms and persists for 8 to 12 weeks until p24 antibody appears. In recent years, p24 antigen testing has been replaced by HIV branched-chain DNA (bDNA) or RNA viral load testing in the acute as well as chronic phase of the illness. Viremia can be detected by PCR or bDNA assays during the period before clinical illness and disappears when p24 antibody becomes detectable (6,8,9,43). PCR or bDNA detection of viremia may be the earliest laboratory confirmation of the diagnosis. In such cases, the overall viral load is usually quite high, that is, more than 100,000 copies/μL. The PCR and bDNA assays are not licensed for diagnosis (as opposed to monitoring), however, in part because low titers (i.e., less than 5,000 copies/μL) may represent false-positive results. Thus, a diagnosis of acute HIV syndrome is highly likely in an enzyme-linked immunosorbent assay (ELISA)-negative individual or if the viral load is more than 100,000 copies/μL but should be viewed with skepticism if the viral load is less than 5,000 copies/μL (6). The magnitude of viremia and the duration of persistence correlate with prognosis. For almost all patients, the results of ELISA and Western blot tests become positive within 2 to 4 months of HIV acquisition. Cases of persistent "seronegativity," with HIV detectable by PCR, bDNA, or co-cultivation, have been reported but are extremely unusual and merit reevaluation by an experienced laboratory (51,52). Some of these cases of persistent seronegativity may represent flawed performance or interpretation of laboratory tests. Antibody to HIV proteins can be detected by Western blot a few days or weeks before the ELISA test becomes positive (6).

It would thus appear that well over half of all persons who acquire HIV infection have a symptomatic acute syndrome. Many do not seek medical attention for this nonspecific syndrome, however. In addition, most health care providers would have no reason to initiate an HIV evaluation for this type of nonspecific disorder unless the patient drew attention to a history of potential HIV exposure. Studies suggest that early intervention with antiretroviral therapy can slow the decline of CD4+ cells and reduce the number of clinical events during the initial several years of infection (6,12,53–58). Whether a strategy of early intervention with antiretroviral therapy at the time an acute syndrome or seroconversion is recognized produces long-term benefit including prolonged survival remains to be adequately determined.

Asymptomatic Stage

After acquisition of HIV infection and resolution of the acute retroviral syndrome, if one occurs, patients are free from life-threatening opportunistic infections or tumors for a median of about 8 years, although life-threatening processes have been documented within a few weeks, months, or years after seroconversion, and acute opportunistic infections occasionally occur as part of the acute retroviral syndrome (59–66). A substantial number of the 800,000 to 900,000 people in the United States who have HIV infection are coming to medical attention before they develop an acquired immunodeficiency syndrome (AIDS)-defining illness or any HIV-related clinical manifestations. They come voluntarily and involuntarily to medical attention because of increased awareness of HIV and its manifestations, by health care practitioners, by organizations that require HIV screening such as correctional facilities or life insurance companies, and by the persons themselves who recognize that they are at high risk. A distressingly large number of individuals, however, are still unaware that their behavior places them in a high-risk category for acquiring HIV infection. A large number have HIV infection that is unknown to them until they develop a serious clinical manifestation or until a sexual partner recognizes that he or she is infected, leading the individual to be tested.

When HIV infection is confirmed, it is important to assess the patient's prognosis, how rapidly these processes cause disease, and what are the precise manifestations of disease for any given patient. Most studies have assessed the rate of progression of HIV infection by measuring the time from seroconversion to the development of AIDS-related complex or AIDS, or death or progression through standardized classification systems. AIDS has been defined by the Centers for Disease Control and Prevention (67–69) and by the World Health Organization (1,70). These classification systems are useful for surveillance purposes and as objective staging systems for research protocols. For assessing the prognosis for an individual patient, however, they are not always ideally suited. For instance, a patient with Kaposi's sarcoma and a high CD4$^+$ cell count and a patient with cytomegalovirus (CMV) retinitis and a low CD4$^+$ cell count both meet the case definition of AIDS, although the two patients have vastly different prognoses. Similarly, some patients with persistent generalized adenopathy may have a low CD4$^+$ cell count and persistent fever and have a much worse prognosis than patients with similar adenopathy but a normal CD4$^+$ cell count and normal temperature curve. Thus, the use of these staging systems in clinical practice may not provide the type of data most useful to the clinician. The CD4$^+$ cell count and HIV viral load are used most commonly to assess prognosis (Table 113.1).

The natural history of HIV infection has been dramatically altered by antiretroviral therapy, better prevention and therapy of opportunistic processes, and improved supportive care. The likelihood of an initial AIDS-defining infection or tumor developing in an untreated person who is HIV seropositive probably averages about 4% to 10% per year after acquisition of HIV infection (31,36–39,42). The rate of transition from asymptomatic infection without AIDS to AIDS is relatively low in the first few years after seroconversion. The incidence curve appears to be steeper thereafter. In a cohort study from San Francisco involving homosexual men who received little antiretroviral therapy or prophylaxis against opportunistic infection, the actuarial progression rate to AIDS during 9 years after seroconversion was 42%; an additional 32% had developed HIV-related disorders that did not meet the definition of AIDS over this period (60). Similar results have been obtained in other studies involving homosexual men and hemophiliac patients (31,37,59,60,65). Rates of progression may differ in other populations of patients, such as parenteral drug users and elderly transfusion recipients. Highly active antiretroviral therapy (HAART) and chemoprophylaxis against opportunistic infections significantly reduce rates of progression (72–74).

Some patients remain clinically well 10 to 20 years after they were first found to be seropositive. A few of these patients have normal or almost normal CD4$^+$ lymphocyte counts. These un-usual patients, termed *long-term nonprogressors*, characteristically have preserved immune function and low viral burdens (39,40). Why they have been able to preserve immune function and what their ultimate outcome will be remain uncertain. A mutation in the CCR5 T-cell receptor, Δ32, will decrease T-cell infection in both heterozygous and homozygous forms and is associated with slower disease progression (38). Not all long-term progressors have a homozygous or heterozygous CCR5 mutation, however. Long-term nonprogressors who are culture positive for HIV never become culture negative without specific therapy, with perhaps a very few exceptions.

Some clinical parameters correlate with the likelihood of progression from an asymptomatic stage to a symptomatic or life-threatening manifestation of HIV. Clinically, the presence of oral candidiasis in a seropositive patient who is not receiving corticosteroids or antibiotics and who does not have diabetes correlates with enhanced likelihood of progression to AIDS, as does the finding of oral hairy leukoplakia (15,18,20). These diagnoses must be arrived at by careful observation, and the inexperienced or hurried health care provider can often mistake saliva or products of poor oral hygiene for these entities. Direct microscopic examination of mucosal scrapings for *Candida* organisms is helpful diagnostically. Biopsy can also be diagnostic but is rarely necessary outside a research setting. Lymphadenopathy and dermatomal zoster correlate with HIV seropositivity but do not appear to correlate with likelihood of disease progression, although some data suggest that the site, extent, severity, or frequency of zoster may have some prognostic significance (36,37,60,71). Fever, night sweats, weight loss, and chronic diarrhea appear to correlate with likelihood of progression to AIDS, especially in early studies.

In terms of laboratory parameters, the absolute peripheral CD4$^+$ lymphocyte count and the percentage of peripheral cells that are CD4$^+$ both correlate best with the likelihood of developing AIDS (42,43,75–80). Retrospective and prospective studies show that the lower the absolute CD4$^+$ lymphocyte count or percentage, the more likely the patient is to develop life-threatening opportunistic infections. For instance, CMV retinitis almost always occurs in patients with an absolute CD4$^+$ lymphocyte count less than 50 cells/mm^3 or less than 5% CD4$^+$ cells (75,78). *Pneumocystis carinii* pneumonia (PCP) usually occurs in patients with a CD4$^+$ lymphocyte count less than 100 to 200 cells/mm^3 or less than 10% (21,75). Some non–life-threatening opportunistic infections, such as oral candidiasis, and some serious opportunistic processes, such as tuberculosis (*Mycobacterium tuberculosis*), often occur at somewhat higher CD4$^+$ ranges than CMV retinitis or PCP, but it is clear that the lower a patient's CD4$^+$ lymphocyte count or percentage, the more likely the patient is to develop an opportunistic infectious process. Neither HAART nor interleukin-2 (IL-2) modifies this relationship between CD4$^+$ cell count and the occurrence of opportunistic infections (66,81).

The percentage of peripheral mononuclear cells that are CD4$^+$ is at least as useful as the absolute number of CD4$^+$ cells for predicting the occurrence of opportunistic infections (75–77). The CD4$^+$ cell percentage is a number measured directly by the fluorescent antibody cell sorter; the absolute number of CD4$^+$ cells is derived by multiplying this percentage by the total lymphocyte count, which is itself the product of the white cell count and differential. The percentage usually fluctuates less than the absolute number, which is an advantage for monitoring, although clinicians are generally more accustomed to following absolute numbers. The CD4$^+$-to-CD8$^+$ ratio also correlates with susceptibility to infection and prognosis, but the correlation is not as strong as with the absolute number or percentage of CD4$^+$ cells, and this ratio is rarely used anymore. In a few situations, the CD4$^+$ percentage is a more accurate predictor of susceptibility

TABLE 113.1. Risk for Progression to AIDS-Defining Illness in a Cohort of Homosexual Men Predicted by Baseline CD4+ T-Cell Count and Viral Load

CD4+ ≤ 200 Plasma viral load (copies/mL)[a]			% AIDS (AIDS-defining complication)[b]		
bDNA	RT-PCR	n	3 yr	6 yr	9 yr
≤500	≤1,500	0[d]	—	—	—
501–3,000	1,501–7,000	3[d]	—	—	—
3,001–10,000	7,001–20,000	7	14.3	28.6	64.3
10,001–30,000	20,001–55,000	20	50.0	75.0	90.0
>30,000	>55,000	70	85.5	97.9	100.0

CD4+ 201–350[c] Plasma viral load (copies/mL)			% AIDS (AIDS-defining complication)		
bDNA	RT-PCR	n	3 yr	6 yr	9 yr
≤500	≤1,500	3[d]	—	—	32.2
501–3,000	1,501–7,000	27	0	20.0	66.2
3,001–10,000	7,001–20,000	44	6.9	44.4	84.5
10,001–30,000	20,001–55,000	53	36.4	72.2	92.9
>30,000	>55,000	104	64.4	89.3	

CD4+ > 350 Plasma viral load (copies/mL)			% AIDS (AIDS-defining complication)		
bDNA	RT-PCR	n	3 yr	6 yr	9 yr
≤500	≤1,500	119	1.7	5.5	12.7
501–3,000	1,501–7,000	227	2.2	16.4	30.0
3,001–10,000	7,001–20,000	342	6.8	30.1	53.5
10,001–30,000	20,001–55,000	323	14.8	51.2	73.5
>30,000	>55,000	262	39.6	71.8	85.0

[a]MACS numbers reflect plasma HIV RNA values obtained by version 2.0 bDNA testing. RT-PCR values are consistently 2–2.5-fold higher than first-generation bDNA values, as indicated. It should be noted that the current generation bDNA assay (3.0) gives similar HIV-1 RNA values as RT-PCR except at the lower end of the linear range (<1,500 copies/mL).
[b]In this study, AIDS was defined according to the 1987 CDC definition and does not include asymptomatic individuals with CD4+ T cells < 200 mm³.
[c]A recent evaluation of data from the MACS cohort by of 231 individuals with CD4+ T cell counts > 200 and < 350 cells/mm³ demonstrated that of 40 (17%) individuals with plasma HIV RNA < 10,000 copies/mL, none progressed to AIDS by 3 years (Alvaro Munoz, personal communication). Of 28 individuals (29%) with plasma viremia of 10,000–20,000 copies/mL 4% and 11% progressed to AIDS at 2 and 3 years, respectively. Plasma HIV RNA was calculated as RT-PCR values from measured bDNA values.
[d]Too few subjects were in the category to provide a reliable estimate of AIDS risk.
MACS, Multi-Center AIDS Cohort Study; bDNA, branched-chain DNA; RT-PCR, reverse transcription polymerase chain reaction; CDC, Centers for Disease Control and Prevention.
Modified from Department of Health and Human Services and Kaiser Family Foundation. *Guidelines for antiretroviral therapy in adults and adolescents.* Available online: *www.aidsinfo.nih.gov,* with permission.

to infection than is the absolute CD4+ count; patients who are pregnant or who have had a splenectomy would be such patients (82).

The relationship of the CD4+ lymphocyte count to the development of opportunistic infectious complications of HIV infection is important in approaching the management of HIV infection. First, HIV infection implies that unless an effective therapeutic intervention is administered, immune function inexorably declines, and infectious complications occur. Second, monitoring the immunologic decline provides the clinician with a means of anticipating certain complications. This anticipation should allow earlier diagnosis of acute complications, thus improving outcome. This anticipation should also allow reduction of the likelihood of certain complications if safe and effective prophylactic regimens can be instituted. Third, the immunologic state measured by CD4+ cell count provides guidance regarding the benefit of antiretroviral therapy: when the CD4+ count falls below 200 cells/μL, effective antiretroviral therapy can clearly improve survival. At higher CD4+ counts, antiretroviral therapy

may improve survival, as discussed later. Fourth, a rise in CD4+ lymphocyte number in response to antiretroviral therapies, and perhaps to certain immunotherapies such as IL-2, predicts clinical benefit of therapeutic intervention (83–86).

Quantitative measurement of plasma viremia, most often performed by quantitative PCR tests or branched-chain DNA assays, provides information that is not only prognostically useful but also useful for documenting a response to antiretroviral therapy and thus improving subsequent prognosis in terms of fewer AIDS-defining illnesses and longer survival (42,43,84–90). When HIV infection is definitely diagnosed and the patient's prognosis is estimated, the health care provider must help the patient find resources to deal with the emotional, spiritual, psychological, and financial aspects of the disease as well as the medical issues. The patient needs to be encouraged to consider how HIV infection and its many ramifications affect family, friends, employment, living accommodations, and finances and to be made aware of issues such as health insurance, medical assistance, durable power of attorney, and wills. Referrals to psychologists, psychiatrists, social workers, support groups, or comprehensive assistance agencies may enhance the quality of the patient's subsequent existence as much as the medical help that is provided. Such referrals may also enhance the patient's success in adhering to a medical regimen that can so dramatically improve survival.

Symptomatic Stage

Symptomatic manifestations of HIV disease can occur at almost any juncture during the immunologic decline that HIV produces. The manifestations that occur as the CD4$^+$ cell count falls from the 800 to 1,200 cells/mm^3 range (normal) to 200 to 250 cells/mm^3 are often not life threatening, although tuberculosis, geographical fungal diseases, oropharyngeal candidiasis, lymphoma, and Kaposi's sarcoma can occur. As CD4$^+$ cell counts fall below 200 to 250 cells/mm^3, the same manifestations can occur, but in addition, many life-threatening opportunistic pathogens (e.g., *P. carinii*, nontuberculous mycobacteria, CMV, cryptosporidia) become frequent causes of morbidity (75,79–83). Which manifestations an individual patient develops or when in the temporal evolution of HIV disease the first manifestation or subsequent ones occur are difficult to predict. For primary and secondary infectious manifestations, the patient's past and present microbial environments, in terms of person-to-person transmission, geographical location, and fortuitous events (e.g., exposure to contaminated food, waste, animals, or aerosols) are important determinants. *M. tuberculosis, Histoplasma capsulatum, Coccidioides immitis, Leishmania chagasi, Penicillium marneffei, Trypanosoma cruzi,* and *Isospora belli* are examples of pathogens with strong geographical predispositions that could cause disease if the patient were exposed to the appropriate source. Some pathogens, such as *P. jiroveci, M. tuberculosis,* and *H. capsulatum,* can be latent for many months or years and cause disease only when the CD4$^+$ cell count declines sufficiently.

As organisms are characterized by more specific laboratory techniques, it is becoming clearer that infectious complications are not all due to reactivation of latent infections. At least some infectious complications are due to recent acquisition of primary infection or to reinfection with a newly acquired strain that is phenotypically or genotypically different from an infecting organism documented previously. Other factors that are not well understood also influence whether and when a patient develops certain manifestations. Chapters 115 through 117 provide details about the diagnosis and therapy of important HIV-related manifestations. As each manifestation occurs and appropriate diagnostic and therapeutic steps are taken, the health care provider needs to reconsider what the occurrence signifies prognostically: First, can the manifestation itself be successfully treated? Second, does therapy of the new manifestation interfere with current therapeutic, suppressive, or prophylactic regimens? Third, what does the occurrence of the manifestation indicate about the immunologic and virologic status of the patient and future clinical events? Appropriate communication with the patient about how these symptomatic episodes alter management and prognosis is in order.

REDUCTION OF COMPLICATIONS

Once it is established that a patient definitely has HIV infection and where in the natural evolution of HIV disease the particular patient is, a major focus of management must be the prevention of complications of HIV disease. Management to reduce the number and frequency of complications and to prolong survival should include (a) antiretroviral therapy; (b) reduction of exposure to pathogens; (c) chemoprophylaxis and immunization; and (d) prompt and aggressive management of infections, tumors, and other complications.

Antiretroviral Therapy

Zidovudine was the first drug licensed by the U.S. Food and Drug Administration (FDA) for therapy of HIV. Trials completed at the time of its approval in 1987 demonstrated that monotherapy with zidovudine produces a modest immunologic benefit (i.e., rise in CD4$^+$ cell count), a modest antiviral effect (i.e., decline in plasma HIV viral load), and a reduction in AIDS-defining events (i.e., fewer cases of opportunistic infection or death) (91). However, the effects of monotherapy with zidovudine were not durable. Within 1 year, most patients had experienced a progressive rise in their viral load and fall in their CD4$^+$ count (92–94). Monotherapy with other nucleosides available in the late 1980s and early 1990s (didanosine, zalcitabine, stavudine) showed only slightly better results. Combination nucleoside therapy had more efficacy than monotherapy, but the impact on long-term survival continued to be modest. Nucleosides had substantial toxicities, and regimens, especially those used in the late 1980s and early 1990s, were difficult to adhere to because of food restrictions and, in some cases, frequent dosing.

Beginning in 1995, new classes of drugs were approved that, when used in combination regimens, provided more potent antiretroviral effect and more durable immunologic and clinical benefit (95–99). These drugs ultimately included protease inhibitors (saquinavir, indinavir, ritonavir, nelfinavir, amprenavir, and the combination ritonavir-lopinavir), nonnucleoside reverse transcriptase inhibitors (nevirapine, delavirdine, and efavirenz), and a nucleotide reverse transcriptase inhibitor (tenofovir) (89). A more potent nucleoside reverse transcriptase inhibitor (abacavir) was also approved. Clinical trials and observational studies clearly showed that combination regimens, usually using at least two different classes of drugs, could reduce plasma HIV viral loads to levels below the limit of detection of currently used assays (50 copies/μL), and could raise CD4$^+$ count by several hundred cells/μL. These effects were associated with protection from HIV-related opportunistic infections and with prolonged survival (95–102). The regimens recommended for initial therapy by the U.S. Public Health Service–Infectious Disease Society of America (USPHS-IDSA) guidelines are listed in Table 113.2. Many different regimens can provide sustained efficacy if patients have a drug-sensitive virus, can adhere to the regimen, can tolerate the regimen, and have access to appropriate health care services.

When should therapy be initiated in the natural history of HIV disease? Therapeutic strategies have evolved during the era of antiretroviral therapy. When there were hopes that the virus could be eradicated by available agents, most clinicians advocated early intervention regardless of the CD4$^+$ count or viral load. As clinicians and patients recognized the difficulties of adhering to the regimens, the substantial toxicities of the drugs and the inability of therapy to eradicate viruses (to date, virtually all patients who have stopped drugs after several years of therapy have had return of viral load to baseline values within 1 to 4 weeks), the strategy of early intervention was reassessed. Risks and benefits of early versus late interaction of antiretroviral therapy are outlined in Table 113.3. Most experts and the USPHS-IDSA guidelines would agree that all symptomatic patients should be treated. Analysis of several databases suggested that long-term outcome was improved if HAART were initiated before the CD4$^+$ count was less than 200 cells/μL. There was no clear benefit in initiating therapy at higher CD4$^+$ counts. Current guidelines recommend that all patients with CD4$^+$ counts

TABLE 113.2. Recommended Antiretroviral Agents for Initial Treatment of Established HIV Infection

This table provides a guide to the use of available treatment regimens for individuals with no prior or limited experience on HIV therapy. In accordance with the established goals of HIV therapy, priority is given to regimens in which clinical trials data suggest the following: sustained suppression of HIV plasma RNA (particularly in patients with high baseline viral load) and sustained increase in CD4$^+$ T-cell count (in most cases over 48 weeks), and favorable clinical outcome (i.e., delayed progression to AIDS and death). Particular emphasis is given to regimens that have been compared directly with other regimens that perform sufficiently well with regard to these parameters to be included in the "Strongly Recommended" category. Additional consideration is given to the regimen's pill burden, dosing frequency, food requirements, convenience, toxicity, and drug interaction profile compared with other regimens.

It is important to note that all antiretroviral agents, including those in the "Strongly Recommended" category, have potentially serious toxic and adverse events associated with their use.

Antiretroviral drug regimens are composed of one choice each from columns A and B. Drugs are listed in alphabetical, not priority, order.

	Column A	Column B
Strongly Recommended	Efavirenz	Didanosine + lamivudine
	Indinavir	Stavudine + didanosine[d]
	Nelfinavir	Stavudine + lamivudine
	Ritonavir + indinavir[a]	Zidovudine + didanosine
	Ritonavir + lopinavir[b]	Zidovudine + lamivudine
	Ritonavir + saquinavir (SGC[c] or HGC[c])	
Recommended as Alternatives	**Column A**	**Column B**
	Abacavir	Zidovudine + zalcitabine
	Amprenavir	
	Delavirdine	
	Nelfinavir + saquinavir-SGC	
	Nevirapine	
	Ritonavir	
	Saquinavir-SGC	
No Recommendation: Insufficient Data[e]	Hydroxyurea in combination with antiretroviral drugs	
	Ritonavir + amprenavir	
	Ritonavir + nelfinavir	
	Tenofovir[h]	
Not Recommended:	All monotherapies, whether from column A or B[f]	
Should Not Be Offered	**Column A**	**Column B**
	Saquinavir-HGC[g]	Stavudine + zidovudine
		Zalcitabine + didanosine
		Zalcitabine + lamivudine
		Zalcitabine + stavudine

[a]Based on expert opinion.
[b]Coformulated as Kaletra.
[c]Saquinavir-SGC, soft-gel capsule (Fortovase); Saquinavir-HGC, hard-gel capsule (Invirase).
[d]Pregnant women may be at increased risk for lactic acidosis and liver damage when treated with the combination of stavudine and didanosine. This combination should be used in pregnant women only when the potential benefit clearly outweighs the potential risk.
[e]This category includes drugs or combinations for which information is too limited to allow a recommendation for or against use.
[f]Zidovudine monotherapy may be considered for prophylactic use in pregnant women with low viral load and high CD4$^+$ T-cell counts to prevent perinatal transmission.
[g]Use of saquinavir-HGC (Invirase) is not recommended, except in combination with ritonavir.
[h]Data from clinical trials are limited to use in salvage. Data from trials of tenofovir as initial therapy may be available in the near future.
Modified from Department of Health and Human Services and Kaiser Family Foundation. *Guidelines for antiretroviral therapy in adults and adolescents.* Available online: www.aidsinfo.nih.gov, with permission.

below 200 cells/μL should be treated and that therapy should be offered to patients with counts of 200 to 350 cells/μL, suggesting less confidence that the latter patients unequivocally benefit from therapy (103,104) (Table 113.4). The guidelines also indicated that therapy should also be offered to patients with CD4$^+$ counts more than 350 cells/μL and high viral loads, that is, viral loads more than 55,000 copies/mL. In many controlled trials where motivated patients are well supervised while taking potent regimens, a substantial fraction of patients (often, 40% to 50%) do not have a sustained virologic response after 48 weeks of therapy (i.e., their viral loads either never fall below the level of assay detection or, more commonly, rise after being below the level of detection for many weeks or months). Health care providers have recognized many reasons for these failures in so many patients.

When most patients initially present for medical therapy, their virus is sensitive to all licensed drugs. However, as individuals acquire infection from patients who have failed their own therapy, the incidence of drug resistance among newly acquired infections is increasing. In some studies, resistance to one or more licensed drugs can be seen in 5% to 10% of patients (14). This suggests that drug susceptibility testing may be useful for certain patients before antiretroviral therapy is initiated. Currently, however, most health care providers do not do such testing unless there is a clear epidemiologic link to a virus that is likely to be resistant, for example, a sexual partner who has failed antiretroviral therapies.

Many patients have difficulty adhering to antiretroviral regimens. Regimens often require multiple pills to be taken several times daily. The absorption of some drugs is improved with food; the absorption of other drugs is better if not taken with food or certain other antiretroviral drugs. Many patients miss a considerable number of drug doses leading to viral exposure to substantial drug levels and the development of resistance. Adherence correlates with regimen efficacy in many studies that have looked at this parameter. These problems with adherence have prompted the development of more convenient once- or twice-daily combinations, sometimes taking advantage

TABLE 113.3. Risks and Benefits of Delayed Initiation of Therapy and of Early Therapy in the Asymptomatic HIV-Infected Patient

Risks and benefits of delayed therapy

Benefits of delayed therapy
- Avoid negative effects on quality of life (i.e., inconvenience)
- Avoid drug-related adverse events
- Delay in development of drug resistance
- Preserve maximum number of available and future drug options when HIV disease risk is highest

Risks of delayed therapy
- Possible risk for irreversible immune system depletion
- Possible greater difficulty in suppressing viral replication
- Possible increased risk for HIV transmission

Risks and benefits of early therapy

Benefits of early therapy
- Control of viral replication easier to achieve and maintain
- Delay or prevention of immune system compromise
- Lower risk for resistance with complete viral suppression
- Possible decreased risk for HIV transmission[a]

Risks of early therapy
- Drug-related reduction in quality of life
- Greater cumulative drug-related adverse events
- Earlier development of drug resistance, if viral suppression is suboptimal
- Limitation of future antiretroviral treatment options

[a]The risk for viral transmission still exists; antiretroviral therapy cannot substitute for primary HIV prevention measures (e.g., use of condoms and safer sex practices).
Modified from Department of Health and Human Services and Kaiser Family Foundation. *Guidelines for antiretroviral therapy in adults and adolescents.* Available online: *www.aidsinfo.nih.gov*, with permission.

of pharmacokinetic interactions to "boost" drug levels, for example, ritonavir plus another protease inhibitor. Before a patient is started on an antiretroviral regimen, the health care provider should ascertain that the patient is committed and capable of adhering to the regimen. Some patients may not have optimal pharmacokinetic profiles to produce a sustained antiretroviral effect. There is considerable interest in assessing the relationships of pharmacokinetic parameters such as peak serum concentration, trough serum concentration, and area under the curve to virologic and immunologic outcome. Therapeutic drug monitoring is being investigated to establish its utility (105). It is not yet standard of practice to do drug monitoring routinely, nor is it clear what pharmacokinetic targets should be sought. It is clear, however, that certain drug interactions can cause substantial alterations in pharmacokinetic profiles, especially drugs that alter the cytochrome P450 system that is responsible for metabolizing the protease inhibitors and nonnucleoside reverse transcriptase inhibitors (106). These alterations in pharmacokinetics can lead to high levels of the antiretroviral agent, that is, when fluconazole or delavirdine are added to a regimen that includes a protease inhibitor. These alterations can lead to levels of a protease inhibitor that are likely to be subtherapeutic, that is, when rifampin or the alternative drugs St. John's wort or garlic capsules are added to a regimen containing a single protease inhibitor (107,108). These interactions can be used for clinical advantage, as when ritonavir is used to boost the levels of other protease inhibitors, and thus permit less frequent dosing. These interactions can also lead to drug failure and the development of viral resistance, however, if appropriate dose alterations are not made.

Patients may have difficulty tolerating regimens because of toxicities. Some drug toxicities are annoying but not life-threatening: diarrhea due to nelfinavir, nausea due to zidovudine, and insomnia due to efavirenz are examples. Antiretroviral

---

TABLE 113.4. Indications for the Initiation of Antiretroviral Therapy in the Chronically HIV-1–Infected Patient

The optimal time to initiate therapy in asymptomatic individuals with more than 200 CD4+ T cells is not known. This table provides general guidance rather than absolute recommendations for an individual patient. All decisions to initiate therapy should be based on prognosis as determined by the CD4+ T-cell count and level of plasma HIV RNA shown in Table 113.1, the potential benefits and risks of therapy shown in Table 113.3, and the willingness of the patient to accept therapy.

Clinical category	CD4+ T-cell count	Plasma HIV RNA	Recommendation
Symptomatic (AIDS, severe symptoms)	Any value	Any value	Treat
Asymptomatic, AIDS	CD4+ T cells < 200/mm³	Any value	Treat
Asymptomatic	CD4+ T cells > 200/mm³ but < 350/mm³	Any value	Treatment should generally be offered, though controversy exists.[a]
Asymptomatic	CD4+ T cells > 350/mm³	>55,000 (by bDNA or RT-PCR)[b]	Some experts would recommend initiating therapy, recognizing that the 3-year risk of developing AIDS in untreated patients is > 30% and that some would defer therapy and monitor CD4+ T-cell counts more frequently.
Asymptomatic	CD4+ T cells > 350/mm³	<55,000 (by bDNA or RT-PCR)[b]	Many experts would defer therapy and observe, recognizing that the 3-year risk of developing AIDS in untreated patients is < 15%.

[a]Clinical benefit has been demonstrated in controlled trial only for patients with CD4+ T cells < 200/mm³. However, most experts would offer therapy at a CD4+ T-cell threshold < 350/mm³. A recent evaluation of data from the Multi-Center AIDS Cohort Study (MACS) cohort of 231 individuals with CD4+ T-cell counts > 200 and < 350 cells/mm³ demonstrated that of 40 (17%) individuals with plasma HIV RNA < 10,000 copies/mL none progressed to AIDS by 3 years (Alvaro Munoz, personal communication). Of 28 individuals (29%) with plasma viremia of 10,000–20,000 copies/mL, 4% and 11% progressed to AIDS at 2 and 3 years, respectively. Plasma HIV RNA was calculated as RT-PCR values from measured bDNA values.
[b]Although there was a 2–2.5-fold difference between RT-PCR and the first bDNA assay (version 2.0), with the current bDNA assay (version 3.0), values obtained by bDNA and RT-PCR are similar except at the lower end of the linear range (<1,500 copies/mL).
bDNA, branched-chain DNA; RT-PCR, reverse transcription polymerase chain reaction.
Modified from Department of Health and Human Services and Kaiser Family Foundation. *Guidelines for antiretroviral therapy in adults and adolescents.* Available online: *www.aidsinfo.nih.gov*, with permission.

drugs can be associated with toxicities that are incapacitating or life threatening: nucleoside-associated peripheral neuropathies and abacavir hypersensitivity reactions are examples of such toxicities. There is growing recognition of more obvious long-term complications, such as fat redistribution syndromes, osteoporosis, osteonecrosis, hypercholesterolemia, hypertriglyceridemia, diabetes, and accelerated atherosclerosis, which are related to antiretroviral drugs and which may necessitate changing the regimen to other classes of drugs (109–112).

One strategy to reduce drug toxicities and drug cost that has been proposed is using periods of "treatment interruption." For this approach, patients are treated for several weeks or months, and then stop therapy for several days or weeks. Such an approach, termed "strategic" or "supervised" treatment interruption, needs to be studied intensively to determine whether toxicity is in fact reduced and to determine whether efficacy is preserved in terms of both long-term virologic response and long-term immune function.

What is the definition of a successful regimen? Optimally, a recommended regimen should reduce the viral load by at least 1 log by 8 weeks and attain a viral load of less than 50 copies/ml by 4 to 6 months (89). Concurrently, these should be a substantial increase in CD4$^+$ count. A failure is defined as clinical disease progression, failure to attain a viral load of less than 50 copies/ml, failure to manifest a CD4$^+$ count rise, or inability to tolerate a drug. In the face of drug failures or tolerance, the health care provider must assess the reason for the failure, considering adherence, viral resistance, pharmacologic factors, and toxicities. Most clinicians would perform drug resistance testing on the patient's virus to guide future choices. Current techniques to assess resistance by genotypic or phenotypic methods should logically provide useful information. Studies have shown that therapy guided by such tests can provide benefit in terms of virologic response over the short term (113–115). Whether these assays, as they are currently interpreted, improve long-term clinical outcome is under investigation.

Immunomodulating Therapies

There has been considerable interest in enhancing the immune system to prevent clinical manifestations of HIV, either as an adjustment to antiretroviral therapy or as a separate therapeutic strategy. IL-2, interferon-α, granulocyte-macrophage colony-stimulating factor, and therapeutic immunization are examples of approaches that have been assessed. IL-2 is the approach that has been most intensively studied. Intermittent IL-2, given subcutaneously for 5 consecutive days over 2 to 3 months, can lead to a substantial rise in CD4$^+$ count and provide long-term clinical protection; whether antiretroviral therapy should be given concurrently remains to be determined (88,116).

Prophylaxis and Suppression of Specific Opportunistic Pathogens

REDUCTION OF EXPOSURE TO PATHOGENS

Patients with HIV infection, like all other humans, are constantly exposed to microorganisms in their environment. Opportunistic pathogens are present in the air (e.g., *P. jiroveci, M. tuberculosis*, and *Streptococcus pneumoniae*), food (e.g., *Cryptosporidium* and *Salmonella* species), and water (e.g., *Cryptosporidium* species). Pathogens can also be acquired by specific activities such as sexual intercourse (e.g., CMV and *Treponema pallidum*), contact with children in day care (e.g., CMV and *Cryptosporidium* and *Salmonella* species), contact with pets (e.g., *Salmonella, Cryptosporidium*, and *Bartonella* species), or working in prisons,

shelters, or hospitals (e.g., *M. tuberculosis*). Patients with HIV infection cannot eliminate exposure to these pathogens, but they can consider whether they wish to modify their behavior to reduce exposure or at least be monitored carefully (e.g., by frequent tuberculin skin tests) to determine whether infection has taken place. Even if patients already have serologic or skin test evidence of prior infection with a particular organism, it may be reasonable to reduce the potential for becoming infected with a different strain, a situation that is known to occur with tuberculosis and may occur with other pathogens.

Patients and their health care providers need to consider jointly whether the inconvenience of behavioral modification is warranted by the magnitude of likely benefit. An HIV-infected patient who is seronegative for CMV, for example, may wish to practice safe sex with an HIV-infected, CMV-seropositive sexual partner, even if the sexual relationship is monogamous. Conversely, if a patient lives in a city with a municipal water supply that conforms to accepted standards, it may not be worthwhile to use boiled or bottled water because the risk for acquiring cryptosporidiosis or other enteric pathogens is likely to be low.

CHEMOPROPHYLAXIS AND IMMUNIZATION OF SPECIFIC PATHOGENS

As long as antiretroviral therapy (and perhaps immunomodulating therapy) can prevent or slow the decline in CD4$^+$ cell counts and such counts remain above 200/μL, the number of serious infectious complications is substantially reduced. Antiretroviral and immunomodulatory strategies have not yet been devised that can prevent this decline indefinitely, however, and thus almost all patients eventually develop a level of immunodeficiency such that they would benefit from the addition of specific chemoprophylaxis or immunization to reduce the frequency of opportunistic infections.

In the last half of the 1990s, a wide and expanding array of drugs and immunizations are available that can reduce the frequency of specific opportunistic infections (66,72–74). In addition, immunizations are available that it is logical to employ, even if their benefit is not proved. Using all the regimens that are available is impractical because of the number of pills required, their interactions, their toxicity, and their cost. Thus, clinicians and patients need to consider all available options and give highest priority to the immunizations and drug regimens that are likely to prevent the most common and most serious processes. For patients with different behavioral risk factors and for different geographical areas, those choices may differ. For instance, prophylaxis against *P. jiroveci* and *Mycobacterium avium* complex is more important in North America than in Brazil, where toxoplasmosis, tuberculosis, and fungal disease are more important. For patients in the United States, the USPHS-IDSA has issued guidelines suggesting prioritization of chemoprophylaxis and immunization (73).

PCP deserves particular attention because it is so frequent and so serious in North America. Before the era of antipneumocystis prophylaxis and antiretroviral therapy, 75% to 80% of patients with HIV infection eventually developed one or more episodes of PCP (21,72–74), which was the most common causes of life-threatening opportunistic infection. Clinical studies have determined when in the natural course of HIV infection PCP occurs and have defined highly effective, convenient, safe, and inexpensive prophylactic regimens. Several studies have convincingly shown a strong survival benefit for patients who receive antipneumocystis prophylaxis, independent of other factors such as antiretroviral regimen and CD4$^+$ cell count (72–74). Thus, it is logical for *P. jiroveci* prophylaxis to be considered standard care and to be at the top of the priority list for chemoprophylactic options.

Antipneumocystis prophylaxis can be expected to reduce the frequency of PCP, although no regimen is 100% effective. Convincing data demonstrate that if prophylaxis is initiated when the CD4$^+$ cell count falls to 200 cells/μL or (regardless of CD4$^+$ cell count) when oral candidiasis, hairy leukoplakia, or perhaps substantial weight loss occurs, most cases of PCP can be prevented. A few cases occur at higher CD4$^+$ cell counts, before any indicator signs, but a larger number of patients would have to receive prophylaxis to prevent these relatively few cases.

A variety of regimens have been shown to have antipneumocystis activity (72–74). Trimethoprim-sulfamethoxazole is the regimen of choice because it is more effective than any other, is inexpensive and convenient, and has activity against other pathogens, including *Toxoplasma gondii*, *S. pneumoniae*, and *Haemophilus influenzae*. Dapsone alone is probably the second choice, although dapsone-pyrimethamine combinations are also effective. Aerosol pentamidine is also effective, as detailed in Chapter 283. The best regimen for an individual patient depends on a complex array of issues, including the patient's ability to tolerate the various regimens, compliance issues, and cost.

Prevention of *M. tuberculosis* disease is also a high priority (73). It is well recognized that clinical disease is likely to occur if patients with HIV infection become infected with *M. tuberculosis* (117–119). In addition, *M. tuberculosis* infection appears to stimulate enhanced retroviral activity. Not only does *M. tuberculosis* cause morbidity and mortality in the infected patient, but also there is a sizable risk for transmission, especially because the patient is likely to habituate areas frequented by other highly susceptible individuals. Acute tuberculosis also stimulates an increase in HIV viral load. Patients with no history of tuberculin reactivity should be retested at least annually and offered prophylaxis if their skin test becomes positive or if the test result is positive with no history of prophylaxis, as detailed in Chapter 265 (73). It may be reasonable to offer tuberculosis prophylaxis to certain individuals at high risk regardless of tuberculin test status. Isoniazid prophylaxis has been shown to provide survival benefit for tuberculin test–positive individuals (119). Thus, it should be clear that chemoprophylaxis for tuberculosis, like that for PCP, should be standard care.

Prevention of bacterial infections is being recognized as a desirable goal to decrease the morbidity of these processes as well as their potential to stimulate HIV replication. The use of immunization is controversial because efficacy has not been proved and because immunization could theoretically produce deleterious effects (73). Some drugs, such as trimethoprim-sulfamethoxazole and macrolides, which are used for other purposes, appear to decrease the frequency of bacterial infections. However, bacterial resistance to these drugs is likely to be an increasing problem.

Other opportunistic pathogens that cause serious complications can be prevented by chemoprophylaxis, including *M. avium* complex [rifabutin or azithromycin or clarithromycin (79,120–122), oral ganciclovir and valganciclovir (123,124)], *Candida* and *Cryptococcus* species (fluconazole) (125), and *Toxoplasma* species (trimethoprim-sulfamethoxazole or dapsone-pyrimethamine) (73,126,127). As other studies are completed, additional regimens will probably be shown to be capable of preventing opportunistic infections. Because each of these regimens is associated with toxicities and cost, several of them cause important drug interactions, and there is a limit to how many drugs an individual can take, a decision to add one or more of these regimens to antipneumocystis and antituberculosis chemoprophylaxis is difficult to standardize in any uniform manner for all patients. Some patients are able to tolerate and afford more pills than others, and they may be receiving other drugs that do not interact with the prophylactic agents. Another consideration, however, is that any of these chronic regimens may promote the development of resistant pathogens. That prospect may be sufficient to warrant declining a primary prophylactic regimen that has not proved to prolong survival or substantially improve quality of life compared with other strategies such as prompt therapy when disease is first recognized or when a surrogate marker such as an antigen or nucleic acid detection system indicates a high likelihood of clinical disease.

For opportunistic infections that are not life threatening, such as oral candidiasis or perirectal herpes simplex, primary prophylaxis is probably not as sensible as a strategy of waiting for the first episode of disease to occur, treating it, and then considering the desirability of chronic prevention. There are reports that reactivation of viruses, such as herpes simplex virus, may stimulate HIV replication, suggesting that suppression may be a desirable strategy to prevent immunologic decline. Until this concept is validated, however, there is no strong evidence on which to base recommendations for therapy.

Secondary prophylaxis needs to be considered after successful therapy for any opportunistic infection in a patient with HIV infection, regardless of whether the infection was merely annoying or life threatening (73). After therapy for any opportunistic pathogen in an HIV-infected patient, with the possible exception of *M. tuberculosis* and common bacterial pathogens, there is a great likelihood that another episode of the disease will occur within weeks or months, often in the same anatomic location as the original disease (e.g., the same locus in the brain for toxoplasmosis, the same locus in the retina for CMV retinitis). In some instances, the subsequent episode is almost certainly a relapse because the original therapy suppressed but did not eradicate the original pathogen. This appears to be the situation with herpes simplex virus, varicella-zoster virus, CMV, *T. gondii*, and *Cryptococcus neoformans* infections, regardless of whether results of immediate posttherapy cultures and titers suggest active infection. Whether more aggressive therapy or more potent agents could eradicate all pathogens and obviate long-term therapy remains to be determined. In other instances, the subsequent episodes may represent relapse or reinfection with another strain; for PCP and candidal infections, it is not known which scenario occurs more commonly. In some situations, secondary prophylaxis might represent long-term suppressive therapy; in other situations, it might represent prevention of reinfection.

Regardless of terminology, a long-term regimen is indicated after acute therapy for most life-threatening opportunistic infections (73). These long-term regimens need to be convenient, inexpensive, effective, and compatible with other drugs taken for long periods, such as antiretroviral agents, if they are to gain widespread use. They do not, however, need to be given lifelong if patients are able to attain a substantial boost in the CD4$^+$ count due to antiretroviral therapy and can meet other criteria specific to each opportunistic disease (73). For non–life-threatening infections, the desirability of secondary prophylaxis or long-term suppression depends on how severe and how frequent the relapses are. For perirectal herpes, for instance, chronic suppression with oral acyclovir might be desirable if relapses occurred predictably within a few weeks of terminating acute-phase therapy. In contrast, if relapse occurs only once or twice a year, it may be more convenient and cost-effective to treat each episode when it occurs, starting therapy promptly when symptoms or signs are first recognized.

Expeditious Treatment of Infections and Tumors

Prompt therapy of opportunistic infections and tumors is an important strategy if complications of host diseases are to be minimized. There is convincing evidence, for example, that early recognition and treatment of PCP minimize the likelihood of respiratory failure or death. It seems reasonable to assume that many of the chronic sequelae of PCP, such as bronchopleural fistulas and severe pulmonary fibrosis, also occur less frequently if therapy is started earlier in the natural history of the infectious process. Similarly, early therapy of CMV colitis would be likely to reduce the frequency of bowel hemorrhage and perforation. Early therapeutic intervention would also be a rational approach to minimizing acute and chronic sequelae of other life-threatening processes, such as toxoplasmosis, cryptococcosis, tuberculosis, histoplasmosis, central CMV retinitis, and salmonellosis. Therapy for many non–life-threatening processes—oral or vaginal candidiasis, perirectal or oral herpes simplex, painful cutaneous or disfiguring Kaposi's sarcoma lesions—is palliative. Because these infectious processes are usually symptomatic, prompt initiation of such therapy is appropriate. It must be recognized, however, that for certain non–life-threatening processes, such as nondisfiguring, painless cutaneous Kaposi's sarcoma, early therapeutic intervention may be inconvenient and toxic without providing clear benefit to the patient. Thus, for some serious but non–life-threatening processes, prompt therapy may not be useful.

For prompt therapy of life-threatening processes to be initiated, both health care providers and patients need to be educated about which subtle signs and symptoms warrant immediate diagnostic evaluation. Both health care providers and patients need to recognize the enhanced urgency of evaluating subtle manifestations if the peripheral CD4$^+$ cell count is below 200 to 250 cells/μL. The increasing availability of diagnostic studies that are noninvasive and inexpensive has enhanced the enthusiasm of health care providers and patients for initiating diagnosis early. Induced sputum examinations for *P. jiroveci*, serum antigen tests for cryptococcal disease, and lysis centrifugation or radiometric culture techniques for mycobacteria and fungi are examples of sensitive and specific outpatient techniques that are less invasive and less costly than approaches used previously. Clinicians need to keep in mind, however, that when the index of suspicion is high for a life-threatening process and results of these screening tests are negative, more sensitive examinations, such as bronchoscopy, lumbar puncture, computed tomography, percutaneous organ biopsy, and even surgical exploration and biopsy, should in many instances be performed even if they are more expensive and more invasive and cause more morbidity.

Empiric Versus Specific Therapy

With any disease process, both health care providers and patients are often enthusiastic about treating a new manifestation empirically and thus avoiding the discomfort, inconvenience, cost, and morbidity of diagnostic procedures. There is a role for empiric therapy for certain complications of HIV disease, but the desirability of empiric therapy depends on four factors: how certain the identity of the pathogen is; how effective the empiric regimen is; how toxic and inconvenient the empiric regimen is; and how difficult it will be to establish the diagnosis later if the empiric regimen is not successful (128).

When a patient with HIV infection develops pneumonia, for example, empiric therapy might be reasonable in certain circumstances. If hypoxemia is mild (e.g., room air partial pressure of oxygen greater than 70 to 80 mm Hg or oxygen saturation greater than 95%), the process is not progressing rapidly, the CD4$^+$ cell count is below 200 cells/μL, the chest radiograph is typical of PCP, the patient is compliant and can tolerate an oral regimen, the patient has not been receiving trimethoprim-sulfamethoxazole prophylaxis, and diagnostic facilities are not readily available,

then an empiric trial of trimethoprim-sulfamethoxazole may be reasonable. In this setting, the most likely treatable cause of pneumonia is *P. jiroveci*. If the patient becomes worse or fails to improve after 4 or 5 days, an induced sputum examination or bronchoalveolar lavage is indicated.

Empiric therapy might also be appropriate for oral thrush, esophagitis, or a contrast-enhancing cerebral lesion. Because few processes mimic oral candidiasis, a clinical diagnosis of this entity can be made with a high degree of confidence by an experienced clinician, and empiric antifungal therapy can be instituted. Most cases of esophagitis are caused by *Candida* species, and these patients respond within several days to topical, oral, or parenteral therapy. Topical nystatin, topical clotrimazole, or preferably oral fluconazole or itraconazole is generally tolerated well. Life-threatening complications of esophagitis caused by CMV, herpes simplex virus, or tumors are unusual. Thus, an empiric course of antifungal therapy for several days is reasonable in patients with clinical esophagitis. If the clinical response is not prompt and complete, the inconvenience, expense, and discomfort of a diagnostic procedure such as endoscopy are warranted.

For cerebral lesions that show contrast enhancement, empiric antitoxoplasmal therapy is also appropriate. Although many infections and neoplastic processes can cause contrast-enhancing cerebral lesions in patients with HIV infection, almost all such masses are due to either *T. gondii* or lymphoma. If lesions represent *Toxoplasma* species, there should be radiographic evidence of a response to pyrimethamine plus sulfadiazine within 2 weeks (129). If the lesions turn out to be due to lymphoma, little harm is likely to come to the patient because cerebral lymphomas usually do not progress dramatically in such a short interval. Moreover, the success of therapy for lymphoma in this setting is modest, and waiting for 2 or 3 weeks is not likely to influence outcome adversely. Thus, empiric therapy is warranted in certain clinical settings for patients with HIV infection. Given the cost, inconvenience, toxicity, and potential drug interactions associated with many therapies, however, empiric therapies need to be chosen judiciously.

CONCLUSION

Since AIDS was first recognized and described in 1981, dramatic progress has been made in understanding its etiology, pathogenesis, and natural history. New information on diagnosis, therapy, prophylaxis, and prognosis is rapidly becoming available. Clinicians need to assess these new approaches promptly but cautiously, so that those that provide clear benefit can be used and those that are not real improvements can be avoided or abandoned. The progress made in the 1980s provided clinicians in the 1990s with opportunities to improve the quality and duration of survival for the growing population of patients with HIV, an infectious process that is becoming increasingly chronic.

The next decade is likely to see a changing array of clinical manifestations of HIV infection. First, the demographics of the HIV-infected populations are shifting, and more women and more drug abusers from lower socioeconomic strata are becoming infected. This shift should accentuate the reduction in frequency of Kaposi's sarcoma that is already occurring because women and heterosexual intravenous drug abusers rarely develop it. In addition, less prosperous socioeconomic groups are more likely to have been exposed to *M. tuberculosis* and thus to develop tuberculosis when their immunity is suppressed. Other complications of poverty and drug abuse will be superimposed on manifestations of HIV in more and more patients. Members of lower socioeconomic groups are also less likely to obtain early medical intervention with antiretroviral therapy or evaluation of acute syndromes; thus, they are likely to come to medical attention with more florid, more advanced disease than was usually the case in the late 1980s. Second, antiretroviral therapy is slowing the progression of clinical disease and perhaps diminishing the severity of clinical complications. Patients will live longer and may ultimately manifest complications, such as cardiomyopathy, pneumonitis, or bowel dysfunction, that have been relatively uncommon so far. Third, the use of specific antiinfective prophylactic agents is having a considerable impact on clinical disease. Prophylaxis for PCP, for instance, allows patients to live longer and ultimately provides an opportunity for more HIV-mediated processes, such as cardiomyopathy, more neoplasms, and previously unrecognized opportunistic infections. Episodes of PCP that do occur may be atypical in their pulmonary manifestations, may be extrapulmonary, and may be more difficult to diagnose and treat. Thus, clinicians caring for HIV-infected patients must remain alert to new and changing clinical manifestations, changes in sensitivity of various diagnostic approaches, and changes in the efficacy of therapeutic and prophylactic approaches.

As newer antiretroviral drugs are widely used and prophylactic antiinfective agents are used more widely and more chronically, drug resistance is likely to become a clinically important phenomenon that must be tested for and that requires alterations in therapeutic regimens. Unless new drugs with novel mechanisms of action continue to be developed for HIV and for opportunistic pathogens, many of the gains of the first 25 years of the epidemic may be eroded.

REFERENCES

1. Available online: *www.unaids.org/epidemic-update*
2. Centers for Disease Control and Prevention. Update AIDS—United States 2000. *MMWR Morb Mortal Wkly Rep* 2002;51(27):592–595.
3. Centers for Disease Control and Prevention. Summary of notifiable diseases, United States, 2001. *MMWR Morb Mortal Wkly Rep* 2003;50(53).
4. Landon BE, Wilson IB, Wenger NS, et al. Specialty training and specialization among physicians who treat HIV/AIDS in the United States. *J Gen Intern Med* 2002;17(1):12–22.
5. Bozzette SA, Joyce G, McCaffrey DF, et al. Expenditures for the care of HIV-infected patients in the era of highly active antiretroviral therapy. *N Engl J Med* 2001;15;344(11):817–823.
6. Daar ES, Little S, Pitt J, et al. Diagnosis of primary HIV-1 infection: Los Angeles County Druncey HIV Infection Recruitment Network. *Ann Intern Med* 2001;134:25–29.
7. Daar ES, Mougdil T, Meyer RD, et al. Transient high level of viremia in patients with primary human immunodeficiency virus type 1 infection. *N Engl J Med* 1991;324:961.
8. Niu MT, Stein DS, Schnittman SM. Primary human immunodeficiency virus type 1 infection: review of pathogenesis and early treatment interventions in humans and animal retrovirus infections. *J Infect Dis* 1993;168:1490.
9. Schacker T, Collier AC, Hughes J, et al. Clinical and epidemiologic features of primary HIV infection. *Ann Intern Med* 1996;125:257.
10. Rustin MHA, Ridely CM, Smith MD, et al. The acute exanthem associated with seroconversion to human T-cell lymphotropic virus III in a homosexual man. *J Infect Dis* 1986;12:161.
11. Zaunders J, Carr A, McNally L, et al. Effect of primary HIV-1 infection on subsets of CD4$^+$ and CD8$^+$ T lymphocytes. *AIDS* 1995;9:561.
12. Kinloch-DeLoes S, Hirschel BJ, Hoen B, et al. A controlled trial of zidovudine in primary human immunodeficiency virus infection. *N Engl J Med* 1995;333:408.
13. Altfeld M, Rosenberg ES, Shankarappa R, et al. Cellular immune responses and viral diversity in individuals treated during acute and early HIV-1 infection. *J Exp Med* 2001;193(2):169–180.
14. Sullivan PS, Buskin SE, Turner JH, et al. Low prevalence of antiretroviral resistance among persons recently affected with human immunodeficiency virus in two US cities. *Int J STD AIDS* 2002;13:554–558.
15. Greenspan D, Greenspan JS, Hearst NG, et al. Relation of oral hairy leukoplakia to infection with the human immunodeficiency virus and the risk of developing AIDS. *J Infect Dis* 1987;155:475.
16. Buchbinder SP, Katz MH, Hessol NA, et al. Herpes zoster and human immunodeficiency virus infection. *J Infect Dis* 1992;166:1153.
17. Rowland RW, Escobar MR, Friedman RB, et al. Painful gingivitis may be an early sign of infection with the human immunodeficiency virus. *Clin Infect Dis* 1993;16:233.
18. Feigal DW, Katz MH, Greenspan D, et al. The prevalence of oral lesions in HIV-infected homosexual and bisexual men: three San Francisco epidemiological cohorts. *AIDS* 1991;5:519.
19. Metroka CE, Cunningham-Rundles S, Pollack MS, et al. Persistent generalized lymphadenopathy in homosexual men. *Ann Intern Med* 1983;99:585.
20. Klein RS, Harris CA, Small CB, et al. Oral candidiasis in high-risk patients as the initial manifestation of the acquired immunodeficiency syndrome. *N Engl J Med* 1984;31:354.
21. Kovacs JA, Hiemenz JW, Macher AM, et al. *Pneumocystis carinii* pneumonia: a comparison between patients with the acquired immunodeficiency syndrome and patients with other immunodeficiencies. *Ann Intern Med* 1984;100:663.
22. Kalb RE, Grossman ME. Chronic perianal herpes simplex in immunocompromised hosts. *Am J Med* 1986;80:486.
23. Kovacs JA, Kovacs AA, Polis M, et al. Cryptococcosis in the acquired immunodeficiency syndrome. *Ann Intern Med* 1985;103:533.
24. Hawkins CC, Gold JWM, Whimbey E, et al. *Mycobacterium avium* complex infections in patients with the acquired immunodeficiency syndrome. *Ann Intern Med* 1986;105:184.
25. DeHovitz JA, Pape JW, Boncy M, et al. Clinical manifestations and therapy of *Isospora belli* infection in patients with acquired immunodeficiency syndrome. *N Engl J Med* 1986;315:87.
26. Janoff EN, Breiman RF, Daley CL, et al. Pneumococcal disease during HIV infection. *Ann Intern Med* 1992;117:314.
27. Koehler JE, Quinn FD, Berger TG, et al. Isolation of *Rochalimaea* species from cutaneous and osseous lesions of bacillary angiomatosis. *N Engl J Med* 1992;327:1625.
28. Luft BJ, Hafner R Korzun AH, et al. Toxoplasmic encephalitis in patients with the acquired immunodeficiency syndrome. *N Engl J Med* 1993;329:995.
29. McCutchan JA. Cytomegalovirus infections of the nervous system in patients with AIDS. *Clin Infect Dis* 1995;20:747.
30. Porter SB, Sande MA. Toxoplasmosis of the central nervous system in acquired immunodeficiency syndrome. *N Engl J Med* 1992;327:1643.
31. Jaffe HW, Darrow WW, Echenberg DF, et al. The acquired immunodeficiency syndrome in a cohort of homosexual men: a six year follow-up study. *Ann Intern Med* 1985;103:210.
32. Thiebaut R, Morlat P, Jacqmin-Gadda H, et al. Clinical progression of HIV-1 infection according to the viral response during the first year of antiretroviral treatment. Groupe d'Epidemiologie du SIDA en Aquitaine (GECSA). *AIDS* 2000;14(8):971–978.
33. Grabar S, Le Moing V, Goujard C, et al. Clinical outcome of patients with HIV-1 infection according to immunologic and virologic response after 6 months of highly active antiretroviral therapy. *Ann Intern Med* 2000;133(6):401–410.
34. Phillips AN, Staszewski S, Weber R, et al. HIV viral load response to antiretroviral therapy according to the baseline CD4 cell count and viral load. *JAMA* 2001;286(20):2560–2567.
35. Miller V, Mocroft A, Reiss P, et al. Relations among CD4 lymphocyte count nadir, antiretroviral therapy, and HIV-1 disease progression: results from the EuroSIDA study. *Ann Intern Med* 1999;130(7):570–577.
36. Moss AR, Bacchetti P, Osmond D, et al. Seropositivity for HIV and the development of AIDS or ARC: three year follow-up of the San Francisco General Hospital cohort. *BMJ* 1988;296:745.
37. O'Brien TR, Blattner WA, Waters P, et al. Serum HIV-1 RNA levels and time to development of AIDS in the Multicenter Hemophilia Cohort Study. *JAMA* 1996;276:105.
38. Samson M, Libert F, Doranz BJ, et al. Resistance to HIV-1 infection in Caucasian individuals bearing mutant alleles of the CCR-5 chemokine receptor gene. *Nature* 1996;382:722.
39. Cao Y, Qin L, Zhang L, et al. Virologic and immunologic characterization of long-term survivors of human immunodeficiency virus type 1 infection. *N Engl J Med* 1995;332:201.
40. Pantaleo G, Menzo S, Vaccarezza M, et al. Studies in subjects with long-term nonprogressive human immunodeficiency virus infection. *N Engl J Med* 1995;332:209.
41. Katzenstein D, Hammer S, Hughes M, et al. The relation of virologic and immunologic markers to clinical outcomes after nucleoside therapy in HIV-infected adults with 200 to 500 CD4 cells. *N Engl J Med* 1996;335:1091.
42. Mellors JW, Rinaldo CR Jr, Gupta P, et al. Prognosis of HIV infection predicted by the quantity of virus in plasma. *Science* 1996;272:1167.
43. Mellors JW, Kingsley LA, Rinaldo CR Jr, et al. Quantitation of HIV-1 RNA in plasma predicts outcome after seroconversion. *Ann Intern Med* 1995;122:573.
44. Stricof RL, Morse DL. HTLV-III/LAV seroconversion following a deep intramuscular needlestick injury. *N Engl J Med* 1986;314:1115.
45. Lorenzo JI, Moscardo F, Lopez-Aldeguer J, et al. Progression to acquired immunodeficiency syndrome in 94 human immunodeficiency virus-positive hemophiliacs with long-term follow-up. *Haematologica* 2001;86(3):291–296.
46. Stein DS, Korvick JA, Vermund SH. CD4$^+$ lymphocyte cell enumeration for prediction of clinical course of human immunodeficiency virus disease: a review. *J Infect Dis* 1992;165:352.
47. Cohen OJ, Paolucci S, Bende SM, et al. CXCR4 and CCR5 genetic polymorphisms in long-term nonprogressive human immunodeficiency virus infection: lack of association with mutations other than CCR5-Delta32. *J Virol* 1998;72(7):6215–6217.

48. Sterling TR, Vlahov D, Astemborski J, et al. Initial plasma HIV-1 RNA levels and progression to AIDS in women and men. *N Engl J Med* 2001;344(10):720–725.

49. Kessler HA, Blauw B, Spear J, et al. Diagnosis of human immunodeficiency virus infection in seronegative homosexuals who present with an acute viral syndrome. *JAMA* 1987;258:1196.

50. Goudsmit J, De Wolf F, Paul DA, et al. Expression of human immunodeficiency virus antigen (HIV Ag) in serum and cerebrospinal fluid during acute and chronic infection. *Lancet* 1986;2:177.

51. Ranki A, Valle S-L, Krohn M, et al. Long latency period precedes overt sero-conversion in sexually transmitted human immunodeficiency virus infection. *Lancet* 1987;2:589.

52. Centers for Disease Control and Prevention. Persistent lack of detectable HIV-1 antibody in a person with HIV infection: Utah, 1995. *MMWR Morb Mortal Wkly Rep* 1996;45:181.

53. Altfeld M, Rosenberg ES, Shankarappa R, et al. Cellular immune responses and viral diversity in individuals treated during acute and early HIV-1 infection. *J Exp Med* 2001;193(2):169–180.

54. Kaufmann GR, Zaunders JJ, Cunningham P, et al. Rapid restoration of CD4 T cell subsets in subjects receiving antiretroviral therapy during primary HIV-1 infection. *AIDS* 2000;14(17):2643–2651.

55. Plana M, Garcia F, Gallart T, et al. Immunological benefits of antiretroviral therapy in very early stages of asymptomatic chronic HIV-1 infection. *AIDS* 2000;14(13):1921–1933.

56. Zaunders JJ, Cunningham PH, Kelleher AD, et al. Potent antiretroviral therapy of primary human immunodeficiency virus type 1 (HIV-1) infection: partial normalization of T lymphocyte subsets and limited reduction of HIV-1 DNA despite clearance of plasma viremia. *J Infect Dis* 1999;180(2):320–329.

57. Lafeuillade A, Poggi C, Tamalet C, et al. Effects of a combination of zidovudine, didanosine, and lamivudine on primary human immunodeficiency virus type 1 infection. *J Infect Dis* 1997;175(5):1051–1055.

58. Malhotra U, Berrey MM, Huang Y, et al. Effect of combination antiretroviral therapy on T-cell immunity in acute human immunodeficiency virus type 1 infection. *J Infect Dis* 2000;181(1):121–131.

59. Saah AJ, Munoz A, Kuo V, et al. Predictors of the risk of development of acquired immunodeficiency syndrome within 24 months among gay men seropositive for human immunodeficiency virus type 1: a report from the Multicenter AIDS Cohort Study. *Am J Epidemiol* 1992;135:1147.

60. Goedert JJ, Kessler CM, Aledort LM, et al. A prospective study of human immunodeficiency virus type 1 infection and the development of AIDS in subjects with hemophilia. *N Engl J Med* 1989;321:1141.

61. Katzenstein DA, Hammer SM, Hughes MD, et al. The relation of virologic and immunologic markers to clinical outcomes after nucleoside therapy in HIV-infected adults with 200 to 500 CD4 cells per cubic millimeter. AIDS Clinical Trials Group Study 175 Virology Study Team. *N Engl J Med* 1996;335(15):1091–1098.

62. Lifson AR, Hessol NA, Rutherford GW. Progression and clinical outcome of infection due to human immunodeficiency virus. *Clin Infect Dis* 1992;14:966.

63. Carne CA, Weller IVD, Loveday C, et al. From persistent generalised lymphadenopathy to AIDS: who will progress?. *BMJ* 1987;294:868.

64. Hoover DR, Saah AJ, Bacellar H. Clinical manifestations of AIDS in the era of *Pneumocystis* prophylaxis. *N Engl J Med* 1993;329:1922.

65. Enger C, Graham M, Peng Y, et al. Survival from early, intermediate, and late stages of HIV infection. *JAMA* 1996;275:1329.

66. Kaplan JE, Hanson D, Dworkin MS, et al. Epidemiology of human immunodeficiency virus-associated opportunistic infections in the United States in the era of highly active antiretroviral therapy. *Clin Infect Dis* 2000;30[Suppl 1]:S5–14.

67. Centers for Disease Control and Prevention. 1993 Revised classification system for HIV infection and expanded surveillance case definition for AIDS among adolescents and adults. *MMWR Morbid Mortal Wkly Rep* 1992;41(RR-17):1.

68. Centers for Disease Control. Revision of the CDC surveillance case definition for acquired immunodeficiency syndrome. *MMWR Morbid Mortal Wkly Rep* 1987;36[Suppl 1]:1S.

69. Centers for Disease Control and Prevention. Current trends update. Acquired immunodeficiency syndrome—United States, 1994. *MMWR Morb Mortal Wkly Rep* 1999;48:29–31.

70. World Health Organization. Interim proposal for a WHO staging system for HIV infection and diseases. *Wkly Epidemiol Rec* 1990;65:221.

71. Melbye M, Grossman RJ, Goedert JJ, et al. Risk of AIDS after herpes zoster. *Lancet* 1987;1:728.

72. Gallant JE, Moore RD, Chaisson RE. Prophylaxis for opportunistic infections in patients with HIV infection. *Ann Intern Med* 1994;120:932.

73. 2001 USPHS/IDSA guidelines for the prevention of opportunistic infections in persons infected with human immunodeficiency virus. Available online: *www.hivatis.org*

74. Kovacs JA, Masur H. Prophylaxis against opportunistic infections in patients with human immunodeficiency virus infection. *N Engl J Med* 2000;342(19):1416–1429.

75. Masur H, Ognibene FP, Yarchoan R, et al. CD4 counts as predictors of opportunistic pneumonias in human immunodeficiency virus infected individuals. *Ann Intern Med* 1989;111:223.

76. Taylor JMB, Fahey JL, Detels R, et al. CD4 percentage, CD4 number, and CD4:CD8 ratio in HIV infection: which to choose and how to use. *J Acquir Immune Defic Syndr* 1989;2:114.

77. Crowe SM, Carlin JB, Stewart KI, et al. Predictive value of CD4 lymphocyte numbers for the development of opportunistic infections and malignancies in HIV-infected persons. *J Acquir Immune Defic Syndr* 1991;4:770.

78. Whitley RJ, Jacobson MA, Friedberg DN, et al. Guidelines for the treatment of cytomegalovirus diseases in patients with AIDS in the era of potent antiretroviral therapy: recommendations of an international panel. International AIDS Society-USA. *Arch Intern Med* 1998;158(9):957–969.

79. Phair J, Munoz A, Detels R, et al. The risk of *Pneumocystis carinii* among men infected with human immunodeficiency virus type 1. *N Engl J Med* 1990;322:161.

80. Chaisson RE, Moore RD, Richman DD, et al. Incidence and natural history of *Mycobacterium avium*-complex infections in patients with advanced HIV disease treated with zidovudine. *Am Rev Respir Dis* 1992;146:285.

81. Miller V, Mocroft A, Reiss P, et al. Relations among CD4 lymphocyte count nadir, antiretroviral therapy, and HIV-1 disease progression: results from the EuroSIDA study. *Ann Intern Med* 1999;130(7):570–577.

82. Zurlo JJ, Wood L, Gaglione MM, et al. Effect of splenectomy on T lymphocyte subsets in patients infected with the human immunodeficiency virus. *Clin Infect Dis* 1995;20(4):768–771.

83. Giorgi JV, Lyles RH, Matud JL, et al. Predictive value of immunologic and virologic markers after long or short duration of HIV-1 infection. *J Acquir Immune Defic Syndr* 2002;29(4):346–355.

84. Kim S, Hughes MD, Hammer SM, et al. Both serum HIV type 1 RNA levels and CD4+ lymphocyte counts predict clinical outcome in HIV type 1-infected subjects with 200 to 500 CD4+ cells per cubic millimeter. AIDS Clinical Trials Group Study 175 Virology Study Team. *AIDS Res Hum Retroviruses* 2000;16(7):645–653.

85. Melbye M, Biggar JR, Ebbesen P, et al. Long-term HTLV-VIII seropositive homosexual men without AIDS develop measurable immunologic and clinical abnormalities: a longitudinal study. *Ann Intern Med* 1986;104:496.

86. Miller V, Staszewski S, Sabin C, et al. CD4 lymphocyte count as a predictor of the duration of highly active antiretroviral therapy-induced suppression of human immunodeficiency virus load. *J Infect Dis* 1999;180(2):530–533.

87. Abrams DI, Bebchuk JD, Denning ET, et al. Randomized, open-label study of the impact of two doses of subcutaneous recombinant interleukin-2 on viral burden in patients with HIV-1 infection and CD4+ cell counts of > or = 300/mm³: CPCRA 059. *J Acquir Immune Defic Syndr* 2002;29(3):221–231.

88. Davey RT Jr, Murphy RL, Graziano FM, et al. Immunologic and virologic effects of subcutaneous interleukin 2 in combination with antiretroviral therapy: a randomized controlled trial. *JAMA* 2000;284(2):183–189.

89. Department of Health and Human Services and Kaiser Family Foundation. *Guidelines for antiretroviral therapy in adults and adolescents.* Available online: *www.hivatis.org*

90. Hammer S, Katzenstein D, Hughes M, et al. A trial comparing nucleoside monotherapy with combination therapy in HIV-infected adults with CD4 counts from 200 to 500 per cubic millimeter. AIDS Clinical Trial Group Study Team. *N Engl J Med* 1996;335:1081.

91. Fischl MA, Richman DD, Grieco MH, et al. The efficacy of azidothymidine (AZT) in the treatment of patients with AIDS and AIDS-related complex. *N Engl J Med* 1987;317:185.

92. D'Aquila RT, Johnson VA, Welles SL, et al. Zidovudine resistance and HIV-1 disease progression during antiretroviral therapy. *Ann Intern Med* 1995;122:401.

93. Fischl M, Richman DD, Causey AM, et al. Prolonged zidovudine therapy in patients with AIDS and advanced AIDS related complex. *JAMA* 1989;262:2405.

94. Fischl MA, Parker CB, Pettinelli C, et al. A randomized controlled trial of a reduced daily dose of zidovudine in patients with the acquired immunodeficiency syndrome. *N Engl J Med* 1990;323:1009.

95. Collier AC, Coombs RW, Schoenfeld DA, et al. Treatment for human immunodeficiency virus infection with saquinavir, zidovudine, and zalcitabine. *N Engl J Med* 1996;334:1011.

96. Markowitz M, Saag M, Powderly WG, et al. A preliminary study of ritonavir, an inhibitor of HIV-1 protease, to treat HIV-1 infection. *N Engl J Med* 1995;333:1534.

97. Gulick RM, Mellors JW, Havlir D, et al. Treatment with indinavir, zidovudine, and lamivudine in adults with human immunodeficiency virus infection and prior antiretroviral therapy. *N Engl J Med* 1997;337(11):734–739.

98. Hammer SM, Squires KE, Hughes MD, et al. A controlled trial of two nucleoside analogues plus indinavir in persons with human immunodeficiency virus infection and CD4 cell counts of 200 per cubic millimeter or less. *N Engl J Med* 1997;337(11):725–733.

99. Cameron DW, Health-Chiozzi M, Danner S, et al. Randomized placebo-controlled trial of ritonavir in advanced HIV-1 disease. The Advanced HIV Disease Ritonavir Study Group. *Lancet* 1998;351(9102):2568–2577.

100. Mocroft A, Vella S, Benfield TL, et al. Changing patterns of mortality across Europe in patients infected with HIV-1. EuroSIDA Study Group. *Lancet* 1998;352(9142):1725–1730.

101. Palella FJ Jr, Delaney KM, Moorman AC, et al. Declining morbidity and mortality among patients with advanced human immunodeficiency virus infection. HIV Outpatient Study Investigators. *N Engl J Med* 1998;338(13):853–860.

102. Vittinghoff E, Scheer S, O'Malley P, et al. Combination antiretroviral therapy and recent declines in AIDS incidence and mortality. *J Infect Dis* 1999;179(3):717–720.

103. Hogg RS, Yip B, Chan KJ, et al. Rates of disease progression by baseline CD4 cell count and viral load after initiating triple-drug therapy. *JAMA* 2001;286(20):2568–2577.

104. Phillips AN, Staszewski S, Weber R, et al. HIV viral load response to antiretroviral therapy according to the baseline CD4 cell count and viral load. *JAMA* 2001;286(20):2560–2567.
105. Burger DM, Aarnoutse RE, Hugen PW. Pros and cons of therapeutic drug monitoring of antiretroviral agents. *Curr Opin Infect Dis* 2002;15(1):17–22.
106. Piscitelli SC, Gallicano KD. Interactions among drugs for HIV and opportunistic infections. *N Engl J Med* 2001;344(13):984–996.
107. Piscitelli SC, Burstein AH, Welden N, et al. The effect of garlic supplements on the pharmacokinetics of saquinavir. *Clin Infect Dis* 2002;34(2):234–238.
108. Piscitelli SC, Burstein AH, Chaitt D, et al. Indinavir concentrations and St John's wort. *Lancet* 2000;355(9203):547–548.
109. Miller KD, Jones E, Yanovski JA, et al. Visceral abdominal-fat accumulation associated with use of indinavir. *Lancet* 1998;351(9106):871–875.
110. Miller J, Carr A, Smith D, et al. Lipodystrophy following antiretroviral therapy of primary HIV infection. *AIDS* 2000;14(15):2406–2407.
111. Miller KD, Masur H, Jones EC, et al. High prevalence of osteonecrosis of the femoral head in HIV-infected adults. *Ann Intern Med* 2002;137(1):17–25.
112. Carr A, Miller J, Eisman JA, et al. Osteopenia in HIV-infected men: association with asymptomatic lactic acidemia and lower weight pre-antiretroviral therapy. *AIDS* 2001;15(6):703–709.
113. Meynard JL, Vray M, Morand-Joubert L, et al. Phenotypic or genotypic resistance testing for choosing antiretroviral therapy after treatment failure: a randomized trial. *AIDS* 2002;16(5):727–736.
114. Torre D, Tambini R. Antiretroviral drug resistance testing in patients with HIV-1 infection: a meta-analysis study. *HIV Clin Trials* 2002;3(1):1–8.
115. Hanna GJ, D'Aquila RT. Clinical use of genotypic and phenotypic drug resistance testing to monitor antiretroviral chemotherapy. *Clin Infect Dis* 2001;32(5):774–782.
116. Kovacs JA, Vogel S, Albert J, et al. Sustained increases in CD4 counts in HIV-infected patients treated with interleukin-2 during a randomized, controlled trial. *N Engl J Med* 1996;335:1350.
117. Beck-Sague C, Dooley SW, Hutton MD, et al. Hospital outbreak of multidrug-resistant *Mycobacterium tuberculosis* infections: factors in transmission to staff and HIV-infected patients. *JAMA* 1992;268:1280.
118. Dooley SW, Villarino ME, Lawrence M, et al. Nosocomial transmission of tuberculosis in a hospital unit for HIV-infected patients. *JAMA* 1992;267:2632.
119. Pape JE Jean SS, Ho JL, et al. Effect of isoniazid prophylaxis on incidence of active tuberculosis and progression of HIV infection. *Lancet* 1993;342:268.
120. Nightingale SD, Cameron DW, Gordin FM, et al. Two controlled trials of rifabutin prophylaxis against *Mycobacterium avium* complex infection in AIDS. *N Engl J Med* 1993;329:828.
121. Havlir DV, Dube MP, Sattler FR, et al. Prophylaxis against disseminated *Mycobacterium avium* complex with weekly azithromycin, daily rifabutin, or both. *N Engl J Med* 1996;335:392.
122. Pierce M, Crampton S, Henry D, et al. A randomized trial of clarithromycin as prophylaxis against disseminated *Mycobacterium avium* complex infection in patients with advanced acquired immunodeficiency syndrome. *N Engl J Med* 1996;335:384.
123. Martin DF, Sierra-Madero J, Walmsley S, et al. A controlled trial of valganciclovir as induction therapy for cytomegalovirus retinitis. *N Engl J Med* 2002;346(15):1119–1126.
124. Spector SA, McKinley GF, Lalezari JP, et al. Oral ganciclovir for the prevention of cytomegalovirus disease in persons with AIDS. *N Engl J Med* 1996;334:1491.
125. Powderly WG, Finkelstein DM, Feinberg J, et al. A randomized trial comparing fluconazole with clotrimazole troches for the prevention of fungal infections in patients with advanced human immunodeficiency virus infection. *N Engl J Med* 1995;332:700.
126. Carr A, Tindall B, Brew BJ, et al. Low-dose trimethoprim-sulfamethoxazole prophylaxis for toxoplasmic encephalitis in patients with AIDS. *Ann Intern Med* 1992;117:106.
127. Mallolas J, Zamora L, Gatell JM, et al. Primary prophylaxis for *Pneumocystis carinii* pneumonia: a randomized trial comparing cotrimoxazole aerosolized pentamidine and dapsone plus pyrimethamine. *AIDS* 1993;7:59.
128. Masur H, Shelhamer J. Empiric outpatient management of HIV-related pneumonia: economical or unwise. *Ann Intern Med* 1996;124:451.
129. Luft BJ, Hafner R, Korzun AH, et al. Toxoplasmic encephalitis in patients with the acquired immunodeficiency syndrome. *N Engl J Med* 1993;329:995.

CHAPTER 114
International Epidemiology of Human Immunodeficiency Virus

Thomas C. Quinn and Richard E. Chaisson

HISTORICAL PERSPECTIVE

In 1981, the first cases of the acquired immunodeficiency syndrome (AIDS) were recognized in previously healthy homosexual men residing in the United States (1–4). During the next few years, additional cases were recognized in members of other high-risk groups, including injecting drug users (IDUs), hemophiliacs, and recipients of blood transfusions (5). By 1984, it was evident that AIDS was already widespread throughout North America, the Caribbean, and parts of Central Africa, Europe, and Oceania (6–10). By the end of the 1980s, it was clear that AIDS had become a global pandemic. Two decades later, more than 65 million people had become infected with the human immunodeficiency virus type 1 (HIV-1), the cause of AIDS (11–14) (Fig. 114.1). By 2003, more than 25 million people had died from AIDS, and it became ranked as one of the leading causes of death throughout the world (12,15–19).

Unfortunately, the disease continues to escalate in many areas of the world. In 2002, 42 million people were infected with HIV, 5 million of whom were newly infected, and in sub-Saharan Africa alone, 3.5 million people became newly infected (12) (Fig. 114.2). Of those newly infected, 50% worldwide were women, the first time that global statistics have indicated this marked increase in HIV among women. Half of all the new infections occurred in young individuals between the ages of 15 and 24 years. Eight hundred thousand children became newly infected in 2002, a time in which mother-to-infant transmission should have been prevented through antiretroviral treatment and prophylaxis. In 2002, 3.1 million people died from AIDS, including 610,000 children (12) (Table 114.1). As in previous years, more than 95% of all new infections and fatalities occurred in developing countries where access to antiretroviral drugs remains limited and, in some cases, not available at all (20–23) (Table 114.2).

EVOLUTION OF THE EPIDEMIC

Temporally, the HIV pandemic has undergone four major phases of evolution during the past three decades (24). These phases can be characterized as emergence, dissemination, escalation, and stabilization. Before AIDS was ever recognized, HIV emerged from remote rural areas, where it might have been endemic at low levels, and disseminated to more populated, urban areas (25). This resulted in rapid spread among high-risk populations, such as female sex workers and their clients in developing countries and homosexual men in industrialized countries (7,26). This first phase of emergence was followed by a phase of dissemination in which the virus quickly spread to various regions of the world primarily through population migration (27). Although rural-to-urban migration and international travel played an important role in dissemination, another factor associated with migration was the enormous social disruption that occurred during this period of urbanization, particularly in sub-Saharan Africa (28). This social disorganization and cultural change directly influenced

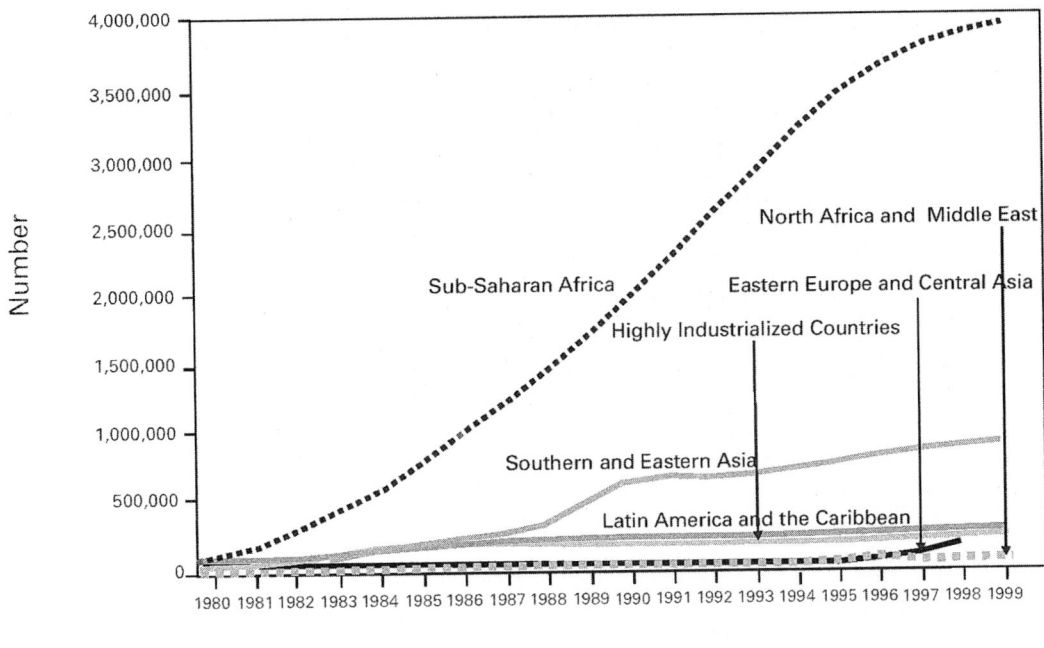

Figure 114.1. Estimated number of new HIV infections, by region and year—worldwide, 1980–1999. (Data from Centers for Disease Control and Prevention. Global HIV and AIDS pandemic. *MMWR Morb Mortal Wkly Rep* 2001:436, with permission.)

vulnerability to HIV. During the next phase of escalation, which occurred in the 1980s, transmission of HIV was further amplified among high-risk populations, including IDUs and heterosexual partners of infected individuals (26,29). This resulted in further spread of HIV from restricted high-risk populations and segments of the general population in some regions. This phase of escalation is most dramatically illustrated in the densely populated regions of Southeast Asia, where it has been estimated that 7 million cumulative HIV infections have occurred within the past 5 years (30–32).

A fourth phase of the HIV pandemic became evident as HIV prevalence and reported AIDS cases appeared to stabilize, particularly in the developed regions of Australia, North America, and Western Europe (12,33). Although such changes might represent a positive development from a prevention perspective, they may also indicate a transition from epidemic HIV to endemic HIV infection (33). Although HIV incidence may have stabilized in many developed countries, such as the United States and Western Europe, the introduction of combination antiretroviral therapy has dramatically reduced HIV- and AIDS-related mortality from 1996 through 2000 (34,35) (Fig. 114.3). From 2000 to 2003, this trend in reduced mortality has leveled, and further declines do not appear to be present. This increase in survival in people living with HIV has led to a steady increase in the total number of people living with HIV in these countries (Fig. 114.3). Thus, although incidence has stabilized, the total number of individuals has markedly increased as a result of the decreased death rate as a benefit of antiretroviral drugs. About 500,000 people in these countries received antiretroviral drugs within the past 2 years. Unfortunately, this benefit in increased survival has not been attained in developing countries because of the high cost and low access to these expensive medications.

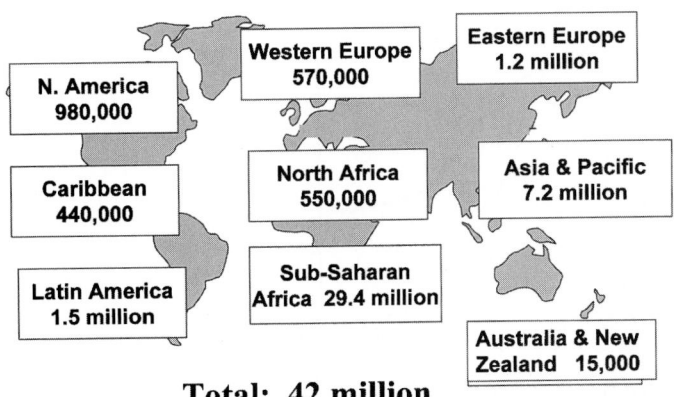

Total: 42 million

Figure 114.2. Estimated distribution of total adult and pediatric HIV infections from 1980 until December 2002. (Data from UNAIDS/WHO. *AIDS epidemic update, December 2002.* Geneva: UNAIDS and WHO, 2002: 1–38, with permission.)

TABLE 114.1. Global Summary of the HIV/AIDS Epidemic, December 2002

Number of people living with HIV/AIDS	
Total	42 million
Adults	38.6 million
Women	19.2 million
Children <15 yr	3.2 million
People newly infected with HIV in 2002	
Total	5 million
Adults	4.2 million
Women	2 million
Children <15 yr	800,000
AIDS deaths in 2002	
Total	3.1 million
Adults	2.5 million
Women	1.2 million
Children <15 yr	610,000

TABLE 114.2.   Regional HIV/AIDS Statistics and Features, End of 2002

Region	Epidemic started	Adults and children living with HIV/AIDS	Adults and children newly infected with HIV	Adult prevalence[a] (%)	HIV-positive adults who are women (%)	Main mode(s) of transmission[b] for adults living with HIV/AIDS
Sub-Saharan Africa	Late 1970s, early 1980s	29.4 million	3.5 million	8.8	58	Heterosexual
North Africa & Middle East	Late 1980s	550,000	83,000	0.3	55	Heterosexual, IDU
South & South-East Asia	Late 1980s	6 million	700,000	0.6	36	Heterosexual, IDU
East Asia & Pacific	Late 1980s	1.2 million	270,000	0.1	24	IDU, heterosexual, MSM
Latin America	Late 1970s, early 1980s	1.5 million	150,000	0.6	30	MSM, IDU, heterosexual
Caribbean	Late 1970s, early 1980s	440,000	60,000	2.4	50	Heterosexual, MSM
Eastern Europe & Central Asia	Early 1990s	1.2 million	250,000	0.6	27	IDU
Western Europe	Late 1970s, early 1980s	570,000	30,000	0.3	25	MSM, IDU
North America	Late 1970s, early 1980s	980,000	45,000	0.6	20	MSM, IDU, heterosexual
Australia & New Zealand	Late 1970s, early 1980s	15,000	500	0.1	7	MSM
TOTALS		42 million	5 million	1.2	50	

[a]The proportion of adults (15 to 49 years of age) living with HIV/AIDS in 2002, using 2002 population numbers.
IDU, injecting drug use; MSM, men who have sex with men.

Stabilization may also mask disproportionate increases in particular modes of transmission such as an increase in heterosexually transmitted HIV or disproportionate increase in new HIV infections among young people as evidenced in the United States and Europe (12,33,36,37). Stabilization of HIV prevalence and reported AIDS cases is simply one more facet of the evolving global nature of HIV infection. These trends of stabilization continue to occur in developed countries, and with escalation continuing in developing countries, it is evident that the major force of the epidemic will be in sub-Saharan Africa, Eastern Europe, and Asia, where more than half of the world's population resides (12,32,38).

The global pandemic of HIV infection consists of many different epidemics, each with its own dynamics, influenced by many factors such as the time of introduction, population density, and cultural and social factors that might increase vulnerability to HIV infection (Fig. 114.1). Even within some regions, the HIV epidemic consists of a multitude of smaller, ongoing epidemics, which, although related, pursue their own course with different velocities (39,40). The spread of the epidemic has varied dramatically between the developed and developing countries, depending on the culture of the regions as well as many other social and behavioral patterns. Incidence rates have been highest in developing countries, where heterosexual transmission is most common, as in sub-Saharan Africa, the Caribbean, and Southeast Asia (12,21,41). In addition to continued spread in already affected areas, HIV is spreading rapidly to communities and countries little affected during the 1980s. Nigeria, once considered an

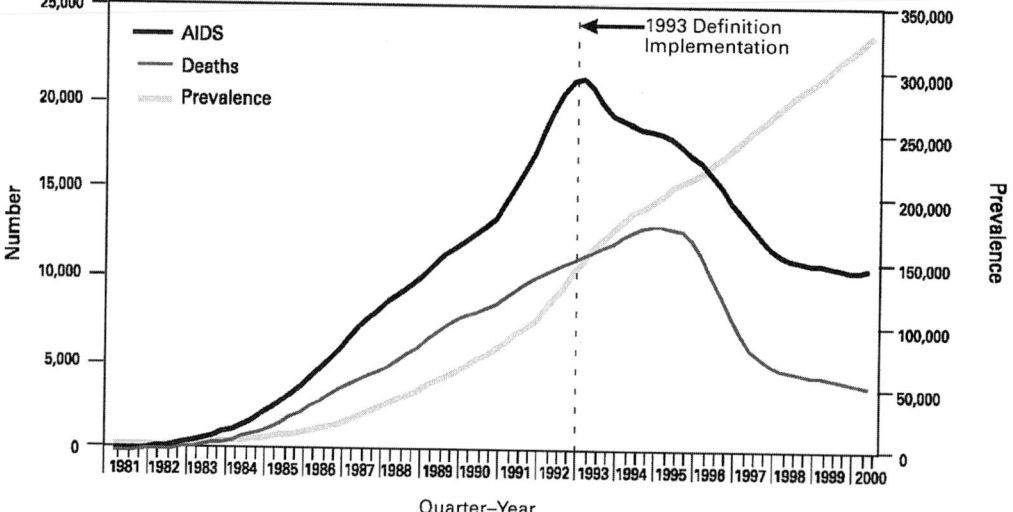

Figure 114.3. Estimated AIDS incidence (*), deaths, and prevalence by quarter year of diagnosis/death for the United States, 1981–2000. (Data from Centers for Disease Control and Prevention. HIV and AIDS in the United States. *MMWR Morb Mortal Wkly Rep* 2001:432, with permission.)

area of minimal HIV activity located between the West African and central African epicenters, now estimates that nearly 6% of the population is infected (12). Similarly, South Africa and Botswana estimate that more than 20% and 35% of the population is infected, respectively. In Southeast Asia, particularly India, Myanmar (Burma), and Thailand, the volatility of the pandemic is most dramatically seen (38,42). With the continued escalation of HIV transmission in Asia and sub-Saharan Africa, it is estimated that nearly 95% of all HIV-infected people reside in these developing countries.

MOLECULAR EPIDEMIOLOGY

The diversity of the global AIDS pandemic is also reflected in the heterogeneity of the viral subtypes, or clades, of HIV. On the basis of genetic sequence data, HIV-1 can be grouped into at least nine distinct genetic subtypes and numerous circulating recombinant forms (43–45). In addition, there are at least five different subtypes of HIV-2, the predominant virus originally identified in West African countries (46). A broad overview of the geographical distribution of HIV strains can be obtained from molecular epidemiologic studies, which can offer clues to how the virus spread between regions and continents (47–49). Global diversity of HIV is most likely affected by the number of infected individuals and the overall rate of transmission. The pattern of global variation and distribution seems to have resulted from accidental trafficking (viral migration) than from diversification (viral mutation) (47). The uniform occurrence of the B subtype in the Americas and Europe represents a "founder" effect. Similarly, a subtype E virus (now referred to as CRFO1_AE) recovered from central Africa quickly emerged as the dominant form of the outbreak in female sex workers in Thailand, and subtype B was found predominantly in IDUs in Thailand, providing evidence for two separate but concurrent epidemics (50–52). Given the chance nature of HIV migrations, it is quite possible that one or more rare viral subtypes could be brought swiftly into ascendance: subtype F, a minor form in Brazil and Africa, has become a major form in Romania; and subtype G, found in central Africa, appears to have been introduced into southern Russia (53).

In some countries in Africa, which were either among the earliest centers of infection or had significant population migration and transmission, at least five viral subtypes are known to be present. Similarly, diversity is now being documented in India and in Brazil, where there is documentation of recombination such as BF recombinants (47,54–56). In some cases, the degree of viral divergence within a given region may also reflect the duration of the epidemic. For example, in Africa, there is already 20% to 30% genetic diversity within a genotype, whereas in Thailand, this diversity is much more limited (51). The immunologic importance of this genetic heterogeneity is not fully understood, but it is clear that any globally effective vaccine will have to induce protective immunity through a broad range of genetic and potentially antigenic subtypes. The low levels of genetic diversity seen in some regions of HIV-1 spread present rapidly closing windows of opportunity for vaccination against still relatively homologous viral challenge. The diversity in HIV subtypes may also have important biologic and immunologic implications. Intrinsic biologic properties of these viruses include infectivity and replication capacities that contribute to different epidemic curves (50). In 1985, a second human retrovirus associated with AIDS, HIV-2, was identified in West Africa (57,58). This virus has been found to have relatively high prevalence among hospitalized patients, female prostitutes, and patients who attend sexually transmitted disease (STD) clinics in several countries of West Africa (46,59–61). Because this virus is spread by

the same modes of transmission as HIV-1, it is likely that similar epidemiologic patterns may be observed for HIV-2 in the near future. Currently, HIV-2 is spread predominantly by heterosexual transmission, similarly to HIV-1 (46,62,63). Systematic surveys for HIV-2 outside West Africa have documented cases in parts of central Africa, Europe, North America, and Brazil.

In comparison with HIV-1, however, HIV-2 is characterized by lower rates of sexual and perinatal transmission, lesser cell killing, lower viral burdens, more gradual $CD4^+$ cell loss, slower rates of progression to AIDS and death, and relative geographical confinement (46,62,64–68). Travers and colleagues (69) demonstrated that HIV-2–infected women in Senegal had a lower incidence of HIV-1 than did the seronegative women and close to a 70% reduction in risk for HIV-1 infection, despite similar high-risk sexual behavior and the same frequency of STDs. These data suggested that the protection observed might be a result of cross-reactive immunity to epitopes conserved between HIV-1 and HIV-2. However, the study also demonstrated for the first time sequential infection with two different HIV subtypes, first with HIV-2 and then with HIV-1. Further studies are urgently needed to determine whether cross-reactive immunity can be induced to epitopes conserved between different strains of the virus.

Molecular techniques have also been used to investigate clusters of HIV infection. For example, in a Florida dental practice, molecular subtyping confirmed that a dentist's HIV-1 infection had been transmitted to several of his patients (70–73). Although the study demonstrated that the patients were infected with the same HIV strain as the dentist, questions persist regarding how the infection occurred and whether new cases of this kind are likely to be encountered. Another case has been studied in southern Russia, where nearly 90 children became infected with the same strain (53,74). It is clear from this cluster and from a series in Australia in which four women were infected with a strain similar to one identified in a patient with AIDS that nosocomial transmission can and does occur, particularly with unsterilized instruments (75).

With molecular typing, it is possible to discern geographical differences in the proportion of cases acquired by one mode of transmission or another, but the three major modes of transmission—sexual, parenteral, and perinatal—remain the major means of acquisition of either HIV-1 or HIV-2. Each of these modes of transmission is discussed in detail, with particular geographical references when appropriate.

MODES OF TRANSMISSION

Sexual Transmission

Sexual transmission probably accounts for more than 85% of HIV-1 infection worldwide. In developed countries, homosexual transmission has been strongly associated with the number of sexual partners and the frequency at which individuals practice receptive anal intercourse (76–78). As the prevalence of HIV-1 infection increased among bisexual men and intravenous drug abusers, an increasing number of women were infected with HIV-1 through heterosexual contact (26,33,79–81). In Africa, the male-to-female ratio is 1:1 (4,7,82,83), and even in the United States and Europe, the greatest proportional increase in AIDS cases has been documented among heterosexual contacts of HIV-1–infected persons (26,84,85). Urban populations with consistently high rates of STDs, prostitution and intravenous drug abuse have the highest rates of HIV-1 infection. In many urban centers of Central Africa, 5% to 20% of sexually active persons are already infected with HIV-1 (27,83,86). Rates of infection among

TABLE 114.3.   Factors that Affect Infectiousness of or Susceptibility to HIV

Infectiousness	Susceptibility
Level of plasma/genital viral load	Genital ulcerations
Acute primary HIV infection	Other sexually transmitted
Advanced clinical stage of HIV	diseases
Genital ulcerations (chancroid,	Lack of male circumcision
syphilis, herpes)	Traumatic sex
Cervical ectopy	Lack of condom use
Antiretroviral therapy (decreased	Anal intercourse
infectiousness)	Sex during menses
Consistent condom use (decreased	
infectiousness)	

some prostitute groups range from 40% in Kinshasa, Zaire, to 80% in Nairobi, Kenya, and 88% in Butari, Rwanda (87–89). Rural areas that are culturally more conservative and, where the incidence of STDs is much lower, appear to have lower rates of HIV-1 infection, although rural rates of HIV infection are rising in some areas of Uganda, Tanzania, and other countries (27). Certain risk factors, such as promiscuity, anal intercourse, sex with an infected person, prostitution, and other behavioral factors, appear to be responsible for increased risk for heterosexual transmission.

Although the relative efficiencies of bidirectional transmission have not been well documented, it is evident that most heterosexual transmission of HIV-1 among sexual partners occurs during vaginal intercourse and that receptive anal intercourse also increases the risk for infection in women (Table 114.3). Variable rates of heterosexual transmission of HIV-1 among sexual partners of infected persons have been documented in studies in the United States, Europe, and Africa (36,90). Reported rates of infection for sexual partners of an infected person range from 15% to 50% and are dependent on the presence or absence of other STDs, which may serve as cofactors for transmission, as well as on the relative infectivity of the infected individual. In studies by Goedert and co-workers (91), the risk for transmission from one person to a sexual partner was greatest among those with CD4$^+$ cell counts of less than 200 cells/mm^3 and those with p24 antigenemia.

In one study in Rakai, Uganda of 415 HIV-serodiscordant couples, 90 (22%) of the HIV-negative partners seroconverted during the course of a 3-year period for an incident rate of 11.8 per 100 person-years (92). The rate of transmission from male to female was identical to the rate of transmission from female to male, with one exception. If the seronegative male partner was circumcised, no seroconversions occurred, in contrast to an incidence of 16.7% among 137 uncircumcised male partners. Although the median age at enrollment was 30 years of age, the highest incidence of seroconversion occurred in couples between the ages of 15 and 19 years, with an incidence of 18.6%. The incidence declined with age of both the HIV-negative and HIV-positive partners. Interestingly, very few behavioral characteristics were associated with transmission within these couples in these rural communities. However, symptoms of STDs in the HIV-infected partner, such as vaginal or urethral discharge or dysuria, were associated with a greater risk for transmission to the uninfected partner. Similarly, the presence of AIDS-defining symptoms or signs was also significantly associated with an increased risk for transmission. The most important variable that predicted transmission and acquisition of HIV in these discordant couples was the viral level of HIV in the infected partner before seroconversion in the HIV-negative partner. Among cou-

ples in which transmission occurred, the mean serum HIV RNA level in the positive index partner was significantly (threefold) higher than in couples in whom no seroconversions occurred. This study demonstrated a significant dose-response effect with respect to both male-to-female transmission and female-to-male transmission. The rate of transmission rose from 2.2% among individuals with viral RNA levels of less than 3,500 copies/mL to 23% at levels more than 50,000 copies/mL. Among the 51 couples in whom the HIV-positive partner had a viral level of less than 1,500 copies/mL, no transmissions occurred. For every log of viral load increase, there was an associated risk for HIV sexual transmission of 2.5. This dose-response relationship is nearly identical to that described between maternal viral burden and vertical transmission from mother to infant (93). As indicated earlier, age was inversely associated with risk for transmission.

The results of this one study had important implications for furthering our understanding of heterosexual HIV transmission and for development of methods to prevent such transmission. Although individuals who have reduced viral levels as a result of antiretroviral drug use may still be infectious to their partner, the relative risk appears to decrease. However, in a separate analysis of the same population in Uganda, it was apparent that the presence of genital ulcers or infection with herpes simplex virus markedly increased the risk for transmission across all viral loads (94). Thus, heterosexual transmission involves a complex interaction between biologic, behavioral, and cultural variables. These studies and others have identified a number of factors associated with risk for transmission, which could potentially be modified to reduce the spread of heterosexual HIV transmission (92,94–96).

An epidemiologic synergy has been demonstrated between HIV and STDs that is related to both behavioral and biologic factors (97). Epidemiologic studies from sub-Saharan Africa, Asia, Europe, and North America have suggested that there is about a fourfold greater risk for becoming HIV-infected in the presence of a genital ulcer caused by syphilis or chancroid and a twofold to threefold greater risk in the presence of other STDs, such as gonorrhea, chlamydial infection, and trichomoniasis (97,98). In a World Health Organization (WHO) report, the prevalence of four curable STDs—gonorrhea, chlamydial infection, syphilis, and trichomoniasis—was estimated to be 333 million individuals (99). The greatest number of these STDs occurred in Southeast Asia and sub-Saharan Africa, the two regions with the highest rates of HIV infection (24).

With the strong association between STDs and HIV infection among heterosexuals, increased attention should be focused on integrated HIV STD services (99,100). The development of programs with an integrated approach to inducing behavior change, promoting condom use, and controlling STDs would inevitably reduce the infectivity of HIV transmitters and the susceptibility of HIV exposed persons. In Kinshasa, Zaire, investigators demonstrated that intensive STD diagnosis and treatment, coupled with a condom distribution program for female sex workers, successfully decreased both the incidence and the prevalence of both STDs and HIV (99). In a national condom promotion campaign in Thailand, the prevalence of STDs declined nationwide, with a subsequent decrease in HIV incidence (101). In another study, investigators demonstrated that a community-based syndromic approach to the treatment of symptomatic STDs led to a 42% decrease in HIV incidence compared with control villages in Mwanza, Tanzania (102). Subsequent to the study in Mwanza, Tanzania, a community-based trial of mass treatment of STDs was undertaken in the Rakai district of Uganda to determine whether a decline in the prevalence of STDs secondary to antibiotic therapy is associated with a decline in HIV incidence

(103). The baseline prevalence of HIV infection in this population was 16%. The investigators were able to demonstrate a decline in syphilis, trichomoniasis, gonorrhea, and chlamydia infection but unfortunately had no impact on the incidence of HIV infection, which remained at 1.5 per 100 person-years in both groups. Thus, in this one study, STD intervention did not have a dramatic impact on incidence of HIV infection. It has been concluded from these two separate studies that the greatest impact of STD intervention on slowing HIV transmission would be in the early phases of the epidemic during the escalation phase. However, once the epidemic becomes well established, as in Rakai, Uganda, such interventions may have an effect that is modest to none. Additional studies are underway to validate these observations, but STD control remains a mainstay, particularly for genital ulcer diseases, in which the risk for the individual is extremely high for HIV transmission or acquisition.

Perinatal Transmission

With increasing evidence of HIV infection among women, perinatal transmission, which may occur *in utero*, during delivery, or postnatally through breast-feeding, continues to increase in areas where heterosexual transmission is most common. Transmission rates have been highly variable in different regions, ranging from 13% to 52% (104,105). Reanalysis of transmission on the basis of an international standard definition has shown that the rates of vertical transmission have much greater consistency within geographical areas than previously reported. Factors associated with increased perinatal transmission include advanced maternal stage of disease, increased viral titers, decreased maternal serum vitamin A levels, chorioamnionitis, maternal anemia, low neutralizing titers to antibody, and titers to antibody to the V3 loop of glycoprotein gp120 of HIV (106–109) (Table 114.4). The more common use of breast-feeding in developing countries may also contribute to increased perinatal transmission compared with that observed in developed countries. Data suggest that up to 15% of infants breast-fed by HIV-infected mothers may become infected through breast-feeding (110). A metaanalysis of several prospective studies indicated

TABLE 114.4. Presumptive Evidence of the Timing of Maternal–Infant Transmission of HIV

In utero
  Identification of HIV in aborted fetal tissue from infected women
  Presence of HIV in peripheral blood in about 50% of infected infants in the first week of life
  Rapid progression of HIV disease in some infants
Peripartum
  Higher transmission rates in first-born twins than in second-born twins
  No detectable circulating virus in about 50% of infected infants in the first week of life
  Decreased transmission with cesarean section
  Lower transmission rates with administration of zidovudine to the mother in late pregnancy[a] and the peripartum period and to the infant in the neonatal period
  Two distinct patterns of disease progression (rapid and less rapid) in infected infants
  Absence of congenital malformations and symptoms and signs of HIV infection at birth

[a]In the AIDS Clinical Trial Group Protocol 076 trial, zidovudine therapy was started at a median of 26 weeks of gestation.

TABLE 114.5. Approaches to Reducing the Transmission of HIV from Mother to Child

Avoidance of breast-feeding
Antiretroviral therapy (for the mother during pregnancy and delivery and for the infant after birth)
  Zidovudine
  Nevirapine
Reduction in peripartum exposure
  Cesarean section
  Avoidance of intrapartum invasive procedures
  Vaginal disinfection
  Treatment of sexually transmitted diseases

that the risk attributable to breast-feeding ranged from 7% to 22%. Although bottle-feeding is recommended for HIV-infected women in developed countries, this would not be appropriate in some countries with high rates of infectious diseases and poor sanitation (111).

Strategies for reducing perinatally acquired HIV include preventing HIV infection among women in general and, for women infected with HIV, avoiding pregnancy or refraining from breast-feeding their infants (112) (Table 114.5). In addition, antiretroviral therapy with zidovudine has been shown to reduce significantly the risk for perinatal transmission from 25.5% to 8.3%, a 67.5% reduction (113). In countries where the cost is prohibitive, trials are underway to examine modified timing and dosing of antiretroviral drugs for pregnant women to find the most cost-efficient method of reducing perinatal transmission (114–117). In a study in Kampala, Uganda, investigators were able to demonstrate the efficacy and cost-effectiveness of nevirapine in preventing mother-to-infant HIV transmission compared with zidovudine. In a population in which more than 95% of the mothers breast-feed, treatment of the mother at delivery and to the baby for the first week after birth with nevirapine had a significant decline in HIV transmission compared with zidovudine (114). At 16 weeks of age, 13.1% of the infants born to nevirapine-treated mothers were infected compared with 25% of mothers and babies treated with zidovudine. This study revolutionized global efforts to prevent mother-to-infant transmission because it did provide a cost-effective method of a single-dose nevirapine regimen to decrease perinatal HIV transmission significantly in resource-poor settings. For example, in a follow-up analysis, the associated cost-effectiveness ratio was $138.00 per case averted, or $5.25, and 25% per disability-adjusted life-year (DALY) for populations with a high prevalence of HIV infection (115). Even at lower prevalence populations, the overall cost would be $11.00 per DALY. Additional studies are underway to determine whether treatment of the infant during the first few weeks of life with nevirapine will be beneficial in the prevention of transmission during breast-feeding. Interventions found to be successful, however, must be affordable and sustainable, particularly in developing countries, where the impact would be greatest (116,117).

Parenteral Transmission

The third mode of infection is parenteral transmission, which includes blood transfusion and exposure to blood through reuse of needles or syringes among IDUs or in health care facilities where sterilization of instruments is inadequate. Transmission among IDUs is a major problem for developed countries and an increasing problem for countries such as those in Southeast Asia, Thailand, India, and Myanmar as well as some countries of Latin America. Seroprevalence among IDUs varies widely but may be as high as 60% to 70% in some regions (118). Although HIV incidence continues to rise among IDUs in some regions of the world, substantial HIV prevention programs targeting IDUs have resulted in stabilization of infection rates and in some cases a decline (119). In a study in New York City, HIV seroprevalence remained stable between 1984 and 1992 at slightly more than 50% (120). Attributes of successful AIDS prevention programs for IDUs have included confidential HIV testing and counseling, outreach and education, successful and appropriate drug abuse treatment, and access to sterile injecting equipment, such as through needle exchange programs (121–125). Previous studies have reported that syringe exchange programs have played a significant role in lowering rates of HIV transmission in IDUs in the Netherlands, Sweden, Australia, the United Kingdom, and some cities of the United States (122,123,126). Other studies have reported that syringe exchange programs have served as sources of referral to social services, medical services, and drug treatment (119,121–123,126).

HIV transmission by blood or blood products has markedly declined in most developed countries because of widespread donor testing and exclusion criteria that were implemented in 1985 (127). The risk for transfusion-transmitted HIV infection in the United States and Europe is about 1 in 225,000 donations (128). However, in many parts of the developing world, HIV screening of the blood supply is still severely limited because of cost factors. Nevertheless, a study in Zambia demonstrated in a cost-benefit analysis that screening of the blood supply cost 3 cents per person, with a cost per case of HIV prevented calculated as $31.62 (129). An estimated 3,625 undiscounted healthy years of life were saved, of which 69% were those of children younger than 6 years, at a cost of $1.32 per year of life saved. In areas where universal screening of blood donations has not been implemented, progress toward a safer supply of blood and blood products can also be achieved through appropriate selection and retention of voluntary, nonremunerated, low-risk donors and through more rational use of blood aimed at decreasing the number of people receiving transfusions as well as using blood substitutes and plasma expanders whenever possible.

The risk for HIV transmission in a health care setting through accidental exposure to HIV-infected blood is estimated to be 0.3%, and the risk after mucocutaneous exposure is much less (130,131). However, the number of parenteral exposures of health care workers is thought to be considerable. In 1990, between 378,000 and 756,000 needlestick injuries were estimated to have occurred among health care workers in the United States. Of these, 1,300 to 8,300 probably involved patients known to be infected with HIV (132). It is hoped that through the use of universal precautions, parenteral, mucous membrane, and nonintact skin exposure of health care workers to infectious blood has been limited (131,133,134).

HIV transmission from an infected health care worker to a patient appears to be extremely rare. With the exception of the documented case of HIV transmission from an infected dentist to six patients, the probability of transmission from an HIV-infected surgeon to a patient is in the range of about 1 in 42,000 procedures to 1 in 20,000 procedures (131,135–137).

Other Modes of Transmission

Household transmission may occur when there is contact with blood or other body secretions or excretions from a person already known to be infected with HIV. Eight instances of HIV transmission in households through direct contact with blood or body secretions have now been reported (138). Consequently, persons who provide nursing and care for HIV-infected persons in home settings should employ similar universal precautions to reduce exposure to blood and other body fluids. Because of the social, economic, and medical benefits of home care, the number of persons with HIV who receive health care outside hospitals is increasing.

REGIONAL EPIDEMICS

Sub-Saharan Africa

Although AIDS has had an enormous medical, cultural, and economic impact on all countries of the world, this disease has taken its greatest toll in the countries of sub-Saharan Africa (21,22,139,140). More than 28 million individuals—7% of the population of the subcontinent—have been infected with HIV (12). About 3.5 million new infections occurred in 2002, and 2 million people died. Ten million young people (15 to 24 years of age) and almost 3 million children younger than 15 years of age are living with HIV. In addition, 11 million children have been orphaned by the premature death of a parent as a result of AIDS. More than half of the infected adults are women, and as many as 6 million African children are estimated to have been infected as a result of mother-to-infant transmission. In some geographical areas, specific population groups are disproportionately affected by the epidemic. Men and women between 20 and 40 years old, people with STDs, and people in certain occupational groups such as long-distance truck drivers, military personnel, and women employed in commercial sex usually have the highest prevalence of infection (7,27,86). HIV prevalence higher than 80% has been reported for female sex workers in East Africa and central Africa. In some areas, HIV infection has now been documented among members of the general population, as evidenced by the initially slow but accelerating spread among pregnant women. Seroprevalence of HIV among pregnant women ranges from 5% to 35%, with the highest rates in urban centers, such in Malawi, Botswana, Zambia, Zimbabwe, and South Africa (104,106,141). In some urban populations, more than 10% of the adults are infected, and the annual incidence is estimated to be 3% (142,143).

About 50% to 65% of HIV infections in Africa have been in East Africa and central Africa, an area that accounts for only 15% of the total population of sub-Saharan Africa. Serologic data indicate that the pandemic has continued to evolve, particularly in western and southern Africa (12). At least 10% of those aged 15 to 49 years are infected in 12 African countries. Seven countries, all in southern Africa, now have a prevalence higher than 20%: Botswana (38.8%), Lesotho (31%), Namibia (22.5%), South Africa (20.1%), Swaziland (33.4%), Zambia (21.5%), and Zimbabwe (33.7%). Women account for the majority of persons living with HIV in sub-Saharan Africa (58%). With increasing rates among women, HIV prevalence in pregnant women also appears to be increasing. For example, in Botswana, median HIV prevalence among pregnant women in urban areas rose from 38.5% in 1997 to 44.9% in 2001, whereas in Zimbabwe, prevalence climbed from 29% in 1997 to 35% in 2000. Prevalence is even higher among specific age groups—as high as 55.6% among 25- to 29-year-old women attending antenatal clinics in Botswana. In Nigeria, a country with more than 117 million inhabitants (20% of sub-Saharan Africa's population), HIV is rapidly spreading among female sex workers and their clients (144,145). Currently, the nationwide prevalence is 5.8%. Similarly, in southern Africa, HIV prevalence of 30% to 40% has been documented among adults in major urban areas of Botswana

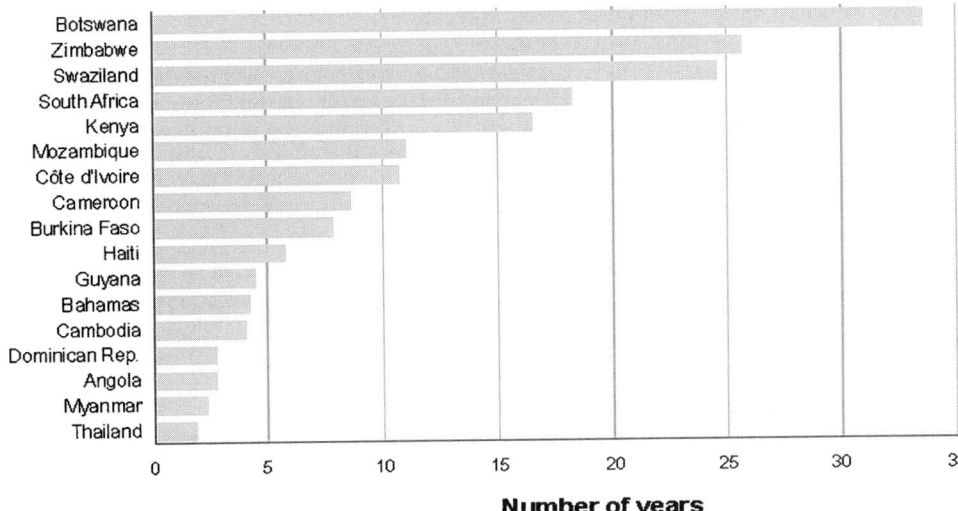

Figure 114.4. Reduction in life expectancy compared to the "no AIDS" scenario in selected countries: 2000–2005. (Data from United Nations Department of Economic and Social Affairs. *World population prospects: the 2000 revision.* Population Division, United Nations: New York, 2001, with permission.)

(12). South Africa witnessed a 10-fold increase in HIV prevalence between 1990 and 2000 in women attending antenatal clinics (146).

AIDS has emerged as the leading cause of adult death in Abidjan, in Kinshasa, and in rural communities in Uganda and Tanzania (13,15,16,147). Excess deaths attributable to HIV are highest in 25- to 34-year-olds, usually a group with low mortality. Nearly 90% of deaths in this age group were in excess of background rates and were attributable to HIV. Because AIDS deaths are concentrated in childhood and young adulthood, their effects are substantial, reducing life expectancy by more than 20 years in several countries (Fig. 114.4). Population growth will decline more rapidly than expected, and the size of the African population in the year 2005 will be smaller than it would have been without AIDS. These additional HIV AIDS cases will put an increasing strain on the health care systems, which are already overburdened, and on individual households, which are trying to manage with limited economic resources. Care and support for children orphaned by AIDS will be a growing concern throughout the region (148), and the social, economic, and demographic impact of AIDS will be enormous. For a country with a current HIV prevalence of 8%, the expected increased demand for health care services ranges from 2.3% to 9.3%, depending on the state of development of its health care sector (139). The strong association of HIV with a burgeoning tuberculosis epidemic (149,150), combined with the excess mortality associated with HIV infection, underscores the critical importance of the HIV epidemic in Africa.

Asia

With more than half of the world's population, Asia is still in the early phases of an explosive HIV AIDS epidemic. Although HIV was introduced much later in Asia than in the rest of the world, it is now estimated that more than 6.0 million people are infected with HIV (12). Asia and the Pacific are now home to more people living with HIV or AIDS than any other region besides sub-Saharan Africa. In India, an estimated 4 million people were living with HIV or AIDS at the end of 2002—more than any other country in the world except South Africa. Moreover, this region's epidemic is spreading into the general population. The median HIV prevalence among women attending antenatal clinics in some areas was higher than 2% and exceeded 1% in several other states of India.

In addition to those in India, major HIV epidemics already exist in Thailand and Myanmar, and the epidemic has begun to emerge in Cambodia, Vietnam, Indonesia, China, Taiwan, Singapore, and the Philippines (32,38,42).

In China, with a fifth of the world's population, there has been a marked rise in HIV infection of more than 67% in 2001. Although surveillance data are sketchy, an estimated 1 million Chinese were living with HIV or AIDS at the end of 2002. Parenteral drug use has been a driving force for some of the epidemics in this region. However, since the early 1990s, tens of thousands of rural villagers have become infected in China through unsafe blood donation procedures. Most of these people live in Henan province in central China, but there are concerns that similar situations are unfolding in other provinces, including Anhui and Shanxi. Serious localized HIV epidemics are also occurring among IDUs in at least seven provinces, with a prevalence higher than 70% among IDUs in areas such as Xinjiang and Yunnan province. Another nine provinces are on the brink of similar HIV epidemics because of very high rates of needle sharing. There are also signs of heterosexually transmitted HIV epidemics in at least three provinces (Guangdong, Guangxi, and Yunnan), where HIV prevalence was as high as 11% among the sex worker population in 2000. Along with the rise in HIV, there are also concerns of increases in STDs, which rose from 430,000 in 1997 to 860,000 in 2000, suggesting that unprotected sex with nonmonogamous partners is increasing in China. In addition, massive population mobility (about 100 million Chinese are temporarily or permanently away from their registered addresses) and increasing social and economic disparities add to the likelihood of HIV spread.

Another concern is the rising HIV epidemic in Indonesia, the world's fourth most populous country. After more than 10 years of negligible HIV prevalence, the infection rates among IDUs, sex workers, and blood donors in some regions are rapidly increasing. At one drug treatment center in Jakarta, HIV prevalence rose from 15.4% in 2000 to more than 40% in mid-2001.

The pattern of HIV spread in Asia appears to be different from that described in other regions. HIV was initially noted among IDUs in Thailand, Myanmar, and India. HIV seroprevalence increased dramatically between 1988 and 1991 from 1.2% to 45% in Thailand (151–153), and in the northeastern state of Manipur, India, it rose from 55% to 80% (30,38,154). In addition, the first evidence of HIV in Yunnan province of China, bordering Burma and Laos and considered part of the "golden triangle" of heroin exportation, demonstrated an alarming HIV prevalence of 43% to 82% in IDUs (155,156). Data from Malaysia and Vietnam show similar increases in HIV levels among IDUs (12).

During this rise of HIV infection among IDUs, HIV infection was noted among female sex workers. Although highly variable by region, HIV prevalence of 30% to 65% has been reported among female sex workers in various cities of Thailand and India (30,38,41). Successive waves of heterosexual transmission from these sex workers to their male clients and subsequently to other sexual partners, including spouses, occurred, resulting in rapid spread of HIV to segments of the general population. Among military recruits in Thailand in 1993, HIV prevalence was 4% overall and 12.4% in recruits from the northern province of Chiang Mai (157,158). Among pregnant women, HIV prevalence rose to 8% in Chiang Mai and Chiang Rai in northern Thailand, and the overall prevalence for pregnant women in the country was estimated as 2% (159). From these data, it was estimated that more than 840,000 persons in Thailand, or 1% of the Thai population, were HIV infected by 1994 (12). If this rate of HIV transmission continues, there will be 2 to 4 million cumulative HIV infections in Thailand alone by the year 2000.

In urban centers in India, the rise in HIV seroprevalence among female sex workers and their sexual contacts has been equally dramatic. In a study of 2,800 attendees of STD clinics in Pune, the overall HIV seroprevalence was 23.4% (160). Among initially seronegative persons, the subsequent HIV incidence was 26.1 per 100 person-years of observation for female sex workers, 9.4 for men, and 8.4 for women who were not sex workers (161). Recurrent genital ulcer disease and urethritis or cervicitis during the follow-up period were independently associated with an increased risk for seroconversion. Given the prevailing sexual practices, large population of HIV-infected female sex workers, low social status of women, male patronage of sex workers, high rates of STDs, low rates of condom use, and high frequency of injecting drug use, a scenario similar to that described for India and Thailand is likely for many other populous countries of Asia (32). For the more developed areas, such as Japan, South Korea, Taiwan, Singapore, and Hong Kong, HIV epidemics may not be as explosive, but there will probably be a slow and steady increase in HIV infections. Throughout Asia, the HIV incidence could exceed 1 million new infections per year within the next few years.

Oceania

About 50,000 cumulative adult HIV infections have occurred in this region, with nearly half in Australia and New Zealand (162). The annual reported number of HIV infections from these last two countries seems to have reached its peak, and since 1987, there has been a downward trend for both countries in the number of HIV infections reported each year. Most of the infections have occurred among homosexual men, and the male-to-female ratio among infected individuals is 7:1, indicating a lower degree of heterosexual transmission than that observed in other regions. The frequency of HIV infection among IDUs in Australia and New Zealand also remains lower than that in Western Europe or North America, probably because of the early availability of sterile injection equipment.

For most other countries of the Pacific region, the cumulative numbers of reported AIDS cases and HIV infections have been too few to allow meaningful analysis by time or mode of transmission. However, despite the low number of cases, there is a great potential for HIV to spread rapidly within this region. Epidemiologic and behavioral studies indicate generally high rates of injecting drug use, unprotected sexual activity including

commercial sex, and a high prevalence of STDs. Moreover, many parts of Asia and the Pacific are undergoing rapid development. As trade, tourism, and migration increase, so may the opportunities for HIV dissemination (162). Papua New Guinea has reported the highest HIV infection rates among the Pacific Island countries and territories. Results of recent studies in the capital of Port Moresby show high HIV prevalence levels among female sex workers (17%) and attendees of STD clinics (7%). The Philippines continues to maintain a low HIV prevalence, although high rates of other STDs among Filipino sex workers, their clients, and men who have sex with men (MSM) indicate low levels of condom use and the potential for a rapid rise in HIV.

The Americas

About 4.5 million cumulative HIV infections have occurred in the countries of the Americas, with more than 1.5 million in North America and 3 million in Latin America and the Caribbean (12). About 250,000 new HIV infections are estimated to occur each year (12,163–168).

The United States has had the highest number of reported AIDS cases in the world, with more than 807,075 cases and 462,653 fatalities (57%) as of late 2001 (33,164–168). At the end of 2001, an estimated total of 362,827 persons in the United States were living with AIDS. After the use of highly active antiretroviral therapy (HAART) became widespread during 1996, sharp declines in AIDS incidence occurred through 1999 (Fig. 114.3). Since then, AIDS incidence began to level, and essentially no changes occurred from 1999 through 2002. Similarly, from 1996 through 1997, the number of deaths among persons with AIDS also declined sharply and continued to decline each year through 2001. As a result, AIDS prevalence has increased steadily over time, and at the end of December 2001, about 362,827 persons in the United States were living with AIDS. By region, 39% of persons living with AIDS lived in the South, 29% in the Northeast, 19% in the West, 10% in the Midwest, and 3% in the U.S. territories. Of persons living with AIDS, 42% were African-American, 37% were white or Caucasian, 20% were Hispanic, 1% were Asian or Pacific Islander, and less than 1% were American Indian or Alaska Native (Fig. 114.5). By risk, 57% were MSM, 24% were IDUs, 9% were exposed through heterosexual contact, and 8% were MSM IDUs (Fig. 114.6). Of the 76,696 adult and adolescent women with AIDS in 2001, 59% were exposed

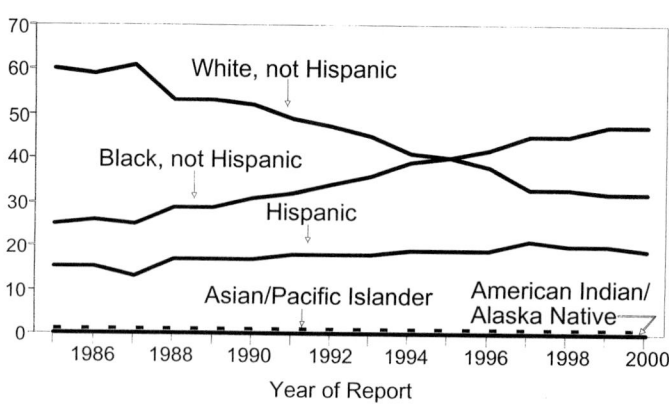

Figure 114.5. Percentage of AIDS cases reported to the Centers for Disease Control and Prevention by race and ethnicity in the United States from 1985 through year 2000. (Data from Centers for Disease Control and Prevention. Update: AIDS—United States, 2000. *MMWR Morb Mortal Wkly Rep* 2002;51:592–595, with permission.)

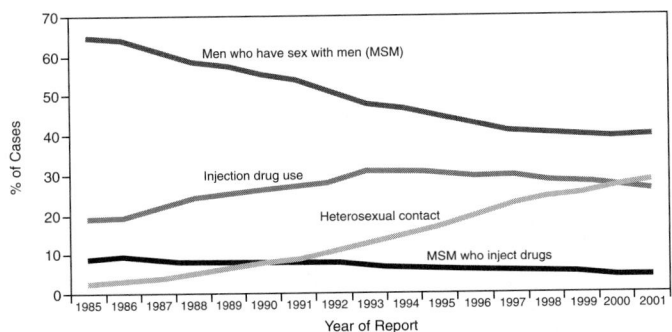

Figure 114.6. Percentage of AIDS cases reported to the Centers for Disease Control and Prevention in men who have sex with men (MSM), injecting drug use (IDU), heterosexual contact, and MSM/IDU from 1985 through year 2000 for the United States. (Data from Centers for Disease Control and Prevention. Update: AIDS—United States, 2000. *MMWR Morb Mortal Wkly Rep* 2002;51:592–595, with permission.)

through heterosexual contact, and 38% were exposed through injecting drug use. The number of AIDS cases in children has markedly declined since the advent of antiretroviral drug use during pregnancy to prevent HIV perinatal transmission. Nevertheless, in 2001, 175 new cases of AIDS were diagnosed in children. Of these, 150 (86%) were attributed to perinatal exposure.

In the United States, the impact of HIV and AIDS in the African American community has been particularly devastating (Fig. 114.5). Representing only an estimated 12% of the total U.S. population, African Americans make up 38% of all AIDS cases reported in the country. Of persons infected with HIV, it is estimated that almost 129,000 African Americans are living with AIDS. In 2000, more African Americans were reported with AIDS than any other racial or ethnic group. Nearly half of all reported AIDS cases in 2000 were among African Americans. Almost two thirds (63%) of all women reported with AIDS were African American, and African American children represented two thirds of all reported pediatric cases. The 2000 rate of reported AIDS cases among African Americans was 58.1 per 100,000 population, more than two times the rate for Hispanics and eight times the rate for whites.

Thus, the HIV and AIDS epidemic in the United States has evolved from a small outbreak among homosexual men in a few cities to a major killer of young adults. Moreover, the epidemic is continuing to evolve. Although there are encouraging reports of decreasing transmission among homosexual and bisexual men in general, data also indicate that new infections are occurring in this population, particularly among younger men. Heterosexual transmission is also becoming an increasingly important part of the U.S. epidemic, with certain groups at a disproportionately high risk. At greatest risk are the young, disadvantaged, and minority populations, particularly women living in the inner cities of the Northeast and in parts of the rural South. A major source of infection for these women has been male IDUs; transmission occurs particularly among women with multiple sexual partners and those who exchange sex for drugs or money. Transmission in these settings has also been facilitated by the presence of other STDs. Persons at highest risk for infection are often those who are the hardest to reach through conventional health education programs. Yet, these persons with their myriad social and economic problems are the individuals who need to be reached most urgently. Finally, the impact on the health care delivery system will be particularly dramatic. HIV seroprevalence in sentinel hospital patients ranged from 0.1% to 5.8% (169). In

one emergency department, the prevalence of HIV among unselected adults rose from 6% to 11.3% during a 4-year period (170).

In Latin America and the Caribbean, the HIV pandemic is also continuing to evolve. Within the past 5 years, there has been evidence of increasing heterosexual transmission, principally among bisexual men and their female sex partners and among female sex workers and their clients (12,163,171). In 2002, about 1.9 million adults and children in Latin America and the Caribbean were living with HIV or AIDS—1.5 million in Latin America and 420,000 in the Caribbean. About 2,000 individuals acquired the virus in 2001. For the region overall, 100,000 AIDS deaths occurred, increasing the number of orphans living in Latin America to 330,000 and to 250,000 in the Caribbean (most in Haiti). Twelve countries in this region, including the Dominican Republic and Haiti and several Central American countries, have an estimated HIV prevalence of 1% or more. In these areas, the epidemic is firmly rooted in the wider population and is driven primarily by heterosexual transmission.

HIV and AIDS are now the leading cause of death in the Caribbean, where adult prevalence is surpassed only by the rates in sub-Saharan Africa (172,173). Haiti's life expectancy in 2000 to 2005 is nearly 6 years less than it would have been in the absence of the AIDS epidemic. In the Bahamas and Guyana, the number of deaths among 15- to 34-year-olds is 2.5 times higher than it would have been in the absence of AIDS. Haiti and the Bahamas are the most affected countries in the Caribbean, where adult HIV prevalence is more than 6% and 3.5, respectively. Recent surveillance data indicate a relatively stable HIV prevalence of 2.5% among the adult population. In Mexico, the adult HIV prevalence is still under 1%, but prevalence is much higher in specific population groups in some parts of the country—up to 6% among injecting drug users and 50% among MSM. Similarly, relatively low national HIV prevalence in most of South and Central American countries mask the fact that the epidemic is firmly lodged among specific population groups such as those described in Mexico. Of note, Brazil's prevention program for IDUs has resulted in a substantial decline of HIV prevalence among this population group in several large metropolitan areas. Furthermore, Brazil has led the region in the provision of antiretroviral drugs to HIV-infected individuals. At the end of 2001, it was estimated that 170,000 people across the region were receiving antiretroviral treatment, including 105,000 in Brazil. For the region of 24 countries surveyed in 2001, 11 have policies regulating or guaranteeing access to antiretroviral therapy. By reducing HIV- and AIDS-related morbidity, Brazil's treatment and care program is now estimated to have avoided 234,000 hospitalizations and to be a cost-savings program. In Brazil, the proportion of reported AIDS cases attributable to heterosexual transmission has markedly increased (12). HIV infections among IDUs are also a growing problem. For example, in Argentina, the prevalence of HIV infection among IDUs ranges from 30% to 50%; in Brazil, it ranges from 20% to 60% (12).

Europe

About 1.5 million individuals are estimated to be HIV infected in Western and Eastern Europe (12). Differences continue to exist in HIV transmission patterns between and even within individual countries (174). The HIV epidemic in Western Europe is the result of a multitude of epidemics that differ in their timing, their scale, and their effects on populations. Overall, the number of new HIV infections transmitted through heterosexual intercourse rose 48% in Western Europe between 1995 and 2000. New infections contracted through needle sharing declined by

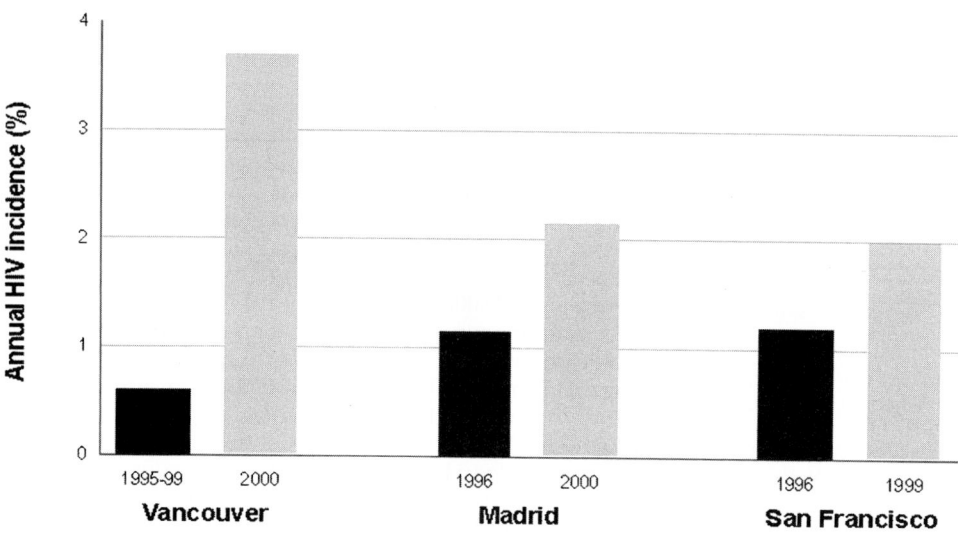

Figure 114.7. HIV incidence among men who have sex with men in Vancouver, Madrid, and San Francisco: 1995–2000. (Data on Vancouver from Hogg RS, Yip B, Chan KJ, et al. Rates of disease progression by baseline CD4 cell count and viral load after initiating triple-drug therapy. *JAMA* 2001;286:2568–2577, with permission; data on Madrid from Del Romero J, Castill J, Garcia S, et al. Time trend in incidence of HIV seroconversion among homosexual men repeatedly tested in Madrid, 1988–2000. *AIDS* 2001;15:1319–1321, with permission; data on San Francisco from Katz MH, Schwarcz SK, Kellogg TA, et al. Impact of highly active antiretroviral treatment on HIV seroincidence among men who have sex with men: San Francisco. *Am J Public Health* 2002;92:388–394, with permission.)

32% within the same period. In Spain, a significant share of HIV infections (24%) is occurring through heterosexual transmission. However, injecting drug use is the main mode of transmission, and reported HIV prevalence in IDUs is estimated at 20% to 30% nationwide, whereas in France, prevalence ranges between 10% and 20%. IDUs constitute two thirds or more of the cases reported in Italy and Spain. Portugal faces a similar serious epidemic among IDUs. More than half of their new HIV infections reported in 2000 were among IDUs. At 37.3 per 100,000 persons, Portugal's rate of reported new infections is the highest among all reporting countries in Western Europe. Similar to the United States, most of the countries of Western Europe have witnessed a marked decrease in AIDS fatality rates and in the reporting of AIDS as a result of the introduction of antiretroviral drugs. Consequently, adult HIV prevalence has risen slightly in these countries, primarily because of antiretroviral therapy keeping HIV-positive people alive longer. This benefit of increased survival, however, has led to a concomitant increase in unsafe sex, triggering higher rates of STDs and in some cases higher HIV incidence among MSM. Rising incidences of STDs among MSM

have been noted in Amsterdam, London, Madrid, Sydney, and several cities in the United States (Fig. 114.7). This widespread risk taking is eclipsing the safer sex ethic promoted so effectively for much of the 1980s and 1990s. In a French study in 2000, 38% of surveyed HIV-positive MSM said they had recently practiced unsafe sex, compared with 26% in 1997.

Eastern Europe and Central Asia are now witnessing the fastest-growing epidemic of HIV in the world. Currently, 1 million people in Eastern Europe and Central Asia are living with HIV or AIDS, more than double the number in 1999 (12). An estimated 300,000 new HIV infections occurred in 2002. The epidemic is relatively new in this region. In 1994, no country in this region was reporting more than a few HIV infections. By 1995, an HIV outbreak had occurred in Ukraine and Belarus. The epidemic then started to increase in Moldova and the Russian Federation, followed by Latvia and then Kazakhstan (Fig. 114.8). In the Russian Federation, new cases of HIV have been doubling annually for several years. The Ukraine remains the most affected country in this region and, in fact, in all of Europe, with an estimated adult HIV prevalence of more than 1%.

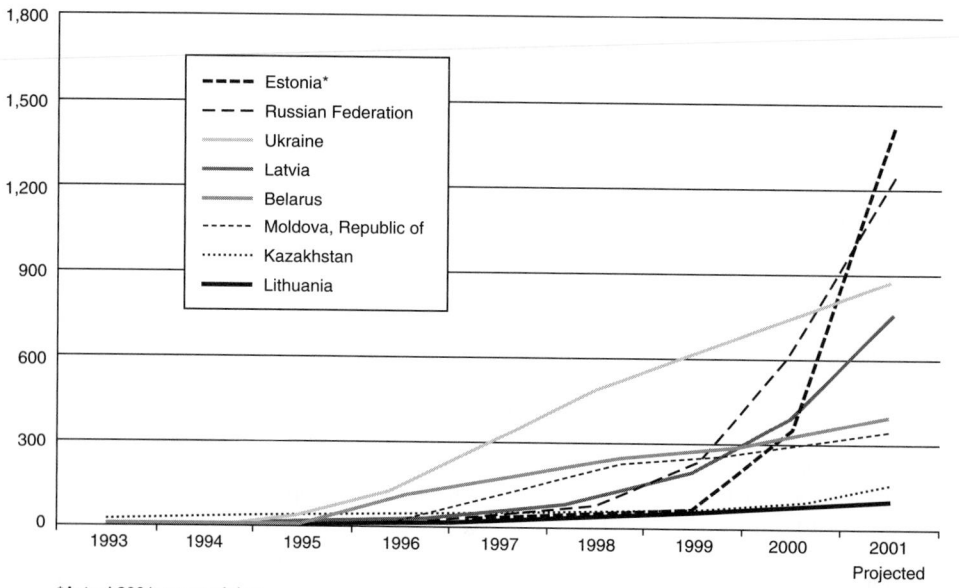

*Actual 2001 year-end data

Figure 114.8. Cumulative reported HIV infections per 1 million population in Eastern European countries: 1993–2001. (From National AIDS Programmes. *HIV/AIDS surveillance in Europe: mid-year report.* 2001, with permission; data compiled by the European Centre for the Epidemiologic Monitoring of AIDS.)

Several factors have contributed to the widespread escalation in the HIV epidemic. Mass unemployment and economic insecurity, along with deterioration in the public health services, appears to have led to a marked increase in STDs and injecting drug use.

Most reported HIV infections are among young people and chiefly those who inject drugs. It is estimated that up to 1% of the population of the commonwealth of independent states are injecting drugs, placing these people and their sexual partners at high risk for infection. Although IDUs are currently responsible for three fourths of HIV infection in Ukraine, the proportion of sexually transmitted HIV infections is also increasing. HIV-infected women primarily acquire HIV through sexual transmission, and more pregnant women are now testing positive for HIV, suggesting a shift of the epidemic into the wider population. Extremely high rates of STDs continue to be documented in Eastern Europe and Central Asia, which further increases the odds of HIV being transmitted through unprotected sex (175–177). For example, in 2000, the number of reported cases of syphilis in the Russian Federation was 157 per 100,000 persons, dramatically higher than the 4.2 per 100,000 in 1987. Similar general trends are visible in other countries of the commonwealth and independent states, in the Baltic states, and in Romania. In the first 6 months of 2002, there were as many new HIV infections in these countries as had been reported in the whole of the previous decade (12). Although there is no reliable method for accurately forecasting the long-term trajectory of the AIDS epidemic in this region, the prospect of Eurasian HIV cases and AIDS deaths in the decades ahead represents a disaster socially, economically, and culturally.

NATURAL HISTORY OF HUMAN IMMUNODEFICIENCY VIRUS TYPE 1 INFECTION

Studies of the natural history of HIV-1 infection in homosexual men, hemophiliacs, and recipients of infected blood transfusions in developed countries have shown an annual progression rate of disease of about 2% to 5% (178–182). Disease progression in HIV-1–infected African heterosexuals appears to be similar to the rate observed in white homosexual men and hemophiliacs. Among HIV-1–seropositive female prostitutes in Nairobi, 6% developed severe illness during a 12-month follow-up period (82). Among African men and women with lymphadenopathy syndrome or AIDS-related complex followed in Brussels, the annual progression rates to AIDS were 1.1% and 20.7%, respectively (82). In Zaire, 6.3% of 56 persons who had become seropositive between 1984 and 1986 had developed AIDS-related conditions by the end of 1986, and 5% had developed AIDS (183,184). Among 91 already seropositive men and women who enrolled in the cohort in 1984, by 1986, a 2-year period, 16.3% had AIDS-related conditions, 3.3% had AIDS, and 11.9% had died with suspected AIDS.

Prognostic factors for disease progression were originally identified in cohort studies in Europe and the United States. A specific loss of immunoglobulin G antibodies against *gag* gene products of HIV-1 (p24) was identified with clinical progression of HIV-1 infection, whereas antibodies to viral *env* glycoproteins (gp41 and gp120/160) remained stable (185–188). In these cohorts, an increase in *gag* viral antigen (p24) was also correlated with progression to AIDS, although p24 antigenemia was found less often in serum from African patients with AIDS than in serum from European or U.S. patients (189,190). These studies underscore the importance of viral RNA levels in predicting disease progression.

Whether microbial infections act as cofactors to enhance HIV-1 infection remains to be determined. Frequent exposure to a wide variety of infections in the developing world, such as malaria, mycobacterial infections, STDs, and infections with other viruses such as cytomegalovirus and herpes simplex virus, has been hypothesized to increase viral replication, thereby enhancing disease progression (191). Co-infection with human T-cell Lymphotropic virus type I, which occurs in many tropical areas, may also influence the natural history of HIV-1 infection, as cohort studies in Trinidad and Brazil demonstrated (192,193).

In addition to its association with STDs, HIV is associated with many other opportunistic infections. Most notable is its association with tuberculosis. Tuberculosis is already one of the leading causes of adult death in many developing countries, killing about 3 million people a year (149,194–197). An alarming increase in cases has been reported in parallel with the AIDS epidemic in many countries (149,198,199). HIV infection is now the most potent biologic risk factor for the development of active tuberculosis (150,197,200). People with latent tuberculosis may readily develop the disease when their immune system has been damaged by HIV. Of individuals who are dually infected, 5% to 10% may develop active tuberculosis each year (201). Moreover, data from the United States indicate that some of the increase in active tuberculosis is attributable to new infections among those with HIV infection who have increased susceptibility to active tuberculosis (202–206). About 30% to 50% of adults in most developing countries have latent tuberculosis infection (149,200).

Projections by the WHO suggest that the annual number of tuberculosis cases worldwide will reach 10.2 million by the year 2000 (194,202). Even though several factors contribute to the increase, HIV infection plays a dominant role in many resource-poor countries. In some African countries heavily affected by the HIV epidemic, the number of tuberculosis cases annually has more than doubled, and the rates of HIV-associated tuberculosis are beginning to increase in parts of Asia. With these trends, tuberculosis control programs in many resource-poor countries are being overburdened. Potential solutions are allocating more resources for tuberculosis control, redistributing some activities to other parts of the health sector, and simplifying tuberculosis control activities so that more cases can be managed with the staff and resources available (201). Underfunding is clearly a major obstacle to progress in the control of tuberculosis. DeCock and Wilkinson (207) have suggested an alternative approach to the treatment of tuberculosis similar to that described for STDs. The traditional etiologically based management of STDs failed at a public health level and is now being replaced by syndromic management aiming for compliance of patients with effective therapy without specific diagnostic confirmation. The new tuberculosis control strategy would incorporate reducing laboratory investigation, using one global regimen, providing all treatment on a directly observed basis, and integrating tuberculosis control program activities better into other health services provided at the district level (207–209). This tuberculosis control strategy aims for maximal public health impact by ensuring adherence to effective therapy after diagnosis, delivered in a simple way, with minimal subsequent investigation. Because the WHO has declared tuberculosis a global emergency, a uniform international response examining these strategies urgently needs to be evaluated (202).

Future Projections

The long-term dimensions of the HIV pandemic cannot yet be forecast with confidence. However, on the basis of available data, the WHO has projected that by the year 2000, there will be a cumulative total of more than 40 million infections in men, women, and children, of which more than 90% will be in developing countries (12). The projected cumulative total of adult AIDS cases will be close to 10 million. By the year 2000, the cumulative number of HIV-related deaths in adults is predicted to rise from its current total of 2 million to more than 8 million individuals. Unless our interventions are more effective, between 15 and 20 million new HIV infections will occur in the next 5 years. In addition, more than 5 million children younger than 10 years will be orphaned as a result of AIDS-related fatalities (210,211). The number of orphans will increase further in the early years of the next century as a result of the deaths of mothers who were infected with HIV in the 1990s. As the epidemic matures in some parts of the world, a large number of young people becoming sexually active will replenish the pool of susceptible people, especially in developing countries, where the base of the age pyramid is quite broad (43). Evidence for a high incidence in young populations compared with older cohorts is already emerging for various countries. In the United States, the number of 13- to 21-year-olds who had become infected with HIV rose by 77% between 1991 and 1993. In sub-Saharan African countries, the highest HIV seroprevalence is in women between 15 and 25 years old (142).

Heterosexual spread of HIV is causing an epidemiologic shift of infection from high-risk populations such as homosexual men and IDUs to populations more reflective of the general population, especially adolescents and young women of childbearing age. As a consequence, the number of persons with AIDS will continue to increase, causing unprecedented personal suffering, high direct costs for medical care, reduced economic output, and a substantial indirect cost to society. The impact of HIV in many countries will be immense.

In conservative projections, the annual number of new AIDS cases in North America and Western Europe during the next two decades is expected to remain fairly constant at close to 100,000. This is because HIV-infected persons will eventually develop AIDS, and the annual HIV incidence in these regions, projected to be close to 100,000, will nearly equal the number of fatalities. In sub-Saharan Africa, the peak occurrence of AIDS, estimated at 750,000 cases per year, will not be reached until the middle of the next decade. However, in Asia, the annual number of AIDS cases will increase steadily in the next decade and will not begin to level off until 2010 at about 850,000 cases per year (32). Although the absolute number of new HIV infections in Asia is equal to the high level found in Africa, the rate of new infections or new cases per year as a percentage of the adult population is still much lower in Asia than in sub-Saharan Africa. This is because the adult population of Asia is more than five times larger than the adult population of sub-Saharan Africa. If unchecked, the rising incidence in Asia will produce an unprecedented number of new cases in that region. On the basis of current data, cumulative HIV infections in Asia are conservatively projected to be more than 10 million (0.46% of the population) in the year 2000 and more than 18 million in 2010. In sub-Saharan Africa, the cumulative number of HIV infections is projected to reach about 15 million in the year 2000 (3%) and about 20 million in 2010 (1.7%). In North America and Western Europe, conservative estimates are about 2 million cumulative HIV infections in the year 2000 (0.23%) and about 2.7 million infections in 2010 (0.17%).

GLOBAL CONTROL OF HUMAN IMMUNODEFICIENCY VIRUS INFECTION

Control of HIV infection has become a public health priority in most countries of the world. With no prospect for an effective vaccine or curative treatment in the near future, prevention is the only effective way to control HIV infection and AIDS. With an estimated 20 million HIV-infected people worldwide, the need for a global program to coordinate control activities was urgently needed. In 1986, the WHO created the Global Programme on AIDS, which developed three primary objectives: to prevent new HIV infections, to provide support and care to those already infected, and to link national and international efforts against AIDS (82,212). The basic tenets of control, including professional and public education on the modes of transmission, risk behavior reduction for persons at high risk, and screening of blood supplies to prevent further transmission by transfusions, are all attainable, but the obstacles to complete control are enormous (213). Information alone is not sufficient motivation to change risk behaviors, and even intervention by screening blood donors has not been implemented in many developing countries owing to economic constraints and lack of adequate blood-banking facilities and appropriate laboratory technology.

The modes of HIV transmission are common to all countries, but the relative importance and characteristics are variable in specific areas. For example, heterosexual transmission among prostitutes and their clients in certain cities in Africa and the Caribbean, homosexual transmission in North America and Europe, and HIV transmission by bisexual males in the Caribbean and South America are all forms of sexual transmission (213), but curbing each requires different educational approaches and interventions. Although it is the most difficult objective in the control of AIDS, preventing HIV transmission by changing sexual behaviors, if successful, would have the greatest impact on the containment of AIDS. It is therefore important to direct educational efforts to persons who exhibit high-risk behavior and to adolescents. Whenever possible, AIDS education should be incorporated in existing health education programs. Reducing the risk for sexual transmission must be accomplished by limiting the number of sexual partners, especially anonymous partners, and increasing condom use. Spermicides containing nonoxinol 9 have been shown in the laboratory to inactivate HIV and may provide additional protection. With increasing evidence that HIV transmission is facilitated by genital ulcers and other STDs, programs to diagnose and treat these disease should be integrated into AIDS control efforts (99,101,102).

The success of programs in preventing STDs depends on the delivery of messages to specific audiences and the provision of support services such as counseling and providing condoms to maximize compliance (214). Because few data on sexual practices are available, surveys of knowledge, attitudes, and practices are needed to identify the culturally appropriate messages for various segments of the population in each country, such as prostitutes, adolescents, homosexual males, and bisexuals. Programs to prevent STDs have been undertaken before, and the success and failure of such programs should be examined so that mistakes made previously can be avoided in AIDS control programs.

Parenteral transmission of HIV remains a major problem, particularly among IDUs in developed countries and recipients of blood transfusions in developing countries where screening has not been implemented (215). As with implementing changes in sexual behavior, the challenge of altering needle-sharing habits among drug users is formidable. Advocating a change of behavior among drug users must be integrated into strategies at current treatment centers, which must be made more widely available (216). Specific recommendations for the control of HIV-1 infection among IDUs include HIV antibody testing, which should be voluntary; free distribution of sterile needles and syringes; methadone maintenance and other drug treatment programs, which should be available on demand for all IDUs as a means of reducing the spread of HIV infection; and educational strategies to prevent persons from starting injecting drug use, which should be broad based and directed at all persons at high risk (217). Among the target populations are IDUs who wish to enter drug treatment programs; current IDUs who do not want treatment for their drug abuse; persons who are not currently IDUs but who are at risk for becoming so; and all young people, especially those who live in areas with high rates of injecting drug use. In addition, sexual partners of staff and inmates of correctional facilities and all health care workers, counselors, and hospital personnel should be specifically educated about the potential risk for acquiring HIV infection through parenteral exposure to blood-contaminated needles and syringes and through sexual contact with an HIV-infected partner (90).

Although transmission by blood transfusion is now rare in most industrialized countries, in some developing countries, blood transfusions are probably the second most important route of HIV transmission, accounting for up to 10% of infections in adults and up to 30% in children. An HIV-free blood supply is an attainable goal with available technology and would have an immediate impact on the spread of AIDS. Major drawbacks have been logistic problems of setting up a blood-bank screening infrastructure in developing countries. Donor deferral or screening of donors on the basis of clinical or epidemiologic criteria is unlikely to protect the blood supply and could drastically reduce the available donor pool; however, an intensive program to educate physicians about the risk for HIV transmission through transfusions and the development of stringent criteria for prescribing transfusions should dramatically decrease the number of blood transfusions (218). Coupled with screening using inexpensive, rapid diagnostic assays, these measures should help prevent further transmission of HIV by blood transfusion, even in remote rural areas.

In some developing countries such as those in Africa, the frequent exposure to blood-contaminated needles and syringes that are reused for medicinal purposes may result in a substantial number of HIV infections. The potential importance of HIV transmission by needle reflects several cultural factors that merit emphasis. Patients often express a strong preference for parenteral rather than oral therapy. Injections, as well as scarifications, may be administered in clinics or nonmedical sites by personnel inadequately trained in aseptic technique. Financial and other practical constraints also lead to reuse of disposable equipment and to inadequate sterilization of needles and instruments. In contrast, the lack of association between HIV seropositivity and childhood vaccination probably reflects the wider use of properly sterilized injection equipment and immunization programs.

Prevention of perinatal transmission of HIV depends primarily on the success of limiting the spread of HIV infection of women of childbearing age and use of antiretroviral drugs, such as zidovudine, in HIV-infected pregnant women. In the developed world, when a mother is HIV infected, the known and potential benefit of breast-feeding for the child should be compared with the incremental risk to the infant of becoming infected through breast-feeding. In developing countries, where safe and effective alternatives for breast-feeding are not generally available, breast-feeding by the biologic mother should continue to be the feeding method of choice, regardless of the mother's HIV infection status. The issues of childbearing, contraception, breast-feeding, and abortion are obviously complex and require different approaches depending on the cultural background of the population.

With the magnitude of the current AIDS epidemic and the continued escalation in spread of HIV infection, it is evident that control and prevention of AIDS will require a sustained long-term commitment. Research is still urgently needed to define the size of the problem in different geographical areas through serosurveys of representative samples of the population. Research is needed to clarify the dynamics of transmission and the possible role of intercurrent infections or other cofactors in increasing the risk for infection or disease. Additional research is also urgently needed to develop effective control programs, which will rely on new studies of patterns of sexual behavior and the evaluation of the efficacy of health education interventions. The overall success of these national programs and the regional and global AIDS control efforts will depend on a unifying international political and societal commitment.

REFERENCES

1. Gottlieb MS, Schroff R, Schanker HM, et al. *Pneumocystis carinii* pneumonia and mucosal candidiasis in previously healthy homosexual men: evidence of a new acquired cellular immunodeficiency. *N Engl J Med* 1981;305:1425.
2. Masur H, Michelis MA, Greene JB, et al. An outbreak of community-acquired *Pneumocystis carinii* pneumonia: initial manifestation of cellular immune dysfunction. *N Engl J Med* 1981;305:1431.
3. Siegal FP, Lopez C, Hammer GS, et al. Severe acquired immunodeficiency in male homosexuals, manifested by chronic perianal ulcerative herpes simplex lesions. *N Engl J Med* 1981;305:1444.
4. Centers for Disease Control and Prevention. Kaposi's sarcoma and *Pneumocystis* pneumonia among homosexual men: New York City and California. *MMWR Morb Mortal Wkly Rep* 1981;30:305.
5. Centers for Disease Control and Prevention. Acquired immunodeficiency syndrome (AIDS) update: United States. *MMWR Morb Mortal Wkly Rep* 1983;32:309.
6. Mann JM, Chin J, Piot P, et al. The international epidemiology of AIDS. *Sci Am* 1988;259(4):82.
7. Quinn TC, Mann JM, Curran JW, et al. AIDS in Africa: an epidemiologic paradigm. *Science* 1986;234:955.
8. Pape J, Johnson WD Jr. AIDS in Haiti: 1982–1992. *Clin Infect Dis* 1993;17[Suppl 2]:S341.
9. Pape JW, Liautaud B, Thomas F, et al. Characteristics of the acquired immunodeficiency syndrome in a heterosexual population in Zaire. *Lancet* 1984;2:65.
10. Piot P, Quinn TC, Taelman H, et al. Acquired immunodeficiency syndrome in a heterosexual population in Zaire. *Lancet* 1984;2:65.
11. Centers for Disease Control and Prevention. The Global HIV and AIDS epidemic, 2001. *MMWR Morb Mortal Wkly Rep* 2001;50:434–439.
12. UNAIDS/WHO. *AIDS epidemic update, December 2002*. Geneva: UNAIDS and WHO, 2002:1–38.
13. Barre-Sinoussi F, Chermann JC, Rey F, et al. Isolation of a T-lymphotropic retrovirus from a patient at risk for acquired immune deficiency syndrome (AIDS). *Science* 1983;220:868.
14. Gallo RC, Salahuddin SZ, Popovic M, et al. Frequent detection and isolation of cytopathic retroviruses (HTLV-III) from patients with AIDS and at risk for AIDS. *Science* 1984;224:500.
15. DeCock KM, Barrere B Diaby L, et al. AIDS: the leading cause of adult death in the West African city of Abidjan, Ivory Coast. *Science* 1990;249:793.
16. Selik RM, Chu SY, Buehler JW. HIV infection as leading cause of death among young adults in U.S. cities and states. *JAMA* 1993;269:2991.
17. Mulder DW, Nunn AJ, Karnali A, et al. Two-year HIV-1-associated mortality in a Ugandan rural population. *Lancet* 1994;343:1021.
18. Sewankambo NK, Wawer MJ, Gray RH, et al. Demographic impact of HIV infection in rural Rakai district, Uganda: results of a population-based cohort study. *AIDS* 1994;8:1707.
19. Centers for Disease Control and Prevention. *Update: AIDS—United States, 2000*. 2002;51:592–595.
20. Stover J, Walker N, Garentt GP, et al. Can we reverse the HIV/AIDS pandemic with an expanded response? *Lancet* 2002;360:73–77.
21. DeCock KM, Mbori-Ngacha D, Marum E. Shadow on the continent: public health and HIV/AIDS in Africa in the 21st century. *Lancet* 2002;360:67–72.
22. Weidle PJ, Mastro TD, Grant AD, et al. HIV/AIDS treatment and HIV vaccines for Africa. *Lancet* 2002;359:2261–2267.
23. Morison L. The global epidemiology of HIV/AIDS. *Br Med Bull* 2001;58:7–18.
24. Quinn TC. Global burden of the HIV pandemic. *Lancet* 1996;348:99.
25. Nzilambi N, De Cock KM, Forthal DN, et al. The prevalence of infection with human immunodeficiency virus over a 10-year period in rural Zaire. *N Engl J Med* 1988;318:276.
26. Curran JW, Jaffe HW, Hardy AM, et al. Epidemiology of HIV infection and AIDS in the United States. *Science* 1988;239:610.
27. Quinn TC. Population migration and the spread of types 1 and 2 human immunodeficiency viruses. *Proc Natl Acad Sci USA* 1994;91:2407.
28. Decosas J, Kane F, Anarfi JK, et al. Migration and AIDS. *Lancet* 1995;346:826.
29. Piot P, Plummer FS, Mhalu JL, et al. AIDS: an international perspective. *Science* 1988;239:573.

30. Bollinger RC, Tripathy SP, Quinn TC. The human immunodeficiency virus epidemic in India. *Medicine (Baltimore)* 1995;74:97.
31. Mertens TE, Burton A, Stoneburner R, et al. Global estimates and epidemiology of HIV infections and AIDS. *AIDS* 1994;8[Suppl 1]:5361.
32. Chin J. Scenarios for the AIDS Epidemic in Asia. *Asia-Pacific population research reports*, No. 2. Honolulu: February 1995.
33. Centers for Disease Control and Prevention and Prevention. HIV and AIDS—United States, 1981–2000. *MMWR Morb Mortal Wkly Rep* 2001;50:430–434.
34. Egger M, May M, Chene G, et al. Prognosis of HIV-1-infected patients starting highly active antiretroviral therapy: a collaborative analysis of prospective studies. *Lancet* 2002;360:119–129.
35. Hogg RS, Yip B, Chan KJ, et al. Rates of disease progression by baseline CD4 cell count and viral load after initiating triple-drug therapy. *JAMA* 2001;286:2568–2577.
36. Haverkos HW, Quinn TC. The third wave: HIV infection among heterosexuals in the United States and Europe. *Int J STD AIDS* 1995;6:227.
37. Centers for Disease Control and Prevention and Prevention. Update: acquired immunodeficiency syndrome—United States, 1994. *MMWR Morb Mortal Wkly Rep* 1995;44:64.
38. Kaldor JM, Sittitrai W, John TJ, et al. The emerging epidemic of HIV infection and AIDS in Asia and the Pacific. *AIDS* 1994;8[Suppl 2]:S165.
39. Mann J, Tarantola D. The state of the HIV/AIDS pandemic. In: Mann J, Tarantola D, Netter J, eds. *AIDS in the world*, Vol II. London: Oxford University Press, 1996.
40. Quinn TC, Zacarias FRK, St. John RK. HIV and HTLV-1 infections in the Americas: a regional perspective. *Medicine (Baltimore)* 1989;68:189.
41. U.S. Bureau of the Census. *HIV/AIDS in Asia*. Washington, DC: U.S. Bureau of the Census, 1995. Research Note 18.
42. Brown T, Xenos P. AIDS in Asia: the gathering storm. In: *Asia-Pacific Issues*, No 16. Honolulu: East-West Center, 1994.
43. Thomson MM, Perez-Alvarez L, Najera R. Molecular epidemiology of HIV-1 genetic forms and its significance for vaccine development and therapy. *Lancet* 2002;2:461–471.
44. Tatt ID, Barlow KL, Nicoll A, et al. The public health significance of HIV-1 subtypes. *AIDS* 2001;15[Suppl 5]:S59–71.
45. Alaeus A. Significance of HIV-1 genetic subtypes. *Scand J Infect Dis* 2000;32:455–463.
46. Marlink R. Biology and epidemiology of HIV-2. In: Essex M, Kalengay M, Kanki P, et al., eds. *AIDS in Africa*. New York: Raven Press, 1994:47–65.
47. Myers G. HIV: between past and future. *AIDS Res Hum Retroviruses* 1994;10:1317.
48. Artenstein AW, Coppola J, Brown AE, et al. Multiple introductions of HIV-1 subtype E into the Western hemisphere. *Lancet* 1995;346:1197.
49. Brodine SK, Mascola JR, Weiss PJ, et al. Detection of diverse HIV-1 genetic subtypes in the U.S.A. *Lancet* 1995;346:1198.
50. Kunanusont C, Foy HM, Kreiss JK, et al. HIV-1 subtypes and male-to-female transmission in Thailand. *Lancet* 1995;345:1078.
51. Weniger BG, Takebe Y, Ou C-Y, et al. The molecular epidemiology of HIV in Asia. *AIDS* 1994;8[Suppl 2]:513.
52. Ou C-Y, Takebe Y, Weiniger BG, et al. Independent introduction of two major HIV-1 genotypes into distinct high-risk populations in Thailand. *Lancet* 1993;341:1171.
53. Bobkov A, Garaev MM, Rzhaninova A. Molecular epidemiology of HIV-1 in the former Soviet Union: analysis of *env* V3 sequences and their correlation with epidemiologic data. *AIDS* 1994;8:619.
54. Louwagie J, Delwart EL, Mullins JL, et al. Genetic analysis of HIV-1 isolates from Brazil reveals presence of two distinct genetic subtypes. *AIDS Res Hum Retroviruses* 1994;10:561.
55. Morgado MG, Sabino EC, Shpaer EG, et al. V3 region polymorphisms in HIV-1 from Brazil: prevalence of subtype B strains divergent from North American/European prototype and detection of subtype F. *AIDS Res Hum Retroviruses* 1994;10:569.
56. Pieniazek D, Janini LM, Ramos A, et al. HIV-patients may harbor viruses of different phylogenetic subtypes: implications for the evolution of the HIV/AIDS pandemic. *Emerg Infect Dis* 1995;1:86.
57. Clavel F, Guetard D, Brun-Vezinet F, et al. Isolation of a new retrovirus from West African patients with AIDS. *Science* 1986;233:343.
58. Kanki PJ, Barin F, M'Boup S, et al. New human T-lymphotropic retrovirus related to simian T-lymphotropic virus type III (STLV-IIIAGM). *Science* 1986;232:238.
59. Clavel F, Mansinho K, Chamaret S, et al. Human immunodeficiency virus type 2 infection associated with AIDS in West Africa. *N Engl J Med* 1987;316:1180.
60. Clavel F. HIV-2, the West African AIDS virus. *AIDS* 1987;1:135.
61. De Cock KM, Adjorlolo G, Ekpini E, et al. Epidemiology and transmission of HIV-2: why there is no HIV-2 pandemic. *JAMA* 1993;270:2083.
62. Kanki P, M'Boup S, Marlink R, et al. Prevalence and risk determinants of human immunodeficiency virus type 2 (HIV-2) and human immunodeficiency virus type 1 (HIV-1) in West African female prostitutes. *Am J Epidemiol* 1992;136:895.
63. Markovitz DM. Infection with the human immunodeficiency virus type 2. *Ann Intern Med* 1993;118:211.
64. DeCock KM, Brun-Vezinet F. Epidemiology of HIV-2 infection. *AIDS* 1989;3[Suppl 1]:S89.
65. Kanki P. Biologic features of HIV-2: an update. *AIDS Clin Rev* 1991;17.
66. Kanki PJ, Travers KU, M'Boup S, et al. Slower heterosexual spread of HIV-2 than HIV-1. *Lancet* 1994;343:943.
67. Adjorlolo-Johnson G, De Cock KM, Ekpini E, et al. Prospective comparison of mother-to-child transmission of HIV-1 and HIV-2 in Abidjan, Ivory Coast. *JAMA* 1994;272:462.
68. Kanki PJ, DeCock KM. Epidemiology and natural history of HIV-2. *AIDS* 1994;8[Suppl 1]:S85.
69. Travers K, Mboup S, Marlink R, et al. Natural protection against HIV-1 infection provided by HIV-2. *Science* 1995;268:1612.
70. Ou C-Y, Ciesielski CA, Myers G, et al. Molecular epidemiology of HIV transmission in a dental practice. *Science* 1992;256:1165.
71. Jaffe HW, McCurdy JM, Kalish ML, et al. Lack of HIV transmission in the practice of a dentist with AIDS. *Ann Intern Med* 1994;121:855.
72. Ciesielski CA, Marianos DW, Schochetman G, et al. The 1990 Florida dental investigation: the press and the science. *Ann Intern Med* 1984;121:886.
73. Ou CY, Ciesielski CA, Myers G, et al. Molecular epidemiology of HIV transmission in a dental practice. *Science* 1992;256:1165.
74. Cheingsong-Popov R, Bobkov A, Garaev MM, et al. Identification of human immunodeficiency virus type 1 subtypes and their distribution in the Commonwealth of Independent States (former Soviet Union) by serologic V3 peptide-binding assays and V3 sequence analysis. *J Infect Dis* 168:292, 1993.
75. Chant K, Lowe D, Rubin G, et al. Patient-to-patient transmission of HIV in private surgical consulting rooms. *Lancet* 1993;342:1548.
76. Kingsley LA, Zhou SYJ, Bacellar H, et al. Temporal trends in human immunodeficiency virus type 1 seroconversion 1984–1989. *Am J Epidemiol* 134:331, 1991.
77. Winkelstein W, Lyman DM, Padian N, et al. Sexual practices and risk of infection by the human immunodeficiency virus: the San Francisco Men's Health Study. *JAMA* 1987;257:321.
78. Kingsley LA, Detels R, Kaslow R, et al. Risk factors for seroconversion to human immunodeficiency virus among male homosexuals. *Lancet* 1987;1:345.
79. Padian NS. Heterosexual transmission of acquired immunodeficiency syndrome: international perspectives and national projections. *Rev Infect Dis* 1987;9:947.
80. Centers for Disease Control and Prevention and Prevention. Heterosexually acquired AIDS—United States, 1993. *MMWR Morb Mortal Wkly Rep* 1994;43:155.
81. Prevots DR, Ancelle-Park RA, Neal JJ, et al. The epidemiology of heterosexually acquired HIV infection and AIDS in Western industrialized countries. *AIDS* 1994;8[Suppl 1]:5109.
82. Piot P, Plummer FA, Mhlau FS, et al. AIDS: an international perspective. *Science* 1988;239:573.
83. Piot P, Goeman J, Laga M. The epidemiology of HIV and AIDS in Africa. In: Essex M, Mboup S, Kanki P, et al., eds. *AIDS in Africa*. New York: Raven Press, 1994:157–172.
84. Piot P, Kreiss JK, Ndinya-Achola JO, et al. Heterosexual transmission of HIV. *AIDS* 1988;2:1.
85. Quinn TC, Fauci AS. The changing demography of AIDS: emergence of heterosexual transmission. In: Isselbacher KJ, Braunwald E, Wilson JD, et al., eds. *Harrison's principles of internal medicine*, Suppl 9. New York: McGraw-Hill, 1994:1–9.
86. Piot P, Kapita BM, Were JBO, et al. AIDS in Africa: the first decade and challenges for the late 1990s. *AIDS* 1991;5:S1.
87. Kreiss JK, Koech D, Plummer FA, et al. AIDS virus infection in Nairobi prostitutes: spread of the epidemic to East Africa. *N Engl J Med* 1986;314:414.
88. Mann JM, Nzilambi N, Piot P, et al. Human immunodeficiency viral infection and associated risk factors in female prostitutes in Kinshasa, Zaire. *AIDS* 1988;2:255.
89. Piot P, Plummer FS, Rey MA, et al. Retrospective seroepidemiology of AIDS virus infection in Nairobi populations. *J Infect Dis* 1987;155:1108.
90. Holmberg SD, Horsburgh CR, Ward JW, et al. Biologic factors in the sexual transmission of human immunodeficiency viruses. *J Infect Dis* 1989;160:116.
91. Goedert JJ, Eyster ME, Bigger RJ, et al. Heterosexual transmission of human immunodeficiency virus: association with severe depletion of T-helper lymphocytes in men with hemophilia. *AIDS Res Hum Retroviruses* 1987;4:355.
92. Quinn TC, Wawer MJ, Sewankambo N, et al. Viral load and heterosexual transmission of human immunodeficiency virus type 1. Rakai Project Study Group. *N Engl J Med* 2002;342:921–929.
93. Garcia PM, Kalish LA, Pitt J, et al. Maternal levels of plasma human immunodeficiency virus type 1 RNA and the risk of perinatal transmission. Women and Infants Transmission Study Group. *N Engl J Med* 199;34:394–402.
94. Gray RH, Wawer MJ, Brookmeyer R, et al. Probability of HIV-1 transmission per coital act in monogamous, heterosexual, HIV-1-discordant couples in Rakai, Uganda. *Lancet* 2001;357:1149–1153.
95. Tovanabutra S, Robison V, Wongtrakul J, et al. Male viral load and heterosexual transmission of HIV-1 subtype E in northern Thailand. *J Acquir Immun Defic Syndr Hum Retrovirol* 2002;29:275–283.
96. Fideli US, Allen SA, Musonda R, et al. Virologic and immunologic determinants of heterosexual transmission of human immunodeficiency virus type 1 in Africa. *AIDS Res Hum Retroviruses* 2001;17:901–910.
97. Wasserheit JN. Epidemiological synergy: interrelationships between human immunodeficiency virus infection and other sexually transmitted diseases. *Sex Transm Dis* 1992;19(2):61–77.
98. Laga M, Diallo MO, Buve A. Inter-relationship of sexually transmitted diseases and HIV: where are we now? *AIDS* 1994;8[Suppl 1]:S119.

99. World Health Organization. *An overview of selected curable sexually transmitted diseases.* Global Programme on AIDS. Geneva: World Health Organization, 1995.

100. Laga M. STD control for HIV prevention: it works. *Lancet* 1995;346:518.

101. Hanenberg RS, Rojanapithayakorn W, Kunasol P, et al. Impact of Thailand's HIV-control programme as indicated by the decline of sexually transmitted diseases. *Lancet* 1994;344:243.

102. Grosskurth H, Mosha F, Todd J, et al. Impact of improved treatment of sexually transmitted diseases on HIV infection in rural Tanzania: Randomised controlled trial. *Lancet* 1995;346:530.

103. Wawer MJ, Sewankambo NK, Serwadda D, et al. Control of sexually transmitted diseases for AIDS prevention in Uganda: a randomized community trial. Rakai Project Study Group. *Lancet* 1999;353:525–535.

104. The Working Group on Mother-to-Child Transmission of HIV. Rates of mother-to-child transmission of HIV-1 in Africa, America, and Europe: results from 13 perinatal studies. *J Acquir Immune Defic Syndr Hum Retrovirol* 1995;8:506.

105. Peckham C, Gibb D. Mother-to-child transmission of the human immunodeficiency virus. *N Engl J Med* 1995;333:298.

106. St. Louis M, Kamenga M, Brown C, et al. Risk for perinatal HIV-1 transmission according to maternal immunologic, virologic, and placental factors. *JAMA* 1993;269:2853.

107. Burns DN, Landesman S, Muenz LR, et al. Cigarette smoking, premature rupture of membranes, and vertical transmission of HIV-1 among women with low CD4+ levels. *J Acquir Immune Defic Syndr Hum Retrovirol* 1994;7:718.

108. Weisner B, Nachman S, Tropper P, et al. Quantitation of human immunodeficiency virus type 1 during pregnancy: relationship of viral titer to mother-to-child transmission and stability of viral load. *Proc Natl Acad Sci USA* 1994;91:8037.

109. Semba RLD, Miotti PG, Chiphangwi JD, et al. Maternal vitamin A deficiency and mother-to-child transmission of HIV-1. *Lancet* 1994;343:1593.

110. Dunn DT, Newell ML, Ades AE, et al. Risk of human immunodeficiency virus type 1 transmission through breast-feeding. *Lancet* 1992;340:585.

111. World Health Organization. Global Programme on AIDS. Consensus statement from the WHO/UNICEF consultation on HIV transmission and breast-feeding. *Wkly Epidemiol Rec* 1992;67:177.

112. Centers for Disease Control and Prevention. U.S. Public Health Service recommendations for human immunodeficiency virus counseling and voluntary testing for pregnant women. *MMWR Morb Mortal Wkly Rep* 1995;44(RR-7):1.

113. Connor EM, Sperling RS, Gelber R, et al. Reduction of maternal-infant transmission of human immunodeficiency virus type 1 with zidovudine treatment. *N Engl J Med* 1994;331:1173.

114. Centers for Disease Control and Prevention. USPHS Task Force recommendations for use of antiretroviral drugs in pregnant HIV-1-infected women for maternal health and interventions to reduce perinatal HIV-1 transmission in the United States. *MMWR Morb Mortal Wkly Rep* 2002;51(RR18):1–38.

115. Centers for Disease Control and Prevention. Successful implementation of perinatal HIV prevention guidelines. 2001;50(RR-06).

116. Fowler MG, Simonds RJ, Roongpisuthipong A. Update on perinatal HIV transmission. *Pediatr Clin North Am* 2002;47:21–38.

117. Mofenson LM. Technical report: perinatal human immunodeficiency virus testing and prevention of transmission. Committee on Pediatric AIDS. *Pediatrics* 2000;106:E88.

118. Des Jarlais DC, Friedman SR Choopanya K, et al. International epidemiology of HIV and AIDS among injecting drug users. *AIDS* 1992;6:1053.

119. Des Jarlais DC, Friedman SR, Friedmann P, et al. HIV/AIDS-related behavior change among injecting drug users in different national settings. *AIDS* 1995;9:611.

120. Des Jarlais DC, Friedman SR, Sotheran JL, et al. Continuity and change within an HIV epidemic: injecting drug users in New York City, 1984 through 1992. *JAMA* 1994;271:121.

121. Waters JK, Estilio MJ, Clark GL, et al. Syringes and needle exchange as HIV/AIDS prevention for injection drug users. *JAMA* 1994;271:115.

122. Lurie P, Reingold AC, Bowser B, et al. *The public health impact of needle exchange programs in the United States and abroad,* Vol 1. Atlanta: Centers for Disease Control and Prevention and Prevention, 1993.

123. Normand J, Vlahov D, Moses LE, eds. *Preventing HIV transmission: the role of sterile needles and bleach.* Washington, DC: National Academy Press, 1995.

124. World Health Organization. *Global Programme on AIDS.* Geneva: World Health Organization, 1995. WHO/GPA/RID/PRS/95.1.

125. Centers for Disease Control and Prevention and Prevention. Syringe exchange programs—United States, 1994–1995. *MMWR Morb Mortal Wkly Rep* 1995;44:684.

126. Des Jarlais DC, Hagan H, Friedman SR, et al. Maintaining low HIV seroprevalence in populations of injecting drug users. *JAMA* 1995;274:1226.

127. Centers for Disease Control and Prevention. Provisional Public Health Service interagency recommendations for screening donated blood and plasma for antibodies to the virus causing acquired immunodeficiency syndrome. *MMWR Morb Mortal Wkly Rep* 1985;34(1):1.

128. Ward JW, Holmberg SD, Allen JR. Transmission of human immunodeficiency virus (HIV) by blood transfusions screened as negative for HIV antibody. *N Engl J Med* 1988;318:473.

129. Foster S, Buve A. Benefits of HIV screening of blood transfusions in Zambia. *Lancet* 1995;346:225.

130. Centers for Disease Control and Prevention. Recommendations for prevention of HIV transmission in health-care settings. *MMWR Morb Mortal Wkly Rep* 1986;36[Suppl 2]:1S.

131. Gerberding JL. Management of occupational exposures to blood-borne viruses. *N Engl J Med* 1995;332:444.

132. Centers for Disease Control and Prevention. Public Health Service statement on management of occupational exposure to human immunodeficiency virus, including considerations regarding zidovudine postexposure use. *MMWR Morb Mortal Wkly Rep* 1990;39(RR-1):1.

133. Centers for Disease Control and Prevention. Guidelines for prevention of transmission of human immunodeficiency virus and hepatitis B virus to health-care and public-safety workers. *MMWR Morb Mortal Wkly Rep* 1989;38[Suppl 6]:1.

134. Centers for Disease Control and Prevention. Update: universal precautions for prevention of transmission of HIV, hepatitis B virus, and other bloodborne pathogens in health-care settings. *MMWR Morb Mortal Wkly Rep* 1988;37:377, 387.

135. Centers for Disease Control and Prevention. Recommendations for preventing transmission of human immunodeficiency virus and hepatitis B virus to patients during exposure-prone invasive procedures. *MMWR Morb Mortal Wkly Rep* 1991;40(RR-8):1.

136. Centers for Disease Control and Prevention. Update: investigations of persons treated by HIV-infected health-care workers—United States. *MMWR Morb Mortal Wkly Rep* 1993;42:329.

137. Robert LM, Chamberland ME, Cleveland JL, et al. Investigations of patients of health care workers infected with HIV. *Ann Intern Med* 1995;122:653.

138. Centers for Disease Control and Prevention and Prevention. Human immunodeficiency virus transmission in household settings—United States. *MMWR Morb Mortal Wkly Rep* 1994;43:347.

139. Buve A, Bishikwabo-Nsarhaza K, Mutangadura G. The spread and effect of HIV-1 infection in sub-Saharan Africa. *Lancet* 2002;359:2011–2017.

140. Gayle HD, Hill GL. Global impact of human immunodeficiency virus and AIDS. *Clin Microbiol Rev* 2001;14:327–335.

141. Miotti PG, Dallabetta G, Ndovi E, et al. HIV-1 and pregnant women: associated factors, prevalence, estimate of incidence and role in fetal wastage in central Africa. *AIDS* 1990;4:733.

142. Wawer M, Sewankambo N, Berkley S, et al. HIV incidence in a rural district of Uganda. *BMJ* 1994;308:171.

143. U.S. Bureau of the Census. *Trends and patterns of HIV and AIDS infection in selected developing countries.* Country profiles: June 1994. Washington, DC: U.S. Bureau of the Census, 1994. Research Note 14.

144. Dada AJ, Oyewole F, Onofowokan R, et al. Demographic characteristics of retroviral infections (HIV-1, HIV-2, and HTLV-1) among female prostitutes in Lagos, Nigeria. *J Acquir Immune Defic Syndr Hum Retrovirol* 1993;269:2853.

145. Olaleye OD, Bernstein L, Ekweozor CC, et al. Prevalence of human immunodeficiency virus types 1 and 2 infections in Nigeria. *J Infect Dis* 1993;167:710.

146. Swanevelder R. Fifth national HIV survey of women attending antenatal clinics, South Africa, October/November 1994. In: Kustner H, ed. *Epidemiological comments,* Vol 22, No 5. Washington, DC: U.S. Department of Health and Human Services, 1995:90–100.

147. Dondero TJ, Curran JW. Excess deaths in Africa from HIV: confirmed and quantified. *Lancet* 1995;343:989.

148. Preble EA. Impact of HIV/AIDS on African children. *Soc Sci Med* 1990;31:671.

149. Harries AD. Tuberculosis and human immunodeficiency virus infection in developing countries. *Lancet* 1990;335:387.

150. DeCock KM, Soro B, Coulibaly I-M, et al. Tuberculosis and HIV infection in sub-Saharan Africa. *JAMA* 1992;268:1581.

151. Weniger BG, Limpakarnjanarat K, Ungchusak K, et al. The epidemiology of HIV infection and AIDS in Thailand. *AIDS* 1991;5[Suppl 2]:S71.

152. Brown T, Sittirai W, Vanichseni S, et al. The recent epidemiology of HIV and AIDS in Thailand. *AIDS* 1994;8[Suppl 2]:S131.

153. Kitayaporn D, Uneklabh C, Weniger BG, et al. HIV-1 incidence determined retrospectively among drug users in Bangkok, Thailand. *AIDS* 1994;8:1443.

154. Naik TN, Sarkar S, Singh HL, et al. Intravenous drug users: a new high-risk group for HIV infection in India. *AIDS* 1991;5:117.

155. Cheng H, Zhang J, Capizzi J, et al. Introduction of HIV-1 subtype E into Yunnan, China. *Lancet* 1994;344:953.

156. Xia M, Kreiss JK, Holmes KK. Risk factors for HIV infection among drug users in Yunnan province, China: association with intravenous drug use and protective effect of boiling reusable needles and syringes. *AIDS* 1994;8:1701.

157. Nelson KE, Celentano DD, Supraset S, et al. Risk factors for HIV infection among young adult men in northern Thailand. *JAMA* 1993;270:955.

158. Kitsiripornchai S. *HIV-1 infection in young men entering the Royal Thai Army: trends and demographic risk factors* [Abstract]. Presented at the Third International Conference on AIDS in Asia and the Pacific, Fifth National AIDS Seminar in Thailand, September 17–21, 1995, Chiang Mai, Thailand.

159. Brown T, Sittirai W. The HIV/AIDS epidemic in Thailand: addressing the impact on children. In: *Asia-Pacific population and policy,* No 35. Honolulu: East-West Center Program on Population, 1995.

160. Rodrigues JJ, Mehendale SM, Shepherd ME, et al. Risk factors for HIV infection in people attending clinics for sexually transmitted diseases in India. *BMJ* 1995;311:283.

161. Mehendale SM, Rodrigues JJ, Brookmeyer RS, et al. Incidence and predictors of human immunodeficiency virus type 1 seroconversion in patients attending sexually transmitted diseases clinics in India. *J Infect Dis* 1995;172:1486.

162. World Health Organization. HIV and AIDS in the western Pacific region. In: *AIDS surveillance report: western Pacific region,* No 5. Geneva: World Health Organization, 1995:1–8.

163. Cahn P, Belloso WH, Murillo J, et al. AIDS in Latin America. *Infect Dis Clin North Am* 2000;14:185–209.

164. Vu MQ, Steketee RW, Valleroy L, et al. HIV incidence in the United States, 1978–1999. *J Acquir Immune Defic Syndr Hum Retrovirol* 2002;31:188–201.

165. Blair JM, Fleming PL, Karon JM. Trends in AIDS incidence and survival among racial/ethnic minority men who have sex with men, United States, 1990–1999. *J Acquir Immune Defic Syndr Hum Retrovirol* 2002;31:339–347.

166. Estrada AL. Epidemiology of HIV/AIDS, hepatitis B, hepatitis C, and tuberculosis among minority injection drug users. *Public Health Rep* 2002;117[Suppl 1]:S126–134.

167. Katz MH, Schwarcz SK, Kellogg TA, et al. Impact of highly active antiretroviral treatment on HIV seroincidence among men who have sex with men: San Francisco. *Am J Public Health* 2002;92:388–394.

168. Centers for Disease Control and Prevention. HIV testing among racial/ethnic minorities—United States, 1999. *MMWR Morb Mortal Wkly Rep* 2001;50:1054–1058.

169. Janssen RS, St. Louis ME, Satten G, et al. HIV infection among patients in U.S. acute-care hospitals: strategies for the counseling and testing of hospital patients. *N Engl J Med* 1992;327:445.

170. Kelen GD, Hexter DA, Hansen KN, et al. Trends in HIV infection among an inner-city emergency department patient population: implications for emergency department based HIV-screening programs. *Clin Infect Dis* 1995;21:867.

171. Sawanpanyalert P, Ungchusak K, Thanprasertsuk S, et al. HIV-1 seroconversion rates among female commercial sex workers, Chiang Mai, Thailand: a multi cross-sectional study. *AIDS* 1994;8:825.

172. Wheeler VW, Radcliffe KW. HIV infection in the Caribbean. *Int J STD AIDS* 1994;5:79.

173. Newton EAC, White FMM, Sokal DC, et al. Modeling the HIV/AIDS epidemic in the English-speaking Caribbean. *Bull Pan Am Health Org* 1994;28:239.

174. The European Study Group. European community concerted action on HIV seroprevalence among sexually transmitted disease patients in 18 European sentinel networks. *AIDS* 1993;7:393.

175. Kozlov AP, Volkova GV, Malykh AG, et al. Epidemiology of HIV infection in St. Petersburg, Russia. *J Acquir Immune Defic Syndr Hum Retrovirol* 1993;6:208.

176. Kalichman SC, Kelly JA, Sikkema KJ, et al. The emerging AIDS crisis in Russia: review of enabling factors and prevention needs. *Int J STD AIDS* 2000;11:71–75.

177. Kazionny B, Wells CD, Kluge H, et al. Implications of the growing HIV-1 epidemic for tuberculosis control in Russia. *Lancet* 2001;358:1513–1514.

178. Melnick SL, Sherer R, Louis TA, et al. Survival and disease progression according to gender of patients with HIV infection. *JAMA* 1994;272:1915.

179. Hogg RS, Strathdee SA, Craib KJP, et al. Lower socioeconomic status and shorter survival following HIV infection. *Lancet* 1994;344:1120.

180. Baltimore D. Lessons from people with nonprogressive HIV infection. *N Engl J Med* 1995;332:259.

181. Osmond D, Charlebois E, Lang W, et al. Changes in AIDS survival time in two San Francisco cohorts of homosexual men, 1983 to 1993. *JAMA* 1994;271:1083.

182. Schrager LK, Young JM, Fowler MG, et al. Long-term survivors of HIV-1 infection: definitions and research challenges. *AIDS* 1994;8[Suppl 1]:S95.

183. Ngaly B, Ryder RW, Kapita B, et al. Human immunodeficiency virus infection among employees in an African hospital. *N Engl J Med* 1988;319:1123.

184. Mann JM, Kapita B, Colebunders RL, et al. Natural history of HIV infection in Zaire. *Lancet* 1986;2:707.

185. Polk BF, Fox R, Brookmeyer R, et al. Predictors of the acquired immunodeficiency syndrome developing in a cohort of seropositive homosexual men. *N Engl J Med* 1987;317:1114.

186. Allain JP, Laurian Y, Paul DA, et al. Long-term evaluation of HIV antigen and antibodies to p24 and gp41 in patients with hemophilia: Potential clinical importance. *N Engl J Med* 1987;317:1114.

187. Spira TJ, Kaplan JE, Feorino PM, et al. Human immunodeficiency virus viremia as a prognostic indicator in homosexual men with lymphadenopathy syndrome. *N Engl J Med* 1987;317:1093.

188. Moss AR, Bacchetti P, Osmond D, et al. Seropositivity for HIV and the development of AIDS or AIDS-related condition: three-year follow-up of the San Francisco General Hospital cohort. *BMJ* 1988;269:745.

189. Baillou A, Barin F, Allain JP, et al. Human immunodeficiency virus antigenemia in patients with AIDS and AIDS related disorders: a comparison between Europe and Central African populations. *J Infect Dis* 1987;156:830.

190. Mellors JW, Kingsley LA, Rinaldo CR Jr, et al. Quantitation of HIV-1 RNA in plasma predicts outcome after seroconversion. *Ann Intern Med* 1995;122:573.

191. Quinn TC, Piot P, McCormick JB, et al. Serologic and immunologic studies in patients with AIDS in North America and Africa: the potential of infectious agents as cofactors in human immunodeficiency virus infection. *JAMA* 1987;257:2617.

192. Bartholomew C, Blattner W, Cleghorn F. Progression to AIDS in homosexual men co-infected with HIV and HTLV-1 in Trinidad [Letter]. *Lancet* 1987;2:1469.

193. Schechter M, Harrison LH, Halsey NA, et al. Coinfection with human T-cell lymphotropic virus type 1 and HIV in Brazil. *JAMA* 1994;271:353.

194. Raviglione MC, Snider DE, Kochi A. Global epidemiology of tuberculosis: morbidity and mortality of a worldwide epidemic. *JAMA* 1995;273:220.

195. Perriens JH, Colebunders RL, Karahunga C, et al. Increased mortality and tuberculosis treatment failure rate among human immunodeficiency virus (HIV) seropositive compared with HIV seronegative patients with pulmonary tuberculosis treated with "standard" chemotherapy in Kinshasa, Zaire. *Am Rev Respir Dis* 1991;144:750.

196. Ackah A, Coulibaly D, Digbeau H, et al. Response to therapy, mortality, and CD4+ lymphocyte counts in HIV-infected persons with tuberculosis in Abidjan, Côte d'Ivoire. *Lancet* 1994;344:1323.

197. Espinal MA, Reingold AL, Koenig E, et al. Screening for active tuberculosis in HIV testing centre. *Lancet* 1995;345:890.

198. Narian JP, Raviglione MC, Kochi A. HIV associated tuberculosis in developing countries: epidemiology and strategies for prevention. *Tuber Lung Dis* 1992;73:311.

199. Garcia Garcia L, Valdespino Gomez JL, Sancho MC, et al. Epidemiology of AIDS and tuberculosis. *Bull Pan Am Health Org* 1995;29:37.

200. DeCock KM, Lucas SB, Lucas S, et al. Clinical research, prophylaxis, therapy, and care for HIV disease in Africa. *Am J Public Health* 1993;83:1385.

201. DeCock KM. Screening for tuberculosis and HIV in resource-poor countries. *Lancet* 1995;345:873.

202. World Health Organization. *WHO report on the tuberculosis epidemic, 1995.* Geneva: World Health Organization, 1995. WHO/TB/95.183.

203. Small PM, Schecter GF, Goodman PC, et al. Treatment of tuberculosis in patients with advanced human immunodeficiency virus infection. *N Engl J Med* 1991;324:289.

204. Centers for Disease Control and Prevention. National action plan to combat multidrug-resistant tuberculosis. *MMWR Morb Mortal Wkly Rep* 1992;41(RR-11):1.

205. Centers for Disease Control and Prevention and Prevention. Tuberculosis morbidity—United States, 1994. *MMWR Morb Mortal Wkly Rep* 1995;44:387.

206. Selwyn PA, Hartel D, Lewis VA, et al. A prospective study of the risk of tuberculosis among intravenous drug users with human immunodeficiency virus infections. *N Engl J Med* 1989;320:545.

207. DeCock KM, Wilkinson D. Tuberculosis control in resource-poor countries: alternative approaches in the era of HIV. *Lancet* 1995;346:675.

208. Alwood K, Keruly J, Moore-Rice K, et al. Effectiveness of supervised, intermittent therapy for tuberculosis in HIV-infected patients. *AIDS* 1994;8:1103.

209. Weis SE, Slocum PC, Blais FX, et al. The effect of directly observed therapy on the rates of drug resistance and relapse in tuberculosis. *N Engl J Med* 1994;330:1179.

210. Chin J. Current and future dimensions of the HIV/AIDS pandemic in women and children. *Lancet* 1990;336:221.

211. Preble EA. Impact of HIV/AIDS on African children. *Soc Sci Med* 1990;31:671.

212. Mann JM, Chin J. AIDS: a global perspective. *N Engl J Med* 1988;319:302.

213. Quinn TC, Zacarias FR, St.John RK. AIDS in the Americas: an emerging public health crisis [Editorial]. *N Engl J Med* 1989;320:1005.

214. Ngugi EN, Plummer FA, Simonsen JN, et al. Prevention of transmission of human immunodeficiency virus in Africa: effectiveness of condom promotion and health education among prostitutes. *Lancet* 1988;2:887.

215. Quinn TC, Kline R, Francis H, et al. Rapid latex agglutination assay using recombinant envelope polypeptide for the detection of antibody to the human immunodeficiency virus. *JAMA* 1988;260:510.

216. Des Jarlais DC, Friedman SR, Stoneburner RL. HIV infection and intravenous drug use: critical issues in transmission dynamics, infection, outcome and prevention. *Rev Infect Dis* 1988;10:151.

217. Brickner PW, Torres RA, Barnes M, et al. Recommendations for control and prevention of human immunodeficiency virus infection in intravenous drug users. *Ann Intern Med* 1989;110:833.

218. Greenberg AE, Nguyen-Dinh P, Mann JM, et al. The association between malaria, blood transfusion, and HIV seropositivity in a pediatric population in Kinshasa, Zaire. *JAMA* 1988;259:545.

CHAPTER 115

Pulmonary Infections in Patients with Human Immunodeficiency Virus Infection

John G. Bartlett

Acquired immunodeficiency syndrome (AIDS) was first identified when an unusual number of cases of *Pneumocystis carinii* pneumonia (PCP) were recognized in homosexual men in California and New York (1,2). Since the first reports of AIDS, the lungs have continued to be a frequent site of disease; PCP, either alone or in combination with other opportunistic processes, was initially the AIDS-defining diagnosis in up to 65% of reported cases (3,4). The frequency of PCP subsequently decreased substantially, first because of PCP prophylaxis and then as a result of highly active antiretroviral therapy (HAART). Nevertheless, this remains the most frequent AIDS-defining diagnosis. In addition, bacterial pneumonia is now as frequent as PCP, and pulmonary tuberculosis has emerged as the most important human immunodeficiency virus (HIV)-associated complication in resource-limited areas (5,6). This chapter summarizes the infectious complications involving the lung in persons with HIV infection.

EFFECTS OF HUMAN IMMUNODEFICIENCY VIRUS INFECTION ON LUNG DEFENSES

The CD4$^+$ lymphocyte plays a critical role in immune-mediated lung defenses because it is crucial to the functioning of alveolar macrophages and natural killer cells, and it conditions the response of B lymphocytes to specific antigens (7). Moreover, HIV is known to infect macrophages and dendritic cells, perhaps interfering with their function; thus, HIV infection has a multifactorial effect on the ability of the lungs to respond to infectious agents (7). The most apparent HIV-induced abnormalities in host defenses involve cell-mediated immunity. The suppression of this arm of the immune system is manifested clinically by reduction in reactivity to intradermally administered antigens such as tuberculin (8,9). Humoral immunity is also impaired, as indicated by the diminished antibody response to pneumococcal or influenza vaccine (10,11). Both cell-mediated and humoral responses are highly dependent on disease stage as indicated by CD4 cell count (8–12) and to a lesser extent to plasma HIV RNA levels (13).

Data from prospective cohort studies have shown that there is an increased frequency of lung disease throughout the course of HIV disease, or at least beginning well before the stage of advanced immunosuppression is reached. In early and midcourse HIV disease, acute bronchitis is the most frequent pulmonary disease encountered (13). Pyogenic bacterial pneumonia and tuberculosis may occur at any point, early or late. Pneumonia caused by *P. carinii*, *Pseudomonas aeruginosa*, or aspergillosis occurs only in patients with advanced immune suppression. The stage of HIV disease at which a given pathogen causes lung disease presumably relates to the virulence or pathogenicity of the organism.

BACTERIAL PNEUMONIA

Multiple studies show high rates of bacterial pneumonia in patients with HIV infection (3–22). Most studies show no clear etiologic pathogen in the majority—an observation that applies to community-acquired pneumonia in immunocompetent patients as well. When a pathogen is detected, the most common in virtually all series is *Streptococcus pneumoniae*. Far less frequent are *Haemophilus influenzae*, *P. aeruginosa*, and *Staphylococcus aureus*. *Legionella* species, *Chlamydia pneumoniae*, and *Mycoplasma pneumoniae* appear to be uncommon in HIV-infected patients (23–25). HAART has had a significant impact on the incidence of bacterial pneumonia that appears independent of its effect on CD4 cell count (26). Mortality rates due to bacterial pneumonia are 10-fold higher than those in immunocompetent patients (17), and chronic lung disease with emphysema is a common sequelae (27,28).

S. pneumoniae is by far the most frequent identifiable pulmonary pathogen in patients with HIV infection. It is estimated that the frequency of pneumococcal bacteremia in patients with HIV infection is increased 100-fold compared with the general population (19,29,30). The increased risk applies to all CD4 strata but increases with progressive decline in CD4 count. All patients are at increased risk, but injection drug users are at a particularly high risk, as they are in the absence of HIV infection (7,15,16,26). The presentation of pneumococcal pneumonia in patients with HIV infection is not distinctive compared with those without HIV infection except for high rates of bacteremia (19,29,30). Cases of extrapulmonary infection, such as pneumococcal meningitis, endocarditis, or septic arthritis, do not appear to be unusually frequent. This complication is usually easy to distinguish from PCP based on common clinical features: acute onset, sputum production, pleurisy, consolidated infiltrate on chest radiography, and a CD4 count that may be above 200 cells/mm^3. Trimethoprim-sulfamethoxazole prophylaxis for PCP significantly reduces the frequency of pneumococcal infection (19); other PCP prophylaxis regimens do not.

Treatment guidelines are analogous to those for other patient populations with pneumococcal pneumonia, although there often needs to be concern about other unusual pathogens when the etiology is unclear, and serious pneumococcal infections require antibiotics selected on the assumption of β-lactam resistance unless sensitivity test results are available. The use of pneumococcal vaccine (Pneumovax) to prevent pneumococcal pneumonia in patients with HIV infection is controversial. An analysis by the Centers for Disease Control and Prevention (CDC) supports efficacy (31), but the vaccination causes a transient increase in HIV viremia (32), patients with CD4 counts less than 200 cells/mm^3 show a poor antigenic response (33), a study in Uganda actually showed this vaccine was associated with a significant increase in risk for pneumococcal infection (34), and others have shown no vaccine benefit (19). The current recommendation is to offer this vaccine to HIV-infected persons with CD4 counts greater than 200 cells/mm^3 (35).

H. influenzae is usually a distant second to *S. pneumoniae* among identified bacterial pathogens in bacterial pneumonia (15,16,18,20,36–38). The frequency of *H. influenzae* bacteremia is increased 100-fold compared with adults without HIV infection (36–38). Most pneumonia cases are caused by nonencapsulated strains (36–38). Most pneumonia cases are caused by nonencapsulated strains (36–38). Like pneumococcal pneumonia, clinical features of *H. influenzae* pneumonia in patients with HIV infection are not unique compared with persons without HIV infection, except for the increased rate of bacteremia, especially in late-stage disease. Management guidelines are also the same. *H.*

influenzae vaccine type B is not recommended because efficacy in this population has not been established, most cases are caused by nontypable strains, and infection rates are relatively low (35).

S. aureus plays an important role in patients with HIV-associated pulmonary infections because of its role in tricuspid valve endocarditis in injection drug users. The CD4 count appears to be important in the risk for endocarditis and for endocarditis outcome (36). Trimethoprim-sulfamethoxazole is active against most strains of community-acquired *S. aureus*, making it potentially useful for endocarditis prophylaxis as well, but efficacy for this is not clearly established. *S. aureus* endocarditis in injection drug users with HIV infection is clinically similar to this complication in patients without HIV infection; most cases involve the tricuspid valve, and patients present with fever, continuous bacteremia, and chest radiographs showing embolic lesions to the lung. Standard treatment is nafcillin-oxacillin with or without gentamicin, or vancomycin with or without gentamicin, for 2 to 4 weeks. The abbreviated 2-week course is commonly advocated for injection drug users with uncomplicated tricuspid valve endocarditis due to *S. aureus*, but the standard 4-week course is recommended in the presence of HIV infection (37). *S. aureus* may also cause pneumonia without endocarditis, but the frequency is low (4,7,14–22), except for nosocomial cases.

P. aeruginosa is a rare cause of community-acquired pneumonia in AIDS patients, except those with late-stage disease, when the CD4 count is less than 50 cells/mm^3 (18). Other risk factors are neutropenia and chronic corticosteroid use. Many of these patients have bacteremia. The prognosis is poor, and the recommendations for therapy are those for any patient with a systemic infection involving *P. aeruginosa*—usually a β-lactam (piperacillin, ticarcillin, ceftazidime, cefepime, imipenem, meropenem), usually in combination with tobramycin. Oral fluoroquinolones are sometimes used to shorten the course of intravenous therapy, but rates of relapse and fluoroquinolone resistance are high.

Atypical agents, including *Legionella* species, *C. pneumoniae*, and *M. pneumoniae*, appear to be relatively uncommon causes of community-acquired pneumonia (23–25). One study showed a 50-fold increase in the frequency of legionellosis in patients with HIV infection, but this is an isolated report not supported by subsequent studies (23). Blatt and colleagues (24) reviewed eight cases of legionellosis in HIV-infected patients and noted that the average CD4 count was 83 cells/mm^3; five cases were nosocomial, and none occurred in patients receiving trimethoprim-sulfamethoxazole prophylaxis. *C. pneumoniae* infection is not associated with immunodeficiency, and HIV-infected patients infrequently have this infection, or they have it based only on tenuous diagnostic criteria (15,18,20,25). One report indicated *C. pneumoniae* in 13 of 319 cases (2.5%) (25). Of the 13 cases, 3 had radiographic changes suggesting PCP. *M. pneumoniae* is also not generally associated with immunosuppression and infrequently appears in HIV-infected patients (15,18,20). With each of these three agents of atypical pulmonary infection, the diagnosis and management are similar for patients with and without HIV infection.

Rhodococcus equi is an uncommon opportunistic pathogen that may cause pneumonia in AIDS patients, usually when the CD4 count is less than 100 cells/mm^3 (39–42). Most patients have bacteremia. Changes in the lung are variable and include nodules, abscess, consolidated pneumonia, and empyema. It may be difficult to distinguish from pulmonary tuberculosis (43). Antibiotics that are most consistently active are erythromycin, rifampin, fluoroquinolones, aminoglycosides, vancomycin, and imipenem. Most patients are treated with at least two agents for at least 6 weeks, although most of this may be with oral agents (44). Some have also suggested patient isolation, although person-to-person transmission has not been convincingly demonstrated (41).

TUBERCULOSIS

Significance

The importance of tuberculosis as an HIV-associated process relates to several features of the infection. First is its frequency, especially in populations from resource-poor countries and in others with a high prevalence of preexisting tuberculous infection (6,45–47). Second, tuberculosis is perhaps the only HIV-associated infection that clearly can be transmitted from person to person, whether the person is HIV infected or not (48). Third, if diagnosed, the disease is easily and effectively treated (45). Fourth, the use of isoniazid preventive therapy and treatment of HIV infection (HAART) each significantly reduces the risk for tuberculosis in patients with latent *Mycobacterium tuberculosis* (49–52). Finally, treatment of active and latent tuberculosis significantly reduces morbidity and mortality in HIV-infected persons (45,51).

Tuberculosis complicating HIV infection has been noted primarily in persons and populations that are known to have relatively high rates of tuberculous infection—intravenous drug users and minority populations in the United States and the general population in persons in resource-limited countries (6,44–47). Thus, the major factors found to determine the likelihood of tuberculosis in a prospective cohort study were the place of residence and the severity of immunocompromise (52). The place of residence presumably served as a proxy for the background prevalence of tuberculosis. In the United States, the risk for active tuberculosis is high for injection drug users with HIV infection, but rates in the pre-HAART era ranged from 0.8 per 100 person-years to 7.9 per 100 person-years (52,53). Rates in these studies were significantly greater among persons with less than 200 CD4$^+$ cells/mm^3 and among those with positive (5 mm or more) tuberculin reactions. Rates were not higher among anergic subjects (52–54).

The full impact of HIV infection on the epidemiology of tuberculosis is substantial, especially in developing countries that show high rates of tuberculosis-related deaths in HIV-infected patients—far more than for PCP or any other opportunistic pathogen (6,45,47). Active tuberculosis is also recognized as a marker for suspect HIV infection in the United States and European countries (46,55).

Clinical Features

The clinical manifestations of tuberculosis in patients with HIV infection vary considerably, depending at what stage of HIV infection tuberculosis develops (52,54). In most series, the majority of tuberculosis diagnoses have antedated the identification of nontuberculous, AIDS-defining disease. Tuberculosis in early-stage HIV infection when the CD4 count is greater than 200 cells/mm^3 generally presents with the usual features of upper-lobe cavitary disease. In late-stage HIV infections, especially when the CD4 count is less than 50 cells/mm^3, there is a high frequency of disseminated or extrapulmonary sites of involvement, unusual radiographic manifestations, and nonreactive tuberculin skin test results. Lymph node involvement, including intrathoracic adenopathy, is frequent, and a variety of unusual manifestations have been noted, including central nervous system involvement with brain abscesses, tuberculomas, and meningitis; osteomyelitis; pericarditis; gastric tuberculosis; tuberculous peritonitis; and scrotal tuberculosis (45,55–59). In addition, *M. tuberculosis* has been frequently cultured from blood as well as from bone marrow (60).

Chest radiographs of HIV-infected patients with low CD4 counts and tuberculosis often show atypical features ranging from lower-zone involvement, diffuse infiltrates that may resemble PCP, or negative radiographs (61). Cavitation has been unusual, and intrathoracic adenopathy, an unusual finding in immunocompetent adults with tuberculosis, has been relatively frequent.

Diagnosis

As would be expected, persons with advanced HIV infection usually react minimally—or not at all—to the tuberculin skin test, but in earlier stages of the infection, reactivity may be sustained (46). The ability to respond to tuberculin is an indicator of the status of cell-mediated immunity, which in turn is an indicator of the stage of HIV infection. Because of the frequency of blunted skin test responses or anergy, it has been recommended that a reaction of at least 5 mm of induration to 5 tuberculin units of purified protein derivative (PPD) be regarded as indicative of tuberculous infection in persons with HIV infection (46). Most reported series indicate that the prevalence of positive sputum smears and cultures in patients with pulmonary tuberculosis is the same among HIV-infected and noninfected persons (52). In some instances, sputum induction or bronchoscopic procedures have been necessary to diagnose pulmonary tuberculosis. In general, the yield with induced sputa or bronchoscopy has not been better than expectorated sputa; thus, these methods are useful when they are done primarily for detection of other pathogens such as *P. carinii* or because there is no sputum production (62). Specimens from any site of infection in patients who have or may have HIV infection should be examined for mycobacteria by smear and culture. Potential high-yield sources include lymph nodes, bone marrow, urine, and blood.

Treatment

With a few notable exceptions, reported series of patients with tuberculosis and HIV infection demonstrate a good response to antituberculosis treatment (45,63), although failures have been reported (55,64,65). Current recommendation for adult patients with HIV infection is treatment that is identical to that for patients without HIV infection: isoniazid, 300 mg per day; rifampin, 600 mg per day (450 mg for persons weighing less than 50 kg); ethambutol, 15–25 mg/kg per day; and pyrazinamide, 20 to 30 mg/kg per day during the first 2 months of therapy. Isoniazid and rifampin should be continued for another 4 months, making the total duration of therapy 6 months (66). The single exception is the rifamycin component, which must be adjusted in form (rifabutin versus rifampin) and dose in patients receiving protease inhibitors or nonnucleoside reverse transcriptase inhibitors (67). Strong consideration should be given to administering therapy under direct observation to ensure adherence to the regimen. This can be facilitated by twice- or thrice-weekly dosing after an initial phase of daily treatment; patients with advanced HIV infection should receive intermittent treatment at least thrice weekly owing to reported rifamycin resistance with less frequent dosing in the initial stage of treatment (68,69).

Findings of at least one study suggested that persons with HIV infection have more adverse reactions to antituberculosis drugs (9); thus, patients with HIV infection should be observed closely with appropriate laboratory and clinical monitoring. Concurrent HAART therapy may be problematic in patients treated for tuberculosis because of the complexity of the regimens, the high frequency of adverse reactions to these drugs, and the frequent problem of drug interactions, as with rifamycin. For patients with previously untreated HIV infection

who have indications for antiretroviral agents, the World Health Organization has made the following recommendations (70):

- Active tuberculosis always takes precedence for immediate treatment due, in part, to the public health issues.
- Treatment of both tuberculosis and HIV should not be started simultaneously because of problems anticipated with seven or eight new drugs with high rates of adverse reactions and drug intolerances.
- With advanced HIV infection with CD4 counts less than 50 cells/mm^3, antiretroviral therapy should begin as soon as antituberculosis treatment is tolerated. With less advanced disease (CD4 counts of 50 to 350 cells/mm^3), the antiretroviral regimen can be delayed for 2 months.

Resistance to primary antituberculosis agents was problematic in HIV-infected patients in the mid-1990s, especially among injection drug users in New York City (71,72). The problem of multidrug-resistant *M. tuberculosis* was largely resolved by implementation of standard public health measures, but the experience serves to remind us about the importance of standard disease control strategies, including the need for adherence to standard regimens with emphasis on directly observed therapy. Multidrug-resistant *M. tuberculosis* remains a concern, especially in some areas of the world where access to drugs is erratic (73).

Response to therapy is generally similar in patients with and without HIV co-infection (65). This includes the time to sputum conversion (74). In general, symptoms should improve within 4 weeks, sputum AFB smear and culture should be negative in 2 to 3 months, and chest radiographs should show improvement in 2 to 3 months. If smears or cultures are positive at 2 to 3 months, there should be concern for noncompliance or resistance. Patients with resistant strains need treatment with at least two active drugs.

Preventive Therapy

Preventive therapy, now considered treatment of latent tuberculosis, has been proved to be widely effective in preventing active tuberculosis among multiple groups of persons with tuberculous infection, including persons infected with HIV. HIV infection represents a greater risk for active tuberculosis than virtually any other risk factor among persons with latent tuberculosis (46). For this reason, tuberculin testing must be a routine part of HIV management. Patients who react with at least 5 mm of induration to 5 tuberculin units of PPD are considered to have tuberculous infection and must be offered preventive therapy. The sensitivity of the PPD skin test approaches 100% in persons who are immunocompetent but is insensitive when the CD4 count is below 200 cells/mm^3, as noted earlier. This observation justifies the need to test in early-stage disease when possible and to repeat these tests with immune reconstitutions in those with negative tests done only in later stages of HIV infection.

The preferred regimens are isoniazid plus pyridoxine for 9 months or rifampin-rifabutin plus pyrazinamide for 2 months. The advantages of the rifampin-rifabutin plus pyrazinamide regimen are that efficacy is established and the regimen can be completed in 2 months, which is a substantial advantage in patients who have a low probability of completing the 9-month course of isoniazid, especially when considering the magnitude of the risk associated with HIV infection. The problem with this 2-month regimen has been cases of severe hepatotoxicity, including six deaths attributed to this combination (75). The decision for rifabutin versus rifampin in this regimen is based on the concurrent use of protease inhibitors or nevirapine because of the profound effect of rifampin-associated drug interactions (67). The potential advantage of the isoniazid regimen is the assumption of better safety and lack of drug interactions with antiretroviral agents; this would be preferred in cases in which compliance with the 9 months of treatment is not problematic, especially if given with directly observed treatment (76). Immune reconstitution is another method that is highly effective in reducing the risk for active tuberculosis in patients with latent infection (49). Another preventive strategy is adequate management of persons placed at risk by exposure to patients with active pulmonary tuberculosis. This is particularly important in health care workers who deal with these patients, although the risk does not appear to be different with exposure to active tuberculosis in patients with or without HIV infection (48). Nevertheless, substantial outbreaks of tuberculosis with HIV-infected patients as the source have been reported (77,78).

MYCOBACTERIA OTHER THAN TUBERCULOSIS

Patients with advanced HIV infection often have disseminated *Mycobacterium avium* infection with involvement of bone marrow, lymph nodes, and multiple other organs. The organism can usually be isolated from blood, bone marrow, and other sites of involvement (79). The lung is infrequently involved in these cases. Much less commonly, *M. avium* complex may produce focal disease limited to the lung or endobronchial lesions may be seen at bronchoscopy.

Except for *M. avium* complex, infections with nontuberculous mycobacteria have been uncommon in patients with HIV infection. However, there are several case reports and small series of infections involving *Mycobacterium kansasii*, *Mycobacterium xenopi*, *Mycobacterium scrofulaceum*, *Mycobacterium szulgai*, *Mycobacterium flavescens*, *Mycobacterium gordonae*, *Mycobacterium asiaticum*, and *Mycobacterium malmoense* (80,81).

FUNGAL INFECTIONS

Pneumocystis carinii Pneumonia

EPIDEMIOLOGY

Serologic studies indicate that most persons have antibody to *P. carinii* by 2 years of age (82). The assumption has been that infection in adults reflects activation of a dormant pathogen when the host is immunosuppressed. More recent data suggest the organism may be transmitted, and exposure may account for a substantial number of cases (83–85) regardless of the mechanism of acquisition. PCP continues to be the most frequent identifiable cause of lung infection among persons with less than 200 CD4$^+$ lymphocytes/mm^3, and this occurs despite wide use of effective PCP prophylaxis and HAART (82). Because *P. carinii* is not a particularly pathogenic organism, severe immune compromise, indicated by a marked reduction in CD4$^+$ lymphocytes, must be present for the organism to proliferate and cause disease. Kovacs and associates (85) found that patients with PCP had a median of 26 CD4$^+$ cells/mm^3 (interquartile range, 12 to 62.5 cells/mm^3). In only 2 of 46 episodes of PCP were the CD4$^+$ cell counts greater than 200 cells/mm^3. Others have reported similar results (86,87).

CLINICAL FEATURES

The most common presenting symptoms of PCP are fever, cough, and dyspnea (5,85–87). The shortness of breath usually progresses from being present only with exertion to being present at rest. Cough is generally nonproductive but may be associated with sputum in patients who smoke and those who have bacterial bronchitis or bacterial pneumonia as well as PCP. At the time evaluation for PCP is undertaken, the respiratory symptoms may be prominent or relatively minor. Antipneumocystis prophylaxis reduces the severity of PCP, so that the presenting symptoms may be subtle. Conversely, patients who have not been under medical care and who do not readily seek medical attention may present with advanced pneumonia and severe symptoms. A highly characteristic feature of PCP in patients with HIV infection is the relatively slow evolution of disease over weeks; this is in sharp contrast to PCP in other patient populations (88) and in patients with bacterial pneumonia.

For patients with PCP, the physical examination is not particularly helpful, except for fever and tachypnea, which are nearly always present. Initial laboratory evaluation shows the CD4 count is usually but not invariably below 200 cells/mm^3 (87), and blood gases or pulse oximetry usually show oxygen desaturation. Chest radiographs most often show diffuse interstitial infiltration involving all portions of the lungs equally (85). Several variations of the basic pattern may be seen, including uneven distribution or a more miliary appearance. Other variations include diffuse and focal airspace consolidation, cystic changes or pneumatoceles (particularly during the healing process), cavitation, and spontaneous pneumothorax. Pleural effusions and intrathoracic adenopathy are uncommon. About 10% to 20% of patients have normal chest radiographs. High-resolution or thin-section computed tomography (CT) in these cases usually shows a characteristic ground-glass appearance (85).

DIAGNOSIS

P. carinii cannot be detected in purulent sputum because the cells and cellular debris preclude detection of the organism. Standard methods for specimen collection are induced sputa and bronchoscopy specimens. The sensitivity of induced sputa is highly variable but usually reported at 60% to 95% (85,89–92). With bronchoscopy, the sensitivity is 95% or greater (85,93). An experimental polymerase chain reaction (PCR) technique may facilitate this diagnosis with a simple method to obtain specimens using an oral wash or gargle (85,94,95). Standard teaching in the past has been that detection of *P. carinii* in a respiratory specimen is diagnostic of PCP; use of PCR technology with oral washes with positive results in the absence of disease has caused skepticism about this dictum (94).

TREATMENT

Empirical treatment remains controversial. On the negative side of the argument, another treatable process may be missed, and such an approach exposes the patient to the risks of therapy, perhaps without benefit. On the positive side, for patients who have classic clinical features, it has been demonstrated that a presumptive diagnosis can be established with a high degree of accuracy by experienced clinicians, it saves the expense and ardor related to obtaining induced sputa or bronchoscopy, and it is especially attractive for patients who are not seriously ill and have very typical symptoms (96,97).

Treatment of PCP in patients with AIDS is essentially the same as for patients with other forms of immunosuppression (see Chapter 283), but several points deserve mention. First, after therapy is instituted, patients with PCP and AIDS may worsen before they improve (98). The response to a specific agent cannot be determined within the first 5 or 6 days of treatment. Second, adverse reactions to antipneumocystis agents are common in AIDS patients and tend to occur between days 5 and 15 of treatment. Third, patients with more severe forms of PCP benefit from corticosteroid therapy (99–101). Despite the advances in HIV management, the mortality rate for PCP remains at 15% to 20% for hospitalized patients treated with standard regimens (102). Changes in treatment are most successful if the reason to change treatment is due to adverse reactions rather than therapeutic failure. However, there are multiple regimens from which to select, all of which have established merit (103). Resistance to standard drugs, including trimethoprim-sulfamethoxazole, appears to either be unprovable or nonexistent (104).

PROPHYLAXIS

Prophylaxis for PCP has proved to be effective and important for persons with HIV infection (105–107). Preventive therapy is indicated for patients who have any of the following: CD4$^+$ lymphocyte count less than 200 cells/mm^3, unexplained and persistent fever, oral candidiasis, or prior PCP. Trimethoprim-sulfamethoxazole is usually considered the prophylactic agent of choice, although dapsone, atovaquone, and aerosolized pentamidine are also effective (105).

Pulmonary Aspergillosis

Aspergillus species accounts for 1% to 4% of pneumonias in patients with AIDS (106–109). Nearly all patients have CD4 counts of less than 50 cells/mm^3, and about half have neutropenia, corticosteroid administration, or both. Other risk factors include marijuana use, structural disease of the lung, and exposure to broad-spectrum antibiotics.

The two clinical forms of aspergillosis in this population are invasive parenchymal disease and tracheobronchial disease. Invasive parenchymal aspergillosis is associated with three types of changes on chest radiograph: cavitary disease usually involving the upper lobe, focal infiltrates that are often pleural based, and bilateral infiltrates that may show a nodular or interstitial pattern (106). The types of tracheobronchial disease include a pseudomembranous form (110) and an ulcerative form (111), or an obstructive form with mucous plugs (112). Patients with the invasive form usually present with fever, cough, and dyspnea that evolves over a period of weeks or months. There may be pleurisy or hemoptysis (106,109). The usual clinical features of tracheobronchial disease are dyspnea, cough, and wheezing accompanied by a chest radiograph that is usually normal or shows atelectasis.

The diagnosis requires the recovery of *Aspergillus* species from a normally sterile site or positive cultures or stains recovered twice from respiratory secretions with a compatible clinical illness, including chest imaging (113,114). Clinical correlations are critical because *Aspergillus* species may colonize airways or represent a laboratory contaminant. The predominant species in AIDS patients with aspergillosis is *Aspergillus fumigatus*.

The overall prognosis is poor, with a median survival time of 3 months (109). Amphotericin B is considered the drug of choice; itraconazole may be effective, but the experience is somewhat limited, and this drug is recommended primarily for long-term follow-up after amphotericin induction (109,115). Also important is treatment directed against underlying defects, including neutropenia and corticosteroid use. HAART with immune reconstitution may represent the best option for long-term control of this pathogen.

Pulmonary Cryptococcosis

Cryptococcosis is a common complication of late-stage HIV infection, usually with meningitis that may be accompanied by pulmonary involvement, or, less commonly, there may be pneumonia without extrapulmonary disease (116–118). The CD4 cell count is usually less than 100 cells/mm^3.

The usual symptoms with pulmonary cryptococcosis are fever, cough, and dyspnea with or without pleurisy that evolves over a period of weeks (116–118). Some patients have completely silent symptoms with lesions detected on radiograph. The chest radiograph usually shows diffuse interstitial infiltrates that often suggest PCP; other radiographic changes include focal infiltrates, cavities, reticulonodular infiltrates, hilar adenopathy, or pleural effusions.

About 90% of patients with cryptococcosis have positive serum antigen assays for *Cryptococcosis neoformans* (119). The antigen may also be detected in respiratory secretions with pulmonary infections (120), but the preferred diagnostic test is recovery of the organism in sputum or bronchoalveolar lavage (BAL) (121). This organism is a relatively rare contaminant, so recovery is virtually diagnostic. All patients with pulmonary cryptococcosis should have a lumbar puncture to determine the concurrent presence of meningitis that may be clinically silent.

The treatment of cryptococcal meningitis usually consists of amphotericin B, followed by lifelong fluconazole as reviewed elsewhere in this book (see Chapter 33). Experience is limited for patients with pulmonary infection without disseminated disease, but most authorities recommend amphotericin B for serious infections and fluconazole for more indolent infections (122). The duration of treatment in the absence of meningitis is ill defined. For follow-up, there should be attention to chest radiograph changes and cultivability of *C. neoformans*; serum cryptococcal antigen assays are not useful (123,124). As with virtually all opportunistic infections, effective antiviral therapy for HIV with immune reconstitution probably plays an important role in controlling this disease.

Histoplasmosis

Histoplasma capsulatum is endemic in the Mississippi, Ohio, and St. Lawrence River valleys. Histoplasmosis has been reported in more than 5% of patients with AIDS living in the endemic area (125). Cases in the endemic area usually represent primary infection with progressive dissemination; patients residing outside the endemic area usually have reactivation of latent infection (126). Serious and disseminated disease is usually a consequence of severe immunosuppression, and most patients have CD4 cell counts below 100 cells/mm^3.

Most patients with histoplasmosis complicating AIDS have disseminated disease, but pulmonary involvement is seen in up to 70% of these patients (125,127). Common pulmonary symptoms include cough, fever, and dyspnea that are usually indolent in onset. Other common features that reflect disseminated disease include typical lesions of the skin and mucosal surfaces, wasting, bone marrow suppression, hepatosplenomegaly, lymphadenopathy, and diarrhea.

The usual changes on chest radiograph are diffuse, interstitial, or reticulonodular infiltrates; other features found less commonly are focal infiltrates, hilar adenopathy, and pleural effusions (125,127).

The preferred diagnostic test is detection of *H. capsulatum* polysaccharide antigen in blood or urine by radioimmunoassay, a test available from reference laboratories. The sensitivity of this test is 85% to 97% among patients with disseminated histoplasmosis; the antigen may also be detected in BAL specimens of up to 90% of patients with pulmonary involvement (128,129). The organism may also be detected by stain and culture of expectorated sputum in about 30% of patients (130,131). Standard serologic tests are relatively insensitive (50% to 70%), and the histoplasmosis skin test is useless (125).

The standard treatment for disseminated histoplasmosis or the progressive pulmonary form is amphotericin B, and this is recommended for patients with severe disease (122,130). Liposomal amphotericin is superior in terms of clinical efficacy and reduced side effects (131). Itraconazole may be used for initial treatment in patients with mild or moderately severe infection and for those with more serious disease after amphotericin B induction (132). Fluconazole is inferior to itraconazole (132). Response to therapy may be monitored by the reduction in titers of *Histoplasma* species capsular antigen in blood and urine (129).

Coccidioidomycosis

Coccidioides immitis is endemic in the southwestern United States and represents a significant risk for patients with HIV infection. The rate in Arizona for 1994 to 1997 was reported at 4% per year for AIDS patients, a 300-fold increase over that seen in the general population (133).

Pulmonary involvement is frequent, and many patients also have extrapulmonary involvement that is most commonly expressed as cutaneous lesions, joint infections, or meningitis. Typical symptoms include cough, fever, and dyspnea, usually with an indolent presentation. The chest radiograph typically shows diffuse or focal infiltrates; less frequent findings are pulmonary nodules, hilar adenopathy, cavity formation, or pleural effusions (134,135). The diagnosis is usually established with serology or stain and culture of respiratory secretions. The skin test is generally not useful in the HIV-infected population.

Patients with diffuse pulmonary disease or disseminated disease have a poor prognosis and should receive aggressive treatment with amphotericin B or an azole (122). A current controversy is the use of prophylactic azoles in patients with AIDS who reside in the endemic area due to the substantial risk for disseminated disease with low CD4 counts (133).

VIRAL INFECTIONS

Although a variety of viral pathogens have been isolated from the lungs of patients with HIV infection, it is difficult to determine the frequency with which these agents actually cause pneumonitis. Members of the herpesvirus family, especially cytomegalovirus (CMV), are found commonly in lung-derived specimens. In general, however, it appears that CMV infection is common but is infrequently the cause of significant lung disease (136). The organism is frequently detected in bronchoscopy specimens, but the significance is often unclear. This diagnosis requires demonstration of typical cytopathic effect or isolation of the virus combined with compatible histologic findings and failure to define an alternative agent. Treatment of CMV pneumonitis in patients with HIV has not proved to be particularly effective, although experience is limited. Ganciclovir and valganciclovir have been useful in treating both retinitis and colitis, and cidofovir and foscarnet are probably equally effective; therefore, any of these agents may be tried in patients with pneumonitis.

Other herpesvirus infections (herpes simplex, varicella-zoster, and Epstein-Barr virus infection) have also been implicated as causing lung disease in patients with HIV infection, but recovery from respiratory secretions is inadequate to establish a pathogenic role. Varicella-zoster virus associated with typical skin lesions, for example, varicella pneumonia, is regarded as a serious infection in AIDS patients that requires rapid institution of intravenous acyclovir and possibly corticosteroids (137).

Influenza virus is a potentially important agent in patients with HIV infection because it is common in all patient populations, it appears to predispose to pneumonia caused by common bacterial pathogens such as *S. pneumoniae*, and one study showed a substantial risk for influenza-related deaths in AIDS patients hospitalized with influenza (138). The current recommendation is for influenza vaccine in all persons with HIV infection (139), although the response rate is low or nil if the CD4 count is less than 100 cells/mm³ and the viral load is greater than 30,000 copies/mL (140). This vaccination may cause a transient (2- to 4-week) increase in HIV viral load, but this finding is inconsistent, and its significance, if real, is unknown (141).

EVALUATION

The differential diagnosis in the HIV-infected patient with a suspected pulmonary infection requires a thoughtful analysis based largely on five variables: geography (developed versus developing countries), temporal evolution (acute versus chronic), CD4 count, extrapulmonary findings, and changes seen on chest radiograph (Tables 115.1 and 115.2). Exposure to antimicrobial agents for treatment and prophylaxis is also important. The CD4 cell count is critical (Table 115.1). Nearly all opportunistic infections are relatively rare in patients with CD4 cell counts exceeding 200 cells/mm³; the major exceptions are pneumococcal pneumonia and tuberculosis. Patients with injection drug use have this as an independent risk factor for pneumococcal pneumonia, tuberculosis, and tricuspid valve endocarditis with septic emboli to the lung. The chest radiograph is critical for establishing pneumonia and for suggesting specific etiologic agents. The differential diagnosis based on chest radiograph changes is summarized in Table 115.2. Nearly all infectious diseases involving the pulmonary parenchyma are associated with demonstrable infiltrates on radiograph, although false-negative radiographs are seen in up to 30% of patients with PCP and in occasional patients with pulmonary tuberculosis, cryptococcosis, or *M. avium* infection. CT scans and high-resolution CT scans are relatively

TABLE 115.1.   Etiologic Agent Based on CD4 Count

CD4 count	Common	Infrequent
>200 cells/mm³	*Streptococcus pneumoniae*	Atypical agents
		Staphylococcus aureus
	Haemophilus influenzae	Endemic fungi
		Pneumocystis carinii
	Mycobacterium tuberculosis	Mycobacteria other than tuberculosis (MOTT)
		Anaerobic bacteria
		Respiratory viruses
50–200 cells/mm³	Above plus	Above plus
	Pneumocystis carinii	Kaposi's sarcoma
		Lymphoma
		Cryptococcosis
		Legionella species infection
		Nocardia species infection
		Rhodococcus equi
		Aspergillus species infection
		Mycobacterium kansasii
<50 cells/mm³	Above	Above plus
		Cytomegalovirus
		Aspergillosis

TABLE 115.2. Differential Diagnosis of Pulmonary Complications Based on Chest Radiograph Changes

Change	Most common agents	Infrequent
Consolidation	Pyogenic bacteria[a] Cryptococcosis Kaposi's sarcoma	*Nocardia* species *M. tuberculosis* *Mycobacterium kansasii* *Bordetella bronchiseptica*
Diffuse interstitial or reticulonodular infiltrates	*Pneumocystis carinii*[a] Miliary tuberculosis Histoplasmosis Coccidioidomycosis Cryptococcosis	Kaposi's sarcoma Lymphocytic interstitial pneumonia *Leishmania donovani* *Toxoplasma gondii*
Nodule	*Mycobacterium tuberculosis* Cryptococcosis Kaposi's sarcoma	
Cavity	*M. tuberculosis* *Pseudomonas aeruginosa* GNB (other) *M. kansasii* Cryptococcosis Histoplasmosis Coccidioidomycosis Aspergillosis *Rhodococcus equi* Anaerobic bacteria *Staphylococcus aureus* (IDU) *Nocardia* species	*Legionella* species *P. carinii* Lymphoma *Mycobacterium avium*
Pleural effusion	Pyogenic bacteria[a] Kaposi's sarcoma *M. tuberculosis* Cryptococcosis *P. carinii* Hypoalbuminemia Septic emboli (IDU) Heart failure	*R. equi* Histoplasmosis Coccidioidomycosis *L. donovani* Lymphoma *M. avium* *Nocardia* species *P. carinii* Aspergillosis
Hilar adenopathy	*M. tuberculosis* Cryptococcosis *M. avium* Histoplasmosis Coccidioidomycosis Kaposi's sarcoma Lymphoma	
Normal radiograph	*P. carinii*[a] *M. tuberculosis*	*Cryptococcus* species *M. avium*

GNB, gram-negative bacteria; IDU, injection drug user.
[a]Most common cause.
Adapted from Bartlett JG. Medical management of HIV infection. Baltimore, JG Bartlett, 1998:247, with permission.

sensitive in terms of detection of subtle lesions and also for defining pathology.

Etiologic Diagnosis

Expectorated sputum for stain and culture remains the preferred diagnostic test for recognition of common bacterial pathogens (other than atypical agents), mycobacteria, and occasional fungal infections; these specimens are useless for detection of noninfectious diseases with pulmonary involvement (lymphoma and Kaposi's sarcoma), members of the herpesvirus group, and *P. carinii*. Induced sputum is an alternative method to obtain lower respiratory tract secretions for detection of *P. carinii* and *M. tuberculosis*; utility for detecting other respiratory tract pathogens is less well established. Bronchoscopy is advocated for enigmatic pulmonary infections, including PCP (with negative induced sputa or no induced sputa) and tuberculosis (with negative tests using alternative specimens). Bronchoscopy with biopsy may be required for patients with selected noninfectious pulmonary conditions (lymphoma, Kaposi's sarcoma) and some fungal infections. Bronchoscopy is not considered superior to expectorated sputum for detection of acid-fast bacilli (AFB) or for detecting conventional bacteria.

Respiratory secretions, when obtained, should have Gram stain and sputum cytology, and specimens suggesting *S. pneumoniae* should preferably have laboratory confirmation with a quellung test. Specialized tests advocated for selective organisms include acid-fast stains for mycobacteria, Gomori methenamine silver stain, potassium hydroxide, and calcofluor white stain for fungi; and direct fluorescent antibody staining for influenza virus, respiratory syncytial virus, adenovirus, and parainfluenza. Conventional media are used for detecting the usual bacteria, and specialized media are required for *Legionella* and most fungi other than *Candida*.

Empirical Treatment

It is often necessary to initiate antibiotic therapy before diagnostic studies become available; even when these tests are available, they are often negative or indecisive. Patients with suspected bacterial pneumonia should be treated according to standard guidelines (136). The recommendation for outpatients is a macrolide, fluoroquinolone, or doxycycline. For hospitalized patients on a general medical ward, the recommendation is for a β-lactam (cefotaxime or ceftriaxone) with or without a macrolide; the alternative is a fluoroquinolone. Patients with clinical features supportive of a diagnosis of PCP must be treated for that disease because of universal lethality without treatment and a mortality rate of 15% to 20% even with treatment. Although empirical treatment is sometimes advocated, most patients merit a diagnostic evaluation, which often means empirical treatment pending results of induced sputum or bronchoscopy. Only a negative bronchoscopy is considered definitive evidence against this diagnosis. The usual treatment is trimethoprim-sulfamethoxazole, but this cannot be considered adequate for concurrent coverage of common bacteria such as *S. pneumoniae* because of high rates of resistance. Patients with suspected pulmonary tuberculosis should be treated empirically with four drugs and placed on appropriate precautions pending results of AFB smears and cultures. Positive AFB smears usually indicate *M. tuberculosis*.

REFERENCES

1. Wallace JM, Hansen NI, Lavange L, et al. Respiratory disease trends in the Pulmonary Complications of HIV Infection study cohort. *Am J Respir Crit Care Med* 1997;155:72.
2. Hirschtick RE, Glassroth J, Jordan MC, et al. Bacterial pneumonia in persons infected with the human immunodeficiency virus. *N Engl J Med* 1995;333:845.
3. Centers for Disease Control and Prevention. *HIV/AIDS Surveillance Report* 1995;7:18.
4. Murray JF, Felton CP, Garay S, et al. Pulmonary complications of the acquired immunodeficiency syndrome. Report of a National Heart, Lung, and Blood Institute Workshop. *N Engl J Med* 1984;310:1682.
5. Beck JM, Rosen MJ, Peavy HH. Pulmonary complications of HIV infection. *Am J Respir Crit Care Med* 2001;164:21.
6. Lanjewar DN, Duggal R. Pulmonary pathology in patients with AIDS: An autopsy study from Mumbai. *HIV Med* 2001;2:266.
7. Wallace JM, Hansen NI, LaVange L, et al. Respiratory disease trends in the pulmonary complications of HIV infection study cohort. *Am J Respir Crit Care Med* 1997;155:72.
8. Markowitz N, Hansen NI, Wilcosky TC, et al. Tuberculin and anergy in HIV seropositive and HIV-seronegative persons. *Ann Intern Med* 1993;119:185.
9. Chaisson RE, Schecter, GF, Theuer CP, et al. Tuberculosis in patients with the acquired immunodeficiency syndrome: clinical features, response to therapy, and survival. *Am Rev Respir Dis* 1987;136:570.
10. Huang BD, Ruben FL, Rinaldo CR, et al. Antibody response after influenza and pneumococcal immunization in HIV-infected homosexual men. *JAMA* 1989;261:245.
11. Nelson KE, Clements ML, Miotti P, et al. The influence of human immunodeficiency virus (HIV) infection on antibody responses to influenza vaccines. *Ann Intern Med* 1988;109:383.
12. USPHS/IDSA Prevention of Opportunistic Infections Working Group: 1997 USPHS/IDSA guidelines for the prevention of opportunistic infections in persons infected with human immunodeficiency virus: disease-specific recommendations. *Clin Infect Dis* 1997;25[Suppl 3]:S313.
13. Wallace JM, Rao AV, Glassroth J, et al. Respiratory illness in persons with human immunodeficiency virus infection. *Am Rev Respir Dis* 1993;148:523.
14. Swindells S, Evans S, Zackin R, et al. Predictive value of HIV-1 viral load on risk of opportunistic infection. *J Acquir Immune Defic Syndr* 2002;30:154.
15. Hirschtick RE, Glassroth J, Jordan MC, et al. Bacterial pneumonia in persons infected with the human immunodeficiency virus. *N Engl J Med* 1995;333:845.
16. Witt DJ, Craven DE, McCabe WR. Bacterial infections in adult patients with the acquired immunodeficiency syndrome (AIDS) and AIDS-related complex. *Am J Med* 1987;82:900.
17. Lin JC, Nichol KL. Excess mortality due to pneumonia or influenza during influenza seasons among persons with acquired immunodeficiency syndrome. *Arch Intern Med* 2001;161:441.
18. Cordero E, Pachon J, Rivero A, et al. Community-acquired bacterial pneumonia in HIV-infected patients: validation of severity criteria. *Am Rev Respir Care Med* 2000;162:2063.
19. Navin TR, Rimland D, Lennox JL, et al. Risk factors for community-acquired pneumonia among persons infected with HIV. *J Infect Dis* 2000;181:158.
20. Park DR, Sherbin VL, Goodman MS, et al. The etiology of community-acquired pneumonia at an urban public hospital: influence of HIV infection and initial severity of illness. *J Infect Dis* 2001;184:268.
21. Cordero E, Pachon J, Rivero A, et al. Usefulness of sputum culture in the diagnosis of bacterial pneumonia in HIV-infected patients. *Eur J Clin Microbiol Infect Dis* 2002;21:362.
22. Benito N, Rano A, Moreno A, et al. Pulmonary infiltrates in HIV-infected patients in the highly active antiretroviral therapy era in Spain. *J Acquir Immune Defic Syndr* 2001;27:35.
23. Stout JE, Yu VL. Legionellosis. *N Engl J Med* 1997;337:682.
24. Blatt SP, Dolan MJ, Hendrix CW, et al. Legionnaires' disease in human immunodeficiency virus-infected patients: eight cases and review. *Clin Infect Dis* 1994;18:227.
25. Comandini UV, Maggi P, Santopadre P, et al. *Chlamydia pneumonia* respiratory infections among patients infected with the human immunodeficiency virus. *Eur J Clin Microbiol Infect Dis* 1997;16:720.
26. Sullivan JH, Moore RD, Keruly JC, et al. Effect of antiretroviral therapy on the incidence of bacterial pneumonia in patients with advanced HIV infection. *Am J Respir Crit Care Med* 2000;162:64.
27. Morris AM, Huang L, Bacchette P, et al. Permanent declines in pulmonary function following pneumonia in HIV-infected persons. *Am J Respir Crit Care Med* 2000;162:612.
28. Diaz PT, King MA, Pacht ER, et al. Increased susceptibility to pulmonary emphysema among HIV seropositive smokers. *Ann Intern Med* 2000;132:369.
29. Nuorti JP, Butler JC, Gelling L, et al. Epidemiologic relation between HIV and invasive pneumococcal disease in San Francisco County, California. *Ann Intern Med* 2000;132:182.
30. McEllistrem MC, Mendelsohn AB, Pass MA, et al. Recurrent invasive pneumococcal disease in individuals with HIV infection. *J Infect Dis* 2002;185:1364.
31. Breiman RF, Keller DW, Phelan MA, et al. Evaluation of effectiveness of the 23-valent pneumococcal capsular polysaccharide vaccine for HIV-infected patients. *Arch Intern Med* 2000;160:2633.
32. Brichacek B, Swindells S, Janoff EN, et al. Increased plasma human immunodeficiency virus type 1 burden following antigenic challenge with pneumococcal vaccine. *J Infect Dis* 1996;174:1191.
33. French N, Naiziyingi J, Carpenter LM, et al. 23-Valent pneumococcal polysaccharide vaccine in HIV-1-infected Ugandan adults: double-blind, randomized and placebo-controlled trial. *Lancet* 2000;355:2106.
34. Dworkin MS, Ward JW, Hanson DL, et al. Pneumococcal disease among human immunodeficiency virus-infected persons: incidence, risk factors, and impact of vaccination. *Clin Infect Dis* 2001;32:794.
35. Center for Disease Control and Prevention. Guidelines for preventing opportunistic infections among HIV-infected persons—2002. Recommendations of the U.S. Public Health Service and the Infectious Diseases Society of America. *MMWR Morb Mortal Wkly Rep* 2002;51;RR-8:1.
36. Cordero E, Pachon J, Rivero A, et al. *Haemophilus influenzae* pneumonia in HIV-infected patients. *Clin Infect Dis* 2000;30:361.
37. Munoz P, Miranda ME, Llacaqueo A, et al. *Haemophilus* species bacteremia in adults. *Arch Intern Med* 1997;157:1869.
38. Steinhart R, Reingold AL, Taylor F, et al. Invasive *Haemophilus influenzae* infections in men with HIV infection. *JAMA* 1992;268:3350.
39. Blatt SP, Dolan MU, Hendrix CW, et al. Legionnaires' disease in human immunodeficiency virus-infected patients: eight cases and review. *Clin Infect Dis* 1994;18:227.
40. Weinstock DM, Brown AE. *Rhodococcus equi*: an emerging pathogen. *Clin Infect Dis* 2002;34:1379.
41. Verville TD, Huycke MM, Greenfield RA, et al. *Rhodococcus equi* in humans: 12 cases and a review of the literature. *Medicine* 1994;73:119.
42. Arlotti M, Zoboli G, Moscatelli G, et al. *Rhodococcus equi* infection in HIV-positive subjects: a retrospective analysis of 24 cases. *Scand J Infect Dis* 1996;28:463.
43. Gray KJ, French N, Lugada E, et al. *Rhodococcus equi* and HIV infection in Uganda. *J Infect* 2000;41:227.
44. Rouquet RM, Clave D, Massip P, et al. Imipenem/vancomycin for *Rhodococcus equi* pulmonary infection in an HIV-positive patient. *Lancet* 1991;337:337.
45. Coleblunders R, Lambert ML. Management of co-infection with HIV and tuberculosis. *BMJ* 2002;324:802.
46. Centers for Disease Control and Prevention. New ATS/CDC guidelines for testing and treatment of latent tuberculosis. *MMWR Morb Mortal Wkly Rep* 2000;49:RR-6.
47. Mwachari CW, Cohen CR, Meier AS, et al. Respiratory tract infection in HIV-1-infected adults in Nairobi, Kenya: evaluation of risk factors and the World Health Organization treatment algorithm. *J Acquir Immune Defic Syndr* 2001;27:365.
48. Zahnow K, Matta JP, Hillman D, et al. Rates of tuberculosis infection in health-care workers providing services to HIV-infected populations. *Infect Control Hosp Epidemiol* 1998;19:829.
49. Badri M, Wilson D, Wood R. Effect of highly active antiretroviral therapy on incidence of tuberculosis in South Africa: a cohort study. *Lancet* 2002;359:2059.
50. Sterling TR, Alwood K, Gachuhi R, et al. Relapse rates after short course (6 months) treatment of tuberculosis in HIV-infected and uninfected persons. *AIDS* 1999;13:1899.
51. Wilkinson D, Squire SB, Garner P. Effect of preventive treatment for

tuberculosis in adults infected with HIV: systematic review of randomized placebo controlled trials. *BMJ* 1998;317:625.

52. Kirk O, Gattell JM, Mocroft A, et al. Infections with *Mycobacterium tuberculosis* and *Mycobacterium avium* among HIV-infected patients after the introduction of highly active antiretroviral therapy. *Am J Respir Crit Care Med* 2000;162:865.

53. Selwyn PA, Hartel D, Lewis VA, et al. A prospective study of the risk of tuberculosis among intravenous drug users with human immunodeficiency virus infection. *N Engl J Med* 1989;320:545.

54. Jones BE, Young SMM, Antoniskis D, et al. Relationship of the manifestations of tuberculosis to CD4 cell counts in patients with human immunodeficiency virus infection. *Am Rev Respir Dis* 1993;148:1292.

55. Sunderam G, McDonald RJ, Maniatis T, et al. Tuberculosis as a manifestation of the acquired immunodeficiency syndrome (AIDS). *JAMA* 1986;256:362.

56. Brody JM, Muller DK, Zeman RK, et al. Gastric tuberculosis: a manifestation of acquired immunodeficiency syndrome. *Radiology* 1986;159:347.

57. Barnes P, Leedon J, Radin DR, et al. An unusual case of tuberculous peritonitis in a man with AIDS. *West J Med* 1986;144:467.

58. Smith MB, Boyars MC, Veasey S, et al. Generalized tuberculosis in the acquired immune deficiency syndrome. *Arch Pathol Lab Med* 2000;124:1267.

59. Saltzman BR, Motyl MR, Friedland GH, et al. *Mycobacterium tuberculosis* bacteremia in the acquired immunodeficiency syndrome. *JAMA* 1986;256:390.

60. Pedro-Botet MFM, Modol JM, Valles X, et al. Changes in bloodstream infections in HIV-positive patients in a university hospital in Spain (1995–1997). *Int J Infect Dis* 2002;6:17.

61. Small PM, Hopewell PC, Schecter GF, et al. Evolution of chest radiographs in treated patients with pulmonary tuberculosis and HIV infection. *J Thorac Imaging* 1994;9:74.

62. Conde MB, Soares SL, Mello FC, et al. Comparison of sputum induction with fiberoptic bronchoscopy in the diagnosis of tuberculosis. *Am J Crit Care Med* 2000;162:2238.

63. Small PM, Schecter GF, Goodman PC, et al. Treatment of tuberculosis, in patients with advanced human immunodeficiency virus infection. *N Engl J Med* 1991;324:289.

64. Iseman MDR. Is standard chemotherapy adequate in tuberculosis patients infected with the HIV infection? *Am Rev Respir Dis* 1987;176:1326.

65. Perriens JH, St. Louis ME, Mukadi JB, et al. Pulmonary tuberculosis in HIV-infected patients in Zaire: a controlled trial of treatment for either 6 or 12 months. *N Engl J Med* 1995;332:779.

66. American Thoracic Society/Centers for Disease Control. Treatment and prevention of tuberculosis and tuberculosis infection in adults and children. *Am J Respir Crit Care Med* 1994;149:1359.

67. Centers for Disease Control and Prevention. Updated guidelines for the use of rifabutin or rifampin in HIV-infected patients receiving antiretroviral agents. *MMWR Morb Mortal Wkly Rep* 2000;49:185.

68. Centers for Disease Control and Prevention. Acquired rifamycin resistance in persons with advanced HIV disease being treated for active tuberculosis with intermittent rifamycin-based regimens. *MMWR Morb Mortal Wkly Rep* 2002;51:214.

69. Pape JW, Jean SS, Ho JL, et al. Effect of isoniazid prophylaxis on incidence of active tuberculosis and progression of HIV infection. *Lancet* 1993;342:268.

70. World Health Organization. *Scaling up antiretroviral therapy in resource-limited settings: guidelines for a public health approach.* Available online: *http://www.who.int/HIV_AIDS/HIV_AIDS_Care/ARV*, August 2002.

71. Freiden TR, Sterling T, Pablo-Mandez A, et al. The emergence of drug-resistant tuberculosis in New York City. *N Engl J Med* 1993;328:521.

72. Salomon N, Perlman DC, Friedmann P, et al. Predictors and outcome of multidrug-resistant tuberculosis. *Clin Infect Dis* 1995;21:1245.

73. Kazionny B, Wells CD, Kluge H, et al. Implications of the growing HIV-1 epidemic for tuberculosis control in Russia. *Lancet* 2001;358:1513.

74. Telzak EE, Fazal BA, Pollard CL, et al. Factors influencing time to sputum conversion among patients with smear-positive pulmonary tuberculosis. *Clin Infect Dis* 1997;25:666.

75. Gordin F, Chaisson RE, Matts JP, et al. Rifampin and pyrazinamide vs. isoniazid for prevention of tuberculosis in HIV-infected persons: An international randomized trial. *JAMA* 2000;283:1445.

76. Chaisson RE, Barnes GL, Hackman J, et al. A randomized controlled trial of intervention to improve adherence to isoniazid therapy to prevent tuberculosis in injection drug users. *Am J Med* 2001;110:610.

77. Di Perri G, Cruciani M, Danzi MC, et al. Nosocomial epidemic of active tuberculosis among HIV-infected patients. *Lancet* 1989;2:1502.

78. Daley CL, Small PM, Schecter GF, et al. An outbreak of tuberculosis with accelerated progression among persons infected with human immunodeficiency virus: an analysis using restriction-fragment-length polymorphisms. *N Engl J Med* 1992;326:231.

79. Akpek G, Lee SM, Gagnon DR, et al. Bone marrow aspiration, biopsy and culture in the evaluation of HIV-infected patients for invasive *Mycobacteria* and *Histoplasma* infections. *Am J Hematol* 2001;67:100.

80. Horsburgh CR, Selik RM. The epidemiology of disseminated nontuberculous mycobacterial infection in the acquired immunodeficiency syndrome (AIDS). *Am Rev Respir Dis* 1989;139:4.

81. Arasteh KN, Cordes C, Ewers M, et al. HIV-related non-tuberculous *Mycobacteria* infection: incidence, survival analysis and associated risk factors. *Eur J Med Res* 2000;5:424.

82. Peglow SL, Smulian AG, Linke MJ, et al. Serologic responses to *Pneumocystis carinii* antigens in health and disease. *J Infect Dis* 1990;161:296.

83. Huang L, Beard CB, Creasman J, et al. Sulfa or sulfone prophylaxis and geographic region predict mutations in the *Pneumocystis carinii* dihydropteroate synthase gene. *J Infect Dis* 2000;182:1192.

84. Morris AM, Swanson M, Ha H, et al. Geographic distribution of HIV-associated *Pneumocystis carinii* pneumonia in San Francisco. *Am J Respir Crit Care Med* 2000;162:1622.

85. Kovacs JA, Gill VJ, Meshnick S, et al. New insights into transmission, diagnosis, and drug treatment of *Pneumocystis carinii* pneumonia. *JAMA* 2001;286:2450.

86. Kovacs JA, Hiemenz JW, Macher AM, et al. *Pneumocystis carinii* pneumonia: a comparison between patients with the acquired immunodeficiency syndrome and patients with other immunodeficiencies. *Ann Intern Med* 1984;100:663.

87. Goldie SJ, Kaplan JE, Losina E, et al. Prophylaxis for HIV-related *Pneumocystis carinii* pneumonia. *Arch Intern Med* 2002;162:921.

88. Santamauro JT, Aurora RN, Stover DE. *Pneumocystis carinii* pneumonia in patients with and without HIV infection. *Compr Ther* 2002;28:96.

89. Kovacs JA, Ng VL, Masur H, et al. Diagnosis of *Pneumocystis carinii* pneumonia: improved detection in sputum with use of monoclonal antibodies. *N Engl J Med* 1988;318:589.

90. Bigby T, Margolskee D, Curtis J, et al. The usefulness of induced sputum in the diagnosis of *Pneumocystis carinii* pneumonia in patients with the acquired immunodeficiency syndrome. *Am Rev Respir Dis* 1986;133:515.

91. Kroe DM, Kirsch CM, Jensen WA. Diagnostic strategies for *Pneumocystis carinii* pneumonia. *Semin Respir Infect* 1997;12:70.

92. Ng VL, Gartner I, Weymouth LA, et al. The use of mucolysed induced sputum for the identification of pulmonary pathogens associated with human immunodeficiency virus infection. *Arch Pathol Lab Med* 1989;113:488.

93. Huang L, Hecht FM, Stansell JD, et al. Suspected *Pneumocystis carinii* pneumonia with a negative induced sputum examination: is early bronchoscopy useful? *Am J Respir Crit Care Med* 1995;151:1866.

94. Sing A, Trebesius K, Roggenkamp A, et al. Evaluation of diagnostic value and epidemiological implications of PCR for *Pneumocystis carinii* in different immunosuppressed and immunocompetent patient groups. *J Clin Microbiol* 2000;38:1461.

95. Fischer S, Gill VJ, Kovacs J, et al. The use of oral washes to diagnose *Pneumocystis carinii* pneumonia: a blinded prospective study of a polymerase chain reaction-based detection system. *J Infect Dis* 2001;184:1485.

96. Miller RF, Millar AB, Weller IVD, et al. Empirical treatment without bronchoscopy for *Pneumocystis carinii* pneumonia in the acquired immunodeficiency syndrome. *Thorax* 1989;44:559.

97. Masur H, Shelhamer J. Empiric outpatient management of HIV-related pneumonia: economical or unwise? *Ann Intern Med* 1996;111:451.

98. Wharton JM, Coleman DL, Wofsy CB, et al. Trimethoprim-sulfamethoxazole or pentamidine for *Pneumocystis carinii* pneumonia in the acquired immunodeficiency syndrome. *Ann Intern Med* 1985;105:37.

99. The National Institutes of Health, University of California Expert Panel for Corticosteroids as Adjunctive Therapy for *Pneumocystis* Pneumonia. Consensus statement on the use of corticosteroids as adjunctive therapy for *Pneumocystis* pneumonia in the acquired immunodeficiency syndrome. *N Engl J Med* 1990;323:1500.

100. Bozette SA, Sattler FR, Chiu J, et al. A controlled trial of early adjunctive treatment with corticosteroids for *Pneumocystis carinii* pneumonia in the acquired immunodeficiency syndrome. *N Engl J Med* 1990;323:1451.

101. Gagnon S, Boota AM, Fischl MA, et al. Corticosteroids as adjunctive therapy for severe *Pneumocystis carinii* pneumonia in the acquired immunodeficiency syndrome. *N Engl J Med* 1990;323:1444.

102. Dworkin MS Nanson DL, Navin TR. Survival of patients with AIDS after diagnosis of *Pneumocystis carinii* pneumonia in the United States. *J Infect Dis* 2001;183:1409.

103. Smego RA Jr, Nagar S, Maloba B, et al. A meta-analysis of salvage therapy for *Pneumocystis carinii* pneumonia. *Arch Intern Med* 2001;161:1529.

104. Navin TR, Beard CB, Huang L, et al. Effect of mutations in *Pneumocystis carinii* dihydropteroate synthase gene on outcome of *P. carinii* pneumonia in patients with HIV-1: a prospective study. *Lancet* 2001;358:545.

105. Simonds RJ, Hughes WT, Feinberg J, et al. Preventing *Pneumocystis carinii* pneumonia in persons infected with human immunodeficiency virus. *Clin Infect Dis* 1995;21[Suppl]:544, 1995.

106. Schneider MME, Hoepelman AIM, Eftnick-Schattenkirk JKM, et al. A controlled trial of aerosolized pentamidine or trimethoprim-sulfamethoxazole as primary prophylaxis against *Pneumocystis carinii* pneumonia in patients with human immunodeficiency virus infection. *N Engl J Med* 1992;327:1836.

107. Bozzette SA, Finkelstein DM, Spector SA, et al. A randomized trial of three antipneumocystis agents in patients with advanced human immunodeficiency virus infection. *N Engl J Med* 1995;332:693.

108. Leoung GS, Feigel DW Jr, Montgomery AB. Pentamidine for prophylaxis against *Pneumocystis carinii* pneumonia: the San Francisco community prophylaxis trial. *N Engl J Med* 1990;323:769.

109. Holding KJ, Dworkin MS, Wan PC, et al. Aspergillosis among people with HIV. *Clin Infect Dis* 2000;31:1253.

110. Pervex NK, Kleinerman J, Kattan M, et al. Pseudomembranous necrotizing bronchial aspergillosis: a variant of invasive aspergillosis in patients with hemophilia and acquired immune deficiency syndrome. *Am Rev Respir Dis* 1985;131:961.

111. Kemper CA, Hostetler JS, Follansbee SE, et al. Ulcerative and plaque-like tracheobronchitis due to infection with Aspergillus in patients with AIDS. *Clin Infect Dis* 1993;17:344.

112. Denning DW. Unusual manifestations of aspergillosis. *Thorax* 1995;50:812.
113. Bowden R, Chandrasekar P, White MH, et al. A double-blind randomized controlled trial of amphotericin B colloidal dispersion versus amphotericin B for treatment of invasive aspergillosis in immunocompromised patients. *Clin Infect Dis* 2002;35:359.
114. Lortholary O, Meyoha MC, Dupont B, et al. Invasive aspergillosis in patients with acquired immunodeficiency syndrome: report of 33 cases. *Am J Med* 1993;95:171.
115. Hebrecht R, Denning DW, Patterson TF, et al. Voriconazole versus amphotericin B for primary therapy of invasive aspergillus. *N Engl J Med* 2002;347:408.
116. Chuck SL, Sande MA. Infections with *Cryptococcus neoformans* in the acquired immunodeficiency syndrome. *N Engl J Med* 1989;321:794.
117. Clark RA, Greer D, Atkinson W, et al. Spectrum of *Cryptococcus neoformans* infection in 68 patients infected with human immunodeficiency virus. *Rev Infect Dis* 1990;12:768.
118. Chechani V, Kamholz SL. Pulmonary manifestations of disseminated cryptococcosis in patients with AIDS. *Chest* 1990;98:1060.
119. Eng RH, Bishburg E, Smith SM, et al. Cryptococcal infections in patients with acquired immunodeficiency syndrome. *Am J Med* 1986;81:19.
120. Baughman RP, Rhodes JC, Dohn MN, et al. Detection of Cryptococcal antigen in bronchoalveolar lavage fluid: a prospective study of diagnostic utility. *Am Rev Respir Dis* 1992;145:1226.
121. Malabonga VM, Basti J, Kamholz SL. Utility of bronchoscopic sampling techniques for cryptococcal disease in AIDS. *Chest* 1991;99:370.
122. American Thoracic Society. Fungal infections in HIV-infected persons. *Am J Respir Crit Care Med* 1995;152:816.
123. Sepkowitz KA. Opportunistic infections in patients with and without acquired immunodeficiency syndrome. *Clin Infect Dis* 2002;34:1293.
124. Alberg JA, Watson J, Segal M, et al. Clinical utility of monitoring serum cryptococcal antigen (sCRAG) titers in patients with AIDS-related cryptococcal disease. *HIV Clin Trials* 2000;1:1.
125. Wheat LJ, Connolly-Stringfield PA, Baker RL. Disseminated histoplasmosis in the acquired immunodeficiency syndrome: clinical findings, diagnosis and treatment, and review of the literature. *Medicine* 1990;69:361.
126. Salzman SH, Smith RL, Aranda CL. Histoplasmosis in patients at risk for the acquired immunodeficiency syndrome in a nonendemic setting. *Chest* 1988;93:916.
127. Sarosi GA, Johnson PC. Disseminated histoplasmosis in patients infected with human immunodeficiency virus. *Clin Infect Dis* 1992;14[Suppl 1]:S60.
128. Wheat LJ, Garringer T, Brizendine E, et al. Diagnosis of histoplasmosis by antigen detection based upon experience at the histoplasmosis reference laboratory. *Diagn Microbiol Infect Dis* 2002;43:29.
129. Wheat LJ. *Histoplasma capsulatum* antigen detection: comparison of the performance characteristics of a new inhibition immunoassay to those of an established antibody sandwich immunoassay. *J Clin Microbiol* 1999;37:2387.
130. Wheat LJ, Cloud G, Johnson PC, et al. Clearance of fungal burden during treatment of disseminated histoplasmosis with liposomal amphotericin B versus itraconazole. *Antimicrob Agents Chemother* 2001;45:2354.
131. Prechter GC, Prakash UBS. Bronchoscopy in the diagnosis of pulmonary histoplasmosis. *Chest* 1989;95:1033.
132. Wheat LJ, Connolly P, Smedema M, et al. Emergence of resistance to fluconazole as a cause of failure during treatment of histoplasmosis in patients with AIDS. *Clin Infect Dis* 2001;33:1920.
133. Woods CW, McKill C, Plikaytis BD, et al. Coccidioidomycosis in human immunodeficiency virus-infected persons in Arizona, 1994–97: incidence, risk factors and prevention. *J Infect Dis* 2000;181:1428.
134. Ampel NM, Dols CL, Galgiani JN. Coccidioidomycosis during human immunodeficiency virus infection: results of a prospective study in coccidioidal endemic area. *Am J Med* 1993;94:235.
135. Fish DG, Ampel NM, Galgiani JN, et al. Coccidioidomycosis during human immunodeficiency virus infection: a review of 77 patients. *Medicine* 1990;69:384.
136. Jacobson MA, Mills J, Rush J. Morbidity and mortality of patients with AIDS and first episode *Pneumocystis carinii* pneumonia is unaffected by concomitant pulmonary cytomegalovirus infection. *Am Rev Respir Dis* 1991;144:6.
137. Popara M, Pendle S, Sacks L, et al. Varicella pneumonia in patients with HIV/AIDS. *Int J Infect Dis* 2002;6:6.
138. Lin JC, Nichol KL. Excess mortality due to pneumonia or influenza during influenza seasons among persons with acquired immunodeficiency virus syndrome. *Arch Intern Med* 2001;161:441.
139. Centers for Disease Control and Prevention, Advisory Council for Immunization Practices. Recommendation for influenza vaccine. *MMWR Morb Mortal Wkly Rep* 2002;51:RR-3:8.
140. Fine AD, Bridges CB, DeGuzman AM, et al. Influenza A among patients with human immunodeficiency virus: an outbreak of infection at a residential facility in New York City. *Clin Infect Dis* 2001;32:1784.
141. Fuller JD, Craven DE, Steger KA, et al. Influenza vaccination of human immunodeficiency virus (HIV)-infected adults: impact on plasma levels of HIV type 1 RNA and determinants of antibody response. *Clin Infect Dis* 1991;28:541.

CHAPTER 116

Gastrointestinal and Nutritional Complications of Human Immunodeficiency Virus Infection

John G. Bartlett

The gastrointestinal tract is highly relevant to the complications and treatment of human immunodeficiency virus (HIV) infection. Patients with advanced disease usually have oral candidiasis. *Candida* species esophagitis is second only to *Pneumocystis carinii* pneumonia (PCP) as the initial acquired immunodeficiency syndrome (AIDS)-defining opportunistic infection. Up to one third of patients develop herpes simplex virus (HSV) perirectal lesions, and 30% to 80% experience chronic or intermittent diarrhea. Nutritional concerns are also important, including wasting with advanced HIV and the dietary complications of highly active antiretroviral therapy (HAART), including diabetes and hyperlipidemia. Gastrointestinal side effects are among the most frequent limitations to advances that have revolutionized disease outcome.

TYPES OF CONDITIONS

Gay Bowel Syndrome

In the 1970s, there was increasing recognition of the gastrointestinal complications of homosexual men, including proctitis, proctocolitis, and enteritis (1,2). Pathogens encountered in these conditions include three groups: (a) enteric pathogens that are commonly recognized in other populations of patients, such as *Shigella* species, *Entamoeba histolytica*, and *Giardia lamblia*; (b) sexually transmitted pathogens, including *Neisseria gonorrhoeae*, HSV, *Chlamydia trachomatis*, and *Treponema pallidum*; and (c) occasional enteric pathogens that may be idiosyncratic in this population of patients, such as *Campylobacter cinaedi* and *Campylobacter fennelliae*. The high prevalence of these pathogens in homosexual men presumably reflects promiscuity, sexual practices, and the high incidence of asymptomatic and untreated infections (1,2). Since the early 1980s, there has been a 10- to 20-fold decrease in rates of gonococcal proctitis and other sexually transmitted pathogens among gay men that presumably reflects modified sexual practices. A concern is a subsequent increase in these conditions as markers of unsafe sexual practices reflecting a perception that HIV is treatable or that it prevents HIV transmission (3).

Oral Lesions

The most common oral lesions are candidiasis (thrush), oral hairy leukoplakia, herpes simplex, aphthous ulcers, and various dental complications (Table 116.1). Less common are Kaposi's sarcoma, CMV infections, and non-Hodgkin's lymphoma.

Thrush is seen as an early manifestation of advanced immunosuppression, usually with CD4 counts of less than 200 cells/mm^3 (4). Early lesions are easily managed with topical

TABLE 116.1.   Oral Lesions in Patients with HIV Infection

Condition	Clinical features	Diagnosis	Stage	Treatment
Candidiasis (thrush)	Pseudomembranous form: white, creamy plaques on inflamed base Erythematous form (atrophic): spotty or confluent red patches Hyperplastic form (*Candida* leukoplakia): white lesions that do not wipe off and respond to azole therapy *Symptoms:* often asymptomatic; oral pain, taste perversion; odynophagia with esophagitis in late-stage disease White fibrillar patches, usually on tongue, especially the lateral surface; do not scrape off	Clinical appearance Oral swab, scraping, or rinse specimen for (a) KOH preparation or Gram stain to show yeast and pseudomycelia and/or (b) culture, primarily to show azole susceptibility	CD4$^+$ cell count <300/mm^3 Promote with antibiotic treatment More common and severe with late-stage disease	Local: clotrimazole troche, nystatin, amphotericin B Systemic: azoles— primarily fluconazole; intravenous (IV) amphotericin B occasionally required
Oral hairy leukoplakia (as in candidiasis)	*Symptoms:* often asymptomatic; pain, altered voice or taste Small painful ulcers or vesicles on an erythematous base, usually on gingiva and palate	Clinical appearance Biopsy: epithelial hyperplasia with "hairs"	CD4$^+$ cell count <300/mm^3	Usually not treated Symptomatic disease: oral acyclovir (high dose) or ganciclovir
Herpes simplex virus (HSV)	*Symptoms:* local pain Small painful ulcers at any location in oral cavity	Clinical appearance Scraping: multinucleated giant cells with Tzanck preparation, culture or fluorescent antibody technique for HSV	Any stage: more common and severe with late-stage disease	Acyclovir by mouth or IV (valacyclovir and famciclovir also effective) Acyclovir resistance: foscarnet
Aphthous ulcers	*Symptoms:* Local pain, often severe with or without voice change or dysphagia Red or purple nodules, usually on palate or gingiva; most have cutaneous lesions also	Clinical appearance plus studies to exclude HSV	May occur at any stage; more severe in late-stage disease	Topical: fluocinonide, lidocaine, dyclonine, or dexamethasone Local injection: corticosteroids Systemic: corticosteroids or thalidomide
Kaposi's sarcoma	*Symptoms:* usually asymptomatic; may be cosmetic concern or disruption of teeth	Clinical appearance Biopsy	CD4$^+$ cell count <300/mm^3	Usually not treated Laser or intralesional vinblastine Large lesions: radiation

agents (clotrimazole or nystatin) or fluconazole, but the late-stage disease can be problematic, especially with resistance complicating extensive exposure to azoles (5). Many cases are asymptomatic; symptoms, when present, consist of mouth pain, taste perversion, and, with *Candida* esophagitis, odynophagia (4–6). The diagnosis is usually made by clinical appearance with characteristic pseudomembranous lesions, which are white, creamy plaques on an inflamed base located on the buccal mucosa, tongue, gingiva, or palate. The plaques are easily removed with scraping. The erythematous or "atrophic" form of thrush shows spotty or confluent red patches and is more elusive to identify (4). The diagnosis may be established with a potassium hydroxide wet mount or Gram stain of an oral swab or scrapings to demonstrate typical yeast and pseudomycelia, but this is usually not necessary. Culture is not generally required except to detect resistant strains. Nearly all lesions found in early-stage disease are due to *Candida albicans*; late-stage disease with prolonged exposure to azoles often results in thrush involving fluconazole-

resistant *C. albicans* or non-albicans *Candida* species that often play an uncertain role in the disease process (5). Treatment consists of topical agents (clotrimazole troches or nystatin) or low-dose fluconazole, but recurrences are frequent (7). Refractory or recurrent disease is often managed with oral fluconazole in higher doses for longer periods, other azoles, or intravenous amphotericin B. Most patients respond well to immunologic reconstitution with HAART (8).

Oral hairy leukoplakia was first described in 1984 (9) and is now reported in 10% to 25% of patients with advanced HIV infection (10). The typical lesion is a nonremovable patch on the tongue, especially the lateral surfaces that tend to show a corrugated texture; close inspection shows fibrillar projections, which account for the name. Electron microscopy and nucleic acid hybridization implicate Epstein-Barr virus (10), an expression of Epstein-Barr virus that appears to be almost uniformly restricted to patients with immunosuppression. The major differential diagnosis is thrush; oral hairy leukoplakia can be distinguished by its anatomic location, difficulty in removing plaques with scraping (in contrast to thrush), a smear that fails to show *Candida* hyphae, lack of response to antifungal therapy, or biopsy with histologic characteristics of oral hairy leukoplakia (11). Most patients are asymptomatic, and this lesion is commonly overlooked with routine inspection of the mouth (12). The usual symptoms are pain, burning, and altered taste; symptoms and lesions resolve with acyclovir or ganciclovir but tend to recur when treatment is discontinued (13).

Oral herpes is common in the general population, but in patients with advanced HIV infection, the lesions are likely to be more extensive, more frequent, more likely to disseminate, and more refractory to treatment (4). The usual appearance is painful vesicles or ulcers 1 to 3 mm in diameter on the lips or oral cavity. The major differential diagnosis is aphthous ulcers; features suggesting HSV include a prior history of typical oral herpetic lesions, positive Tzanck preparation (positive in about 75%), positive cultures for HSV (positive in about 80%), and response to treatment with acyclovir. These lesions may be quite painful and may be extensive, with involvement of the mucous membranes and adjacent skin. The standard treatment is oral acyclovir, famciclovir, or valacyclovir in conventional doses, but high-dose oral treatment or intravenous acyclovir is sometimes required (14). Refractory cases suggest acyclovir resistance and may require foscarnet treatment for severe disease (14).

Aphthous ulcers may not be more common than in the general population, but they appear to be more severe and prolonged in patients with HIV infection. The lesions appear identical to HSV lesions and may be found any place in the oral cavity (4). A biopsy, if done, shows nonspecific inflammation. Symptoms include pain, dysphagia, and altered speech. There are multiple treatments: topical treatment consists of fluocinonide (1:1 with orobase), dexamethasone elixir, and various combinations of lidocaine and steroids or intralesional steroids; severe or refractory cases often require systemic prednisone or thalidomide (15). Other causes of vesicles or ulcers in the mouth include CMV, varicella-zoster virus, and *Molluscum contagiosum*, but all of these are infrequent.

Periodontal disease is frequent in patients with HIV infection and may be severe. The most common form involves gingivitis and periodontitis as found in the general population, but these disorders are more common and more severe with advanced stages of HIV infection (16). The usual presentation is a red gingival margin sometimes referred to as *HIV gingivitis* (4). A less common but distinctive form of disease referred to as *necrotizing ulcerative periodontitis* (formerly HIV-associated periodontitis) is characterized by local pain, spontaneous bleeding, intense erythema, edema, bone loss, and then tooth loss. Recommended treatment consists of débridement, scaling and root planing, and povidone-iodine irrigations, sometimes accompanied by topical chlorhexidine oral rinses and metronidazole.

Esophageal Disease

Esophageal disease is common. The most frequent complaint is odynophagia; the usual causes are candidiasis, CMV, or aphthous ulceration; and nearly all forms are treatable (17) (Table 116.2).

Candida is the most common cause of esophagitis, and *Candida* esophagitis is usually accompanied by thrush. Distinctive features, compared with other forms of esophagitis, are that pain is diffuse, it is associated primarily with swallowing, and fever is unusual. Treatment is usually presumptive, with endoscopy reserved for those who fail to respond, have an atypical presentation, or need *Candida* sensitivity testing (6,18–20). The usual finding with endoscopy is pseudomembranous plaques that

resemble the lesions found with thrush; brushings show yeast and pseudomycelia, and cultures may be done to detect azole-resistant strains. The usual treatment is oral azoles, either ketoconazole or fluconazole (19). Most patients respond, but relapse rates are high, maintenance therapy is often required, and resistance to therapy with or without azole-resistant *Candida* species is common with late-stage disease and excessive azole exposure (5,7,20). The best therapy is immune reconstitution with HAART (8).

Esophageal ulcers are usually caused by CMV or are idiopathic (aphthous ulcers) (21). HSV as a cause is infrequent, is often associated with typical oral herpetic lesions, and is important to recognize because of the ease of effective treatment. All three forms of ulcerative esophagitis may cause severe odynophagia that is focal (rather than diffuse as seen with *Candida* infection) and causes chest pain (rather than pain precipitated only by swallowing). Endoscopy is necessary for detecting these forms of ulcerative esophagitis and is essential for proper management using intravenous ganciclovir for CMV, intravenous acyclovir for HSV, and prednisone for aphthous ulcers (14,22,23). Patients with CMV esophagitis often have relapses requiring maintenance treatment with oral valganciclovir (24) or immune reconstitution; patients with refractory aphthous ulcers may respond to thalidomide (25).

Other diagnostic considerations in patients with dysphagia or odynophagia are drug-induced complications, including those associated with medications such as zidovudine (26), and selected unusual infections for this anatomic location such as *Mycobacterium avium* infection, tuberculosis, cryptosporidia infection, *P. carinii* infection, histoplasmosis, Kaposi's sarcoma, and non-Hodgkin's lymphoma (27). These require endoscopy for detection.

Recommended diagnostic tests depend on symptoms and stage of disease. With CD4+ cell counts greater than 500 cells/mm^3, the patient should be evaluated as in the absence of HIV infection. Essentially all of the HIV-associated complications that have been noted are seen with CD4+ cell counts less than 300 cells/mm^3, and most, other than aphthous ulcers, are seen with median CD4+ cell counts less than 50 cells/mm^3. Barium studies are of limited value. Endoscopy is generally preferred to make the distinctions summarized earlier (Table 116.2). Prior reports indicate that a likely diagnosis can be established by endoscopy in 70% to 95% of cases (28).

Enteric Infection

The frequency of diarrhea in the pre-HAART era was usually reported as 30% to 60% of AIDS patients in developed countries and continues to be 60% to 90% in developing countries (2,29–40). Management recommendations for diagnostic evaluation depend on clinical symptoms, stage of disease, and diagnostic resources. Acute diarrhea is usually caused by common bacterial or viral agents or is a side effect of antiretroviral agents, but may be the early expression of chronic diarrhea associated with late-stage disease (40,41). The most frequent identifiable pathogen with acute diarrhea that reflects immunodeficiency is salmonella. Chronic diarrhea in late-stage AIDS is usually caused by microsporidia, cryptosporidia, *Isospora* species, *M. avium*, or cytomegalovirus (CMV). The relative frequency of these microbes is summarized in Table 116.3 on the basis of multiple studies from developed countries in the pre-HAART era (2,33–40). Diagnostic probabilities depend to a large extent on medications, the CD4+ cell count, the symptoms, and the distinction between acute and chronic diarrhea.

The usual diagnostic evaluation begins with a review of medications to implement appropriate interventions discussed

TABLE 116.2. Esophageal Disease in Patients with AIDS

Characteristic	*Candida* species infection	CMV infection	Aphthous ulcer	HSV infection
Frequency (as cause of esophageal symptoms)	50%–70%	10%–20%	10%–20%	2.5%
Clinical features				
Dysphagia	++	+	+	+
Odynophagia	++	+++	+++	+++
Oral lesions	Thrush—70%	None	None	HSV >50%
Pain localization	Diffuse—esophageal	Focal—chest	Focal—chest	Focal—chest
Fever	None	Usually	None	Variable
Stage	CD4$^+$ cell count <100 cells/mm^3	CD4$^+$ cell count <50 cells/mm^3	CD4$^+$ cell count <50 cells/mm^3	CD4$^+$ cell count <150 cells/mm^3
Diagnosis				
Endoscopy	Usually treated empirically Pseudomembranous plaques	Ulcers—single or multiple discrete Biopsy—required to detect CMV	Ulcers—identical to those in CMV	Ulcers—shallow, small, confluent
Microbiology	Brush—yeast and pseudomycelia Culture for *in vitro* sensitivity test	Histopathology to show intranuclear inclusions; culture is inconclusive	Negative studies for alternative agents	Histopathology showing intracytoplasmic inclusions and multinucleated giant cells; HSV by fluorescent antibody stain or culture
Treatment				
Acute (2–3 wk)	Azoles; usually fluconazole Some require IV amphotericin	Ganciclovir Alternative is foscarnet	Systemic prednisone with or without antifungal prophylaxis Thalidomide	Acyclovir by mouth or intravenously
Maintenance	Fluconazole or other azole only with repeated episodes	Arbitrary—some use only for recurrent disease	None	Arbitrary
Comment	Response to fluconazole: 85%	Should obtain ophthalmologic examination	May be severely debilitating	Relatively rare cause of esophageal ulcer Response to treatment is usually good

CMV, cytomegalovirus; HSV, herpes simplex virus; +, modest; ++, moderate; +++, severe.

later (41). If medications are not implicated and diarrhea is severe or chronic, the workup often starts with culture for enteric pathogens (*Salmonella* species, *Campylobacter jejuni*, *Shigella* species, and, less frequently, *Yersinia* species, *Aeromonas* species, *Escherichia coli* O157:H7, and noncholera *Vibrio* species), stool

TABLE 116.3. Prevalence of Enteric Pathogens in Patients with AIDS with Diarrhea

Pathogen	Mean (%)	Range (%)
Cryptosporidium species	20	7–37
Microsporidia	19	2–39
Cytomegalovirus	20	8–45
Mycobacterium avium	9	2–25
Giardia lamblia	5	2–12
Entamoeba histolytica	3	0–25
Campylobacter jejuni	3	0–11
Clostridium difficile	2	0–7
Salmonella species	2	0–25
Shigella species	2	0–5
Isospora	1	0–4
Enteric viruses	4	2–15

Data from references 33–40.

for ova and parasites (preferably with acid-fast stain for detection of *Cryptosporidium*, *Isospora*, and *Cyclospora* species), and a *Clostridium difficile* toxin assay (preferably with an enzyme immunoassay or tissue culture assay) (35,42). A stool leukocyte examination, preferably using lactoferrin, is a good method for distinguishing inflammatory from secretory causes of diarrhea (43). The common inflammatory causes of diarrhea in patients with HIV infection include bacterial agents (especially *Salmonella* species, *Campylobacter jejuni*, and *C. difficile*), and CMV (42). Protozoan parasites, viruses other than CMV, and *M. avium* are not commonly associated with fecal leukocytes and are classified as agents of secretory diarrhea (33–41). Microsporidia may be detected in stool using a special trichrome stain that is variable in terms of availability and technical expertise (39,44).

Treatment of patients with acute diarrhea when *C. difficile* is unlikely or excluded may include a fluoroquinolone given empirically if symptoms are severe; most treatable bacterial pathogens are susceptible, except *C. difficile* and many *C. jejuni* infections (42). Antiperistaltic agents are often advocated for empirical treatment of acute or chronic diarrhea. Patients with negative stool studies who are unresponsive to empirical therapy and have persistent severe symptoms usually undergo endoscopy (36–38). If the clinical presentation suggests colonic or inflammatory diarrhea (fever, cramps, fecal leukocytes), the usual initial anatomic study is lower endoscopy. If the symptoms suggest secretory diarrhea with malabsorption (large-volume stools, no fecal leukocytes, absence of fever, absence of cramps), there should be consideration of upper endoscopy (35–40). About one third of HIV-infected patients with severe or prolonged diarrhea unrelated to medications have a negative evaluation, including endoscopy. One study with long-term follow-up of such "pathogen-negative" HIV-infected patients with chronic diarrhea showed that most had low-volume diarrhea that resolved spontaneously or was easily controlled with antimotility agents (45). Small bowel biopsies of patients with advanced HIV infection show villus atrophy with crypt hyperplasia, but the consequences of these anatomic changes are unclear because the same histopathologic picture is seen as a manifestation of late-stage HIV infection whether diarrhea is present or absent (36,38,46–48).

Idiopathic diarrhea may be explained by undetected enteric pathogens (especially adenovirus, spirochetosis, adenoadherent *E. coli*, or CMV) (39,46), AIDS enteropathy (as described earlier) because these anatomic changes may be associated with mild malabsorption of carbohydrates (48,49), a direct effect of HIV infection of the gut (50,51), inflammatory mediators such as cytokines, or autonomic neuropathy (52–55).

ACUTE DIARRHEA

The most common infectious agents identified in patients with acute diarrhea are viruses (astroviruses, picobirnavirus, adenovirus, and small round viruses including *Calicivirus* species) (56–58) and selected bacterial pathogens (*Salmonella* species, *C. difficile*, and possibly, enteroadherent *E. coli*) (39,42,56–58). Salmonella is especially common (42,59–63) and may be seen with relatively high CD4$^+$ cell counts, reflecting the virulence of this organism. Many patients present with symptoms of enteric fever without diarrhea, although gastroenteritis is another common presentation. The rate of salmonellosis in patients with HIV infection is estimated to be about 100-fold greater than that of those without HIV infection (60,61). Unusual features of salmonellosis in patients with HIV include the lack of an identifiable source of infection in most patients, high rates of bacteremia, and a propensity of infection to recur after discontinuation of antibiotic treatment (60–63). Although most authorities do not recommend antibiotic treatment for *Salmonella* gastroenteritis, patients with advanced HIV infection should be treated, usually with a fluoroquinolone for at least 3 weeks (42). The frequency of salmonellosis may be modified by the use of zidovudine (which has *in vitro* activity against it) (64) and prophylactic trimethoprim-sulfamethoxazole for *P. carinii*. *C. difficile* is relatively common in patients with HIV infection, but most authorities believe this simply reflects the frequency of antibiotic use in this population rather than any inherent HIV-associated risk (65). Management is similar to that used in other populations (66). Enteroadherent *E. coli* has been implicated as a cause of diarrhea in up to 17% of U.S. patients and 60% to 80% of Zambian patients with advanced HIV infection (46,47). This organism has been detected on histopathologic studies in the right colon or cecum, showing attachment to microvilli or aggregates at sites of damaged epithelium; it is identified by adherence to HEp-2 tissue culture cells (47), but this technology is available only from research laboratories. The suggested treatment is with a fluoroquinolone, but the experience is limited (Table 116.4).

CHRONIC DIARRHEA

The most common pathogens found in chronic diarrhea in nearly all reports are cryptosporidia, microsporidia, *M. avium*, and CMV (29–40,67–70) (Table 116.5). There is a long list of miscellaneous agents, including many of those described as agents of acute diarrhea such as *Salmonella* species, *C. difficile*, enteroadherent *E. coli*, and most of the enteric viral agents summarized earlier. The "big four" are discussed subsequently.

Spore-forming protozoa associated with HIV infection include two that are common, cryptosporidia and microsporidia, and two that are infrequent, *Isospora* and *Cyclospora* species. Shared properties include the following: all are human pathogens that are intracellular pathogens found within enterocytes; spores or oocytes are shed in stool and represent the infecting source; malabsorption and morphologic changes are related to the organism load; they are most common in tropical areas and locations with poor sanitation; the source of acquisition is fecal-oral contamination or contaminated water or food; all may cause asymptomatic infection, self-limited diarrhea, or, in immunodeficient patients, chronic diarrhea; and the diagnosis is based on microscopic examination of stools (68) (Table 116.6). Pathologic changes are similar with all four and are characterized by villus blunting and crypt hyperplasia analogous to changes summarized earlier for AIDS enteropathy. The life cycle starts with ingestion of the spore, followed by invasion of the enterocyte and replication with maturation to produce the infectious agent, the oocyst or spore, which is sloughed in the intestine. Detection is by acid-fast staining of stool with distinction between pathogens based on morphology and the size of oocysts (Table 116.6). The exception is microsporidia, which are 1 to 2 μm and best seen with a modified trichrome or fluorescent stain (44).

CYTOMEGALOVIRUS INFECTION

CMV gastrointestinal disease is found in at least 20% of AIDS patients with chronic diarrhea (39). Nearly all have late-stage HIV infection with CD4$^+$ cell counts less than 50 cells/mm^3. Sites of involvement include virtually any level of the gastrointestinal tract, and the accompanying clinical syndromes reflect the site: dysphagia and retrosternal pain with esophageal involvement; ulcer symptoms that fail to respond to antacids with gastroduodenitis; abdominal pain with malabsorption and with steatorrhea when the small bowel is infected; and chronic diarrhea that may be watery, bloody, or associated with excessive mucus when the colon is involved. Most common is CMV colitis with inflammatory diarrhea, fecal leukocytes, blood, fever, and cramps (71–73). Less common presentations include a solitary intestinal ulcer, toxic megacolon, intestinal perforation, or obstruction caused by mass lesions in the small bowel (74). Typical findings of contrast studies include segmental colitis or pancolitis with mucosal granularity, thickened folds, spasticity, or superficial erosions (75). Colonic involvement may be diffuse, segmental, or restricted to the cecum. Computed tomography usually shows a thickened colonic mucosa with ulcerations, and endoscopy usually shows focal or diffuse inflammatory changes with hemorrhagic plaques and superficial ulcerations. Biopsy and histologic examination of typical lesions show CMV vasculitis with inflammation and hemorrhage in the lamina propria and typical intranuclear inclusions within endothelial cells. The usual treatment is oral valganciclovir (900 mg twice a day) or intravenous ganciclovir (5 mg/kg every 12 hours) for 14 to 28 days. Response with esophagitis is usually good but is less impressive with colitis. A placebo-controlled trial in AIDS patients with CMV colitis showed ganciclovir treatment reduced the number of cultures positive for CMV and improved colonoscopy scores, but there was no significant change in diarrhea, abdominal pain, or fatigue (76). Foscarnet is the alternative agent, and a comparative trial of foscarnet and ganciclovir showed that the two agents were equally effective (77,78).

CRYPTOSPORIDIOSIS

Cryptosporidium parvum is a relatively common cause of infectious diarrhea in AIDS patients, which is more severe and more likely to be chronic compared with immunocompetent patients (67,68,79,80). Common associated symptoms are nausea and

TABLE 116.4. Acute Infectious Diarrhea in Patients with AIDS

Agent	Frequency (%)[a]	Clinical features	Diagnosis	Treatment
Salmonella species	5–15	Watery diarrhea; fever; fecal white blood cells (WBCs) variable: CD4+ cell count variable; increased frequency with low CD4+ cell count	Stool culture Blood culture	Ciprofloxacin (Cipro), 500–750 mg PO b.i.d. for 14 d Trimethoprim-sulfamethoxazole (TMP-SMX), 1–2 double-strength (DS) tablets PO b.i.d. for 14 d Ampicillin, 2 g/d PO or 6 g/d intravenously for 14 d (if sensitive) Third-generation cephalosporin or chloramphenicol Treatment may need to be extended in ≥4 wk
Shigella species	1–3	Watery diarrhea or bloody flux; fever; fecal WBCs common; any CD4+ cell count	Stool culture	Cipro, 500 mg PO b.i.d. for 3 d TMP-SMX, 1 DS tablet PO b.i.d. for 3 d
Campylobacter jejuni	4–8	Watery diarrhea or bloody flux, fever, fecal leukocytes variable; any CD4+ cell count	Stool culture; most laboratories cannot detect *Campylobacter cinaedi*, *Campylobacter fennelli*, and others	Cipro, 500 mg PO b.i.d. for 3–5 d Erythromycin, 500 mg PO q.i.d. for 5 d
Clostridium difficile	10–15	Watery diarrhea; fecal WBCs variable; fever and leukocytosis common; antibacterial agent nearly always—especially clindamycin, ampicillin, and cephalosporins; any CD4+ cell count	Endoscopy: pseudomembranous colitis, colitis, or normal Stool toxin assay: tissue culture of enzyme immunoassay preferred Computed tomographic scan: colitis with thickened mucosa	Metronidazole, 250–500 mg PO q.i.d. for 10–14 d Vancomycin, 125 mg PO q.i.d. for 10–14 d Antiperistaltic agents (diphenoxylate-atropine sulfate [Lomotil] or loperamide) contraindicated
Enteroadherent *Escherichia coli*	10–20	Watery diarrhea; acute, but may be chronic	Adherence to HEp-2 cells (research laboratories only)	Fluoroquinolone
Enteric viruses	15–30	Watery diarrhea acute, but one third of cases become chronic; any CD4+ cell count	Major agents: adenovirus, astrovirus, picobirnavirus, calicivirus,[b] clinical laboratories cannot detect these viruses	Supportive treatment: diphenoxylate-atropine sulfate or loperamide
Idiopathic	25–40	Variable Noninfectious causes—rule out medications, diet, irritable bowel syndrome; any CD4+ cell count	Negative studies including culture, ova and parasites examination, and *C. difficile* toxin assay	Severe acute diarrhea: Cipro, 500 mg PO b.i.d. or ofloxacin, 200–300 mg PO b.i.d. for 5 d with or without metronidazole[c]

[a]Frequency among patients with acute diarrhea defined as three or more loose or watery stools for 3–10 d.
[b]Data from Grohmann GS, Glass RI, Pereira HG, et al. Enteric viruses and diarrhea in HIV-infected patients. *N Engl J Med* 1993;329:14.
[c]Data from Goodman LJ, Trenholme GM, Kaplan RL, et al. Empiric antimicrobial therapy of domestically acquired acute diarrhea in urban adults. *Arch Intern Med* 1990;150:541. Also from Wistrom J, Jertborn M, Ekwall E, et al. Empiric treatment of acute diarrheal disease with norfloxacin. *Ann Intern Med* 1992;117:202.

vomiting. About one third of patients have fever. One study of 128 AIDS patients showed four patterns: asymptomatic carriage (4%); transient, self-limited disease (29%); chronic disease (60%); and fulminant disease (8%) (80). Transmission is by oocysts excreted by humans and large animals such as cows and sheep; it can infect water supplies despite chlorination. Clinical expression with severity and chronicity of symptoms depends largely on the CD4+ cell count; patients with counts less than 50 cells/mm³ may have devastating diarrhea, with fluid losses of 10 to 20 L per day and lifelong persistence of cryptosporidia (68,79–81). Cryptosporidiosis is the most common identifiable cause of chronic diarrhea in AIDS patients, but its frequency has decreased to less than 1% of AIDS patients in the United States in the HAART era; it continues to cause debilitating diarrhea in up to 20% of AIDS patients in developing countries

(29–38,81,82). The usual method of detection is stool exam to demonstrate typical oocysts utilizing modified Ziehl-Neelsen, modified Kinyoun acid-fast, or auramine O fluorescent direct fluorescent antibody (DFA) stains using commercially available monoclonal antibody or enzyme immunoassay (EIA) (67,68, 79–82). Examination of small bowel biopsy specimens shows typical 4-μm circular organisms on the apical membrane of the enterocyte. Associated histologic changes include partial atrophy and distortion of the villi with a mononuclear infiltrate of the lamina propria, predominantly in the ileum and jejunum. Other sites of involvement of the gastrointestinal tract, including the esophagus and colon, have been reported. Biliary infections include a sclerosing cholangitis, acalculous cholecystitis, and pancreatitis (67,68,83,84). Patients with acalculous sclerosing cholangitis present with right upper quadrant pain and

TABLE 116.5. Chronic Infectious Diarrhea in Patients with AIDS

Agent	Frequency (%)[a]	Clinical features	Diagnosis	Treatment
Microsporidia Enterocytozoon bieneusi or Septata intestinalis	15–30	Enteritis; watery diarrhea; no fecal white blood cells (WBCs); fever uncommon; remitting disease over years; malabsorption; wasting; CD4+ cell count <100 cells/mm3	Special trichrome stain described[b] Biopsy—electron microscopy or Giemsa stain	Albendazole, 400–800 mg PO b.i.d. for 4 wk; larger doses may be required; efficacy is not established[c] (available only through Treatment IND) Metronidazole (anecdotal), 500 mg PO b.i.d.[d]
Cryptosporidium species	10–30	Enteritis; watery diarrhea; no fecal WBCs; no fever; malabsorption; wasting; large stool volume with abdominal pain; remitting symptoms for months to years; CD4+ cell count <200 cells/mm3	Acid-fast bacillus smear of stool to show oocyst of 4–6 μm	Paromomycin, 500 mg PO q.i.d. for ≥ 4 wk Octreotide, 50–500 μg subcutaneously or IV t.i.d. (nonspecific) Azithromycin, 1,200 mg PO b.i.d. for 1 d, then 1,200 mg/d for 27 d, then 600 mg/d May require parenteral hyperalimentation
Cytomegalovirus	15–40	Colitis and/or enteritis; fecal WBCs and/or blood; cramps; fever; watery diarrhea and/or blood; may cause perforation; hemorrhage, toxic megacolon, ulceration; CD4+ cell count <50 cells/mm3	Biopsy to show intranuclear inclusion bodies, preferably with inflammation, vasculitis Computed tomography (CT); segmental or pancolitis	Ganciclovir, 5 mg/kg IV b.i.d. Foscarnet, 40–60 mg/kg IV q8h Results of treatment variable[e]; foscarnet and ganciclovir are equally effective[f]
Mycobacterium avium	10–20	Enteritis; watery diarrhea; no fecal WBCs; fever and wasting common; diffuse abdominal pain in late stage; CD4+ cell count <50 cells/mm3	Positive blood cultures for M. avium; biopsy may show changes like Whipple's disease, but with acid-fast bacilli; CT may be supportive; hepatosplenomegaly, adenopathy, and thickened small bowel	Clarithromycin, 500 mg–1 g PO t.i.d. + ethambutol, 15 mg/kg/d; rifampin, 600 mg/d and/or clofazimine, 100 mg/d
Isospora species	1–3	Enteritis; watery diarrhea; no fecal WBCs; no fever; wasting; malabsorption; CD4+ cell count <100 cells/mm3	Acid-fast bacillus smear of stool; oocytes 20–30 μm	Trimethoprim-sulfamethoxazole (TMP-SMX), 3–4 double-strength (DS) tablets/d Pyrimethamine, 50–75 mg/d PO
Entamoeba histolytica	1–3	Colitis; bloody stools; cramps; no fecal WBCs (bloody stools); most patients asymptomatic carriers; any CD4+ cell count	Stool ova and parasites (O&P) examination	Metronidazole, 500–750 mg PO or IV t.i.d. for 5–10 d, then iodoquinol, 650 mg PO t.i.d. for 21 d or paromomycin, 500 mg PO q.i.d. for 7 d
Giardia species	1–3	Enteritis; watery diarrhea and/or malabsorption, bloating; flatulence; any CD4+ cell count	Stool O&P examination	Quinacrine, 100 mg PO t.i.d. for 10 d or metronidazole, 250 mg PO t.i.d. for 10 d
Cyclospora cayetanensis	<1%	Enteritis; watery diarrhea; CD4+ cell count <100 cells/mm3	Stool acid-fast bacillus smear—resembles that of Cryptosporidium species	TMP-SMX, 1 DS b.i.d. for 3 d
Small bowel overgrowth	Not known	Watery diarrhea; malabsorption; wasting; often associated with hypochlorhydria	Hydrogen breath test; quantitative culture of small bowel aspirate	Amoxicillin-clavulanate, 250–500 mg PO t.i.d. Doxycycline, 100 mg PO t.i.d.
Idiopathic	20–30	Watery diarrhea; malabsorption; no fecal WBCs	Biopsy shows villus atrophy, crypt hyperplasia and no identifiable cause despite endoscopy with biopsy and electron microscopy for microsporidia[g]	Supportive care: diphenoxylate-atropine sulfate (Lomotil) or loperamide Nutritional support

[a]Frequency among patients with advanced HIV infection and chronic diarrhea defined as more than two or three loose or watery stools a day for ≥21 d.
[b]Data from reference 168.
[c]Data from reference 195.
[d]Data from Schattenkerk JKME, van Gool T, van Ketel RJ, et al. Clinical significance of small-intestinal microsporidiosis in HIV-infected individuals. Lancet 1991;337:895.
[e]Data from reference 72 and Reed EC, Wolford JL, Kopecky KJ, et al. Ganciclovir for the treatment of cytomegalovirus gastroenteritis in bone marrow transplant recipients. Ann Intern Med 1990;112:505.
[f]Data from reference 78.
[g]Data from reference 37.

TABLE 116.6. Comparison of Intestinal Spore-Forming Protozoa

Characteristic	*Cryptosporidium* species	*Microsporidium* species	*Isospora* species	*Cyclospora* species
Agents—human disease	*Cryptosporidium parvum*	*Enterocytozoon bieneusi* *Septata intestinalis*	*Isospora belli*	*Cyclospora cayetanensis*
Source of infection (suspected or established)	Humans, farm animals Food or water	Humans Food or water	Humans Food or water	Humans Food or water
Frequency in AIDS patients with diarrhea	10%–20%	6%–50% *E. bieneusi/S. intestinalis* (7.1%)	United States: 2% Developing countries: 10%–12%	United States: <1% Haiti: 11%
Clinical expression				
Immunocompetent persons	Self-limited diarrhea (3–25 d)	Nonpathogenic	Self-limited diarrhea	Self-limited diarrhea; may be chronic
AIDS patients	Most: transient or chronic diarrhea; may be devastating	Transient or chronic diarrhea	Transient or chronic diarrhea	Transient or chronic diarrhea
Extraintestinal disease	Biliary infection Negative	Biliary infection Disseminated disease	Biliary infection Negative	Negative Negative
Detection				
Modified acid-fast bacillus (AFB) stain	Positive	Negative	Positive	Positive or negative
Size of oocyst	4–6 μm	1–2 μm	20–30 μm	8–10 μm
Diagnosis	AFB-stool	Trichrome or fluorescent antibody stain	AFB-stool	AFB-stool
Therapy	Paromomycin	*E. bieneusi*—none *E. intestinalis*—albendazole	Trimethoprim-sulfamethoxazole	Trimethoprim-sulfamethoxazole

Adapted from Goodgame RW. Understanding intestinal spore-forming protozoa: cryptosporidia, microsporidia, isospora, and cyclospora. *Ann Intern Med* 1996;124:429–441, with permission.

increasing alkaline phosphatase. Extensive efforts have been made to treat cryptosporidial infections using more than 95 therapeutic agents, but none has proved consistently effective (85). Paromomycin is a nonabsorbable aminoglycoside that is active *in vitro* and effective at high doses in animals with cryptosporidiosis, but clinical trials have given inconsistent results in patients. Consequently, the best treatment is supportive care (loperamide or opiates, rehydration, replacement of electrolyte losses) and immune reconstitution (86). With biliary cryptosporidiosis, uncontrolled studies show response to sphincterotomy, but results are variable, and relief of pain is often temporary (84). The role of cholecystectomy is also unclear (87).

ISOSPOROSIS

Isospora belli is also a protozoan parasite that invades microvilli of the small intestine and may cause severe and protracted secretory diarrhea in patients with AIDS. Histologic changes in the small bowel and diagnostic testing using small bowel biopsies or direct stool examination are analogous to those described for cryptosporidiosis (68,88–90). On stool examination, the organism is readily distinguished from *Cryptosporidium* species on the basis of size (68) (Table 116.6). Isosporosis is relatively rare in AIDS patients in the United States but accounts for 15% to 20% of AIDS-associated diarrheas in patients from Zaire and Haiti (68,91). Treatment with trimethoprim-sulfamethoxazole is highly effective, but the relapse rate is relatively high, suggesting the possible need for long-term maintenance therapy (68,90,91). Trimethoprim-sulfamethoxazole or sulfadoxine-pyrimethamine prevents recurrent disease (91).

MICROSPORIDIOSIS

Microsporidia are intracellular parasites in the phylum *Microsporidia*, which contains more than 1,000 species and 144 gen-

era. They are ubiquitous and cause zoonotic or waterborne diarrhea in compromised hosts, including patients with AIDS with CD4 counts less than 100 cells/mm^3 (33,35–38,92). Two species have been implicated as intestinal pathogens, *Enterocytozoon bieneusi* and *Encephalitozoon (Septata) intestinalis* (93–95). Both cause noninflammatory, usually intermittent, chronic diarrhea without fever; malabsorption studies show severe malabsorption of fat and D-xylose and low zinc levels (34,68). *E. bieneusi* is the more common species involved in diarrheal disease and may cause cholangitis; *E. intestinalis* causes diarrhea, keratoconjunctivitis, and disseminated disease. As the name implies, microsporidia are small parasites (1 to 5 μm) that require stain and adequate magnification ($\times$1,000) for detection. The usual method stains used for stool specimens are Chromotrope 2R, calcofluor white, and Uvitex 2B (35,68,96–100). For small bowel biopsy specimens, the stains advocated for detecting microsporidia in tissue include hematoxylin-eosin, Brown-Hopps, Gram stain, toluidine blue, Warthin-Starry, acid-fast, Chromotrope 2A, and Giemsa stain (68). Asymptomatic infection in the small bowel has been described but is rare (97). In general, three stools with chromotrope and chemofluorescent stains are adequate. With disseminated disease (*E. intestinalis*), exam of urine is also recommended. With regard to therapy, albendazole (400 mg twice a day) is effective for *E. intestinalis* but is not effective for infections involving *E. bieneusi* (98,101,102).

MYCOBACTERIUM AVIUM INFECTION

Prior studies indicated that 40% to 50% of late-stage AIDS patients develop disseminated *M. avium* infection, although this frequency is notably reduced with *M. avium* complex (MAC) prophylaxis and with HAART (103–106). Gastrointestinal involvement reflects disseminated disease with a CD4 count less than 100 cells/mm^3 and is expressed clinically as chronic diarrhea, malabsorption, weight loss, crampy abdominal pain, and fever (34–38,107–109). Pathologic changes noted with colonic involvement include edema, erythema, and friability, and biopsy specimens show typical acid-fast organisms within macrophages and free within the lamina propria (107). With small bowel involvement, the typical pathologic changes are nearly identical to those of Whipple's disease, with foamy macrophages distended by vesicles containing periodic acid–Schiff–positive material in the lamina propria (108). Nearly all patients have *M. avium* bacteremia (109). The organism is commonly detected with acid-fast stains and cultures of stool (112), but this finding simply supports the diagnosis of disseminated infection and does not necessarily indicate invasion of the gut. The usual treatment is with combination antimicrobials, using clarithromycin or azithromycin plus ethambutol, sometimes with the addition of rifabutin or a fluoroquinolone (113,114). Patients should be treated lifelong unless there is immune reconstitution (115,116).

MISCELLANEOUS CONDITIONS

Infections

Patients with HIV infection are subject to the same types of enteric pathogens that are encountered in healthy hosts, although these infections may be unusually severe or prolonged in immunosuppressed persons. For example, AIDS patients with shigellosis often have *Shigella* bacteremia (117) or may have persistent infection (118); infections with *Campylobacter* species may include bacteremia with opportunistic pathogens such as *Campylobacter fetus*, *C. jejuni*, or *C. cinaedi* (119–121). Hemolytic-uremic syndrome and thrombotic thrombocytopenic purpura caused by verocytotoxin-producing *E. coli* have been reported in AIDS patients (123). Parasites other than those reviewed above that are found occasionally include *E. histolytica* and *G. lamblia* (123). Perhaps the most controversial is *Blastocystis hominis,* which has been found in 5% to 15% of healthy persons and 35% to 50% of homosexual men and has occasionally been implicated as an agent of enteric disease in diverse hosts, including those with HIV infection (124). When treatment is deemed appropriate, metronidazole is the preferred agent, but the evidence that this organism is an enteric pathogen is poor. There is no good evidence that *Endolimax nana, Entamoeba coli, Entamoeba hartmanni,* and other nonpathogenic parasites are peculiarly virulent in patients with HIV infection. The most common identified viral pathogens are CMV and HSV, but multiple other enteric viruses have been found in AIDS patients with both acute and chronic diarrhea as summarized earlier (39,56–58). These agents are not detectable with the usual laboratory resources, and there is no specific treatment. Fungi are uncommon causes of enteric infection, although there may be intestinal involvement with disseminated disease caused by histoplasmosis, aspergillosis, or cryptococcosis (125–127). The most common is enteritis with disseminated *Histoplasma capsulatum* (127).

Tumors

Tumors of the gastrointestinal tract associated with HIV infection include Kaposi's sarcoma, non-Hodgkin's lymphoma, cloacogenic carcinoma of the rectum, squamous cell carcinoma of the rectum and anus, squamous carcinoma of the tongue, and Burkitt's lymphoma. The most common, Kaposi's sarcoma, may involve the gut in up to 40% to 50% of patients who have cutaneous lesions (128,129). Most are asymptomatic, although oral lesions may be painful, esophageal lesions may cause dysphagia, and lower gastrointestinal tract involvement may cause diarrhea, subacute intestinal obstruction, protein-losing enteropathy,

or a rectal ulcer. Oral lesions are readily apparent on inspection, and endoscopy may show typical raised, red nodules, with or without central umbilication. Histologic confirmation is difficult owing to the depth of the lesions. In one study, only 7 of 30 lesions observed by endoscopy were confirmed with histologic examination (129). The lymphomas associated with HIV infection are usually extranodal high-grade B-cell lymphomas. The gastrointestinal tract is involved in up to 20% of all HIV-infected patients with lymphomas, and there may be involvement of any site from the oral cavity to the rectum. Anal cancer is significantly more frequent in gay men and in both men and women with HIV infection (130). Nevertheless, the relationship of this cancer to immunosuppression is unclear owing to variable results and the lack of a clear association with CD4 count (130,131).

GASTROINTESTINAL MANIFESTATIONS OF ANTIRETROVIRAL AGENTS

Drugs used in antiretroviral regimens have a high frequency of gastrointestinal adverse reactions that frequently limits compliance (132). Most common are nausea, vomiting, abdominal pain, and diarrhea. Most serious are pancreatitis, hepatotoxicity, and lactic acidosis.

Nausea, vomiting, and abdominal pain are commonly encountered with zidovudine, didanosine, ritonavir, amprenavir, and indinavir, but may be seen with any of these drugs. Management is symptomatic. Many drug effects improve with continued use and some, especially those of zidovudine and ritonavir, improve when administered with food. With protease inhibitors (PIs), the gastrointestinal complications are dose related; hence, tolerance is commonly improved with the lower doses used in PI combinations, as with low-dose ritonavir to boost lopinavir, indinavir, amprenavir, or saquinavir. With respect to diarrhea, nearly all of these drugs may have this as a side effect, but nelfinavir and lopinavir have particularly high rates (133). These patients generally respond well to loperamide (2 mg with each loose stool), calcium (500 mg twice daily), or other common antidiarrheal treatment (134).

Pancreatitis is a serious and potentially life-threatening complication seen most frequently with didanosine and combinations of didanosine and stavudine with or without hydroxyurea; it is less common with stavudine alone and is possibly seen with lamivudine (135–138). The incidence with didanosine is 1% to 9%, with an average fatality rate of 6%. The presumed cause is mitochondrial toxicity, the presentation is similar to pancreatitis in other settings, and management is the same as well. Risk factors include prolonged administration of the nucleosides noted previously and other risk factors for pancreatitis, including alcoholism, hypertriglyceridemia, cholelithiasis, endoscopic retrograde cholangiopancreatography, and concomitant use of stavudine or stavudine plus hydroxyurea (135–137).

Lactic acidosis represents an important and potentially life-threatening complication of nucleosides presumably due to mitochondrial toxicity as reflected by reduced mitochondrial nuclear DNA levels (139,140). Presentation includes gastrointestinal symptoms with abdominal pain, nausea, vomiting, diarrhea, wasting, or hepatic steatosis (139,141,142). The usual laboratory finding is a lactic acid level greater than 5 mmol/mL. Mortality is directly correlated with lactic acid levels (139). It is greater than 40% with levels greater than 10 mmol/mL. The frequency is generally reported at 1.2 to 15 per 1,000 patient-years of exposure to nucleosides; the most frequently implicated agent is stavudine, although all agents in this class have been implicated, and multiple nucleosides in combinations magnify the risk. The combination of stavudine and didanosine appears particularly common. Ribavirin, a nucleoside that is used for hepatitis C rather than HIV, must also be considered a risk when treating hepatitis C virus (HCV) and HIV co-infection (143). Treatment consists of nucleoside withdrawal or substitution with agents in this class that are less frequently implicated; recovery requires weeks or months (140,144).

Hepatotoxicity is another common complication of antiretroviral therapy. All antiretroviral agents have been implicated. Mechanisms are diverse and include mitochondrial toxicity with lactic acidosis and hepatic steatosis with nucleosides, the hypersensitivity from nonnucleoside reverse transcriptase inhibitors (NNRTIs), especially nevirapine, and drug-induced hepatitis as seen with all protease inhibitors. Hepatic damage with nucleosides is characteristically hepatic steatosis in association with hyperlactatemia and characteristic changes on hepatic scans (142,144). This occurs late in the course of therapy and is most common with stavudine or stavudine plus didanosine. The damage may be extensive and lead to late hepatic failure (145). With nevirapine and possibly other NNRTIs, hepatic injury usually occurs in the first 6 to 12 weeks of therapy and may be asymptomatic or combined with other symptoms of hypersensitivity such as rash and fever (145–148). Recommendations for monitoring include frequent measurement of liver function tests, especially during the first 12 weeks of treatment. The frequency of transaminase level increases to more than five times the upper limit of normal (grade 3 toxicity) is reported at 8% to 20% for nevirapine and substantially less with delavirdine and efavirenz (145). All protease inhibitors appear to cause increases in transaminase levels. The reported frequency of alanine transaminase (ALT) levels to more than five times the upper limits of normal (grade 3 toxicity) ranges from zero for nelfinavir to 12% for ritonavir (149). Many patients have preexisting liver disease owing to co-infection with hepatitis B or, more frequently, hepatitis C. The frequency of PI-associated hepatotoxicity is increased in those co-infected with HCV or HBV, although most are asymptomatic (150–152).

NUTRITION AND WASTING

Wasting

The definition of *wasting* as an AIDS-defining diagnosis is the unintentional loss of at least 10% of baseline body weight accompanied by chronic diarrhea or fever. Wasting was second only to *P. carinii* pneumonia as the initial AIDS-defining complication in the pre-HAART era, and it continues to be an important complication (153,154). Contributing factors are anorexia (medication-associated, oral or esophageal lesions), altered metabolism, enteropathy with malabsorption, hypogonadism, active infection, excessive cytokine production, and toxicity of antiretroviral agents such as lactic acidosis (155–159). Interventions need to be individualized based on cause and other patient-related factors.

Appetite Stimulation

Megesterol acetate is a synthetic progestational agent that produces weight gain that is primarily fat (160). In men, the drug is commonly combined with testosterone to maintain sexual function. Dronabinol, the active component of marijuana, is another appetite stimulant used for HIV-associated wasting, but evidence of its efficacy is generally lacking (161).

Anabolic Steroids

Hypogonadism was noted in up to 50% of men with AIDS in the pre-HAART era; this is now decreased as a result of the success of

antiretroviral therapy, but is still reported at 20% (162). Replacement testosterone in this setting has been successful in reversing weight lean body mass (163). Synthetic anabolic agents include oxandrolone, nandrolone, and oxymetholone; these may also be used to increase lean body mass, but testosterone is preferred in hypogonadal men (164). Supraphysiologic doses of testosterone in eugonadal men may also cause increase in lean body mass (165). It is emphasized that hypogonadism is the strongest indication for this treatment, and testosterone in replacement doses is the preferred treatment.

Resistance Exercise Training

Resistance exercise training has been successful in showing significant increases in lean body mass in men (166) and women (167). The main problem has been adherence (167).

Growth Hormone

Pharmacologic doses of growth hormone increase body mass and decrease fat (168), but at substantial cost of the drug and with results that are no better than resistance exercise training.

REFERENCES

1. Quinn TC, Stamm WE, Goodell SE, et al. The polymicrobial origin of intestinal infections in homosexual men. *N Engl J Med* 1983;309:576.
2. Laughon BE, Druckman DA, Vernon A, et al. Prevalence of enteric pathogens in homosexual men with and without AIDS. *Gastroenterology* 1988;94:984.
3. Scheer S, Chu PL, Klausner JD, et al. Effect of highly active antiretroviral therapy on diagnosis of sexually transmitted diseases in people with AIDS. *Lancet* 2001;357:432.
4. Greenspan D, Greenspan JS. HIV related oral disease. *Lancet* 1996;348:729.
5. Maenza JR, Keruly JC, Moore RD, et al. Risk factors for fluconazole-resistant candidiasis in human immunodeficiency virus-infected patients. *J Infect Dis* 1996;173:219.
6. Tavitian A, Raufman J-P, Rosenthal LE. Oral candidiasis as a marker for esophageal candidiasis in the acquired immunodeficiency syndrome. *Ann Intern Med* 1986;104:54.
7. Vasquez JA. Therapeutic options for the management of oropharyngeal and esophageal candidiasis in HIV/AIDS patients. *HIV Clin Trials* 2000;1:47.
8. Arribas JR, Hernandez-Albujar S, Gonzalez-Garcia JJ, et al. Impact of protease inhibitor therapy on HIV-related oropharyngeal candidiasis. *AIDS* 2000;14:979.
9. Greenspan D, Greenspan JS, Conant M, et al. Oral "hairy" leukoplakia in male homosexuals: evidence of association with both papillomavirus and a herpes-group virus. *Lancet* 1984;2:831.
10. Greenspan JS, Greenspan D, Lennette ET, et al. Replication of Epstein-Barr virus within the epithelial cells of oral "hairy" leukoplakia, an AIDS-associated lesion. *N Engl J Med* 1985;313:1564.
11. Aragues M, Sanchez Perez J, Fraga J, et al. Hairy leucoplakia: a clinical, histopathological and ultrastructural study in 33 patients. *Clin Exp Dermatol* 1990;15:335.
12. Paauw DS, Wenrich MD, Curtis JR, et al. Ability of primary care physicians to recognize physical findings associated with HIV infection. *JAMA* 1995;274:1380.
13. Resnick L, Herbst JS, Ablashi D, et al. Regression of oral hairy leukoplakia after orally administered acyclovir therapy. *JAMA* 1988;259:384.
14. Whitley RJ, Roizman B. Herpes simplex virus infections. *Lancet* 2001;357:357.
15. MacPhail LA, Greenspan D, Greenspan JS. Recurrent aphthous ulcers in association with HIV infection: diagnosis and treatment. *Oral Surg Oral Med Oral Pathol* 1992;73:283.
16. Winkler JR, Herrera C, Westenhouse J, et al. Periodontal disease in HIV-infected and uninfected homosexual and bisexual men. *AIDS* 1992;6:1041.
17. Laine L, Bobacini M. Esophageal disease in HIV infection. *Arch Intern Med* 1994;154:1577.
18. Porro GB, Parente F, Cernuschi M. The diagnosis of esophageal candidiasis in patients with acquired immune deficiency syndrome: is endoscopy always necessary? *Am J Gastroenterol* 1989;84:143.
19. Laine L. The natural history of esophageal candidiasis after successful treatment in patients with AIDS. *Gastroenterology* 1994;107:744.
20. Fichtenbaum CJ, Koletar S, Yiannoutsos C, et al. Refractory mucosal candidiasis in advanced HIV infection. *Clin Infect Dis* 2000;30:749.
21. Wilcox CM, Straub RF, Clark WS. Prospective evaluation of oropharyngeal findings in HIV-infected patients with esophageal ulceration. *Am J Gastroenterol* 1995;90:1938.
22. Goodgame RW. Gastrointestinal cytomegalovirus disease. *Ann Intern Med* 1993;119:924.

23. Wilcox CM, Schwartz DA. Comparison of two corticosteroid regimens for the treatment of HIV associated idiopathic esophageal ulcer. *Am J Gastroenterol* 1994;89:2163.

24. Martin DF, Sierra-Madero J, Walmsley S, et al. A controlled trial of valganciclovir as induction therapy for cytomegalovirus retinitis. *N Engl J Med* 2002;346:1119.

25. Paterson DL, Georghiou PR, Allworth AM, et al. Thalidomide as treatment of refractory aphthous ulceration related to human immunodeficiency virus infection. *Clin Infect Dis* 1995;20:250.

26. Edwards P, Turner J, Gold J, et al. Esophageal ulceration induced by zidovudine. *Ann Intern Med* 1990;112:65.

27. Greenspan JS, Greenspan D, eds. *Oral manifestations of HIV infection*. Proceedings of the 2nd International Workshop on the Oral Manifestations of HIV Infection, January 31–February 3, 1993. Carol Stream, IL: Quintessence Publishing, 1995.

28. Wilcox CM. Esophageal disease in acquired immunodeficiency syndrome: etiology, diagnosis, and management. *Am J Med* 1992;92:412.

29. Wilcox CM. Etiology and evaluation of diarrhea in AIDS: a global perspective at the millennium. *World J Gastroenterol* 2000;6:177.

30. Clumeck N, Sonnet J, Taelman H, et al. Acquired immune deficiency syndrome in African patients. *N Engl J Med* 1984;310:492.

31. Piot P, Quinn TC, Taelman H, et al. Acquired immunodeficiency syndrome in a heterosexual population in Zaire. *Lancet* 1984;2:65.

32. Serwadda E, Mugewrwa RD, Sewankambo NK, et al. Slim disease: a new disease in Uganda and its association with HTLV-III infection. *Lancet* 1985;2:849.

33. Kotler DP, Orenstein JM. Prevalence of intestinal microsporidiosis in HIV-infected individuals referred for gastroenterological evaluation. *Am J Gastroenterol* 1994;89:1998.

34. Ullrich R, Heise W, Bergs C, et al. Gastrointestinal symptoms in patients infected with human immunodeficiency virus: relevance of infective agents isolated from gastrointestinal tract. *Gut* 1992;33:1080.

35. Mayer HB, Wanke CA. Diagnostic strategies in HIV-infected patients with diarrhea. *AIDS* 1994;8:1639.

36. Sharpstone D, Gazzard B. Gastrointestinal manifestations of HIV infection. *Lancet* 1996;348:379.

37. Bartlett JG, Belitsos PC, Sears CL. AIDS enteropathy. *Clin Infect Dis* 1992; 15:726.

38. Greenson JK, Belitsos PC, Yardley JH, et al. AIDS enteropathy: occult enteric infections and duodenal mucosal alterations in chronic diarrhea. *Ann Intern Med* 1991;114:366.

39. Orenstein JM, Dieterich DT. The histopathology of 103 consecutive colonoscopy biopsies from 82 symptomatic patients with acquired immunodeficiency syndrome: original and look-back diagnoses. *Arch Pathol Lab Med* 2001;125:1042.

40. Weber R, Ledergerber B, Zbinden R, et al. Enteric infections and diarrhea in human immunodeficiency virus-infected patients. *Arch Intern Med* 1999;159:1473.

41. Sherman DS, Fish DN. Management of protease inhibitor-associated diarrhea. *Clin Infect Dis* 2000;30:908.

42. Guerrant RL, van Gilda T, Steiner TS, et al. Practice guidelines for the management of infectious diarrhea. *Clin Infect Dis* 2001;32:331.

43. Choi SW, Choong HP, Silva TMJ, et al. To culture or not to culture: fecal lactoferrin screening for inflammatory bacterial diarrhea. *J Clin Microbiol* 1996;34:928.

44. van Gool T, Snijders F, Reiss P, et al. Diagnosis of intestinal and disseminated microsporidial infections in patients with HIV by a new rapid fluorescence technique. *J Clin Pathol* 1993;46:694.

45. Wilcox MC, Schwartz DA, Cotsonis G, et al. Chronic unexplained diarrhea in human immunodeficiency virus infection: determination of the best diagnostic approach. *Gastroenterology* 1996;110:30.

46. Kotler DP, Giang TT, Thiim M, et al. Chronic bacterial enteropathy in patients with AIDS. *J Infect Dis* 1995;171:552.

47. Mathewson JJ, Jiang ZD, Zumla A, et al. HEp-2 cell-adherent *Escherichia coli* in patients with human immunodeficiency virus-associated diarrhea. *J Infect Dis* 1995;171:1636.

48. Ullrich R, Zeitz M, Heise W, et al. Small intestinal structure and function in patients infected with human immunodeficiency virus (HIV): evidence for HIV induced enteropathy. *Ann Intern Med* 1989;111:15.

49. Keating J, Bjarnason I, Somasundaram S, et al. Intestinal absorptive capacity, intestinal permeability and jejunal histology in HIV and their relation to diarrhoea. *Gut* 1995;37:623.

50. Fox CH, Kotler D, Tierney A, et al. Detection of HIV-1 RNA in the lamina propria of patients with AIDS and gastrointestinal disease. *J Infect Dis* 1989;159:467.

51. Heise C, Dandekar S, Kumar P, et al. Human immunodeficiency virus infection of enterocytes and mononuclear cells in human jejunal mucosa. *Gastroenterology* 1991;100:1521.

52. MacDonald TT, Spencer J. Evidence that activated mucosal T cells play a role in the pathogenesis of enteropathy in human small intestine. *J Exp Med* 1988;167:1341.

53. Belitsos PC, Greenson JK, Sisler J, et al. Association of chronic wasting diarrhea with gastric hypoacidity and opportunistic enteric infections in patients with acquired immunodeficiency syndrome (AIDS). *J Infect Dis* 1992;166:277.

54. Freeman R, Roberts MS, Friedman LS, et al. Autonomic function and human immunodeficiency virus infection. *Neurology* 1990;40:575.

55. Batman PA, Miller ARO, Sedgwick PM, et al. Autonomic denervation in jejunal mucosa of homosexual men infected with HIV. *AIDS* 1991;5:1247.

56. Kaljot KT, Ling JP, Gold JWM, et al. Prevalence of acute enteric viral pathogens in acquired immunodeficiency syndrome patients with diarrhea. *Gastroenterology* 1989;97:1031.

57. Schmidt W, Schneider T, Heise W, et al. Stool viruses, coinfections, and diarrhea in HIV-infected patients. *J Acquir Immune Defic Syndr Hum Retrovirol* 1996;13:33.

58. Grohmann GS, Glass RI, Pereira HG, et al. Enteric viruses and diarrhea in HIV-infected patients. *N Engl J Med* 1993;329:14.

59. Nelson MR, Shanson DC Hawkins DA, et al. *Salmonella*, Campylobacter and Shigella in HIV-seropositive patients. *AIDS* 1992;6:1495.

60. Mundy LM, Sears CL. Small intestinal infections: *Salmonella* and human immunodeficiency virus-associated enteropathy. *Curr Opin Gastroenterol* 1993;9:77.

61. Gruenewald R, Blum S, Chan J. Relationship between human immunodeficiency virus infection and salmonellosis in 20- to 59-year-old residents of New York City. *Clin Infect Dis* 1994;18:358.

62. Jacobs JL, Gold JWM, Murray HW, et al. *Salmonella* infections in patients with the acquired immunodeficiency syndrome. *Ann Intern Med* 1985;102:186.

63. Smith PD, Macher AM, Bookman MA, et al. *Salmonella typhimurium* enteritis and bacteremia in the acquired immunodeficiency syndrome. *Ann Intern Med* 1985;102:207.

64. Salmon D, Detruchis P, Leport C, et al. Efficacy of zidovudine in preventing relapses of *Salmonella* bacteremia in AIDS. *J Infect Dis* 1991;163:415.

65. Lu SS, Schwartz JM, Simon DM, et al. *Clostridium difficile*–associated diarrhea in patients with HIV positivity and AIDS: a prospective controlled study. *Am J Gastroenterol* 1994;89:1226.

66. Bartlett JG. Antibiotic-associated diarrhea. *N Engl J Med* 2002;346:334.

67. Chen XM, Keithly JS, Paya CV, et al. Cryptosporidiosis. *N Engl J Med* 2002; 346:1723.

68. Goodgame RW. Understanding intestinal spore-forming protozoa: cryptosporidia, microsporidia, isospora, and cyclospora. *Ann Intern Med* 1996;124: 429.

69. Smith PD, Quinn TC, Strober W, et al. Gastrointestinal infections in AIDS. *Ann Intern Med* 1992;116:63.

70. Rabeneck L. Diagnostic workup strategies for patients with HIV-related chronic diarrhea. *J Clin Gastroenterol* 1993;16:245.

71. Dieterich DT, Kotler DP, Busch DF, et al. Ganciclovir treatment of cytomegalovirus colitis in AIDS: a randomized, double-blind, placebo-controlled multicenter study. *J Infect Dis* 1993;167:278.

72. Dieterich DT, Rahmin M. Cytomegalovirus colitis in AIDS: presentation in 44 patients and a review of the literature. *J Acquir Immune Defic Syndr Hum Retrovirol* 1991;4[Suppl 1]:529.

73. Cohen J, West AB, Bini EJ. Infectious diarrhea in HIV. *Gastroenterol Clin North Am* 2001;30:637.

74. Rich JD, Crawford JM, Kazanjian SN, et al. Discrete gastrointestinal mass lesions caused by cytomegalovirus in patients with AIDS: report of three cases and review. *Clin Infect Dis* 1992;15:609.

75. Frager DH, Frager JD, Wolf EL, et al. Cytomegalovirus colitis in acquired immune deficiency syndrome: radiologic spectrum. *Gastrointest Radiol* 1986; 111:241.

76. Chachoua A, Dieterich D, Krasinski K, et al. 9-(1,3-Dihydroxy-2-propoxymethyl) guanine (ganciclovir) in the treatment of cytomegalovirus gastrointestinal disease with the acquired immunodeficiency syndrome. *Ann Intern Med* 1987;107:133.

77. Dieterich DT, Poles MA, Dicker M, et al. Foscarnet treatment of cytomegalovirus gastrointestinal infections in acquired immunodeficiency syndrome patients who have failed ganciclovir induction. *Am J Gastroenterol* 1993;88:542.

78. Blanshard C, Benhamou Y, Dohin E, et al. Treatment of AIDS-associated gastrointestinal cytomegalovirus infection with foscarnet and ganciclovir: a randomized comparison. *J Infect Dis* 1995;172:622.

79. Petersen C. Cryptosporidiosis in patients infected with the human immunodeficiency virus. *J Infect Dis* 1993;15:903.

80. Flanigan T, Whalen C, Turner J, et al. Cryptosporidium infection and CD4 counts. *Ann Intern Med* 1992;116:840.

81. Current WL, Garcia LS. Cryptosporidiosis. *Clin Microbiol Rev* 1991;4:325.

82. Wuhib T, Silva TM, Newman RD, et al. Cryptosporidial and microsporidial infections in human immunodeficiency virus-infected patients in northeastern Brazil. *J Infect Dis* 1994;170:490.

83. Vakil NB, Schwartz SM, Buggy BP, et al. Biliary cryptosporidiosis in HIV-infected people after the waterborne outbreak of cryptosporidiosis in Milwaukee. *N Engl J Med* 1996;334:19.

84. Benhamou Y, Caumes E, Gerosa Y, et al. AIDS-related cholangiopathy: critical analysis of a prospective series of 26 patients. *Dig Dis Sci* 1993;38:1113.

85. White BC Jr, Chappell CL, Hayat CS, et al. Paromomycin for cryptosporidiosis in AIDS: a prospective, double-blind trial. *J Infect Dis* 1994;170:419.

86. Miao YM, Awad-El-Kariem FM, Franzen C, et al. Eradication of cryptosporidia and microsporidia following successful antiretroviral therapy. *J Acquir Immune Defic Syndr* 2000;25:124.

87. French AL, Beaudet LM, Benator DA, et al. Cholecystectomy in patients with AIDS: clinicopathologic correlations in 107 cases. *Clin Infect Dis* 1995;21: 852.

88. DeHovit JA, Pape JW, Boncy M, et al. Clinical manifestations and therapy of *Isospora belli* infection in patients with the acquired immunodeficiency syndrome. *N Engl J Med* 1986;315:87.

89. Soave R, Johnson WD. AIDS commentary: *Cryptosporidium* and *Isospora belli* infections. *J Infect Dis* 1988;157:225.

90. Pape JEW, Liautaud B, Thomas F, et al. The acquired immunodeficiency syndrome in Haiti. *Ann Intern Med* 1985;103:674.
91. Pape JW, Johnson WD Jr. *Isospora belli* infections. *Frog Clin Parasitol* 1991;2:119.
92. Shadduck JA. Human microsporidiosis and AIDS. *Rev Infect Dis* 1989;11:203.
93. Orenstein JM. Microsporidiosis in the acquired immunodeficiency syndrome. *J Parasitol* 1991;77:843.
94. Dascomb K, Clark R, Aberg J, et al. Natural history of intestinal microsporidiosis among patients infected with human immunodeficiency virus. *J Clin Microbiol* 1999;37:3421.
95. Ambroise-Thomas P. Parasitic diseases and immunodeficiencies. *Parasitology* 2001;122:S65.
96. Weber R, Bryan RT, Owen RL, et al. Improved light-microscopical detection of microsporidia spores in stool and duodenal aspirates. The Enteric Opportunistic Infections Working Group. *N Engl J Med* 1992;326:161.
97. Rabeneck L, Gyorkey F, Genta RM, et al. The role of microsporidia in the pathogenesis of HIV-related chronic diarrhea. *Ann Intern Med* 1993;119:895.
98. Weber R, Sauer B, Spycher MA, et al. Detection of *Septata intestinalis* in stool specimens, and coprodiagnostic monitoring of successful treatment with albendazole. *Clin Infect Dis* 1994;19:242.
99. Garcia LS. Laboratory identification of the microsporidia. *J Clin Microbiol* 2002;40:1892.
100. Franzen C, Muller A. Microsporidiosis: human diseases and diagnosis. *Microbes Infect* 2001;3:389.
101. Dieterich DT, Lew EA, Kotler DP, et al. Treatment with albendazole for intestinal disease due to *Enterocytozoon bieneusi* in patients with AIDS. *J Infect Dis* 1994;169:178.
102. Conteas CN, Berlin OG, Ash LR, et al. Therapy for human gastrointestinal microsporidiosis. *Am J Trop Med Hyg* 2000;63:121.
103. Kirk O, Gatell JM, Mocroft A, et al. Infections with *Mycobacterium tuberculosis* and *Mycobacterium avium* among HIV-infected patients after introduction of highly active antiretroviral therapy. *Am J Respir Crit Care Med* 2000;162:865.
104. Benson CA, Williams PL, Cohn DL, et al. Clarithromycin or rifabutin alone or in combination for primary prophylaxis of *Mycobacterium avium* complex disease in patients with AIDS. *J Infect Dis* 2000;181:1289.
105. Masur H, et al. Recommendations on prophylaxis and therapy for disseminated *Mycobacterium avium* complex disease in patients infected with the human immunodeficiency virus. *N Engl J Med* 1993;329:898.
106. El-Sadr WM, Burman WJ, Grant LB, et al. Discontinuation of prophylaxis against *Mycobacterium avium* complex disease in HIV-infected patients who have a response to antiretroviral therapy. *N Engl J Med* 2000;342:1085.
107. Damsker B. *Mycobacterium avium–Mycobacterium intracellulare* from the intestinal tracts of patients with the acquired immunodeficiency syndrome: concepts regarding acquisition and pathogenesis. *J Infect Dis* 1985;151:179.
108. Roth RI, Owen RL, Keren DF. AIDS with *Mycobacterium avium-intracellulare* lesions resembling those of Whipple's disease. *N Engl J Med* 1983;309:1324.
109. Hawkins CC, Gold JWM, Whimbey E, et al. *Mycobacterium avium* complex infections in patients with the acquired immunodeficiency syndrome. *Ann Intern Med* 1986;105:184.
110. Benson CA. Disease due to *Mycobacterium avium* complex in patients with AIDS: epidemiology and clinical syndrome. *Clin Infect Dis* 1994;18:S218.
111. Hellyer TJ, Brown IN, Taylor MB, et al. Gastrointestinal involvement in *Mycobacterium avium-intracellulare* infection inpatients with HIV. *J Infect* 1993;26:55.
112. Kiehn TE, Edwards FF, Brannon P, et al. Infections caused by *Mycobacterium avium* complex in immunocompromised patients: diagnosis by blood culture and fecal examination, antimicrobial susceptibility tests, and morphological and seroagglutination characteristics. *J Clin Microbiol* 1985;21:168.
113. Dunne M, Fessel J, Kumar P, et al. A randomized, double blind trial comparing azithromycin and clarithromycin in the treatment of disseminated *Mycobacterium avium* infection in patients with human immunodeficiency virus. *Clin Infect Dis* 2000;31:245.
114. Cohn DL, Fisher EJ, Peng GT, et al. A prospective randomized trial of four three-drug regimens in the treatment of disseminated *Mycobacterium avium* complex disease in AIDS patients: excess mortality associated with high-dose clarithromycin. *Clin Infect Dis* 1999;29:155.
115. Zeller W, Truffot C, Agher R, et al. Discontinuation of secondary prophylaxis against disseminated *Mycobacterium avium* complex infection and toxoplasmic encephalitis. *Clin Infect Dis* 2002;34:662.
116. Currier JS, Williams PL, Koletar SL, et al. Discontinuation of *Mycobacterium avium* complex prophylaxis in patients with antiretroviral therapy-induced increases in CD4 cell count. *Ann Intern Med* 2000;133:493.
117. Baskin DH, Lax JD, Barenberg D. *Shigella* bacteremia in patients with the acquired immune deficiency syndrome. *Am J Gastroenterol* 1987;82:338.
118. Blaser MJ, Hale TL, Formal SB. Recurrent shigellosis complicating human immunodeficiency virus infection: failure of preexisting antibodies to confer protection. *Am J Med* 1989;86:105.
119. Dworkin B, Wormser GP, Abdoo RA, et al. Persistence of multiply antibiotic-resistant *Campylobacter jejuni* in a patient with the acquired immune deficiency syndrome. *Am J Med* 1986;80:965.
120. Perlman DM, Ampel NM, Schitman RB, et al. Persistent *Campylobacter jejuni* infections in patients infected with human immunodeficiency virus (HIV). *Ann Intern Med* 1988;108:540.
121. Evans TG, Riley D. *Campylobacter laridis* colitis in a human immunodeficiency virus-positive patient treated with a quinolone. *Clin Infect Dis* 1992;15:172.
122. Manfredi R, Calza L, Chiodo F. Enteric and disseminated *Campylobacter* species infection during HIV disease. *Am J Gastroenterol* 2002;97:510.
123. Esforzado N, Poch E, Almiralli J, et al. Hemolytic uremic syndrome associated with HIV infection [Letter]. *AIDS* 1991;5:1041.
124. Lowther SA, Dworkin MS, Hanson DL. *Entamoeba histolytica/Entamoeba dispar* infections in human immunodeficiency virus-infected patients in the United States. *Clin Infect Dis* 2000;30:955.
125. Haggerty CM, Britton MC, Dorman JM, et al. Gastrointestinal histoplasmosis in suspected acquired immunodeficiency syndrome. *West J Med* 1985;143:244.
126. Cappell MS. Extensive gastrointestinal aspergillosis associated with AIDS. *Dig Dis Sci* 1991;36:1500.
127. Wheat LJ, Connolly-Stringfield PA, Baker RL, et al. Disseminated histoplasmosis in the acquired immune deficiency syndrome: clinical findings, diagnosis and treatment, and review of the literature. *Medicine* (Baltimore) 1990;69:361.
128. Lemlich G, Schwam L, Lebwohl M. Kaposi's sarcoma and acquired immunodeficiency syndrome: postmortem findings in twenty-four cases. *J Am Acad Dermatol* 1987;16:319.
129. Friedman S, Wright T, Altman D. Kaposi's sarcoma and the gastrointestinal tract: the San Francisco experience. *Gastroenterology* 1983;84:1160.
130. Selik RM, Byers RH, Dworkin MS. Trends in diseases reported on U.S. death certificates that mention HIV infection 1987–1999. *J Acquir Immune Defic Syndr* 2002;29:378.
131. Gates AE, Kaplan LD. AIDS malignancies in the era of highly active antiretroviral therapy. *Oncology* 2002;16:441.
132. Fellay J, Boubaker K, Ledergerber B, et al. Prevalence of adverse events associated with potent antiretroviral treatment. *Lancet* 2001;358:1322.
133. Raines CP, Flexner C, Sun E, et al. Safety, tolerability and antiretroviral effects of ritonavir-nelfinavir combination therapy administered for 48 weeks. *J Acquir Immune Defic Syndr* 2000;25:322.
134. Sherman DS, Fish DN. Management of protease inhibitor diarrhea. *Clin Infect Dis* 2000;30:908.
135. Dassopoulos I, Ehrenpreis ED. Acute pancreatitis in human immunodeficiency virus-infected patients: a review. *Am J Med* 1999;107:78.
136. Floridia M, Vella S, Seeber AC, et al. A randomized trial (ISS 902) of didanosine versus zidovudine in previously untreated patients with mildly symptomatic human immunodeficiency virus infection. *J Infect Dis* 1997;175:255.
137. Abonlafia DM. Acute pancreatitis: a fatal complication of AIDS therapy. *J Clin Gastroenterol* 1997;25:640.
138. Manodia AP, Sossenheimer M, Martin SP, et al. Prevalence and predictors of severe acute pancreatitis in patients with AIDS. *Am J Gastroenterol* 1999;94:784.
139. Falco V, Rodriguez D, Ribera E, et al. Severe nucleoside-associated lactic acidosis in human immunodeficiency virus-infected patients: report of twelve cases and review of the literature. *Clin Infect Dis* 2002;34:838.
140. Cote HC, Brumme ZL, Craib KJ, et al. Changes in mitochondrial DNA as a marker of nucleoside toxicity in HIV-infected patients. *N Engl J Med* 2002;346:811.
141. John M, Moore CB, James IR, et al. Chronic hyperlactemia in HIV-infected patients taking antiretroviral therapy. *AIDS* 2001;15:717.
142. Miller KD, Cameron M, Wood LV, et al. Lactic acidosis and hepatic steatosis associated with use of stavudine: report of four cases. *Ann Intern Med* 2000;133:192.
143. Lafeuillade A, Hittinger G, Chadapaud S. Increased mitochondrial toxicity with ribavirin in HIV/HCV coinfection. *Lancet* 2001;357:280.
144. Carr A, Cooper DA. Adverse effects of antiretroviral therapy. *Lancet* 2000;356:1423.
145. Carr A, Morey A, Mallon P, et al. Fatal portal hypertension, liver failure and mitochondrial dysfunction after HIV-1 nucleoside analogue-induced hepatitis and lactic academia. *Lancet* 2001;357:1412.
146. Palmon R, Koo BC, Shoultz DA, et al. Lack of hepatotoxicity associated with non-nucleoside reverse transcriptase inhibitors. *J Acquir Immune Defic Syndr* 2002;29:340.
147. Centers for Disease Control and Prevention. Serious adverse events attributed to nevirapine regimens for postexposure prophylaxis after HIV exposures—worldwide, 1997–2000. *MMWR Morb Mortal Wkly Rep* 2001;49:1153.
148. Martinez E, Blanco JL, Amaiz JA, et al. Hepatotoxicity in HIV-1-infected patients receiving nevirapine-containing antiretroviral therapy. *AIDS* 2001;15:1261.
149. Aceti A, Pasquazzi C, Zechini B, et al. Hepatotoxicity development during antiretroviral therapy containing protease inhibitors in patients with HIV. *J Acquir Immune Defic Syndr* 2002;29:41.
150. Nunez M, Lana R, Mendoza JL, et al. Risk factors for severe hepatic injury after introduction of highly active antiretroviral therapy. *J Acquir Immune Defic Syndr* 2001;27:426.
151. Sulkowski MS, Thomas DL, Chaisson RE, et al. Hepatotoxicity associated with antiretroviral therapy in adults infected with human immunodeficiency virus and the role of hepatitis C or B virus infection. *JAMA* 2000;283:74.
152. Monforte AA, Bugarini R, Pezzotti P, et al. Low frequency of severe hepatotoxicity and association with HCV coinfection in HIV-positive patients treated with HAART. *J Acquir Immune Defic Syndr* 2001;28:114.
153. Guenter P, Muurahainen N, Simons G, et al. Relationships among nutritional status, disease progression and survival in HIV infection. *J Acquir Immune Defic Syndr* 1993;6:1130.
154. Wanke C, Silva M, Knox T, et al. Weight loss and wasting remain complications in individuals infected with HIV in the era of highly active antiretroviral therapy. *Clin Infect Dis* 2000;31:803.
155. Grunfield C, Kotler DP, Shigenaga JK, et al. Circulating interferon-α levels and hypertriglyceridemia in the acquired immunodeficiency syndrome. *Am J Med* 1991;90:154.

156. Macallan DC, McNurlan MA, Milne E, et al. Whole body protein turnover from leucine kinetics and the response to nutrition in human immunodeficiency virus infection. *Am J Clin Nutr* 1995;61:818.
157. Macallan DC, Noble C, Baldwin C, et al. Energy expenditure and wasting in human immunodeficiency virus infection. *N Engl J Med* 1995;333:83.
158. Macallan DC, Noble C, Baldwin C, et al. Prospective analysis of patterns of weight change in stage IV human immunodeficiency virus infection. *Am J Clin Nutr* 1993;58:417.
159. Scuba WW. Nutritional support. *N Engl J Med* 1997;336:41.
160. Oster M, Enders S, Samuels S, et al. Megesterol acetate in patients with AIDS cachexia. *Ann Intern Med* 1994;121:400.
161. Timpone JG, Wright DJ, Li N, et al. The safety and pharmacokinetic of single agent and combination therapy with megesterol acetate and dronabinol for treatment of HIV wasting syndrome. *J AIDS* 1997;13:305.
162. Rietshcel P, Corcoran C, Stanley T, et al. Prevalence of hypogonadism among men with weight loss related to human immunodeficiency virus infection who were receiving highly active antiretroviral therapy. *Clin Infect Dis* 2000;31:1240.
163. Grinspoon S, Corcoran C, Askari H, et al. Effects of androgen administration in men with AIDS wasting: a randomized, placebo-controlled trial. *Ann Intern Med* 1998;129:18.
164. Berger J, Pall L, Hall C, et al. Oxandrolone in AIDS-wasting myopathy. *AIDS* 1991;10:1657.
165. Strawford A, Barbieri T, Neese R, et al. Effects of nandrolone decanoate therapy in borderline hypogonadal men with HIV-associated weight loss. *J Acquir Immune Defic Syndr Hum Retrovirol* 1999;20:137.
166. Roubenoff R, McDermott A, Weiss L, et al. Short-term progressive resistance training increases strength and lean body mass in adults infected with HIV. *AIDS* 1999;13:231.
167. Agin D, Kotler DP, Papandreou D. Effects of whey protein and resistance exercise on body composition and muscle strength in women with HIV infection. *Ann N Y Acad Sci* 2000;904:607.
168. Patton N, Newton P, Sharpstone D, et al. Short-term growth hormone administration at the time of opportunistic infections in HIV-positive people. *AIDS* 1999;13:1995.

CHAPTER 117
Cutaneous Infections in Human Immunodeficiency Virus Disease

Carrie Ann Cusack, Marsha L. Chaffins, and Clay J. Cockerell

A wide variety of cutaneous infectious disorders develop in patients infected with the human immunodeficiency virus type 1 (HIV-1). Many of these disorders also occur in immunocompetent patients; however, in HIV-infected hosts, the clinical manifestations are often unusual, severe, or prolonged. Occasionally they may serve as an initial clue to the diagnosis of HIV infection (Table 117.1). Skin or mucosal lesions may reflect the dissemination of an underlying systemic infectious illness or may serve as an acquired immunodeficiency syndrome (AIDS)-defining indicator (Tables 117.2 and 117.3). Furthermore, the development of certain cutaneous disorders can be correlated with the CD4+ lymphocyte counts (Table 117.4). Early recognition and appropriate treatment of cutaneous infections may have a significant impact on lessening morbidity and mortality.

VIRAL INFECTIONS

Acute Exanthem of Human Immunodeficiency Virus Disease

The acute exanthem of HIV infection is an acute reaction that is associated with HIV seroconversion. This phenomenon

TABLE 117.1. Common Cutaneous Infections that Provide Clues to HIV Infection

Cutaneous infection	Clue
Herpes simplex	Ulcerative lesion(s), lasting >1 mo, especially perianal location
Herpes zoster	Involvement of more than one dermatome; recurrent episodes
Verrucae	Multiple periungual lesions; numerous flat warts on face and beard area
Molluscum contagiosum	Multiple lesions on face, especially periorbital location; giant lesions
Impetigo	Axillary, inguinal, or other intertriginous locations
Staphylococcal folliculitis	Plaquelike folliculitis; progression to botryomycosis
Scabies	Hyperkeratotic crusted lesions (Norwegian scabies)
Oral candidiasis	Refractory or recurrent disease
Onychomycosis	Proximal white subungual involvement
Tinea versicolor	Extensive disease

TABLE 117.2. AIDS-Defining Cutaneous Disorders

Chronic herpes simplex ulceration >1 mo duration
Kaposi's sarcoma
Cutaneous cytomegalovirus infection, ulceration
Cutaneous cryptococcosis
Cutaneous lesions secondary to disseminated histoplasmosis, coccidioidomycosis, or mycobacterial infections

TABLE 117.3. Cutaneous Infections that May Predict Progression to AIDS

Disease	Percentage of patients progressing to AIDS
Severe acute HIV infection	78% within 3 yr
Herpes zoster	34% within 3 yr
Oral hairy leukoplakia	83% within 3 yr

TABLE 117.4. Relationship of Cutaneous Infections to CD4+ Cell Count

Cutaneous disease	Average CD4+ cell count at disease presentation (cells/mm³)
Acute exanthem of HIV	Normal
Bacterial folliculitis, impetigo	>500
Tinea	>500
Seborrheic dermatitis	>500
Intraepithelial neoplasia	<500
Oral hairy leukoplakia	<400
Verrucae	500–250
Herpes zoster	500–250
Herpes simplex	500–250
Scabies	<250
Bacillary angiomatosis	<250
Leishmaniasis	<250
Molluscum contagiosum	<250
Oral candidiasis	<250
Cytomegalovirus infection	<200

develops in 10% to 80% of all newly diagnosed cases of HIV infection but is often subclinical (1–4). It generally occurs after an incubation period of 3 to 6 weeks and corresponds to widespread infection of cells with HIV (5). This is thought to lead to release of cytokines and inflammatory mediators that result in the expression of this exanthem. This cutaneous manifestation appears to be more common when HIV infection is transmitted by sexual intercourse rather than intravenously (6).

CLINICAL MANIFESTATIONS

Patients experience a sensation of malaise and develop fever with a temperature that can be 102°F or higher. Night sweats, pharyngitis, fatigue, lymphadenopathy, and a fine morbilliform eruption involving the trunk, chest, back, and upper arms develop within one to several days (1,2) (Fig. 117.1). The cutaneous eruption is similar to that seen with other viral illnesses or drug reactions. The entire syndrome lasts 4 to 14 days and usually resolves without sequelae. Patients are highly infectious during this time, and although the CD4+ cell count may remain perfectly normal, it may fall to as low as 200 cells/mm³. The primary infection and resultant lymphocyte decrease leads to immunosuppression, which may by associated with opportunistic infections seen in AIDS (7).

A severe form of acute HIV infection may develop with persistent HIV p24 antigenemia, recurrent viremia, rapid decline in CD4+ cell numbers, and accelerated disease progression (8). Systemic manifestations include pneumonitis, esophagitis, meningitis, abdominal pain, and melena. Skin manifestations that may be seen include urticaria, perlèche, palatal and esophageal ulcers, enanthemata, and candidiasis (8,9). Herpesvirus infections may also supervene (8). The prognosis for patients who suffer from prolonged symptomatic primary HIV infection is significantly poorer than for those with asymptomatic or mild primary infection (Table 117.3).

DIAGNOSIS

The diagnosis of the acute HIV exanthem is based on the presence of a characteristic clinical picture in an individual with risk factors for the development of HIV infection. The histologic features are somewhat nonspecific, consisting of superficial perivas-

cular dermatitis with occasional necrotic keratinocytes, again similar to those of a drug eruption or other viral exanthem (10). Immunocytochemistry has revealed that most of the infiltrating cells in skin lesions are CD4+ T cells with an admixture of CD8+ cells (10).

Because the eruption occurs around the time of HIV seroconversion, the patient may test negatively for HIV antibody; however, HIV p24 antigen or HIV RNA may be detected. Elevated erythrocyte sedimentation rate, leukopenia, and cerebrospinal fluid lymphocytic pleocytosis are nonspecific findings that may be observed. In the case of fulminant acute HIV infection, laboratory findings of profound immunosuppression as alluded to earlier may be demonstrated (5).

TREATMENT

Zidovudine and other antiviral agents have been administered to patients with the acute HIV viral exanthem without repeatable success (11–13). Early intervention with antiretrovirals may result in preservation of specific anti-HIV immune responses and thus an improved long-term result (14).

Herpesvirus Infections

Infections with human herpesvirus types 1, 2, and 6, varicella-zoster virus, Epstein-Barr virus, and cytomegalovirus (CMV) are commonly encountered with patients infected with HIV. With advanced immunosuppression, the prevalence of infection with these viruses ranges from between 20% and 40% with herpes simplex virus (HSV) to virtually 100% with CMV (15–17).

HERPES SIMPLEX AND VARICELLA-ZOSTER VIRUS INFECTIONS

HSV and varicella-zoster virus are enveloped double-stranded DNA viruses that may produce both primary and recurrent disease and that have long latency periods. In HIV infection, primary infections tend to be more severe and may be life threatening (18). Latent virus may be found in the nervous system and reticuloendothelial system as well as in other tissues such as the skin. With the onset of immunosuppression, the herpesvirus may become reactivated and produce recurrent disease.

The presence of a genital herpetic ulcer is a significant risk factor for the acquisition of HIV infection because the lesions serve as a portal of entry for the virus (19,20). In addition, *in vitro* studies have shown that HSV can potentiate HIV infection (21). Of note, genital herpes is the most common sexually transmitted disease among HIV-positive individuals (22).

CLINICAL MANIFESTATIONS

Herpes Simplex. Lesions of herpes simplex are typically painful grouped vesicles on an erythematous base that rupture, become crusted, and heal within 2 weeks. After significant immune suppression supervenes, lesions caused by HSV may become progressive and manifest as chronic ulcerative mucocutaneous lesions that last for longer than 1 month (23). Tender, painful ulcerative lesions of the penis, perianal area, lip, perioral area, and digits are quite characteristic. Lesions that are untreated may continue to enlarge dramatically and become painful. Persistent herpetic ulcerations may be recognized by their serpiginous, macerated border. Verrucous and hyperplastic changes may also ensue. Infrequently, HSV may present as treatment-resistant facial folliculitis (24).

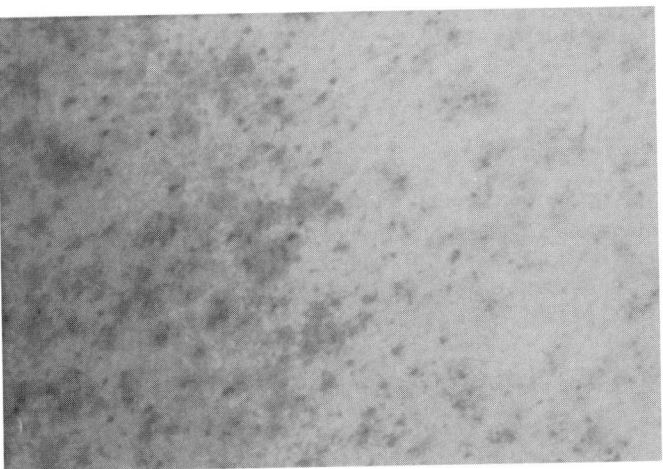

Figure 117.1. Acute exanthem of HIV infection. A widespread eruption of fine macules and papules distributed over the trunk, extremities, and sometimes the head and neck is characteristic.

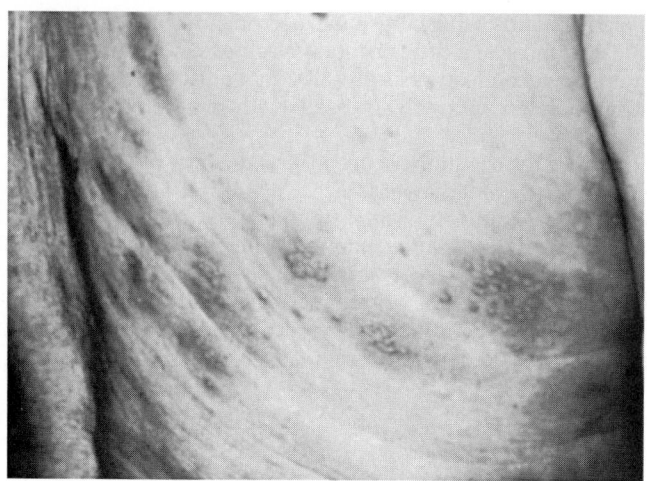

Figure 117.2. Herpes zoster. A linear dermatomal distribution of painful vesicles on erythematous bases is characteristic of herpes zoster.

Varicella-Zoster. Primary varicella lesions in HIV-infected patients appear like those in non–HIV-infected hosts as clear vesicles on a rose-colored base that heal with crusting and occasionally scars. However, in HIV-infected individuals, varicella is more likely to have a prolonged course and to be associated with systemic complications; it may even be fatal (25). In one study, 40% of HIV-positive children who developed primary varicella suffered a complication, and in 5% of these individuals, the outcome was fatal (26).

Zoster presents as tense vesicles on an erythematous base in a dermatomal distribution and is often associated with significant pain (Fig. 117.2). In the HIV-infected host, lesions involving multiple dermatomes or dissemination of lesions over large areas of the skin may occur (27,28). In HIV-infected children, herpes zoster may develop shortly after a course of primary varicella (29). In addition, unusual clinical patterns such as verrucous lesions and crusted, punched-out ulcerations that leave atrophic painful scars have been noted. Postherpetic neuralgia also seems to be more common.

DIAGNOSIS
A diagnosis of HSV or varicella-zoster virus infection can usually be made readily by the performance of the Tzanck smear. Direct fluorescent antigen test may also be performed from a lesional smear. Histopathologic examination of lesions reveals an intraepidermal acantholytic vesicular dermatitis associated with characteristic cytopathic effects in epithelial cells.

TREATMENT
First-line therapy for herpesvirus infections is acyclovir administered orally (Table 117.5). Both famciclovir and valacyclovir are effective for HSV in HIV-positive patients. Acyclovir-resistant strains of HSV can develop, however, and require treatment with intravenous foscarnet sodium or vidarabine (30–32). Cidofovir has been useful for acyclovir-resistant mucocutaneous HSV in AIDS patients (33). On occasion, patients with seemingly resistant HSV or varicella-zoster virus infection may be suffering from atrophic gastritis that prevents absorption of acyclovir; hence, a change to intravenous administration may be necessary. Those suffering from frequent recurrent HSV infections may benefit from prophylactic acyclovir (600 to 800 mg per day) (34). A recent study demonstrated that acyclovir therapy offered a substantial survival benefit to patients with HIV infection (35).

Herpes zoster should be treated with higher doses of acyclovir, 800 mg orally every 4 hours while the patient is awake. Nonsteroidal antiinflammatory agents or narcotics may be necessary to help relieve associated pain. Topical therapy with cool compresses or sitz baths and topical anesthetics may also be helpful. Postherpetic neuralgia often responds poorly to treatment. Topical application of capsaicin-containing compounds, eutectic mixture of local anesthetics (EMLA) cream, low-dose tricyclic antidepressants, carbamazepine, fentanyl patches, nerve blocks, biofeedback, and hypnosis have been reported to be effective in some cases. Varicella immune globulin should be given to HIV-seropositive patients at risk for primary varicella if exposure to the virus occurs (34). Treatment of varicella includes acyclovir, famciclovir, or valacyclovir along with evaluation for systemic diseases. If systemic disease is present, treatment must be administered by the intravenous route (36).

Cytomegalovirus Infections

Despite the high frequency of systemic CMV infections in the HIV-positive population, cutaneous involvement is rarely seen. In fact, some authors question its pathogenic role in most mucocutaneous lesions (37). However, when skin involvement does occur, it usually portends a poor prognosis.

CLINICAL MANIFESTATIONS
Cutaneous lesions of CMV infection that have been reported include localized and diffuse ulcerations, keratotic verrucous lesions, and palpable purpuric papules (38,39) (Fig. 117.3). CMV-associated perianal ulcerations most often represent contiguous spread from the gastrointestinal tract (40). Co-infection with CMV and HSV occurs not infrequently (41,42). CMV has been reported to induce hyperpigmented plaques, diffuse morbilliform eruptions, and vesicular lesions, as well as a bullous toxic epidermal necrolysis-like reaction (39,43–45). Adrenal infection may be associated with diffuse hyperpigmentation. Although no characteristic lesion exists for CMV infection, a persistent ulceration should warrant a search for CMV (46).

DIAGNOSIS
Skin biopsy is necessary for definitive diagnosis of cutaneous disease. CMV characteristically infects dermal fibroblasts and endothelial cells, resulting in ulceration of the epidermis. CMV-infected cells are enlarged to several times their normal diameter and develop purplish intracytoplasmic and intranuclear inclusions that have a somewhat crystalline shape. Immunoperoxidase antibody stains to CMV may be used to confirm the diagnosis. When a biopsy specimen for CMV is evaluated, it is important to search for other pathogens because co-infections are not uncommon (41,42).

TREATMENT
Ganciclovir at a dose of 5 mg/kg per day is needed for the treatment of CMV infection (47). The combination of ganciclovir and foscarnet may be more effective than either agent alone, and continued prophylactic treatment with ganciclovir may be indicated for severely immunocompromised patients (34).

Oral Hairy Leukoplakia

Oral hairy leukoplakia (OHL) is caused by infection with the Epstein-Barr virus; although initially described only in HIV-infected patients, it may be seen in other diseases associated with immunosuppression (48,49). The incubation period from

TABLE 117.5. Treatment of Common Cutaneous Infections in HIV-Infected Patients

Viral infection	Treatment of choice	Comment
Herpes simplex	Acyclovir, 200–600 mg PO q4h while awake Famciclovir, 500 mg PO tid	Higher doses may be required. Acyclovir-resistant cases require foscarnet, vidarabine, or trifluorthymidine.
Primary varicella (? vaccine)	Acyclovir, 200–800 mg q4h while awake	Patients at risk for primary varicella should be given varicella-zoster immune globin within 96 h of known exposure to varicella.
Herpes zoster	Acyclovir, 800–1,000 mg q4h while awake	In severe cases, IV therapy may be required. Topical anesthetics, nonsteroidal antiinflammatory drugs, and narcotics may be needed for pain control. Interferon-α may be helpful in recalcitrant cases.
Verrucae vulgaris	Liquid nitrogen cryotherapy; 16%–20% salicylic acid, liquid or plaster	Recurrences are common.
Flat verrucae	Tretinoin 0.05% cream or 0.01% gel applied bid 5% 5-fluorouracil cream applied bid Light liquid nitrogen cryotherapy	
Condylomata accuminata	Podofilox 0.5% applied bid 3 d of each week for 7 wk Liquid nitrogen cryotherapy	Multiple treatments usually are necessary.
Molluscum contagiosum	Liquid nitrogen cryotherapy Curettage	Topical tretinoin cream or gel is a useful adjunctive therapy. Recurrence is the rule.
Oral hairy leukoplakia	None Topical podophyllum 20% qd Acyclovir, 200–400 mg q4h while awake for 14 d	After discontinuation of therapy, recurrence is usual.
Bacterial folliculitis	Dicloxacillin, erythromycin, or cephalexin, 250–500 mg qid with daily Hibiclens baths	Culture confirmation should be obtained, although most cases are due to *Staphylococcus aureus*. Mupirocin bid to the nares or rifampin 300 mg bid for 10–14 d can decrease carriage.
Impetigo	After culture, dicloxacillin, 250–500 mg q6h for 7–10 d	
Syphilis	Uncomplicated primary and secondary: benzathine penicillin G, 2.4 million units IM qwk × 3; serology checks at 1, 3, 6, 9, and 12 mo; 4 × decrease in titer within 6 mo Primary or secondary with positive lumbar puncture: procaine penicillin G, 2.4 million units IM qd for 10–14 d and oral probenicid 500 mg followed by benzathine penicillin, 2.4 million units IM qwk for 3 wk or 3–4 million units IV aqueous crystalline penicillin G q4h × 10–14 d	Lumbar puncture is advised to rule out neurosyphilis.
Tinea versicolor	Ketoconazole, 200 mg qd for 3–5 d Selenium sulfide 2.5% qd topically, left on 15–20 min	
Dermatophytosis	Topical application of clotrimazole, econazole, cyclopirox, nafitine bid until resolved Griseofulvin, 500 mg bid for 1–2 wk Itraconazole, 100 mg bid for 2 wk	Longer courses of therapy may be required. Should not be used in patients with liver disease or porphyria.
Onychomycosis	Itraconazole, 200 mg qd 1 wk/mo for 4 mo	For all mentioned medications, continued maintenance therapy is often needed.
Oral candidiasis	Miconazole troches four or five times a day Nystatin oral suspension, 100,000 U/mL, gargle and swallow qid Ketoconazole, 200 mg/d Fluconazole, 100 mg/d Itraconazole, 100 mg/d	Fluconazole resistance may emerge.
Scabies	5% permethrin cream or gamma benzene hexachloride applied from neck to toes and left on 8–12 h; repeat application in 1 wk Postscabetic pruritus and nodular scabies: crotamiton (Eurax) lotion applied bid Oral antihistamines q4–6h with topical triamcinolone 0.025% cream applied bid Ivermectin 200 mg/kg once and repeat in 1 wk	Treatment of household contacts is required. Careful laundering of linen and clothing as well as vacuuming is recommended.

primary HIV infection to the detection of OHL varies from 5 to 10 years. Development of this condition is thought to correlate with progression from HIV infection to AIDS (50) (Table 117.3).

CLINICAL MANIFESTATIONS

OHL presents as one or more whitish corrugated plaques usually on the lateral margins of the tongue. These lesions are generally asymptomatic, although rarely they may become verrucous and lead to dysphagia.

DIAGNOSIS

Characteristically, OHL does not rub off when scraped with a tongue depressor, which distinguishes it from candidiasis. Scrapings also yield negative results when examined microscopically

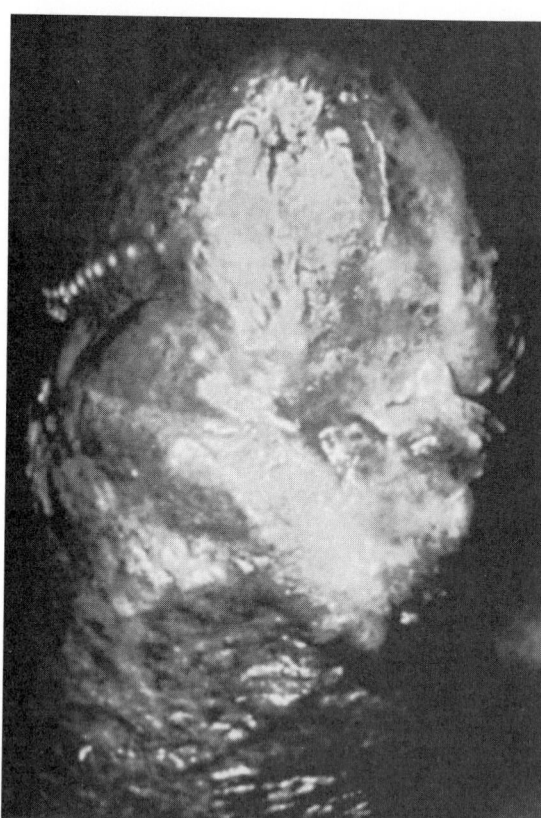

Figure 117.3. Cytomegalovirus (CMV) infection. This nondescript penile ulceration was due to cutaneous CMV infection. Biopsy and cultures are necessary to establish this diagnosis.

after treatment with potassium hydroxide. Histopathologically, OHL is characterized by epithelial hyperplasia with pale-staining, ballooned keratinocytes. The lack of cytologic atypia differentiates it from premalignant leukoplakia. Epstein-Barr virus particles may be demonstrated with electron microscopy and *in situ* hybridization techniques (51,52).

TREATMENT

No treatment of the condition is usually required; however, lesions may respond temporarily to acyclovir at a dosage of 200 to 400 mg five times a day. Topical application of podophyllum resin, 20% in alcohol, two or three times daily also leads to resolution, but recurrence after discontinuation is usual (53,54). Tretinoin gel applied to lesions twice a day may be helpful along with local destructive measures.

Human Papillomavirus Infections

The human papillomavirus (HPV), a double-stranded DNA virus, characteristically infects epithelial cells producing hyperplastic changes. HPV infection is one of the most common viral infections of humans and is transmitted by close repeated contact, which may be sexual in nature (55). After internalization, the virus enters the nucleus, where it either produces productive infection or undergoes latency.

In HIV-infected individuals, HPV infection is quite prevalent. In one study, 48% of HIV-seronegative homosexual men and 54% of homosexual men with AIDS were shown to have evidence of HPV infection (56). Defective cell-mediated immunity and up-regulation of HPV expression induced by HIV Tat protein may be responsible for the high incidence of HPV-induced lesions in HIV-positive patients (57–59).

CLINICAL MANIFESTATIONS

Verrucae vulgaris manifests as skin-colored to reddish verrucous hyperkeratotic papules or plaques that may occur on any surface of the skin. The glabrous skin, especially around the fingers and on the extremities, is commonly involved, although the face, head, and neck are also common sites of involvement. Individual small blackish bleeding points can be seen, correlating with dilated blood vessels and intraepidermal hemorrhage. In HIV-infected individuals, multiple verrucae vulgaris, especially in periungual locations, along with extensive flat and filiform warts on the bearded area of the face are seen commonly. Exuberant cauliflower-like plaques of condylomata acuminata involving the perianal region as well as flexural areas such as the axillae and oral commissures are also common findings. Difficulty with defecation and secondary constipation may result from extensive perianal condylomata. HIV-infected patients have been shown to have higher rates of cervical, anal, and genital cancers.

Epidermodysplasia verruciformis (EDV) has been reported in association with HIV infections (60). A widespread maculopapular eruption of reddish to skin-colored, flat, wartlike lesions involving mostly the sun-exposed areas of the skin is noted. In addition to harboring HPV, individual lesions may be associated with cytologic atypia and may develop into squamous cell carcinoma (see later).

Bowenoid papulosis, related to HPV types 16 and 18, may also be seen in HIV-infected hosts (61,62). This classically presents as multiple 2- to 5-mm red-brown papules involving the shaft of the penis. Bowenoid papulosis of the anus has been reported in association with the development of squamous cell carcinoma of the anus in an HIV-positive patient (62). In addition, extragenital bowenoid papulosis has been reported to occur on the neck in an HIV-positive individual (63).

DIAGNOSIS

Diagnosis of HPV infection is based on clinical features in the context of characteristic histopathologic findings. Verrucae and condylomata are characterized by marked epithelial hyperplasia, papillomatosis, and koilocytosis. EDV is manifest as koilocytic changes in conjunction with keratinocyte atypia that is suggestive of evolving squamous cell carcinoma *in situ*. Histopathologically, bowenoid papulosis demonstrates the features of condyloma acuminatum combined with atypical keratinocytic proliferation involving the full thickness of the epithelium. In difficult cases, immunoperoxidase stains for HPV antigens, DNA *in situ* hybridization, and the polymerase chain reaction (PCR) can be performed to increase the sensitivity of diagnosis (61,64,65).

TREATMENT

In the setting of HIV infection, lesions can be recalcitrant to treatment. Treatment generally consists of destructive measures such as application of topical agents or surgery. Podophyllum resin (20% to 50%) in tincture of benzoin, 20% to 40% trichloroacetic acid, or salicylic acid (6% to 40%) may successfully be used to destroy verruca or condyloma; however, repeated applications are almost always necessary. Podofilox (Condylox) applied twice a day for 3 days a week for 3 to 4 weeks can be used by the patient at home (66). Verruca plana and filiform verrucae may be treated with tretinoin (Retin-A), 0.05% cream or 0.01% gel, or topical 5-fluorouracil cream (Efudex). Cryosurgery with liquid nitrogen, electrodesiccation and curettage, and carbon dioxide laser vaporization are other treatment modalities commonly employed. Intralesional, subcutaneous, and parenteral interferon-α has been shown to be effective against recalcitrant condyloma and acral verruca; however, the use of this agent usually entails repeated visits to the physician and significant cost (67,68). Recent advances include imiquimod and topical cidofovir. Topical imiquimod (Aldara) has been effective in eradicating verrucae, with applications three times per week advancing to once per day. This increase is often limited by erythema and irritation (69,70). Patients receiving highly active antiretroviral therapy (HAART) improved to a greater degree than those not treated with HAART. Moreover, topical cidofovir therapy hastened resolution of verrucae in HIV-infected individuals (71). The lesions of EDV and bowenoid papulosis may respond to 5-fluorouracil cream, cryotherapy, electrodesiccation, or other destructive modalities. Recalcitrant lesions of EDV have been treated successfully with a combination of acitretin and interferon-α2a, as recently reported (72).

Poxvirus Infections

Poxviruses are complex DNA viruses that are transmitted by direct contact. These viruses replicate in the cytoplasm and are adapted to epidermal cells. Molluscum contagiosum develops in 10% to 20% of patients with AIDS (3,73). Most patients who develop widespread molluscum contagiosum are severely immunocompromised at the time of infection, with CD4$^+$ cell counts less than 200 to 250 cells/mm^3 (74).

CLINICAL MANIFESTATIONS
Molluscum contagiosum is characterized by dome-shaped umbilicated translucent 2- to 4-mm papules that may occur on any part of the body but localize especially around the eyes. The number of lesions may exceed 100, with individual lesions becoming quite large, expanding to more than 1 cm in diameter (75). In addition, clusters of lesions may coalesce, forming large plaques. In some cases, molluscum contagiosum may induce a localized dermatitis known as *molluscum dermatitis* (76). In HIV-infected patients, molluscum tends to erupt during a short time, from 2 to 4 weeks, and then persists for months to years. Rare cases of treatment-resistant folliculitis have been noted (77).

DIAGNOSIS
Diagnosis of molluscum is generally established on the basis of clinical appearance. In atypical cases, a biopsy may be necessary to rule out other disorders. Lesions that occur in HIV-positive patients and may appear similar to molluscum include those of cryptococcosis, histoplasmosis, *Penicillium marneffei*, cutaneous pneumocystosis, pyogenic granulomata, keratoacanthoma, and basal cell carcinoma. Histopathologically, molluscum lesions are characterized by a dome-shaped papule with a central crater that arises as a consequence of coalescence of infected keratinocytes. Viral particles fill the cells, forming the pathognomonic molluscum body, which is a pinkish, hyaline-like, oval structure within the cytoplasm of keratinocytes.

Vaccinia is diagnosed on the basis of the clinical appearance of the eruption in the context of a history of exposure to the causative agent. Virtually all cases develop in patients with occupational exposure and in those who have recently been vaccinated for smallpox. Histologically, prominent intraepidermal ballooning and reticular degeneration are seen.

TREATMENT
Treatment of molluscum contagiosum is generally accomplished by using destructive measures similar to those used to treat HPV infection. Cryotherapy, electrosurgery, topical keratolytic preparations, cantharidin, and curettage are standard effective therapies. Tretinoin cream, 0.025%, may be applied to decrease recurrence. Treatment in the setting of HIV infection can be quite challenging, and destructive methods may not be satisfactory.

Imiquimod may be applied topically to hasten the resolution of molluscum that have not responded to destructive measures (78).

Other Viral Infections

There are sporadic reports of other viral infections occurring in HIV-positive patients. Parvovirus B$_{19}$, the cause of erythema infectiosum (fifth disease), has been reported to cause an exanthem in patients with HIV infection and to lead to persistent and occasionally fatal aplastic anemia (79). Paramyxovirus (measles), some coxsackieviruses, and enteroviruses may cause an exanthem in HIV-infected individuals. The clinical course of such infections varies greatly and depends on the background immune status of the host (80,81,82).

BACTERIAL INFECTIONS

Pyogenic Infections

Staphylococcus aureus is the most common cutaneous and systemic bacterial pathogen of the HIV-infected adult. Defective neutrophil chemotaxis and decreased oxidative burst in conjunction with other immune alterations may lead to defective eradication of organisms (83,84). A nasal carriage rate of about 50% has been observed in HIV-infected hosts, which is twice that of HIV-seronegative homosexual and heterosexual men (85). Multiple breaks in the skin from needlesticks, dermatoses, and immunodeficiency are risk factors for the development of *S. aureus* infection. Up to 83% of patients with AIDS may suffer from some form of *S. aureus* infection during the course of their disease (86,87). Infections with gram-negative organisms occur less frequently but still represent a significant proportion of skin infections in HIV disease (88–90).

CLINICAL MANIFESTATIONS

Gram-Positive Infections. Folliculitis is generally manifest as widely distributed acneiform papules and pustules that may be pruritic and excoriated. Although infections are confined to the skin in most cases, sepsis may develop occasionally. In some cases, the bacterial density may increase significantly, leading to botryomycosis or ecthyma, which appear as nondescript verrucous papules or as necrotic, deeply seated chronic ulcerations, respectively (91,92). An atypical form of folliculitis may develop that presents as large violaceous plaques with superficial pustules and crusts occurring in the groin, axilla, or scalp (93).

Soft tissue and deeply seated bacterial infections such as cellulitis, pyomyositis, deep soft tissue abscesses, and necrotizing fasciitis may also develop (86,94). Extreme toxemia is often associated with deeper infections; hence, early recognition is essential. A characteristic infection, streptococcal axillary lymphadenitis, presents as a bilateral diffuse, painful swelling of the axillary lymph nodes (95). Impetigo is manifest as localized or erythematous areas of the skin associated with yellowish surface crusts and, rarely, intact bullae and pustules. In patients with HIV infection, it may be seen in unusual locations such as axillary, inguinal, and other intertriginous locations. Patients with AIDS are often predisposed to developing furunculosis. In addition, secondary infection of other primary dermatoses with *S. aureus* occurs frequently.

Toxin-producing strains of *Streptococcus pyogenes* and *S. aureus* may produce a toxic shock-like syndrome (96,97). Diffuse cutaneous erythema followed by desquamation, fever, and shock is seen.

Gram-Negative Infections. *Pseudomonas aeruginosa* and *Pseudomonas cepacia* may produce clinical conditions similar to those described earlier; thus, culture of lesions is essential (88–90). Abscesses or nodular skin lesions secondary to *P. aeruginosa* have developed in patients with AIDS, who tend to be systemically ill with negative blood cultures (98). Malacoplakia, presenting as red papules, ulcers, or draining abscesses, has also been reported to occur in the setting of HIV (99). An unusual form of cellulitis of the head and neck caused by *Haemophilus influenzae* may develop in patients with HIV infection (100). This infection tends to be aggressive and may become disseminated or involve deeper soft tissues and vital structures. Infections with *Streptomyces*, *Nocardia*, and *Actinomyces* may produce thickened verrucous plaques and chronic draining sinuses (101,102). Deeply seated abscesses caused by *Rhodococcus equi* have been observed on multiple occasions (103). *Corynebacterium diphtheriae* may cause bullous lesions that ulcerate and become covered with a grayish pseudomembrane (104).

DIAGNOSIS

Gram stains and cultures are extremely important in evaluating pyogenic infections in HIV-infected individuals because they often have unusual or mixed infections. A characteristic leukocytosis and "left shift" may not occur in some patients despite significant infections.

Skin biopsy, tissue culture, or both may be needed to establish the diagnosis.

TREATMENT

Treatment of each of the aforementioned disorders is based on accurate diagnosis and identification of causative microorganisms and their sensitivities to antibiotics. Pyogenic bacterial infections generally respond to treatment with dicloxacillin, cephalexin, or ciprofloxacin. Chlorhexidine gluconate washes of the skin and application of topical antibiotics such as polymyxin B sulfate, bacitracin, or mupirocin ointment preparations into the nostrils may help to eradicate bacterial colonization. Unfortunately, in immunocompromised hosts, recurrence is the rule.

Bacillary Angiomatosis

Bacillary angiomatosis is a rare condition caused by rickettsia-like organisms of the species *Bartonella* (formerly *Rochalimaea*) *henselae* and *Bartonella quintana* (105–107). The pathogenesis is not completely known, but it has been postulated that a vasoproliferative factor is produced or is induced as a consequence of bacterial infection. Bacillary angiomatosis is seen in AIDS patients with CD4+ T-cell counts usually less than 200 cells/μL (108). Sound epidemiologic evidence has demonstrated an association between exposure to cats and bacillary angiomatosis (109,110). However, one third of patients have no history of prior feline contact; thus, infection from another source such as the soil may also be important.

CLINICAL MANIFESTATIONS

Small pinpoint reddish to purple papules that resemble angiomata or pyogenic granulomata are the most common lesions. They range in number from one to several thousand and in size from 1 mm to several centimeters. Subcutaneous nodules are seen in about 50% of patients with skin lesions and may be located deep in the subcutis and involve soft tissue and bone (111,112). When bone is involved, lesions are usually osteolytic in nature. Nondescript crusted ulcerations, plaques, and cellulitis may also be seen in 5% to 10% of patients (111). Lesions may be pruritic or tender. Systemic symptoms such as fever, malaise, headache, and weight loss often accompany cutaneous lesions.

Visceral involvement may occur as well. The most common sites of involvement are the liver and spleen, in which dilated blood-filled vascular spaces develop; these conditions are known as *bacillary peliosis hepatis* and *splenis*, respectively (113,114). In addition, patients with bacillary angiomatosis may develop a bacteremic syndrome of fever, weight loss, and night sweats (114,115). Endocarditis has been reported in both immunocompromised and immunocompetent patients (116–118).

DIAGNOSIS

The diagnosis of bacillary angiomatosis can usually be established on the basis of characteristic histopathologic findings along with clinical suspicion. Lesions show a lobular proliferation of capillaries admixed with neutrophils and granular masses of bacteria. Organisms appear as black tangled strands after staining with the Warthin-Starry stain. *B. henselae* can be isolated from blood if lysis centrifugation blood cultures are used while *B. quintana* can be isolated from cutaneous lesions by cocultivation with an endothelial cell monolayer (119,120). Serum may be sent to the Centers for Disease Control and Prevention for determination of antibody titers to the bacillary angiomatosis organisms, whereas a few centers perform PCR analysis on culture or fresh tissue specimens.

TREATMENT

Bacillary angiomatosis responds well to treatment with erythromycin ethylsuccinate at doses of 500 mg taken orally four times a day for 4 weeks to 6 months. A strong tendency to relapse may be substantial, requiring longer durations of treatment (121). Doxycycline hydrochloride, 100 mg taken orally twice a day, is also effective (122). Azithromycin and roxithromycin have also been used with good response (123,124). A Jarisch-Herxheimer–like reaction has been reported to occur with initiation of therapy (125). In addition, surgical excision and local destruction have been useful as adjunctive therapy.

Mycobacterial Infections

The incidence of tuberculosis has increased since the advent of the AIDS epidemic. Skin lesions are seen in up to 10% of patients with systemic mycobacterial infections and may be caused by *Mycobacterium tuberculosis*, *Mycobacterium avium-intracellulare*, and other atypical mycobacteria. A significant percentage of *M. tuberculosis* infections represent reactivation of a preexisting infectious focus. Leprosy has been observed only rarely in patients with HIV infection, the reason for which remains unknown.

CLINICAL MANIFESTATIONS

Mycobacterial skin lesions may assume a number of different appearances. The lesions may present as small papules and pustules that resemble folliculitis, verrucous papules, localized cutaneous abscesses, suppurative lymphadenitis, ulcerations, or sporotrichoid nodules (Fig. 117.4). Tuberculous lymphadenitis, in particular, is a characteristic finding of disseminated tuberculosis in intravenous drug users with AIDS and is manifested as suppurative draining lymph nodes in the neck, axillae, or groin (126). Miliary tuberculosis is reported most commonly in AIDS patients (127). *Mycobacterium marinum* may cause classic swimming pool granulomata in patients with HIV disease manifested as verrucous nodules classically extending up one extremity in a linear arrangement. Nodules, pustules, ulcers, or a cellulitis-like patch may occur from hematogenous dissemination of *M. avium-intracellulare* in AIDS patients (128). *Mycobacterium haemophilum* may cause cutaneous infections in AIDS patients, which

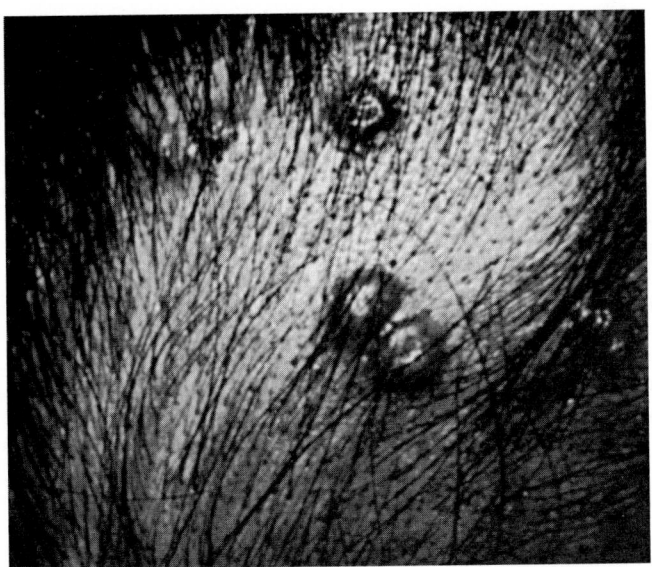

Figure 117.4. Atypical mycobacterial infection. Two draining ulcerations on the leg were caused by *Mycobacterium avium-intracellulare*.

usually present as painful erythematous papules and nodules on the distal extremities and ears (129).

DIAGNOSIS

In cases of suspected mycobacterial infections, cultures and smears for acid-fast organisms should be performed. Biopsy generally shows a suppurative granulomatous infiltrate. Acid-fast stains may be used to identify organisms; however, these stains may be negative even in an ongoing active infection.

TREATMENT

Cutaneous mycobacterial infections demonstrate variable responses to antibiotics; therefore, it is important to determine sensitivities. In general, cutaneous tuberculosis responds to antituberculous regimens of isoniazid and rifampin with or without pyrazinamide. Ethambutol is added if isoniazid resistance is suspected or proved on culture. Multidrug therapy is recommended for all types of tuberculosis. Multidrug-resistant tuberculosis has been described and may not respond to any medication currently available (130). Triple-drug therapy is usually continued for 12 to 24 months in the HIV-positive patient. Clarithromycin, rifabutin (Ansamycin), clofazimine, minocycline, and trimethoprim-sulfamethoxazole all have variable degrees of efficacy in the treatment of atypical mycobacterial infections. Disseminated *M. avium-intracellulare* is treated with multiple therapy—azithromycin or clarithromycin plus rifabutin, ethambutol, clofazimine, and streptomycin or amikacin (128). *M. haemophilum* is usually sensitive to ciprofloxacin and rifampin, but even in cases in which both antibiotics are used, chronic relapse may be noted (129).

Syphilis

Syphilis is common in patients with HIV infection, and of all reported cases of syphilis, 25% occur in HIV-infected hosts (131).

CLINICAL MANIFESTATIONS

Syphilis may occur in a number of forms in patients with HIV infection, ranging from classic papulosquamous forms with involvement of the palms and soles and mucous membranes

to unusual forms such as sclerodermiform lesions, rupial verrucous plaques, extensive oral ulcerations, keratoderma, deep cutaneous nodules, rubeoliform eruptions, and widespread gummata (132). Rapid progression from the primary chancre to gummatous tertiary lues or lues maligna (syphilis with vasculitis) may occur. Central nervous system disease has been noted more frequently and with greater severity (133). In the HIV-infected patient, syphilis may have unusual serologies, such as false-positive results, and a refractory course after appropriate therapy.

DIAGNOSIS

Serology is the most important parameter in establishing a diagnosis of syphilis; however, HIV-positive patients with syphilis may have negative serologic tests for syphilis as well as a negative antibody test despite the presence of active infection. Seronegativity may be due to either a prozone phenomenon or true absence of antibody. In these cases, a skin biopsy may be helpful. Histopathologic examination usually shows a prominent infiltrate of plasma cells arranged around swollen endothelial cells. In about one fourth of cases, plasma cells are few or absent. Warthin-Starry stains can be used to demonstrate the organisms.

TREATMENT

Syphilis responds to penicillin at higher doses and must be continued for longer courses than in immunocompetent hosts. Recommended treatment regimens are summarized in Table 117.5. Lumbar puncture is recommended to rule out concomitant neurosyphilis. Careful follow-up with repeated serologic testing is recommended. In patients who are allergic to penicillin, penicillin desensitization is recommended.

Other Venereal Diseases

Multiple sexually transmitted diseases are commonly seen in association with HIV infection; however, this phenomenon may be decreasing somewhat with improved education about safe sex. In addition to the more common sexually transmitted diseases, less common ones may be encountered in HIV-positive patients.

Chancroid, caused by the gram-negative coccobacillus *Haemophilus ducreyi*, has been reported in a number of patients with HIV infection, especially in those from Africa. Lesions most often present as a solitary, painful penile or labial ulceration with ragged edges and a necrotic base, although widespread ulcerations may develop (134). The ulcers can be accompanied by inguinal adenopathy in 40% to 70% of cases (135). In HIV-positive patients, ulcer number and duration may be longer (136). Granuloma inguinale caused by *Calymmatobacterium granulomatis* may also occur. This disorder is characterized by chronic vegetating beefy-red ulcerations of the penis and vulva associated with pseudobuboes in the inguinal crease. Although uncommon, lymphogranuloma venereum, caused by L1, L2, and L3 immunotypes of *Chlamydia trachomatis*, has also been associated with HIV infection and is manifested as generalized lymphadenopathy accompanied by vulvar or penile edema with ulcerations and erosions. Severe gonococcemia with gonococcal arthritis has also been reported (137).

DIAGNOSIS

Appropriate smears and cultures are important in evaluating these disorders. Granuloma inguinale is characteristically diagnosed by crush preparations of a friable skin lesion followed by histologic examination. Histiocytes with characteristic intracytoplasmic inclusion bodies, Donovan bodies, are noted. Chancroid is diagnosed by microscopic examination of Gram-stained smears of lesions that demonstrate clusters of thin gram-negative rods, the characteristic "schools of fish." Lymphogranuloma venereum is diagnosed by clinical presentation and high complement fixation antibody titers (more than 1:64).

TREATMENT

Chancroid is treated with oral azithromycin, 1 g in a single dose, intramuscular ceftriaxone, 250 mg in a single dose, oral ciprofloxacin, 500 mg twice daily for 3 days, or erythromycin, 500 mg taken orally four time daily for 7 days (138). Close follow-up is mandatory because HIV-infected patients may require longer treatment courses. Lymphogranuloma venereum responds to doxycycline, 100 mg taken orally twice daily for 21 days, along with incision and drainage. Oral erythromycin, 500 mg four times daily for 21 days can also be effective (138). Granuloma inguinale responds to treatment with doxycycline or trimethoprim-sulfamethoxazole; however, intravenous gentamicin should be considered in HIV-infected patients (138). Gonorrhea is treated with regimens generally consisting of penicillin, spectinomycin, or ceftriaxone.

FUNGAL INFECTIONS

Deep Fungal Diseases

The systemic fungal infections associated with HIV infection are summarized in Table 117.6. The most common opportunistic fungal infections to involve the skin are histoplasmosis and cryptococcosis. Nearly 20% of HIV-positive patients with disseminated histoplasmosis, and up to 10% of those with disseminated cryptococcosis develop mucosal or cutaneous lesions. Mucocutaneous lesions associated with systemic fungal infections may assume a number of different features. The most common are pustules and ulcers, although papules and nodules are also frequently observed. Less often, patches, plaques, and verrucous lesions are seen. It is important to recognize that cutaneous lesions caused by disseminated fungi may mimic the appearance of other diseases.

CLINICAL MANIFESTATIONS

Histoplasmosis. In one review, 17% of HIV-positive patients with disseminated histoplasmosis developed cutaneous lesions (139). In addition, oral lesions can be seen on initial presentation with disseminated disease. Clinically, the lesions had highly variable clinical appearances. Cutaneous histoplasmosis commonly presents with cutaneous or mucosal ulcerations, although erythematous macules, papules, nodules, verrucous plaques, ab-

scesses, purpura, and pustules, along with associated erythema nodosum, erythema multiforme, and herpetiform lesions, may also occur (140,141). Histoplasma capsulatum and Kaposi's sarcoma (KS) were found to coexist in a single skin lesion, whereas coexistent psoriasis and histoplasmosis have also been observed (142,143). The possibility of human-to-human transmission of histoplasmosis between two HIV-seropositive individuals by close skin contact has been postulated but not proved (144).

Cryptococcosis. Cryptococcosis develops not uncommonly and is the most common life-threatening fungal infection in HIV-infected individuals. Up to 10% of patients with disseminated cryptococcal infection develop skin involvement. Mucocutaneous lesions of cryptococcosis are polymorphous, appearing as erythematous papules, nodules, pustules, or ulcers as well as cellulitis of the skin and mucosa (Fig. 117.5). The clinical appearance of cutaneous cryptococcosis has been reported to mimic lesions of HSV infection and molluscum contagiosum as well as soft tissue hypertrophic lesions such as rhinophyma and KS (145,146). Cutaneous lesions portend a poor prognosis.

Sporotrichosis. Clinical forms of sporotrichosis include fixed cutaneous, lymphocutaneous, disseminated cutaneous, and systemic. Fixed cutaneous forms consist of a solitary lesion; lymphocutaneous forms are manifest as multiple lesions developing along the lines of lymphatic drainage. Disseminated cutaneous lesions occur over widespread areas (147). Systemic disease may present as either localized pulmonary disease or widespread involvement of numerous organs. Skin lesions may be ulcers, papules, nodules, plaques, or pustules (148).

Less Common Deep Fungal Infections

Penicillium marneffei, a fungus that is endemic in Asia, causes an infection that has been reported with increasing frequency in patients with AIDS in Thailand (149). Systemic manifestations include fever, weight loss, anemia, and lymphadenopathy. Seventy-six percent of affected individuals develop skin disease. The most characteristic lesions are umbilicated papules resembling molluscum contagiosum that tend to occur on the genitalia, face, and extremities. Ecthyma-like lesions, folliculitis, subcutaneous nodules, abscesses, and rare oral lesions may also occur (150). Lesions tend to appear once the CD4+ T-cell count is less than 50 cells/μL (151).

Sporadic reports of disseminated coccidioidomycosis, blastomycosis, and paracoccidioidomycosis with cutaneous involvement in HIV-infected hosts have appeared in the literature. Cutaneous infection with *Coccidioides immitis* is infrequent but has produced leukocytoclastic vasculitis, subcutaneous abscesses,

TABLE 117.6. Summary of Deep Fungal Infections

Disease	Causative organism	Endemic area	Distinctive cutaneous lesion(s)
Cryptococcosis	*Cryptococcus neoformans*	Widespread distribution; found in pigeon excrement	Cellulitis, purpura, molluscum contagiosum–like lesions
Histoplasmosis	*Histoplasma capsulatum*	Central river valleys of United States; in droppings of blackbirds	Acneiform lesions, oral ulcerations
Blastomycosis	*Blastomyces dermatitidis*	Southeastern and south-central North America	Raised plaque with heaped-up border; skin and mucosal ulcerations
Coccidioidomycosis	*Coccidioides immitis*	Lower Sonoran life zones	Verrucous plaques, erythema nodosum
Sporotrichosis	*Sporothrix schenckii*	Tropical or subtropical Americas; found in soil and wood	Linear nodules in line of lymphatic drainage
Paracoccidioidomycosis	*Paracoccidioides brasiliensis*	Latin America, from Mexico to Argentina	Mucosal ulceration, periorificial lesions

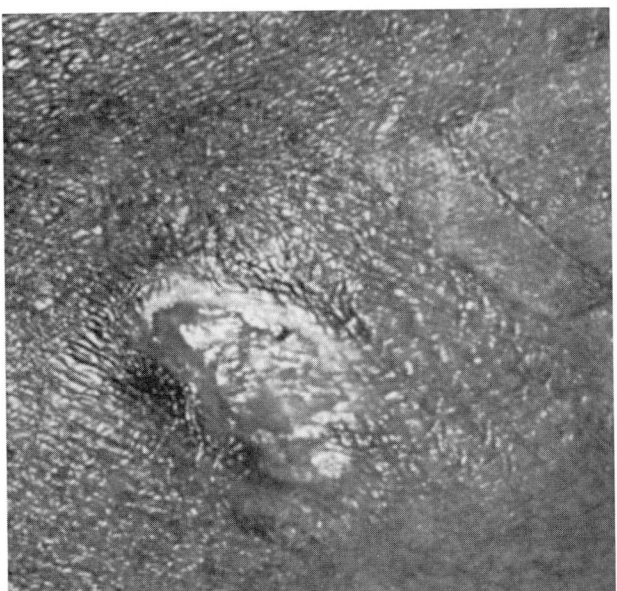

Figure 117.5. Cutaneous cryptococcosis. This somewhat yellowish translucent crusted papule with a nondescript appearance was caused by *Cryptococcus neoformans*. This emphasizes the need to perform biopsies and cultures of virtually any lesion in a patient with HIV infection.

ulcerations, and nodules (152). Prognosis for HIV-positive patients with coccidiomycosis is poor (153). Fatal disseminated blastomycosis with cutaneous pustules, nodules, and ulcers has been observed (154). An HIV-positive patient from Brazil with painful ulcerations of the face and thigh caused by *Paracoccidioides brasiliensis* has been described as well (155). Disseminated *Scedosporium inflatum*, *Pseudallescheria boydii*, and *Microsporum canis* infections have been observed in these patients, as have infections with zygomycotic organisms (156–159). The clinical lesions seen most often in these cases were ulcerations. *Aspergillus* species has been noted to cause cutaneous lesions in AIDS; lesions have resembled inflammatory tinea capitis and molluscum contagiosum (160,161).

DIAGNOSIS

When the possibility is considered that a mucocutaneous lesion in an HIV-infected patient is secondary to dissemination of a systemic fungal infection, a tissue biopsy and potassium hydroxide preparation or tissue smear, as well as culture, should be performed. Biopsies and smears can often yield a more rapid diagnosis than is possible with cultures, which may take up to several weeks. Serologies can be useful in diagnosing histoplasmosis and cryptococcus. Histology characteristically reveals epithelial hyperplasia with suppurative granulomatous inflammation. The number of organisms may vary; thus, special staining for fungi with either periodic acid–Schiff or Gomori methenamine silver stain is necessary. A diligent search for concurrent infectious organisms is warranted because HIV-infected individuals often harbor more than one pathogen.

TREATMENT

Intravenous amphotericin B remains the drug of choice for the treatment of most deep fungal infections and is occasionally combined with 5-fluorocyotsine (162). In most instances, maintenance treatment is required for cryptococcal infections, with fluconazole as the preferred agent (163). Ketoconazole, fluconazole, or itraconazole may be effectively used in the treatment

of sporotrichosis. In some cases, the lymphocutaneous form can be treated successfully with potassium iodide, although careful monitoring is necessary to avoid recurrences; however, it is rarely successful in HIV-positive patients. Fluconazole and itraconazole are promising less toxic alternatives for the initial or maintenance therapy of these systemic fungal infections in HIV-infected patients.

Superficial Fungal Infections

YEAST INFECTIONS

Oral thrush involving the tongue or buccal mucosa is the most common manifestation of candidiasis in HIV-seropositive patients and may be the initial sign of HIV infection in many individuals (164,165) (Fig. 117.6). In fact, the rate of oral carriage of *Candida* species nears 100% in HIV-positive patients (166). Candidal infection may also produce chronic paronychia, onychodystrophy, chronic refractory vaginal candidiasis, distal urethritis, and persistent monilial infection of the axilla, glans penis, groin, or inframammary area. Despite the high prevalence of mucocutaneous candidiasis, disseminated candidiasis is quite rare in this population. Broad-spectrum antibiotics, indwelling catheters, parenteral nutrition and neutropenia are risk factors that predispose one to the development of disseminated disease.

Pityrosporum ovale and *Pityrosporum orbiculare* (*Malassezia furfur*) are normal residents of the hair follicles of the scalp and have been suggested to cause or exacerbate seborrheic dermatitis in patients with HIV infection. In one study, the density of *P. ovale* on the involved skin was found to correlate with the severity of

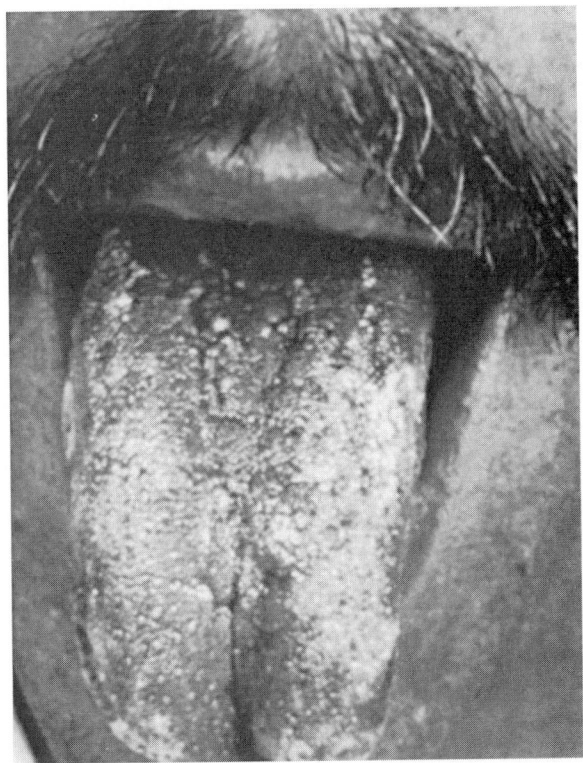

Figure 117.6. Candidiasis. Whitish curdlike exudates present on mucous membranes that are easily scraped off with a tongue depressor are characteristic of candidiasis. This is often associated with candidal esophagitis, which may result in severe dysphagia.

seborrheic dermatitis (167). The severity of seborrheic dermatitis correlates with HIV activity (168). *Pityrosporum* folliculitis, characterized by pruritic papules and pustules on the trunk and extremities, may also develop in HIV-infected hosts. Extensive tinea versicolor, also caused by *P. ovale*, may occur in patients with HIV infection.

DERMATOPHYTE INFECTIONS

Any cornified epithelial surface may be involved by a dermatophyte. In HIV-positive patients, the severity but not the incidence of dermatophyte infections is increased. Tinea pedis and onychomycosis are commonly found in HIV-infected individuals (169). Proximal white subungual onychomycosis of the toenails characteristically occurs in patients with HIV infection, in contrast to the classic form of distal subungual onychomycosis (170). More than 50% of these infections are caused by *Trichophyton rubrum* (169). Extensive widespread tinea corporis should raise the possibility of underlying HIV infection.

Trichosporosis caused by infection with *Trichosporon beigelii* generally causes white piedra, a superficial infection of the hair endemic to tropical and subtropical regions of the world and regions of the southeastern United States. Carriage of this organism has been shown to be increased in homosexual men, and several cases of invasive disease with positive blood and urine cultures have been reported (171).

Dematiaceous fungi can also be a cause of cutaneous fungal infections. *Cladosporium cladosporioides* has been reported to cause pustular nodules in an HIV-infected patient (172). Surgical excision in this case was curative. Cutaneous alternariosis presenting as an eschar on the leg and *Curvularia* phaeohyphomycosis causing a keratotic lesion on the scrotum have both been observed in HIV-infected individuals (173,174).

DIAGNOSIS

Microscopic examination of potassium hydroxide preparations of skin scrapings and cultures should establish the diagnosis in most if not all cases. Cultures from lesions of onychomycosis are often negative despite active clinical infection. In these cases, histopathologic examination of the nail plate may be helpful.

TREATMENT

Appropriate treatment regimens are summarized in Table 117.5. Topical antifungal agents may be effective and are first-line therapy. Many patients require oral medications with continued prophylactic therapy (175–177). Fluconazole-resistant *Candida albicans* is well documented in HIV-positive patients and may necessitate therapy with alternative agents such as itraconazole (178). Onychomycosis is best treated with pulse therapy with itraconazole at doses of 200 mg taken orally twice daily for 1 week per month for 3 to 4 months, or terbinafine at 250 mg taken orally daily for 3 to 4 months. Amphotericin B occasionally in conjunction with 5-fluorocytosine is used for systemic disease.

PARASITIC INFECTIONS AND ECTOPARASITIC INFESTATIONS

Scabies

Scabies, caused by the mite *Sarcoptes scabiei* var. *humanus*, is the most common ectoparasitic infection in HIV-infected individuals, occurring in about 20% of patients (179). Severe infestation with scabies often develops as a consequence of impaired cell-mediated immunity and impaired Langerhans cell function

(180). In immunocompetent hosts, the number of infesting mites ranges from 10 to 20, whereas in HIV-infected patients, they may number in the millions.

CLINICAL MANIFESTATIONS

Clinical manifestations vary, ranging from a few scattered pruritic papules to thick hyperkeratotic plaques covering the palms, soles, extremities, and trunk. The latter variant is commonly referred to as *crusted*, or *Norwegian, scabies*. Characteristic lesions of scabies are localized to intertriginous sites and the genitalia, although typical lesions may not be found in HIV-infected hosts. In addition to the crusted variant, widespread papulosquamous eruptions resembling atopic dermatitis along with scalp and facial scaling resembling seborrheic dermatitis have been reported (179,181). Anergic scabies, a diffuse papular eruption, occurs in patients with CD4$^+$ counts less than 200 cells/μL (182). Associated pruritus is particularly severe at night. In HIV-infected patients, characteristic burrows may be difficult to identify, so that virtually any patient with a scaly persistent pruritic eruption should have skin lesions scraped and examined histologically in search of scabies mites. Once scabies has been treated, persistent pruritic nodules may occur, usually in intertriginous sites (nodular scabies). Severe forms of scabies may be associated with secondary infection, bacteremia, and fatal septicemia, especially in severely immunocompromised hosts (183).

DIAGNOSIS

The diagnosis of scabies depends primarily on the clinical appearance and distribution of the eruption as well as the demonstration of mites on microscopic examination of skin scrapings. In Norwegian scabies, multiple mites are visible in the stratum corneum of the skin biopsy specimen. In nodular scabies, a dense infiltrate in the dermis containing numerous eosinophils is recognized, but the number of mites is few.

TREATMENT

Scabies in HIV-infected individuals often responds poorly to conventional methods. Ivermectin, a semisynthetic macrocyclic lactone, has been shown to eradicate mites at doses of 200 μg/kg or greater (184,185). This is used often concomitantly with 5% permethrin cream to avoid environmental contamination. Keratolytics can be used several days later to enhance scale removal. In other cases, scabies may respond to treatment with lindane lotion or 5% permethrin cream applied from head to toe, left in place for 8 to 12 hours, then washed off and repeated in 1 week. Patients should be given careful instructions to ensure that sites such as under the fingernails are treated and that linens and clothing are laundered. Household contacts should be treated as well. Lindane should be used with caution because of its potential for neurotoxicity. Postscabetic pruritus is common and may be treated with antihistamines such as doxepin, 10 to 25 mg taken orally three to four times a day, along with topical application of corticosteroid preparations to diminish inflammation. Crotamiton 10% (Eurax) lotion has a poor efficacy and is used rarely in the United States; however, it is used in other countries in controlling pruritus and in preventing reinfestation (186).

Less Common Infestations

One hundred fifty cases of leishmaniasis in HIV-infected hosts have been diagnosed in India, Southeast Asia, and the Mediterranean coast (187). The most common agent reported is *Leishmania donovani*. Papular demodicidosis, which is the result of an excess proliferation of *Demodex folliculorum*, has also been reported sporadically in patients with HIV infection (188). Some investigators believe that *Demodex* is a cause of HIV-related eosinophilic folliculitis (189). There are rare reports of cutaneous *Pneumocystis carinii* infection, disseminated strongyloidiasis caused by *Strongyloides stercoralis*, acanthamebiasis caused by *Acanthamoeba castellani*, and disseminated *Toxoplasma gondii* (190–193). *Phthirus pubis* behaves similarly in HIV-infected and non–HIV-infected patients (194).

CLINICAL MANIFESTATIONS

Leishmaniasis usually appears as scaly lichenified plaques with dyspigmentation. Demodicidosis generally consists of a persistent pruritic follicular eruption that may involve the face, trunk, and extremities. *P. carinii* infection of the skin may present as friable reddish papules or nodules seen in the ear canal or the nares. Small translucent molluscum contagiosum–like papules, bluish cellulitic plaquelike lesions, and deeply seated abscesses have also been observed. The one case of toxoplasmosis that has been reported had an appearance of a papular dermatitis, whereas strongyloidiasis gives rise to a rapidly migrating serpiginous urticarial eruption known as *larva currens*. Acanthamebiasis manifests as painful nodular lesions with ulcerations usually on the trunk or extremities.

DIAGNOSIS

In these unusual conditions, the diagnosis rests on histology with confirmatory cultures when possible. Careful inspection of skin biopsy specimens usually reveals the characteristic organism.

TREATMENT

Leishmaniasis is best treated with stibogluconate sodium at a dosage of 20 mg/kg per day for 3 to 4 weeks. Systemic metronidazole at doses of 250 to 750 mg taken orally twice daily should be used to treat amebiasis; however, response to therapy is often quite poor. Demodicosis may be treated with either topical or systemic metronidazole, oral itraconazole, or oral isotretinoin. Oral antihistamines, topical steroids, and ultraviolet B therapy have been used for pruritus (189). Strongyloidiasis requires treatment with thiabendazole, 25 mg/kg twice daily for 4 to 5 days to several weeks. Cutaneous *Pneumocystis* infection responds to usual *Pneumocystis* treatments. *Phthirus pubis* may be treated with permethrin 1% cream rinse, topical lindane shampoo, or pyrethrins with piperonyl butoxide along with bedding and clothing decontamination (194).

CUTANEOUS INFECTIONS IN HUMAN IMMUNODEFICIENCY VIRUS–INFECTED CHILDREN

The spectrum of cutaneous infections that occur in HIV-infected children is similar to that in adults; however, the frequency of some disorders differs between the two populations. For example, cutaneous neoplasms are rarely a manifestation of pediatric HIV infection, but multiple cutaneous infections are commonly seen.

Viral Infections

Herpetic gingivostomatitis and herpes zoster are common in HIV-infected children and may be severe (195,196). Measles without the characteristic rash has been reported with progression to giant cell pneumonia (82). Oral hairy leukoplakia has rarely been reported in children (197). The clinical manifestations of molluscum, condyloma, and verrucae are similar to those in the adult population.

Bacterial Infections

As previously mentioned, HIV-infected children frequently suffer from severe recurrent bacterial infections. This is most likely the result of HIV infection occurring before the development of memory cells to bacterial antigens (195). The most common pathogen is *S. aureus*, and the most common clinical manifestations are impetigo, cellulitis, and folliculitis. Intravenous immune globulin may have some benefit in the treatment of severe recurrent infections, although one large study showed that the overall mortality rate after its administration was unchanged (198–200). For unknown reasons, mycobacterial skin infections and bacillary angiomatosis are rare in HIV-infected children.

Fungal Infections

C. albicans is the most common fungal infection in the pediatric HIV-infected population, with oral thrush or severe diaper dermatitis being the first manifestation of the disease (164,195). In children older than 1 year of age, recalcitrant thrush or diaper dermatitis should raise suspicion of possible HIV infection. Angular cheilitis and onychomycosis secondary to *Candida* may also occur (195). As in adults, disseminated deep fungal infections with cutaneous involvement are extremely uncommon in children. Treatment regimens are similar for adults and children, with appropriate dosage adjustments.

VIRUS-RELATED NEOPLASMS

A variety of different neoplastic disorders may develop in patients with HIV disease, many of which have been associated with a viral agent. Impaired and altered immunity that results from HIV infection may be important in the genesis of these neoplasms, as may be direct interaction between HIV and other viral agents.

Squamous Cell Carcinoma and Other Epithelial Neoplasms

The frequency of intraepithelial neoplasia of both the uterine cervix in women and the anorectal mucosa in homosexual men is markedly increased in HIV-infected individuals (201,202). Women with AIDS have a twofold increased risk for the development of cervical cancer, and cervical cancer is now included as an AIDS-defining illness in women (203). In American patients with AIDS, there is a 40-fold increased risk for the development of anal cancer, with most of the cases occurring in homosexual men (202,204). Cervical and anal cancers have both been associated with infection with HPV types 16, 18, and 31 (202,204). In HIV-infected women, cervical cancer may demonstrate rapid progression and a greater tendency to recurrence; hence, close surveillance and follow-up are particularly important. Less is known concerning the natural history of anal carcinoma, although it might be expected that these lesions would be more aggressive in AIDS patients.

As mentioned previously, epidermodysplasia verruciformis has been associated with immunosuppression, including HIV disease (51,205,206). HPV types 5 and 8 are unique to this disorder and are strongly associated with neoplastic transformation. The combination of oncogenic viral infection, ultraviolet radiation from sun exposure, and altered immune surveillance induces neoplastic epithelial changes.

Kaposi's Sarcoma

EPIDEMIOLOGY AND PATHOGENESIS

KS, first described by Moritz Kaposi in 1872, was observed in a small subset of individuals before the AIDS pandemic. This vascular neoplastic proliferative disorder is the most frequent neoplastic disorder to develop in AIDS patients (207,208). In the early years of the AIDS epidemic, KS was observed in about 50% of the male homosexual AIDS patients in San Francisco (208). Dropping significantly, KS is reported in only 15% of HIV-seropositive patients, mostly homosexual men. This decrease in incidence is attributed to safer sexual practices. In the United States, KS is far less common among all other groups of HIV-positive individuals, including intravenous drug users, women, hemophiliacs, and their sexual partners. In addition to HIV-positive homosexual men, KS has been reported in a group of homosexual men with no HIV infection but with risk factors for it (209). In these patients, a more indolent course, similar to that observed in elderly Italian and Jewish men, is seen.

A unique herpesvirus, human herpesvirus type 8 or KS-associated herpesvirus, closely related to *Herpesvirus saimiri*—a virus of squirrel monkeys—has been identified in lesions of KS and is believed to be the cause of all types of KS (210–214). Altered levels of cytokines, such as transforming growth factor-β, oncostatin M, scatter factor, interleukin-6, tumor necrosis factor-α, and basic fibroblastic growth factor, which can occur in HIV-infected individuals, promote the growth of KS cells (215–219). In addition, HIV Tat protein can stimulate the growth of AIDS-associated KS cells *in vitro* (220). Recent observations demonstrate that HIV is not necessary for KS development, but rather promotes the proper inflammatory environment in which KS may develop. The recent advances with HAART therapy reveal that HAART modifies immunosuppression, not human herpesvirus 8 growth, thus indirectly affecting KS development (221).

CLINICAL MANIFESTATIONS

Clinically, KS skin lesions may be pink, red, brown, or purple macules, patches, or plaques. Purplish to brown-black nodules and tumors may also develop. Lesions are commonly oriented along the lines of skin tension and may spread locally in areas of trauma. Favored sites include mucous membranes, face, lower extremities, and genitalia (222). Internal organ involvement, particularly of the gastrointestinal tract and lymphatics, is common, and as a rule, one internal lesion is present for every five skin lesions. Pulmonary lesions are common as well, with 15% of patients having no mucocutaneous involvement (223). Importantly, KS induction or exacerbation has been demonstrated with corticosteroid therapy (224).

DIAGNOSIS

Diagnosis is based on the characteristic clinical features in conjunction with histopathologic findings. Skin biopsy typically shows a proliferation of spindle-shaped endothelial cells forming irregular jagged vascular slits. There are often associated hemosiderin deposition and an infiltrate of plasma cells. The diagnosis of HIV-related KS should be made with caution in women and children from the United States because the neoplasm occurs only rarely in these populations of patients.

TREATMENT

Treatment of uncomplicated cutaneous KS is performed for cosmesis only. Local destructive measures are generally most effective, including liquid nitrogen cryotherapy for early, flat lesions, along with radiotherapy and laser therapy. Alitretinoin gel 0.1%, a retinoid, has also been effective (225). Intralesional injections of vinblastine, interferon-α (Intron A), and daunorubicin are promising alternatives, as is infusion of liposome-encapsulated daunorubicin and doxorubicin, which localizes to the skin (226–228). Paclitaxel has been used in patients with anthracycline-resistant disease with promising results (229). Systemic chemotherapy is reserved for patients with widespread disease caused by associated immunosuppression. Future treatments under investigation include angiogenesis inhibitors, such as fumagillin and thalidomide, oral alitretinoin, and purified human chorionic gonadotropin (230,231).

T-Cell Leukemia and Lymphoma

Human T-cell lymphotrophic virus type I (HTLV-I) is a retrovirus that is endemic to southern Japan, northern South America, southern North America, and areas of Africa. Less than 1% of carriers develop an aggressive T-cell leukemia that is characterized by multiple skin lesions and lytic bone lesions. Tropical spastic paraparesis may also be a rare complication of infection with this virus. A few patients have been observed who have dual infection with HTLV-I and HIV, and in these patients, the HIV appeared to accelerate the appearance of T-cell leukemia and tropical spastic paraparesis (232–235). In addition, two patients have been reported with dual HTLV-I and HIV infection who developed cutaneous lesions similar to those in mycosis fungoides. Sézary cells were demonstrated in peripheral blood and skin (236).

Human T-cell lymphotrophic virus type II (HTLV-II) is closely related to but distinct from HTLV-I. This virus is found in the Native American and Brazilian Indian populations as well as among intravenous drug users and may rarely be associated with hairy cell leukemia. No cases of hairy cell leukemia have been found in patients with concomitant HTLV-II and HIV infection, although a cutaneous disorder resembling mycosis fungoides has been described (237). The eruption was characterized by extensive scaling, lichenified plaques, peripheral eosinophilia, and dermatopathic lymphadenopathy. Histologically, a dermal infiltrate of CD8$^+$ lymphocytes and giant cells was seen.

Lymphomas, such as immunoblastic, Burkitt's, and diffuse large cell, are usually aggressive B-cell types and tend to occur late in the course of HIV infection, with the risk for development much greater compared with the general population (238,239). The development of lymphoma in AIDS patients is more common in men, whereas all age groups are affected (240). It is unclear at this time what host factors predispose to the development of lymphoma. HAART has not been associated with a decrease in the development of AIDS-related lymphomas. The skin may be involved, but not as frequently as other organ systems.

The effects of concurrent retroviral infections are just beginning to be observed and studied; however, combined adverse effects are expected. *In vitro*, HTLV-I has been shown to promote penetration of HIV into CD4$^+$ cells and to enhance HIV proliferation (240,241). In addition, both HTLV and HIV can activate Epstein-Barr virus (242,243).

CONCLUSIONS

The diagnosis and management of HIV infection have evolved dramatically since its initial recognition. Early diagnosis and prevention of opportunistic infections, as well as treatment of HIV disease itself, have become significant priorities. A wide variety of cutaneous infections occur in HIV disease and can be the source of significant morbidity. By recognizing these signs and symptoms and by performing appropriate diagnostic testing to establish correct diagnoses, these complications can be minimized significantly.

REFERENCES

1. Tindall B, Barker S, Donovan B, et al. Characterization of the acute clinical illness associated with human immunodeficiency virus infection. *Arch Intern Med* 1988;148:945–949.
2. Sinicco A, Palestro G, Caramello P, et al. Acute HIV-1 infection: Clinical and biologic study of twelve patients. *J Acquir Immune Defic Syndr Hum Retrovirol* 1990;3:260–265.
3. Gaines H. Primary HIV infection: clinical and diagnostic aspects. *J Infect Dis* 1989;61[Suppl]:1–46.
4. Ho DD, Sarngadharan MG, Reznick, L, et al. Primary human T-lymphocyte virus type III infection. *Ann Intern Med* 1985;103:880–883.
5. Isaksson B, Albert J, Chiodi F, et al. AIDS two months after primary human immunodeficiency virus infection. *J Infect Dis* 1988;158:866–868.
6. Sinicco A, For AR, Sciandra M, et al. Risk of developing AIDS after primary acute HIV-1 infection. *J Acquir Immune Defic Syndr Hum Retrovirol* 1993;6:575–581.
7. Pedersen C, Lindhart BO, Jensen BL. Clinical course of primary HIV infection: consequences of subsequent course of infection. *BMJ* 1989;299:154–157.
8. Kinlock S, de Saussure PH, Vanhems PH, et al. Primary HIV infection: a prospective and retrospective study. Poster presented at the VIII International Conference on AIDS; July 19–24, 1992; Amsterdam.
9. Rabeneck L, Popovic M, Gartner S, et al. Acute HIV infection presenting with painful swallowing and esophageal ulcers. *JAMA* 1990;263:2318–2322.
10. McMillan A, Bishop PE, Aw D, et al. Immunohistology of the skin rash associated with acute HIV infection. *AIDS* 1989;3:309–312.
11. Henderson DK, Gerberding JL. Prophylactic zidovudine after occupational exposure to the human immunodeficiency virus: an interim analysis. *J Infect Dis* 1989;160:321–323.
12. Looke DFM, Grove DI. Failed prophylactic zidovudine after needle-stick injury [Letter]. *Lancet* 1990;335:1280.
13. Lange J, Boucher CAB, Hollack CEM, et al. Failure of zidovudine prophylaxis after accidental exposure to HIV-1. *N Engl J Med* 1990;322:1375–1377.
14. Rosenberg EC, Altfeld M, Poon SH, et al. Immune control of HIV-1 after early treatment of acute infection. *Nature* 2000;407:523–526.
15. Safran S, Ashley R, Houlihan C, et al. Clinical and serologic features of herpes simplex virus infection in patients with AIDS. *AIDS* 1991;5:1107–1110.
16. Klatt EC, Shibata D. Cytomegalovirus infection in the acquired immunodeficiency syndrome. *Arch Pathol Lab Med* 1988;112:540–544.
17. Masur H. Clinical implications of herpesvirus infections in patients with AIDS. *Am J Med* 1992;92(2A):1S–2S.
18. Corey YL, Spear PG. Infections with herpes simplex viruses (Part II). *N Engl J Med* 1986;314:749–756.
19. Simonson JN, Cameron WD, Gakenya MN, et al. Human immunodeficiency virus infection among men with sexually transmitted diseases: experience from a center in Africa. *N Engl J Med* 1988;319:274–278.
20. Stamm WE, Hansfield HH, Rompalo AM, et al. The association between genital ulcerative disease and acquisition of HIV infection in homosexual men. *JAMA* 1988;260:1429–1433.
21. Lawrence J: Perspective. Molecular interactions among herpes viruses and human immunodeficiency viruses. *J Infect Dis* 1990;162:338–347.
22. O'Farrell N, Tovey SJ. High cumulative incidence of genital herpes amongst HIV-1 seropositive heterosexuals in south London. *Int J STD AIDS* 1994;5:415–418.
23. Siegal FP, Lopez C, Hammer GS, et al. Severe acquired immunodeficiency in male homosexuals, manifested by chronic perianal ulcerative herpes simplex lesions. *N Engl J Med* 1981;305:1439–1444.
24. Jang KA, Kim SH, Choi JH, et al. Viral folliculitis on the face. *Br J Dermatol* 2000;142:555–559.
25. Buchbinder SP, Katz MH, Hessal NA, et al. Herpes zoster and human immunodeficiency virus infection. *J Infect Dis* 1992;166:1153–1156.
26. Leibovitz E, Cooper D, Giurgiutiu D, et al. Varicella-zoster virus infection in Romanian children infected with the human immunodeficiency virus. *Pediatrics* 1993;92:838–842.
27. Cohen PR, Beltranny VP, Grossman ME. Disseminated herpes zoster in patients with immunodeficiency virus infection. *Am J Med* 1988;84:1076–1080.
28. Jura E, Chadwick EG, Josephs HS, et al. Varicella zoster virus infections in children infected with human immunodeficiency virus. *Pediatr Infect Dis J* 1989;8:856–590.
29. Gilson IH, Barnett JH, Conans MA, et al. Disseminated ecthymatous varicella-zoster virus infection in patients with acquired immunodeficiency syndrome. *J Am Acad Dermatol* 1989;20:637–642.
30. Jacobson MA, Berger TG, Fikrig S, et al. Acyclovir-resistant varicella zoster virus infection after chronic oral acyclovir therapy in patients with the acquired immunodeficiency syndrome (AIDS). *Ann Intern Med* 1990;112:187–191.
31. Hardy WD: Foscarnet treatment of acyclovir-resistant herpes simplex virus infection in patients with acquired immunodeficiency syndrome: preliminary results of a controlled, randomized, regimen-comparative trial. *Am J Med* 1992;92:30s–35s.
32. Chatis PA, Miller CH, Schrager LE, et al. Successful treatment with foscarnet of an acyclovir-resistant mucocutaneous infection with herpes simplex virus in a patient with acquired immunodeficiency syndrome. *N Engl J Med* 1989;320:297–300.
33. Lalezari J, Schaker T, Feinberg J, et al. A randomized, double-blind, placebo-controlled trial of cidofovir gel for the treatment of acyclovir-unresponsive mucocutaneous herpes simplex virus infection in patients with AIDS. *J Infect Dis* 1997;176:892–898.
34. Gallant JE, Moore RD, Chaisson RE. Prophylaxis for opportunistic infections in patients with HIV infection. *Ann Intern Med* 1994;120:932–944.
35. Ioannidis JP, Collier AC, Cooper DA, et al. Clinical efficacy of high-dose acyclovir in patients with human immunodeficiency virus infection: a meta-analysis of randomized individual patient data. *J Infect Dis* 1998;178:349–359.
36. Perrone C, et al. Varicella in patients infected with the human immunodeficiency virus. *Arch Dermatol* 1990;126:1033.
37. Dauden E, Fernandez-Buezo G, Fraga J, et al. Mucocutaneous presence of cytomegalovirus associated with human immunodeficiency virus infection: discussion regarding its pathogenetic role. *Arch Dermatol* 2001;137:443–448.
38. Lin CS, Pinha PD, Krishnan MN, et al. Cytomegalic inclusion disease of the skin. *Arch Dermatol* 1981;117:282–284.
39. Feldman PS Walker AN, Baker R. Cutaneous lesions heralding disseminated cytomegalovirus infections. *J Am Acad Dermatol* 1982;7:545–548.
40. Horn TD, Hood AF. Cytomegalovirus is predictably present in perineal ulcers from immunosuppressed patients. *Arch Dermatol* 1990;126:642–644.
41. Lee JY, Peel R. Concurrent cytomegalovirus and herpes simplex virus infections in skin biopsy specimens from two AIDS patients with fatal CMV infection. *Am J Dermatopathol* 1989;11:136–143.
42. Smith KJ, Skelton HG, James WD, et al. Concurrent epidermal involvement of cytomegalovirus and herpes simplex virus in two HIV-infected patients. *J Am Acad Dermatol* 1991;25:500–506.
43. Muehler-Stamou A, Sen HJ, Emodi G. Epidermolysis in a case of severe cytomegalovirus infection. *BMJ* 1974;3:609–611.
44. Minars N, Silverman JF, Escobar NR, et al. Fatal cytomegalic inclusion disease: associated skin manifestations in a renal transplant patient. *Arch Dermatol* 1977;113:1569–1571.
45. Jacobson MA, Mills J. Serious cytomegalovirus disease in the acquired immunodeficiency syndrome (AIDS). *Ann Intern Med* 1988;108:585–594.
46. Dauden E, Fernandez-Buezo G, Fraga J, et al. Mucocutaneous presence of cytomegalovirus associated with human immunodeficiency virus infection: discussion regarding its pathogenetic role. *Arch Dermatol* 2001;137:443–448.
47. Treatment of serious cytomegalovirus infections with 9-(1,3-dihydroxy-2-propoxymethyl)guanine in patients with AIDS and other immunodeficiencies. Collaborative DHPG Treatment Study Group. *N Engl J Med* 1986;314:801–805.
48. Greenspan JS, Greenspan D, Lenette ET, et al. Replication of Epstein-Barr virus within epithelial cells of oral "hairy" leukoplakia and AIDS associated lesion. *N Engl J Med* 1985;313:1564–1571.
49. Itin PH. Oral hairy leukoplakia: 10 years on. *Dermatology* 1993;187:159–163.
50. Greenspan D, Greenspan JS, Overby G, et al. Risk factors for rapid progression from hairy leukoplakia to AIDS: a nested case-control study. *J Acquir Immune Defic Syndr Hum Retrovirol* 1991;4:652–658.
51. Fowler CD, Reed KD, Brannon RB. Intranuclear inclusions correlate with the ultrastructural detection of herpes-type virions in oral hairy leukoplakia. *Am J Surg Pathol* 1989;13:114–119.
52. DeSouza YG, Greenspan D, Feltzen JR, et al. Localization of Epstein-Barr virus DNA in the epithelial cells of oral hairy leukoplakia via in situ hybridization of tissue sac [Letter]. *N Engl J Med* 1989;320:1559.
53. Gaglioti D, De Pietro M, Ficarra G, et al. Oral hairy leukoplakia: clinical appearance and treatment results [Abstract]. Presented at the V International Conference on AIDS, June 4–9, 1989; Montreal; p 473.
54. Schofer H, Ochsendorf FR, Elm EB, et al. Treatment of oral hairy leukoplakia in AIDS patients with vitamin A acid (topically) or acyclovir (systemically) [Letter]. *Dermatologica* 1987;174:150–151.
55. Beutner KR, Becker TM, Stone KM. Epidemiology of HPV infections. *Dermatol Clin* 1991;9:211–218.
56. Palefsky JM, Gonzales J, Greenblatt RM, et al. Anal intraepithelial neoplasia and anal papillomavirus infection among homosexual males with group IV HIV disease. *JAMA* 1990;263:2911–2916.
57. Chardonnet Y, Viac J, Staqnet MJ. Cell mediated immunity to human papillomavirus. *Clin Dermatol* 1985;3:156–161.
58. Doherty R, Tanskanen E, Churchill MJ, et al. Interactions between human immunodeficiency virus and human papillomavirus. Poster presented at the VIII International Conference on AIDS; July 19–24, 1992; Amsterdam.
59. Tornesello ML, Buonaguro FM, Galloway DA, et al. Human immunodeficiency virus type 1 *tat* gene enhances human papillomavirus early gene expression. *Intervirology* 1992;36(2):57–64.

60. Berger TG, Sawchuk WS, Leonardi C, et al. Epidermodysplasia verruciformis-associated papillomavirus infection complicating human immunodeficiency virus disease. *Br J Dermatol* 1991;126:79–83.

61. Braun L Farmer ER, Shah KV. Immunoperoxidase localization of papillomavirus antigen and cutaneous warts in bowenoid papulosis. *J Med Virol* 1983;12:187–193.

62. Rudlinger R, Buchmann P. HPV 16-positive bowenoid papulosis and squamous-cell carcinoma of the anus in an HIV positive man. *Dis Colon Rectum* 1989;32:1042–1045.

63. Fader, D, Stoler M, Anderson T. Isolated extragenital HPV-thirties-group-positive bowenoid papulosis in an AIDS patient. *Br J Dermatol* 1994;131:577–580.

64. Beckmann AM, Myerson D, Daling JR, et al. Detection and localization of human papillomavirus DNA in human genital condylomas by in situ hybridization with biotinylated probes. *J Med Virol* 1985;16:265–273.

65. Shibata KK, Arnheim M, Martin WJ. Detection of human papillomavirus in paraffin-embedded tissue using the polymerase chain reaction. *J Exp Med* 1988;167:225–230.

66. Beutner KR Conant M, Friedman-Kien AE, et al. Patient-applied podofilox for treatment of genital warts. *Lancet* 1989;1:831–838.

67. Lane HC. Interferons in HIV and related diseases. *AIDS* 1994;8:19–23.

68. Friedman-Kien AE, Eron LJ, Conant M, et al. Natural interferon alfa for treatment of condylomata acuminata. *JAMA* 1988;259:533–538.

69. Beutner KR, Spruance SL, Hougham AJ, et al. Treatment of genital warts with an immune-response modifier (imiquimod). *J Am Acad Dermatol* 1998;38:230–239.

70. Conant M. Immunomodulatory therapy in the management of viral infections in patients with HIV infection. *J Am Acad Dermatol* 2000;43:S27–30.

71. Davis M, Gostout B, et al. Large plantar wart caused by human papillomavirus-66 and resolution by topical cidofovir therapy. *J Am Acad Dermatol* 2000;43:340–343.

72. Anadolu R, et al. Treatment of epidermodysplasia verruciformis with a combination of acitretin and interferon alfa-2a. *J Am Acad Dermatol* 2001;45:296–299.

73. Stern RS. Epidemiology of skin disease in HIV infection: a cohort study of health maintenance organization members. *J Invest Dermatol* 1994;102:345–37S.

74. Redfield RR, Wright DC, James WD, et al. Disseminated vaccinia in a military recruit with human immunodeficiency virus (HIV) disease. *N Engl J Med* 1987;316:673–676.

75. Fivenson DP, Weltman RE, Gibson SH. Giant molluscum contagiosum presenting as basal cell carcinoma in an AIDS patient [Letter]. *J Am Acad Dermatol* 1988;19:912–914.

76. Berger TG, Greene I. Bacterial, viral, fungal and parasitic infections in HIV disease and AIDS. *Dermatol Clin* 1991;3:465–492.

77. Jang KA, Kim SH, Choi JH, et al. Viral folliculitis on the face. *Br J Dermatol* 2000;142:555–559.

78. Buckley R, Smith K. Topical imiquimod therapy for chronic giant molluscum contagiosum in a patient with advanced human immunodeficiency virus 1 disease. *Arch Dermatol* 1999;135:1167–1169.

79. Torok TJ. Parvovirus and human disease. *Adv Intern Med* 1992;37:431–455.

80. Ross LA, Kim KS, Comport Z. Successful treatment of disseminated measles in a patient with acquired immune deficiency syndrome: consideration of anti-viral and passive immunotherapy. *Am J Med* 1990;88:313–314.

81. Coldiron BM, Freeman RG, Beaudoing DL. Isolation of adenovirus from a granuloma annulare-like lesion in the acquired immunodeficiency syndrome-related complex. *Arch Dermatol* 1988;124:654–655.

82. Markowitz LE, Chandler FW, Roldan EO, et al. Fatal measles and pneumonia without rash in a child with AIDS. *J Infect Dis* 1988;158:480–483.

83. Ellis M, Gupta S, Gellant S, et al. Neutrophil function in patients with AIDS or AIDS-related complex: a comprehensive evaluation. *J Infect Dis* 1988;158:1268–1276.

84. Pahwa SG, Quilop MT, Lange M, et al. Defective B-lymphocyte function in homosexual men in relation to acquired immune deficiency syndrome. *Ann Intern Med* 1984;101:757–763.

85. Ganesh R, Castle S, Gibbon D, et al. Staphylococcal carriage in HIV infection [Letter]. *Lancet* 2:558, 1989.

86. Nichols SL, Balog K, Silverman M. Bacterial infection and AIDS. Clinical pathologic correlations in a series of autopsy cases. *Am J Clin Pathol* 1989;92:787–790.

87. Raviglione MC, Battan R, Pablos-Mendez A, et al. Infections associated with Hickman catheters in patients with acquired immune deficiency syndrome. *Am J Med* 1989;86:780–786.

88. el Baze P, Thyss A, Vinti H, et al. A study of nineteen immunocompromised patients with extensive skin lesions caused by *Pseudomonas aeruginosa* with and without bacteremia. *Acta Derm Venereol* (Stockh) 1991;71:411–415.

89. Kielhofner M, Atmar RL, Hamill RF, et al. Life-threatening *Pseudomonas aeruginosa* infections in patients with human immunodeficiency virus infection. *Clin Infect Dis* 1992;14:403–411.

90. Sangeorzan JA, Bradley SF, Kaufman CA. Cutaneous manifestation of *Pseudomonas* infection in the acquired immune deficiency syndrome. *Arch Dermatol* 1990;126:832–833.

91. Patterson JW, Kitces EN, Neafie RC. Cutaneous botryomycosis in a patient with acquired immunodeficiency syndrome. *J Am Acad Dermatol* 1987;16:238–242.

92. Weitzner JM, Dhawan SS, Rosen LB, et al. Successful treatment of botryomy-cosis in a patient with acquired immunodeficiency syndrome. *J Am Acad Dermatol* 1989;21:1312–1314.

93. Becker BA, Odom RB, Berger TG. Atypical plaque-like staphylococcal folliculitis in human immunodeficiency virus infected persons. *J Am Acad Dermatol* 1989;21:1024–1026.

94. Gaut P, Wong PK, Meyer RD. Pyomyositis in a patient with the acquired immunodeficiency syndrome. *Arch Intern Med* 1988;148:1608–1610.

95. Janssen F, Zelinsky-Gurung A, Caumes E, et al. Group A streptococcal cellulitis-adenitis in a patient with the acquired immunodeficiency syndrome. *J Am Acad Dermatol* 1991;24:363–365.

96. Kline MW, Dunkle LM. Toxic shock syndrome in the acquired immunodeficiency syndrome. *Pediatr Infect Dis J* 1988;7:736–738.

97. Cipriano J, Feranno J, Ferranti E. Acquired immunodeficiency syndrome in non-menstrual toxic shock syndrome [Letter]. *Ann Intern Med* 1986;105:300.

98. Sangeorzan JA, et al. Cutaneous manifestations of Pseudomonas infection in AIDS. *Arch Dermatol* 1990;126:832.

99. Wittenberg GP, et al. Cutaneous malacoplakia in a patient with AIDS. *Arch Dermatol* 1998;134:244.

100. Steinhart R, Reingold AL, Taylor F, et al. Invasive *Haemophilus influenzae* infections in men with HIV infection. *JAMA* 1992;268:3350–3352.

101. Javaly K, Horowitz HW, Wormser GP. Nocardiosis in patients with human immunodeficiency virus infection. *Medicine* (Baltimore) 1992;71:128–138.

102. Watkins KV, Richmond AS, Langstein IM. Nonhealing extraction site due to *Actinomyces naeslundii* in patients with AIDS. *Oral Surg Oral Med Oral Pathol* 1991;71:675–677.

103. Drancourt M, Bonnet E, Gallais H, et al. *Rhodococcus equi* infection in patients with AIDS. *J Infect* 1992;24:123–131.

104. Patey O, Halioua B, Casciani JP, et al. *Corynebacterium diphtheriae* septicemia in an AIDS patient [Abstract]. Presented at the VIII International Conference on AIDS; July 19–24, 1992; Amsterdam.

105. Cockerell CJ, Whitlow MA, Webster GF, et al. Epithelioid angiomatosis: a distinct vascular disorder in patients with acquired immunodeficiency syndrome or AIDS-related complex. *Lancet* 1987;329:654–656.

106. Relman DA, Loutit JS, Schmidt TM, et al. The agent of bacillary angiomatosis: an approach to the identification of uncultured pathogens. *N Engl J Med* 1990;323:1573–1580.

107. Relman DA, Lepp PW, Sadler KN, et al. Phylogenetic relationships among the agents of bacillary angiomatosis. *Mol Microbiol* 1992;6:1801–1807.

108. Mohle-Boetnai J, Koehler J, Berger T, et al. Bacillary angiomatosis and bacillary peliosis in patients infected with human immunodeficiency virus: clinical characteristics in a case-control study. *Clin Infect Dis* 1996;22:794–800.

109. Tappero JW, Mohle-Boetani JM, Koehler JE, et al. The epidemiology of bacillary angiomatosis and bacillary peliosis. *JAMA* 1993;269:770–775.

110. Koehler JE, Claser CA, Tappero JW. *Rochalimaea henselae* infection: a new zoonosis with the domestic cat as reservoir. *JAMA* 1994;271:531–535.

111. Webster GF, Cockerell CJ, Friedman-Kien AE. The clinical spectrum of bacillary angiomatosis. *Br J Dermatol* 1992;126:535–541.

112. Schinella RA, Alba-Greco M. Bacillary angiomatosis presenting as a soft-tissue tumor without skin involvement. *Hum Pathol* 1990;21:567–569.

113. Perkocha LA, Geaghan SM, Yen TS, et al. Clinical and pathological features of bacillary peliosis hepatis in association with human immunodeficiency virus infection. *N Engl J Med* 1990;323:1581–1586.

114. Welch DF, Pickett DA, Slater LN, et al. *Rochalimaea henselae* sp. nov., a cause of septicemia, bacillary angiomatosis and parenchymal bacillary peliosis. *J Clin Microbiol* 1992;30:275–280.

115. Slater LN, Welch DF, Hensel D, et al. A newly recognized fastidious gram-negative pathogen as a cause of fever and bacteremia. *N Engl J Med* 1990;323:1587–1593.

116. Daly JS, Worthington MG, Brenner DJ, et al. *Rochalimaea elizabethae* sp. nov. isolated from a patient with endocarditis. *J Clin Microbiol* 1993;31:872–881.

117. Draincort M, Mainardi JL, Brouqui P, et al. *Bartonella* (*Rochalimaea*) *quintana* endocarditis in three homeless men. *N Engl J Med* 1995;332:419–423.

118. Spach DH, Kanter AS, Doughtery ML, et al. *Bartonella* (*Rochalimaea*) *quintana* bacteremia in inner-city patients with chronic alcoholism. *N Engl J Med* 1995;332:424–428.

119. Koehler JE, Quinn FD, Berger TG, et al. Isolation of *Rochalimaea* species from cutaneous and osseous lesions of bacillary angiomatosis. *N Engl J Med* 1992;327:1625–1631.

120. Regnery RL, Anderson BE, Clarridge JEI, et al. Characterization of a novel *Rochalimaea* species, *R. henselae* sp. nov., isolated from blood of a febrile human immunodeficiency virus-seropositive patient. *J Clin Microbiol* 1992;30:265–274.

121. Lucey D, Dolan MJ, Moss CW, et al. Relapsing illness due to *Rochalimaea henselae* in immunocompetent hosts: implication for therapy and new epidemiological associations. *Clin Infect Dis* 1992;14:683–688.

122. Mui BSK, Mulligan ME, George WL. Response of HIV-associated disseminated cat-scratch disease to treatment with doxycycline. *Am J Med* 1990;89:229–231.

123. Guierra LG, Neka CJ, Boman D, et al. Rapid response of AIDS-related bacillary angiomatosis to azithromycin. *Clin Infect Dis* 1993;17:264–266.

124. Duong M, Dalao S, Chavanet P, et al. Angiomatose bacillair au tours de l'infection à VIH. Mise au point à propos d'un cas traité par le roxithromycine. *Ann Intern Med* 1992;143:107–112.

125. Koehler JE, Quinn FD, Berger TG, et al. Isolation of *Rochalimaea* species from cutaneous and osseous lesions of bacillary angiomatosis. *N Engl J Med* 1992;327:1625–1631.

126. Barbaro DJ, Orcutt VL, Colder BM: *Mycobacterium avium-intracellulare* infection limited to the skin and lymph nodes in patients with AIDS. *Rev Infect Dis* 1989;11:625–628.

127. Koehler JE, Quinn FD, Berger TG, et al. Isolation of *Rochalimaea* species from cutaneous and osseous lesions of bacillary angiomatosis. *N Engl J Med* 1992;327:1625–1631.

128. Friedman BF, et al. *M. avium-intracellulare*: cutaneous presentations of disseminated disease. *Am J Med* 1988;85:257.

129. Rogers PL, Walker RE, Wayne HC, et al. Disseminated *Mycobacterium haemophilum* infection in two patients with AIDS. *Am J Med* 1988;84:640–642.

130. Geman MD. Treatment of multidrug resistant tuberculosis. *N Engl J Med* 1993;329:784–791.

131. Quinn TC, Cannon RO, Glasser D, et al. The association of syphilis with risk of human immunodeficiency virus in patients attending sexually transmitted disease clinics. *Arch Intern Med* 1990;159:1297–1302.

132. Gregory N, Sanchez M, Buchness MR. The spectrum of syphilis in patients with human immunodeficiency virus infection. *J Am Acad Dermatol* 1990;22:1061–1067.

133. Johns DR, Tierney M, Felsenstein D. Alteration of the natural history of neurosyphilis by concurrent infection with the human immunodeficiency virus. *N Engl J Med* 1987;316:1569–1572.

134. Quale J, Tepletts E, Augenbraun F. Atypical presentation of chancroid in a patient infected with the human immunodeficiency virus. *Am J Med* 1990; 88[Suppl 5]:43–44.

135. Ortiz-Zepeda C, Hernandez-Perez E, Marroquin-Burgos R. Gross and microscopic features in chancroid: a study in 200 new culture-proven cases in San Salvador. *Sex Transm Dis* 1994;21:112–117.

136. King R, Choudhri SH, Nasio J, et al. Clinical and in situ cellular responses to *Haemophilus ducreyi* in the presence or absence of HIV infection. *Int J STD AIDS* 1998;9:531–536.

137. Strongin IS, Kale SA, Raymond MK, et al. An unusual presentation of gonococcal arthritis in an HIV-positive patient. *Ann Rheum Dis* 1991;50:572–573.

138. Centers for Disease Control and Prevention. 1998 Guidelines for the treatment of sexually transmitted diseases. *MMWR Morb Mortal Wkly Rep* 1998; 47(RR-1):1–16.

139. Cohen PR, Grossman ME, Silvers DN. Disseminated histoplasmosis and human immunodeficiency virus infection. *Int J Dermatol* 1991;30:614–622.

140. Hazelhurst JA, Vismer HF. Histoplasmosis presenting with unusual skin lesions in acquired immunodeficiency syndrome (AIDS). *Br J Dermatol* 1985;113:345–348.

141. Bundy AT, Simjee S, Ray M, et al. Psoriatic patient presenting with perioral herpetiform lesions. *Arch Dermatol* 1989;125:1440–1441.

142. Cole MC, Cohen PR, Satra KH, et al. The concurrent presence of systemic disease pathogens and cutaneous Kaposi's sarcoma in the same lesion: *Histoplasma capsulatum* and Kaposi's sarcoma coexisting in a single skin lesion in a patient with AIDS. *J Am Acad Dermatol* 1992;26:285–287.

143. Chaker MB, Cocerell CJ. Concomitant psoriasis, seborrheic dermatitis and disseminated cutaneous histoplasmosis in a patient infected with the human immunodeficiency virus. *J Am Acad Dermatol* 1993;29:311–313.

144. Cohen PR, Held JL, Grossman ME, et al. Disseminated histoplasmosis presenting as an ulcerated verrucous plaque in a human immunodeficiency virus-infected man: report of a case possibly involving human-to-human transmission of histoplasmosis. *Int J Dermatol* 1991;30:104–108.

145. Rico NJ, Penneys NS. Cutaneous cryptococcosis resembling molluscum contagiosum in a patient with AIDS. *Arch Dermatol* 1985;121:901–902.

146. Mares M, Sartori MT, Carretta M, et al. Rhinophyma-like cryptococcal infection as an early manifestation of AIDS in a hemophilia B patient. *Acta Haematol* 1990;84:101–103.

147. Bibler MR, Luber HJ, Glueck HI, et al. Disseminated sporotrichosis in a patient with HIV infection after treatment for acquired factor VIII inhibitor. *JAMA* 1986;256:3125–3126.

148. Shaw JC, Levinson W, Montanara A. Sporotrichosis in the acquired immunodeficiency syndrome. *J Am Acad Dermatol* 1989;21:1145–1147.

149. Borradori L, Schmit J-C, Stetzkowski M, et al. Penicilliosis *marneffei* infection in AIDS. *J Am Acad Dermatol* 1994;31:843–846.

150. Kantipong P, Walsh DS. Oral penicilliosis in a patient with human immunodeficiency virus in Northern Thailand. *Int J Dermatol* 2000;39:926–941.

151. Kantipong R, Panich V, Pongsurachet V, et al. Hepatic penicilliosis in patients without skin lesions. *Clin Infect Dis* 1998;26:1215–1217.

152. Fish DG, Ampel NM, Galgiani JN, et al. Coccidioidomycosis during human immunodeficiency virus infection: a review of 77 patients. *Medicine* (Baltimore) 1990;69:384–391.

153. Galgiani JN, Ampel NM. Coccidiomycosis in human immunodeficiency virus-infected patients. *J Infect Dis* 1990;162:1165–1169.

154. Fraser VJ, Keath EJ, Powderly WG. Two cases of blastomycosis from a common source: Use of DNA restriction analysis to identify strains. *J Infect Dis* 1991;163:1378–1381.

155. Bakos L, Kronfeld M, Hampe S, et al. Disseminated paracoccidioidomycosis with skin lesions in a patient with acquired immunodeficiency syndrome [Letter]. *J Am Acad Dermatol* 1989;20:854–855.

156. Wood GM, McCormack JG, Muir DB, et al. Clinical features of human infection with *Scedosporium inflatum*. *Clin Infect Dis* 1992;14:1027–1033.

157. Scherr GR, Evans SG, Kiyabu MT, et al. *Pseudallescheria boydii* in the acquired immunodeficiency syndrome. *Arch Pathol Lab Med* 1992;116:535–536.

158. Hevia O, Kligman D, Penneys NS. Non-scalp hair infection caused by *Microsporum canis* in a patient with acquired immunodeficiency syndrome. *J Am Acad Dermatol* 1991;24:789–790.

159. Frazer R, Stoole E, et al. Head and neck *Zygomycetes/Aspergillus* infections in patients with AIDS. Poster presented at the IX International Conference on AIDS; June 6–12, 1993; Berlin.

160. Diamond HJ, Phelphs RG, Gordon ML, et al. Combined *Aspergillus* and zygomycotic (*Rhizopus*) infection in a patient with the acquired immunodeficiency syndrome. *J Am Acad Dermatol* 1992;26:1017–1018.

161. Hunt SJ, Nagi C, Gross KG, et al. Primary cutaneous aspergillosis near central venous catheters in patients with the acquired immunodeficiency syndrome. *Arch Dermatol* 1992;128:1229–1232.

162. Chuck SL, Sande MA. Infections with *Cryptococcus neoformans* in the acquired immunodeficiency syndrome. *N Engl J Med* 1989;321:794–799.

163. Powderly WG. A controlled trial of fluconazole or amphotericin B to prevent relapse of cryptococcal meningitis in patients with the acquired immunodeficiency syndrome. *N Engl J Med* 1992;326:793–798.

164. British Society for Antimicrobial Chemotherapy Working Group. Antifungal chemotherapy in patients with acquired immunodeficiency syndrome. *Lancet* 1992;340:648–651.

165. Klein RS, Harris CA, Small CB, et al. Oral candidiasis in high-risk patients as the initial manifestation of the acquired immunodeficiency syndrome. *N Engl J Med* 1984;311:354–358.

166. Durden RM, Elewski B. Fungal Infections in HIV-infected patients. *Semin Cutan Med Surg* 1997;16:200–212.

167. Hing MCY, Henderson CL, Barker DC, et al. Correlation of *Pityrosporum ovale* density with clinical severity of seborrheic dermatitis as assessed by simplified technique. *J Am Acad Dermatol* 1990;23:82–86.

168. Groisser D, Bottone E, Lebwohl M. Association of *Pityrosporum orbiculare* (*Malassezia furfur*) with seborrheic dermatitis in patients with acquired immunodeficiency syndrome. *J Am Acad Dermatol* 1991;20:770–773.

169. Torssander J, Karlsson A, Morfeldt-Manson L, et al. Dermatophytosis and HIV infection: a study in homosexual men. *Acta Derm Venereol* (Stockh) 1988;68:563–565.

170. Noppakun N, Head ES. Proximal white subungual onychomycosis in a patient with acquired immunodeficiency syndrome. *Int J Dermatol* 1986;25:586–587.

171. Lief HL, Semperkopf MS. Invasive trichosporonosis in a patient with AIDS. *J Infect Dis* 1989;160:356–357.

172. Drabick JJ, Gomatos PJ, Solis JB. Cutaneous cladosporiosis as a complication of skin testing in a man positive for HIV. *J Am Acad Dermatol* 1990;22:135–136.

173. Lavy-Clotz B, Badillet G, Cavelier-Balloy B, et al. Alternariose cutanée au cours d'un SIDA. *Arch Derm Venereol* 1985;112:739–740.

174. Duvic M, Lowe L, Rios A, et al. Superficial phaeohyphomycosis of the scrotum in a patient with AIDS [Letter]. *Arch Dermatol* 1987;123:1597–1599.

175. Pons V, Greenspan D, Debruin M. Therapy for oropharyngeal candidiasis in HIV-infected patients: a randomized, prospective multicenter study of oral fluconazole versus clotrimazole troches. *J Acquir Immune Defic Syndr Hum Retrovirol* 1993;6:1311–1316.

176. Odom R. Common superficial fungal infections in immunosuppressed patients. *J Am Acad Dermatol* 1994;31[Suppl]:56–59.

177. Greenspan D. Treatment of oropharyngeal candidiasis in HIV-positive patients. *J Am Acad Dermatol* 1994;31[Suppl]:51–55.

178. Sanguineti A, Carmichael K, Campbell D. Fluconazole-resistant *Candida albicans* after long-term suppressive therapy. *Arch Intern Med* 1993;153:1122–1124.

179. Sadick N, Kaplan MH, Pahwa SG, et al. Unusual features of scabies complicating human T-lymphotrophic virus type III infection. *J Am Acad Dermatol* 1986;15:482–486.

180. Belsito DB, Sanchez MR, Baer RL, et al. Reduced Langerhans' cell Ia antigen and ATPase activity in patients with the acquired immunodeficiency syndrome. *N Engl J Med* 1984;310:1279–1282.

181. Jucowics P, Ramon ME, Donn PC, et al. Norwegian scabies in an infant with acquired immunodeficiency syndrome. *Arch Dermatol* 1989;125:1670–1671.

182. Berger TG. Treatment of bacterial, fungal and parasitic infections in the HIV-infected host. *Semin Dermatol* 1993;112;296–300.

183. Skinner SM, DeVillez RL. Sepsis associated with Norwegian scabies in patients with acquired immunodeficiency syndrome. *Arch Dermatol* 1992;50:213–216.

184. Meinking TL, Taplin D, Hermida J, et al. The treatment of scabies with Ivermectin. *N Engl J Med* 1995;333:26–30.

185. Taplin D, Meinking TL. Treatment of HIV-related scabies with emphasis on the efficacy of ivermectin. *Semin Cutan Med Surg* 1997;16:235–240.

186. Meinking TL, Taplin D. Safety of permethrin vs, lindane for treatment of pediculosis and scabies. *Arch Dermatol* 1996;132:959–962.

187. Montelban C, Martinez-Fernandez R, Calleja JL, et al. Visceral leishmaniasis (kala-azar) as an opportunistic infection in patients with HIV disease in Spain. *Rev Infect Dis* 1989;11:655–660.

188. Dominey A, Roen R, Tschen J. Papulonodular demodicidosis associated with acquired immunodeficiency syndrome. *J Am Acad Dermatol* 1989;20:197–201.

189. Majors MJ, Berger TG, Blauvelt A, et al. HIV-related eosinophilic folliculitis: a panel discussion. *Semin Cutan Med Surg* 1997;16:219–223.

190. Hennessey NP, Parro EL, Cockerell CJ. Cutaneous *Pneumocystis carinii* infection in patients with acquired immunodeficiency syndrome. *Arch Dermatol* 1991;127:1699–1701.

191. Hirschmann JV, Chu AC. Skin lesions with disseminated toxoplasmosis in

a patient with the acquired immunodeficiency syndrome. *Arch Dermatol* 1988;124:1446–1447.

192. Portnoy BL, Micheletti GA. *Acanthamoeba* infection of skin and sinuses in an AIDS patient: diagnosis and treatment [Abstract]. Presented at the VIII International Conference on AIDS; July 19–24, 1992; Amsterdam.

193. Glezerov V, Masci JR. Disseminated strongyloidiasis and other selected unusual infections in patients with acquired immunodeficiency syndrome. *Prog AIDS Pathol* 1990;2:137–142.

194. Czelusta A, Yen-Moore A, et al. An overview of sexually transmitted diseases. Part III. Sexually transmitted diseases in HIV-infected patients. *J Am Acad Dermatol* 2000;43:409–432.

195. Nickles SW. The opportunistic and bacterial infections associated with pediatric human immunodeficiency virus disease. *Acta Paediatr* 1994;[Suppl 400]:46–50.

196. Silverman S Jr, Wara D. Oral manifestations of pediatric AIDS. *Pediatrician* 1989;16:185–187.

197. Greenspan JS, Masrucci, Legott PF, et al. Hairy leukoplakia in a child [Letter]. *AIDS* 1988;2:143.

198. Mofenson LM, Moye J Jr. Intravenous immune globulin for the prevention of infections in children with symptomatic human immunodeficiency virus infection. *Pediatr Res* 1993;33[Suppl]:80–89.

199. The National Institutes of Child Health and Human Development Immunoglobulin Study Group. Intravenous immune globulin for the prevention of bacterial infection in children with symptomatic human immunodeficiency virus infection. *N Engl J Med* 1991;325:73–80.

200. Spector SA, Gelber RD, McGrath N, et al. Results of the ACTG 051: a double blind placebo controlled trial to evaluate intravenous gammaglobulin (IVIG) in children with symptomatic HIV infection receiving zidovudine. Anaheim, CA: Infectious Disease Society of America. *N Engl J Med* 1994;331:1181–1187.

201. Feingold AR, Vermund SK Burk RD, et al. Cervical cytologic abnormalities and papillomavirus in women infected with human immunodeficiency virus. *J Acquir Immune Defic Syndr Hum Retrovirol* 1990;3:896–903.

202. Palefsky JM, Holly EA, Gonzales J, et al. Detection of human papilloma DNA in anal intra-epithelial neoplasia and anal cancer. *Cancer Res* 1991;51:1014–1019.

203. 1993 Revised classification system for HIV infection and expanded surveillance case definition for AIDS among adolescents and adults. *MMWR Morbid Mortal Wkly Rep* 1992;41(RR-17):1–19.

204. Beckmann AM, Daling JR, Sherman KJ, et al. Human papillomavirus infection and anal cancer. *Int J Cancer* 1989;43:1042–1049.

205. Majewski S, Jablonska S. Epidermodysplasia verruciformis as a model of human papillomavirus-induced genetic cancers: the role of local immunosurveillance. *Am J Med Sci* 1992;304:174–179.

206. Lutzner M, Croisant O, Ducasse MF, et al. A potentially oncogenic human papillomavirus (HPV5) found in two renal allograft recipients. *J Invest Dermatol* 1980;75:353–356.

207. Haverkos HW. Factors associated with the pathogenesis of AIDS. *J Infect Dis* 1987;156:251–257.

208. Rutherford GW, Payne SF, Lemp GF, et al. The epidemiology of AIDS-related Kaposi's sarcoma in San Francisco. *J Acquir Immune Defic Syndr Hum Retrovirol* 1990;3[Suppl 1]:S4–S7.

209. Friedman-Kien AE, Saltzman BR, Cao YZ, et al. Kaposi's sarcoma in HIV-negative homosexual men. *Lancet* 1990;335:168–169.

210. Huang YQ, Li JJ, Rush MG, et al. HPV 16-related DNA sequences in Kaposi's sarcoma. *Lancet* 1992;339:515–518.

211. Chang Y, Cesarman E, Pessin MS, et al. Identification of herpes virus-like DNA sequences in AIDS-associated Kaposi's sarcoma. *Science* 1994;266:1865–1869.

212. Su I-J, Hsu Y-S, Chang Y-C, et al. Herpesvirus-like DNA sequences in Kaposi's sarcoma from AIDS and non-AIDS patients in Taiwan (Letter). *Lancet* 1995;345:722–723.

213. Huang Y-Q, Li JJ, Kaplan MH, et al. Human herpesvirus-like nucleic acid in various forms of Kaposi's sarcoma. *Lancet* 1995;345:759–761.

214. Moore PS, Chang Y. Detection of herpesvirus-like DNA sequences in Kaposi's sarcoma in patients with and those without HIV infection. *N Engl J Med* 1995;332:1181–1185.

215. Roth WK. TGF-beta and FGF-like growth factors involved in the pathogenesis of AIDS-associated Kaposi's sarcoma. *Res Virol* 1993;144:105–109.

216. Miles SA, Matrinez-Maza O, Rezai A, et al. Oncostatin M as a potent mitogen for AIDS-related Kaposi's sarcoma-derived cells. *Science* 1992;255:1432–1434.

217. Naidu TM, Rosen EM, Zitnick R, et al. Role of scatter factor in the pathogenesis of AIDS-related Kaposi sarcoma. *Proc Natl Acad Sci U S A* 1994;91:5281–5285.

218. Miles SA, Rezai AR, Salazar Gozalez JF, et al. AIDS Kaposi sarcoma-derived cells produce and respond to interleukin 6. *Proc Natl Acad Sci USA* 1990;87:4068–4072.

219. Samaniego F, Markham PD, Gallo RC, et al. Inflammatory cytokines induce AIDS-Kaposi's sarcoma-derived spindle cells to produce and release basic fibroblast growth factor and enhance Kaposi's sarcoma-like lesion formation in nude mice. *J Immunol* 1995;154:3582–3592.

220. Ensoli B, Barillari S, Salahuddin SZ, et al. Tat protein of HIV-1 stimulates growth cells derived from Kaposi's sarcoma lesions of AIDS patients. *Nature* 1990;345:84–86.

221. Dezube B. The role of human immunodeficiency virus-1 in the pathogenesis of acquired immunodeficiency syndrome-related Kaposi's sarcoma: the importance of an inflammatory and angiogenic milieu. *Semin Oncol* 2000;27:420–423.

222. Dezube BJ. Clinical presentation and natural history of AIDS-related Kaposi's sarcoma. *Hematol Oncol Clin North Am* 1996;10:1023–1029.

223. Huang L, Schnapp LM, Gruden JF, et al. Presentation of AIDS-related pulmonary Kaposi's sarcoma diagnosed by bronchoscopy. *Am J Respir Crit Care Med* 1996;153:1385–1390.

224. Gill PS, Loureiro C, Bernstein-Singer M, et al. Clinical effect of glucocorticoids on Kaposi sarcoma related to the acquired immunodeficiency syndrome. *Ann Intern Med* 1989;110:937–940.

225. Walmsley S, Northfelt DW, Melosky B, et al. Treatment of AIDS-related cutaneous Kaposi's sarcoma with topical alitretinoin (9-cis-retinoic) gel. *J Acquir Immune Defic Syndr Hum Retrovirol* 1999;22:235–246.

226. Serfing U, Hood AF. Local therapies for cutaneous Kaposi's sarcoma in patients with AIDS. *Arch Dermatol* 1991;127:1479–1481.

227. Sturzl M, Zietz C, Eisenburg B, et al. Liposomal doxorubicin in the treatment of AIDS-associated Kaposi's sarcoma: clinical histological and cell biological evaluation. *Res Virol* 1994;145:261–269.

228. Newman S. Treatment of epidemic Kaposi's sarcoma with intralesional vinblastine injection [Abstract]. *Proc Am Soc Clin Oncol* 1988;7:19.

229. Gill PS, Tulpule A, Espina BM, et al. Paclitaxel is safe and effective in the treatment of advanced AIDS-related Kaposi's sarcoma. *J Clin Oncol* 1999;17:1876–1883.

230. Dezube BJ, Von Roenn JG, Holden-Wiltse J. Fumagillin analog in the treatment of Kaposi's sarcoma: a phase I AIDS Clinical Trial Group study. *J Clin Oncol* 1998;16:1444–1449.

231. Gill PS, Lunardi-Iksandar Y, Louie S, et al. The effects of preparations of human chorionic gonadotropin on AIDS-related Kaposi's sarcoma. *N Engl J Med* 1996;335:1261–1269.

232. Harper ME, Kaplan MH, Marselle LM, et al. Concomitant infection of HTLV-I and HTLV III in a patient with TS lymphoproliferative disease. *N Engl J Med* 1986;315:1073–1078.

233. Shibata D, Brynes RK, Rabinowitz A, et al. Human T-cell lymphotropic virus type I (HTLV I)-associated adult T-cell leukemia lymphoma in a patient infected with human immunodeficiency virus type 1 (HIV-1). *Ann Intern Med* 1989;111:871–875.

234. Getchell JP, Heath JL, Hicks DR, et al. Detection of human T cell leukemia virus type I and human immunodeficiency virus in cultured lymphocytes of a Zairian man with AIDS. *J Infect Dis* 1987;155:612–616.

235. vonder Helm K, vonder Helm D, Deinhardt F. Simultaneous infection with the human immunodeficiency virus and HTLV-I in a patient with AIDS [Letter]. *J Infect Dis* 1988;157:205–207.

236. Zucker-Franklin D, Pancake B, Friedman-Kien AE. Cutaneous disease resembling mycosis fungoides in HIV-infected patients whose skin and blood cells also harbor proviral HTLV type I. *AIDS Res Hum Retroviruses* 1994;10:1173–1177.

237. Kaplan MH, Hall WW, Susin M, et al. Syndrome of severe skin disease, eosinophilia and dermatopathic lymphadenopathy in patients with HTLV-II complicating human immunodeficiency virus infection. *Am J Med* 1991;91:300–309.

238. Cote TR, Biggar RJ, Rosenberg PS, et al. Non-Hodgkin's lymphoma among people with AIDS: incidence, presentation, and public health burden. *Int J Cancer* 1997;73:645–650.

239. Levine AM. AIDS related lymphoma. *Blood* 1992;80:8–20.

240. Hartge P, Devesa SS, Fraumeni JF Jr. Hodgkin's and non-Hodgkin's lymphomas. *Cancer Surv* 1994;20:423–453.

241. Siekevitz M, Josephs SF, Dukovich M, et al. Activation of the HIV-1 LTR by T cell mitogens and the transactivator protein of HTLV-I. *Science* 1987;238:1557–1559.

242. Zack JA, Cann AJ, Lugo JP, et al. HIV-I production from infected peripheral blood T cells after HTLV-I mitogenic stimulation. *Science* 1988;240:1026–1028.

243. Pagano JS, Kenny S Markowitz D, et al. Epstein-Barr virus and interaction with human retroviruses. *J Virol Methods* 1988;21:29–39.

CHAPTER 118
Human Immunodeficiency Virus Serology and Viral Burden

John G. Bartlett

Human immunodeficiency virus (HIV) is usually detected with HIV serology, although it is occasionally desirable to use other methods to demonstrate antibody or antigen. There has been interest in and emphasis on measurement of viral concentration in plasma as a measure of viral "burden" to facilitate decisions regarding antiviral therapy.

HUMAN IMMUNODEFICIENCY VIRUS SEROLOGY

Standard criteria for a positive test are a repeatedly positive enzyme-linked immunosorbent assay (ELISA) followed by a positive Western blot (Table 118.1). The Western blot criteria of the Centers for Disease Control and Prevention and the Association of State and Territorial Public Health Laboratory Directors require the following: gp41 and pg120/160 or p24 and pg120/160 (1).

The predictive value depends on seroprevalence rates in the population of patients being tested. False-negative results for a high-prevalence population such as injection drug users with a seroprevalence rate of about 30% occur in 0.3% (1) and for a low-prevalence population such as Red Cross blood donors in 0.001% (2–5). The usual cause of false-negative test results is the window period between the time of viral transmission and seroconversion. The time delay to positive ELISA averages 10 to 14 days from HIV transmission; some do not seroconvert for 3 to 4 weeks, and rarely patients require more than 6 months (1,4). The first antibody to appear is usually anti-p24. Western blot alone has a 2% rate of false-positive results. An occasional cause of false-negative results is related to the subtype of HIV. Subtypes are designated A-H, M, and O on the basis of genetic variation; the distribution varies with geography. The predominant subtypes are B in North America and Europe, B and F in South America, B and F in Asia, and A-H in Africa. The routine serologic test readily detects A-H but does not detect subtype O, found primarily in Cameroon (6,7). Rare cases of subtype O have been found in the United States, and there is concern that this or another genetic variant in the future may reduce the sensitivity of routine HIV serology. HIV type 2 (HIV-2) is another genetic variant with a distinctive serologic pattern and a source primarily in West Africa (8,9). As of 2000, there were about 100 patients in the United States with this strain, and most could be traced to a West African contact (10). About 80% of HIV-2–infected patients have a positive ELISA with routine HIV type 1 (HIV-1) serology and Western blots that are weakly reactive; thus, most are either negative or have indeterminate results (8). Serologic tests for HIV-2 and for combined HIV-1 and HIV-2 are available and routinely used in Red Cross screening (9). Another cause of false-negative results is the presence of agammaglobulinemia.

The frequency of false-positive results in a low-prevalence population is 1 in 135,000, or 0.0007% (11). A single case of a false-positive test ascribed to autoantibodies has been reported for a patient with lupus erythematosus (12). This isolated exception, however, subsequently proved to be a true positive (13). Another patient with two positive tests and two indeterminate tests was found to be HIV negative based on negative culture and polymerase chain reaction (PCR) tests (14). The most common cause of false-positive tests is vaccination. A review of 266 volunteers in vaccine studies showed that 68% had a positive ELISA and 0% to 44% had a positive Western blot, depending on the criteria used for interpretation and the immunogen used for vaccination (15). Occasional patients report factitious positive HIV serology, emphasizing the need to repeat tests for some patients with unverified claims (16).

Results showing a positive ELISA and a single band on a Western blot are usually reported as indeterminate results. Studies with blood donors show that this occurs in about 2 per 10,000. Possible causes are the following: seroconversion is occurring, usually with p24 antibody as the first to appear; there is advanced HIV infection with decreased titers of antibodies, primarily anti-p24; there are cross-reacting alloantibodies from blood transfusions, pregnancy, or organ transplantation; there are autoantibodies as seen with some collagen-vascular diseases, malignancy, or autoimmune diseases; there is infection with subtype O or HIV-2; or there is HIV vaccine exposure. The most important factor in the interpretation of indeterminate results is a careful review of the risk profile. Virtually all low-risk patients, such as those detected with blood donations, are negative with full analysis (17). The cause of the indeterminate results in such cases is usually enigmatic and not indicative of any recognized disease state. The standard recommendation for patients with indeterminate test results is risk assessment: if high-risk behavior, suspect seroconversion in progress; if low risk, suspect that these results are inconsequential. In either event, the test should be repeated in 2 to 3 months (18,19).

ALTERNATIVE HUMAN IMMUNODEFICIENCY VIRUS ANTIBODY DETECTION METHODS

The usual justifications for using alternative techniques for detecting HIV antibody are to improve acceptance by patients, to clarify inconsistent or challenged serologic results, and to decrease the lag time for results.

Home test kits have been developed that show good sensitivity and specificity. These are available in drugstores for about $50 with blood samples submitted on filter strips for enzyme immunoassay and Western blot. The consumer mails the sample to a reference laboratory and obtains results by telephone (20). Acceptance by the public has been good (21), but use is less than expected. The initial experience is that about 1% of samples are positive, and 97% of users called for results (22).

Salivary tests and urine tests have been developed for detection of HIV antibody. The goal here is to improve patients' acceptance of testing by offering an alternative to blood sampling. This may be used for a screening ELISA or more definitive tests using the screening ELISA plus Western blotting (23,24).

Rapid tests are available that provide preliminary results within 10 minutes with accuracy analogous to that of standard serologic tests (25–27). Advantages of these tests are that the specimens for testing may be saliva as well as blood, and the diagnostic strips may be read by the provider to bypass the lab. These tests are attractive for use in clinical settings, where immediate results are often important for management decisions. An example is an occupational needlestick exposure involving a source with unknown HIV serologic status. The rapid test might also be useful for screening in clinical settings in which compliance with

TABLE 118.1.   Tests for Human Immunodeficiency Virus Type 1 and Viral Burden

Assay	CD4$^+$ cell counts	Percentage positive (sensitivity)	Comments
Routine serology	>3 mo after viral transmission	>98	Readily available and inexpensive.
Rapid tests SUDS (Murex)	>3 mo after viral transmission	>98	Advantage is that test results are available in ≤10 min. There are two commercial suppliers of FDA-approved reagents. Specificity is 99.6%, so positive tests should be confirmed. Tests are highly sensitive, so negative tests do not usually require confirmation (18,19).
Plasma RNA viremia	>500/mm^3 <200/mm^3	Rare 75–100	Detection of cell-free virus in plasma indicates active replication; persistence of plasma viremia is a sign of poor prognosis. Rates of recovery are inversely related to CD4$^+$ cell counts. Samples containing >30 pg of p24 antigen by EIA are usually positive.
Peripheral blood mononuclear cell culture	<500/mm^3	95–100	Expensive and labor-intensive. The test is nearly always positive at all stages and during treatment. Quantitative yield correlates with stage: mean titer 20 per 10^6 cells in asymptomatic patients and 2,200 per 10^6 cells in patients with AIDS (21,30). The greatest potential use is for therapeutic monitoring. A 10-fold decrease in titer is significant. Quantitative RNA PCR and bDNA assays are less expensive and generally preferred.
DNA PCR assay	All stages	99–100	Qualitative DNA PCR is used to detect cell-associated proviral DNA; primers are commercially available from Roche Laboratories. Sensitivity approaches 100%, but rigorous quality assurance is necessary. Its main use is in viral detection: acute viral syndrome, neonatal HIV infection, and confused or challenged serologic assays.
Quantitative RNA PCR			RNA PCR to detect proviral RNA shows good reproducibility (≤ twofold differences between laboratories; three- to fourfold changes or 0.5 log considered significant). Threshold for detection is 200–500 copies/mL (34). Most laboratories report titers ranging from 10^2 to 10^6 copies/mL.
Quantitative bDNA			Quantitative bDNA shows reproducibility comparable to that of quantitative RNA PCR. Its major use is for therapeutic monitoring and for staging (21,26). The detection threshold with first-generation tests is 10,000 copies/mL; for second-generation tests, it is about 200 copies/mL; for third-generation tests, it is about 25 copies/mL.

FDA, U.S. Food and Drug Administration; EIA, enzyme immunoassay; PCR, polymerase chain reaction; bDNA, branched-chain DNA; AIDS, acquired immunodeficiency syndrome.

follow-up visits may be difficult to achieve, such as emergency rooms or sexually transmitted disease clinics (28).

VIRAL DETECTION

Alternatives to serology for HIV detection include techniques for detecting HIV antigen, viral isolation, or HIV PCR. These tests are considered inferior to routine serology in terms of sensitivity, specificity, technical requirements, and cost. The usual test is plasma HIV RNA, and the major use for diagnostic purposes in seronegative cases is for detection of the acute HIV syndrome before seroconversion. Other possible uses are when routine serologic tests provide confusing results or results that are challenged, there is a need to clarify indeterminate serology, the patient has a cause for false-negative tests such as agammaglobulinemia, or there is a need for detection of neonatal infection. Viral culture may also be desirable for genetic mapping to determine the source of infection. An important limitation in quantitative plasma HIV RNA level measurements for detection of HIV infection is a 2% to 9% rate of false-positive results (29,30). The alternative in such cases is the p24 antigen assay, which is less expensive and highly specific, but only about 80% sensitive (29). With false-positive quantitative plasma HIV RNA assays, the titers are usually relatively low, usually less than 10,000 copies/mL (29,30). An alternative test for HIV detection in cases where serologic tests are not conclusive is DNA PCR, which is reported to be highly sensitive and specific, but the reagents are

not approved by the U.S. Food and Drug Administration, and techniques are not well standardized (31).

MEASUREMENT OF VIRAL BURDEN

Quantitative plasma HIV RNA measurements have become standard methods to monitor HIV-infected patients, generally using one of these commercially available assay techniques: (a) HIV RNA PCR, (b) branched-chain DNA (bDNA) assays, or (c) nucleic acid sequenced amplification. The currently used reagents for these assays have overcome many prior limitations and now detect and quantify subtypes A through G, show a dynamic range of 100 to 500,000 copies/mL or greater, and can be done on sera samples of 0.2 to 1 mL (32,33).

Reproducibility testing of these assays shows 2 standard deviations of 0.3 to 0.5 log (twofold to threefold) (34,35). Women and men have the same prognosis in terms of longevity from the time of transmission, but women have a lower viral load by about twofold in the early stages of disease (36). This difference does not impact therapeutic decisions based on CD4 counts, which show no gender differences, but would potentially alter therapeutic decisions based on viral load when the CD4 count exceeds 350 cells/mm^3.

Viral load testing has become a standard component of care to determine prognosis, risk for transmission, and response to therapy. For prognosis, the current concept of HIV pathogenesis is that the interaction between the immune system, primarily the

HIV-specific cytotoxic T-lymphocyte cell response, with HIV determines the viral "set point" soon after primary infection (37,38). The level of the set point dictates to a large extent the rate of CD4 cell decline and, consequently, the rate of progression. Thus, the viral load is an important factor in determining prognosis (39).

As with virtually all infectious diseases, the HIV viral load dictates to a large extent the inoculum size with exposures and the probability of transmission (40–42).

The most important clinical use of the viral load test is for therapeutic monitoring (43,44). The major goal of therapy is to reduce the viral load to as low as possible for as long as possible (45). This goal is based theoretically on the assumption that the goal of "no detectable virus" will halt disease progression and eliminate the generation of mutations that are responsible for antiretroviral drug resistance. The experience with highly active antiretroviral therapy appears to justify this goal (45–47).

REFERENCES

1. Mylonakis E, Paliou M, Lally M, et al. Laboratory testing for infection with the human immunodeficiency virus: established and novel approaches. *Am J Med* 2000;109:568.
2. Farzadegan H, Vlahov D, Solomon L, et al. Detection of human immunodeficiency virus type 1 infection by polymerase chain reaction in a cohort of seronegative intravenous drug users. *J Infect Dis* 1993;168:327.
3. Van de Perre P, Simonon A, Msellati P, et al. Postnatal transmission of human immunodeficiency virus type 1 from mother to infant. *N Engl J Med* 1991; 325:593.
4. Morens DM. Serologic screening tests for antibody to human immunodeficiency virus: the search for the perfection in an imperfect world. *Clin Infect Dis* 1997;25:101.
5. Busch MP, Eble BE, Khayam-Bashi H, et al. Evaluation of screened blood donations for human immunodeficiency virus type 1 infection by culture and DNA amplification of pooled cells. *N Engl J Med* 1991;325:1.
6. Loussert-Ajaka I, Ly TD, Chaix ML, et al. HIV-1/HIV-2 seronegativity in HIV-1 subtype O infected patients. *Lancet* 1994;343:1393.
7. De Cock KM, Adjorlolo G, Ekpini E, et al. Epidemiology and transmission of HIV-2: why there is no HIV-2 pandemic. *JAMA* 1993;270:2083.
8. Markovitz DM. Infection with the human immunodeficiency virus type 2. *Ann Intern Med* 1993;118:211.
9. George JR, Rayfield MA, Phillips S, et al. Efficacies of U.S. Food and Drug Administration-licensed HIV-1 screening enzyme immunoassays for detecting antibodies to HIV-2. *AIDS* 1990;4:321.
10. Centers for Disease Control and Prevention. Update: HIV-2 infection among blood and plasma donors—United States, June 1992–June 1995. *MMWR Morb Mortal Wkly Rep* 1995;44:603.
11. Burke DS, Brundage JF, Redfield RR, et al. Measurement of false positive rate in a screening program for human immunodeficiency virus infection. *N Engl J Med* 1988;319:961.
12. Jindal R, Solomon M, Burrows L. False positive tests for HIV in a woman with lupus and renal failure. *N Engl J Med* 1993;328:1281.
13. Povolotsky J, Polsky B, Laurence J, et al. Withdrawal of conclusion: false-positive tests for HIV in a woman with lupus. *N Engl J Med* 1994;331:881.
14. Louria DB, Denny T, Palumbo P, et al. An unusual case of false-positive serology for the human immunodeficiency virus: report from the heterosexual HIV transmission study. *Clin Infect Dis* 1992;15:707.
15. Belshe RB, Clements ML, Keefer MC, et al. Interpreting HIV serodiagnostic test results in the 1990s: social risks of HIV vaccine studies in uninfected volunteers. *Ann Intern Med* 1994;121:584.
16. Craven DE, Steger KA, La Chappelle R, et al. Factitious HIV infection: the importance of documenting infection. *Ann Intern Med* 1994;121:763.
17. Jackson JB, MacDonald KL, Cadwell J, et al. Absence of HIV infection in blood donors with indeterminate Western blot tests for antibody to HIV-1. *N Engl J Med* 1990;322:217.
18. Mylonakis E, Paliou M, Greenbough TC, et al. Report of a false-positive HIV test result and the potential use of additional tests in establishing HIV serostatus. *Arch Intern Med* 2000;160:2386.
19. Rich JD, Dickinson BP, Spaulding A, et al. Interpretation of indeterminate HIV serology results in an incarcerated population. *J Acquir Immune Defic Syndr Hum Retrovirol* 1998;17:376.
20. Bayer R, Stryker J, Smith MD. Testing for HIV infection at home. *N Engl J Med* 1995;332:1296.
21. Phillips KA, Flatt SJ, Morrison KR, et al. Potential use of home HIV testing. *N Engl J Med* 1995;332:1308.
22. Branson BM. Home sample collection tests for HIV infection. *JAMA* 1998; 280:1699.
23. Ishikawa S, Hashida S, Hashinaka K, et al. Diagnosis of HIV-1 infection with whole saliva by detection of antibody IgG to HIV-1 with ultrasensitive enzyme immunoassay using recombinant reverse transcriptase as antigen. *J Acquir Immune Defic Syndr Hum Retrovirol* 1995;10:41.
24. Emmons WW, Paparello SF, Decker CF, et al. A modified ELISA and Western blot accurately determine anti-human immunodeficiency virus type 1 antibodies in oral fluids obtained with a special collecting device. *J Infect Dis* 1995;171:1406.
25. Malone JD, Smith ES, Sheffield J, et al. Comparative evaluation of six rapid serological tests for HIV-1 antibody. *J Acquir Immune Defic Syndr* 1993;6: 115.
26. Kallenborn JC, Price TG, Carrico R, et al. Emergency department management of occupational exposures: cost analysis of rapid HIV test. *Infect Control Hosp Epidemiol* 2001;22:289.
27. Palmer CJ, Dubon JM, Koenig E, et al. Field evaluation of the Determine rapid human immunodeficiency virus diagnostic test in Honduras and the Dominican Republic. *J Clin Microbiol* 1999;37:3698.
28. Kassler WJ, Haley C, Jones WK, et al. Performance of a rapid, on-site human immunodeficiency virus antibody assay in a public health setting. *J Clin Microbiol* 1995;33:2899.
29. Daar ES, Little S, Pitt J, et al. Diagnosis of primary HIV-1 infection. Los Angeles County Primary HIV Infection Recruitment Network. *Ann Intern Med* 2001;134:25.
30. Rich JD, Merriman NA, Mylonakis E, et al. Misdiagnosis of HIV infection by HIV-1 plasma viral load testing: a case series. *Ann Intern Med* 1999;130:37.
31. Owens DK, Holodniy M, Garber AM, et al. Polymerase chain reaction for the diagnosis of HIV infection in adults: a meta-analysis with recommendations for clinical practice and study design. *Ann Intern Med* 1996;124:803.
32. Erice A, Brambilla D, Bremer J, et al. Performance characteristics of the QUANTIPLES HIV-1 RNA 3.0 assay for detection and quantitation of human immunodeficiency virus type 1 RNA in plasma. *J Clin Microbiol* 2000;38: 2837.
33. Shepard RN, Schack J, Robertson K, et al. Quantitation of human immunodeficiency virus type 1 RNA in different biological compartments. *J Clin Microbiol* 2000;38:1414.
34. Brambilla D, Reichelderfer PS, Bremer JW, et al. The contribution of assay variation and biological variation to the total variability of plasma HIV-1 RNA measurements. The Women Infant Transmission Study Clinics. Virology Quality Assurance Program. *AIDS* 1999;13:2269.
35. Paxton WB, Coombs RW, McElrath MJ, et al. Longitudinal analysis of quantitative virologic measures in HIV-infected subjects with >400 CD4 lymphocytes: implications for applying measurements to individual patients. *J Infect Dis* 1997;175:247.
36. Sterling T, Vlahov D, Astemborski J, et al. Initial plasma HIV-RNA levels and progression to AIDS in women and men. *N Engl J Med* 2001;344:720.
37. Fauci AS, Pantaleo G, Stanley S, et al. Immunopathogenic mechanisms of HIV infection. *Ann Intern Med* 1997;124:654.
38. Lyles CM, Dorrucci M, Vlahov D, et al. Longitudinal HIV type 1 load in the Italian seroconversion study: correlates and temporal trends of virus load. *J Infect Dis* 1999;180:1018.
39. Mellors JW, Kingsley LA, Rinaldo CR, et al. Quantitation of HIV-1 RNA in plasma predicts outcome after seroconversion. *Ann Intern Med* 1995;122:573.
40. Quinn TC, Wawer MJ, Sewankambo N, et al. Viral load and heterosexual transmission of HIV. *N Engl J Med* 2000;342:921.
41. Ragni MV, Faruki H, Kingsley LA. Heterosexual HIV-1 transmission and viral load in hemophilic patients. *J Acquir Immune Defic Syndr Hum Retrovirol* 1998;17:42.
42. Pedraza MA, del Romero J, Roldan F, et al. Heterosexual transmission of HIV-1 is associated with high plasma viral load levels and a positive viral isolation in the infected partner. *J Acquir Immune Defic Syndr* 1999;21:120.
43. Havlir DV, Richman DD. Viral dynamics of HIV: implications for drug development and therapeutic strategies. *Ann Intern Med* 1996;124:984.
44. Katzenstein DA, Hammer SM, Hughes MD, et al. The relation of virologic and immunologic markers to clinical outcomes after nucleoside therapy in HIV-infected adults with 200 to 500 CD4 cells per cubic millimeter. *N Engl J Med* 1996;335:1091.
45. Deeks SG, Barbour JD, Martin JN, et al. Sustained CD4 T-cell response after virologic failure of protease inhibitor regimens in patients with HIV infection. *J Infect Dis* 2000;181:946.
46. Carpenter CC, Cooper DA, Fischl MA, et al. Antiretroviral therapy in adults: updated recommendations of the International AIDS Society-USA Panel. *JAMA* 2000;283:381.
47. Ledergerber B, Egger M, Opravil M, et al. Clinical progression and virologic failure on highly active antiretroviral therapy in HIV-1 patients: a prospective cohort study. Swiss HIV Cohort Study. *Lancet* 1999;353:863.

CHAPTER 119
Antiretroviral Treatment

John G. Bartlett

Treatment of human immunodeficiency virus (HIV) infection began with zidovudine [azidothymidine (AZT)] with the demonstration in 1986 that this drug reduced rates of progression to acquired immunodeficiency syndrome (AIDS) and increased survival (1). The next 9 years of drug development and therapeutic trials resulted in a lineage of new drugs in the nucleoside analog class including didanosine, zalcitabine), stavudine, and lamivudine. These drugs provided the foundation for recommendations for antiviral treatment by the expert panel representing guidelines of the U.S. Public Health Service made in June 1993 (2). During the next 3 years, there were dramatic changes that notably altered therapeutic recommendations.

1. Studies of HIV kinetics showed rapid replication of HIV throughout the course of the disease, with an average of approximately 10^{10} new virions daily (3). Conclusions are that the mean half-life of HIV in plasma is 6 hours and the half-life of the infected $CD4^+$ cell is only 1.6 days. The implication is that 99% of viral production is from recently infected cells. Furthermore, each cycle of HIV replication is associated with the production of genetic variants, so high levels of replication result in enormous genetic diversity, including strains that are drug resistant.
2. The second major development was the use of quantitative methods to determine concentrations of HIV ribonucleic acid (RNA) in plasma referred to as *viral load* or *viral burden* (4,5). Using stored serum samples collected during 10 years in a natural history study of HIV, Mellors et al. (4,5) defined the history of HIV infection in terms of viral burden. This work demonstrated that acute HIV infection is associated with high-level HIV viremia in concentrations that often exceed 10^7/mL. After immune response, primarily a cytotoxic T-cell response, the patient establishes a "set point" that remains relatively stable with only gradual increases for a period of years in the absence of treatment (6). The set point appears to dictate the rate of disease progression independently of the $CD4^+$ cell count. The average patient, in the absence of treatment, progresses to an AIDS-defining diagnosis during 9 to 10 years after viral transmission and has an average viral burden of 10^4 to 10^5 copies/mL. Higher concentrations are associated with a more rapid progression, and "chronic nonprogressors" (i.e., patients with a normal $CD4^+$ cell count for 8 years in the absence of treatment) have mean concentrations lower than 10^2/mL. Studies of antiviral agents show significant changes in viral burden within days, and this test is consequently favored for therapeutic monitoring.
3. The third development was the introduction of a new series of drugs for HIV, protease inhibitors (PIs), which became available in late 1995, and then the nonnucleoside reverse transcriptase inhibitors (NNRTIs). These drugs are generally more potent against HIV than nucleoside analogs, especially with combination treatment. By 2002 there were 16 U.S. Food and Drug Administration (FDA)–approved drugs available for HIV infection and a long list of additional drugs in therapeutic trials.
4. Concurrent with the increasing availability of new drugs were several studies demonstrating superiority of combination therapy in terms of viral burden, $CD4^+$ cell slope (the rate of decline of the number of $CD4^+$ cells), and rates of progression. By 1997, mortality rates attributed to HIV infection decreased 47%. In fact, virtually all indicators of HIV progression decreased by 60% to 80%. These include rates of AIDS-defining diagnosis, hospitalizations, and newly reported AIDS cases (7–10). However, in 2002 these declines reached a plateau, and the number of AIDS cases in 2001 increased compared with 2001, the first increase since 1995.
5. The foregoing sequence of events showing benefits was accompanied by disappointments as well. It was quickly learned that the goal of therapy, reduction in viral load to undetectable levels, could be achieved only with complex regimens that were associated with substantial side effects (11). It was also learned that at least 95% of the prescribed doses had to be taken for a 50% probability of achieving no detectable virus, and the price of noncomplete viral suppression is resistance (12). Resistance is particularly problematic because it means reduced treatment options in the individual patient, but it also extracts a societal penalty because resistant strains can be transmitted (13–15).

This evolution of events transformed HIV therapeutics from a simplistic strategy with limited options and modest, if any, benefits to highly complex, though often controversial, treatments involving multiple combinations of drugs with complicated patterns of toxicity, drug interactions, and resistance profiles. Though complicated, the new therapeutic regimens proved to be on the horizon of transforming HIV from an inevitably progressive disease to one in which appropriate therapy offered the probability of clinical stability for sustained periods for most patients.

NATURAL HISTORY

The natural history of HIV is summarized in Figure 119.1, which shows the sequence of events from transmission of virus to death for the average patient in the absence of antiviral therapy. After viral acquisition, there is the acute retroviral syndrome accompanied by high-level viremia and variable expression of symptoms (Table 119.1). This syndrome is an acute febrile illness that is often accompanied by pharyngitis, lymphadenopathy, aphthous ulcers, variable neurologic complications, lymphopenia with a low $CD4^+$ cell count, weight loss averaging 10 pounds, and high-level HIV viremia detected with p24 antigen or quantitative HIV polymerase chain reaction. Standard serologic test results are negative or indeterminate (16,17).

The subsequent course of HIV infection is determined by multiple factors that are independent of antiviral therapy. The major correlates with rate of progression are the baseline HIV plasma concentration that is established at about 6 months after the acute retroviral syndrome and the $CD4^+$ cell slope (18). Large population-based studies show the average $CD4^+$ cell count slope is a reduction of 30 to 60 cells/mm^3 per year and the mean viral burden is stable at 10^4 to 10^5 copies/mL. Lymphoid tissue (e.g., lymph nodes, tonsils, spleen) is the primary site of HIV replication. Virus produced in lymphatic tissue is rapidly transmitted to the plasma compartment, so that quantitative plasma HIV RNA reflects the number of infected cells.

Longitudinal cohort studies, such as the Multicenter AIDS Cohort Study, show that the median time from seroconversion to an AIDS-defining diagnosis in the absence of therapy is 9.1 years; the frequency of a delay of 12 years or more is 32% to 40%, that of a delay of 16 years is 19% to 25%, and that of a delay

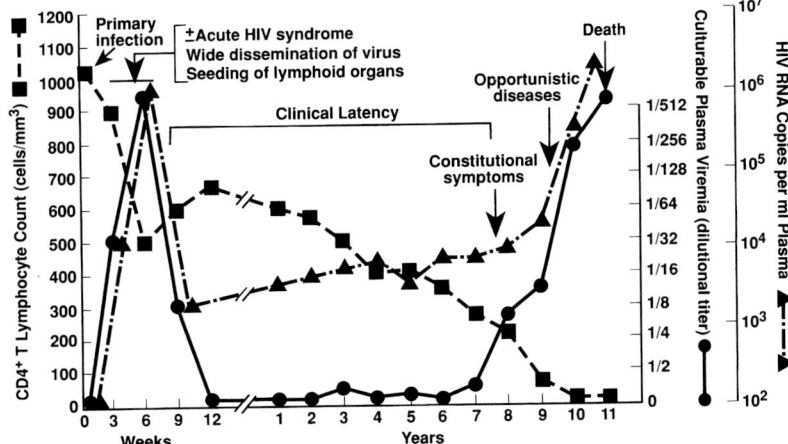

Figure 119.1. Natural history of human immunodeficiency virus (HIV) infection showing CD4+ cell count *(squares)*, plasma HIV ribonucleic acid (RNA) concentrations *(triangles)*, and cultivable plasma viremia *(circles)*. The initial event at 5 to 30 days after virus transmission is the acute retroviral syndrome associated with high concentrations of plasma HIV RNA and a decline in the CD4+ cell count. This is followed by the cytotoxic CD8+ cell response with clinical recovery and a decrease in plasma concentrations of HIV RNA copies. The decline in CD4+ cell count averages 30 to 60/mm³ per year in the absence of antiretroviral treatment. The rate of progression without antiretroviral drugs averages 9.1 years from the time of seroconversion to an acquired immunodeficiency syndrome (AIDS)–defining diagnosis, the median survival after the CD4+ cell count reaches 200/mm³ or less is 2.7 years, and the median survival after an AIDS-defining event is 1.3 years. The viral load reaches a plateau at about 6 months after the acute retroviral syndrome; this concentration, or set point, correlates directly with rates of progression (4). Individual patients show great variation in viral RNA concentrations and rates of progression (19–25) presumably related to variations in HIV virulence (21), immune response (19), genetic determination of receptor sites (22), age (23), and therapy (25). (From Haynes BF, Panteleo G, Fauci AS. Toward an understanding of the correlates of protective immunity to HIV infection. *Science* 1996;271:324–328, with permission.)

of 20 or more years is 10% to 17%. There is no discrete group in this cohort with no eventual CD4+ cell decline, suggesting that virtually all eventually have progressive disease (20). Variables that dictate rates of progression are incompletely understood, although it is known that defective viruses explain slow progression in few patients (21) and genetic variation in susceptibility of receptor sites may play a role (22); the most important factor appears to be the host antiviral immune response (19), which is influenced by age (23), possibly reflecting thymic function. In general, the CD4+ cell slope and the viral burden are independent predictors of progression, but they also show the anticipated correlation with high HIV counts correlated with rapid declines in CD4+ cell slope and low counts correlated with relatively stable CD4+ cell counts. Nevertheless, there are notable exceptions in both directions, referred to as *discordant responses* such as patients with rapid CD4+ cell decline despite relatively low viral burden and those with stable CD4+ cell counts in the presence of a high viral burden.

NUCLEOSIDE ANALOGS

Nucleoside analogs inhibit reverse transcriptase by competitive binding to the reverse transcriptase enzyme and/or act as an

TABLE 119.1.   Clinical Features of Acute Human Immunodeficiency Virus Syndrome

Symptomatic disease: 50% (17) to 89% (16)
Frequency of correct diagnosis with medical consultation: 25% (16)
Incubation period (HIV exposure to onset of symptoms): 2–6 wk (17)
Symptoms and signs (17)[a]

Fever	96%	Diarrhea	32%
Adenopathy	74%	Nausea or vomiting	27%
Pharyngitis	70%	Hepatosplenomegaly	14%
Rash	70%	Thrush	12%
Myalgias	54%	Meningoencephalitis	6%
Headache	32%	Peripheral neuropathy	6%

Duration of symptoms (mean): 1–2 wk
Laboratory tests: p24 antigenemia (1,200–4,200 pg/mL), plasma viremia with high titer (peak of 10^5–10^7 copies per mL), high-titer HIV-1 in peripheral blood mononuclear cells (10^2–10^4 tissue culture infective doses per mL), HIV-1 serologic test negative

[a]Metaanalysis of 209 reported cases.
HIV, human immunodeficiency virus.

TABLE 119.2. Nucleoside Analogs

	Zidovudine (AZT)	Didanosine (ddI)	Zalcitabine (ddC)	Stavudine (d4T)	Lamivudine (3TC)	Abacavir (ABC)	Tenofovir (TDF)
Usual dose	300 mg b.i.d.	>60 kg 400 mg q.d. <60 kg 250 mg q.d.	0.75 mg t.i.d.	>60 kg: 40 mg b.i.d. <60 kg: 30 mg b.i.d.	150 mg b.i.d.	300 mg b.i.d.	300 mg b.i.d.
Intracellular half-life	3 hr	25–40 hr	3 hr	3.5 hr	12 hr	3.3 hr	4 hr
CNS penetration	60%	20%	20%	30%–40%	10%	30%	?
Toxicity	Anemia Neutropenia GI intolerance Headache	Pancreatitis Peripheral neuropathy GI intolerance	Peripheral neuropathy Stomatitis	Peripheral neuropathy	None	Hypersensitivity reactions	None
Drug interactions	None	Methadone ↓ ddI levels 41%	Methadone ↓ d4T levels 27%	None	None	None	None

b.i.d., twice a day; CNS, central nervous system; GI, gastrointestinal; q.d., every day; t.i.d., three times a day.

alternative substrate leading to viral deoxyribonucleic acid (DNA) chain termination (Table 119.2). Drugs in this class are essentially prodrugs that must be metabolically activated by intracellular enzymes to 5′-triphosphates. Variations in intracellular metabolism including variations in affinity for converting enzymes account for some differences in potency and toxicity. Major limitations with nucleoside analogs are the development of resistance, reduced potency, and toxicity (17). Nevertheless, these drugs form the backbone of highly active antiretroviral regimens.

Zidovudine (Retrovir, AZT)

Zidovudine was the first antiviral agent tested for HIV and continues to be one of the most frequently used drugs. The initial clinical trial in 1986 included 282 patients with relatively late-stage disease randomized to receive zidovudine or placebo (1). Analysis of results by the Data and Monitoring Board in September 1986 showed 19 deaths in the placebo group compared with 1 among zidovudine recipients; the trial was discontinued, and all participants were offered zidovudine, and the FDA approved the agent in March 1987.

Zidovudine is well absorbed, but extensive glucuronidization in the liver reduces bioavailability to about 60% (18). The intracellular half-life of active triphosphate is 3 to 4 hours. The dosing recommendation is 600 mg per day in two divided doses. Zidovudine (and other nucleoside analogs) appears to achieve a threshold for efficacy, meaning that doses higher than the recommendation of 600 mg per day do not increase potency. The major toxicity of zidovudine is bone marrow suppression with neutropenia or anemia; these are dose dependent and stage related, with a higher frequency in late-stage disease (20). Both complications are treated with discontinuation of drug, or use of cytokines with erythropoietin for anemia and granulocyte colony-stimulating factor for neutropenia. Other common side effects include gastrointestinal (GI) intolerance (nausea, vomiting, diarrhea, anorexia), myalgias, fatigue, and headache. Few patients develop zidovudine-associated myopathy accompanied by elevated levels of creatine kinase. Most studies show that 10% to 30% of patients are not able to tolerate zidovudine, often because of "nonspecific effects" such as asthenia, insomnia, GI intolerance, and headaches (20).

Zidovudine has established efficacy in properly controlled trials demonstrating the following: decrease in viral burden (mean decrease of approximately 0.5 $\log_{10}$ copies/mL), increase in CD4$^+$ cell count (mean increase of 30–50/mm^3), delay in progression to an AIDS-defining opportunistic infection, prolonged survival (0–6 months), improvement in HIV-associated dementia, increased platelet count in HIV-associated idiopathic thrombocytopenic purpura, prevention of vertical transmission, safety during the second and third trimesters of pregnancy, and reduction in rates of HIV transmission to health care workers after needlestick exposure to HIV (1,24–26).

The benefit of zidovudine monotherapy in therapeutic trials is "time limited," because of the development of resistance (27,28). Resistant phenotypes show site-directed mutations with amino acid substitutions at codons 41, 67, 70, 215, and/or 219 (14). The multiplicity of resistance mutations is especially important. The time of emergence of zidovudine resistance is earlier with late-stage disease and with a high viral burden; in general, resistance is initially seen at 6 months, and about 50% of patients receiving monotherapy have resistant strains at 2 years. The prevalence of one or more mutations associated with zidovudine resistance was noted in 5% to 10% of strains in untreated patients in industrialized countries in 2001 (28).

Didanosine (Videx, Videx EC)

Didanosine is the second nucleoside analog approved by the FDA in October 1991 and has proved to be an effective agent with modest but sustained antiviral activity. The original formulation was acid labile and required buffering; the newer enteric-coated preparation (Videx EC) has the advantages of better tolerance and fewer drug interactions. Both formulations must be administered with an empty stomach. The plasma half-life is about 1.6 hours, but the intracellular half-life is 8 to 24 hours, making once-daily therapy feasible (29,30). Major toxicities include GI intolerance, peripheral neuropathy, and pancreatitis. The neuropathy is reversible if it is recognized early and the drug is discontinued (31). Patients should be warned of this side effect and promptly discontinue the drug when pain or paresthesias is noted, most frequently in the distal lower extremities. Pancreatitis occurs in 4% to 5% of patients, and this frequency of pancreatitis increases with alcohol abuse, a history of episodes of pancreatitis, or the concurrent use of other drugs associated with this complication including stavudine and with late-stage HIV infection (30). Many patients have difficulty with GI intolerance to didanosine.

Zalcitabine (Hivid)

Zalcitabine is the third nucleoside analog approved by the FDA in June 1992 and has been used primarily in combination with zidovudine or PIs. The combination with zidovudine has documented superiority compared with zidovudine monotherapy in zidovudine-naive patients (26,32). Nevertheless, data from clinical trials showing efficacy are limited, and toxicity is an important limitation. The major side effect is peripheral neuropathy that is related to dose and duration of treatment and stage of disease (30).

Stavudine (Zerit, d4T)

Stavudine is the fourth nucleoside analog approved by the FDA in June 1994, it has been proven to have modest antiviral activity, and it is well tolerated (33). The drug is well absorbed with a bioavailability of 90%. The plasma half-life is about 1 hour, and the intracellular half-life of the triphosphate is about 3.5 hours, suggesting that once-daily dosing may be acceptable. The major side effect is peripheral neuropathy. Use in combination with didanosine appears to magnify the frequency of lactic acidosis, pancreatitis, and peripheral neuropathy. This drug selects for thymidine analog mutations (TAMs), which reduce sensitivity to stavudine, AZT, and abacavir. AZT mutations confer stavudine resistance, and these two drugs together cause pharmacological antagonism, so they should not be used together (34,35). Attractive features of stavudine are the twice-daily dosing schedule, low pill burden, and good acceptance by patients. The disadvantages are the frequent implication in lactic acidosis, lipoatrophy, and peripheral neuropathy (35).

Lamivudine (Epivir, 3TC)

Lamivudine is the fifth nucleoside analog approved by the FDA in November 1995. Early studies showed rapid development of high-grade resistance ascribed to a rapid selection of strains with a mutation at codon 184, and this was associated with a 10,000-fold decrease in susceptibility (14). The initial impression was poor, but two subsequent observations rejuvenated substantial interest in this drug: First, the codon 184 mutation is accompanied by enhanced susceptibility to zidovudine, stavudine, and tenofovir (36). Second, this drug is remarkably well tolerated with good oral bioavailability, a relatively long plasma half-life, and a twice-daily dosing recommendation with the anticipated potential for once-daily dosing (37,38). Lamivudine is one of the most potent nucleoside reverse transcriptase inhibitors (NRTIs), and even strains with the 184 codon mutation sustain relatively good activity versus HIV (39). This drug is also highly active against hepatitis B virus (40).

Abacavir (Ziagen, ABC)

Abacavir represents the fifth NRTI approved by the FDA in April 1999 (41). It is the most potent of the NRTIs in terms of HIV viral load reduction, and it is synergistic *in vitro* in combination with zidovudine, lamivudine, and didanosine; it is additive with stavudine, NNRTIs, and PIs (42). Oral bioavailability is good and is not affected by food; central nervous system (CNS) penetration is good. Abacavir is commonly combined with zidovudine and lamivudine as Trizivir to provide the most simplified antiretroviral regimen with potent anti-HIV activity. Abacavir selects for *RT* gene mutations at codons 65, 74, 115, and 184; each results in a twofold to fourfold reduction in abacavir activity. Clinical trials suggest that the 184 codon mutation plus at least three TAMs predicts abacavir failure. The main limitation of the drug is a poorly understood hypersensitivity reaction characterized by fever, skin rash, fatigue, GI symptoms, arthralgias, cough, and/or dyspnea (43). These reactions usually occur in the first 6 weeks of treatment and are noted with a frequency of 2% to 5%. Repeated dosing will predictably result in recurrence of symptoms, and this may be done as a therapeutic trial. Rechallenge after discontinuation may cause a fatal reaction. Abacavir may be used with initial therapy as a component of a triple nucleoside regimen with or without a PI or an NNRTI, or it may be used to intensify (44). It is usually used with zidovudine.

Tenofovir (Viread, TDF)

Tenofovir is a nucleotide that has modest antiretroviral activity with median decreases in HIV RNA levels in plasma of 0.5 $\log_{10}$ copies/mL. Advantages are sparse side effects, activity against most strains that are resistant to nucleosides, and once-daily administration.

NONNUCLEOSIDE REVERSE TRANSCRIPTASE INHIBITORS

NNRTIs make up a category of drugs that also inhibit reverse transcriptase, but by an alternative mechanism compared with nucleoside analogs: The NNRTIs inactivate the enzyme by conformational change (45) (Table 119.3). They do not require cellular processing to become active, whereas nucleosides require cellular phosphorylation. Activity is highly selective for HIV-1, and these drugs are not active versus HIV-2 or other retroviruses. These drugs are associated with relatively high rates of rash reactions, they are active against HIV strains that are resistant to nucleoside analogs and PIs, they are synergistic with nucleosides *in vitro,* and use is complicated by rapid evolution of resistance when they are given with incomplete viral suppression.

TABLE 119.3. Nonnucleoside Reverse Transcriptase Inhibitors

	Nevirapine	Delavirdine	Efavirenz
Daily dose	200 mg q.d. × 14 d then 200 mg b.i.d.	400 mg t.i.d.	600 mg h.s.
Serum half-life	25–30 hr	5.8 hr	40–55 hr
Elimination	Metabolized cytochrome P450	Metabolized cytochrome P450	Metabolized cytochrome P450
Major toxicity	Rash Hepatotoxicity	Rash	CNS "disconnected," Rash

b.i.d., twice a day; CNS, central nervous system; h.s., at bedtime; q.d., every day; t.i.d., three times a day.

Nevirapine (Viramune)

Nevirapine has a bioavailability of more than 90%, it is largely metabolized by cytochrome P450 (CYP), and metabolic products are eliminated primarily in the urine (46). Nevirapine autoinduces metabolism by inducing CYP enzymes so that the half-life is reduced from 45 to 25 hours after 2 to 4 weeks of treatment. This drug also decreases the plasma levels of other drugs that use this metabolic pathway, including PIs. The major side effects are hepatotoxicity with transaminase elevations in 10% to 20% and rash reactions, which develop in about 18% of patients (46–48). Potentially lethal side effects include rare cases of fulminant hepatic failure and Stevens-Johnson syndrome in about 0.5%. A major problem is rapid evolution of high-grade resistance when this drug is used as monotherapy. Within 2 weeks, there is reduced *in vitro* activity ascribed to mutations on the reverse transcriptase gene, primarily at codons 103 and 181, but also 106, 108, 188, and/or 190. By 8 weeks of monotherapy, there is a more than 100-fold decrease in susceptibility, and this may occur with a single mutation. Superior results with profound decreases in viral burden for sustained periods were seen in nucleoside-naive patients treated with combination regimens (49). The advantages of these regimens are the twice-daily dosing regimen, a relatively low pill burden, good tolerance, pronounced antiviral activity in combination therapy, good CNS penetration, relatively few drug interactions, reservation of PI options, and probable reduced frequency of lipodystrophy (50). A single 200-mg dose at onset of labor plus one dose to the infant is significantly better than AZT in preventing perinatal transmission.

Delavirdine (Rescriptor)

Delavirdine was the second NNRTI approved by the FDA, in April 1997. This agent is another potent NNRTI for use in combination with nucleoside analogs. Clinical trials show that delavirdine in combination with zidovudine produced a $0.5 \log_{10}$ copies/mL decrease that persisted more than 1 year and better results with triple therapy including zidovudine, didanosine, and delavirdine. As with nevirapine, rash is the major side effect, noted in 12% to 18% of patients. This usually does not require drug discontinuation. *In vitro* synergy is shown with nucleoside analogs. Bioavailability is good, and the plasma half-life is relatively long. The standard dose is 400 mg three times a day. As with nevirapine, resistance develops rapidly with monotherapy and is high level, but there is no cross-resistance with PIs or with nucleoside analogs. Metabolism is largely by CYP 3A. Drugs that should not be used concurrently include rifabutin, rifampin, terfenadine, astemizole, cisapride, triazolam, midazolam, simvastatin, lovastatin, histamine-2 (H$_2$) blockers, proton pump inhibitors, ergotamine, and St. John's wort.

Efavirenz (Sustiva)

Efavirenz was the third NNRTI and was FDA approved in September 1998. This is a potent NNRTI that showed anti-HIV activity superior to indinavir when each was combined with zidovudine plus lamivudine in treatment-naive patients (51). The drug has a half-life of 40 to 55 hours, permitting once-daily dosing. The major concern is the CNS side effects characterized as "disconnected" changes often with inability to concentrate, vivid dreams, confusion, and dizziness (52). These side effects are unexplained and usually resolve in 2 to 3 weeks. Other side effects include rash and hepatotoxicity, usually in the first 6 weeks of treatment. Resistance usually results from an *RT* gene mutation at codon 103, which confers class NNRTI resistance. This drug both inhibits and induces the CYP 3A4 pathway.

Drugs contraindicated for concurrent use include astemizole, terfenadine, cisapride, midazolam, triazolam, ergotamine, and St. John's wort. The drug should not be used in pregnant women. The main advantages of efavirenz are the good tolerance after the first 3 weeks, good potency, even in treatment-naive patients with baseline viral loads exceeding 100,000 copies/mL, the convenience of once-daily dosing, sparing of PIs, and possibly reduced frequency of lipodystrophy (53,54). Disadvantages are the single-step mutation to high-level resistance, the CNS toxicity in early treatment, and the caution necessary to prevent exposure to pregnant women.

PROTEASE INHIBITORS

Intracellular replication of HIV results in two types of polyproteins: the *gag* gene encodes structural proteins of the viral core, and *gag* and *pol* encode retroviral enzymes including reverse transcriptase, protease, and integrase. These precursor proteins align on the viral envelope and are cleaved by protease to mature structural proteins and enzymes, a critical component of viral maturation. HIV protease is a symmetric homodimer containing 99 amino acids. PIs are peptide derivatives that competitively inhibit HIV protease. This enzyme was characterized by crystallography in 1989 (55), but subsequent development of PIs was hampered by multiple obstacles in drug development: poor oral bioavailability because of poor absorption and/or rapid metabolism by hepatic CYP enzymes, unexpected toxicity, high degree of plasma protein binding, rapid development of resistance, and poor penetration of the CNS (56). To date, six PIs are approved by the FDA and several others are in development (Table 119.4).

Saquinavir (Invirase)

This drug was the first PI approved by the FDA, in November 1995. (57) The first formulation was Invirase, which had only 4% bioavailability. The soft gel formulation of saquinavir, Fortovase, has far better bioavailability and has supplanted the use of Invirase except when combined with ritonavir. Saquinavir is generally well tolerated, although occasional patients have gastrointestinal intolerance or diarrhea. Additional potential advantages compared with other PIs are a limited number of identified codon mutations that impart resistance and the relative lack of demonstrated cross-resistance with other PIs (27,58).

Ritonavir (Norvir)

Ritonavir was approved by the FDA in March 1996, and it is a PI with potent antiviral activity *in vitro* and *in vivo* verses HIV and has a unique pharmacological profile. Oral bioavailability is approximately 70%, the plasma half-life is approximately 1 to 2 hours, and the major mechanism of excretion is hepatic metabolism via the CYP 3A4 isoform (59–61). Ritonavir is an exceptionally potent inhibitor of CYP enzymes and can serve as an inducer of CYP isoforms (59–63). This leads to potent drug interactions when ritonavir is given in combination with agents that are metabolized by CYP enzymes, accounting for a long list of drugs that need to be avoided among recipients of ritonavir (59), but this type of drug interaction may be exploited by combining ritonavir with other PIs to magnify their area under the curve (AUC) to provide a pharmacological barrier to resistance. Ritonavir is now usually used with other PIs in doses of 200 to 400 mg per day ("baby doses"), in which case its only role is the pharmacological interaction (see Table 119.4). Alternatively,

TABLE 119.4. Protease Inhibitors

	Indinavir	Ritonavir	Saquinavir	Nelfinavir	Amprenavir	Lopinavir
Dose Single PI	800 mg q8h	600 mg b.i.d.	1,200 mg t.i.d.	1,250 mg b.i.d.	1,200 mg b.i.d.	400/100 mg b.i.d.
Combined with RTV (mg)	IDV 400+ RTV 400 b.i.d. *or* IDV 800+ RTV 100–200 b.i.d.	—	SQV 400+ RTV 400 b.i.d.	—	APV 600+ RTV 100–200 b.i.d.	Fixed formulation
Half-life	1.5–2 hr	3–5 hr	1–2 hr	3.5–5 hr	7–10 hr	5–6 hr
CNS penetration	Moderate	Poor	Poor	Moderate	Moderate	Moderate
Elimination	CYP 3A4	CYP 3A4, 2D6	CYP 3A4	CYP 3A4	CYP 3A4	CYP 3A4
Toxicity	GI intolerance Renal calculi 10%–20% Hepatitis Lipodystrophy	GI intolerance 20%–40% Circumoral paresthesias Hepatitis Lipodystrophy	GI intolerance 20%–30% Headache Hepatitis Lipodystrophy	Diarrhea 10%–30% Hepatitis Lipodystrophy	GI intolerance Rash 20%–25% Paresthesias Hepatitis Lipodystrophy	GI intolerance Hepatitis Diarrhea Lipodystrophy

APV, amprenavir; b.i.d., twice a day; CNS, central nervous system; CYP, cytochrome P450; IDV, indinavir; RTV, ritonavir; SQV, saquinavir; t.i.d., three times a day.

it may be given in doses of 800 mg per day or more to provide an antiviral effect. The major side effects associated with ritonavir are diarrhea, nausea, and vomiting; all are dose related and many patients have improved tolerance with a graduated dosing regimen and continued use.

Therapeutic trials with ritonavir showed that when it was used in combination with nucleoside analogs or saquinavir, there was a 2- to 3-$\log_{10}$ copies/mL reduction in quantitative HIV RNA that was sustained for up to 2 years (62–64). However, the most use of ritonavir at present is in combination with other PIs that provide high levels and increased AUC of the companion PI. Advantages of this agent include this favorable effect on virtually all PIs except nelfinavir. Disadvantages include a multitude of potentially serious interactions with drugs including several agents that are commonly used by patients with HIV infection and dose-related poor GI tolerance.

Indinavir (Crixivan)

Indinavir is another PI approved by the FDA in March 1996 and is a potent inhibitor of HIV both *in vitro* and *in vivo* when used in combination with nucleoside analogs (65–67). Oral bioavailability is about 60%; when taken on an empty stomach, the half-life is 1.5 to 2.0 hours; and excretion is primarily by hepatic metabolism via the CYP pathway. Indinavir inhibits CYP enzymes, but the inhibition is less profound than that with ritonavir. The major toxicity, nephrolithiasis, noted in 10% to 20% of patients, correlates with peak levels (68). This is dose related and reduced by use of large volumes of oral fluid. Hepatitis, alopecia, keratoconjunctivitis sicca, and GI intolerance are other common side effects (65,69,70). A major concern is the need for thrice-daily dosing, a problem that can be largely obviated by combining indinavir with ritonavir for twice-daily dosing.

Nelfinavir (Viracept)

Nelfinavir was the fourth PI approved by the FDA, which occurred in March 1997. Potency appears similar to that of indinavir and ritonavir with a 2- to 3-$\log_{10}$ copies/mL decrease in plasma HIV RNA levels (71). Like others in this class, nelfinavir is extensively metabolized by CYP and is an inhibitor of CYP 3A4 isoform. The drug is generally well tolerated and can be given twice daily, two factors that made the drug an instant favorite

(71,72). The major side effect is a secretory diarrhea, which can usually be controlled by loperamide hydrochloride or calcium (73).

Amprenavir (Agenerase)

Amprenavir was the fifth PI approved by the FDA, which occurred in April 1999. This drug is another potent inhibitor of HIV, it shows good bioavailability, and the prolonged half-life of 7 to 11 hours permits twice-daily administration (74,75). Like other PIs, the drug is largely metabolized by the CYP mechanism, and the drug inhibits CYP 3A4 to a level comparable to indinavir or nelfinavir. There is great interest in combining amprenavir with ritonavir to extend the half-life and reduce the pill burden, which is 16 pills per day if using standard dosing. The major side effect is a rash, presumably reflecting its structure as a sulfonamide. Nevertheless, prior reactions to sulfonamides do not represent a contraindication to the drug. Other common side effects include GI intolerance, oral paresthesias, and headache.

Lopinavir-Ritonavir (Kaletra)

The combination lopinavir-ritonavir is a PI product approved by the FDA in September 2000 as the sixth PI. The lopinavir-ritonavir combination is the most potent PI and the first to be combined with ritonavir in a single pill formulation. The recommended dose is lopinavir (400 mg) plus ritonavir (100 mg) twice daily. This combination gives a unique pharmacological profile to the drug in terms of potency and sustained levels (76,77).

SIDE EFFECTS

Several adverse effects of antiretroviral agents are idiosyncratic to specific agents, as summarized earlier, but there are also some troubling adverse events that appear to be related to either a class of agents or to any form of highly active antiretroviral therapy (HAART).

Lactic acidosis: This is an adverse effect reported with NRTIs in the early 1990s (78), which is attributed to mitochondrial toxicity, and now reported with increasing frequency.

Patients typically present with fatigue, nausea, vomiting, abdominal pain, weight loss, and/or dyspnea (79). Laboratory evaluation shows elevated lactic acid levels; normal levels are less than 2 mmol/mL, modest evaluations that may or may not be significant are 2 to 5 mmol/mL, levels more than 5 mmol/mL are clearly abnormal, and levels more than 10 mmol/mL are potentially lethal. Other common findings include computed tomography (CT) scan and biopsy evidence of steatosis (79), elevated levels of creatinine phosphokinase, aminotransferase, lactic dehydrogenase, increased anion gap, and low bicarbonate. The frequency of lactic acidosis with NRTI therapy is 1.3 to 10 per 1,000 patient-years. All NRTIs have been implicated, but it is most prevalent with stavudine and didanosine. The only therapy is to discontinue NRTIs or substitute an alternative agent from this class that is less likely to cause lactic acidosis. The response when NRTIs are suspended is very slow, usually requiring 1 to 3 months to return to normal.

Lipodystrophy: Components of lipodystrophy include fat atrophy and/or fat accumulation or "fat redistribution." Lipoatrophy is characterized by atrophy involving the extremities, buttocks, and buccal fat of cheeks. Fat accumulation occurs in the dorsal neck ("buffalo hump"), breasts (gynecomastia in men), visceral or abdominal fat ("protease paunch"), and lipomatosis (80–82). The original impression was that these changes reflect use of PIs in HAART regimens, but several observations have challenged the notion, implicating a single class of drugs or even the conclusion that antiretroviral drugs are essential for these changes. The frequency of these changes among recipients varies from 10% to 30% depending on definition. Nevertheless, it often should be emphasized that this change is largely cosmetic, but it often bothers patients and they should be warned.

Hyperlipidemia: Increases in serum triglyceride and cholesterol levels occur with or without fat redistribution and are often accompanied by insulin resistance (83). The concern is the consequences of glucose intolerance or type 2 diabetes, and/or hyperlipidemia in terms of atherosclerosis with coronary artery disease or stroke. These changes appear most clearly related to PIs, and the National Cholesterol Education Program Treatment (84,85) is advocated for management. The PIs appear more clearly implicated here, changes are usually noted within 3 months of starting treatment, and therapeutic monitoring with a fasting lipid profile is recommended at baseline, at 3 months, and then with a frequency dictated by the results of these tests and other risk factors.

Hepatic injury: All antiretroviral agents are associated with the potential for hepatic injury. With NRTIs, the mechanism appears to be mitochondrial toxicity with steatosis. For other drugs, the mechanism is less clear, although some cases are serious or life threatening (86,87). These reactions are more common in patients with hepatitis B or C coinfection, but this should not limit such patients from access to HAART because most tolerate the drugs well. Monitoring of liver function test results is recommended for recipients of nevirapine, but not for recipients of other antiretroviral agents.

TREATMENT GUIDELINES

The goals of therapy are (a) to reduce HIV viral load as much as possible for as long as possible, (b) to improve quality of life, and (c) to preserve therapeutic options (88,89).

When to Start Therapy

When HAART became available in 1995, the highly quoted goal of therapy was "hit hard and hit early." The assumption was that aggressive treatment in early stage disease had a high probability of cure. Since then, it has been learned that cure is unlikely even with no detectable virus for 50 years (90). Additionally, it was learned that the treatment had associated long-term risks (lipodystrophy, hyperlipidemia, diabetes, osteonecrosis, lactic acidosis, etc.), required at least three drugs to achieve maximum viral suppression, adherence was challenging but critical (12,91), and resistance was the penalty for noncompliance and represents a major public health problem (27,28,92). Added to this tabulation of therapeutic nihilism is the observation that despite hundreds of studies with thousands of patients, there was no evidence of long-term benefit with therapy started before the CD4 count was 200/mm^3; there were large cohort studies that showed that treatment initiated with a CD4 count of less than 200/mm^3 was beneficial and possibly too late. The result of these observations is the recommendation to start therapy when the CD4 count is 350/mm^3, but that some authorities would use the threshold of 200/mm^3, and some would use viral load test results to augment the decision. The other critical component in the recommendation concerns patient acceptance of therapy. Thus, the decision to start antiretroviral agents is complex, and the strength of the recommendation depends on prognosis as dictated primarily by CD4 count and to a lesser extent viral load and patient readiness.

What to Start

Once the decision is made to initiate treatment, the regimen used should provide maximum viral suppression. This is best achieved with one of the following (88,89):

> Generally recommended
> > Two nucleosides and a PI
> > Two nucleosides and an NNRTI
> > Two nucleosides and two PIs
> Possible alternatives
> > Three nucleosides (zidovudine, lamivudine, and abacavir)
> > Two nucleosides, a PI, and an NNRTI
> > (May limit future options)

When to Change

The goal is maximal viral suppression, which is generally defined as a viral load less than 20 to 50 copies/mL after at least 6 months of treatment. The rationale for this goal is that maximal viral suppression means minimal viral replication with evolution of resistance mutations. Nevertheless, it should be acknowledged that (a) opportunistic infections are infrequent with viral loads less than 5,000 copes/mL (93); (b) the threshold for risk of resistance is unclear (94,95); (c) there is benefit to treatment even in the absence of a demonstrable antiviral effect attributed to viral fitness (96); and (d) for many patients, the goal of a viral load of less than 20 to 50 copies/mL is unrealistic, so changes based on this threshold could result in the rapid loss of therapeutic options (97). The conclusion is that the goal of therapy should ideally be "no detectable virus" using an assay with a threshold of 20 to 50 copies/mL, but that several additional considerations include the need to preserve therapeutic options and the benefit of partial suppression (98).

What to Change To

Recommendations for changing therapy are optimally based on resistance testing (88,89,99), although there are some important limitations: (a) These tests measure only the dominant species, so archived strains with resistance can only be predicted based on drug exposure history. (b) Genotypic testing assumes knowledge of the mutations that confer resistance. (c) Phenotypic testing is not well designed to measure resistance of complex combinations, and (d) these tests are better at predicting agents that will not work than at predicting drugs that will work. (e) Clinical correlations to better define thresholds that indicate resistance are not well established.

TREATMENT ISSUES

Monitoring: The major method to determine response to therapy is sequential viral load measurements. Expectations with HAART for treatment-naive patients is a viral load decrease of 1 to 2 $\log_{10}$ copies/mL at 1 to 2 months, viral load less than 400 copies/mL at 12 weeks, and less than 50 copies/mL at 16 to 24 weeks (98). Factors that reduce the likeliness of this response include poor adherence, 12 high baseline viral load (98), prior antiretroviral therapy (100), the potency of the regimen, and the baseline CD4 count (101). The CD4 count is another method to monitor response to therapy and is the most critical measurement for determining vulnerability to HIV-associated complications. In general, the average increase in CD4 count with complete viral suppression is 80 to 100 cells/mm^3 per year. Discordance in the CD4 cell response and the viral load response is seen in up to 30% of patients, about 15% showing a CD4 response with minimal viral response, and 15% showing a good virologic response with no CD4 response (102).

Adherence: This is an obvious but critical component of treatment. It appears that with the standard HAART regimen, the patient must consume more than 95% of prescribed doses to achieve an 80% probability of a viral load of less than 500 copies/mL at 6 months (12,91). With less than 95%, this probability decreases to less than 50%.

Immune-based therapy: Treatment recommendations are directed against the virus with the anticipation of immune reconstitution as indicated by an increase in CD4 response. An alternative method to increase CD4 count is with interleukin-2 (IL-2) therapy, which appears to work, but the optimal response is when it is least needed, with a baseline CD4 count of more than 200/mm^3 (103). Nevertheless, this tactic and therapeutic vaccines to improve immune regulation of HIV are attractive potential developments.

Immune reconstitution: The immune response to HAART is quantitative based on CD4 response and qualitative based on pathogen-specific immune response. The initial CD4 response is an increase in CD38 and MO-positive (memory) cells, which is followed after 6 months by increases in CD38 and MA-positive (naive) cells including naive cells of thymic origin. The biological adequacy of this response is determined by protection against opportunistic infections and ability to discontinue opportunistic infection prophylaxis when the CD4 count returns toward baseline. Studies to date support this concept (104–107), so the current guidelines are to suspend primary and secondary prophylaxis for virtually all opportunistic pathogens with immune recover based on CD4 response (108).

Recommendations to Reduce Perinatal Transmission of Human Immunodeficiency Virus

AIDS Clinical Trials Group (ACTG) 076 was designed to determine the efficacy of zidovudine for reducing vertical transmission of HIV (109). This was a placebo-controlled trial with the following eligibility criteria: pregnancy of 14 to 34 weeks of gestation, no antiretroviral therapy during the current pregnancy, and CD4$^+$ cell count exceeding 300/mm^3. The drug regimen was the following:

Before delivery: zidovudine (100 mg five times a day) initiated at 14 to 34 weeks of gestation and continued to the onset of labor

During labor: intravenously administered zidovudine (loading dose of 2 mg/kg for 1 hour, followed by continuous infusion of 1 mg/kg per hour until delivery)

Infant: zidovudine for the newborn (zidovudine syrup at 2 mg/kg every 6 hours) for the first 6 weeks of life beginning 8 to 12 hours after birth

The rate of transmission was 28% in the placebo group compared with 8% among zidovudine recipients. Further observations included the following: (a) Zidovudine did delay the diagnosis of HIV infection in the infant, (b) there was no significant zidovudine toxicity to pregnant women, (c) there was no evidence in this study of congenital malformations that could be ascribed to zidovudine (109), (d) the only adverse effect observed among infants who received zidovudine was a mild transient anemia, (e) the benefit of AZT appeared to be independent of viral load (110,111), (f) the AZT benefit may be independent of AZT resistance (112), and (g) there is reduction in perinatal transmission even when the baseline viral load is less than 1,000 copies/mL (113). Although the initial study was limited to women with CD4$^+$ cell counts higher than 200/mm^3, subsequent analyses have shown that zidovudine is protective across all CD4$^+$ cell counts (114,115).

Subsequent studies have shown that the probability of perinatal transmission is directly related to the viral load. Specifically, the risk with a maternal viral load of more than 100,000 copies/mL was 41%; with 1,000 to 10,000 copies/mL, it was 17%; and with less than 1,000 copies/mL, it was nil (116). Despite these findings for viral loads less than 1,000 copies/mL, authorities caution that there is no viral load that can be considered "safe" (17). The implication of this work is that the goal of therapy for prevention is a viral load that is as low as possible at the time of highest risk, which is at the time of passage in the birth canal.

The other drug that has been systematically studied for benefit in preventing perinatal transmission is nevirapine using a single 200-mg dose to the mother during labor and a single dose of 2 mg/kg to the infant within the first 72 hours. This regimen proved superior to AZT given at the time of labor but was associated with a risk of HIV resistance due to the K103N mutation (118).

Caesarian section has also proven effective in preventing perinatal transmission. In a large prospective trial in Europe, the rate of perinatal transmission was 1.8% among 170 assigned to elective caesarian section compared with 10.5% among 200 in those with vaginal deliveries (119).

Based on these observations, recommendations for management are the following:

Treatment-Naive Pregnant Women

- Baseline viral load more than 1,000 copies/mL: HAART therapy with AZT and optional delay until the second trimester
- Baseline viral load less than 1,000 copies/mL: AZT monotherapy after 10 to 12 weeks of gestation
- At 36 weeks: caesarian section at 38 weeks offered if viral load more than 1,000 copies/mL
- Presents in labor: options include nevirapine alone, AZT alone, or AZT plus nevirapine

Treatment-Experienced Pregnant Women

- Continue standard therapy, but include AZT if possible; consider discontinuation of HAART during first trimester.

• At 36 weeks of gestation, caesarian section at 38 weeks is offered if viral load is more than 1,000 copies/mL.

Antiretroviral Agents

Available data support the safety of antiretroviral agents in pregnancy with the following exceptions: (a) Efavirenz should be avoided in the first trimester and possibly throughout pregnancy, (b) hydroxyurea should be strictly avoided, and (c) the combination of stavudine plus didanosine has been associated with maternal deaths caused by lactic acidosis (120).

Occupational Exposure of Health Care Workers

As of June 2000, 56 health care workers had been reported to the Centers for Disease Control and Prevention with occupationally acquired HIV confirmed by seroconversion in the context of HIV exposure. An additional 132 cases of probable HIV transmission in the workplace were not confirmed by documented seroconversion. The occupations most at risk were nurses and laboratory technicians. All transmissions involved blood or bloody body fluids except for three laboratory workers who were exposed to HIV cultures. Most transmissions followed needlestick injuries, although five documented cases involved mucocutaneous exposures. Numerous studies indicate that the risk of acquiring HIV with needlestick injury from an HIV-infected source is 0.3% and the risk with mucocutaneous exposure is less than 0.1% (121). Factors associated with increased risk were examined in a retrospective case-control trial of health care workers with occupational percutaneous HIV exposures, including 31 with seroconversion and 679 control subjects (122). Odds ratios for risk are summarized in Table 119.5. This table shows that significant risks were associated with deep injury, visible blood on the device, terminal illness in the source, and needle placement in an artery or vein. These observations are not surprising; they simply verify that the inoculum size of HIV and the depth of challenge correlate with the efficiency of transmission. An additional observation in this study was that zidovudine prophylaxis reduced the risk of transmission by 79%. On the basis of these observations, the U.S. Public Health Service now recommends the use of prophylaxis with antiviral agents for health care workers who have occupational exposures using a two-drug regimen or a three-drug regimen, depending on risk assessment, which includes severity of the injury, inoculum size, and source data (123) (see

Table 119.5). The two-drug regimen consists of two nucleosides, and the three-drug regimen adds a third agent—a PI or an NNRTI other than nevirapine.

REFERENCES

1. Fischl MA, Richman DD, Grieco MH, et al. The efficacy of azidothymidine (zidovudine) in the treatment of patients with AIDS and AIDS-related complex: a double-blind, placebo-controlled trial. N Engl J Med 1987;317:185.
2. Sande MA, Carpenter CCJ, Cobbs CG, et al. Antiretroviral therapy for adult HIV-infected patients: recommendations from a state-of-the-art conference. National Institute of Allergy and Infectious Diseases State-of-the-Art Panel on Anti-Retroviral Therapy for Adult HIV Infected Patients. JAMA 1993;270:2583.
3. Ho DD, Neumann QU, Perelson AS, et al. Rapid turnover of plasma virions and CD4 lymphocytes in HIV-1 infection. Nature 1995;373:123.
4. Mellors JW, Kingsley LA, Rinaldo CR Jr, et al. Quantitation of HIV-1 RNA plasma predicts outcome after seroconversion. Ann Intern Med 1995;122:573.
5. Mellors JW, Rinaldo CR Jr, Gupta P, et al. Prognosis in HIV-1 infection predicted by the quantity of virus in plasma. Science 1996;272:1167.
6. Fauci AS, Pantaleo G, Stanley S, et al. Immunopathogenic mechanisms of HIV infection. Ann Intern Med 1996;124:654.
7. Palella FJ Jr, Delaney KM, Moorman AC, et al. Declining morbidity and mortality among patients with advanced HIV infection. N Engl J Med 1998;338:853.
8. Sendi P, Palmer AJ, Gafni A, et al. Highly active antiretroviral therapy: pharmacoeconomic issues in management of HIV infection. Pharmacoeconomics 2001;19:709.
9. Gebo KA, Diener-West M, Moore RD. Hospitalization rates in an urban cohort after the introduction of highly active antiretroviral therapy. J Acquir Immun Defic Syndr 2001;27:143.
10. Ledergerber B, Egger M, Opravil M, et al. Clinical progression and virological failure on highly active antiretroviral therapy in HIV-1 patients. Lancet 1999;353:863.
11. Martinez E, Moncroft A, Garcia-Viejo MA, et al. Risk of lipodystrophy in HIV-1–infected patients treated with protease inhibitors: a prospective cohort study. Lancet 2001;357:592.
12. Paterson DL, Swindells S, Mohr J. Adherence to protease inhibitor therapy and outcomes in patients with HIV infection. Ann Intern Med 2000;133:21.
13. Fauci AS. Resistance to HIV-1 infection: it's in the genes. Nat Med 1996;2:966.
14. Arts EJ, Wainberg MA. Mechanisms of nucleoside analog antiviral activity and resistance during human immunodeficiency virus reverse transcription. Antimicrob Agents Chemother 1996;40:527.
15. Blower SM, Aschenbach AN, Gershengorn HB, et al. Predicting the unpredictable: transmission of drug-resistant HIV. Nat Med 2001;7:1016.
16. Daar ES, Little S, Pitt J, et al. Diagnosis of primary HIV-1 infection. Ann Intern Med 2001;134:25.
17. Niu MT, Stein D, Schnittman SM. Primary human immunodeficiency virus type 1 infection: review of pathogenesis and early treatment intervention in humans and animal retrovirus infections. J Infect Dis 1993;168:1490.
18. Stein DS, Korvick JA, Vermund SH. CD4+ lymphocyte cell enumeration for prediction of clinical course of human immunodeficiency virus disease: a review. J Infect Dis 1992;165:352.
19. Haynes BF, Panteleo G, Fauci AS. Toward an understanding of the correlates of protective immunity to HIV infection. Science 1996;271:324.
20. Fischl MA, Richman DD, Hansen N, et al. The safety and efficacy of zidovudine (zidovudine) in the treatment of subjects with mildly symptomatic human immunodeficiency virus type 1 (HIV) infection: a double-blind, placebo-controlled trial. Ann Intern Med 1990;112:721.
21. Learmont J, Tindall B, Evans L, et al. Long term symptomless HIV-1 infection in recipients of blood products from a single donor. Lancet 1992;340:863.
22. Weiss RA. HIV receptors and the pathogenesis of AIDS. Science 1996; 272:1885.
23. Mocroft A, Vella S, Benfield TL, et al. Changing patterns of mortality across Europe in patients infected with HIV-1. EuroSIDA Study Group. Lancet 1998;352:1725.
24. Shapiro DE, et al. Effect of zidovudine on perinatal HIV-1 transmission and maternal viral load. Lancet 1999;354:156.
25. Cardo DM, Zulver DH, Ciesielski CA, et al. A case-control study of HIV seroconversion in health care workers after percutaneous exposure. N Engl J Med 1997;337:1485.
26. Hammer SM, Datzenstein DA, Hughes MD, et al. A trial comparing nucleoside monotherapy with combination therapy in HIV-infected adults with CD4 cell counts from 200 to 500 per cubic millimeter. N Engl J Med 1996;335:1081.
27. Richmond DD. Resistance, drug failure and disease progression. AIDS Res Hum Retroviruses 1994;10:901.
28. Re MC, Monari P, Borderi M, et al. Presence of genotypic resistance to antiretroviral drugs in a cohort of therapy naive HIV-1–infected Italian patients. J Acquir Immun Defic Syndr 2001;27:315.
29. Cooley TP, Kunches LM, Saunders CA, et al. Once-daily administration of 2′,3′-dideoxyinosine (ddI) in patients with the acquired immunodeficiency syndrome or AIDS-related complex. results of a phase I trial. N Engl J Med 1990;322:1340.
30. Lipsky JJ. Zalcitabine and didanosine. Lancet 1993;341:30.

TABLE 119.5.   Risk Factors for Human Immunodeficiency Virus Transmission in Health Care Workers with Needlestick Injuries from an Infected Source[a]

Risk	Odds ratio
Deep injury (not further defined)	16.1
Visible blood on the device	5–2
Needle placement in artery or vein	5.1
Source with late-stage disease (died within 2 mo of HIV-related complications)	8.2
Zidovudine prophylaxis	0.2

[a]Case-control retrospective analysis of 31 cases showing seroconversion compared with 679 control subjects who did not seroconvert. The source in all cases and control subjects was known to have HIV infection.
Source: From Centers for Disease Control and Prevention. Update: provisional recommendations for chemoprophylaxis after occupational exposure to human immunodeficiency virus. MMWR Morb Mortal Wkly Rep 1996;45:468–472, with permission.

31. Kieburtz KD, Seidlin M, Lambert JS, et al. Extended follow-up of peripheral neuropathy in patients with AIDS and AIDS-related complex treated with dideoxyinosine. *J Acquir Immun Defic Syndr* 1992;5:60.

32. Fischl MA, Stanley K, Collier K, et al. Combination and monotherapy with zidovudine and zalcitabine in patients with advanced HIV disease. *Ann Intern Med* 1995;122:24.

33. Dudley MN, Graham KK, Kaul S, et al. Pharmacokinetics of stavudine in patients with AIDS or AIDS-related complex. *J Infect Dis* 1992;166:480.

34. Boucher CAB, Lange JMA, Miedema FF, et al. HIV-1 biological phenotype and the development of zidovudine resistance in relation to disease progression in asymptomatic individuals during treatment. *AIDS* 1992;6:1259.

35. Moyle GJ, Gazzard BG. The role of stavudine in the management of adults with HIV infection. *Antivir Ther* 1997;24:207.

36. Larder BA, Kemp SD, Harrigan PR. Potential mechanism for sustained antiretroviral efficacy of AZT-3TC combination therapy. *Science* 1995;269:696.

37. Eron JJ, Benoit SL, Jemsek J, et al. Treatment with lamivudine, zidovudine, or both in HIV positive patients with 200 to 500 CD4$^+$ cells per cubic millimeter. *N Engl J Med* 1995;333:1662.

38. Staszewski S, Loveday C, Picazo JJ, et al. Safety and efficacy of lamivudine-zidovudine combination therapy in zidovudine-experienced patients. *JAMA* 1996;276:111.

39. St. Clair MH, Martin JL, Tudor-Williams G, et al. Resistance to ddI and sensitivity to AZT induced by a mutation in HIV-1 reverse transcriptase. *Science* 1991;253:1557.

40. Lok AS, Heathcote EJ, Hoofnagle JH. Management of hepatitis B: 2000—summary of a workshop. *Gastroenterology* 2001;120:1828.

41. Daluge SM, Good SS, Faletto MB, et al. 1592 succinate—a novel carbocyclic nucleoside analog with potent, selective anti-HIV activity. *Antimicrob Agents Chemother* 1997;14:1082.

42. McMahan D, Lederman M, Haas DW, et al. Antiretroviral activity and safety of abacavir in combination with selected HIV-1 protease inhibitors in therapy-naive HIV-1–infected adults. *Antivir Ther* 2001;6:10.

43. Shapiro M, Ward KM, Stern JJ. A near-fatal hypersensitivity reaction to abacavir: case report and literature review. *AIDS Read* 2001;11:222.

44. Rozenbaum W, Katlama C, Massip P, et al. Treatment intensification with abacavir in HIV-infected patients with at least 12 week previous lamivudine/zidovudine therapy. *Antivir Ther* 2001;6:135.

45. Spence RA, Kati WM, Anderson KS, et al. Mechanism of inhibition of HIV-1 reverse transcriptase by nonnucleoside inhibitors. *Science* 1995;267:988.

46. Havilar D, Cheeseman SH, McLaughlin M, et al. High dose nevirapine: safety, pharmacokinetics and antiviral effect in patients with HIV infection. *J Infect Dis* 1995;171:537.

47. Centers for Disease Control and Prevention. Serious adverse events attributed to nevirapine regimens for postexposure prophylaxis after HIV exposures—worldwide, 1997–2000. *MMWR Morb Mortal Wkly Rep* 2001;79:1153.

48. Das S, Allan PS, Wade AA. Adverse effects of nevirapine. *Lancet* 2001;358:506.

49. D'Aquilla RT, Hughes MD, Johnson VA, et al. Nevirapine, zidovudine, and didanosine compared with zidovudine and didanosine in patients with HIV-1 infection: a randomized, double-blind, placebo-controlled trial. *Ann Intern Med* 1996;124:1019.

50. Martinez E, Conget I, Lozano L, et al. Reversion of metabolic abnormalities after switching from HIV-1-protease inhibitors to nevirapine. *AIDS* 1999;13:805.

51. Staszewski S, Morales-Ramirez J, Tashima KT, et al. Efavirenz plus zidovudine and lamivudine, efavirenz plus indinavir, and indinavir plus zidovudine and lamivudine in the treatment of HIV-1 infection in adults. *N Engl J Med* 1999;341:1865.

52. Blanch J, Martinez E, Rousaud A, et al. Preliminary data of a prospective on neuropsychiatric side effects after initiation of efavirenz. *J Acquir Immun Defic Syndr* 2001;27:336.

53. Rey D, Schmitt MP, Partisani M, et al. Efavirenz as a substitute for protease inhibitors in HIV-1-infected patients with undetectable plasma viral load on HAART. *J Acquir Immun Defic Syndr* 2001;27:459.

54. Albrocht MA, Bosch RJ, Hammer SM, et al. Nelfinavir, efavirenz, or both after the failure of nucleoside treatment of HIV infection. *N Engl J Med* 2001;345:318.

55. Wlodawer A, Miller M, Jaskolski M, et al. Conserved folding in retroviral proteinases: crystal structure of a synthetic HIV-1 protease. *Science* 1989;245:616.

56. Wlodawer A. Rational drug design: the proteinase inhibitors. *Pharmacotherapy* 1994;14:95.

57. Kitchen VS, Skinner C, Ariyoshi K, et al. Safety and activity of saquinavir in HIV infection. *Lancet* 1995;345:952.

58. Vella S. Clinical experience with saquinavir. *AIDS* 1996;9:21.

59. Ritonavir (Norvir) [package insert]. North Chicago, IL: Abbott Laboratories, 1996.

60. Kumar GN, Rodrigues AD, Buko AM, et al. Cytochrome P-450–mediated metabolism of the HIV-1 protease inhibitor ritonavir (ABT 538) in human liver microsomes. *J Pharmacol Exp Ther* 1996;277:423.

61. Saah AJ, Windchell GA, Nessly ML, et al. Pharmacokinetic profile and tolerability of indinavir-ritonavir combinations in healthy volunteers. *Antimicrob Agents Chemother* 2001;45:2710.

62. Markowitz M, Saag M, Powderly WG, et al. A preliminary study of ritonavir, an inhibitor of HIV-1 protease, to treat HIV 1 infection. *N Engl J Med* 1995;333:1534.

63. Danner SA, Carr A, Leonard JM, et al. A short-term study of the safety, phar-macokinetics, and efficacy of ritonavir, an inhibitor of HIV-1 protease. *N Engl J Med* 1995;333:1528.

64. Jacobsen H, Yasargil K, Winslow D, et al. Characterization of human immunodeficiency virus type-1 mutants with decreased sensitivity to proteinase inhibitor Ro31-8959. *Virology* 1995;206:527.

65. Indinavir (Crixivan) [package insert]. West Point, PA: Merck, Sharp and Dohm, 1996.

66. AVANTI 2: randomized double blind trial to evaluate the efficacy and safety of zidovudine plus lamivudine versus zidovudine plus lamivudine plus indinavir in HIV-1–infected antiretroviral-naive patients. *AIDS* 2000;14:367.

67. Gulick RM, Mellors JW, Havlir D, et al. 3-year suppression of HIV viremia with indinavir, zidovudine, and lamivudine. *Ann Intern Med* 2000;133:35.

68. Saltel E, Angel JB, Futter NG, et al. Increased prevalence and analysis of risk factors for indinavir nephrolithiasis. *J Urol* 2000;164:1895.

69. Caeiro JP, Visnegarwala F, Rodriquez-Barradas MC. Gynecomastia-associated with indinavir therapy. *Clin Infect Dis* 1998;27:1539.

70. Bouscarat F, Prevot MH, Matheron S. Alopecia-associated with indinavir therapy. *N Engl J Med* 1999;341:618.

71. Tebas P, Powderly WG. Nelfinavir mesylate. *Expert Opin Pharmacother* 2000;1:1429.

72. Walmsley SL, Becker MI, Zhang M, et al. Predictors of virologic response in HIV-infected patients to salvage antiretroviral therapy that includes nelfinavir. *Antivir Ther* 2001;6:47.

73. Sherman DS, Fish DN. Management of protease inhibitor-associated diarrhea. *Clin Infect Dis* 2000;30:908.

74. Kost RG, Hurley A, Zhang L, et al. Open label phase II trial of amprenavir, abacavir, and fixed dose zidovudine/lamivudine in newly and chronically HIV-infected patients. *J Acquir Immun Defic Syndr* 2001;26:332.

75. Schooley RT, Clumeck N, Habrich R, et al. A dose ranging study to evaluate the antiretroviral activity and safety of amprenavir alone and in combination with abacavir in HIV-infected adults. *Antivir Ther* 2001;6:89.

76. Hurst M, Faulds D. Lopinavir. *Drugs* 2000;60:1371.

77. Lopinavir/ritonavir: a protease inhibitor combination. *Med Lett Drugs Ther* 2001;43:1.

78. Brahams D. Death in U.S. fialuridine trial. *Lancet* 1994;343:1494.

79. Miller KD, Cameron M, Wood LV. Lactic acidosis and hepatic steatosis associated with stavudine: report of four cases. *Ann Intern Med* 2000;133:192.

80. Miller KD, Jones E, Yanovski JA, et al. Visceral abdominal-fat accumulation associated with use of indinavir. *Lancet* 1998;351:871.

81. Carr A, Samaras K, Chisholm DJ, et al. Pathogenesis of HIV-1 protease inhibitor associated peripheral lipodystrophy, hyperlipidemia, and insulin resistance. *Lancet* 1998;352:1881.

82. Martinez E, Moncraft A, Garcia-Viejo MA, et al. Risk of lipodystrophy in HIV-1–infected patients with protease inhibitors: a prospective cohort study. *Lancet* 2001;357:592.

83. Hadigan C, Meigs JB, Corcoran C, et al. Metabolic abnormalities and cardiovascular disease risk factors in adults with HIV infection and lipodystrophy. *Clin Infect Dis* 2001;32:130.

84. Dube MP, Sprecher D, Henry WK, et al. Preliminary guidelines for the evaluation and management of dyslipidemia in adults infected with HIV and receiving antiretroviral therapy. *Clin Infect Dis* 2000;31:1216.

85. Executive summary of the Third Report of The National Education Program (NCEP) Expert Panel on Detection, Education and Treatment of High Blood Cholesterol in Adults. *JAMA* 2001;285:2486.

86. Nunoz M, Lana R, Mendoza JL, et al. Risk factors for severe hepatic injury after introduction of highly active antiretroviral therapy. *J Acquir Immun Defic Syndr* 2001;27:426.

87. Sulkowski MS, Thomas DL, Chaisson RE, et al. Hepatotoxicity associated with antiretroviral therapy in adults infected with immunodeficiency virus and the role of hepatitis C or B virus infection. *JAMA* 2000;283:74.

88. Department of Health and Human Services Panel. Guidelines for the use of antiretroviral agents in HIV-infected adults and adolescents. *Ann Intern Med* 2002;137:381.

89. Carpenter CC, Cooper DA, Fischl MA, et al. Antiretroviral therapy in adults: updated recommendations of the International AIDS Society—USA Panel. *JAMA* 2000;283:381.

90. Zhang L, Ramratnam B, Tenner-Racz K, et al. Quantifying residual HIV-1 replication in patients recovery combination antiretroviral therapy. *N Engl J Med* 1999;340:1605.

91. Anston JH, Demas PA, Farzadegan H, et al. Antiretroviral therapy adherence and viral suppression in HIV-infected drug users: comparison of self-report and electronic monitoring. *Clin Infect Dis* 2001;33:1417.

92. Harrigan PR, Montaner JS, Wegner SA, et al. World wide variation in HIV-1 phenotypic susceptibility in untreated individuals. *AIDS* 2001;15:1671.

93. Williams PL, Currier JS, Sindells S. Joint effects of HIV-1 RNA levels and CD4 lymphocyte cells on the risk of specific opportunistic infections. *AIDS* 1999;13:1035.

94. Havlir DV, Bassett R, Levitan D, et al. Prevalence and predictive value of intermittent viremia with combination HIV therapy. *JAMA* 2001;286:171.

95. Hermankova M, Ray SC, Ruff C, et al. HIV-1 drug resistance profiles in children and adults with viral load of <50 copies/mL receiving combination therapy. *JAMA* 2001;286:196.

96. Deeks SG, Barbour JD, Martin JN. Sustained CD4$^+$ T-cell response after virologic failure of protease inhibitor–based regimens in patients with HIV. *J Infect Dis* 2000;181:946.

97. Lucas GM, Chaisson RE, Moore RD. Highly active antiretroviral therapy in a

large urban clinic: risk factors for virologic failure and adverse drug reactions. *Ann Intern Med* 1999;131:81.

98. Clough LA, D'Agata E, Raffanti S, et al. Factors that predict incomplete virological response to protease inhibitor–based antiretroviral therapy. *Clin Infect Dis* 1999;29:75.

99. Hirsh MS, Brun-Vezinet F, D'Aquila RT, et al. Antiretroviral drug resistance testing in adult HIV-1 infection: recommendations of an AIDS Society—USA Panel. *JAMA* 2000;283:2417.

100. Lederberger B, Egger M, Opravil M, et al. Clinical progression and virologic failure on highly active antiretroviral therapy in HIV-1 patients: a prospective cohort study. *Lancet* 1999;353:863.

101. Erb P, Battegay M, Zimmerli W, et al. Effect of antiretroviral therapy on viral load, CD4 cell count, and progression to AIDS in a community HIV-infected cohort. Swiss Cohort Study. *Arch Intern Med* 2000;160:1134.

102. Grabar S, LeMoing V, Goujard C. Clinical outcome of patients with HIV-1 infection according to immunologic and virologic response after six months of highly active antiretroviral therapy. *Ann Intern Med* 2000;133:401.

103. Levy Y, Capitant C, Houhou S, et al. Comparison of subcutaneous and intravenous interleukin-2 in asymptomatic HIV-1 infection: a randomized controlled trial. *Lancet* 1999;353:1923.

104. Lederberger B, Mocroft A, Reiss P, et al. Discontinuation of secondary prophylaxis against *Pneumocystis carinii* pneumonia in patients with HIV infection who have a response to antiretroviral therapy. *N Engl J Med* 2001;344:168.

105. Lopez Bernaldo d Quiros JC, Miro JM, Pena JM, et al. A randomized trial of the discontinuation of primary and secondary prophylaxis for *Pneumocystis carinii* pneumonia after highly active antiretroviral therapy in HIV infection. *N Engl J Med* 2001;344:159.

106. Currier JS, Williams PL, Koletar SL, et al. Discontinuation of *Mycobacterium avium* complex prophylaxis in patients with antiretroviral therapy-induced increases in CD4 cell count. *Ann Intern Med* 2000;133:493.

107. Furrer H, Opravil M, Benasconi E, et al. Stopping primary prophylaxis in HIV-1–infected patients at high risk of toxoplasma encephalitis. *Lancet* 2000;355:2217.

108. Kaplan JE, Masur H, Holmes KK, et al. Guidelines for preventing opportunistic infections among HIV-infected persons—2002. *Morb Mortal Wkly Rep* 2002;51(RR-8):1.

109. Sperling RS, Shapiro DE, Coombs RW, et al. Maternal viral load, zidovudine treatment, and the risk of transmission of HIV-1 from mother to infant. *N Engl J Med* 1996;335:1621.

110. Mofenson LM, Lambert JS, Stieham ER, et al. Risk factors for perinatal transmission of human immunodeficiency virus type 1 in women treated with zidovudine. *N Engl J Med* 1999;341:385.

111. Wilson D. Effect of zidovudine on perinatal HIV-1 transmission and maternal viral load. *Lancet* 1999;356:156.

112. Welles SL, Pitt J, Colgrove R, et al. HIV-1 genotypic zidovudine drug resistance and the risk of maternal-infant transmission. *AIDS* 2000;14:263.

113. Loannidas JP, Abrams EJ, Ammann A, et al. Perinatal transmission of HIV-1 by pregnant woman with viral loads <1000 copies/mL. *J Infect Dis* 2001;183:539.

114. Wiznia AA, Crane M, Lambert G, et al. Zidovudine use to reduce perinatal HIV type 1 transmission in an urban medical center. *JAMA* 1996;275:1504–1506.

115. Frenkel LM, Wagner LE, Demeter LM, et al. Effects of zidovudine use during pregnancy on resistance and vertical transmission of HIV-1. *Clin Infect Dis* 1995;20:1321.

116. Garcia PM, Kalish LA, Pitt J, et al. Maternal levels of plasma HIV-1 RNA and the risk of perinatal transmission. *N Engl J Med* 1999;341:394.

117. Shaffer N, Roongpisuthipong A, Sinwasin W, et al. Maternal virus load and perinatal HIV-1 subtype E transmission. *J Infect Dis* 1999;179:590.

118. Jackson JB, Becker-Pergola G, Guay LA, et al. Identification of the K103 N resistance mutation in Ugandan woman receiving nevirapine to prevent HIV-1 vertical transmission. *AIDS* 2000;14:F111.

119. Perinatal HIV Group. The mode of delivery and the risk of vertical transmission of HIV-1: meta-analysis of 15 prospective cohort studies. *N Engl J Med* 1999;340:977.

120. Morris AB, Cu-Uvin S, Harwell JI, et al. Multicenter review of protease inhibitors in 89 pregnancies. *J Acquir Immun Defic Syndr* 2000;25:306–311.

121. Henderson DK, Fahey BJ, Willy M, et al. Risk for occupational transmission of human immunodeficiency virus type 1 (HIV 1) associated with clinical exposures: a prospective evaluation. *Ann Intern Med* 1990;113:740–746.

122. Centers for Disease Control and Prevention. Update: provisional recommendations for chemoprophylaxis after occupational exposure to human immunodeficiency virus. *MMWR Morb Mortal Wkly Rep* 1996;45:468–472.

123. Updated U.S. Public Health Service guidelines for the management of occupational exposures to HBV, HCV, and HIV and recommendations for postexposure prophylaxis. *MMWR Morb Mortal Wkly Rep* 2001;50(RR-1):1.

CHAPTER 120

Prevention of Human Immunodeficiency Virus Transmission

Jonathan Zenilman

Human immunodeficiency virus (HIV) prevention efforts are based on altering the known modes of transmission. Because HIV is a dynamic epidemic, effective prevention programs depend on continuous surveillance and an understanding of the risk behaviors that promote HIV transmission.

"Primary" prevention reduces infection risk by eliminating the behavioral risk factor. For example, primary prevention would be the goal of sexual abstinence or preventing intravenous drug use. From a practical perspective, primary prevention is an option only in the long term because drug and sexual behaviors are widespread, are conducted within social situations that are supportive of these behaviors, and are pleasurable (1). Implementing behavior change is a gradual process for most individuals, and maintaining these changes (intervention "maintenance") is equally difficult. Most intervention efforts are therefore designed to reduce risk or harm. Risk reduction can be effected through decreasing frequencies of risky behaviors or by decreasing transmission efficiency of the behavior. Decreasing sexual partner turnover, intercourse frequency, and drug use frequency are examples of decreased risk frequency, analogous to a simplistic dose-response model. Two examples of settings in which behavior frequency remains the same, but transmission efficiency is reduced, are condom use, which reduces the efficiency of sexual transmission, and needle-exchange programs, which decrease transmission among intravenous drug users (IDUs).

A key part of facilitating and maintaining HIV behavioral interventions are structural supports (2,3). Structural factor approaches are based on altering the environment and/or context in which the risk behavior occurs. This can include providing increased access to health care services, strategic efforts to change population-based attitudes such as sex and HIV prevention education, government regulation of activities such as prostitution alcohol or drug use, and even modifying the workplace or social environments to enable health promotion.

Developing comprehensive HIV prevention programs requires a complex menu of services including individual-based interventions, community-wide education, ensuring access to health care services, especially HIV counseling, testing, and treatment services, and providing access to drug treatment services and sexually transmitted disease (STD) diagnostic and treatment services. Interventions must be culturally sensitive and appropriate, a process that often requires initial ethnographic formative research within a targeted community. Unless carefully conceived, intervention programs targeting one risk group have the potential to alienate or marginalize other risk group members from the prevention effort. For example, early HIV intervention programs targeted homosexual men and IDUs. As the epidemic evolved, safer sex messages for gay men and safer injecting practice messages targeted at IDUs often became inappropriate for heterosexuals, and vice versa (Table 120.1).

TABLE 120.1.   Human Immunodeficiency Virus Prevention Strategies: Summary

Transmission mode	Prevention strategy
Blood-borne transmission	• Blood donor screening
Perinatal transmission	• VCT as part of prenatal care
	• Perinatal outreach
	• Peripartum antiretroviral therapy to mother and neonate for HIV-positive women
	• Minimize breast-feeding, if feasible
Sexual transmission	• Counseling and testing
	• Model-based behavioral interventions targeting risky sexual behaviors
	• Changing peer and group sexual norms
	• Identification of structural/community factors and resources
	• Identification of covariates of risky sexual behavior—substance use, mental health
	• Reducing individual level risk number of sexual partners, types of sexual partners
	• Reduction in risky sexual practices—unprotected rectal intercourse
	• Provision and access to condoms and sexual healthy services
	• Sexually transmitted infection diagnosis and treatment
Intravenous drug use	• Access to drug treatment
	• Harm reduction—needle exchange, bleach provision
	• Prevention focused on social networks
	• Counseling to reduce sexual transmission
	• Integration of VCT and behavioral intervention into drug treatment
Special populations, approaches	• Field outreach to marginalized populations
	• Rapid HIV testing for same-visit results
	• Mobile clinic vans to community settings
	• Outreach efforts to occupation core groups (e.g., truck drivers, migrant workers)
	• Intensified screening and prophylaxis in high-STD-risk groups

HIV, human immunodeficiency virus; STD, sexually transmitted disease; VCT, voluntary HIV counseling and testing.

EPIDEMIOLOGIC ISSUES RELEVANT TO PREVENTION

Effective prevention and risk-reduction intervention approaches require a current understanding of HIV epidemiology, in particular the groups at highest risk of infection. Behavioral and risk-reduction interventions designed for one ethnic, cultural, or sexual preference group may be inappropriate or ineffective in other groups, highlighting the need for continuous epidemiologic monitoring and program effectiveness evaluation. Evaluation of intervention effectiveness is often difficult because the HIV epidemic is dynamic.

Through December 2000, of the 774,467 persons diagnosed with AIDS, 448,060 had died: 79% were men, 61% black or Latino; 46% were men who have sex with men (MSM), 25% were IDUs (4). This contrasts with data from 1981 to 1987: Most cases were white; homosexual men accounted for 64% of cases; and women, predominantly infected through heterosexual contact, accounted for 19% of cases (4,5). Acquired immunodeficiency syndrome (AIDS)–defined cases are estimated to account for 24% to 27% (6). Therefore, there are an estimated 1 to 1.2 million HIV-infected persons in the United States. Despite these changes, in the late 1990s, MSMs again reemerged as the group at highest risk for incident HIV, especially young MSMs from minority groups (7). The dynamism of HIV epidemiology is particularly seen in the MSM situation. The initial HIV prevention efforts in gay men resulted in more than 80% reductions of incident infections and risky behaviors by the late 1980s. However, in 1990s (8,9), rectal gonorrhea, syphilis in MSMs, and other markers of high-risk behavior in homosexual men (4,10–14) began to increase substantially in the United States (4,15,16), England, and western Europe (17). This was interpreted by some observers as a cohort effect of younger gay men becoming sexually active, or in some situations, as a reaction of younger gay men to the "safer sex" culture that had developed. HIV prevention programs must therefore be flexible.

BIOLOGIC APPROACHES TO REDUCING DISEASE TRANSMISSION: A BRIEF SUMMARY

Blood and Biologic Product Screening

Universal screening of blood and biologic products has essentially eliminated transmission through transfusion. Although there continues to be concern over the possibility of false-negative results either due to HIV variants or the seroconversion "window" period, the risk has been substantially reduced by the use of new-generation screening tests, the application of stringent blood donor screening procedures, heat treatment of clotting concentrate products, and the accelerated development of recombinant non–human-derived clotting factor replacements. Since implementing comprehensive screening, the estimated risk for infection by screened blood components in Europe and the United States is approximately 1 in 1.6 million [for hepatitis B virus (HBV), hepatitis C virus (HCV), and HIV-1 and HIV-2] transfused blood components. In the future, the safety of blood components may be increased by testing donated blood with nucleic acid amplification techniques and by photochemical decontamination of cellular blood components (18).

A recent Centers for Disease Control and Prevention (CDC) study estimated the HIV risk through blood products as less than 1 in 493,000 (19). Similar procedures have been also instituted to reduce risk through other biologic products, such as allogeneic organ transplantation and artificial insemination. In developing countries, however, testing of blood products is not universal, even in areas with high HIV-seroprevalence rates.

VACCINES

Primary prevention through vaccination is an attractive theoretical option, which will not, however, be realized anytime soon. Developing HIV vaccines has proven to be an enormous technical challenge. The challenges to development include elucidating the protective immune response, the high antigenic variation of the virus, the role of immune modulators, and the rapid neurotropism of the virus. Even if a vaccine were developed, there are difficult epidemiologic issues and ethical problems that are incurred in the clinical trials, which would be necessary.

PREVENTING VERTICAL TRANSMISSION: DEVELOPMENT OF A PHARMACOLOGIC PREVENTION INTERVENTION (20)

Vertical transmission has been demonstrated perinatally or post-natally through breast-feeding (21–23) and is directly related to plasma virus load (24). Without intervention, HIV transmission occurs in 15% to 35% (25–28). Obstetric complications, such as premature rupture of membranes, nearly doubles the transmission risk (29), and one study has suggested that older maternal age increases the transmission risk (30).

When circumstances permit, delivery by cesarean section reduces perinatal infection by 50% (31). Pharmacologic intervention during pregnancy, perinatally, and postnatally has been found to profoundly reduce the vertical transmission rate. Initial studies were performed with zidovudine monotherapy (AIDS Clinical Trials Group Protocol 076), in which the vertical transmission rate was reduced threefold, from 25% to 8% (32). Later studies have focused on simplifying the regimen and found that short courses of nevirapine in the peripartum period had similar effect (33,34). In developing countries, the cost of the medications is prohibitive and will limit implementation. Even when cost is not a factor, and even with new, shorter, and less complex regimens, this intervention requires that women be enrolled in a prenatal care program; that they be offered and accept HIV counseling and testing; that on the basis of a positive HIV test result, they be offered treatment. Successful implementation is therefore dependent on medical care infrastructure access.

There was initial concern over the acceptability of HIV counseling and testing. Studies in the Bronx, New York (35), and in North Carolina (36) found that most pregnant women diagnosed with HIV antenatally accepted the treatment options.

Current CDC testing guidelines emphasize that (37)

- HIV testing is a routine part of prenatal care
- All pregnant women be tested for HIV
- Testing and counseling messages should be clear; pretest counseling is not a barrier to testing
- The consent process should be facilitated and flexible
- Providers explore and address reasons for refusal of testing
- HIV testing and treatment should be given at the time of labor and delivery for women who have not received prenatal testing and considering use of rapid tests

Another problem in developing countries is that the attributable fraction due to breast-feeding is estimated at 22% (38). Reducing breast-feeding poses profound ethical dilemmas, as sanitary and socioeconomic conditions often preclude the availability of safe formula feeding.

These programs have served the vast majority of pregnant women. Between 1998 and 2001, an estimated 93% of American women knew their HIV status before delivery, and many prenatal programs had integrated HIV testing as an "opt-out" procedure, that is, HIV counseling and testing was offered unless specifically refused (39). In Michigan, perinatal antiretrovirals increased from 27% in 1993 to 95% in 1998, resulting in a 93% reduction in perinatal HIV infections (40). In Thailand, a national program in 65 provinces found that 93% of women received HIV counseling and testing services, and 86% and 80% of the 3,865 children born to HIV-infected women received zidovudine and infant formula, respectively, through the program (41).

Postexposure Prophylaxis

With the advent of effective antiretroviral therapy and the success of the perinatal exposure model, there has been an increasing interest in postexposure prophylaxis (PEP) (42–46). The first groups considered for PEP were health care workers who had either a needlestick or mucosal exposure, and PEP has evolved to be the standard of care in the occupational setting. In these incidents, the time of exposure is known and usually the risk of the patient to whom the worker was exposed, i.e., HIV status is either known or can be rapidly determined. More controversial is the role of PEP after risky sexual exposure, especially when serostatus of the partner (or partners) is not known. PEP, to be effective, must be administered within 24 hours after exposure, and there is increasing concern that development of drug-resistant strains as primary HIV isolates necessitates complex PEP regimens. For PEP after sexual exposure to be effective, access to clinical resources is required, especially during nights and weekends. Despite the level of interest, there are major concerns whether PEP is truly effective. Prophylaxis failures, even in the well-managed occupational setting, are well documented, and the sample sizes required to demonstrate regimen effectiveness are enormous, making a clinical trial impossible. These concerns in turn pose policy questions of cost-effectiveness and resource utilization for the role of PEP in a comprehensive HIV prevention program.

BEHAVIORAL INTERVENTION APPROACHES (47–50)

Population-based Mass-media Campaigns

Initial approaches to HIV control used *educational* approaches, with the intervention hypothesis being that provision of accurate information would induce a rational change in individuals' behavior. Included within this were mass-media campaigns and a national mail-out of HIV education materials, school-based HIV prevention information (as opposed to structured interactive curricula), and incorporation of HIV-based themes into the popular media. These efforts increased the knowledge base of the population as measured in national surveys and local studies and may have reduced HIV-related discrimination. There are few data to suggest that these have had an impact on high-risk behaviors related to HIV transmission (51,52). As the epidemic progressed, it also became clear that more-sophisticated approaches were required to develop and evaluate behavioral interventions.

Behavioral Approaches to Human Immunodeficiency Virus Control: Sexual Behavior

SURVEYS OF SEXUAL BEHAVIOR

Designing interventions to reduce high-risk sexual behavior requires an accurate definition of the "baseline" state, without which program effectiveness evaluation would be impossible. Assessment of sexual behavior—behavioral surveillance—is a key tool in this effort, and sexual behavior modules were therefore incorporated into large national health surveys. These surveys have shown both positive and negative trends.

The General Social Survey, which is a national probability sample of 2,896 adults (1988–1990), estimated that 3 to 6 million adults had five or more sex partners in the past year, and that alcohol consumption doubled the incidence of high-risk sexual behavior (53). Similar data were found in the National Survey of Family Growth, which surveys reproductive health issues in women aged 15 to 44 years: 23% of all women surveyed had more than five lifetime sexual partners, and within the past 3 months, 8% of unmarried women had three or more sexual partners (54). Between 1989 and 1995, condom use at last intercourse in never-married women increased from 18% to 34% (55). In the National Survey of Adolescent Males, which is a nationally representative interview study of boys aged 15 to 19 years, the average age at first intercourse was 15.6 years in 1989 to 1991 (56). Although age at first coitus had not changed significantly, the proportion of adolescents who were sexually active decreased from 76% to 68% by 1995 (57) and condom use increased from 57% to 67% ($p < .01$) (58). In the latter part of the decade, the CDC Youth Risk Behavioral Surveillance system showed that sexual activity continued to decrease (59). Positive behavioral trends were particularly evident in African American males, where overall sexual activity decreased by 23%, and more than two thirds in 2001 reported having used condoms at last intercourse, compared with 46% in 1990. Condom use increases have also been documented in other populations, such as college students (60,61). In compilations of national survey data (62) and in the national Behavioral Risk Surveillance System (BRFSS) in 1997, of 33,913 respondents, 11% reported having multiple sex partners during the preceding year, and median prevalence of condom use at last sex was 65% (53%–79%) (63).

More recent behavioral surveillance approaches have focused on demographic groups suspected to be at high risk of HIV infection. Because obtaining behavioral surveillance data is expensive and may take a prolonged period, we can expect these targeted efforts to increase. For example, studies of urban young gay men obtained via community sampling provided data confirming the increased high-risk behaviors in gay men observed in the late 1990s, and that young gay black men were at extraordinary risk. For example, 77% reported anal intercourse, 37% unprotected anal intercourse. Sixteen percent of those tested were HIV positive, and most were not aware of their infection (64). These data have induced development of intervention efforts specific to these communities.

In summary, the behavioral surveys are a useful population-based baseline for the evaluation of HIV prevention interventions directed at sexual behaviors and to a lesser extent drug-using behavior. These surveys also demonstrate the high rate of sexual activity among adolescents, underscoring the need for prevention efforts in these groups. Behavior surveys have evolved as one potential method for evaluating impact of interventions on large proportions of the population.

Adaptation of Behavioral Deterministic Models to Human Immunodeficiency Virus Intervention Efforts

More sophisticated efforts at developing behavioral interventions require a model of human behavior and action (65–67). A behavioral model provides the following:

- A rational explanation of the determinants of behavior. This in turn provides insight into how an intervention should be developed.
- A qualitative and quantitative framework for which to evaluate intervention effectiveness. In HIV prevention interventions, direct measurement of HIV seroincidence is rarely used as an intervention outcome. HIV seroincidence is a relatively rare event (in a statistical sense) and would require a long follow-up. Program evaluation measures often focus on either changes in high-risk behaviors or changes in other correlates (such as attitudes and beliefs). For example, if self-efficacy in using condoms was shown to highly correlate with HIV/STD risk, an intervention may focus its efforts and evaluation on improving condom use self-efficacy. This is especially important because HIV incidence is almost never measurable in an intervention to reduce high-risk sexual behaviors. Additionally, fully controlled studies of sexual behavior interventions, where the control condition receives no intervention, are unethical. Therefore, behavioral models offer a series of behavioral variables that can be evaluated in place of the biologic HIV outcome. No one model is accepted as a standard for HIV risk-reduction interventions, and often, elements of multiple models are blended in an intervention program (66).

In adapting behavior models for HIV interventions, several themes predominate (65). Successful intervention efforts are developed by multidisciplinary teams including physicians, epidemiologists, behavioral scientists, and often anthropologists and social workers. For example, anthropologists can provide crucial information by elucidating deep-seated cultural attitudes toward sexual behaviors and which behaviors are amenable to intervention. In terms of developing intervention approaches, several themes predominate, all of which are interrelated.

Increasing Knowledge Base. Providing accurate information about sexuality, HIV, STDs, and drug use are important. At-risk individuals often have poor access to accurate information. This includes opportunities to explore local beliefs and myths related to sensitive behaviors in a nonjudgmental environment.

Self-esteem. Investigators have focused on developing self-esteem within sexual relationships, and especially how this relates to the decision to have sexual intercourse or use drugs.

Communication Skills. Improving communication and negotiation skills is, especially within the context of sensitive behaviors such as sexual behaviors, important for being able to make one's wishes known to sexual partners. Condom use interventions, for example, have stressed development of negotiating skills (e.g., convincing a partner that a condom should be used), as well as increasing self-esteem (including the ability to refuse sexual intercourse if a condom is not used).

Technical and Self-efficacy. In sexual behavior and condom use interventions, the technical aspects of using condoms or other barrier methods are important. A flaw in many traditional public health approaches is that "use-condom" messages assume that the intended intervention recipients use them correctly (68).

Social Norms. Behaviors occur within a social environment—usually one's peer group (69,70). Individual-based approaches to behavior change are often ineffective if the operative external environment doesn't change. For example, smoking behaviors in the United States between 1960 and 2000 underwent a drastic transformation, from acceptance or promotion in most social settings to a situation in which the behavior is actively discouraged in social group settings and in the environment, such as workplaces, restaurants, and public places. This type of social norm change takes time. The most successful approach to changing social norms for sexual behavior has focused on identifying "peer opinion leaders" to which the group looks for leadership and guidance.

Beliefs. Understanding the relationship between beliefs about health conditions, perceived susceptibility to illness, severity of illness, and ability to implement change.

Recognition of Behavior Change as a Continuum (Stages of Change) (71,72). From a methodologic perspective, intervention studies must be longitudinal and hence are very costly, because short-term relapse is common. Most intervention approaches still consider behavior amenable to rapid intervention. Sexual and drug-using behavioral patterns, however, often develop over long periods and in response to multiple individual-based and community-based stimuli. All of these factors cannot be changed simultaneously. There has been increasing realization that sexual and drug-use behaviors have clinical characteristics more akin to a chronic disease, which can be treated with a long-term "management plan," but which also may go through cycles of remission and relapse. One of the key behavioral concepts that has therefore emerged is that of "maintenance," that is, developing individual and social supports to maintain behavior change and prevent relapse.

Caveats with Behavioral Models

No single behavioral model has been shown to work in all situations. In part, this is due to the cultural diversity of at-risk populations and the need to specifically tailor intervention approaches, making comparisons difficult. There are also problems inherent to the models themselves, including the following:

- The models were derived from research in a variety of health areas, such as treatment of phobias and programs designed to increase compliance with no-smoking campaigns and immunization programs. In contrast, sexual and drug-related behaviors are much more likely to be drive stimulated. Integrated behavioral models, such as the one described in reference 66, incorporate features of several base models.
- The models assume that sexual and drug-use behaviors are rational consequences of a consistent set of determinants, which can be defined. This is not the case.
- Sexual and drug-related behaviors present major problems in measurement. For example, in an STD treatment environment, there is an implicit social desirability to overreport condom use, due to the context of the setting. These settings cannot usually be controlled in the clinical environment, where disease prevention messages are provided through various venues. Measurement of these behaviors is nearly always by self-report. However, because the disease incidence rate is low, the interventions require that outcomes be measured by self-reports in nearly every situation (73).
- The models make a contextual assumption that risky behaviors can be addressed independently irrespective of other needs, such as drug treatment, HIV treatment, medical care, or income maintenance.
- The HIV epidemic is heterogeneous, as are the populations at risk. Each cultural and ethnic group may have different beliefs and customs regarding sexual behavior, which need to be addressed in interventions.
- Behavior occurs within a social context. Nearly all of the behavioral models include "social norms" within one's peer group as a major factor in changing behavior, or in maintaining "safe" behaviors.

SOCIAL NETWORKS AND THEIR IMPORTANCE IN PREVENTION EFFORTS: IMPACT ON PEER NORMS

Social influence, especially by friends, has been found to affect numerous health-related behaviors (74). Social networks include an individual's immediate personal (including sexual) and family relationships. These form the basis of tangible and emotional support and are the basis in many situations for the social norms of behavior. In the context of HIV prevention, social networks include an individual's sexual and drug-using partners but may also include other members of the social groups, such as friends and acquaintances. There has been increasing recognition of the potential importance of social influence in HIV prevention, of the ability to gain access to risky communities, and the public health potential of using social networks to disseminate public health interventions. When HIV and STD epidemics are mapped with partner chains, individuals who are perceived to be at low infection risk (by virtue of their personal behavior profile) may actually be at high HIV transmission risk through the behaviors of their partners (75–77).

For example, in early studies of drug users, friends' HIV infection risk behaviors were the strongest predictors of behavioral change (78). Friends' risk behavior was a stronger determinant of risk reduction than was knowledge about AIDS, education level, or personal knowledge of someone with AIDS. The community-wide risk reduction among gay men in San Francisco suggests that social influence can be an important factor in risk reduction (79). This effect is termed "diffusion of innovation of prevention practices," and understanding the dynamics of this process within these networks has become a major area of prevention research. As a consequence of the social network structure, behavior change in key members of the social networks, or "opinion leaders" (70,80), translates into changing social norms and hence changing behaviors within the group. This approach has the advantage of "leveraging" scarce intervention resources, because the intervention would be primarily focused on changing attitudes, norms, and behaviors of the identified group leaders. This approach has been applied successfully in gay men, drug users, persons with STD exposure, and in adolescents, where peer educators have been used to promote STD/HIV control and contraceptive programs.

A type of social network analysis is the tracing of sexual contacts, which is often done as part of HIV and STD transmission investigations. A key feature in these investigations is demonstrating that individuals who may be self-perceived low personal risk (e.g., because they may be monogamous) are actually at high risk because of their partners' sexual or drug-using behavior. One recent investigation in the rural South demonstrated these aspects (81) (Fig. 120.1) and shows how in an extended sexual network that contains HIV-positive members, HIV can be rapidly transmitted to persons who may not perceive themselves to be at risk.

Core and Bridge Populations

Related to social networks are the concepts of "core" and "bridge" populations. Core populations are defined within networks as groups that have high rates of endemic infection and multiple sexual or needle-sharing contacts, and are therefore able to spread infection to many individuals. Bridge populations, a related concept, are groups who by virtue of demographics or behavior are in a position to spread infection from a highly infected population (i.e., endemic settings) to populations with

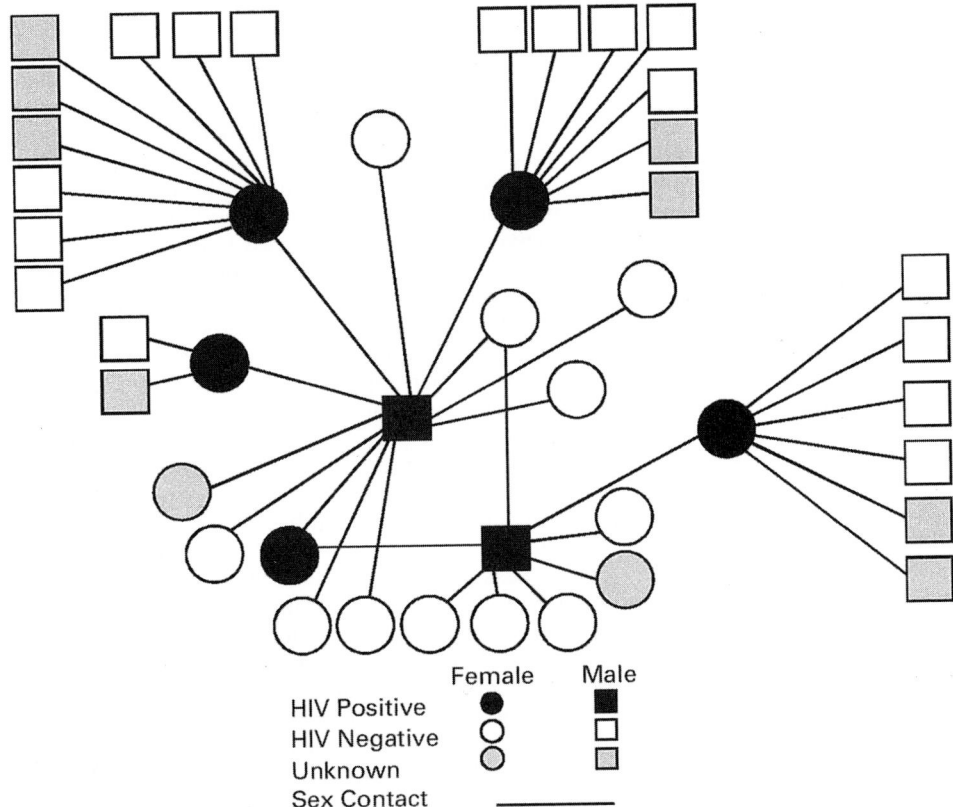

Figure 120.1. A dense heterosexual network from a human immunodeficiency virus outbreak in Mississippi. Note the importance of concurrent multiple partners in spreading the epidemic, and the large number of persons exposed through "bridge" contacts. [From Cluster of HIV-infected adolescents and young adults—Mississippi, 1999. *MMWR Morb Mortal Wkly Rep* 2000;49(38):861–864, with permission.]

Female   Male

HIV Positive

HIV Negative

Unknown

Sex Contact

low infection rates. Heterogeneity in sexual behavior is vital to generate a high sexual activity "core group" within which HIV spreads rapidly. How far out of this core group the virus will spread depends on the patterns of mixing within populations. Interventions to reduce the incidence of HIV have to be targeted at those most likely to spread the virus (82). In practice, core groups are often commercial sex workers (CSWs), homosexual men in areas where there is anonymous sexual exposure, such as bathhouses, and IDUs in high-prevalence areas who practice risky behaviors such as needle sharing and high-risk sexual behaviors (83).

Identification of "core" and "bridge" populations is important in developing intervention strategies, especially in settings where the infection has been recently introduced. For example, in Thailand, men who have sex with CSWs (the highly infected population) and who have spousal partners (the uninfected populations) would be defined as a bridge population. Certain occupational groups, such as long-distance truck drivers in Asia and Africa, are prototypic examples of bridge populations (84). Individuals with multiple simultaneous sexual partners are key elements of core groups for STD and sexual HIV transmission. For example, modeling studies in populations have shown that when one half of the partnerships in a population are concurrent, the size of the epidemic after 5 years is 10 times as large as under sequential monogamy. The primary cause of this amplification is the growth in the number of people connected in the network at any point: the size of the largest "component." Concurrency increases the size of this component, and the result is that the infectious agent is no longer trapped in a monogamous partnership after transmission occurs but can spread immediately beyond this partnership to infect others partners (85). Mixing between the "core" groups and low-prevalence groups, either directly or through bridging partners, is a key factor in increasing HIV transmission (86).

However, the presence of the risk behavior does not necessarily confer infection risk. For example, in some settings, the risk networks may exist without HIV having been introduced, with minimal or no infection present in the network. In these cases, prevention efforts need to be focused on both reducing overall infection risk and preventing introduction. The converse also holds true: For example, in a study on New York drug users, 31 of 80 network components included *no* members who were infected; and a median of the linkages of network member had lasted more than 6 months—termed "islands of seronegatives." Prevention of epidemic outbreaks by small size of connected component can be considered a social network process akin to herd immunity (87).

Sexual networks can also develop through creative mechanisms using technology. For example, the internet has developed as a "meeting place" for sexual partners, in which the "assortative" group characteristic would be the technical capacity to "meet" on-line and arrange for subsequent sexual activity. Because people can use the Internet to solicit sex partners, especially on an anonymous basis, it is a risk environment for STDs (88–90). The potential of this modality for disease transmission was demonstrated in a widely publicized syphilis outbreak among homosexual men, in which partners met over the Internet. In a creative approach, the health department developed on-line strategies and chat-room monitoring to promote health education messages on sites where partners from the outbreak had met (91,92).

APPLYING THE BEHAVIORAL APPROACH

Interventions to Reduce the Risk of Sexual Exposure through Promoting Condom Use

CONDOM EFFICACY

Promoting condom use has been one of the central tenets of the HIV and STD risk-reduction strategy, both in the United States and abroad. Condoms are effective when used correctly and consistently. Studies of HIV discordant heterosexual couples in California (93) and Italy (94,95) have conclusively demonstrated that consistent use in controlled settings results in an approximately sevenfold decrease in HIV seroconversions. Two careful metaanalyses concluded that condoms are 87% (96) to 90% to 95% effective (97) when used consistently; consistent condom users are 10 to 20 times less likely to become infected when exposed to the virus than are inconsistent or nonusers. Condoms are also effective in reducing the risk of bacterial STDs (98,99) and genital herpes simplex (100), which attains an increasing importance as the relationships of STDs as cofactors continue to be elucidated.

The largest observational study that demonstrated condom efficacy was the Uganda Rakai project. This study, which was a large population-based longitudinal clinical trial conducted in southwestern Uganda, was designed to assess whether STD treatment intervention reduced HIV seroincidence (see below). Because of the large sample size (more than 18,000), multiple observational substudies were embedded. Condom usage information was obtained prospectively from 17,264 sexually active individuals aged 15 to 59 years over 30 months. HIV incidence and STD prevalence was determined for consistent and irregular condom users, compared with nonusers. Consistent condom use significantly reduced HIV incidence by 63% and bacterial STDs by 50%, all results that were highly statistically significant (101).

Behavioral studies of condom use have focused on understanding the determinants and issues related to their use, especially considering the low consistent-use rate indicated by the national surveys. Increased condom use is influenced by the appreciation of a perceived benefit (e.g., STD/HIV prevention), the peer group social norms, and sex education with specific instruction in condom use (102–104). Challenges to maintain continued use include the need to continually reinforce the perceived benefit; the result of a successful prevention is that no adverse event occurs, in contrast to other interventions or commercial marketing strategies where self-reinforcement of continued behavior is easier. As with other sex education programs, promoting condom use has not been found to increase sexual activity in adolescents or to result in earlier sexual debut (105). Effective condom promotion requires integration of public health and social marketing efforts. As described in the section on behavioral surveillance ("Surveys of Sexual Behavior"), steady increases in condom use have been observed, especially in heterosexual minority adolescents. Probably the most intensive and successful effort has been implemented in Thailand, where the "100% condom" program (106) has been implemented since 1991 and includes intensive advertising, an infrastructure to purchase and distribute condoms, and linkages in promoting condoms with stakeholders including the Army, provincial and municipality governments, and CSWs. Recent large-scale reductions in HIV seroincidence in Thailand have been in part attributed to this program (107). The Thai program provides a useful model on the development of an effective condom promotion and sexual risk-reduction campaign. The program includes open discussion of HIV prevention and condom promotion, mass-media campaigns, and the active participation of a large variety of "stakeholders" including the military, government, medical community, and even the brothels. In other words, this effective program's major accomplishment was to change the social norms across a broad spectrum of society to encourage condom use.

THEORY-BASED RISK-REDUCTION INTERVENTIONS

Education is often confused with interventions and counseling. *Education* refers to the transmittal of knowledge, in this case, knowledge of HIV transmission patterns, risks, and methods to avoid risk. In contrast, *risk-reduction counseling* entails a dialog between the counselor and the counseled, which may occur in either an individual format or a group format. *Structured behavioral interventions* may include a combination of counseling, education, and attempts to alter group norms. Multiple-session, small-group, and individual counseling are the intervention formats that have been most frequently used and that appear to be the most effective. Although clinic-based interventions are the types most commonly reported, interventions have been integrated into other venues, such as school curricula. For example, one school-based intervention consisted of six interactive sessions conducted in a high school using a traditional classroom environment (108). Other approaches have used student peer educators, street outreach workers, and co-workers in places of employment.

The longitudinal aspect (i.e., multiple session) of these interventions is critical; evaluation of single-session interventions has demonstrated equivocal efficacy at best. Probably the best example of an unintended "single-session" intervention occurred in 1991, when basketball player Magic Johnson announced he was HIV positive and was retiring from basketball. At that time, a multisession, behavioral intervention study was being conducted in high-risk heterosexuals recruited from an STD clinic in Baltimore (109). Evaluation of participants 1 month after the announcement found a one-third reduction in high-risk behavior. Follow-up 1 year later found that the level of high-risk behavior had returned to baseline and the effect of Mr. Johnson's announcement had dissipated. This example illuminates the need for continued "maintenance" and reinforcement of behavioral risk reduction in any intervention context.

Multisession, longitudinal client-focused, and culturally sensitive approaches have demonstrated reductions in self-reported HIV sexual behavior risks in homosexual men, heterosexuals, and adolescents. For example, in 318 African American homosexual men recruited from gay bars and bathhouses, a triple-session intervention reduced the incidence of self-reported rectal intercourse from 45% to 20%, with no change reported in the control groups (110). Heterosexual studies compared multisession educational, counseling, and skill-building sessions (which included self-esteem building and condom use negotiation skills) conducted in San Francisco (95,111), Milwaukee (112), and Philadelphia (113–115). For example, in the San Francisco study, inner-city women were recruited through street outreach. The intervention group had consistent increases in reported condom use and greater measures of sexual communication between partners (negotiating skills). These results are encouraging and suggest that behavioral change can be induced and maintained in high-risk populations.

ISSUES IN BEHAVIORAL INTERVENTION STUDIES

- *Advantages:* Focused interventions are usually conducted in small group settings, using interventions that are developed specifically for the target populations. The more innovative efforts have used community group members as facilitators or team leaders, which many believe enhances the effectiveness.
- *Disadvantages:* There are three major disadvantages of these interventions, which make it difficult to generalize their use.
1. The community-based focus makes these interventions extremely expensive. Sexual and drug-using behaviors occur within a social context, which must be defined for each target group.
2. Intervention effectiveness can be measured only through self-reported change in sexual behavior. Some authorities

believe that this may predispose to reporting bias, that is, that within an intervention setting, there is bias to over-report condom use and safer sex practices. For example, within Baltimore STD clinics, self-reported condom use was found not to correlate with incident STD (116).

3. Intervention efforts require enrollment and participation by the community members in a long-term process. This may be difficult, especially in settings where there is substantive competition for an individual's time, such as employment, child care, and so on.

It appears that focused behavioral interventions may be an option for specific high-risk groups. From a physician's perspective, it may be useful to approach high-risk behavioral reduction, from a chronic disease model, as a gradual incremental improvement when it occurs, requiring continued maintenance, and subject to relapse.

BEHAVIORAL INTERVENTIONS TO REDUCE RISKY SEXUAL BEHAVIOR

Determining efficacy of behavioral interventions is challenging, because of varied populations studied, which limit generalizability, the need for behavioral models, and the measurement issues that have been descried. Because of the immense logistics and expense, only a few randomized trials of behavioral interventions have been performed.

Project LIGHT was a multisession behavioral intervention in which 3,700 participants were recruited form 37 clinical sites. Compared with the 1,855 individuals in the control group, participants assigned to a small-group, seven-session HIV risk-reduction program reported fewer unprotected sexual acts, had higher levels of condom use, and were more likely to use condoms consistently over a 12-month follow-up period. Overall, the reduction in risky sexual behaviors was 25% to 40%, depending on the specific behavior measured (117). Project RESPECT was a five-clinic intervention study conducted at STD clinics, in which more than 5,500 subjects were enrolled. The interventions evaluated included a four-session counseling intervention and a two-session intervention, based on the Theory of Reasoned Action and the Stages of Change Model. Both interventions demonstrated higher rates of consistent condom use and abstinence, compared with the controls (118). Other behavioral randomized controlled trials (RCTs) demonstrating similar results include studies in African American adolescents (119) and Texas minority women (120), both of which used multisession, model-driven skill-building interventions that emphasized skill building and communication skills.

CHALLENGES/BARRIERS TO IMPLEMENTATION OF HUMAN IMMUNODEFICIENCY VIRUS PREVENTION EFFORTS

Community-level Barriers

As demonstrated by the Thai model, effective community-based prevention interventions require a change in social norms and frank open discussion of sensitive behavioral issues such as sexuality and drug use. Persons with HIV or who are at risk of acquiring HIV are often also at risk of being marginalized from society, because of their behaviors. For example, an effective HIV prevention program must include approaches to homosexual men, IDUs, CSWs, adolescents, and minorities.

Patient-level Barriers

Simplistically, implementation of HIV prevention interventions at the personal level requires the perception that one is at risk and the technical efficacy to implement these interventions. Persons connected to risky social networks may not perceive themselves to be at risk but may be so because of their partners' behaviors. These issues are independent of the motivations behind sexual and drug use behavior, which must always be recognized as pleasure seeking and drive oriented. For example, successful implementation of condom use intervention requires the following steps to occur in sequence:

- Recognition that sexual activity is going to occur, and recognizing the need for a condom (judgment)
- Accessibility to a condom (access/availability)
- Negotiation of condom use with partner
- Technical efficacy
  - Removing condom from the package
  - Putting it on correctly
  - Using it during intercourse
  - Removing it correctly

Conditions that could impede the successful completion of these tasks, as well as other behaviorally oriented interventions, include mental illness and substance abuse (see below). *Condom breakage* is occasionally cited as a potential problem, especially among patients attending STD clinics. Studies of breakage rates (121–124) in high-risk patients (i.e., STD clinics) have found the rates to be from 2% to 7%, with higher rates seen in homosexual men and the lowest rates in CSWs (125,126). Condom use is also related to emotional connectedness to partners, especially in gay men where contraception is not an issue (127). *Partner selection* is another factor that could have an impact on effectiveness of condom intervention. In practice, many individuals use condoms selectively. Typically, the pattern is to use condoms with casual sexual partners, but not with regular partners (unless the condom is also being used as a contraceptive method). HIV risk in these situations would be dependent on the HIV seroprevalence in the partner pool with whom the individual is having unprotected intercourse.

MENTAL ILLNESS

Psychiatric problems are extraordinarily common in HIV-infected patients (128). Although these disorders may occur as a response to HIV infection, in many cases they are long standing and probably contribute to the high-risk behaviors that predispose to HIV infection. For example, studies in STD clinic populations, representing persons at *risk* for HIV transmission, have found that up to one third of patients may have diagnosable affective disorder (129). Whether an individual is HIV infected and continues to be sexually active, or whether the individual is at risk of being infected because of depression or other mental illness, implementation of behavioral interventions is not likely to occur unless the underlying psychiatric disorder is treated.

SUBSTANCE USE: GENERAL ISSUES

Substance abuse can impede intervention efforts via two mechanisms. First, substance use may be associated with increased risk-taking behavior, which may include high-risk sexual behavior. Second, substance abuse, especially alcohol, may impede the technical efficacy in implementing risk reduction, which includes the technical steps in placing a condom correctly and negotiating with sexual partners.

Alcohol is increasingly recognized as a risk factor for HIV and high-risk sexual behaviors. Early studies in homosexual men found that heavy alcohol use was associated with general increases in risky sexual behavior (130), decreased condom use, and increased risk to relapse into risky sexual behavior after successful behavioral intervention (131). Contextual substance use (i.e., immediately before sexual activity or being "high" or intoxicated during intercourse) appears to have the highest risk. Similar results have been found in heterosexual populations. Studies in adolescents (132), STD patients (133) in San Francisco, and African American women in Birmingham (134) demonstrated that alcohol use was associated with a twofold to fourfold increased risk of not using condoms at last intercourse decreased. Studies in the Royal Thai Army demonstrated a conclusive link between alcohol use, CSW exposure, and HIV seroconversion (135). As part of the successful Thai Army HIV intervention program, structural interventions were developed to minimize the level of alcohol intake during training and deployments. In combination with the 100% condom program, this intervention resulted in lower levels of alcohol use and sharp decreases in seroconversion rates (136).

HUMAN IMMUNODEFICIENCY VIRUS IN SUBSTANCE ABUSERS: DESCRIPTIVE EPIDEMIOLOGY AND INTERVENTION APPROACHES

The seroprevalence rate in IDUs varies by community. Risks are greatest for those who share injection equipment, the practices associated with sharing injecting equipment or sharing drug preparations ("backloading" and "frontloading"), and those who inject in "shooting galleries (137–139). For noninjectors, such as crack-cocaine smokers, cross-sectional studies have demonstrated that the seroprevalence rate ranges between 0% and 15%, depending on the locality (140), with highest rates in the Northeast and the South. In IDUs, the barriers to prevention implementation are not the pharmacologic effect of drugs, as much as the social milieu. Nevertheless, there are a number of major problems. In a study conducted early in the HIV epidemic, HIV-infected female IDUs in the Bronx were offered intensive counseling and testing and contraceptive counseling. Nevertheless, 24% of the HIV-positive women became pregnant within 2 years, compared with 22% of HIV-negative controls (141). More than 90% of IDUs are sexually active, and more than half identify a primary sexual partner within the previous 6 months. However, studies of condom use have ranged between 9% and 34% for self-reported consistent condom use (142). In a multicity study conducted of IDUs, HIV infection was found to be associated with increased self-reported condom use (143). However, 31% of patients in that study still reported unsafe sexual activity. In a large Baltimore longitudinal study, in which more than 2,000 active IDUs were recruited and whom had an initial seroprevalence rate of 30% for those who used shooting galleries, 23% for those who shared needles, and 16% for those who denied either of these activities, the subsequent seroconversion rate has been 7% to 9% per year, of which half is estimated to be due to sexual transmission.

NON–INJECTION DRUG USE

Non–injection heroin (144) and crack-cocaine use are recognized risk factors for HIV and other STDs in various populations including STD clinic attendees, prenatal populations (145–147), and HIV-infected persons recruited from an urban community (148). For example, in a study of crack-using female CSWs recruited from three U.S. cities, 28% were HIV infected and 38% had positive syphilis serologies (149). HIV transmission in this setting is related to the sexual behavior associated with cocaine use, especially drug-related prostitution activities. Crack-cocaine use was also associated with increased risky sexual behavior in persons diagnosed with HIV, characterized by CSW contact, low condom-use rates (150–152), and increased incidence of other STDs, particularly epidemic genital ulcer diseases such as chancroid, syphilis, and lymphogranuloma venereum, all of which have been associated with facilitated HIV transmission (147,153,154). The term *intersecting* epidemics has been used to describe this constellation of phenomena (155). Based on the aforementioned social network models, non-IDUs form potential bridge populations for disease transmission.

DRUG USE INTERVENTIONS: RISK REDUCTION

Primary prevention of HIV through cessation of drug use or through drug treatment is clearly the most preferable policy option. However, the number of currently active IDUs overwhelms the availability of drug treatment (156), and the medical model of substance abuse recognizes this disorder as a chronic condition that is prone to relapse and exacerbation in many individuals. Therefore, though politically attractive, HIV prevention through cessation of drug use has inherent practical problems. Recognizing this, many public health officials and substance abuse experts have recommended harm-reduction approaches, in other words, acknowledging drug use activity and taking interventions to make injection drug use less likely to promote HIV infection. These interventions were guided by the epidemiologic studies demonstrating that needle sharing and its associated practices were the risks most likely to promote HIV transmission.

Comprehensive Efforts

In 1995, an international group of investigators (157) identified five large cities with large IDU populations, and where HIV seroprevalence remained less than 5% for 5 consecutive years. The three common characteristics were implementation of IDU-directed HIV prevention activities when seroprevalence was low, implementation of a needle-exchange programs or other mechanisms to provide sterile injection equipment, and street-level community outreach efforts. These findings underscore the necessity for a multidisciplinary approach to HIV risk reduction in IDUs, even when comprehensive drug treatment options are not available. Studies of drug users in even severely impacted areas such as New York (158,159) and Bangkok demonstrated that substantial behavior change has taken place among IDUs, particularly regarding injection practices and sharing of needles. These changes were more pronounced in individuals who had increased interpersonal communication (e.g., talked about HIV prevention with their friends), in individuals who had been previously tested for HIV, and depending on individual educational level. Use of "underground" needle exchanges also contributed to decreased high-risk practices. The following information has evolved from these studies:

1. Drug users can adopt prevention behaviors related to HIV.
2. Prevention activities appear to be more focused on drug-use behaviors, although most drug users are sexually active.
3. Drug treatment has a positive impact on implementation of HIV prevention behaviors (160).

4. HIV prevention behaviors are most effectively implemented when in a community context. This argues strongly against the "marginalization" of drug users.

Bleach Distribution

Promoting bleach disinfectant was the initial approach taken and was based on the general infection-control procedures recommended by the CDC and other public health agencies. Initial community-based programs were established to distribute bleach kits to IDUs and their social networks, achieving distribution rates as high as 74%. Bleach distribution is inexpensive. Follow-up process evaluation studies of IDUs found that the majority were aware of the bleach distribution programs. Compliance, however, was variable (161). However, despite the widespread implementation of bleach distribution, effectiveness in preventing HIV has been difficult to demonstrate. In part, this may be due to the multifaceted risks in the target population of IDUs; observational studies cannot control for the myriad social, substance abuse, and sexual risks that may be present. A 1995 review from the Institute of Medicine acknowledged these shortcomings.

Needle Exchange (162)

Syringe-exchange programs (SEPs) or needle-exchange programs as a means of risk reduction have gained increasing popularity and have been subject to considerable political controversy. In the late 1980s, underground (i.e., "illegal") needle-exchange programs developed in a number of large cities. In some areas, these have become legitimatized and are operated by health departments or community groups. The underlying hypothesis of the needle-exchange programs is that access to and provision of clean injection equipment is attractive to IDUs and will result in decreased sharing practices. These arguments were strengthened by findings in diabetic IDUs. In the Baltimore longitudinal IDU study (163), insulin-dependent diabetes was used as a surrogate for the availability of legal injection equipment. Cross-sectional seroprevalence in diabetic drug users was 9.8%, compared with 24.3% in the nondiabetics, despite a similar profile of injection frequency. Diabetics were less likely to share needles and other injection paraphernalia.

Client acceptance rates for SEPs or needle-exchange programs have been consistently high; for example, surveys of IDUs in San Francisco found that 41% were regular users of the needle exchange and that 65% had visited it within the past year (164).

The opposing arguments include the potential to increase initiation of drug use and increase occupational risk to medical and law-enforcement personnel. In addition, senior law enforcement officials and many legislators have opposed needle exchange for legal and moral grounds. Nevertheless, a recent report from the Institute of Medicine, reviewing all the evidence, believed that syringe exchange provided a beneficial health benefit and that the risks cited earlier were minimal (156).

Community-based needle-exchange programs, often illicit, have been operating since the late 1980s. The data from observational studies conducted in a large number of venues in the United States, western Europe, more recently in developing countries strongly suggest that SEPs are associated with decreased HIV seroincidence (165,166), despite methodologic shortcomings. This relationship is biologically plausible. SEPs reduce the amount of syringe sharing, they reduce the circulation time of syringes in a particular drug-using network, and

they reduce the amount of reuse of syringes within a particular drug-using network. SEPs have been proposed to have potential indirect effects, termed either *collateral impact* or *diffusion of innovation* (162,167). These include increased opportunities to reduce sexual risk exposures, provide condoms and instruction on condom use, provide HIV counseling and testing, and provide access to HIV and other health care services to those who desperately need it.

In addition, SEPs have been associated with reducing the length of time until IDUs enter drug treatment (akin to the stages of change model in behavioral science) and diffusing innovation by providing positive benefits to IDUs in the SEP enrollee's social network (i.e., SEPs benefit persons who are not directly exchanging syringes but are exchanging syringes through a third party).

In sum, approaches to reducing risk among drug users need to include the following elements (168):

- Access to drug treatment as definitive intervention
- Harm reduction through bleach provision, needle exchange, and legal access to syringes
- Reduction/elimination of needle sharing
- Reduction of sexual risk
- Access to HIV counseling, testing, and care
- Use of innovative approaches, such as community-based outreach, social network, and diffusion of risk-reduction interventions within the networks

HUMAN IMMUNODEFICIENCY VIRUS COUNSELING AND TESTING APPROACHES: DIAGNOSIS OR INTERVENTION?

Since 1986, HIV testing and counseling programs have been the cornerstones of HIV prevention policies and programs. HIV testing must be accompanied by pretest counseling, to ensure that patients understand the nature of the test and the potential implications of the results. HIV pretest and posttest counseling protocols vary by locality but consist of the following elements.

1. Ensuring that the testing is voluntary. Mandatory testing occurs in only very specific situations, such as the military.
2. Education regarding current concepts of HIV disease. Counselors emphasize that HIV disease is a continuum, that a diagnosis of AIDS represents the late stage of HIV disease. The asymptomatic latent period of HIV disease is stressed, with particular emphasis that disease transmission can occur while asymptomatic.
3. Ensuring that the individual understands the impact of a positive test result including:
   a. That HIV is a chronic lifelong disease
   b. That medical therapy is available, which affects the disease course
   c. In confidential testing, that the case may be reported to local health authorities, depending on local statute
4. Prevention messages, including counseling on safer sexual and drug-using behaviors. Unfortunately, what occurs in most settings is *education*. To be effective, *counseling* requires more time and more client interaction than the circumstances typically allow in an HIV counseling and testing setting.
5. Obtaining informed consent.

In *anonymous* testing, no patient identifiers are used to ensure absolute confidentiality; therefore, patients have to return in person for test results, and no follow-up is possible for those who test positive but do not return. *Confidential* testing is performed in settings where the test result becomes part of the medical record, for example, in STD clinics, tuberculosis clinics, and private physician offices. Follow-up is possible, and many local health departments will use disease intervention outreach personnel to contact individuals who do not return for test results. Interviewing for sex partners and HIV partner notification is often part of confidential testing protocols.

The standard HIV testing algorithm uses one or more enzyme-linked immunosorbent assay (ELISA) screening tests, followed by a Western blot confirmatory test. Laboratory processing of specimens takes a minimum of 2 working days primarily because of the time and interpretation requirements of the Western blot. Because of the laboratory delay, the time between testing and receipt of result is 1 week in optimal settings. In some public health settings, where testing is done in a centralized lab, delays of 2 to 3 weeks are not uncommon. Simple, rapid HIV tests have been developed, in large part in response to demand from the developing world for simple inexpensive tests that can be performed in field settings and where batch processing for ELISA is not practical. These have been evaluated in field settings in developing countries (169) and in emergency department settings (170). However, the impact of these new technologies on behaviors is unknown.

In theory, HIV testing and counseling programs serve three roles: case identification (diagnosis), partner referral, and risk reduction. Through diagnosis, HIV counseling and testing play an important role in facilitating referral for medical care interventions, such as antiretroviral therapy, opportunistic infection prophylaxis, and prenatal therapy for pregnant women. Confidential partner referral is an integral part of the federal counseling and testing program and has been implemented except in states where local statute prohibits reporting of HIV-infected individuals (as opposed to AIDS cases). Of sexual partners interviewed in partner referral programs, 15% will be new previously undiagnosed cases of HIV (171,172). As a preventive intervention, the effectiveness of HIV counseling and testing is more controversial. A large review of 66 studies conducted between 1986 and 1990 found reductions in self-reported risk behaviors among IDUs, homosexual men, and heterosexuals (173). However, the effects and the sample sizes in many of the studies were small. Two studies conducted in STD clinic settings, in Miami (174) and Baltimore (175), found that HIV counseling and testing had little impact on subsequent STD incidence rates, a biologic marker of continued high-risk sexual activity. A more in-depth study conducted in women counseled and tested in Connecticut community health centers also found that HIV counseling and testing have minimal effects on subsequent sexual behaviors (176).

The apparent limited efficacy of HIV counseling and testing in reducing HIV transmission (as opposed to diagnosing cases) is due to a number of factors:

1. Despite the large investment, many HIV-infected individuals remain undiagnosed (177,178). By definition, the large number of undiagnosed individuals, presumably unaware of their seropositive status, are still at risk of infecting others through drug and sexual behaviors.
2. Sexual and drug-related behaviors are complex phenomena, driven by both biologic and social cues. Typically, these behavior patterns have developed over a long period. Therefore, it is unlikely that a single, short counseling session will result in sustained changes of risk-taking behaviors.

In summary, HIV counseling and testing is effective as a means of case diagnosis, which in turn provides entry into clinical care. In terms of behavioral intervention, the data suggest that if it is effective, the impact is only marginal. The behavioral literature suggests that a more intensive and longitudinal approach is required.

KEY CONCEPTS IN DEVELOPING HUMAN IMMUNODEFICIENCY VIRUS PREVENTIONS FOR DRUG AND SEXUAL BEHAVIORS

Des Jarlais has succinctly summarized 15 years of experience in behavioral prevention into 4 principles (1). These include the following:

- Most people will change their behavior in response to behavioral intervention. Behavioral models help define the key determinants of the risk behavior in specific populations.
- Nevertheless, it is rare to achieve 100% compliance, either at an individual level (i.e., 100% condom use) or at a population level. Policy makers and public health clinicians therefore need to define the level of "residual risk" that is tolerable. Residual risk is still a major problem, especially in high-seroprevalence areas.
- Reducing high-risk behavior and maintaining change is difficult, largely because sex and drug-using behaviors are pleasurable. Maintenance of behavioral change therefore requires continued reinforcement.
- Be prepared for unpleasant surprises. Examples are the resurgence of STDs and HIV risk in homosexual men and changes in drug-use patterns, which may either promote or hinder public health prevention efforts.

HUMAN IMMUNODEFICIENCY VIRUS EARLY INTERVENTION: INTERACTION BETWEEN MEDICAL CARE AND PREVENTION

Programmatic approaches to HIV management have typically separated treatment and prevention functions. For example, HIV prevention initiatives are usually coordinated by local health departments, whereas medical care is provided by the hospital system and physicians.

High-risk behaviors often continue after a diagnosis of HIV is made. For example, in Baltimore, 15% of patients who were tested and received posttest counseling for HIV in an STD clinic setting returned within 3 months with a new STD diagnosis (179). In a Los Angeles HIV continuity clinic, 9% of patients reported having unprotected intercourse with an HIV-negative sex partner, and 13% with an HIV-status-unknown sex partner (180). In a Boston intervention study, high-risk behavior was consistently found in HIV-seropositive patients 1 year after diagnosis, and higher rates were found in those individuals with depression or other diagnosable mental illness (181). These findings highlight the need to develop appropriate interventions for HIV-infected patients, targeting behavioral intervention and the need to reduce risk to their sex and drug partners. Traditional medical care programs often neglect behavioral intervention strategies but focus solely on the clinical aspects of medication provision and prophylaxis of opportunistic infection. Nevertheless, many HIV-infected patients, even those with low CD4 counts, continue to be sexually active. From an alternative standpoint, all newly infected individuals contracted the disease from an individual with active infection. Focusing prevention efforts on the already infected may therefore be an efficient, albeit widely neglected, approach.

Reducing transmission through medical treatment was initially proposed by Anderson, Gupta, and May (182) as theoretically attractive. Antiretroviral therapy, by reducing the viral load in blood and secretions, could potentially lower transmission risk by lowering the transmission efficiency. This presumes access and compliance with antiretroviral therapy regimens. There are obvious ethical and practical problems in studying this prospectively, necessitating consideration only of empiric data. A small study of 18 HIV-infected persons treated with highly active antiretroviral therapy (HAART) found that semen viral loads were profoundly reduced (183). Because transmissibility is directly proportional to viral load concentration (184), these findings have stimulated the development of programs to provide HAART therapy not only for primary treatment but also as a mechanism for secondary prevention (185,186).

This concept is not new. *Comprehensive HIV early intervention,* integrating medical care, case management services, and social support, was proposed by Francis, and soon after antiretroviral therapy became available (187,188). This paradigm integrated medical care, case management, and treatment for comorbid conditions, such as mental illness and substance abuse, as well as a focus on preventing secondary spread. Early data from the Baltimore STD clinics found that implementation of HIV early intervention in inner-city patients diagnosed with HIV in an STD clinic setting resulted in a 71% decreased incidence of gonorrhea compared with historical HIV-positive controls (179). Most primary HIV case management interventions, however, are still oriented toward medical management and improving compliance. The advent of HAART in 1996 and funding resources provided by the federal Ryan White Act have made integrated case management the national norm.

Development of effective therapy was accompanied by a number of troubling prevention trends. We saw earlier (see section "Epidemiologic Issues Relevant to Prevention") that in the late 1990s, there was a profound relapse of prevention efforts in homosexual men, with accompanying increases in STD rates and HIV seroconversions. Paradoxically, improved therapies have reduced concerns over unsafe sex, as HIV has evolved into a managed chronic disease (189,190). Studies in a large HIV clinic at Hopkins found that in 691 patients in 1998, 58% reported sexual activity in the past 90 days, 7.4% reported multiple sexual partners in the past month, and 34.6% did not use a condom at last sexual encounter. In addition, 7.5% of those screened had either current or recent (within 1 year) gonococcal or chlamydial infection. The convergence of these phenomena was demonstrated in San Francisco, where in homosexual men seen at the STD clinic, the HIV incidence rate was an extraordinary 5.3% (191) and having a diagnosis of rectal gonorrhea was associated with an even higher rate of 6.7%. Based on the remarkable changed epidemiology of STDs and risky behaviors in HIV-infected persons, CDC has strongly recommended specific outreach and prevention approaches targeting HIV-infected persons, which include the following elements (192):

- Increase the number of HIV-infected persons who know their serostatus
- Increase the use of health care and preventive services
- Increase high-quality care and treatment
- Increase adherence to therapy by individuals with HIV
- Increase the number of individuals with HIV who adopt and sustain HIV/STD risk-reduction behavior

CONTROL OF SEXUALLY TRANSMITTED DISEASES AS A HUMAN IMMUNODEFICIENCY VIRUS PREVENTION INTERVENTION

Epidemiologic Relationships (193–195)

As with an STD, the transmission of HIV is facilitated by the same risky behaviors as those associated with the traditional STDs, for example, having multiple sexual partners, sex with prostitutes, and drug-using sexual partners. Because of these behavioral confounders, establishing the link between STDs and HIV infection has been methodologically difficult. Cross-sectional and prospective studies both in the developed and in the developing world have firmly established that bacterial and viral STDs are biologic cofactors in facilitating HIV transmission. Multiple factors contribute to this biologic relationship including the following (196):

1. Facilitated access to the vascular portal of entry: HIV has been cultured from the base of genital ulcers (197) in persons with coexistent genital ulcer disease and HIV infection. Similarly, mucosal inflammation caused by STDs or increased cervical friability (198) induced by STDs or hormonal contraceptives may reduce the barriers to vascular entry.
2. Recruitment of target cells: STDs such as syphilis and chlamydia induce a lymphocytic response. Theoretically, recruitment of an increased number of CD4 target lymphocytes into areas that are exposed to HIV could facilitate infection.
3. Potentiation of HIV replication: Studies have demonstrated that HIV replication is potentiated by presence of herpes simplex virus (HSV) (viral transactivation). Recent human challenge studies of gonorrhea in HIV-infected men demonstrated that gonococcal infection increases HIV shedding by 2 logs (100-fold increase) (199). Acute bacterial sexually transmitted infection resulted in increased HIV-1 viremia. This may be mediated through increased inflammatory cytokines or through modulation of immune responses that control HIV-1 viremia (200). Similar results are seen in HSV infection (201,202), even in persons who are asymptomatic. These studies suggest that the presence of other STDs may increase the inoculum size, beyond the threshold required for infectivity.
4. HIV subtype: HIV subtype E preferentially infects Langerhans' epithelial cells, which are found in surfaces such as skin. Type E has been found to predominate in areas where heterosexual transmission is common, such as in sub-Saharan Africa. By disrupting the epithelial barrier, STDs may facilitate contact with the Langerhans target cells.
5. STDs and genital inflammation have been shown to increase the number of CCR5 receptors on genital Langerhans' cells and locally recruited CD4 lymphocytes.

Genital Ulcer Disease (203)

HIV prevalence studies demonstrated a threefold to fivefold increased odds ratio for HIV positivity in various patient populations with genital ulcer disease. HIV transmission facilitated by genital ulcers is important, especially in developing countries or in impoverished areas of developed countries. These studies included Baltimore patients with syphilis (204) and Kenyan STD clinic attendees in whom the majority of genital ulcer infections were due to chancroid (205,206). In Nairobi CSWs, the cross-sectional HIV-seroprevalence rate in persons with genital ulcers was 27% to 33%. Baltimore STD clinic patients had HIV seroprevalence rates three to four times that of the general STD clinic population (207). Serologic evidence of genital herpes is associated with a twofold to threefold increased odds ratio for HIV infection (201). In Kenya, where the population-based prevalence rate for persons aged 15 to 44 years is between 10% and 30%, the 6-month seroconversion rate for prostitutes with genital ulcers was 12%. In India, the overall population-based incidence of HIV was 2.6 times higher in CSWs. Prospectively, genital ulcer disease was associated with a seven times increased seroconversion risk (208,209); similar results were found in a large prospective study of Thai army recruits (210). In the United

States, a prospective study conducted in Bronx STD clinics of heterosexual patients during a chancroid outbreak found that HIV-seroconversion risk was three times higher in men with a genital ulcer compared with men without genital ulcer disease (147). Mechanistically, chancroid, lymphogranuloma venereum, and HSV were all associated with increased viral replication and mucosal HIV shedding (211,212).

Gonorrhea and Chlamydia

In Baltimore, a case-control study of HIV seroconverters found a threefold increased risk in patients who had a diagnosis of gonorrhea at their last STD clinic visit before seroconversion (207). Prospective studies in India (209) and Zaire (213) conclusively demonstrated an association between an exudative STD and HIV seroconversion. In the Zaire study, prostitutes were closely followed: Those with chlamydia had a 4.6 relative risk for seroconversion and those with gonorrhea had a relative risk of 3.6; both relationships were stable after controlling for other confounding variables. From a population perspective, gonorrheal and chlamydial infection may be more important because they may be associated with a higher attributable fraction of HIV-seroconversion cases. For example, the Baltimore investigators, whose population included a large number of IDUs, concluded that the adjusted attributable fraction of HIV seroconversions related to coexistent gonococcal infection was 18%.

The relationships between bacterial/viral STDs and HIV transmission have been suspected since the late 1980s. Bacterial vaginosis (BV), an inflammatory condition caused by altered vaginal flora, has been linked to increased HIV susceptibility. BV is especially prevalent in sub-Saharan Africa, afflicting approximately one third of women. Studies in Uganda (214) and in Malawi (215) found that BV was associated with a threefold increase in prevalent HIV, although this does not form a direct causal connection.

Sexually Transmitted Disease Control as a Human Immunodeficiency Virus Intervention

The epidemiologic evidence suggests that control of STDs may reduce HIV seroincidence. Because behavioral change is a long-term and incremental process, this option is increasingly attractive. A large population-based study in Tanzania has demonstrated that this may be a feasible approach (216). In this study, STD clinical facilities were upgraded, and drug treatment regimens were upgraded to be in concordance with World Health Organization guidelines (217). In control communities, no changes were made. This intervention resulted in a 42% decrease in HIV seroconversions after 2 years, despite no change in sexual behavior patterns or condom use rates. Most of the decrease was due to either decreased STD incidence or duration of STD infections. The second large population-based study was a randomized mass treatment trial of STDs as a primary HIV prevention intervention, which was conducted in the Rakai province in Uganda, which was an area with high HIV and STD rates (218). More than 18,000 persons were enumerated, enrolled in a longitudinal trial, and randomized by village into treatment and control groups. The treatment group received mass therapy for treatable STDs every 8 months, using a combination regimen of ciprofloxacin, azithromycin, and metronidazole, which would be effective for gonorrhea, chlamydia, chancroid, trichomoniasis, and BV. Syphilis was also aggressively diagnosed and treated (219). Extensive behavioral surveys and diagnostic evaluation were also conducted at the visit intervals. At study conclusion, the HIV *incidence* rate was similar in both the treatment and the control group, at 1.5 per 100 person-years, although treatment groups demonstrated a substantial reduction in STD burden (220). A number of interpretations and subsequent analyses concluded that the trial failed to demonstrate effect because of two major factors. First, the HIV seroprevalence in the Rakai province was already high, at 14%, and therefore, the proportional impact of STD treatment would have been minimal. In contrast, the HIV prevalence in the successful Tanzanian study was 4%. Second, the prevalence of HSV type 2 seropositivity in the Rakai study population was more than 70%, nearly all genital ulcers were HSV-2 seropositive, and both HSV-2 seropositivity and herpes genital ulcer disease were associated with HIV seroconversion. The antimicrobial regimens used in this study would have had no impact on HSV-2 genital ulcer disease. Furthermore, data from the Rakai study have been invaluable in defining the relationship between plasma viral load and HIV transmission (184), in demonstrating the increased risk of acquisition and transmission in relationships in which the male partner is uncircumcised (221), and in demonstrating the efficacy of condom use in HIV-discordant couples (101).

IMPLEMENTING SEXUALLY TRANSMITTED DISEASE INTERVENTIONS IN FIELD SETTINGS

STD screening tests have been developed that use deoxyribonucleic acid (DNA) amplification technology and that can diagnose gonococcal and chlamydial infection in urine, eliminating the need for invasive procedures and examinations. STD treatment protocols have been developed with a focus on single-dose oral regimens (222). These developments have simplified STD clinical management in the primary care setting. STD control therefore needs to be incorporated as an integral part of HIV prevention efforts. Effective integrated STD/HIV control efforts require the following:

1. Implementation of an effective HIV and STD screening strategy to populations at high risk.
2. HIV counseling and testing offered to individuals evaluated for STD.
3. Rapid access to STD diagnosis and treatment.
4. Effective integration of STD diagnosis and treatment facilities with other components of the medical care system.

PREVENTION ISSUES SPECIFIC TO WOMEN

Women are at higher risk for HIV and STD transmission for both biologic and behavioral factors. During unprotected intercourse, women are potentially exposed to a higher viral inoculum (through ejaculation) than their male partners. Changes in the vaginal and cervical mucosa through inflammation or hormonally induced changes can increase the tissue's friability and therefore its ability to act as a conduit to the host's vasculature. Inflammation occurs most frequently in the setting of lower reproductive tract infection. Hormonal contraceptives, including oral contraceptives, cause an increased proliferation of columnar epithelium in the cervix (ectropion), which is more friable. Hormonal contraceptives have been epidemiologically associated with increased risk of HIV transmission, which coincidentally causes a major policy dilemma in developing countries where overpopulation and the HIV epidemic coexist.

Nevertheless, women are at significant risk. In many sexual relationships, women may not be able to refuse sexual relations or may not be able to require their male partner to use a condom because of either economic circumstance or fear of physical and/or emotional abuse (223,224). For example, CSWs may be at an economic disadvantage if the client's preference is for unprotected intercourse. These issues have intensified the need to develop female-controlled disease-prevention methods.

Female Condoms

Female condoms are one approach and have been approved in the United States since 1993. The female condom is essentially a double-ring latex pouch, with one ring adjacent to the cervix and the other to the introitus, that is inserted before intercourse (225). Evaluations of the device have been mixed. Cost is the major barrier to its increased use, with the per-device cost ranging from $2 to $3 a piece in the United States. Studies of female condom acceptability have found that training in its use is required and that acceptability is higher in women who have previously used intravaginal devices such as tampons (226).

Vaginal Microbicides

Vaginal microbicide methods should demonstrate physical and chemical stability in the vaginal environment, allowing insertion some time before intercourse, should not interfere with sexual intercourse, and should be inexpensive (227). The ideal compound would be cidal to bacterial and viral pathogens while being nontoxic to the host epithelium. Besides the potential toxicity to host epithelium, another consideration is the potential effect on the commensal vaginal microflora and the consequent BV and inflammation. To date, vaginal microbicides have been chemical detergents that are water soluble and can solubilize the lipid membranes of bacteria and spermatozoa, and nonoxynol-9 was the prototype.

Carefully controlled trials of nonoxynol-9 film and gel formulations in developing country settings found that the microbicide-condom arm was associated with higher STD rates than condom control arms (228–231). These were not CSW populations, and the gel actually contained less nonoxynol-9 than in previous studies that used the intravaginal sponge. Even more concerning were studies in West Africa, of 892 CSWs, which found that in women who used nonoxynol-9 more than three times per day, their risk of HIV was doubled. No effect was shown in the women who were occasional users (232). In retrospect and with careful examination, the problem appears to be that nonoxynol-9, chemically a detergent, caused cervical and vaginal microerosions, independent of the presence of STDs (233) and caused profound changes in the vaginal microflora, especially lactobacilli (234). There are a large number of other microbicide candidates in clinical trials, but none has yet been approved for clinical use. Microbicides under development are targeting three potential mechanisms for HIV/STD prevention (235):

- Killing or disabling the pathogen (e.g., surfactants, pH buffers, antibody approaches)
- Preventing attachment of the pathogen to host cell membrane (e.g., peptides and sulfated polysaccharides)
- Preventing pathogenesis after the pathogen has passed the cell membrane, such as anti-HIV drug approaches incorporated into microbicides

There has therefore been increased research interest in developing chemically stable, buffered, nonionic compounds that could be potentially used as vaginal microbicides. Current experimental approaches have included organic polymers, dextran congeners, and incorporation of reverse-transcriptase inhibitors into a biologically inert matrix.

Market survey studies of broad groups of women have found that microbicides would be popular and marketable. Based on a national survey conducted in the mid-1990s, an estimated 21.3 million U.S. women have some potential current interest in using a microbicidal product. Depending on product specifications and cost, as many as 6 million women who are worried about getting an STD would be very interested in current use of a microbicide. These women are most likely to be unmarried and not cohabiting, of low income and less education, and black or Hispanic. They also are more likely to have visited a doctor for STD symptoms or to have reduced their sexual activity because of STDs, to have a partner who had other partners in the past year, to have no steady partner, or to have ever used condoms for STD prevention (236).

HUMAN IMMUNODEFICIENCY VIRUS TRANSMISSION AND CONTRACEPTION

There is an evolving debate over the potential role of hormonal contraception in facilitating HIV transmission. Studies in cohorts in East Africa have demonstrated that women using hormonal contraception are at threefold to fourfold higher risk for HIV acquisition (237–240). Risks are higher in women who are taking progesterone-only injectable contraceptive, who have lower CD4 cell counts, and who have vitamin A deficiencies. This association, however, has been criticized as being confounded by study design issues, and because many of the cohorts studied were sex workers (241). This issue is not yet resolved but would have a tremendous public health impact because many of the areas with highest HIV incidence, such as East Africa, also have unsustainable fertility rates. From a programmatic standpoint, it therefore becomes imperative to stress the utility and feasibility of dual-use methods (e.g., hormonal contraception plus condom use) for contraception and disease prevention.

ESTABLISHMENT OF COMPREHENSIVE HUMAN IMMUNODEFICIENCY VIRUS PREVENTION PROGRAMS

Primary care providers have the opportunity to counsel patients at risk of HIV infection through a large variety of interactions, and HIV testing and counseling has been recommended for pregnant women and all individuals who are homosexual, drug users, or heterosexual with multiple partners (242). Overall, patients feel more comfortable discussing HIV and sexual issues with their physicians than with other individuals (243). Surveys have shown that physicians offer HIV counseling to more than 90% of homosexual men or drug users but offer HIV counseling to only two thirds of heterosexuals with multiple partners and less than half of non-IDUs or sexually active adolescents. Provider education interventions using interactive formats have been found to increase both providers' comfort level in addressing sensitive behavioral issues and increased the compliance with STD and HIV screening recommendations.

One of the impediments to extensive implementation of effective HIV prevention programs within traditional health care settings is time and reimbursement. Effective HIV intervention requires education, counseling, trust, and intensive behavioral intervention, little of which is reimbursable under current payment schemes. This issue will pose a major challenge to the health care system, especially because the financial expense alone of HIV infections is extraordinarily high.

On a community-wide basis, developing and maintaining a comprehensive HIV prevention program necessitates a multidisciplinary approach. From the policy perspective, identification of target populations, behaviors, and defining outcome indicators is an important program component. For example an intervention in a developing country would focus predominantly on heterosexual transmission and STD treatment, whereas in the United States and western Europe, intervention needs of IDUs and homosexual men must be addressed. Guidance in developing large-scale intervention programs has been developed by the World Health Organization (244) and the CDC (245), which can be used to assess program effectiveness while being flexible enough to be adapted to a large variety of operating environments. These program effectiveness guidelines encompass aspects of epidemiologic surveillance, risk assessment, STD and drug treatment, risk reduction, and behavioral intervention—the critical components of effective prevention of HIV infection.

Tailoring the Program to Local Needs

Programmatic approaches to HIV prevention need to account for local epidemic characteristics, intervening factors such as drug use, and local health resources. There are stark differences in needs and planning priorities for developing and developed countries, as well as for specific risk communities within each environment.

In developing countries, HIV intervention approaches need to take into account the health care infrastructure and traditional social attitudes toward sexuality and medical care (246). In most developing country settings, the primary transmission mode is heterosexual, and HIV is often associated with occupations with increased mobility, such as truck drivers or migratory mine workers. Individual-based prevention approaches usually emphasize reducing risky heterosexual behaviors, providing diagnostic and treatment services for STDs, and increasing condom use. Medical interventions emphasize protecting the blood supply and providing prenatal screening and perinatal treatment in areas that do not yet have these services. Successful structural interventions have included regulation of commercial sex, improving the health care infrastructure, political commitment to HIV prevention at all levels of government, and reducing stigma.

In developed countries, the priorities are often different (247,248). The health infrastructures are developed. Personal interventions should be focused on homosexual men and high-risk heterosexuals to reduce risky sexual partnerships and increase condom use. Structural interventions require providing access to drug-abuse prevention and treatment services, including injection equipment. In both settings, providing support for continued maintenance of prevention efforts is a key component. As recent features of the epidemic demonstrate, HIV prevention is an ongoing process that is very akin to that of a chronic disease model and prone to relapse and remission.

REFERENCES

1. Des Jarlais D, Semaan S. HIV prevention research: cumulative knowledge or accumulating studies? An introduction to the HIV/AIDS prevention research synthesis project supplement. *J Acquir Immune Defic Syndr* 2002;30[Suppl 1]: S1–S7.
2. Sumartojo E. Structural factors in HIV prevention: concepts, examples, and implications for research. *AIDS* 2000;14[Suppl 1]:S3–S10.
3. Parker RG, Easton D, Klein CH. Structural barriers and facilitators in HIV prevention: a review of international research. *AIDS* 2000;14[Suppl 1]:S22–S32.
4. HIV and AIDS—United States, 1981–2000. *MMWR Morb Mortal Wkly Rep* 2001; 50(21):430–434.
5. First 500,000 AIDS cases—United States, 1995. *MMWR Morb Mortal Wkly Rep* 1995;44(46):849–853.
6. Diagnosis and reporting of HIV and AIDS in states with HIV/AIDS surveillance—United States, 1994–2000. *MMWR Morb Mortal Wkly Rep* 2002; 51(27):595–598.
7. HIV/AIDS among racial/ethnic minority men who have sex with men—United States, 1989–1998. *MMWR Morb Mortal Wkly Rep* 2000;49(1):4–11.
8. Fox KK, del Rio C, Holmes KK, et al. Gonorrhea in the HIV era: a reversal in trends among men who have sex with men. *Am J Public Health* 2001;91(6):959–964.
9. Centers for Disease Control and Prevention. Increases in unsafe sex and rectal gonorrhea among men who have sex with men—San Francisco, California, 1994–1997. *JAMA* 1999;281(8):696–697.
10. Trends in gonorrhea in homosexually active men—King County, Washington, 1989. *MMWR Morb Mortal Wkly Rep* 1989;38(44):762–764.
11. Stolte IG, Dukers NH, de Wit JB, et al. Increase in sexually transmitted infections among homosexual men in Amsterdam in relation to HAART. *Sex Transm Infect* 2001;77(3):184–186.
12. Hopkins S, Lyons F, Mulcahy F, et al. The great pretender returns to Dublin, Ireland. *Sex Transm Infect* 2001;77(5):316–318.
13. Poulton M, Dean GL, Williams DI, et al. Surfing with spirochetes: an ongoing syphilis outbreak in Brighton. *Sex Transm Infect* 2001;77(5):319–321.
14. Halsos AM, Edgardh K. An outbreak of syphilis in Oslo. *Int J STD AIDS* 2002;13(6):370–372.
15. Whittington WL, Collis T, Dithmer-Schreck D, et al. Sexually transmitted diseases and human immunodeficiency virus-discordant partnerships among men who have sex with men. *Clin Infect Dis* 2002;35(8):1010–1017.
16. Primary and secondary syphilis among men who have sex with men—New York City, 2001. *MMWR Morb Mortal Wkly Rep* 2002;51(38):853–856.
17. Dupin N, Jdid R, N'Guyen YT, Gorin I, et al. Syphilis and gonorrhea in Paris: the return. *AIDS* 2001;15(6):814–815.
18. Vrielink H, Reesink HW. Transfusion-transmissible infections. *Curr Opin Hematol* 1998;5(6):396–405.
19. Schreiber GB, Busch MP, Kleinman SH, et al. The risk of transfusion-transmitted viral infections. The Retrovirus Epidemiology Donor Study. *N Engl J Med* 1996;334(26):1685–1690.
20. Minkoff H. Prevention of mother-to-child transmission of HIV. *Clin Obstet Gynecol* 2001;44(2):210–225.
21. Peckham C, Gibb D. Mother-to-child transmission of the human immunodeficiency virus. *N Engl J Med* 1995;333(5):298–302.
22. Dunn DT, Newell ML, Ades AE, et al. Risk of human immunodeficiency virus type 1 transmission through breastfeeding. *Lancet* 1992;340(8819):585–588.
23. St Louis ME, Kamenga M, Brown C, et al. Risk for perinatal HIV-1 transmission according to maternal immunologic, virologic, and placental factors. *JAMA* 1993;269(22):2853–2859.
24. Hart CE, Lennox JL, Pratt-Palmore M, et al. Correlation of human immunodeficiency virus type 1 RNA levels in blood and the female genital tract. *J Infect Dis* 1999;179(4):871–882.
25. Ryder RW, Nsa W, Hassig SE, et al. Perinatal transmission of the human immunodeficiency virus type 1 to infants of seropositive women in Zaire. *N Engl J Med* 1989;320(25):1637–1642.
26. Blanche S, Rouzioux C, Moscato ML, et al. A prospective study of infants born to women seropositive for human immunodeficiency virus type 1. HIV Infection in Newborns French Collaborative Study Group. *N Engl J Med* 1989; 320(25):1643–1648.
27. Risk factors for mother-to-child transmission of HIV-1. European Collaborative Study. *Lancet* 1992;339(8800):1007–1012.
28. Datta P, Embree JE, Kreiss JK, et al. Mother-to-child transmission of human immunodeficiency virus type 1: report from the Nairobi Study. *J Infect Dis* 1994;170(5):1134–1140.
29. Landesman SH, Kalish LA, Burns DN, et al. Obstetrical factors and the transmission of human immunodeficiency virus type 1 from mother to child. The Women and Infants Transmission Study. *N Engl J Med* 1996;334(25):1617–1623.
30. Mayaux MJ, Blanche S, Rouzioux C, et al. Maternal factors associated with perinatal HIV-1 transmission: the French Cohort Study: 7 years of follow-up observation. The French Pediatric HIV Infection Study Group. *J Acquir Immune Defic Syndr Hum Retrovirol* 1995;8(2):188–194.
31. The mode of delivery and the risk of vertical transmission of human immunodeficiency virus type 1—a meta-analysis of 15 prospective cohort studies. The International Perinatal HIV Group. *N Engl J Med* 1999;340(13):977–987.
32. Connor EM, Sperling RS, Gelber R, et al. Reduction of maternal-infant transmission of human immunodeficiency virus type 1 with zidovudine treatment. Pediatric AIDS Clinical Trials Group Protocol 076 Study Group. *N Engl J Med* 1994;331(18):1173–1180.
33. Guay LA, Musoke P, Fleming T, et al. Intrapartum and neonatal single-dose nevirapine compared with zidovudine for prevention of mother-to-child transmission of HIV-1 in Kampala, Uganda: HIVNET 012 randomised trial. *Lancet* 1999;354(9181):795–802.
34. Dorenbaum A, Cunningham CK, Gelber RD, et al. Two-dose intrapartum/newborn nevirapine and standard antiretroviral therapy to reduce perinatal HIV transmission: a randomized trial. *JAMA* 2002;288(2):189–198.
35. Wiznia AA, Crane M, Lambert G. Zidovudine use to reduce perinatal HIV type 1 transmission in an urban medical center. *JAMA* 1996;275(19):1504–1506.
36. Fiscus SA, Adimora AA, Schoenbach VJ, et al. Perinatal HIV infection and

the effect of zidovudine therapy on transmission in rural and urban counties. *JAMA* 1996;275(19):1483–1488.

37. Revised recommendations for HIV screening of pregnant women. *MMWR Recomm Rep* 2001;50(RR-19):63–85.

38. Van de PP, Simonon A, Msellati P, et al. Postnatal transmission of human immunodeficiency virus type 1 from mother to infant. A prospective cohort study in Kigali, Rwanda. *N Engl J Med* 1991;325(9):593–598.

39. HIV testing among pregnant women—United States and Canada, 1998–2001. *MMWR Morb Mortal Wkly Rep* 2002;51(45):1013–1016.

40. FCenters for Disease Control and Prevention. Progress toward elimination of perinatal HIV infection—Michigan, 1993–2000. *MMWR Morb Mortal Wkly Rep* 2002;51(5):93–97.

41. Kanshana S, Simonds RJ. National program for preventing mother-child HIV transmission in Thailand: successful implementation and lessons learned. *AIDS* 2002;16(7):953–959.

42. Desmond NM, Coker RJ. Should preventive antiretroviral treatment be offered following sexual exposure to HIV? The case for. *Sex Transm Infect* 1998;74(2):144–145.

43. Evans B, Darbyshire J, Cartledge J. Should preventive antiretroviral treatment be offered following sexual exposure to HIV? Not yet! *Sex Transm Infect* 1998;74(2):146–148.

44. Gerberding JL, Katz MH. Post-exposure prophylaxis for HIV. *Adv Exp Med Biol* 1999;458:213–222.

45. Henderson DK. HIV postexposure prophylaxis in the 21st century. *Emerg Infect Dis* 2001;7(2):254–258.

46. Lurie P, Miller S, Hecht F, et al. Postexposure prophylaxis after nonoccupational HIV exposure: clinical, ethical, and policy considerations. *JAMA* 1998;280(20):1769–1773.

47. Auerbach JD, Coates TJ. HIV prevention research: accomplishments and challenges for the third decade of AIDS. *Am J Public Health* 2000;90(7):1029–1032.

48. Elwy AR, Hart GJ, Hawkes S, et al. Effectiveness of interventions to prevent sexually transmitted infections and human immunodeficiency virus in heterosexual men: a systematic review. *Arch Intern Med* 2002;162(16):1818–1830.

49. Kelly JA, Kalichman SC. Behavioral research in HIV/AIDS primary and secondary prevention: recent advances and future directions. *J Consult Clin Psychol* 2002;70(3):626–639.

50. Auerbach JD, Wypijewska C, Brodie HKH. *AIDS and behavior—an integrated approach.* Washington: National Academy Press, 1994.

51. Anderson JE, Wilson R, Doll L, et al. Condom use and HIV risk behaviors among U.S. adults: data from a national survey. *Fam Plann Perspect* 1999;31(1):24–28.

52. Anderson JE, Dahlberg LL. High-risk sexual behavior in the general population. Results from a national survey, 1988–1990. *Sex Transm Dis* 1992;19(6):320–325.

53. Laumann EO, Gagnon J, Michael RT, et al. *The social organization of sexuality.* Chicago: University of Chicago Press, 1994.

54. Kost K, Forrest JD. American women's sexual behavior and exposure to risk of sexually transmitted diseases. *Fam Plann Perspect* 1992;24(6):244–254.

55. Bankole A, Darroch JE, Singh S. Determinants of trends in condom use in the United States, 1988–1995. *Fam Plann Perspect* 1999;31(6):264–271.

56. Ku L, Sonenstein FL, Pleck JH. Young men's risk behaviors for HIV infection and sexually transmitted diseases, 1988 through 1991. *Am J Public Health* 1993;83(11):1609–1615.

57. Ku L, Sonenstein FL, Lindberg LD, et al. Understanding changes in sexual activity among young metropolitan men: 1979–1995. *Fam Plann Perspect* 1998;30(6):256–262.

58. Sonenstein FL, Ku L, Lindberg LD, et al. Changes in sexual behavior and condom use among teenaged males: 1988 to 1995. *Am J Public Health* 1998;88(6):956–959.

59. Trends in sexual risk behaviors among high school students—United States, 1991–2001. *MMWR Morb Mortal Wkly Rep* 2002;51(38):856–859.

60. Peipert JF, Domagalski L, Boardman L, et al. Sexual behavior and contraceptive use. Changes from 1975 to 1995 in college women. *J Reprod Med* 1997;42(10):651–657.

61. Peipert JF, Domagalski L, Boardman L, et al. College women and condom use, 1975–1995. *N Engl J Med* 1996;335(3):211.

62. Catania JA, Canchola J, Binson D, et al. National trends in condom use among at-risk heterosexuals in the united states. *J Acquir Immune Defic Syndr* 2001;27(2):176–182.

63. Prevalence of risk behaviors for HIV infection among adults—United States, 1997. *MMWR Morb Mortal Wkly Rep* 2001;50(14):262–265.

64. Unrecognized HIV infection, risk behaviors, and perceptions of risk among young black men who have sex with men—six U.S. cities, 1994–1998. *MMWR Morb Mortal Wkly Rep* 2002;51(33):733–736.

65. DiClemente RJ, Peterson JL (eds). *Preventing AIDS. Theories and methods of behavioral interventions.* New York: Plenum Press, 1994.

66. Catania JA, Kegeles SM, Coates TJ. Towards an understanding of risk behavior: an AIDS risk reduction model (ARRM). *Health Educ Q* 1990;17(1):53–72.

67. Fishbein M. The role of theory in HIV prevention. *AIDS Care* 2000;12(3):273–278.

68. Murphy DA, Stein JA, Schlenger W, et al. Conceptualizing the multidimensional nature of self-efficacy: assessment of situational context and level of behavioral challenge to maintain safer sex. National Institute of Mental Health Multisite HIV Prevention Trial Group. *Health Psychol* 2001;20(4):281–290.

69. Kelly JA, Murphy DA, Sikkema KJ, et al. Randomised, controlled, community-level HIV-prevention intervention for sexual-risk behaviour among homosexual men in US cities. Community HIV Prevention Research Collaborative. *Lancet* 1997;350(9090):1500–1505.

70. Kelly JA, St Lawrence JS, Diaz YE, et al. HIV risk behavior reduction following intervention with key opinion leaders of population: an experimental analysis. *Am J Public Health* 1991;81(2):168–171.

71. O'Campo P, Fogarty L, Gielen AC, et al. Distribution along a stages-of-behavioral-change continuum for condom and contraceptive use among women accessed in different settings. Prevention of HIV in Women and Infants Demonstration Projects. *J Community Health* 1999;24(1):61–72.

72. Prochaska JO, DiClemente CC, Norcross JC. In search of how people change. Applications to addictive behaviors. *Am Psychol* 1992;47(9):1102–1114.

73. Catania JA, Gibson DR, Chitwood DD, et al. Methodological problems in AIDS behavioral research: influences on measurement error and participation bias in studies of sexual behavior. *Psychol Bull* 1990;108(3):339–362.

74. Gottlieb BH. Social networks and social support: an overview of research, practice, and policy implications. *Health Educ Q* 1985;12(1):5–22.

75. Rothenberg RB, Potterat JJ, Woodhouse DE, et al. Social network dynamics and HIV transmission. *AIDS* 1998;12(12):1529–1536.

76. Klovdahl AS, Potterat JJ, Woodhouse DE, et al. Social networks and infectious disease: the Colorado Springs Study. *Soc Sci Med* 1994;38(1):79–88.

77. Laumann EO, Gagnon JH, Michaels S, et al. Monitoring AIDS and other rare population events: a network approach. *J Health Soc Behav* 1993;34(1):7–22.

78. Friedman SR, Des J, Sotheran JL, et al. AIDS and self-organization among intravenous drug users. *Int J Addict* 1987;22(3):201–219.

79. Dowsett GW. Sustaining safe sex: sexual practices, HIV and social context. *AIDS* 1993;7[Suppl 1]:S257–S262.

80. Rothenberg R, Narramore J. The relevance of social network concepts to sexually transmitted disease control. *Sex Transm Dis* 1996;23(1):24–29.

81. Cluster of HIV-infected adolescents and young adults—Mississippi, 1999. *MMWR Morb Mortal Wkly Rep* 2000;49(38):861–864.

82. Garnett GP. The basic reproductive rate of infection and the course of HIV epidemics. *AIDS Patient Care STDS* 1998;12(6):435–449.

83. Friedman SR, Neaigus A, Jose B, et al. Sociometric risk networks and risk for HIV infection. *Am J Public Health* 1997;87(8):1289–1296.

84. Morris M, Podhisita C, Wawer MJ, et al. Bridge populations in the spread of HIV/AIDS in Thailand. *AIDS* 1996;10(11):1265–1271.

85. Morris M, Kretzschmar M. Concurrent partnerships and the spread of HIV. *AIDS* 1997;11(5):641–648.

86. Service S, Blower SM. HIV transmission in sexual networks: an empirical analysis. *Proc R Soc Lond B Biol Sci* 1995;260(1359):237–244.

87. Friedman SR, Kottiri BJ, Neaigus A, et al. Network-related mechanisms may help explain long-term HIV-1 seroprevalence levels that remain high but do not approach population-group saturation. *Am J Epidemiol* 2000;152(10):913–922.

88. Hospers HJ, Harterink P, Van Den HK, et al. Chatters on the Internet: a special target group for HIV prevention. *AIDS Care* 2002;14(4):539–544.

89. Elford J, Bolding G, Sherr L. Seeking sex on the Internet and sexual risk behaviour among gay men using London gyms. *AIDS* 2001;15(11):1409–1415.

90. Bull SS, McFarlane M. Soliciting sex on the Internet: what are the risks for sexually transmitted diseases and HIV? *Sex Transm Dis* 2000;27(9):545–550.

91. Klausner JD, Wolf W, Fischer-Ponce L, et al. Tracing a syphilis outbreak through cyberspace. *JAMA* 2000;284(4):447–449.

92. McFarlane M, Bull SS, Rietmeijer CA. The Internet as a newly emerging risk environment for sexually transmitted diseases. *JAMA* 2000;284(4):443–446.

93. Padian NS, O'Brien TR, Chang Y, et al. Prevention of heterosexual transmission of human immunodeficiency virus through couple counseling. *J Acquir Immune Defic Syndr* 1993;6(9):1043–1048.

94. Saracco A, Musicco M, Nicolosi A, et al. Man-to-woman sexual transmission of HIV: longitudinal study of 343 steady partners of infected men. *J Acquir Immune Defic Syndr* 1993;6(5):497–502.

95. de V, I. A longitudinal study of human immunodeficiency virus transmission by heterosexual partners. European Study Group on Heterosexual Transmission of HIV. *N Engl J Med* 1994;331(6):341–346.

96. Davis KR, Weller SC. The effectiveness of condoms in reducing heterosexual transmission of HIV. *Fam Plann Perspect* 1999;31(6):272–279.

97. Pinkerton SD, Abramson PR. Effectiveness of condoms in preventing HIV transmission. *Soc Sci Med* 1997;44(9):1303–1312.

98. Weller S, Davis K. Condom effectiveness in reducing heterosexual HIV transmission. *Cochrane Database Syst Rev* 2002;(1):CD003255.

99. Davis KR, Weller SC. The effectiveness of condoms in reducing heterosexual transmission of HIV. *Fam Plann Perspect* 1999;31(6):272–279.

100. Wald A, Langenberg AG, Link K, et al. Effect of condoms on reducing the transmission of herpes simplex virus type 2 from men to women. *JAMA* 2001;285(24):3100–3106.

101. Ahmed S, Lutalo T, Wawer M, et al. HIV incidence and sexually transmitted disease prevalence associated with condom use: a population study in Rakai, Uganda. *AIDS* 2001;15(16):2171–2179.

102. Orr DP, Langefeld CD. Factors associated with condom use by sexually active male adolescents at risk for sexually transmitted disease. *Pediatrics* 1993;91(5):873–879.

103. Cohen DA, Dent C, MacKinnon D, et al. Condoms for men, not women. Results of brief promotion programs. *Sex Transm Dis* 1992;19(5):245–251.

104. Ku LC, Sonenstein FL, Pleck JH. The association of AIDS education and sex education with sexual behavior and condom use among teenage men. *Fam Plann Perspect* 1992;24(3):100–106.

105. Sellers DE, McGraw SA, McKinlay JB. Does the promotion and distribution of condoms increase teen sexual activity? Evidence from an HIV prevention program for Latino youth. *Am J Public Health* 1994;84(12):1952–1959.

106. Rojanapithayakorn W, Hanenberg R. The 100% condom program in Thailand. *AIDS* 1996;10(1):1–7.

107. Nelson KE, Celentano DD, Eiumtrakol S, et al. Changes in sexual behavior and a decline in HIV infection among young men in Thailand. *N Engl J Med* 1996;335(5):297–303.

108. Walter HJ, Vaughan RD. AIDS risk reduction among a multiethnic sample of urban high school students. *JAMA* 1993;270(6):725–730.

109. Sexual risk behaviors of STD clinic patients before and after Earvin "Magic" Johnson's HIV-infection announcement—Maryland, 1991–1992. *MMWR Morb Mortal Wkly Rep* 1993;42(3):45–48.

110. Peterson JL, Coates TJ, Catania J, et al. Evaluation of an HIV risk reduction intervention among African-American homosexual and bisexual men. *AIDS* 1996;10(3):319–325.

111. DiClemente RJ, Wingood GM. A randomized controlled trial of an HIV sexual risk-reduction intervention for young African-American women. *JAMA* 1995;274(16):1271–1276.

112. Kelly JA, Murphy DA, Washington CD, et al. The effects of HIV/AIDS intervention groups for high-risk women in urban clinics. *Am J Public Health* 1994;84(12):1918–1922.

113. Jemmott JB III, Jemmott LS, Fong GT. Abstinence and safer sex HIV risk-reduction interventions for African American adolescents: a randomized controlled trial. *JAMA* 1998;279(19):1529–1536.

114. Jemmott JB III, Jemmott LS, Fong GT, et al. Reducing HIV risk-associated sexual behavior among African American adolescents: testing the generality of intervention effects. *Am J Community Psychol* 1999;27(2):161–187.

115. Jemmott JB III, Jemmott LS, Fong GT. Reductions in HIV risk-associated sexual behaviors among black male adolescents: effects of an AIDS prevention intervention. *Am J Public Health* 1992;82(3):372–377.

116. Zenilman JM, Weisman CS, Rompalo AM, et al. Condom use to prevent incident STDs: the validity of self-reported condom use. *Sex Transm Dis* 1995;22(1):15–21.

117. The NIMH Multisite HIV Prevention Trial: reducing HIV sexual risk behavior. The National Institute of Mental Health (NIMH) Multisite HIV Prevention Trial Group. *Science* 1998;280(5371):1889–1894.

118. Kamb ML, Fishbein M, Douglas JM Jr, et al. Efficacy of risk-reduction counseling to prevent human immunodeficiency virus and sexually transmitted diseases: a randomized controlled trial. Project RESPECT Study Group. *JAMA* 1998;280(13):1161–1167.

119. Jemmott JB III, Jemmott LS, Fong GT. Abstinence and safer sex HIV risk-reduction interventions for African American adolescents: a randomized controlled trial. *JAMA* 1998;279(19):1529–1536.

120. Shain RN, Piper JM, Newton ER, et al. A randomized, controlled trial of a behavioral intervention to prevent sexually transmitted disease among minority women. *N Engl J Med* 1999;340(2):93–100.

121. Steiner M, Trussell J, Glover L, et al. Standardized protocols for condom breakage and slippage trials: a proposal. *Am J Public Health* 1994;84(12):1897–1900.

122. Richters J, Donovan B, Gerofi J. How often do condoms break or slip off in use? *Int J STD AIDS* 1993;4(2):90–94.

123. Rugpao S, Beyrer C, Tovanabutra S, et al. Multiple condom use and decreased condom breakage and slippage in Thailand. *J Acquir Immune Defic Syndr Hum Retrovirol* 1997;14(2):169–173.

124. Lindberg LD, Sonenstein FL, Ku L, et al. Young men's experience with condom breakage. *Fam Plann Perspect* 1997;29(3):128–131, 140.

125. Albert AE, Warner DL, Hatcher RA, et al. Condom use among female commercial sex workers in Nevada's legal brothels. *Am J Public Health* 1995;85(11):1514–1520.

126. Macaluso M, Kelaghan J, Artz L, et al. Mechanical failure of the latex condom in a cohort of women at high STD risk. *Sex Transm Dis* 1999;26(8):450–458.

127. Carballo-Dieguez A, Dolezal C. HIV risk behaviors and obstacles to condom use among Puerto Rican men in New York City who have sex with men. *Am J Public Health* 1996;86(11):1619–1622.

128. Lyketsos CG, Hutton H, Fishman M, et al. Psychiatric morbidity on entry to an HIV primary care clinic. *AIDS* 1996;10(9):1033–1039.

129. Erbelding EJ, Hummel B, Hogan T, et al. High rates of depressive symptoms in STD clinic patients. *Sex Transm Dis* 2001;28(5):281–284.

130. Siegel K, Mesagno FP, Chen JY, et al. Factors distinguishing homosexual males practicing risky and safer sex. *Soc Sci Med* 1989;28(6):561–569.

131. Ekstrand ML, Coates TJ. Maintenance of safer sexual behaviors and predictors of risky sex: the San Francisco Men's Health Study. *Am J Public Health* 1990;80(8):973–977.

132. Shafer MA, Hilton JF, Ekstrand M, et al. Relationship between drug use and sexual behaviors and the occurrence of sexually transmitted diseases among high-risk male youth. *Sex Transm Dis* 1993;20(6):307–313.

133. Weinstock HS, Lindan C, Bolan G, et al. Factors associated with condom use in a high-risk heterosexual population. *Sex Transm Dis* 1993;20(1):14–20.

134. Wingood GM, DiClemente RJ. The influence of psychosocial factors, alcohol, drug use on African-American women's high-risk sexual behavior. *Am J Prev Med* 1998;15(1):54–59.

135. Nopkesorn T, Mock PA, Mastro TD, et al. HIV-1 subtype E incidence and sexually transmitted diseases in a cohort of military conscripts in northern Thailand. *J Acquir Immune Defic Syndr Hum Retrovirol* 1998;18(4):372–379.

136. Celentano DD, Bond KC, Lyles CM, et al. Preventive intervention to reduce sexually transmitted infections: a field trial in the Royal Thai Army. *Arch Intern Med* 2000;160(4):535–540.

137. Chitwood DD, Griffin DK, Comerford M, et al. Risk factors for HIV-1 seroconversion among injection drug users: a case-control study. *Am J Public Health* 1995;85(11):1538–1542.

138. Schoenbaum EE, Hartel D, Selwyn PA, et al. Risk factors for human immunodeficiency virus infection in intravenous drug users. *N Engl J Med* 1989;321(13):874–879.

139. Vlahov D, Munoz A, Anthony JC, et al. Association of drug injection patterns with antibody to human immunodeficiency virus type 1 among intravenous drug users in Baltimore, Maryland. *Am J Epidemiol* 1990;132(5):847–856.

140. Lehman JS, Allen DM, Green TA, et al. HIV infection among non-injecting drug users entering drug treatment, United States, 1989–1992. Field Services Branch. *AIDS* 1994;8(10):1465–1469.

141. Selwyn PA, Schoenbaum EE, Davenny K, et al. Prospective study of human immunodeficiency virus infection and pregnancy outcomes in intravenous drug users. *JAMA* 1989;261(9):1289–1294.

142. Watkins KE, Metzger D, Woody G, et al. Determinants of condom use among intravenous drug users. *AIDS* 1993;7(5):719–723.

143. Des J, Friedman SR, Friedmann P, et al. HIV/AIDS-related behavior change among injecting drug users in different national settings. *AIDS* 1995;9(6):611–617.

144. Sanchez J, Comerford M, Chitwood DD, et al. High risk sexual behaviours among heroin sniffers who have no history of injection drug use: implications for HIV risk reduction. *AIDS Care* 2002;14(3):391–398.

145. Minkoff HL, McCalla S, Delke I, et al. The relationship of cocaine use to syphilis and human immunodeficiency virus infections among inner city parturient women. *Am J Obstet Gynecol* 1990;163(2):521–526.

146. Chirgwin K, DeHovitz JA, Dillon S, et al. HIV infection, genital ulcer disease, and crack cocaine use among patients attending a clinic for sexually transmitted diseases. *Am J Public Health* 1991;81(12):1576–1579.

147. Telzak EE, Chiasson MA, Bevier PJ, et al. HIV-1 seroconversion in patients with and without genital ulcer disease. A prospective study. *Ann Intern Med* 1993;119(12):1181–1186.

148. Rothenberg RB, Long DM, Sterk CE, et al. The Atlanta Urban Networks Study: a blueprint for endemic transmission. *AIDS* 2000;14(14):2191–2200.

149. Jones DL, Irwin KL, Inciardi J, et al. The high-risk sexual practices of crack-smoking sex workers recruited from the streets of three American cities. The Multicenter Crack Cocaine and HIV Infection Study Team. *Sex Transm Dis* 1998;25(4):187–193.

150. Kalichman SC, Rompa D, Cage M. Sexually transmitted infections among HIV seropositive men and women. *Sex Transm Infect* 2000;76(5):350–354.

151. Campsmith ML, Nakashima AK, Jones JL. Association between crack cocaine use and high-risk sexual behaviors after HIV diagnosis. *J Acquir Immune Defic Syndr* 2000;25(2):192–198.

152. Wilson TE, Minkoff H, DeHovitz J, et al. The relationship of cocaine use and human immunodeficiency virus serostatus to incident sexually transmitted diseases among women. *Sex Transm Dis* 1998;25(2):70–75.

153. Gomez MP, Kimball AM, Orlander H, et al. Epidemic crack cocaine use linked with epidemics of genital ulcer disease and heterosexual HIV infection in the Bahamas: evidence of impact of prevention and control measures. *Sex Transm Dis* 2002;29(5):259–264.

154. Bauwens JE, Orlander H, Gomez MP, et al. Epidemic Lymphogranuloma venereum during epidemics of crack cocaine use and HIV infection in the Bahamas. *Sex Transm Dis* 2002;29(5):253–259.

155. Edlin BR, Irwin KL, Faruque S, et al. Intersecting epidemics—crack cocaine use and HIV infection among inner-city young adults. Multicenter Crack Cocaine and HIV Infection Study Team. *N Engl J Med* 1994;331(21):1422–1427.

156. *Preventing HIV infection—the role of sterile needles and bleach.* Washington: National Academy Press, 2003.

157. Des J, Hagan H, Friedman SR, et al. Maintaining low HIV seroprevalence in populations of injecting drug users. *JAMA* 1995;274(15):1226–1231.

158. Des J, Friedman SR, Perlis T, et al. Risk behavior and HIV infection among new drug injectors in the era of AIDS in New York City. *J Acquir Immune Defic Syndr Hum Retrovirol* 1999;20(1):67–72.

159. Des J, Marmor M, Friedmann P, et al. HIV incidence among injection drug users in New York City, 1992–1997: evidence for a declining epidemic. *Am J Public Health* 2000;90(3):352–359.

160. Friedman SR, Jose B, Deren S, et al. Risk factors for human immunodeficiency virus seroconversion among out-of-treatment drug injectors in high and low seroprevalence cities. The National AIDS Research Consortium. *Am J Epidemiol* 1995;142(8):864–874.

161. Knowledge and practices among injecting-drug users of bleach use for equipment disinfection—New York City, 1993. *MMWR Morb Mortal Wkly Rep* 1994;43(24):439, 445–439, 446.

162. Vlahov D, Des J, Goosby E, et al. Needle exchange programs for the prevention of human immunodeficiency virus infection: epidemiology and policy. *Am J Epidemiol* 2001;154(12)[Suppl]:S70–S77.

163. Nelson KE, Vlahov D, Cohn S, et al. Human immunodeficiency virus infection in diabetic intravenous drug users. *JAMA* 1991;266(16):2259–2261.

164. Watters JK, Estilo MJ, Clark GL, et al. Syringe and needle exchange as HIV/AIDS prevention for injection drug users. *JAMA* 1994;271(2):115–120.

165. Bastos FI, Strathdee SA. Evaluating effectiveness of syringe exchange programmes: current issues and future prospects. *Soc Sci Med* 2000;51(12):1771–1782.

166. Diaz T, Chu SY, Weinstein B, et al. Injection and syringe sharing among HIV-infected injection drug users: implications for prevention of HIV transmission. Supplement to HIV/AIDS Surveillance Group. *J Acquir Immune Defic Syndr Hum Retrovirol* 1998;18[Suppl 1]:S76–S81.

167. Gibson DR, Flynn NM, Perales D. Effectiveness of syringe exchange programs in reducing HIV risk behavior and HIV seroconversion among injecting drug users. *AIDS* 2001;15(11):1329–1341.

168. Needle RH, Coyle SL, Normand J, et al. HIV prevention with drug-using populations—current status and future prospects: introduction and overview. *Public Health Rep* 1998;113[Suppl 1]:4–18.

169. Kassler WJ, Alwano-Edyegu MG, Marum E, et al. Rapid HIV testing with same-day results: a field trial in Uganda. *Int J STD AIDS* 1998;9(3):134–138.

170. Kelen GD, Shahan JB, Quinn TC. Emergency department-based HIV screening and counseling: experience with rapid and standard serologic testing. *Ann Emerg Med* 1999;33(2):147–155.

171. Jones JL, Wykoff RF, Hollis SL, et al. Partner acceptance of health department notification of HIV exposure, South Carolina. *JAMA* 1990;264(10):1284–1286.

172. Wykoff RF, Jones JL, Longshore ST, et al. Notification of the sex and needle-sharing partners of individuals with human immunodeficiency virus in rural South Carolina: 30-month experience. *Sex Transm Dis* 1991;18(4):217–222.

173. Higgins DL, Galavotti C, O'Reilly KR, et al. Evidence for the effects of HIV antibody counseling and testing on risk behaviors. *JAMA* 1991;266(17):2419–2429.

174. Otten MW Jr, Zaidi AA, Wroten JE, et al. Changes in sexually transmitted disease rates after HIV testing and posttest counseling, Miami, 1988 to 1989. *Am J Public Health* 1993;83(4):529–533.

175. Zenilman JM, Erickson B, Fox R, et al. Effect of HIV posttest counseling on STD incidence. *JAMA* 1992;267(6):843–845.

176. Ickovics JR, Morrill AC, Beren SE, et al. Limited effects of HIV counseling and testing for women. A prospective study of behavioral and psychological consequences. *JAMA* 1994;272(6):443–448.

177. Berrios DC, Hearst N, Coates TJ, et al. HIV antibody testing among those at risk for infection. The National AIDS Behavioral Surveys. *JAMA* 1993;270(13):1576–1580.

178. Grinstead OA, Peterson JL, Faigeles B, et al. Antibody testing and condom use among heterosexual African Americans at risk for HIV infection: the National AIDS Behavioral Surveys. *Am J Public Health* 1997;87(5):857–859.

179. Golden MR, Rompalo AM, Fantry L, et al. Early intervention for human immunodeficiency virus in Baltimore Sexually Transmitted Diseases Clinics. Impact on gonorrhea incidence in patients infected with HIV. *Sex Transm Dis* 1996;23(5):370–377.

180. Wenger NS, Kusseling FS, Beck K, et al. Sexual behavior of individuals infected with the human immunodeficiency virus. The need for intervention. *Arch Intern Med* 1994;154(16):1849–1854.

181. Cleary PD, Van Devanter N, Steilen M, et al. A randomized trial of an education and support program for HIV-infected individuals. *AIDS* 1995;9(11):1271–1278.

182. Anderson RM, Gupta S, May RM. Potential of community-wide chemotherapy or immunotherapy to control the spread of HIV-1. *Nature* 1991;350(6316):356–359.

183. Sadiq ST, Taylor S, Kaye S, et al. The effects of antiretroviral therapy on HIV-1 RNA loads in seminal plasma in HIV-positive patients with and without urethritis. *AIDS* 2002;16(2):219–225.

184. Quinn TC, Wawer MJ, Sewankambo N, et al. Viral load and heterosexual transmission of human immunodeficiency virus type 1. Rakai Project Study Group. *N Engl J Med* 2000;342(13):921–929.

185. Vernazza PL, Gilliam BL, Flepp M, et al. Effect of antiviral treatment on the shedding of HIV-1 in semen. *AIDS* 1997;11(10):1249–1254.

186. Hosseinipour M, Cohen MS, Vernazza PL, et al. Can antiretroviral therapy be used to prevent sexual transmission of human immunodeficiency virus type 1? *Clin Infect Dis* 2002;34(10):1391–1395.

187. Francis DP, Anderson RE, Gorman ME, et al. Targeting AIDS prevention and treatment toward HIV-1–infected persons. The concept of early intervention. *JAMA* 1989;262(18):2572–2576.

188. Francis DP. Every person infected with HIV-1 should be in a lifelong early intervention program. *Sex Transm Dis* 1996;23(5):351–352.

189. Kalichman SC, Nachimson D, Cherry C, et al. AIDS treatment advances and behavioral prevention setbacks: preliminary assessment of reduced perceived threat of HIV-AIDS. *Health Psychol* 1998;17(6):546–550.

190. Kalichman SC, Schaper PE, Belcher L, et al. It's like a regular part of gay life: repeat HIV antibody testing among gay and bisexual men. *AIDS Educ Prev* 1997;9(3)[Suppl]:41–51.

191. Schwarcz SK, Kellogg TA, McFarland W, et al. Characterization of sexually transmitted disease clinic patients with recent human immunodeficiency virus infection. *J Infect Dis* 2002;186(7):1019–1022.

192. Janssen RS, Holtgrave DR, Valdiserri RO, et al. The Serostatus Approach to Fighting the HIV Epidemic: prevention strategies for infected individuals. *Am J Public Health* 2001;91(7):1019–1024.

193. Fleming DT, Wasserheit JN. From epidemiological synergy to public health policy and practice: the contribution of other sexually transmitted diseases to sexual transmission of HIV infection. *Sex Transm Infect* 1999;75(1):3–17.

194. Wasserheit JN. Epidemiological synergy. Interrelationships between human immunodeficiency virus infection and other sexually transmitted diseases. *Sex Transm Dis* 1992;19(2):61–77.

195. Royce RA, Sena A, Cates W Jr, et al. Sexual transmission of HIV. *N Engl J Med* 1997;336(15):1072–1078.

196. Vernazza PL, Eron JJ, Fiscus SA, et al. Sexual transmission of HIV: infectiousness and prevention. *AIDS* 1999;13(2):155–166.

197. Kreiss JK, Coombs R, Plummer F, et al. Isolation of human immunodeficiency virus from genital ulcers in Nairobi prostitutes. *J Infect Dis* 1989;160(3):380–384.

198. Kreiss J, Willerford DM, Hensel M, et al. Association between cervical inflammation and cervical shedding of human immunodeficiency virus DNA. *J Infect Dis* 1994;170(6):1597–1601.

199. Moss GB, Overbaugh J, Welch M, et al. Human immunodeficiency virus DNA in urethral secretions in men: association with gonococcal urethritis and CD4 cell depletion. *J Infect Dis* 1995;172(6):1469–1474.

200. Anzala AO, Simonsen JN, Kimani J, et al. Acute sexually transmitted infections increase human immunodeficiency virus type 1 plasma viremia, increase plasma type 2 cytokines, and decrease CD4 cell counts. *J Infect Dis* 2000;182(2):459–466.

201. Wald A, Link K. Risk of human immunodeficiency virus infection in herpes simplex virus type 2–seropositive persons: a meta-analysis. *J Infect Dis* 2002;185(1):45–52.

202. Mbopi-Keou FX, Gresenguet G, Mayaud P, et al. Interactions between herpes simplex virus type 2 and human immunodeficiency virus type 1 infection in African women: opportunities for intervention. *J Infect Dis* 2000;182(4):1090–1096.

203. Dickerson MC, Johnston J, Delea TE, et al. The causal role for genital ulcer disease as a risk factor for transmission of human immunodeficiency virus. An application of the Bradford Hill criteria. *Sex Transm Dis* 1996;23(5):429–440.

204. Quinn TC, Cannon RO, Glasser D, et al. The association of syphilis with risk of human immunodeficiency virus infection in patients attending sexually transmitted disease clinics. *Arch Intern Med* 1990;150(6):1297–1302.

205. Plourde PJ, Pepin J, Agoki E, et al. Human immunodeficiency virus type 1 seroconversion in women with genital ulcers. *J Infect Dis* 1994;170(2):313–317.

206. Plourde PJ, Plummer FA, Pepin J, et al. Human immunodeficiency virus type 1 infection in women attending a sexually transmitted diseases clinic in Kenya. *J Infect Dis* 1992;166(1):86–92.

207. Kassler WJ, Zenilman JM, Erickson B, et al. Seroconversion in patients attending sexually transmitted disease clinics. *AIDS* 1994;8(3):351–355.

208. Mehendale SM, Shepherd ME, Divekar AD, et al. Evidence for high prevalence & rapid transmission of HIV among individuals attending STD clinics in Pune, India. *Indian J Med Res* 1996;104:327–335.

209. Rodrigues JJ, Mehendale SM, Shepherd ME, et al. Risk factors for HIV infection in people attending clinics for sexually transmitted diseases in India. *BMJ* 1995;311(7000):283–286.

210. Celentano DD, Nelson KE, Suprasert S, et al. Risk factors for HIV-1 seroconversion among young men in northern Thailand. *JAMA* 1996;275(2):122–127.

211. Behets FM, Brathwaite AR, Hylton-Kong T, et al. Genital ulcers: etiology, clinical diagnosis, and associated human immunodeficiency virus infection in Kingston, Jamaica. *Clin Infect Dis* 1999;28(5):1086–1090.

212. Gadkari DA, Quinn TC, Gangakhedkar RR, et al. HIV-1 DNA shedding in genital ulcers and its associated risk factors in Pune, India. *J Acquir Immune Defic Syndr Hum Retrovirol* 1998;18(3):277–281.

213. Laga M, Manoka A, Kivuvu M, et al. Non-ulcerative sexually transmitted diseases as risk factors for HIV-1 transmission in women: results from a cohort study. *AIDS* 1993;7(1):95–102.

214. Sewankambo N, Gray RH, Wawer MJ, et al. HIV-1 infection associated with abnormal vaginal flora morphology and bacterial vaginosis. *Lancet* 1997;350(9077):546–550.

215. Taha TE, Gray RH, Kumwenda NI, et al. HIV infection and disturbances of vaginal flora during pregnancy. *J Acquir Immune Defic Syndr Hum Retrovirol* 1999;20(1):52–59.

216. Grosskurth H, Mosha F, Todd J, et al. A community trial of the impact of improved sexually transmitted disease treatment on the HIV epidemic in rural Tanzania: 2. Baseline survey results. *AIDS* 1995;9(8):927–934.

217. Hayes R, Mosha F, Nicoll A, et al. A community trial of the impact of improved sexually transmitted disease treatment on the HIV epidemic in rural Tanzania: 1. Design. *AIDS* 1995;9(8):919–926.

218. Wawer MJ, Sewankambo NK, Berkley S, et al. Incidence of HIV-1 infection in a rural region of Uganda. *BMJ* 1994;308(6922):171–173.

219. Wawer MJ, Gray RH, Sewankambo NK, et al. A randomized, community trial of intensive sexually transmitted disease control for AIDS prevention, Rakai, Uganda. *AIDS* 1998;12(10):1211–1225.

220. Wawer MJ, Sewankambo NK, Serwadda D, et al. Control of sexually transmitted diseases for AIDS prevention in Uganda: a randomised community trial. Rakai Project Study Group. *Lancet* 1999;353(9152):525–535.

221. Gray RH, Kiwanuka N, Quinn TC, et al. Male circumcision and HIV acquisition and transmission: cohort studies in Rakai, Uganda. Rakai Project Team. *AIDS* 2000;14(15):2371–2381.

222. Centers for Disease Control and Prevention. Sexually transmitted diseases treatment guidelines 2002. *MMWR Recomm Rep* 2002;51(RR-6):1–78.

223. Padian NS. Prostitute women and AIDS: epidemiology. *AIDS* 1988;2(6):413–419.

224. Rothenberg KH, Paskey SJ. The risk of domestic violence and women with HIV infection: implications for partner notification, public policy, and the law. *Am J Public Health* 1995;85(11):1569–1576.

225. Soper DE, Shoupe D, Shangold GA, et al. Prevention of vaginal trichomoniasis by compliant use of the female condom. *Sex Transm Dis* 1993;20(3):137–139.

226. el Bassel N, Krishnan SP, Schilling RF, et al. Acceptability of the female condom among STD clinic patients. *AIDS Educ Prev* 1998;10(5):465–480.

227. Stein ZA. HIV prevention: the need for methods women can use. *Am J Public Health* 1990;80(4):460–462.

228. Kreiss J, Ngugi E, Holmes K, et al. Efficacy of nonoxynol 9 contraceptive sponge use in preventing heterosexual acquisition of HIV in Nairobi prostitutes. *JAMA* 1992;268(4):477–482.

229. Niruthisard S, Roddy RE, Chutivongse S. Use of nonoxynol-9 and reduction in rate of gonococcal and chlamydial cervical infections. *Lancet* 1992;339(8806):1371–1375.

230. Weir SS, Roddy RE, Zekeng L, et al. Nonoxynol-9 use, genital ulcers, and HIV infection in a cohort of sex workers. *Genitourin Med* 1995;71(2):78–81.

231. Roddy RE, Zekeng L, Ryan KA, et al. Effect of nonoxynol-9 gel on urogenital gonorrhea and chlamydial infection: a randomized controlled trial. *JAMA* 2002;287(9):1117–1122.

232. Van Damme L, Ramjee G, Alary M, et al. Effectiveness of COL-1492, a nonoxynol-9 vaginal gel, on HIV-1 transmission in female sex workers: a randomised controlled trial. *Lancet* 2002;360(9338):971–977.

233. Stafford MK, Ward H, Flanagan A, et al. Safety study of nonoxynol-9 as a vaginal microbicide: evidence of adverse effects. *J Acquir Immune Defic Syndr Hum Retrovirol* 1998;17(4):327–331.

234. Rosenstein IJ, Stafford MK, Kitchen VS, et al. Effect on normal vaginal flora of three intravaginal microbicidal agents potentially active against human immunodeficiency virus type 1. *J Infect Dis* 1998;177(5):1386–1390.

235. McCormack S, Hayes R, Lacey CJ, et al. Microbicides in HIV prevention. *BMJ* 2001;322(7283):410–413.

236. Darroch JE, Frost JJ. Women's interest in vaginal microbicides. *Fam Plann Perspect* 1999;31(1):16–23.

237. Martin HL Jr, Nyange PM, Richardson BA, et al. Hormonal contraception, sexually transmitted diseases, and risk of heterosexual transmission of human immunodeficiency virus type 1. *J Infect Dis* 1998;178(4):1053–1059.

238. Mostad SB, Jackson S, Overbaugh J, et al. Cervical and vaginal shedding of human immunodeficiency virus type 1–infected cells throughout the menstrual cycle. *J Infect Dis* 1998;178(4):983–991.

239. Patterson BK, Landay A, Andersson J, et al. Repertoire of chemokine receptor expression in the female genital tract: implications for human immunodeficiency virus transmission. *Am J Pathol* 1998;153(2):481–490.

240. Mostad SB, Overbaugh J, DeVange DM, et al. Hormonal contraception, vitamin A deficiency, and other risk factors for shedding of HIV-1 infected cells from the cervix and vagina. *Lancet* 1997;350(9082):922–927.

241. Stephenson JM. Systematic review of hormonal contraception and risk of HIV transmission: when to resist meta-analysis. *AIDS* 1998;12(6):545–553.

242. Sox HC Jr. Preventive health services in adults. *N Engl J Med* 1994;330(22):1589–1595.

243. Gerbert B, Maguire BT, Coates TJ. Are patients talking to their physicians about AIDS? *Am J Public Health* 1990;80(4):467–468.

244. Mertens T, Carael M, Sato P, et al. Prevention indicators for evaluating the progress of national AIDS programmes. *AIDS* 1994;8(10):1359–1369.

245. Rugg DL, Heitgerd JL, Cotton DA, et al. CDC HIV prevention indicators: monitoring and evaluating HIV prevention in the USA. *AIDS* 2000;14(13):2003–2013.

246. Ainsworth M, Teokul W. Breaking the silence: setting realistic priorities for AIDS control in less-developed countries. *Lancet* 2000;356(9223):55–60.

247. Coates TJ, Feldman MD. An overview of HIV prevention in the United States. *J Acquir Immune Defic Syndr Hum Retrovirol* 1997;14[Suppl 2]:S13–S16.

248. Coates TJ, Aggleton P, Gutzwiller F, et al. HIV prevention in developed countries. *Lancet* 1996;348(9035):1143–1148.

CHAPTER 121

Pediatric Human Immunodeficiency Virus Infection

Arry Dieudonne and James Oleske

HISTORY

The human immunodeficiency virus (HIV)/acquired immunodeficiency syndrome (AIDS) epidemic has entered its second decade since the initial cases of an unusual syndrome of immunodeficiency in children were described and soon recognized as part of the syndrome seen in adults (1). There have been considerable advances, especially in the last 5 years, in the management of pediatric HIV infection. These have included the development and availability of HIV deoxyribonucleic acid (DNA) polymerase chain reaction (PCR) assays for early diagnosis, the advent of new classes of antiretroviral drugs for use in combination therapy, and better monitoring tools, in particular, HIV ribonucleic acid (RNA) PCR (viral load). With these advances, the prevalence of HIV infection in infants through significant interruption in perinatal HIV transmission has been reduced and changed the epidemiology of pediatric HIV infection in the United States and western European countries from an acutely fatal disease to a chronic, treatable illness. New challenges include the changing care required of children surviving with HIV infection into adulthood and the globalization of the HIV/AIDS epidemic.

As we have learned more about the relationship between clinical symptoms, immune status, and viral load in light of monitoring, the clinical and laboratory definition of HIV infection has undergone several revisions, and guidelines for antiretroviral therapy (ART) and medical management of pediatric HIV infection are being updated on a regular basis (Tables 121.1 through 121.3). This chapter provides an overview of pediatric HIV management in settings with adequate access to medical care. It reflects the continuum of care in pediatric patients as they advance into young adults but does not address many health and social issues of adolescents with adult behavior–acquired HIV infection.

EPIDEMIOLOGY

All the aforementioned advances were preceded in 1994 by the first major prevention breakthrough in the HIV epidemic, Protocol 076, which has demonstrated a reduction rate of perinatal HIV transmission from 25% to 8% with perinatal and infant prophylaxis (2). Guidelines were published by the U.S. Public Health Service for the use of zidovudine (ZDV) to reduce perinatal HIV transmission, and their rapid implementation and acceptance by HIV-infected mothers in the United States have resulted in a dramatic and continued decrease in perinatal HIV transmission for the last 5 years. Follow-up of perinatal transmission rates by other studies such as the nutritional study Pediatric AIDS Clinical Trials Group Protocol 247 (PACTG 247) has demonstrated a decline of perinatal HIV transmission to almost 2% by 2001 in the United States (3).

Through December 2000, 8,908 children younger than 13 years and 4,061 adolescents between 13 and 19 years of age

TABLE 121.1.   1994 Revised Human Immunodeficiency Virus Pediatric Classification System: Clinical Categories

Category N: Not symptomatic
  Children who have no signs or symptoms considered to be the result of HIV infection or who have only one of the conditions listed in category A.

Category A: Mildly symptomatic
  Children with two or more of the following conditions but none of the conditions listed in categories B and C:
  - Lymphadenopathy ($\geq$0.5 cm at more than two sites; bilateral = one site)
  - Hepatomegaly
  - Splenomegaly
  - Dermatitis
  - Parotitis
  - Recurrent or persistent under respiratory tract infection, sinusitis, or otitis media

Category B: Moderately symptomatic
  Children who have symptomatic conditions other than those listed for category A or category C that are attributed to HIV infection. Examples of conditions in clinical category B include but are not limited to the following:
  - Anemia (<8 gm/dL), neutropenia (<1,000/mm^3), or thrombocytopenia (<100,000/mm^3)
  - Bacterial meningitis, pneumonia, or sepsis (single episode)
  - Candidiasis, oropharyngeal (i.e., thrush) persisting for >2 mo in children older than 6 mo
  - Cardiomyopathy
  - Cytomegalovirus infection with onset before age 1 mo
  - Diarrhea, recurrent or chronic
  - Hepatitis
  - HSV stomatitis, recurrent (i.e., more than two episodes within 1 yr)
  - HSV bronchitis, pneumonitis, or esophagitis with onset before age 1 mo
  - Herpes zoster (i.e., shingles) involving at least two distinct episodes or more than one dermatome
  - Leiomyosarcoma
  - LIP or pulmonary lymphoid hyperplasia complex
  - Nephropathy
  - Nocardiosis
  - Fever lasting >1 mo
  - Toxoplasmosis with onset before age 1 mo
  - Varicella, disseminated (i.e., complicated chickenpox)

Category C: Severely symptomatic
  Children who have any condition listed in the 1987 surveillance case definition for acquired immunodeficiency syndrome, with the exception of LIP (which is a category B condition).

HIV, human immunodeficiency virus; HSV, herpes simplex virus; LIP, lymphoid interstitial pneumonia.
Source: From Centers for Disease Control and Prevention. 1994 revised classification system for human immunodeficiency virus infection in children less than 13 years of age. *MMWR Morb Mortal Wkly Rep* 1994;43(RR-12), with permission.

were diagnosed with AIDS in the United States (4,5) (Table 121.4). In addition, 27,232 young adults between 20 and 24 years of age have been registered as having AIDS (4). Given the long clinical latent period until onset of AIDS and the increased survival in the United States due to the use of highly active antiretroviral therapy (HAART), the latter group includes men and women who acquired HIV infection perinatally or during adolescence. In 1985, 89% of reported AIDS cases from this age-group were men. However, as heterosexual contact has accounted for an increasing portion of HIV infection, the proportion of young

TABLE 121.2.   1994 Revised Human Immunodeficiency Virus Pediatric Classification System: Immune Categories Based on Age-specific CD4$^+$ T Cell and Percentage

Immune category	<12 mo		1–5 yr		6–12 yr	
	No./mm^3	(%)	No./mm^3	(%)	No./mm^3	(%)
Category 1: no suppression	$\geq$1,500	($\geq$25%)	$\geq$1,000	($\geq$25%)	$\geq$500	($\geq$25%)
Category 2: moderate suppression	750–1,499	(15%–24%)	500–999	(15%–24%)	200–499	(15%–24%)
Category 3: severe suppression	<750	(<15%)	<500	(<15%)	<200	(<15%)

Source: Modified from Centers for Disease Control and Prevention. 1994 revised classification system for human Immunodeficiency virus infection in children less than 13 years of age. *MMWR Morb Mortal Wkly Rep* 1994;43(RR-12):1–10, with permission.

TABLE 121.3.   Pediatric Human Immunodeficiency Virus Classification for Children Younger than 13 Years

Immune category	Clinical category			
	(N) No symptoms	(A) Mild symptoms	(B)[a] Moderate symptoms	(C)[a] Severe symptoms
(1) No suppression	N1	A1	B1	C1
(2) Moderate suppression	N2	A2	B2	C2
(3) Severe suppression	N3	A3	B3	C3

Note: Using this system children are classified according to three parameters: infection status, clinical status, and immunologic status. The categories are mutually exclusive. Once classified in a more severe category, a child is not reclassified in a less severe category even if the clinical or immunologic status improves. Children whose human immunodeficiency virus infection status is not confirmed are classified by using this grid with a letter *E* (for vertically exposed) placed before the appropriate classification code (e.g., EN2).
[a]Both category C and lymphoid interstitial pneumonitis in category B are reportable to state and local health departments as acquired immunodeficiency syndrome.
Source: From Centers for Disease Control and Prevention. Revised classification system for human immunodeficiency virus infection in children less than 13 years of age. *MMWR Morb Mortal Wkly Rep* 1994;43(RR-12):1–12, with permission.

female adults reported with AIDS has steadily increased. Among children who were infected perinatally and developed AIDS in the United States, the distribution of their mothers' exposure has changed over time. In the early 1980s, most of these women were exposed through injection drug use and a smaller proportion of the women were exposed through heterosexual contact. Through the 1990s, a smaller proportion was attributed to the mother's injection drug use and more to heterosexual contact, trends that are similar to those seen with women with AIDS, especially in the developing world (4–7). HIV infection and AIDS disproportionately affect minorities. The rate of AIDS among black children in 2000 was 1.7 per 100,000, 17 times higher than among white children (0.1/100,000) and more than five times higher than among Hispanic children (0.5/100,000) (4). These rates also reflect the disproportionate racial/ethnic distribution

of HIV/AIDS among women in the United States. The World Health Organization (WHO) assumes that 34.3 million people have been infected with HIV type 1 (HIV-1) and 1.3 million of them are children younger than 15 years (8). More than 1 million children are presumed to be living with HIV and AIDS and 90% of them live in sub-Saharan Africa and the developing countries of Asia (8,9). Efforts to prevent mother-to-child transmission of HIV infection are critical and the success of short-course ZDV and nevirapine therapy offers hope for developing countries to reduce perinatal transmission (10–13). Fortunately, in the United States and other industrialized countries, the transmission rate has decreased to the extent that in the United States, fewer than 200 cases are expected yearly (3).

HIV TRANSMISSION

Vertical transmission, from mother to child, is the predominant source of HIV-1 acquisition in children. The term *perinatal transmission* as proposed by the Centers for Disease Control and Prevention (CDC) describes the route of infection that includes the prenatal intrapartum and the postpartum period. Current data suggest that the majority of transmissions may occur during the intrapartum period. The exposure of the infant's skin/mucous membranes to blood and secretions in the maternal genital tract during delivery play an important role in transmission. Evaluation of the infection status of twins born to HIV-1–infected mothers has shown that the first born has an almost threefold greater risk of infection than the second born, suggesting that relative exposure to birth canal secretion is important in transmission (14). An infant would be considered to have *in utero* infection if the HIV-1 genome could be detected by PCR or be cultured from blood within 48 hours of birth. In contrast, a child would be considered to have intrapartum infection if results of diagnostic assays such as culture, DNA PCR, and serum p24 antigen assay were negative in blood samples obtained during the first week of life but became positive during the period from day 6 to day 90 and the infant has not been breast-fed (15–17). HIV transmission may occur through breast-feeding. The virus has been identified in both cell-free and cell-associated fractions of breast milk (18). A metaanalysis suggested the attributable risk of transmission by breast-feeding to be 14% (19). However, other studies have suggested that the risk may be as high as 32% or as

TABLE 121.4.   AIDS in Children Younger than 13 Years by Exposure Category Reported in 2000 and Cumulative, United States

Exposure category	2000		Cumulative 1982–2000	
	No.	%	No.	%
Perinatally acquired	177	90	8,133	91
Transfusion associated	2	1	382	4
Hemophilia	1	1	237	3
Other/note reported	16	8	156	2
Total	196	100	8,908	100

Note: In 2000, 196 children were reported to the Center for Disease Control and Prevention with acquired immunodeficiency syndrome (AIDS), a marked decrease from 263 in 1999. Ninety percent of these children acquired human immunodeficiency virus (HIV) infection perinatally, that is, from their mother during pregnancy. Since the beginning of the AIDS epidemic, 8,908 children have been reported with AIDS. Again, the majority of these children (91%) were infected perinatally. Another 4% acquired HIV from a transfusion of blood or blood products, and 3% because of their hemophilia. Of the 2% of children with "other or not reported exposure," 141 had an unidentified risk, and the remainder were infected as a result of unusual exposures: 1 was infected following intentional inoculation with HIV-infected blood, 2 were exposed to HIV-infected blood in a household setting, and 12 children had sexual contact with an adult with or at high risk for HIV infection. Nearly all newly infected children acquire HIV perinatally by their mothers.

low as 9% (20,21). It is recommended in the United States and other industrialized countries to avoid breast-feeding given the availability of safe infant formula. The problem is quite opposite in the developing world. Breast milk is an important source to provide maternal antibodies against endemic pathogens. Unsanitary conditions and poor socioeconomic status make the use and availability of infant formula more risky. The benefit of breast-feeding by an infected mother may outweigh the risk of transmission. Therefore, the WHO recommends that infected women in resource-poor countries continue to breast-feed their infants unless there is a mechanism of ensuring access to safe formula (21,22). Ongoing studies to develop strategies to prevent HIV-1 transmission through breast-feeding may help decrease the rate of transmission in developing countries.

The importance of sexual transmission in children and adolescents should not be overlooked, especially when perinatal transmission is ruled out. Sexual abuse should be considered, and the matter must be investigated in close collaboration with social service agencies. In adolescents, the likelihood of engaging in unsafe sex practice may be highest among adolescent homosexual boys. This group may not understand the consequences and the risks of their behavior, especially when alcohol and drug use are included. Another emerging group at risk of transmitting the disease to their sexual partners is the long-term survivors. Since the use of HAART in the United States and other industrialized countries has been established, HIV-infected children live longer and move from childhood to young adulthood. Their sexual identity is just becoming established, which increases the risks of transmitting HIV infection. Sexual issues should be discussed individually or in small peer groups. Condoms should be offered and made available during their clinic visits. Practitioners in health care facilities taking care of HIV-infected adolescents are facing a new challenge when they decide to become sexually active. Procreative rights cannot be denied, although appropriate counseling must be offered, detailing the risk of transmission of HIV infection to their partners and their infants. Adolescents with histories of injection drug use should be counseled about their risks of acquiring HIV infection and hepatitis B and hepatitis C viruses (HBV and HCV). They become a bridge to further spread of infection through their sexual contacts. One has to remember that needle sharing, the primary mechanism of HIV-1 transmission among injection drug users, appears to be associated with younger age, not completing high school, history of prior arrest, being on public assistance, and male-male sexual behavior. It appears that their drug of choice is cocaine and those sharing needles inject drugs more often (23,24). Adolescents with risky behavior of acquiring or transmitting HIV-1 should be enrolled in comprehensive HIV risk-reduction programs including drug treatment, condom distribution, and voluntary testing (25,26).

The period of highest risk of blood product exposure to HIV-1 occurred after 1970 and April 1985 before the availability of HIV-1 antibody–screened blood products. Since 1985, there has been a dramatic decrease in transmission of HIV-1 in the United States because of routine screening of all blood donations for HIV-1 antibody. The risk of HIV-1 transmission through screened blood is estimated at 1 in every 450,000 to 660,000 donations of screened blood (27). Transmission of HIV-1 through organ transplantation has been rare but documented, as has transmission through artificial insemination (28–30). It has been recommended that tissue from living donors not be used until the donor is tested again 6 months later and confirmed to be seronegative (31).

HIV-1 antibody screening of blood products is not available in some of developing countries. It is common practice to give "mini-transfusions" to patients, especially children and pregnant women to treat moderate or severe anemia secondary to malaria, malnutrition, and obstetric-related bleeding. Transmission via transfusion is estimated at about 5% to 10% of all infections in Africa (32). The current antibody test to detect HIV-1 subtype B may not detect the other subtypes, nonclade B, which are more common in Africa. A new assay with the capability of identifying all subtypes of HIV has been developed. Its Food and Drug Administration (FDA) approval in the United States is still pending. The universal use of screened blood donations will dramatically decrease the transmission of HIV infection in the developing world and is an achievable and important goal.

The risk of transmission via nosocomial percutaneous or mucous membrane exposure to HIV-1 is very low. It is estimated to be 0.3% after a single percutaneous exposure of health care workers to blood-borne pathogens through improper use and disposal of sharps used for phlebotomy. The use of barriers, such as gloves, and incorporation of universal precautions are still recommended. Only eight cases of possible household transmission of HIV-1 have been reported, some of which involved children (33–38). HIV-1 transmission through exposure to saliva appears to be extremely low and would require unusually high infectivity to have contact with broken skin or mucosa. Although HIV exposure theoretically can occur in school settings or from children playing together, transmission of HIV-1 by human bites remains unlikely and no well-documented case can be found in the literature (39). Counseling is very important and disclosure issues should be discussed between the families of the children involved. Fortunately, the rate of perinatal transmission can be decreased substantially by therapeutic intervention and HIV education. Potential strategies for intervention are still being developed to minimize perinatal HIV transmission both in the developed and most importantly in the less-developed countries (40).

IMMUNE SYSTEM

The CD4$^+$ lymphocyte is the target cell of HIV infection, and its destruction by the HIV affects all portions of the immune system. This cell plays an important role in the complex interplay of the interlacing network of cells and noncellular mediations that constitute the immune response (41). Because the immune system of the neonate and the young infant is immature, it is not unexpected that the signs and symptoms of HIV infection in that population are more severe compared with those in older children and in the adult population. The development of flow cytometric analysis to study lymphocyte subpopulations has established age-related changes in the numbers of different lymphocyte subgroups (42). Comparison of lymphocyte subsets in HIV-infected versus noninfected children younger than 2 years reveals no difference for absolute CD8$^+$ counts, but clearly decreased levels of CD4$^+$ cell counts (43). Abnormalities in both humoral and cellular immunity are seen in perinatal HIV infection, with humoral immunity dysfunction having repercussions more commonly in children compared with the adolescent or young adult population. Immunodysregulation, reflected by increased levels of immunoglobulins but in some cases hypogammaglobulinemia, and cytokine abnormalities are characteristic of HIV-1 infection in young children and may occur early in life. Early during the epidemic, Bernstein et al. (44) demonstrated abnormalities in both primary and secondary antibody response to both T-cell–dependent antigens and T-cell–independent antigens. Other studies have found an abnormality of at least one immunoglobulin G (IgG) subclass in 85% of a group of 47 HIV-infected children, including some patients who had IgG2, IgG4, or combined IgG2-IgG4 deficiencies without a clear correlation between the incidence of bacterial infections and specific subclass deficiencies (45).

Impaired T-cell immunity occurs later than B-cell dysfunction, even though it is the hallmark of HIV-1 infection. HIV-specific cytotoxic T-lymphocyte (CTL) responses can occur early in infancy; however, they are not as commonly present as seen in adult primary infection. Immune categories in infants, children, and adolescents infected with HIV are based on age-specific CD4$^+$ T-cell number and percentage (46) (Table 121.2). CD4$^+$ lymphocyte levels in healthy uninfected infants are considerably higher than those observed in the adult population; however, a subsequent decline in these levels reaches adult normal values by 6 years of age. There are convincing data supporting the role of CD4$^+$ helper cells based on the associated cytokine responses they produce. Interleukin-2 (IL-2) and IL-12 production is associated with helper T-cell subtype 1 (T$_H$1), whereas helper T-cell subtype 2 (T$_H$2) lymphocytes are associated with the production of IL-4, IL-5, IL-6 and IL-10, and promote T-cell–dependent humoral response. Helper T-cell subtype 0 (T$_H$0) is a clone of cells that produces a composite of helper T-cell subtype 1/2 pattern. A progression of type 1 to a type 0, and type 2 pattern of T-cell function has been hypothesized as associated with disease progression (47,48). Some investigators have proposed that HIV-specific CTL response may be associated with decreased HIV disease progression; however, increase in viral load and decline in CD4$^+$ lymphocyte count has been observed despite the presence of CTL responses (49). Functional defects in other cell lines have been detected during progression of HIV infection in children, especially in the hemophagocytic line where the cells constitute likely reservoirs of persistent virus (50).

DIAGNOSIS

The definitive diagnosis of HIV infection in children older than 18 months is made using the enzyme-linked immunosorbent assay (ELISA) and Western blot assays. These assays provide the serologic evidence of a humoral immune response to the HIV by detecting HIV-specific IgG antibodies. The age-requirement rationale is that passively acquired maternal antibodies to the HIV are no longer present after 18 months, and an infant older than this age has an immune system that is able to mount a humoral immune response. HIV infection can be reasonably excluded with two negative HIV ELISA test results done at 18 months of age or older. HIV viral-specific assays such as HIV viral culture, the standard p24 antigen capture assay, and the immune complex–dissociated p24 antigen capture assay have been used to determine infection status before the age of 18 months. However, HIV DNA PCR has revolutionized the diagnosis of HIV infection in young infants, replacing viral culture as the most effective method of diagnosis.

HIV viral culture is performed on peripheral blood mononuclear cells, co-cultured with uninfected mononuclear cells that can support HIV growth and detect latent HIV-infected cells, by stimulating viral replication. Published data indicate that the sensitivity of this test is age dependent. The sensitivity is 24% during the first week of life, exceeding 90% in infants by 2 to 3 months of age and nearly 100% by 6 months of age (51–52). In a large cohort study, McIntosh et al. (53) had showed that two negative cultures taken between 1 month and 6 months of age had a specificity of 99.2% to 100% in defining an uninfected infant.

The sensitivity and specificity of HIV DNA PCR as a diagnostic tool are similar to those of HIV culture (43,54,55). A meta-analysis of data from 271 infants has revealed that 38% of HIV-infected infants had a positive PCR within the first 48 hours and

93% of infected infants were positive by 14 days of age (43). A presumptive diagnosis of HIV infection can be made with one positive HIV culture or PCR assay on noncord blood and a definitive diagnosis made with a confirmatory test on a different blood sample. HIV infection can be reasonably excluded with two negative HIV culture or PCR results, one obtained at age 1 month or later, the other at age 4 months or later (56). The current standard of care still requires negative HIV ELISA and Western blot results at age 18 months to exclude HIV infection definitely.

The antigen capture assay test/HIV p24 antigen assay is quite specific and can be used to help establish the diagnosis if it is positive after the first week of life. However, its sensitivity is quite low and it cannot be used to exclude HIV infection in the first year of life. The reason for the low sensitivity of the standard p24 antigen assay is that maternal HIV-specific IgG antibody can result in antibody-excess immune complexes that cause a negative result. Immune complex dissociation (ICD) p24 antigen capture was developed, but because of lack of published data on age-specific sensitivity, it should not be used to rule out HIV infection. Currently in the United States, the recommended virologic diagnostic assays are the HIV DNA PCR and HIV culture, with HIV DNA PCR as the preferred one because of its availability, added laboratory safety, and quick turnaround time. In less-developed areas, the ICD p24 antigen assay still has utility due to resource issues.

Detection and quantification of plasma for HIV-1 RNA as it became available has been used by some clinicians to detect the presence of HIV infection in patients with acute HIV infection or in those who have reactive ELISA results and indeterminate Western blots results. The test is not FDA approved for this diagnostic purpose, even though it appears to be quite sensitive for the detection of HIV infection in those circumstances. Developing countries in which HIV DNA PCR or HIV cultures are not available have been using this assay for diagnostic purposes. Clinicians should be cautious about using that test in infants younger than 1 year for diagnostic purposes, because false-positive results usually with low copy numbers have been reported (57).

Rapid HIV tests provide opportunities for persons to learn about their HIV antibody test on the day they are tested. It can be very useful in settings in which pregnant mothers in labor had no prenatal care or in pregnant women who have not been offered HIV counseling and testing during their prenatal care. This improves opportunities to prevent HIV transmission to their newborns by using ZDV and/or nevirapine. Only one FDA-approved rapid HIV test is available, but other second-generation rapid tests are expected soon. Several such assays are being used outside the United States. They require a single step and can be performed on whole blood, serum, secretions, or plasma including a blood sample obtained by simple fingerstick. The sensitivity and the specificity are similar to those of the standard enzyme immunoassay (EIA). Such tests also raise the possibility of implementing strategies such as one recommended by the WHO, whereby specific combinations of different rapid tests might be used to confirm reactive HIV test results on the day a person is tested. The impact of HIV rapid test in pediatric HIV care other than during the prenatal period has yet to be established but may play a role in outreach programs to high-risk adolescents.

INFECTIOUS COMPLICATIONS

The working group has published guidelines for the treatment of specific secondary infections. The use of prophylaxis for opportunistic infections (OIs) and childhood immunization has played a greater role in the decreased incidence of infections in the pediatric population (58–60). (See Table 121.5 for immunization and Tables 121.6 through 121.8 for primary and secondary of prophylaxis of opportunistic disease.)

Signs and symptoms of disease in HIV-infected children may present in three patterns. Infants who are infected intragestationally become symptomatic within the first few months of life because of possibly early disruption in maturation of their immune system. The largest groups of vertically HIV-infected children who are less symptomatic are believed to acquire the disease perinatally. Their immune system seems to be more competent and may mount some immune response that delays the onset of signs and symptoms of HIV infection. Another group of infected children do not develop evidence of disease progression until after 8 to 10 years of age (15,61). Many studies have compared disease-progression rates between infants whose disease was transfusion acquired during the neonatal period and infants with vertically acquired infection. The latter group developed symptomatic disease more rapidly than those who acquired infection via neonatal transfusion (62). Other factors are believed to contribute to the rapidity of clinical progression such as the inherent virulence properties of the transmitted viral strain and/or initial viral burden, genetic factors, such as human leukocyte antigen (HLA) genotype, and the mother's and/or infant's cellular or humoral immune response (41,63–66). There are data supporting that low age-related CD4 lymphocyte count and percentage and rapid $CD4^+$ cell decline correlate with disease progression in older infants and children. Other immunologic markers, such as tumor necrosis factor (TNF), β_2-microglobulin, increased production of IL-4 and IL-10, low or absent titers of HIV-1–specific antibodies, are also associated with disease progression (67–70).

The following sections provide a summary of the most common opportunistic diseases seen in pediatric HIV infection.

Bacterial Infections

Since the defective B-cell function occurs early in life, recurrent and serious bacterial infections such as sepsis, pneumonia, meningitis, and abscesses may be the first indication of perinatal HIV-1 infection (71,72). Bacteremia with or without a focus may occur and is the most reported serious infection (73). Invading pathogens are encapsulated bacteria commonly associated with childhood infections such as *Streptococcus pneumoniae*, *Staphylococcus aureus*, *Neisseria meningitidis*, *Salmonella* species, and *Haemophilus influenzae*. *Staphylococcus epidermidis* is mostly found in hospitalized patients with central venous catheters or who are neutropenic (72–74). Since the beginning of the HIV epidemic, a resurgence of tuberculosis has been observed, especially in the inner cities among HIV-infected adults with subsequent exposure of both HIV-infected and HIV-exposed children. An increase in coinfection with HIV and tuberculosis has been observed in the United States and in Africa (75). The diagnosis of *Mycobacterium tuberculosis* infection is difficult in the HIV-infected pediatric population, as in adults, because of the anergy that is often associated with the disease, leading to a negative tuberculin skin-test result even in the presence of active infection. A tuberculin skin test that results in an induration of five or more is considered "reactive" in any patient with HIV infection regardless of immune status.

Mycobacterium avium complex (MAC) (nontuberculous mycobacteria) in the respiratory or gastrointestinal (GI) tract is common in persons with HIV infection. Most infections remain localized at the portal of entry or in regional lymph nodes. Infants and children will be at risk of developing MAC infection if their $CD4^+$ lymphocyte count is less than 100 cells/mm². Common

clinical manifestations of systemic involvement include recurrent fever, anorexia, failure to gain weight, and weight loss followed by wasting syndrome, persistent/recurrent diarrhea, and severe anemia secondary to bone marrow depression. Blood and tissue culture, including culture of bone marrow aspiration, are used to make the diagnosis. Clinical isolates of MAC usually are resistant to the many approved antituberculosis drugs, including isoniazid. Treatment guidelines recommend the use of at least two drugs, and one of them must be either clarithromycin or azithromycin. Many clinicians have added one or more of the following as a third or fourth agent: rifampin, rifabutin, and/or ciprofloxacin. However, drug interactions are a concern when protease inhibitors (PIs) are used, especially with rifabutin (Table 121.9). Guidelines for MAC prophylaxis recommend the weekly use of azithromycin in children whose CD4 count is less than 100 cells/mm² (60) (Table 121.6). Before the HAART era, MAC infection was a prominent cause of morbidity and mortality in HIV-infected children, but the incidence of this complication has decreased dramatically with combination antiretroviral drug therapy (76).

Viral Infections

Viral infections can cause significant morbidity and mortality in HIV-infected children with altered immune status. Common childhood viral infections can be severe, persistent, and recurrent. Varicella-zoster virus (VZV) infection may be severe, disseminated, prolonged, and complicated by bacterial suprainfections. Zoster follows a more aggressive course with progressive immune deficiency, which may often manifest as recurrent episodes of shingles or an atypical folliculitis-like picture with disseminated lesions (77,78). Resistant strains to standard treatment of the VZV virus may emerge after those recurrences (79,80). Chronic ulcerative stomatitis caused by HSV-1 complicated by dissemination to the esophagus and other organ systems has been described in HIV-infected children (81). Frenkel et al. (82) have reported that cytomegalovirus (CMV) is found in 45% of children with symptomatic HIV infection. Any organ system can be involved when disseminated CMV infection is present. The most common manifestations include retinitis and pneumonitis (82,83). CMV can become resistant to treatment with ganciclovir, necessitating the use of foscarnet or combination regimens (84,85). Infections with respiratory syncytial, influenza, and parainfluenza viruses and adenovirus alone or in combination can also result in rapid and sometimes fatal respiratory compromise and persistent chronic viral shedding or infection may persist for months (86,87). Both HBV and HCV can be transmitted transplacentally. Therefore, infants can be born infected with both HIV and a hepatitis virus. Hepatitis B immunoprophylaxis is the most effective way to prevent HBV transmission. Hepatitis B immunization is recommended for all infants as part of the immunization schedule (Table 121.5). Postexposure immunoprophylaxis with either hepatitis B vaccine and hepatitis B immune globulin or hepatitis B vaccine alone can prevent infection after exposure (88). HIV-infected or HIV-exposed children may also be exposed to HCV. The seroprevalence rate is 0.2% for children younger than 12 years and 0.4% for those 12 to 19 years. Seroprevalence rates vary among individuals according to their associated factors. Mother-to-infant transmission is only 5% (range, 0%–25%). However, maternal complication with HIV has been associated with increased risk of perinatal transmission of HCV. It may depend in part on the HCV genotype and the serum titer of maternal HCV RNA. Immunoprophylaxis is not recommended so far, and maternal HCV infection is not a contraindication to breast-feeding. However, in the United States, breast-feeding is already contraindicated in mothers with HIV

(Text continues on p. 1077.)

TABLE 121.5. Recommended Immunization Schedule for Human Immunodeficiency Virus–Infected Children[a]

Vaccine	Birth	1 mo	2 mo	4 mo	6 mo	12 mo	15 mo	18 mo	24 mo	4–6 yr	11–12 yr	14–16 yr
Recommendations for these vaccines are the same as those for immunocompetent children												
Hepatitis B[b]		Hep B1	Hep B2 →		Hep B3 →						(Hep B)	
Diphtheria, and tetanus toxoids, pertusis[c]			DTaP	DTaP	DTaP	DTaP →				DTaP	Td →	
Haemophilus influenzae type b[d]			Hib	Hib	Hib	Hib						
Inactivated polio[e]			IPV	IPV	IPV →					IPV		
Hepatitis A[f]											Hep A in selected areas	
Recommendations for these vaccines differ from those for immunocompetent children												
Pneumococcus[g]			PCV	PCV	PCV	PCV			PPV23	PPV23 (age 5–7 yr)		
Measles, mumps, rubella[h]		Do not administer to severely immuno-suppressed (category 3) children				MMR				MMR	(MMR)	
Varicella[i]		Administer only to asymptomatic nonimmunosuppressed (category 1) children contraindicated for all other HIV-infected children				Var	Var				(Var)	
Influenza[j]					A dose is recommended every year							

☐ Range of recommended ages for vaccination

⬭ Vaccines to be administered if previously recommended doses were missed or were administered at other than the recommended minimum age

☐ Recommended in selected states or regions

[a]This schedule indicates the recommended ages for routine administration of licensed childhood vaccines as of November 1, 2000, for children aged birth–18 years. Additional vaccines might be licensed and recommended during the year. Licensed combination vaccines might be used whenever any components of the combination are indicated and the vaccine's other components are not contraindicated. Providers should consult the manufacturer's package inserts for detailed recommendations.

[b]Infants born to hepatitis B surface antigen (HBsAg)–negative mothers should receive the first dose of hepatitis B vaccine (Hep B) at birth and no later than age 2 months. The second dose should be administered ≥1 months after the first dose. The third dose should be administered ≥4 months after the first dose and ≥2 months after the second dose, but not before age 6 months. Infants born to HBsAg-positive mothers should receive Hep B and 0.5 mL hepatitis B immune globulin (HBIG) ≤12 hours after birth at separate sites. The second dose is recommended at age 1–2 months and the third dose at age 6 months. Infants born to mothers whose HBsAg status is unknown should receive Hep B ≤12 hours after birth. Maternal blood should be drawn at delivery to determine the mother's HBsAg status; if the HBsAg test is positive, the infant should receive HBIG as soon as possible (no later than age 1 week). All children and adolescents (through age 18 years) who have not been immunized against hepatitis B should begin the series during any visit. Providers should make special efforts to immunize children who were born in, or whose parents were born in, areas of the world where hepatitis B virus infection is moderately or highly endemic.

[c]The fourth dose of diphtheria and tetanus toxoids and acellular pertussis vaccine (DTaP) can be administered as early as age 12 months, provided 6 months have elapsed since the third dose and the child is unlikely to return at age 15–18 months. Vaccination with tetanus and diphtheria toxoids (Td) is recommended at age 11–12 years if ≥5 years have elapsed since the last dose of diphtheria and tetanus toxoids and pertussis vaccine (DTP), DTaP, or diphtheria and tetanus toxoids (DT). Subsequent routine Td boosters are recommended every 10 years.

[d]Three *Haemophilus influenzae* type b (Hib) conjugate vaccines are licensed for infant use. If Hib conjugate vaccine (polyribosylribitol phosphate-meningococcal outer membrane protein [PRP-OMP]) (PedvaxHIB or ComVax [Merck and Company. Inc., Whitehouse Station, New Jersey]) is administered at ages 2 and 4 months, a dose at age 6 months is not required. Because clinical studies among infants have demonstrated that using certain combination products might induce a lower immune response to the Hib vaccine component. DTaP/Hib combination products should not be used for primary immunization among infants at ages 2, 4, or 6 months, unless approved by the Food and Drug Administration for these ages.

[e]An all-inactivated poliovirus vaccine (IPV) schedule is recommended for routine childhood polio vaccination in the United States. All children should receive four doses of IPV at age 2 months, age 4 months, ages 6–18 months, and ages 4–6 years. Oral polliovirus vaccine should not be administered to HIV-infected persons or their household contacts.

[f]Hepatitis A vaccine (Hep A) is recommended for use in selected states or regions and for certain persons at high risk (e.g., those with Hepatitis B or C infection). Information is available from local public health authorities.

[g]Heptavalent pneumococcal conjugate vaccine (PCV) is recommended for all HIV-infected children aged 2–59 months. Children aged ≥2 years should also receive the 23-valent pneumococcal polysaccharide vaccine: a single revaccination with the 23-valent vaccine should be offered to children after 3–5 years. Refer to the Advisory Committee on Immunization Practices recommendations (see CDC. Preventing pneumococcal disease among infants and young children: recommendations of the Advisory Committee on Immunization Practices [ACIP]. *MMWR Morb Mortal Wkly Rep* 2000;49[No. RR-9]:1–38) for dosing intervals for children starting the vaccination schedule after age 2 months.

[h]Measles, mumps, and rubella (MMR) should not be administered to severely immunocompromised (category 3) children. HIV-infected children without severe immunosuppression would routinely receive their first dose of MMR as soon as possible after reaching their first birthdays. Consideration should be given to administering the second dose of MMR at age 1 month (i.e., a minimum of 26 days) after the first dose rather then waiting until school entry.

[i]Varicella-zoster virus vaccine should be administered only to asymptomatic, nonimmunosuppressed children. Eligible children should receive two doses of vaccine with a ≥3-month interval between doses. The first dose can be administered at age 12 months.

[j]Inactivated split influenza virus vaccine should be administered to all HIV-infected children aged ≥6 months each year. For children aged 6 months–<9 years who are receiving influenza vaccine for the first time, two doses administered 1 month apart are recommended. For specific recommendations, see CDC. Prevention and control of influenza: recommendations of the Advisory Committee on Immunization Practices (ACIP). *MMWR Morb Mortal Wkly Rep* 2002;51(No. RR-4):1–32.

TABLE 121.6. Prophylaxis to Prevent First Episode of Opportunistic Disease Infants and Children Infected with Human Immunodeficiency Virus

Pathogen	Indication	Preventive regimens First choice	Alternatives
I. Strongly recommended as standard of care			
Pneumocystis carinii[a]	HIV infected or HIV indeterminate, infants aged 1–12 mo; HIV-infected children aged 1–5 yr with CD4+ count <500/µL or CD4+ percentage <15%; HIV-infected children aged 6–12 yr with CD4+ count <200/µL or CD4+ percentage <15%	Trimethoprim-sulfamethoxazole (TMP-SMX), 150/750 mg/m²/d in 2 divided doses po t.i.w. on consecutive days (AII) Acceptable alternative Dosage schedules: (AII) • Single dose p.o. t.i.w. on consecutive days; • 2 divided doses p.o. q.d.; 2 divided doses p.o. t.i.w. on alternate days	Dapsone (children aged ≥1 mo), 2 mg/kg (max. 100 mg) p.o. q.d. or 4 mg/kg (max. 200 mg) p.o. q.w. (CII); aerosolized pentamidine (children) aged >5 yr), 300 mg q.m. via Respigard II nebulizer (CIII); atovaquone (children aged 1–3 mo and >24 mo, 30 mg/kg p.o. q.d.; children aged 4–24 mo, 45 mg/kg p.o. q.d.) (CII)
Mycobacterium tuberculosis[b] Isoniazid sensitive	TST reaction, ≥5 mm Or, prior positive TST result without treatment/or contact with any case of active tuberculosis regardless of TST result	Isoniazid 1–15 mg/kg (max. 300 mg) p.o. q.d. × 9 mo (all) or 20–30 mg/kg (max. 900) mg p.o. b.i.w. × 9 mo (BII)	Rifampin, 10–20 mg/kg (max. 600 mg) p.o. q.d. × 4–6 mo (BIII)
Isoniazid resistant	Same as above; high probability of exposure to isoniazid-resistant tuberculosis	Rifampin, 10–20 mg/kg (max. 600 mg) p.o. q.d. × 4–6 mo (BIII)	Uncertain
Multidrug (isoniazid and rifampin) resistant	Same as above; high probability of exposure to multidrug-resistant tuberculosis	Choice of drugs requires consultation with public health authorities and depends on susceptibility of isolate from source patient	
Mycobacteriuim avium complex[b]	For children aged ≥6 yr, CD4+ count <50 µL; aged 2–6 yr CD4+ count <75/µL; aged 1–2 yr, CD4+ count <500/µL; aged <1 yr, CD4+ count <750/µL	Clarithromycin 7.5 mg/kg (max. 500 mg) p.o. b.i.d. (AII), or azithromycin, 20 mg/kg (max. 1,200 mg) p.o. q.w. (AII)	Azithromycin, 5 mg/kg (max. 250 mg) p.o. q.d. (AII); children aged ≥6 yr, rifabutin, 300 mg p.o. q.d. (BI)
Varicella-zoster virus[c]	Significant exposure to varicella or shingles with no history of chickenpox or shingles	VZIG, 1 vial (1.25 mL)/10 kg (max. 5 vials) i.m., administered ≤96 hr after exposure, ideally within 48 hr (AII)	None
Vaccine-preventable pathogens[d]	HIV exposure/infection	Routine Immunizations	None
II. Generally recommend			
Toxoplasma gondii[e]	IgG antibody to *Toxoplasma* and severe immunosuppression	TMP-SMX, 150/750 mg/m²/d in 2 divided doses p.o. q.d. (BIII)	Dapsone (children aged ≥1 mo), 2 mg/kg or 15 mg/m² (max. 25 mg) p.o. q.d. plus pyrimethamine, 1 mg/kg p.o. q.d. plus leucovorin, 5 mg p.o. every 3 days (BIII) Atovaquone (aged 1–3 mo) and >24 mo, 30 mg/kg p.o. q.d.; aged 14–24 mo 45 mg/kg p.o. q.d.) (CIII)
Varicella-zoster virus	HIV-infected children who are asymptomatic and not immunosuppressed	Varicella-zoster vaccine (see "Vaccine-preventable pathogens" section of this table) (BII)	None
Influenza virus	All patients (annually, before influenza season)	Inactivated split trivalent influenza vaccine (see "Vaccine-preventable pathogens" section of this table) (BIII)	Oseltamivir (during outbreaks of influenza A or B) for children ≥13 yr, 75 mg p.o. q.d. (CIII); rimantadine or amantadine (during outbreaks of influenza A); aged 1–9 yr, 5 mg/kg in 2 divided doses (max. 150 mg/d) p.o. q.d.; aged ≥10 yr, use adult doses (CIII)
III. Not recommended for most children; indicated for use only in unusual circumstances			
Invasive bacterial infections[f]	Hypogamma-globulinemia (i.e., IgG <400 mg/dL)	IVIG (400 mg/kg every 2–4 wk) (AI)	None
Cryptococcus neoformans	Severe immunosuppression	Fluconazole, 3–6 mg/kg p.o. q.d. (CII)	Itraconazole, 2–5 mg/kg p.o. every 12–24 hr (CII)
Histoplasma capsulatum	Severe immunosuppression, endemic geographic area	Itraconazole 2–5 mg/kg p.o. every 12–24 hr (CIII)	None
Cytomegalovirus (CMV)[g]	CMV antibody positivity and severe immunosuppression	Oral ganciclovir 30 mg/kg p.o. t.i.d. (CII)	None

Note: Information included in these guidelines might not represent Food and Drug Administration (FDA) approval or approved labeling for the particular products or indications in question. Specifically, the terms *safe* and *effective* might not be synonymous with the FDA-defined legal standards for product approval. The Respigard II nebulizer is manufactured by Marquest, Englewood, Colorado. Letters and Roman numerals in parentheses after regimens indicate the strengh of the recommendation and the quality of the evidence supporting it.

[a]Daily TMP-SMX reduces the frequency of some bacterial infections. TMP-SMX, dapsone-pyrimethamine, and possibly atovaquone (with or without pyrimethamine) appear to protect against toxoplasmosis, although data have not been prospectively collected. When compared with weekly dapsone, daily dapsone is associated with lower incidence of *Pneumocystis carinii* pneumonia (PC) but higher hematologic toxicity and mortality (McIntosh K, Cooper E, Xu J, et al. Toxicity and efficacy of daily vs. weekly dapsone for prevention of *Pneumocystis carinii* pneumonia in children infected with HIV. *Ped Infect Dis J* 1999;18:432–439). The efficacy of parenteral pentamidine (e.g., 4 mg/kg q2–4wk) is controversial. Patients receiving therapy for toxoplasmosis with sulfadazine-pyrimethamine are protected against PCP and do not need TMP-SMX.
[b]Significant drug interactions can occur between rifaimycins (rifampin and rifabutin) and protease inhibitors and nonnucleoside reverse transcriptase inhibitors. Consult a specialist.
[c]Children routinely being administered IVIG should receive VZIG if the last dose of IVIG was administered >21 days before exposure.
[d]HIV-infected and HIV-exposed children should be immunized according to the childhood immunization schedule in this report, which has been adapted from the January-December 2001 schedule recommended for immunocompetent children by the Advisory Committee on Immunization Practices, the American Academy of Pediatrics, and the American Academy of Family Physicians. This schedule differs from that for immunocompetent children in that both the conjugate pneumococcal vaccine (PCV-7) and the pneumococcal polysaccharide vaccine (PPV-23) are recommended (BII) and vaccination against influenza (BIII) should be offered. MMR should not be administered to severely immunocompromised children (DIII). Vaccination against varicella is indicated only for asymptomatic nonimmunosuppressed children (BII). Once an HIV-exposed child is determined not to be HIV-infected, the schedule for immunocompetent children applies.
[e]Protection against toxoplasmosis is provided by the preferred antipneumocystis regimens and possibly by atovaquone. Atovaquone may be used with or without pyrimethamine. Pyrimethamine alone probably provides little, if any, protection.
[f]Respiratory syncytial virus (RSV) IVIG (750 mg/kg) not monoclonal RSV antibody, may be substituted for IVIG during the RSV season to provide broad antiinfective protection, if this product is available.
[g]Oral ganciclovir and perhaps valganciclovir results in reduced CMV shedding in CMV-infected children. Acyclovior is not protective against CMV.
b.i.w., twice a week; IVIG, intravenous immune globulin; q.d., daily; q.m., a monthly; t.i.d., three times a day; t.i.w., three times a week; VZIG, varicella-zoster immune globulin.

TABLE 121.7. Prophylaxis to Prevent Recurrence of Opportunistic Disease (after Chemotherapy for Acute Disease) in HIV-Infected Infants and Children

Pathogen	Indication	Preventive regimens	
		First choice	Alternatives
I. Recommended for life as standard of care			
Pneumocystis carinii	Prior *P. carinii* pneumonia	TMP-SMX, 15/750 mg/m²/d in 2 divided doses p.o. t.i.w. on consecutive days (AII) Acceptable alternative schedules for same Single dose p.o. t.i.w. on consecutive days; 2 divided doses p.o. q.d. 2 divided doses p.o. alternate day	Dapsone (children aged ≥1 mo), 2 mg/kg (max 100 mg) po q.d. Or 4 mg/kg (max 200 mg) po q.w. (CII); aerosolized pentamidine dosage: (AII) (children aged ≥5 yr), 300 mg q.m. via Respirgard II nebulizer (CIII); atovaquone (aged 1–3 mo and >24 mo, 30 mg/kg p.o. q.d.; aged 4–24 mo, 45 mg/kg t.i.w. on p.o. q.d.) (CII)
Toxoplasma gondii[a]	Prior toxoplasmic encephalitis	Sulfadiazine, 85–120 mg/kg/d in 2–4 divided doses p.o. q.d. plus pyrimethamine, 1 mg/kg or 15 mg/m² (max. 25 mg) p.o. q.d. plus leucovorin, 5 mg p.o. every 3 days (AI)	Clindamycin, 20–30 mg/kg/d in 4 divided doses p.o. q.d. plus pyrimethamine, 1 mg/kg p.o. q.d. plus leucovorin, 5 mg p.o. every 3 days (BI)
Mycobacterium avium complex[b]	Prior disease	Clarithromycin, 7.5 mg/kg (max. 500 mg) p.o. b.i.d. (AII) plus ethambutol, 15 mg/kg (max. 900 mg) p.o. q.d. (AII); with or without rifabutin, 5 mg/kg (max. 300 mg) p.o. q.d. (CII)	Azithromycin, 5 mg/kg (max. 250 mg) p.o. q.d. (AII) plus ethambutol, 15 mg/kg (max. 900 mg) p.o. q.d. (AII); with or without rifabutin, 5 mg/kg (max. 300 mg) p.o. q.d. (CII)
Cryptococcus neoformans	Documented disease	Fluconazole, 3–6 mg/kg p.o. q.d. (AII)	Amphotericin B, 0.5–1.0 mg/kg i.v. 1–3 times wk (AI); itraconazole, 2–5 mg/kg p.o. every 12–24 hr (BII)
Histoplasma capsulatum	Documented disease	Itraconazole, 2–5 mg/kg p.o. every 12–48 hr (AIII)	Amphotericin B, 1.0 mg/kg i.v. q.w. (AIII)
Coccidioides immitis	Documented disease	Fluconazole, 6 mg/kg p.o. q.d. (AIII)	Amphotericin B, 1.0 mg/kg i.v. q.w. (AIII) Itraconazole, 2–5 mg/kg p.o. every 12–48 hr (AIII)
Cytomegalovirus	Prior end-organ disease	Ganciclovir, 5 mg/kg i.v. q.d.; or foscarnet, 90–120 mg/kg i.v. q.d. (AI)	(For retinitis) Ganciclovir sustained-release implant every 6–9 mo plus ganciclovir, 30 mg/kg p.o. t.i.d. (BIII)
Salmonella species (non typhi)[c]	Bacteremia	TMP-SMX, 150/750 mg/m² in 2 divided doses p.o. q.d. for several months (CIII)	Antibiotic chemoprophylaxis with another active agent (CIII)
II. Recommended only if subsequent episodes are frequent or severe			
Invasive bacterial infections[d]	>2 infections in 1-yr period	TMP-SMX, 150/750 mg/m², in 2 divided doses p.o. q.d. (BI); or IVIG, 400 mg/kg every 2–4 wk (BI)	Antibiotic chemoprophylaxis with another active agent (BIII)
Herpes simplex virus	Frequent/severe recurrences	Acyclovir, 80 mg/kg/d in 3–4 divided doses p.o. q.d. (AII)	
Candida (oropharyngeal)	Frequent/severe recurrences	Fluconazole, 3–6 mg/kg p.o. q.d. (CIII)	
Candida (esophageal)	Frequent severe recurrences	Fluconazole, 3–6 mg/kg p.o. q.d. (BIII)	Itraconazole solution, 5 mg/kg p.o. q.d. (CIII);

Note: Information included in this paper might not represent Food and Drug Administration (FDA) approval or approved labeling for the particular product or indications in question. Specifically, the terms "safe" and "effective" might not be synonymous with the FDA-defined legal standards for product approval. The Respirgard II nebulizer is manufactured by Marquest, Englewood, Colorado. Letters and Roman numerals in parentheses after regimens indicate the strength of the recommendations and the quality of evidence supporting it.

[a]Only pyrimethamine plus sulfadiazine confers protection against PCP as well as toxoplasmosis. Although the clindamycin plus pyrimethamine regimen is recommended in adults, it has not been tested in children. However, these drugs are safe and are used for other infections.

[b]Significant drug interactions might occur between rifabutin and protease inibitors and nonnucleoside reverse transcriptase inhibitors. Consult an expert.

[c]Drug should be determined by susceptibilities of the organism isolated. Alternatives to TMP-SMX include ampicillin, chloramphenicol, or ciprofloxacin. However, ciprofloxacin is not approved for use in persons aged <18 years; therefore, it should be used in children with caution and only if no alternatives exist.

[d]Antimicrobial prophylaxis should be chosen based on the microorganism and antibiotic sensitivities. TMP-SMX, if used, should be administered daily. Providers should be cautious about using antibiotics solely for this purpose because of the potential for development of drug-resistant microorganisms. IVIG might not provide additional benefit to children receiving daily TMP-SMX but may be considered for children who have recurrent bacterial infections despite TMP-SMX prophylaxis. Choice of antibiotic prophylaxis vs. IVIG should also involve consideration of adherence, ease of intravenous access, and cost. If IVIG is used, respiratory syncytial virus (RSV) IVIG (750 mg/kg) not monoclonal RSV antibody, may be substituted for IVIG during the RSV season to provide broad anti-infective protection, if this product is available.

IVIG, intravenous immune globulin; p.o., by mouth; q.d., daily; q.m., monthly; q.w., weekly; t.i.d., three times a day; t.i.w., three times a week; TMP-SMX, trimethoprim-sulfamethoxazole.

TABLE 121.8. Criteria for Starting, Discontinuing, and Restarting Opportunistic Infection Prophylaxis for Adults with Human Immunodeficiency Virus

Opportunistic illness	Criteria for initiating primary prophylaxis	Criteria for discontinuing primary prophylaxis	Criteria for restarting primary prophylaxis	Criteria for initiating secondary prophylaxis	Criteria for discontinuing secondary prophylaxis	Criteria for restarting secondary prophylaxis
Pneumocystis carinii pneumonia	CD4+ <200 cells/µL or oropharyngeal candidiasis (AI) IgG antibody to *Toxoplasma* and CD4+ <100 cells/µL (AI)	CD4+ >200 cells/µL for ≥3 mo (AI) CD4+ >200 cells/µL for ≥3 mo (AI)	CD4+ <200 cells/µL (AIII) CD4+ <100–200 cells/µL (AIII)	Prior *P. carinii* pneumonia (AI) Prior toxoplasmic encephalitis (AI)	CD4+ >200 cells/µL for ≥3 mo (BII) CD4+ >200 cells/µL sustained (e.g., ≥6 mo) and completed initial therapy and asymptomatic for toxo (CIII)	CD4+ <200 cells/µL (AIII) CD4+ <200 cells/µL (AIII)
Disseminated *Mycobacterium avium* complex	CD4+ <50 cells/µL (AI)	CD4+ >100 cells/µL for ≥3 mo (AI)	CD4+ <50–100 cells/µL (AIII)	Documented disseminated disease (AII)	CD4+ >100 cells/µL sustained (e.g., ≥6 mo) and completed 12 mo of MAC therapy and asymptomatic for MAC (CIII)	CD4+ <100 cells/µL (AIII)
Cryptococcosis	None	Not applicable	Not applicable	Documented disease (AI)	CD4+ >100–200 cells/µL sustained (e.g., >6 mo) and completed initial therapy and asymptomatic for cryptococcosis (CIII)	CD4+ <100–200 cells/µL (AIII)
Histoplasmosis	None	Not applicable	Not applicable	Documented disease (AI)	No criteria recommended for stopping	Not applicable
Coccidioidomycosis	None	Not applicable	Not applicable	Documented disease (AI)	No criteria recommended for stopping	CD4+ <100–150 cells/µL (AIII)
Cytomegalovirus retinitis	None	Not applicable	Not applicable	Documented end-organ disease (AI)	CD4+ >100–50 cells/µL sustained (e.g., ≥6 mo) and no evidence of active disease and regular ophthalmic examination (BII)	CD4+ <100–150 cells/µL (AIII)

TABLE 121.9. Drugs Used in Pediatric HIV Infection

Drug	Dosage	Major toxicities	Drug interactions	Special instructions
		Nucleoside analog reverse transcriptase inhibitor agents		
Abacavir (GW 1592U89, ABC) (Ziagen) Preparations: Pediatric oral solution: 20 mg/mL Tablets: 300 mg Tablets in combination with zidovudine and lamivudine: Trizivir: 300 mg zidovudine, 150 mg lamivudine, 300 mg abacavir	Neonatal dose: Not approved for infants <3 mo of age. For infants 1–3 mo of age, a dose of 8 mg/kg b.i.d. is under study Pediatric/adolescent dose: 8 mg/kg body weight b.i.d. max dose 300 mg b.i.d. Adult dose: 300 mg b.i.d. Adult dose Trizivir: 1 tab b.i.d.	Most frequent: nausea, vomiting, fever, headache, diarrhea, rash, anorexia Less common (more severe): Potentially fatal hypersensitivity reaction in 5% of adults and children: flu-like symptoms or respiratory symptoms such as shortness of breath, ulcerated mucous membranes with or without maculopapular or urticarial skin rash. Increased LFTs, CPK and creatinine; occurs in first 6 wk of therapy. Stop ABC when hypersensitivity reaction is suspected. Do not rechallenge. Hypotension and death have occurred upon rechallenge. Lactic acidosis, severe hepatomegaly with steatosis, including fatal cases reported. Rare: Pancreatitis, increased liver enzymes, elevated triglycerides and fatigue	No significant interactions between ABC, ZDV, and 3TC ABC: not metabolized by cytochrome P450 enzymes. No interaction with drug levels or clearance of agents metabolized by this pathway. Ethanol decreases elimination and causes modest increase in drug exposure	No food restrictions. Caution about the risk of serious hypersensitivity reaction. Provide warning card, report all hypersensitivity reaction to the ABC. Hypersensitivity Registry (1-800-270-0425) Consult your physician before interrupting therapy
Didanosine (ddl) (dideoxyinosine) (Videx) Preparations: Pediatric powder for oral solution (when reconstituted as solution containing antacid, 10 mg/mL) Chewable tablets with buffers, 25, 50, 100, and 150 mg, and 200 mg Buffered powder for oral solution, 100, 167, and 250 mg Delayed-release capsules (enteric-coated beadlets): Videx EC-125, 200, 250, and 400 mg	Neonatal dose (infants ≤90 d): 50 mg/m² q12h Pediatric usual dose: in combination with other antiretrovirals, 90 mg/m² q12h Pediatric dosage range: 90–150 mg/m² q12h (Note: may need higher dose in patients with CNS disease) Adolescent/adult dose: ≥60 kg, 200 mg b.i.d. <60 kg, 125 mg b.i.d. May be administered once daily in adolescent/adults to improve compliance; however, twice-daily dosing provides better therapeutic response than once-daily dosing Videx EC: Adolescent/adult dose: body weight >60 kg: 400 mg once daily. Body weight <60 kg: 250 mg once daily	Most frequent: diarrhea, abdominal pain, nausea, vomiting Unusual (more severe): peripheral neuropathy (dose related), electrolyte abnormalities, hyperuricemia Uncommon: pancreatitis (dose related, less common in children than adults); increased liver enzymes, retinal depigmentation Less common (more severe): Lactic acidosis and severe hepatomegaly with steatosis, including fatal cases have been reported	Possible decrease in absorption of ketoconazole, itraconazole, dapsone; administer at least 2 h before or 2 h after ddl Tetracycline and fluoroquinolone antibiotic absorption significantly decreased (chelation of drug by antacid in pediatric powder and tablets); administer 2 hr before or 2 hr after ddl Concomitant administration of ddl and delavirdine (DLV) may decrease the absorption of these drugs; separate dosing by at least 2 hr Administration with protease inhibitor (PI) agents: indinavir (IDV) should be administered at least 1 hr apart from ddl on an empty stomach. Ritonavir (RTV) should be administered at least 2 hr before or after ddl.	ddl formulation contains buffering agents antacids Food decreases absorption; administer ddl on an empty stomach (1 hr before or 2 hr after a meal). Additional evaluation in children regarding administration with meals is under study. For oral solution: shake well and keep refrigerated; admixture stable for 30 days When administering chewable tablets, at least two tablets should be administered to ensure adequate buffering capacity (e.g., the child's dose in 50 mg, administer two 25-mg tablets and not one 50-mg tablet)

Drug/Preparations	Dose	Toxicity	Comments
Lamivudine (3TC) (Epivir) Preparations: Solution, 10 mg/mL Tablets, 150 mg Tablets: Combivir (150 mg lamivudine in combination with 300 mg zidovudine) Tablets in combination with zidovudine: Combivir: 300 mg zidovudine and 150 mg lamivudine Tablets in combination with zidovudine and abacavir: Trizivir: 300 mg zidovudine, 150 mg lamivudine and 300 mg abacavir	Neonatal dose (infants ≤30 d): 2 mg/kg b.i.d. Pediatric dose: 4 mg/kg b.i.d. Adolescent/adult dose: ≥50 kg: 150 mg b.i.d. <50 kg: 2 mg/kg b.i.d. Adolescent/adult dose Combivir: one tablet twice daily Adolescent/adult dose Trizivir: one tablet twice daily	Most frequent: headache, fatigue, nausea, diarrhea, skin rash, abdominal pain Unusual (more severe): pancreatitis (primarily seen in children with advanced HIV infection receiving multiple other medications), peripheral neuropathy, decreased neutrophil count, increased liver enzymes Less common: Lactic acidosis and severe hepatomegaly with steatosis, including fatal cases have been reported	Trimethoprim-sulfamethoxazole (TMP/SMX) increases 3TC blood levels (possibly competes for renal tubular secretion); unknown significance When used with zidovudine (ZDV) may prevent emergence of ZDV resistance, and for ZDV-resistant virus, reversion to phenotypic ZDV sensitivity may be observed	Can be administered with food For oral solution, store at room temperature Decrease dosage in patients with impaired renal function Decrease dosage in patients with impaired renal function
Stavudine (d4T) (Zerit) Preparations: Solution, 1 mg/mL Capsules, 15, 20, 30, and 40 mg	Neonatal dose: Under evaluation in PACTG 332 Pediatric dose: 1 mg/kg q12h (up to body weight of 30 kg) Adolescent/adult dose: ≥60 kg, 40 mg b.i.d. <60 kg, 30 mg b.i.d.	Most frequent: headache, gastrointestinal disturbances, skin rashes Uncommon (more severe): peripheral neuropathy, pancreatitis Other: increased liver enzymes Less common: lactic acidosis and severe hepatomegaly with steatosis, including fatal cases have been reported	Drugs that decrease renal function could decrease clearance Should not be administered in combination with ZDV (poor antiviral effect)	Can be administered with food Need to decrease dose in patients with renal impairment For oral solution: shake well and keep refrigerated; solution stable for 30 days
Zalcitabine (ddC) (Hivid) Preparations: Syrup, 0.1 mg/mL (investigational; available through compassionate-use program) Tablets, 0.375 and 0.75 mg	Neonatal dose: Unknown Pediatric usual dose: 0.01 mg/kg q8h Pediatric dosage range: 0.005–0.01 mg/kg q8h Adolescent/adult dose: 0.75 mg t.i.d.	Most frequent: headache, gastrointestinal disturbances, malaise Unusual (more severe): peripheral neuropathy, pancreatitis, hepatic toxicity, oral ulcers, esophageal ulcers, hematologic toxicity, skin rashes Less common: lactic acidosis and severe hepatomegaly with steatosis, including fatal cases have been reported	Cimetidine, amphotericin, foscarnet, and aminoglycosides may decrease renal clearance of zalcitabine Antacids decrease absorption of zalcitabine Concomitant use with ddI is not recommended because of the increased risk of peripheral neuropathy Intravenous pentamidine increases the risk pancreatitis (do not use concurrently)	Administer on an empty stomach (1 hr before or 2 hr after a meal) Decrease dosage in patients with impaired renal function
Zidovudine (ZDV, AZT) (Retrovir) Preparations: Syrup, 10 mg/mL Capsules, 100 mg Tablets, 300 mg Tablets: Combivir (300 mg zidovudine in combination with 150 mg lamivudine) Concentrate for injection, for intravenous infusion: 10 mg/mL Tablets: Trizivir (300 mg zidovudine in combination with 150 mg lamivudine and 300 mg abacavir)	Dose in premature infants: (standard neonatal dose may be excessive in premature infants) Under study in PACTG 331: Oral or i.v. 1.5 mg/kg q12h from birth to 2 wk of age; then increase to 2 mg/kg q8h after 2 wk of age Neonatal dose: Oral, 2 mg/kg q6h i.v., 1.5 mg/kg q6h Pediatric usual dose: oral, 160 mg/m² q6h Adolescent/adult dose Trizivir: one tablet twice daily i.v. (intermittent infusion), 120 mg/m² q6h i.v. (continuous infusion), 20 mg/m²/hr	Most frequent: hematologic toxicity (including granulocytopenia and anemia), headache Unusual: myopathy, myositis, liver toxicity Unusual (severe): lactic acidosis and severe hepatomegaly with steatosis, including fatal cases have been reported	Increased toxicity may be observed with concomitant administration of the following drugs (therefore, more intensive toxicity monitoring may be warranted): ganciclovir, interferon-α, TMP-SMX, acyclovir, and other drugs that can be associated with bone marrow suppression The following drugs may increase ZDV concentration (and potential toxicity): methadone, atovaquone valproic acid, probenecid, and fluconazole Decreased renal clearance may be observed with coadministration of cimetidine (may be significant in patients with renal impairment).	Can be administered with food, although manufacturer recommends that ZDV be taken 30 min before or 1 hr after a meal Decrease dosage in patients with severe renal impairment Substantial granulocytopenia or anemia may necessitate interruption of therapy until marrow recovery is observed; use of filgrastim, erythropoietin or reduced ZDV dosage may be necessary in some patients Reduced dosage may be indicated in patients with substantial hepatic dysfunction

(continued)

TABLE 121.9. (continued)

Drug	Dosage	Major toxicities	Drug interactions	Special instructions
Nucleoside analog reverse transcriptase inhibitor agents				
	Pediatric dosage range: 90–180 mg/m^2 q6-8h Adolescent/adult dose: 200 mg t.i.d. or 300 mg b.i.d.		Fluconazole interferes with metabolism and clearance of ZDV increases ZDV area under the curve (AUC) ZDV metabolism may be increased with coadministration of rifampin and rifabutin (clinical significance unknown); clarithromycin may decrease concentration of ZDV probably by interfering with absorption (preferably administer 4 hr apart). Ribavirin decreases the intracellular phosphorylation of ZDV (conversion to active metabolite) Phenytoin may increase or decrease ZDV levels Should not be administered in combination with D4T (poor antiretroviral effect).	Infuse i.v. loading dose or intermittent infusion dose over 1 hr. For i.v. solution, dilute with 5% dextrose injection solution to concentration <4 mg/mL; refrigerated diluted solution stable for 24 hr Some working group participants use a dose of 180 mg/m^2 q12h when using in drug combinations with other antiretroviral compounds, but data on the dosing in children are limited
Nonnucleoside analog reverse transcriptase inhibitor agents				
Delavirdine (DLV) (Rescriptor) Preparations: Tablets, 100 mg and 200 mg	Neonatal dose: unknown Pediatric dose: unknown Adolescent/adult dose: 400 mg t.i.d. or 600 mg b.i.d. (investigational)	Most frequent: headache, fatigue, gastrointestinal complaints, rash (may be severe)	Metabolized in part by hepatic cytochrome P450 3A (CYP 3A); potential for multiple drug interactions Before administration, the patient's medication profile should be reviewed carefully for potential drug interactions DLV decreases the metabolism of certain drugs, resulting in increased drug levels and potential toxicity. DLV is not recommended for concurrent use with antihistamines (e.g., astemizole or terfenadine); sedative-hypnotics (e.g., alprazolam, midazolam, or triazolam); calcicium channel blockers (e.g., nifedipine); ergot alkaloid derivatives; amphetamines, cisapride; or warfarin. DLV clearance is increased, resulting in substantially reduced concentrations of DLV, with concurrent use of rifabutin, rifampin, or anticonvulsants (e.g., phenytoin, carbamazepine, or phenobarbital). Concurrent use is not recommended. Decreased absorption of DLV if given with antacids or H$_2$ receptor antagonists.	Can be administered with food Should be taken 1 hr before or 1 hr after ddI or antacids Tablets can be dissolved in water and the resulting dispersion should be taken promptly. The 100 mg tablets can be dissolved in water and the resulting dispersion taken promptly. However, the 200-mg tablets should be taken as intact tablets, because they are not readily dispersed in water

| Nevirapine (NVP) (Viramune) Preparations: Suspension, 10 mg/mL Tablets, 200 mg, scored | Start at a lower dose, increase in stepwise fashion Neonatal dose: (thru age 3 mo) PACTG Protocol 356: 5 mg/kg or 120 mg/m² q12h q.d. for 14 days followed by 120 mg/m² q12h q.d. for 14 d, followed by 200 mg/m² q12h Pediatric dose: 120–200 mg/m² q12h. Note: start with 120 mg/m² (max 200 mg) q.d. for 14 days increased to 120–200 mg/m² q12h (max 200 mg q12h) if no rash or other untoward effects Or 7 mg/kg q12h <8 yr of age 4 mg/kg q12h >8 yr of age Note: Initiate therapy with daily dose for 14 d and increase to full dose if no rash or other untoward effects Adolescent/adult dose: 200 mg q12h Start dose once daily for first 14 d and increase to full dose q12h if no rash or other untoward effects | (Continuous dosing, not single-dose regimens) More common: skin rash (some severe, requiring hospitalization, Stevens-Johnson syndrome and toxic epidermal necrolysis), fever, nausea, headache and abnormal LFTs Less common: hepatitis, and in some cases, fatal liver damage, very rarely fatal liver failure and granulocytopenia. Hypersensitivity reaction (including but not limited to, severe rash or rash accompanied by fever, blisters, oral lesions, conjunctivitis, facial edema, muscle or joint aches, general malaise and/or significant hepatic abnormalities) | Increased trough concentrations of DLV by ~50% if given with ketoconazole, fluoxetine; increased levels of both drugs if DLV given with clarithromycin DLV may increase dapsone and quinidine plasma concentrations Administration with PI agents: decreases metabolism of saquinavir (SQV) and indinavir (IDV), resulting in a significant increase in SQV and IDV concentrations and a slight decrease in DLV concentration Induces hepatic CYP 3A; autoinduction of metabolism occurs in 2–4 wk with a 1.5–2-fold increase in clearance. Potential for multiple-drug interactions. Before administration, the patient's medication profile should be reviewed carefully for potential drug interactions Administration with PI agents: IDV and SQV (hard- and soft-gel formulation) concentrations are decreased significantly (25%–30%) when administered with NVP SQV-HGC is not recommended for use in children and is recommended only in combination with RTV in adults No data on specific dosing adjustment in pediatric patient for both IDV and NFV Antifungals: NVP reduces ketoconazole concentration. Do not coadminister. If indicated, use fluconazole. Rifampin/rifabutin: Rifampin significantly decreases NVP concentration. Do not coadminister. Rifabutin has less than an effect on NVP concentrations Methadone: Possibility of withdrawal symptoms in patient on methadone maintenance when NVP is added to their regimen. If present, increase dose of methadone and titrate to patient response Anticonvulsants and psychotropics: No data available on the extent of drug interactions with phenobarbital, phenytoin, and carbamazepine. Monitor serum concentrations of these agents. Possibility of interaction between psychotropic drugs and NVP since they use the same metabolic pathways. | Can be administered with food May be administered concurrently with didanosine (ddl) NVP-associated skin rash usually occurs within the first 6 wk of therapy. NVP should be discontinued immediately in patients who develop severe rash or a rash accompanied by constitutional symptoms (i.e., fever, oral lesions, conjunctivitis, or blistering). Hepatotoxicity may be severe and life threatening and fatal in some cases, including fulminant and cholestatic hepatic necrosis and hepatic failure. Increased LFTs or history of hepatitis B or C prior to starting NVP are associated with higher risk for hepatic adverse events. Most cases have occurred during first 12 hr of NVP therapy Clinical and laboratory monitoring is mandatory during this time period. Insidious onset with nonspecific prodromal signs or symptoms of hepatitis progressive to hepatic failure has been reported Patients should be instructed to contact the HIV specialist if signs or symptoms develop to determine the need for evaluation. Nevirapine (NVP) should be permanently discontinued and restarted in patients who develop clinical hepatitis For suspension: must be shaken well; stored at room temperature |

(continued)

TABLE 121.9. (continued)

Drug	Dosage	Major toxicities	Drug interactions	Special instructions
Nonnucleoside analog reverse transcriptase inhibitor agents				
			Monitor carefully when coadministered. Oral contraceptives: NVP may reduce plasma concentration of oral contraceptives and other hormonal contraceptives Do not use oral contraceptives as only means of birth control when NVP is used in female reproductive patients	
Efavirenz, DMP-266, EFV (Sustiva) Preparations: Capsules 50, 100, 200 mg	Neonatal dose: unknown Pediatric dose: administered once daily Body weight: 10 to ≤15 kg: 200 mg; 15 to ≤25 kg: 250 mg 25 to ≤37.5 kg: 350 mg 32.5 to ≤40 kg: 400 mg ≥40 kg: 600 mg	More common: skin rash; CNS (somnolence, insomnia, abnormal dreams, confusion, abnormal thinking, impaired concentration, amnesia, agitation, depersonalization, hallucinations, euphoria) primarily reported in adults. Increased AST, ALT levels, teratogenicity in primates. Pregnancy testing in women with childbearing potential before initiating therapy.	Mixed inducer/inhibition of CYP 3A4 enzymes; increased or decreased concentrations of concomitant drugs depending on specific enzyme pathway involved. Not recommended for concomitant use: antihistamines (astemizole or terfenadine), sedative-hypnotic (midazolam or triazolam), cisapride, or ergot alkaloid derivatives. Careful monitoring if coadministered with warfarin (level potentially increased or decreased); ethinyl-estradiol levels potentially increased. A realistic method of barrier contraception should be used in addition to oral contraceptives. Rifampin, rifabutin, phenobarbital and phenytoin may decrease EFV concentrations: clinical significance unknown. Clarithromycin: levels potentially decreased while its metabolites are increased. Consider alternative (azithromycin). No information available on other macrolides Coadministration with PI: decreased level of SQV (AUC decreased by 50%) and IDV (AUC decreased by 31%). Do not administer with SQV as a sole PI. Increase dose of IDV if given with EFV in adults (800–1,000 mg q8h) Increased levels of both RTV and EFV (AUC increased by 20% for both; higher frequency of side effect). Monitor liver enzymes. Increased levels of NFV (AUC increased by 20%). No dose adjustment needed.	No food restriction. Relative bioavailability increased by 50% following a high far meal. Avoid administration with a high fat meal due potential for increased absorption. No safety data available when given above l recommended dose. Peppery taste when capsules are open and to liquids of foods. Use grape jelly to disguise the taste. Bedtime dosing recommended during the 2–4 wk of therapy to improve tolerability of CNS side effects
Protease inhibitor (PI) agents				
Amprenavir (APV) (Agenerase) Preparations: Pediatric oral solution: 15 mg/ml capsule: 50 and 150 mg	Neonatal dose: not recommended in children <3 yr Pediatric/adolescent dose (<50 kg): For children 4–12 yr or 13–16 yr weighing <50 kg: Oral solution: 22.5 mg/kg b.i.d. or 17 mg/kg t.i.d. (max daily dose 2,800 mg).	More common: vomiting, nausea, diarrhea, perioral paresthesias, rash Less common (more severe): life-threatening rash, including Stevens-Johnson syndrome in 1% of patients	Multiple: review patient's medication profile Coadministration of APV and EFV lowers level of APV 39% Do not coadminister with astemizole, bepridil, cisapride, ergot alkaloid, midazolam, rifampin, and triazolam	Do not use APV in children <4 yr. Oral solution and capsule formulation not interchangeable on a mg per mg basis. The oral bioavailability of the oral solution is 14% less than the capsule

Capsules: 20 mg/kg b.i.d. or 15 mg/kg t.i.d. (max daily dose 2,400 mg)
Adult dose: 1,200 mg b.i.d.

Rare: increased cholesterol levels, new onset diabetes mellitus, hyperglycemia, exacerbation of preexisting diabetes mellitus, hemolytic anemia, and spontaneous bleeding in hemophiliacs

Possible interaction with amiodarone, lidocaine, tricyclic antidepressants, quinidine, and warfarin. Monitor concentration of those drugs if APV is administered

Rifampin reduces plasma concentration of APV (decreased AUC 82%). No significant effect on rifampin plasma levels

APV increases the AUC of rifabutin by 193%. Reduce the dose of rifabutin by at least half the recommended dose when given in combination with APV

APV increases plasma concentration of sildenafil (Viagra) which increases the risk of sildenafil-associated adverse events (hypotension, visual changes, priapism)

APV formulation contains 46 IU vitamin E/mL of oral solution and 109 IU vitamin E, 150-mg capsule. Daily recommended dose for vitamin E in children is 10 IU/d and in adults 30 IU/d. Based on the recommended dose of APV, for adults and children, excess ingestion of or administration will occur. Hypervitaminosis E is associated with creatinuria, decreased platelet aggregation, impaired wound healing, hepatomegaly, prolonged PT, potential risk of vitamin K deficiency coagulopathy, increased response to drugs as warfarin and dicumarol. Do not use concurrently oral anticoagulants with vitamin E doses >400 IU/d. Avoid supplemental use of vitamin E in patients taking APV.

APV contains propylene glycol exceeding WHO standard for use in infants. Half life of propylene glycol is prolonged in neonates (16.9 hr compared to 5 hr in adults). High levels have been associated with hyperosmolarity, lactic acidosis, seizures, and respiratory depression.

Reduced efficacy of birth control pills in patients receiving APV, use additional methods of birth control

Possible potential interactions with medications that are substrates or inducers of CYP 3A4

APV is a sulfonamide. Potential for cross sensitivity with the sulfonamide class is unknown. Use with caution in patients with sulfonamide allergy

Take with or without food. Do not administer APV with a high fat meal

Patients taking antacids (ddl) should take at least 1 hr before and after a high-fat meal

(continued)

TABLE 121.9. (continued)

Drug	Dosage	Major toxicities	Drug interactions	Special instructions
Protease inhibitor agents				
Indinavir (IDV)/q (Crixivan) Preparations: Capsules, 200 and 400 mg	Neonatal dose: unknown; because of side effect of hyperbilirubinemia, should not be given to neonates until additional information available Pediatric dose: under study in clinical trials, 500 mg/m² q8h. Patients with small body-surface areas may require lower doses (300–400 mg/m² q8h) Adolescent/adult dose: 800 mg q8h	Most common: nausea, abdominal pain, headache, metallic taste, dizziness, asymptomatic hyperbilirubinemia (10%) Unusual (more severe): nephrolithiasis (4%), and exacerbation of chronic liver disease Rare: spontaneous bleeding episodes in hemophiliacs, hyperglycemia, ketoacidosis, diabetes, and hemolytic anemia. Possible association with fat redistribution with and without serum lipid abnormalities. (Causal association not definitively established.)	CYP 3A4 responsible for metabolism. Potential for multiple drug interactions. Before administration, the patient's medication profile should be reviewed carefully for potential drug interactions. IDV decreases the metabolism of certain drugs, resulting in increased drug levels and potential toxicity. IDV is not recommended for concurrent use with antihistamines (e.g., astemizole or terfenadine); cisapride; ergot alkaloid derivatives; or sedative-hypnotics (e.g., triazolam or midazolam). IDV levels are significantly reduced with concurrent use of rifampin. Concurrent use is not recommended Rifabutin concentrations are increased and a dose reduction of rifabutin to half the usual daily dose is recommended Ketoconazole and itraconazole cause an increase in IDV concentrations (consider reducing adolescent/adult IDV dose to 600 mg q8h) Coadministration of clarithromycin increases serum concentration of both drugs (dosing modification not needed)	Administer on an empty stomach 1 hr before or 2 hr after a meal (or can take with a light meal) Adequate hydration (at least 48 ounces/d in adult patients) required to minimize risk of nephrolithiasis If coadministered with ddl, give at least 1 hr apart on an empty stomach Decrease dose in patients with hepatic insufficiency Capsules are sensitive to moisture and should not be stored in original container with desiccant
Lopinavir/ritonavir (Kaletra, ABT 378, LPV/RTV) Preparations: Pediatric oral solutions: 80 mg LPV/20 mg RTV Capsules: 133.3 mg LPV/33.3 mg/RTV	Neonatal dose: no pharmacokinetic data in children <6 mo For patients whose regimen does not include NVP or EFV: Pediatric dose: 6 mo to 12 yr of age 7 to <15 kg: 12 mg/kg LPV/3 mg RTV b.i.d with food 15–40 kg: 10 mg/kg LPV/2.5 mg/kg RTV b.i.d. with food	More common: diarrhea, headache, asthma and nausea and vomiting. Increase in blood lipids (cholesterol and triglycerides) rash in patients receiving LPV/RTV other ARVs Rare: pancreatitis, hyperglycemia, ketoacidosis, diabetes, hepatitis, spontaneous bleeding episodes in hemophiliacs	Coadministration with NVP may decrease IDV serum concentrations Administration with other PI agents: coadministration with NVP increases concentration of both drugs; coadministration with saquinavir (SQV) increases concentration of SQV Avoid coadministration with antiarrhythmics (flecainide, propafenone, ergot alkaloid derivatives); antihistamines (astemizole, terfenadine); cisapride; neuroleptics (i.e., pimozide); sedative-hypnotics (i.e., midazolam, triazolam); HMG-CO/A; reductase inhibitors (i.e., lovastatin, simvastatin); rifampin and St. John's wort.	Administer with food. High-fat meals increase absorption especially liquid form If coadministered with ddl, give ddl 1 hr before or 2 hr after LPV RTV Keep oral solution capsules refrigerated, kept at room temperature 77° (25°) if used within month

1072

Drug/Preparation	Dose	Adverse Effects	Drug Interactions	Instructions/Comments
	>40 kg: 400 mg LPV/100 mg RTV 3 capsules or 5 mL b.i.d. twice daily with food, or 230 mg/m² LPV/57.5 mg/m² RTV up to a maximum of 400 mg LPV/100 mg RTV. Adult/adolescent dose: 400 mg LPV/100 mg RTV 3 capsules or 5 mL b.i.d. twice daily with food. For individuals receiving concomitant NVP or EFV or treatment experienced patients with susceptibility or suspicion of reduced susceptibility to LPV: Increased dose is required. Pediatric dose: 6 mo to 12 yr of age (with NVP or EFV) 7 to <15 kg: 13 mg/kg LPV/3.25 mg/kg/RTV b.i.d. with food. 15–50 kg: 11 mg/kg LPV/2.75 mg/kg/RTV b.i.d. with food. >50 kg: 533 mg LPV/133 mg RTV 4 capsules or 6.5 mL b.i.d. with food or 300 mg/m² LPV/75 mg/m² RTV b.i.d. with food to a maximum of 533 mg LPV/133 mg RTV. Adult/adolescent dose: 533 mg LPV/133 mg RTV (4 capsules or 6.5 mL) b.i.d. with food.		Increase dose when coadministered with LPV/RTV. Carbamazepine, phenytoin, and phenobarbital increase CYP 3A activity, leading to increased clearance of LPV. Use with caution: Dexamethasone; decreases LPV concentration. LPV/RTV increases clarithromycin serum concentration. Dose adjustment recommended in patients with impaired renal function (CrCl 30–60 mL/min: decrease clarithromycin dose by 50%; CrCl <30 mL/min: decrease clarithromycin dose by 75%). LPV/RTV increases rifabutin and rifabutin metabolite serum concentration: Reduce rifabutin dose by 75%; LPV/RTV increases serum concentration of sildenafil (Viagra), amiodarone, bepridil, lidocaine (systemic), quinidine, cyclosporine, tacrolimus, rapamycin, dihydropyridine calcium channel blockers (i.e., felodipine, nifedipine, nicardipine, ketoconazole, itraconazole). Monitor for toxicity. LPV/RTV decreases serum concentration of methadone. Monitor withdrawal symptoms. LPV/RTV decreases serum concentration of estradiol. Alternative or additional birth-control method should be used. Disulfiram-like reaction when LPV/RTV is administered with metronidazole or disulfiram (contains 42.5% alcohol).	
Nelfinavir (NFV) (Viracept) Preparations: Powder for oral suspension, 50 mg per 1 level scoop (200 mg per 1 level teaspoon) Tablets, 250 mg	Neonatal dose: Under study in PACTG 353: 40 mg/kg body weight q12h. Pediatric dose: Currently under review: 20–30 mg/kg body weight t.i.d. is FDA approved dose. However, doses as high as 45 mg/kg q8h are routinely used. Twice-daily dosing in pediatric patients is under study (50–55 mg/kg/dose) in older children (>6 yr). Adolescent/adult dose: 1,250 mg (5 tablets) b.i.d. or 750 mg (3 tablets) t.i.d. Doses of 1,500 mg (6 tablets) b.i.d. are under study in adults	Most common: diarrhea. Less common: asthenia, abdominal pain rash, and exacerbation of chronic liver disease. Rare: spontaneous bleeding episodes in hemophiliacs, hyperglycemia, ketoacidosis, and diabetes. Possible association with fat redistribution with and without serum lipid abnormalities. (Causal association not definitively established.)	NFV is in part metabolized by CYP 3A4. Potential for multiple-drug interactions. Before administration, the patient's medication profile should be reviewed carefully for potential drug interactions. NFV decreases the metabolism of certain drugs, resulting in increased drug levels and potential toxicity. NFV is not recommended for concurrent use with antihistamines (e.g., astemizole or terfenadine); cisapride; ergot alkaloid derivatives; certain cardiac drugs (e.g., quinidine or amiodarone); or sedative-hypnotics (e.g., triazolam or midazolam).	Administer with food to optimize absorption. If coadministered with ddI, NFV should be administered 2 hr before or 1 hr after ddI. For oral solution: powder may be mixed with water, milk, pudding, or formula (up to 6 hr). Do not mix with any acidic food or juice because of resulting poor taste. Do not add water to bottles of oral powder. A special scoop is provided with oral powder for measuring purposes

(continued)

TABLE 121.9. (continued)

Drug	Dosage	Major toxicities	Drug interactions	Special instructions
		Protease inhibitor agents		
			Rifampin significantly decreases NFV concentrations and should not be coadministered	Tablets disperse readily in water and can be mixed with milk or chocolate milk. Tablets can also be crushed and administered with pudding
			Rifabutin causes less decline in NFV concentrations; if coadministered with NFV, rifabutin should be reduced to half the usual dose	
			Estradiol levels are reduced by NFV, and alternative or additional methods of birth control should be used if coadministering with hormonal methods of birth control	
			Coadministration with DLV increases NFV concentration twofold and decreases DLV concentrations by 50%. There are no data on coadministration with NVP, but some experts use higher doses of NFV if used in combination with NVP.	
			Administration with other PI agents: Concomitant administration of IDV and NFV may increase plasma concentrations of both drugs	
			Concomitant administration of SQV and NFV can result in substantially increased plasma concentrations of SQV with little change in NFV concentrations	
			Concomitant administration of RTV and NFV increases concentration of NFV without change in RTV concentration	
Ritonavir (RTV) (Norvir) Preparations: Oral solution, 80 mg/mL Capsules, 100 mg	Neonatal dose: under study in PACTG 354 Pediatric dose: 400 mg/m² q12h To minimize nausea/vomiting, initiate therapy at 250 mg/m² q12h and increase stepwise to full dose over 5 d as tolerated Pediatric dosage range: 350–400 mg/m² q12h	Most common: nausea, vomiting, diarrhea, headache, abdominal pain, anorexia Less common: circumoral paresthesias, increase in liver enzymes Rare: spontaneous bleeding episodes in hemophiliacs, pancreatitis, increased levels of triglycerides and cholesterol,	RTV is extensively metabolized in the liver by the CYP 3A. Potential for multiple-drug interactions. Before administration, the patient's medication profile should be reviewed carefully for potential drug interactions. Not recommended for concurrent use with analgesics (e.g., meperidine, piroxicam, or propoxyphene);	Administration with food increases absorption If administered with ddl, there should be 2 hr between taking each of the drugs Capsules must be kept refrigerated To minimize nausea, therapy should be initiated at a low dose and increased to full dose over 5 d as tolerated

Drug	Dose	Adverse effects	Drug interactions	Administration
	Adolescent/adult dose: 600 mg q12h (single PI therapy), 400 mg q12h (in combination with SQV) To minimize nausea/vomiting, initiate therapy at 300 mg q12h and increase stepwise to full dose over 5 d as tolerated Pharmacokinetic enhancer: Used at lower doses as pharmacokinetic enhancer of other protease inhibitors. Doses most commonly used in adults are 200 mg q12h to 400 mg q12h when combined with other protease inhibitors	hyperglycemia, diabetes and hepatitis. Possible association with fat redistribution with and without serum lipid abnormalities. (Causal association not definitively established.)	antihistamines (e.g., astemizole or terfenadine); certain cardiac drugs (e.g., amiodarone, bepridil hydrochloride, encainide hydrochloride, flecainide acetate, propafenone, or quinidine); ergot alkaloid derivatives; cisapride; sedative-hypnotics (e.g., alprazolam, clorazepate, diazepam, estazolam, flurazepam hydrochloride, midazolam, triazolam, or zolpidem tartrate); certain psychotropic drugs (e.g., bupropion hydrochloride, clozapine, or pimozide); rifampin; or rifabutin. Estradiol levels are reduced by RTV, and alternative or additional methods or birth control should be used if coadministering with hormonal methods of birth control. RTV increases metabolism of theophylline (levels should be monitored, and dose may need to be increased) RTV increases levels of clarithromycin (dose adjustment may be necessary in patients with impaired renal function); desipramine (dose adjustment may be necessary); and warfarin (monitoring of anticoagulant effect is necessary). RTV may increase or decrease digoxin levels (monitoring of levels is recommended). Drugs that increase CYP 3A activity and can lead to increased clearance and therefore lower levels of ritonavir or RTV include carbamazepine, dexamethasone, phenobarbital, and phenytoin (anticonvulsant levels should be monitored because RTV can affect the metabolism of these drugs as well). Administration with other PI agents: coadministration with SQV and NFV increases concentration of these drugs with little change in RTV concentration	For oral solution, recommended that it be kept refrigerated and stored in original container; can be kept at room temperature if used within 30 d. Techniques to increase tolerance in children: mix oral solution with milk, chocolate milk, vanilla or chocolate pudding, or ice cream; dull the taste buds before administration—chewing ice, giving popsicles or spoonful of partially frozen orange or grape juice concentrates; coat the mouth by giving peanut butter to eat before the dose; administer strong tasting foods such as maple syrup, cheese, or strong flavor chewing gum immediately after dose
Saquinavir (SQV) Invirase (hard-gel capsule) Fortovase (soft-gel capsule) Preparations: Hard gel capsules (HGC), 200 mg Soft gel capsules (SGC), 200 mg	Neonatal dose: unknown Pediatric dose: under study: 50 mg/kg body weight q8h as single protease inhibitor therapy. 33 mg/kg body weight q8h as usual therapy with nelfinavir	Most common: diarrhea, abdominal discomfort, headache and nausea Rare: spontaneous bleeding episodes of hemophiliacs, hyperglycemia and diabetes.	SQV is metabolized by the CYP 3A system in the liver and there are numerous potential drug interactions. Before administration, the patient's medication profile should be reviewed carefully for potential drug interactions.	Administer with a meal or within 2 hr after meal to increase absorption. Concurrent administration of grapefruit juice increases SQV concentration

(continued)

TABLE 121.9. (continued)

Drug	Dosage	Major toxicities	Drug interactions	Special instructions
		Protease inhibitor agents		
Please note that Saquinavir-HGC (Invirase) is not recommended except in combination with ritonavir.	Adolescent/adult dose: Soft-gel capsules, 1,200 mg t.i.d. or 1,600 mg b.i.d.	Possible association with fat redistribution with and without serum lipid abnormalities. (Causal association not definitively established.)	SQV decreases the metabolism of certain drugs, resulting in increased drug levels and potential toxicity. SQV is not recommended for concurrent use with antihistamines (e.g., astemizole or terfenadine); cisapride; ergot alkaloid derivatives; or sedative-hypnotics (e.g., triazolam or midazolam). SQV levels are significantly reduced with concurrent use of rifampin (decreases SQV levels by 80%), rifabutin (decreases SQV levels by 40%), and NVP (decreases SQV levels by 25%) SQV levels are decreased by carbamazepine, dexamethasone, phenobarbital, and phenytoin SQV levels are increased by delavirdine (or DLV) and ketoconazole SQV may increase levels of calcium channel blockers, clindamycin, dapsone, and quinidine. If used concurrently, patients should be monitored closely for toxicity. Administration with other protease inhibitors: co-administration with IDV, RTV, or NFV increases concentration of SQV with little change in concentration of the other drugs.	Sun exposure can cause photosensitivity reactions and sunscreen or protective clothing is recommended. Capsules must be kept refrigerated. Once brought to room temperature, capsules should be used within 3 mo.

infection regardless of HCV infection status. Because the mother-to-infant transmission rate for HCV infection is 5%, children with coexposure to HIV and HCV should be tested. The duration of maternal HCV antibody in infants is unknown, but it has been postulated to be more than 12 months. Therefore, testing for anti-HCV should not be performed until after 12 months of age. If earlier diagnosis is required, PCR for HCV RNA may be performed at or after the infant's first well-child visit at 1 to 2 months of age. Most children with chronic HCV infection are asymptomatic. However, with coinfection with HIV, chronic hepatitis may develop more rapidly, with the risk of developing cirrhosis and the occurrence of hepatocellular carcinoma. Increased liver function test results requiring medication interruption have been anecdotally reported in HIV-infected children and adolescents infected with HCV receiving HAART. Measles with giant cell pneumonia can be severe and often fatal in immunocompromised patients (89). Measles immunization is recommended (Table 121.5) for children with asymptomatic HIV infection and for those with symptomatic infection who are not severely immunocompromised. In general, children with symptomatic HIV infections have poor immunologic response to vaccines. Therefore, when there is a history of exposure to vaccine-preventable disease such as measles or tetanus, it is strongly recommended to consider passive immunization regardless of the history of immunization (88).

Fungal Infections

Oropharyngeal candidiasis, also known as the *white plague* of the immunocompromised host, is the most common fungal infection seen in HIV-infected infants and children. Several functional defects of the myeloid phagocytes have been observed, including impaired bacterial killing, decreased chemotaxis, and decreased phagocytosis of the most common fungi (90–92). Oropharyngeal candidiasis can be severe, chronic, or recurrent and resistant to conventional therapy. It may progress to the esophagus, causing decreased appetite, progressive weight loss, failure to thrive, and wasting syndrome. Esophageal candidiasis may coexist or occur without oropharyngeal candidiasis. The typical retrosternal burning and dysphagia commonly seen in patients with cancer may not be present and is difficult to assess in young infants (93). Deeply invasive candidiasis is an uncommon complication in pediatric HIV infection. It can be seen in critically ill children, and the incidence increases significantly in the presence of an indwelling central venous catheter. Diaper dermatitis caused by *Candida* is often recurrent and requires protracted therapy. Cryptococcal infections are seen less commonly in children. Meningitis is the most common extrapulmonary manifestation (94). HIV-infected children and adolescents with severe immunosuppression presenting with a history of unexplained fever, headache, and altered mental status should be investigated for cryptococcal meningitis. Maintenance therapy with fluconazole is necessary after treatment with amphotericin B with or without flucytosine to prevent recurrence.

Parasitic and Protozoal Infections

The most common OI seen in HIV-1–infected children is *Pneumocystis carinii* pneumonia (PCP). The number of new cases has greatly diminished in young children largely as a result of effective anti-*Pneumocystis* prophylaxis, primarily with trimethoprim-sulfamethoxazole (TMP-SMX), and HAART (56,95). However, PCP is still the most common life-threatening AIDS indicator condition in the United States, especially in young children. The peak incidence of PCP occurs between 3 and 6 months of age presumably representing primary infections. Its presentation is acute in that age-group, although a slower onset may be seen in older children and adolescents.

CD4+ lymphocyte count has no predictive value of PCP risk in infants younger than 12 months, in whom PCP may occur at CD4+ levels higher than those indicative of severe immunosuppression in adults (95). Current prophylaxis guidelines recommend starting prophylaxis in all infants born to HIV-1–infected mothers beginning at 4 to 6 weeks of age, with subsequent discontinuation if it is determined by nonreactive HIV DNA PCR or viral cultures that those children are not infected, and continuation for at least the first year of life in children who are infected (Table 121.6). The clinical presentation of PCP in children can be insidious with gradually worsening cough tachypnea and fever, or it can be acute with emergence of symptoms in hours with some degree of hypoxia. Chest radiographs initially may show no abnormalities, but the radiologic appearance of a diffuse bilateral alveolar-interstitial disease picture is helpful in reaching a diagnosis. Radiologic change may lag behind the clinical presentation, be atypical, or be confounded by the presence of chronic interstitial changes (96).

Other parasitic infections such as *Cryptosporidium, Isospora belli*, microsporidia, or *Giardia* have been described in children infected with HIV and are associated with intractable diarrhea. In addition to standard precautions, recommendations for prevention and control in child care settings have been established, especially for cryptosporidiosis (60,97). Toxoplasmosis in HIV-infected children is acquired congenitally or when immunosuppression leads to reactivation of latent infection. Toxoplasmic encephalitis is an uncommon OI in children compared with adults with HIV infection. It occurs in less than 1% of children diagnosed with AIDS. The use of TMP-SMX in children with severe immunosuppression and avoidance of exposure are the main strategies to prevent toxoplasmosis (60) (Table 121.6).

ORGAN SYSTEM INVOLVEMENT

Respiratory Tract

Early upper respiratory tract disease is manifested with frequent bouts of otitis media and sinusitis. Recurrent episodes of bacterial pneumonia with normal childhood pathogens are common infectious pulmonary complications in infants and children with HIV. However, PCP, as previously discussed as the most common OI, especially in young children, and lymphocytic interstitial pneumonitis/pulmonary lymphoid hyperplasia (LIP/PLH) complex are the two main pulmonary pathologic processes in HIV-infected children. LIP/PLH is a chronic interstitial pulmonary disease of unknown or poorly understood etiology. It is characterized by lymphoid infiltration of the lungs with a predominance of CD8+ lymphocytes on biopsy specimens, focal peribronchiolar infiltration of lymphocytes (PLH) or a more diffuse lymphoid infiltration of the alveolar septa (LIP) has been observed (98). LIP/PLH complex appears to be part of the group of lymphoproliferative disorders that range from hypergammaglobulinemia and generalized lymphadenopathy to malignant non-Hodgkin's lymphoma. Correlation and coinfection with Epstein-Barr virus (EBV) have been postulated because high titers of EBV viral capsid antigen have been found in lung biopsy specimens of children with LIP/PLH complex (99,100). Presumptive radiographic evidence includes a reticulonodular pattern with or without hilar adenopathy persisting for 2 months or more and unresponsive to antimicrobial therapy.

LIP/PLH complex is considered an indication for ART. The use of antiretroviral agents and corticosteroids has been anecdotally reported to be associated with improvement, which needs to be confirmed with a reduction in the pulmonary load of HIV and/or EBV (99,101,102). Prognostic factors in children with LIP/PLH complex seem to be better, as longer survival time and lower prevalence of OIs have been reported (102–104).

Cardiovascular System

There is no definite consensus about the methods of evaluation of HIV-infected children for cardiac disease (105–107). Therefore, there are wide differences in the incidence of cardiac disease in HIV-infected children (14%–93%). A wide range of manifestations has been described. Signs of left and/or right ventricular dysfunction, as well as arrhythmias, can be demonstrated by electrocardiography, but with echocardiography, the most common abnormality found is progressive left ventricular dysfunction, often combined with an increase in ventricular afterload. Cardiac abnormalities seem to be more severe in children with advanced HIV disease. However, Mofenson (41) and Luginbuhl et al. (108) have reported tachycardia, arrhythmia, and even sudden cardiac arrest in children who were mildly symptomatic, particularly in the presence of concomitant LIP. Another intriguing finding that has also been described in several HIV-infected children is the occurrence of arteriopathy in postmortem studies of children who died of HIV infection. Various organs are affected, including cardiac and cerebral vessels. This can lead to the formation of cerebral aneurysms that can result in neurologic and endocrinologic deficits or even sudden death with hemorrhage.

Gastrointestinal Tract

Diarrhea and malabsorption are common problems in children with AIDS, resulting in failure to thrive, growth failure, and wasting syndrome. Both weight and height velocity appear to be affected, either before the onset of HIV-related symptoms (41). The pathogenesis is multifactorial: (a) endocrine dysfunction, (b) impaired GI tract function, (c) altered cytokine production, (d) excessive energy expenditure, and (e) poor oral intake. A number of organisms, as previously described, have been associated with chronic diarrheal syndrome such as *Cryptosporidium*, microsporidia, *Isospora, Blastomyces hominis, Salmonella, Shigella, Campylobacter,* and mycobacteria, including a number of viruses (rotavirus, adenovirus, astrovirus, and calicivirus). *Clostridium difficile* colitis may be seen secondary to repeated or chronic use of antibiotics (109). It has been postulated that the gut-associated lymphoid tissue harbors a larger number of HIV-1 particles, possibly contributing to the syndrome of chronic diarrhea (110). Primary or secondary lactose intolerance is a common finding, but it is not clearly correlated with the presence of chronic diarrhea (111,112). Oropharyngeal candidiasis, oral hairy leukoplakia, and multiple dental caries are described in HIV-infected children and are associated with poor oral intake. Although liver failure is rare, hepatosplenomegaly, cholestasis, and chronic inflammation of the liver, resulting in elevated transaminase levels that can be secondary to antiretrovirals or other agents used in the management of HIV secondary to other infectious agents as CMV, HBV, HCV, and MAC, have been described (113,114). Pancreatitis can be caused by drugs (e.g., didanosine, zalcitabine, and pentamidine) or infection (CMV, MAC) (114,115). It may become chronic and be associated with persistent elevated amylase and lipase levels and intermittent clinical symptoms. Chronic pancreatitis with, at times, severe abdominal pain has become a common problem in older children surviving with perinatal HIV infection. One such adolescent with painful recurrent pancreatitis had dramatic symptomatic impairment following cholecystectomy.

Genitourinary Tract

The etiology of HIV-associated nephropathy is not known. It has been postulated that renal disease in HIV infection may be immunologically mediated (116). It can be characterized by proteinuria and may result in end-stage renal disease. The most common pathologic findings are focal glomerulosclerosis and mesangial hyperplasia (117). Disease progression occurs more slowly than that observed in the HIV-infected adult population. Other histologic lesions like segmental necrotizing glomerulonephritis, minimal change disease, and tubuloreticular inclusions within glomerular endothelial cells have been described (117–120). Several children with renal failure have become candidates for renal transplants and require renal dialysis. Close collaboration between the pediatric nephrologist and the pediatric infectious disease specialist with experience in management of children with HIV infection is strongly recommended.

Hematopoietic System

Hematologic abnormalities are common findings in HIV-infected children and adolescents. Anemia has been reported in an incidence range from 16% to 94% and is by far the most commonly observed hematologic disorder (121,122). The hematologic cytopenias may be secondary to HIV itself, may be drug induced, and may be due to other processes such as bone marrow infiltration by infection or malignancy, immune dysregulation, and malnutrition (41). Lymphopenia characterized by low CD4 count is the hallmark of HIV infection; however, neutropenia and thrombocytopenia have also been described (121–123). Pure red blood cell aplasia secondary to acute or persistent Parvovirus B19 infection and hemolytic anemia, as part of hemolytic-uremic syndrome, an autoimmune process, or a virus-associated hemophagocytic syndrome, have been observed as well (124,125). Neutropenia may be caused by the infection with HIV per se or by some opportunistic pathogens such as CMV, MAC, and adverse drug reactions. Thrombocytopenia is common and can be the initial manifestation of disease. Direct infection of megakaryocytes and platelets with HIV has been reported, and the use of HAART has been suggested in treating HIV-associated thrombocytopenia (126). Coagulation abnormalities secondary to vitamin K–dependent factors may be seen in late-stage disease, possibly because of severe malnutrition and advanced liver dysfunction. The recent report of Legg-Calvé-Perthes disease (LCPD) in HIV-infected children, similar to osteonecrosis seen in HIV-infected adults, may be a complication of thrombophilia seen with HIV disease or its treatment (127).

Proper identification of the underlying causes is the first and major step in managing hematologic complications of HIV infection. In addition to their treatment, use of some adjuvant products such as erythropoietin and granulocyte colony-stimulating factor have shown positive results in managing anemia and neutropenia in HIV infection.

Central Nervous System

Central nervous system (CNS) involvement in infants, children, and adolescents with HIV infection has been divided into three subclasses: (a) children with HIV-associated encephalopathy characterized by progressive, global deterioration, sometimes associated with loss of milestones, analogous to the process seen in adults termed "AIDS-dementia complex"; (b) children with neuropsychological impairment, also termed HIV-associated CNS compromise, or static encephalopathy; and (c) children who appear to be functioning normally (3,128). Even though encephalopathy is common in pediatric HIV infection and is an AIDS-defining diagnosis from the CDC guidelines, its pathogenesis is unclear. It appears that the risk of developing encephalopathy is especially high for infants born to mothers with far advanced or rapidly progressing disease, probably because the immature and developing nervous system may be more vulnerable to infection due to retroviruses (129). Some studies have found that asymptomatic children infected via blood products have minimal differences, if any, in neurodevelopment compared with matched uninfected control children (130). There is some correlation between the stage of HIV disease and the extent of neurodevelopmental insult in HIV-infected children: A cross-sectional multicenter surveillance study has shown that HIV encephalopathy was diagnosed in 23% of perinatally infected children with AIDS compared with 9.8% of perinatally infected children overall (131). Progressive HIV-associated encephalopathy may be one of the first manifestations of HIV disease in infants and young children (41,132). The neurologic findings of progressive encephalopathy consist in a well-defined triad: (a) impaired brain growth, "brain atrophy," (b) progressive motor dysfunction, and (c) plateauing, or an inadequate rate of neurodevelopmental milestones (133). Static encephalopathies are defined as fixed nonprogressive neurologic or neurodevelopmental deficits, often etiologically related to identifiable historical insults, such as intrauterine exposure to toxins or infectious agents, prematurity, genetic factors, or head trauma. HIV-infected children with static encephalopathy may spontaneously improve with time, may follow a static course, or may show evidence of neurologic decline/progressive encephalopathy (134). Some studies have demonstrated that expressive language apparently is significantly more impaired than receptive language (135). Based on the clinical findings, CNS disease in HIV-infected children is a subcortical, diffuse, white matter disease process, pathologically and radiologically proven. The most common findings seen by computed tomography (CT) and magnetic resonance imaging (MRI) include brain atrophy, calcification of the basal ganglia and periventricular white matter, ventricular enlargement, attenuation of signal intensity of the basal ganglia, and deep white matter (41,136). Successful therapy with ZDV has been shown to ameliorate the neuropsychological impairment caused by HIV infection, with improvement of the neurodevelopment assessment and neuroimaging studies (133,137,138). The effect of the other antiretrovirals combined in HAART on static/progressive encephalopathy is still under study concomitantly with the use of antiinflammatory agents and others like calcium channel blockers (139,140).

There are other pathologies such as CMV infection, toxoplasmosis, rubella infection, and drug exposure *in utero* that can cause progressive or static encephalopathy. They should be excluded, especially in young infants and children with signs and symptoms of neurologic impairment.

MALIGNANCIES

The exact incidence of malignancies in the pediatric HIV-infected population has not been established but appears to be several times more common than in normal children. The most common tumors in the immunocompromised host are lymphomas and mainly non-Hodgkin's lymphomas. They present either as systemic disease or as a primary CNS tumor. In contrast to HIV-1 infection in adults, Kaposi's sarcoma is rarely reported in HIV-infected children in industrialized countries (50,141). However, studies performed in Africa have reported an increased incidence of Kaposi's sarcoma in HIV-infected children (142,143). Leiomyoma and leiomyosarcoma are not usually associated with immunodeficiency, but they have been reported in HIV-infected children (144). Apparent correlation with EBV infection and smooth muscle tumors have been well established not only in HIV-infected children but also in patients who developed leiomyomatous tumors after an organ transplantation (145,146). It has been postulated that EBV is capable of transforming normal B lymphocytes into continuously proliferating cell lines *in vitro*. EBV is also associated with other lymphoproliferative disorders such as LIP/PLH complex. Other unusual malignancies such as papillary carcinoma of the thyroid, rhabdomyosarcoma, and hepatocellular carcinoma have been reported in HIV-infected children (147). An increase in the incidence should be expected as the life expectancy of these children is prolonged due to the advances in ART and other supportive care (41).

ANTIRETROVIRAL MANAGEMENT

The Working Group on Antiretroviral Therapy and Medical Management of HIV-infected Infants, Children, and Adolescents has published specific guidelines regarding treatment and prevention of HIV and its complications. They have been updated on a regular basis. Recommendations for initiating and changing ART can be found in Tables 121.10 and 121.11, and drug dosages, interactions, and toxicity are discussed in these guidelines and summarized in Table 121.9.

There are specific issues that should be addressed before starting therapy. Like infants, adolescents who are identified as HIV infected during their early teenage years are in the initial stages of infection and therefore are ideal candidates for early intervention with more potential for long-term response to ART (59). Long-term survivors of perinatal HIV infections and children who acquire the disease via blood products may have different clinical courses, and perinatal exposure to antiretroviral drugs has as yet an unknown impact on subsequent ART (148). Doses for medications for HIV and OIs should be prescribed by weight or body mass for children and for adolescents according to the Tanner staging of puberty and not on the basis of age (149). Our clinical experience with PIs and nonnucleoside inhibitors is still limited, and adverse events to new classes of drugs in adults have delayed approval pending further studies in children.

Adherence

Ensuring adherence to therapy has become the cornerstone in the management of HIV infection in infants, children, and adolescents. The introduction of HAART in children has increased the complexity of therapeutic regimens. Lack of adherence to prescribed regimens and subtherapeutic levels of antiretroviral medication may enhance the development of drug resistance (150). Strategies should be developed to increase education of infected children and adolescents and their caregivers over several visits, to accommodate the administration of drugs, and to increase medication adherence. Infants and children are dependent on their caregivers for administration of medication. Some special and individual adjustments are necessary in many cases, from choosing an appropriate regimen to scheduling administration and suitability of a formulation. Adherence problems with adolescents are patient, family, and environmentally

TABLE 121.10. Recommended Antiretroviral Regimens for Initial Therapy for Human Immunodeficiency Virus Infection in Children

Strongly recommended

Clinical trial evidence of clinical benefit and/or sustained suppression of HIV replication in adults and/or children.

- One highly active protease inhibitors (nelfinavir or ritonavir) plus two nucleoside analog reverse-transcriptase inhibitors.

  Recommended dual NRTI combinations: The most data on use in children are available for the combinations of ZDV and ddI, ZDV and lamivudine (3TC), and stavudine (d4T) and ddI. More limited data are available for the combinations of d4T and 3TC and ZDV and ddC.[a]

- For children who can swallow capsules: the NNRTI efavirenz (Sustiva)[b] plus two NRTIs, or efavirenz (Sustiva) plus nelfinavir and one NRTI.

Recommended as an alternative

Clinical trial evidence of suppression of HIV replication, but (a) durability may be less in adults and/or children than with strongly recommended regimens or may not yet be defined; or (b) evidence of efficacy may not outweigh potential adverse consequences (e.g., toxicity, drug interactions, cost, etc.) (c) experience in infants and children is limited.

- NVP and two NRTIs
- ABC in combination with ZDV and 3TC
- Lopinavir/ritonavir with two NRTIs or one NRTI and NNRTI[c]
- IDV or SQV soft-gel capsule with two NRTIs for children who can swallow capsules.

Offered only in special circumstances

Clinical trial evidence of either (a) virologic suppression that is less durable than for the "strongly recommended or alternative" regimens; or (b) data are preliminary of inconclusive for use as initial therapy but may be reasonably offered in special circumstances.

- Two NRTIs
- APV in combination with two NRTIs or ABC

Not recommended

Evidence against use because (a) overlapping toxicity may occur, and/or (b) use may be virologically undesirable.

- Any monotherapy[d]
- d4T and ZDV
- ddC and ddI
- ddC and d4T
- ddC and 3TC

[a]ddC is not available commercially in a liquid preparation; although, a liquid formulation is available through a compassionate use program of the manufacturer (Hoffman-La Roche, Inc., (www.rocheusa.com), Nutley, New Jersey. ZDV and ddC is a less preferred choice for use in combination with a PI.
[b]EFV is currently available only in capsule form, although a liquid formulation is available through an expanded access program of the manufacturer (Bristol-Myers Squibb Company (www.bms.com). There are currently no data on appropriate dosage of EFV in children under age three years.
[c]The data presented to the Food and Drug Administration for review during the drug approval process provided significant data on the pharmacokinetics and safety in children receiving lopinavir/ritonavir (Kaletra) for 24 weeks. The combination of lopinavir/ritonavir with either two NRTIs or one NRTI and an NNRTI may be moved up to the Strongly Recommended category as experience with this drug is gained by US investigators.
[d]Except for ZDV chemoprophylaxis is administered to HIV-exposed infants during the first 6 weeks of life to prevent perinatal HIV transmission; if an infant is confirmed as HIV-infected while receiving ZDV prophylaxis, therapy should be changed to a combination antiretroviral drug regimen.
ABC, abacavir; HIV, human immunodeficiency virus; IDU, indinavir; NNRTI, nonnucleoside reverse-transcriptase inhibitor; NRTI, nucleoside reverse-transcriptase inhibitor; NVP, nevirapine; SQV, saquinovir; ZDV, zidovudine.

specific and should be dealt with on an individual basis. Treatment regimens for adolescents must balance the goal of prescribing a maximally potent antiretroviral regimen with realistic assessment of existing and potential support systems to facilitate adherence (59,151). There are data demonstrating the problems of nonadherence to prescribed medications in children with a variety of illnesses, including life-threatening conditions such as cancer and renal transplants (152). Experiences from these other chronic life-threatening conditions should be applied to children with HIV infection.

ANTIRETROVIRAL THERAPY

As of February 2001, 15 antiretroviral drugs were approved for use in HIV-infected adults and adolescents; 11 of these have been approved to be used in the management of HIV infection in infants, children, and adolescents younger than 13 years. They are divided in three major classes: nucleoside reverse-transcriptase inhibitors (NRTIs), nonnucleoside reverse-transcriptase inhibitors (NNRTIs), and PIs. All NRTIs except zalcitabine (ddC) and one NNRTI (nevirapine) are available in liquid formulation. Pharmacokinetic studies of a liquid preparation of efavirenz are under way. Three PIs (ritonavir, amprenavir, and lopinavir-ritonavir) are available in liquid formulation. Nelfinavir has a powder preparation that can be diluted and used in the pediatric population.

Multiple clinical trials and the development of therapeutic strategies for antiretroviral drugs have markedly reduced the morbidity and mortality of HIV-infected infants, children, and adolescents younger than 13 years in the United States. Triple-combination therapy with three NRTIs, two NRTIs plus one NNRTI, two NRTIs plus one PI, or one NRTI and NNRTI plus one PI has been proven effective in decreasing the viral burden

TABLE 121.11. Considerations for Changing Antiretroviral Therapy for Human Immunodeficiency Virus–Infected Children

Virologic considerations[a]
- Less than a minimally acceptable virologic response after 8–12 wk of therapy. For children receiving antiretroviral therapy with two NRTIs and a PI, such a response is defined as a less than tenfold (1.0 log_{10}) decrease from baseline HIV RNA levels. For children who are receiving less potent antiretroviral therapy (i.e., dual NRTI combinations), an insufficient response is defined as a less than fivefold (0.7 log_{10}) decrease in HIV RNA levels from baseline.
- HIV RNA not suppressed to undetectable levels after 4–6 mo of antiretroviral therapy.[b]
- Repeated detection of HIV RNA in children who initially responded to antiretroviral therapy with undetectable levels.[c]
- A reproducible increase in HIV RNA copy number among children who have had a substantial HIV RNA response but still have low levels of detectable HIV RNA. Such an increase would warrant change in therapy if, after initiation of the therapeutic regimen, a greater than threefold (0.5 log_{10}) increase in copy number for children 2 years or older and greater than fivefold (0.7 log_{10}) increase is observed for children 2 years or younger.

Immunologic considerations[a]
- Change in immunologic classification.[d]
- For children with CD4+ T-cell percentages of <15% (i.e., those in immune category 3), a persistent decline of five percentiles or more in CD4+ T-cell percentage (i.e., from 15% to 10%).
- A rapid and substantial decrease in absolute CD4+ T-cell count (i.e., >30% decline in less than months).

Clinical considerations
- Progressive neurodevelopmental deterioration.
- Growth failure defined as persistent decline in weight-growth velocity despite adequate nutritional support and without other explanation.
- Disease progression defined as advancement from one pediatric clinical category to another (i.e., from clinical category A to clinical category B).[e]

[a]At least two measurements (taken one week apart) should be performed before considering a change in therapy.
[b]The initial HIV RNA level of the child at the start of therapy and the level achieved with therapy should be considered when contemplating potential drug changes. For example, an immediate change in therapy may not be warranted if there is a sustained 1.5–2.0 log_{10} decrease in HIV RNA copy number, even if RNA remains detectable at low levels.
[c]More frequent evaluation of HIV RNA levels should be considered if the HIV RNA increase is limited (i.e., if when using an HIV RNA assay with a lower limit of detection of 1,000 copies/mL, there is a ≤ 0.7 log_{10} increase from undetectable to approximately 5,000 copies/mL in an infant younger than 2 years).
[d]Minimal changes in CD4+ T-cell percentile that may result in change in immunologic category (i.e., from 26% to 24%, or 16% to 14%) may not be as concerning as a rapid substantial change in CD4+ percentile within the same immunologic category (i.e., a drop from 35% to 25%).
[e]In patients with stable immunologic and virologic parameters, progression from one clinical category to another may not represent an indication to change therapy. Thus, in patients whose disease progression is not associated with neurologic deterioration or growth failure, virologic and immunologic considerations are important in deciding whether to change therapy.
HIV, human immunodeficiency virus; NRTI, nucleoside reverse-transcriptase inhibitor; PI, protease inhibitor; RNA, ribonucleic acid.

and has dramatically changed the clinical outcome of pediatric HIV infection (76,153–156).

Individual Classes of Antiretroviral Drugs

NUCLEOSIDE REVERSE-TRANSCRIPTASE INHIBITORS
ZDV was the first drug available for the treatment of HIV infection. It was followed later by the development and approval of other NRTIs. Eventually, resistance to these agents when used as a single-drug therapy occurs quickly during long-term therapy. However, combination therapy with other drugs may prevent, delay, or reverse the development of resistance (151).

NRTIs may increase the risk of mitochondrial dysfunction due to inhibition of mitochondrial DNA polymerase gamma. It was reported that the relative potency of the NRTIs in inhibiting this enzyme is highest for ddC, followed by didanosine (ddI), stavudine (d4T), lamivudine (3TC), ZDV, and abacavir (ABC). Those data reflect studies in the HIV-infected adult population; pediatric data are still unknown. Other serious but unusual toxicities, such as lactic acidosis, hepatic steatosis, pancreatitis, myopathy, cardiomyopathy, peripheral neuropathy, osteonecrosis, and osteopenia, and hypersensitivity reactions can occur in patients exposed to NRTIs as well as PIs (151,157,158).

NONNUCLEOSIDE ANALOG REVERSE-TRANSCRIPTASE INHIBITORS
Of the three NNRTIs approved for the treatment of HIV infection, only nevirapine has an approved liquid preparation, whereas delavirdine is not approved for use in children. Efavirenz has a liquid formulation under study and is available through an expanded access program. This class is well known for reducing the viral load rapidly. However, the development of drug resistance quickly after initiation of therapy that does not fully suppress viral replication is quite common. The presence of a major codon of resistance (K103N) confers cross-resistance between the drugs. Recent data have shown sustained suppression of viral load in patients treated with a regimen containing an NNRTI with two NRTIs or an NRTI and a PI (151,159–162). In addition to GI tract disturbances, side effects include rash, Stevens-Johnson syndrome, and CNS-related signs and symptoms and are described in Table 121.9.

PROTEASE INHIBITORS
Nelfinavir and ritonavir are strongly recommended PIs for use in combination with two NRTIs as initial therapy in infected children (151) (Table 121.9). The fixed-dose combination of lopinavir-ritonavir (Kaletra) is approved for children older than 6 months and is available in a liquid formulation. It can be used as an

alternative regimen for initiation of therapy and while changing a regimen in drug-experienced HIV-infected children. Amprenavir in combination with two NRTIs may be offered in special circumstances in selected patients as initial ART and may have some utility in antiretroviral-experienced patients (151). Indinavir is recommended for consideration for children who can swallow capsules. Because of limited bioavailability, the hard-gel capsules of saquinavir are not recommended for use with two NRTIs. Current studies are evaluating the use of the soft-gel saquinavir in children (151,163).

NEWER AGENTS

Progress has been focused more recently on the development of additional antiretroviral agents, vaccines, and vaginal microbicides that target HIV-1 entry into cells. Two entry inhibitor categories with novel mechanisms of action are the fusion inhibitors and co-receptor inhibitors; T-20 and T-1249 fusion peptides are now in clinical trials. T-20, a large peptide compound that requires parenteral administration is being studied in a pediatric trial, and T-1249 is being evaluated in an adult phase 1/2 dose-escalation study. Yet, another class of entry inhibitors, the attachment inhibitors, are also advancing in development and include co-receptor inhibitors that target CXCR4 or CCR5 (151).

Altering Treatment Regimen and Resistance Testing

Immunologic and virologic considerations before changing therapy are described in Table 121.11 and are integral parts of therapy monitoring. However, before choosing a new regimen, one must distinguish between the need to change therapy because of drug failure versus drug toxicity and the need to change therapy because of poor adherence to the present regimen. Antiretroviral resistance testing is now part of clinical management in children and adults. If an actual regimen fails to reduce plasma HIV RNA to below detection by the most sensitive assay available, genotypic/phenotypic resistance studies should be considered. Phenotypic resistance assays are the most direct method for determining drug resistance of isolates. They measure the 50% or 90% inhibitory concentrations of a drug against the virus *in vitro*. They can detect the effects of resistance interactions between various drug-selected mutations. However, they require specialized laboratories, are expensive assays, and take several weeks to complete. The results may lag behind genotypic changes and the results may be strain specific.

Genotypic resistance assays detect actual viral genome mutations. They are rapid and inexpensive with a potential for high sensitivity. Their analysis can be quite comprehensive but at this time is difficult to interpret. Genotypic assays do not tell the clinician what antiretrovirals to use and may not detect minority quasispecies. Interaction between mutations is not described and correlation with phenotypic resistance is not universal. Expert clinical interpretation is advised to determine the clinical applications of these resistance assays (151,164).

Adverse Drug Events

Some basic principles should be observed when clinicians face adverse events secondary to antiretroviral agents. The first step is to try to determine whether the adverse event is attributable to antiretroviral agents, to other medications, to progressive HIV infection itself, or to other infections that may complicate the course of HIV infection. One example is the development of neutropenia in a child on PCP prophylaxis and an antiretroviral regimen that includes ZDV (AZT). That episode of neutropenia may be secondary to ZDV, TMP-SMX, or to the HIV infection itself. Unless it is a life-threatening situation, for example, a hypersensitivity reaction to abacavir, therapy should be continued in the presence of non–life-threatening toxicities. Grades of severity of abnormal laboratory test results and adverse clinical events that may reflect common and potentially severe drug toxicities are depicted in Table 121.12 (151). As a rule, attempts should be made to continue ART at effective doses except in the presence of severe (grade 4) or life-threatening toxicities, in which circumstances therapy should be stopped (151). Toxicities for each antiretroviral agent are described in Table 121.9. Monitoring and evaluation

TABLE 121.12. Toxicity Levels Relevant to the Management of Adverse Drug Reactions (for Children Older Than 3 mo)

Parameter	Grade 1	Grade 2	Grade 3	Grade 4
Hematology				
Hemoglobin	10–10.9	7.0–9.9	<7	Cardiac failure secondary to anemia
Abs. neutrophil count	750–1,200	400–799	250–399	<250
Platelets	>75,000	50,000–75,000	25,000–49,999	<25,000 or bleeding
PT	1.0–1.25 × N	1.26–1.5 × N	1.51–3.0 × N	>3 × N
PTT	1.1–1.66 × N	1.67–2.33 × N	2.34–3.0 × N	>3 × N
Gastrointestinal				
Bilirubin	1.1–1.9 × N	2.0–2.9 × N	3.0–7.5 × N	>7.5 × N
AST (SGOT)	1.0–4.9 × N	5.0–9.9 × N	10.0–15.0 × N	>15.0 × N
ALT (SGPT)	1.1–1.9 × N	5.0–9.9 × N	10.0–15.0 × N	>15.0 × N
GGT	1.1–4.9 × N	5.0–9.9 × N	10.0–15.0 × N	>15.0 × N
Pancreatic Amylase	1.1–1.4 × N	1.5–1.9 × N	2.0–3.0 × N	>3.0 × N
Total Amylase + lipase[a]	1.1–1.4 × N	1.5–2.4 × N	2.5–5.0 × N	>5.0 × N
Diarrhea	Soft stools	Liquid stools	Liquid stools and mild dehydration Bloody stools	Dehydration requiring intravenous therapy or hypotensive shock
Constipation	Mild	Moderate	Severe	Distention and vomiting
Nausea	Mild	Moderate–Decreased oral intake	Severe–Little oral intake	Unable to ingest food or fluid for >24 hr

[a]Both amylase and lipase must be elevated to the same grade or higher (i.e., if total amylase is Grade Four, but lipase is only Grade One, the Toxicity Grade is One.

ALT, alanine aminotransferase; AST, aspartate aminotransferase; PT, prothrombin time; PTT, partial thromboplastine; SGOT, serum glutamic-oxaloacetic transaminase; SGPT, serum glutamic-pyruvic transaminase.

are recommended for lower grade toxicities. For moderately severe toxicities (grade 2 and 3), specific interventions should be considered, such as use of erythropoietin for the treatment of anemia, granulocyte colony-stimulating factor for the treatment of neutropenia. Dose reduction should be considered for agents for which a range of effective dosages have been documented (165,166). If there is a need to discontinue ART for an extended period, it is recommended to stop all antiretroviral agents simultaneously rather than continuing one or two agents alone. This is an attempt to minimize the risk of developing drug resistance in the face of potential increased viral replication (151).

The decline in opportunistic diseases and the growing recognition of the need for long-term therapy with drug combinations lead to the potential of long-term side effects. Despite our better knowledge of HIV pathogenesis and therapy, there is no existing consensus regarding how to better use the drugs and decrease the risk of side effects. Lipodystrophy and other metabolic disturbances in patients taking PIs have been well documented and are a major cause for decreased adherence to regimens by negatively impacting self-image in HIV-infected adolescents and young adults. Recommendations for the management of metabolic complications of antiretroviral management have been recently published (167).

OTHER MANAGEMENT ISSUES IN PEDIATRIC HIV INFECTION

Pain Management

Pain management is an especially important but often undertreated clinical problem in HIV-infected infants. Children with AIDS suffer from two types of pain: the pain of the disease, both acute and chronic, and the pain of the multiple diagnostic and therapeutic procedures these children need. Specific barriers to the management of pain in HIV-infected children include (a) the difficulty of assessing pain in young children, (b) the difficulty of assessing pain in children with neurologic impairment, (c) parental denial of their children's disease, (d) resistance to the use of narcotics by families who have a history of drug use, and (e) resistance by clinicians to treating pain in children because of myths such as children lie about pain to get attention; if children deny pain or do not complain, they are not in pain; and children who can fall asleep or who can play cannot be in pain. Vigorous and proactive use of appropriate pain medications using weight-adjusted dosages, including aspirin, acetaminophen, codeine, ibuprofen, morphine, and methadone, is essential to the overall quality of life for HIV-infected children (168). The use of EMLA cream as a local anesthetic for blood drawing can make the difference between an agonizing or enjoyable visit to the doctor for a child with chronic illness. Nonpharmacological approaches to pain management (including relaxation, hypnosis, play therapy, visualization, and distraction) should also be applied in the control of pain, especially when it is related to procedures (169).

Palliative/Hospice Care

Palliative care is comprehensive and multidisciplinary and includes physical, psychological, social, and spiritual care. Palliative care for children with chronic, multisystem, and life-limiting disease, such as HIV, should ensure the child's comfort and maximum function through the course of illness. The use of palliative care within the context of other forms of medical treatment should not be reserved for the end of life (170,171). For children

with HIV disease, palliative care is an important aspect of a comprehensive treatment program from the time of diagnosis (169,172,173). The principles of palliative care, when applied, improve the quality of life of the child with chronic life-limiting illness. Quality of life, defined in large part by the patient and family members, includes the ability of the child to perform activities of daily living with minimal discomfort while receiving treatment for his or her illness. The quality of life of patients should be the main concern of any physician and the driving force throughout chronic illness (174–179).

For HIV-1–infected children during the course of illness, some types of restorative care are also the best palliative care. The use of ART has had a significant impact on quality of life by improving survival, prolonging the time free of OIs, and improving and maintaining immunologic health. However, at end-stage disease, decisions relating to the continuation of ART must be made balancing the ultimate futility of current treatment after a certain point, and side effects of the medications (180–182). Although HIV-1–infected children can show great variability in the clinical course of their disease, end-stage disease is characterized by the progression to CDC class C3 disease (severe clinical disease with substantial immune suppression). At this stage, there is a shift from restorative care to more supportive care; the physician and the family therefore need to recognize when end-stage disease is present and hospice care is an appropriate option (168,174,183–188).

Hospice care is a philosophy of care that promotes dying with comfort and dignity. It is care that incorporates the principles of palliative care used in earlier stages of illness but with an enhanced emphasis on easing the burden of end-of-life care for the patient and family. The focus is on comfort care while limiting or withdrawing life-sustaining measures. Hospice care is most often provided in the home setting but can be offered in hospitals, nursing homes, and free-standing facilities. As part of the continuum of palliative care, hospice services maximize patient dignity and allow for a transition to appropriate family and staff bereavement (174,189–197).

Providing comprehensive, individualized palliative and terminal care services for children with HIV and their families is unquestionably important yet presents a significant challenge to health care providers and social support systems. Access to appropriate programs varies greatly in different geographical areas, and availability of immediate health care support, a critical part of hospice services, is not available in some disadvantaged areas (198). A goal to support palliative and end-of-life care for HIV-affected children and families is to strengthen access to these services (199).

Nutritional Issues in Children with HIV Infection

Nutrition is an important part of supportive care and a critical component in health maintenance while adding to quality of life. Weight loss and failure to thrive can occur very early in life in HIV-infected children. HIV infection frequently results in nutritional deficiencies that can cause growth failure and wasting syndrome. Failure to thrive and malnutrition are due to a number of factors, including (a) decreased intake resulting from oral and GI tract pathology (MAC, candidal, herpes, and CMV infections) that causes nausea, anorexia, and pain resulting in ineffective swallowing mechanisms; (b) impaired absorption resulting from HIV-related enteropathy and GI tract infections; (c) increased metabolic requirements secondary to the chronic HIV-related inflammatory illness; and (d) decreased intake resulting from side effects and toxicities (such as nausea, anorexia, vomiting, hepatitis, and pancreatitis of various medications used to treat HIV infections and complications) (51,151,200).

Specific nutritional deficiencies of selenium, iron, zinc, vitamin B_6, vitamin A, and vitamin E may result in neurologic or cardiac abnormalities and contribute to the rashes and cytopenias commonly seen in HIV infection (51,201). An aggressive approach to nutritional support is justified in that situation and should include (a) periodic nutritional assessment; (b) diagnosis and treatment of the underlying causes; and (c) aggressive nutritional replacement. Oral supplementation should be tried first with nutritional supplements and adequate diet. In case of failure or persistent anorexia, a more aggressive approach starting with nasogastric tube feeding or gastrostomy tube feeding should be considered before attempting alimentation through a central venous catheter.

The use of parenteral hyperalimentation is often complicated by the occurrence of line sepsis and tunnel infections, especially in immunocompromised patients. Parental education and nursing supervision may help in preventing those infections that sometimes can be severe and cause fulminant sepsis. Appetite stimulants, the use of Megace and dronabinol should be considered at some point.

Nutritional care of HIV-infected children must be individualized and is sometimes culture sensitive. Constitutional growth should be considered because a great number of those children are under the care of extended family members or part of the foster care system and their biological parents cannot be interviewed. Nutritional assessment should include a detailed dietary intake history, including anthropomorphic measurements and sometimes home visits by the nutritionists.

The use of HAART has brought drastic changes in the growth velocity of children infected with HIV. However, it should not undermine the need for adequate nutritional counseling and careful observation of the growth parameters at each physician visit. Nutritional promotion and education in developing countries affected by the AIDS epidemic are essential to prevent growth failure and wasting syndrome, because access to antiretroviral agents is not as available as it is in the United States and other industrialized countries.

SOCIAL ISSUES IN THE DELIVERY OF CARE

The epidemiological data on pediatric HIV disease make it clear that in the United States, there has been a disproportionate impact on the poor and people of color. The health care needs of these people have traditionally been underserved, and previous contact with public agencies may predispose them toward distrust and discourage them from seeking timely medical care (202). Often one of the first relationships of trust that affected families develop is with the health care providers who treat their children. Health care professionals should attempt to establish a partnership with the family rather than reinforcing the more traditional role of passivity and dependence (203).

The conditions of poverty, including inadequate housing, may interfere with the delivery of optimal health care. Mothers are typically the strongest advocates for their children, but this advocacy may be hindered by the fact that the mothers of HIV-infected children are often single parents and poor. In some cases, symptomatic HIV infection or drug use may interfere with a mother's ability to care properly for her child; more often, however, mothers are assertive in seeking care for their children while neglecting their own care needs. The general shortage of openings in drug treatment programs is especially severe for women who are HIV infected, pregnant, or have children. All of these socioeconomic conditions have to be addressed in designing effective health care systems for families with HIV infection. Similar difficulties are encountered by HIV-infected adolescents, who traditionally have not received adequate health care.

Families can also benefit from psychosocial support in dealing with many aspects of an HIV diagnosis in a child. The diagnosis may be the first evidence that a parent is infected and may give rise to guilt or anger, leading to further disruption of the family unit. Apparently resolved emotional issues may require periodic reexamination, as, for example, when parents are confronted repeatedly by the differences between a child who is developmentally delayed and healthy peers (204). Decisions about the disclosure of an HIV diagnosis may arise on multiple occasions as different audiences are encountered such as family, friends, siblings of the infected child, the child, day care workers, school nurses, and teachers. Many parents choose to disclose the diagnosis on a need-to-know basis. However, children and their siblings often find it less stressful to know the diagnosis than to be left in the dark about something unnamed but apparent. Counseling may help parents to decide whether and how to disclose the diagnosis, which should be done in a developmentally appropriate way. Clinical experience suggest that under the proper circumstances, it is beneficial for children with normal cognitive development to have the opportunity to discuss aspects of their illness with trusted adults (205). The issue of disclosure of diagnosis is particularly pressing as perinatally infected children live into mid and late adolescence. Uninfected, but HIV-affected, siblings often have mental health needs as well, especially when they face the eventual loss of siblings and one or both parents. The failure to deal successfully with psychosocial issues may impede families from seeking to obtain optimal medical care for their children.

CONCLUSION

Current research strategies to reduce the risk of prenatal HIV transmission are underway. Since 1994, various modifications of the AIDS Clinical Trials Group Protocol 076 ZDV regimen have been implemented in developing countries. Short-course regimens using ZDV and the use of nevirapine have been reported with positive outcomes. Infant feeding practice and vitamin A supplementation are being evaluated, especially in African countries, as a method of reduction of HIV transmission. Active and passive immunization and vaccine studies targeting the adult population are currently in different stages of development and need to be aggressively applied to children. Important complementary information is expected from those strategies to determine appropriate and more effective methods to reduce HIV transmission from mother to infant. In addition to advances made through clinical trials and research, HIV awareness should be promoted particularly in underprivileged areas of the world. Other challenges have emerged with advances in ART, in particular, long-term adverse drug reactions, and difficulty with adherence to lifelong antiretroviral regimens. Management of adverse events, adherence, and societal issues are essential to address, to increase the long-term survival rate of infants, children, and adolescents infected with HIV with hopes of preventing spread of HIV to vulnerable populations, such as women and children.

ACKNOWLEDGMENTS

This chapter is supported in part by a cooperative agreement between the National Pediatric & Family HIV Resource Center and the HIV/AIDS Bureau of the Health Resources and Services

Administrative (project no. U69HA00038-03-02), the Francois-Xavier Bagnoud Endowed Chair in Pediatrics, and the UMDNJ Foundation.

Special thanks to Marie Stallings for technical skills in the preparation of this document.

REFERENCES

1. Oleske J, Minnefor A, Cooper R, et al. Immune deficiency syndrome in children. *JAMA* 1983;249:2345–2349.
2. Connor EM, Sperling RS, Gelber R, et al. Reduction of maternal infant transmission of immunodeficiency virus type-1 with zidovudine treatment. *N Engl J Med* 1994;331:1173–1180.
3. Oleske J, Winter H, McKinney R, et al. Prospective monitoring of perinatal HIV transmission and infant mortality in Pediatric AIDS Clinical Trials Group (PACTG) Protocol 247: How low can we go? Paper presented at the XIII International AIDS Conference; Durban, South Africa; July 2000 (PO no. MoPe2210).
4. Centers for Disease Control and Prevention. US HIV and AIDS cases through December 2000. *HIV/AIDS Surveillance Report.* September 12, 2001.
5. Lindegren ML, Byers RH, Thomas P, et al. Trends in perinatal transmission of HIV AIDS in the United States. *JAMA* 1999;282:531–538.
6. Lindegren ML, Hanson C, Miller K, et al. Epidemiology of human immunodeficiency virus infection in adolescents, United States. *Pediatr Infect Dis* 1994;13:525–535.
7. Centers for Disease Control and Prevention. US HIV and AIDS cases reported through December 1995. *HIV/AIDS Surveillance Report.* Year-end edition 1996;7:1–38.
8. UN/AIDS/WHO: Joint United Nations Programme on HIV/AIDS (UN/AIDS) World Health Organization. Report on the global HIV/AIDS epidemic. June 1998.
9. Lindegren ML, Steinberg S, Byers RH. Epidemiology of HIV/AIDS in children. *Pediatr Clinics North Am* 2000;47(1):1–20.
10. Shaffer N, Chuachoowong R, Mock PA, et al. Short-course zidovudine for perinatal HIV-1 transmission in Bangkok, Thailand: a randomized controlled trial. Bangkok Collaborative Perinatal HIV Transmission Study Group. *Lancet* 1999;353(9155):773–780.
11. Administration of zidovudine during late pregnancy and delivery to prevent perinatal HIV transmission-Thailand 1996–1998. *MMWR Morb Mortal Wkly Rep* 1998;47(8):151–154.
12. Shaffer N, Bulterys M, Simonds RJ. Short courses of ZDV and perinatal transmission of HIV. *N Engl J Med* 1999;340(13):1041–1042.
13. Eshleman SH, Becker-Pergola G, Deseyve M, et al. Impact of human immunodeficiency virus type 1 (HIV-1) subtype on women receiving single-dose nevirapine prophylaxis to prevent hiv-1 vertical transmission (HIV network for prevention trials 012 study). *J Infect Dis* 2001;184(7):914–917.
14. Duliege AM, Amos CI, Felton S, et al. Birth order delivery route, and concordance in the transmission of HIV-1 from mothers to twin. *J Pediatr* 1995;126:625–632.
15. Bryson YJ, Luzuriaga K, Sullivan JL, et al. Proposed definition for in utero versus intrapartum transmission of HIV-1. *N Engl J Med* 1992;327:1246–1247.
16. Douglas GC, King BF. Maternal-fetal transmission of human immunodeficiency virus: a review of possible routes and cellular mechanisms of infection. *Clin Infect Dis* 1992;15:678–691.
17. Mofenson LM. A critical review of studies evaluating the relationship of mode delivery of perinatal transmission of human immunodeficiency virus. *Pediatr Infect Dis J* 1995;14:169–177.
18. Ruff AJ, Coberley J, Halsey, NA, et al. Prevalence of HIV-1 DNA and p24 antigen in breast milk and correlation with maternal factors. *Pediatr Infect Dis* 1995;14:522–526.
19. Dunn DT, Newell ML, Ades AE, et al. Risk of HIV type-1 transmission through breast feeding. *Lancet* 1992;340:585–588.
20. Datta P, Embree JE, Kreiss JK, et al. Mother to child transmission of HIV type-7: report of the Nairobi Study. *J Infect Dis* 1994;170:1134–1140.
21. Van de Pierre. Post natal transmission of HIV type 1: the breast feeding dilemma. *Am J Obstet Gynecol* 1995;173:483–485.
22. Nicoll A, Newel ML, Van Praag E, et al. Infant feeding policy in the presence of HIV infection. *AIDS* 1995;9:107–119.
23. Centers for Disease Control and Prevention. US HIV and AIDS cases reported through June 1995. *HIV/AIDS Surveillance Report.* Mid-year edition, 1995;7:1–34.
24. Randell W, Vlahov D, Latkin C, et al. Correlates of needle sharing among injection drug users. *Am J Public Health* 1994;84:920–923.
25. DesJarlous DC, Coopanya K, Vanichseni S, et al. AIDS risk reduction and HIV seroconversion among injection drug users in Bangkok. *Am J Public Health* 1994;84:452–455.
26. Van Ameigen EJC, Van de Hoek AJA, Coutenho RA. Injecting risk behavior among drug users in Amsterdam, 1986–1992 and its relationship to AIDS prevention program. *Am J Public Health* 1994;84:275–281.
27. Lackritz EM, Salten G, Alberle-Grasse J, et al. Estimated risk of transmission of HIV by screened blood in the United States. *N Engl J Med* 1995;333:1721–1725.
28. Araneta MR, Mascola L, Ellen A, et al. HIV transmission through artificial donor insemination. *JAMA* 1995;273:854–858.
29. Erice A, Rhame FS, Heussner RC, et al. HIV infection in patients with solid organ transplants: report of five cases and review. *Rev Infect Dis* 1991;13:537–547.
30. Li CM, Ho YR, Liu YC. Transmission of HIV through bone transplantation: a case report. *J Formos Med Assoc* 2001;100(5):350–351.
31. Simonds RJ, Holmberg SD, Hurwitz RL, et al. Transmission of HIV type 1 from a seronegative organ and tissue donor. *N Engl J Med* 1992;326:726–732.
32. Foster B, Buve A. Benefits of HIV screening in Zambia. *Lancet* 1995;346:225–227.
33. Centers for Disease Control and Prevention. Guidelines: apparent transmission of human T-lymphocyte virus type III/lymphadenopathy-associated virus from a child to a mother providing care. *MMWR Morb Mortal Wkly Rep* 1986;35:76–79.
34. Centers for Disease Control and Prevention. HIV infection in two brothers receiving intravenous therapy for hemophilia. *MMWR Morb Mortal Wkly Rep* 1992;41:228–231.
35. Centers for Disease Control and Prevention. HIV transmission between two brothers with hemophilia. *MMWR Morb Mortal Wkly Rep* 1993;42:948–951.
36. Centers for Disease Control and Prevention. HIV transmission in household settings: US. *MMWR Morb Mortal Wkly Rep* 1994;43:347–353.
37. Fitzgibbon JE, Gaun S, Frenkel LD, et al. Transmission from one child to another of HIV-1 with a zidovudine-resistance mutation. *N Engl J Med* 1993;329:1835–1841.
38. Wahn V, Kramer HH, Voit T, et al. Horizontal transmission of HIV infection between two siblings. *Lancet* 1986;2:694.
39. Richman KM, Rickman LS. The potential of transmission of HIV through human bites. *J Acquir Immune Defic Syndr* 1993;6:402–406.
40. Mofenson LM. Epidemiology and determinants of vertical HIV transmission. *Semin Pediatr Infect Dis* 1994;5:252–265.
41. Mofenson LM. Human retroviruses. In: Feigin RD, Cherry JD, eds. *Textbook of pediatric infectious diseases*, 4th ed. Philadelphia: W.B. Saunders, 1998:2169–2226.
42. Denny T, Yogev R, Gelman R, et al. Lymphocyte subsets in healthy children using the first 5 years of life. *JAMA* 1992;267:1484–1488.
43. Dunn DT, Brandt CD, Krivine A, et al. The sensitivity of HIV-1 DNA polymerase chain reaction in the neonatal period and the relative contributions of intrauterine and intra-partum transmission. *AIDS* 1995;9:F7–F11.
44. Bernstein LJ, Krieger BZ, Novick B, et al. Bacterial infection in the acquired immunodeficiency syndrome of children. *Pediatr Infect Dis J* 1985;4:472–475.
45. Roilides E, Black C, Reimer C, et al. Serum immunoglobulin G subclasses in children infected with HIV-type 1. *Pediatr Infect Dis J* 1991;10:134–139.
46. Centers for Disease Control and Prevention. Revised classification system for HIV infection in children less than 13 years of age. *MMWR Morb Mortal Wkly Rep* 1994;43(RR-12):1–12.
47. Clerci M, Shearer GM. A T_H-1 T_H-2 switch is a critical step in the etiology of HIV infection. *Immunol Today* 1993;14:107–122.
48. Jason J, Sleeper LA, Donfield SM, et al. Evidence from a shift from type-1 lymphocyte pattern with HIV disease progression. *J Acquir Immune Defic Syndr* 1995;19:471–476.
49. Aldhous MC, Watret KC, Mok JY, et al. Cytotoxic T-lymphocyte activity and CD8 subpopulation in children at risk for HIV infection. *Clin Exp Immunol* 1994;97:61–67.
50. Dalle JH, Dolfus C, Courpotin C, et al. HIV-associated hemophagocytic syndrome in children [Letter]. *Pediatr Infect Dis J* 1994;13:1159.
51. Grubman S, Oleske J. HIV infection in infants, children and adolescents. In: Wormser, Gary P, eds. *AIDS and other manifestations of HIV infection*. Philadelphia: Lippincott–Raven Publishers, 1998:349–371.
52. Report on a concensus workshop, Siena, Italy, Italy, January 17–18, 1992. Early diagnosis of HIV infection in infants. *J Acquir Immune Defic Syndr* 1992;5:1169–1178.
53. McIntosh K, Pitt J, Brambilla D, et al. Blood culture in the first 6 months of life for the diagnosis of vertically transmitted human immunodeficiency virus infection. *J Infect Dis* 1994;170:996–1000.
54. Chadwick EG, Yogev R, Kwok S, et al. Enzymatic amplification of the human immunodeficiency virus in peripheral blood mononuclear cells from pediatric patients. *J Infect Dis* 1989;160:954–959.
55. Krivine A, Yakudima A, Le May M, Pena-Cruz V, Huang AS, McIntosh K. A comparative study of virus isolation, polymerase chain reaction, and antigen detection in children of mothers infected with human immunodeficiency virus. *J Pediatr* 1990;116:372–376.
56. Grubman S, Oleske J, Simonds RJ, et al. Revised guidelines for prophylaxis against *Pneumocystis carinii* pneumonia for children infected with or perinatally exposed to human immunodeficiency virus. *MMWR* 1995;44:RR-4.
57. Brown AE, Jackson B, Fuller SA, et al. Viral RNA in the resolution of HIV-type 1 diagnostic serology. *Transfusion* 1997;35:1284.
58. Luzuriaga K, Sullivan J. The changing faces of pediatric HIV-1 infection. *N Engl J Med* 2001;345(21):1568–1569.
59. Working Group on Antiretroviral Therapy and Medical Management of Pediatric HIV-Infection: National Pediatric HIV Resource Center. Antiretroviral therapy and medical management of pediatric HIV infection. *Pediatrics* 1998;104(4):1005–1062.
60. U.S. Public Health Service (USPHS) and Infectious Diseases Society of America (IDSA). *2001 USPHS/ISA Guidelines for the prevention of opportunistic*

infections in persons infected with human immunodeficiency virus. November 28, 2001. Available at *www.aidsinfo.nih.gov*

61. Pizzo PA, Wilfert CM, and the Pediatric AIDS Siena Workshop II. Report of a consensus workshop, Siena, Italy, June 4–6, 1993. Markers and determinants of disease progression in children with HIV infection. *J Acquir Immune Defic Syndr* 1995;8:30–44.

62. Frederick T, Mascola L, Ellen A, et al. Progression of HIV disease among infants and children infected perinatally with HIV or through neonatal blood transfusion. *Pediatr Infect Dis J* 1994;13:1091–1097.

63. Tovo P-A, deMarlino M, Gabiano C, et al. AIDS appearance is associated with the velocity of disease progression in their mothers. *J Infect Dis* 1994;170:806–807.

64. Just JJ, Abrams E, Louie LG, et al. Influence of host genotype on progression to AIDS among children infected with HIV type 1. *Pediatrics* 1995;127:544–549.

65. Ljunggren K, Moschese V, Broliden PA, et al. Antibodies mediating cellular cytotoxicity and neutralization correlate with a better clinical stage in children born to HIV-infected mothers. *J Infect Dis* 1990;161:198–202.

66. Van de Perre P, Sumonon A, Zepage P, et al. Biologic markers associated with prolonged survival in African children maternally infected by the HIV type 1. *AIDS* 1992;8:435–442.

67. Vigano A, Principi N, Villa M, et al. Immunologic characterization of children vertically infected with human immunodeficiency virus, with slow or rapid disease progression. *J Pediatr* 1995;126:368–374.

68. Duliege A-M, Messiah A, Blanche S, et al. Natural history of human immunodeficiency virus type 1 infection in children: prognostic value of laboratory tests on the bimodal progression of the disease. *Pediatr Infect Dis* 1992;11:630–635.

69. Ellaurie M, Rubinstein A. Tumor necrosis factor-α in pediatric HIV-1 infection. *AIDS* 1992;6:1265–1268.

70. Roilides E, Clerici M, DePalma L, et al. Helper T-cell responses in children infected with human immunodeficiency virus type 1. *J Pediatr* 1991;118:724–730.

71. Principi N, Marchisio P, Tornaghi R, et al. Occurrences of infections in children with HIV. *Pediatr Infect Dis J* 1991;10:190–193.

72. Andiman WA, Mezger J, Shapiro E. Invasive bacterial infections in children born to women infected with HIV type 1. *J Pediatr* 1994;124:846–852.

73. Ruiz-Anheras J, Ramos JT, Hernandez-Sampelayo T, et al. Sepsis in children with HIV infections. *Pediatr Infect Dis J* 1995;14:522–526.

74. Roilides E, Marshall D, Verdon D, et al. Bacterial infections in HIV type 1 infected children. The impact of central versus catheters and antiretroviral agents. *Pediatr Infect Dis J* 1991;10:813–819.

75. Bakshi SS, Alvarez D, Hilfer CL, et al. Tuberculosis in HIV-infected children: a family infection. *Am J Dis Child* 1993;147:320–324.

76. DeMartino M, Tovo P-A, Balducci M, et al. Reduction in mortality with availability of antiretroviral therapy for children with perinatal HIV-1 infection. *JAMA* 2000;284:190–197.

77. Srugo I, Israele V, Witteck AE, et al. Clinical Manifestations of varicella-zoster virus infection in HIV-infected children. *Am J Dis Child* 1993;147:742–745.

78. Jura E, Chadwick EG, Josepha SH, et al. Varicella virus infections in children infected with HIV. *Pediatr Infect Dis* 1989;58:586–590.

79. Pahwa S, Biron K, Lim W, et al. Continuous varicella-zoster infection associated with acyclovir resistance in a child with AIDS. *JAMA* 1988;260:2879–2882.

80. Hirsch MS, Schooley RT. Resistance to antiviral drugs: The end of innocence. *N Engl J Med* 1989;320:313–314.

81. Jue S, Whitley RJ. Herpes virus infections in children with HIV. In: Pizzo PA, Wilfert CM, eds. *The challenge of HIV infection in infants, children and adolescents,* 2nd ed. Baltimore: Williams & Wilkins, 1994:345–363.

82. Frenkel LM, Gaur S, Tsolera M, et al. Cytomegalovirus infection in children with HIV type 1 infection. *Arch Pediatr Adolesc Med* 1994;148:57–60.

83. Gungor T, Frink M, Linde R, et al. Cytomegalovirus myelitis in perinatally (HIV infection) acquired HIV. *Arch Dis Child* 1993;68:399–401.

84. Walton RC, Whitcup SM, Mueller BV, et al. Combined intravenous ganciclovir and foscarnet for children with recurrent cytomegalovirus retinitis. *Ophthalmology* 1995;102:1865–1870.

85. Butler KM, DeSmet MD, Husson RN, et al. Treatment of aggressive cytomegalovirus retinitis with ganciclovir in combination with foscarnet in a child infected with HIV. *J Pediatr* 1992;120:483–486.

86. King JC, Burke AR, Clemens JD, et al. Respiratory syncytial virus illness in HIV-infected and non infected children. *Pediatr Infect Dis J* 1993;12:733–739.

87. Chandwani S, Borkowsky W, Krasinski K, et al. Respiratory syncytial virus infection in HIV-infected children. *J Pediatr* 1990;117:251–254.

88. American Academy of Pediatrics. Hepatitis B. In: Pickering LK, ed. *Red book: report of the committee on infectious diseases,* 25th ed. Elk Grove Village, IL: American Academy of Pediatrics, 2000:289–302.

89. Centers for Disease Control and Prevention. Measles in HIV-infected children. *MMWR Morb Mortal Wkly Rep* 1988;37:183–186.

90. Elles M, Gupta S, Galant S, et al. Impaired neutrophil function with AIDS on AIDS related complex: a comprehensive evaluation. *J Infect Dis* 1988;158:1268–1276.

91. Roilides E, Mertins S, Eddy J, et al. Impairment of neutrophil chemotactic and bactericidal function in children infected with HIV type 1 and partial reversal after in vitro exposure to granulocyte-macrophage colony stimulating factor. *J Pediatr* 1990;117:531–540.

92. Roilides E, Holmes A, Blake C, et al. Impairment of neutrophil antifungal

93. Walsh TJ. Fungal infections complicating pediatric HIV infection. In: Pizzo PA, Wilfert CM, eds. *Pediatric AIDS. The challenge of HIV infection in infants, children and adolescents.* Baltimore: Williams & Wilkins, 1994:321–347.

94. Leggiadro RJ, Kline MW, Hughes WT. Extrapulmonary cryptococcoses in children with AIDS. *Pediatr Infect Dis J* 1991;10:658–662.

95. Simonds RJ, Lindegren ML, Thomas P, et al. Prophylaxis against *Pneumocystis carinii* pneumonia among children with perinatally acquired human immunodeficiency virus infection in the United States. *N Engl J Med* 1995;332:786–790.

96. Connor E, Bagarazzi M, McSherry G, et al. Clinical and laboratory correlates of *Pneumocystis carinii* pneumonia in children infected with HIV. *JAMA* 1991;265:1693–1697.

97. Cordell RL, Addeso DG. Cryptosporidiosis in child care settings. A review and recommendation for prevention and control. *Pediatr Infect Dis J* 1994;13:310–317.

98. Connor EM, Marquis J, Oleske JM. Lymphoid interstitial pneumonia. In: Pizzo PA, Wilfert CM, eds. *Pediatric AIDS. The challenge of HIV infection in infants, children and adolescents.* Baltimore: Williams & Wilkins, 1994:343–354.

99. Andiman WA, Shearer WT. Lymphoid interstitial pneumonitis. In: Pizzo PA, Wilfert CM, eds. *Pediatric AIDS. The challenge of HIV infection in infants, children and adolescents.* Baltimore: Williams & Wilkins, 1994:323–334.

100. Rubinstein A, Morecki R, Silverman B, et al. Pulmonary disease in children with the acquired immunodeficiency and AIDS related complex. *J Pediatr* 1986;108:498–503.

101. Principi N, Marchisio P, Tornaghi R, et al. Effect of zidovudine in HIV-infected children with lymphocytic interstitial pneumonitis. *AIDS* 1991;5:468–469.

102. Rubinstein A, Bernstein LJ, Charyhan M, et al. Corticosteroid treatment for pulmonary lymphoid hyperplasia in children with AIDS. *Pediatr Pulmonol* 1998;4:13–17.

103. Scott GB, Hutto C, Makuch RW, et al. Survival in children with perinatally acquired immunodeficiency virus type-1 infection. *N Engl J Med* 1989;321:1791–1796.

104. Italian Multicentre Study. Epidemiology, clinical features and prognostic factors in pediatric HIV infection. *Lancet* 1988:1043–1046.

105. Lipshultz SE, Chanock S, Sanders, SP, et al. Cardiovascular manifestations of HIV infection in infants and children. *Am J Cardiol* 1989;63:1489–1497.

106. Steinherz LJ, Brochstein JA, Robins J. Cardiac involvement in congenital acquired immunodeficiency syndrome. *Am J Dis Child* 1989;140:1241–1244.

107. Lane-McAuliffe EM, Lipshultz SE. Cardiovascular manifestations of pediatric HIV infection. *Nurs Clin North Am* 1995;30:291–316.

108. Luginbuhl LM, Orav J, McIntosh K, et al. Cardiac morbidity and related mortality in children with HIV infection. *JAMA* 1993;269:2869–2875.

109. Kotloff KL, Johnson JP, Nair P, et al. Diarrheal morbidity during the first 2 years of life among HIV-infected infants. *JAMA* 1994;271:448–452.

110. Yolken RH, Li S, Perman J, et al. Persistent diarrhea and fecal shedding of retroviral nucleic acids in children infected with HIV. *J Infect Dis* 1991;164:61–66.

111. Yolken RH, Hart W, Oung I, et al. Gastrointestinal dysfunction and disaccharide intolerance in children infected with HIV. *J Pediatr* 1991;118:359–363.

112. Miller TL, Orav EJ, Martin SR, et al. Malnutrition and carbohydrate malabsorption in children with vertically transmitted HIV infection. *Gastroenterology* 1991;100:1296–1302.

113. Persaud D, Bangaru B, Greco A, et al. Cholestatic hepatitis in children infected with HIV. *Pediatr Infect Dis J* 1993;12:497–498.

114. Della Negra M, Queiroz W, Taveras RCJ, et al. Liver disorders in pediatric AIDS patients. *Pediatr AIDS HIV Infect Fetus Adolesc* 1993;4:222–226.

115. Miller TL, Winter HS, Luginbuhl LM, et al. Pancreatitis in pediatric HIV infection. *J Pediatr* 1992;120:223–227.

116. Hart CC. Aerosolized pentamidine and pancreatitis [Letter]. *Ann Intern Med* 1989;111:691.

117. Connor E, Gupta S, Joshi V, et al. Acquired immunodeficiency syndrome associated renal disease in children. *J Pediatr* 1988;113:39–44.

118. Zilleruelo G, Strauss J. HIV nephropathy in children. *Pediatr Clin North Am* 1995;42:1469–1485.

119. Ingulli E, Tejani A, Fikrig S, et al. Nephrotic syndrome associated with AIDS in children. *J Pediatr* 1991;119:710–716.

120. Strauss J, Abitol C, Zilleruelo G, et al. Renal disease in children with the acquired immunodeficiency syndrome. *N Engl J Med* 1989;321:625–630.

121. Mueller BU, Tannenbaum S, Pizzo PA. Bone marrow aspirates and biopsies in children with HIV infection. *J Pediatr Hematol Oncol* 1996;18:266–271.

122. Hilgartner M. Hematologic manifestations in HIV-infected children. *J Pediatr* 1991;119:547–549.

123. Hoots WK, O'Brien NC. Hematologic manifestations of pediatric HIV infection. *Semin Pediatr Infect Dis* 1990;1:77–81.

124. Griffin TC, Squires JE, Timmons CF, et al. Chronic human Parvovirus B$_{19}$–induced erythroid hypoplasia as the initial manifestation of HIV infection. *J Pediatr* 1991;118:899–901.

125. Parmentier L, Boucary D, Salmon D. Pure red cell aplasia in an HIV-infected patient. *AIDS* 1992;6:234–235.

126. Sakaguchi M, Salo T, Cooperman JE. HIV infection of megakaryotic cells. *Blood* 1991;77:481–485.

127. Gaughan DM, Mofenson LM, Hughes MD, et al. Osteonecrosis of the Hip (Legg-Calvé-Perthes Disease) in HIV-infected children. *Pediatrics* 2002;109:E74.

128. Blanche S, Mayaux MJ, Rouzioux C, et al. Relation of the course of HIV infection in children to the severity of the disease in their mothers at delivery. *N Engl J Med* 1994;330:308–312.

129. Brouwers P, Belman AL, Epstein L. Central nervous system involvement: manifestations, evaluation, and pathogenesis. In: Pizzo PA, Wilfert CM, eds. *Pediatrics AIDS: The challenge of HIV infection in infants, children and adolescents,* 2nd ed. Baltimore: Williams & Wilkins, 1994:433–455.

130. Bale JF, Contant CF, Garg B, et al. Neurologic history and examination results and their relationship to H IV type-1 serostatus in hemophiliac subjects: results of the hemophilia growth and development study. *Pediatrics* 1993;91:736–741.

131. Lobato MN, Caldwell MB, Ng P, et al. Antibodies: encephalopathy in children born to HIV-infected mothers. *J Pediatr* 1995;126:710–715.

132. Working Group of the American Academy of Neurology AIDS Task Force. Nomenclature and research case definitions for neurologic manifestations of HIV-type-1 infection. *Neurology* 1991;41:778–785.

133. Mintz M. Clinical comparison of adult and pediatric neuro AIDS. *Adv Neurol Immunol* 1994;4:207–221.

134. Epstein LG, Sharer LR, Oleske JM, et al. Neurologic manifestations of HIV infection in children. *Pediatrics* 1986;78:678–687.

135. Wolters PL, Brouwers P, Moss MA, et al. Adaptive behavior of children with symptomatic HIV infection before and after zidovudine. *J Pediatr Psychol* 1994;19:47–61.

136. Haller JO, Cohen HL. Pediatric HIV infection: An imaging update. *Pediatr Radiol* 1994;24:224–230.

137. Brouwers D, DeCarli C, Civitello L, et al. Correlation between computed tomographic brain scan abnormalities and new psychological function in children such as symptomatic HIV disease. *Arch Neurol* 1995;52:39–44.

138. DeCarli C, Fugate L, Falloon J, et al. Brain growth and cognitive improvement in children with HIV-induced encephalopathy after 6 months of continuous infusion zidovudine therapy. *J Acquir Immune Defic Syndr* 1991;4:585–592.

139. St. Louis ME, Kamenga M, Brown C, et al. Prednisone improves HIV encephalopathy in children. *Pediatr Infect Dis J* 1992;11:49–50.

140. Brouwers P, Tudor-Williams G, DeCarli C, et al. Quinolinic acid in the cerebrospinal fluid of children with symptomatic human immunodeficiency virus type 1 disease: relationship to clinical status and therapeutic responses. *AIDS* 1995;9:713–720.

141. Epstein LG, DiCarlo FJ, Joshi VV, et al. Primary lymphoma of the central nervous system in children with AIDS. *Pediatrics* 1988;82:355–363.

142. Athale WH, Patill PS, Chintu C, et al. Influence of HIV epidemic on the incidence of Kaposi's sarcoma in Zambian children. *Acquir Immune Defic Syndr Hum Retrovir* 1995;8:96–100.

143. Ziegler JL, Katongole-Mbidde E. Kaposi's sarcoma in childhood. An analysis of 100 cases from Uganda and relationship to HIV infection. *Int J Cancer* 1996;65:200–203.

144. Mueller BW, Butler KA, Higham MC, et al. Smooth muscle tumors in children with HIV. *Pediatrics* 1992;90:460–463.

145. McClain KL, Leach CT, Jenson HB, et al. Association of Epstein-Barr virus with leiomyosarcomas in young people with AIDS. *N Engl J Med* 1995;332:12–18.

146. Lee ES, Locker J, Nalesnik M, et al. The association of EBV with smooth muscle tumors occurring after organ transplantation. *N Engl J Med* 1995;332:19–25.

147. Diamond FB, Price L, Nelson PP. Papillary carcinoma of the thyroid in a 7 year old HIV positive child. *Pediatr AIDS HIV Infect Fetus Adol* 1994;5:232–235.

148. Ammann AJ, Cowan MJ, Wara D, et al. Acquired immunodeficiency in an infant: possible transmission by means of blood products. *Lancet* 1983;1:956–958.

149. El Sadr W, Oleske JM, Agins BD. *Evaluation and management of early HIV infection. Clinical Practice Guideline No. 7.* Rockville, MD: Agency for Health Care Policy and Research, Public Health Service, U.S. Department of Health and Human Services; January 1994. AHCPR publication no. 94-0572.

150. Williams A, Friedland G. Adherence, compliance and HAART. *AIDS Clin Care* 1997;9:51–54, 58.

151. The Working Group on Antiretroviral Therapy and Medical Management of HIV-Infected Children convened by the National Pediatric and Family HIV Resource Center. *Guidelines for the use of antiretroviral agents in pediatric HIV infection.* Revised December 14, 2001. Available at *www.hivatis.org.*

152. Matsui DM. Drug compliance in pediatrics clinical and research issues. *Pediatr Clin North Am* 1997;44:1–14.

153. Van Rossum AMC, Niesters HGM, Geelen SPM, et al. Clinical and virologic response to combination treatment with indinavir, zidovudine and lamivudine in children with human immunodeficiency virus type-1 infection: a multicenter study in the Netherlands. *J Pediatr* 2000;136:780–788.

154. Gortmaker SL, Hughes M, Cervia J, et al. Effect of combination therapy including protease inhibitors on mortality among children and adolescents infected with HIV-1. *N Engl J Med* 2001;345:1522–1528.

155. Starr SE, et al. Combination therapy with efavirenz, nelfinavir, and nucleoside reverse-transcriptase inhibitors in children infected with human immunodeficiency virus type-1. *N Engl J Med* 1999;341:1874–1881.

156. Saez-Llorens X, Nelson RP, Emmanuel P, et al. A randomized, double-blind study of triple nucleoside therapy of abacavir, lamivudine, and zidovudine versus lamivudine and zidovudine in previously treated human immunodeficiency virus type-1–infected children. *Pediatrics* 2001;107. Available at *www.pediatrics.org/cgi/content/full/107/1/e4.*

157. John M, Moore CB, James IR, et al. Chronic hyperlactatemia in HIV-infected patients taking antiretroviral therapy. *AIDS* 2001;15:717–723.

158. Bogner JR, Vielhauer V, Beckman RA, et al. Stavudine versus zidovudine and the development of lipodystrophy. *J Acquir Immune Defic Syndr* 2001;27(3):237–244.

159. Luzuriaga K, McManus M, Catalina M, et al. Early therapy of vertical human immunodeficiency virus type 1 (HIV-1) infection: control of viral replication and absence of persistent HIV-1–specific immune responses. *J Virol* 2000;74:6984–6991.

160. Wiznia A, Stanley K, Krogstad P, et al. Combination nucleoside analogue reverse transcriptase inhibitor(s) plus nevirapine, nelfinavir or ritonavir in stable antiretroviral-experienced HIV-infected children: week 24 results of a randomized controlled trial—PACTG 377. *AIDS Res Human Retroviruses* 2000;16:1113–1121.

161. Luzuriaga K, Bryson Y, Krogstad P, et al. Combination treatment with zidovudine, didanosine and nevirapine in infants with human immunodeficiency virus type 1 infection. *N Engl J Med* 1997;336:1343–1349.

162. Luzuriaga K, Wu H, McManus M, et al. Dynamics of human immunodeficiency virus type 1 replication of vertically-infected infants. *J Virol* 1999;73:1343–1349.

163. Kline MW, et al. A randomized trial of combination therapy with Saquinavir soft gel capsules (SQV) in HIV-infected children. In: Programs and abstracts of the 8th conference on Retroviruses and Opportunistic Infections; Chicago, Illinois; February 4–8, 2001. Abstract no. 683.

164. Hanna GJ, D'Aguila RT. Clinical use of phenotypic and genotypic drug resistance testing to monitor antiretroviral chemotherapy. *Clin Infect Dis* 2001;32(5):774–782.

165. Hermans P, Rosenbaum W, Jou A, et al. Filgrastin to treat neutropenia and support myelosuppressive medication dosing in HIV infection G-CSF 92105 Study Group. *AIDS* 1996;10(4):1627–1633.

166. Volberding P. Consensus statement: anemia in HIV infection—current trends, treatment options, and practice strategies. *Clin Ther* 2000;22(9):1003, 1004–1020.

167. Wanke CA, Falutz JM, Shevita A, et al. Clinical evaluation and management of metabolic and morphologic abnormalities associated with human immunodeficiency virus. *Clin Infect Dis* 2002;34:248–259.

168. Czarniecki L, Boland M, Oleske JM. Pain in children with HIV disease. *PAAC Notes* 1993;5:492–495.

169. Ferris F, Flannery J, eds. *A comprehensive guide for the care of persons with HIV disease—module 4: palliative care.* Toronto: Mount Sinai Hospital/Casey House, 1995.

170. Frager G. Pediatric palliative care: building the model, bridging the gaps. *J Palliat Care* 1997;12(3):9–12.

171. Frager G, Shapiro B. Pediatric palliative care and pain management. In: Holland JC, ed. *Psycho-Oncology.* New York: Oxford Press, 1998.

172. Boland M, Burr C, Harvey D. Pediatric AIDES revisited: family, social and legal issues. *Semin Pediatr Infect Dis* 1995;6:40–45.

173. Oleske JM, Ruben-Hale A. Enhancing supportive care and promoting quality of life: clinical practice guidelines. *Pediatr AIDS HIV Infect Fetus Adolesc* 1995;6:187–203.

174. Attig T. Beyond pain: the existential suffering of children. *J Palliat Care* 1996;12:20–23.

175. Lewis SY, Haiken HJ, Hoyt LG. Living beyond the odds: a psychosocial perspective of long-term survivors of pediatric human immunodeficiency virus infection. *J Dev Behav Pediatr* 1994;15:S12–S17.

176. Liben S. Pediatric palliative medicine: Obstacles to overcome. *J Palliat Care* 1996;12:24–28.

177. Fleischman AR, Nolan K, Dubler NN, et al. Caring for gravely ill infants and children. *Pediatrics* 1994;94:433–439.

178. Robinson WM, Ravilly S, Berde C, et al. End of life care in cystic fibrosis. *Pediatrics* 1996;100:205–209.

179. Walco GA, Cassidy RC, Schechter NL. The ethics of pain control in infants and children. *N Engl J Med* 1994;331:541–544.

180. Oleske JM, Rothpletz-Puglia PM, Winter H. Historical perspectives on the evolution in understanding the importance of nutritional care in pediatric HIV infection. *J Nutr* 1996;126:2616S–2619S.

181. Oleske JM. *Preventing disability and providing rehabilitation for infants, children, and youths with HIV/AIDS.* Bethesda, MD: US Department of Health and Human Services/National Institute of Child Health and Human Development; January 1995. NIH publication no. 95-3850.

182. Paris JJ, Schrieber MD. Physicians' refusal to provide life-prolonging medical interventions. *Clin Perinatol* 1996;23:563–571.

183. Committee on Bioethics on the American Academy of Pediatrics. Guidelines for forgoing life-sustaining medical treatment. *Pediatrics* 1994;93:532–536.

184. Institute of Medicine. *Approaching death: improving care at the end of life.* Washington, DC: National Academy Press, 1997.

185. McQuillan R, Finlay I. Facilitating the care of terminally ill children. *J Pain Symp Manage* 1996;12:320–324.

186. Meyers HI. Spiritual care in pediatric hospice. *Am J Hospice Care* 1989;May/June:12.

187. Nelson LJ, Nelson RM. Ethics and the provision of futile, harmful or burdensome treatments to children. *Crit Care Med* 1992;20:427–433.

188. Rothpletz-Puglia PM. Perspectives in practice. Case report of children infected with HIV. *Topics Clin Nutr* 1997;12:69–77.

189. Martinson IM. Hospice care for children: Past, present and future. *J Pediatr Oncol Nurs* 1993;10:93–98.

190. American Academy of Pediatrics, Committee on Psychosocial Aspects of Child and Family Health. The pediatrician and childhood bereavement. *Pediatrics* 1992;89:516–518.

191. Davies B, Clarke D, Connaughty S, et al. Caring for dying children: nurses' experiences. *Pediatr Nurs* 1996;22(6):500–507.

192. Faulkner KM, Armstrong-Dailey A. Care of the dying child. In: Pizzo P, Poplack D, eds. *Principles and practice of pediatric oncology,* 3rd ed. Philadelphia, PA: Lippincott–Raven Publishers, 1997:1349–1351.

193. Goldman A. Home care of the dying child. *J Palliat Care* 1996;12:16–19.

194. Lauer M, Carmitta B. Home care for dying children: a nursing model. *J Pediatr* 1980;97:1032–1035.

195. Martinson IM, Moldow DG, Armstrong GO, et al. Home care for children dying of cancer. *Res Nurs Health* 1986;9:11–16.

196. Martinson IM. Pediatric hospice nursing. *Ann Rev Nurs Res* 1995;13:195–214.

197. Stevens MM, Jones P, O'Riordan E. Family responses when a child with cancer is in palliative care. *J Palliat Care* 1996;12:51–55.

198. Koocher GP, Gudas LJ. Terminal and life threatening illness in childhood. In: Levine MD, Carey WB, Crocker AC, et al, eds. *Developmental-behavioral pediatrics.* Philadelphia: WB Saunders, 1992:327–336.

199. Oleske JM, Czarniecki L. Continuum of palliative care: lessons from caring for children infected with HIV-1. *Lancet* 1999;354:1287–1290.

200. Bentler M, Stanish M. Nutritional support of the pediatric patient with AIDS. *J Am Diet Assoc* 1987;87:488–491.

201. Kavanaugh-MacHugh AL, Ruff A, Perlman E, et al. Selenium deficiency and cardiomyopathy in acquired immunodeficiency syndrome. *J Parenter Enter Nutr* 1991;15:347–349.

202. Boyd-Franklin N, Aleman J. Black, inner-city families and multigenerational issues: the impact of AIDS. *Psychology* 1990;40:14–17.

203. Boland MG, Mahan-Rudolph P, Evans P. Special issues in the care of the child with HIV infection/AIDS. In: Martin B, ed. *Pediatric hospice care: what helps.* Los Angeles: Los Angeles Children's Hospital, 1989:116–144.

204. Jessop DJ, Stein REK. Meeting the needs of individuals and families. In: Stein R, ed. *Caring for children with chronic illness.* New York: Springer-Verlag, 1989:63–74.

205. Lipson M. Disclosure of diagnosis to children with human immunodeficiency syndrome. *Dev Behav Pediatr* 1994;15:S61–S65.

CHAPTER 122
Human T-Cell Lymphotropic Virus Type I and Neurologic Diseases

Richard T. Johnson

Human T-cell lymphotropic virus type I (HTLV-I) is the only retrovirus known to cause human cancer, acute T-cell leukemia, and lymphoma (1). The virus has also been causally related to chronic myelopathies and weakly implicated in several other neurologic conditions.

In 1985, a French research group performing a seroprevalence survey on Martinique noted that nearly 60% of patients with endemic tropical spastic paraparesis (TSP) had antibodies to HTLV-I virus, whereas only 4% of the general population had these antibodies (2). Within months a similar association of antibody to HTLV-I was shown in patients with TSP in Jamaica and Colombia, and intrathecal synthesis of antibody was also found in cerebrospinal fluid (CSF) (3). The following year, patients with HTLV-I infections and chronic myelopathy were reported in the nontropical island of Kyushu, where the prevalence of antibody against HTLV-I is very high (4,5). This chronic myelopathy, named HTLV-I–associated myelopathy (HAM), is now recognized as the same disease as TSP (HAM/TSP). Similar patients were found among Caribbean immigrants to England and local populations of Africa, North America, South America, Europe, and the Seychelles (6). The demonstration of abnormal lobulated lymphocytes in the CSF, the recovery of virus from CSF, and the demonstration of HTLV-I sequences in affected spinal cord provided further evidence for the association of HTLV-I with many cases of chronic spastic paraparesis (5,7–9).

ETIOLOGY

HTLV-I virus belongs to the oncovirus family. It is a positive-sense, single-stranded ribonucleic acid (RNA) virus with an icosahedral nucleocapsid and an envelope with viral-coded glycoproteins. Like other retroviruses, it has a diploid genome. Using a reverse transcriptase, a deoxyribonucleic acid (DNA) copy is made, which can integrate into the host genome. Unlike animal retroviruses that have an *onc* gene responsible for the cellular transformation, HTLV-I has no *onc* gene, and a regulatory gene, *tax*, is thought to be related to oncogenesis.

HTLV-I viruses recovered from patients with spastic paraparesis and proviral DNAs found in peripheral blood and CSF lymphocytes of these patients appear to be the same as those recovered from acute T-cell leukemia and asymptomatic carriers (10). In HTLV-I–induced neoplasms, however, the integration site in an individual patient is the same in all malignant T cells, indicating a monoclonal origin of the leukemia or lymphoma. The pathogenesis of HAM/TSP is obviously different, with HTLV-I provirus integrated at random sites (11) (Table 122.1).

EPIDEMIOLOGY

The modes of transmission of HTLV-I include (a) from mother to child either across the placenta or from breast milk; (b) sexual transmission, with the higher prevalence of antibody in women indicating greater transmissibility from men to women; and (c) from direct inoculation by blood transfusions or contaminated needles and syringes.

The distribution of HTLV-I virus is worldwide with 10 to 20 million persons infected. Seroprevalence is greater in the southern islands of Japan, the Caribbean, the Seychelles, the Pacific coast of Colombia, Brazil, and areas of Africa. It is rare in North America and is exceedingly rare in China and Korea. Specific isolated ethnic groups, such as immigrants from Surinam to Holland, Ethiopian Jews in Israel, and a Jewish population from Marhad, Iran, have higher prevalence rates of antibody. Rates worldwide vary between 0.1% and 30% in adults. In general, the distribution of TSP/HAM reflects the distribution of HTLV-I.

Conversely, among patients with all forms of chronic spastic paraparesis, the role of HTLV-I varies with geography. For example, none of 29 Canadian patients with chronic myelopathy had antibodies to HTLV-I (12), about half of similar patients in Peru had antibodies (personal observation), and in the areas of high HTLV-I antibody prevalence, the virus is implicated in 75% to 90% patients with chronic myelopathy.

PATHOLOGY AND PATHOGENESIS

Autopsy studies show gross atrophy of the lateral columns of the thoracic spinal cord, and microscopic studies show chronic inflammatory lesions accompanied by degeneration of both axons and myelin. Some perivascular collections of mononuclear cells, which are predominately T cells, are spread throughout the neuraxis, but inflammation and tissue destruction are most intense in the midthoracic spinal cord level. In the cord, fibrous thickening of vessel walls and pia is often noted, suggesting preceding intense inflammation (13). In a patient who had a spinal cord biopsy during the first year of symptoms, a more intense

TABLE 122.1. Human T-cell Lymphotropic Virus Type I–Associated Leukemia or Lymphoma and Myelopathy

Observation	Leukemia or lymphoma	Myelopathy
Demographic		
Male/female ratio	1.4:1	1:1.4
Mean age at onset (yr)	40–60	40–45
Place of birth	Southern Japan	
	Seychelles	
	Caribbean basin	Same
	Equatorial Africa	
	Southeastern United States	
Risk factors		
Lifetime risk in seropositives	5%	0.3%–2%
Blood transfusion of HTLV-1$^+$ blood	No observed effect	Increases risk to 20%
Disease	Aggressive: mean survival 10 mo	Indolent: long life expectancy
Virology		
Viral DNA	CD4$^+$ lymphocytes	CD4$^+$ lymphocytes
Integration	At same site in malignant cells of individual (clonal origin)	Random site (polyclonal)
Immune responses	Immunosuppression	Enhanced humoral and some cellular responses to HTLV-I

inflammatory response was found, including the infiltration of many inflammatory cells into thickened vessel walls. This active vasculitis was associated with severe necrosis of the thoracic spinal cord (14).

The host cell of HTLV-I is the CD4$^+$ cell, and in sections of spinal cord, these cells have consistently been shown to be the site of infection, although some early studies implicated limited infection of astrocytes as well (9). It is thought that infected T cells cross into the cord preferentially at a midthoracic level, a watershed zone with slower blood flow. CD8$^+$ cytotoxic T cells directed primarily against the Tax protein expressed by the host cells are the effector cells causing collateral damage to neural cells.

Virus load, immune responses, and host genetics all appear to influence the development of HAM/TSP. Healthy carriers have provirus in 0.1% to 1.0% of peripheral blood lymphocytes; patients with HAM/TSP have up to 30% of monocytes infected. Healthy carriers with higher proviral loads appear at higher risk of disease (15,16). Patients with HAM/TSP have more abundant anti–HTLV-I cytotoxic T cells; these cells are chronically activated, and most recognize a single viral protein, Tax. Increased proviral load and expansion of Tax-specific CD8$^+$ cells also are found in CSF of patients with HAM/TSP (17). Finally, presence of the major histocompatability complex allele HLA-A*02 appears to reduce the risk of HAM/TSP by half (15).

CLINICAL MANIFESTATIONS

Onset is usually in the third and fourth decades of life, although it has been described in children as young as 6 years. TSP/HAM is twice as frequent in women as in men, consistent with the greater female prevalence of HTLV-I antibody. The onset is usually subacute and insidious but occasionally is abrupt. Fever or systemic symptoms are absent. Initial symptoms are heaviness, stiffness, and weakness in the lower extremities and urgency and frequency of urination. Impotence develops in most men. Dysesthesias may be distressing but are usually limited to the lower part of the trunk and legs; occasionally a bandlike sensation involves thoracic dermatomes, similar to the dysesthesias in acute transverse myelitis.

Physical findings are weakness of the legs with spasticity, hyperreflexia, and extensor-plantar responses. Strength in the arms is relatively spared, but deep tendon reflexes tend to be brisk in the upper extremities with a brisk jaw jerk. Despite frequent sensory symptoms, sensory findings are usually limited. Some loss of position and vibratory sense in the lower extremities may be evident, but a profound sensory loss or sensory level is rare. Some patients have loss of the ankle deep tendon reflexes, which suggests peripheral nerve involvement. Cranial nerve function is usually normal, but a few patients have been reported with retrobulbar neuritis, nerve deafness, seizures, or cerebellar ataxia. The disease may be asymmetric at onset, with one leg more affected than the other. Progression is most rapid during the first year and then tends to stabilize, and most patients retain functional use of spastic arms and normal cognition after many years (18).

Peripheral blood studies show no abnormalities except for the presence of lobulated nuclei that may be found in some lymphocytes. Early in disease, CSF usually shows a mononuclear cell pleocytosis and may contain abnormal cells. The CSF protein level is usually moderately elevated; immunoglobulin G (IgG) is increased, and oligoclonal bands are present. Levels of antibody to HTLV-I virus in the CSF are higher than can be accounted for by increased permeability of the blood–brain barrier. Oligoclonal bands of IgG are directed against polypeptides of HTLV-I (19).

In most patients, some subcortical bright foci on T2-weighted images are found. They are not solely artifacts of an aging population, because 60% of patients in their 40s have lesions (20). Foci are only rarely found in a periventricular distribution typical of multiple sclerosis. Magnetic resonance imaging (MRI) of the spinal cord usually fails to show lesions with discrete margins presumably because of the diffuse nature of inflammation and scarring.

DIAGNOSIS

Diagnosis of HAM depends on the typical clinical findings and the demonstration of antibody to HTLV-I in serum and excessive levels of antibody in CSF. Finding abnormal lobulated nuclei and lymphocytes in blood and CSF may assist in this diagnosis, and virus may be cultured from the CSF or detected by polymerase chain reaction (PCR).

Differential diagnosis includes nutritional and toxic myelopathies, as well as meningovascular syphilis, which was for many years thought to be the major cause of TSP. In temperate zones, the major differential diagnosis is multiple sclerosis, and the chronic spinal forms of that disease may be quite similar to HAM/TSP. HAM/TSP associated with retrobulbar neuritis or cerebral lesions on MRI may mimic progressive multiple sclerosis. The vacuolar myelopathy of human immunodeficiency virus infections produces similar clinical findings, and dual infections are well known. Other infections including spinal cysticercosis, tuberculosis, *Brucella melitensis* infections, and *Borrelia* infections; vascular disease including anterior spinal artery occlusions and arterial venous malformations; and spinocerebellar degenerations and neoplasms enter in the differential diagnosis.

TREATMENT

In uncontrolled clinical trials, mild improvements in motor disability scores have been recorded in more than 40% of patients given oral or intravenous steroids or plasmapheresis or lymphocytapheresis. Azathioprine proved less effective or ineffective (21). Transient improvements with steroids seem more evident early in the course of disease, when rapid progression and a more striking pleocytosis is found.

OTHER NEUROLOGIC DISEASES

Polymyositis

In a serologic survey of other neurologic diseases in Jamaica, 7% to 18% of persons showed antibody to HTLV-I, which is the expected frequency for that geographic area, but seven of seven patients with polymyositis were found to have antibodies (22). A recent study of 38 adult Jamaicans with polymyositis 63% were seropositive, and their disease showed a more insidious onset and less responsiveness to corticosteroid therapy (23). Japanese studies have shown a less convincing correlation.

Multiple Sclerosis

In 1985 antibody to p24 protein of HTLV-I and PCR detection of sequences of HTLV-I were reported in blood cells from patients with multiple sclerosis (24). Most subsequent studies have failed to confirm these findings (25).

REFERENCES

1. Johnson JM, Harrod R, Franchini G. Molecular biology and pathogenesis of the human T-cell leukaemia/lymphotropic virus Type-1 (HTLV-1). *Int J Exp Pathol* 2001;82:135–147.
2. Gessain A, Barin F, Vernant JC, et al. Antibodies to human T-lymphotropic virus type I in patients with tropical spastic paraparesis. *Lancet* 1985;2:407–409.
3. Rodgers-Johnson P, Gajdusek DC, Morgan OS, et al. HTLV-I and HTLV-III antibodies and tropical spastic paraparesis [Letter]. *Lancet* 1985;2:1247–1248.
4. Osame M, Usuku K, Izumo S, et al. HTLV-I–associated myelopathy, a new clinical entity. *Lancet* 1986;1:1031–1032.
5. Osame M, Matsumoto M, Usuku K, et al. Chronic progressive myelopathy associated with elevated antibodies to human T lymphotropic virus type I and adult T-cell leukemia-like cells. *Ann Neurol* 1987;21:117–122.
6. Montgomery RD. The epidemiology of myelopathy associated with human T-lymphotropic virus 1. *Trans R Soc Trop Med Hyg* 1993;87:154–159.
7. Hirose S, Uemura Y, Fujishita M, et al. Isolation of HTLV-I from cerebrospinal fluid of a patient with myelopathy. *Lancet* 1986;2:397–398.
8. Hara H, Morita M, Iwaki T, et al. Detection of human T lymphotrophic virus type I (HTLV-I) proviral DNA and analysis of T cell receptor Vβ CDR3 sequences in spinal cord lesions of HTLV-I–associated myelopathy/tropical spastic paraparesis. *J Exp Med* 1994;180:831–839.
9. Lehky TJ, Fox CH, Koenig S, et al. Detection of human T-lymphotropic virus type I (HTLV-I) tax RNA in the central nervous system of HTLV-I–associated myelopathy/tropical spastic paraparesis patients by in situ hybridization. *Ann Neurol* 1995;37:167–175.
10. Nishimura M, McFarlin DE, Jacobson S. Sequence comparisons of HTLV-I from HAM/TSP patients and their asymptomatic spouses. *Neurology* 1993;43:2621–2624.
11. Greenberg SJ, Jacobson S, Waldmann TA, et al. Molecular analysis of HTLV-I proviral integration and T cell receptor arrangement indicates that T cells in tropical spastic paraparesis are polyclonal. *J Infect Dis* 1989;159:741–744.
12. Rice GPA, Armstrong HA, Bulman DE, et al. Absence of antibody to HTLV-I and III in sera of Canadian patients with multiple sclerosis and chronic myelopathy. *Ann Neurol* 1986;20:533–534.
13. Izumo S, Umehara F, Osame M. HTLV-I–associated myelopathy. *Neuropathology* 2000;20:S65–S68.
14. Johnson RT, Griffin DE, Arregui A, et al. Spastic paraparesis and HTLV-I in Peru. *Ann Neurol* 1988;23:5151–5155.
15. Bangham CRM. HTLV-I infections. *J Clin Pathol* 2000;53:581–586.
16. Nagai M, Jacobson S. Immunopathogenesis of human T cell lymphotropic virus type 1-associated myelopathy. *Curr Opin Neurol* 2001;14:381–386.
17. Nagai M, Yamano Y, Brennal MB, et al. Increased HTLV-I proviral load and preferential expansion of HTLV-I tax-specific CD8+ T cells in cerebrospinal fluid from patients with HAM/TSP. *Ann Neurol* 2001;50:807–812.
18. Araujo AdeQ-C, Leite ACCB, Dultra SV, et al. Progression of neurological disability in HTLV-I–associated myelopathy/tropical spastic paraparesis (HAM/TSP). *J Neurol Sci* 1995;129:147–151.
19. Grimaldi LME, Roos RP, Devare SG, et al. HTLV-I–associated myelopathy: oligoclonal immunoglobulin G bands contain anti–HTLV-I p24 antibody. *Ann Neurol* 1988;24:727–731.
20. Nakagawa M, Izumo S, Ijichi S, et al. HTLV-I–associated myelopathy: analysis of 213 patients based on clinical features and laboratory findings. *J Neurovirol* 1995;1:50–61.
21. Nakagawa M, Nakahara K, Maruyama Y, et al. Therapeutic trials in 200 patients with HTLV-I–associated myelopathy/tropical spastic paraparesis. *J Neurovirol* 1995;2:345–355.
22. Mora CA, Garruto RM, Brown P. Seroprevalance of antibodies to HTLV-I in patients with chronic neurological disorders other than tropical spastic paraparesis. *Ann Neurol* 1988;23:S192–S195.
23. Gilbert DT, Morgan O, Smikle MF, et al. HTLV-1 associated polymyositis in Jamaica. *Acta Neurol Scand* 2001;104:101–104.
24. Koprowski H, DeFreitas EC, Harper ME, et al. Multiple sclerosis and human T-lymphotropic retroviruses. *Nature* 1985;318:154–160.
25. Ehrlich GD, Glaser JB, Vryz-Gronia B, et al. Multiple sclerosis, retroviruses, and PCR. *Neurology* 1991;41:335–343.

CHAPTER 123

Human Immunodeficiency Virus Infection in Women

Deborah Cotton

EPIDEMIOLOGY

Worldwide, women now comprise more than half of all newly diagnosed cases of acquired immunodeficiency syndrome (AIDS) and most have been infected heterosexually. The vast majority of human immunodeficiency virus (HIV)–positive women live in sub-Saharan Africa. Reported cases of AIDS in women in South America, eastern Europe, India, China, and Southeast Asia are rising dramatically and AIDS is now one of the leading causes of death in women globally (1–3).

In the United States, women comprise nearly one fourth of newly reported cases of AIDS and the epidemiology of HIV infection has changed markedly in recent years. Although still heavily concentrated in urban areas of the eastern seaboard where most cases are attributed to intravenous drug use, the incidence in women is rising rapidly in the south. Heterosexual transmission is now the dominant route of infection throughout the nation, except in the northeast.

The incidence of HIV infection in women begins to rise in adolescence, and most women with AIDS are in their childbearing years at the time of diagnosis. Among adolescents with AIDS, girls outnumber boys. This gender disparity may be due in part to girls acquiring infection from older male partners. In addition, cervical ectopy, common in adolescents or other biologic modifiers, may increase the risk of HIV acquisition during the teenage years (6). An estimated 7,000 HIV-positive women give birth in the Untied States each year (4,5).

Heterosexual Transmission

Male-to-female HIV transmission is much more efficient than female-to-male transmission (7–10). The risk of infection to women through heterosexual contact depends the specific type of sexual contact, with receptive anal intercourse conferring greater risk than vaginal intercourse for the female partner. Oral sex has been shown to confer a small but measurable risk of HIV infection among men who have sex with men; it is presumed that this also holds true for women. There are only a few reported cases of HIV transmission between women who are exclusively lesbian; however, lesbians self-report sexually transmitted disease (STD) and the risk may not be negligible (11,12).

Reported risk factors for acquisition of HIV infection by women include sex with an uncircumcised male partner, viral load in the male partner, and trauma during intercourse, intercourse occurring during menses, cervical ectopy, STDs and genital ulcers, and pelvic inflammatory disease (PID) (13–18). Some but not all epidemiologic studies have found an association between oral contraceptive use and acquisition of HIV (19,20). Possible risk factors for transmission from infected women to uninfected men include genital ulcers, high viral load, lower CD4 cell count, and cervical ectopy.

STDs are a major factor in HIV transmission, both by permitting direct viral entry and through immune activation leading to up-regulation of HIV in the genital track. Bacterial vaginosis (BV), an imbalance of vaginal flora that alters vaginal pH level, is common in HIV-negative and HIV-positive women and is postulated to induce expression of HIV by increasing the level of cytokines and other factors (21–28).

Our understanding of the earliest events in the pathogenesis of heterosexually transmitted HIV is limited, and the immunology and virology of the cervical-vaginal compartment are areas of intense research interest. Recently, it has been reported that dendritic cells, plentiful in the vaginal and cervical mucosa, have a specific receptor for HIV and can transport virus from the genital mucosa to lymphoid cells. Animal studies have suggested that progesterone may reduce HIV infectability through inhibition of chemokine receptor expression and that estrogen may protect against HIV transmission (30,31).

Most studies have found a direct correlation between the amount of HIV in genital tract fluids and the amount in plasma (32–35). Lowered plasma HIV viral burden from highly effective combination antiretroviral therapy (ART) may be correlated with decreased HIV viral burden in genital secretions (36). However, HIV has been isolated from cervical secretions in women with undetectable plasma viral load, and significant genotypic differences have been reported in virus from plasma and the vagina (37). These data suggest that the female genital tract may represent a separate compartment or even reservoir of HIV. There are conflicting data on whether the level of HIV in female genital secretions is influenced by the menstrual cycle (38–40).

Perinatal Transmission

In the absence of ART, about 15% to 30% of children of HIV-positive pregnant women are infected perinatally. Both *in utero* and peripartum infection occur. Although there are documented cases of fetuses infected early in pregnancy, there is no specific embryopathy associated with HIV infection. A recent model of perinatal transmission (41) based on clinical trials of prophylaxis with variable treatment duration has estimated that of 100 pregnancies at risk, 1 fetus will be infected before 14 weeks of gestation, 4 from 14 to 36 weeks, 12 from 36 weeks through labor, and 8 intrapartum. Maternal factors that have been associated with increased risk of vertical transmission include high viral load, HIV env diversity, low CD4 count, high maternal weight, anemia, clinical vaginosis, hepatitis C coinfection, and drug use (42–53). Although it has been surmised that seroconversion during pregnancy results in very high maternal viral load, one study did not find any difference in perinatal outcomes between mothers who were already HIV positive at the time of pregnancy and those who had acute infection during pregnancy (54).

Transmission has been observed across the entire range of maternal HIV ribonucleic acid (RNA) levels including undetectable levels, and the predictive value of RNA copy number for transmission in an individual untreated woman has been relatively poor. Similarly, although there is an indirect correlation between risk of transmission with CD4 count, infections have been documented in women with CD4 counts of more than 1,000 cells/mL. Obstetric factors that have been associated with transmission include prolonged rupture of membranes, chorioamnionitis, and fetal exposure to maternal blood and secretions during invasive procedures such as the insertion of scalp electrodes. Cesarean section has been associated with a reduced risk of vertical transmission in both a large clinical trial and a formal metaanalysis (55–57). Fetal factors associated with increased risk include prematurity and male sex. Absence of the CCR5 receptor in infants has been associated with decreased transmission from mothers with relatively low viral loads (58).

Breast-feeding is also a very efficient means of HIV transmission to babies. The risk from breast-feeding has been shown to occur with colostrum and breast milk. Reported risk factors for increased transmission postnatal include higher maternal viral load, low CD4 count, maternal nipple lesions, mastitis, maternal seroconversion while breast-feeding, oral thrush in the infant during the first 6 months of life, and breast-feeding longer than 15 months (59–63). In developing countries, infant mortality appears to be lower in the first few months in breast-fed babies; this is likely due to the competing risk of infant diarrhea from poorly prepared and stored formula. By 6 months of age, the situation reverses, with mortality lower in formula-fed babies. In one study, babies fed by the breast exclusively for 3 months or more had similar risk of postpartum transmission than those babies who were never breast-fed, but babies who had mixed feeding using both breast and formula had the highest risk (64).

NATURAL HISTORY

In cross-sectional studies, at any given CD4 count, women have a lower viral load than men, but there does not appear to be a difference in time to AIDS or in rate of progression to AIDS (65,66). In longitudinal studies, women appear to have a lower viral "set point" than men soon after seroconversion. This difference diminishes with time, and among patients with advanced HIV infection, there appears to be no gender difference in viral load (67–71). Possible confounding effects of race and ethnicity on these results are being explored (71,72).

Early studies reported shorter survival among women with AIDS compared with men; however, such differences were likely due to confounding variables such as age, race, and ethnicity, as well as poorer access to care and less use of aggressive antiretroviral and supportive therapy (73–75). Pregnancy does not adversely affect survival in HIV-infected women, with the possible exception of women who are in very advanced stages of disease (76,77).

Overall, women have similar risks and patterns of opportunistic infections (OIs) and other complications of HIV infection. However, women are at substantially less risk of Kaposi's sarcoma than men, although when it occurs, it may be more aggressive (78,79). They also appear to have a greater risk of esophageal candidiasis, bacterial pneumonia, and perhaps refractory herpes simplex virus (HSV) infection (80–82). Women do not appear to be at increased risk of non-Hodgkin's lymphoma compared with men; however, as the number of HIV-infected women increases, this complication is being reported more frequently (83). There is no evidence that HIV-infected women are at greater risk for breast cancer (84,85), although HIV-infected women may have a significantly increased risk of lung cancer compared with the general population (86). Women with HIV infection have an increased risk of osteopenia due to weight loss, relative androgen deficiency, and changes in body composition including decreased muscle mass (87,88).

Recurrent vaginal candidiasis is often the presenting manifestation of women with HIV infection (89). PID is relatively common in HIV-infected women, and when it occurs, it is more likely to result in tuboovarian abscess (90–101). A number of menstrual abnormalities have also been reported HIV-infected women including amenorrhea, polymenorrhea, menometrorrhagia, cycle variability, and pelvic pain (102–104). Not all of these have been found in well-controlled studies to be associated with HIV infection though.

Cervical squamous intraepithelial lesions (CSILs), believed to be a precursor of cervical cancer, has been strongly associated with human papillomavirus (HPV) infection. In predominately cross-sectional studies, women with HIV infection are more likely to have CSILs than HIV-negative women, and there is an inverse relationship of both HPV presence and persistence with CD4 count. HIV may increase the risk of cervical dysplasia in women infected with HPV through its association with increased expression of HPV and multiple HPV infections. Studies of risk of cervical dysplasia in HIV-infected women have been limited, because most did not correct for the presence of HPV infection (105–112). Cigarette smoking has been associated with cervical dysplasia (113).

Independent risk factors for abnormal cervical cytology in a multivariate analysis from a large cohort study included HIV infection, lower CD4 cell count, and higher plasma HIV RNA level, as well as presence of HPV in cervicovaginal lavage specimens (114). A recent study of both HIV-positive and HIV-negative adolescent girls showed that HPV infection was common in both groups but statistically significantly a more common occurrence in HIV-positive girls, who also were more likely to be infected with HPV subtypes most strongly associated with invasive squamous cell cancer. HIV-positive girls were more likely to have abnormal cytologic findings despite that they were felt to be early in infection with well-preserved immune function (115).

Although women with HIV infection have an increased risk of HPV infection and low-grade CSILs, there is a low prevalence of high-grade CSILs, and to date there has not been an "epidemic" of this cancer among HIV-infected women, as had been predicted in the early 1990s. However, this may reflect the long latency time of this disease. Some studies have concluded that when cervical cancer occurs in HIV-infected women, it is more likely to be multifocal, rapidly progressive, and refractory to standard therapy. Development of vulvovaginal and perianal condyloma acuminatum and intraepithelial neoplasia was significantly higher in HIV-positive women than in matched HIV-negative controls in a recent study, and thus such women may be at increased risk of future development of invasive vulvar carcinoma (116).

The incidence of anal cancer is increasing in the United States. Anal HPV infection is associated with anal squamous intraepithelial lesions (ASILs), thought to be a precursor of anal cancer, and there is an association between the HPV types common in cervical cancer and those associated with anal cancer. In a recent study, anal HPV infection was common in both HIV-positive (76%) and high-risk HIV-negative women (42%) and was significantly more common than cervical HPV infection in both groups. Although there was a clear association between HPV at the cervical and anal sites and overall the spectrum of HPV types was the same in the cervical and anal specimens, most women had different HPV types found in the cervix and anus at the same visit (117).

DIAGNOSIS OF HUMAN IMMUNODEFICIENCY VIRUS INFECTION IN WOMEN

Major impediments to optimal medical care of HIV-infected women include failure to consider the diagnosis and poor access to early intervention (118). Women have also had poor access to clinical trials, although this may be improving (119,120). Older women and black women are more likely to be diagnosed late in the course of disease (121). Women who present with a history of STD, a large number of sexual partners, or illicit drug use should be considered at high risk, even if these risks were in the distant past. Women who do not have known risks but who live in communities where HIV infection is prevalent should also be offered testing regardless of known personal risk factors.

Any woman who presents with recurrent pneumonia, tuberculosis, recurrent vaginal candidiasis without known predisposing cause, cervical dysplasia, severe genital herpes, shingles, diffuse adenopathy, or unexplained weight loss should also be considered possibly HIV infected. HIV infection should also be included in the differential diagnosis of fever of unknown origin, interstitial pulmonary infiltrates, and non-Hodgkin's lymphoma. The possibility of acute HIV seroconversion should be considered in the workup of all women presenting with mononucleosis-like illnesses or viral meningitis.

Finally, because ART has been shown to dramatically lessen the risk for perinatal transmission of HIV, it has been recommended by the Institute of Medicine and the American College of Obstetrics and Gynecology that all pregnant women in the United States be offered HIV antibody testing. Women with unexpected positive results or with an indeterminate Western blot result should have further testing performed, because the overall prevalence in the United States among pregnant women is low and because multiparous women can have antibodies to human leukocyte antigens that cross-react in some enzyme-linked immunosorbent assays and all Western blot kits.

Management of the Nonpregnant HIV-infected Woman

Women who are found to be HIV infected should have a detailed baseline history and physical examination including pelvic examination. Routine immunizations including pneumococcal and influenza vaccines should be given as appropriate, and tuberculin skin test should be performed.

A baseline CD4 cell count and viral load should be obtained, and ART and prophylaxis against OIs should be prescribed as indicated by results. Because women appear to have a lower viral load than men when matched for CD4 count, current guidelines for the initiation of combination ART according to viral load, derived from studies largely done in men, may not be applicable and therapy must be individualized.

Ascertainment of cytomegalovirus (CMV) serostatus is useful in the event that transfusion is needed, in which case CMV-negative or leukocyte-filtered blood should be given if the woman is seronegative, or for future reference should the patient become pregnant. Women with young children or who work in day care or health care settings should have good hand-washing practices reinforced to prevent acquisition of CMV in these high-risk settings. Toxoplasma serostatus, both immunoglobulin G (IgG) and immunoglobulin M (IgM), should be ascertained, and prevention should be stressed again because women are usually the family members responsible for preparation of meals and care of pets. Similarly, women need to be counseled about the risks for infection from other sources of food and water, both for themselves and for other HIV-positive family members. Smoking should be discouraged because smoking may be a cofactor in HIV disease progression and risk for lung cancer may be greater in HIV-positive women than the general population (86,123). Women with wasting may benefit from androgen replacement (124).

Despite some controversy Papanicolaou (Pap) smear screening appears to be a sensitive and specific screening test in HIV-infected women as long as findings of atypical squamous cells of undetermined significance (ASCUS), often dismissed in women, are considered abnormal and patients with this finding referred for colposcopy (125,126). Two cytologies should be obtained in the first year of diagnosis and then a yearly Pap smear obtained. A recent study has suggested that a targeted strategy in which HPV screening is added to the initial cytologic screening after diagnosis and the frequency of Pap smears is increased to every 6 months in HPV-positive women is both clinically effective and cost-effective (127).

Low-grade CSIL in HIV-infected women usually has a slow rate of progression and a significant rate of regression without specific therapy. A recent trial of isotretinoin in such women showed no benefit over placebo (128). In women with high-grade cervical dysplasia, recurrence may be increased after standard surgical therapies (129). Intravaginal 5-fluorouracil (5-FU) after standard surgery reduced recurrence and was well tolerated (130). A variety of surgical approaches to cervical dysplasia have been employed and conization may have a higher rate of recurrence in HIV-infected women (131). Potent combination ART against HIV has been reported to slow progression of cervical dysplasia and even result in regression of such lesions (132). Currently there are few guidelines regarding detection and treatment of anal dysplasia and few providers are skilled in anal cytologic assessment, limiting aggressive disease detection and treatment.

Recurrent vaginal candidiasis can usually be managed with topical therapy of recurrences or with low maintenance doses of fluconazole, a little as 100 mg every week (133). Overall, most studies suggest that HIV-positive women with PID can be managed with standard drug regimens (134). However, tuboovarian abscess is more common, and early ultrasound is indicated in patients with persistent fever and pain despite adequate antibiotic therapy (135).

ANTIRETROVIRAL THERAPY IN THE NONPREGNANT WOMAN

Outside of studies of perinatal transmission prophylaxis, participation of women in clinical trials has generally been too low to permit statistically valid subgroup analyses. This has restricted attempts to discern any gender-associated differences in antiretroviral efficacy and toxicity. Few studies to date have suggested that there may be important gender differences in time to viral suppression, the risk of progression to clinical end points, and drug toxicity (136,137).

Hyperlactatemia, sometimes leading to life-threatening lactic acidosis, has been reported with many reverse-transcriptase inhibitors. Stavudine, with or without didanosine (ddI) appears to be the most likely drug in this class to cause this disorder (138,139). Women, especially those who are obese, may be more susceptible to this drug toxicity.

Recently, life-threatening hepatic failure in several health care workers receiving nevirapine as part of occupational postexposure prophylaxis regimens has been reported (140). Nevirapine should be avoided for all postexposure prophylaxis, a common reason for use of ART in women, who constitute the largest number of health care workers at risk of occupational exposure and who also often receive prophylaxis in the setting of sexual exposure. Rash resulting from nevirapine use appears to be significantly more common in HIV-positive women than men (141).

Overall, women appear to have similar benefit and toxicity from protease inhibitors (PIs) compared with men. Metabolic complications of lipodystrophy including lipidemias, insulin resistance, and the occurrence of peripheral fat wasting, buffalo hump, and mesenteric fat deposition have all been reported in women and men, as have osteonecrosis and osteopenia (142). Studies of these complications have been only modestly successful in including women; hopefully this will improve and permit gender analysis of these often treatment-limiting complications.

Because most women with HIV infection are of childbearing age, the possibility of pregnancy occurring on all regimens must be considered. While preconceptual counseling would permit the tailoring of antiretroviral regimens in HIV-infected women to maximize interruption of perinatal transmission while avoiding fetal toxicity, many if not most HIV-positive women have unplanned pregnancies and may even first learn of their infection in prenatal care. Thus, it is imperative that all HIV-positive women of childbearing age be explicitly informed concerning both pregnancy prevention and early detection at the time that ART is prescribed and that choice of drugs be informed by the woman's pregnancy plans. Efavirenz is teratogenic in monkeys; and use of this agent in women who may become pregnant should be limited to situations where there are no alternatives (143). Combination therapy with stavudine and ddI should be avoided in any woman who is at risk of pregnancy because fatalities have occurred in pregnant women on this regimen (144).

Monitoring during Pregnancy

Women who are seeking to become pregnant or who present for prenatal care should be assessed both by standard guidelines for health maintenance during pregnancy and for HIV-specific concerns. Antibodies against *Toxoplasma gondii* (both IgG and IgM) and CMV should be obtained. A purified protein derivative (PPD) of tuberculin should be placed, or if the patient is known to be PPD positive, a chest radiograph should be obtained prepregnancy or after the first trimester. For pregnant women with a positive tuberculin skin-test reaction or at high risk of having acquired tuberculosis, isoniazid should be begun after the first trimester.

Salmonella and *Listeria* are pathogens that may pose a special threat to women who are both pregnant and HIV infected; patients should be strongly advised to avoid raw eggs, soft cheeses, and all raw milk products during pregnancy and to take care when cooking eggs and poultry.

Normal pregnancy is accompanied by mild immunosuppression, but most studies have not found a lasting decline postpartum (145,146). A CD4 cell count should be obtained during the first trimester or at the first pregnancy visit and repeated during the third trimester. At present, the same CD4 cell count thresholds as in the nonpregnant state should be used to determine risk of opportunistic infection.

ANTIRETROVIRAL THERAPY AND OTHER MEASURES IN PREGNANT HIV-INFECTED WOMEN

HIV-positive women may receive ART during pregnancy solely to prevent perinatal transmission, for their own health, or most commonly in developed countries, for both of these indications simultaneously. The use of multidrug regimens is increasing rapidly in pregnant women (146a). In addition, HIV-negative pregnant women may receive postexposure prophylaxis with antiretroviral agents in the setting of occupational exposure, sexual assault, or "morning-after" prophylaxis for consensual sex. In all of these situations, the overriding principle when choosing therapy should be that maternal health and well-being are optimized. Revised federal guidelines for antiretroviral treatment of pregnant women with HIV infection have recently been released as a "living document" *(www.hivatis.org/trtgdlns.html#Perinatal)* and should be consulted for detailed information and management advice.

If a woman would meet current criteria for combination antiretroviral treatment if not pregnant, than she should in almost all cases receive such therapy while she is pregnant. New guidelines for nonpregnant adults *(www.hivatis.org/trtgdlns.html#AdultAdolescent)* are in general more conservative than those published just a few years ago in light of increasing recognition of the problems of adherence, toxicity, and resistance associated with complex antiretroviral regimens. Thus, a greater number of women may now fall into the category of "watchful waiting" in regard to their own need for therapy.

According to these guidelines, "decisions regarding the use and choice of an antiretroviral regimen should be individualized based on discussion with the woman about (a) her risk for disease progression and the risks and benefits of delaying initiation of therapy; (b) possible benefit of lowering viral load for reducing perinatal transmission; (c) potential drug toxicities and interactions with other drugs; (d) the need for strict adherence to the prescribed drug schedule to avoid the development of drug resistance; (e) unknown long-term effects of *in utero* drug exposure on the infant; and (f) preclinical, animal, and clinical data relevant to use of the currently available antiretrovirals during pregnancy. Due to the evolving and complex nature of the management of HIV-1 infection, a specialist with experience in the treatment of HIV-infected pregnant women should be involved in their care."

Although most studies of ART to prevent perinatal transmission have used zidovudine (ZDV) monotherapy or ZDV in combination with lamivudine, these regimens are no longer used in the developed world for nonpregnant patients because of lack of efficacy and emergence of resistance (42,147–151). Moreover, potent combination antiretroviral regimens appear to provide enhanced protection against perinatal transmission without obvious fetal toxicity (152,153). Thus, most experts now favor use

of potent combination regimens during pregnancy because of these considerations, even when the mother does not meet current guidelines for initiation of therapy in her own right. Initiation of therapy is deferred until the second trimester in previously untreated women. Women already on ART at the time pregnancy is established should in general have that therapy continued during the first trimester, although the risk/benefit ratio of such therapy for mother and fetus must be considered on an individual basis.

The mechanism by which ZDV reduces transmission is not known and its effect cannot be completely explained by reduction in maternal viral load (154). Protection is likely multifactorial and probably includes prophylaxis of the infant by passage of ZDV across the placenta, leading to inhibitory levels of the drug in the fetus during the birth process. Other antiretroviral drugs have variable transplacental passage. Thus, given these theoretical considerations and its proven track record, ZDV should be included as a component of combination antenatal therapy whenever possible. If a woman does not receive ZDV antenatally as part of her regimen, or if she has not been treated at all, intrapartum and newborn ZDV or nevirapine should still be given. An observational study in New York has concluded that even in the absence of maternal therapy, therapy of the newborn within 48 to 72 hours substantially reduces risk of perinatal HIV infection (155).

Use of PIs with their now well-known metabolic side effects requires careful monitoring of patients. Hyperglycemia, presumably due to insulin resistance, is common, and because pregnancy itself can result in hyperglycemia, pregnant women receiving PIs should have blood glucose level monitored frequently.

Recent concerns have been raised that the hepatic steatosis and lactic acidosis associated with administration of reverse-transcriptase inhibitors, which are frequently life threatening and may occur with increased frequency in HIV-infected women, especially those who are obese, may be yet more common and severe in pregnant HIV-positive women. These disorders are similar to the HELLP syndrome (i.e., hemolysis, elevated liver function, and low platelets), a condition described in the third trimester of pregnancy in previously healthy, HIV-negative women that can be fatal (156). Recently Bristol-Myers Squibb reported three maternal deaths in women receiving stavudine and ddI, in combination with either PIs or nevirapine (144,157). Both drugs, as well as zalcitabine (not currently widely in use), are known to interfere with mitochondrial replication to a greater degree than other nucleoside analogs, although all drugs of this class do so to some degree. Use of stavudine and ddI in combination during pregnancy should be avoided unless there are no therapeutic alternatives and the mother's own health requires treatment. In all pregnant women receiving ART, liver enzymes and electrolytes should be monitored frequently, especially during the third trimester; some experts also recommend routine determination of serum lactate in this setting.

Eight cases of HIV-negative infants with *in utero* and/or neonatal exposure to either ZDV-lamivudine (four infants) or ZDV alone (four infants) who developed evidence of mitochondrial dysfunction have been reported from France (158). Two of these infants who had received ZDV-lamivudine developed severe neurologic disease and died. However, review of a large database that included 223 deaths in more than 20,000 children with and without antiretroviral drug exposure who were born to HIV-infected women followed prospectively in the United States revealed no similar deaths, although few had received the combination of ZDV and lamivudine (159). Similarly, an African perinatal trial that compared three regimens of ZDV-lamivudine showed no increased risk of neurologic events observed in those babies treated with ZDV-lamivudine compared with babies receiving placebo (150).

Efavirenz (Sustiva), a nonnucleoside reverse-transcriptase inhibitor (NNRTI), has been associated with serious embryopathy in monkeys and is contraindicated for use during pregnancy (143). Women on this drug who become pregnant should have it discontinued. Use of other NNRTIs should also be approached with caution because of possible maternal side effects. Recently nevirapine has been associated with hepatic failure in health care workers who received this drug for occupational exposure prophylaxis. To date, this severe adverse outcome has not been associated with therapeutic use in HIV-infected individuals. However, nevirapine has been associated with rash (141), which may be more severe in women and with hypersensitivity reactions including cases of Stevens-Johnson syndrome and must be gradually phased in by giving a half dose for the first 2 weeks of use.

Although small studies concluded that rates of prematurity were higher in HIV-infected women who received PIs (160), in a recent study of 89 pregnant women who received combination ART including PIs, the rate of prematurity was 19%, which is consistent with the incidence in untreated HIV-infected women, and in a multivariate analysis, only cocaine use and prolonged rupture of membranes were associated with prematurity (161). Similar results were found in an Italian study (162).

A large clinical trial and a metaanalysis of several observational studies have concluded that elective cesarean section reduces the risk of perinatal transmission; this protective effect is seen even in women with low viral loads who are receiving ART (163). Several studies have suggested that although maternal morbidity is low after cesarean section in HIV-infected women, it is still substantially higher than that seen in HIV-negative women who have this surgery, and opinion is divided on the efficacy of cesarean section in further reducing an already low risk of vertical transmission in women on combination ART with undetectable viral loads (163–168).

An observational, nonexperimental registry sponsored by pharmaceutical companies that make and market antiretroviral drugs has been created. The registry does not use patient names, and registry staff members obtain birth outcome follow-up from the reporting physician. Providers for pregnant women receiving antiretroviral drugs are urged to register their patients (Antiretroviral Pregnancy Registry, 1410 Commonwealth Drive, Wilmington, NC 28403; telephone 800-258-4263; fax 800-800-1052; website www.apregistry.com).

In the United States and other countries where infant formula is readily available, breast-feeding is highly discouraged, to reduce the incidence of HIV transmission to babies. However, the situation is far more complex in those parts of the world where more than 95% of HIV-infected women reside. In those countries, formula is scarce and expensive and often results in increased infant mortality due to diarrheal disease. Further, because breast-feeding is nearly universal, use of bottle-feeding can reveal that a mother is HIV-infected, leading to her being stigmatized and ostracized and in some cases resulting in physical violence. Nonetheless, a recent study demonstrated that the benefit of short-term antiretroviral regimens in decreasing perinatal HIV infection is significantly lessened over time in a breast-feeding population and has largely disappeared by 18 months of life (150). Studies of the efficacy of early weaning in the prevention of pediatric HIV infection are underway in Africa.

Prophylaxis against Opportunistic Pathogens during Pregnancy

For almost all drugs used for prophylaxis against OIs associated with HIV infection, there are few data on use in pregnancy, including information on teratogenicity. Because the blood plasma volume is increased in pregnancy, drug concentrations tend to be lower than in the nonpregnant state, and doses of drugs at the high end of recommended ranges should generally be used in prophylactic regimens. Guidelines have been published that address pregnancy-related issues in prophylaxis of HIV-related OIs (169–171).

Prophylaxis for *Pneumocystis carinii* pneumonia (PCP) should be started when the $CD4^+$ cell count is less than $200/mm^3$ in an asymptomatic pregnant woman or less than $250/mm^3$ in women who have had recurrent oral or vaginal candidiasis, shingles, or other clinical manifestations of HIV infection. Trimethoprim-sulfamethoxazole is preferred throughout pregnancy, even at term, despite theoretical concerns regarding neonatal kernicterus as it has efficacy superior to other agents in preventing PCP and has the added advantage of providing prophylaxis against toxoplasmosis. The higher maintenance dose of one double-strength tablet daily should be used during pregnancy. In pregnant women who are allergic to trimethoprim-sulfamethoxazole or cannot tolerate it, dapsone is thought to be both effective and safe, although data are limited. There are no controlled data on the use of atovaquone in pregnancy. Aerosolized pentamidine is clearly inferior to other prophylactic agents and should be limited to those who cannot tolerate systemic regimens. When used, it does have the advantage of low teratogenic potential because there is no systemic absorption.

For recurrent oral or vaginal candidiasis requiring systemic therapy, the lowest dose and frequency of fluconazole to control disease should be used; for many women, 100 mg per week orally of fluconazole prevents recurrent vaginal candidiasis (133). Orally administered ganciclovir is not recommended during pregnancy for prevention of CMV retinitis or other CMV disease. Women with advanced HIV infection should have a dilated ophthalmologic examination during pregnancy. In asymptomatic women with less than 50 CD4 cells/mm^3 or in those women with less than 100 CD4 cells/mm^3 who have had an AIDS-defining OI, the risk for development of *Mycobacterium avium* complex infection during the subsequent year and the devastating consequences of such an infection for both mother and fetus warrant the use of prophylactic therapy. Clarithromycin and azithromycin are closely related to erythromycin, which is considered safe in pregnancy. If it is feasible, initiation of prophylaxis should be delayed until after the first trimester.

Treatment of Opportunistic Infection during Pregnancy

For women who develop OIs during pregnancy, the risk from the infection itself, almost always life threatening, usually outweighs any real or theoretical risk from adverse drug effects for either mother or fetus. The same philosophy holds for most instances in which maintenance therapy is needed to prevent a recurrence of OIs. The least teratogenic drugs should be chosen of those that are effective.

PCP is the most common OIs in women with AIDS and carries a high mortality during pregnancy (172). High-dose Bactrim is the drug of choice in this setting despite theoretical concerns regarding neonatal kernicterus. There is limited experience with pentamidine in pregnancy, but no fetal malformations have been reported. Trimetrexate is contraindicated because it is a folate antagonist; it should be used only when there are no alternatives.

A special issue is raised by primary or recurrent toxoplasmosis during pregnancy. Pyrimethamine, a mainstay of therapy in combination with sulfadiazine, is considered teratogenic by the Food and Drug Administration. Although there are isolated case reports of use during pregnancy without ill effects on the fetus, no larger studies have been reported (173,174). However, acute and reactivation toxoplasmosis in HIV-infected patients usually occurs in the setting of advanced immune suppression and is often fatal even with optimal therapy. In this life-threatening situation, pyrimethamine should not be withheld, but the mother should be given all relevant data.

For induction and maintenance therapy for systemic mycoses, some experts favor avoiding fluconazole at least during the first trimester because it has been reported to cause fetal osseous abnormalities and fetal loss in rats because of inhibition of estrogen synthesis. However, these effects have not been reported in women treated with fluconazole (175,176), and because fluconazole has been shown to be superior to amphotericin B in controlled clinical trials in the acute treatment and secondary prophylaxis of cryptococcal meningitis, it is the drug of choice for this disease in the second and third trimesters (177).

PREVENTION OF HIV INFECTION IN WOMEN

Although the widespread use of combination ART in developed countries has resulted in decreased death rates from HIV infection, no known current therapies can eradicate HIV or cure AIDS. Attempts at prevention of HIV infection thus must still be paramount. Even more compelling is the case for prevention in those parts of the world where HIV infection is decimating entire societies and where effective therapies are tragically not yet available.

Although regular condom use can dramatically lower HIV infection rates, this approach is unavailable to many women worldwide who are unable to determine when and with whom they have sexual relations, let alone compel the use of a condom by their male partners. Only if biomedical approaches to prevention are coupled with overall improvement in the economic status of women and recognition of their human rights will there be any real chance of success in stemming the onslaught of this disease.

A female condom has been developed, which consists of a ring that covers the cervix attached to a ring that covers the introitus by a latex sheath (178). Although many women at risk are successfully using this device, it is expensive and cumbersome. Microbicides promise an ideal method that would be woman controlled, could be used well before sexual contact, and would be more likely to be accepted by male partners or to be unknown to male partners (179). Unfortunately, microbicides tested to date have not been found to be effective in reducing risk of either STDs or HIV acquisition by women. Products containing nonoxynol-9, a spermicide long used as a contraceptive that effectively kills HIV *in vitro*, have been especially disappointing in this regard and are also commonly associated with subjective and objective toxicities of chemical irritation. There is concern that vaginal microabrasions caused by nonoxynol-9 may increase rather than decrease the risk of HIV transmission (180). Several promising new candidate microbicides are now in clinical trials (181–183). Ideal products would include both spermicidal and nonspermicidal formulations, allowing women to separate competing needs to prevent HIV acquisition while permitting pregnancy. Disappointingly, recent trials in Africa of aggressive diagnosis and management of STDs in women and men have failed to show any benefit in reducing HIV transmission (184,185).

In addition to barrier methods, a current focus of prevention is on the use of testing to prevent transmission. Only a minority of HIV-infected persons in the United States are aware of their serostatus; prevention efforts are now being targeted to HIV-positive individuals including women. However, pregnant women make up the only group in the United States, apart from the military, in whom routine HIV testing has become the norm.

REFERENCES

1. Fowler MG, Melnick SL, Mathieson BJ. Women and HIV. Epidemiology and global overview. *Obstet Gynecol Clin North Am* 1994;24(4):705–729.
2. AIDS epidemic faster in Eastern Europe than in rest of world. *Int J Epidemiol* 2002;31(1):277.
3. Bollinger RC, Tripathy SP, Quinn TC. The human immunodeficiency virus epidemic in India. Current magnitude and future projections. *Medicine (Baltimore)* 1995;74(2):97–106.
4. Gayle H. An overview of the global HIV/AIDS epidemic, with a focus on the United States. *AIDS* 2000;14[Suppl 2]:S8–S17.
5. Rogers MF. Epidemiology of HIV/AIDS in women and children in the USA. *Acta Paediatr Suppl* 1997;421:15–16.
6. Glynn JR, Carael M, Auvert B, et al. Why do young women have a much higher prevalence of HIV than young men? A study in Kisumu, Kenya and Ndola, Zambia. *AIDS* 2001;15[Suppl 4]:S51–S60.
7. Padian N, Marquis L, Francis DP, et al. Male-to-female transmission of human immunodeficiency virus. *JAMA* 1987;258:780–790.
8. Padian NS, Shiboski SC, Jewell NP. Female-to-male transmission of human immunodeficiency. virus. *JAMA* 1991;25:1664–1667.
9. European Study of the Heterosexual Transmission of HIV. Comparison of female to male to male to female transmission of HIV in 563 stable couples. *BMJ* 1992;304:809–813.
10. Padian NS, Shiboski SC, Glass So, et al. Heterosexual transmission of human immunodeficiency virus (HIV) in northern California: results from a ten-year study. *Am J Epidemiol* 1997;146:350–357.
11. Bauer GR, Welles SL. Beyond assumptions of negligible risk: sexually transmitted diseases and women who have sex with women. *Am J Public Health* 2001;91(8):1282–1286.
12. Marrazzo JM, Koutsky LA, Stine KL, et al. Genital human papillomavirus infection in women who have sex with women. *J Infect Dis* 1998;178(6):1604–1609.
13. Quinn TC, Wawer MJ, Sewankambo N, et al, and the Rakai Project Study Group. Viral load and heterosexual transmission of human immunodeficiency virus type 1. *N Engl J Med* 2000;342:921–929.
14. Tovanabutra S, Robison V, Wongtrakul J, et al. Male viral load and heterosexual transmission of HIV-1 subtype E in northern Thailand. *J Acquir Immune Defic Syndr* 2002;29(3):275–283.
15. Moss GB, Clemetson D, D'Costa L, et al. Association of cervical ectopy with heterosexual transmission of human immunodeficiency virus: results of a study of couples in Nairobi, Kenya. *J Infect Dis* 1991;164(3):588–591.
16. Gray RH, Wawer MJ, Brookmeyer R, et al, and the Rakai Project Team. Probability of HIV-1 transmission per coital act in monogamous, heterosexual, HIV-1 discordant couples in Rakai, Uganda. *Lancet* 2001;357:1149–1153.
17. Plourde PJ, Pepin J, Agoki E, et al. Human immunodeficiency virus type 1 seroconversion in women with genital ulcers. *J Infect Dis* 1994;170(2):313–317.
18. Clemetson DB, Moss GB, Willerford DM, et al. Detection of HIV DNA in cervical and vaginal secretions. Prevalence and correlates among women in Nairobi, Kenya. *JAMA* 1993;269:2860–2864.
19. Mati JK, Hunter DJ, Maggwa BN, et al. Contraceptive use and the risk of HIV infection in Nairobi, Kenya. *Int J Gynaecol Obstet* 1995;48:61–67.
20. Wang CC, Reilly M, Kreiss JK. Risk of HIV infection in oral contraceptive pill users: a meta-analysis. *J Acquir Immune Defic Syndr* 1999;21(1):51–58.
21. Al-Harthi L, Roebuck KA, Olinger GG, et al. Bacterial vaginosis-associated microflora isolated from the female genital tract activates HIV-I expression. *J Acquir Immune Defic Syndr* 1999;21(3):194–202.
22. Warren D, Klein RS, Sobel J, et al, and the HIV Epidemiology Research Study Group. A multicenter study of bacterial vaginosis in women with or at risk for human immunodeficiency virus infection. *Infect Dis Gynecol* 2001;9(3):133–141.
23. Hasherni FB, Ghasserni M, Roebuck KA, et al. Activation of human immunodeficiency virus type 1 expression by *Gardnerella* vaginalis. *J Infect Dis* 1999;179(4):924–930.
24. Martin HL, Richardson BA, Nyange PIvI, et al. Vaginal lactobacilli, microbial flora, and risk of human immunodeficiency virus type 1 and sexually transmitted disease acquisition. *J Infect Dis* 1999;180(6):1863–1868.
25. Hasherni FB, Ghasserni M, Faro S, et al. Induction of human immunodeficiency virus type 1 expression by anaerobes associated with bacterial vaginosis. *J Infect Dis* 2000;181(5):1574–1580.
26. Royce RA, et al. Bacterial vaginosis associated with HIV infection in pregnant women from North Carolina. *J Acquir Immune Defic Syndr Hum Retrovirol* 1999;20(4):382–386.
27. Olinger GG, Hashemi FB, Sha BE, et al. Association of indicators of bacterial vaginosis with a female genital tract factor that induces expression of HIV-I. *AIDS* 1999;13(14):1905–1912.
28. Sturrm-Ramirez K, Gaye-Diallo A, Eisen G, et al. High levels of tumor necrosis factor-alpha and interleukin-1 beta in bacterial vaginosis may increase susceptibility to human immunodeficiency virus. *J Infect Dis* 2000;182(2):467–473.

29. Geijtenbeek TB, Kwon DS, Torensma R, et al. DC-SIGN, a dendritic cell-specific HIV-1–binding protein that enhances trans-infection of T cells. *Cell* 2000;100(5):587–597.

30. Vassiliadou N, Tucker L, Anderson DJ. Progesterone-induced inhibition of chemokine receptor expression on peripheral blood mononuclear cells correlates with reduced HIV-1 infectability *in vitro*. *J Immunol* 1999;162(12):7510–7518.

31. Smith SM, Baskin GB, Marx PA. Estrogen protects against vaginal transmission of simian immunodeficiency virus. *J Infect Dis* 2000;182(3):708–715.

32. Goulston C, McFarland W, Katzenstein D. Human immunodeficiency virus type 1 RNA shedding in the female genital tract. *J Infect Dis* 1998;177(4):1100–1103.

33. Hart CE, Lennox JL, Pratt-Palmore M, et al. Correlation of human immunodeficiency virus type 1 RNA levels in blood and the female genital tract. *J Infect Dis* 1999;179(4):871–882.

34. Rasheed S, et al. Presence of cell-free human immunodeficiency virus in cervicovaginal secretions is independent of viral load in the blood of human immunodeficiency virus-infected women. *Am J Obstet Gynecol* 1996;175(1):122–129.

35. Kovacs A, Wasserman SS, Burns D, et al, and the DATRI Study Group (WIHS Study Group). Determinants of HIV-1 shedding in the genital tract of women. *Lancet* 2001;358(9293):1593–1601.

36. Ellerbrock TV, Lennox JL, Clancy KA, et al. Cellular replication of human immunodeficiency virus type 1 occurs in vaginal secretions. *J Infect Dis* 2001;184(1):28–36.

37. Lawn SD, Subbarao S, Wright TC, et al. Correlation between human immunodeficiency virus type 1 RNA levels in the female genital tract and immune activation associated with ulceration of the cervix. *J Infect Dis* 2000;181(6):1950–1956.

38. Mostad SB, Jackson S, Overbaugh J, et al. Cervical and vaginal shedding of human immunodeficiency virus type 1-infected cells throughout the menstrual cycle. *J Infect Dis* 1998;178(4):983–991.

39. Reichelderfer PS, Coornbs RW, Wright DJ, et al. Effect of menstrual cycle on HIV-I levels in the peripheral blood and genital tract. WHS 001 Study Team. *AIDS* 2000;14(14):2101–2107.

40. Villanueva JM, Ellerbrock TV, Lennox JL, et al. The menstrual cycle does not affect human immunodeficiency virus type 1 levels in vaginal secretions. *J Infect Dis* 2002;185(2):170–177.

41. Kourtis AP, Bulterys M, Nesheim SR, et al. Understanding the timing of HIV transmission from mother to infant. *JAMA* 2001;285(6):709–712.

42. Connor EM, Sperling RS, Gelber R, et al. Reduction of maternal-infant transmission of human immunodeficiency virus type 1 with zidovudine treatment. Pediatric AIDS Clinical Trials Group Protocol 076 Study Group. *N Engl J Med* 1994;331(18):1173–1180.

43. Garcia PM, Kalish LA, Pitt J, et al. The Women and Infants Transmission Study Group. Maternal levels of plasma human immunodeficiency virus type 1 RNA and the risk of perinatal transmission. *N Engl J Med* 1999;341(6):394–402.

44. Shapiro DE, Sperling RS, Mandelbrot L, et al. Risk factors for perinatal human immunodeficiency virus transmission in patients receiving zidovudine prophylaxis. Pediatric AIDS Clinical Trials Group protocol 076 Study Group. *Obstet Gynecol* 1999;94(6):897–908.

45. Dickover RE, Garratty EM, Herman SA, et al. Identification of levels of maternal HIV-1 RNA associated with risk of perinatal transmission. Effect of maternal zidovudine treatment on viral load. *JAMA* 1996;275(8):599–605.

46. Mwanyumba F, Gaillard P, Inion I, et al. Placental inflammation and perinatal transmission of HIV-1. *J Acquir Immune Defic Syndr* 2002;29(3):262–269.

47. Fawzi W, Msamanga G, Renjifo B, et al. Predictors of intrauterine and intrapartum transmission of HIV-1 among Tanzanian women. *AIDS* 2001;15(9):1157–1165.

48. John GC, Nduati RW, Mbori-Ngacha DA, et al. Correlates of mother-to-child human immunodeficiency virus type 1 (HIV-1) transmission: association with maternal plasma HIV-1 RNA load, genital HIV-1 DNA shedding, and breast infections. *J Infect Dis* 2001;183(2):206–212.

49. Cao Y, Krogstad P, Korber BT, et al. Maternal HIV-1 viral load and vertical transmission of infection: the Ariel Project for the prevention of HIV transmission from mother to infant. *Nat Med* 1997;3(5):549–552.

50. Shapiro DE, Sperling RS. Coombs effect of zidovudine on perinatal HIV-1 transmission and maternal viral load. Pediatric AIDS Clinical Trials Group 076 Study Group. *Lancet* 1999;354(9173):156–158.

51. Panther LA, Tucker L, Xu C, et al. Genital tract human immunodeficiency virus type 1 (HIV-1) shedding and inflammation and HJV-1 env diversity in perinatal HIV-1 transmission. *J Infect Dis* 2000;181(2):555–563.

52. Welles SL, Pitt J, Colgrove R, et al. HIV-1 genotypic zidovudine drug resistance and the risk of maternal—infant transmission in the women and infants transmission study. The Women and Infants Transmission Study Group. *AIDS* 2000;14(3):263–271.

53. Hershow RC, Riester KA, Lew J, et al. Increased vertical transmission of human immunodeficiency virus from Hepatitis C coinfected mothers. *J Infect Dis* 1997;176:414–420.

54. Roongpisuthipong A, Siriwasin W, Simonds RJ, et al. HIV seroconversion during pregnancy and risk for mother-to-infant transmission. *J Acquir Immune Defic Syndr* 2001;26(4):348–351.

55. Landers DV, Duarte G, Beckerman KP, et al, and the International Perinatal HIV Group. Mode of delivery and the risk of vertical transmission of HIV-1. *N Engl J Med* 1999;341:205–207.

56. The International Perinatal HIV Group. The mode of delivery and the risk of vertical transmission of human immunodeficiency virus type 1—a meta-analysis of 15 prospective cohort studies. *N Engl J Med* 1999;340:977–987.

57. Riley LE, Greene MF. Elective cesarean delivery to reduce the transmission of HIV. *N Engl J Med* 1999;340:1032–1033.

58. Ometto L, Zanchetta M, Mainardi M, et al. Co-receptor usage of HIV-1 primary isolates, viral burden, and CCR5 genotype in mother-to-child HIV-1 transmission. *AIDS* 2000;14(12):1721–1729.

59. Embree JE, Njenga S, Datta P, et al. Risk factors for postnatal mother-child transmission of HIV-1. *AIDS* 2000;14(16):2535–2541.

60. John GC, Richardson BA, Nduati RW, et al. Timing of breast milk HIV-1 transmission: a meta-analysis. *East Afr Med J* 2001;78(2):75–79.

61. Bulterys M. Breastfeeding in women with HIV. *JAMA* 2000;284(8):956.

62. Nduati R, Mbori-Ngacha D, John G, et al. Breastfeeding in women with HIV. *JAMA* 2000;284(8):956–957.

63. Semba RD. Mastitis and transmission of human immunodeficiency virus through breast milk. *Ann N Y Acad Sci* 2000;918:156–162.

64. Coutsoudis A, Pillay K, Kuhn L, et al. Method of feeding and transmission of HIV-1 from mothers to children by 15 months of age: prospective cohort study from Durban, South Africa. *AIDS* 2001;15(3):379–387.

65. Rezza G, Lepri AC, Monforte A, et al. Plasma viral load concentrations in women and men from different exposure categories and with known duration of HIV infection. *J Acquir Immune Defic Syndr* 2000;25(1):56–62.

66. Rompalo AM, et al. Comparison of clinical manifestations of HIV infection among women by risk group, CD4+ cell count, and HIV-1 plasma viral load. HER Study Group. HIV Epidemiology Research. *J Acquir Immune Defic Syndr Hum Retrovirol* 1999;20(5):448–454.

67. European Collaborative Study. Level and pattern of HIV-1-RNA viral load over age: differences between girls and boys? *AIDS* 2002;16(1):97–104.

68. Sterling TR, et al. Sex differences in longitudinal human immunodeficiency virus type 1 RNA levels among seroconverters. *J Infect Dis* 1999;180(3):666–672.

69. Evans JS, Nims T, Cooley J, et al. Serum levels of virus burden in early-stage human immunodeficiency virus type 1 disease in women. *J Infect Dis* 1997;175(4):795–800.

70. Sterling TR, Vlahov D, Astemborski J, et al. Initial plasma HIV-1 RNA levels and progression to AIDS in women and men. *N Engl J Med* 2001;344:720–725.

71. Kalish LA, Collier AC, Flanigan TP, et al. Plasma human immunodeficiency virus (HIV) type 1 RNA load in men and women with advanced HIV-1 disease. *J Infect Dis* 2000;182(2):603–606.

72. Anastos K, Gange SJ, Lau B, et al. Association of race and gender with HIV-1 RNA levels and immunologic progression. *J Acquir Immune Defic Syndr* 2000;24(3):218–226.

73. Lemp G, Hiroza A, Cohen J, et al. Survival for women and men with AIDS. *J Infect Dis* 1992;166:74–79.

74. Whyte B, Swanson C, Cooper D. Survival of patients with the acquired immunodeficiency syndrome in Australia. *Med J Aust* 1989;150:358–362.

75. Chaisson RE, Keruly JC, Moore RD. Race, sex, drug use, and progression of human immunodeficiency virus disease. *N Engl J Med* 1995;333(12):751–756.

76. French R, Brocklehurst P. The effect of pregnancy on survival in women infected with HIV: a systematic review of the literature and meta-analysis. *Br J Obstet Gynaecol* 1998;105(8):827–835.

77. Weisser M, Rudin C, Battegay M, et al. Does pregnancy influence the course of HIV infection? Evidence from two large Swiss cohort studies. *J Acquir Immune Defic Syndr Hum Retrovirol* 1998;17(5):404–410.

78. Cooley TP, Hirschhorn LR, O'Keane JC. Kaposi's sarcoma in women with AIDS. *AIDS* 1996;10(11):1221–1225.

79. Nasti G, Serraino D, Ridolfo A, et al. AIDS-associated Kaposi's sarcoma is more aggressive in women: a study of 54 patients. *J Acquir Immune Defic Syndr Hum Retrovirol* 1999;20(4):337–341.

80. Feldman C, Glatthaar M, Morar R, et al. Bacteremic pneumococcal pneumonia in HIV-seropositive and HIV-seronegative adults. *Chest* 1999;116(1):107–114.

81. Flanigan TP, et al. Self-reported bacterial infections among women with or at risk for human immunodeficiency virus infection. *Clin Infect Dis* 1999;29(3):608–612.

82. Fleming PL, Ciesielski CA, Byers RH, et al. Gender differences in reported AIDS-indicative diagnoses. *J Infect Dis* 1993;168(1):61–67.

83. Levine AM, Seneviratne L, Espina BM, et al. Evolving characteristics of AIDS-related lymphoma. *Blood* 2000;96(13):4084–4090.

84. Amir H, Kaaya EE, Kwesigabo G, et al. Breast cancer before and during the AIDS epidemic in women and men: a study of Tanzanian cancer. Registry Data 1968 to 1996. *J Natl Med Assoc* 2000;92(6):301–305.

85. Amir H, Makwaya C, Mhalu F, et al. Breast cancer during the HIV epidemic in an African population. *Oncol Rep* 2001;8(3):659–661.

86. Phelps RM, Smith DK, Heilig CM, et al. HER Study Group Cancer incidence in women with or at risk for HIV. *Int J Cancer* 2001;94(5):753–757.

87. Huang JS, Wilkie SJ, Sullivan MP, et al. Reduced bone density in androgen-deficient women with acquired immune deficiency syndrome wasting. *J Clin Endocrinol Metab* 2001;86(8):3533–3539.

88. Grinspoon S, Corcoran C, Miller K, et al. Body composition and endocrine function in women with acquired immunodeficiency syndrome wasting. *J Clin Endocrinol Metab* 1997;82(5):1332–1337.

89. Rhoads JL, Wright DC, Redfield RR, et al. Chronic vaginal candidiasis in women with HIV infection. *JAMA* 1987;257:3105–3107.

90. Barbosa C, Macasaet M, Brockmann S, et al. Pelvic inflammatory disease and human immunodeficiency virus infection. *Obstet Gynecol* 1997;89(1):65–70.

91. Hoegsberg B, Abulafia O, Sedlis A, et al. Sexually transmitted diseases and human immunodeficiency virus infection among women with pelvic inflammatory disease. *Am J Obstet Gynecol* 1990;1135–1139.

92. Irwin KL, Moorman AC, O'Sullivan MJ, et al. Influence of human immunodeficiency virus infection on pelvic inflammatory disease. *Obstet Gynecol* 2000;95(4):525–534.

93. Jamieson DJ, Duerr A, Macasaet MA, et al. Risk factors for a complicated clinical course among women hospitalized with pelvic inflammatory disease. *Infect Dis Obstet Gynecol* 2000;8(2):88–93.

94. Safrin S, Dattel B, Haver L, et al. Seroprevalence and epidemiologic correlates of infection in women with acute pelvic inflammatory disease. *Obstet Gynecol* 1990;75:666–670.

95. Safrin S, Dattel B, Haver L, et al. Seroprevalence and epidemiologic correlates of infection in women with acute pelvic inflammatory disease. *Obstet Gynecol* 1990;75:666–670.

96. Barbosa C, Macasaet M, Brockmann S, et al. Pelvic inflammatory disease and human immunodeficiency virus infection. *Obstet Gynecol* 1997;89(1):65–70.

97. Cu-Uvin S, et al. Prevalence of lower genital tract infections among human immunodeficiency virus (HIV)–seropositive and high-risk HIV-seronegative women. *Clin Infect Dis* 1999;29(5):1145–1150.

98. Hoegsberg B, Abulafia O, Sedlis A, et al. Sexually transmitted diseases and human immunodeficiency virus infection among women with pelvic inflammatory disease. *Am J Obstet Gynecol* 1990;1135–1139.

99. Irwin KL, Moorman AC, O'Sullivan MJ, et al. Influence of human immunodeficiency virus infection on pelvic inflammatory disease. *Obstet Gynecol* 2000;95(4):525–534.

100. Jamieson DJ, Duerr A, Macasaet MA, et al. Risk factors for a complicated clinical course among women hospitalized with pelvic inflammatory disease. *Infect Dis Obstet Gynecol* 2000;8(2):88–93.

101. Sobel JD. Gynecologic infections in human immunodeficiency virus-infected women. *Clin Infect Dis* 2000;31(5):1225–1233.

102. Clark RA, Mulligan K, Stamenovic E, et al. Frequency of anovulation and early menopause among women enrolled in selected adult AIDS clinical trials group studies. *J Infect Dis* 2001;184:1325–1327.

103. Harlow SD, Schuman P, Cohen M, et al. Effect of HIV infection on menstrual cycle length. *J Acquir Immune Defic Syndr* 2000;24:68–75.

104. Chirgwin KD, Feldman J, Muneyyirci-Delale O, et al. Menstrual function in human immunodeficiency virus-infected women without acquired immunodeficiency syndrome. *J Acquir Immune Defic Syndr Hum Retrovirol* 1996;12(5):489–494.

105. Henry M, Stanley M, Cruikshank S, et al. Association of human immunodeficiency virus-induced immunosuppression with human papillomavirus infection and cervical intraepithelial neoplasia. *Am J Obstet Gynecol* 1989;160:52–53.

106. Schrager LK, Friedland GH, Maude D, et al. Cervical and vaginal squamous cell abnormalities in women infected with human immunodeficiency virus. *J Acquir Immune Defic Syndr* 1989;2(6):570–575.

107. Maiman M, Fruchter R, Serur E, et al. Human immunodeficiency virus and cervical neoplasia. *Gynecol Obstet* 1990;38:377–382.

108. Vermund SH, Kelley KF, Klein RS, et al. High risk of human papillomavirus infection and cervical squamous : intraepithelial lesions among women with symptomatic human immunodeficiency virus infection. *Am J Obstet Gynecol* 1991;165(2):392–400.

109. Safrin S, Dattel BJ, Hauer L, et al. High frequency of latent and clinical human papillomavirus cervical infections in immunocompromised human immunodeficiency virus–infected women. *Obstet Gynecol* 1992;79(3):321–327.

110. Ellerbrock TV. Human papillomavirus infection in human immunodeficiency virus-seropositive women. *Obstet Gynecol* 1995;85(5)[pt 1]:680–686.

111. Klein RS, Ho GYF, Vermund SH, et al. Risk factors for squamous intraepithelial lesions on pap smear in women at risk for human immunodeficiency virus infection. *J Infect Dis* 1994;(6):1404–1409.

112. Ahdieh L, Klein RS, Burk R, et al. Prevalence, incidence, and type-specific persistence of human papillomavirus in human immunodeficiency virus (HIV)–positive and HIV-negative women. *J Infect Dis* 2001;184(6):682–690.

113. Kanetsky PA, Gammon MD, Mandelblatt J, et al. Cigarette smoking and cervical dysplasia among non-Hispanic black women. *Cancer Detect Prev* 1998;22(2):109–119.

114. Stratton P, Gupta P, Riester K, et al. Cervical dysplasia on cervicovaginal Papanicolaou smear among HIV-1–infected pregnant and nonpregnant women. Women and Infants Transmission Study. *J Acquir Immune Defic Syndr Hum Retrovirol* 1999;20(3):300–307.

115. Moscicki AB, Ellenberg JH, Vermund SH, et al. Prevalence of and risks for cervical human papillomavirus infection and squamous intraepithelial lesions in adolescent girls: impact of infection with human immunodeficiency virus. *Arch Pediatr Adolesc Med* 2000;154(2):127–134.

116. Conley LJ, Ellerbrock TV, Bush TJ, et al. HIV-1 infection and risk of vulvovaginal and perianal condylomata acuminata and intraepithelial neoplasia: a prospective cohort study. *Lancet* 2002;359(9301):108–113.

117. Palefsky JM, Holly EA, Ralston ML, et al. Prevalence and risk factors for anal human papillomavirus infection in human immunodeficiency virus (HIV)– positive and high-risk HIV-negative women. *J Infect Dis* 2001;183(3):383–391.

118. Mocroft A, Gill MJ, Davidson W, et al. Are there gender differences in starting protease inhibitors, HAART, and disease progression despite equal access to care? *J Acquir Immune Defic Syndr* 2000;24(5):475–482.

119. Cotton DJ, Feinberg J, Finkelstein D. Participation of women in a large multicenter HIV/AIDS clinical trials program in the United States. *J Acquir Immune Defic Syndr* 1993;6:1322–1328.

120. Gifford AL, Cunningham WE, Heslin KC, et al. Participation in research and access to experimental treatments by HIV-infected patients. *N Engl J Med* 2002;346(18):1373–1382.

121. Hu DJ, Byers R Jr, Fleming PL, et al. Characteristics of persons with late AIDS diagnosis in the United States. *Am J Prev Med* 1995;11(2):114–119. MA A. Stoto, Almario D, McCormick MC. Committee on Perinatal Transmission of HIV. *Reducing the odds: preventing perinatal transmission of HIV in the United States.* Washington, DC: National Academy Press, 1998

122. Guidelines for using antiretroviral agents among HIV-infected adults and adolescents. Recommendations of the Panel on Clinical Practices for Treatment of HIV. *MMWR Morb Mortal Wkly Rep* 2002;51(RR-7):1–55.

123. Page-Shafer K, Delorenze GN, Satariano WA, et al. Comorbidity and survival in HIV-infected men in the San Francisco Men's Health Survey. *Ann Epidemiol* 1996;6(5):420–430.

124. Miller K, Corcoran C, Armstrong C, et al. Transdermal testosterone administration in women with acquired immunodeficiency syndrome wasting: a Pilot study. *J Clin Endocrinol Metab* 1998;83(8):2717–2725.

125. Goodman A, Chaudhuri PM, Tobin-Enos NJ, et al. The false negative rate of cervical smears in high risk HIV seropositive and seronegative women. *Int J Gynecol Cancer* 2000;10(1):27–32.

126. Holcomb K, Abulafia O, Matthews RP, et al. The significance of ASCUS cytology in HIV-positive women. *Gynecol Oncol* 1999;75(1):118–121.

127. Goldie SJ, et al. The costs, clinical benefits, and cost-effectiveness of screening for cervical cancer in HIV-infected women. *Ann Intern Med* 1999;130(2):97–107.

128. Robinson WR, Andersen J, Darragh TM, et al. Isotretinoin for low-grade cervical dysplasia in human immunodeficiency virus-infected women. *Obstet Gynecol* 2002;99(5):777–784.

129. Tate DR, Anderson RJ. Recrudescence of cervical dysplasia among women who are infected with the human immunodeficiency virus: a case-control analysis. *Am J Obstet Gynecol* 2002;186(5)[Pt 1]:880–882.

130. Maiman M, Watts DH, Andersen J, et al. Vaginal 5-fluorouracil for high-grade cervical dysplasia in human immunodeficiency virus infection: a randomized trial. *Obstet Gynecol* 1999;94(6):954–961.

131. Holcomb K, Matthews RP, Chapman JE, et al. The efficacy of cervical conization in the treatment of cervical intraepithelial neoplasia in HIV-positive women. *Gynecol Oncol* 1999;74(3)428–431.

132. Minkoff H, Ahdieh L, Massad LS, et al. The effect of highly active antiretroviral therapy on cervical cytologic changes associated with oncogenic HPV among HIV-infected women. *AIDS* 2001;15(16):2157–2164.

133. Schuman P, Capps L, Peng G, et al. Weekly fluconazole for the prevention of mucosal candidiasis in women with HIV infection. A randomized, double-blind, placebo-controlled trial. Terry Beirn Community Programs for Clinical Research on AIDS. *Ann Intern Med* 1997;126(9):689–696.

134. Bukusi EA, Cohen CR, Stevens CE, et al. Effects of human immunodeficiency virus 1 infection on microbial origins of pelvic inflammatory disease and on efficacy of ambulatory oral therapy. *Am J Obstet Gynecol* 1999;181(6):1374–1381.

135. Cohen CR, Sinei S, Reilly M, et al. Effect of human immunodeficiency virus type 1 infection upon acute salpingitis: a laparoscopic study. *J Infect Dis* 1998;178(5):1352–1358.

136. Currier JS, Spino C, Grimes J, et al. Differences between women and men in adverse events and CD4$^+$ responses to nucleoside analogue therapy for HIV infection. The AIDS Clinical Trials Group 175 Team. *J Acquir Immune Defic Syndr* 2000;24(4):316–324.

137. Moore AL, Mocroft A, Madge S, et al. Gender differences in virologic response to treatment in an HIV-positive population: a cohort study. *J Acquir Immune Defic Syndr* 2001;26(2):159–163.

138. Boubaker K, Flepp M, Sudre P, et al. Hyperlactatemia and antiretroviral therapy: the Swiss HIV Cohort Study. *Clin Infect Dis* 2001;33(11):1931–1937.

139. Miller KD, Cameron M, Wood LV, et al. Lactic acidosis and hepatic steatosis associated with use of stavudine: report of four cases. *Ann Intern Med* 2000;133(3):192–196.

140. Cattelan AM, Erne E, Salatino A, et al. Severe hepatic failure related to nevirapine treatment. *Clin Infect Dis* 1999;29(2):455–456.

141. Antinori A, Baldini F, Girardi E, et al. Female sex and the use of anti-allergic agents increase the risk of developing cutaneous rash associated with nevirapine therapy. *AIDS* 2001;15(12):1579–1581.

142. Hadigan C, Miller K, Corcoran C, et al. Fasting hyperinsulinemia and changes in regional body composition in human immunodeficiency virus–infected women. *J Clin Endocrinol Metab* 1999;84(6):1932–1937.

143. Notice on efavirenz and pregnancy. *AIDS Treat News* 3 Apr 1998;292:7.

144. Sarner L, Fakoya A. Acute onset lactic acidosis and pancreatitis in the third trimester of pregnancy in HIV-1 positive women taking antiretroviral medication. *Sex Transm Infect* 2002;78(1):58–59.

145. Brettle RP, Raab GM, Ross A, et al. HIV infection in women: immunological markers and the influence of pregnancy. *AIDS* 1995;9(10):1177–1184.

146. Temmerman M, Nagelkerke N, Bwayo J, et al. HIV-1 and immunological

changes during pregnancy: a comparison between HIV-1–seropositive and HIV-1–seronegative women in Nairobi, Kenya. *AIDS* 1995;9(9):1057–1060.

146a. Minkoff H, Ahdieh L, Watts H, et al. The relationship of pregnancy to the use of highly active antiretroviral therapy. *Am J Obstet Gynecol* 2001;184(6):1221–1227.

147. Lallemant M, Jourdain G, Le Coeur S, et al. A trial of shortened zidovudine regimens to prevent mother-to-child transmission of human immunodeficiency virus type 1. Perinatal HIV Prevention Trial (Thailand) Investigators. *N Engl J Med* 2000;343(14):982–991.

148. Shaffer NR, Chauchoowong PA, Mock C, et al. Short-course zidovudine for perinatal transmission of HIV-1 transmission in Bangkok, Thailand: a randomised controlled trial. *Lancet* 1999;353:773–780.

149. Jackson JB, Becker-Pergola G, Guay LA, et al. Identification of the K103N resistance mutation in Ugandan women receiving nevirapine to prevent HIV-1 vertical transmission. *AIDS* 2000;14(11):F111–F115.

150. Efficacy of three short-course regimens of zidovudine and lamivudine in preventing early and late transmission of HIV-1 from mother to child in Tanzania, South Africa, and Uganda (Petra study): a randomised, double-blind, placebo-controlled trial. *Lancet* 2002;359(9313):1178–1186.

151. Brocklehurst P, Volmink J. Antiretrovirals for reducing the risk of mother-to-child transmission of HIV infection (Cochrane Review). *Cochrane Database Syst Rev* 2002;(1):CD003510.

152. Cooper ER, Charurat M, Mofenson L, et al. Combination antiretroviral strategies for the treatment of pregnant HIV-1–infected women and prevention of perinatal HIV-1 transmission. *J Acquir Immune Defic Syndr* 2002;29(5):484–494.

153. Bucceri AM, Somigliana E, Matrone R, et al. Combination antiretroviral therapy in 100 HIV-1–infected pregnant women. *Hum Reprod* 2002;17(2):436–441.

154. Sperling RS, Shapiro DE, Coombs RW, et al. Pediatric AIDS Clinical Trials Group Protocol 076 Study Group. Maternal viral load, zidovudine treatment, and the risk of transmission of human immunodeficiency virus type 1 from mother to infant. *N Engl J Med* 1996;335(22):1621–1629.

155. Wade NA, Birkhead GS, Warren BL, et al. Abbreviated regimens of zidovudine prophylaxis and perinatal transmission of the human immunodeficiency virus. *N Engl J Med* 1998;339(20):1409–1414.

156. Wolf JL. Liver disease in pregnancy. *Med Clin North Am* 1996;80(5):1167–1187.

157. Warning for pregnant women on HIV therapy. *FDA Consum* 2001;35(3):5.

158. Blanche S, Tardieu M, Rustin P, et al. Persistent mitochondrial dysfunction and perinatal exposure to antiretroviral nucleoside analogues. *Lancet* 1999;354:1084–1089.

159. Bulterys M, Nesheim S, Abrams EJ, et al, and the Perinatal Safety Review Working Group. Lack of evidence of mitochondrial dysfunction in the offspring of HIV-infected women. Retrospective review of perinatal exposure to antiretroviral drugs in the Perinatal AIDS Collaborative Transmission Study. *Ann N Y Acad Sci* 2000;918:212–221.

160. Lorenzi P, Spicher VM, Laubereau B, et al. Antiretroviral therapies in pregnancy: maternal, fetal and neonatal effects. Swiss HIV Cohort Study, the Swiss Collaborative HIV and Pregnancy Study, and the Swiss Neonatal HIV Study. *AIDS* 1998;12(18):F241–F247.

161. Morris AB, Cu-Uvin S, Harwell JI, et al. Multicenter review of protease inhibitors in 89 pregnancies. *J Acquir Immune Defic Syndr* 2000;25(4):306–301.

162. Bucceri AM, Somigliana E, Matrone R, et al. Combination antiretroviral therapy in 100 HIV-1–infected pregnant women. *Hum Reprod* 2002;17(2):436–441.

163. Ioannidis JP, Abrams EJ, Ammann A, et al. Perinatal transmission of human immunodeficiency virus type 1 by pregnant women with RNA virus loads <1000 copies/mL. *J Infect Dis* 2001;183(4):539–545.

164. Read JS, Tuomala R, Kpamegan E, et al. Mode of delivery and postpartum morbidity among HIV-infected women: the women and infants transmission study. *J Acquir Immune Defic Syndr* 2001;26(3):236–245.

165. Tscherning-Casper C, Dolcini G, Mauclere P, et al. Maternal complications after caesarean section in HIV infected women. *Eur J Obstet Gynecol Reprod Biol* 2000;90(1):73–76

166. Riley LE, Greene MF. Elective cesarean delivery to reduce the transmission of HIV. *N Engl J Med* 1999;340:1032–1033.

167. Vimercati A, Greco P, Loverro G, et al. Maternal complications after caesarean section in HIV infected women. *Eur J Obstet Gynecol Reprod Biol* 2000;90(1):73–76.

168. Grubert TA, Reindell D, Kastner R, et al. Complications after caesarean section in HIV-1–infected women not taking antiretroviral treatment. *Lancet* 1999;354(9190):1612–1613.

169. 1999 USPHS/IDSA guidelines for the prevention of opportunistic infections in persons infected with HIV: part II. Prevention of the first episode of disease. U. S. Department of Health and Human Services, Public Health Service, Centers for Disease Control and Prevention. U. S. Public Health Service/Infectious Diseases Society of America. *Am Fam Physician* 2000;61(2):441–442.

170. 1999 USPHS/IDSA guidelines for the prevention of opportunistic infections in persons infected with HIV: part III. Prevention of disease recurrence. United States Public Health Service/Infectious Diseases Society of America. *Am Fam Physician* 2000;61(3):771–778.

171. 1999 USPHS/IDSA guidelines for the prevention of opportunistic infections in persons infected with HIV: part I. Prevention of exposure. *Am Fam Physician* 2000;61(1):163–174.

172. Ahmad H, Mehta NJ, Manikal VM, et al. *Pneumocystis carinii* pneumonia in pregnancy. *Chest* 2001;120(2):666–671.

173. Deen JL, von Seidlein L, Pinder M, et al. The safety of the combination artesunate and pyrimethamine-sulfadoxine given during pregnancy. *Trans R Soc Trop Med Hyg* 2001;95(4):424–428.

174. Hedriana HL, Mitchell JL, Brown GM, et al. Normal fetal outcome in a pregnancy with central nervous system toxoplasmosis and human immunodeficiency virus infection. A case report. *J Reprod Med* 1993;38(9):747–750.

175. Sorensen HT, Nielsen GL, Olesen C, et al. Risk of malformations and other outcomes in children exposed to fluconazole in utero. *Br J Clin Pharmacol* 1999;48(2):234–238.

176. Jick SS. Pregnancy outcomes after maternal exposure to fluconazole. *Pharmacotherapy* 1999;19(2):221–222.

177. Saag MS, Graybill RJ, Larsen RA, et al. Practice guidelines for the management of cryptococcal disease. Infectious Diseases Society of America. *Clin Infect Dis* 2000;30(4):710–718.

178. Gollub EL. The female condom: tool for women's empowerment. *Am J Public Health* 2000;90(9):1377–1381.

179. Blocker ME, Cohen MS. Biologic approaches to the prevention of sexual transmission of human immunodeficiency virus. *Infect Dis Clin North Am* 2000;14(4):983–999.

180. Centers of Disease Control and Prevention. CDC statement on study results of product containing nonoxynol-9. *JAMA* 2000;284(11):1376.

181. Mayer KH, Peipert J, Fleming T, et al. Safety and tolerability of BufferGel, a novel vaginal microbicide, in women in the United States. *Clin Infect Dis* 2001;32(3):476–482.

182. Msellati P, Meda N, Leroy V, et al. Safety and acceptability of vaginal disinfection with benzalkonium chloride in HIV infected pregnant women in west Africa: ANRS 049b phase II randomized, double blinded placebo controlled trial. DITRAME Study Group. *Sex Transm Infect* 1999;75(6):420–425.

183. van De Wijgert J, Fullem A, Kelly C, et al. Phase 1 trial of the topical microbicide BufferGel: safety results from four international sites. *J Acquir Immune Defic Syndr* 2001;26(1):21–27.

184. Wawer MJ, Sewankambo NK, Serwadda D, et al, and the Rakai Project Study Group. Control of sexually transmitted diseases for AIDS prevention in Uganda: a randomised community trial. *Lancet* 1999;353(9152):525–535.

185. Gray RH, Wabwire-Mangen F, Kigozi G, et al. Randomized trial of presumptive sexually transmitted disease therapy during pregnancy in Rakai, Uganda. *Am J Obstet Gynecol* 2001;185(5):1209–1217.

Immunocompromised Hosts

CHAPTER 124

Approach to the Immunocompromised Patient

Michael H. Grieco

The first step in approaching management of an immunodeficient patient is to recognize what defects are likely to be present in a host. This exercise is useful in forming a basis for the second step: deducing the probability of infectious complications. The third step involves the selection of empiric therapy for patients presumed to be infected.

CLASSIFICATION OF IMMUNODEFICIENCY DISORDERS

Immunodeficiency disorders include abnormalities involved in the development of antigen-specific primary or secondary

TABLE 124.1. Congenital, Acquired, and Drug-induced Inflammatory and Immunodeficiency Disorders

Phagocytes (neutrophils, monocytes)	Complement components	Antibody-mediated immunity	Cell-mediated immunity
Defense mechanisms			
Chemotactic responsiveness	Kinin activity, C4	Interfere with adherence, SIgA	Delayed-type hypersensitivity
Adherence	Viral neutralization, C1, C4	Neutralization of viruses, SIgA	(CD4$^+$ T$_H$1 lymphocyte)
Vacuole formation	Opsonization, C3b	Microbicidal, IgG, IgM	Direct cytotoxicity (CD8$^+$ T
Degranulation	Chemotaxis, C3a, C5a	Immune adherence, IgG, IgM	lymphocyte)
Microbicidal activity	Anaphylatoxin, C3a, C5a	Antibody-dependent cellular	CD16$^+$/56$^+$ NK cells
	Neutrophil activation, C5a	cytotoxicity, IgG (NK cell,	CD3$^+$ and CD16$^+$/56$^+$ NKT cells
	Cytolysis, C5b-9	macrophage, neutrophil,	$\gamma\delta$ TCR$^+$ T cells
		eosinophil)	
Congenital or hereditary Disorders			
Neutropenia	C3, AR	Reticular dysgenesis, U	Reticular dysgenesis, AR
Infantile genetic agranulocytosis	C5, AR	SCID (thymic dysplasia), AR,	SCID (thymic dysplasia), AR, XLR
Autoimmune neutropenia	C6, AR	occasionally XLR	SCID with ADA deficiency, AR
Isoimmune neonatal	C7, AR	SCID with ADA deficiency, AR	SCID with ZAP-70 deficiency, AR
neutropenia	C8, AR	SCID with ZAP-70 deficiency, AR	SCID with Jak3 deficiency, AR
Kostmann's syndrome	Factor I, AR	SCID with Jak3 deficiency, AR	DiGeorge syndrome, V
Abnormal chemotaxis	Properdin, XLR	X-linked agammaglobuhnemia,	Nezelof syndrome, U
Chédiak-Higashi, AR	CR3 (LAD), AR	XLR	Chronic mucocutaneous
Lazy leukocyte, U		CVID, U	candidiasis, V
Hyper-IgE, U		Congenital hypogamma-	Wiskott-Aldrich syndrome, XLR
Abnormal digestion		globulinemia, AR	Ataxia-telangiectasia, AR
Griscelli's syndrome,		IgA deficiency, V	Cartilage-hair hypoplasia, AR
actin-myosin dysfunction,		IgM deficiency, U	CVID, U
AR		Hyper-IgM, XLR	Nucleoside phosphorylase
Abnormal microbicidal			deficiency, U
Chédiak-Higashi, AR			X-linked recessive
CGD, XLR (70%), AR (30%)			lymphoproliferative syndrome,
MPD, AR			Duncan's syndrome, XLR
G6PD, XLR			MHC class I deficiency, AR
Abnormal adhesion			MHC class II deficiency, AR
LAD type 1, AR			
LAD type 2, AR			
Acquired Disorders			
Neutropenia	Factor B	Multiple myeloma	Hodgkin's disease
Acute leukemia	Splenectomy	Macroglobulinemia	Sézary's syndrome
Chronic leukemia	Sickle cell disease	Heavy chain diseases	Organ transplantation
Alcoholism	Hypocomplementemia	Non-Hodgkin's lymphoma	Bone marrow transplantation
Nutritional deficiency (vitamin	SLE	Chronic lymphatic leukemia	Stem cell transplantation
B$_{12}$, folate)			
Infectious diseases (e.g., HIV-1)	Protein-calorie	AIDS	AIDS
	malnutrition		
Bone marrow transplant-related			
suppression			
Abnormal chemotaxis			
Intrinsic			
Diabetes mellitus			
Rheumatoid arthritis, Felty			
syndrome, SLE			
Acute infections			
Burn injuries			
Alcoholism (chronic)			
Job syndrome			
Circulating inhibitor to CFs			
Renal disease			
Hepatic cirrhosis			
Hodgkin's disease			
Lepromatous leprosy			
Sarcoidosis			
Circulating inhibitor to cells			
Hepatic cirrhosis			
Sarcoma			
Carcinoma			
Anergy			

(continued)

| | TABLE 124.1. *(continued)* | | |

Phagocytes (neutrophils, monocytes)	Complement components	Antibody-mediated immunity	Cell-mediated immunity
Abnormal granulocyte adherence			
Alcoholism (acute)			
Abnormal phagocytosis			
Rheumatoid arthritis			
Acute infections			
Hyperosmolar states			
Abnormal microbicidal			
Malakoplakia			
Felty's syndrome			
Drug-induced disorders		Cyclophosphamide (alkylating agent)	Cyclophosphamide (alkylating agent)
Neutropenia		Azathioprine (antimetabolite)	Azathioprine (antimetabolite)
Cytoxic drugs (e.g., cyclophosphamide)			Corticosteroids
Noncytotoxic drugs (chloramphenicol)			Cyclosporine
Abnormal phagocytosis			Tacrolimus
Colchicine			Sirolimus (Rapamycin)
Tetracycline			Mycophenolate mofetil
Cyclophosphamide			Daclizumab (monoclonal antibody)
Abnormal granulocyte adherence			Basiliximab (monoclonal antibody)
Corticosteroids			
Aspirin			
Abnormal microbicidal			
Phenylbutazone			
Chloramphenicol			

ADA, adenosine deaminase; AIDS, acquired immunodeficiency syndrome; AR, autosomal recessive; basiliximab, chimeric monoclonal antibody to CD25 IL-2Rα chain; CFs, chemotactic factors; CGD, chronic granulomatous disease; CVID, common variable immunodeficiency; daclizumab, humanized monoclonal antibody to CD25 IL-2Rα chain; G6PD, glucose-6-phosphate dehydrogenase deficiency; HIV, human immunodeficiency virus; IgA, IgE, IgG, IgM, immunoglobulins A, E, G, M; Jak3, Janus-associated kinase 3; LAD, leukocyte adhesion disorder; MHC, major histocompatibility complex; MPD, myeloperoxidase deficiency; NK, natural killer cells; NKT, natural killer T lymphocytes; SCID, severe combined immunodeficiency disease; SIgA, secretory IgA; SLE, systemic lupus erythematosus; U, unknown; V, variable; XLR, X-linked recessive; ZAP-70, CD3 zeta chain-associated protein.
Source: Adapted from Grieco MH. Introduction to the abnormal host and complicating infections. In: Grieco MH, ed. *Infections in the abnormal host.* New York: Yorke Medical Books, 1980, with permission.

immune responses and aberrations of inflammatory cells functioning in effector mechanisms. Table 124.1 outlines some of the major defects of phagocytes, complement, antibody formation, and cell-mediated immunity and associated categories of congenital and/or hereditary, acquired, and drug-induced clinical disorders (1,2).

Phagocytic Disorders

After the natural barriers of the skin or the mucociliary apparatus have been penetrated, the phagocyte system, including neutrophils, monocytes, and macrophages, constitutes the next line of defense (3,4). Neutropenia, resulting from inadequate production or excessive destruction, is the most frequent abnormality that leads to complicating infections. Reduction of the number of circulating granulocytes to less than $400/mm^3$ is associated with increased rates of infection, but a critical decrease to less than $100/mm^3$ is associated with bacteremia. Abnormalities of chemotaxis, adherence, and phagocytosis and bactericidal disorders are common manifestations of several metabolic, inflammatory, and neoplastic diseases listed in Table 124.1 and may also contribute to secondary infections.

Phagocytic deficiency states result in infections that are often recurrent and respond poorly to antibiotic therapy. As can be seen in Table 124.1, a wide variety of disorders are associated with compromise of phagocyte function.

Complement Disorders

Complement activity results from the sequential interaction of more than 30 proteins in plasma and cell surfaces (5). Three pathways of complement activation are recognized: the classical, mannose-binding lectin, and the alternative. Antigen-antibody complexes or antibody-coated particles activate the classical pathway, and antibodies or cell surface carbohydrates or proteins binding C3b activate the alternative pathway. Bacterial cell surface mannose groups bind mannose-binding lectin complexes (a pattern-recognition component of the innate immune system) in a manner similar to C1s. All three pathways form C3 convertases, which cleave the C3 component of complement, a key protein used in common. The three pathways then proceed in identical fashion to bind late-acting components to form a membrane attack complex (MAC) (C5b-9) that results in target cell lysis.

Inherited disorders of complement may result in a propensity for infection. Typically, only deficiencies of C3 and of late-acting components and some nonregulatory components of the alternative pathway are associated with infectious sequelae. Recurrent pyogenic infections are associated with inherited deficiency of C3, properdin, factor D, and factor I, whereas recurrent disseminated meningococcal infections are reported with deficiencies of alternative pathway properdin and late complement components C5, C6, C7, and C8. Patients with late complement component deficiencies have intact complement-enhanced phagocytosis. This may account for the low case-fatality rate of 2.9% with the latter, which contrasts with the 64% rate associated with infection in properdin-deficient persons (6). Laboratory tests of total hemolytic complement activity, if results are normal, do not exclude alternative pathway deficiency, evaluation for which requires a specific assay.

Patients with leukocyte adhesion deficiency type 1 have a hereditary disorder involving the β_2 leukocyte integrins including leukocyte function–associated antigen 1, CR3/MAC-1, and p150,95, which function as adhesion molecules on neutrophils. This is a rare disorder in which β-chain synthesis is abnormal and interferes with expression of these three heterodimers on neutrophil and monocyte membrane surfaces. Both CR3 and p150,95 contain CR3 moieties, so that binding to iC3b is defective and may contribute to clinical infections. Patients with this disorder have markedly depressed inflammatory responses, recurrent bacterial and fungal infections, retarded healing, and severe gingivitis and periodontal disease (3). Complement disorders associated with infection are principally hereditary and thus relatively infrequent.

Antibody Disorders

Antibody deficiency reduces the host's resistance to infection through lack of a secretory antibody, which favors mucosal attachment by pathogens and by reduced circulatory antibodies that provide protective neutralizing, microbicidal, phagocytic, and cytotoxic actions. Respiratory and gastrointestinal (GI) tract infections predominate. Agammaglobulinemia and hypogammaglobulinemia result primarily from congenital hereditary disorders and from some hematologic malignancies, such as chronic lymphatic leukemia. Drug-induced hypogammaglobulinemia is rarely of clinical importance.

Cell-mediated Immunity Disorders

Monocytes, lymphocytes, and natural killer cells play critical roles in the control of intracellular pathogens (7). This category of protective mechanisms accounts for many infectious sequelae associated with modern immunosuppressive medical therapy and includes bacterial, fungal viral, and protozoan infections. Both primary pathogenic and opportunistic pathogens are incriminated. The organisms that cause disseminated infection in these circumstances are able to proliferate within cells, including monocytes, and are protected from cytolytic destruction by cytotoxic T cells and natural killer cells, as well as from lymphokines that would normally activate monocytes to control intracellular infections that are less susceptible to the effects of serum factors such as antibody and complement.

INFECTIOUS SYNDROMES AND INFECTIOUS AGENTS

Categorization of the underlying disorder or disorders is important in assessment because of the associations with various infectious syndromes and agents. In other chapters, inherited immunodeficiency states, acquired malignancy, and organ and bone marrow transplantation, as well as the infectious complications of therapy with corticosteroid and immunosuppressive agents, are discussed. Here I attempt to summarize the types of infections seen in association with various immunodeficiencies (Table 124.2).

Phagocytic Disorders

Functional or quantitative defects of neutrophils result in complicating infections with pyogenic bacteria, including *Streptococcus pneumoniae*, *Staphylococcus aureus*, *Staphylococcus epidermidis*, *Klebsiella pneumoniae*, *Enterobacter cloacae*, *Pseudomonas aeruginosa*, and *Acinetobacter baumannii*. There is some variation among the primary phagocytic disorders, depending on the particular stage of impairment of granulocyte function; however, a wide variety of infections may result. A case in point is chronic granulomatous disease (CGD), a group of rare disorders (incidence of 1 in 1 million persons) of phagocytic cell superoxide production that lead to recurrent infections with catalase-positive organisms and chronic inflammation. CGD is transmitted by X-linked inheritance in 70% and by autosomal recessive inheritance in 30%. Neutrophils from most patients with X-linked CGD have a mutation of a 91-kd glycoprotein component of membrane-associated cytochrome b_{558} that is required for production of superoxide. Some variants lack cytosolic components of the NADPH (reduced form of nicotinamide adenine dinucleotide phosphate) oxidase system. It is now clear that CGD is a disorder resulting from defects in any one of four subunits of NADPH oxidase, an enzyme involved in the generation of hydrogen peroxide. Most of the identified infectious agents are catalase-positive, oxidase-negative microorganisms capable of destroying hydrogen peroxide, most commonly *S. aureus* (16%). Less frequent infectious agents occur with *Aspergillus* species, *Chromobacterium violaceum*, *Burkholderia cepacia*, *Nocardia* species, and *Serratia marcescens*. Infections resulting from catalase-negative microorganisms are unusual (3).

Patients with neoplastic diseases often develop neutropenia complicated by bacterial and fungal infections. Neutropenic patients usually become infected with their endogenous flora, most often bacteria from the GI tract. The most common sites identified are the lungs, urinary tract, wounds, and perineum and perirectal areas. Bacteremia is present in approximately 16% to 20% of patients with neutrophil counts less than $100/mm^3$ (3,8). Gram-positive aerobic bacteria now predominate in the United States and western Europe and include coagulase-negative staphylococci, viridans streptococci, *S. aureus*, and enterococci. Aerobic gram-negative bacilli, especially *Escherichia coli*, *K. pneumoniae*, and *P. aeruginosa*, and fungi are important pathogens as well. The increasing incidence of aerobic gram-positive coccal infections has influenced substantially the recommendations for empiric therapy of fever and presumed infections in immunocompromised patients, especially with regard to the use of glycopeptides such as vancomycin (8–10).

Complement Disorders

Primary deficiencies of late complement components have been linked to infectious sequelae, but this has been rare with acquired defects. C3 is positioned at a critical point for the classical, mannose-binding lectin complex and alternative complement pathways. A deficiency of C3 is associated with serious recurrent infection with *S. pneumoniae* and *Neisseria meningitidis*.

Deficiencies of the later acting components, C5, C6, C7, and C8, as well as of properdin, are linked to life-threatening infections with *N. meningitidis* and *Neisseria gonorrhoeae* (11). The neisserial infections are usually in the meninges, associated with bacteremia. Pneumonia, otitis media, pyelonephritis, and endocarditis have been reported infrequently. Homozygotic late component deficiencies are complicated by neisserial infections at some time in more than 40% of subjects (mean of 17 years of age at the time of neisserial infection). Mortality resulting

TABLE 124.2. Common Infectious Complications of Inflammatory and Immunodeficiency Disorders

Microbe	Phagocytes (neutrophils, monocytes)	Complement components	Antibody-mediated immunity	Cell-mediated immunity
Bacteria				
Enterobacteriaceae	+++	+	+	
Gram-positive cocci	+++	++	+++	
Haemophilus influenzae	+	+	+++	
Pseudomonas aeruginosa	+++	+	+	+
Bartonella henselae				++
Bartonella quintana				++
Campylobacter jejuni				+
Legionella species				+
Listeria monocytogenes				++
Mycobacterium avium complex				++
Mycobacterium tuberculosis				+
Nocardia asteroides				++
Rhodococcus bronchialis				++
Salmonella species				+
Fungi				
Aspergillus species	+++			
Candida species				
Systemic	++			+
Chronic mucocutaneous				+
Fusarium species	++			
Mucor, Absidia, Rhizopus	+++			+
Coccidioides immitis				++
Cryptococcus neoformans				+
Histoplasma capsulatum				++
Penicillium marneffei				
Viruses				
Adenoviruses			+	+
Cytomegalovirus				++
Enteroviruses			++	+
Hepatitis B virus			++	++
Hepatitis C virus				+
Herpes simplex virus type 1			+	+
Herpes simplex virus type 2			+	+
Influenza virus				+
Papovaviruses				+
Respiratory syncytial virus			+	+
Rotavirus				
Rubella virus				+
Vaccinia virus				+
Varicella-zoster virus				
Parasites				
Cryptosporidium parvum			+	+
Cyclospora cayetanensis				+
Giardia lamblia			++	+
Isospora belli			+	+
Microsporida (Enterocytozoon species, Encephalitozoon species, Septata species)			+	
Pneumocystis carinii[a]			++	++
Toxoplasma gondii				++
Strongyloides stercoralis				+

[a] Now reclassified with fungi.
Source: Adapted from Grieco MH. Introduction to the abnormal host and complicating infections. In: Grieco MH, ed. *Infections in the abnormal host.* New York: Yorke Medical Books, 1980, with permission.

from meningococcal infection is higher in properdin deficiency than in disorders of the late complement components (11). Recurrent pyogenic infections with encapsulated bacteria complicate other alternative complement pathway deficiencies, such as diminished C3 in partial lipodystrophy and chronic membranoproliferative nephritis and low titer of factor B in newborns. Mannose-binding lectin deficiency has been described in young children with recurrent pyogenic infections and failure to thrive (12).

Antibody Disorders

Table 124.2 lists bacterial, viral, and parasitic agents associated with antibody deficiencies that produce respiratory tract, diarrheal, and central nervous system (CNS) syndromes.

RESPIRATORY SYNDROMES

In patients with X-linked agammaglobulinemia, infections with encapsulated pneumococci and *Haemophilus influenzae,* and to a

TABLE 124.3. Infectious Syndromes and Organisms Associated with Defective Cell-Mediated Immunity

Syndrome	Common pathogens	Less common pathogens
Mucocutaneous infections	Herpes simplex virus *Candida albicans*	Varicella-zoster virus
Esophagitis	*C. albicans*	Cytomegalovirus
Enteritis	*Cryptosporidium parvum*	Herpes simplex virus *Campylobacter* species *Giardia lamblia* *Isospora belli* Microsporida *Salmonella* species *Shigella* species *Strongyloides stercoralis*
Pneumonia	Cytomegalovirus *Pneumocystis carinii*	*Coccidioides immitis* *Crytococcus neoformans* *Histoplasma capsulatum* *Legionella* species *Mycobacterium avium* complex *Mycobacterium* tuberculosis *Rhodococcus bronchialis* *S. stercoralis*
Meningitis Encephalpathy	*Cryptococcus neoformans* *Toxoplasma gondii*	*Listeria monocytogenes* *Aspergillus* species Cytomegalovirus HIV-1, HIV-2 *Mucor, Absidia, Rhizopus* *Nocardia asteroides* Papovavirus
Retinitis	Cytomegalovirus	Herpes simplex virus Herpes zoster virus *T. gondii* *Treponema pallidum*
Septicemia	*Mycobacterium avium* complex *Salmonella* species	*L. monocytogenes*

lesser extent streptococci and staphylococci, result in pneumonia, recurrent otitis media, purulent sinusitis, meningitis, and furunculosis. Subjects with common variable immunodeficiency have been noted to have pneumonia (87%), sinusitis (60%), and bronchiectasis (53%).

DIARRHEAL SYNDROMES

Chronic diarrhea, the second most important sequela of antibody deficiency, may result from rotavirus and enterovirus infections, from parasites such as *Cryptosporidium parvum, Isospora belli, Giardia lamblia, Cyclospora cayetanensis,* and Microsporida (13,14), as well as from gram-negative bacteria such as *Salmonella* and *Campylobacter.*

CENTRAL NERVOUS SYSTEM SYNDROMES

Viral infections of the CNS are severe infectious sequelae of hypogammaglobulinemia. Patients with X-linked agammaglobulinemia are susceptible to chronic echovirus infection of the CNS and less frequently to infections with other viruses, including herpes simplex virus, coxsackievirus, and adenovirus (15). In addition, these patients are more likely to develop paralytic poliomyelitis after live poliovirus vaccination. CNS syndromes rarely complicate common variable immunodeficiency.

OTHER SYNDROMES

Other infections described in association with severe hypogammaglobulinemia include progressive vaccinia, disseminated adenovirus infection, and *Pneumocystis carinii* pneumonia.

Cell-mediated Immunity Disorders

A wide variety of infectious agents, bacteria, fungi, viruses, and parasites cause disease in patients with defective cell-mediated immunity (see Table 124.2). Most of these agents are sequestered in intracellular sites, where they are protected from the effects of serum factors such as antibody and complement.

In adults, acquired immunodeficiency syndrome is complicated by infectious syndromes that are primarily the result of defective cell-mediated immunity, and this syndrome serves as a model that is readily applicable to other conditions of immune suppression such as neoplastic diseases, primary immunodeficiency disorders, and drug- and radiation-induced suppression, as for transplant recipients. Some infectious syndromes and implicated organisms are outlined in Table 124.3.

EMPIRIC THERAPY IN THE CASE OF PRESUMED INFECTION

Neutropenia

EMPIRIC MULTIPLE ANTIMICROBIAL AGENT THERAPY

In immunosuppressed patients with neutropenia, less than 60% of episodes of fever are ever associated with bacterial infection, but rapid institution of antibiotic programs improves these patients' prognosis. More than a decade ago, combination therapy with carbenicillin (5 g every 4 hours), gentamicin, and cephalothin or cephapirin (2 g every 4 hours) was used to cover likely gram-negative and gram-positive bacteria. Later, results of large prospective comparative trials suggested that three-drug combination therapy might not be necessary (16,17). The Infectious Diseases Society of America (IDSA) has published very useful guidelines in 1997 for the use of antimicrobial agents in neutropenic patients with unexplained fever (8). All febrile patients with neutrophil counts less than 500/mm^3 or with counts expected to fall to such levels should be treated with broad-spectrum bactericidal antibiotics. Oral vitamin K may be advisable because of antibiotic-associated hypothrombinemia and bleeding resulting from suppression of intestinal flora that usually produce menaquinones. Pizzo (18) has emphasized the value of distinguishing low-risk patients (i.e., those with solid tumors receiving less intensive chemotherapy with neutropenia for no more than 10 days) from high-risk patients (i.e., those with neutropenia for more than 10 days) who are much more vulnerable to acute bacterial infections and multiple infections.

Gram-positive infections account for 60% to 70% of microbiologically documented infections associated with neutropenia in the United States and western Europe. In the presence of fever of 38.3°C or higher and neutropenia less than 500/mm^3, the initial issue to be addressed is the necessity for vancomycin. The glycopeptide is indicated in the presence of severe mucositis, quinolone prophylaxis, known colonization with gram-positive β-lactam–resistant organisms, clear evidence of catheter-related infection, or hypotension. Vancomycin should be discontinued after 3 to 4 days if a gram-positive β-lactam–resistant bacterium is not identified. The combination of vancomycin and ceftazidime was recommended for initial empiric therapy based on extensive study, broad-spectrum coverage, and wide margin of safety (8,19). However, based on individual clinical circumstances, the combination of vancomycin with imipenem-cilastatin, cefepime, or meropenem would be reasonable alternative regimens.

In the absence of an indication for vancomycin, both monotherapy and dual-therapy regimens appear to be equally efficacious as empiric therapy (20,21). The guidelines indicate that monotherapy can be considered a standard of therapy (8). Treatment with either ceftazidime or imipenem-cilastatin has been recommended with the caveat that cefepime or meropenem may be as effective. It is important to note that quinolone monotherapy was not recommended for empiric initial therapy.

The recommended dual therapy is an aminoglycoside (gentamicin, tobramycin, or amikacin) with an antipseudomonal β-lactam including a carboxy penicillin (ticarcillin) or ureidopenicillin (azlocillin, mezlocillin or piperacillin) or cephalosporin such as ceftazidime (8). Imipenem-cilastatin, cefepime, and meropenem are appropriate alternatives for dual therapy. The side effects of aminoglycosides should be considered with regard to nephrotoxicity, ototoxicity, and hypokalemia, and suitable precautions should be taken to avoid additive toxic effects in combination with other drugs or renal or electrolyte disorders.

One of the most important developments in the treatment of serious gram-negative infections is the establishment of the relationship of elevated trough levels of aminoglycosides to nephrotoxicity. Aminoglycoside properties of dose-dependent killing and postantibiotic suppression of bacterial growth remain valuable. Several clinical trials using once-daily dosing of aminoglycosides, rather than more frequent conventional dosing, have shown that once-daily aminoglycoside therapy appears to be as effective as standard therapy and is associated with reduced toxicity (22,23). Once-daily dosing of amikacin and ceftriaxone appeared to be as effective as and no more toxic than multiple daily doses of amikacin and ceftazidime for the empiric therapy of infection in patients with cancer and granulocytopenia (23).

Holleran, Wilbur, and DeGregorio (24) have summarized empiric amphotericin B therapy trials. Blood cultures for fungi give positive results in only 12% to 34% of cases of acute leukemia with documented fungal infection, usually *Candida* or *Aspergillus*. Although criteria for initiating empiric therapy with amphotericin B have varied, it would appear reasonable to add this drug for patients who remain febrile with neutropenia (cell count less than 500/mm^3) and after receiving 7 days of multidrug bactericidal combination therapy. Amphotericin B should not be used in initial therapy, but it is advisable to consider this drug in high-risk patients not responding at 1 week. In such patients, infection with *Candida* or *Aspergillus* is a likely cause of infection in approximately one third (25). An azole such as fluconazole may be an alternative for patients intolerant to amphotericin B (8).

Complement Disorders

Primary deficiencies of complement components are relatively rare. Patients with known disorders of properdin, factor B, C3b, and the later acting components should be treated for presumed pyogenic infections, including *N. meningitidis* and *N. gonorrhoeae*, before culture identification is complete, especially for life-threatening infections such as meningitis. Ampicillin should be instituted immediately if there is a history of severe recurrent infection with encapsulated organisms.

The principal modality of management is education of the patient with regard to prevention and early treatment of infection. If the deficient person is younger than 2 years at the time of diagnosis, it is reasonable to administer antibiotics to prevent infections with *N. meningitidis*, *S. pneumoniae*, and *H. influenzae*, at least until an age when vaccines are likely to be effective. Similarly, early treatment of infectious complications is extremely important. Vaccines effective against *S. pneumoniae* and *H. influenzae* should be administered as is currently recommended for all children and meningococcal vaccine added for patients with a defect of one of the components of the complement terminal attack complex (26).

Antibody-mediated Immune Disorders

Conventional antibiotic therapy directed against probable encapsulated pneumococci and *H. influenzae* is usually indicated soon after the onset of clinical signs of respiratory tract infection. Replacement γ-globulin therapy, as well as prophylactic antibiotics, usually decreases the severity and frequency of these infections. Therapy of diarrheal syndromes usually depends on the initial identification of an agent.

Devastating CNS echovirus infections are usually not responsive to γ-globulin replacement, because the blood–brain barrier prevents accumulation of high concentrations of antibody in the cerebrospinal fluid. Control of CNS infection has been reported with intraventricular administration of immune serum globulin via a permanent Ommaya reservoir (27).

Cell-mediated Immune Disorders

In general, therapy is dependent on identification of a specific agent by culture, stain, or serologic or histopathologic examination (28,29). There are at least three situations in which empiric therapy is indicated before there is a definitive diagnosis. Therapy should be initiated presumptively whenever it is likely that a patient may have pneumonitis caused by *P. carinii*, encephalitis caused by *Toxoplasma gondii*, or retinitis caused by cytomegalovirus. Early treatment of these infections has been associated with improved clinical outcome in immunodeficient patients, including those who have acquired immunodeficiency syndrome (30–33).

REFERENCES

1. Grieco MH, ed. *Infections in the abnormal host.* New York: Yorke Medical Books, 1980.
2. Grieco MH. Introduction to the abnormal host and complicating infections. In: Grieco MH, ed. *Infections in the abnormal host.* New York: Yorke Medical Books, 1980:2–3.
3. Lekstrom-Himes JA, Gallin JI. Immunodeficiency diseases caused by defects in phagocytes. *N Engl J Med* 2000;343:1703.
4. Cohen MS. Molecular events in the activation of human neutrophils for microbial killing. *Clin Infect Dis* 1994;18[Suppl 2]:S170.
5. Walport MJ. Complement. *N Engl J Med* 2001;344:1058, 1140.
6. Densen P, Weiler JM, McLeod Griffiss J, et al. Familial properdin deficiency and fatal meningococcemia. Correction of the bactericidal defect by vaccination. *N Engl J Med* 1987;316:922.
7. Buckley RH. Primary immunodeficiency diseases due to defects in lymphocytes. *N Engl J Med* 2000;343:1313.
8. Hughes WT, Armstrong D, Bodey GP, et al. 1997 guidelines for the use of antimicrobial agents in neutropenic patients with unexplained fever. *Clin Infect Dis* 1997;25:551.
9. Feld R. Vancomycin as part of initial empirical antibiotic therapy for febrile neutropenia in patients with care: pros and cons. *Clin Infect Dis* 1999;29:503.
10. Rolston KVI. New trends in patient management: risk-based therapy for febrile patients with neutropenia. *Clin Infect Dis* 1999;29:515.
11. Ross SC, Densen P. Complement deficiency states and infection: epidemiology, pathogenesis, and consequences of neisserial and other infections in an immune deficiency. *Medicine (Baltimore)* 1984;63:243.
12. Soothill JF, Harvey BA. Defective opsonization: a common deficiency. *Arch Dis Child* 1976;51:91.
13. Weber R, Bryan RT, Schwartz DA, et al. Human microsporidial infections. *Clin Microbiol Rev* 1994;7:426.
14. Shadduck JA. Human microsporidiosis and AIDS. *Rev Infect Dis* 1989;11:203.
15. Stiehm ER, Chin TW, Haas A, et al. Infectious complications of the primary immunodeficiencies. *Clin Immunol Immunopathol* 1986;40:69.
16. European Organization for Research on Treatment of Cancer. Three antibiotic regimens in the treatment of infection in febrile granulocytopenic patients with cancer. *J Infect Dis* 1987;137:14.
17. Wade JC, Petty BF, Conrad G, et al. Cephalothin plus an aminoglycoside is more nephrotoxic than methicillin plus aminoglycoside. *Lancet* 1978;2:604.
18. Pizzo PA. Fever in immunocompromised patients. *N Engl J Med* 1999;341:893.
19. European Organization for Research and Treatment of Cancer (EORTC) International Antimicrobial Therapy Cooperative Group and the National Cancer Institute of Canada-Clinical Trials Group. Vancomycin added to empirical combination antibiotic therapy for fever in granulocytopenic cancer patients. *J Infect Dis* 1991;163:951.
20. Pizzo PA, Hathorn JW, Hiemenz J. A randomized trial comparing ceftazidime alone with combination antibiotic therapy in cancer patients with fever and neutropenia. *N Engl J Med* 1986;315:552.
21. Sanders JW, Powe NR, Moore RD. Ceftazidime monotherapy for empiric treatment of febrile neutropenic patients: a meta-analysis. *J Infect Dis* 1991;164:907.
22. Prins JM, Bueller HR, Kuijper EJ, et al. Once versus thrice daily gentamicin in patients with serious infections. *Lancet* 1993;341:335.
23. International Antimicrobial Therapy Cooperative Group of the European Organization for Research and Treatment of Cancer. Efficacy and toxicity of single daily doses of amikacin and ceftriaxone versus multiple daily doses of amikacin and ceftazidime for infection in patients with cancer and granulocytopenia. *Ann Intern Med* 1993;119:584.
24. Holleran WM, Wilbur JR, DeGregorio WM. Empiric amphotericin B therapy in patients with acute leukemia. *Rev Infect Dis* 1989;7:619.
25. Pizzo PA, Robichaud RJ, Gill FA. Duration of empiric antibiotic and antifungal therapy for cancer patients with prolonged fever and granulocytopenia. *Am J Med* 1982;72:101.
26. Frank MM. Complement deficiencies. *Pediatr Clin North Am* 2000;47:1339.
27. Erlendsson K, Swartz T, Dwyer JM. Successful reversal of echovirus encephalitis in X-linked hypogammaglobulinemia by intraventricular administration of immunoglobulin. *N Engl J Med* 1985;312:351.
28. Glatt AE, Chirgwin K, Landesman SH. Treatment of infections associated with human immunodeficiency virus. *N Engl J Med* 1988;318:1439.
29. Young LS. Treatable aspects of infections due to human immunodeficiency virus. *Lancet* 1987;2:1503.
30. Sattler FR, Cowan R, Nielsen DM, et al. Trimethoprim-sulfamethoxazole compared with pentamidine for treatment of *Pneumocystis carinii* pneumonia in AIDS. *Ann Intern Med* 1988;109:280.
31. Luft BJ, Brooks RG, Conley FK, et al. Toxoplasmic encephalitis in patients with AIDS. *JAMA* 1984;252:913.
32. Drew WL. Cytomegalovirus infection in patients with AIDS. *J Infect Dis* 1988;158:449.
33. Reed EC, Bowden RA, Dandliker PS, et al. Treatment of CMV pneumonia with ganciclovir and intravenous CMV immunoglobulin in patients with bone marrow transplants. *Ann Intern Med* 1988;109:783.

CHAPTER 125

Infections Associated with Malignancy

Gerald P. Bodey

Once effective therapy became available for malignant diseases, it became apparent that appropriate management of infectious complications was of critical importance in the care of these patients. Although substantial progress has been made in the treatment of these infections during the past three decades, they continue to be a major cause of morbidity and mortality. The introduction of broader spectrum and more potent antimicrobial agents has reduced the mortality rates from many bacterial infections, but this has been offset by the use of more aggressive and toxic antitumor regimens that have resulted in an increase in fungal and viral infections, which often are more difficult to diagnose and treat. Also, the extensive use of antibacterial and antifungal agents for prophylaxis and therapy has led to the emergence of organisms that are resistant to many commonly prescribed antimicrobial regimens.

FACTORS ASSOCIATED WITH INFECTION IN CANCER PATIENTS

Common factors predisposing to infection in cancer patients are listed in Table 125.1. Some, such as obstruction, gastrointestinal (GI) tract ulcerations, or tumor necrosis, are the direct consequence of local tumor masses. Impairment of normal host defenses such as monocytopenia, neutropenia, impaired cellular immunity, and hypogammaglobulinemia has systemic consequences. Chemotherapeutic agents have profound effects on the patient, causing oral mucositis, GI tract ulceration, neutropenia, impaired macrophage function, and depletion of $CD4^+$ helper T lymphocytes, making patients susceptible to a variety of infectious complications (1). The use of implantable devices, such as cerebrospinal fluid (CSF) shunts, orthopedic devices, and especially intravascular catheters, has had a major impact on the frequency of some infections.

Neutropenia

Neutropenia is the most significant predisposing factor for infection in cancer patients. Most episodes of neutropenia are due to the myelosuppressive effects of antitumor agents on normal bone marrow; thus, with conventional therapeutic regimens, neutropenia is usually neither severe nor of long duration. Severe and prolonged neutropenia occurs most often during remission induction chemotherapy of acute leukemia, bone marrow transplantation, and intensive chemotherapy for potentially curable lymphomas and solid tumors. The frequency and severity of infection was first demonstrated to be related to the degree and duration of neutropenia in patients with acute leukemia (2). The frequency of infection begins to increase when the neutrophil count falls to less than 1,000 cells/mm³ and increases substantially at levels less than 500 cells/mm³. In that study, all patients with a neutrophil count of less than 100 cells/mm³ for a period of 3 weeks became infected. Subsequently, similar correlations have been found in patients receiving chemotherapy for breast carcinoma, but the frequency of infection at each level of neutropenia

TABLE 125.1. Factors Predisposing to Infection in Cancer Patients

Factor	Cause	Associate infections
Neutropenia	Acute leukemia, myelodysplatic syndromes, chemotherapy	Gram-positive organisms, gram-negative bacilli, *Aspergillus, Candida*
Monocytopenia	Hairy cell leukemia	Mycobacteria, *Toxoplasma, Pneumocystis*
Impaired cellular immunity	Hodgkin's disease, lymphoma, chemotherapy	*Listeria,* mycobacteria, *Cryptococcus, Toxoplasma, Brucella*
Impaired macrophage function	Adrenal corticosteroids	Molds (especially *Aspergillus*), *Pneumocystis*
Deficient CD4+ helper T lymphocytes	Chemotherapy (fludarabine)	*Pneumocystis, Listeria,* varicella-zoster, cytomegalovirus
Hypogammaglobulinemia	Multiple myeloma, chronic lymphocytic leukemia	Gram-positive cocci
Mucositis	Chemotherapy	Herpes simplex, oral bacterial flora, *Candida*
Gastrointestinal ulceration	Chemotherapy, tumor involvement	Gram-negative bacilli, anaerobes
Bronchial obstruction	Bronchogenic carcinoma	Gram-positive cocci, gram-negative bacilli, anaerobes
Splenectomy	Hematological malignancies	*Pneumococcus, meningococcus, Haemophilus, Babesia, Capnocytophaga*
Vascular catheters	—	Gram-positive and gram-negative bacilli

is lower than in patients with acute leukemia. The frequency of bacteremia associated with local infections, such as pneumonia also is related to the degree of neutropenia. Furthermore, the frequency of response to effective therapy is related to recovery from neutropenia (3).

CLINICAL FEATURES AND MICROBIOLOGY

Because antibiotics are administered promptly when fever occurs, the presence of infection as the cause of fever often cannot be documented. Hence, infection is clinically documented in only about 50% of febrile episodes and the infecting organism is determined in only 50% of clinically documented infections. About 60% of infections are caused by gram-positive cocci and 35% by gram-negative bacilli. Anaerobic infections are uncommon in neutropenic patients.

Problem Infections. Respiratory tract infections are common and often difficult to treat. Sinus infections may be caused by bacteria but often are due to *Aspergillus* species or other molds. Because these fungi cause thrombosis of blood vessels and infarction of tissues, they can cause extensive local destruction or erode through the skull and infect the brain. Pneumonia is a common cause of infectious death in neutropenic patients. These patients are unable to produce adequate sputum specimens and bronchoscopy with bronchoalveolar lavage often fails to provide a diagnosis. Percutaneous needle or open lung biopsies are usually contraindicated, and the diagnostic yield is too low to justify the risk of bleeding in many of these patients who usually have thrombocytopenia. Empiric antibacterial regimens are often ineffective because an undetected fungus or virus is the cause of infection.

Necrotizing enterocolitis and perianal infections are unique problems in severely neutropenic patients (4). Necrotizing enterocolitis may be confined to the cecum (typhlitis) or involve extensive areas of the intestines, causing fever, abdominal pain, and diarrhea. Associated bacteremia due to aerobic gram-negative bacilli or *Clostridium septicum* is common. Patients may respond to broad-spectrum antibiotics and supportive measures, although surgery is sometimes necessary if the disease is localized. Perianal infections are especially common in patients with acute monocytic leukemia but are a potentially life-threatening complication in any patient with prolonged severe neutropenia (5). They are associated with hemorrhoids and anal fissures, cause considerable discomfort, and may result in bacteremia. Antibacterial agents and supportive therapy are usually effective, but surgery has been beneficial in some patients, despite the absence of abscess formation.

Problem Pathogens. Though recently less common, *Pseudomonas aeruginosa* remains a threat to patients with acute leukemia because of the potential fulminant nature of the infection (6). The prompt administration of potent antipseudomonal agents has resulted in response rates exceeding 70%. About 15% of bacteremias caused by α-hemolytic streptococci, most often by *Streptococcus mitis* and *Streptococcus sanguis*, are fulminant infections associated with renal failure, septic shock, adult respiratory distress syndrome, or rapid death (7). Predisposing factors include mucositis, high-dose cytarabine therapy, and fluoroquinolone prophylaxis. Because some organisms are tolerant or resistant to penicillin G, vancomycin is the preferable therapy. *Clostridium perfringens* and *Clostridium septicum* occasionally cause fulminant and rapidly fatal infections, predominantly in patients with acute leukemia, but also in patients with tumors of the GI or genitourinary tract, which are the source of most of these infections.

Patients with prolonged neutropenia are susceptible to infections caused by *Candida* species, *Aspergillus* species, and less frequently *Trichosporon beigelii, Blastoschizomyces capitatus,* and *Fusarium* species. Thrush and esophagitis are the most frequent candidal infections, but acute disseminated candidiasis occurs in

10% to 30% of patients with prolonged neutropenia (8). Because the organism may not be recovered from multiple blood culture specimens in at least 30% of patients with disseminated candidiasis, antifungal therapy often must be administered without a definitive diagnosis. Response to antifungal therapy is unusual in patients with persistent neutropenia. Chronic disseminated candidiasis is a unique infection that is usually diagnosed when a patient has persistent fever after recovery from a prolonged period of neutropenia (9). The patient has anorexia, weight loss, and debilitation sometimes associated with hepatosplenomegaly or right upper quadrant abdominal pain. Typically, the serum alkaline phosphatase level becomes highly elevated and multiple small lesions are detected in the liver and spleen on ultrasonography or computed tomography (CT). Fluconazole and lipid formulations of amphotericin B appear to be the most effective therapies, but signs of response may require several weeks of treatment.

Aspergillus infections predominantly originate in the sinuses and lungs, but occasionally in the skin (at catheter sites) and the GI tract (10). Because the organisms invade blood vessels causing thrombosis and infarction, about 30% of patients with pulmonary infection present with signs and symptoms of an acute pulmonary embolism. About 30% of infections disseminate and the brain is usually involved. The organism is seldom cultured from infected patients (except in skin and sinus infections), but many patients with pulmonary infection have characteristic abnormalities on CT scan of the lung. Lipid formulations of amphotericin B are probably the preferred therapy, but neutropenic patients rarely respond in the absence of neutrophil recovery. Surgical excision of residual lesions is often appropriate in patients who have responded to therapy.

EMPIRIC THERAPY OF FEVER IN NEUTROPENIC PATIENTS

Because neutropenic patients are unable to mount an adequate inflammatory response, the only sign of infection may be fever. For example, fewer than 10% of severely neutropenic (less than 100 cells/mm^3) patients produce purulent sputum when they develop pneumonia and more than 30% of patients with neutropenia (less than 1,000 cells/mm^3) have a normal chest roentgenogram at the onset of gram-negative pneumonia (11). Untreated infection in neutropenic patients can progress rapidly if not treated promptly. This is especially true for infections caused by most gram-negative bacilli, whereas infections caused by some gram-positive organisms are more indolent and respond even if optimum therapy is delayed for a few days. It is the accepted practice to administer antibiotics promptly at the onset of fever after collection of appropriate culture specimens.

Single-agent therapy with potent broad-spectrum β-lactam antibiotics (e.g., cefepime, imipenem-cilastatin, or meropenem) is as effective as antimicrobial combinations (12). These agents or piperacillin-tazobactam, ticarcillin-clavulanate, or ceftazidime may be combined with an aminoglycoside or fluoroquinolone. Fluoroquinolones may be preferable to aminoglycosides in combination regimens because of their greater efficacy as single agents in neutropenic patients. Aminoglycosides should not be relied on as single agents for the treatment of infections in neutropenic patients (3). The selection of an empiric regimen must be based on the predominant pathogens and antibiotic-susceptibility patterns at the local hospital, as well as the patient's organ function and potential toxicities of other drugs being administered.

Many gram-positive organisms, including *Corynebacterium jeikeium*, *Bacillus* species, and many coagulase-negative staphylococci, are susceptible only to vancomycin or teicoplanin. Whereas infections caused by these organisms are usually indolent, others caused by α-hemolytic streptococci or methicillin-

resistant *Staphylococcus aureus* can be fulminant, and delays in administration of appropriate therapy can cause unnecessary fatalities. The decision to use vancomycin in the initial regimen depends on the frequency of these infections at each hospital. However, vancomycin usually should be included for patients with catheter site infections or severe mucositis or for those who have received ciprofloxacin prophylaxis, but it should be discontinued within 3 days if there is no evidence to support its use (12). Colonization and infection with vancomycin-resistant enterococci have become a serious problem in some hospitals, especially where vancomycin has been used extensively.

Patients whose fever persists for more than 3 days require careful reexamination and reassessment. The most common causes of persistent fever are listed in Table 125.2. The oropharynx, gums, axilla, groin, and perianal areas, as well as catheter sites, should receive special attention. CT scans of the sinuses, chest, and abdomen should be considered, depending on the patient's symptoms and physical findings and repeated culture specimens should be collected as well as appropriate serologic studies. If no specific cause can be determined, it is appropriate to administer antifungal therapy empirically because of the high frequency of undetected fungal infections in these patients.

Impairment in Cell-mediated Immunity

Diseases that are associated with deficiencies in cellular immunity include lymphomas, Hodgkin's disease, chronic lymphocytic leukemia (CLL), and hairy cell leukemia. Important components of cellular immunity include the CD4$^+$ helper T lymphocyte, monocyte, and macrophage. Two types of helper T lymphocytes are recognized; type 1, which are associated with intense phagocytic activity, and type 2, which suppress phagocytosis (13). The activities of these cells are complex and beyond the scope of this discussion. Patients with malignancies are prone to type 2 responses at the expense of type 1 responses. Patients with hairy cell leukemia have monocytopenia in addition to neutropenia.

Antitumor agents interfere with cellular immunity, with different agents having different effects (1). Some of these effects occur at doses that do not cause myelosuppression. Alkylating agents such as cyclophosphamide interfere with various stages of cellular immune response, including antigen processing, blastogenesis, and antibody production. Purine analogs, such as fludarabine, have important specific effects on host defenses. Fludarabine causes profound and prolonged deficiencies of CD4$^+$ helper T lymphocytes, causing recipients to be susceptible to a variety of pathogens, including *Listeria monocytogenes*, *Pneumocystis carinii*, varicella-zoster, and cytomegalovirus (CMV). Adrenal corticosteroids have multiple effects on host defenses, including interference with macrophage function. Because macrophages are a primary defense against *Aspergillus* spores, patients receiving these drugs are at risk of developing aspergillosis.

TABLE 125.2. Causes of Persistent Fever in Neutropenic Patients

1. Slowly resolving infection due to persistent severe neutropenia, foreign body, necrotic tissue, etc.
2. Bacterial pathogen resistant to therapeutic regimen
3. Superinfection with a resistant bacterial organism
4. Fungal or viral infection
5. Drug allergies
6. Tumor fever

CLINICAL FEATURES AND MICROBIOLOGY

Patients with impaired cellular immunity are susceptible to infections caused by a wide variety of pathogens, many of which are intracellular pathogens (Table 125.3). Because of this diversity, the primary focus is on establishing the diagnosis so appropriate therapy will be selected, as opposed to the use of empiric therapy in neutropenic patients. Nevertheless, it is critical to establish the diagnosis expeditiously because untreated infection can progress rapidly, if not treated promptly. In addition to collecting culture specimens, other diagnostic modalities, such as serologic tests, special stains of clinical specimens, and tissue biopsies, are an important component of the evaluation. For example, lung biopsy is more likely to yield a diagnosis than in neutropenic patients.

Problem Pathogens. Patients with impaired cellular immunity are especially susceptible to serious infections by several bacterial pathogens, although they do not occur often. Gastroenteritis accounts for about 50% of *Salmonella* infections, but the remainder are more serious and include septicemia, pneumonia, osteomyelitis, meningitis, and urinary tract infection. Few patients have recurrent episodes despite appropriate therapy. *L. monocytogenes* infection causes septicemia and meningitis in these patients. Some patients with meningitis may not have meningismus and occasionally the CSF is not abnormal. *L. monocytogenes* may be difficult to culture from the CSF or misidentified as diphtheroids. *Nocardia* infection has been associated with lymphoma and Hodgkin's disease but also occurs in patients with solid tumors undergoing chemotherapy. Most *Nocardia* infections involve the brain or lung and sometimes may be mistaken for metastatic tumors.

Patients with Hodgkin's disease and lymphoma, as well as pulmonary and head and neck malignancies, are susceptible to tuberculosis (14). Patients with Hodgkin's disease and lymphoma are more likely to develop acute pneumonia or disseminated tuberculosis that is associated with a high mortality rate. The diagnosis may be difficult to establish because the symptoms may be attributed to the malignancy and the patient is often anergic. Reactivation of latent infection may occur in patients undergoing cancer chemotherapy. Elderly patients with evidence of prior tuberculosis should receive isoniazid prophylaxis. Atypical mycobacterial infections also occur in these patients and in some series have been as common as tuberculosis. Patients with hairy cell leukemia are particularly prone to developing disseminated infection caused by *Mycobacterium avium-intracellulare* complex.

Cryptococcosis is the most common fungal infection in cancer patients with impaired cellular immunity. Because the fungus is a respiratory tract pathogen, infection begins in the lung, where it may remain asymptomatic (15). Some patients may develop an acute, rapidly progressive pulmonary infection that may terminate fatally despite therapy. Disseminated infection is common in these patients and may involve the skin, bone, CNS, lymph nodes, kidneys, prostate, and liver. Patients with disseminated infection most often present with signs and symptoms of acute, subacute, or chronic meningitis. Patients exposed to the pathogenic fungi, *Histoplasma capsulatum* or *Coccidioides immitis* are at risk of developing fulminant pneumonia or disseminated infection. Patients who have residual lesions from infection contracted when their host defenses were normal may experience reactivation and dissemination of the infection. Patients with deficient numbers of CD4+ helper T lymphocytes are susceptible to superficial candidal infections of the oropharynx and esophagitis.

A variety of viral infections are prevalent in patients with impaired cellular immunity. Infections caused by herpes simplex virus (HSV) are the most common viral infections in patients with lymphoma but also occur in patients with acute leukemia and bone marrow transplant recipients. Lesions occur on the lips and oral mucosa and sometimes the genitalia. They may progress to large painful ulcerations and can become superinfected, especially with *S. aureus*. Some patients develop HSV esophagitis that may be confused with candidal infection. This infection may spread to involve the larynx and trachea. Few patients develop pneumonia or disseminated infection that may involve the CNS, liver, spleen, kidneys, pancreas, and GI tract.

Varicella is a potentially serious infection in children undergoing cancer chemotherapy, and because the virus is highly contagious, epidemics have occurred on pediatric cancer units. About 30% of these children develop serious complications during varicella infection and the fatality rate approaches 10%. The characteristic vesicular rash becomes hemorrhagic and necrotic in thrombocytopenic patients, and bacterial superinfection occurs in about 10% of infected children. Infection may disseminate to internal organs causing pneumonia, fulminant encephalitis, or focal necrosis of the liver, pancreas, or adrenal glands. Herpeszoster occurs most often in patients with lymphoproliferative disorders (16). The infection is characterized by a unilateral vesicular rash involving one or two adjacent sensory dermatomes, most often in the cervical, thoracic, or lumbar area. Few patients develop generalized infection. In cancer patients, infection often arises at sites where tumor is in proximity to a nerve trunk or at sites of previous irradiation. Varicella infection may progress to necrotic lesions that heal slowly and lead to scarring in these immunocompromised patients. Rarely, visceral dissemination may occur, causing hepatitis, pneumonitis, pancreatitis, or meningoencephalitis. Also, postherpetic neuralgia and motor paralysis are more prevalent in immunocompromised patients.

CMV infection is a special problem among bone marrow transplant recipients. It appears to be increasing in frequency

TABLE 125.3. Organisms Causing Infection in Patients with Impaired Cellular Immunity

Bacteria	Fungi	Viruses	Parasites
Brucella species	*Cryptococcus neoformans*	Cytomegalovirus	*Toxoplasma gondii*
Mycobacterium species	*Histoplasma capsulatum*	Herpes simplex	*Strongyloides stercoralis*
Listeria monocytogenes	*Coccidioides immitis*	Varicella-zoster	
Legionella species	*Aspergillus* species	Creutzfeldt-Jakob disease[a]	
Nocardia species	*Candida* species		
Salmonella species	*Pneumocystis carinii*		

[a]Considered to be caused by a prion rather than a virus.

among patients with acute leukemia and occurs in patients with CLL who are treated with purine analogs (17). Some patients develop a relatively benign viremia that is associated with fever and sometimes elevations in liver function test results. Other patients develop a mononucleosis syndrome or have delayed bone marrow recovery. The most serious infections are pneumonia and colitis. Rarely, patients develop hepatitis, myocarditis, retinitis, or encephalitis. The risk of CMV infection in bone marrow transplant recipients has been reduced by the screening of recipients, donors, and blood products and preemptive use of ganciclovir based on the detection of CMV antigenemia in the blood or detection of CMV in bronchoalveolar lavage fluid.

Community respiratory tract viruses can cause serious pulmonary infections in immunocompromised hosts (18). Most of these infections have been recognized in bone marrow transplant recipients and patients undergoing therapy for acute leukemia. Although these patients are neutropenic, it is most probable that deficiencies of other host defenses are responsible for these infections. Respiratory syncytial virus (RSV) infection has caused epidemics on bone marrow transplant and leukemia units. In some patients, the infection remains limited to the upper respiratory tract, but if the infection progresses to the tracheobronchial tree and the lung, most patients will die if not treated promptly with aerosolized ribavirin. Strict infection-control measures during the RSV season are important in preventing epidemics. Influenza and parainfluenza also can cause fatal pneumonia in these patients.

Most *P. carinii* infection occurs in patients with impaired cellular immunity and is especially prevalent among children receiving maintenance therapy for acute leukemia. It is also being diagnosed more often among some patients with solid tumors. Most episodes probably represent reactivation of latent infection, but some are new infections, as evidenced by occasional patient-to-patient transmission. *P. carinii* may be insidious in onset or progress rapidly. The most common presenting symptoms are fever, nonproductive cough, and dyspnea on exertion. As the disease progresses, patients develop tachypnea, cyanosis, and tachycardia. Auscultatory findings are minimal even when the chest roentgenogram reveals extensive pulmonary involvement. Microscopic examination of specially stained sputum or bronchoalveolar lavage fluid usually will establish the diagnosis.

Toxoplasmosis is an uncommon infection in cancer patients and 50% of cases occur in patients with Hodgkin's disease. Infection may be newly acquired or represent reactivation of a latent infection. Infection may be acquired from ingestion of undercooked meat products or from blood transfusions. CNS infection accounts for 60% of infections in patients with Hodgkin's disease and may present as encephalopathy, diffuse meningoencephalitis, or with focal neurologic defects. *Toxoplasma gondii* also causes lymphadenitis, myositis, myocarditis, hepatitis, or pneumonitis. The diagnosis is established by serologic tests for the detection of antibodies or from examination of tissue biopsies.

Hypogammaglobulinemia

Deficiencies in the production of normal immunoglobulins are characteristic of multiple myeloma and Waldenström's macroglobulinemia but also occur in CLL and some lymphomas. Most patients with CLL will develop severe, permanent hypogammaglobulinemia as their disease progresses. Patients may have a predominant immunoglobulin A deficiency that is associated with an increased frequency of upper respiratory tract infections, including chronic sinusitis. Pathogens that have classically been associated with impaired humoral immunity are the encapsulated bacteria, *Streptococcus pneumoniae, Haemophilus*

influenzae and *Neisseria meningitidis*. These organisms can cause fulminant septicemia, resulting in a fatal outcome despite appropriate therapy. Because more intensive chemotherapy is being used for these diseases, the toxicities of these drugs, such as neutropenia and CD4$^+$ helper T lymphocytopenia, have a greater impact on the types of infection occurring in these patients.

Other Predisposing Factors

Tumors and their therapy may facilitate infectious complications. Bronchogenic carcinoma may cause bronchial obstruction, resulting in postobstructive pneumonia, which often fails to respond to antimicrobial therapy unless the obstruction can be removed. Likewise, tumors of the genitourinary tract and adjacent structures can obstruct urinary tract drainage, resulting in infection. Ulcerated or necrotic tumor masses of the skin and soft tissue structures or of the GI tract may become infected. These infections often cannot be treated successfully and become superinfected with increasingly resistant bacteria and sometimes fungi. Extensive surgical excision is the only effective therapy but may not be possible. Heavily irradiated skin sites may break down and become infected and are difficult to treat. CSF shunts, biliary tract and urinary tract stents, ileal bladders, and other devices are subject to infection that is difficult to manage.

Some chemotherapeutic agents cause extensive mucosal damage of the oropharynx and GI tract. Ulcerations of the lower GI tract may become the site of origin of multiple organism bacteremias and candidemias. Oral mucositis may be severe and lead to local infection or to bloodstream invasion by organisms making up the oral flora. These include α-hemolytic streptococci, *Capnocytophaga* species, *Stomatococcus mucilaginosus*, and *Candida albicans*. *S. mucilaginosus* can cause serious infections with septic shock, pneumonia, meningitis, and adult respiratory distress syndrome.

Surgically implanted intravascular catheters or other devices or long-line silastic catheters are used for nearly all cancer patients undergoing chemotherapy. A variety of organisms may cause catheter-related infections including *S. aureus, Staphylococcus epidermidis, Bacillus* species, *Enterococcus* species, *P. aeruginosa, Stenotrophomonas maltophilia, Acinetobacter* species, *Mycobacterium chelonae*, and *Candida* species (19). Some of these organisms, especially *S. aureus*, can cause serious complications such as endocarditis, septic emboli, and septic thrombophlebitis. Untreated or inadequately treated catheter-related candidemias can result in ophthalmitis or osteomyelitis. Infections with many of these organisms will recur despite appropriate therapy unless the catheter is removed.

Splenectomy is used in the management of some malignant diseases. Splenectomized patients are susceptible to fulminant septicemias caused by *S. pneumoniae, H. influenzae*, or *N. meningitidis*. They are also susceptible to babesiosis and *Capnocytophaga canimorsus* infections. Pneumococcal and *H. influenzae* immunization should be given before splenectomy, and pneumococcal immunization should be repeated at about 5-year intervals. These patients should be instructed to self-administer an antibiotic such as amoxicillin-clavulanate or one of the new fluoroquinolones and seek immediate medical attention if they develop a febrile illness with rigors or prostration.

PROPHYLAXIS OF INFECTION

Various measures have been used to prevent infection in cancer patients. Antibacterial agents (fluoroquinolones, trimethoprim-sulfamethoxazole), antifungal agents (fluconazole, itraconazole), and antiviral agents (acyclovir, ganciclovir, valacyclovir, famciclovir) are used for prophylaxis in neutropenic patients. The decision to use these agents depends on the anticipated frequency and severity of infections in the population at risk, toxicities, and potential for acquisition of resistant organisms. For example, ciprofloxacin has been effective in reducing gram-negative bacillary infections but has been associated with an increase in gram-positive infections and emergence of resistance among gram-negative bacilli. Intravenous γ-globulin reduces the frequency of infection in patients with hypogammaglobulinemia, but antibacterial agents are more effective and less expensive. Laminar airflow rooms, high-efficiency particular air filters, and cooked-food diets reduce the exposure to potential pathogens for severely compromised patients. The administration of growth factors (granulocyte colony-stimulating factor and granulocyte-macrophage colony-stimulating factor) shortens the duration of chemotherapy-induced neutropenia but is of value only in marrow transplant recipients and malignancies requiring intensive chemotherapy for long-term remissions or cure. Careful attention to dental care and immunizations are important, as well as simple infection-control measures such as meticulous hand washing.

REFERENCES

1. Bodey GP, Hersh EM, Valdivieso M, et al. Effects of cytotoxic drugs and immunosuppressive agents on the immune system. *Postgrad Med* 1975;58:67–74.
2. Bodey GP, Buckley M, Sathe YS, et al. Quantitative relationships between circulating leukocytes and infection in patients with acute leukemia. *Ann Intern Med* 1966;64:328–340.
3. Bodey GP. Antibiotics in patients with neutropenia. *Arch Intern Med* 1984;144:1845–1851.
4. Dosik GM, Luna M, Valdivieso M, et al. Necrotizing colitis in patients with cancer. *Am J Med* 1979;67:646–656.
5. Vanhueverzwyn R, Delannoy A, Michaux JL, et al. Anal lesions in hematologic diseases. *Dis Colon Rectum* 1980;23:310–312.
6. Chatzinikolaou I, Abi-Said D, Bodey GP, et al. Recent experience with Pseudomonas aeruginosa bacteremia in patients with cancer. Retrospective analysis of 245 episodes. *Arch Intern Med* 2000;160:501–509.
7. Bochud PY, Calandra T, Francioli P. Bacteremia due to viridans streptococci in neutropenic patients: a review. *Am J Med* 1994;97:256–264.
8. Bodey GP. Hematogenous and major organ candidiasis. In: Bodey GP, ed. *Candidiasis: pathogenesis, diagnosis, and treatment.* New York: Raven Press, 1992:279–329.
9. Haron E, Feld R, Tuffnell P, et al. Hepatic candidiasis: an increasing problem in immunocompromised hosts. *Am J Med* 1987;83:17–26.
10. Bodey GP, Vartivarian S. Aspergillosis. *Eur J Clin Microbiol Infect Dis* 1989;8:413–437.
11. Sickles EA, Greene WH, Wiernik PH, et al. Clinical presentation of infection in granulocytopenic patients. *Arch Intern Med* 1975;135:715–719.
12. Hughes WT, Armstrong D, Bodey GP, et al. 1997 guidelines for the sue of antimicrobial agents in neutropenic patients with fever. *Clin Infect Dis* 1997;25:551–573.
13. Spellberg B, Edwards JE Jr. Type 1/type 2 immunity in infectious diseases. *Clin Infect Dis* 2001;32:76–102.
14. Kaplan MH, Armstrong D, Rosen P. Tuberculosis complicating neoplastic disease. A review of 201 cases. *Cancer* 1974;33:850–858.
15. Zimmerman LE, Rappoport H. Occurrence of cryptococcosis in patients with malignant disease of the reticuloendothelial system. *Am J Clin Pathol* 1954;24:1050.
16. Schimpff S, Serpick A, Stoler B, et al. Varicella-zoster infection in patients with cancer. *Ann Intern Med* 1972;76:241–252.
17. Mera JR, Whimbey E, Elting L, et al. Cytomegalovirus pneumonia in adult nontransplantation patients with cancer: review of 20 cases occurring from 1964 through 1990. *Clin Infect Dis* 1996;22:1046–1050.
18. Whimbey E, Bodey GP. Viral pneumonia in the immunocompromised adult with neoplastic disease: the role of common community respiratory viruses. *Semin Respir Infect* 1992;7:122–131.
19. Groeger JS, Lucas AB, Thaler HT, et al. Infectious morbidity associated with long-term use of venous access devices in patients with cancer. *Ann Intern Med* 1993;19:1168–1174.

CHAPTER 126
Infections in Organ Transplant Recipients

Nina E. Tolkoff-Rubin and Robert H. Rubin

The transformation of organ transplantation from an interesting experiment in human immunobiology to the most practical means of rehabilitating patients with end-stage renal, cardiac, hepatic, and lung disease has to be viewed as one of the great accomplishments of twentieth century medicine. Today, at transplant centers around the world, rates of 1-year allograft survival of more than 90% are being achieved regularly for the first three of these forms of transplantation, with lung transplantation having a success rate of about 75% at many centers. These accomplishments have been achieved because of advances in a number of areas: tissue typing and cross-matching of donor and recipient; increased skill in the technical management of the transplant operation and postoperative care; and the more expert deployment of the drugs that make up the *therapeutic prescription* for the transplant recipient. This last area has two components: an immunosuppressive program to prevent and treat allograft rejection and an antimicrobial program that is closely linked to the nature of the immunosuppressive program required, to make immunosuppressive therapy as safe as possible. There has never been and likely never will be an immunosuppressive program that does not promote infection; the responsibility of the clinician is to understand the particular forms of infection associated with a given immunosuppressive program and to devise preventive strategies to limit the impact of these infections. Despite great progress in this area, infection remains the leading cause of death for transplant recipients, and it is estimated that at least two thirds of allograft recipients will suffer at least one episode of significant infection posttransplantation (1–4).

The risk of infection, particularly opportunistic infection, in transplant recipients is largely determined by the interaction of three factors: the presence of *technical/anatomic abnormalities* related to operative or perioperative misadventures; the *epidemiologic exposures* the patient has encountered; and the patient's *net state of immunosuppression*. The technical/anatomic problems of importance include the following: the presence of devitalized tissue or fluid collections (be they blood, lymph, urine, or bile); the prolonged requirement for drains and catheters that traverse or injure the primary mucocutaneous barrier to infection; and difficulties with the management of the endotracheal tube, vascular access devices, and a variety of drains and catheters. A general rule is that any technical/anatomic problem is almost always complicated by invasive infection, and the correction of any such problem before microbial invasion is an important rule of clinical management. The incidence of such problems is largely determined by the complexity of the operation and the general condition of the transplant recipient immediately preoperatively and postoperatively. Thus, technical/anatomic problems leading to infection are most common in liver allograft recipients and least common among kidney allograft recipients (1,4,5).

The epidemiologic exposures of importance to the transplant recipient can be divided into two general categories: those occurring in the community and those occurring within the hospital (Table 126.1). In the community, recent and remote exposures to the geographically restricted systemic mycoses, tuberculosis,

TABLE 126.1.   Classification of Infections Occurring in Transplant Recipients

Infections related to technical complications[a]
    Transplantation of a contaminated allograft
    Anastomotic leak or stenosis
    Wound hematoma
    Intravenous line contamination
    Iatrogenic damage to the skin
    Mismanagement of endotracheal tube leading to aspiration
    Infection related to biliary, urinary, and drainage catheters
Infections related to excessive nosocomial hazard
    Aspergillus species
    Legionella species
    Pseudomonas aeruginosa and other gram-negative bacilli
    Nocardia asteroides
Infections related to particular exposures within the community
    Systemic mycotic infections in certain geographic areas
        Histoplasma casulatum
        Coccidoides immitis
        Blastomyces dermatitidis
    Strongyloides stercoralis
    Community-acquired opportunistic infection resulting from
        ubiquitous saprophytes in the environment[b]
        Cryptococcus neoformans
        Aspergillus species
        N. asteroides
        Pneumocystis carinii
    Respiratory tract infections circulating in the community
        Mycobacterium tuberculosis
        Influenza
        Adenoviruses
        Parainfluenza
        Respiratory syncytial virus
    Infections acquired by the ingestion of contaminated food/water
        Salmonella species
        Listeria monocytogenes
    Viral infections of particular importance in transplant patients
        Herpes group viruses
        Hepatis viruses
        Papillomavirus
        Human immunodeficiency virus

[a]All lead to infection with gram-negative bacilli, *Staphylococcus* species (see reference 5) and/or *Candida* species.
[b]The incidence and severity of these infections, and to a lesser extent the other infections listed, are related to the net state of immunosuppression present in a particular patient.
Source: From Rubin R. Infection in the organ transplant recipient. In: Rubin RH, Young LS, eds. *Clinical approach to infection in the immunocompromised host,* 4th ed. New York: Kluwer Academic/Plenum Publishing, 2002:573–679, with permission.

and *Strongyloides stercoralis* can have an important effect post-transplantation. As far as the systemic mycoses and tuberculosis are concerned, three patterns of disease are observed: reactivation of old foci with secondary dissemination; progressive primary disease, with post primary dissemination; and superinfection, in which patients who had been rendered immune by previous infection have this immunity attenuated by posttransplantation immunosuppression, and on reexposure develop an illness akin to progressive primary disease, again with a particular emphasis on dissemination (2,4,5).

In the case of *Strongyloides,* a unique autoinfection cycle can maintain asymptomatic gastrointestinal (GI) tract carriage of the organism for decades after the patient has left the endemic site of acquisition. Posttransplantation, two clinical syndromes can occur with the initiation of immunosuppressive therapy: a hyperinfestation syndrome with hemorrhagic pneumonia and/or hemorrhagic enterocolitis; or a disseminated infection in which

trophozoites leave the GI tract and invade other tissues, usually accompanied by gut bacteria, so that the presenting syndrome can be gram-negative bacteremia and/or meningitis unresponsive to antibacterial therapy. Because of the grave nature of these syndromes, screening for this infection serologically or by duodenal intubation is advocated before the transplantation, with preemptive therapy carried out before the initiation of immunosuppressive therapy (2,5).

Other community-acquired infections of importance include the respiratory viruses [e.g., influenza, respiratory syncytial virus (RSV), parainfluenza, and so on], which are associated with a higher rate of pneumonia and bacterial superinfection than that noted in nonimmunosuppressed individuals with similar infections. Finally, more opportunistic pathogens such as *Aspergillus, Nocardia,* and *Cryptococcus* can be acquired in the general community with exposures related to such activities as construction and gardening, when an aerosol of organisms is created and inhalational disease results (1,5).

As important as community-acquired exposures are, nosocomial exposures have an even greater impact. Nosocomial infections are usually acquired when immunosuppressed transplant recipients are exposed to air or potable water that is contaminated with infectious agents such as *Aspergillus* species, *Legionella* species, and gram-negative organisms such as *Pseudomonas aeruginosa.* Two epidemiologic patterns are observed: *domiciliary* and *nondomiciliary.* Domiciliary exposures occur on the ward where the patient is housed and are relatively easy to detect because of clustering of cases in time and space. The risk of domiciliary exposures is greatly decreased by providing high-efficiency particular air filtration to patients' rooms. In contrast, nondomiciliary exposures occur when patients are exposed to contaminated air at central locations in the hospital, such as radiology or operating suites, where they are taken for special procedures. These exposures are probably more common than domiciliary exposures but are more difficult to detect because of a lack of clustering of cases in time and space. The leading clue to this entity is the occurrence of opportunistic infection at a point when the net state of immunosuppression is not great enough to allow this to occur in the absence of an excessive exposure. One additional form of nosocomial infection that bears mention is the person-to-person spread of such antimicrobial-resistant organisms as methicillin-resistant *Staphylococcus aureus,* vancomycin-resistant enterococci, and azole-resistant *Candida* species on the hands of hospital personnel, particularly physicians who ignore hand-washing directives (1,4–7).

The net state of immunosuppression is a complex function determined by the interaction of a number of factors (Table 126.2). Although the major driving force is the dose, duration, and temporal sequence in which immunosuppressive therapy is deployed, the importance of other factors in determining the net state of immunosuppression is underlined by the following observations: Such metabolic factors as protein-calorie malnutrition, hyperglycemia, and uremia contribute to the net state of immunosuppression. For example, the risk of life-threatening infection in transplant recipients is increased 10-fold if the serum albumin level is 2.5 g/dL or less. Perhaps the most important lesson in this area is the recognition that certain viral infections [most notably cytomegalovirus (CMV), Epstein-Barr virus (EBV), human herpesvirus-6 (HHV-6), hepatitis B virus and hepatitis C virus (HBV and HCV), and the human immunodeficiency virus (HIV)] markedly increase the risk of opportunistic infection. Thus, more than 90% of opportunistic infections occur in patients with ongoing infection with one or more of these viruses. Indeed, the 10% of exceptions are usually shown to be due to an excessive environmental exposure (2,4,5).

TABLE 126.2. Factors that Determine the Net State of Immunosuppression in an Organ Transplant Recipient

- Immunosuppression caused by the underlying disease
- Dose, duration, and temporal sequence of immunosuppressive therapy
- Neutropenia
- Technical/anatomic abnormalities that compromise the primary mucocutaneous barrier to microbial invasion
- Metabolic disturbances
  - Protein-calorie malnutrition
  - Uremia
  - Hyperglycemia
  - ? other
- Immunomodulating Viral Infection
  - Cytomegalovirus
  - Epstein-Barr virus
  - Human herpesvirus-6
  - Hepatitis viruses (B and C)
  - Human immunodeficiency virus
- Age younger than 1 and older than 65 years
- ? race

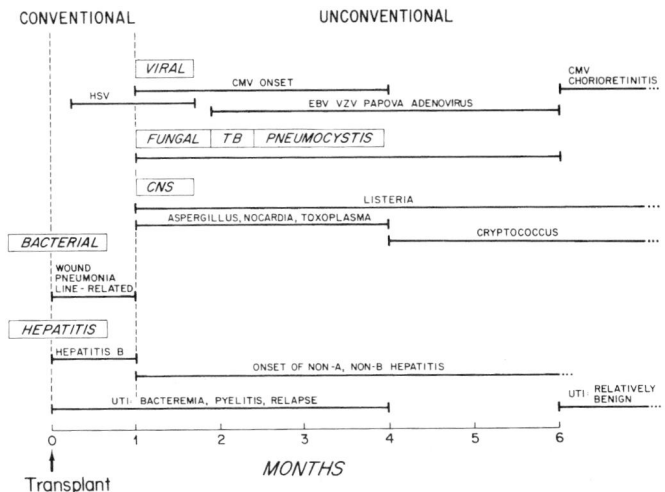

Figure 126.1. Expected timetable of infection in organ transplant recipients.

Finally, recent observations raise the possibility that racial heritage may play a role in determining the net state of immunosuppression. African Americans have an increased rate of allograft rejection and a decreased risk of infection while being treated with the same immunosuppressive regimen as white patients. This suggests that more intensive immunosuppressive regimens can be safely and beneficially used in African Americans without a dangerous increase in the net state of immunosuppression (2,4,8,9).

EXPECTED TIMETABLE OF INFECTION IN ORGAN TRANSPLANT RECIPIENTS

The immunosuppressive programs used to prevent and treat allograft rejection are very similar in all transplant recipients, consisting of a calcineurin inhibitor (cyclosporine or tacrolimus), a purine antagonist (mycophenolate or azathioprine), and prednisone. Antilymphocyte antibody therapy can be used in two different ways: as *induction* therapy initially, a particularly useful strategy if ischemia-reperfusion injury of the kidneys (i.e., acute tubular necrosis) is an issue; and as *antirejection* therapy for steroid-resistant rejection. In addition, sirolimus (rapamycin) and anti–interleukin-2 (anti–IL-2) receptor antibodies are being used in an effort to limit the dose of both steroid and calcineurin inhibitor required. In any case, from an infectious disease point of view, these standardized regimens that are virtually identical in all forms of organ transplantation result in a very stereotyped temporal pattern of infection, that is, a timetable of infection can be defined. What this means is that such infectious disease syndromes as pneumonia can occur at any point in the posttransplantation course, but the cause of the pneumonia is very different at different time points. The timetable (Figure 126.1) is useful to the clinician in three ways: in constructing the differential diagnosis in a patient who presents with an infectious disease syndrome; in devising focused, cost-effective antimicrobial preventive strategies; and as a useful means of assessing environmental hazards as part of infection-control efforts (exceptions to the timetable are usually due to unexpected environmental hazards, often within the hospital environment). The posttransplantation course can be divided into three distinct time periods: the first month after transplantation, first 1 to 6 months

after transplantation, and the late period, which is more than 6 months after transplantation (2,4,5,10).

Infection in the First Month after Organ Transplantation

Three categories of infection should be considered in transplant recipients who present with clinical syndromes of possible infectious origin: (a) Infection that was present in the transplant recipient before the transplantation and that is exacerbated by the operation, anesthesia, or the institution of immunosuppressive therapy. This is a particular problem with liver and cardiac transplant candidates, who may require life support systems, with all of the infectious disease problems inherent with such intensive care before transplantation. Thus, aspiration pneumonia, vascular access device infections, left ventricular assist device–related infections, and spontaneous bacterial peritonitis are of major concern. (b) Infection can be transmitted with a contaminated allograft (usually due to an undetected bloodstream infection in the donor). This renders the vascular anastomoses at risk of microbial seeding and the subsequent development of mycotic aneurysms that undergo catastrophic rupture. (c) More than 95% of the infections that occur during this time are the same bacterial or candidal infections of the surgical wound, lungs, urine, vascular access, or drainage catheters observed in nonimmunosuppressed patients undergoing comparable forms of surgery, although the consequences in transplant recipients can be much greater. Although appropriate antimicrobial prophylaxis offers some protection against these infections, the major determinant is the technical skill with which the surgery is performed and the various invasive lines and catheters are managed. Because of the particular technical demands associated with liver and lung transplantation, these transplant recipients are at greatest risk of developing this form of infectious complication (2,3,5,11,12).

Prevention of infection during this time begins with technically impeccable surgery and perioperative management of the endotracheal tube, vascular access, drains, and catheters. In addition, perioperative antimicrobial prophylaxis will provide some further protection. Particularly in the case of renal transplantation, low dose trimethoprim-sulfamethoxazole (TMP-SMX) (or fluoroquinolone) prophylaxis has been shown to essentially eliminate the risk of urosepsis (without such prophylaxis, the incidence of urinary tract infection has been reported to be as high as 60% among renal transplant recipients) (2,13–15).

Noteworthy by their absence in this period are opportunistic infections. Even though the daily doses of immunosuppressive drugs are at their highest in the first month posttransplantation, the duration of this therapy (the "area under the curve") has not been sufficient to produce a net state of immunosuppression such that opportunistic infection can occur without an unusually intense exposure. Indeed, the occurrence of opportunistic infection in the first month posttransplantation should be taken as strong evidence of the presence of a significant environmental hazard requiring correction (2,4,5).

Infection 1 to 6 Months after Transplantation

The infections occurring from 1 to 6 months after transplantation can be divided into two general categories: (a) The most common causes of symptomatic infection are the immunomodulating viruses—CMV, EBV, HHV-6, HBV, HCV, and HIV. CMV itself is the cause of approximately two thirds of infections occurring during this time. (b) The combination of sustained immunosuppressive therapy and immunomodulating viral infection creates a net state of immunosuppression great enough for opportunistic infection caused by such organisms as *Pneumocystis carinii*, *Listeria monocytogenes*, and *Aspergillus fumigatus* to occur without a particularly intense environmental exposure. Prevention of these infections then has three major components: low-dose TMP-SMX prophylaxis, an effective antiviral strategy (particularly aimed against CMV), and continued vigilance against environmental hazards (2,4,5,10).

Infection More than 6 Months after Transplantation

Organ transplant recipients who continue to receive immunosuppression to maintain functioning allografts more than 6 months after transplantation can be divided into three groups in terms of their infectious disease risks: (a) the 80% or more of transplant recipients who have had a good result from transplantation—good allograft function, minimal maintenance immunosuppression, and no chronic viral infection. These individuals are at risk of such community-acquired infections as those caused by the respiratory viruses (e.g., influenza, parainfluenza, RSV, etc.), food-borne infections such as *Salmonella*, *Listeria*, and *Campylobacter* and inhalation of endemic or opportunistic fungi when aerosols are created due to construction, gardening, or environmental cleanup activities. As a general rule, avoidance of these risks is the best policy, because the incidence of complications with these infections is much higher with these patients than with the general population. Of these community-acquired infections, the respiratory viruses are especially important, with complicating pneumonia being particularly common. (b) The 10% with chronic hepatitis virus infection will have an accelerated course progressing to end-stage liver disease and/or hepatocellular carcinoma resulting from immunosuppression unless effective antiviral therapy can be delivered. (c) The 10% of patients who have had a poor result from transplantation—poor allograft function, too much acute and chronic immunosuppression, and often chronic viral infection; we have termed "chronic n'er do wells." These are the transplant recipients at highest risk of opportunistic infection with such pathogens as *P. carinii*, *Cryptococcus neoformans*, *L. monocytogenes*, and *Nocardia asteroides*. These must be maintained on TMP-SMX prophylaxis indefinitely and considered for such other preventive treatments as fluconazole (2,4,5,10,16–22).

INFECTIONS OF SPECIAL IMPORTANCE IN ORGAN TRANSPLANT RECIPIENTS

From the preceding comments, it is clear that infection of transplant recipients can be divided into four major categories: those related to technical complications, those related to particular epidemiologic exposures, those caused by certain viruses, and opportunistic infections caused by organisms that are essentially nonpathogenic for normal hosts (see Table 126.2). Although viruses are the single most important group of microbial pathogens for transplant recipients, bacterial, fungal, and parasitic infections must be considered as well, because their occurrence is much influenced by technical and epidemiologic factors, as well as the immunomodulating effects of certain viruses (2,4,5,10).

Viral Infections

The most important form of infection affecting organ transplant recipients is that caused by viruses. The potential clinical impact of viral infections for these patients is much broader than for immunocompetent hosts. Viral infections can directly cause clinical syndromes such as fever, pneumonia, and hepatitis. In addition, because of the elaboration of cytokines, chemokines, and growth factors by the host in response to viral replication, there are a series of *indirect* effects that expand the impact of the particular virus on the host: (a) They can produce a global state of immunosuppression that makes possible superinfections with a variety of opportunistic pathogens such as *P. carinii*, *L. monocytogenes*, and a variety of fungal organisms. (b) They can initiate a series of pathogenic events that damage the allograft by mechanisms other than those of classic allograft rejection. (c) Finally, in persons whose immune function is permanently suppressed, a virus can contribute to the development of malignancies. The viruses of greatest importance for the transplant recipient include the following: the herpesviruses (especially CMV and EBV), the hepatitis viruses, the respiratory viruses, the hepatitis viruses, and the papovaviruses (2,4,5,10–12).

HERPESVIRUSES
The HHVs share several characteristics that make them particularly well adapted for causing significant disease in transplant recipients.

Latency
Once infected with a herpesvirus, an individual forever harbors nonreplicating virus that is capable of being reactivated by exogenous factors in the host. Serologic positivity in the absence of replicating virus is the laboratory marker of latent infection. Latency appears to be quite stable with CMV, varicella-zoster virus (VZV), and HHV-6, HHV-7, and HHV-8, requiring specific events for reactivation and the potential of significant disease occurring. In contrast, EBV and herpes simplex virus types 1 and 2 (HSV-1 and HSV-2) not only respond to similar stimuli as the other herpesviruses, but also will spontaneously reactivate, thus explaining some of the clinical events associated with these viruses (2,5,10,11).

Cell Association
Herpesviruses spread from cell to cell by direct contact, rendering neutralizing antibody relatively inefficient and cell-mediated immunity of great importance in the control of these viruses. In particular, the key host defense is major histocompatibility complex (MHC)–restricted, virus-specific, cytotoxic T cells—just that

element of host defense most affected by currently employed immunosuppressive programs. It is not surprising that these viruses are spread from individual to individual by intimate contact, through organ transplantation, and the transfusion of viable leukocyte-containing blood products from seropositive donors (2,5,10,11).

Oncogenicity

All herpesviruses should be considered potentially oncogenic, although EBV-induced posttransplantation lymphoproliferative disorder (PTLD) is the only clearcut example of this phenomenon. Of great interest is the observation that the incidence of EBV-induced PTLD is increased about 10-fold by the occurrence of symptomatic CMV disease, an effect thought to be mediated by the cytokine milieu induced by the CMV infection (2,23,24).

Cytomegalovirus. CMV is the single most important infectious agent affecting organ transplant recipients: At least two thirds of them manifest evidence of viral replication posttransplantation. The critical first step in the pathogenesis of CMV is the reactivation of the virus from latency, whether from endogenous sites within the recipient or from the allograft. There are three signaling pathways that can be involved in this reactivation process: the first and most important is triggered by tumor necrosis factor (TNF) in the circulation. Binding of TNF to the TNF receptor of latently infected cells activates a signaling pathway that results in the production of nuclear factor-κB (NF-κB), the nuclear transcription factor that initiates CMV replication. It is not surprising then that replicating CMV with the potential for causing clinical disease can be identified in any circumstance in which TNF release occurs, including the following: allograft rejection, the use of such drugs as the antilymphocyte antibodies (OKT3 and antithymocyte globulin) and amphotericin B, and systemic sepsis. Indeed, a "second-wave" phenomenon can be defined after significant infections of a variety of types; for example, 2 to 3 weeks after a patient presents with such infections as pneumococcal sepsis, urosepsis, or gram-negative pneumonia, not only can replicating CMV be identified, but a second wave of fever, now due to CMV, is often present (2,25–32).

The other two pathways for reactivating CMV result in the formation of cyclic adenosine monophosphate (cAMP), which also can activate this virus. The triggers for these signaling pathways are the catecholamines, epinephrine and norepinephrine, and proinflammatory prostaglandins (2,25).

There are three patterns of transmission of CMV in the organ transplant recipient, each with a different incidence of clinical disease (2,4,11,33–40).

1. **Primary infection:** When cells from a latently infected (seropositive) donor are transferred into a seronegative recipient. Although those cells can be leukocytes in a blood product, most transplant centers prevent this form of transmission by using seronegative blood products or by using leukocyte filters when giving the patient a blood transfusion. Currently, more than 95% of primary infection is due to the transplantation of an allograft from a seropositive donor into a seronegative recipient (D+R−). These individuals have a 50% to 65% incidence of symptomatic disease (direct manifestations) (33–36).

2. **Reactivation infection:** When endogenous latent infection in a seropositive allograft recipient is reactivated (D+/−R+). These individuals have a 10% to 20% incidence of symptomatic disease (33–36).

3. **Superinfection:** When an allograft from a seropositive donor is transplanted into a seropositive recipient, and the virus that

is reactivated is of donor origin (D+R+). These individuals have a 15% to 25% incidence of symptomatic disease (2,37–40).

The direct clinical effects of CMV replication and invasion are outlined in Table 126.3 and are similar in all forms of organ transplantation, with one notable exception: A transplanted organ is more affected by the virus than a native organ. Thus, CMV hepatitis is only a clinical issue in liver transplant, myocarditis in a cardiac transplant, pancreatitis in a pancreas transplant, and so on. It should be emphasized that CMV itself is the predominant cause of infectious disease syndromes in the second through the sixth month after transplantation. When prophylaxis with an antiviral agent is carried out and it fails, the usual effect is to extend the incubation period so the CMV that is observed occurs 6 to 12 months posttransplant (2,4,5,10).

In addition to the direct causation of infectious disease syndromes, CMV, like other herpesviruses, can cause indirect effects, these being mediated by cytokines, chemokines, and growth factors elaborated by the allograft recipient in response to CMV replication and invasion. CMV, as previously noted, contributes significantly to the net state of immunosuppression, thus predisposing to infection with *P. carinii, L. monocytogenes,* a variety of fungi, and gram-negative bacteria. In addition, CMV infection has been linked not only to an increased incidence of PTLD but also to a significant increase in the hepatitis C viral load. Finally, CMV has been linked to acute and chronic allograft injury, particularly the occurrence and extent of bronchiolitis obliterans in lung transplant recipients and accelerated coronary artery disease (CAD) in heart transplant recipients (2,4,5,10). Prophylaxis trials of valacyclovir and oral ganciclovir have demonstrated a significant decrease in the incidence of rejection among recipients of the antiviral drug. In addition, a 1-month course of intravenously administered ganciclovir that prevented symptomatic CMV was associated with a decrease in posttransplant CAD in the heart allograft over an observational period of 7 to 10 years. Studies in transplant recipients, as well as in animal models, have suggested that the array of mediators (chemokines, cytokines, and growth factors) produced in response to CMV or during rejection are essentially identical, and that rejection and

---

TABLE 126.3. Effects of Cytomegalovirus on the Organ Transplant Recipient

A. Direct manifestations
- Fever
- Mononucleosis
- Pneumonia
- Hepatitis
- Gastrointestinal ulceration, with bleeding, perforation, or both
- Leukopenia
- Thrombocytopenia
- Encephalitis[a]
- Transverse myolitis[a]
- Cutaneous vasculitis[a]
- Progressive chorioretinitis[b]

B. Indirect manifestations
- Contributes to net state of immunosuppression, leading to opportunistic superinfection
- Can cause acute and/or chronic allograft injury
- Increase the incidence of posttransplant lymphoproliferative disease

[a]Rare events.
[b]A late manifestation of cytomegalovirus infection (>6 mo posttransplant).

CMV infection are synergistic in terms of their long-term impact (2,4,5,10,41–48).

The different immunosuppressive drugs have differing effects on the pathogenesis of CMV: In terms of reactivating the virus from latency, antithymocyte globulin and OKT3 are potent reactivators of the virus (undoubtedly because of the large amounts of TNF released in response to these agents); cytotoxic drugs (e.g., azathioprine and mycophenolate) have moderate reactivating effects; and cyclosporine, tacrolimus, rapamycin, and prednisone have no ability to reactivate the virus. However, once small amounts of replicating virus are present, the use of steroid pulses or the calcineurin inhibitors (cyclosporine and tacrolimus) will up-regulate the level of virus produced, thus resulting in increasing viral loads. Indeed, we refer to these drugs as "in vivo polymerase chain reactions" (PCRs) for CMV. These observations explain several clinical observations: Whereas seropositive recipients of transplants immunosuppressed with standard three-drug immunosuppression (a calcineurin inhibitor, azathioprine or mycophenolate, and prednisone) have a 10% to 15% incidence of symptomatic disease, if an antilymphocyte antibody is given to treat rejection, then this incidence rises to about 65%; whereas in the precyclosporine era, relapsing CMV disease was essentially unheard of; today this is not an uncommon occurrence, particularly in those with primary disease, a high viral load, a foreshortened course of treatment, and a six-antigen histocompatibility mismatch between donor and recipient. Further, although primary resistance to ganciclovir is essentially unknown, relapsing infection is a situation in which this can develop. What is thought to be operative here is that small amounts of replicating virus that are not eliminated by the combination of host response and antiviral therapy will be amplified by the ongoing need for immunosuppression with cyclosporine or tacrolimus ("the PCR effect" at work) (2,4,5).

The diagnosis of CMV infection can be accomplished in one of two ways: biopsy of a tissue that shows evidence of an inflammatory lesion (e.g., the lung in a patient with pneumonitis, the liver in the face of hepatic dysfunction, or the gut in the face of ulceration and/or inflammation) or the demonstration of virus in accessible bodily fluids (urine, respiratory tract secretions, and blood). Serial blood tests to measure anti-CMV antibody posttransplantation do not provide timely enough information in this era of antiviral chemotherapy. The traditional approach to viral diagnosis has involved the growth of virus in tissue culture, with a characteristic cytopathic effect being noted after several weeks in culture. Again, such an approach does not permit informed therapeutic decision making. The first major advance in this regard was the development of the shell vial technique. This methodology involves the centrifugation of the clinical specimen onto a fibroblast monolayer, which assists adsorption of any virus present, resulting in a fourfold increase in sensitivity, with no sacrifice in specificity. After incubation for 24 to 48 hours, at a time when there is no visible evidence of viral growth, the monolayer is stained with a monoclonal antibody to the major immediate early protein of CMV by immunofluorescence. This works particularly well for tissue, urine, and respiratory tract secretions. Unfortunately, this approach has a sensitivity of 50% or less for detecting viremia, which is the most reliable laboratory marker for significant CMV replication. Because of the importance of viremia in CMV diagnosis, two other techniques have become the standard for the care of transplant recipients: an antigenemia assay and quantitative PCR assays (carried out, often, after qualitative PCR has been shown to be positive). These latter two tests have delineated the importance of viral load in understanding both the clinical syndromes emerging and the response to therapy. In addition, the fact that these assays are usually posi-

tive 4 to 7 days before the onset of clinical symptoms has allowed the development of a preemptive approach to CMV disease prevention (2,4,5,45).

The standard of care for symptomatic CMV disease remains intravenously administered ganciclovir, at a dose of 5 mg/kg twice daily, which is continued until viremia is cleared (which usually takes 2–3 weeks). Because of the concerns regarding relapse, particularly in patients with primary infection, this is usually followed by a 2- to 3-month course of oral therapy. It is likely that as more experience with oral valganciclovir is gained, this oral drug will be substituted for intravenously administered ganciclovir once control of the clinical syndrome has been achieved (2,4,5,49,50).

A variety of preventive strategies have been developed to limit the occurrence of the direct manifestations of CMV disease. The use of either valacyclovir and valganciclovir prophylactically for about 3 months has been shown to be quite effective in preventing CMV disease, especially in the seropositive recipient not receiving antilymphocyte antibody therapy (2,5,46). Alternatively, two forms of preemptive therapy have been shown to be useful: If a seropositive individual receives antilymphocyte antibody therapy in the treatment of rejection, the risk of symptomatic CMV disease rises from 10% to 15% to 50% to 75%. If ganciclovir is administered at a dose of 5 mg/kg intravenously for the duration of the antilymphocyte antibody therapy, this risk falls to about 20%; and if an oral ganciclovir is given for an additional 2 to 3 months, the risk falls to near zero. The second form of preemptive therapy is to monitor patients at regular intervals for the presence of presymptomatic viremia by antigenemia or PCR assays, and then treating preemptively when it turns positive. For those at risk of primary disease, we advocate prophylaxis; for seropositive individuals, preemptive therapy, if logistically feasible, is our approach of choice. It must be emphasized, however, that the data available only address the direct manifestations of CMV; there are currently few data available regarding the efficacy of one or another preventive program in the prevention of the indirect effects of CMV or other viruses (2,4,5,51,52).

Before the advent of cyclosporine-based immunosuppression, relapsing CMV infection was essentially unknown. Now, it occurs at a rate of 20% to 30%, particularly in those with primary disease. It is in the context of relapsing infection that ganciclovir-resistant infection may appear. Factors contributing to this occurrence include the following: 6-antigen MHC mismatch between donor and recipient; high viral load; an inadequate course of antiviral therapy (both dose and duration being important); a history of more than one relapse; and the requirement for augmented immunosuppression during and after the antiviral treatment. Infection with a resistant isolate of CMV can be treated with foscarnet (with significant risk of renal toxicity), either alone or in an innovative protocol in which half-dose foscarnet is combined with half-dose ganciclovir (2,4, 5,52–56).

Epstein-Barr Virus. In both normal and immunosuppressed persons, EBV infection produces clinical effects quite similar to those of CMV, and it is likely that in transplant recipients, EBV contributes to the net state of immunosuppression and to the causation of a mononucleosis-like syndrome. A more detailed understanding of the importance of this virus for transplant recipients has been handicapped by the ubiquity of CMV infection. One aspect of EBV infection in organ transplant recipients is uniquely important: Its role in the pathogenesis of EBV-associated PTLD. This entity, which has the histologic appearance of a polymorphic B-cell lymphoma, commonly presents with invasion of the central nervous system (CNS), nasopharynx, liver, small bowel, heart, or allograft in addition to lymphoid tissue [a computed tomographic (CT) scan that fails to reveal adenopathy does not rule out PTLD]. It appears that EBV-associated lymphoproliferative disease represents a continuum of clinical disease ranging from benign EBV-dependent polyclonal B-cell hyperplasia to malignant EBV-independent monoclonal B-cell lymphoma. Indeed, this entire continuum can be represented simultaneously in the same patient, greatly complicating the staging of patients and in evaluating the effects of different forms of therapy (2,57–61).

The incidence of PTLD is in part related to the EBV viral load, with at least two situations defined in which this is particularly high: primary EBV infection and when excessive amounts of immunosuppression have been used. The current concept of pathogenesis is as follows: In healthy immunocompetent persons who have latent EBV infection (and are thus EBV seropositive), circulating cytotoxic T lymphocytes specific for EBV antigens on the surface of infected B lymphocytes prevent the outgrowth of virally induced, transformed cells that are believed to initiate the oncogenic process that culminates in lymphoproliferative disease. In immunosuppressed patients, especially those with primary infection, this defense system is defective. Thus, drugs such as cyclosporine and tacrolimus will inhibit the recipient's ability to eliminate the outgrowth of EBV-transformed B lymphocytes in a dose-related fashion. In contrast, antilymphocyte antibodies exert their primary effect by increasing the amount of virus that has been reactivated and is actively replicating, thus increasing the level of transformed B lymphocytes. Accordingly, the occurrence of EBV-related PTLD should be regarded as a consequence of the net state of immunosuppression. As a further example of this, the occurrence of symptomatic CMV disease increases the incidence of PTLD by a factor of 7 to 10 (2,23,24,57,60–69).

The optimal treatment of EBV-associated PTLD remains to be defined. All patients should have a major reduction of immunosuppressive therapy (with complete cessation in kidney transplant recipients who can be maintained on dialysis); most centers prescribe high-dose acyclovir or ganciclovir as well, although it is unclear what role such therapy plays because antivirals have no effect on the episomal form of the virus present in the infected B cells. Approximately one third of patients respond to these maneuvers. Patients with residual local disease, particularly of the gut, have responded well to surgical extirpation. For the remainder of patients, a wide variety of approaches have been taken: anti–B-cell antibody therapy usually being the next treatment used, followed by such approaches as adoptive immunotherapy with the infusion of T cells directed against specific EBV antigens, lymphoma chemotherapy, interferon plus immunoglobulin G (IgG), anti–IL-6 monoclonal antibody, and others. At present, the optimal therapy has yet to emerge (2,70–77).

Other Herpesviruses. Of the remaining herpesviruses, the one that has received the most attention is HHV-6, which has considerable genetic homology with CMV. Evidence of HHV-6 viremia, often in conjunction with CMV, can be found in an estimated 35% of transplant recipients, although the consequences of HHV-6 viremia have not been completely elucidated. In an occasional patient, HHV-6 can cause bone marrow dysfunction, encephalitis, hepatitis, interstitial pneumonia, and/or a mononucleosis syndrome. In addition, it is likely that active infection with both CMV and HHV-6 simultaneously may induce a greater amount of disease than either virus by itself. A role for HHV-6 in the pathogenesis of allograft injury, in adding to the net state of immunosuppression, and in extending hospital stay is quite likely. Fortunately, HHV-6 appears to be sensitive to ganciclovir. There is much more to be learned about the importance of this

virus, HHV-7, and even HHV-8 (the cause of Kaposi's sarcoma) in the organ transplant recipient (2,78–87).

Reactivation VZV infection, in the form of dermatomal zoster, affects at least 10% of organ transplant recipients. Visceral dissemination of VZV in these patient is quite uncommon. Therapy with valacyclovir or famciclovir shortens the duration of the clinical syndrome. In contrast to the benignity of reactivation VZV infection in the transplant recipient, primary VZV infection is a rapidly lethal visceral infection characterized by pneumonia, pancreatitis, hepatitis, encephalitis, and disseminated intravascular coagulation. Large doses of intravenously administered acyclovir (10–12 mg/kg thrice daily, with dosage adjustments for renal dysfunction) can be life saving in the management of these patients, provided it is initiated early in the course. The VZV serologic status of all transplant candidates should be determined before transplantation, and varicella vaccine should be offered to all seronegative individuals. Proof of seroconversion should be obtained after immunization. For seronegative transplant recipients, vaccine should also be offered posttransplantation, with close follow-up of the consequences of the vaccine (possible varicella, which requires therapy) or failure to seroconvert. For seronegative individuals who are exposed to VZV, immediate varicella-zoster immune globulin (VZIG) prophylaxis is essential, with close clinical follow-up to detect failures, who will require antiviral intervention. It is important to recognize that the failures of VZIG prophylaxis (an estimated 10%–25% of patients) may have attenuation of trivial aspects of the infection while developing lethal visceral infection. Thus, the typical varicella rash, the most easily recognizable part of the syndrome, may be absent in patients who are succumbing to visceral disease post-VZIG prophylaxis (2,87–90).

Reactivated HSV-1 and HSV-2 infection is quite common after organ transplantation, especially with intensive antirejection therapy. Localized mucocutaneous infection of either the oral or the anogenital area is the usual result, although the lesions, especially in the anogenital area, often have an atypical appearance, with ulcers being more common that vesicles. Rare instances of disseminated primary infection, probably transmitted with the allograft, have been described, with a clinical syndrome akin to visceral VZV infection resulting. Other uncommon manifestations of HSV infection in transplant recipients that have been described include (a) tracheal (and even bronchopulmonary) and esophageal infection, which almost invariably is due to the combination of a nasogastric or endotracheal tube traumatizing these sites in the face of active oral HSV infection in any transplant recipient but with a particular impact on the lung transplant recipients and their bronchial anastomosis; (b) eczema herpeticum (also called Kaposi's varicelliform eruption), a disseminated skin infection without visceral involvement in patients with such underlying dermatologic conditions as eczema; (c) meningoencephalitis due to HSV-2 in patients with anogenital infection; and (d) a zosteriform dermatomal rash akin to that of VZV. HSV is quite sensitive to both acyclovir and ganciclovir, so either drug may be used either prophylactically or therapeutically, depending on the clinical situation (2).

HEPATITIS VIRUSES

The prevalence of chronic liver disease in organ transplant recipients is approximately 10%, with virtually all of it caused by HBV and HCV [hepatitis A virus (HAV) can lead to acute hepatic failure requiring, uncommonly, liver transplantation but does not recur posttransplant; in contrast, HCV rarely, if ever, causes acute hepatic failure but commonly recurs]. The impact of these viruses on the transplant recipient is twofold: (a) both HBV and HCV are immunomodulating viruses that contribute significantly to transplant recipients' net state of immunosuppression, increasing the risk of opportunistic infection, and (b) the course of these viruses is exacerbated by immunosuppression, and over a 10-year period a significant proportion of patients who have not responded to antiviral therapy progress to end-stage liver disease and/or hepatocellular carcinoma. Because of this risk, we advocate liver biopsy before kidney, heart, and lung transplantation in patients who have serologic markers of active viral replication (2,4,5).

The efficiency of transmission of HBV with organ transplantation from an infected donor approaches 100%, with a relatively high rate of acute, fulminant hepatitis associated with the acquisition of HBV in the peritransplant period. Accordingly, every effort should be made to screen both organ and blood donors to prevent this event. In addition to donors who are hepatis B surface antigen (HBsAg) positive, those with antibody to hepatitis B core antibody may transmit the virus, with as many as 20% to 30% liver allografts, although it is very uncommon for this to occur with the other organs (2,5,91–93).

Patients who come to transplantation with chronic HBV infection will exhibit an increase in the level of HBV replication because of the exogenous immunosuppressive therapy, particularly corticosteroids, and the possibility of an acceleration of the course of hepatitis. CMV and presumably other immunomodulating viruses will likewise cause an increase in the viral load. This effect is noteworthy in that 10 years after transplantation, 42% of patients with chronic HBV infection now had cirrhosis and 54% had died of either chronic liver disease or hepatocellular carcinoma (in contrast, HCV had a 20% incidence of such events 10 years after transplantation) (2,94).

HBV infection is well managed with lamivudine therapy; however, 1 to 3 years after initiating such therapy, resistant mutants appear. Liver transplant recipients benefit from the combination of HBV immune globulin and lamivudine, and the question of whether such combination therapy would be useful in kidney transplant recipients is currently under study. Fortunately, there are additional anti-HBV drugs in clinical trial that appear quite promising, as it is likely that a therapeutic strategy akin to that used against HIV will be needed—multiple drugs to overcome the development of resistance (2,95–108).

HBV is far more virulent than HCV in terms of the progression to end-stage liver disease or cancer. However, therapy is becoming available, and the prognosis is reasonably good because of this. In contrast, HCV is more desultory, but the therapy currently available (ribavirin plus interferon) is far less effective, with no other drugs on the horizon (2).

HCV is responsible for more than 80% of the chronic liver disease that occurs in transplant recipients. The biggest issue regarding HCV in transplantation involves the approach to possible organ donors who are anti-HCV positive (1%–5% of the potential donor pool). The risk of transmitting the virus with transplantation of an organ from an anti-HCV–positive donor is about 50%. If the PCR assay for HCV RNA in the serum of the donor is positive, the rate of transmission with transplantation approaches 100%. Given the relatively slow course of HCV in the transplant recipient and the chronic shortage of organs, there has been considerable argument over the appropriate approach to such donors. Our own policy is to reserve organs from anti-HCV–positive donors for critically ill candidates or for older individuals, with the belief that the several years necessary for HCV to become clinically apparent after transplantation offers a trade-off that is acceptable for these two population groups (2,109–113).

COMMUNITY-ACQUIRED RESPIRATORY VIRUSES IN THE ORGAN TRANSPLANT RECIPIENT

Transplant recipients are particularly susceptible to infection with the respiratory viruses that circulate in the community.

The severity of these illnesses is greater than that in the general population. Both viral pneumonia and bacterial superinfection resulting in pneumonia due to such organisms as *Streptococcus pneumoniae, Haemophilus influenzae, S. aureus,* and gram-negative bacilli are far more common in transplant recipients than in the normal population. Trials of influenza vaccine in renal transplant recipients have shown a lack of toxicity or adverse effects, but a disappointing level of efficacy. Unfortunately, there is little information on the efficacy of amantadine or the neuraminidase inhibitors in this setting. Thus, avoidance of influenza exposures is exceedingly important in preventing this infection and its consequences (2,5).

RSV infection of a particularly virulent nature, causing an increased rate of pneumonia and mortality, has been observed in both pediatric and adult transplant recipients with acute respiratory failure. Because there are some anecdotal reports suggesting that aerosolized ribavirin therapy may have therapeutic efficacy for this infection, an aggressive approach to diagnosis is appropriate (2,4,5).

Other respiratory viruses noted to cause serious disease in transplant recipients include adenoviruses, parainfluenza, and rhinovirus. Because our therapies are relatively primitive for this class of infection, and because transplant recipients have a significantly higher rate of complications than the general population, it is worth a special effort to isolate them from such exposures throughout their posttransplantation course (2).

PAPOVAVIRUSES

The papovaviruses are DNA viruses with oncogenic potential that are divided into two genera: the polyomaviruses and the papillomaviruses. The polyomaviruses, BK and JC (BKV and JCV), are acquired in most individuals in childhood, with no particular clinical syndrome being associated with this acquisition. Structurally and antigenically, these viruses are closely related to the oncogenic virus SV40. Posttransplantation immunosuppression results in reactivation of these viruses such that the great majority of organ transplant recipients excrete one or both of these viruses and/or a rise in specific antibody levels. BKV in the renal transplant recipient has been linked to the occurrence of ureteral strictures since it was isolated more than 30 years ago. Of greater importance, BKV in the renal transplant recipient can cause a tubulointerstitial nephritis that is an important cause of allograft failure. The effects of BKV on recipients of other organs have not been established. JCV is the cause of progressive multifocal leukoencephalopathy (PML), a subacute, progressive, demyelinating disease of the CNS (2).

The incidence of BKV-related interstitial nephritis has risen significantly in the past decade (an incidence as high as 5% among renal transplant recipients), linked to intensive immunosuppressive therapy, particularly regimens that include tacrolimus and mycophenolate. Although asymptomatic BKV replication can be found in 40% of renal transplant recipients, kidney biopsies from patients with invasive disease reveal the following: viral cytopathic changes with necrosis and particular involvement of the tubular epithelium, plus an intense inflammatory infiltrate that can contain numerous plasma cells. Differential diagnostic considerations include rejection and calcineurin inhibitor toxicity. Definitive diagnosis can be made by immunoperoxidase staining of a renal biopsy with a monoclonal antibody specific for BKV or by electron microscopy of ultrathin sections from the biopsy. The patient's urine can be screened for BKV by cytologic examination of by electron microscopic examination of negatively stained urine specimens. Negative results of a urine screen essentially rule out BKV interstitial nephritis. Positive results, in the setting of renal dysfunction, merit a biopsy. BKV nephritis has a poor prognosis, with the only management strategy available being a major decrease in immunosuppression. Serial biopsies are often necessary to steer a course between rejection and nephritis (2,5,114–117).

JCV was first isolated from the brain of a patient with PML. Since then, it has been shown to be the cause of this illness (a demyelinating disease of the white matter of the brain, characterized by the development of progressive motor and sensory deficits, dementia, and death within 3–6 months). Management of this entity demands a marked decrease in immunosuppression. Unfortunately, no drugs that have been studied thus far have convincing activity against JCV (2).

The most noticeable effect of papillomavirus infection in the organ transplant recipient is the production of warts, which may be extensive enough to be disfiguring. The level of warts in these patients is determined in large part by the intensity of the immunosuppression prescribed. The clinical importance of these warts goes well beyond the cosmetic. Particularly in sun-exposed areas, these warts can undergo malignant transformation, which is thought to be due to the combined effects of the virus, immunosuppression, and ultraviolet irradiation. A particular subgroup of papillomaviruses, the epidermodysplasia verruciformis-associated types, has been linked to the pathogenesis of cutaneous and anogenital squamous cell carcinomas in these patients. Finally, cervical papillomavirus, likewise, is more extensive in transplant recipients, is similarly modulated by the intensity of immunosuppressive therapy, and has been linked to the development of cervical cancer in both normal and immunosuppressed individuals (2,118–121).

Bacterial Infections in the Organ Transplant Recipient

Bacterial infections affecting the organ transplant recipient can be divided into four general categories (2):

1. Infection conveyed via a contaminated allograft. Although an uncommon problem, when present the vascular suture line is quite vulnerable, with the potential for the development of a mycotic aneurysm that is at risk for catastrophic rupture.
2. Infection related to technical/anatomic abnormalities created by misadventures in the operating room and/or the management of vascular access devices, an endotracheal tube, as well as drains and catheters that abridge or attenuate the protection provided by an intact mucocutaneous surface. Not surprisingly, conventional bacteria, particularly the Enterobacteriaceae, *P. aeruginosa*, *S. aureus*, as well as such antimicrobial-resistant organisms as methicillin-resistant staphylococci, vancomycin-resistant enterococci, and resistant gram-negative bacilli, are the major problem here.
3. Infection related to conditions present in the patient that lead to infection in any individual, but with greater impact on the transplant recipients. For example, the most important forms of GI tract bacterial infection occurring in transplant patients is *Clostridium difficile* colitis and diverticulitis. *C. difficile* colitis is both more common and more severe in the transplant recipients. Diverticulitis is very common, with a high rate of perforation and abscess formation. Whereas immunologically normal individuals with diverticulitis are usually treated medically with a first episode, surgical extirpation under coverage of appropriate antibiotics is the correct approach in the transplant recipient. In addition, the GI tract of transplant recipients is particularly susceptible to invasion by nontyphoidal salmonellae and *L. monocytogenes*. Both infections can present as acute diarrheal syndromes that progress to bacteremia, plus or minus metastatic infection quite quickly.
4. Infection caused by such atypical bacteria as *Nocardia* species and *Mycobacterium* species. Nocardial infection usually presents as a subacute chronic pulmonary syndrome, although it may be recognized first on the basis of such metastatic sites of infection as the skin, skeletal system, and the brain. In this respect, nocardial infection resembles the vascular invasive fungi (e.g., *Aspergillus, Fusarium, and Mucor*); dissemination is the rule, not the exception, and a careful metastatic workup is obligatory. Early diagnosis and therapy with high-dose TMP-SMX for a minimum period of 4 to 6 months has significant benefits for those individuals.

Mycobacterial infection remains a significant problem in organ transplant recipients for several reasons. It is much more common in these patients than in the general population. Antituberculosis therapy with the mycobacterial agents, isoniazid, rifampin, and pyrazinamide, which permit relatively short course therapy, is often difficult because of hepatic dysfunction and the effects of these agents on the metabolism of cyclosporine and tacrolimus. Unusual regimens (e.g., ofloxacin plus ethambutol) for longer durations (e.g., 2–3 years) will often be required in this population of patients. As with other forms of serious infection in transplant recipients, the attenuation of signs and symptoms due to the immunosuppressive (and antiinflammatory) drugs leads to more advanced disease and a higher microbial burden than in the general population. Also, the incidence of disseminated tuberculosis is far higher and should be carefully searched for. Clearly, active tuberculosis must be sought and aggressively treated; more controversial is the appropriate management of asymptomatic patients with positive tuberculin skin-test results. Our approach is not to use prophylaxis for patients whose only evidence of mycobacterial infection is a long-standing positive skin-test result and who can be followed closely clinically. Prophylaxis is prescribed for patients who have other risk factors such as non-white racial status, another immunosuppressing illness, protein-calorie malnutrition, a clearly abnormal chest radiograph, or a history of active tuberculosis.

Atypical mycobacterial infection has also been observed in transplant recipients: pulmonary, skin, skeletal, and disseminated infection due to *Mycobacterium kansasii*; pulmonary infection due to *Mycobacterium avian*; or isolated skin infection (usually after injury to the skin, often water immersion) by any of a variety of relatively less virulent mycobacterial species, including *Mycobacterium marinum, Mycobacterium haemophilum,* and *Mycobacterium chelonae*. Management of such infections often requires a combination approach: decreasing the dose of immunosuppressive drugs, surgical excision, and appropriate chemotherapy.

Fungal Infection

Two principal types of fungal infections affect transplant recipients: disseminated primary or reactivated infection with one of the geographically restricted systemic mycoses (histoplasmosis, blastomycosis, and coccidioidomycosis) and invasive infection by the opportunistic pathogens *Candida* species, *Aspergillus* species, *C. neoformans*, the Mucoraceae, and a group of fungi that are termed "new and emerging pathogens" (e.g., *Fusarium, Scedosporium,* and *Trichosporon*). Clinical syndromes that suggest the first category (in persons with a history of recent or remote epidemiologic exposure) include subacute respiratory illness, with focal, disseminated, or military infiltrates on chest radiographs; a nonspecific systemic febrile illness; unexplained pancytopenia; and an illness in which metastatic aspects of the infection predominate (e.g., mucocutaneous manifestations in histoplasmosis and blastomycosis or CNS manifestations in coccidioidomycosis or histoplasmosis). The management of one of the endemic mycoses has become standardized in recent years: induction therapy with an amphotericin preparation to "gain control" of the infection followed by long-term consolidation therapy with an azole administered orally. Presently available evidence shows that itraconazole is the azole of choice for the consolidation therapy of histoplasmosis and blastomycosis, with fluconazole being the choice for coccidioidomycosis. One caution that must be emphasized is that significant adjustment of cyclosporine and tacrolimus dosages will be required when the azole therapy is initiated, with an average decrease in dose of 75% or more required to keep blood levels in the therapeutic range and avoid nephrotoxicity and overimmunosuppression (2,4,5).

Far more common is infection with one of the opportunistic fungi. The following types of opportunistic fungal infection are observed in transplant recipients (2,5):

1. *P. carinii* pneumonia is the most common form of life-threatening fungal infection occurring in transplant recipients, with a frequency of 10% to 15% unless prophylaxis is administered to patients at high risk for this infection. High-risk groups for *Pneumocystis* infection include patients 1 to 6 months posttransplantation, especially those with immunomodulating viral infection; and the *chronic* n'er do wells more than 6 months after transplantation. In both these groups, low-dose TMP-SMX prophylaxis essentially eliminates not only this infection but also nocardiosis, listeriosis, urosepsis, and toxoplasmosis.

2. Infection with *Candida* species are extremely common in transplant recipients, ranging from relatively trivial mucocutaneous infections to bloodstream infections with potential for causing disseminated disease. The following syndromes merit special attention: bloodstream invasion, which carries a risk of more than 50% of metastatic seeding; secondary infection of fluid collections, whether these be blood, lymph, urine, or bile, and areas of devitalized tissue (all of these merit both systemic antifungal therapy in conjunction with drainage of these fluid collections and/or extirpation of the devitalized, infected tissue; candiduria, which, particularly in those with impaired bladder emptying, can lead to obstructing fungal balls at the ureteral-vesical junction, ascending infection, and pyelonephritis; and esophageal infection, which can be present in the absence of visible oropharyngeal infection. Each of these entities merit aggressive systemic antifungal treatment. In contrast, the identification of *Candida* species in the sputum does not connote either respiratory tract invasion or the need for antifungal therapy. Indeed, the biggest danger from respiratory tract colonization is that a greater density of organisms will be found on the skin, contributing to the occurrence of bloodstream infection through contamination of vascular access devices. The one exception to this observation occurs in lung transplantation, where respiratory tract candidal colonization poses a danger for the bronchial suture line and as a result merits aggressive treatment.

3. Invasive primary infection, usually of the lungs, but also the nasal sinuses and damaged skin, with *Aspergillus* species and such other vasculotropic molds as *Mucor, Scedosporium,* and *Fusarium.* The clinical effects of such invasion are largely due to the vascular tropism of these organisms, resulting in three events that are the hallmarks of these infections: infarction, hemorrhage, and bloodstream dissemination. *Aspergillus* species, particularly *Aspergillus fumigatus,* account for more than 90% of these infections, with a mortality rate higher than 50% being present among organ transplant recipients, largely due to delays in diagnosis such that 50% or more of these patients have disseminated disease at diagnosis. A variation on this theme is infection due to *C. neoformans,* which also has a pulmonary portal of entry, with spread to the brain and subarachnoid space being extremely common (*C. neoformans* infection is a much blander process than the other fungi listed, but clearly can produce metastatic infection not only to the CNS, but also to the skin, prostate gland, and skeletal system).

4. Sequential and concurrent secondary infections of technically compromised wounds and operative sites, the lungs, or infected vascular access with *Candida* or *Aspergillus* species.

The first principle of antifungal therapy is early diagnosis and treatment. Even better is to prevent infection with either prophylaxis or preemptive therapy. Recently, considerable progress has been made in the use of a fungal antigen-detection test and a PCR approach for monitoring patients for early infection, and then instituting preemptive therapy (2).

After many decades of being restricted to amphotericin therapy for serious infection, a number of new agents have been introduced that offer the promise of increased efficacy and fewer side effects. Thus, lipid-associated amphotericin products decrease the incidence and severity of both the initial fever and chills (the "cytokine storm") and the progressive renal dysfunction that occurs as a result of rejection. Efficacy among the various amphotericin preparations appears to be relatively the same, but with significant differences in price. Two new drugs have now been approved that hold significant promise for the

TABLE 126.4. Antifungal Drugs in the Treatment of Invasive Fungal Infection in the Organ Transplant Recipient

Type of infection	Initial (induction) therapy[a]	Consolidation therapy
Invasive candidiasis	Fluconazole (or amphotericin)	Fluconazole
Invasive aspergillosis	voriconazole	Voriconazole
Mucormycosis	Ultrahigh-dose amphotericin B[b]	Amphotericin B
Fusarium	Amphotericin B[b] or voriconazole	Voriconazole
Scedisporium	Amphotericin B[b] or voriconazole	Voriconazole
Coccidioidomycosis	Amphotericin B[b]	Fluconazole
Blastomycosis	Amphotericin B[b]	Itraconazole
Histoplasmosis	Amphotericin B[b]	Itraconazole
Cryptococcosis	Amphotericin + flucytosine	Fluconazole

[a]"Induction therapy" is initial therapy to "gain control" of the infection; it is always followed by oral consolidation therapy.
[b]Amphotericin B deoxycholate and lipid-associated amphotericin are currently thought to be equivalent in terms of efficacy, but with the lipid formulations having far less toxicity. Doses range from 0.75–1.0 mg/kg for candidal infection to 1.0–1.25 mg/kg for the rest of the infections, with the exception of mucormycosis in which the dose should be 1.5 mg/kg/d in conjunction with surgery.

management of fungal disease. Voriconazole, in a head-to-head comparison to amphotericin, was comparable in efficacy to AmBisome when used for empiric therapy in leukemic patients (122). Even more impressive was the clearcut improvement in patient survival seen in patients with invasive aspergillosis being treated with voriconazole, as opposed to amphotericin (123). Finally, caspofungin, the first of the echinocandins, has come to market. Although scant information has been developed, caspofungin appears promising for the treatment of both candidal and *Aspergillus* infection. Its mechanism of action (inhibition of the synthesis of the fungal cell wall through inhibition of glucan synthetase). Specific recommendations for antifungal therapy are delineated in Table 126.4.

Parasitic Infections

Two types of parasitic infection are of particular importance to the organ transplant recipient: the previously discussed *S. stercoralis* and toxoplasmosis. Although disseminated toxoplasmosis has been reported in recipients of kidney and liver transplants, it is a particular problem with heart transplantation. Transplantation of a heart from a donor who is seropositive for toxoplasmosis (connoting latent infection with this organism, particularly in the heart muscle) into a seronegative recipient is associated with a rate of disseminated toxoplasmosis in recipients. Such a syndrome has a particular clinical impact on the heart (myocarditis, which has been mistakenly diagnosed and treated as rejection, with disastrous consequences) and the brain (focal abscesses or diffuse encephalitis). It is now accepted practice to screen heart donors and recipients serologically for toxoplasmosis, and to give prophylaxis treatment to those patients at risk of primary disease with either TMP-SMX or the more traditional antitoxoplasmosis program of pyrimethamine and sulfasoxazole for a period of 3 to 6 months (2,4,5).

CONCLUSION

Considerable change has occurred in the field of transplant infectious disease over the past decade, and considerable change is on the horizon. The following summary statements should help us to approach the contemplated changes:

1. The interaction between epidemiologic exposures and the net state of immunosuppression will remain the basis for the clinician's approach to the infectious disease problems of the organ transplant recipient. The integration of these factors is well represented by the timetable of infection.
2. Whenever a new immunosuppressive program or agent is introduced, its effects on the incidence, severity, and nature of infection must be delineated with an eye for preventive strategies.
3. Antimicrobial therapy decisions in the organ transplant population are complex. In the future, there will be increasing interest in novel preemptive and therapeutic strategies, as opposed to empirical and prophylactic strategies.
4. The link between infection and rejection remains very strong, with cytokines and other mediators being the effectors of this link. New targeted strategies aimed at this link will be brought into clinical practice.
5. The future of transplantation will include donor-specific tolerance and xenotransplantation, each of which will encompass new infectious disease problems.
6. Most important, the rewards of caring for such courageous patients with a multidisciplinary team of colleagues remain unchanged. Insights gained in the care of these patients will continue to illuminate our thinking in other groups of patients, immunosuppressed and nonimmunosuppressed. To quote Winston Churchill, "It is not the beginning of the end; it is the end of the beginning."

REFERENCES

1. Hariharan S, Johnson CP, Bresnahan BA, et al. Improved graft survival after renal transplantation in the United States, 1988 to 1996 [see Comments]. *N Engl J Med* 2000;342:605–612.
2. Rubin R. Infection in the organ transplant recipient. In: Rubin RH, Young LS, eds. *Clinical approach to infection in the compromised host*, 4th ed. New York: Kluwer Academic/Plenum Publishers, 2002:573–679.
3. Sharing UNfO. Annual report, the U.S. Scientific Registry of Transplant Recipients and the Organ Procurement and Transplantation Network, 1999:7–8.
4. Rubin R, Ikonen T, Gummert J, et al. The therapeutic prescription for the organ transplant recipient: the linkage of immunosuppression and antimicrobial strategies. *Trans Infect Dis* 1999;1:29–39.
5. Fishman JA, Rubin RH. Infection in organ-transplant recipients [see Comments]. *N Engl J Med* 1998;338:1741–1751.
6. Rubin R. Infectious disease problems. In: Maddrey W, ed. *Current topics in gastroenterology: transplantation of the liver*. New York: Elsevier Science Publishing (in press).
7. Hopkins CC, Weber DJ, Rubin RH. Invasive aspergillus infection: possible non-ward common source within the hospital environment. *J Hosp Infect* 1989;13:19–25.
8. Rubin RH, Tolkoff-Rubin NE. Antimicrobial strategies in the care of organ transplant recipients. *Antimicrob Agents Chemother* 1993;37:619–624.
9. Rubin RH. Infectious disease complications of renal transplantation [Clinical Conference]. *Kidney Int* 1993;44:221–236.
10. Rubin RH, Wolfson JS, Cosimi AB, et al. Infection in the renal transplant recipient. *Am J Med* 1981;70:405–411.
11. Meier-Kriesche HU, Friedman G, Jacobs M, et al. Infectious complications in geriatric renal transplant patients: comparison of two immunosuppressive protocols. *Transplantation* 1999;68:1496–1502.
12. Meier-Kriesche HU, Ojo A, Magee JC, et al. African-American renal transplant recipients experience decreased risk of death due to infection: possible implications for immunosuppressive strategies. *Transplantation* 2000;70:375–379.
13. Tolkoff-Rubin N, Cosimi A, Russell P, et al. A controlled study of trimethoprim-sulfamethoxazole prophylaxis of urinary tract infections in renal transplant recipients. *Rev Infect Dis* 1982;4.
14. Fox BC, Sollinger HW, Belzer FO, et al. A prospective, randomized, double-blind study of trimethoprim-sulfamethoxazole for prophylaxis of infection in renal transplantation: clinical efficacy, absorption of trimethoprim-sulfamethoxazole, effects on the microflora, and the cost-benefit of prophylaxis. *Am J Med* 1990;89:255–274.
15. Maki DG, Fox BC, Kuntz J, et al. A prospective, randomized, double-blind study of trimethoprim-sulfamethoxazole for prophylaxis of infection in renal transplantation. Side effects of trimethoprim-sulfamethoxazole, interaction with cyclosporine. *J Lab Clin Med* 1992;119:11–24.
16. Sable CA, Hayden FG. Orthomyxoviral and paramyxoviral infections in transplant patients. *Infect Dis Clin North Am* 1995;9:987–1003.
17. Rabella N, Rodriguez P, Labeaga R, et al. Conventional respiratory viruses recovered from immunocompromised patients: clinical considerations. *Clin Infect Dis* 1999;28:1043–1048.
18. Krinzman S, Basgoz N, Kradin R, et al. Respiratory syncytial virus–associated infections in adult recipients of solid organ transplants. *J Heart Lung Transplant* 1998;17:202–210.
19. McGrath D, Falagas ME, Freeman R, et al. Adenovirus infection in adult orthotopic liver transplant recipients: incidence and clinical significance. *J Infect Dis* 1998;177:459–462.
20. Bridges ND, Spray TL, Collins MH, et al. Adenovirus infection in the lung results in graft failure after lung transplantation. *J Thorac Cardiovasc Surg* 1998;116:617–623.
21. Simsir A, Greenebaum E, Nuovo G, et al. Late fatal adenovirus pneumonitis in a lung transplant recipient. *Transplantation* 1998;65:592–594.
22. Ghosh S, Champlin R, Couch R, et al. Rhinovirus infections in myelosuppressed adult blood and marrow transplant recipients [see Comments]. *Clin Infect Dis* 1999;29:528–532.
23. Basgoz N, Hibberd P, Tolkoff-Rubin N, et al. Possible role of cytomegalovirus disease in the pathogenesis of post-transplant lymphoproliferative disorder. Paper presented at the American Society of Transplant Physicians, 12th Annual Meeting; Houston; 1993.
24. Manez R, Breinig MC, Linden P, et al. Posttransplant lymphoproliferative disease in primary Epstein-Barr virus infection after liver transplantation: the role of cytomegalovirus disease. *J Infect Dis* 1997;176:1462–1467.
25. Reinke P, Prosch S, Kern F, et al. Mechanisms of human cytomegalovirus (HCMV) (re)activation and its impact on organ transplant patients. *Trans Infect Dis* 1999;1:157–164.
26. Fietze E, Prosch S, Reinke P, et al. Cytomegalovirus infection in transplant recipients. The role of tumor necrosis factor. *Transplantation* 1994;58:675–680.

27. Stein J, Volk HD, Liebenthal C, et al. Tumour necrosis factor alpha stimulates the activity of the human cytomegalovirus major immediate early enhancer/promoter in immature monocytic cells. *J Gen Virol* 1993;74:2333–2338.

28. Prosch S, Staak K, Stein J, et al. Stimulation of the human cytomegalovirus IE enhancer/promoter in HL-60 cells by TNF-alpha is mediated via induction of NFκB. *Virology* 1995;208:107–116.

29. Docke WD, Prosch S, Fietze E, et al. Cytomegalovirus reactivation and tumour necrosis factor. *Lancet* 1994;343:268–269.

30. Mutimer D, Mirza D, Shaw J, et al. Enhanced (cytomegalovirus) viral replication associated with septic bacterial complications in liver transplant recipients. *Transplantation* 1997;63:1411–1415.

31. Mutimer DJ, Shaw J, O'Donnell K, et al. Enhanced (cytomegalovirus) viral replication after transplantation for fulminant hepatic failure [see Comments]. *Liver Transpl Surg* 1997;3:506–512.

32. Kutza AS, Muhl E, Hackstein H, et al. High incidence of active cytomegalovirus infection among septic patients [see Comments]. *Clin Infect Dis* 1998;26:1076–1082.

33. Betts RF, Freeman RB, Douglas RG Jr, et al. Transmission of cytomegalovirus infection with renal allograft. *Kidney Int* 1975;8:385–392.

34. Ho M, Suwansirikul S, Dowling JN, et al. The transplanted kidney as a source of cytomegalovirus infection. *N Engl J Med* 1975;293:1109–1112.

35. Suwansirikul S, Rao N, Dowling JN, et al. Primary and secondary cytomegalovirus infection. *Arch Intern Med* 1977;137:1026–1029.

36. Naraqi S, Jackson GG, Jonasson O, et al. Prospective study of prevalence, incidence, and source of herpesvirus infections in patients with renal allografts. *J Infect Dis* 1977;136:531–540.

37. Chou SW. Acquisition of donor strains of cytomegalovirus by renal-transplant recipients. *N Engl J Med* 1986;314:1418–1423.

38. Grundy JE, Super M, Lui S, et al. The source of cytomegalovirus infection in seropositive renal allograft recipients is frequently the donor kidney. *Transplant Proc* 1987;19:2126–2128.

39. Grundy JE, Lui SF, Super M, et al. Symptomatic cytomegalovirus infection in seropositive kidney recipients: reinfection with donor virus rather than reactivation of recipient virus. *Lancet* 1988;2:132–135.

40. Rubin R, Colvin R. The impact of CMV infections on renal transplantation. In: Racusen L, Solez K, Burdick J, eds. *Kidney transplant rejection.* New York: Marcel Dekker, 1998:605–626.

41. Rubin R, Kemmerly S, Conti D, et al. Prevention of primary cytomegalovirus disease in organ transplant recipients. *Trans Infect Dis* 2000;2:112–117.

42. Rubin RH. The indirect effects of cytomegalovirus infection on the outcome of organ transplantation. *JAMA* 1989;261:3607–3609.

43. Rubin RH. Cytomegalovirus disease and allograft loss after organ transplantation [Editorial; Comment]. *Clin Infect Dis* 1998;26:871–873.

44. Grattan MT, Moreno-Cabral CE, Starnes VA, et al. Cytomegalovirus infection is associated with cardiac allograft rejection and atherosclerosis. *JAMA* 1989;261:3561–3566.

45. Tolkoff-Rubin NE, Rubin RH. Recent advances in the diagnosis and management of infection in the organ transplant recipient. *Semin Nephrol* 2000;20:148–163.

46. Lowance D, Neumayer HH, Legendre CM, et al. Valacyclovir for the prevention of cytomegalovirus disease after renal transplantation. International Valacyclovir Cytomegalovirus Prophylaxis Transplantation Study Group [see Comments]. *N Engl J Med* 1999;340:1462–1470.

47. Valantine HA, Gao SZ, Menon SG, et al. Impact of prophylactic immediate posttransplant ganciclovir on development of transplant atherosclerosis: a post hoc analysis of a randomized, placebo-controlled study. *Circulation* 1999;100:61–66.

48. Valantine H. Role of CMV in transplant coronary artery disease and survival after heart transplantation. *Transpl Infect Dis* 1999;25–30.

49. Pescovitz MD, Pruett TL, Gonwa T, et al. Oral ganciclovir dosing in transplant recipients and dialysis patients based on renal function. *Transplantation* 1998;66:1104–1107.

50. Pescovitz M. Oral ganciclovir and pharmacokinetics of valganciclovir in liver transplant recipients. *Transpl Infect Dis* 1999;1[Suppl 1]:31–34.

51. Hibberd PL, Tolkoff-Rubin NE, Cosimi AB, et al. Symptomatic cytomegalovirus disease in the cytomegalovirus antibody seropositive renal transplant recipient treated with OKT3. *Transplantation* 1992;53:68–72.

52. Fishman JA, Doran MT, Volpicelli SA, et al. Dosing of intravenous ganciclovir for the prophylaxis and treatment of cytomegalovirus infection in solid organ transplant recipients. *Transplantation* 2000;69:389–394.

53. Turgeon N, Fishman JA, Basgoz N, et al. Effect of oral acyclovir or ganciclovir therapy after preemptive intravenous ganciclovir therapy to prevent cytomegalovirus disease in cytomegalovirus seropositive renal and liver transplant recipients receiving antilymphocyte antibody therapy. *Transplantation* 1998;66:1780–1786.

54. Kruger RM, Shannon WD, Arens MQ, et al. The impact of ganciclovir-resistant cytomegalovirus infection after lung transplantation. *Transplantation* 1999;68:1272–1279.

55. Bienvenu B, Thervet E, Bedrossian J, et al. Development of cytomegalovirus resistance to ganciclovir after oral maintenance treatment in a renal transplant recipient. *Transplantation* 2000;69:182–184.

56. Alain S, Honderlick P, Grenet D, et al. Failure of ganciclovir treatment associated with selection of a ganciclovir-resistant cytomegalovirus strain in a lung transplant recipient. *Transplantation* 1997;63:1533–1536.

57. Tanner J, Alfieri C. The Epstein-Barr virus and post-transplant lymphoproliferative disease: interplay of immunosuppression, EBV, and the immune system in disease pathogenesis. *Transpl Infect Dis* 2001;3:60–69.

58. Herbert D, Sullivan E. Malignancy and post-transplant lymphoproliferative disorder (PTLD) in pediatric renal transplant recipients: a report of the North American Pediatric Transplant Cooperative Study Group (NAPRTCS). *Pediatr Transplant* 1998;2:57.

59. Stephaman E, Gruber S, Dunn D, et al. Posttransplant lymphoproliferative disorders. *Transplant Rev* 1991;5:120–129.

60. Mutimer D, Kaur N, Tang H, et al. Quantitation of Epstein-Barr virus DNA in the blood of adult liver transplant recipients. *Transplantation* 2000;69:954–959.

61. Preiksaitis J. Epstein-Barr virus infection and malignancy in solid organ transplant recipients: strategies for prevention and treatment. *Transpl Infect Dis* 2001;3:56–59.

62. Preiksaitis JK, Diaz-Mitoma F, Mirzayans F, et al. Quantitative oropharyngeal Epstein-Barr virus shedding in renal and cardiac transplant recipients: relationship to immunosuppressive therapy, serologic responses, and the risk of posttransplant lymphoproliferative disorder. *J Infect Dis* 1992;166:986–994.

63. Harris NL, Jaffe ES, Stein H, et al. A revised European-American classification of lymphoid neoplasms: a proposal from the International Lymphoma Study Group [see Comments]. *Blood* 1994;84:1361–1392.

64. Harris NL, Ferry JA, Swerdlow SH. Posttransplant lymphoproliferative disorders: summary of Society for Hematopathology Workshop. *Semin Diagn Pathol* 1997;14:8–14.

65. Nalesnik M. The diverse pathology of post-transplant lymphoproliferative disorder: importance of a standardized approach. *Transpl Infect Dis* 2001;3:88–96.

66. Green M, Reyes J, Webber S, et al. The role of viral load in the diagnosis, management, and possible prevention of Epstein-Barr virus–associated post-transplant lymphoproliferative disease following solid organ transplantation. *Transpl Infect Dis* 2001;3:97–103.

67. Rowe D, Webber S, Shauer E, et al. Epstein-Barr virus load monitoring: its role in the prevention and management of post-transplant lymphoproliferative disease. *Transpl Infect Dis* 2001;3:79–87.

68. Crawford DH, Sweny P, Edwards JM, et al. Long-term T-cell–mediated immunity to Epstein-Barr virus in renal-allograft recipients receiving cyclosporin A. *Lancet* 1981;1:10–12.

69. Bird AG, McLachlan SM, Britton S. Cyclosporin A promotes spontaneous outgrowth in vitro of Epstein-Barr virus–induced B-cell lines. *Nature* 1981;289:300–301.

70. Oertel SH, Ruhnke MS, Anagnostopoulos I, et al. Treatment of Epstein-Barr virus–induced posttransplantation lymphoproliferative disorder with foscarnet alone in an adult after simultaneous heart and renal transplantation. *Transplantation* 1999;67:765–767.

71. Green M, Reyes J, Webber S, et al. The role of antiviral and immunoglobulin therapy in the prevention of Epstein-Barr virus infection and post-transplant lymphoproliferative disease following solid organ transplantation. *Transpl Infect Dis* 2001;3:97–103.

72. Hanto DW, Frizzera G, Gajl-Peczalska KJ, et al. Epstein-Barr virus–induced B-cell lymphoma after renal transplantation: acyclovir therapy and transition from polyclonal to monoclonal B-cell proliferation. *N Engl J Med* 1982;306:913–918.

73. Pirsch JD, Stratta RJ, Sollinger HW, et al. Treatment of severe Epstein-Barr virus–induced lymphoproliferative syndrome with ganciclovir: two cases after solid organ transplantation. *Am J Med* 1989;86:241–244.

74. Rooney CM, Smith CA, Ng CY, et al. Use of gene-modified virus–specific T lymphocytes to control Epstein-Barr virus–related lymphoproliferation. *Lancet* 1995;345:9–13.

75. Oertel SH, Anagnostopoulos I, Bechstein WO, et al. Treatment of posttransplant lymphoproliferative disorder with the anti-CD20 monoclonal antibody rituximab alone in an adult after liver transplantation: a new drug in therapy of patients with posttransplant lymphoproliferative disorder after solid organ transplantation? *Transplantation* 2000;69:430–432.

76. Durandy A. Anti-B cell and anti-cytokine therapy for the treatment of posttransplant lymphoproliferative disorder: past, present, and future. *Transpl Infect Dis* 2001;3:104–107.

77. Fischer A, Blanche S, Le Bidois J, et al. Anti–B-cell monoclonal antibodies in the treatment of severe B-cell lymphoproliferative syndrome following bone marrow and organ transplantation. *N Engl J Med* 1991;324:1451–1456.

78. Singh N. Human herpesviruses-6, -7, and -8 in organ transplant recipients. *Clin Microbial Infect* 2000;6:453–459.

79. Agut H. Puzzles concerning the pathogenicity of human herpesvirus 6 [Editorial; Comments]. *N Engl J Med* 1993;329:203–204.

80. Flamand L, Gosselin J, Stefanescu I, et al. Immunosuppressive effect of human herpesvirus 6 on T-cell functions: suppression of interleukin-2 synthesis and cell proliferation [published erratum in *Blood* 1995;85:1263–1271]. *Blood* 1995;86(1):418.

81. Carrigan DR, Knox KK. Human herpesvirus 6 (HHV-6) isolation from bone marrow: HHV-6–associated bone marrow suppression in bone marrow transplant patients [see Comments]. *Blood* 1994;84:3307–3310.

82. Oren I, Sobel JD. Human herpesvirus type 6: review. *Clin Infect Dis* 1992;14:741–746.

83. McCullers JA, Lakeman FD, Whitley RJ. Human herpesvirus 6 is associated with focal encephalitis. *Clin Infect Dis* 1995;21:571–576.

84. Ward KN, Gray JJ, Efstathiou S. Brief report: primary human herpesvirus 6 infection in a patient following liver transplantation from a seropositive donor. *J Med Virol* 1989;28:69–72.

85. Singh N, Paterson DL. Encephalitis caused by human herpesvirus-6 in transplant recipients: relevance of a novel neurotropic virus. *Transplantation* 2000;69:2474–2479.

86. Dockrell DH, Smith TF, Paya CV. Human herpesvirus 6. *Mayo Clin Proc* 1999; 74:163–170.

87. Griffiths PD, Ait-Khaled M, Bearcroft CP, et al. Human herpesviruses 6 and 7 as potential pathogens after liver transplant: prospective comparison with the effect of cytomegalovirus. *J Med Virol* 1999;59:496–501.

88. Lynfield R, Herrin JT, Rubin RH. Varicella in pediatric renal transplant recipients. *Pediatrics* 1992;90:216–220.

89. McGregor RS, Zitelli BJ, Urbach AH, et al. Varicella in pediatric orthotopic liver transplant recipients. *Pediatrics* 1989;83:256–261.

90. Cohen JI, Brunell PA, Straus SE, et al. Recent advances in varicella-zoster virus infection. *Ann Intern Med* 1999;130:922–932.

91. Scullard GH, Smith CI, Merigan TC, et al. Effects of immunosuppressive therapy on viral markers in chronic active hepatitis B. *Gastroenterology* 1981;81:987–991.

92. Marinos G, Rossol S, Carucci P, et al. Immunopathogenesis of hepatitis B virus recurrence after liver transplantation. *Transplantation* 2000;69:559–568.

93. Huang CC, Lai MK, Fong MT. Hepatitis B liver disease in cyclosporine-treated renal allograft recipients. *Transplantation* 1990;49:540–544.

94. Rao KV, Andersen RC. Long-term results and complications in renal transplant recipients. Observations in the second decade. *Transplantation* 1988;45:45–52.

95. Jarvis B, Faulds D. Lamivudine. A review of its therapeutic potential in chronic hepatitis B [published erratum in *Drugs* Oct1999;58(4):587]. *Drugs* 1999; 58:101–141.

96. Ben-Ari Z, Shmueli D, Mor E, et al. Beneficial effect of lamivudine in recurrent hepatitis B after liver transplantation. *Transplantation* 1997;63:393–396.

97. Rostaing L, Henry S, Cisterne JM, et al. Efficacy and safety of lamivudine on replication of recurrent hepatitis B after cadaveric renal transplantation. *Transplantation* 1997;64:1624–1627.

98. Al Faraidy K, Yoshida EM, Davis JE, et al. Alteration of the dismal natural history of fibrosing cholestatic hepatitis secondary to hepatitis B virus with the use of lamivudine. *Transplantation* 1997;64:926–928.

99. Jain A, Demetris AJ, Manez R, et al. Incidence and severity of acute allograft rejection in liver transplant recipients treated with alfa interferon. *Liver Transpl Surg* 1998;4:197–203.

100. Andreone P, Caraceni P, Grazi GL, et al. Lamivudine treatment for acute hepatitis B after liver transplantation. *J Hepatol* 1998;29:985–989.

101. Nery JR, Weppler D, Rodriguez M, et al. Efficacy of lamivudine in controlling hepatitis B virus recurrence after liver transplantation. *Transplantation* 1998;65:1615–1621.

102. Gauthier J, Bourne EJ, Lutz MW, et al. Quantitation of hepatitis B viremia and emergence of YMDD variants in patients with chronic hepatitis B treated with lamivudine. *J Infect Dis* 1999;180:1757–1762.

103. Seehofer D, Rayes N, Berg T, et al. Lamivudine as first- and second-line treatment of hepatitis B infection after liver transplantation. *Transpl Int* 2000; 13:290–296.

104. Puchhammer-Stockl E, Mandl CW, Kletzmayr J, et al. Monitoring the virus load can predict the emergence of drug-resistant hepatitis B virus strains in renal transplantation patients during lamivudine therapy. *J Infect Dis* 2000; 181:2063–2066.

105. Fontaine H, Thiers V, Chretien Y, et al. HBV genotypic resistance to lamivudine in kidney recipients and hemodialyzed patients. *Transplantation* 2000;69:2090–2094.

106. Malkan G, Cattral MS, Humar A, et al. Lamivudine for hepatitis B in liver transplantation: a single-center experience. *Transplantation* 2000;69:1403–1407.

107. Yoshida EM, Erb SR, Partovi N, et al. Liver transplantation for chronic hepatitis B infection with the use of combination lamivudine and low-dose hepatitis B immune globulin. *Liver Transpl Surg* 1999;5:520–525.

108. Bain V. Hepatitis B in transplantation. *Transpl Infect Dis* 2000;2:153–165.

109. McCaughan G, Zekry A. Effects of immunosuppression and organ transplantation on the natural history and immunopathogenesis of hepatitis C virus infection. *Transpl Infect Dis* 2000;2.

110. Liang TJ, Rehermann B, Seeff LB, et al. Pathogenesis, natural history, treatment, and prevention of hepatitis C. *Ann Intern Med* 2000;132:296–305.

111. Charlton M, Seaberg E, Wiesner R, et al. Predictors of patient and graft survival following liver transplantation for hepatitis C. *Hepatology* 1998;28:823–830.

112. Rosen HR, Chou S, Corless CL, et al. Cytomegalovirus viremia: risk factor for allograft cirrhosis after liver transplantation for hepatitis C. *Transplantation* 1997;64:721–726.

113. Bizollon T, Palazzo U, Ducerf C, et al. Pilot study of the combination of interferon alfa and ribavirin as therapy of recurrent hepatitis C after liver transplantation [see Comments]. *Hepatology* 1997;26:500–504.

114. Cheeseman SH, Black PH, Rubin RH, et al. Interferon and BK Papovavirus—clinical and laboratory studies. *J Infect Dis* 1980;141:157–161.

115. Hogan TF, Borden EC, McBain JA, et al. Human polyomavirus infections with JC virus and BK virus in renal transplant patients. *Ann Intern Med* 1980;92:373–378.

116. Narayan O, Penney JB Jr, Johnson RT, et al. Etiology of progressive multifocal leukoencephalopathy. Identification of papovavirus. *N Engl J Med* 1973;289:1278–1282.

117. Howell DN, Smith SR, Butterly DW, et al. Diagnosis and management of BK polyomavirus interstitial nephritis in renal transplant recipients. *Transplantation* 1999;68:1279–1288.

118. Wolfson JS, Sober AJ, Rubin RH. Dermatologic manifestations of infections in immunocompromised patients. *Medicine (Baltimore)* 1985;64:115–133.

119. Ostrow RS, Bender M, Niimura M, et al. Human papillomavirus DNA in cutaneous primary and metastasized squamous cell carcinomas from patients with epidermodysplasia verruciformis. *Proc Natl Acad Sci U S A* 1982;79:1634–1638.

120. Hopfl R, Bens G, Wieland U, et al. Human papillomavirus DNA in nonmelanoma skin cancers of a renal transplant recipient: detection of a new sequence related to epidermodysplasia verruciformis associated types. *J Invest Dermatol* 1997;108:53–56.

121. Arends MJ, Benton EC, McLaren KM, et al. Renal allograft recipients with high susceptibility to cutaneous malignancy have an increased prevalence of human papillomavirus DNA in skin tumours and a greater risk of anogenital malignancy. *Br J Cancer* 1997;75:722–728.

122. Walsh TJ, Pappas P, Winston DJ, et al. Voriconazole compared with liposomal amphotericin B for empirical antifungal therapy in patients with neutropenia and persistent fever. *N Engl J Med* 2002;346:225–234.

123. Herbrecht R, Denning DW, Patterson TF. Randomized comparison of voriconazole and amphotericin B in primary therapy of invasive aspergillosis. *N Engl J Med* 2002;347:408–415.

CHAPTER 127

Infections Associated with Bone Marrow Transplantation

Joan Mannick and Richard T. Ellison, III

Bone marrow transplantation with intravenous infusion of bone marrow stem cells was first attempted in humans in 1939 and was successfully performed in the 1960s (1). As knowledge developed regarding the supportive and immunosuppressive approaches necessary for success, bone marrow transplantation became an established clinical therapy in the 1970s. Now approximately 15,000 transplantations are performed yearly (2). Three basic forms of bone marrow transplantation are performed. *Syngeneic* transplantation involves the infrequent circumstance of transplantation of bone marrow from a genetically identical twin and is a preferred option when feasible. *Autologous* transplantation involves the transplantation of the recipient's own bone marrow that has been harvested before the patient has undergone bone marrow ablative treatment. This therapeutic approach allows the administration of otherwise lethal doses of chemotherapy and radiation therapy for the treatment of different forms of neoplasia. *Allogeneic* transplantation involves the transplantation of bone marrow from a human leukocyte antigen (HLA)–matched nonidentical donor. Whenever possible, allogenic transplantation is performed with an HLA-matched sibling donor to decrease the risk of graft-versus-host disease (GVHD). Less desirable options are transplantation from an unrelated closely HLA-matched donor or from a relative with a partial HLA match.

There are significant differences in the relative risks of autologous and allogenic transplantation. Because there is no risk of GVHD, the degree of immunosuppression is less with autologous transplantation. GVHD is the most serious complication arising from allogenic transplantation. This primarily presents with skin disease, gastrointestinal (GI) tract disease, and hepatitis (Table 127.1). However, GVHD is also accompanied by

TABLE 127.1. Clinical Classification of Acute Graft-versus-Host Disease

	Organ injury		
Level of injury	Skin	Liver (bilirubin)	Gastrointestinal tract
1	Maculopapular rash on <25% of body surface	2–3 mg/dL	500–1,000 mL liquid stool per day
2	Maculopapular rash on 25%–50% of body surface	>3–6 mg/dL	>1,000 and <1,500 mL liquid stool per day
3	Generalized erythroderma	>6–15 mg/dL	>1,500 mL liquid stool per day
4	Generalized erythroderma with formation of bullae and desquamation	>15 mg/dL	Severe abdominal pain with or without ileus

	Level of injury		
Clinical grade[a]	Skin	Liver	Gastrointestinal tract
I	1 or 2	0	0
II	1–3	1	1
III	2 or 3	2 or 3	2 or 3
IV	2–4	2–4	2–4

[a]A grade of II or higher requires skin injury plus liver or intestinal injury or both. A grade of IV requires an extreme decrease in performance status.
Source: Adapted from Armitage SO. Bone marrow transplantation. *N Engl J Med* 1994;330:827–838, with permission.

profound immunosuppression and increases the risk of infectious complications.

The risk of infection for the transplant recipient follows directly from the loss and reconstitution of various components of host defenses (1,3). The sequence of immune injury and gradual recovery gives a temporal pattern to the infectious and noninfectious complications of transplantation (Table 127.2).

INFECTION DURING THE IMMEDIATE TRANSPLANT PERIOD

Patients undergoing transplantation are typically at some risk of developing systemic or localized infection based on their underlying disease. Once the transplantation procedure is initiated, all bone marrow transplant recipients are at significantly increased risk of infection during a period of profound leukopenia

TABLE 127.2. Temporal Pattern of Infectious and Noninfectious Complications of Bone Marrow Transplantation

	Preengraftment (0–30 days)	Early postengraftment (31–100 days)	Late postengraftment (100+ days)
Host defense defect	Neutropenia, mucositis, indwelling venous catheters	Acute GVHD, defects in humoral and cell-mediated immunity, indwelling venous catheters	Chronic GVHD, delay in development of humoral and cell-mediated immunity
Bacterial infections	*Staphylococcus aureus, Pseudomonas aeruginosa,* viridans streptococci	Coagulase-negative staphylococci	Encapsulated bacteria (*S. pneumoniae, H. influenzae*)
Fungal infections	*Candida* species *Aspergillus* species *Candida glabrata*[a] *Mucorales* species *Fusanum* species[a] *Pityrosporum* species[a]	*Candida* species *Aspergillus* species *Cryptococcus neoformans*[a] *Histoplasma capsulatum*[a] *Coccidioides immitis*[a]	*Candida* species *Aspergillus* species
Viral infections	HSV Adenovirus[a] Rotavirus[a] Coxsackie virus[a]	CMV HSV[a] Adenovirus[a] BK virus[a] Respiratory syncytial virus[a] Parainfluenza virus[a]	Varicella-zoster virus
Other infections		*Pneumocystis carinii* toxoplasmosis Nocardiosis	

[a]Uncommon pathogens that may occur in these time periods.
CHV, cytomegalovirus; GVHD, graft-versus-host disease; HSV, herpes simplex virus.

with both absolute neutropenia and lymphocytopenia. The duration of leukopenia will depend on the conditioning regimen used, the use of *ex vivo* marrow treatments to prevent GVHD, and whether colony-stimulating factors are used (4,5). It typically lasts approximately 3 to 4 weeks. The major risk of infection begins to resolve as the neutrophil count increases. Still, *in vitro* studies have shown that qualitative defects in neutrophil and macrophage function persist even though there is a quantitative recovery in circulating cells (3,6,7). Additionally, B-cell and CD4$^+$ T-lymphocyte cell number and function appear to remain dysfunctional for up to a year after the transplantation (3,8).

Other major predisposing factors for infection in this period include the presence of indwelling intravenous catheters and damage to the oropharyngeal and GI tract mucosal surfaces, arising as a complication of conditioning radiation and chemotherapy. Xerostomia, increased mucus production, and reactivated herpes simplex infections also contribute to oral mucosal injury, which occurs in approximately 70% of allogenic transplant recipients (2).

Bacterial Infections

During this period of severe immunodeficiency, the major infectious complications are bacteremia, fungal infections with *Candida* and *Aspergillus,* and recurrent herpes infections. Bacterial infections are the most common identified illnesses, and the spectrum of pathogens is comparable to other neutropenic hosts. They consist predominantly of Enterobacteriaceae and *Pseudomonas aeruginosa* from the GI tract, and gram-positive organisms (*Staphylococcus aureus*, coagulase-negative staphylococci, and viridans streptococci) from the skin, indwelling catheters, and oropharynx. The exact spectrum of organisms and their patterns of antimicrobial susceptibility vary significantly from one institution to another, and selection of empiric antimicrobial therapy should be based on the epidemiology of the individual transplant center. Infection caused by anaerobic organisms is infrequent, as are bacterial pneumonias in the absence of bacteremia (9). Infectious gastroenteritis may occur due to adenovirus, rotavirus, coxsackievirus, and *Clostridium difficile* (10). These gastroenteric infections can be quite prolonged and are associated with an increased mortality rate.

The general approach to management of bacterial infections is comparable to that of other neutropenic patients, with empiric antibiotic therapy directed against the predominant pathogens initiated after the collection of appropriate samples for microbiologic cultures. During the past several years, there has been both a decrease in the incidence of bacteremia and a shift from a predominance of infections with *S. aureus* and gram-negative bacilli to disease caused by coagulase-negative staphylococci and viridans streptococci (2,11). These shifts appear to be related to improved supportive care, the general use of prophylactic antibiotic therapy, and the greater reliance on indwelling catheters. A number of different empiric antibiotic regimens can be used when patients have fever and there are no localizing signs or symptoms. Appropriate regimens that have been found to be effective include (a) an aminoglycoside and an antipseudomonal β-lactam antibiotic (e.g., mezlocillin, azlocillin, piperacillin, or ceftazidime); (b) monotherapy with ceftazidime or imipenem-cilastatin; (c) vancomycin plus an aminoglycoside and an antipseudomonal penicillin (or third-generation cephalosporin); and (d) the use of an antipseudomonal ureidopenicillin and an antipseudomonal third-generation cephalosporin (12). The choice of any specific regimen should be based on knowledge of a center's own microbiologic epidemiology. If a patient continues to be febrile for 3 days, a reevaluation of the patient should take place and modification of antibiotic therapy considered. If unexplained fever persists for 7 days, then amphotericin B therapy should be initiated to treat for occult fungal disease (12).

Fungal Infections

Infections caused by fungi also often occur in this immediate posttransplantation period before engraftment, predominantly due to *Candida* or *Aspergillus* species. Hepatosplenic candidiasis is an increasingly recognized complication arising from seeding of the portal circulation with *Candida* after GI tract mucosal injury. This syndrome presents with fever, hepatosplenomegaly, and an elevated alkaline phosphatase level as the neutrophil count begins to normalize (13). Multiple round defects are demonstrable in the liver and spleen by hepatic ultrasound or computed tomographic (CT) evaluation. Fluconazole has been shown to be an alternative agent for the treatment of candidemia in the nonimmunocompromised patient, but its therapeutic efficacy for this infection remains undefined in the transplant recipient (14). *Aspergillus* is the other fungus commonly causing infection during periods of profound neutropenia; less commonly, infections occur with Mucorales (including *Mucor* and *Rhizopus*), *Fusarium, Trichosporon, Pityrosporum,* and other soil saprophytic fungi (15–18). The incidence of invasive *Aspergillus* increases greatly in patients with neutropenia persisting longer than 21 days; infection usually involves the sinuses, lungs, or central nervous system (CNS) and blood cultures are rarely positive (2,19). Voriconazole is now the drug of choice for treatment of invasive fungal disease even though the use of cyclosporine and other nephrotoxic drugs complicates treatment in allogenic transplant recipients (19a). Amphotericin B can also be used to treat invasive aspergillosis, although the mortality rate associated with this infection remains high (19,20).

Viral Infections

Before the use of acyclovir prophylaxis, there was a 75% incidence of herpes simplex virus (HSV) reactivation in seropositive marrow transplant recipients during the early posttransplantation period, correlating with suppression in HSV-specific immunity (2,21). Reactivation characteristically occurred with oral or genital lesions, although the appearance was often atypical. HSV reactivation could be complicated by HSV esophagitis, HSV pneumonitis, or bacterial superinfection. The incidence of these complications is substantially decreased by routine acyclovir prophylaxis (200 mg orally three times a day) (22,23).

During this period, serious infections can also develop due to community-acquired respiratory viruses (CRVs) including influenza A and B, respiratory syncytial virus (RSV), parainfluenza, and adenoviruses (24,25). Illness can progress from mild upper respiratory tract infections to diffuse interstitial pneumonia. Because potentially effective therapy exists for influenza and RSV disease, efforts should be undertaken to define the precise cause of these infections with viral culture of upper respiratory tract secretions, and as necessary pulmonary secretions. The neuraminidase inhibitors oseltamivir and zanamivir have activity against both influenza A and B, and rimantadine and amantadine are active against influenza A. Uncontrolled studies suggest that aerosolized ribavirin given in conjunction with RSV hyperimmunoglobulin may have efficacy against RSV pneumonia (26).

Antimicrobial Prophylaxis

Several modalities have been used to prevent infection in marrow transplant recipients in this time period with varying results (5). Prophylactic oral and systemic antibiotics are used commonly. Trimethoprim-sulfamethoxazole (160/800 mg orally daily or three times weekly in adults) during the time of immunosuppression will decrease the risk of *Pneumocystis carinii* pneumonia (27). Oral quinolone prophylaxis may reduce bacteremia rates but has not been shown to decrease mortality (28,29). In a randomized placebo-controlled trial, fluconazole given 400 mg per day from the time of transplantation until day 75 increased survival, decreased gut GVHD, and protected against disseminated candidal infections and candidiasis-related death (30). In selected institutions where fluconazole prophylaxis has been used routinely, there has been the emergence of infections due to fluconazole-resistant organisms including *Candida krusei* and fluconazole-resistant *Candida albicans*. Fluconazole prophylaxis does not protect against *Aspergillus* infection, which has become the fungal infection found most often at autopsy in bone marrow transplant recipients (31). Chemoprophylaxis with rimantadine for influenza A only or a neuraminidase inhibitor could be considered during community-acquired influenza outbreaks, although the safety and efficacy of this approach remain undefined (23).

INFECTION EARLY AFTER TRANSPLANT ENGRAFTMENT (DAYS 30 TO 100)

Host Defense Defects

Once marrow engraftment occurs, the risk of infection associated with leukopenia decreases significantly, as does the incidence of serious HSV mucosal infection. However, there are still profound abnormalities in host defense mechanisms, and the kinetics of immune reconstitution follow normal immune ontogeny (3,9). The more general early immune mechanisms such as cytotoxic and phagocytic cells recover first, followed by the more specialized humoral and cell-mediated immune systems. Multiple defects exist in the function of effector and accessory cells, as well as in cytokine regulation. There are prolonged delays in the development of antibody production to specific antigens, as well as in the development of antigen-specific T-cell responses. The response to some antigens appears to require reexposure in the form of active infection for reconstitution (21). Another major factor that influences the rate of full immunologic recovery is the occurrence of acute GVHD, which directly prolongs the period of immunosuppression. Moreover, all of the therapeutic interventions used to treat GVHD suppress the cell-mediated immune response (16,32). The damage that acute GVHD does to the integrity of the skin and GI tract mucosa further predisposes the patient to bacterial and fungal infection. In addition, acute GVHD appears to alter neutrophil function (6).

Bacterial, Fungal, and Parasitic Infections

Infections caused by bacteria, fungi, protozoa, and viruses can all occur during this period after transplantation. Bacterial disease typically occurs either as a complication of indwelling central venous catheters or a complication of GVHD-mediated skin or GI tract damage. The same spectrum of nosocomial bacterial pathogens that cause illness during the neutropenic period can produce illness early in this period, although overwhelming infection is unusual except in patients with severe GVHD, graft rejection, or graft failure (9). Fungal infections continue to be common with the predominant pathogens remaining, *Candida* and *Aspergillus* species. Systemic aspergillosis usually arises slightly later in the course than candidal disease; the median onset is 6 to 8 weeks after transplant (9). Aspergillosis occurs more commonly in allogenic than autologous transplant recipients, related to the greater degree of immunosuppression. Infections with *Cryptococcus neoformans* and the focally endemic fungi *Histoplasma capsulatum* and *Coccidioides immitis* also occur occasionally. *P. carinii* pneumonia can occur in this period, but its incidence has decreased dramatically with the standard use of prophylaxis with trimethoprim-sulfamethoxazole (27). Cerebral toxoplasmosis can also be seen less commonly in patients with severe acute GVHD; it typically presents as an intracranial lesion with headache, focal neurologic findings, and an intracerebral ring-enhancing lesion on CT or magnetic resonance imaging studies.

Viral Infections

Infections with deoxyribonucleic acid (DNA) viruses also become a significant concern early after transplant engraftment. Cytomegalovirus (CMV) is the most common cause of severe viral disease in the transplant recipient (33). The patients at highest risk of CMV disease are the CMV-positive recipients, followed by the CMV-negative recipients with a CMV-seropositive donor. The clinical manifestations of CMV infection are quite diverse in the transplant recipient and include persistent unexplained fever, leukopenia, thrombocytopenia, esophagitis, gastroenteritis, retinitis, hepatitis, polyarthritis, CNS disease, and pneumonia. Of these syndromes, the most serious is CMV pneumonia. Despite advances in therapy, the mortality rate of this illness remains approximately 50%. It develops in 15% to 25% of seropositive allogenic transplant recipients and 1% to 2% of autologous transplant recipients, and it may be more common in seropositive patients receiving antithymocyte globulin (34,35). The high frequency of CMV pneumonia in transplant recipients with GVHD in comparison to its rarity in patients with the acquired immunodeficiency syndrome (AIDS) has suggested that the pulmonary disease is mediated by an aberrant immunopathogenic response and not by direct viral injury (36). In support of this premise, treatment of CMV pneumonia with ganciclovir therapy alone has little effect, whereas combined therapy with both ganciclovir and intravenous CMV immune globulin has reduced mortality from 85% to 50% (37). Foscarnet is a second antiviral agent effective for treatment of CMV disease, but its relative utility in the management of transplant recipients remains undefined except for the treatment of ganciclovir-resistant CMV infection.

CMV is the most common cause of severe gastroenteritis after marrow transplantation, usually presenting with protracted nausea, vomiting, or diarrhea; esophageal involvement is characterized by dysphagia and retrosternal pain. However, the incidence of CMV colitis, retinitis, and CNS infection is lower than that in patients with AIDS.

To prevent CMV disease in seronegative patients, CMV-seronegative or leukocyte-filtered blood products should be used (38). In addition, preemptive or prophylactic ganciclovir therapy (5 mg/kg per dose every 12 hours for 7–14 days, then 5 mg/kg per day) reduces the rate of symptomatic CMV disease in seropositive allogenic marrow transplant recipients, although the treatment is complicated by neutropenia (23,39–41). The beneficial effect of ganciclovir therapy may be enhanced by the concurrent administration of granulocyte or granulocyte-macrophage colony-stimulating factor or by targeting preemptive ganciclovir therapy to patients who are CMV pp65 antigen positive or CMV polymerase chain reaction (PCR) positive (23,39,40,42). Neutropenic patients should not be screened by PCR because patients must have circulating leukocytes for the antigenemia test to be reliable (43).

Infections with herpes-zoster virus, Epstein-Barr virus, human herpesvirus-6 (HHV-6), BK polyoma virus (hemorrhagic cystitis), CRVs, and adenoviruses also occur during the early transplant period (44–49). Varicella-zoster occurs in approximately 30% of seropositive transplant recipients who do not receive any antiviral prophylaxis. Most of these infections are cutaneous, although disseminated disease can be seen with severe GVHD. Treatment of herpes-zoster is with acyclovir.

Reactivation of Epstein-Barr virus is usually noted through asymptomatic shedding or seroconversion. HHV-6 infection occasionally causes acute febrile illness with rash and continued bone marrow suppression; the value of antiviral treatment for this complication is unknown (45,46). BK virus and adenovirus have both been associated with the development of hemorrhagic cystitis. Adenovirus has also been associated with pneumonia, renal insufficiency, gastroenteritis, and hepatitis. No definitive therapy for these last two viral pathogens is available.

Interstitial Pneumonitis

In addition to these defined infectious processes, diffuse interstitial pneumonitis is a significant complication of allogenic marrow transplant that occurs from approximately 3 to 7 weeks after the transplantation. Although its incidence has decreased, it still occurs in 7% to 12% of transplant recipients (50–52). It is defined as the presence of tachypnea, hypoxemia, and interstitial pulmonary infiltrates in the absence of obvious bacterial or fungal infection, pulmonary edema, or pulmonary hemorrhage. Approximately half of these pneumonias are due to CMV, and CRVs may also present with this syndrome; the majority of the remainder being classified as idiopathic. Risk factors for this complication include methotrexate therapy, older age, severe GVHD, a prolonged period after diagnosis and before transplant, and a poor performance status before transplantation (50–52). Unfortunately, this complication continues to have a high mortality rate.

INFECTION LATE AFTER TRANSPLANT ENGRAFTMENT (AFTER DAY 100)

Chronic Graft-versus-Host Disease

After 100 days following engraftment, there has usually been resolution of both the leukopenic period and the immunosuppression of acute GVHD. The major risks of infection relate to the development of chronic GVHD and delays in the development of antigen-specific humoral and T-cell–mediated immunity. The majority of syngeneic, autologous, and allogeneic transplant recipients without chronic GVHD will experience only one or two late infections other than recurrent herpes-zoster (53). Chronic GVHD arises in approximately 30% to 60% of allogeneic transplant recipients either as a continuation of acute GVHD or *de novo*. It resembles a mixed autoimmune disease with multiorgan involvement, predominantly of the immune system, skin, mucous membranes, liver, and bone marrow. Immunologic abnormalities include impaired proliferation of B cells, decreased antibody production to specific antigens, and a decrease in the number and function of $CD4^+$ T cells (32). Skin and mucous membrane changes can be limited to mild dermatitis or evolve

into a scleroderma-like pattern with severe destruction of dermal appendages and a sicca syndrome. A cholestatic hepatitis can develop and progress to cirrhosis. Hematopoietic involvement is characteristically manifest as thrombocytopenia. Further, most patients with chronic GVHD appear to be functionally asplenic.

Viral, Bacterial, and Fungal Infections

Infections that arise in patients during this late phase reflect breaches in anatomic host defenses and the defects in humoral and cell-mediated immunity. The most common infection seen in this period is recurrent varicella-zoster caused by reactivation of latent virus. The median time to onset is 5 months after transplantation, with 80% of episodes occurring within 9 months (44). Most of these episodes appear as zoster, but 15% of the episodes are varicella and 35% of the episodes of zoster are associated with dissemination. Acyclovir treatment has demonstrated efficacy in treating zoster in this population; newer antiviral agents (e.g., ganciclovir, famciclovir, and foscarnet) are also likely to be effective, but their use in treating varicella-zoster virus has not been well studied in transplant recipients. The risk of severe CRV disease also persists in patients with chronic GVHD. Bacterial infections that occur are predominantly sinusitis and pneumonia due to encapsulated organisms (*Streptococcus pneumoniae* and *Haemophilus influenzae*) related to abnormalities associated with chronic GVHD and immunoglobulin A deficiency. Systemic pneumococcal infection can occur and is associated with an inability to produce opsonizing antibody, even after systemic infection (54). Patients with significant skin and mucous membrane damage from chronic GVHD also suffer cutaneous infection with *S. aureus* and group A streptococci. Severe fungal disease is less common at this stage, but impaired cell-mediated immunity contributes to continued problems with oropharyngeal or vaginal candidiasis.

Prevention of Infection

Prophylactic measures can lower the incidence of late infectious complications. Oral acyclovir will prevent recurrent HSV and varicella-zoster virus disease as long as patients receive therapy, although routine prophylactic therapy during this period is not routinely recommended (21,55). The use of oral trimethoprim-sulfamethoxazole chemoprophylaxis has lowered the incidence of bacterial infections caused by *S. pneumoniae* and *H. influenzae* while providing prophylaxis against late cases of *P. carinii* pneumonia (56). Prophylaxis has been recommended in allogeneic transplant recipients with chronic GVHD for as long as therapy for GVHD is administered (23).

Transplantation leads to a significant decline in antibody titers against vaccine-preventable diseases. Therefore, it is recommended that between 12 and 24 months after transplantation, recipients should be immunized again against diphtheria, tetanus, pertussis, *H. influenzae* type B, polio, measles, mumps, and rubella (23).

REFERENCES

1. Armitage JO. Bone marrow transplantation. *N Engl J Med* 1994;330:827–838.
2. Sable CA, Donowitz GR. Infections in bone marrow transplant recipients. *Clin Infect Dis* 1994;18:273–281.
3. Lum LG. The kinetics of immune reconstitution after human marrow transplantation. *Blood* 1987;69:369–380.
4. Nemunaitis J, Rabinowe SN, Singer JW, et al. Recombinant granulocyte-macrophage colony-stimulating factor after autologous bone marrow transplantation for lymphoid cancer. *N Engl J Med* 1991;324:1773–1778.

5. Petersen F, Thornquist M, Buckner C, et al. The effects of infection prevention regimens on early infectious complications in marrow transplant patients: a four armed randomized study. *Infection* 1988;16:199–208.

6. Clark RA, Johnson FL, Klebanoff SJ, et al. Defective neutrophil chemotaxis in bone marrow transplant recipients. *J Clin Invest* 1976;58:22–31.

7. Storb R, Prentice RL, Buckner CD, et al. Graft-versus-host disease and survival in patients with aplastic anemia treated by marrow grafts from HLA-identical siblings. Beneficial effect of a protective environment. *N Engl J Med* 1983;308:302–307.

8. Mackall CL, Fleisher TA, Brown MR, et al. Age, thymopoiesis, and CD4+ T-lymphocyte regeneration after intensive chemotherapy. *N Engl J Med* 1995; 332:143–149.

9. Meyers JD. Infections associated with bone marrow transplantation. In: Gorbach SL, Bartlett JG, Blacklow NR, eds. *Infectious diseases*. Philadelphia: WB Saunders, 1992:1047–1050.

10. Yolken RH, Bishop CA, Townsend TR, et al. Infectious gastroenteritis in bone-marrow transplant patients. *N Engl J Med* 1982;306:1009–1012.

11. Bochud P-Y, Eggiman P, Calandra T, et al. Bacteremia due to viridans streptococcus in neutropenic patients with cancer: clinical spectrum and risk factors. *Clin Infect Dis* 1994;18:25–31.

12. Hughes WT, Armstrong D, Bodey GP, et al. Guidelines for the use of antimicrobial agents in neutropenic patients with unexplained fever. *J Infect Dis* 1990;161:381–396.

13. Thaler M, Pastakia B, Shawker TH, et al. Hepatic candidiasis in cancer patients: the evolving picture of the syndrome. *Ann Intern Med* 1988;108:88–100.

14. Rex JH, Bennett JE, Sugar AM, et al. A randomized trial comparing fluconazole with amphotericin B for the treatment of candidemia in patients without neutropenia. *N Engl J Med* 1994;331:1325–1330.

15. Goodman JL, Winston DJ, Greenfield RA, et al. A controlled trial of fluconazole to prevent fungal infections in patients undergoing bone marrow transplantation. *N Engl J Med* 1992;326:845–851.

16. Pirsch JD, Maki DG. Infectious complications in adults with bone marrow transplantation and T-cell depletion of donor marrow. Increased susceptibility to fungal infections. *Ann Intern Med* 1986;104:619–631.

17. Blazar BR, Hurd DD, Snover DC, et al. Invasive *Fusarium* infections in bone marrow transplant recipients. *Am J Med* 1984;77:645–651.

18. Bufill JA, Lum LG, Caya JG, et al. *Pityrosporum* folliculitis after bone marrow transplantation. *Ann Intern Med* 1988;108:560–563.

19. Wingard JR, Beals SU, Santos GW, et al. *Aspergillus* infections in bone marrow transplant recipients. *Bone Marrow Transplantation* 1987;2:175–181.

19a. Herbrecht R, Denning DW, Patterson TF, et al. Voriconazole versus amphotericin B for primary therapy of invasive aspergillosis. *N Engl J Med* 2002;347:408–415.

20. Denning DW, Lee JY, Hostetler JS, et al. NIAID mycoses study group multicenter trial of oral itraconazole therapy for invasive aspergillosis. *Am J Med* 1994;97:135–144.

21. Meyers JD, Flournoy N, Thomas ED. Infection with herpes simplex virus and cell-mediated immunity after marrow transplant. *J Infect Dis* 1980;142:338–346.

22. Ringden O, Heimdahl A, Lonnqvist B, et al. Decreased incidence of viridans streptococcal septicaemia in allogenic bone marrow transplant recipients after the introduction of acyclovir. *Lancet* 1984;1:744.

23. Guidelines for preventing opportunistic infections among hematopoietic stem cell transplant recipients. Recommendations of CDC, the Infectious Disease Society of America, and the American Society of Blood and Marrow Transplantation. *MMWR Morb Mortal Wkly Rep* 2000;49:1–125.

24. Sable CA, Hayden FG. Orthomyxoviral and paramyxoviral infections in transplant patients. *Infect Dis Clin North Am* 1995;9:987–1003.

25. Whimbey E, Champlin R, Couch RB, et al. Community respiratory virus infections among hospitalized adult bone marrow transplant recipients. *Clin Infect Dis* 1996;22:778–782.

26. Hall CB. Respiratory syncytial virus and parainfluenza virus. *N Engl J Med* 2001;344:1917–1928.

27. Tuan IZ, Dennison D, Weisdorf DJ. *Pneumocystis carinii* pneumonitis following bone marrow transplantation. *Bone Marrow Transplantation* 1992;10:267–272.

28. Cruciani M, Rampazzo R, Malena M, et al. Prophylaxis with fluoroquinolones for bacterial infections in neutropenic patients: a meta-analysis. *Clin Infect Dis* 1996;23:795–805.

29. Murphy M, Brown AE, Sepkowitz KA, et al. Fluoroquinolone prophylaxis for the prevention of bacterial infections in patients with cancer—is it justified? *Clin Infect Dis* 1997;25:346–348.

30. Marr KA, Seidel K, Slavin MA, et al. Prolonged fluconazole prophylaxis is associated with persistent protection against candidiasis-related death in allogenic marrow transplant recipients: long-term follow-up of a randomized, placebo-controlled trial. *Blood* 2000;96:2055–2061.

31. van Burik JH, Leisenring W, Myerson D, et al. The effect of prophylactic fluconazole on the clinical spectrum of fungal disease in bone marrow transplant recipients with special attention to hepatic candidiasis. An autopsy study of 355 patients. *Medicine (Baltimore)* 1998;77:246–254.

32. Ferrara JLM, Deeg HJ. Graft-versus-host disease. *N Engl J Med* 1991;324:667–674.

33. Meyers JD. Prevention of cytomegalovirus infection after marrow transplantation. *Rev Infect Dis* 1989;11[Suppl 7]:S1691–S1705.

34. Meyers JD, Flournoy N, Thomas ED. Risk factors for cytomegalovirus infection after human marrow transplantation. *J Infect Dis* 1986;153:478–488.

35. Wingard JR, Chen DY, Burns WH, et al. Cytomegalovirus infection after autologous bone marrow transplantation with comparison to infection after allogeneic bone marrow transplantation. *Blood* 1988;71:1432–1437.

36. Grundy JE, Shanley JD, Griffiths PD. Is cytomegalovirus interstitial pneumonitis in transplant recipients an immunopathological condition? *Lancet* 1987;2: 996–999.

37. Reed EC, Bowden RA, Dandliker PS, et al. Treatment of cytomegalovirus pneumonia in marrow transplant patients with ganciclovir and intravenous cytomegalovirus immunoglobulin. *Ann Intern Med* 1988;109:783–788.

38. Sayers MH, Anderson KC, Goodnough LT, et al. Reducing the risk for transfusion-transmitted cytomegalovirus infection. *Ann Intern Med* 1992;116: 55–62.

39. Goodrich JM, Bowden RA, Fisher L, et al. Ganciclovir prophylaxis to prevent cytomegalovirus disease after allogenic marrow transplant. *Ann Intern Med* 1993;118:173–178.

40. Winston DJ, Ho WG, Bartoni K, et al. Ganciclovir prophylaxis of cytomegalovirus infection and disease in allogeneic bone marrow transplant recipients. Results of a placebo-controlled, double-blind trial. *Ann Intern Med* 1993;118:179–184.

41. Schmidt GM, Horak DA, Niland JC, et al. A randomized, controlled trial of prophylactic ganciclovir for cytomegalovirus pulmonary infection in recipients of allogeneic bone marrow transplants. *N Engl J Med* 1991;324:1005–1011.

42. Einsele H, Ehninger G, Hebart H, et al. Polymerase chain reaction monitoring reduces the incidence of cytomegalovirus disease and the duration and side effects of antiviral therapy after bone marrow transplantation. *Blood* 1995;86:2815–2820.

43. van Burik JA, Weisdorf DJ. Infections in recipients of blood and marrow transplantation. *Hematol Oncol Clin North Am* 1999;13:1065–1089.

44. Locksley RM, Flournoy N, Sullivan KM, et al. Varicella zoster virus infection after marrow transplantation. *J Infect Dis* 1985;152:1172.

45. Yoshikawa T, Suga S, Asano Y, et al. Human herpesvirus-6 infection in bone marrow transplantation. *Blood* 1991;78:1381–1384.

46. Drobyski WR, Dunne WM, Burd EM, et al. Human herpesvirus-6 (HHV-6) infection in allogenic bone marrow transplant recipients: evidence of a marrow-suppressive role for HHV-6 in vivo. *J Infect Dis* 1993;167:735–739.

47. Russell SJ, Vowels MR, Vale T. Haemorrhagic cystitis in paediatric bone marrow transplant patients: an association with infective agents, GVHD and prior cyclophosphamide. *Bone Marrow Transplantation* 1994;13:533–539.

48. Arthur RR, Shah KV, Baust SJ, et al. Association of BK viruria with hemorrhagic cystitis in recipients of bone marrow transplants. *N Engl J Med* 1986;315:230–234.

49. Shields AF, Hackman RC, Fife KH, et al. Adenovirus infections in patients undergoing bone marrow transplantation. *N Engl J Med* 1985;312:529–533.

50. Weiner RS, Bortin MM, Gale RP, et al. Interstitial pneumonitis after bone marrow transplantation. *Ann Intern Med* 1986;104:168–175.

51. Clark JG, Hansen JA, Hertz MI, et al. Idiopathic pneumonia syndrome after bone marrow transplantation. *Am Rev Respir Dis* 1993;147:1601–1606.

52. Kantrow SP, Hackman RC, Boeckh M, et al. Idiopathic pneumonia syndrome. Changing spectrum of lung injury after marrow transplantation. *Transplantation* 1997;63:1079–1086.

53. Atkinson K, Farewell V, Storb R, et al. Analysis of late infections after human bone marrow transplantation: role of genotypic nonidentity between marrow donor and recipient and of nonspecific suppression cells in patients with chronic graft-versus-host disease. *Blood* 1982;60:714–720.

54. Winston DJ, Schiffman G, Wang DC, et al. Pneumococcal infections after human bone-marrow transplantation. *Ann Intern Med* 1979;91:835–841.

55. Ljungman P, Wilczek H, Gahrton G, et al. Long-term acyclovir prophylaxis in bone marrow transplant recipients and lymphocyte proliferation responses to herpes virus antigens *in vitro*. *Bone Marrow Transplantation* 1986;1:185–192.

56. Wingard JR, Santos GW, Saral R. Late-onset interstitial pneumonia following allogeneic bone marrow transplantation. *Transplantation* 1985;39: 21–23.

CHAPTER 128
Infections Associated with Corticosteroids and Immunosuppressive Therapy

Neil L. Barg and Robert Fekety

In this chapter, we focus on infections in immunocompromised hosts that result not from factors inherent in their underlying disease but instead from the immunosuppressive effects of treatment of those diseases. The chapter concerns iatrogenic infectious diseases, or so-called diseases of medical progress, which result from violations, albeit well intentioned, of a fundamental tenet of therapy: "Above all, do no harm." These diseases illustrate all too well that many therapeutic measures are undertaken despite their striking an uncertain compromise between risks and benefits. As the costs of keeping such immunosuppressed persons alive escalate, medical scientists and society as a whole will have to make difficult choices about who will live and who will die; these decisions will, unfortunately, be based on financial considerations as often as on humanitarian principles.

Infections in immunosuppressed hosts have many features that overlap with infections in compromised hosts such as patients with the acquired immune deficiency syndrome, but the latter may suffer from even broader and more diverse derangements in host defenses. Infections in immunosuppressed hosts most often result from treatment-induced reductions in granu-

locyte numbers or function or both or from impairment of cellular immunity related to effects on lymphocytes, monocytes, or macrophages. In addition, immunocompromised patients may have deficiencies in immunoglobulins, the complement system, and other key defensive mechanisms. Significantly, these patients are also subject to infections related to the presence of catheters, prostheses, other foreign bodies, tissue damage, obstruction, and bleeding from the underlying disease. Whereas in clinical practice problems associated with granulocytopenia and impaired cellular immunity are even more complex than the terms imply, it is useful to consider them here as isolated problems. More details concerning the diagnosis and management of the specific infections seen in these patients are provided in other chapters of this book.

INFECTIONS IN PATIENTS RECEIVING GLUCOCORTICOSTEROID THERAPY

Short- or long-term administration of adrenal glucocorticosteroids results in a wide range of dose-related negative effects on inflammatory and immune defenses against infections. The most important mechanism by which steroids suppress inflammation and enhance susceptibility to infection is by impairing the mobilization, migration, and function of neutrophils and mononuclear cells at sites of primary lodgment of microorganisms in tissues. Thus, even though corticosteroids may cause leukocytosis, these patients actually have a risk of infection similar to that of neutropenic patients but with three important additional features. First, these deficiencies in neutrophil mobilization may persist for long periods if steroid therapy is continued. Second, neutrophil deficiencies (decreased killing of organisms contained by phagocytosis) are often accompanied by lymphopenia, monocytopenia, or deficiencies in monocyte, macrophage, and lymphocyte function, with resultant impairment of important cellular immune mechanisms that are normally effective in preventing infections with certain pathogens (Table 128.1). Third, these patients often have all the infection-related risks of the anatomic abnormalities of the underlying disease and also those resulting from treatment with immunosuppressive or cytostatic agents, radiation, implantation of foreign bodies, and surgical procedures. Intensive treatment leads to infection with pyogenic bacteria and increased risk of surgical site infections. Prolonged treatment with corticosteroids (greater than 21 days) results in prolonged suppression of T cell function and leads to opportunistic infections. Consequently, multiple sequential infections or polymicrobial infections frequently afflict these patients, especially those undergoing organ transplantation (1). Corticosteroid administration may also lead to reactivation of latent infections such as tuberculosis or endemic fungi. Therefore, patients administered corticosteroids for more than 1 month at a dose of 15 mg/kg or greater should receive isoniazid if they have a positive tuberculin skin test result (2). For patients with a history of infection with endemic fungi, consider co-administration of an antifungal agent if prolonged corticosteroid therapy is necessary.

FEVER AND INFECTION IN NEUTROPENIC PATIENTS

With the increasing use of myelosuppressive and immunosuppressive agents or radiation for the treatment of neoplastic diseases and in transplantation, infections in granulocytopenic patients have become more common. Experience has shown that appropriate empiric therapy must be started early during the

---

TABLE 128.1. Pathogens That Often Cause Infections in Patients with Deficiencies of Cell-Mediated Immunity

Bacteria
  Legionella pneumophila
  Listeria monocytogenes
  Mycobacterium tuberculosis
  Mycobacterium avium-intracellulare
  Nocardia asteroides
  Pseudomonas species
  Salmonella species
Viruses
  Cytomegalovirus
  Herpes simplex virus
  Varicella-zoster virus
  Epstein-Barr virus
Fungi
  Aspergillus
  Blastomyces dermatitidis
  Candida species
  Coccidioides immitis
  Cryptococcus neoformans
  Histoplasma capsulatum
  Zygomycetes (Mucor)
Protozoa
  Toxoplasma gondii
  Giardia lamblia
  Entamoeba histolytica
Helminths
  Strongyloides stercoralis

course of infections in neutropenic patients if a fatal outcome is to be prevented (3). Antibiotics should not be withheld because the infection and its pathogens have not been documented precisely. Unfortunately, the usual manifestations of infection typically are absent during the early stages in patients with marked neutropenia, for whom a temperature higher than 101.5°F, erythema, local pain, and tenderness are often the only signs of infection (4). The frequency of infections during neutropenia is inversely proportional to the absolute neutrophil count (Fig. 128.1). They begin to increase when the neutrophil count falls below 500/mm^3, and both the frequency and severity of infection increase steadily as the granulocyte count approaches zero. Severe infections with bacteremia tend to occur when the granulocyte count is below 100 to 200/mm^3. Because corticosteroid therapy impairs granulocyte mobilization and function (5), the risk of infection at a given level of granulocytopenia further increases when these patients are also treated with corticosteroids. The frequency of infectious complications of steroid therapy rises with doses of prednisone equivalents of more than 20 mg per day, or a total of more than 700 mg, and with treatment for longer than 30 days. Susceptibility may be reduced by using alternate-day dosing and by keeping the dose as small as possible (5–7). The duration of the neutropenic state also is directly related to the infection rate; neutropenia is usually sustained longer and infections are more frequent after treatment of leukemia or after bone marrow transplantation (approximately 2 to 4 weeks) than after treatment of most carcinomas and solid tumors, in which profound neutropenia usually lasts only 7 to 10 days on average.

Pathogens

Although many different kinds of organisms have been isolated from the blood and infected sites of neutropenic patients, certain organisms are more common than others (Table 128.2). Most of

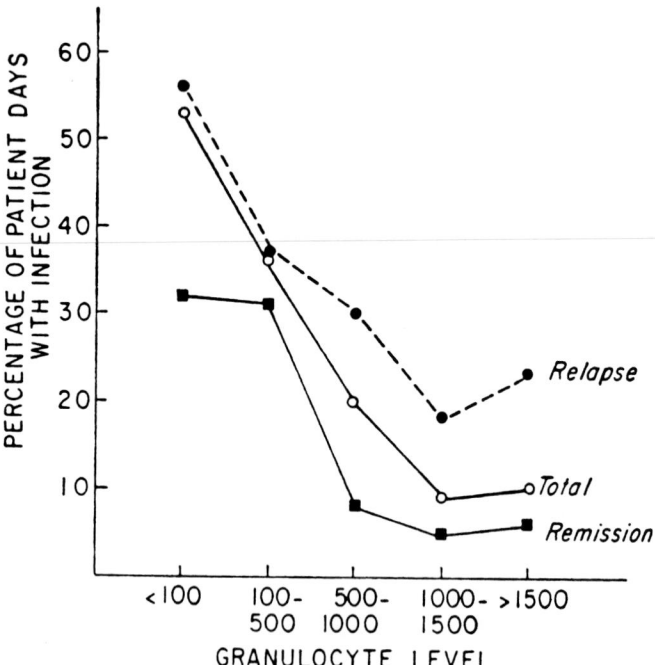

Figure 128.1. Quantitative relationship between various degrees of neutropenia and infection. (From Bodey GP, Buckely M, Sathe YS, Freireich EJ. Quantitative relationships between circulating leukocytes and infection in patients with acute leukemia. *Ann Intern Med* 1966;64:328–340, with permission.)

TABLE 128.2. Pathogens That Most Often Infect Granulocytopenic Patients

Bacteria
  Gram-negative bacilli
    Common: *Escherichia coli, Pseudomonas aeruginosa, Klebsiella pneumoniae, Enterobacter cloacae, Enterobacter aerogenes, Proteus* species
    Less common: *Serratia marcescens, Aeromonas, Bacteroides, Capnocytophaga* species
  Gram-positive cocci and bacilli
    Common: *Staphylococcus aureus, Staphylococcus epidermidis, Enterococcus faecalis*
    Less common: corynebacteria JK, *Bacillus* species, *Clostridium* species
Polymicrobial infections of yeasts and molds
    Common: *Candida, Aspergillus,* zygomycetes (Mucor, *Rhizopus*) species
    Less common: *Fusarium, Trichosporon* species, *Pseudallescheria boydii*

these organisms normally colonize areas adjacent to the site of infection. Although they may be considered part of the normal flora, they have often been acquired nosocomially and are also resistant to antibiotics, especially if the patient received broad-spectrum antibiotic therapy before the onset of the infection (8). In addition, a shift of the normal oropharyngeal flora toward more resistant gram-negative organisms has correlated with increasing severity of the underlying diseases, use of nasogastric tubes, and use of antacid medications, even in the absence of antibiotic exposure. Suppression of the "colonization resistance" normally provided by intestinal anaerobes also favors a shift in the intestinal flora toward pathogenic, antibiotic-resistant aerobes; this is usually the result of treatment with antibiotics that have good activity against colonic anaerobes. Fungal infections typically occur as complications or as superinfections that follow successful treatment of bacterial infections in these patients. On occasion, fungal organisms may cause primary infection.

Increasingly, unusual organisms, recognized now primarily because of their isolation from patients with acquired immunodeficiency syndrome, cause infections in neutropenic patients and patients treated for prolonged periods with corticosteroids. For example, atypical mycobacteria (9), the fungus *Fusarium solani* (10,11), Prototheca (12), *Bartonella henselae* (the agent of bacillary angiomatosis and cat-scratch disease) (13), and *Rhodococcus equi* (14) have been isolated from blood, catheters, or wounds in transplant patients.

Sites of Infection

In most studies of infection in febrile neutropenic patients, approximately 20% of patients are found to have bacteremia, often from perirectal infection, an intravascular line, or an inapparent source in the gastrointestinal tract; 20% have microbiologically defined infections at a site such as the lungs, skin, oral cavity, or urinary tract; 20% have a recognizable probable site of infection but a specific bacterial pathogen cannot be determined; 20% have fever caused by factors unrelated to infection; and the remaining 20% have fever of unknown cause. Common viruses probably cause many of the last. Infections of the oral cavity, sinuses, skin, or perirectal area are often minor in appearance and are thus overlooked, but they are important nonetheless in neutropenic patients (15). Oral mucositis in association with cytarabine therapy seems uniquely associated with a high frequency of viridans streptococcal bacteremia and especially with *Streptococcus mitis,*

Streptococcus sanguis, and *Streptococcus oralis.* Fortunately, these organisms are usually susceptible to the antimicrobials in the usual regimens started empirically for neutropenic fever (16).

Diagnosis

Culture plates should be propagated with blood, material from intravenous access sites, and exudate from sites of infection as soon as possible after infection is suspected; aspirate or biopsy specimens from cutaneous lesions should also be cultured. Chest radiography should be performed even if there are no pulmonary symptoms, because minimal infiltrates may be an early clue to pneumonitis and serve as a baseline in patients with prolonged neutropenia. High-resolution computed tomography may depict infiltrates when the conventional chest radiograph appears normal (17). Routine surveillance cultures from asymptomatic body sites do not appear to be worthwhile as a guide to empiric therapy, because it is common for many organisms to be isolated, which makes selecting the probable opportunistic pathogen difficult, and because of the expense and inherent delay in obtaining results of these cultures (18).

More rapid and sensitive tools have become available with use of polymerase chain reaction-based techniques for diagnosis of toxoplasmosis (19) and for infections with viruses such as cytomegalovirus (CMV) (20), *Parvovirus* (21), and hepatitis C virus (22). Assays, for C-reactive protein, I16, I18, and procalcitonin have been proposed as tests to assist in the diagnosis of infection. The consensus at this time suggests that elevations of these substances are not associated closely enough with infection and bacteremia to be useful (23).

Therapy

EMPIRIC THERAPY

Because bacteremia is relatively common in neutropenic patients, empiric therapy should be instituted promptly for patients with fever (greater than 101°F or greater than 100.4°F for longer than 1 hour) after blood cultures have been obtained, especially if the granulocyte count is lower than 500/mm^3 or if the patient appears to be in a toxic state. If there is a suspected site of infection, therapy should be based on knowledge of the normal flora at contiguous areas and on the results of Gram staining or other stain examination when exudate is available. Previous antibiotic therapy and hospitalization favoring selection of resistant organisms should be considered.

Because both gram-positive (in many institutions, between 60% and 70% of documented infections) and gram-negative organisms are common causes of these infections, empiric therapy should be broad and designed to cover both kinds of organisms. In high-risk patients, two antimicrobial drugs are usually given simultaneously, one primarily for gram-positive organisms and another for gram-negative organisms. Many different regimens have been studied and recommended, and in general none is clearly superior. In individual patients and in specific places, some regimens may be clearly better than others (24). Unless intravascular lines are the probable source of the infection or Gram stain examination suggests staphylococci, many experts prefer to direct empiric therapy primarily toward gram-negative aerobic or facultative anaerobic pathogens to limit the use of vancomycin because of the emergence of vancomycin-resistant gram-positive strains. Infections with strict anaerobes do occur, but they are both rare and rarely associated with signs of severe sepsis in neutropenic patients unless there are localizing findings that suggest intraabdominal or necrotizing infection. Therefore, current empiric therapy often ignores the possibility of obligate anaerobes as the etiologic agents. Some prefer, in fact, to use drugs with poor activity against anaerobic organisms (such as aztreonam or ceftazidime), because they may preserve colonization resistance in the intestines, thus reducing the likelihood of sepsis caused by gram-negative enteropathogens. Therapy should be bactericidal if possible, because granulocytes present in small numbers cannot be relied on to kill bacteria. This means that large doses of parenteral antibiotics designed to achieve bactericidal serum levels may be needed. Combination antibiotic therapy employing an antipseudomonal β-lactam agent plus an aminoglycoside is favored by most experts because it may result in synergistic or at least additive effects and reduce the emergence of antibiotic-resistant strains (25). Neutropenic patients who exhibit bacteremia or are in shock as a result of infection (which is relatively uncommon in neutropenic patients) have better response rates when treated with a synergistic combination of antimicrobials (26,27). Other experts prefer to use an antipseudomonal β-lactam or carbapenem alone initially for febrile neutropenic patients who do not appear to be in a toxic condition or severely ill; aminoglycosides, vancomycin, or antifungal therapy is added later as needed, on the basis of culture results, clinical findings, and the course of the illness. Vancomycin should be added to the regimen when methicillin-resistant coagulase-positive or coagulase-negative staphylococci are either definitely implicated or strongly suspected. Serum levels of aminoglycosides and vancomycin, as well as renal function, may need to be monitored to minimize toxicity and maximize therapeutic responses. After the infecting organisms and their susceptibility patterns have been determined and the patient's condition begins to improve, it may be possible, and in fact desirable, to discontinue aminoglycosides or other unnecessary antibiotics or to reduce the dosage so as to minimize toxicity. The antimicrobials used most often for these infections are listed in Table 128.3.

TABLE 128.3. Antibiotics Most Often Used In Combination for Empirical Therapy of Suspected Infection in Granulocytopenic Patients

Antibacterial agents (usually initial therapy is with an antipseudomonal β-lactam plus an aminoglycoside)

Penicillins	Cephalosporins
Ticarcillin	Ceftazidime
Timentin	Cefotaxime
Piperacillin	Cefoperazone
Azlocillin	Ceftizoxime
Mezlocillin	Monobactams
Carbapenems	Aztreonam
Imipenem-cilastatin	

Aminoglycosides
  Gentamicin
  Tobramycin
  Amikacin
  Netilmicin
Agents usually added in special circumstances
  Vancomycin (methicillin-resistant *Staphylococcus aureus,*
    Staphylococcus epidermidis, enterococci, corynebacteria JK)
  Erythromycin (*Legionella*)
  Ciprofloxacin, ofloxacin (*Pseudomonas*)
  Metronidazole (anaerobes)
  Ampicillin-sulbactam (anaerobes)
  Trimethoprim-sulfamethoxazole (*Pneumocystis carinii*)
    Antifungal agents

Amphotericin B	Itraconazole
Flucytosine	Fluconazole
Ketoconazole	Miconazole

Some studies of empiric therapy for neutropenic fever indicate that results with single agents (usually a β-lactam such as ceftazidime) are as good as those with a combination of drugs. Most of these studies can be criticized on the grounds that they have included too few cases of either documented gram-negative bacteremia or sustained neutropenia (because such patients are at greatest risk of a bad outcome) or because they included too many patients with minor infections or no proven infection or patients with only brief episodes of neutropenia, because this last group has done relatively well even when given no antibiotic therapy. In one well-controlled study by the European Organization for Research and Treatment of Cancer that compared empiric combination therapy of febrile neutropenic patients with amikacin given for either 3 or 9 days in addition to ceftazidime given to both groups for 9 days, the overall response rate was 64% in 266 patients given amikacin for 3 days and 68% in 368 patients given amikacin for 9 days, an insignificant difference (28). However, in the 80 patients with documented gram-negative bacteremia, the response rate was only 48% in those given amikacin for 3 days but 81% in those given amikacin for 9 days. The difference favoring the longer course of amikacin in patients with bacteremia was seen with each of the most frequent specific organisms (*Escherichia coli, Klebsiella pneumoniae,* and *Pseudomonas aeruginosa*). Although a comparison of short-course versus long-course therapy with an aminoglycoside is not entirely relevant to the issue of combination therapy versus monotherapy, these results do demonstrate the importance of analyzing data according to specific pathogens and sites instead of looking only at overall results. Conversely, in another study that is often cited to support monotherapy with ceftazidime for neutropenia and fever, a large proportion of patients eventually required modification of monotherapy to achieve a good response (for example, vancomycin may have been added because a gram-positive infection was documented). Patients who required such a modification of therapy were not considered treatment failures by the investigators, as they survived despite delayed initiation of appropriate therapy (29). Unfortunately, only a relatively small number of patients in this study had documented bacteremia, and the number was too small to permit valid statistical tests to determine significant differences in outcome. Because imipenem-cilastatin (Primaxin) has a broad spectrum of activity and is resistant to inducible β-lactamases, it has been considered attractive for monotherapy (18). In one study, imipenem-cilastatin yielded as good results as the double β-lactam combinations studied for comparison, but it produced seizures when given in a dose of 1.0 g intravenously every 6 hours (30). Finally, resistant organisms are reported to emerge more rapidly with monotherapy (31), and combination therapy may be better in that regard (3,32–34). Current recommendations support the use of monotherapy for febrile neutropenic patients without evidence of complications of infection or other underlying illnesses. The best agents provide excellent activity against gram positive and gram-negative bacteria. Cefepime, imipenem-cilastin, meropenem, piperacillin/tazobactam, have all been used successfully (23).

For initial therapy of high-risk febrile neutropenic patients, most experts recommend an aminoglycoside plus an antipseudomonal β-lactam or carbapenem antimicrobial drug. Quinolones are an alternative second antimicrobial, but only when these agents have not been used for prophylaxis of infection in afebrile neutropenic patients. No single combination of antibiotics seems clearly superior to other popular ones when response rates, toxicity, and cost are taken into consideration (26,33). When neutropenic patients are given appropriate antibiotics for a documented infection, it usually takes at least 3 or 4 days for a good response to become evident; therefore, unless new diagnoses are made, antibiotic regimens should probably not be altered more often than that if fever persists. When modifications are indicated during the course of empiric therapy, anaerobic coverage should be added when necrotizing gingivitis, perirectal cellulites, typhlitis or neutropenic colitis is present. Vancomycin should be added when methicillin-resistant *Staphylococcus aureus* or *Staphylococcus epidermidis* infection is identified. Initial use of vancomycin should be limited to patients with suspected catheter-related infection or blood cultures yielding gram-positive bacteria, patients known to be colonized or infected with methicillin-resistant *Staphylococcus aureus* or β-lactam–resistant pneumococcus, patients with severe stomatitis or clinical evidence of sepsis. Likely pathogens and local susceptibility patterns should be considered. Neutropenic patients with catheter related infections could be treated without removal of the catheter if there is no involvement of the tunnel or infusion-port pocket, coagulase negative staphylococci are the cause of infection, and a rapid clinical response is observed (35). Catheters may require removal if *P. aeruginosa*, gram-positive bacteria resistant to multiple antibiotics, or fungi have infected the device. Some experts have begun to cautiously treat low-risk patients with neutropenic fever as outpatients, using agents such as oral quinolones alone or in combination with amoxicillin/clavulanic acid, clindamycin, aztreonam, ceftriaxone, or once-daily aminoglycosides (36–39). Most of these patients do not have serious, culture proven, bacterial infections. The best candidates for such therapy are those with low risk and recovering white blood cell counts. Low risk patients include those with neutrophil and monocyte counts greater than 100 cells/mm^3, a normal chest radiograph, no evidence of catheter-related infection, fever less than 39°C and no significant findings of clinical disease (40,41). Although some patients did not respond to such therapy and later required admission to the hospital for more aggressive anti-infective therapy, the overall results were surprisingly good and mortality rates were low (2%). Advantages included lower costs, lower exposure to nosocomial organisms, fewer superinfections, and improved quality of life. A variant of this that is becoming popular is the early discharge from the hospital of patients with neutropenic fever who are doing well, whose cultures and other diagnostic studies do not reveal anything alarming, and who are reliable and able to take antibiotics orally or parenterally at home.

Controversies in the Treatment of Neutropenic Patients

Prophylaxis of infection in neutropenic patients has been tried. Both trimethoprim-sulfamethoxazole (TMP-SMX) and fluoroquinolones have been used as prophylaxis against infection in afebrile, neutropenic patients. Although effective at reducing the frequency of febrile episodes, the use of TMP-SMX resulted in increased isolation of antibiotic resistant bacteria, an increased rate of fungal colonization and prolongation of neutropenia. TMP-SMX is effective at prevention of *Pneumocystis* pneumonia in patients at risk for this infection (42). The use of fluoroquinolone prophylaxis in patients with neutropenic fever has been reported to reduce the duration and amount of antibiotic therapy required but is likely to select for quinolone-resistant organisms, particularly α-hemolytic streptococci such as *S. mitis, S. oralis,* and *S. sanguis* (16). Vancomycin prophylaxis of catheter-related infections is not recommended because of the likelihood of the emergence of vancomycin-resistant gram-positive bacteria. Fluconazole may be useful in treatment of fungal infections and reduce the need for treatment with amphotericin B, but both therapy and prophylaxis with fluconazole have been followed by the emergence of fluconazole-resistant *Candida* species; consequently, most authorities discourage the use of fluconazole prophylaxis during neutropenic fever. Detailed discussions of the advantages and disadvantages of various popular regimens have been published (33,34). Current guidelines do not recommend the use for fluconazole prophylaxis in neutropenic patients (23). Another still controversial area in the management of neutropenic fever concerns the use of so-called double β-lactam therapy, that is two β-lactam drugs given simultaneously, such as ceftazidime plus piperacillin or aztreonam plus cefoperazone. Double β-lactam combinations are used most often in the hope of achieving better coverage against *Pseudomonas* and other resistant gram-negative pathogens without incurring the toxicity risks of aminoglycosides. Reasons for *not* using double β-lactam therapy include possible antagonism, undesirable alterations in fecal anaerobic flora (43), the possibility of promoting resistance (because two β-lactamase inducers are present or because more penicillin binding sites are blocked), the possibility of greater frequency of coagulation defects, more frequent side effects such as rash, and increased expense (32,44,45).

Granulocyte colony-stimulating factor and granulocyte-macrophage colony-stimulating factor are being used with increasing frequency to produce early return of granulocytes in the peripheral blood of patients with neutropenic fever. This is an expensive innovation and one that has not yet been clearly shown to reduce mortality rates, the duration of fever, or the use of antimicrobials, even though the duration of neutropenia, and hospitalization is shortened during their use (46,47). At this time, the use of these agents is not recommended for the treatment of fever in patients with uncomplicated neutropenia (48).

MODE OF ADMINISTRATION OF ANTIBIOTICS

Although some experts prefer to give aminoglycosides by continuous infusion, evidence supports the notion that the efficacy of aminoglycosides in immunocompromised patients is related more to peak concentrations than to sustained concentrations and that the reverse is true for βlactams, possibly because they have a brief postantibiotic effect. Thus, it has been recommended that β-lactams be given to neutropenic patients by continuous infusion and that aminoglycosides be given intravenously, either once or more times per day or continuously (49).

DURATION OF THERAPY

Whatever empiric regimen is used, it is clear that persistent profound granulocytopenia is associated with substantially lower favorable response rates than those seen in patients with rising granulocyte counts. In a study that compared three β-lactam plus aminoglycoside combinations, only 27% of patients with persistent granulocytopenia had good responses, whereas 73% of those whose granulocyte counts rose during therapy responded well (50). Patients who respond and become afebrile and whose neutropenia resolves need not be treated longer than 10 days in most cases. The proper duration of therapy for persistently neutropenic patients whose disease has responded to antimicrobial agents is still controversial. Most authorities recommend therapy for 10 to 14 days or for 1 week after the fever subsides. In contrast, others advocate continuing therapy until neutropenia resolves, as determined by the granulocyte count rising to 500 to 1,000/mm^3, despite the attendant risks of possibly increased

toxicity, antibiotic resistance, and expense. Still others believe that therapy should be discontinued despite persistent neutropenia after 7 to 10 afebrile days if the patient has no other significant complaints or problems and that diagnostic studies and therapy should be reinstituted if fever returns or the patient's clinical status deteriorates (40,51,52). Patients with expected prolonged neutropenia that become afebrile and are clinically stable and without mucositis may stop antimicrobials after 2 weeks with the addition of a prophylaxis regimen.

Prophylaxis with oral quinolones or trimethoprim-sulfamethoxazole, with or without antifungal prophylaxis with itraconazole or fluconazole, is frequently given instead of continued treatment to afebrile but persistently neutropenic patients, particularly those who have leukemia, who tend to have more profound and prolonged neutropenia than that induced by drugs in patients with solid tumors (26,53,54). A regimen of oral ciprofloxacin or ofloxacin and amphotericin may provide better results than other prophylactic regimens, with less risk of emergence of resistant strains (53). Intensive gut decontamination regimens employing oral drugs such as vancomycin, erythromycin, neomycin, colistin, framycetin, nystatin, or amphotericin B with or without a parenteral third-generation cephalosporin can also be effective in preventing infection during persistent neutropenia (27), but they are no longer used at most centers unless patients are also in a total protective environment designed to limit exposure to resistant organisms. In addition, such regimens are likely to favor the emergence and spread of antibiotic-resistant organisms.

Persistent Fever and Neutropenia Despite Broad Antibacterial Therapy

When fever persists more than 3 to 5 days in neutropenic patients despite treatment and despite failure to diagnose a specific infection, consider infection caused by antibiotic resistant bacteria, an abscess or catheter-related infection or a non-bacterial infection. Other possibilities for persistent fever include inadequate doses of antimicrobial agents and drug allergy. After a thorough clinical evaluation, most physicians recommend changing antibiotics to include bacteria resistant to the first chosen agents or the selection of new agents to treat infection at a new site suggested by clinical examination. Finally, consider adding antifungal therapy with amphotericin B or fluconazole, even though this practice may not increase survival rates (55). Liposomal preparations of amphotericin B are not superior in this instance but have less toxicity (56,57). Fluconazole can be used if there is no clinical evidence of a mold infection, that is no evidence of sinusitis and no infiltrates observed on chest radiograph. Itraconazole, which is active against many molds, has been used successfully in this setting (58). Empiric antibacterial therapy is also continued in most cases, but superinfections are common in this setting. Table 128.4 is a modification of a published algorithm for managing persistent neutropenia and fever in the presence of empiric therapy (59). Granulocyte transfusions are no longer used as often in these cases, although they may be given when patients with documented gram-negative bacteremia or fungal infections that fail to respond to intensive and appropriate antimicrobial therapy (60,61).

Fungal Infections

The diagnosis of invasive fungal infection in an immunosuppressed host is often difficult, and dissemination may occur while therapy is being withheld for fear of the toxicity of

TABLE 128.4. Modifications of Therapy That May Be Required in Cases of Persistent Fever and Neutropenia

Clinical problem	Suggested modification
Persistent unexplained fever and neutropenia	After 4–7 d, add antifungal therapy and continue antibiotics.
Breakthrough bacteremia	Add vancomycin if isolate is gram-positive. Switch to new, more intensive regimen if isolate is gram-negative.
Intravenous catheter-related infection	Add vancomycin or gram-negative coverage if not already being given. Add amphotericin B or fluconazole if there is evidence of *Candida* retinitis, pyelonephritis, fungemia, or skin infection.
Severe oral mucositis or gingivitis	Add coverage specific for anaerobes if not already being given.
Perianal tenderness or infection	Add specific anaerobe coverage if not already being given.
Esophagitis	Add oral clotrimazole, amphotericin, or fluconazole.
Pneumonitis	
New infiltration	Watch and wait if granulocyte count is rising and patient is otherwise doing well. If granulocyte count is not rising, obtain sputum or biopsy sample and add amphotericin or fluconazole while awaiting results.
Diffuse or interstitial infiltrates	Add trimethoprim-sulfamethoxazole and erythromycin.

Adapted from Pizzo PA. After empiric therapy: what to do until the granulocyte comes back. *Rev Infect Dis* 1987; 9:214–219.

amphotericin B or while awaiting a definitive diagnosis (8). *Candida* ophthalmitis is a definite indication for therapy with parenteral amphotericin or parenteral fluconazole, and these agents are often used for *Candida* pyelonephritis or fungemia with cutaneous lesions. As is the case with bacterial infections, the outcome of treatment of fungal infections in neutropenic patients is improved with early therapy. Earlier antifungal therapy may become more popular as confidence increases in the efficacy of oral antifungals, especially fluconazole. Once begun, amphotericin B therapy should be continued for a total dose of 500 mg or more for 10 to 14 days unless there is toxicity or the granulocytopenia resolves provided imaging studies fail to document invasive disease. Patients with documented invasive or disseminated fungal infection should be treated according to the usual guidelines, generally with 1 to 2 g of amphotericin B. In patients without neutropenia or major immunodeficiency, parenteral fluconazole, given as 400 mg/d for at least 14 days after the last positive culture result, has also been reported to be effective (62).

FOCAL HEPATIC AND SPLENIC CANDIDIASIS

Focal hepatic and splenic *Candida* infection has been recognized with increasing frequency in neutropenic patients (63,64). Patients usually present with persistent fever of unknown origin that is not responsive to antibiotic therapy. The syndrome usually does not occur until the neutrophil count has returned to normal. It most often affects patients with leukemia but has also been associated with neutropenia and solid tumors or aplastic anemia. There is usually a history of *Candida* infection during the neutropenic period, but there is little or no evidence of an active *Candida* infection when the syndrome is recognized. Abdominal pain and enlargement of the liver and spleen may occur, along with leukocytosis and an elevated serum alkaline phosphatase level. Characteristic lesions are seen in the liver at ultrasonography (bull's eye, or target, lesions) or computed tomography (Fig. 128.2). Liver biopsy examination shows yeasts or pseudohyphae in the center of granulomatous lesions; surprisingly,

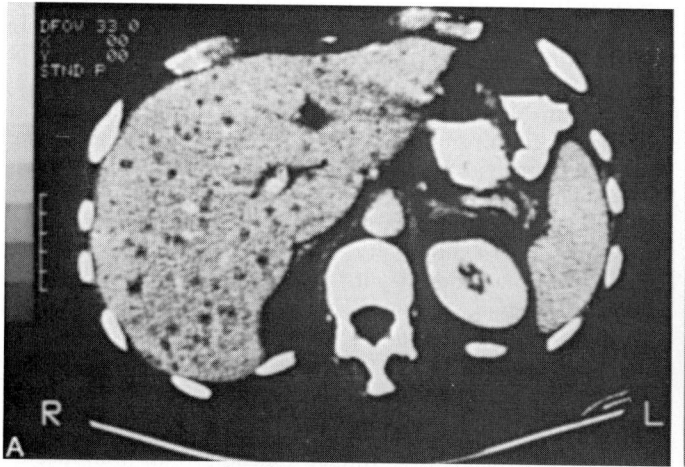
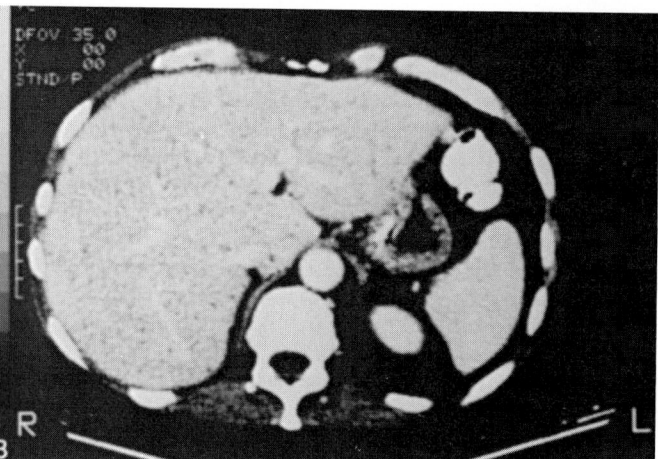

Figure 128.2. Computed tomographic scan of the liver of a patient with hepatic candidiasis after recovery from neutropenia. **A,** At time of diagnosis. **B,** One month later, after treatment with intravenous amphotericin B.

cultures of the biopsy specimen and blood are usually sterile, especially if the patient was previously treated with antifungal therapy. *Candida albicans* is most often implicated. Treatment is frequently unsuccessful unless it is aggressive: more than 2 g of amphotericin B (with or without flucytosine) is given to most patients. Multiple biopsy examinations and scans and multiple courses of therapy are frequently required because of treatment failure or relapse. Liposomal amphotericin B may prove superior to ordinary amphotericin because of enhanced delivery of liposomes to the sites of infection in the liver and spleen as well as reduced toxicity. Some patients who failed to respond to amphotericin or suffered toxicity were treated successfully with fluconazole, 200 to 400 mg per day for 6 to 12 months (65). Both the increasing efficacy of therapy of leukemia or solid tumors and the availability of ultrasonography and computed tomography have probably combined to increase.

INFECTIONS IN ORGAN TRANSPLANTATION

Infections and organ rejection after solid organ transplantation persist as the major complications despite advances in surgical technique and improvements in immunosuppressive therapy. The incidence and the type of infection are related to the level of immunosuppression. The degree of immune system compromise is determined by the dose, the duration, and the sequence of administration of the immunosuppressive agents (66). Immunosuppression used for organ transplantations causes primarily a decrease in cell-mediated immunity and to a lesser extent, reduced antibody responses. As a result, these patients have increased susceptibility to intracellular pathogens such as *Toxoplasmosis, Listeria,* and Herpesviruses. In many instances, infections caused by these agents can be prevented by antimicrobial prophylaxis, infection control measures, and risk avoidance. Infecting organisms may be acquired from the patients' immediate environment, the reactivation of latent infection, and transmission from the transplanted organ. As in neutropenic patients, the signs and symptoms of infection are diminished or eliminated by immunosuppression.

Donor and recipient exposure histories and serologic screening assist in identifying potential infections. Protocols for these screenings are published (67). Time after transplant helps to predict the type of infection as well. In the first month, most infections are a results of surgical complications or other nosocomially acquired infections. In the next 5 months, reactivation of endogenous infections such as herpes, tuberculosis, and fungi usually occurs. At this time, transplant-associated infections are most likely to develop such as infection caused by CMV, *Pneumocystis, Aspergillis, Nocardia, Toxoplasmosis,* and *Listeria.*

Infections and Renal Transplantation

A retrospective review of infections in 162 renal allograft recipients studied before 1976 at the University of Michigan showed that 83% of patients developed an infection during the first year after transplantation (during which the mean daily dose of prednisone was 50 mg), and infection was an important contributory cause in 73% of deaths (6). Urinary tract, pulmonary, surgical wound, blood stream, meningeal, and shunt infections were most common. *S. aureus,* enteric bacteria, *Pseudomonas,* and *Candida* species were most frequently implicated, but a wide variety of conventional and opportunistic pathogens were detected. *Cryptococcus neoformans* was the most common cause of meningitis, which often presented as a chronic or subacute illness characterized by headache and low-grade fever. The fre-

quency of fatal infections after renal transplantation has declined markedly because lower maintenance doses (less than 20 mg of prednisone per day) of steroids are now used, because of less frequent production of neutropenia by cytotoxic immunosuppressive agents, and because of less frequent use of vigorous immunosuppressive therapy designed to save the kidney from being rejected at all costs. Also, the newer immunosuppressive agents may be more effective at preventing rejection. The effect on the incidence of infections varies. Tacrolimus is associated with a higher incidence of infections, whereas Neoral may reduce the incidence of infection associated with immunosuppression (68). The use of mycophenolate for immunosuppression is associated with a lower incidence of *Pneumocystis* pneumonia (69,70).

In recent years, conventional bacterial infections, in particular urinary tract infections are the most common infections. Twenty-five percent of these infections may originate from contamination of the transplanted cadaveric kidney (71). Risks are increased if there has been long-term pretransplant dialysis. Post transplant, the incidence of urinary tract infections have decreased dramatically with the use of TMP-SMX during the first year (72). Although the incidence of urinary tract infection has been reduced, infection at this site is still the cause of 50% of bacteremia in renal transplant patients. *Pseudomonas,* enterococci and enteric gram-negative bacilli are the most common organisms isolated (73). Bacteremias from non-typhi salmonella infections are more common in renal transplant patients than the general population. Salmonella infections are associated with anti-rejection therapy and are often recurrent (74). Opportunistic bacteria, *Nocardia, Listeria,* and *Legionella* also cause infections among renal transplant patients. *Legionella* and *Listeria* (75) have caused nosocomial outbreaks. *Nocardia* most commonly caused pneumonia and brain abscess but is relatively rare in renal transplants. Skin involvement with *Nocardia* is common and infection in almost any other organ site has been reported (67).

Fungal infections, particularly from candidal species still occur but infections caused by Aspergillus are least often seen in renal transplant patients. When present, *Aspergillus* infections have a high mortality. Multiple instances of infections with the phaeohyphomycosis group also termed dematiaceous fungi have been reported in renal transplant patients and usually respond to antifungal treatment with itraconazole plus surgical debridement (76,77). Occasionally *Cryptococcus* may present in forms more commonly associated with other organisms, such as necrotizing fasciitis (78).

Newer pathogens, such as *Rhodococcus equi,* and *Bartonella* species, first recognized in patients with acquired immunodeficiency syndrome, are being reported in patients with renal transplants (79). Rhodococcus is a gram-positive coccus resistant to most antibiotics except vancomycin and rifampin, and infections with it are usually associated with cavitary pulmonary lesions (80). Bartonella may cause bacillary angiomatosis as in patients with acquired immunodeficiency syndrome. Tuberculosis, usually reactivation, is also seen in renal transplant patients, particularly after a period of intensive immunosuppression. Twenty-five percent of infections were disseminated on presentation in one report (81). Atypical mycobacteria also cause infection but disease is usually localized and presents as a cutaneous nodule, or as infection of bone, joint or tendon sheath.

It is noteworthy that the acquired immunodeficiency syndrome was a recognized complication of renal transplantation. Human immunodeficiency virus has usually been transmitted along with the transplanted kidney, which has generally shown remarkably little evidence of rejection. Acquired immunodeficiency syndrome usually pursues a rapid course in these patients (82). This complication has become uncommon after routine testing for human immunodeficiency virus of all organ donors and of blood for transfusion.

CMV infections are important in renal transplant recipients, partly because primary CMV infection in a transplant recipient is associated with doubling of the rate of rejection, although causality has not been proved. Several studies have shown that CMV infection is more likely to occur after therapy for rejection with antilymphocyte preparations such as OKT3 or antilymphoblast globulin (83). Preemptive therapy with ganciclovir may prevent severe CMV infection in this setting (84). Primary CMV infection tends to be more serious than reactivation of a latent infection in these patients. Its major manifestations, in addition to rejection, are fever of unknown origin and leukopenia (85). Administration of prophylactic anti-CMV immunoglobulin has been shown to prevent severe CMV related disease in seronegative recipients of grafts from seropositive donors, even when they are being treated for rejection (86). Ganciclovir may also be useful in treatment of these infections when they are documented early during rejection (87). Recently, persistent infection caused by resistance to ganciclovir has been reported in patients receiving high-dose immunosuppression for a prolonged course (88). Other viral infections that are common in renal transplant patients include hepatitis B, C, and *Parvovirus* infections. Since the advent of screening for hepatitis B, most cases are associated with progressive worsening of preexisting infections in the recipient after immunosuppression (89). After CMV, hepatitis C virus is the next most common cause of hepatitis in transplant patients. Approximately 25% of patients have positive tests for hepatitis C by 1 year after transplantation (90). Their illness is often mild and may not cause elevated transaminase values. However, its progression may be insidious and patients with elevated transaminase levels are at increased risk of complications (91). Infections with other herpes viruses, herpes simplex virus (HSV), varicella-zoster virus (VZV), and Epstein-Barr virus (EBV) occur. HSV is spread person to person and from the allograft. Pneumonitis is the most serious form and is often fatal. HSV also may cause disseminated disease. There is an association of HSV pneumonia and endotracheal intubation in the presence of oral herpetic lesions. VZV infection most often causes dermatomal disease (shingles) but may disseminate and involve deep organs with high dose immunosuppression. Both HSV and VZV infections may respond to treatment with acyclovir. EBV infection is also associated with the post-transplant lymphoproliferative syndrome. EBV related lymphomas are treated by reduction of immunosuppression. HHV8 and Kaposi's sarcoma may result and represent reactivation of latent virus with immunosuppression or be acquired from the transplanted organ. HHVS also causes bone marrow failure (92,93). *Parvovirus* can cause red blood cell aplasia and unresponsive anemia in immunosuppressed transplant patients, especially if they are children or young adults (94,95). There is an absence of reticulocytes during infection. Unless treated with intravenous immunoglobulin, *Parvovirus* infection may be fatal. An outbreak of *Parvovirus* has been reported in a renal transplant unit, perhaps related to prolonged shedding of the virus 96. Other viruses such as JC virus, the cause of progressive multifocal leukodystrophy, BK virus associated with urethral stricture, worsening renal function, and chronic rejection and adenovirus, a cause of hemorrhagic cystitis, have been detected in renal transplant patients.

Infections and Liver Transplantation

Although mortality rates associated with serious infections in patients with liver transplants have declined, such infections are still common and occur in 50% of transplanted patients.

Their frequency is related directly to operative time and difficulties with this surgical procedure involving clean-contaminated sites. The most serious infections are polymicrobial peritonitis, cholangitis, and hepatic or other intraabdominal abscesses and are associated with anastomotic leakage of bacteria from the intestinal tract, leakage of bile, or fungal superinfections. Cholangitis due to stricture or instrumentation of the biliary tract may resemble rejection clinically. Most bacterial infections occur within two to three weeks post-transplant. Gram-positive bacteremias (especially with *S. aureus* and *Enterococcus*) are notably more common in patients with liver transplants than in patients with other solid organ transplants (97). Gram-positive bacteremias are primarily associated with catheter-related infections. Multiple antibiotic-resistant strains of the bacteria are commonly isolated from infected liver transplant patients. In one review, 25% of *S. aureus* were methicillin-resistant and caused bacteremia in 68% of those infected with these strains (98). *S. aureus* caused not only catheter-related infections and surgical site infections, but in addition, intra-abdominal infections, and pneumonia. There was a high mortality associated with the deep infections caused by antibiotic-resistant gram-positive cocci. Vancomycin-resistant enterococci have been isolated with increasing frequency as well, ranging from one-third to two-thirds of the patients with bacteremia (99). Treatment of infections with vancomycin-resistant enterococci is limited to the streptogramin antibiotic combination quinupristin-dalfopristin or the oxazolidine antibiotic linezolid. Bacteremia from gram-negative bacilli is associated with biliary stricture and liver abscess.

Bacterial infections within the first post transplantation month are often mixed, along with fungal infection (100). Unusual bacteria may be isolated because of the nature of the surgery. Roux-en-Y anastomoses may permit easy bacterial access to the biliary tree, and concomitant treatment with vancomycin may select for vancomycin-resistant organisms such as lactobacilli (101), and vancomycin-resistant enterococci. Perioperative administration of antibiotics has been effective in reducing postoperative infections in liver transplant patients. Use of granulocyte colony-stimulating factor for 7 to 10 days postoperatively to keep the total leukocyte count between 10,000 and 20,000/mm^3 has been reported to reduce significantly the incidence of sepsis and sepsis-related deaths as well as the rate of rejection, even though these patients were never neutropenic (102).

Aspergillus infections are relatively frequent after liver transplantation and may cause fungemia, infection of the central nervous system, or severe wound infections within the first 2 to 4 weeks after transplant (103). *Aspergillus* causes the majority of brain abscesses that occur in liver transplant patients (104). Mycotic aneurysm caused by either *Aspergillus* or *Candida* is a cause of intracerebral hemorrhage in these patients. Concomitant diabetes is an associated risk factor (105). Other risks for *Aspergillus* infection include decreased function of the transplanted liver, severe renal insufficiency requiring dialysis and retransplantation (106). Mortality of patients infected with *Aspergillus* remains very high. Recovery of this mold from sputum culture or bronchoalveolar lavage (BAL) cultures should raise suspicion of pulmonary infection. Various prophylaxis strategies have been tried, itraconazole, low dose amphotericin B and liposomal preparations of amphotericin but none appear too generally effective (107). *Aspergillus* infections have been reported despite the prophylactic postoperative administration of amphotericin B (0.5 mg/kg) (108). The incidence of postoperative fungal infections may be reduced by the administration of liposomal amphotericin B to patients with liver transplants (109). The cost of administration of the liposomal preparations to all transplant patients, however, could be prohibitive. Identification of patients at high risk and early institution of appropriate therapy is currently, the best approach. Treatment of identified or suspected cases of *Aspergillus* infection may be superior using liposomal preparations (110).

Candida infections have decreased with better surgical practices but remain an important cause of post-transplant infections. With use of fluconazole for prophylaxis or treatment of fungal infections, the incidence of azole resistant non-albicans species causing infection in transplant patients has increased. Prophylaxis with fluconazole does decrease the incidence of cutaneous infections but does not prevent serious candidal infections (111). Use of fluconazole may increase the rate of infections caused by *Aspergillus* in liver transplant patients (112). Prolonged treatment with ciprofloxacin appears to be a risk factor for developing candidal infections (97). Other fungi cause infection as well. Cryptococcus has also been reported to cause severe cellulitis indistinguishable from bacterial skin and soft tissue infections in these patients (113). As with renal transplant patients, dematiaceous molds primarily cause cutaneous and soft tissue infections in liver transplant patients. Brain abscess caused by these fungi has also been reported and may be more amenable to treatment than *Aspergillus* central nervous system infections (114).

Pneumocystis carinii pneumonia, a late infection after liver transplantation, has been effectively prevented by the prophylactic administration of trimethoprim-sulfamethoxazole (115).

Almost all of the viral infections that occur after liver transplantation represent relapses of infection acquired before the transplantation (116). Acute severe viral hepatitis is frequent after a patient with chronic active hepatitis B receives a liver transplant, even when hyperimmune globulin is also given. Hepatitis C is also seen in liver transplant patients and is surpassed in frequency only by CMV infection. Pretransplantation screening for hepatitis C can identify the patients at risk for this complication. As in renal transplant patients, the infection may be indolent, and severe liver damage may result (91).

Acquisition of primary CMV infection is substantially worse in transplant patients when compared to reactivated disease, although complications are produced from either type of infection. Mortality caused by CMV infection of liver transplant patients may be decreased by early diagnosis and treatment. With infection there is increased risk of rejection and hepatic artery thrombosis, analogous to early coronary artery disease in cardiac transplantation (117). Early diagnosis in high-risk patients is afforded by the shell vial culture or the more sensitive CMV antigen assay for a 63-Kd viral protein. Elevated levels of CMV antigen correlate with early infection.

An association has been noted between CMV hepatitis, rejection, and the need for retransplantation. An increased risk of CMV infection is also associated with the use of OKT3 (118). CMV infection is also more likely to occur in patients that have reactivated HHV6 infection (119).

Because clinical infection carries substantial risks, preemptive therapy has been successful at reducing complications of infection in patients that might develop clinical illness. Not all high-risk patients will succumb to CMV infection. For those identified as high risk, that is, seropositive patients or seronegative patients receiving a seropositive organ, CMV status can be monitored using the CMV antigen assay. When this assay shows elevated levels treatment with IV ganciclovir or oral ganciclovir has been effective (120). Patients in whom a positive CMV antigen assay does not develop do not experience CMV clinical disease (121,122). Valganciclovir, an oral form with bioavailability similar to intravenous ganciclovir will likely provide an alternative to intravenous treatment. Other Herpesviruses, HHV6 and HHV8, are recognized as pathogens in liver transplant patients as well. HHV6, the agent of exanthem subitum, reactivates in transplant

patients, occurring in 20% to 40% of liver transplants within the first 2 weeks after transplant. Activated infection presents as a fever of unknown origin (123).

HHV6 is also transmitted from infected organs. HHV6 affects immune function and increases the risks of infection from fungus and CMV. Active HHV6 infection can be diagnosed using a shell vial assay. This virus is susceptible to ganciclovir and foscarnet. Like HHV6, HHV8 or Kaposi's sarcoma, herpes viruses reactivate and are seen more often in liver transplants in comparison to other solid organ transplants (124). Kaposi's sarcoma lesions may be seen when this virus has reactivated.

Infections and Heart and Heart-Lung Transplantation

Infections are a major cause of morbidity and mortality after heart transplantation, and in some centers more than half of early deaths have resulted from infection. Infecting organisms may be transmitted via the graft, transfused blood, direct contact, or from environmental reservoirs. Additional infections are caused by bacteria originating in the patient's endogenous flora or acquired during earlier infections. Most of the nosocomial bacterial infections are encountered principally in the first 30 to 60 days after transplantation, and their frequency appears to be reduced by perioperative antibiotic prophylaxis; no single regimen is widely applicable, but one popular regimen used at Stanford consists of cefazolin plus erythromycin and the administration of an nonabsorbable oral antifungal (125). Opportunistic infections with relatively less virulent pathogens usually do not occur during this early period unless the patient has been treated for acute rejection. The frequency of infection after the first month or two is directly related to the intensity of the immunosuppressive therapy required to prevent rejection. The use of antilymphocyte preparations for the treatment of rejection is also associated with increased severity of infections in the first 3 months postoperatively (126). Heart transplant recipients who require mechanical support with an intraaortic balloon pump, a left ventricular assist device, or a total artificial heart are at higher risk for severe infection and death. Most often, mediastinal infections occur in this time period, half of which are caused by staphylococci. Cases of mediastinitis in which the initial cultures were negative have been found to be caused by atypical mycobacteria or *Legionella*. Protective isolation has not been shown to have a favorable effect on morbidity or mortality resulting from infection of these patients.

Protocols using cyclosporines to prevent rejection have been associated with a lowering of rates of severe infection. A multicenter report of patients who underwent transplantation in the cyclosporine era indicated that 58% of 384 patients developed infection, but there were only 20 infection-related deaths (5%) (126). All classes of organisms were involved, but the most frequent pathogens were *Staphylococcus*, gram-negative enterics, *Nocardia, Aspergillus, Cryptococcus*, CMV, other herpesviruses, *P. carinii*, and *Toxoplasma gondii*. A recent review of 620 transplants identified a bacterial pathogen in 44% of infected patients, 41% were viral in origin and 10% were fungal. The remaining infections were caused by *P. carinii* and parasites (125). Pulmonary infections are more common and more serious after heart or heart-lung transplantation than with other organ allografts. Lung transplantation is associated with the highest incidence of pulmonary infection among solid organ transplants and the lung is the most common site of infection in this patient group. The donor lung may be the source of infection in 25% of pneumonia cases (127). *Pseudomonas* is the most common bacterial cause of pneumonia while *Aspergillus* causes largest proportion of fungal pneumonias. Most infections with *Aspergillus* in heart transplant patients occur about 1 month post procedure (128). BAL cultures yielding *Aspergillus* are suspicious for pulmonary infection, but as many as one third of cases will have negative BAL cultures (129). Almost one third of *Aspergillus* pneumonia will disseminate, and is the single greatest cause of mortality from infection in one series (125). Routine use of prophylaxis with TMP-SMX postoperatively has markedly reduced the incidence of *Pneumocystis* pneumonia; similarly, the prophylactic administration of pyrimethamine has reduced the incidence and severity of Toxoplasma infection (130,131). In fact, *P. carinii* pneumonia occurs only in patients not taking TMP-SMX prophylaxis (125). Two thirds of *Pneumocystis* infections occur in the first six months, most of the remaining cases occur more than 1 year after transplant. Toxoplasmosis usually causes pneumonia and disseminated disease in donor-positive, recipient-negative patients who are not receiving prophylaxis. This infection is uniformly fatal once it occurs.

Pulmonary infections in heart transplant recipients frequently disseminate and are associated with a high rate of intracranial infection with opportunistic pathogens (Table 128.5). *Nocardia* and *Aspergillus* infections have been noted to cause intracranial abscesses with poorly developed capsules and extensive tissue necrosis in heart transplant recipients; the cerebrospinal fluid is usually normal in these patients. Infections of the nervous system tend to occur within the first 3 months after transplantation and in association with treatment of episodes of rejection. Viral infections are implicated in the same proportion of patients as bacterial infections. HSV stomatitis and shingles together comprise 50% of the infections. CMV, however causes most of the morbidity. CMV pneumonia, and more often in heart transplants, gastritis and colitis, are common sites of involvement. Retinitis is less common. CMV may also be associated with gastrointestinal bleeding in heart transplant patients; this may present with abdominal pain and refractory nausea. This infection does respond to treatment with ganciclovir (132). Decreased rates of CMV infection, as with other solid organ transplants, seems to be associated with increased graft survival and a lower incidence of other severe infections such as disseminated or pulmonary *Aspergillosis*.

A syndrome of unexplained fever, hepatitis, interstitial pneumonitis, leukopenia, and atypical lymphocytosis is common in heart transplant patients with primary CMV infection. Accelerated coronary atherosclerosis has been linked to CMV infection in a group of young transplant patients, especially if infection occurs within the first year (133,134). It appears that preemptive treatment of CMV infections in patients undergoing solid organ transplant has resulted in decreased morbidity and mortality. Prophylactic treatment would require prolonged therapy in a larger number of patients. Prolonged time of administration has been associated with the emergence of ganciclovir resistant CMV (135,136).

A comprehensive approach to prophylaxis can be taken by transplant centers to minimize the risk of acquisition and development of bacterial and opportunistic infections. The Stanford center uses perioperative cefazolin plus erythromycin and an oral topical antifungal to diminish early post-operative infections. Aerosolized amphotericin B is administered for the remainder of the post-operative hospital stay to prevent *Aspergillus* pneumonia. TMP-SMX (double strength) twice daily three times weekly, is given to prevent PCP and also prevents *Toxoplasmosis* and *Listeria* infections. When CMV is detected in the recipient, IV ganciclovir is administered 5 mg/kg twice daily for 2 weeks, then 6 mg/kg for 4 weeks. When the donor is CMV positive and the recipient is negative, 2 additional weeks of ganciclovir are administered in conjunction with a 16-week course of CMV immunoglobulin. For donor-positive/recipient-negative toxoplasmosis, pyrimethamine is added at 25 mg per day for 4 to 6 weeks (25).

Infections and Bone Marrow Transplantation

See Chapter 128.

REFERENCES

1. Korvick J, Yu VL. Simultaneous infection with *Cryptococcus neoformans* and *Legionella pneumophila*. In vivo expression of common defects in cell-mediated immunity. *Respiration* 1988;53:132.
2. Klein NC, Go CH, Cunha BA. Infections associated with steroid use. *Infect Dis Clin North Am* 2001;15:423.
3. Schimpff SC. Overview of empiric therapy for the febrile neutropenic patient. *Rev Infect Dis* 1985;7(Suppl 4):5734.
4. Sickles EA, Greene WH, Wernik PH. Clinical presentation of infection in granulocytopenic patients. *Arch Intern Med* 1975;135:715.
5. Fauci AS, Dale DC, Balow JE. Glucocorticosteroid therapy: mechanisms of action and clinical considerations. *Ann Intern Med* 1976;84:304.
6. Murphy JF, McDonald FD, Dawson M, et al. Factors affecting the frequency of infection in renal transplantation recipients. *Arch Intern Med* 1976;136:670.
7. Stuck AE, Minder CE, Frey FJ. Risk of infectious complications in patients taking glucocorticoids. *Rev Infect Dis* 1989;11:954.
8. Whimbey E, Kiehn TE, Brannon P, et al. Bacteremia and fungemia in patients with neoplastic disease. *Am J Med* 1987;82:723.
9. Ingram CW, Tanner DC, Durack DT, et al. Disseminated infection with rapidly growing mycobacteria. *Clin Infect Dis* 1993;16:463.
10. Bushelman SJ, Callen JP, Roth DN, et al. Disseminated *Fusarium solani* infection. *J Am Acad Dermatol* 1995;32:346.
11. Ammari LK, Puck JM, McGowan KL, et al. Catheter-related *Rusarium solani* fungemia and pulmonary infection in a patient with leukemia in remission. *Clin Infect Dis* 1993;16:148.
12. Tsuji K, Hirohara J, Fukui Y, et al. Prototothecosis in a patient with systemic lupus erythematosus. *Intern Med* 1993;32:540.
13. Koeler JE, Glaser CA, Tappero JW. *Rochalimaea henselae* infection. A new zoonosis with the domestic cat as reservoir. *Infection* 1994;16:186.
14. Novak RM, Polisky EL, Janda WM, et al. Osteomyelitis caused by *Rhodococcus equi* in a renal transplant recipient. *Infection* 1988;16:186.
15. Glenn J, Cotton D, Wesley R, Pizzo P. Anorectal infections in patients with malignant diseases. *Rev Infect Dis* 1988;10:42.
16. Richard P, Amador Del Valle G, Moreau P, et al. Viridans streptococcal bacteraemia in patients with neutropenia. *Lancet* 1995;345:1607.
17. Heussel CP, Kauczor HU, Heussel GE, et al. Pneumonia in febrile neutropenic patients and bone marrow and blood stem cell transplant recipients: use of high resolution computed tomography. *J Clin Oncol* 1999;17:796–805.
18. Daw MA, Munnely P, McCann SR, et al. Value of surveillance cultures in the management of neutropenic patients. *Eur J Clin Microbiol Infect Dis* 1998;7:742.
19. Holliman J, Johnson D, Savva D, et al. Diagnosis of toxoplasma infection in cardiac transplant recipients using the polymerase chain reaction. *J Clin Pathol* 1992;45:9331.
20. Drouet I, Michelson S, Denoyel G, Colimon R. Polymerase chain reaction detection of human cytomegalovirus in over 2000 blood specimens correlated with virus isolation and related to urinary virus excretion. *J Virol Methods* 1993;45:259.
21. Heegaard ED, Hornsleth A. Parvovirus: the expanding spectrum of disease. *Acta Paediatr* 1995;84:109.
22. Wright TL, Donegan E, Hsu HH, et al. Recurrent and acquired hepatitis C viral infection in liver transplant recipients. *Gastroenterology* 1992;103:317.

TABLE 128.5.   Causes of Central Nervous System Infection in Transplant Patients

Cryptococcus neoformans
Listeria monocytogenes
Toxoplasma gondii
Nocardia asteroides
Zygomycetes (Mucor)
Aspergillus fumigatus
Candida species
Varicella-zoster virus
Progressive multifocal leukoencephalopathy

23. Hughes WT, Armstrong D, Bodey GP, et al. 2002 guidelines for the use of antimicrobial agents in neutropenic patients with cancer. *Clin Infect Dis* 2002;34:730–751.

24. Bodey GP. Infection in cancer patients. A continuing association. *Am J Med* 1986;81:11.

25. Gaya H. Combination therapy and monotherapy in the treatment of severe infection in the immunocompromised host. *Am J Med* 1986;80(Suppl 6B):149.

26. Young LS. Antimicrobial prophylaxis in the neutropenic host: lessons of the past and perspectives for the future. *Eur J Microbiol Infect Dis* 1988;7:93.

27. Gava H. Rational basis for the choice of regimens for empirical therapy of sepsis in granulocytopenia patients. *Clin Hematol* 1984;13:573.

28. Group TEIATC. Ceftazidime combined with a short or long course of amikacin for empirical therapy of gram-negative bacteremia in cancer patients with granulocytopenia. *N Engl J Med* 1987;317:1692.

29. Pizzo PA, Hawthorn JW, Hiemenz J, et al. A randomized trial comparing ceftazidime along with combination antibiotic therapy in cancer patients with fever and neutropenia. *N Engl J Med* 1986;315:552.

30. Mortimer J, Millar S, Black D, et al. Comparison of cefoperazone and mezlocillin with imipenem as empiric therapy in febrile neutropenic cancer patients. *Am J Med* 1988;851:17.

31. Gribble MJ, Chow AW, Naiman SC, et al. Prospective randomized trial of piperacillin monotherapy versus carboxypenicillin/aminoglycoside combination regimens in the empirical treatment of serious bacterial infections. *Antimicrob Agents Chemother* 1983;24:388.

32. Brown AE. Management of the febrile neutropenic patient with cancer: therapeutic considerations. *J Pediatr* 1985;106:1035.

33. Wade JS. Antibiotic therapy for the febrile granulocytopenic patient: combination therapy vs monotherapy. *Rev Infec Dis* 1989;11(Suppl 7):S1572.

34. Young LS. Neutropenia: antibiotic combinations for empiric therapy. *Eur J Clin Microbiol Infec Dis* 1989;8:118.

35. Douard MC, Arlet G, Longuet P, et al. Diagnosis of venous access port-related infections. *Clin Infect Dis* 1999;29:1197.

36. Rolston KVI. New trends in patient management: risk-based therapy for febrile patients with neutropenia. *Clin Infect Dis* 1999;29:515.

37. Freifeld A, Marchigiani D, Walsh T, et al. A double-blind comparison of empirical oral and intravenous antibiotic therapy for low-risk febrile patients with neutropenia during cancer chemotherapy. *N Engl J Med* 1999;341:305.

38. Garcia-Carbonero R, Cortes-Funs H. Outpatient therapy with oral ofloxacin for patients with low risk neutropenia and fever: a prospective, randomized clinical trial. *Cancer* 1999;85:213.

39. Malik IA, Khan WA, Karim M, et al. Feasibility of outpatient management of fever in cancer patients with low-risk neutropenia: results of a prospective randomized trial. *Am J Med* 1995;98:224.

40. Talcott JA, Siegel RD, Finberg R, et al. Risk assessment in cancer patients with fever and neutropenia: a prospective, two-center validation of a prediction rule. *J Clin Oncol* 1992;10:316.

41. Klastersky J, Paesmans M, Rubenstein EB, et al. The multinational association for supportive care in cancer: a multinational scoring system for identification of low-risk febrile neutropenic cancer patients. *J Clin Oncol* 2000;18:3038.

42. Hughes WT, Rovera GK, Schell MJ, et al. Successful intermittent chemoprophylaxis for Pneumocystis carinii pneumonitis. *N Engl J Med* 1987;316:1627.

43. Meijer-Severs GJ, Joshi JH. The effect of new broad-spectrum antibiotics on faecal flora of cancer patients. *J Antimicrob Chemother* 1989;24:605.

44. Anaissie EJ, Fainstein V, Bodey GP, et al. Randomized trial of beta-lactam regimens in febrile neutropenic cancer patients. *Am J Med* 1988;84:581.

45. Jones P, Body GP, Rolston K, et al. Cefoperazone plus mezlocillin for empiric therapy of febrile cancer patients. *Am J Med* 1988;85:3.

46. Mayordomo JI, Rivera F, Diaz-Puente MT, et al. Improving treatment of chemotherapy-induced neutropenic fever by administration of colony-stimulating factors. *J Natl Cancer Inst* 1995;87:803.

47. Riikonen P, Saarinen UM, Makipernaa A, et al. rhGM-CSF in the treatment of fever and neutropenia: A double-blind placebo controlled study in children with malignancy. *Proc Annu Meet Am Soc Clin Oncol* 1993;12:Al 1532.

48. Ozer H, Armitage JO, Bennett CL, et al. 2000 update of recommendations for the use of hematopoietic colony-stimulating factors: evidence-based clinical practice guidelines. *J Clin Oncol* 2000;18:3558.

49. Bakker-Woudenberg IAJM, Roossendaal R. Impact of dosage regimens on the efficacy of antibiotics in the immunocompromised host. *J Antimicrob Chemother* 1988;21:145.

50. Klastersky J, Glauser MP, Schimpff SC, et al. Prospective randomized comparison of three antibiotic regimens for empirical therapy of suspected bacteremic infection in febrile granulocytopenic patients. *Antimicrob Agents Chemother* 1986;29:263.

51. DiNubile MJ. Stopping antibiotic therapy in neutropenic patients. *Ann Intern Med* 1988;108:289.

52. Talbot GH, Provencher M, Cassileth PA. Persistent fever after recovery from granulocytopenia in acute leukemia. *Arch Intern Med* 1988;148:2561.

53. Dekker AW, Rosenberg-Arska M, Verhoef J. Infection prophylaxis in acute leukemia: a comparison of ciprofloxacin with trimethoprim-sulfamethoxazole and colistin. *Ann Intern Med* 1987;106:1.

54. Karp JE, Merz WG, Hendricksen C, et al. Oral norfloxacin for prevention of gram-negative bacterial infections in patients with acute leukemia and granulocytopenia. *Ann Intern Med* 1987;106:1.

55. EORTC Cooperative Group. Empiric antifungal therapy in febrile granulocytopenic patients. *Am J Med* 1989;86:668.

56. Fleming RV, Kantarjian HM, Husni R, et al. comparison of amphotericin B lipid complex (ABLC) vs. AmBisome in the treatment of suspected or documented fungal infections in patients with leukemia. *Leuk Lymph* 2001;40:511–20.

57. Wingard JR, White MH, Anaissie E, et al. A randomized, double-blind comparative trial evaluating the safety of liposomal amphotericin B versus amphotericin B lipid complex in the empirical treatment of febrile neutropenia. L Amph/ABLC Collaborative Study Group. [see comments]. *Clin Infect Dis* 2000;31:1155.

58. Boogaerts M, Winston DJ, Bow EJ, et al. Itraconazole Neutropenia Study G. Intravenous and oral itraconazole versus intravenous amphotericin B deoxycholate as empirical antifungal therapy for persistent fever in neutropenic patients with cancer who are receiving broad-spectrum antibacterial therapy. A randomized, controlled trial. *Ann Intern Med* 2001;135:412.

59. Pizzo PA. After empiric therapy: what to do until the granulocyte comes back. *Rev Infect Dis* 1987;9:124.

60. Dignani MC, Anaissie EJ, Hester JP, et al. Treatment of neutropenia-related fungal infections with granulocyte colony-stimulating factor-elicited white blood cell transfusions: a pilot study. *Leukemia* 1997;11:1621.

61. Hubel K, Dale DC, Engert A, Liles WC. Current status of granulocyte (neutrophil) transfusion therapy for infectious diseases. *J Infect Dis* 2001;183:321.

62. Rex JH, Bennett JE, Pappas PG, et al. A randomized trial comparing fluconazole with amphotericin B for the treatment of candidemia in patients without neutropenia. *N Engl J Med* 1994;331:1325.

63. Tashjian LS, Ambramson JS, Peacock JE. Focal Hepatic candidiasis. A distinct clinical variant of candidiasis in immunocompromised patients. *Rev Infect Dis* 1984;6:689.

64. Thaler M, Pastakian B, Shawku TH, et al. Hepatic candidiasis in cancer patients. The evolving picture of the syndrome. *Ann Intern Med* 1988;108:88.

65. Kauffman CA, Bradley SR, Ross SS, Weber DR. Hepatosplenic candidiasis: Successful treatment with fluconazole. *Am J Med* 1991;91:137.

66. Rubin RH. *Infection in the organ transplant recipient*, 3rd ed. New York: Plenum, 1994;629.

67. Patel R, Paya CV. Infections in solid-organ transplant recipients. *Clin Microbiol Rev* 1997;10:86.

68. Ghasemian SR, Light JA, Currier C, Sasaki TM, Aquino A. Tacrolimus vs neoral in renal and renal/pancreas transplantation. *Clin Transplant* 1999;13:123.

69. Anonymous. A blinded, randomized clinical trial of mycophenolate mofetil for the prevention of acute rejection in cadaveric renal transplantation. The Tricontinental Mycophenolate Mofetil Renal Transplantation Study Group. *Transplantation* 1996;61:1029.

70. Anonymous. Mycophenolate mofetil for the treatment of refractory, acute, cellular renal transplant rejection. The Mycophenolate Mofetil Renal Refractory Rejection Study Group. *Transplantation* 1996;61:722.

71. Wyner LM. The evaluation and management of urinary tract infections in recipients of solid-organ transplants. *Semin Urol* 1994;12:134.

72. Fox BC, Sollinger HW, Belzer FO, Maki DG. A prospective, randomized, double-blind study of trimethoprim-sulfamethoxazole for prophylaxis of infection in renal transplantation: clinical efficacy, absorption of trimethoprim-sulfamethoxazole, effects on the microflora, and the cost-benefit of prophylaxis. *Am J Med* 1990;89:255.

73. Wagener MM, Yu VL. Bacteremia in transplant recipients: a prospective study of demographics, etiologic agents, risk factors, and outcomes. *Am J Infect Control* 1992;20:239.

74. Dhar JM, al-Khader AA, al-Sulaiman M, al-Hasani MK. Non-typhoid *Salmonella* in renal transplant recipients: a report of twenty cases and review of the literature. *Q J Med* 1991;78:235.

75. Reek C, Tenschert W, Elsner HA, Kaulfers PM, Huland H. Pulsed-field gel electrophoresis for the analysis of *Listeria monocytogenes* infection clusters after kidney transplantation. *Urol Res* 2000;28:93.

76. Lussier N, Laverdiere M, Delorme J, Weiss K, Dandavino R. *Trichosporon beigelii* funguria in renal transplant recipients. *Clin Infect Dis* 2000;31:1299.

77. Halaby T, Boots H, Vermeulen A, et al. Phaeohyphomycosis caused by *Alternaria infectoria* in a renal transplant recipient. *J Clin Microbiol* 2001;39:1952.

78. Marcus JR, Hussong JW, Gonzalez C, Dumanian GA. Risk factors in necrotizing fasciitis: a case involving *Cryptococcus neoformans*. *Ann Plast Surg* 1998;40:80.

79. Cline MS, Cummings OW, Goldman M, et al. Bacillary angiomatosis in a renal transplant recipient. *Transplantation* 1999;67:296.

80. Lezama JA, Garcia-Arenzana JM, Viedma PI, Aznar MS. Pulmonary infection caused by *Phodococcus equi* in renal transplant recipient. *Med Clin (Barc)* 1992;99:143.

81. Hall CM, Willcox PA, Swanepoel CR, et al. Mycobacterial infection in renal transplant recipients. *Chest* 1994;106:435.

82. Briner V, Zimmerli W, Cathomas G, et al. HIV infection caused by kidney transplant: case report and review of 18 published cases. *Schweiz Med Wochenschr* 1989;119:1046.

83. Bailey TC, Powderly WG, Storch GA, et al. Symptomatic cytomegalovirus infection in renal transplant recipients given either Minnesota antilymphoblast globulin (MALG) or OKT3 for rejection prophylaxis. *Am J Kidney Dis* 1993;21:196.

84. Hibberd PL, Rubin RH. Renal transplantation and related infections. *Semin Resp Infect* 1993;8:216.

85. Bosch RH, Hoctsma AL, Janssen HP, et al. Cytomegalovirus infection and diseases in renal transplant patients treated with cyclosporine. A prospective study. *Transplant Int* 1989;2:92.

86. Metselaar JJ, Rothbart PH, Browwer RM, et al. Prevention of cytomegalovirus-related death by passive immunization. A double-blind placebo-controlled

study in kidney transplant recipients treated for rejection. *Transplantation* 1989; 48:264.

87. Turgeon N, Fishman JA, Basgoz N, et al. Effect of oral acyclovir or ganciclovir therapy after preemptive intravenous ganciclovir therapy to prevent cytomegalovirus disease in cytomegalovirus seropositive renal and liver transplant recipients receiving antilymphocyte antibody therapy. *Transplantation* 1998;66:1780.

88. Limaye AP, Corey L, Koelle DM, et al. Emergence of ganciclovir-resistant cytomegalovirus disease among recipients of solid-organ transplants. *Lancet* 2000;356:645.

89. Hamada T, Kumashiro MR, Koga Y, et al. Fatal acute hepatitis B virus infection while receiving immunosuppressants after renal transplantation. *Intern Med* 1993;32:547.

90. Brunson ME, Lau JY, Davis GL, et al. Non-A, non-B hepatitis and elevated serum aminotransferases in renal transplant patients. Correlation with hepatitis C infection. *Transplantation* 1993;56:1364.

91. Chan TM, Wu PC, Lau JY, et al. Clinicopathologic features of hepatitis C virus infection in renal allograft recipients. *Transplantation* 1994;58:996.

92. Farge D, Lebbe C, Marjanovic Z, et al. Human herpes virus-8 and other risk factors for Kaposi's sarcoma in kidney transplant recipients. Groupe Cooperatif de Transplantation d' Ile de France (GCIF). *Transplantation* 1999;67:1236.

93. Luppi M, Barozzi P, Schulz TF, et al. Bone marrow failure associated with human herpesvirus 8 infection after transplantation. *N Engl J Med* 2000; 343:1378.

94. Rao SP, Miller ST, Cohen BJ. B 19 parvovirus infection in children with malignant solid tumors receiving chemotherapy. *Med Pediatr Oncol* 1994;22(255).

95. Uemura N, Ozawa K, Tani K, et al. Pure red cell aplasia caused by parvovirus B 19 infection in a renal transplant recipient. *Eur J Haematol* 1995;54:68.

96. Lui SL, Luk WK, Cheung CY, Chan TM, Lai KN, Peiris JS. Nosocomial outbreak of parvovirus B19 infection in a renal transplant unit. *Transplantation* 2001;71:59–64.

97. Wade JJ, Rolando N, Hayllar K, et al. Bacterial and fungal infections after liver transplantation: an analysis of 284 patients. *Hepatology* 1995;21:1328.

98. Singh N, Paterson DL, Chang FY, et al. Methicillin-resistant *Staphylococcus aureus:* the other emerging resistant gram-positive coccus among liver transplant recipients. *Clin Infect Dis* 2000;30:322.

99. Papanicolaou GA, Meyers BR, Meyers J, et al. Nosocomial infections with vancomycin-resistant Enterococcus faecium in liver transplant recipients: risk factors for acquisition and mortality. *Clin Infect Dis* 1996;23:760.

100. Barkholt L, Erizon BG, Tollemar J, et al. Infections in human liver recipients: Different patterns early and late after transplantation. *Transplant Int* 1993;6:77.

101. Patel R, Cockerill FR, Porayko MK, et al. Lactobacillemia in liver transplant patients. *Clin Infect Dis* 1994;18:207.

102. Foster PF, Mital D, Sankary HN, et al. The use of granulocyte colony-stimulating factor after liver transplantation. *Transplantation* 1995;59:1557.

103. Pla MP, Berenguer J, Arzuaga JA, et al. Surgical wound infection by *Aspergillus fumigatus* in liver transplant recipients. *Diagn Microbiol Infec Dis* 1992;15:703.

104. Selby R, Ramirez CB, Singh R, et al. Brain abscess in solid organ transplant recipients receiving cyclosporine-based immunosuppression. *Arch Surg* 1997;132:304.

105. Wijdicks EF, de Groen CF, Wiesner RH, Drom RA. Intracerebral hemorrhage in liver transplant recipients. *Mayo Clin Proc* 1995;70:443.

106. Paterson DL, Singh N. Invasive aspergillosis in transplant recipients. *Medicine* 1999;78:123.

107. Singh N. The current management of infectious diseases in the liver transplant recipient. *Clin Liv Dis* 2000;4:657–73, ix.

108. Singh N, Meiles L, Yu VL, Gayowski T. Invasive aspergillosis in liver transplant recipients: association with candidemia and consumption coagulopathy and failure of prophylaxis with low-dose amphotericin B. *Clin Infect Dis* 1993;17:906.

109. Tollemar J, Hockerstedt K, Ericzon BG, et al. Liposomal amphotericin B prevents invasive fungal infections in liver transplant recipients. A randomized, placebo-controlled study. *Transplantation* 1995;59:45.

110. White MH, Anaissie EJ, Kusne S, et al. Amphotericin B colloidal dispersion vs. amphotericin B as therapy for invasive aspergillosis. *Clin Infect Dis* 1997;24:635.

111. Lumbreras C, Cuervas-Mons V, Jara P, et al. Randomized trial of fluconazole versus nystatin for the prophylaxis of *Candida* infection following liver transplantation. *J Infect Dis* 1996;174:583.

112. Fortun J, Lopez-San Roman A, Velasco JJ, et al. Selection of *Candida glabrata* strains with reduced susceptibility to azoles in four liver transplant patients with invasive candidiasis. *Eur J Clin Microbiol Infect Dis* 1997;16:314.

113. Singh N, Rihs JD, Gayowski T, Yu VL. Cutaneous cryptococcosis mimicking bacterial cellulitis in a liver transplant recipient: case report and review in solid organ transplant recipients. *Clin Transplant* 1994;8:365.

114. Singh N, Chang FY, Gayowski T, Marino IR. Infections due to dematiaceous fungi in organ transplant recipients: case report and review [review]. *Clin Infect Dis* 1997;24:369.

115. Hayes MJ, Torzillo PJ, Sheil AG, McCaughan GW. *Pneumocystis carinii* pneumonia after liver transplantation in adults. *Clin Tranplant* 1994;8:499.

116. Weinstein JS, Poterucha JJ, Zein N, et al. Epidemiology and natural history of hepatitis C infections in liver transplant recipients. *J Hepatol* 1995;22:154.

117. Pastacaldi S, Teixeira R, Montalto P, Rolles K, Burroughs AK. Hepatic artery thrombosis after orthotopic liver transplantation: a review of nonsurgical causes. *Liver Transplant* 2001;7:75.

118. Stratta RJ, Shaeffer MS, Markin RS, et al. Cytomegalovirus infection and disease after liver transplantation. An overview. *Dig Dis Sci* 1992;37:673.

119. Dockrell DH, Prada J, Jones MF, et al. Seroconversion to human herpesvirus 6 following liver transplantation is a marker of cytomegalovirus disease. *J Infect Dis* 1997;176:1135.

120. Gane E, Saliba F, Valdecasas GJ, et al. Randomised trial of efficacy and safety of oral ganciclovir in the prevention of cytomegalovirus disease in liver-transplant recipients. The Oral Ganciclovir International Transplantation Study Group. *Lancet* 1997;350:1729.

121. Conti DJ, Freed BM, Gruber SA, et al. Impact of retransplant status on delayed graft function: an analysis of paired cadaver kidneys. *Transplant Proc* 1995;27:1070.

122. Verdonck LF, Dekker AW, Rozenberg-Arska M, van den Hock MR. A risk-adapted approach with a short course of ganciclovir to prevent cytomegalovirus (CMV) pneumonia in CMV-seropositive recipients of allogeneic bone marrow transplants. *Clin Infect Dis* 1997;24:901.

123. Singh N, Carrigan DR. Human herpesvirus-6 in transplantation: an emerging pathogen [review]. *Ann Intern Med* 1996;124:1065.

124. Farge D. Kaposi's sarcoma in organ transplant recipients. The Collaborative Transplantation Research Group of Ile de France. *Eur J Med* 1993;2(6):339–343.

125. Montoya JG, Giraldo LF, Efron B, et al. Infectious complications among 620 consecutive heart transplant patients at Stanford University Medical Center. *Clin Infect Dis* 2001;33:629.

126. Grossi P, De Maria R, Caroli A, et al. Infections in heart transplant recipients: the experience of the Italian heart transplantation program. Italian Study Group on Infections in Heart Transplantation. *J Heart Lung Transplant* 1992;11:847.

127. Low DE, Kaiser LR, Haydock DA, et al. The donor lung: infectious and pathologic factors affecting outcome in lung transplantation. *J Thorac Cardiovasc Surg* 1993;106:614.

128. Miller LW, Naftel DC, Bourge RC, et al. Infection after heart transplantation: a multiinstitutional study. Cardiac Transplant Research Database Group. *J Heart Lung Transplant* 1994;13:381.

129. Guillemain R, Lavarde V, Amrein C, et al. Invasive aspergillosis after transplantation. *Transplant Proc* 1995;27:1307.

130. Wreghitt TG, Gray GG, Pavel P, et al. Efficacy of pyrimethamine for the prevention of donor-acquired *Toxoplasma gondii* infection in heart and heart-lung transplant patients. *Transplant Int* 1992;5:187.

131. Keating MR, Wilhelm MP, Walker RC. Strategies for prevention of infection after cardiac transplantation. *Mayo Clin Proc* 1992;67:676.

132. Arabia FA, Rosade LJ, Huston CC, et al. Incidence and recurrence of gastrointestinal cytomegalovirus infection in heart transplantation. *Ann Thorac Surg* 1993;55:8.

133. Dummer S, Lee A, Breinig MK. Investigation of cytomegalovirus infection as a risk factor for coronary atherosclerosis in the explanted hearts of patients undergoing heart transplantation. *J Med Virol* 1994;44:305.

134. Koskinen PK, Nieminen MS, Krogerus LA, et al. Cytomegalovirus infection accelerates cardiac allograft vasculopathy: correlation between angiographic and endomyocardial biopsy findings in heart transplant patients. *Transplant Int* 1993;6:341.

135. Baldanti F, Simoncini L, Sarasini A, et al. Ganciclovir resistance as a result of oral ganciclovir in a heart transplant recipient with multiple human cytomegalovirus strains in blood. *Transplantation* 1998;66:324.

136. Kruger RM, Shannon WD, Arens MQ, et al. The impact of ganciclovir-resistant cytomegalovirus infection after lung transplantation. *Transplantation* 1999;68:1272.

BIBLIOGRAPHY

Bodey GP, Buckely M, Sathe YS, Freireich EH: Quantitative relationships between circulating leukocytes and infection in patients with acute leukemia. *Ann Intern Med* 64:328, 1966.

Goering P, Berlinger NT, Weisdorf DJ: Aggressive combined modality treatment of progressive sinonasal fungal infections in immunocompromised patients. *Am J Med* 85:619, 1988.

Hertz MI, Englund JA, Snover D, et al: Respiratory syncytial virus-induced acute lung injury in adult patients with bone marrow transplants: A clinical approach and review of the literature. *Medicine (Baltimore)* 68:269, 1989.

Linder J: Infection as a complication of heart transplantation. *J Heart Transplant* 7:390, 1988.

Melewski DJ, Higby DJ, Reese PA: Infectious complications in neutropenic patients. Clinical-laboratory correlations. *J Med* 19:1, 1988.

Meyers JD, Leszczynski J, Zaia JA, et al: Prevention of cytomegalovirus infection by cytomegalovirus immune globulin after marrow transplantation. *Ann Intern Med* 98:442, 1983.

van der Meer JWM, Guiot HFL, van den Broek PJ, van Furth R: Infections in bone marrow recipients. *Semin Hematol* 21:123, 1984.

Watson JG: Problems of infection after bone marrow transplantation. *J Clin Pathol* 36:683, 1983.

Winston DJ, Ho WG, Lin CH, et al: Intravenous immune globulin for prevention of cytomegalovirus infection and interstitial pneumonia after bone marrow transplantation. *Ann Intern Med* 106:12, 1987.

CHAPTER 129

Treatment and Prevention of Infections in Immunocompromised Hosts

Stephen H. Zinner

The acquired immunodeficiency syndrome (AIDS) epidemic has highlighted the critical role of the intact immune system in the prevention of infection. This chapter focuses on a general approach to the treatment of infection in patients with immune defects (other than AIDS and human immunodeficiency virus [HIV] infection) and reviews the several methods reported to prevent infection in such patients.

SPECIFIC DEFECTS PREDICT INFECTING ORGANISMS

The approach to the treatment of infections in the immunocompromised patient depends on an understanding of the specific immune defect. The nature of the immune defect roughly predicts the most likely infecting organisms (Table 129.1).

The white blood cell is critically important in maintaining an infection-free state. A variety of conditions may impair white blood cell number and function. Neutropenia is among the most common defects in host response. It may be found in patients with leukemia, AIDS, carcinoma metastatic to the bone marrow, and tuberculosis or other infections involving the marrow-forming elements. Neutropenia may also occur in patients receiving cytotoxic chemotherapy or radiation therapy. Many drugs may cause granulocytopenia, including anticonvulsants (carbamazepine, phenytoin), antibiotics (penicillins, cephalosporins, chloramphenicol, sulfonamides and trimethoprim-sulfamethoxazole, rifampin), nonsteroidal and other anti-inflammatory drugs, antidepressants, phenothiazines, clozapine, antithyroid drugs (carbimazole, methimazole, propylthiouracil) and many others; however, these effects are usually or often reversible on discontinuation of the agent or in response to colony stimulating factors if needed (1,2).

The risk of infection increases as the granulocyte count falls below 1,000 cells/mm^3, but the most severe risk occurs at counts below 100/mm^3, especially if prolonged for several days or weeks (3,4). Patients with prolonged neutropenia are subject to bacterial infections; *Escherichia coli, Klebsiella pneumoniae, Pseudomonas aeruginosa, Staphylococcus aureus,* and *Staphylococcus epidermidis* used to be isolated most frequently (5,6). Over the last decade gram-positive cocci have become more frequent than Gram-negative rods, and viridans streptococci, coagulase-negative staphylococci, *Streptococcus* sp., and *Enterococcus* sp. play a major role (7–10). Factors responsible for this shift include mucositis produced by intensive chemotherapy regimens (especially those containing cytosine arabinoside), long-term indwelling vascular cannulas, fluoroquinolone and other antibiotic prophylaxis, and perhaps the use of histamine type 2 blockers (10). Shock and the acute respiratory distress syndrome have been associated with bacteremia caused by viridans streptococci (11). Bacteremia caused by gram-negative rods continues to occur, and may be on the increase again. Organisms such as *Stenotrophomonas* (formerly *Xanthomonas*) *maltophilia* may be

particularly difficult to eradicate. Some organisms described in neutropenic patients include *Legionella* sp., *Leptotrichia buccalis, Capnocytophaga* sp., *Corynebacterium jeikeium, Stomatococcus mucilaginosus, Leuconostoc* sp., *Rhodococcus equi,* and *Bartonella henselae* (12). A recent report suggests that special cultures for cell wall–deficient bacteria might be productive (13).

The emergence of antibiotic-resistant bacteria has impacted infections in neutropenic patients. Penicillin and cephalosporin resistance is increasing among viridans streptococci (14) and quinolone resistance is becoming more prevalent among *E. coli* (15). Outbreaks of vancomycin-resistant enterococci have been described in oncology units (16). Physicians caring for immunocompromised patients should be aware of local rates of methicillin-resistant *Staphylococcus aureus* (MRSA), penicillin-resistant *Streptococcus pneumoniae* (PRSP), and antibiotic resistant gram-negative bacilli.

Neutropenic patients are also subject to infections with fungi such as *Candida* and *Aspergillus* spp., often after antibiotic therapy. Unusual fungal infections with *Drechslera, Trichosporon, Fusarium,* and *Geotrichum* spp., among others, may occur in patients with malignancies (17,18). *Fusarium* sp. infections are particularly troublesome and may present with erythematous or purpuric papules, which may become necrotic. Although high dose Amphotericin B may have some activity against the organism, disseminated fusariosis is often fatal (19).

Defects in the ability of granulocytes to move to sites of infection may also be associated with various bacterial infections (20,21). Defective chemotactic activity is described in patients with diabetes mellitus (22), alcoholism (23), chronic renal failure (24), systemic lupus erythematosus, paroxysmal nocturnal hemoglobinuria (an acquired defect in pluripotential stem cells associated with acute hemolysis) (25), Hodgkin's disease, C3A or C5A deficiency, Chédiak-Higashi syndrome, neutrophil actin dysfunction, Job syndrome, corticosteroid therapy, as well as in a variety of congenital immunodeficiencies including IgG deficiency, properdin deficiency, congenital ichthyosis, lazy leukocyte syndrome, and hyperimmunoglobulinemia E or A (20,21). Defective chemotaxis is associated with infections of the skin and respiratory system, usually caused by staphylococci, streptococci, and yeasts (20,21). Patients with rare leukocyte adhesion deficiencies lack the ability to form pus and are subject to recurrent bacterial infections despite neutrophilia (21).

In the presence of normal numbers of neutrophils, defects in the ability of the neutrophil to kill ingested bacteria are well described in chronic granulomatous disease (26), myeloperoxidase deficiency (27), and sometimes Down syndrome (28). Neutrophils from patients with chronic granulomatous disease (CGD) are unable to produce toxic oxygen radicals with their resultant microbicidal activity. In X-linked CGD, this may be due to the absence of cytochrome *b*-558, which is responsible for activation of the intracellular respiratory burst, and phagocytic membrane defects also occur (21,29). These patients have subcutaneous, lung, and bone infections with organisms that produce catalase or are unable to generate hydrogen peroxide, such as *S. aureus, E. coli,* other gram-negative rods, and *Candida albicans* (26). Patients with a defect in the lysosomal enzyme myeloperoxidase are frequently infected with *Candida* spp. and staphylococci. A premature infant with myeloperoxidase deficiency and severe fungal infection has been reported recently (30). Patients with Chédiak-Higashi syndrome suffer from repeated pyogenic infections, due to decreased chemotaxis and bactericidal activity (21).

Several conditions affect the number and function of B-lymphocytes responsible for the production of specific

TABLE 129.1.   Specific Defects in Host Response and the Likely Infecting Organisms

Defects	Conditions	Associated infecting organisms
Neutropenia	Leukemia, cytotoxic chemotherapy, AIDS, systemic lupus erythematosus, Felty syndrome, drugs	*Escherichia coli, Klebsiella pneumoniae, Pseudomonas aeruginosa, Staphylococcus aureus, Staphylococcus epidermidis,* streptococci, yeasts, *Aspergillus* spp, and other fungi
Defective chemotaxis	Diabetes, alcoholism, renal failure, systemic lupus erythematosus, Hodgkin's disease, trauma, lazy leukocyte syndrome, paroxysmal nocturnal hemoglobinuria	Staphylococci, streptococci, yeasts
Defective neutrophil killing	Chronic granulomatous disease, Down syndrome, myeloperoxidase deficiency, Chédiak-Higashi syndrome	Catalase-positive bacteria (e.g., *S. aureus, E. coli, Candida* spp.)
B-lymphocyte defects	Congenital and acquired agammaglobulinemia, burns, enteropathies, myeloma, lymphocytic leukemia	Encapsulated organisms, e.g., *Streptococcus pneumoniae, Haemophilus influenzae, Neisseria* spp.; also *Salmonella* and *Campylobacter* spp.
T-lymphocyte defects	Congenital immunodeficiencies, HIV infection and AIDS, lymphoma, sarcoidosis, Epstein-Barr virus infection, systemic lupus erythematosus, cytomegalovirus infections	Intracellular infections with bacteria, mycobacteria, viruses, parasites, fungi
Complement components	Congenital absence	Miscellaneous bacterial infections

AIDS, Acquired immunodeficiency syndrome; HIV, human immunodeficiency virus.

immunoglobulin antibodies and are associated with hypogammaglobulinemia. These disorders include congenital agammaglobulinemias; primary immunodeficiencies of the major immunoglobulins G, A, and M (IgG, IgA, and IgM); multiple myeloma; chronic lymphocytic leukemia; nephrotic syndrome; severe burns; and protein-losing enteropathies. Humoral immunity may also be deficient after splenectomy. Patients with B-cell deficiency states and hypogammaglobulinemia are subject to pyogenic infections, especially those caused by *Streptococcus pneumoniae, Haemophilus influenzae,* and *Neisseria meningitidis* (31), although infections with *Neisseria gonorrhoeae* and *Salmonella* and *Campylobacter* spp. may occur (32,33). IgM deficiency is associated with infections caused by encapsulated bacteria. *Giardia* spp. infections may be particularly difficult for patients with selective IgA deficiency. Deficiencies in IgG subclasses may result in recurrent infections with *S. pneumoniae* and *H. influenzae* (especially if also associated with IgA deficiency) (20). A new approach to children with subclass deficiencies has been published recently (34).

Defective T-lymphocyte–mediated immunity may occur in several congenital immunodeficiency states, including congenital thymic aplasia, combined immunodeficiency, Swiss type agammaglobulinemia, adenosine deaminase deficiency, nucleoside phosphorylase deficiency, ataxia-telangiectasia, and DiGeorge syndrome (28). Some of these conditions also cause humoral immune defects. Acquired defects in T-cell numbers or function include HIV infection and AIDS; sarcoidosis; Hodgkin's disease; systemic lupus erythematosus; non-Hodgkin's lymphoma; cytomegalovirus (CMV) and Epstein-Barr virus infections; pregnancy; and immunosuppressive therapy with corticosteroids, cyclophosphamide, cyclosporine, azathioprine, and antilymphocyte globulin.

Patients with defective T-cell-mediated immunity are subject to a broad spectrum of infection with intracellular pathogens, including such bacteria as *Mycobacterium tuberculosis* and other less virulent mycobacteria, *Salmonella* spp., *Listeria monocytogenes,* and *Bacillus* and *Nocardia* spp. These patients are not infrequently infected with herpesviruses, including herpes simplex virus, varicella-zoster virus, and CMV. Patients with

T-cell defects are also subject to fungal infections, including cryptococcal meningitis, candidal esophagitis, and disseminated candidiasis. *Pneumocystis carinii, Toxoplasma gondii, Isospora belli,* and *Cryptosporidium* spp. cause serious infections in these patients.

The complement system is critically important in mediating humoral defense mechanisms (35). The complement system may be activated via the classical pathway by viruses and gram-negative rods, the alternative pathway by bacterial products in the absence of specific immune responses and other organisms including fungi and viruses, and the mannose-binding lectin pathway by microbes that express terminal mannose groups on their surface. Specific defects of many complement components have been described that predispose patients to bacterial infections. Deficiencies in the terminal complement components C5 through C8 are associated with *Neisseria* infection (35,36). Defects in the early components are associated with serious pneumococcal infections. Some enteric pathogens and C3 deficiencies commonly lead to recurrent respiratory and skin infections with pneumococci, streptococci, some enteric bacteria, and *H. influenzae* (37).

As mentioned in Chapter 127, the patient undergoing bone marrow transplantation for the treatment of leukemia or other malignant diseases has several infectious risks. These risks vary with time since transplantation and duration of immunosuppressive therapy.

APPROACH TO THE TREATMENT OF INFECTIONS IN THE IMMUNOCOMPROMISED PATIENT

According to the cause and extent of immunosuppression, an immunocompromised patient may have infection in any of several sites. The skin may be the focus of recurrent pyogenic infections such as furuncles caused by staphylococci, cellulitis associated with streptococci, or zoster caused by reactivation of varicella-zoster virus in a dermatomal distribution. Disseminated herpesvirus infection may occur in severely immunocompromised patients and extensive or confluent warts caused by human papillomavirus are not uncommon in these patients, especially after renal transplantation (38). Mucocutaneous candidiasis or necrotizing superficial erosive infections with *Mucor* spp. or other fungi may develop. Solitary or multiple cryptococcal lesions may occur on the skin (38), and these may antedate systemic infection (39). Prototheccosis (infection caused by the algae *Prototheca* sp.) may present as vesicobullous, nodular, or ulcerative skin lesions; or as bursitis, gastroenteritis, or disseminated disease (40). Aspiration, biopsy, and/or direct culture from the lesion should be used to diagnose skin conditions in the immunocompromised host.

Respiratory infections are common in the immunocompromised patient, including otitis media, pharyngitis, bronchitis, and pneumonia. Interstitial infiltrates may be due to *P. carinii*, CMV, or less commonly *T. gondii*. Bronchopneumonia and lobar pneumonia may be due to pyogenic bacteria, including *S. pneumoniae, S. aureus, P. aeruginosa, Legionella pneumophila*, and *M. tuberculosis*. Extensive multilobar bronchopneumonia and necrotizing pneumonitis may occur with *C. albicans, Aspergillus* spp., or other fungi. *Nocardia asteroides* may produce lobar or segmental infiltrates with nodular densities and ultimately may form thick-walled abscess cavities. Solitary nodules may be seen with *Cryptococcus neoformans, Nocardia* spp., and so forth. A review of pulmonary disease in immunocompromised patients with excellent radiologic images has been published recently (41).

When possible, coughed or induced sputum should be examined for the usual bacterial pathogens; however, fiberoptic bronchoscopy with washings and biopsies may be necessary to establish a diagnosis. However, simply finding an organism in washings or sputum specimens does not make the diagnosis of pulmonary infection; tissue is often required (42). Transthoracic needle aspiration or biopsy is quite useful for peripheral lung lesions and is relatively safe if at least 75,000 platelets per mm^3 are present (28). Open-lung biopsy remains controversial; however, Rubin and Green effectively argued that this and other aggressive or invasive procedures are most likely to be successful and useful in patients whose underlying disease prognosis is good (e.g., renal transplantation, Hodgkin's disease, collagen vascular diseases) but not necessarily in patients with advanced leukemia or AIDS (42–45). Fiberoptic bronchoscopy with high resolution computed tomography may prove useful in these patients with normal chest X-ray examinations (46).

The gastrointestinal tract may be involved with a variety of pathogenic organisms including *Salmonella* and *Shigella* spp. and *Strongyloides stercoralis*. Disseminated infection may occur with any of these organisms. Cytomegalovirus, *Clostridium difficile*, rotavirus, adenovirus, *Isospora belli* and *Cryptosporidium* spp. are not infrequent causes of infection in severely immunocompromised patients (47). Infections of the upper gastrointestinal tract occur, including esophagitis caused by herpes simplex virus, CMV, or *Candida* spp. and other fungi. Hepatitis may be due to CMV or the hepatitis viruses. Fungal and mycobacterial infections may disseminate and involve the liver. Biopsy may be necessary to establish the diagnosis (47).

Central nervous system infections include meningitis caused by *Listeria monocytogenes, C. neoformans*, and other more usual causes of meningitis (e.g., *S. pneumoniae, N. meningitidis*) also may occur in immunocompromised patients (48). Meningoencephalitis may be caused by herpes simplex virus; varicella-zoster virus; *T. gondii*; tuberculous and nontuberculous mycobacteria; human polyomavirus (progressive multifocal leukoencephalopathy) and disseminated infections with *Candida, Aspergillus*, or other fungal species. Lumbar puncture may establish a diagnosis in some of these conditions, but brain scans, computed tomography with use of contrast medium, magnetic resonance imaging, and brain biopsy may be required.

FEVER IN THE NEUTROPENIC PATIENT

Neutropenic patients spend approximately 50% of their hospital days with fever (31). Fever may be the only manifestation of infection in a granulocytopenic patient (32).

Fever in the neutropenic patient (Table 129.2) is associated with a microbiologically documented infection in approximately 40% of patients; bacteremia accounts for about half of these (5,6). Clinically documented infections such as pneumonia without definitive microbiologic identification account for another 20% of fevers, and possible infections for another 20%. Only 20% of fevers in neutropenic patients are presumed to be due to the underlying disease or to other noninfectious causes, although the specific cause of the febrile episode is frequently not identified.

The diagnosis of infection in a severely granulocytopenic patient may be difficult because of the lack of typical physical findings. Classic signs of fluctuance, calor, rubor, and lymphadenopathy are found less frequently in neutropenic than in nonneutropenic patients, although pain may be a presenting symptom (51,52). Neutropenic patients with pneumonia may not show an initial infiltrate on a chest radiograph. Frequent radiographs may be needed to localize infection to the lung. Exudates may be less common in pharyngeal infections, and patients with urinary infections may not have pyuria. Even in some meningitides, the meningeal reaction may be limited by the inability to mobilize granulocytes to the site of infection.

In evaluating a febrile granulocytopenic patient, frequent physical examinations should emphasize examination of mucosal sites, including the perianal area. The examination should also include the liberal use of blood, urine, and sputum cultures, if available, as well as cerebrospinal fluid cultures when symptoms point to the nervous system (52,53). Routine lumbar punctures are not recommended, especially in the presence of thrombocytopenia.

The organisms usually responsible for bacterial infections in the febrile, neutropenic patient include *E. coli, K. pneumoniae, P. aeruginosa*, and *S. aureus*. However, in the last decade most centers noted a dramatic increase in the relative frequency of gram-positive coccal bacteremia (7–10) including infections with viridans streptococci, pneumococci, *S. pyogenes, Enterococcus* spp., and staphylococci. Many other organisms have been described as new etiologic agents in these patients (12). Overall infection-attributable mortality has decreased over the past two decades.

Over the years, much has been written about the optimal treatment of febrile neutropenic patients (52,55–57). There is clearly

---

TABLE 129.2. Causes of Fever in Neutropenic Patients

Condition	Approximate rate (%)
Bacteremia	15–29
Microbiologically documented infections	6–20
Clinically documented infections	20–26
Possible infection	20–39
Infection doubted	15–25

Based on several therapeutic trials by the European Organization for Research and Treatment of Cancer's International Antimicrobial Therapy Cooperative Group (see references 6, 8, 9, 63, 64).

no single drug or drug combination of choice. Most investigators agree with early empiric institution of antibiotics after obtaining specimens for culture (50). Formerly, most authorities instituted treatment with a combination of an aminoglycoside plus a β-lactam compound, such as an antipseudomonal penicillin or a cephalosporin (50,57). Several drugs have been used for this purpose (Table 129.3). Double β-lactam combinations, such as a penicillin and a cephalosporin (e.g., piperacillin plus ceftazidime cephalothin plus carbenicillin) (58–60) may be used; however, these combinations may not have optimal activity against *S. aureus* (especially MRSA) and *P. aeruginosa*, and they might induce β-lactamase production in gram-negative rods.

Aminoglycosides provide rapid bactericidal activity against most gram-negative rods, and patients with persistent profound granulocytopenia and gram-negative rod bacteremia respond better to two antimicrobial agents that are active or synergistically active against the infecting organism (60–62); therefore, aminoglycoside-containing combinations are still useful. In a trial of ceftazidime plus amikacin, neutropenic patients with gram-negative rod bacteremia did better with a full course of both antibiotics than when the aminoglycoside was discontinued after three days (63). This finding was most prominent in patients with profound and prolonged granulocytopenia. Susceptibility to the β-lactam is an important determinant of outcome in gram-negative rod bacteremia treated with an aminoglycoside-containing regimen (64). Depending on local susceptibility patterns, reasonable initial drug combinations include ceftazidime, cefepime, imipenem, meropenem or piperacillin-tazobactam plus an aminoglycoside. If gram-negative rod bacteremia is not documented, the aminoglycoside can be discontinued.

Several studies of single-drug empiric therapy have been performed (65–67), and the current Infectious Diseases Society of America (IDSA) guidelines include monotherapy with ceftazidime, cefepime, imipenem, or meropenem (53). These broad-spectrum active drugs might be as effective as aminoglycoside–β-lactam combinations, but some patients require additional specific therapy (e.g., vancomycin) if staphylococci or other gram-positive cocci are isolated from blood. Aminoglycosides may be required for bacteremia with *P. aeruginosa* and other gram-negative rods, especially in profoundly neutropenic patients (63). In a study comparing ceftazidime with imipenem as monotherapy, both drugs were effective with similar modifications of initial therapy in both groups (66). Meropenem also has been used to treat febrile neutropenic patients and in one study compared favorably to ceftazidime plus amikacin (67). Recent data support the use of piperacillin-tazobactam alone especially in patients with expected short-term granulocytopenia and no evidence for gram-negative rod bacteremia (68).

Centers with large numbers of *S. aureus* infections might consider starting with a vancomycin-containing regimen (69), but several studies support the later addition of this drug if lack of response to empiric antibiotics is due to gram-positive coccal infection (70,71). Current IDSA guidelines suggest the use of initial empiric vancomycin in the presence of penicillin-resistant or tolerant viridans streptococci, severe mucositis, serious intravascular catheter infection, fluoroquinolone prophylaxis and known colonization with methicillin-resistant staphylococci or penicillin-resistant pneumococci (53).

One study reported the clinical equivalence of single daily doses of ceftriaxone plus amikacin and multiple daily dosing of ceftazidime plus amikacin (72). The single daily dose of amikacin was given as an intravenous infusion of 20 mg/kg during 1 hour. The regimens had similar associated nephrotoxicity (2% to 3%), but nephrotoxicity was associated with additional nephrotoxic agents and occurred later in patients receiving single daily doses. In another trial, piperacillin-tazobactam plus single daily doses of amikacin was more effective than ceftazidime plus amikacin (8). A recent study investigated whether ceftazidime plus aminoglycoside is still effective empiric therapy and concluded in the affirmative but warned about increasing resistance (73).

The duration of empiric therapy for fever in the granulocytopenic patient is also controversial (53,58,74,75). If the patient responds, therapy can continue until the granulocyte count has increased above 500 cells/mm^3 (53,74,75). Some authors treat documented gram-negative rod bacteremia for 10 to 14 days, regardless of the granulocyte count (57). Pizzo and colleagues showed that rebound infection, shock, or both developed in patients who remain granulocytopenic and febrile who had antibiotics discontinued after 7 days (74,75). Young suggested that antibiotics could be stopped in febrile patients with no bacterial diagnosis after seven days if the granulocyte count exceeds 500/mm^3 for 2 days (57). However, if further chemotherapy or profound granulocytopenia is expected, antibiotic use should continue. Concern must be given to the potential for invasive fungal infections during prolonged antibiotic treatment. Recommended duration of therapy is included in the IDSA guidelines (53).

Patients with documented bacteremia generally respond to appropriate antimicrobial agents within 4 to 5 days. However, failure to respond should prompt a search for loculated infections such as perirectal, intraabdominal, or subcutaneous abscesses. Antimicrobial activity can be adjusted to increase serum bactericidal activity, and granulocyte transfusions can be considered. Patients without documented bacterial sepsis who remain febrile after 4 to 7 days of empiric antibiotics should be considered for empiric antifungal therapy with amphotericin B (74–76). Fluconazole is useful in the treatment of candidal infections in the immunocompromised host. Some species, notably *Candida krusei* and *Candida glabrata*, may be resistant. Leukemic patients with hepatosplenic candidiasis have been successfully treated with fluconazole (77). This infection should be suspected if patients

---

TABLE 129.3. Current Antibiotics Used as Empirical Therapy for Fever in Granulocytopenic Patients

Combinations[a]		Single-drug therapy[a,b]
Azlocillin		Ceftazidime
Carbenicillin		Imipenem
Mezlocillin		Meropenem
Piperacillin		Cefepime
Ticarcillin[c]	plus aminoglycoside[d]	
Ceftazidime[e]		
Cefoperazone[c]		
Piperacillin-tazobactam		
Meropenem		
Ceftazidime plus piperacillin		
Azlocillin plus ceftazidime		
Ciprofloxacin plus amoxicillin/clavulanate[f]		

[a]Some authors have also used a cephalosporin plus a penicillin plus an aminoglycoside. Vancomycin is often added.
[b]Trials with piperacillin-tazobactam as a single agent are in progress.
[c]With or without clavulanate or sulbactam.
[d]Amikacin, gentamicin, netilmicin, tobramycin.
[e]Other cephalosporins such as ceftriaxone, cefotaxime, ceftizoxime and the cefamycin moxalactam have been used, but they have no activity against *P. aeruginosa*.
[f]For use in low-risk out-patients.
From Hughes WT, Armstrong D, Bodey GP, et al. Guidelines for the use of antimicrobial agents in neutropenic patients with unexplained fever. *Clin Infect Dis* 1997;5:551–573, with permission.

become febrile as or after the granulocyte count has normalized. A recent comparative trial of empiric fluconazole versus amphotericin B in febrile neutropenic patients showed equivalent results with both drugs (67% to 68% satisfactory responses) but warned that patients at risk of aspergillosis or resistant *Candida* infections required special diagnostic attention and might benefit from amphotericin B (78). Fewer adverse effects were reported in fluconazole-treated patients. New lipid preparations of amphotericin B have been introduced and are effective in neutropenic patients (79). In one study itraconazole compared favorably to amphotericin B as empiric antifungal therapy in neutropenic patients (80), but published experience with documented invasive fungal infection in these patients is limited. Two new antifungal drugs, caspofungin and voriconazole, have been introduced and are being evaluated for use in these patients.

Although enthusiasm had been raised for adjunctive treatments with antiendotoxin antibodies, antibodies to tumor necrosis factor, and interleukin-1 receptor antagonist, results of clinical trials have been disappointing (57–59). Further investigation of the molecular biology of endotoxin should reveal potentially useful interventions for sepsis in neutropenic and other patients. Several authors have reviewed their approaches to the treatment of febrile neutropenic patients (52,84–86).

Although granulocyte colony-stimulating factor (G-CSF) and granulocyte-macrophage colony-stimulating factor (GM-CSF) have been studied as adjunctive therapy in febrile neutropenic patients with documented bacterial infection, results are contradictory. A recent recommendation of the American Society of Clinical Oncology (ASCO) states that although CSFs might be considered for some febrile neutropenic patients at high risk of infection associated complications and poor outcome (profound neutropenia, hypotension, severe underlying disease, multiorgan failure, etc.), the benefits have not been proven (87). These drugs are not routinely recommended as adjuncts to antibiotics, but they may shorten the duration of neutropenia, antibiotic treatment and hospitalization (88).

The role of granulocyte transfusions as adjuncts to antibiotics in febrile neutropenic patients is controversial. A recent review summarizes the mixed results reported in studies over the past 10 years (89). G-CSF–stimulated donor transfusions might be useful in severely neutropenic patients with sepsis who do not respond to appropriate antibiotics (90). The long-term safety of G-CSF donor stimulation has not been established (89).

Several biologic markers have been suggested as possible predictors of bacterial infection in febrile neutropenic patients. These include C-reactive protein (CRP), amyloid A, protein C, tumor necrosis factor-α (TNF-α), several interleukins (IL-1, IL-6, IL-8), soluble TNF receptors, soluble IL-2 receptors, interferon (IFNγ), soluble adhesion molecules (ICAM-1, VCAM-1, soluble E-selectin), and procalcitonin. Although there are some intriguing data, a recent review suggested that there were not enough data to strongly support a predictive role for these markers in neutropenic patients (91–93).

Risk factor analyses have been used to identify patients at highest risk for bacteremia (and therefore needing aggressive intravenous treatment with potent antibiotics) and those who probably would be neutropenic for a short time and have a lower risk of serious infection. In patients at high risk, duration of granulocytopenia before fever, low platelet counts, high fever, shock, and clinical evidence of localized infection are some of the predictive factors that have been identified. Similarly, patients at low risk for bacteremia, excluding those with resistant bacterial infections, abnormal hepatic function, shock, hypercalcemia, altered mental state, tachypnea and hyponatremia, have been safely treated at home with intravenous or oral therapy. Two scoring systems to assess risk have been proposed and tested, the Talcott Score and the Multinational Association for Supportive Care in Cancer risk index (94,95).

Using similar estimates of low-risk, two recent trials of oral antibiotics to treat febrile patients with expected duration of granulocytopenia less than 10 days have been reported (96,97). Both studies reported that oral therapy with ciprofloxacin plus amoxicillin-clavulanate provided acceptable results. Although still somewhat controversial, a recent review suggests that low-risk children can be identified for home treatment with either oral or intravenous regimens with considerable success (98).

PREVENTION OF INFECTION IN THE IMMUNOCOMPROMISED PATIENT

Prevention of infection in immunosuppressed patients depends in part on the specific host defect and the likely source of infection. For example, neutropenic patients are primarily infected with organisms that colonize body sites, including the oropharynx, gastrointestinal tract, and skin (4,99,100). Most of the approaches to infection prevention have been developed for granulocytopenic patients, and some also apply to other immunosuppressed patients (Table 129.4).

Attempts should be made to improve or eliminate the defect in host defenses. Patients who are hypogammaglobulinemic can be treated effectively with maintenance doses of intravenous immunoglobulins (101,102). Patients with leukemia can be treated to achieve remission, rendering them non-neutropenic and lowering their risk of infection.

Methods for improving nutritional status are worthwhile. Careful attention should be paid to adequate protein, vitamin, and calorie intake. Peripheral hyperalimentation may be necessary in some circumstances, but this carries its own risk of infection (103).

Although vaccinations are effective in preventing a variety of infectious diseases in immunocompetent patients, many immunocompromised patients are less able to respond appropriately (104). Pneumococcal vaccination and *H. influenzae* type b

---

TABLE 129.4. General Considerations for Infection Prevention in Immunocompromised Patients

I. Improve host defenses
  A. Treat underlying disease
  B. Improve nutrition, protein, vitamin, and calorie intake
  C. Vaccines: influenza, pneumococcal, hepatitis B, varicella-zoster virus, varicella-zoster immune globulin on exposure
  D. Immunomodulators: lithium, intravenous immune globulin, GM-CSF, G-CSF
II. Minimize invasive procedures and maximize care for indwelling intravenous and bladder catheters
III. Reduce acquisition of new pathogens
  A. Hand washing and cleansing of patient's skin
  B. Low-bacterial foods and fluids; avoid fresh flowers
  C. Housekeeping
  D. Laminar airflow and other infection control methods
IV. Reduce colonizing bacterial load
  A. Nonabsorbable oral antibiotics, antifungal agents, antiseptics
  B. Absorbable antibiotics
  C. Selective gastrointestinal bacterial suppression
  D. Systemic antibacterial prophylaxis
  E. Local or systemic antifungal prophylaxis
  F. Acyclovir prevention of dissemination of herpesvirus infections

G-CSF, granulocyte colony-stimulating factor; GM-CSF, granulocyte macrophage colony-stimulating factor.

vaccination is useful if given at least two weeks before splenectomy. Influenza vaccine might minimize risk of this disease, and hepatitis B vaccine also has a role (105,106). An excellent review of immunizations in transplant recipients has been published recently (107). CMV pneumonia has been prevented with anti-CMV-IgG and seronegative blood products in some but not all bone marrow transplant recipients (108,109).

Many attempts at modifying the immune defect have been studied. Lithium has been used to stimulate the bone marrow (110) and recombinant GM-CSF and granulocyte colony-stimulating factor have been widely used to minimize the period of neutropenia after cancer chemotherapy and to reduce granulocytopenia-associated infection. These cytokines are frequently used to elevate peripheral granulocyte counts after treatment for lymphomas and solid tumors, but the new ASCO guidelines recommend their routine use in these patients only in those who have received previous chemotherapy or who might be at extremely high risk for infection (87). They are not recommended for all patients with cancer who receive chemotherapy.

Although CSFs after induction chemotherapy for acute myeloid leukemia decrease marrow recovery time, hospitalization, and antibiotic use, they do not have major effects on response rates, transfusion requirements or survival (87). In addition, reduction in antibiotic-requiring infections after consolidation therapy is reported with G-CSF (87). Other than this latter effect, CSFs are only recommended in acute myeloid leukemia treatment if the reduced hospitalization benefits outweigh CSF cost (87). Although data are incomplete, the ASCO guidelines recommend that G-CSF can be used after or during initial chemotherapy for acute lymphoblastic leukemia with expected reductions in the duration of neutropenia of up to 1 week (87); response rates might be improved, but no effect on survival should be expected. GM-CSF also raises peripheral blood leukocyte counts in neutropenic patients with AIDS (111). Intravenous IgG has been used successfully to protect chronic lymphocytic leukemia patients from bacterial infection (112).

It is important to minimize invasive procedures and maximize care of indwelling intravenous and urinary catheters. Use of Hickman, Broviac, and Port-A-Cath long-term indwelling devices for patients with hematologic and other malignancies is increasing, and these devices have a real potential for infection. Guidelines for the management of infections associated with intravenous devices have been published recently (113).

Several measures are useful for reducing the acquisition of new pathogenic bacteria. Obviously, careful hand washing is required. Skin cleansing with soap and antiseptic solutions is recommended for the patient. An often-overlooked area of infection prevention is the provision of low-bacterial food and fluids. Foods such as natural cheeses, uncooked vegetables, raw meats or salads, cold soups, and uncooked herbs and spices are notoriously high in bacteria. These are well tolerated by immunocompetent hosts but are potential sources of infection for neutropenic patients (114). Fresh flowers should not be permitted in these patients' rooms. Laminar airflow units are clearly effective in providing a low-particle-count atmosphere for patients (115,116) and are essential for patients undergoing bone marrow transplantation. Patients are usually also treated with antibiotics (discussed in following paragraphs) (116).

Although there is a large literature on antibacterial prophylaxis in these patients, the most recent IDSA guidelines do not recommend routine antibacterial prophylaxis for all neutropenic patients (37). When bacterial infection prevention is used it is directed at a reduction of bacterial colonization of the gastrointestinal tract. Several methods are available, including use of nonabsorbable or absorbable antibiotics, selective microbial suppression, or partial antimicrobial decontamination (116–121). Compliance of patients is critical for success of these regimens (121). The efficacy of prophylactic regimens can be measured in terms of reduction of infection, with its associated morbidity and mortality, and the degree to which additional cancer chemotherapy can be administered (122). Although no preventive approach is perfect, well-tolerated regimens, such as those using trimethoprim-sulfamethoxazole (TMP-SMX) or an oral fluoroquinolone, are used most frequently.

Nonabsorbable oral antibiotics include combinations of gentamicin, vancomycin plus nystatin, and neomycin plus colistin and nystatin (117). Treatment also may include the application of antimicrobial ointments to the vagina or rectum, nares, auditory canals, and gums. Povidone-iodine and chlorhexidine are used as douches, swabs, or mouthwashes. Although some studies have shown dramatic reductions in infection rates with oral nonabsorbable antibiotics, side effects of nausea, vomiting, and abdominal cramps limit compliance and patients' acceptance. Rebound overgrowth and infection have been reported after discontinuation of these regimens, and the gastrointestinal tract may be colonized with resistant bacteria (117,123). These regimens are not widely used now, except in conjunction with protective environment units; they are not recommended for sporadic use in most neutropenic patients.

Several studies have compared TMP-SMX with placebo or with other regimens (121,123–126). Hughes and colleagues (125) observed that TMP-SMX reduced bacterial infections in patients with acute leukemia during prophylaxis against *P. carinii* pneumonia. In a large number of granulocytopenic patients with solid tumors, leukemia, and lymphomas, Pizzo and coworkers (121) showed a reduction in febrile episodes and infection in totally compliant recipients of TMP-SMX plus erythromycin.

TMP-SMX is not without dermatologic side effects. Also it has been reported to prolong granulocytopenia, delay marrow engraftment, and result in the emergence of resistant organisms (123,127). A randomized, double-blind comparative trial of bone marrow transplant patients showed similar prophylactic efficacy of TMP-SMX and ciprofloxacin, but TMP-SMX recipients had more *Clostridium difficile* colitis, slightly more gram-negative rod infections, and a trend for prolonged granulocytopenia (128).

Another approach has been to individualize antibiotic prophylaxis and eliminate susceptible enteric flora while preserving the anaerobic flora, with its property of colonization resistance. Antibiotics such as TMP-SMX, colistin, neomycin, and nalidixic acid have been used (119,120,126,129).

Several studies of prophylaxis with fluoroquinolone drugs have been reported. Two meta-analyses of the extant studies have been published (130,131). Although slightly different inclusion criteria were used, both reported that fluoroquinolone prophylaxis reduced gram-negative rod infections but did not reduce gram-positive infections (unless a specific gram-positive agent such as penicillin is added (132). The effect on febrile morbidity was variable and fluoroquinolone prophylaxis did not affect mortality. Fungal infections were not increased. Both authors raise concerns about increasing fluoroquinolone resistance, especially among *E. coli*, and this has been reported from cancer centers with heavy prophylactic fluoroquinolone use (133,134). The new broader spectrum fluoroquinolones such as gatifloxacin and moxifloxacin have not been effectively studied for prophylactic use in neutropenic patients. The use of prophylactic acyclovir was shown to reduce bacteremia during acute leukemia induction therapy, possibly through the prevention of ulcerative herpes simplex lesions (135). In a retrospective study of 3,002 febrile neutropenic patients in four trials of the International Antimicrobial Therapy Cooperative Group, patients who received antifungal prophylaxis were at increased risk of bacteremia (136).

Although no mechanism was proven to explain this association, it was somewhat stronger with absorbable antifungal agents.

Prevention of Fungal Infections

Invasive fungal infections are major problems in immunocompromised patients. Despite advances in antifungal chemotherapy, the overall prognosis remains poor for profoundly neutropenic patients infected with fungi. Several approaches to prevent these infections in immunocompromised patients have met with variable success and antifungal prophylaxis remains controversial. A recent review of antifungal agents for prophylaxis suggests that oral antifungals provide some benefit in patients with hematologic malignancies (137). Although the IDSA guidelines do not routinely recommend antifungal prophylaxis (53), they do find them appropriate in institutions with high rates of fungal infections. A recent review of antifungal prophylaxis for solid organ transplant patients suggest that prophylaxis against invasive aspergillosis and candidiasis is indicated, however available evidence does not support the efficacy of oral itraconazole or amphotericin B in liver transplant recipients (138). Intravenous itraconazole might be more effective.

The polyenes nystatin and amphotericin B have been evaluated as oral antifungal prophylactic agents, but they are not substantially absorbed from the gastrointestinal tract, and colonization and invasive candidiasis have been reported despite varying doses (139). Oral polyenes and the imidazole ketoconazole do not reduce *Aspergillus* infection; however, aerosolized amphotericin B has been studied with some success (140,141).

Administration of clotrimazole troches every four hours while the patient is awake minimizes oropharyngeal candidiasis. However, this does not prevent disseminated fungal infection. Fluconazole, an oral triazole antifungal agent, reduced superficial fungal infections in bone marrow transplant recipients from 33% to 8.4% (*P* value less than .001) and systemic fungal infections from 15.8% to 2.8% (*P* value less than .001) when administered at 400 mg/d compared with placebo (142). In a similar trial in patients with acute leukemia not undergoing bone marrow transplantation, fluconazole reduced fungal colonization and superficial infection with *Candida* sp. but not invasive fungal infection, use of amphotericin B, or death (143). A recent placebo controlled study reported reduced candidal gastrointestinal colonization and invasive fungal infections (primarily candidal) in neutropenic patients with leukemia and BMT recipients who received 400 mg daily oral fluconazole (144,145). The benefit was seen most clearly in acute myeloid leukemic patients who received intensive cytotoxic chemotherapy. Fluconazole prophylaxis has been associated with increased infection with *C. krusei, C. glabrata,* and other resistant yeasts (145–147).

Although itraconazole absorption may be erratic and patient adherence may be difficult, it reduced proven invasive fungal infection relative to placebo or historical controls (148,149). These and other approaches in bone marrow transplant patients have been reviewed recently (150). Itraconazole and amphotericin B oral solutions were recently found statistically similar as prophylactic agents but the azole appeared to reduce the need for systemic antifungal therapy (151). New antifungal agents such as candicidins and voriconazole are currently under study.

Antiviral Prophylaxis

With the introduction of acyclovir, effective antiviral prophylactic therapy is available. Acyclovir is used intravenously (250 mg/m² every 8 hours) and orally (200 mg four times daily) to prevent herpes simplex virus infections in patients undergoing bone marrow or kidney transplantation or high-dose cancer chemotherapy (152). Varicella-zoster virus infection in immunocompromised patients can be minimized within 72 hours of exposure with varicella-zoster immune globulin, one vial (1.25 mL)/10 kg up to a maximum of five vials (6.25 mL), intramuscularly (153).

Vidarabine and acyclovir prevent dissemination of zoster in compromised patients (154,155). In a recent study in 151 patients undergoing allogeneic marrow transplantation, varicella-zoster infection did not develop in patients who received either ganciclovir (5 mg/kg i.v. three times a week) or acyclovir (1200 mg orally or 750 mg intravenously daily) (156). Viral infections were seen promptly after these drugs were discontinued. Intravenous acyclovir (10 to 12 mg/kg intravenously three times a day for 7 days) is used to treat chickenpox in immunocompromised patients (157,158). Oral therapy is also used. A live varicella-zoster virus vaccine resulted in seroconversion in children with acute leukemia who were in remission. This vaccine may modify disease (154) and is now licensed for use. It is recommended for pretransplant patients who are seronegative, but it not recommended after transplantation (107).

Oral acyclovir is effective in preventing CMV infections in bone marrow and kidney transplant recipients, although it is ineffective as therapy for CMV infections (159). Although intravenous immunoglobulin reduced non-CMV viral infections, it did not add prophylactic activity for CMV infection to that obtained with the use of CMV-seronegative blood products alone (160). Ganciclovir at 2.5 mg/kg every 8 hours for the week before transplantation followed by 6 mg/kg per day for 5 days per week after transplantation reduces the incidence and severity of CMV infection in bone marrow transplant recipients (161). Ganciclovir also reduces CMV disease in CMV-positive recipients but concern is raised by its myelosuppressive potential (156). Late CMV infections may develop after discontinuation of antiviral drugs.

SUMMARY

In summary, each center must develop an organized approach to the prevention of infection in immunocompromised patients. General measures include awareness of infection control techniques, proper hand washing, vaccines where applicable, use of appropriate food, and reduction of bacterial colonization. Because specific antimicrobial agents are developed against the usual causes of infection in immunocompromised hosts, careful studies to evaluate their prophylactic role are necessary. Continuing attention must be paid to changes in local antimicrobial resistance and physicians must be aware of new drugs that have activity against these organisms. Large and careful controlled studies of new antimicrobials in compromised patients are needed before they are included for routine prophylactic or therapeutic use. Physicians should remain alert to new seemingly non-pathogenic microbes that cause infections in severely immunocompromised patients.

REFERENCES

1. Kaufman DW, Kelly JP, Jurgelon J, et al. Drugs in the aetiology of agranulocytosis and aplastic anemia. *Eur J Haematol* 1996;57(suppl 60):23–30.
2. Dale DC. Neutropenia and neutrophilia. In: Buetler E, Lichtman MA, Coller BS, Kipps TJ, and Seligsohn U, eds. *Williams hematology,* 6th ed. New York: McGraw-Hill, 2001:832–834.
3. Bodey GP, Buckley M, Sathe YS, et al. Quantitative relationships between circulating leukocytes and infection in patients with acute leukemia. *Ann Intern Med* 1966;64:328–340.

4. Schimpff SC, Hahn DM, Brouillet MD, et al. Infection prevention in acute leukemia: comparison of basic infection prevention techniques with standard room reverse isolation or with reverse isolation plus added air filtration. *Leuk Res* 1978;2:231–240.

5. Schimpff SC, Young VM, Greene WH, et al. Origin of infection in acute nonlymphocytic leukemia: significance of hospital acquisition of potential pathogens. *Ann Intern Med* 1972;77:707–714.

6. The EORTC International Antimicrobial Therapy Project Group. Three antibiotic regimens in the treatment of infection in febrile granulocytopenic patients with cancer. *J Infect Dis* 1978;137:14–29.

7. Gibson J, Johnson L, Snowdon L, et al. Trends in bacterial infection in febrile neutropenic patients: 1986–1992. *Aust NZ J Med* 1994;24:374–377.

8. Cometta A, Zinner S, deBock R, et al. Piperacillin-tazobactam versus ceftazidime plus amikacin as empiric therapy for fever in granulocytopenic patients with cancer. *Antimicrob Agents Chemother* 1995;39:445–452.

9. EORTC International Antimicrobial Therapy Cooperative Group and the National Cancer Institute of Canada-Clinical Trials Group. Vancomycin added to empirical combination antibiotic therapy for fever in granulocytopenic cancer patients. *J Infect Dis* 1991;163:951–958.

10. Elting LS, Bodey GP, Keefe BH. Septicemia and shock syndrome due to viridans streptococci: a case-control study of predisposing factors. *Clin Infect Dis* 1992;14:1201–1207.

11. Marron A, Carratalà J, González-Barca E, et al. Serious complications of bacteremia caused by viridans streptococci in neutropenic patients with cancer. *Clin Infect Dis* 2000;31:1126–1130.

12. Zinner SH. New pathogens in neutropenic patients with cancer: an update for the new millennium. *Int J Antimicrob Agents* 2000;16:97–101.

13. Woo PC, Wong SS, Lum PN, et al. Cell-wall-deficient bacteria and culture-negative febrile episodes in bone-marrow-transplant recipients. *Lancet* 2001;357:675–679.

14. Doern GV, Ferraro MJ, Brueggemann AB, et al. Emergence of high rates of antimicrobial resistance among viridans streptococci in the United States. *Antimicrob Agents Chemother* 1996;40:891–894.

15. Cometta A, Calandra T, Bille J, et al. *Escherichia coli* resistant to fluoroquinolones in patients with cancer and neutropenia. *N Engl J Med* 1994;330:1240–1241.

16. Gray JW, George RH. Experience of vancomycin-resistant enterococci in a children's hospital. *J Hosp Infect* 2000;45:11–18.

17. Anaissie E, Bodey GP, Kantarjian H, et al. New spectrum of fungal infections in patients with cancer. *Rev Infect Dis* 1989;11:369–378.

18. Walsh TJ, Hiemenz JW, Anaissie E. Recent progress and current problems in treatment of invasive fungal infections in neutropenic patients. *Infect Dis Clin North Am* 1996;10:365–400.

19. Musa MO, Al Eisa A, Halim M, et al. The spectrum of *Fusarium* infection in immunocompromised patients with haematological malignancies and non-immunocompromised patients: a single institution experience over 15 years. *Br J Haematol* 2000;108:544–548.

20. Van der Meer JWM: Defects in host-defense mechanisms. In: Rubin RH, Young LS, eds. *Clinical approach to infections in the compromised host,* 3rd ed. New York: Plenum, 1994:33–66.

21. Boxer LA. Neutrophil disorders: qualitative abnormalities of the neutrophil. In: Buetler E, Lichtman MA, Coller BS, Kipps TJ, Seligsohn U, eds. *Williams hematology,* 6th ed. New York: McGraw-Hill, 2001:835–852.

22. Mowat A, Baum J. Chemotaxis of polymorphonuclear leukocytes from patients with diabetes mellitus. *N Engl J Med* 1971;284:621–627.

23. Brayton RG, Stokes PE, Schwartz MS, et al. Effect of alcohol and various diseases on leukocyte mobilization, phagocytosis and intracellular bacterial killing. *N Engl J Med* 1970;282:123–128.

24. Salant DJ, Glover AM, Anderson R, et al. Depressed neutrophil chemotaxis in patients with chronic renal failure and after renal transplantation. *J Labor Clin Med* 1976;88:536–545.

25. Gonzalez Moraleja J, Rubio Perez P, Cabello Carro J, et al. Recurrent infections, severe neutropenia and neutrophil chemotaxis defect in paroxysmal nocturnal hemoglobinuria. *Anal Med Intern* 1994;11:490–492.

26. Johnston RB Jr, Baehner RL. Chronic granulomatous disease: correlation between pathogenesis and clinical findings. *Pediatrics* 1971;48:730–739.

27. Lanza F. Clinical manifestation of myeloperoxidase deficiency. *J Mol Med* 1998;76:676–681.

28. Rosner F, Kozinn PJ, Jervis GA. Leukocyte function and serum immunoglobulins in Down's syndrome. *NY State J Med* 1973;73:672–675.

29. Clark RA. Activation of the neutrophil respiratory burst oxidase. *J Infect Dis* 1999;179(Suppl 2):S309–S317.

30. Chiang AKS, Chan GCF, Ma SK, et al. Disseminated fungal infection associated with myeloperoxidase deficiency in a premature neonate. *Pediatr Infect Dis J* 2000;19:1025–1027.

31. Ochs HD, Wedgwood RJ. Disorders of the B-cell system. In: Stiehm ER, ed. *Immunologic disorders in infants and children.* Philadelphia: WB Saunders, 1989:226–256.

32. Christenson JC, Hill HR. Infections complicating congenital immunodeficiency syndromes. In: Rubin RH, Young LS, eds. *Clinical approach to infection in the compromised host,* 3rd ed. New York: Plenum, 1994:521–549.

33. Rosen FS, Cooper MD, Wedgewood RJP. The primary immunodeficiencies. *N Engl J Med* 1984;311:235–242.

34. Lawton AR. IgG Subclass deficiency and the day-care generation. *Pediatr Infect Dis J* 1999;18:462–466.

35. Walport, MJ. Complement. *N Engl J Med* 2001;344:1058–1066.

36. Petersen BH, Lee JJ, Snyderman RJ, et al. *Neisseria meningitidis* and *Neisseria gonorrhoeae* bacteremia associated with C6, C7 or C8 deficiency. *Ann Intern Med* 1979;90:917–920.

37. Alper CA, Colten HA, Gear JSS, et al. Homozygous human C3 deficiency: the role of C3 in antibody production in C1s induced vasopermeabilty and cobra venom-induced passive hemolysis. *J Clin Invest* 1976;57:222–229.

38. Kaye ET, Johnson RA, Wolfson JS, Sober AJ. Dermatologic manifestations of infection in the compromised host. In: Rubin RH, Young LS, eds. Clinical approach to infection in the compromised host, 3rd ed. New York: Plenum, 1994:105–119.

39. Kerkering TM, Duma RJ, Shadomy S. The evolution of pulmonary cryptococcosis: clinical implications from a study of 41 patients with and without compromising host factors. *Ann Intern Med* 1981;94:611–618.

40. Wirth FA, Passalacqua J-A, Kao G. Disseminated cutaneous protothecosis in an immunocompromised host: a case report and literature review. *Cutis* 1999;63:185–188.

41. Conces DJ Jr. Lung disease in immunocompromised patients, Part II. *J Thorac Imaging* 1999;14:1–73.

42. Cunha BA. Pneumonias in the compromised host. *Infect Dis Clin North Am* 2001;15:591–612.

43. Rubin RH, Green R. Clinical approach to the compromised host with fever and pulmonary infiltrates. In: Rubin RH, Young LS, eds. Clinical approach to infection in the compromised host, 3rd ed. New York: Plenum, 1994:121–161.

44. Cockerill FR III, Wilson WR, Carpenter HA, et al. Open lung biopsy in immunocompromised patients. *Arch Intern Med* 1985;145:1398–1404.

45. Cheson BD, Samlowski WE, Tang TT, et al. Value of open lung biopsy in 87 immunocompromised patients with pulmonary infiltrates. *Cancer* 1985;55:453–459.

46. Ramila E, Sureda A, Martino R, et al. Bronchoscopy guided by high-resolution computed tomography for the diagnosis of pulmonary infections in patients with hematologic malignancies and normal plain chest X-ray. *Haematologica* 2000;85:961–966.

47. Baden LR, Maguire JH. Gastrointestinal infections in the immunocompromised host. *Infect Dis Clin North Am* 2001;15:639–670.

48. Cunha BA. Central nervous system infections in the compromised host: a diagnostic approach. *Infect Dis Clin North Am* 2001;15:567–590.

49. Gurwith MJ, Brunton JL, Lank BA, et al. Granulocytopenia in hospitalized patients.1. Prognostic factors and etiology of fever. *Am J Med* 1978;64:121–126.

50. Schimpff S, Satterlee W, Young VM, et al. Empiric therapy with carbenicillin and gentamicin for febrile patients with cancer and granulocytopenia. *N Engl J Med* 1971;284:1061–1065.

51. Sickles EA, Greene WH, Wiernik PH. Clinical presentation of infection in granulocytopenic patients. *Arch Intern Med* 1975;135:715–719.

52. Pizzo PA. Fever in immunocompromised patients. *N Engl J Med* 1999;341:893–900.

53. Hughes WT, Armstrong D, Bodey, GP, et al. 1997 Guidelines for the use of antimicrobial agents in neutropenic patients with unexplained fever. *Clin Infect Dis* 1997;5:551–573.

54. Viscoli C, Castagnola E. Planned progressive antimicrobial therapy in neutropenic patients. *Br J Haematol* 1998;102:879–888.

55. Bodey GP. Antibiotics in patients with neutropenia. *Arch Intern Med* 1984;144:1845–1851.

56. Anaissie E, Rolston K, Bodey GP. Treatment of gram-negative bacteremia in patients with neutropenia and cancer (letter). *N Engl J Med* 1988;318:1694–1695.

57. Young LS. Fever and septicemia. In: Rubin RH, Young LS, eds. *Clinical approach to infections in the compromised host,* 3rd ed. New York: Plenum, 1994:67–104.

58. Bodey GP, Valdivieso M, Feld R, et al. Carbenicillin plus cephalothin or cefazolin as therapy for infections in neutropenic patients. *Am J Med Sci* 1977;273:309–318.

59. Young LS. Double beta-lactam therapy in the immunocompromised host. *J Antimicrob Chemother* 1985;16:4–6.

60. Joshi JH, Newman KA, Brown BW, et al. Double beta-lactam regimen compared to an aminoglycoside/beta-lactam regimen as empiric antibiotic therapy for febrile granulocytopenic cancer patients. *Supportive Care Cancer* 1997;1:186–194.

61. DeJongh CA, Joshi JH, Newman KA, et al. Antibiotic synergism and response in gram-negative bacteremia in granulocytopenic cancer patients. *Am J Med* 1986;80(Suppl 5C):96–100.

62. Klastersky J, Zinner SH. Synergistic combinations of antibiotics in gram-negative bacillary infections. *Rev Infect Dis* 1982;4:294–301.

63. The EORTC International Antimicrobial Therapy Cooperative Group. Ceftazidime combined with a short or long course of amikacin for empirical therapy of gram-negative bacteremia in cancer patients with granulocytopenia. *N Engl J Med* 1987;317:1692–1698.

64. Klastersky J, Glauser MP, Schimpff SC, et al. European Organization for Research on Treatment of Cancer Antimicrobial Therapy Project Group: prospective randomized comparison of three antibiotic regimens for empirical therapy of suspected bacteremic infection in febrile granulocytopenic patients. *Antimicrob Agents Chemother* 1986;29:263–270.

65. Bodey GP, Alvarez ME, Jones PG, et al. Imipenem-cilastatin as initial therapy for febrile cancer patients. *Antimicrob Agents Chemother* 1986;30:211–214.

66. Freifeld AG, Walsh T, Marshall D, et al. Monotherapy for fever and neutropenia in cancer patients: a randomized comparison of ceftazidime versus imipenem. *J Clin Oncol* 1995;13:165–176.

67. Cometta A, Calandra T, Gaya H, et al. Monotherapy with meropenem versus combination therapy with ceftazidime plus amikacin as empiric therapy for fever in granulocytopenic patients with cancer. *Antimicrob Agents Chemother* 1996;50:1108–1115.

68. Cometta A, Kern WV, DeBock R, et al. An EORTC-IATG double-blind trial of vancomycin (Van) versus placebo (Pla) for persistent fever in neutropenic cancer patients (NCP) given piperacillin/tazobactam (PT) monotherapy. Abstracts of the 41st Interscience Conference on Antimicrobial Agents and Chemotherapy. Chicago, IL, Sept. 2001. Washington DC, American Society for Microbiology, abstract no. 79.

69. Shenep JL, Hughes WT, Roberson PK, et al. Vancomycin, ticarcillin, and amikacin compared with ticarcillin-clavulanate and amikacin in the empirical treatment of febrile neutropenic children with cancer. *N Engl J Med* 1988;319:1053–1058.

70. Rubin M, Hathorn JW, Marshall D, et al. Gram-positive infections and the use of vancomycin in 550 episodes of fever and neutropenia. *Ann Intern Med* 1988;108:30–35.

71. Ramphal R, Bolger M, Oblon DJ, et al. Vancomycin is not an essential component of the initial empiric treatment regimen for febrile neutropenic patients receiving ceftazidime: A randomized prospective study. *Antimicrob Agents Chemother* 1992;36:1062–1067.

72. International Antimicrobial Therapy Cooperative Group of the EORTC. Efficacy and toxicity of single daily dose of amikacin and ceftriaxone versus multiple daily doses of amikacin and ceftazidime for infection in patients with cancer and granulocytopenia. *Ann Intern Med* 1993;119:584–593.

73. Fanci R, Paci C, Martinez RL, et al. Management of fever in neutropenic patients with acute leukemia: current role of ceftazidime plus amikacin as empiric therapy. *J Chemother* 2000;12:232–239.

74. Pizzo PA, Robichaud KJ, Gill FA, et al. Duration of empiric antibiotic therapy. *Am J Med* 1979;67:194–200.

75. Pizzo PA, Robichaud KJ, Gill FA, et al. Empiric antibiotic and antifungal therapy for cancer patients with prolonged fever and granulocytopenia. *Am J Med* 1982;72:101–111.

76. EORTC International Antimicrobial Therapy Cooperative Group. Empiric antifungal therapy in febrile granulocytopenic patients. *Am J Med* 1989;86:668–672.

77. Flannery MT, Simmons DB, Saba H, et al. Fluconazole in the treatment of hepatosplenic candidiasis. *Arch Intern Med* 1992;152:406–408.

78. Winston DJ, Hathorn JW, Schuster MG, et al. A multicenter, randomized trial of fluconazole versus amphotericin B for empiric antifungal therapy of febrile neutropenic patients with cancer. *Am J Med* 2000;108:282–289.

79. Walsh TJ, Finberg RW, Arndt C, et al. Liposomal amphotericin B for empirical therapy in patients with persistent fever and neutropenia. *N Engl J Med* 1999;340:764–771.

80. Boogaerts M, Garber G, Winston D, et al. Itraconazole (IT) compared with amphotericin B (AMB) as empirical therapy for persistent fever of unknown origin (FUO) in neutropenic patients (PTS). *Bone Marrow Transplant* 1999;340:764–771.

81. Calandra T, Glauser MP, Schellekens J, et al. Treatment of gram negative septic shock with human IgG antibody to *Escherichia coli* J5: a prospective, double-blind randomized trial. *J Infect Dis* 1988;158:312–319.

82. Ziegler EJ, Fisher CJ Jr, Sprung CL, et al. Treatment of gram-negative bacteremia and septic shock with HA-1A human monoclonal antibody against endotoxin—a randomized, double-blind, placebo-controlled trial. The HA1A Sepsis Study Group. *N Engl J Med* 1991;324:429–436.

83. Greenman RL, Schein RM, Martin MA, et al. A controlled clinical trial of E5 murine monoclonal IgM antibody to endotoxin in the treatment of gram-negative sepsis. *JAMA* 1991;266:1097–1102.

84. Klastersky J. Empirical treatment of sepsis in neutropenic patients. *Int J Antimicrob Agents* 2000;16:131–133.

85. Glauser MP. Neutropenia: clinical implications and modulation. *Intens Care Med* 2000;26:S103–S110.

86. Viscoli C, Castagnola E. Planned progressive antimicrobial therapy in neutropenic patients. *Br J Haematol* 1998;102:879–888.

87. Ozer H, Armitage JO, Bennett CL, et al. 2000 update of recommendations for the use of hematopoietic colony-stimulating factors: evidence-based, clinical practice guidelines. *J Clin Oncol* 2000;18:3558–3585.

88. Garcia-Carbonero R, Mayordomo JI, Tornamira MV, et al. Granulocyte colony-stimulating factor in the treatment of high-risk febrile neutropenia: a multicenter randomized trial. *J Natl Cancer Inst* 2000;93:31–38.

89. Hübel, K, Dale DC, Liles WC. Granulocyte transfusion therapy: update on potential clinical applications. *Curr Opin Haematol* 2001;8:161–164.

90. Peters C, Minkov M, Matthes-Martin S, et al. Leukocyte transfusions from rhG-CSF or prednisolone stimulated donors for treatment of severe infections in immunocompromised neutropenic patients. *Br J Haematol* 1999;106:689–696.

91. Südhoff T, Giagounidis A, Karthaus M. Evaluation of neutropenic fever: value of serum and plasma parameters in clinical practice. *Chemother* 2000;46:77–85.

92. Fleischhack G, Kambeck I, Cipic D, et al. Procalcitonin in paediatric cancer patients: its diagnostic relevance is superior to that of C-reactive protein, interleukin 6, interleukin 8, soluble interleukin 2 receptor and soluble tumour necrosis factor receptor II. *Br J Haematol* 2000;111:1093–1102.

93. Mesters RM, Helterbrand J, Utterback BH, et al. Prognostic value of protein C concentrations in neutropenic patients at high risk of severe septic complications. *Crit Care Med* 2000;28:2209–2216.

94. Talcott JA, Siegel RD, Finberg R, et al. Risk-assessment in cancer patients with fever and neutropenia: a prospective, two-center validation of a prediction rule. *J Clin Oncol* 1992;10:316–322.

95. Klastersky J, Paesmans M, Rubenstein EB, et al. The Multinational Association for Supportive Care in Cancer risk index: a multinational scoring system for identifying low-risk febrile neutropenic cancer patients. *J Clin Oncol* 2000;18:3038–3051.

96. Freifeld A, Marchigiani D, Walsh T, et al. A double-blind comparison of empirical oral and intravenous antibiotic therapy for low-risk febrile neutropenia during cancer chemotherapy. *N Engl J Med* 1999;341:305–311.

97. Kern WV, Cometta A, deBock R, et al. Oral versus intravenous empirical antimicrobial therapy for fever in patients with granulocytopenia who are receiving cancer chemotherapy. *N Engl J Med* 1999;341:312–318.

98. Mullen CA. Which children with fever and neutropenia can be safely treated as outpatients? *Br J Haematol* 2001;112:832–837.

99. Newman KA, Schimpff SC, Young VM, et al. Lessons learned from surveillance cultures from patients with acute nonlymphocytic leukemia: usefulness for epidemiologic prevention and therapeutic research. *Am J Med* 1981;70:423–431.

100. Cohen ML, Murphy MT, Counts GW, et al. Prediction by surveillance cultures of bacteremia among neutropenic patients treated in a protective environment. *J Infect Dis* 1983;147:789–793.

101. Eibl MM, Cairns L, Rosen FS. Safety and efficacy of a monomeric, functionally intact intravenous IgG preparation in patients with primary immunodeficiency syndromes. *Clin Immunol Immunopathol* 1984;31:151–160.

102. Bjorkander J, Wadsworth C, Hanson LA. 1040 prophylactic infusions with an unmodified intravenous immunoglobulin product causing few side effects in patients with antibody deficiency syndromes. *Infection* 1985;13:102–110.

103. Shamberger RC, Pizzo PA, Goodgame JT, et al. The effect of total parenteral nutrition on chemotherapy induced myelosuppression: a randomized study. *Am J Med* 1983;74:40–48.

104. Siber GR, Weitzman SA, Aisenberg AC, et al. Impaired antibody response to pneumococcal vaccine after treatment for Hodgkin's disease. *N Engl J Med* 1978;299:442–448.

105. Ortbals DW, Liebhaber H, Presant CA, et al. Influenza immunization of adult patients with malignant diseases. *Ann Intern Med* 1977;87:552–557.

106. Dienstag JL, Katkov WN. Viral hepatitis in the compromised host. In: Rubin RH, Young LS, eds. *Clinical approach to infection in the compromised host*, 3rd ed. New York: Plenum, 1994:355–377.

107. Molrine DC, Hibberd PL. Vaccines for transplant recipients. *Infect Dis Clin North Am* 2001;15:273–305.

108. Meyers JD, Leszczynski J, Zaia JA, et al. Prevention of cytomegalovirus infection by cytomegalovirus immune globulin after marrow transplantation. *Ann Intern Med* 1983;98:442–446.

109. Bowden RA, Sayers M, Fluornoy N, et al. Cytomegalovirus immune globulin and seronegative blood products to prevent primary cytomegalovirus infection after marrow transplantation. *N Engl J Med* 1986;314:1006–1010.

110. Stein RS, Beamon C, Ali MY, et al. Lithium carbonate attenuation of chemotherapy-induced neutropenia. *N Engl J Med* 1977;297:430–431.

111. Groopman JE, Mitsuyasu RT, DeLeo MJ, et al. Effect of recombinant human granulocyte-macrophage colony-stimulating factor on myelopoiesis in the acquired immunodeficiency syndrome. *N Engl J Med* 1987;317:593–598.

112. Cooperative Group for the Study of Immunoglobulin in Chronic Lymphocytic Leukemia. Intravenous immunoglobulin for the prevention of infection in chronic lymphocytic leukemia: a randomized, controlled clinical trial. *N Engl J Med* 1988;319:902–907.

113. Mermel, LA, Farr BM, Sherertz RJ, et al. Guidelines for the management of intravascular catheter-related infections. *Clin Infect Dis* 2001;1249–1272.

114. Remington JS, Schimpff SC. Please don't eat the salads. *N Engl J Med* 1981;304:433–435.

115. Bodey GP, Johnson D. Microbiological evaluation of protected environment during patient occupancy. *Appl Microbiol* 1971;22:828–836.

116. Levine AS, Siegel SE, Schreiber AD, et al. Protected environments and prophylactic antibiotics: a prospective controlled study of their utility in the therapy of acute leukemia. *N Engl J Med* 1973;288:477–483.

117. Schimpff SC, Greene WH, Young VM, et al. Infection prevention in acute nonlymphocytic leukemia: laminar air flow room reverse isolation with oral, nonabsorbable antibiotic prophylaxis. *Ann Intern Med* 1975;82:351–358.

118. Schimpff SC. Infection prevention during profound granulocytopenia: new approaches to alimentary canal microbial suppression. *Ann Intern Med* 1980;93:358–361.

119. Hargadon MT, Young VM, Schimpff SC, et al. Selective suppression of alimentary tract microbial flora as prophylaxis during granulocytopenia. *Antimicrob Agents Chemother* 1981;20:620–624.

120. Sleijfer DTH, Mulder NH, de Vries-Hospers HG, et al. Infection prevention in granulocytopenic patients by selective decontamination of the digestive tract. *Eur J Cancer* 1980;16:859–869.

121. Pizzo PA, Robichaud KJ, Edwards BK, et al. Oral antibiotic prophylaxis in patients with cancer: a double-blind randomized placebo-controlled trial. *J Pediatr* 1983;102:125–133.

122. Pizzo PA, Schimpff SC. Strategies for the prevention of infection in the myelosuppressed or immunosuppressed cancer patient. *Cancer Treat Rep* 1983;67:223–234.

123. Wade JC, Schimpff SC, Hargadon MT, et al. A comparison of trimethoprim-sulfamethoxazole plus nystatin with gentamicin plus nystatin in the prevention of infection in acute leukemia. *N Engl J Med* 1981;304:1057–1062.

124. EORTC International Antimicrobial Therapy Project Group. Trimethoprim-sulfamethoxazole in the acute nonlymphocytic leukemia: a double-blind, placebo-controlled study. *J Infect Dis* 1984;150:372–379.

125. Hughes WT, Kuhn S, Chaudhary S, et al. Successful prophylaxis for *Pneumocystis carinii* pneumonitis. *N Engl J Med* 1977;297:1419–1426.

126. Wade JC, de Jongh CA, Newman KA, et al. Selective antimicrobial modulation as prophylaxis against infection during granulocytopenia: trimethoprim-sulfamethoxazole vs. nalidixic acid. *J Infect Dis* 1983;147:624–634.

127. Wilson JM, Guiney DG. Failure of oral trimethoprim-sulfamethoxazole prophylaxis in acute leukemia: isolation of resistant plasmids from strains of *Enterobacteriaceae* causing bacteremia. *N Engl J Med* 1982;306:16–20.

128. Lew MA, Kehoe K, Ritz J, et al. Ciprofloxacin versus trimethoprim/sulfamethoxazole for prophylaxis of bacterial infections in bone marrow transplant recipients: a randomized controlled trial. *J Clin Oncol* 1995;13:239–250.

129. Bow EJ, Rayner E, Scott BA, et al. Selective gut decontamination with nalidixic acid or trimethoprim-sulfamethoxazole for infection prophylaxis in neutropenic cancer patients: relationship of efficacy to antimicrobial spectrum and timing of administration. *Antimicrob Agents Chemother* 1987;31:551–557.

130. Cruciani M, Rampazzo R, Malena M, et al. Prophylaxis with fluoroquinolones for bacterial infections in neutropenic patients: a meta-analysis. *Clin Infect Dis* 1996;23:795–805.

131. Engels EA, Lau J, Barza M. Efficacy of quinolone prophylaxis in neutropenic cancer patients: a meta-analysis. *J Clin Oncol* 1998;16:1179–1187.

132. International Antimicrobial Therapy Cooperative Group of the European Organization for Research and Treatment of Cancer. Reduction of fever and streptococcal bacteremia in granulocytopenic patients with cancer: a trial of oral penicillin V or placebo combined with pefloxacin. *JAMA* 1994;272:1183–1189.

133. Cometta A, Calandra T, Bille J, et al. *Escherichia coli* resistant to fluoroquinolones in patients with cancer and neutropenia. *N Engl J Med* 1994;330:1240–1241.

134. Yoo, J-H, Huh D-H, Choi J-H, et al. Molecular epidemiological analysis of quinolone-resistant *Escherichia coli* causing bacteremia in neutropenic patients with leukemia in Korea. *Clin Infect Dis* 1997;25:1385–1391.

135. Lonnqvist B, Palmblad J, Ljungman P, et al. Oral acyclovir as prophylaxis for bacterial infections during induction therapy for acute leukaemia in adults. The Leukemia Group of Middle Sweden. *Supportive Care Cancer* 1993;1:139–144.

136. Viscoli C, Paesmans M, Sanz M, et al. Association between antifungal prophylaxis and rate of documented bacteremia in febrile neutropenic cancer patients. *Clin Infect Dis* 2001;32:1532–1537.

137. Prentice AG, Donnelly P. Oral antifungals as prophylaxis in haematological malignancy. *Blood Rev* 2001;15:1–8.

138. Singh N. Antifungal prophylaxis for solid organ transplant recipients: seeking clarity amidst controversy. *Clin Infect Dis* 2000;31:545–553.

139. Meunier F. Prevention of mycoses in immunocompromised patients. *Rev Infect Dis* 1987;9:408–416.

140. Reichenspurner H, Gamberg P, Nitschke M, et al. Significant reduction in the number of fungal infections after lung, heart-lung, and heart transplantation using aerosolized amphotericin B prophylaxis. *Transplant Proc* 1997;29:627–628.

141. Beyer J, Barzen G, Risse G, et al. Aerosol amphotericin B for prevention of invasive pulmonary aspergillosis. *Antimicrob Agents Chemother* 1993;37:1367–1369.

142. Goodman JL, Winston DH, Greenfield RA, et al. A controlled trial of fluconazole to prevent fungal infections in patients undergoing bone marrow transplantation. *N Engl J Med* 1992;326:845–851.

143. Winston DJ, Chandrasekar PH, Lazarus HM, et al. Fluconazole prophylaxis of fungal infections in patients with acute leukemia: results of a randomized placebo-controlled, double-blind, multicenter trial. *Ann Intern Med* 1993;118:495–503.

144. Rotstein C, Bow EJ, Laverdiere M, et al. Randomized placebo-controlled trial of fluconazole prophylaxis for neutropenic cancer patients: benefit based on purpose and intensity of cytotoxic therapy. *Clin Infect Dis* 1999;28:331–340.

145. Laverdière M, Rotstein C, Bow EJ, et al. Impact of fluconazole prophylaxis on fungal colonization and infection rates in neutropenic patients. *J Antimicrob Chemother* 2000;46:1001–1008.

146. Wingard JR, Merz WG, Rinaldi MG, et al. Increase in *Candida krausei* infection among patients with bone marrow transplantation and neutropenia treated prophylactically with fluconazole. *N Engl J Med* 1991;325:1274–1277.

147. Wingard JR, Merz WG, Rinaldi MG, et al. Association of *Torulopsis glabrata* infections with fluconazole prophylaxis in neutropenic bone marrow transplant patients. *Antimicrob Agents Chemother* 1993;37:1847–1849.

148. Menichetti F, Del Favero A, Martino P, et al. Itraconazole oral solution as prophylaxis for fungal infections in neutropenic patients with hematologic malignancies: a randomized, placebo-controlled, double-blind multicenter trial. *Clin Infect Dis* 1999;28:259–255.

149. Glasmacher A, Molitor E, Hahn C, et al. Antifungal prophylaxis with itraconazole in neutropenic patients with acute leukemia. *Leukemia* 1998;12:1338–1343.

150. Wilkin A, Feinberg J. Prophylaxis against fungal infections and cytomegalovirus disease after bone marrow transplantation. *Oncology* 2000;13:1701–1708.

151. Harousseau JL, Dekker AW, Stamatoullas-Bastard A, et al. Itraconazole oral solution for primary prophylaxis of fungal infections in patients with hematological malignancy and profound neutropenia: a randomized, double-blind, double-placebo, multicenter trial comparing itraconazole and amphotericin B. *Antimicrob Agents Chemother* 2000;44:1887–1893.

152. Gold D, Corey L. Acyclovir prophylaxis for herpes simplex virus infection. *Antimicrob Agents Chemother* 1987;31:361–367.

153. Anonymous. Varicella-zoster immune globulin: United States. *MMWR* 1981;30:15–16.

154. Straus SE, Ostrove JM, Inchauspe G, et al. NIH conference. Varicella-zoster virus infections. Biology, natural history, treatment, and prevention. *Ann Intern Med* 1988;108:221–237.

155. Balfour HH Jr, Bean B, Laskin OL, et al. Acyclovir halts progression of herpes zoster in immunocompromised patients. *N Engl J Med* 1983;308:1448–1453.

156. Steer CB, Szer J, Sasadeusz J, et al. Varicella-zoster infection after allogeneic bone marrow transplantation: incidence, risk factors and prevention with aciclovir and ganciclovir. *Bone Marrow Transplant* 2000;25:657–664.

157. Shepp DH, Dandliker PS, Meyers JD. Treatment of varicella-zoster virus infection in severely immunocompromised patients: a randomized comparison of acyclovir and vidarabine. *N Engl J Med* 1986;314:208–212.

158. Balfour HH Jr. Varicella zoster virus infections in immunocompromised hosts: a review of the natural history and management. *Am J Med* 1988;85(Suppl. 2A):68–73.

159. Balfour HH Jr, Chace BA, Stapleton JT, et al. A randomized placebo-controlled trial of oral acyclovir for the prevention of cytomegalovirus disease in recipients of renal allografts. *N Engl J Med* 1989;320:1381–1387.

160. Winston DJ, Ho WG, Bartoni K, et al. Intravenous immunoglobulin and CMV-seronegative blood products for prevention of CMV infection and disease in bone marrow transplant recipients. *Bone Marrow Transplant* 1993;12:283–288.

161. Winston DJ, Ho WG, Bartoni K, et al. Ganciclovir prophylaxis of cytomegalovirus infection and disease in allogeneic bone marrow transplant recipients: results of a placebo-controlled, double-blind trial. *Ann Intern Med* 1993;118:179–184.

Skin and Soft Tissue

CHAPTER 130
Approach to the Patient with Skin or Soft Tissue Infection

David S. Feingold and Jan V. Hirschmann

Because the skin is the major interface between humans and their environment, it is not surprising that bacterial, fungal, and viral infections of the skin and the underlying soft tissues are the most common human infections. A knowledge of the anatomy of the skin and soft tissues is central to understanding their vulnerability to infection and their defenses against it (Fig. 130.1).

The skin is composed of the epidermis, the dermis, and subcutaneous fat. The epidermis is an avascular, proliferating layer that generates on its surface a constantly renewing tough barrier of protein and lipid, the stratum corneum. The stratum corneum, a protective sheath all over the body, is both an important permeability barrier and a wall that excludes most environmental pathogens. The epidermis is, on average, the thickness of a piece of paper.

The dermis, deep to the epidermis, contains blood vessels and lymphatics as well as fibroblasts, which synthesize the collagen and elastic tissue that impart strength and resilience to the skin. The skin "appendages," that is, eccrine sweat glands, sebaceous

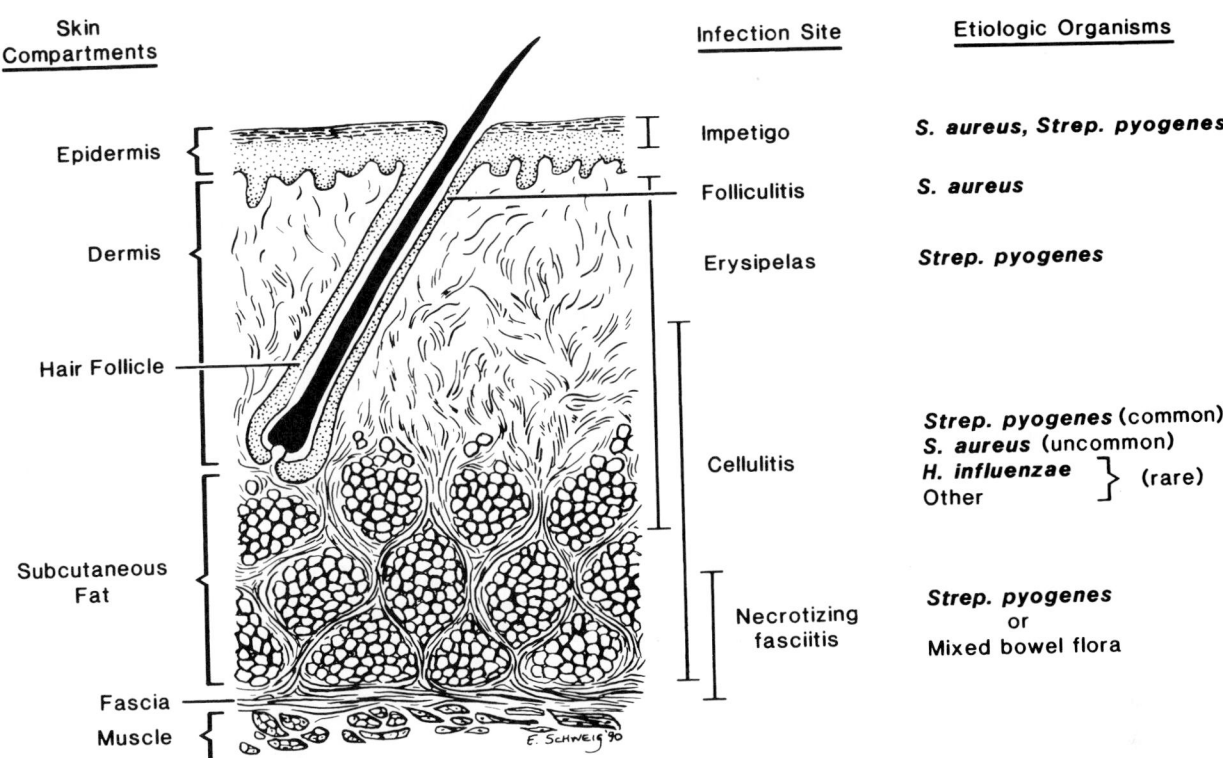

Figure 130.1. Cutaneous anatomy, sites of infection, and infecting organisms.

glands, and hair follicles, originate in the dermis. The skin appendages may harbor organisms of the normal skin microbial flora but also are susceptible to invasion by pathogens because they create gaps in the protective stratum corneum. The subcutaneous fat is of variable thickness over the body. It is both an effective cushion and an energy storage reserve; for better or worse, its distribution sculpts our appearance. Beneath the subcutaneous fat, the superficial fascia, which must be penetrated by all the important vessels and nerves, separates the skin from underlying muscle. All these layers may become infected, often by predictable microorganisms, causing distinct syndromes.

Specific infections may involve one or more layers of soft tissue. For example, impetigo is restricted to the epidermis; folliculitis involves hair follicles; erysipelas is a superficial cellulitis of the dermis that spreads along the dermal lymphatics; acute cellulitis affects the subcutaneous fat and the dermis; and necrotizing fasciitis centers in the superficial fascia; and myositis involves muscle. Pyoderma is a general term referring to bacterial infections of the skin caused by pyogenic organisms.

Table 130.1 lists factors to consider when bacterial infection of the soft tissues is suspected clinically. Primary cutaneous infections of the skin originate in grossly healthy skin. They usually have a characteristic morphologic appearance and are caused by

a single organism. The portal of entry for the pathogen is often not obvious, although minor trauma is suspected. Secondary infections develop in preexisting lesions, which serve as portals of entry for the organisms.

Atopic dermatitis and other eczematous lesions are the most common cutaneous lesions that become secondarily infected. Various lesions that interrupt the integrity of the stratum corneum, for example, surgical or traumatic wounds, burns, insect bites, and ulcers, are prone to secondary infection. Secondary infections are frequently polymicrobial and more likely to be caused by organisms less pathogenic for the normal soft tissues.

When a patient has impaired phagocytic or immune defenses, secondary infections are much more likely to develop and to progress rapidly. Thus, in leukopenic or immunosuppressed patients or in poorly controlled diabetic persons, scrupulous skin care to minimize portals for pathogen entry and aggressive treatment of early infections are indicated.

Most cutaneous infections in the normal host are self-limited. Early treatment is indicated when the tempo of extension is rapid or when associated fever or chills suggest a failure to contain the infection. It is always important to try to establish a specific etiology of the infection but even more so in this instance; blood cultures as well as local cultures and Gram stains are indicated before initiating antibiotic therapy.

Knowledge of recent environmental exposure may be critical to making a correct etiologic diagnosis. There are many examples of zoonoses or environmental contamination with pathogens. For example, one must consider *Aeromonas hydrophila* when severe cellulitis follows traumatic exposure to fresh water (1) and *Pasteurella multocida* infection after bites or scratches by dogs or cats (2). Probably most important in making a prompt etiologic diagnosis is recognition of a characteristic localization and morphologic appearance of a specific lesion. For example, erysipelas often involves the face, causing erythema that expands rapidly, often with raised margins and central clearing; this is almost

---

TABLE 130.1. Some Considerations in Managing Bacterial Skin and Soft Tissue Infections

Primary versus secondary
Infection, portal of entry
Impaired host defenses against infection
Associated signs and symptoms
Localization and morphology of lesion
Recent environmental exposure

always caused by streptococci, usually group A. Acute ascending lymphangitis, characterized by a centrally extending red streak, also is almost invariably caused by hemolytic streptococci. Impetigo may be caused by *Staphylococcus aureus* or *S. pyogenes*. It is characterized by honey-colored crusting lesions, is usually seen in children, and involves areas that are subject to epidermal trauma. A paronychia, when acute, is usually caused by *S. aureus*. When paronychia is chronic, *Pseudomonas aeruginosa* or *Candida albicans* is usually the cause.

Cutaneous infection may not originate in the skin but may be a manifestation of systemic infection, making possible prompt diagnosis of often occult infection. Cutaneous signs in systemic disease are not always suppurative but may represent a hypersensitivity response or possibly a vasculitis, as may be seen in patients with subacute bacterial endocarditis. Some of the cutaneous manifestations of systemic infection are listed in Table 130.2.

Although the clinical picture may suggest the etiology of soft tissue infections, definitive diagnosis rests on culture. In impetigo, culture under a crust usually yields the offending *S. aureus* or *S. pyogenes*. In lesions having a purulent focus, as in folliculitis or cutaneous abscesses, culture of the pus is usually helpful. In cellulitis, cultures of tissue aspirate specimens from the lesion have been productive in a minority of the cases, unless a primary focus was present, when the culture usually yielded a pathogen and agreed with a positive aspirate result, if obtained (3,4). In a prospective study of erysipelas and cellulitis of the leg reported from France in 1989, direct immunofluorescence assays were positive for group streptococcal antigen in 29 of the 42 cases. In combination with culture, direct immunofluorescence studies identified a causative agent in 37 of the cases (5). Search for bacterial antigen in tissue is an experimental procedure but some day may become a clinically useful diagnostic test. Amplification in vitro of microbial DNA from tissue using the polymerase chain reaction also has potential for sensitive, specific etiologic diagnosis of cellulitis (6).

In summary, when there is an open or a purulent cutaneous lesion, culture is usually productive. Aspiration of inflammatory lesions has a low yield. Because of the increasing problem of methicillin-resistant *S. aureus* in pyodermas, isolation of organisms has become more important, especially in areas where methicillin resistance is common. Identification of the causative pathogen is especially important in immunosuppressed patients with acquired immunodeficiency syndrome or other diseases, in whom unusual organisms are common. For aggressive soft tissue infections, such as necrotizing fasciitis or myositis, it is often mandatory to aspirate or biopsy the involved tissue surgically to confirm the diagnosis and guide appropriate treatment.

TABLE 130.2. Some Cutaneous Signs in Systemic Infection

Noninfectious
  Erythema nodosum
  Erythema multiforme
  Necrotizing vasculitis
  Osler nodes
  Janeway lesions
  Disseminated intravascular coagulation
Infectious
  Purulent petechiae in meningococcemia
  Cutaneous abscesses in staphylococcal sepsis
  Ecthyma gangrenosum in *Pseudomonas* sepsis
  Cellulitis in *Vibrio vulnificus* septicemia
  Erythema migrans in Lyme disease (*Borrelia burgdorferi*)

The preceding discussion applies mainly to bacterial soft tissue infections. Specific soft tissue tropisms and morphologic patterns of infection also occur with viral and fungal infections. These are discussed in other chapters. They are important to recognize, because patients with acquired immunodeficiency syndrome or other forms of deficient host defenses frequently have a variety of viral and fungal cutaneous problems that look different from those seen in normal hosts.

REFERENCES

1. Hanson PG, Standridge J, Jarrett F, et al. Freshwater wound infection due to *Aeromonas hydrophila. JAMA* 1977;238:1053.
2. Weber DJ, Wolfson JS, Swartz MN, et al. *Pasteurella multocida* infections, report of 34 cases and review of the literature. *Medicine (Baltimore)* 1984;63:133.
3. Hook EW III, Hooton TM, Horton CA, et al. Microbiologic evaluation of cutaneous cellulitis in adults. *Arch Intern Med* 1986;146:295.
4. Duvanel T, Auckenthaler R, Rohrer P, et al. Quantitative cultures of biopsy specimens from cutaneous cellulitis. *Arch Intern Med* 1989;149:293.
5. Bernard P, Bedane C, Mounier M, et al. Streptococcal cause of erysipelas and cellulitis in adults: a microbiologic study using direct immunofluorescence technique. *Arch Dermatol* 1989;125:779.
6. Fredricks DN, Relman DA. Application of polymerase chain reaction to the diagnosis of infectious diseases. *Clin Infect Dis* 1999;29:475.

CHAPTER 131
Normal Cutaneous Flora and Infections They Cause

Jan V. Hirschmann and David S. Feingold

The normal cutaneous flora (1–3) is a teeming population of microorganisms comprising relatively few species. Aerobes vary in density from $10^2/cm^2$ on dry skin to $10^7/cm^2$ in moist areas such as the axilla and toe web spaces. Anaerobes, infrequent in other sites, reach concentrations of 10^4 to $10^6/cm^2$ in areas rich in sebaceous glands. The sweat glands and ducts are ordinarily sterile, but anaerobes populate the deeper parts of the hair follicles and sebaceous glands. Table 131.1 lists the resident cutaneous flora and the skin diseases associated with each.

The permanent cutaneous flora persists primarily because the organisms can attach to skin cells and reproduce there. "Transients," organisms found only temporarily on the skin, usually originate from the environment or from adjacent, non-cutaneous surfaces such as mucous membranes, but do not adhere well to cutaneous cells and cannot thrive or reproduce on the skin for sustained periods. A third subpopulation of cutaneous organisms includes temporary residents or nomads. Often because of changes in the environment or the population of the permanent residents, these microbes can briefly attach to skin cells and multiply for short periods.

Several factors other than epithelial cell adherence limit the normal flora to only a few species and prevent colonization and invasion by pathogens. Probably most important is an intact stratum corneum. Its overlapping cells form a barricade that impedes entry of microorganisms into the epidermis below, and its dryness discourages growth of many microbes, such as gram-negative bacilli and *Candida* species, that require moisture to thrive. The cell remnants in the stratum corneum constantly shed, discouraging most organisms from establishing permanent residence. Another factor inhibiting the growth of many

TABLE 131.1. Resident Cutaneous Flora and Associated Skin Disorders

Organisms	Associated cutaneous disorder
Gram-positive cocci	
Staphylococcus aureus	Bullous and non-bullous impetigo, ecthyma, blistering distal dactylitis, pustules, folliculitis, cutaneous abscesses
Coagulase-negative staphylococci	—
Micrococcus species	
M. sedentarius	Pitted keratolysis
Gram-positive bacilli	
Corynebacterium species	Trichomycosis axillaris, dermatophytosis complex, axillary odor, erythrasma, pitted keratolysis
C. minutissimum	
Brevibacterium species	Cheesy foot odor
Propionibacterium species	—
P. acnes	Acne
Gram-negative bacilli	
Acinetobacter species	—
Fungi	
Pityrosporum orbiculare (ovale)	Tinea (pityriasis) versicolor, Seborrheic dermatitis, *Pityrosporum* folliculitis

microbes is the low pH of normal skin (about 5.5), which results from the resident cutaneous flora's ability to produce acids from the lipids of sebum. The host's immune system also seems important, because defects in cell-mediated immunity, granulocyte function, or secretion of antibodies (ordinarily present in sweat as immunoglobulins A and G) may predispose to recurrent, severe cutaneous infection. In addition, the resident flora itself may reduce colonization with other microorganisms by occupying binding sites, exhausting nutrients, or elaborating antimicrobial substances.

IDENTITY OF THE NORMAL FLORA

Gram-positive Cocci

Staphylococcus aureus usually does not colonize the skin, but up to 20% of normal people harbor it in the intertriginous areas, especially the perineum, and approximately 20% to 40% carry the bacterium in the anterior nares. In contrast, coagulase-negative staphylococci are the most numerous organisms of the skin flora. Prominent among these is *Staphylococcus epidermidis*, which tends to colonize the upper body and represents more than half of the resident staphylococci. Other *Staphylococcus* species include *S. hominis*, *S. haemolyticus*, *S. capitis*, *S. warneri*, *S. cohnii*, *S. simulans*, and *S. saprophyticus*, which is often a resident of the perineum and a common cause of urinary tract infections in females.

Other gram-positive cocci commonly residing on the skin are *Micrococcus* species, primarily *M. luteus* and *M. varians*. The anaerobic staphylococcus *Peptococcus saccharolyticus* is part of the normal flora in 20% of the population, especially on the forehead and in the antecubital fossa.

Streptococci are not members of the normal skin flora, although oral streptococci may reside transiently on the perioral skin. The cutaneous pathogen *Streptococcus pyogenes* (group A

streptococcus) usually dies quickly on normal, intact skin; disruption of the stratum corneum is necessary for infection to occur. In some normal hosts, however, it can survive for a few days, but many develop impetigo shortly afterward (4).

Gram-positive Bacilli

The coryneforms are gram-positive pleomorphic bacilli that include primarily *Corynebacterium* and *Brevibacterium* species. *Corynebacterium* species are lipophilic—they thrive in areas of high lipid content—and are a major component of the normal flora, particularly in moist areas, including the interdigital toe spaces. Group JK coryneforms are antibiotic-resistant *Corynebacterium* species that colonize intertriginous areas, especially in immunocompromised hosts. *Brevibacterium* species inhabit the skin of many normal people, primarily in moist areas. They are frequently isolated from the toe webs, particularly in patients with tinea pedis, and probably cause the cheesy odor of sweaty feet.

Propionibacterium species, which normally inhabit hair follicles and sebaceous glands, are the most common anaerobes of the permanent cutaneous flora. *Propionibacterium acnes*, present in almost all adults, is most numerous on the scalp, forehead, and back; its density correlates directly with the quantity of sebum present. Other *Propionibacterium* species are *P. granulosum*, present in small numbers at all skin sites, and *P. avidum*, usually found in moist areas, especially the anterior nares, axilla, and perineum.

Gram-negative Bacilli

In part because they flourish best only in moist areas, gram-negative bacilli are unusual in the normal flora, although they occasionally become residents in intertriginous sites. The most common of these is *Acinetobacter* species, found in up to 25% of the population. They are especially prevalent in summer, probably because increased sweating provides a moist milieu hospitable for their growth.

Fungi

Pityrosporum orbiculare, *Malassezia furfur*, and *Pityrosporum ovale*, synonyms for the same organism, are lipophilic yeasts that are most dense on the back and chest, areas of greatest sebum excretion. *Candida* species, although common in the oral cavity and elsewhere in the alimentary tract, rarely reside on the normal skin.

RESIDENT FLORA AS CUTANEOUS PATHOGENS

Coryneforms

Erythrasma is a common, usually asymptomatic superficial cutaneous infection apparently caused by *Corynebacterium* species, possibly including *C. minutissimum* (5). It especially affects intertriginous areas such as the groin, axillae, and toe webs. In tropical climates, extensive disease can occur anywhere on the body. In its most common form, scaling, fissuring, and maceration occur in the toe webs, especially the fourth interspace. In other areas the lesions are scaly, slightly brown or red patches that are irregular in shape but have well-delineated borders. In all locations, the involved skin fluoresces red to pink with ultraviolet light from a Wood lamp because the organisms produce porphyrins. This procedure is the major diagnostic test. Treatments include vigorous washing with soap; topical azoles, such as miconazole (6), which have antibacterial (gram-positive) as well as antifungal activity; oral erythromycin; and topical erythromycin or clindamycin (7).

Trichomycosis axillaris is the presence of yellow, red, or black nodules on the axillary hair, caused by large colonies of *Corynebacterium* species of several biochemical types forming on the outside of the hair shaft (7). Because the bacteria can invade the cuticle, the hair may become brittle. The same process may affect the pubic or facial hair (8). Increased sweating, poor hygiene, and failure to use an axillary deodorant are predisposing factors. Shaving the hair eliminates the disease, although topical clindamycin or erythromycin may also be effective (8).

Pitted keratolysis consists of multiple pitted erosions of the soles that measure 1 to 7 mm in diameter or, occasionally, collarettes on the palms. The lesions become more prominent if soaked in water for 10 to 15 minutes (9). Usually asymptomatic, pitted keratolysis seems to occur in settings of increased moisture from such factors as excessive sweating, occlusive footwear, or frequent contact with water. An intense malodor of the feet is common, and reddened plaques, scaling, pruritus, and tender soles may develop in some patients. Some studies suggest coryneform bacteria as the cause; organisms are recovered from the erosion or pit rather than the adjacent normal skin. The bacteria may produce enzymes that digest keratin and create excavations of the stratum corneum (9). One investigation found both *C. minutissimum* and *Micrococcus sedentarius* in all cases of pitted keratolysis. The authors reproduced the disease experimentally in a volunteer by using *M. sedentarius* in pure culture under occlusion over the surface of the heel (10). Coryneform bacteria and *M. sedentarius* may be synergistic, or each organism may be able to produce the disorder independently. Several treatments are effective, including topical imidazoles such as miconazole and clotrimazole, topical erythromycin and clindamycin, antiseptics such as glutaraldehyde and formaldehyde, and systemic erythromycin (9).

The term dermatophytosis complex applies to dermatophyte infection combined with bacterial overgrowth in the moist, partially occluded interdigital toe spaces (11). Scaling produced by the fungal infection, combined with occlusion, maceration, and wetness, promotes the growth of coryneforms, especially *Brevibacterium* species. The result is white maceration, soggy scaling, pruritus, and malodor in the interdigital space. Redness, tenderness, edema, and fissuring may occur in severe cases. The dermatophytes, forced lower in the stratum corneum, become more difficult to isolate from superficial scrapings, but are detectable on biopsy of the deepest portion of the stratum corneum. Effective antimicrobial therapy requires agents active against both the fungi and the bacteria, such as the azoles (e.g., clotrimazole or miconazole). Drying of the area by removing the shoe, separating the interspaces with soft pads, and applying astringents such as aluminum chloride are also useful measures.

Propionibacterium Species

The presence of *P. acnes* in the sebaceous follicle is a critical element in the development of acne vulgaris. This organism produces certain extracellular factors that may initiate the inflammatory phase of acne. Papules and pustules result from rupture of the follicular wall and inflammation of the surrounding dermis. Therapies for acne involve decreasing one or more of the three basic pathogenetic elements: sebum production, hyperkeratosis of the follicular duct, and the *P. acnes* population. Diminishing the number of *P. acnes* organisms can be accomplished with oral antibiotics such as tetracycline or topical antibiotics such as

erythromycin or clindamycin, which are therapeutically equivalent to the oral agents (12). Other topical antibacterial substances such as benzoyl peroxide are also effective (12).

Pityrosporum Species

Certain factors cause *P. orbiculare* (*P. ovale* or *Malassezia furfur*) to transform from a saprophyte into a pathogen, a process often, but not always, accompanied by a morphologic change from yeasts to hyphal forms. These conditions include high temperature and humidity, increased sweating, occlusive clothing, greasy skin, and certain systemic conditions such as depressed cellular immunity and excessive exogenous or endogenous corticosteroids (13). When the hyphal form of *P. orbiculare* involves the stratum corneum, tinea (or pityriasis) versicolor results. This condition is usually asymptomatic, but pruritus sometimes occurs. Mildly scaly macules or large patches of hypopigmented or hyperpigmented skin develop, predominantly on the trunk but also on the neck, and upper arms. Occasionally the perineum, genitalia, axillae, and thighs may be involved. The lesions may be white, red, or yellowish-tan to brown. On white skin they tend to be hyperpigmented, but on tanned or dark skin the lesions are paler than the surrounding skin. With ultraviolet light from the Wood's lamp, the lesions may show pale yellow-green fluorescence. The diagnosis is established by finding hyphae and yeast ("spaghetti and meatballs") on potassium hydroxide preparations. Treatment is topical application of selenium sulfide left on for a few minutes to several hours and then washed off. This program is repeated daily for one week, then periodically as necessary. Propylene glycol, 50% in water twice daily, is also effective, as are the topical azoles, such as ketoconazole. For extensive disease or in patients unable to apply the topical treatments, oral azoles are effective, including a single 400-mg dose of ketoconazole or fluconazole or itraconazole 200 mg for 5 to 7 days. Relapses are common, but may be averted by monthly prophylaxis using single applications of topical agents or single doses of an oral azole.

P. orbiculare can also cause an itchy folliculitis, usually on the upper back, chest, and upper arms and usually in adults 30 years of age or older (14). The lesions are small, dome-shaped follicular papules or pustules. Lesions are occasionally present on the forearms, hands, legs, and face. Direct microscopy of material examined with potassium hydroxide, methylene blue, or Gram stain shows budding yeasts, which are also visible by skin biopsy. Topical therapy is effective, consisting of selenium sulfide for 30 minutes daily for 3 days then once weekly; propylene glycol, 50% in water twice daily for 3 weeks; or a topical azole, such as ketoconazole, daily for 1 week, followed by treatment once a week for several months (13). Oral azoles also clear the infection, for example, itraconazole 200 mg every day for 7 days (15).

P. orbiculare probably causes seborrheic dermatitis, a scaly erythematous disorder that involves the scalp, face, sternal and interscapular regions of the chest, and intertriginous areas. The scale tends to have a greasy appearance and may form crusts. The scalp lesions usually respond to treatment with selenium sulfide, although a potent corticosteroid such as fluocinolone may be necessary. Lesions on the face, ears, and groin are controlled by hydrocortisone; those on the trunk may require more potent corticosteroids. The evidence that *Pityrosporum* species cause the seborrheic dermatitis consists not only of the regular isolation of the organism from lesions but also of the successful treatment of this disorder with topical miconazole and oral or topical ketoconazole (16–18). Corticosteroids are superior to topical ketoconazole, however, in controlling the disease (19), which tends to be chronic and relapsing.

REFERENCES

1. Noble WC. *Microbiology of human skin,* 2nd ed. London: Lloyd Luke, 1981.
2. Leyden JJ, McKinley KJ, Nordstrom KM, et al. Skin microflora. *J Invest Dermatol* 1987;88:65s.
3. Roth RR, James WD. Microbiology of the skin: resident flora, ecology, infection. *J Am Acad Dermatol* 1989;20:367.
4. Ferrieri P, Dajani AS, Wannamaker LW, et al. Natural history of impetigo. I. Site sequence of acquisition and familial patterns of spread of cutaneous streptococci. *J Clin Invest* 1972;51:2851.
5. Sarkany I, Taplin D, Blank H. The etiology and treatment of erythrasma. *J Invest Dermatol* 1961;37:283.
6. Pitcher DG, Noble WC, Seville RH. Treatment of erythrasma with miconazole. *Clin Exp Dermatol* 1979;4:453.
7. Freeman RG, McBride ME, Know JM. Pathogenesis of trichomycosis axillaris. *Arch Dermatol* 1969;100:95.
8. White SW, Smith J. Trichomycosis pubis. *Arch Dermatol* 1979;115:444.
9. Zaias N. Pitted and ringed keratolysis: a review and update. *J Am Acad Dermatol* 1982;7:787.
10. Nordstrom KM, McGinley KJ, Capiello L, et al. Pitted keratolysis: the role of *Micrococcus sedentarius. Arch Dermatol* 1987;123:1320.
11. Leyden JJ, Kligman AM. Interdigital athlete's foot. *Arch Dermatol* 1988;114: 1691.
12. Hirschmann JV. Topical antibiotics in dermatology. *Arch Dermatol* 1989;14: 1466.
13. Sunenshine PJ, Schwartz RA, Janniger CK. Tinea versicolor. *Int J Dermatol* 1998; 37:648.
14. Back O, Faergemann J, Homqvist R. *Pityrosporum* folliculitis: a common disease of the young and middle-aged. *J Am Acad Dermatol* 1985;12:56.
15. Parsad D, Saini R, Negi KS. Short-term treatment of *Pityrosporum* folliculitis: a double blind placebo-controlled study. *J Eur Acad Dermatol Venereol* 1998;11:188.
16. Ford GP, Farr PM, Ive FA, et al. The response of seborrheic dermatitis to ketoconazole. *Br J Dermatol* 1984;111:603.
17. Faergemann J. Seborrheic dermatitis and *Pityrosporum orbiculare*: treatment of seborrhoeic dermatitis of the scalp with miconazole-hydrocortisone (Daktacort), miconazole and hydrocortisone. *Br J Dermatol* 1986;114:695.
18. Skinner RB, Noah PW, Taylor RM, et al. Double-blind treatment of seborrheic dermatitis with 2% ketoconazole cream. *J Am Acad Dermatol* 1985;12:852.
19. Stratigos JD, Antoniou C, Katsambas A, et al. Ketoconazole 2% cream versus hydrocortisone 1% cream in the treatment of seborrheic dermatitis: a double-blind comparative trial. *J Am Acad Dermatol* 1988;19:850.

CHAPTER 132

Staphylococcal and Streptococcal Skin or Soft Tissue Infections

Jan V. Hirschmann and David S. Feingold

Cutaneous pyogenic infections usually occur when inflammation, trauma, maceration from excessive moisture, or other factors disrupt the protective stratum corneum of the skin. Although the normal resident flora can sometimes cause the ensuing infectious complications, especially cutaneous abscesses, organisms acquired from elsewhere are usually responsible, particularly *Staphylococcus aureus* and *Streptococcus pyogenes* (group A streptococcus).

S. aureus is present in the anterior nares of 20% to 40% of the normal population (1). From this reservoir it can cause persistent skin colonization in some people and, occasionally, a predisposition to recurrent staphylococcal skin infections. The rate of colonization of the anterior nares and skin may be increased in intravenous drug abusers, diabetics requiring insulin, hospital workers, patients receiving allergy injections, and those undergoing hemodialysis (2). The bacterium frequently resides on areas damaged by dermatitis. The degree of colonization directly correlates with the severity of exudation. *S. aureus* is present on the skin of most patients with atopic dermatitis, nummular eczema, and lichen simplex chronicus. It is present in approximately 20% of those with seborrheic dermatitis and, in low numbers, in approximately 50% of patients with psoriasis (3). *S. aureus* can spread from person to person, but in previously un-colonized people it typically appears first in the nose and only later on normal skin. It usually colonizes the skin before causing cutaneous infection.

In contrast, *S. pyogenes* rarely persists on mucocutaneous surfaces. It is usually acquired from others whose skin is infected or briefly colonized with the organism. In those who develop cutaneous infection, it typically appears on the skin first and only later spreads to the respiratory tract, which is opposite to the order of spread in *S. aureus* infection (4).

IMPETIGO

S. pyogenes and *S. aureus*, independently or together, cause several types of skin infections. Their clinical appearance depends on the depth and anatomic location of the inflammation. The most superficial of these is impetigo, which involves the formation beneath the stratum corneum of vesicles and pustules containing numerous neutrophils and occasional gram-positive cocci. In the bullous variety the fluid collection is also below the stratum corneum, but it often contains few or no neutrophils. Other histologic features of impetigo are neutrophilic and lymphocytic inflammation of the upper dermis and epidermal edema (spongiosis).

In nonbullous impetigo, thin-walled vesicles and pustules form on an erythematous base. They rupture and release their liquid contents, which dry to create yellow-brown ("honey-colored") scabs. Most common on the face and extremities, the lesions usually occur on skin that is damaged by minor trauma, such as cuts, abrasions, and insect bites. The crusts later separate from the underlying skin, which does not scar because the infection is so superficial. Impetigo may be pruritic and regional lymph node enlargement may occur, but systemic manifestations such as fever are rare.

In bullous impetigo, superficial flaccid bullae form. When they rupture, the released liquid dries to become a thin, brown covering resembling lacquer. Lesions several centimeters wide may occur through coalescence of many smaller areas.

Impetigo may complicate underlying dermatitis, particularly atopic eczema. The clinical distinction between an exudative dermatitis and superimposed impetigo may be difficult, because a weeping, crusted skin surface may be present in both. The diagnosis of superinfections is most convincing when pustules, surrounding cellulitis, contiguous lymphangitis, or regional lymphadenitis is present, in addition to positive skin culture results for *S. aureus* or *S. pyogenes*.

Poor personal hygiene, crowded living conditions, and hot, humid climates predispose to impetigo, which can occur in outbreaks among family members or populations in closed institutions. Carriers of *S. pyogenes* or *S. aureus* and those with infected skin may transmit the organism to others, in whom the bacteria reside briefly on normal skin. Minor trauma such as insect bites, often complicated by scratching, disrupts the cutaneous surface, allowing the bacteria to enter the skin. In nonbullous impetigo, either *S. pyogenes* or *S. aureus* can be the initial pathogen, but combined infection with both organisms is frequent. Bullous impetigo, however, is a primary infection with certain strains of *S. aureus*, usually group II phage. These organisms produce a toxin, exfoliatin, that causes cleavage beneath the stratum corneum. The same toxin is responsible for the staphylococcal

TABLE 132.1. Systemic Antibiotic Therapy for Streptococcal and Staphylococcal Pyoderma

Agent	Usual adult dose
Benzathine penicillin	1.2 million units IM as single dose
Penicillin V	250 mg PO qid
Cloxacillin, dicloxacillin	250 mg PO qid
Nafcillin, oxacillin	500 mg IV qid
Cephradine, cephalexin	250 mg PO qid
Cefazolin	500 mg IV tid
Clindamycin	150 mg PO qid
Erythromycin	500 mg PO qid

IM, Intramuscularly; IV intravenously, PO, orally; qid, four times a day; tid, three times a day; bid, twice a day.

scalded skin syndrome. Impetigo complicating eczema and other skin disorders is typically staphylococcal, but *S. pyogenes* is sometimes present.

The definitive diagnosis of the various forms of impetigo requires isolation of *S. pyogenes* or *S. aureus* from cultures of the involved skin. Microbiologic studies, however, are frequently unnecessary in clinically obvious cases.

Although impetigo may resolve spontaneously, treatment is indicated to relieve symptoms more rapidly, halt the formation of new lesions, and prevent potentially serious infectious complications, such as cellulitis. Whether antimicrobial therapy decreases the risk of poststreptococcal glomerulonephritis, a rare immunologic reaction provoked by certain "nephritogenic" strains of *S. pyogenes*, is uncertain. Often, the renal disorder is already evident when the patient comes to medical attention (5).

Nonbullous impetigo of limited extent may respond well to topical antibiotics (6). Mupirocin is the best topical agent, and, when applied to the lesions three times a day for 7 to 8 days, it is as effective as oral erythromycin (7). Unlike systemic antimicrobials, however, topical agents are inconvenient to use with widespread disease or simultaneous infection of several family members, and they are not very effective in bullous impetigo. Furthermore, they do not eradicate streptococci in the respiratory tract, an important reservoir for spread of infection to others, especially during epidemics or when nephritogenic strains are involved. In these circumstances, systemic antibiotics are indicated to minimize contagion.

When systemic antimicrobials are warranted (Table 132.1), an agent effective against both streptococci and staphylococci is advisable because penicillin-resistant *S. aureus* is now usually the predominant or sole pathogen isolated in nonbullous impetigo. Two studies demonstrated the superiority of such an approach (8,9). Dicloxacillin is a good choice. In patients allergic to penicillin, clindamycin is an acceptable alternative for susceptible strains, or, if the allergy is not life-threatening, an oral cephalosporin is reasonable. Erythromycin is usually successful, but in some locales *S. aureus* is often resistant to it. The duration of oral therapy for impetigo with any of these agents should be approximately 1 week. When the risk of impetigo is high, such as for young children living in a hot, humid climate, prophylactically applying topical neomycin-bacitracin to areas of minor trauma, such as insect bites and abrasions reduces the frequency of subsequent impetigo (10).

ECTHYMA

Ecthyma is a streptococcal or staphylococcal infection causing dermal ulceration that often occurs in patients with preceding trauma, malnutrition, or poor hygiene. In alcoholics, the lesions have sometimes been labeled "wine sores." Like impetigo, it begins with vesicles that form crusts, but the infection causes ulceration beneath the adherent scabs. Ecthyma usually occurs on the lower extremities, appearing as single or multiple erythematous ulcerations with overlying crusts. Because of the deeper level of infection, ecthyma, unlike impetigo, causes scarring. Appropriate therapy should be an antibiotic that is effective against both *S. aureus* and *S. pyogenes*, such as dicloxacillin (11).

BLISTERING DISTAL DACTYLITIS

Blistering distal dactylitis, an infection with *S. pyogenes*, or less commonly *S. aureus*, usually occurs in children (12). A superficial, tender or nontender bulla with an erythematous base appears over the anterior fat pad of the distal phalanx of a finger, thumb, or toe and may extend to the nail folds. Gram staining of the blister fluid demonstrates gram-positive cocci in chains or clusters. Clusters yield *S. pyogenes* or *S. aureus*. Incision and drainage are appropriate for painful lesions. When *S. pyogenes* is responsible, penicillin is the drug of choice; for *S. aureus* an antistaphylococcal agent such as dicloxacillin is indicated.

FOLLICULITIS

Folliculitis is an inflammation of the ostium of a hair follicle. The pathogenesis apparently involves a combination of ostial occlusion and superficial follicular inflammation, which may be caused by bacteria, fungi, chemicals, or other agents. Among the many causes of folliculitis is *S. aureus*, sometimes in children but rarely in adults, in whom other causes of folliculitis predominate. Erythematous papules or pustules develop around individual hairs, often in crops and usually on the scalp or extremities. They tend to subside rapidly with systemic antistaphylococcal antibiotics.

FURUNCLES AND CARBUNCLES

S. aureus can cause infections of the hair follicle. Inflammation extends deeper than in folliculitis to involve the dermis. There is an inflammatory nodule surmounted by a pustule through which the hair emerges. Discrete lesions, whether single or multiple, are called furuncles. They are called carbuncles when the infection affects several adjacent follicles, producing a coalescent inflammatory mass with pus draining from multiple follicular orifices. Furuncles can occur anywhere on hairy skin. Carbuncles tend to develop on the back of the neck. For small furuncles, moist heat, which seems to promote drainage, is satisfactory. Larger furuncles and carbuncles require incision and drainage. Systemic antistaphylococcal antibiotics are usually unnecessary unless extensive surrounding cellulitis or fever occurs.

RECURRENT STAPHYLOCOCCAL SKIN INFECTIONS

Some patients have recurrent episodes of furunculosis or other staphylococcal skin infections. Diabetes mellitus, chronic hemodialysis, and intravenous drug abuse are predisposing factors. Occasionally, a disorder of immune or granulocytic function is present, but most victims are apparently healthy. These patients are usually chronic nasal carriers of *S. aureus*, and they probably repetitively inoculate the organism onto the skin from this nasal reservoir.

Many topical antibiotics applied to the anterior nares eliminate *S. aureus* during use; however, once the drug is discontinued, the organism quickly returns. Mupirocin is the most effective topical agent and can eradicate nasal carriage for a protracted period, but resistant *S. aureus* has emerged during its use (5). Nevertheless, in nasal staphylococcal carriers prone to repeat staphylococcal skin infections, the use of nasal mupirocin the first 5 days of each month decreased the incidence of subsequent episodes (13).

Oral therapy with penicillinase-resistant penicillins such as dicloxacillin is not effective alone. Rifampin by itself or combined with an antistaphylococcal penicillin is successful, and eradication can persist for many weeks after drug discontinuation. With rifampin alone, however, development of resistance is common. The quinolones, such as ciprofloxacin, may be effective, but resistance is again a concern (14). Clindamycin appears to be the most useful oral antimicrobial for if the staphylococci are susceptible to it. In a controlled trial of 150 mg daily for 3 months, clindamycin eliminated recurrent staphylococcal skin infections in 82% of patients with a previous history of them, whereas 64% of those receiving placebo continued to have infections (15). Furthermore, most of those receiving clindamycin had no recurrent infections for at least 9 months after discontinuation of the drug. This suggests long-term eradication of nasal carriage, although nasal cultures were not performed.

ERYSIPELAS AND CELLULITIS

Infection involving the dermal lymphatics produces erysipelas, that affecting the deeper dermis and subcutaneous fat causes cellulitis. The clinical manifestations are rapidly spreading areas of edema, redness, and heat, sometimes accompanied by lymphangitis, regional lymphadenitis, and systemic signs of fever, tachycardia, confusion, and hypotension. Vesicles, bullae, and cutaneous hemorrhage may occur in the inflamed skin, whose edematous surface with numerous pits in the area of the hair follicles resembles an orange peel (*peau d'orange*). On the face the infection typically involves one or both cheeks and the nasal bridge. Erysipelas has a more sharply demarcated, elevated border than cellulitis, but the distinction between the two, often difficult to discern on examination, is clinically unimportant. Furthermore, because practitioners use the terminology inconsistently, "cellulitis" and "erysipelas" are best considered to be clinically synonymous.

These infections may complicate pre-existing skin infections such as impetigo or ecthyma, but more commonly they arise from minor, often inapparent, breaks in the skin. Important predisposing factors include edema from such disorders as venous insufficiency and lymphatic obstruction; disruption of the cutaneous barrier by ulceration, wound, fissured toe webs, or other inflammatory dermatoses, such as eczema; obesity; and skin previously damaged by such trauma as burns, radiation therapy, and surgery, particularly sites of previous saphenous venectomy (16,17). The most common locations are the legs and face.

Blood cultures and needle aspirations or punch biopsies of the inflamed skin usually fail to yield an organism. The available evidence, including studies using immunofluorescent antibodies, indicate that the vast majority of these infections arise from streptococci, often group A, but also other groups such as B, C, or G (18,19). The source of these organisms is frequently unclear, but in many infections of the lower extremities the responsible streptococci are present in the interdigital toe spaces, emphasiz-

ing the importance of detecting and treating tinea pedis and other causes of toe web maceration and fissuring in these patients (20). Occasionally, the reservoir is in the anal canal (21). Staphylococci occasionally cause cellulitis, usually in patients with a cutaneous abscess or penetrating trauma, including injection sites of illicit drug use. Special circumstances should suggest other infectious agents. Cellulitis complicating cat or dog bites is commonly due to *Pasteurella* species; *Aeromonas hydrophila* may cause infection following immersion injuries in fresh water; and cases after salt water immersion may arise from *Vibrio vulnificus*. *Pseudomonas aeruginosa* or other gram-negative bacilli may produce cellulitis in neutropenic hosts. In patients with deficient cell-mediated immunity *Cryptococcus neoformans* can cause infection.

Treatment for the usual case of erysipelas or cellulitis should include an antibiotic active against streptococci, such as penicillin G, although many clinicians cover the possibility of staphylococci as well. Reasonable parenteral therapy is nafcillin or oxacillin or a first-generation cephalosporin such as cefazolin. Appropriate oral agents include dicloxacillin or cephalexin. Treatment is usually for 5 to 7 days. Cutaneous inflammation and systemic toxicity may worsen after initiating therapy, presumably because the abrupt killing of organisms releases potent enzymes responsible for many of the clinical manifestations. Systemic corticosteroids may attenuate the inflammatory reaction and hasten resolution: a trial of an 8-day tapering oral course beginning with approximately 40 mg of prednisone accelerated improvement in hospitalized patients, allowing a switch to oral therapy earlier and a more rapid hospital discharge (22). Another important, and often neglected therapeutic maneuver, is elevating the affected area, which encourages gravity drainage of the edema and inflammatory substances.

Repeated episodes may permanently damage lymphatics, leading to lymphedema, sometimes severe enough to cause elephantiasis. Measures to reduce recurrences include controlling edema with diuretics and mechanical methods, such as elevation of the extremity, compressive stockings or pneumatic pressure pumps; treatment of tinea pedis; and, for those with frequent infections, prophylactic antibiotics. Options include monthly or semi-monthly benzathine penicillin injections or twice-daily oral therapy with 250 mg of penicillin or erythromycin (23,24).

REFERENCES

1. Roth RR, James WD. Microbiology of the skin: resident flora, ecology, infection. *J Am Acad Dermatol* 1989;20:367.
2. Sheagren JN. *Staphylococcus aureus*: the persistent pathogen. *N Engl J Med* 1984; 310:1368.
3. Leyden JJ, McGinley KJ, Nordstrom KM, et al. Skin microflora. *J Invest Dermatol* 1987;88:65s.
4. Ferrieri P, Dajani AS, Wannamaker LW, et al. Natural history of impetigo. I. Site sequence of acquisition and familial patterns of spread of cutaneous streptococci. *J Clin Invest* 1972;51:2851.
5. Hirschmann JV. Topical antibiotics in dermatology. *Arch Dermatol* 1988;124: 1691.
6. Dillon HC. The treatment of streptococcal skin infections. *J Pediatr* 1970;76:676.
7. Barton LL, Friedman AD, Sharkey AM, et al. Impetigo contagiosa. III. Comparative efficacy of oral erythromycin and topical mupirocin. *Pediatr Dermatol* 1989;6:134.
8. Barton LL, Friedman AD. Impetigo: a reassessment of etiology and therapy. *Pediatr Dermatol* 1987;4:185.
9. Dagan R, Bar-David Y. Comparison of amoxicillin and clavulanic acid (augmentin) for the nonbullous impetigo. *Am J Dis Child* 1989;143:916.
10. Maddox JS, Ware JC, Dillon HC. The natural history of streptococcal skin infection: prevention with topical antibiotics. *J Am Acad Dermatol* 1985;13:207.
11. Musher DM, McKenzie SO. Infections due to *Staphylococcus aureus*. *Medicine (Baltimore)* 1977;56:383.
12. Norcross ML Jr, Mitchell DF. Blistering distal dactylitis caused by *Staphylococcus aureus*. *Cutis* 1993;51:353.
13. Raz R, Miron D, Colodner R, et al. A 1-year trial of nasal mupirocin in the prevention of recurrent staphylococcal nasal colonization and skin infection. *Arch Intern Med* 1996;156:1109–1112.

14. Chow JW, Yu VL. *Staphylococcus aureus* nasal carriage in hemodialysis patients: its role in infection and approaches to prophylaxis. *Arch Intern Med* 1989;149:1258.

15. Klempner MS, Styrt B. Prevention of recurrent staphylococcal skin infections with low-dose oral clindamycin therapy. *JAMA* 1988;260:2682.

16. Dupuy A, Bndchikhi H, Roujeau JC, et al. Risk factors for erysipelas of the leg (cellulitis): case-control study. *BMJ* 1999;318:1591.

17. Dan M, Heller K, Shapira I, et al. Incidence of erysipelas following venectomy for coronary artery bypass surgery. *Infection* 1987;2:107.

18. Bernard P, Bedane C, Mounier M, et al. Streptococcal cause of erysipelas and cellulitis in adults. A microbiologic study using a direct immunofluorescent technique. *Arch Dermatol* 1989;125:779.

19. Eriksson B, Jorup-Rönström C, Karkkonen K, et al. Erysipelas: clinical and bacteriologic spectrum and serological aspects. *Clin Infect Dis* 1996;23:1091.

20. Semel JD, Goldin H. Association of athlete's foot with cellulitis of the lower extremities: diagnostic value of bacterial cultures of ipsilateral interdigital space samples. *Clin Infect Dis* 1996;23:1162.

21. Eriksson BKG. Anal colonization of group G β-hemolytic streptococci in relapsing erysipelas of the lower extremity. *Clin Infect Dis* 1999;29:1319.

22. Bergkvist PI, Sjöbeck K. Antibiotic and prednisolone therapy of erysipelas: a randomized, double blind, placebo-controlled study. *Scand J Infect Dis* 1997;29:377.

23. Wang JH, Liu YC, Cheng DL, et al. Role of benzathine penicillin G in prophylaxis for recurrent streptococcal cellulitis of the lower legs. *Clin Infect Dis* 1997;25:685.

24. Kremer M, Zuckerman R, Avraham Z, et al. Long-term antimicrobial therapy in the prevention of recurrent soft-tissue infections. *J Infect* 1991;22:37.

CHAPTER 133
Gram-Negative Bacillary Skin or Soft Tissue Infections

David S. Feingold and Jan V. Hirschmann

Pseudomonas aeruginosa causes several characteristic cutaneous infections. The organism is common in moist environmental niches and colonizes moist areas of the body. Typical *Pseudomonas* infections include external otitis or swimmer's ear, paronychia, and erosive interdigital infections in patients whose hands are frequently in water, and folliculitis associated with hot tub use. Drying the skin and eliminating the exposure are often adequate to cure these infections.

Malignant (sometimes called invasive) external otitis is a serious, locally invasive *Pseudomonas* infection that typically occurs in elderly diabetic patients (1,2). Reported predisposing factors in addition to diabetes include chronic external otitis and ear trauma, as may be seen in hearing aid users or with irrigation for cerumen impaction. Severe otalgia is the regular presenting complaint of malignant external otitis. Purulent drainage and granulation tissue in the external auditory canal are usually found on examination. Local cellulitis and bone destruction are best documented by radiographic imaging techniques. Extension to the central nervous system may cause neurologic deficit and even death.

In the past, successful treatment of malignant external otitis required prolonged hospitalization of at least 6 weeks for débridement and parenteral antipseudomonal therapy. The availability of the fluoroquinolone antibiotics with excellent antipseudomonal activity and tissue penetration after oral administration has obviated prolonged hospitalization and parenteral therapy with the associated complications. A series of 23 consecutive patients with malignant external otitis treated with oral ciprofloxacin (usually 750 mg twice daily) and local surgical débridement was reported from Israel (3). Twenty-one patients were cured. Ciprofloxacin therapy was continued for at least 6 weeks, but hospitalization averaged only 17 days.

P. aeruginosa may colonize the soles of used, not new, shoes; nail puncture wounds may cause inoculation of the organism into the foot, with resultant cellulitis and osteomyelitis (4). Surgical débridement and antibiotics are required. A distinctive acute eruption of tender papules on the feet from wading pools containing high concentrations of *P. aeruginosa* has been described (5). Removal from the source of the organism and symptomatic treatment brought resolution within 2 weeks.

During *Pseudomonas* sepsis, usually in impaired hosts, skin lesions that yield the organism on culture occasionally occur. Four types have been described: vesicles and bullae, gangrenous cellulitis, macular or papular lesions, and ecthyma gangrenosum (a black eschar with surrounding erythema) (6). These lesions may be important clues for the diagnosis of *Pseudomonas* sepsis. Of the gram-negative bacilli, *Pseudomonas* spp. show a tropism for the skin during sepsis that is rarely seen with other gram-negative organisms. In typhoid fever, rose-colored spots may occur on the skin. In systemic *Vibrio vulnificus* infection, metastatic areas of cutaneous cellulitis are common (7). Also in the differential diagnosis of metastatic cutaneous lesions in sepsis are *Escherichia coli* (rare), *Neisseria meningitidis*, *Neisseria gonorrhoeae*, and fungi of the *Aspergillus* and *Rhizopus* groups.

V. vulnificus and *Aeromonas hydrophila* are waterborne organisms that cause cutaneous infection. *V. vulnificus* is commonly found in seawater and fish, especially in the southern United States but as far north as New England in the summer (8). Two types of *V. vulnificus* cutaneous involvement occur (7). Wounds incurred in seawater may become contaminated and culminate in aggressive *V. vulnificus* cellulitis. Areas of cutaneous cellulitis may also develop as part of a life-threatening sepsis that occurs when susceptible patients, particularly those with liver disease, ingest *Vibrio*-contaminated seafood. Therapy with tetracyclines or other appropriate antibiotics based on sensitivities is mandatory. *A. hydrophila* grows in fresh or brackish water. It may contaminate preexisting wounds or traumatic wounds incurred in water. The severe cellulitis that may occur requires aggressive antibiotic treatment.

Pasteurella multocida is a normal inhabitant of the oral flora of dogs and cats. Many cases of localized soft tissue or bone infection have occurred after dog or cat bites or scratches (9). Generalized sepsis is rare. Penicillin is the treatment of choice.

Before widespread immunization against *Haemophilus influenzae* type b, this organism was a common cause of infection in young children (10). One characteristic form of this infection is a facial cellulitis, presumably because the respiratory tract is the source of the organism. The lesions may be violaceous, but in most patients, *H. influenzae* cellulitis is difficult to distinguish from that due to streptococci or other causes. Because bacteriologic testing often yields no pathogen, it is wise to treat facial cellulitis in children with an antibiotic regimen that is effective against *H. influenzae*.

Gram-negative folliculitis is seen mostly by dermatologists as a complication of antibiotic therapy for acne. When acne patients receiving antimicrobial agents (usually tetracyclines) develop worsening "acne" with pustular lesions, superinfection of the follicles with gram-negative bacilli, including *E. coli* or *Klebsiella* and *Pseudomonas* spp., may have occurred. The diagnosis depends on history, Gram stain, and culture. At times, discontinuing the antibiotic may allow spontaneous clearing of the infection, but more often, appropriate antimicrobial agents, based on sensitivity tests, are indicated.

REFERENCES

1. Chandler JR. Malignant external otitis. *Laryngoscope* 1968;78:1257.
2. Dorughaji RM, Nadol JB, Hyslop NE Jr, et al. Invasive external otitis. *Am J Med* 1981;71:603.
3. Lang R, Goshan S, Kitzes-Cohen R, et al. Successful treatment of malignant external otitis with oral ciprofloxacin: report of experience with 23 patients. *J Infect Dis* 1990;161:537.
4. Fisher MC, Goldsmith JF, Gilligan PH. Sneakers as a source of *Pseudomonas aeruginosa* in children with osteomyelitis following puncture wounds. *J Pediatr* 1985;106:607.
5. Fiorillo L, Zucker M, Sawyer D, et al. The *Pseudomonas* hot-foot syndrome. *N Engl J Med* 2001;345:335.
6. Weinberg AN, Swartz MN. Gram-negative coccal and bacillary infections. In: Fitzpatrick TB, et al, eds. *Dermatology in general medicine*, 3rd ed. New York: McGraw-Hill, 1987:2127.
7. Hill MK, Sanders CV. Localized and systemic infection due to *Vibrio* species. *Infect Dis Clin* 1987;1:687.
8. Oliver JD, Warner RA, Deland DR. Distribution of *Vibrio vulnificans* and other lactose fermenting vibrios in the marine environment. *Appl Environ Microbiol* 1983;45:985.
9. Weber DJ, Wolfson JJ, Swartz MN, Hooper DC. *Pasteurella multocida* infections: report of 34 cases and review of the literature. *Medicine (Baltimore)* 1984;63:133.
10. Dajani AS, Asmar BI, Thirumoorthi MC. Systemic *Haemophilus influenzae* disease: an overview. *J Pediatr* 1979;94:355.

CHAPTER 134
Cutaneous Abscesses and Ulcers

Jan V. Hirschmann and David S. Feingold

ABSCESSES

Staphylococcus aureus can cause cutaneous abscesses, but it is isolated, usually in pure culture, in only about 25% of all cases (1). The location of the abscess is the most important determinant of the infecting flora. *S. aureus* is present in half or more of axillary abscesses (1–3), finger paronychia (4), and breast abscesses in puerperal women (5). It is isolated in about 20% to 40% of toe paronychia (4) and breast abscesses in nonpuerperal women (5). It is present in about the same percentage of abscesses of the trunk, extremities, hands, buttocks, and inguinal regions. This organism is less frequent in abscesses of the head and neck, vulvovaginal, scrotal, and perianal areas (1,2,6,7).

When *S. aureus* is not the cause, the usual infecting bacteria are anaerobes alone or a mixture of aerobic and anaerobic organisms. These organisms may constitute the normal regional skin flora or include transient bacteria from adjacent mucous membranes. Abscesses on the head, neck, and trunk, for example, commonly contain *Staphylococcus epidermidis* and *Propionibacterium* and *Peptococcus* spp., all part of the resident skin bacteria of those areas (1). Perineal abscesses involving the vulvovaginal, inguinal, scrotal, perianal, and buttocks regions, by contrast, typically yield cultures containing fecal flora, such as *Bacteroides* spp., anaerobic gram-positive cocci, and α-hemolytic or nonhemolytic streptococci (1,2,6,7). *S. aureus* and β-hemolytic streptococci (isolated commonly only in hand abscesses) are clearly capable of causing disease by themselves. The other aerobic and anaerobic organisms grown from most cutaneous abscesses possess little virulence individually. When several of these species together are inoculated into the dermis or subcutaneous tissue by trauma or other mechanisms, however, they can produce inflammation and purulence.

Cutaneous abscesses are usually painful, tender, fluctuant, erythematous nodules, often with a pustule on top. In some cases, extensive surrounding cellulitis, lymphangitis, lymphadenitis, and fever may be present. Evacuation of the pus by incision and drainage ordinarily provides effective therapy (1). Some clinicians leave the incision open, others pack the cavity with gauze for a few days, and still others suture the incision immediately after drainage. In any event, Gram stain and culture of the pus are usually unnecessary, as are systemic antibiotics (1,8), unless extensive surrounding cellulitis, cutaneous gangrene, seriously impaired host defenses, or systemic manifestations of infection are present.

ULCERS

Some organisms, such as mycobacteria, can cause primary cutaneous ulcers; more commonly, however, bacteria colonize or infect ulcers of noninfectious causes. Most frequent in clinical practice are those due to pressure (decubitus ulcers or bedsores), neuropathic changes (e.g., diabetic ulcers), or vascular insufficiency from venous or arterial disease. In all these types of ulcers, bacteria, often of several different species, flourish.

In ulcers due to venous insufficiency, *S. aureus* and various gram-negative bacilli alone or in combination are the usual isolates (9,10). The flora of an individual ulcer generally remains constant, regardless of local therapy or systemic antibiotics, until healing occurs. The species and concentration of the bacteria do not correlate well with either the degree of purulence or the rate of healing (9). In two randomized trials, oral antibiotic treatment of the organisms isolated from the ulcers did not accelerate resolution of the ulcers compared to control groups receiving no antimicrobial therapy (10,11). The use of antimicrobial therapy, however, encouraged the emergence of bacteria resistant to the agents used (11). These findings indicate that routine cultures of venous ulcers are unrewarding and that purulent exudation in the wound by itself does not warrant antimicrobial therapy, which should be reserved for ulcers complicated by extensive surrounding cellulitis, lymphangitis, or systemic signs of infection.

Diabetic foot ulcers and decubitus ulcers are the subject of the following chapter (see Chapter 135).

REFERENCES

1. Meislin HW, Lerner SA, Graves MH, et al. Cutaneous abscesses: anaerobic and aerobic bacteriology and outpatient management. *Ann Intern Med* 1977;87:145.
2. Ghoneim ATM, McGoldrick J, Blick PWH, et al. Aerobic and anaerobic bacteriology of subcutaneous abscesses. *Br J Surg* 1981;68:498.
3. Leach RD, Eykyn SJ, Phillips I, et al. Anaerobic axillary abscess. *BMJ* 1979;2:5.
4. Whitehead SM, Eykyn SJ, Phillips I. Anaerobic paronychia. *Br J Surg* 1981;68:420.
5. Leach RD, Eykyn SJ, Phillips I, et al. Anaerobic subareolar breast abscess. *Lancet* 1979;1:35.
6. Whitehead SM, Leach RD, Eykyn SJ, et al. The aetiology of perirectal sepsis. *Br J Surg* 1982;69:166.
7. Whitehead SM, Leach RD, Eykyn SJ, et al. The aetiology of scrotal sepsis. *Br J Surg* 1982;69:729.
8. Macfie J, Harvey J. The treatment of acute superficial abscesses: a prospective clinical trial. *Br J Surg* 1977;64:264.
9. Erickson G, Eklund AE, Kallinger LO. The clinical significance of bacterial growth in venous leg ulcers. *Scand J Infect Dis* 1984;16:175.
10. Alinovi A, Bassissi P, Pini M. Systemic administration of antibiotics in the management of venous ulcers: a randomized clinical trial. *J Am Acad Dermatol* 1986;15:186.
11. Huovinen S, Kotilainen P, Jarvinen H, et al. Comparison of ciprofloxacin or trimethoprim therapy for venous leg ulcers: results of a pilot study. *J Am Acad Dermatol* 1994;31:279.

CHAPTER 135

Foot Infections in the Diabetic Patient and Infections Associated with Pressure Sores

Francisco L. Sapico

FOOT INFECTIONS IN THE DIABETIC PATIENT

The economic, social, and personal costs of foot infections in diabetic patients are considerable. In the United States, at least 20% of hospital admissions among diabetic patients are for foot problems. Fifty percent to 70% of all nontraumatic amputations are performed on patients with diabetes (1–3). This increased susceptibility to foot infection has been attributed to several factors: immune dysfunction, neuropathy, and vascular insufficiency. The same factors also play important roles in the poor healing often observed in this population of patients.

Pathogenesis and Microbiology

Minor foot trauma and improperly fitting footwear contribute to the initiation and perpetuation of early lesions. Early lesions are characterized by local cellulitis, non-foul-smelling drainage, and poorly healing tissue defects without tissue necrosis and gangrene. These infections are usually monomicrobial in origin (i.e., *Staphylococcus aureus,* coagulase-negative staphylococci, enterococci, and aerobic streptococci) (4,5). Moderate-to-severe infections (especially when tissue necrosis or gangrene is present) are usually characterized by polymicrobial picture generally with a mixture of aerobic, as well as anaerobic, organisms (6,7). The most common organisms isolated from blood cultures in diabetic patients with foot infections have been *Bacteroides fragilis* and *S. aureus* (8).

Collection of specimens for culture necessitates removal of superficial necrotic tissue overlying the base of the ulcer (usually by sharp débridement). Bits of tissue can be obtained from the underlying surface using dermal curette or a scalpel for aerobic and anaerobic cultures using appropriate transport media (9). Pus obtained by needle aspiration is excellent for culture, but results obtained after injection of nonbacteriostatic normal saline and subsequent reaspiration have been disappointing (7).

Certain variants of necrotizing soft tissue infections are more prevalent in diabetic patients. Necrotizing fasciitis (usually polymicrobial), nonclostridial anaerobic myonecrosis, spontaneous (hematogenous) clostridial myonecrosis (usually caused by *Clostridium septicum*), as well as crepitant anaerobic cellulitis have been observed to occur with increased frequency in the diabetic (10).

Diagnostic Evaluation

The status of the neurologic and vascular systems should be evaluated thoroughly in diabetic patients with foot infections. Noninvasive tests, such as Doppler ultrasonography with waveform analysis and transcutaneous oximetry can help assess the vascular status. Plain radiographs, computed tomographic scans, technetium bone and gallium scans, and white blood cell scans

have problems with lack of sensitivity and/or specificity for the diagnosis of osteomyelitis. Enthusiasm for magnetic resonance imaging has been generated by some studies (11,12). Another promising diagnostic modality is the use of monoclonal antibody scan (13).

Management

Antimicrobial therapy should be directed at the most likely organisms involved. Milder cases of localized cellulitis or infected ulcers (without gangrene, tissue necrosis, or foul smell) generally necessitate therapy directed primarily at gram-positive aerobic cocci (i.e., *S. aureus*). A first-generation cephalosporin such as cefazolin may be used if there are no contraindications. Moderate to more severe infections may require broader spectrum coverage such as parenteral ampicillin-sulbactam (14), ticarcillin-clavulanate, or piperacillin-tazobactam (15), or imipenem (13). Vancomycin may be added if there is good probability of oxacillin-resistant staphylococcus. The presence of vancomycin-resistant enterococci may necessitate quinupristin-dalfopristin or of linezolid. The antimicrobial regimen may be changed on the basis of the culture results. The reliability of anaerobic cultures depends on the techniques of culture collection and may vary from one laboratory to another and the presence of gangrene, tissue necrosis, and/or foul-smelling discharge strongly suggests the presence of anaerobes regardless of culture results. The length of therapy can vary depending on the severity of infection, from 7 to 10 days for mild cellulitis to several weeks for more severe infections. The presence of osteomyelitis dictates longer therapy if complete ablation of infected bone is not performed. A minimum of 4 weeks of parenteral therapy or a combination of parenteral and oral therapy totaling 10 weeks has been suggested for osteomyelitis (16).

Surgical removal of necrotic, devitalized tissue and drainage of pus are essential. Limited ablative surgery removing all infected bone and soft tissue (e.g., toe amputation, metatarsal ray resection) may shorten the course of antibiotic therapy, and hospital stay (17). The level of surgical amputation is dictated by the extent of soft tissue and bone involvement, as well as the vascular status of the extremity. Vascular reconstruction may be necessary in the presence of vascular insufficiency, and healing of some persistent ulcers may be accelerated by this surgical procedure.

There appears to be no clear-cut superiority of any form of local therapy. Normal saline wet-to-dry dressings following surgical débridement, and removal of external pressures plus avoidance of dependent position will accelerate wound healing.

Other modalities of treatment have included the use of hyperbaric oxygen, bioengineered tissue grafts, and recombinant platelet-derived growth factors (18). More controlled studies, especially in infected wounds, are needed for these modalities of treatment.

INFECTED PRESSURE SORES

It has been estimated that more than 1 million patients in hospitals and nursing homes in the United States suffer from pressure sores and that at least 3% of patients in acute care hospitals are similarly afflicted (19,20).

The pathophysiology of pressure sore formation involves an interplay of pressure, shearing forces, friction, excess moisture, local spasticity, and local blood supply deficiency (19–21). Because more than 90% of pressure sores are located on the lower part of the body (usually sacral, trochanteric, and ischial), and especially since patients are often fecally incontinent, these sores are colonized by a variety of microorganisms. Continued worsening of tissue necrosis may lead to soft tissue infection, osteomyelitis, and septic complications.

Microbiology

Moderate to severely infected pressure sores show polymicrobial flora similar to that seen in infected feet in diabetic patients (22–24). The dominant microorganisms constitute fecal flora. *Escherichia coli* and *Proteus mirabilis* are the most common gram-negative aerobic enteric bacilli seen. Among the gram-positive aerobic cocci, *S. aureus*, *Enterococcus* spp., and coagulase-negative staphylococci are the most common. Anaerobes, such as *Bacteroides* and *Peptostreptococcus* spp. are clearly dominant organisms in this disease entity, especially when the sores are close to the perianal area (24).

Bacteremic sepsis associated with infected pressure sores is most often associated with *B. fragilis, P. mirabilis, Peptostreptococcus* spp., and *S. aureus* (22,25). As the pressure sore heals and necrotic and gangrenous tissue is eliminated, anaerobic microorganisms gradually disappear, but gram-negative bacilli and gram-positive cocci may persist. When the sore is almost healed and a smaller lesion with healthy granulation tissue remains, fewer microorganisms may be seen, primarily *P. aeruginosa* and *Enterococcus* spp. (23).

Proper anaerobic culture collection using proper transport media includes submission of material such as aspirated pus or deep tissue or bone obtained after overlying superficial necrotic tissue is removed.

Diagnostic Evaluation

Pressure sores may be classified into four stages. Stage I represents nonblanchable erythema of intact skin, stage II involves partial-thickness skin loss involving epidermis and/or dermis, stage III involves full-thickness skin loss with damage or necrosis of subcutaneous tissue down to but not through underlying fascia, and stage IV represents extensive destruction with damage to muscle, bone, or supporting structures (26).

As with the evaluation for osteomyelitis in foot infections, plain radiographs may be limited in sensitivity and specificity. Lack of specificity has also hampered radionuclide scans, and more is needed with magnetic resonance imaging for this disease entity. Bone biopsy for histologic examination is still considered to be the "gold standard" for the diagnosis of osteomyelitis (27–29). Quantitative microbiology of bone was disappointing in one study (29).

Management

Surgical removal of dead, necrotic tissue is of paramount importance in the management of infected pressure sores. These surgical procedures may have to be performed repeatedly to keep up with continuing advance of tissue necrosis. Liquid purulent material should be drained as completely as possible. Infected bone should be surgically removed until healthy bone is encountered.

Empiric antimicrobial coverage before culture results should address the potential presence of polymicrobial flora. The choice of antimicrobial agents for moderate-to-severe infections would be similar to the choice in the case of moderate to severe foot infections in diabetic patients. The antimicrobial regimen can be changed later depending on the culture results. The presence of tissue gangrene, necrosis, and foul smell strongly suggests the presence of anaerobes. There is no consensus on the length of antimicrobial therapy. One study found no necessity to treat longer than 3 weeks as long as there is thorough surgical removal of infected bone (28). Another recommended 6 weeks of antimicrobial therapy (29).

There is also no clear consensus on the most efficacious type of local therapy (30). As with diabetic foot ulcers, normal saline wet-to-dry dressings are often used. Recently, the use of silver sulfadiazine has achieved some popularity (31). Frequent turning, proper positioning, pressure dispersion, and the use of specialized beds and mattresses are of paramount importance in the prevention and therapy of pressure sores. Control of muscle spasticity and surgical release of flexion contractures are likewise important measures in preventing, as well as alleviating, pressure sores.

Besides removal of necrotic tissue, infected bone, and bony prominences, surgical management includes the use of a variety of myocutaneous flaps once the wound is clean and shows healthy granulation tissue (32,33).

Other innovative, or unconventional modalities of management have included those discussed in diabetic foot ulcer management, the use of vacuum sealing technique, and the use of maggot therapy (34,35). More studies are needed for the vacuum seal technique. Patient and physician acceptance of the maggot therapy are limiting factors for widespread adoption of the latter modality.

REFERENCES

1. Sapico FL. Foot infections in patients with diabetes mellitus. *J Am Podiatr Med Assoc* 1989;79:482–485.
2. Levin ME, O'Neal LW, eds. Preface. In: *The diabetic foot,* 4th ed. St. Louis: CV Mosby, 1988:ix–x.
3. Gibbons GW, Eliopoulos GM. Infections of the diabetic foot. In: Kozak GP, Hoar CS, Rawbottom JL, et al, eds. *Management of diabetic foot problems.* Philadelphia: WB Saunders, 1984:97.
4. Leslie CA, Sapico FL, Ginunas VJ, et al. Randomized, controlled trial of topical hyperbaric oxygen for the treatment of diabetic foot ulcers. *Diabetes Care* 1988;11:111–115.
5. Lipsky BA, Pecoraro RE, Larson SA, et al. Outpatient management of uncomplicated lower-extremity infections in diabetic patients. *Arch Intern Med* 1990;150:790–797.
6. Sapico FL, Canawati HN, Witte JL, et al. Quantitative aerobic and anaerobic bacteriology of infected diabetic feet. *J Clin Microbiol* 1980;12:413–420.
7. Sapico FL, Witte JL, Canawati HN, et al. The infected foot of the diabetic patient: quantitative microbiology and analysis of clinical features. *Rev Infect Dis* 1984;6(Suppl 1):171–176.
8. Sapico FL, Bessman AN, Canawati HN. Bacteremia in diabetic patients with infected lower extremities. *Diabetes Care* 1982;5(2):101–104.
9. Louie TJ, Bartlett JG, Tally FP, et al. Aerobic and anaerobic bacteria in diabetic foot ulcers. *Ann Intern Med* 1976;85:461–463.
10. Leslie CA, Sapico FL, Bessman AN. Infections in the diabetic host. *Comp Ther* 1989;15(7):23–32.
11. Yuh WTC, Corson JD, Baraniewski HM, et al. Osteomyelitis of the foot in diabetic patients: evaluation with plain film, ^{99m}Tc-MDP bone scintigraphy, and MR imaging. *AJR* 1989;152:795–800.
12. Wang A, Weinstein D, Greenfield L, et al. MRI and diabetic foot infections. *Magn Reson Imaging* 1990;8:805–809.
13. Hakki S, Harwood SJ, Morisey MA, Camblin JG, Laven DL, Webster WB Jr. Comparative study of monoclonal antibody scan in diagnosing orthopaedic infection. *Clin Orthop Rel Res* 1997;335:275–285.
14. Grayson ML, Gibbons GW, Habershaw GM, et al. Use of ampicillin/sulbactam versus imipenem/cilastatin in the treatment of limb-threatening foot infections in diabetic patients. *Clin Infect Dis* 1994;18:683–693.
15. Tan JS, Wishnow RM, Talan DA, et al. Treatment of hospitalized patients with complicated skin and skin structure infections: double-blind randomized multicenter study of piperacillin-tazobactam versus ticarcillin-clavulanate. *Antimicrob Agents Chemother* 1993;37:1580–1586.
16. Bamberger DM, Dans GP, Gerding DN. Osteomyelitis in the feet of diabetic patients: long-term results, prognostic factors, and the role of antimicrobial and surgical therapy. *Am J Med* 1987;83:653–660.
17. Tan JS, Miller C, File TM, et al. Can aggressive therapeutic intervention of diabetic foot infection reduce the length of hospitalization? *Clin Infect Dis* 1994;23:286–291.
18. Millington JT, Norris TW. Effective treatment strategies for diabetic foot wounds. *J Fam Pract* 2000;49:S40–S48.

19. Reuler JB, Cooney TG. The pressure sore: pathophysiology and principles of management. *Ann Intern Med* 1981;94:661–666.
20. Allman RM, Laprade CA, Noel LB, et al. Pressure sores among hospitalized patients. *Ann Intern Med* 1986;105:337–342.
21. Cooney TG, Reuler JB. Pressure sores. *West J Med* 1984;940:622–624.
22. Galpin JE, Chow AW, Bayer AS, et al. Sepsis associated with decubitus ulcers. *Am J Med* 1975;61:345–350.
23. Sapico FL, Ginunas VJ, Thornhill-Joynes M, et al. Quantitative microbiology of pressure sores in different stages of healing. *Diagn Microbiol Infect Dis* 1986;5:31–38.
24. Brook I. Microbiological studies of decubitus ulcers in children. *J Pediatr Surg* 1991;26:207–209.
25. Bryan CS, Dew CE, Reynolds KL. Bacteremia associated with decubitus ulcers. *Arch Intern Med* 1983;143:2093–2095.
26. Pressure ulcer prevalence, cost and risk assessment: consensus development conference statement—The National Pressure Ulcer Advisory Panel. *Decubitus* 1989;2:24–28.
27. Sugarman B, Hawes S, Musher DM, et al. Osteomyelitis beneath pressure sores. *Arch Intern Med* 1983;143:683–688.
28. Thornhill-Joynes M, Gonzales F, Stewart CA, et al. Osteomyelitis associated with pressure sores. *Arch Phys Med Rehab* 1986;67:314–318.
29. Darouiche RO, Landon GF, Klima M, et al. Osteomyelitis associated with pressure sores. *Arch Intern Med* 1994;154:753–758.
30. DeLisa JA, Mikulic MH. Pressure ulcers: what to do if preventive management fails. *Postgrad Med* 1985;77:209–220.
31. Kucan JO, Robson MC, Heggers JP, et al. Comparison of silver sulfadiazine povidone-iodine and physiologic saline in the treatment of chronic pressure ulcers. *J Am Geriatr Soc* 1981;29:232–235.
32. Mathes SJ, Nahai F. *Clinical applications for muscle and musculocutaneous flaps.* St. Louis: CV Mosby, 1982.
33. Rubayi S, Cousins S, Valentine WA. Myocutaneous flaps. *AORN J* 1990;52:40–55.
34. Müllner T, Mrkonjic L, Kwasny O, Vecsei V. The use of negative pressure to promote the healing of tissue defects: a clinical trial using the vacuum sealing technique. *Br J Plast Surg* 1997;50(3):194–199.
35. Sherman RA. A new dressing design for use with maggot therapy. *Plast Reconstr Surg* 1997;100(2):451–456.

CHAPTER 136
Fungal Infections of the Skin

Jill R. Rosenthal

Some of the material in this chapter has previously been published by the author in *Current Opinion in Pediatrics* (Rosenthal JR: Pediatric fungal infections from head to toe: What's new? *Curr Opin Pediatr* 1994;6:435–441).

Cutaneous fungal infections are common in all age groups worldwide; the superficial mycoses include infections caused by dermatophytes, *Candida* species, *Pityrosporum* yeasts, several nondermatophyte molds, and the agents of black and white piedra. Other conditions include infections caused by dematiaceous fungi, which cause chromoblastomycosis, phaeohyphomycosis, and mycetoma (see Chapter 274). Candidiasis and deep infections caused by other agents, including cryptococcosis, aspergillosis, histoplasmosis, coccidioidomycosis, sporotrichosis, blastomycosis, paracoccidioidomycosis, and the phycomycoses, are covered elsewhere.

DERMATOPHYTOSES

Dermatophytes are extremely common causes of infection in humans. They are aerobic fungi that produce proteases that digest keratin, allowing colonization, invasion, and infection of the stratum corneum of the skin, the hair shaft, and the nail (1). Many can infect multiple cutaneous structures, causing a variety of

clinical syndromes; similarly, a given skin structure or site may be infected by more than one species. For example, hair infections can be caused by *Microsporum* and *Trichophyton* species, nail infections by *Trichophyton* and *Epidermophyton* species, and skin infections by fungi of all three genera. In addition, different species predominate as causes of each clinical type of infection in different parts of the world; even in a given geographic location, species predominance may change in time (1–8). For these reasons, dermatophytoses are classified by anatomic site rather than by species.

Dermatophytes are preferentially distributed in certain habitats and, depending on the species (Table 136.1), may be found in the soil (geophilic), on animals (zoophilic), or on humans (anthropophilic). Anthropophilic species are transmitted from person to person and often cause chronic infections, but geophilic and zoophilic dermatophytes are more frequently acquired as sporadic, incidental infections and often tend to produce more inflammatory host responses than their anthropophilic counterparts (9). This difference in host response appears to be due in part to differences in protease production by zoophilic dermatophytes, depending on the keratin source on which the fungus is growing (10). There are approximately 40 dermatophyte species (10). However, most infections are caused by 11 species, and within the continental United States, most infections are caused by six species (11). The spread of anthropophilic species is more common in the presence of close contact, such as the transmission of tinea capitis due to *Trichophyton tonsurans* within the family unit or in conditions of social crowding; this is paralleled in the animal kingdom, where dermatophyte infections are more commonly seen in social animals that live together than in species that tend to be solitary (11).

Diagnosis of dermatophyte infections is made by microscopic examination of scrapings from the involved site, placed in potassium hydroxide (KOH) solution, which allows visualization of fungal hyphae and spores. In culture, structures such as macroconidia, microconidia, and specialized vegetative structures such as pectinate or spiral hyphae are seen, which along with nutritional requirements and morphologic features in culture allow species identification. However, these specialized structures are not present in keratinized tissues, and thus precise identification of dermatophyte species cannot be based on KOH microscopy alone (12).

DERMATOPHYTE INFECTIONS OF THE HAIR

Tinea Capitis

Tinea capitis (ringworm of the scalp), caused by *Microsporum* and *Trichophyton* species, is by far the most common pediatric dermatophyte infection worldwide, accounting for up to 92.5% of dermatophytoses in children younger than 10 years; the disease is rare in adults (2,6,13,14). In the United States, tinea capitis is most common in school-age African-American males and is usually caused by *T. tonsurans*, although all races and age groups can be affected (4). The age predilection is thought to be due to the presence of *Pityrosporum orbiculare* (also known as *Pityrosporum ovale*), part of the normal flora, and the fungistatic properties of short and medium chain saturated fatty acids in postpubertal sebum (5,15–17). Fatty acids present in hair oils commonly applied in India are thought to contribute to the low frequency of tinea capitis there (18). Some authors postulate that tinea capitis is more common in boys with short hair than in girls because the stratum corneum is relatively more accessible for the initial colonization (11).

TABLE 136.1. Classification of Dermatophytes

Anthropophilic	Zoophilic	Geophilic
Microsporum audouinii	Trichophyton verrucosum	Microsporum vanbreuseghemii
Epidermophyton floccosum	Microsporum persicolor	Microsporum fulvum
Trichophyton megninii	Trichophyton mentagrophytes	Microsporum gypseum
Trichophyton gourvilii	var. mentagrophytes	Microsporum racemosum
Trichophyton soudanense	Trichophyton mentagrophytes	Trichophyton ajelloi
Trichophyton yaoundei	var. erinacei	Microsporum nanum
Trichophyton violaceum	Trichophyton mentagrophytes	Trichophyton terrestre
Trichophyton concentricum	var. quinckeanum	Microsporum cookei
Microsporum ferrugineum	Microsporum canis	
Trichophyton mentagrophytes	Microsporum distortum	
var. interdigitale	Microsporum (?Trichophyton)	
	gallinae	
Trichophyton rubrum	Trichophyton equinum	
Trichophyton schoenleinii	Trichophyton verrucosum	
Trichophyton tonsurans	Trichophyton simii	

During the second half of this century, *T. tonsurans* has replaced *Microsporum audouinii* and *Microsporum canis* as the most common cause of tinea capitis in the United States; it now causes more than 90% of cases of tinea capitis (4). However, in other parts of the world, other species still predominate, including zoophilic species such as *M. canis,* usually because of acquisition by direct contact with infected animals, in particular with stray cats, which in some areas are the source for 70% of infections (2,6,16,19). In other areas, *Trichophyton violaceum, Trichophyton rubrum, Trichophyton schoenleinii,* and *M. audouinii* are more common, varying by country (2). In Africa, *Trichophyton soudanense, Trichophyton yaoundei,* and *Trichophyton gourvilii* predominate (20).

The clinical presentation varies from a mildly scaly noninflammatory dermatosis with patchy or diffuse seborrheic dermatitis-like scaling with variable alopecia, to black-dot tinea capitis (in which the infected hairs fracture, leaving the infected dark stubs visible in the follicular orifices), to a more inflammatory pattern with pustules and oozing, to the highly inflammatory boggy mass known as a kerion (Fig. 136.1; see also Color Figure 136.1). Cervical lymphadenopathy is common. The host's response is thought to determine the degree of inflammation, in part influenced by the infecting species, but the possible role of secondary bacterial infection has been postulated by some authors (21,22). Permanent scarring alopecia may result, particularly with more inflammatory presentations such as kerion.

Inflammatory pustules and kerions have in general been presumed to be the result of the host's immune response to the fungus. Although bacteria may sometimes be cultured, it is not clear whether they represent contamination, colonization, or secondary infection or whether they are actually pathogenic (14). Cultures from 44 patients with kerions grew *Staphylococcus aureus* in 50% of cases and gram-negative rods in 27% (21). However, addition of oral antibiotics and oral steroids to griseofulvin in the treatment of kerions does not hasten flattening of kerions, although it may help to decrease scaling and pruritus (22). Because griseofulvin monotherapy cures almost all cases of tinea capitis, and the addition of oral antibiotics does not hasten this, it remains to be seen whether *S. aureus* or gram-negative organisms, when present, play a pathogenic role (14). Similarly, whether steroids decrease the extent or frequency of permanent scarring alopecia in patients with kerion remains to be proved, but given the relative safety of a 1- or 2-week course of oral steroids in an otherwise healthy young person, it is appropriate to consider oral steroid therapy in this setting (14,23).

Tinea capitis has also been reported in other age groups. Both tinea capitis and tinea faciei due to *M. canis* have occurred in infants as young as 16 days old, acquired from mothers and siblings; dermatophyte infections have also been reported in even younger infants (24–28). A nosocomial outbreak of *M. canis* tinea capitis and tinea corporis in six premature infants in a level II intermediate care nursery was traced to a nurse; what is most striking about this report is that the infections were acquired from an asymptomatic human carrier of this zoophilic fungus, which is usually acquired by direct contact with infected animals (29). A more typical nosocomial outbreak is exemplified by one involving the anthropophilic dermatophyte *T. tonsurans* in nine hospital staff and one family member who cared for a child with tinea capitis and tinea corporis before a diagnosis of dermatophyte infection was made (30).

Although tinea capitis in adults is more common in women than in men, possibly caused by increased exposure to infected children and hormonal factors, a healthy 52-year-old African-American man acquired tinea capitis caused by *T. tonsurans* from contaminated haircutting instruments (5). *T. rubrum* tinea capitis was reported in a 67-year-old African-American woman with systemic lupus erythematosus after treatment with topical and intralesional corticosteroids; *T. rubrum* rarely causes scalp infections in the United States but is the most commonly isolated cause of tinea capitis in Benghazi, Libya, and in Bangkok, Thailand (15). Several children with Langerhans cell histiocytosis were noted to have secondary infections with tinea capitis, and it should be kept in mind that the clinical appearance may be similar, potentially delaying the diagnosis of either condition (31).

Endothrix infections, in which arthrospores are present within the hair shaft, involve hairs in both anagen and telogen phases, contributing to the chronicity of these infections. *T. tonsurans,* the most common cause of tinea capitis in the United States, belongs to this group, along with *T. violaceum* and other *Trichophyton* species. Endothrix infection begins in the surface stratum corneum, followed by follicular invasion and colonization of the hair cortex. As the hair grows out, the hyphae break up into arthrospores; the cortex is replaced by spores and swells, and the hair weakens and fractures as it emerges from the scalp. The swollen cortex forms a coiled plug in the infundibulum, producing the clinically visible black dot (3). Hair invasion in ectothrix infections produces arthrospores both within the hair shaft and on its surface. Wood light fluorescence occurs in the ectothrix infections caused by *M. audouinii, M. canis, Microsporum distortum,* and *Microsporum ferrugineum* as well as in favus caused by *T. schoenleinii.*

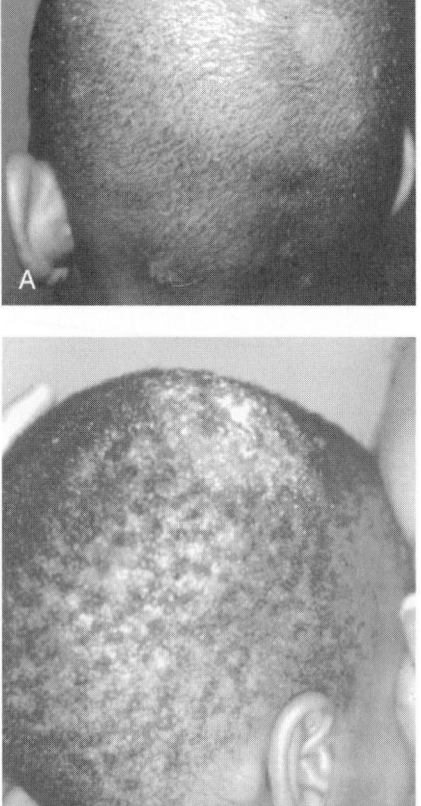

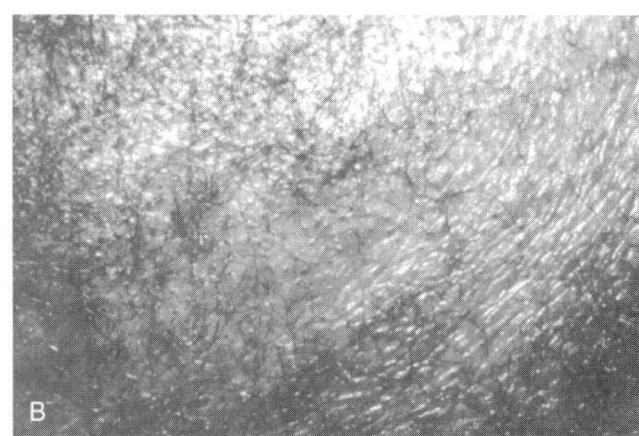

Figure 136.1. (See also Color Figure 136.1.) Tinea capitis. **A:** Multiple scaly alopecic plaques. **B:** Black-dot tinea capitis. **C:** Kerion with visibly enlarged postauricular lymph node.

Historically, when tinea capitis was more commonly caused by *M. audouinii* and *M. canis,* Wood lamp examination could be used to rapidly screen large numbers of children in schools for infection, but this is no longer useful now that *T. tonsurans,* a nonfluorescing endothrix infection, is responsible for most tinea capitis in the United States. Rapid diagnosis of tinea capitis is made by KOH examination of infected hairs (visible as black dots) and surrounding scale—a sensitive and specific examination in the hands of an experienced practitioner—or by culture on Sabouraud agar, which takes several weeks. Samples for KOH examination or culture may be obtained with a sterile toothbrush, a moistened cotton swab or gauze pad, or a no. 15 blade (14,32). Because oral therapy for at least 8 weeks is required, it is important to document the presence of fungal infection.

The differential diagnosis of tinea capitis includes other scalp dermatoses characterized by scaling, alopecia, or pustule formation. Depending on the clinical presentation, these may include seborrheic dermatitis, atopic dermatitis, psoriasis, alopecia areata, bacterial folliculitis, trichotillomania, lichen planopilaris, discoid lupus erythematosus, secondary syphilis, and Langerhans cell histiocytosis. However, most of these can often be ruled out on clinical grounds, and definitive diagnosis of tinea can usually be documented with KOH examination or culture.

Treatment of dermatophyte infections of the hair and nails requires systemic therapy. Griseofulvin remains the treatment of choice, given for 8 to 12 weeks, although longer courses are occasionally necessary. The usual adult dosage is 500 mg micro-crystalline orally twice a day or 250 mg ultramicrosized orally twice a day. Children should be treated with 15 to 20 mg/kg per day microcrystalline or 7.5 to 10 mg/kg per day ultramicrosized, usually given as a single daily dose with a fatty meal to increase enteric absorption and decrease the risk of gastrointestinal side effects. Higher doses are occasionally necessary (33). Other adverse effects may include headache in 10% to 15% of patients (usually only for the first few days of therapy), photosensitivity, and exacerbation of systemic lupus erythematosus and porphyrias.

Shampooing twice weekly with a sporicidal shampoo containing selenium sulfide 2.5%, zinc pyrithione, or ketoconazole may help to decrease contagion by lowering spore counts. However, topical therapy alone is inadequate to treat tinea capitis, and oral ketoconazole is less effective than is griseofulvin in the treatment of tinea capitis. A few reports suggest that fluconazole and itraconazole may be useful in some patients with tinea capitis who cannot tolerate or fail to respond to griseofulvin (20,34–36). Oral terbinafine also appears promising as a potential therapy, although additional studies with larger numbers of patients are necessary to document safety in children and efficacy against *T. tonsurans* tinea capitis (37–41). Itraconazole at 5 mg/kg per day for 6 weeks also appears effective in the treatment of tinea capitis in children (42). If kerion is present, oral or intralesional steroid use should be considered; when secondary bacterial infection is present, appropriate cultures should be performed, and antibiotic therapy may be added to the antifungal regimen (23).

Even when the presentation is inflammatory, *T. tonsurans* frequently causes chronic infections that do not necessarily resolve after puberty, as *M. audouinii* infections may; adults may thus be infected or colonized and may serve as carriers (4,43). The carriage rate in family members of all ages can be high; 48% of 31 children with *T. tonsurans* tinea capitis had at least one additional family member from whom *T. tonsurans* could be cultured (4). Positive culture results were found in 20 (63%) of 32 siblings and 5 (14%) of 35 adult family members. Twenty-five percent of the culture-positive siblings and 80% of the culture-positive adults were asymptomatic—important because asymptomatic carriers of *T. tonsurans* may transmit this anthropophilic fungus to other persons. Family members of affected children should be examined if at all possible, and consideration should be given to possible culture and treatment of these individuals; whether asymptomatic carriers should be treated with oral griseofulvin or with ketoconazole shampoo requires further study (4,16). Sharing of combs, brushes, hats, and other fomites should be avoided until the infection has cleared.

Favus

Favus is a severe, chronic scalp ringworm caused by *T. schoenleinii*, characterized by yellow cup-shaped crusts called scutula that surround the hair follicles. Rarely, it may be caused by *T. violaceum* or *Microsporum gypseum*. The name comes from the Latin word for honeycomb. Infection begins with a small yellow-red papule that develops surrounding erythema and scaling, spreading to give a patchy distribution. Scarring alopecia may result. Favus is seen mostly in Africa, the Mediterranean, and the Middle East, with rare cases in North and South America, usually in descendants of immigrants from endemic areas. It is generally acquired early in life and tends to cluster in families. Diagnosis is made by the clinical appearance, mousy odor, dull fluorescence on Wood light examination, KOH preparation, and culture. Treatment consists of long-term griseofulvin.

Tinea Barbae

Tinea barbae refers to infections of the beard and mustache hair in adult men. It is most commonly caused by *Trichophyton verrucosum* or *Trichophyton mentagrophytes*, which produce a large-spore ectothrix infection similar to that seen in tinea capitis caused by the same organisms. *T. verrucosum* infection is especially common in dairy farmers and cattle ranchers, who may acquire an intensely inflammatory zoophilic infection from infected cows, but the infection can also be acquired from horses or dogs.

Tinea barbae presents clinically as an inflammatory pustular folliculitis in the beard or mustache area, often with exudate and crusting and sometimes with draining sinuses. It may be accompanied by systemic symptoms such as fever, malaise, and regional lymphadenopathy. Occasionally, the lesions are less inflammatory, consisting of scaling red plaques with broken-off hairs (Fig. 136.2). Tinea barbae may heal with scarring.

The differential diagnosis includes sycosis barbae (caused by *S. aureus*), bacterial folliculitis, acne, rosacea, pseudofolliculitis barbae, actinomycosis, and herpes simplex. A history of animal contact should raise the index of suspicion for tinea barbae. As with tinea capitis, diagnosis is made by the demonstration of Arthroconidia in involved hairs and pus with a KOH preparation or culture. Treatment consists of oral griseofulvin, in regimens similar to those used for tinea capitis, and epidemiologic control of infection in the animal population. As with tinea capitis, itraconazole, fluconazole, or terbinafine may be considered alternative therapies (23).

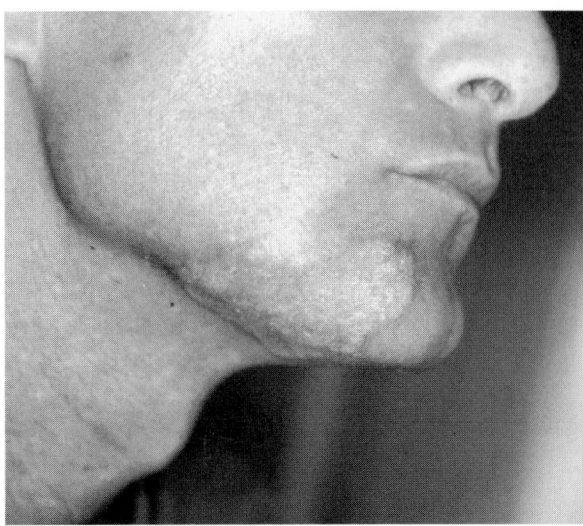

Figure 136.2. Tinea barbae. Pink scaly plaque with raised red border in the beard area.

DERMATOPHYTE INFECTIONS OF THE SKIN

Tinea Corporis

Tinea corporis (ringworm) refers to dermatophyte infections of the glabrous skin other than specialized sites such as the scalp, groin, palms, and soles. It may be caused by any species of *Trichophyton*, *Microsporum*, or *Epidermophyton*, but the most common agents are *T. rubrum*, *T. mentagrophytes*, *Epidermophyton floccosum*, and *M. canis*. Infections are common worldwide but may be more common in hot, humid areas and may be acquired by humans from other people, animals, fomites, or soil. The species most frequently acquired from animals are *M. canis* and *T. mentagrophytes*. Inflammatory infections with *T. verrucosum* or *Trichophyton equinum* may result from exposure to infected cattle or horses (44,45).

In tinea corporis, infection is limited to the top layer of the epidermis, the stratum corneum, but involvement of follicles may lead to persistent or recurrent infection. Infection begins with inoculation of fungal spores or hyphae from an infected person, animal, fomite, or soil or from lesions elsewhere on the body. Lesions begin as pruritic erythematous papules that spread outward to form sharply marginated annular plaques, usually with central clearing and red, raised scaly borders (Fig. 136.3; see also Color Figure 136.3). Central postinflammatory hyperpigmentation or hypopigmentation is common. Vesicles or pustules are sometimes seen at the border in more inflammatory lesions (Fig. 136.4). Frankly bullous lesions of tinea corporis from which *M. canis* was cultured were reported in a 63-year-old woman who also had classic annular lesions (46). Thicker psoriasiform or granulomatous lesions may occasionally be seen, and verrucous lesions may occur in immunocompromised hosts; a deeper form, tinea profunda, which is analogous to kerion formation on the scalp, also exists (11). Lesions may coalesce to form larger lesions with serpiginous borders. More inflammatory lesions may be seen with zoophilic or geophilic species, although the infected animal may have disease that is inconspicuous or even subclinical (47).

A granulomatous perifollicular form of tinea corporis known as Majocchi granuloma may be seen on the lower legs in women as the result of shaving. This appears as multiple inflammatory follicular papules coalescing into irregular plaques. It may also be seen if lesions of tinea corporis are occluded or treated

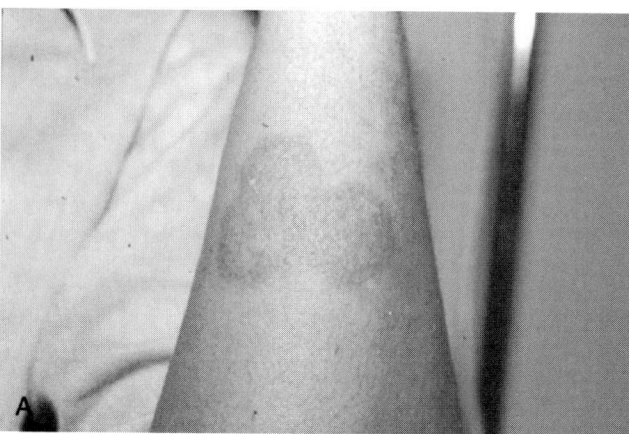
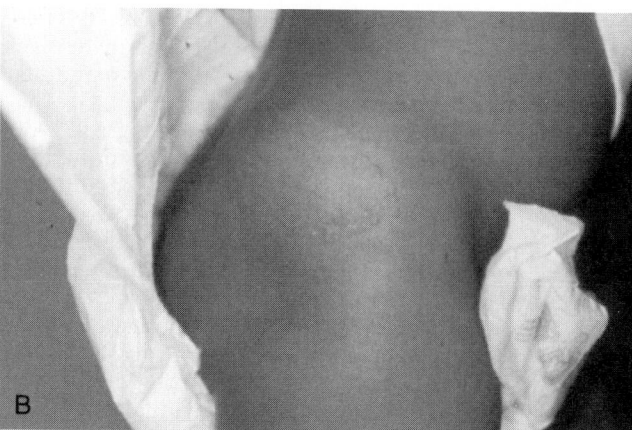

Figure 136.3. (See also Color Figure 136.3.) Tinea corporis. **A:** Coalescing scaly annular plaques on the forearm. **B:** Annular erythematous plaque on an infant's hip, occluded by the diaper.

with topical corticosteroids. A suppurative folliculitis with rupture of the follicles results in release of fungal elements into the dermis, causing a granulomatous inflammatory response (41) (Fig. 136.5). Majocchi granuloma is usually caused by *T. violaceum, T. rubrum, E. floccosum,* or *T. mentagrophytes* (48). A deep form may be seen in patients treated with systemic steroids or other immunosuppressive medications and in patients with acquired immunodeficiency syndrome (AIDS) (49).

The differential diagnosis depends on the body site and morphologic features of the lesions but may include contact dermatitis, nummular dermatitis, the herald patch of pityriasis rosea, seborrheic dermatitis, *Candida* infection, psoriasis, and other skin diseases. The diagnosis of tinea corporis is established by KOH examination of infected scale scraped with a No. 15 blade from the active border of the lesion (Fig. 136.6). Culture of infected material may also be performed on Sabouraud agar with antibiotics to suppress bacterial overgrowth.

Tinea corporis may be treated with a variety of topical antifungal agents; oral therapy should be considered for patients with extensive disease or infections that are resistant to therapy (50). If the infection was acquired from a zoonotic source, the infected animal should also be treated. Therapy is discussed in more detail later.

Tinea Corporis Gladiatorum

Epidemics of tinea corporis and tinea capitis in wrestlers, caused by *T. tonsurans* or *T. verrucosum,* have been termed tinea corporis gladiatorum (51–55). Lesions are typically seen on the shoulders, face, neck, and scalp—areas that are frequently abraded and may be inoculated by direct contact with opponents' skin; contact with wrestling mats or sharing of headgear may also contribute to the spread of infection but this mode of transmission is less likely (51,52,55). Control of tinea corporis gladiatorum requires regular screening of wrestlers and participants in other contact sports for signs of dermatophyte infection and exclusion of infected athletes from practice and competition, analogous to precautions taken for herpes simplex gladiatorum. As for all dermatophyte infections, therapy is determined by the site and extent of infection; most patients can be treated topically, although scalp infections must obviously be treated with oral griseofulvin.

Tinea Imbricata

Tinea imbricata (tokelau ringworm) is a distinctive infection caused by the anthropophilic dermatophyte *Trichophyton*

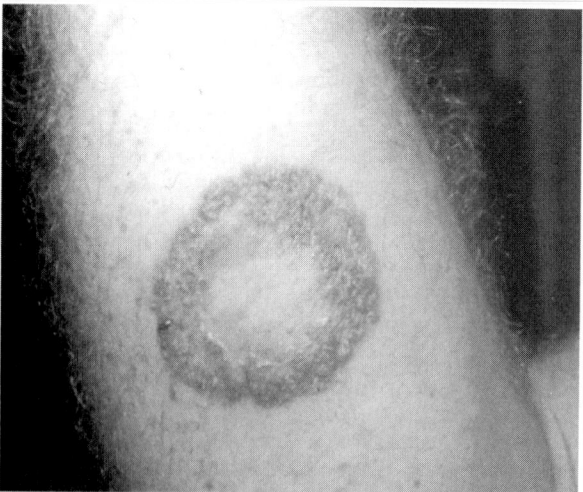

Figure 136.4. Tinea corporis. Inflammatory annular plaque with vesicular border on the forearm.

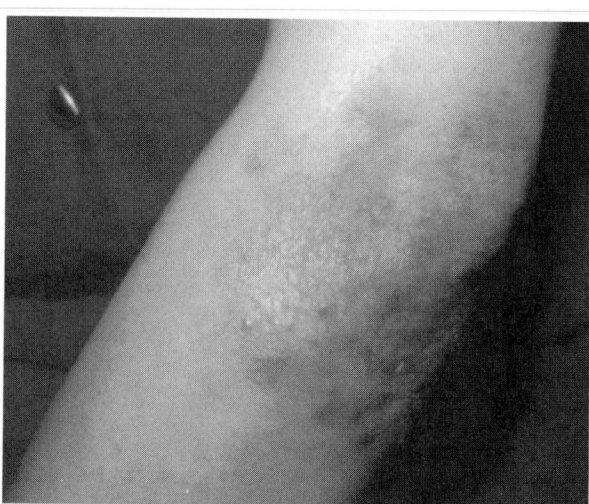

Figure 136.5. Majocchi granuloma. Coalescing plaques with follicular papules on the elbow.

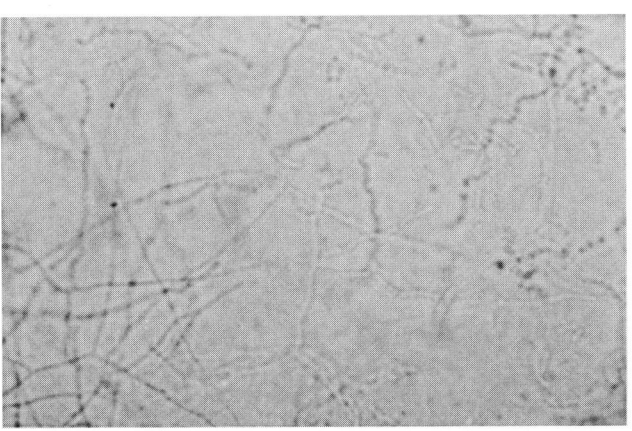

Figure 136.6. KOH preparation. Dermatophyte hyphae visualized on microscopic examination in KOH. (Courtesy of Victor Newcomer, MD, Santa Monica, CA.)

concentricum seen only in the Pacific Islands, Southeast Asia, and Central and South America. Multiple concentric brownish scaly rings are seen, resembling the rings of a tree. There appears to be a genetic predisposition, probably inherited as an autosomal recessive trait. Relapses after treatment are common and may be characterized by the intense pruritus and inflammation normally seen only in the early stages of infection. Systemic terbinafine seems slightly superior to itraconazole in the treatment of tinea imbricata (56).

Tinea Faciei

Tinea corporis of the face, excluding the beard and mustache area of adult men, is known as tinea faciei. The usual causative agents are *T. mentagrophytes* and *T. rubrum*; infections with *M. canis* acquired from kittens are not uncommon. Tinea faciei tends to be erythematous but much less scaly than other forms of tinea corporis, leading to frequent misdiagnosis (Fig. 136.7). In addition to seborrheic dermatitis, tinea faciei has been mistaken for lupus erythematosus, polymorphous light eruption, rosacea, and perioral dermatitis. A history of animal contact, particularly with kittens, should raise the clinical suspicion for tinea and prompt a careful search for fungal elements on a KOH scraping. Successful treatment is usually accomplished with topical antifungal agents.

Tinea Cruris

Tinea cruris (jock itch, dhobie itch) refers to dermatophyte infection of the groin, perineum, or perianal area; infection also commonly spreads to the buttocks. Infection is seen almost exclusively in adolescent and adult men. *E. floccosum, T. rubrum,* and *T. mentagrophytes* are the most commonly isolated agents, presumably because they are also the usual causes of tinea pedis, which is often the source of infection. Tinea cruris presents with pruritic, well-demarcated scaly erythematous and hyperpigmented plaques with central clearing and scalloped borders and tends to involve the inner thighs and inguinal creases but spares the scrotum and penis, unlike *Candida* infections. Diagnosis and treatment are the same as for tinea corporis.

In infants, diaper dermatitis due to dermatophyte infection is rare. However, cases due to *T. rubrum* and *E. floccosum*; which commonly cause tinea cruris in adults, and also *T. verrucosum* in an infant whose father was a cattle farmer (57), have been reported.

Tinea Manuum

Tinea manuum refers to dermatophyte infection of the palmar surfaces, although infection may also occur on the dorsal hands. It is most commonly seen in association with tinea pedis, and therefore the most common pathogen is *T. rubrum,* followed by *E. floccosum* and *T. mentagrophytes* var. *interdigitale*. It frequently presents in a two-feet-one-hand distribution, for unknown reasons. Lesions most commonly consist of dry, powdery, hyperkeratotic scale accentuated in the creases; there is usually little to no erythema, although inflammatory and vesicular forms occasionally occur (Fig. 136.8). One or more fingernails may be involved as well. The differential diagnosis includes xerosis, irritant contact dermatitis, other forms of hand dermatitis, and palmar keratodermas. The presence of a unilateral hand dermatitis should prompt a search for tinea, especially if the feet are also involved. Diagnosis and treatment are the same as for tinea pedis, consisting of KOH examination, culture, and topical antifungal agents; oral therapy is occasionally required.

Tinea Pedis

Tinea pedis (athlete's foot) is the most common fungal infection in adults. The most common etiologic agents are *T. rubrum, T. mentagrophytes* var. *interdigitale,* and *E. floccosum*. Tinea pedis is

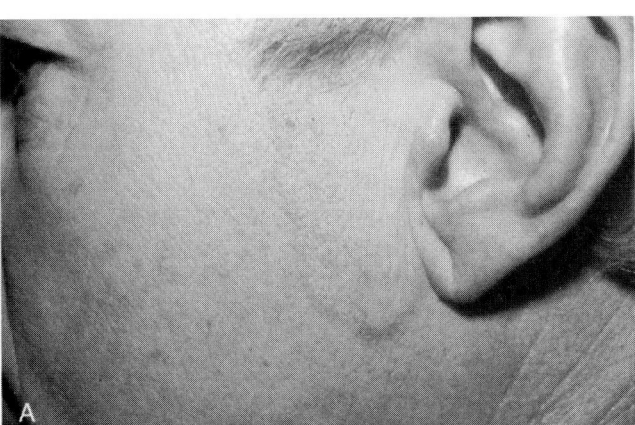
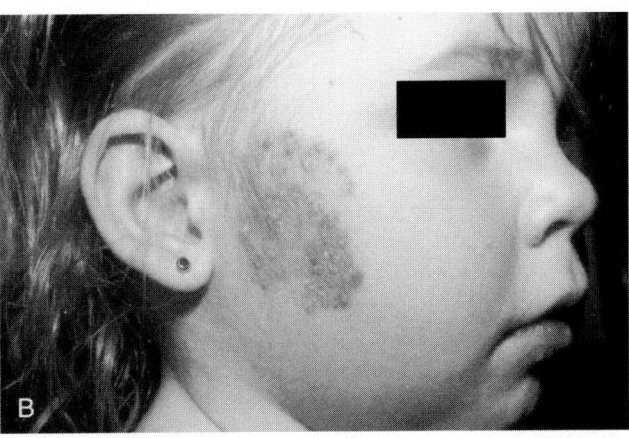

Figure 136.7. Tinea faciei. **A:** Erythematous annular plaque in the left preauricular area. Note the relative absence of scale. **B:** Inflammatory, erythematous, slightly scaly plaques and papules on the face of a 2-year-old girl.

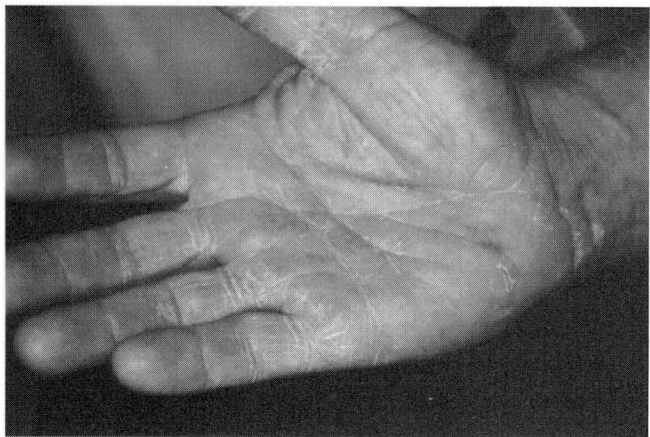

Figure 136.8. Tinea manuum. (Courtesy of Nellie Konnikov, MD, New England Medical Center Hospital, Boston, MA.)

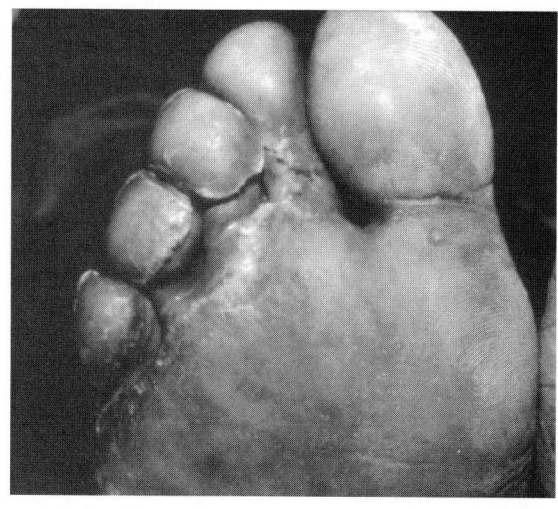

Figure 136.10. Dermatophytosis complex. Mixed infection with dermatophytes and bacteria.

primarily a dermatosis of shoe-wearing populations, illustrating the importance of local factors such as maceration, heat, moisture, and occlusion. Acquisition of tinea pedis commonly occurs at communal athletic and bathing facilities, locker rooms, and swimming pools, where infected individuals walk barefoot and floors are frequently wet (58,59).

Fungal infections of the feet and nails occur less frequently in children than in adults, the incidence rising with age. However, foot and nail infections are not uncommonly observed in children and seem to occur with some frequency in children with trisomy 21, as do other chronic dermatophytoses (14,60–62). Clearly, tinea must be considered in the differential diagnosis of children with foot dermatitis. Twenty-five percent of cases of childhood tinea pedis are associated with a positive family history, usually in a parent, suggesting genetic as well as environmental factors (63).

There are three main clinical types of tinea pedis. The most common is an infection limited to the interdigital web spaces, most commonly involving only the fourth web space, between the fourth and fifth toes (Fig. 136.9). This area is thought to be predisposed because it lacks sebaceous glands that produce fungistatic lipids, which help to prevent infection in other areas. Tinea pedis presents clinically with peeling, maceration, erythema, and fissuring and is often pruritic. The differential diagnosis of interdigital tinea pedis includes candidiasis, bacterial

infections, and erythrasma. Normally a mild infection, this type, known as dermatophytosis simplex, may, in the setting of occlusion and secondary bacterial growth, develop into dermatophytosis complex, a mixed infection characterized by maceration, pruritus, and malodor produced by various bacterial products (14,64) (Fig. 136.10). Bacterial superinfection due to *S. aureus, Micrococcus sedentarius, Brevibacterium epidermidis, Corynebacterium minutissimum, Pseudomonas,* and *Proteus* may occur, which may mask the underlying fungal infection both clinically and when cultures are performed because of production of antifungal sulfur compounds, which may allow the gradual conversion from fungal to bacterial infection (64). Similarly, the bacteria are frequently antibiotic resistant owing to prior exposure to antibiotic substances produced by the fungi (64,65). In addition to antifungal and antibacterial therapy, treatment requires agents that dry the web space, such as aluminum chloride, gentian violet, or Castellani paint (14). Ciclopirox olamine and terbinafine are two antifungal agents that also have antibacterial properties *in vitro* and *in vivo* against gram-positive and gram-negative organisms, making them useful in the treatment of mixed fungal and bacterial infections such as interdigital dermatophytosis complex (66).

The second type of tinea pedis is the acute vesicular type, a pruritic eruption characterized by erythema and vesicles

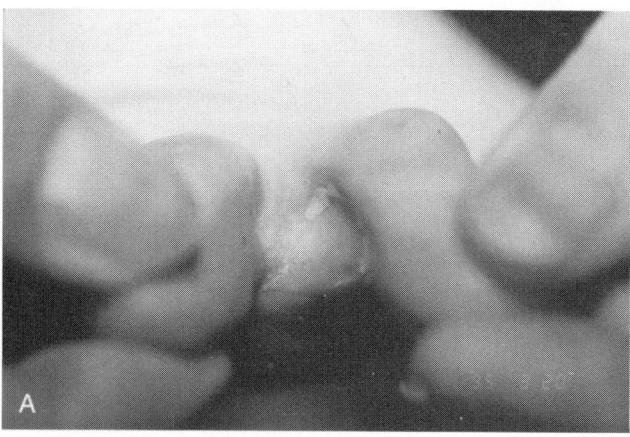

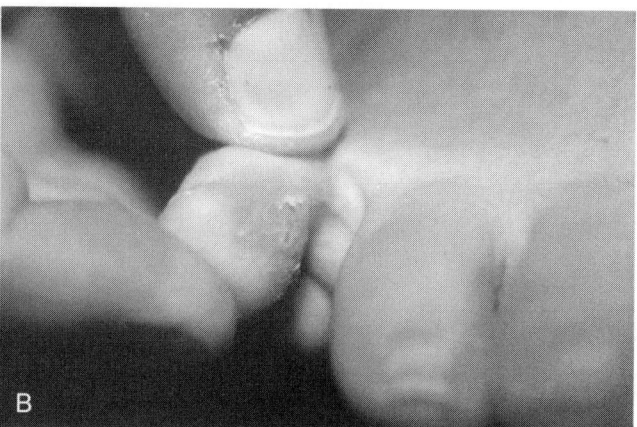

Figure 136.9. Tinea pedis. **A:** Interdigital maceration and scaling. (Courtesy of Nellie Konnikov, MD, New England Medical Center Hospital, Boston, MA.) **B:** Interdigital maceration and scaling.

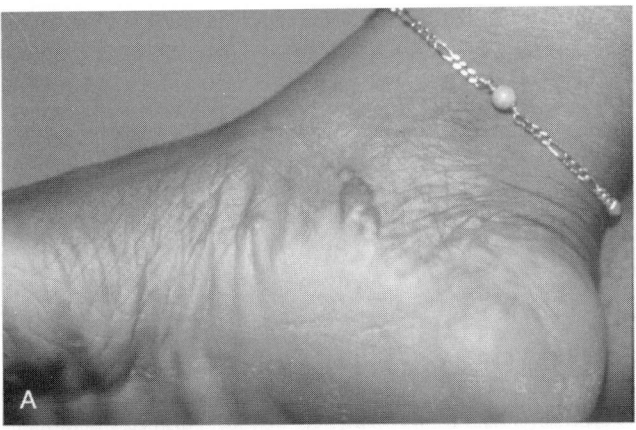

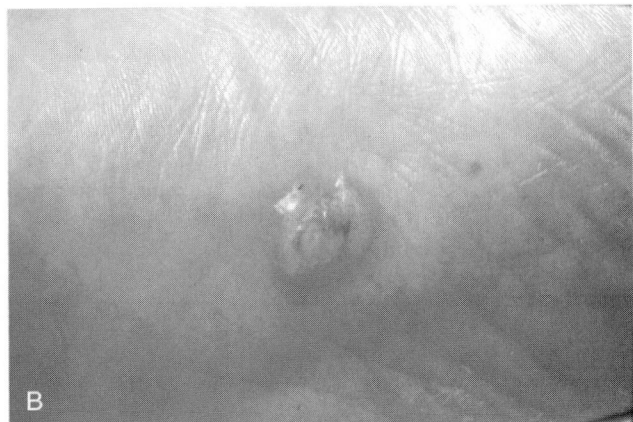

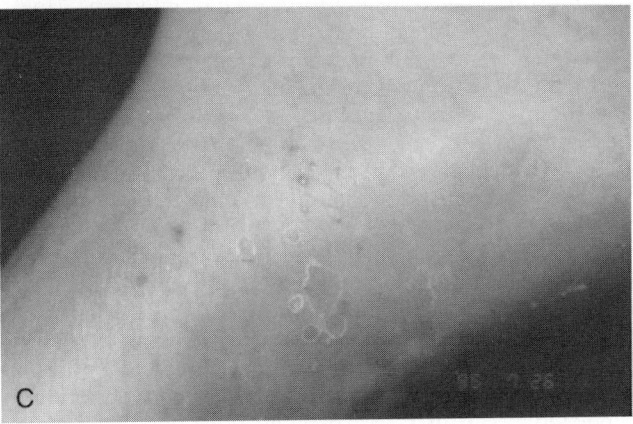

Figure 136.11. Vesicular tinea pedis. **A:** Scattered and coalescing vesicles. **B:** Coalescing vesicles. **C:** Multiple small vesicles and peeling collarettes.

commonly seen on the instep of the foot (Fig. 136.11). Diagnosis is established by demonstration of fungal hyphae on the undersurface of the blister roof on a KOH examination or by fungal culture. Treatment is as for other types of tinea pedis.

The third type of tinea pedis is the chronic hyperkeratotic form, often called moccasin-type tinea pedis because of its distribution. Dry hyperkeratotic scale and variable erythema are present on the soles and along the sides of the feet and toes (Fig. 136.12). This infection is usually caused by *T. rubrum*. Recurrences are common and are the rule when nail involvement

is present, as it frequently is. Interestingly, almost all chronic dermatophyte infections involving the skin and nails are due to *T. rubrum*. Several reasons are postulated that may help to explain this phenomenon. First, *T. rubrum* cell wall mannan inhibits the immune response; second, in some people, *T. rubrum* does not elicit a cell-mediated response adequate to clear the infection but rather preferentially activates specific suppressor T cells; third, the fungus is nonaggressive and remains in the stratum corneum, rather than attempting to invade the dermis where it might encounter complement, neutrophils, and other immune defenses; and finally, it is stable in the environment in a spore form for long periods (67).

Tinea Incognito

Tinea that has been treated with topical corticosteroids is known as tinea incognito because of the suppression of the usual inflammatory response, resulting in an altered morphologic appearance. In addition to making the diagnosis more difficult clinically, the steroid use, by blunting the immune response, potentiates the underlying infection. The patient is frequently led to believe that the steroid is treating the condition because inflammation and pruritus appear to subside, but when treatment is discontinued, the rash recurs. Corticosteroid-treated lesions tend to be less raised and less scaly; scaling is one of the host defenses by which the infectious organisms are normally shed (Fig. 136.13). The appearance may be further modified by the development of steroid side effects, such as atrophy and telangiectasia, or by the development of perioral dermatitis on the face. Diagnosis is made by KOH examination, which may be easier to perform a few days after the steroid is discontinued, when scaling resumes (12).

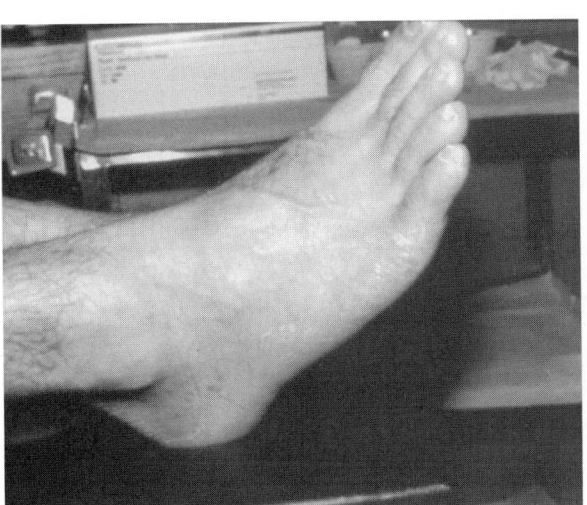

Figure 136.12. Chronic moccasin-type tinea pedis.

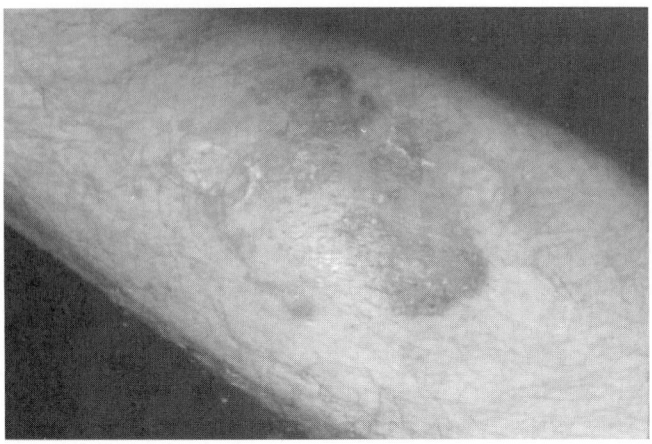

Figure 136.13. Tinea incognito. Tinea corporis previously treated with hydrocortisone. Note the clinical similarity to tinea in an immunosuppressed patient with AIDS (see Fig. 136.21).

Treatment consists of discontinuing steroid use and implementing appropriate topical antifungal therapy. If infection has invaded the follicles under the influence of the steroid, leading to the development of Majocchi granuloma, oral therapy may be required to eradicate infection. Combination agents containing both antifungal and corticosteroid medications should be avoided; permanent scars may result from the exacerbation of tinea corporis due to such agents (68). The potential risks of using potent topical steroids, and the potential decreased efficacy of the antifungal agent in the presence of steroid-impaired host defenses, make it difficult to justify use of these combination agents in the treatment of dermatophyte infections. In cases in which it is unclear whether a lesion is fungal or inflammatory, it is preferable to document fungal infection with a KOH examination and employ specific antifungal treatment once an accurate diagnosis has been made (69).

Dermatophytid Reactions

Dermatophytids, also known as id reactions, are uncommon cutaneous allergic responses to dermatophyte infections, usually occurring in the setting of inflammatory tinea. The id reaction occurs at a site distant from the infection, and cultures of the lesions are negative. The classically described id reaction consists of a pompholyx-like vesicular hand dermatitis in response to tinea pedis; the id reaction resolves when the underlying infection is treated. Many children with tinea capitis will develop a pruritic eruption of pinpoint lichenoid papules over the face and upper body when therapy for the tinea is initiated (Fig. 136.14; see also Color Figure 136.14). This reaction is self-limited and appears to be an immune response to fungal antigens; it is important to continue treatment and not to misdiagnose it as a drug eruption due to griseofulvin. True allergy to griseofulvin is rare (33).

DERMATOPHYTE INFECTIONS OF THE NAILS

Onychomycosis refers to any fungal infection of the nails; tinea unguium refers specifically to those nail infections caused by dermatophytes. Fungal nail infections are chronic and respond poorly to therapy, although newer agents that persist in the nail plate, some of which are fungicidal, are proving useful. Onychomycosis may cause a great deal of morbidity in terms of discomfort, functional impairment, and psychological distress (59). Nail infection is relatively uncommon in children in general but appears common in children with trisomy 21 (Fig. 136.15).

Tinea unguium is usually seen in association with tinea pedis or tinea manuum and is most commonly caused by *T. rubrum* or *T. mentagrophytes* var. *interdigitale,* with some cases caused by *E. floccosum. Microsporum* species do not invade the nail. Infection usually starts in one nail and may spread to involve others over a period of years. Although many saprophytic nondermatophyte molds can also cause nail infections, and *Candida* can produce onychomycosis in patients with chronic mucocutaneous candidiasis, there are three clinical types of true dermatophyte nail infection.

Distal Subungual Onychomycosis

Distal subungual onychomycosis is the most common type of tinea unguium and is characterized by distal subungual hyperkeratosis, onycholysis, and thickening of the nails (Fig. 136.16). Infection begins in the keratin of the hyponychium and spreads proximally to the nail bed and nail plate. Subungual hyperkeratosis, the nail equivalent to scaling as an attempt to rid the body of infection, ultimately results in the lifting up of the nail plate from the nail bed (onycholysis). The nail may become thickened

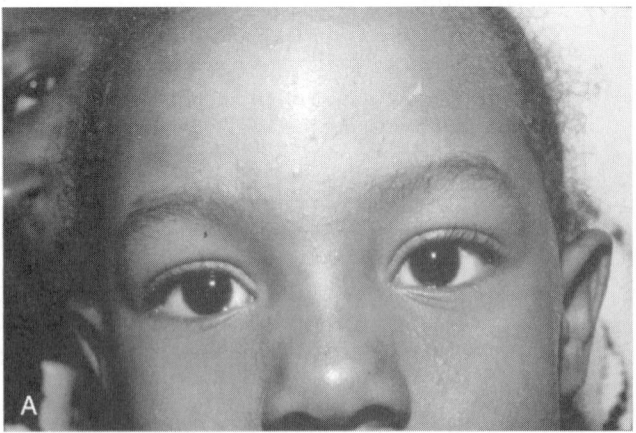
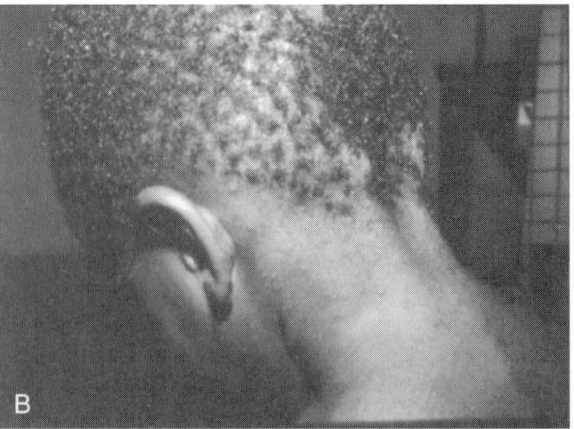

Figure 136.14. (See also Color Figure 136.14.) Id reaction. **A:** Fine papular eruption on the face in a 3-year-old girl with tinea capitis. **B:** Tinea capitis with fine papular id reaction on the neck.

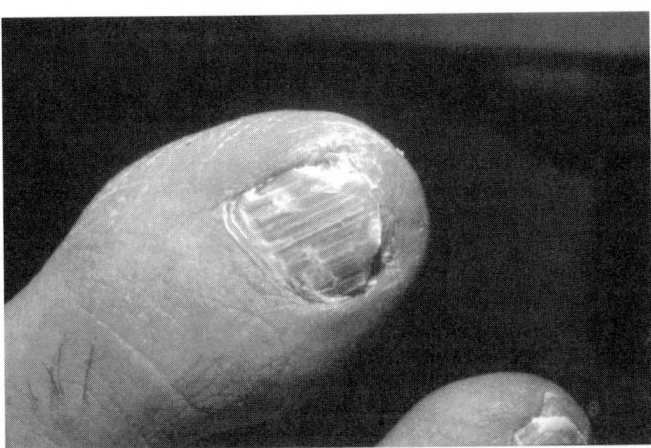

Figure 136.15. Onychomycosis in a patient with trisomy 21.

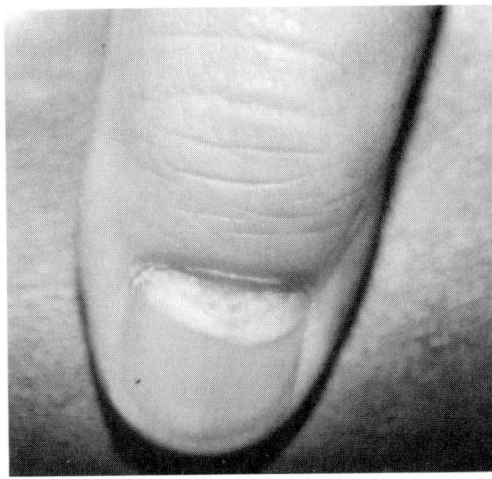

Figure 136.17. Proximal subungual onychomycosis. This type of onychomycosis occurs more commonly in AIDS. (Courtesy of Nellie Konnikov, MD, New England Medical Center Hospital, Boston, MA.)

and crumbly; secondary infection with bacteria or nondermatophytic fungi may also occur. The dystrophic nail that results may be painful when shoes are worn.

Proximal Subungual Onychomycosis

Proximal subungual onychomycosis is the rarest type of tinea unguium. The organism invades under the cuticle, and infection involves the ventral surface of the nail, creating irregular white spots under the nail that begin proximally and spread distally with the nail (Fig. 136.17). This type of tinea unguium appears to occur more commonly in patients with human immunodeficiency virus (70). It may occur without involvement of the skin and is usually caused by *T. rubrum*, although *T. schoenleinii*, *Trichophyton megninii*, and *E. floccosum* have also been reported (71).

Superficial White Onychomycosis

Superficial white onychomycosis occurs in toenails and is usually caused by *T. mentagrophytes*, which directly infects the nail plate. Other etiologic agents may include nondermatophyte molds such as *Acremonium* spp., *Fusarium oxysporum*, and *Aspergillus terreus* (72,73). Involved nails develop dull opaque superficial white patches, which may be focal or may involve the entire nail (Fig. 136.18). In patients with human immunodeficiency virus, *T. rubrum* may cause superficial white onychomycosis (70).

Onychomycosis Caused by Nondermatophyte Molds

Nondermatophyte molds that commonly cause onychomycosis include *Acremonium*, *Aspergillus*, and *Fusarium* species and *Onycochola canadensis*, *Scopulariopsis brevicaulis*, *Hendersonula toruloidea* (*Scytalidium dimidiatum*), and *Scytalidium hyalinum* (73,74). *Scytalidium* is an especially important pathogen in tropical and subtropical countries (74). It is important to distinguish these agents by culture because they do not respond to the agents usually used to treat dermatophyte infections of the skin and nails. Clues to the diagnosis of nail infections with nondermatophyte molds may include the involvement of only one nail, frequently after trauma because these agents tend to invade only previously damaged nails, or the presence of brown or black pigmentation of the nail (59). Some of these agents may respond to long-term oral terbinafine (75). Onychomycosis caused by *Aspergillus flavus* has been successfully treated with itraconazole (76).

Diagnosis

The differential diagnosis of tinea unguium includes psoriasis, traumatic nail dystrophy, fungal infections other than those caused by dermatophytes, congenital deformities such as pachyonychia congenita, and nail changes due to systemic diseases.

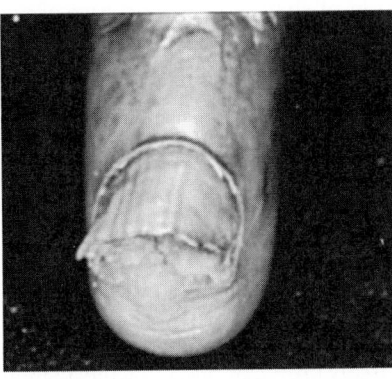

Figure 136.16. Distal subungual onychomycosis. Note the distal subungual hyperkeratosis.

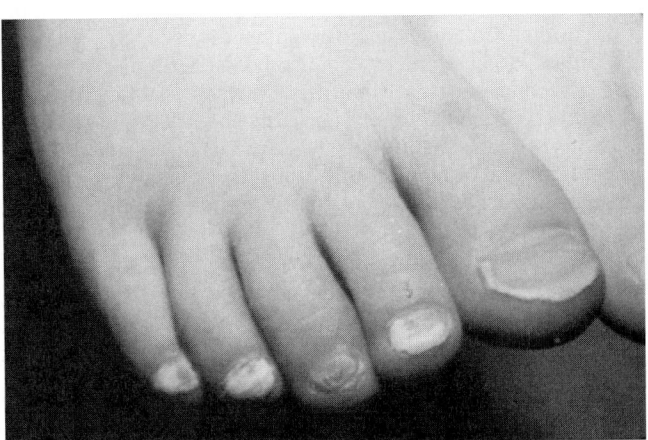

Figure 136.18. Superficial white onychomycosis.

KOH examination, culture, or both are required to confirm a diagnosis of tinea unguium. An alternative diagnostic method involves clipping a piece of the involved nail and sending it for histologic mounting and periodic acid-Schiff or silver staining to identify fungal elements. If necessary, nail biopsy may be performed.

Treatment

Tinea unguium cannot be cured with topical agents currently available, although amorolfine and tioconazole are under investigation and may prove useful in the treatment of mild to moderate infections in which the lunula and matrix remain uninvolved (77–79). Although they are not curative, ciclopirox olamine and naftifine appear to have some nail penetration and may be helpful in some patients (80). Surgical avulsion or chemical avulsion may be a useful adjunctive therapy in some patients in combination with topical or oral therapy (81).

Oral agents that can be used include griseofulvin, ketoconazole, fluconazole, and itraconazole (72). Griseofulvin must be given for 6 to 12 months for fingernail infections and for 12 to 18 months for toenail involvement, because the agent is fungistatic and nails grow so slowly. Griseofulvin is also limited by its effectiveness only against dermatophytes, because other fungi may also infect nails, either alone or coinfecting with dermatophytes (82). Ketoconazole use is limited by the risk for hepatotoxicity. Itraconazole and fluconazole are active against a broad spectrum of fungi and can be used to treat nail infections caused by dermatophytes, *Candida, Aspergillus,* and other species (80,83). Both, particularly itraconazole, may be prescribed in pulsed-dose regimens, as well as continuous ones, because they persist in the nail plate (84). Adverse effects of itraconazole and fluconazole include gastrointestinal symptoms, headache, rashes, and hepatotoxic reactions, although the last appear to be less common with the triazoles than with ketoconazole; drug interactions are common with all three agents because they work by interfering with the cytochrome P-450 system, which many other drugs depend on for their metabolism (42,85,86).

The most promising breakthrough will probably be oral terbinafine, because it is fungicidal and persists for long periods in the nail (see later) (14,84). Either terbinafine, 250 mg daily, or itraconazole, 200 mg daily, achieves rapid penetration and prolonged persistence in nails, enabling treatment periods to be shortened to as little as 6 weeks for fingernails and 12 weeks for toenails; the fungicidal nature of terbinafine also enables shortened treatment schedules (83). Mycologic cure rates of about 80% and low relapse rates of about 10% at 12 months after short courses of these two drugs appear to be much better than those for previously available therapies for the treatment of tinea unguium and chronic moccasin-type tinea pedis (83,87). Intermittent, pulsed-dose regimens can also be used. Some patients require a second course of treatment (88). It is anticipated that terbinafine will be extremely useful in the treatment of fungal infections of the hair and nails (89). Studies in several countries indicate that oral terbinafine is the most cost-effective therapy for dermatophyte infections of both toenails and fingernails (90,91).

SUPERFICIAL MYCOSES CAUSED BY NONDERMATOPHYTES

Piedra

Piedra refers to a rare infection of hair characterized by the presence of localized nodules consisting of fungal spores or hyphae attached to the hair shaft. There are two forms, each produced by different organisms, neither of which is a dermatophyte.

White piedra is caused by *Trichosporon beigelii,* a fungus that may be isolated from soil, air, and skin in endemic areas. It is usually seen in South America, central and eastern Europe, and Japan but has rarely been reported in the United States. Infection may involve the scalp but more commonly affects beard, mustache, axillary, or pubic hairs and produces white to tan, red, brown, or greenish nodules up to 1 mm in diameter that are easily detached from the hairs. Eyebrow and eyelash hairs may also be involved. Because the fungus grows inside and outside the hair shaft, the hair is weakened and may fracture. Diagnosis is made by KOH examination, which will distinguish white piedra from trichomycosis axillaris or pubis caused by several *Corynebacterium* species. Pruritus and the distinctive shape and adherence of nits should help to distinguish pediculosis from white piedra. Microscopic examination also rules out trichorrhexis nodosa.

In the past decade, the role of *T. beigelii* as a sole pathogen in white piedra has come into question. There appears to be an increased rate of carriage of bacteria, in particular of coryneform bacteria distinct from those causing trichomycosis axillaris, in hairs infected with *T. beigelii;* it has been proposed that white piedra results from a synergistic infection of *T. beigelii* and a specific type III coryneform bacterium, a newly characterized species of *Brevibacterium* called *Brevibacterium mcbrellneri* (92–95).

T. beigelii has also been reported to cause onychomycosis in healthy adults and systemic opportunistic infection in immunocompromised hosts (93,96–99). Culture media without cycloheximide are necessary for the isolation of this organism (96).

Black piedra is characterized by adherent, hard, gritty black nodular concretions on the hair shaft; these concretions may vary in size from microscopic to more than 1 mm in diameter. Invasion of the shaft may result in hair breakage. Black piedra usually involves the scalp but may involve other sites, such as the mustache, beard, and pubic area. It is caused by *Piedraia hortae,* another soil fungus, and is rare in the United States, occurring mainly in tropical areas of South America and Southeast Asia, the Pacific Islands, and Africa.

Treatment of piedra consists primarily of shaving or cutting the affected hair. Terbinafine has been reported as a successful treatment for black piedra, with demonstration of *in vitro* susceptibility of the isolate corresponding to the clinical and mycologic cure (92,100). Treatment of white piedra is difficult. In addition to shaving the affected hairs, reported treatments have included topical and oral imidazoles, ciclopirox olamine, selenium sulfide, bichloride of mercury, benzoic acid, salicylic acid, 3% to 6% precipitated sulfur ointment, chlorhexidine, Castellani paint, zinc pyrithione, amphotericin B lotion, 2% to 10% glutaraldehyde, and 2% formalin (92,101). In view of the location of infection within and on the hair, and the likely involvement of both *T. beigelii* and *B. mcbrellneri,* consideration should be given to a combination of shaving, oral and topical antifungal therapy, and topical antibacterial soaps or topical antibiotics effective against coryneform bacteria.

TINEA NIGRA

Although it is not a dermatophyte infection, tinea nigra is included in this discussion because it is another superficial fungal infection involving only the stratum corneum. The disease is caused by *Exophiala werneckii* and occurs sporadically throughout the world but most commonly in tropical and subtropical areas. It presents as a well-demarcated but irregularly shaped superficial nonscaly brown or black macule, usually on the palm but occasionally on the sole and rarely on other body sites. The differential diagnosis includes melanoma, junctional nevus, lentigo, postinflammatory hyperpigmentation, and chemical staining. Diagnosis is easily made when the KOH preparation reveals pigmented septate hyphae or budding forms, and culture on Sabouraud glucose agar can be done to confirm the diagnosis. Treatment consists of scraping of the lesion, followed by application of a topical imidazole or a keratolytic agent such as benzoic acid or salicylic acid.

NONDERMATOPHYTE MOLDS

H. toruloidea (*S. dimidiatum*) and *S. hyalinum* are nondermatophyte molds that may cause infections clinically identical to tinea pedis, tinea manuum, and tinea unguium. A patient with a tinea capitis-like infection due to *H. toruloidea* has also been described (102). These infections are technically referred to as dermatomycoses. *H. toruloidea* has been found in the southeastern United States and the western states; outside the United States, it has been found in Canada, South America, the Caribbean, Africa, India, and the Far East, and most infections have been reported in these areas (103). Clinical presentations of tinea pedis due to these agents include interdigital and moccasin types. Mixed infections with true dermatophytes are common. Microscopic examination with KOH reveals narrow, septate, branching hyphae that are similar to those of the dermatophytes. Because these infections fail to respond to conventional antifungal agents, they must be distinguished from true tinea. Growth of these agents is inhibited by cycloheximide, so it is important to perform cultures on cycloheximide-free media in addition to the traditional dermatophyte media that contain cycloheximide to eliminate overgrowth of contaminants (103). A positive finding on the KOH examination, coupled with a negative culture on cycloheximide-containing agar (e.g., dermatophyte test medium, Mycosel Mycobiotic) should raise the clinical suspicion for one of these agents, especially with a history of treatment failure or living in or visiting an endemic area (74,103). Terbinafine, amorolfine, tioconazole, econazole, or benzoic acid (Whitfield ointment) may be effective topical therapies, but to date there is no one reliable agent for treating these dermatomycoses (12,59,104–106).

PITYROSPORUM INFECTIONS

Pityrosporum ovale (*P. orbiculare, Malassezia furfur*) is a lipophilic yeast present as normal postpubertal skin flora in the hair follicles in sites rich in sebaceous glands, such as the face, scalp, and upper trunk. The amount of *P. ovale* present in different age groups seems to correlate with variations in sebum production that are age-dependent (107). Under certain host conditions, however, it causes diseases such as tinea versicolor (pityriasis versicolor) and *Pityrosporum* folliculitis and appears to be involved in the pathogenesis of seborrheic dermatitis (16). It has also been postulated to play a role in some patients with atopic dermatitis and in confluent and reticulated papillomatosis of Gougerot and Carteaud, although the latter association has come into question (107,108). Finally, *Pityrosporum* is rarely the cause of disseminated infection (16,101,109,110).

Tinea Versicolor

Tinea versicolor is a common scaling dermatosis that occurs when *Pityrosporum* overgrowth extends from the follicles to adjacent skin, resulting in hyperpigmented or hypopigmented, thin, finely scaly 0.5- to 1-cm papules that may coalesce to form larger plaques, usually on the upper trunk and proximal upper extremities (Fig. 136.19A). Lesions on tanned skin tend to be

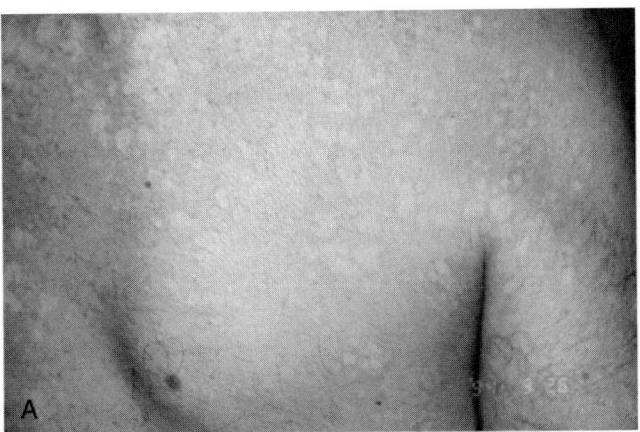

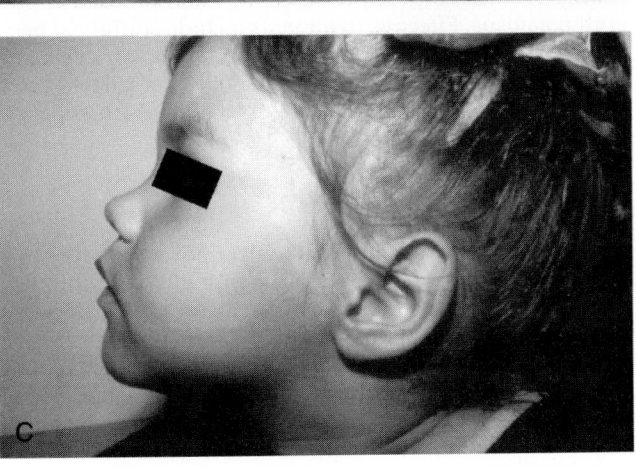

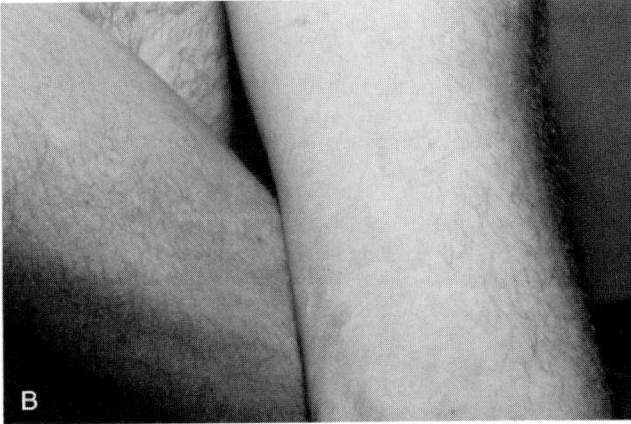

Figure 136.19. Tinea versicolor. **A:** innumerable finely scaly hypopigmented thin papules on the trunk and proximal extremities. **B:** Hypopigmented and hyperpigmented lesions in the same patient. The lesions on the sun-exposed dorsal forearms were hypopigmented, whereas those on the relatively sun-protected volar forearms were hyperpigmented compared with normal skin. **C:** Hypopigmented finely scaly papules extending onto the face of a 3-year-old child.

hypopigmented, and both hyperpigmented and hypopigmented lesions may be seen in the same patient in different locations (Fig. 136.19B). In children, involvement occasionally extends onto the face and scalp, especially in tropical climates (Fig. 136.19C). In early cases, the lesions may be seen to be perifollicular in origin. It is occasionally pruritic but is often asymptomatic.

Hot, humid environments favor the development of tinea versicolor, and the disease is more common in tropical and subtropical climates than in temperate ones, where it may appear only during the summer and may be quiescent during the winter months. Heredity, glucocorticosteroid medications, hyperhidrosis, greasy skin, and exogenously applied oils can also be predisposing factors (107,111,112). Tinea versicolor occurs most commonly in adolescents and young adults, in whom sebum production is higher than that in other age groups, and seems to correlate with increased colonization by *Pityrosporum* with increasing age (5% to 15% in 0- to 10-year-old children compared with 56% to 90% for 11- to 20-year-old individuals) (108). Because tinea versicolor is a disease produced by normal flora, it is not contagious.

The diagnosis of tinea versicolor is usually straightforward, but in some cases the differential diagnosis may include pityriasis alba, seborrheic dermatitis, tinea corporis, vitiligo, or postinflammatory hyperpigmentation or hypopigmentation. Diagnosis is confirmed by the classic "spaghetti and meatballs" appearance of abundant short stubby hyphae and spores seen on KOH microscopic examination of scrapings. Culture is not routinely performed because special oil-containing medium is required.

Treatment consists of topical agents such as selenium sulfide lotion applied for 10 to 20 minutes nightly to the trunk and proximal extremities for 1 to 2 weeks. Other topical therapies include the imidazoles, ciclopirox olamine, zinc pyrithione, sulfur or salicylic acid preparations, propylene glycol, benzoyl peroxide, sodium hyposulfite, and the allylamines naftifine and terbinafine, which work topically but not orally to treat tinea versicolor (87,111,112). Extensive cases, or those in which lesions extend into the hairline, may be treated with brief courses of oral ketoconazole, itraconazole, or fluconazole (111,112). One or two weekly oral doses of ketoconazole 400 mg, or itraconazole 200 mg daily for 5 days, is an effective regimen in the treatment of tinea versicolor (42,113). Ketoconazole should be taken with breakfast, including an acidic juice, and the patient should avoid bathing for at least 12 hours because the drug is delivered to the skin primarily in the sweat. Griseofulvin is effective only for treatment of dermatophyte infections and cannot be used to treat tinea versicolor. Because the disease is caused by endogenous flora, recurrence is common but may be prevented or delayed with once-monthly prophylactic topical treatment.

Pigment alteration may take months to resolve after treatment, especially for patients with hypopigmented forms. Hypopigmentation is thought to result from the organism's production of azelaic acid, which interferes with melanin synthesis; the cause of hyperpigmentation is unknown but does not appear to involve the production of melanin (112,114).

Pityrosporum Folliculitis

P. ovale may cause a folliculitis characterized by pruritic follicular erythematous papules and pustules on the trunk, especially on the back (Fig. 136.20). Like tinea versicolor, it occurs more frequently in hot, humid environments (107). It appears to be more common in diabetic patients, in immunocompromised hosts, in circumstances where skin is occluded, and after systemic steroid or antibiotic therapy (107). The differential diagnosis includes bacterial folliculitis due to *S. aureus* or gram-negative organisms such as in hot tub folliculitis due to *Pseudomonas* eosinophilic

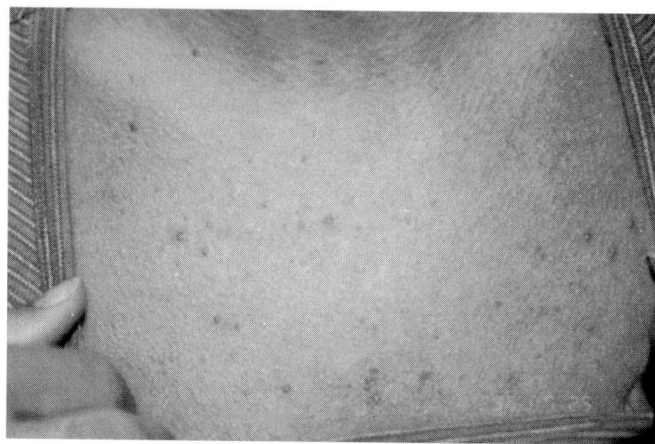

Figure 136.20. *Pityrosporum* folliculitis. Monomorphous pinpoint papulopustules.

folliculitis, and acne vulgaris. It is possible that steroid acne is a variant of *Pityrosporum* folliculitis. Diagnosis is usually made by skin biopsy with use of special stains to demonstrate the presence of budding yeast forms in the follicle, but the organism can occasionally be identified by a KOH examination of the contents of a pustule. Treatment is as for tinea versicolor, but oral therapy, at least initially, may be required. Topical amphotericin B can also be used.

Seborrheic Dermatitis

P. ovale has been implicated in both infantile and adult seborrheic dermatitis. 16 Characterized by orange-red to dull red plaques with greasy scale, seborrheic dermatitis typically involves the scalp and hairline, ears and retroauricular folds, forehead, glabella, eyebrows, nasolabial folds, and beard and mustache areas. Blepharitis may be seen, and fissuring below the earlobe is common when this site is involved. The central chest and back and the axillae and groin may also be involved. Cultures have repeatedly demonstrated increased carriage of *Pityrosporum* in patients with seborrheic dermatitis compared with unaffected patients, and topical agents such as ketoconazole are efficacious in treating the disease (73). The condition is also seen with increased frequency and severity in patients with acquired immunodeficiency syndrome. It is believed that abnormal host immune response to *Pityrosporum* causes the aberrant inflammatory reaction and dermatitis, possibly through the alternative pathway of complement activation (71,101,107).

The differential diagnosis of seborrheic dermatitis includes psoriasis, tinea corporis, tinea capitis, and occasionally lupus erythematosus. Effective treatments include antifungal preparations such as ketoconazole cream and shampoo, selenium sulfide, and zinc pyrithione; keratolytics such as salicylic acid and sulfur; and tars and mild topical steroids, which suppress inflammation.

Atopic Dermatitis

Evidence that *Pityrosporum* may be an important allergen in some patients with atopic dermatitis is mounting. In both children and young adults with atopic dermatitis, there appears in general to be increased sensitization to *P. ovale*; in particular, sensitization to *P. ovale* appears to correlate with atopic dermatitis involving the face, scalp, neck, and upper back of adults. Whether hypersensitivity to *P. ovale* is pathogenic or is merely an epiphenomenon due to altered skin barrier function leading to increased sensitization has not yet been determined (108). Reports of clearance of dermatitis with ketoconazole treatment suggest that *P. ovale* may be pathogenic (107). In addition, although colonization is not increased in patients with atopic dermatitis, specific immunoglobulin E antibodies to *P. ovale* are found only in atopic individuals and occur more frequently in children with atopic dermatitis than in patients with other forms of atopy (14,108). Positive skin prick test responses to *P. ovale* are also seen only in patients with atopic dermatitis, primarily in adolescents and adults (107,108).

Confluent and Reticulated Papillomatosis

Confluent and reticulated papillomatosis of Gougerot and Carteaud is characterized by the presence of hyperpigmented thin scaly or hyperkeratotic papules that become confluent centrally, with a reticulated pattern peripherally, primarily over the chest and central back. It is usually seen in adolescents and young adults. The clinical appearance, coupled with reports of patients with this condition in whom *M. furfur* was demonstrated on biopsy and who responded to ketoconazole or other treatments for tinea versicolor, has led to speculation by some authors that this condition may be caused by *P. ovale* or by an abnormal host response to this normal inhabitant of the skin (107,115). However, in most patients, the presence of *Pityrosporum* cannot be demonstrated and treatment directed against this agent is unsuccessful. On the basis of histologic and electron microscopic data as well as response to retinoids and other agents that work by altering keratinization, numerous reports have suggested that this disease is instead a disorder of abnormal keratinization (116–121). Possibly, abnormal keratinization predisposes patients with this condition to infection with *Pityrosporum*, leading to the early hypothesis that it was causative.

Disseminated Infections

Pityrosporum, presumably because of its lipophilic nature, has been reported as a cause of sepsis in premature neonates and adults with underlying gastrointestinal disease, associated with intravenous intralipid feeding (16,101[p. 157],109,110,122,123). It presents with fever, leukocytosis, and thrombocytopenia, sometimes with pulmonary infiltrates; lipid-rich culture media are necessary for the isolation of the organism from blood cultures (101,109,110,122). Yeast may sometimes be visualized on Gram stain of the buffy coat from central venous blood specimens (110). When blood specimens are drawn from patients receiving parenteral lipids, consideration should be given to the possibility of sepsis with a lipophilic fungus such as *M. furfur,* and special lipid-supplemented media should be employed to assist in the isolation of such organisms; Sabouraud medium covered with a thin layer of sterile olive oil may suffice (109,110). Treatment consists of removal of the infected catheter, withdrawal of intralipid therapy, and chemotherapy with azoles or amphotericin B (109,110).

HOST IMMUNE RESPONSE AND PATHOPHYSIOLOGY

Various factors contribute to the host's resistance to dermatophyte infection. The local environment may be made less hospitable by medium chain free fatty acids on the skin surface, which potentiate the growth of *Pityrosporum* and inhibit that of dermatophytes; these free fatty acids may also interfere with fungal adhesion to keratinocytes (16). However, it is primarily the host's cell-mediated immunity that clears the skin of dermatophyte infections, in part by producing keratinocyte proliferation, epidermal thickening, and scaling, leading to desquamation of infected skin, perhaps mediated by lymphocyte or monocyte cytokines (9,14,16,124). Immunophenotyping of dermal cellular infiltrates in two studies of biopsy specimens of tinea revealed helper T lymphocytes, with some Langerhans cells and macrophages, but essentially no B cells (125,126).

Nonspecific host immune defenses also play a role. Unsaturated transferrin (serum inhibitory factor) in sweat and serum produces inhibition of fungal growth by binding iron and making it unavailable to the fungus (16,124,127). Growth is also inhibited by complement activation through the alternative pathway by products in fungal cell walls (127). Neutrophil adhesion to opsonized and unopsonized hyphae also results in fungal growth inhibition but does not necessarily cause fungal killing (127). Polymorphonuclear leukocyte activation and inhibition of fungal growth may occur even in the absence of cell-mediated immunity and appears to involve the myeloperoxidase-hydrogen peroxide-halide system (127). Similarly, although dermatophytes will invade viable epidermis in tissue culture, they do not do so *in vivo*, even in the absence of cell-mediated immunity, possibly because of this complement activation and neutrophil attack (124).

Fungal substances such as cell wall mannans appear to suppress the host's immune response, preventing eradication of infection or predisposing to reinfection. Mannans inhibit turnover of the stratum corneum and *in vitro* suppress the immune response in several ways, possibly inhibiting lymphoproliferation by interfering with antigen presentation (124,128). Interestingly, *T. rubrum* mannans produce greater *in vitro* suppression of cell-mediated immune responses than do mannans from zoophilic dermatophytes (124). This correlates clinically with the observation that zoophilic dermatophytes tend to produce inflammatory responses, whereas *T. rubrum,* an anthropophilic fungus, tends to produce chronic, noninflammatory infections such as moccasin-type tinea pedis. *T. rubrum* mannans may enable infections with other dermatophytes, because inoculation of the usually highly inflammatory *T. mentagrophytes* into patients chronically infected with *T. rubrum* produces only slight inflammation (129). However, this could be due either to suppression by *T. rubrum* mannan or to an inherent host unresponsiveness that allowed chronic infection in the first place (14).

An example of the give and take between dermatophyte and host is illustrated by tinea pedis due to *T. mentagrophytes,* which may consist of chronic low-grade scaling punctuated by acute episodes of vesicular tinea pedis. When local environmental factors tip the balance in favor of the fungus and proliferation and penetration into the stratum corneum lead to contact of the epidermis with fungal antigens, T-cell–mediated immune response is triggered, resulting in a vesicular dermatitis analogous to allergic contact dermatitis; the blistering and scaling serve to shed the fungus from the skin (64).

Studies of such inflammatory infections show that clearing of experimental *T. mentagrophytes* infections in previously uninfected individuals is associated with the development of cell-mediated immunity, acute inflammatory reaction, and conversion to a positive response to the trichophytin intradermal test; subsequent reinfection requires a much larger inoculum and clears spontaneously (124,129). In contrast, chronic infections are associated with immunodeficiency, atopy, or predisposing local cutaneous environmental factors (124). Poor cell-mediated immunity, the presence of an immunoglobulin E response, and negative trichophytin test result tend to be associated with chronic infections, requiring treatment, both in humans and in athymic rats (129).

Specific immunoglobulin E antibodies to dermatophytes may block interactions between T cells and antigen-presenting cells, thus interfering with the development of delayed hypersensitivity (129). Th1 cells produce interferon-γ, which promotes the development of delayed hypersensitivity and cell-mediated immunity; Th2 cells produce interleukin-4, which promotes immunoglobulin E production; preferential sensitization or response of either cell type may determine whether dermatophyte infections will be quickly cleared or will result in an immunoglobulin E host response and chronic infection (14,129). Interferon-γ, interleukin-2, and granulocyte-macrophage colony-stimulating factor were detected in the culture supernatant after incubation of trichophytin with peripheral blood mononuclear cells obtained from a patient with a dermatophyte infection; the authors postulated that these cytokines may play a role in the development of delayed-type hypersensitivity to trichophytin (130).

IMMUNOCOMPROMISED HOSTS

Extensive, severe, recalcitrant dermatophyte infections may be seen in the setting of abnormal T-cell function, such as in patients with AIDS or other T-cell immune deficiencies (16,131). The sites and organisms are the same as those involved in normal patients, but infections are often more extensive and more chronic, and the appearance may be atypical; superficial fungal infections occur early in the clinical course of human immunodeficiency virus infection and affect almost all patients with advanced disease (71,73,132) (Fig. 136.21). Even dermatophytes as nonaggressive and noninvasive as *T. rubrum* may cause atypical, aggressive infections such as deep folliculitis, granuloma formation, and even abscesses in neutropenic or otherwise immunocompromised patients; other dermatophytes reported to cause local invasion in immunocompromised patients include *M. audouinii*, *T. schoenleinii*, *T. violaceum*, and *E. floccosum* (70,133). Dermatophyte infections in human immunodeficiency virus-positive patients, especially infections of a deep type, may require systemic oral therapy as well as topical treatment (70). Patients treated with immunosuppressive agents for organ transplantation or hematologic malignant neoplasms, or those receiving systemic corticosteroids, may be at risk for extensive dermatophyte infections (Fig. 136.22). These may culminate in dermal invasion, usually presenting with erythematous papules or nodules within an area of chronic *T. rubrum* infection but sometimes appearing as

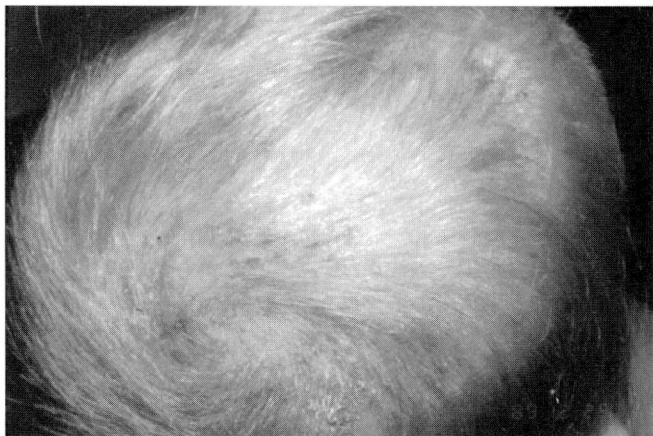

Figure 136.22. Tinea capitis in a 6-year-old girl receiving chemotherapy for Wilms tumor.

firm or fluctuant dusky or hemorrhagic nodules (134). Long-term topical steroid therapy or radiation therapy can also predispose to locally invasive disease (135). The dematiaceous fungi can also cause abscesses in such hosts (133). Invasive dermatophyte infections may occur while patients are receiving systemic therapy with amphotericin B, which, although it has *in vitro* activity against dermatophytes, is not effective *in vivo* against dermatophytes because it is not secreted in sweat or sebum and minimal tissue levels are obtained in the stratum corneum by passive diffusion. Consideration should be given to combined therapy with fluconazole and topical agents in such infections (133). Candidal infections of various types are also common.

Organisms such as *P. ovale* and *T. beigelii*, which ordinarily cause benign superficial infections (tinea versicolor and white piedra, respectively), have been reported to cause systemic opportunistic infections in immunocompromised patients as well as in a neutropenic murine model (16,97–99,136). Opportunistic infections with *T. beigelii* occur most commonly in neutropenic patients with underlying neoplasms but have also been reported in patients with AIDS and in those with a history of intravenous drug use, organ transplantation, and chronic active hepatitis (97,137). Infection often involves the lungs, kidneys, liver, spleen, and heart as well as the skin in approximately 30% of patients (137). *T. beigelii* septic arthritis has been reported in a patient with acute leukemia (138). The prognosis for disseminated trichosporosis is poor (97). Several authors have found an increased frequency of rectal carriage of *T. beigelii* in homosexual men, as high as 15.5% compared with 3.1% for other hospitalized patients, raising the possibility of sexual transmission of this organism; not surprisingly, white piedra has also been reported to be sexually transmitted in heterosexuals (97,136,139–141). *T. beigelii* has been found to colonize normal perigenital skin in approximately 12% of patients, more commonly in men than in women (142).

Hosts who otherwise have normal immune systems but who have abnormal skin may also be predisposed to dermatophyte infections, which may be more difficult to diagnose because of the underlying skin disease. These include patients with various types of ichthyosis (143–146). The apparent increased occurrence in patients with trisomy 21 may in part be due to the retention hyperkeratosis commonly seen in these patients, which provides a thickened stratum corneum that the fungus may invade. Increased occurrence has also been noted in hereditary palmoplantar keratodermas, in which the amount of keratin was considered the most important factor for dermatophyte affinity for the palms and soles (147).

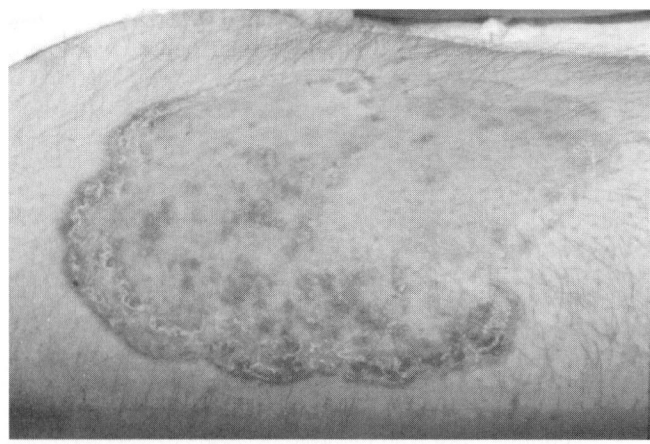

Figure 136.21. Tinea corporis on the thigh of a patient with AIDS. Large scaling erythematous plaque with numerous papules within it.

Nondermatophyte infections of many types are also common in immunocompromised patients, including candidiasis, which may involve multiple mucocutaneous sites, and disseminated fungal infections, including histoplasmosis, cryptococcosis, coccidioidomycosis, sporotrichosis, aspergillosis, and other infections that are covered elsewhere. As a general rule, however, fungal infections in patients with AIDS and other immunocompromised patients may present with atypical findings; therefore, the index of suspicion must be high and the threshold for biopsy and culture low.

ANTIFUNGAL AGENTS AND THERAPY FOR DERMATOPHYTOSES

The choice of therapeutic agents in the treatment of dermatophyte infections is influenced by site affected, pathogen, severity, extent of infection, drug spectrum and efficacy, drug safety profile, potential drug interactions, dosage schedule and drug pharmacokinetics, patient's compliance, and cost. Required duration of therapy may also be a factor and varies with the agent, its antifungal mechanism, and the site of infection. For example, therapy with fungistatic drugs must be continued until the infected tissue has been shed, resulting in longer treatment courses for infections of the hair and nails than are required for infections involving only the skin. This can cause problems with the patient's compliance even in treating skin infections, because patients frequently discontinue therapy once symptoms have improved but before the infection has been adequately treated, increasing the risk for recurrence (148,149). For similar reasons, negative cultures generally precede negative results of the KOH examination by several weeks because of the delay in stratum corneum turnover (150).

Routine fungal sensitivity testing is generally not available but may be of potential clinical use in the treatment of selected patients. Methods of assessing *in vitro* susceptibility of dermatophytes to antifungal agents include a simple disk diffusion method that measures growth inhibition zones and the more complicated dilution method for measuring minimal inhibitory concentrations (151,152). Staining with neutral red can also be used as an in vitro method of assessing the viability of fungal cells after exposure to antifungal agents (153). In areas where routine testing is not available, awareness of patterns of drug susceptibility may help to guide therapy.

Many classes of antifungal agents are active against dermatophytes, and most are fungistatic and appear to work by interfering in fungal cell wall synthesis. The azoles include both the older imidazoles, such as clotrimazole, miconazole, and ketoconazole, and the newer triazoles itraconazole, terconazole, and fluconazole. These drugs inhibit cytochrome P-450 14-α-demethylase, blocking demethylation of lanosterol in membrane ergosterol biosynthesis (42). The triazoles are slightly more specific for inhibition of fungal sterols compared with human sterols than are the original azole compounds (105). Other types of compounds include the thiocarbamide tolnaftate, which inhibits squalene epoxidase and is active only against growing dermatophytes; ciclopirox olamine, which blocks membrane protein synthesis; and griseofulvin, which inhibits microtubule polymerization (42). Griseofulvin is normally administered orally and delivered to the stratum corneum by sweat, but a few studies of this agent against experimentally induced *T. mentagrophytes* and various dermatophytes in tinea pedis and tinea corporis suggested that topical use may also be possible (154,155). Nystatin and amphotericin B are polyene antibiotics, which bind to ergosterol and disrupt fungal cell membrane transport and are generally active only against yeasts (80). Newer classes of drugs that are fungicidal include the dimethylmorpholines (amorolfine) and the allylamines (naftifine, terbinafine). Dimethylmorpholines inhibit ergosterol synthesis at two steps, 14-reduction and 7-8-isomerization, causing accumulation of ignosterol and depletion of ergosterol in the fungal cell membrane. 42 Allylamines are broad-spectrum fungicidal agents; without inhibiting the host's cytochrome P-450, they inhibit squalene epoxidase, the enzyme that catalyzes the conversion of squalene to squalene-2,3-epoxide in the ergosterol synthetic pathway (148). Interference with cell wall structure, and presumably function, by naftifine and terbinafine has been demonstrated by scanning electron microscopy, which revealed structural abnormalities of *E. floccosum* cell walls after treatment with these drugs (156). In addition, some naturally occurring products, such as azelaic acid, have been shown to have *in vitro* activity against dermatophytes and several other fungi and may deserve further investigation (14,157).

Topical therapies currently available in the United States include the imidazoles, ciclopirox olamine, the allylamines, and tolnaftate, which is somewhat less effective. Most infections of the skin can be treated with these agents. In part because it is fungicidal, topical terbinafine produces high clinical and mycologic cure rates in brief treatment courses for interdigital tinea pedis, tinea cruris, tinea corporis, and chronic moccasin-type tinea pedis, with more rapid attainment of a higher cure rate and a lower relapse rate than traditional longer courses with clotrimazole (149,150,158–162). One study suggested that terbinafine cream may be effective after a single application in the therapy of tinea pedis (163). With moccasin-type tinea pedis, higher cure rates and lower relapse rates are obtained in patients without onychomycosis, because reinfection tends to occur owing to seeding from infected nails (150). The other allylamine, naftifine, is also usually fungicidal and is frequently superior to other agents; however, a report of naftifine failure in two children with tinea corporis due to *T. tonsurans* suggested the need for additional *in vivo* studies in children with *T. tonsurans* infections (164,165). Another promising topical agent is amorolfine, not yet available in the United States, which is active against molds and *Candida* as well as dermatophytes; it produces excellent results in all types of tinea pedis, including infections with yeasts, mixed infections, and dermatophyte infections, including chronic *T. rubrum* moccasin-type tinea pedis (166).

Oral therapy for dermatophyte infections is necessary for treatment of infections that involve the hair, nails, extensive areas of the skin, or multiple inoculation sites and often in recalcitrant infections such as chronic moccasin-type tinea pedis, although topical allylamines may suffice in the latter (148). Griseofulvin is currently the treatment of choice for tinea capitis, although itraconazole, fluconazole, and oral terbinafine may become useful. Griseofulvin can also be used for extensive cutaneous infections, although it has a lower rate of clinical and mycologic cure and a higher relapse rate than oral terbinafine or itraconazole after a 2-week course (167–169). Once-weekly doses of fluconazole for 1 to 4 weeks are also effective as therapy for tinea corporis and tinea cruris and slightly less so for tinea pedis (170–172). The possible utility of oral ketoconazole for cutaneous dermatophyte infections is usually outweighed by the potential risk for hepatotoxic effects, even more so when the long treatment course necessary for nail infections is considered, but once-weekly dosing of 400 mg for 3 to 8 weeks can be used for dermatophyte infections of the skin (42,82,173). Itraconazole in a dosage regimen of 100 mg daily for 2 weeks, or 200 mg daily for 1 week, is extremely effective in the treatment of tinea corporis and tinea cruris; tinea pedis can be treated with 200 mg twice daily for 1 week (174–177).

Terbinafine, the newest allylamine, is lipophilic and keratinophilic and achieves excellent and persistent penetration into sebum and keratin, including nails; it is also rapidly fungicidal and highly active (37). The drug persists in stratum corneum, nails, hair, and sebum for months after discontinuation of a 4-week oral course of 250 mg daily (178). It is fungicidal against dermatophytes, molds, dimorphic fungi, and some yeasts but not against *Candida albicans*, and it is highly effective in the treatment of dermatophyte infections of the hair and nails (38,89). These characteristics allow brief treatment schedules that may enhance the patient's compliance. Although oral therapy would obviously be unnecessary for most patients with skin infections, terbinafine is also highly effective in 1- to 2-week courses for the treatment of tinea corporis, tinea cruris, and tinea pedis, and some patients may prefer the convenience of a brief course of oral medication to the use of a topical agent (42,179). Terbinafine may be slightly more effective than itraconazole in the treatment of tinea pedis and has a much lower relapse rate than griseofulvin in this condition (180,181). Adverse effects occur in about 10% of patients treated with oral terbinafine but tend to be mild; these effects include abdominal pain, nausea, rash, pruritus, headache, dizziness, fatigue, and anorexia (38,87).

Oral steroids may help to reduce the risk for and extent of permanent alopecia in the treatment of kerion, but the use of topical corticosteroids should be avoided in the treatment of dermatophyte infections. Combination products containing both a topical antifungal medication and a potent topical steroid have been advocated by some for treatment of inflammatory tinea to provide more rapid symptomatic relief. However, there is ample evidence that the steroid agents frequently impair the host's natural cell-mediated immunity to the point that the ability of the antifungal agent to eradicate the infection is overwhelmed (68,182). This may be even more of a problem with organisms that are less sensitive to the antifungal agent, as in the case of *M. canis* and clotrimazole (182). In these cases, substitution of the identical antifungal ingredient without the steroid is often adequate to clear the infection, although when the infection has progressed to Majocchi granuloma, oral therapy may be required.

REFERENCES

1. Macura AB. Dermatophyte infections. *Int J Dermatol* 1993;32:313.
2. Al-Fouzan AS, Nanda A. Dermatophytosis of children in Kuwait. *Pediatr Dermatol* 1992;9:27.
3. Lee JYY, Hsu ML. Pathogenesis of hair infection and black dots in tinea capitis caused by *Trichophyton violaceum*: a histopathological study. *J Cutan Pathol* 1992;19:54.
4. Vargo K, Cohen BA. Prevalence of undetected tinea capitis in household members of children with disease. *Pediatrics* 1993;92:155.
5. Hayes AG, Buntin DM, Wible LO. Black dot tinea capitis in a man. *Int J Dermatol* 1993;32:740.
6. Venugopal PV, Venugopal TV. Tinea capitis in Saudi Arabia. *Int J Dermatol* 1993;32:39.
7. Rippon JW. Forty-four years of dermatophytes in a Chicago clinic (1944-1988). *Mycopathologia* 1992;119:25.
8. Rogers M, Muir D, Pritchard R. Increasing importance of *Trichophyton tonsurans* in childhood tinea in New South Wales. The pattern of childhood tinea in New South Wales, Australia, 1979-1988: The emergence of *Trichophyton tonsurans* as an important pathogen in tinea capitis in white children. *Aust J Dermatol* 1993;34:5.
9. Odom R. Pathophysiology of dermatophyte infections. *J Am Acad Dermatol* 1993;28:S2.
10. Aly R. Ecology and epidemiology of dermatophyte infections. *J Am Acad Dermatol* 1994;31:S21.
11. Rippon JW. Dermatophytosis and dermatomycosis. In: Rippon JW, ed. *Medical mycology: the pathogenic fungi and the pathogenic actinomycetes*, 3rd ed. Philadelphia: WB Saunders, 1988:175–177.
12. Hay RJ, Roberts SOB, MacKenzie DWR. Mycology. In: Champion RH, Burton JL, Ebling FJG, eds. *Textbook of dermatology*, 5th ed. Boston: Blackwell Scientific, 1992:1127–1216.
13. Venugopal PV, Venugopal TV. Superficial mycoses in Saudi Arabia. *Aust J Dermatol* 1992;33:45.
14. Rosenthal JR. Pediatric fungal infections from head to toe: what's new? *Curr Opin Pediatr* 1994;6:435.
15. Stiller MJ, Rosenthal SA, Weinstein AS. Tinea capitis caused by *Trichophyton rubrum* in a 67 year old woman with systemic lupus erythematosus. *J Am Acad Dermatol* 1993;29:257.
16. Hay RJ. Fungal skin infections. *Arch Dis Child* 1992;67:1065.
17. Garg AP, Muller J. Fungitoxicity of fatty acids against dermatophytes. *Mycoses* 1993;36:51.
18. Garg AP, Muller J. Inhibition of growth of dermatophytes by Indian hair oils. *Mycoses* 1992;35:363.
19. Lunder M, Lunder M. Is *Microsporum canis* infection about to become a serious dermatological problem? *Dermatology* 1992;184:87.
20. López-Gómez S, Del Palacio A, Van Cutsem J, et al. Itraconazole versus griseofulvin in the treatment of tinea capitis: a double-blind randomized study in children. *Int J Dermatol* 1994;33:743.
21. Honig PJ, Caputo GL, Leyden JJ, et al. Microbiology of kerions. *J Pediatr* 1993;123:422.
22. Honig PJ, Caputo GL, Leyden JJ, et al. Treatment of kerions. *Pediatr Dermatol* 1994;11:69.
23. American Academy of Dermatology. Guidelines of care for superficial mycotic infections of the skin: tinea capitis and tinea barbae. In: *Dermatology world/guidelines* (supplement). Schaumburg, IL: American Academy of Dermatology, 1995:39–43.
24. Gondim-Goncalves HM, Mapurunga ACP, Melo-Monteiro C, et al. Tinea capitis caused by *Microsporum canis* in a newborn. *Int J Dermatol* 1992;31:367.
25. Virgili A, Corazza M, Zampino MR. Atypical features of tinea in newborns. *Pediatr Dermatol* 1993;10:92.
26. Cabon N, Moulinier C, Taieb A, et al. Tinea capitis and faciei caused by *Microsporon langeronii* in two neonates. *Pediatr Dermatol* 1994;11:281.
27. Hiruma M, Kukita A. Tinea faciei caused by *Microsporum canis* in a newborn. *Dermatologica* 1988;176:130.
28. Johnson ML, Anderson LL. Papulosquamous plaques in a mother and newborn son. *Pediatr Dermatol* 1995;12:281.
29. Snider R, Landers S, Levy ML. The ringworm riddle: an outbreak of *Microsporum canis* in the nursery. *Pediatr Infect Dis J* 1998;12:145.
30. Arnow PM, Houchins SG, Pugliese G. An outbreak of tinea corporis in hospital personnel caused by a patient with *Trichophyton tonsurans* infection. *Pediatr Infect Dis J* 1991;10:355.
31. Pakula AS, Paller AS. Langerhans cell histiocytosis and dermatophytosis. *J Am Acad Dermatol* 1993;29:340.
32. Hubbard TW, de Triquet JM. Brush-culture method for diagnosing tinea capitis. *Pediatrics* 1992;90:416.
33. Frieden IJ, Howard R. Tinea capitis: epidemiology, diagnosis, treatment, and control. *J Am Acad Dermatol* 1994;31:542.
34. Gatti S, Marinaro C, Bianchi L, et al. Treatment of kerion with fluconazole. *Lancet* 1991;338:1156.
35. Elewski B. Tinea capitis: itraconazole in *Trichophyton tonsurans* infection. *J Am Acad Dermatol* 1994;31:65.
36. Legendre R, Escola-Macre J. Itraconazole in the treatment of tinea capitis. *J Am Acad Dermatol* 1990;23:559.
37. Haroon TS, Hussain I, Mahmood A, et al. An open clinical pilot study of the efficacy and safety of oral terbinafine in dry noninflammatory tinea capitis. *Br J Dermatol* 1992;126(Suppl 39):47.
38. Terbinafine for dermatophytes in skin and nail. *Drug Ther Bull* 1992;30:47.
39. Derrick EK, Voyce ME, Price ML. *Trichophyton tonsurans* kerion in an elderly woman. *Br J Dermatol* 1994;130:683.
40. Gordon PM. Rapid clearing of kerion ringworm with terbinafine. *Br J Dermatol* 1993;129:503.
41. Goulden V, Goodfield MJD. Treatment of childhood dermatophyte infections with oral terbinafine. *Pediatr Dermatol* 1995;12:53.
42. Degreef HJ, De Doncker PRG. Current therapy of dermatophytosis. *J Am Acad Dermatol* 1994;31:S25.
43. DeHart DJ. Tinea capitis. *N Engl J Med* 1993;329:849.
44. Halasz CLG. Successful treatment with fluconazole of tinea corporis caused by *Trichophyton verrucosum* (barn itch). *Cutis* 1994;54:207.
45. Shwayder T, Andreae M, Babel D. *Trichophyton equinum* from riding bareback: first reported U.S. case. *J Am Acad Dermatol* 1994;30:785.
46. Terragni L, Marelli MA, Oriani A, et al. Tinea corporis bullosa. *Mycoses* 1993;36:135.
47. Katoh T, Maruyama R, Nishioka K, et al. Tinea corporis due to *Microsporum canis* from an asymptomatic dog. *J Dermatol* 1991;18:356.
48. Janniger CK. Majocchi's granuloma. *Cutis* 1992;50:267.
49. Radentz WH, Yanase DJ. Papular lesions in an immunocompromised patient. *Arch Dermatol* 1993;129:1189.
50. American Academy of Dermatology. Guidelines of care for superficial mycotic infections of the skin: tinea corporis, tinea cruris, tinea faciei, tinea manuum, and tinea pedis. In: *Dermatology world/guidelines* (Supplement). Schaumburg, IL: American Academy of Dermatology, 1995:22–26.
51. Stiller MJ, Klein WP, Dorman RI, et al. Tinea corporis gladiatorum: an epidemic of *Trichophyton tonsurans* in student wrestlers. *J Am Acad Dermatol* 1992;27:632.
52. Cohen BA, Schmidt C. Tinea gladiatorum. *N Engl J Med* 1992;327:820.
53. Werninghaus K. Tinea corporis in wrestlers (letter). *J Am Acad Dermatol* 1993;28:1022.
54. Cohen D, Foa H, Sangueza OP. Trichophytosis gladiatorum (letter). *J Am Acad Dermatol* 1993;28:1022.
55. Beller M, Gessner BD. An outbreak of tinea corporis gladiatorum on a high school wrestling team. *J Am Acad Dermatol* 1994;31:197.

56. Budimulja U, Kuswadji K, Bramono S, et al. A double-blind, randomized, stratified controlled study of the treatment of tinea imbricata with oral terbinafine or itraconazole. *Br J Dermatol* 1994;130(Suppl 43):29.
57. Baudraz-Rosselet F, Ruffieux P, Mancarella A, et al. Diaper dermatitis due to *Trichophyton verrucosum*. *Pediatr Dermatol* 1993;10:368.
58. Education called best means of controlling tinea pedis. *Mycology Observer* 1995;13:4.
59. Elewski B, Hay RJ. International Summit on Cutaneous Antifungal Therapy. Boston, Nov. 11–13, 1994. *J Am Acad Dermatol* 1995;33:816.
60. Roberts DT. Prevalence of dermatophyte onychomycosis in the United Kingdom: results of an omnibus survey. *Br J Dermatol* 1992;126(Suppl 39):23.
61. Williams HC. The epidemiology of onychomycosis in Britain. *Br J Dermatol* 1993;129:101.
62. Kearse HL, Miller OF. Tinea pedis in prepubertal children: does it occur? *J Am Acad Dermatol* 1988;19:619.
63. McBride A, Cohen BA. Tinea pedis in children. *Am J Dis Child* 1992;146:844.
64. Leyden JL. Tinea pedis pathophysiology and treatment. *J Am Acad Dermatol* 1994;31:531.
65. Leyden JJ. Progression of interdigital infections from simplex to complex. *J Am Acad Dermtol* 1993;28:S7.
66. Nolting S, Bräutigam M. Clinical relevance of the antibacterial activity of terbinafine: a contralateral comparison between 1% terbinafine cream and 0.1% gentamicin sulphate cream in pyoderma. *Br J Dermatol* 1992;126(Suppl 39):56.
67. Dahl MV, Grando SA. Chronic dermatophytosis: what is special about *Trichophyton rubrum*? *Adv Dermatol* 1994;9:97–99, discussion 110.
68. Reynolds RD, Boiko S, Lucky AW. Exacerbation of tinea corporis during treatment with 1% clotrimazole/0.05% betamethasone dipropionate (Lotrisone). *Am J Dis Child* 1991;145:1224.
69. Amantea MA, Drutz DJ, Rosenthal JR. Antifungals: a primary care primer. *Patient Care* 1990;24:58.
70. Elmets CA. Management of common superficial fungal infections in patients with AIDS. *J Am Acad Dermatol* 1994;31:560.
71. Odom RB. Common superficial fungal infections in immunosuppressed patients. *J Am Acad Dermatol* 1994;31:S56.
72. American Academy of Dermatology. Guidelines of care for superficial mycotic infections of the skin: onychomycosis. In: *Dermatology world/guidelines* (Supplement). Schaumburg, IL: American Academy of Dermatology, 1995:27–32.
73. Diagnosis and management of cutaneous fungal infections: *Pityrosporum* infections, onychomycosis, common superficial fungal infections in patients with HIV infections. In: *Clinical mycology update.* Fairlawn, OH: Research Center, 1995:1–7.
74. Midgley G, Moore MK, Cook JC, et al. Mycology of nail disorders. *J Am Acad Dermatol* 1994;31:S68.
75. Nolting S, Bräutigam M, Weidinger G. Terbinafine in onychomycosis with involvement by non-dermatophytic fungi. *Br J Dermatol* 1994;130(Suppl 43):16.
76. Scher RK, Barnett JM. Successful treatment of *Aspergillus flavus* onychomycosis with oral itraconazole. *J Am Acad Dermatol* 1990;23:749.
77. Lauharanta J. Comparative efficacy and safety of amorolfine nail lacquer 2% versus 5% once weekly. *Clin Exp Dermatol* 1992;17(Suppl 1):41.
78. Reinel D. Topical treatment of onychomycosis with amorolfine 5% nail lacquer: comparative efficacy and tolerability of once and twice weekly use. *Dermatology* 1992;184(Suppl 1):21.
79. Haria M, Bryson HM. Amorolfine. A review of its pharmacological properties and therapeutic potential in the treatment of onychomycosis and other superficial fungal infections. *Drugs* 1995;49:103.
80. Goldgeier MH. Fungal infections of the skin, hair, and nails. *Pediatr Ann* 1993;22:253.
81. Cohen PR, Scher RK. Topical and surgical treatment of onychomycosis. *J Am Acad Dermatol* 1994;31:574.
82. Piérard GE, Arrese-Estrada J, Piérard-Franchimont C. Treatment of onychomycosis: traditional approaches. *J Am Acad Dermatol* 1993;29:541.
83. Roseeuw D, De Doncker P. New approaches to the treatment of onychomycosis. *J Am Acad Dermatol* 1993;29:545.
84. Roberts DT. Oral therapeutic agents in fungal nail disease. *J Am Acad Dermatol* 1994;31:578.
85. Systemic antifungal drugs. *Med Lett Drugs Ther* 1994;36:16.
86. Bickers DR. Antifungal therapy: potential interactions with other classes of drugs. *J Am Acad Dermatol* 1994;31:S87.
87. Villars VV, Jones TC. Special features of the clinical use of oral terbinafine in the treatment of fungal diseases. *Br J Dermatol* 1992;126(Suppl 39):61.
88. Watson A, Marley J, Ellis D, et al. Terbinafine in onychomycosis of the toenail: a novel treatment protocol. *J Am Acad Dermatol* 1995;33:775.
89. Tüzün Y, Kotogyan A, Oguz O. Terbinafine: efficacy and safety in the treatment of dermatophytosis. *Int J Dermatol* 1992;31:720.
90. Arikian SR, Einarson TR, Kobelt-Nguyen G, et al. A multinational pharmacoeconomic analysis of oral therapies for onychomycosis. The onychomycosis study group. *Br J Dermatol* 1994;130(Suppl 43):35.
91. Einarson TR, Arikian SR, Shear NH. Cost-effectiveness analysis for onychomycosis therapy in Canada from a government perspective. *Br J Dermatol* 1994;130(Suppl 43):32.
92. American Academy of Dermatology. Guidelines of care for superficial mycotic infections of the skin: piedra. In: *Dermatology world/guidelines* (Supplement). Schaumburg, IL: American Academy of Dermatology, 1995:33–35.
93. Kalter DC, Tschen JA, Cernoch PL, et al. Genital white piedra: epidemiology, microbiology, and therapy. *J Am Acad Dermatol* 1986;14:982.
94. Ellner KM, McBride ME, Kalter DC, et al. White piedra: evidence for a synergistic infection. *Br J Dermatol* 1990;123:355.
95. McBride ME, Ellner KM, Black HS, et al. A new *Brevibacterium* sp. isolated from infected genital hair of patients with white piedra. *J Med Microbiol* 1993;39:255.
96. Fusaro RM, Miller NG. Onychomycosis caused by *Trichosporon beigelii* in the United States. *J Am Acad Dermatol* 1984;11:747.
97. Nahass GT, Rosenberg SP, Leonardi CL, et al. Disseminated infection with *Trichosporon beigelii*. *Arch Dermatol* 1993;129:1020.
98. Hospenthal D, Belay T, Lappin P, et al. Disseminated trichosporonosis in a neutropenic murine model. *Mycopathologia* 1993;122:115.
99. El-Ani AS, Castillo NB. Disseminated infection with *Trichosporon beigelii*. *NY State J Med* 1984;84:457.
100. Gip L. Black piedra: the first case treated with terbinafine (Lamisil®). *Br J Dermatol* 1994;130(Suppl 43):26.
101. Rippon JW. Superficial infections. In: Rippon JW, ed. *Medical mycology: the pathogenic fungi and the pathogenic actinomycetes*, 3rd ed. Philadelphia: WB Saunders, 1988:154–168.
102. Frankel DH, Rippon JW. *Hendersonula toruloidea* infection in man. Index cases in the non-endemic North American host, and a review of the literature. *Mycopathologia* 1989;105:175.
103. Elewski BE, Greer DL. *Hendersonula toruloidea* and *Scytalidium hyalinum*: review and update. *Arch Dermatol* 1991;127:1041.
104. Gupta AK, Sauder DN, Shear NH. Antifungal agents: an overview. Part II. *J Am Acad Dermatol* 1994;30:911.
105. Hay RJ. Antifungal drugs on the horizon. *J Am Acad Dermatol* 1994;31:S82.
106. Clayton YM. Relevance of broad-spectrum and fungicidal activity of antifungals in the treatment of dermatomycoses. *Br J Dermatol* 1994;130(Suppl 43):7.
107. Faergemann J. *Pityrosporum* infections. *J Am Acad Dermatol* 1994;31:518.
108. Broberg A, Faergemann J, Johansson S, et al. *Pityrosporum ovale* and atopic dermatitis in children and young adults. *Acta Derm Venereol (Stockh)* 1992;72:187.
109. Garcia CR, Johnston BL, Corvi G, et al. Intravenous catheter-associated *Malassezia furfur* fungemia. *Am J Med* 1987;83:790.
110. Long JG, Keyserling HL. Catheter-related infection in infants due to an unusual lipophilic yeast-*Malassezia furfur*. *Pediatrics* 1985;76:896.
111. American Academy of Dermatology. Guidelines of care for superficial mycotic infections of the skin: pityriasis (tinea) versicolor. In: *Dermatology world/guidelines* (Supplement). Schaumburg, IL: American Academy of Dermatology, 1995:36–38.
112. Fungal infections. In: Arndt KA, Bowers KE, Chuttani AR, eds. *Manual of dermatologic therapeutics*, 5th ed. Boston: Little, Brown, 1995:75–89.
113. Delescluse J. Itraconazole in tinea versicolor: a review. *J Am Acad Dermatol* 1990;23:551.
114. Galadari I, El Komy M, Mousa A, et al. Tinea versicolor: histologic and ultrastructural investigation of pigmentary changes. *Int J Dermatol* 1992;31:253.
115. Griffiths WAD, Leigh IM, Marks R. Disorders of keratinization. In: Champion RH, Burton JL, Ebling FJG, eds. *Textbook of dermatology*, 5th ed. Boston: Blackwell Scientific, 1992:1390.
116. Lee MP, Stiller MJ, McClain SA, et al. Confluent and reticulated papillomatosis: response to high-dose oral isotretinoin therapy and reassessment of epidemiologic data. *J Am Acad Dermatol* 1994;31:327.
117. Hodge JA, Ray MC. Confluent and reticulated papillomatosis: response to isotretinoin. *J Am Acad Dermatol* 1991;24:654.
118. Barnette DJ Jr, Yeager JK. A progressive asymptomatic hyperpigmented papular eruption. Confluent and reticulated papillomatosis (CRP) of Gougerot and Carteaud. *Arch Dermatol* 1993;129:1608.
119. Baalbaki SA, Malak JA, Al-Khars MAA. Confluent and reticulated papillomatosis. Treatment with etretinate. *Arch Dermatol* 1993;129:961.
120. Jimbow M, Talpash O, Jimbow K. Confluent and reticulated papillomatosis: clinical light and electron microscopic studies. *Int J Dermatol* 1992;31:480.
121. Lee SH, Choi EH, Lee WS, et al. Confluent and reticulated papillomatosis: a clinical, histopathological, and electron microscopic study. *J Dermatol* 1991;18:725.
122. Redline RW, Redline SS, Boxerbaum B, et al. Systemic *Malassezia furfur* infections in patients receiving intralipid therapy. *Hum Pathol* 1985;16:815.
123. Powell DA, Aungst J, Snedden S, et al. Broviac catheter-related *Malassezia furfur* sepsis in five infants receiving intravenous fat emulsions. *J Pediatr* 1984;105:987.
124. Dahl MV. Suppression of immunity and inflammation by products produced by dermatophytes. *J Am Acad Dermatol* 1993;28:519.
125. Brasch JB, Sterry W. Immunophenotypical characterization of inflammatory cellular infiltrates in tinea. *Acta Derm Venereol (Stockh)* 1992;72:345.
126. Szepes E, Magyarlaki M, Battyani Z, et al. Immunohistochemical characterization of the cellular infiltrate in dermatophytosis. *Mycoses* 1993;36:203.
127. Dahl MV. Dermatophytosis and the immune response. *J Am Acad Dermatol* 1994;31:534.
128. Blake JS, Dahl MV, Herron MJ, et al. An immunoinhibitory cell wall glycoprotein (mannan) from *Trichophyton rubrum*. *J Invest Dermatol* 1991;96:657.
129. Jones HE. Immune response and host resistance of humans to dermatophyte infection. *J Am Acad Dermatol* 1993;28:512.

130. Koga T, Ishizaki H, Matsumoto T, et al. Cytokine production of peripheral blood mononuclear cells in a dermatophytosis patient in response to stimulation with trichophytin. *J Dermatol* 1993;20:441.

131. Ohashi DK, Crane JS, Spira TJ, et al. Idiopathic CD4+ T-cell lymphocytopenia with verrucae, basal cell carcinomas, and chronic tinea corporis infection. *J Am Acad Dermatol* 1994;31:889.

132. Smith KJ, Skelton HG, Yeager J, et al. Cutaneous findings in HIV-1-positive patients: a 42-month prospective study. *J Am Acad Dermatol* 1994;31:746.

133. Elewski BE, Sullivan J. Dermatophytes as opportunistic pathogens. *J Am Acad Dermatol* 1994;30:1021.

134. Grossman ME, Pappert AS, Garzon MC, et al. Invasive *Trichophyton rubrum* infection in the immunocompromised host: report of three cases. *J Am Acad Dermatol* 1995;33:315.

135. Cohen PR, Maor MH. Tinea corporis confined to irradiated skin: radiation port dermatophytosis. *Cancer* 1992;70:1634.

136. Walzman M, Leeming JG. White piedra and *Trichosporon beigelii*: the incidence in patients attending a clinic in genitourinary medicine. *Genitourin Med* 1989;65:331.

137. Walsh TJ. Trichosporonosis. *Infect Dis Clin North Am* 1989;3:43.

138. McWhinney PH, Madgwick JC, Hoffbrand AV, et al. Successful surgical management of septic arthritis due to *Trichosporon beigelii* in a patient with acute myeloid leukemia. *Scand J Infect Dis* 1992;24:245.

139. Grainger CR. White piedra: a case with evidence of spread by contact. *Trans R Soc Trop Med Hyg* 1986;80:87.

140. Torssander J, Carlsson B, Von Krogh G. *Trichosporon beigelii*: increased occurrence in homosexual men. *Mykosen* 1985;28:355.

141. Stenderup A, Schonheyder H, Ebbesen P, et al. White piedra and *Trichosporon beigelii* carriage in homosexual men. *J Med Vet Mycol* 1986;24:401.

142. Ellner K, McBride ME, Rosen T, et al. Prevalence of *Trichosporon beigelii*. Colonization of normal perigenital skin. *J Med Vet Mycol* 1991;29:99.

143. Moreno-Giménez JC. Infections by *Trichophyton rubrum* (letter). *J Am Acad Dermatol* 1991;24:323.

144. Sheetz K, Lynch PJ. Ichthyosis and dermatophyte fungal infection (letter). *J Am Acad Dermatol* 1991;24:321.

145. Shelley ED, Shelley WB, Schafer RL. Generalized *Trichophyton rubrum* infection in congenital ichthyosiform erythroderma. *J Am Acad Dermatol* 1989;20:1133.

146. Agostini G, Geti V, Difonzo EM, et al. Dermatophyte infection in ichthyosis vulgaris. *Mycoses* 1992;35:197.

147. Nielsen PG. Hereditary palmoplantar keratoderma and dermatophytosis in the northernmost county of Sweden (Norrbotten). *Acta Derm Venereol Suppl (Stockh)* 1994;188:1.

148. Smith EB. Topical antifungal drugs in the treatment of tinea pedis, tinea cruris, and tinea corporis. *J Am Acad Dermatol* 1993;28:524.

149. Berman B, Ellis C, Leyden J, et al. Efficacy of a 1-week, twice-daily regimen of terbinafine 1% cream in the treatment of interdigital tinea pedis. *J Am Acad Dermatol* 1992;26:956.

150. Savin R, Atton AV, Bergstresser PR, et al. Efficacy of terbinafine 1% cream in the treatment of moccasin-type tinea pedis: results of placebo-controlled multicenter trials. *J Am Acad Dermatol* 1994;30:663.

151. Macura AB. In vitro susceptibility of dermatophytes to antifungal drugs: a comparison of two methods. *Int J Dermatol* 1993;32:533.

152. Venugopal PV, Venugopal TV. Disk diffusion susceptibility testing of dermatophytes with allylamines. *Int J Dermatol* 1994;33:730.

153. Nishikawa T, Naka W. Evaluation of antifungal effects of terbinafine and itraconazole using neutral red staining. *Br J Dermatol* 1994;130(Suppl 43):4.

154. Aly R, Bayles CI, Oakes RA, et al. Topical griseofulvin in the treatment of dermatophytoses. *Clin Exp Dermatol* 1994;19:43.

155. Macasaet EN, Pert P. Topical (1%) solution of griseofulvin in the treatment of tinea corporis (letter). *Br J Dermatol* 1991;124:110.

156. Butty P, Mallie M, Bastide JM. Antifungal activity of allylamines on *Epidermophyton floccosum*: scanning electron microscopy study. *Mycopathologia* 1992;120:147.

157. Brasch J, Christophers E. Azelaic acid has antimycotic properties in vitro. *Dermatology* 1993;186:55.

158. Zaias N, Berman B, Cordero CN, et al. Efficacy of a 1-week, once-daily regimen of terbinafine 1% cream in the treatment of tinea cruris and tinea corporis. *J Am Acad Dermatol* 1993;29:646.

159. Evans EGV, Dodman B, Williamson DM, et al. Comparison of terbinafine and clotrimazole in treating tinea pedis. *BMJ* 1993;307:645.

160. Bergstresser PR, Elewski B, Hanifin J, et al. Topical terbinafine and clotrimazole in interdigital tinea pedis: a multicenter comparison of cure and relapse rates with 1- and 4-week treatment regimens. *J Am Acad Dermatol* 1993;28:648.

161. Elewski BE, Bergstresser PR, Hanifin J, et al. Long-term outcome of patients with interdigital tinea pedis treated with terbinafine or clotrimazole. *J Am Acad Dermatol* 1995;32:290.

162. Evans EG. A comparison of terbinafine (Lamisil) 1% cream given for one week with clotrimazole (Canesten) 1% cream given for four weeks, in the treatment of tinea pedis. *Br J Dermatol* 1994;130(Suppl 43):12.

163. Evans EGV, Seaman RAJ, James IGV. Short-duration therapy with terbinafine 1% cream in dermatophyte skin infections. *Br J Dermatol* 1994;130:38.

164. Rabinowitz L, Esterly NB. Naftifine (Naftin) in pediatrics. *Pediatrics* 1992;90:652.

165. Turkish Multicenter Dermatophytosis Study Group. Naftifine treatment for dermatophytosis: multicenter clinical investigations in Turkey. *Int J Dermatol* 1992;31:247.

166. Nolting S, Reinel D, Semig G, et al. Amorolfine spray in the treatment of foot mycoses (a dose-finding study). *Br J Dermatol* 1993;129:170.

167. Voravutinon V. Oral treatment of tinea corporis and tinea cruris with terbinafine and griseofulvin: a randomized double blind comparative study. *J Med Assoc Thai* 1993;76:388.

168. Lachapelle JM, De Doncker P, Tennstedt D, et al. Itraconazole compared with griseofulvin in the treatment of tinea corporis/cruris and tinea pedis/manus: an interpretation of the clinical results of all completed double-blind studies with respect to the pharmacokinetic profile. *Dermatology* 1992;184:45.

169. Katsambas A, Antoniou C, Frangouli E, et al. Itraconazole in the treatment of tinea corporis and tinea cruris. *Clin Exp Dermatol* 1993;18:322.

170. Suchil P, Gei FM, Robles M, et al. Once-weekly oral doses of fluconazole 150 mg in the treatment of tinea corporis/cruris and cutaneous candidiasis. *Clin Exp Dermatol* 1992;17:397.

171. Montero-Gei F, Perera A. Therapy with fluconazole for tinea corporis, tinea cruris, and tinea pedis. *Clin Infect Dis* 1992;14(Suppl 1):S77.

172. Stengel F, Robles-Soto M, Galimberti R, et al. Fluconazole versus ketoconazole in the treatment of dermatophytoses and cutaneous candidiasis. *Int J Dermatol* 1994;33:733.

173. Segal R, Trattner A, Alteras I, et al: Once-weekly treatment with oral ketoconazole for superficial fungal infections. *J Am Acad Dermatol* 1993;28:126.

174. Decroix J. Tinea pedis (moccasin-type) treated with itraconazole. *Int J Dermatol* 1995;34:122.

175. Pariser DM, Pariser RJ, Ruoff G, et al. Double-blind comparison of itraconazole and placebo in the treatment of tinea corporis and tinea cruris. *J Am Acad Dermatol* 1994;31:232.

176. Ketele A, Moens M, Stoops K, et al. International Registration File R 51211/86. Titusville, NJ: Janssen Pharmaceutica, 1987.

177. Parent D, Decroix J, Heenen M. Clinical experience with short schedules of itraconazole in the treatment of tinea corporis and/or tinea cruris. *Dermatology* 1994;189:378.

178. Faergemann J, Zehender H, Denouël J, et al. Levels of terbinafine in plasma, stratum corneum, dermis-epidermis (without stratum corneum), sebum, hair and nails during and after 250 mg terbinafine orally once per day for four weeks. *Acta Derm Venereol (Stockh)* 1993;73:305.

179. Farag A, Taha M, Halim S. One-week therapy with oral terbinafine in cases of tinea cruris/corporis. *Br J Dermatol* 1994;131:684.

180. De Keyser P, De Backer M, Massart DL, et al. Two-week oral treatment of tinea pedis, comparing terbinafine (250 mg/day) with itraconazole (100 mg/day): a double-blind, multicentre study. *Br J Dermatol* 1994;130(Suppl 43):22.

181. Hay RJ, Logan RA, Moore MK, et al. A comparative study of terbinafine versus griseofulvin in 'dry-type' dermatophyte infections. *J Am Acad Dermatol* 1991;24:243.

182. Rosen T, Elewski B. Failure of clotrimazole-betamethasone dipropionate cream in treatment of *Microsporum canis* infections. *J Am Acad Dermatol* 1995;32:1050.

Viral Exanthems and Localized Viral Skin Infections

CHAPTER 137
Measles

Michael A. Gerber and Gilbert M. Schiff

The epidemiology of measles (rubeola) in developed countries has been altered dramatically by the introduction of effective vaccines (1). Before licensure of the measles vaccine in 1963, approximately 500,000 cases and 500 deaths were reported annually in the United States. In 1999, a total of 100 confirmed cases of measles were reported (2). Most of these cases were imported from countries in Europe and Asia or were linked to imported cases. Available data strongly suggest that measles is no longer endemic in the United States (2). In contrast, in developing areas of the world, measles has high attack rates among children younger than 12 months of age and is associated with case fatality rates as high as 25%.

CLINICAL MANIFESTATIONS

The incubation period for measles, during which the patient is usually asymptomatic, is 10 to 11 days, although it may be longer in adults (Fig. 137.1). The illness is ushered in by the appearance of fever and malaise, probably coinciding with the secondary viremia; these findings are accompanied within 24 hours by coryza, conjunctivitis, and cough. These clinical findings gradually increase in severity and peak with the appearance of the exanthem on the fourth day. The typical case of measles lasts 7 to 10 days.

There is usually a stepwise increases in temperature until the fifth or sixth day of illness. The maximal temperature coincides with the peak of the eruption and then rapidly falls to normal over the next 24 hours. In some patients, the temperature may peak by the end of the first day and remain elevated at 39.5°C to 40.5°C for the next 5 to 6 days. Fever that persists for more than 3 days after the onset of the rash should raise suspicion of a complication.

Respiratory findings are similar to those seen with a severe common cold. Coryza begins with frequent sneezing followed by nasal congestion and a copious, mucopurulent discharge, which becomes most prominent at the peak of the exanthem. The cough has a brassy quality, and although there is usually marked improvement when the eruption subsides, a mild cough may persist for several weeks.

The degree of conjunctivitis can be quite variable, but marked inflammation of the conjunctivae may be associated with edema of the lids and caruncles. There is increased lacrimation. Photophobia is common and may be severe in older patients. The conjunctivitis disappears shortly after the fever has subsided.

Koplik spots, the pathognomonic enanthem of measles, are faint, white 1- to 2-mm elevated lesions on an erythematous background located on the buccal mucosa. They usually appear opposite the lower molars 2 days before the onset of rash. By the end of the second day of the rash, the spots begin to fade rapidly, and, by the end of the third day of rash, the mucous membranes appear normal.

The rash of measles appears about the 14th or 15th day after exposure, and 4 days after the onset of illness. The erythematous maculopapular eruption begins at the hairline and involves the area behind the ears, the forehead, and the upper part of the neck. It then spreads downward, and, by the third day, the face, neck, trunk, upper extremities, buttocks, and lower extremities are involved. The soles of the feet and the palms of the hands are not involved. The initial lesions are light pink and discrete, but they become confluent at the earliest involved sites. Those on the extremities remain fairly discrete. The exanthem begins to fade by the third day, following the same sequence as its appearance. The initial color of the rash is red, and the lesions blanch with pressure. After 3 to 4 days, as the rash begins to fade, it assumes a brownish coppery appearance. This brownish discoloration does not clear with pressure and probably represents staining of the skin as a result of capillary hemorrhages. The exanthem typically lasts 5 to 6 days; its end is marked by a fine desquamation usually involving the confluent areas.

Malaise and anorexia are common during the febrile period, and young children may occasionally have diarrhea, vomiting, and abdominal pain. Measles may be associated with enlarged cervical, postauricular, and occipital lymph nodes. In moderate-to-severe cases, there may be generalized lymphadenopathy. Most patients with measles also have varying degrees of laryngotracheitis, bronchitis, bronchiolitis, and pneumonitis caused by the primary viral infection.

At the height of the illness, usually the second day of the rash, the patient appears to be quite miserable with a diffuse rash, high temperature, malaise, copious nasal discharge, cough, and conjunctivitis. However, within the next 24 to 36 hours the

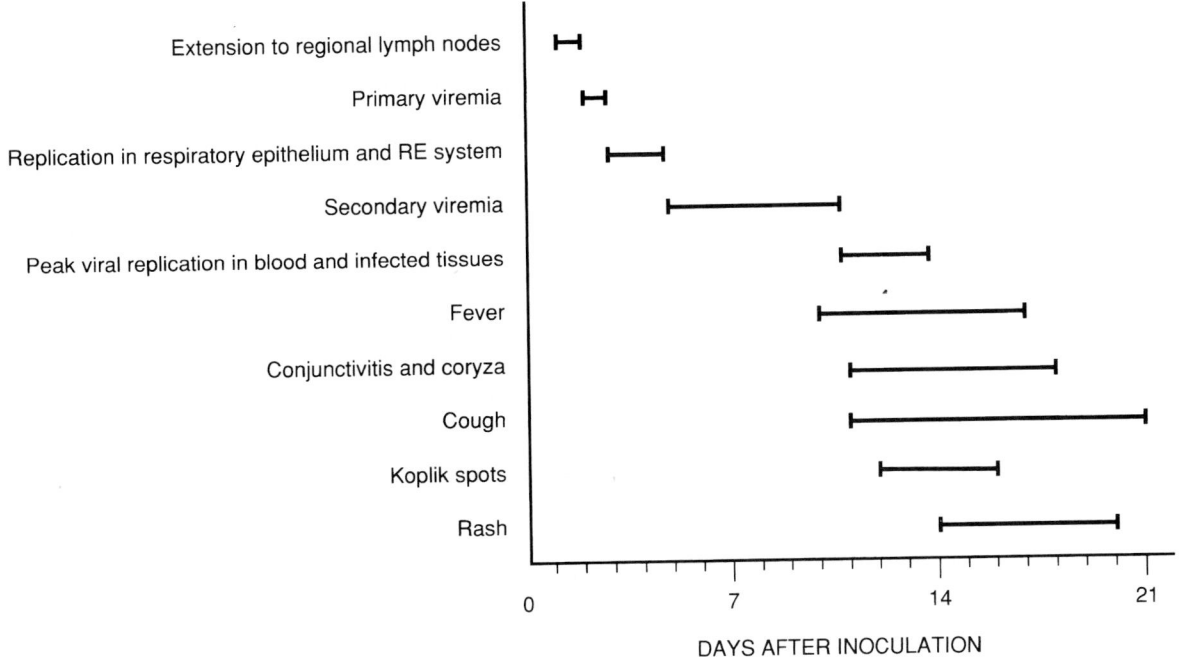

Figure 137.1. After inoculation of the epithelial surface of the nasopharynx, this sequence of events takes place during uncomplicated measles. RE, Reticuloendothelial.

temperature falls, the coryza and conjunctivitis clear, and the cough decreases in severity, and within a few days the child is well. Although nutritional status and age are commonly thought of as the major risk factors for severe infections, some investigators have suggested that overcrowding and intensive exposure may be more important factors (3).

Atypical Measles

In 1965, Rauh and Schmidt reported a severe, atypical form of measles occurring in children who had received inactivated measles vaccine 2 to 4 years before exposure to wild-type measles (4). Although far more common after administration of inactivated measles vaccine, a similar atypical syndrome has been reported in children who had received live measles vaccine (5).

The incubation period of atypical measles is similar to that of typical measles, but the prodromal period is marked by the acute onset of high fever and headache. The exanthem usually appears after a prodrome of 1 to 3 days. In contrast to the rash of typical measles, the rash of atypical measles begins peripherally and progresses in a cephalad direction. The rash is usually maculopapular but can be urticarial, petechial, or purpuric; it is most prominent on the ankles and wrists and may involve the palms and soles. In some cases, the rash becomes vesicular and may resemble the exanthem of varicella. Although coryza and conjunctivitis are less prominent than in typical measles, respiratory distress is common. Radiographic evaluation reveals pulmonary involvement in virtually all cases and patients are frequently severely ill with high fever. The illness may last 2 weeks or more.

Modified Measles

Modified measles is a mild form that occurs in partially immune individuals. Partial immunity can result from the presence of maternally-derived, transplacental antibody (infants younger than 9 months old), the administration of serum immune globulin (IG) to exposed, susceptible children, or the administration of live measles vaccine. Modified measles may also rarely occur as a reinfection in those with documented previous measles (6).

The symptoms of modified measles are similar to, but milder than, those of typical measles. The incubation period may be longer (14 to 21 days) and the prodromal period slightly shorter. Cough, coryza, conjunctivitis, and fever are minimal and Koplik spots are few in number or absent. Similarly, the exanthem follows the same progression as that in typical measles but is milder and confluence of lesions rarely occurs.

MEASLES IN IMMUNOCOMPROMISED PATIENTS

Measles infections in patients who are immunocompromised either by chemotherapy or by inherited or acquired disorders of cell-mediated immunity (e.g., severely malnourished children) are usually severe and often fatal (7,8). One of the more common complications of measles in immunocompromised patients, and the one responsible for the largest number of deaths, is giant cell pneumonia (7,8). A unique form of measles encephalitis has also been described in patients with deficits in cell-mediated immunity (9). This encephalitis is chronic and resembles subacute sclerosing panencephalitis (SSPE), but has an incubation period of only 5 weeks to 6 months.

HUMAN IMMUNODEFICIENCY VIRUS INFECTION

Reports have emphasized the severe nature of measles infection in children infected with HIV (9,10). As in other patients with impaired T-cell immunity, HIV-infected children can develop fatal measles infection in the absence of a rash (11).

MEASLES IN PREGNANT WOMEN

Unlike rubella, measles during pregnancy does not appear to cause congenital malformations. However, measles in a pregnant woman can lead to spontaneous abortion, prematurity, and stillbirth (12).

COMPLICATIONS

Complications of measles may be due to an extension of the inflammation caused by the virus, secondary bacterial infection, or a combination of both. The sudden appearance of a leukocytosis or the prolonged presence of fever should alert the physician to the possibility of complications.

Otitis media is the most common complication of measles and the most common cause of a persistent fever. It is more common in infants, those with previous episodes of otitis media, and those with severe measles. The usual pathogens responsible for otitis media are involved.

Some pulmonary involvement occurs in the majority of cases of measles and pneumonia is the leading cause of measles-related deaths. The pneumonia may result from an extension of the viral infection, a superimposed bacterial infection, or a combination of both. Pulmonary complications should be considered in any child with measles in whom respiratory distress associated with persistent or recurrent fever develops.

Neurologic complications of measles can be acute or chronic (see the section on RNA viruses in Part VII and Chapter 244). Acute encephalomyelitis occurs in approximately 0.1% of measles cases. Examination of the cerebrospinal fluid usually reveals a pleocytosis with a lymphocytic predominance, elevated protein level, and a normal glucose level. Symptoms of encephalitis usually develop between the second and sixth days after the onset of the rash. However, they occasionally appear either before or after the presence of the rash (13). The course of the encephalomyelitis may be extremely variable; however, approximately 60% of patients recover completely, 15% die, and 25% have residual brain damage (e.g., mental retardation, recurrent seizures, deafness, hemiplegia, and paraplegia). The cause of the acute encephalomyelitis is not clear. Although measles virus can rarely be recovered from these patients (14), the encephalomyelitis is considered by most investigators to be an autoimmune demyelinating disease (15).

Other central nervous system complications of measles include retrobulbar neuritis, hemiplegia, and cerebellar ataxia. The rare condition of SSPE can be considered a late complication of measles, with an incidence of approximately 1 per 100,000 cases (see Chapter 244).

DIAGNOSIS

The diagnosis of typical measles in an epidemic setting is straightforward and is based on history and physical findings. Sporadic cases in a highly immunized population may be more difficult to diagnose and laboratory tests may be of value in this situation. Virus isolation or rapid detection of measles antigens in nasopharyngeal secretions can be attempted, but these techniques are difficult and not readily available (16). Therefore, laboratory confirmation of measles is usually accomplished by serologic tests that document a significant rise in antibody titer (16). The hemagglutination inhibition assay has been the most commonly used test but is now being replaced by the enzyme-linked immunosorbent assay (ELISA) (17). Acute and convalescent serum samples showing a significant rise in immunoglobulin G antibody confirm the diagnosis, while a positive ELISA test result for immunoglobulin M antibody on a single serum specimen is diagnostic (17).

The differential diagnosis of measles should include all illnesses associated with an erythematous maculopapular rash. The brown discoloration and intensity of the measles rash—in the presence of a history of typical febrile prodrome with cough, coryza, conjunctivitis, and caudal progression of the rash—make differentiation from rubella, erythema infectiosum, roseola infantum, and enteroviral infection relatively simple. A history of possible exposure should always be sought. The exanthems produced by Epstein-Barr virus and *Mycoplasma pneumoniae* infections, and by drug eruptions may be the most difficult to differentiate from measles. The presence of Koplik spots is considered pathognomonic. Modified measles may cause more difficulty in the diagnosis because of the generally milder nature of the illness and the usual absence of Koplik spots. The differential considerations in atypical measles include Rocky Mountain spotted fever, anaphylactoid purpura, *M. pneumoniae* infections, and drug eruptions.

TREATMENT

No specific antiviral drugs or agents have been shown to be effective for the treatment of measles or for the viral complications of measles. Ribavirin is active against measles virus in vitro, and intravenous ribavirin has been used in the treatment of immunocompromised patients with measles pneumonia and encephalitis (18). However, it has not been evaluated in controlled clinical trials. High doses of vitamin A appear to reduce the morbidity and mortality of young children hospitalized with measles in developing countries (19). The World Health Organization has, therefore, recommended vitamin A treatment of children with measles in communities where vitamin A deficiency is a recognized problem and where mortality related to measles is 1% or greater. In the United States, vitamin A supplementation should be considered for patients 6 months to 2 years of age hospitalized with measles and for patients older than 6 months of age with measles and specific risk factors for vitamin A deficiency (20). Antibiotics are indicated when secondary bacterial infection occurs.

PREVENTION

Effective methods (passive and active prophylaxis) are available for the prevention of measles. Exposure to measles is not a contraindication to immunization; if given within 72 hours of exposure, measles vaccine will provide protection in some cases. Vaccine is the intervention of choice for control of measles outbreaks in child care centers and schools.

Passive Immunization

Immune globulin administered to susceptible persons within 6 days of exposure has been shown to be effective in prevent-

ing or modifying measles (20). The usual recommended dose is 0.25 mL/kg given intramuscularly; immunocompromised patients should receive 0.5 mL/kg (maximum dose in either situation is 15 mL). Immune globulin is indicated for susceptible household contacts of patients with measles, particularly contacts less than 1 year of age, pregnant women, and immunocompromised persons for whom the risk of complications is highest. If active disease is prevented by the administration of IG, follow-up active immunization should be given if not contraindicated provided that the child is at least 12 months old. The measles vaccine should be administered at least 5 months after administration of IG (if the dose was 0.25 mL/kg) or 6 months (if the dose was 0.5 mL/kg).

Active Immunization

Highly effective and safe vaccines have been available to prevent measles since 1963. Initially, both inactivated and attenuated live measles vaccines were developed. The inactivated vaccines required a series of inoculations, and the early live attenuated vaccines were administered simultaneously with IG to reduce the high rate of side effects. In 1965, further attenuated live measles vaccines were developed. When used properly, these vaccines are 90% to 95% effective. Factors that must be considered at the time of vaccination include patient's age and immune status, interval since use of IG or other blood products, concurrent illness, and storage conditions.

In 1989, the American Academy of Pediatrics recommended that two doses of measles-containing vaccine be given to all children after their first birthday. The first dose was to be given at 15 months of age (which was subsequently revised to 12 to 15 months) and the second dose was to be given at around 12 years of age. In 1989, the US Public Health Service also recommended two doses of measles vaccine, but the second dose was to be given at 4 to 6 years of age. In 1998, the AAP revised the age for routine administration of the second dose of measles-containing vaccine to 4 to 6 years of age (21). Regardless of the age when given, a second dose of measles-containing vaccine is highly effective in inducing immunity in the 2% to 5% of children who did not have a response to the first dose. Although there have been isolated reports of secondary vaccine failures, most vaccine failures in the United States are primary vaccine failures; the second dose of vaccine is designed to provide protection for children who have experienced a primary vaccine failure.

Hypersensitivity reactions to measles-containing vaccines occur rarely and usually are minor. These reactions have been attributed to trace amounts of gelatin or neomycin, or some other component in the vaccine formulation. Most neomycin allergies manifest as contact dermatitis, which is not a contraindication to receiving measles-containing vaccine. Measles vaccine is produced in chick embryo cell culture but does not contain a significant amount of egg white (ovalbumin) cross-reacting proteins. Children with egg allergy are at low risk for anaphylactic reactions to measles-containing vaccines and skin testing of these children is not predictive of reactions to measles-containing vaccines (20). Pregnancy, recent administration of IG, and certain immunodeficiency conditions are contraindications for receiving measles-containing vaccines.

In the absence of contraindications, all 12 to 15 month old children, as well as recipients of killed vaccine, those who received live vaccine before their first birthday, those who were born after 1957 who have no history of measles or vaccination, those who received an unknown type of measles vaccine from 1963 to 1967 or received an unknown type of vaccine and simultaneous IG, those who were immunized before 1979, and all known susceptible individuals exposed to measles within the past 72 hours should receive measles vaccine.

The available data suggest that many children infected with human immunodeficiency virus (HIV) can be vaccinated safely (22). Measles immunization is recommended at the usual age for persons with asymptomatic HIV infections and for those with symptomatic infection who are not severely immunocompromised. Severely immunocompromised, HIV-infected persons should not receive measles-containing vaccines because vaccine-related pneumonia has been reported in such patients (23). Regardless of their immunization status, all HIV-infected children who are exposed to measles should receive IG prophylaxis because immunization may not provide protection (20).

There has been the recent suggestion, based on a report by Wakefield and colleagues, that immunization with MMR vaccine may be related to the development of autism (24).

Although this report generated great interest and appeared to provide a biologic mechanism by which MMR vaccine could cause autism, the British Medical Research Council and others, found the evidence unconvincing because of a number of serious methodologic flaws (25) and there has never been independent corroboration of their laboratory findings by other investigators in other populations. Furthermore, several comprehensive, epidemiological studies in Great Britain and Sweden could find no temporal relationship between immunization with MMR and the onset of regressive symptoms or between increased reporting of autism and increased use of MMR (26,27). A recent analysis by the California Department of Health Services comparing Developmental Services data with MMR vaccination coverage of children born between 1980 and 1994 found no evidence to support an association between MMR immunization and autism (28). A recent Institute of Medicine Immunization Safety Review Committee and a special review panel commissioned by the American Academy of Pediatrics both concluded that the hypothesis that MMR vaccine may cause autism has little support, and the current scientific evidence argues against a causal association (29,30).

REFERENCES

1. Markowitz LE, Preblud SR, Orenstein WA, et al. Patterns of transmission in measles outbreaks in the United States 1985–1986. N Engl J Med 1989;320:75.
2. Centers for Disease Control. Summary of notifiable diseases, United States, 1999. MMWR 2001;48:1.
3. Aaby P. Malnutrition and overcrowding/intensive exposure in severe measles infection: review of community studies. Rev Infect Dis 1988;10:478.
4. Rauh LW, Schmidt R. Measles immunization with killed virus vaccine: serum antibody titers and experience with exposure to measles epidemic. Am J Dis Child 1965;109:232.
5. Cherry JD, Feigin RD, Lobes LA Jr, et al. Atypical measles in children previously immunized with attenuated measles virus vaccines. Pediatrics 1972;50:712.
6. Cherry JD, Feigin RD, Lobes LA Jr, et al. Urban measles in the vaccine era: a clinical, epidemiologic, and serologic study. J Pediatr 1972;81:217.
7. Meadow SR, Weller RO, Archibald RWR. Fatal systemic measles in a child receiving cyclophosphamide for nephrotic syndrome. Lancet 1969;2:876.
8. Katz M, Stiehm ER. Host defense in malnutrition. Pediatrics 1977;59:490.
9. Krasinski K, Borkowsky W. Measles and measles immunity in children infected with human immunodeficiency virus. JAMA 1989;261:2512.
10. Centers for Disease Control. Epidemiologic notes and reports: measles in HIV infected children, United States. MMWR 1988;37:183.
11. Markowitz LE, Chandler FW, Roldan EO, et al. Fatal measles pneumonia without rash in a child with AIDS. J Infect Dis 1988;158:480.
12. Atmar RL, Englund JA, Hammill H. Complications of measles in pregnancy. Clin Infect Dis 1992;14:217.
13. LaBoccetta AC, Tornay AS. Measles encephalitis: report of 61 cases. Am J Dis Child 1964;107:247.
14. Meulen VT, Kackell Y, Muller D, et al. Isolation of infectious measles virus in measles encephalitis. Lancet 1972;2:1172.
15. Johnson RT, Griffin DE, Hirsch RL, et al. Measles encephalomyelitis: clinical and immunologic studies. N Engl J Med 1984;310:137.
16. Salmi AA. Measles virus. In: Murray PR, ed. Manual of clinical microbiology, 7th ed. Washington DC: ASM Press, 1999:951–958.
17. Rossier E, Miller H, McCulloch B, et al. Comparison of immunofluorescence and enzyme immunoassay for detection of measles-specific immunoglobulin M antibody. J Clin Microbiol 1991;9:1069.
18. Forni AL, Schluger NW, Roberts B. Severe measles pneumonitis in adults. Evaluation of clinical characteristics and therapy with intravenous ribavirin. Clin Infect Dis 1994;19:454.
19. Hussey GD, Klein M. A randomized controlled trial of vitamin A in children with severe measles. N Engl J Med 1990;323:160.
20. Pickering LK, ed. Report of the committee on infectious diseases (2000 red book). In: Measles, 25th ed. Elk Grove Village, IL: American Academy of Pediatrics, 2000:385–396.
21. Committee on Infectious Diseases, American Academy of Pediatrics. Age for routine administration of the second dose of measles-mumps-rubella vaccine. Pediatrics 1998;101:129.
22. Centers for Disease Control and Prevention. Measles, mumps, and rubella - vaccine use and strategies for elimination of measles, rubella and congenital rubella syndrome and control of mumps: recommendations of the Advisory Committee on Immunization Practices (ACIP). MMWR 1998;47(RR-8):21.
23. Centers for Disease Control and Prevention. Measles pneumonitis following measles-mumps-rubella vaccination of a patient with HIV infection. MMWR 1996;45:603.
24. Wakefield AJ, Murch SH, Anthony A, et al. Ileal-lymphoid-nodular hyperplasia, non-specific colitis, and pervasive developmental disorder in children. Lancet 1998;351:637.
25. Medical Research Council. Report of the Strategy Development Group Subgroup on Research Into Inflammatory Bowel Disorders and Autism. London, England: Medical Research Council; 2000. Available at www.mrc.ac.uk/Autism_report.html.
26. Taylor B, Miller E, Farrington CP, et al. Autism and measles, mumps, and rubella vaccine: no epidemiological evidence for a causal association. Lancet 1999;353:2026.
27. Gillberg C, Heijbel H. MMR and autism. Autism 1998;2:423.
28. Dales L, Hammer SJ, Smith NJ. Time trends in autism and in MMR immunization coverage in California. JAMA 2001;285:1183.
29. Halsey NA, Hyman SL, and the Conference Writing Panel. Measles-mumps-rubella vaccine and autistic spectrum disorder: report from the new challenges in childhood immunizations conference convened in Oak Brook, Illinois, June 12-13, 2000. Pediatrics 2001;107(5):e84.
30. Stratton K, Gable A, Shetty P, McCormick M, eds. Immunization safety review: measles-mumps-rubella vaccine and autism. Washington DC: National Academy Press, 2001.

CHAPTER 138

Rubella (German Measles)

Hans M. L. Spiegel and John L. Sever

BACKGROUND

Postnatal rubella infection is usually a mild self-limited illness with few relatively rare complications. The major interest in rubella, and in the development of vaccines against it, has originated in the concern to prevent the devastating consequences that congenital rubella infection of the mother can have for the infant.

EPIDEMIOLOGY

Rubella is a ubiquitous infection that is still present throughout the world. Different epidemiologic patterns have been observed. For developed countries such as the US, and Europe, the incidence of rubella infection is low (88,89). For populous developing countries, childhood infection is common and women of childbearing age have a low rate of seronegativity. However since rubella epidemics have characteristically followed a cyclic pattern, exposure varies over the years, and the number of women of childbearing age who are susceptible to rubella can increase (90).

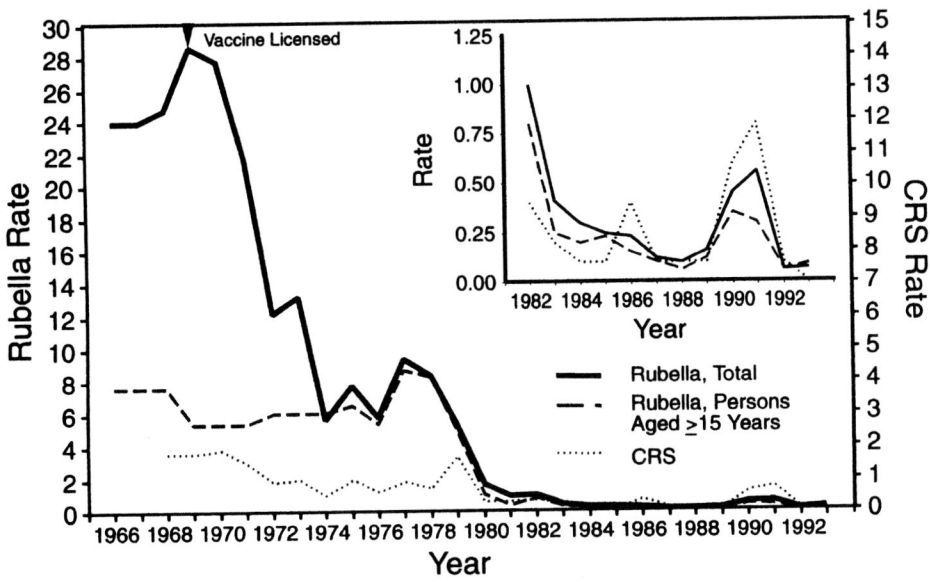

Figure 138.1. Incidence rates of rubella* and CRS†. United States, 1966 to 1993. (From Rubella and congenital rubella syndrome—United States, January 1, 1991–May 7, 1994. *MMWR* 1994;43:391, 397–401, with permission.)

*Cases reported to the National Notifiable Disease Surveillance System per 100,000 population.
†Cases reported to the National CRS Registry per 100,000 live births.

In some rural areas of developing countries, and island countries, seroprevalence is low between epidemics, with more than half of women of childbearing age remaining seronegative (24). Since the licensing of the first rubella vaccine in the United States in 1969, the incidence of rubella has decreased significantly, from 0.45 per 100,000 in 1990 to 0.1 per 100,000 in 1999. During the same time period, the annual median number of reported rubella cases in the United States has been 232, with a range of 128 to 1,412 (89), and the average number of confirmed congenital rubella syndrome (CRS) cases has been 6 infants born with CRS per year, which constitutes a significant decrease compared to the pre-vaccination era (Fig. 138.1).

According to Centers for Disease Control and Prevention statistics, the vast majority of acquired and congenital rubella cases seen in the United States in the past few years were confined to either a small, unimmunized population (such as the Amish) or recent immigrants or visitors from countries that do not have or have only recently instituted a national rubella vaccination program (89,91). This is reflected in the higher rate of confirmed and probable CRS cases of 3.1 per 10,000 live births in a predominantly Hispanic immigrant population, as compared to the current overall rate of 0.01 to 0.08 per 10,000 live births in the United States (92). Since its inception in 1969, the National Congenital Rubella Syndrome Registry (NCRSR) tracks all US-born infants with CRS. For the years 1990 through 1999, a total of 117 cases of CRS have been reported, 110 (94%) of the cases were confirmed CRS and 7 (6%) probable CRS. More than half of all patients were born in the years 1990 and 1991 and the infection of one third of all CRS cases was associated with two cluster outbreaks, the multi-county rubella outbreak in southern California in 1989 and the 1991 rubella outbreak among an Amish community in Pennsylvania (93,94).

Transmission

Human beings appear to be the only natural host for the rubella virus, although certain animals can be infected in the laboratory setting. The mode of transmission for acquired cases is respiratory. Prolonged exposure to an infected person is required, with a single, brief exposure to an infected person appearing to be relatively inefficient in transmitting disease (5). In closed populations of susceptible people, such as military recruits and prisoners, the infection rate has been as high as 90% to 100% (6). In individuals with a history of either infection or appropriate vaccination, re-infection can occur, after prolonged or repeated exposures.

Congenitally infected infants can serve as a potential reservoir of infectious virus, because they cannot fully neutralize the virus for prolonged periods. Up to half of the infants shed virus until the sixth month of life, and some of these infants are found to be actively shedding virus up to 1 year of age (7). However, the overall contribution of these infants to the spread of infection is considered minimal.

PATHOGENESIS AND PATHOLOGY

Acquired Infection

The portal of entry for the virus appears to be the upper respiratory tract. From there, via the lymphatic system and/or by transient viremia, the virus spreads to lymph nodes, where replication occurs (23,24). Approximately 7 to 9 days after exposure, the virus disseminates by the hematogenous route and may infect multiple tissues, including the placenta. The peak of viremia occurs between 10 and 17 days after exposure, and this is followed by the onset of rash on postexposure days 16 to 18 (23,25). The virus is cleared from the serum a few days later, as neutralizing antibody titers rise, which become first detectable usually 2 to 3 days after rash onset and peak within a month of exposure (95). Rubella virus may persist in peripheral blood lymphocytes and monocytes for 1 to 4 weeks (1,26). Virus excretion occurs from the nasopharynx, kidneys, cervix, and gastrointestinal tract starting on postexposure days 9 to 11. Nasopharyngeal virus shedding, usually copious, typically persists for 2 weeks, with the highest rate of nasopharyngeal excretion and risk of virus transmission being from 5 days before to 6 days after the appearance of rash. The etiology of the rash is unclear. Some investigators speculate that the rash may result from circulating immune complexes. However, rubella virus has been isolated from both involved and uninvolved skin, and circulating immune complexes containing rubella virus antigen are detectable in only 16% of patients (27).

Immune mechanisms may play a role in the development of arthralgias and arthritis. The incidence of arthritis and arthralgias varies considerably among different studies. The rates of both arthralgias and arthritis after natural infection are higher in females, suggesting a hormonal influence on their development. Other studies have shown the presence of virus in joint fluid, leading to the possibility that an active infection or an immune mechanism is the actual cause of the arthritis or arthralgia (28–34).

The immune response after natural infection is considered to confer complete protection from reinfection, but cases of reinfection with rubella have occurred and have been attributed to incomplete primary immune response and high attack rate due to exposure in closed environments (1). The immune response to RV is likely involved in the development of acute rubella encephalitis and in the late complication of diabetes mellitus after natural rubella infection (20). The pathogenesis of rubella has been studied in animal models, particularly primates and small animals (35,36). Because of the frequently benign course of acquired rubella, little pathologic experience exists. Lymphoreticular tissues demonstrate mild edema, nonspecific follicular hyperplasia, and some loss of follicular morphology. Examination of brain tissue of patients with encephalitis reveals diffuse swelling, nonspecific degeneration, and little meningeal or perivascular infiltration (46).

CONGENITAL INFECTION

Rubella virus is transmitted in utero to the fetus via the placenta during primary maternal infection (37). There are rare reports of maternal re-infection leading to fetal infection, but the rate of risk in such cases is considered to be exceptionally low (38,39). With primary maternal infection during the first trimester, regardless of whether presenting symptomatic or asymptomatic, fetal infection rates were 40% to 90%, with the higher rate observed when more sensitive isolation methods were used (96). In a large study (97), a significantly lower incidence of fetal infection was found (10% of cases), when the maternal primary infection occurred past the 8th week of gestation. Similar frequencies were observed in other studies, with a 90% infection rate for primary rubella infection prior to 11 weeks of gestation, a 39% infection

rate for exposure during the second trimester, and an increased rate of 53% for the third trimester (131,132). Persistent placental infection can be detected in general twice as frequently as fetal infection (98). Congenital infection may give rise to multiple outcomes (39,40): no fetal evidence of infection, resorption of the embryo if infection occurs early, spontaneous abortion, stillbirth, isolated placental infection without involvement of the fetus, and involvement of both fetus and placenta. Outcomes of infected infants may also range from severe multiorgan involvement to apparent absence of disease. A variable outcome is further demonstrated by viral infection of one monozygotic twin that leaves the other twin unaffected.

It has long been recognized that the younger the gestational age at the time of infection, the higher the risk of congenital anomalies (15). These defects are more severe and more likely to involve multiple organs if acquired during the first 8 weeks of gestation (Table 138.1).

Infants born with congenital rubella who were exposed after the first trimester, usually do not have apparent defects and therefore long-term follow up is necessary to detect late sequelae. In children with serologically confirmed CRS, the frequency of CRS-associated defects at the 6 to 8 year follow-up has been shown to be 75% for maternal infection before 8 weeks of gestation; 52%, between 9-12 weeks of gestation; and 18%, between 13-20 weeks; while no defects where noted in children with infection past 20 weeks of gestation. (99). Rubella virus is known to persist in congenitally infected infants, and the virus can be found throughout gestation (43) and for many months postnatally. By 1 year of age, up to 10% of infants still shed virus and virus shedding may continue beyond 2 years of age (25). Virus can most consistently be recovered from the nasopharynx, but as well from urine, conjunctival fluid, stool, cerebrospinal fluid, bone marrow, and peripheral leukocytes (44). Because of these two mechanisms of damage, clinical manifestations can be divided into transient, permanent, and late emerging (20,45) (Table 138.2). Transient features, including low birth weight, thrombocytopenia, hepatitis, and in some instances meningoencephalitis, and permanent features, including cardiac defects (such as atrial septal defects and pulmonary pulmonic stenosis), eye lesions, and sensorineural deafness, appear to be caused by either the first mechanism of damage or a combination of the two. Late-emerging features, such as sensorineural deafness, endocrine abnormalities, and progressive panencephalitis, appear to be secondary to

TABLE 138.1.   Fetal Infection Rates After Confirmed Maternal Rubella Infection

Gestational age (wk)	Fetal infection, no. infected/no. exposed (%)	Rubella-associated defects/seropositive infants, no./no. (%)	Overall risk[a]
2–3	4/13 (31)	NA	NA
4–6	10/10 (100)	11/11 (100)	100
7–10	9/9 (100)	24/29 (83)	83
11–12	8/13 (62)	20/25 (80)	55
13–14	16/25 (64)	16/31 (52)	33
15–16	24/46 (52)	17/38 (45)	23
17–20	13/33 (39)	2/33 (6)	2
21–23	6/35 (17)	0/16 (0)	0
24–30	19/63 (30)	(0)	0
31–36	15/25 (60)	(0)	0
>36	8/8 (100)	(0)	0

[a]The overall risk was calculated as follows: % seropositive fetuses with defects ×% infants infected.
NA, Not available.
From Ghidini A, Lynch I. Prenatal diagnosis and significance of fetal infections. *West J Med* 1993;159:370, with permission.

TABLE 138.2.   Congenital Rubella: Transient (T), Permanent (P), and Developmental (D) Manifestations

Common		Uncommon or rare	
Low birth weight	T	Jaundice	T
Thrombocytopenic purpura	T	Dermatoglyphic	P
Hepatosplenomegaly	T	"abnormality"	
Bony "lesions"	T	Glaucoma	P
Large anterior fontanelle	T	Cloudy cornea	T
Meningoencephalitis	T	Severe myopia	P, D
Hearing loss	P, D	Myocardial abnormalities	P
Cataract (and microphthalmia)	P	Hepatitis	T
Retinopathy	P	Generalized lymphadenopathy	T
Patent ductus arteriosus	P	Hemolytic anemia	T
Pulmonic stenosis	P, D	Rubella pneumonitis	T
Mental retardation	P, D	Diabetes mellitus	P, D
Behavior disorders	P, D	Thyroid disorders	D, P
Central language disorders	P, D	Seizure disorders	D
Cryptorchidism	P	Precocious puberty	D
Inguinal hernia	P	Degenerative brain disease	D
Splastic diplegia	P		
Microcephaly	P		

From Cooper LZ. Congenital rubella in the United States. In: Krugman S, Gershon A, eds. *Infections of the fetus and the newborn infant.* New York: Alan R. Liss, 1975. Copyright © 1975 Wiley-Liss. Reprinted by permission of Wiley-Liss, a subsidiary of John Wiley & Sons, Inc.

persistence of virus. In fact, more than half of all newborn infants with congenital rubella syndrome appear normal at birth and may still develop late-emerging deficits years later (20). In a recent large retrospective series of serologically confirmed CRS cases from Mexico, major manifestations of CRS were common, such as ocular lesions (74%), neurologic lesions (66%), and congenital heart disease (67%); however only 21% of all women had experienced a rash during pregnancy (100).

Much more is known of the histopathologic appearance of congenital infection than of acquired infection. Predominantly normal tissue cells are interspersed with small foci of infected cells (47) and cellular necrosis and secondary inflammation are minimal. However, a generalized vasculitis is present. Virtually every organ is involved to some degree, and hypoplasia is a characteristic finding (48). Owing to the nature of a chronic, persistent infection, the pathologic process is progressive. Both healing and new lesions can be found in the same specimen. Perivascular calcifications in the brain, giant cell hepatitis, and micronecrosis in autopsy specimens have been reported. Embryos infected early in the first trimester do not seem to have identifiable cellular or humoral immunologic responses. Compared to other congenital infections, inflammation in fetal tissues in CRS cases at any time is minimal, consisting of a low-level infiltration of small lymphocytes (1). Despite this lack of apparent immune response, the infection rate is only 1 cell in 10^3 to 2.5×10^5 cells of the fetus. Rubella virus generally spreads through the vascular system of the infected fetus, and the observed end-organ pathology as well as the generalized growth retardation may be due to the focal cytopathic effect on the blood vessel wall. The lens pathology seems to be due to a direct cytopathic effect and mitotic arrest, while the protective lens capsule has not yet been formed (101). The cytopathologic studies in infected fetal tissues further suggest necrosis and/or apoptosis, and inhibition of cell division of critical precursor cells involved in organogenesis, to be involved in the pathway by which RV infection causes teratogenesis (102). The termination of susceptibility to teratogenesis in the second trimester is consistent with development of the fetal immune response and increased transfer of maternal IgG (101).

The placenta typically shows hypoplasia, inflammatory foci, granulomatous changes, mild edema, focal hyalinization and necrosis, and an extensive necrotizing angiopathy in the chorion (49). Placental infections appear to be more extensive when infection occurs in the last trimester of pregnancy. The decreased risk of embryonic infection and increased risk during the first and third trimesters of pregnancy are presumably due to unspecified changes in the placenta (101).

CLINICAL MANIFESTATIONS

Acquired Infection

Rubella is typically a mild disease with few complications. Symptoms are typically more pronounced in adults than in children. The ratio of subclinical to clinical presentation varies based on intensity of exposure and can be as high as 7:1 (50,51). The incubation period for the virus infection is usually 16 to 18 days, but it can be 14 to 21 days (48). For children, the first symptom is typically the rash. In adults, the rash is preceded by 1 to 5 days of prodromal symptoms, such as low-grade fever, headache, malaise, anorexia, mild conjunctivitis, coryza, pharyngitis, cough, and lymphadenopathy (suboccipital, postauricular, and/or cervical nodes) (48). Once the rash becomes apparent, and it is usually pruritic in adults, the prodromal symptoms subside. An enanthema (Forchheimer spots) consisting of small, red macules on the soft palate occasionally precedes or accompanies the rash. The rash itself can last 1 to 5 days or longer but frequently may not be present. The rash is morbilliform, but with more coalescence than is seen with rubeola, and typically begins on the face and behind the ears, spreading downward during the next 1 or 2 days. Peeling of affected skin usually does not occur. The tip of the spleen is often palpable, and a transient hepatitis can occur. This hepatitis peaks 3 to 10 days after the onset of rash and in one study was noted in 7.5% of 241 children with acute rubella infection (52).

There are a number of possible complications of acquired rubella infection, with arthralgias and arthritis being the most common ones. Complications are more common in adults, particularly in young women. The joint manifestations can appear at any time from when the rash subsides up to several weeks later. The arthritis or arthralgias last from 5 to 10 days in the majority of affected subjects. This has raised interest in the possible role of rubella virus in chronic rheumatic disease in children, but no definitive ties have been described (53).

Other, very rare complications of acquired rubella infection include thrombocytopenia (less than 1 in 3,000 cases; may persist up to 6 months), myocarditis, Guillain-Barré syndrome, relapsing encephalitis, optic neuritis, and bone marrow aplasia (20). Acute postrubella encephalitis (1 in 5,000 to 6,000 cases) is clinically similar to postmeasles encephalitis (20). Unlike the findings in postmeasles encephalitis, demyelination of nerves is not seen.

Congenital Infection

In 1941, Norman Gregg, an Australian ophthalmologist, reported congenital defects, which included eye cataracts, cardiac defects, and low birth weight, in infants born to mothers who had had clinically apparent rubella in the early months of pregnancy (57). Subsequently, CRS was described as a collection of defects, including cardiac, eye, and hearing abnormalities, with or without mental retardation and microcephaly. The most common manifestations, in descending frequency are (20,58): Auditory nerve deafness (80% to 90%), intrauterine growth retardation (50% to 85%), eye cataracts (35%), retinopathy (35%), patent ductus arteriosus (30%), in utero death (10% to 30%), pulmonary arterial hypoplasia (25%), mental retardation, meningoencephalitis, behavioral disorders, hepatosplenomegaly and bone radiolucencies all at about a frequency of 10% to 20%.

However, the time at which these various defects manifest themselves varies. In fact, silent infections, which may become clinically apparent later, are more common than early symptomatic cases. Of congenitally infected neonates who appeared normal, manifestations of infections developed in 71% during the first 5 years of life (59). In addition, existing defects may progress or become manifest at any time throughout life because of continued active infection. Defects associated with CRS can be categorized into three groups (45): transient manifestations, permanent manifestations, and delayed manifestations (Table 138.3).

Transient manifestations are seen in neonates and infants and in some circumstances may represent circulating immune complexes in the presence of active infection (40). These findings usually resolve within days to weeks, and most have little prognostic significance. However, in the presence of extreme prematurity, several of these manifestations can be life-threatening (60). Included in this group are gross cardiac defects or myocarditis with congestive heart failure, progressive hepatitis, extensive meningoencephalitis, and interstitial pneumonitis (40). In general, transient manifestations of CRS can include hepatitis, hepatosplenomegaly, jaundice, thrombocytopenia with petechiae, violaceous lesions of dermal erythropoiesis ("blueberry muffin" lesions), chronic rubelliform rash, hemolytic anemia, hypogammaglobulinemia, lymphadenopathy, meningoencephalitis, large anterior fontanelle, interstitial pneumonitis, myositis, myocarditis, chronic diarrhea, cloudy cornea, and osteopathy (40). Intrauterine growth retardation is present in more than half of all cases (20).

Permanent manifestations may be present at birth or develop during the first year of life and represent defects in organogenesis (except for the case of deafness); thus, they are uncommon if infection occurred after the eighth week of gestation. Included in this group, in decreasing order of frequency, are hearing prob-

TABLE 138.3. Summary of Centers for Disease Control and Prevention Criteria for the Classification of Congenital Rubella Syndrome Cases

CRS confirmed
  Presence of defects and at least one of the following:
   A. Isolation of rubella virus
   B. Detection of rubella-specific IgM antibodies
   C. Rubella-specific HI titer in the infant persisting beyond the period expected from that of passively transferred maternal antibodies
CRS compatible
  Insufficient laboratory data for confirmation of diagnosis and any two complications from A or one from A and one from B:
   A. Cataracts or congenital glaucoma, congenital heart disease, hearing loss, pigmentary retinopathy
   B. Purpura, splenomegaly, jaundice, radiolucent bone disease, meningoencephalitis, microcephaly, mental retardation
CRS possible
  Presence of some compatible clinical findings but insufficient criteria for either the confirmed or compatible categories
Congenital rubella infection only
  No defects are present, but laboratory evidence of infection is found
Stillbirths
  Stillbirths believed to be a consequence of maternal rubella infection
Not CRS
  At least one of the following inconsistent laboratory findings in an immunocompetent child:
   A. Absence of rubella-specific HI titer in a child younger than 2 yr of age
   B. Absence of rubella-specific HI titer in the mother
   C. Decline in rubella-specific HI titer in an infant in a manner consistent with what is expected from passively transferred maternal antibodies (a twofold dilution drop per month)

CRS, Congenital rubella syndrome.
From Freij BJ, South MA, Sever JL. Maternal rubella and the congenital rubella syndrome. *Clin Perinatol* 1988;15:247–257, with permission.

lems, central nervous system disorders, ocular defects, and cardiovascular system defects (20,21,40,61).

Deafness is the most common manifestation of CRS (occurring in 80% to 90% of subjects), and it is usually bilateral (40,62). Deafness can occur alone, with no other stigmata of congenital rubella infection, and can develop at any point in an affected subject's life. Thus, the true incidence of deafness related to congenital rubella infection was not appreciated in the past. The deafness is due to either central or peripheral neurologic damage, with the organ of Corti being specifically affected. The hearing loss is usually across all frequencies, and asymptomatic vestibular dysfunction can accompany it.

Central nervous system abnormalities are also common, and approximately three fourths of children with confirmed CRS attend special schools (17). These abnormalities can manifest themselves at any time during life, but the vast majority are noted in the first year after birth. Included among central nervous system abnormalities are microcephaly, psychomotor retardation, behavioral and psychiatric disorders, including autism, spastic diplegia, meningoencephalitis, and chronic encephalitis (63,103). Psychomotor retardation is common, and there is a strong correlation between the magnitude of cognitive defects and the degree of growth failure (64). It appears that the most profoundly affected children are those infected early in the first trimester, suggesting an organogenesis defect, but active and persistent rubella infection can also play a major role, as seen in the manifestations of both meningoencephalitis and chronic encephalitis (20,61). The most common ocular findings are cataracts and retinopathy, both of which are usually present at birth, although the cataracts may not appear until several months of age in some cases (20). The retinopathy has a characteristic pigmentary "salt-and-pepper" appearance and is non-progressive (46,65,66). The retinopathy usually involves only one eye, except when cataracts are also present, in which case the retinopathy tends to be bilateral. Cataracts are bilateral half of the time and are often associated with microphthalmos. Glaucoma does not appear to affect a cataractous eye and is an uncommon manifestation of CRS (65).

Cardiovascular defects are frequently associated with other major organ defects, and this is related to the time of infection. Cardiac defects are rare in infants infected after the first trimester but are present more than 50% of the time in children infected in the first 8 weeks of gestation, the time of major organogenesis (20). The most common cardiovascular defects are patent ductus arteriosus and pulmonary arterial hypoplasia, including supravalvular stenosis, valvular stenosis, and peripheral branch stenosis. Other structural cardiovascular defects are rare, with atrial septal defects, ventricular septal defects, aortic stenosis, and tetralogy of Fallot each occurring 2% to 5% of the time (20). The presence of a significantly higher frequency of RV-RNA has been detectable by reverse transcriptase polymerase chain reaction in the myocardium of patients with congenital heart disease, while it was absent in controls (104). Up to 10% of newborns with CRS can present with transient myocarditis, which is indicative of active rubella infection (67).

Developmental or delayed manifestations of congenital rubella infection usually appear later in childhood and are progressive in nature (68). The etiology of these defects appears to be continued subacute active rubella infection leading to direct cytopathic effects, vascular insufficiency, and triggering of autoimmune mechanisms. This group of manifestations includes endocrinopathies, deafness, ocular damage, and central nervous system disease progression. Of these endocrinopathies, in particular insulin-dependent diabetes mellitus and thyroid dysfunction are the most common. Insulin-dependent diabetes mellitus has been reported to occur in as many as 20% of CRS patients by age 35 years (61,69). The risk of developing it is approximately 100 to 200 times that observed for the general population. The exact etiology of insulin-dependent diabetes mellitus development is not clear, but it can occur in all congenitally infected patients, regardless of the timing of infection. Recently it has been associated with possibly glutamic acid decarboxylase (GAD) 65 protein specific CD4[+] and CD8[+] T-cell responses with DRB1*0404-A11 and/or a tandem of DRB1*0404-B35 restriction (105). Approximately 5% of CRS patients develop thyroid dysfunction, which can be manifest as hyperthyroidism, hypothyroidism, or thyroiditis, and this is believed to be secondary to autoantibody production (70).

With regard to deafness, hearing deficits can increase over time and acute-onset sensorineural deafness can occur years after birth. In infants and children up to 3 years of age, hearing loss was confirmed in 50% of the children born to mothers with rubella (106). Late-onset ocular defects include myopia, glaucoma, keratic precipitates, keratoconus, corneal hydrops, spontaneous lens absorption, and delayed visual defects caused by subretinal neovascularization (65). Rubella virus can be reactivated in the central nervous system, and this leads to a progressive rubella panencephalitis, which clinically resembles the subacute sclerosing panencephalitis seen with measles (68). The number of patients who have developed this devastating and fatal delayed manifestation is less than twenty (71). In these cases, ataxia and loss of intellectual function were the first manifestations, usually occurring in the second decade of life, progressing to a vegetative state and eventually death (71).

In a large series of late adolescents with CRS, three patterns of growth were observed: normal growth, growth consistently below the 5th percentile, and growth within the normal range or slightly below the fifth percentile followed by early cessation of growth and final height usually below the fifth percentile. No significant cognitive deficits were present in patients with normal growth patterns (107).

DIAGNOSIS

Suspicion

Because acquired rubella infection often presents sub-clinically and is no longer a common illness in the United States, a high index of suspicion is needed. In older children and young adults, a clinical picture consisting of prodromal symptoms followed by postauricular or occipital lymphadenopathy and/or a rash (usually pruritic) should lead one to suspect rubella, especially in high-risk populations such as recent immigrants or visitors from countries where mass immunization against rubella is not practiced. In children, the prodromal symptoms are not seen as often, and the postauricular or occipital lymphadenopathy and coalescing, morbilliform rash originating on the head may be the only clinical clues to an active rubella infection.

In children who present with sensorineural deafness, especially if bilateral, or with ocular signs such as cataracts, congenital rubella infection should be considered as a possible etiology. In general, the most important information needed in case of a suspected rubella infection, be it acquired or congenital, is the immunization status of either the subject (for acquired) or the mother (for congenital).

Differential Diagnosis

It was believed that postauricular or occipital lymphadenopathy occurring together with a rash is pathognomonic for acquired rubella infection. However, enteroviruses, adenoviruses, and human parvovirus B19 can cause a similar clinical picture (20,21). In addition, mild cases of measles, scarlet fever, and allergic reactions can present with a rash similar to that seen in patients with acquired rubella infection. In smaller children, Kawasaki disease (mucocutaneous lymphadenopathy syndrome) must also be considered when the patient has occipital or postauricular lymphadenopathy and a rash.

CRS can be similar to the clinical picture seen with other congenital infections such as syphilis, toxoplasmosis, herpes simplex, and cytomegalovirus infection, all of which can lead to intrauterine growth retardation, deafness, mental retardation, and thrombocytopenic purpura. In addition, several of the enteroviruses can cause an acute hepatitis and thrombocytopenia in the affected neonate.

SPECIFIC DIAGNOSIS

Acquired Infection

Because the presentation of infection may be either subclinical or nonspecific, laboratory diagnosis is essential to the diagnosis of acquired rubella infection. Routine laboratory tests are of little value, as a low to normal leukocyte count is the norm. Plasma cells and atypical lymphocytes are frequently noted, but these are nonspecific findings. Thus, more specific laboratory techniques are required to diagnose acquired rubella infection. Methods used are outlined in the following sections.

VIRUS ISOLATION

Virus isolation is the least used method for diagnosis of acquired rubella infection, because it is generally not readily available and further because of the limited time of virus shedding. When it is utilized, specimens are preferably obtained from the throat or nasopharynx, for inoculation of primary cell cultures, such as African green monkey kidney tissue culture or of continuous cell lines such as RK-13 or Vero cell lines, when the cytopathic effect needs to be assessed (e.g., for virus neutralization assays). Virus shedding usually stops several days after the attenuation of the rash, so cultures must be obtained during the acute illness to be of good sensitivity (20). However a microtiter plate system using different cell lines inoculated in suspension has been used as the screening culture system instead of the conventional roller tube monolayer cultures, showing improved sensitivity. With this system, isolation of RV has been possible in RMK, E6-vero, and additionally in BGM cells (108).

SEROLOGIC DIAGNOSIS

The majority of rubella infections are now diagnosed serologically. Initially developed were the hemagglutination inhibition (HI) and neutralization tests (72,73). The neutralization test determines the capacity of rubella virus antibody to prevent rubella virus infectivity. It is a sensitive test but expensive, time-consuming, and not available in most clinical laboratories. Thus, the HI test became the gold standard initially (72,73). This assay is based on the ability of rubella virus to hemagglutinate erythrocytes from specific animal sources. If specific rubella virus antibodies are present, hemagglutination does not occur in the test specimen. Like the neutralization test, it is sensitive but also time-consuming and difficult to perform and to standardize. Among the other available serologic methods, complement fixation tests are not used frequently because of lower sensitivity, since complement fixation antibodies appear later in the course of the infection (72–74). Passive agglutination tests are difficult to quantitate and rarely used for the diagnosis of recent rubella infection. The present standard technique for the serologic diagnosis of rubella infection is the ELISA. Rubella IgM antibody can be detected by ELISA from early after the onset of illness through the peak at 7 to 10 days and for up to 4 weeks after the appearance of rash. Thus, a single serum specimen obtained within this period, if results are positive, can be viewed as serologic confirmation of a clinically suspected rubella infection. However, the IgM determination may yield false-positive results, especially if there is concomitant exposure to cytomegalovirus or parvovirus B19 (20,72–75). Also, in some laboratories, a false-positive result can be obtained if the ELISA technique used does not avoid nonspecific reactions caused by complexes with rheumatoid antibody (76).

The other way to confirm a suspected rubella infection serologically is to measure acute- and convalescent-phase IgG levels using the ELISA technique. A single measurement is not helpful, because up to 15% of the normal population may have a high baseline IgG level by this method (11). The acute-phase serum should be collected within 7 days of appearance of the rash, and the convalescent-phase serum should be obtained 10 to 14 days later. The serum samples should be tested in tandem (48).

There are several new developments in serologic testing for rubella virus. A major problem with currently available ELISAs is the difficulty of obtaining rubella virus antigens of reliable quality. Rubella virus is both difficult to grow and difficult to purify of cellular debris. Thus, false-positive reactions of immunoglobulins with nonviral contaminants have been reported (72–75). Several studies have compared the use of a synthetic peptide-based EIA with that of the traditional rubella virus lysate-based EIA in detecting rubella antibodies, and the results have been promising (109). Also, tests that use saliva or urine to determine the presence of rubella antibody have been developed and show good reliability (77,78,110).

RUBELLA VIRUS RIBONUCLEIC ACID REVERSE TRANSCRIPTASE–POLYMERASE CHAIN REACTION

Reverse transcriptase–polymerase chain reaction (RT-PCR) has been used directly on the clinical specimen or as second step after short-term viral culture (111–113). Direct RT-PCR on amniotic fluid samples showed 100% sensitivity and specificity for the diagnosis of prenatal rubella infection and provides results 24 to 48 hours after sampling (112). Culture-RT-PCR was able to confirm the results obtained by the direct RT-PCR and by 7 to 10 days after RV infection 96% of cell cultures tested positive, whereas by the same time RV was isolated in less than half of the cell cultures (113).

Rubella virus RNA was further detected by PT-PCR in pharyngeal swabs from patients with serologically confirmed rubella and in 100% agreement with virus culture results (114).

Congenital Infection

A diagnosis of CRS should be considered for any infant born with stigmata consistent with intrauterine rubella infection. The Centers for Disease Control and Prevention have formulated case definitions (47) for either confirmed or compatible cases of CRS (see Table 138.3).

VIRUS ISOLATION

Rubella virus can be isolated from congenitally infected infants and may persist in the majority of such patients for up to 1 year. The virus may be isolated from the nasopharynx and less reliably from conjunctival secretions, cerebrospinal fluid, or urine. However RV isolation is not routinely available in the clinical virology laboratory.

SEROLOGIC DIAGNOSIS

As with acquired rubella infection, the majority of congenital infections are determined by serologic studies. Serologic diagnosis may be made by determining the rubella-specific IgM titer in cord serum (11,79). However, there is a risk of false negative results. If the maternal infection occurred late in the pregnancy, there may not have been sufficient time for the neonate to mount an immune response. Also, IgM is not present in fetuses until approximately the fifth month in utero, so the determination of IgM levels before this time leads to negative results for in utero diagnosis (79). Still, the determination of antirubella virus IgM by EIA is currently an accepted and available way of diagnosing congenital rubella infection in the newborn (79). For any IgM antibody assay, the presence of rheumatoid factor can cause false-positive results. Solid–phase IgM capture assays however are not affected by rheumatoid factor (115).

An alternative method is to follow sequential IgG levels. Because levels of maternally transferred IgG drop, as the infant becomes older, the persistence or rise of specific antirubella virus IgG would be consistent with congenital infection (11).

More challenging is the diagnosis of congenital rubella infection in patients who present with delayed manifestations, such as sensorineural deafness. Positive RV specific IgG levels are not diagnostic, when routine rubella vaccination has been received at 12 to 15 months of life. Investigational serologic assays of potential use are the protein-denaturing enzyme immunoassay measuring the avidity of specific IgG (116). Primary infection of the mother seems to result in primarily low-affinity IgG, while reinfection seems to be associated with high-avidity IgG (1).

The nonreducing Rubella-Immunoblot and the Rubella-IgG-Peptide-Enzyme Immunoassay (EIA) are used to determine the presence of antibodies directed to rubella proteins E1, E2 and C (109,117). While newborns infected later than week 10 of gestation showed normal levels of antibodies, a lack of antibody responses was detectable in infants with CRS.

Polymerase Chain Reaction for Detection of Congenital Rubella Virus Infection

Different RT-PCRs for the detection of rubella virus in prenatal and postnatal samples have been developed (79,112,118,119). These techniques have as well been used for retrospective detection of rubella virus in placental and fetal tissues obtained after termination of pregnancy following primary rubella or rubella virus re-infection. High concordance rates were seen in comparison with virus culture. Rubella virus is detectable with these methods in chorionic villus samples as early as 15 weeks of gestation, however test results did not always correctly predict fetal rubella virus infection (79,118,119). The specificity for direct fetal sampling was very high (79,112,119). Further prenatal sampling techniques that have been used in connection with the RV RT-PCR include amniocentesis and cordocentesis (79).

PREVENTION AND MANAGEMENT

Immunization

In 1969, three live attenuated rubella vaccines were licensed for use in the United States: the HPV-77 (DE-5 and DK-12) vaccines and the Cendehill vaccine (20). In 1979, the RA 27/3 vaccine was licensed, and it is currently the only vaccine used (80). It appears that one dose of vaccine already produces high levels of long-lasting immunity; 92% of vaccinees who had originally seroconverted after a dose of the RA 27/3 vaccine had serologic evidence of immunity up to 18 years after receipt of the vaccine (20). Although primary rubella vaccine failures have not been a major problem, the potential consequences of rubella vaccine failure are substantial (i.e., congenital rubella), and thus an additional dose of rubella vaccine is recommended (11,75). With the current measles, mumps and rubella (MMR) combination vaccine, trivalent immunity is achieved in greater than 90% of subjects immunized (120). It is currently recommended that MMR vaccine be administered when a child is 12 to 15 months of age, with a second dose being given in the early school-age years (75). Special emphasis must continue to be placed on the immunization of postpubertal males and females, especially those living in closed settings, such as in the military or in a college. In general, for this age group, immunization should be performed unless documented evidence of rubella immunization or serologic evidence of naturally acquired immunity is provided. A history of acquired rubella infection is not adequate, as studies have shown a poor correlation between recollection of a rubella infection and confirmation via serologic tests (11).

For the postpubertal population, the Red Book Committee of the American Academy of Pediatrics published the following specific recommendations (121):

1. Postpubertal females, who are not known to be immunized to rubella and are not pregnant, should be immunized. Pregnancy should be avoided for 3 months after vaccination.
2. Premarital serologic screening for rubella immunity is encouraged.
3. Prenatal or antepartum serologic screening for rubella immunity should be routinely undertaken, and rubella vaccine should be administered to susceptible women in the immediate postpartum period before discharge. Receipt of $Rh_0(D)$ immune globulin is not a contraindication to vaccination, however women should be tested 8 or more weeks later to determine whether an active antibody response has developed. Further, breast-feeding is not a contraindication to postpartum vaccination. While transmission of the vaccine virus to breast-fed infants has been documented, these infants remained asymptomatic.
4. Special efforts should be undertaken to vaccinate all individuals who are likely to be exposed to or spread rubella (e.g. staff in educational institutions, childcare centers, health care facilities).
5. Routine serologic testing before immunization is unnecessary. However a prevaccination blood specimen should be held for at least 3 months. When the vaccinee becomes pregnant within 3 months of the immunization, already present immunity can possibly be established by serologic testing of the prevaccination sample. There is no evidence that rubella vaccination after exposure prevents rubella, nor has it been shown that vaccination of individuals incubating rubella is harmful. No international standard exists for the level of antibody considered to be protective. Current recommendation based on available evidence indicates that any appropriately measured detectable antibody level can be considered as evidence of either past natural infection or vaccine-induced immunity (75).

CONTRAINDICATIONS

Pregnancy

Rubella vaccine should not be given to pregnant women because of a theoretical risk of the occurrence of congenital rubella, especially if the vaccine is given in the first trimester (75). As of the present, none of the infants born to women who received the RA 27/3 vaccine during the first trimester have congenital defects. Of these infants, 2% had asymptomatic infection (as shown by serologic determinations), which led the Centers for Disease Control and Prevention to estimate a maximal theoretical risk of 1.6% (based on the standard deviation from zero) for the occurrence of congenital rubella after administration of the presently used vaccine during the first trimester (11,75). While vertical transmission of the RA27/3 live-attenuated rubella vaccine virus can occur in cases of inadvertent vaccination and can led to persistent fetal infection with prolonged virus shedding for more than 8 months, no symptoms compatible with the congenital rubella syndrome or late onset disease have been observed in any of these children (122).

Recent Receipt of Immune Globulin

Because of the potential for antibodies to neutralize the vaccine virus, it is recommended that rubella vaccine not be given in the 2 weeks before or the 3 months after the administration of immune globulin or blood transfusion (75).

Altered Immunity

Patients with immunodeficiency diseases (except human immunodeficiency virus infection) or who are receiving immunosuppressive therapy or large, systemic doses of corticosteroids, alkylating agents, antimetabolites, or radiation should not be recipients of the rubella vaccine (75). It is recommended that patients with human immunodeficiency virus infection receive rubella vaccine, and several studies have shown that these patients have the highest rate of serologic conversion to the rubella component of the measles-mumps-rubella vaccine (81–83). For patients who are receiving immunosuppressive therapy (such as for leukemia or lymphoma), the interval between cessation of such therapy and rubella vaccine receipt should be approximately 3 months to allow the immune system to be properly restored (75). Mild febrile childhood illnesses (such as upper respiratory infections) should not be perceived as contraindications to measles-mumps-rubella vaccine administration. If the fever is a manifestation of a more serious condition, the vaccine should be withheld until recovery (75).

ADVERSE EVENTS

By day 5 to 7 after vaccination, virus may be detected in peripheral blood lymphocytes, and thus the main complications of a naturally acquired rubella infection can occur (63). All complications secondary to rubella vaccine are more common in adults than in children and most common in women older than 25 years. Overall, the vaccine is safe and complications after vaccination are but a percentage of those seen after natural infection.

Fever, rash, and/or lymphadenopathy can develop in 5% to 15% of children who receive the vaccine, and the rate is higher in adults. Joint pain, usually affecting small peripheral joints in children, is seen in 0.5% of child vaccine recipients (75). However, in women, this adverse event is more frequent, most commonly presenting as joint pain, and with up to 10-20% having arthritis-like signs and symptoms (54–56,75). Other rare complications include transient peripheral neuritic complaints, central nervous system manifestations, including acute disseminated encephalomyelitis, responding to steroid therapy (123), and thrombocytopenia, although a causal relationship to vaccine receipt has not been firmly established for the last two (75,124). A country wide surveillance study of adverse events in Finland found a possible or indeterminate causal relation with MMR vaccination at a rate of 5.3 per 100,000 vaccinees or 3.2 per 100,000 vaccine doses (124).

RUBELLA ERADICATION

When a random sample of viruses isolated in the 1990s was analyzed along with viruses from the 1960s and 1970s, the resulting phylogenetic tree revealed that viruses isolated prevaccination are more similar to one another than they are to viruses isolated in the 1990s. However considerable stability of the E1 surface protein has been shown for pre- and postvaccination isolates, with only 3% amino acid sequence variation over a 36-year interval, not indicating significant viral escape (1,125).

Effective prevention strategies to eliminate CRS and rubella infection in the United States require improvement in the surveillance of CRS, particularly through augmented laboratory capabilities to identify infants with CRS, and studies of methods to identify high-risk populations and geographic areas for rubella and CRS. The case definition for CRS must be revised to reflect the current scientific information available (89,126) Mathematic modeling of the effect of different rubella vaccination strategies, in particular with respect to the herd effect, is available (88,127,128). Possible strategies for eradication of CRS in developed countries are the universal MMR vaccination at 12 to 18 months and 4 to 12 years and vaccination of adolescents and adults at any opportunity. Possible strategies for eradication of CRS in developing countries are the increased universal immunization with MR or MMR at 9 to 12 months of age, mass vaccination campaigns of children 1 to 14 years of age with MR or MMR and vaccination of female adolescents and adults at any opportunity (129).

Chemotherapy

Chemotherapy is rarely needed in acquired infection, considering the typical uncomplicated clinical course seen with rubella infection. For patients with chronic arthritis secondary to natural infection, there has been some success with systemic steroid therapy, but this course of therapy is not routinely recommended (20,55,56).

For patients with CRS, the experience with chemotherapeutic agents is also limited. Trials of amantadine or interferon therapy did not show an improvement in clinical outcome (86,87) and at present the number of children affected by CRS is so small that future clinical trials may be difficult to conduct.

Large doses of immunoglobulin have been used for the prevention or modification of rubella in susceptible pregnant women who were exposed to the infection, and did not wish to interrupt their pregnancy. However, it has been shown that immune globulin may suppress symptoms but does not necessarily prevent viremia. Also, most commercially available immunoglobulins have varying concentrations of antibody to rubella, and thus the use of immune globulin is not recommended (11,75).

Immunoglobulin therapy has however successfully been used in CRS patients with dysgammaglobulinemia, where improvement of the immunoglobulin abnormalities correlated with correction of CD154 expression on peripheral blood mononuclear cells (130).

Isolation Procedures

Patients with acquired rubella infection continue to shed virus for 5 to 7 days after the onset of rash and thus should be isolated from susceptible subjects, especially women of childbearing age. In addition, hospitalized exposed patients should be placed under contact isolation until the 21st day after exposure. Only health care workers with serologically proven immunity should work with patients infected or potentially infected with rubella. Infants with CRS can shed virus for the first year of life and occasionally even longer. Thus, these infants should be considered potentially infectious until results of repeated nasopharyngeal and urine viral cultures are negative. Until that time, appropriate isolation measures should be used.

Clinical Management of Congenitally Infected Infants

Owing to the chronic, persistent nature of congenital rubella infection, patients must be viewed as having a continually evolving disease. A multidisciplinary approach is often needed because of the broad range of potential problems, and defects must be looked for aggressively and repeatedly in infants known to have become infected in utero (20). Children in whom congenital rubella infection was not suspected but who develop a delayed manifestation should also be examined thoroughly for other potential defects.

Hearing disability is the most common abnormality seen after congenital rubella infection, with more than 80% of infants having some degree of hearing disability. Proper hearing is paramount to language and communication development, and thus hearing should be tested definitively as soon as possible in the infant suspected to have had congenital rubella infection (20). Unfortunately, many physicians believe that hearing cannot be adequately tested in infants. However, in proper centers specific audiometric testing of infants can be performed, and infants found to be severely affected should be enrolled in specially designed programs of education. Also, children should be fitted with hearing aids and visual aids, including contact lenses. Even though congenital rubella infection can lead to a decrease in intelligence, at times an infant's lack of or delayed development is secondary to hearing or vision defects, and thus a full ophthalmologic examination is also indicated. Children should further receive speech, language, physical and occupational therapy as needed. In the United States, most patients with documented or suspected CRS are eligible for early intervention and rehabilitation services, based on the Federal Individuals with Disabilities Education Act of 1997.

SUMMARY

Rubella, in its acquired form, is a rather benign infection. However, congenital infection can lead to devastating consequences and thus it is imperative to eliminate it through continued mandatory immunization of infants and aggressive immunization of postpubertal individuals who have no documentation of rubella immunity. Since 1969, when the first rubella vaccines were introduced, there has been a remarkable decrease in the number of both acquired and congenital rubella infections; however coverage by vaccination is not complete and the remaining susceptibility of women of child bearing age requires vigilance. With universal MMR vaccination of children and vaccination of adolescents and adults, in particular immigrants, at all possible occasions, eradication of rubella in the United States and in the future internationally is now a realistic public health policy objective.

REFERENCES

1. Centers for Disease Control and Prevention. Rubella and congenital rubella syndrome—United States, Jan 1, 1991-May 7, 1994. *MMWR* 1994;43:391.
2. Assad R, Ljungars-Esteves K. Rubella—world impact. *Rev Infect Dis* 1985;7(Suppl 1):S29.
3. Bart KJ, Ortenstein NA, Preblud SR, et al. Universal immunization to interrupt rubella. *Rev Infect Dis* 1985;7(Suppl 1):S177.
4. Centers for Disease Control. Update: changes in notifiable disease surveillance data—United States, 1992-1993. *MMWR* 1993;42:824.
5. Marcy SM, Jordan MC. Rubella. In: Hoeprich PD, Jordan MC, eds. *Infectious diseases: a modern treatise of infectious processes*, 4th ed. Philadelphia: JB Lippincott, 1989:866.
6. Pollard RB, Edwards EA. Epidemic survey of rubella in a military recruit population. *Am J Epidemiol* 1975;101:435.
7. Garner JS, Simmons BP. CDC guidelines for isolation precautions in hospitals. *Infect Control* 1983;4:245.
8. Witte JJ, Karchmer AW Case G, et al. Epidemiology of rubella. *Am J Dis Child* 1969;118:107.
9. Preblud SR, Serdual MK, Frank JA Jr, et al. Rubella vaccination in the United States: a ten-year review. *Epidemiol Rev* 1980;2:171.
10. Jackson B, Payton T, Horst G, et al. An epidemiologic investigation of a rubella outbreak among the Amish of northeastern Ohio. *Public Health Rep* 1993;108:436.
11. The American College of Obstetricians and Gynecologists (ACOG). Rubella and pregnancy: ACOG technical bulletin number 171 - August 1992. *Int J Gynecol Obstet* 1993;42:60.
12. Condon RJ, Bower C. Rubella vaccination and congenital rubella syndrome in Western Australia. *Med J Aust* 1993;158:379.
13. Ostlere LS, Stevens HP, Dillon MJ, et al. Chronic rash associated with congenital rubella. *J R Soc Med* 1994;87:242.
14. Ghidini A, Lynch L. Prenatal diagnosis and significance of fetal infections. *West J Med* 1993;159:366.
15. Miller E, Cradock-Watson JE, Pollock TM. Consequences of confirmed maternal rubella at successive stages of pregnancy. *Lancet* 1982;2:781.
16. Enders G, Nickerl-Pacher U, Miller E, Cradock-Watson JE. Outcome of confirmed periconceptional maternal rubella. *Lancet* 1988;1:1445.
17. Munro ND, Sheppard S, Smithells RW, et al. Temporal relations between maternal rubella and congenital defects. *Lancet* 1987;2:201.
18. Grillner L, Forsgren M, Barr B, et al. Outcome of rubella during pregnancy with special reference to the 17th-24th weeks of gestation. *Scand J Infect Dis* 1983;15:321.
19. Grangeot-Keros L. Rubella and pregnancy. *Pathol Biol (Paris)* 1992;40:706.
20. Cherry JD. Rubella. In: Feigin RD, Cherry JD, eds. *Textbook of pediatric infectious diseases*, 4th ed. Philadelphia: WB Saunders, 1998:1922–1941.
21. Gershon A. Rubella virus (German measles). In: Mandell G, Bennett J, Dolin R, eds. *Principles and practice of infectious diseases*, 5th ed. Philadelphia: Churchill Livingstone, 2000:1708–1714.
22. Cradock-Watson JE, Ridehalgh MKS, Anderson MJ, et al. Fetal infection resulting from maternal rubella after the first trimester of pregnancy. *J Hyg (Lond)* 1980;83:381.
23. Green RH, Balsame MR, Giles JP, et al. Studies of the natural history and prevention of rubella. *Am J Dis Child* 1965;110:348.
24. Halstead SB, Diwan AR, Oda AI. Susceptibility to rubella among adolescents and adults in Hawaii. *JAMA* 1969;210:1881.
25. Sever JL, Monif G. Limited persistence of virus in congenital rubella. *Am J Dis Child* 1965;110:452.
26. O'Shea S, Mutton D, Best JM. In vivo expression of rubella antigens on human leukocytes: detection by flow cytometry. *J Med Virol* 1988;25:297.
27. Ziola B, Lund G, Meurman O, et al. Circulating immune complexes in patients with acute measles and rubella virus. *Infect Immun* 1983;41:578.
28. Tingle AJ, Allen M, Petty RE, et al. Rubella associated arthritis. Comparative study of joint manifestations associated with natural rubella infection and RA 27/3 rubella immunization. *Ann Rheum Dis* 1986;45:110.
29. Graham R, Armstrong R, Simmons NA, et al. Isolation of rubella virus from synovial fluid in five cases of seronegative arthritis. *Lancet* 1981;2:649.
30. Phillips CA, Behbehani AM, Johnson LW et al. Isolation of rubella virus: an epidemic characterized by rash and arthritis. *JAMA* 1965;191:615.
31. Ogra PL, Herd JK. Arthritis associated with induced rubella infection. *J Immunol* 1971;107:810.
32. Smith CA, Petty RE, Tingle AJ. Rubella virus and arthritis. *Rheum Dis Clin North Am* 1987;13:265.
33. Graham R, Armstrong R, Simmons NA, et al. Chronic arthritis associated with the presence of intrasynovial rubella virus. *Ann Rheum Dis* 1983;42:2.
34. Chantler JK, Ford DK, Tingle AJ. Persistent rubella infection and rubella-associated arthritis. *Lancet* 1982;1:1323.
35. Parkman PD, Phillips PE, Kirchstein RL, et al. Experimental rubella virus infection in the rhesus monkey. *J Immunol* 1965;95:743.
36. Fabiyi A, Gitnick GL, Sever JL. Chronic rubella infection in the ferret (*Mustela putorius fero*) puppy. *Proc Soc Exp Biol Med* 1967;125:766.
37. Rawls WE, Desmyter J, Melnick JL. Serologic diagnosis and fetal involvement in maternal rubella. *JAMA* 1968;203:627.
38. Grangeot-Keros L, Nicolas JC, Bricout F, et al. Rubella reinfection and the fetus. *N Engl J Med* 1985;313:1547.
39. Weber B, Enders G, Schlosser R, et al. Congenital rubella syndrome after maternal reinfection. *Infection* 1993;21:118.
40. Hanshaw JB, Dudgeon JA. Rubella. In: Hanshaw JB, Dudgeon JA, Marshall WC, eds. *Viral diseases of the fetus and newborn*, 2nd ed. Philadelphia: WB Saunders, 1985:13.
41. Thompson KM, Tobin J. Isolation of rubella virus from abortion material. *BMJ* 1970;2:264.
42. Nusbacher J, Hirschhorn K, Cooper LZ. Chromosomal studies on congenital rubella. *N Engl J Med* 1967;276:1409.
43. Krugman S. Rubella symposium. *Am J Dis Child* 1965;110:345.
44. Schiff GM, Dine MS. Transmission of rubella from newborns. A controlled study among young adult women and report of an unusual case. *Am J Dis Child* 1965;110:447.
45. Cooper LZ. Congenital rubella in the United States. In: Krugman S, Gershon A, eds. *Infections of the fetus and the newborn infant*. New York: Alan R Liss, 1975:1–22.
46. Cherry JD. Rubella. In: Feigin RD, Cherry JD, eds. *Textbook of pediatric infectious diseases*, 2nd ed. Philadelphia: WB Saunders, 1987:1810.
47. Freij BJ, South MA, Sever JL. Maternal rubella and the congenital rubella syndrome. *Clin Perinatol* 1988;15:247.
48. Cooper LZ, Alford CA Jr. Rubella. In: Remington JS, Klein JO, eds. *Infectious diseases of the fetus and newborn*, 5th ed. Philadelphia: WB Saunders, 2001:347–388.
49. Garcia AGP, Marques RLS, Lobato YY, et al. Placental pathology in congenital rubella. *Placenta* 1985;6:281.
50. Horstmann DM, Leibhaber H, LeBouvier GL, et al. Rubella. Reinfection of vaccinated and naturally immune persons exposed in an epidemic. *N Engl J Med* 1970;283:771.
51. Brody JA. The infectiousness of rubella and the possibility of reinfection. *Am J Public Health* 1966;56:1082.
52. Sugaya N, Nirasawa M, Mitamura K, et al. Hepatitis in acquired rubella infection in children (letter). *Am J Dis Child* 1988;142:817.
53. Chantler JK, Tingle AJ, Petty RE. Persistent rubella virus infection associated with chronic arthritis in children. *N Engl J Med* 1985;313:1117.
54. Howson CP, Howe CJ, Fineberg HV, eds. *Adverse effects of pertussis and rubella vaccine*. Washington DC: Institute of Medicine, National Academy Press, 1991:195–197.
55. Tingle AJ, Chantler JK, Pot KH. Postpartum rubella immunization: association with development of prolonged arthritis, neurological sequelae, and chronic rubella viremia. *J Infect Dis* 1985;152:606.
56. Mitchell LA, Tingle AJ, Shukin R, et al. Chronic rubella vaccine-associated arthropathy. *Arch Intern Med* 1993;153:2268.
57. Gregg NM. Congenital cataracts following German measles in the mother. *Trans Ophthalmol Soc Aust* 1941;3:35.
58. South MA, Sever JL. Teratogen update: the congenital rubella syndrome. *Teratology* 1985;31:297.
59. Schiff GM, Sutherland J, Light L. Congenital rubella. In: Thalhamer O, ed. *Prenatal infections*. International Symposium of Vienna, September 2–3, 1970. Stuttgart: Georg Thieme, 1971:31.
60. Cooper LZ. The history and medical consequences of rubella. *Rev Infect Dis* 1985;7(Suppl 1):51.
61. Williams LL, Shannon BT, Leguire LE, et al. Persistently altered T cell

immunity in high school students with the congenital rubella syndrome and profound hearing loss. *Pediatr Infect Dis J* 1993;12:831.

62. Kobayashi H, Suzuki A, Nomura Y. Unilateral hearing loss following rubella infection in an adult. *Acta Otolaryngol Suppl (Stockh)* 1994;514:49.

63. Cooper LZ, Buimovici-Klein E. Rubella. In: Fields BN, Knipe DM, eds. *Virology.* New York: Raven Press, 1985:1005.

64. Chiriboga-Klein S, Oberfield SE, Castillo AM, et al. Growth in congenital rubella syndrome and correlation with clinical manifestations. *J Pediatr* 1989; 115:251.

65. Arnold JJ, McIntosh EDG, Martin FJ, et al. A fifty-year follow-up of ocular defects in congenital rubella: late ocular manifestations. *Aust NZ J Ophthalmol* 1994;22:1.

66. Yoser SL, Forster DJ, Rao NA. Systemic viral infections and their retinal and choroidal manifestations. *Surv Ophthalmol* 1993;37:339.

67. Baley JE, Goldfarb J. The immune system, viral infections. In: Fanaroff AA, Martin RJ, eds. *Neonatal-perinatal medicine, diseases of the fetus and infant,* 5th ed. St. Louis: Mosby-Year Book, 1992:113–117.

68. Sever JL, South MA, Shaver KA. Delayed manifestations of congenital rubella. *Rev Infect Dis* 1985;7(Suppl 1):5164.

69. Menser MA, Forrest JM, Bransby RD, et al. Long-term observation of diabetes and the congenital rubella syndrome in Australia. In: Mimura G, Baba S, Goto Y, et al, eds. *Clinicogenetic genesis of diabetes mellitus.* Amsterdam: Excerpta Medica, 1982:221.

70. Rubenstein P, Walker ME, Fedun B, et al. The HLA system in congenital rubella patients with and without diabetes. *Diabetes* 1982;31:1088.

71. Waxham MN, Wolinsky JS. Rubella virus and its effect on the nervous system. *Neurol Clin* 1984;2:367.

72. Zrein M, Joncas JH, Pedneault L, et al. Comparison of a whole-virus enzyme immunoassay (EIA) with a peptide-based EIA for detecting rubella virus immunoglobulin G antibodies following rubella vaccination. *J Clin Microbiol* 1993;31:1521.

73. Pedneault L, Zrein M, Robillard L, et al. Comparison of novel synthetic peptide-based DETECT-RUBELLA enzyme immunoassays with Enzygnost and IMx for detection of rubella-specific immunoglobulin G. *J Clin Microbiol* 1994;32:1085.

74. Condorelli F, Ziegler T. Dot immunobinding assay for simultaneous detection of specific immunoglobulin G antibodies to measles virus, mumps virus, and rubella virus. *J Clin Microbiol* 1993;31:717.

75. Committee on Infectious Diseases of the American Academy of Pediatrics. *Report of the committee on infectious diseases (the red book),* 23rd ed. Elk Grove Village, IL: American Academy of Pediatrics, 1994:406–412.

76. Meurman OH, Ziola BR. IgM-class rheumatoid factor interference in the solid-phase immunoassay of rubella-specific IgM antibodies. *J Clin Pathol* 1978;31:483.

77. Thieme T, Piacentini S, Davidson S, et al. Determination of measles, mumps, and rubella immunization status using oral fluid samples. *JAMA* 1994;272:219.

78. Perry KR, Brown DWG, Parry JV, et al. Detection of measles, mumps, and rubella antibodies in saliva using antibody capture radioimmunoassay. *J Med Virol* 1993;40:235.

79. Valente P, Sever JL. In utero diagnosis of congenital infections by direct fetal sampling. *Isr J Med Sci* 1994;30:416.

80. Wharton M, Cochl SL, Williams WW. Measles, mumps, and rubella vaccines. *Infect Dis Clin North Am* 1990;4:47.

81. Frenkel LM, Nielsen K, Garakian A, et al. A search for persistent measles, mumps, and rubella vaccine virus in children with human immunodeficiency virus type I infection. *Arch Pediatr Adolesc Med* 1994;148:57.

82. Sprauer MA, Markowitz LE, Nicholson JKA, et al. Response of human immunodeficiency virus-infected adults to measles-rubella vaccination. *J Acquir Immune Defic Syndr* 1993;6:1013.

83. Brena AE, Cooper ER, Cabral HJ, et al. Antibody response to measles and rubella vaccine by children with HIV infection. *J Acquir Immune Defic Syndr* 1993;6:1125.

84. Ou D, Chong P, Tingle AJ. Mapping T-cell epitopes of rubella virus structural proteins E1, E2, and C recognized by T-cell lines and clones derived from infected and immunized populations. *J Med Virol* 1993;40:175.

85. Hobman TC, Lundstrom ML, Mauracher CA, et al. Assembly of rubella virus structural proteins into virus-like particles in transfected cells. *Virology* 1994;202:574.

86. Arvin AM, Schmidt NJ, Cantell K, et al. Alpha interferon administration to infants with congenital rubella. *Antimicrob Agents Chemother* 1982;21:259.

87. Plotkin SA, Klaus RM, Whitely JA. Hypogammaglobulinemia in an infant with congenital rubella syndrome. *J Pediatr* 1966;69:1085.

88. Edmunds WJ, Gay NJ, Kretzschmar M, Pebody RG, Wachmann H. The pre-vaccination epidemiology of measles, mumps and rubella in Europe: implications for modelling studies. *Epidemiol Infect* 2000;125:635–650.

89. Reef SE, Frey TK, Theal K, et al. The changing epidemiology of rubella in the 1990s. on the verge of elimination and new challenges for control and prevention. *JAMA* 2002;287:4.

90. Seth P, Manjunath N, Balaya S. Rubella infection: the indian scene. *Rev Infect Dis* 1985;7(Suppl. 1).:S64–68.

91. Centers for Disease Control and Prevention. Control and prevention of rubella: evaluation and management of suspected outbreaks, rubella in pregnant women, and surveillance for congenital rubella syndrome. *MMWR* 2001;50(RR12):1–23.

92. Zimmerman L, Reef SE. Incidence of congenital rubella syndrome at a

hospital serving a predominantly hispanic population, El Paso, Texas. *Pediatrics* 2001;107:E40.

93. Lee SH, Ewert DP, Frederick PD, Mascola L. Resurgence of congenital rubella syndrome in the 1990s: report on missed opportunities and failed prevention policies among women of childbearing age. *JAMA* 1992;267:2616–2620.

94. Mellinger AK, Cragan JD, Atkinson WL, et al. High incidence of congenital rubella syndrome after a rubella outbreak. *Pediatr Infect Dis J* 1995;4:573–578.

95. Green RH, Balsame MR, Giles JP, et al. Studies of the natural history and prevention of rubella. *Am J Dis Child* 1965;110:348.

96. Rawls WE, Desmyter J, Melnick JL. Serologic diagnosis and fetal involvement in maternal rubella. *JAMA* 1968;203:627.

97. Alford CA Jr. Congenital rubella: a review of the virologic and serologic phenomena occurring after maternal rubella in the first trimester. *South Med J* 1966;59:745.

98. Alford CA, Neva FA, Weller TH. Virologic and serologic studies on human products of conception after maternal rubella. *N Engl J Med* 1964;271:1275.

99. Peckham GS. Clinical and laboratory study of children exposed in utero to maternal rubella. *Arch Dis Child* 1972;47:571.

100. Solorzano-Santos F, Lopez-Kirwan A, Alvarez y Munoz MT, et al. [In Process Citation]. *Gac Med Mex* 2001;137:105–109.

101. Webster WS. Teratogen update: congenital rubella. *Teratology* 1998;58:13–23.

102. Lee JY, Bowden DS. Rubella virus replication and links to teratogenicity. *Clin Microbiol Rev* 2000;13:571–587.

103. Trottier G, Srivastava L, Walker CD. Etiology of infantile autism: a review of recent advances in genetic and neurobiological research. *J Psychiatry Neurosci* 1999;24:103–115.

104. Wang X, Zhang GC, Han M. [Detection of TORCH genome in the cardiac tissue of congenital heart disease]. *Zhonghua Shi Yan* 2001;15:176–178.

105. Ou D, Jonsen LA, Metzger DL, Tingle AJ. CD4+ and CD8+ T-cell clones from congenital rubella syndrome patients with IDDM recognize overlapping GAD65 protein epitopes. Implications for HLA class I and II allelic linkage to disease susceptibility. *Hum Immunol* 1999;60:652–664.

106. Niedzielska G, Katska E, Szymula D. Hearing defects in children born of mothers suffering from rubella in the first trimester of pregnancy. *Int J Pediatr Otorhinolaryngol* 2000;54:1–5.

107. Chiriboga-Klein S, Oberfield SE, Casullo AM et al. Growth in congenital rubella syndrome and correlation with clinical manifestations. *J Pediatr* 1989; 115:251–255.

108. O'Neill HJ, Russell JD, Wyatt DE, McCaughey C, Coyle PV. Isolation of viruses from clinical specimens in microtitre plates with cells inoculated in suspension. *J Virol Methods* 1996;62:169–178.

109. Nedeljkovic J, Jovanovic T, Oker-Blom C. Maturation of IgG avidity to individual rubella virus structural proteins. *J Clin Virol* 2001;22:47–54.

110. Terada K, Niizuma T, Kataoka N, Niitani Y. Testing for rubella-specific IgG antibody in urine. *Pediatr Infect Dis J* 2000;19:104–108.

111. Eggerding FA, Peters J, Lee RK, Inderlied CB. Detection of rubella virus gene sequences by enzymatic amplification and direct sequencing of amplified DNA. *J Clin Microbiol* 1991;29:945–952.

112. Revello MG, Baldanti F, Sarasini A, Zavattoni M, Torsellini M, Gerna G. Prenatal diagnosis of rubella virus infection by direct detection and semiquantitation of viral RNA in clinical samples by reverse transcription-PCR. *J Clin Microbiol* 1997;35:708–713.

113. Revello MG, Sarasini A, Baldanti F, Percivalle E, Zella D, Gerna G. Use of reverse-transcription polymerase chain reaction for detection of rubella virus RNA in cell cultures inoculated with clinical samples. *New Microbiol* 1997; 20:197–206.

114. Bosma TJ, Corbett KM, O'Shea S, Banatvala JE, Best JM. PCR for detection of rubella virus RNA in clinical samples. *J Clin Microbiol* 1995;33:1075–1079.

115. Krech U, Wilhelm JA. A solid-phase immunosorbent technique for the rapid detection of rubella IgM by haemagglutination inhibition. *J Gen Virol* 1979;44:281.

116. Herne V, Hedman K, Reedik P. Immunoglobulin G avidity in the serodiagnosis of congenital rubella syndrome. *Eur J Clin Microbiol Infect Dis* 1997;16:763–766.

117. Meitsch K, Enders G, Wolinsky JS, et al. The role of rubella-immunoblot and rubella-peptide-EIA for the diagnosis of the congenital rubella syndrome during the prenatal and newborn periods. *J Med Virol* 1997;51:280–283.

118. Ho-Terry L, Terry GM, Londesborough P. Diagnosis of foetal rubella virus infection by polymerase chain reaction. *J Gen Virol* 1990;71:1607–1611.

119. Bosma TJ, Corbett KM, Eckstein MB, et al. Use of PCR for prenatal and postnatal diagnosis of congenital rubella. *J Clin Microbiol* 1995;33:2881–2887.

120. Sarno MJ, Blase E, Galindo N, Ramirez R, Schirmer CL, Trujillo-Juarez DF. Clinical immunogenicity of measles, mumps and rubella vaccine delivered by the Injex jet injector: comparison with standard syringe injection. *Pediatr Infect Dis J* 2000;19:839–842.

121. Red Book Committee of the American Academy of Pediatrics. *Report of the committee on infectious diseases (red book 2000),* 25th ed. Elk Grove Village, IL: American Academy of Pediatrics, 2000.

122. Hofmann J, Kortung M, Pustowoit B, Faber R, Piskazeck U, Liebert UG. Persistent fetal rubella vaccine virus infection following inadvertent vaccination during early pregnancy. *J Med Virol* 2000;61:155–158.

123. Tsuru T, Mizuguchi M, Ohkubo Y, Itonaga N, Momoi MY. Acute disseminated encephalomyelitis after live rubella vaccination. *Brain Dev* 2000;22:259–261.

124. Patja A, Davidkin I, Kurki T et al. Serious adverse events after measles-mumps-rubella vaccination during a fourteen-year prospective follow-up. *Pediatr Infect Dis J* 2000;19:1127–1134.
125. Frey TK, Marr LD. Sequence of the region coding for virion proteins C and E2 and the carboxy terminus of the nonstructural proteins of rubella virus: comparison with alphaviruses. *Gene* 1988;62:85.
126. Reef SE, Plotkin S, Cordero JF, et al. Preparing for elimination of congenital Rubella syndrome (CRS): summary of a workshop on CRS elimination in the United States. *Clin Infect Dis* 2000;31:85–95.
127. Watson JC, Hadler SC, Dykewicz CA, Reef S, Phillips L. Measles, mumps, and rubella—vaccine use and strategies for elimination of measles, rubella, and congenital rubella syndrome and control of mumps: recommendations of the Advisory Committee on Immunization Practices (ACIP). *MMWR* 1998;47:1–57.
128. Cutts FT, Vynnycky E. Modelling the incidence of congenital rubella syndrome in developing countries. *Int J Epidemiol* 1999;28:1176–1184.
129. Plotkin SA. Rubella eradication. *Vaccine* 2001;19:3311–3319.
130. Kawamura N, Okamura A, Furuta H, et al. Improved dysgammaglobulinaemia in congenital rubella syndrome after immunoglobulin therapy: correlation with CD154 expression. *Eur J Pediatr* 2000;159:764–796.
131. Miller E, Cradock-Watson JE, Pollock TM. Consequences of confirmed maternal rubella at successive stages of pregnancy. *Lancet* 1982;2:781.
132. Cradock-Watson JE, Ridehalgh MKS, Anderson MJ, et al. Fetal infection resulting from maternal rubella after the first trimester of pregnancy. *J Hyg (London)* 1980;85:381.

CHAPTER 139
Varicella and Herpes Zoster

John A. Zaia and Charles Grose

HISTORICAL BACKGROUND

Varicella is the vesicular exanthem caused by primary infection with varicella-zoster virus (VZV), commonly termed chickenpox. Herpes zoster is the clinical syndrome of segmental vesicular exanthem and pain associated with reactivation of latent VZV infection in a nerve ganglion, commonly termed shingles.

The history and epidemiology of varicella have been reviewed in detail (1,2). The documented record of varicella dates from the ninth century AD, when the Persian physician Rhazes noted the mild pustular skin eruption that was not protective against smallpox (3). It was formally differentiated in the medical literature from scarlet fever in the 16th century but was not distinguished from smallpox until the late 17th century (2,3). The vernacular term chickenpox seems to derive from the Old English *gican*, meaning "to itch" or "to scratch" (4), although other derivations from folklore have been suggested (5). The itching rash of chickenpox was termed varicella in the mid-18th century, formally distinguishing it from the severe morbidity of variola (2). More than a century later, varicella became epidemiologically linked to herpes zoster.

Herpes zoster has been recognized from antiquity as the creeping eruption that girdles the body; from this characteristic feature, the common name shingles is derived (Latin *cingulum*, a "girdle") (1). It was not until 1892, however, that the observation was made by von Bokay that varicella can develop after exposure to shingles (6). Subsequently, varicella was observed to occur after inoculation of susceptible children with zoster vesicle fluid (7). In addition, the histopathology of these two entities was noted to be virtually identical (8). It was later suggested by Garland (9) that this relationship reflected the reactivation of a latent virus. Not until Weller (10) and co-workers demonstrated the method for isolation and serial propagation of VZV were these two clinical syndromes conclusively shown to be due to the same viral agent. Viral isolates obtained from varicella

and from zoster were demonstrated to be identical on the basis of cytopathic effect (11), antigen reactivity (12), viral morphology (13,14), identity of deoxyribonucleic acid (DNA) molecular weight (15), and restriction fragment length polymorphism (16–18).

EPIDEMIOLOGY

Transmission and Communicability

The spread of infectious VZV is by air droplets from nasopharyngeal secretions; this usually requires face-to-face exposure but can also occur without direct contact through air currents to susceptible individuals (19). The period of infectivity is generally considered to be between 48 hours before and 4 days after appearance of the exanthem; this is derived from published observations of varicella in cohorts of children quarantined for other infections. In this setting, it was rare to observe spread of varicella from a child who exposed other wardmates more than 2 days before the onset of rash (20,21). Although there is a single report that infectivity could occur 4 days before exanthem (22), this case is suspect and would be the exception to the common experience, which suggests that exposure more than 1 day before exanthem is unlikely to be infectious (20,21). The recommendation of the Centers for Disease Control and Prevention is to consider the period of infectivity 48 hours before rash until the skin lesions are crusted (23).

Herpes zoster is spread by direct contact or by exposure to airborne infectious material (24,25). The incubation period for chickenpox after exposure to zoster (24) is the same as that after exposure to varicella (21) (median time, 15 days; range, 10 to 21 days). The clinical varicella attack rate after household zoster, however, is only 15% among history-negative children (24), compared with an attack rate of 87% after exposure to household chickenpox (26). This difference is thought to be due to a shorter infectious period (approximately 2 days) in herpes zoster.

Incidence and Morbidity Data

Prior to the use of VZV vaccine, there were approximately 3.5 million cases of varicella and 300,000 cases of herpes zoster in the United States per year (27). The age-specific epidemiologic analysis is shown in Table 139.1. More than 90% of all cases of varicella occurred in persons younger than 15 years, and nearly half of all cases in children occurred between the ages of 5 and 9 years. On the basis of public records, the incidence of herpes zoster was constant for each age group through middle adulthood. Thereafter, the incidence of zoster increased with age, such that persons in their 80s had a 1 in 100 chance per year of developing zoster (28). When it is adjusted for prior occurrence of varicella, the incidence of zoster in younger children was also higher, a known association in children who have acquired varicella before their first year of life (29).

Data from population-based studies of hospital discharges in the pre-vaccine era showed a relatively constant rate of serious varicella-related complications for each age group up to 14 years, but the rate increased by more than tenfold for persons older than 20 years. The types of complications that led to hospitalization in VZV infection have been reviewed (2,27,30–32) and are summarized in Table 139.2. Bacterial skin infections and bacterial pneumonias occurred in the youngest groups, and before the antibiotic era, severe bacterial infections, including osteomyelitis, were not uncommonly associated with varicella. With the development of antibiotics, however, the major complications of VZV infection in childhood included encephalitis

TABLE 139.1.   Pre-VZV Vaccine Era Epidemiologic Data for Varicella and Herpes Zoster in the United States

	Varicella					Herpes zoster[e]		
Age (y)	Susceptibility[a] (%)	Incidence[b]	Total cases (%)	Hospitalization rate[c]	Mortality[d]	Age (y)	General incidence[b]	Incidence after varicella[f]
<1	100	3,377	3.3	10	7.2			
1–4	97	8,214	32.3	9	1.4	<5	20	110
5–9	64	9,027	49.9	8	1.4	5–9	30	51
10–14	18	1,753	11.1	12	1.4	10–14	59	69
15–19	10	291	1.9	42	1.4	15–19	63	70
>20	8	33	1.5	127	1.3	20–50	42	68
					30.9			

[a]Based on serologic surveys and comparison to incidence rates.
[b]Incidence = cases per 100,000 persons per year.
[c]Hospitalization per 10,000 varicella cases.
[d]Mortality = deaths per 100,000 varicella cases. From Preblud SR: Varicella: Complications and costs. P 78(Suppl):728–735,1986; ages 1 to 4 combined.
[e]Based on published data from Ragozzino MW, Melton LJ 3d Kurland LT, et al. Population-based study of herpes and its sequelae. *Medicine (Baltimore)* 1982;61:310–316, and Guess HA, Broughton DD, Melton LJ III, Kurland LT. Epidemiology of herpes zoster in children and adolescents: a population-based study. *Pediatrics* 1985;76:512–517.
[f]Incidence = cases per 100,000 persons per year with prior varicella.
Modified from population-based data in Guess HA, Broughton DD, Melton LJ III, Kurland LT. Population-based studies of varicella complications. *Pediatrics* 1986;78[Suppl]:723–727, Guess HA, Broughton DD, Melton LJ III, Kurland LT. Chickenpox hospitalizations among residents of Omsted County, Minnesota, 1962 through 1981, A population based study. *Am J Dis Child* 1984;138:1055–1057, and Meyer PA, Seward JF, Jumaan AO, Wharton M. Varicella mortality trends before vaccine licensure in the United States, 1970–1994. *J Infect Dis* 2000;182:383–90.

and Reye's syndrome. Encephalitis occurred in approximately 1 in 11,000 cases in the group aged 5 to 14 years and is described below. Reye's syndrome was associated with the use of aspirin during varicella and had been observed to occur at a rate as high as 1 in 6,600 cases in certain regions of the United States (30). The occurrence of Reye's syndrome is now rare because of the recommendation that aspirin be avoided in children with varicella (27,33).

In older teenagers and adults, the primary complications are encephalitis and varicella pneumonia (30). Encephalitis occurs in approximately 1 in 3,000 cases of varicella in persons older than 15 years. Varicella pneumonia occurs at a constant rate in those aged 15 to 19 years, but thereafter the pneumonia rate is much higher. Clinically significant disease is seen in 1 in 375 cases of varicella, and asymptomatic disease with radiographic changes is common, occurring in as many as 16% of adults (34).

TABLE 139.2.   Pre-VZV Vaccine Era Age-Specific Complication Rate of Varicella in the United States

Age (y)	Complication	Rate
<5	Bacterial skin infections	1:3,800[a]
	Pneumonia	1:7,700
5–9	Encephalitis	1:11,100
	Reye's syndrome	1:16,700[b]
10–14	Encephalitis	1:11,100
	Reye's syndrome	1:6,700[b]
15–19	Encephalitis	1:3,400
	Varicella pneumonia	1:4,100
>20	Encephalitis	1:3,000
	Varicella pneumonia	1:375

[a]Hospitalization rate per number of varicella cases.
[b]Rates calculated before 1982 and exceed currently reported rates (see text).
Modified from Preblud SR. Varicella: complications and costs. *Pediatrics* 1986;78[Suppl]:728–735, and Guess HA, Broughton DD, Melton LJ III, Kurland LT. Population-based studies of varicella complications. *Pediatrics* 1986;78[Suppl]:723–727.

Mortality and Estimated Cost

The case reports to public health agencies of deaths due to varicella had indicated a range slightly below 100 fatalities per year in the United States. It is possible that this rate was falling with the increased ability to treat the infection (27). The mortality rate for all cases of chickenpox in normal children 1 to 14 years of age was estimated to be 0.0014% (1.4 per 100,000 cases), and the estimated rate was 31 per 100,000 in normal adults (27). Pregnant women were at increased risk for complications during varicella (35,36). The two highest risk groups for lethal complications of varicella were susceptible immunosuppressed persons and neonates born within 5 days of onset of maternal varicella; these groups are discussed in detail later.

The cost of hospitalization for VZV infections was estimated to be $17 million per year (27). However, the more significant cost of this infection in an industrialized society was lost wages by parents for home care of their sick children. In the United States, this totaled approximately $380 million per year (27). The major cost of VZV infection, therefore, was not related to the severity of disease but to lost income in affected families.

PATHOPHYSIOLOGY

Primary Infection: Varicella

CLINICAL FEATURES

In most healthy children, the clinical features of VZV infection appear at a median time of 15 days after exposure (21,24,26) and present as a mild exanthem often associated with prodromal malaise, pharyngitis, and rhinitis. The rash is characterized as a vesicular eruption that emerges in successive crops during the first 3 to 4 days of illness, usually with concomitant enanthema. Each skin vesicle appears on an erythematous base—hence the simile "a dewdrop on a rose petal" to describe this lesion (Fig. 139.1). However, it is difficult to see this stage of infection because of the rapid progression of the skin changes. Within 12 hours, this lesion becomes an umbilicated papule (Fig. 139.2);

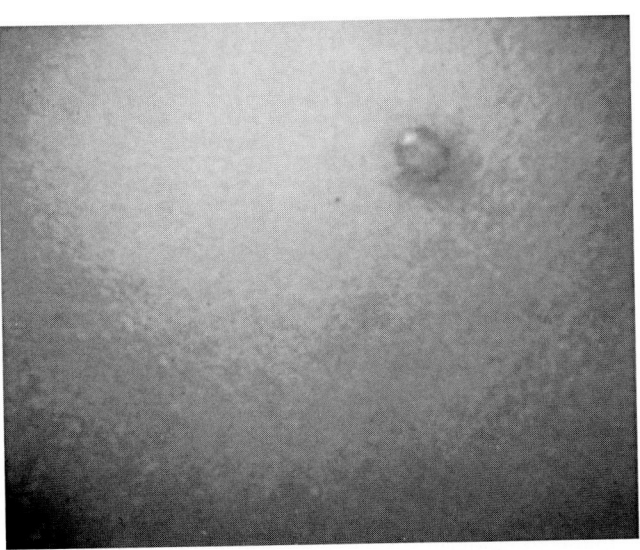

Figure 139.1. Initial vesicular lesion of varicella, appearing as a dewdrop on a rose petal.

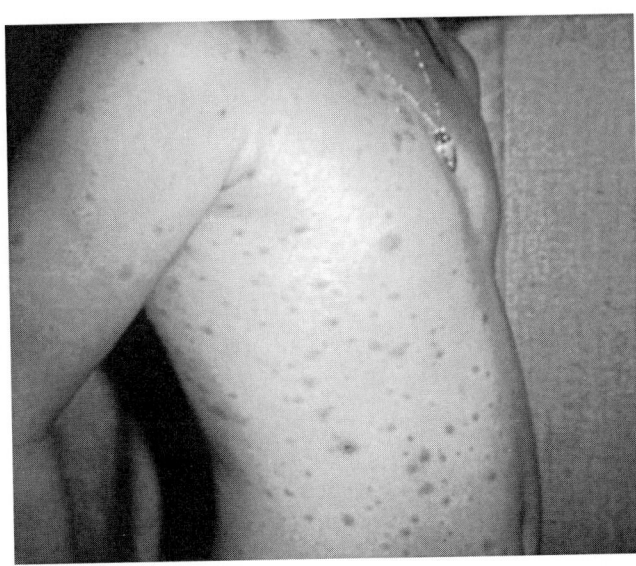

Figure 139.3. Varicella, day 2; note truncal distribution and lesions in multiple stages of development.

the involved area then undergoes leukocytic infiltration and develops into a pustule, which evolves into a hardened, crusted papule. This rapid progression from stage to stage characterizes the clinical syndrome of varicella and enables it to be distinguished from certain other vesicular eruptions. The exanthem usually begins on the head and quickly progresses to the trunk and arms, finally appearing on the legs (Figs. 139.3 and 139.4). Because of the rapid progression of individual lesions, it is common to see all stages of the exanthem, including macules, vesicles, papules, and crusts, in the same region of the skin. The most definitive clinical description of varicella was made by Ross (26), and a summary of the fever and rash of chickenpox is shown in Table 139.3. Fever can be expected to be elevated for the first 4 days of the exanthem. Much of the morbidity is associated with the extent of the cutaneous exanthem. The average number of pox per child is variable, apparently depending on the child's age and on whether the infection occurred as a secondary case within a family (26).

PATHOGENESIS

The events leading to the clinical syndrome of varicella are thought to be similar to those that were first proposed by Fenner (37) to explain an animal model of viral exanthem. In this schema, virus enters the host from an exogenous source, spreads locally to a site of initial augmentation, and then, by a primary viremia, spreads to a location of subsequent viral growth (Fig. 139.5). After several days of replication, the virus spreads by means of a second viremia to the skin and mucosal surfaces, where the exanthem and enanthema occur (37). The time course for such virus replication and spread varies from 10 to 21 days, the range observed for the incubation period of varicella (21,24,26). The existence of the primary viremia has not been documented, but the secondary viremia is well described (38). Virus spreads to endothelial cells of the skin and then infects the basal and deep malpighian layers of the epidermis. Here "ballooning degeneration" of these cells occurs, and local collection of extracellular

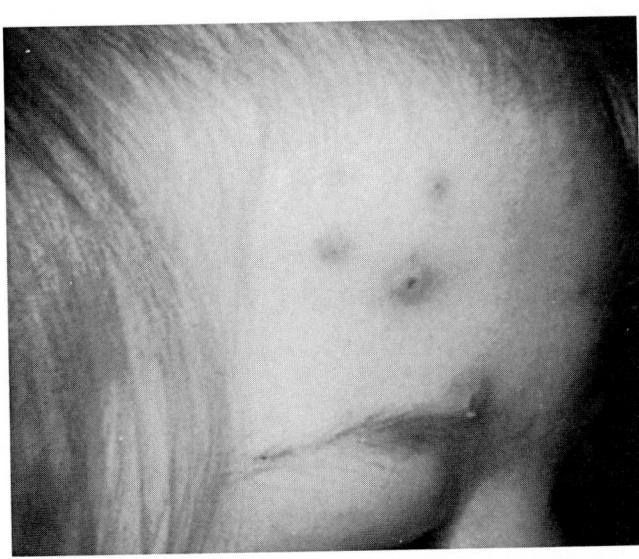

Figure 139.2. Vesiculopustular lesions of varicella.

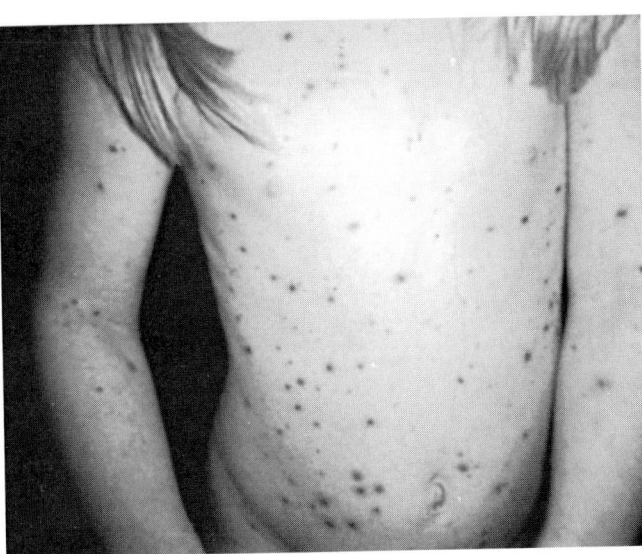

Figure 139.4. Varicella, day 4; note crusting of lesions in the same patient as in Figure 139.3.

TABLE 139.3.   Clinical Course of Varicella in Children

Group	T_{max} (°F)[a]			Pox count	
	Day 2	Day 4	Day 6	<5 Years	>5 Years
Primary infection[b]	101.0	100.2	99.3	207	258
Secondary infections[c]	100.8	100.5	99.4	310	510

[a]Average maximal daily temperature.
[b]Primary infection was defined as the first case of varicella in a child having clinically well siblings.
[c]Secondary infections were all subsequent cases of varicella in siblings of the primary case.
Modified from Ross AH. Modification of chicken pox in family contacts by administration of gamma globulin. *N Engl J Med* 1962;267:369–376.

edema results in unilocular and multilocular vesicles (1,8) (Fig. 139.6). In addition to swelling of infected cells, multinucleation occurs, forming the basis for the Tzanck assay, and condensation of viral proteins within the nuclei results in intranuclear inclusions.

Reactivation Infection: Herpes Zoster

CLINICAL FEATURES

The initial symptom of herpes zoster is pain, which is usually localized to a single spinal nerve dermatome. In 1900, Head and Campbell (39) described the anatomic pathology of this syndrome and its precise localization to single dermatomes, which permitted a mapping of the cutaneous distribution of the spinal nerves. The clinical morbidity of herpes zoster is determined largely by the involved dermatome, cranial nerve syndromes being particularly severe. The distribution mimics that of varicella, with thoracolumbar dermatomes being most frequently involved, followed by cranial dermatomes, and then by cervical and lumbar dermatomes (39–41).

Histopathologic studies have shown that the dorsal spinal ganglion is the site of intense inflammation, often with hemorrhagic necrosis of nerve cells and eventual destruction of portions of the ganglion. There is intense inflammatory response to the site of VZV reactivation, and this results in nerve dam-

age manifested clinically as meningitis or encephalitis, with or without paresis of limbs, face, gut, or urinary bladder (42–49). In addition, there can be considerable inflammation and scarring of the involved epidermis (Figs. 139.7 and 139.8), resulting in loss of epidermal appendages, corneal clouding, and vascularization of ophthalmic structures (46). In addition to severe inflammation, it is associated with postherpetic neuralgia, which occurs with increasing frequency in older persons and can be a significant problem lasting for many months (28,41,49). VZV-associated central nervous system (CNS) complications observed with varicella and herpes zoster are compared in Table 139.4. Varicella complications present equally as cerebral or cerebellar abnormalities, the latter being a more benign disease (45,50,51). Rarer CNS disorders, such as granulomatous angiitis, have been observed after herpes zoster, but these are poorly understood syndromes that have not been etiologically related to reactivation of VZV infection (52). In immunodeficient persons, CNS disease is an important problem in herpes zoster, as with varicella, and progressive CNS disease occurs in persons with human immunodeficiency virus type 1 infection (53,54).

As with varicella, zoster-related neurologic disease can occur either before or after the acute infection (55,56) and can occur

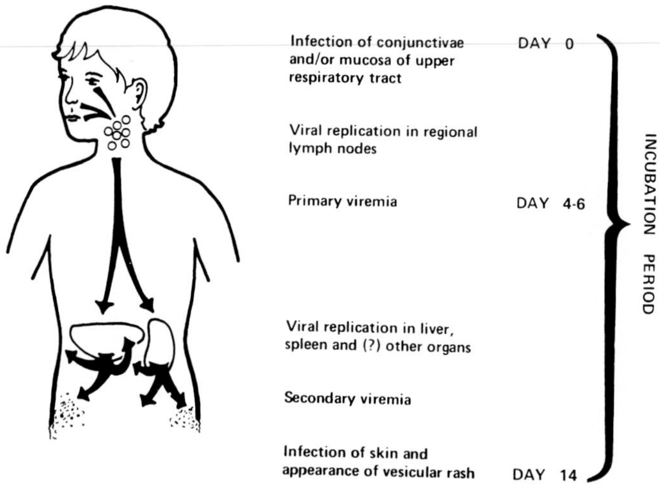

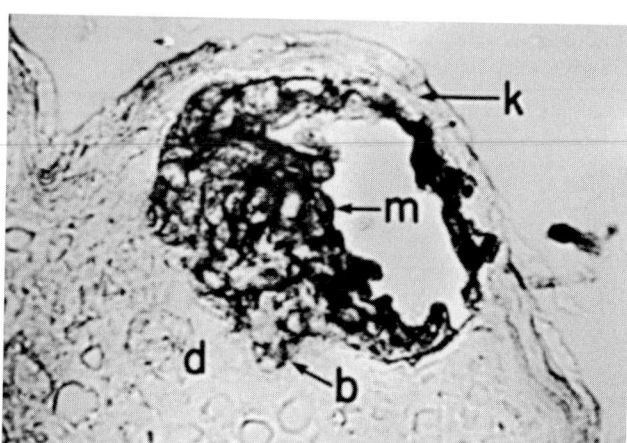

Figure 139.6. Location of VZV-specific antigen in a herpes zoster vesicle. Thin sections of a vesicle biopsy specimen were examined by indirect staining with a murine VZV immune globulin-specific monoclonal antibody and a peroxidase-conjugated rabbit antiserum to mouse immunoglobulin G. VZV antigens appear as black areas throughout the basal (*b*) and malpighian (*m*) layers of the epidermis. The outer granular and keratin (*k*) layers overlying the emergent vesicle and the inner dermis (*d*) were negative for VZV-specific antigens. (From Weigle KA, Grose C. Common expression of varicella-zoster viral glycoprotein antigens in vitro and in chickenpox and zoster vesicles. *J Infect Dis* 1983;148:630–638, with permission.)

Infection of conjunctivae and/or mucosa of upper respiratory tract — DAY 0

Viral replication in regional lymph nodes

Primary viremia — DAY 4-6

INCUBATION PERIOD

Viral replication in liver, spleen and (?) other organs

Secondary viremia

Infection of skin and appearance of vesicular rash — DAY 14

Figure 139.5. Schema for the pathogenesis of varicella. It is assumed to involve a biphasic course during the incubation period consisting of a primary and secondary viremia before appearance of the exanthem. (From Grose C. Variation on a theme by Fenner: the pathogenesis of chickenpox. *Pediatrics* 1981;68:735–737, with permission.)

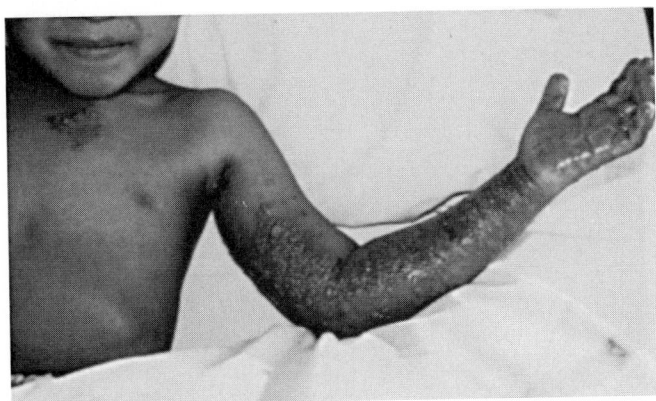

Figure 139.7. Herpes zoster in an otherwise healthy child. Note the dermatomal distribution of this unusually severe form, which required skin grafts to restore full range of motion.

TABLE 139.4. Clinical Features of Varicella-Zoster Virus-Associated Neurologic Complications

Feature	Varicella (%)[a] (N = 52)	Herpes zoster (%)[b] (N = 39)
Mild confusion	7	18
Altered sensorium or hallucinations	15	46
Stupor, semicoma	30	15
Meningismus	26	10
Headache	32	13
Ataxia	48	10
Seizure	17	10
Cranial nerve palsies	5	10
Extracranial nerve palsies	0	21
Cerebrospinal fluid findings		
Glucose	Normal	Normal
Protein	5.2–76 mg/dL	48–123 mg/dL
Cells	0–260	20–800

[a]Modified from Johnson R, Milboum PE. Central nervous system manifestations of chickenpox. *Can Med Assoc J* 1970;102:831–834.
[b]Modified from Jemsek J, Greenberg SB, Taber L, et al. Herpes zoster-associated encephalitis: Clinicopathologic report of 12 cases and review of the literature. *Medicine (Baltimore)* 1983;62:81–97.

with VZV reactivation in the absence of skin eruption, an entity called *zoster sine herpete* (57). Several CNS syndromes, including aseptic meningitis, polyneuropathy, myelitis, and encephalitis, have been observed in normal persons in association with otherwise occult VZV infection (58).

PATHOGENESIS

Two factors important in the pathogenesis of herpes zoster are recognized: VZV becomes latent in dorsal spinal ganglia after primary VZV infection (14,59,60), and clinical zoster presents after reactivation of this latent infection (43,61). But the additional factors involved in controlling this reactivation are not understood. The virus is thought to reactivate in either the ganglion cell or the perineuronal cells (62). The disease process involves demyelination as well as active replication of virus (63). When reactivation occurs, the virus spreads within the ganglion and within the distribution of that spinal nerve.

Because of its tropism for nervous tissue, in persons with profound immunodeficiency, VZV can spread transsynaptically within specific neuronal systems, producing necrosis of brain (64). In general, however, the immune system generates intense

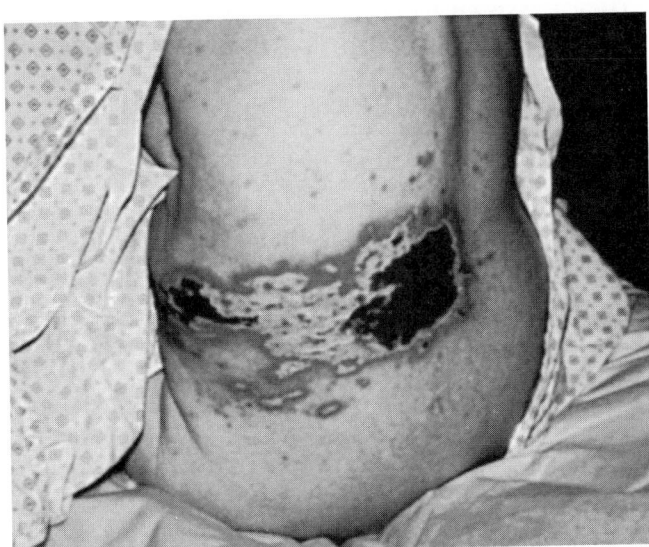

Figure 139.8. Herpes zoster in same patient as in Figures 139.10 and 139.11, day 18. Note necrosis and scarring of skin of this person, in whom postherpetic neuralgia developed.

inflammation at the initial site of virus reactivation, and the tissue reaction leads to nerve damage with pain syndrome and to damage in the epidermal structures with functional abnormalities. A generalized vesicular rash appears during the first week of herpes zoster in approximately 10% of normal adults (40,41,65,66), suggesting that failure to control the virus at the initial site of reactivation permits spread in a manner similar to that of varicella. This rash consists of a single crop of vesicles, which lack the polymorphism of varicella unless continued dissemination occurs (66). Furthermore, in recipients of bone marrow transplantation, disseminated vesicular exanthem without primary dermatomal skin eruption can follow reactivation (67). This and the observation of frequent subclinical VZV viremia in marrow transplant recipients (68) suggest that VZV latency might occur in sites other than dorsal spinal ganglia and that reactivation at extraneuronal sites could lead to viremia and generalized spread.

Varicella-Zoster Virus Infection in the Immunocompromised Host

CLINICAL FEATURES OF PROGRESSIVE VARICELLA-ZOSTER VIRUS INFECTION

With the initiation of anticancer therapy and the use of immunosuppressive agents, progressive VZV infection has been observed (69). Here, severe skin eruption occurs with or without hemorrhage (Fig. 139.9). There is high fever with dissemination of infection to visceral organs, producing hepatitis, pneumonitis, pancreatitis, small bowel obstruction, and encephalitis (70,71). A major manifestation of visceral dissemination in addition to fever is severe abdominal or back pain (72). In the pre-antiviral era, visceral dissemination occurred in 30% of children with chickenpox while they were receiving active cancer therapy (70). Pneumonitis occurred between 3 and 7 days after onset of varicella in 25% of such patients. Without antiviral therapy, the overall mortality in such cases is approximately 7%. In placebo-controlled trials of antiviral agents in similar patients, a fatal outcome occurred

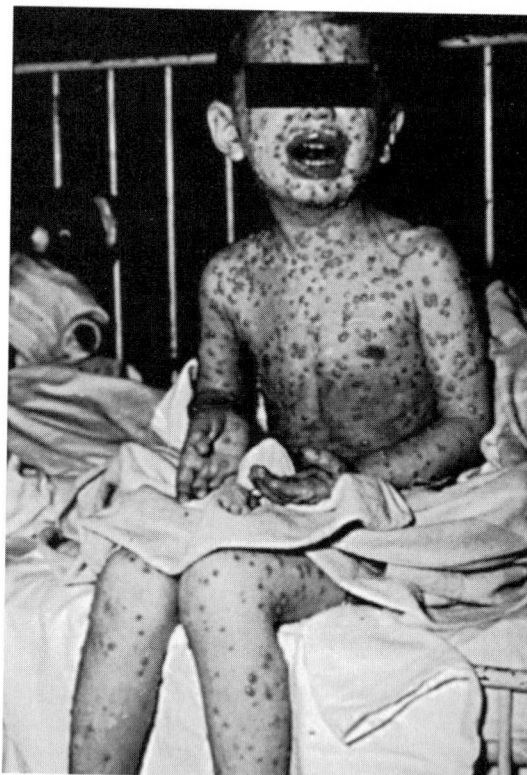

Figure 139.9. Disseminated varicella in child with leukemia receiving chemotherapy in 1950s. (Courtesy of Dr. Thomas Weller, Harvard University School of Public Health, Boston.)

in 17% and visceral dissemination in 52% of the placebo groups (73–75). In addition to virus dissemination, bacterial superinfection was a problem, and bacteremia accounted for significant morbidity during VZV dissemination (70).

The severity of herpes zoster is less predictable in patients receiving immunosuppressive agents (Fig. 139.10). Persons undergoing treatment for cancer are at higher risk for developing herpes zoster than are others. Certain of these patients, such as those with Hodgkin's disease and those undergoing bone mar-

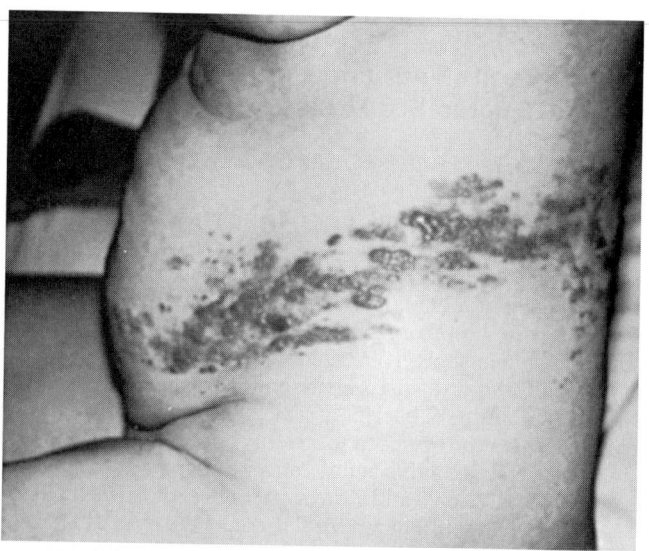

Figure 139.10. Herpes zoster in immunosuppressed adult, day 3.

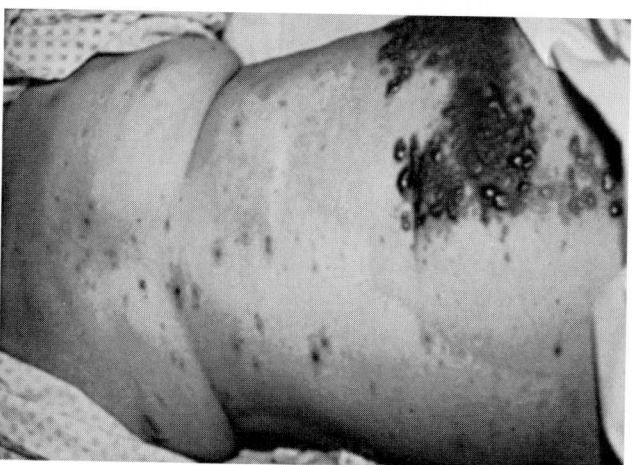

Figure 139.11. Herpes zoster in same patient as in Figure 139.10, day 8; note cutaneous dissemination of vesicular rash and hemorrhage into dermatomal lesion.

row transplantation, experience reactivation of VZV in 35% to 50% of cases during the first year of treatment (67,76–79). In the pre-antiviral era, the significant feature of herpes zoster was interruption of cancer therapy and further hospitalization. In general, mortality was low compared with disseminated VZV infection occurring during varicella; yet in the immunosuppressed person, herpes zoster can be associated with prolonged infection, delayed healing, and chronic postherpetic neuralgia. General cutaneous dissemination of virus will occur in 30% to 50% of these patients (Fig. 139.11), and although most can be expected to have a relatively benign illness, in certain groups, up to 10% will have significant visceral involvement with hepatitis, pneumonitis, and occasionally encephalitis (76,78,79). In addition, in the neutropenic patient, bacterial superinfection and staphylococcal sepsis can be a particular threat (77). The mortality rate for immunosuppressed patients with disseminated herpes zoster was 3% to 5% in the pre-antiviral era (76,77). Antiviral therapy significantly reduces this morbidity and, when it is used early in reactivation, can usually eliminate mortality (74,80,81).

PATHOGENESIS OF VARICELLA-ZOSTER VIRUS DISSEMINATION

The relationship between immunosuppression and VZV reactivation supports the view that the host's immune function controls both reactivation and dissemination of VZV infections. The explanation for this control is poorly understood. It has been observed that herpes zoster occurs in children when primary VZV infection has occurred in the first year of life (29) and in the elderly (28,49) at times when immune regulation may not be completely functional (82). The reactivation associated with bone marrow transplantation occurs between 3 and 9 months after the initial radiochemotherapy for bone marrow transplantation; this interval suggests that immune factors involved in control of reactivation are lost after marrow engraftment (67,68). It is recognized that humoral factors can influence blood-borne virus dissemination (83), but declining humoral immunity in the bone marrow transplant recipient probably does not account for the reactivation of herpes zoster. Furthermore, children with hypogammaglobulinemia usually have no difficulty controlling primary VZV infection and have no recognized increased incidence of herpes zoster (84). Progressive VZV dissemination is observed in children with primary cell-mediated immune deficiency (85) and in children and adults with acquired

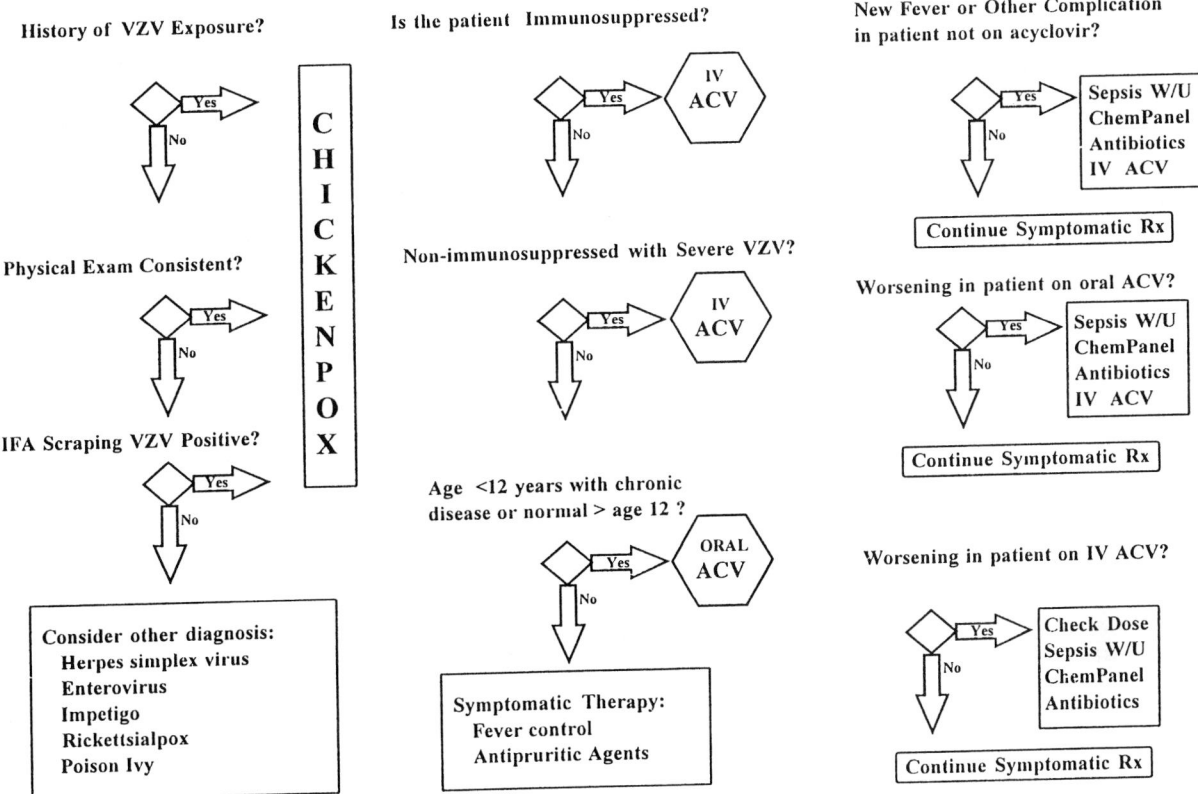

1. Diagnosis

History of VZV Exposure?

Physical Exam Consistent?

IFA Scraping VZV Positive?

CHICKENPOX

Consider other diagnosis:
Herpes simplex virus
Enterovirus
Impetigo
Rickettsialpox
Poison Ivy

2. Initial Assessment

Is the patient Immunosuppressed?

IV ACV

Non-immunosuppressed with Severe VZV?

IV ACV

Age <12 years with chronic disease or normal > age 12 ?

ORAL ACV

Symptomatic Therapy:
Fever control
Antipruritic Agents

3. Secondary Assessment

New Fever or Other Complication in patient not on acyclovir?

Sepsis W/U
ChemPanel
Antibiotics
IV ACV

Continue Symptomatic Rx

Worsening in patient on oral ACV?

Sepsis W/U
ChemPanel
Antibiotics
IV ACV

Continue Symptomatic Rx

Worsening in patient on IV ACV?

Check Dose
Sepsis W/U
ChemPanel
Antibiotics

Continue Symptomatic Rx

Figure 139.12. Flowchart for guiding the management of chickenpox. The three steps include establishing the diagnosis, making the initial assessment of the patient, and then making secondary assessments, as described in text. IFA, Indirect fluorescent antibody assay; IV ACV, intravenous acyclovir; W/U, work-up. (From Zaia JA. Varicella-zoster virus. In: Schlossberg D, ed. *Current therapy of infectious disease.* Philadelphia: Mosby-Year Book, 1995:501, with permission.)

immunodeficiency syndrome (53,54,86,87). It appears that VZV antibody can moderate the extent or duration of viremia and that cellular immunity is required to prevent VZV replication (83–89). In the elegant studies of Arvin and co-workers (89), it was shown that severity of disease is a function of decreased T-cell activation, as indicated by proliferative responses *in vitro*. In addition, interferon-α production can play a role in limiting virus spread (73,90); immunosuppressed children with severe varicella have been shown to have diminished production of interferon-α and significantly reduced lymphocyte proliferative response to VZV antigen (89).

MANAGEMENT

Diagnosis

The diagnosis of VZV infection is discussed in Chapter 234. The primary reason for documenting this diagnosis is to confirm the need for antiviral therapy or for control of nosocomial infection. Basically, the diagnosis of VZV infection rests on three pieces of information: (a) the history of exposure and the clinical appearance of exanthem; (b) the presence of virus, viral antigens, or virus-associated cytopathic effect within the lesion; and (c) the subsequent documentation of antibody production to VZV From a practical standpoint, the diagnosis can often be made on clinical grounds, and this is especially true for secondary cases of varicella and for herpes zoster. However, because other vesicular

exanthems, such as streptococcal impetigo, poison ivy, and coxsackievirus infections, can mimic VZV infection, it is sometimes necessary to document the diagnosis of infection more exactly (Fig. 139.12).

Antiviral Therapy

GENERAL APPROACH

The initial assessment of the patient with VZV infection should include (a) determination of diagnosis by history, physical examination, and laboratory tests; (b) determination of whether the individual is at higher than normal risk for severe infection; and (c) characterization of current status of the infection (see Fig. 139.12). Once a tentative diagnosis is established, the critical information on which antiviral therapy hinges is whether there is risk for complications of infection and whether there is existing evidence of virus dissemination. Persons at risk for complications[1] are those receiving immunosuppressive medication or those who are immunodeficient from previous medication or radiation therapy; those with congenital or acquired immunodeficiency, including acquired immunodeficiency syndrome; adults with varicella; and premature infants with varicella or neonates with varicella acquired from a maternal source (Table 139.5). Because the increased risk is not easy to assess in many persons,

[1] See references 23,27,30,67,69,65,70,76,78,83,86,87.

TABLE 139.5. Groups at Risk for Complications of Varicella-Zoster Virus Infection[a]

Susceptible persons receiving immunosuppressive therapy[b]
Persons with congenital cellular immunodeficiency
Persons with an acquired immunodeficiency, including acquired immunodeficiency syndrome
Persons older than 20 y
Newborn infants exposed to onset of maternal varicella <5 d before or shortly after birth
Premature infants[c]

[a]Susceptible (antibody-negative) persons exposed to VZV by indoor face-to-face contact with an infected person less than 2 d before or anytime during vesiculopustular stage of varicella rash are at highest risk.
[b]In general, all types of cytoreductive therapy and radiotherapy are considered immunosuppressive. The dose of prednisone that is immunosuppressive can vary in individual cases but is in the range of 1 mg/kg/d.
[c]The risk for complications of VZV infection in this group is poorly defined and is based on the likelihood of protective maternal antibody versus gestational age at birth.

especially in normal adults with varicella or with cutaneous dissemination of zoster, it is necessary to base the clinical decision to treat with an antiviral agent on the course of infection. In doing this, it is necessary to determine the progression of the illness using parameters such as fever, continued development of new vesicles on skin, change in hepatic enzyme levels, pulmonary examination and chest radiographic findings, and physical and laboratory evidence of specific organ involvement. Fever several days into the course of infection, especially in association with abdominolumbar pain, can be an indication of visceral dissemination (72). Hepatic enzyme levels will be mildly elevated in most cases of varicella, even in nonimmunodeficient persons (91), but can be useful to observe disease progression. Certain organ involvement, such as eye, lung, or brain, should always be treated with antiviral medication.

RECOMMENDED USE OF ANTIVIRAL AGENTS

The commercially available antiviral drugs that are approved for treatment of VZV infection include acyclovir, famciclovir, and valacyclovir. In the United States, acyclovir is the only agent approved for the treatment of chickenpox or for disseminated VZV infection in immunosuppressed persons (73–75,80,81,92–95). For the treatment of zoster, acyclovir, famciclovir and valacyclovir are approved agents (96–99). Acyclovir accelerates the time to healing (96). Famciclovir also improves the time to healing and appears to improve the occurrence of postherpetic neuralgia (97,98). Valacyclovir is similar to famciclovir in enhancing the resolution of zoster-associated pain and postherpetic neuralgia (99). Resistance of VZV to acyclovir and related drugs has been observed, and use of foscarnet is recommended in treatment failure, particularly in patients with acquired immunodeficiency syndrome (92).

The recommended dosage of acyclovir is 10 mg/kg (or 500 mg/m^2) given intravenously every 8 hours in a 1-hour infusion for 7 days (Table 139.6). Because of the risk for crystallization of drug in the renal tubule, it is recommended that serum creatinine levels be obtained every 3 days, and dosage modification is necessary for renal failure (see Table 139.6). To minimize the occurrence of renal complications during therapy, it is useful to give a volume of intravenous fluid equal to the volume of acyclovir, if tolerated, to initiate a diuresis before the infusion of acyclovir, and acyclovir should be infused in a concentration of 4 mg/mL or less.

Acyclovir (800 mg five times daily), famciclovir (500 mg three times daily) and valacyclovir (1 g three times daily) have been licensed in the United States for administration by oral route for the treatment of herpes zoster in otherwise healthy adults (96–99). Oral acyclovir can lessen the fever and the number and duration of skin lesions and is licensed for the treatment of chickenpox (100). However, the American Academy of Pediatrics does not recommend that it be used for this indication in otherwise healthy children younger than 12 years. It recommends, instead,

TABLE 139.6. Antiviral Treatment of Chickenpox and Zoster

Agent	Indication	Creatinine clearance (mL/min/1.73 M^2)	Dose	Dosing interval	Duration
Oral acyclovir	Chickenpox >age 12 Zoster	>25	20 mg/kg up to 800 mg	q6h	5 days
		10–25	Same	q8h	5 days
		0–10[a]	Same	q12h	5 days
IV acyclovir	Life-threatening VZV Infection	>50	500 mg/M^2 or 10 mg/kg[b,c]	q8h	7 days
		25–50	Same	q12h	7 days
		10–25	Same	q24h	7 days
		0–10[a]	250 mg/M^2	q24h	7 days
Famciclovir	Zoster > age 18	>60	500 mg	q8h	7 days
		40–59	500 mg	q12h	7 days
		20–39	500 mg	q24h	7 days
Valacyclovir	Zoster > age 18	>50	1,000 mg	q8h	7 days
		29–49	1,000 mg	q12h	7 days
		10–29	1,000 mg	q24h	7 days
		<10	500 mg	q24h	7 days
Foscarnet	Acyclovir-resistant VZV[d]	>100[e]	60 mg/kg	q8h	7–10 days

See package insert for recommended dose adjustment of all drugs.
[a]An additional dose is recommended after each hemodialysis treatment.
[b]To minimize renal toxicity an adequate urine output is required. This can be assured if the acyclovir is infused at a concentration of approximately 4 mg/ml over 1 hour and the same volume of fluid is given over the next hour prior to the acyclovir.
[c]Use ideal body weight for height to calculate dose in obese person: M^2, square meter of body surface area.
[d]Foscarnet is recommended by experts for treatment of life-threatening acyclovir-resistant VZV infection, but this is not an FDA-approved indication for foscarnet use. Appropriate informed consent should be obtained before such use.
[e]Foscarnet is nephrotoxic, and dosage should be based on creatinine clearance. Guidelines for doseage adjustment are listed in the package information.

that oral acyclovir be used to treat chickenpox in those with chronic cutaneous or pulmonary disorders, in those receiving chronic salicylate therapy, in those receiving short or intermittent courses of corticosteroids or aerosolized corticosteroids, and in otherwise healthy persons older than 12 years (101). Some experts recommend the use of oral acyclovir for secondary household cases in which the disease usually is more severe (101). The use of oral acyclovir for chickenpox in immunodeficient persons is not generally recommended because of the poor absorption of the oral formulation. However, as noted by the American Academy of Pediatrics, with case-by-case evaluation of risk versus benefit and with assurance of follow-up, oral acyclovir is used by some experts for treatment of chickenpox in selected immunosuppressed persons (101).

For herpes zoster, the risk for postherpetic neuralgia is related to the patient's age, the rash severity, and the acute pain severity and can be lessened by the early use of antiviral agents, particularly famciclovir and valacyclovir (97–99). The pathogenesis of postherpetic neuralgia is not understood (102), yet, on the basis of the likelihood that the inflammation produces neuronal changes necessary for pain induction, anti-inflammatory agents have been used to treat herpes zoster. Because these studies have yielded variable results, no clear recommendation can be made regarding the use of corticosteroids for zoster (96,103–105).

Management of Specific Problems

SYMPTOMATIC TREATMENT

Because itching is the major symptom of chickenpox, topical antipruritic agents such as cold calamine lotion with diphenhydramine (Benadryl) are often helpful. Warm baths containing baking soda (⅓ cup per tub of water) can temporarily relieve pruritus and should be combined with use of oral antihistamines. Antipyretics should be given to reduce fever, but aspirin must be avoided because of the association with Reye's syndrome (105,106). In herpes zoster and disseminated VZV infection, pain is a major symptom and must be treated with vigorous and effective analgesia; however, narcotic analgesics must be used at reduced dosage in the presence of hepatitis.

BACTERIAL INFECTION

Pyoderma is the most frequently observed bacterial complication of varicella (2,31) and causes the poxlike scars associated with varicella. This problem can be minimized by attention to good hygiene, including daily bathing with bacteriostatic soap, trimming of children's fingernails to minimize excoriation of itchy skin, and early recognition and treatment of superinfection. Bacterial infection should be treated with appropriate oral antibiotics, usually either erythromycin or a β-lactamase-resistant semisynthetic penicillin. Because of the persistence of infection beneath crusted lesions, débridement with salt solution soaks can be helpful.

RESPIRATORY TRACT INFECTION

Laryngitis and laryngotracheobronchitis can occur during varicella and may require treatment with analgesics and humidification of air. Bacterial superinfection can also involve the lower respiratory tract, producing pneumonia and bronchitis, and pneumonia in the otherwise healthy child with varicella is usually due to the respiratory pathogens, including *Streptococcus pneumoniae*, *Haemophilus influenzae*, and *Staphylococcus aureus* (31).

MUCOSITIS

Varicella is a generalized infection involving all epithelial areas including mucosal surfaces of respiratory, alimentary, and genitourinary systems. Involvement of the bladder and urethra can result in severe dysuria with functional bladder obstruction. Urinary analgesics and, occasionally, bladder drainage may be required.

GASTROINTESTINAL COMPLICATIONS AND REYE'S SYNDROME

Some of the most serious complications of VZV infection occur in the gastrointestinal system. Vomiting is not usually part of the clinical course, and this symptom should alert the physician to abdominal or CNS complications. As with other viral infections, surgical emergencies such as appendicitis and intussusception can occur during varicella. Mild hepatic involvement is seen in a majority of children with varicella and is usually manifested by asymptomatic elevation of hepatic enzyme values, for which no treatment is necessary (91). As noted earlier, Reye's syndrome has been described in association with varicella, often with concomitant use of aspirin in the child older than 5 years (105,106). Reye's syndrome and other metabolic diseases must be excluded in any child with varicella in whom there is vomiting and changes in mental status (107). Since 1980, when the use of aspirin during respiratory infections was actively discouraged, the incidence of postvaricella Reye's syndrome has decreased so significantly that its presence should suggest an inborn error of metabolism as the primary diagnosis (107).

ENCEPHALITIS OR MYELITIS

VZV infection involving the CNS is of two types: cerebellar or cerebral complications during varicella, and cranial or peripheral nerve complications during herpes zoster (see Table 139.4). Cerebellar ataxia is the most common syndrome associated with varicella encephalitis. It is generally a benign entity that is thought to be due to postinfectious demyelination (50,51,63). Cerebral involvement is more serious, although it, too, has a favorable outcome in the normal child. However, in the immunosuppressed patient, cerebral involvement with seizures and altered mental status occurs and has a grave prognosis. Antiviral therapy is indicated in patients with CNS syndromes in which there is reason to suspect continued replication of virus, such as in any immunosuppressed person, any person with congenital or acquired immunodeficiency, and anyone in whom there is clinical evidence of continued new cutaneous vesicular lesions. From a practical standpoint, any major disorder of cerebral function occurring in association with acute VZV infection should be treated with acyclovir until diagnostic evaluation indicates that there is another explanation for the disease.

THROMBOCYTOPENIA AND BLEEDING DISORDERS

Bleeding disorders can occur during varicella and are due to disseminated intravascular coagulation, vasculitis, or idiopathic thrombocytopenia. The syndrome of purpura fulminans must be treated with supportive and antibiotic therapy until sepsis is ruled out. Anaphylactoid purpura can follow an otherwise uncomplicated case of varicella and must be managed with appropriate attention to the status of renal function and the possibility of occult intraabdominal hemorrhage. Idiopathic thrombocytopenic purpura can occur during active infection or during convalescence. Mild hemorrhage into vesicles during active infection does not require specific treatment, but excessive hemorrhage and profound thrombocytopenia should be treated with platelet infusions, intravenous immune globulin, and antiviral therapy.

MATERNAL, CONGENITAL, AND PERINATAL VARICELLA-ZOSTER VIRUS INFECTION

The most significant danger of VZV infection during pregnancy is to the health of the mother, who has nearly a 10% risk for severe pneumonia (36). Therefore, antiviral therapy should be instituted immediately if the pregnant woman develops any signs of respiratory distress. Early induction of labor, if appropriate, should be a consideration in the management of this infection. In addition, there is a risk of VZV infection to the unborn infant; this can be in the form of either congenital teratogenic infection (36,108–110) or perinatal infection (36,111). If maternal varicella occurs less than 5 days before or shortly after delivery, there is an increased mortality associated with subsequent VZV infection in the infant (111). The risk of severe VZV infection appears to be a function of the level of transplacental maternal antibody to VZV in the infant (111,112). It is recommended that such high-risk neonates exposed to maternal varicella, as well as premature infants likely to lack such maternal antibody, be given passive immunization with varicella-zoster immune globulin (VZIG) (23). Maternal herpes zoster presents no significant risk to mother or infant (36).

A pregnant woman with significant exposure to VZV infection should be evaluated for susceptibility to VZV with appropriate antibody assay (see Chapter 234) if she has a negative or unknown history of having had varicella as a child. Seronegative women should receive passive immunization with VZIG (23).

Intrauterine VZV infection can occur after maternal varicella in all trimesters of gestation, but teratogenic or developmental damage results from infection before the third trimester (36,110). The rate of transplacental infection is 24%, but clinically apparent disease is approximately 3% for maternal varicella in early pregnancy (36). The stigmata of early fetal infection include defects of the extremities, skin, and *eyes* as well as microcephaly, hydrocephalus, and brain calcifications (108,109). The abnormalities of the extremities derive from hypoplasia during development and appear as limb shortening and deformity. The characteristic cutaneous manifestations are deep cicatricial scarring, often in association with the limb abnormalities. The eye defects include microphthalmos, cataracts, and chorioretinitis. Virtually all the defects can be attributed to an interruption in the developing neurologic system of the fetus; the period of greatest risk for severe disease is the first trimester, when the fetal limb muscles are formed and innervated by nerves from the developing spinal cord. This represents a process in which the known neurotropism of the virus manifests itself in its most virulent form (110).

Approach to the Immunocompromised Host

GENERAL MANAGEMENT
In the pre-antiviral era, the management of the immunocompromised child focused on the prevention of exposure to VZV infection. This strategy relied on awareness by parents, friends, and school personnel of the importance of early notification of possible varicella contagion. This system aimed at passive immunization of high-risk groups, but because it depended on timely reaction to exposure, it was less than optimal and resulted in prolonged absences from school. With the introduction of antiviral therapy and active immunization, we are closer to the elimination of VZV as a cause of morbidity and mortality in immunosuppressed children, and there is less emphasis on the importance of varicella awareness. The VZV vaccine is not indicated for routine use in immunosuppressed persons, but children with acute lymphoblastic leukemia can and should receive this form of protection by use of an investigational protocol available from the manufacturer. Parents and school personnel must continue to be aware of exposure to VZV and of the importance

of actual VZV rash in unvaccinated high-risk children so that VZIG or early antiviral treatment can be given in the most timely fashion.

USE OF VARICELLA-ZOSTER IMMUNE GLOBULIN
It has been recognized for decades that convalescent serum from persons with VZV infection could protect from severe clinical disease (21). Ross demonstrated that immune serum globulin would modify infection in otherwise healthy children (26). Subsequently, it was shown that the effective administration of passive antibody to immunosuppressed persons failed unless convalescent antibody was used (113). With the development of efficient screening procedures for selection of high-titer outdated donor blood units (114), VZIG became commercially available. VZIG has been demonstrated to be effective for the prevention of severe varicella in the immunosuppressed person (83). Any susceptible person at risk for complications of varicella (see Table 139.5) should receive passive immunization if exposure to VZV was adequate and occurred within approximately 4 days. VZIG should not be used in the person with prior history of varicella; sensitive serologic testing for VZV antibody, using an enzyme immunoassay, a fluorescent antibody assay, or a rapid slide agglutination test, is available to make this distinction.

ANTIVIRAL THERAPY
The specific use of antiviral agents was described earlier, but management of individual patients may be less straightforward. Chickenpox in immunosuppressed persons should be treated with intravenous acyclovir until progression of disease is controlled, and then oral anti-VZV agents can be substituted. The use of intravenous acyclovir is particularly recommended for groups in which the risk of disseminated infection is particularly high or unpredictable, for example, varicella in children receiving treatment for leukemia, varicella in profound immunodeficiency states, and herpes zoster in the first 6 months after bone marrow transplantation (67,101,115). Although famciclovir and valacyclovir have not been licensed for use in immunosuppressed persons nor in children, some experts recommend use of these agents when intravenous acyclovir is not required.

Management of Nosocomial Infections

Nosocomial VZV infection is a well-recognized problem, particularly in tertiary care centers for immunosuppressed patients (116,117). Clusters of varicella can be difficult to eradicate from chronic care facilities for children and frequently affect paramedical staff from foreign countries where the rate of susceptibility among adults is higher than in the United States (118). Interestingly, herpes zoster cases have been described after exposure to VZV infection; there is no explanation for these occurrences (24,119).

Control of nosocomial infections involves three actions: (a) surveillance of susceptibility and use of VZV vaccine in susceptible or history-negative hospital staff, (b) adequate isolation of contagious VZV infections, and (c) rapid evaluation and response to reported VZV exposure. Hospitals that care for immunodeficient patients should screen staff at the time of employment for susceptibility. This can be done efficiently by performing antibody tests on those who have a negative or unknown history of prior varicella. Susceptible employees should be excluded from care of patients with VZV infection. Recommended isolation procedures for varicella are respiratory precautions, including double-door isolation, with gown, gloves, and mask for persons in the patient's room (120,121). Recommended isolation procedures for herpes zoster vary on the basis of a report that airborne spread of VZV can be associated with reactivated virus infection. However, for practical reasons in cancer centers, contact precautions are sufficient unless there is a threat of viral dissemination due to the presence of VZV pneumonia (116,117).

VARICELLA VACCINE

A live attenuated VZV vaccine was developed by Takahashi and co-workers in 1974; since that time there has been extensive experience with live virus vaccination for prevention of VZV infection (122). This vaccine was prepared by attenuation of a VZV isolate (Oka strain) in human embryonic cells, and then in human diploid fibroblasts (123). The vaccine virus is biologically different from wild VZV in its growth characteristics and DNA restriction enzyme profile (124).

This vaccine has been used extensively in Japan in healthy children and has been demonstrated to be effective for the prevention of varicella after exposure and for curtailment of outbreaks of VZV infection (122,126). A live attenuated VZV vaccine (Varivax®) was approved in the United States in 1995 (125). A single dose of vaccine results in seroconversion in 97% of susceptible children 1 to 12 years old, in 79% of children 13 to 17 years old, and in 82% of adults. Two doses of vaccine result in seroconversion in 94% of adults (126–128). VZV vaccine is recommended for all healthy children 12 months to 12 years of age in chickenpox history-negative persons, especially healthcare and daycare workers, college students, prisoners, military recruits, nonpregnant women of childbearing age, and international travelers. For adolescent and adult patients serotesting for VZV antibody is usually cost effective before vaccination (129,130). The vaccine is not recommended for infants younger than 1 year; for immunosuppressed persons; for those receiving salicylate therapy; for pregnant women; or for persons allergic to components of the vaccine, including neomycin, gelatin, and monosodium glutamate.

The effectiveness of the varicella vaccine has been reported in long term follow up studies (126–128). Vaccine effectiveness in preventing chickenpox is approximately 85% and the effectiveness for preventing severe disease is approximately 97%. Breakthrough varicella occurs in approximately 20% of vaccinees after household exposure, and the risk factors for such breakthrough are close contact with varicella, age 14 months or younger at vaccination, and receipt of low titre vaccine (131). In this regard, subjects with low serologic immune response to the vaccine appear to reactivate the vaccine virus resulting in persistent increasing serum antibody titers, suggesting that the vaccine virus persisted in vivo and reactivates in the presence of antibody titers (132). If this is true, the vaccination should result in long-term immunity.

Herpes zoster due to vaccine strain virus is very rare but does occur (133). Chickenpox has been contracted from a sibling who developed zoster 5 months after immunization with VZV vaccine (134). Despite this, it has been shown that immunization of HIV-infected children with varicella vaccine is safe in those who are mildly infected by HIV (135). Other immunosuppressed individuals such as solid organ transplant recipients who are on continuous iatrogenic immunosuppression are not recommended for receipt of VZV vaccine, and it is unlikely that these patients will have an effective immune response to the vaccine (136). However, in children with leukemia studied in the United States, vaccination given to those in remission produced a 5-year seropositivity of 70% and an attack rate of chickenpox after household exposure to VZV of only 14% (131,132). The protection from varicella exposure requires use of VZV vaccine in health care workers and the safe use of this vaccine in this population has been described (137). Other aspects of VZV vaccine have recently been reviewed. (138)

Acknowledgments

The authors express their gratitude to Ms. Suzanne Kelly for her assistance in the preparation of the manuscript.

REFERENCES

1. Taylor-Robinson D, Caunt AE. *Varicella virus.* Vienna: Springer-Verlag, 1972.
2. Gordon JE, Ingalls TH. Chickenpox: an epidemiologic review. *Am J Med Sci* 1962;244:362.
3. Bett WR. *A short history of some common diseases.* London: Oxford University Press, 1934.
4. Scott-Wilson JH. Why 'chicken' pox? [Letter]. *Lancet* 1978;1:1152.
5. Lerman SJ. Why is chickenpox called chickenpox? *Clin Pediatr* 1981;20:1111.
6. von Bokay J. Das Auftreten von Varizellen unter Eigentumlichen. *Magy Orvosi Arch* November 3, 1892. As cited in Blatt ML, Zeldes M, Stein AF. Chickenpox following contact with herpes zoster. *J Lab Clin Med* 1940;25:951.
7. Lipschutz B, Kundratit K. Über die Aetiologie des Zoster und uber seine Beziehungen zu Varizellen. *Wien Klin Wochenschr* 1925;38:499.
8. Tyzzer EE. The histology of the skin lesions in varicella. *J Med Res* 1906;14:361.
9. Garland J. Varicella following exposure to herpes zoster. *N Engl J Med* 1943;1228:336.
10. Weller TH. Serial propagation in vitro of agents producing inclusion bodies derived from varicella and herpes zoster. *Proc Soc Exp Biol* 1953;83:340.
11. Weller TH, Witton HM, Bell EJ. The etiologic agents of varicella and herpes zoster: isolation, propagation, and cultural characteristics in vitro. *J Exp Med* 1958;108:843.
12. Weller TH, Coons AH. Fluorescent antibody studies with agents of varicella and herpes zoster propagated in vitro. *Proc Soc Exp Biol Med* 1954;86:789.
13. Kimura A, Tosaka K, Nakao T. An electron microscopic study of varicella skin lesions. *Arch Gesamte Virusforsch* 1972;36:1.
14. Esiri MM, Tomlinson AH. Herpes zoster—demonstration of virus in trigeminal nerve and ganglion by immunofluorescence and electron microscopy. *J Neurol Sci* 1972;15:35.
15. Iltis JP, Oakes JE, Hyman RW, Rapp F. Comparison of the DNAs of varicella-zoster viruses isolated from clinical cases of varicella and herpes zoster. *Virology* 1977;82:345.
16. Richards JC, Hyman RW, Rapp F. Analysis of the DNAs from seven varicella-zoster virus isolates. *J Virol* 1979;32:812.
17. Pichini B, Ecker JR, Grose C, Hyman RW. DNA mapping of paired varicella-zoster virus isolates from patients with shingles. *Lancet* 1983;2:1223.
18. Straus SE, Reinhold W, Smith HA, et al. Endonuclease analysis of viral DNA from varicella and subsequent zoster infections in the same patient. *N Engl J Med* 1984;311:1362.
19. Leclair JM, Zaia JA, Levin MJ, et al. Airborne transmission of chickenpox in a hospital. *N Engl J Med* 1980;302:450.
20. Thomson FH, Aberd CM. The aerial conveyance of infection. *Lancet* 1916;1:341.
21. Gordon JE, Meader FM. The period of infectivity and serum prevention of chickenpox. *JAMA* 1929;93:2013.
22. Evans P, Mane MB. An epidemic of chickenpox. *Lancet* 1940;2:339.
23. Centers for Disease Control and Prevention. Prevention of varicella: recommendations of the advisory committee on immunization practices (ACIP). *MMWR* 1996;45:1.
24. Seiler HE. A study of herpes zoster particularly in its relationship to chickenpox. *J Hyg* 1949;47:253.
25. Josephson A, Gombert ME. Airborne transmission of nosocomial varicella from localized zoster. *J Infect Dis* 1988;158:238.
26. Ross AH. Modification of chickenpox in family contacts by administration of gamma globulin. *N Engl J Med* 1962;267:369.
27. Preblud SR. Varicella: complications and costs. *Pediatrics* 1986;78[Suppl]:728.
28. Hope-Simpson RE. Herpes zoster in the elderly. *Geriatrics* 1967;22:151.
29. Brunell PA, Kotchmar GS. Zoster in infancy: failure to maintain virus latency following intrauterine infection. *J Pediatr* 1981;98:71.
30. Guess HA, Broughton DD, Melton LJ III, Kurland LT. Population-based studies of varicella complications. *Pediatrics* 1986;78[Suppl]:723.
31. Bullowa JGM, Wishik SM. Complications of varicella: I. Their occurrence among 2,534 patients. *Am J Dis Child* 1935;49:923.
32. Preblud SR. Age-specific risks of varicella complications. *Pediatrics* 1981;68:14.
33. Barret MJ, Hurwitz ES, Schonberger LB, Rogers MR. Changing epidemiology of Reye syndrome in the United States. *Pediatrics* 1986;77:598.

34. Weber DM, Pellechia JA. Varicella pneumonia: study of prevalence in adult men. *JAMA* 1965;192:572.

35. Pearson HE. Parturition varicella-zoster. *Obstet Gynecol* 1964;23:21.

36. Paryani SG, Arvin AM. Intrauterine infection with varicella-zoster virus after maternal varicella. *N Engl J Med* 1986;314:1542.

37. Grose C. Variation on a theme by Fenner: the pathogenesis of chickenpox. *Pediatrics* 1981;68:735.

38. Ozaki T, Ichikawa T, Matsui Y, et al. Viremic phase in nonimmunocompromised children with varicella. *J Pediatr* 1984;104:85.

39. Head H, Campbell AW. The pathology of herpes zoster and its bearing on sensory localization. *Brain* 1900;23:353.

40. Hope-Simpson RE. The nature of herpes zoster: a long-term study and a new hypothesis. *Proc R Soc Med* 1965;58:9.

41. Burgoon DF Jr, Burgoon JS, Baldridge GD. The natural history of herpes zoster. *JAMA* 1957;164:265.

42. Denny-Brown D, Adams RD, Fitzgerald PJ. Pathologic features of herpes zoster—a note on "geniculate herpes." *Arch Neurol Psychol* 1944;51:216.

43. Gold E. Serologic and virus-isolation studies of patients with varicella or herpes-zoster infection. *N Engl J Med* 1966;274:181.

44. Jellinek EH, Tulloch WS. Herpes zoster with dysfunction of bladder and anus. *Lancet* 1976;2:1219.

45. Jemsek J, Greenberg SB, Taber L, et al. Herpes zoster-associated encephalitis: clinicopathologic report of 12 cases and review of the literature. *Medicine (Baltimore)* 1983;62:81.

46. Womack LW, Liesegang TJ. Complications of herpes zoster ophthalmicus. *Arch Ophthalmol* 1983;101:42.

47. Winkelmann RK, Perry HO. Herpes zoster in children. *JAMA* 1959;171:376.

48. Guess HA, Broughton DD, Melton LJ III, Kurland LT. Epidemiology of herpes zoster in children and adolescents: a population-based study. *Pediatrics* 1985;76:512.

49. Ragozzino ME, Melton LJ III, Kurland LT, et al. Population-based study of herpes zoster and its sequelae. *Medicine (Baltimore)* 1982;61:310.

50. Johnson R, Milbourn PE. Central nervous system manifestations of chickenpox. *Can Med Assoc J* 1970;102:831.

51. Underwood EA. The neurological complications of varicella—a clinical and epidemiologic study. *Br J Child Dis* 1935;32:83,177,241.

52. Blue MC, Rosenblum WI. Granulomatous angiitis of the brain with herpes zoster and varicella encephalitis. *Arch Pathol Lab Med* 1983;107:126.

53. Cole EL, Meister DM, Calabrese LH, et al. Herpes zoster ophthalmicus and acquired immune deficiency syndrome. *Arch Ophthalmol* 1984;102:1027.

54. Gilden DH, Murray RS, Wettish M, et al. Chronic progressive varicella-zoster virus encephalitis in an AIDS patient. *Neurology* 1988;38:1150.

55. Goldston AS, Millichap JG, Miller RH. Cerebellar ataxia with preeruptive varicella. *Am J Dis Child* 1963;106:111.

56. McCarthy JT, Amer J. Postvaricella acute transverse myelitis: a case presentation and review of the literature. *Pediatrics* 1978;62:202.

57. Lewis GW. Zoster sine herpete. *BMJ* 1958;2:418.

58. Mayo DR, Booss J. Varicella zoster-associated neurologic disease without skin lesions. *Arch Neurol* 1989;46:313.

59. Hyman RW, Ecker JR, Tenser RB. Varicella-zoster virus RNA in human trigeminal ganglia. *Lancet* 1983;2:814.

60. Gilden DH, Rozenman Y, Murray R, et al. Detection of varicella-zoster virus nucleic acid in neurons of normal human thoracic ganglia. *Ann Neurol* 1987;22:377.

61. Pichini B, Ecker JR, Grose C, Hyman RW. DNA mapping of paired varicella-zoster virus isolates from patients with shingles. *Lancet* 1983;2:1223.

62. Croen KD, Ostrove JM, Dragovic LJ, Straus SE. Patterns of gene expression and sites of latency in human nerve ganglia are different for varicella-zoster and herpes simplex viruses. *Proc Natl Acad Sci USA* 1988;85:9773.

63. McCormick WF, Rodnitzky RL, Schochet SS, McKee AP. Varicella-zoster encephalomyelitis. *Arch Neurol* 1969;26:559.

64. Rostad SW, Olson K, McDougall J, et al. Transsynaptic spread of varicella zoster virus through the visual system: a mechanism of viral dissemination in the central nervous system. *Hum Pathol* 1989;20:174.

65. Oberg G, Svedmyr A. Varicelliform eruption in herpes zoster-Some chemical and serological observations found. *Scand J Infect Dis* 1969;1:47.

66. Hutton PW. Bilateral zoster and zoster varicellosus. *Lancet* 1935;2:302.

67. Locksley RM, Flournoy N, Sullivan KM, Meyers JD. Infection with varicella-zoster virus after marrow transplantation. *J Infect Dis* 1985;152:1172.

68. Wilson A, Sharp M, Koropchak CM, et al. Subclinical varicella-zoster viremia, herpes zoster, and T lymphocyte immunity to varicella-zoster viral antigens after bone marrow transplantation. *J Infect Dis* 1992;165:119.

69. Cheatham WJ, Weller TH, Dolan TF Jr, et al. Varicella: report of 2 fatal cases with necroscopy, virus isolation, and serologic studies. *Am J Pathol* 1956;32:1015.

70. Feldman S, Hughes WT, Daniel CB. Varicella in children with cancer: seventy-seven cases. *Pediatrics* 1975;56:388.

71. David DS, Tegtmeier BR, O'Donnell MR, et al. Visceral varicella-zoster after bone marrow transplantation: report of a case series and review of the literature. *Am J Gastroenterol* 1998;93:810–813.

72. Simmons RL, Balfour HH Jr. Complication of disseminated varicella-zoster infection. *Surgery* 1978;83:486.

73. Arvin AM, Kusher JH, Feldman S, et al. Human leukocyte interferon for treatment of varicella in children with cancer. *N Engl J Med* 1982;306:761.

74. Prober DG, Kirk LE, Keeney RE. Acyclovir therapy of chickenpox in immunosuppressed children—a collaborative study. *J Pediatr* 1982;101:622.

75. Whitley RJ, Hilty M, Haynes R, et al. Vidarabine therapy of varicella in immunosuppressed patients. *J Pediatr* 1982;1:125.

76. Feldman S, Hughes WT, Kim HY. Herpes zoster in children with cancer. *Am J Dis Child* 1973;126:178.

77. Schimpff SC, Fortner WH, Greene WH, Wiernik P. Cytosine arabinoside for localized herpes zoster in patients with cancer: failure in a controlled trial. *J Infect Dis* 1974;130:673.

78. Schimpff S, Serpick A, Stoler B, et al. Varicella-zoster infection in patients with cancer. *Ann Intern Med* 1972;76:241.

79. Sokol JE, Firat D. Varicella-zoster infection in Hodgkin's disease. *Am J Med* 1965;39:452.

80. Balfour HH Jr, Bean B, Laskin OL, et al. Acyclovir halts progression of herpes zoster in immunocompromised patients. *N Engl J Med* 1983;308:1448.

81. Shepp DH, Dandliker PS, Meyers JD. Treatment of varicella-zoster virus infection in severely immunocompromised patients—a randomized comparison of acyclovir and vidarabine. *N Engl J Med* 1986;314:208.

82. Hayward AR, Herberger M. Lymphocyte responses to varicella zoster virus in the elderly. *J Clin Immunol* 1987;7:174.

83. Zaia JA, Levin MJ, Preblud SR, et al. Evaluation of varicella-zoster immune globulin - protection of immunosuppressed children after household exposure to varicella. *J Infect Dis* 1983;147:737.

84. Good RA, Zak SJ. Disturbances in gamma globulin synthesis as "experiments of nature." *Pediatrics* 1956;18:109.

85. Lux SE, Johnston RB, August CS, et al. Chronic neutropenia and abnormal cellular immunity in cartilage-hair hypoplasia. *N Engl J Med* 1970;282:231.

86. Giller RH, Bowden RA, Levin MJ, et al. Reduced cellular immunity to varicella zoster virus during treatment for acute lymphoblastic leukemia of childhood: in vitro studies of possible mechanisms. *J Clin Immunol* 1986;6:472.

87. Hayward AR, Cosyns M, Jones M, et al. Cytokine production in varicella-zoster virus-stimulated cultures of human blood lymphocytes. *J Infect Dis* 1998;178[Suppl 1]:s95–98.

88. Arvin AM, Koropchak CM, Williams BRG, et al. Early immune response in healthy and immunocompromised subjects with primary varicella-zoster virus infection. *J Infect Dis* 1986;154:422.

89. Torigo S, Ihara T, Kamiya H. IL-12, IFN-gamma, and TNF-alpha released from mononuclear cells inhibit the spread of varicella-zoster virus at an early stage of varicella. *Microbiol Immunol* 2000;44:1027–1031.

90. Pitel PA, McCormick KL, Fitzgerald E, Orson JM. Subclinical hepatic changes in varicella infection. *Pediatrics* 1980;65:631.

91. Pahwa S, Biron K, Lim W, et al. Continuous varicella-zoster infection associated with acyclovir resistance in a child with AIDS. *JAMA* 1988;260:2879.

92. Crumpacker CS, Schnipper LE, Zaia JA, Levin MJ. Growth inhibition by acycloguanosine of herpesviruses isolated from human infections. *Antimicrob Agents Chemother* 1979;15:642.

93. Merigan TC, Rand KH, Pollard RB, et al. Human leukocyte interferon for the treatment of herpes zoster in patients with cancer. *N Engl J Med* 1978;298:981.

94. Winston DJ, Eron LJ, Ho M, et al. Recombinant interferon alpha-2a for treatment of herpes zoster in immunosuppressed patients with cancer. *Am J Med* 1988;85:147.

95. McKendrick MW, McGill JI, White JE, Wood MJ. Oral acyclovir in acute herpes zoster. *BMJ* 1986;293:1529.

96. Whitley RJ, Weiss H, Gnann JW, et al. Acyclovir with and without prednisone for the treatment of herpes zoster. A randomized, placebo-controlled trial. The National Institute of Allergy and Infectious Diseases Collaborative Antiviral Study Group. *Ann Intern Med* 1996;125:376–383.

97. Tyring S, Barbarash RA, Nahlik JE, et al. Famciclovir for the treatment of acute herpes zoster: effects on acute disease and postherpetic neuralgia. A randomized, double-blind, placebo-controlled trial. Collaborative Famciclovir Herpes Zoster Study Group. *Ann Intern Med* 1995;123:89–96.

98. Dworkin RH, Boon RJ, Griffin DR, et al. Postherpetic neuralgia: Impact of famciclovir, age, rash severity, and acute pain in herpes zoster patients. *J Infect Dis* 1998;178[Suppl 1]:S76–S80.

99. Tyring SK, Beutner KR, Tucker BA, et al. Antiviral therapy for herpes zoster: randomized, controlled clinical trial of valacyclovir and famciclovir therapy in immunocompetent patients 50 years and older. *Arch Fam Med* 2000;9:863–869.

100. Balfour HH, Kelly JM, Suarez CS, et al. Acyclovir treatment of varicella in otherwise healthy children. *J Pediatr* 1990;116:633.

101. American Academy of Pediatrics. Varicella-zoster infections. In: Pickering LK, ed. *2000 red book: report of the committee on infectious diseases,* 25th ed. Elk Grove Village, IL: American Academy of Pediatrics, 2000:624–628.

102. Schon F, Mayer ML, Kelly JS. Pathogenesis of post-herpetic neuralgia. *Lancet* 1987;2:366.

103. Eaglstein WH, Katz R, Brown JA. The effects of early corticosteroid therapy on the skin eruption and pain of herpes zoster. *JAMA* 1970;211:1681.

104. Esmann V, Kroon S, Peterslund NA, et al. Prednisolone does not prevent postherpetic neuralgia. *Lancet* 1987;2:126.

105. McGowan JE Jr, Chesney PJ, Crossley KB, LaForce FM. Guidelines for the use of systemic glucocorticoids in the management of selected infections. *J Infect Dis* 1992;165:1.

106. Hurwitz ES, Barrett MJ, Bregman D, et al. Public health service study of Reye syndrome and medications: report of the main study. *JAMA* 1987;257:1905.

107. Rowe PC, Valle D, Bruislowo SW. Inborn errors of metabolism in children referred with Reye's syndrome: a changing pattern. *JAMA* 1988;260:3168.

108. Laforet EG, Lynch CL. Multiple congenital defects following maternal varicella. *N Engl J Med* 1947;236:534.

109. Schulze A, Deitzsch HJ. The natural history of varicella embryopathy: a 25-year follow-up. *J Pediatr* 2000;137:871–874.
110. Grose C, Itani O. Pathogenesis of congenital infection with three diverse viruses: varicella-zoster virus, human parvovirus, and human immunodeficiency virus. *Semin Perinatol* 1989;13:278.
111. Meyers JD. Congenital varicella in term infants: risk reconsidered. *J Infect Dis* 1974;129:215.
112. Gershon AA, Raker R, Steinberg S, et al. Antibody to varicella-zoster virus in parturient women and their offspring during the first year of life. *Pediatrics* 1976;58:692.
113. Gershon AA, Steinberg S, Brunell PA. Zoster immunoglobulin: a further assessment. *N Engl J Med* 1974;290:243.
114. Zaia JA, Levin MJ, Wright GG, Grady GF. A practical method for the preparation of varicella-zoster immune globulin. *J Infect Dis* 1978;137:601.
115. Balfour HH Jr. Intravenous acyclovir therapy for varicella in immunocompromised children. *J Pediatr* 1984;104:134.
116. Preblud SR. Nosocomial varicella: worth preventing, but how? *Am J Public Health* 1983;78:13.
117. Myers MG, Rasley DA, Hierholzer WJ. Hospital infection control for varicella zoster virus infection. *Pediatrics* 1982;70:199.
118. Sinha DP. Chickenpox - a disease predominantly affecting adults in rural West Bengal, India. *Int J Epidemiol* 1976;5:367.
119. Berlin BS, Campbell T. Hospital-acquired herpes zoster following exposure to chickenpox. *JAMA* 1970;211:1831.
120. Garner JS, Simmons BP. Guideline for isolation precautions in hospitals. *Infect Control* 1983;4[Suppl 4]:245.
121. Zaia JA. Varicella-zoster virus. In: Mayhall CG, ed. *Hospital epidemiology and infection control,* 2nd ed. Philadelphia: Lippincott Williams & Williams, 1999:543–553.
122. Takahashi M. Clinical overview of varicella vaccine: development and early studies. *Pediatrics* 1986;78[Suppl]:736.
123. Takahashi M, Okuno Y, Otsuka T, et al. Development of a live attenuated varicella vaccine. *Biken J* 1975;18:25.
124. Loparev VN, Argaw T, Krause PR, et al. Improved identification and differentiation of varicella-zoster virus (VZV) wild-type strains and an attenuated varicella vaccine strain using a VZV open reading frame 62-based PCR. *J Clin Microbiol* 2000;38:3156–3160.
125. Prevention of varicella. Update recommendations of the advisory committee on immunization practices (ACIP). *MMWR* 1999;48:1–5.
126. Ozaki T, Nishimura N, Kajita Y. Experience with live attenuated varicella vaccine (Oka strain) in healthy Japanese subjects; 10-year survey at pediatric clinic. *Vaccine* 2000;18:2375–2380.
127. Vazquez M, LaRussa PS, Gershon AA, et al. The effectiveness of the varicella vaccine in clinical practice. *N Engl J Med* 2001;344:955–960.
128. Vessey SJ, Chan CY, Kuter BJ, et al. Childhood vaccination against varicella: persistence of antibody, duration of protection, and vaccine efficacy. *J Pediatr* 2001;139:297–304.
129. Harel Z, Ipp L, Riggs S, et al. Serotesting versus presumptive varicella vaccination of adolescents with a negative or uncertain history of chickenpox. *J Adolesc Health* 2001;28:26–29.
130. Smith KJ, Roberts, MS. Cost effectiveness of vaccination strategies in adults without a history of chickenpox. *Am J Med* 2000;108:723–729.
131. Lim YJ, Chew FT, Tan AY, et al. Risk factors for breakthrough varicella in healthy children. *Arch Dis Child* 1998;79:478–480.
132. Krause PR, Klinman DM. Varicella vaccination: evidence for frequent reactivation of the vaccine strain in healthy children. *Nat Med* 2000;6:451–454.
133. Liang MG, Heidelberg KA, Jacobson RM, et al. Herpes zoster after varicella immunization. *J Am Acad Dermatol* 1998;38:761–763.
134. Brunell PA, Argaw T. Chickenpox attributable to a vaccine virus contracted from a vaccinee with zoster. *Pediatrics* 2000;106:E28.
135. Levin MJ, Gershon AA, Weinberg A, et al. Immunization of HIV-infected children with varicella vaccine. *J Pediatr* 2001;139:305–310.
136. Donati M, Zuckerman M, Dhawan A, et al. Response to varicella immunization in pediatric liver transplant recipients. *Transplantation* 2000;70:1401–1404.
137. Burgess MA, Cossart YE, Wilkins TD, et al. Varicella vaccination of health-care workers. *Vaccine* 1999;17:765–769.
138. Gershon A. Live-attenuated varicella vaccine. *Infect Dis Clin North Am* 2001;15:65–81.

CHAPTER 140
Smallpox

John Noble and Joseph J. Esposito

Smallpox is one of the most dreaded diseases of humans. It raged in epidemic and endemic forms for over 3000 years. Smallpox "... exerted a singular influence on human history through the ages before its extinction in 1977—suddenly removing or temporarily indisposing leaders of nations, destroying armies, disrupting cities, and laying waste to ordinary citizens, devastating virgin populations and influencing fateful decisions ..." (1).

The high mortality of smallpox caused an average of 10% of all deaths each year in towns and cities where the disease was endemic. Mortalities up to 100% were recorded in the devastating epidemics of smallpox that swept through Native American populations of North, Central, and South America (2). The disease continued into the 20th century; there were 65 cases with 20 deaths in Seattle in 1945, 12 cases with two deaths in New York City in 1947, and 8 cases with one death in Texas in 1949. These were the last reported cases of smallpox in the United States.

The World Health Organization (WHO) established an Intensified Smallpox Eradication Program in 1966, with the goal of attaining global eradication of smallpox in 10 years. At that time, smallpox was reported in 41 countries, extending from Afghanistan to Malaysia and Indonesia, throughout most of Africa south of the Sahara, and including Brazil, Argentina, and other dispersed locations. National eradication campaigns were conducted in more than 80 countries between 1966 and 1977. Using standardized potent vaccine in well-organized vaccination campaigns, intensive surveillance for smallpox outbreaks, and extensive public education, this program eradicated smallpox. The last case of naturally occurring smallpox was reported in Somalia in October 1977. This remarkable accomplishment, the first disease to be eradicated, was comprehensively chronicled by Fenner and colleagues (3). The threat of bioterror attacks with variola virus has recently brought considerable attention to smallpox, its prevention, control, and treatment. The Centers for Disease Control and Prevention (CDC) and the WHO web sites, *www.cdc.gov* and *www.who.ch*, contain much information on smallpox.

Variola virus, a member of genus *Orthopoxvirus,* causes smallpox. Biologic and molecular biologic features of members of the family *Poxviridae* have recently been reviewed (4,5). The deoxyribonucleic acid and neutralizing antibodies of variola viruses show many similarities to other orthopoxviruses, including cowpox, monkeypox and vaccinia viruses, which can infect humans, and ectromelia, taterapox, and camelpox viruses. Variola virus is a strictly human virus, with no known non-human reservoir of disease. A narrow range of laboratory animals are susceptible to experimental infection. By clinical and epidemiologic criteria and laboratory tests, two subspecies were apparent that produced illness of varying severity and mortality—variola major virus caused a 5% to 25% case-fatality rate and variola minor (alastrim) virus produced 1% or less deaths. A fatality rate of 5% to 15% was typical in Africa and Indonesia, suggesting an *intermedius* subspecies, but extensive laboratory testing finally did not support establishing this viral subclass.

The clinical illness variola major varies in prognosis, differential diagnosis, and transmissibility (Table 140.1). Ordinary smallpox is transmitted by the aerosol route through droplet nuclei, dust, and by fomites. Inadvertent or deliberate (variolation) skin

TABLE 140.1.   A Classification of Clinical Types of Variola Major

Ordinary	Raised pustular skin lesions presenting as three subtypes: Confluent: confluent rash lesions on face and forearms Semiconfluent: confluent rash lesions on face, discrete elsewhere on the body Discrete: areas of normal skin between pustules on the body, including the face
Modified	Similar to the ordinary type but with an accelerated course
Variola sine eruptione	Fever without rash caused by variola virus; serologic confirmation required
Flat	Pustules remained flat; usually confluent or semiconfluent
Hemorrhagic	Widespread hemorrhages in skin and mucous membranes; two subtypes: Early, with purpuric rash; always fatal Late, with hemorrhages into base of pustules; usually fatal

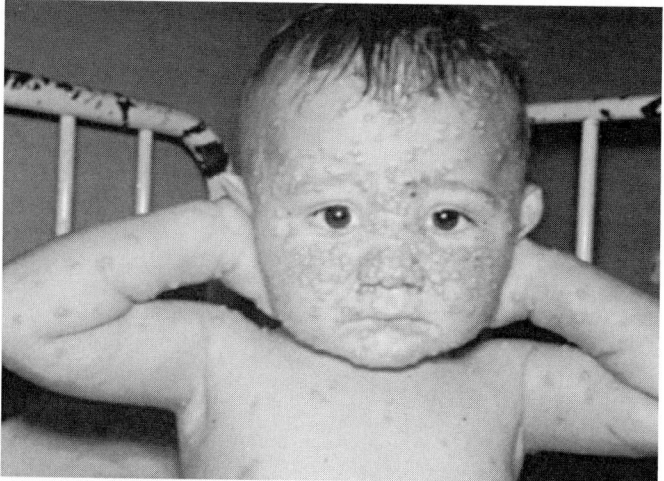

Figure 140.1. Appearance of the rash of smallpox on day 6 and 7. All of the lesions are in the same stage of development.

infection may produce less morbidity and mortality than infection by aerosol.

The virus is shed in large quantities in nasal and oropharyngeal secretions at the end of a 12- to 14-day incubation period, which is followed by production of skin lesions that evolve from macular to papular to vesicular pustules. Infectious virus is found in the vesicular fluids of the clinical lesions and the scabs and it can be readily cultured from bed linen and clothing. Scabs are associated with less viral transmissibility than aerosol droplets. The capacity for the virus to spread through convection currents of air within buildings and by contaminated articles and clothing was the basis for the repeated widespread epidemics that occurred throughout history until 1977.

The site of initial infection is usually the oropharynx, nasopharynx, or lower respiratory tract. Virus proliferates in macrophages and spreads to lymph nodes during the primary viremic phase, which is followed by diffuse involvement of the reticuloendothelial system and a secondary viremic phase that transits virus to capillaries for migration into the dermis.

Patients become febrile and often develop severe constitutional symptoms at the end of the incubation period, the prodromal phase, commonly with splitting headache, backache, and malaise. Vomiting and colicky abdominal pain, occasionally suggestive of appendicitis, often occur and a few patients may develop seizures. A diffuse erythematous "allergic" rash may be seen in some fair-skinned patients in the preeruptive phase. Lesions on mucous membranes in the oropharynx and the upper and lower airway appear first (*enanthema*). Then the true maculopapular rash (*exanthema*) of smallpox begins 2 to 3 days after the onset of the prodrome, at a time when the patient is defervescing. Skin lesions develop uniformly and appear predominantly on the head, torso, and extremities in a centrifugal distribution. The reason for this distinctive pattern of involvement and for the dermotropism of the variola virus is unknown.

The rash of smallpox becomes apparent within 2 to 4 days. Early-stage lesions may be confused with those of chickenpox, which usually crop up non-uniformly. Although smallpox lesions on the face are often more advanced than those on the legs, all of the lesions in an area of the body evolve as a single crop (Fig. 140.1). Most patients have lesions on the palms and soles, which is uncharacteristic of chickenpox. Papules evolve into vesicles by day 3 or 4 and into pustules by day 5 or 6 of the rash. The lesions are firm to the touch, domed, or umbilicated

(dimpled); when extensive, they often coalesce, becoming confluent. Pustules reach their maximum size on or about the ninth day of the rash. Fever returns during the pustular stage and persists until the lesions have become inspissated, scabbed over, and sloughed off. By the 20th day, all of the scabs are usually separated except for those embedded in the thick corneum stratum of the palms and soles. Depigmentation persists at the base of skin lesions for 3 to 6 months after illness. Smallpox leaves permanent scars depressed 1 to 2 mm below the surface of the skin. Such pockmarks result from fibrosis in the dermis and sebaceous glands. Scarring is usually most extensive on the face.

Smallpox, especially variola major, produces a rapidly fatal toxemic illness in some patients, suggesting severe cytokine imbalance. Diagnosis had been difficult when death occurred from hemorrhagic complications before the appearance of the rash. Pneumonia, dehydration, and septicemia secondary to denuded, sloughed skin are other serious complications (Fig. 140.2). Conjunctivitis, corneal ulceration, and blepharitis occur,

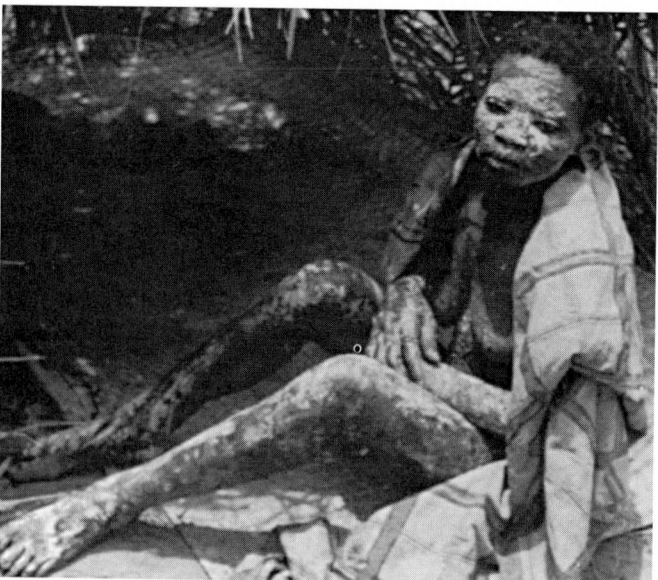

Figure 140.2. Denuded areas of skin produced by the sloughing of confluent smallpox lesions.

producing corneal opacity in 1.0% to 4.4% of cases. Osteomyelitis variolosa is a rare complication that produces deformities in children, afflicting the elbows more often than other joints.

DESTRUCTION OF VARIOLA VIRUS STOCKS AND SMALLPOX BIOTERRORISM PREPAREDNESS

There has been a recent surge to prepare for the potential of smallpox by bioterror (6,7), although its emergence otherwise, for example, by a laboratory accident or from graves in the permafrost, has been an issue for some time (8). In the early 1980s, following the World Health Assembly (WHA) sanction of a Global Commission report proclaiming smallpox had been eradicated, WHO undertook a program to implement the Commission's posteradication recommendations, including calling for global cessation of routine smallpox vaccination, which was realized by 1983, except for certain militaries that continued for several years. The Commission also advised countries to destroy their live variola virus samples or send them to a WHO-authorized repository, which made WHO responsible for ensuring the security of the remaining samples and overseeing their final fate. Thus, a repository was created at the CDC, which by 1983 held specimens from British, Japanese and Dutch reference laboratories, in addition to the Centers for Disease Control (CDC), U.S. Army, and American Type Culture Collection samples. The repository at CDC contains about 450 samples, mostly cultures of lesion material from selected smallpox cases around the end of the eradication era, with some viral isolate overlap in the collections. A repository of about 120 samples, with minor overlap to those at CDC, was established at the Moscow Research Institute for Viral Preparations. However, at some point, the Russian government transferred the samples (without WHO sanction) to the State Research Center for Virology and Biotechnology, Koltsovo, Novosibirsk Region. Nevertheless, in 1994, WHO inspected and approved the new site.

The fate of the remaining samples has been and remains controversial. Several reports for or against destruction appeared in the 1990s. Prodestructionists argued, for example, that the stocks represent an unwarranted biohazard or a terrorist target that may lead to reappearance of smallpox; that because variola was a strictly human virus, no other living system would provide precise data on its pathogenesis; that it would be best to focus antiviral research on preventing postvaccinal complications because if smallpox reappeared, the vaccine would be used and not a drug unproved against the human illness; and that harboring or using the virus is a crime against humanity. But then, antidestructionists contended that the virus could be safely manipulated in proper containment; that if the virus is held by terrorists or rouge states, then comprehensive knowledge of its properties will provide the best ways of averting catastrophe associated with an outbreak; and that enormous health benefits could come from biomolecular studies of viral dynamics in animals and cultures, considering the virus uniquely mediates human cellular death and survival mechanisms, including within the immune system.

In 1990, 1994, and 1999, the samples were formally proposed for destruction by a WHO ad hoc Committee on Orthopoxvirus Infections, and subsequently in May 1999 by the 52nd WHA. However, before the WHA meeting, President William J. Clinton ordered temporary retention of the samples at CDC for continued research aimed at saving lives should smallpox reappear. The order followed a U.S. Executive Office review that included an assessment by the National Academy of Sciences, Institute of Medicine (IOM) of the scientific needs for live variola virus. The IOM reported that the virus was required for development of effective and safe antivirals (the highest priority) and new vaccines to protect against high-dose aerosol infections, and a smallpox animal model for testing antivirals and vaccines. More, the virus was needed to understand its genetic diversity and pathogenesis and modernize laboratory diagnostics and environmental detection. In light of the changed U.S. position, the 1999 WHA resolution provided for retention of the samples no later than (Dec. 31) 2002, essentially for the studies indicated by the IOM, but under peer review of a WHO Advisory Committee on Variola Virus Research. Such a review would enable WHO to counsel the WHA on whether or not the research results sufficiently justified destruction.

Overriding the scientific and public health debate, a revelation that secret stores of variola virus may exist came from British and U.S. intelligence agencies. By the mid-1990s, they described that in the early 1980s, following USSR endorsement of the 1972 Biological and Toxin Weapons Treaty (BTW), the former Soviet Union had accelerated bioweapons programs, including producing multi-ton amounts of variola virus for use in ballistic missiles. The Soviet reasoning was that smallpox would be a more effective weapon once vaccination ended and world immunity waned. Russia claimed the material was destroyed soon after the USSR breakup. However, the knowledge that such amounts existed fostered fears at official levels that the virus may have made it into maleficent hands or rogue countries, or as a paradigm that other nations or individuals may have also produced the virus for malicious use.

Soon after the terrorist destruction of the World Trade Center in 2001, considering the remote but potentially devastating prospect that clandestinely held variola virus could be used for bioterror or in war against the U.S., President George W. Bush ordered retention of the samples at CDC—until better vaccine measures and at least two smallpox antivirals are developed, particularly for immunocompromised persons. In this light, in December 2001, the WHO reviewers advised that destruction should be postponed for completion of key studies under WHO auspices and the work should be time-limited and focused on particular outcomes, a status WHO accepted in January 2002.

The intelligence reports stirred differences of opinion on destruction between the Department of Health and Human Services (HHS), which considered the public health impact should the virus escape containment, and the Department of Defense (DOD), which considered research needs to reduce the potential of smallpox use in bioterror or biowar. In the climate of the 1995 Tokyo subway gassing by the Aum Shinrikyo and the bombing of the Murra Building in Oklahoma City, HHS and DOD were directed to form a Joint Coordinating Group to institute a U.S. smallpox research agenda that included studying variola virus to develop antivirals and improved vaccines and diagnostics and animal model(s) of smallpox, essentially the studies later suggested by the IOM and expanded into international collaborations under WHO auspices.

U.S. smallpox research efforts were established before enactment of the 1996 Defense Against Weapons of Mass Destruction Act (which followed on the 1991 Conventional Forces In Europe Treaty Implementation Act) to support ways (e.g., the Cooperative Threat Reduction Program (CTR)) to help former Soviet countries reduce weapons of mass destruction, including bioweapons, and comply with BTW. An outcome of CTR has been HHS implementation, with other agency support, of a Biotechnology Engagement Program (BTEP) to facilitate collaboration, through an International Science and Technology Center, between U.S. scientists focusing on bioterrorism preparedness and former Soviet bioweapons researchers.

Following the 2001 World Trade Center attack and creation of the Office of Homeland Security, which implements plans to help secure the U.S. from terrorism, HHS created an Office of Public Health Preparedness (OPHP). Under aegis of OPHP, NIH pursues basic studies relative to bioterrorism preparedness and CDC serves as the lead agency to respond to bioterror. CDC presently provides epidemiologists to detect, investigate and diagnose cases in support of state and local health departments, stockpiles of materials and treatments, and a health alert network for state and local health departments. More, CDC efforts focus on strengthening the public health infrastructure, improving epidemiologic and surveillance practices, developing information and communication systems, and providing policy and evaluation for a deft national readiness and response. CDC efforts to deal with smallpox include providing vaccinia immunoglobulin (VIG) and vaccine stockpiles for emergency use, including updating the Immunization Practices Advisory Committee recommendations for vaccinia vaccination; implementing a smallpox clinical education program for medical professionals and other first responders; providing protocols for clinical specimen triage and laboratory testing using standard methods to identify and differentiate human orthopoxviruses and varicella virus (chickenpox may be confused with smallpox); and continuing smallpox research.

Within the preparedness effort, a Laboratory Response Network (LRN) was developed by the CDC, Federal Bureau of Investigation (FBI), and Association of Public Health Laboratories (APHL), which is now implemented as a CDC-APHL joint program of county, city, state, and national public health laboratories to respond to bioterror. LRN laboratories can accept clinical specimens and other samples from hospitals, clinics, the FBI, and other law enforcement groups, emergency medical services, the military, and other agencies.

Presently, CDC is the only site for Biosafety Level 4 laboratory for receipt and manipulation of live variola virus. All suspect smallpox cases should be referred through local and state channels to CDC. It is crucial for safety and security that chickenpox is ruled out clinically so that non-CDC laboratories do not propagate variola virus, potentially spreading infection to nonvaccinated staff using lower biosafety levels.

CDC has purchased, for emergency use, over 250 million doses of a new cell culture based smallpox vaccine, which is in clinical trials at this writing. Deciding to administer the vaccine, which contains vaccinia not variola virus, to the U.S. public is not a simple task, also considering estimates (B. Schwartz, CDC, pers. comm.) that 1% to 2% of the U.S. population is immunocompromised by transplants, genetics, infection, cancer, leukemia, certain medications, autoimmunity, etc., thus contraindicated for this vaccine. Even in apparently healthy persons, live vaccinia vaccines are not absolutely effective or entirely safe. Morbidity and mortality rates of vaccination were key factors for ceasing smallpox vaccination. Adverse postvaccinal reactions following primary vaccination have included generalized vaccinia, encephalitides, eczema vaccinatum, vaccinia necrosum, and autoinoculation that may lead to severe eye or fetal infections. Timely use of VIG intramuscularly may clear certain side effects (the U.S. Army is seeking approval for an intravenous VIG formulation). Over 32,000 VIG doses may be needed to treat complications if the vaccine stockpile is used extensively.

Timely use of VIG or some antiviral drugs may also be effective against smallpox. Cidofovir, a drug for treating certain herpesvirus infections, has shown promise as a poxvirus antiviral. Vaccinia vaccination within 4 days of exposure may be effective for treating variola virus infection, in which case use of VIG or Cidofovir must be weighed against compromising the vaccination. During the eradication era, antivirals such as thiosemicarbazones and nucleotide arabinosides were tried but were ineffective.

CDC has produced an Interim Smallpox Response Plan and Guidelines (available at *www.cdc.gov*) that will be updated as necessary. The Plan is presently organized into sections that provide criteria for implementing plan, procedures for notification of suspect cases, and the responsibilities and activities of CDC, state and local agencies, including emergency planning and mobilization of vaccine and personnel. In addition, the Plan contains guidelines and annexes to assist federal, state, and local health officials to implement activities essential for managing a smallpox emergency and containing an outbreak. The guidelines define a suspected smallpox case as a fever of at least 101°F, followed by a rash with firm, deep-seated bumps on the body, in a patient whose illness cannot be explained otherwise. Medical personnel should first notify their local and state public health authorities of a suspected case of smallpox. The CDC Bioterrorism Preparedness and Response Program can be reached by contacting the CDC by telephone.

The recent national debate on smallpox is summarized in a series of publications (9).

REFERENCES

1. Hopkins DR. *Princes and peasants: smallpox in history.* Chicago, University of Chicago Press, 1983.
2. Duffy J. Smallpox and the indians of the american colonies. *Bull Hist Med* 1951;25:324–341.
3. Fenner F, Henderson DA, Arita I, Jezek Z, Ladnyi ID. *Smallpox and its eradication.* Geneva: World Health Organization, 1988.
4. Esposito JJ, Fenner F. Poxviruses. In: Knipe DM, Howley PM, Griffin DE, et al, eds. *Fields virology,* 4th ed, vol 2. Philadelphia: Lippincott, Williams & Wilkins, 2001:2885–2921.
5. Moss B. *Poxviridae*: the viruses and their replication. In: Knipe DM, Howley PM, Griffin DE, et al, eds. *Fields virology,* 4th ed, vol 2. Philadelphia: Lippincott, Williams & Wilkins, 2001:2849–2883.
6. Miller J, Engelberg S, Broad W. *Germs: biological weapons and america's secret war.* New York: Simon & Schuster, 2001.
7. Tucker JH. *Scourge: the once and future threat of smallpox.* New York: Atlantic Monthly Press, 2001.
8. World Health Organization. Smallpox eradication: destruction of variola virus stocks. *Week Epidemiol Rec* 1999;74:185–192.
9. Mack T. A different view of smallpox and vaccination. *N Engl J Med* 2003;348:460–463. Related letters 348:1920–1925.

CHAPTER 141
Mumps

Adriano Arguedas, Hillel Janai, and Melvin I. Marks

Mumps is an acute, contagious, generalized viral disease that usually causes painful enlargement of the salivary glands, most commonly the parotid glands.

HISTORY

Mumps was first described as a clinical entity by Hippocrates in 500 BC. The viral origin was firmly established in 1934 when Johnson and Goodpasture (1) successfully reproduced the disease in monkeys. In 1945, the virus was grown in hen eggs, and the viral property of hemagglutination was described. Subsequently, the virus was successfully attenuated in 1960, and the live mumps virus vaccine was prepared in chick embryo tissue culture by Hilleman and Buynack in 1966 (2).

MICROBIOLOGY

Mumps is caused by a member of the paramyxovirus group. The virus particle contains a single-stranded ribonucleic acid enclosed in an envelope of protein and lipid. The viral envelope contains three proteins: (a) HN protein, which has both hemagglutinin and neuraminidase activity; (b) F protein, which has hemolytic and cell fusion activity; and (c) M protein, which forms the inner layer of the viral envelope. There is only one known serotype. For more information, refer to the mumps virus chapter.

EPIDEMIOLOGY

Mumps is endemic in heavily populated areas but may occur in epidemic areas when susceptible individuals are crowded together. The virus is spread from its human reservoir by direct contact through infected saliva and urine. Incidence peaks occur in late winter and early spring.

The disease has a worldwide distribution and affects both sexes equally. Infection is uncommon during the early months of life owing to infrequent exposure and to protection conferred by transplacental passage of maternal antibodies. Although the majority of cases occur in children younger than 15 years (85%), there are rare reports of neonatal cases (3), and an increase in the number of cases in adolescents between 15 and 19 years of age was noticed from 1986 to 1987. This phenomenon was attributed to a failure in the vaccination programs between 1968 and 1977 (4). The source of infection is not always found because 20% of mumps infections are asymptomatic and an additional 40% to 50% may have only mild, nonspecific symptoms (5,6).

It is not known how long a patient may be infectious. However, transmission does not seem to occur longer than 24 hours before the appearance of the swelling or later than 3 days after it has subsided. Virus has been isolated from saliva as long as 7 days before and 8 days after the appearance of salivary swelling. Urine cultures have shown the presence of the virus from 1 to 14 days after the onset of the salivary gland swelling (7). Lifelong immunity is usually achieved after a clinical or subclinical infection.

PATHOGENESIS

Humans are the only reservoir for mumps virus, and person-to-person contact is essential for spreading to occur. The mumps virus initially attaches to the epithelial cells of the respiratory tract, producing, in both immune and nonimmune individuals, upper (e.g., common cold and pharyngitis) and lower (e.g., bronchopneumonia, croup, and bronchiolitis) respiratory symptoms. This virus-epithelial cell interaction induces local immunologic responses characterized by secretion of secretory immunoglobulin A, edema, lymphocyte infiltration, and increased vascular permeability (8). After the initial multiplication in the respiratory tract (12 to 25 days), the virus is bloodborne to many tissues and glands (e.g., salivary glands). Viremia usually lasts for 3 to 5 days.

Infection with mumps virus stimulates humoral and cell-mediated immune responses. Levels of immunoglobulins G and M as well as interferon and local immunoglobulin A are increased in patients after mumps infection (9). Lymphocyte proliferation to mumps antigen has been documented in response to cutaneous hypersensitivity (10).

Parotid swelling is produced by interstitial edema. The main changes occur in the salivary ducts, ranging from mild epithelial swelling with sparse polymorphonuclear cell infiltration to complete desquamation of the epithelium resulting in dilated lumens choked with debris.

Changes in the brain may occur in acute viral meningoencephalitis. These include neuronal destruction and inflammation with lymphocyte infiltration, perivascular edema, and vasculitis. After the acute process, perivascular demyelination and glial reaction follow recovery. Occasionally, mumps meningoencephalitis may cause hydrocephalus due to aqueductal stenosis secondary to scarring at the sites of necrotic ependymal cells (11).

In orchitis, there are massive interstitial edema and perivascular lymphocyte exudate. The histologic changes are characterized by a patch destruction of the epithelium of some seminiferous tubules; the Leydig cells are usually both histologically normal and functional. These changes are usually focal and unilateral (80% to 90%), accompanied by epididymitis in 85% of cases (12).

Rarely, acute self-limited inflammation of the pancreas (less than 10%), thyroid, joints (0.4%), or labyrinth may develop (13). On histologic examination, there is an acute inflammatory response in the interstitium consisting of mononuclear cells with edema and swelling.

Intrauterine infection with mumps virus has been associated with multiple anomalies, including endocardial fibroelastosis; imperforate anus; spina bifida; auditory, optic, and urogenital deformities; and abortions (14). Animal studies have suggested the possible association between mumps infection during pregnancy and congenital hydrocephalus, probably secondary to obstructive lesions in the spinal canal (15).

CLINICAL MANIFESTATIONS OF PAROTITIS

The incubation period of mumps ranges from 14 to 25 days, most commonly 14 to 18 days. In children, prodromal symptoms and signs are rare and may be manifested by 2 to 3 days of malaise, anorexia, headache, muscle pain, and fever. Orchitis or meningitis may precede parotitis or may be the sole manifestation of mumps. Approximately 20% to 30% of all mumps infections are subclinical. This group of patients represents a significant risk for spread of the disease.

The onset of illness is usually characterized by pain and swelling in one or both parotid glands (Fig. 141.1). The parotid swelling begins by filling the space between the posterior border of the mandible and the mastoid and then extends downward and forward, being limited above by the zygoma. Local heat and erythema are absent. The swollen tissues push the earlobe upward and outward as the angle of the mandible is no longer visible. Swelling is usually maximal during a 2- to 3-day period and disappears by 7 to 10 days. Redness and swelling are commonly noted around the opening of the Stensen or Wharton duct. Because salivary gland ducts may be partially occluded by inflammation, pain can be experienced on exposure to acid drinks and other stimulants of salivary secretion.

Swelling of the sublingual and submaxillary glands is frequently associated with mumps. In 10% to 15% of patients, only the submandibular gland is swollen. The inflammation is usually an ovoid enlargement extending forward and downward from the angle of the mandible. Submandibular infection is usually not as painful as when the parotid is involved, but the swelling subsides more slowly. Less commonly, only the sublingual glands may be infected. The infection is usually bilateral and noted in the submental region and on the floor of the mouth.

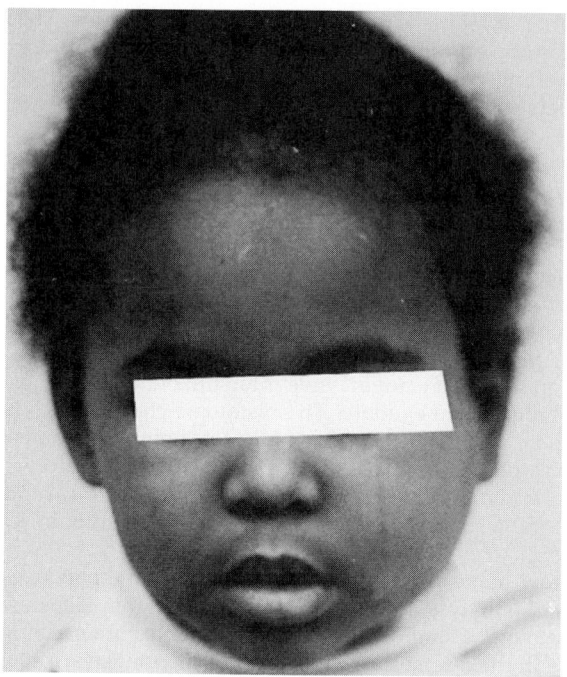

Figure 141.1. Female patient with swelling of left parotid gland due to parotitis. Note the difference with the right parotid gland. (Courtesy of Dr. A. Deveikis, Memorial Miller Children's Hospital and Health System, Long Beach, CA.)

COMPLICATIONS

Complications of mumps virus infection can occur during the acute, convalescent, or post-convalescent phase. Viremia, early in the infection, is the route of infection in organs other than the salivary glands (Table 141.1). The frequency of mumps-related complications is higher in the postpubertal population than in the prepubertal group. It is also higher in males than in females (16).

TABLE 141.1.   Complications of Mumps

Neurologic	Hematologic
Meningoencephalitis	Thrombocytopenia
Guillain-Barré syndrome	Hemolysis
Myelitis	Leukemoid reaction
Neuropathies	Paroxysmal cold hemoglobinuria
Deafness	Splenomegaly
Labyrinthitis	Other
Hydrocephalus	Pancreatitis
Diabetes insipidus	Thyroiditis
Facial Palsy	Mastitis
Ocular	Hepatitis
Conjunctivitis	Polyarthritis
Scleritis	Myocarditis
Keratitis	Laryngitis
Optic neuritis	Psychosis
Iritis	Teratogenicity
Iridocyclitis	
Dacryoadenitis	
Genitourinary	
Orchitis	
Epididymitis	
Oophoritis	
Nephritis	
Prostatitis	

Acute meningoencephalitis is the most frequent complication in childhood. The true frequency is difficult to estimate, but clinical central nervous system involvement during the infection occurs in 15% of cases reported to the Centers for Disease Control and Prevention in the United States (17). The mortality rate is about 2%, and males are affected three to five times more frequently than females are (16). A case of chronic mumps encephalitis with mental deterioration and recurrent seizures that may have responded to antiviral therapy was reported (18).

In most cases, central nervous system signs become evident 1 to 6 days after the onset of parotitis and are characterized by fever (94%), vomiting (84%), nuchal rigidity (71%), lethargy (69%), parotid swelling (47%), headache (47%), convulsions (18%), and delirium (6%) (19). The cerebrospinal fluid usually contains less than 500 cells/mm^3, almost exclusively lymphocytes; the protein concentration is slightly elevated, and the glucose concentration is usually normal. However, hypoglycorrhachia has been reported in some patients with mumps meningitis (20). Mumps virus can be isolated from the cerebrospinal fluid in the illness. The prognosis is favorable in most cases, although permanent sequelae, such as unilateral (rarely bilateral) nerve deafness or facial paralysis, may result (21,22). The incidence of deafness after mumps is approximately 1 in 20,000, but findings suggest that because of diagnostic problems it may be higher (13). The pathogenesis is not completely understood but appears to be secondary to hematogenous viral invasion of the labyrinth (23,24). Other unusual central nervous system manifestations include acute cerebellar ataxia, transverse myelitis, and polyneuritis (25,26). Ependymitis appears to be a common finding in patients with central nervous system involvement. Ependymal cells and cytoplasmic inclusions of viral nucleocapsid-like material are usually found in the cerebrospinal fluid of these patients and have been implicated in the pathogenesis of hydrocephalus (11).

Orchitis is a complication that is most commonly observed during adolescence and young adulthood. About 20% to 50% of postpubertal male patients develop orchitis (5). It is usually unilateral, and therefore sterility is rare (12); however, approximately 50% of patients with orchitis have some degree of testicular atrophy. Bilateral involvement has been reported to occur in 17% to 38% of cases (27,28). Orchitis may occur before or in the absence of parotitis, but the majority of cases become clinically apparent 3 to 7 days after the parotid swelling has subsided (29). The onset is usually abrupt with a rise in temperature, chills, headache, nausea, vomiting, and lower abdominal pain. Within 12 to 24 hours, the affected gonad displays an inflammatory reaction characterized by marked swelling, warmth, and pain. The average duration of illness is 4 days. The risk for testicular neoplasia has been found to be higher for men with history of mumps orchitis (30). Despite the rare complications of sterility and neoplasia, the course of mumps orchitis is generally self-limited. Appropriate therapy includes use of analgesics and adequate support of the testes. Steroids are not effective and may potentiate the parotitis or increase the rate of secondary infection (29). Nerve blocks should be reserved for patients with intractable pain.

Oophoritis may be a complication of mumps infection and is noted in about 5% to 7% of postpubertal female patients. The clinical manifestations are less dramatic than in orchitis, and, similar to patients with an acute appendicitis, the main complaints are usually pelvic pain and tenderness in the lower abdominal quadrants. There is no evidence of impairment of fertility after infection.

Mumps-induced pancreatitis has been reported in less than 10% of patients and is usually a late effect of the infection, developing days or weeks after the parotid swelling. Approximately one third of the cases have occurred in the absence of parotitis (29). It is more common in young adults. Nausea, vomiting, fever, chills, and epigastric pain are usually the main complaints. These symptoms disappear in 1 week, and most of the patients recover completely. Serum amylase determination is not a helpful diagnostic tool in the early onset cases because it is normally elevated with parotitis in the absence of pancreatic inflammation. Serum lipase determination may be more helpful. Epidemiologic and serologic correlations between mumps and type I diabetes mellitus have been suggested; however, controlled studies have failed to confirm this association (31–34).

Thyroid inflammation has been reported to occur approximately 1 week after the onset of parotitis. Although it is uncommon in children, the appearance of a diffuse, tender, swollen thyroid is suggestive of this complication.

Arthritis has been observed in 0.4% of patients with mumps (35). Arthritic complaints are more common in men during the third decade of life, usually starting 10 to 14 days after parotid swelling and persisting an average of 12 days (36). The large joints (e.g., knees, ankles, and shoulders) are most frequently involved, but any joint can be affected. The arthritic pain is migratory and self-limited, resolving after a few days without any residual joint damage or recurrence (37).

Mumps myocarditis is a rare complication. However, fatal cases have been reported in the literature (38).

Viruria has frequently been noted. The frequency of renal involvement in children is unknown, but the virus is isolated from the urine of 72% of patients during the first 5 days of mumps parotitis (39,40). Cases of symptomatic nephritis after mumps are unusual, but fatal cases have been reported (41).

Recently a case report from Japan described a 3-year-old male who developed facial palsy after mumps suggesting that this association should be consider in the evaluation of pediatric patients with facial palsy (43).

Rare complications of mumps virus include mastitis, prostatitis, dacryoadenitis, transient abnormalities in liver function tests, and thrombocytopenic purpura.

DIAGNOSIS

Diagnosis of clinical cases during an epidemic is simple, based on the epidemiologic condition, the history, and the physical examination. When clinical manifestations are limited to one of the less common sites of infection, or when the case is sporadic, the diagnosis is more difficult to establish.

Swelling of the parotid or other salivary glands due to mumps virus must be distinguished from other causes of parotid swelling. Infectious, noninfectious, and nonparotid causes of swelling should always be excluded (Table 141.2).

Routine laboratory tests are usually nonspecific. The white blood cell count is usually within the normal range, although leukopenia with lymphocytosis may occur. A polymorphonuclear leukocytosis is more commonly present with extraparotid involvement.

The serum amylase value is above normal in mumps and usually parallels the parotid swelling, reaching its peak in 1 week and returning to normal in the course of the next 2 weeks. Serum and urine amylase values can be used to differentiate between parotid and non-parotid swelling. Both values are increased when parotid involvement is present and are normal when the swelling is due to extraparotid disease.

The definitive diagnosis of mumps is established by a positive viral culture or by serologic methods (42). For details, refer to Chapter 243.

TABLE 141.2. Differential Diagnosis of Parotid Swelling

Infectious
  Mumps
  Influenza
  Cytomegalovirus infection
  Coxsackievirus infection
  Lymphocytic choriomeningitis
  Echovirus infection
  Bacterial abscess
  Actinomyces infection
  Mycobacterial infection
  Cat-scratch disease
  Toxoplasmosis
  HIV infection
Noninfectious
  Drug hypersensitivity
  Sarcoidosis
  Tumors, mixed
  Hemangioma, lymphangioma
  Sialectasis
  Sjögren syndrome
  Mikulicz syndrome
  Recurrent idiopathic parotitis
  Pneumoparotitis
  Trauma
  Sialolithiasis
  Foreign body
  Cystic fibrosis
  Waldenström macroglobulinemia
  Reiter syndrome
  Amyloidosis
Nonparotid swelling
  Hypertrophy of masseter muscle
  Lymphadenopathy
  Rheumatoid mandibular joint swelling
  Tumors of jaw
  Infantile cortical hyperostosis

TREATMENT AND PREVENTION

Treatment of parotitis and the majority of its complications is entirely symptomatic. Bed rest may help reduce discomfort, and diet should be adjusted according to the ability of the patient to chew. As mentioned previously, patients may have difficulty with acid foods; therefore, diet should be light, with generous offering of fluids to preserve good hydration.

Analgesics, such as acetaminophen, may be used for headache and general malaise. Potent analgesics, such as morphine, are sometimes useful for orchitis or pancreatitis. Patients with orchitis require bed rest. Measures to minimize testicular tension, such as supporting the scrotum in a sling on an adhesive tape bridge between the thighs, and applying ice packs often help relieve pain. Pancreatic inflammation is treated with bed rest, withholding of oral feeding for 48 to 72 hours, and intravenous administration of dextrose and saline solutions. Electrolyte imbalance and metabolic alkalosis should be suspected when vomiting is severe. Headaches associated with meningoencephalitis may be relieved by oral analgesics; in intractable cases, lumbar puncture may be considered.

The patient should remain in isolation until glandular swelling subsides. Usually, patients can be considered noncontagious 9 days after the onset of parotid swelling. Susceptible contacts should be observed closely from 14 to 28 days after exposure. Mumps immune globulin and immune serum globulin are not helpful in preventing the disease.

Live mumps virus vaccine (5000 TCID$_{50}$ [median tissue culture infective dose]/dose) is the agent of choice for active immunization. The commercially available mumps vaccines are administered in a single subcutaneous injection of 0.5 mL, either alone or in combination with measles and rubella vaccines. The vaccines are immunogenic in 93% to 98% of subjects and has a protective efficacy of approximately 95% (6). Mumps vaccine should be routinely given after the first birthday. Simultaneous administration of mumps with measles and rubella at 13 to 15 months of life, with a booster at ages between 4 to 10 years of life, is safe and has been shown, if properly used, to reduce the number of mumps cases and related diseases (44–46).

Currently there are three mumps strains used in different vaccine preparations; the Jeryl Lynn strain, the Urabe Am 9 strain and the RIT 4385 strain. Although these three mumps strains are inmunogenic and highly effective, the Urabe Am 9 mumps strain have been associated with a high risk (1:11,000) of benign cases of post-vaccine aseptic meningitis and therefore, its use have been suspended in countries were alternative vaccines are available (47,48).

Serologic and epidemiologic evidence suggests that vaccine-induced immunity is long lasting and may be lifelong. Vaccine-induced antibody may develop slowly (14 to 28 days) and, therefore, may not prevent infection during the first few weeks after vaccination.

Adverse reactions attributed to live mumps vaccine are extremely rare (49). The vaccine may produce a noncommunicable, subclinical infection and may induce reactions in patients allergic to the egg protein or neomycin (vaccine contains 25 μg of neomycin). In view of the possible teratogenic effect of all live virus vaccines, mumps vaccines are contraindicated in pregnancy. As indicated previously, vaccines containing the Urabe Am 9 mumps strain have been associated with cases of aseptic meningitis.

Recently, the results of a small clinical trial designed to compare the inmunogenicity and reactogenicity of a measles, mumps and rubella (MMR) vaccine delivered by a new needle-free jet injector with the standard needle syringe administration were published (50). Although the needle free devise reported less vaccine associated adverse events and a similar immune response than the one detected with the vaccine administer by a syringe, the results of this preliminary trial need to be confirmed by larger clinical trials.

Any of the mumps vaccines should be given within 3 months after administration of immune globulin or blood transfusion because of the possible neutralization of the vaccine; it should also not be given to immunosuppressed patients. It is recommended, however, for patients with symptomatic human immunodeficiency virus infection. Rare complications after administration of mumps vaccine include nerve deafness, purpura, and orchitis (6,7).

REFERENCES

1. Johnson CD, Goodpasture EW. An investigation of the etiology of mumps. *J Exp Med* 1934;59:1–20.
2. Hilleman MR, Buynack EB, Weibel RE, et al. Live attenuated mumps-virus vaccine. *N Engl J Med* 1968;278:227–233.
3. Lacour M, Maherzi M, Vienny H, et al. Thrombocytopenia in a case of neonatal mumps infection: evidence of further clinical presentations. *Eur J Pediatr* 1993;152:739–741.
4. Cochi SL, Preblud SR, Orenstein WA. Perspectives on the relative resurgence of mumps in the United States. *Am J Dis Child* 1988;142:499–507.
5. Brunell PA. Mumps. In Feigin RD, Cherry JD, eds. *Textbook of pediatric infectious diseases*. Philadelphia: WB Saunders, 1987:1628–1632.
6. Marks MI. Mumps. In: Braude AI, Davis CE, Fierer J, eds. *Infectious diseases and medical microbiology*, 2nd ed. Philadelphia: WB Saunders, 1986:776–782.
7. Tolipn MD, Schauf V. Mumps virus. In: Belshe RB, ed. *Textbook of human virology*. Littleton, MA: PSG Publishing, 1985:311–331.
8. Friedman MG. Salivary IgA antibodies to mumps virus during and after mumps. *J Infect Dis* 1981;143:617.
9. Glikmann G, Mordhorst CH. Serological diagnosis of mumps and parainfluenza type-1 virus infections by enzyme immunoassay, with a comparison of two different approaches for detection of mumps IgG antibodies. *Acta Pathol Microbiol Immunol Scand* 1986;94:157–166.
10. Chiba Y, Dzierba JL, Morag A, et al. Cell-mediated immune response to mumps virus infection in man. *J Immunol* 1976;116:12–15.
11. Herndon RM, Johnson RT, Davis LE, et al. Ependymitis in mumps virus meningitis. *Arch Neurol* 1974;30:475–479.
12. Tsvetkov D. Spermatological disorders in patients with post mumps orchitis. *Akush Ginekol (Sofiia)* 1990;29:46–49.
13. Yamamoto M, Watanabe Y, Mizukoshi K. Neurotological findings in patients with acute mumps deafness. *Acta Otolaryngol Suppl (Stockh)* 1993;504:94–97.
14. Garcia AGP, Pereira JMS, Vidigal N, et al. Intrauterine infection with mumps virus. *Obstet Gynecol* 1980;156:756–759.
15. London WT, Ken SG, Palmer AE, et al. Induction of congenital hydrocephalus with mumps virus in rhesus monkeys. *J Infect Dis* 1979;139:324–328.
16. Donald PR, Burger PJ, Becker WB. Mumps meningoencephalitis. *S Afr Med J* 1987;71:283–285.
17. Centers for Disease Control. Mumps vaccine. *MMWR* 1977;26:393–394.
18. Ito M, Go T, Okuno T, et al. Chronic mumps virus encephalitis. *Pediatr Neurol* 1991;7:467–470.
19. Azimi PH, Cramblett HG, Haynes RE. Mumps meningoencephalitis in children. *JAMA* 1969;207:509–512.
20. Wilfert CM. Mumps meningoencephalitis with low cerebrospinal-fluid glucose, prolonged pleocytosis and elevation of protein. *N Engl J Med* 1969;280:855–859.
21. Kirk M. Sensorineural hearing loss and mumps. *Br J Audiol* 1987;21:227–228.
22. Yanagita N, Nakashima T, Ohno Y, et al. Estimated annual number of patients treated for sensorineural hearing loss in Japan. Results of a nationwide epidemiological survey in 1987. *Acta Otolaryngol Suppl (Stockh)* 1994;514:9–13.
23. Izushima N, Murakami Y. Deafness following mumps: the possible pathogenesis and incidence of deafness. *Auris Nasus Larynx* 1986;1:S55–S57.
24. Fukuda S. Experimental viral labyrinthitis - an immunohistochemical investigation of the cochlear lesion. *Hokkaido Igaku Zasshi* 1986;61:58–71.
25. Nussinovitch M, Brand N Frydman M, et al. Transverse myelitis following mumps in children. *Acta Paediatr* 1992;81:183–184.
26. Cohen HA, Ashkenazi A, Nussinovitch M, et al. Mumps-associated acute cerebellar ataxia. *Am J Dis Child* 1992;146:930–931.
27. Beard CM, Benson RC, Kelalis PP, et al. The incidence and outcome of mumps orchitis in Rochester, Minnesota, 1935 to 1974. *Mayo Clin Proc* 1977;52:3–7.
28. Philip RN, Reinhard KR, Lackman DB. Observations on a mumps epidemic in a "virgin" population. *Am J Hyg* 1959;69:91–111.
29. Lerner AM. Guide to immunization against mumps. *J Infect Dis* 1970;122:116–121.
30. Swerdlow AJ, Huttly SR, Smith PG. Testicular cancer and antecedent diseases. *Br J Cancer* 1987;55:97–103.
31. Levy NL, Notkins AL. Viral infections and diseases of the endocrine system. *J Infect Dis* 1971;124:94–103.
32. Schulz B, Michaelis D, Hildmann W, et al. Islet cell surface antibodies (ICSA) in subjects with a previous mumps infection - a prospective study over a 4 year period. *Exp Clin Endocrinol* 1987;90:62–70.
33. Ratzman KP, Jahr H, Richter KV. Complement-mediated cytotoxic effects of islet cell surface antibodies in non-diabetic subjects with antecedent mumps infection and diabetic risk. *Exp Clin Endocrinol* 1988;91:176–182.
34. Toniolo A, Conaldi PG, Garzelli C, et al. Role of antecedent mumps and reovirus infections on the development of type 1 (insulin-dependent) diabetes. *Eur J Epidemiol* 1985;1:172–179.
35. Gold HE, Boxerbeum B, Leslie HJ. Mumps arthritis. *Am J Dis Child* 1968;116:547–548.
36. Caranasos GJ, Felker JR. Mumps arthritis. *Arch Intern Med* 1967;119:394–398.
37. Hyer FH, Gottlied NL. Rheumatic disorders associated with viral infection. *Semin Arthritis Rheum* 1978;8:17–31.
38. Brown NJ, Richmond SJ. Fatal mumps myocarditis in an 8-month old child. *BMJ* 1980;281:356–357.
39. Eknoyan G, Dillman RO. Renal complications of infectious disease. *Med Clin North Am* 1978;52:979–1002.
40. Lin CY, Chen WP, Chiang H. Mumps associated with nephritis. *Child Nephrol Urol* 1990;10:68–71.
41. Hughes WT, Steigman AJ, Delong HF. Some implications of fatal nephritis associated with mumps. *Am J Dis Child* 1966;111:297–301.
42. Perry KR, Brown DN, Parry JV, et al. Detection of measles, mumps and rubella antibodies in saliva using antibody capture radioimmunoassay. *J Med Virol* 1993;40:235–240.
43. Endo A, Izumi H, Miyashita M, et al. Facial palsy associated with mumps parotitis. *Pediatr Infect Dis J* 2001;20:815–816.
44. Kanesaki T, Baba K, Tsuda N, et al. Protection of mumps in children with various underlying diseases: application of a live attenuated mumps and trivalent measles-rubella-mumps vaccines in these children. *Biken J* 1986;29:63–71.
45. Peltola H, Heinonen OP, Valle M, et al. The elimination of indigenous measles, mumps, and rubella from Finland by a 12-year, two-dose vaccination program. *N Engl J Med* 1994;331:1397–1402.
46. CDC. Measles, mumps and rubella–vaccine use and strategies for elimination

of measles, rubella and congenital rubella syndrome and control of mumps: recommendations of the advisory committee on immunization practices (ACIP). *MMWR* 1998;47(RR-8):1–57.

47. Usonis V, Bakasenas V, Kaufhold A, et al. Reactogenicity and immunogenicity of a new live attenuated combined measles, mumps and rubella vaccine in healthy children. *Pediatr Infect Dis J* 1999;18:42–48.

48. Block HL, Usonis V, Arguedas A, et al. Review of recent developments in MMR vaccination and practices in Latin America. *Rev Med Cir* 1999;1:39–49.

49. Patja A, Davidkin I, Kurki T, et al. Serious adverse events after measles-mumps-rubella vaccination during a fourteen-year prospective follow up. *Pediatr Infect Dis J* 2000;19:1127–1134.

50. Sarno MJ, Blasé E, Galindo N, et al. Clinical immunogenicity of measles, mumps and rubella vaccine delivered by the Injex jet injector: comparison with standard syringe infection. *Pediatr Infect Dis J* 2000;19:839–842.

CHAPTER 142
Human Papillomaviruses and Warts

Mathijs H. Brentjens, Kimberly A. Yeung-Yue, Patricia C. Lee, and Stephen K. Tyring

Condyloma acuminata have been documented since the time of Hippocrates, but it was not until the late 18th century that the infectious nature of genital warts became known. Payne first recognized that cutaneous warts were transmissible in 1891. In 1901, Heidingsfeld described transmission of condyloma acuminata through sexual contact. Strauss et al isolated the infectious agent responsible for genital warts in 1949, the human papillomavirus (HPV) (1).

Human papillomavirus infection has been associated with both benign and malignant lesions. In addition to the benign lesions of condyloma acuminata, human papillomaviruses are responsible for non-sexually transmitted infections such as common warts (verruca vulgaris), plantar warts, lesions of the mouth nose and throat, conjunctival papillomatosis, cervical intraepithelial neoplasias, and the lesions found in epidermodysplasia verruciformis. Human papillomaviruses are also found in malignant diseases such as anogenital cancers, squamous cell carcinomas, and cervical cancer.

Although there is currently no definitive therapy for HPV infection, recent treatment modalities offer promise for both improved control of HPV infection, and possible prevention of HPV infection. This chapter reviews the structure of HPV, the pathogenesis of wart formation, classification of HPV types, clinical manifestations of warts, and their treatment.

STRUCTURE

Human papillomaviruses belong to the family Papillomaviridae, which includes HPV and papillomaviruses affecting other species. They were previously classified as Papovaviridae, which have now been replaced by two families: Papillomaviridae and Polyomaviridae (2). These viruses show remarkable species specificity and are not known to affect species other than their natural hosts (3).

Human papillomaviruses are double-stranded deoxyribonucleic acid (DNA) viruses with icosahedral structural symmetry. Seventy-two proteins (consisting of minor and major capsid proteins) form the outer coat. The genome consists of a circular double-stranded DNA of approximately 8 Kb. It encodes nine genes and contains a single control region. The genome is separated into early and late genes. Early genes (E1-E7) are involved with regulation of viral replication and transcription. They are also involved in oncogenic transformation in certain high-risk HPV types. Late genes encode the proteins that comprise the outer capsid.

Human papillomavirus E1 and E2 proteins are both involved in promoting viral replication and inhibiting viral integration into the host genome. In fact, it has been demonstrated that E1 and E2 proteins are both necessary and sufficient to promote HPV replication in host cells (4,5). The HPV E2 gene also has a role in viral transcription. This protein has been extensively studied in bovine papillomaviruses, and produces three separate proteins that function to either enhance or repress viral transcription (6). In high-risk oncogenic HPV types, full-length E2 transcripts have been shown to prevent cell growth *in vitro* (7). This suggests that E2 plays a large role in prevention of oncogenic transformation in infected cells. HPV E4 protein has been associated with collapse of the cellular cytokeratin network, enhancing virus exit from the cell (8). Modification of cellular growth factor pathways by the E5 protein apparently promotes oncogenic transformation (9). It forms complexes with platelet-derived and epidermal growth factor receptors, resulting in constitutional receptor activation (10). The oncogenic potential of HPV is largely related to expression of E6 and E7 proteins. These proteins inhibit tumor suppressor genes P53 and RB respectively (11–13). In high-risk types, the E6 protein binds to P53 with great affinity, thereby significantly enhancing its degradation. E7 binds to RB in a similar manner, both promoting the release of E2F (which stimulates cell cycle progression), and the degradation of RB. E6 and E7 together down-regulate expression of interferon (IFN) responsive genes and limit host immune response to HPV (14,15). Numerous other mechanisms have been proposed to explain the oncogenic potential of E6 and E7.

PATHOGENESIS

HPV infects squamous epithelial cells. After gaining access through traumatized epithelium, HPV then enters the basal epithelial cells, where early gene transcription and translation occur. As these cells mature and move toward the skin surface, late genes encoding capsid proteins undergo transcription and translation. Viral DNA packaging and capsid formation take place in terminally differentiated cells in the upper epidermal layers. Viral particles are then released on the skin surface.

Infection with HPV may take one of three clinical paths: latent infection (where no histopathological or clinical evidence of disease is apparent), subclinical infection (where there is microscopic but no clinical evidence of disease), and clinically apparent disease. Most HPV infections follow latent or subclinical paths (16). Manifestations of clinically apparent HPV infection (i.e., warts) include epidermal thickening, hyperplasia of the stratum spinosum, and hyperkeratosis. In the absence of treatment, clinically apparent lesions may undergo spontaneous regression, persist, or transform to more atypical lesions (neoplasias) (17,18). Although the exact mechanism producing progression of HPV-induced lesions is not yet understood, the integration of HPV DNA into host genetic material appears to play an important role. The locus of integration into the host genome is non-specific, but HPV DNA often breaks in the E1-E2 region of the genome (19). The loss of E1 and E2 gene products subsequently leads to decreased transcriptional control of other early (potentially oncogenic) HPV genes.

CLASSIFICATION

HPV typing is determined by genetic homology to previously identified strains. The 1995 International Papillomavirus Conference defined novel HPV types as having less than 90% genetic homology in the L1 open reading frame (ORF) with known types. Currently more than 100 HPV types are recognized (20). In addition to genetic HPV typing, two more clinically significant classification systems are often used.

HPV types may be classified according to their tissue tropism. This classification divides HPV into dermatotropic or mucosotropic groups. Lesions induced by dermatotropic types generally affect non-genital cutaneous tissues, while types described as mucosotropic affect genital and mucosal tissues. The most common dermatotropic HPV types include 1 to 4, which are responsible for common warts (verruca vulgaris), plantar warts, and flat warts (21). The most common mucosotropic types are 6 and 11 (which cause most cases of condyloma acuminata), and 16 and 18 (which cause genital neoplasias) (3,22). A table of common dermatotropic and mucosotropic types may be found elsewhere in this text.

The other clinically relevant classification system divides HPV types according to their potential for oncogenic transformation. In this classification, HPV are characterized as either high-risk or low-risk. By far, the most common high-risk types are 16 and 18, which are found in 68% to 78% of all cervical cancer specimens positive for HPV DNA (23,24). Further classification of common high-risk and low-risk types may be found in the chapter on HPV in this text.

Finally, there are HPV types not typically found in otherwise healthy individuals (see the chapter on HPV in this text). Instead, they infect immunocompromised individuals and individuals with a rare genetic disorder affecting cell-mediated immunity called epidermodysplasia verruciformis (EV). Oncogenic transformation of warts is much more common in immunocompromised patients and those with EV.

CLINICAL MANIFESTATIONS

Human papillomaviruses are responsible for a wide variety of benign non-genital cutaneous lesions. These tend to be more common in a younger population and include verruca vulgaris, plantar warts, and flat warts (25,26). Transmission of HPV associated with these lesions is by physical contact of traumatized epithelium with infected surfaces, either the wart itself or fomites (surfaces that have been in contact with a lesion, such as toys). Most often, warts are self-limited and regress spontaneously within 2 years (27).

Verruca vulgaris (common warts) represent the most frequent clinical manifestation of cutaneous HPV infections. They are found on the dorsal surfaces of the hands (especially periungual regions), although they may also be found on the face, palms, plantar aspects of the feet, and indeed on virtually any skin surface. HPV types often associated with common warts include types 2 and 4. Meat handlers such as butchers and abattoir workers can present with warts on their hands caused by HPV type 7 (butcher's warts) (28). Although the exact relationship between these warts and the occupational hazards of meat workers is not currently known, it is thought that these lesions may occur as a result of factors found in the handled meat products (29). Common warts may initially present as flesh-colored papules, but eventually develop into a typical hyperkeratotic nodule with a brown-gray appearance. The differential diagnosis includes corns as well as molluscum contagiosum. Common warts typically demonstrate punctate hemorrhagic or thrombosed vessels within the lesion after debridement of the wart surface, thereby distinguishing it from corns or molluscum (30). As with other cutaneous manifestations of HPV infections, the diagnosis is most often made clinically. However, common warts do present a relatively unique histologic picture. Prominent papillomatosis, focal parakeratosis, and clarified granular cells containing keratohyaline granules are usually noted on light microscopy (31).

Plantar warts (myrmecia warts or verrucae plantaris) are often painful and occur on the soles of the feet and toes, usually in weight-bearing areas. A variant of plantar warts, mosaic warts present on the plantar surfaces of the foot as multiple confluent lesions with a polygonal outline. In contrast to typical plantar warts, they are often painless (32). Plantar warts are frequently associated with HPV type 1 and occur most often in teenagers (30). The differential diagnosis includes foreign body reaction, lichen planus, fibrokeratomas, and common warts. Clinically, plantar warts are characterized by endophytic growth, with a horny, hyperkeratotic surface. After debridement of the surface, a central depression is characteristically present. As with verruca vulgaris, punctate bleeding and stippling from entrapped capillaries may occur after debridement. Plantar warts may be distinguished from verrucae vulgaris by the associated pain of plantar warts (common warts are not typically painful), and the fact that plantar warts usually occur as single lesions (common warts often present as multiple lesions). The diagnosis is again usually made clinically, but plantar warts also have notable histologic features. On light microscopy, endophytic epidermal growth is noted with large eosinophilic cytoplasmic inclusions. The upper epidermal layer contains basophilic parakeratotic cells with nuclear basophilic inclusions noted in other cells (32).

Flat warts are the least common cutaneous warts, noted in only 4% of people with warts (30). HPV types 3 and 10 are usually found in these lesions. They are most often found on the face or dorsum of the hands in children. In adults, they are found in areas that are shaved, such as legs in women and beards in men. Clinically, flat warts appear as small (usually less than 5 mm) flat-topped papules with smooth or mildly hyperkeratotic surfaces. Scratching at the lesions may result in the development of a series of flat warts arranged in a linear pattern (known as the Koebner phenomenon). Flat warts should be distinguished from common warts. Histologic features of planar warts include a basket weave appearance of the stratum corneum and vacuolization of spinous and granular cells.

Other non-malignant lesions associated with HPV include keratoacanthomas, actinic keratoses, and seborrheic keratoses (33–36). Although HPV DNA has been found in some of these lesions, there is currently no evidence supporting a causal role for papillomaviruses. One recent study also found HPV DNA in 88% of clinically diagnosed skin tags (37).

Basal cell carcinomas (BCC) and squamous cell carcinomas (SCC) have also been tentatively linked with HPV infections. Although causality has not been proven, this association is especially strong for SCC in both immunocompromised hosts and EV patients (38–41).

Benign genital-mucosal lesions induced by HPV include papillomas of the upper airway as well as genital warts (condyloma acuminata). Condyloma acuminata are of great clinical interest currently since genital lesions caused by HPV are closely associated with malignancies, including cervical cancer. As mentioned previously, HPV types 6, 11, 16, and 18 are most frequently associated with genital-mucosal lesions.

Mucosal lesions of the upper respiratory tract induced by HPV include nasal, oral, and laryngeal papillomas. These lesions typically present as pedunculated fleshy lesions and are often asymptomatic. However, they may result in dangerous clinical symptoms. Obstruction of the airway may occur, particularly in children. Although these lesions most often spontaneously regress, they also may recur after treatment. It is thought that recurrence after surgical excision may be due to residual HPV in clinically normal tissue surrounding the lesion. There is also evidence linking HPV infection with the development of squamous cell carcinoma of the oropharynx (42). Involvement of the pulmonary parenchyma in these lesions is associated with frequent complications (43).

Condyloma acuminata represent one of the most frequent viral sexually transmitted diseases in the world (16). In males, they occur most frequently on the foreskin of uncircumcised patients or on the glans penis. In homosexual males, the perianal region is frequently involved. In females, external genital warts involving the vulva are common, but lesions of the vaginal walls and cervix also occur. Cervical HPV infection is of particular interest since virtually all cervical carcinomas are associated with HPV infection (discussed elsewhere in this text). Warts of the anal canal are often found in homosexual and bisexual men (44). Condyloma acuminata may also be found in the urethra. Clinically, anogenital HPV infections may present as cauliflower-like lesions, smooth fleshy papules, lesions resembling flat warts, or hyperkeratotic lesions. The appearance of these lesions relates to the type of epithelial tissue involved. They most often regress spontaneously, but may persist even with treatment. Recurrences after treatment are also common. Histologically, condylomas demonstrate hyperplasia with mild thickening of the stratum corneum, significant acanthosis, thickening and branching of the rete ridges, and occasional mitotic figures. These lesions may be differentiated from squamous cell carcinoma by a discrete border between the hyperplastic epithelium and dermis, and an orderly arrangement of epithelial cells. Of diagnostic significance is the presence of perinuclear vacuolization extending deep into the epithelium. The dermis may appear edematous and show a moderately dense chronic infiltrate (31). Condyloma acuminata should be distinguished from other viral infections that may present in the anogenital area (such as molluscum contagiosum) as well as malignancies.

TREATMENT

No single therapy has proven uniformly successful in the treatment of warts. Most have high recurrence rates. Side effects, cost, or treatment requirements also limit the usefulness of some therapeutic modalities. Recent research has largely concentrated on the treatment of condyloma acuminata, although there are also case reports and smaller studies evaluating some promising new therapies for non-genital warts.

Non-Genital Warts

The most commonly used cytodestructive therapy for non-genital warts is cryotherapy. This procedure uses liquid nitrogen to freeze the warts and some of the surrounding tissue. The resulting necrosis of the warts is bloodless but can result in significant pain for the patient. Cryotherapy appears to be less effective than either surgical excision or laser therapy. In one study, 24 of 25 patients treated for plantar warts with cryotherapy were still observed to harbor HPV DNA on repeat biopsies of lesion sites (45). Patients also often need multiple doctor visits to achieve acceptable results.

Surgical excision remains one of the modalities for the treatment of cutaneous warts. However, since clinically unaffected tissue surrounding these warts still often harbors HPV, the recurrence rate is very high. Scar formation, bleeding from the excision site, and secondary infection remain significant side effects.

Laser ablation has also been used in the treatment of both cutaneous and oropharyngeal HPV induced lesions. This therapy has demonstrated promising results in controlling oropharyngeal papillomas (46). However, recurrence rates remain high. HPV DNA has also been found in the smoke plume of carbon dioxide lasers, leading to the potential for respiratory infections of the operator (47). The cost of laser therapy and the specific operator skills necessary make it impractical for widespread use in cutaneous or oropharyngeal HPV infections.

Newer therapies for cutaneous and oropharyngeal warts are also being explored. Cidofovir, an antiviral nucleoside has shown promising results as a topical therapy in case reports and preliminary studies. These studies have concentrated on using cidofovir in immunocompromised patients, a population with HPV-induced lesions (both cutaneous and genital) that are particularly refractory to standard therapies (50–53). Intralesional injection of *Candida* and mumps skin test antigens may also be effective in treatment of refractory cutaneous warts (54,55). Finally, although not approved for the primary treatment of cutaneous warts, dermatologists often prescribe the immunomodulators, imiquimod (see below and Fig. 142.1), after cytodestructive therapy. Imiquimod may prevent recurrence after primary treatment of cutaneous warts by other methods.

Genital Warts

The cytodestructive and antiviral therapies described above are still frequently used in the treatment of anogenital warts with variable success, but other treatments also have been extensively studied. Although they may also be used as therapy for

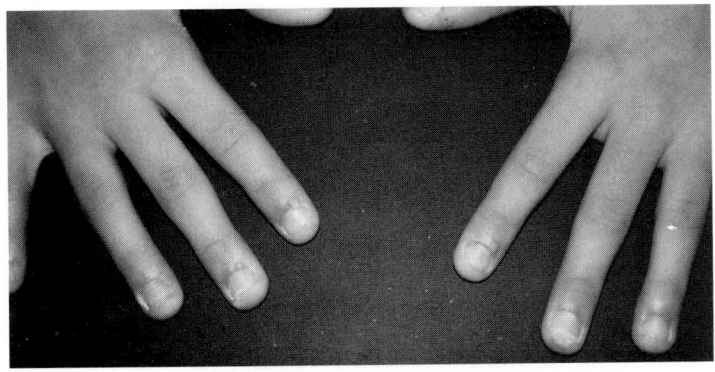
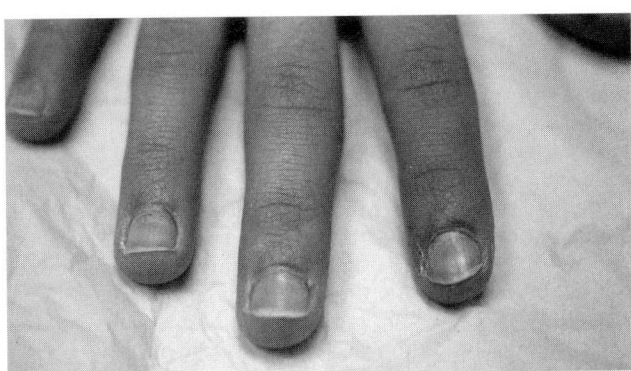

A   B

Figure 142.1.   A: Extensive periungual warts in an 8-year-old girl. **B:** Resolution of warts after 8 weeks of monotherapy (three times a week) with imiquimod.

non-genital warts, most clinical trials have focused on anogenital HPV infections. Some of the newer treatments are becoming more popular because of a favorable side effect profile and lower recurrence rates.

Other chemical cytodestructive methods used in the treatment of genital warts include trichloroacetic acid, bichloracetic acid, salicylic acid, podophyllin, and podophyllotoxin. Podophyllin is a solution that comes in concentrations of 10% or 25%. However, this compound is not standardized and therefore has variable efficacy (48). Furthermore, at least two chemical mutagens are found in this solution (49). Recurrence rates are high. Podophyllotoxin has been identified as the active ingredient in podophyllin and has the advantage of being approved for patient self-application (the only therapy apart from imiquimod that has this advantage). Additionally, podophyllotoxin has increased clearing rates with respect to podophyllin. Side effects of these two treatments include burning, erosions, pain, and inflammation. At least two deaths have been attributed to the application of topical podophyllin.

The antimetabolite 5-fluorouracil (5-FU) may be applied either topically or intralesionally. This drug acts to disrupt cell division by inhibiting DNA synthesis. Trials of topical 5-FU have had mixed results with respect to efficacy, while intralesional 5-FU has been found to be significantly more effective than placebo (56–59). Side effects of topical 5-FU are usually minor, with local inflammation and irritation. Intralesional 5-FU may result in pain, erythema, and ulceration at the site of the wart (58).

Immunomodulatory medications include interferons and imiquimod. These compounds act to enhance a patient's own immune responses.

Interferons α, β, and γ have all been extensively studied as topical, intralesional and systemic therapies for genital warts. Topical therapy with interferon has resulted in response rates from 42% to 90% with only mild side effects in some studies (60–64). Intralesional therapies appear to have the greatest efficacy, with complete clearances between 35% and 80% (65–70). Recurrence rates are relatively low, but systemic side effects commonly occur. Intralesional injections of warts in the anogenital area may also lead to objections from patients. Systemic interferon therapy appears to have little value in treating warts and the systemic side effects can be significant (including headaches, fevers, and flu-like syndromes). Cost of therapy limits the use of interferon in everyday practice. One recent cost-effectiveness analysis estimated that interferon therapy would cost as much as 20 times more than surgical excision (71).

Imiquimod is another immune response modifier and has been approved for self-application on external anogenital warts. Applied overnight three times a week, this medication enhances immune function by increasing cytokine production and stimulating cell-mediated immunity to HPV. A recent study demonstrated that imiquimod application to genital warts results in significant increases of local levels of interferon α, β, and γ as well as tumor necrosis factor (72). Imiquimod has demonstrated complete responses in over 50% of patients treated with 5% imiquimod cream (published studies show complete response ranges between 24% and 79%) (72–77). This therapy also resulted in a significant reduction of total wart area even in those who did not demonstrate complete responses (72–76). The recurrence rate is very low, with 87% of complete responders wart-free after 12 weeks (75). Side effects of imiquimod are typically mild, with local irritation being the most frequent complaint. Other side effects include erythema, pruritus, and rare erosions at the site of application. Imiquimod is becoming increasingly popular in the treatment of anogenital warts because of its effectiveness, minimal side effects, suitability for patient self-application, and a very low recurrence rate in comparison with other therapies.

Finally, vaccine candidates have recently been developed and are undergoing clinical trials both for prevention and possible treatment of HPV infections. HPV vaccine research is currently focused on preventing and/or treating high-grade neoplastic lesions and carcinomas induced by high risk HPV types 16 and 18 and are discussed elsewhere in this text.

CONCLUSION

Non-malignant HPV infections remain a great source of morbidity. Recurrent or persistent infections are difficult to treat, especially in immunocompromised hosts. Recent advances in therapy for warts are promising, but to date no single treatment has proved uniformly effective in eradicating HPV infections. Treatment of both cutaneous and anogenital warts requires patience on the part of the clinician and patient, and may require the use of multiple modalities before a satisfactory treatment is found.

REFERENCES

1. Syrjanen K, Syrjanen S. Historical overview of papillomavirus research. In: *Papillomavirus infections in human pathology*. Chichester, NY: John Wiley & Sons, 2000:1–10.
2. Butel J. Papovaviruses. In: Baron S, ed. *Medical microbiology*. Galveston, TX: The University of Texas Medical Branch at Galveston, 1996:799–811.
3. Beutner KR, Tyring S. Human papillomavirus and human disease. *Am J Med* 1997;102:9–15.
4. Chiang CM, Ustav M, Stenlund A, et al. Viral E1 and E2 proteins support replication of homologous and heterologous papillomaviral origins. *Proc Natl Acad Sci USA* 1992;89:5799–5803.
5. Ustav M, Stenlund A. Transient replication of BPV-1 requires two viral polypeptides encoded by the E1 and E2 open reading frames. *Embo J* 1991;10:449–457.
6. Hubbert NL, Schiller JT, Lowy DR, et al. Bovine papilloma virus-transformed cells contain multiple E2 proteins. *Proc Natl Acad Sci USA* 1988;85:5864–5868.
7. Dowhanick JJ, McBride AA, Howley PM. Suppression of cellular proliferation by the papillomavirus E2 protein. *J Virol* 1995;69:7791–7799.
8. Doorbar J, Ely S, Sterling J, et al. Specific interaction between HPV-16 E1-E4 and cytokeratins results in collapse of the epithelial cell intermediate filament network. *Nature* 1991;352:824–827.
9. DiMaio D, Petti L, Hwang E. The E5 Transforming proteins of the papillomaviruses. *Semin Virol* 1994;5:369–379.
10. Cohen BD, Goldstein DJ, Rutledge L, et al. Transformation-specific interaction of the bovine papillomavirus E5 oncoprotein with the platelet-derived growth factor receptor transmembrane domain and the epidermal growth factor receptor cytoplasmic domain. *J Virol* 1993;67:5303–5311.
11. Boyer SN, Wazer DE, Band V. E7 protein of human papilloma virus-16 induces degradation of retinoblastoma protein through the ubiquitin-proteasome pathway. *Cancer Res* 1996;56:4620–4624.
12. Gu J, Rubin RM, Yuan ZM. A sequence element of p53 that determines its susceptibility to viral oncoprotein-targeted degradation. *Oncogene* 2001;20:3519–3527.
13. Hengstermann A, Linares LK, Ciechanover A, et al. Complete switch from Mdm2 to human papillomavirus E6-mediated degradation of p53 in cervical cancer cells. *Proc Natl Acad Sci USA* 2001;98:1218–1223.
14. Lee SJ, Cho YS, Cho MC, et al. Both e6 and e7 oncoproteins of human papillomavirus 16 inhibit IL-18-induced IFN-gamma production in human peripheral blood mononuclear and NK cells. *J Immunol* 2001;167:497–504.
15. Nees M, Geoghegan JM, Hyman T, et al. Papillomavirus type 16 oncogenes downregulate expression of interferon-responsive genes and upregulate proliferation-associated and NF-kappaB-responsive genes in cervical keratinocytes. *J Virol* 2001;75:4283–4296.
16. Koutsky L. Epidemiology of genital human papillomavirus infection. *Am J Med* 1997;102:3–8.
17. Carr J, Gyorfi T. Human papillomavirus. Epidemiology, transmission, and pathogenesis. *Clin Lab Med* 2000;20:235–255.
18. Liaw KL, Glass AG, Manos MM, et al. Detection of human papillomavirus DNA in cytologically normal women and subsequent cervical squamous intraepithelial lesions. *J Natl Cancer Inst* 1999;91:954–960.
19. Barbosa MS. The oncogenic role of human papillomavirus proteins. *Crit Rev Oncog* 1996;7:1–18.
20. Gharizadeh B, Kalantari M, Garcia CA, et al. Typing of human papillomavirus by pyrosequencing. *Lab Invest* 2001;81:673–679.
21. Syrjanen K, Syrjanen S. HPV infections of the skin. *Papillomavirus infections in human pathology*. Chichester, NY: John Wiley & Sons, 2000:315–340.

22. Grce M, Husnjak K, Skerlev M, et al. Detection and typing of human papillomaviruses by means of polymerase chain reaction and fragment length polymorphism in male genital lesions. *Anticancer Res* 2000;20:2097–2102.
23. Munoz N. Human papillomavirus and cancer: the epidemiological evidence. *J Clin Virol* 2000;19:1–5.
24. Pilch H, Gunzel S, Schaffer U, et al. The presence of HPV DNA in cervical cancer: correlation with clinico-pathologic parameters and prognostic significance: 10 years experience at the Department of Obstetrics and Gynecology of the Mainz University. *Int J Gynecol Cancer* 2001;11:39–48.
25. Larsson PA, Liden S. Prevalence of skin diseases among adolescents 12–16 years of age. *Acta Derm Venereol* 1980;60:415–423.
26. Rubben A, Kalka K, Spelten B, et al. Clinical features and age distribution of patients with HPV-induced common warts. *Arch Dermatol Res* 1997;289:337–340.
27. Brady M. Common viral skin problems of childhood: warts and molluscum. *J Pediatr Health Care* 1988;2:208–210.
28. Jablonska S, Obalek S, Golebiowska A, et al: Epidemiology of butchers' warts. *Arch Dermatol Res* 1988;280:S24–S28.
29. Keefe M, al-Ghamdi A, Coggon D, et al: Cutaneous warts in butchers. *Br J Dermatol* 1994;130:9–14.
30. Plasencia JM: Cutaneous warts: diagnosis and treatment. *Prim Care* 2000;27:423–434.
31. Lever W, Schaumberg-Lever G. *Histopathology of the skin.* Philadelphia: Lippincott, 1990.
32. Jablonska S, Majewski S, Obalek S, et al. Cutaneous warts. *Clin Dermatol* 1997;15:309–319.
33. Hsi ED, Svoboda-Newman SM, Stern RA, et al. Detection of human papillomavirus DNA in keratoacanthomas by polymerase chain reaction. *Am J Dermatopathol* 1997;19:10–15.
34. Lu S, Syrjanen K, Havu VK, et al. No evidence of human papillomavirus DNA in actinic keratosis. *Arch Dermatol Res* 1995;287:649–651.
35. Stockfleth E, Rowert J, Arndt R, et al. Detection of human papillomavirus and response to topical 5% imiquimod in a case of stucco keratosis. *Br J Dermatol* 2000;143:846–850.
36. Tsambaos D, Monastirli A, Kapranos N, et al. Detection of human papillomavirus DNA in nongenital seborrhoeic keratoses. *Arch Dermatol Res* 1995;287:612–615.
37. Dianzani C, Calvieri S, Pierangeli A, et al. The detection of human papillomavirus DNA in skin tags. *Br J Dermatol* 1998;138:649–651.
38. London NJ, Farmery SM, Will EJ, et al. Risk of neoplasia in renal transplant patients. *Lancet* 1995;346:403–406.
39. Leigh IM, Glover MT. Skin cancer and warts in immunosuppressed renal transplant recipients. *Rec Results Cancer Res* 1995;139:69–86.
40. Majewski, S, Jablonska S. Epidermodysplasia verruciformis as a model of human papillomavirus-induced genetic cancer of the skin. *Arch Dermatol* 1995;131:1312–1318.
41. Harwood CA, Surentheran T, McGregor JM, et al. Human papillomavirus infection and non-melanoma skin cancer in immunosuppressed and immunocompetent individuals. *J Med Virol* 2000;61:289–297.
42. Moore CE, Wiatrak BJ, McClatchey KD, et al: High-risk human papillomavirus types and squamous cell carcinoma in patients with respiratory papillomas. *Otolaryngol Head Neck Surg* 1999;120:698–705.
43. Blackledge FA, Anand VK. Tracheobronchial extension of recurrent respiratory papillomatosis. *Ann Otol Rhinol Laryngol* 2000;109:812–818.
44. Breese PL, Judson FN, Penley KA, et al. Anal human papillomavirus infection among homosexual and bisexual men: prevalence of type-specific infection and association with human immunodeficiency virus. *Sex Transm Dis* 1995;22:7–14.
45. El-Tonsy, MH, Anbar TE, El-Domyati M, et al. Density of viral particles in pre and post Nd: YAG laser hyperthermia therapy and cryotherapy in plantar warts. *Int J Dermatol* 1999;38:393–398.
46. Dedo HH, Yu KC. CO(2) laser treatment in 244 patients with respiratory papillomas. *Laryngoscope* 2001;111:1639–1644.
47. Gloster HM, Jr., Roenigk RK. Risk of acquiring human papillomavirus from the plume produced by the carbon dioxide laser in the treatment of warts. *J Am Acad Dermatol* 1995;32:436–441.
48. Longstaff E, von Krogh G. Condyloma eradication: self-therapy with 0.15-0.5% podophyllotoxin versus 20-25% podophyllin preparations—an integrated safety assessment. *Regul Toxicol Pharmacol* 2001;33:117–137.
49. Petersen CS, Weismann K. Quercetin and kaempherol: an argument against the use of podophyllin? *Genitourin Med* 1995;71:92–93.
50. Zabawski EJ Jr, Sands B, Goetz D, et al. Treatment of verruca vulgaris with topical cidofovir. *JAMA* 1997;278:1236.
51. Calista D. Topical cidofovir for severe cutaneous human papillomavirus and molluscum contagiosum infections in patients with HIV/AIDS. A pilot study. *J Eur Acad Dermatol Venereol* 2000;14:484–488.
52. Calista D. Resolution of recalcitrant human papillomavirus gingival infection with topical cidofovir. *Oral Surg Oral Med Oral Pathol Oral Radiol Endod* 2000;90:713–715.
53. Matteelli A, Beltrame A, Graifemberghi S, et al. Efficacy and tolerability of topical 1% cidofovir cream for the treatment of external anogenital warts in HIV-infected persons. *Sex Transm Dis* 2001;28:343–346.
54. Johnson SM, Roberson PK, Horn TD. Intralesional injection of mumps or Candida skin test antigens: a novel immunotherapy for warts. *Arch Dermatol* 2001;137:451–455.
55. Signore RJ. Candida immunotherapy of warts. *Arch Dermatol* 2001;137:1250–1251.
56. Holmes MM, Weaver SH 2nd, Vermillion ST. A randomized, double-blind, placebo-controlled trial of 5-fluorouracil for the treatment of cervicovaginal human papillomavirus. *Infect Dis Obstet Gynecol* 1999;7:186–189.
57. Davila GW, Shroyer KR. Topical 5-fluorouracil in the treatment of cervical human papillomavirus infection. *Gynecol Obstet Invest* 1996;41:275–277.
58. Swinehart JM, Skinner RB, McCarty JM, et al. Development of intralesional therapy with fluorouracil/adrenaline injectable gel for management of condylomata acuminata: two phase II clinical studies. *Genitourin Med* 1997;73:481–487.
59. Swinehart JM, Sperling M, Phillips S, et al. Intralesional fluorouracil/epinephrine injectable gel for treatment of condylomata acuminata. A phase 3 clinical study. *Arch Dermatol* 1997;133:67–73.
60. Schneider A, Grubert T, Kirchmayr R, et al. Efficacy trial of topically administered interferon gamma-1 beta gel in comparison to laser treatment in cervical intraepithelial neoplasia. *Arch Gynecol Obstet* 1995;256:75–83.
61. Stentella P, Frega A, Di Renzi F, et al: Topic and systemic administration of natural alfa interferon in the treatment of female and male HPV genital infections. *Clin Exp Obstet Gynecol* 1996;23:29–36.
62. Syed TA, Lundin S, Cheema KM, et al. Human leukocyte interferon-alpha in cream, for the treatment of genital warts in Asian women: a placebo-controlled, double-blind study. *Clin Investig* 1994;72:870–873.
63. Syed TA, Cheema KM, Khayyami M, et al. Human leukocyte interferon-alpha versus podophyllotoxin in cream for the treatment of genital warts in males. A placebo-controlled, double-blind, comparative study. *Dermatology* 1995;191:129–132.
64. Syed TA, Ahmadpour OA. Human leukocyte derived interferon-alpha in a hydrophilic gel for the treatment of intravaginal warts in women: a placebo-controlled, double-blind study. *Int J STD AIDS* 1998;9:769–772.
65. Eron LJ, Judson F, Tucker S, et al. Interferon therapy for condylomata acuminata. *N Engl J Med* 1986;315:1059–1064.
66. Friedman-Kien A. Management of condylomata acuminata with Alferon N injection, interferon alfa-n3 (human leukocyte derived). *Am J Obstet Gynecol* 1995;172:1359–1368.
67. Friedman-Kien AE, Eron LJ, Conant M, et al. Natural interferon alfa for treatment of condylomata acuminata. *JAMA* 1988;259:533–538.
68. Monsonego J, Cessot G, Ince SE, et al: Randomised double-blind trial of recombinant interferon-beta for condyloma acuminatum. *Genitourin Med* 1996;72:111–114.
69. Penna, C, Fallani MG, Gordigiani R, et al. Intralesional beta-interferon treatment of cervical intraepithelial neoplasia associated with human papillomavirus infection. *Tumori* 1994;80:146–150.
70. Vance JC, Bart BJ, Hansen RC, et al. Intralesional recombinant alpha-2 interferon for the treatment of patients with condyloma acuminatum or verruca plantaris. *Arch Dermatol* 1986;122:272–277.
71. Alam M, Stiller M. Direct medical costs for surgical and medical treatment of condylomata acuminata. *Arch Dermatol* 2001;137:337–341.
72. Tyring SK, Arany I, Stanley MA, et al. A randomized, controlled, molecular study of condylomata acuminata clearance during treatment with imiquimod. *J Infect Dis* 1998;178:551–555.
73. Beutner KR, Spruance SL, Hougham AJ, et al. Treatment of genital warts with an immune-response modifier (imiquimod). *J Am Acad Dermatol* 1998;38:230–239.
74. Beutner KR, Tyring SK, Trofatter KF Jr, et al. Imiquimod, a patient-applied immune-response modifier for treatment of external genital warts. *Antimicrob Agents Chemother* 1998;42:789–794.
75. Edwards L, Ferenczy A, Eron L, et al. Self-administered topical 5% imiquimod cream for external anogenital warts. HPV study group. Human papillomavirus. *Arch Dermatol* 1998;134:25–30.
76. Fife KH, Ferenczy A, Douglas JM Jr, et al. Treatment of external genital warts in men using 5% imiquimod cream applied three times a week, once daily, twice daily, or three times a day. *Sex Transm Dis* 2001;28:226–231.
77. Wagman FA, Estape RE, Angioli R, et al. Self-administered topical 5% imiquimod cream for external anogenital warts in adolescent girls. *Obstet Gynecol* 2001;97:S14.

CHAPTER 143
Erythema Infectiosum, Roseola, and Enteroviral Exanthems

Walter W. Tunnessen, Jr.*

ERYTHEMA INFECTIOSUM

Fifth disease (erythema infectiosum) is the only exanthem that retains the numerical eponym assigned to it during the late 1800s and early 1900s. This distinctive exanthem was first described by Tschamer in 1886, and the label erythema infectiosum was applied by Stricker in 1899 (1). The first report in the American literature appeared in 1905, but the cases described were actually seen in Vienna (2). Herrick's careful description of 74 cases provided the first record of a large outbreak in the United States.

The cause of erythema infectiosum defied discovery until 1984, when the sera of 36 children involved in an outbreak of this exanthem were tested for the presence of specific immunoglobulin M (IgM) antibody to human parvovirus (HPV) and all showed significant titers (3). A number of reports confirmed this association (4–6).

HPV-B19 was discovered in 1975 in blood obtained from adult donors who were asymptomatic or had mild symptoms during an evaluation of hepatitis B detection tests (7). HPV-B19 has since then been incriminated as the cause of aplastic crises in persons with hemolytic anemias; it has been found to be a cause of acute arthritis in some adults; it has been associated with spontaneous abortions, stillbirths, and hydrops fetalis; and it may lead to chronic marrow hypoplasia from persistent red blood cell precursor lysis in immunocompromised patients who develop persistent infections (8).

Epidemiology

The mode of spread of HPV is presumed to be person to person through the respiratory tract. Erythema infectiosum has a worldwide distribution. It tends to occur in epidemics, most commonly in the late winter and early spring. The exanthem seems to be fairly well confined to school-age children. Herrick found all but four of his 74 cases in the 6- to 15-year age bracket (1). Ager and co-workers similarly observed the peak attack rate between 5 and 14 years, with 80% of 364 patients younger than 15 years (9). School attack rates during epidemics have varied between 13% and 43.9% (3,10,11). The attack rate in household contacts is approximately 50%. (12) Antibody to HPV increases with age. Almost 20% of children 10 to 14 years of age, 35% of adults 30 to 39 years of age, and 50% of persons older than 50 years will demonstrate antibody (4). This suggests that adults may acquire the infection but frequently do not manifest the exanthem.

Pathogenesis

Healthy adult volunteers inoculated intranasally with HPV obtained from an asymptomatic blood donor demonstrated a two-phase illness. A week after inoculation, during intense viremia, the volunteers had a mild illness with fever, malaise, myalgia,

and itching. At 17 to 18 days, the second phase occurred when a fine maculopapular rash and arthralgias that lasted 3 to 4 days developed in three of four volunteers (13). During the latter phase, viral secretion was absent, suggesting that infected persons are not contagious when the rash appears. The appearance of the rash coincided with high titers of IgM antibodies to HPV, suggesting an immune-mediated rash.

Clinical Manifestations

The most characteristic feature of erythema infectiosum is the striking erythematous eruption on the face, which creates a "slapped cheek" appearance. The borders of the erythema are sharp, and the eruption is often raised. The malar areas and chin are usually involved, and the bright red color fades to a violet hue in a few days. The second stage occurs about 1 day later, when an erythematous, maculopapular rash erupts on the trunk, buttocks, and extremities. This rash is less characteristic and has been described as morbilliform, confluent, circinate, or annular (9). The individual lesions measure 2 mm to as much as 30 mm in diameter. This stage lasts for a few days to 1 week.

The third stage of the rash is perhaps the most pathognomonic. The eruption on the trunk fades, but it persists on the extremities, particularly the thighs and forearms (Fig. 143.1). Areas of clearing develop in the macular confluence, creating a reticular or lacy appearance. An unusual feature of this stage is the rash's tendency to fade and reappear. Whereas the rash disappears in the majority of cases in less than 10 days, it persists or recurs in 15% for more than 20 days and in 1% for longer than 80 days. The longest reported case lasted 95 days (9). The evanescent character of the rash is observed in about one

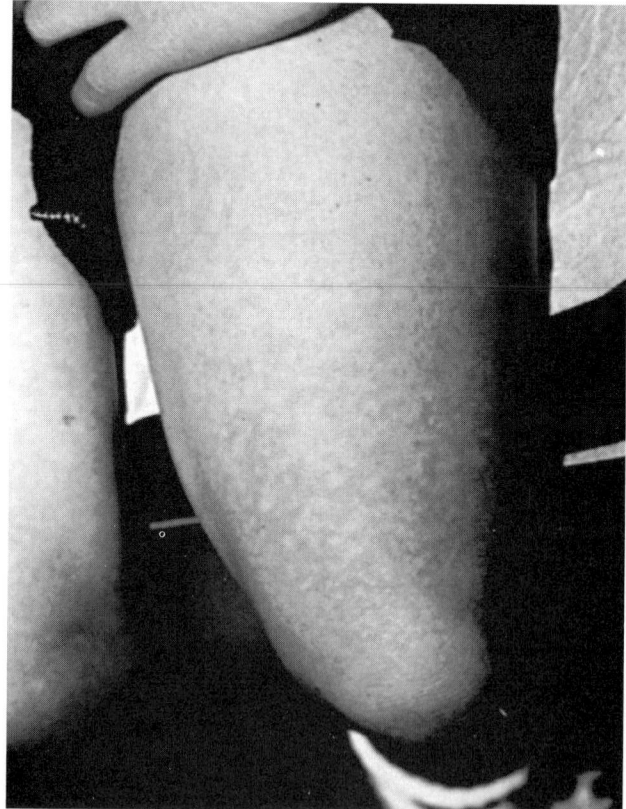

Figure 143.1. A lacy or reticular pattern of erythema, as evident on the thigh, is characteristic of erythema infectiosum.

* Deceased.

TABLE 143.1. Signs and Symptoms of Erythema Infectiosum

Sign or symptom	Reported frequency (%)
Rash	
Face	52–87
Arms	78–87
Legs	74–77
Chest	48–71
Pruritus	46–71
Fever	20–44
Headache	23–51
Sore throat	8–44
Nasal stuffiness	3–44
Cough	8–32
Anorexia	13–24
Arthralgia	5–77
Joint swelling	3–60

Compiled from references 3, 9, 10, 11.

third of cases. The reappearance is often precipitated by chilling, sunlight, bathing, exercise, or emotional stress. An enanthema consisting of macular areas of erythema is occasionally described. Papular, vesicular, and purpuric variants of the rash have also been described (14,15).

Erythema infectiosum is most often a mild illness. A prodrome consisting of malaise, low-grade fever, sore throat, and nasal stuffiness may herald the appearance of the rash. Table 143.1 summarizes the signs and symptoms associated with erythema infectiosum. The frequency of many symptoms, particularly arthralgia and arthritis, varies with the age of the infected person. Whereas Ager and colleagues found that 77.2% of adults 20 years and older complained of joint pain and 59.6% had joint swelling, only 5.1% of children 9 years or younger complained of joint pain and 2.8% had joint swelling (9). Similarly, in the 10- to 19-year age group, 11.5% and 5.3%, respectively, had these complaints.

Complications of erythema infectiosum are uncommon. Two children have been reported who developed an encephalopathy with erythema infectiosum, one with persistent neurologic sequelae (15,16). Children with chronic hemolytic anemias who develop erythema infectiosum rarely develop aplastic crises (17).

Two different cutaneous eruptions attributed to HPV-B19 are worth noting. One is a purpuric, petechial, and pseudopustular rash involving the buttocks and wrists, followed by the development of a morbilliform rash and Koplik spots in the mouth. The other is a petechial glove and sock rash with the hallmarks of fever, pruritic edema followed by pain, and petechial rash of the hands and feet with sharp demarcation at the wrist and ankle and an enanthema consisting of petechiae and oral erosions (18,19).

Diagnosis

Serologic testing for HPV IgG and IgM antibodies by use of indirect immunofluorescence is more readily available than are nucleic acid hybridization probes to detect B19 DNA. HPV-B19 IgM antibody can be detected by the third day of symptoms of erythema infectiosum or transient aplastic crisis and can persist for 2 to 3 months after infection. IgG antibody is usually present by the seventh day of illness and persists for years. Routine laboratory tests provide no specific clues to the diagnosis. The differential diagnosis of erythema infectiosum includes rubella, which should easily be separated on the basis of its short duration, and scarlet fever, which shares the slapped cheek appearance.

Treatment and Prevention

No antiviral therapy for or immunization against erythema infectiosum is available. Because the disease is benign, often lasts for weeks, and is probably not communicable a few days after the rash appears, there is no reason to exclude infected persons from school or work.

ROSEOLA

Zahorsky (20) is credited with separating roseola from other exanthems with which it previously had been included; however, the first description may have been more than 100 years earlier, in 1809, in a book written by Robert Willan, a British dermatologist (21). The benign nature of this disease and its frequent occurrence were soon recognized. In 1921, Veeder and Hempelmann suggested the name exanthem subitum (sudden) to separate roseola from rubella (22). Although this distinctive exanthematous disorder has received many appellations, including sixth disease, roseola is the name most often used. The discovery of a viral cause for roseola in 1988 has finally completed the etiologic identification of the numbered exanthems.

Microbiology

The agent responsible for roseola had eluded investigators for years. The exanthem was thought to be a hypersensitivity response to a number of different viruses, because roseolalike rashes were identified with several echoviruses and coxsackieviruses. In 1988, Yamanishi and coworkers (23) isolated a virus from cultured lymphocytes from four infants with roseola. The virus was cultured in cord blood lymphocytes and shown to be antigenically related to human herpesvirus 6 (HHV-6). The morphologic features of the virus on thin-section electron microscopy resembled those of the herpesvirus group, and convalescent serum samples demonstrated seroconversion against HHV-6. In a subsequent report, antibody titers to HHV-6 developed in 11 of 12 infants observed serologically, seven of whom had documented roseola within 9 months of birth (24). An infant who had typical roseola at 6 months had a second roseola-like illness at age 13 months. Seroconversion to HHV-7 was found (25). In Japan, HHV-7 was found to be responsible for 10% to 31% of roseola-like illness (26).

Although HHV-6, a human B lymphotropic virus, was first isolated in 1986 (27), it is interesting that both Breese (28) and Kempe (29), 60 and 50 years ago, considered herpes simplex virus the possible agent of roseola.

Epidemiology

It was suspected early in the history of roseola that the agent responsible was ubiquitous, because adults and older children rarely developed the disease and most children affected were younger than 3 years but older than 4 months. It was also noted that cases were almost always sporadic with rare outbreaks in hospitals or foundling homes, which suggested carriage of the infectious agent by healthy adults or older children (30). Serum from an 18-month-old infant with roseola injected intravenously into a 6-month-old infant produced the typical disease course 9 days later (29). Three of 14 infants injected intramuscularly with blood from persons with typical cases of roseola developed a similar illness 6 to 9 days later (31).

Roseola is thought to be the most common infectious exanthem affecting children in the first 2 years of life. Breese observed

70 newborn infants in his practice for 1 year and found that roseola developed in 16% (28). He concluded that approximately 30% of children eventually contract clinical roseola. Of 1,653 children presenting to an emergency department with an acute febrile illness 10% of those up to 2 years of age and 21% of those 6 to 12 months of age had documented HHV-6 infections. A rash developed in only 17% of these HHV-6–infected children (32). One third of children younger than 2 years who suffered febrile seizures were HHV-6 positive. The majority of infants affected are between 6 months and 2 years of age, with 80% younger than 2 years and 90% younger than 3 years. The reduced frequency in infants younger than 6 months suggests protection from transmitted maternal antibodies. Rare cases have been reported in older children (22,33).

The illness may occur at any time of year, although late winter to early spring and fall seem to produce more cases. The incubation period appears to average 10 days, ranging from 5 to 15 days (30).

Clinical Manifestations

The typical clinical picture is the abrupt onset of fever in a young child; the temperature remains elevated for 3 to 5 days, then rapidly falls to normal and is followed by the appearance of the rash. Children with roseola usually have little or no prodrome. They may have mild malaise. The fever starts suddenly, and temperature generally ranges from 38.8°C to above 40°C. It tends to be constant rather than intermittent. Despite the fever, affected infants do not act ill. They may be more listless or irritable during peak fever, but appetite is not severely affected. Infants may occasionally have some vomiting, diarrhea, or mild cough and coryza.

Early in the illness, the physical examination is not of much diagnostic help. Palpebral edema has been reported in some infants early in the illness, but rarely later than day 3 (34). An occasional child may have a bulging fontanel (35). Mild inflammation of the pharynx and tonsils and erythematous macules on the soft palate are sometimes seen. The presence of uvulo-palatoglossal ulcers may be of predictive value, up to 95.3%, of roseola before the appearance of the rash (36). The tympanic membranes may be mildly injected. Some observers have noted posterior occipital, auricular, and cervical adenopathy in infants with roseola (20,33,37).

The frequency of signs and symptoms in infants with virologically confirmed exanthem subitum is shown in Table 143.2 (38).

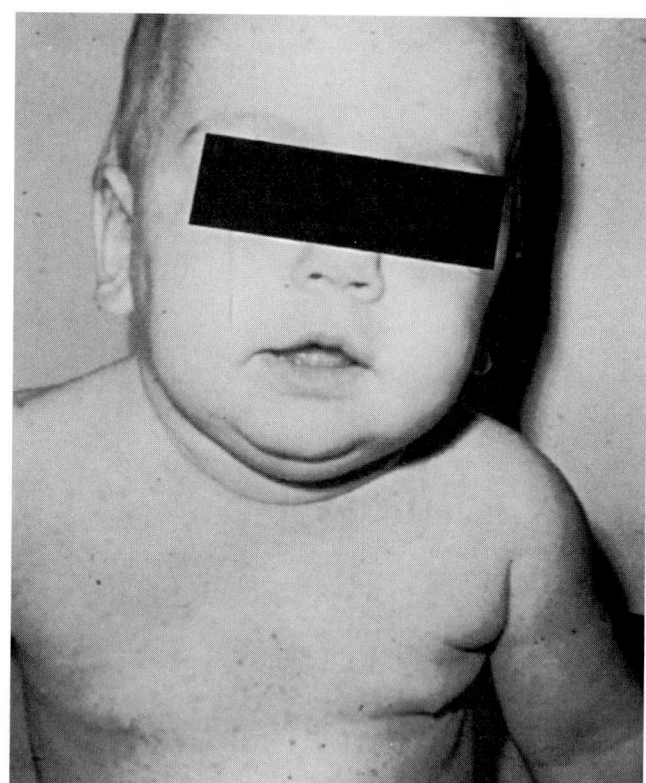

Figure 143.2. The scattered maculopapular rash of roseola is most evident on the trunk, the face being relatively spared.

The fever falls to normal rapidly (crisis) in about half the cases and more gradually (lysis) in the other half (30). The rash, which consists of discrete 1- to 5-mm pink macules, may appear just before the fever breaks or within 12 hours after it disappears. The rash is frequently sparse and is first noted on the neck and back. It rapidly spreads to the chest and extremities, the face and feet almost always being spared (Fig. 143.2). The lesions are occasionally papular and frequently have a whitish halo. The duration of the rash may be as short as a few hours or as long as 2 days.

Diagnosis

The diagnosis of roseola is a clinical one. There are no helpful laboratory tests. The white cell count is usually elevated (in the range of 12,000 to 15,000/mm^3) in the first 24 to 36 hours of illness; by the third day, there is definite leukopenia and relative lymphocytosis (39). Rarely, cerebrospinal fluid may show a mild lymphocytic pleocytosis. IgG antibody to HHV-6 may be determined by indirect immunofluorescent antibody assay. Polymerase chain reaction techniques may also be used for identification of this virus.

Complications of roseola are uncommon. Febrile convulsions are the most common adverse association, but their frequency varies with practice or hospital-based reports. Hemiplegia, sometimes persistent, has been reported (40,41).

The caveat in the diagnosis of roseola is possible confusion with a drug eruption. The fever and mild tympanic injection in young infants often prompt prescription of antibiotics. The appearance of the rash may be mistaken for a drug eruption. Rubella is unlikely to be associated with such a high fever, and the rash is more diffuse and longer lasting. Rubeola is readily differentiated by its prodrome and course.

TABLE 143.2. Frequency of Signs and Symptoms in Infants with Virologically Confirmed Exanthem Subitum

Sign or symptom	Frequency (%)
Fever	98
Rash	98
Diarrhea, mild	68
Erythematous pharyngeal papules	65
Cough	50
Edematous eyelids	30
Mild cervical lymphadenopathy	31
Bulging fontanelle	26
Seizures	8

Adapted from Asano Y, Yoshikawa T, Suga S, et al. Clinical features of infants with primary human herpesvirus 6 infection (exanthem subitum, roseola infantum). *Pediatrics* 1994;93:104, with permission.

Treatment and Prevention

There is no specific therapy for roseola. Antipyretic agents, such as acetaminophen, may help make the infant more comfortable during the high fever. No active or passive immunizations are currently available. Lifelong immunity seems to result from active disease.

ENTEROVIRAL EXANTHEMS

The enteroviruses of which more than 30 have been associated with rashes, are common causes of exanthematous disease in childhood. Unlike measles, rubella, erythema infectiosum, and other classic exanthems, enteroviral rashes, with the exception of hand-foot-and-mouth disease and herpangina, are not distinctive or specific enough to allow differentiation on clinical grounds, and one virus type may produce various rashes.

Epidemiology

The enteroviruses gain entrance to their human host through the oropharynx, replicate in the epithelial and lymphoid cells of the intestinal tract, and spread to other organ sites through the blood stream. They are shed from the oropharynx and urine for 1 week but in the feces for as long as 1 month (42). Although they can be disseminated from the respiratory tract, the intestinal route by manual transmission is most common. The incubation period for these viruses appears to be short, 4 to 7 days.

The diseases associated with enteroviruses tend to occur in epidemics, and most appear in the summer months or early fall in temperate climates. There is no seasonal pattern in tropical climates. Crowded conditions and poor hygiene encourage their spread.

Pathogenesis

Direct invasion of the skin or mucous membranes through the blood stream is the most likely mechanism for the production of the vesicular or ulcerative lesions seen in hand-foot-and-mouth disease and herpangina. The more prevalent maculopapular exanthems are probably the result of the skin's reacting with circulating or cell-mediated immune factors. Unfortunately, accurate histologic definition of the viral exanthems is sparse.

Clinical Manifestations

Hand, foot, and mouth disease, anatomically describing the most common sites of the vesicles and ulcers associated with this illness, is the most readily recognized and distinctive enteroviral exanthem. The first recognized outbreak of this disease occurred in Toronto in 1957 (43). The appellation hand-foot-and-mouth disease was given after an epidemic in Birmingham, England, in 1959 (44). Since then, the disease has occurred worldwide, most often in the summer and early fall.

Coxsackievirus A16 is responsible for the majority of cases of hand, foot, and mouth disease, but this exanthem has also been described with coxsackievirus types A5, A7, A9, A10, B2, and B5. The virus is highly contagious. Whereas up to 100% of infected preschool-age children develop a rash, only 38% of school-age children and 11% of infected adults have cutaneous manifestations (45).

The most common presentation is the complaint of a sore throat or mouth, usually without prodrome. The enanthema is vesicular but rapidly ulcerates. Usually, five to ten oral lesions are present; as opposed to herpangina, they may occur anywhere in the mouth (46). The exanthem, primarily consisting of hand

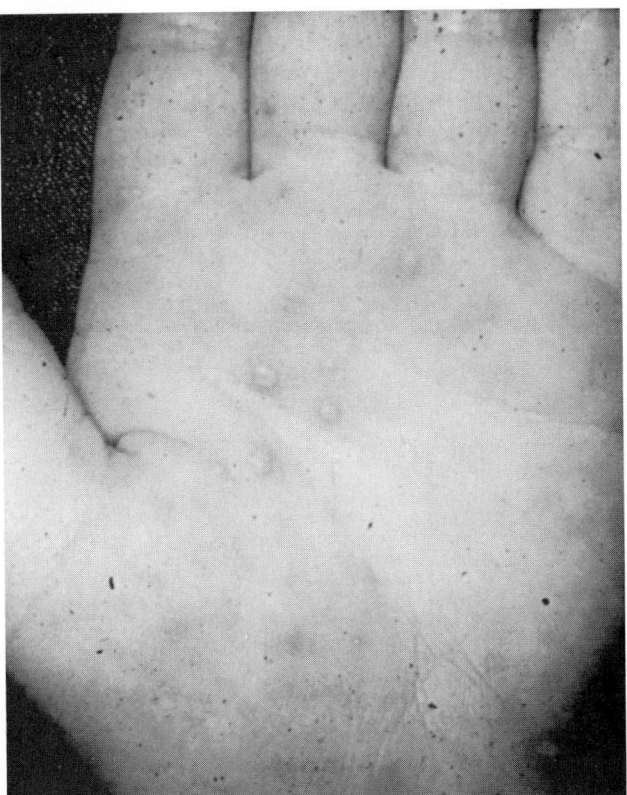

Figure 143.3. Multiple vesicles of hand, foot, and mouth disease are present on the palm.

and foot lesions, follows shortly after the oral lesions. The vesicles generally measure 3 to 7 mm and are set on an erythematous base (Fig. 143.3). Frequently, the vesicles take on linear or arcuate forms. The vesicular fluid contains the virus and provides a mode of spread through contact. The vesicles can be found in other body areas, but sparingly. The buttocks are most frequently involved besides the typical sites.

Hand-foot-and-mouth disease usually runs a benign course lasting approximately 1 week. Rarely, a more severe chronic or relapsing course is seen (47). The differential diagnosis of hand, foot, and mouth disease is limited because of the characteristic rash. When oral ulcerations are found, the hands and feet should be inspected for vesicles before a diagnosis of herpes simplex, aphthous stomatitis, or herpangina is assigned.

Herpangina is caused by several enteroviruses, including coxsackieviruses A1 through A10, A16, and A22, and less commonly by coxsackieviruses B and echoviruses. The characteristic feature of this infection is the presence of small (2- to 4-mm) vesicles or ulcers on the tonsillar pillars, soft palate, or uvula. The lesions are usually few in number (two to six), but they are associated with a sore throat and pain on swallowing. The illness may be heralded by the abrupt onset of fever, vomiting, headache, and myalgia.

Echovirus 16 is best known as the cause of the Boston exanthem, named for the site of the first recorded epidemic in 1951 (48). A subsequent epidemic occurred in Pittsburgh in 1954 (49). The illness is often described as resembling roseola. In children, a temperature of 102°F (39°C) for 24 to 36 hours is common, and associated symptoms are mild. Sore throat is occasionally present, and punched-out ulcers of the soft palate may occur. The exanthem, which consists of pink or salmon-colored, discrete, 0.5- to 1.5-cm macules and maculopapules, appears as the fever declines (42). The rash almost always involves the face (roseola does not) and lasts 1 to 5 days.

TABLE 143.3.   Enteroviral Exanthems

Maculopapular
  Rubelliform: echovirus 9, also 2, 4, 11, 19, 25 and coxsackievirus
    A9; size: 1-3 mm
  Roseola-like: echovirus 16 (Boston exanthem); also echovirus 11,
    25 and coxsackievirus B1, B5; size: 5-15 mm
Vesicular
  Hand-foot-and-mouth: coxsackievirus A16, also A5, A7, A9, A10,
    B2, B5
  Herpangina: coxsackievirus A22, also A1-10, A16
  Insect bite-like: coxsackievirus A4, crops, last 1-2 wk (52)
  Non-pustule forming: coxsackievirus A9; also echovirus 11, 30 (53)
Petechial
  Coxsackievirus B5, A9; echovirus 9
  Problem separating from meningococcemia
Hemangioma-like
  Transient, sparse: echovirus 25, 32 (54, 55)
Papular acrodermatitis
  Coxsackievirus A16

Children are much more likely to develop an exanthem with this illness than are adults; adults are generally sicker than children, with higher fever, prostration, muscle aches, and crampy abdominal pain. A small outbreak was described in the summer of 1974 in ten children, five of whom were neonates (50). Aseptic meningitis was associated in six of the ten.

Echovirus 9 has been described as causing a rubelliform eruption in children and adults and is particularly troublesome when it occurs in pregnant women (51). Fever, headache, and nuchal rigidity are common in affected persons. The rash consists of discrete maculopapules 1 to 5 mm in diameter, which appear first on the face and neck shortly after the onset of fever. The exanthem lasts 3 to 5 days and is much more prominent in children, occurring in 57% of those younger than 4 years, 41% of 5- to 9-year-old children, and only 8% of adults. The rash may take on a petechial component, resembling meningococcemia.

Table 143.3 summarizes the most common of the types of rashes associated with coxsackievirus and echovirus infections. Note the diversity of lesions and the different types of rashes caused by the same virus. Exanthems occurring in children during the summer and fall are most likely caused by these viruses.

REFERENCES

1. Herrick TP. Erythema infectiosum. *Am J Dis Child* 1926;31:486.
2. Shaw HLK. Erythema infectiosum. *Am J Med Sci* 1905;6.
3. Anderson MJ, Lewis E, Kidd IM, et al. An outbreak of erythema infectiosum associated with human parvovirus infection. *J Hyg (Camb)* 1984;93:85.
4. Nunoue T, Okochi K, Mortimer PP, et al. Human parvovirus (B19) and erythema infectiosum. *J Pediatr* 1985;107:38.
5. Okabe N, Koboyashi S, Tatsuzawa O, et al. Detection of antibodies to human parvovirus in erythema infectiosum (fifth disease). *Arch Dis Child* 1984;59:1016.
6. Plummer FA, Hammond GW, Forward K, et al. An erythema infectiosum-like illness caused by human parvovirus infection. *N Engl J Med* 1985;313:74.
7. Cossart YE, Cant B, Field AM, et al. Parvovirus-like particles in human sera. *Lancet* 1975;1:72.
8. Anderson LJ. Role of parvovirus B19 in human disease. *Pediatr Infect Dis J* 1987;6:711.
9. Ager EA, Chin TDY, Poland JD. Epidemic erythema infectiosum. *N Engl J Med* 1966;275:1326.
10. Brass C, Elliott LM, Stevens DA. Academy rash. *JAMA* 1982;248:568.
11. Lauer BA, MacCormack JN, Wilfert C. Erythema infectiosum. An elementary school outbreak. *Am J Dis Child* 1976;130:252.
12. Chorba T, Coccia P, Holman RC, et al. The role of parovirus B 19 in aplastic crisis and erythema infectiosum (fifth disease). *J Infect Dis* 1986;154:383.
13. Anderson MJ, Higgins PG, Davis LR, et al. Experimental parvoviral infection in humans. *J Infect Dis* 1985;152:257.
14. Condon FJ. Erythema infectiosum: report of an area-wide outbreak. *Am J Public Health* 1959;49:528.
15. Balfour HH Jr, Schiff GM, Bloom JE. Encephalitis associated with erythema infectiosum. *J Pediatr* 1970;77:133.
16. Hall CB, Homer FA. Encephalopathy with erythema infectiosum. *Am J Dis Child* 1977;131:65.
17. Nunoue T, Koike T, Koike R, et al. Infection with human parvovirus (1319), aplasia of the bone marrow, and a rash in hereditary spherocytosis. *J Infect* 1987; 14:67.
18. Evans LM, Grossman ME, Gregory W. Koplik spots and a purpuric eruption associated with parvovirus B19 infection. *J Am Acad Dermatol* 1992;27:466.
19. Halasz CLG, Cormier D, Den M. Petechial glove and sock syndrome caused by parvovirus B19. *J Am Acad Dermatol* 1992;27:835.
20. Zahorsky J. Roseola infantum. *JAMA* 1913;16:1446.
21. Altshuler EL. Oldest description of roseola and implications for the antigenicity of human herpesvirus 6. *Pediatr Infect Dis J* 2000;19:903.
22. Veeder BS, Hempelmann TO. A febrile exanthem occurring in childhood (exanthem subitum). *JAMA* 1921;77:1787.
23. Yamanishi K, Okuno T, Shiraki K, et al. Identification of human herpesvirus 6 as a causal agent for exanthem subitum. *Lancet* 1988;1:1065.
24. Takahashi K, Sonoda S, Kawakami K, et al. Human herpesvirus 6 and exanthem subitum. *Lancet* 1988;1:1463.
25. Asano Y, Suga S, Yoshikawa T, et al. Clinical features and viral excretion in an infant with primary human herpesvirus 7 infection. *Pediatrics* 1995;95: 187.
26. Leach CT. Human herpesvirus-6 and -7 infection in children: agents of roseola and other syndromes. *Curr Opin Pediatr* 2000;12:269.
27. Salahuddin SZ, Ablashi DV, Markham PD, et al. Isolation of a new virus, HBLV in patients with lymphoproliferative disorders. *Science* 1986;234:596.
28. Breese BB Jr. Roseola infantum (exanthem subitum). *NY State J Med* 1941;41: 1854.
29. Kempe CH, Shaw EB, Jackson JR, et al. Studies on the etiology of exanthem subitum. *J Pediatr* 1950;37:561.
30. Barenberg LH, Greenspan L. Exanthem subitum (roseola in fantum). *Am J Dis Child* 1939;58:983.
31. Hellstrom B, Vahlquist B. Experimental inoculation of roseola infantum. *Acta Paediatr* 1951;40:189.
32. Hall CB, Long CE, Schnabel KC, et al. Human herpesvirus-6 infection in children. *N Engl J Med* 1994;331:432.
33. Letchner A. Roseola infantum: a review of fifty cases. *Lancet* 1955;1:1163.
34. Berliner BC. A physical sign useful in diagnosis of roseola in fantum before the rash. *Pediatrics* 1960;25:1034.
35. Oski FA. Roseola infantum. Another cause of bulging fontanel. *Am J Dis Child* 1961;101:376.
36. Chua KB. The association of uvulo-palatoglossal junctional ulcers with exanthem subitum: a 10-year paediatric outpatient study. *Med J Malaysia* 1999;54:58.
37. McEnery JT. Postoccipital lymphadenopathy as a diagnostic sign in roseola infantum (roseola subitum). *Clin Pediatr* 1970;9:512.
38. Asano Y, Yoshikawa T, Suga S, et al. Clinical features of infants with primary human herpesvirus 6 infection (exanthem subitum, roseola infantum). *Pediatrics* 1994;93:104.
39. Berenberg W, Wright S, Janeway CA. Roseola infantum (exanthem subitum). *N Engl J Med* 1949;241:253.
40. Burnstine RC, Paine RS. Residual encephalopathy following roseola infantum. *Am J Dis Child* 1959;98:144.
41. Holliday PB Jr. Preemptive neurological complications of the common contagious diseases—rubella, rubeola, and varicella. *J Pediatr* 1950;36:185.
42. Lerner AM, Klein JO, Cherry JD, et al. New viral exanthems. *N Engl J Med* 1963;269:678.
43. Robinson CR, Doane FW, Rhodes AJ. Report of an outbreak of febrile illness with pharyngeal lesions and exanthem: Toronto, summer 1957-isolation of group A coxsackievirus. *Can Med Assoc J* 1958;79:615.
44. Alsop J, Flewett TH, Foster JR. "Hand-foot-and-mouth disease" in Birmingham in 1959. *BMJ* 1960;2:1708.
45. Cherry JD. Viral exanthems. *Curr Probl Pediatr* 1983;13:1.
46. Tindall JP, Callaway JL. Hand-foot-and-mouth disease. It's more common than you think. *Am J Dis Child* 1972;124:372.
47. Evans AD, Waddington E. Hand, foot and mouth disease in South Wales, 1964. *Br J Dermatol* 1967;79:307.
48. Neva FA, Enders JF. Cytopathogenic agents isolated from patients during unusual epidemic exanthem. *J Immunol* 1954;72:307.
49. Neva FA, Feemster RF, Gorback IJ. Clinical and epidemiologic features of unusual epidemic exanthem. *JAMA* 1954;155:544.
50. Hall CB, Cherry JD, Hatch MH, et al. The return of the Boston exanthem. *Am J Dis Child* 1977;131:323.
51. Bell EJ, Ross CAC, Grist NR. Echo 9 infection in pregnant women with suspected rubella. *J Clin Pathol* 1975;28:267.
52. Rouchouse B, Bonnefoy M, Pallot B, et al. Acute generalized exanthematous pustular dermatitis and viral infection. *Dermatologica* 1986;173:180.
53. DeChamps C, Peigue-Lafeville HH, Laveran H, et al. Four cases of vesicular lesions in adults caused by enterovirus infections. *J Clin Microbiol* 1988;26: 2182.
54. Guidotti MB. An outbreak of skin rash by echovirus 25 in an infant home. *J Infect* 1983;6:67.
55. Cherry JD, Bobinski JE, Horvath FL, et al. Acute hemangioma-like lesions associated with ECHO viral infection. *Pediatrics* 1969;44:498.

Bones and Joints

CHAPTER 144
Osteomyelitis

Francis A. Waldvogel and Daniel P. Lew

DEFINITIONS

Osteomyelitis is an infectious process involving the various components of bone, namely, periosteum, medullary cavity, and cortical bone. The disease is characterized by progressive inflammatory destruction of bone, necrosis, and new bone apposition.

Acute osteomyelitis evolves during several weeks; the term *acute* is used in opposition to *chronic* osteomyelitis, a disease characterized by long-standing infection that evolves during months or even years and by the persistence of microorganisms, low-grade inflammation, the presence of dead bone (sequestra) and foreign material, and fistulous tracks. The terms acute and chronic do not have a sharp demarcation and are often used somewhat loosely. Nevertheless, they are useful clinical concepts in infectious disease, because they describe two different patterns of the same disease due to the same microorganisms but with different clinical presentations and pathogenic factors, different evolutions (1), and different responses to therapy.

Osteomyelitis secondary to bacteremia has to be distinguished from septic arthritis, a condition in which the inflammatory reaction resides in the joint synovium with little bone participation, for instance, as in *Neisseria gonorrhoeae* bacteremia. Occasionally, as in neonates, both the joint and the adjacent bone are involved in the septic process, a condition for which the term *osteoarthritis* has been coined.

PATHOPHYSIOLOGY AND PATHOLOGY

For many years, most of our information about osteomyelitis was obtained from pathologic observations obtained during surgery or at autopsy. Microscopic examination in the area of acute osteomyelitis has demonstrated an acute suppurative inflammation in which bacteria are embedded. A variety of phlogistic factors, and possibly leukocytes themselves, contribute to the tissue necrosis, the destruction of bone trabeculae, and the removal of bone matrix. Vascular channels are obliterated by the inflammatory process, further contributing to bone necrosis (2). Segments of bone devoid of blood supply can become separated to form sequestra. Meanwhile, bone apposition occurs, sometimes exuberantly, causing periosteal apposition and new bone formation in a mosaic pattern similar to that of Paget's disease.

Experimental Models

New experimental models of bone infection have established with accuracy the time course of these events and the necessity of producing profound bone trauma (i.e., with morrhuate sodium or other sclerosing agents) to initiate the disease (3). Intravenous injection of bacteria has consistently produced osteomyelitis in chickens without trauma (4); abscesses were most commonly observed in the metaphyseal area of long bones within 24 hours of bacterial inoculation, bordering on the epiphyseal growth plate. Sequestra could be observed within 8 days after inoculation (5). Furthermore, it has been shown that in this area of bone growth, the vascular endothelium is discontinuous, allowing bacteria to escape into adjacent tissue—a valid explanation why bacteremic osteomyelitis so frequently occurs before puberty.

FAVORING FACTORS AND ROLE OF FOREIGN BODY

Most cases of osteomyelitis are of bacterial origin. Favoring factors are numerous and include trauma or the presence of foreign material such as implants and orthopedic devices (6). Major contributors to the development of infection in this setting include a striking phagocytic defect of resident polymorphonuclear leukocytes in the vicinity of a foreign body (6) and strong adhesion of bacteria, mostly *Staphylococcus aureus* and coagulase-negative staphylococci, on the inflammatory tissue or foreign body surface through a ligand interaction of the bacterial surface with host proteins such as fibrinogen, fibronectin, and others coating the foreign body (7). Within a few days, bacteria accumulate on their cell surface a thick layer of extracellular molecules called either slime or glycocalyx, which probably interferes with many host immune functions (8). Many additional local factors are probably operational in favoring the development and the persistence of infections under these conditions (9).

Other general contributing conditions to the development of osteomyelitis deserve further study. Patients with sickle cell disease develop, besides intraosseous sickling crises, osteomyelitis due to *Salmonella* species (10). Patients with diabetes often suffer from microvascular disease and are at risk for developing osteomyelitis of the lower extremities, mostly due to *S. aureus* or to anaerobic organisms. Finally, patients with congenital defects of phagocyte function are frequently observed to develop *S. aureus* osteomyelitis. Thus, the presence of a competent phagocytic axis, good vascular supply to bone, and absence of foreign and necrotic material are important determinants in the clearing of small bacterial inocula within bone structures.

CLINICAL MANIFESTATIONS AND CHARACTERISTICS OF THE PATHOGEN

From a practical point of view, it is useful to distinguish three types of osteomyelitis, which are described separately. Hematogenous osteomyelitis follows bacteremic spread, is seen mostly in prepubertal children and in elderly patients, and is characterized by local multiplication of bacteria within bone during septicemia. In most cases, infection is located in the metaphyseal area of long bones or in the spine. Osteomyelitis secondary to a contiguous focus of infection follows trauma or an orthopedic procedure. It implies a first infection, which by continuity gains access to bone. By definition, it can occur at any age and can involve any bone. Osteomyelitis secondary to vascular insufficiency is one of the consequences of poor blood supply, usually to the lower extremities. Often associated with diabetes, this disease entity is difficult to analyze as to its most important contributing factors; diabetes and its metabolic consequences, bone ischemia, neuropathy, and infection probably all contribute to bone destruction.

Hematogenous Osteomyelitis

Historically, hematogenous osteomyelitis has been described in children. It involves mostly the metaphysis of long bones (particularly the tibia and femur), usually as a single focus. Although rare in adults, it most frequently involves the vertebral bodies (1).

Bacteria responsible for hematogenous osteomyelitis reflect essentially their bacteremic incidence as a function of age, so the organisms most frequently encountered in neonates include *S. aureus* and group B streptococci; in infants, the majority of infections are due to *S. aureus,* coagulase-negative staphylococci, various streptococci, and *Haemophilus influenzae.* Later in life, *S. aureus* predominates; in elderly persons, who are frequently subject to gram-negative bacteremias, most cases of vertebral osteomyelitis are due to gram-negative rods and more rarely to *S. aureus.*

The clinical features of hematogenous osteomyelitis in long bones are typical: chills, fever, and malaise reflect the bacteremic spread of microorganisms; pain and local swelling are the hallmarks of the local infectious process. Toxic shock, with its characteristic rash, may occasionally occur if *S. aureus* produces the corresponding toxin. Pneumonia, empyema, endocarditis, or subcutaneous abscesses may reflect widespread staphylococcal disease. Microorganisms responsible for acute hematogenous osteomyelitis are summarized in Table 144.1. Their respective frequency depends on the age of the patient. *S. aureus* and *Staphylococcus epidermidis* still account for the majority of these infections (more than 50%) and can be isolated from the bloodstream in a large percentage of cases. Not specifically mentioned in Table 144.1 is fungal osteomyelitis, a complication of intravenous device infections or of immunodeficiency; *Pseudomonas aeruginosa* hematogenous osteomyelitis is often seen in drug addicts and has a predilection for the spine. Viral osteomyelitis is currently almost nonexistent.

Osteomyelitis Secondary to a Contiguous Infection

The situation and the clinical picture are more complex in cases of osteomyelitis associated with a contiguous focus of infection, for example, as a complication of the insertion of a total hip prosthesis. After a few days' pain that follows surgery, the situation improves and the patient is progressively mobilized. During that period, pain reappears, mostly on weight bearing. The patient is mildly febrile, and the wound is slightly erythematous, sometimes with discharge. No other clinical signs point toward the diagnosis of osteomyelitis, and no radiographic examination is fully diagnostic. Under such conditions, careful probing of the wound or arthrocentesis followed by Gram stain and quantitative cultures are the only diagnostic procedures of immediate help.

Similar clinical reasoning has to be used to diagnose osteomyelitis secondary to a contiguous infection such as a comminuted fracture, which can become contaminated by the contiguous wound infection. Any other prosthetic material can become contaminated during surgery and produce signs of infection during the ensuing weeks. Exceptionally, prosthetic material may become seeded by the bacteremic spread from a distant infectious focus.

Acute purulent frontal sinusitis can lead to bone involvement, with a characteristic edema of the forehead (Pott puffy tumor). Dental root infection can lead to local bone destruction. Finally, deep-seated decubitus ulcers can lead to local bone destruction, usually of the sacrum (11). Under all these conditions, the inflammatory reaction may be mild, and the bone destruction difficult to assess, unless the wound is probed and aspirated and the material adequately stained and cultured.

What organisms are responsible for this type of osteomyelitis? In the past, *S. aureus* and coagulase-negative staphylococci were most frequently the culprits. In more recent years, other microorganisms have been isolated: various types of streptococci; *Propionibacterium acnes*; Enterobacteriaceae; and even *P. aeruginosa*, mostly in the setting of chronic osteomyelitis, comminuted fractures, and puncture wounds to the heel. Finally, osteomyelitis of the mandible, secondary to decubitus ulcers, and due to bites, frequently contains anaerobic flora.

Osteomyelitis Secondary to Vascular Insufficiency

Osteomyelitis secondary to vascular insufficiency is a special entity observed in patients with diabetes or vascular impairment and is located almost exclusively on the lower extremities. The disease starts insidiously in a patient who has complained of intermittent claudication in an area of previously traumatized skin. Cellulitis may be kept at a minimum, and infection progressively burrows its way to the underlying bone (e.g., toe, metatarsal head, tarsal bone). Physical examination elicits either no pain (in case of advanced neuropathy) or excruciating pain if bone destruction has been acute; an area of cellulitis may or may not be present; crepitus can be felt occasionally, which points toward the presence of either anaerobes or Enterobacteriaceae. Physical examination includes a careful assessment of the vascular supply to the affected limb and the evaluation of a concomitant neuropathy. Here again, the whole gamut of human pathogenic bacteria can be isolated, often in multiple combinations. *S. aureus* still predominates, but any other gram-positive or gram-negative, aerobic or anaerobic bacteria deserve close consideration and treatment, because infection is often the only reversible process in this multifactorial disease.

DIAGNOSTIC PROCEDURES

In osteomyelitis of any kind, it is of paramount importance to isolate the offending organisms; this can be done by blood cultures (40% hematogenous cases of disease yield a positive result, particularly *S. aureus*) or by isolation via direct biopsy of the involved bone. This procedure sometimes has to be performed under regional or general anesthesia, but its importance cannot be overstated (12). Isolation of microorganisms from material taken from an open sinus track by swab will give conflicting results because of possible contamination by nonpathogenic microorganisms (13).

Second in importance are radiographic procedures (Fig. 144.1). The sequence of events observed in hematogenous

---

TABLE 144.1.   Microorganisms Responsible for Acute Hematogenous Osteomyelitis of Long Bones

Organisms	Comments
Staphylococcus aureus, *Staphylococcus epidermidis*	Most frequent isolates in any age The use of foreign material
Group B streptococci	Mostly in neonates
Candida species	Mostly following prolonged use of intravenous devices/parenteral therapy
Gram-negative bacilli	Rare, in elderly patients, associated with urinary tract infection

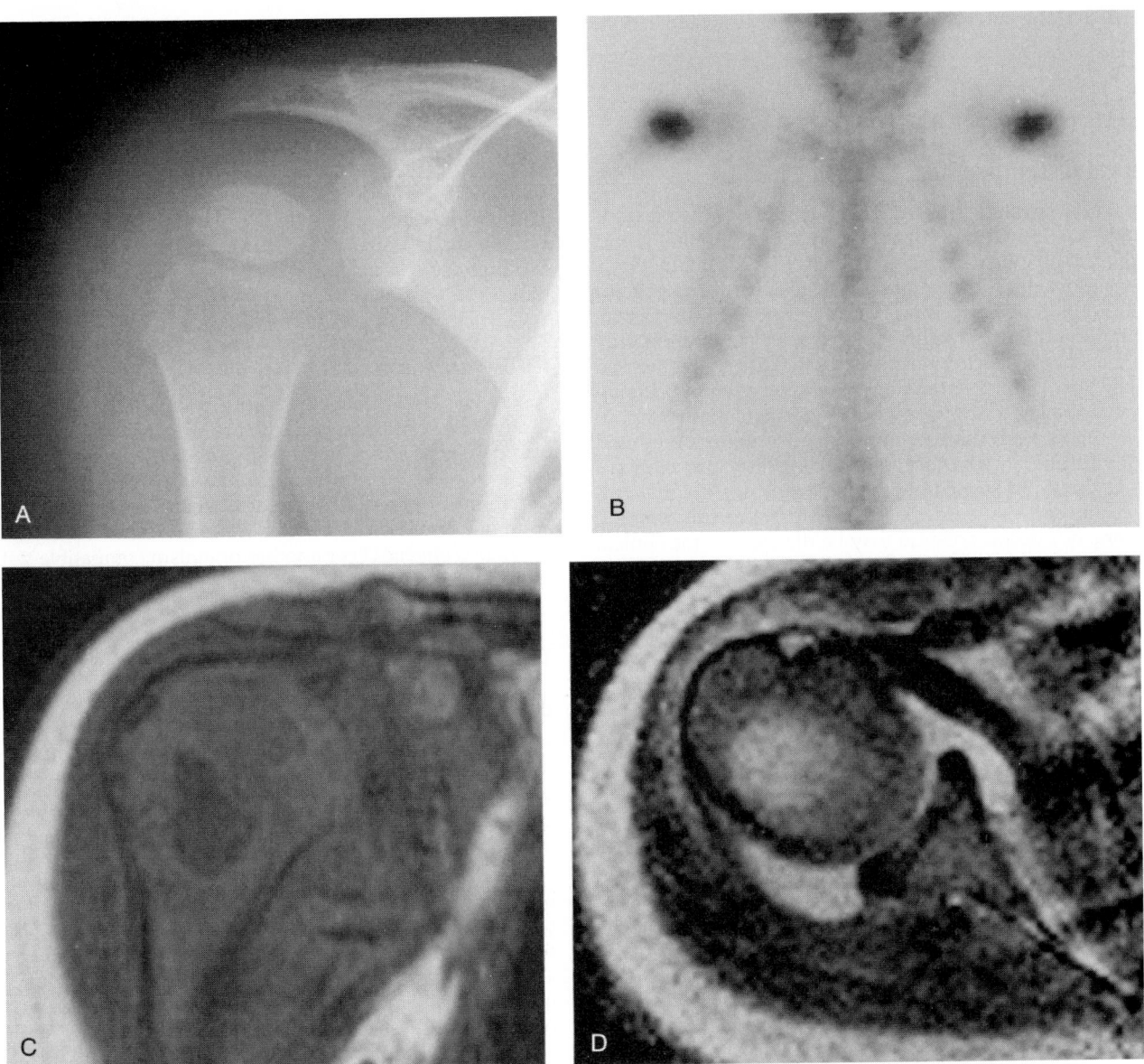

Figure 144.1. Acute hematogenous osteomyelitis in a 20-month-old child presenting with mild fever and impotence of the right shoulder. **A:** The conventional radiographs on admission do not show major bone modifications. **B:** Technetium scan on the same day demonstrates symmetric uptake of the two shoulder areas. **C:** Nuclear magnetic resonance imaging performed 4 days later is more explicit, showing in a clear metaphyseal ovoid hypointense area on a T1-weighted image. **D:** The transverse section on a T2-weighted image of the same area shows hyperintensity similar to subcutaneous fat tissue. There is also an effusion in the same joint.

osteomyelitis is well described and includes irregular bone destruction followed by new bone apposition and end-stage sclerosis. These events extend for a period of many weeks and months, in asynchrony with the clinical evolution; the x-ray appearance is often normal during the acute phase of the disease, whereas "apparent bone destruction" is sometimes observed during the treatment phase. Computed tomography is of little additional help, except for identifying complications such as an intramedullary abscess, a sequestrum, or an early subcutaneous abscess (14). Intramedullary complications and early edema—a nonspecific but sometimes useful sign—are best seen by magnetic resonance imaging, as are infectious lesions of the spine (15). Technetium scintigraphy is helpful as well because it also shows early, localized changes while plain films are still normal (1,12).

In osteomyelitis secondary to adjacent infection or to impaired blood supply, the problem is complicated not only by the insensitivity of the radiographic procedures but also by their lack of specificity, because prior surgery, bone reaction in the vicinity of foreign material, and aseptic bone necrosis can mimic infection. Radiographic changes consistent with extensive involvement of a joint, progressive bone destruction, or bilateral loosening of foreign material usually point toward an infectious process (16). Although not yet routinely accepted, leukocyte scanning procedures may be of help under particular conditions.

Other laboratory tests are of little value; the erythrocyte sedimentation rate or C-reactive protein may be helpful in assessing the progression or regression of the disease; calcium, phosphate, and alkaline phosphatase values are invariably normal, as opposed to the values in metastatic or some metabolic bone diseases.

SPECIFIC CLINICAL CONDITIONS

Vertebral Osteomyelitis

Vertebral osteomyelitis is most frequently of the hematogenous type and usually involves the lower dorsal and lumbar spine; occasional involvement of the cervical spine has been described. The disease usually presents in an adult as a febrile lumbago or torticollis (12). Radiographs are usually normal on admission, and abnormality in technetium scintigraphy may be the only clue to the diagnosis; later, narrowing of the disk space, mottled destruction of adjacent vertebral plateaus, and anterior bridging may occur. Owing to the many organisms potentially responsible for this type of disease, needle biopsy under computed tomographic guidance has become the diagnostic procedure of choice. Complications, including paraspinal abscess, cord compression, and soft tissue extension, have to be carefully sought, and emergency decompression may be dictated by the clinical and radiographic findings (12,16).

Osteomyelitis in Other Unusual Locations

Involvement of the sternoclavicular joint area has been described in intravenous drug abusers and in patients with indwelling intravenous devices. Sacral involvement has to be carefully sought in patients with decubitus ulcers of the overlying area. Osteomyelitis of the calcaneus, often due to *P. aeruginosa*, follows apparently innocent puncture wounds. Osteomyelitis of the sternum may follow cardiac surgery; frequently due to coagulase-negative staphylococci, it is difficult to differentiate from delayed healing after sternotomy. Another interesting clinical presentation consists of the development of multiple, well-delineated areas of bone destruction. As documented radiographically, in association with skin disorders such as acne conglobata or palmoplantar pustulosis, acute multifocal osteomyelitis is characterized by negative bone cultures and by spontaneous healing in a period of several months (17).

Anaerobic Osteomyelitis

Osteomyelitis due to anaerobic organisms has been described in a variety of clinical situations (18). It may be due to deep inoculation during a human bite, it may follow deep tooth socket infection or radiation therapy to the mandible, and finally it can be observed in diabetic foot infection.

Osteomyelitis in Sickle Cell Anemia

Patients with homozygous sickle cell disease, who under all circumstances are subject to severe *Salmonella* infections, often suffer from osteomyelitis due to this organism. The disease, which presents either acutely or subacutely, is sometimes difficult to differentiate from bone infarction due to the underlying disease (10).

Osteomyelitis in Drug Addicts

Septic arthritis and osteomyelitis of long bones are frequently found in drug addicts. Infection usually occurs by the hematogenous route and is often due to *S. aureus* and *P. aeruginosa*. Of note is the frequent absence of fever in these cases (19).

Tuberculosis

Osteomyelitis of long bones due to *Mycobacterium tuberculosis* has become a rarity in industrialized countries but still has to be considered in patients with the combination of localized bone destruction, fistula, and negative bone cultures. Still important is the concept of spinal involvement by *M. tuberculosis*; this entity is characterized by low fever, a subacute course, slow bone destruction, and absence of periosteal reaction. Abscess formation can sometimes be visualized by computed tomography, and spine compression is a surgically correctable but feared complication (20).

Brodie Abscess

Brodie abscess is characterized by bone pain, low-grade fever, if any, and a radiographic picture of central destruction surrounded by sclerosis. Seventy-five percent of cases occur in the lower extremities, usually in patients under 20 years of age. The differential diagnosis encompasses many inflammatory lesions and bone tumors; diagnosis is best resolved by biopsy and isolation of *S. aureus* (1) or another organism compatible with this type of infection.

TREATMENT

Basic Principles

The many pathogenic factors, modes of contamination, and clinical presentations of osteomyelitis have precluded a scientific approach to therapy, with well-controlled, statistically valid studies. However, experimental models have helped us to understand some basic principles of antibiotic therapy. Thus, except for the fluoroquinolones, which penetrate well into bone, bone antibiotic levels 3 to 4 hours after administration usually do not exceed 20% to 30% of the peak serum levels (21). Second, antibiotic treatment has to be given for several weeks to achieve an acceptable cure rate. Third, early antibiotic treatment, given before extensive bone destruction has occurred, produces the best results (22). Finally, a combined antimicrobial and surgical approach should at least be discussed in all cases; whereas at one end of the spectrum (e.g., hematogenous osteomyelitis) surgery is usually unnecessary, at the other end (a consolidated infected fracture) cure may be achieved with minimal antibiotic treatment provided that the foreign material is removed.

Antimicrobial Therapy

Single-agent chemotherapy is usually adequate for the treatment of osteomyelitis of any type. A conventional choice of antimicrobial agents for the most commonly encountered microorganisms is given in Table 144.2. As a general principle, these antibiotics should be given for 4 to 6 weeks if possible by the intravenous route. Results of serum bactericidal tests, which are notoriously difficult to standardize, have been proposed to monitor therapy efficacy, particularly for patients treated orally, and trough levels at a dilution higher than 1:2 are associated with a higher cure rate (23). If signs of infection do not abate after 1 week, possible complications should be sought; such as the presence of a subcutaneous, subperiosteal, or intramedullary abscess; the formation of sequestra; or the presence of foreign material. Most of the time, a surgical intervention solves this problem more radically than the switch to other antibiotics, provided

TABLE 144.2. Parenteral Antibiotic Treatment of Hematogenous Osteomyelitis in Adults

Microorganisms isolated	Treatment of choice	Alternatives
S. aureus Penicillin sensitive	Penicillin G (4 million units, every 6 h)	A cephalosporin II[a], clindamycin (600 mg, every 6 h) or vancomycin
Penicillin-resistant	Nafcillin[b] (2 g, every 6 h)	A cephalosporin II, clindamycin (600 mg, every 6 h) or vancomycin
Methicillin-resistant	Vancomycin (1 g, every 12 h)	Teicoplanin[c] (400 mg every 24 h, first day every 12 h)
Various streptococci (group A or B β-hemolytic; *S. pneumoniae*)	Penicillin G (3 million units every 4–6 h)	Clindamycin (600 mg, every 6 h), erythromycin (500 mg, every 6 h) or vancomycin
Enteric gram-negative rods	Quinolone (ciprofloxacine, 500–750 mg every 12 h, i.v. or oral)	A cephalosporin III[d]
Serratia species *P. aeruginosa*	Piperacilline[e] (2–4 g, every 4 h) and gentamycin (1.5 mg/kg/day)	A cephalosprin III[e] or a quinolone (with aminoglycoides)
Anaerobes	Clindamycin (600 mg, every 6 h)	Amoxicillin-clavulanic acid (2.2 g every 8 h) or Metronidazole for gram-negative anaerobes (500 mg every 8 h)
Mixed infection (aerobic and anaerobic microorganisms)	Amoxicillin-clavulanic acid (2.2 g every 8 h)	Imipenem[f] (500 mg every 6 h)

[a]II, second generation.
[b]Flucloxacillin in Europe.
[c]Teicoplanin is presently only available in Europe.
[d]III, third generation.
[e]Depends on sensitivities; piperacillin/tazobactam and imipenem are useful alternatives.
[f]In cases of aerobic gram-negative microorganisms resistant to amoxicillin-clavulanic acid.
i.v., intravenously.

that adequate microbiologic results have led to appropriate chemotherapy.

New approaches to antimicrobial therapy have been developed experimentally and validated clinically. Thus, in hematogenous osteomyelitis of childhood, short parenteral administration of antibiotics may be followed with an equal success rate by oral therapy for several weeks, provided that the organism is known, the clinical signs abate rapidly, the patient's compliance is good, and the serum antibiotic levels can be monitored (24,25). This approach has now also been validated in adults (25,26). Another approach that has gained acceptance because of its reduced cost is parenteral administration of antibiotics, first in the hospital, then on an outpatient basis; effective as it is for hematogenous osteomyelitis, the question remains open whether this mode can be used for postsurgical osteomyelitis. Long-term oral therapy extending for years is aimed at palliation of acute flare-ups of chronic, refractory osteomyelitis. Local administration of antibiotics, either by instillation or by gentamicin-laden beads, has its advocates both in the United States and in Europe, but it has not been submitted to a critical, controlled study; antibiotic diffusion is limited in time and space but may be of some additional benefit in osteomyelitis secondary to a contiguous focus of infection. Finally, the fluoroquinolones have been shown to be efficient in experimental infections and in selected cases in adults. Whereas their efficacy in the treatment of most gram-negative osteomyelitis seems undisputed, their advantage over conventional therapy in osteomyelitis due to *S. aureus* or *Pseudomonas* species remains to be demonstrated except for their ease of administration (27,28).

SURGICAL APPROACHES

It is beyond the scope of this chapter to describe and discuss the many orthopedic procedures used in the treatment of osteomyelitis, and only some general principles are discussed (12). In hematogenous osteomyelitis, the help of the surgeon is required mainly for the treatment of complications such as ab-

scesses and sequestra. In osteomyelitis secondary to a contiguous focus of infection, the help of the surgeon is almost always required. In acute infection after total hip arthroplasty, for instance, the surgeon delineates the depth of the septic process and evaluates the indication for removal of the prosthesis (29). Under other conditions, when infection occurs without consolidation of a fracture, removal of the foreign material is mandatory; if consolidation is already present, full mechanical recovery can be achieved in spite of sepsis, and the fixation material may be removed later, complemented by a short course of antibiotics. Finally, under conditions in which foreign material has to remain in place, at least for a certain time, combination therapy with rifampin and quinolones shows promising results (30–32).

PREVENTION

Under many circumstances in which implantation of prosthetic material is necessary, infection should be avoided by all possible means. This is particularly the case in clean orthopedic procedures, such as the implantation of artificial joints. Besides laminar airflow, cleansing techniques, and other general procedures to avoid nosocomial infections, the empiric use during the operating time of an antibiotic directed against gram-positive organisms (a semisynthetic penicillin or a cephalosporin) has been associated with a reduced risk for infection. Although criticized and not considered to be applicable to all patients, such a short course of antibiotics is justified in a high-risk population, such as patients with diabetes, rheumatoid arthritis, previous orthopedic surgery, or another favoring factor such as a foreign body.

REFERENCES

1. Waldvogel FA, Medoff G, Swartz MN. Osteomyelitis: a review of clinical features, therapeutic considerations, and unusual aspects. *N Engl J Med* 1970;282: 198, 260, 316.

2. Trueta J. The three types of acute hematogenous osteomyelitis: a clinical and vascular study. *J Bone Joint Surg Br* 1959;41:671.

3. Norden CW. Experimental osteomyelitis. II. Therapeutic trials and measurement of antibiotic levels in bone. *J Infect Dis* 1971;124:565.

4. Emslie KR, Nade S. Pathogenesis and treatment of acute hematogenous osteomyelitis: evaluation of current views with reference to an animal model. *Rev Infect Dis* 1986;8:841.

5. Elek SD, Conen PE. The virulence of *Staphylococcus pyogenes* for man: a study of the problems of wound infection. *Br J Exp Pathol* 1957;38:573.

6. Zimmerli W, Lew PD, Waldvogel FA. Pathogenesis of foreign body infection. Evidence for a local granulocyte defect. *J Clin Invest* 1984;73:1191.

7. Vaudaux P, Waldvogel FA, Morgenthaler JJ, et al. Adsorption of fibronectin onto polymethylmethacrylate and promotion of *Staphylococcus aureus* adherence. *Infect Immun* 1984;45:768.

8. Mayberry-Carson KJ, Tober-Meyer B, Smith JK, et al. Bacterial adherence and glycocalyx formation in osteomyelitis experimentally induced with *Staphylococcus aureus. Infect Immun* 1984;43:825.

9. Bisno AL Waldvogel FA, eds. *Infections associated with indwelling medical devices.* Washington, DC: American Society for Microbiology, 1989.

10. Barrett-Conner E. Bacterial infection and sickle cell anemia: an analysis of 150 infections in 166 patients and a review of the literature. *Medicine (Baltimore)* 1971;50:97.

11. Sugarman B, Hawes S, Musher DM, et al. Osteomyelitis beneath pressure sores. *Arch Intern Med* 1983;143:683.

12. Waldvogel FA, Vasey H. Osteomyelitis: the past decade. *N Engl J Med* 1980;303:360.

13. Mackowiak PA, Jones SR, Smith JW. Diagnostic value of sinustract cultures in chronic osteomyelitis. *JAMA* 1978;239:2772.

14. Kuhn JP, Berger PE. Computed tomographic diagnosis of osteomyelitis. *Radiology* 1979;130:503.

15. Smith FW, Runge V, Permezel M, et al. Nuclear magnetic resonance (NMR) imaging in the diagnosis of spinal osteomyelitis. *Magn Reson Imaging* 1984; 2:53.

16. Eftekhar NS. The infected total hip. *AAOS Instruct Course Lect* 1977;26: 66–74.

17. Meller Y, Yagupsky P, Elitsur Y, et al. Chronic multifocal symmetrical osteomyelitis. *Am J Dis Child* 1984;138:349.

18. Raff MJ, Melo JC. Anaerobic osteomyelitis. *Medicine (Baltimore)* 1978;57:83.

19. Chandrasekar PH, Narula AP. Bone and joint infections in intravenous drug abusers. *Rev Infect Dis* 1986;8:904.

20. Hodgson AR, Yau A, Kwon JS, et al. A clinical study of 100 consecutive cases of Pott's paraplegia. *Clin Orthop* 1964;36:128.

21. Auckenthaler R, Waldvogel FA. Bone and synovial fluid. In: Ristuccia AM, Cunha BA, eds. *Antimicrobial therapy.* New York: Raven, 1984:505–512.

22. Emslie KR, Nade S. Acute hematogenous staphylococcal osteomyelitis: evaluation of cloxacillin therapy in an animal model. *Pathology* 1984;16:441.

23. Weinstein MP, Stratton CW, Hawley HB, et al. Multicenter collaborative evaluation of a standardized serum bactericidal test as a predictor of therapeutic efficacy in acute and chronic osteomyelitis. *Am J Med* 1987;83:218.

24. Tetzlaff TR, McCracken GH, Nelson JD. Oral antibiotic therapy for skeletal infections of children. II. Therapy of osteomyelitis and suppurative arthritis. *J Pediatr* 1978;92:485.

25. Gentry LO. Oral antimicrobial therapy for osteomyelitis [Editorial; see comments]. *Ann Intern Med* 1991;114:986.

26. Black J, Hunt TL, Godley PJ, et al. Oral antimicrobial therapy for adults with osteomyelitis or septic arthritis. *J Infect Dis* 1987;155:968.

27. Waldvogel FA. Use of quinolones for the treatment of osteomyelitis and septic arthritis. *Rev Infect Dis* 1989;11(suppl 5):1259.

28. Lew DP, Waldvogel FA. Use of quinolones for treatment of osteomyelitis and septic arthritis. In: Hooper DC, Wolfson JS, eds. *Quinolone antimicrobial agents.* Washington, DC: American Society for Microbiology, 1993:371–379.

29. Fitzgerald RH Jr, Nolan DR, Ilstrup DM, et al. Deep wound sepsis following total hip arthroplasty. *J Bone Joint Surg Am* 1977;59:693.

30. Drancourt M, Stein A, Argenson JN, et al. Oral rifampin plus ofloxacin for treatment of *Staphylococcus*-infected orthopedic implants. *Antimicrob Agents Chemother* 1993;37:1214.

31. Zimmerli W, Widmer AF, Blatter M, et al. Role of rifampin for treatment of orthopedic implant-related staphylococcal infections: a randomized controlled trial. Foreign-Body Infection (FBI) Study Group. *JAMA* 1998;279:1575.

32. Stein A, Drancourt M, Raoult D. Ambulatory management of infected orthopedic implants. In: Waldvogel F, ed. *Infections associated with indwelling medical devices,* 3rd ed. Washington, DC: American Society for Microbiology, 2000:211.

CHAPTER 145
Infectious Arthritis

Nancy Y. Liu and David F. Giansiracusa

Acute bacterial arthritis, the most common cause of joint infection, is a medical emergency due to the potential for joint destruction (1) and even mortality if diagnosis and treatment are delayed, particularly in elderly individuals and in patients with preexisting arthritis (2–9). In the majority of cases, bacteria gain access to the joints by hematogenous spread (2,9–11). Skin flora is the most common source of microorganisms, but the respiratory, gastrointestinal, and genitourinary systems may also be sources. Less frequently, joint sepsis results from penetrating injury; diagnostic and therapeutic procedures, including arthroscopy (12–14); or extension from contiguous osteomyelitis, cellulitis, soft tissue abscesses, tenosynovitis, or septic bursitis (11). Factors that increase vulnerability to septic arthritis include underlying joint disease and seeding of a joint by trauma or intraarticular injection. Predisposing factors affect the types and numbers of joints involved, the nature of the infecting organisms, and the clinical outcomes (11). Table 145.1 lists the microbiology of bacterial arthritis in relationship to the patient's age (15).

NONGONOCOCCAL BACTERIAL ARTHRITIS

Nongonococcal bacterial infections are generally the most serious type of septic arthritis because of the potential for cartilage damage within 1 to 2 days (1,16). Gram-positive aerobic bacteria comprise about 80% of infecting microorganisms. In adults, *Staphylococcus aureus* is the most common cause of primary septic arthritis and of septic arthritis associated with intraarticular injection, trauma, or debilitating illness such as diabetes mellitus, rheumatoid arthritis, or systemic lupus erythematosus (17). Nearly all strains of *S. aureus* are resistant to penicillin, and some strains are resistant to methicillin (17,18). Approximately 15% of infecting gram-positive bacteria are group A β-hemolytic streptococci, and 3% are *Streptococcus pneumoniae* (2). Group B streptococcus is the predominant cause of joint infection in diabetic adults (9). Fifteen percent to 20% of bacterial infections are caused by gram-negative and anaerobic organisms. These bacteria are an increasing cause of joint infection in debilitated patients, parenteral drug abusers, elderly persons, young children, and immunocompromised hosts (2,10,19). Anaerobic joint infections occur in patients with postoperative wound infections, especially joint replacements and extremity wounds, and in the setting of gastrointestinal malignant neoplasms (20).

Pathophysiology

Within hours of entry into a joint, hematologic seeding with bacteria of the highly vascular synovial membrane results in bacterial trapping and multiplication in the subsynovium and phagocytosis by polymorphonuclear leukocytes (PMNs) and synovial lining cells (21,22). Neovascularization, synovial proliferation, and growth of granulation tissue develop. Proteolytic enzymes released from synovial lining cells and PMNs (particularly when the synovial fluid white cell counts exceed 50,000/mm³) and increased intracavitary pressure from accumulation of purulent synovial fluid cause necrosis of synovium and cartilage. Vascular plugging of granulation tissue by inflammatory cells and bacteria may also cause necrosis of bone (20). Proinflammatory

TABLE 145.1. Microbiology of Bacterial Septic Arthritis Related to Age of Patient

Organism	Children (6 mo to 5 yr)	Young adult	Adult	Elderly
Staphylococcus aureus	10%–20%	15%–20%	60%–70%	45%–65%
Streptococci	5%–10%	1%–5%	15%–20%	10%–15%
Gram-negative bacteria	1%–5%	Rare	10%–15%	15%–35%
Haemophilus influenzae	30%–50%	1%–5%	1%–5%	Rare
Neisseria gonorrhoeae	1%–5%	60%–80%	1%–5%	Rare

Percentages were compiled from several studies.
From Zimmermann B, Lally EV, Liu NY. Infectious agents and the musculoskeletal system. In: Noble J, Greene H, Levinson W, et al., eds. *Primary care and general medicine,* 2nd ed. St. Louis: Mosby-Year Book, 1996:1187, with permission.

cytokines such as interleukin-1 and tumor necrosis factor-α also contribute to joint injury. The degree of synovial, cartilage, and bone destruction is a function of the size of the inoculum, the virulence of the infecting microorganisms, the host response to the infection, and the rapidity of diagnosis and treatment (23–25).

Clinical Presentation

Eighty percent to 90% of bacterial arthritis affects one joint; the knees, hips, and shoulders (in decreasing frequency) are the most commonly involved sites. Less frequently involved joints are the elbows, wrists, ankles, and small joints of the hands and feet, although any joint may be affected, including facet joints of the spine (2,10,23,25–29). Repeated trauma to the knee may be the explanation for the frequency of involvement (30). The hip is particularly vulnerable to secondary osteonecrosis of the femoral head (2,11). Infection may also spread to the diaphysis of the bone, especially in children under 7 years of age (11).

Most patients with septic arthritis present with chills, fever, malaise, and the acute onset of monarticular and less frequently polyarticular arthritis (23,31). Localized signs of inflammation and severe, even incapacitating, pain are usually present (11). However, in elderly, severely ill, bedridden, or immunocompromised patients, symptoms and findings may be subtle (16,29,32).

In cases of polyarticular septic arthritis, the causative bacterium is also *S. aureus* in approximately 80% of cases and streptococcal species in 4% (3). In one study, approximately one fourth of the patients with polyarticular septic arthritis were not febrile on presentation, and nearly half (10 of 25 patients) had a peripheral white cell count of less than 10,000/mm³. Concurrent rheumatic disease, generally advanced, long-standing rheumatoid arthritis (33), was present in 52% of the patients (in patients with rheumatoid arthritis, superficial infection of rheumatoid nodules or of ulcerated calluses on feet was the major source of bacteria; joint prostheses were a major site of joint sepsis) (3). Other studies have also indicated that affected patients with rheumatoid arthritis tend to have long-standing, erosive, destructive joint disease, often in the setting of receiving chronic corticosteroid or cytotoxic drug therapy or intraarticular steroid injections (11,24,34,35). Mortality secondary to the infection or its consequences was 32% in the 25 patients with polyarticular septic arthritis and as high as 49% in those with rheumatoid arthritis compared with a mortality rate of 4% for 95 cases of monarticular septic arthritis (3). In other studies of polyarticular septic arthritis, the mortality rate among patients with rheumatoid arthritis has ranged from 20% to 56% (33,36).

Other host risk factors for developing polyarticular septic arthritis include intravenous drug abuse, cirrhosis, diabetes mellitus, other chronic diseases, and immunosuppression (3).

Prompt arthrocentesis for bacterial cultures and examination of synovial fluid should be performed on all inflamed joints (4,37).

Age may also affect clinical presentation. Bacterial arthritis is infrequently observed in neonates and infants (38–40). Infections may be community or hospital acquired. Although joints may rapidly become swollen, warm, and erythematous (41), such signs may not be present, and the child may simply cry and refrain from moving the affected extremity. Systemic features of high fevers rather than local symptoms and signs may predominate, possibly resulting in a delay of diagnosis (39). Severely ill neonates and infants may develop polyarticular joint sepsis and infection of soft tissues and bone (42,43). *S. aureus* and other gram-positive organisms, particularly group B streptococcal species, are the pathogens in the majority of cases (approximately 80%); gram-negative organisms, including *Pseudomonas aeruginosa* and other coliform microorganisms, constitute a smaller proportion. The severely ill infant may develop polymicrobial joint infections (41).

In children 6 months to 2 years of age, *Haemophilus influenzae* is the most common isolate causing joint sepsis (41,44,45). The *H. influenzae* vaccine may significantly reduce the frequency of *H. influenzae* septic arthritis. Urinary tract infection rather than meningitis is the common source of *H. influenzae* in about half of the children (30,41).

In children 2 years of age and older, the organisms causing septic arthritis and the joints affected are similar to those in adults (26,30,41). As in adults, knees and hips are the most frequently affected joints (26,30,41). Osteomyelitis and adjacent soft tissue infection may accompany septic arthritis, particularly in children under 10 years of age.

Predisposing Factors

PROSTHETIC JOINTS

Prosthetic joint infection is a rare but devastating complication of total joint arthroplasties and contributes to loosening and failure of the prosthetic joint. Infections occurring within 3 to 6 months of surgery are categorized as early, those 6 months postoperatively as late. The incidence of early infections has decreased to less than 2% with the advent of improved surgical techniques and prosthetic hardware, identification of high-risk patients, and use of perioperative antibiotics. Late infections occur at an annual rate of 0.18% to 0.60% (46). The mechanism of early infection is usually wound contamination or seeding from another infected site, such as the urinary tract, lungs, or dental caries. Late infections are presumed to be secondary to hematogenous seeding from a distant source, usually identifiable if sought.

Gram-positive organisms (*S. aureus, Staphylococcus epidermidis,* and *Streptococcus*) remain the most common bacteria identified in both early and late infections, with gram-negative and anaerobic organisms constituting the remainder (47,48). Fungal infections comprise less than 1% of the cases. Recommendations for antibiotic prophylaxis in the setting of prosthetic joints has evolved to target hosts at greatest risk (those with inflammatory arthropathies, with immunosuppressing diseases or therapy, with type I diabetes mellitus, with hemophilia, with malnourishment, with previous prosthetic infection, or with joint replacement within 2 years), dental procedures with bleeding, and other procedures with high incidence of bacteremia (49,50). Treatment with appropriate intravenous antibiotics is similar to that of native septic joints except that surgical intervention with exploration and débridement of the prosthetic joint is usually necessary (27,48), followed by an excision arthroplasty or revision arthroplasty (29).

INTRAVENOUS DRUG ABUSE

S. aureus is the most frequent cause of septic arthritis in intravenous drug abusers, but gram-negative infections also occur, particularly due to P. aeruginosa. In addition to the commonly infected joints, the sternoclavicular, sacroiliac, and manubriosternal joints and the symphysis pubis may be infected (11,23,39,51,52). Sternoclavicular septic arthritis may present with pain on shoulder motion and a paucity of swelling, warmth, or erythema. Infection at this site may spread to the thoracic wall or into the anterior mediastinum and may require aggressive medical and surgical treatment (53,54). Sacroiliac involvement produces poorly localized pain in the buttocks, abdomen, or hip and may cause sciatic pain. Although motion of the ipsilateral hip may be full, the FABER maneuver (hip flexion, abduction, external rotation) often elicits or aggravates pain in the region of the sacroiliac joint, as may direct palpation of the joint or pelvic compression of the lateral iliac wings. Purulent drainage from the sacroiliac joints may extend into the retroperitoneal space and into the psoas muscle (55).

IMMUNOCOMPROMISED STATES

Immunocompromised hosts, including young or old individuals with multiorgan system disease, patients with human immunodeficiency virus (HIV) infection (56), transplant recipients (29), and patients treated with immunosuppressant therapy for malignant and nonmalignant (including collagen-vascular or autoimmune) disease (57), present an increasing population of individuals susceptible to polyarticular polymicrobial bacterial arthritis. Patients with HIV infection may have numerous rheumatic manifestations, but septic arthritis is generally caused by the same bacteria that infect joints of immunocompetent hosts (58–61) as well as by opportunistic microbials (19).

Diagnosis

Arthrocentesis through noncellulitic skin for synovial fluid cultures, smears, and analysis is the single most important diagnostic procedure in the evaluation of possible septic arthritis. In cases of polyarticular involvement, all inflamed joints should be aspirated. Synovial fluid should be sent for Gram stain, culture, white blood cell count, and differential. In S. aureus arthritis, bacteria may be identified on Gram stain in 50% to 75% and cultured in more than 90% of cases (28). Gram stains are less frequently positive in identifying gram-negative organisms (10). If synovial fluid is not grossly purulent, Gram stain of the centrifuged synovial fluid pellet may increase the yield of positive findings (2,26,45,62). Synovial fluid samples should be cultured for aerobic and anaerobic organisms in appropriate media. Bacterial antigen determinations by counterimmunoelectrophoresis

may be performed in cases of partially treated bacterial arthritis, but these studies are not routinely done (2,26). Cultures of blood and of all suspected extraarticular sites of infection should also be performed. The positive growth of blood cultures in patients with nongonococcal bacterial arthritis occurs in about 50% of cases (2,41). Synovial fluid white blood cell counts generally exceed $50,000/mm^3$ with more than 90% PMNs (2,23,25,26,31,41). However, such high cell counts and predominance of PMNs may also occur in rheumatoid arthritis, crystal-induced arthritis, Reiter syndrome (reactive arthritis), and psoriatic arthritis (28,63,64). Synovial fluid glucose and protein levels have not proved helpful in distinguishing septic from noninfectious causes of inflammatory joint disease (65).

Imaging studies include conventional radiographs, which are rarely diagnostic but provide a baseline status of the joint and adjacent bone and may identify a focus of osteomyelitis. Rarefaction and erosion of subchondral bone may not be present for several (2 to 4) weeks after the onset of joint symptoms (66). Scintigraphy (radionuclide scans) with technetium diphosphonate reflects the presence of inflammation but does not define a specific cause. Such studies may be particularly helpful in evaluating for inflammation of sacroiliac, sternoclavicular, and facet joints (67). Indium- or technetium diphosphonate–labeled leukocyte scans may help localize sites of bone and joint infections, but these are much more expensive and of no greater usefulness than radioiodinated monoclonal antigranulocyte antibody studies when such are available (11). Computed tomography is useful to evaluate sacroiliac and sternoclavicular joints for erosive bone changes and to localize retroperitoneal, intrapsoas, and mediastinal abscesses (53,68,69). Fluoroscopic or computed tomographic guidance is helpful for aspiration of the sacroiliac joints (55). Magnetic resonance imaging is the method of choice for evaluating deep-seated bone and joint disease because it can demonstrate synovitis, joint effusions, osteonecrosis (avascular-ischemic necrosis of bone), and marrow space edema (11,29,70,71).

Differential Diagnosis

The differential diagnosis of septic arthritis depends on the presence of monarticular versus polyarticular joint involvement and the age of the patient. Monarticular arthritis in children or adults may be due to juvenile rheumatoid arthritis (in children), Lyme disease, or a spondyloarthropathy. Polyarticular arthritis in children and adults may be caused by rheumatoid arthritis, systemic lupus erythematosus, a spondyloarthropathy, acute rheumatic fever, Kawasaki syndrome, and viral illnesses (particularly parvovirus infection, rubella, and hepatitis B). In older adults, crystal-induced arthritis, "pseudoseptic" rheumatoid arthritis (64,72), reactive arthritis (9), neuropathic arthropathy (63), and infectious arthritis caused by other microorganisms including mycobacteria and fungi are in the differential diagnosis of septic (bacterial) arthritis (11).

Treatment

Treatment of bacterial arthritis consists of adequate joint drainage, joint rest and mobilization, and antibiotics (2,23,25, 26,41,45,62). Drainage of the affected joints should be performed daily until synovial fluid is sterile and minimal effusion is evident. Rapid reaccumulation of synovial effusions may indicate resistance to antibiotics, the presence of more than one microorganism, or loculation of synovial fluid in the joint cavity (11). Methods of joint drainage include percutaneous needle aspiration, arthroscopic surgical drainage, and open surgical drainage.

TABLE 145.2.   Initial Antibiotic Therapy for Presumed Bacterial Arthritis in an Adult (Pathogen Unknown)

Gram stain	Presumed organism	Antibiotic
Positive		
Gram-positive cocci	*Staphylococcus aureus*	Oxacillin or nafcillin (alternative: cefazolin or vancomycin)
Gram-positive cocci (prosthetic joint)	*Staphylococcus epidermidis*	Vancomycin ($\pm$ rifampin)
Gram-negative cocci	*Neisseria gonorrhoeae*	Ceftriaxone or cefotaxime (alternative: a fluroquinolone)
Gram-negative bacilli	*Escherichia coli, Serratia marcescens,* other Enterobacteriaceae	Third-generation cephalosporin, or imipenem, or aztreonam, or a fluroquinolone (and in cases of bacteremia or severe infection, the addition of an aminoglycoside)
Gram-negative bacilli (thin)	*Pseudomonas aeruginosa*	Ceftazidime (or piperacillin, or imipenem, or aztreonam) plus tobramycin or a fluroquinolone
Negative		
Noncompromised host	*Staphylococcus aureus,* Enterobacteriaceae	Nafcillin plus gentamicin, or alternatively a third-generation cephalosporin (ceftriaxone or cefotaxime) or a fluroquinolone plus vancomycin
Compromised host	*Staphylococcus aureus,* Enterobacteriaceae, and *Pseudomonas aeruginosa*[a]	Nafcillin plus gentamicin, or alternatively (ceftazidime or aztreonam) plus vancomycin, or alternatively imipenem plus (tobramycin or a fluroquinolone)

Ciprofloxacin and levofloxacin are available for parenteral use.
[a]Treatment for both gram-positive and gram-negative pathogens must be continued until cultures return.
Modified from Upchurch KS, Giansiracusa DF. Rheumatic diseases in the intensive care unit. In: Rippe JM, Irwin RS, Fink MP, et al., eds. *Intensive care medicine,* 3rd ed. Boston: Little, Brown, 1996:2397, with permission.

Percutaneous needle drainage is the procedure of choice for accessible joints in the absence of underlying joint disease such as rheumatoid arthritis. Indications for surgical drainage include all cases of septic arthritis of the hip (23,39–41,73), failure of percutaneous aspiration (generally after 5–7 days) (2,74), and appropriate antibiotics, suspected synovial fluid loculations, and joints anatomically altered by underlying joint diseases. Arthroscopic surgery offers the opportunity to débride and lavage the joint with less extensive surgery than an open procedure. The choice of arthroscopic versus open surgical drainage is generally best made cooperatively by the rheumatologist and orthopedic surgeon (75–78).

Antibiotic therapy is initially determined by results of the synovial fluid Gram stain and by the clinical setting, for example, the presence of an extraarticular focus such as gram-negative urinary tract infection. If the Gram stain is unrevealing, judicious antibiotics to cover the most likely organisms should be started as soon as appropriate cultures have been obtained. Table 145.2 lists general initial antibiotic recommendations in the setting of the pathogens not being known. Table 145.3 lists antibiotic choices and alternatives in the cases of known bacterial pathogens (79,80).

Treatment of bacterial arthritis of hand joints as a result of human or animal bites should include antibiotics effective against oral flora, such as ampicillin or ampicillin-sulbactam. Ceftriaxone and doxycycline are alternatives for the penicillin-allergic patient (9).

Parenteral antibiotics should be continued for at least 4 weeks at adequate bactericidal blood levels to ensure eradication of the bacteria (11). Other authorities recommend 2 weeks of parenteral antibiotics for septic arthritis due to *H. influenzae,* streptococci, or gram-negative cocci and 3 weeks for staphylococcal or gram-negative bacillary septic arthritis (9). Sterilization of synovial fluid within 5 days of antibiotic therapy generally indicates a good response to treatment (9). Home intravenous therapy may be an alternative to long-term hospitalization, particularly in

TABLE 145.3.   Antibiotic Therapy for Acute Bacterial Arthritis in the Critically Ill Adult (Known Pathogen)

Organism	Antibiotic choice	Alternatives
Staphylococcus aureus	Nafcillin, 9–12 g/day (every 4 h), or oxacillin, 9–12 g/day (every 4 h)	Cefazolin, 4.5–6 g/day (every 8 h), or vancomycin, 2 g/day (every 12 h)
Staphylococcus aureus, methicillin resistant	Vancomycin, 2 g/day	None
Streptococcus pyogenes, Streptococcus pneumoniae	Penicillin G, 12–18 million units/day (every 4 h)[a]	Cefazolin or vancomycin
Neisseria gonorrhoeae	Ceftriaxone, 1–2 g/day (every 12 h), or cefotaxime, 3–6 g/day (every 8 h)	Tetracycline, or a fluroquinolone or penicillin G if sensitive
Pseudomonas aeruginosa	Piperacillin, 12 g/day (every 4 h), plus tobramycin, 4–5 mg/kg/day (every 4 h)	Ceftazidime, 6 g/day (every 8 h), or imipenem-cilastatin, 2–3 g/day, or ciprofloxacin[b] plus tobramycin or gentamicin
Enterobacteriaceae	Third-generation cephalosporin, plus gentamicin, 4–5 mg/kg/day (every 8 h)	Aztreonam, 3 g/day (every 8 h), or a fluoroquinolone plus gentamicin or amikacin

[a]Modify therapy for *Streptococcus pneumoniae* depending on susceptibility of the isolate to penicillin.
[b]Ciprofloxacin and levofloxacin are available for parenteral use.
Modified from Upchurch KS, Giansiracusa DF. Rheumatic diseases in the intensive care unit. In: Rippe JM, Irwin RS, Fink M, eds. *Intensive care medicine,* 3rd ed. Boston: Little, Brown, 1996:2397, with permission.

the patient with involvement of a non–weight-bearing joint and a good initial response to antibiotics and drainage. Long-term oral antibiotic therapy may be necessary for protracted bone and prosthetic joint infections (48,81).

As a result of experimental studies of septic arthritis in animals indicating that prolonged immobilization is detrimental, immobilization is now recommended only for incapacitatingly painful joints and joints treated with surgical drainage. Passive joint mobilization and functional splinting for the severely ill patient and passive and active range of motion for the less ill patient are recommended to prevent joint contractures and to preserve joint function (11).

The prognosis of septic arthritis is affected by a number of variables. In general, the sooner the diagnosis is established and appropriate therapy instituted, the better the outcome (23,25,39, 41,45,62). Factors indicating poor prognosis include (a) age over 60 years; (b) comorbid conditions, such as preexisting rheumatoid arthritis; and (c) hip, shoulder, or polyarticular involvement (9). The infecting organism (specifically *S. aureus* and gram-negative bacteria) (15), persistence of positive synovial fluid cultures after 7 days of appropriate antibiotics, and host-microbial interactions may also adversely influence the outcome.

Major changes in the past decade in nongonococcal bacterial arthritis have been (a) the longer life expectancy, thus increasing the number of elderly patients and those with comorbid conditions; (b) the increased frequency of methicillin-resistant *S. aureus* joint infections; (c) the increased use of arthroscopy, which poses a risk for postprocedure infection as well as being a surgical option for draining septic joints; (d) the increased number of patients with prosthetic joints; and (e) the increasing frequency of septic arthritis in patients infected with HIV (11).

GONOCOCCAL ARTHRITIS

Gonococcal arthritis is the most common form of septic arthritis among sexually active young adults (2,82), constituting up to 66% of the cases of septic arthritis and tenosynovitis in this population (83). Disseminated gonococcal infection (DGI) may also occur in children and in the elderly (84,85), in patients with systemic rheumatic diseases, and in patients with HIV infection (86,87). The prevalence of DGI varies from 0.5% to 3% (88). DGI occurs four times as frequently in women as in men. The risk for dissemination increases during menstruation and pregnancy and in the immediate postpartum period. Approximately one half of women who develop DGI do so in association with one of these risk factors (89–91). In men, risk factors for dissemination include homosexual activity with asymptomatic rectal or pharyngeal involvement (92). Less common risk factors for DGI include inherited terminal complement component deficiencies (C5 through C8, especially C8) (93) and more rarely deficiencies of the third and fourth components of complement (83). Humans are the only known source of the organism, *Neisseria gonorrhoeae*. Disseminated disease occurs only after mucous membrane infection of the endocervix, urethra, pharynx, or rectum. Most cases of DGI result from asymptomatic primary gonococcal infection of the genitourinary tract that has been sexually transmitted days to months previously. Symptomatic genitourinary infection including urethral or vaginal discharge, urethritis, urinary frequency, and dysuria is rarely present (83).

Clinical Features

DGI is characterized by the acute onset of oligoarthralgias or polyarthralgias, which may have a diffuse, migratory, or additive pattern generally progressing to a maximum during several days (83). Constitutional symptoms with chills and fever, which may be low to moderate, are common. Two thirds of patients develop tenosynovitis, most frequently involving the wrists, fingers, ankles, and toes, with or without the presence of an arthritis. Less than half of patients with DGI develop a true arthritis that is generally monarticular but can be oligoarticular or polyarticular. The most commonly affected joints are the knees, wrists, hands, and ankles (94–96), although any joint may be involved, including the hip (97).

Skin involvement occurs in approximately two thirds of patients with DGI. Most lesions are painless and may go unnoticed by the patient. The most common lesions are macules, papules, or pustules on an erythematous base. Lesions may progress to central necrosis. Vesicular lesions and lesions resembling bullae, erythema nodosum, and erythema multiforme have also been described. Lesions are few in number, occurring mostly on the extremities, sometimes on the trunk, and rarely on face, palms, and soles (82,88,96). Skin lesions develop simultaneously with tenosynovitis and arthritis, continue to evolve for 48 hours, and then resolve, even if untreated (98).

DGI may present in one of two forms, a bacteremic form and a suppurative form. The bacteremic form, which is more common, presents as tenosynovitis, dermatitis, chills, fever, and a true arthritis with joint effusions that are typically culture negative. In the suppurative form, arthritis is the major clinical manifestation. Joint effusions tend to be large and purulent. Some patients present with both clinical forms (90).

Differential Diagnosis

The differential diagnosis of DGI includes those conditions manifested by arthritis, dermatitis, and often fever. These include Reiter syndrome (reactive arthritis), nongonococcal bacterial arthritis, bacterial endocarditis (99), meningococcal arthritis, chronic meningococcal septicemia, hepatitis B and C, rheumatic fever, Lyme disease, systemic lupus erythematosus, rheumatoid arthritis, and Still disease (66). Of these, acute and subacute bacterial endocarditis can be particularly difficult to distinguish from DGI because patients with endocarditis and DGI may present with arthralgias accompanied by tenosynovitis followed by arthritis. The synovitis in both may be sterile unless hematogenous spread of organisms to the synovium has occurred. Skin lesions, particularly pustules and pustulonecrotic lesions, may occur in both (82,83). Splinter hemorrhages, Osler nodes, Janeway lesions, rheumatoid factor, and positive blood cultures help to establish the diagnosis of endocarditis, as does the finding of valvular vegetations. Acute and chronic meningococcemia may also have clinical features resembling DGI. Helpful features in distinguishing meningococcemia are the presence of a greater number of skin lesions and a positive throat culture for the organism. Definitive diagnosis of meningococcemia is established by identification of the organisms in blood or synovial fluid (82,83).

Diagnosis

The diagnosis of DGI and gonococcal arthritis is based on an appropriate clinical presentation and positive cultures. A definite diagnosis of DGI is established by positive cultures of *N. gonorrhoeae* or identification of the organism by Gram stain in samples of synovial fluid, blood, or skin lesions. The majority of patients presenting with DGI will have elevated peripheral white cell counts and elevated erythrocyte sedimentation rates. Synovial fluid from joints affected with gonococcal arthritis will frequently contain 30,000 to 100,000 white blood cells per mm^3, with a PMN predominance, but counts may be much lower (89,94). The majority of Gram stain examinations of synovial fluid specimens fail to reveal organisms. Yield may be increased by Gram staining the pellet of centrifuged synovial fluid. Cultures of synovial fluid fail to yield growth in more than 50% of cases, even when they are carefully performed (100). Fluid from patients with the suppurative form is more likely to yield growth (almost 50% of cases) than is fluid from patients with the bacteremic form (82,88,90). Gram stain and cultures of skin lesions rarely yield positive results (94). Blood culture positivity occurs in less than 30% of patients, with positive yield being more likely in patients with dermatitis and tenosynovitis (83,88,96,101).

The highest yields of culture positivity for gonococci are from genitourinary tract samples (100). In women, cultures of cervical swabs yield growth in 80% to 90% of cases. In men, Gram stain and culture of urethral discharge, or of urethral swab in the absence of a discharge, yield positive results in 50% to 70% of cases (89,94). To maximize yield of positive cultures, all potentially infected mucosal sites, including pharynx and rectum, should be sampled. In some situations, all cultures of the presenting patient will be negative, but cultures of the sexual partner may yield growth of the organisms. To maximize culture yields, samples from the urethra, endocervix, rectum, and pharynx should be cultured on chocolate agar containing antibiotics (modified Thayer-Martin media); samples of joint fluid, blood, and skin lesions are cultured on plain chocolate agar (83).

In most patients, a diagnosis of DGI or gonococcal arthritis is made indirectly by the presence of positive urethral, endocervical, rectal, or pharyngeal cultures in patients with appropriate clinical features. A presumptive diagnosis may be made by the typical presentation and rapid response to appropriate antibiotics (83).

Treatment of Disseminated Gonococcal Infection and Gonococcal Arthritis

Patients should be educated regarding the sexual mode of gonococcal transmission, identification of sexual partners, and risk for other sexually transmitted diseases. Serologic testing for syphilis should be done and testing for HIV infection encouraged and for hepatitis B if high-risk behaviors are practiced.

Initial hospitalization is recommended for management of DGI, particularly if (a) the diagnosis is in question, (b) compliance is uncertain, (c) purulent effusions are present (requiring repeated joint aspirations), and (d) complications of endocarditis, meningitis, or myopericarditis are suspected (82,83).

With regard to antibiotic therapy, because a significant number of the infecting strains are penicillin (β-lactamase) resistant (100,102–104), initial treatment in the penicillin-tolerant (nonallergic) patient should consist of a third-generation β-lactamase–resistant cephalosporin (82). Antibiotic therapy for the patient tolerant of penicillins is listed in Table 145.4. Antibiotic therapy for the penicillin-allergic patient is listed in Table 145.5.

Unless *Chlamydia* diagnostic testing is available and yields negative results for coinfection, patients, in addition to being treated for gonococcal infection, should be treated with a 7-day course of doxycycline, 100 mg twice daily, or the pregnant woman is treated with azithromycin, 1 g, as one dose or erythromycin base, 500 mg four times daily for 7 days (82).

With appropriate antibiotics, signs and symptoms of DGI generally improve within 48 hours, and dermatitis and arthralgias resolve within 5 days, but joint pain may persist for several weeks. Mean duration of hospitalization in one study was 5.8 days (100). Management for large, purulent synovial effusions with regard to drainage and immobilization or exercise is

similar to that for nongonococcal bacterial arthritis, although the response is generally more rapid in the case of gonococcal arthritis, and the eventual outcome is generally excellent (100). Although the clinical features of gonococcal arthritis have changed little in the past few decades, patients presenting with gonococcal arthritis may more commonly have an underlying condition such as intravenous drug abuse or systemic lupus erythematosus and be infected with a penicillin-resistant gonococcal organism (100).

After completion of antibiotics, patients should be reevaluated, including undergoing repeated sampling of sites that previously yielded positive cultures. Serologic testing for syphilis

---

TABLE 145.4. Antibiotic Treatment of Disseminated Gonococcal Infection in Penicillin-Tolerant (Nonallergic) Patients

Parenteral therapy
  Ceftriaxone, 1 g intramuscularly or intravenously (i.v.) every 24 h
    or
  Cefotaxime, 1 g i.v. every 8 h
  Continue parenteral therapy until signs and symptoms of infection resolve or clinical improvement is evident (usually 2–4 days)
Oral therapy (to complete total of 7 days of antibiotics)
  Amoxicillin, 500 mg, plus clavulanate, 125 mg, three times daily
    or
  Cefixime, 400 mg twice daily
    or
  Ciprofloxacin, 500 mg twice daily (in the nonpregnant patient)
    or
  Ofloxacin 400 mg orally twice daily
Concurrent treatment of *Chlamydia trachomatis*
  Doxycycline, 100 mg orally twice daily for 7 days
    or
  Azithromycin, 1 g (one dose)
    or
  Erythromycin base, 500 mg 4 times daily for 7 days

From Centers for Disease Control and Prevention. Guidelines for treatment of sexually transmitted diseases. *MMWR* 1998;47(RR-1):1–111, with permission.

TABLE 145.5. Antibiotic Treatment of Disseminated Gonococcal Infection in β-lactam–Allergic Patients

Parenteral therapy (until clinical improvement)
  Spectinomycin, 2 g intramuscularly every 12 h
  In the nonpregnant patient
    Ciprofloxacin 500 mg i.v. every 12 h
      or
    Ofloxacin 400 mg i.v. every 12 h
Oral therapy (to complete a 7-day course of antibiotics)
  In the nonpregnant patient
    Ciprofloxacin, 500 mg twice daily
      or
    Ofloxacin 400 mg twice daily
  In the pregnant patient
    Erythromycin base, 500 mg 4 times a day for 7 days
Concurrent therapy for *Chlamydia trachomatis*
  In the nonpregnant patient
    Doxycycline, 100 mg twice daily for 7 days
  In the pregnant patient
    Azithromycin, 1 g as one dose
      or
    Erythromycin base, 500 mg 4 times a day for 7 days

From Centers for Disease Control and Prevention. Guidelines for treatment of sexually transmitted diseases. *MMWR* 1998;47(RR-1):1–111, with permission.

should be repeated 4 to 6 weeks after completion of antibiotic therapy.

SEPTIC BURSITIS

Infections of the subcutaneous bursae (olecranon, prepatellar, and infrapatellar) are common owing to their superficial location and susceptibility to trauma resulting in the percutaneous inoculation of bacteria. The infection may remain contained within the bursal cavity, lined by a thin layer of synovial cells, or may rupture into surrounding soft tissues and clinically resemble cellulitis. Deep bursal infections of the subacromial, trochanteric, and iliopsoas bursae are rare and usually result from hematogenous seeding or underlying joint infection.

The gram-positive bacteria are the primary causative organisms, with S. aureus contributing to over 80% of all septic bursitis and the various streptococcal species responsible for 5% to 30% in large reported series (105,106). However, gram-negative and polymicrobial bacterial infections may occur, especially in immunocompromised or chronically debilitated patients. Fungal and mycobacterial bursitis have also been reported.

Clinical presentations may vary from minimal erythema and bursal swelling to systemic symptoms of malaise, fevers, and severe pain in the involved area. On physical examination, discrete swelling over the olecranon or prepatellar areas is often present but extensive peribursal cellulitis extending beyond the borders of the bursa occurs in other cases.

The diagnosis of septic bursitis is based on aspiration and analysis of bursal fluid for total white cell count, culture, and crystals. In contrast to septic joint fluid, the bursal white cell counts may be low, often less than 10,000/mm³ with a range from 920 to 300,000/mm³, but PMNs will predominate (106). Confirmation of infection is based on positive bursal fluid cultures. Because crystalline bursitis may occur simultaneously with a septic process, infection is not excluded until final cultures are negative.

Treatment of septic bursitis requires appropriate antibiotics, serial closed needle drainage, and immobilization of the joint. In otherwise healthy patients, septic olecranon and prepatellar bursitis are treated in the outpatient setting with oral antibiotics. The usual length of treatment is 5 days beyond the first sterile bursal fluid with a typical course of 10–14 days (107). For chronically debilitated or immunocompromised patients, initial hospital admission with intravenous antibiotics for 4 to 7 days with documentation of response can be followed by an additional 7 to 14 days of oral or intravenous antibiotics as outpatient may be more appropriate and prudent. Septic bursitis that fails to respond to outpatient therapy may require inpatient management. Risk factors for poor outcome include prepatellar location, delay in treatment, prior bursal infection, underlying disease of the bursa, extension of infection beyond the bursal sac, and bacteremia (106). Rarely, surgical incision and drainage or débridement of the bursa is required if (a) serial cultures remain positive despite appropriate antibiotics, (b) loculations or abscesses develop that are inaccessible to closed needle drainage, or (c) foreign or necrotic material is present. Immobilization of the knee is an important adjunct of treatment for prepatellar bursitis accompanied by isometric strengthening exercises within a few days of immobilization.

FUNGAL ARTHRITIS

Fungal arthritis is relatively rare and was previously described in patients with endemic mycoses: histoplasmosis, blastomyco-

sis, or coccidioidomycosis. With emergence of a larger number of immunocompromised patients, including patients with acquired immunodeficiency syndrome and those treated with immunosuppressive drugs for malignant and nonmalignant disorders, mycotic joint infections including unusual organisms have become more frequent. Maintenance on home total parenteral nutrition or intravenous administration of antibiotics also poses a risk for development of fungal infection.

The most common musculoskeletal fungal infections in immunocompetent hosts include those due to Coccidioides immitis, Blastomyces dermatitidis, Histoplasma capsulatum, Sporothrix schenckii, and Cryptococcus neoformans (108). A hypersensitivity reaction with associated polyarthralgias, polyarthritis, and erythema nodosum accompanies primary infections of H. capsulatum (0%–34%) and C. immitis (30%) (108). The symptoms are often migratory, self-limited, and without sequelae. Disseminated (or secondary) fungal infections commonly affect the skeletal system with C. immitis (10%–50%), B. dermatitidis (25%–60%), and C. neoformans (5%) (108). Septic arthritis typically results from extension of contiguous osteomyelitis (109). Hematogenous seeding rarely occurs. Although C. immitis and C. neoformans arthritis appear more chronic and indolent with physical findings of monarthritis, B. dermatitidis arthritis is often associated with systemic symptoms and may be polyarticular. The knee is the most commonly involved joint, followed by ankle, elbow, and wrist. Synovial fluid is moderately inflammatory, with a predominance of mononuclear cells, but in B. dermatitidis infection, purulent fluid with an elevated number of PMNs is typical. S. schenckii infection, in contrast, develops secondary to direct inoculation from trauma. Chronic monarticular or polyarticular arthritis in the hands, wrist, knee, or feet, tenosynovitis, and bursitis are the usual musculoskeletal manifestations with accompanying systemic features.

In immunocompromised or chronically ill patients, Candida, Aspergillus (particularly Aspergillus fumigatus), Cryptococcus, and Histoplasma are the most common fungi associated with skeletal infections. The pathogenesis and manifestations of bone and joint disease are similar to those of patients who are immunocompetent.

Candida arthritis develops by direct inoculation or hematogenous seeding, each of which is equally common. Direct inoculation occurs when Candida is introduced into osteoarthritic or rheumatoid joints by repeated aspirations or corticosteroid injections. The corticosteroids may alter host defense in an already abnormal joint. Direct inoculation may also occur during prosthetic joint replacement or other surgical procedures. In all these situations, patients are typically healthy but have a pathologic process in the knee, hip, or shoulder. Some patients may be immunocompromised from their rheumatoid arthritis, concomitant corticosteroid therapy, or other immunosuppressive therapy. The arthritis develops insidiously, often without associated systemic symptoms. The course is indolent, and the diagnosis is often delayed. Synovial fluid analysis reveals a variable degree of inflammatory fluid with predominantly PMNs and an associated low glucose level. Blood cultures are usually negative. The diagnosis is established by positive fluid or synovial tissue culture for the fungus. The most common species include Candida parapsilosis and Candida albicans; Candida tropicalis and Candida guilliermondii are rare (110). Radiographs may reveal changes of the underlying joint disease and, in the case of a prosthetic joint, loosening, sometimes accompanied by osteomyelitis.

Disseminated candidiasis with associated septic arthritis is primarily reported in the pediatric population under 6 months of age. These infants are usually hospitalized and have underlying illnesses. Joint infection is usually associated with osteomyelitis. In adults, septic arthritis secondary to disseminated candidiasis is associated with immunocompromised states, prolonged systemic antibiotics, indwelling catheters, and intravenous drug abuse. In contrast to direct inoculation, the majority of patients (66%) with hematogenously seeded joints are acutely ill; 33% of patients may have an insidious onset (111). Monarthritis of the knee is most common, although polyarticular infection can occur and is frequently observed in infants. Other joints involved include the hip, ankle, shoulder, or elbow. *C. albicans* is identified in 70% of the cases; *C. tropicalis*, *C. parapsilosis*, and *C. guilliermondii* (in order of decreasing frequency) are less common (111). In intravenous drug abusers, the infection has a predilection for the fibrocartilaginous joints (sacroiliac, costochondral, sternoclavicular, and intervertebral disks).

Aspergillus infections similarly have a predisposition for the vertebral disc spaces and rarely involve the joint. *C. immitis* musculoskeletal infections occur with dissemination and are relatively rare (112).

Diagnosis of fungal arthritis is often delayed but is established by examination of synovial fluid or, more commonly, synovial tissue and bone biopsy specimens for identification of various fungal morphologic phases by culture, histopathology, or cytology. Aside from synovial fluid, *Candida* may be cultured from multiple sites (blood, cerebrospinal fluid, urine, pharynx, stool, catheter tips, bone marrow) in patients with hematogenous dissemination. *C. immitis* and *B. dermatitidis* may have cutaneous lesions such as ulcerations or draining sinus tracks from which fungus may be cultured. Serodiagnosis provides additional confirmation of infection, but discussion of the various methods and their sensitivity and specificity is beyond the scope of this section (refer to Part X of this book).

Amphotericin B alone or in combination with flucytosine or an azole derivative has been the primary treatment of fungal arthritis (please refer to Chapter 33 for details of therapy). In *Candida* arthritis, current recommendations include initial course of amphotericin B for 2 to 3 weeks followed by fluconazole for 6 to 12 months or combination intravenous amphotericin B and fluconazole therapy (113). Itraconazole may be the primary therapy for sporotrichosis, blastomycosis, and coccidioidomycosis as alternatives to amphotericin B (114–116). In cryptococcal infections, specific studies on musculoskeletal infections are not available. The optimal drug regimen depends on evidence of CNS involvement as well as immune status of the patient. Recommended regimens range from oral azoles or amphotericin B alone to induction/consolidation therapy with amphotericin B, flucytosine, and then fluconazole if CNS disease or an immunocompromised state exists (117).

As an adjunct to antifungal therapies, surgical drainage, débridement, or synovectomy may be necessary in cases of prosthetic joint infection, loculated joint effusions, or failure to respond to medical therapy. Removal of the prosthesis is necessary in the majority of patients with prosthetic *Candida* arthritis (111).

VIRAL ARTHRITIS

Various viral infections have been associated with acute arthritis or persistent arthropathy. The pathogenesis includes direct synovial infection, immune complex–mediated inflammation, and mechanisms as yet to be defined. Although most of the viral arthritides are self-limited and present in the prodromal state, rubella and parvovirus may cause chronic arthritis.

Rubella, by natural infection or immunization with attenuated virus, is the most common form of viral arthritis. The pathogenesis of the arthritis is direct infection and viral replication within the joint. A frequency has been reported of 52% in female patients compared with 8.7% in male patients who developed polyarthritis after natural rubella infection. Nearly 50% of adult women developed joint disease after immunizations, with 30% of nonimmune women developing acute arthropathy after immunization with live, attenuated rubella vaccine, RA 27/3 (118). Polyarthritis of small joints, knees, wrist, ankles, and elbows occurs within 1 week of the rash in natural infections and within 2 to 3 weeks of immunization. The arthritis is typically self-limited, but persistent symptoms beyond 1 year have been described in up to 30% of adult women (119,120).

Human parvovirus B19 (HPV-B19) infection, also known as erythema infectiosum, is a common self-limited childhood disease that can cause arthralgias and arthritis in both children and nonimmune adults. Joint symptoms follow the viremic phase of the infection and coincide with the development of the IgM antibody response.

In the 8% of children who develop arthritis with HPV-B19 infection, the joint pattern typically is asymmetric and pauciarticular, and predominantly involves large joints. Symptoms resolve within 4 months, but approximately 25% of children had persistent arthritis for up to 13 months (121). In contrast, up to 60% to 80% of infected adults develop joint symptoms, with women affected much more than men (59% vs. 30%) (122). Most joint symptoms were brief, but persistent polyarticular arthritis (defined as greater than 2 months) occurred in 20% of the women for up to 7 months (123). Long-term follow-up at 5 years, however, revealed no persistent joint swelling or limitation (124). The pattern of joint involvement clinically resembles rheumatoid arthritis, with symmetric polyarthritis of the proximal interphalangeal and metacarpophalangeal joints and prolonged morning stiffness. However, despite the chronicity and persistent symptoms, neither erosive changes nor rheumatoid factor develop. Arthroscopic findings reveal normal synovium without cartilage damage. Findings on synovial histologic examination are essentially normal (125). Although the persistence of B19-specific DNA sequences has been demonstrated in bone marrow aspirates and the synovium of some patients with chronic HPV-B19 arthropathy or classic rheumatoid arthritis, other studies have not supported the theory that parvovirus B19 is the cause of rheumatoid arthritis or other forms of chronic arthropathy (126–128).

Hepatitis B–associated arthritis due to antigen-antibody complexes develops during the prodromal phase. The patients typically have polyarthralgias with or without frank polyarthritis. The arthritis usually resolves with the onset of jaundice. Chronic arthritis and other rheumatic syndromes (essential mixed cryoglobulinemia, polyarteritis nodosa, and glomerulonephritis) may develop in the setting of chronic active hepatitis.

Musculoskeletal manifestations including myalgias, arthralgias, arthritis, and fibromyalgia occur in 31% of patients with hepatitis C virus (HCV) infection. Polyarthralgias may occur in 9% of patients while frank arthritis was reported in only 4% (129). No consistent pattern of joint involvement has been described although patients with HCV-related mixed cryoglobulinemia typically have intermittent monarticular or pauciarticular medium or large joint involvement (130). Erosive disease has not been described. Etiopathogenesis of HCV-associated arthritis remains unclear. Interferon-α may improve rheumatic symptoms but incompletely.

The most common retroviral infection associated arthritis is HIV-1 (131). Arthritis is characterized as asymmetric, large joint involvement characteristic of spondyloarthropathies but not associated with HLA-B27. Humans infected with human T cell leukemia virus (HTLV)-I may develop a polyarthritis resembling rheumatoid arthritis (132). Transgenic mice bearing HTLV-I genes have developed inflammatory polyarthritis (133).

Other viruses that may infrequently produce acute joint inflammation include Epstein-Barr virus (134), varicella virus

(135), mumps virus (136), coxsackievirus B (137), herpes simplex virus type 1, and cytomegalovirus (138). The six arthropod-borne alpha viruses (chikungunya, o'nyong-nyong, Sindbis, Mayaro, Barmah Forest, and Ross River) produce distinct febrile polyarthritis syndromes in endemic regions.

MYCOBACTERIAL INFECTIONS

The increased frequency of *Mycobacterium tuberculosis* and some of the other atypical mycobacterial infections has been closely associated with the rise in prevalence of HIV infections. Similar to fungal infections, mycobacterial involvement of bone and joints is typically insidious, evolves slowly, and is often not associated with systemic symptoms.

Bone and joint involvement occurs in approximately 2% of all cases of tuberculosis (139). Osteoarticular involvement typically develops secondary to hematogenous and lymphatic dissemination of tuberculosis, but local extension from an infected site may occur. Initial osteoarticular infection is often silent and remains dormant for a variable time before active symptoms develop. Tuberculosis has a predilection for the axial skeleton and weight-bearing joints, but case reports of numerous other joints, bursae, or tendons exist. Infection of vertebral disk space and the anterior vertebral bodies in the lower thoracic and upper lumbar regions, also known as Pott's disease, account for 50% to 60% of musculoskeletal tuberculosis (140). Progressive infection results in disk space narrowing and anterior vertebral body collapse, producing kyphosis. Paravertebral abscesses and neurologic compromise may complicate spinal tuberculosis. Peripheral arthritis is usually monarticular and involves, in order of decreasing frequency, the knee, hip, and ankle (141). The monarthritis is clinically indistinguishable from other forms of chronic infection or chronic inflammatory arthropathies such as the seronegative spondyloarthropathies or rheumatoid arthritis. Poncet's disease, an aseptic, reactive inflammatory polyarthritis involving large joints, occurs concomitantly with active pulmonary infection. Its pathogenesis may be secondary to immunologic cross-reactivity between components of *M. tuberculosis* heat shock protein and articular cartilage (140).

Index of suspicion must be high in patients with acute or persistent monarthritis with or without prior history of tuberculosis or other risk factors for atypical infections. Chest x-rays may reveal evidence of pulmonary disease in 50% of cases, but only 20% will have active disease. Purified protein derivative test results will be positive 90% of the time (140). Synovial fluid analysis is variably inflammatory, with synovial fluid leukocytes averaging 10,000 to 20,000/mm^3 but ranging from 1,000 to 100,000/mm^3 (142). Synovial fluid acid-fast stain is positive in only 20%, while synovial fluid cultures are positive in 80%; the highest yield is synovial tissue biopsy smears and cultures, ranging from 70% to 95% (142). Biopsies often reveal caseating or noncaseating granulomatous synovitis, but nonspecific inflammatory changes are reported as well. Radiographs of late-stage peripheral joint infection may reveal subchondral erosions before articular cartilage narrowing develops. Computed tomographic scans are the most accurate imaging technique for visualizing the posterior vertebral elements; magnetic resonance imaging is most useful for delineating soft tissue or extradural involvement (143).

The U.S. Food and Drug Administration has approved direct amplification tests (DAT) using polymerase chain reaction (PCR) for *Mycobacterium tuberculosis* in the diagnosis of pulmonary tuberculosis in acid-fast positive sputum samples. However, the utility of DAT in osteoarticular tuberculosis remains to be clarified since specificity was approximately 83% in the specimens tested (144).

Chemotherapy is the primary form of treatment for osteoarticular tuberculosis (refer to Chapter 34). Extrapulmonary tuberculosis treatment is identical to regimens for pulmonary tuberculosis. A 6-month course of combination therapy with isoniazide (INH), rifampin, and pyrazinamide for the first 2 months followed by INH and rifampin for the remaining 4 months is recommended for immunocompetent patients, and the duration can be extended to a 12-month course in immunosuppressed patients. At this time, no reports of skeletal multidrug-resistant *M. tuberculosis* exist. Surgical débridement is a necessary adjunct to chemotherapy if neurologic compromise, spinal instability, large abscesses, proliferative pannus, or loose bodies in peripheral joints develop.

Atypical mycobacterial skeletal infections are rare and primarily involve tendon sheaths and bursae; less commonly, they cause monarthritis of wrist, finger, and knee joints. The pathogenesis is usually through percutaneous inoculation of atypical mycobacteria, which are ubiquitous in soil, water, or animals. Hematogenous seeding is rare and usually occurs in the immunocompromised host. The most common organisms include *Mycobacterium marinum*, *Mycobacterium avium-intracellulare*, and *Mycobacterium kansasii*. *M. marinum* typically involves the metacarpophalangeal, proximal interphalangeal, and wrist joints or tendon sheaths of healthy individuals with vocational or avocational contact with fish or water activities. *M. avium-intracellulare* similarly involves the tenosynovia or bursae and rarely involves bones and joints. *M. kansasii* typically infects joints with preexisting abnormalities or immunocompromised hosts (145). Case reports of other mycobacterial infections have included *Mycobacterium haemophilum*, *Mycobacterium fortuitum*, *Mycobacterium chelonae*, and *Mycobacterium terrae* (146,147).

Diagnosis of atypical mycobacterial infection is based on isolation of the organism from synovial fluid or tissue samples. Histologic appearance is similar to that of *M. tuberculosis* infection. The sensitivity of granulomata on pathologic examination was 60%, whereas that of acid-fast staining was only 30% (148). PCR-based DAT for atypical mycobacterium has been reported, but application of these techniques to clinical practice remains unclear. Treatment is primarily with combined chemotherapeutic agents (refer to Chapter 34). Surgical débridement or excision is often necessary.

REFERENCES

1. Riegels-Nielson P, Frimodt-Moller N, Jensen JS. Rabbit model of septic arthritis. *Acta Orthop Scand* 1987;58:14.
2. Goldenberg DL, Reed JI. Bacterial arthritis. *N Engl J Med* 1985;312:764.
3. Dubost JJ, Fis I, Denis P, et al. Polyarticular septic arthritis. *Medicine (Baltimore)* 1993;72:296.
4. Gardner GC, Weisman MH. Pyarthrosis in patients with rheumatoid arthritis: a report of 13 cases and a review of the literature from the past 40 years. *Am J Med* 1990;88:503.
5. Cooper C, Cawley MI. Bacterial arthritis in an English health district: a 10 year review. *Ann Rheum Dis* 1986;45:458.
6. Cooper C, Cawley MI. Bacterial arthritis in the elderly. *Gerontology* 1986;32:222.
7. Newman ED, Davis DE, Harrington TM. Septic arthritis due to gram-negative bacilli: Older patients with good outcome. *J Rheumatol* 1988;15:659.
8. Mateo Soria L, Nolla Sole JM, Rozadilla Sacanell A, et al. Infectious arthritis in patients with rheumatoid arthritis. *Ann Rheum Dis* 1992;51:402.
9. Smith JW, Piercy EA. Infectious arthritis. *Clin Infect Dis* 1995;20:225.
10. Baker DG, Schumacher HR. Acute monoarthritis. *N Engl J Med* 1993;329:1013.
11. Mikhail IS, Alarcon GS. Nongonococcal bacterial arthritis. *Rheum Dis Clin North Am* 1993;19:311.
12. Ajemian E, Andrews L, Hryb K, et al. Hospital acquired infections after arthroscopic knee surgery. A probable environmental source. *Am J Infect Control* 1987;15:159.

13. D'Angelo GL, Ogilvie-Harris DJ. Septic arthritis following arthroscopy with cost/benefit analysis of antibiotic prophylaxis. *Arthroscopy* 1988;4:10.
14. Toye B, Thomson J, Karsh J. *Staphylococcus epidermis* septic arthritis post arthroscopy. *Clin Exp Rheumatol* 1987;5:165.
15. Zimmermann B, Lally EV, Liu NY. Infectious agents and the musculoskeletal system. In: Noble J, Greene H, Levinson W, et al., eds. *Primary care and general medicine*, 2nd ed. St. Louis: Mosby-Year Book, 1996:1186–1199.
16. Sharp JT, Lidsky MD, Duffy J, et al. Infectious arthritis. *Arch Intern Med* 1979;139:1125.
17. Espersen F, Frimodt-Moller, Rosdahl VT, et al. Changing pattern of bone and joint infections due to *Staphylococcus aureus*: study of cases of bacteremia in Denmark, 1959–1988. *Rev Infect Dis* 1991;13:347.
18. Ang-Fonte GZ, Rozboril MB, Thompson GR. Changes in nongonococcal septic arthritis: drug abuse and methicillin-resistant *Staphylococcus aureus*. *Arthritis Rheum* 1985;28:210.
19. Belzunegui J, DeDois JR, Intxausti JJ, et al. Septic arthritis caused by *Stenotrophomonos maltophilia* in a patient with acquired immunodeficiency syndrome [Letter]. *Clin Exp Rheumatol* 2000;18:265.
20. Hale BB, Rosenblatt JE, Fitzgerald RH Jr. Anaerobic septic arthritis and osteomyelitis. *Orthop Clin North Am* 1984;15:505.
21. Mahowald ML. Animal models of infectious arthritis. *Clin Rheum Dis* 1986;12:403.
22. Mahowald ML, Peterson J, Raskind DA, et al. Antigen-induced experimental septic arthritis in rabbits after intraarticular injection of *Staphylococcus aureus*. *J Infect Dis* 1986;54:273.
23. Esterhai JL Jr, Gelb I. Adult septic arthritis. *Orthop Clin North Am* 1991;22:503.
24. Riegels-Nielson P, Frimodt-Moller N, Sorensen M, et al. Antibiotic treatment insufficient for established septic arthritis. *Staphylococcus aureus* experiments in rabbits. *Acta Orthop Scand* 1989;60:113.
25. Schmid FH. New developments in bacterial arthritis. *Bull Rheum Dis* 1992;41:1.
26. Goldenberg DL. The evaluation of patients with nongonococcal bacterial arthritis. In: Espinoza L, Goldenberg DL, Arnett FC, et al., eds. *Infections in the rheumatic diseases: a comprehensive review of microbial relations to rheumatic diseases*. Orlando, FL: Grune & Stratton, 1988:9.
27. Ho G Jr. Bacterial arthritis. *Curr Opin Rheumatol* 1992;4:509.
28. Finals RS. Polyarthritis and fever. *N Engl J Med* 1994;330:769.
29. Ho G Jr. Bacterial arthritis. *Curr Opin Rheumatol* 2001;13:310–314.
30. Sequeira W, Swedler WI, Skosey JL. Septic arthritis in childhood. *Ann Emerg Med* 1985;14:1185.
31. Goldenberg DL. Pathophysiology—nongonococcal bacterial arthritis. In: Espinoza L, Goldenberg DL, Arnett FC, et al., eds. *Infections in the rheumatic diseases: a comprehensive review of microbial relations to rheumatic diseases*. Orlando, FL: Grune & Stratton, 1988:3.
32. Yoshikawa TT. Geriatric infectious diseases: an emerging problem. *J Am Geriatr Soc* 1983;31:34.
33. Nolla JM, Gomez-Vaquero C, Fiter J, et al. Pyarthrosis in patients with rheumatoid arthritis: a detailed analysis of 10 cases and a literature review. *Semin Arthritis Rheum* 2000;30:121–126.
34. Von Essen R, Savolainen HA. Bacterial infection following intraarticular injection. A brief review. *Scand J Rheumatol* 1989;18:7.
35. Goldenberg DL. Infectious arthritis complicating rheumatoid arthritis and other chronic rheumatic disorders. *Arthritis Rheum* 1989;32:496.
36. Epstein JH, Zimmermann B III, Ho G Jr. Polyarticular septic arthritis. *J Rheumatol* 1986;13:1105.
37. Ho G Jr. Bacterial arthritis. In: McCarty DJ, Koopman WJ, eds. *Arthritis and allied conditions: a textbook of rheumatology*, 12th ed, Vol. 2. Philadelphia: Lea & Febiger, 1993:2003–2023.
38. Peltola H, Vahvanen V. Acute purulent arthritis in children. *Scand J Infect Dis* 1983;15:75.
39. Wang CH, Huang FY. Septic arthritis in early infancy. *Acta Paediatr Sin* 1990;31:69.
40. Welkon CH, Long SS, Fisher MC, et al. Pyogenic arthritis in infants and children: a review of 95 cases. *Pediatr Infect Dis* 1986;5:669.
41. Fink CW, Nelson JD. Septic arthritis and osteomyelitis in children. *Clin Rheum Dis* 1986;12:423.
42. Deshpande PG, Wagle SU, Mehta SD, et al. Neonatal osteomyelitis and septic arthritis. *Ind Pediatr* 1990;27:453.
43. Morrissy RT. Bone and joint infection in the neonate. *Pediatr Ann* 1989;18:33.
44. Spesier JC, Moore TL, Osborn TG, et al. Changing trends in pediatric septic arthritis. *Semin Arthritis Rheum* 1985;15:132.
45. Blackburn WD Jr. Gram-negative septic arthritis. In: Espinoza L, Goldenberg DL, Arnett FC, et al., eds. *Infections in the rheumatic diseases: a comprehensive review of microbial relations to rheumatic diseases*. Orlando, FL: Grune & Stratton, 1988:21.
46. Blackburn WD, Alarcon GS. Prosthetic joint infections: a role for prophylaxis. A review. *Arthritis Rheum* 1991;34:110.
47. Inman RD, Gallegos KV, Brause BD, et al. Clinical and microbial features of prosthetic joint infection. *Am J Med* 1984;77:47.
48. Kleshinski J, Georgiades GM, Duggan JM. Group C streptococcus infection in a prosthetic joint. *South Med J* 2000;93:1217–1220.
49. American Dental Association, American Academy of Orthopaedic Surgeons Advisory Statement. Antibiotic prophylaxis for dental patients with total joint replacement. *JADA* 1997;128:1004–1008.
50. Tong DC, Rothwell BR. Antibiotic prophylaxis in dentistry; a review and practice recommendations. *JADA* 2000;131:366–374.
51. Brancos MA, Peris P, Miro JM, et al. Septic arthritis in heroin addicts. *Semin Arthritis Rheum* 1991;21:81.
52. Chandrasekas PH, Narula AP. Bone and joint infections in intravenous drug abusers. *Rev Infect Dis* 1986;8:904.
53. Pollack MS. Staphylococcal mediastinitis due to sternoclavicular pyarthrosis. CT appearance. *J Comput Assist Tomogr* 1990;14:924.
54. Wohlgethan JR, Newberg AH, Reed JI. The risk of abscess from sternoclavicular septic arthritis. *J Rheumatol* 1988;15:1302.
55. Hodgson BF. Pyogenic sacroiliac joint infection. *Clin Orthop* 1989;246:146.
56. Bleasel JF, York JR, Rickard KA. Septic arthritis in human immunodeficiency virus infected haemophiliacs. *Br J Rheumatol* 1990;29:494.
57. Steinberg AD Jr. Principles in the use of immunosuppressive agents. In: Schumacher HR, ed. *Primer on the rheumatic diseases*, 9th ed. Atlanta: Arthritis Foundation, 1988:288.
58. Zimmermann B III, Erickson AD, Mikolich DJ. Septic acromioclavicular arthritis and osteomyelitis in a patient with acquired immunodeficiency syndrome. *Arthritis Rheum* 1989;32:1175.
59. Berman A, Espinoza LR, Diaz JD, et al. Rheumatic manifestations of human immunodeficiency virus infection. *Am J Med* 1988;85:59.
60. Calabrese LH. The rheumatic manifestations of infection with human immunodeficiency virus. *Semin Arthritis Rheum* 1989;18:225.
61. Fernandez SM, Cardenal A, Balsa A, et al. Rheumatic manifestations in 556 patients with human immunodeficiency virus infection. *Semin Arthritis Rheum* 1991;21:30.
62. Goldenberg DL. Gram-positive, anaerobic, and mixed bacterial arthritis. In: Espinoza L, Goldenberg DL, Arnett FC, et al. *Infections in the rheumatic diseases: a comprehensive review of microbial relations to rheumatic diseases*. Orlando, FL: Grune & Stratton, 1988:17.
63. Louthrenoo W, Ostrov BE, Park YS, et al. Pseudoseptic arthritis: an unusual presentation of neuropathic arthropathy. *Ann Rheum Dis* 1991;50:717.
64. Singleton JD, West SG, Nordstrom DM. "Pseudoseptic" arthritis complicating rheumatoid arthritis. A report of six cases. *J Rheumatol* 1991;18:1319.
65. Shmerling RH, Delbanco TL, Tosteson AN, et al. Synovial fluid tests. What should be ordered? *JAMA* 1990;264:1009.
66. Mitchell M, Howard B, Haller J, et al. Septic arthritis. *Radiol Clin North Am* 1988;26:1295.
67. Kim EE, Haynie TP, Podoloff DA, et al. Radionuclide imaging in the evaluation of osteomyelitis and septic arthritis. *Crit Rev Diagn Imaging* 1989;29:257.
68. Hatfield MK, Gross BH, Glazer GM, et al. Computed tomography of the sternum and its articulations. *Skel Radiol* 1984;11:197.
69. Morgan GJ, Schlegelmilch JG, Spiegel PK. Early diagnosis of septic arthritis of the sacroiliac joint by use of computerized tomography. *J Rheumatol* 1981;18:979.
70. Stoller DW, Genant HK, Helms CA, eds. *Magnetic resonance imaging in orthopaedics and rheumatology*. Philadelphia: JB Lippincott, 1989:220–229, 239–243, 259–262.
71. Hickey NAJ, White PG. Septic arthritis of a lumbar facet joint causing multiple abscesses. *Clin Radiol* 2000;55:481–483.
72. Fuchs HA. Polyarticular pseudosepsis in rheumatoid arthritis. *South Med J* 1992;85:381.
73. Broy SB, Schmid FR. A comparison of medical drainage (needle aspiration) and surgical drainage (arthrotomy or arthroscopy) in the initial treatment of infected joints. *Clin Rheum Dis* 1986;12:501.
74. Rosenthal J, Bole GG, Robinson WD. Acute non-gonococcal infectious arthritis. Evaluation of risk factors, therapy, and outcome. *Arthritis Rheum* 1980;23:889.
75. Broy SB, Stulberg SD, Schmid FR. The role of arthroscopy in the diagnosis and management of the septic joint. *Clin Rheum Dis* 1986;12:489.
76. Ohl MD, Kean JR, Steensen RN. Arthroscopic treatment of septic arthritic knees in children and adolescents. *Orthop Rev* 1991;20:894.
77. Parisien JS, Shaffer B. Arthroscopic management of pyarthrosis. *Clin Orthop* 1992;275:243.
78. Theiry JA. Arthroscopic drainage in septic arthritides of the knee: a multicenter study. *Arthroscopy* 1989;5:65.
79. Sanford JP. *Guide to antimicrobial therapy 1992*. Dallas: Antimicrobial Therapy, 1992.
80. Symonds J, Geddes AM. Cephalosporins in gram-positive infections. *Drugs* 1987;34(suppl 2):121.
81. Dickie AS. Current concepts in the management of infection in bones and joints. *Drugs* 1986;32:458.
82. Cucurull E, Espinoza LR. Gonococcal arthritis. *Rheum Dis Clin North Am* 1998;24:305–322.
83. Scopelitis E, Martinez-Osuna P. Gonococcal arthritis. *Rheum Dis Clin North Am* 1993;19:363.
84. Fink CW. Gonococcal arthritis in children. *JAMA* 1965;194:123.
85. Shapira O, Bar-On E, Sagiv S, et al. Disseminated gonococcal infection. *J Am Geriatr Soc* 1990;38:678.
86. Rowe IF, Forster SM, Seifert MH, et al. Rheumatologic lesions in individuals with human immunodeficiency virus infection. *Q J Med* 1989;272:1167.
87. Strogin IS, Kale SA, Raymond MK, et al. Unusual presentation of gonococcal arthritis in an HIV positive patient. *Ann Rheum Dis* 1991;50:572.
88. Holmes KK, Counts GW, Beaty HN. Disseminated gonococcal infection. *Ann Intern Med* 1971;74:979.
89. Masi AT, Eisenstein BI. Disseminated gonococcal infection and gonococcal arthritis (GCA). II. Clinical manifestations, diagnosis, complications, treatment, and prevention. *Semin Arthritis Rheum* 1981;10:173.

90. Keiser H, Ruben FL, Wolinsky E, et al. Clinical forms of gonococcal arthritis. *N Engl J Med* 1968;279:234.
91. Zbella EA, Deppe G, Elrad H. Gonococcal arthritis in pregnancy. *Obstet Gynecol Surg* 1984;39:8.
92. Wilson J, Zaman AG, Simmon AV. Gonococcal arthritis complicated by acute pericarditis and pericardial effusion. *Br Heart J* 1990;63:134.
93. Peterson BH, Lee TJ, Snyderman R, et al. *Neisseria meningitides* and *Neisseria gonorrhoeae* bacteremia associated with C₆, C₇, or C₈ deficiency. *Ann Intern Med* 1979;90:917.
94. O'Brien JP, Goldenberg DL, Rice PA. Disseminated gonococcal infection: a prospective analysis of 49 patients and a review of the pathophysiology and immune mechanisms. *Medicine (Baltimore)* 1983;62:395.
95. Grippo GN, Genovese MN, Piccora R. Monarthric gonococcal arthritis involving the calcaneocuboid joint. *J Am Podiatr Med Assoc* 1990;80:91.
96. Brogadir SP, Schimmer BM, Myers AR. Spectrum of the gonococcal arthritis-dermatitis syndrome. *Semin Arthritis Rheum* 1979;8:177.
97. Lee AH, Chin AE, Ramanujam T, et al. Gonococcal septic arthritis of the hip. *J Rheumatol* 1991;18:1932.
98. Koss PG. Disseminated gonococcal infection. The tenosynovitis-dermatitis and suppurative arthritis syndromes. *Cleve Clin Q* 1985;52:161.
99. Gonzalez-Juanatey C, Gonzalez-Gay MA, Llorca J, et al. Rheumatic manifestations of infective endocarditis in non-addicts: a 12 year study. *Medicine* 2001;80:9–19.
100. Wise CM, Morris CR, Wasilauskas BL, et al. Gonococcal arthritis in an era of increasing penicillin resistance. *Arch Intern Med* 1994;154:2690.
101. Gelfand SC, Masi AT, Gardia-Kutzbach A. Spectrum of gonococcal arthritis. Evidence for sequential stages and clinical subgroups. *J Rheumatol* 1975;2:83.
102. Jaffe HW, Biddle JW, Johnson SR, et al. Infections due to penicillinase producing *Neisseria gonorrhoeae* in the United States 1976–1980. *J Infect Dis* 1981;144:191.
103. Centers for Disease Control and Prevention. Sentinel surveillance for antimicrobial resistance in *Neisseria gonorrhoeae*—United States 1988–1991. *MMWR* 1993;43(NSS-3):29.
104. Faruki H, Kohmescher RN, McKinney WP, et al. A community-based outbreak of infection with penicillin-resistant *Neisseria gonorrhoeae* not producing penicillinase (chromosomally mediated resistance). *N Engl J Med* 1985;313:607.
105. Canoso JJ, Barza M. Soft tissue infections. *Rheum Dis Clin North Am* 1993;19:293.
106. Zimmermann B 3d, Mikolich DJ, Ho G Jr. Septic bursitis. *Semin Arthritis Rheum* 1995;24:391.
107. Ho G, Su EY. Antibiotic therapy of septic bursitis. *Arthritis Rheum* 1981;24:905.
108. Cuellar ML, Silveira LH, Citera G, et al. Other fungal arthritides. *Rheum Dis Clin North Am* 1993;19:439.
109. MacDonald PB, Black GB, MacKenzie R. Orthopedic manifestations of blastomycosis. *J Bone Joint Surg Am* 1990;72:860.
110. Cuende E, Barbadillo C, E-Mazzucchelli R, et al. *Candida* arthritis in adult patients who are not intravenous drug addicts: report of three cases and review of the literature. *Semin Arthritis Rheum* 1993;22:224.
111. Silveira LH, Cuellar ML, Citera G, et al. *Candida* arthritis. *Rheum Dis Clin North Am* 1993;19:427.
112. Kushwaha VP, Shaw BA, Gerardi JAL. Musculoskeletal coccidiomycosis: a review of 25 cases. *Clin Orthop* 1996;332:190.
113. Rex JH, Walsh TJ, Sobel JD, et al. Practice guidelines for the treatment of candidiasis. *Clin Infect Dis* 2000;30:662.
114. Chapman SW, Bradsher RW, Campbell GD, et al. Practice guidelines for the management of patients with blastomycosis. *Clin Infect Dis* 2000;30:679.
115. Galgiani JN, Ampel NM, Catanzaro A, et al. Practice guidelines for the treatment of coccidioidomycosis. *Clin Infect Dis* 2000;30:658.
116. Kauffman CA, Hajjeh R, Chapman SW, et al. Practice guidelines for the management of patients with sporotrichosis. *Clin Infect Dis* 2000;30:684.
117. Saag MS, Graybill RJ, Larsen RA, et al. Practice guidelines for the management of cryptococcal disease. *Clin Infect Dis* 2000;30:710.
118. Tingle AJ, Mitchell LA, Grace M, et al. Randomized double-blind placebo controlled study on adverse effects of rubella immunization in seronegative women. *Lancet* 1997;349:1277.
119. Howson CP, Katz M, Johnston RB, et al. Chronic arthritis after rubella vaccination. *Clin Infect Dis* 1992;15:307.
120. Mitchell LA, Tingle AJ, Shukin R, et al. Chronic rubella vaccine-associated arthropathy. *Arch Intern Med* 1993;153:2268.
121. Nocton JJ, Miller LC, Tucker LB, et al. Human parvovirus B19–associated arthritis in children. *J Pediatr* 1993;122:186.
122. Torok T. Parvovirus B19 and human disease. *Adv Intern Med* 1992;37:431.
123. Woolf A, Campion G, et al. Clinical manifestations of human parvovirus B19 infection in adults. *Arch Intern Med* 1989;149:1153.
124. Speyer I, Breedveld FC, Dijkmans BAC, et al. Human parvovirus B19 infection is not followed by inflammatory joint disease during long-term follow-up: a retrospective study of 54 patients. *Clin Exp Rheumatol* 1998;16:576.
125. Naides SJ. Rheumatic manifestations of parvovirus B19 infection. *Rheum Dis Clin North Am* 1998;24:457.
126. Foto F, Saag KG, Scharosch LL, et al. Parvovirus B19–specific DNA in bone marrow from B19 arthropathy patients: evidence for B19 virus persistence. *J Infect Dis* 1993;167:744.
127. Cassinotti P, Siegl G, Michel BA, et al. Presence and significance of human parvovirus B19 DNA in synovial membranes and bone marrow from patients with arthritis of unknown origin. *J Med Virol* 1998;56:199.
128. Takahashi Y, Murai C, Shibata S, et al. Human parvovirus B19 as a causative agent for rheumatoid arthritis. *Proc Natl Acad Sci USA* 1998;95:8227.
129. Buskila D, Shnaider A, Neumann L. Musculoskeletal manifestations and autoantibody profile in 90 hepatitis C infected Israeli patients. *Semin Arthritis Rheum* 1998;28:107.
130. Rivera J, Farcia-Monforte A, Pineda A, et al. Arthritis in patient with chronic hepatitis C virus infection. *J Rheumatol* 1999;26:420.
131. Itescu S. Adult immunodeficiency and rheumatic disease. *Rheum Dis Clin North Am* 1996;22:53.
132. Nishioka K, Nakajima T, Hasunuma T, et al. Rheumatic manifestation of human leukemia virus infection. *Rheum Dis Clin North Am* 1993;19:489.
133. Iwakura Y, Saijo S, Kioka Y, et al. Autoimmunity induction by human T cell leukemia virus type 1 in trangenic mice that develop chronic inflammatory arthropathy resembling rheumatoid arthritis in humans. *J Immunol* 1995;155:1588.
134. Ray GC, Gall EP, Minnich LL, et al. Acute polyarthritis associated with active Epstein-Barr virus infection. *JAMA* 1982;248:2990.
135. DiLiberti JH, Bartel SJ, Humphrey TR, et al. Acute monoarticular arthritis in association with varicella: a case report. *Clin Pediatr* 1977;16:663.
136. Gordon SC, Lauter CB. Mumps arthritis: a review of the literature. *Rev Infect Dis* 1984;6:338.
137. David JJ, Dietz FR, Jones MM. Coxsackie-B monarthritis with hepatitis. *J Bone Joint Surg Am* 1993;75:1685.
138. Friedman HM, Pincus T, Gibilisco P, et al. Acute monoarticular arthritis caused by herpes simplex virus and cytomegalovirus. *Am J Med* 1980;69:241.
139. Meier JL. Mycobacterial and fungal infections of bone and joints. *Curr Opin Rheum* 1994;6:408.
140. Kramer N, Rosenstein E. Rheumatologic manifestations of tuberculosis. *Bull Rheum Dis* 1998;46(3):5.
141. Evanchick CC, Davis DE, Harrington TM. Tuberculosis of peripheral joints: an often missed diagnosis. *J Rheumatol* 1986;13:187.
142. Garrido G, Gomez-Reino JJ, Fernandez-Dapica P. A review of peripheral tuberculous arthritis. *Semin Arthritis Rheum* 1988;18:142.
143. Hoffman EB, Crosier JH, Cremin BJ. Imaging in children with spinal tuberculosis: a comparison of radiography, computed tomography, and magnetic resonance imaging. *J Bone Joint Surg Br* 1993;75:233.
144. Harrington J. The evolving role of direct amplification tests in diagnosing osteoarticular infections caused by mycobacteria and fungi. *Curr Opin Rheum* 1999;11:289.
145. Glickstein SL, Nashel DJ. *Mycobacterium kansasii* septic arthritis complicating rheumatic disease: case report and review of the literature. *Semin Arthritis Rheum* 1987;16:231.
146. Wallace RJ, O'Brien R, Glassroth J, et al. Diagnosis and treatment of disease caused by nontuberculous mycobacteria. *Am Rev Respir Dis* 1990;142:940.
147. Strauss WL, Ostroff SM, Jernigan DB, et al. Clinical and epidemiologic characteristics of *Mycobacterium haemophilum*, an emerging pathogen in immunocompromised patients. *Ann Intern Med* 1994;120:118.
148. Kozin S, Bishop A. Atypical mycobacterial infections of the upper extremity. *J Hand Surg* 1994;19:480.

Eye and Paranasal Sinuses

CHAPTER 146
Infections of the Eye

Jules Baum and Michael Barza

INFECTIONS OF THE ANTERIOR EYE AND ADNEXAE

Most ocular infections involve tissues that are visible to the naked eye, and many have a characteristic appearance that suggests the diagnosis. Additional information may be gained by viewing the external ocular structure with magnification. Whereas the ophthalmologist routinely uses a slit lamp for this purpose,

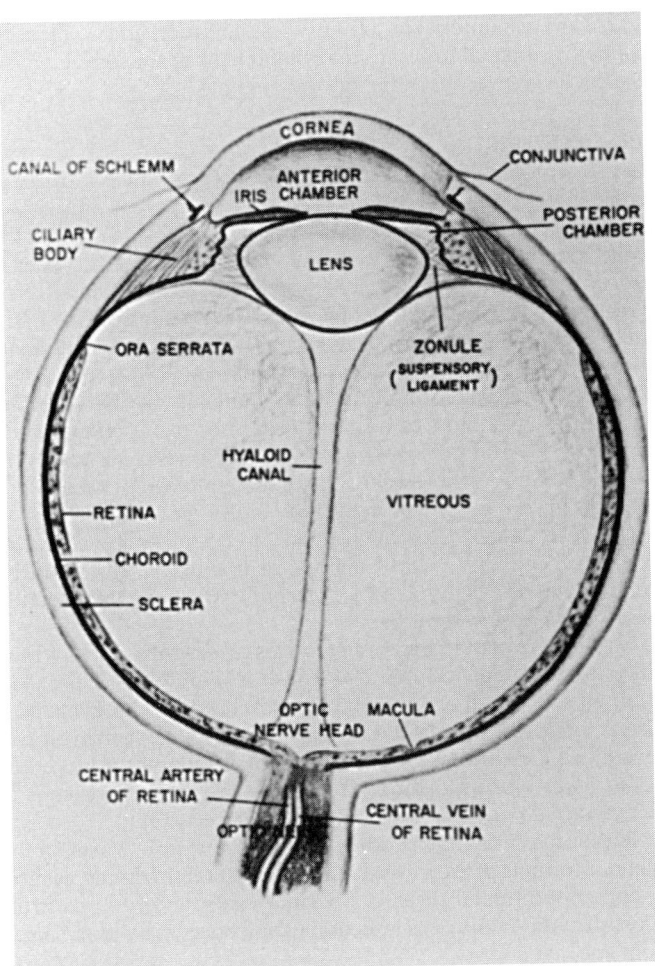

Figure 146.1. Schematic diagram of the eye. (From Barza M, Baum J. Treatment of bacterial infections of the eye. *Curr Clin Top Infect Dis* 1980;158: 159, with permission.)

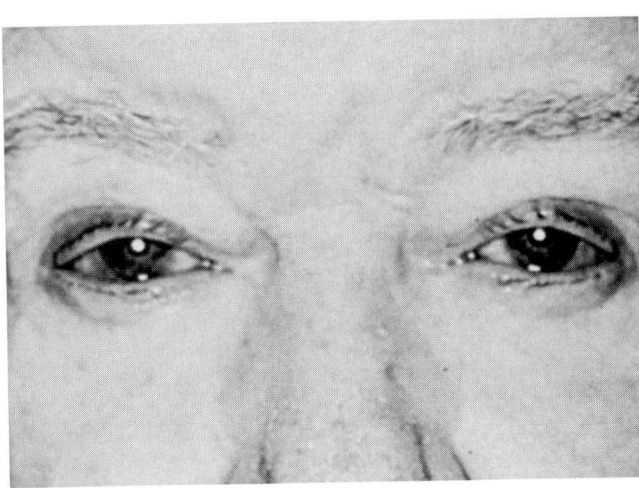

Figure 146.2. Staphylococcal blepharitis. Note erythema of lid margins.

other physicians may use a penlight and hand magnifier or loupe to see, for example, the molluscum nodule partially concealed by the eyelash, follicles on the palpebral conjunctiva suggestive of viral or chlamydial conjunctivitis, or the characteristic dendrite of herpes simplex epithelial keratitis after staining with fluorescein. This chapter provides an overview of a variety of infections of the eyelid, conjunctiva, cornea, and lacrimal apparatus and also of the deeper structures (endophthalmitis). For a more detailed treatment, the reader may consult more comprehensive publications (see refs. 1–4). Figure 146.1 provides a schematic diagram of the structure of the eye for purposes of orientation.

Eyelid Infections

BACTERIAL INFECTIONS

Staphylococcal blepharitis (Fig. 146.2) is among the most common bacterial infections of the eyelids. Because coagulase-negative staphylococci may be grown in cultures from the lids and conjunctiva of as many as 70% of normal persons and *Staphylococcus aureus* may be cultured from these sites in up to 40% of normal persons (5), it has been difficult to establish the role of these species in the disease. The diagnosis is made on clinical grounds. The disease rarely may be acute, but characteris-

tically it is chronic and bilateral, lasting months to years if not effectively treated. It is often seen in association with rosacea, seborrheic blepharitis, or keratoconjunctivitis sicca. The patient usually has only mild discomfort. The eyelid margins of patients with chronic symptoms are diffusely injected, and flakes of keratinized epithelium cling to the lashes. Fibrin exudate is commonly seen at the base of the lashes, often forming a characteristic "collarette." Eyelid margins may be thickened and irregular with telangiectasia, misdirected lashes, and sparse and whitened (poliosis) lashes.

Treatment consists of topical antibiotic applications and local hygiene, in some instances for many months. Compliance for this long period is often difficult to obtain, but it is important. Bacitracin ophthalmic ointment is applied to the lid margin with a cotton-tipped applicator after dried exudate has been wiped off. Depending on the severity of the condition, bacitracin may be applied two to four times a day initially for 1 to 2 weeks; the frequency may then be reduced gradually to once a night at bedtime for 4 to 8 weeks. Treatment should be continued for 1 month after all signs of inflammation have disappeared (6). If antibiotic therapy is discontinued too soon after a supposed cure, the process may be reactivated. Erythromycin or gentamicin ophthalmic ointment may be used if clinical resistance or a reaction to bacitracin develops. Vancomycin eyedrops, 1%, may be used when methicillin-resistant staphylococci are encountered, but the eyedrops must be formulated individually because there is no such commercial product. Topical ciprofloxacin or ofloxacin, 0.3%, or levofloxacin, 0.5% eyedrops, may be of use in this circumstance.

When staphylococcal blepharitis is seen in association with rosacea, oral tetracycline is suggested for treatment, because the tetracyclines are thought to be concentrated in the meibomian glands. An initial dose of 250 mg four times daily for 1 to 2 weeks can be reduced to 250 mg once daily for some months, until it is found by trial and error that treatment can be discontinued without reactivation of the disease. Doxycycline, 100 mg orally once or twice daily, is another option. Lid hygiene is an important component of therapy. Moist cotton-tipped applicators are used to keep the eyelids clean and to apply a mild baby shampoo twice a week to the base of the eyelashes. The contents of congested meibomian glands should be expressed periodically by compressing the lid margins between the tips of two applicators, one placed on the inner and one on the outer lid margin, after application of a drop of topical anesthesia. Hordeolum (stye), acute meibomitis, and chalazion, which may occur independently or in association with staphylococcal blepharitis, are described in the following sections.

HORDEOLUM AND CHALAZION

Hordeola (styes) are of two types. An external hordeolum, the more common variety, is a staphylococcal microabscess of one of the glands of Zeis, a series of superficial sebaceous glands at the base of the eyelashes. An acute infection produces localized pain, redness, and swelling. Within a day or two, the 1- to 2-mm milk-white abscess points at the lid margin. Almost invariably, it ruptures and drains spontaneously, but resolution and relief of pain are hastened if the lesion is pierced with a sterile needle. No antibiotic therapy is required.

An internal hordeolum, a staphylococcal cellulitis-like infection of a meibomian gland, appears clinically as a painful focal area of swelling and induration of the eyelid. The signs and symptoms are more severe than those of a chalazion (see later). Meibomian glands are a series of sebaceous glands whose orifices are visible along the length of the lid margin. We believe, as do others, that acute meibomitis is a better term than internal hordeolum for this minor infection. Because the meibomian glands lie buried in the tarsus, a cartilaginous support of the lid, the abscess of acute meibomitis cannot drain easily, as a stye can. An oral preparation of an antistaphylococcal antibiotic is often used to eradicate the infection.

A chalazion (Fig. 146.3) is a granulomatous nodule that develops in a meibomian gland, often in association with staphylococcal blepharitis. It is not clear why the granuloma forms, but it may be as a response to lipid retained in the gland. Initial mild pain for 24 to 72 hours is followed by the development of a painless lump within the lid. Untreated, 80% of chalazia resolve within a month (7). For those that persist, the commercial preparation of triamcinolone acetonide, 10 mg/mL, is diluted to 5 mg/mL, and 0.1 mL of the dilute solution is injected into the lesion (8). A second injection may be necessary 3 to 7 days later. This treatment eradicates or greatly reduces the size of the nodule in more than one half of cases. Surgical excision may be necessary for lesions that do not respond to corticosteroid injection. Antibiotic treatment is ineffective. Multiple chalazia that develop at different locations in the same lid within a period of several months generally should be treated as if they were staphylococcal blepharitis.

Angular blepharitis is a minor infection of the skin at the lateral canthus. The infection may persist indefinitely without treatment, but it responds rapidly to topical antibiotic therapy. *Moraxella lacunata*, a gram-negative bacillus, had been the major cause, especially among derelicts (9). For reasons that are not clear, *Moraxella* infections are now less common and *S. aureus* is the major cause. Rarely, angular blepharitis is caused by anaerobic bacteria, mycobacteria, or other agents.

VIRAL BLEPHARITIS

Herpes simplex virus, usually type 1, may produce a primary ocular infection in children. It is clinically apparent only 4% of the time. Typically, a cluster of umbilicated vesicles forms on the eyelid together with acute follicular conjunctivitis. The cornea is rarely involved in a primary infection, whereas it is often affected in recurrent disease in adults. The blepharitis usually heals without treatment in 1 to 2 weeks. In severe cases, ulcerative blepharitis and dendritic keratitis may develop. In such instances, acyclovir ophthalmic ointment (not commercially available in the United States) should be administered four or five times daily for 10 days. Alternatively, treatment may consist of acyclovir, 200 to 400 mg four times daily (pediatric solution or tablets), or famciclovir, 250 mg three times daily orally for 10 days.

Varicella-zoster virus may infect the upper or lower eyelid when, respectively, the ophthalmic or maxillary branch of the trigeminal nerve is involved. For treatment, see the later section on varicella-zoster keratitis.

Molluscum contagiosum, a poxvirus disease, produces white, often umbilicated nodules 2 to 3 mm in diameter on the skin of an eyelid. Small lesions may be obscured by the eyelashes. Characteristic cytoplasmic eosinophilic bodies are seen in biopsy specimens. Cryotherapy, curettage, or incision of the nodule sufficient to produce bleeding often cures the infection except in HIV-positive patients, in whom it is often recurrent.

Papillomavirus may produce single or multiple warts on the eyelid. Products of the infection may cause conjunctival injection or corneal epithelial disease. Vaccinia virus, another poxvirus, may infect the eyelid; this infection usually occurs by inoculation from another site.

PARASITIC INFECTIONS

Phthirus pubis, the crab louse, may affect the eye, usually after pubic infestation. The major symptom is itching. The transparent adult lice, which are attached to the lashes, are difficult to see, even with magnification, but the nits (eggs) are more readily visible. A bland ophthalmic ointment such as sterile petrolatum may be applied to smother the lice, and the nits can be removed mechanically. In refractory cases, lindane cream, 1%, may be used cautiously on the eyelid margins as a single application, avoiding contact with the eyes. Family members and sexual contacts should also be examined and, if necessary, treated. Permethrin 5% cream is preferred over lindane for other scabies infections but is irritating to the eyes and should not be used for ocular infection.

FUNGAL INFECTIONS

In warm climates as many as 22% of healthy persons harbor fungi along their eyelid margins (10), yet fungal infections of the eyelids are unusual. Dermatophytes (ringworm) may produce superficial infection of the eyelids. Fungi that produce systemic infection, such as *Candida albicans* and *Blastomyces dermatitidis*, may cause ulcers and granulomata of the lids.

Infections of the Conjunctiva

Clinical features that help to distinguish bacterial, viral, and chlamydial conjunctivitis are presented in Table 146.1, and features that distinguish conjunctivitis from keratitis and iritis are presented in Table 146.2. Conjunctival infections are almost always bilateral. In otherwise healthy patients they are also usually

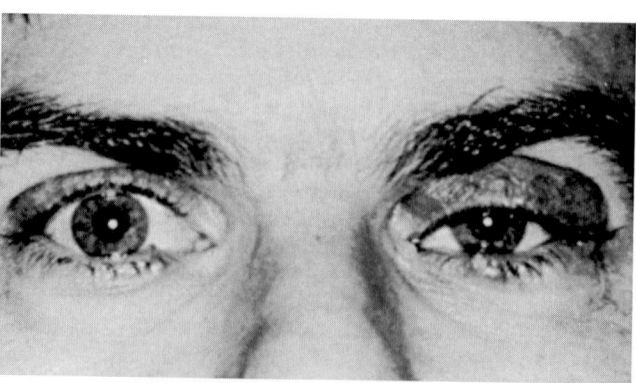

Figure 146.3. Multiple bilateral chalazia.

TABLE 146.1. Features that Distinguish Bacterial from Viral and Chlamydial Conjunctivitis

Feature	Bacterial conjunctivitis	Viral conjunctivitis	Chlamydial conjunctivitis
Conjunctival injection	Moderately severe	Minimal	Absent or minimal
Exudate	Moderate to profuse (polymorphonuclear)	Minimal (usually mononuclear)	Minimal in adults, copious in newborns
Sticking of lids on awakening	Yes	No	Absent in adults, present in newborns
Palpebral conjunctival lesions	Papillae	Follicles	Papillae may be present in adults or newborns, follicles in adults only
Preauricular lymphadenopathy	No	Yes	Present in adults, absent in newborns
Response to antibiotic therapy	Yes	No	Yes
Duration of untreated disease	Up to several weeks	Several weeks	Persistent

Modified from Barza M, Baum J. Ocular infections. *Med Clin North Am* 1983;67:131–152, with permission.

self-limited, except for chlamydial and staphylococcal conjunctivitis.

In developed countries most conjunctival infections are caused by viruses. The most common viral agent of conjunctivitis is adenovirus. The infection usually abates spontaneously within several weeks. Follicles (foci of lymphoid hyperplasia that appear as translucent grains of sand on the palpebral conjunctiva) and preauricular lymphadenopathy are the hallmarks of viral conjunctivitis. If follicular conjunctivitis persists longer than 1 month in adults, and especially if the follicles appear relatively large, chlamydial infection should be suspected. Infants with chlamydial conjunctivitis do not exhibit follicles because their lymphoid system is underdeveloped. Conversely, older children with fever for any reason may develop conjunctival follicles as part of a generalized lymphatic response even in the absence of ocular infection.

Bacterial conjunctivitis produces a papillary rather than a follicular conjunctival response. Papillae appear as opaque grains of sand on the palpebral conjunctiva. With magnification, a central blood vessel is seen in each papilla, whereas blood vessels surround a follicle but none are seen centrally.

Infectious conjunctivitis is usually a bilateral disease and is usually transferred to the second eye via fingers, towels, or other objects. Patients should be cautioned about infecting the other eye and other persons. Adenoviral conjunctivitis is especially contagious.

BACTERIAL CONJUNCTIVITIS

Bacterial conjunctivitis may be classified by the duration of the illness as acute or chronic and by the nature of the exu-

TABLE 146.2. Features that Distinguish Conjunctivitis from Keratitis or Iritis

Feature	Conjunctivitis	Keratitis or iritis
Vision	Normal	May be reduced
Pain	Gritty sensation	Frank pain
Conjunctiva	Diffuse injection	Ciliary flush
Exudate	Minimal to profuse	Usually none
Mattering of lids (dried exudate)	May be present	Absent
Photophobia	Absent	Present
Lacrimation	Usually absent	Present
Pupillary diameter	Normal	Usually small

Modified from Barza M, Baum J. Ocular infections. *Med Clin North Am* 1983;67:131–152, with permission.

date as purulent or mucopurulent. Historically, the names hyperpurulent and purulent conjunctivitis have been used interchangeably, as have the terms acute catarrhal and mucopurulent conjunctivitis.

In this chapter, we use the shorter terms, purulent and mucopurulent. A purulent or mucopurulent discharge and the presence of papillae on the palpebral conjunctiva are the diagnostic signs of bacterial conjunctivitis. The tendency for the eyelids to be stuck together on awakening, which reflects purulence of the exudate, is usually associated with bacterial, not viral, conjunctivitis. Although the grossly visible inflammatory reaction is not a precise indicator from which the cause of conjunctivitis may be inferred, purulent reactions suggest infection by *Neisseria gonorrhoeae* or *Neisseria meningitidis* or chlamydiae in neonates, whereas most other forms of bacterial conjunctivitis are mucopurulent. Chronic conjunctivitis is most often caused by staphylococci or gram-negative bacilli. Chronic conjunctivitis with blepharitis suggests infection by staphylococci or by *M. lacunata*.

Acute Conjunctivitis

Most cases of acute bacterial conjunctivitis are caused by gram-positive cocci, but when the conjunctiva is abnormal as a result of exposure (e.g., thyroid exophthalmos, coma) or keratinization (e.g., after irradiation), gram-negative bacilli may cause infection.

Different pathogens characteristically produce different degrees of purulence in the secretions. Purulent conjunctivitis with copious exudate is most frequently caused by *N. gonorrhoeae* and less commonly by *N. meningitidis*. Gonococcal infection most often appears in newborns, being acquired during passage through the birth canal. The infection becomes clinically apparent 2 to 5 days after birth. The exudate may become trapped beneath swollen eyelids, causing pressure necrosis of the corneal epithelium. Devitalization of the epithelium renders the cornea more prone to infection. Adults acquire purulent gonococcal conjunctivitis through sexual contact.

Mucopurulent conjunctivitis, known to the laity as "pinkeye," is usually caused by *S. aureus, Streptococcus pyogenes, Streptococcus pneumoniae* (in colder climates), or *Haemophilus influenzae* (in warmer climates).

True membranous conjunctivitis is caused by *Corynebacterium diphtheriae* infection but is rarely seen today. Pseudomembranes derived from inflammatory debris and fixed loosely to the palpebral conjunctiva occur in β-hemolytic streptococcal and adenoviral conjunctivitis. Conjunctival petechiae may be seen in conjunctivitis caused by streptococci and *H. influenzae. Haemophilus aegyptius*, a close relative of *H. influenzae*, is the cause of Brazilian hemorrhagic fever; the conjunctivitis antedates the generalized illness by 3 to 15 days (11). Other species of gram-negative bacteria, including *Pseudomonas* and *Escherichia coli,* may produce conjunctivitis, especially when the conjunctiva is abnormal. Such gram-negative infections are sometimes difficult to eradicate.

Chronic Conjunctivitis

Chronic bacterial conjunctivitis is most often caused by coagulase-positive staphylococci. It is frequently associated with staphylococcal blepharitis and at times is accompanied by a noninfectious keratitis. As stated earlier, chronic gram-negative bacillary conjunctivitis is seen in patients with devitalized conjunctiva. *M. lacunata* organisms produce both chronic blepharitis and conjunctivitis, most frequently in derelicts; these infections are rare today. Whereas most organisms that cause conjunctivitis do not affect the skin simultaneously, *Moraxella* and staphylococcal organisms can both be involved in chronic conjunctivitis and may simultaneously affect the skin, the lid margin, and the conjunctiva.

Treatment of Bacterial Conjunctivitis

Some general principles for treatment of conjunctivitis should be kept in mind. Although most cases of bacterial conjunctivitis resolve spontaneously within a week or two, appropriate antibiotic therapy shortens the course of the infection. (Exceptions are *Staphylococcus* and *Moraxella* infections, which may become chronic if not adequately treated.) As a rule, conjunctival cultures are not performed, and acute bacterial conjunctivitis is treated empirically. Eyedrops generally are preferred over ointments for adults because ointments blur vision. By contrast, ointments are preferred for infants and children because eyedrops are squeezed out and diluted during crying. Ointments are acceptable for adults at bedtime and are useful because they are eliminated slowly, so their action persists during sleep. Eyedrops containing fluoroquinolones (ciprofloxacin, ofloxacin, or levofloxacin), aminoglycosides (gentamicin, tobramycin), a combination of neomycin, gramicidin, and polymyxin B, or a combination of trimethoprim and polymyxin B, applied every 2 to 4 hours while the patient is awake, are commonly used, as are ointments containing gentamicin, tobramycin, or bacitracin with polymyxin B, applied three to four times a day. Physicians treating acute bacterial conjunctivitis empirically should remember that aminoglycosides are weakly active against streptococci. Vancomycin eyedrops at 5 mg/mL (not available commercially) may be used for methicillin-resistant staphylococcal infections. Although adverse effects of topically applied medications are rare, neomycin may induce a dose-related epithelial keratitis, and chloramphenicol applied topically has caused fatal bone marrow aplasia (12).

Gonococcal conjunctivitis in neonates is treated primarily by the parenteral route because the swelling of the eyes often makes it difficult to instill drops. Almost all other forms of bacterial conjunctivitis are treated exclusively by the topical route. Although topical antibiotics were often part of the standard treatment of gonococcal conjunctivitis in the past, they are probably unnecessary if the patient is receiving treatment by the parenteral route. A suggested regimen for the treatment of gonococcal conjunctivitis in adults is a single dose of ceftriaxone 1 g intramuscularly. The infected eye should be lavaged with saline once. For neonates, ceftriaxone should be given in a single dose of 25 to 50 mg/kg intravenously (IV) or intramuscularly, not to exceed 125 mg (13). The mother and her sexual partner should also be evaluated and, if necessary, treated. A neonate born to a mother with proven gonococcal infection should be given the same dosage of ceftriaxone for prophylaxis as for treatment of proven neonatal gonococcal conjunctivitis. Saline irrigation of the eyes is also suggested (13). Other regimens for the treatment

of genital and disseminated gonococcal infections are described in Chapter 103. Their efficacy in gonococcal conjunctivitis has not been well established. Patients with gonococcal eye infection, like patients with other gonococcal infections, should be evaluated for coinfection with *Chlamydia trachomatis.* The issue of routine topical prophylaxis for neonates is discussed in the section on inclusion conjunctivitis.

CHLAMYDIAL CONJUNCTIVITIS

Inclusion conjunctivitis and trachoma are caused by various serotypes of chlamydiae, which are grouped under the acronym TRIC (trachoma-inclusion conjunctivitis) agent. Trachoma, caused mainly by serotypes A, B, and C, is the leading cause of blindness in the world, whereas inclusion conjunctivitis, caused mainly by serotypes D through K, is almost invariably a benign, self-limited condition.

TRACHOMA

The prevalence of trachoma throughout the world has decreased as a result of improved personal hygiene and sanitation, but millions of people, largely in developing countries, are still afflicted. The disease is spread by person-to-person contact, by fomites, and by flies that carry the chlamydiae from human excrement to the eye and then from eye to eye. Young children in endemic areas are at high risk.

The incubation period is 5 to 14 days. Discomfort is minimal. Follicles develop on the palpebral conjunctiva and may also appear at the limbus. Healed limbal follicles leave the diagnostic scars called Herbert pits. Papillae as well as follicles develop on the palpebral conjunctiva. In short order the cornea is affected with punctate epithelial and subepithelial keratitis. With persistence of the low-grade inflammation for months to years, conjunctival cicatrization develops, along with in-turned eyelashes (trichiasis) and eyelid margins (entropion), obliteration of lacrimal gland ducts, and destruction of conjunctival goblet cells. These abnormalities combine to produce a dry eye, which, along with an abrasive effect from the scarred palpebral conjunctiva, create corneal scarring and vascularization (pannus). These changes eventually lead to blindness. Secondary bacterial keratitis further increases the risk for blindness. Unfortunately, in endemic areas, reinfection is common among patients successfully treated for the initial infection. Laboratory diagnosis of the infection is made most often by fluorescent antibody examination of conjunctival cells obtained by a scraping.

Treatment of Acute Trachoma

ADULTS

Azithromycin has been shown to be effective in a single oral dose of 20 mg/kg (14). Doxycycline may be given 100 mg orally twice daily, or tetracycline, 250 mg four times daily orally for 2 weeks.

PREGNANT WOMEN

Tetracycline or erythromycin ointment may be given two or three times daily for 2 months, or erythromycin, 500 mg orally every 8 hours for 3 to 4 weeks, or a combination of these.

CHILDREN YOUNGER THAN 8 YEARS

A single dose of azithromycin, 20 mg/kg, appears to be as effective as repetitive treatment with an eye ointment containing tetracycline and polymyxin, and compliance is easier to achieve (15). Nevertheless, as with all regimens, persistence of infection and reinfection is common. The traditional alternative is tetracycline or erythromycin ophthalmic ointment twice daily for 2 months.

The treatment of chronic trachoma is complicated and is best left to those with wide experience. The eradication of trachoma from endemic areas depends less on antibiotic treatment than on improvements in hygiene, including the availability of fresh running tap water.

INCLUSION CONJUNCTIVITIS

Inclusion conjunctivitis in adults is the most common sexually transmitted ocular disease in the United States. Clinically, the disease in adults and neonates is quite different. Adults have bilateral, low-grade, chronic follicular conjunctivitis that produces only mild discomfort and little or no exudate. Follicles larger than those of viral conjunctivitis are characteristically seen on the inferior palpebral conjunctiva (Fig. 146.4). The follicles persist for months without therapy, whereas follicles associated with viral infection resolve in a few weeks. Disease in neonates usually appears 7 to 10 days (range 5 to 13) after birth. A copious purulent exudate is typically seen, but no follicles form because the newborn has yet to develop a lymphoid system. If the disease smolders untreated for some months, epithelial keratitis may ensue and pannus (superficial corneal blood vessels) may form. Ten percent to 20% of infected infants develop chlamydial pneumonitis, typically 3 to 6 weeks after birth, as the result of spread of the TRIC agent to the respiratory tract through the lacrimal outflow system. Otitis media is less common.

The differential diagnosis of conjunctivitis in the newborn (ophthalmia neonatorum) includes a number of infections that may be distinguished by the interval until onset of signs or symptoms: gonococcal conjunctivitis (2–5 days), chlamydial conjunctivitis (7–10 days), infection produced by other bacteria and herpes simplex virus (any time), and chemical conjunctivitis secondary to prophylactic instillation of silver nitrate (day 1).

Treatment

NEONATES
Erythromycin may be given at 50 mg/kg per day, orally, in four doses for 2 weeks.

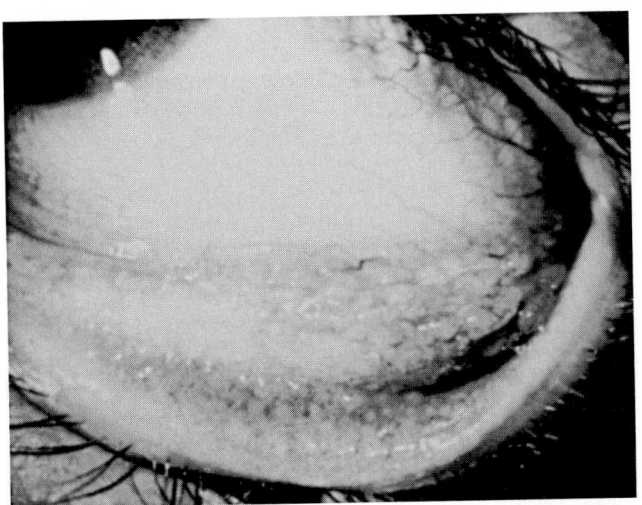

Figure 146.4. Large follicles on the inferior palpebral conjunctiva, typically seen in adult chlamydial (inclusion) conjunctivitis.

ADULTS
Doxycycline may be given at 100 mg orally, twice daily, for 7 days or azithromycin at 1 g orally once.

PREGNANT WOMEN
Erythromycin base may be given at 500 mg orally four times daily for 7 days.

Prophylaxis of Ophthalmia Neonatorum

All infants should receive routine topical prophylaxis, in a single application, to prevent ophthalmia neonatorum.

Silver nitrate 1% drops (Credé method) is the traditional prophylactic agent for neonatal conjunctivitis. After instillation of the drops, the eyes should not be irrigated. Silver nitrate is active against gonococci but not against the TRIC agent. Because chlamydial conjunctivitis is more common in the United States than is gonococcal infection, some authorities have advocated the use of tetracycline or erythromycin ointment instilled within 1 hour of birth for prophylaxis; however, these two antibiotics are only partially effective in preventing neonates' conjunctivitis, either chlamydial or gonococcal. Povidone-iodine 2.5% eyedrops were shown to be more effective than either silver nitrate or erythromycin for prophylaxis against *C. trachomatis* and as effective as the other two agents against *N. gonorrhoeae* (16). Povidone-iodine was also less toxic and is less expensive than the other two agents.

OTHER CONJUNCTIVAL INFECTIONS
Lymphogranuloma venereum, another sexually transmitted chlamydial infection, may cause Parinaud oculoglandular conjunctivitis. The ocular manifestations are usually unilateral. If the disease is not treated, both the conjunctiva and cornea may become scarred.

Parinaud oculoglandular conjunctivitis is a unilateral chronic granulomatous process; typically there is severe enlargement of the ipsilateral preauricular lymph node. Cat-scratch disease is by far the most common cause of the syndrome in the United States. Other causes include tuberculosis, syphilis, lymphogranuloma venereum, chancroid, tularemia, infectious mononucleosis, mumps, and various fungal infections.

VIRAL CONJUNCTIVITIS

Adenoviral Conjunctivitis
In the United States, viral conjunctivitis is more common than either bacterial or chlamydial conjunctivitis. The most common viral cause of conjunctivitis is adenovirus. Adenoviral infection usually presents clinically as epidemic keratoconjunctivitis (EKC) or pharyngoconjunctival fever.

EKC, usually caused by adenovirus serotype 8 or 19, is an acute, usually bilateral infection that often affects persons 20 to 40 years of age. It is highly infectious and typically is seen in epidemics. Patients, their contacts, and school personnel should be educated about the substantial risk from contact with infected persons, contaminated objects, and swimming pools. The virus survives on dry surfaces for long periods. Infections are contagious for about 2 weeks.

The clinical hallmarks are a moderately severe follicular conjunctivitis with preauricular lymphadenopathy. Subconjunctival hemorrhages may also appear. A minority of patients develop keratitis 1 week after the onset of the conjunctivitis. The keratitis causes pain, photophobia, and increased lacrimation. Characteristic focal subepithelial corneal infiltrates are seen on slit-lamp examination (Fig. 146.5).

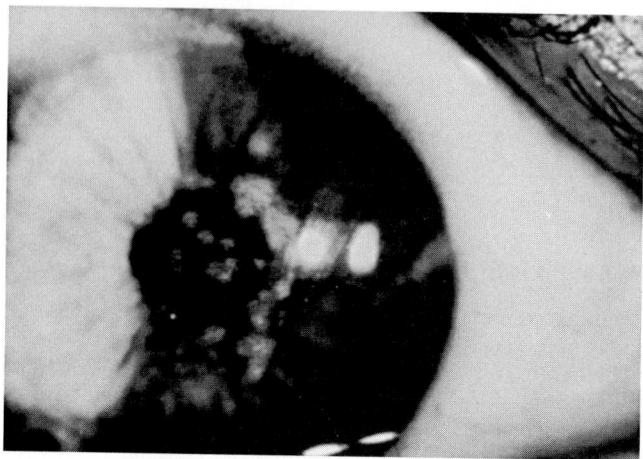

Figure 146.5. Subepithelial corneal infiltrates in a patient with epidemic keratoconjunctivitis (adenovirus).

These corneal infiltrates usually resolve without scarring after a few weeks, but occasionally they persist, either symptomatically or asymptomatically. The conjunctivitis usually abates spontaneously after 2 to 3 weeks. Its course may be prolonged, however, by the development of a pseudomembrane on the palpebral conjunctiva. A topical corticosteroid eyedrop may be considered if the pseudomembrane or keratitis is severe, but such treatment may also prolong the keratitis.

Pharyngoconjunctival fever is principally a disease of children under 10 years of age. Epidemics are usually caused by adenovirus serotypes 3 and 7 and sporadic cases by serotype 4. Typically the conjunctivitis is accompanied by malaise, sore throat, and fever. The ocular findings are similar to those of EKC, but the cornea is involved much less often. The issues of communicability are similar to those for EKC. There is no specific therapy.

Other Viral Causes of Conjunctivitis

Acute hemorrhagic conjunctivitis was pandemic in the 1970s but is uncommon at present, for reasons unknown. The first outbreaks were caused by an enterovirus of serotype 70, but subsequent outbreaks were caused by coxsackievirus A24 and adenovirus 11. Typically there is fulminating bilateral conjunctivitis with severe eyelid edema, chemosis, extensive subconjunctival hemorrhage, and copious mucoid exudate. A follicular reaction and preauricular lymphadenopathy occur. Some patients develop punctate keratitis with photophobia, and there may be features suggestive of systemic involvement, including sore throat, malaise headache, and myalgia. Rarely, Bell's palsy and paralysis of the legs may develop. Ocular signs and symptoms generally resolve spontaneously within 2 weeks. There is no specific treatment.

Viruses that produce blepharitis, including herpes simplex virus, varicella-zoster virus, papillomavirus (the agent of molluscum contagiosum), and vaccinia virus, may also produce conjunctivitis. Other viruses that cause conjunctivitis include Epstein-Barr virus, cytomegalovirus, and the agents of measles, mumps, influenza, rubella, smallpox, and Newcastle disease (paramyxovirus). Measles keratitis, a punctate keratitis, resolves spontaneously but may be followed by secondary *H. influenzae* conjunctivitis; this is especially common in developing countries.

Corneal Infections

Corneal infections pose a serious risk of permanent loss of vision and perforation of the globe. Inflammation of the cornea (kerati-

tis) often causes corneal scarring and opacification, and enzymes from microorganisms (e.g., metalloproteinases) and neutrophils act to thin the corneal matrix. In developed countries the most common cause of infectious keratitis is herpes simplex virus; in developing countries bacteria and fungi are the usual agents. These latter types of infections are often secondary to trauma and trachoma. Keratitis caused by bacteria is usually more fulminant than infection caused by other agents and requires prompt diagnosis and treatment to reduce the threat to vision and the risk for perforation.

BACTERIAL KERATITIS

The cornea is resistant to bacterial infection, in large part owing to the protective effect of the epithelium. Corneal epithelial drying, trauma, or hypoxia increase the susceptibility of the cornea to infection. Drying may occur from increased evaporation, as in lagophthalmos or exophthalmos, or from decreased tearing, as in keratoconjunctivitis sicca. Hypoxia of the corneal epithelium may occur in patients who wear soft contact lenses for prolonged periods or during sleep. Diabetes and the use of corticosteroids and immunosuppressive drugs are other risk factors for corneal infection.

The most common bacterial agents of corneal ulcers are *S. aureus* and *Staphylococcus epidermidis*. Other frequently encountered pathogens are *S. pneumoniae*, α- and β-hemolytic streptococci, *Pseudomonas aeruginosa*, and *Bacillus cereus*. An association has been observed between the wearing of extended-wear soft contact lenses and the development of corneal ulcers caused by *P. aeruginosa*; indeed, more than 50% of corneal ulcers in wearers of extended-wear soft contact lenses are caused by *P. aeruginosa*.

P. aeruginosa keratitis must be addressed promptly, as the organisms produce a proteoglycanase that can cause corneal perforation within a few days (17). *B. cereus* keratitis is perhaps the most fulminant of corneal infections; it typically occurs in rural areas after trauma (18). Less common pathogens include *Serratia marcescens,* other gram-negative bacilli, *Neisseria* species, *M. lacunata* (in derelict populations), *Mycobacterium fortuitum* and *Mycobacterium chelonae,* and anaerobic species of bacteria.

In a typical case of bacterial corneal ulcer, the patient experiences ocular pain, lacrimation, and photophobia. The eye is red and there is a milk-white corneal infiltrate. The surrounding cornea is hazy (edematous; Fig. 146.6), the eyelids are swollen, and the pupil is miotic. A hypopyon may be present.

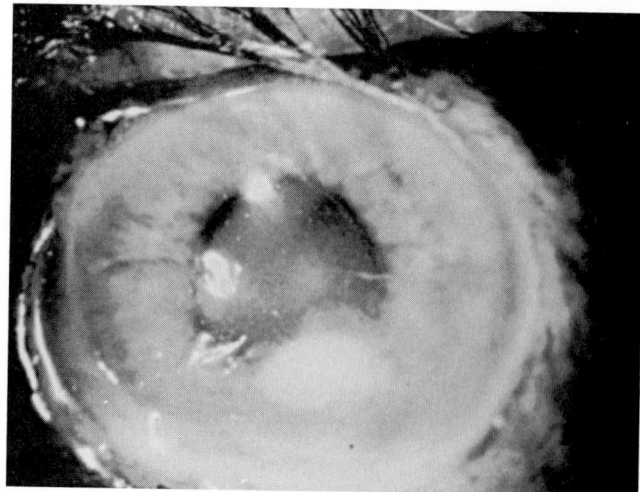

Figure 146.6. Bacterial corneal ulcer. Note stromal infiltrate.

Approach to the Management of Corneal Ulcer

Identification of the Specific Agent. Before fluoroquinolone eyedrops became commercially available, it was the practice routinely to attempt to determine the causative agent of keratitis. The infiltrated area of the cornea would be scraped with a platinum spatula or a calcium alginate swab to obtain material for Gram stain, as well as Grocott methenamine silver stain to detect fungi (19), and would be cultured before therapy was begun. Because most of the pathogens responsible for microbial keratitis are susceptible to the fluoroquinolones, laboratory diagnosis is now used by many clinicians only for the more severe and central ulcers and for those that fail to respond to initial therapy.

Empiric Treatment. We advocate an empiric approach because treatment must be started promptly and there is a relatively poor correlation between the results of Gram stain and culture (20) (Table 146.3). In the past, we recommended two antibiotics, for example, cefazolin and gentamicin, in order to assure activity against the most likely pathogens. In place of a combination of drugs, we now suggest a topical fluoroquinolone eyedrop as initial therapy for the less severe and more peripheral infiltrates unless *Pseudomonas aeruginosa* is the suspected pathogen (e.g., if the patient has used a soft contact lens, especially one worn overnight, or if the ulcers commence in the intensive care unit). For the more severe or centrally located lesions, the use of two antibiotics that cover both gram-positive and gram-negative pathogens commonly encountered is recommended.

Topical fluoroquinolones are likely to be highly effective against the more commonly encountered gram-positive and gram-negative corneal pathogens, except that streptococcal infections occasionally fail to respond. Third-generation cephalosporins also are highly active against the usual bacterial pathogens. Cefazolin plus either gentamicin or tobramycin commonly has been used (21). If *P. aeruginosa* infection is suspected initially, tobramycin plus piperacillin, ticarcillin, or ceftazidime is suggested (21,22).

Topical Treatment by Frequent Administration of Fortified Antibiotic Eyedrops. Except for the fluoroquinolones, antibiotic eyedrops that are available commercially are not likely to be as effective as the more concentrated solutions that hospital pharmacists can prepare (6). For initial treatment, eyedrops are usually instilled every 15 to 30 minutes around the clock for 2 or 3 days. Another method, perhaps less fatiguing to the patient, hospital staff, and family, is to administer one antibiotic, one drop every minute for five doses, to wait for 5 minutes, and then to instill the second antibiotic in a similar manner. The process is repeated every hour. It should be remembered that an eye can hold only one drop and that a 5-minute interval should be allowed between the administration of different preparations of eyedrops to avoid a washout effect. Animal studies have verified that when concentrated antibiotic eyedrops are instilled frequently, bactericidal corneal drug levels are achieved and bacterial counts are sharply and promptly reduced (23,24).

In studies in animals, subconjunctival injections have been found to be no more effective than frequently administered concentrated antibiotic eyedrops (23,24). These injections are now used principally when compliance is in doubt or to treat infections in infants and small children, who frequently squeeze out the eyedrops and dilute them as they cry. Orally or parenterally administered antibiotics produce only modest corneal concentrations and probably offer little or no benefit to patients who are being treated with intensive topical applications of concentrated eyedrops. In special circumstances, however, as in gonococcal keratitis, or when the cornea has perforated, or the infection has spread to involve the sclera, parenteral as well as topical therapy is suggested.

FUNGAL KERATITIS

The incidence of fungal keratitis is lower than that of either bacterial or viral keratitis. Fungal keratitis is more common in warmer climates and in rural areas. It often follows trauma to the cornea, especially by vegetable matter or objects contaminated by soil. Topical application of corticosteroids may predispose to fungal

---

TABLE 146.3. Antimicrobial Treatment of Bacterial Corneal Ulcers

A. Initial empirical therapy for suspected bacterial corneal ulcers (see text)
  1. Low suspicion of *Pseudomonas aeruginosa*[a]
    Topical: Fluoroquinolone (commercially available eyedrops of ciprofloxacin or ofloxacin or levofloxacin)
    or
    Aminoglycoside (commercially available eyedrops of gentamicin or tobramycin), plus cefazolin[b]
    In patients allergic to β-lactam drugs, vancomycin[b] or bacitracin[b] eyedrops can be substituted for cefazolin[b] eyedrops.
    Subconjunctival (see text for indications): cefazolin[c], or vancomycin[a]; combined with gentamicin[c] or tobramycin[c]
  2. High suspicion of *P. aeruginosa* (see text)
    Topical: Tobramycin[b], combined with one of the following: ticarcillin[b], piperacillin[b] or ceftazidime[b] eyedrops
    Subconjuntival (see text for indications): tobramycin combined with either piperacillin[c] or ceftazidime[c]
B. Antibiotic choices for defined pathogen. Change treatment only if pathogen is resistant *in vitro* to the antibiotics being administered and there is a poor clinical response.
  1. *Staphylococcus* (oxacillin susceptible)
    Topical: vancomycin[b] or bacitracin[b] eyedrops
    Subconjunctival (see text for indications): cefazolin[c], oxacillin[c], or vancomycin[c]
  2. *Streptococcus*
    Topical and subconjunctival
    Similar to treatment for staphylococcus
  3. Gram-negative
    Topical: aminoglycoside[b] or fluoroquinolone[b]
    Subconjunctival (see text for indications): gentamicin[c] or tobramycin[c], possibly with ticarcillin[c] or piperacillin[c] or ceftazidime[c]

[a]For severe ulcers, even if low suspicion of *Pseudomonas aeruginosa*, may consider fortified drops and subconjunctival injections.
[b]Fortified eyedrops (prepared by pharmacist): bacitracin 10,000 units/mL; cefazolin 50 mg/mL; ceftazidime 50 mg/mL; gentamicin 10–20 mg/mL; piperacillin 6–20 mg/mL; ticarcillin 6–20 mg/mL; tobramycin 10–20 mg/mL; vancomycin 33 mg/mL.
[c]Subconjunctival injections (prepared by ophthalmologist): total dosages, delivered in 0.5 mL are cefazolin, 100 mg; ceftazidime, 100 mg; gentamicin, 40 mg; oxacillin, 100 mg; piperacillin, 100 mg; ticarcillin, 100 mg; tobramycin, 40 mg; vancomycin, 25 mg.
Modified from Glaser DB, Baum J. Bacterial keratitis. In: Stenson SM, ed. *Surgical management of external eye disease.* New York: Igaku-Shoin, 1995;127, with permission.

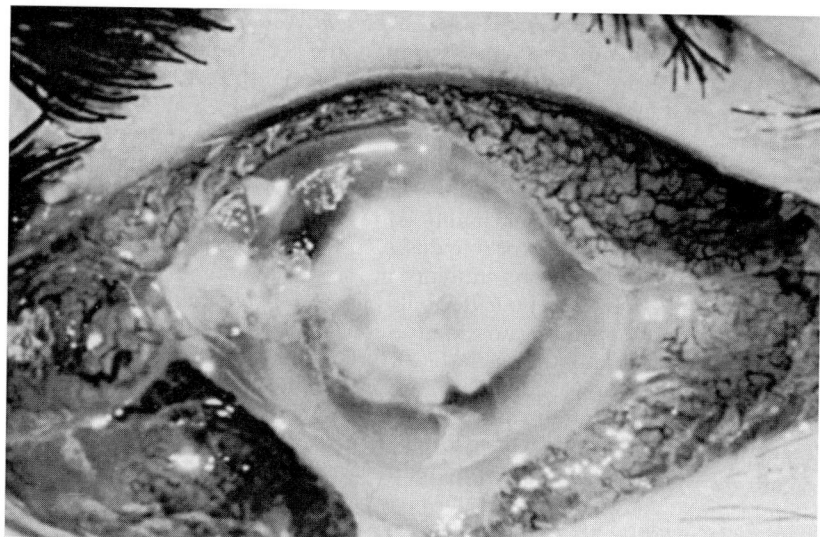

Figure 146.7. Fungal ulcer of the cornea. Note satellite lesions.

keratitis (25). Unlike most nonocular fungal infections, many fungal corneal infections are due to filamentous species, particularly the nonpigmented *Fusarium solani*. This species often causes infection after minor trauma to the cornea. In northern climates and in immunosuppressed patients whose corneal epithelium has been compromised by decreased sensation, exposure, or drying, *Candida albicans* infection is not uncommon. Less frequent causes of infection include *Aspergillus fumigatus* and *Alternaria, Curvularia,* and *Acremonium* species.

A corneal fungal infiltrate typically enlarges slowly during a period of weeks and has characteristic fine feathery margins, heaped-up edges, and adjacent satellite lesions (Fig. 146.7). The clinical diagnosis is confirmed by scraping material from the lesion and observing fungal elements with methenamine silver stain (19) and by culture of material in Sabouraud medium without cyclohexamide, an inhibitor to growth of filamentous species. Sometimes the scraping fails to demonstrate the pathogen, which may reside in the posterior corneal stroma, in which case examination of a corneal biopsy specimen may be necessary to prove the diagnosis.

The outcome of treatment of fungal keratitis has often been poor. The laboratory may be slow to identify the pathogen, which delays treatment; in some instances cultures fail to yield the organism, so specific treatment is not given. In the past, it was usual to administer amphotericin B in eyedrops in a concentration of 1% to 5% (26). However, the high concentration of the desoxycholate solubilizer makes such solutions irritating, and they may damage the cornea. Noncompliance may also have contributed to the unsatisfactory results with these eyedrops. Studies suggest that treatment with eyedrops containing much lower concentrations of amphotericin B (0.05%–0.15%) produces a good clinical response in keratitis caused by a variety of species of fungi and is tolerated well (27). Amphotericin B eyedrops usually are given at the rate of one drop each hour while the patient is awake. Treatment should be continued for 3 to 6 weeks if there is improvement, after which time the frequency of administration is gradually reduced. Oral flucytosine has been used on occasion to supplement therapy with amphotericin B in the treatment of *Candida* keratitis. Natamycin eyedrops, in the form of a 5% suspension, are effective in the treatment of superficial *Fusarium* keratitis but less effective for deeper corneal infections because the drug penetrates the corneal stroma poorly. The imidazoles are variably effective against a wide range of pathogens. Ketoconazole, 200 to 400 mg per day orally for adults or as a 2%

eyedrop suspension every 30 to 60 minutes for 3 to 6 weeks, has in large part replaced miconazole. Fluconazole may be an even better choice. Very preliminary experience suggests that some of the newer azole drugs such as voriconazole or posaconazole, applied topically, may have utility as well. Despite the availability of a number of agents and pending more information about the newer azoles, at present we prefer dilute preparations of amphotericin B eyedrops for the treatment of fungal keratitis.

VIRAL KERATITIS

Of all forms of infectious keratitis in developed countries, herpes simplex keratitis is unquestionably the most prevalent and carries the highest rate of morbidity (28). This section addresses herpes simplex and herpes zoster keratitis. Other viral diseases that sometimes affect the cornea but primarily affect the conjunctiva were discussed earlier in the section on viral conjunctivitis.

Herpes Simplex Keratitis

The pathogenesis of herpes simplex keratitis is complex and continues to be the subject of extensive basic investigation. Most clinically significant episodes of herpes keratitis occur in adults, but they are thought to be sequelae of subclinical primary infections that occur quite early in life, perhaps in infancy (29). Humans are the only natural host for the virus. After the primary infection, the virus becomes dormant in nervous tissue (e.g., trigeminal or ciliary ganglion) for years. Various stimuli— sunlight, fever, trauma, other infection, and stress—can trigger the dormant virus to produce infectious particles, which travel from ganglia through nerves to the cornea to produce recurrent corneal infection. Investigations have raised the additional possibility that latent virus resides in corneal stromal cells and that recurrent corneal disease follows reactivation from this source (30). This hypothesis perhaps better explains recurrent corneal infection but not the recurrent infections in other ocular tissues that are innervated by branches of the trigeminal nerve. There is some evidence to suggest that certain strains of herpes simplex virus are more likely than others to lead to recurrent infection and that infection with a strain with a low potential for recurrence may be protective against infection by a strain with a high potential for recurrence (29). Evidence also suggests that properties of the individual strain determine the number and shape of the dendritic epithelial lesions and that both the virus and the host response determine the stromal manifestations (29).

Herpes simplex virus type 1 accounts for the majority of infections seen in children and for the vast majority of those in adults. By contrast, type 2 strains are responsible for most illness in neonates, who are infected during passage through the birth canal.

In children and neonates, clinically evident primary herpes simplex virus infection of the eye characteristically involves the eyelid and conjunctiva but only rarely the cornea. The process is usually benign and self-limited, is most often unilateral, and generally lasts 1 to 2 weeks. The corneal epithelium, when involved, displays punctate lesions or typical dendrites with fluorescein staining. Stromal involvement is rare, possibly because it is immunologically mediated and the immune response to the virus is not well developed at the time of primary infection. By contrast, recurrent herpes simplex keratitis in adults may affect all corneal layers and the uveal tract and almost always is monocular. Typically, the initial attack of keratitis in the adult produces infectious dendritic figures (Fig. 146.8). Early on, the dendritic figures are thin and often terminate in bulbs. The epithelium is hypoesthetic. With effective antiviral therapy, the dendrites resolve within 1 to 2 weeks but sometimes leave a subepithelial "ghost" imprint, which fades during a period of weeks. Especially in adults, the stroma may be involved in an immune reaction, displaying either a ground-glass appearance due to edema or appearing densely white because of a cellular infiltrate. Stromal involvement is more serious than epithelial involvement, being more intractable, and scarring of the stroma may result in permanent loss of vision.

The major component of herpetic stromal disease is thought to be a manifestation of delayed hypersensitivity. Viral antigens have been found in the stromal matrix and in stromal keratocytes (31). Stromal edema (disciform keratitis) develops when sensitized lymphocytes are activated by viral antigen. In addition to stimulating delayed hypersensitivity, particles may trigger complement-mediated damage in the form of corneal infiltrates and "immune rings" (30). Even with optimal treatment, there is a 25% to 50% incidence of stromal reactivation within 2 years of an attack, and often the stromal recurrence may last

weeks to months. The development of keratic precipitates on the endothelium, flare and cells in the aqueous humor, and elevated intraocular pressure are manifestations of corneal endothelial and uveal tract involvement.

The treatment of herpes simplex keratitis may be divided into two components: a regimen for epithelial disease, which is relatively easy to treat, and stromal involvement, for which treatment is difficult and multifactorial. Epithelial dendritic keratitis without stromal involvement typically responds well to topical antiviral therapy. Trifluridine (trifluorothymidine), which is available as an eyedrop, initially is given nine times daily for 10 to 14 days. It appears to be slightly more effective than vidarabine, which is available topically only as an ointment and is usually given five times a day. Most patients show a good response to treatment as manifested by relief of symptoms and the beginning of resolution of the dendrites within 48 hours. Topical acyclovir, not yet commercially available in the United States, has proved to be at least as effective as trifluridine (28) in the treatment of herpes simplex keratitis and is the least toxic of all the antiviral agents. Orally administered drugs are also effective in treating herpes simplex epithelial keratitis (e.g., acyclovir, 400 mg three times a day, or famciclovir, 250 mg twice daily for 7-10 days) (28). In patients whose response is poor, epithelial débridement is usually undertaken to reduce the viral load. Stromal keratitis, a refractory infection with a tendency to recur, is usually treated with topical corticosteroids and a topical antiviral agent. The addition of oral acyclovir to this regimen appears to offer no benefit for active stromal disease but is of prophylactic value when given orally, 400 mg twice daily for 1 year or longer (28,32).

Varicella-Zoster Keratitis

Recurrent (recrudescent) varicella-zoster virus infection of the eye occurs primarily along the distribution of the ophthalmic division of the trigeminal nerve. Approximately 60% of patients with involvement of the skin in the distribution of the ophthalmic division of the trigeminal nerve develop varicella-zoster virus keratitis. Severe ocular pain may precede signs of ocular and cutaneous infection. Ocular manifestations involve principally the cornea. In immunocompromised patients, most often those with lymphoma, other ocular tissues and cranial nerves may be involved. Even patients who are not immunocompromised may develop iridocyclitis and glaucoma, either subsequently or concomitantly, as a result of varicella-zoster virus keratitis.

The corneal manifestations of recrudescent varicella-zoster virus infection are varied. The epithelium may develop punctate staining or dendrites (which differ from those of herpes simplex keratitis in that the processes are fewer, shorter, and wider, lack end bulbs, and usually disappear within a few days, even without therapy). However, the most common site of ocular involvement is the corneal stroma, and involvement of this site has the most serious consequences for vision. The stroma may develop edema and infiltrates, which may eventually lead to scarring and permanent loss of vision. Endothelial involvement is suggested by the development of diffuse stromal edema and keratic precipitates. The cornea often becomes permanently anesthetic (neurotrophic keratitis), in which case the corneal epithelium, if abraded, reepithelializes poorly. Perforation of the cornea may occur unless the process is recognized and arrested.

Acyclovir is effective in treating the cutaneous components of the infection, but its value in treating varicella-zoster keratitis is uncertain. A dose of 800 mg orally, five times a day for 10 days, reduces virus shedding and pain, provided that treatment is started within 3 days of the appearance of the skin lesion. Famciclovir, 500 mg, or valacyclovir, 1 g orally three times a day

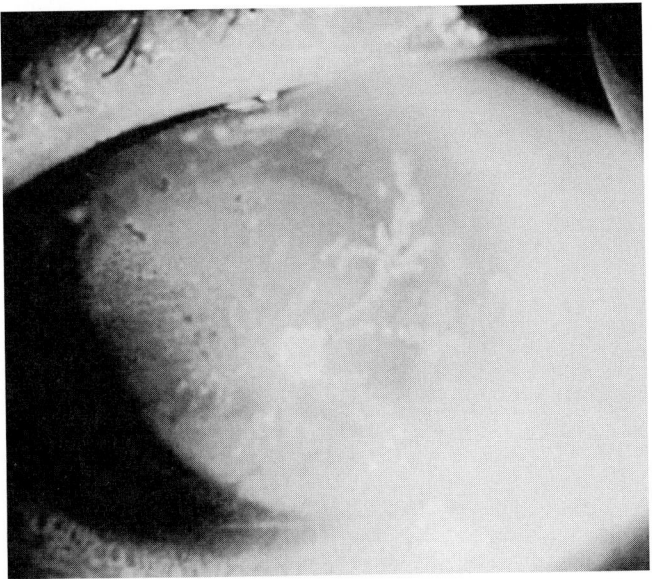

Figure 146.8. Dendritic figures (stained with fluorescein) characteristic of herpes simplex dendritic (epithelial) keratitis.

for 7 to 10 days, is as effective as acyclovir in acute disease and may be more effective in preventing postherpetic neuralgia. Desipramine or other tricyclic antidepressants given orally are also effective in inhibiting development of long-term pain (33).

ACANTHAMOEBA KERATITIS

It has been almost 30 years since the first reports were published of *Acanthamoeba* keratitis (34,35). In the past, the disease was often misdiagnosed as herpes simplex keratitis. Many authorities suspect that the disease is more common than the number of reports would suggest.

Acanthamoeba organisms are free-living protozoa commonly found in soil, air, and water. They are hardy and survive extremes of temperature ($-20°$ to $42°C$). Under adverse conditions, the trophozoites revert to an inactive cyst form, both in the cornea and in the environment. *Acanthamoeba polyphaga* and *Acanthamoeba castellani* are the most common isolates from corneal infections.

The risk factors for *Acanthamoeba* keratitis are trauma to the corneal epithelium, which may result from wearing soft contact lenses, and exposure to the parasite, which may occur through swimming or the use of hot tubs or contaminated contact lens solutions. Clinically, the earliest sign of corneal infection is an atypical "abrasion," in which the epithelium appears shaggy and does not heal quickly. At this stage, the prompt institution of appropriate therapy has the greatest likelihood of a nonsurgical cure. Without specific therapy, the process waxes and wanes but gradually worsens. A foreign body sensation gives way to intense pain that is out of proportion to the signs. The epithelium cyclically heals and breaks down and the corneal stroma becomes hazy. Typically, an arc-like or annular stromal infiltrate develops (Fig. 146.9) many weeks after the onset of the disease, and there is severe iritis with or without hypopyon.

The diagnosis is confirmed by placing the scraped fragments of infected tissue on a microscope slide, staining the material with calcofluor white, and visualizing the characteristic cysts under a fluorescence microscope (36,37). Confocal microscopy is a useful *in vivo* technique for the visualization of intrastromal cysts (38). Material may be cultured on nonnutrient agar (e.g., agar seeded with a gram-negative bacterium such as *Escherichia coli*).

The earlier treatment is begun, the greater is the potential for cure by drug therapy. At an early stage, when the amebal load is largely restricted to the corneal epithelium, epithelial débridement is suggested to both decrease the load and increase drug delivery. If treatment is delayed, the results of all therapies are usually disappointing but a combination of surgical treatment and chemotherapy appears to be the most effective approach (39). Although dozens of drugs are active against the protozoa *in vitro*, most produce a poor response in patients.

Until recent years, standard therapy consisted of 0.1% propamidine isothionate eyedrops, and 5% neomycin eyedrops (or the commercially available combination of neomycin-gramicidin-polymyxin B eyedrops) (40). Two newer agents, polyhexamethylene biguanide (41,42) 0.02% and chlorhexidine 0.02% (42,43), appear to be more effective than other therapies. The former agent is sold in the United States as Bacquicil (ICI Americas, Wilmington, DE, U.S.A.), a swimming pool disinfectant. Whichever drugs are used, they are alternated every 15 to 60 minutes for 5 to 7 days, after which the frequency of instillation is decreased gradually during a period of weeks as the clinical condition stabilizes and then improves. It has been suggested that treatment be given for 5 to 9 months in an attempt to sterilize the infection (44,45). If medical therapy fails, a penetrating keratoplasty followed by additional drug therapy has proved effective (39). Eyedrops of 1% clotrimazole have also been shown to be effective clinically (46). The efficacy of topical miconazole or paromomycin and of oral ketoconazole has yet to be clearly defined. The value of topical corticosteroid therapy is still undetermined.

Infection of the Lacrimal Apparatus

DACRYOADENITIS

The anatomy of the lacrimal system is shown in Fig. 146.10. Infection of the lacrimal gland, dacryoadenitis, is usually caused by bacteria, but occasionally by viruses, fungi, or parasites. Fungal and parasitic infections are rare in developed countries. The most common bacterial cause is *S. aureus*. Less common infecting agents are streptococci, gonococci, *Mycobacterium tuberculosis*, and *Treponema pallidum*. The most common viral causes of dacryoadenitis are mumps virus and Epstein-Barr virus.

Acute dacryoadenitis caused by staphylococci and streptococci produces swelling, pain, and tenderness over the lateral

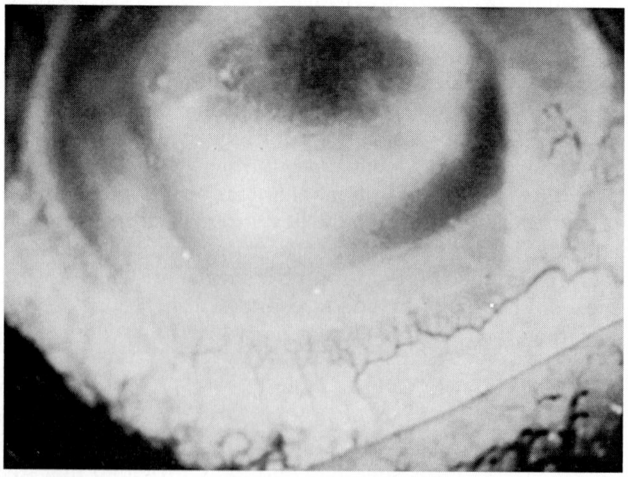

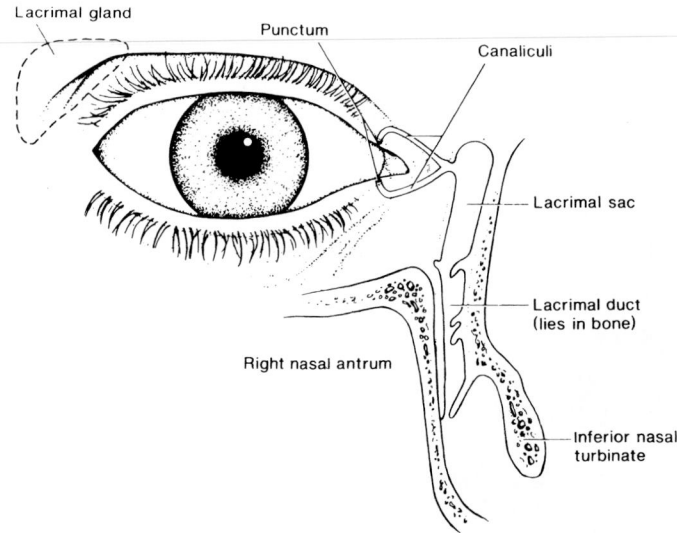

Figure 146.10. Schematic diagram of the lacrimal apparatus. (From Barza M, Baum J. Ocular infections. *Med Clin North Am* 1983;67:131–152, with permission.)

Figure 146.9. *Acanthamoeba* keratitis. Note typical anular appearance with less dense central area.

portion of the upper lid. Fever and malaise are often present. The other microorganisms characteristically produce subacute or chronic disease, with swelling of the gland but few other symptoms. Treatment is usually empiric, because the pathogen is often sequestered in deeper tissue and not evident in conjunctival cultures; however, material for Gram stain examination and culture may be obtained by inserting a fine needle into the gland and aspirating fluid. Treatment should be started immediately after the clinical diagnosis has been made. Acute bacterial infections should be treated for 4 to 7 days with parenteral antibiotics that are active against *S. aureus* and streptococci. If there is an abscess, hot packs should be used and surgical incision may be required.

CANALICULITIS

Infection of the small ducts that carry tears from the eye to the lacrimal sac is termed canaliculitis. The most common cause is *Actinomyces israelii*. Fungi (*Candida, Aspergillus*), bacteria (streptococci), viruses (herpes simplex virus, varicella-zoster virus), and TRIC agents are occasional causes of canaliculitis. Stasis within the outflow tract, which may occur in infants because of congenital pouches, increases the risk for infection.

Pain, swelling, and erythema at the inner third of the upper or lower eyelid accompanied by tearing are present in varying degrees. In some instances, mucopurulent exudate can be expressed through an abnormally dilated lacrimal punctum by finger pressure against the skin overlying the lacrimal sac. When *A. israelii* is the pathogen, cheesy white concretions can often be expressed. The ophthalmologist treats *A. israelii* infection by irrigating the outflow tract with 10% sulfacetamide eyedrops introduced through the punctum using a cannula attached to a syringe. Penicillin G, in a concentration of 100,000 units/mL or clindamycin, 10 mg/mL, are alternative antibiotics.

DACRYOCYSTITIS

Infection of the lacrimal sac, or dacryocystitis, is the most common infection of the lacrimal system. The most common agents are gram-positive bacteria, especially *S. pneumoniae* and *S. aureus*. Other pathogens include *H. influenzae, P. aeruginosa,* and *Proteus mirabilis*. Fungi such as *C. albicans* and *Aspergillus* species are less frequent causes. As with canaliculitis, stasis within the lacrimal outflow tract increases the risk for infection.

Infection of the lacrimal sac may be either acute or chronic. With acute infection, the patient experiences localized pain and tearing. The lacrimal sac and overlying tissues are erythematous, swollen, and tender. With chronic infection, as is usually the case in newborns, symptoms are typically absent except for tearing. The lacrimal sac area usually looks normal but may be swollen. Clues to chronic infection include a dilated lacrimal punctum and regurgitation of exudate from the punctum after finger pressure applied to the skin overlying the lacrimal sac. When the disease is acute, the organisms are located in the wall of the sac and the infection is best treated by parenteral or oral administration of antibiotics. When the disease is chronic, the organisms reside in the lumen of the sac and are most effectively eradicated by irrigation of antibiotics through the punctum.

ENDOPHTHALMITIS

Endophthalmitis means inflammation within the eye. In common usage, the term denotes an intraocular infection involving the vitreous humor. In this chapter, both exogenous and endogenous (metastatic) bacterial and fungal endophthalmitis are discussed. Infections that primarily affect the retina and choroid but not the vitreous humor, such as HIV, cytomegalovirus infection,

and toxoplasmosis, are not addressed. For a more comprehensive review of bacterial endophthalmitis, the reader is referred elsewhere (47,48). References are also provided for retinal infection from HIV and cytomegalovirus (49–52).

Most cases of bacterial endophthalmitis are exogenous and occur after ocular surgery or accidental trauma. A smaller number are endogenous (i.e., result from hematogenous spread from an infection elsewhere) (53,54). Endophthalmitis almost never occurs as a complication of periorbital infection and only rarely is the result of bacterial conjunctivitis, mainly meningococcal conjunctivitis. Endophthalmitis is among the most injurious of ocular infections and is the one with the poorest prognosis for vision.

Most cases of postoperative endophthalmitis follow cataract extraction. Older studies reported an incidence of bacterial endophthalmitis of approximately 0.1% to 0.5% after cataract extraction (55–57), but more recent data yield an incidence of 0.07% (58). The incidence after other forms of intraocular surgery (secondary lens implantation, pars plana vitrectomy, glaucoma filtering surgery) has been reported as 0.3% to 0.6% (58). By contrast, the incidence of endophthalmitis after traumatic penetration of the globe was higher, 2% and 3%, in two series (59,60).

Exogenous Bacterial Endophthalmitis

Table 146.4 shows a comparison of the bacterial species isolated from patients with exogenous endophthalmitis after various forms of surgical and nonsurgical trauma based on a retrospective analysis. In endophthalmitis after cataract extraction, *S. epidermidis* is the most common bacterial isolate, followed by *S. aureus*, streptococcal species, and a variety of gram-negative organisms, including *Pseudomonas* and *Proteus* species and *H. influenzae, S. marcescens,* and *E. coli* (61). Data from the Endophthalmitis Vitrectomy Study (62,63), a prospective study of endophthalmitis after cataract extraction, show a similar distribution of pathogens but an even greater preponderance of gram-positive cocci, especially coagulase-negative staphylococci. Among the 70% of patients in that study with "confirmed" growth from the eye, the major infecting species were coagulase-negative staphylococci (70%), *S. aureus* (10%), and streptococcal species (9%); gram-negative species were found in about 6% (63). There was no confirmed instance of fungal infection among 420 patients.

Patients with filtering blebs after surgery for glaucoma are at special risk for streptococcal and *H. influenzae* endophthalmitis, in part because the thin wall of the bleb facilitates penetration of the globe by these encapsulated pathogens (64) and in part because of the common postoperative prophylactic use of topical aminoglycosides, which have limited activity against streptococci. The most common pathogen in endophthalmitis associated with accidental trauma is *B. cereus*, followed by other *Bacillus* species; staphylococci, especially *S. epidermidis*; *Streptococcus* species; various gram-negative species; and anaerobes (65,66). Except following accidental trauma, endophthalmitis caused by obligately anaerobic bacteria is rare. In a series of 18 cases of endophthalmitis caused by anaerobes, *Propionibacterium acnes* was isolated in 14 cases, and in 10 it was the only pathogen isolated (66). In the remaining cases, it was part of a polymicrobial infection. Again, except following accidental trauma, polymicrobial infection is uncommon.

Endogenous Bacterial Endophthalmitis

Endogenous (metastatic, hematogenous) bacterial endophthalmitis is now much rarer than in the preantibiotic era.

TABLE 146.4.   Microbiology of Endophthalmitis

Organism	Postoperative infections (%) (n = 63)	Bleb-associated infections (%) (n = 30)	Traumatic infections (%) (n = 30)
Staphylococcus epidermidis	38	0	20
Staphylococcus aureus	21	7	0
Streptococcus species	11	57	13
Bacillus species	0	0	27
Haemophilus influenzae	3	23	0
Other gram-negative species	13	7	20
Fungi	8	3	17
Other	6	3	3
Mixed flora	2	0	11

Modified from Forster RK. Endophthalmitis. In: Tasman W, Jaeger EA, eds. *Clinical ophthalmology.* Vol. 4. Philadelphia: Lippincott Williams & Wilkins, 1994:11, with permission.

Furthermore, the clinical characteristics of patients with this form of endophthalmitis are different from those before the advent of antibiotics (53,54). Two risk factors, immunosuppression and IV drug abuse, which were rare 50 years ago, are contributing factors today. The infection is presumed to have occurred by hematogenous spread, although in some patients bacteremia cannot be demonstrated. Tables 146.5 and 146.6 compare the sites of primary infection and the pathogens for the years 1935 to 1975 and 1976 to 1985. In the preantibiotic era, meningitis was the most common primary infection associated with endogenous endophthalmitis, and *N. meningitidis* was the most common infecting organism. The pattern has changed, and a wide variety of sources and infecting organisms have been reported (53,54). A striking association is a fulminant endophthalmitis caused by *B. cereus* in injection drug users. In one more recent series, not shown in the tables, diabetes mellitus was the most common underlying medical disorder, streptococcal species were the most common infecting group of organisms (although *S. aureus* was the most common single species), and endocarditis and the gastrointestinal tract were the most common sources of infection (54). Vitreous cultures and blood cultures are each positive in about 70% of patients (53,54). Because the ocular symptoms (decreased vision, floaters, redness, discharge, eye pain, headache) and systemic symptoms are usually vague, at least initially, the diagnosis of endogenous endophthalmitis is often made relatively late (54). About 80% of infections are unilateral, and the right eye is somewhat more likely to be infected than the left, probably because of the shorter, more direct arterial route from the carotid artery to the right eye. The overall visual prognosis for endogenous endophthalmitis is poor. There is a suggestion that early treatment with intravitreal injection of antibiotics and vitrectomy may be of some benefit (54). Treatment of the primary infection, usually with antibiotics administered intravenously, is also indicated.

Fungal Endophthalmitis

Fungal endophthalmitis is much less common than bacterial endophthalmitis. In contrast to bacterial endophthalmitis, fungal endophthalmitis is more often endogenous than exogenous. The most common pathogen is *C. albicans. Aspergillus* species are the second most common isolates, *A. fumigatus* being more commonly found than *Aspergillus flavus* (67,68). A variety of other fungi occasionally are seen.

The incidence of endogenous fungal endophthalmitis has increased in the past few decades, in large part owing to the increased use of total parenteral nutrition, hemodialysis, urinary and intravenous catheters, and immunosuppressive agents, and to an increase in the incidence of immunosuppressive diseases, such as acquired immunodeficiency syndrome, all of which are risk factors for fungal infection. The increased frequency of injection drug use, with the potential for injection of contaminated

TABLE 146.5.   Site of Primary Infection in Patients Developing Metastatic Bacterial Endophthalmitis

Primary infections	108 Patients 1935–1975		72 Patients 1976–1985	
	n	%	n	%
Meningitis	59	55	19	26
Endocarditis	1–2	—	10	14
Urinary tract	7	6	10	14
Gastrointestinal tract or abdomen	—	—	8	11
Skin	12	11	5	7
Lungs	9	8	4	6
Puerperium	6	6	—	—
Other	15[a]	14	16	22

[a] Including endocarditis.
Data from Shammas (52a), and Greenwald et al. (53)

TABLE 146.6.   Pathogens in Metastatic Bacterial Endophthalmitis in Two Time Periods

Organism	1935–1975		1976–1985	
	n	%	n	%
Streptococcus pneumoniae	14	13	2	3
Streptococcus species	9	8	10	14
Staphylococcus aureus	11	10	7	10
Bacillus cereus	1		11	15
Listeria monocytogenes	1		3	4
Clostridium perfringens	1		—	
Neisseria meningitidis	56	52	8	11
Haemophilus influenzae	—		7	
Actinobacillus species	—		2	
Escherichia coli	4	3.7	5	7
Klebsiella pneumoniae	1		5	
Serratia species	—		3	4
Salmonella species	—		3	
Pseudomonas aeruginosa	2		2	
Proteus species	2		—	
Nocardia asteroides	6	5.5	3	
Unidentified	—		1	

Data from Shammas (52a), and Greenwald et al. (53)

material, is another important risk factor. In an extensive review of the literature on endogenous *Candida* endophthalmitis, blood cultures were found to be positive in 41 of 100 patients (67).

Exogenous fungal endophthalmitis is most frequently seen after cataract surgery. The pathogens include *Candida, Aspergillus, Cephalosporium, Penicillium,* and *Curvularia* species, among others. Contaminated lots of solutions containing commercial intraocular lenses have been responsible for the two largest series of cases. Thirteen cases of *Paecilomyces lilacinus* (69) and 15 cases of *Candida parapsilosis* infection (70) followed use of contaminated solutions to store intraocular lenses or to adjust the pH of lenses immediately before implantation.

Clinical Manifestations

Although the clinical presentation of bacterial endophthalmitis is influenced by a variety of factors, including the virulence of the infecting pathogen, symptoms typically begin 2 to 5 days after surgery, at which time the patient may experience decreased vision, ocular pain, and headache. There are no systemic symptoms except in cases involving *B. cereus,* when fever and malaise may be present. Ocular signs include lid edema, increasing conjunctival injection, corneal haze, increasing flare and cells in the anterior chamber with or without hypopyon, and, most importantly, increasing haziness of the vitreous humor with a decreased or absent red reflex because of infiltration by polymorphonuclear leukocytes. Organisms of low virulence, such as *S. epidermidis* and *P. acnes* (71–73), have been associated with a delayed onset of initial signs and symptoms. Of special note are reports of *P. acnes* endophthalmitis appearing as a smoldering process as long as 10 months after extracapsular cataract extraction (66,74,75). The bacteria seem to be sequestered in residual lens cortex. The onset of the clinical infection may, at times, be triggered by subtle events such as laser therapy. By contrast, a short interval between trauma and onset of clinical infection, averaging 1.5 days, was reported in seven patients with *B. cereus* endophthalmitis (18).

The usual presentation of fungal endophthalmitis is an insidious, slowly progressive loss of visual acuity with little or no pain.

In the case of exogenous infection, symptoms usually begin from a week to several months after surgery or a penetrating injury to the eye. Whitish fungus balls are seen in the vitreous humor. By contrast, in endogenous infection the route of entry is the retinal vasculature, and small whitish lesions are seen around the retinal vessels. During some days to weeks they increase in number and size, becoming fluffier and finally extending into the vitreous humor. Patients sometimes perceive the vitreous material as floaters.

Laboratory Diagnosis

Because the damage caused by endophthalmitis and the difficulty of eradicating the infection increase sharply the longer treatment is delayed, early diagnosis and treatment are crucial. Clinical studies confirm that the most fruitful source of material for culture is the vitreous humor (61,71). This is true even with exogenous endophthalmitis and whether or not the lens is present (the lens serving as a barrier to passage of the pathogen from aqueous to vitreous), suggesting that vitreous humor is a better culture medium than aqueous humor. Nevertheless because on rare occasions the aqueous humor may yield organisms when the vitreal sample does not (61,71), both aqueous humor and vitreous humor should be harvested for culture. If a vitrectomy has been performed, the contents of the vitrectomy cassette should also be cultured, for example, by culture of a membrane through which the fluid has been filtered (71). Individual drops of each specimen are placed on culture media, which include chocolate agar and liquid thioglycolate. In the Endophthalmitis Vitrectomy Study, fewer than half of all ocular samples had a positive Gram stain result. Vitrectomy did not produce significantly more positive cultures than material obtained by aspiration or vitreous biopsy and should not be done purely for diagnostic purposes (71). If a fungal infection is suspected, culture material is also plated on Sabouraud agar and some of the sample is stained with Grocott methenamine silver. There is a greater chance of obtaining fungi for culture if a vitrectomy unit is used or if the needle point is placed into a vitreal fluffball under direct observation. When endogenous endophthalmitis is suspected, blood cultures should be obtained. Except in endophthalmitis secondary to an infected bleb, culturing the lids or conjunctiva is unrewarding and is likely to yield organisms not responsible for the infection.

Treatment

PHARMACOLOGIC PRINCIPLES

Major barriers impede delivery of antibiotic to the vitreous humor, the principal site of infection in endophthalmitis (76,77) (Fig. 146.11). The corneal epithelial barrier, the lens-iris apparatus, and the diluting effect of flow of the aqueous humor combine to prevent topically applied drugs from accumulating in therapeutic concentrations in the vitreous. Most antimicrobial agents are not very lipid soluble. Studies in animals and some data in humans have also established that, for these drugs, therapeutic intravitreal antibiotic concentration cannot be achieved after subconjunctival or parenteral administration (77).

Drugs given by subconjunctival injection pass fairly readily through the sclera but do not traverse the barrier of the retinal pigment epithelium and are largely absorbed into the sys-

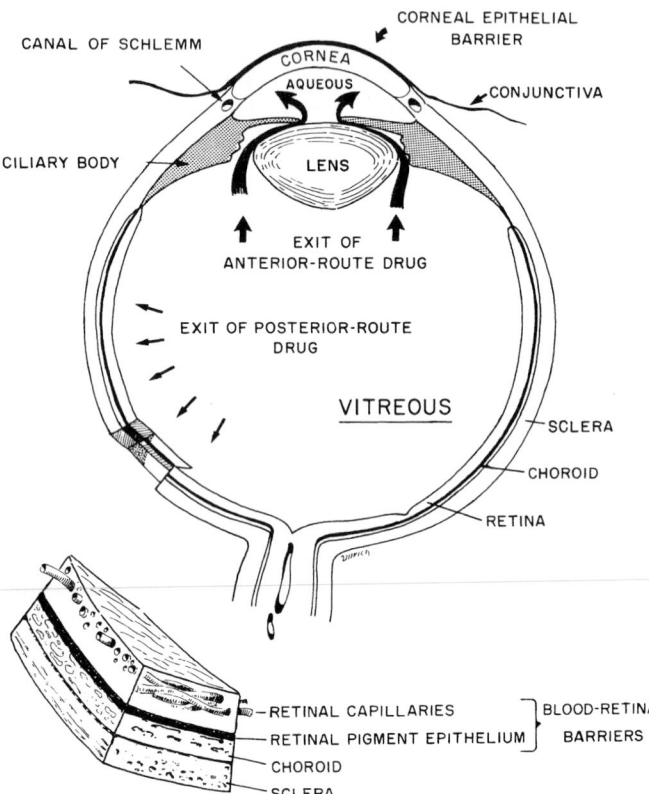

Figure 146.11. The major pharmacokinetic features of the eye. There are three barriers to ocular penetration: (1) the corneal epithelium, which, when intact, prevents topically applied agents from passing through the cornea into the aqueous humor; (2) the retinal pigment epithelium, which, by its tight junctions, prevents drug given by subconjunctival injection from entering the vitreous humor; and (3) the blood-retinal barriers. The outer blood-retinal barrier is in the retinal pigment epithelium; the inner one lies in the tight junctions of the retinal capillaries. The blood-retinal barrier contains an active transport pump for organic anions. Anterior-route drugs (aminoglycosides) leave the vitreous by way of the aqueous humor and canal of Schlemm. Posterior-route drugs (penicillins, cephalosporins) leave by active transport across the retina. (From Barza M. Pharmacokinetics of antibiotics. In: Sabath LD, ed. *Action of antibiotics in patients.* Bern, Switzerland: Hans Huber, 1982:11–39, with permission.)

temic circulation through the uveal vessels. The third-generation cephalosporins were thought possibly to achieve higher vitreous concentrations than older drugs after subconjunctival injection, especially because their vitreous half-life is longer, but this did not prove to be the case in studies in rabbits (78,79). Moreover, in a study of ceftriaxone and ceftazidime in humans with uninfected eyes, vitreous concentrations of ceftriaxone and ceftazidime after a single subconjunctival injection were generally undetectable. Vancomycin was also undetectable in the vitreous in that study (78).

Most drugs injected systemically do not traverse the tight junctions of the nonfenestrated retinal capillaries and do not reach high vitreal concentrations. Therapeutic intravitreal levels of antibiotics can probably be achieved after subconjunctival or parenteral administration of drugs that are quite lipid soluble, such as rifampin, metronidazole, chloramphenicol, minocycline, and sulfamethoxazole. However, these are not drugs of first choice for most strains of bacteria that cause endophthalmitis. Vancomycin, given in a dose of 1 g intravenously to patients with postoperative endophthalmitis, produced vitreous concentrations 1 to 5 hours later that were only 0.4 to 4.5 μg/mL and were not bactericidal *in vitro*. By contrast, intravitreal injection of 1 mg produced concentrations that, even 44 to 72 hours later, ranged from 25 to 182 μg/mL (80). Repeated oral administration of trimethoprim-sulfamethoxazole or ciprofloxacin to a few patients with uninfected eyes produced concentrations in the vitreous that were similar to those in the serum after 48 hours (M. Barza and B. Doft, unpublished data). Although this degree of penetration may be useful in some circumstances, it cannot compare with the high intraocular concentrations achievable promptly and with certainty after intravitreal injection and is not a substitute for intravitreal injection in the initial treatment of bacterial endophthalmitis.

There are two principal routes of egress of antimicrobial agents from the vitreous humor (Fig. 146.11). The aminoglycosides and vancomycin are eliminated by diffusion from the vitreous humor into the aqueous humor and through the canal of Schlemm; this is called the anterior route. Because the route is long and relatively confined, the vitreal half-life of anterior-route drugs is comparatively long, about 24 hours in the normal rabbit eye (Table 146.7). Because of the larger volume of the human eye, the half-life of anterior-route drugs is about twice as long in humans as in rabbits (76). In inflamed eyes the half-life is reduced by about 50%, presumably because the eyes are more "leaky." The half-life is also shortened by extraction of the lens, perhaps because the lens-iris barrier is violated.

The second major route of elimination from the vitreous humor is the so-called posterior, or retinal, route (Fig. 146.11). This is the route taken by most penicillins and cephalosporins, and probably clindamycin. The retinal route consists of an active transport system (81) that removes weak organic acids from the vitreous humor and transports them into the circulation. Because of the short diffusion distances and the active transport system, drugs eliminated by the retinal route have a relatively short vitreal half-life (Table 146.7). The active transport pump is probably located in the retinal pigment epithelium, the retinal capillaries, or both sites (82,83). Probenecid, even when given systemically, inhibits the pump and prolongs the half-life of β-lactam drugs in the vitreous humor (84). Inflammation has at least two effects on transport by the retinal route from the vitreous humor: it impairs the function of the transport pump, which reduces drug elimination, but it makes the eye leaky, which enhances drug elimination from the vitreous humor. The net effect is little change in the vitreal half-life of retinal-route drugs as a result of inflammation.

TABLE 146.7. Regimens for Intravitreal Injection in Humans (Pharmacokinetic Data Estimated from Data in Rabbits)

Drug	Dose (μg)	Peak vitreal concentration (μg/mL)	Estimated half-life (hours) in vitreous humor of humans		Days for concentration to fall by eightfold or three half-lives[a]	
			Uninflamed eye	Inflamed eye	Uninflamed eye	Inflamed eye
Anterior route						
Gentamicin	200–400	40–80	40–60 (less with aphakia)	20–40	6	3
Tobramycin	200–400	40–80	Presumably, as for gentamicin		Presumably, as for gentamicin	
Amikacin	400	40	Presumably, as for gentamicin		Presumably, as for gentamicin	
Vancomycin	1,000–2,000	200–400	40–60	48	6	6
Retinal route						
Penicillin G	600 units	120	8	—	1	—
Carbenicillin	2,000	400	6–8	10	1	1
Cefazolin	2,000	400	10–12	18	1.5	2
Ceftizoxime	Not known		10	15	1.5	4.5
Ceftriaxone	3,000	600	15	22	2	3
Ceftazidime	2,000	400	30	38	4	5
Clindamycin	1,000	200	6	—	1	—

[a]Calculated by multiplying the half-life in rabbits by 2.0 for anterior-route drugs and by 1.7 for retinal-route drugs.
Data from Barza (77) and Maurice (76).

The effect of protein binding on the ocular pharmacokinetics of antibiotics has not been studied well (85). On theoretical grounds, one would predict that a high degree of serum protein binding would restrict the passage of drug from the systemic circulation into the ocular tissues and fluids.

Prognosis for Vision

Before the early 1970s, when most treatment was administered by the systemic route, the visual outcome for patients with bacterial endophthalmitis was dismal. In approximately 75% of patients, the final visual acuity in the affected eye was no better than "light perception" (56). Intravitreal injections of drug and vitrectomy (86) have improved somewhat the prognosis for the restoration of vision. In one series, factors associated with a poor visual result (worse than 20/400) included infection by virulent organisms, poor visual acuity at outset of treatment, and infection secondary to accidental trauma (87). In the Endophthalmitis Vitrectomy Study, at the start of treatment risk factors for a poor outcome included poor vision, a corneal infiltrate or ring ulcer, and absence of a red reflex (62). In many instances, poor initial visual acuity is related to a long interval between onset of infection and initiation of therapy; presumably, the delay allows bacteria to multiply in the vitreous humor, resulting in large inocula and in considerable retinal damage. A long interval before onset of treatment has also been shown experimentally to be associated with a poor bactericidal effect of various classes of antimicrobial agents (88).

Among the common infections, *S. epidermidis* infection has the best prognosis for recovery of vision (47,88,89). This probably results from the relatively low virulence of this species. In one review of *S. epidermidis* infection following cataract extraction, 78% of patients had a final visual acuity of 20/400 or better and 33%, 20/40 or better (89). In the Endophthalmitis Vitrectomy Study, in which 70% of microbiologically confirmed infections were caused by coagulase-negative staphylococci, 53% of patients achieved a final visual acuity of 20/40 or better and 74% achieved 20/100 or better (62). Infection caused by other species or in settings other than cataract surgery has a poorer prognosis. In posttraumatic bacterial endophthalmitis caused by *Bacillus* species (60), anaerobic infections caused by species other than

P. acnes (66), and endophthalmitis associated with filtering blebs in which streptococci and *H. influenzae* are often the cause (64), the final visual acuity for most infected eyes is less than 20/200, qualifying as legal blindness.

With endogenous bacterial endophthalmitis, the chance of having useful vision is even worse than with the exogenous variety because the pathogen is often more virulent, there is a high incidence of immune compromise, and retinal ischemia sometimes occurs as a result of septic embolic occlusion of the central retinal artery (53). In addition, there is often a delay to recognition and treatment of the infection (54). Data on fungal endophthalmitis are meager. The outcome of postoperative fungal infection is better than with the endogenous type, presumably because the latter usually occurs in a setting of poor host defense mechanisms; however, the prognosis for vision recovery in fungal endophthalmitis is guarded because recognition and treatment are often delayed, owing to the insidious nature of the infection and to the problem of delivering high concentrations of effective antifungal agents to the infection site without causing toxicity to the retina.

Treatment of Bacterial Endophthalmitis

As soon as the clinical diagnosis of bacterial endophthalmitis is made, the patient should be brought to the operating room for a diagnostic tap of the vitreous and aqueous humor, intravitreal administration of antibiotics, and, possibly, vitrectomy. Speed is essential because a delay in treatment is associated with poorer visual outcome. Experimental (90) and clinical (91) studies attest to the value of corticosteroids in the treatment of this infection, although debate continues on the timing and routes of administration of the drug (92,93).

A plan for initial empirical therapy of postoperative bacterial endophthalmitis when no specific pathogen is implicated is outlined in Table 146.8. Even if the Gram stain examination suggests certain pathogens, it is recommended that initial treatment involve a regimen that is active against the most common gram-positive and gram-negative pathogens, to reduce the likelihood of inadequate treatment resulting from misinterpretation of the Gram stain. The most popular regimens currently involve a combination of vancomycin and either amikacin or

TABLE 146.8.   Initial Empirical Therapy Used in the Endophthalmitis Vitrectomy Study (62) for Postoperative Bacterial Endophthalmitis

Immediately after diagnosis and aspiration of vitreous and aqueous humor for diagnostic purposes, begin therapy as follows:

Intravitreal injection: amikacin, 0.4 mg (400 μg), or ceftazidime, 2.25 mg, in 0.1 mL, and vancomycin, 1.0 mg (1,000 μg) in 0.1 mL of normal saline solution.

Periocular injection: vancomycin, 25 mg in 0.5 mL, and ceftazidime, 100 mg in 0.5 mL. (If allergic to ceftazidime, substitute amikacin 25 mg in 0.5 mL.) Dexamethasone 6 mg in 0.25 mL.

Systemic administration: generally not necessary (see text).

Topical administration (if evidence of wound infection or leak): vancomycin 50 mg/mL alternating with amikacin, 20 mg/mL) drops, one drop every 1–4 h

Systemic corticosteroids: Prednisone, 30 mg twice daily orally for 5–10 days

TABLE 146.10.   Maximal Nontoxic Dose of Antibiotic and Antifungal Agents for Vitrectomy Infusion Fluid for Endophthalmitis

Agent	Maximal nontoxic dose (μg/mL)
Chloramphenicol	10
Clindamycin	9
Amikacin	10
Tobramycin	10
Gentamicin	8
Ceftazidime	100
Netilmicin	4
Methicillin	20
Oxacillin	10
Penicillin	80
Amphotericin B methyl ester	75[a]

[a]Recommended dose is 10 μg/mL.
Modified from Peyman GA, Schulman JA. *Intravitreal surgery: principles and practice*, 2nd ed. Norwalk, CT: Appleton-Century-Crofts, 1994:905, and Peyman GA, personal communication, regarding ceftazidime, with permission.

ceftazidime. The vancomycin is directed at strains of staphylococci (coagulase negative and positive) (94) and streptococci (64) (including *Enterococcus faecalis*) and, in posttraumatic infections, *B. cereus* (60). The drug is well tolerated (95), and its intravitreal half-life is long. Amikacin is preferred over gentamicin or tobramycin because, in experimental animals, it is less toxic to the retina (96,97). Because of concerns about rare instances of macular infarction possibly attributable to the intravitreal or subconjunctival injection of aminoglycosides (98), some ophthalmologists prefer ceftazidime to amikacin. Nevertheless, because of the broad experience with amikacin, and because aminoglycosides, but not ceftazidime, show concentration-dependent killing and synergy *in vitro* with vancomycin against many common intraocular pathogens, the Endophthalmitis Vitrectomy Study elected to use amikacin for postoperative endophthalmitis (99). Only 1 patient of 420 treated in this manner was observed to have a macular infarction, and relation of that infarction to the intravitreal injection of amikacin could not be determined.

Table 146.9 lists the intravitreal doses of various antibiotics when given by intravitreal injection, and Table 146.10 suggests

TABLE 146.9.   Intravitreal Antibiotic Injection

Antibiotic	Intravitreal dose (mg)	Duration of therapeutic level in vitreous (h)
Aminoglycosides		
Gentamicin	0.4	48–72
Tobramycin	0.4	48–72
Amikacin	0.4	48–72
Penicillins and cephalosporins		
Oxacillin	0.5	24
Ampicillin	5.0	24
Carbenicillin	2.0	16–24
Cefazolin	2.0	24
Ceftazidime	2.25	36–48
Miscellaneous		
Clindamycin	1.0	16–24
Vancomycin	1.0	72
Antifungal antibiotic		
Amphotericin B	5–10 μg	120–168

Modified from Baum J. Antibiotic use in ophthalmology. In: Tasman W, Jaeger EA, eds. *Duane's clinical ophthalmology*. Vol. 4. Philadelphia: Lippincott Williams & Wilkins, 1997, with permission.

drug concentrations for instances in which the antibiotics are incorporated into the vitrectomy infusion fluid rather than being given by direct intravitreal injection. In addition to the drugs (vancomycin and either amikacin or ceftazidime) suggested for initial empiric treatment in postoperative endophthalmitis, the tables provide data for other antibiotics that may be used in circumstances in which the pathogen and its susceptibility happen to be known, for example, reinjection of an eye from which cultures have already been taken. These dosages recommended for intravitreal injection or infusion in humans are generally intended to produce a peak vitreal concentration equal to 10% of the lowest concentration that produces retinal toxicity in the rabbit eyes. Any antibiotic solution for intraocular administration is best prepared by the hospital pharmacist. For *Bacillus cereus* infection, clindamycin or vancomycin is preferred. If an anaerobic infection is suspected or documented, penicillin or clindamycin is the drug of choice (66). Metronidazole would probably be highly effective for infection by strict anaerobes. There are no data for its use by intravitreal injection but, because it is so lipid soluble, it would probably penetrate well by systemic routes. Vancomycin is recommended in infection by *P. acnes* (75).

The role of vitrectomy in the initial treatment of endophthalmitis has been controversial. The procedure has the theoretical advantage of decreasing the infective inoculum and of removing destructive toxins and enzymes, thereby reducing the morbidity of the disease. In addition, by reducing the vitreal opacification, vitrectomy enhances visualization of the retina. Some reports suggested that the procedure improves the final visual acuity (100), whereas others concluded that the effect is harmful. However, the studies were retrospective and subject to marked allocation bias. Likewise, it has not been shown that antibiotics administered intravenously are necessary in patients receiving antibiotics by intravitreal and periocular injection for endophthalmitis occurring after cataract extraction (101). Because of these uncertainties, the Endophthalmitis Vitrectomy Study was undertaken (62). This was a multicenter, randomized trial of both immediate vitrectomy and (in a separate randomization) of intravenous antibiotics (ceftazidime and amikacin) in the treatment of endophthalmitis after cataract extraction or secondary lens implantation. All patients received intravitreal injections of vancomycin and amikacin, as well as subconjunctival and topical antibiotics and corticosteroids. The results showed that immediate vitrectomy (as opposed to no or delayed vitrectomy—which was done only in eyes in which the response to initial treatment was poor) offered no benefit except in the subgroup of patients whose initial presenting visual acuity was no better than light perception. Eleven percent of eyes that did not undergo immediate vitrectomy and 7% of eyes that underwent immediate vitrectomy later met criteria for vitrectomy or another surgical procedure; 8% and 7%, respectively, had a repeat intravitreal injection of antibiotics. Thus, most eyes in both groups did not require a subsequent procedure. Intravenously administered antibiotics afforded no benefit to the total group or any subgroup in this study. Some have objected that the results may be biased because the intravenous regimen did not include vancomycin but, as noted above, vancomycin given by this route barely penetrates into the vitreous even of the inflamed eye (80), and the levels would be trivial compared with those afforded by intravitreal injection. In summary, in this prospective study of endophthalmitis after cataract extraction, in which most eyes were infected by coagulase-negative staphylococci, immediate vitrectomy was beneficial only in eyes with poor vision at the time of initial presentation. Intravenous antibiotics were of no benefit, and most patients required only a single intravitreal injection of antibiotics. The results of the EVS study cannot necessarily be generalized to other forms of endophthalmitis, such as endogenous or posttraumatic endophthalmitis, chronic indolent endophthalmitis, or endophthalmitis due to unusual organisms (48).

In refractory cases of bacterial endophthalmitis, repeat intravitreal injections may be needed. If so, an interval of about 3 days between successive injections may be suggested for many of the agents based on limited human data (80,102) and by extrapolation (Table 146.7) from the half-life of various antimicrobial agents in rabbit eyes.

Treatment of Fungal Endophthalmitis

Potential approaches to the treatment of fungal endophthalmitis include the systemic route, intravitreal injection, or both. The choice depends on the site of the lesions (confined to the retina, or involving the vitreous humor) and the pharmacologic characteristics of the drug (103). Most of the available information is based on experience with *Candida* species and with the drugs amphotericin B and fluconazole: there is far less experience with infection by other genera of fungi and very little information on the vitreous penetration of the newer azoles and echinocandins.

Early in endogenous (hematogenous) endophthalmitis, lesions tend to be restricted to the area within and immediately around the retinal vessels. The infection may be better described as chorioretinitis than endophthalmitis. At this stage, systemic administration of either amphotericin B, or one of its lipid formulations, or fluconazole (presuming the infecting species is susceptible), is likely to be effective. Itraconazole, a bulkier molecule than fluconazole, may not penetrate the vitreous as well as fluconazole, which does so readily (104). A dosage of fluconazole of 100 to 200 mg per day orally for about 2 months has been effective (105), but a dosage of 400 mg per day might now be preferred (103). The efficacy of treatment can be monitored by the ophthalmologist via slit-lamp examination. If the disease is not extensive, vitrectomy may not be of value (unless needed for diagnosis). The duration of treatment is difficult to specify and may be influenced by the need for treatment of systemic infection, if one is present. In general, one would tend to continue treatment until all active ocular lesions detectable by slit lamp had resolved.

For infection extending into the vitreous humor (exogenous infection and later-stage endogenous infection), and infection by fluconazole-resistant species, the treatment of choice is amphotericin B given by intravitreal injection (103). The drug is generally well tolerated in dosages of 5 μg in the eyes of rabbits and 10 to 20 μg in the eyes of primates (106,107). Accordingly, a dose of 5 to 10 μg in 0.1 mL is suggested in humans (47,103). Although liposomal amphotericin B is tolerated in even higher dosages than amphotericin B desoxycholate (106), there is no evident advantage to the liposomal formulations. The half-life of amphotericin B in the vitreous is more than 2 days (108,109), so repeat injections, if necessary, should be spaced at least a few days apart. For infection restricted to the eye, it is not clear that intravenous administration of amphotericin B adds any value to intravitreal injection of the drug.

Early vitrectomy is advisable for eyes with substantial vitreous involvement to remove the bulk of the infectious and inflammatory debris, facilitate examination by the ophthalmologist, and, perhaps, aid drug diffusion within the eye. Amphotericin B can be injected intravitreally at the time of vitrectomy. In some patients with endogenous endophthalmitis, there is no evidence of systemic infection once the endophthalmitis has occurred: intravitreal injection alone, possibly with vitrectomy, may suffice to cure such infections (103).

REFERENCES

1. Tasman W, Jaeger E, eds. Duane's clinical ophthalmology. Vol. 4. Philadelphia: Lippincott Williams & Wilkins, 2000.
2. Tabbara KF, Hyndiuk RA. *Infections of the eye,* 2nd ed. Boston: Little, Brown. 1996:xvi, 741.
3. Pepose JS, Holland GN, Wilhelmus KR. *Ocular infection & immunity.* St. Louis: CV Mosby, 1996:xl, 1552.
4. Pavan-Langston D. Viral disease of the cornea and external eye. In: Albert D, Jakobiec F, eds. *Principles and practice of ophthalmology.* Philadelphia: WB Saunders, 2000:846–892.
5. Barza M, Baum J. Ocular infections. *Med Clin North Am* 1983;67(1):131–152.
6. Baum J. Antibiotic use in ophthalmology. In: Tasman W, Jaeger E, eds. *Duane's clinical ophthalmology.* Philadelphia: Lippincott Williams & Wilkins, 1997:1–33.
7. Perry HD, Serniuk RA. Conservative treatment of chalazia. *Ophthalmology* 1980;87(3):218–221.
8. Pizzarello LD, et al. Intralesional corticosteroid therapy of chalazia. *Am J Ophthalmol* 1978;85(6):818–821.
9. Baum J, Fedukowicz HB, Jordan A. A survey of Moraxella corneal ulcers in a derelict population. *Am J Ophthalmol* 1980;90(4):476–480.
10. Wilson LA, et al. Fungi from the normal outer eye. *Am J Ophthalmol* 1969;67(1):52–56.
11. Brazilian purpuric fever: epidemic purpura fulminans associated with antecedent purulent conjunctivitis. Brazilian Purpuric Fever Study Group. *Lancet* 1987;2(8562):757–761.
12. Fraunfelder FT, Bagby GC Jr, Kelly DJ. Fatal aplastic anemia following topical administration of ophthalmic chloramphenicol. *Am J Ophthalmol* 1982;93(3):356–360.
13. Centers for Disease Control and Prevention. 1993 sexually transmitted diseases treatment guidelines. *MMWR* 1993;42(RR-14):1–102.
14. Bailey RL, et al. Randomised controlled trial of single-dose azithromycin in treatment of trachoma. *Lancet* 1993;342(8869):453–456.
15. Dawson CR, et al. A comparison of oral azithromycin with topical oxytetracycline/polymyxin for the treatment of trachoma in children. *Clin Infect Dis* 1997;24(3):363–368.
16. Isenberg SJ, Apt L, Wood M. A controlled trial of povidone-iodine as prophylaxis against ophthalmia neonatorum. *N Engl J Med* 1995;332(9):562–566.
17. Kreger AS, Griffin OK. Physicochemical fractionation of extracellular cornea-damaging proteases of *Pseudomonas aeruginosa. Infect Immun* 1974;9(5): 828–834.
18. O'Day DM, et al. The problem of bacillus species infection with special emphasis on the virulence of *Bacillus cereus. Ophthalmology* 1981;88(8):833–838.
19. Forster RK, et al. Methenamine-silver-stained corneal scrapings in keratomycosis. *Am J Ophthalmol* 1976;82(2):261–265.
20. Jones D. A plan for antimicrobial therapy in bacterial keratitis. *Trans Am Acad Ophthalmol Otolaryngol* 1975;79:95–103.
21. Baum JL. Initial therapy of suspected microbial corneal ulcers. I. Broad antibiotic therapy based on prevalence of organisms. *Surv Ophthalmol* 1979;24(2): 97–105.
22. Kremer I, et al. The effect of topical ceftazidime on pseudomonas keratitis in rabbits. *Cornea* 1994;13(4):360–363.
23. Baum J, Barza M. Topical vs subconjunctival treatment of bacterial corneal ulcers. *Ophthalmology* 1983;90(2):162–168.

24. Leibowitz HM, Ryan WJ Jr, Kupferman A. Route of antibiotic administration in bacterial keratitis. *Arch Ophthalmol* 1981;99(8):1420–1423.

25. Koenig S. Fungal keratitis. In: Tabbara KF, Hyndiuk RA, eds. *Infections of the eye.* Boston: Little, Brown, 1986:331–342.

26. Jones BR. Principles in the management of oculomycosis. XXXI Edward Jackson memorial lecture. *Am J Ophthalmol* 1975;79(5):719–751.

27. Wood TO, Tuberville AW, Monnett R. Keratomycosis and amphotericin B. *Trans Am Ophthalmol Soc* 1985;83:397–409.

28. Pavan-Langston D. Herpes simplex of the ocular anterior segment. *Curr Clin Top Infect Dis* 2000;20:298–324.

29. Rayfield M, Kaufman HE. Pathogenicity and strain specificity of herpes simplex virus. In: Duane T, Jaeger E, eds. *Foundations of clinical ophthalmology.* Philadelphia: JB Lippincott, 1988:1–17.

30. Sabbaga EM, et al. Detection of HSV nucleic acid sequences in the cornea during acute and latent ocular disease. *Exp Eye Res* 1988;47(4):545–553.

31. Meyers-Elliott RH, Pettit TH, Maxwell WA. Viral antigens in the immune ring of herpes simplex stromal keratitis. *Arch Ophthalmol* 1980;98(5):897–904.

32. Barron BA, et al. Herpetic Eye Disease Study. A controlled trial of oral acyclovir for herpes simplex stromal keratitis. *Ophthalmology* 1994;101(12):1871–1882.

33. Pavan-Langston D. Ophthalmic zoster. In: Watson C, Gershon A, eds. *Herpes zoster and postherpetic neuralgia.* Amsterdam: Elsevier Science, 2001:119–129.

34. Jones DB, Visvesvara GS, Robinson NM. *Acanthamoeba polyphaga* keratitis and *Acanthamoeba* uveitis associated with fatal meningoencephalitis. *Trans Ophthalmol Soc UK* 1975;95(2):221–232.

35. Naginton J, et al. Amoebic infection of the eye. *Lancet* 1974;2(7896):1537–1540.

36. Epstein RJ, et al. Rapid diagnosis of *Acanthamoeba* keratitis from corneal scrapings using indirect fluorescent antibody staining. *Arch Ophthalmol* 1986;104(9):1318–1321.

37. Silvany RE, Luckenbach MW, Moore MB. The rapid detection of Acanthamoeba in paraffin-embedded sections of corneal tissue with calcofluor white. *Arch Ophthalmol* 1987;105(10):1366–1367.

38. Pfister DR, et al. Confocal microscopy findings of *Acanthamoeba* keratitis. *Am J Ophthalmol* 1996;121:119–128.

39. Auran JD, Starr MB, Jakobiec FA. *Acanthamoeba* keratitis. A review of the literature. *Cornea* 1987;6(1):2–26.

40. Wright P, Warhurst D, Jones BR. *Acanthamoeba* keratitis successfully treated medically. *Br J Ophthalmol* 1985;69(10):778–782.

41. Larkin DF, Kilvington S, Dart JK. Treatment of *Acanthamoeba* keratitis with polyhexamethylene biguanide. *Ophthalmology* 1992;99(2):185–191.

42. Lindquist TD. Treatment of *Acanthamoeba* keratitis. *Cornea* 1998;17(1):11–16.

43. Seal D, et al. Successful medical therapy of *Acanthamoeba* keratitis with topical chlorhexidine and propamidine. *Eye* 1996;10(Part 4):413–421.

44. Cohen EJ, et al. Medical and surgical treatment of *Acanthamoeba* keratitis. *Am J Ophthalmol* 1987;103(5):615–625.

45. Moore MB. *Acanthamoeba* keratitis. *Arch Ophthalmol* 1988;106(9):1181–1183.

46. Driebe WT Jr, et al. *Acanthamoeba* keratitis. Potential role for topical clotrimazole in combination chemotherapy. *Arch Ophthalmol* 1988;106(9):1196–1201.

47. Forster RK. Endophthalmitis. In: Tasman W, Jaeger E, eds. *Duane's clinical ophthalmology.* Philadelphia: Lippincott Williams & Wilkins, 1994.

48. Doft BH, Barza M. Optimal management of postoperative endophthalmitis and results of the Endophthalmitis Vitrectomy Study. *Curr Opin Ophthalmol* 1996;7(3):84–94.

49. Tay-Kearney ML, Jabs DA. Ophthalmic complications of HIV infection. *Med Clin North Am* 1996;80(6):1471–1492.

50. Holland GN. New strategies for the management of AIDS-related CMV retinitis in the era of potent antiretroviral therapy. *Ocul Immunol Inflamm* 1999;7(3–4):179–188.

51. Davis JL, et al. Effect of potent antiretroviral therapy on recurrent cytomegalovirus retinitis treated with the ganciclovir implant. *Am J Ophthalmol* 1999;127(3):283–287.

52. Whitcup SM. Cytomegalovirus retinitis in the era of highly active antiretroviral therapy. *JAMA* 2000;283(5):653–657.

52a. Shammas, HF. Endogenous *E. coli* endophthalmitis *Surv Ophthalmol* 1977;21:429–435.

53. Greenwald MJ, Wohl LG, Sell CH. Metastatic bacterial endophthalmitis: a contemporary reappraisal. *Surv Ophthalmol* 1986;31(2):81–101.

54. Okada AA, et al. Endogenous bacterial endophthalmitis. Report of a ten-year retrospective study. *Ophthalmology* 1994;101(5):832–838.

55. Christy NE, Lall P. Postoperative endophthalmitis following cataract surgery. Effects on subconjunctival antibiotics and other factors. *Arch Ophthalmol* 1973;90(5):361–366.

56. Allen HF, Mangiaracine AB. Bacterial endophthalmitis after cataract extraction. II. Incidence in 36,000 consecutive operations with special reference to preoperative topical antibiotics. *Arch Ophthalmol* 1974;91(1):3–7.

57. Fahmy JA. Endophthalmitis following cataract extraction. A study of 24 cases in 4,498 operations. *Acta Ophthalmol (Copenh)* 1975;53(4):522–536.

58. Kattan HM, et al. Nosocomial endophthalmitis survey. Current incidence of infection after intraocular surgery. *Ophthalmology* 1991;98(2):227–238.

59. Barr CC. Prognostic factors in corneoscleral lacerations. *Arch Ophthalmol* 1983;101(6):919–924.

60. Affeldt JC, et al. Microbial endophthalmitis resulting from ocular trauma. *Ophthalmology* 1987;94(4):407–413.

61. Forster RK. Etiology and diagnosis of bacterial postoperative endophthalmitis. *Ophthalmology* 1978;85(4):320–326.

62. Results of the Endophthalmitis Vitrectomy Study. A randomized trial of immediate vitrectomy and of intravenous antibiotics for the treatment of postoperative bacterial endophthalmitis. Endophthalmitis Vitrectomy Study Group. *Arch Ophthalmol* 1995;113(12):1479–1496.

63. Han DP, et al. Spectrum and susceptibilities of microbiologic isolates in the Endophthalmitis Vitrectomy Study. *Am J Ophthalmol* 1996;122(1):1–17.

64. Mandelbaum S, et al. Late onset endophthalmitis associated with filtering blebs. *Ophthalmology* 1985;92(7):964–972.

65. Brinton GS, et al. Posttraumatic endophthalmitis. *Arch Ophthalmol* 1984;102(4):547–550.

66. Ormerod LD, et al. Anaerobic bacterial endophthalmitis. *Ophthalmology* 1987;94(7):799–808.

67. Brod RD, Flynn HW Jr, Miller D. *Endogenous fungal endophthalmitis.* In: Tasman W, Jaeger E, eds. *Duane's clinical ophthalmology.* Philadelphia: Lippincott Williams & Wilkins, 2001:1–29.

68. Doft BH, et al. Endogenous *Aspergillus* endophthalmitis in drug abusers. *Arch Ophthalmol* 1980;98(5):859–862.

69. Pettit TH, et al. Fungal endophthalmitis following intraocular lens implantation. A surgical epidemic. *Arch Ophthalmol* 1980;98(6):1025–1039.

70. Stern WH, et al. Epidemic postsurgical *Candida parapsilosis* endophthalmitis. Clinical findings and management of 15 consecutive cases. *Ophthalmology* 1985;92(12):1701–1709.

71. Barza M, et al. Evaluation of microbiological diagnostic techniques in postoperative endophthalmitis in the Endophthalmitis Vitrectomy Study. *Arch Ophthalmol* 1997;115(9):1142–1150.

72. Bode DD Jr, Gelender H, Forster RK. A retrospective review of endophthalmitis due to coagulase-negative staphylococci. *Br J Ophthalmol* 1985;69(12):915–919.

73. Ficker L, et al. Chronic bacterial endophthalmitis. *Am J Ophthalmol* 1987;103(6):745–748.

74. Meisler DM, Mandelbaum S. *Propionibacterium*-associated endophthalmitis after extracapsular cataract extraction. Review of reported cases. *Ophthalmology* 1989;96(1):54–61.

75. Winward KE, et al. Postoperative *Propionibacterium* endophthalmitis. Treatment strategies and long-term results. *Ophthalmology* 1993;100(4):447–451.

76. Maurice D. Injection of drugs into the vitreous body. In: Leopold I, Burns R, eds. *Symposium on ocular therapy.* New York: John Wiley & Sons, 1976:59–72.

77. Barza M. Antibacterial agents in the treatment of ocular infections. *Infect Dis Clin North Am* 1989;3(3):533–551.

78. Barza M, Doft B, Lynch E. Ocular penetration of ceftriaxone, ceftazidime, and vancomycin after subconjunctival injection in humans. *Arch Ophthalmol* 1993;111(4):492–494.

79. Meredith TA. Antimicrobial pharmacokinetics in endophthalmitis treatment: studies of ceftazidime. *Trans Am Ophthalmol Soc* 1993;91:653–699.

80. Ferencz JR, et al. Vancomycin concentration in the vitreous after intravenous and intravitreal administration for postoperative endophthalmitis. *Arch Ophthalmol* 1999;117(8):1023–1027.

81. Forbes M, Becker B. The transport of organic anions by the rabbit eye. II. *In vivo* transport of iodopyracet (Diodrast). *Am J Ophthalmol* 1960;50:867–875.

82. Ficker L, et al. Cefazolin levels after intravitreal injection. Effects of inflammation and surgery. *Invest Ophthalmol Vis Sci* 1990;31(3):502–505.

83. Cunha-Vaz J. The blood-ocular barriers. *Surv Ophthalmol* 1979;23(5):279–296.

84. Barza M, Kane A, Baum J. Pharmacokinetics of intravitreal carbenicillin, cefazolin, and gentamicin in rhesus monkeys. *Invest Ophthalmol Vis Sci* 1983;24(12):1602–1606.

85. Barza M, Baum J. Penetration of ocular compartments by penicillins. *Surv Ophthalmol* 1973;18:71–82.

86. Stern GA, Engel HM, Driebe WT Jr. The treatment of postoperative endophthalmitis. Results of differing approaches to treatment. *Ophthalmology* 1989;96(1):62–67.

87. Bohigian GM, Olk RJ. Factors associated with a poor visual result in endophthalmitis. *Am J Ophthalmol* 1986;101(3):332–341.

88. Rowsey JJ, et al. Endophthalmitis: current approaches. *Ophthalmology* 1982;89(9):1055–1066.

89. Driebe WT Jr, et al. Pseudophakic endophthalmitis. Diagnosis and management. *Ophthalmology* 1986;93(4):442–448.

90. Baum JL, et al. The effect of corticosteroids in the treatment of experimental bacterial endophthalmitis. *Am J Ophthalmol* 1975;80(3 Part 2):513–515.

91. Baum JL, Rao G. Treatment of post-cataract bacterial endophthalmitis with periocular and systemic antibiotics and corticosteroids. *Trans Am Acad Ophthalmol Otolaryngol* 1976;81(5):952.

92. Meredith TA, et al. Intraocular dexamethasone produces a harmful effect on treatment of experimental *Staphylococcus aureus* endophthalmitis. *Trans Am Ophthalmol Soc* 1996;94:241–252.

93. Shah GK, et al. Visual outcomes following the use of intravitreal steroids in the treatment of postoperative endophthalmitis. *Ophthalmology* 2000;107(3):486–489.

94. Davis JL, et al. Coagulase-negative staphylococcal endophthalmitis. Increase in antimicrobial resistance. *Ophthalmology* 1988;95(10):1404–1410.

95. Pflugfelder SC, et al. Intravitreal vancomycin. Retinal toxicity, clearance, and interaction with gentamicin. *Arch Ophthalmol* 1987;105(6):831–837.

96. D'Amico DJ, et al. Comparative toxicity of intravitreal aminoglycoside antibiotics. *Am J Ophthalmol* 1985;100(2):264–275.

97. Talamo JH, D'Amico DJ, Kenyon KR. Intravitreal amikacin in the treatment of bacterial endophthalmitis. *Arch Ophthalmol* 1986;104(10):1483–1485.

98. Campochiaro PA, Lim JI. Aminoglycoside toxicity in the treatment of endophthalmitis. The Aminoglycoside Toxicity Study Group. *Arch Ophthalmol* 1994;112(1):48–53.

99. Doft BH, Barza M. Ceftazidime or amikacin: choice of intravitreal antimicrobials in the treatment of postoperative endophthalmitis. *Arch Ophthalmol* 1994;112(1):17–18.

100. Cottingham AJ Jr, Forster RK. Vitrectomy in endophthalmitis. Results of study using vitrectomy, intraocular antibiotics, or a combination of both. *Arch Ophthalmol* 1976;94(12):2078–2081.

101. Pavan PR, et al. Exogenous endophthalmitis initially treated without systemic antibiotics. *Ophthalmology* 1994;101(7):1289–1296; discussion 1296–1297.

102. Cobo LM, Forster RK. The clearance of intravitreal gentamicin. *Am J Ophthalmol* 1981;92(1):59–62.

103. Barza M. Treatment options for candidal endophthalmitis [Editorial; comment]. *Clin Infect Dis* 1998;27(5):1134–1136.

104. O'Day DM, et al. Ocular uptake of fluconazole following oral administration. *Arch Ophthalmol* 1990;108(7):1006–1008.

105. Akler ME, et al. Use of fluconazole in the treatment of candidal endophthalmitis. *Clin Infect Dis* 1995;20(3):657–664.

106. Barza M, et al. Ocular toxicity of intravitreally injected liposomal amphotericin B in rhesus monkeys. *Am J Ophthalmol* 1985;100(2):259–263.

107. Axelrod AJ, Peyman GA, Apple DJ. Toxicity of intravitreal injection of amphotericin B. *Am J Ophthalmol* 1973;76(4):578–583.

108. Wingard LB Jr, et al. Intraocular distribution of intravitreally administered amphotericin B in normal and vitrectomized eyes. *Invest Ophthalmol Vis Sci* 1989;30(10):2184–2189.

109. Tremblay C, et al. Reduced toxicity of liposome-associated amphotericin B injected intravitreally in rabbits. *Invest Ophthalmol Vis Sci* 1985;26(5):711–718.

Nervous System

CHAPTER 147
Approach to the Patient with Infection of the Central Nervous System

David N. Irani and Diane E. Griffin

Central nervous system (CNS) infections are relatively infrequent, accounting for less than 1% of all hospital admissions. When encountered, however, such infections require prompt diagnosis and treatment. In these situations, the potential for rapid progression and permanent neurologic injury lends greater urgency than occurs with many other types of infectious disease.

CNS infections take a great variety of forms, ranging from acute but benign forms of viral meningitis to rapidly fatal bacterial meningitis to the slowly progressive mental deterioration caused by fungal, mycobacterial, or persistent viral infection (Table 147.1). The most common of these diseases are viral and bacterial meningitis, with 2.3% of men and 1.5% of women developing either condition some time before age 80 (1). The outcome from bacterial infections of the CNS is determined by a number of factors, including age, the virulence of the invading organism, and the speed and appropriateness of therapy (2–5). Indeed, most deaths from these infections occur within the first 48 hours of hospitalization (6). For this reason, bacterial infections of the CNS must be recognized early and the probable infecting agent determined as rapidly as possible. Proper initial assessment of the patient requires a careful history with attention to the tempo of the disease, exposures to infectious agents, and host factors that may increase susceptibility to certain infections. The physical examination is directed toward an anatomic localization of the neurologic process and a search for evidence of systemic infection. These efforts are supplemented by examination of the cerebrospinal fluid (CSF) and, when indicated, imaging studies of the CNS.

ANATOMIC CONSIDERATIONS

The CNS is relatively protected from infection. The scalp, skull, and meninges help to prevent spread of infection from external sources, while the blood-brain barrier excludes most circulating pathogens. When infection of the CNS is suspected, much of the initial evaluation should be directed at determining the anatomic site of infection. This helps to narrow the differential diagnosis, determine the necessary therapy, and predict the eventual outcome. Although some infections of the CNS spread to involve more than one neuroanatomic site, most characteristically localize to one particular region or compartment.

Dura

The dura overlying the brain is relatively adherent to the skull in many places. In the spine, however, the dura is not adherent to bone and the epidural space with its rich vascular network can more easily be invaded by infectious pathogens. Between the dura and the arachnoid is a potential space with few restraining structures, allowing subdural abscesses to become relatively large, space-occupying lesions (7,8). Infections in both of these parameningeal locations are usually associated with direct invasion by microorganisms secondary to trauma, catheters, neurosurgical procedures, or spread from nearby sites of disease. Occasionally, blood-borne organisms may seed the spinal epidural space from a distant site of infection (3,9).

Leptomeninges

The pia and arachnoid overlying the brain and spinal cord are usually involved together in infectious processes. Viruses, mycoplasmas, rickettsia, bacteria, mycobacteria, fungi, and parasites are all capable of causing leptomeningitis when they invade the subarachnoid space. While recirculation of CSF in this compartment may disseminate infection throughout the neuraxis, inflammation often collects at the base of the brain, causing cranial nerve palsies, hydrocephalus (due to obstructed CSF flow), and even vascular involvement with ensuing stroke. Organisms are usually carried to the subarachnoid space via hematogenous dissemination (10), causing acute, subacute, or chronic disease, depending on the infecting agent and the immune status of the host.

Parenchyma

Infection of the brain parenchyma may result via the local spread of organisms from a contiguous source of infection (usually resulting in a single lesion) or by hematogenous spread (often resulting in multiple lesions) (11,12). Bacterial infections usually begin as a localized cerebritis with focal softening, necrosis, inflammation, and edema of the brain. As the process continues, fibroblasts may proliferate at the periphery to encapsulate the infected area (13). Symptoms may result from the local destruction of tissue, but most often are due to surrounding edema and mass effect from the expanding lesion. Viral infection of the brain parenchyma causes encephalitis, which may be either focal or diffuse. Most viruses that cause encephalitis reach the brain from the bloodstream. These pathogens directly infect neurons and

TABLE 147.1. Incidence and Mortality Rate for Central Nervous System Infections from 1950 to 1981, in Olmsted County, Minnesota

Infection	Incidence (per 100,000 person-years)	Mortality (%)
Aseptic meningitis	10.9	0.0
Bacterial meningitis	8.6	10.0
Viral encephalitis	7.4	3.8
Brain abscess	1.1	37.5
Chronic meningitis	0.4	43.4

Adapted from Nicolosi A, Hauser WA, Beghi E, et al. Epidemiology of central nervous system infections in Olmsted County Minnesota, 1950–1981. *J Infect Dis* 1986;154:399, with permission.

TABLE 147.2. Organisms that Most Often Cause Central Nervous System Infection in Immunocompromised Hosts

Deficiencies in complement and antibody production
   Streptococcus pneumoniae
   Neisseria meningitidis
   Haemophilus influenzae
   Enteroviruses
Deficiencies in cellular immunity
   Cryptococcus
   Toxoplasma
   Nocardia
   Listeria
   JC virus (progressive multifocal leukoencephalopathy)
   Human immunodeficiency virus
   Cytomegalovirus

glial cells, leading to seizures, paralysis, and changes in mental status (14).

EPIDEMIOLOGIC CONSIDERATIONS

Many viral, rickettsial, and bacterial infections have distinct seasonal and geographic variations that help to narrow the differential diagnosis. Arthropod-borne infections occur in locations where their insect vectors are present and at the times of the year when the vectors are active. Tick-borne infections, such as Rocky Mountain spotted fever, tick-borne encephalitis, and Lyme disease, are most common in spring and early summer (15,16). Mosquito-borne diseases such as eastern equine, La Crosse, St. Louis, and West Nile virus encephalitides occur during the summer and early fall, often in particular regions of the country (17). Enteroviral infections, the most common cause of viral meningitis and encephalitis, also have their highest incidence during the late summer and fall months (18–20). Bacterial meningitis peaks in the winter and may occur in outbreaks (6,21–23).

HOST CONSIDERATIONS

Host factors are important determinants of susceptibility to CNS infection. A history of recent open trauma, surgery, or severe burn suggests the possibility of infection with staphylococcal or gram-negative organisms from the environment and skin (4,8,24,25). Head trauma resulting in a basilar skull fracture and subsequent CSF leak is strongly associated with pneumococcal meningitis (26). The majority of individuals with spinal epidural abscesses have some degree of underlying degenerative spine disease (3). Brain abscesses occur more frequently in persons with chronic sinusitis or otitis, congenital heart disease, recent esophageal procedures, or other conditions that produce bac-

teremia (11,12). CSF shunts, reservoirs, and catheters most often become infected with staphylococci (27).

Immune defenses against CNS invasion of organisms from the bloodstream are compromised by abnormalities of cellular immunity, antibody formation, complement production, and phagocytosis. This is because prevention of spread to the CNS depends on prompt clearance of pathogens from both tissue and blood. Different types of immune compromise are preferentially associated with certain types of CNS infections. Genetic and acquired deficiencies in phagocytosis (e.g., sickle cell disease, traumatic or surgical asplenia, Fc receptor deficiency), in antibody synthesis, or in circulating levels of complement specifically predispose to CNS infections with encapsulated bacteria (28–30). Hypogammaglobulinemia also predisposes to chronic enteroviral infection (31). Genetic and acquired deficiencies of cellular immunity, resulting in inadequate clearance of organisms from tissue and diminished control of latent or persistent organisms, mainly predispose to CNS infection by fungi and obligate or facultative intracellular pathogens such as viruses, *Listeria, Norcardia,* mycobacteria, and parasites (32–40) (Table 147.2).

Age is an important host factor in considering the cause and predicting the outcome of CNS infection (2,4,6,10,19–21,24,41) (Table 147.3). Meningitis (both bacterial and viral) and encephalitis are most common in childhood. Infants, possibly because of their immature immune status, are highly susceptible to CNS infection caused by *Listeria,* gram-negative bacilli, group B streptococci, enteroviruses, and herpesviruses (19,23,42–45). As maternal antibody levels wane but *de novo* production of antibodies against bacterial polysaccharides lags, young children become susceptible to bacterial pathogens such as *Haemophilus, Pneumococcus,* and *Meningococcus* (4,45). Routine vaccination against *H. influenzae* type b has dramatically reduced the risk of bacterial meningitis in children 1 month to 5 years of age (45). With advancing age, susceptibility to gram-negative organisms increases (45), accounting for nearly one fourth of all CNS infections in

TABLE 147.3. Organisms that Most Often Cause Central Nervous System Infection in Immunologically Normal Hosts at Different Ages

<1 Month	1 Month to 5 years	6–59 Years	>60 Years
Gram-negative bacilli	Enteroviruses	Enteroviruses	*S. pneumoniae*
Group B streptococci	*N. meningitidis*	*N. meningitidis*	Gram-negative baci
Listeria	*S. pneumoniae*	*S. pneumoniae*	*Listeria*
Herpes simplex virus		Herpes simplex virus	

persons over 65 years of age (46). Overall mortality from bacterial infections of the CNS is highest in patients over age 60 (24).

CLINICAL ASSESSMENT

Headache or backache are common, but not universal, indicators of CNS infection. Fever generally accompanies most acute CNS infections but may be absent in chronic infections. Physical examination should seek evidence of cranial trauma and include careful assessment of mental status and level of consciousness. Cranial nerve palsies, focal motor or sensory deficits, meningismus, and evidence of increased intracranial pressure should also be sought.

Subdural or epidural infections that have spread from contiguous or distant areas of involvement are likely to present with localized pain in the head or spine. Spinal epidural abscesses typically progress, at a variable pace, from localized back pain to pain along nerve root distributions to overt paralysis below the level of the lesion. A sensory level and disturbed bowel and bladder function are common occurrences as well (3,9).

Infections limited to the leptomeninges usually begin with signs and symptoms of meningeal irritation. Inflammation of the meninges causes reflex paraspinous muscle spasm, which is reflected in opisthotonic posturing (particularly in children), nuchal rigidity, inability to straighten a raised leg, and flexion of the leg when the neck is flexed (47). Most patients with acute bacterial meningitis beyond the neonatal period have signs of meningeal irritation at the time of presentation (6,10,24,48). Those adults without such signs are more likely to be elderly and to have gram-negative meningitis (46). Neonates usually exhibit listlessness and seizures, but may not otherwise have obvious CNS signs on examination (49). Chronic meningeal inflammation may localize to the base of the brain, resulting in cranial nerve palsies, hydrocephalus (headache, nausea and vomiting, mental deterioration) or even localized infarction secondary to vasculitis involving branches off the circle of Willis.

Infection within the brain parenchyma may result in seizures, altered level of consciousness, acute changes in personality or behavior, or focal neurologic deficits. Such focal signs can include aphasia, hemiparesis, hemisensory loss, and visual field deficits. Patients with viral encephalitis typically progress from lethargy to confusion, stupor, and coma. Signs of meningeal inflammation may or may not be present. The hypothalamic-pituitary axis may be involved, causing severe hyper- or hypothermia and diabetes insipidus (14). Signs of bizarre behavior, hallucinations, and aphasia are common in herpes simplex encephalitis, given the strong propensity of that infection to localize within the temporal and inferior frontal lobes of the brain (50). Brain abscesses usually present with headache of increasing severity followed by nausea and vomiting. Fever is often absent, particularly in older patients and those with temporal lobe abscesses (11,12). Increased intracranial pressure can cause papilledema, third and sixth cranial nerve palsies, and progressive obtundation.

Myelitis can occur with or without encephalitis. Transverse myelitis, resulting in para- or quadraparesis, a sensory level, and loss of bowel and bladder function, may be caused by either intra- or extramedullary spinal cord lesions. Local back pain strongly suggests the latter type of process. Anterior spinal artery occlusion secondary to infectious vasculitis usually spares position and vibration sense below the level of the lesion. Ascending myelitis is characterized by early bowel and bladder involvement, flaccid paralysis, and ascending sensory loss. The classic poliomyelitis picture, in which anterior horn cells are primarily involved, presents with flaccid paralysis and muscle pain without significant sensory involvement.

A search should be made for foci of infection outside the CNS as well as for physical signs that suggest a specific microbial cause. Meningitis in the setting of pneumonia suggests pneumococcal infection (6). The presence of petechiae may suggest meningococcal infection or Rocky Mountain spotted fever (51). Exanthems are also found with varicella, herpes zoster, and typhus, and occasionally with *Haemophilus influenzae, Streptococcus pneumoniae, Mycoplasma,* coxsackievirus and echovirus infections, Lyme disease, and syphilis.

Evidence of CNS infection may be masked by other disease processes, especially in elderly individuals (46,52). Fever may be attributed to a recognized infection elsewhere, such as pneumonia, cellulitis, endocarditis, otitis, or sinusitis. Nuchal rigidity may be falsely interpreted as degenerative disease of the cervical spine. Altered CNS function may be blamed on intoxication, head trauma, stroke, brain tumor, subarachnoid hemorrhage, or various metabolic abnormalities (46,52). Treatable CNS infections, particularly bacterial meningitis, must still be ruled out in such patients. This is usually achieved through a strong clinical index of suspicion and a low threshold to perform a lumbar puncture.

LABORATORY STUDIES

Examination of the CSF is an essential part of the diagnostic approach to suspected CNS infection. Careful consideration should be given to the type of information desired and to what supplemental information (such as peripheral glucose values) may be necessary to interpret the results. Normal CSF is crystal clear; it contains less than five mononuclear cells per cubic millimeter; has a protein content less than 4.5 g/L, of which 14% or less is γ-globulin; has a glucose concentration about two thirds of serum levels (except in diabetic patients and those individuals who have recently received intravenous glucose); and is under pressure of less than 180 mm water (53).

CNS infection usually produces detectable changes in the CSF (Table 147.4). These may include accumulation of leukocytes, an increased protein concentration, and a decreased glucose concentration. Total and differential white blood cell counts should always be performed. Mononuclear cells usually predominate in mycobacterial, fungal, rickettsial, spirochetal, and viral infections, whereas polymorphonuclear cells predominate in other bacterial and amebic infections. One polymorphonuclear leukocyte or more than five mononuclear cells per microliter of uncentrifuged CSF is considered abnormal. However, there may be no increase in cells during the earliest stages of any of these diseases, and polymorphonuclear cells may be present in large numbers early in viral infections. Thus, repeat examination of the CSF in 8 to 24 hours often is useful (54). Severely immunocompromised persons may also fail to mount an inflammatory response at any stage of CNS infection (33,37,39). Conversely, a pleocytosis may be found in subacute bacterial endocarditis, after prolonged seizures, during systemic viral infections such as measles, or after treatment with anti-CD3 antibody for graft rejection that may simulate CNS infection (53). Significant numbers of erythrocytes in the CSF may be found during herpesvirus infections and in postinfectious and amebic encephalitis (55).

CSF should be stained and cultured for suspected infectious agents. Furthermore, because CNS infections frequently are complications of systemic disease, other relevant body fluids (e.g., blood, stool, throat swabs, sputum, urine) should be examined and cultured as well. Short-term antibiotic treatment before admission does not significantly alter the total or differential white cell count in the CSF, but it does reduce the frequency of a diagnostic Gram strain and bacterial growth on culture

TABLE 147.4.   Typical Cerebrospinal Fluid Findings in Various Types of Central Nervous System Infections

Infection	Cells/mm^3	Cell types	Protein level	Glucose level	Culture
Meningitis					
Bacterial	500–10,000	PMNs	High–very high	Low–very low	Positive
Viral	50–1,000	Monocytes	Slightly elevated	Normal	Positive
Tuberculous	50–1,000	Monocytes	High	Low	Positive
Parenchymal					
Brain abscess	5–100	PMNs, monocytes	High–very high	Normal	Negative
Viral encephalitis	5–100	Monocytes	Normal-high	Normal	Negative
Parameningeal					
Epidural	5–100	PMNs, monocytes	High–very high	Normal	Negative
Subdural	5–100	PMNs, monocytes	High	Normal	Negative

PMNs, polymorphonuclear leukocytes.

(6,56). Antigens released by certain microbes (e.g., *Cryptococcus, Haemophilus, Pneumococcus,* and *Meningococcus*) may be detected by rapid immunodiagnostic techniques, thus providing a mechanism to identify the infecting organism in previously treated persons (56–58). Polymerase chain reaction is increasingly useful for diagnosis of CNS viral infections (39,43,59,60).

CSF protein levels increase with most CNS infections, and in chronic infections an increased proportion of this protein may be locally synthesized immunoglobulin. The relative increase in CSF protein concentration may be slight with viral compared to bacterial, fungal, or tuberculous infections. An increased protein value may be the only CSF abnormality found in brain abscesses and parameningeal infections. The immunoglobulins present in CSF are often reactive against the infecting agent and may be a means to diagnose acute (IgM) and chronic (IgG) viral and spirochetal infections (14,61). A diagnosis of arboviral (e.g., West Nile, Japanese encephalitis, and St. Louis encephalitis viruses) encephalitis, in particular, depends on the detection of virus-specific IgM in the serum and CSF (62,63).

The CSF glucose value is usually low in untreated bacterial meningitis, and is frequently low in fungal, amebic, and tuberculous meningitis. In most persons, the CSF glucose value can be interpreted only if the plasma glucose level is measured at approximately the same time. The CSF glucose value, usually normal during viral or rickettsial infections of the CNS (14,19,51), may be depressed in some viral encephalitides (particularly those caused by mumps and lymphocytic choriomeningitis viruses), CNS sarcoid, tumors, and subarachnoid hemorrhage (53).

The major risk in performing a lumbar puncture occurs when there is increased intracranial pressure due to a mass lesion within the cranial vault. With removal of CSF from the lumbar region, the changing intracranial pressure dynamics may predispose to downward shifting of the brain through the tentorial notch or foramen magnum. This is particularly likely when there is a large, asymmetric, supratentorial mass or a mass in the posterior fossa (64,65). In contrast, herniation is almost never seen with diffuse increases in pressure throughout the subarachnoid space as occurs with generalized infection or meningitis. If a mass lesion is suspected based on the history or physical examination, or if increased intracranial pressure is evident on funduscopic examination, then computed tomography (CT) or magnetic resonance imaging (MRI) of the brain should precede the lumbar puncture. In all other situations the lumbar puncture should not be delayed, because information gained from examining the CSF is crucial for diagnosis and the early institution of treatment. The practice of performing routine CT before lumbar puncture imposes a significant and unnecessary delay in the treatment of bacterial meningitis (66).

IMAGING STUDIES

Plain radiographs of the skull or spine are only useful in situations involving trauma. CT with infusion of contrast material may or may not confirm meningeal inflammation, particularly in chronic meningitis (67), but it is useful in the diagnosis of epidural, subdural, or parenchymal brain abscess and takes less time than MRI (11–13). Cranial MRI, however, is much more sensitive for identifying parenchymal infections–progressive multifocal leukoencephalopathy, herpes simplex encephalitis, human immunodeficiency virus–associated dementia white matter lesions, and bacterial cerebritis before the development of the capsule (68–70). In the spine, MRI has replaced myelography as the standard means to identify and characterize both epidural and intramedullary lesions.

INITIAL MANAGEMENT

The first steps in the management of suspected CNS infection are dictated by the type and location of the infectious process. For viral infections, the most important steps are aimed at diagnosis (collection of "acute-phase serum" and cultures from appropriate sites), supportive care (control of seizures, optimization of fluid and electrolyte balance, respiratory assistance) if needed, and initiation of antiviral therapy if herpes simplex virus encephalitis is suspected (14,59). It should be remembered that herpes simplex virus causes less than 10% of all cases of viral encephalitis in the United States each year.

Stereotactic biopsy of focal lesions may be useful (71), and for focal parenchymal bacterial infections, the most important initial step is surgical drainage if there is threat of abscess rupture or evidence of mass effect compromising neurologic function. Prompt drainage is also imperative for subdural empyemas and spinal epidural abscesses under almost all circumstances. Appropriate antibiotic therapy alone can be sufficient for the treatment of intraparenchymal bacterial abscesses if drainage is not necessary to relieve pressure (72).

For suspected bacterial meningitis, bactericidal antibiotics that penetrate the CNS (e.g., ampicillin, ceftriaxone, or cefotaxime) should be initiated as soon as blood and CSF cultures have been obtained (4,10). If there is an unavoidable delay in obtaining CSF for culture, antibiotic therapy should be initiated (56,66). The antibiotic regimen selected should include coverage for organisms suspected on the basis of CSF Gram stain and antigen detection tests, but should also cover all likely possibilities until a definitive diagnosis has been made (4). In children, routine adjunctive therapy with dexamethasone is controversial now that *H. influenzae* infection occurs infrequently (73). If clinical presentation or epidemiologic considerations suggest rickettsial disease, chloramphenicol or tetracycline should be included in the therapeutic regimen.

REFERENCES

1. Nicolosi A, Hauser WA, Beghi E, et al. Epidemiology of central nervous system infections in Olmsted County Minnesota, 1950–1981. *J Infect Dis* 1986;154:399.
2. Mauser HW, Van Houwelingen HC, Tullekin CAF. Factors affecting the outcome in subdural empyema. *J Neurol Neurosurg Psychiatry* 1987;50:1136.
3. Danner RL, Hartman BJ. Update of spinal epidural abscess: 35 cases and review of the literature. *Rev Infect Dis* 1987;9:265.
4. Quagliarello VJ, Scheld WM. Treatment of bacterial meningitis. *N Engl J Med* 1997;336:708.
5. Bonsu BK, Harper MB. Fever interval before diagnosis, prior antibiotic treatment, and clinical outcome for young children with bacterial meningitis. *Clin Infect Dis* 2001;32:566.
6. Geiseler PJ, Nelson KE, Levin S, et al. Community-acquired purulent meningitis: a review of 1316 cases during the antibiotic era, 1954–1976. *Rev Infect Dis* 1980;2:725.
7. Kaufman DM, Mitler MH, Steigbigel NH. Subdural empyema: analysis of 17 recent cases and review of the literature. *Medicine (Baltimore)* 1975;54:485.
8. Dill SR, Cobbs CG, McDonald CK. Subdural empyema: analysis of 32 cases and review. *Clin Infect Dis* 1995;20:372.
9. Auletta JJ, John CC. Spinal epidural abscesses in children: a 15-year experience and review of the literature. *Clin Infect Dis* 2001;32:9.
10. Quagliarello V, Scheld WM: Bacterial meningitis: pathogenesis, pathophysiology, and progress. *N Engl J Med* 1992;327:864.
11. Chun CH, Johnson JD, Hofstetter M, et al. Brain abscess: a study of 45 consecutive cases. *Medicine (Baltimore)* 1986;65:415.
12. Mathisen GE, Johnson JP. Brain abscess. *Clin Infect Dis* 1997;25:763.
13. Britt RH, Enzmann DR. Clinical stages of human brain abscesses on serial CT scans after contrast infusion: computerized tomographic, neuropathological, and clinical correlations. *J Neurosurg* 1983;59:972.
14. Griffin DE. Viral infections of the central nervous system. In: Galasso GJ, Whitley RJ, Merigan TC, eds. *Antiviral agents and viral diseases of man*, 4th ed. Philadelphia: Lippincott-Raven, 1997:493–531.
15. Wilfert CM, MacCormack JN, Kleeman K, et al. Epidemiology of Rocky Mountain spotted fever as determined by active surveillance. *J Infect Dis* 1984;150:469.
16. Surveillance for Lyme disease—United States, 1992–1998. *MMWR* 2000;49:1.
17. Arboviral infections of the central nervous system—United States, 1989. *MMWR* 1990;39:407.
18. Deibel R, Barron A, Millian S, et al. Central nervous system infections in New York State. *N Y State J Med* 1974;74:1929.
19. Berlin LE, Rorabaugh ML, Heldrich F, et al. Aseptic meningitis in infants <2 years of age: diagnosis and etiology. *J Infect Dis* 1993;168:888.
20. Koskiniemi M, Rautonen J, Lehtokoski-Lehtiniemi E, et al. Epidemiology of encephalitis in children: A 20-year study. *Ann Neurol* 1991;29:492.
21. Schlech WF, Ward JI, Band JD, et al. Bacterial meningitis in the United States, 1978 through 1981: the national bacterial meningitis surveillance study. *JAMA* 1985;253:1749.
22. Greenwood BM. Selective primary health care: strategies for control of disease in the developing world. XIII. Acute bacterial meningitis. *Rev Infect Dis* 1984;6:374.
23. Linnan MJ, Mascola L, Lou XD, et al. Epidemic listeriosis associated with Mexican-style cheese. *N Engl J Med* 1988;319:823.
24. Durand ML, Calderwood SB, Weber DJ, et al. Acute bacterial meningitis in adults: a review of 493 episodes. *N Engl J Med* 1983;328:21.
25. Winkelman MD, Galloway PG. Central nervous system complications of thermal burns: a postmortem study of 139 patients. *Medicine (Baltimore)* 1992;71:271.
26. Pappas DG Jr, Hammerschlag PE, Hammerschlag M. Cerebrospinal fluid rhinorrhea and recurrent meningitis. *Clin Infect Dis* 1993;17:364.
27. Morissette I, Gourdeau M, Francoeur J. CSF shunt infections: a fifteen-year experience with emphasis on management and outcome. *Can J Neurol Sci* 1993;20:118.
28. Cullingford GL, Watkins DN, Watts AD, et al. Severe late postsplenectomy infection. *Br J Surg* 1991;78:716.
29. Fijen CAP, Kuijper EJ, te Bulte MT, et al. Assessment of complement deficiency in patients with meningococcal disease in the Netherlands. *Clin Infect Dis* 1999;28:98.
30. Platonov AE, Shipulin GA, Vershinina IV, et al. Association of human FcγRIIa (CD32) polymorphism with susceptibility to and severity of meningococcal disease. *Clin Infect Dis* 1998;27:746.
31. McKinney RE Jr, Katz SL, Wilfert CM. Chronic enteroviral meningoencephalitis in agammaglobulinemic patients. *Rev Infect Dis* 1987;9:334.
32. Salaki JS, Louria DB, Chmel H. Fungal and yeast infections of the central nervous system: a clinical review. *Medicine (Baltimore)* 1984;63:108.
33. Luft BJ, Remington JS. Toxoplasmic encephalitis in AIDS. *Clin Infect Dis* 1992;15:211.
34. Peterson PK. Host defense abnormalities predisposing the patient to infection. *Am J Med* 1984;76:2.
35. Wong B. Parasitic diseases in immunocompromised hosts. *Am J Med* 1984;76:479.
36. Stamm AM, Dismukes WE, Simmons BP, et al. Listeriosis in renal transplant recipients: report of an outbreak and review of 102 cases. *Rev Infect Dis* 1982;4:665.
37. Powderly WG. Cryptococcal meningitis and AIDS. *Clin Infect Dis* 1993;17:837.
38. Mischel PS, Vinters HV. Coccidioidomycosis of the central nervous system: neuropathological and vasculopathic manifestations and clinical correlates. *J Infect Dis* 1995;20:400.
39. McCutchan JA. Cytomegalovirus infections of the nervous system in patients with AIDS. *Clin Infect Dis* 1995;20:747.
40. Lerner PI. Nocardiosis. *Clin Infect Dis* 1996;22,891.
41. Wenger JD, Hightower AW, Facklam RR, et al. Bacterial meningitis in the United States, 1986: report of a multistate surveillance study. *J Infect Dis* 1990;162:1316.
42. Dillon HC Jr, Khare S, Gray BM. Group B streptococcal carriage and disease: a 6 year prospective study. *J Pediatr* 1987;110:31.
43. Rotbart HA. Enteroviral infections of the central nervous system. *Clin Infect Dis* 1995;20:971.
44. Whitley RJ, Hutto C. Neonatal herpes simplex virus infections. *Pediatr Rev* 1985;7:119.
45. Schuchat A, Robinson K, Wenger JD, et al. Bacterial meningitis in the United States in 1995. *N Engl J Med* 1997;337:970.
46. Behrman RE, Meyers BR, Mendelson MH, et al. Central nervous system infections in the elderly. *Arch Intern Med* 1989;149:1596.
47. Verghese A, Gallemore G. Kernig's and Brudzinski's signs revisited. *Rev Infect Dis* 1987;9:1187.
48. Metersky ML, Williams A, Rafanan AL. Retrospective analysis: are fever and altered mental status indications for lumbar puncture in a hospitalized patient who has not undergone neurosurgery? *Clin Infect Dis* 1997;25:285.
49. Rorabaugh ML, Berlin LE, Heldrich F, et al. Aseptic meningitis in infants younger than 2 years of age. Acute illness and neurologic complications. *Pediatrics* 1993;92:206.
50. Whitley RJ, Soong S-J, Linneman C Jr, et al. Herpes simplex: clinical assessment. *JAMA* 1982;247:317.
51. Thorner AR, Walker DH, Petri WA. Rocky mountain spotted fever. *Clin Infect Dis* 1998;27:1353.
52. Quaade F. Meningitis in the aged. *Geriatrics* 1963;18:860.
53. Fishman RS. *Cerebrospinal fluid in diseases of the nervous system*, 2nd ed. Philadelphia: WB Saunders, 1992.
54. Feigin RD, Shackelford PG. Value of repeat lumbar puncture in the differential diagnosis of meningitis. *N Engl J Med* 1973;289:571.
55. Koskiniemi M, Vaheri A, Taskinen E. Cerebrospinal fluid alterations in herpes simplex virus encephalitis. *Rev Infect Dis* 1984;6:608.
56. Talan DA, Hoffman JR, Yoshikawa TT, et al. Role of empiric antibiotics prior to lumbar puncture in suspected bacterial meningitis: state of the art. *Rev Infect Dis* 1988;10:365.
57. Granoff DM, Murphy TV, Ingram DL, et al. Use of rapidly generated results in patient management. *Diagn Microbiol Infect Dis* 1986;4(suppl):157.
58. Wilson CB, Smith AL. Rapid tests for the diagnosis of bacterial meningitis. *Curr Clin Top Infect Dis* 1986;7:134.
59. Whitley RJ, Lakeman F. Herpes simplex virus infections of the central nervous system: therapeutic and diagnostic considerations. *Clin Infect Dis* 1995;20:414.
60. Lakeman F, Whitley RJ, and the NIAID Collaborative Antiviral Study Group. Diagnosis of herpes simplex encephalitis: application of polymerase chain reaction to cerebrospinal fluid from brain-biopsied patients and correlation with disease. *J Infect Dis* 1995;171:857.
61. Schutzer SE, Coyle PK, Krupp LB, et al. Simultaneous expression of Borrelia OspA and OspC and Igm response in cerebrospinal fluid in early neurologic Lyme disease. *J Clin Invest* 1997;100:763.
62. Asnis DS, Conette R, Teixeira AA, et al. The West Nile Virus outbreak of 1999 in New York: The Flushing Hospital experience. *Clin Infect Dis* 2000;30:413.
63. Burke DS, Nisalak A, Ussery MA, et al. Kinetics of IgM and IgG responses to Japanese envephalitis virus in human serum and cerebrospinal fluid. *J Infect Dis* 1985;151:1093.
64. Garfield J. Management of supratentorial intracranial abscess: a review of 200 cases. *BMJ* 1969;2:7.
65. Duffy GP. Lumbar puncture in the presence of raised intracranial pressure. *BMJ* 1969;1:407.
66. Bryan CS, Reynolds KL, Crout L. Promptness of antibiotic therapy in acute bacterial meningitis. *Ann Emerg Med* 1986;15:544.
67. Ogawa SK, Smith MA, Brennessel DJ, et al. Tuberculous meningitis in an urban medical center. *Medicine (Baltimore)* 1987;66:317.
68. Berger JR, Kaszovitz B, Post JD, et al. Progressive multifocal leukoencephalopathy associated with human immunodeficiency virus infection: a review of the literature with a report of sixteen cases. *Ann Intern Med* 1987;107:78.
69. Walot I, Miller BL, Chang L, et al. Neuroimaging findings in patients with AIDS. *Clin Infect Dis* 1996;22:906.
70. Buff BL Jr, Mathews VP, Elster AD. Bacterial and viral parenchymal infections of the brain. *Top Magn Reson Imaging* 1994;6:11.
71. Gildenberg PL, Gathe JC, Kim JH. Stereotactic biopsy of cerebral lesions in AIDS. *Clin Infect Dis* 2000;30:491.
72. Rousseaux M, Lesoin F, Destee A, et al. Developments in the treatment and prognosis of multiple cerebral abscesses. *Neurosurgery* 1985;16:304.
73. Schaad UB, Kaplan SL, McCracken GH Jr. Steroid therapy for bacterial meningitis. *Clin Infect Dis* 1995;20:685.

CHAPTER 148
Acute Bacterial Meningitis

Morton Swartz

Bacterial meningitis is a rapidly evolving inflammatory process, affecting the arachnoid, the pia mater, and the intervening cerebrospinal fluid (CSF), that results from invasion by pyogenic bacteria. Onset is usually acute and most often the infection is associated with a predominantly polymorphonuclear pleocytosis. Uncommonly, bacterial meningitis is caused by nonpyogenic bacteria, such as *Mycobacterium tuberculosis, Francisella tularensis, Brucella* species, *Borrelia burgdorferi, Treponema pallidum,* and *Leptospira interrogans,* or unusual meningeal pathogens such as *Nocardia asteroides,* and *Actinomyces* species and *Tropherema whippelii.* In these processes the clinical picture is usually subacute or chronic and the pleocytosis is (in the first six instances) lymphocytic.

The incidence of bacterial meningitis in the United States in the 1970s and 1980s had been estimated to be 20,000 to 30,000 cases annually (1). The overall attack rate for bacterial meningitis during the period 1978 to 1981 in the United States was 3.0 per 100,000 population per year, but this figure likely represents underreporting by 60% (2). In many cases initial examination of CSF does not provide identification of the infecting microorganism. Since 1990 in the United States the annual attack rate for bacterial meningitis has declined as a result of a sharp decrease in the incidence of invasive infections with *Haemophilus influenzae.* Classification of bacterial meningitis into categories is helpful, because the relative frequency of individual bacterial species varies among the categories, which are related to age (neonatal, childhood, adult) and setting (community acquired, nosocomial).

BACTERIOLOGY

In the past the three most frequent bacterial pathogens of community-acquired meningitis (*H. influenzae, Neisseria meningitidis, Streptococcus pneumoniae*) have been responsible for about 80% of reported cases in the United States (Table 148.1). Until the 1990s *H. influenzae* had been the leading cause of bacterial meningitis, accounting for almost 50% of cases. When age-specific attack rates have been examined, the highest rate, 76.7 per 100,000 population per year, has been among children under 1 year of age (2). The dominant position of *H. influenzae* as the leading cause of bacterial meningitis in infants and young children has been altered dramatically by the widespread use since the late 1980s of *H. influenzae* type b (Hib) conjugate vaccines. In children under 5 years of age in the United States in the mid-1980s, the rate of Hib meningitis had been about 40 per 100,000, but by 1993 it had dropped to about 2 per 100,000 (3). As a result, the relative frequencies of *S. pneumoniae* and *N. meningitidis* have increased. For example, at one urban children's hospital the number of cases of bacterial meningitis seen annually had decreased by 66% between the periods 1985 to 1987 and 1991 to 1992, primarily as a result of a decline in Hib meningitis. During the same two time periods, the percentage of cases of community-acquired childhood bacterial meningitis caused by *S. pneumoniae* and *N. meningitidis* in the aggregate increased from a mean of 31% to 73% (4). The other common bacterial causes have been group B streptococci, *Listeria monocytogenes,* and enteric gram-negative bacilli. Whereas formerly

Escherichia coli and other gram-negative bacilli were the principal agents of meningitis in infants during the first months of life, they have been superseded by group B streptococci (2). *L. monocytogenes* has assumed an increasing role in bacterial meningitis, owing to the increasing numbers of immunocompromised and otherwise vulnerable persons at risk (e.g., transplant recipients, patients receiving hemodialysis, patients with liver disease) and possibly to changes in dairy food production methods. At Massachusetts General Hospital, *L. monocytogenes* increased about ninefold (0.5%–4.5%) in relative frequency among bacterial causes of meningitis between the 1950s and the 1980s. At the same institution, gram-negative bacilli accounted for about 4.5% of cases of bacterial meningitis in the 1950s, whereas more recently they accounted for close to 10%. In series of cases of bacterial meningitis, 6% to 10% of cases are of unknown cause (2,5–7).

The frequencies of the various bacterial species in community-acquired meningitis are strikingly age related (8) (Table 148.2). Surveillance data for the United States in 1995 for neonatal meningitis show group B streptococci as the predominant (70%) etiology followed by *L. monocytogenes* (20%), but *E. coli* and other enteric gram-negative bacilli are not included in this tabulation (8). From the ages of 1 to 23 months the leading etiology is *S. pneumoniae* (45%), followed by *N. meningitidis* (30%) and group B streptococci (20%). During childhood and adolescence (ages 2–18 years), *N. meningitidis* is predominant (60%), followed by *S. pneumoniae.* In the adult years *S. pneumoniae* is the major etiology (60%–69%), followed by *N. meningitidis* (20%) in the group 19 to 59 years of age and *L. monocytogenes* (23%) in those 60 years of age and older. From surveillance data for the five leading causes of community-acquired bacterial meningitis in the United States (the above four plus *H. influenzae*), the total number of cases of bacterial meningitis in the community in 1995

TABLE 148.1. Pathogens of Bacterial Meningitis in the United States, 1978–1981

Organism	Cases n	Cases %	Case-fatality rate (%)
Haemophilus influenzae	6,756	48.3	6
Neisseria meningitidis	2,742	19.6	10.3
Streptococcus pneumoniae	1,865	13.3	26.3
Group B streptococci	476	3.4	22.5
Listeria monocytogenes	265	1.9	28.5
Other	1,043	7.5	33.7
Escherichia coli	115	0.8	
Staphylococcus aureus	84	0.6	
Klebsiella-Enterobacter-Serratia	61	0.4	
Streptococci, unspecified	43	0.3	
Staphylococcus species	35	0.3	
Staphylococcus epidermidis	27	0.2	
Streptococcus, group A	25	0.2	
Pseudomonas species	25	0.2	
Haemophilus species	24	0.2	
Viridans streptococci	20	0.2	
Salmonella and *Arizona* species	18	0.1	
Miscellaneous species	76	0.5	
Unidentified species	470	3.3	
Unknown	827	5.9	16.4
Total	13,974	99.9	

Modified from Schlech WF III, Ward JI, Band JD, et al. Bacterial meningitis in the United States, 1978 through 1981. *JAMA* 1985;253:1749–1754, with permission.

TABLE 148.2. Frequencies of Pathogens in Community-Acquired Bacterial Meningitis

Pathogen	Age <1 month[a] (%)	Age 1–23 months (%)	Age 2–18 years (%)	Age 19–59 years (%)	Age ≥60 years (%)
Streptococcus pneumoniae	10	45	27	60	69
Neisseria meningitidis	—	30	60	20	2
Listeria monocytogenes	20	—	2	8	23
Haemophilus influenzae	—	5	8	10	4
Group B streptococci	70	20	3	2	2
	100	100	100	100	100

[a]Meningitis due to *Escherichia coli* or other enteric organisms among infants younger than 1 month of age is not included in surveillance.
Modified from Suchat A, Robinson K, Wenger JD, et al. Bacterial meningitis in the United States in 1995. *N Engl J Med* 1997;337:970–976, with permission.

has been estimated to be 5,800, representing a 55% decline from the comparable estimate (12,900 cases) made in 1986 (8).

Between the two time periods 1978 to 1981 and 1995, surveillance data in the United States has shown a tendency to reduction of case fatality rates for the leading causes of community-acquired bacterial meningitis (2,8). That for *S. pneumoniae* has been reduced from 26% to 21%; for *N. meningitidis*, from 10% to 3%; for *L. monocytogenes*, from 28% to 15%; for group B streptococci, from 22% to 7%; and for *H. influenzae*, it has remained unchanged at 6%.

In adults with bacterial meningitis treated in large hospitals, cases of nosocomial as well as community origin are not infrequently seen, and the infecting organisms may be more varied (9,10). Among community-acquired cases, *S. pneumoniae*, *N. meningitidis*, and *L. monocytogenes* are the leading causes, accounting for about 40%, 15%, and 10% of cases, respectively (Table 148.3). In contrast, among nosocomial cases, gram-negative bacilli, various streptococcal species (group B occurring with increasing frequency recently in adults over 50 years of age), *S. aureus*, and coagulase-negative staphylococci are the principal infecting microorganisms, accounting for about 40%, 10%, 10%, and 10% of cases, respectively. Gram-negative bacillary meningi-

tis is commonly a postneurosurgical (nosocomial) complication but may be spontaneous (in hospitalized patients or in the community setting). The incidence of both categories is increasing: the former as a result of more frequent and extensive neurosurgical procedures, the latter as a result of a larger population at risk for gram-negative bacillary bacteremia (11–16). *E. coli* and *Klebsiella* infections account for more than half of the cases of gram-negative bacillary meningitis in adults (Table 148.4).

S. aureus is the pathogen in 1% to 9% of cases of bacterial meningitis overall (2,17). Cases occur in several categories, based on predisposing circumstances: central nervous system (CNS) disorders (usually involving prior neurosurgery) in about 50%, endocarditis in about 20%, and bacteremia from other sites of infection (often in the setting of diabetes, cancer, or alcoholism) in about 25%.

Obligate anaerobic bacteria rarely cause meningitis (18). Such infections usually occur in the setting of leakage of a brain abscess into the ventricular system, recent neurosurgery or trauma, chronic otitis media (19), or bacteremia from abdominal infections. The principal organisms involved are anaerobic streptococci, *Fusobacterium necrophorum*, *Prevotella melaninogenica*, and *Bacteroides fragilis*. *Clostridium perfringens* meningitis has been reported in 16 patients, usually in association with penetrating head injury, recent neurosurgery, or bacteremia after gastrointestinal or genitourinary operations (20).

TABLE 148.3. Causative Organisms in Episodes (Nonrecurrent) of Bacterial Meningitis in Adults at a Tertiary Care Hospital,[a] 1962–1989

Organism	Community acquired (%) (n = 253)	Nosocomial (%) (n = 151)
Streptococcus pneumoniae	38	5
Gram-negative bacilli	4	38
Neisseria meningitidis	14	1
Streptococci[b]	7	9
Listeria monocytogenes	11	3
Staphylococcus aureus	5	9
Coagulase-negative staphylococci	0	9
Mixed bacterial species	2	7
Haemophilus influenzae	4	4
Enterococci	0	3
Other[c]	2	3
Culture-negative	13	11

[a]Massachusetts General Hospital.
[b]Including groupable and nongroupable streptococci.
[c]Including micrococci, anaerobes, *Neisseria* species, and diphtheroids.
Modified from Durand ML, Calderwood SB, Weber DJ, et al. Acute bacterial meningitis in adults. A review of 493 episodes. *N Engl J Med* 1993;328:21–28, with permission.

TABLE 148.4. Agents of Gram-Negative Bacillary Meningitis in Adults

Organism	Cases (n)	%
Escherichia coli	99	33
Klebsiella species	74	24
Pseudomonas species	35	12
Enterobacter species	27	9
Serratia species	20	7
Acinetobacter species	15	5
Salmonella species	8	3
Proteus species	11	4
Pasteurella multocida	3	1
Citrobacter species	4	1
Aeromonas species, Flavobacterium species	2	1
Mixed	6	2
Total	304	102

Compilation of 221 cases from eight reported series spanning the period 1961–1997 (9–16). *Haemophilus influenzae* and gram-negative anaerobic bacilli are not included.

About 1% of cases of bacterial meningitis are polymicrobial infections (21). Before the antibiotic era, most cases of mixed bacterial meningitis were associated with otitis media or pharyngeal infection. Subsequently, the common predisposing factors for mixed bacterial meningitis have become CSF fistulas, neoplasms in proximity to the CNS, such as carcinoma of the rectosigmoid eroding through the sacrum to the subarachnoid space, and contiguous sites of infection. Mixtures of Enterobacteriaceae, obligate anaerobes (*B. fragilis*, *Clostridium* species, *peptostreptococci*), *S. aureus*, *Pseudomonas* species, and *H. influenzae* have been involved most often (21).

Rarely, unusual bacterial species of zoonotic importance may produce meningitis in humans, and epidemiologic considerations may provide clues to diagnosis. Ingestion of imported (unpasteurized) cheese, travel to Mexico or the Mediterranean littoral, work in an abattoir or as a veterinarian, or work in a bacteriology laboratory might raise suspicion of *Brucella* meningitis (22). Rarely, meningitis due to *Francisella tularensis* follows exposure to an infected rabbit, squirrel, or cat, although such meningitis usually follows an episode of one of the more typical forms of tularemia and is characterized by a predominantly mononuclear pleocytosis (23). *Streptococcus suis* is carried by healthy swine and is the cause of meningitis in young pigs. About 60 cases of *S. suis* meningitis have occurred, principally in pig breeders and abattoir workers (24).

EPIDEMIOLOGY

Meningococcal meningitis is the major form of meningococcal infection, and the one form of bacterial meningitis capable of producing epidemic disease. Meningococcal infection also occurs as the asymptomatic carrier state, the frequency of which varies with age (0.5%–1.0% for children 3 to 48 months of age, 5% for those 14 to 17 years of age, and 20%–40% for young adults), endemic disease (sporadic cases), or hyperendemic disease (cyclic waves of increased incidence). The annual attack rate for meningococcal meningitis in the United States is 0.6 cases per 100,000 population (as high as 13 per 100,000 in the first year of life, thereafter reaching the level of 0.2–0.6 per 100,000 for adults) (2). Group B (particularly of one clonal complex) and C meningococci have been associated in recent decades with endemic or hyperendemic disease in industrial countries. Epidemic meningococcal disease occurs on all continents, is commonly due to type A strains, and tends to recur at 20- to 30-year intervals. Major epidemics in the past 25 years have occurred in Finland (1973), Brazil (1974), northern Nigeria (1977), and Nepal (1983). Annual attack rates may be extremely high: 370 per 100,000 in Sao Paulo, Brazil, in 1974. A unique combination of endemic, hyperendemic, and epidemic meningococcal disease is present in the "meningitis belt" of sub-Saharan Africa, where major outbreaks occur in approximately 10-year cycles. A large epidemic due to serogroup A occurred in 1987 at the Hajj in Mecca, and since then pilgrims at this crowded annual gathering have been at increased risk.

Concentration of large numbers of persons from different geographic origins in proximity, as occurs in training of military recruits, may result in heightened rates of meningococcal transmission via aerosol dispersion and eventuate in outbreaks of meningitis. Under similar conditions of crowding in an elementary school classroom with reduced seat-to-seat distances, an outbreak of five cases of group C meningococcal disease occurred in a 6-day period (25). In the United States, such outbreaks in the military during World War II were due to group A strains and during the mid-1960s to group B and C strains. This is no longer a problem in the military since introduction of the meningococcal vaccine (groups A, C, Y, W-135), and the demonstrated prophylactic efficacy of newer antimicrobials in eradicating the meningococcal carrier state.

Nasopharyngeal carriage of *N. meningitidis*, the usual means of acquiring immunity, produces an increase in bactericidal antibody within 5 to 12 days. Complement is an important component of serum bactericidal activity. Isolated congenital late complement component (C5, C6, C7, or C8) deficiency, a rare occurrence, has been associated with repeated *Neisseria* infections (26). Recurrent episodes of meningococcal meningitis have occurred in patients with such complement deficiencies. Congenital (late component) complement, acquired complement (C1, C3, C4), and properdin deficiencies appear to be risk factors for development of initial episodes of endemic meningococcal meningitis and meningococcemia (27,28).

In the endemic setting, household contacts of index cases of meningococcal infection in the United States are at greater risk (up to 1,000-fold) for contracting the disease than the general population (29,30). Other high-risk groups include those living in close quarters such as in freshman college dormitories (meningococcal vaccine now advised for this group), in day care centers, and in jail.

Before the introduction of Hib conjugate vaccines, more than 85% of all invasive *H. influenzae* disease occurred in children under 5 years of age, and 95% of disease in this age group was caused by Hib (31). Most Hib meningitis occurred before 18 months of age. Host factors that may contribute to bacteremic Hib disease and meningitis include sickle cell disease, immunoglobulin deficiencies, history of splenectomy, and CSF fistula.

Unimmunized household contacts under 4 years of age of an index case of *H. influenzae* meningitis are at risk for invasive *H. influenzae* disease (32). In the 30 days after onset of Hib meningitis in an index case, the age-adjusted risk is 585 times greater for household contacts than for the general population. The aforementioned data applied to household contacts in the United States in the 1970s and 1980s (before widespread use of Hib conjugate vaccines in children under 6 months of age) and are applicable currently to populations elsewhere where such immunization is not yet administered.

H. influenzae is an infrequent cause (1%–4%) of meningitis in adults. The leading predisposing factor in 119 cases was head trauma (20% of cases) (33). Other important predisposing factors were sinusitis (15%), otitis (13%), pneumonia, diabetes, alcoholism, immunodeficiency, and asplenia.

PATHOGENESIS

General Features

The usual sequence of events in the development of meningitis due to the three common bacterial species (*H. influenzae*, *N. meningitidis*, *S. pneumoniae*), all encapsulated organisms, consists of initial mucosal colonization, followed by bloodstream invasion, penetration of the blood-brain barrier, and multiplication within the CSF.

Fimbriae, or pili, are involved in the binding of *N. meningitidis* to nonciliated mucosal epithelial cells, the initial step in colonization or invasive infection, but for *H. influenzae* the expression of pili does not appear to be required for such attachment (34). Such adherence is facilitated by prior damage to nearby ciliated cells by smoking or respiratory viral infections. All three major pathogens (*S. pneumoniae*, *N. meningitidis*, and *H. influenzae*) in community-acquired bacterial meningitis produce immunoglobulin A proteases, cleaving immunoglobulin

A antibody in the hinge region and inactivating this early mucosal defense. The invasion routes taken by these pathogens on their ingress from the mucosal surface differ (35). For example, meningococci enter nonciliated epithelial cells via endocytosis and are carried in membrane-bound vacuoles to the abluminal sides; *H. influenzae*, on the other hand, invades intercellularly by creating gaps in the apical tight junctions between the columnar epithelial cells. In the absence of specific antibody, the factors that determine whether initial exposure to these encapsulated species eventuates in benign nasopharyngeal carrier state or bacteremic invasion are unclear. Undefined strain-specific virulence factors or prior respiratory viral infections may play a role.

The incubation period from nasopharyngeal to invasive infection with *N. meningitidis* is less than 10 days and often only 1 to 4 days. Among prospectively studied military recruits, only about 20% of those whose secretions were cultured within 7 days preceding hospitalization for meningococcal disease were carriers of the implicated strain.

A polysaccharide capsule is a feature of each of the principal meningeal pathogens: *H. influenzae, N. meningitidis, S. pneumoniae, E. coli* K1 (the predominant *E. coli* serotype in neonatal meningitis), and *Streptococcus agalactiae* (group B streptococcus). Such encapsulation inhibits phagocytosis by neutrophils and antibody-independent complement-mediated bactericidal activity in different ways (34). The capsular sialic acid of *N. meningitidis* facilitates binding of complement factor H to Cab, and this interferes with factor B binding and alternative pathway activation. In the case of *S. pneumoniae*, factor B binds poorly to Cab on its capsular surface, and the polyribosyl phosphate capsule of Hib is not able to serve as an acceptor for covalent C3 deposition.

In monkeys under 2 months of age, meningitis after intranasal inoculation of Hib develops within hours of bacteremia, reaching a level of 10^6 colony-forming units per milliliter (36). The initial site of Hib entry into the CNS is the vascular choroid plexus, which shows the earliest histopathologic evidence of inflammation. After egress from the inflamed plexus capillaries, the organisms enter the lateral ventricles and the subarachnoid space. Once infection is introduced into the CSF, bacteria multiply rapidly because of inadequate local defenses: lack of complement-mediated lysis (37), opsonizing antibody, and neutrophil phagocytosis.

Specific Predisposing Factors

The most common route of entry of bacteria into the CSF is hematogenous, but bacterial meningitis may also result from spread of infection from a contiguous structure or via a CSF fistula. The principal barriers to hematogenous spread to the meninges are circulating antibody and complement-mediated bactericidal activity. Immunoglobulin deficiencies predispose to invasive infection, particularly by encapsulated organisms (*S. pneumoniae, H. influenzae, N. meningitidis*). Complement deficiencies predispose to systemic infections with *N. meningitidis*. Complement deficiency may also predispose to meningitis caused by unencapsulated *N. meningitidis* and by *Neisseria*-related bacteria such as *Moraxella* species and *Acinetobacter* species (38). In patients with decreased spleen function, increased susceptibility to systemic infections with encapsulated organisms occurs, attributed to reduced clearance of intravascular organisms because of lower levels of complement components and decreased antibody formation.

Infection of a parameningeal structure may lead to bacterial penetration into the subarachnoid space. The organisms involved are representative of those involved in the primary parameningeal infection (e.g., anaerobic bacteria and microaerophilic streptococci in the setting of chronic sinusitis or leakage of a brain

TABLE 148.5. Predisposing Factors in Pneumococcal Meningitis

Predisposing factor	Frequency (%)
Otitis media or mastoiditis[a]	30
Sinusitis[b]	3
Previous head trauma[c]	10
CSF rhinorrhea[c]	4
Pneumonia[d]	20
Neoplastic disease, collagen-vascular disease, or immunosuppression	5
Alcoholism	9
Diabetes mellitus	2

Compilation from four series of cases occurring between 1956 and 1976 (5–7, 38).
[a]Based on data from a total of 459 cases.
[b]Based on data from a total of 119 cases.
[c]Based on data from a total of 281 cases.
[d]Based on data from a total of 234 cases.

abscess into the ventricular system; *S. pneumoniae, H. influenzae*, or *S. aureus* in acute frontal sinusitis; *S. aureus* or gram-negative bacilli in vertebral body or cranial osteomyelitis; *S. epidermidis* or *S. aureus* in infections of CSF shunts).

Meningitis complicating CSF fistulas (congenital, traumatic, or postsurgical) is associated with species that vary with the site of the abnormal communication (e.g., pneumococci with leaks about the cribriform plate and air sinuses, *S. aureus* and facultative gram-negative bacilli with congenital dermal sinuses or meningomyeloceles along the spine, and members of the Enterobacteriaceae and anaerobic intestinal flora with erosion of colonic neoplasms into the lumbosacral subarachnoid space).

Predisposing factors for pneumococcal meningitis are varied (39) (Table 148.5). Antecedent acute otitis media is the most common predisposing factor. In this instance, meningitis follows bacteremia rather than direct invasion through the mastoid. In occasional cases of chronic otitis media in which cultures of drainage have consistently grown *P. aeruginosa* or *Proteus* species, acute meningitis caused by *S. pneumoniae* has developed. CSF rhinorrhea has been noted in 4% of cases of pneumococcal meningitis (Table 148.5); however, this is probably an underestimate, because in this compilation a quarter of the cases with head injury had skull fractures (and were likely to have had CSF leaks as well). Also, CSF rhinorrhea is likely to be a more frequent predisposing factor (12%) for pneumococcal meningitis in adults (5).

At least 18 cases of mixed bacterial-viral meningitis have been reported (7,40). Most cases have involved children; the bacterial pathogens have been principally Hib, *N. meningitidis*, and *Salmonella* organisms; and the most frequent viruses have been echovirus, coxsackievirus, and herpes simplex virus. Whether viral aseptic meningitis preceded and predisposed to subsequent bacterial invasion is unknown.

PATHOPHYSIOLOGY

A multitude of pathophysiologic changes develop as a consequence of bacterial meningitis and involve the brain, its linings, cranial nerves, meningeal and other intracranial blood vessels, and the spinal cord. In experimental animal models, specific bacterial subcapsular components (for *S. pneumoniae*, peptidoglycan or lipoteichoic acid; for Hib, lipopolysaccharide) are the major inducers of the meningeal inflammation that follows bacterial entry and multiplication in the CSF (34). Ampicillin-induced lysis of pneumococci in the CSF results in a transient increase in polymorphonuclear pleocytosis, consistent with the release of cell wall debris (41). This inflammatory response is caused by the release into the subarachnoid space of various proinflammatory cytokines such as interleukin-1 and tumor necrosis factor from meningeal cells. These cytokines elicit increased adherence and transendothelial movement of neutrophils by induction of several families of adhesion molecules on endothelium that interact with corresponding leukocytic receptors. These include (a) the selectin family, for example, endothelial-leukocyte adhesion molecule and CD62, and (b) the immunoglobulin superfamily, for example, intercellular adhesion molecules (ICAM-1, ICAM-2). The integrin (CD18) subfamily of adhesion molecules is expressed only on leukocytes and can be increased rapidly by chemoattractants. Another leukocyte adhesion molecule (LAM-1), belonging to the selectin family, mediates adhesion to endothelium even under conditions of flow; its binding affinity for its endothelial receptor is increased by exposure to cytokines (tumor necrosis factor, granulocyte-macrophage colony-stimulating factor), thus furthering neutrophil trafficking into the subarachnoid space.

Once within the subarachnoid space, activated neutrophils release prostaglandins and toxic oxygen metabolites that increase vascular permeability and may cause neurotoxicity. Early in the course of meningitis in animal models, changes occur in meningeal and cerebral capillaries. These vessels, which by virtue of their tight intercellular endothelial junctions constitute the blood-brain barrier, undergo morphologic changes (opening of tight junctions, enhanced pinocytosis) and become permeable to proteins (42). In experimental Hib meningitis, the increase in permeability in the blood-brain barrier appears to correlate with the bacterial titer in the CSF but is augmented by increasing pleocytosis (43).

A variety of mediators of the inflammatory response, such as interleukin-1, tumor necrosis factor, complement components, and arachidonate metabolites, probably contribute to the breakdown of the blood-brain barrier and the cerebral manifestations of bacterial meningitis (44). The major physiologic consequence of altered vascular permeability is (vasogenic) cerebral edema.

Brain edema may also have cytotoxic (from inflammatory mediators and hypoxia) and interstitial (impaired CSF absorption due to arachnoid villus blockage by fibrin and leukocytes) components (45). Increased intracranial pressure (ICP) due to cerebral edema and reduced CSF resorption produce vomiting and obtundation. In extreme instances cerebral edema produces temporal lobe or cerebellar herniation with brainstem compression and respiratory arrest.

Cerebral blood flow appears enhanced in early stages of meningitis but declines subsequently, reflecting the severity of the inflammatory process. Focal areas of marked hypoperfusion (attributable to local vasculitis or thrombosis) can occur in patients with overall normal blood flow. In some patients, impaired autoregulation of cerebral blood flow may contribute to development of cerebral edema or ischemia by altering cerebral perfusion pressure.

With spread of the meningeal inflammation over the cerebral hemispheres and into the basal cisterns, superficial pial arteries and veins may be subject to thrombosis. Decreased cerebral blood flow due to cerebral edema or vascular thrombosis, plus any hypoxia due to pneumonia or respiratory insufficiency, results in enhanced glucose metabolism via the anaerobic glycolytic pathway, with ensuing lactate accumulation in brain and CSF. This central lactic acidosis may contribute considerably to the obtundation and coma of patients with severe meningitis (46).

Cranial nerve palsies may be the consequence of accumulation of basilar exudate about these nerves in their course through the subarachnoid space. Seizures may result from a variety of pathophysiologic changes in meningitis: fever (and hypoglycemia) in infants and young children, hyponatremia secondary to increased release of antidiuretic hormone (47), and cerebral infarction due to arteritis or cortical venous thrombophlebitis. Hydrocephalus probably results from choroid plexus necrosis and aqueductal occlusion (obstructive hydrocephalus) or from impaired CSF resorption due to obstruction by exudate of the arachnoid villi. Focal signs of cerebral dysfunction such as hemiparesis, dysphasia, and visual field defects are probably a consequence of arterial vasculitis or venous infarction from cortical thrombophlebitis.

Brain abscess is a rare complication of meningitis; more often, bacterial meningitis is a complication of a brain abscess leaking into the ventricular system. When meningitis is complicated by brain abscess it occurs in the neonate and almost invariably is caused by *Citrobacter diversus* (48). Brain abscess has developed in 41 of 53 cases (77%) of *C. diversus* neonatal meningitis.

CLINICAL MANIFESTATIONS

History

In community-acquired bacterial meningitis, antecedent upper respiratory tract infection is common (40%); another 10% to 15% of patients have an ill-defined prior illness (often diagnosed as otitis media) (7). Between 25% and 75% of patients have a rapid onset (within 24 hours) of headache, lethargy, and confusion. Other patients have more prolonged (1–7 days) respiratory tract or ear symptoms, and meningeal symptoms develop and progress more slowly. In patients with *L. monocytogenes* meningitis, the prodromal symptomatic period tends to be longer than in patients with other types of pyogenic meningitis; indeed, in about 15% of patients the premonitory symptoms may be present for 7 or more days before hospitalization. Rarely, patients have had meningeal symptoms that predate hospitalization by several weeks. In such instances, parental neglect and, in one case, complement deficiency (49) have been factors.

Fever, vomiting, irritability, lethargy, and headache are features in most patients. Neck stiffness is a symptom in less than half of patients, but nuchal rigidity is noted as a sign in more than 80%. Myalgias (especially in meningococcal disease) and backache occur less frequently. Photophobia is more often associated with viral meningitis.

In young infants, manifestations of meningitis may be difficult to recognize. Fever and vomiting, features common to many types of infections, may be the only abnormalities noted by parents. Nuchal rigidity may be absent on examination of the infant. Bulging of the fontanelle and diastasis of the sutures may suggest the diagnosis but may be absent early in meningitis or if the infant is markedly dehydrated. Occasionally, lumbar puncture performed in the absence of overt signs has revealed a clear CSF without even minor pleocytosis, and the infant has been treated with antipyretic measures and sent home only to return some hours later because of parental concern or a seizure. Another CSF examination may then show pleocytosis, and in the next 24 hours bacteria, usually Hib, are isolated from the initial CSF culture.

General Physical Findings

Drowsiness, reduced cognitive function, stiff neck, and Kernig and Brudzinski signs—all manifestations of meningeal inflammation—are usually present along with fever. These findings may be overlooked or misinterpreted in patients who are obtunded because of other illness or in elders, particularly those with pneumonia or congestive failure.

A petechial or purpuric rash, predominantly on the extremities, in a patient with meningeal signs almost always indicates a meningococcal cause and requires immediate treatment because of the rapidity with which this type of infection can advance. About 50% of patients with meningococcal meningitis have such skin lesions. Occasionally a maculopapular rash is seen in patients with meningococcal meningitis. In more severe infections, large purpuric areas with gunmetal gray necrotic or vesicular centers (suggillations) develop, usually accompanying hypotension or shock and evidence of disseminated intravascular coagulation. Although such lesions may provide an initial clue to bacteriologic diagnosis, rarely they occur in meningitis caused by *S. pneumoniae* or *H. influenzae.* Quite rarely, petechial and purpuric skin lesions occur in patients with acute *S. aureus* endocarditis who have meningeal signs and pleocytosis (due to either staphylococcal meningitis or cerebral embolic infarction). In this setting, one or two of the purpuric lesions often contain a purulent center, and aspirated material reveals staphylococci on Gram stain examination. Macular and petechial skin lesions accompanied by meningeal signs may occur with enteroviral aseptic meningitis in summer outbreaks. The presence of an initial pleocytosis of up to several hundred cells, with neutrophils predominating at first, enhances the mimicry of meningococcal disease.

Neurologic Findings and Complications

Confusion, stupor, or delirium is common in bacterial meningitis, but about 20% to 40% of patients are noted on admission to the hospital to have normal consciousness (5,10,39).

CRANIAL NERVE DYSFUNCTION

Ten percent to 20% of patients with bacterial meningitis have cranial nerve dysfunction. Cranial nerves III, VI, and VIII are most often involved. Prospective studies using brainstem evoked potentials indicate that neurosensory deafness affects about 10% of infants and young children with bacterial meningitis (50). The highest frequency is associated with *S. pneumoniae* meningitis. About 20% of those children who become deaf during Hib meningitis recover their hearing by the time of hospital discharge (51,52). Unfortunately, for the remaining children deafness is permanent. Vasculitis-induced infarction of cranial nerve VIII and necrosis of cells in the organ of Corti may be responsible for such permanent deafness. In studies of an animal model of pneumococcal meningitis, hearing loss could be detected as early as 12 hours after infection; it progressed rapidly,

and the severity of meningogenic hearing loss correlated with the degree of inflammation observed on cochlear histopathologic study and the inflammatory changes in CSF (53,54). Involvement of the inner ear is not a result of direct extension of infection from the middle ear (55). Rather, contiguous infection is represented by extension of the process from the subarachnoid space to the inner ear via the cochlear aqueduct. This view is supported by studies in infant rats with Hib meningitis produced by intraperitoneal or intranasal inoculation. In seven adults with acute bacterial meningitis and complicating hearing loss, high-resolution MRI of the inner ear showed contrast enhancement in five (56). The clinical and MRI findings showed correlation: all nine ears with cochlear enhancement were deaf, whereas that was not the case for the five ears with normal MRI findings.

SEIZURES

Early seizures occur in 15% to 30% of cases (5,6,10,57). Seizures may be focal or generalized. In adult meningitis, *S. pneumoniae* was the cause in a greater percentage of patients who had seizures than of patients who did not, but alcoholism was a confounder (10). Seizures occurring early in hospitalization do not herald the onset of a permanent seizure disorder, but those that persist beyond the first few days or develop later during hospitalization may.

FOCAL CEREBRAL SIGNS

Focal cerebral signs (hemiparesis, quadriparesis, visual field defects, disorders of conjugate gaze, dysphasia) occur in 10% to 20% of patients with meningitis, more frequently with pneumococcal than with other types of community-acquired meningitis (5,6,10) (Table 148.6). They may appear early in the course of meningitis, or, less frequently, later in the course of the disease due to cortical arteritis or phlebitis. Postictal hemiparesis (Todd's paralysis) must be distinguished from persisting focal cerebral signs. The postictal changes, however, may last several hours.

In the adult the most frequent neurologic complications of bacterial meningitis are cerebrovascular ones, occurring in about 37% of patients with intracranial complications, followed in frequency by brain swelling (34%) detected by computed tomography (CT) and hydrocephalus (29%) (58). These figures are derived from a study of 86 adults with bacterial meningitis in whom cerebral arteriography was performed on those who had focal deficits either clinically or at cranial CT (or both) and in those with persistent coma without apparent cause after 3 days of antimicrobial therapy. The spectrum of cerebrovascular changes includes (a) narrowing and spasm of major arteries at the base of the brain, such as the supraclinoid portion of the internal carotid artery; (b) irregularities or focal aneurysmal dilatations

TABLE 148.6.   Focal Cerebral Signs and Seizures in Community-Acquired Bacterial Meningitis in Adults

Time of onset of findings	Episodes of meningitis (%)					
	Hemiparesis	Aphasia	Visual field defect	Gaze preference	Seizures	Other[a]
Early (≤24 h)	9	6	3	10	15	5
Late (>24 h)	2	1	0.3	0	8	1
Total[b]	11	7	2.3	10	23	6

[a]These findings included ataxia, dysmetria, nystagmus, monoparesis, hemianesthesia, and central seventh nerve palsy.
[b]Percentage of 279 episodes in which individual finding occurred.
Modified with permission from Durand ML, Calderwood SB, Weber DJ, et al. Acute bacterial meningitis in adults: review of 493 episodes. *N Engl J Med* 1993;328:21–28, with permission.

of medium-sized arteries; (c) occlusions of distal branches of the middle cerebral artery with or without retrograde flow; (d) focal abnormal parenchymal blush; (e) marked prolongation of circulation time; and (f) thrombosis of cortical veins or the superior sagittal sinus, or both.

BRAIN SWELLING

Cerebral edema can occur in acute bacterial meningitis. Manifestations include obtundation and coma, third nerve palsies (including dilated, poorly reactive, or nonreactive pupils), abnormal reflexes, hypertension, decerebrate posturing, abnormal respiratory pattern, and bradycardia. Brain edema causes increased ICP, which in older infants has been shown to result in reduced cerebral blood flow velocity (59). Impairment of cerebral blood flow autoregulation, as measured by transcranial Doppler ultrasonography of the middle cerebral artery, causing cerebral blood flow to correspond directly with mean arterial blood pressure with attendant hyper- or hypoperfusion of the brain, occurs in the early phase of acute bacterial meningitis. This may account for some of the reversible changes (due to hypoperfusion and ischemia) that occur early in the process (60). On recovery, the capacity of the cerebral vasculature to maintain a constant level of perfusion (autoregulation) is restored. Such decreased cerebral perfusion is another potential cause of brain injury. Papilledema is rare because of the relatively brief duration of the meningeal process and increased CSF pressure. In one study of 279 episodes of community-acquired meningitis in adults, only 1% of patients had findings of "blurred optic disc margins" and "early papilledema" along with extremely high CSF pressures of 440 mm H_2O or higher (10). Its presence should suggest the possibility of another suppurative intracranial process, such as brain abscess or subdural empyema. Rarely, rhombencephalitis due to *L. monocytogenes* may accompany listerial meningitis, or occur in the absence of overt meningitis (61). Its histologic characteristics are those of a suppurative encephalitis with vasculitis and hemorrhages in the pons and medulla.

Markedly increased ICP due to meningitis may lead to impending herniation. Signs of herniation include (a) bradycardia and abnormal respiratory patterns; (b) mid-position, nonreactive pupils; (c) unequal or dilated, nonreactive pupils; (d) skew deviation or dysconjugate eye movements; and (e) decorticate or decerebrate posturing.

Marked hyperpnea sometimes occurs in patients with severe bacterial meningitis: CSF acidosis, due mainly to increased lactic acid levels, provides much of the respiratory drive. Persistent or late-developing obtundation without focal findings might suggest any of several anatomically distinct processes: cerebral swelling (with or without herniation), subdural effusion (particularly in young infants, where it may cause enlargement of the head and abnormal transillumination findings), hydrocephalus, loculated ventriculitis or ventricular empyema, or rarely, subdural empyema or superior sagittal sinus thrombosis. Minor or extensive arteritis or cortical vein thrombophlebitis may be responsible for obtundation, focal cerebral deficits (62), and seizures as a result of cortical infarction. Rarely, arteritis complicating meningitis involves a spinal or radicular artery and causes paraplegia with a sensory level. The pathologic basis of the neurologic complications (including cerebral vasculitis) in meningitis is provided in the classic study of Adams and co-workers (63) of fatal cases of *H. influenzae* meningitis.

LATE NEUROLOGIC SEQUELAE

The long-term prognosis for neurologic complications has been evaluated mainly in childhood meningitis. In a prospective study of 185 infants and children with acute bacterial meningitis between 1973 and 1977 (mean follow-up of 8.9 years), the per-

centage of patients with significant neurologic abnormalities decreased from 37% 1 month after the meningitis to 14% with permanent deficits (64). Only 10% of the study group had permanent sensorineural hearing loss, and other major permanent neurologic deficits such as hemiparesis, quadriparesis, mental retardation, or blindness were present in another 5%. Seizures were noted in 31% of patients during acute bacterial meningitis. Late-onset epilepsy occurred principally in patients with clinical evidence of permanent cerebral dysfunction. Normal results of neurologic examination shortly after meningitis indicate an excellent prognosis for full neurologic recovery.

Children who had recovered from *H. influenzae* meningitis 6 to 8 years earlier were found to perform as well as their comparably aged siblings in spelling, reading, and arithmetic, despite having slightly lower IQ scores and mild deficits in neuropsychological testing (65).

Persons who have meningitis as neonates or young infants more frequently have long-term sequelae. Among survivors in a study of group B streptococcal meningitis, only half were judged to be functioning normally when evaluated for long-term sequelae at mean age of 6 years (66).

Recurrent Meningitis

About 8% of adults seen in a large urban general hospital with bacterial meningitis had recurrent episodes, and about 16% of episodes of meningitis in this setting were recurrent (10). The interval between recurrences is usually months to years. Predisposing circumstances for the development of recurrent bacterial meningitis are generally either anatomic defects, which allow direct ingress of bacteria into the subarachnoid space while circumventing the usual immune defenses of circulating immunoglobulins, or immunodeficiencies (Table 148.7). The principal predisposing factor, CSF leak, is identifiable in about 75% of patients with recurrent meningitis.

The bacteriologic findings in recurrent meningitis differ for community-acquired and nosocomial varieties. *S. pneumoniae* is the agent of about 33% of episodes of the former but less than 5% of the latter (10). Overall, about two thirds of episodes of community-acquired recurrent meningitis are due to bacterial species that can normally be found in the upper respiratory tract (*S. pneumoniae*, other streptococcal species, meningococci, *H. influenzae*). In adults, *H. influenzae* is the agent of only 4% of cases of bacterial meningitis, yet about two thirds of such patients have CSF leaks. In recurrent episodes of nosocomial meningitis,

---

TABLE 148.7. Predisposing Factors to Recurrent Bacterial Meningitis

Anatomic defects
    CSF fistulae (leak at cribriform plate, leak into nasal air sinus or middle ear, empty sella syndrome)
    Head injury (with CSF otorrhea or rhinorrhea)
    Mastoid erosion by osteomyelitis or cholesteatoma
    Neurosurgical complication (with dural tear)
Immunoglobulin deficiency
Asplenia
Complement deficiencies (congenital deficiencies of late-acting components or acquired deficiencies of early-acting components, predisposing to recurrent *Neisseria* infections and rarely to recurrent meningococcal meningitis)
Failure (rare) to mount specific immune response to *Haemophilus influenzae* type b after *H. influenzae* type b meningitis in an infant

CSF, cerebrospinal fluid.

gram-negative bacilli (other than *H. influenzae*) are the cause in about 45% of cases and staphylococci (coagulase-positive and -negative), another 20% to 25%.

Clinical Course of Infection

Untreated acute bacterial meningitis rapidly progresses to a fatal outcome. With early diagnosis and appropriate therapy the case-fatality rate for meningitis due to *H. influenzae* is 6%; for *N. meningitidis*, 10%; for *L. monocytogenes*, 15%; and for *S. pneumoniae*, 21% (8). In adults, the overall meningitis-related case-fatality rate is 19%; for gram-negative bacillary meningitis, 20% to 25% (10). There has been a decrease in the case-fatality rate for gram-negative bacillary meningitis in the past two decades compared with the two prior decades, but the case-fatality rate for pneumococcal meningitis has not changed. The overall case-fatality rate for recurrent community-acquired bacterial meningitis is about one fifth that of nonrecurrent community-acquired bacterial meningitis.

Nonneurologic Complications

SHOCK

Shock may develop early in the course of acute bacterial meningitis, usually as a consequence of intense bacteremia, as can occur in meningococcemia-meningitis or in pneumococcal bacteremia in asplenic patients. In these instances the major acute impact of the illness stems from the high-grade bacteremia.

COAGULOPATHIES

In patients with meningitis, coagulation disorders may complicate bacteremias and hypotension. The coagulopathy may be mild and consist only of thrombocytopenia, but in patients with more profound bacteremia the clinical features and laboratory findings may be typically those of disseminated intravascular coagulation.

SEPTIC COMPLICATIONS

Early treatment of pneumococcal meningitis or its initiating infection and bacteremia has made acute bacterial endocarditis an uncommon complication of this form of meningitis. In the rare instance in which endocarditis develops, it usually involves the aortic valve. It may not become evident (recrudescence of fever, a new aortic diastolic murmur) until a few days after conclusion of a course of antibiotic therapy for meningitis. Pyogenic arthritis due to the common agents of community-acquired meningitis may complicate the bacteremia occurring early in the course of CNS infection.

IMMUNE-MEDIATED MANIFESTATIONS

In about 10% of patients with meningococcal meningitis, a serum sickness–like syndrome develops 4 to 10 days after initiation of antimicrobial therapy, when the meningitis is clearly responding to treatment. Fever, arthritis, and pericarditis are the principal features, but occasionally pleuritis and new papulobullous skin lesions appear. The synovial and pericardial fluids are serosanguineous and sterile, unlike the purulent infected effusions that sometimes occur at these sites during the first 2 or 3 days of meningococcal meningitis. Usually, such late-onset pericardial effusions are not hemodynamically significant, but nonetheless they warrant careful monitoring of cardiovascular status. Symptomatic relief is afforded by salicylates and nonsteroidal anti-inflammatory agents. A likely role for immune complex formation in the pathogenesis of these sterile processes has been suggested.

PROLONGED FEVER

Most patients with the common types of community-acquired bacterial meningitis become afebrile within 2 to 5 days of initiation of appropriate antimicrobial therapy. Occasionally, fever persists for 8 to 10 days or longer or recurs after initial defervescence. Such a febrile course accompanied by persisting headache, stiff neck, depressed sensorium, and focal cerebral signs suggests that antimicrobial therapy has been inadequate or that a neurologic complication—cortical vein thrombophlebitis and arteritis, ventriculitis, ventricular empyema, subdural effusion or empyema, or sagittal sinus thrombosis—has supervened. Reevaluation of CSF findings, particularly Gram-stained smears and cultures, is of paramount importance; appearance of new focal cerebral signs would be an indication for cranial CT or MRI. Drug fever or a serum sickness–like syndrome should be considered in a patient with persistent fever whose clinical course and CSF findings show continued improvement.

Laboratory Findings

CEREBROSPINAL FLUID EXAMINATION

CSF values characteristic of acute pyogenic meningitis include pleocytosis of 100 to 5,000 cells per mm^3 (predominantly neutrophils), elevated opening pressure, elevated protein level, and Gram-stained smear of centrifuged CSF that shows the infecting agent in 60% to 90% of cases (Table 148.8). The frequency of a positive CSF Gram stain in untreated bacterial meningitis is somewhat dependent on the infecting microorganism: *S. pneumonia*, 70% to 90%; *H. influenzae*, about 80%; *N. meningitidis*, 50% to 80%; and group B streptococcus, 60% to 85% (67). However, in community-acquired meningitis in adults, in which 13% of cases are "culture negative," the overall frequency of positive Gram stains on initial CSF examination is 60% (10). More common misinterpretations of Gram-stained smears include mistaking pneumococci for *H. influenzae*, because of bipolar gram-positive staining of the organism due to inadequate decolorizing, or mistaking *Listeria* for pneumococci. *Enterococcus* species in the CSF may be mistaken for *S. pneumoniae*. *Acinetobacter baumannii* or *Pasteurella multocida* may sometimes suggest on Gram stain a mixture of *H. influenzae* and *N. meningitidis*.

Initial CSF opening pressures may be markedly elevated (450–500 mm H$_2$O or more) in about 5% of patients (Table 148.8). Clear

---

TABLE 148.8.   Cerebrospinal Fluid Findings in Bacterial Meningitis

Pleocytosis (831 episodes between 1963 and 1984)

Cell count	Prevalence (%)
0–100	15
101–1,000	27
1,001–5,000	33
5,001–10,000	14
10,001–50,000	9
>50,000	1

Glucose (681 evaluable episodes) <40 mg/dL or <40% of level of simultaneous blood glucose in 52% of episodes

Opening pressure (354 evaluable episodes)

mm H$_2$O	Prevalence (%)
≤200	36
>200–300	32
>300–450	20
>450–500	6
>500	6

Episodes of meningitis at Massachusetts General Hospital.

CSF with less than 40 to 50 cells per mm^3 may occasionally be seen in early bacterial meningitis, particularly in young infants, or in neutropenic patients. Among 261 cases of meningitis in infants, 2.7% had less than 10 leukocytes per mm^3 of CSF, but *H. influenzae, S. pneumoniae, N. meningitidis* and group B streptococci were isolated on initial cultures (68). Rarely, the CSF of a patient who is not neutropenic will be grossly cloudy but contain only a few neutrophils. In this instance the turbidity is due to myriad pneumococci, and the prognosis is poor. Although most patients with pyogenic meningitis have brisk pleocytosis, the cell count in 75% of patients with *L. monocytogenes* meningitis is 1,000/mm^3 or less. Although two thirds of patients with *Listeria* meningitis have neutrophilic pleocytosis of more than 70%, about 10% (usually neonates, neutropenic children or adults, or rarely a nonneutropenic adult) have mononuclear pleocytosis of about 80%. Rarely, lymphocytic pleocytosis is observed in a nonneutropenic child with meningitis due to one of the common bacteria, such as *H. influenzae.*

The CSF protein level is elevated in 95% of patients with bacterial meningitis—in 50%, 200 mg/dL or higher. Latex particle agglutination and other rapid tests to detect bacterial antigens can be used as an adjunct to Gram stain examination and culture, particularly in the patient who received prior parenteral antibiotic therapy. However, in view of the sensitivity of the CSF Gram stain and culture in patients who have not received prior parenteral antibiotics, it has been suggested that CSF antigen testing be deferred (with the initial CSF sample stored at 2° to 8°C) for 48 hours until CSF and blood cultures are determined to be negative (69). The sensitivity of latex particle agglutination in detecting antigen of the common species of bacteria implicated in community-acquired meningitis varies among organisms. *H. influenzae* antigen can be detected in 95% of cases, including some with negative Gram stain findings (67); *N. meningitidis* in 64% to 78% of cases; and *S. pneumoniae* in 67% of cases. PCR techniques can detect bacterial DNA in CSF of patients with meningitis, but its use in routine diagnostic laboratories has been limited by its time-consuming and technically demanding nature.

A variety of chemical and enzymatic changes have been noted in the CSF of patients with acute bacterial meningitis. Determination of these values has been suggested as a means of distinguishing acute bacterial from aseptic meningitis. The tests include levels of C-reactive protein (70), lactate (67,70), lactate dehydrogenase (71), special profiles of fatty acids and carbohydrate metabolites as detected by gas-liquid chromatography (70), and endotoxin (67). C-reactive protein levels higher than 100 ng/mL of CSF or a qualitative latex slide agglutination test had a sensitivity (for bacterial meningitis) of about 95% in patients with pleocytosis greater than 10 leukocytes per mm^3 but a somewhat lower specificity of 86%. The value of the test is limited by the fact that some patients fail to mount a prompt response and that it provides no information on the nature of the infecting bacteria. Levels of CSF lactate above 3.9 mM are usually observed in bacterial meningitis, and levels are generally lower in patients with aseptic meningitis. Occasional patients with bacterial meningitis have normal values, and the level can be elevated independently in the presence of cerebral ischemia, cerebral edema, or brain tumor. Recently, elevated serum concentrations of procalcitonin have been found as a marker of acute bacterial meningitis and have been used to distinguish bacterial from viral meningitis (72).

The Limulus amebocyte lysate test for detection of endotoxin of gram-negative bacteria in CSF can provide additional bacteriologic information. It has an overall sensitivity of 99% (100% for *H. influenzae* and *N. meningitidis* meningitis but only 67% for other types of gram-negative bacillary meningitis) (73). The value of this test lies only in its capacity to identify a meningeal pathogen as a gram-negative bacterium.

Models using a combination of discriminating values for CSF glucose, protein, total leukocyte, and PMN counts have been used to distinguish bacterial from viral meningitis (74), but experienced physicians usually reach the same conclusion clinically as with the statistical approach.

OTHER LABORATORY STUDIES

Blood cultures from patients with community-acquired meningitis often reveal the pathogen: 90% of *H. influenzae,* 80% of *S. pneumoniae,* and 90% of *N. meningitidis* (75). Culture of the nasopharynx cannot be used to identify the cause in a patient with pyogenic meningitis.

Bacteremic skin lesions associated with highly invasive organisms may reveal the agent on Gram-stained smear. Thus, aspiration of the whitish center of the purulent purpura associated with *S. aureus* bacteremia may reveal the pathogen. The petechial lesions in bacterial meningitis, however, are unlikely to be revealing on Gram stain examination.

Gram stain examination and culture of fluid aspirated from a middle-ear effusion may provide a bacteriologic clue when findings of CSF smear examination are equivocal. The peripheral leukocyte count is commonly elevated in patients with bacterial meningitis, 14,000 to 24,000 cells per mm^3 and generally higher in pneumococcal and meningococcal than in *H. influenzae* disease (76).

Hyponatremia in the course of meningitis is due either to complications of inappropriate antidiuretic hormone secretion (SIADH) or to inappropriate fluid administration.

RADIOGRAPHIC FINDINGS

Chest radiography should be performed to discover any predisposing pulmonary portal of infection. Films of the air sinuses and mastoids should be taken at an appropriate time after commencing antimicrobial therapy if history or findings suggest infection of these structures.

When the history, clinical setting, or physical signs (papilledema, focal cerebral findings) suggest a suppurative intracranial collection, cranial CT should be carried out without delay—and before lumbar puncture (but after blood cultures have been taken and therapy with appropriate antimicrobials for meningitis of unknown bacterial cause has been instituted). In the absence of focal neurologic findings or a history suggestive of an intracranial mass lesion in a patient suspected of having community-acquired meningitis, performance of a diagnostic lumbar puncture should not be deferred pending a head CT examination. In a recent study of 301 adults with suspected meningitis admitted to an urban hospital emergency department, 235 underwent head CT prior to lumbar puncture; 24% of the scans were abnormal, but evidence of a mass effect was present in only 5% (77). Among clinical features in those with abnormal CT findings were age over 60 years, history of central nervous system disease, abnormal level of consciousness, seizure within the prior week, visual field abnormalities, aphasia, and limb drift. In contrast, among the 96 patients with none of these clinical features who had CT scans, 97% of the scans were normal and only one showed a mass effect (mild, hydrocephalus), indicating that clinical features can be used to identify those who are unlikely to show CT abnormalities. In this study the mean time from emergency department admission to lumbar puncture was significantly delayed for patients who first underwent CT (5.3 vs. 3.0 hours).

A variety of abnormalities detectable by head CT may occur during bacterial meningitis (58,78,79): contrast enhancement of the leptomeninges and ventricular lining, cerebral edema, widening of the subarachnoid space, patchy areas of diminished density in the cerebrum from cerebritis or necrosis, multifocal enhancing lesions consistent with cerebral infarcts, subdural effusion, subdural empyema, ventriculomegaly or hydrocephalus, and ventricular empyema. The rare complication of sagittal sinus thrombophlebitis can be detected by MRI.

Patients with bacterial meningitis rarely have clinically significant CT findings without concomitant focal neurologic abnormalities (10,78,79). In a prospective study of head CT in 43 children with acute bacterial meningitis, abnormalities were noted in 30%. In the two patients who died within 72 hours of admission, CT showed generalized cerebral edema. Focal infarction was seen in five of the eight patients who developed hemiparesis (78). In the course of community-acquired meningitis in children, CT is most valuable when persistent focal neurologic findings occur, when CSF cultures remain positive, or when meningitis is recurrent (80). In about 30% of adults with community-acquired meningitis, CT shows abnormalities related to meningitis or its complications (10). Cerebral edema and dural enhancement are abnormalities seen on early scans within 72 hours of admission, whereas cerebral infarcts are seen on later scans. Although subdural effusions are often found in infants with meningitis, they are uncommon in adults (in only 2 of 87 adults with meningitis undergoing CT) (10). Ventriculomegaly is the most common CT abnormality in adult meningitis: 15% of all cases, 15% of which require a shunting procedure. In this study of adult meningitis, of the 48 patients with nonfocal findings, only 8 (17%) had CT abnormalities. Thus, CT in meningitis should not be routine but should be used as indicated by the clinical setting, neurologic findings, and clinical course.

DIFFERENTIAL DIAGNOSIS

The clinical manifestations of meningeal inflammation (headache, fever, stiff neck, obtundation) are common to various other types of meningitis (viral, fungal, rickettsial, mycobacterial, treponemal, borrelial, parasitic, hypersensitivity) as well as to acute pyogenic bacterial meningitis and to parameningeal infections. Analysis of CSF findings is central to the development of the differential diagnosis (see Chapter 147).

Enteroviral aseptic meningitis usually can be distinguished from bacterial meningitis by its seasonal incidence, somewhat more gradual onset, occasional occurrence in outbreaks, occasional accompanying maculopetechial rash, and a lymphocytic pleocytosis without hypoglycorrhachia. Echovirus 9 aseptic meningitis may produce an initial pleocytosis of up to 500 to 1,000 cells per mm^3, with up to 60% neutrophils, shifting in the next 12 to 36 hours to predominance of lymphocytes. The CSF glucose level is usually above 40 mg/dL but may be slightly reduced in rare patients if the pathogen is the virus of lymphocytic choriomeningitis, mumps, or herpes simplex. Aseptic meningitis may be associated with the acute human immunodeficiency virus mononucleosis-like syndrome, but it is readily distinguished from acute bacterial meningitis by associated risk factors, lymphadenopathy, truncal maculopapular rash, and lymphocytic pleocytosis (81). Acute herpes simplex virus type 2 aseptic meningitis, often recurrent, occurs in sexually active persons and may be distinguished from bacterial meningitis by the presence of clustered vesicular lesions in the genital area or in the L1, L2, or S3–5 dermatomes, and by its lymphocytic pleocytosis.

Meningococcal meningitis might be suggested by the fever, maculopetechial rash, and headache of Rocky Mountain spotted fever, but the geographic and seasonal predilections of the latter can provide clues. About 10% of patients hospitalized with Rocky Mountain spotted fever have CSF cell counts of at least 100/mm^3 ($\geq$70% PMNs) and are thus thought to have bacterial meningitis.

To provide greater accuracy in discriminating between acute bacterial and viral meningitis, retrospective analysis of the predictive value of initial clinical and laboratory observations was performed in 422 patients with meningitis seen between 1969 and 1980 (82). Five CSF values were found to be individual predictors of bacterial infection with 99% or greater certainty: (a) CSF glucose level less than 1.9 mM (34 mg/dL), (b) CSF/blood glucose ratio of less than 0.23, (c) CSF protein level greater than 2.2 g/L, (d) greater than 2,000/mm^3 CSF leukocytes, or (e) greater than 1,180/mm^3 CSF neutrophils. Although any one of the foregoing tests could rule in bacterial meningitis with a high likelihood, none could exclude it.

Diagnosis of acute syphilitic meningitis would be suggested by a history of a recent chancre, maculopapular rash or generalized lymphadenopathy, lymphocytic pleocytosis (with or without mildly depressed CSF glucose level), and positive Venereal Disease Research Laboratory (VDRL) tests of serum and CSF. The aseptic meningitis picture of neuroborreliosis can be distinguished from acute pyogenic meningitis by its more subacute onset, exposure to an area endemic for Lyme disease, history of erythema chronicum migrans, lymphocytic pleocytosis, and positive serologic test result for Lyme disease. Leptospiral meningitis might be suggested by a biphasic illness, conjunctivitis, and lymphocytic pleocytosis occurring in a person exposed to rodents, dogs, or cows. Diagnosis is usually made serologically. Tuberculous meningitis occurs in a setting of either past tuberculous infection (meningeal tuberculoma) or recently acquired infection with miliary dissemination to the meninges. The onset of tuberculous meningitis is less abrupt than that of acute pyogenic meningitis. Characteristic CSF changes are lymphocytic pleocytosis, hypoglycorrhachia, and elevated protein level. Bilateral palsies of cranial nerve VI suggest a basilar meningitis and with the aforementioned CSF formula strongly suggest tuberculous meningitis.

Fungal meningitides are almost always more subacute in onset than bacterial meningitis, produce a lymphocytic pleocytosis with hypoglycorrhachia, and are suggested by epidemiologic clues. Fungal meningitides most commonly present the clinical picture of chronic meningitis and are diagnosed by culture and antigen detection (*Cryptococcus neoformans*) in the CSF or by CSF and serum antibody determination. Rarely, chronic meningitis may be characterized by a predominantly neutrophilic CSF formula, and several bacterial and mycotic agents are responsible (83).

Parameningeal infections (particularly brain abscess, subdural empyema, and cranial and spinal epidural abscess) should be considered in the differential diagnosis of acute bacterial meningitis. These processes might be suspected in a patient with features of meningeal inflammation who also has a chronic ear, sinus, or lung infection. Focal cerebral signs and neurologic symptoms antedating the onset of the acute meningitis suggest a space-occupying intracranial infection, such as a brain abscess. In a patient with presumed bacterial meningitis whose CSF formula shows an atypical neutrophilic pleocytosis, a normal glucose level, and no demonstrable organisms on a Gram-stained smear, parameningeal infections warrant particular attention in the differential diagnosis. Isolation of anaerobic bacteria from CSF, especially in mixed culture, suggests parameningeal infection.

Rarely, a fulminant, acute, and usually fatal purulent meningitis is caused by *Naegleria fowleri*, a species of free-living ameba. This diagnosis would be considered when the patient had recently swum in warm freshwater. Early symptoms may include an altered sense of smell and taste. In addition to a neutrophilic pleocytosis with a low to normal glucose level, the CSF often contains numerous red blood cells. Diagnosis is made by finding motile amebic trophozoites on fresh preparations of unspun CSF.

The clinical picture of acute meningitis may develop in bacterial endocarditis. It may represent true bacterial meningitis due to pyogenic organisms (e.g., *S. pneumoniae, Staphylococcus aureus*), or it may result from cerebral embolic infarctions in endocarditis produced by nonpyogenic organisms such as viridans streptococci. Heart murmurs or peripheral signs of endocarditis suggest this pathogenesis for the meningeal process. CSF findings of cerebral infarction in the latter setting include pleocytosis of several hundred cells, with varying numbers of neutrophils, a normal glucose level, and absence of bacteria. In occasional patients with meningeal symptoms due to small cerebral embolic infarctions in acute *S. aureus* endocarditis, the diagnosis may sometimes be made by examination of Gram-stained smears of cutaneous lesions of purulent purpura.

Chemical meningitis occasionally results from leakage into the subarachnoid space of debris from an intracranial tumor, commonly a craniopharyngioma or an epidermoid tumor of the posterior fossa. This may produce the picture of recurrent meningitis. CSF findings include an initial neutrophilic (or lymphocytic) pleocytosis, with or without hypoglycorrhachia. Birefringent material (keratinized debris) from an epidermoid tumor or a craniopharyngioma may be observed under polarized light microscopy.

Occasionally, meningitis may be the principal manifestation of hypersensitivity to drugs such as sulfonamides and nonsteroidal antiinflammatory agents. The pleocytosis may be predominantly neutrophilic or lymphocytic, and some eosinophils may be present, but the glucose level in CSF is normal. Another rare, noninfectious cause of meningitis is systemic lupus erythematosus. The CSF formula is usually a lymphocytic pleocytosis with normal glucose, but rarely, numerous neutrophils and hypoglycorrhachia are features. Antinuclear antibodies are present in high titers in the serum. Rarely, acute, recurrent episodes of meningitis of unknown cause occur in Behçet's syndrome, Mollaret's meningitis, or familial Mediterranean fever. Hypopyon, orogenital lesions, and pathergic skin changes would be indicative of Behçet's syndrome. Mollaret's meningitis, characterized by episodes of fever, meningeal findings, mononuclear pleocytosis (sometimes neutrophilic at inception), and the presence in the CSF of unusual cells variously described as "epithelial" or "endothelial," has been associated in some instances with underlying herpes simplex virus type 1 infections (84) or with CNS epidermoid cysts (85).

TREATMENT

Essential for prompt treatment of meningitis is early recognition in the community of meningeal signs, particularly the transition from a predisposing illness, such as otitis media, which may have been responsible for earlier fever and headache. In the hospital emergency department there is need for timely triage of patients with symptoms suggestive of meningitis, rapid contact with a physician, early lumbar puncture in the absence of suspicion of a mass lesion, and prompt delivery of appropriate antimicrobial(s). In a study at two urban children's hospitals, the median time from triage in an emergency department until administration of parenteral antibiotics was 2.0 hours; only 16% of the children with bacterial meningitis received antibiotics within

1 hour, and only 1% within 30 minutes or less after presentation (86).

Therapy of acute bacterial meningitis involves (a) rapid identification of the pathogen, (b) prompt institution of an appropriate antimicrobial, when it can be defined on initial CSF examination, or institution of treatment directed at meningitis of unknown cause (utilizing clues provided by the age of the patient and clinical setting) pending definitive culture information, (c) management of neurologic and systemic complications, and local predisposing conditions (e.g., mastoiditis), and (d) study of predisposing factors, such as CSF fistulas, in the patient with recurrent bacterial meningitis.

General Aspects of Antimicrobial Treatment

The efficacy of antimicrobial therapy in bacterial meningitis depends on a variety of factors: antimicrobial susceptibility of the organism, bactericidal activity of the antimicrobial, capacity of the drug to penetrate the blood-brain barrier, and effectiveness of various modes of antibiotic administration in achieving desired concentrations of the drug in CSF. In view of the lack of intrinsic opsonic and bactericidal activity in CSF early in bacterial meningitis, bactericidal rather than bacteriostatic agents are needed (37). CSF concentrations of β-lactam antibiotics or aminoglycosides must be 10 to 20 times higher than the minimal bactericidal concentration for the infecting organism for optimal bactericidal effects (87). The low pH and abundance of nucleic acids in purulent CSF inhibit bacterial killing by aminoglycosides.

Antagonism by a bacteriostatic drug, chloramphenicol, of the early bactericidal effect of penicillin in experimental canine pneumococcal meningitis and of the bactericidal activity of gentamicin in experimental *Proteus mirabilis* meningitis in rabbits has been demonstrated (88). Little clinical information relating to humans on this point is available. There is evidence of antagonism between chlortetracycline and penicillin in the treatment of pneumococcal meningitis (89).

Most antibiotics used in the treatment of bacterial meningitis, with the exception of chloramphenicol and rifampin, do not readily penetrate the normal blood-brain barrier. β-lactam antibiotics penetrate to only 0.5% to 2.0% of peak serum concentrations (88), but higher levels are achieved when the meninges are inflamed. Clindamycin, erythromycin, and first- and second-generation cephalosporins should not be used to treat bacterial meningitis because effective bactericidal levels cannot be obtained. For antimicrobial drugs such as β-lactams, aminoglycosides, and vancomycin, which poorly penetrate even inflamed meninges, intermittent bolus parenteral administration is preferable to continuous administration.

Specific Antimicrobial Therapy

Acute bacterial meningitis requires prompt antimicrobial treatment based on examination of a Gram-stained smear of the spun sediment of CSF (Table 148.9). When clinical evaluation suggests a parameningeal suppurative mass lesion and head CT is needed before performance of a lumbar puncture, antibiotic therapy should be instituted, directed toward meningitis of unknown cause (Table 148.10), after blood cultures have been obtained. If in this situation CT has excluded a mass lesion and the subsequent CSF examination shows bacterial types not treated by the initial empirical program, antimicrobial therapy can be altered. Such initial therapy is unlikely to prevent identification of the pathogen if CSF is sampled within 2 or 3 hours.

TABLE 148.9. Antimicrobial Therapy of Community-Acquired Bacterial Meningitis of Known Cause

Organism	Preferred therapy			Alternative therapy		
	Antimicrobial	Adults, 24-hour dose	Children, 24-hour dose	Antimicrobial	Adults, 24-hour dose	Children, 24-hour dose
Streptococcus pneumoniae Penicillin MIC < 0.1 µg/mL	Penicillin G *or* Ampicillin	24 million units i.v., every 4 h aliquots 12 g i.v., every 4 h aliquots	300,000 units/kg i.v., every 4 h aliquots 200–300 mg/kg i.v., every 4 h aliquots	Cefotaxime *or* Ceftriaxone[a] *or* Vancomycin *or* Chloramphenicol	12 g i.v., every 4 h aliquots 4 g i.v., every 12 h aliquots 2 g i.v., every 8–12 h aliquots[b] (4–6 g i.v., every 6 h aliquots)	200 mg/kg i.v., every 4–6 h aliquots 100 mg/kg i.v., every 12 h aliquots 50–60 mg/kg i.v., every 6 h aliquots (100 mg/kg i.v., every 6 h aliquots)
Penicillin MIC 0.1–1.0 µg/mL	Ceftriaxone[a] *or* Cefotaxime	4 g i.v., every 12 h aliquots 12 g i.v., every 4 h aliquots	100 mg/kg i.v., every 12 h aliquots[a] 200–300 mg/kg i.v., every 4–6 h aliquots	Vancomycin[b] *or* Meropenem[c]	2 g i.v., every 8–12 h aliquots 6 g i.v., every 8 h aliquots	50–60 mg/kg i.v., every 6 h aliquots 120 mg/kg i.v., every 8 h aliquots
Penicillin MIC > 1.0 µg/mL	Vancomycin[b,d] plus Cefotaxime *or* Ceftriaxone as above	2 g i.v., every 8–12 h aliquots[b]	60 mg/kg i.v., every 6 h aliquots	Meropenem[c]	6 g i.v., every 8 h aliquots	120 mg/kg i.v., every 8 h aliquots
Neisseria meningitidis	Penicillin G Ampicillin	24 million units i.v., every 4 h aliquots 12 g i.v., every 4 h aliquots	300,000 units/kg i.v., every 4 h aliquots 200–400 mg/kg i.v., every 4 h aliquots	Ceftriaxone[a] *or* Cefotaxime *or* Chloramphenicol	Dose as above Dose as above 4 g i.v., every 6 h aliquots	80–100 mg/kg i.v., every 12 h aliquots 200 mg/kg i.v., every 4–6 h aliquots 100 mg/kg i.v., every 6 h aliquots
Haemophilus influenzae β-lactamase-negative	Ampicillin	12 g i.v., every 4 h aliquots	200–300 mg/kg i.v., every 4 h aliquots	Third-generation cephalosporin[e] or chloramphenicol	Dose as above	Dose as above
β-lactamase-positive	Ceftriaxone[a] *or* Cefotaxime	4 g i.v., every 12 h aliquots 12 g i.v., every 4 h aliquots	100 mg/kg i.v., every 12 h aliquots 200 mg/kg i.v., every 4–6 h aliquots	Chloramphenicol	Dose as above	100 mg/kg i.v., every 6 h aliquots
Listeria monocytogenes	Ampicillin[f] *or* Penicillin G[f]	12 g i.v., every 4 h aliquots 24 million units i.v., every 4 h aliquots	200–400 mg/kg i.v., every 4 h aliquots 300,000 units/kg i.v., every 4 h aliquots	TMP-SMX	10–20 mg/kg i.v.,[g] every 6–8 h aliquots	15–20 mg/kg i.v.,[g] every 6 h aliquots

Dosages are those for patients with normal renal and hepatic function.

[a]Maximal daily dose is 4 g.

[b]Monitoring of peak and trough serum levels is advisable; cerebrospinal fluid levels may need to be monitored if the patient is not responding well and, if low, the daily dose may need to be increased temporarily by 0.5–1.0 g in adults or adjuvant intrathecal vancomycin added as in treatment of methicillin-resistant *S. aureus* meningitis (see text).

[c]Use may be associated with an increased incidence of seizures.

[d]Addition of rifampin should be considered. Consider intrathecal (or intraventricular) vancomycin (5–20 mg/day) if not responding to intravenous therapy.

[e]Ceftriaxone or cefotaxime.

[f]Addition of intravenous gentamicin might be considered.

[g]Dosage is based on the trimethoprim component of the combination.

i.v., intravenously; TMP-SMX, trimethoprim-sulfamethoxazole.

TABLE 148.10. Initial Therapy for Community-Acquired Purulent Meningitis of Unknown Cause

Age or condition	Likely pathogens	Preferred drugs	Alternative drugs
0–4 wk	Group B streptococci, *Escherichia coli*, *Listeria monocytogenes*	Ampicillin + cefotaxime	Ampicillin + aminoglycoside[a]
4–12 wk	Group B streptococci, *E. coli*, *L. monocytogenes*, *Haemophilus influenzae*, *Streptococcus pneumoniae*	Ampicillin + either cefotaxime or ceftriaxone	Ampicillin + vancomycin + chloramphenicol
Immunocompetent			
3 mo through 17 yr	*S. pneumoniae*, *Neisseria meningitidis*, *H. influenzae*	Cefotaxime or ceftriaxone + vancomycin	Ampicillin + chloramphenicol or meropenem
18–50 yr	*S. pneumoniae*, *N. meningitidis*	Cefotaxime or ceftriaxone + vancomycin	Meropenem
>50 yr	*S. pneumoniae*, *N. meningitidis*, *L. monocytogenes*	Cefotaxime or ceftriaxone + ampicillin + vancomycin	Trimethoprim-sulfamethoxazole + meropenem
Impaired cellular Immunity	*L. monocytogenes*, gram negative bacilli, *S. aureus*	Ampicillin + ceftazidime + vancomycin	Trimethoprim-sulfamethoxazole + meropenem
Basilar skull fracture or CSF leak	*S. pneumoniae*, various streptococci, *H. influenzae*, *N. meningitidis*	Cefotaxime or ceftazidime + vancomycin	Vancomycin + chloramphenicol or meropenem
CSF mechanical Shunt	*Staphylococcus aureus*, coagulase-negative staphylococci, *Pseudomonas aeruginosa*, Enterobacteriaceae	Vancomycin + ceftazidime	Meropenem + vancomycin

[a]Gentamicin or tobramycin (or amikacin in hospitals where gentamicin-resistant enteric organisms are common).

COMMUNITY-ACQUIRED MENINGITIS

Streptococcus pneumoniae

Penicillin G and ampicillin have been the drugs of choice for meningitis due to penicillin-susceptible *S. pneumoniae*. Formerly, *S. pneumoniae* was universally susceptible to penicillin *in vitro* [minimal inhibitory concentration (MIC) ≤ 0.06 μg/mL], but in the past two decades, relatively resistant (MIC 0.1–1.0 μg/mL) and very resistant (MIC 1.0–2.0 μg/mL or more) strains have been isolated from patients (88). Such resistance in these strains is chromosomal in origin (alterations in penicillin-binding proteins). In other parts of the world (South Africa, Hungary, parts of South America, and Spain), as many as 40% to 50% of strains show moderate or high degrees of resistance (90–92). Although reports of isolation of penicillin-resistant pneumococci, sometimes resistant as well to other drugs (tetracycline, erythromycin, chloramphenicol, clindamycin), from abroad appeared as early as the 1970s, only 0.02% of isolates of *S. pneumoniae* in a nationwide surveillance program between 1979 and 1987 in the United States showed high-level resistance to penicillin (93). Subsequent studies of both children and adults in a variety of regions indicate that the percentage of penicillin-resistant isolates among invasive *S. pneumoniae* ranged from 2% to 17%. Most disturbing is the finding, in a 1994 survey of *S. pneumoniae* isolates from more than 400 patients with invasive infection in the Atlanta area, of resistance to penicillin in 25% (7% high level) (94). Multiple antimicrobial resistance was common among the penicillin-resistant isolates: 75% resistant to trimethoprim-sulfamethoxazole; 41% to erythromycin; 34% to cefotaxime; 24% to tetracycline; 23% to imipenem; and 12% to chloramphenicol. Among all the 431 isolates analyzed, 9% were resistant to cefotaxime, a proportion identical to that in Barcelona, Spain (95). Molecular fingerprinting has indicated that a multidrug-resistant clone of *S. pneumoniae* serotype 23F, related to multidrug-resistant isolates from Spain and South Africa, has spread to the United States and become widely disseminated (96,97).

The increasing prevalence of penicillin resistance (and multidrug resistance) among strains of *S. pneumoniae* mandates susceptibility testing of any isolate from blood or normally sterile body sites. In view of the increase in prevalence of penicillin resistance in *S. pneumonia*, penicillin should not be used as the drug of choice in the empiric treatment of pyogenic meningitis when *S. pneumoniae* is a likely pathogen. Even with "meningeal dosages" of penicillin it is difficult to achieve, during the first and subsequent days, CSF concentrations greater than 1 μg/mL. In view of the prevalence of relatively penicillin resistant strains in the 1980s, third-generation cephalosporins such as cefotaxime or ceftriaxone in high dosage have been used as initial treatment when *S. pneumoniae* was a suspected cause (98,99). During the past 10 years in the United States the occurrence of meningitis caused by strains of *S. pneumoniae* intermediately susceptible (MIC 1 μg/mL) (11% of isolates) and resistant (MIC ≥ 2 μg/ml) (9% of isolates) to third-generation cephalosporins has presented a new therapeutic problem (100); reports of patients with such infecting strains who have been unsuccessfully treated with such cephalosporins have appeared (101,102). Such treatment failures attributed to cephalosporins have led to recommendations for the use of vancomycin (to which all strains of *S. pneumoniae* remain susceptible) in addition to a third-generation cephalosporin for initial empiric treatment of meningitis where *S. pneumoniae* may be a cause in both children (103) and adults (104). In an analysis of 109 cases of pneumococcal meningitis in three cities in the United States from 1994 to 1996, a period when combination therapy with a β-lactam with vancomycin (29% received vancomycin on admission; 52% within 48 hours) was becoming standard for suspected pneumococcal meningitis, clinical outcomes were similar for those with cefotaxime-nonsusceptible (9% mortality) and those with susceptible (15% mortality) strains (100).

Vancomycin has been used successfully, alone or in combination with other drugs such as rifampin, in the treatment of a small number of patients with meningitis who were unsuccessfully treated initially with cefotaxime or ceftriaxone and whose infecting strains of *S. pneumoniae* had MIC values for these third-generation cephalosporins of 2 to 8 μg/mL (102).

In a study of the pharmacodynamics of vancomycin treatment of experimental penicillin- and cephalosporin-resistant pneumococcal meningitis, the level of penetration of vancomycin into CSF was approximately 20% of concurrent serum levels, and the peak CSF concentrations in CSF were 4- to 8-fold higher than the minimum bactericidal concentration and were adequate for bacterial clearance (105). The coadministration of dexamethasone in the same study reduced the penetration of vancomycin into the CSF by 29% and lowered the rate of bacterial elimination. Higher doses of vancomycin with steroid use allowed therapeutic peak antibiotic concentrations in CSF, suggesting the possibility of circumventing the effect of corticosteroids by use of larger doses of vancomycin (105). In one series of 11 patients with pneumococcal meningitis (three strains with a penicillin MIC of 1 μg/mL, four strains with an MIC of 2–4 μg/mL) treated with intravenous vancomycin, and adjunctive intravenous dexamethasone, 10 were eventually cured, but 4 required a shift to other drugs because of failure of vancomycin (106). Possible causes of therapeutic failure, because vancomycin resistance has not been observed among pneumococci, include inadequate serum levels of vancomycin and poor penetration of the drug into the CSF, possibly abetted by the antiinflammatory effect of adjunctive dexamethasone therapy. At present, vancomycin together with rifampin is the most reasonable therapy for meningitis due to highly penicillin- and cephalosporin-resistant *S. pneumoniae*. Intrathecal or intraventricular vancomycin (5–20 mg/day without preservative) may be added in management if the response to intravenous vancomycin is unsatisfactory (107). In this situation, measurement of CSF levels may be helpful.

For several decades, chloramphenicol has been the alternative treatment for pneumococcal meningitis in the highly β-lactam–allergic patient. Although only 3% of 431 isolates of *S. pneumoniae* from Atlanta in 1994 showed resistance to chloramphenicol (MIC $\geq$8 μg/mL), 12% of penicillin-resistant isolates were also resistant to chloramphenicol (94). In a South African study of pneumococcal meningitis due to strains that were both penicillin resistant and chloramphenicol susceptible, 80% of children who were treated initially with chloramphenicol had an unsatisfactory outcome (death, neurologic deficit, poor clinical response) (108). In contrast, adverse outcomes occurred in only 33% of children with meningitis due to penicillin-susceptible strains who were treated with penicillin. The penicillin-resistant strains were more likely to have had a higher chloramphenicol minimal bactericidal concentration (4 μg/mL or more), suggesting that the poor clinical results might have been attributable to inadequate bactericidal activity of chloramphenicol against penicillin-resistant strains. In view of the increasing frequency of penicillin-resistant strains in *S. pneumoniae* meningitis, initial treatment of the highly β-lactam allergic patient with suspected pneumococcal meningitis should consist of vancomycin along with rifampin or chloramphenicol, but not chloramphenicol alone as in the past. Vancomycin (with or without the addition of rifampin) is the drug of choice for treatment of meningitis caused by highly penicillin- and cephalosporin-resistant pneumococci.

Neisseria meningitidis

Penicillin or ampicillin remains the antimicrobial of choice for treatment of meningitis caused by *N. meningitidis*. Strains (55%) intermediately resistant to penicillin (MIC 0.1–1.0 μg/mL) due to reduced affinity for penicillin-binding protein 2 have been frequently observed (55%) among clinical isolates in Spain (109), but rarely observed (3%) in the United States (110). Worldwide, there have been only five penicillin-resistant (β-lactamase–producing) isolates, and none from the United States. Sporadic penicillin-resistant strains have been reported from elsewhere in Europe, South Africa, and Canada. They have belonged to serogroup B or C, and the DNA fingerprints containing the penicillin-binding protein 2 gene of these strains have shown considerable diversity when compared with penicillin-susceptible strains (111). In treating such infections, cefotaxime or ceftriaxone are the drugs of choice (112).

Haemophilus influenzae

Although ampicillin was the drug of choice in the treatment of Hib meningitis from the late 1960s to the mid-1970s, the emergence and increasing prevalence of β-lactamase–producing strains (approximately 30% of isolates in the United States) (113) have required a change in therapy. Thus, ceftriaxone or cefotaxime have become the drugs of choice for treatment of Hib meningitis.

Resistance of *H. influenzae* to ceftriaxone or cefotaxime has not yet been reported as a problem. Cefuroxime, a second-generation cephalosporin, was used in the mid-1980s in the initial treatment of childhood meningitis. However, subsequent trials comparing cefuroxime and ceftriaxone in the treatment of childhood bacterial meningitis, although showing no difference in mortality (no deaths in either group), did demonstrate a delay in sterilization of the CSF at 18 to 36 hours with cefuroxime and an increased incidence of sensorineural hearing loss (17% vs. 4%). Thus, cefuroxime should not be considered as an initial choice for treatment of childhood meningitis or known Hib meningitis.

ACUTE BACTERIAL MENINGITIS OF UNDEFINED CAUSE

Initial antimicrobial treatment of acute bacterial meningitis of unknown cause is based on coverage of the likely pathogens, as suggested by the age of the patient and the clinical setting (community or nosocomial origin, compromised host; Table 148.10). In adults, *S. pneumoniae*, *N. meningitidis*, various streptococci, and *L. monocytogenes* are responsible for most cases of community-acquired meningitis (10). The combination of high-dose ceftriaxone or cefotaxime with vancomycin (with or without rifampin) is mandated as initial therapy because of the prevalence of penicillin resistance among *S. pneumoniae* (94,95,114,115). The role of *H. influenzae* and Enterobacteriaceae in 5% to 10% of episodes of community-acquired meningitis in adults further supports the use of ceftriaxone or cefotaxime in initial combination therapy. The likelihood of *L. monocytogenes* as the cause of meningitis is increased in patients over 50 years of age, in the presence of immunosuppression or pregnancy, and in the setting of liver disease. In view of the relative insusceptibility of *Listeria* to third-generation cephalosporins, there is a need for the addition of ampicillin to the combination of ceftriaxone (or cefotaxime) and vancomycin in initial treatment of the aforementioned categories of patients (61). In the penicillin-allergic patient, an alternative antimicrobial for treatment of *L. monocytogenes* meningitis is trimethoprim-sulfamethoxazole (TMP-SMX), which is bactericidal *in vitro* against this organism (116). In an epidemic of 57 cases of listeriosis in adults (almost 80% with meningitis or meningoencephalitis), 7 patients with CNS infection were treated with TMP-SMX and survived (117). The addition of gentamicin to penicillin or ampicillin might be considered, in view of synergism *in vitro* and enhanced killing in animal models, in culture-proven cases of severe infection caused by *L. monocytogenes* or if such infections failed to respond to treatment.

NOSOCOMIAL MENINGITIS

The principal agents of nosocomial bacterial meningitis are gram-negative bacilli (including *Pseudomonas*), *S. aureus*, and *S. epidermidis* (Tables 148.11 and 148.12). Accordingly, for initial treatment of nosocomial meningitis prior to bacteriologic confirmation, vancomycin and a cephalosporin with good activity against *Pseudomonas* such as ceftazidime, should be used (114). A third-generation cephalosporin is the treatment of choice for meningitis caused by Enterobacteriaceae; for *P. aeruginosa* meningitis, intravenous ceftazidime in combination with an aminoglycoside such as tobramycin is the treatment of choice. Among 24 patients with *Pseudomonas* meningitis treated

TABLE 148.11.   Antimicrobial Therapy of Nosocomial Bacterial Meningitis of Known Cause

| Organism | Preferred therapy | | Alternative therapy |
	Antimicrobial	Adjunctive intrathecal therapy	Antimicrobial
Staphylococcus aureus			
Methicillin susceptible	Nafcillin or oxacillin ± rifampin	—	Vancomycin
Methicillin resistant	Vancomycin ± rifampin	Vancomycin, if needed, 5–20 mg/day[a]	Linezolid; trimethoprim-sulfamethoxazole + rifampin
Coagulase-negative *Staphylococcus*	Vancomycin ± rifampin	Vancomycin, if needed, 5–20 mg/day[a]	Linezolid
Enterobacteriaceae	Cefotaxime or ceftriaxone	—	Meropenem; aztreonam; trimethoprim-sulfamethoxazole
Pseudomonas aeruginosa	Ceftazidime + tobramycin or gentamicin	Gentamicin, if needed, 2–4 mg/day[b]	Meropenem, aztreonam, piperacillin + tobramycin or gentamicin
Streptococcus agalactiae (group B Streptococcus)	Ampicillin or penicillin G	—	Cefotaxime or ceftriaxone; vancomycin
Enterococcus species	Ampicillin or penicillin G + gentamicin	Gentamicin, if needed, 2–4 mg/day[b]	Vancomycin + gentamicin; linezolid ± gentamicin; ? chloramphenicol[c]; ?quinupristin/dalfopristin[d]
Empiric therapy for specific settings (nosocomial)			
After neurosurgery or head trauma	Vancomycin + ceftazidime	—	—
Immunocompromised host	Vancomycin + ceftazidime + ampicillin	—	—

[a]Intrathecal vancomycin has been used as adjunctive therapy when response to intravenous vancomycin was unsatisfactory. For intrathecal use it should be free of preservative.

[b]Without preservative, in 5–10 mL of cerebrospinal fluid (CSF) or in a volume of sterile saline (without preservative, comparable to the 5–10 mL of CSF removed from an adult for analysis). Injection should be administered slowly for 10 minutes.

[c]If other antimicrobials ineffective or cannot be used.

[d]For vancomycin-resistant *E. faecium* only.

with ceftazidime alone or in combination with an aminoglycoside, 19 (79%) were cured (118). Cefepime, a broad-spectrum, fourth-generation cephalosporin with good activity against the common causes (including penicillin-resistant pneumococci) of community-acquired meningitis is also active against many gram-negative bacilli (*E. coli, K. pneumoniae, P. aeruginosa*) (114). It shows excellent CSF penetration in the experimental meningitis model (119). These characteristics would make it a useful alternative drug for many types of bacterial meningitis, but clinical experience is limited as yet.

With the ready penetration of ceftazidime and other third-generation cephalosporins into CSF in the presence of meningeal inflammation, intrathecal or intraventricular aminoglycoside is not needed for meningitis caused by Enterobacteriaceae or *P. aeruginosa*. It may be considered, however, when patients do not respond to parenteral therapy, particularly when access to intraventricular administration is available from prior neurosurgery.

Limited experience indicates that other drugs may be available as alternatives should a third-generation cephalosporin prove ineffective in gram-negative bacillary meningitis. Meropenem, which penetrates the inflamed blood-brain barrier to about 10%, has been effective in treatment of meningitis in children caused by *S. pneumoniae, H. influenzae*, and *N. meningitidis* (120). Meropenem has been used to treat sepsis caused by many strains of gram-negative bacilli, and it is active against most strains of *P. aeruginosa*. Aztreonam, which readily penetrates the blood-brain barrier, has been effective in the treatment of a small number of cases of meningitis caused by susceptible aerobic gram-negative bacilli (121). Although some fluoroquinolones readily penetrate the CSF in the presence of meningitis (10%–90% of simultaneous serum levels), there are as yet only few

data on their use in bacterial meningitis. Fluoroquinolones have been used successfully in the treatment of some patients with gram-negative bacillary meningitis (122,123). Their place in the therapy of meningitis is limited at present to the treatment of infections caused by multidrug-resistant gram-negative bacilli that are susceptible to ciprofloxacin. Newer, broad-spectrum fluoroquinolones (moxifloxacin, gatifloxacin, grepafloxacin) with high activity against gram-positive bacteria showed good penetrance into CSF and effectiveness in the experimental model of meningitis due to highly penicillin-resistant *S. pneumoniae* (124–126). Data on clinical effectiveness of these newer fluoroquinolones in the treatment of meningitis due to highly penicillin- and cephalosporin-resistant *S. pneumoniae, S. aureus* and coagulase-negative staphylococci are not available.

Stenotrophomonas maltophilia is increasingly important as a nosocomial pathogen and is often resistant to third-generation cephalosporins and meropenem but susceptible to TMP-SMX. On the basis of *in vitro* susceptibilities and experience in treatment of several cases of *S. maltophilia* meningitis after neurosurgery, TMP-SMX appears to be the treatment of choice (127).

Treatment of nosocomial meningitis due to *Enterobacter* species with third-generation cephalosporins may be complicated by the development of resistance to the third-generation cephalosporin during the course of therapy, and by clinical failure. In a study of 12 patients with *Enterobacter* meningitis at one hospital, resistance to the third-generation cephalosporin used developed in 4 of 10 patients who received initial therapy with the cephalosporin (128). TMP-SMX appears to be a useful drug when such resistance develops or when *Enterobacter* is isolated from CSF even when the initial CSF isolate is susceptible to third-generation cephalosporins. *A. baumannii* has been involved increasingly in the past decade with outbreaks of

TABLE 148.12. Dosages for Antimicrobial Agents in Treatment of Nosocomial Meningitis in Adults

Antimicrobial agent	Total daily dose[a]	Frequency of doses
Third-generation cephalosporins		
Cefotaxime	12 g	Every 4 h
Ceftriaxone	4 g	Every 12 h
Ceftazidime	6 g	Every 6–8 h
Penicillins		
Penicillin G	24 million units	Every 4 h
Ampicillin	12 g	Every 4 h
Nafcillin	9–12 g	Every 4 h
Oxacillin	9–12 g	Every 4 h
Piperacillin	24 g	Every 4 h
Aminoglycosides[b]		
Gentamicin	3–5 mg/kg	Every 8–12 h
Tobramycin	3–5 mg/kg	Every 8–12 h
Amikacin	15 mg/kg	Every 8–12 h
Vancomycin[c]	2 g	Every 8–12 h
Chloramphenicol[d]	4–6 g	Every 6 h
Rifampin	600 mg	Every 24 h
Aztreonam	6–8 g	Every 6–8 h
Ciprofloxacin	1,200 mg	Every 8 h
Trimethoprim-sulfamethoxazole[e]	20 mg/kg	Every 6–12 h
Meropenem[f]	6 g	Every 8 h
Linezolid (for VRE)	1,200 mg	Every 12 h
Quinupristin/darupristin	22.5 mg/kg	Every 8 h

All dosages are for intravenous administration.
[a]Dosages are for adults with normal renal and hepatic function.
[b]Aminoglycoside peak and trough serum levels should be monitored for dosage regulation.
[c]Vancomycin peak and trough serum levels should be monitored for dosage regulation.
[d]Chloramphenicol serum levels may need to be monitored for dosage regulation.
[e]Dosage refers to trimethoprim component.
[f]May induce seizure activity.

nosocomial infections, including meningitis after invasive neurosurgical procedures (129). Treatment with a combination of an extended-spectrum ureidopenicillin (mezlocillin, piperacillin) and an aminoglycoside (amikacin, tobramycin) has been successful. Because of variable antimicrobial susceptibilities, other drugs may be required. Most clinical isolates have shown susceptibility to imipenem or meropenem, ciprofloxacin, ceftazidime, and minocycline (129). As in treatment of other resistant gram-negative bacillary meningitides, use of intrathecal as well as parenteral aminoglycosides may be indicated.

Treatment of *S. aureus* meningitis involves the use of intravenous nafcillin or oxacillin. For meningitis caused by methicillin-resistant *S. aureus*, or when such methicillin-resistant organisms are likely, or for patients who are allergic to penicillin, vancomycin is the alternative of choice (16). The addition of rifampin to either nafcillin or vancomycin should be considered when the therapeutic response has been inadequate, or, from the beginning, when the infection is severe. Because coagulase-negative staphylococci are the most frequent causes of CSF shunt infections (and complicating meningitis), and because two thirds of such nosocomial strains are methicillin resistant, vancomycin is the initial drug of choice, although its penetration is limited in the absence of marked meningeal inflammation. If the response to treatment is unsatisfactory, rifampin (which readily penetrates the CSF) might be added.

Enterococci are uncommon causes of meningitis. Rarely, but increasingly, vancomycin-resistant *Enterococcus faecium* (VREF),

is the cause of nosocomial meningitis and presents therapeutic problems. Linezolid penetrates readily into CSF and has been used successfully in treatment of several cases of VREF meningitis (130).

Meningitis in the presence of an infected CSF shunt requires initial therapy directed by findings on Gram stain of CSF. In the absence of the finding of a likely pathogen on an initial Gram-stained smear, initial antimicrobial treatment should be directed at the most likely pathogens (*S. aureus*, coagulase-negative staphylococci, and aerobic gram-negative bacilli such as Enterobacteriaceae and *P. aeruginosa*) until culture results become available (131). All components of the infected shunt should be removed at the onset of antimicrobial therapy. External ventriculostomy is recommended at the same time to reduce ventriculitis and for observation of CSF changes (132). Ventricular irrigation with an antibiotic solution has been used in the treatment of severe or difficult to eradicate infections, with amikacin (30 μg/mL) or gentamicin (15 μg/mL) solutions (without preservative) in a continuous flow through a functioning ventriculostomy (132). Intraventricular antibiotic administration may be used for distribution through the ventricular system and CSF in the absence of external ventriculostomy, to overcome the problem of poor CSF penetration after intravenous administration of drugs such as gentamicin and vancomycin (132–135). When an aminoglycoside is used intraventricularly for treatment of an aerobic gram-negative bacillary infection, it should be combined with a parenteral drug (e.g., a third-generation cephalosporin or an extended-spectrum ureidopenicillin) as well as with a parenteral aminoglycoside.

ADJUNCTIVE INTRATHECAL THERAPY

Intrathecal therapy is unnecessary for the common types of community-acquired meningitis. Third-generation cephalosporins, which achieve CSF levels that are bactericidal for many of the gram-negative bacilli involved in nosocomial meningitis, have eliminated the need for intrathecal aminoglycosides in most situations. Occasionally, with refractory meningitis caused by gram-negative bacilli, adjunctive use of intrathecal (or intraventricular) aminoglycosides might be considered.

The adjunctive use of intrathecal gentamicin occasionally might be indicated in the treatment of enterococcal (*E. faecalis*) meningitis when the response to initial treatment with intravenous penicillin (or ampicillin) and gentamicin has not been satisfactory. Adjuvant intrathecal vancomycin is occasionally used in the treatment of meningitis (or CSF shunt infections) caused by methicillin-resistant *S. aureus* or coagulase-negative staphylococci that does not respond satisfactorily to intravenous vancomycin. Intrathecal, preservative-free vancomycin, in doses up to 20 mg daily for adults (or approximately 0.5 mg/kg for children), is administered slowly or by barbotage after dilution in CSF or preservative-free physiologic diluent (107).

Adjunctive intraventricular gentamicin has been administered in a daily dosage of 4 to 8 mg in adults (1–2 mg in infants) (132,134). Adjunctive intraventricular vancomycin has been given in doses of 4 to 10 mg daily (132,135,136).

DURATION OF ANTIMICROBIAL THERAPY

Treatment of meningococcal meningitis for 7 days (for 5 days after the patient becomes afebrile) is adequate. Treatment of *H. influenzae* meningitis should continue for 7 to 10 days (for 7 days after the patient becomes afebrile). However, studies have shown that 7 days' treatment of childhood meningitis with ceftriaxone is generally effective and the results are comparable with results from 10 days' treatment (137). Indeed, in a recent small study of childhood meningitis (mainly caused by *H. influenzae*, *N. meningitidis*, and *S. pneumoniae*) in Chile, the results of 7 days and 4 days of treatment with ceftriaxone, in children with rapid initial recovery, appeared comparable (138). It would seem more prudent, in the case of pneumococcal meningitis, to treat longer (for 10–14 days), because of the occurrence of strains with penicillin/ceftriaxone resistance, the not infrequent presence of a predisposing otitis media and mastoiditis, and because of possible metastatic foci of infection. More prolonged therapy is needed in the presence of an accompanying parameningeal infection.

Repeated CSF examination at the conclusion of a course of antimicrobial therapy for *H. influenzae* and *N. meningitidis* meningitis is unnecessary in most instances when there has been a prompt and satisfactory clinical recovery (139). Follow-up examination should be done for pneumococcal meningitis at the completion of therapy, because of occasional relapse from an associated parameningeal site of infection and because of therapeutic problems with *S. pneumoniae* strains that are relatively or highly resistant to penicillin. In the patient who has not shown satisfactory improvement in the first 24 to 48 hours of treatment, CSF examination should be repeated to determine whether viable bacteria persist. This would apply particularly when the antibiotic used (e.g., vancomycin) enters the CSF in limited concentrations and when simultaneous use of corticosteroids may reduce its penetrance by attenuating meningeal inflammation.

Treatment of nosocomial meningitis, usually associated with neurosurgical procedures, is more prolonged than that of community-acquired meningitis, because of the associated anatomic changes (subgaleal collections, CSF fistulas) and the antimicrobial resistance patterns of the causative organisms. Gram-negative bacillary meningitis requires treatment for 3 weeks or more because of the frequent association of an infected subgaleal collection communicating with the subarachnoid space.

Management of Acute Brain Swelling and Markedly Heightened Cerebrospinal Fluid Pressure

Markedly elevated CSF pressures (at least 500 mm H_2O) are observed in about 5% of cases of acute bacterial meningitis in the absence of any complicating mass lesion. Such elevated pressure is usually the result of acute cerebral edema; complicating cerebral herniation has been reported in bacterial meningitis in children (140) and adults (10). Of 27 adults with community-acquired bacterial meningitis who died within the first week of illness, 30% had evidence of temporal lobe herniation with prominent cerebral edema (10). In the majority, clinical deterioration occurred within several hours of performance of a lumbar puncture that had shown markedly elevated CSF pressure. Herniation has occurred in occasional cases of bacterial meningitis in the absence of a proximate lumbar puncture. Although the relationship is unproved by controlled study, it would seem reasonable to exercise the following precautions in the patient whose CSF pressure is 450 to 500 mm H_2O or higher: (a) removal of only the amount of CSF in the manometer (sufficient for Gram stain, cell count, culture); (b) intravenous infusion of 20% mannitol solution (0.25–0.5 g/kg; higher doses with evidence of herniation) during 20 to 30 minutes; and (c) continued control of increased ICP, if needed, with subsequent infusions of dexamethasone (10 mg intravenously, followed by 4 mg every 6 hours) or mannitol. Direct measurement of CSF pressure by an ICP monitoring device may be helpful in the treatment of patients with bacterial meningitis who have clinical (stupor, coma) or neuroimaging signs of markedly increased ICP (141–143). ICP greater than 20 mm Hg is abnormal and should be treated to forestall herniation and brainstem injury. Treatment of ICP levels even of greater

than 15 mm Hg may be warranted to avoid greater elevations or "plateau waves," sustained elevations of ICP that may develop spontaneously or as a consequence of small increments in cerebral blood volume produced by fever, hypoxia, or intratracheal suctioning (141,144,145). The increase in ICP associated with intubation may be blocked by preceding use of succinyl choline and opioids, with possible use of adjunctive intravenous lidocaine. Subsequent transient increases associated with hyperactive airway reflexes can be lessened by intratracheal instillation of lidocaine before vigorous suctioning.

If signs suggesting marked increase in ICP or impending herniation develop, a variety of measures may be used to reduce ICP such as (a) elevation of the head of the bed 30 degrees to assist venous drainage; (b) intubation and hyperventilation to maintain the partial pressure of arterial carbon dioxide between 25 and 32 mm Hg to induce vasoconstriction and reduce cerebral blood volume; and (c) intravenous mannitol (1.0 g/kg over 10–15 minutes in an adult; 0.5–2.0 g/kg over 30 minutes in a child) (145). Reduction of the partial pressure of arterial carbon dioxide to 20 mm Hg or below should be avoided to prevent resultant cerebral ischemia. Hyperventilation becomes less effective with duration of use and may have little effect after 48 hours of use.

Initial fluid management of the patient with bacterial meningitis involves careful evaluation of the state of hydration. Hypovolemia or shock requires fluid replacement to maintain systemic blood pressure and sustain cerebral perfusion. In children with meningitis, hyponatremia has been observed and attributed to SIADH (low serum sodium level, urine concentrated inappropriately for the degree of hyponatremia or serum hypotonicity, absence of dehydration, normal renal and adrenal function) (146). Studies in the past have shown elevated plasma levels of arginine vasopressin in children with bacterial meningitis (147). The SIADH might then be expected to be associated with excessive free water retention and contribute to the development of cerebral edema. The frequency of SIADH reported in bacterial meningitis varies widely, from 4% to 88% (148,149). This led to conservative fluid administration early in the treatment of meningitis. The hyponatremia sometimes observed in patients with meningitis may be the result of a negative sodium balance (fever, vomiting) rather than representing dilutional hyponatremia due to water retention as occurs in SIADH. A randomized study of children with meningitis comparing the effect on plasma arginine vasopressin concentrations of giving maintenance fluid requirements plus replacement of any deficit with restricting fluids to two thirds of maintenance for 24 hours supports this hypothesis. Plasma arginine vasopressin concentrations were significantly lower at the end of 24 hours in the children who received maintenance plus replacement fluids than after fluid restriction (150). Further support for this concept is provided by a prospective study in India examining the effect of fluid restriction on body water and the outcome of children with acute meningitis (151). Routine fluid restriction did not improve the outcome; in fact, a decreased volume of extracellular water at 48 hours increased the possibility of an adverse outcome. Thus, rather than routine fluid restriction (e.g., 800–1,000 mL/m^2 per day) in a patient with meningitis without obvious shock or dehydration, maintenance plus replacement fluids can be administered in the initial 24 to 48 hours, but with subsequent monitoring for SIADH.

Other Aspects of Treatment

Patients with acute bacterial meningitis require constant nursing attention in an intensive care unit to prevent aspiration and hypoxia and to allow prompt recognition and treatment of seizures.

Diazepam (Valium; 5–10 mg for adults; 0.3 mg/kg for children to a maximum of 10 mg) should be administered slowly over several minutes for acute control of a seizure. Maintenance anticonvulsant therapy is continued subsequently with intravenous phenytoin until the medication can be given by mouth. Routine use of sedation should be avoided.

Surgical drainage of an associated pyogenic focus such as mastoiditis should be deferred until full recovery from meningitis. In the rare instance when a mastoid infection is hyperacute (e.g., Bezold abscess), early drainage may be necessary after 48 to 72 hours' antibiotic treatment, when the acute meningeal process will have abated somewhat.

When shock develops early in bacterial meningitis it is usually a consequence of the accompanying bacteremia (meningococcemia) rather than the meningitis itself. Management involves the standard measures used to treat septic shock (see Chapter 61).

Coagulopathies may occur in patients with meningitis, particularly with the meningococcemia-meningitis syndrome. Clinical and laboratory features of disseminated intravascular coagulation may develop in more severely ill patients. These abnormalities alone do not warrant consideration of heparin therapy unless active bleeding supervenes.

Role of Corticosteroids

Corticosteroids reduce the intense leukocyte responses, CSF outflow resistance, and development of brain edema in experimental models of pneumococcal meningitis (87). In another study of Hib meningitis in a rabbit model, adjunctive dexamethasone with ceftriaxone caused a lowering of CSF tumor necrosis factor concentrations (over the reduction with ceftriaxone alone), a significant decrease in neutrophilic pleocytosis, and a trend toward earlier improvement in CSF levels of glucose, protein, and lactate, but without any evident decrease in *in vivo* bacterial killing within the CSF (152).

In 1988, a double-blind placebo-controlled study evaluated 4 days' adjunctive dexamethasone therapy (with either cefuroxime or ceftriaxone) in 200 infants and children with bacterial meningitis (153). Only one death occurred among the 200, and that was in the placebo group. Those receiving dexamethasone became afebrile more rapidly than those receiving placebo, and they had a more rapid increase in CSF glucose and decrease in CSF lactate and protein levels after 24 hours' treatment. Those treated with dexamethasone developed moderate to severe bilateral sensorineural hearing loss less frequently (3.3% vs. 15.5%). The benefit of reduced sensorineural hearing loss was significant only in patients receiving cefuroxime and not ceftriaxone, but the former is now known to be inferior to ceftriaxone in treatment of childhood bacterial meningitis. Gastrointestinal bleeding requiring blood transfusions occurred in two patients receiving adjunctive dexamethasone.

In a subsequent randomized, placebo-controlled, double-blind trial, infants and children in Costa Rica received cefotaxime with either placebo or dexamethasone administered 15 to 20 minutes before the antibiotic (154). Those receiving adjunctive dexamethasone had a decreased incidence of neurologic sequelae, principally ataxia, but only a trend toward reduction of sensorineural hearing loss. There were no differences in mortality between those receiving cefotaxime with and without dexamethasone.

A metaanalysis of all the randomized trials to evaluate dexamethasone therapy in childhood bacterial meningitis, 11 in number and including approximately 1,100 patients, carried out between 1988 and 1996 involved mainly cases caused by *H. in-*

fluenzae (62%) (155). Mortality in this metaanalysis did not differ significantly between those receiving dexamethasone and the controls. Dexamethasone treatment (for 2 or 4 days) provided a significant benefit in reducing severe hearing loss from *H. influenzae* meningitis (3.1% vs. 11.6%). Benefit did not depend on the specific antibiotic employed (all were active against the infecting strains), and it was independent of the timing (before, at the same time, or after the first antibiotic dose) (155,156). For *S. pneumoniae* meningitis the difference was not significant statistically, although there was a trend in favor of dexamethasone (152,153). Evaluation of neurologic deficits other than hearing loss (seizures, cranial nerve palsies, ataxia, hydrocephalus, psychomotor retardation) in 757 children showed a suggestive but nonsignificant benefit in favor of the group receiving dexamethasone. The only adverse event significantly more frequent in the corticosteroid group was recurrence of fever (38.7% vs. 26.7%). While overall gastrointestinal tract bleeding was not significantly increased (2.3% vs. 0.5%), it was significantly more frequent (2.8%) with 4 days of corticosteroid treatment compared with 2 days (0.8%).

A general consensus has emerged for the use of adjunctive dexamethasone (0.15 mg/kg every 6 hours intravenously) to reduce the frequency of neurologic and audiologic complications in infants and children with Hib meningitis, particularly those patients with elevated ICP, coma, and high concentrations of bacteria in the CSF. On the basis of animal models and clinical trials, dexamethasone is best administered either 15 minutes before or simultaneously with antimicrobial therapy to lessen the inflammatory response in the CSF to bacterial lysis. Evidence indicates that a 2-day course is comparable in efficacy to one of 4 days and may reduce the possibility of complicating gastrointestinal bleeding (157). Several caveats should be borne in mind in considering the use of adjuvant corticosteroids in treatment of bacterial meningitis:

1. Clinical data as yet do not support the routine use of adjuvant dexamethasone in the treatment of community-acquired bacterial meningitis in adults, although it can be helpful in the management of cerebral edema and high CSF pressure. A small European multicenter, randomized study of adjuvant dexamethasone, reported subsequent to the previously mentioned metaanalysis, involved 60 adults with community-acquired bacterial meningitis (31 *S. pneumoniae*; 18 *N. meningitidis*) and failed to show any difference statistically in the rate of cured patients without neurologic sequelae (158). However, this study used intravenous amoxicillin as initial antimicrobial therapy and was stopped prematurely when the increasing frequency of penicillin-resistant *S. pneumoniae* mandated initial antibiotic therapy with a third-generation cephalosporin and vancomycin. An ongoing Dutch study (results anticipated soon) of dexamethasone in community-acquired meningitis in adults is expected to fill this gap (155,159).

2. Benefit from adjunctive dexamethasone, although shown for treatment of Hib meningitis in infants and children, has not been demonstrated as yet in the treatment of meningitis due to *S. pneumoniae*. However, the American Academy of Pediatrics recently recommended that adjunctive dexamethasone treatment be considered for *S. pneumoniae* meningitis (160).

3. Immunization of infants with Hib polysaccharide-protein conjugate vaccines has dramatically reduced the incidence of meningitis caused by *H. influenzae* in this age group and has given *S. pneumoniae* an ascendant position as the cause.

4. Initial favorable clinical response to ceftriaxone and adjuvant dexamethasone in meningitis caused by *S. pneumoniae* with decreased susceptibility to the third-generation

cephalosporins may be misleading in that the apparent response may be due to the antiinflammatory effects of dexamethasone rather than to the expected antibiotic effect (161). This masking effect of the corticosteroid may delay performance of another lumbar puncture (revealing continuing bacterial presence) that would have been mandated earlier by virtue of an unsatisfactory clinical response.

5. Adjunctive dexamethasone may not be beneficial, indeed may be detrimental, in the treatment of meningitis caused by highly penicillin resistant *S. pneumoniae* by decreasing meningeal inflammation, reducing vancomycin levels in CSF, and thus delaying bacterial killing (162).

6. There have been no clinical studies performed demonstrating benefits to the use of adjuvant dexamethasone in the treatment of meningitis caused by gram-negative bacilli (other than *H. influenzae*) or to other microorganisms often involved in nosocomial meningitis or meningitis in immunocompromised hosts.

Use of dexamethasone after initial infusions of mannitol to control brain swelling in patients with bacterial meningitis (caused by highly antibiotic-susceptible organisms) and markedly heightened CSF pressure is appropriate on the basis of experimental animal studies and extrapolation from its use in cerebral edema of other causes.

Management of Bacterial Meningitis Associated with a Cerebrospinal Fluid Fistula

Congenital defects along the cerebrospinal axis, particularly persistent dermal sinuses or meningoceles, may predispose to meningitis, especially in neonates or young children. In older children and adults, fistulas occur about the cribriform plate, paranasal sinuses, and temporal bone, resulting from accidental or surgical trauma or from erosion by tumor, sequestrum, or cholesteatoma (163,164).

Such a fistula should be suspected in any patient who has recurrent bacterial meningitis, a history of skull fracture or clear rhinorrhea, or a midline dermal sinus. CSF rhinorrhea commonly originates from a defect in the cribriform plate or a paranasal sinus, but it may result from a defect in the temporal bone that allows fluid to pass into the middle ear and down the eustachian tube into the nasopharynx (paradoxic rhinorrhea). CSF otorrhea occurs with a leak into the middle ear. The most common cause of CSF rhinorrhea is trauma, and rhinorrhea complicates 1% to 2% of blunt head injuries (163,164). The incidence of CSF rhinorrhea is highest (approximately 25%) when blunt trauma has produced fractures involving the paranasal sinuses.

With the onset of acute bacterial meningitis, CSF rhinorrhea may cease as a result of the increased viscosity of the purulent CSF. Thus, it is important to check all patients with pyogenic meningitis (particularly pneumococcal, especially if recurrent) for CSF rhinorrhea by history and physical examination at the onset of illness and again after recovery. A history of a salty taste and frequent swallowing (due to extra fluid entering the pharynx from above) suggests CSF rhinorrhea. Anosmia might suggest cribriform plate leakage. On examination with the head in the brow-down position, fluid from CSF rhinorrhea may flow from one or both nostrils and, unlike nasal mucus, does not stiffen a handkerchief on drying. Collection of several drops in a test tube for determination of glucose and chloride levels is the preferred method for determining whether a clear nasal secretion is CSF. CSF normally has a glucose content of 50 to 75 mg/dL and a chloride level of about 120 mEq/L. Identification by electrophoresis and immunofixation of a specific isoform of transferrin, present only in CSF, in clear nasal fluid can help define a CSF leak (165).

Rhinorrhea of an otic or sphenoid origin may be noted with the patient in the lateral decubitus or prone position, respectively. If the tympanic membrane is intact, fluid and air bubbles may be seen behind the eardrum. Visual fields should be evaluated because they are frequently abnormal when the cause of CSF rhinorrhea is a pituitary cyst or tumor. Visual fields are normal in the atrophic type of empty sella syndrome, which also can be associated with CSF leakage.

Studies to define an anatomic defect are indicated in patients with CSF rhinorrhea and bacterial meningitis, or in patients with repeated episodes of bacterial meningitis. Head CT should be performed for most accurate anatomic definition of the site of leakage (skull fracture, opacification or air-fluid levels in an air sinus or in mastoid air cells, or pneumocephalus), particularly in the case of a nontraumatic leak, when an intracranial mass lesion may be responsible. Contrast cisternography (with iopamidol or iohexal preferred to metrizamide as a contrast agent) may be confirmatory but requires an active CSF leak at the time of testing (163).

Direct confirmation of the leak exit site is essential for surgical correction. Radiolabeled (iodine 131 or technetium 99m) albumins are used to determine sites of CSF leakage; Cottonoid strips are placed into the sphenoid-ethmoid recess, in the region of the middle meatus, into the anterior superior nasal cavity, and into the ear canal to detect leakage after lumbar injection of the radionuclide. Fluorescein (0.5 mL of 10% fluorescein solution in 10 mL of physiologic diluent injected slowly during 3–5 minutes into the lumbar sac) is preferred by some physicians (164) because it can be visualized directly and promptly. Also, fluorescein stains the tympanic membrane in CSF otorrhea, and it can be used intraoperatively to allow direct visualization of the origin of the leak.

Recurrent meningitis is most commonly associated with a CSF leak (10). The organisms responsible for recurrent meningitis vary depending on whether the episodes are community acquired or nosocomial (Table 148.13). Thus, the setting provides some direction for selection of initial antimicrobial therapy.

Posttraumatic rhinorrhea or otorrhea usually subsides within several weeks of the trauma. Such acute CSF rhinorrhea is treated expectantly with head elevation at 45 degrees and, if required,

TABLE 148.13. Causative Organisms in Recurrent Meningitis in Adults at Massachusetts General Hospital, 1962–1988

Organism	Community-acquired (%) (38 episodes)	Nosocomial (%) (41 episodes)
Streptococcus pneumoniae	34	2
Gram-negative bacilli[a]	0	46
Neisseria meningitidis	8	0
Streptococci[b]	11	2
Staphylococcus aureus	3	15
Haemophilus influenzae	11	0
Mixed bacterial species	0	5
Coagulase-negative staphylococci	0	7
Other	5	2
Culture-negative	29	20

[a]Exlcusive of *H. influenzae*.
[b]Mainly α-hemolytic, nongroupable strains.
Modified with permission from Durand ML, Calderwood SB, Weber DJ, et al. Acute bacterial meningitis in adults. A review of 493 episodes. *N Engl J Med* 1993;328: 21–28, with permission.

a spinal drain; this usually eliminates the rhinorrhea within 5 to 7 days (163). Indications for surgical correction include prior leak and one or more episodes of bacterial meningitis, profuse leakage that does not abate in the 2 weeks after the trauma; and persistent leakage for longer than 6 weeks after the trauma (164). Prospective study of the value of prophylactic antibiotics (e.g., penicillin) in preventing bacterial meningitis in patients with a CSF leak has not been performed. In a retrospective study of 1,192 patients with basilar skull fractures reported in eight non-randomized series between 1970 and 1988, 8% of 803 patients receiving prophylactic antibiotics and 3% of 389 patients not receiving antibiotic prophylaxis developed meningitis (difference not statistically significant) (166). In the subset of 117 patients with basilar skull fractures who developed obvious CSF otorrhea or rhinorrhea, prophylactic antibiotics did not protect against development of meningitis. In another retrospective study of CSF fistulas (mainly traumatic) from a neurosurgical unit in England, which compared the incidence of meningitis among 106 patients treated with prophylactic antibiotics with 109 patients who were untreated, antibiotic prophylaxis did not reduce the risk for meningitis significantly (167). Prolonged use of prophylactic antibiotics increases the likelihood of involvement of a resistant organism if meningitis does develop. For example, posttraumatic meningitis caused by *S. aureus* and gram-negative bacilli has developed in patients receiving penicillin prophylaxis. At present, routine prophylactic antibiotic use is not recommended for patients with a traumatic CSF leak. However, this is a considerable problem and merits a large multiinstitutional prospective, randomized trial.

The type of surgical repair used for CSF fistulas depends on the nature of the fistula. Nontraumatic high-pressure fistulas are usually secondary to obstructive hydrocephalus resulting from posterior fossa tumors or basilar arachnoiditis. After treatment of any complicating meningitis, initial neurosurgical management involves CSF shunting or removal of obstruction to CSF flow. For nontraumatic normal-pressure leaks, large CSF leaks, or posttraumatic leaks that persist for 4 to 6 weeks, surgical repair by obliteration of the leak site is indicated. Transsinus approaches have been used successfully by skilled otolaryngologists to repair leaks through the cribriform plate and sphenoid and frontal sinuses (163,164).

PREVENTION

Meningococcal Disease

The risk of meningococcal disease for household contacts of an initial case is 500 to 800 times greater than the endemic rate for meningococcal disease in the general population. Chemoprophylaxis is indicated for close contacts (e.g., household or day care center; medical personnel in close direct contact before institution of respiratory precautions) of a patient with meningococcal disease. Rifampin, 80% to 90% effective in eliminating asymptomatic nasopharyngeal carriage, is the recommended drug for chemoprophylaxis in a dose of 600 mg orally every 12 hours for 2 days for adults (10 mg/kg every 12 hours for children over 1 month of age, and 5 mg/kg every 12 hours for children under 1 month of age). Because the carrier state may recur shortly after discontinuation of treatment with high doses of penicillin, rifampin should also be administered to patients with meningococcal disease before discharge from hospital if penicillin, rather than a third-generation cephalosporin, was used in treatment.

Single-dose oral ciprofloxacin, 500 or 750 mg in the adult, is about 90% effective in eradicating pharyngeal carriage (168,169).

Ciprofloxacin is the alternative of choice for rifampin for prophylaxis in adults and may replace it as the drug of choice if rifampin resistance should become widespread among meningococci (170). Owing to potential side effects on growing cartilage, it would not be recommended for children or pregnant women. Ceftriaxone (250 mg intramuscularly in adults and 125 mg in children) eliminated the carriage of serogroup A meningococci in more than 90% of patients for up to 2 weeks. In pregnant patients and young infants, ceftriaxone is probably the safest alternative to rifampin for prophylaxis. Recently, in a small study in adults in Egypt, single-dose (500 mg) azithromycin was found to be as effective (93%) in eradicating nasopharyngeal carriage of *N. meningitidis* as rifampin (171).

In the United States, immunoprophylaxis of meningococcal disease currently involves use of a quadrivalent (A/C/Y/W-135) polysaccharide vaccine only in the military, in college freshmen living in dormitories, in travelers to countries with hyperendemic or epidemic disease, in aborting outbreaks due to serogroups in the vaccine, in developing countries and as a complement to prophylactic chemotherapy in neighborhood or school outbreaks, and for persons at high risk such as asplenic patients or those who have terminal complement component deficiencies.

Haemophilus influenzae Disease

The risk for secondary spread of invasive Hib infection to non-immunized household contacts under 4 years of age is 2% to 6% during the 30-day period after exposure. The highest rate occurs in contacts under 1 year of age. The majority of secondary cases occur within a week of onset of disease in the index case.

Rifampin is effective in eliminating nasopharyngeal carriage of Hib. If another child (whether previously given Hib vaccine or not) under 4 years of age resides in the household, rifampin prophylaxis is recommended for all household contacts, including adults (except pregnant women), of an index case: 20 mg/kg orally once daily for 4 days (maximal daily dose 600 mg) (170,172). Because nasopharyngeal carriage may reappear after discontinuation of antimicrobial therapy for systemic infection, the index patient should receive rifampin before hospital discharge. Ceftriaxone in treatment of *H. influenzae* meningitis has eliminated nasopharyngeal carriage during treatment. Thus, it is reasonable to assume that it would be a suitable alternative to rifampin in Hib chemoprophylaxis, but this has not been established by direct study (170).

Whether contacts of patients in day care centers outside the home are at greater risk for secondary spread of infection is debatable. Risk may vary from region to region and depends on the age of the exposed children. Children under 2 years of age are at higher risk than those over 2 years of age. If two or more cases occur within 60 days in a day care center, rifampin prophylaxis should be given to all contacts, including adults (except pregnant women). Whether such prophylaxis is indicated after a single case is controversial, but it does seem warranted if any of the exposed classroom contacts is younger than 2 years. Widespread use of Hib polysaccharide-protein conjugate vaccines in infancy in the United States has sharply reduced this as a problem in the past decade.

REFERENCES

1. Centers for Disease Control and Prevention. Bacterial meningitis and meningococcemia—United States, 1978. *MMWR* 1979;28:277.
2. Schlech WF III, Ward JI, Band JD, et al. Bacterial meningitis in the United States, 1978 through 1981. *JAMA* 1985;253:1749.

3. Adams WG, Deaver KA, Cochi SL, et al. Decline of childhood *Haemophilus influenzae* type b (Hib) disease in the Hib vaccine era. *JAMA* 1993;269:221.

4. Buchanan GA, Darville T. Impact of immunization against *Haemophilus influenzae* type b (HIB) on the incidence of HIB meningitis treated at Arkansas Children's Hospital. *South Med J* 1994;87:38.

5. Swartz MN, Dodge PR. Bacterial meningitis—a review of selected aspects. *N Engl J Med* 1965;272:725.

6. Carpenter RR, Petersdorf RG. The clinical spectrum of bacterial meningitis. *Am J Med* 1962;33:262.

7. Geiseler PJ, Nelson KE, Levin S, et al. Community-acquired purulent meningitis: a review of 1,316 cases during the antibiotic era, 1954–1976. *Rev Infect Dis* 1980;2:726.

8. Schuchat A, Robinson K, Wenger JD, et al. Bacterial meningitis in the United States in 1995. *N Engl J Med* 1997;337:970.

9. Cherubin CE, Marr JS, Sierra MF, et al. *Listeria* and gram-negative bacillary meningitis in New York City, 1972–1979. *Am J Med* 1981;71:199.

10. Durand MI, Calderwood SB, Weber DJ, et al. Acute bacterial meningitis in adults: a review of 493 episodes. *N Engl J Med* 1993;328:21.

11. Crane LIZ, Lerner AM. Nontraumatic gram-negative bacillary meningitis in the Detroit Medical Center, 1964–1974. *Medicine (Baltimore)* 1978;57:197.

12. Buckwold FJ, Hand R, Hansebout RR. Hospital-acquired bacterial meningitis in neurosurgical patients. *J Neurosurg* 1977;46:494.

13. Mancebo J, Domingo P, Blanch L, et al. Postneurosurgical and spontaneous gram-negative bacillary meningitis in adults. *Scand J Infect Dis* 1986;18:533.

14. Gower DJ, Barrows AA III, Kelly DL Jr, et al. Gram-negative bacillary meningitis in the adult: review of 39 cases. *South Med J* 1986;79:1499.

15. Berk SL, McCabe WR. Meningitis caused by gram-negative bacilli. *Ann Intern Med* 1980;93:253.

16. Harder E, Møller K, Skinhoj P. Enterobacteriaceae meningitis in adults: a review of 20 consecutive cases 1977–97. *Scand J Infect Dis* 1999;31:287.

17. Schlesinger LS, Ross SC, Schaberg DR. *Staphylococcus aureus* meningitis: a broad-based epidemiologic study. *Medicine (Baltimore)* 1987;66:148.

18. Swartz MN. Central nervous system infections. In: Finegold SM, George WL, eds. *Anaerobic infections in humans.* San Diego: Academic, 1989:155–212.

19. Tärnvik A. Anaerobic meningitis in children. *Eur J Clin Microbiol* 1986;5:271.

20. Long JG, Preblud SR, Keyserling HL. *Clostridium perfringens* meningitis in an infant: case report and literature review. *Pediatr Infect Dis J* 1987;6:752.

21. Downs NJ, Hodges GR, Taylor SA. Mixed bacterial meningitis. *Rev Infect Dis* 1987;9:693.

22. Bouza E Garcia de la Torre M, Parras F, et al. *Brucella* meningitis. *Rev Infect Dis* 1987;9:810.

23. Lovell VM, Cho CT, Lindsey NJ, et al. *Francisella tularensis* meningitis: a rare clinical entity. *J Infect Dis* 1986;154:916.

24. Arends JP, Zanen HC. Meningitis caused by *Streptococcus suis* in humans. *Rev Infect Dis* 1988;10:131.

25. Feigin RD, Baker CJ, Herwaldt LA, et al. Epidemic meningococcal disease in an elementary school classroom. *N Engl J Med* 1982;307:1255.

26. Merino J, Rodriques-Valverde V, Lamelas JA, et al. Prevalence of deficits of complement components in patients with recurrent meningococcal infections. *J Infect Dis* 1983;148:331.

27. Ellison RT, Kohler PH, Curd JG, et al. Prevalence of congenital or acquired complement deficiency in patients with sporadic meningococcal disease. *N Engl J Med* 1983;308:913.

28. Griffis JM, Brandt BL. Nonepidemic (endemic) meningococcal disease: pathogenic factors and clinical features. *Curr Clin Top Infect Dis* 1986;7:27.

29. Meningitis Disease Surveillance Group. Household chemoprophylaxis for meningococcal disease: observations on the meningococcal secondary attack rate and the practice of chemoprophylaxis in the United States. *JAMA* 1976;235:261.

30. DeWSals P, Hertoghe L, Borlée-Grimée, et al. Meningococcal disease in Belgium. Secondary attack rate among household, day-care nursery and preelementary school contacts. *J Infect* 1981;3(suppl 1):53.

31. Wenger JD, Ward JI, Broome CV. Prevention of *Haemophilus influenzae* type b disease: vaccines and passive prophylaxis. *Curr Clin Top Infect Dis* 1989;10:306.

32. Ward JI, Fraser DW, Baraff LJ, et al. *Haemophilus influenzae* meningitis. A national study of secondary spread in household contacts. *N Engl J Med* 1979;301:122.

33. Spagnuolo PJ, Ellner JJ, Lerner PI, et al. *Haemophilus influenzae* meningitis: the spectrum of disease in adults. *Medicine (Baltimore)* 1982;61:74.

34. Quagliariello V, Scheld WM. Bacterial meningitis: pathogenesis, pathophysiology and progress. *N Engl J Med* 1992;327:864.

35. Stephens DS, Farley MM. Pathogenic events during infection of the human nasopharynx with *Neisseria meningitidis* and *Haemophilus influenzae*. *Rev Infect Dis* 1991;13:22.

36. Smith AL, Daum RS, Scheifele D, et al. Pathogenesis of *Haemophilus influenzae* meningitis. In: Sell SH, Wright PF, eds. *Haemophilus influenzae*: epidemiology, immunology and prevention of disease. New York: Elsevier, 1982:89–109.

37. Simberkoff M, Moldover H, Rahal J Jr. Absence of detectable bactericidal and opsonic activities in normal and infected cerebrospinal fluids: a regional host defense deficiency. *J Lab Clin Med* 1980;95:362.

38. Fijen CA, Kuijper EJ, Tjia HG, et al. Complement deficiency predisposes for meningitis due to nongroupable meningococci and *Neisseria*-related bacteria. *Clin Infect Dis* 1994;18:780.

39. Bohr V, Hansen B, Jessen O, et al. Eight hundred and seventy-five cases of bacterial meningitis. Part I of a three-part series: clinical data, prognosis, and the role of specialized hospital departments. *J Infect* 1983;7:21.

40. Sferra TJ, Pacini DL. Simultaneous recovery of bacterial and viral pathogens from cerebrospinal fluid. *Pediatr Infect Dis J* 1988;7:552.

41. Tuomanen E, Hengstler B, Rich R, et al. Nonsteroidal antiinflammatory agents in the therapy for experimental pneumococcal meningitis. *J Infect Dis* 1987;155:985.

42. Quagliariello VJ, Long WJ, Scheld M. Morphologic alterations of the blood-brain barrier with experimental meningitis in the rat. *J Clin Invest* 1986;77:1084.

43. Lesse AJ, Moxon ER, Zwahlen A, et al. Role of cerebrospinal fluid pleocytosis and *Haemophilus influenzae* type b capsule on blood brain barrier permeability during experimental meningitis in the rat. *J Clin Invest* 1988;82:102.

44. Tuomanen E. Partner drugs: A new outlook for bacterial meningitis. *Ann Intern Med* 1988;109:690.

45. Scheld WM, Dacey R, Winn R, et al. Cerebrospinal fluid outflow resistance in rabbits with experimental meningitis. Alterations with penicillin and methylprednisolone. *J Clin Invest* 1980;66:243.

46. Posner JB, Plum F. Spinal fluid pH and neurologic symptoms in systemic acidosis. *N Engl J Med* 1967;277:605.

47. Kaplan SL, Feigin RD. The syndrome of inappropriate secretion of antidiuretic hormone in children with bacterial meningitis. *J Pediatr* 1978;92:758.

48. Kline MW. *Citrobacter* meningitis and brain abscess in infancy: epidemiology, pathogenesis, and treatment. *J Pediatr* 1988;113:430.

49. Rosen MS, Lorber B, Myers AR. Chronic meningococcal meningitis. An association with C5 deficiency. *Arch Intern Med* 1988;148:1441.

50. Dodge PR, Davis H, Feigin RD, et al. Prospective evaluation of hearing impairment as a sequela of acute bacterial meningitis. *N Engl J Med* 1984;311:869.

51. Vienny H, Despland PA, Liitschz J, et al. Early diagnosis and evolution of deafness in childhood bacterial meningitis: a study using brainstem auditory evoked potentials. *Pediatrics* 1984;73:579.

52. Ozdamar O, Kraus N, Stein L. Auditory brainstem responses in infants recovering from bacterial meningitis: audiologic evaluation. *Arch Otolaryngol* 1983;109:13.

53. Bhatt SM, Halpin C, Hsu W, et al. Hearing loss and pneumococcal meningitis: an animal model. *Laryngoscope* 1991;101:1285.

54. Bhatt SM, Lauretano A, Cabellos C, et al. Progression of hearing loss in experimental pneumococcic meningitis: correlation with cerebrospinal fluid cytochemistry. *J Infect Dis* 1993;167:675.

55. Eavey RD, Gao YZ, Schuknecht HF, et al. Otologic features of bacterial meningitis of childhood. *J Pediatr* 1985;106:402.

56. Dichgans M, Jäger L, Mayer MD, et al. Bacterial meningitis in adults: demonstration of inner ear involvement using high-resolution MRI. *Neurology* 1999;52:1003.

57. Bohr VA, Rasmussen N. Neurologic sequelae and fatality as prognostic measures in 875 cases of bacterial meningitis. *Dan Med Bull* 1988;35:92.

58. Pfister H-W, Borasio GD, Dirnagl U, et al. Cerebrovascular complications of bacterial meningitis in adults. *Neurology* 1992;42:1497.

59. McMenamin JB, Volpe JJ. Bacterial meningitis in infancy: effects on intracranial pressure and cerebral blood flow velocity. *Neurology* 1984;34:500.

60. Möller K, Larsen FS, Qvist J, et al. Dependency of cerebral blood flow on mean arterial pressure in patients with acute bacterial meningitis. *Crit Care Med* 2000;28:1027.

61. Bartt R. *Listeria* and atypical presentations of *Listeria* in the central nervous system. *Semin Neurol* 2000;20:361.

62. DiNubile MJ, Boom WH, Southwick FS. Septic cortical thrombophlebitis. *J Infect Dis* 1990;161:1216.

63. Adams RD, Kubik CS, Bonner FJ. The clinical and pathological aspects of influenzae meningitis. *Arch Neurol* 1984;65:354, 408.

64. Pomeroy SL, Holmes SJ, Dodge PR, et al. Seizures and other neurological sequelae of bacterial meningitis in children. *N Engl J Med* 1990;323:1651.

65. Feldman HM, Michaels RH. Academic achievement in children 10 to 12 years after *Haemophilus influenzae* meningitis. *Pediatrics* 1988;81:339.

66. Edwards MS, Reuch MA, Haffar AAM, et al. Long-term sequelae of group B streptococcal meningitis in infants. *J Pediatr* 1985;106:717.

67. Wilson CW, Smith AL. Rapid tests for the diagnosis of bacterial meningitis. *Curr Clin Top Infect Dis* 1986;7:134.

68. Polk BP, Steele RW. Bacterial meningitis presenting with normal cerebrospinal fluid. *Pediatr Infect Dis J* 1987;6:1040.

69. Maxson S, Lewno MJ, Schutze GE. Clinical usefulness of cerebrospinal fluid bacterial antigen studies. *J Pediatr* 1994;125:235.

70. Komorowski RA, Farmer SG, Knox KK. Comparison of cerebrospinal fluid C-reactive protein and lactate for diagnosis of meningitis. *J Clin Microbiol* 1986;24:982.

71. Abramson JS, Hampton KD, Babu S. The use of C-reactive protein from cerebrospinal fluid for differentiating meningitis from other central nervous system diseases. *J Infect Dis* 1985;151:854.

72. Nathan BR, Scheld WM. The potential role of C-reactive protein and procalcitonin concentrations in the serum and cerebrospinal fluid in the diagnosis of bacterial meningitis. *Curr Clin Top Infect Dis* 2002;22:125.

73. Saubolle MA, Jorgenson JH. Use of the Limulus amebocyte lysate test as a cost-effective screen for gram-negative agents of meningitis. *Diagn Microbiol Infect Dis* 1987;7:177.

74. Baty V, Viel JF, Schuhmacher H, et al. Prospective validation of a diagnosis model as an aid to therapeutic decision making in acute meningitis. *Eur J Clin Microbiol Infect Dis* 2000;19:422.

75. Bohr V, Rasmussen N, Hansen B, et al. Eight hundred seventy-five cases of bacterial meningitis: diagnostic procedures and the impact of preadmission antibiotic therapy. *J Infect* 1983;7:193.

76. Valmari P. White blood count, erythrocyte sedimentation rate and serum C-reactive protein in meningitis: magnitude of the response related to bacterial species. *Infection* 1984;12:328.

77. Hasbrun R, Abrahams J, Jekel J, et al. Computed tomography of the head before lumbar puncture in adults with suspected meningitis. *N Engl J Med* 2001;345:1727.

78. Cabral DA, Flodmark O, Farrell K, et al. Prospective study of computed tomography in acute bacterial meningitis. *J Pediatr* 1987;111:201.

79. Bodino J, Lylyk P, Del Volle M, et al. Computed tomography in purulent meningitis. *Am J Dis Child* 1982;136:495.

80. Kline MK, Kaplan SL. Computed tomography in bacterial meningitis of childhood. *Pediatr Infect Dis J* 1988;7:855.

81. Ho DD, Sarngadharan MG, Resnick L, et al. Primary human T-lymphotropic virus type III infection. *Ann Intern Med* 1985;103:880.

82. Spanos A, Harrell FE, Durack DT. Differential diagnosis of acute meningitis. An analysis of the predictive value of initial observations. *JAMA* 1989;262:2700.

83. Peacock JE Jr, McGinnis MR, Cohen MS. Persistent neutrophilic meningitis: report of four cases and review of the literature. *Medicine (Baltimore)* 1984;63:379.

84. Yamamoto LY, Tedder DG, Ashley R, et al. Herpes simplex virus type 1 DNA in cerebrospinal fluid of a patient with Mollaret's meningitis. *N Engl J Med* 1991;325:1082.

85. Crossly GH, Dismukes WE. Central nervous system epidermoid cyst: a probable etiology of Mollaret's meningitis. *Am J Med* 1990;89:805.

86. Meadow WL, Lantos J, Tanz RR, et al. Ought "standard care" be the "standard of care"? A study of the time to administration of antibiotics in children with meningitis. *Am J Dis Child* 1993;147:40.

87. Scheld WM, Sande MA. Bactericidal versus bacteriostatic antibiotic therapy of experimental pneumococcal meningitis in rabbits. *J Clin Invest* 1983;71:411.

88. Tunkel AR, Wispelwey B, Scheld WM. Bacterial meningitis: recent advances in pathophysiology and treatment. *Ann Intern Med* 1990;112:610.

89. Lepper MH, Dowling HF. Treatment of pneumococcic meningitis with penicillin compared with penicillin plus aureomycin. *Arch Intern Med* 1951;88:489.

90. Friedland IR, McCracken GH Jr. Management of infections caused by antibiotic-resistant *Streptococcus pneumoniae*. *N Engl J Med* 1994;331:337.

91. Tomasz A. Multiple-antibiotic resistant pathogenic bacteria—a report on the Rockefeller University workshop. *N Engl J Med* 1994;330:1247.

92. Appelbaum PC. Antimicrobial resistance in *Streptococcus pneumoniae*: an overview. *Clin Infect Dis* 1992;15:77.

93. Spika JS, Facklam RR, Plikaytis BD, et al. Antimicrobial resistance of *Streptococcus pneumoniae* in the United States, 1979–1987. *J Infect Dis* 1991;163:1273.

94. Hofman J, Cetron MS, Farley MM, et al. The prevalence of drug-resistant *Streptococcus pneumoniae* in Atlanta. *N Engl J Med* 1995;333:481.

95. Pallares R, Liñares J, Vadillo M, et al. Resistance to penicillin and cephalosporin and mortality from severe pneumococcal pneumonia in Barcelona Spain. *N Engl J Med* 1995;333:474.

96. McDougal LK, Facklam R, Reeves M, et al. Analysis of multiply antimicrobial-resistant isolates of *Streptococcus pneumoniae* from the United States. *Antimicrob Agents Chemother* 1992;36:2176.

97. Tomasz A. The pneumococcus at the gates. *N Engl J Med* 1995;333:514.

98. Viladrich PF, Gudiol F, Liñares J, et al. Characteristics and antibiotic therapy of adult meningitis due to penicillin-resistant pneumococci. *Am J Med* 1988;84:839.

99. Friedland IR, Istre GR. Management of penicillin-resistant pneumococcal infections. *Pediatr Infect Dis J* 1992;11:433.

100. Fiore AE, Moroney JF, Farley MM, et al. Clinical outcomes of meningitis caused by *Streptococcus pneumoniae* in the era of antibiotic resistance. *Clin Infect Dis* 2000;30:71.

101. Friedland IR, Shelton S, Paris M, et al. Dilemmas in diagnosis and management of cephalosporin-resistant *Streptococcus pneumoniae* meningitis. *Pediatr Infect Dis J* 1993;72:196.

102. Tan TQ, Schutze GE, Mason EO Jr, et al. Antibiotic therapy and acute outcome of meningitis due to *Streptococcus pneumoniae* considered intermediately susceptible to broad-spectrum cephalosporins. *Antimicrob Agents Chemother* 1994;38:918.

103. American Academy of Pediatrics. Therapy for children for invasive pneumococcal infections. *Pediatrics* 1997;99:289.

104. Quagliarello VJ, Scheld WM. Treatment of bacterial meningitis. *N Engl J Med* 1997;336:708.

105. Ahmed A, Jafri H, Lutsar I, et al. Pharmacodynamics for vancomycin for the treatment of experimental penicillin- and cephalosporin-resistant pneumococcal meningitis. *Antimicrob Agents Chemother* 1999;43:876.

106. Viladrich PF, Gudiol F, Liñares J, et al. Evaluation of vancomycin for therapy of adult pneumococcal meningitis. *Antimicrob Agents Chemother* 1991;35:2467.

107. Gump DW. Vancomycin for treatment of bacterial meningitis. *Rev Infect Dis* 1981;3(suppl):289.

108. Friedland IR, Klugman KP. Failure of chloramphenicol therapy in penicillin-resistant pneumococcal meningitis. *Lancet* 1992;339:405.

109. Arreaza L, de la Fuente L, Vásquez JA. Antibiotic susceptibility patterns of *Neisseria meningitidis* isolates from patients and asymptomatic carriers. *Antimicrob Agents Chemother* 2000;44:1705.

110. Rosenstein NE, Stocker SAA, Popovic T, et al. Antimicrobial resistance of *Neisseria meningitidis* in the United States. *Clin Infect Dis* 2000;30:212.

111. Zhang Q-Y, Jones DM, Saez Nieto JA, et al. Genetic diversity of penicillin-binding protein 2 genes of penicillin-resistant strains of *Neisseria meningitidis* revealed by fingerprinting of amplified DNA. *Antimicrob Agents Chemother* 1990;34:1523.

112. Latorre C, Gené A, Juncosa T, et al. *Neisseria meningitidis*: evolution of penicillin resistance and phenotype in a children's hospital in Barcelona, Spain. *Acta Paediatr* 2000;89:661.

113. Jorgensen JH. Update on mechanisms and prevalence of antimicrobial resistance in *Haemophilus influenzae*. *Clin Infect Dis* 1992;14:1119.

114. The choice of antibacterial drugs. *Med Lett* 2001;43(1111–1112):70.

115. Ahmed A. A critical evaluation of vancomycin for treatment of bacterial meningitis. *Pediatr Infect Dis J* 1997;16:895.

116. Levitz RE, Quintiliani R. Trimethoprim-sulfamethoxazole for bacterial meningitis. *Ann Intern Med* 1984;100:881.

117. Bula CJ, Bille J, Glauser MP. An epidemic of food-borne listeriosis in western Switzerland: description of 57 cases involving adults. *Clin Infect Dis* 1995;20:66.

118. Fong IW, Tomkins KB. Review of *Pseudomonas aeruginosa* meningitis with special emphasis on treatment with ceftazidime. *Rev Infect Dis* 1985;7:604.

119. Gerber CM, Cottagnoud M, Neftel K, et al. Evaluation of cefepime alone and in combination with vancomycin against penicillin-resistant pneumococci in the rabbit meningitis model and *in vitro*. *J Antimicrob Chemother* 2000;45:63.

120. Odio CM, Ping JR, Feris JM, et al. Prospective, randomized, investigator-blinded study of the efficacy and safety of meropenem vs. cefotaxime therapy in bacterial meningitis in children. *Pediatr Infect Dis J* 1999;18:581.

121. Kilpatrick M, Girgis N, Farid Z, et al. Aztreonam for treating meningitis caused by gram-negative rods. *Scand J Infect Dis* 1991;23:125.

122. Tunkel AR, Scheld WM. Treatment of bacterial meningitis. In: Wolfson JS, Hooper DC, eds. *Quinolone antimicrobial agents*. Washington, DC: American Society for Microbiology, 1993:481–495.

123. Lipman J, Allworth A, Wallis SC. Cerebrospinal fluid penetration of high doseas of intravenous ciprofloxacin in meningitis. *Clin Infect Dis* 2000;31:1131.

124. Østergaard C, Sørensen TK, Knudsen JD, et al. Evaluation of moxifloxacin, a new 8-methoxyquinolone, for treatment of meningitis caused by a penicillin-resistant pneumococcus in rabbits. *Antimicrob Agents Chemother* 1998;42:1706.

125. Lutsar I, Friedland IR, Wubbel L, et al. Pharmacodynamics of gatifloxacin in cerebrospinal fluid in experimental cephalosporin-resistant pneumococcal meningitis. *Antimicrob Agents Chemother* 1998;42:2650.

126. Gerber CM, Tovar L, Cottagnoud M, et al. Grepafloxacin against penicillin-resistant pneumococci in the rabbit meningitis model. *J Antimicrob Chemother* 2000;46:249.

127. Nguyen MH, Muder RR. Meningitis due to *Xanthomonas maltophilia*: case report and review. *Clin Infect Dis* 1994;19:325.

128. Wolff MA, Young CL, Ramphal R. Antibiotic therapy for *Enterobacter* meningitis: a retrospective review of 13 episodes and review of the literature. *Clin Infect Dis* 1993;16:772.

129. Siegman-Igra Y, Bar-Yosef S, Avram J. Nosocomial *Acinetobacter* meningitis secondary to invasive procedures: report of 25 cases and review. *Clin Infect Dis* 1993;17:843.

130. Gardner P, Leipzig T, Sadigh M. Infections of mechanical cerebrospinal fluid shunts. *Curr Clin Top Infect Dis* 1988;9:185.

131. Zeana C, Kubin CJ, Della-Latta P, et al. Vancomycin-resistant *Enterococcus faecium* meningitis successfully managed with linezolid: case report and review of the literature. *Clin Infect Dis* 2001;33:477.

132. Kaufman BA, McLone DG. Infections of cerebrospinal fluid shunts. In: Scheld WM, Whitley RJ, Durack DT, eds. *Infections of the central nervous system*. New York: Raven, 1991:561–585.

133. McLaurin RL. Infected cerebrospinal fluid shunts. *Surg Neurol* 1973;1:191.

134. Wald SL, McLaurin RL. Cerebrospinal fluid antibiotic levels during treatment of shunt infections. *J Neurosurg* 1980;52:41.

135. Paul AK, Smego RA, Fisher MA. Intraventricular vancomycin: observations of tolerance and pharmacokinetics in two infants with ventricular shunt infections. *Pediatr Infect Dis J* 1986;5:93.

136. Reesor C, Chow AW, Kureishi A, et al. Kinetics of intraventricular vancomycin in infections of cerebrospinal fluid shunts. *J Infect Dis* 1988;158:1142.

137. Lin TY, Chrane DF, Nelson JD, et al. Seven days of ceftriaxone therapy is as effective as ten days' treatment for bacterial meningitis. *JAMA* 1985;253:3559.

138. Roine I, Ledermann W, Foncea LM, et al. Randomized trial of four vs seven days of ceftriaxone treatment for bacterial meningitis in children with rapid initial recovery. *Pediatr Infect Dis J* 2000;19:219.

139. Durack DT, Spanos A. End-of-treatment spinal tap in bacterial meningitis. Is it worthwhile? *JAMA* 1982;248:75.

140. Horwitz SJ, Boxerbaum B, O'Bell J. Cerebral herniation in bacterial meningitis in childhood. *Ann Neurol* 1980;7:524.

141. Dacey RG. Monitoring and treating increased intracranial pressure. *Pediatr Infect Dis J* 1987;6:1161.

142. Lyons MK, Meyer FB. Cerebrospinal fluid physiology and the management of increased intracranial pressure. *Mayo Clin Proc* 1990;65:684.

143. Ashwal S, Perkin RM, Thompson JR, et al. Bacterial meningitis in children: current concepts of neurologic management. *Curr Probl Pediatr* 1994;24:267.

144. Roos KL, Scheld WM. The management of fulminant meningitis in the intensive care unit. *Crit Care Clin* 1988;4:375.

145. Roos L, Tunkel AR, Scheld WM. Acute bacterial meningitis in children and adults. In: Scheld WM, Whitley RJ, Durack DT, eds. *Infections of the central nervous system.* New York: Raven, 1991:335–409.

146. Brown LB, Feigin RD. Bacterial meningitis: fluid balance and therapy. *Pediatr Ann* 1994;23:93.

147. Kaplan SL, Feigin RD. The syndrome of inappropriate secretion of antidiuretic hormone in children with bacterial meningitis. *J Pediatr* 1978;92:758.

148. Feigin RD, Kaplan SL. Inappropriate secretion of antidiuretic hormone in children with bacterial meningitis. *Am J Clin Nutr* 1977;30:1482.

149. Prince AS, Neu HC. Fluid management of *Haemophilus influenzae* meningitis. *Infection* 1980;8:5.

150. Powell KR, Sugarman LI, Eskenazi AE, et al. Normalization of plasma arginine vasopressin concentrations when children with meningitis are given maintenance plus replacement fluid therapy. *J Pediatr* 1990;117:515.

151. Singhi SC, Singhi PD, Srinivas B, et al. Fluid restriction does not improve the outcome of acute meningitis. *Pediatr Infect Dis J* 1995;14:495.

152. Mustafa MM, Ramilo O, Mertsola J, et al. Modulation of inflammation and cachectin activity in relation to treatment of experimental *Haemophilus influenzae* type b meningitis. *J Infect Dis* 1989;160:818.

153. Lebel MH, Frey BJ, Syrogiannopoulos GA, et al. Dexamethasone therapy for bacterial meningitis. Results of two double-blind, placebo-controlled trials. *N Engl J Med* 1988;319:964.

154. Odie CM, Faingezicht I, Paris M, et al. The beneficial effects of early dexamethasone administration in infants and children with bacterial meningitis. *N Engl J Med* 1991;324:1525.

155. McIntyre PB, Berkey CS, King SM, et al. Dexamethasone as adjunctive therapy in bacterial meningitis: a meta-analysis of randomized clinical trials since 1988. *JAMA* 1997;278:925.

156. Coyle PK. Glucocorticoids in central nervous system bacterial infection. *Arch Neurol* 1999;56:796.

157. Syrogiannopoulos GA, Lourida AN, Theodoridou MC, et al. Dexamethasone therapy for bacterial meningitis in children: 2- versus 4-day regimen. *J Infect Dis* 1994;169:853.

158. Thomas R, Le Tulso Y, Bouget J, et al. Trial of dexamethasone treatment for severe bacterial meningitis in adults. *Intensive Care Med* 1999;25:475.

159. Enting R. Dexamethasone in bacterial meningitis: we need the answer. *Lancet* 1997;349:1179.

160. American Academy of Pediatrics Committee on Infectious Diseases. Therapy for children with invasive pneumococcal infections. *Pediatrics* 1997;99:289.

161. Paris MM, Hickey SM, Uscher MI, et al. Effect of dexamethasone on therapy of experimental penicillin- and cephalosporin-resistant pneumococcal meningitis. *Antimicrob Agents Chemother* 1994;38:1320.

162. Bradley JS. Dexamethasone therapy in meningitis: potentially misleading antiinflammatory effects in central nervous system infections. *Pediatr Infect Dis J* 1994;13:823.

163. Pappas DG, Hammerschlag PE, Hammerschlag M. Cerebrospinal fluid rhinorrhea and recurrent meningitis. *Clin Infect Dis* 1993;17:364.

164. Hyslop NE Jr, Montgomery WM. Diagnosis and management of meningitis associated with cerebrospinal fluid leaks. *Curr Clin Top Infect Dis* 1982;3:254.

165. Rouah E, Rogers BB, Buffone GJ. Transferrin analysis by immunofixation as an aid in the diagnosis of cerebrospinal fluid otorrhea. *Arch Pathol Lab Med* 1987;111:756.

166. Rathore MH. Do prophylactic antibiotics prevent meningitis after basilar skull fracture? *Pediatr Infect Dis J* 1991;10:87.

167. Eljamel MS. Antibiotic prophylaxis in unrepaired CSF fistulae. *Br J Neurosurg* 1993;7:501.

168. Dworzak DL, Sanders CC, Horowitz EA, et al. Evaluation of single-dose ciprofloxacin in the eradication of *Neisseria meningitidis* from nasopharyngeal carriers. *Antimicrob Agents Chemother* 1988;32:1740.

169. Gaunt PN, Lambert BE. Single-dose ciprofloxacin for the eradication of pharyngeal carriage of *Neisseria meningitidis*. *J Antimicrob Chemother* 1988;21:489.

170. Peltola H. Prophylaxis of bacterial meningitis. *Infect Dis Clin North Am* 1999;13:685.

171. Girgis N, Sultan Y, Frenck RW, et al. Azithromycin compared with rifampin for eradication of nasopharyngeal colonization by *Neisseria meningitidis*. *Pediatr Infect Dis J* 1998;17:816.

172. Lieberman JM, Greenberg DP, Ward JI. Prevention of bacterial meningitis. Vaccines and chemoprophylaxis. *Infect Dis Clin North Am* 1990;4:703.

CHAPTER 149
Acute Viral Meningitis and Encephalitis

Stephen G. Baum and Brian Koll

Acute viral meningitis is a subset of the group of central nervous system (CNS) infections known as aseptic meningitis. This latter term antedates the science of virology and signifies syndromes that involve infection of the subarachnoid space and meninges in which no etiologic bacterial pathogen can be isolated or otherwise identified.

If a specific virus can be isolated or identified by molecular biologic techniques from the cerebrospinal fluid (CSF) of a patient with aseptic meningitis syndrome, the physician is entirely justified in diagnosing viral meningitis. Unfortunately, owing to the pathophysiology of many viral infections, the relative inaccessibility and expense of viral isolation procedures, and a lack of interest in pursuing etiologic diagnoses in non–life-threatening illnesses, diagnosis often rests primarily on clinical grounds, substantiated, in retrospect, by serologic responses.

The term *encephalitis* defines a condition in which there is inflammation in brain tissue, as opposed to *meningitis*, which involves only the covering of the brain. The sine qua non for the diagnosis of encephalitis is an altered state of consciousness. Although there are noninfectious causes of encephalitis that include allergic reactions and toxins, by far the most common cause is viral infection. A number of viruses are capable of infecting the brain as part of a multiorgan disease such as measles and mumps. These viruses often cause meningoencephalitis, and grouping for discussion under either site of CNS infection versus the other may be helpful, but is artificial. Other viruses, primarily the arboviruses, selectively target the brain and neural tissue during infection. This probably is due to receptor specificity, because initial infection may be at some distance from the CNS. Appropriate chapters of this book should be consulted for complete descriptions of each virus and the diseases it causes.

Owing to advances in molecular biologic techniques such as the polymerase chain reaction (PCR), and the use of monoclonal antibodies and enzyme-linked immunosorbent assays, we are about to enter an exciting era in the rapid and accurate diagnosis of viral infections of the CNS.

MENINGITIS

Epidemiology

Many viruses can cause acute meningitis, and the epidemiology of specific syndromes differs with the etiologic agent (Table 149.1). The principal viruses identified with acute meningitis include the enteroviruses (coxsackievirus, echovirus, and poliovirus), the herpesviruses [herpes simplex virus types 1 and 2 (HSV-1 and HSV-2) and varicella-zoster virus], the flaviviruses (which cause St. Louis encephalitis), paramyxoviruses (which cause mumps), bunyaviruses (California group, La Crosse), morbillivirus (which causes measles), arenaviruses (which cause lymphocytic choriomeningitis), and adenoviruses. Less common causative viruses include other herpesviruses (e.g., Epstein-Barr virus and cytomegalovirus) and hepatitis B virus.

Enteroviruses, of which there are more than 70 serotypes (1,2), cause more than one half of the cases of acute meningitis in which

TABLE 149.1. Epidemiology of Acute Viral Meningitis

Season	Patient's age (yr)	Patient's sex	Risk factor	Suggested viral agent
		Epidemiologic factors[a]		
Summer–fall	Infant	—	Infected mother	Coxsackievirus B
	1–15	—	Swimming pools, closed communities	Enteroviruses
			Geographic area: California, southeastern United States	California serogroup virus
Winter	1–15	—	School exposure	Varicella virus, measles virus
		Male/female 3:1		Mumps virus
	16–21	—	College exposure	Measles virus
		Male/female 3:1		Mumps virus
		—		Epstein-Barr virus (mononucleosis)
	Any	—	Mice, rats, hamsters	Lymphocytic choriomeningitis virus
	Adults	—	Varicella-zoster	Varicella-zoster virus
Any	Any	—	Immunocompromise	Adenovirus
		—	Acquired immunodeficiency syndrome	Human immunodeficiency virus

[a]Epidemiologic factors are suggestive but should not be used to exclude diagnoses in individual cases.

a specific viral agent is identified (3), and probably an even greater proportion of unproven cases. As would be expected from the viruses involved, which most often cause infectious diseases in childhood, the majority of cases of acute viral meningitis occur in infants, young children, and adolescents; however, no age group is spared. In infants, eight of the serotypes (five echoviruses and three type B coxsackieviruses) cause about 80% of the cases (4). In neonates over 7 days of age, the enteroviruses would appear to be the most common cause of meningitis, accounting for one third of cases (5). The mode of spread depends on the agent involved. Enteroviruses are transmitted both by fecal-oral and respiratory routes from person to person; lymphocytic choriomeningitis is transmitted to humans through direct contact with rodents; adenovirus can be spread by the respiratory route or can cause meningitis in immunocompromised persons by reactivation of latent infection. The enteroviruses cause infection during the summer and fall in temperate climates, whereas mumps, measles, and varicella-zoster meningitides peak in the winter and spring months.

Pathogenesis

Involvement of the meninges in the course of viral infection, whether caused by enteroviruses or by one of the other virus groups, is probably secondary to hematogenous dissemination from the primary focus of infection. This has been demonstrated in the case of poliovirus (6), and is suggested by the fact that infection with genital HSV-2 rather than oronasal HSV-1 is more often associated with meningitis (7). Viremic spread remains hypothetic in other diseases because of a lack of totally applicable animal models and the fact that in humans the viruses that cause meningitis are rarely isolated from the bloodstream. The factors that predispose to meningitis as a complication of common viral infections are unclear. In poliomyelitis, involvement of particular segments of the spinal cord appears to relate to limbs that were exercised during the viremic phase of the illness (8). An analysis of meningitis cases in seven outbreaks of enteroviral illness among high school students showed a statistically relevant increased attack rate of meningitis among football players (9). These findings suggest that increased blood flow or minor trauma might predispose to meningitis. Because most viral meningitides have low mortality rates when not complicated by encephalitis, the pathologic changes and the nature of the inflammatory response can be surmised only from the cell

content of the CSF. Here, lymphocytes predominate after a 24- to 48-hour polymorphonuclear response. The CSF lymphocytes have been identified as T cells (10), and one study has shown that suppressor T cells bearing the OKT8 marker predominate (11). This study found that cell-free CSF from patients with aseptic meningitis could inhibit B-cell generation *in vitro*.

Lymphocytes of the B-cell line are probably also involved in the CNS immune response, because virus-specific antibody has been detected in the CSF of patients with viral meningitis in excess of the concentration seen in serum (12,13). There is controversy surrounding this point, there being some indication that in acute viral meningitis all virus-specific antibody in the CSF derives from loss of the integrity of the blood-brain barrier and leakage of serum (14). In fatal cases of enteroviral meningitis in infants or in cases in which encephalitis does supervene, the leptomeninges show inflammation, with involvement of the pons, cerebrum, and cerebellum manifested by increased number of microglial cells and perivascular cuffing (15). Both white matter and gray matter show marked cellular destruction. In these cases of encephalitis compounding meningitis, it is the former involvement that most probably leads to death. In fatal cases, myocarditis often is found, as is inflammation of the liver and lungs (15). The mortality rate of acute viral meningitis in the absence of brain and other systemic involvement is probably 1% or less.

Diagnosis

Etiologic diagnosis usually rests on clinical and epidemiologic criteria. Features common to cases of acute viral meningitis include headache, fever (usually temperature lower than 102°F), photophobia, mild to moderate meningismus, and irritability. These may be accompanied by findings that are more specific for a given disease, such as parotitis in mumps, a zosteriform eruption in zoster, a typical multiphasic vesiculopustular eruption in varicella, asymmetric paralysis in poliomyelitis and enterovirus type 71 infection, gastrointestinal disturbance and rash in other enteroviral illness, and pharyngitis with diffuse adenopathy and psychosis (16) in mononucleosis (Table 149.2). In most cases, however, these helpful concomitant findings are absent.

Signs and symptoms of meningitis should prompt the clinician to perform lumbar puncture. The most important elements of CSF analysis are a search for bacteria or fungal elements and

TABLE 149.2. Clinical and Laboratory Findings in Viral Meningitis*

Clinical presentation	Suggestive laboratory findings		Suggested viral agent
	CSF	Other	
Parotitis, orchitis	Glucose ↓	Amylase ↑	Mumps virus
Diffuse rash, gastroenteritis, upper respiratory tract infection	—	—	Enteroviruses
Herpangina (soft palate enanthem)	—	—	Coxsackievirus A
Hand- and-foot-mouth rash	—	—	Coxsackievirus A
Pleurisy, orchitis, carditis	—	—	Coxsackievirus B
Orchitis, influenza-like syndrome	>2000 lymphocytes/mm^3, glucose ↓	Leukopenia, thrombocytopenia	Lymphocytic choriomeningitis virus
Zosteriform rash	—	—	Varicella-zoster virus
Encephalitis with focal neurologic signs	Erythrocytes	—	Herpes simplex virus
Pneumonia, immunocompromise	—	—	Adenovirus
Lymphadenopathy, splenomegaly, pharyngitis, Psychosis	—	Atypical lymphocytes, monospot	Epstein-Barr virus

*These findings may be present in only a minority of cases but are nevertheless helpful.
CSF, cerebrospinal fluid.

enumeration and differential count of any leukocytes present. The absence of bacteria should be assessed by examination of a Gram-stained preparation of the CSF sediment obtained by centrifuging 1 to 10 mL of CSF in a laboratory centrifuge for 5 minutes. A drop of CSF sediment should be allowed to air dry on a slide, after which it is heat fixed and stained. The presence or absence of fungi (primarily *Cryptococcus neoformans*) is assessed initially by adding another drop of CSF sediment to a drop of India ink and examining the wet preparation under the microscope. The cryptococci are seen as budding yeast forms in about 50% of proven cases. Cryptococcal antigen assay should be ordered, and results are usually available in 4 to 12 hours. This test has a sensitivity of more than 90%.

The cell count in viral meningitis is variable but usually does not exceed 1,000 white blood cells per mm^3. In most cases the count is less than 200 white blood cells per mm^3. Although the classic finding in viral meningitis is a predominance of small lymphocytes, polymorphonuclear leukocytes may predominate for the first 24 to 48 hours. The protein content of the CSF is usually normal but may be elevated to about 200 mg/dL. The glucose concentration also is usually normal (at least 50 mg/dL or at least 50% of the value in a simultaneously drawn sample of blood), but hypoglycorrachia has been reported in cases of meningitis due to mumps (17) and lymphocytic choriomeningitis (18) infection. Of the many viruses that cause meningitis, only some of the enteroviruses can be cultured readily from the CSF. Isolation of some type A coxsackieviruses requires inoculation of newborn mice. These isolations are rarely attempted, however, except as part of a virus surveillance study. Most often, if confirmation of the clinical diagnosis is sought, it is through finding a fourfold increase in antibodies to the suspected virus. In the case of enteroviruses, which may be ubiquitous in the oropharynx and stool of children, a diagnostic increase in antibody to the virus isolated from these sites must be demonstrated to ensure a causal relationship. Other specific diagnostic measures are discussed below, and clinical and laboratory findings suggestive of a specific cause are given in Table 149.2. A number of researchers have indicated that levels of lactate dehydrogenase (19), lactate (20), and other nonspecific acute-phase reactants can be used to differentiate viral from bacterial meningitis. It appears that concentrations of these substances vary directly with the number of leukocytes present and so contribute little

additional helpful information. A most promising addition to the diagnostic armamentarium is the application of PCR technology to this problem. Using PCR, several laboratories have demonstrated high degrees of sensitivity and specificity in finding nucleic acid sequences of enteroviruses in CSF with a single pair of oligonucleotide primers that detect the highly conserved 5′ end of the enterovirus sequence (21–24). This technology not only should improve the epidemiologic accuracy of detecting enteroviral disease but will do so quickly enough to have a major impact on treatment by allowing withdrawal of antimicrobials and discharge from the hospital.

Differential Diagnosis

The most significant decision one can make in evaluating meningitis is whether or not the infection will respond to specific antimicrobial therapy. Once pyogenic bacterial and fungal meningitides are excluded, there remain several causes of the aseptic meningitis syndrome that require specific treatment. These include tuberculosis, syphilis, leptospirosis, Lyme disease, and far less commonly, protozoal meningitis. In addition, and perhaps more common than any of these, is pyogenic bacterial meningitis in a patient who received some antibiotic treatment before the lumbar puncture. In these cases, bacteria may not be evident on Gram stain, and the initial polymorphonuclear response may have shifted to a mononuclear lymphocytic one. Although assays for bacterial antigens in the CSF, including counterimmunoelectrophoresis and latex agglutination, were developed to assist in just such cases, it has been our experience, substantiated by numerous personal communications, that these assays are no more sensitive than is Gram stain. In other words, it is highly unlikely that results of bacterial antigen tests will be positive if there is a negative Gram stain. One must take careful and sometimes repeated histories to exclude casual prior antibiotic use at the onset of symptoms.

Specific Meningitis Syndromes

Although viral meningitis syndromes are often nonspecific, sometimes a specific viral cause is suggested by the accompanying signs, symptoms, and laboratory findings.

ENTEROVIRUSES

The enteroviruses cause a multiplicity of syndromes in children and young adults. The most common clinical presentation is a febrile illness associated with mild respiratory or gastrointestinal symptoms. Exanthems or enanthemas may be associated with particular virus groups. Herpangina, painful vesicular and ulcerative lesions on the soft palate and tonsillar fauces, is associated with coxsackievirus A, as is the hand-foot-and-mouth syndrome consisting of isolated vesicles on an erythematous base in the aforementioned locations. Type B coxsackieviruses can be associated with pleuritis (pleurodynia, devil's grip), pericarditis, myocarditis, and orchitis. Echovirus infection, as well as other coxsackievirus infections, can be associated with a generalized macular or vesicular exanthem. Coxsackievirus B infection may be fatal to infants (15). Enterovirus type 71 can cause a paralytic syndrome in young children that is indistinguishable from that caused by poliovirus. This virus has also been associated with Guillain-Barré syndrome, aseptic meningitis, and encephalitis (25).

Mumps Virus

In the prevaccine era, mumps virus was the most common cause of meningoencephalitis in the United States and accounted for up to 10% of cases of this syndrome. Parotitis, the cardinal sign of mumps, was absent in up to one half of cases, and affected males outnumbered females by three to one (26). With the advent of live mumps vaccine in 1967, the incidence of mumps and its associated syndromes diminished dramatically; however, a significant number of children born in the late 1960s and early 1970s were not vaccinated. Because of herd immunity, these children had little chance of contracting natural infection. We recently witnessed a marked upsurge in the incidence of mumps among young adults, which stimulated college immunization programs. In nonimmunized adults, we may see a reappearance of mumps-related CNS syndromes that are more common in older age groups. This infection should be suspected in males who develop aseptic meningitis in winter or spring. Evidence of parotitis and epididymoorchitis should be sought, and an elevated serum amylase level may be found even in the absence of overt parotitis (26).

HERPESVIRUS

Although HSV-1 and HSV-2 can cause CNS infection, data from several studies indicate that HSV-2 is more likely than HSV-1 to cause aseptic meningitis (7). HSV involvement of the CNS can be the result of either primary or recurrent herpesvirus infection, although it appears to be more common as a complication of primary infection. One study showed that 36% of women and 13% of men with primary genital HSV-2 infection had stiff neck, photophobia, and headache (7). The absence of herpetic lesions does not exclude the possibility of HSV involvement of the CNS. Herpetic meningitis has a much better prognosis than encephalitis and is almost invariably self-limited and without sequelae. There have been several intriguing reports implicating HSV-2 as a cause of the benign recurrent lymphocytic meningitis syndrome (Mollaret's). This association, made possible by the use of PCR, would be entirely consistent with the recurring nature of HSV infections (27,28). Varicella-zoster virus, another member of the herpesvirus family, can cause meningitis. This can occur during the course of childhood or adult chickenpox as a rare complication, or in adult patients with zoster of any dermatome (29,30). CSF pleocytosis without meningeal signs or symptoms is probably quite common in zoster (30). Occasionally,

the CNS involvement antecedes the rash in either condition. If there is no encephalitic component, the illness is usually mild and self-limited (29).

LYMPHOCYTIC CHORIOMENINGITIS VIRUS

Lymphocytic choriomeningitis virus causes sporadic meningitis. Mice and other rodents are colonized with this organism and excrete it in their urine and feces. The peak incidence may occur any time except summer months, and disease occurs in localized areas of the United States and Europe.

The only clue to the diagnosis of this infection is a history of exposure to rodents. Forty years ago, pet Syrian hamsters were shown to be a source of epidemic human infection, and both a nonmeningitic influenza-like syndrome, accompanied in some cases by orchitis, and meningitic illness have been reported (18,31). Exposure to chronically infected nude mice, or mouse tissues, has been shown to transmit the disease to laboratory workers (32). CSF findings are nonspecific, but elevated protein concentration and lymphocytosis of up to 2,000 cells per mm^3 are common. Hypoglycorrachia occurs in about 30% of cases.

ADENOVIRUS

In patients who are immunocompromised as a result of kidney or bone marrow transplantation, adenovirus has been found to be a relatively common cause of CNS infection. Typically, this takes the form of meningoencephalitis and is often associated with acute adenovirus pneumonia. Types 7, 12, and 32 have been implicated (see Chapter 229).

Therapy

There is no effective antiviral therapy for viral meningitis. Adenine arabinoside and acyclovir, which have proved somewhat useful in treating herpes simplex and varicella-zoster encephalitis, are probably not necessary in cases of uncomplicated meningitis.

Prevention

Vaccines are available for the prevention of measles, mumps, varicella, and poliomyelitis. There are no commercially available vaccines for any of the other viruses discussed in this chapter. Spread of the enteroviruses is so ubiquitous during the summer and fall that infection control measures are of little use. One study group has recommended that women in the third trimester of pregnancy avoid swimming in pools to prevent enteroviral vaginal colonization (33).

ENCEPHALITIS

Epidemiology

There are two distinct epidemiologic patterns in viral encephalitis. One is identical to that previously described for the meningitides and involves respiratory or oral person-to-person transmission as exemplified by measles virus, mumps virus, enteroviruses, and herpesviruses, including varicella-zoster virus. The other, typical of the arboviral diseases, requires inoculation of the virus into the human bloodstream through the bite of an infected insect, usually a mosquito (Flaviviridae, Togaviridae, and Bunyaviridae) or tick (tick-borne encephalitis virus). In the case of rabies virus and monkey herpesvirus B, direct inoculation into neural tissue by the bite of an infected animal is the mode of transmission. Table 149.3 gives the taxonomic grouping

TABLE 149.3. Grouping and Mode of Transmission of Encephalitis Viruses

Family	Member virus	Transmission (vector)
Flaviviridae	Japanese encephalitis	
	St. Louis encephalitis	
	Murray Valley encephalitis	*Culex* mosquitos
	West Nile encephalitis	
	Powassan	*Ixodes* ticks
	Tick-borne encephalitis	
Togaviridae (alphaviruses)	Eastern equine encephalitis	
	Western equine encephalitis	
	Venezuelan equine encephalitis	*Culex* mosquitos
Bunyaviridae	California group	
	La Crosse	*Aedes* mosquitos
	Jamestown Canyon	
Herpesviridae	HSV-1 > HSV-2	Person to person
	Cytomegalovirus	Person to person
	Varicella-zoster	Person to person
	Monkey B	Monkey bite
Retroviridae	Human immunodeficiency virus type 1	Person to person

and vectors of some of the viruses that most commonly cause encephalitis.

The epidemiology of arboviral encephalitis is extremely complex and represents highly specialized adaptation of the virus to replication in a given species of mosquito or tick vector, as well as availability of that insect's preferred blood meal source. These intermediate animal hosts are usually birds or horses. Humans are often incidental and "dead-end" hosts of infection. For these reasons, there is specific geographic localization of the arboviral syndromes based on the presence of insect vector and animal reservoir. On the other hand, the viruses transmitted from person to person, and the diseases they cause, are found worldwide. Table 149.4 summarizes some of the epidemiologic and diagnostic factors useful in assessing the cause of encephalitis in a given patient.

The incidence of viral encephalitis varies greatly with the specific virus, season, geographic location, and climatic conditions (Table 149.4). Epidemiologic reporting is both deficient and inaccurate, so many cases probably go unreported. In the United States, the most common cause is herpesvirus type 1, of which there are about 1,000 cases reported annually. The next most common agents are the arboviruses, especially St. Louis encephalitis virus or California virus, although in any given year other arboviruses such as eastern equine encephalitis virus may predominate (34–36). The total number of arbovirus cases per year in the United States usually does not exceed 1 to 200; however, there were 3,000 cases of St. Louis encephalitis in 1933 (34), and Japanese encephalitis virus is responsible for tens of thousands of cases in Southeast Asia annually (37,38). Postinfectious encephalitis (von Economo encephalitis), has been seen after influenza, but never to the extent seen after the 1918 epidemic attributed to infection with swine influenza virus.

The number of complications associated with the acquired immunodeficiency syndrome (AIDS) is ever growing. Included in these are a multiplicity of CNS syndromes caused by various opportunistic agents such as *Toxoplasma gondii*, *Mycobacterium tuberculosis*, cytomegalovirus, and *Treponema pallidum*. It is now clear that the human immunodeficiency virus, which is the cause of AIDS, can itself infect neural tissue to produce

TABLE 149.4. Epidemiologic Characteristics and Laboratory Diagnosis of Viral Encephalitis

Virus	Recent travel	Risky habitat	Month of exposure[a]	Patients age	Diagnostic test	Research laboratory
St. Louis encephalitis	United States	Unscreened home	JJA	Older	IgM ELISA	CDC
Japanese encephalitis	Asia	Rice fields	MJJAS	Any	IgM ELISA	WRAIR
Eastern equine encephalitis	Western North America, South America	Agroecosystems in Western United States	JJAS	Any	IgM ELISA	CDC
Eastern equine encephalitis	Eastern United States	Coastal marshland	JJA	<10, >55 yr	IgM ELISA	CDC
Venezuelan equine encephalitis	South America to Texas	Rural	Rainy months	Adult men	IgM ELISA CSF	CDC
Tick-borne encephalitis	Central Europe and Asia	Woodlands	JJA	Any	IgM ELISA CSF	
Herpes simplex	Anywhere	None	Any	Any	Brain biopsy	U. Vienna
California encephalitis	Western United States	Rural areas	JJASO	Children	IgM ELISA	CDC
Murray Valley encephalitis	Southern Australia	River valley area	JFMAM	Any	IgM ELISA	CDC
West Nile encephalitis	North Africa, eastern and southern Asia	Rice areas	JJAS	Any	ELISA Virus isolation	WRAIR
	East Coast of United States	New York City Metropolitan Area	JJAS	Any	PCR, virus isolation	Most
Powassan	North Central United States, southern Canada	Rural areas	JJAS	<20 or >50 yr	HAI, CF	CDC
La Crosse	Midwestern United States	Woodlands	JJAS	Boys <19 yr	ELISA	CDC
Rocio	Sao Paulo Brazil	Poor rural areas	FMAMJJ	Young men	HAI, ELISA	CDC
Jamestown Canyon	New York and Westward	Rural areas	JJAS	Children	CF, NT	
Human immunodeficiency virus type 1	Worldwide	All	Any	Undefined	ELISA Immunoblot	Most
B virus		Monkey colony	Any	Adult	Virus isolation	SFBR

ELISA, enzyme-linked immunosorbent assay; PCR, polymerase chain reaction; HAI, hemagglutination inhibition; CF, complement fixation; NT, neutralization test; IgM, immunoglobulin M; CDC, Fort Collins, CO (303-221-6407); WRAIR, Department of Viral Diseases, Walter Reed Army Institute of Research, Washington, DC (202-576-2054); U. Vienna, University of Vienna, Vienna, Austria; SFBR, Southwest Foundation for Biomedical Research, San Antonio, TX.
[a]Initial of months in most cases; the first J refers to June in all entries, the first M to March.

meningoencephalitis (39). Diagnosis of this condition rests on excluding the other potential causes of CNS infection. In fact, involvement of the CNS is perhaps the only direct result of human immunodeficiency virus infection, the other elements of AIDS being indirect results of damaged immunity. This involvement, with the attendant requirement that anti-AIDS drugs penetrate brain tissue, represents one of the major stumbling blocks to effective treatment of AIDS.

Pathogenesis

In herpesvirus B infection and rabies, the virus travels from the bite site along peripheral nerves to the CNS. In the arboviral encephalitides and in mumps and measles, viremia is the source of infection of the CNS (40–42). Encephalitis viruses are neurotropic and apparently replicate in neurons, thereby lysing them. In addition, later in infection there may be an immune inflammatory component to neuronal damage (43,44). Histologically, there is perivascular infiltration by both mononuclear and polymorphonuclear cells. Neuronal cells degenerate and are phagocytosed.

Disease Manifestations

Incubation periods in cases other than those caused by animal bite are difficult to calculate precisely. In cases of arboviral encephalitis the incubation period may vary from several days to 2 weeks (34,37). The vast majority (greater than 90%) of arboviral infections result in mild disease resembling an influenza-like illness. If encephalitis occurs, the syndrome generally consists of fever, headache, malaise, and abnormal mental state progressing over several days to stupor and coma. This syndrome may be accompanied by nuchal rigidity and seizures. After the first week, either flaccid or spastic paralysis may occur. Many patients exhibit electrolyte imbalance caused by the syndrome of inappropriate secretion of antidiuretic hormone. Once signs and symptoms are present, they progress for 1 to 2 weeks, at which time the patient either dies or begins to show signs of recovery. Because of the damage to neurons, which are incapable of regeneration, there are often severe sequelae of infection. Patients may be left with cognitive and cranial nerve deficits, including dysarthria, as well as paralysis and aphasia. Parkinsonian tremors have been noted after recovery from Japanese and postinfluenzal encephalitis.

There are differences in the propensity to develop clinical disease and in the severity of disease after arboviral infection that vary with the virus and with the age and underlying condition of the host. St. Louis encephalitis tends to cause most severe disease in the elderly, especially in black persons and people with hypertension, whereas Japanese B encephalitis and California virus encephalitis are most common in children. The case-fatality rate in Japanese encephalitis and eastern equine encephalitis is in excess of 30%, whereas St. Louis encephalitis has a 7% mortality rate in young adults and a 20% mortality rate in the elderly. Most other arboviral encephalitides carry a mortality rate of less than 1% (34,37,45). Herpesvirus B infection and untreated rabies are almost universally fatal; herpes simplex encephalitis has an inherent mortality rate of 70% to 80%, which has been reduced to less than 30% with the early use of acyclovir (46).

Diagnosis

The encephalitis syndrome itself provides little clue in any given case as to the cause. Although localization of neurologic signs to the temporal lobe is probably most common in HSV encephalitis, the absence of this localization does not rule out an HSV cause, and other encephalitides may affect the temporal lobe. The most important factor in establishing a probable cause of encephalitis is the taking of a careful history, including habitation or travel in an area endemic for a particular disease (arboviruses); exposure to animals such as rodents (lymphocytic choriomeningitis), dogs, bats, raccoons, skunks (rabies), and monkeys (herpesvirus B); and the presence of concomitant illness (measles, mumps, varicella, or zoster).

Routine laboratory investigation is not usually helpful. The peripheral white blood cell count is elevated in most cases, with a relative lymphocytosis present. Examination of the CSF reveals a mild to moderate pleocytosis (25–250 white blood cells per mm^3). Although polymorphonuclear cells may predominate early in infection, by the second or third day of symptoms the majority of cells in the CSF are mononuclear. Protein levels may be slightly elevated and the glucose concentration is usually normal (see the earlier section on meningitis for exceptions). The presence of 100 to 200 erythrocytes per mm^3 in the CSF is more common in HSV encephalitis than in other encephalomeningitides. These are essentially the CSF findings in aseptic meningitis, and attempts should be made to exclude treatable causes of this syndrome before assuming that one is dealing with viral encephalitis. Such treatable causes would include tuberculosis, cryptococcal meningitis, toxoplasmosis in the patient with AIDS, and partially treated bacterial meningitis.

CSF also can be cultured for the presence of specific arboviruses, which grow quite well on a variety of monkey cell cultures, but attempts to culture CSF for HSV have been unsuccessful. One can also assay CSF for the presence of immunoglobulin M antibodies to specific etiologic agents. Although the specificity of these assays is high, antibodies may not be present at the outset of disease, thereby yielding a false-negative result. Because of the importance of arboviral outbreaks, attempts should be made to arrive at specific diagnoses of suspected arboviral encephalitis even if such results would not help the care of the patient at hand. In appropriate geographic locations, state health agencies should be able to provide diagnostic help. Further information can be obtained from the Centers for Disease Control and Prevention, Vector-Borne Diseases Laboratory, Fort Collins, Colorado.

The greatest hope for rapid and accurate etiologic diagnoses in cases of viral encephalitis lies in the commercially available application of the PCR. This test can reveal infinitesimal amounts of nucleic acid with great specificity in CSF and other body fluids. PCR has already been successfully applied experimentally to the diagnosis of HSV, enteroviral, and arboviral CNS diseases (22,24,37,47).

Ancillary tests may help to confirm a diagnosis of encephalitis, but they do not establish the cause. Electroencephalography is probably the most sensitive early in infection and may show focal slow waves over the affected area of the brain and diffuse delta activity indicating thalamic involvement. Computed tomography is insensitive early, but magnetic resonance imaging has been used successfully to reveal early brain involvement (47,48).

Treatment

The only form of viral encephalitis for which effective treatment exists is that caused by the herpesviruses. HSV encephalitis responds well to early (before coma) institution of therapy with acyclovir. The drug is given intravenously at a dose of 30 mg/kg per day in three divided doses for at least 14 days. Before the advent of acyclovir, it was recommended that brain biopsy be performed to obtain tissue for HSV testing by immunofluorescence and electron microscopy. The relative nontoxicity of acyclovir makes this procedure unnecessary in our opinion, unless there is no response to therapy, and one is searching for the presence of another causative agent. It is probably worthwhile to initiate therapy with acyclovir in cases of herpesvirus B encephalitis (49). Although no controlled studies have been done, patients with zoster encephalitis appear to benefit from treatment with acyclovir. Cytomegalovirus more often causes meningitis than encephalitis in patients with AIDS. However, these patients often have an encephalopathy of undetermined cause. Human immunodeficiency virus encephalopathy may also improve after therapy with zidovudine.

Prevention

Because there is no effective therapy for most causes of viral encephalitis, vaccines would be desirable in protecting against infection. Vaccines have been developed against Japanese B, Venezuelan, and tick-borne encephalitides, but only the first of these (JE-VAX, Aventis Pasteur, Swiftwater, Pennsylvania) is commercially available in the United States. Visitors to endemic areas of Asia should consider obtaining the Japanese B vaccine. However, in Australia, where the vaccine is available, there have been several reports of vaccine-associated severe allergic reactions (44). Perhaps the best advice would be to take all measures available to prevent exposure to the mosquito or tick vectors.

Mumps and measles vaccinations have decreased markedly the incidence of encephalitis due to these two diseases. The newer rabies vaccine is effective in preventing disease even after the bite of an infected animal.

West Nile Virus Encephalitis in North America

West Nile virus, a mosquito-borne flavivirus closely related to St. Louis encephalitis and Japanese encephalitis viruses, is endemic to Africa, the Middle East, and southwest Asia. The virus is transmitted between *Culex* mosquitos and wild birds, with incidental infections occurring in humans. In late August 1999, the first recognized occurrence of West Nile virus in the Western Hemisphere was recognized when an outbreak in New York City resulted in 62 cases of acute encephalitis. Seven patients died, and mortality among horses and birds was substantial (50,51). Infected *Culex* mosquitos were the only known vectors in this outbreak. Fifty-nine patients with meningoencephalitis were hospitalized with West Nile virus meningoencephalitis during the summer of 1999.

Most patients were at least 50 years old, had encephalitis, and presented with fever, weakness, nausea, vomiting, headache, and altered mental status. Twenty percent of the patients had an erythematous macular, papular, or morbilliform eruption involving some combination of the neck, trunk, and arms and legs. Decreased muscle strength and hyporeflexia were noted in a third of the cases. Older age was associated with a substantially higher risk of more severe neurologic disease. An age of 75 years or older was the factor most strongly associated with death. The presence of diabetes mellitus was also significantly associated with death. The overall case fatality rate was 12% (52).

Several clues should alert one to the possibility of this disease. First, unexpected deaths in bird or horse populations are likely to be sentinel events that precede the infection of humans. Second, although West Nile virus infects persons of all ages, the risk for meningoencephalitis increases by a factor of more than 20 in those over age 50. Third, the West Nile virus has some clinical features, including the pattern of weakness and the presence of neu-

ropathy, that are unusual in other forms of encephalitis. Lastly, a significant proportion of patients had an erythematous rash, and many had lymphocytopenia, both relatively unusual features in viral encephalitis. The presence of any of these features should raise the suspicion of West Nile virus and prompt definitive diagnostic testing (53). A PCR test or viral culture of the CSF are the preferred diagnostic tests. There is currently no known effective antiviral therapy or vaccine, although high doses of ribavarin have been found to inhibit West Nile virus replication and cytopathogenicity in human neural cells *in vitro* (54).

The initial outbreak followed a pattern more characteristic of recent outbreaks of encephalitis in areas where the virus is not endemic and where the level of immunity of the population to the West Nile virus is lower (e.g., Romania and Russia). In these outbreaks, recognized illness was characterized by severe neurologic disease that affected primarily older adults. In areas where the virus is endemic, outbreaks of milder febrile illness usually occur (52).

Since the 1999 outbreak, West Nile virus has been isolated from birds and mosquitos throughout 44 states and the District of Columbia in the United States, and in the province of Ontario, Canada. In addition, several new modes of transmission, including transmission via transplanted organs or blood products from infected donors, via breast milk from a nursing mother to a newborn infant, and via the placenta from a pregnant mother to a fetus, have been documented (55).

ACKNOWLEDGMENT

This chapter is affectionately dedicated to the memory of Bernard N. Fields, M.D.—friend, colleague, and virologist.

REFERENCES

1. Schmidt NJ, Lennette EH, Ho HH. An apparently new enterovirus isolated from patients with disease of the central nervous system. *J Infect Dis* 1974; 129:304.
2. Matthews REF. Fourth report of the International Committee on Taxonomy of Viruses. *Intervirology* 1982;17:1.
3. Centers for Disease Control and Prevention. Enterovirus surveillance—United States, 1983. *MMWR* 1983;32:535.
4. Berlin LE, Rorabaugh ML, Heldrick F, et al. Aseptic meningitis in infants <2 years of age: diagnosis and etiology. *J Infect Dis* 1993;168:888.
5. Shattuck KE, Chonmaitree T. The changing spectrum of neonatal meningitis over a fifteen-year period. *Clin Pediatr* 1992;31:130.
6. Bodian D. Emerging concepts of poliomyelitis infection. *Science* 1955;122:105.
7. Corey L, Adams HG, Brown ZA, et al. Genital herpes simplex virus infections: clinical manifestations, course and complications. *Ann Intern Med* 1983;98:958.
8. Horstmann DM. Acute poliomyelitis. Relation of physical activity at the time of onset to the course of the disease. *JAMA* 1950;142:236.
9. Moore M, Baron RC, Filstein MR, et al. Aseptic meningitis and high school football players. *JAMA* 1983;249:2039.
10. Naess A, Solberg CO, Tonder O. Granulocyte and lymphocyte membrane receptors in aseptic meningitis, infectious mononucleosis and other viral infections. *Acta Pathol Microbiol Immunol Scand* 1985;93:37.
11. Bertotto A, Stagni G, Fabietti GM. Plasma cell generation inhibition in lymphocyte cultures containing cerebrospinal fluid from children with central nervous system viral infections. *Microbiologica* 1985;8:11.
12. Forsberg P, Fryden A, Link H, et al. Viral IgM and IgG antibody synthesis within the central nervous system in mumps meningitis. *Acta Neurol Scand* 1986;73:372.
13. Ichimura H, Shimase K Tamura I, et al. Neutralizing antibody and interferon-α in cerebrospinal fluids and sera of acute aseptic meningitis. *J Med Virol* 1985;15:231.
14. Siemes H, Siegert M. Immune response in the CSF in viral infections. *Frog Brain Res* 1983;59:133.
15. Kaplan MH, Klein SW, McPhee J, et al. Group B coxsackie infections in infants younger than three months of age: a serious childhood illness. *Rev Infect Dis* 1983;5:1019.
16. Grose CF. Neurologic complications of infectious mononucleosis. In: Schlossberg D, ed. *Infectious mononucleosis.* New York: Springer-Verlag, 1989: 49–68.

17. Wilfert CM. Mumps meningoencephalitis with low cerebrospinal fluid glucose, prolonged pleocytosis and elevation of protein. *N Engl J Med* 1969;280:855.
18. Biggar RJ, Woodall JP, Walter PD, et al. Lymphocytic choriomeningitis outbreak associated with pet hamsters: fifty-seven cases from New York State. *JAMA* 1975;232:494.
19. Martin WJ. Rapid and reliable techniques for the laboratory detection of bacterial meningitis. *Am J Med* 1983;75:119.
20. Jordan GW, Statland B, Halsted C. CSF lactate in disease of the CNS. *Arch Intern Med* 1983;143:85.
21. Rotbart HA. Diagnosis of enteroviral meningitis with the polymerase chain reaction. *J Pediatr* 1990;117:85.
22. Sawyer MH, Holland D, Aintablian N, et al. Diagnosis of enteroviral central nervous system infection by polymerase chain reaction during a large community outbreak. *Pediatr Infect Dis* 1994;13:177.
23. Schlesinger Y, Sawyer MH, Storch GA. Enteroviral meningitis in infancy: potential role for polymerase chain reaction in patient management. *Pediatrics* 1994;94:157.
24. Rotbart HA, Sawyer MH, Fast S, et al. Diagnosis of enteroviral meningitis by using PCR with a colorimetric microwell detection assay. *J Clin Microbiol* 1994;32:2590.
25. Alexander JP, Baden L, Pallansch MA, et al. Enterovirus 71 infections and neurologic disease-United States, 1977–1991. *J Infect Dis* 1994;169:905.
26. Baum SG, Litman N. Mumps virus. In: Mandell GL, Douglas RG Jr, Bennett JE, eds. *Principles and practice of infectious diseases,* 4th ed. New York: John Wiley & Sons, 1995:1496–1501.
27. Tedder DG, Ashley R, Tyler K, et al. Herpes simplex infection as a cause of benign recurrent lymphocytic meningitis. *Ann Intern Med* 1994;121:334.
28. Picard FJ, Dekaban GA, Silva J, et al. Mollaret's meningitis associated with herpes simplex type 2 infection. *Neurology* 1993;43:1722.
29. Johnson R, Milbourne PE. Central nervous system manifestations of chickenpox. *Can Med Assoc J* 1970;102:831.
30. Barnes DW, Whitley RJ. CNS disease associated with varicella zoster virus and herpes simplex infection. *Neurol Clin* 1986;4:265.
31. Baum SG, Lewis AM Jr, Rowe WP, et al. Epidemic nonmeningitic lymphocytic choriomeningitis virus infection. *N Engl J Med* 1966;274:934.
32. Dykewicz CA, Dato VM, Fisher-Hock SP. Lymphocytic choriomeningitis outbreak associated with nude mice in a research institute. *JAMA* 1992;267:1349.
33. Reyes MP, Zalenski D, Smith F, et al. Coxsackievirus-positive cervices in women with febrile illnesses during the third trimester in pregnancy. *Am J Obstet Gynecol* 1986;–155:159.
34. Tsai TF. Arboviral infections in the United States. *Infect Dis Clin North Am* 1991;1:73.
35. Centers for Disease Control and Prevention. Arboviral disease—United States, 1991. *MMWR* 1992;41:545.
36. Centers for Disease Control and Prevention. Arboviral diseases—United States, 1992. *MMWR* 1993;42:467.
37. Vaughn DW, Hoke CH. The epidemiology of Japanese encephalitis: prospects for prevention. *Epidemiol Rev* 1992;14:197.
38. Thisyakom U, Thisyakom C. Diseases caused by arboviruses—Dengue hemorrhagic fever and Japanese B encephalitis. *Med J Aust* 1994;160:22.
39. Gabuzda DH, Hirsch MS. Neurologic manifestations of infection with human immunodeficiency virus. *Ann Intern Med* 1987;107:383.
40. Tsiang H. Pathophysiology of rabies virus infection of the nervous system. *Adv Virus Res* 1993;42:375.
41. Dupont JR, Earle KM. Human rabies encephalitis: a study of forty-nine fatal cases with a review of the literature. *Neurology* 1965;15:1023.
42. Weigler BJ. Biology of B virus in macaque and human hosts: a review. *Clin Infect Dis* 1992;14:555.
43. de la Monte S, Castro F, Bonilla NJ. The systemic pathology of Venezuelan equine encephalitis virus infection in humans. *Am J Trop Med Hyg* 1985;34:194.
44. Johnson RT. The pathogenesis of acute viral encephalitis and post infectious encephalomyelitis. *J Infect Dis* 1987;155:359.
45. Ohtaki E, Murakami Y, Komori H, et al. Acute disseminated encephalomyelitis after Japanese B encephalitis vaccination. *Pediatr Neurol* 1992;8:137.
46. Whitley RJ, Alford CA, Hirsch MS, et al. Vidarabine versus acyclovir therapy in herpes simplex encephalitis. *N Engl J Med* 1986;314:144.
47. Schlesinger Y, Buller RS, Brunstrom JE, et al. Expanded spectrum of herpes simplex encephalitis in childhood. *J Pediatr* 1995;126:234.
48. Misra UK Kalita J, Jain SK, et al. Radiological and neurophysiological changes in Japanese encephalitis. *J Neurol Neurosurg Psychiatry* 1994;57:1484.
49. Centers for Disease Control and Prevention. B-virus infection in humans—Pensacola, Florida. *MMWR* 1987;36:289.
50. Outbreak of West Nile—like viral encephalitis—New York, 1999. *MMWR* 1999;48:845.
51. Asnis DS, Conetta R, Teixeira AA, et al. The West Nile virus outbreak of 1999 in New York. *Clin Infect Dis* 2000;30:413.
52. Nash D, Mostashari F, Fine A, et al. The outbreak of West Nile virus infection in the New York City area in 1999. *N Engl J Med* 2001;344:1807.
53. Tyler KL. West Nile virus encephalitis in America. *N Engl J Med* 2001;344:1858.
54. Jordan I, Briese T, Fischer N, et al. Ribavirin inhibits the West Nile virus replication and cytopathic effect in neural cells. *J Infect Dis* 2000;182:1214.
55. Iwamoto M, Jernigan DB, Guasch A, et al. Transmission of West Nile Virus from an organ donor to four transplant recipients. *N Engl J Med* 2003;348:2196.

CHAPTER 150
Chronic Meningitis

John C. Pottage, Jr., and Alan A. Harris

Chronic meningitis is defined as a constellation of signs and symptoms of meningeal irritation for greater than 4 weeks with an associated cerebrospinal fluid (CSF) pleocytosis (1). Included in this syndrome is meningitis with an acute onset in which the signs, symptoms, and CSF pleocytosis fail to resolve in the presence of appropriate antibacterial therapy and negative bacterial cultures. Characteristically, the patient remains symptomatic and progressively deteriorates over days to weeks until specific treatment is given. In contrast, relapsing meningitis has asymptomatic periods with normal CSF, even without therapy. Chronic meningitis is less commonly observed than acute pyogenic or viral meningitis. Despite an extensive body of literature on specific causes, data on the syndrome as a whole are sparse (1), reflecting the difficulty in diagnosis, the small number of cases seen at a single institution, and the vast number of possible causes.

History and physical examination are the major tools for focusing the diagnosis. Symptoms of global dysfunction such as headache or alteration in consciousness help in pointing to encephalitis, whereas clues such as cranial nerve deficits or seizures suggest localized cortical, meningeal, or vascular involvement. Evidence of systemic illness, such as neoplasm, collagen-vascular disease, oral or genital ulceration, sarcoid, exposure to tuberculosis, or the use of immunosuppressive drugs, should be sought. Multiple sexual contacts or a history of other venereal diseases suggest human immunodeficiency virus (HIV) infection, syphilis, or recurrent herpes simplex infection. Travel to areas endemic for illnesses such as Lyme disease, histoplasmosis, blastomycosis, coccidioidomycosis, and parasitic infection suggests important tests that may otherwise be omitted. Unusual exposures, such as ingestion of unpasteurized dairy products, may suggest mycobacterial disease or brucellosis. Symptoms at extraneural sites, such as ears, mouth, and chest, should be elicited. Medications should be documented, including over-the-counter drugs such as ibuprofen, as should surgical procedures or trauma involving the spine or head.

The physical examination should evaluate any focal neurologic findings, particularly cranial neuropathy. Radiculopathy or mononeuritis may suggest spirochetal disease, systemic lupus erythematosus, or sarcoidosis. The ears and nose should be examined for masses or obstruction, the teeth for abscess or cavities, and the sinuses for tenderness or decreased transillumination. Careful examination of the lumbar area and less commonly the occiput may reveal congenital dermal sinuses or fistulas communicating to the subarachnoid space. A detailed ophthalmologic examination should be conducted to assess for papilledema, granulomatous uveitis, choroidal tubercles, cytoid bodies, and Roth spots. Evaluation of the lymphoreticular, skin, and musculoskeletal systems is necessary, because these areas readily lend themselves to biopsy and specific diagnosis. Skin examination may reveal erythema nodosum, vasculitis, septic embolization, or a specific infectious lesion.

Laboratory confirmation of the suspected diagnosis is frequently difficult to achieve. Optimally, CSF cultures will be positive or serologic studies will suggest local antibody production. Because these results may be delayed and are frequently not diagnostic, extensive evaluation for extraneural disease should be quickly initiated and the results should help guide early

TABLE 150.1.   Diagnostic Evaluation of Patients with Chronic Meningitis

Suggested for all patients
  Complete blood count
  Chemistry panel, with attention to diabetes insipidus
  Cultures of blood, urine, and sputum if possible
  Chest radiograph
  CT of head with infusion
  ANA, rheumatoid factor, erythrocyte sedimentation rate
  Serum serology for histoplasmosis, coccidioidomycosis, syphilis, and Lyme disease
  Skin test with 5 TU of PPD (second-strength PPD and anergy profile if intermediate test is negative)
  CSF. For glucose, protein, cell count, India ink; culture for bacteria, fungus, and AFB; cryptococcal antigen and antibody; CSF VDRL; cytology
Additional studies as indicated
  CSF serology for histoplasmosis, coccidioidomycosis, *Borrelia*, aspergillosis, sporotrichosis, brucellosis
  CSF, blood, and urine for *Histoplasma* antigen
  CSF for TB-PCR, tuberculous antigens or antibodies, immunoglobulin G/albumin ratio
  Cultures of serum and CSF for *Brucella*
  MRI of head and spine to evaluate for parameningeal and parenchymal lesions
  Electroencephalography
  Lymph node biopsy of enlarged node
  Bone marrow and liver biopsy for pathologic study and culture
  Skin and muscle biopsy for vasculitis or sarcoid
  Cerebral angiography

CT, computed tomography; ANA, antinuclear antibodies; PPD, purified protein derivative; AFB, acid-fast bacillus; CSF VDRL, cerebrospinal fluid Venereal Disease Research Laboratory; TU, tuberculin units; MRI, magnetic resonance imaging.
Modified from Wilhelm C, Ellner JJ. Chronic meningitis. *Neurol Clin* 1986;4:115–141, with permission.

presumptive therapy. A laboratory evaluation is suggested in Table 150.1 (2). The CSF formula, comprising cell count and differential, glucose, and protein, does not provide the etiology but prioritizes the differential diagnosis and assists in guiding early empirical therapy. The predominant CSF cell type is the basis for categorization of the clinical entities discussed here and in Table 150.2 (3).

LYMPHOCYTIC OR MONONUCLEAR CELL PREDOMINANCE

Tuberculosis

Mycobacterium tuberculosis meningitis remains the most common cause of chronic meningitis (4). CSF inflammation occurs due to breakdown of a meningeal focus that developed at the time of primary dissemination. This breakdown may occur soon after primary spread in children. In 50% of adults, reactivation is associated with an immunocompromising condition such as chemotherapy, alcoholism, diabetes mellitus, gastrectomy, malnutrition, or pregnancy (5). Only half of all cases have a documented exposure to tuberculosis (6). Other conditions that depress T-cell immunity, such as sarcoidosis, Hodgkin's disease, measles, organ transplantation, and HIV infection, predispose to dissemination and therefore meningitis. All patients with a new diagnosis of tuberculosis, regardless of which organ systems are involved, should have a serologic test for HIV. "Atypical" mycobacteria have been documented to cause meningitis (7) but are extremely rare in non–HIV-infected patients. In HIV-infected patients, the most commonly seen organism is *Mycobacterium avium* complex. Although *M. avium* complex infection is common in patients with advanced HIV infection who are not being treated

TABLE 150.2.   Differential Diagnoses of Chronic Meningitis by Predominant Cerebrospinal Fluid Inflammatory Cell Type

Etiology	Lymphocytic	Neutrophilic	Eosinophilic
Viral	Lymphocytic choriomeningitis; mumps; herpes simplex; herpes zoster; arbovirus, flavivirus, and echovirus infections; HIV	Herpes simplex, cytomegalovirus infection	
Bacterial	Tuberculosis, brucellosis, tularemia, syphilis, Lyme disease, leptospirosis, recurrent fever, nocardiosis, actinomycosis, listeriosis, subacute bacterial endocarditis	Tuberculosis, nocardiosis, actinomycosis, brucellosis, meningococcal infection in complement deficiency	Tuberculosis, syphilis
Fungal	Cryptococcosis; coccidioidomycosis; histoplasmosis; blastomycosis; *Candida, Aspergillus,* Zygomycetes, and *Pseudallescheria boydii* infections	*Candida* infection; coccidioidomycosis; histoplasmosis; blastomycosis; *Aspergillus,* dematiaceous fungi, Zygomycetes, and *P. boydii* infections	Coccidioidomycosis
Parasitic	Cysticercosis, paragonimiasis, schistosomiasis, *Fasciola hepatica* infection, echinococcosis, trichinosis, visceral larva migrans		*Angiostrongylus cantonensis* infection, cysticercosis, *Gnathostoma spinigerum* infection, paragonimiasis, schistosomiasis, echinococcosis, trichinosis, *Fasciola hepatica* infection, visceral larva migrans
Protozoal	Toxoplasmosis; *Acanthamoeba* infection; Trypanosomiasis	*Naegleria* infections	
Noninfectious	Solid neoplasm, lymphoma leukemia, sarcoidosis, vasculitis, collagen-vascular disease, Behçet's disease, Vogt-Koyanagi-Harada syndrome	Foreign body in the central nervous system, sarcoidosis, drug induced, chemical induced, solid neoplasm	Foreign body in the central nervous system, sarcoidosis, lymphoma
Other	Parameningeal focus, benign chronic lymphocytic meningitis	Parameningeal focus	

with highly active antiretroviral therapy (HAART), spread to the CNS is uncommon. In addition, most patients have evidence of *M. avium* complex infection elsewhere in the body (8).

Clinical manifestations are not specific. The presentation can be acute, but classically it is subacute, usually spanning weeks. The duration of symptoms is usually less than a month before a physician is contacted. Fever of varying degree is almost always present (9). Headache, nausea, and vomiting occur in 70% of cases. In a minority of cases, palsies of cranial nerves II, III, IV, VI, and VII are present, suggesting involvement of the basilar meninges. Diabetes insipidus is nonspecifically associated with tuberculous meningitis and with sarcoidosis. Choroidal tubercles are rare but aid significantly in early diagnosis and should be aggressively sought. Manifestations of hydrocephalus and focal neurologic findings from infarction increase with disease progression.

Culturing *M. tuberculosis* from CSF makes a definitive diagnosis. Smears for acid-fast bacilli are positive in only 10% to 40% of patients (10). Yield may be improved by extensive examination of an auramine-rhodamine fluorochrome stain for 20 to 60 minutes, by obtaining multiple specimens, or by centrifuging the CSF. Up to 80% of CSF samples will be positive by culture (11), but results may require 2 to 8 weeks. Automated systems with lysis centrifugation can indicate growth within 1 to 2 weeks. DNA probes can be used to identify *M. tuberculosis* once the organism is growing in culture (12). Polymerase chain reaction (PCR)-based assays and the detection of mycobacterial antigen with a dot immunobinding assay have been shown to have better sensitivity than smears, but false-negative results still occur (13,14).

CSF hypoglycorrhachia is present in 70% to 85% of patients on admission (11,15) and will be present in 98% of patients some time during hospitalization (11). Fungal meningitis is also associated with a low CSF glucose level, but this finding does exclude most viral processes. With CSF lymphocytosis and an appropriate syndrome, patients with hypoglycorrhachia warrant empirical antituberculous therapy as the workup continues. Daily fluctuations in the CSF formula may be a clue to tuberculous meningitis. This same variability limits the value of sequential analysis of CSF in monitoring the early response to therapy.

Tests for extraneural disease are important. Chest radiographs reveal evidence of past or present tuberculosis in at least 50% of patients (9). Sputum analysis is warranted, because 10% to 20% of patients have active pulmonary disease. Results of skin testing with an intermediate-strength purified protein derivative will be negative in many patients. Results of tests with second-strength purified protein derivative (250 tuberculin units) will be positive in 80% of patients (16), but a lack of specificity at this concentration limits its usefulness. A negative second-strength test result in the absence of anergy does not exclude tuberculous meningitis.

Outcome is strongly associated with the severity of neurologic symptoms at presentation and any delay in initiation of therapy in the presence of CSF lymphocytosis and hypoglycorrhachia (5,17). When the organism is susceptible, initial treatment consists of isoniazid, rifampin, and a third or fourth antituberculous drug such as ethambutol, pyrazinamide, or ethionamide. In such situations, standard 6- and 9-month regimens for pulmonary and extrapulmonary disease have been deemed acceptable, but data are limited. When isoniazid resistance in an area exceeds 4%, four drugs should be used initially. When a patient has tuberculosis resistant to isoniazid and rifampin, the best therapy is unknown, but three drugs to which the organism is susceptible should be used. Six- and 9-month regimens cannot currently be recommended in the presence of isoniazid or rifampin resistance.

In a "trial of therapy," rifampin should be used cautiously because its broad spectrum against bacteria, fungi, and spirochetes may partially treat other infections. A response to treatment may take 2 to 4 weeks. Daily fluctuations in neurologic status and CSF abnormalities do not require alteration in treatment. In the absence of an alternative diagnosis, once initiated, antituberculous therapy should be continued for at least 12 months.

The mortality rate associated with tuberculous meningitis is 10% to 30%, and 40% of patients have persisting neurologic deficits. Mental retardation, paralysis and paresis, sphincter incontinence, and seizure disorders may be lasting residua. Severe disease has been associated with cerebral infarctions caused by an arteritis at the circle of Willis (18). Corticosteroids have been advocated for children with infarction as well as for hydrocephalus. With corticosteroids, CSF abnormalities may resolve more quickly and the risk of herniation may be decreased (19). However, evidence of decreased morbidity and mortality is lacking, and we do not support their general use. When the patient is receiving therapy and computed tomography (CT) demonstrates stable or progressive obstructive hydrocephalus and increased intracranial pressure, steroids should be used. If there is no response, shunting has resulted in decreased morbidity compared with historical controls (20).

Fungal Meningitis

CRYPTOCOCCOSIS

Meningitis caused by *Cryptococcus neoformans* is difficult to distinguish from tuberculous meningitis, but subtle clues are available (21). The onset is more gradual, taking up to 20 years from onset to diagnosis. Headache is the most common presenting symptom. Mental status changes and nuchal rigidity occur only half as often as in tuberculous meningitis. Abnormal hosts account for 50% to 80% of patients with *C. neoformans*, and this is the most common cause of subacute and chronic meningitis in this population. Most patients are immunosuppressed as a result of corticosteroids, cytotoxic drugs, lymphoreticular hematologic malignancies, or transplants. HIV infection is the major risk factor in many centers. Today, HIV testing is warranted for all patients despite a known alternative immunocompromising condition. Physical findings, especially cranial nerve abnormalities, are less common than in tuberculous meningitis, except for optic nerve invasion with subsequent papilledema and vision loss (2). Disease outside the CSF is frequently present but may not be clinically apparent. The chest radiograph is helpful, although less commonly than with tuberculosis. Cultures are positive from extrapulmonary sites such as skin, bone marrow, lymph nodes, and prostate in greater than one third of patients (21).

Early diagnosis is facilitated by positive CSF India ink smear. The sensitivity of the test is unfortunately less than 50%, and false-positive results are common in less experienced laboratories. Cryptococcal antigen in the CSF is present in 85% of patients, and more than 90% of patients have the presence of either CSF or serum cryptococcal antigen. CSF cryptococcal antigen assay is at least 80% specific and is more sensitive than culture. A patient with a CSF cryptococcal antigen titer greater than 1:8 should be treated despite negative cultures (22). Neither hypoglycorrhachia nor other routine CSF tests help in establishing an etiologic diagnosis (23). No skin testing is available. CSF white blood cell counts of greater than $20/mm^3$ in patients with altered mental status have been a favorable prognostic sign (24). Hypoglycorrhachia, a positive India ink smear, high CSF cryptococcal antigen titers and low CSF white blood cell counts portend a poor outcome. Elevated CSF pressure may also be associated with a poor outcome. Aggressive therapy to reduce elevated CSF pressure has been associated with improved outcome (25).

The standard treatment for cryptococcal meningitis in non–HIV-infected patients is intravenous amphotericin B (0.7–1.0 mg/kg per day) plus oral flucytosine (100 mg/kg per day). The duration of therapy is 4 to 6 weeks (25,26). As an alternative form of therapy, a 14-day course of amphotericin B and flucytosine (at standard dose regimens) followed by at least a 10 week course of fluconazole, 400 mg orally once daily, has been proposed (25,26). Treatment with a more prolonged course of fluconazole may be necessary. A fluconazole consolidation course may be associated with a reduced relapse rate (26). Treatment with intrathecal or intraventricular amphotericin B may be needed in severe cases. Although intraventricular amphotericin B given via an Ommaya reservoir is usually unnecessary, it results in earlier clearing of infection (27) and possibly reduced occurrence of relapse (21). The lipid formulations of amphotericin B are useful if the patient has underlying renal disease (25).

Initial therapy for cryptococcal meningitis in HIV-infected patients consists of amphotericin B with flucytosine at the same dose regimen as that used for treatment of non–HIV-infected patients (25,28,29). After successful initial therapy, maintenance therapy with fluconazole (200–400 mg orally, once daily) is begun and continued for the remainder of the patient's life (25,30). Patients who have been successfully treated with initial therapy for cryptococcal disease and have responded to HAART with a sustained elevation of their CD4 T-lymphocyte count above 100 to 200 cells/μL for greater than 6 months can discontinue maintenance therapy (31,32). The combination of fluconazole and flucytosine as well as the newer azole antifungal agents is investigational (33).

COCCIDIOIDOMYCOSIS

Coccidioides immitis is a common cause of fungal pulmonary disease in the southwestern United States, Mexico, and Central America. High skin test positivity rates in local residents indicate self-limited or subclinical infection in most persons. Meningitis may follow a prolonged latent period. Therefore, the diagnosis must be considered in a patient with a prior history of travel to an endemic area. Two thirds of patients have no risk factors for dissemination. One third of patients with meningitis are already known to have disease in other organs, but in two thirds the symptoms of meningitis are the presenting complaints (34).

Headache, lethargy, disorientation, confusion, and coma are common and may reflect the propensity of this organism to cause hydrocephalus. Constitutional manifestations are usually present. Nodular, ulcerative, and subcutaneous skin lesions should be sought. The chest radiograph is usually abnormal, but sputum and blood cultures are rarely positive. CSF cultures are positive in only one third of patients, and smears are rarely positive. Diagnosis rests on finding elevated titers of coccidioidal complement-fixing antibodies in serum or CSF (34). Skin testing may falsely elevate the titers and should not be used diagnostically. Hypoglycorrhachia is usually present, but the CSF profile is not distinguishable from that of other fungal or mycobacterial causes of chronic meningitis.

The standard initial therapy for *Coccidioides* meningitis is either fluconazole or itraconazole (35,36). For severe cases, intrathecal amphotericin B can be added (37). Placement of an Ommaya reservoir is preferable to minimize arachnoiditis. However, complications such as obstruction occur in up to 85% of reservoirs (34). Drug-induced arachnoiditis may limit treatment and also makes pleocytosis uninterpretable as a reliable indicator of therapeutic response. Therapeutic response can be assessed clinically and by the disappearance of CSF antibody. The relapse rate is high, and chronic therapy is frequently required.

INFREQUENT FUNGAL CAUSES

Less common fungal meningitides caused by *Candida* species, *Blastomyces dermatitidis*, *Histoplasma capsulatum*, and *Sporothrix schenckii* are associated with predominantly lymphocytic meningitis. The clinical presentation is indistinguishable from that of the previously discussed infections. Although dissemination with these organisms is rare, meningitis is common in disseminated disease. *Candida* is an exception as it disseminates often but is an unusual cause of meningitis. *Candida* meningitis can have an acute presentation and is found in debilitated hospitalized patients with central venous catheters receiving hyperalimentation or corticosteroids. Intravenous drug addicts and premature infants are also at risk (38). Most patients have received prior antibacterial therapy. CSF cultures are usually positive, with *Candida albicans* being the most frequent isolate. When cultures are negative, the diagnosis is rarely made antemortem. The role of serology has yet to be defined.

B. dermatitidis has been reported in the CNS in as many as 33% of patients with disseminated disease (39,40). A few patients with blastomycosis have concurrent disease due to *M. tuberculosis* or malignancy. Demonstrating the organism in skin, sputum, prostatic secretions, or joints makes the diagnosis. CSF cultures are rarely positive, and serology is unreliable (39,40). *Blastomyces* is an unusual pathogen in HIV-infected patients. However, disseminated blastomycosis in the setting of advanced HIV infection is frequently associated with CNS disease (41).

Histoplasma meningitis occurs in a population of patients similar to blastomycosis. Like cryptococcal meningitis, it may be present for years before detection. Culturing the organism from bone marrow, blood, liver, lymph nodes, sputum, or urine makes the diagnosis (42,43). One half of patients have positive CSF cultures. Detection of *H. capsulatum* polysaccharide antigen is also useful. Tests for antigen should be performed on CSF, blood, and urine (43). CSF antibodies are diagnostically useful, with a sensitivity of almost 90% (44); however, there is cross-reactivity with other fungi. CNS sporotrichosis is also rare. The organism is difficult to culture but local CSF antibody production can be used to make the diagnosis (45).

In all CNS fungal infections except for *Candida* infections, the diagnostic yield of cultures is thought to be augmented by sampling large volumes of CSF or by obtaining CSF from the ventricles. A mainstay of antemortem diagnosis is documentation of extraneural infection. Standard therapy is systemic amphotericin B, and the prognosis is related to the patient's status at the time of therapeutic intervention. Recently, liposomal amphotericin B has been reported to be more effective and less toxic than conventional amphotericin B in patients with acquired immunodeficiency syndrome who have disseminated histoplasmosis (46). Local therapy is usually unnecessary. If blastomycotic meningitis occurs as frequently as has been suggested, lumbar puncture will be necessary in all patients with blastomycosis, because azoles may not predictably treat asymptomatic subclinical meningitis. We currently do not recommend routine lumbar puncture in all patients with blastomycosis.

Patients with HIV infection usually use lifelong maintenance therapy to prevent relapse of disease caused by susceptible fungi. Itraconazole is effective therapy to prevent relapse in histoplasmosis (47). The preferred agent to prevent relapse in patients with blastomycosis or coccidioidomycosis remains to be determined. In patients with advanced HIV infection (≤50 CD4+ cells per mm³) who live in endemic areas, primary prophylaxis with azoles may be warranted (31).

Chronic Bacterial Meningitis

Chronic bacterial infections can mimic tuberculous and fungal meningitis. Meningitis with these infections may be more common than appreciated, because antibiotic therapy given for systemic manifestations in the absence of CSF examination may treat subclinical meningitis. If initial treatment is suboptimal for CNS infection, localized chronic infection can develop.

The classic manifestations of systemic brucellosis are night sweats, fever, adenopathy, and hepatosplenomegaly. Neural involvement occurs in less than 5% of patients. However, one third of patients with neurobrucellosis present with an isolated meningitis syndrome (48). Cranial nerve abnormalities, seizures, hydrocephalus, radiculopathy, and peripheral neuropathy are frequently present. The key to diagnosis is obtaining a history of exposure to unpasteurized dairy products, travel to an endemic area such as the Mediterranean or South or Central America, or previous infection (48). The CSF formula is abnormal but nonspecific. Hypoglycorrhachia and increased protein level are present in more than 90% of patients but do not narrow the differential diagnosis. Cultures of blood and CSF require special media and incubation of 2 to 4 weeks, and are usually negative. The diagnosis can be established by use of blood or CSF agglutination titers. Although brucellosis is rarely lethal, cure is difficult and usually requires two drugs for at least 6 weeks. Tetracycline or doxycycline with rifampin or streptomycin has been effective. Trimethoprim-sulfamethoxazole may also be effective.

Meningitis caused by *Francisella tularensis* is clinically similar to brucellosis meningitis but is rare. In the setting of chronic meningitis and an appropriate zoonotic exposure, the diagnosis should be attempted by culture or serology (49). The laboratory should be alerted of your concern to avoid potentially fatal pneumonia in a laboratory worker. The usual treatment is chloramphenicol. *Listeria monocytogenes* and *Neisseria meningitidis* cause acute meningitis in normal hosts. Rarely, they cause a chronic meningitis, possibly with lymphocytic preponderance, in the immunocompromised host. Isolation of one of these pathogens in association with a benign or prolonged disease course warrants an evaluation for occult immunodeficiency, for example, HIV infection with *Listeria* (50) or terminal complement deficiency with *N. meningitidis* (51). Bacterial encephalitis due to *Tropheryma whippelii* (Whipple's disease) or *Bartonella henselae* (cat-scratch disease) may cause chronic progressive neurologic deficits with minimal meningeal involvement. Because these disorders are treatable, diagnostic brain biopsy should be performed in patients with a compatible syndrome.

A prolonged clinical course may occur when meningeal irritation is due to the gradual expansion of a parameningeal focus. Patients manifest meningismus and a sterile CSF with pleocytosis. Purulent meningitis occurs if a parameningeal abscess ruptures into the subarachnoid space. The entire neuraxis needs to be evaluated with CT or magnetic resonance imaging (MRI) because spinal epidural (52) or subdural abscess can also cause CSF pleocytosis. Thorough evaluation includes investigation for dental (53), otic (54), and sinus disease.

Spirochetal Meningitis

All spirochetes have a neurotropism resulting in varied and numerous clinical manifestations (Table 150.3). After inoculation, these organisms disseminate hematogenously with meningeal seeding. Because host defenses have not yet developed, CSF cultures may be positive at a time when patients have no CSF pleocytosis, have other CSF abnormalities, or have only systemic manifestations. This occurs in 30% of patients with syphilis (55). Classic manifestations of secondary disease occur when an active host response develops. Relapses of secondary manifestations occur in syphilis and relapsing fever because *Treponema pallidum* and *Borrelia recurrentis* alter cell surface antigens, resulting in periodic development of an immune response to new antigens.

SYPHILIS

Meningitis may occur in all spirochetal infections. Syphilitic meningitis usually appears within 2 years of infection. The rash of secondary syphilis is present only 10% of the time (56). Fever may not be present. Abnormalities of cranial nerves VI, VII, and VIII are common. Patients may present with hydrocephalus in association with papilledema unrelated to optic neuritis (57). Syphilitic meningitis may be chronic, self-limited, or present as an acute medical emergency. A CSF pleocytosis with high protein and hypoglycorrhachia occurs, but the fluid characteristics may also mimic a viral process. The diagnosis is suggested by a positive serum treponemal test (e.g., fluorescent treponemal antibody absorption) and a positive CSF Venereal Disease Research Laboratory (VDRL) test result. Although the serum VDRL result is almost always positive in patients with active syphilitic meningitis, it may be negative in tertiary disease. Appropriate therapy is a 10- to 14-day course of high-dose penicillin G (18–24 million units per day intravenously) (58). With suboptimal therapy, symptoms may resolve while CNS infection persists. The development of tertiary complications, tabes dorsalis, general paresis, or gummata in a 10- to 30-year period can be considered sequelae of long-term chronic meningitis (59).

LYME DISEASE

Lyme disease, caused by *Borrelia burgdorferi*, is a cause of chronic meningitis. In Europe, Bannwarth's syndrome, or lymphocytic meningoradiculitis, is probably the same disease. About 15% of patients who contract Lyme disease develop symptomatic

TABLE 150.3.   Spirochetal Infections Commonly Associated with Neurologic Manifestations

Disease	Exposure	Primary lesion	Secondary neurologic manifestation	Tertiary neurologic manifestation
Syphilis	Sexual	Chancre	Meningitis	Meningovascular infarcts Tabes dorsalis General paresis
Lyme disease	*Ixodes* ticks (deer, mice, birds)	Erythema chronicum migrans	Meningitis	Multiple sclerosis-like syndrome Psychiatric changes Chronic fatigue syndrome
Leptospirosis Relapsing fever	Rodents, dogs Ticks, lice	Leptospiremia	Meningitis Meningitis	None None

meningitis (60). This occurs in the second stage of the disease, several months after tick exposure and initial infection; hence, there is preponderance in late summer and early fall. Patients usually present with headache. Two thirds have symptoms of radiculopathy, usually in a distribution associated with the antecedent tick bite. Cranial and peripheral nerve abnormalities are common, Bell's palsy being the most frequent (61).

Lyme disease should be considered in the differential diagnosis of any aseptic meningitis. Many patients cannot give a history of tick bite or the characteristic rash, erythema chronicum migrans. Therefore, history of exposure in an endemic area needs to be sought. The CSF formula varies widely. Most patients have CSF pleocytosis and elevated protein level; 15% have hypoglycorrhachia (61). A false-positive CSF VDRL test result can occur, but false-positive treponemal test results do not. Local CSF antibody production occurs, but serologic studies lack sensitivity. Twelve percent of patients are negative on tests from both serum and CSF (61). Early treatment may confound serodiagnosis without eradicating infection. The recommended treatment for patients with CNS disease is intravenous therapy with ceftriaxone, 2 g, once daily for 2 to 4 weeks. Intravenous penicillin G or cefotaxime are alternative antibiotics (62). Successful therapy with doxycycline has also been reported (63). It should be noted that the response to antimicrobial therapy might be slow. Repeat or prolonged therapy is generally not recommended. Later in the infection, patients may have other neurologic manifestations such as chronic fatigue or psychiatric symptoms (64) (Table 150.3). The pathogenesis of these symptoms is not well understood, but when present, meningeal symptoms or CSF pleocytosis is rare.

OTHER SPIROCHETES

Other spirochetal infections also present as acute or subacute meningitis. In 24% of patients hospitalized with Weil's disease, clinical meningitis occurs concomitantly with other systemic manifestations of leptospirosis (65). Dog, animal, or natural water exposures are the epidemiologic clues. Relapsing fever caused by *Borrelia recurrentis* is associated with CNS manifestations in 8% of tick-borne and 30% of louse-borne disease (66). Cranial nerve abnormalities are common. The CSF formula in both these conditions is similar to that observed in other spirochetal diseases. There are no chronic sequelae, and the illnesses are usually self-limiting. Both respond to appropriate treatment, but evidence that therapy alters long-term neurologic outcome is limited. Any spirochetal illness may be associated with a Jarisch-Herxheimer reaction. Patients should be closely observed for several hours after initiation of therapy.

Viral Central Nervous System Infection

Viral CNS infection usually presents as encephalitis or meningoencephalitis with altered levels of consciousness. CSF pleocytosis may be present. Although the CSF glucose level is usually normal, hypoglycorrhachia has been observed with mumps, lymphocytic choriomeningitis, and herpesvirus infection (67). What was previously considered slow virus disease, chronic viral infections causing kuru, or Creutzfeldt-Jakob disease is actually disease due to prions. Subacute sclerosing panencephalitis is a chronic infection due to abnormal measles virus. Human T-cell lymphotropic virus type I (68) and HIV (69) have become significant causes of encephalitis manifested by a chronic CSF pleocytosis without meningeal symptoms. Immune defects can predispose to chronic infection. Malignancy, organ transplantation, and acquired immunodeficiency syndrome have been associated with progressive multifocal leukoencephalopathy (70).

Agammaglobulinemia predisposes to chronic echovirus or coxsackievirus meningoencephalitis spanning months to years (71). Some of the above-mentioned diagnoses can be made serologically, but often brain biopsy is necessary. Biopsy is generally diagnostic if directed toward regions of abnormality as seen by electroencephalography or MRI. Blind biopsy has a low yield.

Central Nervous System Infection Due to Protozoa

Protozoa as a cause of a chronic meningitis syndrome are unusual. Protozoa that are associated with central nervous system disease usually cause meningoencephalitis or CNS mass lesions.

In an immunocompromised patient, *Toxoplasma gondii* causes a meningoencephalitis, usually associated with multiple mass lesions in the brain. A lymphocytic pleocytosis may be present in the CSF. CSF IgG antibodies may be helpful in securing the diagnosis. Free-living amebae are associated with a meningoencephalitis syndrome. *Naegleria* meningoencephalitis, associated with freshwater exposure, runs an acute fulminant course. Disseminated *Acanthamoeba* may cause a chronic meningoencephalitis syndrome in an immunocompromised patient. Evidence of *Acanthamoeba* is usually seen elsewhere in the body, particularly in the skin. *Entamoeba histolytica* is associated with a brain abscess. West African trypanosomiasis can cause a chronic meningoencephalitis. An important clue to this diagnosis is travel or residence in the endemic area.

Carcinomatous Meningitis

Chronic meningitis occurs without infection. Metastatic malignancy presenting as meningitis before detection of the primary tumor occurs with carcinoma of the breast and lung, lymphoma, and melanoma. Leukemic infiltration also occurs, especially in acute lymphocytic leukemia. Clinical suspicion is increased by noncontiguous focal deficits suggestive of multiple areas of involvement, and by a greater severity of signs and symptoms (72). Headache, change in mental status, and back or radicular pain are frequently observed. Fever is rare. On presentation, 52% of patients have mental status changes and 60% have absent reflexes in an extremity (72). Cranial nerve abnormalities and pareses are common. The CSF formula is nondiagnostic. Pleocytosis may be absent but the profile is rarely normal. Elevation of CSF lactate dehydrogenase is suggestive of malignancy (73). Cytology is positive in half of initial lumbar punctures, and examining multiple specimens increases the yield to 80%. The yield in CSF lymphoma is much lower. Imaging studies demonstrate lesions corresponding to cranial or spinal nerve deficits. CT, MRI, and metrizamide myelography are the procedures of choice. Long-term prognosis is poor, but neurologic function can be improved with treatment (74).

Meningitis due to Disorders of Unknown Etiology

SARCOIDOSIS

Sarcoidosis has neurologic manifestations in 5% to 15% of cases, and in half of these they are the presenting manifestations (75). Bell's palsy or other cranial nerve deficits are typical. Decreased visual acuity, hydrocephalus, diabetes insipidus, and seizures may occur. Single or multiple brain masses can involve any area of the neuraxis. When granulomatous involvement of the basal meninges predominates, the disease is indistinguishable from tuberculous meningitis (76). There is chest or eye involvement in 88% and 55% of patients, respectively (75). The CSF findings are normal in half of the patients with neurologic signs or symptoms.

Hypoglycorrhachia is associated with diffuse meningeal sarcoidosis (77). CSF eosinophilia has been reported with neurosarcoidosis (77).

Diagnosis is by exclusion of infectious and neoplastic diseases and demonstration of noncaseating granulomata on biopsy. Extraneural tissues such as lung, lymph nodes, conjunctiva, or liver are usually available for biopsy. With isolated CNS disease, the diagnosis may require biopsy of abnormal areas detected by head CT or MRI. Peripheral or spinal nerve biopsy results may be positive. Elevation of serum angiotensin-converting enzyme is characteristic but not pathognomonic. Steroids are recommended in neurosarcoidosis, although the response to therapy is variable. Controlled studies of steroids have not been reported. Because of the similarity of sarcoidosis, tuberculosis, and fungal meningitis, steroids should not be given until these other diagnoses have been excluded (77,78).

SYSTEMIC VASCULITIS

Systemic vasculitides, with the exception of giant cell arteritis, have caused meningeal inflammation with abnormal CSF. Symptoms and signs are usually due to focal ischemia or infarction, but diffuse meningoencephalitis also occurs (79). Polyarteritis nodosa is characterized by peripheral neuropathies. Hepatitis B surface antigen is present in at least 15% of patients. Muscle biopsy, sural nerve biopsy, or renal angiography may establish the diagnosis (80). In contrast, Wegener granulomatosis, lymphomatoid granulomatosis, isolated CNS angiitis, and granulomatous angiitis have cranial nerve or focal findings. However, clinical overlap is great. In suspected Wegener's and lymphomatoid granulomatosis, head CT frequently reveals hypodense lesions consistent with infarction (79). A thorough search must be made for the expected sites of extraneural disease: lungs, sinuses, and kidneys. If no extraneural disease is present, cerebral angiography will be necessary. A beaded pattern is characteristic (81). Caution is necessary because many infectious diseases previously discussed can cause a similar arteriographic pattern. If the evaluation is not diagnostic, brain biopsy will be necessary before making a decision to initiate steroids or cytotoxic therapy (79). During treatment, patients must be monitored for the emergence of disseminated tuberculosis or fungal infection.

Collagen-vascular disease can present with CNS vasculitis associated with CSF pleocytosis (82). Complement levels, circulating immune complexes, and serologic evaluation for systemic lupus erythematosus, Sjögren's syndrome, and rheumatoid arthritis should be performed. CNS vasculitis has also been present in cat-scratch disease, herpes encephalitis, and Hodgkin's disease. Atrial myxoma and subacute bacterial endocarditis may be associated with immune complex disease and vasculitis. Blood cultures, electrocardiography, and cardiac ultrasonography are warranted to evaluate these processes.

BEHÇET'S DISEASE

Behçet's disease usually manifests as the triad of oral and genital ulcers, skin lesions, and uveitis. Twenty-five percent of patients develop meningoencephalitis. Neurologic symptoms are nonspecific but are almost always associated with a flare-up of oral or genital ulcers (83). These lesions are frequently asymptomatic, necessitating a thorough examination. Ophthalmologic findings occur later in the disease. The CSF usually shows a pleocytosis and increased protein level, even in patients without neurologic symptoms. The CSF glucose value is normal. The clinical course is notable for episodes of deterioration, sometimes acute, alternating with periods of stability but not spontaneous resolution (83). Most manifestations improve with corticosteroid or cytotoxic therapy.

VOGT-KOYANAGI-HARADA SYNDROME

Vogt-Koyanagi-Harada syndrome is a rare disease characterized by meningoencephalitis, skin lesions, and uveitis. People with darker pigmentation appear more susceptible. Photophobia, headache, ocular pain, bilateral visual impairment, and intracranial hypertension are common (84). The ophthalmic and neurologic symptoms usually present within days of each other and persist for several weeks. Sensorineural deafness, diabetes insipidus, or other focal findings usually follow meningitis (85). Alopecia, poliosis (whitened eyebrows and lashes), and vitiligo occur in one third of patients and also typically follow the meningitis (84). The severity of sequelae does not correlate with the severity of the initial symptoms. On presentation, 81% of patients have a CSF pleocytosis. The diagnosis is primarily clinical but is supported by the ophthalmologic findings of granular inflammation of the iris, ciliary body, and retina. Treatment is with corticosteroids or cytotoxic drugs.

NEUTROPHILIC PREDOMINANCE

Chronic neutrophilic meningitis is a syndrome with persistent CSF neutrophils for greater than 1 week, negative bacterial cultures, and no response to routine antibacterial therapy (86). Prolonged CSF neutrophilic pleocytosis is occasionally seen in patients with more typical lymphocytic meningeal processes, including candidiasis (38), brucellosis, tuberculosis, blastomycosis, histoplasmosis, and coccidioidomycosis (Table 150.2). This usually occurs early in the illness but can be perpetuated by treatment (87). However, several chronic meningitides are associated with a preponderance of CSF neutrophils throughout the course of the illness.

Bacterial Meningitis

Actinomyces and *Nocardia* species are bacterial causes of this syndrome. Actinomycosis usually occurs in a normal host with a portal of entry (88). The source is typically the mouth, where the organism is normal flora. There may be an otic focus. A primary pulmonary process may result from aspiration. CNS involvement occurs by direct invasion or hematogenous seeding. Although typically associated with abscess formation, 13% of neural actinomycosis was found to be meningitis or meningoencephalitis (88).

In the absence of trauma, nervous system nocardiosis is associated with disseminated disease in normal patients or those with depressed cell-mediated immunity, typically after transplantation or steroid therapy. Persons with pulmonary alveolar proteinosis, Cushing's disease, and systemic lupus erythematosus are at specific risk. As with actinomycosis, intracerebral abscess formation is a classic finding and should be prospectively sought with CNS imaging studies. Isolated meningitis does occur and the diagnosis can be made by CSF culture (89).

FUNGAL MENINGITIS

Fungal causes of neutrophilic pleocytosis typically present in an indolent fashion. The fungal diseases that typically present with a neutrophilic predominance include *Aspergillus* infections, *Zygomycetes*, and *Pseudallescheria boydii* infections. CNS infection caused by *Aspergillus* species is usually associated with disseminated disease in a neutropenic patient. Zygomycosis (mucormycosis) is associated with oral, nasal, or facial disease in a diabetic or acidotic host. Altered mental status, stroke syndromes, or symptoms due to space-occupying lesions are the typical presentation. There may be meningitis without mass effect, particularly if they follow surgery of the neural axis (86). *P. boydii* and other dematiaceous fungi can also cause meningitis without a demonstrable brain mass (90). These are common soil fungi inoculated after penetrating injuries to the cranial vault or orbit. Disseminated disease occurs in immunosuppressed persons, typically renal or bone marrow transplant recipients. *P. boydii* is important to consider, as patients do not respond predictably to amphotericin B (91). Treatment with miconazole has been associated with successful outcomes (91). More recently, there have been successful treatment outcomes of both *P. boydii* meningitis and brain abscess with voriconazole (92,93). Difficulty in establishing disease caused by these fungi is related to the low yield of CSF culture and a lack of sensitive or specific serologic tests (86). Diagnoses can be made by isolating the organism from an extraneural site such as sinuses, ears, lungs, or wounds. Skin lesions should be sought and biopsies performed. A search for mass lesions along the neuraxis should be done with CT and MRI. If a lesion is seen, surgery will likely be required for diagnosis and therapy.

VIRAL MENINGITIS

A cytomegalovirus (CMV)-induced polyradiculopathy in patients with advanced HIV infection presents with weakness and sensory loss coupled with a neutrophilic predominant CSF (94,95). The diagnosis can be confirmed with viral cultures. PCR techniques are useful in establishing the diagnosis quickly. Early treatment with ganciclovir may be beneficial (96). The incidence of CMV disease associated with HIV infection has declined markedly with increased use of HAART (97).

DRUG-INDUCED MENINGITIS

Meningitis associated with systemic medications is usually neutrophilic and acute in onset. Common causes include isoniazid, sulfonamides, γ-globulin, and OKT3 monoclonal antibody. Patients with underlying collagen-vascular disease, especially mixed connective tissue disease, appear predisposed to this syndrome associated with nonsteroidal antiinflammatory agents. Occasionally, the disease course is subacute or chronic. Chronic neutrophilic meningitis is more typical when due to contrast myelography or methylprednisolone injections (76). Other substances used in intrathecal injection, such as antibiotics, methotrexate, or contaminating disinfectants, have also caused neutrophilic meningitis.

EOSINOPHILIC PREDOMINANCE

Eosinophilic meningitis is rare (98) (Table 150.2). Peripheral and CSF eosinophilia is well described in coccidioidomycosis. While described with mycobacterial, other fungal, and noninfectious causes of chronic meningitis, helminthic infections predominate within this differential diagnosis. Worldwide, the most frequent cause is *Angiostrongylus cantonensis*, the rat lung worm. This is acquired by ingesting raw fish, mollusks, and snails in the Far East and Pacific Islands, including Hawaii (99). Patients present subacutely with symptoms of meningitis and fever without other findings. The diagnosis is primarily clinical, based on CSF eosinophilia with an appropriate exposure history. Serologic tests are being developed (99). In Southeast Asia, *Gnathostoma spinigerum* also presents as eosinophilic meningitis but in association with painful radiculopathy, subarachnoid hemorrhage, and symptoms of visceral and cutaneous larva migrans (100).

Cysticercosis is the other parasitic infection that usually presents with isolated CNS findings. Seizures or symptoms associated with increased intracranial pressure and space-occupying lesions are classic, but meningitis occurs (101). Eosinophilia is present in half of early inflammatory cases and is helpful in suggesting the diagnosis if there has been exposure in an endemic region. The characteristic lesions are usually present at CT or MRI. Diagnosis is assisted by serology (102). Even with space-occupying lesions, the prognosis is good if hydrocephalus is not present. Praziquantel and albendazole have been shown to be efficacious (103). Steroids are used at the onset of therapy when there are ocular or intraventricular cysts.

Other parasitic infections associated with eosinophilic meningitis usually have manifestations outside the CNS, and the diagnosis is based on extraneural identification. Fresh stool for ova and parasite examination should be obtained on at least three occasions when a patient has unexplained CSF eosinophilia. Despite an absence of eosinophilia, parasites such as *Schistosoma*, *Paragonimus westermani*, and *Echinococcus* warrant consideration if patients with unexplained chronic meningitis have traveled to endemic regions. In immunocompromised patients, disseminated strongyloidiasis and strongyloides meningitis occur without eosinophilia (104). Strongyloidiasis should be considered as a source of persistent or relapsing gram-negative bacteremia or gram-negative bacterial meningitis.

APPROACH TO THE PATIENT

Despite a thorough evaluation for CNS or extraneural diseases, a pathogen will not be identified in 30% to 50% of patients with subacute or chronic meningitis (4). Many patients respond to empiric antituberculous treatment, particularly children and patients from endemic areas (4). In a normal host, CSF lymphocytosis with hypoglycorrhachia should prompt therapy for tuberculosis until an alternative diagnosis is established. In a patient with an underlying cellular immunodeficiency, this CSF formula is more likely to be caused by cryptococcal disease. Undiagnosed patients with CSF pleocytosis and without spontaneous resolution of symptoms may receive empirical treatment with antituberculous therapy, even in the absence of hypoglycorrhachia. Empirical therapy should be continued until an alternative diagnosis is established or cultures are negative and the patient has not responded clinically. Initiation of empiric therapy should not delay continued diagnostic evaluation. This includes CT or MRI of the entire neural axis, cerebral angiography if vasculitis is suspected, and, when feasible, brain biopsy of any lesions seen on these studies. Blind biopsy has a much lower yield and is not generally recommended (2,4). If the patient progresses on antituberculous therapy, empiric intravenous amphotericin B should be initiated if there has been a previous exposure to an area endemic for histoplasmosis, blastomycosis, or coccidioidomycosis. Negative serologic evaluation does not preclude a trial of amphotericin B. At least several weeks are needed to assess a response. Combinations of empirical therapy become confusing when a beneficial response occurs. In the presence of clinical improvement, empiric antibiotics should be continued for a full course unless a definitive alternative diagnosis is made.

Trials of steroids may be warranted in the progressively declining patient, but we rarely recommend their empirical use, and then only when the patient is simultaneously receiving antituberculous treatment and amphotericin B. Patients with undiagnosed tuberculosis and fungal infections may progress despite a transient clinical response or improved CSF pleocytosis associated with steroid therapy. Patients with diseases requiring steroid therapy may need indefinite treatment to prevent relapse. More likely they will subsequently tolerate steroid tapering and withdrawal (4).

Some patients may have chronic benign lymphocytic meningitis. This entity consists of minimal localizing symptoms, normal CSF glucose value, and a lymphocytic pleocytosis that gradually decreases and resolves without therapy (105). The cause is presumed to be similar to other aseptic meningitides, but with a prolonged resolution. This diagnosis of exclusion can be made only if the patient has recovered without receiving antimicrobial therapy and has had an exhaustive diagnostic evaluation. If a patient has already received antibiotics, a full course will be necessary because a therapeutic response is indistinguishable from this benign self-limited condition.

RECURRENT MENINGITIS

Recurrent meningitis is a distinct syndrome in which episodes are separated by asymptomatic periods with normal CSF. Recurrent infection with *N. meningiditis* suggests a terminal complement deficiency. Skin flora such as *Staphylococcus epidermidis* or *Propionibacterium acnes* suggests an epidermal fistula. Recurrent *Streptococcus pneumoniae* (106) or *Haemophilus influenzae* (107) meningitis suggests a CSF communication to the ears or nasopharynx. Localization of CSF leaks may require an arduous search by metrizamide cisternography, radioiodinated albumin studies, technetium scans with pledgets in the nose and ears, gadolinium MRI, or any combination of these. Other infectious causes of recurrent meningitis include *Brucella, M. tuberculosis, Cryptococcus,* viruses, and hydatid cysts. Noninfectious diseases include migraine, systemic lupus erythematosus, sarcoidosis, Behçet's disease, and Vogt-Koyanagi-Harada syndrome (108). The intermittent rupture of a dermoid cyst or intracranial tumor can cause an episodic sterile reactive meningitis, which is usually neutrophilic and diagnosed only by thorough physical examination, CT, or MRI. The CSF cholesterol may be elevated when a cyst ruptures into the subarachnoid space.

Mollaret's meningitis is a condition frequently considered a chronic meningitis but one that actually has a recurrent presentation. The onset is abrupt and includes transient focal neurologic findings such as seizures, delirium, cranial nerve dysfunction, and abnormal reflexes (108). The CSF is characterized by pleocytosis, including cells termed "endothelial" by Mollaret but that are actually large monocytes. Both the symptoms and the CSF abnormalities resolve in several days with or without treatment. The cause is unknown, but patients have been reported with polymerase chain reaction evidence of herpes simplex virus type 1 and, more commonly, herpes simplex virus type 2 (109,110). Indeed, herpes simplex virus is the most common cause of relapsing lymphocytic meningitis. Acyclovir should be given for acute treatment and possibly for prophylaxis. Further study is needed (110).

REFERENCES

1. Ellner JJ, Bennett JE: Chronic meningitis. *Medicine (Baltimore)* 1976;55: 341–369.
2. Wilhelm C, Ellner JJ. Chronic meningitis. *Neurol Clin* 1986;4:115–141.
3. Swartz MN. "Chronic meningitis"—many causes to consider. *N Engl J Med* 1987;317:957–959.
4. Anderson NE, Willoughby EW. Chronic meningitis without predisposing illness—a review of 83 cases. *Q J Med* 1987;63:283–295.
5. Klein NC, Damsker B, Hirschman SZ. Mycobacterial meningitis: retrospective analysis from 1970 to 1983. *Am J Med* 1985;79:29–34.
6. Kennedy DH, Fallon RJ. Tuberculous meningitis. *JAMA* 1979;241:264–268.
7. Lincoln EM, Gilbert LA. Diseases in children due to mycobacteria other than *Mycobacterium tuberculosis. Am Rev Respir Dis* 1972;105:683–714.
8. Benson CA. Disease due to the *Mycobacterium avium* complex in patients with AIDS: epidemiology and clinical syndrome. *Clin Infect Dis* 1994;18(suppl 3):S218–S222.
9. Ogawa SK, Smith MA, Brenuessel DJ, et al. Tuberculous meningitis in an urban medical center. *Medicine (Baltimore)* 1987;66:317–326.
10. Root TE, Harris AA, Levin S. Diagnosis and treatment of tuberculous and fungal meningitis. In: Klawans HL, ed. *Clinical neuropharmacology.* Vol. 2. New York: Raven, 1977:151–177.
11. Lepper MH, Spies HW. The present status of the treatment of tuberculosis of the central nervous system. *Ann N Y Acad Sci* 1963;106:106–123.
12. Peterson EM, Lu R, Floyd C, et al. Direct identification of *Mycobacterium tuberculosis, Mycobacterium avium,* and *Mycobacterium intracellulare* from amplified primary cultures in BACTEC media using DNA probes. *J Clin Microbiol* 1989;27:1542–1547.
13. Bonington A, Strang JIG, Klapper PE, et al. Use of Roche AMPLICOR *Mycobacterium tuberculosis* PCR in early diagnosis of tuberculosis meningitis. *J Clin Microbiol* 1998;36:1251–1254.
14. Sumi MG, Mathai A, Ruben S, et al. A comparative evaluation of dot immunobinding assay (Dot-Iba) and polymerase chain reaction (PCR) for the laboratory diagnosis of tuberculosis meningitis. *Diagn Microbiol Infect Dis* 2002;42:35–38.
15. Hinman AR. Tuberculous meningitis at Cleveland Metropolitan General Hospital, 1959 to 1963. *Am Rev Respir Dis* 1967;95:670–673.
16. Steiner P, Portugaleza C. Tuberculous meningitis in children. *Am Rev Respir Dis* 1973;107:22–29.
17. Freiman I, Geefhuysen J. Evaluation of intrathecal therapy with streptomycin and hydrocortisone in tuberculous meningitis. *J Pediatr* 1970;76:895–901.
18. Leiguarda R, Berthier M, Starkstein S, et al. Ischemic infarction in 25 children with tuberculous meningitis. *Stroke* 1988;19:200–204.
19. O'Toole RD, Thornton GF, et al. Dexamethasone in tuberculous meningitis. *Ann Intern Med* 1969;70:39–47.
20. Bulloch MR, Van Dellen JR. The role of cerebrospinal fluid shunting in tuberculous meningitis. *Surg Neurol* 1982;18:274–277.
21. Stockstill MT, Kauffman CA. Comparison of cryptococcal and tuberculous meningitis. *Arch Neurol* 1983;40:81–85.
22. Snow RM, Dismukes WE. Cryptococcal meningitis: diagnostic value of cryptococcal antigen in cerebrospinal fluid. *Arch Intern Med* 1975;134: 1155–1157.
23. Butler WT, Alling DW, Spickard A, et al. Diagnostic and prognostic value of clinical and laboratory findings in cryptococcal meningitis. *N Engl J Med* 1964;270:59–67.
24. Dismukes WE, Cloud G, Gallis HA, et al. Treatment of cryptococcal meningitis with combination amphotericin B and flucytosine for four as compared with six weeks. *N Engl J Med* 1987;317:334–341.
25. Saag MS, Graybill JR, Larsen RA, et al. Practice guidelines for the management of cryptococcal disease. *Clin Infect Dis* 2000;30:710–718.
26. Pappas PG, Perfect JR, Cloud GA, et al. Cryptococcosis in human immunodeficiency virus-negative patients in the era of effective azole therapy. *Clin Infect Dis* 2001;33:690–699.
27. Polsky B, Depman MR, Gold JWM, et al. Intraventricular therapy of cryptococcal meningitis via a subcutaneous reservoir. *Am J Med* 1986;81:24–28.
28. Larsen RA, Leal MAE, Chan LS. Fluconazole compared with amphotericin B plus flucytosine for cryptococcal meningitis in AIDS: a randomized trial. *Ann Intern Med* 1990;113:183–187.
29. Saag MS, Powderly WG, Cloud GC, et al. Comparison of amphotericin B with fluconazole in the treatment of acute AIDS-associated cryptococcal meningitis. *N Engl J Med* 1992;326:83–89.
30. Powderly WG, Saag MS, Cloud GA, et al. A controlled trial of fluconazole or amphotericin B to prevent relapse of cryptococcal meningitis in patients with the acquired immunodeficiency syndrome. *N Engl J Med* 1992;326: 793–798.
31. Centers for Disease Control and Prevention. Guidelines for preventing opportunistic infections among HIV-infected persons—2002. *MMWR* 2002;51:1–51.
32. Aberg JA, Price RW, Heeren DM, et al. A pilot study of the discontinuation of antifungal therapy for disseminated cryptococcal disease in patients with acquired immunodeficiency syndrome following immunologic response to antiretroviral therapy. *J Infect Dis* 2002;185:1179–1182.
33. Larsen RA, Bozzette SA, Jones BE, et al. Fluconazole combined with flucytosine for treatment of cryptococcal meningitis in patients with AIDS. *Clin Infect Dis* 1994;19:741–745.
34. Bouza E, Dreyer JS, Hewitt WL, et al. Coccidioidal meningitis: an analysis of thirty-one cases and review of the literature. *Medicine (Baltimore)* 1981;60: 139–172.
35. Galgiani JN, Ampel NM, Catanzaro A, et al. Practice guidelines for the treatment of coccidioidomycosis. *Clin Infect Dis* 2000;30:658–661.
36. Deresinski SC. Coccidioidomycosis: efficacy of new agents and future prospects. *Curr Opin Infect Dis* 2001;14:693–696.
37. Labadie EL, Hamilton RH. Survival improvement in coccidioidal meningitis by high-dose intrathecal amphotericin B. *Arch Intern Med* 1986;146: 2013–2018.
38. Bayer AS, Edwards JE, Seidrl JS, et al. *Candida* meningitis: report of seven cases and review of the English literature. *Medicine (Baltimore)* 1976;55:477–486.
39. Kravitz GR, Davies SF, Eckman MR, et al. Chronic blastomycotic meningitis. *Am J Med* 1981;71:501–505.
40. Gonyea EF. The spectrum of primary blastomycotic meningitis: a review of central nervous system blastomycosis. *Ann Neurol* 1978;3:26–39.
41. Pappas PG, Pottage JC Jr, Powderly WG, et al. Blastomycosis in patients with the acquired immunodeficiency syndrome. *Ann Intern Med* 1992;116: 847–853.

42. Karalakulasingam R, Arora KK, Adams G, et al. Meningoencephalitis caused by *Histoplasma capsulatum. Arch Intern Med* 1976;136:217–220.

43. Wheat LJ, Batteiger BE, Sathapatayavongs B. *Histoplasma capsulatum* infections of the central nervous system: a clinical review. *Medicine (Baltimore)* 1990;69:244–260.

44. Wheat LJ, French M, Batteiger B, et al. Cerebrospinal fluid histoplasma antibodies in central nervous system histoplasmosis. *Arch Intern Med* 1985;145:1237–1240.

45. Scott NE, Kaufman L, Brown AC, et al. Serologic studies in the diagnosis and management of meningitis due to *Sporothrix schenckii. N Engl J Med* 1987;317:935–940.

46. Johnson PC, Wheat LJ, Cloud GA, et al. Safety and efficacy of liposomal amphotericin B compared with conventional amphotericin B for induction therapy of histoplasmosis in patients with AIDS. *Ann Intern Med* 2002;137:105–109.

47. Wheat LJ, Hafner R, Wulfsohn M, et al. Prevention of relapse of histoplasmosis with itraconazole in patients with the acquired immunodeficiency syndrome. *Ann Intern Med* 1993;118:610–616.

48. Bouza E, de la Torre MG, Parras F, et al. Brucellar meningitis. *Rev Infect Dis* 1987;9:810–822.

49. Lovell VM, Cho CT, Lindsey NJ, et al. *Francisella tularensis* meningitis: a rare clinical entity. *J Infect Dis* 1986;154:916–918.

50. Harvey RL, Chandrasekar PH. Chronic meningitis caused by *Listeria* in a patient infected with human immunodeficiency virus. *J Infect Dis* 1988;157:1091–1092.

51. Rosen MS, Lorber B, Myer AR. Chronic meningococcal meningitis: an association with C5 deficiency. *Arch Intern Med* 1988;148:1441–1442.

52. Danner RL, Hartman BJ. Update of spinal epidural abscess: 35 cases and review of the literature. *Rev Infect Dis* 1987;9:265–274.

53. Hedstrom SA, Nord CE, Ursing B. Chronic meningitis in patients with dental infections. *Scand J Infect Dis* 1980;12:117–121.

54. Habib RG, Girgis NI, Abu El Ella AH, et al. The treatment and outcome of intracranial infection of otogenic origin. *J Trop Med Hyg* 1988;91:83–86.

55. Lukehart SA, Hook EW. Invasion of the central nervous system by *Treponema pallidum*: Implications for diagnosis and treatment. *Ann Intern Med* 1988;109:855–862.

56. Simon RP. Neurosyphilis. *Arch Neurol* 1985;42:606–613.

57. Trenholme GM, Harris AA. Syphilitic meningitis with papilledema. *South Med J* 1977;70:1013–1014.

58. Centers for Disease Control and Prevention. Sexually transmitted diseases treatment guidelines 2002. *MMWR* 2002;51(RRG):1–79.

59. Hotson JR. Modern neurosyphilis: a partially treated chronic meningitis. *West J Med* 1981;135:191–200.

60. Pachner AR. Spirochetal diseases of the CNS. *Neurol Clin* 1986;4:207–222.

61. Stierstedt G, Gustafsson R. Clinical manifestations and diagnosis of neuroborreliosis. *Ann N Y Acad Sci* 1988;539:46–55.

62. Wormser GP, Nadelman RB, Dattwyler RJ, et al. Practice guidelines for the treatment of Lyme disease. *Clin Infect Dis* 2000;31(suppl 1):51–54.

63. Dotevall L, Hagberg L. Successful oral doxycycline treatment of Lyme disease–associated facial palsy and meningitis. *Clin Infect Dis* 1999;28:569–574.

64. Finkel MF. Lyme disease and its neurologic complications. *Arch Neurol* 1988;45:99–104.

65. Lecour H, Miranda M. Human leptospirosis—a review of 50 cases. *Infection* 1989;17:8–12.

66. Southern PM, Sanford JP. Relapsing fever: a clinical and microbiologic review. *Medicine (Baltimore)* 1969;48:129–149.

67. Fishman RA. Cerebrospinal fluid in diseases of the nervous system. Philadelphia: WB Saunders, 1980:269–272.

68. Yokota T, Yamada M, Furukawa T, et al. HTLV-I associated meningitis. *J Neurol* 1988;235:129–130.

69. McArthur JC, Cohen BA, Farzedegan H, et al. Cerebrospinal fluid abnormalities in homosexual men with and without neuropsychiatric findings. *Ann Neurol* 1988;23(suppl):34–37.

70. Richardson EP. Progressive multifocal leukoencephalopathy 30 years later. *N Engl J Med* 1988;318:315–317.

71. McKinney RE, Katz SL, Wilfert CM. Chronic enteroviral meningoencephalitis in agammaglobulinemic patients. *Rev Infect Dis* 1987;9:334–356.

72. Olson ME, Chernik NL, Posner JB. Infiltration of the leptomeninges by systemic cancer. *Arch Neurol* 1974;30:122–137.

73. Twijnstra A, Van Zanten AP, Hart AAM, et al. Serial lumbar and ventricle cerebrospinal fluid lactate dehydrogenase activities in patients with leptomeningeal metastases from solid and haematological tumours. *J Neurol Neurosurg Psychiatry* 1987;50:313–320.

74. Wasserstrom WR, Glass JP, Posner JB. Diagnosis and treatment of leptomeningeal metastases from solid tumors: experience with 90 patients. *Cancer* 1982;49:759–772.

75. Stern BJ, Krumholz A, Johns C, et al. Sarcoidosis and its neurological manifestations. *Arch Neurol* 1985;42:909–917.

76. Reik L. Disorders that mimic CNS infections. *Neurol Clin* 1986;4:223–248.

77. Vinas FC, Rengachary S. Diagnosis and management of neurosarcoidosis. *J Clin Neurosci* 2001;8:505–513.

78. Cahill DW, Salcman M. Neurosarcoidosis: a review of the rarer manifestations. *Surg Neurol* 1981;15:204–211.

79. Moore PM, Cupps TR. Neurological complications of vasculitis. *Ann Neurol* 1983;14:155–167.

80. Smith C, Rae SA, Berry H. Polyarteritis nodosa presenting as meningoencephalitis. *J R Soc Med* 1987;80:704–705.

81. Calabrese LH, Malleh JA. Primary angiitis of the central nervous system: report of 8 new cases, review of the literature, and proposal for diagnostic criteria. *Medicine (Baltimore)* 1988;67:20–39.

82. Sigal LH. The neurologic presentation of vasculitic and rheumatologic syndromes: a review. *Medicine (Baltimore)* 1987;66:157–180.

83. Alema G. Behçet's disease. In: Vinken RJ, Bruyn GW, Klawans HL, eds. *Handbook of clinical neurology.* Vol. 34. Amsterdam: Elsevier, 1978:475–512.

84. Manor RS. Vogt-Koyanagi-Harada syndrome and related diseases. In: Vinken PJ, Bruyn GW, Klawans HL, eds. *Handbook of clinical neurology.* Vol. 34. Amsterdam: Elsevier, 1978:513–544.

85. Pattison EM. Uveomeningoencephalitis syndrome (Vogt-Koyanagi-Harada). *Arch Neurol* 1965;12:197–205.

86. Peacock JE, McGinnis MR, Cohen MS. Persistent neutrophilic meningitis: report of four cases and review of the literature. *Medicine (Baltimore)* 1984;63:379–395.

87. Teoh R, O'Mahony G, Yeung VTF. Polymorphonuclear pleocytosis in the cerebrospinal fluid during chemotherapy for tuberculous meningitis. *J Neurol* 1986;233:237–241.

88. Smego RA. Actinomycosis of the central nervous system. *Rev Infect Dis* 1987;9:855–865.

89. Buggy BP. *Nocardia asteroides* meningitis without brain abscess. *Rev Infect Dis* 1987;9:228–231.

90. Kershaw P, Freeman R, Templeton D, et al. *Pseudallescheria boydii* infection of the central nervous system. *Arch Neurol* 1990;47:468–472.

91. Lutwick LI, Rytel MW, Yanez JP, et al. Deep infections from *Petriellidium boydii* treated with miconazole. *JAMA* 1979;241:272–273.

92. Nesky MA, McDougal EC, Peacock Jr JE. *Pseudallescheria boydii* brain abscess successfully treated with voriconazole and surgical drainage: case report and literature review of central nervous system Pseudallescheriasis. *Clin Infect Dis* 2000;31:673–677.

93. Poza G, Montoya J, Redondo C, et al. Meningitis caused by *Pseudallescheria boydii* treated with voriconazole. *Clin Infect Dis* 2000;30:981–982.

94. Behar R, Wiley C, McCutchan JA. Cytomegalovirus polyradiculopathy in acquired immunodeficiency syndrome. *Neurology* 1987;37:557–561.

95. Said G, LaCroix C, Chemouilli P, et al. Cytomegalovirus neuropathy in acquired immunodeficiency syndrome: a clinical and pathological study. *Ann Neurol* 1989;29:139–146.

96. Miller RG, Storey J, Greco C. Ganciclovir treatment of lumbosacral polyradiculopathy in AIDS. *Lancet* 1990;334:48–49.

97. Baril L, Jouan M, Agher R, et al. Impact of highly active antiretroviral therapy on the onset of *Mycobacterium avium* complex infection and cytomegalovirus in patients with AIDS. *AIDS* 2000;14:2593–2596.

98. Kuberski T. Eosinophils in the cerebrospinal fluid. *Ann Intern Med* 1979;91:70–75.

99. Koo J, Pien F, Kliks MM. *Angiostrongylus (Parastrongylus)* eosinophilic meningitis. *Rev Infect Dis* 1988;10:1155–1161.

100. Schmutzhard E, Boongird P, Vejjajiva A. Eosinophilic meningitis and radiculomyelitis in Thailand, caused by CNS invasion of *Gnathostoma spinigerum* and *Angiostrongylus catonensis. J Neurol Neurosurg Psychiatry* 1988;51:80–87.

101. Sotelo J, Guerrero V, Rubio F. Neurocysticercosis: a new classification based on active and inactive forms: a study of 753 cases. *Arch Intern Med* 1985;145:442–445.

102. Scharf D. Neurocysticercosis: two hundred thirty-eight cases from a California hospital. *Arch Neurol* 1988;45:777–780.

103. Takayangni OM, Jardim E. Therapy for neurocysticercosis: comparison between albendazole and praziquantel. *Arch Neurol* 1992;49:290–294.

104. Belani A, Leptrone D, Shands JW. *Strongyloides* meningitis. *South Med J* 1987;80:916–918.

105. Hopkins AP, Harvey PKP. Benign chronic lymphocytic meningitis. *J Neurol Sci* 1973;18:443–453.

106. Levin S, Nelson KE, Spies HW, et al. Pneumococcal meningitis: the problem of the unseen cerebrospinal fluid leak. *Am J Med Sci* 1972;264:319–327.

107. Bol P, Spanjaard L, van Alphen L, et al. Epidemiology of *Haemophilus influenzae* in patients more than six years of age. *J Infect Dis* 1987;15:81–94.

108. Hermans PE, Goldstein NP, Wellman WE. Mollaret's meningitis and differential diagnosis of recurrent meningitis: report of case with review of the literature. *Am J Med* 1972;52:128–140.

109. Yamamoto LJ, Tedder D, Ashley R, et al. Herpes simplex virus type 1 DNA in cerebrospinal fluid of a patient with Mollaret's meningitis. *N Engl J Med* 1991;325:1082–1085.

110. Picard FJ, Dekaban GA, Silva J, et al. Mollaret's meningitis associated with herpes simplex type 2 infection. *Neurology* 1993;43:1722–1727.

CHAPTER 151
Central Nervous System Shunt Infections

Majid Sadigh, Pierce Gardner, and Thomas J. Leipzig

The early Greeks described hydrocephalus (from the Greek *hydro*, "water," and *kephale*, "head") and recognized its poor prognosis. Although more than 20 causes of hydrocephalus have been described, the physiologic end result is an abnormal accumulation of cerebrospinal fluid (CSF) in the cerebral ventricles. Hydrocephalus is classified as either communicating (no obstruction between the ventricles and the subarachnoid space) or noncommunicating (obstruction between the ventricles and the subarachnoid space). In the United States, nearly 70,000 yearly hospital admissions are for hydrocephalus (1).

Attempts to reduce CSF production (normally about 500 mL per day regardless of age) (2) by using drugs such as acetazolamide offer only short-term benefits (3). Surgical decompression is the definitive treatment of hydrocephalus (4). Shunting has dramatically extended the life span of infants and children with hydrocephalus; survival rates now range from 70% to 85%. Approximately 30% to 40% of patients maintain normal intelligence (4,5), and an equal number show no physical abnormalities, but only 20% suffer no mental and physical handicaps (4,5).

Many variations for the surgical diversion of CSF from the ventricular system to other anatomic compartments have been tried, but currently more than 95% of CSF shunts drain into either the peritoneal cavity [ventriculoperitoneal (VP) shunts] or right atrium [ventriculoatrial (VA) shunts] (6). The standard shunt system consists of a proximal ventricular catheter, a reservoir, a one-way valve, and a distal peritoneal or right atrial catheter (Fig. 151.1). The usual catheter material is barium-impregnated Silastic (6).

This chapter focuses on infections of CSF shunts placed for the treatment of adult and pediatric hydrocephalus. The principles in the diagnosis and treatment of these infections apply to any permanent or temporary CSF diversionary apparatus. The continued difficulty with infectious and mechanical complications of these devices has led to a resurgence of other strategies, such as endoscopic third ventriculostomy to treat noncommunicating hydrocephalus (7).

EPIDEMIOLOGY

Incidence

In the United States more than 125,000 individuals have CSF shunts (8). Yearly, over 36,000 shunt-related procedures are performed; 33,000 procedures are for placement of a shunt, of which 14,000 are for revision. Approximately 18,000 new CSF shunts are placed annually in the United States (8). The frequency of shunt infection varies from 1.5% to 39% (average, 10%–15%) (5,9–11). Compared with series reporting infection rates per procedure (with relatively short periods of follow-up), the rates are higher in series measuring an individual patient's lifelong risk for infection (9,12,13). Improved shunt materials, shorter operating time, fewer invasive preoperative tests, and other factors have contributed to the lower infection rates (generally 3%–10%) in more recent reports (9,10–12,13–15).

Host Factors

Infection rates do not appear to vary by the type, severity, underlying cause of hydrocephalus, or the patient's sex or race (9–11). Age, however, is a significant risk factor; infection rates exceed 50% in low-birth-weight infants who require shunts before 3 months of age (9–10). The increased infection rates observed in neonates may be due to a greater density of colonization with coagulase-negative staphylococci, which have high bacterial adherence properties (16). Higher infection rates are also reported in elderly patients (17).

Skin conditions that favor bacterial proliferation are associated with shunt infections by skin microflora. Likewise, the risk for shunt infection is increased by intercurrent infection at other sites or by a history of a previous shunt infection (10,11).

Patients with CSF shunts appear to have an increased risk for bacterial meningitis caused by traditional meningitis pathogens (*Haemophilus influenzae*, *Streptococcus pneumoniae*, and *Neisseria meningitidis*) (9,18,19). This suggests that the presence of a shunt may facilitate the entry of organisms into the CSF during bacteremia. The meninges, rather than the shunt, appear to be the focus of infection in this situation as evidenced by the high rate of success with antibiotic therapy without shunt revision (18,19).

Technical Factors

Rates of infection do not appear to vary with the type of valve used (9,20), although favorable experience has been reported with one-piece shunt systems (21). Surgical technique and the experience of the neurosurgeon are important determinants of infection rates (22). A significantly higher risk for infection has been associated with increased touching of the shunt intraoperatively by inadvertently breached surgical gloves and the presence of a postoperative CSF leak (1).

Microbiology

Although a wide variety of microorganisms have been reported to infect CSF shunts (23–27) (Table 151.1), the majority of VP and VA shunt infections are caused by *Staphylococcus epidermidis* (36%–80%). *Staphylococcus aureus* accounts for approximately 25% of shunt infections, and gram-negative enteric bacteria cause another 5% to 10% (9,13,17). Anaerobic skin flora (mainly *Propionibacterium* species) alone or in mixed culture have been isolated from 2% to 35% of shunt infections (29).

PATHOGENESIS

There are three principal ways by which CSF shunts become infected: (a) organisms directly colonize the shunt, usually at the time of surgery (4,9,22); (b) organisms reach the CSF and shunt by hematogenous spread (9,18,19); and (c) organisms travel in a retrograde fashion from the contaminated distal end of the catheter (9,25). The observation that 70% of cases become manifest within 2 months of surgery and are caused by skin microflora suggests that the majority of infections are due to seeding of the wound in the perioperative period (9–11). An important pathogenic factor in infection by staphylococci is their ability to produce an exopolysaccharide slime, or glycocalyx (Fig. 151.2). This slime not only promotes binding of the organisms to the catheter material but also protects the organisms from local host defenses by inhibiting neutrophil phagocytosis, chemotaxis, and oxidative metabolism, suppressing mononuclear cell lymphoproliferative responses and natural killer cell toxicity (30,31) and reducing antibiotic penetration (30–32). The clinical impact of slime

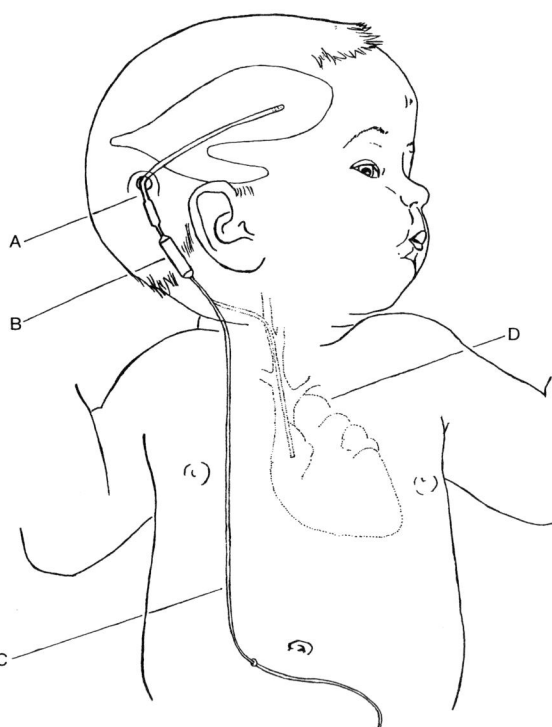

Figure 151.1. Schematic diagram of a typical cerebrospinal fluid shunt system. The shunt is composed of three components: a ventricular catheter **(A),** a unidirectional flow valve **(B),** and a distal catheter directed into the peritoneum **(C)** or the atrium **(D).** A reservoir may be located in-line as demonstrated in this diagram. (From Gardner P, Leipzig T, Phillips P. Infections of central nervous system shunts. *Med Clin North Am* 1985;69:297–314, with permission.)

TABLE 151.1.	Pathogens Associated with Cerebrospinal Fluid Shunt Infections

Gram-positive organisms	Gram-negative organisms
Bacillus subtilis	*Achromobacter* species
Bacillus cereus	*Acinetobacter* species
Corynebacterium jeikeium	*Alcaligenes* species
Corynebacterium striatum	*Bacteroides fragilis*
Enterococci	*Brucella melitensis*
Listeria monocytogenes	*Enterobacter* species
Micrococcus luteus	*Escherichia coli*
Oerskovia xanthineolytica	*Francisella tularensis*
Peptococci	*Flavobacterium*
Propionibacterium acnes	*Haemophilus influenzae*
Rhodococcus equi	*Hafnia* species
Staphylococcus aureus[a]	*Klebsiella pneumoniae*
Coagulase-negative	*Moraxella bovis*
staphylococci[b]	*Neisseria gonorrhoeae*
Staphylococcus citreus	*Neisseria meningitidis*
Staphylococcus epidermidis	*Pseudomonas aeruginosa*
Streptococci	*Salmonella* species
α-Hemolytic	*Serratia marcescens*
Viridans streptococci	Mycobacteria
β-Hemolytic, group A and B	*Mycobacterium aquae*
Streptococcus pneumoniae	*Mycobacterium fortuitum*
	Mycobacterium tuberculosis
	Fungi
	Candida albicans
	Candida glabrata
	Candida stellatoides
	Coccidioides immitis
	Histoplasma capsulatum
	Paecilomyces variotii
	Trichosporon beigelii
	Polymicrobial (including anaerobes)

[a]Accounts for about 25% of shunt infections.
[b]Accounts for 36%–80% of shunt infections.

production includes more frequent shunt obstruction and refractory response to antibiotic therapy (32). Host factors (including fibronectin, fibrinogen, vitronectin, and activated complement factor C9) may also foster the ability of bacteria to adhere to and persist on polymer surfaces (32,33).

Thirty percent of shunts become infected more than 2 months following insertion (9,11,13). In these instances, the route of inoculation usually differs with the type of shunt. For VA shunts, seeding of the distal atrial end by blood-borne organisms is the rule (9,11,13,34). Accordingly, blood cultures offer better diagnostic yield than cultures of CSF obtained by lumbar puncture. In late-onset VP shunt infections, enteric bacteria, presumably of intestinal origin, constitute a greater proportion of the infecting organisms (9,29).

CLINICAL MANIFESTATIONS

The clinical presentations of CSF shunt infection are varied and often subtle and nonspecific. Only a minority of patients present with signs and symptoms that are clearly indicative of meningeal inflammation (severe headache, lethargy, meningismus, photophobia) (9). Almost all patients have a temperature greater than 100°F, and a majority of patients are febrile to 102°F or more (9,13,17). Shunt infection commonly presents as shunt malfunction. Therefore it is recommended that any catheter material removed during revision or replacement be cultured (9,17).

Shunt infections in the early postoperative period often show signs of inflammation along the course of the catheter (9,13,17). Initially, infection is usually established in the distal part of the shunt, and the local and regional complications associated

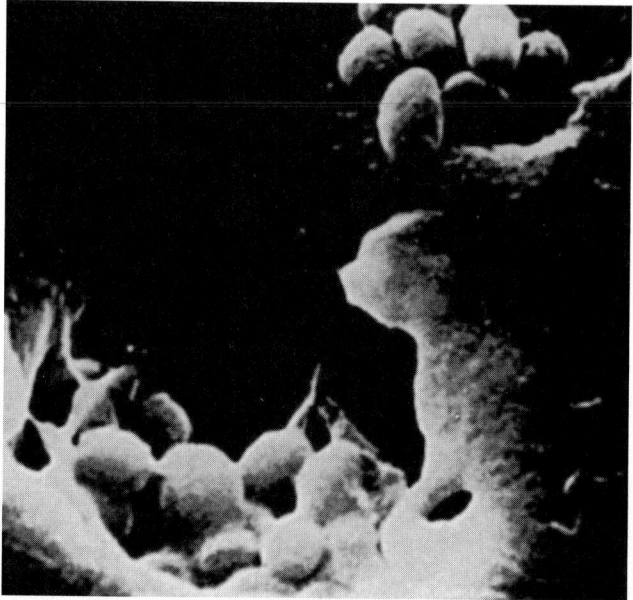

Figure 151.2. Scanning electron micrograph of *Staphylococcus aureus* cells attached to a cerebrospinal fluid shunt. (From Guevara JA, Zuccaro G, Trevisan A, et al. Bacterial adhesion to cerebrospinal fluid shunts. *J Neurosurg* 1987;67:438–445, with permission.)

with each type of shunt may differ. Approximately one third of patients with VP shunts present primarily with abdominal symptoms (29,35,36). Predictably, but infrequently, VP shunts are associated with serious intraabdominal complications, including peritonitis, bowel obstruction or perforation, and peritoneal cysts (35,36). Patients with infections of VA shunts may manifest signs of chronic bacteremia with immune complex nephritis (37,38,39), hypocomplementemia (39), and septic pulmonary emboli (40). Surprisingly, the frequency of right-sided endocarditis does not appear to be increased in patients with VA shunts. Fortunately, the clinical manifestations of shunt infection are usually reversible with successful treatment (37,38,41).

DIAGNOSIS

The diagnosis of shunt infection requires a high index of suspicion and a willingness to aggressively collect appropriate specimens for evaluation and culture. Common clinical presentations of shunt infections are listed in Table 151.2, together with suggestions for the appropriate diagnostic evaluations. Because infection is best established in the distal (nonventricular) catheter, culture of lumbar CSF has a lower yield than does culture of blood in VA shunt infections (9,42) or needle aspirate of inflamed areas along the distal catheter path in VP shunt infections (9). However, for any type of shunt infection, culture of CSF obtained by needle aspiration of the shunt reservoir yields a microbial diagnosis in more than 90% of cases (9,42,43). The high diagnostic yield, the ease of the procedure, and the low rate of complications make aspiration of the reservoir the single most useful diagnostic test in the evaluation of a possible shunt infection (43). In patients with shunt infections, the peripheral white cell count is characteristically elevated, but it is below 10,000/mm³ in 25% of cases (9).

The CSF cellular reaction to shunt infection is usually less than 200 cells per mm³ (11). The proportion of segmented neutrophils, and in some series eosinophils, is characteristically elevated (11,44). Gram-stained smears are usually positive in patients with an active CSF inflammatory response (42,44,45). Positive cultures may be obtained in the absence of CSF pleocytosis (9,43,45) but, in general, the more inflammatory cells in the CSF, the higher the yield of culture. The presence of more than 100 white blood cells per mm³ of CSF correlates with a 90% yield of pathogens by culture (42,45). When the white blood cell count is less than 20 per mm³, fewer than half of CSF cultures grow pathogens (42,45). CSF protein level is usually high, but hypoglycorrhachia is not a consistent feature and is often mild when present (43). In future, for early diagnosis of central nervous system shunt infection, the presence of some of the CSF cytokines may become a valuable diagnostic test (46).

Elevated levels of serum lactate dehydrogenase and C-reactive protein are common but rarely have significant diagnostic value (47). A variety of radiographic studies are useful for evaluating the size of the ventricular system and the location, configuration, and functional status of the shunt (43), or for assessing potential intraabdominal complications of a VP shunt (48).

TREATMENT

Variables that influence therapeutic choices for shunt infections include the patency of the shunt system, the necessity for uninterrupted ventricular drainage, the presence of ventriculitis, the infecting pathogen and its antimicrobial susceptibility pattern, and the presence of clinical complications such as bowel obstruction or perforation (49).

Complete replacement of the shunt system with intensive antibiotic therapy delivered in a dosage and route that will produce effective CSF drug levels consistently yields excellent results and is the therapeutic gold standard (4,5,9,29,50–52). The antibiotics most commonly used are vancomycin by the intraventricular (as well as systemic) route and β-lactam agents (Table 151.3). When ventriculitis is present, ventricular drainage and intraventricular

---

TABLE 151.2.   Clinical Presentation of Shunt Infection and Suggested Diagnostic Steps

Clinical presentation	Major diagnostic steps
Shunt malfunction	Assessment of shunt malfunction by pumping reservoir
	Needle aspiration of reservoir (shunt tap)
	Computed tomography of brain and abdomen, if indicated
	Contrast radiographic studies of shunt
Wound or shunt track inflammation	Culture of aspirate of inflamed area, shunt tap, lumbar puncture (if no mass present)
Infection of proximal site: meningitis, ventriculitis, brain abscess	Computed tomography of brain, shunt tap, lumbar puncture (if no mass present)
Infection of distal site	
Ventriculoatrial shunt	
Bacteremia (acute or chronic)	Blood culture, shunt tap, evaluation for right-sided endocarditis
Septic thrombophlebitis	Blood culture, shunt tap
Septic pulmonary embolism	Blood culture, chest radiograph, sputum Gram stain and culture, shunt tap
Circulating immune complex–related diseases: nephritis and arthritis	Blood culture, shunt tap, serum complement, circulating immune complexes, urine sediment examination
Ventriculoperitoneal shunt	
Acute abdomen, peritonitis, obstruction or perforation of bowel, intraabdominal abscess, liver abscess, peritoneal cyst	Shunt tap, aspiration of inflammation along distal catheter, evaluation for surgical abdomen clinically and radiographically

Adapted from Gardner P, Leipzig TJ, Sadigh M. Infections of mechanical cerebrospinal fluid shunts. *Clin Top Infect Dis* 1988;9:198–214, with permission.

TABLE 151.3.   Antimicrobial Treatment of Common Cerebrospinal Fluid Shunt Pathogens

Organism	Systemic antibiotics	Route	Remarks	Intraventricular or intrashunt antibiotics
Staphylococci (β-lactam resistant)	Vancomycin, 2 g/day Children: 40 mg/kg/day ± Rifampin, 10–20 mg/kg/day	i.v. p.o.	Keep the serum vancomycin level at 10–20 μg/mL Keep the cerebrospinal fluid vancomycin level at 10–20 μg/mL	Vancomycin, 10–20 mg/day Children: 0.5 mg/kg/day
	or based on susceptibility: Trimethoprim, 10–20 mg/kg/day and Sulfamethoxazole, 50–100 mg/kg/day + Rifampin, 10–20 mg/kg/day	i.v.	Keep the serum sulfamethoxazole level at 75–150 μg/mL	
Staphylococci (β-lactam susceptible)	Nafcillin, 12 g/day Children: 300 mg/kg/day or based on susceptibility:	i.v.		Nafcillin 1–4 mg/kg/day not to exceed 50 mg/day
	Trimethoprim 10–20 mg/kg/day and Sulfamethoxazole, 50–100 mg/kg/day + Rifampin, 10–20 mg/kg/day	i.v. p.o.	Keep the serum sulfamethoxazole level at 75–150 μg/mL	
Streptococcus pneumoniae *Neisseria meningitidis* *Proprionibacterium* species	Penicillin G, 24 million units/day Children: 250,000 units/kg/day	i.v.	If *Streptococcus pneumoniae* is resistant to penicillin then ceftriaxone or vancomycin according to susceptibility pattern	
Haemophilus influenzae Gram-negative enteric bacilli *Pseudomonas aeruginosa*	Ceftriaxone, 2 g every 12 h Children: 50–100 mg/kg/day An anti-*Pseudomonas* β-lactam agent, e.g., ceftazidime, 2 g every 8 h Children: 150 mg/kg/day +	i.v. i.v.		
	An aminoglycoside, e.g., gentamicin, 2 mg/kg loading dose then 1.5 mg/kg every 8 h	i.v.	Keep the serum peak gentamicin level at 4–8 μg/mL	Gentamicin, 4–8 mg/day Children: 1–2 mg/day

i.v., intravenously; p.o., orally.

TABLE 151.4.   Standard Treatment of Central Nervous System Shunt Infection

Step	Procedure
I[a]	Removal of the entire infected shunt
II	Placement of external ventricular drainage
III	Administration of effective systemic antibiotics (refer to Table 151.3)
IV[b]	Administration of effective intraventricular antibiotics through external ventricular drainage once or twice daily (refer to Table 151.3)
V	Removal of external ventricular drainage and discountinuation of intraventricular antibiotics, after 3–5 days when ventricular infection is clinically improved
VI	Placement of a new shunt preferably in a site different from the previously removed infected shunt
VII	Continuation of systemic antibiotics for 7–10 days after removal of the infected shunt

[a]Alternatively, the distal part of the infected shunt can be externalized, followed by steps III to VII.
[b]Clamp the drain for 30 minutes after dosage administration.

TABLE 151.5. Alternative Treatment of Uncomplicated Functioning Shunt Infections Caused by Non–Slime-Producing Organisms

Step	Procedure
I	Externalization of the distal part of infected shunt
II	Administration of effective systemic antibiotics (refer to Table 151.3)
III[a]	Administration of effective intraventricular antibiotics once or twice daily (refer to Table 151.3) retrograde through the reservoir
IV	Continuation of systemic and intrashunt antibiotic regimen for 2–3 wk
V	Revision and replacement of the distal shunt

[a]Clamp the drain for 30 minutes after dosage administration.

TABLE 151.6. Suggested Prophylactic Antibiotic Regimens for Prevention of Central Nervous System Shunt Infection

Start antibiotics 1 h before operation and continue for 24–48 h
1. Antistaphylococcal β-lactam agents
   Nafcillin: 2 g intravenously (i.v.) every 6 h (children: 25 mg/kg i.v. every 6 h)
   ±
   Rifampin: 5–10 mg/kg every 12 h orally (p.o.)
[a]2. Vancomycin: 1 g i.v. every 12 h (children: 20 mg/kg every 12 h i.v.)

[a]Dosage adjustment according to renal function is necessary.
i.v., intravenously.

antibiotic administration are indicated. Although immediate replacement of the entire infected shunt has good cure rates and avoids the risks associated with external ventricular drainage, it can be technically difficult and carries a slightly higher risk for subsequent shunt infection. Therefore, it is preferable either to place a temporary external ventricular catheter or to externalize the distal portion of the infected shunt system to drain the ventricle and to provide easy access for administration of antibiotics. Antibiotics can be given in a retrograde fashion once or twice daily, with the drain clamped for 30 minutes after dosage administration. To prevent superinfection, the external drainage system (ventricular catheter or old infected shunt) should be removed within 3 to 5 days after the infection has been controlled, and a new shunt should be placed at a different site (4,51,53–55) (Table 151.4). For patients with functioning shunts infected by non–slime-producing organisms susceptible to bactericidal antibiotics and who have neither active ventricular infection nor other complications requiring surgery (e.g., bowel perforation), it is often possible to cure the infection without completely removing the shunt. The most successful regimen consists of externalization of the distal catheter followed by intraventricular and systemic antimicrobial therapy for 2 to 3 weeks with subsequent replacement of the distal shunt (41) (Table 151.5). Meningitis due to organisms that reach the CSF through the bloodstream (e.g., *H. influenzae, S. pneumoniae, N. meningitidis*) can usually be treated without shunt revision or removal (18,19).

PROGNOSIS

Retrospective studies indicate that shunt infections cause deterioration of cognitive function and are associated with increases in both short-term and long-term mortality (5,9,17,34).

PREVENTION

Efforts to prevent shunt infections have focused on technical improvements in shunt materials, insertion techniques, and antibiotic prophylaxis during the perioperative period (56). Although the new valve designs have not reduced the incidence of shunt infection (20), the use of an antibiotic-impregnated catheter has shown promise (57). Studies of systemic and topical antibiotic prophylaxis in the perioperative period have yielded conflicting results (15,58–63). Two of the more recent metaanalyses have suggested a benefit from antibiotic prophylaxis (64,65). Therefore, prophylaxis with a β-lactam antibiotic with or without rifampin,

vancomycin, or trimethoprim-sulfamethoxazole has become the standard protocol (9,62) (Table 151.6). Antibiotic prophylaxis is recommended for patients with VA shunts who must undergo dental or other procedures that may cause bacteremia (66,67). The value of prophylaxis for patients with VP shunts undergoing similar procedures is not clear. However, when peritoneal infection (e.g., ruptured appendix or diverticulum) is suspected in patients with VP shunts, antibiotic prophylaxis should be given. It would also seem logical to avoid placing VP shunts in women who have a history of recurrent pelvic inflammatory disease or an intrauterine contraceptive device in place.

REFERENCES

1. Kulkarni AV, Drake JM, Lamberti-Pasculli M. Cerebrospinal fluid shunt infection: a prospective study of risk factors. *J Neurosurg* 2001;94:195.
2. McComb JG. Recent research into the nature of cerebrospinal fluid formation and absorption. *J Neurosurg* 1983;59:369.
3. Matson DD. Hydrocephalus. *N Engl J Med* 1964;271:1360.
4. Keucher TR, Mealey J. Long-term results after ventriculoatrial and ventriculoperitoneal shunting for infantile hydrocephalus. *J Neurosurg* 1979;50:179.
5. Overton MC, Snodglass SR. Ventriculovenous shunts for infantile hydrocephalus: a review of five years' experience with this method. *J Neurosurg* 1965;23:517.
6. Post EM. Currently available shunt systems: a review. *Neurosurgery* 1985;16:257.
7. Murshid WR. Endoscopic third ventriculostomy: towards more indications for the treatment of non-communicating hydrocephalus. *Minim Invasive Neurosurg* 2000;43:75.
8. Bondurant CP, Jiminez DF. Epidemiology of cerebrospinal fluid shunting. *Pediatr Neurosurg* 1995;23:254.
9. Schoenbaum SC, Gardner P, Schillito J. Infections of cerebrospinal fluid shunts: epidemiology, clinical manifestations and therapy. *J Infect Dis* 1975;131:543.
10. Renier D, Lacombe J, Pierre-Kahn A, et al. Factors causing acute shunt infection; computer analysis of 1174 operations. *J Neurosurg* 1984;61:1072.
11. Spanu G, Karussos G, Achinolfi D, et al. An analysis of cerebrospinal fluid shunt infections in adults. A clinical experience of twelve years. *Acta Neurochir (Wien)* 1986;80:79.
12. Younger JJ, Simmons JCH, Barrett FF. Operative related infection rates for ventriculoperitoneal shunt procedures in a children's hospital. *Infect Control* 1987;8:67.
13. Kontny U, Hofling B, Gutjahr P, et al. CSF shunt infections in children. *Infection* 1993;21:89.
14. Morissette I, Gourdeau M, Francoeur J. CSF shunt infections: a fifteen-year experience with emphasis on management and outcome. *Can J Neurol Sci* 1993;20:118.
15. Choux M, Genitori L, Lang D, et al. Shunt implantation: reducing the incidence of shunt infection. *J Neurosurg* 1992;77:875.
16. Pople IK, Bayston R, Hayward RD. Infection of cerebrospinal fluid shunts in infants: a study of etiological factors. *J Neurosurg* 1992;77:29.
17. George R, Leibrock L, Epstein M. Long-term analysis of cerebrospinal fluid shunt infections: a 25 year experience. *J Neurosurg* 1979;51:804.
18. Petrak RM, Pottage JC, Harris AA, et al. *Haemophilus influenzae* meningitis in the presence of a cerebrospinal fluid shunt. *Neurosurgery* 1986;18:79.
19. Leggiardo RJ, Atluru VL, Katz SP. Meningococcal meningitis associated with cerebrospinal fluid shunts. *Pediatr Infect Dis* 1984;3:489.
20. Drake JM, Kestle JR, Milner R, et al. Randomized trial of cerebrospinal fluid shunt valve design in pediatric hydrocephalus. *Neurosurgery* 1998;43:294–303.

21. Haase J, Bang F, Tange M. Danish experience with the one-piece shunt. A long-term follow-up. *Childs Nerv Syst* 1987;3:93.

22. Bayston R, Lari J. A study of the sources of infection in colonized shunts. *Dev Med Child Neurol* 1974;16(suppl 32):16.

23. Angel-Moreno A, Frances A, Granado JM, et al. Ventriculoperitoneal shunt infection by *Candida glabrata* in an adult. *J Infect* 2000;41:178–179.

24. Montero A, Romero J, Vargas JA, et al. *Candida* infection of cerebrospinal fluid shunt devices; report of two cases and review of the literature. *Acta Neurochir (Wien)* 2000;141:67–74.

25. Morgan DF, Falconi L, Canady AI, et al. Gonococcal infection in cerebrospinal fluid and the presence of a ventriculoperitoneal shunt. *J Pediatr Adolesc Gynecol* 1997;10:93–94.

26. Scotton PG, Tonon E, Giobbia M, et al. *Rhodococcus equi* nosocomial meningitis cured by levofloxacin and shunt removal. *Clin Infect Dis* 2000;30:223–224.

27. Midani S, Rathore MH. *Mycobacterium fortuitum* infection of ventriculoperitoneal shunt. *South Med J* 1999;92:705–707.

28. Westergren H, Westergren V, Forsum U. *Proprionebacterium acnes* in cultures from ventriculoperitoneal shunts; infection or contamination? *Acta Neurochir (Wien)* 1997;139:33–36.

29. Brook I, Johnson N, Overturf GD, et al. Mixed bacterial meningitis: a complication of ventriculo- and lumboperitoneal shunts. *J Neurosurg* 1977;47:961.

30. Gray ED, Peters G, Verstegen M, et al. Effect of extracellular slime substance from *Staphylococcus epidermidis* on the human cellular immune response. *Lancet* 1984;1:365.

31. Diaz Mitoma F, Hardking G, Hoban DJ, et al. Clinical significance of a test for slime production in ventriculoperitoneal shunt infections caused by coagulase-negative staphylococci. *J Infect Dis* 1987;156:555.

32. Hermann M, Vaudaux PE, Pittet D, et al. Fibronectin, fibrinogen, and laminin act as mediators of adherence of clinical staphylococcal isolates to foreign material. *J Infect Dis* 1988;158:693.

33. Lundberg F, Li DQ, Falkenback D, Lea T, et al. Presence of vitronectin and activated complement factor C9 on ventriculoperitoneal shunts and temporary ventricular drainage catheters. *J Neurosurg* 1999;90:101–108.

34. Forrest DM, Cooper DGW. Complications of ventriculoatrial shunts: a review of 455 cases. *J Neurosurg* 1968;29:506.

35. Grosfeld JL, Cooney DR, Smith J, et al. Intraabdominal complications following ventriculoperitoneal shunt procedures. *Pediatrics* 1974;54:791.

36. Salomao JF, Leibinger RD. Abdominal pseudocysts complicating CSF shunting in infants and children. Report of 18 cases. *Pediatr Neurosurg* 1999;31:274–278.

37. Wakabayashi Y, Kobayashi Y, Shigematsu H. Shunt nephritis: histological dynamics following removal of the shunt. *Nephron* 1985;40:111.

38. Haffner D, Schindra F, Aschoff A, et al. The clinical spectrum of shunt nephritis. *Nephrol Dial Transplant* 1997;12:1143–1148.

39. Strife CF, McDonald BM, Ruley EJ, et al. Shunt nephritis: the nature of the serum cryoglobulins and their relation to the complement profile. *J Pediatr* 1976;88:403.

40. Gibney RTN, Donovan F, Fitzgerald MX. Recurrent symptomatic pulmonary embolism caused by an infected Pudenz cerebrospinal fluid shunt device. *Thorax* 1978;33:662.

41. McLaurine RL, Frame PT. Treatment of infections of cerebrospinal fluid shunts. *Rev Infect Dis* 1987;9:595.

42. Odio C, McCracken GH, Nelson JD. CSF shunt infections in pediatrics: a seven-year experience. *Am J Dis Child* 1984;138:1103.

43. Noetzel MJ, Baker RP. Shunt fluid examination: risks and benefits in the evaluation of shunt malfunction and infection. *J Neurosurg* 1984;61:328.

44. Wiersbitzky SK, Ahrens N, Becker T, et al. The diagnostic importance of eosinophilic granulocytes in the CSF of children with ventriculoperitoneal shunt systems. *Acta Neurol Scand* 1998;97:201–203.

45. Forward KR, Fewer HD, Stiver HG. Cerebrospinal fluid shunt infections: a review of 35 infections in 32 patients. *J Neurosurg* 1983;59:725.

46. Asi-Bautista MC, Heidemann SM, Meert KL, et al. Tumor necrosis factor-alpha, interleukin 1 beta, and interleukin 6 concentrations in cerebrospinal fluid predict ventriculoperitoneal shunt infection. *Crit Care Med* 1997;25:1713–1716.

47. Bayston R. Serum c-reactive protein test in diagnosis of septic complications of cerebrospinal fluid for hydrocephalus. *Arch Dis Child* 1979;54:545.

48. Agha FP, Amendola MA, Shirazi KK, et al. Abdominal complications of ventriculoperitoneal shunts with emphasis on the role of imaging methods. *Surg Gynecol Obstet* 1983;156:473.

49. Walters BC. Cerebrospinal fluid shunt infection. *Neurosurg Clin North Am* 1992;3:387.

50. Garvey G. Current concepts of bacterial infections of the central nervous system: bacterial meningitis and bacterial brain abscess. *J Neurosurg* 1983;59:725.

51. James HE, Walsh JW, Wilson HD, et al. The management of cerebrospinal fluid shunt infections: a clinical experience. *Acta Neurochir (Wien)* 1981;59:157.

52. James HE, Walsh JW, Wilson HD. Prospective randomized study of therapy in cerebrospinal fluid shunt infections. *Neurosurgery* 1980;7:459.

53. Mori K, Raimondi AJ. An analysis of external ventricular drainage as a treatment for infected shunts. *Childs Brain* 1975;1:243.

54. James HE, Wilson HD, Connor JD, et al. Intraventricular cerebrospinal fluid antibiotic concentrations in patients with intraventricular infections. *Neurosurgery* 1982;10:50.

55. Jacobs F, Delecluse F, Raftopoulos C, et al. Intraventricular vancomycin in CSF shunt infections. *Neurosurgery* 1987;21:112.

56. Venes JL. Control of shunt infection: report of 150 consecutive cases. *J Neurosurg* 1976;45:311.

57. Bayston R, Lambert E. Duration of protective activity of cerebrospinal fluid shunt catheters impregnated with antimicrobial agents to prevent bacterial catheter related infection. *J Neurosurg* 1997;87:247–251.

58. Bullock R, van Dellen JR, Ketelbey W, et al. A double-blind placebo-controlled trial of perioperative prophylactic antibiotics for elective neurosurgery. *J Neurosurg* 1988;69:687.

59. Haines SJ, Taylor F. Prophylactic methicillin for shunt operations: effects on incidence of shunt malfunction and infection. *Childs Brain* 1982;9:10.

60. Slight PH, Gundling K, Plotkin SA, et al. A trial of vancomycin for prophylaxis of infection after neurosurgical shunts. *N Engl J Med* 1985;312:921.

61. Schmidt K, Gjerris F, Osgaard O, et al. Antibiotic prophylaxis in cerebrospinal fluid shunting. A prospective randomized trial in 152 hydrocephalic patients. *Neurosurgery* 1985;17:1.

62. Goran C, Blomstedt MD. Results of trimethoprim-sulfamethoxazole prophylaxis in ventriculostomy and shunting procedures. A double-blind randomized trial. *J Neurosurg* 1985;62:694.

63. Whitby M, Johnson BC, Atkinson RL, et al. The comparative efficacy of intravenous cefotaxime and trimethoprim/sulfamethoxazole in preventing infection after neurosurgery; a prospective randomized study. Brisbane Neurosurgical infection Group. *Br J Neurosurg* 2000;14:13–18.

64. Langley JM, LeBlanc JC, Drake J, et al. Efficacy of antimicrobial prophylaxis in placement of cerebrospinal fluid shunts: meta-analysis. *Clin Infect Dis* 1993;17:98.

65. Haines SJ, Walters BC. Antibiotic prophylaxis for cerebrospinal fluid shunts: a meta-analysis. *Neurosurgery* 1994;34:87–92.

66. Croll TP, Greiner DG, Schut L. Antibiotic prophylaxis for the hydrocephalic dental patient with a shunt. *Pediatr Dent* 1979;1:81.

67. Monfared AH, Kee SK, Apuzzo MLJ, et al. Obstetric management of pregnant women with extracranial shunts. *Can Med Assoc J* 1979;120:562.

CHAPTER 152
Brain Abscess

Staci A. Fischer and Alan A. Harris

Brain abscesses remain uncommon, accounting for approximately 1 in 10,000 hospital admissions in the United States. Unlike focal infections in other anatomic sites, brain abscesses often present insidiously, with few systemic signs of infection, mimicking tumors (1–18). Pneumoencephalography, arteriography, and myelography, invasive procedures relied upon for diagnosis of brain abscesses in the past, have been replaced by computed tomography (CT) and magnetic resonance imaging (MRI), which may detect small or multiple central nervous system (CNS) lesions and may identify the underlying cause of abscess formation (e.g., chronic otic and sinus abnormalities). As a result of such advances, abscesses may be diagnosed at an earlier stage and surgically approached more safely and accurately. In the past two decades, the prevalence of cryptogenic abscesses has decreased from 35% to less than 20% (15). The collaboration of neurosurgical and infectious disease disciplines remains critical to successful treatment of the patient with brain abscess (19–22). Our therapeutic armamentarium continues to expand with additional bactericidal agents with penetration into abscess cavities and surrounding brain tissue. The attributable mortality from brain abscesses has declined in the last two decades, likely as a result of advances in diagnosis and treatment, yet significant morbidity and mortality persist. Prognosis continues to depend on the age and immune function of the patient as well as neurologic function and mental status at the time of diagnosis.

PATHOGENESIS

In the 1970's, the association of brain abscess with cyanotic heart disease (15,23–25) and pulmonary arteriovenous malformations (24,26,27) provided early pathophysiologic clues that areas of microscopic ischemia or macroscopic infarction were more vulnerable to the development of brain abscess. These foci (particularly at the gray-white matter junction) comprise a *locus minoris resistentiae* susceptible to bacteremic seeding, facilitated by organisms bypassing the pulmonary filtering process via right-to-left shunting. Bacteremia remains the most common underlying cause of brain abscesses diagnosed in developed countries.

Abscesses may also develop as a result of direct extension from continuous foci of infection, including otic or sinus infection. Abscesses subsequent to open head trauma in humans and to direct inoculation of bacteria in some animal models demonstrate that otherwise normal brain is vulnerable to abscess formation (28).

Clearly, organisms vary in their capability to induce brain abscess. In a rat model, inoculation of *Escherichia coli* was more infective than *Pseudomonas* species, *Staphylococcus aureus*, or *Streptococcus pyogenes*. *E. coli* strains with K1 capsules were more infective than unencapsulated forms (29,30). *Citrobacter diversus*, a major cause of meningitis-associated brain abscess in neonates, demonstrated strain variation in its ability to cause abscess by either hematogenous spread or inoculation (31). *Streptococcus milleri*, the most commonly identified bacterial cause of brain abscess in most series, characteristically produces purulence at any site of infection.

Host factors are also important considerations. The immunocompromised host is at risk for infection with opportunistic pathogens and may demonstrate altered clinical and radiographic presentations of brain abscess. In canine studies, the effect of immunosuppression with azathioprine or prednisone on CT monitoring of abscess formation has been evaluated. Immunosuppression retarded abscess formation, with a diminution of surrounding edema and mass effect, although eventually the abscess became larger than in the immunocompetent control animals (32). Corticosteroids clearly retard the inflammatory response to infection and delay encapsulation, important components in the evolution of brain abscesses with consequent therapeutic implications.

PREDISPOSING FACTORS

Brain abscess occurs most often in males in the second through fourth decades of life (13,15,16,33). The overall incidence of infection is 0.18% to 1.3% in autopsy studies. Despite advances in diagnostic technology, cryptogenic abscesses still occur in 15% to 20% of cases (15).

Ischemia, infarction, and contusion likely provide a fertile soil for inoculation or bacteremic seeding of organisms and resultant brain abscess in humans. Brain abscess rarely complicates bacteremia from pyelonephritis, pneumonia, cellulitis, and vascular catheter sepsis. Bacterial endocarditis, while associated with multiple neurologic complications, rarely results in brain abscess formation (15,34). Abscess formation in these patients is usually accompanied by microemboli or cerebrovascular disease, resulting in locally decreased oxygenation or perfusion (35). In watershed areas with little collateral flow, sludging or vascular stasis associated with conditions such as hyperviscosity, cryoglobulinemia, or altered red blood cell rheology may also create an environment conducive to bacterial seeding.

Systemic or localized vascular disorders have been associated with brain abscess. Pulmonary arteriovenous malformations (AVMs) comprise an extracardiac right-to-left shunt from which paradoxic emboli may be propagated to the brain and hypoxemia may develop. Eighty percent of patients with pulmonary AVMs have underlying hereditary hemorrhagic telangiectasia (Osler-Weber-Rendu disease), which may also cause cerebral AVMs at risk for infection (23,24,36–40). Five to ten percent of patients with this disorder develop brain abscesses, a risk approximately 1,000 times that of the general population (26,37,38,40,41). As brain abscess may be the initial presentation of hereditary hemorrhagic telangiectasia, this condition should be suspected whenever a patient has more than one apparently cryptogenic brain abscess during his or her lifetime (42). Cyanotic congenital heart disease may similarly predispose to brain abscess formation; it is estimated that 3% to 5% of patients with such malformations will develop brain abscesses over the course of their lifetimes (37). Carotid endarterectomy and preeclampsia have been complicated by intracranial hemorrhage with subsequent hematogenous seeding and development of staphylococcal brain abscess (43,44).

Brain abscesses may develop from contiguous infection in the middle ear, paranasal sinuses, and mastoids, either via direct spread through cranial osteitis or osteomyelitis or retrograde spread from thrombophlebitic emissary or diploic veins (13,14,16,17,45–55). Brain abscess complicates chronic otitis media or mastoiditis four to eight times more frequently than their acute counterparts (15,56). Cholesteatomas are an additional risk factor, particularly in adults, in whom they have been associated with more than 50% of otogenic brain abscesses (57,58). Otogenic infections most commonly produce temporal lobe or cerebellar abscesses and are often polymicrobial, involving anaerobes and gram-negative bacilli (53,54). Thrombosis of the sigmoid sinus or lateral sinus may complicate otogenic abscesses. Abnormalities or infections of the paranasal sinuses predispose to abscess formation in predictable locations: with ethmoid and frontal sinuses, the frontal lobes, and with sphenoid sinuses, the pituitary and sella turcica area. Superior sagittal sinus thrombosis may accompany brain abscess from the paranasal sinuses. Because hematogenous spread may occur with otic or sinus infections, the presence of multiple abscesses or lesions in noncontiguous sites does not rule out these underlying processes (18,59). In the individual patient, it is difficult to reliably identify the predisposing source based solely on the anatomic location of the abscess.

When clinical and radiographic evaluation does not reveal evidence of otic, sinus, or mastoid infection, more occult sources of underlying infection should be considered. Dental infection with spread of anaerobic bacteria through valveless intracranial veins and even the cavernous sinus has been estimated to cause up to 10% of brain abscesses, usually in the frontal or temporal lobes (15,18,60–62). With hematogenous spread, multiple lesions may be seen.

Although intracranial neurosurgical procedures may be complicated by wound infections, bone flap osteomyelitis, subdural empyema, or meningitis, brain abscess is rare, occurring in less than 0.2% of clean procedures (18). Localized intraparenchymal abscesses may develop secondary to deep wound infection or extension of a superficial infection through a dural rent, particularly in the patient with preceding trauma. Surgical procedures such as submucous resection of the nasal septum (63), ventriculostomy (1), or placement of cranial traction with Crutchfield tongs or halo orthoses (64–67) have been complicated by intracranial abscesses (68). Postoperative brain abscess of uncertain cause should raise concern for an unsuspected source of bacteremia or a microscopic communication between the ears or sinuses and the cranial vault.

Posttraumatic brain abscess may follow penetrating cranial injuries produced by numerous objects, including missiles (e.g., gunshot wounds), spears, lawn darts, and pencil tips (69–72). While staphylococcal species are most frequently isolated, with soil contamination, enteric gram-negative bacteria, anaerobes, and fungi may be involved as well. The presence of foreign bodies, including bone fragments within the brain parenchyma, may predispose to abscess formation presenting years after trauma (72–74). Cerebellar abscesses have complicated congenital occipital dermal sinuses and epidermoid cysts (75,76).

Meningitis caused by group B streptococci, the most common cause of neonatal meningitis, is rarely followed by brain abscess. Several important meningitis pathogens in the neonate are notable for their association with abscess formation. *Citrobacter diversus* causes necrotizing vasculitis and abscess formation in more than 70% of infants with meningitis and is associated with a high mortality rate (15,77,78). Similarly, premature neonates and infants with *Enterobacter sakazakii* meningitis may develop brain abscesses; bacteremia with the same organism has not resulted in CNS infection in adults (79).

Multiple series attest to the rarity of brain abscess as a sequela of adult community-onset meningitis caused by *Streptococcus pneumoniae, Haemophilus influenzae,* and *Neisseria meningitidis* in adults. Meningitis due to *Listeria monocytogenes* is complicated by abscess formation in 3% to 10% of patients; the frontal and parietal lobes are most commonly involved (80–82). Two to three percent of patients with listeriosis have brain abscess without concurrent meningitis. Infection generally occurs in patients with underlying defects in cell-mediated immunity, including transplantation, hematologic malignancies, third trimester of pregnancy and, less commonly, HIV infection (78). *Haemophilus aphrophilus* and *Haemophilus paraphrophilus,* frequent causes of "culture negative" endocarditis associated with large vegetations with a tendency to embolize, have resulted in brain abscess secondary to meningitis or bacteremia (83–86). Certain opportunistic fungi such as *Cryptococcus neoformans* and *Coccidioides immitis* may be associated with meningitis and subsequent abscess formation, along with several other pathogens discussed later.

Hematogenous spread of extraneural infection to the CNS may occur in patients presenting with skin and soft tissue infection, osteomyelitis, intraabdominal infection, pleuropulmonary infection, or pelvic infection (15,33). Multiple abscesses may be seen, frequently at the gray matter–white matter junction in the distribution of the middle cerebral artery. Dilatation of esophageal strictures and sclerosis of esophageal varices have been complicated by bacteremia and subsequent development of brain abscess, frequently involving a multitude of oropharyngeal bacteria (87–90).

MICROBIOLOGY

In light of the pathophysiologic considerations above, a plethora of bacterial, fungal, and protozoal pathogens may be isolated from abscess contents (Tables 152.1 and 152.2). Polymicrobial flora is to be expected when the abscess is formed by contiguous spread, especially from otic or sinus infections; in some series, 30% to 60% of brain abscesses are polymicrobial (13).

Streptococci—aerobic, anaerobic, and microaerophilic—are isolated in up to 70% of brain abscesses, with *S. milleri* the most commonly identified aerobic organism (1–10,13,15,17,33,91,92). *Prevotella* and *Bacteroides* species, including *Prevotella melaninogenica* (formerly *Bacteroides melaninogenicus*), *Prevotella oralis* (formerly *Bacteroides oralis*), and *Bacteroides fragilis,* are found in up to 40% of cases (13). *Fusobacterium* species are anaerobic oral flora and may be associated with extensive tissue necrosis; *Actinomyces, Eikenella, Veillonella,* and *Clostridium* species may be involved in brain abscesses as well, frequently as part of mixed infections (13,24,33,51,93). Infection with *Actinomyces* results from spread from pulmonary or cervicofacial foci, either by direct ex-

TABLE 152.1. Bacterial Pathogens Isolated from Brain Abscesses

Class	Organism
Aerobes	*Streptococcus* species
	S. milleri–S. intermedius group
	Other viridans streptococci
	Group C streptococci
	S. pneumoniae
	Staphylococcus aureus
	Coagulase-negative *Staphylococcus*
	Proteus mirabilis
	Klebsiella pneumoniae
	Klebsiella ozaenae
	Escherichia coli
	Citrobacter diversus
	Enterobacter species
	Haemophilus species
	Salmonella species
	Listeria monocytogenes
	Streptobacillus moniliformis
	Nocardia asteroids
	Brucella melitensis
	Pseudomonas aeruginosa
	Abiotrophia species
Anaerobes	*Bacteroides fragilis*
	Prevotella melaninogenica
	Prevotella (formerly *Bacteroides*) *oralis*
	Peptostreptococcus speices
	Clostridium species
	Actinomyces israelii
	Fusobacterium species
	Eikenella species
	Veillonella species
	Prevotella species
	Desulfovibrio species

tension or by hematogenous dissemination; it is often the sole pathogen isolated in these patients (93). Abscesses complicating bacteremia or bacterial meningitis are usually caused by a single agent. Posttraumatic or postneurosurgical abscesses may be monomicrobial (staphylococci) or polymicrobial. *S. aureus,* once a major cause of brain abscess, has diminished in frequency over the years. It is usually secondary to bacteremia, including acute endocarditis, or complicates local cranial wound infection or neurosurgical procedures. Its diminished frequency likely reflects the use of early broad-spectrum antimicrobial therapy and improved microbiologic techniques to detect other pathogens, especially anaerobes.

Enterobacteriaceae and *Pseudomonas* species may be isolated in up to 30% to 40% of cases, complicating bacteremia (*E. coli* or *Proteus* species), trauma, or neurosurgery. Chronic otic conditions are usually associated with *Pseudomonas* or *Proteus* species as well as anaerobic flora (94). *Klebsiella* and *Enterobacter* are observed less frequently in these settings. *C. diversus* and *Proteus mirabilis* are important considerations in the neonate with brain abscess and meningitis.

Salmonella species, important causes of community-onset bacteremia, exhibit tropism for endothelial surfaces. Systemic disease most frequently involves bones, joints, atherosclerotic aneurysms, and heart valves, but meningitis and brain abscess may occur (95). *Salmonella* species, including *Salmonella typhi,* have been reported to cause brain abscess during, years after, or in the absence of gastrointestinal disease (96,97). Lesions are most commonly located in the temporal or parietal lobes and have been reported to superinfect glioblastoma multiforme lesions (98). *Klebsiella ozaenae,* a cause of atrophic rhinitis or ozena

TABLE 152.2. Predominant Pathogens Associated with Specific Conditions that are Occasionally Followed by Brain Abscess

Predisposing conditions	Pathogens
Otitis, mastoiditis, invaded paranasal sinus, lung abscess, empyema	Usually polymicrobial—anaerobic and microaerophilic streptococci, *Bacteroides, Prevotella, Fusobacterium, Pseudomonas, Proteus* species, other Enterobacteriaceae[a]
Noninvaded paranasal sinus, dental	Usually polymicrobial—anaerobic and microaerophilic streptococci, *Bacteroides, Prevotella, Fusobacterium* species
Trauma or neurosurgery	Monomicrobial or polymicrobial—*Staphylococcus aureus,* Enterobacteriaceae, *Pseudomonas* species
Meningitis (not surgical or traumatic)	*Listeria monocytogenes, Citrobacter diversus*
Bacteremia	
Without apparent source	*Salmonella* species, *S. aureus, Listeria monocytogenes*
Genitourinary or gastrointestinal source	Enterobacteriaceae
Wound source	*S. aureus,* Enterobacteriaceae
Endocarditis	Viridans streptococci, enterococci, *S. aureus, Haemophilus aphrophilus, Candida, Aspergillus* species

The extent of the microbiologic evaluation should be dictated by epidemiologic concerns about the potential pathogen. In addition to routine Gram stain, and aerobic and anaerobic cultures, prolonged incubation, special media, and evaluation by smear and culture for mycobacteria, fungi, and *Nocardia* organisms may be appropriate for specific patients.

[a] *Escherichia, Proteus, Klebsiella, Enterobacter, Serratia, Salmonella, Shigella, Arizona, Citrobacter, Edwardsiella, Hafnia, Morganella, Providencia, Yersinia,* and *Erwinia* species.

and a nasal colonizer, has also caused brain abscess, presumably through contiguous spread (99). Infection with *Legionella pneumophila* is commonly associated with encephalopathy, and rarely with brain abscess (100).

The immunocompromised host is at risk for infection from a variety of opportunistic pathogens. In the transplant population, *Aspergillus* species cause the majority of brain abscesses, so empiric therapy for abscess in the transplant recipient should include antifungal therapy (101). Concurrent lung lesions are detected in up to 90% of these patients; abscesses are most commonly located in the frontal or parietal lobes (101). The zygomycetes and a growing number of ubiquitous dematiaceous fungi have been isolated in brain abscesses in this population, often following intensive rejection treatment and concurrent with pulmonary colonization or infection. *Actinomyces* and *Mucorales* species colonize the upper respiratory tract and may cause brain abscess secondary to local invasion (90). Brain abscess caused by *Pseudoallescheria boydii* complicating near drowning, intravenous catheter infections, and open head trauma has also been described (103–105). *Nocardia asteroides* causes a lung-brain syndrome, with nodular or cavitary pulmonary infiltrates and mass lesions in the brain. A diagnosis of systemic nocardiosis warrants investigation for intracerebral lesions, even if overt clinical signs or symptoms are absent. Cerebral mass lesions caused by *Mycobacterium tuberculosis* or *C. neoformans* typically accompany systemic disease; however, atypical mycobacteria may cause cerebral involvement secondary to trauma, disseminated disease, and cranial wound infection. Table 152.3 lists the additional infectious and noninfectious causes of CNS mass lesions in the immunocompromised host.

The anatomic location of an abscess may suggest an underlying contiguous infection, thereby directing early diagnostic procedures and antibiotic therapy. Cultures of superficial wound drainage do not always correlate with the organism responsible for deep wound infection. The underlying source of bacteremia resulting in brain abscess may be cryptic or only historically apparent at the time the abscess becomes clinically evident.

CLINICAL MANIFESTATIONS

Signs and symptoms depend on the stage of the abscess, its anatomic location, and the patient's ability to communicate. The classic triad of fever, headache, and focal neurologic deficits is present in less than half of all affected patients, with fever present in only 40% to 50% (13,15,106). Consequently, the clinical findings in the patient with brain abscess are not specific for infection, with most patients presenting with signs of an expanding mass lesion in the brain. Most patients present with a less than 2-week history of symptoms, with headache present in approximately 75% of cases; nausea, vomiting, altered level of consciousness, and seizures are variably present (1,15,107). If present, fever is frequently of low grade. Localizing signs or symptoms may be noted, with ataxia and nystagmus in the patient with cerebellar abscess, hemiparesis in the patient with basal ganglia or thalamic involvement, and altered personality in the patient with a frontal lobe lesion (33,108). In neonates, a rapid increase in head circumference has been noted (109). If posttraumatic in nature, brain abscesses may be accompanied by localized scalp erythema, swelling, and tenderness, possibly with purulent wound drainage. Should the abscess be juxtaposed to meningeal surfaces, there may be commensurate meningeal irritation with nuchal rigidity or meningismus. If the clinical picture initially suggests a focal lesion but rapid deterioration occurs with fever, headache, and stiff neck, rupture of an abscess into the subarachnoid or intraventricular space should be considered; these patients may develop brain herniation within hours, which would pose a true neurologic emergency (110,111). The vagueness of neurologic signs and symptoms demands consideration of brain abscess in the differential diagnosis of malignancy, aneurysm, infarction, vasculitis, embolism, and a multitude of meningoencephalitides, including herpes simplex encephalitis (1–10,13).

TABLE 152.3. Causes of Mass Lesions of the Brain in the Immunocompromised Host

Type of organism	Infectious causes: organism	Noninfectious causes
Bacteria	*Streptococcus* species and other typical pathogens (see Table 152.1)	Neoplasm
	Pseudomonas aeruginosa	Primary
	Listeria monocytogenes	Metastatic
	Enterobacteriaceae	Infraction
	Nocardia asteroides	Aneurysm
	Stenotrophomonas maltophilia	Vascular malformation
	Gordona terrae	Radiation necrosis
	Salmonella typhi	
	Rhodococcus equi	
Fungi	*Aspergillus* species	
	Mucorales	
	Candida species	
	Cryptococcus neoformans	
	Coccidiodes immitis	
	Fusarium oxysporum	
	Pseudoallescheria boydii	
	Fonsecaea pedrosoi	
	Cladosporium trichoides	
	Absidia species	
	Scopulariopsis species	
	Bipolaris species	
	Curvularia species	
	Acremonium species	
	Acrophialophora fusispora	
Mycobacteria	*Mycobacterium tuberculosis*	
	Mycobacterium kansasii	
	Mycobacterium avium complex	
Protozoa	*Toxoplasma gondii*	
	Strongyloides stercoralis	
	Acanthamoeba species	
Viruses	Progressive multifocal leukoencephalopathy (JC virus)	
	Cytomegalovirus	

Peripheral leukocytosis is uncommonly noted, but if present it is generally mild (total white cell count less than 15,000/mm^3) and does not help differentiate infection from neoplastic, immune-mediated, or vascular processes in the differential diagnosis (33). Absence of fever or leukocytosis should not eliminate brain abscess from diagnostic consideration. Erythrocyte sedimentation rates are usually elevated, but this finding is nonspecific. Blood cultures are likely to be negative unless the brain abscess is associated with septic embolization from an intravascular endothelial infection such as endocarditis, arteriovenous malformation, or aneurysm. Hyponatremia may be seen, concomitant with the syndrome of inappropriate secretion of antidiuretic hormone.

DIAGNOSIS

Despite its essential role in diagnosing other CNS infections, lumbar puncture is often contraindicated when brain abscess is suspected, due to the risk for herniation, which carries a mortality rate in excess of 25% to 30% (13,112).

Children with cyanotic congenital heart disease or lead poisoning have suffered herniation after lumbar puncture even in the absence of obvious space-occupying lesions. If performed, lumbar puncture rarely reveals specific information; cultures are usually negative (13,15). CSF demonstrates a pleocytosis of less than 500 cells per mm^3 in 60% to 70% of cases; lymphocytes usually predominate, although polymorphonuclear cells (PMNs) may be seen (15). A CSF leukocyte count in excess of 1,000/mm^3 with a predominance of PMNs in the setting of brain abscess suggests meningitis secondary to rupture of the abscess into the ventricular or subarachnoid space. In general, lumbar puncture yields little diagnostic information and carries a significant risk for morbidity and mortality in the patient with brain abscess and should be avoided unless intraventricular rupture has already occurred (112).

Advances in radiologic techniques have aided the diagnosis and management of CNS infections (113). More invasive techniques such as myelography and pneumoencephalography are rarely necessary or indicated. Arteriography may still be required to help distinguish tumor, abscess, and ruptured aneurysm, but has been supplanted by magnetic resonance angiography (MRA) in many centers. Importantly, gas noted on skull films or CT scans may result from infection with gas-producing organisms or indicate extracranial communication (51,114). Electroencephalography and ultrasonography may be helpful in neonates with suspected brain abscess, but are rarely of value in adults (115–117). Indium-111 leukocyte scans, while of use in detecting abscesses in the abdomen and elsewhere, are only 50% to 60% sensitive in the setting of brain abscesses; false-positive scans may be seen with infarcts, tumors, and hematomas (25,33,118–124). They are of little to no value in the evaluation of a space-occupying lesion.

COMPUTED TOMOGRAPHY

The development of CT scanning revolutionized the diagnosis and care of patients with brain abscesses. CT has been studied extensively in animal models and has been correlated with pathologic findings in the evolution of brain abscess formation (125–130). An additional advantage of CT scanning is that it allows for detection of underlying sinusitis or mastoiditis with the use of dedicated bone windows (131).

Inoculation of brain parenchyma with mixed aerobic and anaerobic flora has been followed by pathologic correlation with CT findings in a number of animal studies (128,129,132). Histopathologic examination at surgery and autopsy indicates that humans go through a similar staging process (130). Abscesses progress from early cerebritis (days 1–3) to late cerebritis (days 4–9) after inoculation of bacteria. Capsule formation begins at days 10 to 13, with well-formed capsules present after day 14 in the untreated patient (133). The early cerebritis stage is marked radiographically by poorly delineated areas of low attenuation on CT, with little to no contrast enhancement. As the capsule begins to form, peripheral enhancement may be noted, with a characteristic diffusion of contrast media into the center of the lesion on delayed (e.g., 60-minute) scanning. As the lesion becomes more encapsulated, this centripetal enhancement is lost, signaling the development of a necrotic center with limited vascular supply (a concept with important clinical implications, as noted below). Typically, there is smooth ring enhancement when contrast material is used in conjunction with CT, but enhancement may be irregular, especially with smaller lesions, making it difficult to exclude a neoplastic process. Capsules tend to form more readily and to be thicker on the side adjacent to gray matter, which is better vascularized than the white matter (33). Concurrent antibiotic therapy, steroids, radiation, immunosuppression, or neutropenia may alter the expected radiographic progression. Steroid therapy may reduce the thickness of the capsule and the degree of ring enhancement present; importantly, capsule size may increase after the discontinuation of steroids, often without clinical deterioration or evidence of abscess expansion. In following the progression of disease and effect of therapy, the size of the enhancing capsule has been recommended as a general guide (130).

None of the CT findings are pathognomonic for brain abscess, especially in the early cerebritis stage. Other CNS processes, such as primary or metastatic tumor, infarction, resolving hematoma, and radiation necrosis, may produce ring-enhancing lesions, further complicating definitive diagnosis (13,33,134,135). Brain abscess and neoplastic processes may coexist.

MAGNETIC RESONANCE IMAGING

The improved sensitivity and soft tissue resolution of MRI has revolutionized the diagnosis, treatment, and follow-up of brain abscesses in recent years. Studies of humans have corroborated the findings of animal studies of enhanced and earlier sensitivity, leading some authorities to suggest that MRI is now the diagnostic procedure of choice in brain abscess (136–140). The use of contrast enhancement with gadolinium-pentetic acid allows for evaluation of tissue perfusion and disruption of the blood-brain barrier (Fig. 152.1). Additional advantages include the ability to better evaluate edema, atrophy, and hemorrhage as intraparenchymal complications of infection. Bone detail and calcification, however, are more difficult to evaluate by MRI than by CT, limiting its usefulness in evaluating underlying cranial abnormalities (137,141). With the use of venography or MRV, thrombotic complications in the venous sinuses may be diagnosed via this technique.

Cerebritis appears as an area of high signal intensity on T2-weighted MRI images; the subsequent capsule appears as a ring-like area of low signal intensity (140,142). As with CT, infection progression and resolution may be followed by using the size

of the enhancing rim as a guide. Recent studies using diffusion-weighted MRI have suggested that this modality may help differentiate purulent material within the brain parenchyma from cystic fluid associated with some tumors (142–144) (Fig. 152.2). Additional investigation is needed to confirm these initial findings in animal models as well as humans.

Definitive diagnosis of brain abscess and identification of its microbiologic cause can be obtained only by examination and culture of surgically acquired tissue or fluid. The procedures available are discussed below.

TREATMENT

Surgical Therapy

Before the advent of antibiotics, surgery was the only therapy available. Potential procedures included aspiration, external tube drainage, excision, and marsupialization (145). Surgery reduced the nearly 100% mortality rate to approximately 60%. With advances in diagnosis and antimicrobial agents, the overall mortality rate has declined to 10% to 20% (33,146). Surgery remains a mainstay of therapy, with aspiration or excision combined with prolonged antibiotic courses the most common treatment approach (147). With stereotactic techniques available, surgical therapy has become more precise and less dangerous (52,148–150).

By the early 1950s, it became apparent that aspiration was often as effective as excision and that early antibiotic therapy might diminish the size of a lesion, obviating the need for surgical intervention. Aspiration of a lesion is often necessary for diagnostic purposes and is helpful therapeutically, especially in patients with deep-seated abscesses (e.g., in the cerebellum, brainstem, or thalamus) (52,151–153). Removal of purulent material provides a more favorable local environment for antimicrobial activity, in addition to allowing definitive identification of the etiologic organisms involved. The most common complication of this procedure is intracranial hemorrhage, due to parenchymal bleeding during the cerebritis stage or from the vascularized capsule of a well-formed abscess (13,25,154). A decision to proceed with aspiration and antibiotics, or occasionally with antibiotics alone, demands close clinical observation and sequential CT or MRI studies at intervals dictated by the clinical course. Deterioration of neurologic status or enlargement of the abscess warrants a more extensive procedure with repeat cultures (155).

Excision of an abscess (with removal of the abscess contents and capsule) is often required for the treatment of posttraumatic brain abscess, to débride the area and remove bone fragments or other foreign bodies that may predispose to relapse of infection. In addition, multiloculated abscesses, which are difficult to treat medically and to aspirate effectively, may require excision for effective treatment. Clinical failures or relapses have been noted in treatment of fungal abscesses with medical and aspiration therapy; the presence of fungal elements within the capsule itself suggests that surgical excision is a more effective means of treatment. If mastoiditis is the cause of an abscess, mastoidectomy should be performed to prevent relapse.

Ultrasonography has been minimally useful in the preoperative diagnosis of intraparenchymal lesions in adults, but intraoperative ultrasonography has assisted in localizing and draining small lesions, minimizing potential damage to surrounding normal brain tissue (156,157). Instillation of saline microbubbles at the time of surgical aspiration provides sonographic contrast, which may identify a loculation that requires drainage (158). Brain abscesses in neonates have been aspirated using intraoperative ultrasonography through the fontanels (159).

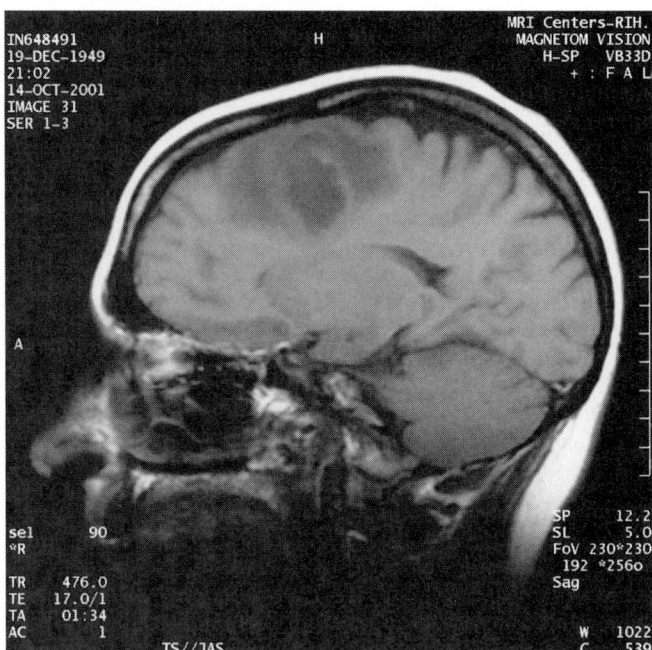

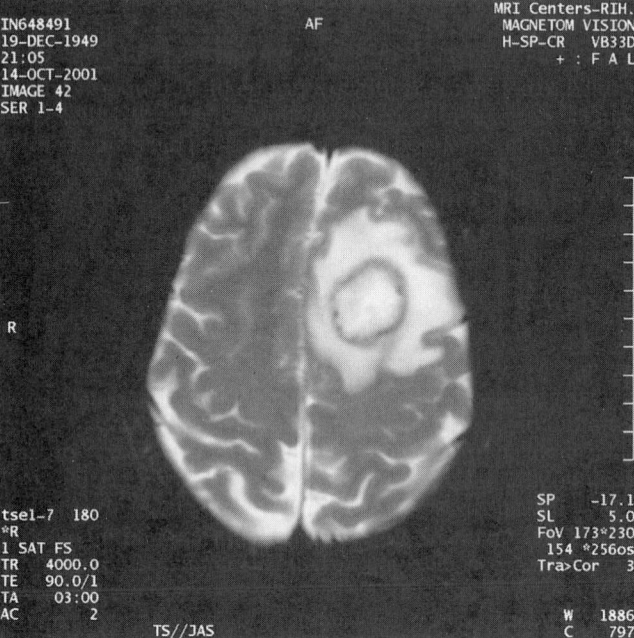

Figure 152.1. Radiographs of a previously healthy 51-year-old woman who presented with a 2-month history of fatigue and generalized weakness, with a 1-week history of worsening confusion, and a 24-hour history of aphasia and severe headache. **A:** T1-weighted magnetic resonance image demonstrates a 7.5-cm ring-enhancing lesion in the left frontal lobe with associated vasogenic edema and midline shift. **B:** T1-weighted sagittal view demonstrates a septated or loculated lesion. **C:** T2-weighted view suggests hemorrhage into the lesion wall. A stereotactic aspiration was performed and cultures grew *Streptococcus anginosus* (*Streptococcus milleri*) in pure culture. She received 6 weeks of intravenous penicillin with complete clinical and radiologic resolution.

A comparison of aspiration and surgical excision in the treatment of brain abscess is difficult because no randomized, controlled trials have been performed and selection bias may confound the available retrospective studies. Overall, there appears to be no difference in survival between the two procedures. However, some researchers have reported the occurrence of seizures and focal neurologic deficits to be increased in patients undergoing complete excision (25,159,160). Conversely, it has been suggested that aspiration may be associated with a higher relapse rate (8% vs. 0% in one study) (73). As further advances in stereotactic techniques are made and newer antimicrobial agents become available, the efficacy, complications, and role of the many surgical approaches available to treat brain abscess will need to be reassessed.

Direct instillation of antibiotics into the abscess has been suggested for therapy of pathogens that are particularly viru-lent or difficult to treat, such as *Pseudomonas* and many fungi (15,161). This approach has been limited by the epileptogenic properties of certain instilled antibiotics (e.g., high doses of β-lactam agents) and, when performed during the early cerebritis stage, potential spread of infection (25,106,162). Of note, there is no evidence that local instillation of antibiotics improves outcome, although rigorous studies have not been performed.

A surgical procedure should be considered part of the definitive diagnostic and therapeutic approach to any patient with brain abscess (163,164). Improved surgical technique, early diagnosis, and antibiotic therapy have diminished acute surgical mortality from approximately 15% to a rare event (165–167). Surgery will reduce mass effect, establish a diagnosis, and usually define the etiologic agent and its susceptibility pattern (168). Although both the available antimicrobial agents and the dosage

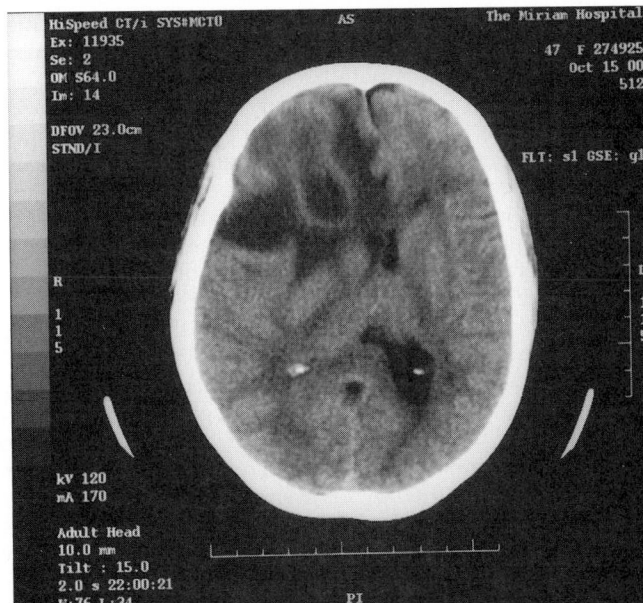

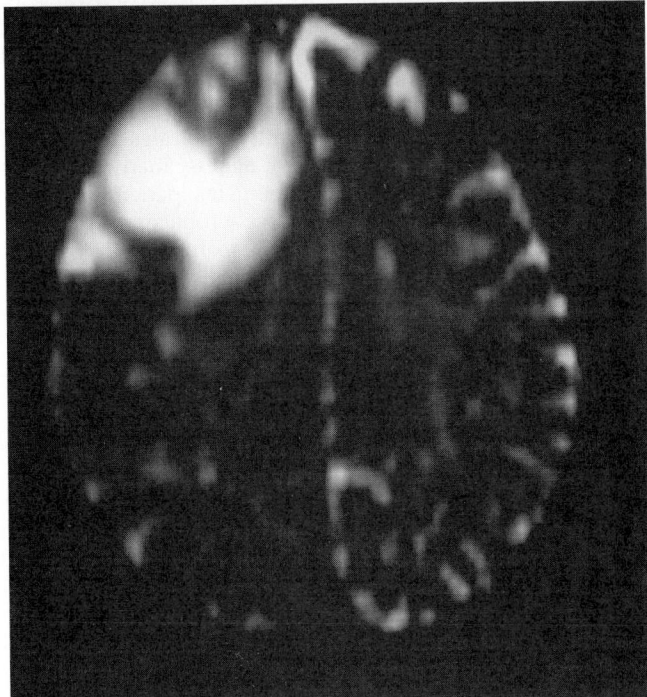

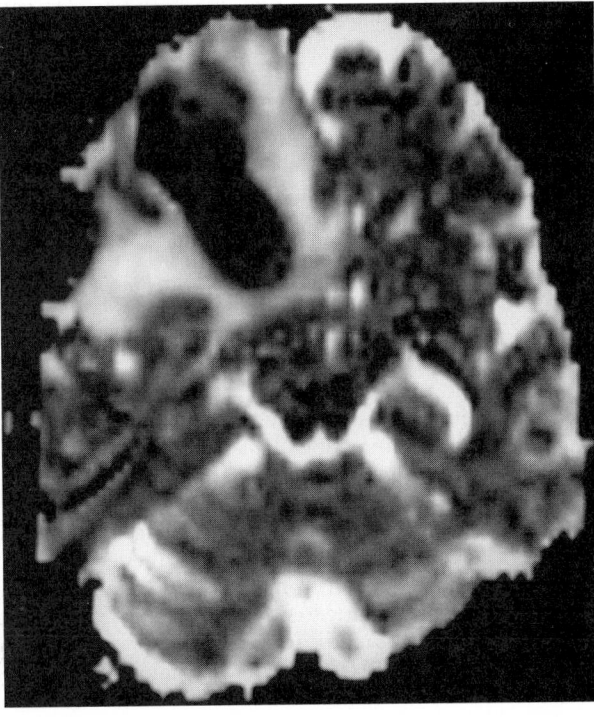

Figure 152.2. Diffusion-weighted images on the patient described in Fig. 152.1. Diffusion gradients (rates of diffusion of water within a mass visualized on magnetic resonance imaging) are measured in multiple orthogonal directions, and an apparent diffusion coefficient (*ADC*) is calculated. **A:** Noncontrast computed tomography scan of a 47-year-old woman with a history of alcohol and drug abuse who presented with headache and right-sided weakness without fever. **B:** Markedly increased signal within the lesion on trace-weighted, diffusion-weighted imaging. **C:** ADC map image demonstrating markedly decreased signal relative to cerebrospinal fluid within the mass; mean ADC was 0.52 mm^2/s. A stereotactic biopsy revealed gross pus; cultures grew *Streptococcus milleri*.

used have expanded over time, use of antibiotic therapy for brain abscess was not initially associated with decreased morbidity or mortality. Because ring enhancement on CT occurs during late cerebritis and does not necessarily indicate capsule formation (21,169,170), reported responses to antibiotic therapy alone may be due partially to therapy of cerebritis rather than to well-defined brain abscess (20). At surgery, susceptible organisms have been isolated from brain abscess even in the presence of therapeutic antimicrobial levels (162). Abscesses smaller than 3 to 4 cm in diameter have been found to respond to antibiotics alone, whereas larger ones are likely to require excision or drainage (73,159,171).

At a minimum, we recommend a diagnostic aspiration with Gram stain and aerobic and anaerobic culture to facilitate antimicrobial decision making. The use of special stains and cultures for mycobacteria, fungi, or other unusual pathogens should be dic-

tated by the clinical setting. Historically, patients who were not candidates for surgery because of general condition, age, or number, location, or size of the lesions have been treated with antibiotic therapy alone (12,172–174). Observational studies have indicated that the possibility of cure with antibiotics alone is higher during the early cerebritis stage (before capsule formation) than in later stages of abscess development. It remains unclear which patients should be treated with aspiration and antimicrobials or antimicrobials alone. Clearly in the immunocompromised host, where opportunistic pathogens are likely involved, aspiration with cultures is indicated (25).

Antimicrobial Therapy

Antibiotics used to treat brain abscess should be intravenous, preferably bactericidal and effective against the likely pathogens

TABLE 152.4.   Antibiotic Selection Based on Condition Predisposing to Brain Abscess

Focus	Antibiotic
Otic Mastoid Paranasal sinus (operated on or irrigated) Empyema Lung abscess	Third- or fourth-generation cephalosporin[a] and metronidazole
Dental Paranasal sinus (not operated on or irrigated) Bacteremia	Penicillin[b] and metronidazole
Gastrointestinal origin	Third- or fourth-generation cephalosporin[a] and metronidazole
Urinary tract origin	Third- or fourth-generation cephalosporin[a]
Endocarditis	As for the pathogen causing endocarditis

Wounds
  Use Gram stain for early decision
  Pure gram-negative or mixed flora
	Third- or fourth-generation cephalosporin[a] and metronidazole

Gram-positive cocci	Penicillinase-resistant antistaphylococcal penicillin[b]

Use maximal daily doses with adjustments as dictated by renal and hepatic function. Therapy should eventually be tailored to results of culture and susceptibility tests. Remember that anaerobes may take weeks to grow.
[a]Ceftriaxone, ceftazidime, cefotaxime, ceftizoxime, cefepime. Carbapenems such as meropenem or imipenem are alternatives, although the lowering of serizure threshold in the presence of these agents may complicate care.
[b]Vancomycin should be used for penicillin-allergic patients or when methicillin-resistant *Staphylococcus aureus* is a concern. Vancomycin should be the drug of choice when the gram-*positive* cocci are from a surgical wound.

involved. In addition, they should penetrate the abscess as well as any underlying site of infection (Table 152.4).

Penicillin G, administered at doses of 20 million units in divided doses each day, remains active against many oral anaerobes and streptococci. However, resistance in gram-negative rods precludes its use as single-agent empiric therapy of brain abscess. Chloramphenicol (50–100 mg/kg divided daily), which penetrates CSF and brain tissue extremely well relative to other antibiotics, is active against many gram-positive, gram-negative, and anaerobic bacteria (175). Although its toxicity decreases its attractiveness, as does its bacteriostatic effects on many bacteria, it remains an alternative treatment in the patient with penicillin allergy. Metronidazole (7.5 mg/kg given intravenously every 6 hours) penetrates abscess cavities at levels comparable with that in serum. It is bactericidal and effective at acid pH in the presence of pus or neutropenia, but it provides no aerobic coverage, and its activity against *Peptococcus* and *Peptostreptococcus* may be marginal (176–178). Therefore, metronidazole must usually be used in conjunction with a second agent, such as penicillin or a third- or fourth-generation cephalosporin (33). Clindamycin, while effective *in vitro* against many of the anaerobes and gram-positive bacteria causing brain abscesses, penetrates the blood-brain barrier poorly and the blood-CSF barrier worse, even in the presence of meningeal inflammation, limiting its usefulness in the treatment of brain abscesses (179). Ceftriaxone, cefotaxime, ceftizoxime, cefepime, and ceftazidime have been used in many patients with brain abscess; they penetrate the CNS well and cover many methicillin-susceptible *S. aureus*, streptococci, Enterobacteriaceae, and *Pseudomonas*

species (13,15,180). In combination with intravenous metronidazole, these agents provide broad-spectrum empirical coverage in many patients with bacterial brain abscess (181). None of the cephalosporins have activity against *L. monocytogenes,* a cause of both meningitis and brain abscess. The carbapenems (e.g., imipenem/cilastatin and meropenem) penetrate the blood-brain barrier, although CNS toxicity, particularly in the form of seizures, theoretically limits their usefulness as drugs of choice for brain abscess (182). Fluoroquinolones are active against a range of gram-negative aerobes and variably penetrate CSF; their CNS toxicity profile may be prohibitive in some cases. There are no controlled studies of the use of these agents in brain abscesses.

Expanded-spectrum penicillins, including nafcillin and oxacillin, have proven efficacious when given in high doses (e.g., 12–18 g per day of nafcillin) (33,183). Traditionally, the aminoglycosides (gentamicin, tobramycin, and amikacin) have been the gold standard of therapy for systemic infections caused by Enterobacteriaceae and *Pseudomonas aeruginosa.* Aminoglycosides penetrate the blood-brain and blood-CSF barriers poorly, although they are safely and effectively administered intraventricularly in the treatment of gram-negative meningitis and ventriculitis. The decreased activity of aminoglycosides at acidic pH levels present within an abscess, as well as the renal toxicity and ototoxicity of these agents, further limit their usage in the treatment of brain abscesses (175).

Aztreonam is a monocyclic β-lactam with activity against gram-negative aerobic bacilli and penetrates CSF effectively. The tetracyclines, while effective against many gram-positive and anaerobic gram-negative organisms, penetrate CSF poorly. Vancomycin, effective against most aerobic gram-positive cocci and an alternative therapy in the patient with β-lactam allergy, penetrates abscesses well, with levels 60% to 80% of concomitant serum levels (175,184). Data on the use of oxazolidinones (i.e., linezolid) in the treatment of brain abscess are not available.

EMPIRIC ANTIBIOTIC THERAPY IN THE PATIENT WITH BRAIN ABSCESS

Selection of empiric antibiotics in the patient with brain abscess should reflect presumed underlying etiologies. Secretions or drainage from any underlying focus should be obtained for Gram stains and culture if at all possible. Rarely, the organism will have already been isolated from underlying abscess, blood, sinus, empyema, or wound specimens, and initial antimicrobial therapy can be based on known susceptibility. Otherwise, empiric therapy is dictated by the anatomic location of the brain abscess and a suspected underlying cause.

When otic, paranasal sinus, or mastoid infection is the underlying etiology, coverage of Enterobacteriaceae, *P. aeruginosa,* aerobic streptococci, and anaerobes is paramount, so that metronidazole and a third- or fourth-generation cephalosporin are appropriate. An abscess of dental origin dictates a β-lactam with anaerobic activity for streptococci, *Eikenella* and *Prevotella* species potentially present. An obvious source of bacteremia dictates coverage of the likely organisms involved (e.g., gram-negative organisms from the abdomen or urinary tract; staphylococcal or streptococcal species from wounds).

The therapy of infections caused by methicillin-susceptible *S. aureus* is best accomplished with a narrow-spectrum β-lactamase–stable penicillin, such as oxacillin or nafcillin. These are preferable to broader spectrum antistaphylococcal β-lactam antibiotics and are more active on a weight basis. Any antistaphylococcal β-lactamase–stable penicillin should be given in intravenous doses of 12 g per day or more (183). Vancomycin is generally reserved for the therapy of methicillin-resistant *S. aureus*, clinically significant *Staphylococcus epidermidis*, and other gram-positive coccal infections in penicillin-allergic patients (184).

Adjunctive therapy of brain abscess has included mannitol, hyperventilation, and corticosteroids, which have been used to reduce intracranial swelling and cerebral edema. The osmotic effect of mannitol has been associated with an increase in gentamicin concentrations in the abscess and surrounding tissue.

The effect of corticosteroids on the clinical course and radiographic appearance of brain abscesses has been addressed in several animal models. In rats with *E. coli* abscesses, steroids increase bacterial organism load, delay capsule formation and decrease macrophage and glial response, all associated with diminished survival (33,185–187). Despite the suspicion that steroids would decrease antibiotic penetration into abscesses, no consistent changes in antibiotic delivery have been noted in animal studies (33,185–187). In patients with bacterial meningitis, the use of steroids has been associated with decreased antibiotic concentrations in CSF while also improving outcomes in some settings. When *P. melaninogenica* was inoculated stereotactically to produce abscess, concomitant use of corticosteroids significantly reduced the local concentrations of benzyl penicillin, but not of metronidazole (188). Methylprednisolone has been found to decrease collagen deposition 8 days after inoculation of organisms, but no effect on capsule thickness was apparent by 18 days after inoculation (189). In studies involving only a handful of patients, steroids decrease ring enhancement and are associated with overall clinical improvement (190). After discontinuation of steroids, enhancement increases and clinical conditions deteriorate. Corticosteroids have no impact on survival, neurologic sequelae, or length of hospital stay (1,186). When steroids are indicated to decrease cerebral edema and elevated intracranial pressure, their duration should be limited. If brain abscess is suspected, these agents should not be given without concurrent appropriate antimicrobial therapy.

Duration of antibiotic therapy should be 4 to 6 weeks for most pathogens. In the immunocompromised host, more prolonged antibiotic courses may be necessary, based on the organisms involved and the specific immunosuppressed state of the host. If the abscess is excised completely, a shorter course may be appropriate. The use of selected oral antibiotics once abscesses have been drained has been addressed in several small studies (191,192). If an oral agent is prescribed, documentation of high therapeutic serum levels is recommended. CT or MRI has been recommended in addition to clinical follow-up to document abscess resolution (73,193). It should be noted, however, that ring-enhancing lesions may persist for as long as 3 to 4 months on CT scans, even in the setting of complete, appropriate antibiotic therapy (25). Therefore, duration of antiinfective therapy should not be based solely on the persistence of radiographic signs. Surgical intervention is indicated if, either during or after completion of therapy, symptoms recur or progress, or the lesion enlarges.

PROGNOSIS

Relapses occur in 5% to 10% of patients, usually within 6 weeks of completion of antibiotic therapy (14,25). Occasional cases of recurrent infection have been noted years after presumed adequate therapy. Relapses may be related to inadequate antimicrobial therapy (e.g., ineffective agents, poor abscess penetration at doses prescribed, development of resistance), failure to aspirate a lesion or treat the underlying cause, or the presence of a foreign body or persistent extracranial communication. The patient with recurrent abscess should undergo an extensive search for and eradication of the underlying cause of treatment failure.

Morbidity related to brain abscess may be substantial (25,160). Since the advent of CT and MRI, patients are more alert and have fewer lesions and a better-defined surgical site at the time of diagnosis. Postoperative complications such as relapse, hemorrhage, and cerebral edema are more specifically and easily identified by CT or MRI (194). Focal neurologic sequelae are usually minor and infrequently observed but have occurred in up to 24% of patients. The prevalence of mental retardation has averaged about 16% and is correlated with disease in childhood and underlying cyanotic congenital heart disease (160,195). Seizures have been reported in 10% to 72% of patients, with mean onset in the third year after abscess treatment (25,160,196). Electroencephalographic abnormalities have not correlated directly with overall prognosis (197). Meningiomas and gliosarcomas have been reported to develop in the patient previously treated for brain abscess (198–200).

Mortality from brain abscesses remains approximately 10% (16,33,165–167,201). The presence of multiple lesions, deep-seated lesions, abscess rupture, and age older than 40 years portend higher risk for death, although in many studies the only factor predictive of mortality or sequelae is level of consciousness at presentation (107,189,202–204). The prognosis is poorer with diminishing state of consciousness at presentation—from lethargy to obtundation, stupor, and coma (159,205).

Brain abscess remains a disease of low frequency but significant morbidity and mortality. With further advances in surgical and neuroradiologic techniques as well as antimicrobial therapy and delivery systems, the prognosis of these infections will hopefully continue to improve.

REFERENCES

1. Chun CH, Johnson JD, Hofstetter M, et al. Brain abscess: a study of 45 consecutive cases. *Medicine (Baltimore)* 1986;65:415.
2. Harris LF, Maccubbin DA, Triplett JN, et al. Brain abscess: recent experience at a community hospital. *South Med J* 1985;78:704.
3. Garvey G. Current concepts of bacterial infections of the central nervous system. Bacterial meningitis and bacterial brain abscess. *J Neurosurg* 1983;59:735.
4. Renier D, Flandin C, Hirsch E, et al. Brain abscesses in neonates: a study of 30 cases. *J Neurosurg* 1988;69:877.
5. Sutton DL, Ouvrier RA. Cerebral abscess in the under 6 month age group. *Arch Dis Child* 1983;58:901.
6. Theophilo F, Markakis E, Theophilo L, et al. Brain abscess in childhood. *Childs Nerv Syst* 1985;1:324.
7. Hegde AS, Venkataramana NK, Das BS. Brain abscess in children. *Childs Nerv Syst* 1986;2:90.
8. Tavora L, Antunes JL. Brain abscesses and ischemic necrotic lesions during early childhood. *Neurosurgery* 1987;21:923.
9. Small M, Dale BA. Intracranial suppuration 1968–1982—a 15 year review. *Clin Otolaryngol* 1984;9:315.
10. Molavi AA, Dinubile MJ. Brain abscess. In: Harris AA, ed. *Handbook of clinical neurology.* Amsterdam: Elsevier, 1988:143–166.
11. Samson DS, Clark K. A current review of brain abscesses. *Am J Med* 1973;54:201.
12. Donald FE, Firth JL, Holland IM, et al. Brain abscess in the 1980's. *Br J Neurosurg* 1990;4:265.
13. Wispelwey B, Scheld WM. Brain abscess. *Semin Neurol* 1992;12:273.
14. Beller AJ, Sahar A, Praiss I. Brain abscess: review of 89 cases over a period of 30 years. *J Neurol Neurosurg Psychiatry* 1973;36:757.
15. Wispelwey B, Scheld WM. Brain abscess. *Clin Neuropharmacol* 1987;10:483.
16. Lakshmi V, Rao RR, Dinakar I. Bacteriology of brain abscess—observations on 50 cases. *J Med Microbiol* 1993;38:187.
17. Richards J, Sisson PR, Hickman JE, et al. Microbiology, chemotherapy and mortality of brain abscess in Newcastle-upon-Tyne between 1979 and 1988. *Scand J Infect Dis* 1990;22:511.
18. Kangsanarak J, Fooanant S, Ruckphaopunt K, et al. Extracranial and intracranial complications of suppurative otitis media. Report of 102 cases. *J Laryngol Otol* 1993;107:999.

19. Hervas JA, Ciria L, Henales V, et al. Nonsurgical management of neonatal multiple brain abscesses due to *Proteus mirabilis. Helv Paediatr Acta* 1987; 42:451.

20. Neuwelt EA, Lawrence MS, Blank NK. Effect of gentamicin and dexamethasone on the natural history of the rat *Escherichia coli* brain abscess model with histopathological correlation. *Neurosurgery* 1984;15:475.

21. Mathisen GE, Meyer RD, George WL, et al. Brain abscess and cerebritis. *Rev Infect Dis* 1984;6:5101.

22. Boom WH, Tuazon CU. Successful treatment of multiple brain abscesses with antibiotics alone. *Rev Infect Dis* 1985;7:189.

23. Kagawa M, Takeshita M, Yato S, et al. Brain abscess in congenital cyanotic heart disease. *J Neurosurg* 1983;58:913.

24. Coroli M, Arienta C, Rampini PM, et al. Recurrence of brain abscess associated with asymptomatic arteriovenous malformation of the lung. *Neurochirurgia* 1992;35:167.

25. Osenbach RK, Loftus CM. Diagnosis and management of brain abscess. *Neurosurg Clin North Am* 1992;3:403.

26. Hall WA. Hereditary hemorrhagic telangiectasia (Rendu-Osler-Weber disease) presenting with polymicrobial brain abscess: case report. *J Neurosurg* 1994;81:294.

27. Roman G, Fisher M, Perl DP, et al. Neurological manifestations of hereditary hemorrhagic telangiectasia (Rendu-Osler-Weber disease): report of two cases and review of the literature. *Ann Neurol* 1978;4:130.

28. Kurzydlowski H, Wollenschlager C, Venezio FR, et al. Reevaluation of an experimental streptococcal canine brain abscess model. *J Neurosurg* 1987; 67:717.

29. Costello GT, Heppe R, Winn HR, et al. Susceptibility of brain to aerobic, anaerobic, and fungal organisms. *Infect Immun* 1983;41:535.

30. Enzmann DR, Britt RR, Obana WB, et al. Experimental *Staphylococcus aureus* brain abscess. *AJNR* 1986;7:395.

31. Kline MW, Kaplan SL, Hawkins EP, et al. Pathogenesis of brain abscess formation in an infant rat model of *Citrobacter diversus* bacteremia and meningitis. *J Infect Dis* 1988;157:106.

32. Obana WB, Britt RH, Placone RC, et al. Experimental brain abscess development in the chronically immunosuppressed host. *J Neurosurg* 1986;65:382.

33. Kaplan K. Brain abscess. *Med Clin North Am* 1985;69:345.

34. Kanter MC, Hart RG. Neurologic complications of infective endocarditis. *Neurology* 1991;41:1015.

35. Lerner PI. Neurologic complications of infective endocarditis. *Med Clin North Am* 1985;69:385.

36. Gelfand MS, Stephens DS, Howell El, et al. Brain abscess: association with pulmonary arteriovenous fistula and hereditary hemorrhagic telangiectasia: report of three cases. *Am J Med* 1988;85:719.

37. Dong SL, Reynolds SF, Steiner IP. Brain abscess in patients with heredity hemorrhagic telangiectasia: case report and literature review. *J Emerg Med* 2001;20:247.

38. Swanson KL, Prakash UB, Stanson AW. Pulmonary arteriovenous fistulas: Mayo clinic experience, 1982–1997. *Mayo Clin Proc* 1999;74:671.

39. Summers LE, Mascott CR, Tompkins JR, et al. Frontal sinus osteoma associated with cerebral abscess formation: a case report. *Surg Neurol* 2001;55:235.

40. Press OW, Ramsey PG. Central nervous system infections associated with hereditary hemorrhagic telangiectasia. *Am J Med* 1984;77:86.

41. Hall WA. Hereditary hemorrhagic telangiectasia (Rendu-Osler-Weber disease) presenting with polymicrobial brain abscess. *J Neurosurg* 1994;81:294.

42. Gibbons JR, McIlrath TE, Bailey IC. Pulmonary arteriovenous fistula in association with recurrent cerebral abscess. *Thorac Cardiovasc Surg* 1984;33: 319.

43. Biller J, Baker WH, Quinn JP, et al. Intracranial hematoma with subsequent brain abscess after carotid endarterectomy. *Surg Neurol* 1984;23:605.

44. Biller J, Adams HP Jr, Godersky JC, et al. Preeclampsia complicated by cerebral hemorrhage and brain abscess. *J Neurol* 1985;232:378.

45. Gower D, McGuirt WF. Intracranial complications of acute and chronic infectious ear disease: a problem still with us. *Laryngoscope* 1983;93:1028.

46. Gower DJ, McGuirt WF, Kelley DL Jr. Intracranial complications of ear disease in a pediatric population with special emphasis on subdural effusion and empyema. *South Med J* 1984;78:429.

47. Bradley PJ, Manning KP, Shaw MD. Brain abscess secondary to otitis media. *J Laryngol Otol* 1984;98:1185.

48. Samuel J, Fernandes CM, Steinberg JL. Intracranial otogenic complications: a persisting problem. *Laryngoscope* 1986;96:272.

49. Venezio FR, Naidich TP, Shulman ST. Complications of mastoiditis with special emphasis on venous sinus thrombosis. *J Pediatr* 1982;101:509.

50. Nunez DA, Browning GG. Risks of developing an otogenic intracranial abscess. *J Laryngol Otol* 1990;104:468.

51. Jurado R, Garcia-Herola A, Garcia-Lazaro M, et al. Brain abscess with intracranial gas formation: case report. *Clin Infect Dis* 1994;19:219.

52. Kondziolka D, Duma CM, Lunsford LD. Factors that enhance the likelihood of successful stereotactic treatment of brain abscesses. *Acta Neurochir* 1994;127:85.

53. Cohen JT, Hochman II, DeRowe A, et al. Complications of acute otitis media and sinusitis. *Curr Infect Dis Rep* 2000;2:130.

54. Kurien M, Job A, Mathew J, et al. Otogenic intracranial abscess: concurrent craniotomy and mastoidectomy—changing trends in a developing country. *Arch Otolaryngol Head Neck Surg* 1998;124:1353.

55. Osma U, Cureoglu S, Hosoglu S. The complications of chronic otitis media: report of 93 cases. *J Laryngol Otol* 2000;114:97.

56. Sennaroglu L, Sozeri B. Otogenic brain abscess: review of 41 cases. *Otolaryngol Head Neck Surg* 2000;123:751.

57. Mathews TJ. Acute and acute-on-chronic mastoiditis (a five year experience at Groote Schuur Hospital). *J Laryngol Otol* 1988;102:115.

58. Nalbone VP, Kuruvilla A, Gacek RR. Otogenic brain abscess: the Syracuse experience. *Ear Nose Throat J* 1992;71:238.

59. Kratimenos G, Crockard HA. Multiple brain abscess: a review of fourteen cases. *Br J Neurosurg* 1991;5:153.

60. Li X, Tronstad L, Olsen I. Brain abscesses caused by oral infection. *Endod Dent Traumatol* 1999;15:95.

61. Aldous JA, Powell GL, Stensaas SS. Brain abscess of odontogenic origin: report of case. *J Am Dent Assoc* 1987;115:861.

62. Ingham, HR, Kalbag RM, Tharagonnet D, et al. Abscesses of the frontal lobe of the brain secondary to covert dental sepsis. *Lancet* 1978;2:497.

63. Haddad FS, Hubballa J, Zaytoun G, et al. Intracranial complications of submucous resection of the nasal septum. *Am J Otolaryngol* 1985;6:443.

64. Celli P, Palatinsky E. Brain abscess as a complication of cranial traction. *Surg Neurol* 1985;23:594.

65. Martinez-Lage JF, Perez-Espejo MA, Masegosa J, et al. Bilateral brain abscesses complicating the use of Crutchfield tongs. *Childs Nerv Syst* 1986;2:208.

66. Goodman ML, Nelson PB. Brain abscess complicating the use of a halo orthosis. *Neurosurgery* 1987;20:27.

67. Williams FH, Nelms DK, McGaharan KM. Brain abscess: a rare complication of halo usage. *Arch Phys Med Rehabil* 1992;73:490.

68. Blomstedt GC. Infections in neurosurgery: a retrospective study of 1143 patients and 1517 operations. *Acta Neurochir* 1985;78:81.

69. Tay JS, Garland JS. Serious head injuries from lawn darts. *Pediatrics* 1987;79:261.

70. Foy P, Sharr M. Cerebral abscesses in children after pencil-tip injuries. *Lancet* 1980;2:662.

71. Bank DE, Carolan PL. Cerebral abscess formation following ocular trauma: a hazard associated with common wooden toys. *Pediatr Emerg Care* 1993; 9:285.

72. Lee JH, Kim DG. Brain abscess related to metal fragments 47 years after head injury. *J Neurosurg* 2000;93:477.

73. Rosenblum ML, Mampalam TJ, Pons VG. Controversies in the management of brain abscesses. *Clin Neurosurg* 1986;33:603.

74. Pancek TL, Burchiel KJ. Delayed brain abscess related to a retained foreign body with culture of *Clostridium bifermentans*. Case report. *J Neurosurg* 1986;64:813.

75. Schijman E, Monges J, Cragnaz R. Congenital dermal sinuses, dermoid and epidermoid cysts of the posterior fossa. *Childs Nerv Syst* 1986;2:83.

76. Martens F, Ectors P, Noel P, et al. Unusual cause of cerebellar abscess. Occipital dermal sinus and dermoid cyst. *Neuropediatrics* 1987;18:107.

77. Morgan MG, Stuart C, Leanord AT, et al. *Citrobacter diversus* brain abscess: case reports and molecular epidemiology. *J Med Microbiol* 1992;36:273.

78. Curless RG. Neonatal intracranial abscess: two cases caused by *Citrobacter* and a literature review. *Ann Neurol* 1980;8:269.

79. Lai KK. *Enterobacter sakazakii* infections among neonates, infants, children, and adults: case reports and a review of the literature. *Medicine* 2001;80:113.

80. Dee RR, Lorber B. Brain abscess due to *Listeria monocytogenes*: case report and literature review. *Rev Infect Dis* 1986;8:968.

81. Eckburg PB, Montoya JG, Vosti KL. Brain abscess due to *Listeria monocytogenes*: five cases and a review of the literature. *Medicine* 2001;80:223.

82. Mylonakis E, Hohmann EL, Calderwood SB. Central nervous system infection with listeria monocytogenes: 33 years' experience at a general hospital and review of 776 episodes from the literature. *Medicine* 1998;77:313.

83. Abla AA, Maroon JC, Slifkin M. Brain abscess due to *Haemophilus aphrophilus*: possible canine transmission. *Neurosurgery* 1986;19:123.

84. Jensen KT, Hojbjerg T. Meningitis and brain abscess due to *Haemophilus paraphrophilus. Eur J Clin Microbiol* 1985;4:419.

85. Habib M, Fosse T, Pellissier JF, et al. Metastatic cerebral abscesses due to *Haemophilus paraphrophilus. Arch Neurol* 1984;41:1290.

86. Pajeau AK, Yu PK, Ebersold MJ. *Haemophilus paraphrophilus* frontal lobe abscess: case report. *Neurosurgery* 1988;23:643.

87. Schlitt M, Mitchem L, Zorn G, et al. Brain abscess after esophageal dilation for caustic stricture: report of three cases. *Neurosurgery* 1985;17:947.

88. Cohen FL, Koerner RS, Taub SJ. Solitary brain abscess following endoscopic injection sclerosis of esophageal varices. *Gastrointest Endosc* 1985;31:331.

89. Algoed L, Boon P, De Vos M, et al. Brain abscess after esophageal dilatation for stenosis. *Clin Neurol Neurosurg* 1992;94:169.

90. Robert JY, Raoul JL, Bretagne JF, et al. Unusual presentation of a case of brain abscess after endoscopic injection sclerotherapy of esophageal varices. *Endoscopy* 1991;23:237.

91. Ariza J, Casanova A, Fernandez Viladrich P, et al. Etiological agent and primary source of infection in 42 cases of focal intracranial suppuration. *J Clin Microbiol* 1986;24:899.

92. Su TM, Lin YC, Lu CH, et al. Streptococcal brain abscess: analysis of clinical features in 20 patients. *Surg Neurol* 2001;56:189.

93. Smego RA. Actinomycosis of the central nervous system. *Rev Infect Dis* 1987;9:855.

94. Gupta SK, Mohanty S, Tandon SC, et al. Brain abscess: with special reference to infection by *Pseudomonas. Br J Neurosurg* 1990;4:279.

95. Rodriguez RE, Valero V, Watanakunakorn C. *Salmonella* focal intracranial infections: review of the world literature (1884–1984) and report of an unusual case. *Rev Infect Dis* 1986;8:31.

96. Iplikcioglu AC, Kokes F, Bayar MA, et al. Brain abscess caused by *Salmonella typhimurium:* case report and review of the literature. *J Neurosurg Sci* 1991; 35:165.
97. Hanel RA, Araujo JC, Antoniuk A, et al. Multiple brain abscesses caused by *Salmonella typhi:* case report. *Surg Neurol* 2000;53:86.
98. Noguerado A, Cabanyes J, Vivancos J, et al. Abscess caused by *Salmonella enteritidis* with a glioblastoma multiforme. *J Infect* 1987;15:61.
99. Strampfer MJ, Schoch PE, Cunha BA. Cerebral abscess caused by *Klebsiella ozaenae. J Clin Microbiol* 1987;25:1553.
100. Andersen BB, Sogaard I. Legionnaire's disease and brain abscess. *Neurology* 1987;37:333.
101. Singh N, Husain S. Infections of the central nervous system in transplant recipients. *Transplant Infect Dis* 2000;2:101.
102. Couch L Theilen F, Mader JT. Rhinocerebral mucormycosis with cerebral extension successfully treated with adjunctive hyperbaric oxygen therapy. *Arch Otolaryngol Head Neck Surg* 1988;14:791.
103. Perez RE, Smith M, McClendon J, et al. *Pseudallescheria boydii* brain abscess. Complication of an intravenous catheter. *Am J Med* 1988;84:359.
104. Nesky MA, McDougal EC, Peacock JE. *Pseudallescheria boydii* brain abscess successfully treated with voriconazole and surgical drainage: case report and literature review of central nervous system pseudallescheriasis. *Clin Infect Dis* 2000;31:673.
105. Dworzack DL, Clark RB, Borkowski WJ Jr, et al. *Pseudallescheria boydii* brain abscess: association with near-drowning and efficacy of high-dose, prolonged miconazole therapy in patients with multiple abscesses. *Medicine* 1989; 68:218.
106. Yang SY. Brain abscess: a review of 400 cases. *J Neurosurg* 1981;55:794.
107. Bidzinski J, Koszewski W. The value of different methods of treatment of brain abscess in the CT era. *Acta Neurochir* 1990;105:117.
108. Brydon HL, Hardwidge C. The management of cerebellar abscess since the introduction of CT scanning. *Br J Neurosurg* 1994;8:447.
109. Lahat E, Livneh M, Schiffer J, et al. Rapidly growing head circumference as an isolated presenting symptom of brain abscesses in an infant. *Clin Neurol Neurosurg* 1987;89:269.
110. Takeshita M, Kawamata T, Izawa M, et al. Prodromal signs and clinical factors influencing outcome in patients with intraventricular rupture of purulent brain abscess. *Neurosurgery* 2001;48:310.
111. Ferre C, Ariza J, Viladrich P, et al. Brain abscess rupturing into the ventricles or subarachnoid space. *Am J Med* 1999;106:254.
112. Nielsen H. Cerebral abscess in children. *Neuropediatrics* 1983;14:76.
113. Sarwar M, Falkoff G, Naseem M. Radiologic techniques in the diagnosis of CNS infections. *Neurol Clin* 1986;4:41.
114. Young RF, Frazee J. Gas within intracranial abscess cavities: an indication for surgical excision. *Ann Neurol* 1984;16:35.
115. Kawamura H Umezawa Y, Amano K, et al. EEG topographic changes of brain abscesses in children. *No Shinkei Geka* 1987;15:381.
116. Frank JL. Sonography of intracranial infection in infants and children. *Neuroradiology* 1986;28:440.
117. Gray PH, O'Reilly C. Neonatal *Proteus mirabilis* meningitis and cerebral abscess: diagnosis by real-time ultrasound. *J Clin Ultrasound* 1984;12:441.
118. Rehncrona S, Brismar J, Holtas S. Diagnosis of brain abscesses with indium-111–labeled leukocytes. *Neurosurgery* 1985;16:23.
119. Bellotti C, Aragno MG, Medina M, et al. Differential diagnosis of CT-hypodense cranial lesions with indium-111-oxine–labeled leukocytes. *J Neurosurg* 1986;64:750.
120. Dudiak CM, Ali A, Dickerson M, et al. Acute tentorial subdural hematoma as a false-positive in indium-111 leukocyte scintigraphy. *Clin Nucl Med* 1985;10:513.
121. Balachandran S, Husain MM, Adametz JR, et al. Uptake of indium-111–labeled leukocytes by brain metastasis. *Neurosurgery* 1987;20:606.
122. Shih WJ, DeLand FH. Equivocal findings on cranial CT but apparent cerebral lesion(s) on conventional radionuclide imaging. *Clin Nucl Med* 1987;12:219.
123. Palestro CJ, Swyer AJ, Kim CK, et al. Role of In-111 labeled leukocyte scintigraphy in the diagnosis of intracerebral lesions. *Clin Nucl Med* 1991;16:305.
124. Whelan MA, Hilal SK. Computed tomography as a guide in the diagnosis and follow-up of brain abscesses. *Radiology* 1980;135:663.
125. Enzmann DR, Placone RC, Britt RH. Dynamic computed tomographic scans in experimental brain abscess. *Neuroradiology* 1984;26:309.
126. Enzmann DR, Britt RH, Placone R. Staging of human brain abscess by computed tomography. *Radiology* 1983;146:703.
127. Weisberg LA. The role of CT in the evaluation of patients with intracranial CNS infectious-inflammatory disorder. *Comput Radiol* 1984;8:29.
128. Britt RH, Enzmann DR, Yeager AS. Neuropathological and computerized tomographic findings in experimental brain abscess. *J Neurosurg* 1981;55: 590.
129. Enzmann DR, Britt RH, Yeager AS. Experimental brain abscess evolution: computed tomographic and neuropathologic correlation. *Radiology* 1979;133:113.
130. Enzmann DR, Britt RH, Placone R. Staging of human brain abscess by computed tomography. *Radiology* 1983;146:703.
131. Carter BL, Bankoff MS, Fisk JD. Computed tomographic detection of sinusitis responsible for intracranial and extracranial infections. *Radiology* 1983;147:739.
132. Britt RH, Enzmann DR, Placone RC Jr, et al. Experimental anaerobic brain abscess: computerized tomographic and neuropathological correlations. *J Neurosurg* 1984;60:1148.
133. Britt RH, Enzmann DR. Clinical stages of human brain abscesses on serial CT scans after contrast infusion. Computerized tomographic, neuropathological, and clinical correlations. *J Neurosurg* 1983;59:972.
134. Piszczor M, Thornton G, Bia FJ. The evaluation of contrast-enhancing brain lesions: pitfalls in current practice. *Yale J Biol Med* 1985;58:19.
135. Berry AD III, Reintjes SL, Kepes JJ. Intracranial malignant fibrous histiocytoma with abscess-like tumor necrosis. Case report. *J Neurosurg* 1988;69:780.
136. Sze G, Zimmerman RD. The magnetic resonance imaging of infections and inflammatory diseases. *Radiol Clin North Am* 1988;26:839.
137. Davidson HD, Steiner RE. Magnetic resonance imaging in infections of the central nervous system. *AJNR* 1985;6:499.
138. Schroth G, Kretzschmar K, Gawehn J, et al. Advantage of magnetic resonance imaging in the diagnosis of cerebral infections. *Neuroradiology* 1987;29:120.
139. Bertorini TE, Laster RE, Thompson BF, et al. Magnetic resonance imaging of the brain in bacterial endocarditis. *Arch Intern Med* 1989;149:815.
140. Enzmann DR. Magnetic resonance imaging update on brain abscess and central nervous system aspergillosis. *Curr Clin Top Infect Dis* 1993;13:269.
141. Gooding CA, Brasch RC, Lallemand DP, et al. Nuclear magnetic resonance imaging of the brain in children. *J Pediatr* 1984;104:509.
142. Kollias SS, Bernays RL. Interactive magnetic resonance imaging—guided management of intracranial cystic lesions by using an open magnetic resonance imaging system. *J Neurosurg* 2001;95:15.
143. Ketelslegers E, Duprez T, Ghariani S, et al. Time dependence of serial diffusion-weighted imaging features in a case of pyogenic brain abscess. *J Comput Assist Tomogr* 2000;24:478.
144. Tung GA, Evangelista P, Rogg J, et al. Diffusion-weighted MR imaging of rim-enhancing brain masses: is markedly decreased water diffusion specific for brain abscess? *AJR* 2001;177:709.
145. Stephanov S. Surgical treatment of brain abscess. *Neurosurgery* 1988;22:724.
146. Habib AA, Mozaffar T. Brain abscess. *Arch Neurol* 2001;58:1302.
147. Garfield J. Management of supratentorial intracranial abscess: a review of 200 cases. *BMJ* 1969;2:7.
148. Itakura T, Yokote H, Ozaki F, et al. Stereotactic operation for brain abscess. *Surg Neurol* 1987;28:196.
149. Stephanov S. Surgical treatment of brain abscess. *Neurosurgery* 1988;22:724.
150. Whittle IR, Denholm SW, Elshunnar K. CT-guided stereotactic neurosurgery using the Brown-Roberts-Wells system: experience with 125 procedures. *Aust N Z J Surg* 1991;61:919.
151. Coin CG, Hucks-Folliss AG, Mahegan CC. Computed-tomographically guided percutaneous transmastoid drainage of a cerebellar abscess. *Surg Neurol* 1980;20:387.
152. Hollander D, Villemure JG, Leblanc R. Thalamic abscess: a stereotactically treatable lesion. *Appl Neurophysiol* 1987;50:168.
153. Nauta HJ, Briner RP, Eisenberg HM. Computed tomogram-guided stereotactic brain biopsy in the pediatric patient. *Pediatr Neurosci* 1985–1986;12:63.
154. Stroobandt G, Zech F, Thauvoy C, et al. Treatment by aspiration of brain abscesses. *Acta Neurochir* 1987;85:138.
155. Johnson DL, Markle BM, Wiedermann BL, et al. Treatment of intracranial abscesses associated with sinusitis in children and adolescents. *J Pediatr* 1988;113:15.
156. Knake JE, Bowerman RA, Silver TM, et al. Neurosurgical applications of intraoperative ultrasound. *Radiol Clin North Am* 1985;23:73.
157. Pery M, Borovich B, Kaftori JK, et al. Intraoperative ultrasonography in cystic brain lesions. *Isr J Med Sci* 1988;24:405.
158. Theophilo F, Burnett A, Juca Filho G, et al. Ultrasound-guided brain abscess aspiration in neonates. *Childs Nerv Syst* 1987;3:371.
159. Leys D, Christiaens JL, Derambure P, et al. Management of focal intracranial infections: is medical treatment better than surgery? *J Neurol Neurosurg Psychiatry* 1990;53:472.
160. Nielsen H, Harmsen A, Gyldensted C. Cerebral abscess: a long-term follow-up. *Acta Neurol Scand* 1983;67:330.
161. Adler DE, Milhorat TH, Miller JI. Treatment of rhinocerebral mucormycosis with intravenous, interstitial, and cerebrospinal fluid administration of amphotericin B: case report. *Neurosurgery* 1998;42:644.
162. Black P, Graybill JR, Charache P. Penetration of brain abscess by systemically administered antibiotics. *J Neurosurg* 1973;38:705.
163. De Louvois J. The bacteriology and chemotherapy of brain abscess. *J Antimicrob Chemother* 1978;4:395.
164. Choudhury AR, Taylor JC, Whitaker R. Primary excision of brain abscess. *BMJ* 1977;2:1119.
165. Mampalam TJ, Rosenblum ML. Trends in the management of bacterial brain abscesses: a review of 102 cases over 17 years. *Neurosurgery* 1988;23:451.
166. Freeman J. Changing concepts in the management of otitic intracranial infection: use of computerized axial tomography in early detection and monitoring of cerebritis. *Laryngoscope* 1984;94:907.
167. Patrick CC, Kaplan SL. Current concepts in the pathogenesis and management of brain abscesses in children. *Pediatr Clin North Am* 1988;35:625.
168. Villar LA, Massanari RM, Koontz FP. Brain abscess due to penicillin- and clindamycin-resistant *Bacteroides melaninogenicus. Surg Neurol* 1983;20: 453.
169. Rennels MB, Woodward CL, Robinson WL, et al. Medical cure of apparent brain abscesses. *Pediatrics* 1983;72:220.
170. Dobkin JF, Healton EB, Dickinson PC, et al. Nonspecificity of ring enhancement in "medically cured" brain abscess. *Neurology* 1984;34:139.
171. Petit H, Rousseaux M, Lesoin F, et al. Primacy of medical treatment of cerebral abscesses (19 cases). *Rev Neurol (Paris)* 1983;139:575.

172. De Louvois J, Gortvai P, Hurley R. Antibiotic treatment of abscesses of the central nervous system. *BMJ* 1977;2:985.

173. Yoshikawa TT, Goodman SJ. Brain abscess—teaching conference. University of California, Los Angeles, and Harbor General Hospital, Torrance (Specialty Conference). *West J Med* 1974;121:207.

174. Daniels SR, Price JK, Towbin RB, et al. Nonsurgical cure of brain abscess in a neonate. *Childs Nerv Syst* 1985;1:346.

175. Saez-Llorens XJ, Umana MA, Odio CM, et al. Brain abscess in infants and children. *Pediatr Infect Dis* 1989;8:449–458.

176. Barling RWA, Selkon JB. The penetration of antibiotics into cerebrospinal fluid and brain tissue. *J Antimicrob Chemother* 1978;4:203.

177. Warner JF, Perkins RL, Cordero L. Metronidazole therapy of anaerobic bacteremia, meningitis, and brain abscess. *Arch Intern Med* 1979;139:167.

178. Ingham HR, Selkon JB, Roxby CM. Bacteriological study of otogenic cerebral abscesses: chemotherapeutic role of metronidazole. *BMJ* 1977;2:991.

179. Panzer JD, Brown DC, Epstein WL, et al. Clindamycin levels in various body tissues and fluids. *J Clin Pharmacol* 1972;12:259.

180. Sjolin J, Eriksson N, Arneborn P, et al. Penetration of cefotaxime and desacetyl-cefotaxime into brain abscesses in humans. *Antimicrob Agents Chemother* 1991; 35:2606.

181. Sjolin J, Lilja A, Eriksson N, et al. Treatment of brain abscess with cefotaxime and metronidazole: prospective study on 15 consecutive patients. *Clin Infect Dis* 1993;17:857.

182. Carton JA, Perez F, Maradona JA, et al. Successful treatment of recurrent cerebral empyema and brain abscesses with imipenem. *Eur J Clin Microbiol* 1987;6:578.

183. Fong IW. Staphylococcal central nervous system infections treated with cloxacillin. *J Antimicrob Chemother* 1983;12:607.

184. Levy RM, Gutin PH, Baskin DS, et al. Vancomycin penetration of a brain abscess: case report and review of the literature. *Neurosurgery* 1986;18: 632.

185. Neuwelt EA, Baker DE, Pagel MA, et al. Cerebrovascular permeability and delivery of gentamicin to normal brain and experimental brain abscess in rats. *J Neurosurg* 1984;61:430.

186. McGowan JE, Chesney PJ, Crossley KB, et al. Guidelines for the use of systemic glucocorticosteroids in the management of selected infections. *J Infect Dis* 1992;165:1.

187. Seydoux C, Francioli P. Bacterial brain abscesses: factors influencing mortality and sequelae. *Clin Infect Dis* 1992;15:394.

188. Kourtopoulos H, Holm SE, Norrby SR. The influence of steroids on the penetration of antibiotics into brain tissue and brain abscesses. An experimental study in rats. *J Antimicrob Chemother* 1983;11:245.

189. Schroeder KA, McKeever PE, Schaberg DR, et al. Effect of dexamethasone on experimental brain abscess. *J Neurosurg* 1987;66:264.

190. Black KL, Farhat SM. Cerebral abscess: loss of computed tomographic enhancement with steroids. Case report. *Neurosurgery* 1984;14:215.

191. Smith AL. Oral antibiotic therapy for serious infections. *Annu Rev Med* 1988;39:171.

192. Skoutelis AT, Gogos CA, Maraziotis TE, et al. Management of brain abscesses with sequential intravenous/oral antibiotic therapy. *Eur J Clin Microbiol Infect Dis* 2000;19:332.

193. Rousseaux M, Lesoin F, Destee A, et al. Developments in the treatment and prognosis of multiple cerebral abscesses. *Neurosurgery* 1985;16:304.

194. Rosenblum ML, Hoff JT, Norman D, et al. Decreased mortality from brain abscesses since advent of computerized tomography. *J Neurosurg* 1978; 49:658.

195. Hirsch JF, Roux FX, Sainte-Rose C, et al. Brain abscess in childhood. A study of 34 cases treated by puncture and antibiotics. *Childs Brain* 1983;10:251.

196. Legg NJ, Gupta PC, Scott DF. Epilepsy following cerebral abscess: a clinical and EEG study of 70 patients. *Brain* 1973;96:259.

197. Mises J, Daviet F, Moussalli-Salefranque F, et al. Brain abscess in the newborn infant (27 cases: initial electroclinical study, course). *Rev Electroencephalogr Neurophysiol Clin* 1987;17:301.

198. Reid PM, Barber PC. Gliosarcoma developing in close relationship to an abscess cavity injected with Thorotrast. *Surg Neurol* 1988;29:67.

199. Prager J, Zaret BS, Davidson R, et al. Gliosarcoma at the site of a surgically treated *Actinomyces* cerebral abscess. *Neurosurgery* 1984;15:868.

200. Reichenthal E, Rubenstein AB, Shevach I, et al. Meningioma presenting at a site of previously aspirated brain abscess. *Acta Neurochir* 1991;109:142.

201. Jefferson AA, Keogh AJ. Intracranial abscesses: a review of treated patients over 20 years. *J Med* 1977;183:389.

202. Dohrmann PJ, Elrick WL. Observations on brain abscess. Review of 28 cases. *Med J Aust* 1982;2:81.

203. Karandanis D, Shulman JA. Factors associated with mortality in brain abscess. *Arch Intern Med* 1975;135:1145.

204. Witzmann A, Beran H, Bohm-Jurkovic H, et al. Brain abscess. Prognostic factors. *Dtsch Med Wochenschr* 1989;20:114.

205. Mampalam TJ, Rosenblum ML. Trends in the management of bacterial brain abscesses: a review of 102 cases over 17 years. *Neurosurgery* 1988;23: 451.

CHAPTER 153
Slow Viral Infections of the Central Nervous System

David M. Asher

Several neurologic diseases once considered to be degenerative are caused by infections with asymptomatic incubation periods of months or years and durations of overt clinical illness that may also be quite long. Although the infectious agents may be latent in other organs of the body, pathologic changes are found only in the nervous system. Sigurdsson (1–3) studied such diseases of sheep and coined the term *slow infection* to describe them. Some slow infections—the spongiform encephalopathies (Chapter 264)—are caused by unique infectious agents of unknown structure, called *prions* (4) or transmissible spongiform encephalopathy (TSE) agents (5). Other slow infections of the human nervous system are caused by viruses with conventional physical properties—viruses that more often cause acute self-limited illnesses. This chapter reviews five such slow viral infections of humans (Table 153.1): progressive multifocal leukoencephalopathy (PML), subacute sclerosing panencephalitis (SSPE), rubella panencephalitis (RPE), tropical spastic paraparesis (TSP; also called human T-lymphotrophic virus–associated myelopathy [HAM]), and chronic tick-borne encephalitis (TBE). Other viral infections causing human neurologic diseases after prolonged latent periods with human immunodeficiency virus (HIV), cytomegalovirus, herpes simplex virus, varicella-zoster virus, and rabies virus are considered elsewhere in this book (Chapters 255, 235, 230, 234, and 262, respectively).

HISTORY

Progressive Multifocal Leukoencephalopathy

PML (6) is a progressive demyelinating disease of the nervous system caused by activation of a latent infection with the JC papovavirus (7,8) in immunosuppressed subjects, for whom it is invariably fatal. PML was first recognized complicating leukemia and Hodgkin's disease (6). It is now most often recognized as an opportunistic infection with acquired immunodeficiency syndrome (AIDS) in adults (9) and rarely children (10). In 1969, structures resembling virions of papovaviruses (Fig. 153.1) were detected by electron microscopy in oligodendrocytes of patients with PML (7). Two years later the causative agent, the JC virus (JCV), was isolated in cultures of fetal spongioblasts (glial precursor cells) (8).

Subacute Sclerosing Panencephalitis

SSPE is caused by a persistent measles virus infection. It was first clearly described by Dawson (11), who postulated its viral etiology. Bouteille et al. (12) observed that brain cells of patients with SSPE contained tubular structures (Fig. 153.2) similar to those seen in cells infected with measles virus, and Connolly, Allen, and Hurwitz (13) showed that patients with SSPE had high levels of antibodies to measles virus in serum and cerebrospinal fluid (CSF) and measles viral antigens in brain cells. Measles virus was isolated from brains of patients with SSPE in 1969 (14–17).

TABLE 153.1.   Slow Infections of the Human Nervous System Caused by Conventional Viruses

	Causative virus	Virus genus and family	Virus size and morphology	Viral nucleic acid
Progressive multifocal leukoencephalopathy (PML)	JC	Polyomavirus, Papovaviridae	45 nm, spherical, nonenveloped	dsDNA, circular, 5 kbp
Subacute sclerosing panencephalitis (SSPE)	Measles	Morbillivirus, Paramyxoviridae	150–300 nm, spherical/ filamentous (pleomorphic), enveloped	ssRNA, negative sense, 16 kb
Rubella panencephalitis (RPE)	Rubella	Rubivirus, Togaviridae	60–70 nm, spherical, enveloped	ssRNA, positive sense, 10 kb
Tropical spastic paraparesis (TSP)/ HTLV0I-associated myelopathy (HAM)	Human T-lymphotropic virus type I (HTLV-I)	Deltaretrovirus, Retroviridae	80–100 nm, spherical enveloped	ssRNA, positive sense, homodimer, 9 kb
Kozhevnikov epilepsy and other chronic forms of tick-borne encephalitis (TBE)	Tick-borne encephalitis (Russian spring-summer encephalitis)	Flavirus, Flaviviridae	45–60 nm, spherical, enveloped	ssRNA, positive sense, 10.7 kb

Note: Deltaretrovirus is a new genus.
ss, single stranded; ds, double stranded; kb, kilobase; kbp, kilobase pairs.
Source: From Goff SP. Retroviridae: the retroviruses and their replication. In: Knipe DM, Howley PM, eds. *Fields virology,* 4th ed.
Philadelphia: Lippincott Williams & Wilkins, 2001:1871–1940, with permission.

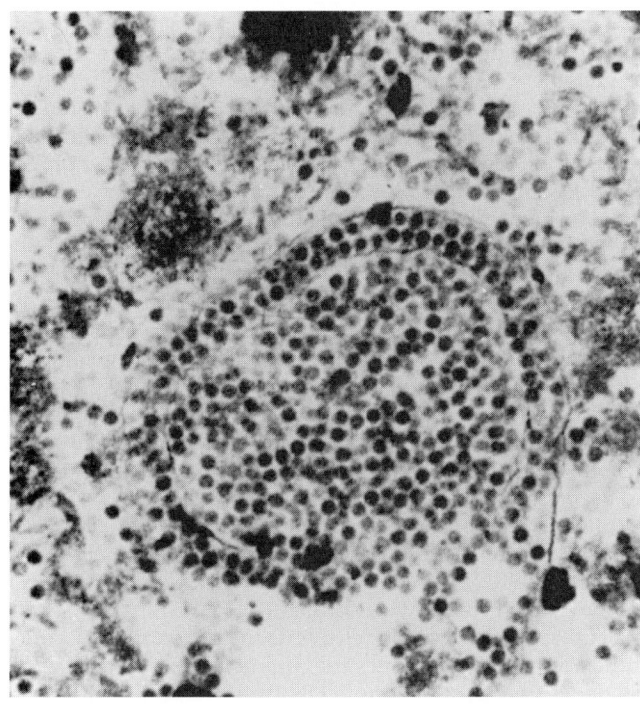

Figure 153.1. Progressive multifocal leukoencephalopathy. Crystalloid array of JC virus particles in the nucleus of an oligodendrocyte. (Courtesy of Dr. E. O. Major, National Institutes of Health, Bethesda, MD. From Major EO, Amemiya K, Tornatore CS, et al. Pathogenesis and molecular biology of progressive multifocal leukoencephalopathy, the JC virus-induced demyelinating disease of the human brain. *Clin Microbiol Rev* 1992;5:4973, with permission.)

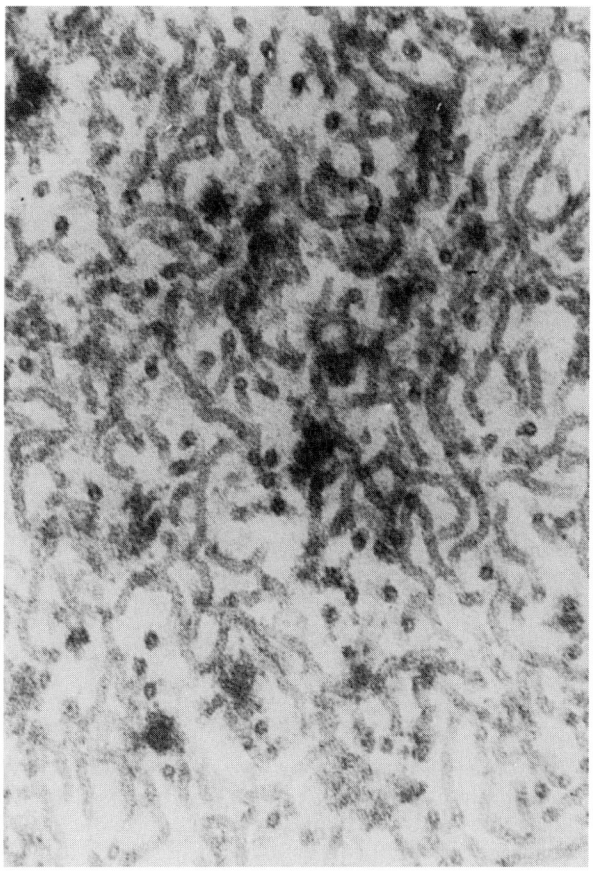

Figure 153.2. Measles nucleocapsids in the nucleus of a cell from the brain of a patient with subacute sclerosing panencephalitis. (Courtesy of Dr. Jerzy Kulczycki, Institute of Psychiatry and Neurology, Warsaw, Poland.)

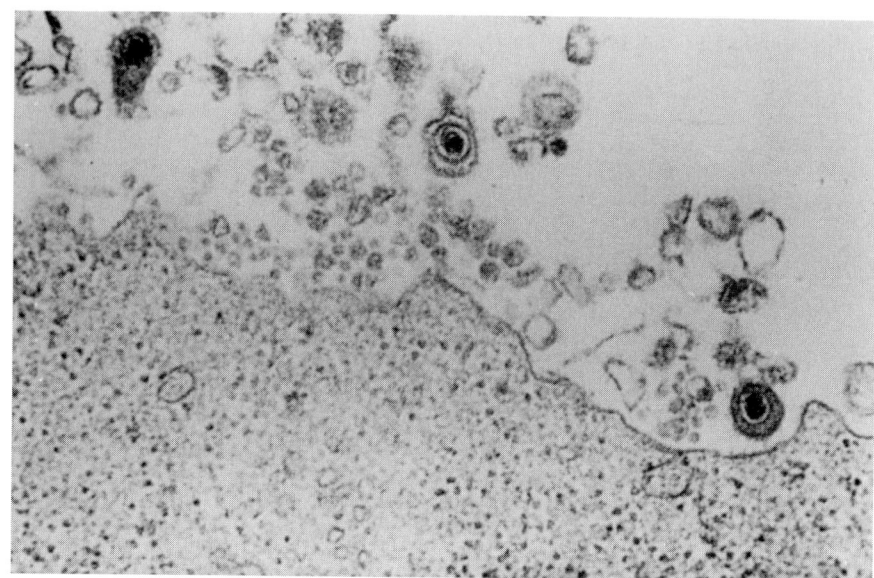

Figure 153.3. Tropical spastic paraparesis/human T-lymphotrophic virus type I–associated myelopathy (TSP/HAM). Extracellular particles of HTLV-I from the spinal cord of a patient with TSP/HAM, cultured in normal human peripheral blood cells. (Courtesy of the late Dr. C. J. Gibbs, Jr., National Institutes of Health, Bethesda, Maryland.)

Rubella Panencephalitis

RPE was first described in 1974 by Lebon and Lyon (18) affecting a boy with typical congenital rubella syndrome, an association that suggested that rubella virus might be the causative agent. Rubella virus was isolated from the brain of a patient with RPE by Cremer et al. in 1975 (19).

Tropical Spastic Paraparesis

TSP was long known as a chronic neurologic disease affecting the spinal cord in adolescents and adults living in several tropical regions. A serologic study on the island of Martinique led Gessain et al. (20) to recognize that most subjects with TSP had antibodies to the oncogenic retrovirus human T-lymphotrophic virus type I (HTLV-I), whereas normal subjects and those with other neurologic diseases rarely did. That finding was confirmed for patients with TSP in other tropical populations and in patients with a similar condition in Japan, where the condition was designated *HAM.* Soon afterward, Hirose et al. (21) isolated HTLV-I from the CSF of a patient with HAM/TSP (Fig. 153.3).

Chronic Tick-borne Encephalitis

Chronic progressive neurologic diseases have been described in patients who recovered from acute TBE in Europe and Asia (22), and limited evidence suggests that the syndromes may be associated with persistence of virus in the central nervous system (CNS) (23).

MICROBIOLOGY

Properties of the viruses are summarized in Table 153.1. JCV is a member of the family Papovaviridae in the genus *Polyomavirus*—a small double-stranded circular deoxyribonucleic acid (DNA) with unenveloped icosahedral nucleocapsid sharing some antigens with other members of that genus (9). JCV strains causing PML are heterogeneous and presumably generated from ordinary archetypal strains during asymptomatic persistence (24), rather than from especially neurovirulent progenitors. JCV isolates from brain shared certain similarities in DNA sequences and differed from strains found in kidney (25,26), especially in

the noncoding region of the genome, prompting the hypothesis that mutations in regulatory genes play an important role in establishing viral latency and reactivation in the nervous system (27). A synergy was demonstrated between a host protein that activates promoters of JCV, expressed on oligodendrocytes, and the JCV large-tumor antigen (28), suggesting another potential mechanism by which lytic infection of those cells might be established.

Measles virus is a Morbillivirus of the family Paramyxoviridae a negative-sense enveloped ribonucleic acid (RNA) virus that forms pleomorphic spherical and filamentous particles (29). The genomes of strains of measles virus isolated from patients with SSPE contain multiple mutations (30). No consistent genomic abnormalities have been identified in strains of measles virus isolated from brains of SSPE patients (one cluster of SSPE cases suggestive of a point-source outbreak caused by a strain of special virulence has been described) (31,32). Complete measles virus particles are not found in the brains of patients with SSPE, and the matrix (M) protein required for the final assembly and budding of virus from the host cells is reduced or missing, not only from brain tissues of patients but also from cells cultured from their brains; however, the full complement of genetic material needed to code for all proteins, including M protein, is present and functional, and when infected brain cells are cultivated together with permissive cells, complete measles virus often emerges. Mutations in other genes of measles virus have also been associated with SSPE (29).

Rubella virus is the sole member of the genus *Rubivirus* in the family Togaviridae, a group of small spherical enveloped positive-sense RNA viruses. Nothing is known about the mechanism by which rubella virus causes RPE (33,34).

HTLV-I, the first human retrovirus to be identified, occurs as spherical enveloped particles containing homodimers of single-stranded RNA (35), as well as in DNA transcripts integrated into host genomic DNA. No molecular changes in HTLV-I associated with neurotropism are known. The distantly related virus HTLV-II has not been associated with neurologic disease. Leukemias and other diseases caused by these viruses are described elsewhere (Chapter 255).

TBE virus is a flavivirus of the family Flaviviridae—a group of antigenically related small spherical enveloped viruses, mostly arthropod-borne, with single-stranded positive-sense genomes. A mutation in the envelope gene of attenuated yellow fever vaccine virus distantly related to TBE virus appears to cause acute encephalitis in humans (36), and the same region of the genome may encode neurovirulence of the TBE virus for mice (37,38). Strains of TBE virus that cause delayed onset of chronic movement disorders in monkeys have been isolated (23), but the molecular basis is unknown.

EPIDEMIOLOGY

JCV most often causes silent infections in normal children and adolescents (39,40); about 75% of normal adults have antibodies to the virus (9). PML occurs many years after those initial infections, affecting primarily adults with immune systems compromised for a variety of reasons—congenital syndromes or AIDS, leukemias and lymphomas, immunosuppressive therapy for tumors or transplantation, miliary tuberculosis, sarcoidosis, and others. A few patients have PML without any other diagnosis (27,41). Possibly because of the lower prevalence of latent infections with JCV in the early years of life, only a few cases of PML have been recognized in children with congenital immunodeficiencies (41) and AIDS (10,42), in whom it may represent a primary infection (9). The epidemiology of PML reflects that of its underlying conditions; the spread of AIDS resulted in a dramatic increase in cases of PML recognized, as well as a reduction in mean age of patients (from the sixth to the fifth decade of life) and relative increase in proportion of men affected (43). Although PML remains rare overall, it is a common opportunistic infection among patients with AIDS, affecting more than 4% in some series (44).

SSPE occurs throughout the world. Data for the United States have been compiled for cases with onset in 1956 or later by the USA/International SSPE Registry (45) (maintained by Dr. Paul R. Dyken, Institute of Research in Childhood Neurodegenerative Diseases, Mobile, Alabama) (46). The disease has been diagnosed in patients younger than 1 year (47) to those older than 30 years (48), but it affects primarily children and young adolescents. More than 85% of cases in the National Registry had onset between 5 and 15 years of age (45). The average age at onset of SSPE in patients reported before 1980 was about 10 years; between 1980 and 1984, it rose to almost 14 years. Since 1990 almost all cases reported to the National Registry were among immigrant children (46). Acquisition of measles before the age of 18 months increased the risk of SSPE substantially (47).

Mean annual incidence rates of SSPE in the United States fell markedly from 0.61 case per million persons younger than 20 years in 1960 to an estimated 0.06 case in 1980 (45). After 1982, fewer than five new cases were registered each year from the entire United States—only two or three each year since 1990 (46). This decrease presumably resulted from the decline in measles cases after the introduction of live attenuated measles vaccine in 1963. The risk of SSPE was estimated as 8.5 SSPE cases per million cases of measles for a 6-year period during which the estimated risk after measles vaccination was only 0.7 case per million doses of vaccine. Of the patients with SSPE reported to the National Registry since 1969, only 14% had a history of measles vaccination without also having clinically apparent measles, and a roughly equal number had no history of either acute measles illness or receiving vaccine (49). SSPE has never been demonstrated to result from persistent infection with measles vaccine virus; more likely, SSPE in vaccinated subjects resulted from undiagnosed wild-type measles infection either preceding vaccination or after unsuccessful immunization. Lack of measles vaccination itself constituted a highly significant risk factor in one study of SSPE (49). In a survey of England and Wales, the overall risk of SSPE after measles was 29 compared with that after measles

vaccination, and the relative risk for children who had measles before the age of 1 year was more than 100 (50,51). An increased incidence of SSPE has been attributed to a transient resurgence of measles in the United States from 1989 to 1991, most cases infected with the D3 genotype of virus; the rate of SSPE in that cohort has been estimated at 1 case for every 10 thousand cases of measles—far exceeding rates seen in the prevaccination era (52). In none of the cases studied was the viral RNA of vaccine origin.

RPE (33,34) is exceedingly rare; since its first description in 1974 (16), fewer than 20 cases have been reported. All patients were males 8 to 21 years old; most had typical stigmata of the congenital rubella syndrome, including cataracts, deafness, and mental retardation, but several had recovered completely from childhood rubella (18,53,54). Cases of RPE may be expected where rubella still occurs (55).

TSP/HAM has been recognized most often in the West Indies, Colombia, and other countries of Central and South America, West Africa, the Seychelles, and southern Japan, as well as in migrants from those areas (56); the asymptomatic carriage rate of HTLV-I is quite high in affected populations. The overall prevalence of HTLV-I antibodies among healthy blood donors in the United States was estimated to be 0.025%. The estimated lifetime risk of myelopathy among those infected is less than 1%—substantially lower than the risk of leukemia. Mechanisms of transmission of HTLV-I are similar to those for HIV: from mother to child in breast milk, sexually, by transfusion, and by use of shared needles. Unlike HIV, HTLV-I appears to be transmitted only by infected cells. Transfusion-acquired cases of TSP/HAM had relatively short incubation periods, probably because of the large infecting dose of virus. Women are more often affected by TSP/HAM than men, and adults more often than children. The distantly related virus HTLV-II, with similar epidemiology, has not been recognized to cause myelopathy.

Most cases of chronic progressive TBE have been reported from Russia (57), affecting mainly young adults from rural villages, especially in Siberia (23,58). Two typical patients were described in Japan (59). In most areas, the chronic illness is an uncommon late complication of acute TBE, although in some clinical series as many as 20% of patients recovering from acute encephalitis were reported to develop new signs of neurologic disease months or years later (23). TBE virus is spread by tick bites or less commonly by ingesting milk from infected animals (60).

PATHOLOGY AND PATHOGENESIS

The histopathologic picture of PML (61) is characterized by diffusely scattered demyelinated lesions, variable in size and distribution—generally most numerous in the cerebral hemispheres (Fig. 153.4), less in brainstem and cerebellum, and tending to spare the spinal cord. Myelin sheaths within the lesions are degenerated and replaced by lipid-bearing phagocytes, leaving neuronal axis cylinders. Oligodendroglial cells at the margins of lesions are abnormal, with enlarged degenerated nuclei and intranuclear eosinophilic inclusions. Astrocytes are enlarged with abnormal or multiple nuclei. Perivascular lymphocytic cuffing occurs. In electron micrographs from AIDS patients with PML, virions of papovavirus are observed not only in oligodendrocytes and astroglial cells but also in macrophages and neurons (62,63). The histopathologic findings of PML complicating AIDS are the same as those with other predisposing conditions (64). JCV has been found in kidneys and circulating B lymphocytes of asymptomatically infected subjects (65). One hypothesis holds

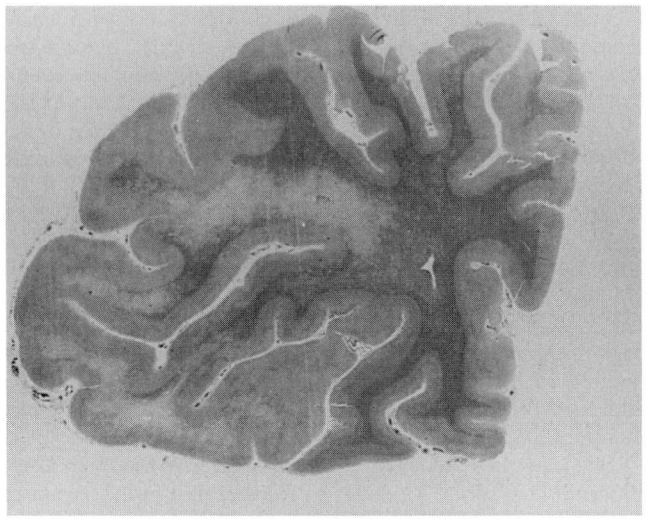

Figure 153.4. Patchy demyelination in the cerebrum of a patient with progressive multifocal leukoencephalopathy. (Courtesy of the late Dr. C. J. Gibbs, Jr., National Institutes of Health, Bethesda, Maryland.)

that latently infected B lymphocytes are activated during immune suppression and carry JCV from the blood into the brain to infect oligodendrocytes and astrocytes, causing loss of myelin and functional impairments of neurons (27). Lymphocytes, primarily T cells, found in the brains of patients with PML in areas of inflammation are reported to contain JCV consistently, but only rarely are they infected with HIV, opportunistic viruses other than JCV, or *Toxoplasma* (66). Phagocytosis of papovaviral particles by macrophages has been observed (63). The role of those cells and of JCV-infected neurons (62) in the pathogenesis of PML remains uncertain.

The histopathologic characteristics of SSPE include inflammation, necrosis, and repair (46,67). Brain biopsy performed in the early stages of SSPE shows mild inflammation of meninges and a panencephalitis involving cortical and subcortical gray matter and white matter, with cuffs of plasma cells and lymphocytes around blood vessels (Fig. 153.5), and increased numbers of glial cells throughout. Neuronal loss may not be marked until later in the course of illness. Loss of myelin secondary

to neuronal degeneration may be apparent (67). Intranuclear Cowdry type A inclusion bodies surrounded by clear halos (Fig. 153.6), noted by Dawson (11) in his original description, may be seen in hematoxylin-eosin–stained sections within the nuclei of neurons, astrocytes, and oligodendrocytes, but they are sometimes difficult to find. By electron microscopy, the inclusions are found to contain tubular structures (12) (see Fig. 153.2) typical of paramyxoviral nucleocapsids. Measles viral antigens can be demonstrated by labeled antibody techniques within the inclusions and in cells without inclusions. Lesions may be unevenly distributed throughout the brain, so biopsy is not always diagnostic, particularly when small samples of tissue are obtained. The same findings of inclusion body panencephalitis are generally present in the brain at autopsy; however, late in disease it may be difficult to find typical areas of inflammation, and the main histopathologic changes are necrosis and gliosis. SSPE is believed to begin in the cortical gray matter, subsequently progressing to white matter and subcortical gray matter and, finally, to lower structures (46). (Myoclonus probably results from extrapyramidal involvement.) Although persistent infection of lymphoid tissues with measles virus has been claimed (68–70), those tissues show no pathologic changes. Cerebral vascular endothelial cells may be infected without showing structural abnormalities (71–73) (Fig. 153.7) and might constitute a portal of entry into the CNS for measles virus. The increased risk in children who had measles as infants implies that either their immunologic immaturity or low levels of residual maternal antibodies predisposes them to SSPE. The frequent finding in the nucleic acid sequences of measles virus isolated from SSPE of mutations in the M gene, with reduced expression of M protein, or of other mutations interfering with viral assembly and budding suggests that the progressive encephalitis may result from intracellular accumulation of incomplete measles virus not cleared by antibodies or cell-mediated immunity. A recent report of elevated levels of antibodies to the CD9 glycoprotein expressed in a variety of normal cells, including several types in the nervous system, suggests an additional mechanism for the progressive brain damage typical of SSPE (74).

Histopathologic changes in brains of patients with RPE (75, 76) are similar to those in SSPE, with cuffs of lymphocytes and plasma cells around blood vessels, glial nodules in the cortex, some loss of neurons, and an increase in numbers of astrocytes

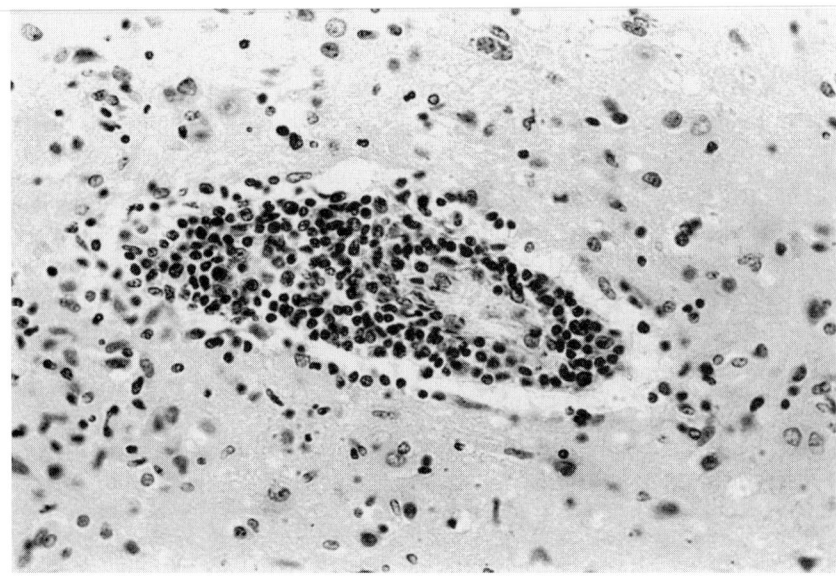

Figure 153.5. A cuff of inflammatory cells surrounding a blood vessel in the cerebral cortex of a child with subacute sclerosing panencephalitis. (Courtesy of Dr. P. Swoveland, University of Maryland, Baltimore, Maryland. From Asher DM. Slow viral infections. In: Scheld WM, Whitley RJ, Durack DT, eds. *Infections of the nervous system,* 2nd ed. New York: Raven Press, 1997:199–221, with permission.)

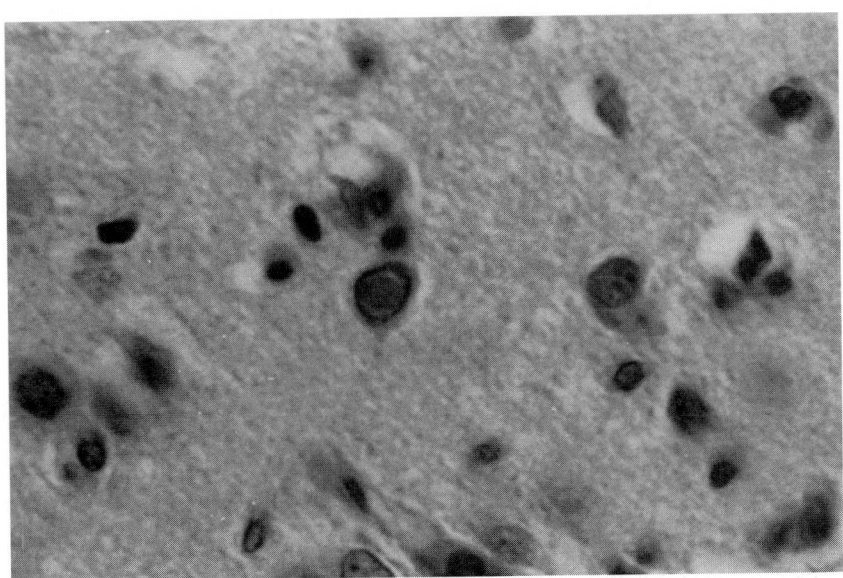

Figure 153.6. An intranuclear inclusion in the cerebral cortex of a child with subacute sclerosing panencephalitis. (Courtesy of Dr. P. Swoveland, University of Maryland, Baltimore, Maryland. From Asher DM. Slow viral infections. In: Scheld WM, Whitley RJ, Durack DT, eds. *Infections of the nervous system,* 2nd ed. New York: Raven Press, 1997:199–221, with permission.)

throughout gray matter and white matter. The histopathologic picture of RPE differs from that of SSPE in two important respects: No inclusion bodies have been recognized in RPE and deposits of amorphous material stained by the periodic acid–Schiff reaction are found around vessels in subcortical white matter.

The histopathologic changes in spinal cords (and, to a lesser extent, brains) of patients with TSP/HAM from Jamaica and from Japan are similar: chronic inflammation (Fig. 153.8), perivascular cuffing with mononuclear cells, loss of neurons, and proliferation of astrocytes and microglial cells (77). Inflammatory changes in spinal cords of TSP patients who survived for many years were minimal, but there was a vacuolar myelopathy resembling that seen in AIDS (78).

Although patients with TSP/HAM generally have no other evidence of leukemia, atypical T cells resembling those in adult T-cell leukemia have been observed in their blood and CSF (56). One study suggested that 1 or 2 in 10,000 peripheral blood lymphocytes from patients with TSP/HAM contained viral transcripts (79), somewhat less than previously thought. These cells may be the progeny of a few infected founder cells (80). Infected lymphocytes are predominantly CD4+, although CD4 is not a receptor for HTLV-I (56). Virus-infected lymphocytes from patients with TSP/HAM express activation markers on their surfaces and proliferate spontaneously in culture. The role of infected lymphocytes in the pathogenesis of TSP/HAM is not yet understood; they have been postulated to provoke an autoimmune demyelinating process. Uninfected CD8+ lymphocytes, common in the CSF of patients with TSP/HAM, are cytotoxic to HTLV-I–infected cells and might cause demyelination by killing of infected glial cells, although it remains unclear whether neurons and glial cells are actually infected (56).

Brain tissues from biopsies of patients with Kozhevnikov's epilepsy (81) and progressive bulbar paralysis (59) after TBE contained perivascular cuffs and parenchymal infiltrates of inflammatory cells, with loss of neurons and sclerosis; no inclusion bodies were described.

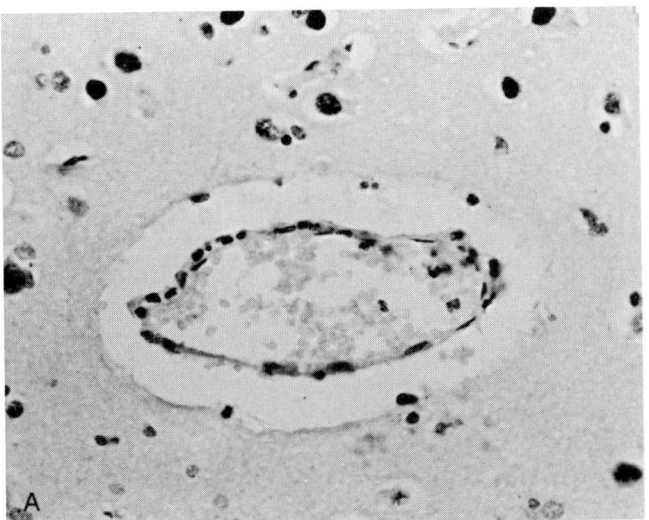
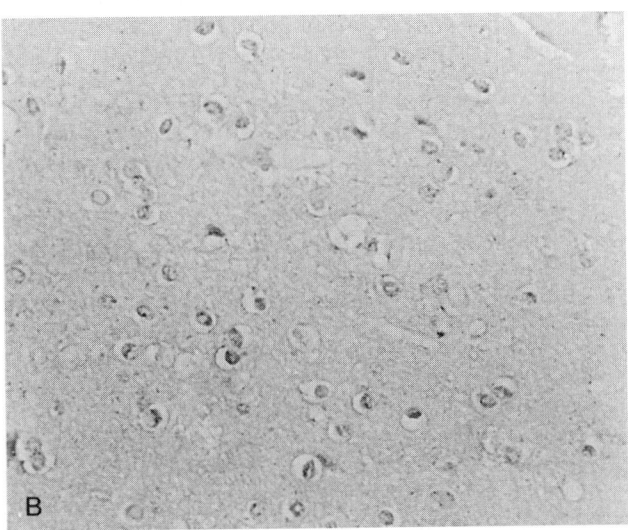

Figure 153.7. In situ reverse-transcriptase polymerase chain reaction and labeled-probe hybridization followed by immunostaining (72) from formalin-fixed, paraffin-embedded sections of brain. **A:** Measles virus–infected neurons, oligodendrocytes, astrocytes, and vascular endothelial cells in subacute sclerosing panencephalitis are stained. **B:** A section from a control patient shows no staining.

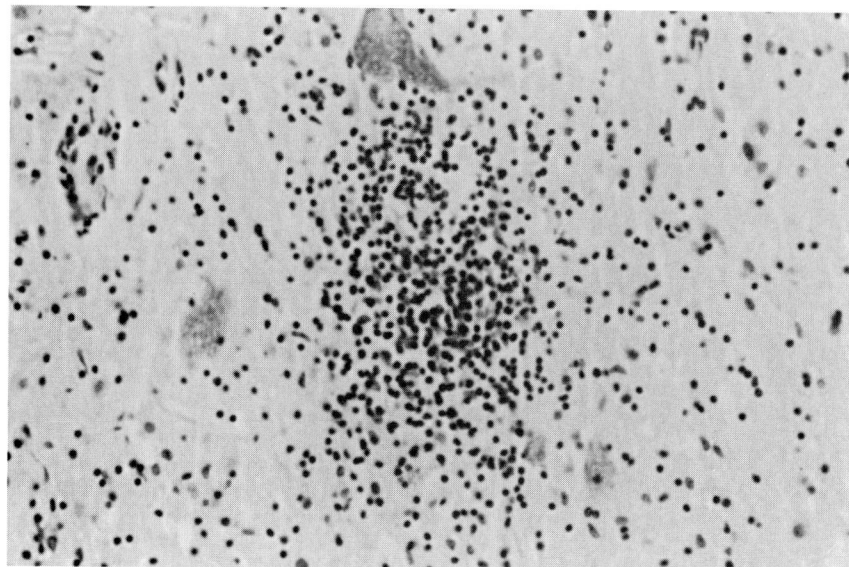

Figure 153.8. Tropical spastic paraparesis/human T-lymphotrophic virus type I–associated myelopathy: an infiltrate of inflammatory cells in the spinal cord. (Courtesy of the late Dr. C. J. Gibbs, Jr., National Institutes of Health, Bethesda, Maryland.)

CLINICAL MANIFESTATIONS

PML causes a variety of clinical abnormalities, reflecting the multifocal distribution of lesions; findings include pareses, sensory deficits, seizures, dementia, dysarthria and other bulbar signs, and cerebellar signs. Progression is relatively rapid. Average survival in one series of AIDS patients was less than 3 months after onset of PML (44). Although most patients with PML live less than a year, few patients with PML have survived longer (82).

Most children with SSPE recovered from typical measles several years before the onset of neurologic disease. Measles may not have been especially severe. Some patients with SSPE had measles pneumonia, but none had a history of typical measles encephalitis. The mean interval between measles and onset of SSPE in the United States was formerly about 7 years (83), later increasing to 12 years (45). The National SSPE Registry divided the clinical course of typical SSPE into four stages marked by the onset and disappearance of myoclonic jerks and the degree of disability, with several patterns of progression depending on degree of chronicity and occurrence of remissions. Most cases were classified as acute, subacute, or chronic progressive, and only a few were remitting. The onset of SSPE is usually insidious, marked by subtle changes in behavior and deterioration of schoolwork, followed by more overtly bizarre behavior and eventually by frank dementia (Fig. 153.9). There is no fever, photophobia, or other finding of acute encephalitis except for an occasional complaint of headache. Diffuse neurologic disease becomes progressively more severe. The appearance of massive repetitive myoclonic jerks generally symmetric, especially involving the axial musculature and occurring at 5- to 10-second intervals, marks the onset of the second clinical stage of SSPE. True convulsions may also appear at any stage of illness. In addition to myoclonic jerks, which tend to disappear as disease progresses, a variety of other abnormal movements and dystonias have been observed. Cerebellar ataxia may be noted as well (45,46,84). Retinopathy and optic atrophy may occur at any time, sometimes preceding behavioral changes (85); cortical blindness has also been described (86). Dementia progresses to stupor and coma, sometimes with autonomic insufficiency. Patients may be rigid or spastic with decorticate postures or may be flaccid. The rate of progression is highly variable, but most often the course is inexorable and relatively rapid. Total duration of illness may be as short as a few

months, but most patients live more than a year after diagnosis, with a mean survival of about 18 months (45,46,67). A few patients show some spontaneous improvement and have lived for more than 10 years. In the mid-1980s, the few patients diagnosed with SSPE in the United States had a relatively long survival, perhaps because of improvements in long-term care. Patients with SSPE have the usual secondary complications associated with incapacitating neurologic diseases, including pneumonia and decubitus ulcers.

The onset of RPE resembles that of SSPE (75,87), with insidious changes in behavior and deterioration of intellectual performance. Those are followed by dementia and other signs of multifocal brain disease, including seizures, cerebellar ataxia, and spastic weakness. Myoclonus and other abnormal movements

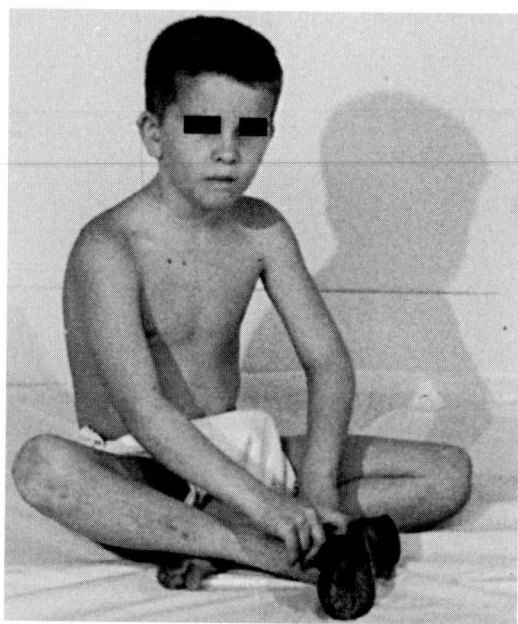

Figure 153.9. An 8-year-old boy became ill with subacute sclerosing panencephalitis 7 years after having an uneventful recovery from typical measles. He was incontinent, confused, and ataxic and could not put on his slipper.

may occur (87,88), but those are not as common as in SSPE. Retinopathy (similar to that of acute rubella) and optic atrophy may be found (87,89,90). The course of RPE is similar to that of SSPE, with progression to coma, spasticity, brainstem involvement, and death in 2 to 5 years.

TSP/HAM also begins insidiously with progressive weakness and spasticity of the lower limbs and sometimes of the upper limbs as well, usually more marked proximally than distally; sensory changes—loss of position and vibration sense, dysesthesias, radiating back pain—may also occur (56,77). Bladder and bowel dysfunction with constipation and impaired sexual function are common complaints. Various cerebral and cerebellar lesions occur less often, as do myositis, uveitis, and other nonneurologic involvement. Progression of disease is typically indolent, and some patients remain relatively stable or even improve over long periods (91).

Chronic TBE most often begins with relatively sudden onset of epilepsia partialis continua (Kozhevnikov's epilepsy)—repetitive clonic jerking of the extremities or of face or neck—in a person who previously recovered from acute encephalitis, with or without residual paralysis; the condition may also begin with major motor seizures, or those may appear later. The course of illness is variable, and some patients with Kozhevnikov's epilepsy after TBE have apparently made sufficient recovery to lead reasonably normal lives (92). Progressive ("progredient") paralytic disease after TBE more often begins insidiously and runs a long but inexorable course; in one typical case, progressive deafness and tinnitus appeared 13 years after recovery from acute TBE, followed soon after by hallucinations and other mental changes and later by diplopia, optic atrophy, ataxia, and intention tremor, scanning speech, and a variety of other signs of cerebral, cerebellar, and bulbar involvement that progressed during a 10-year period (59).

DIAGNOSIS

The diagnosis of PML is suggested by signs of multifocal neurologic disease in an immunodeficient patient. Cranial imaging typically reveals the presence in various areas of the brain of multiple noncompressing lesions (93) that enlarge as disease progresses (41). Measurement of serum antibodies to JCV in AIDS patients was of no value in diagnosing PML (94). JCV genomic sequences were successfully amplified by polymerase chain reaction (PCR) from specimens of CSF of patients with PML (95–98), although that did not always provide a sensitive diagnostic test. One study demonstrated papovavirus particles in CSF of patients by electron microscopy (99). Isolation of virus from the brain, requiring human fetal brain cultures, is rarely available. Negative-stain electron microscopy augmented by incubation with immune serum was useful for detecting JCV particles in suspensions of brain tissue (100). JCV is now most easily detected by amplification of viral DNA using PCR (9,27,101–103).

The diagnosis of SSPE should be suspected in young patients with progressive encephalopathy and a history of measles or residence in measles-endemic areas. The electroencephalogram (EEG) is useful in supporting the diagnosis of SSPE (Fig. 153.10), although early in disease it may be normal or show only moderate nonspecific slowing (104). In the myoclonic stage, most patients with SSPE have episodes of "suppression-burst" high-amplitude slow and sharp waves recurring at intervals of 3 to 5 seconds on a slow background; however, that pattern is not unique to SSPE (105). Later in the illness the EEG becomes increasingly disorganized, with high-amplitude random dysrhythmic slowing; in terminal disease, the amplitude may fall

(45,46,84). Computed tomograms or magnetic resonance images of patients with SSPE may show variable cortical atrophy and ventricular enlargement, and there may be focal or multifocal low-density lesions in white matter. Those studies may also be normal, especially early in the disease (106).

The blood of patients with SSPE has elevated titers of antibodies to measles virus; antibodies are of the immunoglobulin G (IgG) and immunoglobulin M (IgM) classes and are directed against all the component proteins of measles virus except the M protein. Examination of the CSF has been most useful for establishing the diagnosis of SSPE. Cell content of the CSF is generally normal, although stained sediments were reported to show plasma cells. Total protein content of the CSF is generally normal or only slightly elevated; however, the globulin fraction is greatly elevated, usually constituting at least 20% of total protein in CSF, resulting in a paretic type of colloidal gold curve. When the CSF is examined by electrophoresis or isoelectric focusing, "oligoclonal" bands of immunoglobin are usually observed. IgG and IgM antibodies to measles virus, not normally found in unconcentrated CSF, make up most of the immunoglobulin, and these may often be detected in dilutions of 1:8 or higher. Complement fixation, hemagglutination inhibition, immunofluorescence, and other serologic tests, including enzyme-linked immunosorbent assay, demonstrate increased levels of measles antibodies in the CSF. The normal ratio of titer in serum to titer in CSF is reduced (below 200) for measles antibodies, whereas serum/CSF ratios are normal for other viral antibodies and for albumin, indicating that the increased amounts of measles antibodies in CSF of patients with SSPE result from synthesis within the nervous system and that the blood–brain barrier is normal (107).

Brain biopsy should not ordinarily be needed to diagnose SSPE. When performed, it often shows the typical histopathologic findings described earlier. Examination of frozen sections by immunostaining techniques may demonstrate the presence of measles viral antigens. Measles virus was isolated from brain tissue by co-cultivating viable brain cells together with cells susceptible to measles virus and then propagating the mixed cultures for several serial passages (14–17). Persistence of measles virus infection in cultures can be demonstrated by labeled antibody techniques before complete virus appears. Even in highly experienced laboratories, many specimens failed to yield complete virus, although measles antigens were demonstrated in cultures (108).

PCR (109) detected various regions of the measles virus genome by reverse transcription of RNA in extracts of brain from patients with SSPE (105,110) (Fig. 153.11); in situ reverse-transcription PCR with labeled-probe hybridization demonstrated the measles virus genome in formalin-fixed paraffin-embedded brain of patients with SSPE (72,73) (see Fig. 153.7).

In the diagnosis of SSPE and other slow viral infections, potentially treatable illnesses, such as bacterial infections and tumors, must be excluded. Various cerebral storage diseases and non-storage poliodystrophies, leukodystrophies, and demyelinating diseases of childhood can also produce progressive dementia with seizures and paralysis resembling SSPE (106). Early in the course of illness, SSPE must be distinguished from atypical acute viral encephalitides (111–113). Other slow infections, such as Creutzfeldt-Jakob disease and RPE, should be considered. The presence of a typical EEG pattern is suggestive of SSPE, as are unusually high levels of measles antibodies in serum. The diagnosis is confirmed if elevated levels of measles antibodies are detected in unconcentrated CSF.

The presence of stigmata of congenital rubella syndrome or a history of German measles in a young male patient with progressive neurologic disease suggests the diagnosis of RPE. EEGs

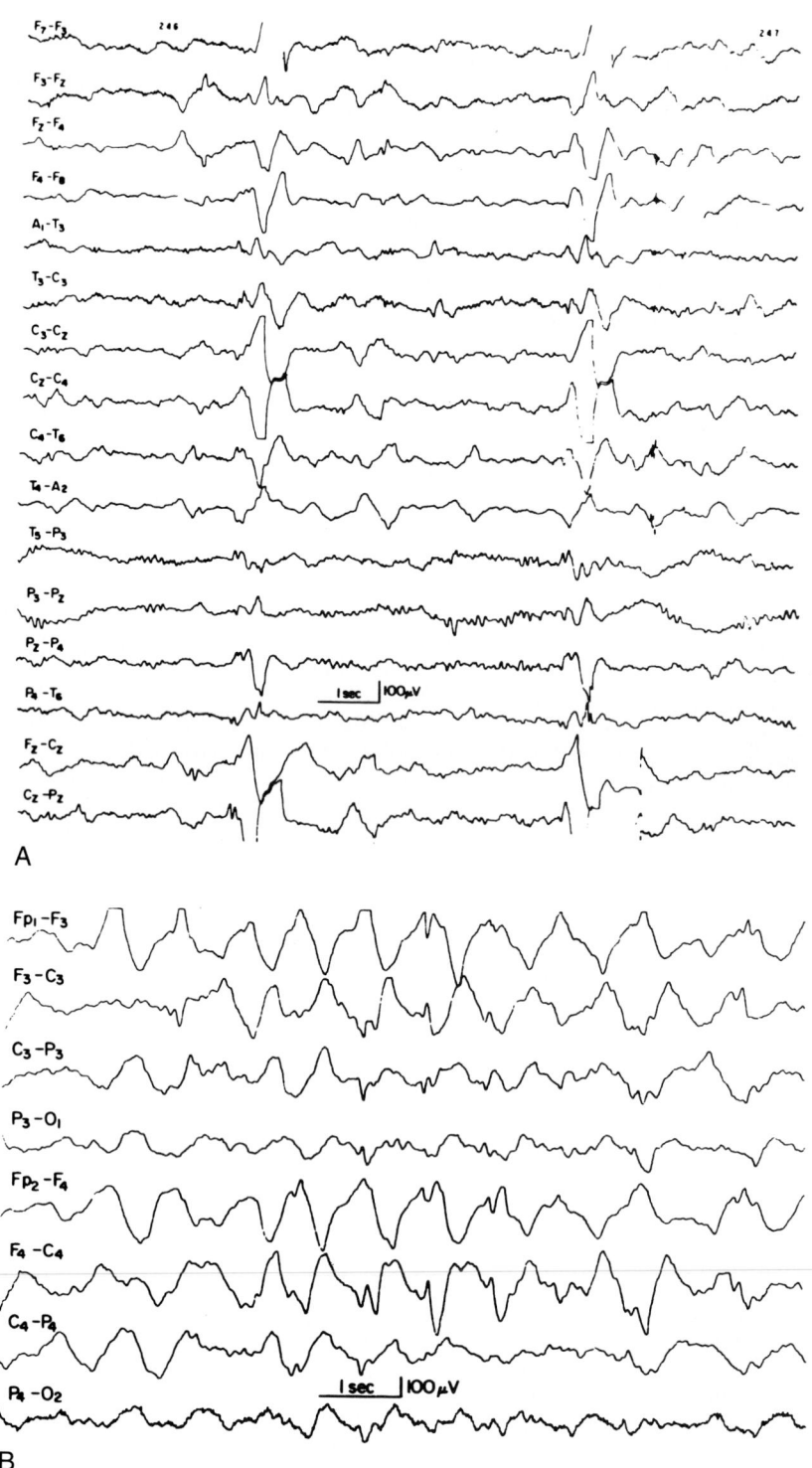

A

B

Figure 153.10. Electroencephalograms from several patients with subacute sclerosing panencephalitis. (Courtesy of Drs. E. Niedermeyer and E. Vining, Johns Hopkins University School of Medicine, Baltimore, Maryland. From Asher DM. Slow viral infections. In: Scheld WM, Whitley RJ, Durack DT, eds. *Infections of the nervous system*, 2nd ed. New York: Raven Press, 1997:199–221, with permission.)

show generalized slowing with occasional high-voltage activity, but the suppression-burst pattern of SSPE has not been seen in progressive RPE. Encephalograms may show enlargement of ventricles (especially the fourth) with cerebellar atrophy. The peripheral blood is normal in progressive RPE, except for elevated titers of antibodies to rubella virus. The CSF shows normal or slightly elevated cell content; the CSF protein level is slightly elevated, with marked increase in globulin, which may make up more than 50% of total protein (54,75). Oligoclonal electrophoretic bands of globulin are found in CSF of patients with progressive RPE; the bands resemble those in SSPE but consist

of antibodies to rubella virus antigens (90). Antibodies to rubella virus are readily detectable in CSF, often at dilutions of 1:8 or higher. Complement fixation, hemagglutination inhibition, and enzyme-linked immunosorbent assay should be satisfactory for testing CSF. Most of the rubella antibodies are IgG, although IgM antibodies have also been detected early in the course of RPE; the serum/CSF ratio of antibody titers to rubella virus is reduced (90), whereas ratios of titers to measles and other viruses are normal. The presence of elevated levels of antibodies to rubella virus in the CSF (and reduction of normal serum/CSF ratio for rubella antibodies) establishes the diagnosis. Isolation of rubella virus

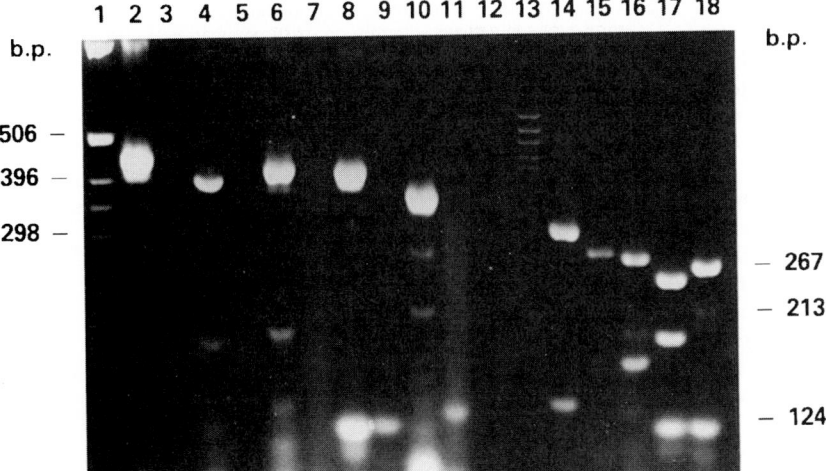

Figure 153.11. Electrophoresis in agarose gel, stained with ethidium bromide and visualized under ultraviolet light, showing products amplified by polymerase chain reaction with complementary deoxyribonucleic acid (DNA) transcribed from ribonucleic acid (RNA) extract of brain from a patient with subacute sclerosing panencephalitis (lanes 2, 4, 6, 8, and 10). RNA from the brain of a control patient (lanes 3, 5, 9, and 11) was included in the same study. Lanes 1 and 13 contain nucleic acid–size markers (b.p., number of base pairs). Pairs of oligonucleotide primers amplifying five regions of measles viral genes were selected. Digestion of the complementary DNA products displayed in lanes 2, 4, 6, 8, and 10 with restriction enzyme AluI or AvaII yielded smaller fragments of sizes predicted for measles viral genome (lanes 141 through 148), confirming identity as measles. Lane 12 is blank. (From Godec MS, Asher DM, Masters CL, et al. Detection of measles virus genomic sequences in SSPE brain tissue. *J Med Virol* 1990;30:237–244, with permission.)

from blood lymphocytes may be attempted. Brain biopsy should not be required.

In patients with clinical illnesses suggestive of TSP/HAM, oligoclonal immunoglobulin bands and antibodies to HTLV-I in CSF are highly suggestive of TSP/HAM (56). Infection with HTLV-I can be confirmed by the presence of serum antibodies (see Chapter 255), detected by enzyme-linked immunosorbent assay or gel agglutination test; specificity of antibodies (to core and envelope antigens of HTLV-I) should be demonstrated by immunoblotting or a comparable assay. Specialized laboratories can isolate HTLV-I and distinguish it from HTLV-II by PCR amplification.

Chronic TBE may be suspected in patients with Kozhevnikov's epilepsy or progressive paralytic syndrome who were potentially exposed to infected ticks or milk in Europe or Asia. Most patients have a history of recovering from acute encephalitis with onset in the spring or summer. The serum should contain antibodies to TBE virus. In one case, well studied in Japan, elevated levels of antibodies to TBE virus were found in the CSF (59). Chronic TBE has not been recognized in the United States.

PREVENTION, TREATMENT, AND PRECAUTIONS

Prevention of the underlying predisposing immunodeficiency state is the most promising approach to control of PML. Results of therapy for PML, even after early diagnosis, have been discouraging (44), although reports suggested that treatment with interferon-α, with or without cytarabine, was followed by clinical improvement (114,115). No special precautions are indicated for PML, although they may be for the underlying conditions.

As noted earlier, not only does successful immunization prevent measles, it also protects children from SSPE (46). A variety of treatments have been reported to produce some improvement in SSPE, although none is curative. It has been reported that treatment of SSPE with inosiplex increased the number of patients with prolonged survival and some clinical improvement in degree of disability (45,84). Several groups claimed to have slowed progression of SSPE after intrathecal or intraventricular injections of interferon-α (116–120). However, in other trials no improvement in CSF abnormalities in SSPE followed treatment with inosiplex alone (31) or with inosiplex plus interferon (121). One report claimed to have stabilized the rate of clinical deterioration in SSPE by immunomodulation with cimetidine (122). A single attempt to treat SSPE by immune reconstitution using

transfused cells from an unaffected sibling failed (123). At the moment, combined therapy with oral isoprinosine and intrathecal interferon-α appears to be the therapy most often offered (67), although it may not be without adverse effect (124). Information on current therapeutic trials may be sought through the USA/International SSPE Registry (46).

The persistent measles infection in SSPE produces no complete virus particles. Patients with SSPE should pose no hazard of infecting others, and no special precautions need ordinarily be taken. Claims that measles virus was present in blood of SSPE patients were not confirmed (125). In any case, universal blood and body fluid precautions should be observed for all patients (126), including those with SSPE.

Immunization with currently recommended measles-mumps-rubella vaccine probably protects children against RPE and SSPE. No successful therapy has been reported. Patients with RPE should pose no substantial risk of infection to others, although isolation of rubella virus from separated blood lymphocytes of a patient with RPE has been claimed (54). Rubella virus has not been detected in urine of patients with panencephalitis, and their secretions have apparently never been studied.

TSP/HAM may be prevented by interfering with transmission of HTLV-I, screening and discarding potentially infected blood and blood products, discouraging infected mothers from breast-feeding (where social conditions allow that to be done), and promoting the same methods used to reduce sexual and drug-related spread of HIV. Although there is no specific therapy for TSP/HAM, some patients may benefit from corticosteroid treatments (56); other therapies have also been attempted (91). Blood precautions should be observed.

Infection with TBE virus can be prevented by immunization with inactivated vaccines (60), as well as by preventing exposure to infected ticks and milk. There is no documented effective therapy for the acute or chronic encephalitis. Patients with chronic TBE syndromes should not pose any risk of infecting others.

OTHER POSSIBLE SLOW INFECTIONS OF THE HUMAN CENTRAL NERVOUS SYSTEM: RASMUSSEN ENCEPHALITIS

Patients with chronic encephalitis not associated with known viral infection have been recognized throughout the world. In the United States, a syndrome of seizures (especially epilepsia partialis continua), spastic paralysis, and mental retardation associated with chronic encephalitis was described by Rasmussen et al. (127–133) in children, adolescents, and young adults. Patients had no history of preceding acute encephalitis. Computed tomograms of patients with Rasmussen's encephalitis show cerebral cortical atrophy and ventricular dilation, and when brain tissue was resected, a panencephalitis without inclusion bodies or without virus-like particles was found. Later reports implicated the Epstein-Barr virus in two cases of Rasmussen's encephalitis (134,135) and cytomegalovirus in several other cases of the disease (136,137); those findings remain unconfirmed (138). Efforts to isolate viruses from brains of patients with Rasmussen's encephalitis were unsuccessful (23). A report that chronic encephalitis with seizures was produced in experimental animals immunized with a glutamate receptor and that patients with Rasmussen's syndrome had antibodies to glutamate receptor in their serum suggests that the disease may be autoimmune and not caused by a persistent infection (139).

A variety of other chronic neurologic diseases—multiple sclerosis best known among them—have been postulated to be caused by slow infections, but in spite of a variety of intriguing but unconfirmed preliminary reports (140), their etiology remains unknown (35,141).

REFERENCES

1. Sigurdsson B. Observations on three slow infections of sheep. 1. Maedi, a slow progressive pneumonia of sheep: an epizootological and a pathological study. Br Vet J 1954;110(7):255–270.
2. Sigurdsson B. Observations on three slow infections of sheep. 2. Paratuberculosis (Johne's disease) of sheep in Iceland. Immunological studies and observations on its mode of spread. Br Vet J 1954;110(6):307–322.
3. Sigurdsson B. Observations on three slow infections of sheep. 3. Rida, a chronic encephalitis of sheep, with general remarks on infections which develop slowly and some of their special characteristics. Br Vet J 1954;110(9):341–354.
4. Prusiner SB. Shattuck lecture—neurodegenerative diseases and prions. N Engl J Med 2001;344(20):1516–1526.
5. Chesebro B. Prion protein and the transmissible spongiform encephalopathy diseases. Neuron 1999;24(3):503–506.
6. Aström K, Mancall EL, Richardson EP. Progressive multifocal leukoencephalopathy. A hitherto unrecognized complication of chronic lymphatic leukemia and Hodgkin's disease. Brain 1958;81:93–111.
7. Zu Rhein GM. Association of papova-virions with a human demyelinating disease (progressive multifocal leukoencephalopathy). Prog Med Virol 1969;11:185–247.
8. Padgett BL, Zu Rhein GM, Walker DL, et al. Cultivation of papova-like virus from human brain with progressive multifocal leukoencephalopathy. Lancet 1971;1:1257–1260.
9. Major EO. Human polyoma viruses. In: Knipe DM, Howley PM, eds. Fields virology, 4 ed. Philadelphia: Lippincott Williams & Wilkins, 2001:2175–2196.
10. Vandersteenhoven JJ, Dbaibo G, Boyko OB, et al. Progressive multifocal leukoencephalopathy in pediatric acquired immunodeficiency syndrome. Pediatr Infect Dis J 1992;11(3):232–237.
11. Dawson JR. Cellular inclusions in cerebral lesions of lethargic encephalitis. Am J Pathol 1933;9:7–16.
12. Bouteille M, Fontaine C, Verenne C, et al. Sur un cas d'encephalite subaigue a inclusions. Etude anatamoclinique et ultrastructurale. Rev Neurol (Paris) 1965;118:454.
13. Connolly JH, Allen IV, Hurwitz LJ. Measles-virus antibody and antigen in subacute sclerosing panencephalitis. Lancet 1967;1:542–544.
14. Chen TT, Watanabe I, Zeman W, et al. Subacute sclerosing panencephalitis: Propagation of measles virus from brain biopsy in tissue culture. Science 1969;163:1193–1194.
15. Horta-Barbosa L, Fuccillo DA, Sever JL, et al. Subacute sclerosing panencephalitis: Isolation of measles virus from a brain biopsy. Nature 1969;221:974.
16. Horta-Barbosa L, Fuccillo DA, London WT, et al. Isolation of measles virus from brain cell cultures of two patients with subacute sclerosing panencephalitis. Proc Soc Exp Biol Med 1969;132:272–277.
17. Payne FE, Baublis JV, Itabashi HH. Isolation of measles virus from cell cultures of brain from a patient with subacute sclerosing panencephalitis. N Engl J Med 1969;281:585–589.
18. Lebon P, Lyon G. Non-congenital rubella encephalitis. Lancet 1974;2:468.
19. Cremer NE, Oshiro LS, Weil ML, et al. Isolation of rubella virus from brain in chronic progressive panencephalitis. J Gen Virol 1975;29:143–153.
20. Gessain A, Barin F, Vernant JC, et al. Antibodies to human T-lymphotropic virus type-I in patients with tropical spastic paraparesis. Lancet 1985;2(8452):407–410.
21. Hirose S, Uemura Y, Fujishita M, et al. Isolation of HTLV-I from cerebrospinal fluid of a patient with myelopathy. Lancet 1986;2(8503):397–398.
22. Mickiene A, Laiskonis A, Gunther G, et al. Tickborne encephalitis in an area of high endemicity in Lithuania: disease severity and long-term prognosis. Clin Infect Dis 2002;35(6):650–658.
23. Asher DM, Gajdusek DC. Virologic studies in chronic encephalitis. In: Andermann F, editor. Chronic encephalitis and epilepsy: Rasmussen's syndrome. Boston: Butterworth-Heinemann, 1991:147–158.
24. Iida T, Kitamura T, Guo J, et al. Origin of JC polyomavirus variants associated with progressive multifocal leukoencephalopathy. Proc Natl Acad Sci U S A 1993;90(11):5062–5065.
25. Ault GS, Stoner GL. Two major types of JC virus defined in progressive multifocal leukoencephalopathy brain by early and late coding region DNA sequences. J Gen Virol 1992;73:2669–2678.
26. Ault GS, Stoner GL. Human polyomavirus JC promoter/enhancer rearrangement patterns from progressive multifocal leukoencephalopathy brain are unique derivatives of a single archetypal structure. J Gen Virol 1993;74:1499–1507.
27. Major EO, Amemiya K, Tornatore CS, et al. Pathogenesis and molecular biology of progressive multifocal leukoencephalopathy, the JC virus-induced demyelinating disease of the human brain. Clin Microbiol Rev 1992;5(1):49–73.
28. Renner K, Leger H, Wegner M. The POU domain protein Tst-1 and papoviral large tumor antigen function synergistically to stimulate glia-specific gene expression of JC virus. Proc Natl Acad Sci U S A 1994;91:6433–6437.
29. Griffin DE. Measles virus. In: Knipe DM, Howley PM, eds. Fields virology, 4th ed. Philadelphia: Lippincott Williams & Wilkins, 2001:1558–1564.
30. Cattaneo R, Schmid A, Billeter MA, et al. Multiple viral mutations rather than host factors cause defective measles virus gene expression in a subacute sclerosing panencephalitis cell line. J Virol 1988;62(4):1388–1397.
31. Beersma MF, Galama JM, Van Druten HA, et al. Subacute sclerosing panencephalitis in The Netherlands—1976–1990. Int J Epidemiol 1992;21(3):583–588.
32. Sie TH, Weber W, Freling G, et al. Rapidly fatal subacute sclerosing panencephalitis in a 19-year-old man. Eur Neurol 1991;31(2):94–99.
33. Frenkel LM, Nielsen K, Garakian A, et al. A search for persistent rubella virus infection in persons with chronic symptoms after rubella and rubella immunization and in patients with juvenile rheumatoid arthritis. Clin Infect Dis 1996;22(2):287–294.
34. Wolinsky JS. Subacute sclerosing panencephalitis, progressive rubella panencephalitis, and multifocal leukoencephalopathy. Res Publ Assoc Res Nerv Ment Dis 1990;68:259–268.
35. Green PL, Chen ISY. Human T-cell leukemia viruses types 1 and 2. In: Knipe DM, Howley PM, eds. Fields virology, 4th ed. Philadelphia: Lippincott Williams & Wilkins, 2001:1941–1969.
36. Jennings AD, Gibson CA, Miller BR, et al. Analysis of a yellow fever virus isolated from a fatal case of vaccine-associated human encephalitis. J Infect Dis 1994;169(3):512–518.
37. Pletnev AG, Bray M, Lai CJ. Chimeric tick-borne encephalitis and dengue type 4 viruses: effects of mutations on neurovirulence in mice. J Virol 1993;67(8):4956–4963.
38. Pletnev AG, Karganova GG, Dzhivanyan TI, et al. Chimeric Langat/Dengue viruses protect mice from heterologous challenge with the highly virulent strains of tick-borne encephalitis virus. Virology 2000;274(1):26–31.
39. Taguchi F, Kajioka J, Miyamura T. Prevalence rate and age of acquisition of antibodies against JC virus and BK virus in human sera. Microbiol Immunol 1982;26(11):1057–1064.
40. Padgett BL, Walker DL. Prevalence of antibodies in human sera against JC virus, an isolate from a case of progressive multifocal leukoencephalopathy. J Infect Dis 1973;127(4):467–470.
41. Katz DA, Berger JR, Hamilton B, et al. Progressive multifocal leukoencephalopathy complicating Wiskott-Aldrich syndrome. Report of a case and review of the literature of progressive multifocal leukoencephalopathy with other inherited immunodeficiency states. Arch Neurol 1994;51(4):422–426.
42. Berger JR, Scott G, Albrecht J, et al. Progressive multifocal leukoencephalopathy in HIV-1–infected children. AIDS 1992;6(8):837–841.
43. Stoner GL, Walker DL, Webster HD. Age distribution of progressive multifocal leukoencephalopathy. Acta Neurol Scand (Copenh) 1988;78(4):307–312.
44. Karahalios D, Breit R, Dal Canto MC, et al. Progressive multifocal leukoencephalopathy in patients with HIV infection: lack of impact of early diagnosis by stereotactic brain biopsy. J AIDS 1992;5(10):1030–1038.
45. Dyken PR, Cunningham SC, Ward LC. Changing character of subacute sclerosing panencephalitis in the United States. Pediatr Neurol 1989;5(6):339–341.
46. Dyken PR. Neuroprogressive disease of post-infectious origin: a review of a resurging subacute sclerosing panencephalitis (SSPE). Ment Retard Dev Disabil Res Rev 2001;7(3):217–225.
47. Modlin J, Halsey N, Eddins D, et al. Epidemiology of subacute sclerosing panencephalitis. J Pediatr 1979;94:231–236.
48. Cape CA, Martinez AJ, Roberston JT, et al. Adult onset of subacute sclerosing panencephalitis. Arch Neurol 1973;28:124–127.
49. Halsey NA, Modlin JF. Subacute sclerosing panencephalitis. Pediatr Neurol 1991;7(2):151.

50. Miller C, Farrington CP, Harbert K. The epidemiology of subacute sclerosing panencephalitis in England and Wales 1970–1989. *Int J Epidemiol* 1992;21(5):998–1006.

51. Farrington CP. Subacute sclerosing panencephalitis in England and Wales: transient effects and risk estimates. *Stat Med (Chichester)* 1991;10(11):1733–1744.

52. Bellini W, Rota J, Katz R, et al. *Increased incidence of subacute sclerosing panencephalitis stemming from the 1989 to 1991 resurgence of measles in the United States [abstract W19-2]. In American society for virology, 21st Annual Meeting; 2002 20–24 July 2002. Lexington, Kentucky: ASM, 2002:99.*

53. Dayras JC, Lyon G, Ponsot G, Allemon MC. Progressive chronic rubella encephalitis. Report of a personal case [in French]. *Dem Hôp Paris* 1980;56:1703–1708.

54. Wolinsky JS, Dau PC, Buimovici-Kleine E, et al. Progressive rubella panencephalitis: immunological studies and results of isoprinosine therapy. *Clin Exper Immunol* 1979;35:397–404.

55. Guizzaro A, Volpe E, Lus G, et al. Progressive rubella panencephalitis. Follow-up EEG study of a case. *Acta Neurol* 1992;14(4-6):485–492.

56. Hollsberg P, Hafler DA. Seminars in medicine of the Beth Israel Hospital, Boston. Pathogenesis of diseases induced by human lymphotropic virus type I infection. *N Engl J Med* 1993;328(16):1173–1182.

57. Brody JA, Hadlow WJ, Hotchin J, et al. Soviet search for viruses that cause chronic neurologic diseases. *Science* 1965;147:1114–1116.

58. Asher DM. Persistent tick-borne encephalitis infection in man and monkeys: relation to chronic neurological diseases. In: Kurstak E, ed. *Arctic and tropical arboviruses*. New York: Academic Press, 1979:179–195.

59. Ogawa M, Okubo H, Tsuji Y, et al. Chronic progressive encephalitis occurring 13 years after Russian spring-summer encephalitis. *J Neurol Sci (Amsterdam)* 1973;19:363–373.

60. Burke DS, Monath TP. Flaviviruses. In: Knipe DM, Howley PM, eds. *Fields virology*, 4th ed. Philadelphia: Lippincott Williams & Wilkins, 2001:1043–1125.

61. Richardson EP. Pathology of progressive multifocal leukoencephalopathy. *N Engl J Med* 1961;265:815.

62. Boldorini R, Cristina S, Vago L, et al. Ultrastructural studies in the lytic phase of progressive multifocal leukoencephalopathy in AIDS patients. *Ultrastructural Pathol* 1993;17(6):599–609.

63. Mesquita R, Parravicini C, Bjorkholm M, et al. Macrophage association of polyomavirus in progressive multifocal leukoencephalopathy: an immunohistochemical and ultrastructural study. Case report. *APMIS (Copenh)* 1992;100(11):993–1000.

64. Kuchelmeister K, Gullotta F, Bergmann M, et al. Progressive multifocal leukoencephalopathy (PML) in the acquired immunodeficiency syndrome (AIDS). A neuropathological autopsy study of 21 cases. *Pathol Res Pract* 1993;189(2):163–173.

65. Tornatore C, Berger JR, Houff SA, et al. Detection of JC virus DNA in peripheral lymphocytes from patients with and without progressive multifocal leukoencephalopathy. *Ann Neurol* 1992;31(4):454–462.

66. Hair LS, Nuovo G, Powers JM, et al. Progressive multifocal leukoencephalopathy in patients with human immunodeficiency virus. *Human Pathol* 1992;23(6):663–667.

67. Garg RK. Subacute sclerosing panencephalitis. *Postgrad Med J* 2002;78(916):63–70.

68. Brown HR, Goller NL, Rudelli RD, et al. Postmortem detection of measles virus in non-neural tissues in subacute sclerosing panencephalitis. *Ann Neurol* 1989;26(2):263–268.

69. Fournier JG, Tardieu M, Lebon P, et al. Detection of measles virus RNA in lymphocytes from peripheral-blood and brain perivascular infiltrates of patients with subacute sclerosing panencephalitis. *N Engl J Med* 1985;313:910–915.

70. Fournier JG, Gerfaux J, Joret AM, et al. Subacute sclerosing panencephalitis: detection of measles virus sequences in RNA extracted from circulating lymphocytes. *Br Med J Clin Res* 1988;296:684.

71. Kirk J, Zhou AL, McQuaid S, et al. Cerebral endothelial cell infection by measles virus in subacute sclerosing panencephalitis: ultrastructural and in situ hybridization evidence. *Neuropathol Applied Neurobiol* 1991;17(4):289–297.

72. Isaacson SH, Asher DM, Gajdusek DC, et al. Detection of RNA viruses in archival brain tissue by in situ RT-PCR amplification and labeled-probe hybridization. *Cell Vision J Analyt Morphol* 1994;1(1):25–28.

73. Isaacson SH, Asher DM, Godec MS, et al. Widespread, restricted low-level measles virus infection of brain in a case of subacute sclerosing panencephalitis. *Acta Neuropathol (Berl)* 1996;91(2):135–139.

74. Shimizu T, Matsuishi T, Iwamoto R, et al. Elevated levels of anti-CD9 antibodies in the cerebrospinal fluid of patients with subacute sclerosing panencephalitis. *J Infect Dis* 2002;185(9):1346–1350.

75. Townsend JJ, Baringer JR, Wolinski JS, et al. Progressive rubella panencephalitis: late onset after congenital rubella. *N Engl J Med* 1975;292:990–993.

76. Townsend JJ, Wolinsky JS, Baringer JR. The neuropathology of progressive rubella panencephalitis of late onset. *Brain* 1976;99(1):81–90.

77. Rodgers-Johnson PEB, Ono SG, Asher DM. Tropical spastic paraparesis and HTLV-I myelopathy: clinical features and pathogenesis. In: Waksman BH, ed. *Immunologic mechanisms in neurologic and psychiatric disease*. New York: Raven Press, 1990:117–130.

78. Petito CK, Navia BA, Cho ES, et al. Vacuolar myelopathy pathologically resembling subacute combined degeneration in patients with the acquired immunodeficiency syndrome. *N Engl J Med* 1985;312(14):874–879.

79. Levin MC, Fox RJ, Lehky T, et al. PCR-in situ hybridization detection of human T-cell lymphotropic virus type 1 (HTLV-1) tax proviral DNA in peripheral blood lymphocytes of patients with HTLV-1–associated neurologic disease. *J Virol* 1996;70(2):924–933.

80. Utz U, Banks D, Jacobson S, et al. Analysis of the T-cell receptor repertoire of human T-cell leukemia virus type 1 (HTLV-1) Tax-specific CD8+ cytotoxic T lymphocytes from patients with HTLV-1–associated disease: evidence for oligoclonal expansion. *J Virol* 1996;70(2):843–851.

81. Omorokov LI. Kozhevnikov's epilepsy in Siberia. *Zh Nevropatol Psikhiatr* 1927;20:13–24.

82. Berger JR, Mucke L. Prolonged survival and partial recovery in AIDS-associated progressive multifocal leukoencephalopathy. *Neurology* 1988;38(7):1060–1065.

83. Control CfD. Subacute sclerosing panencephalitis surveillance—United States. *MMWR Morb Mortal Wkly Rep* 1982;31(43):585–588.

84. Dyken PR, Swift A, Durant RH. Long-term follow up of patients with subacute sclerosing panencephalitis treated with inosiplex. *Ann Neurol* 1982;11:359–364.

85. Johnston HM, Wise GA, Henry JG. Visual deterioration as presentation of subacute sclerosing panencephalitis. *Arch Dis Child* 1980;55:899–901.

86. Kabra SK, Bagga A, Shankar V. Subacute sclerosing panencephalitis presenting as cortical blindness. *Trop Doctor* 1992;22(2):94–95.

87. Weil ML, Itabashi HH, Cremer NE, et al. Chronic progressive panencephalitis due to rubella virus simulating subacute sclerosing panencephalitis. *N Engl J Med* 1975;292:994–998.

88. Abe T, Nukada T, Hatanaka H, et al. Myoclonus in a case of suspected progressive rubella panencephalitis. *Arch Neurol* 1983;40(2):98–100.

89. Wolinsky JS, Berg BO, Maitalnd CH. Progressive rubella panencephalitis. *Arch Neurol* 1976;33(10):722–723.

90. Wolinsky JS. Progressive rubella panencephalitis. In: Bruyn GW, ed. *Handbook of clinical neurology*. Amsterdam: Elsevier North Holland, 1978:331–341.

91. Kuroda Y, Yukitake M, Kurohara K, et al. A follow-up study on spastic paraparesis in Japanese HAM/TSP. *J Neurol Sci* 1995;132(2):174–176.

92. Asher DM. Persistent tick-borne encephalitis infection in man and monkeys: relation to chronic neurologic disease. In: Kurstak E, ed. *Arctic and tropical arboviruses*. New York: Academic Press, 1979:179–195.

93. Whiteman ML, Post MJ, Berger JR, et al. Progressive multifocal leukoencephalopathy in 47 HIV-seropositive patients: neuroimaging with clinical and pathologic correlation. *Radiology* 1993;187(1):233–240.

94. Gillespie SM, Chang Y, Lemp G, et al. Progressive multifocal leukoencephalopathy in persons infected with human immunodeficiency virus, San Francisco, 1981–1989. *Ann Neurol* 1991;30(4):597–604.

95. Gibson PE, Knowles WA, Hand JF, et al. Detection of JC virus DNA in the cerebrospinal fluid of patients with progressive multifocal leukoencephalopathy. *J Med Virol* 1993;39(4):278–281.

96. Henson J, Rosenblum M, Armstrong D, et al. Amplification of JC virus DNA from brain and cerebrospinal fluid of patients with progressive multifocal leukoencephalopathy. *Neurology* 1991;41(12):1967–1971.

97. Moret H, Guichard M, Matheron S, et al. Virological diagnosis of progressive multifocal leukoencephalopathy: detection of JC virus DNA in cerebrospinal fluid and brain tissue of AIDS patients. *J Clin Microbiol* 1993;31(12):3310–3313.

98. Telenti A, Marshall WF, Aksamit AJ, et al. Detection of JC virus by polymerase chain reaction in cerebrospinal fluid from two patients with progressive multifocal leukoencephalopathy. *Eur J Clin Microbiol Infect Dis* 1992;11(3):253–254.

99. Orefice G, Campanella G, Cicciarello S, et al. Presence of papova-like viral particles in cerebrospinal fluid of AIDS patients with progressive multifocal leukoencephalopathy. An additional test for *in vivo* diagnosis. *Acta Neurol* 1993;15(5):328–332.

100. Weiner LP, Narayan O, Penney JB Jr, et al. Papovavirus of JC type in progressive multifocal leukoencephalopathy. Rapid identification and subsequent isolation. *Arch Neurol* 1973;29(1):1–3.

101. Aksamit AJ Jr. Nonradioactive in situ hybridization in progressive multifocal leukoencephalopathy. *Mayo Clin Proc* 1993;68(9):899–910.

102. von Einsiedel RW, Fife TD, Aksamit AJ, et al. Progressive multifocal leukoencephalopathy in AIDS: a clinicopathologic study and review of the literature. *J Neurol* 1993;240(7):391–406.

103. Buckle GJ, Godec MS, Rubi JU, et al. Lack of JC viral genomic sequences in multiple sclerosis brain tissue by polymerase chain reaction. *Ann Neurol* 1992;32(6):829–831.

104. Gimenez-Roldan S, Martin M, Mateo D, et al. Preclinical EEG abnormalities in subacute sclerosing panencephalitis. *Neurology* 1981;31(6):763–776.

105. Gloor P, Kalabay O, Giard N. The electroencephalogram in diffuse encephalopathies: electroencephalographic correlates of grey and white matter lesions. *Brain* 1968;91:779–801.

106. Duda E, Huttenlocher P, Patronas N. CT of subacute sclerosing panencephalitis. *Am J Neuroradiol* 1980;1:35–38.

107. Tourtellotte WW, Ma BI, Brandes DB, et al. Quantification of de novo central nervous system IgG measles antibody synthesis in SSPE. *Ann Neurol* 1981;9(6):551–556.

108. Katz M, Koprowski H. The significance of failure to isolate infectious viruses in cases of subacute sclerosing panencephalitis. Brief report. *Arch Gesamte Virusforsch* 1971;41(4):390–393.

109. Saiki RK, Gelfand DH, Stoffel S, et al. Primer-directed enzymatic amplification of DNA with a thermostable DNA polymerase. *Science* 1988;239:487–491.

110. Godec MS, Asher DM, Swoveland PT, et al. Detection of measles virus genomic sequences in SSPE brain tissue. *J Med Virol* 1990;30:237–244.
111. Whitley RJ. Viral encephalitis. *N Engl J Med* 1990;323(4):242–250.
112. Whitley RJ, Kimberlin DW. Viral encephalitis. *Pediatr Rev* 1999;20(6):192–198.
113. Whitley RJ, Gnann JW. Viral encephalitis: familiar infections and emerging pathogens. *Lancet* 2002;359(9305):507–513.
114. Colosimo C, Lebon P, Martelli M, et al. Alpha-interferon therapy in a case of probable progressive multifocal leukoencephalopathy. *Acta Neurol Belgica* 1992;92(1):24–29.
115. Steiger MJ, Tarnesby G, Gabe S, et al. Successful outcome of progressive multifocal leukoencephalopathy with cytarabine and interferon. *Ann Neurol* 1993;33(4):407–411.
116. Anlar B, Yalaz K, Imir T, et al. The effect of inosiplex in subacute sclerosing panencephalitis: a clinical and laboratory study. *Eur Neurol* 1994;34(1):44–47.
117. Gascon GG, Yamani S, Cafege A, et al. Treatment of subacute sclerosing panencephalitis with alpha interferon. *Ann Neurol* 1991;30(2):227–228.
118. Miyazaki M, Hashimoto T, Fujino K, et al. Apparent response of subacute sclerosing panencephalitis to intrathecal interferon alpha. *Ann Neurol* 1991;29(1):97–99.
119. Steiner I, Wirguin I, Morag A, et al. Intraventricular interferon treatment for subacute sclerosing panencephalitis. *J Child Neurol* 1989;4:20–23.
120. Wirguin I, Steiner I, Brenner T, et al. Intraventricular interferon treatment for subacute sclerosing panencephalitis. *Ann Neurol* 1991;30(2):227.
121. Mehta PD, Kulczycki J, Patrick BA, et al. Effect of treatment on oligoclonal IgG bands and intrathecal IgG synthesis in sequential cerebrospinal fluid and serum from patients with subacute sclerosing panencephalitis. *J Neurol Sci* 1992;109(1):64–68.
122. Anlar B, Gucuyener K, Imir T, et al. Cimetidine as an immunomodulator in subacute sclerosing panencephalitis: a double blind, placebo-controlled study. *Pediatr Infect Dis J* 1993;12(7):578–581.
123. Bakheit AM, Behan PO. Unsuccessful treatment of subacute sclerosing panencephalitis treated with transfusion of peripheral blood lymphocytes from an identical twin. *J Neurol Neurosurg Psychiatry* 1991;54(4):377–378.
124. Caksen H, Odabas D, Atas B. Seizures in a boy with subacute sclerosing panencephalitis during high-dose intrathecal interferon-alpha therapy. *Pediatr Neurol* 2002;27(1):75.
125. Schneider-Schaulies S, Kreth HW, et al. Expression of measles virus RNA in peripheral blood mononuclear cells of patients with measles, SSPE, and autoimmune diseases. *Virology* 1991;182(2):703–711.
126. Labor OSaHAUSDo. Occupational exposure to bloodborne pathogens; final rule (29 CFR Part 1910.1030). *Fed Reg* 1991;56:64175.
127. Rasmussen T, Olszewski J, Lloyd-Smith D. Focal seizures due to chronic localized encephalitis. *Neurology* 1958;8:435–445.
128. Aguilar M, Rasmussen T. Role of encephalitis in pathogenesis of epilepsy. *Arch Neurol* 1960;2:663–676.
129. Rasmussen T, McCann W. Clinical studies of patients with focal epilepsy due to "chronic encephalitis." *Trans Am Neurol Assoc* 1968;93:89–94.
130. Rasmussen T. Further observations on the syndrome of chronic encephalitis and epilepsy. *Appl Neurophysiol* 1978;41:1–12.
131. Rasmussen T. Hemispherectomy for seizures revisited. *Can J Neurol Sci* 1983;10:89–94.
132. Rasmussen TB. Chronic encephalitis and seizures: historical introduction. In: Andermann F, ed. *Chronic encephalitis and epilepsy: Rasmussen's syndrome.* Boston: Butterworth-Heinemann, 1991:1–4.
133. Andermann F. Epilepsia partialis continua and other seizures arising from the precentral gyrus: high incidence in patients with Rasmussen syndrome and neuronal migration disorders. *Brain Dev* 1992;14(5):338–339.
134. Walter GF, Renella RR, Hori A, et al. Detection of Epstein-Barr viruses in Rasmussen's encephalitis. Report of 2 cases. *Nervenarzt* 1989;60(3):168–170.
135. Walter GF, Renella RR. Epstein-Barr virus in brain and Rasmussen's encephalitis. *Lancet* 1989;1(8632):279–280.
136. Power C, Poland SD, Blume WT, et al. Cytomegalovirus and Rasmussen's encephalitis. *Lancet* 1990;336(8726):1282–1284.
137. McLachlan RS, Girvin JP, Blume WT, et al. Rasmussen's chronic encephalitis in adults. *Arch Neurol* 1993;50(3):269–274.
138. Farrell MA, Cheng L, Cornford ME, et al. Cytomegalovirus and Rasmussen's encephalitis. *Lancet* 1991;337(8756):1551–1552.
139. Rogers SW, Andrews PI, Gahring LC, et al. Autoantibodies to glutamate receptor GluR3 in Rasmussen's encephalitis. *Science* 1994;265(5172):648–651.
140. Haas AT. Slow virus infections of the central nervous system. In: Gorbach SL, Bartlett JG, Blacklow NR, eds. *Infectious diseases.* Philadelphia: WB Saunders, 1992:1206–1216.
141. Taller AM, Asher DM, Pomeroy KL, et al. Search for viral nucleic acid sequences in brain tissues of patients with schizophrenia using nested polymerase chain reaction. *Arch Gen Psychiatry* 1996;53(1):32–40.

CHAPTER 154
Infectious Diseases of the Spinal Cord and Peripheral Nervous System

Newton E. Hyslop, Jr., and Rodrigo Hasbun

In this chapter, we review common infectious diseases associated with neurologic findings arising from damage to either the spinal cord or its radicles, plexuses, and peripheral nerves.

Infectious disorders affecting the cord include spinal epidural abscess, spinal subdural empyema, several patterns of myelitis, and intramedullary abscess. Infectious disease affecting peripheral nerves include direct infection, toxins produced by organisms, and "postinfection" syndromes (1).

The clinical patterns of these diseases are a combination of the location of the process within the nervous system itself and the other manifestations of the specific infectious agent. Familiarity with the *neuropathic syndromes* shown in Tables 154.1 through 154.7 allows the clinician to categorize the possible infectious causes. A suggested approach to the patient with bilateral neurologic deficits that could be compatible with spinal cord or peripheral nerve disorders (Figure 154.3) concludes this discussion. A neurology text should be consulted to encompass complete differential diagnoses, because patterns seen with infectious causes *may also be* produced by nutritional deficiencies, toxic metals and drugs, diabetes mellitus, malignancies, metabolic diseases, trauma, reaction to vaccines, and other causes. Furthermore, details of special studies that may pinpoint the anatomic site of the disease process, such as nerve conduction velocity and electromyography (EMG), are not discussed, because they are the province of experts in these technologies (1–3).

PERIPHERAL NERVOUS SYSTEM INFECTIONS

Mononeuropathies and Polyneuropathies

Diseases of the peripheral nervous system (PNS) are clinically complex because a wide range of genetic and acquired disorders acting at several potential target sites produce a limited spectrum of clinical findings. Hence, the expression of clinical disorders is limited to *isolated nerve palsies* (mononeuropathies), *unilateral plexus lesions,* combinations of *cranial palsies,* and *asymmetric* and *symmetric polyneuropathies.* For simplicity, we consider diseases affecting the cranial nerves (CNs) as a subdivision of those affecting peripheral nerves originating from the spinal cord.

Infectious agents are known or suspected causes within each clinical pattern and operate by several mechanisms (1–3). They may act by local compression or destruction of a nerve itself; through toxic effects on Schwann cells; by immune complex damage of the vasa nervorum; by inflammatory injury to sensory ganglia and nerve roots, accompanied by cells in the cerebrospinal fluid (CSF); by perivenous lymphocytic demyelination of ventral and dorsal columns of the cord, causing interruption of neuronal transmission along exiting and entering nerve fibers; or finally, by irreversible cytopathic damage to nerve cells located in anterior or lateral horns of cord, dorsal root ganglia, or sympathetic ganglia.

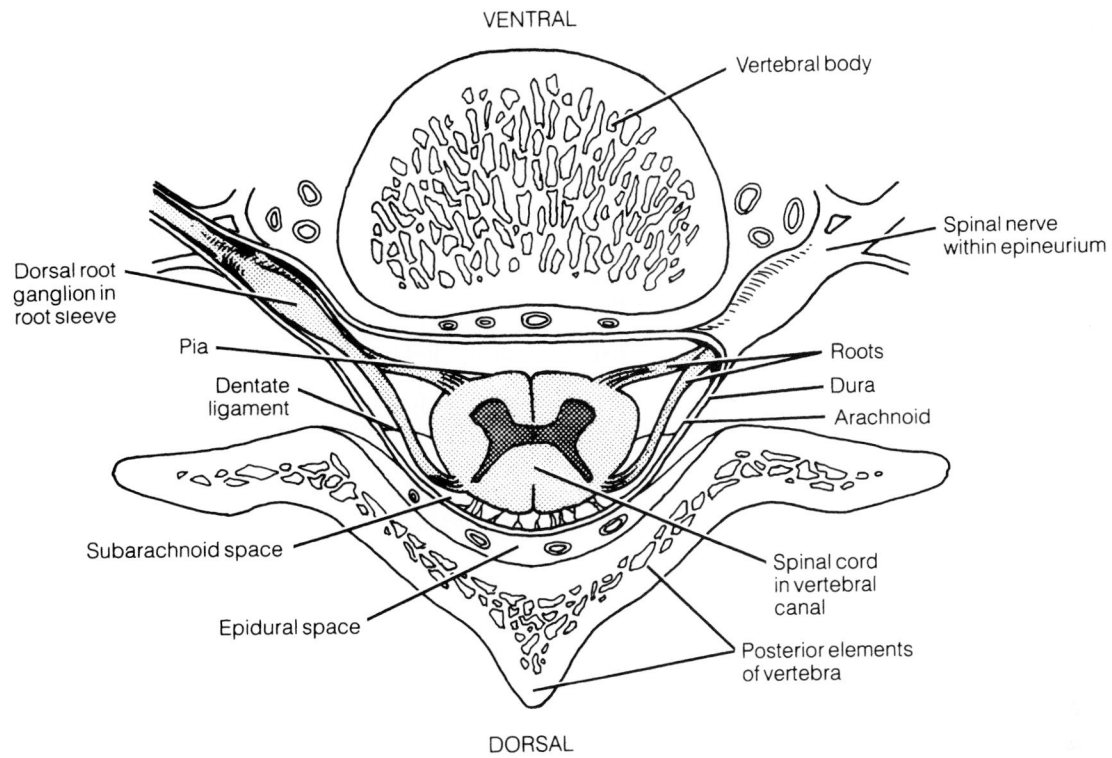

Figure 154.1. Diagram of relations of cord, roots, and cerebrospinal fluid.

ANATOMY

The nervous system is separated anatomically into *central, peripheral,* and *autonomic* categories. The central nervous system (CNS) consists of the brain and spinal cord and is covered by the pia-arachnoid membrane. The PNS consists of all nervous structures lying outside the pia-arachnoid with the exception of the optic nerves and olfactory bulbs, which are considered extensions of the brain. Hence, the PNS comprises CNs III through XII, the brachial, crural, and lumbosacral plexuses, and all other spinal nerves, including their sensory and motor roots and their ganglia.

The peripheral nerves arise as *pairs of roots* from brainstem and cord (Fig. 154.1). The dorsal *(sensory)* roots carry axonal processes of ganglion cells located in the cranial and spinal ganglia. Sensory ganglion cell axons project peripherally (to sensory organs) and centrally (via sensory tracts in cord and brainstem) to the brain. The ventral *(motor)* roots consist of axon processes emerging from brainstem and from the anterior and lateral horn cells of the cord.

After traversing the subarachnoid space, bathed in CSF and covered only by a thin layer of arachnoid, each pair of roots is joined by unmedullated fibers from autonomic ganglia. At the exit point, fibers that are to be myelinated are now enveloped by *Schwann cells,* which produce and maintain the *myelin,* and the neural bundle is then wrapped in a thick supportive sheath of well-vascularized *perineurium* and *epineurium* as it passes to the periphery.

The autonomic nervous system (ANS) is anatomically distinct from the PNS. However, the ANS receives and sends impulses to the CNS via the PNS through the white and gray *communicating rami,* which intersect the anterior roots and spinal nerves, respectively.

PATHOGENESIS

Infectious causes of peripheral nerve injury fall into five main categories:

1. Focal external compression or invasion of a nerve by *infection in adjacent structures,* usually after producing a unique constellation of findings (e.g., Gradenigo's CNs V and VI syndrome and tuberculoid leprosy mononeuropathy)
2. Interruption of nutrient blood supply by *vasculitis involving the vasa nervorum* (e.g., polyarteritis nodosa and granulomatous arteritis)
3. *Demyelination* by lymphocytic invasion (e.g., polyneuritis) or toxic injury to Schwann cells (e.g., diphtheria)
4. *Direct invasion* and proliferation within *nerve sheaths* (e.g., lepromatous leprosy)
5. Inflammatory injury to *ganglion* and associated sensory and motor roots in response to viral *replication in a cranial or spinal ganglion* (e.g., herpes zoster)

Certain *drugs* commonly used in treating infectious diseases are also capable of producing symptoms and signs of peripheral neuropathy. Some interfere with normal metabolic processes required to maintain myelin (e.g., isoniazid), whereas others may produce their effect by interference with axonal transport (e.g., the antivirals dideoxycytosine, dideoxyinosine): In both instances, symptoms arise first in areas served by the longest nerves, and thus initially cause stocking-glove patterns of sensory and motor dysfunction. Antibiotics that produce concentration-dependent neuromuscular blockade (e.g., aminoglycosides and polymyxins) may closely mimic the polyneuropathy syndromes (see Table 154.1).

CLINICAL FEATURES

Although motor dysfunction or paralysis ultimately dominates the signs of most peripheral nerve disorders, usually *sensory disturbances* herald its onset. Characteristic symptoms are *paresthesia* (tingling, electric, numb feelings, or alternatively, aching, cutting, crushing pains) and *dysesthesias* (e.g., burning, tingling provoked by light touch). Spontaneous *unprovoked pain* and *perversion of sensation* are particularly characteristic of tabes dorsalis

TABLE 154.1.   Polyneuropathy Syndromes of Infectious Etiology or Complicating Antimicrobial Therapy

A. Acute ascending motor paralysis with variable sensory dysfunction

1. Acute inflammatory demyelinating polyneuritis: Guillain-Barré syndrome (GBS)

	Symptoms	Signs	Diagnosis

Idiopathic	Preceding nonspecific viral-like illness or stressful event (e.g., surgery) occurs in >50%
	Progressive ascending symmetric weakness involving distal then proximal limbs, truncal and cranial muscles over 10–14 days
	Paresthesias common
	Autonomic dysfunction variable: cardiovascular, gastrointestinal
		Hypotonia without atrophy (initially)
		Facial diplegia (50%)
		  No sphincteric paralysis
		Areflexia
		Sensory loss: minimal to variable
		Respiratory failure - 30%
		Variant forms: c, 10%
		  (1) Descending paralysis
		  (2) Complete ophthalmoplegia, ataxia and areflexia without progression (Miller-Fisher syndrome)
		  (3) Chronic inflammatory demyelinating polyneuritis (CIDP)
			CSF:
			  Cells: 0–5 lymphocytes (90%), 10–50 (10%)
			  Protein: elevated, peak at 4–6 weeks
			  Antibody studies: negative
			  PCR: negative
			Nerve conduction: slowed
			CT and MRI:
			  Absence of myelitis, intramedullary or extramedullary mass
			  Enhancement with gadolinium on MRI:
			    Spinal and cranial nerve roots
			    Spinocerebellar tract in Miller-Fisher variant
			    Correlates with location of symptoms

Infection-associated
  Viral:
    EBV (infectious mononucleosis)
    CMV
    HCV (viral hepatitis)
    HIV
  Other:
    Brucellosis
    Campylobacter jejuni
    Mycoplasma
    Lyme borreliosis
    Psittacosis
	Symptoms and signs of primary illness precede onset of neurologic symptoms
	Gastroenteritis
	Respiratory tract infection
	Other
	Progressive ascending symmetrical weakness: over 10–14 days:
	  Distal→ proximal limbs
	  Truncal→ cranial muscles
	Paresthesias common
		Acute ascending sensorimotor paralysis and variant forms: Indentical to idiopathic GBS	CSF:
			  Cells:
			    0–200 lymphocytes
			    B cells (primarily)
			    IgM positive early in disease
			  Protein: elevated
			    Oligoclonal banding on electrophoresis
			    IgM, IgG increased
			  Specific antibody:
			    ELISA positive in many infections
			    IgM early, then IgG
			    Immunoblot: positive if antibody in high titer
			  Direct identification of organism:
			    PCR: for specific DNA (where available)
			    Culture: insensitive
			Blood serology:
			  Diagnostic of primary infection - acute and sera 10–14 days apart
			Stool culture - *Campylobacter jejuni* found in 20%
			CT and MRI:
			  Same as idiopathic form

2. Diphtheritic polyneuropathy

	Symptoms	Signs	Diagnosis
Prodromal infection:	Pharyngitis: usual Cutaneous: less commonly produces neuropathy Wound infection: rare	Diphtheritic membrane in throat Ulcers in skin or external auditory canal	Culture: *Corynebacterium diphtheriae* (toxin producing)

Early local findings:	Incubation period after onset of primary infection:
	1–2 weeks:
	  Nasal voice
	  Nasal regurgitation
	  Dysphagia
	  Numb lips
	2–3 weeks:
	  Blurred vision
		"Bulbar" symptoms:
		  (if pharyngitis is site of infection)
		  Laryngeal, pharyngeal, and palatal paralysis
		Ciliary paralysis:
		  Loss of accommodation
			CSF:
			  Cells: 0–5
			  Protein: 50–200
			Blood serology:
			  Absent antitoxin titer in early disease
			Culture:
			  C. diphtheriae primary infection site remains positive for weeks

Later systemic findings:	Acute or subacute progression
	5–8 weeks:
	  Ascending, symmetric progressive weakness (Descending pattern also occurs)
	  Paresthesias in extremities
	  Weakness, dyspnea
		Motor weakness:
		  Extremities and trunk
		  Paralysis variable if site of primary infection not in throat
		Sensory loss
		  Distal proprioceptive loss
		  Vibration and position sense
		Carditis:
		  Resting tachycardia
		  Congestive heart failure
			EMG:
			  Mixed pattern
			Nerve conduction:
			  Abnormal
			ECG:
			  Abnormal conduction
			Echo:
			  Cardiomyopathy (20%)

(continued)

TABLE 154.1. (continued)

B. Acute descending motor paralysis with preserved sensory function

	Symptoms	Signs	Diagnosis
Botulism	Prodrome: Gastroenteritis In food-borne source only: 12–36 hours before onset of paralysis Neurologic phase: Descending paralysis Early: Blurred vision, diplopia Dry mouth, painful tongue Nasal voice Hoarseness, dysphagia Dysarthria Later: Rapid progression (2–4 days) of symmetric weakness, including muscles of respiration No paresthesias or numbness	Autonomic dysfunction: Dry mouth: no saliva Beefy red, tender tongue Constipation Dilated pupils Ptosis Early bulbar signs: Extraocular muscles weak Bulbar paralysis Motor weakness: progressive Myasthenia-like fatigability Respiratory insufficiency Absent tendon reflexes Sensation intact	CSF: Normal EMG: Characteristic Nerve conduction: Normal Microbiology: Toxin identification in food source, serum or stool *C. botulinus* culture: in wound or stool Vital capacity: Reduced in severe cases
Neuromuscular blockade by antibiotics Concentration-dependent Reversible Aminoglycosides Polymixins	Generalized myasthenia-like weakness Circumoral paresthesias	Progressive motor fatigue: On repetitive movement Progressing to paralysis at high blood levels of drug Sensation intact	CSF: Normal EMG: Characteristic Nerve conduction: Normal Blood level of drug: Toxic

C. Subacute sensorimotor paralysis

	Symptoms	Signs	Diagnosis
Neurotoxic antiinfectives Chloramphenicol Isoniazid Didanosine (ddI) Dideoxycytosine (ddC) Nitrofurantoin Metronidazole Stavudine (d4T)	Symmetric, distal pattern Sensory loss Distal paresthesia: tingling, aching, burning of toes and feet Hyperesthesia Motor weakness Follows sensory symptoms Footdrop, weakness of hands and wrist	Minimal objective loss in early stages Loss of ankle jerk Distal weakness: Appears first in lower then upper extremities	CSF: Normal EMG: Normal Nerve conduction: Abnormal
Vasculitis Infections associated with circulating immune complexes HIV-associated vasculitis Polyarteritis nodosa Wegener's granulomatosis	Asymmetric, mononeuritis multiplex pattern Distribution: Two or more nerves, Cranial or peripheral Tempo: Abrupt onset Sequential attacks Symptoms: Pain or numbness Weakness	Matched motor and sensory deficits: Distribution of specific peripheral nerve(s)	CSF: Normal Serology: Immune complexes may be present EMG: Abnormal in distribution of specific peripheral nerves Nerve conduction: Abnormal in distribution of specific peripheral nerves Biopsy: Muscle is normal Vasculitis of vasa vasorum: rarely seen

D. Chronic sensorimotor polyneuropathy

	Symptoms	Signs	Diagnosis
Leprosy Lepromatous polyneuritis	Symmetric, proximal and distal pattern: Cutaneous anesthesia: initially in limited areas but eventually symmetric Trophic dyshidrotic changes in skin	Objective anesthesia to pain and temperature in "cooler" areas: Nose Pinnae of ears Dorsum of forearms and hands Anterolateral legs and feet Loss of sweating in affected areas	Skin biopsy or skin-slit technique: High-yield areas: anesthetic site(s), macules AFB stain: positive Culture for mycobacteria: negative PCR for *M. leprae*: positive CSF: Normal

(continued)

TABLE 154.1. (continued)

D. Chronic sensorimotor polyneuropathy

	Symptoms	Signs	Diagnosis
Lepromatous polyneuritis *(continued)*	Relative sparing of motor functions Slow progression Over years Unrecognized cutaneous injury Burns, abrasions, and infections	Motor loss restricted to muscles innervated by nerves close to skin (e.g., ulnar nerve, common peroneal) Tendon reflexes intact (unique feature of leprosy)	NCS and EMG: Abnormal Nerve biopsy: Not needed: if done, avoid motor nerves (skin biopsy shows organisms in Schwann cells of cutaneous nerve fibers) Abnormal: diffuse involvement of all fascicles in large nerves in later stages
Indeterminate leprosy neuritis Borderline states and reversal reactions	Asymmetric pattern: Anesthetic hypopigmented macules or papules Multiple nerves can be affected Large, mixed sensorimotor nerves Painful nerves at times of spontaneous or treatment-induced reversal reactions Active skin lesions with reversal reactions	Selective sensory loss: Loss of pain and temperature sensation Tender swollen sensorimotor nerves in exposed areas with reversal reactions Rapid progression of functional loss	Skin biopsy: Highest yield: anesthetic site(s), macules AFB stain: positive, but paucibacillary Culture for mycobacteria: negative PCR for *M. leprae:* positive if granuloma in specimen CSF: Normal NCS and EMG: Abnormal Nerve biopsy: Abnormal: avoid motor nerves
Tuberculoid leprosy neuritis	Early sign of disease Rapid progression without treatment Asymmetric pattern: Limited number of nerves affected Weakness of muscles innervated by ulnar, median, peroneal, posterior tibial, or facial nerves Anesthetic skin lesions	Palpable subcutaneous sensory and sensorimotor nerves (Localized areas: e.g., greater auricular, common peroneal at fibula, ulnar at elbow) Limited sensory and motorloss: Only in distribution of involved nerves Claw hands: fourth and fifth digits (ulnar claw): ulnar nerve All digits: median and ulnar nerve Wrist drop: radial nerve Claw toe, flat arch: posterior tibial nerve (most common) Lagophthalmia (weak lid levators): facial nerve Conjunctival and corneal anesthesia: trigeminal nerve	Skin biopsy: Highest Yield: anesthetic site(s), macules AFB stain: negative commonly Culture for mycobacteria: negative PCR for *M. leprae:* positive if granuloma in specimen CSF: Normal NCS and EMG: Abnormal Nerve biopsy: Abnormal: avoid motor nerves

and postzoster neuralgia, both of which are associated with inflammatory changes predominantly in the dorsal root. Inflammation always extends into the dorsal column in tabes and may be a factor in the pathogenesis of postzoster neuralgia.

Seemingly paradoxic *dissociations of sensory losses* may be helpful in evaluating the site of lesion. When the disease process mainly targets *myelin,* pain and temperature sensation are spared, but deep tendon reflexes (DTRs) and proprioceptive functions (pressure-touch, vibration, joint-pressure sensations, and two-point discrimination) are abnormal. Conversely, *when nerve itself is invaded* and if invasion is limited by the organism's requirement for localizing in *superficial nerves* (e.g., lepromatous leprosy), proprioceptive functions and tendon reflexes remain intact in the presence of widespread cutaneous anesthesia. *Sensory ataxia* (brusque, flinging, slapping movements, especially of legs) results when motor function is relatively spared, which is characteristic of tabes dorsalis. *Trophic skin changes* (e.g., alteration of color, turgor, temperature, and nail structure) are a sign of cutaneous anesthesia and associated autonomic dysfunction. Anesthesia also increases susceptibility to injuries and infections, which further disfigure anesthetic sites.

Loss of tendon reflexes, especially out of proportion to weakness, is an invariable sign of peripheral nerve disease, with one exception: lepromatous neuritis, which usually spares the muscular nerves. *Motor weakness or paralysis with areflexia* is less discreetly localizing to peripheral nerves but always signifies either *segmental demyelination, axonal interruption,* or *destruction of motor neurons.*

An *abnormal CSF* test result can be an important clue to a possibly treatable cause, because meningeal inflammation often accompanies infections involving peripheral nerves (e.g., Lyme neuroborreliosis, syphilis, herpes viruses).

CLASSIFICATION

Peripheral neuropathies, whatever their etiology, are classified anatomically as focal *(mononeuropathies),* multifocal *(mononeuritis multiplex), plexitis,* and *polyneuropathies* (1–3). Polyneuropathies exhibit several clinical patterns that differ in rate of onset and type of paralysis (see Table 154.1). Because many causes may produce one or more of these syndromes, the most important causes are considered individually.

Included for comparison are two neurologic syndromes caused by toxin-producing organisms—tetanus and botulism—

that affect PNS function but do not cause neuropathy. Polyneuropathies caused by ingestion of neurotoxins from shellfish *(saxitoxin)*, puffer fish *(tetrodotoxin)*, and tropical fish *(ciguatera toxin)* are not discussed, but must be considered in the differential diagnosis of acute polyneuropathy.

Specific Diseases

DIRECT INVASION

Leprosy

Cause. Leprosy (or Hansen's disease) is a chronic mycobacterial infection in which *Mycobacterium leprae* primarily affects the PNS and secondarily involves skin and other tissues (4). *M. leprae* is shed from skin and mucous membranes and transmitted from person to person by prolonged physical contact. The three characteristics of leprosy are anesthetic skin lesions, palpably enlarged peripheral nerves, and in lepromatous patients only, visible acid-fast bacilli (AFB) visible in skin biopsy or slit-skin smear that do not grow in conventional mycobacteriologic cultures.

Epidemiology. See Chapter 158.

Pathogenesis. See Chapter 158.

Clinical Features. Although skin lesions have a variable appearance, anesthesia of the involved skin is the one consistent feature in typical leprosy. Lepromatous leprosy usually results in symmetric anesthesia of the "colder" areas of the body (e.g., pinnae and dorsa of hands and feet), whereas nerve involvement in indeterminate and tuberculoid leprosy is typically asymmetric. Involvement of the ANS supplying the skin results in anhidrosis with impaired sweat response. Eye involvement causes denervation of the iris and reduced intraocular pressure (5).

Anesthetic skin lesions, one of the cardinal clinical manifestations of *tuberculoid leprosy*, exhibit blunting of sensation to touch, temperature, and pain. Light tactile sensation may remain intact. Normally an early finding, this differential loss of sensation may be difficult to elicit in facial lesions because of the generous supply of sensory nerves to the face. In *borderline leprosy* with more varied skin lesions, anesthesia is not always a feature, but there is usually evidence of nerve involvement, such as polyneuropathy or asymmetric multiple nerve pathology. In *lepromatous* leprosy, there is nerve thickening and associated sensory or motor dysfunction, depending on the nerve involved (4).

In the *mononeuritis and mononeuritis multiplex patterns*, early nerve damage consists of thickening of the most superficial (and therefore coolest) nerves, such as the great auricular nerves in the neck, the supraclavicular nerves, the ulnar nerves above the elbow, the radial and median at the wrist, the superficial femoral, the lateral popliteal around the neck of fibula, and the superficial peroneal in the ankle.

Two other patterns may occur: *sensory polyneuropathy*, more common in lepromatous leprosy, and *neuralgia*. Three types of neuralgia are recognized: One is associated with nerve swelling, especially in *nerve reactions*; a second type is dull pain in the extremities and trigeminal territory in *disease-arrested* patients; and the third type is *phantom-pain* neuralgia at the site of *artificial limbs*, which is not unique to leprosy (6).

Diagnosis. The *peripheral nerves most commonly involved* are the ulnar, median, common peroneal, and posterior tibial nerves. The *CNs involved* are the facial and trigeminal. Superficial nerves, such as the ulnar and posterior auricular nerves, are readily accessible to palpation and are often enlarged and tender (5,7).

Sensory impairment manifests as loss of light touch, pain, and temperature. The ability to distinguish between hot and cold is usually the first modality to be lost. Vibration and position senses can be conserved until a later stage.

In facial nerve involvement, the temporal and zygomatic branches of the facial nerve are affected most commonly as they cross the zygoma, resulting in lagophthalmos or inability to close the eye. Unlike Bell's palsy, paralysis of the buccal, mandibular, and cervical branches is uncommon and when present is usually limited to the upper branches, producing loss of facial expression, and inability to close the lips. Trigeminal nerve involvement appears to be limited to the fine nerve endings and causes anesthesia of the face and most importantly of the cornea and conjunctiva (7).

Damage to motor nerves manifests by weakness and paralysis (facial palsy, claw hand, ape hand, dropped foot). Retention of DTRs is a unique feature and relates to the differential susceptibility of deep and superficial nerves to invasion by *M. leprae* (8).

Neurophysiologic studies are helpful in preliminary diagnosis, but in the absence of skin lesions, nerve biopsy of a nonmotor branch of the nerve is often necessary for precise diagnosis (6,7).

When leprosy is suspected, skin biopsies or fluid from slit-skin smears should be stained for AFB. In areas of the world where the disease is rare, such as the United States, *skin biopsy* should be performed (7). Slit-skin smears are performed by making small incisions into the dermis at multiple sites and then collecting fluid for staining. AFB stains of skin biopsies and slit-skin smears are usually positive in lepromatous and borderline lepromatous leprosy, but typically negative in the paucibacillary states of tuberculoid and borderline tuberculoid disease. AFB cultures of smear-positive specimens by definition are negative, because the organism cannot be cultured *in vitro* with conventional methods (7). The organism may be identified by polymerase chain reaction (PCR).

Skin testing with conventional lepromin is not useful in diagnosis, but positive reactions correlate with the presence of cellular immunity. Newer reagents made from *M. leprae* membrane proteins are under investigation (9).

Treatment. See Chapter 158.

NEUROPATHIES DUE TO BACTERIAL TOXINS

Diphtheria, tetanus, and botulism are neurologic disorders caused by bacterial toxins elaborated by metabolically active bacteria. Diphtheria toxin causes direct damage to Schwann cells, affecting conduction, whereas botulinus and tetanus toxins act on nerve–nerve and neuromuscular junctions to interrupt normal function.

Tetanus neurotoxin (TeNT) and botulinum neurotoxins (BoNTs) are produced by *Clostridia* and share certain molecular characteristics despite their disparate clinical features. Both bind to nerve cells, penetrate the cytosol, are internalized, and release zinc proteases, which cleave key components in the protein complex controlling the docking of synaptic vesicles with the cell membrane processes critical to exocytosis of neurotransmitters. Both neurotoxins consist of two polypeptide chains: one contains the metalloendopeptidase activity specific to the toxin and its subtype, and the other determines the tropism for specific neural cells, such that TeNT acts mainly at CNS synapses, whereas the seven BoNTs subtypes act peripherally (10,11). The remarkable specificity of BoNTs is exploited in the treatment of human diseases characterized by a hyperfunction of cholinergic terminals (11).

Botulism

Cause and Pathogenesis. *Clostridium botulinum* is a ubiquitous, spore-forming, anaerobic gram positive rod that lives in soil and aquatic habitats. It produces a potent neurotoxin, termed BoNT, capable of binding irreversibly and blocking acetylcholine release at the neuromuscular junction. Following germination of spores, BoNT is synthesized as a single inactive protein and released during lysis of bacterial cells. Activation of the prototoxin requires proteolytic cleavage into the biologically active dimer composed of a disulfide-linked light and heavy chain.

BoNT is readily destroyed by boiling, but *C. botulinum* spores require superheating to 121°C (250°F) (12). Toxin production has also been identified in other *Clostridium* species (*Clostridium barati* and *Clostridium butyricum*) associated with toxicoinfectious botulism (13,14). *Clostridium argentinense* produce type G BoNT but have not yet been associated with outbreaks.

Eight subtypes of toxin are known: A, B, C_1, C_2, D, E, F, and G (15). Human disease usually results from ingestion of toxin-containing contaminated food and rarely from contamination of a wound (16). Types A, B, E, and F are the toxins most often implicated in human disease (17,18), and a trivalent antitoxin (type ABE) is available in the United States for treatment. Purified BoNT has been mass produced for aerosol use in biological warfare (13) and for medical treatment of dystonias through selective injection of toxin (19,20).

Epidemiology. See Chapter 212.

Prevention. Prevention of food-borne botulism depends on destroying all *C. botulinum* spores in food as it is preserved and/or creating a milieu that will not allow growth of any organisms that survive the preservation procedures or are introduced thereafter (21,22). Heating to 121°C or higher, though usually sufficient to destroy spores, requires a pressure cooker. Other methods for inhibiting growth of *C. botulinum* include adjusting the acidity or salt content of the food item or boiling fruits and certain vegetables whose high sugar content will not support growth (23). Because contamination may occur before and after commercially processed food products are in use, antimicrobial growth inhibitors or acidifying agents are commonly added to products capable of providing an anaerobic environment supportive of germination of ubiquitous *C. botulinum* spores (24). Information about methods for home food preservation readily available from public service and governmental agencies was formerly routinely incorporated into school curricula.

Use of botulinus toxoids as vaccines, studied for more than 40 years and used effectively for high-risk laboratory personnel (23), has once again become a subject of interest in developed countries as a result of the emergence of bioterrorism.

Clinical Features. Neuromuscular symptoms of botulism vary with the age of the patient; whether the exposure is the result of ingestion of preformed prototoxin or from active toxin production following colonization of gut or wound; and by toxin type (17). *Infants* first develop constipation, then hypotonia ("floppy baby syndrome") and ophthalmoplegia (25).

In the *adult* form, most patients present as a "descending" symmetric form of paralysis, because the eye and facial muscles are relatively more sensitive than skeletal muscles to any form of neuromuscular blockade. Clinical features include symmetric cranial neuropathies (e.g., drooping eyelids, diplopia, weakened jaw clench, and difficulty speaking and swallowing), autonomic dysfunction (blurred vision and dry mouth), symmetric descending weakness in a proximal to distal pattern, and respiratory tract dysfunction from respiratory tract paralysis or airway obstruction. Sensory examination is always normal. Wound botulism has the same clinical pattern as food botulism.

If the source is food, there is a predictable interval from exposure to onset of disease. Sixteen to sixty hours after ingestion, signs of autonomic dysfunction (abdominal cramps, dry mouth, blurred vision, inability to accommodate, abnormal pupillary reflexes, urinary difficulty, and diarrhea or constipation) are followed by descending muscle weakness, first in the ocular and bulbar musculature, then in the whole body. In severe disease, paralysis involves the diaphragm and other muscles of respiration (26) (see Table 154.1). Because neurologic effects are dose dependent, members of groups with a common-source exposure will exhibit differing degrees of neurologic findings depending on the amount of prototoxin ingested. Toxin type also affects rate and extent of progression of symptoms (17). Type E has the shortest incubation period, but type A produces more severe illness and requires intubation more often (67%).

Diagnosis. CSF results are normal. The edrophonium bromide (Tensilon) test for myasthenia gravis is negative. Electrophysiologic testing is helpful in distinguishing this disorder from other causes of *motor weakness with preserved sensation* (27). Infants with sudden onset of weakness, respiratory failure, and constipation should undergo immediate electrophysiologic testing, because delay in diagnosis of infantile botulism is associated with higher mortality and morbidity (28).

Diagnosis can be confirmed by measuring toxin in serum (15 to 20 mL in adults), feces (25 to 50 g), gastric contents or vomitus, and if available in the food source (29,30). Stool cultures may contain the organism in infant botulism and sporadic adult cases but rarely in food-borne disease (12,31). Any suspicious wounds should be evaluated with Gram stain and cultured aerobically and anaerobically, and tissues and exudates collected for toxin analysis (32).

Public health authorities should always be notified immediately of any suspected case (33). Attending physicians should immediately notify their state health department or the Centers for Disease Control and Prevention (CDC) when there is suspicion of botulism so appropriate action can be taken to establish the diagnosis, initiate treatment, and investigate the potential outbreak.

Treatment. See Chapter 212.

Diphtheria

Cause and Pathogenesis. *Corynebacterium diphtheriae* can be isolated from nasopharynx and skin, which represent reservoirs for its spread (34). Only strains containing the bacteriophages carrying the *tox* gene, which encodes for *C. diphtheriae* exotoxin, produce severe systemic effects from focal infections. Both toxin-positive and toxin-negative strains are capable of producing locally invasive infections (34). Neurologic, cardiac, and renal complications of diphtheria are due to the elaboration by the microorganism of the extremely potent protein toxin, which acts on the elongation factor, a critical protein needed for mammalian protein synthesis (35). The two major fragments (A and B) of the toxin secreted by *C. diphtheriae* are excluded by the blood–brain barrier, which explains the preferential involvement of peripheral nerves and CNs (36).

The organism remains localized, either in the nose (anterior nasal diphtheria), throat (faucial diphtheria), larynx (laryngeal diphtheria), or cutaneous wounds (skin diphtheria), releasing its toxin for local and systemic effects. The toxin causes a noninflammatory demyelination of the CN and peripheral nerves through its toxic effect on Schwann cells (37).

Corynebacterium ulcerans, which causes respiratory tract diphtheria and mastitis in cattle, and *Corynebacterium pseudotuberculosis* also harbor the diphtheria toxin gene and can produce high levels of toxin. *C. ulcerans* has been implicated in human cases clinically identical to faucial diphtheria (38).

Epidemiology. See Chapter 187.

Prevention. See Chapter 187.

Clinical Features. Disease can affect any mucous membrane and altered skin. Specific clinical manifestations are several: (a) anterior nasal diphtheria, characterized by mucopurulent nasal discharge and a white membrane on the nasal septum; (b) pharyngeal and tonsillar diphtheria or faucial diphtheria, with sore throat, fever, and progressive expansion over days of blue-white adherent membrane, which may turn black after bleeding; (c) laryngeal diphtheria, with hoarseness and barking cough; and (d) cutaneous diphtheria, where scaling, rash, and ulceration may be present and even confined to discreet areas, such as the external auditory canal. *C. diphtheriae* isolates from skin infections are often nontoxigenic.

The most common form is faucial diphtheria, an upper respiratory tract illness characterized by sore throat, dysphagia, lymphadenitis, low-grade fever, malaise, headache, and frequently a nasopharyngeal adherent membrane that may cause airway obstruction. In severe diphtheria, classic features include an extensive membrane, diffuse cervical lymphadenopathy, and soft tissue swelling ("bull-neck" appearance) (39). In the absence of treatment of the primary localized diphtheria infection, the incidence of neurologic complications is about 15% (15,40).

In faucial diphtheria, local production of toxin in the pharynx causes early paralysis of the pharyngeal and laryngeal muscles, and the earliest neurologic manifestation is palatal weakness. The patient speaks with a nasal voice and complains of dysphagia and nasal regurgitation. Within days the trigeminal, facial, vagal, and hypoglossal nerves are affected *(bulbar phase).* By the third week, ciliary paralysis with loss of accommodation and blurring of vision is evident. On occasion, paralysis of the extraocular muscles occurs. Echocardiographic evidence of abnormal contractility in diphtheritic myocarditis is not detectable until 3 weeks after electrocardiographic changes (41).

The onset of sensorimotor polyneuropathy of the trunk and extremities *(systemic paralysis)* is delayed and usually appears 2 to 3 months after the primary infection (see Table 154.1). The polyneuropathy may occur simultaneously in all extremities or it may descend. Occasionally respiratory tract paralysis develops (1–3,15,42). Sensory findings include paresthesias; loss of superficial joint and position senses; and impaired or lost tendon reflexes. Severity of motor weakness varies from a mild deficit with maximal distal involvement to a rapidly ascending paralysis.

Systemic paralysis with diphtheritic polyneuropathy is associated with high morbidity and mortality. A review of 50 hospitalized patients found ventilator-dependent respiratory failure in 20%, persistent neurologic morbidity at 1 year in 80%, and a 16% death rate, half from diphtheritic cardiomyopathy and half from multiple organ failure (40).

Diagnosis. The initial diagnosis is primarily clinical. The receiving laboratory should be notified immediately of suspected diphtheria. In respiratory tract diphtheria, cultures from nasopharynx and from the underside of the removed membrane are useful for culture, staining and *tox* PCR. Swabs and/or aspirated material are helpful in wound diphtheria. To ensure maintenance of viable bacteria, swabs should be brought immediately to the laboratory or transported in semisolid media (34).

The diagnosis is established by recovering the organism from the source (from throat culture in pharyngitis or from wound in the case of cutaneous diphtheria) or by detection of circulating *C. diphtheriae* exotoxin in the blood, which is now the definitive test (43). Isolation of *C. diphtheriae* from blood cultures indicates possible endocarditis (44,45). If exotoxin testing is not available, assays for circulating antitoxin antibody support the diagnosis when the level is nonprotective (less than 0.01 IU/mL) (42). CSF is normal except for an elevated protein level, comparable to that with Guillain-Barré syndrome (GBS). All suspected diphtheria cases should also be reported to local and state health departments.

Treatment. See Chapter 187.

Tetanus

Cause. Tetanus is caused solely by the toxic action on the nervous system of the potent neurotoxin, tetanospasmin, or TeNT, produced by the anaerobic spore-forming rod *Clostridium tetani,* which is widely distributed in nature (46). *C. tetani* is usually introduced into tissues as a spore. Disease develops only if anaerobic conditions are present, which permits growth of the toxin-producing vegetative form. TeNT is synthesized as a single biologically inactive, polypeptide chain. Upon lysis of *C. tetani,* the toxin is cleaved by an intrinsic protease to produce a dimer, consisting of a light and a heavy chain linked by a disulfide bond (47,48). Tetanus toxin is the next most potent toxin after botulinum toxin. Like BoNT, TeNT is a protein with three domains endowed with different functions: neurospecific binding, membrane translocation, and proteolysis for specific components of the neuroexocytosis apparatus.

Pathogenesis. Following inoculation of organisms or spores into the tissues, the incubation period in humans is usually 3 to 21 days, but depending on inoculum size and local microenvironment, may be as short as 1 day or as long as several months (46).

TeNT binds to the presynaptic membrane of the neuromuscular junction, is internalized, and is transported retroaxonally to the spinal cord. It is taken up distally by motor, sensory, and autonomic nerve terminals and is carried to the spinal cord and brainstem before transsynaptic transfer to presynaptic terminals in the neuropil of the ventral horn. The mode of toxin transport to the CNS explains the variable onset of symptoms: the shorter the axon, the earlier the involvement (49).

A significant amount of toxin remains bound to nerve terminals at the neuromuscular junction in the infected site, which interferes with acetylcholine release by means indistinguishable from botulinum toxin.

The tetanic syndrome originates from the toxin's disinhibitory action on spinal reflex arcs (47). TeNT acts within the CNS, in contrast to the specific action of BoNT on the PNS. The heavy chain of TeNT targets and binds to neuronal cells, whereas the light chain, acting as a zinc endopeptidase, binds to protein components of the neuroexocytotic apparatus and inhibits exocytosis of the neurotransmitter γ-aminobutyric acid within the CNS. The spastic paralysis induced by the toxin is due to the blockade of neurotransmitter release from spinal inhibitory interneurons. When inhibitory impulses to the motor neurons are blocked, the uninhibited firing of motor nerve transmissions continues, resulting in prolonged muscle spasms of both flexor and extensor muscles that can persist for weeks.

TeNT's effects on the spinal cord are similar to strychnine and lead to dysfunction of polysynaptic reflexes that involve inhibition of antagonists (46,47). Disturbances of the sympathetic nervous system occur, including labile hypertension, cardiac tachyarrhythmias, peripheral vasoconstriction, and profuse sweating. Neuronal cell death may occur from unopposed excitation (50).

The brain is minimally affected, except in cephalic tetanus where instead of spasm, there is initially paralysis of muscles closest to the site of injury but spasm affecting adjacent muscles. Paralysis, which gives way to spasm during the recovery phase, is considered to be due to higher concentrations of toxin in the brainstem, which cause paralysis instead of abolishing inhibition. Correspondingly, the paralytic phase is associated with electrophysiologic findings of lower motor neuron injury, such as denervation potentials, hyperirritability, loss of motor units, and marginally increased latencies (49,51).

Epidemiology.   See Chapter 211.

Prevention.   See Chapter 211.

Clinical Features.   There are three alternative presentations: (a) local tetanus with muscular contraction at the site of injury, which may persist or progress to the generalized form; (b) cephalic tetanus affecting CNs, mostly the VII pair; and (c) generalized tetanus with lockjaw, reflex spasms easily provoked by external stimuli, opisthotonos, and risus sardonicus (1,2,3).

In *localized tetanus,* a mild form of the disease, unyielding rigidity of muscle groups close to the injury site may persist for weeks or months, finally disappearing without residua (46). Sometimes localized tetanus precedes the generalized form. Localized disease may occur in a partially immune individual (52) or when a nonimmune individual sustaining a wound at high risk for growth of *C. tetani* receives hyperimmune serum at a protective rather than a therapeutic dosage.

In *generalized tetanus,* the most common form of the disease, trismus is the presenting complaint in more than 50% of cases. Associated or alternative initial complaints are restlessness, irritability, neck stiffness, abdominal rigidity, dysphagia, or preexisting localized tetanus. Tonic contractions of muscles of jaw, face, neck, abdomen, and back are common, and abdominal and lumbar muscles may become rigid. Opisthotonos results from viselike persistent constriction of chest and back muscles. The typical *tetanic seizure* is characterized by a sudden burst of tonic contraction of muscle groups causing opisthotonos, flexion and adduction of the arms, clenching of the fists on the thorax, and extension of the lower extremities. The patient is completely conscious during such episodes and experiences intense pain. Glottal or laryngeal spasm and urinary retention may occur. Autonomic involvement results in generalized sympathetic overactivity with hypertension, tachycardia, and arrhythmias (46,53). Spasms are most prominent in the first 2 weeks. Autonomic disturbance follows some days later and peaks during the second week. Rigidity may outlast both spasms and autonomic disturbance. Severe rigidity and muscle spasm necessitate therapeutic paralysis for prolonged periods. If intensive care is not available, death occurs from spasm in respiratory tract muscles (54).

Cephalic tetanus, an unusual form of the disease that is characterized by local muscle paralysis after injuries of the head or otitis media, commonly has an incubation period of only 1 or 2 days. Muscle paralysis is maximal close to the site of injury, whereas spasm is evident at more distal sites. As paralysis recedes with time, it is succeeded by spasm before the muscle returns to normal. Lockjaw is the usual presenting symptom, associated with hemifacial spasm, weakness, paresis, or paralysis. Although CN VII is the one most commonly affected, depending on the site of the infected wound, nerves IX, X, and XII may be affected singly or in combination. Extraocular movements generally are unaf-

fected (55). Cephalic tetanus generally has a good prognosis if treatment is begun early.

Several prognostic scoring systems [Phillips (56), Dakar (57), and Udwadia (58)] incorporate the incubation period, period of onset, entry site, state of protective immunity, presence or absence of spasms, fever, and tachycardia, and other complicating factors in staging clinical tetanus. The incubation period is the time from inoculation to the first symptom and reflects the quantity of toxin released and distance traveled to the CNS. The period of onset, also referred to as the *invasion period* in older literature (52), is the time between the first symptom and start of spasms and reflects rate of progression of neurologic disease.

The most important prognostic factor for generalized tetanus is not the incubation period, but the rate of progression from onset of symptoms to full development of disease (52). The shorter this interval, the higher the mortality, especially where sophisticated intensive care is not available. This point is illustrated by a recent review of 8,697 tetanus cases in India, where case-fatality rate overall was 48%, for neonatal tetanus was 86%, but in the large subgroup not yet progressed to spasm (n = 2,100), mortality was only 2% (59).

Diagnosis.   Diagnosis is based on clinical criteria and is confirmed by the characteristic neurophysiologic findings and absence of serum antitetanus antibody. The CSF is normal. Gram stain and anaerobic cultures of the wound may or may not reveal the organism (52,54).

Treatment.   See Chapter 211.

INFLAMMATORY DEMYELINATING POLYNEUROPATHIES: POLYNEURITIS

Two syndromes of inflammatory polyneuritis are recognized, based on differences in tempo and persistence of paralysis: *acute* inflammatory demyelinating polyneuropathy (AIDP), or Guillain-Barré syndrome (GBS), and *chronic* inflammatory demyelinating polyneuropathy (CIDP). Both syndromes are characterized by an ascending or descending generalized sensorimotor demyelinating polyneuropathy, with elevated protein level and variable lymphocytosis in the CSF (see Table 154.1). Most cases are classified as "idiopathic" and are treated empirically, either with plasmapheresis or intravenous concentrated immune globulin (IVIG). However, AIDP has well-known associations with certain infectious agents, such as its occurrence after infection with *Campylobacter jejuni* (60) and during the seroconversion period of acute HIV infection (61).

Acute Inflammatory Demyelinating Polyneuropathy or the Guillain-Barré Syndrome

Causes and Epidemiology.   GBS is the most common cause of acute paralytic illness in young adults (62). In the United States, the incidence is 9.5 cases per million. It occurs worldwide with a slightly greater prevalence in men and has no seasonal preference (63–65). Incidence peaks between ages 16 to 25 years with a second smaller peak at ages 45 to 60 years.

GBS has a well-known association with various *infectious diseases,* such as herpes viruses cytomegalovirus (CMV) and Epstein-Barr virus (EBV) (66), HIV, hepatitis C virus (67), *Mycoplasma pneumoniae, Chlamydia psittaci, Borrelia burgdorferi* (Lyme disease), and particularly with *C. jejuni* (60,66,68–70).

Whether the occurrence of GBS during HIV infection represents a causal or merely a chance relationship is unknown (61,71–73). GBS in HIV disease typically develops early in the seroconversion period of acute HIV infection and before the onset of advanced immunosuppression (61,71). The course of the illness is very similar to that found in HIV-negative patients, except for the finding of up to 50 white blood cells (WBCs) in the CSF and a higher frequency of coexisting CNS dysfunction (74). However, the illness responds to standard therapy, and prognosis is generally favorable (73).

More often, the acute polyneuritis is *idiopathic*, although in many instances it appears after a precipitating factor. The precipitating factors, or antecedent events, of this *acute idiopathic inflammatory demyelinating polyneuropathy* are numerous: infections other than those mentioned earlier, vaccinations, malignancy, surgery, solid organ transplantation (75), and other stressful events (76). Patients having an antecedent event often mention a viral-like illness: respiratory (58%), gastrointestinal (GI) (22%), or both (10%) (76,77). According to the U.S. national GBS surveillance conducted in the early 1980s before the impact of the HIV epidemic, the "event," always diagnosed in retrospect, usually occurred within 1 to 2 months preceding the syndrome and was present in approximately 80% of patients (76).

In a carefully studied cohort of 229 patients, *C. jejuni,* often isolated from patients with the GI prodrome, was identified as associated with up to 23% of cases of GBS (60,66), CMV with 8%, and EBV with 2%. Specific infectious agents were not linked to specific subtypes of clinical, neurophysiologic, and immunologic features of these cases, reaffirming the importance of host factors in determining disease patterns (66).

Pathogenesis. Two types of lesions have been observed (78). The most common is infiltration by lymphocytic and monocytic inflammatory cells within roots and nerves of the PNS, followed by widespread segmental demyelination, with sparing of axons and of the CNS (79). Remyelination then slowly takes place by Schwann cell proliferation. Nerve biopsies show subperineural edema, macrophage infiltration, and complete demyelination of axon with intratubal macrophages, all characteristics of primary demyelination rather than axonal degeneration (80). The intensity of the inflammatory infiltrate varies according to duration of disease, with more leucocytes and T cells in the endoneurium in the first month than later (81).

The second type of lesion is dominated by macrophages and early marked inflammation, suggestive of antibody-mediated immune destruction. It may be the hallmark of the less common form of GBS, which combines both demyelination and severe axonal degeneration and results in severe residual disability (82). Both types of lesions are seen in the experimental allergic neuritis (EAN) animal model.

A third mechanism is suggested by rare patients who have extensive axonal degeneration, indicating either "innocent bystander" injury by inflammation or a direct attack on axons. A search for viral genomes in the myelin sheaths of affected nerves and in infiltrating cells in biopsies from typical GBS cases has failed to reveal CMV or any other suspects (83,84).

Antibodies to neural antigens, including tubulin (85) and the ganglioside antigens G_{M1}, G_{M1b}, G_{D1a}, GalNAc-G_{D1a}, G_{T1a}, and G_{Q1b} (86) have been detected in the serum of patients with GBS and CIDP. Variation in their prevalence among clinical subtypes may explain the different clinical presentations of a disease with a common pathogenetic mechanism (86,87). The genesis of high titers of antibody to G_{M1} and G_{D1a} in patients with GBS with recent evidence of infection with *C. jejuni* is presumed to be the lipopolysaccharide of *C. jejuni*, which shares similar ganglioside motifs with neural ganglioside antigens. This postinfectious autoimmune response appears to be a unique characteristic of patients with *C. jejuni*–associated GBS, because it normally does not occur after *C. jejuni* gastroenteritis (88).

Searchs for genetic markers predictive of susceptibility to GBS have failed to find significant differences between patients and controls, including studies of genetic polymorphisms of HLA and T-cell receptors (89), but interesting differences have been noted in immunoglobulin G (IgG) receptor IIa alleles on leukocytes (90).

Clinical Features. GBS is a rapidly progressive and slowly reversible *motor neuropathy* and usually follows an ascending pattern, although descending and other variant patterns occur (see Table 154.1). The common ascending pattern starts with progressive and often symmetric weakness in the distal lower limbs, ascends over the entire body within days and may progress for up to a month, often resulting in respiratory tract failure. Facial weakness is often present. Tendon reflexes are usually absent.

Patients at entry can be easily divided into three functional groups: those who can walk, with or without aid, but not run, or who can stand up unaided (mild); those unable to stand up unaided (moderate); and those who need mechanical ventilation (severe) (91).

Approximately 90% of untreated patients reach maximal impairment within 4 weeks, whereas the remainder fluctuate for up to 8 weeks. The progressive paralytic phase is followed by a plateau phase and then a variable period of recovery (92).

Sensory symptoms are mild and do not usually progress, although transient paresthesias and pain in the back and legs are common complaints. Objective sensory loss is variable and when present tends to affect deep sensibility more than superficial (93). *Autonomic involvement* (e.g., hypotension or hypertension, cardiac arrhythmias, abnormalities of sweating, and gastric atony) is not uncommon. Constitutional symptoms are usually absent.

There are three distinctive variant forms of acute idiopathic inflammatory demyelinating polyneuropathy: the *Miller-Fisher syndrome* (acute ophthalmoplegia, ataxia, and generalized areflexia) (94); *polyneuritis cranialis,* where only CNs are involved; and those destined to have *CIDP,* by definition those who do not reach the nadir at 4 weeks but continue to deteriorate (see section "Chronic Inflammatory Demyelinating Polyneuropathy"). In a retrospective analysis of 266 cases of inflammatory polyneuropathy covering 33 years, 84% had typical GBS, 13% CIDP, 1.5% polyneuritis cranialis, and 0.8% each of Miller-Fisher syndrome and predominantly sensory neuropathy (95). Undoubtedly some of these cases represented undiagnosed neuroborreliosis, which is a relatively recently recognized infectious cause of a GBS-like polyneuritis pattern. In one recent prospective study, variant presentations accounted for 10% of cases, meeting the GBS case definition (96).

Clinical risk factors at entry for inability to walk by 48 weeks or for death include age older than 50 years, initial findings of diarrhea, severe arm weakness, inexcitable nerves on electrodiagnostic studies, and laboratory findings of high circulating levels of soluble IL-2 receptor (sIL-2R) and absence of IgM antibody to G_{M1} (66).

Diagnosis. The laboratory hallmark of GBS is called in French "dissociation albumino-cytologique:" a rise in CSF protein (which can be normal during the first days of illness) with minimal concomitant rise of CSF WBCs, although lymphocytosis is not uncommon in the earliest phase of disease (70). CSF protein values peak at 3 to 4 weeks. The protein consists of elevated concentrations of albumin, IgG, IgA, and IgM without unique kappa/lambda ratios, suggesting that the elevated immunoglobulin levels may not be due to intrathecal synthesis (97). The absence of significant lymphocytosis in the CSF is a major distinction between idiopathic GBS and the known infectious causes of polyneuritis (see Table 154.1).

Elevated immunoglobulin levels and increasing numbers of immunoblasts circulate in the blood in the acute phase; reductions in immunoblasts seem to correlate with recovery.

Antimyelin, antitubulin, and antiganglioside antibodies are present in the serum of many acute cases. Findings include circulating immune complexes (98).

MRI has found increasing application in diagnosis of acute and chronic inflammatory demyelinating polyneuropathies. T1-weighted spinal magnetic resonance imaging (MRI) scans show characteristic enhancement of the pial lining of involved nerve roots, cauda equina, and conus medullaris. In Miller-Fisher variant, nerve enhancement is confined to the CNs but may also involve the spinocerebellar tracts in the lower medulla and demonstrate other findings compatible with brainstem encephalitis (99,100).

MRI demonstrates greater involvement than is apparent from symptoms or electrodiagnostic studies (101,102), correlates well with stage and presentation of disease (103), and changes with its progression and remission (104). Enhancement of nerve roots and cord structures is not unique to idiopathic GBS, however, and has been documented in AIDS-related polyradiculopathy associated with CMV (105) and with neuroborreliosis (see section "Neuroborreliosis (Lyme Borreliosis)"). Early electrodiagnostic findings are essential aspects of diagnostic evaluation (106).

Differential Diagnosis.   Idiopathic GBS must be distinguished from the known causes of acute polyneuritis, such as neuroborreliosis, from other neurologic illnesses (such as myasthenia gravis), and from uncommon infectious diseases that mimic polyneuropathy: botulism, diphtheria, poliomyelitis, and the polyradiculitis and myelitis of advanced HIV infection due to herpesviruses and neurosyphilis. Acute flaccid paralysis has also been observed to occur in as many as one third of patients presenting with West Nile fever viral meningoencephalitis but is neither ascending nor descending in its onset. In botulism, the pupillary reflexes are lost early in the illness and are accompanied progressively by other significant autonomic dysfunctions (e.g., bradycardia, dry mouth, abdominal cramps, urinary difficulty). Polio presents with meningeal symptoms, fever, and an asymmetric paralysis. Diphtheria should be considered when bulbar paralysis precedes descending paralysis and is accompanied by fever and pharyngitis.

Concomitant HIV infection extends the range of possible causes. Herpesvirus radiculitis and myelitis typically is subacute, ascending and asymmetric, occurs only in advanced immunosuppression (CD4 less than 50), and has CSF changes of acute inflammation mimicking bacterial infection. Neurosyphilis in HIV infection has a neurologic pattern similar to the subacute onset of herpesvirus infection (107), but the CSF contains lymphocytes instead of neutrophils, and blood and CSF usually test positive for reaginic antibodies [ART, Venereal Disease Research Laboratory (VDRL)]. When CSF VDRL is negative, but treponema-specific blood serology points to prior syphilis, the patient should be treated empirically for neurosyphilis, because HIV infection irrespective of CD4 count may contribute to an unacceptably high number of treatment failures of primary and secondary syphilis with conventional therapy.

Other disorders to consider in patients initially presenting only with symptoms of weakness are hypokalemia, tick paralysis, porphyria, toxic neuropathies, including antibiotic toxicity, and food-source toxins from shellfish, puffer fish and tropical fish, and botulism. In tick paralysis, symptoms begin 2 to 4 days after tick attachment and feeding, and recovery begins within 24 hours of tick removal (108,109). Variants of chronic inflammatory demyelinating neuropathy initially may be indistinguishable from GBS but declare themselves in their relenting or relapsing fashion (110,111).

Treatment.   Immediate hospitalization and surveillance of respiratory tract function (vital capacity, arterial blood gases, cough reflex, swallowing) are required, because the patient's condition can deteriorate rapidly regardless of entry at the mild or moderate functional stage (112). Approximately 30% will require intubation and mechanical ventilation (113). Fluid management, parenteral feeding, prevention of deep venous thrombosis, and physical therapy are usually required. Nosocomial pneumonia, urinary tract infection, and pulmonary emboli are significant complications of the illness.

Therapy of idiopathic GBS consists of respiratory support as necessary, and early immunomodulatory treatment by plasma exchange (69,70,91,110,111,114) or by infusion of IVIG preparations (113,115–119). No advantage is gained by the combination of plasma exchange (PE) followed by IVIG (117).

Early PE showed significant benefit in 70% of patients in controlled collaborative trials, which also showed the optimal number of PEs to be related to functional stage of the patient at the time of presentation. In a study of 556 patients with GBS, those with mild disease needed only two PEs, whereas those with moderate or severe disease required four PEs (91). No further gain was seen with up to six PEs (91,114). PE remains the current recommended treatment of choice for most patients.

IVIG is equally effective as PE (115,117) and is generally reserved for those who cannot tolerate plasmapheresis because of bleeding diathesis, hypotension, hypovolemia, or sepsis (119,120). In GBS clinical trials, the number of doses of IVIG (0.4 g/kg of body weight infused per day) has ranged from three to six infusions administered over 8 to 13 days (117,119). Three treatments appears sufficient for patients with mild and moderate disease at presentation, but severe cases (ventilator dependent) need five or six doses (117,119). IVIG has potential for inducing renal failure, especially in high-risk patients with preexisting renal disease, diabetes mellitus, age older than 60 years, those receiving concurrent nephrotoxic medications, or who are hypovolemic (121). One proposed mechanism is osmotic injury to tubules from disaccharides used as stabilizers for the concentrated immunoglobulin. Recommended doses and infusion rates should not be exceeded (121).

After initial stabilization with either PE or IVIG, treatment-related fluctuations and relapses requiring re-treatment occur in approximately 10% (122). Risk factors include prior gastroenteritis, clinical findings of initial predominant distal weakness, progression to acute motor neuropathy, prolonged course, and absence of anti-G_{M1} antibodies (122). Glucocorticosteroids alone are not beneficial in GBS, based on several well-controlled trials (123,124), but do have a well-established role in CIDP as part of stabilization therapy after initial clinical response to PE or IVIG (see below).

With immunomodulatory therapy and supportive care, about 80% of patients have a complete recovery, but the fatality rate remains at 5% to 13% even when specialized care is available (62,92). Two thirds of patients recover within a year, and the other third usually have mild residual disability (125) including long-term sensory residua (126). The overall long-term relapse rate is approximately 3%.

Cumulative probabilities for progression and outcome, drawn from a large well-studied GBS cohort, indicate that 73% of patients will reach the nadir, or plateau of symptoms, by 1 week and 98% by 4 weeks (92). Improvement will start by 1 week in 36% and reach 85% by 4 weeks. Cumulative rates of clinical recovery climb from 4% at 1 week to 24% at 4 weeks, and to 57% at 6 months, then slow to 70% at 12 months and 82% at 24 months. Choice of primary therapy did not affect rates of progression or recovery (92).

Chronic Inflammatory Demyelinating Polyneuropathy

Causes and Epidemiology. CIDP occurs spontaneously at all ages (127). Unlike GBS, there are no clear associations with prior infection, except the form seen in the early stage of patients infected with HIV (74) (see below). Monoclonal gammopathy of undetermined origin may be found in up to 30% of cases (128).

Clinical Findings. Like GBS (AIDP), CIDP presents primarily as weakness, with variable sensory loss. Physical examination reveals proximal muscle weakness of both the upper and the lower extremities. Weakness of the neck flexors is particularly suspicious (129).

Two major clinical phenotypes of generalized CIDP are recognized: chronic progressive and chronic relapsing (130). Type distribution varies with age (127). Most patients older than 60 years show chronic insidious progression and have sensorimotor neuropathy (127). Approximately half of juvenile patients have a relapsing and remitting form, with initial subacute progression and motor-dominant neuropathy. However, demyelinating and axonal degeneration pathologic types are found in all age-groups (127).

Variant forms distinctive from generalized CIDP (G-CIDP) include upper limb predominant multifocal CIDP (UL-CIDP), in which initial complaints are predominantly sensory symptoms restricted to specific nerves serving one or both hands, or arms. On electrodiagnostic testing, conduction block is found in the forearms (131).

Diagnosis. As in GBS, CSF analysis is remarkable for elevated protein level and the absence of cells. The presence of cells should raise the suspicion of concurrent HIV infection (132). MRI enhancement of involved roots, especially lumbosacral roots, is similar to findings in GBS (133). Electrodiagnostic studies may show relapsing cycles of demyelination and remyelination (106,129). When electrodiagnostic studies are not consistent with demyelination, but clinical findings are suspicious for CIDP, sural nerve biopsy with specialized histopathology may be helpful in diagnosis (134).

Treatment. Steroids, PE, and IVIG have each been used therapeutically (74). Several small, well-controlled clinical trials have shown PE (135) and IVIG (136) to be clinically effective in improving the functional status of patients with either chronic relapsing or chronic progressive CIDP. In the larger trials, PE was performed 10 times over 4 weeks, whereas IVIG (0.4 g/kg of body weight) was given daily on five consecutive days. IVIG (2 g/kg total dose over 1 to 2 days) and prednisone (6 weeks, 60 mg tapering to 10 mg) have also been compared for initial treatment of CIDP, and results from a small study suggest nearly equivalent short-term effects on function (136).

IVIG is the current treatment of choice for initial treatment of most patients with CIDP (137), but unlike GBS, dosing remains unstandardized. Induction regimens have used two to five total doses with daily doses ranging from 0.4 to 2.0 g/kg of body weight. A regimen of 1 g/kg on days 1, 2, and 21 as initial treatment of previously untreated patients with CIDP showed continued benefit through 6 weeks (138). Both CIDP and GBS patients with underlying renal disease are at increased risk of renal failure following IVIG treatment (74,121).

In both chronic progressive and chronic remitting CIDP, once improvement is established by PE or IVIG, maintenance of functional gains requires concurrent corticosteroid, in contrast to GBS (137). Subsequent relapses in both clinical phenotypes respond to IVIG or PE, but multiple PEs are required for match-equivalent effects of one dose of IVIG.

HUMAN IMMUNODEFICIENCY VIRUS TYPE 1–ASSOCIATED NEUROPATHIES

Neuropathy is one of the most common disorders associated with HIV disease (71,72,139). Symptomatic neuropathies affect approximately 15% of all patients and are associated with significant morbidity (61).

HIV-associated neuropathies have six distinctive patterns: (a) distal sensory polyneuropathy, (b) isolated CN palsies, (c) acute, and (d) chronic inflammatory demyelinating polyradiculoneuropathies, (e) progressive polyradiculopathy, (f) mononeuropathy multiplex, and (g) subclinical ANS involvement (140).

Each pattern has multiple potential causes, including treatable infectious agents (140) (Table 154.2). Certain causes produce overlap syndromes by affecting brain, cord, and ganglia. In evaluating individual HIV-infected patients, it is well to remember that two or more causes may be combining to cause the particular clinical syndrome presented by the patient (141).

Early onset neuropathy, an uncommon complication of acute HIV infection, occurs during the early weeks after exposure. This initial clinical manifestation of the infection may be limited to unilateral or bilateral involvement of the facial nerve (Bell's palsy) (142) or present as classic AIDP, or GBS (143). Some cases will progress to CIDP. The rarest form of HIV-associated neuropathy is associated with the diffuse infiltrative lymphocytosis syndrome in which there is intensive CD8 infiltration into nerves in conjunction with abundant HIV infection of macrophages.

TABLE 154.2. Etiology of Neuropathic Syndromes in HIV Infection

Immune-mediated response to HIV
  Bell's palsy
  Acute inflammatory demyelinating neuropathy (Guillain-Barré syndrome)
  Chronic inflammatory demyelinating neuropathy
Vasculitis
  Bell's palsy
  Ataxic dorsal radiculopathy
  Mononeuritis multiplex: HBV-associated cryoglobulinemia
Opportunistic invasive herpesvirus infections
  Cytomegalovirus (CMV)
    Polyradiculopathy
    Multiple mononeuropathy
  Herpes simplex virus type 2
    Polyradiculopathy
  Varicella-zoster virus (VZV)
    Herpes zoster
    Polyradiculopathy
Meningitis
  Cryptococcal
  Neurosyphilitic
  Tuberculous
Malignancy
  Lymphoma
Nutritional
  Multiple vitamin deficiencies: folate, pyridoxine
  Vitamin B_{12} deficiency
Drug toxicity from concurrent anti-infectives
  Antiretroviral nucleoside analogs:
    Dideoxycytosine (ddC)
    Dideoxyinosine (ddI)
    D4T
  Niacin analogs: isoniazid (INH) without B_6
Idiopathic
  Predominantly sensory neuropathy of AIDS

AIDS, acquired immunodeficiency syndrome; HBV, hepatitis B virus; HIV, human immunodeficiency virus.

Late-onset neuropathy is a common feature of advanced immunosuppression, where it is nearly universal at the time of death (74). However, in advanced disease, the presence of neuropathy is often overshadowed by the more striking direct effects on the CNS of HIV infection (vacuolar myelopathy and AIDS dementia complex) or by opportunistic infections and malignancies invading the CNS, such as toxoplasmic encephalitis, CMV myelitis and encephalitis, progressive multifocal leukoencephalopathy, and lymphoma. CMV replication has been consistently demonstrated in peripheral nerve in both progressive polyneuropathy and mononeuritis multiplex (140). Neuropathy also results from neurotoxic side effects of certain drugs used in highly active antiretroviral therapy (HAART) or in treatment of the complications of advanced immunodeficiency.

Predominantly Sensory Neuropathy

Cause and Pathogenesis. Predominantly sensory neuropathy is one of the most common and most debilitating aspects of advanced HIV infection (73,74). Its exact cause is unclear, although immune complex vasculitis has been suggested by pathologic studies (71,74,144). Pathologic findings include macrophage infiltration in peripheral nerves and dorsal root ganglia, degeneration of long axons in distal regions, and loss of unmyelinated fibers (145). Because HIV replication is limited to a small percentage of the macrophages, pathologic destruction is presumed to be mediated by proinflammatory signals amplified by reactive glial elements within the nerve, similar to the proposed mechanism of damage causing HIV encephalopathy (140). Sensory neuropathy usually develops late in advanced HIV infection, at which point multiple factors, including vitamin deficiency and drug toxicity, may contribute to the process.

Clinical Findings. Patients usually complain of painful paresthesias, burning dysesthesias, and hypersensitivity of the distal extremities, beginning with the soles of the feet (74). On examination, only patients with advanced HIV neuropathy will have demonstrable decreased sensation and atrophy of the intrinsic muscles of the feet. DTRs of the ankles are eventually lost, but patellar reflexes may be exaggerated if there is coexisting myelopathy.

Diagnosis. Diagnosis in the early phase is based on characteristic symptoms and absence of objective neurologic findings. When ankle reflexes become affected, nerve conduction studies will demonstrate abnormalities consistent with distal axonal degeneration (74). Because these findings are not unique to HIV sensory polyneuropathy, reversible causes of neuropathy should be excluded before attributing the cause to HIV.

Treatment. Treatment of HIV-associated predominantly sensory neuropathy is generally unsatisfactory (71,73,74). For patients experiencing symptoms of sensory neuropathy before beginning antiretrovirals, HAART regimens should avoid agents with dose-dependent neurotoxicity, such as ddI, ddC, and d4T. Persons receiving these agents regardless of HIV stage should also be monitored regularly for development of clinical neuropathy (73,74,146). Symptomatic medical therapy with antidepressants and carbamazepine may be employed, but significant improvement is unusual. Placebo-controlled trials comparing palliative effects of amitriptyline versus mexiletine are underway, as are therapeutic protocols using human nerve growth factor, lamotrigine (147), and topical capsaicin (148).

Isolated Cranial Neuropathies

Causes. Cranial neuropathies, particularly involving the facial nerve, may occur at any stage of HIV infection (73). Bell's palsy usually occurs early in HIV infection and often is associated with a lymphocytic meningitis (73). In advanced HIV infection, the differential diagnosis of cranial neuropathies includes CNS opportunistic infections such as neurosyphilis, cryptococcosis, acute herpes zoster, and meningeal lymphomatosis (73), as well as disorders seen in healthy hosts, such as neuroborreliosis.

Polyradiculopathy

Causes and Pathogenesis. Polyradiculopathy, the most dramatic of syndromes caused by herpesvirus invasion in advanced HIV diseases, is caused by CMV more often than by other herpesviruses (140,149,150). Essentially unknown before AIDS, CMV invasion of the CNS and PNS in advanced HIV disease is the consequence of systemic infection and is often associated with evidence of active infection in other systems, particularly retinitis (107). The capacity of CMV to invade both endothelial and Schwann cells accounts for its varied clinical manifestations (74), which range from mononeuritis multiplex to acute inflammatory polyradiculitis and ascending myelitis.

Clinical Findings. Like GBS, polyradiculitis is characterized by a subacute onset of ascending motor weakness, areflexia, incontinence/urinary retention, paresthesias, and variable sensory dysfunction (107). Patients often complain of pain in the back and legs (74). Neurologic findings are usually more asymmetric than in GBS.

Diagnosis. The CSF mirrors the intense neutrophilic inflammation of the lumbar nerve roots and dorsal root ganglia, and later the spinal cord, and yields characteristic CSF findings mimicking bacterial meningitis: polymorphonuclear predominance (up to 90%), hypoglycorrhachia, and elevated protein level (74,107). CSF WBC counts can vary from less than 50 to more than 3,000 cells.

Magnetic resonance postcontrast enhancement of lumbosacral plexus and cauda equina has been noted in multiple cases of polyradiculopathy due to CMV and other herpesviruses, as well as a wide range of other causes of polyneuritis, and has shown improvement after specific therapy (105,151).

CMV inclusions have been seen in cytology of CSF and in biopsy specimens (74). Specific herpesviruses have been successfully identified in CSF by PCR, but except for herpes simplex virus (HSV), viral cultures are generally negative (152).

Treatment. If diagnosed and treated early, some cases of CMV polyradiculopathy have responded partially to early treatment with ganciclovir (GCV) at dosages of 5 mg/kg intravenously twice daily for 2 weeks, followed by a maintenance dose of 5 mg/kg every day (107), or oral valganciclovir (valGCV). If GCV resistance is suspected because of prior use of GCV or persistent CSF abnormalities on GCV, foscarnet, or cidofovir are options (150,151).

Pharmacokinetic studies have demonstrated that CSF concentrations, relative to plasma, vary between 24% to 70% for GCV and 13% to 68% for foscarnet (153). Common dose-dependent side effects of GCV and valGCV are leukopenia and thrombocytopenia and require frequent monitoring. Leukopenia can be treated with granulocyte colony-stimulating factor (filgrastim) at doses appropriate to maintain the absolute granulocyte count at 1,000 cells/mm³ or greater. Using standard dosing for CMV retinitis, foscarnet's primary toxicity is renal failure.

Differential Diagnosis. Other causes of subacute polyradiculopathy in HIV infection include *Treponema pallidum* and two other herpesviruses, HSV-2, and *Varicella-zoster* virus (VZV) (74). HSV and VZV cause an acute inflammatory radiculomyelitis in patients with AIDS that may be confused with CMV polyradiculopathy, whereas neurosyphilis has a lymphocytic profile. These agents are discussed in more detail elsewhere in this chapter (see the sections "Acute Inflammatory Demyelinating Polyneuropathy or the Guillain-Barré Syndrome," "Primary and Secondary Myelitis," and "Polymorphic Infections").

Mononeuropathy Multiplex

Causes. Mononeuritis multiplex is characterized by patchy and asymmetric motor and sensory nerve dysfunction, possibly the result of ischemic injury from viral infection of the endothelium of the *vasa nervorum* (74). Mononeuritis multiplex may be seen early in HIV infection even before immunosuppression has occurred. Some cases are associated with cryoglobulinemia in persons dually infected with hepatitis B, in which the course is often benign and generally does not require specific therapy (73,154). In patients with advanced HIV infection and CD4 counts less than 50 cells/mm³, CMV is the most likely cause, and CMV replication in peripheral nerve is demonstrable (140).

Clinical Findings. Mononeuropathy multiplex is defined as a simultaneous or sequential neuropathy of noncontiguous nerve trunks evolving over days to years (1–3).

Diagnosis. Definitive diagnosis requires biopsy, although the characteristic histologic lesions may be missed because of their patchy distribution (73,74). CSF abnormalities, if present, probably reflect a coexisting pathologic process (73). Nerve conduction studies show asymmetric axonal loss rather than demyelination, although considerable overlap does occur (74,107,149,155).

Treatment. Treatment depends on identifying a specific cause. In 47 patients with advanced HIV disease in which mononeuritis multiplex was suspected of being caused by CMV, intravenous GCV was used successfully, but the prognosis, in general, is poor (74) without successful immune reconstitution on HAART.

Autonomic Neuropathy

HIV-associated autonomic neuropathy may occur at any stage of HIV infection. Asymptomatic disease is detected as pupillary autonomic neuropathy (PANP) by measuring the maximal pupillary area. Symptomatic disease is primarily orthostatic hypotension due to cardiovascular autonomic neuropathy (CANP) (156), a disorder seen in advanced HIV with an estimated prevalence of 15%.

POSTINFECTIOUS PERIPHERAL NEUROPATHY

The term *postinfectious* indicates that neurologic findings usually follow the appearance of the characteristic nonneurologic clinical features of the disease and may occur in only a small proportion of infected patients. Further, although the pathogenesis of these lesions usually involves inflammation in the nervous system, the causative agent is not always identifiable in the lesions. GBS is the principal "postinfectious" peripheral neuropathy syndrome recognized and was discussed earlier in this chapter (see the section "Acute Inflammatory Demyelinating Polyneuropathy or the Guillain-Barré Syndrome").

PARAMENINGEAL INFECTIONS: CRANIAL NERVE SYNDROMES

Bacterial and fungal infections of the skull produce characteristic groupings of CN involvement, usually unilateral because of their origin in air sinuses or middle ear. The cause of nerve dysfunction is a combination of inflammatory damage to vasa vasorum and nerve, and invasion by organisms. Bacterial and fungal infections are the most common causes and often occur in persons with diabetes or immunosuppression as part of the syndrome of *rhinocerebral infections*. See Table 154.3.

Causes and Pathogenesis. Bacterial and fungal infections of the *ethmoid–sphenoid* complex of air sinuses that extend into the adjacent *cavernous venous sinuses* cause two characteristic unilateral CN syndromes depending on the extent of invasion: the *Tolosa-Hunt* and the *Foix-Jefferson* syndrome

Bacterial infections of the *middle ear* or postoperative infections of the temporal (petrous) bone also have two patterns of CN involvement. Gradenigo's syndrome (CNs V and VI) results when the *apex of the temporal bone* is the site of inflammation. A peripheral seventh nerve palsy results when inflammation in the *attic of the middle ear* invades the seventh nerve as it passes through the thin bony roof of the middle ear—the tegmen tympani.

Infections involving the *base of the skull* produce two unique patterns of CN palsies. When *malignant otitis externa* or *mastoiditis* extend subperiosteally (Bezold's abscess) and into the soft tissues beneath the temporal bone, extension to the jugular foramen affects CNs IX, X, and XI (Vernet's syndrome). If the location of the infection is in the retropharyngeal tissues (*retropharyngeal abscess* or *retroparotid lymphadenitis*), CNs XII and the cervical sympathetic nerve outflow as well as CNs IX, X, and XI are affected (Villaret's syndrome). Table 154.4 presents the more common unilateral CN syndromes that may be caused by localized infections.

Diagnosis and Treatment. Diagnosis and treatment are discussed in Chapters 44 and 45.

SPINAL CORD INFECTIONS

Primary and Secondary Myelitis

Infections involving the spinal cord may be subdivided into those that directly attack cord structures (primary myelitis) and those that begin as adjacent infections but progress to alter cord function and may ultimately produce irreversible damage (secondary myelitis) (1,2).

ANATOMY

The anatomic relationship between the spinal cord and its coverings explains the classification of spinal cord infections (see Fig. 154.1). The spinal cord lies in the vertebral canal and is protected by three layers of membranous meninges. The outermost layer is the *dura mater*. The *epidural* or extradural space is the potential space between the fibrous dura and the bony vertebral column. The *subdural* space is also a potential space and is located between the dura and the thin *arachnoid* membrane. The arachnoid is separated from the *pia mater*, the innermost layer, by the *subarachnoid* space, which contains the CSF. The pia closely surrounds the spinal cord and extends into Virchow's spaces together with the vessels nourishing the cord. The pia mater also covers the ventral and dorsal roots branching from the cord until they are covered by the perineurium and epineurium of the peripheral nerves.

PATHOLOGY

Primary myelitis refers to either infectious or noninfectious inflammation of the spinal cord. Inflammation involving only the gray matter is referred to as *poliomyelitis* and as *leukomyelitis* if it is confined to the white matter (2a). *Transverse myelitis* is defined as inflammation of an entire cross section of the spinal cord,

TABLE 154.3. Cranial Nerve Syndromes

	Functions	Distribution	Neuronal location	Peripheral nerves or divisions	Signs of peripheral nerve dysfunction	Common infectious causes of abnormalities
III Oculomotor	Somatic motor	Superior, inferior, and medial rectus muscles Inferior oblique muscle Levator of lid	Brainstem	Oculomotor	Abducted eye at rest Inability to rotate eye up, down, or medially Ptosis	Herpes zoster (gasserian) Meningitis Mononeuritis Cavernous sinus syndrome
	Visceral motor	Sphincter pupillae Ciliary body			Dilated nonreactive pupil Paralysis of accommodation	
IV Trochlear	Motor	Superior oblique muscle	Brainstem	Trochlear	Extortion of eye Weak downward gaze	Herpes zoster (gasserian) Meningitis Cavernous sinus syndrome
V Trigeminal	Sensory	Skin: face, scalp (anterior two thirds) Mucosa: nose, mouth, cornea, conjunctiva	Gasserian ganglion	Ophthalmic nerve Maxillary nerve Mandibular nerve	Pain	Herpes zoster Petrositis Cavernous sinus syndrome
	Motor	Masseter muscles Pterygoid muscles	Midpons	Mandibular nerve	Trismus	Central: tetanus Local: adjacent Inflammation
VI Abducens	Motor	External rectus muscles	Brainstem	Abducens	Paralysis of abduction Partially abducted eye at rest	Herpes zoster (gasserian) Meningitis Mononeuritis Cavernous sinus syndrome Petrositis
VII Facial	Sensory	Tongue (anterior two thirds): taste Ear (anterior wall, external auditory canal): all sensations	Geniculate ganglion	Nervus intermedius and branches: Lingual nerve Mandibular nerve	Loss of taste on hemitongue	Herpes zoster (Ramsey-Hunt Syndrome)
	Secretomotor	Lacrimal gland Sublingual glands Submaxillary glands	Brainstem	Chorda tympani nerve	Reduced lacrimation Reduced salivary mucus	Herpes zoster (Ramsey-Hunt syndrome)
	Motor	Facial muscles Stylomastoid muscle Posterior belly, digastric muscle Stapedius muscle	Brainstem (adjacent to VI nerve nuclei)	Facial nerve and branches	Facial palsy or paralysis Eyelids will not close, eye rolls up Creaseless brows Recovery: Weeks to months Late complications: Hemifacial spasm Crocodile tears	Otitis media, Mastoiditis Bell's palsy pattern (no vesicles) Mononeuritis or bilateral Brucellosis Cat-scratch disease HIV Lyme borreliosis Relapsing fever
VIII Cochleovestibular	Sensory	Spiral organ of Corti Semicircular canal	Spiral ganglion (in cochlea)	Cochlear nerve	Deafness Vertigo	Otitis media Meningitis Mastoiditis
		Saccule Utricle	Scarpa's vestibular ganglion (internal auditory meatus)	Vestibular nerve	Nystagmus Absent response to caloric stimulation	Mastoiditis Meningitis
IX Glossopharyngeal	Sensory	Tonsils, soft palate, posterior pharynx	Petrosal ganglion Superior ganglion	Glossopharyngeal nerve	Anesthetic posterior pharynx	Herpes zoster (rare)
	Secretory	Pharyngeal mucosa	Medulla		Palatal paralysis (deviation) Hoarseness	Herpes zoster (rare) Meningitis
	Motor	Pharyngeal striated muscle	Medulla		Dysphagia Weakness upper trapezoid and sternomastoid	Skull-base infections
X Vagus	Sensory	Ear (posterior wall of canal, concha, and pinna)	Jugular ganglion	Posterior auricula	Decreased sensation in auditory canal and back of pinna	Herpes zoster (infrequent)
		Pharynx, larynx, trachea, esophagus	Nodose ganglion	Pharyngeal branch of vagus nerve	Loss of gag reflex (affected side)	
	Somatic motor	Thoracic and abdominal viscera Larynx, pharynx and palate (striated muscle)	Medulla	Thoracoabdominal branch of vagus nerve Pharyngeal branch of vagus nerve	Palatal paralysis: complete Loss of curtain movement of lateral pharyngeal walls Nasal regurgitation Voice nasal, hoarse Abducted vocal cord	Herpes zoster (infrequent) Skull-base infections: petrositis, Bezold's abscess
	Visceral motor	Heart, other thoracic organs Abdominal viscera	Medulla	Thoracoabdominal branch of vagus nerve		
XI Accessory	Motor	Sternocleidomastoid muscle Trapezius muscle	High cervical cord (C1–5)	Accessory nerve	Partial paralysis: trapezius and sternocleidomastoid muscles Wing scapula	Skull-base infections: petrositis, Bezold's abscess
XII Hypoglossal	Motor	Tongue muscles: Genioglossus Styloglossus Hypoglossus	Medulla	Hypoglossal nerve	Hemiparalysis of tongue (deviation to affected side) Progression to wrinkling, atrophy, fibrillary twitches	Basilar meningitis Skull-base infections: petrositis, Bezold's abscess

TABLE 154.4.   Unilateral Cranial Nerve Syndromes Caused by Cranial and Extracranial Focal Infections

Site of lesion	Eponym	Cranial nerve involved	Clinical signs and symptoms	Infectious cause

Cavernous sinus
Lateral wall
	Tolosa-Hunt	III, IV, VI
		Ophthaimic V
			Orbital pain
			Sensory loss over upper face
			Ophthalmoparesis
			Then ophthalmoplegia and
			  exophthalmos develop
				Sinusitis (ethmoid-sphenoid
				  complex)
				Rhinocerebral mycosis

Cavernous sinus invasion	Foix-Jefferson	III, IV, VI Ophthalmic V Maxillary V ± Mandibular V	Same complex plus More extensive area of sensory loss	Sinusitis (ethmoid sphenoid) Rhinocerebral mycosis
Petrous bone Apex	Gradinego	V, VI	Facial neuralgia Double vision Abducens palsy	Petrositis complicating otitis
Middle ear	—	VII	Facial paresis, palsy Ear pain ± drainage Deafness	Otitis media

Jugular foramen
Base of skull
	Vernet	IX, X, XI	Dysphagia
			Paralysis curtain motion of lateral
			  pharyngeal wall
			Oropharyngeal sensory loss:
			  Posterior tongue
			  Soft palate
			  Pharynx
			  Larynx
			Hoarseness
			Weak sternocleidomastoid and
			  trapezius
				Bezold's subperiosteal abscess
				Complication of
				Otitis externa and/or
				  mastoiditis

Posterior retroparotid space (retropharyngeal syndrome)
Base of skull
	Villaret	IX, X, XI, XII
		and
		Cervical sympathetic
		nerves
			Jugular foramen syndrome
			  plus
			Loss of normal tongue mobility
			  and
			Horner's syndrome
			  Ipsilateral ptosis, miosis and
			  enophthalmos
				Retroparotid lymphadenitis
				or
				Retropharyngeal abscess

although it is not necessarily limited to one spinal segment (2). Inflammatory diseases of the spinal cord that also involve adjacent nerve roots and meninges are referred to as *radiculomyelitis* and *meningomyelitis*, respectively (1,2,224). The spinal cord pathology in primary myelitis depends on the cause and ranges from isolated injury to motor neurons, with or without cytolysis, to predominating demyelination associated with focal inflammatory infiltrates, and to more severe diffuse destruction, as shown in Figure 154.2.

CLASSIFICATION

Three relatively discreet clinical patterns of *primary myelitis* are based on the type and location of cord lesions: the syndromes of (a) *anterior poliomyelitis*, (b) *leukomyelitis*, and (c) *transverse myelitis* (1). Whereas anterior poliomyelitis is almost invariably due to acute infection with poliovirus, the cause of the other syndromes varies and in many cases may remain unknown.

Secondary myelitis arises from focal infections located either inside or outside the subarachnoid space. Two infections located within the subarachnoid space commonly have some degree of inflammatory involvement of adjacent cord: infection of the *dorsal root ganglion* in *herpes-zoster* syndrome, caused by *VZV*, and infection of *posterior roots* in the *tabes dorsalis* syndrome, caused by *T. pallidum*. Although neurologists call these disorders more properly infections of the PNS, inflammatory responses to these infections do directly affect the cord. *Spinal intramedullary ab-*

scesses are focal inflammatory responses to hematogenous or posttraumatic infection of the cord, or infection in a congenital dermal sinus.

Infections arising outside the subarachnoid space that secondarily affect the cord include (a) *spinal subdural empyema*, (b) *spinal epidural abscess or granulations*, and (c) *vertebral osteomyelitis*. Extraarachnoid infections affect cord function by a combination of mass effect and by interference with venous and arterial circulation, causing edema and tissue hypoxia. These focal infections are usually caused by bacteria and less commonly by *Mycobacterium tuberculosis*, but *opportunistic fungi* are important causes in immunocompromised patients. If therapy is delayed or unsuccessful, the ultimate sequela is permanent cord injury. *Spinal subdural empyemas* mainly affect cord function by secondary vasospasm and thrombosis of the cord's venous and arterial circulation, including *anterior spinal artery thrombosis*, but may extend into the cord to create an *intramedullary abscess*. Epidural *abscess or granulations* compress cord and interfere with venous and arterial circulation. Vertebral osteomyelitis can be complicated by pathologic vertebral fracture that traumatizes the cord by *dislocation of bony fragments* into the spinal canal.

CLINICAL PATTERNS

The several patterns of clinical findings associated with primary and secondary cord injury caused by infections are described in Tables 154.5 and 154.6. Some authors group leukomyelitis and transverse myelitis together (1,2,157), whereas other believe it useful to make the distinction because of the difference in pace and type of onset, and possible difference in pathogenesis and prognosis (1). Not included in this discussion is multiple sclerosis (158), which may ultimately prove to be infectious in etiology (159). Newer imaging techniques, especially contrast-enhanced MRI, allow precise determination of extent of involvement (160,161).

Specific Diseases

PRIMARY MYELITIS

The enteroviruses are well-known causes of infectious myelitis, of which poliovirus is the most common worldwide (162,163). In developed nations, polio is now unusual, but sporadic cases of myelitis caused by other enteroviruses still occur (e.g., Coxsackie A and B, Echovirus, and other enteroviruses) (163,164). Myelitis caused by the nonpolio enteroviruses is generally less severe than that caused by poliovirus and presents with weakness rather than paralysis. At present, 66 types of enteroviruses are recognized, including the three poliovirus serotypes. Although nonpolio enteroviruses are the most common cause of aseptic meningitis in children, most cases have no neurologic sequelae (165).

Recent application of PCR technology to search for viral sequences in CSF of patients with myelitis has demonstrated that the flavivirus West Nile virus (WNV) and the herpesviruses CMV, EBV, HSV, and VZV are causative agents of myelitis in immunocompetent and in severely immunosuppressed persons. Self-limited outbreaks in healthy populations of subacute myeloopticoneuropathy (SMON), a disorder first seen in Japan and most recently in Cuba, have been associated with the isolation from CSF of the weakly cytopathic Inoue-Melnick virus (166).

Primary myelitis may be associated with several classes of infectious agents besides viruses. Of particular note are *Chlamydia* (psittacosis), *Mycoplasma, spirochetes* (Lyme neuroborreliosis, relapsing fever, neurosyphilis), and *parasites* embolizing to cord (ova of schistosomes, toxoplasma and *Taenia* species) (157,158,167). Some of these agents affect peripheral nerves and CNs in addition to cord and therefore are discussed in the section "Polymorphic Infections."

Etiologic diagnosis of primary myelitis is possible for several agents. Enteroviruses can be recovered in the CSF, as well as from blood, pharynx, and stool, and acute infection can be established by comparison of specific antibody titers in acute and convalescent sera. The presence of virus in the CSF is supportive of direct viral invasion. The ability to detect more difficult to grow organisms in CSF by PCR and to measure locally produced antibodies by enzyme-linked immunosorbent assay (ELISA) and

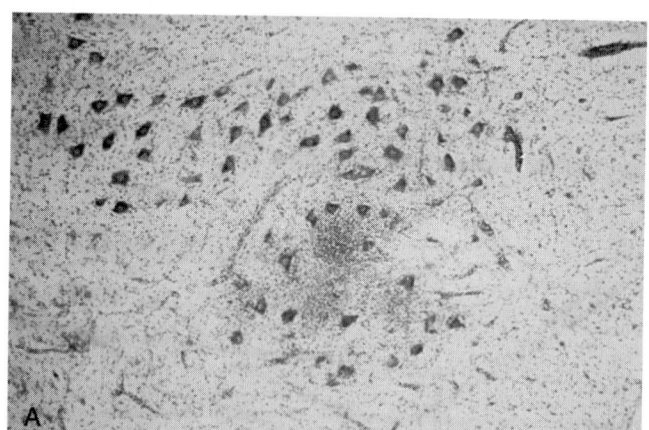
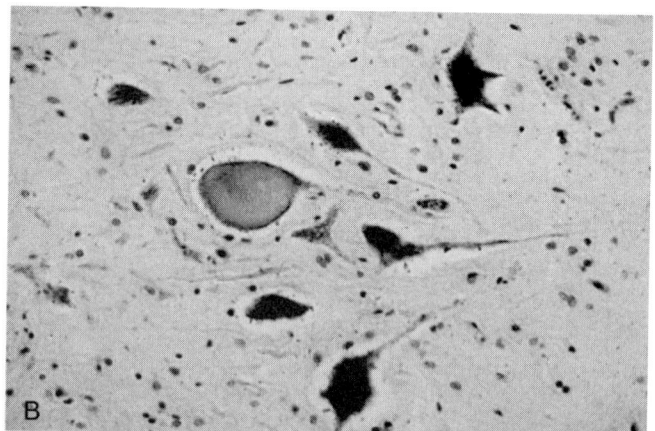
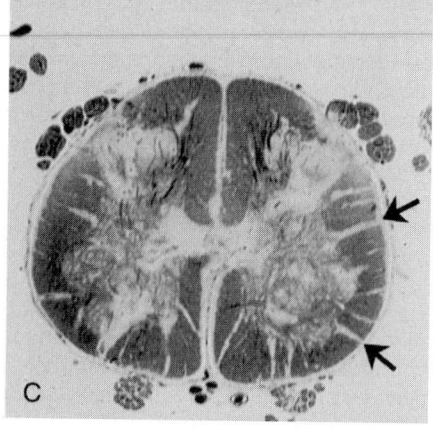
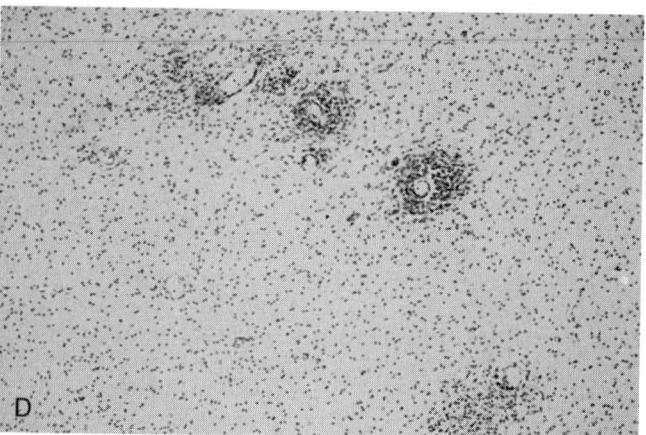

Figure 154.2. Pathology of infectious and postinfectious myelitis. Polio: Direct irreversible injury of cells infected by poliovirus and reversible demyelination from perivascular lymphocytic infiltration. **A:** Anterior horn: neuronophagia and lymphocytic perivascular cuffing in postcapillary venules (×40). **B:** Motor neurones: central chromatolysis of acutely infected cells (×100). Acute disseminated encephalomyelitis: Postinfectious (measles): Demyelination follows pattern of perivascular invasion by lymphocytes and macrophages. **C:** Myelin stain of cord: Pale linear streaks follow radiating postcapillary venules in white matter (×10). **D:** Dense clusters of perivenular lymphocytes and macrophages (×40).

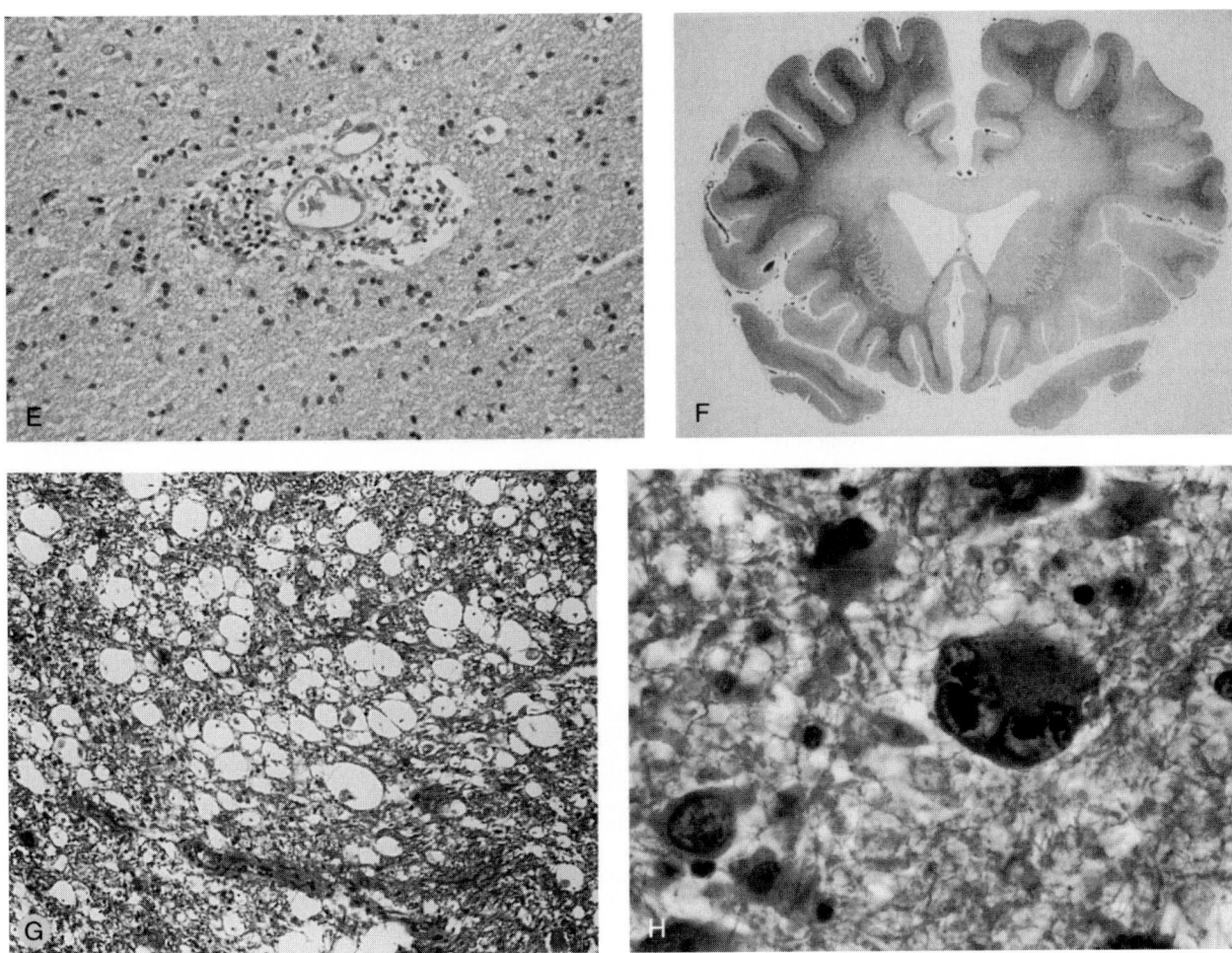

Figure 154.2. (*continued*) **E:** Detail of perivascular infiltrate in postcapillary venule (×100). Human immunodeficiency virus–associated encephalomyelopathy: Demyelination is symmetric and in spinal cord is associated with vacuolar degeneration of myelin with paucity of inflammation. **F:** Myelin stain of whole brain: extensive loss of normal staining pattern (×1). **G:** Myelin stain of cord: vacuolization of white matter (×40). Cytomegalovirus myelitis and radiculitis: Viral replication within several cell types produces direct cytopathic effects and stimulates acute inflammation. **H:** Single and multinucleated cells with intranuclear inclusions (×100). (**A–E:** Courtesy E. P. Richardson, Department of Neuropathology, Harvard Medical School and Massachusetts General Hospital; **F–H:** Courtesy Drs. F. Aydin and S. Mitruka, Department of Pathology, Tulane University School of Medicine.)

immunoblot assays has significantly improved the ability to assign specific causes to cases of primary myelitis. Routine use of PCR screening panels for herpesviruses are especially useful in recognizing their presence (168). In some cases of primary myelitis, it may be difficult to distinguish between immune-mediated postinfectious cord injury and focal destruction by the organism.

Enteroviral Myelitis
Acute Poliomyelitis.

CAUSE. Poliomyelitis is a *clinicopathologic syndrome* caused primarily by enteroviruses (see Table 154.5), although acute flaccid paralysis is also a feature in some patients with infections of the central nervous system by the flavivirus WNV. Within a few days of the onset of an acute febrile illness, it presents with varying degrees of flaccid paralysis, usually asymmetric, of various striated muscles. The poliomyelitis syndrome can be caused by the three types of polioviruses (type 1, Brunhilde; type 2, Lansing; and type 3, Leon), by Coxsackie A and B viruses, Echoviruses, and by the enterovirus types 70 and 71 (the so-called "new" enteroviruses). During the years of epidemic polio in the

United States before polio vaccine, about 85% of the persistent paralytic cases and most of the epidemics over the years were caused by poliomyelitis type 1 (164). As a result of the successful poliovirus eradication programs, in recent years wild-type poliovirus isolates worldwide have been nearly evenly divided between type 1 and type 2 (44%). Among 2,584 cases of poliomyelitis worldwide during 1999 and 2000, 55% were attributed to type 1, 44% to type 3, and only 1.2% to either type 2 (11 cases) or mixed type 1 and 3 (21 cases) (169).

PATHOGENESIS. See Chapter 248.

IMMUNITY. See Chapter 248.

EPIDEMIOLOGY. See Chapter 248.

PREVENTION. See Chapter 248.

DEMOGRAPHIC PATTERNS. There are three demographic patterns of poliomyelitis:

1. The *endemic pattern* is seen in areas with limited sanitation and without vaccine programs. This is the true *infantile paralysis* syndrome that is seen sporadically. In these countries, virtually all children older than 4 years are naturally immune. Because passive immunity is transferred from mother

TABLE 154.5.   Primary Myelitis Syndromes

A. Acute anterior poliomyelitis

Etiology: Enteroviruses
   Usual cause: Polioviruses 1, 2, 3. Rarely a complication of the live vaccine itself (1 case per 2.6 million doses administered) or revertent mutants
   Milder disease: Coxsackie A, B; Echovirus; enterovirus types 70 and 71; and West Nile fever virus may cause flaccid paralysis.
   Poliomyelitis identical to disease caused by wild-type poliovirus occurs in two vaccine-related settings: (a) rarely following administration of oral
      poliovirus vaccine (OPV) to normals or inadvertently to immunodeficient persons [vaccine-associated paralysis (VAPP)]; (b) from rare outbreaks due to
      revertent, pathogenic strains of circulating vaccine-derived poliovirus (cVDPV) among nonimmune, unimmunized susceptibles. As wild-type
      poliovirus is eradicated worldwide, more cases of poliomyelitis will be OPV vaccine–associated or from outbreaks of cVDPV in susceptible
      populations due to incomplete vaccine coverage, or will be due to non–polio enteroviruses.
Pathogenesis: Cord changes include combined irreversible cytolytic destruction of lower motor neurons and reversible inflammatory damage to anterior
   and intermediate horns associated with cytokine release from lymphocytes located in perivenular cuffs. Lesions are not always confined to cord but
   may occur in hypothalamus, thalamus, motor nuclei of brainstem and reticular formation, vestibular nuclei and roof nuclei of cerebellum.
Clinical pattern: Biphasic disease

	Symptoms	Neurologic findings	Laboratory

Viremia phase: "minor illness" (lasts 3–4 days)	"Flu"-like syndrome
	   Listlessness
	   Fever (38–40°C)
	   Sore throat
	   Anorexia, nausea, vomiting
	   Generalized headache
	   Muscle stiffness, aching
		Normal exam	Virus:
			   Isolatable from
			      Blood
			      Throat washings
			      Stool (positive for weeks)

CNS Phase: "major illness" (evolves over 5–7 days)			

A. Nonparalytic stage: Aseptic meningitis	Recrudescence of headache and
	   fever after asymptomatic
	   period (3–5 days) following
	   "minor illness";
	   Otherwise headache intensifies
	Pain in back and neck
	Muscles tender, painful
		Encephalopathic signs:
		   Irritable
		   Restless
		   Emotionally labile
		Meningeal signs
		   Positive Kernig's and Brudzinski's
		      signs
		Muscle spasm
		   (e.g., tight hamstring)
			CSF:
			   Cells:
			      Pleocytosis: PMNs initially,
			         then lymphocytes
			   Glucose:
			      Normal
			   Protein:
			      Elevated
			   PCR: positive for virus
			Serology:
			   ELISA positive for IgM, IgG
			   Neutralizing and CF antibody
			      present: four-fold rise in titer in
			      paired sera (10 days apart)
			Virus
			   Isolatable from blood, throat
			      washings, stool, and CSF (except
			      polioviruses infrequently isolated
			      from CSF)

B. Paralytic stage: Meningomyeloencephalitis	Weakness:
	   Rapid, progressive onset of
	      weakness that continues until
	      afebrile for 48 hr
	Extent of weakness:
	   Dependent on age of patient:
	      Infants: trunk and extremities
	      Children <5: often one leg
	         only
	      Older children: arm and
	         both legs
	      Adolescents and adults:
	         Asymmetric weakness of
	            all four extremities
		"Spinal paralysis" pattern:
		   Muscles:
		      Coarse fasciculations initially
		         (transient-days)
		      Atrophy detectable within 3 wk
		         (permanent)
		   Reflex losses:
		      Abdominal musculature:
		         Cremasteric and abdominal
		            reflexes
		      Limbs: DTRs
		   Subjective paresthesias
		      Objective exam normal
		"Bulbar paralysis" pattern
		   Hiccough
		   Dysphagia, dysphonia, aspiration
		   Respiratory insufficiency;
		      irregular respiration
		   Dysregulation of blood pressure
		      (hyper-, hypotension)
			CSF:
			   Cells:
			      Lymphocytosis
			   Glucose:
			      Normal
			   Protein:
			      Elevated
			      Normalizes over 4–5 wk
			   PCR: positive for virus
			Virus
			   Isolatable from blood, throat
			      washings, stool, and CSF (except
			      polioviruses infrequently isolated
			      from CSF)
			   Stool remains culture-positive for
			      weeks

(continued)

TABLE 154.5. *(continued)*

B. Leukomyelitis

Etiology: *Acute invasive infections:* CMV, EBV, HSV in normals and in advanced immunosuppression (from HIV or immunosuppressive medications); monkey B virus; *Mycoplasma pneumoniae; Chlamydia psittaci;* "postinfectious"; "postvaccinial"
  Subacute with variable chronic meningitis: HIV-associated vacuolar myelopathy; HTLV-1; Inoue-Melnick virus associated subacute myeloopticoneuropathy (SMON), brucellosis; Lyme neuroborreliosis; relapsing fever; neurosyphilis
Associations: *Postinfectious:* influenza, mumps, rubella, rubeola, varicella, variola, WEE, cat-scratch disease (Bartonella henslae)
  Postvaccinial: Japanese B encephalitis vaccine, vaccinia virus, Pasteur rabbit cord rabies vaccine
Pathogenesis: Lesions in cord involve necrosis and demyelination of white matter tracts. Only demyelination is potentially reversible.
  In reactivation of latent infection, herpesviruses ascend axons of neurons, replicate in myelin, necrotize white matter; acute cellular infiltration.
  In diffuse lymphoctic infiltration syndrome (DILS), HIV is found abundantly in phagocytic mononuclear cells associated with myelin destruction.
  In HIV-associated vacuolar myelopathy, degraded myelin is phagocytosed by macrophages without inflammation. In HTLV-I, CD4 cells infiltrate cord.
  Postinfectious and postvaccine pathology is characterized by perivenular demyelination with lymphocytic cuffing.

Symptoms	Neurologic findings	Diagnosis

Prodromal event or risk factors: (Potential associations include host factors)
 Travel or residence in endemic area
 Tick bite or louse bite
 Macaque monkey exposure: (bite, or wound contamination with tissues, conjunctival splash)
 Unpasteurized dairy products
 STD risk
 Exanthem
   For example, erythema chronica migrans within 2 mo
 Advanced immunosuppression (HIV, transplant)
 Vaccine (neurotropic) administration recently (e.g., Japanese B encephalitis vaccine; tenth through twentieth day of serial Pasteur vaccinations)
 Onset over days:
   Weakness in legs, feet
   Numbness in legs, feet (bilateral): may extend to trunk
   Difficulty voiding
 Monophasic course if postinfectious or postvaccine
   Single attack
   Several weeks duration
   Variable recovery
   No relapse
 Rapidly progressive course if herpesvirus
   Encephalomyelitis: can begin with radiculitis; ascends cord, tracts to brain
 Slowly progressive course
   HTLV-1: progressive spastic paraparesis
   HIV vacuolar myelopathy: progression from gait disorder to spastic paraparesis
	Ascending paralysis
	   until reaches spinal sensory and motor level:
	     All function below abolished
	     Progressive sensory and motor weakness
	       Beginning in sacral level
	       Progressing to lumbar then thoracic level
	     Bladder paralysis
	     Spinal shock (flaccid areflexia) may occur initially
	 Progression to encephalopathy or encephalitis, uncommon in normal hosts
	   Normals
	     Monkey B virus
	     Neurobruceliosis
	     Neuroborreliosis
	     Neurosyphilis
	   Immunocompromised
	     Herpesviruses
	 Variants
	   Spastic paraparesis predominantly
	     HTLV-I
	     HIV-associated vacuolar myelopathy
		CT
		   No block or external mass
		 MRI
		   T1 images: enhancement with gadolinium of involved spinal roots and meninges
		   T2 images: bright signals in involved areas of cord
		   Variable swelling of cord
		 CSF:
		   Acute invasive form
		     Cells:
		       Lymphocytes and PMNs
		       B cells: IgM dominantly
		     Glucose:
		       Low or normal
		     Protein:
		       Normal or elevated
		       Oligoclonal banding (on electrophoresis)
		       Immunoglobulins: IgM then IgG
		     Microbial identification
		       Cultures (routine and viral): Negative
		       PCR: positive (viruses, *Borrelia* species)
		       CSF serology: some positive (*Borrelia* species, *Mycoplasma* species)
		   Subacute form
		     Cells:
		       Lymphocytosis
		       B cells: IgG
		     Glucose: Normal
		     Protein:
		       Normal or slightly elevated
		       Oligoclonal banding on electrophoresis
		       Immunoglobulins: IgG
		       CSF serology: some positive (*Borrelia* species)
		     Microbial identification
		       Cultures (routine and viral): negative
		       PCR: positive (viruses, *Borrelia* species)
		       CSF serology: some positive (HTLV-I)
		 Blood serology:
		   Paired sera useful in retrospective diagnosis of new infections, but not reliable in diagnosing reactivation infections

C. Transverse myelitis

Etiology: Agents causing leukomyelitis (herpesviruses; *Mycoplasma; Chlamydia psittaci,* spirochetes) and "postinfectious" and "postvaccine" causes
  Infarction complicating meningococcal meningitis, or delayed treatment of epidural abscess
  Intramedullary spinal cord abscess (frequently *Staphylococcus aureus,* or bacteria of respiratory origin; tuberculoma; brucella granuloma)
  Protozoan reactivation in AIDS (*Toxoplasma gondii*); hematogenous larval encystment (neuroschistosomiasis)
Pathology: Inflammatory injury to white and gray matter in spinal cord at segmental level; Infarct following arteriospasm or thrombosis of anterior spinal artery often spares posterior columns

(continued)

TABLE 154.5. *(continued)*

Symptoms	Neurologic findings	Diagnosis
Prodromal event: (Potential associations: related to primary illness) Lyme borreliosis: prior erythema chronicum migrans Leptospirosis: hepatitis Meningococcal meningitis: early phase Relapsing fever: pattern of periodic fevers Schistosomiasis: acute illness weeks to months after infected Zoster: single or multidermatomal skin eruption AIDS: prior or concomitant cerebral toxoplasmosis Recent immunization or vaccination Vertebral osteomyelitis Rapid onset of sensorimotor level: Loss of voluntary movement Loss of sensation No recovery	Flaccid motor paralysis of extremities related to level: C4–5: complete C5–6: arms, abduct, flex C6–7: arms intact, except hands Below C7, above conus: legs only Conus medullaris syndrome Weak muscles lower legs Sphincteric paralysis only (bladder, bowel) Lax anal sphincter Sacral dermatome sensory loss Absent sphincteric sensory reflexes Sensory level: parallels motor level "Spinal shock": Initial loss (related to level) of reflexes Visceral, genital, cutaneous and deep tendon reflexes Vasomotor tone Return of reflex activity in 1–6 wk ["minimal reflex activity"] Later progression to hyperreflexia below level: Babinski flexion reflexes Tendon reflexes Reflex urination, defecation, sweating Mass reflex responses	CSF Cells: Lymphocytosis Glucose: Normal Protein: Normal or slightly elevated CSF serology: some positive (*Borrelia* species) Microbial identification Cultures (routine and viral): Negative PCR: positive (herpesviruses, *Borrelia* species, *Mycoplasma*) CSF: Dependent on infectious cause PCR: positive if herpesvirus, Mycoplasma CT No block or external mass MRI: sagittal views most useful Intraspinal abscess, or schistosomiasis: T2 images; intramedullary collection with high signals T1 images; well-defined low-density lesions and peripheral contrast enhancement with adjacent medullary edema Variable swelling of cord Holocord abscesses (extend entire lenght of cord) are rare Transverse myelitis: T2 images; uniform area of high signal at area of involvement Variable swelling of cord Serology: Helpful in certain cases (e.g., leptospirosis, neurosyphilis, schistosomiasis, toxoplasmosis) Blood cultures Positive for some conditions associated with bacterial causes

to offspring, many infants experience poliovirus infection while still partially protected by maternal antibodies. Consequently, the ratio of inapparent to apparent infection is highest in infants and young children, and paralytic disease is relatively rare despite common exposure to wild-type virus.

2. The *epidemic pattern* was seen during the first half of the twentieth century in many areas of temperate zones with good standards of community and household hygiene and before vaccine became available. A generally accepted explanation is that improved sanitation and hygiene reduced opportunities for infection among the very young. Thus, increasing numbers of persons encountered poliovirus for the first time in *later childhood or adult* life when infection is more likely to take the paralytic form. This pattern has also been seen in developing countries with rising levels of sanitation before vaccine programs reach high levels of immunity.

3. The *postvaccination* pattern in which isolated cases and outbreaks of polio occur in a vaccinated population. These occur primarily in individuals exposed to oral poliovirus vaccine (OPV) with unique host defense defects that are permissive for vaccine-associated paralytic polio (VAPP). The other cases occur in unvaccinated, nonimmune susceptibles as a result of exposure to introduced wild-type virus or to revertant pathogenic vaccine-derived poliovirus (VDPV) (170).

CLINICAL MANIFESTATIONS. Approximately 90% to 95% of infected persons have an inapparent infection (1,2). Only 4% to 8% of patients have what has been called *minor illness*, non-CNS symptoms and signs such as sore throat, headache, nausea, vomiting, anorexia, and abdominal pain, which generally last 1 to 4 days. Only 1% to 2% of these individuals develop the so-called *major illness* consisting of aseptic meningitis. They present with fever, meningeal signs, paresthesias, neck and back pains, and have an associated CSF pleocytosis with normal or slightly elevated CSF protein and normal CSF glucose level (see Table 154.5).

The *paralytic disease* is occasionally preceded by the minor illness and usually by the major illness. In most cases, the meningitic phase lasts for a day or two before the first signs of paralysis are seen. Severe *muscle pain* and *spasms* precede or accompany onset of paralysis in the extremities. Fasciculation and hyperactive DTRs are transient and are followed by loss of reflexes and flaccid paralysis, progressing usually from 1 to 4 days. In the *spinal form*, there is asymmetric weakness or paralysis of muscle groups of the extremities or trunk. Transient urinary retention also occurs in about 30% of patients. In the *bulbar form*, there is weakness or

TABLE 154.6.   Myelitis Secondary to Adjacent Intrathecal Infection

A. Dorsal root ganglion infection: herpes-zoster syndrome

Etiology: Varicella zoster virus (VZV) primarily; HSV (especially Type 2) rarely
Pathogenesis: Inflammatory injury to (a) isolated cranial or spinal sensory ganglia which is site of recrudescent VZV replication; (b) related spinal cord segment, especially posterior gray matter and dorsal roots; (c) leptomeninges of involved cord segment and roots; and (d) spinal roots and peripheral nerve contiguous to involved ganglia

	Symptoms and signs	Neurologic findings	Diagnosis
General features	Constitutional symptoms 　Fever, malaise Prodromal segmental dysesthesias 　Itching, tingling, burning Radicular pain: 　Onset 72–96 hr before eruption 　Persists 1–4 wk in 70–80%; 　Chronic pain, hypersensitivity in 　　remainder Skin lesions: 　Vesicles on erythematous base 　　Progress to pustules, then crusts 　Surrounding inflammation 　　Tenderness 　　Dermal swelling, can be extensive 　　Hemorrhagic necrosis, in severe cases 　Distribution: 　　Confined to segmental dermatome(s) 　　Unilateral 　　　Recognizes branches of cranial 　　　　nerve V 　　　First division: scalp, forehead, 　　　　lids 　　　Second division: cheek, perioral 　　　Third division: low third of face 　　　　and upper neck Mucous membrane lesions: 　Aphthous-like clusters of unroofed 　　vesicles 　Unilateral distribution 　Only occur with ganglia supplying 　　mucosa: 　　Gasserian (cranial nerve V): 　　　First division: conjunctival and 　　　　corneal 　　　Second division: buccal 　　Geniculate (cranial nerve VII): 　　　Tongue 　　　Anterior palate 　　Cranial nerve IX and X: 　　　Posterior soft palate 　　　Pharynx 　　Sacral: bladder	Segmental, ipsilateral distribution of: 　Vesicles (variable numbers): large 　　numbers correlate with increased 　　risk for pain and postherpetic 　　zoster syndrome 　Superficial sensory loss (common) 　Motor weakness (c. 5%) Patterns: 　Thoracic zoster, 65%: 　　Single dermatome when 　　　immunocompetent 　　Between T5 and T10 most 　　　common 　Craniocervical, 20% 　　One or more adjacent dermatomes 　　Motor involvement frequent 　　Adjacent cranial nerves without 　　　ganglia affected by inflammation 　　　(e.g., III, IV, VI) 　Limb 　　One or more adjacent dermatomes 　Sacral 　　Bladder paralysis, with hematuria 　Disseminated 　　Multiple scattered lesions with one 　　　or more dermatomes heavily 　　　involved 　　　　or 　　Generalized, varicella-like 　　　eruption Premyelitis prodromal symptoms 　Ipsilateral with side of skin lesions: 　　Motor dysfunction, weakness of 　　　extremity 　　Sensory abnormalities: 　　　Spinothalamic, radiating pain 　　　Posterior column, abnormal 　　　　proprioception	Vesicle: scrape base or biopsy 　Tzanck prep: multinicleated giant 　　cells 　DFA: positive with anti-VZV 　EM: positive [not usually done] 　Viral culture: often negative 　　Yield affected by quality of 　　　specimen and handling Blood serology: 　ELISA - anamnestic response noted if 　　patient is immunocompetent 　　(requires paired sera 10 days apart) 　Check HIV status CSF: 　Cells: 　　Lymphocytosis in 40% 　Glucose: 　　Normal 　Protein: 　　Elevated 　Culture: 　　Negative for virus 　Antibody: 　　ELISA and immunobiot: positive for 　　　VZV antibody 　PCR: 　　Positive for VZV 　　(HSV is positive if sensory radiculitis 　　　is not zoster but complication of 　　　genital herpes, or inoculation 　　　herpes) MRI: 　T1 images: gadolinium enhancement 　　in involved roots and ganglia 　T2 images: hyperintense signal in 　　involved cord correlates with risk 　　for postherpetic neuralgia syndrome
Cranial syndromes	Ophthalmic zoster 　(Zoster Ophthalmicus) 　Gasserian (V) ganglion—Ist division Frequency: 10–15% of all zoster Skin lesions: limited to 　Anterior scalp 　Forehead 　Periorbital skin 　Nose tip (nasociliary branch) Mucous membrane lesions: 　Conjunctiva	Pain in scalp, forehead If nasociliary branch has vesicles, at 　risk for corneal lesions, iridocyclitis, 　and peripheral outer retinal necrosis 　(PORN) Ipsilateal cranial neuritis: 　Commonly associated ipsilateral 　　cranial nerve palsies when III, 　　IV, and VI motor roots and/or 　　brainstem involved: 　　Extraocular paresis 　　Ptosis 　　Mydriasis	Eye: 　Slit-lamp exam 　　Corneal and ciliary evaluation 　　Retinal exam MRI: 　T1 images: gadolinium enhancement 　　in involved roots and ganglia 　T2 images: hyperintense signal in 　　brainstem correlates with risk for 　　postherpetic neuralgia syndrome
	Geniculate zoster 　(Ramsey Hunt Syndrome) 　Geniculate (VIIth) ganglion Skin lesions: 　External auditory canal 　Pinna and adjacent scalp (variable) Mucous membrane lesions: 　hemitongue, ipsilateral	Pain in ear canal, pinna, and adjacent 　scalp Ipsilateral cranial neuritis: variable 　VII: Facial nerve palsy (common) 　VIII: Auditory-vestibular 　　involvement: tinnitus, vertigo, 　　deafness 　IX, X Dysphagia	ENT exam 　Exam external auditory canal exam for 　　vesicles and posterior aurical area 　　for vesicles Audiogram MRI: 　T1 images: gadolinium enhancement 　　in involved roots and ganglia

(continued)

TABLE 154.6. (continued)

Cranial syndromes (continued)	Neurologic symptoms: variable tinnitus, vertigo, deafness		T2 images: hyperintense signal in brainstem correlates with risk for postherpetic neuralgia syndrome
	Vagal and glossopharyngeal zoster IX and X ganglia Mucous membrane lesions only: Ipsilateral Soft palate Posterior pharynx	Pain in throat Dysphagia	ENT exam: Evaluate for unilateral mucosal lesions MRI: T1 images: gadolinium enhancement in involved roots and ganglia T2 images: hyperintense signal in brainstem correlates with risk for postherpetic neuralgia syndrome
	Upper cervical zoster (herpes occipitocollaris) C1, C2 ganglia Skin lesions Retroauricular and occipital	Pain in occiput	Vesicles: Evaluate as above MRI: T1 images: gadolinium enhancement in involved roots and ganglia T2 images: hyperintense signal in involved cord correlates with risk for postherpetic neuralgia syndrome

B. Posterior root infection: tabes dorsalis syndrome

Etiology: *Treponema pallidum*
Pathology: Form of neurosyphilis—thinning of posterior roots of lumbosacral cord, with dominant secondary destruction of proprioceptive fibers in radicular nerves and associated degeneration of posterior columns in cord

	Symptoms and signs	Neurologic findings	Diagnosis
Cardinal features	Lightning (lancinating) pains Legs especially Repetitive over hours to days Ataxia: Broad based gait Flinging movements of legs Urinary incontinence	Sensory ataxia Impaired vibration and position sense in feet and legs Positive Romberg's test Intact muscle power and mass Absent knee and ankle reflexes	CSF: Lymphocytosis common Abnormal protein Normal glucose VDRL: usually positive if previously untreated PCR: not commercially available Blood serology: Reaginic test (ART, RPR) variable, but usually positive Specific antibody tests (TPHA and FTAbs) positive
Other common findings	Visceral crises: Epigastric pain Nausea Vomiting Constipation	Neuro-ophthalmologic abnormalities: Abnormal pupils in 90%, including Argyll-Robertson Ophthalmoplegia - variable Optic atrophy Ptosis Insensitive hypotonic bladder Overflow incontinence Megacolon Secondary trophic ulcers Advanced osteoarthritis: Charcot's joints: 1–10% Hips, knees and ankles	MRI Meningeal enhancement Nonspecific white matter lesions Atrophy of medial temporal lobe correlates with general paresis

paralysis of the soft palate, pharynx, and vocal cords. Peripheral facial paralysis and transient oculomotor palsies (rarely) may be seen. There can be disturbances of breathing and circulation resulting from neuronal damage in the respiratory and vasomotor centers of the medulla.

Paralysis remains fixed for a period of days or weeks, after which improvement slowly follows: 60% of eventual recovery is achieved by 3 months and 80% by 6 months (1,2). Minimal further improvement continues over 18 months to 2 years, probably mostly because of learning more effective use of weakened muscles.

During acute polio, there are also rare cases of encephalitis and a variable degree of autonomic disturbance with regional hyperhidrosis or hypohidrosis, transient urinary retention, constipation, labile hypertension, and gastric atony (1,2).

The so-called *postpolio syndrome* of return of weakness or paralysis in later life after childhood or adolescent polio, and in the same distribution as the original attack, is not due to relapse or reacquisition of poliovirus infection, but to gradual loss of the compensatory neuronal and muscle activities that mark the muscle retraining and recovery process (157,171). As postpolio patients age and become increasing sedentary, physical capacity may be even further reduced because of cardiorespiratory deconditioning and weight gain (172).

DIAGNOSIS. In early poliomyelitis, the CSF contains an excess of cells (neutrophils in the first 72 hours, then lymphocytes) and slightly more protein than normal. Virus can usually be grown in tissue culture from pharyngeal swabs or throat washings in the first week of the acute stage of the illness. It can be recovered from the feces for at least 3 weeks and often longer. Although most enteroviruses are readily grown from CSF, poliovirus may not be isolated because of low viral content at the time of clinical presentation but can be recognized by PCR (164). Outbreaks of West Nile fever have been associated with cases of flaccid paralysis but usually have other findings consistent with coexisting encephalitis (173,173a–d). Diagnosis can also be made retrospectively by demonstrating a fourfold or greater rise in specific antibodies in the convalescent serum or by PCR identification of West Nile virus.

In certifying *acute flaccid paralysis* cases as poliomyelitis, the standard World Health Organization case definition permits any of four criteria to confirm the diagnosis, including isolation of poliovirus from a stool specimen (174).

TREATMENT. The treatment of the paralytic form is entirely supportive.

Herpesvirus Myelitis

Macaque Monkey B Virus (*Herpesvirus simiae*) Myelitis

CAUSE. Cercopithecine herpesvirus 1 (B virus), *Herpesvirus simiae*, was first isolated in 1933 from the brain and spinal cord of a researcher who died of rapidly progressive meningoencephalitis after being bitten by a macaque (175). B virus occurs naturally among primates of the genus *Macaca*. It is the biologic counterpart of HSV in humans and usually causes minimal or undetectable morbidity in its natural host (176). No other Old World and no New World monkeys are known to harbor B virus. Indeed, infections in several non-Macaca species cause fatal disease, as in humans.

PATHOGENESIS. Studies in mice on the pathogenesis of B virus infection of the nervous system indicate that route of inoculation controls mode of spread to CNS. Virus introduced *intramuscularly* in the leg ascends the ipsilateral dorsal column, the bilateral spinothalamic and spinoreticular systems, and central autonomic pathways. *Subcutaneous* inoculation spares the dorsal column, but virus otherwise follows the same routes. However, virus introduced *intraperitoneally* spreads in the cord bilaterally, mainly along the spinothalamic and central autonomic pathways. Ascent to the brain in mice is mainly orthograde along ascending systems, regardless of method of inoculation. In brain, virus first accumulates in thalamus, hypothalamus, and motor cortex, and then spreads retrograde along the pyramidal tract and central autonomic systems (177). MRI findings suggest a similar pattern of spread in human cases (175).

EPIDEMIOLOGY. The prevalence of infection is low among immature macaques but reaches more than 80% as animals reach sexual maturity. Latently infected monkeys shed virus only intermittently in conjunctiva, buccal mucosa, and genital areas and primarily during the breeding season or when ill, stressed (e.g., after transport, anesthesia, or invasive procedures), or immunocompromised. Macaques are native to Asia and northern Africa, but thousands are housed in research facilities and zoos and are kept as pets in private homes throughout the world (175). Persons at risk are those experiencing macaque-related injuries and laboratory workers exposed to B-virus–contaminated primary rhesus monkey cells cultures.

Seroprevalence studies among primate handlers indicate that asymptomatic infection does not occur (175). Monkey-related injuries at U.S. research facilities have been monitored closely since 1987. From 1987 to 1994, although several hundred persons following high-risk injuries were treated empirically for B virus infection, only eight infections were confirmed. Infection with B virus must be considered an uncommon result of macaque-related human injuries, because disease is rare despite the annual occurrence of several thousand monkey-inflicted bites, scratches, and other exposures (175).

More than 25 proven cases have been described in persons who handled monkeys or their tissues, including a fatal case after mucocutaneous inoculation from a splash of body fluids into the eye (178). Infection in untreated persons has a fatality rate of approximately 70% (175). One human-to-human transmission has been identified.

PREVENTION. Fortunately, human infections with B virus remain an uncommon result of macaque-related injuries, and thus optimal diagnostic and therapeutic approaches are unclear (176). Experimental evidence suggests that early therapy with acyclovir or postexposure chemoprophylaxis should decrease morbidity and mortality. Clinical experience with acyclovir postexposure chemoprophylaxis and treatment of early disease has been encouraging (179), but a recent case of failure of acyclovir begun shortly after onset of clinical findings of focal infection in the eye indicates outcome may also be influenced by route of virus inoculation, viral virulence, or timing of initiation of treatment (178).

Guidelines established by the CDC for prevention and treatment of B-virus infections in exposed persons include standard operating procedures and quality-control interventions for institutions handling macaques, and instructions for physicians evaluating and treating persons with potential B virus exposure (175). Updated information and any changes in the guidelines are available from the Division of Viral and Rickettsial Diseases at the National Center for Infectious Diseases, CDC, Atlanta (176).

Persons suspected of infection with Cercopithecine herpesvirus 1 (B virus), *H. simiae*, should be placed on contact isolation to avoid human-to-human transmission. Laboratory testing of specimens for viral isolation should not be performed in routine laboratories because of the risk of contamination of health care workers but should be processed at special regional laboratories as designated by the local State Department of Public Health or the CDC (178). See Chapters 159 and 161 for further details of management of asymptomatic exposed persons.

CLINICAL FEATURES. In well-documented human cases, the incubation period between exposure and onset of clinical disease has ranged from 2 to 30 days (175,178). Humans infected with B virus have a prodromal illness of early then intermediate manifestations before progression to *aseptic meningitis* and *rapidly ascending encephalomyelitis*. *Early manifestations* when present are vesicular eruptions or ulcerations at or near the exposure site, often accompanied by severe pain or itching and regional lymphadenopathy. *Intermediate manifestations* include local development of numbness, paresthesia or other neuresthesias, which progress proximally with associated muscle weakness, plus findings compatible with viremia (fever, conjunctivitis) and early brainstem involvement (persistent hiccough). *Late manifestations*, which are generally avoidable if therapy begins early, include sinusitis and central neurologic involvement. Meningitis (headache, stiff neck) progresses to encephalitis, manifested initially as brainstem and cerebellar findings before evidence of cortical involvement (altered mentation, seizures, hemiparesis, hemiplegia, coma, respiratory failure, and urinary retention) (175).

DIAGNOSIS. Human B virus infections are diagnosed by viral culture and serology. These studies must be performed in certified laboratories because of the dangers of viral cultivation, which requires Biosafety Level IV facilities, and the potential for incorrect interpretation of serologic results, due to the cross-reaction of human antibodies to HSV with B virus. Serology is performed on paired acute and convalescent sera, separated by 2 to 3 weeks. False-positive results are reduced by using the monoclonal competitive radioimmunoassay, or by ELISA combined with Western blot (175).

Viral isolation is required for definitive diagnosis. Serial cultures of high-risk asymptomatic and symptomatic exposed persons is recommended. If the initial postinjury wound cultures from an *asymptomatic* person turn positive for B virus, or if shedding was documented in the source monkey exposure of a *symptomatic* person, regardless of results of initial wound cultures, additional swab specimens should be collected for viral cultures from the individual's wound, oropharynx, conjunctiva, and the bases of any papular, vesicular, or ulcerative herpes-like lesions. If after 5 days the first set of cultures is still negative for B virus, at least two additional sets of cultures should be obtained. Detailed instructions for collecting and sending specimens for viral culture are described in published guidelines (175).

CSF in patients with neurologic symptoms contains rising titers of specific antibody, which precedes appearance of detectable serum antibody. Antibody in CSF may inhibit virus recovery, but its presence can be detected by PCR assay for B virus (175).

MRI has proved helpful in diagnosing involvement of meninges and cord, as well as early brainstem encephalitis. The ascending nature of B-virus infections, characterized by preferential early involvement of cerebellum, hypothalamus, thalamus, brainstem, medulla, and pons, may be detected as enhancing lesions by MRI. By contrast, HSV encephalitis localizes early in the temporal lobe (175).

In a case of human ocular exposure, the first clinical findings occurred after 14 days and consisted of conjunctivitis, periorbital swelling, regional lymphadenopathy, and vesicular eruptions in the distribution of the first and second branches of the fifth CN, similar to herpes-zoster cranialis (178). Initial MRI scans were normal. On treatment with intravenously administered acyclovir, the vesicles resolved. However, while still on parenteral therapy 2 weeks later, rapid onset of ascending myelitis was associated with MRI abnormalities extending from the cervical to upper thoracic cord. Within days, the abnormalities extended from the cord to midbrain in conjunction with progressive neurologic deterioration (178).

DIFFERENTIAL DIAGNOSIS. When B virus is not isolated from either a monkey or a high-risk exposed person, neurologic symptoms may still reflect undetected B virus infection. However, other diseases must be considered, such as reactivated HSV infection, herpes zoster, or in severely immunocompromised persons, CMV infection. When serial specimens fail to yield B virus from monkey or patient, definitive diagnosis of encephalitis requires brain biopsy for proper treatment, and especially when there is temporal lobe involvement, because an alterative diagnosis may be found in up to 20% of suspected cases of B virus infection (175).

TREATMENT. The CDC recommends that *asymptomatic* persons with an initially positive wound site culture for B virus be treated with oral acyclovir (800 mg five times daily) and that aggressive efforts be made to confirm evidence of active infection, because an initial positive culture could indicate viral contamination of the site. Absence of continued viral shedding or of clear-cut seroconversion permit cessation of therapy after 14 days. However, the individual should remain under medical supervision to detect recurrence of viral shedding, late seroconversion, or onset of clinical disease (175).

All *symptomatic individuals* should be hospitalized for medical evaluation and for isolation with barrier precautions. Treatment of symptomatic patients should begin empirically while awaiting culture and serology results. Recommended dosages, routes, and duration on admission are related to *risk for encephalitis. Low-risk* individuals are those with herpetiform lesions limited to the trunk or extremities, and only peripheral neurologic symptoms and signs. *High-risk* persons are those with herpetiform lesions on the head or neck or who have signs or symptoms of CNS involvement.

Dosing of acyclovir, the current drug of choice, should be adjusted for renal function, and the intravenous route should always be used in initial therapy of symptomatic persons. Recommended for those at low risk is moderate-dose intravenously administered acyclovir (at least 10 mg/kg per 8 hours, if renal function is normal). High-risk patients should receive maximal dosing intravenously (15/mg/kg per 8 hours). Intravenous treatment should continue until symptoms resolve, and until serial viral cultures for viral shedding are consistently negative for 14 days. Thereafter, oral acyclovir (800 mg five times daily) may be used, with serial monitoring for B virus shedding after the change in route and dose. When viral cultures are negative, the patient can be discharged.

Long-term chronic suppressive therapy and continued intermittent monitoring for viral shedding are recommended (175). The roles of oral valacyclovir, famciclovir, and adjuvant therapies, such as interferon-α, have not been established. Acyclovir-resistant strains of B virus have not yet been described.

Human Herpesviruses (CMV, EBV, HSV, VZV) Myelitis

CAUSES AND EPIDEMIOLOGY. *Acute transverse myelitis* caused by human herpes viruses, once a rare manifestation, is of increasing etiologic importance in the era of AIDS and immunodeficiencies associated with transplantation of bone marrow and solid organs. Immunocompromised persons with a history of prior CMV retinitis or herpes zoster are at high risk for viral reactivation within the CNS (180). CMV (181–184), EBV (185), HSV-1 and HSV-2 (186–191), and VZV (192–195) have all been associated with myelitis, usually in immunocompromised patients. Mixed herpesvirus infections have also been observed (196). Herpesviruses also cause CNS infections in immunocompetent persons, as is increasingly demonstrated through the routine application of the PCR technology to the diagnosis of inflammatory diseases of the CNS (168).

PATHOGENESIS. Myelitis caused by herpesviruses may occur as one of several manifestations of primary infection, especially in younger persons. In older and immunosuppressed persons, the CNS may be one target during systemic reactivation of latent herpesvirus infections. In both primary and recrudescent infection, even when viral cultures are negative, viremia, high viral loads in circulating peripheral blood monocytes, and virus in CSF can be documented by PCR (197). In immunocompetent individuals, specific antibody to viral antigens is produced systemically and intrathecally.

CMV, EBV, HSV-1 and HSV-2, and VZV are each capable of attacking multiple sites in the neuraxis, including peripheral nerves (198), and CMV, HSV, and VZV can invade the retina and optic nerve (180,199). In any one patient, sites of viral replication and injury may be limited or may be multiple and, like monkey B virus, may progressively involve peripheral nerves and plexuses, sensory ganglia, cord, and specific structures in brainstem and cerebral hemispheres. Viral inclusion bodies and cytopathic effects in multiple cell types are found in tissues, together with injury from inflammatory responses when patients retain some level of immune responsiveness (198).

CLINICAL FEATURES. Patients with symptomatic myelitis usually present with fever and progressive neurologic symptoms or deficits. Although findings compatible with severe *ascending necrosis* of the cord appear to be most typical, the patterns of myelitis associated with herpesviruses are often indistinguishable from other causes (200). Further, neurologic findings may be protean because of the herpesviruses ability to invade any site in the neuraxis, causing myelitis to appear in various combinations with meningitis, radiculitis, and encephalitis (201). Clinical findings can be further complicated by infarction of cord or brain from thrombosis in small and large vessels undergoing necrotizing vasculitis (199,202).

Associated clinical findings of concurrent CMV retinitis, peripheral outer retinal necrosis, or active skin lesions characteristic of herpes simplex or zoster are helpful in suggesting CMV, HSV, or VZV, but the absence of these findings does not exclude them (180,203–205).

DIAGNOSIS. The CSF in acute myelitis caused by herpesviruses usually shows a lymphocytic pleocytosis, elevated protein level, and normal glucose level. The predominance of lymphocytosis contrasts with the polymorphonuclear predominance commonly seen with herpesvirus plexitis and/or polyneuritis.

Specific IgM and IgG antibody can be detected in CSF, except in patients with advanced immunodeficiency (206). Patients with active CMV infections may have detectable pp65 antigenemia in peripheral leukocytes.

PCR tests reliably detect the presence of virus in CSF (168,207,208) and can be used to measure viremia (197). Unlike cultures of CSF for enteroviruses, yields for herpesviruses are low compared with detection of virus by PCR (168). Viral culture of CSF is worthwhile, however, because any herpesvirus isolated can be assessed for resistance to antivirals, particularly in previously treated patients.

MRI findings are similar to the range described for evolving B virus infection (178,209). T1-weighted images with contrast may show enhancement in meninges, plexuses, and areas of involved cord. Hyperintense signals seen on T2-weighted images in involved areas of cord and brain are reversible when treatment is effective (210,211). Hyperintense signals in corresponding areas on both noncontrast T1- and T2-weighted images suggest hemorrhagic necrosis. Findings of periventricular abnormalities and contrast enhancement of ependymal cells are particularly associated with CMV or VZV encephalitis and ventriculitis (211).

TREATMENT. In acute ascending or sudden-onset transverse myelitis of unknown etiology, early empiric treatment for possible herpesvirus infection is warranted, because treatment while awaiting laboratory confirmation may preserve cord function. Although immunocompromised patients remain at highest risk of herpesvirus myelitis, the disease also occurs in immunocompetent individuals.

Wild-type EBV, HSV, and VZV, though having different MIC$_{50}$ values *in vitro* for susceptibility to acyclovir, are all inhibited *in vivo* at attainable parenteral doses, but CMV is not. Immunocompromised patients presenting with acute myelitis of unknown etiology and with a history or current findings of CMV retinitis should receive early empiric therapy with GCV or foscarnet pending definitive diagnosis (212).

Viral response to therapy for herpesviruses is reflected in reversion of CSF from positive to negative PCR for viral DNA, reversal of viral load in plasma and peripheral blood leukocytes (197), reversion of abnormalities seen on MRI, and gradual clinical recovery (180,213,214). Length of treatment and the role of adjuvant therapies [e.g., interferons, steroids, plasmapheresis (215)] have not been standardized. Clinical and virologic relapses have been described, especially in patients with concomitant AIDS, who may require long-term suppressive therapy.

Once a definitive diagnosis of EBV, HSV, or VZV myelitis is established, parenteral acyclovir should be continued until there is evidence of clinical and radiologic response. Although the bioavailability of oral acyclovir at 50% is inferior to that of valacyclovir and famciclovir, their role in continuing therapy remains to be established. CMV myelitis in immunodeficient persons requires long-term suppression.

Human Retroviral Myelitis

Causes. Two human lymphotropic retroviruses have been clearly associated with myelitis. HIV-1 has been reported to cause *acute myelopathy* (216) and *acute peripheral neuropathy* in primary infection (see section "Human Immunodeficiency Virus Type 1–associated Neuropathies"). *Chronic vacuolar myelopathy* with spastic paralysis commonly precedes or accompanies the AIDS dementia syndrome (217).

Human T-lymphotropic virus type I (HTLV-I) is associated with a syndrome characterized by slowly progressive paralysis and is called either *tropical spastic paraparesis (TSP)* or, in Japan, *HTLV-I–associated myelopathy (HAM)* (218).

Laboratory Diagnosis. HIV-1 may be isolated from the spinal fluid of some *asymptomatic* individuals, whereas HTLV-I is primarily cell associated. Specific diagnosis of retroviral myelitis requires demonstration of viral-specific oligoclonal immunoglobulins in CSF or detection of retrovirus in tissue by nucleic acid probes (219). Although risk for a retroviral cause in cases of myelitis may be assessed by detecting serum antibodies with standard serologic tests, caution must be observed in using serology alone to diagnose myelitis in populations with a high seroprevalence for HIV-1 and/or HTLV-I infection. HTLV has a very low incidence of myelitis among HTLV-I–infected persons, and HIV-1–infected persons are at risk for several other causes of myelitis (220).

Human Immunodeficiency Virus Type 1 Vacuolar Myelopathy

PATHOLOGY. Vacuolar myelopathy is associated with advanced HIV infection and has been found in up to 50% of patients with AIDS undergoing autopsy (221). Pathologically, the white matter of the cord is vacuolated, primarily in the thoracic segments, with a cellular infiltrate of myelin-containing macrophages. Autopsy studies have failed to show evidence of direct involvement by HIV, CMV, papovaviruses, or human foamy virus (222).

CLINICAL FEATURES. In severe cases, patients develop spastic paraparesis of the lower extremities with or without involvement of the arms. The weakness may be asymmetric and evolves over weeks. Coexisting neuropathy is often present. A discrete sensory level is unusual, and sphincter dysfunction occurs later in the course of the disease. It is also commonly associated with HIV dementia (223).

DIAGNOSIS. Vacuolar myelopathy remains a histopathologic diagnosis and is a diagnosis of exclusion. CSF findings are nonspecific, and the spinal fluid examination is often normal. MRI does not show the enhancement characteristic of acute ascending myelitis. Treatable causes of spinal cord diseases should be excluded, including myelitis caused by herpesviruses or syphilis, epidural abscess, tumor, and vitamin B$_{12}$ deficiency (157,158,224).

TREATMENT. There is no known effective treatment, and long-term prognosis is poor.

Human T-lymphotropic Type I–associated Myelopathy and Tropical Spastic Paraparesis.
TSP and HAM are synonyms for an inflammatory myelopathy characterized by chronic spastic paraparesis or paraplegia with sphincter disturbance and minimal sensory loss.

CAUSE. HTLV-I is the retrovirus associated with both adult T-cell leukemia and TSP/HAM (225). HTLV-II, a related retrovirus commonly transmitted by the same routes and not associated with TSP/HAM, has been reported in one series to cause a TSP-like illness (226).

EPIDEMIOLOGY. See Chapter 255.

PATHOGENESIS. See Chapter 122.

CLINICAL FINDINGS. Patients typically complain of bilateral weakness and stiffness of the lower extremities but may also complain of difficulty ambulating and pain in the back. Later in the disease, neurogenic bladder may develop. Physical examination shows spastic paraparesis, hyperreflexia, and extensor-plantar reflexes. Vibratory sensation and proprioception are reduced. Typically, the disease is slowly progressive, although the upper extremities are usually not affected. Sometimes autonomic neuropathy, manifested by impotence and incontinence, is also present.

DIAGNOSIS. The CSF demonstrates a lymphocytic pleocytosis, elevated CSF IgG and oligoclonal banding on protein electrophoresis. Anti–HTLV-I antibodies are also demonstrable in the CSF on Western blot analysis. Diagnosis is established by the presence of HTLV-I seropositivity in conjunction with characteristic CSF and neurologic findings.

MRI findings on T2-weighted sagittal images may include cord swelling and fusiform regions of increased signal intensity, in contrast to the lack of cord swelling and multiple discreet areas of increased signal intensity characteristic of multiple sclerosis. However, cord swelling and diffuse increased signal intensity are not unique to TSP/HAM but are seen with other causes of acute inflammatory myelitis, including infectious and postvaccine associations (227). Brain lesions consisting of discreet punctate and nodular foci of hyperintensity in periventricular and subcortical white matter without mass effect may be seen in some patients but are of uncertain relationship to HTLV infection.

The differential diagnosis includes multiple sclerosis, syphilitic meningomyelitis, and adhesive arachnoiditis. Because the virus is also associated with polymyositis, weakness secondary to myopathy must also be excluded. Because risk factors for HTLV-I infection overlap with those of HIV and HTLV-II, patients should also be tested for coexisting HIV and HTLV-II infections.

TREATMENT. See Chapter 122.

Postinfectious and Postvaccine Myelitis

Myelitis has been reported following rubeola, varicella, influenza, and mumps (postinfectious) and following certain vaccines (postvaccinial), especially after several vaccines no longer in general use (vaccinia virus, Pasteur-type rabbit cord rabies vaccine). These delayed reactions usually take the form of leukomyelitis or transverse myelitis (Table 154.6), depending on the severity and extent of inflammatory response (157,158,228).

SECONDARY MYELITIS

Infections of Dorsal Root Ganglion and Posterior Spinal Root

The syndromes of *herpes zoster* and *tabes dorsalis* commonly involve the spinal cord and therefore represent *mixed root and cord disorders* (Table 154.6). Because of the multiple target sites of *T. pallidum* in the CNS, tabes dorsalis is discussed in the section "Polymorphic Infections."

Herpes Zoster (Varicella-Zoster Virus). VZV causes disease of sensory nerves through its attack on the dorsal ganglia. It can also affect motor functions of *CNs* and *peripheral nerves* and is a cause of *polyneuritis*. In HIV-infected asymptomatic persons, zoster is usually the first opportunistic infection, and in those with far-advanced disease, it can cause *myelitis* and *encephalitis* (180,199).

PATHOGENESIS. See Chapter 139.

CLINICAL MANIFESTATIONS. The first sign of *sensory radiculitis* is pain in the affected dermatome with focal cutaneous inflammation and maculopapular rash preceding the typical vesicles. The lesions are characteristically, but not exclusively, unilateral and usually limited to a single dermatome. Among 116 patients in one series (229), the most common location of zoster infection was in the thoracic area (53%), followed by cervical (22%), lumbar (18%), facial (15%), and sacral (8%) locations, which closely parallel data from Adams and Victor (1) shown in Table 154.6. Zoster involving sacral plexus outflow may produce vesicles in bladder wall mucosa and symptomatic cystitis with hematuria.

Motor deficits when present usually involve only the motor root from the same segment as the sensory ganglion, except that ipsilateral nerves without sensory ganglia may be affected in cranial neuritis. Motor symptoms may be delayed and not develop until 2 weeks after onset of the rash.

Zoster may directly involve sensory ganglia of the fifth, seventh, eighth, ninth, and tenth CNs, producing the cranial syndromes shown in Tables 154.3 and 154.6. *Cranial neuritis* caused by VZV most commonly involves the gasserian ganglion of CN V; if the ophthalmic branch of the first division (V_1) is affected, the eye is susceptible to the complications of corneal ulcer, necrotizing angiitis, and uveitis. Involvement of the eighth nerve produces deafness or vestibular symptoms. Multiple ipsilateral CNs may be affected in geniculate ganglion zoster (*Ramsay Hunt* syndrome), especially the seventh, eighth, and ninth CNs (*zoster oticus*). Cranial neuritis may be complicated by giant-cell arteritis of great vessels, thrombosis, and stroke (199).

Myelitis occurs in immunocompetent patients but more commonly in *immunosuppressed patients,* and especially those with AIDS and a history of localized herpes zoster (180,199,210). Prodromal neurologic symptoms consist of motor dysfunction and disturbances attributable to spinothalamic and posterior column involvement ipsilateral to the skin eruption. Without antiviral treatment, symptoms precede onset of myelitis by 12 days, after which myelitis progresses another 10 days to maximal deficit (230). In immunosuppressed patients, the cord may be extensively involved by recrudescent VZV: segmental paralysis may develop rapidly and, depending on the extent and level of cord involvement, may occur with diaphragmatic paralysis, neurogenic bladder, and hypotonia (203–205,210). VZV myelitis may precede cutaneous eruption or may never develop skin lesions (202).

Complications in patients with advanced immunosuppression include encephalitis and acute retinal necrosis. Low CD4 counts are associated with multifocal disease, persistent neurologic sequelae, and death despite treatment (180).

DIAGNOSIS. In most patients, the combination of dermatomal sensory disturbances followed by vesicular eruption is the primary clue to diagnosis of herpes zoster. Laboratory confirmation is usually based on immunodiagnosis of VZV in scrapings from the base of the lesions and lack of growth of HSV in cultures.

The CSF in uncomplicated zoster contains lymphocytes in two thirds of patients, with elevated protein, normal glucose, and IgG antibody to VZV. Viral cultures are infrequently positive, but VZV is readily detectable with PCR (168,199).

MRI demonstrates enhancement of involved nerve roots. In uncomplicated zoster of peripheral nerves, findings may include focal swelling of adjacent spinal cord. With CN zoster, focal brainstem lesions may be found even in immunocompetent persons (210). In immunocompromised patients, extensive involvement of the neuraxis, including meningitis, myelitis, encephalitis, and ventriculitis, may be found on MRI (180).

TREATMENT. See Chapter 139.

Intraspinal Abscess and Infections of Subdural and Epidural Spaces

Intraspinal (Intramedullary) Abscess

CAUSES AND PATHOGENESIS. Intramedullary abscess is a rare condition and was usually a necropsy discovery until the advent of MRI and computed tomographic (CT) imaging technology (3,231). Abscesses occur most often in the thoracic segment of the cord and usually involve two or three spinal segments. Holocord abscesses, extending the full length of the cord, are extremely rare (232). Abscess may be limited to only the filum terminale (233).

Half of intramedullary spinal abscesses are believed to be of *hematogenous* origin (3). Subacute endocarditis and vertebral osteomyelitis are common concomitant complications. *Staphylococcus aureus* is the most common pathogen isolated (234). Other pathogens reported include *Brucella* species, *Listeria monocytogenes*, mycobacteria (*M. tuberculosis* and atypicals) (235), various streptococci (including pneumococci), reactivation toxoplasmosis in AIDS, and the larval encystment of cysticercosis and schistosomiasis (167,236). Congenital dermal sinuses, known causes of recurrent bacterial meningitis, are also associated with intramedullary abscess (234,237,238).

At risk for neuroschistosomiasis are travelers, expatriates, and immigrants who have a history of freshwater exposure in schistosomiasis-endemic areas and CNS abnormalities, even in the absence of classic signs and symptoms of acute schistosomiasis (e.g., fever, nausea, vomiting, abdominal pain, diarrhea, and hematuria). Neuroschistosomiasis can occur several months after exposure to infested water and in low-intensity infections in which eggs may be undetectable or difficult to identify in urine or stool (236).

CLINICAL FINDINGS. The symptoms of spinal abscess are indistinguishable from those of epidural abscess (239). Back pain and/or radicular pain is common, but fever and other signs of infection may be absent in more than 50% (234). Neurologic findings depend on the location and extent of the lesion in the cord. A history of prior or recurrent meningitis and new onset of transverse myelitis is suggestive of congenital dermal sinus with intramedullary abscess.

DIAGNOSIS AND TREATMENT. Diagnosis is most easily made with contrast-enhanced MRI. MRI studies show an intramedullary collection with high signals on T2-weighted images, well-defined low-density lesions on T1-weighted images, and peripheral contrast enhancement with adjacent medullary edema (240). When intramedullary lesions are well defined and round, contrast uptake by adjacent periependymal gray matter is suggestive of infectious etiology (241).

Treatment of suppurative abscess includes surgical drainage and prolonged antibiotic therapy (232,234). In acute abscess formation, early surgical intervention is essential to preserve neurologic function and prevent death (234).

Schistosomiasis is treated medically with a combination of corticosteroids and praziquantel, unless praziquantel resistance is anticipated, in which case oxamniquine is indicated (167). Sensitive and specific serologic tests for diagnosing schistosomiasis are available through the CDC's Parasitic Diseases Branch, National Center for Infectious Diseases (telephone 404-488-4050) (236).

Treatment with a single dose of praziquantel (40 to 60 mg/kg of body weight) is safe and effective therapy against the adult worms of the three major species of schistosomes infecting humans (*Schistosoma hematobium, Schistosoma mansoni,* and *Schistosoma japonicum*). Corticosteroids are often useful in neuroschistosomiasis to reduce edema and inflammation. Although CNS schistosomiasis is rare, substantial morbidity from this condition is preventable by early diagnosis and rapid treatment (322).

Spinal Epidural Abscess

CAUSE. Although epidural abscess is a rarely diagnosed condition (0.2 to 1.2 cases per 10,000 admissions in a large tertiary care hospital), the high morbidity and mortality from this infection necessitate familiarity with its presentation, because it warrants prompt diagnosis and immediate medical and surgical attention (242,243). *S. aureus* has been implicated in half of the cases. Other pathogens include coagulase-negative staphylococci, gram-negative bacteria (*E. coli, Pseudomonas* species, *Salmonella typhi*); pneumococci (244), microaerophilic [*Streptococcus milleri* (245)] and anaerobic streptococci; gram-negative anaerobic bacteria (*Fusobacterium necrophorum*); actinomycetes [*Actinomyces israeli* (246)]; *Nocardia asteroides* (247); mycobacteria [*M. tuberculosis* (248)]; and fungi, especially *Aspergillus* species, which remain important pathogens in immunocompromised patients (249). Echinococcal cysts may mimic the symptoms and findings of chronic epidural abscess (250).

EPIDEMIOLOGY. Risk factors for epidural abscess are bacteremias and fungemias complicating injection-drug use (251) or from skin, soft tissue, or respiratory tract infections occurring in persons with defective host defenses, such as diabetes mellitus, alcoholism, immunodeficiency, and immunosuppression from medications (252,253). Sources of nosocomial sepsis include line infections from indwelling intravenous catheters and hemodialysis shunt infections (254). Other risk factors include associated vertebral osteomyelitis, recent spinal surgery, and complications of long-term epidural catheters or of other local procedures.

PATHOGENESIS. Epidural abscesses are most commonly the result of hematogenous infection of contiguous vertebral body or disc space, rather than directly inoculated infection. Epidural abscesses are located predominantly either *anterior* or *posterior* to the cord, depending on pathogenesis (255). Abscesses in the anterior location are usually complications of vertebral osteomyelitis or of intervertebral disc space infections and have varying degrees of purulence and associated granulation tissue depending on the causative organism and host responsiveness.

Posterior epidural abscesses usually do not involve bone, unless they are postsurgical. They are usually hematogenous in origin, often associated with intravenous drug use, or prior trauma, and possible hematoma formation. They are more common in children than adults and extend over a longer length of epidural space than anterior epidural abscesses (256).

CLINICAL FINDINGS. Signs and symptoms of epidural abscess relate to the location of the abscess (cervical, thoracic, lumbar, sacral) and to the underlying cause, which influences the tempo of the process. Table 154.7 describes the findings of *radicular, cord,* and *cauda equina* syndromes that accompany symptomatic spinal epidural abscess.

Classically, *acute* disease progresses in four stages: (a) spinal ache, (b) pain, (c) weakness, bowel, and bladder dysfunction, and (d) paralysis, unless the cause is recognized and treated surgically and medically (257). Patients with *acute* epidural abscess may develop complete paralysis in less than 2 hours (258). *Subacute* and *chronic* forms may follow the same sequence but over weeks to months, and the pathologic findings may be dominated by granulation tissue rather than frank abscess (259).

DIAGNOSIS. Leukocytosis and other signs of acute infection are common in acute epidural abscess but are often absent in chronic cases (252). Erythrocyte sedimentation rate is almost always uniformly elevated. CSF examination usually shows evidence of a parameningeal irritation: Elevated protein level and pleocytosis are common. CSF glucose level, Gram stain, and culture should be normal unless the abscess is entered inadvertently. Blood cultures are often positive at the time of diagnosis of abscess but if negative may have been documented during an earlier septic episode (244,254).

TABLE 154.7. Secondary Myelitis Syndromes

Spinal epidural abscess or granulations: syndromes of radicular spinal cord and cauda equina compression

Etiology: determined by risk factors for (a) associated initial hematogenous osteomyelitis [from community-acquired primary site of infections, injecting drug use, nosocomial bacteremia related to indwelling vascular lines, urosepsis]; (b) immunosuppression or immunodeficiency disorders [diabetes mellitus, organ or bone marrow transplant recipient, AIDS]; (c) reactivation of latent spinal tuberculous or fungal infection; (d) contaminated hardware or contamination of operative field in back surgery; (e) contaminated LP needles [now rare]; (f) residence or travel to endemic area for echinococcosis

Pathogenesis: Bacterial, fungal, mycobacterial or parasitic infection accessing epidural space from (a) adjacent vertebral disc space or osteomyelitis vertebrae and extending secondarily into epidural space (= anterior epidural abscess), then encroaching on root and cord by mass effect and interference with venous return, with potential involvement of anterior spinal artery producing focal infarction; (b) hematogenous seeding of epidural blood clot (most commonly in posterior location)

Site of core compression	Symptoms	Neurologic findings	Diagnosis

Radicular spinal cord syndrome with irritative root: Between C1 and L1 vertebrae	Constitutional symptoms
	  Weight loss: variable
	  Fever: variable
	  Chills: variable
	Segmental (root) symptoms initially:
	  "Spinal ache": at site
	  Pain: knifelike, dull ache
	    Intensified by cough, sneeze, movement
	    Radiates away from spine distally
	  Paresthesias: same distribution
	Onset of cord signs below lesion
	  Difficulty walking
	  Muscle weakness below level of lesion
	  Sphincteric weakness (especially bladder)
		Local findings
		  Involved area of vertebral spine
		  Limited range of motion
		  Paravertebral muscle spasm
		  Spine tender to palpation or percussion
		Progressive segmental abnormalities
		  Limited to root distribution, rarely bilateral
		  Deep tendon reflexes: reduced/lost
		  Muscle groups: decreased tone and strength; fasciculation, then atrophy
		Sensory:
		  Pin prick, touch impaired
		  Posterior column dysfunction: Position, vibration sense, Romberg's sign
		  Sensory level (pain, temperature) on trunk
		Paraparesis: asymmetric spastic weakness
		  Arms and legs: cervical lesions
		  Legs only: thoracolumbar lesion
		Progression to paralysis
			CSF:
			  Protein: elevated
			  Glucose: normal
			  Cells: lymphocytes or PMNs, depending on cause
			  Culture: Negative
			  Pressure: Dynamic block (Queckenstead test) may be present
			CT and MRI:
			  Anterior lesion: epidural mass
			    Disc space infection
			    Vertebral osteomyelitis ± dislocated vertebral bone fragment
			  Posterior lesion: epidural mass
			MRI (T1 and T2 images)
			  Epidural mass: enhances with gadolinium
			  Cord: variable edema
			  Vertebral spine (if anterior abscess): adjacent inflammatory disease
			CT (± myelogram):
			  Spinal stenosis; ± block
			Microbiology:
			  Blood cultures: detect acute bacterial causes only
			  Tissues:: from operation (decompression or laminectomy) and/or CT-guided needle biopsy should be examined for:
			    Bacteria (aerobic and anaerobic)
			    Fungi
			    Mycobacteria

Cauda equina syndrome: Between T10 and L1 (with mixed cord signs) or Below L1 (cord terminus)	Legs and buttocks:
	  Pain
	  Paresthesias: on standing, walking, heavy exertion: relieved by laying down
	  Muscle fatigue: tiredness, Sphincteric dysfunction
		Asymmetric findings below waist
		  Radicular sensory loss
		  Progressive motor loss:
		    Atrophy
		    Areflexia
		    Paralysis (late)
			Lumbar puncture:
			  May yield pus if posterior epidural abscess is as low as L3-L5 level
			Radiologic findings: as above
			Microbiology:
			  Tissues: from aspiration or operation (decompression or laminectomy) should be cultured for:
			    Bacteria (aerobic and anaerobic)
			    Fungi
			    Mycobacteria

MRI has superseded CT for initial evaluation, because it permits detection of smaller abscesses not seen on CT. Both avoid the risk of lumbar puncture and contamination of the subarachnoid space by inadvertent entry into abscess (260,261). Air may be visualized in the abscess if organisms are gas forming.

In cases of epidural and spinal abscess complicating vertebral osteomyelitis, MRI is especially helpful in detecting extension of infection into the pedicles, the presence of extradural fluid, edema of the cord or myelitis, myelomalacia, and any syrinx formation proximal or distal to the cord (262). If meningitis is present, MRI may not be able to demonstrate epidural collections, whereas CT can (259).

CT as a complementary study to MRI is advantageous when preexisting vertebral osteomyelitis is the source of epidural abscess, because CT may identify bony changes not well visualized on routine spinal films or MRI. CT-guided aspiration of epidural abscesses to obtain specimens for microscopic examination and culture is appropriate when acute surgical intervention is not required (254).

TREATMENT AND PROGNOSIS. *Acute epidural abscess* adjacent to the cord normally mandates simultaneous intravenous antibiotic therapy and immediate surgical decompression by bilateral laminectomy (253). Before cultures become available, initial therapy should include an antistaphylococcal agent effective against methicillin-resistant *S. aureus* and coagulase-negative staphylococci, such as vancomycin, and coverage for gram-negative rods (e.g., third-generation cephalosporin plus aminoglycoside), plus additional anaerobic coverage (e.g., metronidazole). Tuberculous and fungal epidural abscesses are more likely to present in a more indolent fashion.

Antibiotic treatment is then adjusted on the basis of results of pretreatment blood cultures and cultures taken at operation. Therapy should last 4 to 6 weeks at a minimum and longer if there is associated osteomyelitis (253).

When vertebral osteomyelitis is present, attention must be given to prevention of posterior displacement of vertebral fragments into the spinal canal. Immobilization of the affected segment of spine is usually sufficient, but anterior vertebrectomy and external and internal bracing may be necessary (253).

Outcome of treatment in acute epidural abscess strongly correlates with severity of neurologic involvement at the initiation of therapy, hence the importance of early diagnosis. In a review of 35 patients (252), all those with *normal* neurologic function at the time of diagnosis and treatment recovered. Of 12 patients with *radicular pain only,* 10 recovered completely and 2 died. Of 12 patients with *weakness,* 6 recovered completely, 4 had residual weakness, and 2 died. Of eight patients who had *paralysis,* none recovered completely, four improved partially, three remained paralyzed, and one died. Functional improvement was closely related to duration of deficit duration; only 2 of 11 patients with weakness or paralysis lasting more than 1.5 days improved (252). These data emphasize the necessity of rapid diagnosis and surgical intervention in epidural abscess, although in selected instances consideration may be given to antibiotic treatment alone (263).

Chronic epidural abscess and/or mass effect from *granulation tissue* are more characteristic of brucellosis, fungal, and tuberculous infections, in which once the etiology is clarified, surgical intervention can be guided by the rate of progression of symptoms and signs. Unexpected reversal of long-standing myelopathic signs by judicious surgical removal of granulation tissues has been reported in tuberculous epidural masses that were unresponsive to antituberculous therapy (264).

Spinal Subdural Empyema.

CAUSES AND PATHOGENESIS. Spinal subdural empyema is an uncommon condition with many similarities to spinal epidural abscess in pathogenesis, microbiology, and clinical findings (265–267). It is often a complication of retropharyngeal abscess, vertebral osteomyelitis, intravenous drug use, or surgery (260,268). *S. aureus, S. pneumoniae,* and *Streptococcus viridans* have been reported pathogens, although anaerobes and microaerophilic organisms from respiratory sources should also be suspected.

DIAGNOSIS AND THERAPY. Diagnosis and therapy are similar to epidural abscess. MRI is the most sensitive technique for diagnosis. Unlike epidural abscesses, which remain relatively localized, subdural infection tends to extend longitudinally, producing the appearance of *multiple defects on examination with MRI or CT myelography,* a diagnostic finding highly suggestive of

subdural empyema (269,270). Prognosis depends on duration and extent of neurologic impairment before initiation of combined medical and surgical therapy. Nonoperative therapy may be appropriate for certain cases (271–273).

POLYMORPHIC INFECTIONS THAT AFFECT CORD, PERIPHERAL, AND CRANIAL NERVES

Causes

Several infectious agents affect two or more parts of the nervous system, producing findings in any given individual in which disorders of either the PNS, the cord, or the brain may dominate, or in which all three are sequentially or simultaneously involved to different degrees. *Normal hosts* infected by either of two spirochetal infections—*B. burgdorferi* and *T. pallidum*—often have polymorphic involvement of the nervous system, whereas symptomatic invasion of the nervous system by *Brucella* species and *M. pneumoniae* is rare. Other organisms of note not discussed here, but that in normal hosts often involve the PNS, cord, and/or brain, are *Chlamydia* (psittacosis) (274), louse-borne (275,276) and tick-borne relapsing fever (277), and murine typhus (278,279). Both normal and immunosuppressed persons are susceptible to polymorphic infections by VZV. In severely *immunosuppressed hosts,* polymorphism is particularly characteristic of opportunistic infections by several herpesviruses, as discussed in the section "Human Herpesviruses (CMV, EBV, HSV, VZV) Myelitis." This section focuses on patterns of polymorphic infections seen in normal hosts.

Neuroborreliosis (Lyme Borreliosis)

CAUSE

Lyme disease, caused by the spirochete *B. burgdorferi,* was initially recognized in 1976 after an outbreak in Old Lyme, Connecticut. Subsequently it was recognized that *B. burgdorferi* infection can result in acute and chronic peripheral neuropathies and other neurologic patterns, leading to its designation as the great imitator (280–282). The Lyme disease spirochetes, *B. burgdorferi* sensu lato, have been divided into three species: *B. burgdorferi* sensu stricto, *Borrelia garinii,* and *Borrelia afzelii.* These genospecies vary in geographic distribution and may have different phenotypic expressions in infected humans (283). For surveillance purposes, Lyme disease is defined by the CDC as the presence of a erythema migrans rash of more than 5 cm in diameter or at least one late manifestation of musculoskeletal, neurologic, or cardiovascular disease with laboratory confirmation of *B. burgdorferi* infection (284).

EPIDEMIOLOGY
See Chapter 214.

PREVENTION
See Chapter 214.

PATHOGENESIS
See Chapter 214.

CLINICAL FEATURES
Lyme disease is a multisystem, multistage, inflammatory disease (285). The *primary disease* is characterized by an early skin lesion called *erythema chronicum migrans,* which develops at the site of a tick bite over days to 1 month (median 7 to 10 days). Early erythema migrans has homogenous or central redness before developing the characteristic central partial clearing (286). Associated flu-like symptoms include low-grade fever, headache,

neck stiffness, arthralgia, or fatigue (286). Multiple skin lesions, which occur in 20%, are considered a sign of disseminated borreliosis (287,288). Several weeks to months thereafter, the *second stage* of neurologic and cardiac manifestations occurs (289). Instances of neurologic disease without initial skin lesions have been recorded (290). The later *third stage* is marked by arthritis (285). The spirochete invades the eye early but remains dormant until later onset of keratitis and neuroretinitis (291).

Acute neuroborreliosis is usually characterized by *peripheral and/or cranial neuropathies,* with or without *meningoencephalitis,* and usually occurs within 4 to 12 weeks after tick bite (292). Acute infection may also present as *myelitis* (293,294). Unilateral or bilateral facial palsies, the result of chronic basilar meningitis, are the most common neurologic manifestations and may be seen in 50% of patients (295). The most common findings in one series were *aseptic meningitis* (89%), *encephalitis* (29%), *unilateral facial palsy* (32%), *bilateral facial palsy* (18%), *abducens nerve palsy* (3%), and *peripheral neuropathy* (32%). Peripheral nerve involvement is typically asymmetric and usually presents as either a motor, a sensory, or a mixed radiculoneuropathy and is expressed in patterns of *mononeuropathy multiplex* and *radiculitis.* Brachial and crural radiculitis—also called *plexitis*—cause paralysis of muscles in arms and legs, respectively. In contrast to GBS, paralysis caused by plexitis of neuroborreliosis is usually accompanied by sensory loss (285).

Months to years after infection, *chronic Lyme borreliosis* can cause intermittent distal paresthesias and radicular pain. Physical examination may be normal, but nerve conduction studies demonstrate axonal neuropathy.

DIFFERENTIAL DIAGNOSIS

Other infectious causes of the neurologic syndromes associated with neuroborreliosis include the known causes of GBS (see the previous section "Acute Inflammatory Demyelinating Polyneuropathy or the Guillain-Barré Syndrome"), Bell's palsy (see Table 154.4), and HIV-associated disorders (see Table 154.2).

Diagnosis

The CSF formula in neuroborreliosis is that of an aseptic meningitis, with lymphocytosis, increased protein level, and normal glucose level. Proof of diagnosis and determination of stage of disease has been evaluated by several groups. Acute disease is characterized by elevated CSF cell count with predominance of T lymphocytes, large amounts of plasma cells, and IgM-positive B lymphocytes, *B. burgdorferi*–specific IgM antibody by ELISA, and a high specific-antibody index (ratio of CSF titers to blood, corrected for albumin content) (296,297). The CSF of untreated past disease, by contrast, contains IgG-bearing B cells and IgG-specific antibody.

Patients with disseminated disease may have anicteric hepatitis, splenomegaly, and an associated myositis visible by gallium-67 nuclear imaging and located near an involved joint or localized neuropathy (298).

Presumptive diagnosis of active neuroborreliosis may be based on clinical and epidemiologic criteria, following recommendations from the American Academy of Neurology (299,300). Specific diagnosis of early or late-stage infection is made most reliably by serology, because culture is cumbersome, and current molecular identification methods by PCR, though increasingly sensitive, are not standardized. Although sensitivity of PCR in CSF is low (18%) in proven neuroborreliosis, positive CSF antibody is almost universal in patients with Lyme

meningitis and other manifestations of acute neuroborreliosis (285,301–304). Serologic diagnosis requires initial testing with a sensitive screening assay, either an ELISA or immunofluorescent assay, followed by standardized Western blot testing for recognition of *B. burgdorferi* antigens by IgM and IgG. Patients with suspected disease in the early stages (first 4 weeks of symptoms) but negative serology should be retested, and acute and convalescent sera run in parallel. Sera from persons with disseminated disease or late-stage disease almost always have a strong IgG-specific immune response that recognizes multiple *B. burgdorferi* antigens on Western immunoblot (305). To distinguish newly acquired infections among persons previously immunized with the OspA vaccine, an ELISA test using recombinant OspA-free *Borrelia* antigens (rNon-OspA) has been developed recently, which can distinguish between populations of naturally infected and OspA-vaccinated persons (306).

TREATMENT

See Chapter 214.

Neurobrucellosis

CAUSE

Brucella melitensis, Brucella abortus, and *Brucella suis* are all capable of producing neurologic disease in humans (307–309). *Brucella* organisms can also cause spondylitis (310), which may progress to epidural abscess (311).

EPIDEMIOLOGY

See Chapter 202.

PATHOLOGY

A systemic infection, brucellosis can involve any organ of the body (309). *Brucella* species replicate intracellularly in macrophages and monocytes, are widely distributed in the reticuloendothelial system, and may be associated with inflammatory lesions in liver, spleen, lymph nodes, bone marrow, joints, and epididymis. The type of inflammatory response evoked varies from granulomata to abscess formation depending on the infecting species. *B. abortus* characteristically elicits a sarcoid-like noncaseating epithelioid granuloma, and *B. melitensis* a more heterologous response, including loose granulomata. *B. suis* is associated with abscess formation, which commonly occurs in liver and spleen. Leukoclastic vasculitis, thrombocytopenia, and splenomegaly are common findings in children with brucellosis.

In neurobrucellosis, the intrathecal roots of CNs and spinal roots may be invaded by granulomatous reactions complicating vertebral osteomyelitis, producing radiculopathy and polyneuritis, which commonly involve the lumbosacral roots (311).

Direct infection of the CNS by hematogenous spread results in encephalitis and/or myelitis. Myelopathy typically involves the corticospinal tracts and produces a pure upper motor neuron syndrome without sensory findings. Vasculitis may result in infarction and formation of mycotic aneurysms (312).

CLINICAL FINDINGS

Approximately 2% to 5% of patients with brucellosis develop a wide array of neurologic complications, often with considerable clinical overlap (312). Neurologic involvement is often subacute or chronic and encompasses *encephalitis, myelitis, meningitis,* and *radiculitis* (313–315). Meningitis is the most common neurologic presentation and may result in *CN palsies* and *vasculitis.* Intracerebral *mycotic aneurysms* may be complicated by stroke and intracerebral hemorrhage.

Fever, with or without arthritis, is a consistent feature of bacteremic brucellosis, occurring in 86% of cases in one study in an endemic area (316). Clinical features of murine typhus may be confused with brucellosis (279).

DIAGNOSIS

CSF usually reveals a lymphocytic pleocytosis, elevated protein level, and hypoglycorrhachia, comparable to findings in fungal and mycobacterial meningitis (309). Specific antibodies are detectable in CSF with the serum agglutination test (SAT). When CSF is cultured without special provision for isolation of fastidious organisms, CSF cultures are positive in fewer than 50% of cases. PCR methodology is reportedly more sensitive than cultures for tissue specimens (317) and can be performed on serum samples (318).

Presumptive diagnosis of systemic brucellosis is based on rising titers of specific antibody in the serum, generally assessed with the SAT, together with fractionation of any specific antibody into IgM and IgG components. False-negative results caused by the prozone phenomenon can occur in infection by *B. melitensis*, *B. abortus*, and *B. suis* if the SAT is performed on inadequately diluted high-titered sera (more than 1:160). A falsely negative SAT result will also occur on the rare occasion when the infecting agent is *Brucella canis*, which cannot be detected by the SAT (309).

Proof of diagnosis requires isolation of *Brucella* species from blood, bone marrow, liver, or other tissue. Cultures of blood and tissue fluids may become positive in 2 to 4 days with modern automated liquid culture systems, particularly when specimens are first processed to release intracellular organisms (319,320). Otherwise, prolonged incubation (14 to 21 days) may be required with nonradiometric liquid culture detection systems (321,322) and more than 4 weeks with enriched solid media (*Brucella* agar) (323). Depending on method used, sensitivity of blood cultures can be as low as the 38% positivity rate seen for 545 cases of brucellosis in one study in Saudi Arabia (316).

The laboratory receiving specimens for culture should be alerted to the provisional diagnosis to avoid misidentification of isolates as *Moraxella* or *Haemophilus* species and because *Brucella* species constitute an important biohazard for laboratory-acquired infections (324,325).

TREATMENT

See Chapter 202.

Neurosyphilis

CAUSE AND PATHOLOGY

Four types of *spinal cord involvement* are associated with *T. pallidum* infections: (a) *tabes dorsalis*, a form of chronic meningoradiculitis that affects the posterior root predominantly; (2) *syphilitic meningomyelitis* (often called *Erb's spastic paraplegia*), a chronic fibrosing meningitis in which myelinated fibers are lost due to bilateral involvement of the corticospinal tract; (c) *anterior spinal artery syndrome* caused by meningovascular syphilis; and (d) *gummata* of the spinal meninges and cord (326,327). Because of its varied pathogenesis, syphilis should be considered in the differential diagnosis of nearly all diseases of the spinal cord (328,329).

CLINICAL FEATURES

The clinical features of *tabes dorsalis* include lightning (lancinating) pains, especially in the legs and repetitive over hours to days; broad-based gait with flinging movements of legs (sensory ataxia); visceral crises (e.g., epigastric pain, nausea, and vomiting); and urinary incontinence. Neurologic findings include absent knee and ankle reflexes, impaired vibration and position sense in feet and legs, positive Romberg's test, intact muscle power and mass, abnormal pupils in 90% (e.g., Argyll-Robertson), ptosis, variable ophthalmoplegia, optic atrophy, insensitive hypotonic bladder with overflow incontinence, megacolon, secondary trophic ulcers, and advanced osteoarthritis in hips, knees, and ankles (Charcot's joints 1% to 10%) (327).

DIAGNOSIS

Diagnosis is by evidence of active infection in the CNS (pleocytosis in CSF, usually with positive VDRL test result), together with serologic evidence of prior syphilis (positive treponema hemagglutination, or treponema fluorescent antibody). The CSF usually shows a lymphocytic pleocytosis, elevated protein level, and normal glucose level. CSF VDRL test is specific but generally insensitive. More recently, CSF assays measuring local production of antitreponema antibody have been advocated. IgM immunoblotting is both sensitive and specific but not widely available. The intrathecal *T. pallidum* antibody index is a ratio comparing CSF and serum IgG levels and is more widely used. Methods for identification of *T. pallidum* by PCR have not been standardized (327).

Neuroradiologic studies with MRI, though relatively insensitive in recognizing meningovascular syphilis involving the cord, may demonstrate cerebral infarcts, nonspecific white matter lesions, and meningeal enhancement (330). MRI findings of medial temporal lobe atrophy correlate clinically with the syndrome of general paresis and explain the failure of antibiotics to reverse behavioral changes (331). Magnetic resonance angiography or conventional angiography may detect arteritis in large vessels, such as reversible spasm of the carotid siphon in acute syphilitic basilar meningitis but does not disclose the small-vessel obliterative endarteritis characteristic of syphilitic leptomeningitis (332).

TREATMENT

See Chapter 105.

Neurologic Syndromes Associated with Mycoplasma Infection

CAUSE

CNS complications of *M. pneumoniae* infection are probably the most frequent extrapulmonary manifestation of this disease, but they are rare (333). Although *encephalitis* is the most common neurologic complication, *meningitis, polyradiculitis,* and *myelitis* have also been reported (334–336).

PATHOGENESIS

The exact pathogenesis of CNS disease is unknown but may be secondary to direct invasion, elaboration of neurotoxins, autoimmune complexes, or vasculitis associated with development of antiphospholipid antibodies (337).

DIAGNOSIS

A history of recent or concurrent respiratory tract infection, especially in a child or young adult, should suggest the diagnosis (338). Serologic diagnosis requires a fourfold increase in antibody titer in paired sera or a single titer greater than 1:64. Acute titers may in fact be greater than convalescent levels, because neurologic disease may present several weeks after respiratory symptoms have resolved. Standard complement fixation assays for *M. pneumoniae* are nonspecific and can cross-react with a variety of other antigens. *M. pneumoniae* can be detected in CSF specimens by PCR, but the test is not widely available (336).

TREATMENT

If active infection is present, antibiotic therapy may be effective. Tetracycline penetrates the CNS more effectively than erythromycin or other macrolides, such as azithromycin, but is usually contraindicated in children younger than 8 years because of permanent dental discoloration (339). Steroids and plasmapheresis have also been advocated but remain controversial. About 15% of patients have a poor outcome with little or no improvement in neurologic deficits.

Whipple's Disease

Whipple's disease is a systemic illness characterized by fever, systemic lymphadenopathy, malabsorption, and variable neurologic manifestations (340).

CAUSE AND PATHOGENESIS

The etiologic agent of Whipple's disease is thought to be *Tropheryma whippelii*, a gram-positive actinomycete originally identified in clinical specimens by molecular techniques and subsequently grown in human fibroblast tissue cultures (341–343). In tissues, the organism can be seen only with electron microscopy. They are located intracellularly inside the periodic acid–Schiff (PAS)–positive material that fills tissue macrophages and that is characteristic of the condition.

The pathogenesis of associated focal cranial and peripheral neuropathies is not clear, because PAS-positive material has been found only in the CNS and not in peripheral nerve biopsies (344).

EPIDEMIOLOGY

The illness affects predominantly white men and has a mean age at onset of 51 years. There are no known risk factors (345).

CLINICAL FINDINGS

Several neuropathic syndromes may accompany Whipple's diseases, including instances of *peripheral neuropathy* preceding other signs of the disease (345). Other neurologic manifestations include progressive *dementia, myoclonus* of face and arms, *ophthalmoplegia, nystagmus,* and *ataxia.* Cognitive changes, supranuclear gaze palsy, and altered level of consciousness are the most common neurologic manifestations, often with a distinctive oculomasticatory and oculofacial-skeletal myorhythmias (346). The associated *polyneuropathy* is possibly related to vitamin deficiencies secondary to malabsorption.

DIAGNOSIS AND TREATMENT

Guidelines for diagnosis and treatment of CNS Whipple's disease have been outlined by Louis et al. (346). Diagnosis is suggested by diarrhea, weight loss, and lymphadenopathy, as well as finding PAS-positive macrophages in jejunal biopsy. PCR-based molecular probes can detect the Whipple's agent in blood, other fluids (342), and tissue biopsies (341).

MRI findings of multiple gadolinium-enhancing lesions in white matter and in the gray matter–white matter junction have been reported in a biopsy-proven case of Whipple's disease with dementia (347).

Diagnosis and treatment of Whipple's disease are discussed in Chapter 79.

APPROACH TO THE PATIENT

Clinical Evaluation

The cardinal features that distinguish disorders affecting peripheral nerve, plexus, root, and cord from symptoms and signs resulting from cerebral lesions are as follows:

1. Distribution and nature of *abnormal sensations,* when present
2. *Hyporeflexia or areflexia* in the presence of weakness or flaccid paralysis, which is characteristic of all plexus, nerve, and root lesions but occurs only in the initial stages of cord injury ("spinal shock")
3. Distribution and nature of *abnormal tendon* reflexes

DISTRIBUTION OF MOTOR FUNCTION ABNORMALITIES
Examination of motor function should answer the following questions:

1. *Symmetry:* Is the weakness or paralysis symmetric or asymmetric? If asymmetric, is there evidence of bilateral lesions (crossover)?
2. *Distribution:* Is the weakness or paralysis distal or generalized ("systemic")? If generalized, did its onset begin in the lower extremities (ascending) or initially with bulbar signs (descending)? If ascending, is there evidence of involvement of the trunk, the neck, and the muscles of respiration?
3. *Anatomic correlations:* If distal, does weakness or paralysis follow anatomic patterns compatible with a spinal segment (or adjacent segments) or root; a plexus (brachial or crural), the cauda equina; or of a peripheral nerve or CN or their branches?
4. *Reflex and autonomic function:* What are the activity levels (absent, depressed, normal, hyperactive) of DTRs and other reflex responses (Babinski's response to noxious stimuli; anogenital and abdominal responses to cutaneous stimuli)? Is there sphincter dysfunction or paralysis of bladder or bowel?
5. *Spasticity or flaccidity:* Is there evidence of denervation (e.g., fasciculation, atrophy, or fatigue on repetitive effort)?

DISTRIBUTION AND TYPE OF SENSORY ABNORMALITIES
Somatic sensory symptoms (pain vs. numbness and anesthesia; dysesthesias, such as tingling, numbness, burning) may be the only abnormality reported by the patient in the early phase of several disorders and may precede objectively demonstrable sensory loss. In such cases, diminished or absent DTRs in the same distribution as sensory symptoms may be the only objective neurologic finding despite disabling symptoms.

Examination should evaluate separately responses to light touch (cotton wisp), pain (pinprick), temperature (cold or hot), and proprioception (vibration, joint position, Romberg's test) and answer the following questions:

1. *Presence or absence of sensory involvement:* Is sensation normal by history and examination?
2. *Distribution of objective findings:* If symptomatic, are objective abnormalities present? If so, are all modalities affected or only selective defects? Do they match the distribution of symptoms? Do they match the distribution of any motor weakness or paralysis?

3. *Symmetry:* Are the symptoms and signs symmetric or asymmetric? Are they distal or generalized? If generalized, are they ascending or descending? If symmetric, is there a sensory level on the trunk?

4. *Pain evaluation:* Is pain one of the sensory symptoms? Are there predictable aggravating factors (certain movements; percussion or palpation tenderness over focal areas of the spine), or is the pain constant or unpredictably intermittent?

5. *Anatomic correlation:* Does the distribution of pain and/or sensory defect follow anatomic patterns compatible with a cranial or spinal segment or root; a plexus; the cauda equina; the conus medullaris; or a peripheral nerve or CN or their branches?

6. *Associated skin and mucous membrane findings:* Are there skin lesions in the area of abnormal sensation (macules, vesicles; trophic changes; ulcers)? If complaints are of a painful unilateral cranial neuropathy, do those areas served by the nerve contain ipsilateral cutaneous vesicles (scalp, face, external auditory canal) or mucosal ulcerations (conjunctiva, tongue, palate, pharynx) that do not cross the midline?

Figure 154.3 uses the answers to these questions in the evaluation of a patient as an example of application of the neurologic data to determine possible infection-related causes of the syndrome.

CLUES TO NEUROPATHY

Neuropathy refers to injury to one or more nerves at any level along their pathways and is termed *cranial* or *peripheral* based on the nerve involved. When the level of nerve injury is proximal, the pathogenic process usually involves nerve roots and sensory ganglia. It may also extend to involve adjacent CNS structures, producing overlap syndromes in which peripheral neuropathy accompanies myelitis and/or meningitis.

Causes of neuropathy—both infectious and noninfectious—often prefer one of four anatomic patterns, as described in Table 154.1, and are further classified based on the type of functional nerve involvement: purely motor, sensory or autonomic or mixed with one functional type predominating. Although motor dysfunction is the most obvious sign of peripheral nerve disease, sensory disturbances often herald its onset. When the level of nerve injury is proximal, involving either nerve roots,

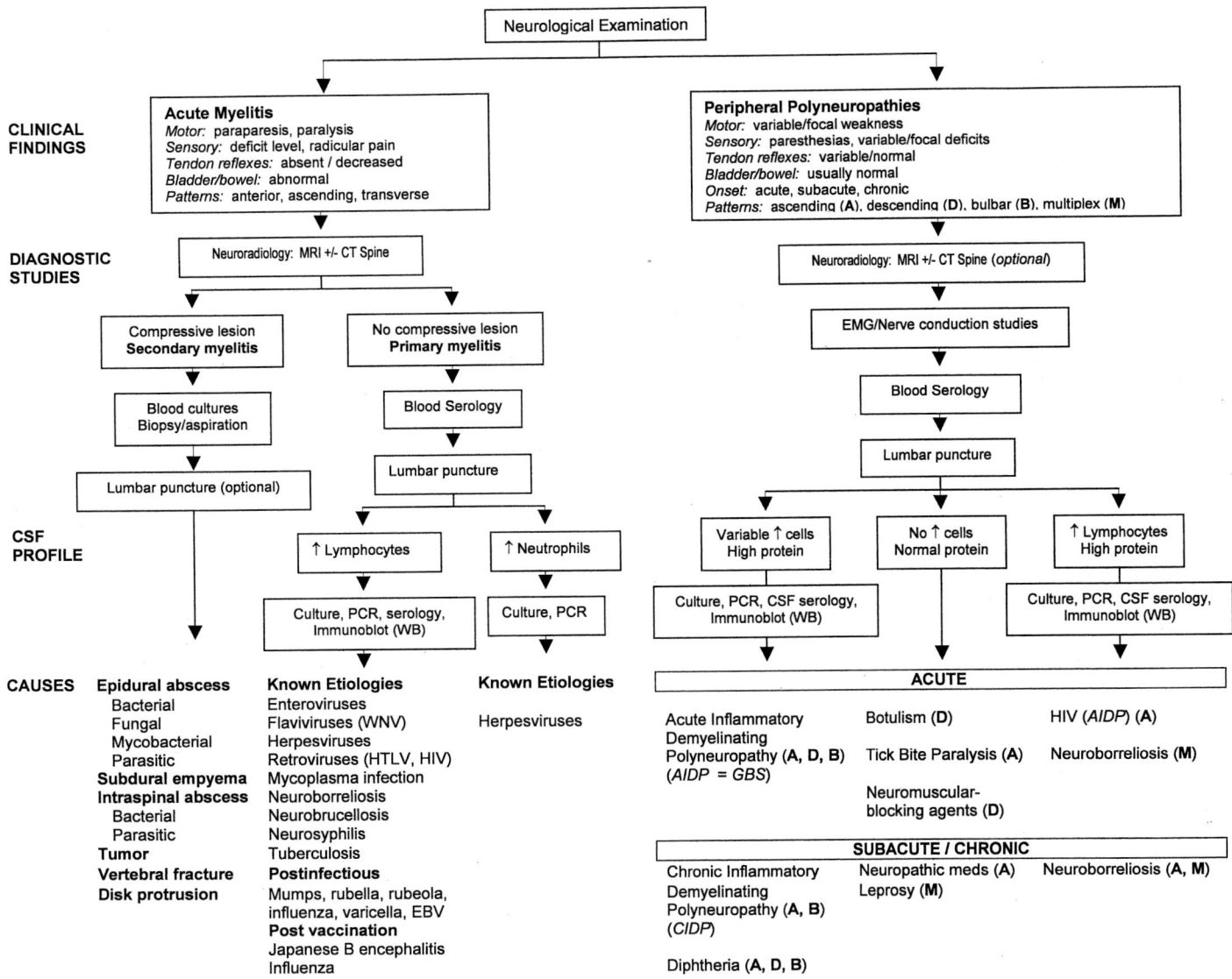

Figure 154.3. Approach to diagnostic evaluation of the patient.

APPENDIX: Diagnosis of Specific Agents Causing Infections of the Peripheral Nervous System and Spinal Cord

Organism	Neurologic disease	Isolation or detection		Antibody detection		Comments
		CSF	Blood	CSF	Blood	
Mycobacteria M. Leprae	Lepromatous and tuberculoid neuritis	Normal	Negative	Negative	N.D.	Skin and/or sensory nerve biopsy for AFB stain and PCR
Actinomycetes Tropheryma whippelii	Peripheral neuropathy, dementia, myoclonus of face and arms, ophthalmoplegia, nystagmus, and ataxia	PCR	PCR detects agent in blood, other fluids and tissues	N.D.	N.D	PAS-positive macrophages in jejunal biopsy and mesenteric lymph nodes
Spirochetes Borrelia burgdorferi	Cranial and/or peripheral neuropathies, meningitis, radiculitis in acute disease	PCR: in development	PCR: in development	Positive ELISA (IgM converts to IgG) with high specific-antibody ratio	Positive ELISA (usually IgG by stage II disease)	Organism can be isolated from blood and CSF in research labs. Serologic tests still being standardized
Treponema pallidum	Tabes dorsalis, syphilitic meningomyelitis, anterior spinal artery syndrome, and gummata of meninges and cord	PCR: in development	Negative	Positive FTA or TPHA, with confirmatory ITPA Index. IgM immunoblot VDRL (positive 50%)	Positive FTA or TPHA. Reaginic test (ART, VDRL) may be negative	Cannot be grown on artificial media; inoculation of laboratory animals is effective but insensitive
Bacteria Brucella species	Meningitis, radiculitis, myelitis, cranial neuropathy	50% positive PCR: in development	Positive	ELISA positive. Agglutinins may be undetectable	Serum agglutinin test (SAT) is positive, except B. canis	Fastidious organism: requires special isolation techniques. Positive serologic tests should be confirmed at reference lab.
Clostridium botulinum	Infant botulism, food-borne botulism, wound botulism, toxico-infectious botulism	Negative	Negative	Negative	Absent at onset of disease	Toxin detection and organism in food source and/or from GI tract in toxico-infectious and floppy baby syndrome. Anaerobic culture of site positive in wound botulism
Clostridium tetani	Local tetanus, cephalic tetanus, generalized tetanus	Negative	Negative	Negative	Absent at onset of disease	Organism often isolatable from wound (anaerobic culture)
Corynebacterium diphtheriae	Bulbar palsy (if throat is source of toxin) precedes systemic paralysis	Negative	Negative	Negative	Absent at onset of disease	Organism isolatable from throat or wound
Mycoplasma M. pneumoniae	Encephalitis, meningitis, polyradiculitis and myelitis.	N.D. PCR: positive	Special culture techniques required.	Positive	Fourfold increase in antibody titer in paired sera or a single titer greater than 1:64.	Complement fixation assays for M. pneumoniae are nonspecific and can cross react with a variety of other antigens. Acute titers may be greater than convalescent levels, because neurologic disease occurs weeks after respiratory symptoms.

Virus	Clinical syndrome					Comments
Enteroviruses						
Poliovirus	Aseptic meningitis, bulbar and/or spinal paralysis (poliomyelitis)	Low yield in viral cultures PCR positive	Positive	Positive	Positive rise in type-specific neutralization titer	Virus is isolatable from stool and throat washings
Flaviviruses						
West Nile virus (WNV)	Aseptic meningitis, acute flaccid paralysis	Positive culture PCR positive	PCR positive	Positive	Positive IgM within 8 days of illness onset	Most WNV infections are mild and often clinically inapparent. Severe disease not confined to any age group. Virus transmitted by mosquito bite, transfusions, transplanted tissues, and breast milk of asymptomatic infected persons.
Herpes viruses						
B virus	Aseptic meningitis, ascending encephalomyelitis	Low yield in viral cultures PCR under development	Negative	Positive before serum	ELISA with Western blot, or RIA	Virus isolation is dangerous! Isolatable from wound site, and/or mucous membranes and pustules
Cytomegalovirus (CMV)	Radiculitis, ascending myelitis, acute transverse myelitis, encephalitis	Low yield in viral cultures PCR positive	Viral antigen detectable by FAB (pp65) PCR positive and measures viral load	Positive if immunocompetent	Positive rise unless severely immuno-suppressed	Virus isolatable from buffy coat of peripheral blood cells in chronic disseminated CMV. CSF cytology positive in some cases.
Epstein-Barr virus (EBV)	Radiculitis, ascending myelitis, acute transverse myelitis	Low yield in viral cultures PCR positive	N.D.	Positive if immunocompetent	Positive rise unless severely immuno-suppressed	EBV also expressed in AIDS-associated B-cell lymphomas of CNS
HSV-1 and 2	Radiculitis, ascending myelitis, acute transverse myelitis, encephalitis	Positive often PCR positive	N.D.	Positive if immunocompetent	Positive rise unless severely immunosuppressed	Virus isolatable from skin lesions. Skin scraping/biopsy positive for immunodiagnosis.
Varicella-zoster virus	Radiculitis, ascending myelitis, acute transverse myelitis, cranial neuritis, encephalitis	Low yield PCR positive	N.D.	Positive if immunocompetent	Positive rise unless severely immuno-suppressed	Skin scraping/biopsy positive for immunodiagnosis.
Retroviruses						
HIV-1	Early: aseptic meningitis, cranial neuropathies, GBS Late: sensory neuropathy, mononeuropathy multiplex, vacuolar myelopathy	Early: p24 antigen and vRNA Late: variable	Positive cultures from PBMs Plasma vRNA	Early: rising ELISA titer Late: low level titers	Positive ELISA and confirmatory test	HIV-1 isolatable from CSF of some asymptomatic persons. CD4 count correlates with stage of disease
HTLV-1	Chronic meningitis, spastic paraparesis	Positive PCR positive	Positive cultures from PBMs	Oligoclonal banding ELISA and Western blot positive	ELISA and Western blot positive	Diagnosis must include other laboratory findings besides positive HTLV-1 serology

N.D. = no data

dorsal ganglia, or the course of the nerve within the subarachnoid space, the composition of the CSF will usually reflect the method of injury.

In classifying the neuropathy, the physical examination should attempt to answer the following questions: Does the involvement include more than one functional nerve type? Is involvement symmetric or asymmetric, distal, or generalized; ascending or descending? Is there a sensory level on the trunk? Do motor and sensory deficits overlap and do they match subjective complaints? What are the activity levels of the DTRs and other reflexes (e.g., Babinski's, genitoanal, and abdominal responses)? Is sphincter function normal? Is there evidence of denervation (e.g., fasciculation, atrophy, fatigability)? Are any nerves palpable? Are there skin lesions associated with the nerve deficits (e.g., anesthetic macules)?

The underlying cause determines the characteristic time course and associated clinical findings. To identify the pattern of disease, the history should focus on the rate of progression of neuropathic symptoms and their relation to antecedent or comorbid illnesses. An *acute onset* is highly suggestive of an infectious etiology, as most neuropathies resulting from infectious diseases will present acutely or subacutely. *Chronic neuropathies* of infectious etiology are less common but do occur, as exemplified by leprosy and Lyme borreliosis.

Diagnostic clues of an infectious etiology in PNS disorders may be suggested by finding risks from inadequate immunizations (diphtheria, tetanus); a recent or current systemic illness (e.g., pharyngitis in diphtheritic neuropathy); *Campylobacter* gastroenteritis (GBS); lymphadenopathy with malabsorption (Whipple's disease); epidemiologic exposures, such as tick bites (Lyme disease, tick paralysis) or consumption of unpasteurized dairy products (brucellosis) or of home-canned or salted foods (botulism); and risks for sexually transmitted diseases (syphilis, HIV, HTLV) or for autoinfection from self-injecting drugs (wound botulism, tetanus). The travel and residence history is of great diagnostic importance in suggesting geographically focused etiologies (Lyme borreliosis, brucellosis).

In general, an acute onset suggests a more favorable prognosis and should prompt a timely search for the underlying etiology to prevent permanent neurologic sequelae. By establishing the rate of onset and anatomic pattern of illness, the neuropathic syndrome can be identified and appropriate studies obtained to diagnose the cause.

CLUES TO MYELITIS

The *five cardinal manifestations of spinal cord disease* are pain, motor deficits, sensory deficits, abnormalities of reflexes/muscle tone, and bladder dysfunction. The distribution of neurologic deficits depends on the spinal segment(s) affected. Local pain occurs at the site of the lesion and can assume a radicular quality if the nerve roots are involved. Paresthesias also occur and have greater localizing value than radicular pain. Weakness is present in virtually all disorders of the spinal cord and, in myelitis, may progress over a period of hours, days, or weeks. Paraplegia and spinal shock can develop and are characterized by areflexia, atonia, and absent plantar reflexes. More slowly progressive lesions are associated with hyperreflexia and hypertonia. Bladder dysfunction is usually not an early sign of spinal cord disease, although if spinal shock develops, flaccid bladder paralysis ensues with urinary retention and overflow incontinence. Chronic myelopathies cause a small spastic bladder and result in urgency, frequency, and incontinence.

The history should explore risks for immunosuppression (low CD4 count in HIV, chronic suppression for transplantation), for hematogenous infections (intravenous drug use), recent exposure to Macaque monkeys (B virus), and travel to areas endemic for Lyme disease, West Nile virus, schistosomiasis, or cysticercosis. A history of distant and recent vaccinations should be obtained to assess the risk for poliovirus infection and possible postvaccinial myelitis or encephalitis, now uncommon since discontinuation of the older rabies and cowpox vaccines. The history or other clinical findings may suggest infectious agents known either to cause or to be associated with acute or chronic *primary myelitis,* such as skin lesions (human or simian herpesviruses, syphilis, Lyme borreliosis). An immediately preceding illness may suggest mycoplasma myelitis or postinfectious transverse myelitis, an uncommon complication of rubeola, varicella, rubella, influenza, and mumps, which is more common in younger patients.

Secondary myelitis due to inflammatory and compressive infections, such as epidural abscess, spinal subdural empyema, and intraspinal abscess, must be distinguished from primary myelitis of infectious etiology. MRI with or without enhancement contrast should be performed early to exclude an operable compressive lesion (348).

DIFFERENTIAL DIAGNOSIS

As weakness or paralysis may also arise from disorders affecting the neuromuscular junction (e.g., myasthenia gravis, neurotoxins, and drugs) or from disease of muscle itself, measurement of nerve conduction velocity and EMG is required to assess whether symptoms and signs are due to demyelination or result from degeneration, neuromuscular blockade, or primary muscle disease. Noninfectious myelopathies include tumor and other causes of myelitis, such as multiple sclerosis or systemic lupus erythematosus.

The differential diagnosis of neurologic symptoms and signs requires consultation with a neurologist. However, the precise location of peripheral lesions and possible infectious causes can be surmised by careful examination of the patient, analysis of CSF, and use of relevant imaging techniques, as indicated in the appendix.

ACKNOWLEDGMENT

We gratefully acknowledge assistance in prior editions by Pierre DeJace, MD (1992), Timothy Leach, MD, MPH&TM (1997) (349), Poh-Lian Lim, MD, MPH&TM (1999) (350), and the many years of stimulation and encouragement by Morton N. Swartz, MD, Raymond D. Adams, MD, C. Miller Fisher, MD, and other colleagues at the Massachusetts General Hospital.

REFERENCES

1. Victor M, Ropper AH, eds. *Principles of neurology,* 7th ed. New York: McGraw Hill, 2001.
2. *Merritt's neurology.* Philadelphia: Lippincott Williams & Wilkins, 2000.
2a. Graham DI, Lantos PL, eds. *Greenfield's neuropathology,* 7th ed. New York: Oxford University Press, 2002.
3. Menezes AH, Graf CJU, Perret GE. Spinal cord abscess; a review. *Surg Neurol* 1977;8:461.
4. Jopling WH, McDougall AC. *Handbook of leprosy.* Oxford: Butterworth–Heinemann, 1988.
5. Jacobson RR. Leprosy (Hansen's disease). In: Rakel RE, ed. *Cohn's current therapy,* 52nd ed. Philadelphia: WB Saunders, 2000:91–94.
6. Haimanot RT, Melaku Z. Leprosy. *Curr Opin Neurol* 2000;13(3):317–322.
7. Bryceson A, Pfaltxgraff RE. Leprosy. In: *Medicine in the tropics,* 3rd ed. Edinburgh: Churchill Livingstone, 1990:1–239.
8. Ramadan W, Mourad B, Fadel W, et al. Clinical, electrophysiological, and immunopathological study of peripheral nerves in Hansen's disease. *Lepr Rev* 2001;72(1):35–49.
9. Brennan PJ. Skin testing development in leprosy: progress with first-generation skin test antigens, and approach to the second generation. *Lepr Rev* 2000;71[Suppl]:S50–S54.

10. Montecucco C, Schiavo G. Structure and function of tetanus and botulinum neurotoxins. *Q Rev Biophys* 1995;28(4):423–472.
11. Pellizzari R, Rossetto O, Schiavo G, et al. Tetanus and botulinum neurotoxins: mechanism of action and therapeutic uses. *Philos Trans R Soc Lond B Biol Sci* 1999;354:258–268.
12. Allen SD, Emery CL, Siders JA. *Clostridium*. In: Murray PR, Baron EJ, Pfaller MA, et al, eds. *Manual of clinical microbiology*, 7th ed. Washington, DC: ASM Press, 1999:654–671.
13. Arnon SS, Schecter R, Inglesby TV, et al. Botulinum toxin as a biological weapon: medical and public health management. *JAMA* 2001;285(8):1059–1070.
14. Gimenez JA, Gimenez MA, DasGupta BR. Characterization of the neurotoxin isolated from a *Clostridium barati* strain implicated in infant botulism. *Infect Immun* 1992;60:518–522.
15. Salazar-Grueso EF, Arnason BGW. Peripheral nerve disease caused by infection, toxins and post infectious syndromes. In: Schlossberg D, ed. *Clinical topics in infectious diseases: infections of the nervous system*. New York: Springer-Verlag, 1990:192–206.
16. Thorne FL, Kropp RJ. Wound botulism: a life-threatening complication of hand injuries. *Plast Reconstr Surg* 1983;71:548.
17. Woodruff BA, Griffin PM, McCroskey LM, et al. Clinical and laboratory comparison of botulism from toxin types A, B, and E in the United States, 1975–1988. *J Infect Dis* 1992;166:1281–1286.
18. Shapiro RL, Hatheway C, Swerdlow DL. Botulism in the United States: a clinical and epidemiological review. *Ann Intern Med* 1998;129(3):221–228.
19. Carduso F, Jankovic J. Clinical use of botulinum neurotoxins. *Curr Top Microbiol Immunol* 1995;195:55–75.
20. Figgitt DP, Noble S. Botulinum toxin B: a review of its therapeutic potential in the management of cervical dystonia. *Drugs* 2002;62:705–722.
21. Centers for Disease Control and Prevention. Type B botulism associated with roasted eggplant in oil—Italy, 1993. *MMWR Morb Mortal Wkly Rep* 1995;44(2):33–36.
22. Townes JM, Cieslak PR, Hatheway CL, et al. An outbreak of type A botulism associated with a commercial cheese sauce. *Ann Intern Med* 1996;125(7):558–563.
23. Terranova T. *Botulism*. In: Evans AS, Feldman HA, eds. *Bacterial infections of humans: epidemiology and control*. New York: Plenum Publishing, 1982:105–118.
24. Brown KL. Control of bacterial spores. *Br Med Bull* 2000;56:158–171.
25. Suranyi A, Milano M. Infantile botulism: clinical and laboratory observations of a rare neuroparalytic disease. *J Paediatr Child Health* 2000;36(2):193–195.
26. Hughes JM, Blumenthal JR, Merson JM, et al. Clinical features of type A and B botulism. *Ann Intern Med* 1981;95:442.
27. Cherington M. Clinical spectrum of botulism. *Muscle Nerve* 1998;21:701–710.
28. Sheth RD, Lotz BP, Hecox KE, et al. Infantile botulism: pitfalls in electrodiagnosis. *J Child Neurol* 1999;14(3):156–158.
29. Hatheway CL. Laboratory procedures for cases of suspected infant botulism. *Rev Infect Dis* 1979;1:647.
30. Lindstrom M, Keto R, Markkula A, et al. Multiplex PCR assay for detection and identification of *Clostridium botulinum* types A, B, E, and F in food and fecal material. *Appl Environ Microbiol* 2001;67:5694–5699.
31. Chia JK, Clark JB, Ruan CA, et al. Botulism in an adult associated with food-borne intestinal infection with *Clostridium botulinum*. *N Engl J Med* 1986;315:239.
32. Centers for Disease Control and Prevention. Diagnosis and Management of foodborne illness. A primer for physicians. *MMWR Morb Mortal Wkly Rep* 2001;50(RR-2):1–20.
33. Centers for Disease Control and Prevention. Wound botulism—California 1995. *MMWR Morb Mortal Wkly Rep* 1995;44:889–892.
34. Funke G, Bernard K. Coryneforme Gram-positive rods. In: Murray PR, Baron EJ, Pfaller MA, et al, eds. *Manual of clinical microbiology*, 7th ed. Washington, DC: ASM Press, 1999:319–345.
35. Efstratiou A, George RC. Laboratory guidelines for the diagnosis of infections caused by *Corynebacterium diphtheriae* and *C. ulcerans*. World Health Organization. *Commun Dis Public Health* 1999;2(4):250–257.
36. Holmes RK. Biology and molecular epidemiology of diphtheria toxin and the *tox* gene. *J Infect Dis* 2000;181[Suppl]:67.
37. Hadfield TL, McEvoy P, Polotsky Y, et al. The pathology of diphtheria. *J Infect Dis* 2000;181[Suppl]:20.
38. Centers for Disease Control and Prevention. Respiratory diphtheria caused by *Corynebacterium ulcerans*—Terre Haute, Indiana, 1996. *MMWR Morb Mortal Wkly Rep* 1997;46(15):330–332.
39. Bisno AL. Acute pharyngitis. *N Engl J Med* 2001;344:205–211.
40. Logina I, Donaghy M. Diphtheritic polyneuropathy: a clinical study and comparison with Guillain-Barré syndrome. *J Neurol Neurosurg Psychol* 1999;67(4):433–438.
41. Groundstroem KW, Molnar G, Lumio J. Echocardiographic follow-up of diphtheritic myocarditis. *Cardiology* 1996;87:79–81.
42. Farizo KM, Strebel PM, Chen RT, et al. Fatal respiratory disease due to *Corynebacterium diphtheriae*: case report and review of guidelines for management, investigation and control. *Clin Infect Dis* 1993;16:59–88.
43. Efstratiou A, Engler KH, Mazurova IK, et al. Current approaches to the laboratory diagnosis of diphtheria. *J Infect Dis* 2000;181[Suppl 1]:S138–S145.
44. Booth LV, Ellis C, Wale MC, et al. An atypical case of *Corynebacterium diphthe-*

riae endocarditis and subsequent outbreak control measures. *J Infect* 1995;31:63–65.
45. Pennie RA, Malik AS, Wilcox L. Misidentification of toxigenic *Corynebacterium diphtheriae* as a *Corynebacterium* species with low virulence in a child with endocarditis. *J Clin Microbiol* 1996;34:1275–1276.
46. Weinstein L. Current concepts: tetanus. *N Engl J Med* 1973;289:1293.
47. Allen SD, Emery CL, Siders JA. Clostridium. In: Murray PR, Baron EJ, Pfaller MA, et al, eds. *Manual of clinical microbiology*, 7th ed. Washington, DC: ASM Press, 1999:654–671.
48. Pellizzari R, Rossetto O, Schiavo G, et al. Tetanus and botulinum neurotoxins: mechanism of action and therapeutic uses. *Philos Trans R Soc Lond B Biol Sci* 1999;354:259–268.
49. Fernandez JM, Ferrandiz M, Larrea L, et al. Cephalic tetanus studied with single fibre EMG. *J Neurol Psychol Neurosurg* 1983;46:862–866.
50. Bagetta G, Nistico C. T⸻⸻⸻⸻⸻⸻⸻⸻⸻⸻⸻dy mechanisms of neuron⸻⸻⸻⸻⸻⸻⸻⸻⸻⸻acol Ther 1994;62:29–39.
51. Bennett J, Ma J, Tra⸻⸻⸻⸻⸻⸻⸻⸻⸻⸻th topical umbilical ghee; co⸻⸻⸻⸻⸻⸻⸻⸻⸻(6):1172–1175.
52. Faust RA, Vickers ⸻⸻⸻⸻⸻⸻⸻⸻⸻⸻t Charity Hospital. *J Trauma* ⸻⸻⸻⸻⸻⸻⸻⸻
53. Wesley AG, Haripa⸻⸻⸻⸻⸻⸻⸻⸻⸻reatment of sympathetic ner⸻⸻⸻⸻⸻⸻⸻243.
54. Farrar JJ, Yen LM,⸻⸻⸻⸻⸻⸻⸻⸻*Psychiatry* 2000;69:292–301.
55. Dastur FD, Shahan⸻⸻⸻⸻⸻⸻⸻⸻nstration of a dual lesion. *J N*⸻⸻⸻⸻⸻⸻
56. Phillips LA. A classification of tetanus. *Lancet* 1967;1:1216–1217.
57. Veronesi R, Gocaccia R. The clinical picture. In: Veronesi R, ed. *Tetanus: important new concepts*. Amsterdam: Excerpta Medica, 1981:183–210.
58. Udwadia FE. *Tetanus*. New York: Oxford University Press, 1994.
59. Patel JC, Mehta BC. Tetanus: study of 8,697 cases. *Indian J Med Sci* 1999;53(9):393–401.
60. Ropper AH. Current concepts: the Guillain-Barré syndrome. *N Engl J Med* 1992;326:1130–1136.
61. Verma A. Epidemiology and clinical features of HIV-1 associated neuropathies. *J Peripher Nerv Syst* 2001;6:8–13.
62. Rees J. Guillain-Barré syndrome. Clinical manifestations and directions for treatment. *Drugs* 1995;49:912–920.
63. Schoenberger LB, Hurwitz ES, Katona P, et al. Guillain-Barré syndrome: its epidemiology and associations with influenza vaccines. *Ann Neurol* 1981;9[Suppl]:31.
64. Govoni V, Granieri E. Epidemiology of the Guillain-Barré syndrome. *Curr Opin Neurol* 2001;14:605–613.
65. Cuadrado JI, de Pedro-Cuesta J, Ara JR, et al. Guillain-Barré syndrome in Spain, 1985–1997: epidemiological and public health views. *Eur Neurol* 2001;46:83–91.
66. Hadden RD, Karch H, Hartung HP, et al. Preceding infections, immune factors, and outcome in Guillain-Barré syndrome. *Neurology* 2001;56:758–765.
67. De Klippel N, Hautekeete ML, De Keyser J, et al. Guillain-Barré syndrome as the presenting manifestation of hepatitis C infection. *Neurology* 1993;43:2143–2145.
68. De Klippel N, Hautekeete ML, De Keyser J, et al. Guillain-Barré syndrome as the presenting manifestation of hepatitis C infection. *Neurology* 1993;43:2143–2145.
69. Feasby TE. Inflammatory-demyelinating polyneuropathies. *Neurol Clin* 1992;10(3):651–670.
70. Ropper AH. *Campylobacter* diarrhea and Guillain-Barré syndrome. *Arch Neurol* 1988;45:655–656.
71. Parry GJ. Peripheral neuropathies associated with human immunodeficiency virus infection. *Ann Neurol* 1988;23[Suppl]:S49–S53.
72. Miller RG, Kipriv DD, Barry G, et al. Peripheral nervous system dysfunction in acquired immunodeficiency syndrome. In: Dr MLR, Levey RM, Bredesen ED, eds. *AIDS and the nervous system*. New York: Raven Press, 1988:65–78.
73. Lange DJ. AAEM Minimonograph no. 41: neuromuscular diseases associated with HIV-1 infection. *Muscle Nerve* 1994;17:16–39.
74. Griffin JW, Wesselingh, Griffin DE, et al. Peripheral nerve disorders in HIV infection. Similarities and contrasts with CNS disorders. In: Price RW, Perry SW, eds. *HIV, AIDS and the Brain*. New York: Raven Press, 1994:159–182.
75. El-Sabrout RA, Radovancevic B, Ankoma-Sey V, et al. Guillain-Barré syndrome after solid organ transplantation. *Transplantation* 2001;71:1311–1316.
76. Hurwitz ES, Holman RC, Nelson DB, et al. National surveillance for Guillain-Barré syndrome. *Neurology* 1983;33:150.
77. Guillain-Barré Syndrome Study Group. Guillain-Barré syndrome: an Italian multicentre case-control study. *Neurol Sci* 2000;21:229–234.
78. Chowdhury D, Arora A. Axonal Guillain-Barré syndrome: a critical review. *Acta Neurol Scand* 2001;103:267–277.
79. Prineas JB. Pathology of the Guillain-Barré syndrome. *Ann Neurol* 1981;9[Suppl]:6.
80. Hall SM, Hughes RA, Atkinson PF, et al. Motor nerve biopsy in severe Guillain-Barré syndrome. *Ann Neurol* 1992;31:441–444.
81. Honavar M, Tharakan JK, Hughes RA, et al. A clinicopathologic study of the Guillain-Barré syndrome. Nine cases and literature review. *Brain* 1991;114:1245–1269.

82. Feasby TE, Hahn AF, Brown WF, et al. Severe axonal degeneration in acute Guillain-Barré syndrome: evidence of two different mechanisms? *J Neurol Sci* 1993;116:185–192.

83. Hughes R, Atkinson P, Coates P, et al. Sural nerve biopsies in Guillain-Barré syndrome: axonal degeneration and macrophage-associated demyelination and absence of CMV genome. *Muscle Nerve* 1992;15:568–575.

84. Hughes RA, Hadden RD, Gregson NA, et al. Pathogenesis of Guillain-Barré syndrome. *J Neuroimmunol* 1999;100(1-2):74–97.

85. Connolly AM, Pestronk A. Anti-tubulin autoantibodies in acquired demyelinating polyneuropathies. *J Infect Dis* 1997;176[Suppl 9].

86. Koga M, Yuki N, Hirata K. Antiganglioside antibody in patients with Guillain-Barré syndrome who show bulbar palsy as an initial symptoms. *J Neurol Neurosurg Psychiatry* 1999;66:513–516.

87. Kuwubara S, Yuki N, Koga M, et al. IgG anti-G_{M1} antibody is associated with reversible conduction failure and axonal degeneration in Guillain-Barré syndrome. *Ann Neurol* 1998;44:202–208.

88. Nachamkin I, Engberg J, Gutacker M, et al. Molecular population genetic analysis of *Campylobacter jejuni* HS:19 associated with Guillain-Barré syndrome and gastroenteritis. *J Infect Dis* 2001;184:221–226.

89. Ma JJ, Nishimura M, Mine H, et al. HLA and T-cell receptor gene polymorphisms in Guillain-Barré syndrome. *Neurology* 1998;51:379–384.

90. Van der Pol WL, van den Berg LH, Scheepers RH, et al. IgG receptor IIa alleles determine susceptibility and severity of Guillain-Barré syndrome. *Neurology* 2000:1661–1665.

91. The French Cooperative Group on Plasma Exchange in Guillain-Barré Syndrome. Appropriate number of plasma exchanges in Guillain-Barré syndrome. *Ann Neurol* 1997;41:298–306.

92. The Italian Guillain-Barré Study Group. The prognosis and main prognostic indicators of Guillain-Barré syndrome. A multicentre prospective study of 297 patients. *Brain* 1996;119:2053–2061.

93. Oh SJ, LaGanke C, Claussen GC. Sensory Guillain-Barré syndrome. *Neurology* 2001;56:82–86.

94. Sauron B, Bouche P, Cathala HP, et al. Miller-Fisher syndrome: clinical and electrophysiological evidence of peripheral origin in 10 cases. *Neurology* 1984;34:953.

95. Gibbels E, Giebisch U. Natural course of acute and chronic monophasic inflammatory demyelinating polyneuropathies (IDP). A retrospective analysis of 266 cases. *Acta Neurol Scand* 1992;85:282–291.

96. Emilia-Romagna Study Group on Clinical and Epidemiological Problems in Neurology. Guillain-Barré syndrome variants in Emilia-Romagna, Italy, 1992–3: incidence, clinical features, and prognosis. *J Neurol Neurosurg Psychiatry* 1998;65:218–224.

97. Araga S, Kagimoto H, Adachi A, et al. Kappa/lambda ratios of IgG, IgA and IgM in the cerebrospinal fluid of patients with Guillain-Barré syndrome. *Jpn J Med* 1991;30:118–122.

98. Cook SD, Doling PC. The role of autoantibodies and immune complexes in the pathogenesis of Guillain-Barré syndrome. *Ann Neurol* 1981;9:70.

99. Petty RK, Duncan R, Jamal GA, et al. Brainstem encephalitis and the Miller-Fisher syndrome. *J Neurol Neurosurg Psychol* 1993;56:201–203.

100. Urushitani M, Udaka F, Kameyama M. Miller-Fisher-Guillain-Barré overlap syndrome with enhancing lesions in the spinocerebellar tracts. *J Neurol Neurosurg Psychol* 1995;58:241–243.

101. Fulbright RK, Erdum E, Sze G, et al. Cranial nerve enhancement in the Guillain Barre syndrome. *Am J Neuroradiol* 1995;16[Suppl 4]:923–925.

102. Georgy BA, Chong B, Chamberlain M, et al. MR of the spine in Guillain-Barré syndrome. *Am J Neuroradiol* 1994;15:300–301.

103. Patel H, Garg BP, Edwards MK. MRI of Guillain-Barré syndrome. *J Comput Assist Tomogr* 1993;17:651–651.

104. Crino PB, Zimmerman R, Laskowitz D, et al. Magnetic resonance imaging of the cauda equina in Guillain-Barré syndrome. *Neurology* 1994;44:1334–1336.

105. Talpos D, Tien RD, Hesselink JR. Magnetic resonance imaging of AIDS-related polyradiculopathy. *Neurology* 1991;41:1995–1997.

106. Gordon PH, Wilbourn AJ. Early electrodiagnostic findings in Guillain-Barré syndrome. *Arch Neurol* 2001;58:913–917.

107. Cohen BA, McArthur JC, Grohman S, et al. Neurologic prognosis of cytomegalovirus polyradiculopathy in AIDS. *Neurology* 1993;43:493–499.

108. Kincaid JC. Tick bite paralysis. *Semin Neurol* 1990;10:32.

109. Centers for Disease Control and Prevention. Tick paralysis—Washington, 1995. *MMWR Morb Mortal Wkly Rep* 1996;45(16):325–326.

110. Hartung HP, Kieseier BC, Kiefer R. Progress in Guillain-Barré syndrome. *Curr Opin Neurol* 2001;14:597–604.

111. Lindenbaum Y, Kissel JT, Mendell JR. Treatment approaches for Guillain-Barré syndrome and chronic inflammatory demyelinating polyradiculoneuropathy. *Neurol Clin* 2001;19(1):187–204.

112. Lawn ND, Fletcher DD, Henderson RD, et al. Anticipating mechanical ventilation in Guillain-Barré syndrome. *Arch Neurol* 2001;58:893–898.

113. Sater RA, Rostami A. Treatment of Guillain-Barré syndrome with intravenous immunoglobulin. *Neurology* 1998;51[Suppl 5]:15.

114. Esperou H, Jars-Guincestre MC, Bolgert F, et al. Cost analysis of plasma-exchange therapy for the treatment of Guillain-Barré syndrome. French Cooperative Group on Plasma Exchange in Guillain-Barré syndrome. *Intensive Care Med* 2000;26:1094–1100.

115. Van der Meche FGA, Schmitz PIM, and the Dutch Guillain-Barré Study Group. A randomized trial comparing intravenous immune globulin and plasma exchange in Guillain-Barré syndrome. *N Engl J Med* 1992;326:1123–1129.

116. van Doorn PA, Brand A, Strengers PFW, et al. High-dose intravenous immunoglobulin treatment in chronic inflammatory demyelinating polyneuropathy: a double blind, placebo-controlled, cross-over study. *Neurology* 1992;40:209–212.

117. Plasma Exchange/Sandoglobulin Guillain-Barré Syndrome Trial Group. Randomized trial of plasma exchange, intravenous immunoglobulin, and combined treatments in Guillain-Barré syndrome. *Lancet* 1997;349:225–230.

118. Kuwarbara S, Mori M, Ogawara K, et al. Intravenous immunoglobulin therapy for Guillain-Barré syndrome with IgG anti-G_{M1} antibody. *Muscle Nerve* 2001;24:54–58.

119. Raphael JC, Chevret S, Harboun M, et al. The French Guillain-Barré Syndrome Cooperative Group. Intravenous immune globulins in patients with Guillain-Barré syndrome and contraindications to plasma exchange: 3 days versus 6 days. *J Neurol Psychiatry* 2001;71:235–238.

120. Wollinsky KH, Hulser PJ, Brinkmeir H, et al. CSF filtration is an effective treatment of Guillain-Barré syndrome: a randomized clinical trial. *Neurology* 2001;57:774–780.

121. Centers for Disease Control and Prevention. Renal insufficiency and failure associated with immune globulin intravenous therapy, 1985–1998. *MMWR Morb Mortal Wkly Rep* 1999;48:518–521.

122. Visser LH, van der Meche FG, Meulstee J, et al. Risk factors for treatment related clinical fluctuations Guillain-Barré syndrome. Dutch Guillain-Barré study group. *J Neurol Neurosurg Psychiatry* 1998;64:242–244.

123. Guillain-Barré Syndrome Steroid Trial Group. Double-blind trial of intravenous methylprednisolone in Guillain-Barré syndrome. *Lancet* 1993;341:586–590.

124. Hughes RA, van Der Meche FG. Corticosteroids for treating Guillain-Barré syndrome. *Cochrane Database Syst Rev* 2000;(3):CD001446.

125. Dowling PC, Blumberg GM, Cook SD. Guillain-Barré syndrome. In: *Handbook of clinical neurology*. Amsterdam: Elsevier, 1987:239.

126. Bernsen RA, Jager AE, Schmitz PI, et al. Long-term sensory deficit after Guillain-Barré syndrome. *J Neurol* 2001;248:483–486.

127. Hattori N, Misu K, Koike H, et al. Age of onset influences clinical features of chronic inflammatory demyelinating polyneuropathy. *J Neurol Sci* 2001:57–63.

128. Sghirlanzoni A, Solari A, Ciano C, et al. Chronic inflammatory demyelinating polyradiculopathy: long-term course and treatment of 60 patients. *Neurol Sci* 2000;21:31–37.

129. Mendell JR. Chronic inflammatory demyelinating polyradiculopathy. *Annu Rev Med* 1993;44:211–219.

130. Hahn AF, Bolton CF, Zochodne D, et al. Intravenous immunoglobulin treatment in chronic inflammatory demyelinating polyneuropathy. A double-blind, placebo controlled cross-over study. *Brain* 1996:1067–1077.

131. Gorson KC, Ropper AH, Weinberg DH. Upper limb predominant, multifocal chronic inflammatory demyelinating polyneuropathy. *Muscle Nerve* 1999:758–765.

132. Koguchi Y, Yamada T, Kuwabara S, et al. Increased CD4 in demyelinating neuropathy indicates radicular involvement. *Acta Neurol Scand* 1995;91:58–61.

133. Bertorini T, Halford H, Lawrence J, et al. Contrast-enhanced magnetic resonance imaging of the lumbosacral roots in the dysimmune inflammatory polyneuropathies. *J Neuroimaging* 1995;5:9–15.

134. Haq RU, Fries TJ, Pendlebury WW, et al. Chronic inflammatory demyelinating polyradiculopathy: a study of proposed electrodiagnostic and histologic criteria. *Arch Neurol* 2000;57:1745–1750.

135. Hahn AF, Bolton CF, Chalk C, et al. Plasma-exchange therapy in chronic inflammatory demyelinating polyneuropathy. A double-blind, sham-controlled, cross-over study. *Brain* 1996;119:1055–1066.

136. Hughes R, Bensa S, Willison H, et al. Randomized controlled trial of intravenous immunoglobulin versus oral prednisolone in chronic inflammatory demyelinating polyradiculopathy. *Ann Neurol* 2001;50:195–201.

137. Hahn AF. Treatment of chronic inflammatory demyelinating polyneuropathy with intravenous immunoglobulin. *Neurology* 1998;51:[Suppl 5]:21.

138. Mendell JR, Barohn RJ, Freimer ML, et al. Randomized controlled trial of IVIg in untreated chronic inflammatory demyelinating polyradiculopathy. *Neurology* 2001;56:445–449.

139. Dalakas MC, Pezeshkpour GH. Neuromuscular diseases associated with human immunodeficiency virus infection. *Ann Neurol* 1988;23[Suppl]:S38–S48.

140. Kolson DL, Gonzalez-Scarano F. HIV-associated neuropathies: role of HIV-1, CMV and other viruses. *J Peripher Nerv Syst* 2001;6:2–7.

141. Miller RG, Kipriv DD, Barry G, et al. Peripheral nervous system dysfunction in acquired immunodeficiency syndrome. In: Miller RG, Levey RM, Bredesen ED, eds. *AIDS and the nervous system*. New York: Raven Press, 1988:65–78.

142. Brew BJ, Sidtis JJ, Petito CK, et al. The neurologic complications of AIDS and human immunodeficiency virus. In: Plum F, ed. *Advances in contemporary neurology*. Philadelphia: FA Davis, 1988.

143. McArthur JC. Neurologic manifestations of AIDS. *Medicine* 1987;66:407.

144. Lipkin WI, Parry G, Kiprov D, et al. Inflammatory neuropathy in homosexual men with lymphadenopathy. *Neurology* 1985;35:1479.

145. Pardo CA, Mc Arthur JC, Griffin JW. HIV neuropathy: insights into the pathology of HIV peripheral nerve disease. *J Peripher Nerv Syst* 2001;6:21–27.

146. Guidelines for the use of antiretroviral agents in HIV-infected adults and adolescents: living document 2002. Available at: *hivatis.org/trtgdlns.html*.

147. Simpson DM, Olney R, McArthur JC, et al. A placebo-controlled trial of lamotrigine for painful HIV-associated neuropathy. *Neurology* 2000;54:2115–2119.

148. Paice JA, Ferrans CE, Lashley FR, et al. Topical capsaicin in the management of HIV-associated peripheral neuropathy. *J Pain Symptom Manage* 2000;19:45–52.

149. Morgello S, Simpson DM. Multifocal cytomegalovirus demyelinative polyneuropathy associated with AIDS. *Muscle Nerve* 1994;17:176–182.

150. Said G, Lacroix C, Chemouilli P, et al. Cytomegalovirus neuropathy in acquired immunodeficiency syndrome: a clinical and pathological study. *Ann Neurol* 1991;29:139–146.

151. Karmochkine M, Molina J-M, Scieux C, et al. Combined therapy with ganciclovir and foscarnet for cytomegalovirus polyradiculomyelitis in patients with AIDS. *Am J Med* 1994;97:196–197.

152. Gozlan J, Salord J-M, Roullet E, et al. Rapid detection of cytomegalovirus DNA in cerebrospinal fluid of AIDS patients with neurologic disorders. *J Infect Dis* 1992;166:1416–1421.

153. Hayden FG. Antiviral agents. In: Mandell GL, Bennett JE, Dolin R, eds. *Principles and practice of infectious diseases*, 4th ed. New York: Churchill Livingstone, 1995:411–450.

154. Simpson DM, Olney RK. Peripheral neuropathies associated with human immunodeficiency virus infection. *Neurol Clin* 1992;10(3):685–711.

155. Gilchrist JM. AAEM Case report no. 26: seventh cranial neuropathy. *Muscle Nerve* 1993;16:447–452.

156. Gluck T, Degenhardt E, Scholmerich J, et al. Autonomic neuropathy in patients with HIV: course, impact of disease stage, and medication. *Clin Autonom Res* 2000;10:17–22.

157. Nordli DR, Bello JA, DeVivo DC. Myelitis. In: Schlossberg D, ed. *Clinical topics in infectious diseases: infections of the nervous system*. New York: Springer-Verlag, 1990:179–191.

158. Jeffrey DR, Mandler RN, Davis LE. Transverse myelitis. Retrospective analysis of 33 cases, with differentiation of cases associated with multiple sclerosis and parainfectious events. *Arch Neurol* 1993;50:532–535.

159. Stoner GL. Implications of progressive multifocal leukoencephalopathy and JC virus for the etiology of MS. *Acta Neurol Scand* 1991;83:20–33.

160. Cumming WJ. Myelitis and toxic, inflammatory and infectious disorders. *Curr Opin Neurol Neurosurg* 1992;5:549–553.

161. Corboy JR, Price RW. Myelitis and toxic, inflammatory and infectious disorders. *Curr Opin Neurol Neurosurg* 1993;6:564–570.

162. Graber D, Fossoud C, Grouteau E, et al. Acute transverse myelitis and coxsackie A9 virus infection. *Pediatr Infect Dis* 1990;13:77.

163. Modlin JF. Coxsackie viruses, echoviruses and newer enteroviruses. In: Mandell GL, Bennett JE, Dolin R, eds. *Principles and practice of infectious diseases*, 4th ed. New York: Churchill Livingstone, 1995:1620–1636.

164. Rotbart HA. Enteroviruses. In: Murray PR, Baron EJ, Pfaller MA, et al. *Manual of clinical microbiology*, 7th ed. Washington, DC: ASM Press, 1999:990–998.

165. Centers for Disease Control and Prevention. Enterovirus surveillance—United States, 1997–1999. *MMWR Morb Mortal Wkly Rep* 2000;49(40):913–916.

166. Ito M, Nishibe Y, Inoue YK. Isolation of Inoue-Melnick virus from cerebrospinal fluid of patients with epidemic neuropathy in Cuba. *Arch Pathol Lab Med* 1998;122:520–522.

167. Pitella JE. Neuroschistosomiasis. *Brain Pathol* 1997;7:649–662.

168. Kleinschmidt-DeMasters BK, DeBiasi RL, Tyler KL. Polymerase chain reaction as a diagnostic adjunct in herpesvirus infections of the nervous system. *Brain Pathol* 2001:452–464.

169. Centers for Disease Control and Prevention. Apparent global interruption of wild poliovirus type 2 transmission. *MMWR Morb Mortal Wkly Rep* 2001;50(12):222–224.

170. Centers for Disease Control and Prevention. Public health dispatch: Acute flaccid paralysis associated with circulating vaccine-derived poliovirus—Philippines, 2001. *MMWR Morb Mortal Wkly Rep* 2001;50(40);874–571.

171. Ramlow J, Alexander M, LaPorte R, et al. Epidemiology of the post-polio syndrome. *Am J Epidemiol* 1992;136:769–786.

172. Stanghelle JK, Festvag LV. Postpolio syndrome: a 5 year follow-up. *Spinal Cord* 1997;35:503–508.

173. Chowers MY, Lang R, Nassar F, et al. West Nile virus: clinical characteristics of the West Nile fever outbreak, Israel, 2000. *Emerg Infect Dis* 2001;7:675–678.

173a. Centers for Disease Control and Prevention. Acute flaccid paralysis syndrome associated with West Nile virus infection—Mississippi and Louisiana, July–August 2002. *MMWR Morb Mortal Wkly Rep* 2002;51(37):825–828.

173b. Petersen LR, Martin AA. West Nile virus: a primer for clinicians. [Review] *Annals Int Med* 2002;137:173–179.

173c. Centers of Disease Control and Prevention. Intrauterine West Nile virus infection—New York, 2002. *MMWR Morb Mortal Wkly Rep* 2002;51(50):1135–1136.

173d. Iwamoto M. Transmission of West Nile virus from an organ donor to four transplant recipients. *New Engl J Med* 2003;348:2196–2203.

174. Centers for Disease Control and Prevention. Progress toward global poliomyelitis eradication, 1985–1994. *MMWR Morb Mortal Wkly Rep* 1995;44:273–281.

175. Holmes GP, Chapman LE, Stewart JA, et al, and the B Virus Working Group. Guidelines for the prevention and treatment of B-virus infections in exposed persons. *Clin Infect Dis* 1995;20:421–439.

176. Centers for Disease Control and Prevention. Publication of guidelines for the prevention and treatment of B virus infections in exposed persons. *MMWR Morb Mortal Wkly Rep* 1995;45:96–97.

177. Gosztonyi G, Falke D, Ludwig H. Axonal and transsynaptic (transneuronal) spread of *Herpesvirus simiae* (B virus) in experimentally infected mice. *Histol Histopathol* 1992;7:63–74.

178. Centers for Disease Control and Prevention. Fatal Cercopithecine herpesvirus 1 (B virus) infection following a mucocutaneous exposure and interim recommendations for worker protection. *MMWR Morb Mortal Wkly Rep* 1998;47(49):1073–1083.

179. Artenstein AW, Hicks CB, Goodwin BS Jr, et al. Human infection with B virus following a needle stick injury. *Rev Infect Dis* 1991;13:288–291.

180. De La Blanchardiere A, Rozenberg F, Caumes E, et al. Neurological complications of varicella-zoster in adults with human immunodeficiency virus infection. *Scand J Infect Dis* 2000;32:262–269.

181. Miles C, Hoffman W, Lai C-W, et al. Cytomegalovirus-associated transverse myelitis. *Neurology* 1993;43:2143–2145.

182. Holland NR, Power C, Mathews VP, et al. Cytomegalovirus encephalitis in acquired immunodeficiency syndrome (AIDS). *Neurology* 1994;44:507–514.

183. Barohn RJ, Bazan C, Jackson CE. Cytomegalovirus radiculomyelitis [Letter]. *Neurology* 1993;43:2421.

184. Tyler KL, Gross RA, Cascino GD. Unusual viral causes of transverse myelitis: hepatitis A and cytomegalovirus. *Neurology* 1986;36:855–858.

185. Caldas C, Bernicker E, Dal Nogare A, et al. Case report: transverse myelitis associated with Epstein-Barr virus infection. *Am J Med Sci* 1994;307:45–48.

186. Folpe A, Lapham LW, Smith HC. Herpes simplex myelitis as a cause of acute necrotizing myelitis syndrome. *Neurology* 1994;44:1955–1957.

187. Farkkila M, Koskiniemi M, Vaheri A. Clinical spectrum of neurologic herpes simplex infection. *Acta Neurol Scand* 1993;87:325–328.

188. Ellie E, Rozenberg F, Dousset V, et al. Herpes simplex type 2 ascending myeloradiculitis: MRI findings and rapid diagnosis by the polymerase chain method. *J Neurol Neurosurg Psychiatry* 1994:869–870.

189. Iwamasa T, Yoshitake H, Sakuda H, et al. Case report. Acute ascending necrotizing myelitis in Okinawa caused by herpes simplex virus type 2. *Virchows Arch A Pathol Anat* 1991:418:71–75.

190. Shyu W-C, Lin J-C, Chang B-C, et al. Recurrent ascending myelitis: an unusual presentation of herpes simplex virus type 1 infection. *Ann Neurol* 1993;34:625–627.

191. Ahmed I. Survival after herpes simplex type 2 myelitis. *Neurology* 1988;38:1500.

192. Barnes DW, Whitley RJ. CNS diseases associated with varicella zoster virus and herpes simplex infection. Pathogenesis and current therapy. *Neurol Clin* 1986;4(1):265–283.

193. Gray F, Belec L, Lescs MC, et al. Varicella-zoster virus infection of the central nervous system in the acquired immune deficiency syndrome. *Brain* 1994;117:987–999.

194. Rosenfeld J, Taylor CL, Atlas SW. Myelitis following chickenpox: a case report. *Neurology* 1993;43:1834–1836.

195. Gilden DH, Beinlich BR, Rubinstein EM, et al. Varicella-zoster virus myelitis: an expanding spectrum. *Neurology* 1994;44:1818–1823.

196. Tucker T, Dix RD, Katzen C, et al. Cytomegalovirus and herpes simplex ascending myelitis in a patient with AIDS. *Ann Neurol* 1985;18:74.

197. Meerbach T, Grunh B, Egerer R, et al. Semiquantitative PCR analysis of Epstein-Barr virus DNA in clinical samples of EBV-associated diseases. *J Med Virol* 2001;65:348–357.

198. Kleinschmidt-DeMasters BK, Gilden DH. The expanding spectrum of herpesvirus infections of the nervous system. *Brain Pathol* 2002;11:440–451.

199. Kleinschmidt-DeMasters BK, Gilden DH. Varicella-zoster infections of the nervous system: clinical and pathological correlates. *Arch Pathol Lab Med* 2001;125:770–780.

200. Dawson DM, Potts F. Acute nontraumatic myelopathies. *Neurol Clin* 1991;9(3):585–603.

201. Majid A, Galeta SL, Sweeney CJ, et al. Epstein-Barr virus myeloradiculitis and encephalomyeloradiculitis. *Brain* 2002;125:1–65.

202. Kenyon LC, Dulaney E, Montone KT, et al. Varicella-zoster ventriculoencephalitis and spinal cord infarction in a patient with AIDS. *Acta Neuropathol* 1996;92:202–205.

203. Heller HM, Carnevale NT, Steigbigel RT. Varicella zoster virus transverse myelitis without cutaneous rash. *Am J Med* 1990;88:550–551.

204. Gomez-Tortosa E, Gadea I, Gegundez MI, et al. Development of myelopathy before herpes zoster rash in a patient with AIDS. *Clin Infect Dis* 1994;18:810–812.

205. Devinsky O, Cho E-S, Petito CK, et al. Herpes zoster myelitis. *Brain* 1991;114:1181–1196.

206. Gilden DH, Bennett JL, Kleinschmidt-DeMasters BK, et al. The value of cerebrospinal fluid antiviral antibody in the diagnosis of neurologic disease produced by varicella zoster virus. *J Neurol Sci* 1998;159:140–144.

207. Studahl M, Hagberg L, Rekabdar E, et al. Herpesvirus DNA detection in cerebral spinal fluid: differences in clinical presentation between alpha-, beta- and gamma-herpesviruses. *Scand J Infect Dis* 2000;32:237–248.

208. Nakajima H, Furutama D, Kimura F, et al. Herpes simplex virus myelitis: clinical manifestations and diagnosis by the polymerase chain reaction method. *Eur Neurol* 1998;39:163–167.

209. Whiteman ML, Dandapani BK, Shebert RT, et al. MRI of AIDS-related polyradiculomyelitis. *J Comput Assist Tomogr* 1994;18:7–11.

210. Haanpaa M, Dastidar P, Weinberg A, et al. CSF and MRI findings in acute herpes zoster. *Neurology* 1998;52:1404–1411.

211. Burke DG, Leonard DG, Imperiale TF, et al. The utility of clinical and radiological features in the diagnosis of cytomegalovirus central nervous system disease in AIDS patients. *Mol Diagn* 1999;4:37–43.

212. Anduze-Faris BM, Fillet AM, Gozlan J, et al. Induction and maintenance therapy of cytomegalovirus central nervous system infection in HIV-infected patients. *AIDS* 2000;14:517–524.

213. Lionnet F, Pulik M, Genet P, et al. Myelitis due to varicella-zoster virus in two patients with AIDS: successful treatment with acyclovir. *Clin Infect Dis* 1996;22:138–140.

214. Hirai T, Korogi Y, Hamatake S, et al. Case report: varicella-zoster myelitis— serial findings. *Br J Radiol* 1996;69:1187–1190.

215. Kushuhara T, Nakajima M, Inoue H, et al. Parainfectious encephalomyelo-radiculitis associated with herpes simplex virus 1 DNA in cerebrospinal fluid. *Clin Infect Dis* 2002;34:1999–1205.

216. Denning DA, Anderson J, Rudge P, et al. Acute myelopathy associated with primary infection with human immunodeficiency virus. *Br Med J* 1987;294:143.

217. Petito CK, Naviax BA, Cho ES, et al. Vacuolar myelopathy pathologically resembling subacute combined degeneration in patients with AIDS. *N Engl J Med* 1985;312:874.

218. Blattner WA. Human T-lymphotropic viruses and diseases of long latency. *Ann Intern Med* 1989;111:4.

219. Rogers-Johnson PEB, Ono S, Gibbs CJ Jr, et al. Tropical spastic paraparesis and HTLV-I-associated myelopathy: clinical and laboratory diagnosis. In: Blattner WA, ed. *Human retrovirology*. New York: Raven Press, 1990:205–212.

220. Brew BJ, Sidtis JJ, Petito CK, et al. The neurologic complications of AIDS and human immunodeficiency virus. In: Plum F, ed. *Advances in contemporary neurology*. Philadelphia: FA Davis, 1988.

221. Dal Pan GJ, Glass JD, McArthur JC. Clinicopathologic correlations of HIV-1-associated vacuolar myelopathy: an autopsy-based case control study. *Neurology* 1994;44:2159–2164.

222. Shepherd EJ, Brettle R, Liberski PP, et al. Spinal cord pathology and viral burden in homosexuals and drug users with AIDS. *Neuropathol Appl Neurobiol* 1999;25:2–10.

223. Berger JR, Levy RM. The neurologic complications of human immunodeficiency virus infection. *Med Clin North Am* 1993;77(1):1–23.

224. Woolsey RM, Young RR. The clinical diagnosis of disorders of the spinal cord. *Neurol Clin* 1991;9(3):573–583.

225. Stoeckle MY. Type C oncoviruses including human T-cell lymphotropic viruses types I and II. In: Mandell GL, Bennett JE, Dolin R, eds. *Principles and practice of infectious diseases*, 4th ed. New York: Churchill Livingstone, 1995:1579–1584.

226. Murphy EL, Glynn SA, Fridley J, et al. Increased incidence of infectious diseases during prospective follow-up of human T-lymphotropic virus type II-and I-infected blood donors. Retrospective Epidemiology Donor Study. *Arch Intern Med* 1999;159:1485–1491.

227. Isoda H, Ramsey RG. MR imaging of acute transverse myelitis (myelopathy). *Radiat Med* 1998;16:179–186.

228. Centers for Disease Control and Prevention. Guidelines for preventing opportunistic infections among hematopoietic stem cell transplant recipients. Recommendations of the CDC, the Infectious Diseases Society of America and the American Society of Blood and Bone Marrow Transplantation. *MMWR Morb Mortal Wkly Rep* 2002;49(RR-10):1–20.

229. Brunell PA. Varicella zoster virus. In: Mandell GL, Gordon Douglas R, Bennett J, eds. *Principles and practice of infectious diseases*, 2nd ed. New York: Wiley, 1985.

230. Devinsky O, Cho ES, Petito CK, et al. Herpes zoster myelitis. *Brain* 1991;114: 1181–1196.

231. Heindel CC, Fergerson JP, Kumarasamy T. Spinal subdural empyema complicating pregnancy. Case report. *J Neurosurg* 1974;40:654–656.

232. Desai KI, Muzumdar DP, Goel A. Holocord intramedullary abscess: an unusual case with review of the literature. *Spinal Cord* 1999;37:866–870.

233. Thome C, Krauss JK, Zevgaridis D, et al. Pyogenic abscess of the filum terminale. Case report. *J Neurosurg* 2001;95[Suppl 1]:4.

234. Chan CT, Gold WL. Intramedullary abscess of the spinal cord in the antibiotic era: clinical features, microbe etiologies, trends in pathogenesis, and outcomes. *Clin Infect Dis* 1998;27:619–626.

235. Bingol A, Yucemen N, Meco O. Medically treated intraspinal (Brucella) granuloma. *Surg Neurol* 1999;52:570–576.

236. Centers for Disease Control and Prevention. Schistosomiasis in U.S. Peace Corps Volunteers—Malawi, 1992. *MMWR Morb Mortal Wkly Rep* 1993; 42(29):565–570.

237. Morandi X, Mercier P, Fournier HD, et al. Dermal sinus and intramedullary spinal cord abscess. Report of two cases and review of the literature. *Childs Nerv Syst* 1999;15:202–206.

238. Maurice-Williams RS, Pamphilon D, Coakham HB. Intramedullary abscess: a rare complication of spinal dysraphism. *J Neurol Neurosurg Psychiatry* 1980;43:1045.

239. DiTullio MV Jr. Intramedullary spinal abscess: a case report with review of 53 previously described cases. *Surg Neurol* 1977;7:351–354.

240. Murphy KJ, Brunberg JA, Quint DJ, et al. Spinal cord infection: myelitis and abscess formation. *Am J Neuroradiol* 1998;19:341–348.

241. Condette-Auliac S, Lacour JC, Anxionnat R, et al. MRI aspects of spinal cord abscesses. Report of 5 cases and review of the literature. *J Neuroradiol* 1998;25: 189–200.

242. Darouiche RO, Hamill RJ, Greenberg SB, et al. Bacterial spinal epidural abscess. Review of 43 cases and literature review. *Medicine* 1992;71:369–385.

243. Nussbaum ES, Rigamonti D, Standiford H, et al. Spinal epidural abscess: a report of 40 cases and review. *Surg Neurol* 1992;38:225–231.

244. Turner DP, Weston VC, Ispahani P. *Streptococcus pneumoniae* spinal infection in Nottingham, United Kingdom: not a rare event. *Clin Infect Dis* 1999;28:873–888.

245. Gelfand MS, Bakhtian BJ, Simmons BP. Spinal sepsis due to *Streptococcus milleri*: two cases and review. *Rev Infect Dis* 1991;13:559–563.

246. Brian JE, Westerman GR, Chadduck WM. Septic complications of chemonucleolysis. *Neurosurgery* 1989;15:730.

247. Saio P, McCabe P, Yagnik P. Nocardial spinal epidural abscess. *Neurology* 1989;39:996.

248. Kaufman DM, Kaplan JG, Littman N. Infectious agents in spinal epidural abscess. *Neurology* 1980;30:844.

249. Hershkowitz S, Link R, Lipons K. Spinal empyema in Crohn's disease. *J Clin Gastroenterol* 1990;12:67–69.

250. Rayport M, Wisoff HS, Zaiman H. Vertebral echinococcosis: report of case of surgical and biological therapy with review of the literature. *J Neurosurg* 1969;21:647.

251. Koppel BS, Tuchman AJ, Mangiardi JR, et al. Epidural spinal infection in intravenous drug abusers. *Arch Neurol* 1988;45:1331–1337.

252. Danner RL, Hartman BJ. Update of spinal epidural abscess: 35 cases and review of the literature. *Rev Infect Dis* 1987;9:265.

253. Boner FA, Garland DE, Zigler JE. Spinal infections in the immunocompromised host. *Orthop Clin North Am* 1996;27:37–46.

254. Obrador GT, Levenson DJ. Spinal epidural abscess in hemodialysis patients: report of three cases and a review of the literature. *Am J Kidney Dis* 1996;27:75–83.

255. Feldenzer JA, McKeever PE, Schaberg DR, et al. The pathogenesis of spinal epidural abscess: microangiographic studies in an experimental model. *J Neurosurg* 1988;69:110–114.

256. Auletta JJ, John CC. Spinal epidural abscess in children: a 15 year experience and review of the literature. *Clin Infect Dis* 2001;32:9–16.

257. Schmutzhard E, Aichner F, Dierckx RA, et al. New perspectives in acute spinal epidural abscess. *Acta Neurochir (Wien)* 1986;80:105.

258. Baker AS, Ojemann RG, Swartz MN, et al. Spinal epidural abscess. *N Engl J Med* 1975;293:463.

259. DiNubile MJ. Spinal epidural abscess. In: Schlossberg D, ed. *Clinical topics in infectious diseases: infections of the nervous system*. New York: Springer-Verlag, 1990:171–178.

260. Post EM, Modesti LM. Subacute postoperative subdural empyema. *J Neurosurg* 1981;55:761–767.

261. Post MJD, Quencer RM, Montalvo BM, et al. Spinal infection: evaluation with MR imaging and intraoperative ultra sound. *Radiology* 1988;169:765–771.

262. Jain AK, Jena A, Dhammi IK. Correlation of clinical course with magnetic resonance imaging in tuberculous myelopathy. *Neurol India* 2000;48:132–139.

263. Lees D, Lesoin F, Viaud C, et al. Decreased morbidity from acute bacterial spinal epidural abscesses using computed tomography and non surgical treatment in selected patients. *Ann Neurol* 1985;17:350–355.

264. Janssens JP, de Haller R. Spinal tuberculosis in a developed country. A review of 26 cases with special emphasis on abscesses and neurologic complications. *Clin Orthop* 1990;257:67–75.

265. Harrier-Jones R, Hernandez-Bronchud M, Anslow P, et al. Meningitis and spinal subdural empyema as a complication of sinusitis. *J Neurol Neurosurg Psychiatry* 1990;58:441.

266. Dill SR, Cobbs CG, McDonald CK. Subdural empyema: analysis of 32 cases and review. *Clin Infect Dis* 1995;20:372–386.

267. Levy ML, Wieder BH, Schneider J, et al. Subdural empyema of the cervical spine: clinicopathological correlates and magnetic resonance imaging. Report of three cases. *J Neurosurg* 1993;79:929–935.

268. Lownie SP, Fergerson GG. Spinal subdural empyema complicating cervical discography. *Spine* 1989;14:1415–1417.

269. Knudsen LL, Volby B, Stagaard M. Computed tomographic myelography in spinal subdural empyema. *Neuroradiology* 1987;29:99.

270. Theodotou B, Woosley RE, Whaley RA. Spinal subdural empyema: diagnosis by spinal computed tomography. *Surg Neurol* 1984;21:610–612.

271. Obana WG, Rosenblum ML. Nonoperative treatment of neurosurgical infections. *Neurosurg Clin North Am* 1992;3:359–373.

272. Sathi S, Schwartz M, Cortez S, et al. Spinal subdural abscess: successful treatment with limited drainage and antibiotics in a patient with AIDS. *Surg Neurol* 1994;42:425–427.

273. Bartels RH, de Jong TR, Grotenhuis JA. Spinal subdural abscess. Case report. *J Neurosurg* 1992;76:307–311.

274. Williams W, Sunderland R. As sick as a pigeon: psittacosis myelitis. *Arch Dis Child* 1989;64:1626.

275. Seboxa T, Rahlenbeck SI. Treatment of louse-borne relapsing fever with low dose penicillin or tetracycline: a clinical trial. *Scand J Infect Dis* 1995;27:29–31.

276. Borgnolo G, Hailu B, Ciancarelli A, et al. Louse-borne relapsing fever. A clinical and epidemiological study of 389 patients in Asella Hospital, Ethiopia. *Trop Geo Med* 1993;45:66–69.

277. Rawlings JA. An overview of tick-borne relapsing fever with emphasis on outbreaks in Texas. *Tex Med* 1995;91:56–59.

278. Samara Y, Saked Y, Maier MK. Delayed neurologic display in murine typhus. Report of two cases. *Arch Intern Med* 1989;149:949.

279. Carter CN, Ronald NC, Steele JH, et al. Knowledge-based patient screening for rare and emerging infectious/parasitic diseases: a case study of brucellosis and murine typhus. *Emerg Infect Dis* 1997;3:73–76.

280. Halperin JJ. Neurologic manifestations of lyme disease. In: Schlossberg D, ed.

Clinical topics in infectious diseases: infections of the nervous system. New York: Springer-Verlag, 1990:304–314.

281. Belman AL, Iyer M, Coyle PK, et al. Neurologic manifestations in children with North American Lyme disease. *Neurology* 1993;43:2609–2614.

282. Steere AC. Medical progress. Lyme disease. *N Engl J Med* 1989;321:586–596.

283. Schwan T, Burgdorfer W, Rosa PA. Borrelia. In: Murray PR, Baron EJ, Pfaller MA, et al, eds. *Manual of clinical microbiology,* 7th ed. Washington, DC: ASM Press, 1999:746–758.

284. Centers for Disease Control and Prevention. Lyme disease—United States, 1999. *MMWR Morb Mortal Wkly Rep* 2001;50(10):181–185.

285. Steere AC. Lyme disease. *N Engl J Med* 2001;345:115–125.

286. Smith RP, Schoen RT, Rahn DW, et al. Clinical characteristics and treatment outcome of early Lyme diseases in patients with microbiologically confirmed erythema migrans. *Ann Intern Med* 2002;136:421–428.

287. Nadelman RB, Wormser GP. Erythema migrans and early Lyme disease. *Am J Med* 1995;98:15S–23S.

288. Dattwyler RJ, Luft BJ, Kunkel MJ, et al. Ceftriaxone compared with doxycycline for treatment of acute disseminated Lyme disease. *N Engl J Med* 1997;337:289–294.

289. Pachner AR. Neurologic manifestations of Lyme disease, the new "great imitator." *Rev Infect Dis* 1989;11:S1482.

290. Reik L, Burgdorfer W, Donaldson JD. Neurologic abnormalities of Lyme disease without erythema chronicum migrans. *Am J Med* 1986;81:73.

291. Lesser RL. Ocular manifestations of Lyme disease. *Am J Med* 1995;98:60S–62S.

292. Pfister H-W, Wilske B, Weber K. Lyme borreliosis: basic science and clinical aspects. *Lancet* 1994;343:1013–1016.

293. Vallat JM, Hugon J, Lubeau M, et al. Tick-bite meningoradiculitis: clinical, electrophysiologic and histologic findings in 10 cases. *Neurology* 1987;7:749–753.

294. Garcia-Monco JC, Beldarrain MG, Estrade L. Painful lumbosacral plexitis with increased ESR and *Borrelia burgdorferi* infection. *Neurology* 1993;43:1269.

295. Pachner AR. Early disseminated Lyme disease: Lyme meningitis. *Am J Med* 1995;98:30S–37S.

296. Tumani H, Nolker G, Reiber H. Relevance of cerebrospinal fluid variables for early diagnosis of neuroborreliosis. *Neurology* 1995;45:1663–1670.

297. Sindern E, Malin JP. Phenotypic analysis of cerebrospinal fluid cells over the course of Lyme meningoradiculitis. *Acta Ctytol* 1995;39:73–75.

298. Ilowite NT. Muscle, reticuloendothelial, and late manifestations of Lyme disease. *Am J Med* 1995;98:638–688.

299. Halperin JJ, Logigian EL, Finkel MF, et al. Practice parameters for the diagnosis of patients with nervous system Lyme borreliosis (Lyme disease). Quality Standards Subcommittee of the American Academy of Neurology. *Neurology* 1996;46:619–627.

300. Practice parameter: diagnosis of patients with nervous system Lyme borreliosis (Lyme disease—Summary statement). Report of the quality standards Subcommittee of the American Academy of Neurology. *Neurology* 1996;46:881–882.

301. Centers for Disease Control and Prevention. Recommendations for the use of Lyme disease vaccine, recommendations of the Advisory Committee on Immunization Practices. *MMWR Morb Mortal Wkly Rep* 1999;48(RR-7):1–17, 21–25.

302. Lebech AM, Hansen K, Brandrup F, et al. Diagnostic value of PCR for detection of *Borrelia burgdorferi* in clinical specimens from patients with erythema migrans and Lyme neuroborreliosis. *Mol Diagn* 2000;5:139–150.

303. Dumler JS. Molecular diagnosis of Lyme disease: review and meta-analysis. *Mol Diagn* 2001;6:1–11.

304. Lebech AM. Polymerase chain reaction in the diagnosis of *Borrelia burgdorferi* infections and studies on taxonomic classification. *APMIS* 2002;105[Suppl]:1–40.

305. Centers for Disease Control and Prevention. Recommendations for test performance and interpretation from the Second National Conference on Serologic Diagnosis of Lyme Disease. *MMWR Morb Mortal Wkly Rep* 1995;44(31):590–591.

306. Gomes-Solecki MJ, Wormser GP, Schriefer M, et al. Recombinant assay for serodiagnosis of Lyme disease regardless of OspA vaccination status. *J Clin Microbiol* 2002;40:193–197.

307. Shakir RA, Al-Din AS, Araj GF, et al. Clinical categories of neurobrucellosis. *Brain* 1987;110:213.

308. Pascual J, Combarros O, Polo JM, et al. Localized CNS brucellosis: report of 7 cases. *Acta Neurol Scand* 1988;78:282.

309. Young EJ. *Brucella* species. In: Mandell GL, Bennett JE, Dolin R, eds. *Principles and practice of infectious diseases,* 4th ed. New York: Churchill Livingstone, 1995:2053–2060.

310. Ariza J, Pujol M, Valverde J, et al. Brucellar sacroiliitis: findings in 63 episodes and current relevance. *Clin Infect Dis* 1993;16:761–765.

311. Colmenero JD, Jiminez-Mejoias ME, Sanchez-Lora FJ, et al. Pyogenic, tuberculous, brucellar vertebral osteomyelitis: a descriptive and comparative study of 219 cases. *Ann Rheum Dis* 1997;56:709–715.

312. McLean DR, Russell N, Khan MY. Neurobrucellosis: clinical and therapeutic features. *Clin Infect Dis* 1992;15:582–590.

313. Habeeb YK, Al-Najdi AK, Sadek SA, et al. Paediatric neurobrucellosis: case report and literature review. *J Infect* 1998;37:59–62.

314. Kochar DK, Agarwal N, Jain N, et al. Clinical profile of neurobrucellosis—a report on 12 cases from Bikaner. *J Assoc Phys India* 2000;48:376–380.

315. Gokul BN, Hussein PA. Neurobrucellosis. *Saudi Med J* 2000;21:577–580.

316. Memish Z, Mah MW, Al Mahmoud S, et al. Brucella bacteremia: clinical and laboratory observations in 160 patients. *J Infect* 2000;40:59–63.

317. Morata P, Queipo-Ortuno MI, Reguera JM, et al. Diagnostic yield of a PCR assay in focal complications of brucellosis. *J Clin Microbiol* 2001;39:3743–3746.

318. Zerva L, Bourantas K, Mitka S, et al. Serum is the preferred clinical specimen for diagnosis of human brucellosis by PCR. *J Clin Microbiol* 2001;39:1661–1664.

319. Navas E, Guerrero A, Cobo J, et al. Faster isolation of *Brucella* spp. From blood by isolator compared with BACTEC NR. *Diagn Microbiol Infect Dis* 1993;16:79–81.

320. Sumerkan B, Gokahetoglu S, Esel D. Brucella detection in blood: comparison of the BacT/Alert standard aerobic bottle, BacT/Alert FAN aerobic bottle and BacT/Alert enhanced FAN aerobic bottle in simulated culture. *Clin Microbiol Infect* 2001;7;369–372.

321. Gamazo C, Vitas AI, Lopez-Goni I, et al. Factors affecting detection of *Brucella melitensis* by BACTEC. NR730, a nonradiometric system for hemocultures. *J Clin Microbiol* 1993;31:3200–3203.

322. Yagupsky P. Detection of *Brucella melitensis* by BACTEC NR660 blood culture system. *J Clin Microbiol* 1994;31:1899–1901.

323. Shapiro DS, Wong JD. Brucella. In: Murray PR, Baron EJ, Pfaller MA, et al, eds. *Manual of clinical microbiology,* 7th ed. Washington, DC: ASM Press, 1999:625–631.

324. Stszkiewicz J, Lewis CM, Colville J, et al. Outbreak of *Brucella melitensis* among microbiology laboratory workers in a community hospital. *J Clin Microbiol* 1991;29:287–290.

325. Boschiroli ML, Foulonge V, O'Callaghan D. Brucellosis: a worldwide zoonosis. *Curr Opin Microbiol* 2001;4:58–64.

326. Goodman LJ, Karakosis PU. Neurosyphilis. In: *Handbook of clinical neurology.* Amsterdam: Elsevier, 1988:231.

327. Tramont EC. *Treponema pallidum* (syphilis). In: Mandell GL, Bennett JE, Dolin R, eds. *Principles and practice of infectious diseases,* 4th ed. New York: Churchill Livingstone, 1995:2117–2133.

328. Harrigan EP, McLaughlin TJ, Feldman RG. Transverse myelitis due to meningovascular syphilis. *Arch Neurol* 1984;41:337–338.

329. Strom T, Schneck SA. Syphilitic meningomyelitis. *Neurology* 1991;41:325–326.

330. Harris DE, Enterline DS, Tien RD. Neurosyphilis in patients with AIDS. *Neuroimag Clin North Am* 1997;7:215–221.

331. Kodama K, Okada S, Komatsu N, et al. Relationship between MRI findings and prognosis for patients with general paresis. *J Neuropsychol Clin Neurosci* 2000;12:246–250.

332. Brightbill TC, Ihmeidan IH, Post MJ, et al. Neurosyphilis in HIV-positive and HIV-negative patients: neuroimaging findings. *Am J Neuroradiol* 1995;16:703–711.

333. Koskiniemi M. CNS Manifestations associated with *Mycoplasma pneumoniae* infections: summary of cases at the University of Helsinki and review. *Clin Infect Dis* 1993;17[Suppl 1]:S52–S57.

334. Mills RW, Schoolfield L. Acute transverse myelitis associated with *Mycoplasma pneumoniae* infection: a case report and review of the literature. *Pediatr Infect Dis* 1992;11:228–231.

335. Heller L, Keren O, Mendelson L, et al. Transverse myelitis associated with *Mycoplasma pneumoniae:* case report. *Paraplegia* 1990;28:522–525.

336. Socan M, Ravnik I, Bencina D, et al. Neurological symptoms in patients whose cerebrospinal fluid is culture- and/or polymerase chain reaction-positive for *Mycoplasma pneumoniae. Clin Infect Dis* 2001;32(2):E31–E35.

337. Yanez A, Cedilla L, Neyrolles O, et al. *Mycoplasma penetrans* bacteremia and primary antiphospholipid syndrome. *Emerg Infect Dis* 1999;5:164–167.

338. Case Records of the Massachusetts General Hospital. *N Engl J Med* 1994;331:1437–1444.

339. Klausner JD, Passaro D, Rosenberg J, et al. Enhanced control of an outbreak of *Mycoplasma pneumoniae* pneumonia with azithromycin prophylaxis. *J Infect Dis* 1998;177:161–166.

340. Dobbins WO III. The diagnosis of Whipple's disease. *N Engl J Med* 1995;332:390–396.

341. Relman DA, Schmidt TM, MacDermott RP, et al. Identification of the uncultured bacillus of Whipple's diseases. *N Engl J Med* 1992;327:293–301.

342. Lowsky R, Archer GL, Fyles G, et al. Brief report: diagnosis of Whipple's disease by molecular analysis of peripheral blood. *N Engl J Med* 1994;331:1343–1346.

343. Raoult D, Birg ML, La Scola B, et al. Cultivation of the bacillus of Whipple's disease. *N Engl J Med* 2000;342:620–625.

344. Knox DL, Green WR, Troncoso JC, et al. Cerebral-ocular Whipple's disease: a 62-year odyssey from death to diagnosis. *Neurology* 1995;45:617–625.

345. Halperin JJ, Dennis DMD, Kleinman GM. Whipple's disease of the nervous system. *Neurology* 1982;32:612.

346. Louis ED, Lynch T, Kaufman P, et al. Diagnostic guidelines in central nervous system Whipple's disease. *Ann Neurol* 1996;40:561–568.

347. Erdem E, Carlier R, Delvalle A, et al. Gadolinium-enhanced MRI in cerebral Whipple's disease. *Neuroradiology* 1993;35:581–583.

348. Smith AS, Blaser SI. MR of infectious and inflammatory diseases of the spine. *Crit Rev Diagn Imag* 1991;32:165–189.

349. Hyslop NE Jr, Leach TS. Infections of the spinal cord and peripheral nervous system. In: Gorbach S, Bartlett JG, Blacklow N, eds. *Infectious diseases,* 2nd ed. Philadelphia: WB Saunders, 1998:1456–1500.

350. Lim PL, Hyslop NE Jr. Myelitis and peripheral neuropathy. In: Schlossberg D, ed. *Current therapy of infectious disease.* St. Louis: Mosby–Year Book, 2001:286–295.

CHAPTER 155
Reye's Syndrome

John R. La Montagne

First described in 1929 (1), Reye's syndrome, originally known as *encephalopathy* with fatty degeneration of the viscera—actually a triad of postinfectious encephalopathy, microvesicular fat infiltration of hepatic parenchyma, and elevated serum transaminase values—was thought to be a rare event until the reports by Reye, Morgan, and Baral in 1963 (2) and later by Johnson, Scurleyis, and Carroll (3). Reye's group reported a series of cases of fatal encephalopathy with associated fatty degeneration of the liver that occurred in 21 Australian children. This report focused on the pathologic manifestations of this clinical presentation and gave rise to the term *Reye's syndrome.* (Although the preferred term is *Reye's syndrome,* it has also been called *Reye syndrome* and *Reye-Johnson syndrome.*) The report by Johnson, Scurleyis, and Carroll (3) in 1970 analyzed a cluster of 16 cases of this syndrome that occurred during an outbreak of influenza B in a community in North Carolina and focused attention on the potential role of epidemic viral infections as important triggering factors in the etiology of Reye's syndrome. In the days after an uncomplicated viral infection, these cases developed an acute onset of persistent, intractable vomiting and dehydration, and the development of neurologic signs and symptoms, including encephalopathy and coma. One of the important early observations was that the disease almost always occurred in children who were otherwise healthy and were in the recovery period after an influenza virus infection, although only a small proportion of influenza virus–infected children (1/20,000) developed this complication (4).

EPIDEMIOLOGY

After the description of this syndrome by Reye, Morgan, and Baral (2) in 1963, there was a dramatic increase in reporting of Reye's syndrome cases to the Centers for Disease Control and Prevention (CDC) during the 1970s (5–11), particularly during influenza B epidemics (12,13). During the epidemic of influenza in 1976, a large number of Reye's syndrome cases was reported to the CDC. Of the 379 cases reported that year, 83% occurred over a 2-month period during an epidemic of influenza type B/Hong Kong/5/72. An increase in Reye's syndrome reports also occurred in 1977 and 1980, 454 and 555 cases, respectively, both coincident with significant influenza B epidemics (7). Although influenza A had been identified as a risk factor for Reye's syndrome in 1967 (14), this association was further strengthened by the appearance of a cluster of 85 cases linked to influenza virus A(H1N1) activity during the winter of 1978 to 1979 (6). Subsequent reports also confirmed the association of Reye's syndrome with influenza A virus, varicella-zoster virus, rotavirus, and dengue virus (15–19).

Because of its association with both influenza and varicella, Reye's syndrome exhibits a distinct seasonal pattern and most cases occur during the winter and spring months. Reye's syndrome principally affects children 18 years and younger, although it has been reported in adults (20–24).

In 1981, the U.S. Public Health Service Task Force on Reye's Syndrome initiated and reviewed a series of retrospective case-control studies and demonstrated that of the medications commonly used to treat influenza or chickenpox, aspirin was sig-nificantly associated with the development of Reye's syndrome (25,26). Since the publication of the results of the U.S. Public Health Service study and the development and dissemination of recommendations against the use of aspirin in children in the setting of a presumed viral infection (27), the incidence of Reye's syndrome has decreased dramatically in the United States (5,8–10,27). The number of cases of Reye's syndrome in the United States each year from 1994 to 1997 continues to be extremely small (5). Since then, reports to the CDC have dropped substantially, with an average of fewer than 20 reports per year, although clusters continue to occur (9,11) (Table 155.1). The decline in cases is attributed to effective dissemination of information on the association of Reye's syndrome with the use of aspirin in children (27).

In the United Kingdom, nationwide Reye's syndrome surveillance was initiated in 1981. During the 1980s, the annual incidence ranged between 0.16 and 0.61 per 100,000 (5) in children younger than 16 years (28–30). A similar pattern in the reduction of reported Reye's syndrome cases was noted in the United Kingdom after both a public education campaign highlighting the risk of aspirin in children after viral illnesses and the withdrawal of children's aspirin formulations. In the United Kingdom and the United States, men and women are equally affected; however, in the United Kingdom, the age distribution of cases is younger (33 to 54 months of age) than that observed in the United States (6 to 8 years of age), a feature attributed in part to differences in the investigation and reporting of inborn errors of metabolism as Reye's syndrome.

Despite this marked decline in cases of Reye's syndrome in the United States, cases do continue to occur, either as isolated cases or in clusters. An unusual cluster of cases was recently reported from northern India (31). This cluster was associated with an ongoing outbreak of measles in the community, as well as the widespread use of insecticides to control mosquitoes. The influenza H5N1 outbreak in Hong Kong in 1998 was brought to light in part because the index case died of Reye's syndrome (32).

A recent comparison of the CDC surveillance data with national hospital admission data suggests that the CDC surveillance system captures about one half of all the cases (48 cases reported to the CDC compared with 93 reported in the hospital database) (33). More and more of the cases that are reported are identified as cases in which there is a genetic defect in metabolism, most commonly glycogen storage diseases, urea cycle defects, carnitine deficiency, propionic acidemia, hereditary fructose intolerance, methylmalonic acidemia, and 3-hydroxy-3-methylglutaric acidemia (34–36). Since the initial reports of Reye's syndrome, improved diagnosis of inborn errors of metabolism with the increased availability of gas chromatography and mass spectrometry may have facilitated a more accurate accounting of Reye's syndrome cases (37,38). Since 1985, 25% of cases initially meeting the case definition of Reye's syndrome were subsequently reclassified as having an inborn error of metabolism (39). Although the reduction in the number of cases of Reye's syndrome has been largely attributed to the significant reduction in the use of aspirin for treatment of fever during influenza and varicella-zoster infection, not all groups have been able to demonstrate this association (40,41).

Two long-term follow-up studies of patients with Reye's syndrome have recently been completed, one in the United Kingdom (30) and one in Australia (41). Both studies report significant long-term sequelae. In the British study, survivors of Reye's syndrome who had the illness before they were 1 year of age had significantly poorer outcomes. In the Australian study in which the 49 original cases first studied by Reye were reexamined, only 26 were available for reexamination (42). Of these 26, 18 were diagnosed with other metabolic diseases, chiefly

TABLE 155.1. Reye's Syndrome in the United States: 1974–1993

Year	Influenza strain	Total	Varicella[a]	Incidence[b]	Case-fatality rate (%)
1974	B	379	NA	0.6	41
1977	B	454	73	0.7	42
1978	A(H3N2)	236	69	0.4	29
1979	A(H1N1)	389	113	0.6	32
1980	B	555	103	0.9	23
1981	A(H3N2)	293	73	0.5	28
1982	B	211	45	0.3	33
1983	A(H3N2)	199	28	0.3	29
1984	A(H1N1)/B	203	26	0.3	24
1985	A(H3N2)	95	15	0.2	29
1986	B	100	5	0.2	25
1987	A(H1N1)	36	7	0.1	31
1988	A(H3N2)	25	4	<0.1	40
1989	A(H1N1)/B	25	3	<0.1	40
1990	A(H3N2)	19	3	<0.1	53
1991	B	15	3	<0.1	40
1992	A(H3N2)/A(H1N1)	13	1	<0.1	46
1993	B/ A(H3N2)	19	1	<0.1	56

[a]Number of Reye's syndrome cases associated with varicella, by year.
[b]Incidence per 100,000 persons younger than 18 years.
NA, not available.
Source: Courtesy Dr. J. Bresee, Centers for Disease Control and Prevention, Atlanta, Georgia, 1995.

medium-chain acylcoenzyme-A dehydrogenase deficiency, suggesting that their metabolic abnormality made them especially susceptible to the development of Reye's syndrome during the infection and reinforcing the need to carefully examine any patient with Reye's syndrome for the presence of an underlying metabolic anomaly.

ETIOLOGY

The temporal association of Reye's syndrome with influenza and varicella prompted speculation that viral factors are important, but none has been identified. Studies aimed at identifying influenza or varicella virus variants that exhibit hepatotropic properties were fruitless (43). The use of common medications, particularly aspirin, was suggested by many workers (44–47). Through epidemiologic studies, the U.S. Public Health Service Task Force demonstrated a statistically significant association between Reye's syndrome and the use of aspirin or salicylate medications. Several reports that examined the possible role of environmental toxins in Reye's syndrome, especially in areas of the world where contamination of foods with toxins such as aflatoxin B1 (48) and pesticides (49) is more common, were unable to demonstrate consistently that they were risk factors for this syndrome. However, several toxins have been noted to produce similar pathologic changes in the liver, including hypoglycin a poisoning (Jamaican vomiting sickness after the ingestion of akee apples) and salicylate intoxication (23,50).

PATHOLOGY AND PATHOGENESIS

Given the severity of the clinical syndrome, the absence of inflammatory changes in the liver is the most striking feature of this disorder (41). There is a panlobular, microvesicular infiltration of the hepatocytes and hepatic mitochondria are swollen with a diffuse matrix, an absence of dense bodies, and few cristae on ul-

trastructural examination. The nature of this injury and its cause have been the subject of many reports (42–49). These changes are not limited to hepatocytes, as mitochondria from the pancreas and muscle have also been shown to exhibit similar structural abnormalities (50). Correlating with these ultrastructural abnormalities, mitochondrial function is also affected with reduced activity of inner membrane and internal mitochondrial enzymes, whereas outer membrane and cytosolic enzyme activities are preserved (50). Elevated levels of aspartate and alanine aminotransferases are characteristic in patients with Reye's syndrome, and levels of mitochondrial isozymes are specifically elevated (51). In addition, liver mitochondria are depleted of adenosine triphosphate relative to hepatocyte cytosol, suggesting that the level of endogenous biochemical activity in the mitochondria is low. This is also supported by the increase in serum levels of known mitochondrial substrates, such as lactate, pyruvate, alanine, and free fatty acids. The mitochondrial injury appears to be completely reversible. In general, the severity with which mitochondria are affected is directly related to the clinical manifestations of Reye's syndrome; the hepatic mitochondrial changes in patients in coma are substantially greater than those among patients with less severe clinical manifestations.

Neuropathologic examination is most consistent with secondary effects from the metabolic derangements and features cerebral edema and anoxic neuronal degeneration without evidence of inflammatory changes, although these changes may be related to a generalized mitochondrial insult (52).

The pathogenesis of Reye's syndrome is complex and is incompletely understood. The lack of inflammatory changes and the profound metabolic changes (Table 155.2) that result in hepatic encephalopathy appear to be more consistent with a toxin than the direct result of an infection. However, the consistent association of Reye's syndrome with antecedent viral infections and concomitant treatment with salicylate-containing medications has led to the hypothesis that the infection acts in some way to predispose to this syndrome, possibly by uncoupling of oxidative phosphorylation and a blockade of beta-oxidation leading to a buildup of short-chain and medium-chain acylcoenzyme A

TABLE 155.2. Metabolic and Pathologic Findings in Reye's Syndrome

Morphologically abnormal mitochondria in liver, muscle, and pancreas
Panlobar microvesicular infiltration of hepatocytes
Hepatomegaly
Ammonemia
Hypoglycemina (especially in young infants)
Elevated levels of aspartate and alanine aminotransferase, usually
Three times the limit of normal
Elevated serum levels of lactate, pyruvate, alanine, and free fatty acids

---

esters that trap free coenzyme A within the mitochondria and interrupt mitochondrial metabolic pathways and respiration (20,30,53,54).

The possible role of mitochondrial toxins in the pathogenesis of Reye's syndrome was first suggested by Aprille (53–56), who used a bioassay of rat liver mitochondria to search for substances in the serum of patients with Reye's syndrome that affected mitochondrial respiration. It was noted that serum from patients with Reye's syndrome stimulated stage IV mitochondrial respiration in their isolated rat liver mitochondria. Segalman and Lee (57) later showed that this stimulation was only transitory and was followed by inhibition of respiration. Subsequent studies suggested that the injury to the mitochondria in Reye's syndrome may be due to the presence of allantoin (58,59). They also showed that calcium ions were important in this process, as the toxic effect of allantoin on mitochondrial respiration could be specifically inhibited by adding inhibitors of calcium transport across the mitochondrial membrane or chelating agents with high affinity for calcium such as ethylene glycol-*bis* (*β*-aminomethyl ether)-*N*,*N'*-tetraacetic acid (egtazic acid, EGTA). Allantoin is an intermediate of purine degradation that is highly toxic and not normally present in human serum, because uric acid is the final product of purine metabolism. Other species of mammals produce allantoin from uric acid by the action of uricase. The source of allantoin in the serum of patients with Reye's syndrome is not known, but Segalman and Lee (57) showed that allantoin could be generated by the direct oxidation of urate by cytochrome c_3 in their mitochondrial assay system *in vitro*.

CLINICAL MANIFESTATIONS

Usually Reye's syndrome develops in the days after a child's recovery from an uncomplicated viral infection, in most instances influenza or varicella. The child is usually afebrile and not jaundiced, although hepatomegaly is common (61). Initial manifestations of the disorder include nausea and 1 to 2 days of intractable vomiting, which may lead to dehydration and contribute to

hypoglycemia, particularly in children younger than 4 years. Although featured in the initial description of patients with Reye's syndrome, profound hypoglycemia is uncommon and more likely to be attributed to the underlying metabolic stress, as normal glucose levels are easily maintained by use of glucose-containing intravenous fluids (62). Increased lethargy, confusion, combativeness, drowsiness, and sleepiness usually follow (63,64). The child may become increasingly difficult to arouse and may eventually lapse into coma. The staging system (Table 155.3) developed for Reye's syndrome is a prognostic indicator (62,65). In general, the more profound the coma, the worse the prognosis, with a mortality rate from 10% to 60% (12,16,20,37,66,67). Although complete neurologic recovery can be expected, neurologic sequelae can be severe, especially in those who develop seizures or decerebrate posturing hospitalization, although all other organ systems appear to recover fully among survivors (58,59).

DIFFERENTIAL DIAGNOSIS

Many inborn errors of metabolism, especially those associated with elevated serum ammonia levels and/or neurologic manifestations (e.g., ornithine transcarbamylase deficiency, carnitine deficiency, and glutaric aciduria), can complicate the diagnosis (4,70,71). These should be considered, especially in situations in which Reye's syndrome appears to be recurrent or has been seen previously in a sibling. Therefore, initial diagnostic investigations should include tests that can establish the diagnosis of an inborn error of metabolism and Reye's syndrome, including a urine specimen for organic acid analysis, plasma for acylcarnitine analysis, and skin biopsy specimens for fibroblast culture and enzyme analysis (37,39). The most common mimics of Reye's syndrome are listed in Table 155.4 (72–77).

DIAGNOSIS

The CDC's case definition of Reye's syndrome (Table 155.5) was developed as an epidemiologic tool for surveillance and reporting (10). The clinical diagnosis of Reye's syndrome is based on the clinical manifestations and medication history of the child, liver biopsy, cerebrospinal fluid examination, and biochemical markers. Reye's syndrome should be actively considered when an afebrile child presents in a state of altered consciousness after a period of intractable vomiting in the setting of a recent febrile illness treated with aspirin or salicylate-containing products. A clinical diagnosis is more difficult in children younger than 1 year, because respiratory disturbances such as hyperventilation or apneic episodes and seizures occur more often. Elevations of serum transaminase (aspartate and alanine aminotransferases) and ammonia levels occur, and the bilirubin value may be only mildly elevated but is often normal. Other laboratory

---

TABLE 155.3. Staging of Reye's Syndrome

Sign	Stage I	Stage II	Stage III	Stage IV	Stage V
Level of consciousness	Lethargy, but follows verbal commands	Combative or stuporous; verbalizes inappropriately	Coma	Coma	Coma
Posture	Normal	Normal	Decorticate	Decerebrate	Flaccid
Response to pain	Purposeful, brisk	Purposeful or nonpurposeful	Decorticate	Decerebrate	None
Pupillary reaction	Normal	Sluggish	Sluggish	Sluggish	None
Oculocephalic (doll's eye reflex)	None	Conjugate deviation	Conjugate deviation	Inconsistent or absent	None

TABLE 155.4. Metabolic Disorders that may Mimic Reye's Syndrome

Disorders of ureagenesis
Ornithine transcarbamylase deficiency
Carbamoylphosphate synthetase deficiency
Argininosuccinic acid synthetase deficiency
Lysinuric protein intolerance
Disorders of branched chain amino acid catabolism
Propionyl-CoA carboxylase deficiency
Methylmalonyl-CoA mutase deficiency
Methylmalonyl-CoA racemase deficiency
Isovaleryl-CoA dehydrogenase deficiency
Disorders of ketogenesis
Various acyl-CoA dehydrogenase deficiencies
3-Hydroxy-3 methyglutaryl-CoA lyase deficiency
Systematic carnitine palmitoyltransferase deficiency
Disorders of carbohydrate metabolism fructose-1,6-diphosphatase
  deficiency
Intoxications
Salicylate or amiodarone intoxication
Jamaican vomiting sickness
Dipropyl acetate

CoA, coenzyme A.

abnormalities, which may include elevations of creatine kinase and lactate dehydrogenase values, as well as decreased prothrombin activity, are supportive of the diagnosis but not definitive. Hypoglycemia may occur in infants, but glucose levels are usually normal in children older than 4 years. The cerebrospinal fluid usually supports the clinical impression of encephalopathy rather than encephalitis or meningoencephalitis, and protein and glucose concentrations are normal, except in cases with concurrent hypoglycemia. Serum should also be analyzed for levels of salicylate and acetaminophen. Liver biopsy is usually not necessary and should be considered only in infants and children with recurrent or familial Reye's syndrome for a more definitive diagnosis of the underlying hepatic pathologic condition.

TREATMENT

Therapy for Reye's syndrome is primarily supportive and closely tied to the stage of coma (see Table 155.3). As with all patients with severe metabolic derangements and altered consciousness,

TABLE 155.5. Reye's Syndrome: Case Definition

According to the Centers for Disease Control and Prevention's case definition, the following conditions must be met for consideration as a Reye's syndrome case:
1. Acute noninflammatory encephalopathy documented by
  a. Alteration in the level of consciousness and, if available, a record of cerebrospinal fluid containing <8 leukocytes/mm³ or
  b. Histologic specimen demonstrating cerebral edema without perivascular or meningeal inflammation
2. Hepatopathy documented either by a liver biopsy or autopsy considered to be diagnostic of Reye's syndrome or by a threefold or greater rise in the levels of serum aspartate aminotransferase, serum alanine aminotransferase, or serum ammonia and
3. No more reasonable explanation for the cerebral and hepatic abnormalities

Source: From Reye syndrom—United States, 1985. *MMWR Morb Mortal Wkly Rep* 1986;35:66, with permission.

hemodynamic monitoring, including careful monitoring of fluid and electrolyte balance, is crucial, as are ventilatory support and protection of the airway, when appropriate. Although continuous monitoring of blood gas values has been recommended (67), anecdotally reported attempts to reverse the metabolic derangements typical of Reye's syndrome by heroic interventions such as hypothermic total-body washout, exchange transfusions, dialysis, barbiturate coma, bowel sterilization, charcoal hemoperfusion plasmapheresis, amino acid and phosphate infusions, and insulin administration have not been demonstrated to be efficacious (4,78,79). However, a report of the experimental effect of interferon-α in prevention of mitochondrial swelling induced by acetylsalicylates suggests that this may offer a specific therapy in the treatment of Reye's syndrome (80). With progressive neurologic deterioration, administration of intravenous fluids should be adjusted to minimize episodes of hypotension and to sustain organ function while not exacerbating the potential of increased intracranial pressure that results from cerebral edema. Intracranial pressure should be carefully monitored because it is the principal contributor to the mortality of Reye's syndrome, and aggressive efforts must be made to control it with mannitol or glycerol or controlled hyperventilation (81).

PREVENTION

The results of the U.S. Public Health Service study clearly demonstrated that aspirin use was significantly related to development of Reye's syndrome (82). The wide publicity that this study received has resulted in a dramatic reduction in the use of aspirin in children and in a parallel drop in cases of Reye's syndrome (82,83) (see Table 155.1). It is clear from this experience that Reye's syndrome can be effectively prevented by avoiding aspirin and acetylsalicylate-containing medications in the treatment of symptoms during a typical viral infection. Nevertheless, children who receive aspirin routinely for treatment of various connective tissue diseases appear to be at an increased risk of Reye's syndrome (84,85), including children with juvenile rheumatoid arthritis. A CDC analysis demonstrated that since 1990, 39% of Reye's syndrome cases were linked to antecedent aspirin use, with most cases in children without chronic underlying conditions that would necessitate the use of aspirin during periods in which influenza and varicella are epidemic, by substituting non–aspirin-containing medications, or by immunizing these children against influenza or varicella (9). Although the number of varicella-associated cases has been insignificant during the past decade, increasing use of the varicella vaccine should continue to minimize the risk that this may contribute to overall Reye's syndrome morbidity and mortality.

REFERENCES

1. Brain WR, Hunter D, Turnbull HM. Acute meningoencephalomyelitis of childhood. *Lancet* 1929;1:221.
2. Reye RDK, Morgan G, Baral J. Encephalopathy and fatty degeneration of the viscera: a disease entity in childhood. *Lancet* 1963;2:749.
3. Johnson GM, Scurleyis TD, Carroll NB. A study of 16 fatal cases of encephalitis-like disease in North Carolina children. *North C Med J* 1970;24:464.
4. Keating JP. Reye syndrome. In: Feigin RD, Cherry JD, eds. *Textbook of pediatric infectious diseases*, 3rd ed. Philadelphia: WB Saunders, 1992:705–708.
5. Belay ED, Bresee JS, Holman RC, et al. Reye's syndrome in the United States from 1981 through 1997. *N Engl J Med* 1999;340:1377–1382.
6. Centers for Disease Control and Prevention. Reye syndrome—United States. *MMWR Morb Mortal Wkly Rep* 1979;28:97.
7. Reye syndrome surveillance—United States, 1989. *MMWR Morb Mortal Wkly Rep* 1991;40:88.
8. Reye syndrome surveillance—United States, 1986. *MMWR Morb Mortal Wkly Rep* 1986;36:689.

9. Bresee JS, Khan AS, Strine T, et al. *Reye syndrome surveillance—United States. Sixty-third annual meeting of the Society for Pediatric Research; May 1994; Seattle, Washington.* 110A.

10. Reye syndrome—United States, 1985. *MMWR Morbi Mortal Wkly Rep* 1986;35:66.

11. Poss WB, Vernon DD, Dean JM. A reemergence of Reye's syndrome. *Arch Pediatr Adolesc Med* 1994;148:89.

12. Corey L, Rubin RJ, Hattwick MAE, et al. A nationwide outbreak of Reye's syndrome: its relationship with influenza B. *Am J Med* 1976;61:615.

13. Corey L, Rubin RJ, Bregman D, et al. Diagnostic criteria for influenza B–associated Reye's syndrome: clinical vs. pathologic criteria. *Pediatrics* 1977;60:602.

14. Hall BD, Hughes WT, Kmetz D. Reye's syndrome: an association with influenza A infection. *J Ky Med Assoc* 1967;4:269.

15. Linnemann CC, Shea L, Partin JC, et al. Reye's syndrome: epidemiological and viral studies, 1963–1974. *Am J Epidemiol* 1975;101:517.

16. Lichetenstein PK. Heubi JE, Caughety CC, et al. Grade I Reye's syndrome: a frequent cause of vomiting and liver dysfunction after varicella and upper respiratory-tract infections. *N Engl J Med* 1983;309:133.

17. Iyngkaran N, Yadav M, Harun F, et al. Augmented tumour necrosis factor in Reye's syndrome associated with dengue virus. *Lancet* 1992;340:1466.

18. Hukin J, Junker AK, Thomas EE, et al. Reye syndrome associate with subclinical varicella zoster virus and influenza A infection. *Pediatr Neurol* 1993;9:134.

19. Devulapulli CS. Rotavirus gastroenteritis possibly causing Reye syndrome. *Acta Paediatr* 2000;89:613–619.

20. Varma RR, Riedel DR, Komorowski RA, et al. Reye's syndrome in nonpediatric age groups. *JAMA* 1979;242–1373.

21. Peters LJ, Wiener GJ, Gilliam J, et al. Reye's syndrome in adults, a case report and review of literature. *Arch Intern Med* 1986;146:2401.

22. Atkins JN, Haponik EF. Reye's syndrome in the adult patient. *Am J Med* 1979;67:672.

23. Al-Tikriti SA, Rowe PA, Munro AJ. Adult Reye's syndrome. *J R Soc Med* 1984;77:694.

24. Chan D. Reye's syndrome in a young adult. *Mil Med* 1993;158:65.

25. Hurwiitz ES, Barrett MJ, Bergman D, et al. Public Health Service study on Reye's syndrome and medications: report of the pilot phase. *N Engl J Med* 1985;313:849.

26. Hurwits ES, Barrett MJ, Bregman D, et al. Public Health Service study of Reye's syndrome and medications. *JAMA* 1987;257:1905.

27. Surgeon General's advisory on the use of salicylates and Reye syndrome. *MMWR Morb Mortal Wkly Rep* 1982;31:289.

28. Monto AS. The disappearance of Reye's syndrome—a public health triumph [Editorial]. *N Engl J Med* 1999;340:1423–1424.

29. Porter JDH, Robinso PH, Glasgow JFT, et al. Trends in the incidence of Reye's syndrome and the use of aspirin. *Arch Dis Child* 1990;65:826.

30. Hall SM, Lynn R. Reye's syndrome [Letter]. *N Engl J Med* 1999;341:845.

31. Ghosh D, Dhadwal D, Aggarwal A, et al. Investigation of an epidemic of Reye's syndrome in northern region of India. *Indian Pediatr* 1999;36:1097–1106.

32. Ku ASW, Chan LTW. The first case of H5N1 avian influenza infection in a human with complications of adult respiratory distress syndrome and Reye's syndrome. *J Paediatr Child Health* 1999;35:207–209.

33. Sullivan KM, Belay ED, Durbin RE, et al. Epidemiology of Reye's syndrome, United States, 1991-94: comparison of CDC surveillance and hospital admission data. *Neuroepidemiology* 2000;19:338–344.

34. Chang PF, Huang SF, Hwu WI, et al. Metabolic disorders mimicking Reye's syndrome. *Formos Med Assoc* 2000;99(4):295–299.

35. Yang TY, Chen HL, Ni YH, et al. Hereditary fructose intolerance presenting as Reye's syndrome: report of one case. *Acta Paediatr Taiwan* 2000;41(4):218–220.

36. Nyhan WL, Bay C, Beyer EW, et al. Neurologic nonmetabolic presentation of propionic academia. *Arch Neurol* 1999;56(9):1143–1147.

37. Glasgow JFT, Moore R. Current concepts in Reye's syndrome. *Br J Hosp Med* 1993;50:599.

38. Green A, Hall SM. Investigation of metabolic disorders resembling Reye's syndrome. *Arch Dis Child* 1992;67:1313.

39. Glasgow JFT, Moore R. Reye's syndrome 30 years on. *BMH* 1993;307:950.

40. Centers for Disease Control and Prevention. Reye syndrome surveillance—United States, 1987 and 1988. *MMWR Morb Mortal Wkly Rep* 1989;38:325.

41. Orlowski JP, Campbell P, Goldstein S. Reye's syndrome: a case control study of medication used and associated viruses in Australia. *Cleve Clin J Med* 1990;57:323.

42. Meekin SL, Glasgow JFT, McClusker CG, et al. A long-term follow-up of cognitive, emotional, and behavioural sequelae to Reye syndrome. *Dev Med Child Neurol* 1999;41:549–553.

43. Orlowski JP. Whatever happened to Reye's syndrome? Did it ever really exist? *J Inherit Metab Dis* 1999;22(4):488–502.

44. La Montagne JR. Summary of a workshop on disease mechanisms and prospects for prevention of Reye's syndrome. *J Infect Dis* 1983;148:943.

45. Mortimer EA Jr, Lepow ML. Varicella with hypoglycemia possibly due to salicylate use. *Am J Dis Child* 1962;103:583.

46. Starko KM, Ray CG, Dominguez LB, et al. Reye's syndrome and salicylate use. *Pediatrics* 1980;66:859.

47. Waldman RJ, Hall WN, McGee N, et al. Aspirin as a risk factor in Reye's syndrome. *JAMA* 1982;247:3089.

48. Halpin TJ, Holtzhauer FJ, Campbell RJ, et al. Reye's syndrome and medication use. *JAMA* 1982;248:687.

49. Bourgeois CH. Encephalopathy and fatty viscera: a possible response to acute aflatoxin poisoning. In: Pollack JD, ed. *Reye's syndrome.* New York: Grune & Stratton, 1975:131–134.

50. Rozee KR, Laltoo M, Lee SHS, et al. Emulsifiers as enhancement factors in virus virulence. In: Crocker JFS, eds. *Reye's syndrome II.* New York: Stratton, 1979:443–457.

51. Makela AL, Lang H, Kopella P. Toxic encephalopathy with hyperammonemia during high-dose salicylate therapy. *Acta Neurol Scand* 1980;61:146.

52. Chaves-Carballo E, Gomez, MR, Sharbrough FW. Encephalopathy and fatty infiltration of the viscera (Reye-Johnson syndrome): a 17-year experience. *Mayo Clin Proc* 1975;50:209.

53. Aprille JR. Reye's syndrome: patient serum alters mitochondrial function and morphology *in vitro. Science* 1977;197:908.

54. Aprille JR, Austin J, Costello C, et al. Identification of the Reye's syndrome "serum factor." *Biochem Biophys Res Commun* 1980;94:381.

55. Aprille JR. Salicylate has several effects on mitochondrial function. *J Natl Reyes Syndr Found* 1981;2:56.

56. Asimakis GK, Aprille JR. Reye's syndrome: the effect of patient serum on mitochondrial respiration *in vitro. Biochem Biophys Res Commun* 1977;79:1222.

57. Segalman TY, Lee CP. Reye's syndrome: plasma-induced alteration in mitochondrial structure and function. *Arch Biochem Biophys* 1982;214:522.

58. Martens ME, Lee CP. Reye's syndrome: salicylates and mitochondrial functions. *Biochem Pharmacol* 1984;33:2869.

59. Martens ME, Chang CH, Lee CP. Reye's syndrome: mitochondrial swelling and Ca^{2+} release induced by Reye's plasma, allantoin, and salicylate. *Arch Biochem Biophys* 1986;244:773.

60. Martens ME, Storey BT, Lee CP. Generation of allantoin from the oxidation of urate by cytochrome *c* and its possible role in the Reye's syndrome. *Arch Biochem Biophys* 1987:252–291.

61. Thaler MM. Clinical and enzymatic indices of hepatic dysfunction in Reye's syndrome. In: Crocker JFS, ed. *Reye's syndrome II.* New York: Grune & Stratton, 1979:443–457.

62. The diagnosis and treatment of Reye's syndrome. *Natl Inst Health Consensus Dev Conf Summ* 1981;4(1):7.

63. Deshmukh DR, Maassab HF, Mason M. Interactions of aspirin and other potential etiologic factors in an animal model of Reye's syndrome. *Proc Natl Acad Sci USA* 1982;79:755.

64. Corkey BE, Hale DE, Glennon MC, et al. Relationship between unusual hepatic acyl coenzyme A profiles and the pathogenesis of Reye's syndrome. *J Clin Invest* 1988;88:782.

65. Corey L, Rubin RJ, Hatwick MAW. Reye's syndrome: clinical progression and evaluation of therapy. *Pediatrics* 1977;60:708.

66. Smith AL. Ammonia disposal in Reye's syndrome. *N Engl J Med* 1976;294:855.

67. Consensus Development Conference. Diagnosis and treatment of Reye's syndrome. *JAMA* 1982;247:3089.

68. Benjamin PY, Levinsohn M, Drotar D, et al. Intellectual and emotional sequelae of Reye's syndrome. *Crit Care Med* 1982;10:583.

69. Brunner RL, O'Grady DJ, Partin JC, et al. Neuropsychologic consequences of Reye syndrome. *J Pediatr* 1979;95:706.

70. Chapoy PR, Amgelini C, Brown WJ, et al. Systemic carnitine deficiency: a treatable inherited lipid-storage disease presenting as Reye's syndrome. *N Engl J Med* 1990;303:1389.

71. Rowe PC, Valle D, Brusilow SW. Inborn error of metabolism in children with Reye's syndrome. *JAMA* 1988;260:3167.

72. Greene CL, Blitzer MF, Sahpira E. Inborn errors of metabolism and Reye syndrome: differential diagnosis. *J Pediatr* 1988;113:156.

73. Rowe PC, Valle D, Brusilow SW. Inborn errors of metabolism in children referred with Reye's syndrome: a changing pattern. *JAMA* 1988;260:3167.

74. Jones DB, Mullick FG, Hoofnagle JH, et al. Reye's syndrome-like illness in a patient receiving amiodarone. *Am J Gastroenterol* 1988;83:967.

75. Noda S, Umezaki H, Yamamoto K, et al. Reye-like syndrome following treatment with the pantothenic acid antagonist, calcium hopantenate. *J Neurol Neurosurg Psychiatry* 1988;51:582.

76. Shahar E, Brand N, Shapira Y, et al. Familial carnitine deficiency: further evidence for autosomal recessive transmission with variable expression. *J Neurol Neurosurg Psychiatry* 1988;51:298.

77. Treem WR, Witzleben CA, Picolli DA, et al. Medium chain and long chain acyl CoA dehydrogenase deficiency: clinical, pathologic and ultrastructural differentiation from Reye's syndrome. *Hepatology* 1986;6:1270.

78. Hottenlocher RP. Reye's syndrome: relation of outcome to therapy. *J Pediatr* 1970;80:845.

79. Trey C, Burns DG, Saunder SJ. Treatment of hepatic coma by exchange blood transfusion. *N Engl J Med* 1966;294:473.

80. Tomoda T, Takeda K, Kurashige T, et al. Experimental study on Reye's syndrome: inhibitory effect of interferon alfa on acetylsalicylate-induced injury to rat liver mitochondria. *Metabolism* 1992;41:887.

81. Kindt GW, Waldman J, Kohl S, et al. Intracranial pressure in Reye's syndrome: monitoring and control. *JAMA* 1975;231:822.

82. Pinksy PF, Hurwitz ES, Schonberger LB, et al. Reye's syndrome and aspirin: evidence for a dose-response effect. *JAMA* 1988;260–657.

83. Khan AS, Kent J, Schonberger LB. Aspirin and Reye's syndrome. *Lancet* 1993;341:968.

84. Sullivan KM, Remington PL, Hurwitz ES, et al. Reye's syndrome among patients with juvenile rheumatoid arthritis. *JAMA* 1988;260:3434.

85. Rennebohm RM, Heubi JE, Daugherty CC. Reye syndrome in children receiving salicylate therapy for connective tissue disease. *J Pediatr* 1985;107:877.

Tuberculosis and Leprosy

CHAPTER 156
Tuberculosis

Kevin P. Fennelly and Jerrold J. Ellner

Tuberculosis (TB) is a preventable and curable disease, yet it continues to be a major cause of mortality, morbidity, and disability, disproportionately affecting poor individuals and countries. The purpose of this chapter is to review the clinical epidemiology, presentations, diagnosis, and management of TB. The global epidemiology, microbiology, pathogenesis, prevention, and control of TB are discussed in Chapter 265. Specific information about antituberculous drugs is provided in Chapter 34, and additional perspectives on TB in patients co-infected with human immunodeficiency virus (HIV) can be found in Chapter 115.

CLINICAL EPIDEMIOLOGY

Risk factors for active TB include conditions that either increase the chance of new infection resulting from exposure to individuals with infectious TB or increase the risk of progression from infection to disease by adversely altering the host immune response, as summarized in Table 156.1. The risk of acquiring a new infection probably increases from infancy to early adulthood (1) and is greater for men than women (2). Both observations have been attributed to the increased risk of exposure. The peak incidence of active disease is in young and middle-aged adults, with another peak after the age of 70 years with the waning of cell-mediated immunity. Most adult cases of TB occur as a result of reactivation of latent infection, whereas most pediatric TB occurs as a result of primary or recent infection with more rapid progression to disease than in adults. Immunocompetent infants with untreated infection have a 40% risk of developing disease that is more often extrapulmonary and more often fatal when compared to adults (3). The risk of developing disease for an immunocompetent adult after infection with *Mycobacterium tuberculosis* is highest in the first 2 years after infection (4). In a British study of 2,550 unvaccinated tuberculin skin-test (TST) converters, 121 (4.7%) developed active TB within 15 years of follow-up; 54% of these occurred during the first year and 82% by the second. TST-positive persons with silicosis have a 30-fold increased risk of developing active TB, and there is an increased risk among those who are underweight or are immunosuppressed by diabetes mellitus, chronic renal failure and hemodialysis, gastrectomy, jejunoileal bypass, solid organ transplantation, carcinomas of the head, neck, and lung, lymphomas and leukemias, and alcoholism (4). A high index of suspicion is paramount because of the serious consequences of misdiagnosis, especially for individuals who are immunosuppressed or who live in congregate settings where they may infect others.

Tuberculosis and Human Immunodeficiency Virus Infection

The epidemiology and natural history of *M. tuberculosis* infection has been dramatically altered by HIV (5). The reduction of cellular immunity by HIV infection is the strongest risk factor for progression of a tuberculous infection to frank TB. In HIV-infected individuals, a 4% to 8% yearly risk for development of reactivation TB contrasts sharply with a 5% to 10% lifetime risk in immunologically intact subjects (4). TB generally occurs earlier in the course of immunodeficiency than other opportunistic infections, especially in developing countries. The clinical presentation of TB depends on the stage of HIV infection. Early on, often before the occurrence of another acquired immunodeficiency syndrome (AIDS)–defining condition and when the CD4 cell count is still high (more than 200), 75% to 100% of TB manifests as pulmonary disease, whereas 25% to 70% of patients who develop TB late in the course of HIV infection when the CD4 count is low (less than 200) have extrapulmonary involvement (6). Unusual radiographic features, such as lower lung field involvement, diffuse infiltration, noncavitary disease, intrathoracic adenopathy, and pleural effusions, are more often seen in this setting (7). Symptoms may be indistinguishable from those of other opportunistic infections. In HIV-infected patients with extrapulmonary TB, active pulmonary TB (PTB) is also likely. The yield of positive sputum smears varies but is typically lower in HIV-infected tuberculous patients, particularly if nonfluorescent stains are used (8). High-yield sources for establishing the diagnosis of disseminated TB include lymph node, blood, bone marrow, and urine samples. There have been conflicting data regarding the infectiousness of HIV-infected compared with non–HIV infected patients, and data from a recent metaanalysis suggested that there is probably no overall difference between the two groups (9). Additional studies are needed to determine the mechanisms underlying the observed variability in infectiousness. Results of TSTs may be negative in up to 60% of patients. The response to therapy is in general good; however, instances of progression of infection or relapse have been reported. Whether maintenance therapy to prevent recurrence of *M. tuberculosis* infection is necessary after completion of successful treatment is not known.

CLINICAL PRESENTATIONS

Pulmonary Tuberculosis

The lungs are the predominant portal of entry and the major target organ for *M. tuberculosis,* which is almost always acquired by inhalation of airborne bacilli. More than 80% of patients with PTB manifest pulmonary findings, and the spectrum of pathology ranges from normal histology despite the presence of bacillary deoxyribonucleic acid (DNA) (10) to severe cavitary disease with fatal exsanguinating hemorrhage (11). Clinical features of PTB in different hosts are summarized in Table 156.2.

Primary pulmonary TB, (i.e., newly acquired infection with inhaled tubercle bacilli) is most often asymptomatic and is identified only by development of skin-test reactivity to tuberculin purified protein derivative (PPD). Occasionally and more commonly in children, fever, a nonproductive cough, and shortness of breath develop. Physical examination may reveal rales or signs of consolidation. Chest radiographs are normal in most patients with primary TB, perhaps because films are obtained after the pulmonary process has resolved. Infiltration without cavitation, in the anterior segment of the upper lobes or in the

TABLE 156.1.   Risk Factors for Progressing from Latent to Active Tuberculosis

	TST criteria for treatment of LTBI (mm induration)
Increased risk due to recent exposure and infection	
Close contacts of newly diagnosed patients with infectious pulmonary tuberculosis	5
HIV infection	5
Recent (<2 yr) TST converters	10
Foreign-born persons (and their families) from high-prevalence areas who have entered the United States within the past 2 yr	10
Children <5 yr	10
Homeless persons	10
Injection drug users	10
Residents and employees of high-risk congregate facilities, such as, health care and long-term care facilities, prisons, homeless shelters, residential facilities for patients with acquired immunodeficiency syndrome	10
Increased risk of reactivation due to host factors	
HIV infection	5
Therapies directed against tumor necrosis factor α	5[a]
Pulmonary fibrotic lesions on radiographs	5
Solid organ transplantation	5
Prolonged immunosuppressive therapy	5
Silicosis	10
Underweight ≤10% ideal	10
Gastrectomy, jejunoileal bypass	10
Chronic renal failure/hemodialysis	10
Diabetes mellitus	10
Carcinoma of head, neck, or lung	10
Lymphoma or leukemia	10

[a]This is our recommendation based on observed cases of reactivation in patients receiving anti-TNFα therapies, but we are not aware of published guidelines or recommendations.
HIV, human immunodeficiency virus; LTBI, latent tuberculosis infection; TST, tuberculin skin test.

TABLE 156.2.   Clinical Features of Pulmonary Tuberculosis in Various Patient Populations

Category	Infants and children <4–6 yr	Older children and immunocompetent adults		HIV-infected older children and adults	
		Early PTB	Late PTB	Early HIV (>300 CD4 cells/mm³)	Late HIV (<200 CD4 cells/mm³)
Symptoms	50% asymptomatic. ~50% weight loss, failure to thrive, cough (102,103)	"Catarrhal" phase; fatigue and fever (~50%–80%) Cough and weight loss (~55%–75%) Hemoptysis (20%)	Early symptoms + dyspnea, chest pain	Fever (95%–100%) (104,105) Weight loss (82%) Cough (49%) Hemopytis (15%)	
Chest radiograph	LAN (90%–100%) (106) Normal in 10% (102,103)	LAN (11%–35%) May be normal in 10%–15% (107,108) Consolidation (50%) Pleural effusions (24%) (108)	LAN (11%) Upper lobe cavitary disease (45%–91% cavitary) (108,109) Pleural effusions (18%–30%) (104) (108) Fibrosis (108)	LAN (13%) Upper lobe cavitary disease (20%–76%) (109) Pleural effusions (27%) (110)	LAN (36%) Upper lobe cavitary disease (0%–33%) (109) Pleural effusions (10%) (110) Mid- and lower-field infiltrates, interstitial patterns/normal (111)
Sputum smear Sputum culture	Usually not done Gastric aspirates +39%–43% (102,103)	+20%–40% (112) 72%–100% (103)	+65%–95% (112)	+56 (110) 100% in most studies by definition (if obtained)	+62%–74% (110,113) +93% (110,113)
Tuberculin skin test	+41% (102)	+80%–96% (67,114)		+75%–91% (110,115)	+0%–61% (110,115)
Extrapulmonary TB	47%	20% without and 8% with pulmonary disease in total population		Same as immunocompetent	59%–62%

HIV, human immunodeficiency virus; LAN, lymphadenopathy; PTB, pulmonary tuberculosis.

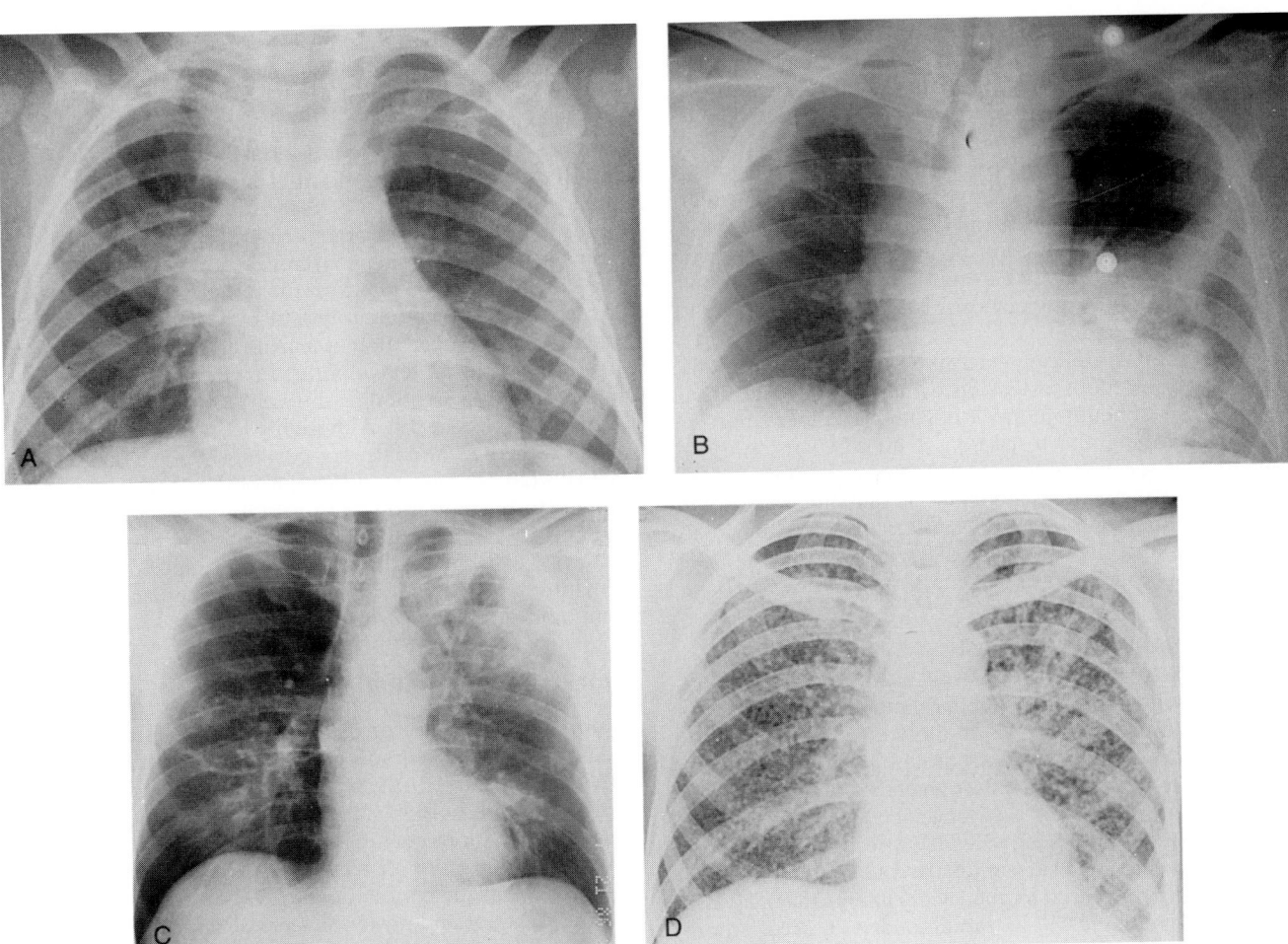

Figure 156.1. Chest radiographs of different presentations of tuberculosis. **A:** Primary tuberculosis in a child (note the right-sided hilar adenopathy, right-sided lower lobe infiltrates, and volume loss). **B:** Lower lung field tuberculosis infiltration and cavity with air-fluid level in lingula. **C:** Reactivated tuberculosis, far-advanced disease with bronchogenic spread. **D:** Miliary tuberculosis.

middle or lower lobes, pleural effusion(s), and unilateral hilar, or paratracheal adenopathy occurs more often in children. In the 15% of patients with radiographic abnormalities, there is mediastinal adenopathy that is often bilateral. Massive hilar adenopathy can lead to atelectasis, commonly involving the anterior segment of the right upper lobe or the medial segment of the right middle lobe. Calcification of both the lymph node lesion and the parenchymal lesion is known as the *Ghon complex.* Primary TB is paucibacillary. Bacteriologic confirmation by culture of sputum or bronchoalveolar lavage can be achieved in 25% to 30% of cases. At times, allergic nonpulmonary manifestations are the only evidence of a primary infection, such as erythema nodosum, scrofular conjunctivitis, or a sterile polyarthritis (12). Tuberculous pleuritis occurs months after primary infection, primarily because of the immune response. Lymph hematogenous dissemination occurs more commonly in children younger than 4 to 6 years, resulting in miliary and meningeal disease.

Progressive primary TB results from the failure of the timely development of a sufficient immune response to limit bacillary growth, so primary infection progresses to the chronic destructive phase of TB within a relatively short time. Presentation is similar to that of patients with reactivation TB. Chest radiographs show upper lobe apical and posterior segment disease, often cavitary, and at times concomitant evidence of primary disease, such as hilar adenopathy. Lower lobe TB, usually a

manifestation of progressive primary disease, constitutes 10% of all PTB (13). There may be endobronchial lesions (14). It is more common in elderly persons and in patients with diabetes mellitus. Chest radiographs sometimes show a single cavity, which may have an air-fluid level (Fig. 156.1). Diagnosis may be particularly difficult in cases in which there is a low bacillary load.

CHRONIC PULMONARY TUBERCULOSIS

Most cases of chronic PTB in adults are probably due to reactivation of bacilli at foci of hematogenous dissemination after a period of "dormancy" or persistence, although some are due to exogenous reinfection (15). In the apices of the lungs, small tubercles or fibrotic areas (Simon's foci), occasionally seen on chest radiographs, are the sites of development of disease. Factors associated with attenuation of the host cellular immune response favor reactivation of TB in latent foci. The onset of symptoms is insidious. Fever, night sweats or chills, fatigue, anorexia, weight loss, cough, chest pain, and sputum production are common. Twenty percent, however, lack such symptoms. Hemoptysis is reported in 25% of cases, usually occurring in advanced disease. Physical examination most often reveals elevated temperature and cachexia. Lung examination may be normal or nonspecific. Clubbing suggests severe or chronic disease (16). Hoarseness or frequent or strong coughing may be signs of associated laryngeal involvement that is usually more infectious.

Chest radiography typically demonstrates a patchy or confluent consolidation with increased linear densities extending to the ipsilateral hilum and thick-walled cavities without air-fluid levels (see Fig. 156.1). The apical or posterior segments of the upper lobes or the superior segments of the lower lobes are commonly involved. With bronchogenic spread, multiple alveolar densities can be seen. Lymph node enlargement is rare. Fibrosis with loss of volume and calcification can be seen in chronic disease. Laboratory abnormalities include a normochromic, normocytic anemia; normal to minimally elevated white blood cell count; and, in 20% of patients, monocytosis. Elevated serum globulin values may be observed.

Empyema may complicate extensive parenchymal cavitary TB, either by contiguous extension or as a result of a bronchopleural fistula. Pneumothorax is uncommon. Pleural fibrosis may lead to trapping and restriction of lung expansion. Massive hemoptysis secondary to the erosion of a pulmonary vessel by a cavity (Rasmussen's aneurysm) is rare but can be fatal. Hemoptysis, moderate to massive, may occur secondary to an aspergilloma in a healed tuberculous cavity. Mild hemoptysis may result from bronchiectasis, a complication of healed TB.

EXTRAPULMONARY TUBERCULOSIS

In the United States, 20% of TB cases in 2000 were extrapulmonary alone, with another 7.6% both pulmonary and extrapulmonary (17). Extrapulmonary TB in the United States has declined more slowly than PTB (18). Although the reasons are not fully understood, this may be a reflection of the disproportionate occurrence of extrapulmonary TB in special populations, such as foreign-born persons and those with HIV infection. In addition, there has been a change in sites of reported extrapulmonary involvement, with a decreased frequency of genitourinary TB and an increase in lymphatic TB. Extrapulmonary TB occurs more often in women for unknown reasons.

Tuberculous Pleuritis

Involvement of the pleural space in TB most commonly results from rupture of a subpleural caseous focus, although it may occur in disseminated disease. It usually several months after a primary infection; however, it may occur any time in the course of TB. Delayed hypersensitivity responses may result in an exudative pleural effusion and systemic symptoms. Overall, pleuritis occurs in 10% of those infected if untreated. In areas of the world where exposure to *M. tuberculosis* is common, tuberculous pleuritis affects a younger population; in the United States, it is seen more often in middle-aged and older persons.

Two thirds of patients with tuberculous pleurisy have symptoms of less than 1 month's duration, at times mimicking acute bacterial pneumonia. Fever, pleuritic chest pain, and a nonproductive cough are present. In one series, 14% of the patients had no fever (19). Weight loss, malaise, and night sweats are usually seen in patients who present with a more chronic illness. Up to 30% of TST results are negative or less than 5 mm of induration early in disease; however, by 2 months, virtually all patients have TST-positive reactions. Effusions are usually moderate in volume, involving between one third and two thirds of a hemithorax in most patients (20). They are unilateral in more than 90% of cases and occur more often in the right hemithorax. Parenchymal disease may be evident in 30%, especially in older patients. The pleural fluid is an exudate with an abundance of lymphocytes; however, polymorphonuclear leukocytes may predominate initially. A small number of mesothelial cells (less than 5%) is consistent with the diagnosis of TB; fluid examination must be performed by an expert cytologist, however. The pleural fluid glucose value is depressed (below 50 mg/dL) in

20% of cases. A pleural fluid pH value below 7.3 favors the diagnosis of TB over malignant effusion. Acid-fast bacilli (AFB) is rarely identified in pleural fluid; mycobacterial cultures, however, are positive in 20% to 50% of cases, especially when larger volumes are cultured. Pleural biopsy often establishes the diagnosis. Granulomatous pleuritis is seen in more than 60% of biopsy specimens, and AFB is seen in the material in 5% to 18%. Tissue cultures yield the organism in 55% of cases but less commonly in biopsy specimens that reveal nonspecific inflammation. The diagnosis can be made on the initial pleural biopsy in 69% of cases and in more than 95% if two or more specimens are procured (21). Tuberculous pleuritis commonly resolves spontaneously within 2 to 4 months; however, there is a considerable risk for reactivation or miliary TB during the first 5 years of follow-up (65%) (19). Although adenosine deaminase (ADA) levels in pleural fluid may support or exclude a diagnosis of TB pleuritis (20,22), they are difficult to obtain in many laboratories. In one study comparing ADA activity to polymerase chain reaction (PCR) of pleural fluid, ADA was slightly more sensitive (88% vs. 74%), but PCR was slightly more specific (90% vs. 86%) (23). Interferon-γ (IFN-γ) levels had intermediate sensitivity but were more specific (97%) (23).

Tuberculous Lymphadenitis

Historically a disease of children, tuberculous lymphadenitis (LAN) presently occurs in adults 20 to 40 years of age. Most patients are Asian or African American, and there is a 2:1 female-to-male predilection. In clinical presentation, more than 90% of cases of tuberculous adenitis involve the lymph nodes of the head and neck, a reflection of recrudescence of TB in areas infected during generalized lymphatic spread of a primary pulmonary infection. Anterior and posterior cervical, supraclavicular, or submandibular nodes and occasionally submental and preauricular lymph nodes are involved. Although mediastinal nodes are the primary regional draining sites for pulmonary infection, only 5% of lymphatic TB is characterized by such involvement. Multiple nodes within a group are involved, and bilateral involvement is common (25%). Generalized lymphadenopathy and hepatosplenomegaly occur in less than 5% of cases. About 20% of patients with lymphadenitis have constitutional symptoms. When an extremity is infected, such as by primary cutaneous inoculation, axillary or inguinal lymph nodes may be involved. The enlargement of the nodes is usually painless but may be painful and rarely ulcerate. Airway compromise secondary to enlarging and eroding parabronchial or paratracheal nodes in young children may lead to paroxysmal cough, wheezing, dyspnea, and finally respiratory distress. In adults, however, mediastinal involvement is commonly asymptomatic. Uncommon presentations include progressive jaundice due to biliary obstruction (24), dysphagia due to cervical adenitis (25), and chyluria due to obstruction of the thoracic duct (26). Physical examination may reveal discrete, rubbery, nontender lymph nodes. TSTs are positive in more than 90% of cases, and chest radiographs are abnormal in 30% of adults and most children younger than 6 years. Biopsy and culture of the involved node are necessary to differentiate adenitis due to *M. tuberculosis* from that due to mycobacteria other than *M. tuberculosis* (MOTT), a more common problem in children (27). In one U.K. series of children with a mean age of 4.86 years, *Mycobacterium avium* complex was isolated in 11 (69%) of 16 culture-proven cases of lymphadenitis due to MOTT (28).

The clinical presentation is dramatically different in HIV-infected patients; two thirds have constitutional symptoms, and almost all have abnormalities on chest radiographs. The adenopathy may be painful and may cause acute abdominal pain. In one study, mean CD4$^+$ cell counts were less than

50 cells/mm³, and all patients were anergic (29). More recent reports suggest that LAN may be exacerbated by highly active antiretroviral therapy (HAART). In HIV-infected patients, fine needle aspiration of the involved node is often diagnostic. Management of adenitis caused by *M. tuberculosis* requires antituberculous chemotherapy, and excisional surgery should be reserved for cases that do not respond to chemotherapy.

Miliary Tuberculosis

Miliary TB results from the hematogenous dissemination of large numbers of tubercle bacilli within a brief period, leading to heavy seeding of tissues and the emergence of innumerable small lesions widespread throughout the body. The frequency of organ involvement in miliary disease parallels blood flow, the most common sites being (in order) the spleen, liver, lungs, bone marrow, kidney, adrenals, and eyes. In the past, the highest prevalence was among children, and this is still the case in developing countries. In the United States, cases occur at all ages, including 30% after age 65 years.

The presentation of miliary TB is often indolent, with a low-grade intermittent or continuous fever, anorexia, weight loss, fatigue, and weakness. Cough is present in up to 60%, but dyspnea and hemoptysis are less common. Headache occurs in 15% and usually indicates meningeal involvement. Hepatomegaly occurs in 30%. Lymphadenopathy and splenomegaly are common in children. Choroidal tubercles may be the only manifestations of extrapulmonary TB (30). They are usually bilateral and from 1 to 10 occur per eye. The classic chest film pattern of diffuse, bilateral, pinpoint 2- to 3-mm densities may be absent at presentation (30%) but may become evident only after repeated examinations (31), on retrospective reviews of initial radiographs, or on chest computed tomography (CT) scans. Bilateral pleural effusions in a patient with TB suggest disseminated disease. Cultures from urine and gastric aspirates are positive for *M. tuberculosis* in 10% to 20% of cases. Histologic examination of the bone marrow is positive in 35% of cases of miliary TB, and the yield is higher with biopsy material than with aspirate, especially in patients with hematologic abnormalities (32). Histologic examination of liver biopsy material reveals granulomata, most often noncaseating, in 50% to 90% of cases. In 20% of liver biopsy specimens, AFB is detected, and sometimes cultures are positive even when granulomata are not demonstrable (33). Fiberoptic bronchoscopy with transbronchial biopsy is diagnostic in approximately 85% of cases (34,35). Mortality in miliary TB remains high; in one series, 26 of 109 patients died within 6 days of starting treatment (35). Meningitis, extremes of age, severe underlying disease, rapid development of symptoms, and delay in diagnosis are associated with poor outcome.

Tuberculosis of Bones and Joints

Skeletal TB affects the vertebral column most often (50%) and is known as *Pott's disease*. On pathologic examination, the disease is a combination of osteomyelitis and arthritis. The thoracic and lumbar vertebrae are most often involved. Patients present with the insidious onset and progression of back pain, sometimes with fever, weight loss, weakness, and numbness. In the thoracic spine, destruction can lead to severe kyphosis. Paraplegia and paraparesis may occur in 4% to 38% of cases (36). Criteria for surgical intervention include neurologic deficit, spinal instability/deformity, unresponsiveness to medical treatment, or a nondiagnostic biopsy (37).

The hip and knee are the next most commonly involved, but virtually any skeletal site may be infected. Tenosynovitis was formerly more common (38). Diagnosis requires biopsy and cul-

ture of the bone. Tuberculous arthritis presents as an indolent monarticular arthritis with swelling, pain, and limitation of motion. One fourth of patients report history of antecedent trauma. Synovial fluid has 25,000 to 100,000 white blood cells/mm³, only about 30% mononuclear cells, and a low glucose value. Culture of synovial fluid grows the organism in up to 80% of cases, whereas AFB can be seen in less than 20%. Histologic examination and culture of synovial biopsy material establish the diagnosis in 95% of cases.

Central Nervous System Tuberculosis

Tuberculous involvement of the brain occurs as a result of hematogenous dissemination, although direct extension from a nearby focus may occur, for example, from tuberculous otitis or spondylitis. The meninges may be seeded during bacillemia, forming Rich's foci, which may in turn seed the subarachnoid space and cause meningitis, tuberculomas, spinal meningitis with transverse myelitis, or a toxic encephalopathy. Tuberculous meningitis (TBM) is characterized by a basilar, exudative inflammation, entrapping the cranial nerves, and a severe arteriolitis, with subsequent thrombosis, most commonly of the branches of the middle and anterior cerebral arteries (39). A prodrome of vague symptoms and feeling ill for 2 weeks is common. Patients may have slight clouding of consciousness; without treatment, stupor, coma, cranial nerve palsies, and convulsions may occur. Acute onset of symptoms has been reported in 50% of cases in children, whereas the disease is more often indolent in adults. Fever is usually present.

The cerebrospinal fluid may initially show predominance of granulocytes; however, on serial examinations, a shift to mononuclear cells and a drop in the glucose level occur. Smears of cerebrospinal fluid reveal AFB in 10% to 20% of cases. Repeated examinations may increase the yield to more than 80%. CT detects meningeal enhancement in 60% to 86% of cases and tuberculomas in less than half of patients. Both meningeal enhancement and tuberculomas (especially less than 1 cm) are, however, more commonly seen by magnetic resonance imaging (40). Hydrocephalus appears to increase with duration of illness and portends a poor prognosis. Mortality in TBM is adversely affected by a delay in instituting therapy, extremes of age, and the degree of mental status alteration on presentation. Moderate evidence favors the use systemic corticosteroid therapy for TBM in addition to antituberculous therapy (41).

Intracranial tuberculomas occasionally mimic pyogenic brain abscesses, and symptoms and signs are due to the mass effects of the lesions, including seizures. Antituberculous therapy, as opposed to surgical resection, is the treatment of choice (42). Corticosteroids may be helpful if brain edema is present.

Gastrointestinal Tuberculosis

Tuberculous enteritis appears to occur concurrently with PTB in endemic areas. Its frequency correlates with the severity of lung disease: 1% with minimal disease and 25% with extensive pulmonary disease (43). However, primary tuberculous enteritis occurs in 20% of all cases of gastrointestinal (GI) tract TB. The resistance of mycobacteria to digestion allows organisms to reach and invade bowel mucosa. The most common site of disease is the ileum; the cecum, jejunum, colon, rectum, and anus are infected less often. Anorexia, weight loss, abdominal pain, nausea, vomiting, night sweats, and diarrhea or constipation are reported; however, 15% of patients with GI tract involvement remain asymptomatic and their disease is discovered at autopsy or during surgery for other reasons.

The onset of illness may be acute, with bowel perforation or obstruction, but more often it is indolent. Physical examination is usually not helpful in diagnosis. Tuberculous enteritis may be complicated by formation of fistulas to adjacent organs and by GI tract hemorrhage. Barium radiographic studies of the GI tract commonly reveal a nodular or ulcerated mucosa, bowel wall edema, and abnormal motility, but such findings are non-specific. Colonoscopy is of limited usefulness in establishing the diagnosis because tuberculous granulomata are commonly sub-mucosal, as opposed to the mucosal location of granulomata in Crohn's disease. Caseating granulomata are found in a minority of patients, and growth of mycobacteria from bowel specimens is uncommon. The response to antituberculous therapy supports the diagnosis of enteric TB. Abdominal TB in HIV-infected patients is almost invariably a manifestation of disseminated disease and is associated with significant mortality (44). Tuberculous peritonitis is a rare manifestation of TB attributed to rupture of a caseous mesenteric node infected during hematogenous dissemination (45).

Pericardial Tuberculosis

Involvement of the pericardium is rare; however, it is associated with mortality of 30% to 40%, despite chemotherapy. The patient presents with cough, dyspnea, orthopnea, chest pain, and weight loss. Fever, tachycardia, hepatomegaly (60%), peripheral edema (50%), distant heart sounds, and jugular venous distention are present on examination. Pericardial rub is heard in 35% of patients, and pulsus paradoxus is found in 23% of cases. Chest radiographs reveal cardiomegaly and often a left-sided pleural effusion. Electrocardiograms may have nonspecific ST-T wave changes, but ST-segment elevation is seen in only 10% of patients. Echocardiography should be performed if pericardial disease is suspected, and hemodynamic monitoring may be indicated for those at risk of tamponade (46). Pericardial biopsy may establish the diagnosis in 10% of patients (47), and cultures of pericardial fluid can be positive in 50% of cases (48). Hemodynamic compromise is present in half of patients and may occur acutely, and recurrent tamponade is common after pericardiocentesis. Surgical drainage and creation of a pericardial window is usually indicated in addition to antituberculous therapy. Without treatment, mortality exceeds 80%. Adjunctive corticosteroids may be necessary to curtail signs of inflammation and control associated arrhythmias.

Endocrine Disease

The most common endocrine complication of TB is adrenal insufficiency. TB, in fact, is the most common cause of adrenal insufficiency worldwide (49). At least 7 of the 11 patients first described by Addison had adrenal TB. Among 871 autopsies of patients with active TB in Hong Kong, 52 (6%) had adrenal involvement (50). Hyponatremia secondary to the syndrome of inappropriate antidiuretic hormone secretion is seen occasionally but is rarely symptomatic. Hypercalcemia is present in up to 25% of patients with active PTB and disappears with treatment of the infection. As in other granulomatous diseases, hypercalcemia in TB is associated with high serum calcitriol (1,25-dihydroxycholecalciferol) levels (51).

Tuberculosis and Cancer

Recent epidemiologic studies have confirmed associations between a history of prior PTB and lung cancer in both Asia (52) and the United States (53), but the mechanisms underlying these associations are mostly unknown. In one series, TB was associated with lung carcinoma in 29 (13%) of 220 cases (54). Among these cases, there were seven "scar carcinomas," two of which arose in scars associated with TB. Poor clearance of carcinogens in scarred areas of the lung is a postulated mechanism. PTB may also complicate other neoplasias due to reactivation (55).

DIAGNOSIS

The gold standard for the diagnosis of active TB remains the demonstration of AFB in clinical specimens, confirmed by growing the organisms in culture. For microscopy, fluorescence staining is preferable because it is more sensitive and less time consuming. Although sputum smears for AFB are criticized for having a variable and poor sensitivity as low as 45%, use of a minimum sputum volume of 5 mL was found to improve sensitivity from 73% to 92% at one center (56). Early growth detection using the BACTEC system and use of highly specific and sensitive nucleic acid amplification (NAA) tests can aid in the diagnosis and identification of *M. tuberculosis* in both smear-positive and smear-negative specimens (57–59). The GenProbe NAA test identified *M. tuberculosis* in 21% of cultures within 1 week and in 66% of cultures within 2 weeks. The radiometric procedure has also been applied to drug susceptibility testing of *M. tuberculosis* and may be superior to conventional susceptibility testing using solid media because of its rapidity (60). A promising approach for rapid drug susceptibility testing is the use of luciferase reporter mycobacteriophages to infect *M. tuberculosis*. In the presence of added substrate (luciferin), only metabolizing (live) organisms produce light, which can then be measured by a liminometer (61). Other methods such as molecular beacons are being developed to rapidly detect drug resistance (62,63).

PTB is most often diagnosed using sputa specimens. If the patient cannot produce a sputum specimen spontaneously, sputum can be induced by inhalation of hypertonic saline. Because these specimens often appear more watery than spontaneously produced ones, they should be labeled as such so that laboratory staff do not mistake the specimen for saliva. The yield of three induced sputa samples was similar to bronchoalveolar lavage in one study (64). The cumulative yield for AFB on smear and culture increased from 64% and 70% on one induced sputum to 98% and 100% on four induced samples (64). When sputa specimens are smear negative, fiberoptic bronchoscopy can establish the diagnosis. Among 41 patients whose spontaneous sputa was smear negative, AFB smears of the bronchoscopic washings were positive in 39 (95%) (65). Postbronchoscopy sputa may be the only specimens that are positive in about 12% of cases (65,66). Bronchoscopy and biopsy may be most helpful in evaluating miliary TB or endobronchial TB. Morning gastric aspirates can also be obtained before the patient arises from bed if sputum is not available. A positive smear of gastric aspirate, particularly if it shows multiple AFB, is suggestive of TB; however, it may indicate only ingested nontuberculous mycobacteria.

Approximately 50% of patients with miliary disease and 25% of those with PTB have a negative TST result (67), so TSTs should not be relied on for the diagnosis of TB disease. However, in low-prevalence settings, a positive TST may suggest a diagnosis of TB. Chest radiography may provide supportive data but cannot provide a definitive diagnosis. Reliance on only posteroanterior views may miss cavities, as illustrated in Figure 156.2. Chest CT is usually not needed, but it may be especially helpful in evaluating possible miliary or cavitary disease, for example, in considering adjunctive resection surgery in multidrug-resistant TB

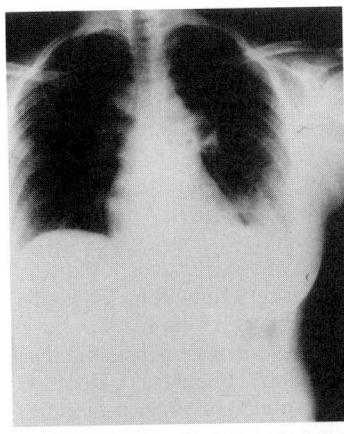
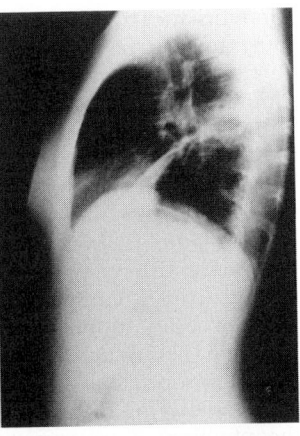

A

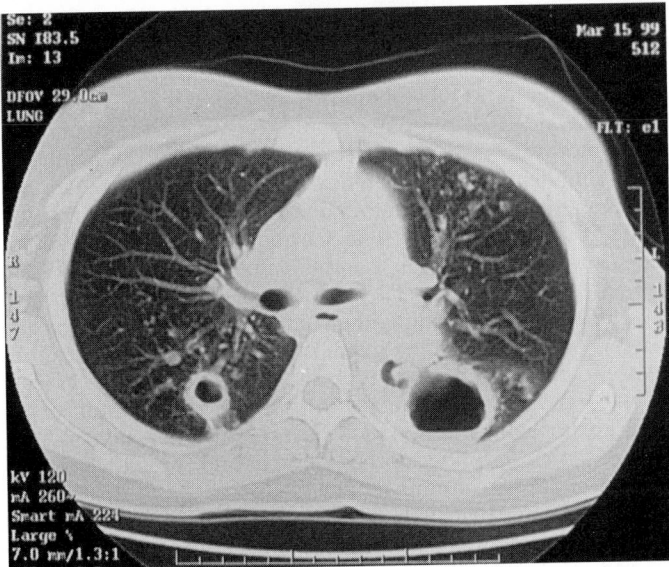

B

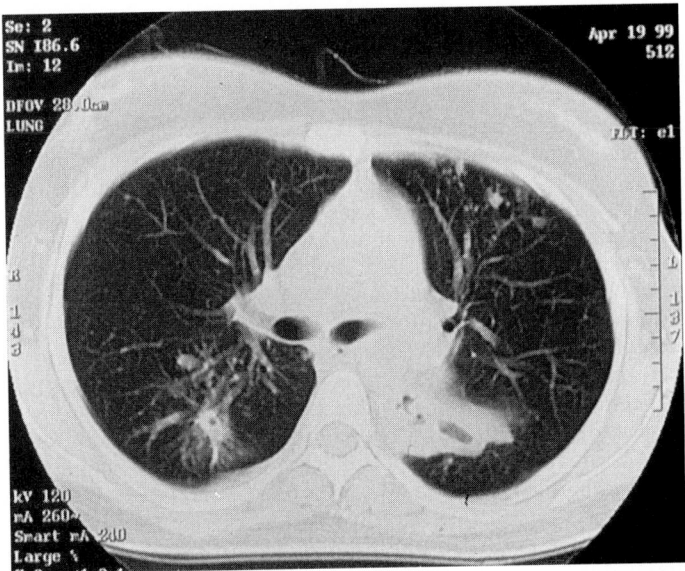

C

Figure 156.2. Chest radiograph (**A**) and computed tomography (CT) scan (**B**), the latter of which more clearly demonstrates two cavitary lesions. A repeated CT scan (**C**) showed improvement after 1 month of treatment in a young woman with primary multidrug-resistant tuberculosis.

(MDR-TB) (68). Magnetic resonance imaging has proven most useful in spinal and soft tissue disease (69).

Differential Diagnosis

The major entity to be distinguished from PTB is carcinoma of the lung. The two may be present concurrently, and in such cases, delayed radiographic evidence of healing despite antituberculous therapy necessitates further diagnostic workup. Bacterial lung abscesses can usually be differentiated from tuberculous infection by their lower lobe distribution and the presence of air-fluid levels in cavities and the common presence of putrid odor indicating anaerobic infection. Other granulomatous infections of the lung can be similar to TB clinically and radiographically. Mimics of TB include fungal processes, such as histoplasmosis, coccidioidomycosis, blastomycosis, and occasionally cryptococcosis; other mycobacterioses, such as *Mycobacterium kansasii* and *M. avium* complex infections; or infections caused by unusual agents, such as *Burkholderia pseudomallei* from Southeast Asia.

Diagnosis of Latent Tuberculosis Infection

Most individuals infected with TB never develop active disease, but treatment of them can decrease the risk of reactivation in the future. Revised U.S. guidelines emphasize the concept that a decision to use the TST should be a decision to treat if the test is positive, with the exception of surveillance of workers in high-risk settings, such as hospitals or prisons (4). In general, testing should be targeted to persons at increased risk of recent infection or at risk of reactivation of latent infection due to immunosuppression or comorbid conditions. (See Table 156.1.)

The diagnosis of latent tuberculosis infection (LTBI) is made using the Mantoux method for tuberculin skin testing in which 5 tuberculin units (TU) of PPD is placed intradermally on the volar forearm, and the diameter of induration is read at 48 to 72 hours. The cut point for a positive TST result is dependent on both the amount of induration and the risk category of the patient. Cross-reactions are due to infection with MOTT and vaccination with bacille Calmette-Guérin (BCG) (70). In general, the larger the induration, the greater the probability of infection with *M. tuberculosis*. Using 15 mm of induration as the cutoff point increases the specificity to diagnose infection with *M. tuberculosis*, but at the cost of decreased sensitivity. A reaction larger than 5 mm should be considered positive in persons who have recently had close contact with a patient with TB, in persons whose chest radiographs are consistent with TB, and in immunosuppressed persons who are likely to show blunted response to the organism, such as HIV-infected persons. Recommended criteria for treating LTBI based on the amount of induration are summarized in Table 156.1 (4).

Waning of skin-test reactivity can occur with advancing age, at a rate of approximately 5% per year. However, delayed hypersensitivity can be restimulated by repeated tests, referred to as boosting. In situations in which repeated skin testing is expected (e.g., yearly testing of hospital employees), a second skin test should be done 1 week after a negative initial test result to establish a baseline with a reduced risk of boosting. False-negative tuberculin reactions are associated with cellular immune hyporesponsiveness, as may occur in concurrent viral infections (HIV infection, measles, varicella), lymphoreticular malignant neoplasms, malnutrition, sarcoidosis, immunosuppressive drugs, chronic renal failure, and severe illness of any kind. Given the limitations of the TST (71), there is a need for better methods to diagnose LTBI. One promising tool is the whole-blood IFN-γ assay, which appears to be less affected by BCG vaccination or exposures to nontuberculous mycobacteria (72).

TREATMENT OF TUBERCULOSIS

The approach to treatment of TB is based on several principles that have evolved over the last four decades (73). First, spontaneous, random, chromosomal mutations that confer resistance to each antituberculous drug proscribe against the use of a single agent for treatment. Treatment with more than one drug is necessary to prevent acquired drug resistance in all cases except when the number of bacilli is very low, for example, in the treatment of latent infection. Second, modern treatment is theoretically aimed at heterogeneous populations of organisms: (a) extracellular bacilli undergoing rapid proliferation, (b) slowly replicating bacilli, perhaps retarded by necrotic conditions, (c) sporadically multiplying or active bacilli, and (d) nonreplicating, "dormant," or persistent bacilli not vulnerable to antibiotic drug actions (74,75). Isoniazid has the best "early bactericidal activity" (EBA) against the rapidly dividing population, whereas pyrazinamide and rifampin are more active against the more slowly dividing bacilli. The third guiding principle is that treatment must be continued for at least 6 months to prevent relapse (76–78). The fourth and most recently learned principle is that directly observed therapy is almost always indicated for effective treatment, although there is not universal agreement (79). The most effective treatment balances efficacy, toxicity, acceptability, deliverability, prevention of resistance, and prevention of relapse (73). Because relapse usually occurs during the first 12 months after completion of therapy, patients should continue to be observed medically during this period.

HIV-infected patients with TB have been found to respond favorably to short-course chemotherapy. Therefore, the same treatment regimens are recommended except for changes due to drug–drug interactions and for extension of the duration of therapy to 9 months if the microbiologic response is slow, for example, the sputum cultures were positive at 2 months (80). The most common drug interactions are between the rifamycins and the protease inhibitors and the nonnucleoside reverse-transcriptase inhibitors (81). Clinicians are advised to consult updated guidelines regarding such therapies. Reconstitution of the immune response with HAART may produce a "paradoxical response" in which patients appear to worsen clinically. In some studies, relapse rates were higher among HIV-infected patients with TB.

Although available data on pretreatment susceptibility testing in initial treatment of TB indicate a marginal impact on the outcome of therapy, such testing should be employed where it is available, such as in the United States. Susceptibility testing is indicated for patients suspected of having drug-resistant TB, those who suffer relapse, those whose sputum smears are still positive

2 months after treatment, and those whose acid-fast sputa stains revert to positive while they are receiving treatment.

The first-line agents in the treatment of TB (isoniazid, rifampin, pyrazinamide, ethambutol, and streptomycin) are potent drugs, associated with relatively little toxicity, and highly effective in combination in most cases. The initial regimen of choice is usually isoniazid, rifampin, pyrazinamide, and ethambutol, which can all be administered orally (82). An alternative to ethambutol is streptomycin, which has the disadvantages of being administered parenterally and of auditory, vestibular, and renal toxicity. Rifampin has many drug interactions associated with its ability to induce hepatic enzymes. Patients should be counseled about such interactions in addition to increasing doses when appropriate (e.g., prednisone should usually be doubled) or to monitoring drug levels (e.g., anticoagulation parameters, theophylline). If drug resistance is ruled out, the ethambutol or streptomycin can be discontinued, although in reality these results are often not available until the end of the 2-month intensive phase. At this time, the regimen can be narrowed to isoniazid and rifampin for another 4 months. A second regimen includes isoniazid and rifampin for 9 months, again using ethambutol or streptomycin until drug susceptibility studies are available. These regimens are equally efficacious, with no failures and relapse rates of 1.5%. The first regimen is less expensive and may be slightly less toxic to the liver. Current guidelines suggest that the fourth drug to initiate therapy is not necessary if there is a very low risk of drug resistance. However, this is often difficult to ascertain, and we recommend including the fourth drug for this reason. When the combination of isoniazid and rifampin cannot be used, the duration of therapy should be extended to at least 12 to 18 months, because data with other regimens for shorter periods are not available. Success of any regimen depends on compliance, so close follow-up is advisable and directly observed therapy should be administered when possible.

Given the age distribution of TB, it disproportionately affects pregnant women in whom it probably causes excessive morbidity and mortality (83). The benefit of treatment outweighs the risk of toxicity to the fetus (84). In the United States, the recommended treatment is isoniazid, rifampin, and ethambutol. Although pyrazinamide has not been documented to cause teratogenicity, its use is discouraged in the use because of inadequate safety data. However, the use of pyrazinamide during pregnancy is recommended in the United Kingdom (85). Streptomycin is contraindicated because of considerable auditory toxicity among exposed infants. Of the second-line drugs, ciprofloxacin has the best safety profile (83).

Tuberculin-reactive patients with chest radiographic patterns consistent with TB (pleural residues, pulmonary infiltrates, and hilar adenopathy) who have at least three smear- and culture-negative sputa can be treated with isoniazid alone for 9 months or isoniazid-rifampin for 4 months (86). Successful treatment of extrapulmonary TB involving the meninges, lymph nodes, and genitourinary system with 9 to 12 months of isoniazid-rifampin has been well documented (87); however, bone and joint involvement requires longer therapy (88). The regimens currently recommended for the treatment of TB in HIV-infected and HIV-uninfected patients are similar. However, in the presence of HIV infection, assessment of bacteriologic and clinical responses is critical and the duration of treatment is based on the rapidity of optimal response.

When drug-resistant isolates are identified, or when patients cannot tolerate first-line agents, second-line agents (p-aminosalicylic acid, ethionamide, cycloserine, capreomycin, kanamycin, amikacin, thiacetazone, clarithromycin, and the quinolones) must be used. These agents have a narrower therapeutic index than the first-line drugs, that is, they are usually more toxic and less efficacious. Most clinicians have little experience with these drugs, which are often administered for unusually long durations lasting 2 years or more. For these reasons, some experts have recommended that these patients be referred to specialized centers with expertise with these drugs (89). Patients who received at least part of their treatment at one referral center had significantly higher completion rates than those treated as outpatients alone (79% vs. 48%.) (90). Although the role of monitoring drug concentrations with pharmacokinetic studies may have limited public health value in drug-susceptible TB (91), a reasonable argument is made for its case in drug-resistant TB given the narrow therapeutic index of these agents combined with the long duration of therapy (92).

At a referral center in the United States from 1973 to 1982, only 56% of patients with MDR-TB responded to intensive medical therapy (93). At the same center from 1983 to 1993, the overall success rate improved to 81% after increasing surgical resection from 5.3% to 57%, using fluoroquinolone antibiotics, and implementing pharmacokinetic drug monitoring (89). Improved outcomes have been noted at other centers without the addition of surgery, such as one multicenter report from New York City in which 24 (96%) of 25 showed clinical and microbiologic responses at a median of 91 weeks. However, this patient population was younger, had drug resistance to fewer drugs, and had a markedly shorter duration of disease than the Denver population. An overall success rate in treating MDR-TB of 77% was achieved at a center in Turkey, with surgical intervention in 23% (94). A poor outcome was independently associated with older age and previous treatment with ofloxacin. A similar cure rate (81%) was achieved at a center in Hong Kong (95). Poor outcomes were associated with the presence of cavitation and resistance to ofloxacin. These data suggest that adjunctive surgical resection of cavities may improve outcomes in MDR-TB, but clinical trials are needed to better define the selection of patients and to assess the benefits versus the surgical risks.

Hepatotoxicity is the major adverse effect of therapy with the first-line antituberculous drugs. Patients must be advised of symptoms (e.g., nausea, anorexia, and jaundice) and instructed to promptly discontinue treatment and inform their physician when they occur. Deaths due to isoniazid hepatotoxicity are associated with continuation of the drug despite symptoms. Although about 10% of patients have abnormal results on liver function tests, only 1% develop clinical hepatitis. Hepatitis usually occurs 4 to 8 weeks after the start of therapy. The rate of occurrence of hepatitis increases with age and is nil for patients younger than 20 years. Daily use of alcohol is a risk factor for development of hepatitis. In general, adverse drug effects are best detected clinically by health care providers at monthly visits rather than by routine monitoring of laboratory values in the absence of symptoms. Though rare, optic toxicity with ethambutol can be devastating, and patients should be informed and advised to report symptoms of any visual changes and should have baseline eye examinations. Monthly visits and periodic eye examinations are also helpful in detecting early toxicity so therapy can be discontinued. GI toxicity is most common with the second-line drugs, occurring in 100% of 60 patients treated for MDR-TB in a community-based program in Peru (96). It is clear that new drugs are needed to treat MDR-TB with greater effectiveness and less toxicity.

Corticosteroids may be beneficial in the initial management of PTB in some patients with hypoxemia, hypoalbuminemia, persistent fever, and weight loss (97). Daily doses of 20 to 60 mg of prednisone have been well tolerated without complications as long as the patient is treated with appropriate chemotherapy. The use of corticosteroids in tuberculous constrictive pericarditis has been associated with better survival, normalization

of rhythm, and fewer requirements for pericardiectomy (98). In TBM and tuberculomas, corticosteroids may promote reduction of cerebral edema, vasculitis, and cranial nerve entrapment. Given the important protective role of IFN-γ, the early finding of improved microbiologic responses to inhaled IFN among patients with MDR-TB (99) suggested that this may be a beneficial immunomodulatory therapy. The future of immunomodulatory therapies is challenging given the paradox of immune stimulation and suppression observed in TB, and well-designed clinical trials are needed.

Treatment of Latent Tuberculosis Infection

Formerly known as *chemoprophylaxis* or *preventive therapy,* treatment of LTBI is intended to decrease the risk of reactivation. Daily isoniazid remains the most highly recommended treatment, but the optimal duration has been extended to 9 months (4). Based on data supporting the use of rifampin and pyrazinamide for a markedly shorter duration of treatment of LTBI in HIV-infected individuals, new guidelines included such regimens as an alternative in all persons regardless of HIV status if necessary because of problems with adherence to the longer regimen or to intolerance of isoniazid (4). However, these recommendations were recently revised because of unexpected hepatotoxicity in HIV-uninfected persons, including five deaths from liver failure, in patients treated with rifampin and pyrazinamide for 2 months (100). The 2-month rifampin-pyrazinamide treatment may be used for the HIV-infected patient, but it should be used with great caution in those not infected with HIV, especially if there is any history of alcoholism, liver disease, or use of hepatotoxic medication. Closer observation and monitoring are recommended (100). Alternative regimens include 4 months of daily rifampin or 3 months of daily rifampin-isoniazid (85). The latter provided sustained protection from active TB for up to 3 years in HIV-infected persons in Uganda, whereas the protection offered by the 6-month regimen of daily isoniazid was less than 1 year (101). The preferred treatment for pregnant women is daily or twice-weekly isoniazid with pyridoxine supplementation.

CONCLUSION

The future holds great promise as the mysteries of TB are unraveled. As cases of active disease decline in developed countries, the major challenge will be to maintain clinical suspicion of TB and to more effectively detect and treat latent infection. In contrast, the challenge in developing nations with limited resources is to provide more rapid diagnosis and more effective treatment of active disease to large numbers of patients.

ACKNOWLEDGMENT

Dr. Fennelly was supported in this work by a National Institutes of Health Career Development Award (1K23AI01676-03).

REFERENCES

1. Sutherland I, Fayers PM. The association of the risk of tuberculous infection with age. Tuberculosis Surveillance Research Unit report no. 3. *Bull Int Union Tuberc* 1975;50:70–81.
2. Holmes CB, Hausler H, Nunn P. A review of sex differences in the epidemiology of tuberculosis. *Int J Tuberc Lung Dis* 1998;1998:96–104.

3. Munoz FM, Starke JR. Tuberculosis in children. In: Reichman LB, Hershfield ES, eds. *Tuberculosis: a comprehensive international approach.* New York: Marcel Dekker, 2000:553–595.

4. American Thoracic Society, Centers for Disease Control and Prevention. Targeted tuberculin testing and treatment of latent tuberculosis infection. *Am J Respir Crit Care Med* 2000;161:S221–S247.

5. Shafer RW, Edlin BR. Tuberculosis in patients infected with human immunodeficiency virus: perspective on the past decade. *Clin Infect Dis* 1996;22:683.

6. Barnes PF, Bloch AB, Davidson PT, et al. Tuberculosis in patients with human immunodeficiency virus infection. *N Engl J Med* 1991;324:1644–1650.

7. Hopewell PC. Tuberculosis and human immunodeficiency virus infection. *Semin Respir Infect* 1989;4:111–122.

8. Long R, Scalcini M, Manfreda J, et al. The impact of HIV on the usefulness of sputum smears for the diagnosis of tuberculosis. *Am J Public Health* 1991;81:1326–1328.

9. Cruciani M, Malena M, Bosco O, et al. The impact of human immunodeficiency virus type 1 on infectiousness of tuberculosis: a meta-analysis. *Clin Infect Dis* 2001;33:1922–1930.

10. Hernandez-Pando R, Jeyanathan M, Mengistu G, et al. Persistence of DNA from *Mycobacterium tuberculosis* in superficially normal lung tissue during latent infection. *Lancet* 2000;356:2133–2137.

11. Rasmussen V, Moore WD. Hemoptysis, especially when fatal, in its anatomical and clinical aspects. *Edinb Med J* 1968;14:385.

12. Dall L, Long L, Stanford J. Poncet's disease: tuberculous rheumatism. *Rev Infect Dis* 1989;11:105–107.

13. Stead WW, Kerby GR, Schlueter DP, et al. The clinical spectrum of primary tuberculosis in adults. *Ann Intern Med* 1968;68:731–745.

14. Chang S, Lee P, Perng R. Lower lung field tuberculosis. *Chest* 1987;91:230.

15. Stead WW. Pathogenesis of a first episode of chronic pulmonary tuberculosis in man: recrudescence of residuals of the primary infection or exogenous reinfection. *Am Rev Respir Dis* 1967;95:729–745.

16. Reeve PA, Harries AD, Nkhoma WA, et al. Clubbing in African patients with pulmonary tuberculosis. *Thorax* 1987;42:986–987.

17. Centers for Disease Control and Prevention, Division of TB Elimination. Reported tuberculosis in the United States, 2000.

18. Rieder HL, Snider DEJ, Cauthen GM. Extrapulmonary tuberculosis in the United States. *Am Rev Respir Dis* 1990;141:347–351.

19. Berger HW, Mejia E. Tuberculous pleurisy. *Chest* 1973;63:88–92.

20. Valdes L, Alvarez D, San Jose E, et al. Tuberculous pleurisy: a study of 254 patients. *Arch Intern Med* 1998;158:2017–2021.

21. Levine H, Metzger W, Lacera W, et al. Diagnosis of tuberculous pleurisy by culture of pleural biopsy specimen. *Arch Intern Med* 1970;126:269–271.

22. Light RW. Establishing the diagnosis of tuberculous pleuritis. *Arch Intern Med* 1998;158:1967–1968.

23. Villegas MV, Labrada LA, Saravia NG. Evaluation of polymerase chain reaction, adenosine deaminase, and interferon-gamma in pleural fluid for the differential diagnosis of pleural tuberculosis. *Chest* 2000;118:1355–1364.

24. Kohen MD, Altman KA. Jaundice due to rare causes: tuberculous lymphadenitis. *Am J Gastroenterol* 1973;59:48–53.

25. Case records of the Massachusetts General Hospital weekly clinicopathological exercise: case 7-1977. *N Engl J Med* 1977;296:384–389.

26. Wilson RS, White RJ. Lymph node tuberculosis presenting as chyluria. *Thorax* 1976;31:617–620.

27. Appling D, Miller RH. Mycobacterial cervical lymphadenopathy: 1981 update. *Laryngoscope* 1981;91:1259–1266.

28. Evans MJ, Smith NM, Thornton CM, et al. Atypical mycobacterial lymphadenitis in childhood—a clinicopathological study of 17 cases. *J Clin Pathol* 1998;51:925–927.

29. Artenstein AW, Kim JH, Williams WJ, et al. Isolated peripheral tuberculous lymphadenitis in adults: current clinical and diagnostic issues. *Clin Infect Dis* 1995;20:876–882.

30. Mansour AM, Haymond R. Choroidal tuberculomas without evidence of extraocular tuberculosis. *Graqefes Arch Clin Exp Opthalmol* 1990;228:382–383.

31. Munt PW. Miliary tuberculosis in the chemotherapy era: with a clinical review in 69 American adults. *Medicine (Baltimore)* 1972;51:139–155.

32. Berger HW, Samortin TG. Miliary tuberculosis: diagnostic methods with emphasis on the chest roentgenogram. *Chest* 1970;58:586–589.

33. Cucin RL, Coleman M, Eckhardt JJ, et al. The diagnosis of miliary tuberculosis: utility of peripheral blood abnormalities, bone marrow, and liver biopsy. *J Chronic Dis* 1973;26:355–361.

34. Willcox PA, Potgieter PD, Bateman ED, et al. Rapid diagnosis of sputum negative miliary tuberculosis using the flexible fiberoptic bronchoscope. *Thorax* 1986;41:681–684.

35. Maartens G, Willcox PA, Benatar SR. Miliary tuberculosis: rapid diagnosis, hematologic abnormalities, and outcome in 109 treated adults. *Am J Med* 1990;89:291–296.

36. Gorse GJ, Pais MJ, Kusske JA, et al. Tuberculous spondylitis. A report of six cases and a review of the literature. *Medicine (Baltimore)* 1983;62:178–193.

37. Rezai AR, Lee M, Cooper PR, et al. Modern management of spinal tuberculosis. *Neurosurgery* 1995;36:87–98.

38. Jackson RH, King JW. Tenosynovitis of the hand: a forgotten manifestation of tuberculosis. *Rev Infect Dis* 1989;11:616–618.

39. Verdon R, Chevret S, Laissy JP, et al. Tuberculous meningitis in adults: review of 48 cases. *Clin Infect Dis* 1996;22:982–988.

40. Gupta RD, Gupta S, Singh D, et al. MR imaging and angiography in tuberculous meningitis. *Neuroradiology* 1994;36:87–92.

41. McGowan JEJ, Chesney PJ, Crossley KB, et al. Guidelines for the use of systemic glucocorticosteroids in the management of selected infections. *J Infect Dis* 1992;165:1–13.

42. Bagga A, Kaira V, Ghai OP. Intracranial tuberculoma: evaluation and treatment. *Clin Pediatr* 1988;27:487–490.

43. Thoeni RF, Margulis AR. Gastrointestinal tuberculosis. *Semin Roentgenol* 1979;14:283–294.

44. Fee MJ, Oo MM, Gabayan AE, et al. Abdominal tuberculosis in patients infected with human immunodeficiency virus. *Clin Infect Dis* 1995;20:938–944.

45. Singh M, Bhargave AN, Jain KP. Tuberculous peritonitis. An evaluation of pathogenetic mechanisms, diagnostic procedures and therapeutic measures. *N Engl J Med* 1969;231:1091–1094.

46. Heurich AE, Quale JM, Burack JH. Pericardial tuberculosis. In: Rom WN, Garay S, eds. *Tuberculosis.* Boston: Little, Brown and Company, 1996:531–540.

47. Fredriksen RT, Cohen LS, Mullins CB. Pericardial windows or pericardiocentesis for pericardial effusions. *Am Heart J* 1971;82:158–162.

48. Rooney JJ, Crocco JA, Lyons HA. Tuberculous pericarditis. *Ann Intern Med* 1970;72:73–81.

49. Lowy J. Endocrine and metabolic manifestations of tuberculosis. In: Rom WN, Garay SM, eds. *Tuberculosis.* New York: Little, Brown, and Company, 1996:669–674.

50. Lam KY, Lo CY. A critical examination of adrenal tuberculosis and a 28-year autopsy experience of active tuberculosis. *Clin Enocrinol (Oxf)* 2001;54:633–639.

51. Abbasi AA, Chanplavil JK, Farah S, et al. Hypercalcemia in active pulmonary tuberculosis. *Ann Intern Med* 1979;90:324–328.

52. Brenner AV, Wang Z, Kleinerman RA, et al. Previous pulmonary diseases and risk of lung cancer in Gansu Province, China. *Int J Epidemiol* 2001;30:118–124.

53. Wu A, Fontham ET, Reynolds P, et al. Previous lung disease and risk of lung cancer among lifetime nonsmoking women in the United States. *Am J Epidemiol* 1995;141:1023–1032.

54. Dacosta NA, Kinare SG. Association of lung carcinoma and tuberculosis. *J Postgrad Med* 1991;37:185–189.

55. Flance IJ. Scar cancer of the lung. *JAMA* 1991;266:2003–2004.

56. Warren JR, Bhattacharya M, De Almeida KN, et al. A minimum 5.0 ml of sputum improves the sensitivity of acid-fast smear for *Mycobacterium tuberculosis.* *Am J Respir Crit Care Med* 2000;161:1559–1562.

57. Centers for Disease Control and Prevention. Update: nucleic acid amplification tests for tuberculosis. *MMWR Morb Mortal Wkly Rep* 2000;49:593–594.

58. Heifets LB, Good RC. Current laboratory methods for the diagnosis of tuberculosis. In: B.R. Bloom, ed. *Tuberculosis: pathogenesis, protection, and control.* Washington, D.C.: ASM Press, 1994:85–110.

59. Ellner PD, Kiehn TE, Cammarata R, et al. Rapid detection and identification of pathogenic mycobacteria by combining radiometric and nucleic acid probe methods. *J Clin Microbiol* 1988;26:1349–1352.

60. Heifets L. Qualitative and quantitative drug susceptibility tests in mycobacteriology. *Am Rev Respir Dis* 1988;137:1217–1222.

61. Jacobs WR, Barletta RG, Udani R, et al. Rapid assessment of drug susceptibilities of *Mycobacterium tuberculosis* by means of luciferase reporter phages. *Science* 1993;260:819–822.

62. Riska PF, Su Y, Bardarov S, et al. Rapid film-based determination of antibiotic susceptibilities of *Mycobacterium tuberculosis* strains by using a luciferase reporter phage and the Bronx Box. *J Clin Microbiol* 1999;37(4):1144–1149.

63. Piatek AS, Tyagi S, Pol AC, et al. Molecular beacon sequence analysis for detecting drug resistance in *Mycobacterium tuberculosis.* *Nat Biotechnol* 1998;16(4):359–363.

64. Al Zahrani K, Al Jahdali H, Poirere L, et al. Yield of smear, culture, and amplification tests from repeated sputum induction for the diagnosis of pulmonary tuberculosis. *Int J Tuberc Lung Dis* 2001;5:855–860.

65. Danek SJ, Bower JS. Diagnosis of pulmonary tuberculosis by flexible fiberoptic bronchoscopy. *Am Rev Respir Dis* 1979;119:677–679.

66. Wallace JM, Deutsch AL, Harrell JH, et al. Bronchoscopy and transbronchial biopsy in evaluation of patients with suspected active tuberculosis. *Am J Med* 1981;70:1189–1194.

67. Nash DR, Douglass JE. Anergy in active pulmonary tuberculosis. A comparison between positive and negative reactors and an evaluation of 5 TU and 250 TU skin test doses. *Chest* 1980;77:32–37.

68. Lee KS, Hwang JW, Chung MP, et al. Utility of CT in the evaluation of pulmonary tuberculosis in patients without AIDS. *Chest* 1996;110:977–984.

69. Soler R, E. R, Remuinan C, Santos M. MRI of musculoskeletal extraspinal tuberculosis. *J Comput Assist Tomogr* 2001;25:177–183.

70. von Reyn CF, Horsburgh CR, Olivier KN, et al. Skin test reactions to *Mycobacterium tuberculosis* purified protein derivative and *Mycobacterium avium* sensitin among health care workers and medical students in the United States. *Int J Tuberc Lung Dis* 2001;5:1122–1128.

71. Huebner RE, Schein MF, Bass JBJ. The tuberculin skin test. *Clin Infect Dis* 1993;17:968–975.

72. Mazurek GH, LoBue PA, Daley CL, et al. Comparison of a whole-blood interferon gamma assay with tuberculin skin testing for detecting latent *Mycobacterium tuberculosis* infection. *JAMA* 2001;286:1740–1747.

73. Iseman M. Tuberculosis chemotherapy, including directly observed therapy. In: *A clinician's guide to tuberculosis.* Philadelphia: Lippincott, Williams & Wilkins, 2000:271–321.

74. Fox W, Mitchison DA. Short-course chemotherapy for pulmonary tuberculosis. *Am Rev Respir Dis* 1975;111:325–353.

75. Mitchison D. Mechanisms of action of drugs in the short course chemotherapy. *Bull Int Union Tuberc* 1985;60:36–40.

76. Controlled clinical trial of five short-course (4-month) chemotherapy regimens in pulmonary tuberculosis. Second report of the 4th study. East African/British Medical Research Councils Study. *Am Rev Respir Dis* 1981; 123:165–170.

77. Bass JBJ, Farer LS, Hopewell PC. Treatment of tuberculosis and tuberculosis infection in adults and children: American Thoracic Society and the Centers for Disease Control and Prevention. *Am J Respir Crit Care Med* 1994;149(5):1359–1374.

78. Tripathy SP. Controlled clinical trial of a 3 month and two 5 month regimens in pulmonary tuberculosis: second study of the short-term treatment administered in Madras. *Bull Int Union Tuberc* 1983;38:97–101.

79. Ogden J. The resurgence of tuberculosis in the tropics: improving tuberculosis control-social science inputs. *Trans R Soc Trop Med Hyg* 2000;94:135–140.

80. Centers for Disease Control and Prevention. Prevention and treatment of tuberculosis among patients infected with human immunodeficiency virus: principles of therapy and revised recommendations. *MMWR Morb Mortal Wkly Rep* 1998;47(RR-20):1–51.

81. Centers for Disease Control and Prevention. Updated guidelines for the use of rifabutin or rifampin for the treatment and prevention of tuberculosis among HIV-infected patients taking protease inhibitors or nonnucleoside reverse transcriptase inhibitors. *MMWR Morb Mortal Wkly Rep* 2000;49:185–189.

82. American Thoracic Society, Centers for Disease Control and Prevention/IDSA. Diagnostic standards and classification of tuberculosis in adults and children. *Am J Respir Crit Care Med* 2000;161:1376–1395.

83. Bothamley G. Drug treatment for tuberculosis during pregnancy: safety considerations. *Drug Safety* 2001;24:553–565.

84. Snider DE, Layde RM, Johnson MW, et al. Treatment of tuberculosis during pregnancy. *Am Rev Respir Dis* 1980;122:65–79.

85. Joint Tuberculosis Committee of the British Thoracic Society. Chemotherapy and management of tuberculosis in the United Kingdom: recommendations 1998. *Thorax* 1998;53:536–548.

86. Dutt AK, Moers D, Stead WW. Smear- and culture-negative pulmonary tuberculosis: four-month short course chemotherapy. *Am Rev Respir Dis* 1989; 139:867.

87. Dutt AK, Moers D, Stead WW. Short-course chemotherapy for extrapulmonary tuberculosis: nine years' experience. *Ann Intern Med* 1986;104:7.

88. Dutt AK, Moers D, Stead WW. Results of therapy in tuberculosis of bones and joints. *Am Rev Respir Dis* 1988;137:24A.

89. Iseman MD. Drug-resistant tuberculosis. *A clinician's guide to tuberculosis.* Philadelphia: Lippincott, Williams & Wilkins, 2000:323–353.

90. Narita M, Alonso P, Lauzardo M, et al. Treatment experience of multidrug-resistant tuberculosis in Florida, 1994–1997. *Chest* 2001;120:343–348.

91. Narita M, Hisada M, Thimmappa B, et al. Tuberculosis recurrence: multivariate analysis of serum levels of tuberculosis drugs, human immunodeficiency virus status, and other risk factors. *Clin Infect Dis* 2001;32:515–517.

92. Peloquin C. Tuberculosis drug levels. *Clin Infect Dis* 2001;33:584–585.

93. Goble M, Iseman MD, Madsen LA, et al. Treatment of 171 patients with pulmonary tuberculosis resistant to isoniazid and rifampin. *N Engl J Med* 1993;328:527–532.

94. Tahaoglu K, Torum T, Sevim T, et al. The treatment of multidrug-resistant tuberculosis in Turkey. *N Engl J Med* 2001;345:170–174.

95. Yew WY, Chan CK, Chau CH, et al. Outcomes of patients with multidrug-resistant pulmonary tuberculosis treated with ofloxacin/levofloxacin-containing regimens. *Chest* 2000;117:744–751.

96. Furin JJ, Mitnick CD, Bayona J, et al. Occurrence of serious adverse effects in patients receiving community-based therapy for multidrug-resistant tuberculosis. *Int J Tuberc Lung Dis* 2001;5:648–655.

97. Alzeer AH, FitzGerald JM. Corticosteroids and tuberculosis: risks and use as adjunct therapy. *Tuberc Lung Dis* 1993;74:6–11.

98. Strang JI, Kakasa HH, Gibson DG, et al. Controlled trial of prednisolone as adjuvant in treatment of tuberculous constrictive pericarditis in Transkei. *Lancet* 1987;2:1418–1422.

99. Condos R, Rom WN, Schluger NW. Treatment of multidrug-resistant pulmonary tuberculosis with interferon-gamma via aerosol. *Lancet* 1997;349:1513–1515.

100. Centers for Disease Control and Prevention. Update: fatal and severe liver injuries associated with rifampin and pyrazinamide for latent tuberculosis infection, and revisions in American Thoracic Society/CDC recommendations—United States, 2001. *MMWR Morb Mortal Wkly Rep* 2001;50:733–735.

101. Johnson JL, Okwera A, Hom DL, et al. Duration of efficacy of treatment of latent tuberculosis infection in HIV-infected adults. *AIDS* 2001;15:2137–2147.

102. Schaaf HS, Beyers N, Gie RP, et al. Respiratory tuberculosis in childhood: the diagnostic value of clinical features and special investigations. *Pediatr Infect Dis J* 1995;14:189–194.

103. Starke JR, Taylor-Watts KT. Tuberculosis in the pediatric population of Houston, *Texas Pediatr* 1989;84:28–35.

104. Shafer RW, Kim DS, Weiss JP, et al. Extrapulmonary tuberculosis in patients with human immunodeficiency virus infection. *Medicine* 1991;70:384–397.

105. Eriki PP, Okwera A, Aisu T, et al. The influence of human immunodeficiency virus infection on tuberculosis in Kampala, Uganda. *Am Rev Respir Dis* 1991;143:185–187.

106. Leung AN, Muller NL, Pineda PR, et al. Primary tuberculosis in children: radiographic manifestations. *Radiology* 1992;182:87–91.

107. Marciniuk DD, McNab BD, Martin WT, et al. Detection of pulmonary tuberculosis in patients with a normal chest radiograph. *Chest* 1999;115:445–452.

108. Woodring JH, Vandiviere HM, Fried AM, et al. Update: The radiographic features of pulmonary tuberculosis. *AJR Am J Roentgenol* 1986;146:497–506.

109. Iseman MD. Tuberculosis in relation to HIV and AIDS. *A clinician's guide to tuberculosis.* Philadelphia: Lippincott, Williams & Wilkins, 2000:199–252.

110. Jones BE, Young SM, Antoniskis D, et al. Relationship of the manifestations of tuberculosis to the CD4 cell counts in patients with human immunodeficiency virus infection. *Am J Respir Crit Care Med* 1993;150:595–596.

111. Post FA, Wood R, Pillay GP. Pulmonary tuberculosis in HIV infection: radiographic appearance is related to CD4+ count. *Tuberc Lung Dis* 1995;76:518–521.

112. Kim TC, Blackman RS, Heatwole KM, et al. Acid-fast bacilli in sputum smears of patients with pulmonary tuberculosis. *Am Rev Respir Dis* 1984;129:264–268.

113. Small PM, Schecter GF, Goodman PC, et al. Treatment of tuberculosis in patients with advanced human immunodeficiency virus infection. *N Engl J Med* 1991;324:289–294.

114. Edwards LB, Palmer CE, Edwards PQ. Further studies of geographic variation in naturally acquired tuberculin sensitivity. *Bull WHO* 1955;12:63–83.

115. Mukadi Y, Perriens JH, St.Louis ME, et al. Spectrum of immunodeficiency in HIV-1–infected patients with pulmonary tuberculosis in Zaire. *Lancet* 1993;342:143–146.

CHAPTER 157

Environmental Mycobacterial Infections

Michael D. Iseman and Mary Ann DeGroote

Mycobacteria are slender, raylike aerobic bacilli; they are tinctorially characterized by retention of dyes despite exposure to the potent decolorizing agent acid alcohol, an attribute that gives rise to the informal designation as acid-fast bacilli (AFB). The most widely recognized human pathogens among the genus are *Mycobacterium tuberculosis*, the bacillus that causes the classic pulmonary and extrapulmonary diseases referred to collectively as "tuberculosis" (TB), and *Mycobacterium leprae* or Hansen's bacillus, the microbe that causes the cutaneous and neural disorder known as leprosy. In this chapter, we deal with the other mycobacterial species that are associated with human disease, both pulmonary and extrapulmonary. Controversy exists over the aggregate designation of these organisms. In the past, they have variously been referred to as anonymous, environmental, unclassified, or atypical. More recently, there have been movements in favor of using the term *nontuberculous mycobacteria* or *mycobacteria other than TB* (MOTT). As an adjective, *nontuberculous* is fundamentally inaccurate, because these organisms typically do elicit gross and histologic "tubercles" in infected tissues. The designation "MOTT" is substantially correct and inclusive; however, it has not found wide acceptance. Hence, in a departure from our prior practice, these organisms will be referred to as "environmental mycobacteria" (EM) in this chapter.

The term *TB* is reserved for disease due to *M. tuberculosis*; mycobacterial infections caused by the EM, including *Mycobacterium bovis*, are referred to as *mycobacterioses*. Although *M. bovis* is part of the TB complex, because the usual sources and modes of transmission are not human to human, we prefer to continue this practice. Recent reports have documented an epidemic involving human-to-human transmission, primarily among human immunodeficiency virus (HIV)–infected persons, with an organism identified genetically as *M. bovis* (1–3). However, this was a highly anomalous organism including a heretofore undescribed 11-drug resistance pattern. Though exceedingly rare, this outbreak highlights the relatedness of some *M. bovis* strains to *M. tuberculosis* (4).

Unlike *M. tuberculosis* and *M. leprae*, EM are generally found free in the water and/or soil. Falkinham (5) has published a thorough and informative review of the environmental sources, biology, and clinical epidemiology of these organisms. It is widely held that they are contracted from these environmental sources and not from other infected humans. Typically, there are demonstrable abnormalities in local host defenses or deficits of immunity associated with the development of EM disease. Indeed, we now evaluate all patients with pulmonary EM disease on the assumption that there are risk factors that have predisposed them to such illness.

EPIDEMIOLOGY

Whereas each species should be considered separately, some observations on the prevalence and distribution of EM disease in the aggregate may be made. Because reporting of EM infections is not mandatory, comprehensive data comparable to those for *M. tuberculosis* are not available. However, national surveys done in the 1980s from the United States (6), Japan (7), and Switzerland (8) showed remarkably similar profiles of EM disease with case prevalences of approximately 1 per 100,000 population. Yet, there are wide variations in the regional distribution of EM pathogens; for example, in one area *Mycobacterium avium* complex (MAC) is predominant, whereas in others *Mycobacterium kansasii* (Mk), *Mycobacterium xenopi* (Mx), or other EM species may be more prevalent (8–12).

One of the more striking features of the recent epidemiology of EM disease in the United States is the consistently high proportion of white patients. In a recent series, the proportion of whites has ranged from 81% to 100% (6,13–15). TB, the prototypic mycobacterial lung infection, is far more prevalent among persons of color than the white population in the United States. Although this finding is readily understood to be due to the human-to-human transmission pattern, higher rates of latent infection in these populations, and various socioeconomic factors, this model does not address the apparent lack of EM disease in persons of color. If the EM are ubiquitous and all races/nationalities are comparably vulnerable, there should be a distribution of EM disease roughly proportionate to the current U.S. demographics. The underrepresentation of persons of color among these recent series needs to be considered. Perhaps it reflects differences in access to health care, less aggressive diagnostic assessment, environmental variables, or constraints on referrals. Or, it could be due to a protective effect of TB infection versus EM (infection with TB "vaccinates" against EM). Rather, though, we suspect that it represents in large measure significant differences in biologic vulnerability, presumably related to the inherited conditions noted in Table 157.1 or other disorders/polymorphisms that are yet to be identified.

The other epidemiological anomaly is the overwhelming majority of women among series of nodular bronchiectatic MAC disease: 17 (81%) of 21, 29 (94%) of 31, 12 (75%) of 16, 13 (76%) of 17, 29 (83%) of 35, 22 (91%) of 24, and 71 (91%) of 78 were women among reports from the United States over the last decade (13,14,16–20). Japanese investigators have also recognized this epidemiological shift; a recent report described pulmonary MAC patients without evident predispositions, of whom 48 (91%) of 53 were women (21). By contrast, men comprised two thirds to 100% of patients with pulmonary MAC reported between 1973 and 1991 (22–26).

Although the *extent* of this shift from male- to female-dominant case series might be disputed, the validity of the trend seems indisputable to those working in this field (27). A variety of explanations for this pattern have been put forward. Voluntary cough suppression or Lady Windemere's syndrome has been proposed by Reich and Johnson (28); however, we are quite dubious about this concept (29,30). One Japanese group proposed that this was related to estrogen deficiency in the postmenopausal population (31). Using a murine model of intratracheal instillation, they demonstrated higher numbers of MAC in the lungs of mice that had undergone ovariectomy, noting that estrogen repletion led to normalization of the mycobacterial burden. They then showed that estrogen enhanced the capacity of bone marrow–derived macrophages, augmented with interferon-γ (IFN-γ), to inhibit intracellular growth of MAC; this was associated with enhanced production of reactive nitrogen intermediates. It might be argued that in addition to postmenopausal individuals, vulnerability to MAC among slender women might be related to the relative paucity of circulating estrogens in this population (32–34). However, these findings do *not* explain the recent predilection of women versus men for MAC. One theory we are considering is the relatively anabolic effects of androgens versus the antiproliferative properties of estrogens on connective tissue (see section "Slender Body Habitus," later in this chapter). Studies among a limited number of women in the Stanford series (13) failed to show relationships with the NRAMP1 or IFN-γR1 genes (35).

Given the ambiguities of the data, it is difficult to offer a precise assessment of the extent of the EM, but it seems probable that there has been an increase in both the absolute and the relative (to TB) incidence of disease due to MAC and the rapidly growing mycobacteria (RGM). Note that these increases are *not* due to the impact of HIV infection; they occurred before and independently of the appearance of acquired immunodeficiency syndrome (AIDS). An overall upward trend for Mk disease is not apparent, although in some communities, it has become the dominant mycobacterial pathogen (36). Sporadic cases or focal endemicity of the other mycobacterioses are the rule.

DISEASE FORMS

For the purposes of this chapter, pulmonary disease, localized extrapulmonary infection, and disseminated or multifocal extrapulmonary disease are discussed separately.

Pulmonary Environmental Mycobacterial Disease

Lung infections caused by EM range in severity from rapidly progressive, destructive pneumonic disease to indolent disorders with minimal clinical findings manifest over the short term. Predisposing conditions or discrete precipitating events may be identified in many cases. Therapy is generally far less predictable than with disease caused by *M. tuberculosis* because of substantially greater levels of drug resistance and underlying lung disorders.

The risk factors that we have identified as predispositions for pulmonary disease caused by the EM are displayed in Table 157.1. They were originally recognized in relation to MAC disease; however, we have recently seen increasing numbers of cases in which RGM are seen in persons with these conditions. In some cases, we have seen simultaneous "mixed" infections with MAC, whereas in others the infections are metachronous, typically with the RGM following MAC disease.

TABLE 157.1. Predisposing Factors for Environmental Mycobacterial Lung Disease

A. Traditional lung disorders
1. Chronic bronchitis and emphysema (chronic obstructive pulmonary disease)
2. Inorganic dust pneumoconioses
3. Fibrosis associated with ankylosing spondylitis or rheumatoid arthritis
4. Radiation lung injury, alveolar proteinosis, pulmonary embolism
B. Heritable conditions
1. α_1-Antitrypsin deficiency
2. Cystic fibrosis
3. Disordered ciliary motility
4. Tracheobronchomegaly
C. Slender body habitus
1. Women: pectus excavatum, scoliosis, mitral valve prolapse
2. Men: history of spontaneous pneumothorax
D. Prior lung infections
1. Tuberculosis
2. Histoplasmosis
3. Coccidioidomycosis
E. Aspiration
1. Gastroesophageal reflux disease
2. Achalasia
3. Abnormalities of deglutition
F. Aerosol exposure/hypersensitivity pneumonitis/bronchiolitis obliterans organizing pneumonia (BOOP)
1. Indoor hot tubs
2. Industrial

Among a large consecutive case population seen from 1996 to 2000 at National Jewish Medical and Research Center (Denver, Colorado) for either MAC or RGM disease, we found the following prevalences for these putative predisposing factors: cystic fibrosis (CF) 16%, abnormal α_1-antitrypsin anomalies 23%, and among those tested, esophageal reflux or dysmotility 72% to 83% (20). It is important to note that this population clearly does not reflect the entire "universe" of such patients in the United States. We acknowledge that referral bias surely results in selection of patients, particularly women, who do not have obvious explanations for their EM disease.

TRADITIONAL LUNG DISORDERS

Early reports of pulmonary disease caused by MAC infection stressed the relationship between cigarette-induced chronic obstructive pulmonary disease (COPD), particularly in men (22–24,26,37). The geographic distribution of these cases in the United States from 1960 to 1980 was mainly in the south and southeastern states (38).

Other conditions that appeared to predispose to EM lung infections include inorganic dust pneumoconioses, most notably silicosis (22,23,26); pulmonary fibrosis associated with ankylosing spondylitis or rheumatoid arthritis (22,39); radiation lung injury, typically related to therapeutic x-irradiation (40) for breast cancer or lymphoma (unpublished data); alveolar proteinosis (41); or prior pulmonary embolism (unpublished data).

HERITABLE CONDITIONS

α_1-Antitrypsin Deficiency.
While α_1-antitrypsin deficiency is commonly associated with premature emphysema, quantitative (or functional) deficiencies of this serum protein appear to predispose to EM infections/disease.

This antiproteolytic compound inhibits a variety of enzymes, but its main *in vivo* substrate is thought to be neutrophil elastase (42–44). It is composed of 394 amino acids and is coded for by a single gene on chromosome 14. It is produced by hepatocytes and released into the serum. α_1-Antitrypsin is an acute-phase reactant, typically rising in the presence of inflammatory events.

Mutations in this chromosome may result in impaired release from hepatocytes, leading in some cases to liver damage and cirrhosis. However, more importantly, homozygous mutations result in impaired capacity to inhibit neutrophil elastases released in the lungs, which may cause precocious and severe emphysema.

Normal alleles are referred to as "M." Persons with the MM phenotype have normal protease inhibitory capacity and normal circulating levels of α_1-antitrypsin. The most common mutation results in the Z allele. Persons homozygous for the Z allele (protease inhibition phenotype Pi-ZZ) have very low circulating levels of the protein and if they are smokers, typically develop emphysema early in their life. The next most common mutation results in the allele S; other rare alleles have been described.

Racial variations in α_1-antitrypsin deficiency may also be relevant to the epidemiology of EM disease in the United States. Northern European whites have far higher rates of Pi-Z mutations than those of African or Asian descent. This may explain, in part, the clear predominance of whites in EM disease series.

The biologic importance of heterozygous alleles such as MZ or MS is controversial. In some surveys, there appear to be minimal or no disturbances of pulmonary function in these persons. However, other reports suggest the heterozygous patients are more vulnerable to airflow obstruction and accelerated declines in pulmonary function (45). In addition, under inflammatory stress, heterozygous patients mount attenuated acute-phase responses (46,47). We believe that the heterozygous states among our patients represent clinically relevant predispositions.

With regard to EM infections, α_1-antitrypsin deficiency has been reported to predispose to bronchiectasis and emphysema (48–52). We originally believed that the airway damage that led to bronchiectasis occurred through the same mechanism as emphysema, the elastase–antielastase model. This may be so, but recent evidence suggests an alternative or complementary mechanism. Shapiro, Pott, and Ralston (53) have called attention to the central role of α_1-antitrypsin in inhibiting the growth of the HIV in whole blood; α_1-antitrypsin, among various effects, inhibits entry of HIV into cells. Perhaps there is an analogous effect on intracellular access for the mycobacteria. Lieberman (54) noted that 56 of 74 α_1-antitrypsin deficiency patients who had received Prolastin repletion therapy and perceived benefit from it thought this was due to fewer infections. This is consistent with the observation that α_1-antitrypsin repletion was associated with fewer hospitalizations (55) and that aerosolized Prolastin suppressed *Pseudomonas aeruginosa* proliferation in a chronic infection rat model (56).

Thus, we now believe that α_1-antitrypsin deficiencies, heterozygous or homozygous, predispose to EM lung disease and bronchiectasis through both inadequate inhibition of neutrophil elastases and vulnerability to recurrent respiratory tract infections through mechanisms not yet defined.

Cystic Fibrosis.
CF an autosomal recessive inherited disorder that typically becomes clinically apparent in infants and children. CF is associated with chronic airflow obstruction, recurrent/chronic respiratory tract infections, and exocrine pancreatic insufficiency.

There are numerous mutations of a single gene on chromosome 7 that influence the disordered physiology and severity of CF. This gene encodes for a membrane protein called the *cystic fibrosis transmembrane regulator* (CFTR). The CFTR regulates primarily chloride channels but also has variable effects on other ions.

Like α_1-antitrypsin deficiency, CF mutations are much more common among whites than Native American, African, or Asian populations. Clinical CF was seen in approximately 1 of 2,500 white (57), 1 of 17,000 black (58), and 1 of 90,000 Asian infants born in Hawaii (59).

Fundamentally, CF mutations result in disordered movement of sodium, chloride, and water across epithelial surfaces, causing abnormally thickened mucus and sweat. Indeed, elevated concentrations of chloride in sweat have been the gold standard for diagnosis.

However, it appears as though some of the mutations that result in less severe dysfunction may produce milder varieties of CF-like disease without an abnormal sweat chloride test (60–62). The most common and functionally profound mutation is the ΔF508; it is found in roughly two thirds of patients with CF, particularly those of northern European ancestry. However, with the advent of genetic analyses of the CF genome, it is apparent that there are several hundred distinctive mutations that can affect the CFTR protein (63,64).

The relationship of "heterozygosity" and clinical dysfunction has recently emerged. Formerly, it was believed that an individual with a single mutation, typically ΔF508, represented a clinically benign carrier state. However, as the number of other recognized mutations has expanded, it has become apparent that some of these "heterozygotes" have abnormalities involving both alleles. In other cases, patients have functionally less severe mutations involving both alleles. Indeed, a small percentage of patients who meet the clinical criteria for the diagnosis of CF have only one identified mutation (63,64). Whether this represents an unrecognized mutation of the other allele, a profound effect of the single mutation or other genetic factors is not yet clear (65,66).

In any case, we believe that CF, typically milder variants, results in increased vulnerability to EM disease among our group of patients. Such infection has been recognized previously among patients with early onset CF (67–69). However, we are seeing CF-related EM disease, usually associated with bronchiectasis, sinusitis, and chronic airflow obstruction, in middle-aged and elderly subjects. Whether the pathogenesis involves dysfunctionally thickened mucus or enhanced adhesion of microbes to airway epithelium, the effects of CF on "defensins" function or other mechanism are yet to be clarified.

Disordered Ciliary Motility. Dysfunctional cilia, either "immotile" or "disordered," predispose to chronic respiratory tract infections and bronchiectasis; we have seen a modest number of cases in which such patients developed EM infections, primarily MAC disease. The typical cases have been young women with a lifelong history of sinusitis, otitis, and bronchitis/pneumonia; infertility is common. They usually present in their 20s or 30s with severe lower lobe bronchiectasis; the middle lobes or lingula are less severely involved and upper lung zones are spared. Rarely do these patients have classic Kartagener's syndrome involving (immotile cilia with absent dynein arms on electron microscopy and *situs inversus universalis* (70); rather, they have morphologically normal cilia that beat in an uncoordinated manner, "disordered ciliary motility" (71,72).

Tracheobronchomegaly. Rare inherited disorders that predispose to EM disease include tracheobronchomegaly. Mounier-Kuhn syndrome (73) or Williams-Campbell syndrome (74) result in grossly dilated central airways and distal bronchiectasis. Such patients present with chronic and recurrent respiratory tract infections from childhood. Among the pathogens that may afflict these patients are the EM (unpublished data).

SLENDER BODY HABITUS

The propensity for slender persons to develop TB goes back to Hippocrates when such individuals were designated as "phthisical," from the Greek for wasting away or consumptive. Modern surveys from the U.S. Navy (75) and Norway (76) document that the slender or asthenic habitus generally antedated the active TB, indicating that it is both a risk factor for TB and a consequence.

We originally noted in 1991 that slender women with varying combinations of pectus excavatum, scoliosis, straight-back syndrome, and/or mitral valve were prominently overrepresented among a series of pulmonary MAC patients seen at National Jewish (77).

As we have come to recognize the roles of α_1-antitrypsin deficiency and CF as risk factors for EM disease, it has become apparent that there is some overlap between these heritable disorders and the aforementioned habitus. However, in the majority of instances, neither of these conditions is present in our slender female patients. Thus, we continue to speculate that by itself, this slender phenotype designates some particular vulnerability to EM disease. Notable, perhaps, is that persons with Marfan's syndrome are typically slender, narrow chested, more likely to have pectus excavatum, and/or scoliosis, apt to have mitral valve prolapse (MVP) (as well as aortic value insufficiency), and at increased risk of spontaneous pneumothorax (78). The presence of these features in many patients with MAC raises the question of whether there might be an abnormality of connective tissue analogous to the fibrillin defects related to Marfan's disorder. A recent report of a large cohort from Belgium referred for suspected Marfan's syndrome described a wide array of physical findings associated with various mutations of the fibrillin-1 gene, FBN1 (78). Hypothetically, diminished tensile strength of the airways and airspaces could result in cystic anomalies in the lungs. These might make patients vulnerable to lower respiratory tract infections, and the coughing that ensued could result in dilation of the airways or bronchiectasis.

The apparently greater risk among women for this process is not evident by analogy to Marfan's syndrome, which is an autosomal dominant disorder. However, it is feasible that the androgenic effects of testosterone may partially compensate for this putative connective tissue weakness. The protective effects of androgens might also be related to the accelerated rate of decline of pulmonary function in women with α_1-antitrypsin Pi-MZ phenotype (45), the increased susceptibility to severe, early onset COPD (79), or earlier deaths among women than men with CF in the United States; median ages at death in 1990 were 25 and 30 years, respectively (80).

An alternative explanation has been put forward in the form of "Lady Windemere's syndrome" (28). This is predicated on the notion that slender, delicate women have been acculturated to voluntarily suppress their cough in an effort to be lady like, thus leading to accumulated secretions. We think this unlikely but do concede that the thoracic anomalies noted may lead to ineffectual cough, perhaps due to airway collapse.

Although the male patients we see with EM lung disease generally are of slender body habitus, smoking-related COPD or inorganic dust pneumoconioses are more prominent risk factors. However, we have noted that among slender, young men with EM disease, there often is a history of recurrent spontaneous pneumothoraces in adolescence and early adulthood. However, scoliosis, pectus excavatum, straight-back syndrome, and MVP are uncommon among these patients.

PRIOR LUNG INFECTIONS

Consistent with the premise that EM generally invade persons with compromised lung defenses, MAC disease has previously been described in persons with prior TB, typically involving regions of the lungs previously damaged (22,23). Recently we reported a series of patients with MAC infection whose residential histories and computed tomographic (CT) scan evidence of hilar/peribronchial/mediastinal/splenic calcifications strongly suggested antecedent histoplasmosis (81). Also, we have seen occasional patients with prior coccidioidomycosis who subsequently develop MAC. In most of these cases, prior chest x-ray films or CT scans indicate that the EM invades the lung zones previously infected; this suggests that the vulnerability to EM occurs through prior damage, not simply because of primary susceptibility to mycobacterial or fungal infections.

ESOPHAGEAL DYSFUNCTION/ASPIRATION

The role of aspiration as an inciting factor for EM pulmonary disease is not well defined, but we believe that it contributes in both a primary and a secondary role to these lung infections. A relationship between achalasia and RGM lung disease has been suggested by an earlier report (82); it has been assumed that the patulous, distended esophagus becomes colonized by RGM, which are then aspirated into the lungs. However, we do not believe this to be the mechanism in most patients.

Our focus on the potential roles of other disorders of esophageal function was initiated by the frequency with which we observed dilation and/or thickening of the esophagus on thoracic CT scans done to evaluate lung disease with or without an evident hiatal hernia. In some cases, patients gave histories consistent with gastroesophageal reflux disease (GERD), but in others, such symptoms ("heartburn") could not be elicited. However, performing contrast studies and/or pH probes on a subset of our patients, most of whom did not have other apparent predispositions, we noted a 83% prevalence of abnormal motility and 72% prevalence of GERD among patients with bronchiectasis and NTM disease. In most of the cases, it has not been possible to establish a direct relationship between the esophageal disorder and the pathogenesis of the NTM lung disease. The extremely high prevalence of the esophagogastric disturbances, though, far exceeds that expected; it is estimated that the prevalence of symptomatic esophagitis occurs in less than 10% of the U.S. adult population daily and less than 20% weekly (83–85).

Some cases appear to reflect nonspecific dysfunction typical in older persons, so-called *presbyesophagus*. However, the pathogenesis in other cases is obscure. The various esophageal motility disorders were recently reviewed (86). It is feasible that chronic cough related to the infection may compromise the integrity of the lower esophageal sphincter (LES) mechanism, possibly by distending the diaphragmatic crura or the phrenoesophageal ligament (87). Certainly the high frequency with which GERD is seen in patients with chronic asthma (88–90), COPD (91), or interstitial pulmonary fibrosis (92) suggests that chronic cough or otherwise altered mechanics of breathing leads to dysfunction of the LES mechanism. In some cases, it may be related to the effects on the LES of various medications employed in these disorders including theophylline, β agonists, anticholinergics, or corticosteroids (93). Or, if our hypothesis regarding relative weakness of the connective tissue in these slender women is correct, this might alter the function and morphology of the esophagus or diaphragm. The high frequency of GERD in children with tracheomalacia (87) is interesting in this regard. We should note that esophageal disturbances also occur in persons with the other predisposing conditions noted earlier, suggesting a secondary role in these cases.

Regarding a mechanistic relationship, we reason that in most instances recurrent aspiration results in injury to the airways or airspaces, making them vulnerable on subsequent exposure to the EMs. This EM exposure might occur by inhalation (see section "*Mycobacterium Avium* Complex") or less likely by inclusion in the aspirated material.

In addition to reflux, aspiration in some cases was related to disordered deglutition. Mechanisms involved with swallowing disturbances include brain or brainstem disorders including Parkinson's disease.

AEROSOL EXPOSURES/HYPERSENSITIVITY PNEUMONITIS/BRONCHIOLITIS OBLITERANS ORGANIZING PNEUMONIA (BOOP)

As noted, we believe that most EM lung infections are acquired by the aerogenic route. However, in contrast to the usual scenario that we posit (inhalation by individuals with predisposing conditions of a relatively small number of mycobacteria suspended in the air), we and others have recently recognized a distinctive syndrome in which it appears that high concentrations of EM are abruptly inhaled inducing a hypersensitivity reaction rather than the usual invasive infection. Settings in which this has been described include indoor hot tubs (94,95), indoor environments with water damage, or industrial situations in which immersion of hot metal or other processes generate aerosols (96–100). In these cases, the EM, perhaps abetted by other waterborne microbes, act more like an organic antigen than a classic invasive pathogen (101).

The patients commonly present with escalating dry cough, dyspnea, obstructive lung dysfunction, and hypoxia, often severe. Early chest x-ray films may be normal or hyperinflated; later, focal opacification/consolidation may appear and fever, malaise, and other constitutional symptoms emerge (102).

CT scan of the lungs is quite useful, revealing various combinations of cellular bronchiolitis ("tree-in-bud" pattern), air-trapping with mosaicism, and/or airspace filling with air bronchograms.

The histopathology of the lung tissue commonly entails bronchiolitis obliterans, features of hypersensitivity pneumonitis including granulomas, and organizing pneumonia. Eosinophilia is rare. Mycobacteria may or may not be demonstrable on stain. The EM may be recovered from respiratory tract secretions, bronchoalveolar lavage, or biopsy specimens. Species most commonly recovered include MAC and the RGM.

Optimum management has not been determined, but we advocate the following. First and most importantly, exposure must be terminated. Hot tubs should be drained and covered; "decontamination" and refilling has not been proven safe. Other environmental (water-damaged walls or rugs) or industrial exposure should be avoided. For patients with substantial symptomatic, physiologic, or radiographic disease, systemic corticosteroids predictably result in improvement, but for those with long-standing or more severe dysfunction, only partial reversal may be seen. Although the mycobacteria are ostensibly acting as organic antigens, we have elected to administer antimicrobial therapy for 3 to 6 months as the corticosteroids are being given. Others, however, have chosen only to break exposure and give steroids with no complications noted to date (94) (C. Rose, personal communication, 2002).

MYCOBACTERIUM AVIUM COMPLEX

Episodic cases of human disease due to *M. avium* infection were described in Europe and North America in the middle part of this century. A series of patients with pulmonary disease was reported from the Battey Hospital in Georgia in 1957 (103); the organism responsible in this group was subsequently named *Mycobacterium intracellulare*, or informally, the Battey bacillus. Bacteriologists found these organisms, *M. avium* and *M. intracellulare*, to be almost indistinguishable by routine laboratory criteria (colonial morphology, biochemical testing, drug-resistance patterns). Distinguishing various strains by their animal virulence and thermal adaptability, Schaefer (104) developed a carbohydrate antigen rabbit antiserum typing system that for years was the primary arbiter of species. In the original Schaefer schema, serotypes 1, 2, and 3 were regarded as *M. avium*, whereas serotypes 4 and higher were deemed *M. intracellulare*. Molecular biologic genetic analyses have allowed rapid and clear distinction of species; such testing has revealed that serotypes 1 through 6 and 8 through 11 are *M. avium* strains (105). Both species are clearly capable of producing severe illness in both healthy and impaired hosts (106). However, for unclear reasons, people with AIDS who develop disseminated mycobacterial disease are much more likely to be infected with *M. avium*, whereas HIV-negative persons with pulmonary disease are modestly more likely to harbor *M. intracellulare* (107). Recently, Falkinham, Norton, and LeChevallier (108) observed that *M. avium* and *M. intracellulare* typically occupy different niches within domestic potable water systems (108); this may bear on epidemiology patterns.

Communications with physicians and laboratories from virtually all of the United States including Alaska and Hawaii have indicated to us that there are increasing numbers of cases of pulmonary MAC in many diverse regions. Whether this is an accurate representation may be debated.

The appearance of an emerging epidemic of MAC lung disease may be deceiving for various reasons. Increased clinician awareness may have led to more aggressive evaluation of typical candidates. CT lung scans, which are the means by which bronchiectasis is recognized, are done with increased frequency with each passing year; on recognizing bronchiectasis, mycobacterial cultures are more likely to be ordered. In addition, the switch from using Lowenstein-Jensen culture medium as the standard recovery system to agar media favors the recovery of more EM; liquid media such as 7H-12 BACTEC medium is particularly favorable for the recovery of these mycobacteria.

While conceding the potential contributions of these factors, we do believe that the number of cases has increased dramatically over the past 20 to 25 years and that the geographic distribution has shifted considerably. Basically, our hypothesis relates to alterations in our human "ecosystem." Elements in this model include the following:

- Before the 1970s, home and institutional water heaters maintained water at approximately 140°F and 165°F, respectively, lethal temperatures for most microorganisms. However, to save energy, lessen deposits in water heaters, and avoid scalding accidents, these heaters are now capped at around 120°F. Many EM strains, including MAC, tolerate the lower temperature quite well (likewise, *Legionella* species).
- During the modern era, many cast iron pipes have been replaced by polyvinyl chloride (PVC); the PVC pipes are associated with more extensive biofilm development (109). Biofilms foster the proliferation of various slime organisms including avirulent amebae such as *Acanthamoeba castellani* (110). *A. castellani* provides a nurturing environment for intracellular microbes including legionella (111), chlamydia (112), and MAC. Indeed, MAC strains grown within *A. castellani* have been found to grow more robustly and be more virulent in a mouse model than strains grown on conventional media (110).
- Surveys indicate that the concentration of MAC in natural or preprocessed water is quite low and that after processing, MAC is virtually undetectable, but that water from institutional taps or reservoirs have variable but substantially greater numbers of MAC (108). These data are indicative of chronic contamination and proliferation of EM within potable water systems

(113,114). This probably is related to the increased resistance to sterilizing agents of microbes embedded in biofilm.
- During the past four decades, Americans have switched from tub bathing to showering. And, progressively, these showers have been taken within enclosed stalls where aerosols might be concentrated. The first evidence that EM might be transmitted via showers came from the West Haven, Connecticut Veterans Administration Hospital (VAH); individuals who were admitted to the VAH for COPD exacerbations subsequently developed diffuse lung infections with Mx (115). Later, it was found that the shower water at the hospital was laced with Mx.

Our model presumes that most of the U.S. population is sporadically exposed to MAC—and possibly RGM—on a regular basis. Most experience no sequelae, but those with the predispositions noted in Table 157.1 (plus others with yet-to-be-recognized conditions) are prone to become first colonized, then invaded, then diseased from the EM.

DIAGNOSTIC CRITERIA

Active or invasive disease due to MAC (or any of the EM) is more difficult to diagnose than TB, because recovery of the *M. tuberculosis* organism from respiratory tract secretions or tissue is tantamount to the diagnosis of disease. Given the wide distribution of MAC in nature, it is vital that clinicians realize that MAC recovered from any nonsterile space may reflect colonization. Considerable effort must be made to distinguish a saprophytic state from invasive disease. Failure to appreciate active disease and withholding therapy puts a patient at risk of progressive lung damage and even death; on the other hand, an erroneous assumption of disease commits a patient to extended use of medication, which entails predictable side effects, significant risk for toxic effects, and a considerable financial burden. Because MAC pulmonary disease generally advances slowly, there is a tendency for clinicians who see patients during a short span, even up to 3 to 6 months, to fail to appreciate that there is progressive damage. Alternatively, the disease does not advance in a linear manner but stepwise, with periods of indolence followed by a spate of activity. What should be appreciated is that there is considerable morbidity and even mortality from untreated or inadequately treated pulmonary MAC disease.

Criteria for the diagnosis of active disease usually include clinical signs and symptoms, sputum bacteriology, and chest radiography. The spectrum of symptoms includes the classic findings of cough, sputum production, malaise, chills, night sweats, hemoptysis, pleuritic, and nonpleuritic chest pain. Dyspnea, weight loss, and fever are common as the disease progresses. Early in the course of MAC disease, however, there may be minimal manifestations, such as a chronic nonproductive cough and mild malaise (described as just not feeling well or lack of energy). A possible source of confusion is the predisposing diseases associated with MAC vulnerability. Chronic bronchitis or emphysema, chronic bronchiectasis, pneumoconiosis, and various other diseases may mimic these manifestations, so the clinician must seek recent quantitative changes in symptoms to discern the contribution of MAC.

The 1997 American Thoracic Society (ATS) statement regarding diagnosis and management of "nontuberculous mycobacteria" was a thoughtful but complex and sometimes confusing document (116). The summary of the microbiologic criteria for diagnosis is contained in Table 157.2. Although the logic in this system is evident, it is rather unwieldy, and it is our impression that it has not enjoyed wide use among clinicians.

Although we agree that the diagnosis of invasive EM lung disease is more secure in the presence of large numbers of

TABLE 157.2. American Thoracic Society Summary Statement on Nontuberculous Mycobacteria Diagnosis

Diagnostic criteria of NTM lung disease in HIV-seropositive and HIV-seronegative hosts.

The following criteria apply to symptomatic patients with infiltrate, nodular, or cavitary disease, or a high-resolution CT scan that shows multifocal bronchiectasis and/or multiple small nodules.

A. If three sputum/bronchial wash results are available from the previous 12 mo:
  1. Three positive cultures with negative AFB smear results *or*
  2. Two positive cultures and one positive AFB smear

B. If only one bronchial wash is available:
  1. Positive culture with a 2+, 3+, or 4+ AFB smear or 2+, 3+, or 4+ growth on solid media

C. If sputum/bronchial wash evaluations are nondiagnostic or another disease cannot be excluded:
  1. Transbronchial or lung biopsy yielding a NTM or
  2. Biopsy showing mycobacterial histopathologic features (granulomatous inflammation and/or AFB) and one or more sputa or bronchial washings are positive for an NTM even in low number

Note: These criteria fit best with *Mycobacterium avium* complex, *Mycobacterium abscessus,* and *Mycobacterium kansasii.* Too little is known of other NTM to be certain how applicable these criteria will be.
At least three respiratory samples should be evaluated from each patient. Other reasonable causes for the disease should be excluded. Expert consultation should be sought when diagnostic difficulties are encountered.
AFB, acid-fast bacilli; CT, computed tomography; HIV, human immunodeficiency virus; NTM, nontuberculous mycobacteria.

mycobacteria on cultivation and/or multiple positive cultures, we think a simpler model will suffice. Our approach is represented in Table 157.3.

Pulmonary MAC disease produces a wide spectrum of radiographic abnormalities. In 1995, Lynch et al. (117) published an excellent review of these findings. A substantial proportion of pulmonary MAC patients' chest films are suggestive of classic TB: unilateral or bilateral upper lobe, apical posterior, fibronodular, partially consolidated, cavitary shadowing (Fig. 157.1). A subset of MAC patients have a distinct radiographic pattern, mainly lower zone, nodular subpleural shadowing, typically bilateral (Fig. 157.2); this is more common among women. On thin-section, high-resolution CT scans, scattered fine nodules, "tree in bud," representing cellular bronchiolitis may be seen (these findings are not unique to MAC but are broadly associated with infectious bronchiolitis). In addition to a number of patients with this pattern, we have encountered women who presented with the predominant abnormality of coarse, saccular bronchiectasis of both the lingula and the right middle lobe (Fig. 157.3). Although patchy abnormalities were typically scattered elsewhere, the most dramatic findings were restricted to these regions. By history, it was not possible to determine absolutely whether the bronchiectasis antedated or was caused by the MAC; but in the absence of a clear history of remote recurrent infections in these patients, we believe that MAC plays a major role in the pathogenesis of such bronchiectasis. Regardless of a primary or secondary role, once established, MAC definitely is part of the ongoing clinical illness with which these patients present.

TREATMENT

Medical Management. Our understanding of the optimal treatment for pulmonary MAC disease is evolving. Because of the extraordinary number of variables involved, randomized trials have been difficult. The results of recent therapy trials for pulmonary MAC are displayed in Table 157.4. One of the really

troublesome issues is that there are no "natural history" data against which to compare the utility of treatment. For patients with cavitary TB-like disease, a strong impression exists that without adequate treatment, these patients will experience rapid (months to years) progression of respiratory tract and constitutional symptoms, compromising quality of life and survival (26,118). For those with primarily bronchiectatic disease, the natural course and treatment benefits are less well understood; however, limited data suggest increased mortality (16). We presume that referral bias results in selection of patients with more progressive or problematic infection for visits to our institution. However, among these patients, we believe the vast majority enjoy clinical, physiologic, and bacteriologic benefits from the management plans described later.

The role of drug susceptibility testing in selecting a regimen for a MAC patient is disputed. Unlike the situation with TB, for which a wealth of experience has shown a correlation between susceptibility testing results *in vitro* and response to treatment, only two studies have shown such an association with pulmonary MAC disease. In an earlier series of 76 patients from the National Jewish Center, there was a statistically significant association between the initial bacteriologic response and the administration of drugs to which patients' MAC strains were sensitive *in vitro* (119). Similarly, Tsukamura (120) in Japan studied 26 patients with pulmonary MAC. Seven patients were considered treatment failures, and six of these had highly resistant strains of MAC. Nine patients were rendered culture negative, and all had been treated with regimens that included drugs to which their MAC strain was relatively susceptible. This study also revealed that during treatment minimum inhibitory concentrations (MICs) of the drugs employed drifted upward, indicating killing of vulnerable populations.

However, the 1997 ATS statement states that the only *in vitro* susceptibility testing that is justifiable is for clarithromycin (or, by extension, azithromycin) (116). The NCCLS 2000 guidelines suggest that the following pulmonary MAC isolates undergo *in vitro* testing for clarithromycin susceptibility: "clinically significant isolates that are from patients receiving prior [sic] macrolide therapy," " . . . from patients who experienced a relapse while receiving macrolide therapy," or "initial isolates . . . from clinically significant respiratory samples . . . to establish baseline values" (121).

Truly, the picture is confusing with MAC (and some other EM, including Mx) when comparing *in vitro* susceptibility and response to treatment. Some studies suggested that "standard" anti-TB regimens may be more effective than tailored regimens using second-line medications selected on the basis of *in vitro* susceptibility (122–124). These results, though, may have been confounded by nonadherence with some of the more toxic second-line drugs like ethionamide and cycloserine. Synergy between rifampin (RIF) and ethambutol (EMB) may partially explain failure of single-drug *in vitro* susceptibility to predict response (125,126), but there remain puzzling findings that imply that *in vitro* testing, even MIC determination, does not provide infallible guidance. A recent British Thoracic Society trial compared 2 years of RIF and EMB with RIF, EMB, and isoniazid (INH), an agent to which MAC shows nearly universal *in vitro* resistance (127). The number of patients was too small to provide statistically meaningful data, but the patients who received RIF-EMB-INH had slightly lower failures and relapses (4 and 2 of 38) than the patients who received RIF-EMB (7 and 8 of 37). Yet, for the MAC patients, as well as the *Mycobacterium malmoense* (Mm) and Mx groups, deaths attributed to mycobacterial disease were higher among INH recipients (overall, 9/111 in the INH-containing regimens versus 1 of 112 in the other arms). Although the authors downplay the utility of *in vitro* susceptibility

TABLE 157.3. Diagnostic Criteria for Pulmonary Disease Caused by Environmental Mycobacteria—National Jewish Model

Symptoms/signs
  First-degree findings
  • Cough
  • Phlegm and/or a sense of congestion
  • Diminished energy with episodic malaise
  Second-degree findings
  • Feverishness with occasional night sweats
  • Fatigue which, on occasion, may be disabling
  • Diminished appetite with gradual weight loss
  • Hemoptysis, usually scant and intermittent
  • Dyspnea with exercise limitation
Radiographic findings
  Tuberculosis-like findings
  • Upper lobes or superior segments of lower lobes
  • Apical pleural thickening/scalloping
  • Variable consolidation
  • Cavitation typically in apical-posterior segments of upper lobes
  • N.B., pleural effusion extremely rare
  Bronchiectasis
  • Medium and small airways involved
  • Cylindrical, varicoid, and saccular variants
  • Small and medium nodules interspersed
  • Cellular bronchiolitis on CT scan
  • RML and lingula prominently involved, typically with associated volume loss (partial atelectasis)
  • Upper zones more involved in cystic fibrosis
  • Lower lobe disease predominant with ciliary disorders
Microbiologic criteria
  Cavitary disease: Patients with overtly cavitary disease caused by EM commonly produce copious secretions that are positive on both smear and culture for the mycobacterial pathogen. Failure to recover mycobacteria in such cases should suggest alternative processes, such as lung abscess, fungal pneumonia, or necrotic lung cancer.
  Bronchiectatic disease: Early in the illness, secretions may be sparse requiring sputum induction or bronchoscopy to recover organisms. The American Thoracic Society criteria (see Table 157.2) are too stringent, in our estimation. Recovery of EM on culture, even in low numbers, on two or more specimens strongly suggests invasive disease in subjects with typical signs and radiographic findings.

Note: Among patients with the predisposing conditions and typical symptomatology and radiographic findings, recovery of EM on two or more specimens strongly suggests invasive disease. Obviously, we should consider alternative pathogens, but among the bronchiectasis patients, co-pathogens may *share* responsibility for the morbidity, particularly gram-negative rods, *Aspergillus* species and other EM species.
CT, computed tomography; EM, environmental mycobacteria; RML, right middle lobe.

testing, their own data demonstrate a trend toward a predictive relationship: Among pooled data from all three mycobacterial groups, adverse treatment outcomes (failures/relapses) were lower among patients with strains susceptible rather than resistant to RIF (14% vs. 21%) and susceptible rather than resistant to EMB (15% vs. 24%).

As we confront the current dilemmas in MAC chemotherapy, we would agree that *in vitro* testing for clarithromycin is indicated at a minimum. Perhaps it is justified to empirically initiate therapy with one of the "standard" regimens represented in Table 157.5. However, for patients with more extensive disease and/or intolerance to or toxicity from the usual drugs, we feel that quantitative *in vitro* data (MICs) are appropriate to select alternative regimens.

The various medications that are routinely employed in the treatment of MAC and other slow-growing EM infections are listed in Table 157.6. Pyrazinamide is not included because of widespread resistance of the EM to this agent. INH is included because there are some data suggesting clinical efficacy despite the general appearance of marginal activity *in vitro*.

The management plan for patients with pulmonary EM infection begins with the question to give antimicrobials or not. We believe that the overwhelming majority of patients with typical symptoms and radiographic abnormalities whose respiratory tract secretions contain MAC (or other commonly pathogenic EM) are *diseased, not colonized*. However, it is not unreasonable among patients with mild or limited bronchiectatic disease to attempt management with nonspecific bronchial hygiene measures. However, if one does choose to treat with inhaled β agonists, Flutter or Pep valves, and short courses of broad-spectrum antibiotics, it is incumbent on the clinician to regularly monitor for progression of symptoms, radiographic abnormalities, and mycobacterial burden.

In general, we attempt to tailor therapy according to the extent and type of disease, the patient's age and general health, historical or current tolerance/intolerance of medications, home support systems, and sadly their insurance coverage (it is possible to wreak financial havoc on individuals and families with such modalities as home intravenous or inhaled antibiotic therapy).

For younger, generally healthy patients with extensive, obviously progressive disease, we employ three or more oral agents with an initial 2- to 6-month course of an aminoglycoside, typically amikacin; regimens appropriate for pulmonary MAC (or other slow-growing EM) are represented in Table 157.5. In such cases, if there is unilateral disease, we are inclined to consider surgery (see the section "Surgery in Pulmonary *Mycobacterium avium* Complex Disease").

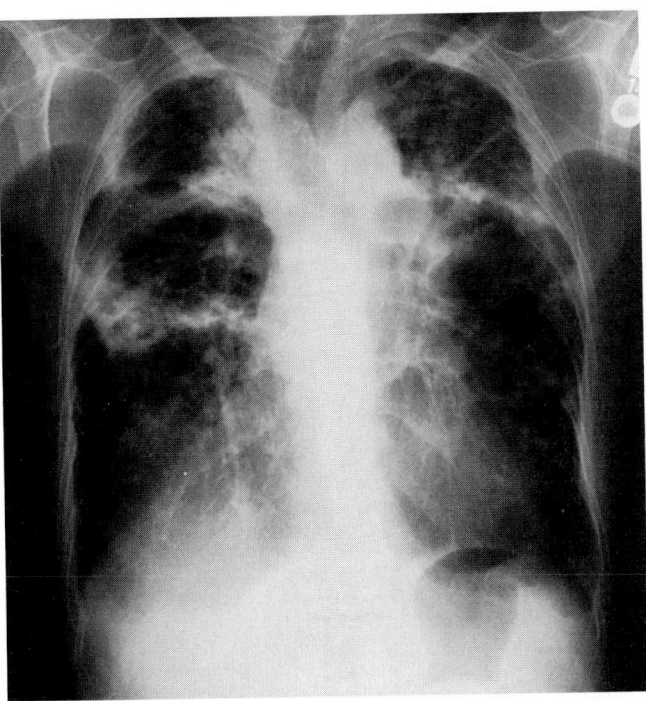

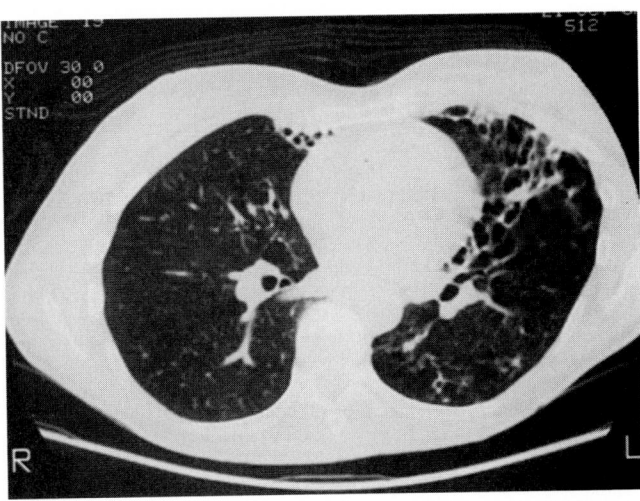

Figure 157.3. A computed tomographic lung scan of a 43-year-old woman, a nonsmoker, with cystic saccular bronchiectasis associated with *Mycobacterium avium* complex involving the inferior segment of the lingula, abutting the heart and to a lesser extent, the medial segment of the right middle lobe, also abutting the heart. This pattern, lingular and middle lobe focal bronchiectasis, is virtually pathognomonic of mycobacterial disease in our experience. In addition, this patient had mild scoliosis, pectus excavatum, and mitral valve prolapse.

Figure 157.1. An anteroposterior view in a 60-year-old woman with 50 pack-years of cigarette abuse and underlying chronic obstructive pulmonary disease. Necrotizing cavitary destruction of both upper lobes with atelectasis and bronchiectasis of the right middle lobe is seen. The patient has oxygen dependency and pulmonary hypertension.

For older patients who are apt to be less tolerant of such aggressive therapy and who stand to lose fewer years of quality life, our approach is to suppress the infection without suppressing the host. However, we do use aminoglycoside therapy among elderly patients if other therapy is insufficient and circumstances merit.

For patients with bronchiectatic MAC, we use very aggressive bronchial hygiene. And, we feel that inhaled aminoglycosides are more effective with this airway-centered disease than with cavitary disease. Monitoring for superinfection with gram-negative rods (such as *P. aeruginosa*, *Alcaligenes xylosoxidans*, or *Stenotrophomonas maltophilia*), *Aspergillus* or even other species of EM are an important element of ongoing care.

Surgery in Pulmonary Mycobacterium avium Complex Disease. Refractoriness to drug therapy led to aggressive use of surgical resection in the early experience at the Battey Hospital in Georgia, where the first large group of pulmonary MAC cases was reported (128). In this series, the operative mortality rate was 7% and major morbidity rate was 24%, including prolonged air leakage requiring thoracoplasty. This series commenced in the 1950s, when surgical approaches were evolving, anesthesia techniques were less safe, and postoperative intensive care was far less sophisticated. As these elements improved, both morbidity and mortality rates diminished during the later years of the series. A later series of patients who underwent surgical resection was reported from Duke University; of 175 pulmonary MAC patients, 37 were selected to undergo surgery (129). Elements in selection included localized disease, freedom from major complicating diseases, and younger age. Among these patients, 33 were available for long-term follow-up; 2 who had relapse responded to re-treatment. There were no operative deaths or serious morbidity in this series. We have regularly employed resection for pulmonary MAC disease over the past 20 years at the National Jewish Center (130). Broadly, there are three groups of patients for whom we feel surgery may be indicated: those with (a) destroyed lungs, (b) extensively cavitated or destroyed lobes, and (c) severe bronchiectasis with or without atelectasis, typically

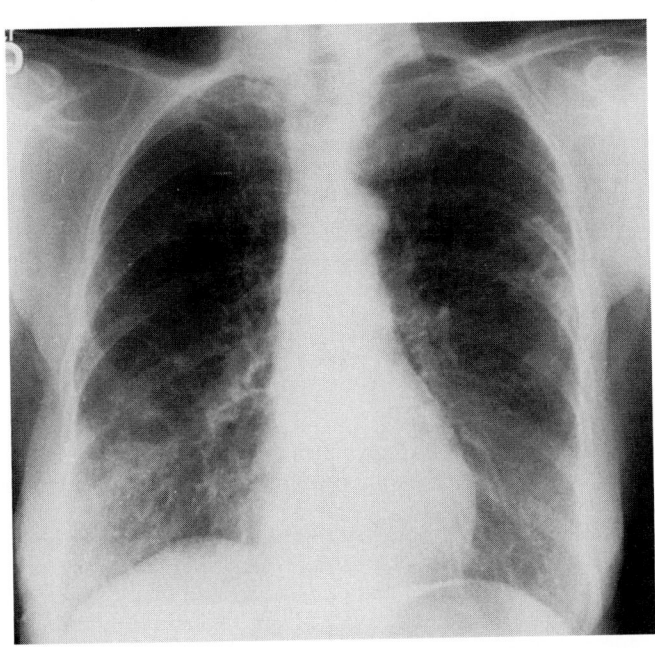

Figure 157.2. An anteroposterior view in a 47-year-old woman, a nonsmoker, with bilateral lower zone patchy infiltrates. Early cavitary formation is seen in the right lower lobe and left upper lobe. A computed tomographic scan confirmed extensive bronchiectasis in the right middle lobe with scattered nodular shadowing. This less distinctive pattern is being seen with increasing frequency among patients, especially women, referred to our institution.

TABLE 157.4. Results of Recent Trials of Chemotherapy for Pulmonary *Mycobacterium avium* Complex

I. Clarithromycin-based regimens

Regimen	Response rate	Comments
A. Clarithromycin monotherapy, 500 mg b.i.d., for 4 mo (270)	11 (58%) of 19 became culture negative; 18 (95%) of 19 had improved cultures and/or chest radiographs	Mostly elderly men with COPD with more extensive disease; only 3 (16%) of 19 developed *in vitro* resistance
B. Clarithromycin, 500 b.i.d.; ethambutol, 25 mg/kg q.d. for 2 mo, then 15 mg/kg; rifampin, 600 mg q.d. (if culture positive at 6 mo, switch to rifabutin, 600 mg q.d.); SM i.v. b.i.w. for 2 mo (if unable to give SM, give Cipro, 750 mg b.i.d.) (271)	36 (92%) of 39 who completed >5 mo of therapy converted; no relapses through 1–3-year follow-up	All isolates were susceptible; authors favored low-dose rifabutin (150 or 300 mg q.d.) over rifampin or higher dose rifabutin
C. Clarithromycin, 10 mg/kg plus rifampin and ethambutol daily for 24 mo; initial kanamycin followed by fluoroquinolone (272)	Overall, 28 (72%) of 39 converted to negative; 26 (84%) of 31 of those with clarithromycin susceptibility converted	Resistance to clarithromycin predicted poor response; kanamycin did not show clear benefit; response rates poor with cavitary disease
D. Clarithromycin, 1,000 mg; ethambutol, 25 mg/kg; and rifabutin, 300–600 mg t.i.w. (273)	Of 41 who completed 6-month therapy, 32 (78%) converted	Adverse reactions to rifabutin were common; for 41%, doses were reduced or stopped; overall, similar in efficacy to daily therapy with clarithromycin or azithromycin

II. Azithromycin-based regimens

Regimen	Response rate	Comments
A. Azithromycin monotherapy, 600 mg q.d. for 4 mo (274)	9 (35%) of 23 of patients with MAC susceptible *in vitro* to azithromycin converted sputum to negative	Mostly smokers; 45% with cavitary disease; GI side effects in 76% and altered hearing in 41% suggest excessive dose; none developed *in vitro*® on treatment
B. Azithromycin thrice weekly, for 6 mo, in two different regimens (275)		
B.1. Azithromycin, 600 t.i.w.; ethambutol, 15 mg/kg q.d.; rifabutin, 300 mg q.d.; SM t.i.w./b.i.w. for 2 mo (1)	19 of 21 completed regimen; 14 (74%) converted; 17 (89%) improved	Some patients with more extensive disease underwent surgery; GI side effects common; patients with prior therapy had higher failure rates
B.2. Azithromycin, 600 t.i.w.; ethambutol, 25 mg/kg t.i.w.; rifabutin, 600 mg t.i.w.; SM b.i.w. or t.i.w. for 2 mo	39% of 47 completed regimen; 24 (62%) converted; 30 (77%) improved	Some patients with more extensive disease underwent surgery; GI side effects common; patients with prior therapy had higher failure rates

III. Nonmacrolide regimens

Regimen	Response rate	Comments
A. Rifampin-ethambutol for 2 years: rifampin, 600 mg (450 if <50 kg) q.d.; ethambutol, 15 mg/kg q.d. (127)	7 (19%) of 37 failures; 8 (47%) of 30 relapse; overall, 59% favorable response	Unexpected benefit from isoniazid, but unexplained higher mortality in isoniazid recipients; after 5 years, only 23 (31%) of 75 "alive and cured" Note trend toward improved outcomes with *in vitro* susceptibility to rifampin and/or ethambutol
B. Isoniazid-rifampin-ethambutol for 2 years; isoniazid, 300 q.d.; rifampin, 600 (450 if <50 kg) q.d.; ethambutol, 15 mg/kg q.d. (127)	4 (11%) of 38 failure; 2 (6%) of 34 relapse; 3 deaths ascribed to MAC; overall, 84% favorable response	

b.i.d., twice a day; b.i.w., twice a week; COPD, chronic obstructive pulmonary disease; GI, gastrointestinal; i.v., intravenously; MAC, *Mycobacterium avium* complex; q.d., every day; t.i.w., three times a week.

involving the right middle lobe, the lingular segment of the left upper lobe, or lower lobes.

Curiously, in contradistinction to *M. tuberculosis*, patients with EM infection are more prone to present with destruction of the right lung. Our early experience with right pneumonectomies met with high rates of complications (130), but innovations in technique have resulted in improved outcomes. Extirpation of the bronchiectatic right middle lobe, lingular segment, or lower lobe(s) is usually justified by extremely poor drainage of these regions leading to relentless infection and nearly continuous symptoms; these procedures have proven generally well tolerated, safe, and efficacious.

Neither we nor others have randomized controlled experience with surgical resection for MAC or other mycobacterial infections. We have regularly revisited this issue but have been unable to visualize or design a protocol that would embrace all of the important variables and generate statistically meaningful information.

Finally, it is vital to note that this type of surgery is extremely complicated because of obliterated or distorted anatomic landmarks, extensive fibrosis that entails highly difficult sharp dissection, very challenging bronchial closure caused by diseased or infected airways, and postoperative "space problems" caused by the limited ability of the remaining lung to undergo compensatory hyperinflation. We maintain that such surgery should be done only in centers with considerable experience in this area.

MYCOBACTERIUM KANSASII

Mk is a prominent cause of EM pulmonary disease in the southern and central United States (6,25,131,132), Britain (9,133),

TABLE 157.5. Suggested Drug Regimens for Slow-Growing Environmental Mycobacteria

I. MAC and other less common slow-growing EM

Regimen	Duration	Comments
A. CLARI-EMB-RIF ± AK q.d. or t.i.w. B. CLARI-EMB-CFZ ± AK q.d. or t.i.w. C. RIF-EMB-CFZ ± AK; ± Cipro q.d. D. CLARI-EMB ± CFZ q.d. or t.i.w.	18–24 mo is usual; may treat for shorter duration in elderly or those for whom treatment is highly onerous	• Can substitute AZI for CLARI if intolerant • Use AK in more extensive disease or in those who do not respond well to oral regimen • t.i.w. therapy is probably comparable in efficacy to q.d.; advantages include economy and lessened toxicity • RBU does not accelerate the elimination of CLARI as RIF does but has other drawbacks • AZI pharmacokinetics are not affected by RIF • Regimen C for cases resistant or intolerant of macrolides; use Cipro if active *in vitro* • *Regimen D for less extensive disease in elderly patient for whom suppression is the objective*

II. *Mycobacterium kansasii*

Regimen	Duration	Comments
RIF-EMB-INH ± AK, q.d. RIF-EMB, q.d. RIF-EMB-CLARI or AZI, q.d. RIF-EMB-AK, q.d.	15–18 mo 9 mo 9 mo 9 mo	The RIF-EMB-INH regimen is the 1997 American Thoracic Society–recommended regimen; AK is advocated for those with more extensive disease; the BTA has shown utility with a 9-mo RIF-EMB regimen; adding CLARI for 2 mo should strengthen regimen
CLARI-EMB-CIP ± AK	15 mo	Use in cases of resistance to or intolerance of RIF-RBU

Note: There are modestly adequate data supporting these regimens for MAC. Disease due to *M. kansasii* is relatively more responsive to chemotherapy; the regimens advocated for this pathogen have been demonstrated to generate 90% or better cure rates. The therapeutic experiences with slow-growing EM disease other than MAC or *M. kansasii* are too limited to define optimal management. Therefore, for patients with *Mycobacterium xenopi, Mycobacterium malmoense, Mycobacterium szulgai, Mycobacterium simiae,* or other less common pathogens of this nature, we employ MAC-like regimens, based on limited clinical observations and *in vitro* susceptibility profiles.
AK, amikacin; AZI, azithromycin; BTA, British Thoracic Association; CFZ, clofazimine; CIP, ciprofloxacin; CLARI, clarithromycin; EM, environmental mycobacteria; EMB, ethambutol; INH, isoniazid; MAC, *Mycobacterium avium* complex; q.d., every day; RBU, rifabutin; RIF, rifampin; t.i.w., three times a week.

and gold miners in South Africa (134). Historically, it has been found mainly in men with predisposing lung disorders including smoking-related COPD and inorganic dust exposure (132,135,136). Recent surveys have shown a modest predisposition among HIV-infected persons for Mk lung disease (137,138). However, Mk is well recognized to produce pulmonary disease in persons without obvious predisposing pulmonary or systemic disorders (25,136). Curiously, neither we nor others have described Mk disease among persons with the heritable conditions listed in Table 157.1 or among slender women with bronchiectasis.

Mk tends to be recovered from water samples more than soil (5,139,140). It is presumed, reasonably, that infection with Mk is acquired from the environment. Although case clusters raise the issue of human-to-human transmission (135,138,141), they might as well be explained by common environmental exposure. Yet it should be made clear that the possibility of such spread has *not* been excluded. The extremely high prevalence among South African gold miners suggests, among other considerations, that the water employed for dust suppression in the mines might be chronically contaminated with Mk (138).

Clinically, patients with Mk lung disease present with various combinations of cough, hemoptysis, feverishness, sweats, weight loss, and chest pain (132,136). Recovery of Mk from respiratory tract secretions in such patients is strongly associated with disease, for example, Mk is less commonly found to be a saprophyte or contaminant than other EM.

Chest radiographic findings among patients with Mk disease are similar to those with TB. However, one series from Britain found a trend toward more unilateral disease, more upper zone involvement, less consolidation, and smaller cavities with Mk compared with TB (142). An earlier report from the United States identified thin-walled cavitation as more typical of Mk disease (143). Though suggestive, such findings are not diagnostic.

Tuberculin skin testing does not allow identification of persons with Mk disease or distinction of those with Mk from those with TB.

Sputum smears are generally positive in patients with cavitary extensive disease. Although Mk grown on culture medium forms longer more filamentous rods than tubercle bacilli, the organisms seen in respiratory tract secretions cannot reliably be distinguished from tubercle bacilli.

Chemotherapy. The typical strain of Mk shows resistance to low concentrations of INH and streptomycin; high-level resistance to pyrazinamide and *p*-aminosalicylic acid is the rule. A standard regimen of INH, RIF, and EMB for 18 months was found effective in 100% of pulmonary Mk cases in Texas (144). This same group later reported that the addition of streptomycin, 1 g thrice weekly for the initial 3 months, resulted in cures for 40 of 41 patients with only 12 months of total therapy (145). The British Thoracic Society published a study in 1994 of a regimen that featured 9 months of therapy with RIF and EMB; of note, most of these patients received additional unspecified medications for the initial few months before the mycobacterial species was identified (146). Of the initial 173, 154 patients completed 9 months of chemotherapy, with 87 patients completing 5 years of follow-up. At the completion of the 5-year follow-up, 15 patients (9.7%) were noted to have relapsed with positive cultures. Favorable results were also described in a series of patients with

TABLE 157.6.   Medications Routinely Used in the Therapy of Slow-Growing Environmental Mycobacterial Disease

Medication and dosage	Side-effects/toxicity	Comments
I. Macrolides/azolides		
CLARI, 500–750 mg q.d. 500 mg b.i.d. 750 mg t.i.w.	Metallic bitter taste; anorexia; griping abdominal distress; loose stools; tinnitus; high-frequency hearing loss	May be given t.i.w.; CYP enzyme inhibitor; durg interactions
AZI, 250–500 q.d./500 t.i.w.	Fewer GI effects than CLARI; tinnitus; high-frequency hearing loss	Long half-life favors intermittent use; but in comparison (see Table 157.4), is moderately less active than CLARI; minimal effects on CYP system
No experience with ketolides		
II. Ethambutol		
EMB, 25 mg/kg q.d. for 2 mo, then 15 mg/kg q.d. 25–30 mg/kg t.i.w.	Optic neuritis with potential for vision impairment or blindness; rash; rare peripheral neuropathy; GI distress; mild hyperuricemia	Has predictable additive effect with CLARI or AZI; may be synergistic with rifamycin. Must monitor vision and reduce dose with renal insufficiency
III. Rifamycins		
RIF, 600 mg q.d. if ≥50-kg body weight, 450 if ≤50 kg; 600 mg t.i.w.	Hepatitis, thrombopenia, mild GI upset, rash	Additive or synergistic with ethambutol vs. many MAC strains; potent CYP system inducer; major effect, lowering CLARI bioavailability
RBU, 150–300 mg q.d.; 300 mg t.i.w.	Hepatitis; neutropenia and thrombopenia more common than with RIF	Additive/synergistic effects comparable to RIF; less effect on CYP (may be advantageous with CLARI). N.B. CLARI slows catabolism of RBU; use lower dose of RBU
No experience with rifapentine		
IV. Fluoroquinolones		
CIP, 500–750 mg b.i.d., 750 mg q.d., 750 mg t.i.w.	Tremors, insomnia, bad dreams; GI upset; rare hepatitis; very rare, Achilles rupture	CIP and LQN usually active vs. *Mycobacterium kansasii;* variable vs. MAC and RGMs; CIP, an inhibitor of CYP
LQN, 500–750 mg q.d.; 750 mg t.i.w.	Less CNS stimulation than CIP; GI upset; very rare, Achilles rupture	Higher maximum concentration and longer half-life than CIP; but slightly higher MICs vs. MAC than CIP
No experience with third-generation FQNs		
V. Aminoglycosides		
AK 12–15 mg/kg i.v. q.d. 15–22 mg/kg i.v. t.i.w.	High-frequency hearing loss; tinnitus; less vestibular toxicity than streptomycin; renal impairment (may be amplified by NSAIDs)	AK or KM probably preferred agents vs. MAC, *M. kansasii,* or other slow-growing EM; may be given i.m., but this may be problematic in slender patients with much soft tissue
KM 12–15 mg/kg i.v. q.d. 15–22 mg/kg i.v. t.i.w.	Similar to AK	More painful than AK when given i.m.
VI. Miscellaneous		
INH, 300–600 mg q.d.; 600 mg t.i.w.	Hepatitis; dysphoria, loss of concentration; lupus syndrome	We have largely abandoned INH for EM; but, in some studies, INH-containing regimens have apparently been effective
Cycloserine 250 mg b.i.d. 500 mg q.d. No experience with t.i.w. regimen	Loss of concentration, impaired cognition, depression, psychosis, violent behavior; tremors, minor and major seizures; rare, peripheral neuritis	Primarily used versus MAC; side effects/toxicity are generally drug concentration and duration dependent; pharmacokinetic monitoring extremely helpful
Clofazimine, 100 mg q.d. until skin pigmentation appears; then 50 mg q.d.; may reduce to 50 mg t.i.w. after skin bronzing is present	GI distress tends to develop several months into use; long tissue half-life (70–90 days) means that side effects persists long after medicine is stopped; reduce dose with skin pigmentation to avoid pruritus and scaling ("alligator skin"), as well as GI complications	
Ethionamide, 250 mg b.i.d., 500 mg q.d. No experience with t.i.w. regimen	Severe metallic taste, even worse than CLARI; GI distress; depression; arthralgias, "frozen shoulder"; hypothyroidism	Probably the least well tolerated of these durgs; used uncommonly in recent era

AK, amikacin; AZI, azithromycin; b.i.d., twice a day; CIP, ciprofloxacin; CLARI, clarithromycin; CYP, cytochrome P450; EM, environmental mycobacteria; EMB, ethambutol; FQN, fluoroquinolones; GI, gastrointestinal; i.m., intramuscularly; INH, isoniazid; i.v., intravenously; KM, kanamycin; MAC, *Mycobacterium avium* complex; MIC, minimum inhibitory concentration; LQN, levofloxacin; NSAIDs, nonsteroidal antiinflammatory drugs; q.d., every day; RBU, rifabutin; RGM, rapidly growing mycobacteria; RIF, rifampin; t.i.w., three times a week.

pulmonary Mk treated with RIF, EMB, and INH for less than 1 year (136).

On the basis of these studies, we would suggest a hybrid regimen that incorporates various features of previously reported experience (see Table 157.5). In many cases, the patients have been treated on the presumption of *M. tuberculosis* disease, probably with a four-drug regimen including INH, RIF, pyrazinamide, and either EMB or streptomycin. If the patient is responding well to this regimen (with subsiding symptoms, diminishing bacillary load, and improving chest radiographs), we would discontinue the INH and pyrazinamide. If the fourth drug is streptomycin and not EMB, we would add EMB while continuing the streptomycin through 2 to 3 months. Depending on the extent of disease and rate of improvement, we would employ RIF and EMB for 10 to 12 months. If, on the other hand, the patient has been started on an empirical EM regimen that contains clarithromycin or azithromycin, a rifamycin, and EMB, we would stop the macrolide/azolide after 2 months and treat for 9 months with RIF-rifabutin and EMB.

Chemotherapy of the usual case of Mk pulmonary disease is relatively straightforward. However, drug toxicity or acquired drug resistance can substantially complicate management. Loss of RIF is the biggest hurdle because this agent is the keystone in treatment. In the situation of toxicity from or resistance to RIF, careful selection of a regimen is critical, lest further drug resistance evolve. Early experience from Texas showed response to sulfonamide-containing regimens (147). A more recent report from Texas described an aggressive regimen for the management of RIF-resistant Mk disease: INH, 900 mg daily, EMB, 25 mg/kg daily, sulfamethoxazole, 1,000 mg three times a day; and an initial course of amikacin or streptomycin (148). Although this regimen was apparently successful in this small series, we have misgivings about the prolonged use of these agents in such high doses. Ciprofloxacin and clarithromycin also have excellent *in vitro* activity against most strains of Mk; these drugs are generally well tolerated and are thus attractive alternative agents (148). Other agents with activity against the usual strain of Mk include ethionamide and cycloserine (147).

In cases of extensive drug resistance or toxic effect, it is appropriate to consider surgical resection for localized disease. Although experience with surgery for Mk is limited, we recommend that these broad principles should be observed: remove cavities and grossly devitalized tissue; do lobectomies or pneumonectomies; avoid wedge or segmental resections; and perform the surgery only under optimal antimicrobial coverage (130).

PULMONARY DISEASE DUE TO OTHER SLOW-GROWING MYCOBACTERIA

Various other slow-growing mycobacteria have been noted to cause pulmonary disease; some of these microbes are clustered regionally or are associated with sporadic, infrequent disease without geographic patterns. Those organisms with sufficient morbidity to be described in formal reports are discussed below.

Mycobacterium xenopi. Pulmonary disease due to Mx has been a chronic or endemic problem in Britain (149,150) and the region of Paris, France (151,152). In a reference laboratory that services southeast England, Mx was the most commonly recovered EM between 1973 and 1993: 23.4% of all isolates versus 12% and 12.3% for Mk and MAC, respectively (9). It was prominent among a series of patients with EM lung disease in Ontario in the 1980s (10).

Clinically and radiographically, Mx disease may be considered generally similar to TB-like MAC or Mk. The usual strain

of Mx shows *in vitro* resistance only to INH and pyrazinamide; susceptibility is the rule to RIF and EMB. However, the response to chemotherapy is often poor with persistently positive cultures and persistence or even worsening of the radiographic abnormalities (149,150). This clearly is a situation of dissociation between susceptibility of the microbes in an artificial culture medium and the response *in vivo*.

An outbreak of pulmonary Mx disease at the West Haven VAH in the 1970s is instructive in several regards (115). The epidemic occurred among 19 patients who had previously been admitted to the hospital, typically with exacerbations of COPD. Following these admissions, 12 of the patients developed new respiratory tract symptoms and radiographic abnormalities; the chest x-ray films ranged from cavitary disease to diffuse nodular abnormalities. Ultimately it was found that these patients had all been exposed to a shower on the ward that yielded substantial growth of Mx. It was strongly inferred that this represented inhalational infection related to contaminated shower water. These patients appeared to respond to various regimens, which were not stipulated.

By contrast, Mx patients in the recent British treatment trial (noted above under MAC therapy) had poor response and survival rates (127). Of the 42 patients treated with either RIF-EMB or RIF-EMB-INH, only 7 patients were alive and cured at 5 years. Although only 7 of the patients were designated failures or relapses, 24 (57%) of the 42 had died from "all causes." Notably, 34 (81%) of the 42 patients with Mx infection had cavitary disease. From these data, we can deduce whether poor response to Mx therapy, comorbid conditions, or both contributed to the striking mortality in these patients (by contrast, mortality was only 25% in the Mm and 31% in the MAC patients).

Because of the absence of useful trial data, we have elected to treat patients with new Mx disease with aggressive regimens typically consisting of RIF, EMB, clarithromycin, or azithromycin and if cavitary disease is present an initial 2- to 4-month course of amikacin. In younger patients with localized disease and without extensive comorbidity, we consider surgical resection if the response to medical treatment is not prompt and substantial (150); however, as signaled by the French experience (151), this is a challenging procedure.

Mycobacterium malmoense. Disease resulting from Mm infection is considerably more prevalent in Europe than in the United States. First described in 1977 in four patients from Malmo, Sweden (153), the initial case reported in the United States was in 1984 (154). Small case series were reported from Scotland (155), northeast England (156), and Wales (123,157). A 1985 review in Britain suggested that Mm cases had begun to increase in frequency around 1980 (158). This review also observed that unlike MAC, Mm had not been recovered from the environment. A 1994 report of 221 cases from Sweden noted that Mm had become the second most common EM infection in that country (159); 170 of the cases were pulmonary, mainly occurring in persons with underlying lung disease.

Clinically and radiographically, Mm disease presents with a chronic or subacute TB-like illness. The chest radiograph usually reveals an upper zone fibronodular, partially confluent pattern with cavitation commonly present.

Treatment results are better than with MAC but far from predictable. Treatment regimens have usually consisted of INH, RIF, and EMB. The recent British trial compared RIF-EMB with RIF-EMB-INH and found no advantage to the INH-containing regimen (127). Of the 111 patients entered, there were 3 failures and 8 relapses; 44 of the 106 were alive and cured after 5 years.

An analysis of *in vitro* susceptibility for 22 strains of pathogenic Mm revealed a discouraging lack of activity for the standard anti-TB agents when tested alone: 21 (95%) of 22 were resistant to 0.25 mg/L of RIF, 100% were resistant to 5 mg/L of EMB or 4 mg/L of amikacin (160). By contrast, 19 (86%) of 22 were susceptible to 4 mg/L of clarithromycin. (We note that the concentrations of RIF, EMB, and amikacin studied here are lower than those used in our laboratory.) Encouraging, though, were the results of combined or synergy testing: When combined with EMB, many of the strains showed additive or synergistic vulnerability to the rifamycins, ciprofloxacin, and/or amikacin.

Based on these fragmentary data, we advocate initial therapy with clarithromycin, rifabutin or RIF, EMB, and amikacin (during the early months). If there is intolerance to these agents, ciprofloxacin might be substituted. For younger patients with localized disease and without substantial comorbidity, surgical resection should be considered.

Others. Other slow-growing mycobacteria that are sporadically associated with pulmonary disease include *Mycobacterium simiae* (161,162), *Mycobacterium szulgai* (163–166), *Mycobacterium gordonae* (167), *Mycobacterium asiaticum* (168), *Mycobacterium shimoidei* (169), and *Mycobacterium terrae* (170). Because clinical experience is very limited, we typically employ a MAC-like regimen in these cases influenced by the *in vitro* susceptibility profile of the isolate. Newly identified mycobacterial pathogens were recently reviewed (171).

PULMONARY DISEASE DUE TO RAPID-GROWING MYCOBACTERIA

Lung disease associated with RGM, particularly *M. abscessus* and *M. chelonae*, appears to have increased in prevalence in the United States over the past decade. Again, hindered by a lack of systematic reporting, we can only speculate about the true frequency of disease. However, in the 1980s, we noted that fewer than 10% of EM cases referred to National Jewish had RGM disease. However, over the past 2 years, 24% of our referred EM patients were infected with RGM. Certainly, this could reflect diminished referrals for patients with MAC disease as physicians, conditioned by their experience treating disseminated MAC (DMAC) in persons with AIDS, became more comfortable managing such infections. It is clear though that the absolute number of RGM cases has increased as well. From 1993 to 1994, approximately 415 RGM isolates were referred to our laboratory; by 1996 to 1997, this number had increased to 450; and by 1992 to 2000, the number had increased to roughly 540 isolates (L. Heifets, unpublished data, 2002).

RGM are widely distributed in water and soil (5), and we presume that most cases of pulmonary disease result from inhalation of aerosols generated either in potable water systems, in natural settings, or in industrial settings. An association between RGM pneumonia and achalasia has suggested aspiration of esophageal contents overgrown by the mycobacteria (82,172,173). It is our impression that RGM disease is more common in the southeast United States, but cases are reported in all 48 contiguous states, plus Alaska and Hawaii.

Clinically most of the cases referred are among women with various combinations of risk factors noted in Table 157.1. Neither we nor others have observed a relationship between HIV/AIDS and pulmonary or disseminated disease caused by the RGM. Most patients have typical nodular bronchiectatic disease including a predilection for the right middle lobe and/or lingula; in addition, focal cavitary lesions are relatively common. Other patients have TB-like disease with lobar or sublobar cavitation and/or destruction. Cough, sputum, malaise, and diminished energy are frequent complaints; feverishness, chills, sweats, and

weight loss seem less prominent in patients with RGM disease than among patients with MAC or TB.

Sputum microscopy is negative or only weakly positive in most cases, except those with frankly cavitary lesions. Cultures may or may not become positive at 1 week on Middlebrook agar, but for specimens with such early positivity, it is virtually always an RGM.

Treatment of RGM lung disease is typically frustrating for patients and physicians alike. No controlled studies have been performed. Chemotherapy regimens are selected on the basis of *in vitro* studies, but the optimal numbers of medications, dosages, and duration of therapy remain empirical. We and others predicate management on the basic principles of TB treatment: multiple drugs to prevent or slow the emergence of resistance, multiple drugs for additive/synergistic effects, and therapy well after sputum conversion in the effort to prevent or delay recurrence (however, we must note that the overwhelming majority of *M. abscessus/M. chelonae* cases do relapse). Surgery is considered in cases with localized disease and manageable comorbidity; however, surgical resection for RGM disease entails a singularly high risk of infection of the thoracic incision by the RGM (Marvin Pomerantz, unpublished data, 2002).

The agents most commonly employed against RGM infections are represented in Table 157.7. The ideal methods of *in vitro* susceptibility testing are not well established, as only limited information supports the correlation between *in vitro* results and response to treatment. The broth microdilution technique is the presently preferred methodology (174). A recent study that examined the comparability and interinstitutional reliability of E-test strips and broth dilution found the former method unacceptable (175). Few laboratories in the United States are capable of performing optimal testing for the RGMs.

We employ pharmacokinetic data to calculate appropriate doses. If the approximate MIC is known for a drug, we attempt to tailor dosing and scheduling to obtain maximal effects for that agent. For example, with a cell wall β-lactam agent, we attempt to achieve extended periods in which the drug concentration exceeds the MIC. By contrast, with aminoglycosides we attempt to deliver the maximum levels of that agent that are safe and tolerable, allowing for an extended washout period to lessen toxicity.

In general, the duration of therapy is constrained by side effects, toxicity, and too often expenses. In view of the almost universal relapses seen with *M. abscessus/M. chelonae* disease, it may be more appropriate to consider the bronchiectatic RGM disease as analogous to *P. aeruginosa* in patients with CF. Rather than pursuing curative treatment, one might choose to episodically suppress the RGM infection when indicated by symptomatic, radiographic, and/or physiologic deterioration. In this setting, the therapeutic armamentarium, which is typically scant, should be carefully husbanded to minimize the risks of acquired resistance or toxicity, which precludes usage.

Regimens that have been employed against RGM disease are noted in Table 157.7. The use of aminoglycosides in elderly patients is problematic because of increased risk for auditory or renal toxicity. Inhaled aminoglycosides including amikacin or tobramycin may be efficacious while lessening the risks of toxic reactions, but such treatment requires sophisticated home health services, may result in laryngitis or asthmatic reactions, can produce eighth nerve toxicity, and is predictably quite expensive.

For patients whose RGM has *in vitro* susceptibility to medications that can be given orally, we may treat with an intensive phase of intravenous medication, then attempt long-term suppression with an oral regimen. Although there are reports of successful monotherapy of cutaneous disease with

TABLE 157.7. Agents Used in the Therapy of Rapidly Growing Mycobacterial Infections

Agent	Side effects/toxicity	Comments
Cefoxitin, 2 g, i.v., q8–12h (or continuous infusion)	Diarrhea; *Clostridium difficile* enterocolitis; rash; fever/hypersensitivity; neutropenia and thrombopenia; anemia	Note that cefoxitin cannot be replaced by other second or third generation cephalosporins; its activity is unique
Imipenem, 1 g i.v. q12h	Nausea and vomiting; seizures; hepatitis, usually mild	Risk of seizures increased with impaired renal function and/or prior CNS disease
Amikacin 12–15 mg/kg i.v. q12h	Hearing loss, vestibular dysfunction, tinnitus, renal impairment (↑ risk with NSAIDs); neuromuscular blockade	Lower dose with age and/or impaired renal function. Possible need for high dosing for CF patients. Alert: beware of family history of aminoglycoside-induced hearing loss
Tobramycin 2.5 mg/kg q12h	Hearing loss, vestibular dysfunction, tinnitus, renal impairment (↑ risk with NSAIDs); neuromuscular blockade	Lower dose with age and/or impaired renal function. Possible need for high dosing in CF patients. Alert: beware of family history of aminoglycoside-induced hearing loss
Clarithromycin 500 mg p.o. b.i.d.	Dysgeusia, nausea, anorexia, loose stools, tinnitus	Note: drug-interactions. Limited experience with azithromycin
Ciprofloxacin 500–750 mg p.o. b.i.d.	Nausea, vomiting, anorexia, anxiety, insomnia, arthralgias, Achilles rupture, hepatitis, and thrush	Note: diminished absorption with antacids or foods. Activities of newer FQNs not well studied
Doxycycline 100 mg p.o. b.i.d. × 2, then 50 mg p.o. b.i.d.	Nausea, vomiting, GI distress; hepatitis, enterocolitis	Note: absorption impaired by antacids. Minocycline with similar activity but ↑ CNS effects
Linezolid 600 mg i.v. b.i.d.	Myelosuppression, peripheral neuritis	Active *in vitro* against 94% of *Mycobacterium chelonae* isolates (276), this agent has been reported in only one case (277)

b.i.d., twice daily; CF, cysticfibrosis; CNS, central nervous system; i.v., intravenously; FQN, fluoroquinolones; GI, gastrointestinal; NSAIDs, nonsteroidal antiinflammatory drugs.

clarithromycin (176), we are very reluctant to do this lest resistance to this agent evolve.

Extrapulmonary Environmental Mycobacterial Disease

Other than head and neck lymphadenitis, extrapulmonary infection historically has constituted a relatively small percentage of all EM disease. But with the appearance of AIDS and the extraordinary prevalence of disseminated mycobacterial infections in these patients, a substantial portion of EM disease came to involve organs outside the lungs. However, with the widespread use of prophylactic therapy and antiretroviral treatment, DMAC infections had fallen from a peak incidence of more than 20 per 100 person-years in 1994 to 1995 to approximately 2 from 1997 to 1998 (177). Among persons with AIDS who are receiving potent antiretroviral therapy, prophylaxis against MAC is no longer recommended.

Localized Environmental Mycobacterial Disease

In large measure, localized EM infections reflect direct-inoculation soft tissue/skeletal infection or lymphadenitis, presumably resulting from spread from contamination of the oropharynx.

SOFT TISSUE AND SKELETAL INFECTION

Environmental mycobacteria may cause localized infection when introduced directly into skin, soft tissues, bone, or joints. This may occur through accidental trauma or iatrogenically through either contamination of medical devices or disruption of defense barriers by invasive procedures.

Mx-related spinal infections after microsurgery for herniated disc were found in 58 patients among approximately 3,000 exposed subjects at one hospital in Paris (152). These cases extended over a decade and appeared related to one particular technique, sequential operations during a day, and chronic contamination of the hospital's water system with Mx.

M. terrae, an organism similar to Mm has been reported in association with tenosynovitis of the hands, typically following puncture wounds (178); the topic was well reviewed in a 2000 article (170).

RGM, including *M. chelonae, M. fortuitum,* and *M. abscessus,* have a striking propensity for iatrogenic infections; they have been associated with corneal abrasions and ulcerations after ophthalmic procedures (179), hypodermic infection site abscesses, monarticular arthritis after intraarticular steroid injections, mastitis after silicone implant mammaplasty (180), otitis media after placement of tympanotomy tubes (181), skin infection after cosmetic surgery in which the gentian violet used to outline the incisions was contaminated (182), injection of contaminated preparations of adrenocortical extract prescribed by alternative healers (183), abscesses after liposuction therapy (184), cellulitis after intravenous therapy (185), mastitis after body piercing (186), contamination of epicardial pacemaker wires (187), and soft tissue infection with osteitis following acupuncture (188). In addition, there have been a variety of infections after open heart surgery (including sternal osteomyelitis, mediastinitis, and endocarditis) (189). Cases of both native valve (190) and prosthetic valve (191) endocarditis resulting from *M. fortuitum* infection have been recently reported. A unique case of meningitis caused by *M. abscessus* infection following a stab wound to the neck was recently reported (192). *Mycobacterium smegmatis*, an organism similar to *M. fortuitum*, has been reported in association with various soft tissue, bone, and other infections (193); in several instances, it appeared to be iatrogenic in origin. In an excellent review of nosocomial infections caused by EM, Phillips and von Reyn (194) document that the great majority of these cases are due to RGM.

Mk can produce both nodular (sporotrichoid) and diffuse (cellulitic) cutaneous disease (195). Most of these cases appear in persons who have impaired immunity, related either to an immunosuppressive disease or to medications. Diagnosis may be delayed by failure of the hosts to form distinctive granulomata. Treatment entails antibiotics, reduction of immunosuppressive therapy, local heat, and when localized débridement.

Mycobacterium marinum infections—swimming pool granulomata, fish-handler's nodules, surfer's nodules—are acquired principally in natural settings. These cases are primarily reported in coastal areas of North America or among individuals who through hobby or employment are exposed to fish tanks or fishing paraphernalia. A report from a coastal county abutting the Chesapeake Bay offered useful insights into this infection (196); there was a strong preponderance of men, and the primary involvement was cutaneous, although joints and tendons were included in some cases. A series of 31 cases seen in Kaiser-Permanente centers in northern California offered useful observations regarding diagnosis and management (197); the upper extremities were involved in 90% of cases, lymphatic or local spread was seen in 81% of the patients, and granulomata were seen in only 63% of biopsies. Unlike the Maryland series, 52% of the patients were women; this may be related to the primary risk factor in this series: More than half of the cases were related to fish tanks. In an uncontrolled manner, treatment with RIF and EMB appeared more effective than minocycline. The incubation period from exposure to overt infection was found in a literature review to be a median of 21 days (198); one third of the cases involved more than 30 days of incubation. A previous report in which *M. marinum* infections were acquired from a mineral springs pool documented a high percentage of patients with substantial reactions to purified protein derivative (PPD) tuberculin skin testing (199).

"Buruli ulcer" is a necrotizing cutaneous disease caused by *M. ulcerans*. Originally described in Australia in 1948 (200), the disease became associated with the Buruli district of Uganda (201). The disease was sporadic—endemic in Central West Africa and Australia during the 1960s and 1970s. Initially seen as cause of concern only for the few individuals afflicted, case numbers have soared recently. According to the World Health Organization, Buruli ulcer is now the third most prevalent mycobacterial disease, soon to exceed leprosy in clinical and public health importance (202). Cases have now been noted throughout sub-Saharan Africa (203), South Central America, India, Southeast Asia, and Papua, New Guinea (204–207), and there have been cases noted in Europe, Japan, and the United States among travelers to those regions (205,208,209).

The incubation period for Buruli ulcer is usually less than 3 months (210). The illness is marked by slowly progressive, necrotizing skin lesions; inflammation with redness and swelling is present early but recedes with chronicity (202). The margins of the ulcers are typically very "clean." Constitutional symptoms or regional lymphadenitis are not reported. Generalized or disseminated infection has not been noted, even in persons with AIDS. Especially among children, extensive soft tissue destruction can result in compromise of joint function, impaired lymph flow with edema, and stunted limb growth (203). Osteomyelitis has also been described (202).

The histopathology of the Buruli ulcer lesions is quite distinctive with prominent extracellular bacilli and extensive necrosis in the skin and fat. For a comprehensive discussion of the histopathology and pathogenesis, see recent reviews

(202,211,212). Currently available evidence suggests that Buruli ulcer causes tissue destruction by elaboration of toxins that result in necrosis with virtually no purulent reaction (212). A soluble toxin, a polyketide named *mycolactone* has been found to be both cytotoxic (213,214) and immunosuppressive (215).

Striking regarding Buruli ulcer is the reported lack of utility of antimicrobial therapy. Aggressive surgical débridement followed by skin grafting appears to be the primary mode of management. RIF has some efficacy (216), but *in vitro* studies suggest that clarithromycin might have more activity (217). Raising the temperature of the affected limb by topical heat appears also to have utility (216). Bacille Calmette-Guérin (BCG) has been shown to offer modest protection versus Buruli ulcer (218,219).

Monarticular arthritis and localized tenosynovitis have also been reported with MAC, *M. terrae* (220), *M. marinum* (221), and as noted RGM (222). In some instances, it seems probable that the process began as a noninfectious condition and was complicated by the iatrogenic introduction of the mycobacteria, often during steroid injections. Because of the immense potential for iatrogenic morbidity, this issue is worth amplification. We have seen a considerable number of cases in which it appears probable that MAC or less commonly RGM had been introduced into wrists, hands, or bursae during steroid injections. In other cases, the infection may have been initiated with a puncture wound resulting in local spread to the joint or tendinous structure.

In other instances, no discrete inciting event can be identified, raising the question of transient mycobacteremia with seeding of a single site (220). Mycobacterial infection that localized to vertebrae following blunt external trauma was reported in three patients infected with *M. abscessus*, MAC, and *M. bovis* BCG (223). In these cases, it appeared as though falls or a motor vehicle accident had either caused compression fractures or hematomas that were then seeded by mycobacteria in the lymphatics or bloodstream, the principle of *locus minoris resistentiae*.

Because in general patients with single-site extrapulmonary EM disease *do not* have deficits of immunity, initial screening including serologic testing for HIV is not indicated unless the patient comes from a high-risk group. Management usually consists of chemotherapy and surgical extirpation or débridement with careful attention to the removal of foreign matter. If the species and susceptibility pattern are known, drugs may be selected as noted in the section "Pulmonary Environmental Mycobacterial Disease." If the species is not yet known or susceptibility has not been determined, one may be forced to begin empirical therapy. Broadly speaking, much empirical therapy might best consist of a macrolide or RIF, EMB, and ciprofloxacin; amikacin should be included in cases in which major joints or vital sites are involved. Such a regimen should be reasonably active against such a diverse group of mycobacteria. We believe that careful quantitative susceptibility testing should be performed to aid in the management of these tenacious infections.

LYMPHADENITIS

EM infection of lymph nodes is primarily a disease of children aged 1 to 5 years; rarely is it seen in adults (224). MAC is by far the most common pathogen, in contrast to earlier reports with higher percentages of Mk or *Mycobacterium scrofulaceum* (225,226). Of note, a recent analysis of MAC serovars that produced cervical adenitis in healthy children and disseminated infection in those with AIDS found that a limited number of strains were involved among patients from Boston, Los Angeles, and Miami (227). Typically, the lymphadenitis presents as unilateral, anterior cervical, preauricular, or submandibular erythematous swelling in an asymptomatic child with a normal chest radiograph (224,226).

In contrast, lymphadenitis caused by *M. tuberculosis* more commonly involves lymph nodes, that drain from intrathoracic sites, the supraclavicular or low cervical nodes. Occasionally, the nodes drain spontaneously or ulcerate. Biopsy typically demonstrates granulomata with or without caseation; in some early lesions, a dimorphic response (mixed granulomatous and pyogenic) is seen. AFB stains are positive in only about half the cases.

Skin testing is a problem. In earlier studies, most children have reacted to EM antigens; however, these are no longer available. Because of cross-reactivity, a portion of EM patients react to PPD-T or S, the antigen of *M. tuberculosis.* Indeed, in the series by Wolinsky series (226), 35% of children showed induration of 10 mm or more to this antigen; conversely, 29% showed reactivity of 0 to 5 mm. Thus, neither a positive nor a negative reaction to PPD-T has much sensitivity or specificity in the etiologic diagnosis of cervical adenitis. Perhaps the most meaningful result of tuberculin skin testing is an intense reaction (20 mm or more of induration) that points toward TB rather than EM infection, but this is not infallible.

Culture of lymph node biopsy material is vital, because the management of adenitis caused by EM is vastly different from that of disease caused by *M. tuberculosis* infection. Unlike *M. tuberculosis* infection of children or adults, which definitely merits chemotherapy, the local EM infection may entail only careful observation or it may be sufficiently controlled with excisional surgery. Although chemotherapy has been administered to many children with EM adenitis, it is not clear that it was beneficial (224–226). Indeed, it is common for inflammation and swelling to persist for many months with or without medical therapy. If a biopsy is performed and demonstrates histopathologic features consistent with mycobacterial lymphadenitis, it may be appropriate to initiate chemotherapy until cultures distinguish between EM and TB. This is especially true for persons with a high-risk epidemiological profile, such as Hispanic, African American, or Asian children. If the culture is positive for EM, therapy may be terminated, or if a distinctly favorable clinical response has been seen, chemotherapy may be continued. If it grows nothing and there are insufficient grounds to rule out TB, therapy might be continued for 9 months. Until TB has been excluded, empirical agents of choice are INH and RIF; EMB is an excellent EM agent in general, but it is difficult to monitor children who cannot comply with standard tests for visual impairment. However, available experience suggests that when clearly indicated, EMB can be given to children with reasonable expectations for safety (228). If MAC is identified, clarithromycin or azithromycin—because of the likelihood of *in vitro* activity and generally benign toxicity profiles—might be employed. Because of the paucibacillary disease and negligible risk of disseminated infection, monotherapy is justified in our opinion. Neither the ideal duration nor proof of efficacy of this approach has been established.

Disseminated or Multifocal Extrapulmonary Environmental Mycobacterial Disease

Given the relatively limited virulence of the EM, we should regard all patients with simultaneous infection in multiple organs as suffering some form of immunologic impairment. The most dramatic example of this is HIV infection/AIDS, but there are other forms of naturally occurring deficiency states associated with disseminated EM, including congenital defects related to IFN-γ or interleukin-12 (IL-12) and/or tumor necrosis factor-α (TNF-α) (229–236). Although a recent report from Thailand described disseminated RGM disease including diffuse lymphadenopathy in a cluster of 16 "immunocompetent hosts" (237),

the unique nature of these cases belies that description. The patients' histories of prior infections strongly suggests an abnormality of cellular immunity.

DISSEMINATED ENVIRONMENTAL MYCOBACTERIAL DISEASE IN PERSONS WITHOUT AIDS

Throughout the latter half of the twentieth century, there were sporadic reports of multifocal or disseminated EM, typically involving younger persons who may or may not have had evidence of otherwise impaired immunity (238–243). Clinicians in these reports inferred disturbances of cellular immunity, describing various anomalies of histopathology, circulating lymphocytes, or responsiveness to antigens. More recently, Holland at the National Institutes of Health (229) and investigators working in Mediterranean Europe (230–232) have described patients with a variety of disseminated EM infections. Sophisticated studies have identified several deficits in these patients variably involving IFN-γ, IL-12, and TNF-α (234–236,244,245). To put these conditions in perspective, authors have published excellent reviews of immunodeficiency states resulting from defects in lymphocytes (246) and phagocytes (247).

Clinically, these patients typically present with illness in infancy and childhood; clinical manifestations include various combinations of failure to thrive, fever, sweats, splenomegaly, lymphadenopathy, diarrhea, and weight loss. Other organ involvement includes pneumonia, sinusitis, enteritis, osteomyelitis, hepatitis, mycobacteremia, cutaneous lesions, and pleural and pericardial disease. Depending on the severity of the deficits or other anomalies of immunity, some of the patients did not manifest illness until adulthood, whereas others had vulnerability to infection other than mycobacteria. Mycobacteria involved included MAC, *M. chelonae, M. fortuitum,* Mk, *M. bovis,* BCG, and *M. smegmatis.*

Disseminated mycobacterial infections have also been seen in children or adults with cyclic neutropenia (C. Kirkpatrick, personal communication, 1986), intestinal lymphangiectasia (C. Kirkpatrick, personal communication, 1982), or chronic granulomatous disease (248). In addition, as noted earlier, a cluster of 16 cases of disseminated disease due to RGM including *M. chelonae-abscessus, M. abscessus,* and *M. fortuitum* was reported from northeastern Thailand (237). These patients presented with bilateral cervical lymphadenopathy and variable involvement of skin, sinuses, lungs, liver, spleen, bone and joint, and toenails. Leukocytosis and anemia were common; all of the subjects were seronegative for HIV. Half of the patients had prior opportunistic infections. The authors described Sweet's syndrome (fever, leukocytosis, and erythematous skin plaques with neutrophilic infiltrates) in 9 of the 16. Treatment with amikacin and a macrolide appeared beneficial in seven patients. Although the authors were unable to identify discrete abnormalities of immunity in these subjects, it is highly probable that they represent a novel deficiency, more likely acquired than inherited (249).

The cases from Thailand are distinctly different from those in a 1993 report and review from Duke (250). They described two patients without identified immune disturbances who presented with disseminated infection caused by *M. fortuitum* and *M. chelonae.* Both men, 56 and 61 years of age, were notable for their presentation with fever of unknown origin, hepatosplenomegaly, no skin lesions, and widespread granulomata.

Other patients in whom disseminated EM disease is likely to occur are those with iatrogenic immune suppression including organ transplantation (251), cancer and antineoplastic chemotherapy (250), or collagen-vascular/vasculitis corticosteroid-cytotoxic therapy (250). Disseminated EM diseases have also been noted in patients with hairy cell leukemia (252–254); notably, in one case the mycobacteriosis involuted spontaneously with treatment of the leukemia with IFN-α (255). Presumably this represented an immune deficit related directly to the malignancy.

DISSEMINATED ENVIRONMENTAL MYCOBACTERIAL INFECTION IN PERSONS WITH AIDS

DMAC was the most common systemic bacterial infection in patients early in the AIDS epidemic in the United States; up to 20% of patients with AIDS developed DMAC before death (256). At highest risk were those individuals with $CD4^+$ T-lymphocyte counts of less than 50 cells/μL. In the absence of chemoprophylaxis, the yearly rate of development of MAC bacteremia was 20%, following an initial AIDS-defining opportunistic infection and a decline in the $CD4^+$ T-lymphocyte count to less than 100 cells/μL (257). With the advent of highly effective antiretroviral therapy, the frequency of DMAC has declined rapidly. However, cases of DMAC continue to appear among persons with AIDS. In an inner-city clinic in Atlanta, the epidemiology of these infections during the 1990s had shifted toward greater involvement of women, blacks, and those who had acquired HIV infection via means other than homosexual contact (258). Clinical findings associated with DMAC in AIDS patients include constitutional symptoms (fever, sweats, inanition), diffuse peripheral lymphadenitis, massive retroperitoneal and mesenteric lymphadenitis, mediastinal or hilar lymphadenitis, infiltrative hepatosplenomegaly, anemia, and cytopenia secondary to infiltration of the bone marrow, and refractory diarrhea due to massive infiltration of intestinal and colonic mucosa by mycobacteria-laden macrophages. Laboratory findings routinely but nonspecifically found in DMAC include anemia, neutropenia, and an elevated serum alkaline phosphatase level.

HIV-infected individuals rarely have clinically significant pulmonary disease secondary to MAC. One report found pulmonary MAC disease in only 2.5% of 200 patients with DMAC (259). When MAC is associated with pulmonary disease, parenchymal infiltrates or nodules are typically seen. Cavitary lesions are uncommon. Airway compromise secondary to endobronchial MAC lesions has been seen.

Isolation of the organism from blood is the most reliable method for the diagnosis of DMAC in patients with AIDS. Isolation of MAC organisms from bone marrow or other normally sterile sites (lymph node, liver, spleen, cerebrospinal fluid) may precede recovery from the blood; recovery from such sites should be interpreted as indicative of disseminated disease. Cultures of either respiratory tract secretions or stool specimens that yield MAC organisms are not diagnostic of disseminated disease.

Untreated DMAC is associated with reduced survival in patients with AIDS, and new antimicrobial agents have afforded clinical and microbiologic responses and improved survival in most patients. Current recommendations for the treatment of DMAC entail either clarithromycin or azithromycin combined with one or more additional agents. In a direct comparison, clarithromycin-EMB was more potent than azithromycin-EMB (260). Note that there is universal agreement on establishing *in vitro* susceptibility to the macrolides. EMB has the advantage of predictably additive activity with clarithromycin and azithromycin (261); as well, EMB may show synergistic or additive effects with RIF or rifabutin (262). And, in an animal model, EMB delayed the evolution of resistance to clarithromycin (263). Adding RIF to a clarithromycin-containing regimen results in a significant reduction in the bioavailability of the macrolide (264,265). One could either accept this result, increase the dose of clarithromycin, or substitute azithromycin, which is not affected by RIF, or alternatively one could use rifabutin, which

has a considerably lesser effect on hepatic cytochrome induction (264). However, the drug–drug interaction between clarithromycin and rifabutin may result in greatly increased serum concentrations of the rifabutin, up to 700% above the usual levels (S. Berning, personal communication, 2001). These high concentrations of rifabutin have proven quite toxic producing uveitis, "pink-man syndrome," neutropenia and/or thrombopenia, and "lupus syndrome" (266). Thus, if clarithromycin and rifabutin are used together, a low dose of rifabutin, 150 mg daily, should be used. Our limited experience suggests that a regimen of azithromycin, EMB, and rifabutin would be well tolerated and effective. It is vital to note that RIF is not compatible with most antiretroviral agents (267). For persons for whom antiretroviral therapy is not feasible (because of unwillingness, toxicity, or loss of efficacy), prophylaxis should be given to those with CD4 counts less than 50 cells/μL (268,269). Azithromycin, 1,200 mg orally *once weekly*, has proven effective and tolerable. Clarithromycin or rifabutin have been demonstrated to have efficacy but are less convenient and effective than azithromycin.

REFERENCES

1. Rivero A, et al. High rate of tuberculosis reinfection during a nosocomial outbreak of multidrug-resistant tuberculosis caused by *Mycobacterium bovis* strain B. *Clin Infect Dis* 2001;32:159–161.
2. Long R, et al. Transcontinental spread of multidrug-resistant *Mycobacterium bovis*. *Am J Respir Crit Care Med* 1999;159:2014–2017.
3. Palenque E, et al. Transmission of multidrug-resistant Mycobacterium bovis to an immunocompetent patient. *Clin Infect Dis* 1998;26:995–996.
4. Sreevatsan S, et al. Restricted structural gene polymorphism in the Mycobacterium tuberculosis complex indicates evolutionarily recent global dissemination. *Proc Natl Acad Sci USA* 1997;94:9869–9874.
5. Falkinham JO. Epidemiology of infection by nontuberculous mycobacteria. *Clin Microbiol Rev* 1996;9(2):177–215.
6. O'Brien RJ, Geiter LJ, Snider DE Jr. The epidemiology of nontuberculous mycobacterial diseases in the United States. Results from a national survey. *Am Rev Respir Dis* 1987;135:1007–1014.
7. Tsukamura M, et al. Epidemiologic studies of lung disease due to mycobacteria other than Mycobacterium tuberculosis in Japan. *Rev Infect Dis* 1981;3(5):997–1006.
8. Debrunner M, et al. Epidemiology and clinical significance of nontuberculous mycobacteria in patients negative for human immunodeficiency virus in Switzerland. *Clin Infect Dis* 1992;15:330–345.
9. Yates MD, et al. Isolation of environmental mycobacteria from clinical specimens in south-east England: 1973–1993. *Int J Tuberc Lung Dis* 1997;1(1): 75–80.
10. Contreras MA, et al. Pulmonary infection with nontuberculous mycobacteria. *Am Rev Respir Dis* 1988;137:149–152.
11. Choudhri S, et al. Clinical significance of nontuberculous mycobacteria isolates in a Canadian tertiary care center. *Clin Infect Dis* 1995;21:128–133.
12. Henriques B, et al. Infection with *Mycobacterium malmoense* in Sweden: report of 221 cases. *Clin Infect Dis* 1994;18:595–600.
13. Huang JH, et al. *Mycobacterium avium-intracellulare* pulmonary infection in HIV-negative patients without preexisting lung disease. Diagnostic and management limitations. *Chest* 1999;115:1033–1040.
14. Kennedy TP, Weber DJ. Nontuberculous mycobacteria. An underappreciated cause of geriatric lung disease. *Am J Respir Crit Care Med* 1994;149:1654–1658.
15. Reich JM, Johnson RE. *Mycobacterium avium* complex pulmonary disease. Incidence, presentation, and response to therapy in a community setting. *Am Rev Respir Dis* 1991;143:1381–1385.
16. Prince DS, et al. Infection with *Mycobacterium avium* complex in patients without predisposing conditions. *N Engl J Med* 1989;321(13):863–868.
17. Wallace RJ Jr, et al. Polyclonal *Mycobacterium avium* complex infections in patients with nodular bronchiectasis. *Am J Respir Crit Care Med* 1998;158:1235–1244.
18. Hartman TE, Swensen SJ, Williams DE. *Mycobacterium avium*-intracellulare complex: evaluation with CT. *Radiology* 1993;187:1–4.
19. Swensen SJ, Hartman TE, Williams DE. Computed tomographic diagnosis of *Mycobacterium avium-intracellulare* complex in patients with bronchiectasis. *Chest* 1994;105:49–52.
20. DeGroote MA, et al. Retrospective analysis of aspiration risk and genetic predisposition in bronchiectasis patients with and without non-tuberculous mycobacteria infection. *Am J Respir Crit Care Med* 2001;163(5):A763.
21. Kubo K, et al. *Mycobacterium avium-intracellulare* pulmonary infection in patients without known predisposing lung disease. *Lung* 1998;176:381–391.
22. Davidson P, et al. Treatment of disease due to *Mycobacterium intracellulare*. *Rev Infect Dis* 1981;3(5):1052–1059.

23. Rosenzweig DY. Pulmonary mycobacterial infections due to *Mycobacterium intracellulare-avium* complex. Clinical features and course in 100 consecutive cases. *Chest* 1979;75:115–119.
24. Ahn CH, et al. A four-drug regimen for initial treatment of cavitary disease caused by *Mycobacterium avium* complex. *Am Rev Respir Dis* 1986;134:438–441.
25. Ahn GH, et al. A demographic study of disease due to *Mycobacterium kansasii* or *M. intracellulare-avium* in Texas. *Chest* 1979;75:120–125.
26. Yeager H Jr, Raleigh JW. Pulmonary disease due to *Mycobacterium intracellulare*. *Am Rev Respir Dis* 1973;108:547–552.
27. Wallace RJ Jr. *Mycobacterium avium* complex lung disease and women. Now an equal opportunity disease. *Chest* 1994;105(1):6–7.
28. Reich J, Johnson NR. *Mycobacterium avium* complex pulmonary disease presenting as isolated lingular or middle lobe pattern: the Lady Windermere syndrome. *Chest* 1992;101:1605–1609.
29. Iseman MD. That's no lady [Letter]. *Chest* 1996;109:1411.
30. Iseman MD. That's no lady, revisited [Letter]. *Chest* 1997;111:255.
31. Tsuyuguchi K, et al. Effect of oestrogen on *Mycobacterium avium* complex pulmonary infection in mice. *Clin Exp Immunol* 2001;123:428–434.
32. Frisch RE. Fatness, menarche, and female fertility. *Perspect Biol Med* 1985;28:611–633.
33. Frisch RE. Body fat, menarche, fitness and fertility. *Prog Reprod Biol Med* 1990;14:1–26.
34. Bates GW, Whitworth NS. Effects of body weight on female reproductive function. In: Givens JR, ed. *The hypothalamus*. Chicago: Year Book Medical, 1984:97–115.
35. Huang JH, et al. Analyses of the NRAMP1 and IFN-gR1 genes in women with *Mycobacterium avium-intracellulare* pulmonary disease. *Am J Respir Crit Care Med* 1998;157:377–381.
36. Bittner M, et al. Emergence of *Mycobacterium kansasii* as the leading mycobacterial pathogen isolated over a 20-year period at a Midwestern Veterans Affairs Hospital. *Clin Infect Dis* 1996;22:1109–1110.
37. Bates JH. A study of pulmonary disease associated with mycobacteria other than *Mycobacterium tuberculosis*: clinical characteristics. *Am Rev Respir Dis* 1967;96:1151–1157.
38. Good RC, Snider DE Jr. Isolation of nontuberculous mycobacteria in the United States, 1980. *J Infect Dis* 1982;146(6):829–833.
39. Strimlan CV. Incidence of pleuropulmonary symptoms in ankylosing spondylitis. *Chest* 2001;120:320.
40. Movsas B, et al. Pulmonary radiation injury. *Chest* 1997;111:1061–1076.
41. Witty LA, Tapson VF, Piantadosi CA. Isolation of mycobacteria in patients with pulmonary alveolar proteinosis. *Medicine* 1994;73:103–109.
42. Lee WL, Downey GP. Leukocyte elastase. Physiological functions and role in acute lung injury. *Am J Respir Crit Care Med* 2001;164:896–904.
43. Crystal RG. α_1-Antitrypsin deficiency, emphysema, and liver disease. *J Clin Invest* 1990;85:1343–1352.
44. Vogelmeier C, et al. Anti-neutrophil elastase defense of the normal human respiratory epithelial surface provided by the secretory leukoprotease inhibitor. *J Clin Invest* 1991;87:482–488.
45. Sandford AJ, et al. Susceptibility genes for rapid decline of lung function in the lung health study. *Am J Respir Crit Care Med* 2001;163:469–473.
46. Meyer KC, et al. Neutrophils, unopposed neutrophil elastase, and alpha 1-antiprotease defenses following human lung transplantation. *Am J Respir Crit Care Med* 2001;164:97–102.
47. Sandford AJ, et al. α_1-antitrypsin geneotypes and the acute-phase response to open heart surgery. *Am J Respir Crit Care Med* 1999;159:1624–1628.
48. Longstreth GF, et al. Bronchiectasis and homozygous alpha-1-antitrypsin deficiency. *Chest* 1975;67(2):233–235.
49. Scott JH, et al. Alpha-1-antitrypsin deficiency with diffuse bronchiectasis and cirrhosis of the liver. *Chest* 1977;71(4):535–538.
50. Jones DK, Godden D, Cavanagh P. Alpha-1-antitrypsin deficiency presenting as bronchiectasis. *Br J Dis Chest* 1985;79:301–303.
51. Shin MS, Ho K-J. Bronchiectasis in patients with a1-antitrypsin deficiency. A rare occurrence? *Chest* 1993;104:1384–1386.
52. Rodriguez-Cintron W, Guntupalli K, Fraire AE. Bronchiectasis and homozygous (P₁ZZ) α1-antitrypsin deficiency in a young man. *Thorax* 1995;50:424–425.
53. Shapiro L, Pott GB, Ralston AH. Alpha-1-antitrypsin inhibits human immunodeficiency virus type 1. *FASEB J* 2001;15(1):115–122.
54. Lieberman J. Augmentation therapy reduces frequency of lung infections in antitrypsin deficiency. A new hypothesis with supporting data. *Chest* 2000;118:1480–1485.
55. Barker AF, et al. Replacement therapy for hereditary alpha-1-antitrypsin deficiency. A program for long-term administration. *Chest* 1994;105:1406–1410.
56. Cantin AM, Woods DE. Aerosolized Prolastin suppresses bacterial proliferation in a model of chronic *Pseudomonas aeruginosa* lung infection. *Am J Respir Crit Care Med* 1999;160:1130–1135.
57. Tsui L-C, Buchwald M. Biochemical and molecular genetics of cystic fibrosis. *Adv Hum Genet* 1991;20:153–266.
58. Kerem E, et al. The relation between genotype and phenotype in cystic fibrosis—analysis of the most common mutation (delta F508). *N Engl J Med* 1990;323(22):1517–1522.
59. FitzSimmons SC. CFF Patient Registry. 1997 Annual Data Report. Bethesda, MD: Cystic Fibrosis Foundation, 1998.
60. Desmarquest P et al. Genotype analysis and phenotypic manifestations of children with intermediate sweat chloride test results. *Chest* 2000;118:1591–1597.
61. Highsmith WE, et al. A novel mutation in the cystic fibrosis gene in patients with pulmonary disease but normal sweat chloride concentrations. *N Engl J Med* 1994;331(15):974–980.
62. Stern RC, et al. Intermediate-range sweat chloride concentration and *Pseudomonas* bronchitis: a cystic fibrosis variant with preservation of exocrine pancreatic function. *JAMA* 1978;239:2676–2680.
63. Stern RC. The diagnosis of cystic fibrosis. *N Engl J Med* 1997;336(7):487–491.
64. Rosenstein BJ, Zeitlin PL. Cystic fibrosis. *Lancet* 1998;351:277–282.
65. Aron Y, et al. HLA class II polymorphism in cystic fibrosis. A possible modifier of pulmonary phenotype. *Am J Respir Crit Care Med* 1999;159:1464–1468.
66. Noone PG, et al. Lung disease associated with the IVS8 5T allele of the CFTR gene. *Am J Respir Crit Care Med* 2000;162:1919–1924.
67. Smith MJ, et al. Mycobacterial isolations in young adults with cystic fibrosis. *Thorax* 1984;39:369–375.
68. Olivier KN, Yankaskas JR, Knowles MR. Nontuberculous mycobacterial pulmonary disease in cystic fibrosis. *Semin Respir Infect* 1996;11(4):272–284.
69. Oliver A, et al. Nontuberculous mycobacteria in patients with cystic fibrosis. *Clin Infect Dis* 2001;32:1298–1303.
70. Afzelius BA. A human syndrome caused by immotile cilia. *Science* 1976;193:317–319.
71. Rayner CFJ, et al. Ciliary disorientation alone as a cause of primary ciliary dyskinesia syndrome. *Am J Respir Crit Care Med* 1996;153(3):1123–1129.
72. de Iongh RU, Rutland J. Ciliary defects in healthy subjects, bronchiectasis, and primary ciliary dyskinesia. *Am J Respir Crit Care Med* 1995;151:1559–1567.
73. Lazzarini-de-Oliveira LC, et al. A 38-year-old man with tracheomegaly, tracheal diverticulosis, and bronchiectasis. *Chest* 2001;120:1018–1020.
74. Williams H, Campbell P. Generalized bronchiectasis associated with deficiency of cartilage in the bronchial tree. *Arch Dis Child* 1960;35:182–191.
75. Palmer C, Jablon S, Edwards P. Tuberculosis morbidity of young men in relation to tuberculin sensitivity and body build. *Am Rev Tuberc Pulm Dis* 1957;76:517–534.
76. Tverdal A. Height, weight, and incidence of tuberculosis. *Bull Int Union Tuberc Lung Dis* 1988;63:16–17.
77. Iseman MD, Buschman DL, Ackerson LM. Pectus excavatum and scoliosis: thoracic anomalies associated with pulmonary disease due to *M. avium* complex. *Am Rev Respir Dis* 1991;144:914–916.
78. Loeys B, et al. Genotype and phenotype analysis of 171 patients referred for molecular study of the fibrillin-1 gene FBN1 because of suspected Marfan syndrome. *Arch Intern Med* 2001;161:2447–2454.
79. Silverman EK, et al. Gender-related differences in severe, early-onset chronic obstructive pulmonary disease. *Am J Respir Crit Care Med* 2000;162:2152–2158.
80. FitzSimmons SC. The changing epidemiology of cystic fibrosis. *J Pediatr* 1993;122:1–9.
81. Chan ED, Iseman MD. Potential association between calcified thoracic lymphadenopathy due to previous *Histoplasma capsulatum* infection and pulmonary *Mycobacterium avium* complex disease. *South Med J* 1999;92(6):572–576.
82. Varghese G, et al. Fatal infection with *Mycobacterium fortuitum* associated with oesophageal achalasia. *Thorax* 1988;43:151–152.
83. Nebel OT, Fornes MF, Castell DO. Symptomatic gastroesophageal reflux: incidence and precipitating factors. *Am J Dig Dis* 1976;21:953–956.
84. Locke GR, et al. Prevalence and clinical spectrum of gastroesophageal reflux: a population-based study in Olmsted County, Minnesota. *Gastroenterology* 1997;112:1448–1456.
85. Kahrilas PJ. Gastroesophageal reflux disease. *JAMA* 1996;276:983–988.
86. Richter C, et al. Predictive markers of survival in HIV-seropositive and HIV-seronegative Tanzanian patients with extrapulmonary tuberculosis. *Tuberc Lung Dis* 1995;76:510–517.
87. Bibi H, et al. The prevalence of gastroesophageal reflux in children with tracheomalacia and laryngomalacia. *Chest* 2001;119:409–413.
88. Field SK, et al. Prevalence of gastroesophageal reflux symptoms in asthma. *Chest* 1996;109:316–322.
89. Harding SM, Guzzo MR, Richter JE. 24-h esophageal pH testing in asthmatics: respiratory symptom correlation with esophageal acid events. *Chest* 1999;115:654–659.
90. Sontag SJ, et al. Prevalence of oesophagitis in asthmatics. *Gut* 1992;33:872–876.
91. Mokhlesi B, et al. Increased prevalence of gastroesophageal reflux symptoms in patients with COPD. *Chest* 2001;119(4):1043.
92. Tobin RW, et al. Increased prevalence of gastroesophageal reflux in patients with idiopathic pulmonary fibrosis. *Am J Respir Crit Care Med* 1998;158:1804–1808.
93. Lagergren J, et al. Association between medications that relax the lower esophageal sphincter and risk for esophageal adenocarcinoma. *Ann Intern Med* 2000;133:165–175.
94. Embil J, et al. Pulmonary illness associated with exposure to *Mycobacterium-avium* complex in hot tub water. Hypersensitivity pneumonitis or infection? *Chest* 1997;111:813–816.
95. Mangione EJ, et al. Nontuberculous mycobacterial disease following hot tub exposure. *Emerg Infect Dis* 2001;7(6):1039–1042.
96. Bernstein DI, et al. Machine operator's lung. A hypersensitivity pneumonitis disorder associated with exposure to metalworking fluid aerosols. *Chest* 1995;108:636–641.
97. Muilenburg ML, Burge HA, Sweet T. Hypersensitivity pneumonitis and exposure to acid-bast bacilli in coolant aerosols [Abstract 683]. *J Allergy Clin Immunol* 1993;91:311.

98. Kreiss K, Cox-Ganser J. Metalworking fluid-associated hypersensitivity pneumonitis: a workshop summary. *Am J Ind Med* 1997;32:423–432.

99. Zacharisen MD, et al. The spectrum of respiratory disease associated with exposure to metal working fluids. *J Occup Environ Med* 1998;40:640–647.

100. Shelton BG, Flanders WD, Morris GK. *Mycobacterium* sp. as a possible cause of hypersensitivity pneumonitis in machine workers. *Emerg Infect Dis* 1999;5(2):270–273.

101. Schuyler M, Cormier Y. The diagnosis of hypersensitivity pneumonitis [Editorial]. *Chest* 1997;111:534–536.

102. Scully RE, et al. Case records of the Massachusetts General Hospital: weekly clinicopathological exercises. *N Engl J Med* 1996;334(8):521–526.

103. Crowe HE, et al. A limited clinical, pathologic, and epidemiologic study of patients with pulmonary lesions associated with atypical acid-fast bacilli in the sputum. *Am Rev Tuberc* 1957;75:199–222.

104. Schaefer W. Type-specificity of atypical mycobacteria in agglutination and antibody absorption test. *Am Rev Respir Dis* 1967;96:1165–1168.

105. Baess I. Deoxyribonucleic acid relationships between different serotypes of *Mycobacterium avium, Mycobacterium intracellulare,* and *Mycobacterium scrofulaceum. Acta Pathol Microbiol Immunol Scand (B)* 1983;91:201–203.

106. Maesaki S, et al. A clinical comparison between *Mycobacterium avium* and *Mycobacterium intracellulare* infections. *Chest* 1993;104:1408–1411.

107. Guthertz LS, et al. *Mycobacterium avium* and *Mycobacterium intracellulare* infections in patients with and without AIDS. *J Infect Dis* 1989;160(6):1037–1041.

108. Falkinham JO III, Norton CD, LeChevallier MW. Factors influencing numbers of *Mycobacterium avium, Mycobacterium intracellulare,* and other mycobacteria in drinking water distribution systems. *Appl Environ Microbiol* 2001;67(3):1225–1231.

109. Schulze-Röbbecke R, Janning B, Fischeder R. Occurrence of mycobacteria in biofilm samples. *Tuberc Lung Dis* 1992;73:141–144.

110. Cirillo JD, et al. Interaction of *Mycobacterium avium* with environmental amoebae enhances virulence. *Infect Immun* 1997;65(9):3759–3767.

111. Tyndall RL, Domingue EL. Cocultivation of *Legionella pneumophila* and free-living amoebae. *Appl Environ Microbiol* 1982;44:954–959.

112. Essig A, et al. Infection of *Acanthamoeba castellanii* by *Chlamydia pneumoniae. Appl Environ Microbiol* 1997;63:1396–1399.

113. duMoulin GC, et al. Concentration of *Mycobacterium avium* by hospital hot water systems. *JAMA* 1988;260(11):1599–1601.

114. von Reyn CF, et al. Persistent colonisation of potable water as a source of *Mycobacterium avium* infection in AIDS. *Lancet* 1994;343:1137–1141.

115. Costrini AM, et al. Clinical and roentgenographic features of nosocomial pulmonary disease due to *Mycobacterium xenopi. Am Rev Respir Dis* 1981;123:104–109.

116. American Thoracic Society. Diagnosis and treatment of disease caused by nontuberculous mycobacteria. *Am J Respir Crit Care Med* 1997;156:S1–S25.

117. Lynch DA, et al. CT features of pulmonary *Mycobacterium avium* complex infection. *J Comput Assist Tomogr* 1995;19(3):353–360.

118. Rosenzweig DY, Schlueter DP. Spectrum of clinical disease in pulmonary infection with *Mycobacterium avium-intracellulare. Rev Infect Dis* 1981;3(5):1046–1051.

119. Horsburgh CR, et al. Response to therapy of pulmonary *Mycobacterium avium intracellulare* infection correlates with results of *in vitro* susceptibility testing. *Am Rev Respir Dis* 1987;135:418–421.

120. Tsukamura M. Diagnosis of disease caused by *Mycobacterium avium* complex. *Chest* 1991;99(3):667–669.

121. Woods GL. Susceptibility testing for mycobacteria. *Clin Infect Dis* 2000;31:1209–1215.

122. Hunter AM, et al. Treatment of pulmonary infections caused by mycobacteria of the *Mycobacterium avium-intracellulare* complex. *Thorax* 1981;36:326–329.

123. Banks J, Jenkins PA, Smith AP. Pulmonary infection with *Mycobacterium malmoense*—a review of treatment and response. *Tubercle* 1985;66:197–203.

124. Etzkorn ET, et al. Medical therapy of *Mycobacterium avium-intracellulare* pulmonary disease. *Am Rev Respir Dis* 1986;134:442–445.

125. Heifets LB. Synergistic effect of rifampin, streptomycin, ethionamide, and ethambutol on *Mycobacterium intracellulare. Am Rev Respir Dis* 1982;125:43–48.

126. Heifets LB. Susceptibility testing of *Mycobacterium avium* complex isolates. *Antimicrob Agents Chemother* 1996;40:1759–1767.

127. Research Committee of the British Thoracic Society. First randomised trial of treatments for pulmonary disease caused by *M. avium intracellulare, M. malmoense,* and *M. xenopi* in HIV negative patients: rifampicin, ethambutol and isoniazid versus rifampicin and ethambutol. *Thorax* 2001;56:167–172.

128. Corpe RF. Surgical management of pulmonary disease due to *Mycobacterium avium intracellulare. Rev Infect Dis* 1981;3:1064–1067.

129. Moran JF, et al. Long-term results of pulmonary resection for atypical mycobacterial disease. *Ann Thorac Surg* 1983;35(6):597–604.

130. Pomerantz M, et al. Surgical management of resistant mycobacterial tuberculosis and other mycobacterial pulmonary infections. *Ann Thorac Surg* 1991;52:1108–1112.

131. Good RC, for the Centers for Disease Control and Prevention. Isolation of nontuberculous mycobacteria in the United States, 1979. *J Infect Dis* 1980;142(5):779–783.

132. Lillo M, et al. Pulmonary and disseminated infection due to *Mycobacterium kansasii:* a decade of experience. *Rev Infect Dis* 1990;12(5):760.

133. Banks J, et al. Pulmonary infection with *Mycobacterium kansasii* in Wales, 1970–9: review of treatment and response. *Thorax* 1983;38:271–274.

134. Corbett EL, et al. Nontuberculous mycobacteria. Defining disease in a prospective cohort of South African miners. *Am J Respir Crit Care Med* 1999;160:15–21.

135. Bloch KC, et al. Incidence and clinical implications of isolation of *Mycobacterium kansasii:* results of a 5-year, population-based study. *Ann Intern Med* 1998;129:698–704.

136. Evans SA, et al. Pulmonary *Mycobacterium kansasii* infection: comparison of the clinical features, treatment and outcome with pulmonary tuberculosis. *Thorax* 1996;51:1248–1252.

137. Levine B, Chaisson RE. *Mycobacterium kansasii:* a cause of treatable pulmonary disease associated with advanced human immunodeficiency virus (HIV) infection. *Ann Intern Med* 1991;114:861–868.

138. Corbett EL, et al. The impact of HIV infection on *Mycobacterium kansasii* disease in South African gold miners. *Am J Respir Crit Care Med* 1999;160:10–14.

139. Joynson DHM. Water: the natural habitat of *Mycobacterium kansasii? Tubercle* 1979;60:77–81.

140. Engel HWB, Berwald LG, Havelaar AH. The occurrence of *Mycobacterium kansasii* in tapwater. *Tubercle* 1980;61:21–26.

141. Onstad GD. Familial aggregations of group I atypical mycobacterial disease. *Am Rev Respir Dis* 1969;99:426–429.

142. Evans AJ, et al. Pulmonary *Mycobacterium kansasii* infection: comparison of radiological appearances with pulmonary tuberculosis. *Thorax* 1996;51:1243–1247.

143. Zvetina J, et al. Pulmonary cavitations in *Mycobacterium kansasii:* distinctions from *M. tuberculosis. AJR Am J Roentgenol* 1984;143:127.

144. Ahn CH, et al. Chemotherapy for pulmonary disease due to *Mycobacterium kansasii:* efficacies of some individual drugs. *Rev Infect Dis* 1981;3:1028–1034.

145. Ahn CH, et al. Short-course chemotherapy for pulmonary disease caused by *Mycobacterium kansasii. Am Rev Respir Dis* 1983;128:1048–1050.

146. British Thoracic Society. *Mycobacterium kansasii* pulmonary infection: a prospective study of the results of nine months of treatment with rifampicin ethambutol. *Thorax* 1994;49:442–445.

147. Ahn CH, et al. Sulfonamide-containing regimens for disease caused by rifampin-resistant *Mycobacterium kansasii. Am Rev Respir Dis* 1987;135:10–16.

148. Wallace RJ Jr, et al. Rifampin-resistant *Mycobacterium kansasii. Clin Infect Dis* 1994;18:736–743.

149. Smith MJ, Citron KM. Clinical review of pulmonary disease caused by *Mycobacterium xenopi. Thorax* 1983;38:373–377.

150. Banks, J, et al. Pulmonary infection with *Mycobacterium xenopi:* review of treatment and response. *Thorax* 1984;39:376–382.

151. Parrot RG, Grosset JH. Post-surgical outcome of 57 patients with *Mycobacterium xenopi* pulmonary infection. *Tubercle* 1988;69:47–55.

152. Astagneau P, et al. Mycobacterium xenopi spinal infections after discovertebral surgery: investigation and screening of a large outbreak. *Lancet* 2001;358:747–751.

153. Schröder KH, Juhlin I. *Mycobacterium malmoense* sp. nov. *Int J Syst Bacteriol* 1977;27:241–246.

154. Warren NG, et al. Pulmonary disease due to *Mycobacterium malmoense. J Clin Microbiol* 1984;20:245–247.

155. France AJ, et al. *Mycobacterium malmoense* infections in Scotland: an increasing problem. *Thorax* 1987;42:593–595.

156. Connolly MJ, Magee JG, Hendrick DJ. *Mycobacterium malmoense* in the northeast of England. *Tubercle* 1985;66:211–217.

157. Roberts C, Clague H, Jenkins PA. Pulmonary infection with *Mycobacterium malmoense:* a report of 4 cases. *Tubercle* 1985;66:205–209.

158. Jenkins PA. *Mycobacterium malmoense. Tubercle* 1985;66:193–194.

159. Henriques B, et al. Infection with *Mycobacterium malmoense* in Sweden: report of 221 cases. *Clin Infect Dis* 1994;18:596–600.

160. Hoffner SE, Hjelm U, Källenius G. Susceptibility of *Mycobacterium malmoense* to antibacterial drugs and drug combinations. *Antimicrob Agents Chemother* 1993;37(6):1285–1288.

161. Valero, et al. Clinical isolates of *Mycobacterium simiae* in San Antonio, Texas. *Am J Respir Crit Care Med* 1995;152:1555–1557.

162. Rynkiewicz DL, et al. Clinical and microbiological assessment of *Mycobacterium simiae* isolates from a single laboratory in southern Arizona. *Clin Infect Dis* 1998;26:625–630.

163. Marks J, Jenkins PA, Tsukamura M. *Mycobacterium szulgai.* A new pathogen. *Tubercle* 1972;53:210–214.

164. Schaefer WB, et al. *Mycobacterium szulgai:* a new pathogen: serologic identification and report of five new cases. *Am Rev Respir Dis* 1973;108:1320–1326.

165. Maloney JM, et al. Infections caused by *Mycobacterium szulgai* in humans. *Rev Infect Dis* 1987;9:1120–1126.

166. Tortoli E, et al. Pulmonary infection due to *Mycobacterium szulgai,* case report and review of the literature. *Eur Respir J* 1998;11:975–977.

167. Eckburg PB, et al. Clinical and chest radiographic findings among persons with sputum culture positive for *Mycobacterium gordonae.* A review of 19 cases. *Chest* 2000;117:96–102.

168. Blacklock ZM, et al. *Mycobacterium asiaticum* as a potential pulmonary pathogen for humans. A clinical and bacteriologic review of five cases. *Am Rev Respir Dis* 1983;127:241–244.

169. Mayall B, et al. Identification of *Mycobacterium shimoidei* by molecular techniques: case report and summary of the literature. *Int J Tuberc Lung Dis* 1999;3(2):169–173.

170. Smith DS, et al. *Mycobacterium terrae:* case reports, literature review, and *in vitro* antibiotic susceptibility testing. *Clin Infect Dis* 2000;30:444–453.

171. Hale YM, Pfyffer GE, Salfinger M. Laboratory diagnosis of mycobacterial infections: new tools and lessons learned. *Clin Infect Dis* 2001;33:834–846.

172. Griffith DE, Girard WM, Wallace RJ Jr. Clinical features of pulmonary disease

caused by rapidly growing mycobacteria. An analysis of 154 patients. *Am Rev Respir Dis* 1993;147:1271–1278.

173. Burke DS, Ullian RB. Megaesophagus and pneumonia associated with *Mycobacterium chelonei*. A case report and a literature review. *Am Rev Respir Dis* 1977;116:1101–1107.

174. Brown BA, Swenson JM, Wallace RJ Jr. Broth microdilution MIC test for rapidly growing mycobacteria. In: Isenberg HD, ed. *Clinical microbiology procedures handbook*. Washington, DC: American Society for Microbiology, 1994.

175. Woods GL, et al. Multisite reproducibility of Etest for susceptibility testing of *Mycobacterium abscessus, Mycobacterium chelonae,* and *Mycobacterium fortuitum*. *J Clin Microbiol* 2000;38(2):656–661.

176. Wallace RJ Jr, et al. Clinical trial of clarithromycin for cutaneous (disseminated) infection due to *Mycobacterium chelonae*. *Ann Intern Med* 1993;119:482–486.

177. Palella FJ, et al. Declining morbidity and mortality among patients with advanced human immunodeficiency virus infection. *N Engl J Med* 1998;338:853–860.

178. Dijkmans BAC, Mouton RP, Macfarlane JD. Bacterial arthritis caused by *Mycobacterium terrae*. *Infection* 1981;9:204–207.

179. LaFlamme MY, Poisson M, Chehade N. *Mycobacterium chelonei* keratitis following penetrating keratoplasty. *Can J Ophthalmol* 1987;22:178–180.

180. Clegg HW, et al. Infection due to organisms of the *Mycobacterium fortuitum* complex after augmentation mammaplasty: clinical and epidemiologic features. *J Infect Dis* 1983;147:427–433.

181. Lowry PW, et al. *Mycobacterium chelonae* causing otitis media in an ear-nose-and-throat practice. *N Engl J Med* 1988;319:978–982.

182. Safranek TJ, et al. *Mycobacterium chelonae* wound infections after plastic surgery employing contaminated gentian violet skin-marking solution. *N Engl J Med* 1987;317(4):197–201.

183. Centers for Disease Control and Prevention. Infection with *Mycobacterium abscessus* associated with intramuscular injection of adrenal cortex extract—Colorado and Wyoming, 1995–1996. *MMWR Morb Mortal Wkly Rep* 1996;45(33):713–715.

184. Centers for Disease Control and Prevention. Rapidly growing mycobacterial infection following liposuction and liposculpture—Caracas, Venezuela, 1996–1998. *MMWR Morb Mortal Wkly Rep* 1998;47(49):1065–1067.

185. Jongevos SF, Prens EP, Habets JMW. Successful triple-antibiotic therapy for cutaneous infection due to *Mycobacterium chelonae*. *Clin Infect Dis* 1999;28:145–146.

186. Trupiano JK, et al. Mastitis due to *Mycobacterium abscessus* after body piercing. *Clin Infect Dis* 2001;33:131–134.

187. Cutay AM, et al. Infection of epicardial pacemaker wires due to *Mycobacterium abscessus*. *Clin Infect Dis* 1998;26:520–521.

188. Woo PCY, et al. Acupuncture mycobacteriosis. *N Engl J Med* 2001;345(11):842–843.

189. Robisek F, et al. Rapidly growing nontuberculous mycobacteria: a new enemy of the cardiac surgeon. *Ann Thorac Surg* 1988;46:703.

190. Spell DW, et al. Native valve endocarditis due to *Mycobacterium fortuitum* biovar *fortuitum*: case report and review. *Clin Infect Dis* 2000;30:605–606.

191. Vail G, et al. Successful treatment of *Mycobacterium fortuitum* prosthetic valve endocarditis: case report. *Clin Infect Dis* 2000;30:629–630.

192. Maniu CV, et al. Failure of treatment for chronic *Mycobacterium abscessus* meningitis despite adequate clarithromycin levels in cerebrospinal fluid. *Clin Infect Dis* 2001;33:745–748.

193. Wallace RJ Jr, et al. Human disease due to *Mycobacterium smegmatis*. *J Infect Dis* 1988;158:52.

194. Phillips MS, von Reyn CF. Nosocomial infections due to nontuberculous mycobacteria. *Clin Infect Dis* 2001;33:1363–1374.

195. Breathnach A, et al. Cutaneous *Mycobacterium kansasii* infection: case report and review. *Clin Infect Dis* 1995;20:812–817.

196. Jõe L, Hall R. *Mycobacterium marinum* disease in Anne Arundel County: 1995 update. *Md Med J* 1995;24(12):1043–1046.

197. Edelstein H. *Mycobacterium marinum* skin infections. Report of 31 cases and review of the literature. *Arch Intern Med* 1994;154:1359–1364.

198. Jernigan JA, Farr BM. Incubation period and sources of exposure for cutaneous *Mycobacterium marinum* infection: case report and review of the literature. *Clin Infect Dis* 2000;31:439–443.

199. Judson FN, Feldman RA. Mycobacterial skin tests in humans 12 years after infection with *M. marinum*. *Am Rev Respir Dis* 1974;109:544–547.

200. MacCallum P, et al. A new mycobacterial infection in man. *J Pathol Bacteriol* 1948;60:93–122.

201. Clancey JK. Mycobacterial skin ulcers in Uganda: description of a new mycobacterium (*Mycobacterium buruli*). *J Pathol Bacteriol* 1964;88:174–187.

202. van der Werf TS, et al. *Mycobacterium ulcerans* infection. *Lancet* 1999;354:1013–1018.

203. Marston BJ, et al. Emergence of Buruli ulcer disease in the Daloa region of Cote d'Ivoire. *Am J Trop Med Hyg* 1995;52:219–224.

204. Johnson PDR, et al. The emergence of *Mycobacterium ulcerans* infection near Melbourne. *Med J Aust* 1996;164:76–78.

205. Yamousoukro. *World Health Organization targets untreatable ulcer: report from the first international conference on Buruli ulcer control and research*. Yamousoukro (Cote d'Ivoire): Inter Press Service, 1998.

206. Horsburgh CR Jr, Meyers WM. Buruli ulcer. In: Horsburgh CR Jr, Nelson AM, eds. Pathology of emerging infections. Washington: American Society for Microbiology Press, 1997:119–126.

207. Igo JD, Murthy DP. *Mycobacterium ulcerans* infection in Papua New Guinea. *Papua New Guinea Med J* 1988;17:150–156.

208. Dawson JF, Allen GE. Ulcer due to *Mycobacterium ulcerans* in Northern Ireland. *Clin Exp Dermatol* 1985;10:572–576.

209. Kozin SH, Bishop AT. Atypical mycobacterial infections of the upper extremity. *J Hand Surg* 1994;19:480–487.

210. Hayman J. Clinical features of *Mycobacterium ulcerans* infection. *Aust J Dermatol* 1985;26:67–73.

211. Dobos KM, et al. Emergence of a unique group of necrotizing mycobacterial diseases. *Emerg Infect Dis* 1999;5(3):367–378.

212. Gomez A, et al. Biochemical and genetic evidence for phospholipase C activity in *Mycobacterium ulcerans*. *Infect Immun* 2000;68(5):2995–2997.

213. George KM, et al. Partial purification and characterization of biological effects of a lipid toxin produced by *Mycobacterium ulcerans*. *Infect Immun* 1998;66(2):587–593.

214. George KM, et al. Mycolactone: a polyketide toxin from *Mycobacterium ulcerans* required for virulence. *Science* 1999;283:854–857.

215. Pimsler M, Sponsler TA, Meyers WM. Immunosuppressive properties of the soluble toxin from *Mycobacterium ulcerans*. *J Infect Dis* 1988;157(3):577–580.

216. Meyers WM, Shelly WM, Connor DH. Heat treatment of *Mycobacterium ulcerans* infections without surgical excision. *Am J Trop Med Hyg* 1974;23:924–929.

217. Portaels F, et al. *In vitro* susceptibility of *Mycobacterium ulcerans* to clarithromycin. *Antimicrob Agents Chemother* 1998;42(8):2070–2073.

218. Uganda Buruli Group. BCG vaccination against *Mycobacterium ulcerans* infection (Buruli ulcer). *Lancet* 1969;1:111–115.

219. Smith PG, et al. The protective effect of BCG against *Mycobacterium ulcerans* disease: a controlled trial in an endemic area of Uganda. *Trans R Soc Trop Med Hyg* 1977;70:449–457.

220. Petrini B, et al. Tenosynovitis of the hand caused by *Mycobacterium terrae*. *Eur J Clin Microbiol Infect Dis* 1989;8:722.

221. Jones MW, Wahid IA, Matthews JP. Septic arthritis of the hand due to *Mycobacterium marinum*. *J Hand Surg* 1988;13:333–334.

222. Wallace RJ Jr. The clinical presentation, diagnosis, and therapy of cutaneous and pulmonary infections due to the rapidly growing mycobacteria, *M. fortuitum* and *M. chelonae*. *Clin Chest Med* 1989;10:419.

223. Chan ED, et al. Vertebral osteomyelitis due to infection with nontuberculous *Mycobacterium* species after blunt trauma to the back: 3 examples of the principle of Locus Minoris Resistentiae. *Clin Infect Dis* 2001;32:1506–1510.

224. Lai KK, et al. Mycobacterial cervical lymphadenopathy. Relationship of etiologic agents to age. *JAMA* 1984;251:1286–1288.

225. Schaad UB, et al. Management of atypical mycobacterial lymphadenitis in childhood: a review based on 380 cases. *J Pediatr* 1979;95:356.

226. Wolinsky E. Mycobacterial lymphadenitis in children: a prospective study of 105 nontuberculous cases with long-term follow-up. *Clin Infect Dis* 1995;20:954–963.

227. Hazra R, et al. Related strains of *Mycobacterium avium* cause disease in children with AIDS and in children with lymphadenitis. *J Infect Dis* 2000;181:1298–1303.

228. Trébucq, A Should ethambutol be recommended for routine treatment of tuberculosis in children? A review of the literature. *Int J Tuberc Lung Dis* 1997;1(1):12–15.

229. Holland SN, et al. Treatment of refractory disseminated nontuberculous mycobacterial infection with interferon gamma. *N Engl J Med* 1994;330:1348–1355.

230. Levin M, et al. Familial disseminated atypical mycobacterial infection in childhood: a human mycobacterial susceptibility gene? *Lancet* 1995;345:79–83.

231. Jouanguy E, et al. Interferon-γ-receptor deficiency in an infant with fatal bacille Calmette-Guérin infection. *N Engl J Med* 1996;335(26):1956–1961.

232. Newport MJ, et al. A mutation in the interferon-g-receptor gene and susceptibility to mycobacterial infection. *N Engl J Med* 1996;335:1941–1949.

233. Pierre-Audigier C, et al. Fatal disseminated *Mycobacterium smegmatis* infection in a child with inherited interferon γ receptor deficiency. *Clin Infect Dis* 1997;24:982–984.

234. Holland SM, et al. Abnormal regulation of interferon-γ, interleukin-12, and tumor necrosis factor-α in human interferon-γ receptor 1 deficiency. *J Infect Dis* 1998;178:1095–1104.

235. Jouanguy E, et al. A human IFNGR1 small deletion hotspot associated with dominant susceptibility to mycobacterial infection. *Nat Genet* 1999;21:370.

236. Jouanguy E, et al. In a novel form of IFN-γ receptor 1 deficiency, cell surface receptors fail to bind IFN-γ. *J Clin Invest* 2000;105:1429–1436.

237. Chetchotisakd P, et al. Disseminated infection due to rapidly growing mycobacteria in immunocompetent hosts presenting with chronic lymphadenopathy: a previously unrecognized clinical entity. *Clin Infect Dis* 2000;30:29–34.

238. Engbaek HC. Three cases in the same family of fatal infection with *M. avium*. *Acta Tuberc Scand* 1964;45:105–117.

239. Schonell ME, et al. Disseminated infection with *Mycobacterium avium*, I: clinical features, treatment and pathology. *Tubercle* 1968;49:12–30.

240. Lincoln EM, Gilbert LA. Disease in children due to mycobacteria other than *Mycobacterium tuberculosis*. *Am Rev Respir Dis* 1972;105:683–714.

241. Metcalf JF, et al. Mycobacterium fortuitum pulmonary infection associated with an antigen-selective defect in cellular immunity. *Am J Med* 1981;71:485–492.

242. Gardner JD, et al. Mycobacterium fortuitum infection: evidence of bactericidal defect due to hyperactive antigen-specific suppressor cells. Correction *in vitro* and *in vivo* by cholinergic agonist and indomethacin. *Am J Med* 1982;73:756–764.

243. Ridgway D, et al. Indomethacin-sensitive monocyte killing defect in a child with disseminated atypical mycobacterial disease. *J Clin Immunol* 1991;11(6):357.

244. Villella A, et al. Recurrent *Mycobacterium avium* osteomyelitis associated with a novel dominant interferon gamma receptor mutation. *Pediatrics* 2001;107(4).
245. Dupuis S, et al. Impairment of mycobacterial but not viral immunity by a germline human STAT1 mutation. *Science* 2001;293:300–303.
246. Buckley RH. Primary immunodeficiency diseases due to defects in lymphocytes. *N Engl J Med* 2000;343:1313–1324.
247. Lekstrom-Hines JA, Gallin JI. Immunodeficiency diseases caused by defects in phagocytes. *N Engl J Med* 2000;343:1703–1714.
248. Winkelstein JA, et al. Chronic granulomatous disease. Report on a national registry of 368 patients. *Medicine* 2000;79:155–169.
249. Griffith DE. The challenge and opportunity of new clinical infectious entities. *Clin Infect Dis* 2001;32:432–435.
250. Ingram CW, et al. Disseminated infection with rapidly growing mycobacteria. *Clin Infect Dis* 1993;16:463–471.
251. Patel R, et al. Infections due to nontuberculous mycobacteria in kidney, heart, and liver transplant recipients. *Clin Infect Dis* 1994;19:263–273.
252. Mackowiak PA, et al. Infections in hairy cell leukemia. Clinical evidence of a pronounced defect in cell-mediated immunity. *Am J Med* 1980;68:718–724.
253. Weinstein RA, et al. Hairy cell leukemia: association with disseminated atypical mycobacterial infection. *Cancer* 1981;48:380–383.
254. Lembersky BC, Golomb HM. Hairy cell leukemia: clinical features and therapeutic advances. *Cancer Metastasis Rev* 1987;6:283–300.
255. Maziarz RT, et al. Reversal of infection with *Mycobacterium avium* intracellulare by treatment with alpha-interferon in a patient with hairy cell leukemia. *Ann Intern Med* 1988;109:292–294.
256. Horsburgh CR Jr, Selik RM. The epidemiology of disseminated nontuberculous mycobacterial infection in the acquired immunodeficiency syndrome (AIDS). *Am Rev Respir Dis* 1989;139:4–7.
257. Nightingale SD, et al. Two controlled trials of rifabutin prophylaxis against *Mycobacterium avium* complex infection in AIDS. *N Engl J Med* 1993;329:828–833.
258. Horsburgh CR Jr, et al. Disseminated *Mycobacterium avium* complex disease among patients infected with human immunodeficiency virus, 1985–2000. *Clin Infect Dis* 2001;33:1938–1943.
259. Kalayjian RC, et al. Pulmonary disease due to infection by *Mycobacterium avium* complex in patients with AIDS. *Clin Infect Dis* 1995;20:1186–1194.
260. Ward TT, et al. Randomized, open-label trial of azithromycin plus ethambutol vs. clarithromycin plus ethambutol as therapy for *Mycobacterium avium* complex bacteremia in patients with human immunodeficiency virus infection. *Clin Infect Dis* 1998;27:1278–1285.
261. Heifets LB, Lindholm-Levy PJ, Comstock RD. Clarithromycin minimal inhibitory and bactericidal concentrations against *Mycobacterium avium*. *Am Rev Respir Dis* 1992;145:856–858.
262. Heifets LB, Lindholm-Levy PJ, Flory MA. Bactericidal activity *in vitro* of various rifamycins against *Mycobacterium avium* and *Mycobacterium tuberculosis*. *Am Rev Respir Dis* 1990;141:626–630.
263. Bermudez LE, et al. Effect of ethambutol on emergence of clarithromycin-resistant *Mycobacterium avium* complex in the beige mouse model. *J Infect Dis* 1996;174:1218–1222.
264. Wallace RJ Jr, et al. Reduced serum levels of clarithromycin in patients treated with multidrug regimens including rifampin or rifabutin for *Mycobacterium avium-Mycobacterium intracellulare* infection. *J Infect Dis* 1995;171:747–750.
265. Peloquin CA, Berning SE. Evaluation of the drug interaction between clarithromycin and rifampin. *J Infect Dis Pharmacother* 1996;2(2):19–31.
266. Berning SE, Iseman MD. Rifamycin-induced lupus syndrome. *Lancet* 1997;349:1521–1522.
267. Burman WJ, Jones BE. Treatment of HIV-related tuberculosis in the era of effective antiretroviral therapy. *Am J Respir Crit Care Med* 2001;164:7–12.
268. US Public Health Service/IDSA. Prevention of Opportunistic Infections Working Group, 1999. USPHS/IDSA guidelines for the prevention of opportunistic infections in persons infected with human immunodeficiency virus. *Clin Infect Dis* 2000;30:S29–S65.
269. Centers for Disease Control and Prevention. 1999 USPHS/IDSA guidelines for the prevention of opportunistic infections in persons infected with human immunodeficiency virus. *MMWR Morb Mortal Wkly Rep* 1999;48:1–59.
270. Wallace RJ Jr, et al. Initial clarithromycin monotherapy for *Mycobacterium avium-intracellulare* complex lung disease. *Am J Respir Crit Care Med* 1994;149:1335–1341.
271. Wallace RJ Jr, et al. Clarithromycin regimens for pulmonary *Mycobacterium avium* complex. *Am J Respir Crit Care Med* 1996;153:1766–1772.
272. Tanaka E, et al. Effect of clarithromycin regimen for *Mycobacterium avium* complex pulmonary disease. *Am J Respir Crit Care Med* 1999;160:866–872.
273. Griffith, DE, et al. Early results (at 6 months) with intermittent clarithromycin-inducing regimens for lung disease due to *Mycobacterium avium* complex. *Clin Infect Dis* 2000;30:288–292.
274. Griffith DE, et al. Azithromycin activity against *Mycobacterium avium* complex lung disease in patients who were not infected with human immunodeficiency virus. *Clin Infect Dis* 1996;23:983–989.
275. Griffith DE, et al. Initial (6-month) results of three-times-weekly azithromycin in treatment regimens for *Mycobacterium avium* complex lung disease in human immunodeficiency virus–negative patients. *J Infect Dis* 1998;178:121–126.
276. Wallace RJ Jr, et al. Activities of linezolid against rapidly growing mycobacteria. *Antimicrob Agents Chemother* 2001;45(3):764–767.
277. Brown-Elliott BA, et al. Successful treatment of disseminated *Mycobacterium chelonae* infection with linezolid. *Clin Infect Dis* 2001;33:1433–1434.

CHAPTER 158
Leprosy

Diana N. J. Lockwood and
Keith P. W. J. McAdam

Leprosy is a chronic granulomatous disease caused by *Mycobacterium leprae*. The principal manifestations of disease are anesthetic skin lesions and peripheral neuropathy with peripheral nerve thickening. The clinical form of the disease in any individual depends on the degree of cell-mediated immunity expressed by that individual toward *M. leprae*. High levels of cell-mediated immunity with elimination of leprosy bacilli produce the tuberculoid form of disease (TT), whereas absent cell-mediated immunity results in lepromatous leprosy (LL). The medical complications of leprosy are due to nerve damage, immunologic reactions, and bacillary infiltration. Nerve damage accompanying leprosy is a particularly serious complication because this will remain with the patient for the rest of his or her life and causes considerable morbidity. Currently available drug treatments are highly effective in clearing viable bacilli but do not prevent nerve damage. Leprosy has a long history as a deforming disease and patients with leprosy are often stigmatized and ostracized. Words such as *leper* should be avoided and naming the disease Hansen's disease may reduce stigmatization.

EPIDEMIOLOGY

About 4 million people have or are disabled by leprosy. The apparent decrease in registered patients from 12 million in 1988 to 0.82 million on treatment in 1999 hides an intriguing picture. Prevalence has decreased because of a combination of effective antibiotic therapy and a change in case definition. Incidence, however, remains stable at around 800,000 new cases annually, with high rates of childhood cases (1). Intensive leprosy elimination campaigns held in 1998 and 1999 detected large numbers of new cases. A week-long campaign in Nepal found 11,696 new cases, which doubled the national case load.

GEOGRAPHIC DISTRIBUTION

India dominates the global picture, with 70% of the world's leprosy cases; 86% of patients with leprosy reside in six countries (India, Brazil, Indonesia, Myanmar, Madagascar, and Nepal) (2). Leprosy has not always been a tropical disease; it was endemic in Norway until the early twentieth century. In North America, small foci of infection are still found in Texas and Louisiana. Nearly all new cases now seen in Europe and North America have acquired their infection abroad (3).

Leprosy is a chronic disease with a long incubation period. An average incubation time of 2 to 5 years has been calculated for tuberculoid cases and 8 to 12 years for lepromatous cases. American military people who developed leprosy after serving in the tropics presented up to 20 years after their presumed exposure (4).

Although leprosy is rarely a primary cause of death, patients have a standardized death rate at least twice that of the general population because of the indirect secondary effects of the disease (5). It is estimated that 1 million disability-adjusted life-years (DALYs) are lost globally each year because of leprosy, with 6.3 years of healthy life being lost per patient.

Age, sex, household contact, and bacille Calmette-Guérin (BCG) vaccination are important determinants of leprosy risk; leprosy incidence reaches a peak at ages 10 to 14 years (6), and an excess of male cases has regularly been found, although this may be because women are reluctant to see health workers because of skin lesions (7). Clustering of cases is well recognized, particularly in low endemic areas (8). Although poor nutritional status was thought to predispose to leprosy, no good evidence substantiates this. Improved socioeconomic conditions, extended schooling, and good housing reduce the risk of leprosy (9).There are weak human leukocyte antigen (HLA) associations with leprosy: HLA-DR2 and HLA-DR3 occur at a higher frequency in patients with TT than in patients with LL/borderline lepromatous (BL) in at least two populations (10), whereas HLA-DQ1 is associated with susceptibility to BL/LL leprosy in three countries (11). In South India, an association has been found between paucibacillary leprosy and a locus on chromosome 10p13 (12).

Studies from Malawi (13), Uganda (14), Mali, and South India (15) have not shown human immunodeficiency virus (HIV) infection to be a risk factor for leprosy. HIV/leprosy–co-infected patients have typical skin lesions and typical leprosy histology and granuloma formation even with low circulating CD4 counts (16).

Subclinical infection with *M. leprae* is probably common, but the development of established disease is rare. There is no reliable test for determining whether a person has encountered *M. leprae* and mounted a protective immune response. In contacts of patients with leprosy, there is often evidence of specific sensitization to *M. leprae* using markers of infection such as serum antibody levels, *in vitro* lymphocyte transformation tests, and skin-test responses to soluble *M. leprae* antigen (17). Contacts of an untreated elderly man with BL leprosy in a British residential home showed that 23 of 30 and 25 of 30 had positive Mitsuda skin-test and positive lymphocyte transformation test responses to *M. leprae* sonicate, but only two contacts had positive antibody [immunoglobulin M (IgM) persistent generalized lymphadenopathy (PGL)] responses (18). Self-healing often occurs in early monomacular tuberculoid cases (19). Leprosy is probably analogous to tuberculosis (TB) in which only 10% of infections manifest as clinical disease (20).

TRANSMISSION

Leprosy is an almost exclusively human disease, with human cases being the only important source and reservoir of infection. Leprosy occurs naturally in nine-banded armadillos in the southern United States and transmission to armadillo handlers has been reported, but this is a small unimportant source of infection (21,22). An untreated patient with LL may discharge up to 6.8×10^{10} acid-fast bacilli (AFB) in a single nose blow. The importance of the nasal discharge in excreting AFB into the environment was recognized in 1898 by Schaffer, who demonstrated that patients with leprosy shed large numbers of AFB while coughing and sneezing (23). In 1960 Shepard showed that the AFB in nasal washings from lepromatous patients were viable in mouse footpad inoculation and the growth pattern resembled that of *M. leprae* (24). Lepromatous granulomata and abundant macrophages containing AFB have been demonstrated in the larynx (25). In Indonesia and Ethiopia, *M. leprae* deoxyribonucleic acid (DNA) has been detected in nasal swabs in 5% of the population (26).

Infection probably also occurs through the nose. *M. leprae* is inhaled, multiplies on the inferior turbinates, and has a brief bacteremic phase before binding to Schwann cells and macrophages.

The turbinates are consistently involved in early lepromatous disease (27). Experimental transmission via the nasal mucosa in nude mice is improved if the mucosa is lightly abraded (28).

The skin is unimportant in leprosy transmission. Bacilli are not excreted by the skin and are rarely found in the epidermis. The only evidence of bacilli entering via the skin comes from case reports of direct inoculation. Leprosy has been transmitted to nude mice through pricks from infected cactus thorns (29). There is no evidence that biting arthropods transmit leprosy. It is surprising that in contrast to TB, there are few documented cases of leprosy occurring in both the medical and the nonmedical attendants of patients with leprosy.

PATHOLOGY

There are four important aspects to the pathogenesis of leprosy: the host immune response, the bacterial load, nerve damage, and immune-mediated reactions. Peripheral nerves and skin are the organs principally affected by leprosy. The most common sites of early infection with *M. leprae* are Schwann cells, subepidermal cells, and superficial perivascular skin macrophages. A mild lymphocytic infiltrate is seen in early lesions, which may resolve spontaneously when bacilli die. If the bacilli persist and multiply, an inflammatory reaction occurs with granuloma formation (30) (Fig. 158.1). Once an infection is established, the host immune response determines not only the histologic picture but also the clinical features of disease and the prognosis. The concept of a spectrum of responses to *M. leprae* was developed by Ridley and Jopling in 1966 (31).The two poles of the spectrum are TT (paucibacillary) and LL (multibacillary). At the tuberculoid pole, well-expressed cell-mediated immunity and delayed hypersensitivity control bacillary multiplication with the formation of epithelioid cell granulomata; in the lepromatous form, there is cellular anergy toward *M. leprae* with abundant bacillary multiplication and inactivated macrophages. Between these two poles is a continuum, varying from the patient with moderate cell-mediated immunity [borderline tuberculoid (BT)] through borderline (BB) to the patient with little cellular response, BL. Figure 158.1 shows the possible routes in the evolution of infection in an untreated person. The polar groups (TT, LL) are stable but within the central groups (BT, BB, BL) downgrading toward the lepromatous pole will occur without treatment and upgrading (reversal reactions) toward the tuberculoid pole may occur before, during, or after treatment. Table 158.1 lists the histologic features seen in biopsies across the spectrum. Figures 158.2 through 158.5 show typical skin biopsies from patients at various points on the spectrum.

NEUROPATHOLOGY

Nerve damage occurs in small dermal nerves in skin lesions and peripheral nerve trunks. In early leprosy, nerve conduction studies are abnormal in tuberculoid (32) and lepromatous patients with a histologic picture of small fiber loss with segmental demyelination and remyelination (33,34). In established tuberculoid disease, there is gross destruction with a heavy lymphocytic infiltrate producing a fibrosed epineurium and replacement of the endoneurium with epithelioid granulomata (35). In lepromatous neuropathy, there is quiet asymptomatic bacillation of Schwann cells with late foamy degeneration. Demyelination, damage, and destruction of the axis cylinder are prominent features, and later wallerian degeneration occurs (36). Despite heavy bacillation, there is only a small inflammatory response,

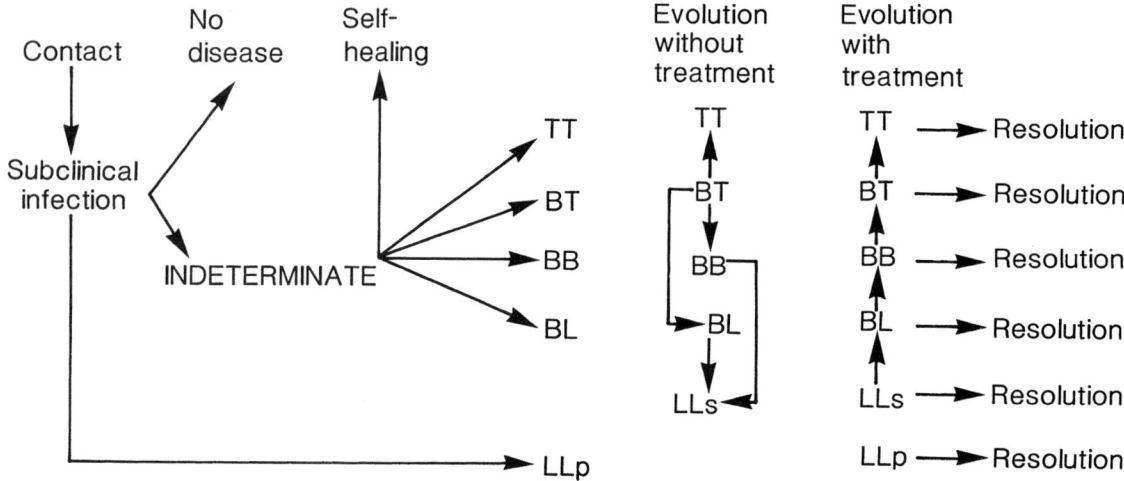

Figure 158.1. The evolution of leprosy infection in untreated patients and after treatment. (From Ridley DS, ed. *Pathogenesis of leprosy and related diseases.* London: Wright, 1988, with permission.)

later the nerve fibroses and is hyalinized (37,38). The formation of small granulomata is characteristic of BL, and granulomatous regions may abut strands of normal-looking but heavily bacillated Schwann cells (39). The combination of lepromatous bacillation and a tuberculoid tissue damaging response produces widespread nerve damage in BL. Acute neuritis occurs particularly during reversal reactions, and edema of the epithelioid cell granuloma compresses the remaining Schwann cells, causing rapid functional loss in an already compromised nerve. The damage may be compounded by new granuloma formation.

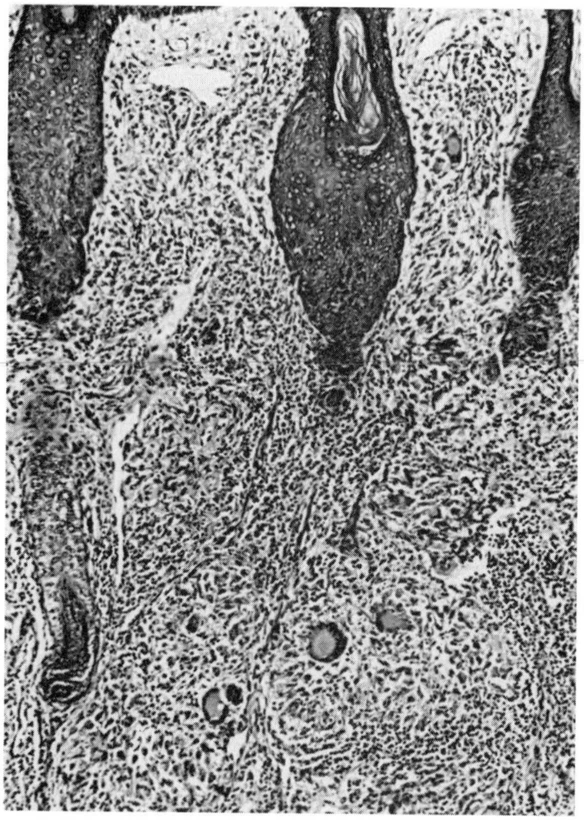

IMMUNOLOGY

Both T cells and macrophages play important roles in the processing, recognition, and response to *M. leprae* antigens. The T-cell response to mycobacteria is initiated with the presentation of processed *M. leprae* antigens in association with HLA class II molecules on the macrophage cell surface to the cellular immune system. The HLA *M. leprae* antigen complex is then recognized by CD4 lymphocytes bearing the α/β T-cell receptor. Binding of the antigen-specific T-cell receptor to the *M. leprae* peptide/HLA class II complex leads to activation and proliferation of α/β T cells with release of interleukin-2 (IL-2). This cytokine amplifies the local response, producing recruitment and activation of T cells. In addition, IL-2 stimulates the expansion of α/β CD8 T cells and antigen nonspecific natural killer cells in the lesion. All three types of cell can produce interferon-γ (IFN-γ), the major cytokine responsible for activating bactericidal mechanisms within the parasitized macrophage (40).

This model of the *M. leprae*–T-cell interaction has as its end point establishment of protective immunity to *M. leprae* with the elimination of *M. leprae* and the establishment of immunologic memory at a T-cell level. In those who develop clinical leprosy, this series of immunologic events is in some way impaired. In tuberculoid leprosy, there is good evidence of a strong cell-mediated immune response. Tests of T-cell function such as lymphocyte transformation tests show that patients with tuberculoid leprosy recognize and respond to *M. leprae* antigens with whole *M. leprae*, separated *M. leprae* antigens (41), and cloned antigens such as the 18 kd (42) and the 65 kd (45). Skin tests with Lepromin, a soluble *M. leprae* sonicate preparation, are strongly positive in these patients. Staining of skin biopsies from tuberculoid lesions with T-cell markers show highly organized granulomata composed predominantly of CD4 cells and macrophages with a peripheral mantle of suppressor/cytotoxic CD8 cells (44).

Patients with LL have no cell-mediated immune responses to *M. leprae*. Lymphocytes from patients with LL respond poorly or not at all in LTT to whole *M. leprae* and cloned antigens. Patients with LL are anergic on Lepromin skin testing. This anergy

Figure 158.2. Skin biopsy: tuberculoid (TT) leprosy. There is a heavy dermal infiltrate with numerous granulomata in the deep dermis. No Bacilli are visible (hematoxylin-eosin stain ×100). (Courtesy Professor Sebastian Lucas.)

TABLE 158.1.   Major Histologic and Immunologic Features of the Disease Spectrum in Leprosy

Characteristics	TT	BT	BB	BL	LL
Histologic and microbial					
Epithelioid cells, mature	++	±	−	−	−
Epithelioid cells, immature	+	++	++	±/−	−
Langhans giant cells, large	++	±/−	−	−	−
Macrophages	−	−	±	++	++
Lymphocytes	+/±	++/±	±	++	±
Bacterial index	0	0–2	3–4	4–5	5–6+
Bacilli in nasal smears	−	−	−	±	++
Immunologic					
Lepromin, Fernandez reaction	++/−	++/−	+/−	−	−
Lepromin, Mitsuda reaction	++/±	++/+	−	−	−
LTT, percent lymphocyte transformation	10	5.7	2.0	0.4	0.2
Antibody, anti–*M. leprae*	−/+	−/++	++	+++	+++

TT, Tuberculoid leprosy; BT, borderline tuberculoid leprosy; BB, borderline leprosy; BL, borderline lepromatous leprosy; LL, lepromatous leprosy; LTT, lymphocyte transformation test; +++, strongly positive; +, positive; ±, indeterminate; −, negative.

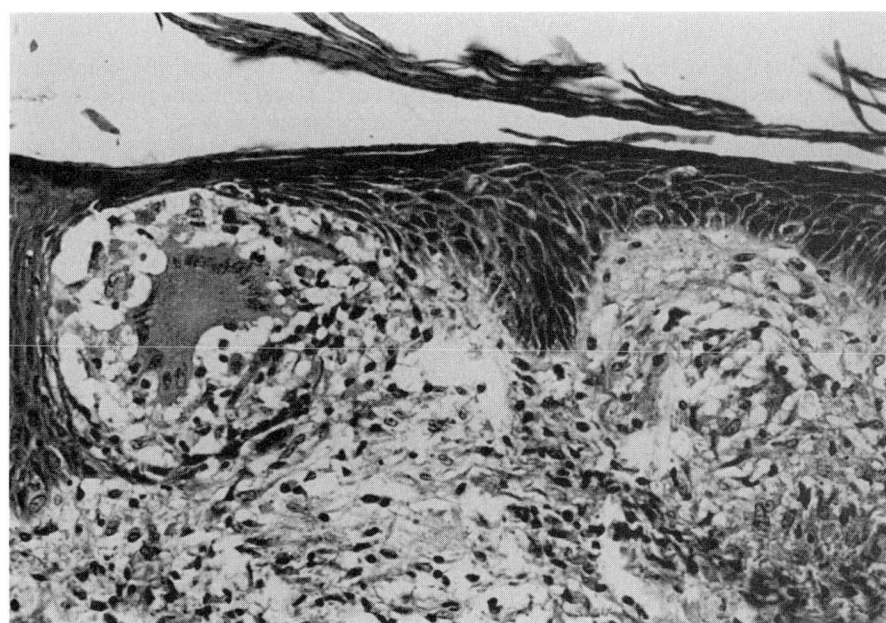

Figure 158.3. Skin biopsy: borderline tuberculoid (BT) leprosy in reversal reaction. New active, edematous granulomata are visible and are eroding the epidermal and subepidermal zones (hematoxylin-eosin stain ×400). (Courtesy Professor Sebastian Lucas.)

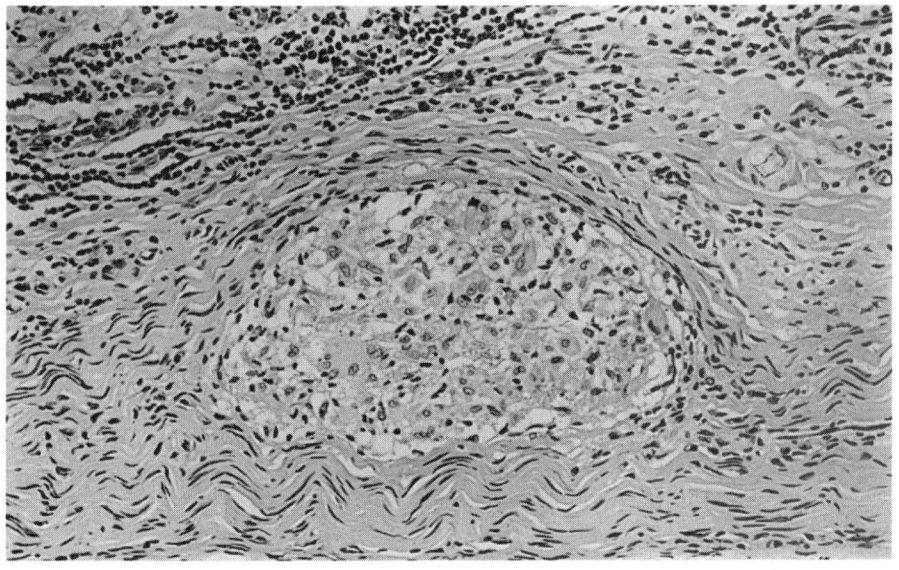

Figure 158.4. Nerve biopsy: borderline tuberculoid (BT) leprosy. This large granuloma in a peripheral nerve is distorting the normal neural architecture, a perineural lymphocytic infiltrate is also present (hematoxylin-eosin ×600). (Courtesy Professor Sebastian Lucas.)

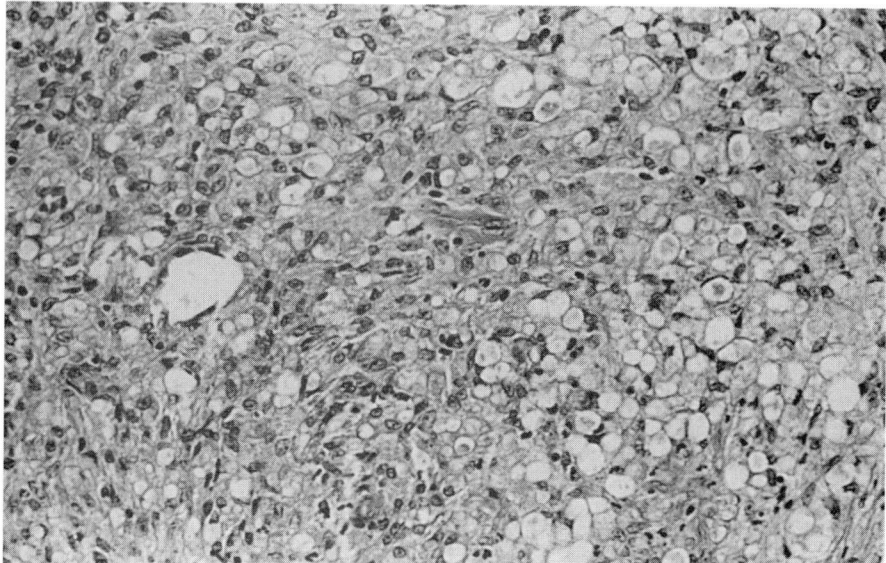

Figure 158.5. Skin biopsy: lepromatous (LL) leprosy. Numerous rounded foamy macrophages with few lymphocytes and no granulomata (hematoxylin-eosin stain ×400). (Courtesy Professor Sebastian Lucas.)

of the lepromatous patient is striking because it is specific for the leprosy mycobacterium, and patients with LL can respond to other mycobacterial antigens such as *M. tuberculosis,* both in *in vitro* lymphocyte studies and in skin tests using other mycobacterial antigens (45). Identification of cell types in LL granulomata shows them to be disorganized with a random admixture of macrophages and T cells; in the latter group CD8 cells predominate (46).

Both T-cell and macrophage dysfunction occurs in lepromatous patients. Because lepromatous patients may convert from being Lepromin skin-test negative to Lepromin positive after prolonged antileprosy drug therapy (47), it seems likely that either clonal anergy or active suppression by *M. leprae* antigens cause the T-cell defect in LL.

Defects in cytokine production have been demonstrated in lepromatous patients; addition of IL-2 to T-cell culture media restored the proliferative response to *M. leprae* (48), and giving

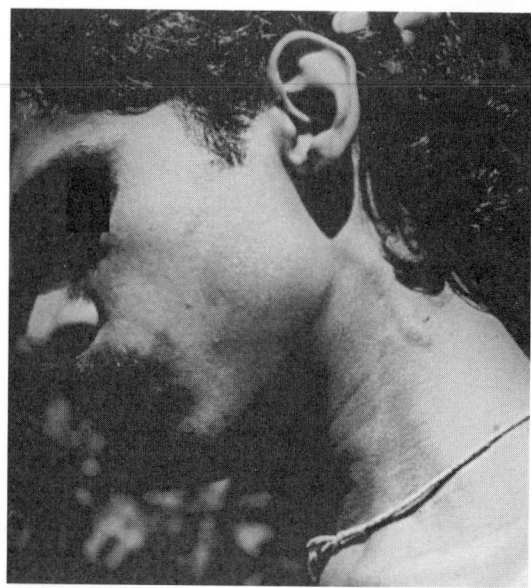

Figure 158.6. Visible thickening of the great auricular nerve.

lepromatous patients intralesional injections of recombinant IL-2 leads to a reconstitution of the local immune response with elimination of *M. leprae* from macrophages (49).

Several macrophage defects have been described in LL disease, including defective antigen presentation and recognition, defective IL-1 production, a failure of macrophages to kill *M. leprae,* and a macrophage suppression of the T-cell response (50) (Fig. 158.6).

Studies of circulating cytokines in patients with leprosy and cytokine production in skin lesions show that tuberculoid patients have a T_H1-type response to *M. leprae* with predominant IL-2 and IFN-γ production, whereas lepromatous patients have a response characterized by T_H2-type cytokines.

Lepromin skin testing assesses *in vivo* responses to a heat-killed suspension of *M. leprae.* This test can be read at 48 to 72 hours (the Fernandez reaction) and again at 21 to 28 days (the Mitsuda reaction). Both tests reflect the patient's cellular response to *M. leprae,* with the Fernandez response being a delayed hypersensitivity reaction to the soluble components of Lepromin and the Mitsuda reaction being a granulomatous response to mycobacterial antigens. Both tests are positive in tuberculoid and negative in lepromatous patients. Neither test is diagnostic because both may be positive in people with no evidence of leprosy.

SEROLOGY

Antibody responses correlate with the number of bacilli present, with the highest antibody levels in patients with LL and the lowest in patients with TT (51). All patients with leprosy mount appropriate antibody responses to bacterial vaccines such as typhoid. Lepromatous patients produce a range of autoantibodies both organ specific (directed against thyroid, nerve, testis, and gastric mucosa) and nonspecific such as rheumatoid factors, anti-DNA, cryoglobulins, and cardiolipin. None of these antibodies plays a role in the elimination of *M. leprae.*

Specific anti–*M. leprae* antibodies are produced against LAM, PGL, and the protein antigens of *M. leprae.* Unfortunately, none of these have been suitable for developing specific serological tests for confirming disease and detecting early subclinical infection (see Chapter 266).

REACTIONS

Leprosy reactions are superimposed on the Ridley-Jopling spectrum. Borderline (BT, BB, BL) patients are immunologically unstable and are at risk of reversal (type 1) reactions. These are delayed hypersensitivity reactions against *M. leprae* antigens in skin and nerve. They are characterized by enhanced T-cell proliferation toward *M. leprae* antigens, increased numbers of CD4[+] cells in granulomata and local production of cytokines such as IFN-γ, IL-12, inducible nitric oxide synthase (iNOS), and tumor necrosis factor-α (TNF-α) (52). Reversal reactions are associated with an overproduction of T_H1 cytokines. Although the end result is an elimination of mycobacteria, this is achieved only at the expense of severe local tissue damage particularly in nerves.

Type 2 reactions, erythema nodosum leprosum (ENL), are partly due to immune complex deposition and occur in patients with BL or LL who produce antibodies and have a large antigen load. Local vasculitis is present with lesional immunoglobulin, complement, and polymorphs and circulating immune complexes (54). There is also enhanced T-cell activity, with increased CD8 cells, increased circulating IL-2 receptors and high levels of circulating TNF-α (55,56). Lepromatous patients revert to a state of immunologic unresponsiveness after an episode.

CLINICAL FEATURES

Patients commonly present with skin lesions, weakness, or numbness because of a peripheral nerve lesion or a burn or an ulcer in an anesthetic hand or foot. Borderline patients may present in reaction with nerve pain, sudden palsy, multiple new skin lesions, pain in the eye, or a systemic febrile illness.

Cardinal Signs

- Typical skin lesions, anesthetic at the tuberculoid end of the spectrum
- Thickened peripheral nerves
- AFB on skin smears or biopsy

Presenting Symptoms

EARLY LESIONS
Indeterminate lesions are slightly hypopigmented or erythematous macules, a few centimeters in diameter, with poorly defined margins. Hair growth and nerve function are unimpaired.

A biopsy may show the perineurovascular infiltrate and only scant AFB. The indeterminate phase may last for months or years before resolving or developing into one of the determinate types of leprosy

Skin. The most common skin lesions are macules or plaques; more rarely papules and nodules are seen. In lepromatous leprosy, a diffuse infiltration of the skin often occurs. Tuberculoid patients have few hypopigmented lesions, and lepromatous patients have numerous sometimes confluent lesions. The few tuberculoid lesions are usually asymmetric, and more numerous lesions are likely to be distributed symmetrically.

Anesthesia. Anesthesia may occur in skin lesions when dermal nerves are involved or in the distribution of a large peripheral nerve. In skin lesions, the small dermal sensory and autonomic nerve fibers supplying dermal and subcutaneous structures are damaged, causing local sensory loss and loss of sweating within that area.

Peripheral Neuropathy

Peripheral nerve trunks are vulnerable at sites where they are superficial or are in fibroosseous tunnels. At these points, a small increase in nerve diameter leads to raised intraneural pressure with consequent neural compression and ischemia. Damage to peripheral nerve trunks produces characteristic signs with dermatomal sensory loss and dysfunction of muscles supplied by that peripheral nerve. The sites for predilection for peripheral nerve involvement are ulnar (at the elbow), median (at the wrist), radial, radial cutaneous (at the wrist), common peroneal (at the knee), posterior tibial and sural nerves at the ankle, facial nerve as it crosses the zygomatic arch, and great auricular in the posterior triangle of the neck (see Fig. 158.6).

CLASSIFICATION OF DISEASE

Classifying patients according to the Ridley-Jopling scale is clinically useful. Borderline tuberculoid leprosy may be associated with rapid severe nerve damage, whereas lepromatous disease is associated with chronicity and long-term complications. Borderline disease is unstable and may be complicated by reactions. There is also a simpler field classification of paucibacillary/multibacillary (Table 158.2), which guides the length of treatment.

TABLE 158.2. Modified World Health Organization–Recommended Multidrug Therapy Regimens

Type of leprosy	Drug treatment		Duration of treatment
	Monthly supervised	Daily self-administered	
Paucibacillary	Rifampicin, 600 mg	Dapsone, 100 mg	6 mo
Multibacillary	Rifampicin, 600 mg	Clofazimine, 50 mg	24 mo
	Clofazimine, 300 mg	Dapsone, 100 mg	
Paucibacillary single lesion	Rifampin-ofloxacin-minocycline (600, 400, and 100 mg, respectively)		Single dose

World Health Organization classification for field use when slit-skin smears are not available:

- Paucibacillary single lesion-leprosy (one skin lesion)
- Paucibacillary (two to five skin lesions)
- Multibacillary (more than five skin lesions)

In this field classification, the World Health Organization recommends treatment of MB patients for 12 months only.

In the United States the National Hansen's Disease Program recommends rifampin 600 mg daily for all patients in the above regimens.

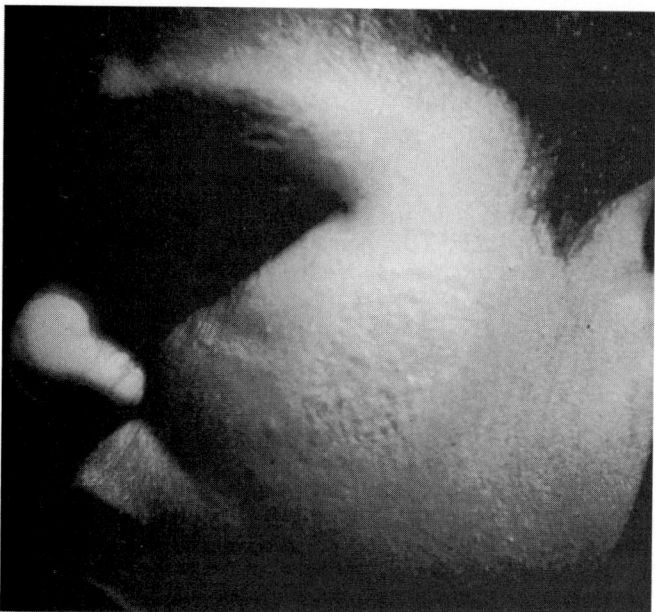

Figure 158.7. Tuberculoid (TT) skin lesion.

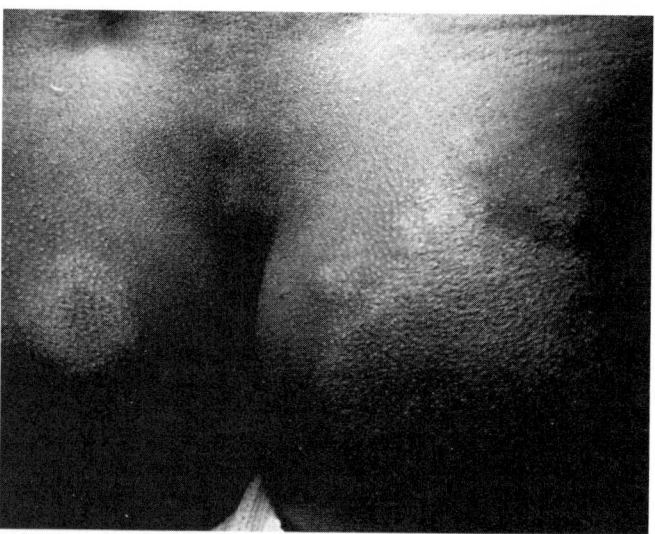

Figure 158.9. Borderline leprosy (BB) lesion.

Tuberculoid Leprosy

Infection is localized and asymmetric. The skin lesions are few and hypopigmented, and they have sharp borders (Fig. 158.7). Anesthesia and loss of sweating are found in the lesion. If peripheral nerve trunk involvement is present, usually only one nerve trunk is enlarged. No *M. leprae* are found in the skin, and the Lepromin test is strongly positive. True tuberculoid leprosy has a good prognosis, with many infections resolving without treatment, and peripheral nerve trunk damage is limited.

Borderline Tuberculoid

The skin lesions of BT are similar to those of TT leprosy but are larger and more numerous. The margins are less well defined and there may be satellite lesions (Fig. 158.8). Damage to

peripheral nerves may be widespread and severe, with several thickened nerve trunks. It is important to recognize BT leprosy because these patients are prone to reversal reactions, leading to rapid deterioration in nerve function and the risk of developing deformities.

Borderline Leprosy

BB disease is the most unstable part of the spectrum and patients usually downgrade toward LL if they are not treated or upgrade toward TT as part of a reversal reaction. There are numerous skin lesions that may be macules, papules, or plaques and vary in size, shape, and distribution. Annular lesions with a broad, irregular edge and a sharply defined punched out center are characteristic of BB disease (Fig. 158.9). Nerve damage is variable.

Borderline Lepromatous Leprosy

BL leprosy is characterized by widespread variable asymmetric skin lesions (Fig. 158.10). There may be erythematous or

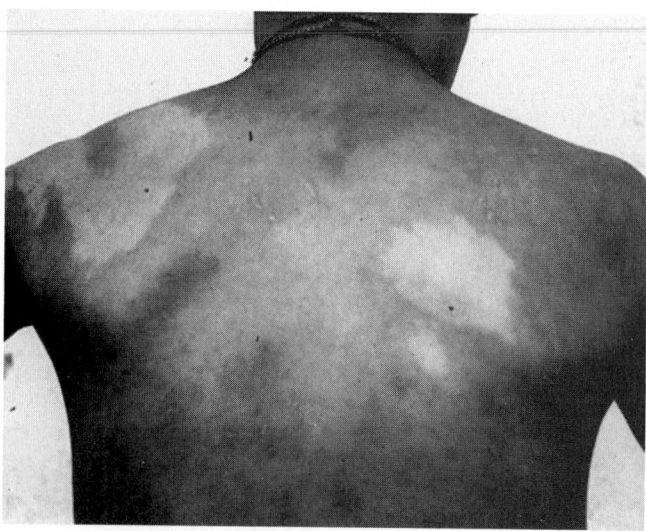

Figure 158.8. Borderline tuberculoid (BT) skin lesion.

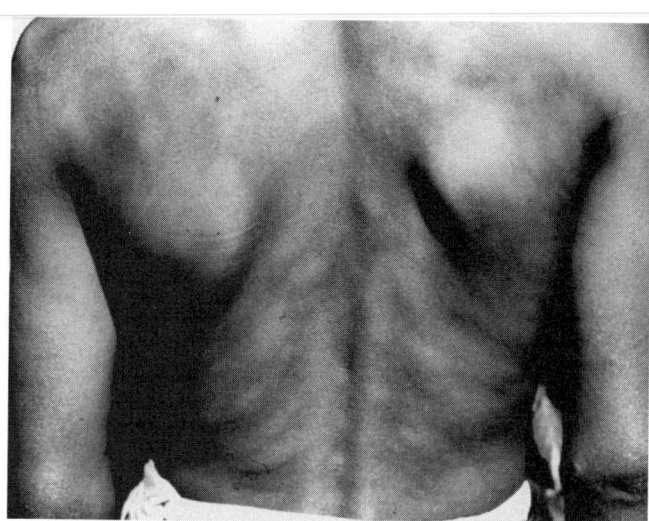

Figure 158.10. Borderline lepromatous (BL) leprosy.

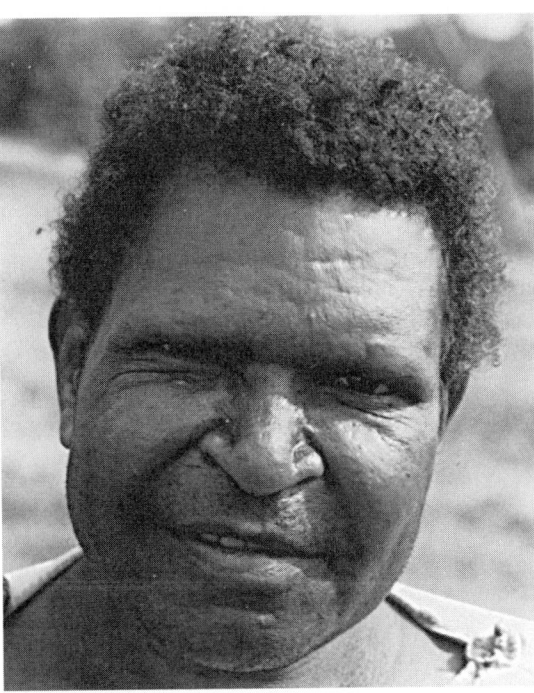

Figure 158.11. Moderately advanced lepromatous (LL) leprosy. There is symmetric infiltration of the face with particular involvement of the eyebrows, nose, and cheek creases. Eyebrow loss (madarosis is also present).

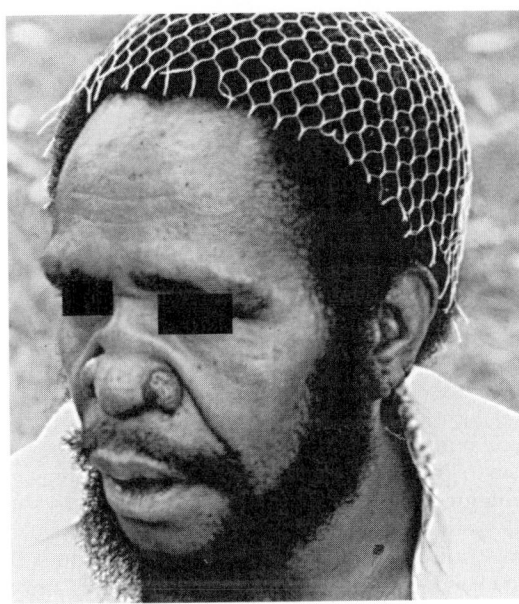

Figure 158.12. Advanced lepromatous leprosy with collapse of the nasal septum.

hyperpigmented papules, succulent nodules or plaques, and sensation in the lesions may be normal. Peripheral nerve involvement is widespread but not as symmetric as in LL disease. Both reversal and ENL reactions may complicate BL disease.

Lepromatous Leprosy

The patient with polar LL may be carrying 10^{11} leprosy bacilli. The onset of disease is often insidious, with the earliest lesions being ill-defined, shiny erythematous macules. Gradually the skin becomes infiltrated and thickened and nodules develop; facial skin thickening causes the characteristic leonine facies (Fig. 158.11). Hair is lost, especially the lateral third of the eyebrows (madarosis). Dermal nerves are destroyed and sensory loss (light touch, pain, and temperature) extends in a glove-and-stocking distribution. Sweating is lost, which can cause profound discomfort in a tropical climate because massive compensatory sweating occurs in the remaining intact areas. Damage to peripheral nerves is symmetric and occurs late in disease.

Nasal symptoms (stuffy nose, nosebleeds, loss of sense of smell) can often be elicited early in the disease, and 80% of newly diagnosed lepromatous cases have invasion of the nasal mucosa (27). Septal perforation may occur. The pathognomic collapse of the bridge of the nose is secondary to bacillary destruction of the bony nasal spine (Fig. 158.12). Bone involvement is common, with osteoporosis and fractures. Testicular atrophy results from diffuse infiltration and the acute orchitis that occurs with ENL reactions. The consequent loss of testosterone leads to azoospermia and gynecomastia.

The Eye in Leprosy

Blindness resulting from leprosy, which occurs in at least 2.5% of patients (57), is a devastating complication for a patient who probably already has sensory loss caused by anesthesia of the hands and feet. Eye damage results from both nerve damage and bacillary invasion. Lagophthalmos results from paresis of the orbicularis oculi because of involvement of the zygomatic and temporal branches of the facial (VII) nerve. These superficial branches are particularly at risk in borderline cases when facial skin lesions are present. In lepromatous disease, lagophthalmos occurs later and is usually bilateral. Damage to the ophthalmic branch of the trigeminal (V) nerve causes anesthesia of the cornea and conjunctiva, which results in drying of the cornea and a reduction in blinking and leaves the cornea at risk of minor trauma and ulceration. Lepromatous infiltration may occur in corneal nerves, producing punctate keratitis and corneal lepromas. Invasion of the iris and ciliary body makes them extremely susceptible to reactions.

Other Forms of Leprosy

There are three variant forms of leprosy: histoid, pure neuritic, and Lucio's leprosy. Histoid lesions are distinctive nodules occurring in lepromatous cases that have relapsed because of dapsone resistance or noncompliance with chemotherapy. Pure neuritic leprosy presents with asymmetric involvement of peripheral nerve trunks and no visible skin lesions. Lucio's leprosy is a form of LL found only in Latin Americans, with a uniform, diffuse, shiny skin infiltration (58).

DIAGNOSIS

Leprosy should be considered as a possible diagnosis in anyone with peripheral nerve or skin lesions who has lived in a leprosy-endemic area. The diagnosis is essentially a clinical one based on finding one or more of the cardinal signs of leprosy and supported by the finding of AFB on slit-skin smears. Histologic examination of a skin or nerve biopsy is essential for accurate classification. Serologic and polymerase chain reaction (PCR)–based diagnostic tests are not yet clinically useful (see Chapter 266).

TABLE 158.3. Bacterial Index	
Score	Bacilli per field
6+	Many clumps (1,000) in an average field
5+	100–1,000 bacilli in an average field
4+	10–100 bacilli in an average field
3+	1–10 bacilli in an average field
2+	1–10 bacilli in 10 fields
1+	1–10 bacilli in 100 fields

Skin examination: It is important to inspect the whole body in a good light so lesions are not missed, particularly on the buttocks in borderline disease. Skin lesions should be tested for anesthesia to light touch, pinprick, and temperature.

Neurologic examination: The peripheral nerves should be palpated systematically, looking for enlargement and tenderness. Nerve function should be assessed by testing the small muscles of the hands and feet. Sensation on the hands and feet can be assessed and monitored using Semmes-Weinstein monofilaments. These are now widely used in leprosy and diabetic clinics (59).

Slit-skin Smears: The AFB load of a patient is determined by modified Ziehl-Neelsen staining of slit-skin smears. Suspect lesions and sites commonly affected in LL should be sampled (forehead, earlobes, chin, extensor surface of the forearm, buttocks, and trunk).

The density of bacilli is scored using the logarithmic scale in Table 158.3. A mean score, the bacterial index (BI), is derived by adding the scores from each site and dividing by the number of sites sampled. In untreated LL, the BI is 5+ or 6+ and 0 in TT disease. Slit-skin smears detect bacilli present at a concentration of more than 10^4/g of tissue only and so cannot be used as a test of microbiologic cure. Slit-skin smears should be repeated annually to assess response to treatment.

Outside leprosy-endemic areas, doctors often fail to consider the diagnosis of leprosy. Of new patients seen from 1995 to 1999 at the Hospital for Tropical Diseases, London diagnosis had been delayed in more than 80% of cases (60). Patients had been misdiagnosed by dermatologists, neurologists, orthopedic surgeons, and rheumatologists. A common problem was failure to consider leprosy as a cause of peripheral neuropathy in patients from leprosy-endemic countries. These delays had serious consequences for patients, with more than half of them having nerve damage and disability.

DIFFERENTIAL DIAGNOSIS

Skin: The variety of leprosy skin lesions means that many skin conditions are in the differential diagnosis. In suspect tuberculoid lesions, the absence of lesional anesthesia is crucial in differentiating leprosy from fungal infections, vitiligo, and eczema. In lepromatous lesions, the presence of AFB in smears differentiates leprosy nodules from onchocerciasis, Kaposi's sarcoma, and post–kala azar dermal leishmaniasis.

Nerves: Peripheral nerve thickening is rarely seen except in leprosy. Hereditary sensory motor neuropathy type III is associated with palpable peripheral nerve hypertrophy. Amyloidosis, which can also complicate leprosy, causes thickening of peripheral nerves. Charcot-Marie-Tooth disease is an inherited neuropathy that causes distal atrophy and weakness. The causes of other polyneuropathies such as HIV, diabetes, alcoholism, vas-

culitides, and heavy-metal poisoning should all be considered when appropriate.

TREATMENT

The treatment of leprosy has six main components: chemotherapy, monitoring and treating nerve damage, management of reactions and neuritis, patient education, prevention of disability, and social and psychological support.

Chemotherapy

All patients with leprosy should be given an appropriate multidrug combination. In the hospital setting where skin smears and skin biopsies can be combined with clinical data, patients can be classified into paucibacillary (skin-smear negative tuberculoid and BT) and multibacillary (skin-smear–positive BT, all BB, BL, and LL). The first-line antileprosy drugs are rifampicin, clofazimine, and dapsone. Table 158.2 gives the drug combinations, doses, and duration of treatment. Multibacillary patients with an initial BI of more than 4 will need longer treatment and the duration should be guided by their clinical status and BI.

Rifampin

Rifampin is a potent bactericidal for *M. leprae.* Four days after a single 600-mg dose, bacilli from a previously untreated multibacillary patient are no longer viable in a mouse footpad test (61). It acts by inhibiting DNA-dependent ribonucleic acid (RNA) polymerase. Because *M. leprae* resistance to rifampin can develop, as a one-step process rifampin should always be given in combination with other antileprotics (62). There is no evidence that daily rifampin treatment is superior to monthly dosing, and the latter has fewer side effects.

Dapsone

Dapsone [4,4-diaminodiphenylsulfone (DDS)] acts by blocking folic acid synthesis. It is only weakly bactericidal. Oral absorption is good and it has a long half-life, averaging 28 hours. It commonly causes mild hemolysis but rarely anemia. Glucose-6-phosphate dehydrogenase deficiency is rarely a problem. The "DDS syndrome," rarely seen in leprosy, starts 6 weeks after commencing DDS and manifests as exfoliative dermatitis associated with lymphadenopathy, hepatosplenomegaly, fever, and hepatitis (63). Agranulocytosis, hepatitis, and cholestatic jaundice occur rarely with DDS therapy.

Clofazimine

Clofazimine has a weakly bactericidal action, the mechanism of which is unknown. It also has an antiinflammatory effect, which has reduced the incidence of ENL reactions. Skin discoloration is the most troublesome side effect, ranging from red to purple-black. The pigmentation usually fades slowly after stopping clofazimine. Clofazimine also produces a characteristic ichthyosis on the shins and forearms.

Ten million patients have been treated successfully with multidrug treatment. Clinical improvement has been rapid and toxicity rare. The treatment duration has been shortened. Monthly supervision of the rifampin component has been crucial to success. The three drugs used for multidrug treatment are donated by the drug manufacturers free of charge for distribution by the World Health Organization (WHO), the Nippon

Foundation, and the International Federation of Anti-Leprosy Associations. At the end of 6 months of treatment of borderline disease, there may still be signs of inflammation, which should not be mistaken for active infection. The distinction between relapse and reaction may be difficult. WHO studies have reported a cumulative relapse rate of 1.07% for paucibacillary leprosy and 0.77% for multibacillary leprosy at 9 years after completion of multidrug treatment (64). *M. leprae* is such a slow-growing organism that relapse occurs only after many years. However, patients with a high bacterial load may be at greater risk of relapse. Data from West Africa (65) and India show that patients with a high initial bacterial load (BI more than 4+) treated with 2 years of rifampicin, clofazimine, and dapsone had a relapse rate of 8 per 100 person-years, whereas patients treated to smear negativity had a relapse rate of 2 per 100 person-years (66,67). These patients may form a subgroup who need treating to skin-smear negativity. Susceptibility testing of *M. leprae* strains from relapsed multibacillary patients have shown them to remain drug sensitive.

Short-course chemotherapy regimens have been tested for paucibacillary leprosy using either rifampin in weekly doses or single-dose chemotherapy using a combination of currently used drugs. So far all of these regimens have had higher relapse rates than the current WHO paucibacillary regimen (68). The fluoroquinolones (pefloxacin and ofloxacin) and the macrolide minocycline are all highly active against *M. leprae*, but because of cost, these are rarely used in field programs. Multicenter trials of daily rifampin-ofloxacin are being conducted by the WHO and afford the possibility of considerably shortening the duration of multidrug treatment.

MONITORING AND TREATING NERVE DAMAGE

Nerve damage occurs before diagnosis and during and after multidrug treatment. It may occur during a reaction or without overt signs of nerve inflammation (silent neuropathy). In field cohort studies, 16% to 56% of newly diagnosed patients have nerve damage (69). In a Bangladeshi study, 25% of multibacillary patients developed nerve damage during treatment (70). Monitoring sensation and muscle power in patients' hands, feet, and eyes should be part of the routine follow-up so new nerve damage is detected early. Any new damage should be treated with a course of oral steroids starting with prednisolone at 40 mg and reducing by 5 mg per day each month. Response rates vary depending on the severity of initial damage but even promptly treated nerve damage will improve only in 60% cases (71).

MANAGEMENT OF REACTIONS AND NEURITIS

Reversal Reactions (Type 1)

These manifest clinically with erythema, edema of skin lesions (Fig. 158.13), and tender painful peripheral nerves. Loss of nerve function can be dramatic, with footdrop occurring overnight secondary to lateral popliteal nerve involvement (72). Nerve pain and tenderness is a prominent and distressing symptom, most commonly affecting the ulnar nerve (73) (Fig. 158.14). Severe reactions may be accompanied by fever, malaise, and anorexia. Awareness of the early symptoms of reversal reactions by both patient and physician is important because if left untreated, severe nerve damage may develop. The peak time for reversal reactions is in the first 2 months of treatment. Patients should be warned about reactions because the sudden appearance of

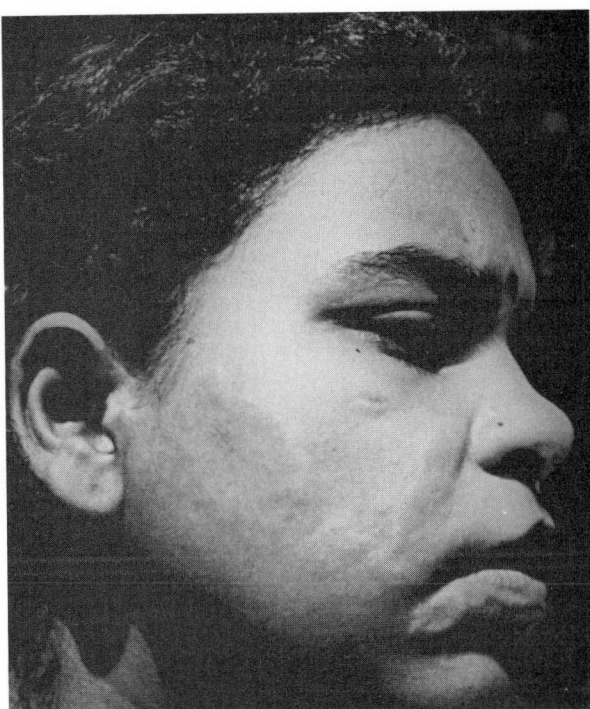

Figure 158.13. Reversal reaction lesions. This lady with BL leprosy suddenly developed erythema and edema of her previously quiescent facial lesions 6 weeks after delivery.

reactional lesions after starting treatment is distressing and undermines confidence. The treatment of reactions is aimed at controlling acute inflammation, easing pain, reversing nerve and eye damage, and reassuring the patient. Multidrug therapy should be continued.

Simple antiinflammatory drugs are rarely sufficient to control symptoms. If there is any evidence of neuritis (nerve tenderness, new anesthesia, and/or motor loss), corticosteroid treatment should be started: prednisolone, starting at 40 to 60 mg daily, reducing to 40 mg after a few days and then by 5 mg every 2 to 4 weeks (74). Patients with BT leprosy in reaction commonly need 2 to 4 months of steroid therapy, whereas BL reactions may need 6 months.

Erythema Nodosum Leprosum Type 2 Reactions

The complication ENL occurs in about 20% of LL and 10% of BL patients. Skin lesions are the most common, with crops of small pink nodules on the face and the extensor surfaces of the limbs (Fig. 158.15). New crops appear as old lesions subside, and a chronic painful panniculitis may develop. Iritis and episcleritis are common and should be treated promptly. The patient is usually unwell with malaise and fever. Other accompanying signs are acute lymphadenitis, orchitis, bone pain, dactylitis, arthritis, and proteinuria. Neuritis may occur but is less dramatic than that seen in reversal reactions. ENL usually starts during the second year of chemotherapy and despite treatment may continue on a relapsing and remitting course for several years.

This is a difficult condition to treat and often requires treatment with high-dose steroids (80 mg daily, tapered down rapidly) or thalidomide. Because ENL frequently recurs, steroid dependency can easily develop. Thalidomide (400 mg daily) is superior to steroids in controlling ENL and is the drug of choice for young men with severe ENL (75). Women with severe ENL

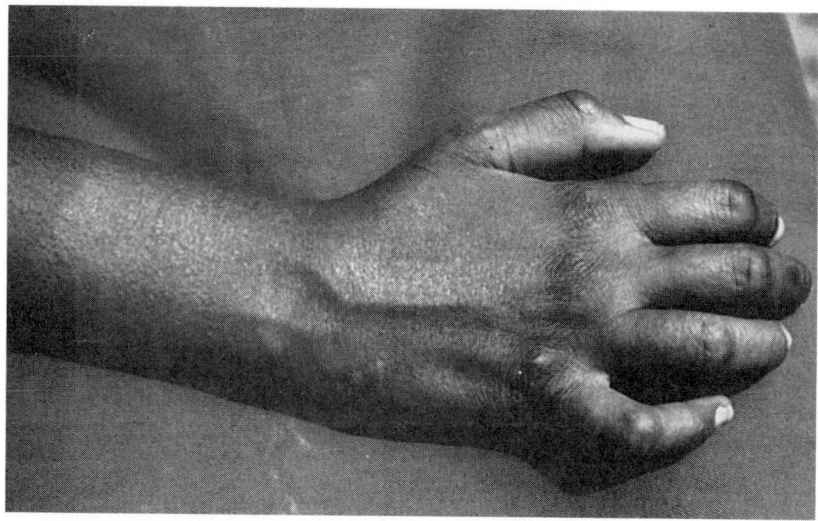

Figure 158.14. Reversal reaction acute neuritis.

may benefit from thalidomide treatment. This is a difficult decision for the woman and her physician and needs careful discussion of the benefits and risks (phocomelia in the offspring when thalidomide is taken in the first trimester). Women should use double contraception and report immediately if menstruation is delayed. Unfortunately, the problems with thalidomide mean that it is unavailable in several leprosy-endemic countries despite its undoubted value. Clofazimine has a useful antiinflammatory effect in ENL and can be used at 300 mg per day for several months. Low-grade chronic erythema nodosum, with iritis or neuritis, will require long-term suppression, preferably with thalidomide or clofazimine. Acute iridocyclitis is treated with 4-hourly instillation of 1% hydrocortisone eyedrops and 1% atropine drops twice daily.

Neuritis

Silent neuritis should be treated similarly to reversal reactions: prednisolone, 40 mg daily and reducing slowly over a period of months. Cyclosporin A has been shown to have a steroid-sparing effect in the treatment of steroid-dependent ENL reactions, but this requires further evaluation (76).

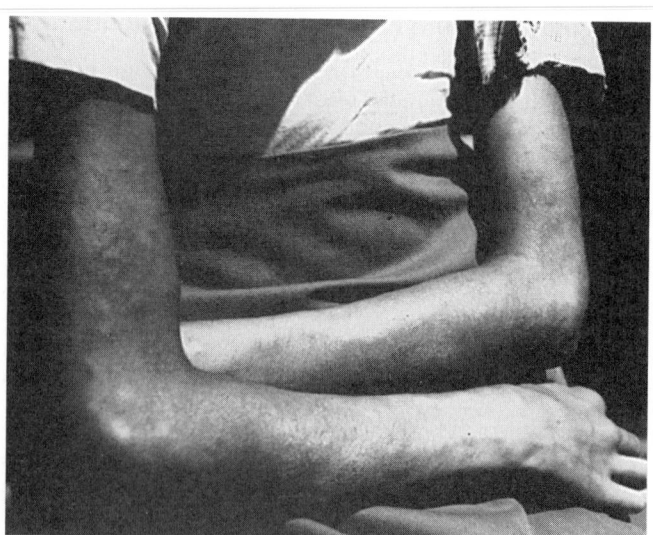

Figure 158.15. Typical cutaneous lesions of erythema nodosum leprosum.

PATIENT EDUCATION

Educating patients with leprosy about their disease is the key to successful management. Patients must be reassured that within a few days of chemotherapy, they will not be infectious and can lead a normal social life. A clear explanation of the disease and refutation of myths about leprosy will help patients come to terms with their diagnosis and may well improve compliance. It is important to emphasize that gross deformities are not the inevitable end point of disease, and that care and awareness of their limbs is as important as chemotherapy.

Prevention of Disability

The morbidity and disability associated with leprosy is secondary to nerve damage (Fig. 158.16). A major goal in prevention of disability is to create patient self-awareness so damage is minimized. The patient with an anesthetic hand or foot needs to understand the importance of daily self-care, especially protection when doing potentially dangerous tasks and inspection for trauma. It is helpful to identify for each patient potentially dangerous situations, such as cooking, car repairs, or smoking. Soaking dry hands and feet followed by rubbing with oil keeps the skin moist and supple.

An anesthetic foot needs the protection of an appropriate shoe. For anesthesia alone, a well-fitting "trainer" with firm soles and shock-absorbing inners will provide adequate protection. Once there is deformity, such as clawing, shoes must be made specially to ensure protection of pressure points and even weight distribution.

The patient should be taught to question the cause of an injury so the risk can be avoided. Plantar ulceration occurs secondary to increased pressure over bony prominences. Ulceration is treated by rest. Unlike ulcers in diabetic or ischemic feet, ulcers in leprosy heal if they are protected from weight bearing. No weight bearing is permitted until the ulcer has healed. Appropriate footwear should be provided to prevent recurrence.

Physiotherapy exercises should be taught to maximize function of weak muscles and prevent contracture. Contractures of hands and feet, footdrop, lagophthalmos, entropion, and ectropion are amenable to surgery.

Reconstructive Surgery

Reconstructive surgery has a role in both improving function and appearance. Lagophthalmos can be ameliorated by either

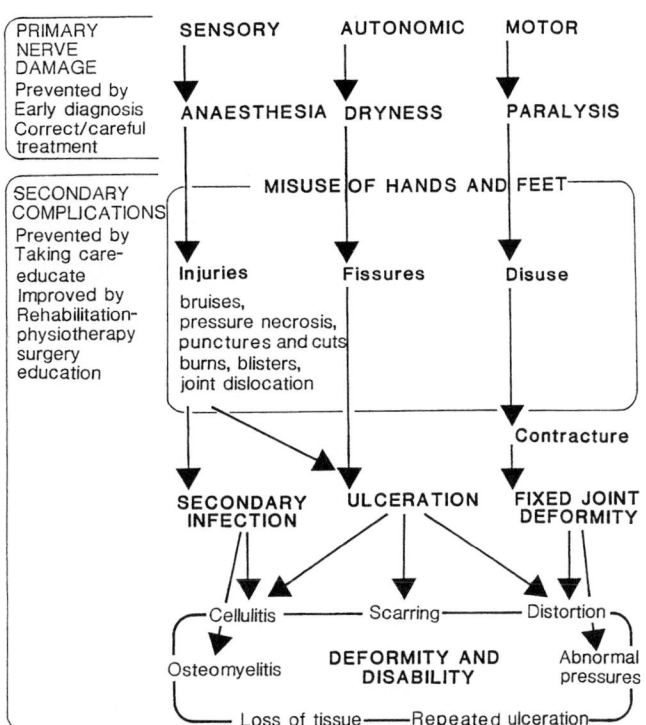

SENSORY AUTONOMIC MOTOR

PRIMARY
NERVE
DAMAGE
Prevented by
Early diagnosis
Correct/careful
treatment

ANAESTHESIA DRYNESS PARALYSIS

SECONDARY
COMPLICATIONS
Prevented by
Taking care-
educate
Improved by
Rehabilitation-
physiotherapy
surgery
education

MISUSE OF HANDS AND FEET

Injuries Fissures Disuse

bruises,
pressure necrosis,
punctures and cuts
burns, blisters,
joint dislocation

Contracture

SECONDARY
INFECTION ULCERATION FIXED JOINT
DEFORMITY

Cellulitis Scarring Distortion

Osteomyelitis **DEFORMITY AND
DISABILITY** Abnormal
pressures

Loss of tissue Repeated ulceration

The pathogenesis of disability following nerve damage in leprosy.

Figure 158.16. The interaction of factors producing deformities in leprosy. (From Bryceson A, Pfaltzgraff RE, eds. *Leprosy.* Edinburgh: Churchill Livingstone, 1979, with permission.)

tarsorrhaphy or temporalis muscle transfer. Appropriate tendon transfers can reduce the effects of ulnar and median nerve paralysis and improve dropfoot and claw toes. Cosmetic surgery, in particular eyebrow replacement, nasal reconstruction, and reduction of gynecomastia, is important in the rehabilitation of severely deformed patients.

Social, Psychological, and Economic Rehabilitation

The social and cultural background of the patient determine the nature of many of the problems that may be encountered. The patient may have difficulty in coming to terms with leprosy. The community may reject the patient. Education, gainful employment, confidence from family, friends, and doctor, and plastic surgery to correct stigmatizing deformity all have a role to play.

PROPHYLAXIS AGAINST LEPROSY

In nonendemic areas, it is very unusual to see leprosy in contacts of patients with leprosy. The last case of secondary transmission in the United Kingdom was in 1923. Household contacts of new patients should be examined for clinical signs of leprosy and advised to report any new skin lesions promptly and to tell their physicians that they have had contact with a known case of leprosy. In the United Kingdom, BCG vaccination is given to contacts who are younger than 12 years. Close contacts of lepromatous patients younger than 12 years are given prophylaxis with rifampicin, 15 mg/kg once a month for 6 months (78).

WOMEN AND LEPROSY

Women with leprosy are in double jeopardy, because they may not only develop postpartum nerve damage but are at particular risk of being socially ostracized with rejection by spouses and family (79). There is little good evidence that pregnancy causes new disease or relapse. However, there is a clear temporal association between parturition and the development of type 1 reactions and neuritis when CMI returns to prepregnancy levels (80). In an Ethiopian study, 42% of pregnancies in BL patients were complicated by a type 1 reaction during the postpartum period. In the same cohort, LL patients experienced ENL reactions throughout pregnancy and lactation. ENL in pregnancy is associated with early loss of nerve function compared with nonpregnant individuals. Pregnant and newly delivered women should have regular neurologic examination and steroid treatment instituted for neuritis. Rifampin, dapsone, and clofazimine are safe during pregnancy. Clofazimine crosses the placenta and babies may be born with mild clofazimine pigmentation. Reactions can be managed with the steroid regimens given earlier, but with a more rapid reduction in dose. Women should be warned before becoming pregnant of the risk of reactions after delivery. Ideally, pregnancies should be planned when leprosy is well controlled.

The WHO started the 1990s with the bold slogan of "Eliminating Leprosy as Public Health Problem by 2000." This initiative galvanized leprosy-control programs worldwide, but the unique biology of *M. leprae* and its interaction with the human host meant that the target was unattainable. As the millennium approached, the slogan was quietly dropped, to the disappointment of many leprosy workers and governments. Leprosy is a bacterial disease with challenging immunologic complications and will be a global and individual problem for many decades. It is unlikely to be eradicated until there is considerable improvement in general health, wealth, living conditions, and education.

In the United States advice on patient management may be obtained from the National Hansen's Disease Programs, 1770 Physicians Park Drive, Baton Rouge, LA 70816.

REFERENCES

1. Weekly Epidemiological Record. Leprosy—Global situation. 2000;75:226–231.
2. Noordeen SK. Epidemiology and control of leprosy—a review of progress over the last 30 years. *Trans R Soc Trop Med Hyg* 1993;87:515–517.
3. Noordeen SK. Elimination of leprosy as a public health problem. *Int J Lepr Other Mycobact Dis* 1994;62:279–283.
4. Brubaker ML, Binford CH, Trautman JR. Occurrences of leprosy in US veterans after service in endemic areas abroad. *Public Health Rep* 1969;84:1057.
5. Noordeen SK. Mortality in leprosy. *Indian J Med Res* 1972;60:439.
6. Fine PEM. The epidemiology of a slow bacterium. *Epidemiol Rev* 1982;4:161.
7. Noordeen SK. The epidemiology of leprosy. In: Hastings RC, ed. *Leprosy.* Edinburgh: Churchill Livingstone, 1994.
8. Feldman RA, Sturdivant M. Leprosy in Louisiana 1855–1970. An epidemiologic study of long term trends. *Am J Epidemiol* 1975;102:303–310.
9. Ponnighaus JM, Fine PEM, Sterne JAC, et al. Extended schooling and good housing conditions are associated with reduced risk of leprosy in rural Malawi. *Int J Lepr Other Mycobact Dis* 1994;62:345–352.
10. Ottenhoff THM, Converse PJ, Bjune G, et al. HLA antigens and neural reversal reactions in Ethiopian borderline tuberculoid leprosy patients. *Int J Lepr Other Mycobact Dis* 1987;55:261–266.
11. de Vries RR. Genetic control of immunopathology induced by *Mycobacterium leprae. Am J Trop Med Hyg* 1991;44:12–16.
12. Siddiqui MR, et al. A major susceptibility locus for leprosy in India maps to chromosome 10p13. *Nat Genet* 2001;27439–441.
13. Ponnighaus JM, Mwanjasi JL, Fine PEM, et al. Is HIV infection a risk factor for leprosy? *Int J Lepr Other Mycobact Dis* 1991;59:221–228.
14. Kawuma HJS, Bwire R, Adatu-Engwau F. Leprosy and infection with the human immunodeficiency virus in Uganda; a case control study. *Int J Lepr Other Mycobact Dis* 1994;62:521–526.
15. Sekar B, Jayasheela M, Chattopadhya D, et al. Prevalence of HIV infection and high-risk characteristics among leprosy patient of south India; a case control study. *Int J Lepr Other Mycobact Dis* 1994;62:527.

16. Sampaio EP, Caneshi JRT, Nery JAC, et al. Cellular immune response to *Mycobacterium leprae* infection in human immunodeficiency virus infected individuals. *Infect Immun* 1995;63:1848–1854.
17. Godal T. Immunological detection of subclinical infection in leprosy. *Lepr Rev* 1974;45:22.
18. Dockrell HM, Eastcott H, Young SK, et al. Possible transmission of *Mycobacterium leprae* in a group of UK leprosy contacts. *Lancet* 1991;338:739–743.
19. Scott GC, Russell DA, Boughton CR, et al. Untreated leprosy: Probability for shifts in Ridley-Jopling classification. Development of "flares" or disappearance of clinically apparent disease. *Int J Lepr Other Mycobact Dis* 1976;44:110.
20. Rees RJW, Meade T. Comparison of the modes of spread and transmission of leprosy and TB. *Lancet* 1974;7:47.
21. Lumpkin LRI, Cox GF, Wolf JE. Leprosy in five armadillo handlers. *Am J Epidemiol* 1983;9:899–903.
22. Truman RW, Shannon EJ, Hagstad HV, et al. Evaluation of the origin of *Mycobacterium leprae* in the wild armadillo, *Dasypus novemcinctus*. *Am J Trop Med Hyg* 1986;35:588–593.
23. Schaffer X. On the spread of leprosy bacilli from the upper parts of the respiratory tract. *Arch Dermatol Syph* 1898;44:159.
24. Shepard CC. Acid-fast bacilli in nasal excretions in leprosy and results of inoculation of mice. *Am J Hyg* 1960;71:147.
25. Desikan KV, Job CK. A review of postmortem findings in 37 cases of leprosy. *Int J Lepr Other Mycobact Dis* 1968;36:32.
26. De Wit MYL, Douglas JT, McFadden J, et al. Polymerase chain reaction for detection of *Mycobacterium leprae* in nasal swab specimens. *J Gen Microbiol* 1993;31:502–506.
27. Barton RPE. A clinical study of the nose in lepromatous leprosy. *Lepr Rev* 1974;45:135.
28. McDermott-Lancaster RD, McDougall AC. Mode of transmission and histology of *M. leprae* infection in nude mice. *Int J Exp Pathol* 1990;71:689.
29. Job CK, Chehl SK, Hastings RC. Transmission of leprosy in nude mice through thorn pricks. *Int J Lepr Other Mycobact Dis* 1994;62:395–398.
30. Job CK The pathology of leprosy. In: Hastings RC, ed. *Leprosy.* Edinburgh: Churchill Livingstone, 1994.
31. Ridley DS, Jopling WH. Classification of leprosy according to immunity. *Int J Lepr Other Mycobact Dis* 1966;34:255–273.
32. Dastur DK. Cutaneous nerves in leprosy: the relationship between histopathology and cutaneous sensibility. *Brain* 1955;78:615–633.
33. Antia NH, Mehta LN, Shetty VP, et al. Clinical, electrophysiological, quantitative, histologic and ultrastructural studies of the index branch of the radial cutaneous nerve in leprosy. 1. Preliminary report. *Int J Lepr Other Mycobact Dis* 1975;43:106–113.
34. Mehta LN, Shetty VP, Antia NH, et al. Quantitative, histologic and ultrastructural studies of the index branch of the radial cutaneous nerve in leprosy and its correlation with electrophysiologic study. *Int J Lepr Other Mycobact Dis* 1975;43:256–264.
35. Shetty VP, Mehta LN, Irani PF, et al. Study of the evolution of nerve damage in leprosy. Part 1: lesions of the index branch of the radial cutaneous nerve in early leprosy. *Indian J Lepr* 1980;52:5–18.
36. Pearson JMH, Weddell AGM. Perineurial changes in untreated leprosy. *Lepr Rev* 1975;46:51–67.
37. Job CK, Desikan KV. Pathologic changes and their distribution in peripheral nerves in lepromatous leprosy. *Int J Lepr Other Mycobact Dis* 1968;36:257–270.
38. Job CK. Pathology of peripheral nerve lesions in lepromatous leprosy—a light and electron microscopic study. *Int J Lepr Other Mycobact Dis* 1993;39:251–268.
39. Job CK. Mechanism of destruction in tuberculoid-borderline leprosy. An electron-microscopic study. *J Neurol Sci* 1973;20:25–38.
40. Britton WJ. Immunology of leprosy. *Trans R Soc Trop Med Hyg* 1993;87:508–514.
41. Lee SP, Stoker NG, Grant KA, et al. Cellular immune responses of leprosy contacts to fractionated *Mycobacterium leprae* antigens. *Infect Immun* 1989;57:2475–2480.
42. Dockrell HM, Stoker NG, Lee SP, et al. T-cell recognition of the 18-kilodalton antigen of *Mycobacterium leprae*. *Infect Immun* 1989;57:1979–1983.
43. Ilangumaran S, Shanker-Narayanan NP, Ramu G, et al. Cellular and humoral responses to recombinant 65KD antigen of *Mycobacterium leprae* in leprosy patients and healthy controls. *Clin Exp Immunol* 1994;96:79.
44. Modlin RL, Hofman FM, Horwitz DA, et al. *In situ* identification of cells in human leprosy granulomas with monoclonal antibodies to interleukin 2 and its receptors. *J Immunol* 1984;132:3085–3090.
45. Paul RC, Stanford JL, Carswell JW. Multiple skin testing in leprosy. *J Hyg Camb* 1975;75:57–68.
46. Modlin RL, Rea TH. Immunopathology of leprosy granulomas. *Springer Semin Immunopathol* 1988;10:359–374.
47. Waters MFR, Ridley DS, Lucas SB. Positive Mitsuda lepromin reactions in long term treated lepromatous leprosy. *Lepr Rev* 1990;61:347–352.
48. Haregewoin A, Godal T, Mustafa AS, et al. T-cell conditioned media reverse T-cell unresponsiveness in lepromatous leprosy. *Nature* 1983;303:342–344.
49. Kaplan G, Kiessling R, Teklemariam S, et al. The reconstitution of cell-mediated immunity in the cutaneous lesions of lepromatous leprosy by recombinant interleukin 2. *J Exp Med* 1989;169:893–907.
50. Birdi TJ, Antia NH. The macrophage in leprosy: a review on the current status. *Int J Lepr Other Mycobact Dis* 1989;57:511–516.
51. Yoder L, Naafs B, Harboe M. Antibody activity against *M. leprae* antigens in leprosy: studies on variation in antibody content throughout the spectrum and on the effect of DDs treatment and relapse in BT leprosy. *Lepr Rev* 1979;50:113.
52. Khanolkar Young S, et al. Tumour necrosis factor-alpha (TNF-alpha) synthesis is associated with the skin and peripheral nerve pathology of leprosy reversal reactions. *Clin Exp Immunol* 1995;99:196–202.
53. Khanolkar Young S, et al. Immunocytochemical localization of inducible nitric oxide synthase and transforming growth factor-beta (TGF-beta) in leprosy lesions. *Clin Exp Immunol* 1998;113:438–442.
54. Wemambu SNC, Turk JL, Waters MFR. Erythema nodosum leprosum: a clinical manifestation of the Arthus phenomenon. *Lancet* 1969;2:933–935.
55. Dharma Rao T, Ramchander Rao P. Enhanced cell-mediated immune responses in erythema nodosum leprosum reactions of leprosy. *Int J Lepr Other Mycobact Dis* 1987;55:36–42.
56. Filley E, Andreolli A, Steele J, et al. A transient rise in a galactosyl IgG correlating with free interleukin-2 receptors during episodes of erythema nodosum. *Clin Exp Immunol* 1989;76:343–348.
57. Anon. Ocular complications of leprosy. *Lancet* 1992;340:642–643.
58. Latapi L, Chevez Zamora A. The "spotted" leprosy of Lucio (la lepra "manchada" de Lucio). An introduction to its clinical and histological study. *Int J Lepr* 1948;16:421–429.
59. Bell-Krotoski JA. Repeatability of the Semmes-Weinstein monofilaments. *J Hand Surg* 1987;12A:155–161.
60. Lockwood DN, Reid AJ. The diagnosis of leprosy is delayed in the United Kingdom. *Q J Med* 2001;94:207–212.
61. Shepard CC, Levy L, Fasal P. Further experience with the rapid bactericidal effect of rifampin on *Mycobacterium leprae*. *Am J Trop Med Hyg* 1974;23:1120–1124.
62. Jacobson RR, Hastings RC. Rifampicin-resistant leprosy. *Lancet* 1976;2:1304.
63. Frey HM, Gershon AA, Borkowsky W, et al. Fatal reaction to dapsone during treatment of leprosy. *Ann Intern Med* 1981;94:777.
64. Grosset JH. Progress in the chemotherapy of leprosy. *Int J Lepr Other Mycobact Dis* 1994;62:268–277.
65. Jamet P, Ji B, and the Marchoux Chemotherapy Study Group. Relapse after long-term follow-up of multibacillary patients treated by WHO multidrug regimen. *Int J Lepr Other Mycobact Dis* 1995;63:195–201.
66. Girdhar BK, et al. Relapses in multibacillary leprosy patients: effect of length of therapy. *Lepr Rev* 2000;71:144–153.
67. Ji B. Does there exist a subgroup of MB patients at greater risk of relapse after MDT? *Lepr Rev* 2001;72:3–8.
68. Daumerie D. Current World Health Organization–sponsored studies in the chemotherapy of leprosy. *Lepr Rev* 2000;71[Suppl]:S88–S90.
69. Van Brakel WH. Peripheral neuropathy in leprosy and its consequences. *Lepr Rev* 2000;71:S146–S153.
70. Croft RP, et al. Nerve function impairment in leprosy: design, methodology, and intake status of a prospective cohort study of 2664 new leprosy cases in Bangladesh (the Bangladesh Acute Nerve Damage Study). *Lepr Rev* 1999;70:140–159.
71. Croft RP, et al. Incidence rates of acute nerve function impairment in leprosy: a prospective cohort analysis after 24 months (the Bangladesh Acute Nerve Damage Study). *Lepr Rev* 2000;71:18–33.
72. Rose P, Waters MFR. Reversal reactions in leprosy and their management. *Lepr Rev* 1991;62:113–121.
73. Lockwood DNJ, Vinayakumar S, Stanley JNA, et al. Clinical features and outcome of reversal (type 1) reactions in Hyderabad, India. *Int J Lepr Other Mycobact Dis* 1993;60:8–15.
74. Kiran KU, Stanley JNA, Pearson JMH. The outpatient treatment of nerve damage in patients with borderline leprosy using a semi-standardised steroid regime. *Lepr Rev* 1985;56:127–134.
75. Jakeman P, Smith WCS. Thalidomide in leprosy reaction. *Lancet* 1994;343:432–433.
76. Miller RA, Shen J, Rea TH, et al. Treatment of chronic erythema nodosum leprosum with cyclosporine A produces clinical and immunohistologic remission. *Int J Lepr Other Mycobact Dis* 1987;55:441–449.
77. Srinivasan H. *Prevention of disabilities in patients with leprosy: a practical guide.* Geneva: World Health Organization, 1993.
78. Department of Health and the Welsh Office. *Memorandum on leprosy.* HMSO, 1997.
79. Morrison A. A woman with leprosy is in double jeopardy. *Lepr Rev* 2000;71:128–143.
80. Lockwood DN, Sinha HH. Pregnancy and leprosy: a comprehensive literature review. *Int J Lepr Other Mycobact Dis* 1999;67:6–12.

Zoonoses

CHAPTER 159
Approach to the Patient with Zoonotic Infection

David R. Stone

Zoonoses are infectious agents, usually seen in animal hosts, that can on occasion cross the species barrier and spread to humans. Animals may or may not become ill as a result of these infections. The severity of disease in humans depends on the virulence of the organism, the organ or organs affected, and the human host's natural immunity to the infection.

Epidemics due to the emergence of newly discovered zoonotic pathogens as well as the recrudescence of more established zoonotic pathogens have drastic effects on the lives of people both in developing and industrialized nations. Exploration, deforestation, and manipulation of wetlands bring people in contact with organisms rarely encountered (1).

War, poverty, lack of sanitation, and overcrowding lead to spread of these infections within the population. International commerce and ease of international travel play a major role in the worldwide dissemination of these new diseases in both animals and humans. The emergence of West Nile virus in the Western Hemisphere is a good example. Isolates from a 1999 outbreak in New York closely resemble those isolated from birds and people in Israel (2). This outbreak could have crossed the Atlantic by a number of sources, including infected humans, mosquitoes, birds, or animals. Once established in the United States, the virus was and continues to be spread widely by infected migratory birds (3).

Our increasing infatuation with pets, including exotic pets obtained throughout the world, puts us at risk for a number of different pathogens. Despite regulations prohibiting importation of nonhuman primates, people still obtain them as pets. Bites from pet macaques can transmit *Herpesvirus simiae* (4). Meningoencephalitis from the virus can occur in humans with a mortality rate as high as 79% (5). Infections with *Bartonella* species can lead to illnesses ranging from cat-scratch disease to endocarditis (6,7). This organism may cause bacteremia without obvious symptoms in cats (8).

Because of increasing human population growth rates, we need to herd large populations of farm animals for food. Farming has become mechanized in many parts of the world. This greatly facilitates the exposure of zoonoses to humans, especially when corners are cut to maximize production. Outbreaks of *Salmonella* species and *Escherichia coli* 0157-H7 infection are now commonly encountered in industrialized nations (9). In addition, antibiotics used in animal feed has led to drug resistance in bacteria such as salmonella and enterococci (10–15).

The spread of zoonotic infections due to farming and processing is best exemplified by the recent discovery of bovine spongiform encephalopathy and variant Creutzfeldt-Jakob disease (16–18). The introduction and spread of prions within a population of cattle in the United Kingdom was associated with the use of animal feed derived from cattle and other ruminants (sheep) that were improperly rendered. The spread from cattle to humans has been observed and most likely is associated with the ingestion of infected meat or milk products.

Severe acute respiratory syndrome (SARS), caused by a newly discovered coronavirus, originated in the Guangdong province of China. It had spread worldwide by the spring of 2003, and has engendered great fear and economic harm in the areas most affected (18a). It possibly was spread to humans who prepared civets or other small mammals for food.

Many other emerging zoonotic infections have a substantial mortality but have gotten far less publicity. Nipah virus, which causes encephalitis in humans, has been associated with swine. An outbreak in pig farmers in Malaysia led to more than 100 deaths in 1998 and 1999 alone (19).

Not all zoonotic outbreaks are unfortunate occurrences of nature. Recently, we have all become aware of the risk of large-scale biological terrorism using zoonotic organisms such as anthrax (20,21). In the fall of 2001, an outbreak of human cutaneous and inhalation anthrax in Florida and the Northeast United States was associated with the delivery of spore-laden mail. Other zoonotic organisms that have been feared to be possible weapons for biological terrorism include plague, tularemia, and hemorrhagic fever viruses such as Ebola (22,23). A new field of biodefense has been established because of this threat.

Zoonotic infections may not necessarily be bad, and knowledge of them is important in the prevention of disease. In the eighteenth century, Jenner noticed that milkmaids had protection against smallpox infection. Vaccination with cowpox and subsequently vaccinia led to the eradication of smallpox in the twentieth century (24).

Humans are not totally to blame for the emergence of zoonoses. Mutation, recombination, and reassortment of genetic material, especially in viruses, have led some organisms to become either more virulent or more amenable to crossing the species barrier to infection.

Environmental factors out of our control, such as excessive rainfall or global warming, may have led some organisms to infect species of animals or arthropods never known to be affected previously. Changes in the arthropod vector populations, in part due to environmental changes, play a very important role in the dissemination of these diseases. Mosquitoes, thought to have been blown by wind currents, have led to the introduction of Japanese encephalitis virus into Australia (25). Ticks containing *Ehrlichia* species have been associated with migrating birds (26). A new strain of influenza A virus has been associated with a recombination event within the poultry markets in Hong Kong. In 1998, the strain H5N1 appeared to have been spread to people directly from infected birds (27–30). Fortunately, the virus was unable to spread from person to person.

Human immunodeficiency virus (HIV) has enabled less virulent zoonotic organisms to spread through segments of this vulnerable immunodeficient population. Infections with *Mycobacterium avium* and *Cryptococcus, Cryptosporidium, Toxoplasma, Bartonella, Salmonella*, and *Rhodococcus* species have been well described in the acquire immunodeficiency syndrome (AIDS) population. People at risk need to take special precautions when dealing with livestock and pets (31).

Zoonotic diseases have been well described throughout recorded history; more than 200 have been documented. They include viral, bacterial, mycotic, protozoan, and helminthic infections along with arthropod infestations. They are transmitted to humans either directly through skin contact, bite or scratch, inhalation, and ingestion, or indirectly through an arthropod intermediate host. In addition, the fear of infections derived from xenotransplants has recently been reviewed (32). Humans usually serve as an accidental host for zoonotic infections; however, on occasion, humans serve along with animals as a reservoir for disease (e.g., yellow fever virus, pneumonic plague). HIV-1 and HIV-2 originated in primates and technically are zoonotic infections (33). Transmission of these simian retroviruses from animals to humans is likely a very rare occurrence at this time. Infection transmitted to laboratory workers from animals has been documented in research institutions where nonhuman primates are kept (34,35).

To understand, control, and possibly prevent these zoonotic diseases, we need the expertise of a team of scientists, including molecular biologists, ecologists, entomologists, epidemiologists, public health officials, and veterinarians.

In this chapter, we highlight some of the unique aspects that need to be considered when zoonotic infections are evaluated. We categorize some of the more common zoonoses by their modes of transmission and discuss preventive measures that can be used to avoid infection.

Questions about zoonoses are usually presented to the clinician in one of three contexts. In the first instance, an animal was known to have been ill, and the question arises as to whether humans can become ill because of contact with that animal. This is clearly a question that should be addressed by a veterinarian. Animals may develop many diseases that are not transmitted to humans.

In the second situation, an ill person has a history of contact with animals or insects (bites), and the question arises as to whether the illness could be related to that contact. In this instance, we should first consider the age of the patient. Children are often intimate and careless in their contact with pets. Their failure to wash hands before eating puts them at risk for developing zoonotic infections transmitted by the fecal-oral route, for example, with *Toxocara canis* and *Toxocara cati* (visceral larva migrans), *Ancylostoma caninum* (dog hookworm), and *Salmonella* and *Campylobacter* species (36–38). In adults, occupational hazards must be considered. Examples include anthrax in wool sorters, leptospirosis in dairy farmers and sewer workers, tularemia in trappers and hunters, psittacosis in pet store workers, and erysipeloid in fishers. The species of the contact animal is important. Some zoonoses are highly host specific (e.g., *Taenia solium* in swine), whereas others have a broad range of hosts (e.g., salmonellosis in reptiles, birds, and mammals). Some monkey species (e.g., *Macaca* species) in the wild are assumed to be infected with herpes B virus and are excluded from general research unless proper precautions can be taken. Whenever possible, a description or identification of an arthropod that bit someone should be obtained for help in anticipating or diagnosing zoonotic illness. A febrile illness after an *Ixodes dammini* tick bite in the northeastern United States would make one consider the possibility of Lyme disease, babesiosis, or ehrlichiosis (39). If the tick were *Dermacentor variablis* (dog tick), one would be concerned about Rocky Mountain spotted fever or tularemia.

Zoonotic infections are often limited to certain geographic areas; hence, a travel history is pertinent. For example, *Taenia saginata*, the beef tapeworm, is commonly transmitted in East Africa but is rare in cattle in the United States. *Trypanosoma cruzi*, the etiologic agent of Chagas' disease, is found in South and Central America. It is rarely found in the United States. Glanders, a disease caused by *Pseudomonas mallei*, was once common throughout the world but is now found only in a few countries in Asia and Africa. It is necessary to inquire where the animal came from and whether it was quarantined. Pet stores, zoos, laboratories, and livestock dealers import animals from foreign countries. Import regulations do not guarantee that the animals are free of exotic zoonoses. Outbreaks of Marburg and Ebola virus infections, transmitted from imported nonhuman primates, have been documented (40,41). Wild and domestic canids from regions enzootic for hydatid disease may carry adult *Echinococcus* tapeworms in their gut and become an imported source of human disease (42).

It should be determined whether the animal has been vaccinated or tested for specific diseases. Dogs and cats should be vaccinated for rabies. Cattle are routinely tested for tuberculosis and brucellosis. It is pertinent to inquire about the health of the contact animal before, during, and after human exposure. Signs of illness may be similar in humans and animals (e.g., skin lesions in ringworm, neurologic signs in rabies). In such situations, demonstration of similar lesions or clinical history in the animal and person may help establish the diagnosis. It is also important to inquire as to whether the animal has given birth recently and whether there was a stillbirth, illness in the newborn, or evidence of an infected placenta (e.g., Q fever, *Leptospirosis* and *Brucella* species infections). For some diseases, the signs of illness may be totally different in humans and animals. For example, a cow transmitting bovine tuberculosis through her milk might have mastitis, whereas the infected person might have tuberculous spondylitis. Many animals with the potential to transmit zoonoses to humans may not appear ill at all. For example, in cats, *Bartonella henselae* bacteremia or *Toxoplasma gondii* infections are usually subclinical.

The third zoonotic context occurs when a patient or a population is documented to have a zoonotic illness and it is necessary to trace the origin of the disease and to institute control and preventive measures. This often requires the cooperation of officials in agriculture or public health at the municipal, state, or federal level. An outbreak of cryptosporidiosis in Milwaukee affecting more than 400,000 people was caused by contamination of the water supply and the failure of authorities to monitor the turbidity of water in one of the city's water treatment plants (43). In the southwestern United States, an outbreak of respiratory failure with a high mortality rate was traced within months to a new strain of *Hantavirus* (44). Using polymerase chain reaction technology, molecular biologists were able to determine that the virus was transmitted by aerosolized excreta from local field mice (45).

TRANSMISSION OF ZOONOSES

Discussion of zoonoses according to their route of transmission is useful in establishing occupational preventive medicine programs, for example, in zoos, veterinary hospitals, stockyards, and laboratories. It is also important in establishing public health guidelines in matters such as the care of animals and the inspection and preparation of food. Tables 159.1 through 159.7 are organized by means of transmission, with some examples and appropriate preventive measures.

TABLE 159.1. Zoonoses Transmitted by Bite or Scratch

Bacteria	Viruses	Fungi
Pasteurella multocida	Rabies virus	*Sporothrix*
Bartonella henselae	Lymphocytic	*schenckii*
Spirillum minus	choriomeningitis	
Streptobacillus	virus	
moniliformis		
Francisella tularensis		
Yersinia pestis		
Capnocytophaga		
carnimorsus		

Prevention:
1. Reduce risk with proper animal-handling techniques.
2. Wash all bites and scratches as soon as possible.
3. Animal workers or travelers at risk need rabies preexposure prophylaxis and checks of serum immunity every other year.

TABLE 159.2.   Zoonoses Transmitted by Direct Contact or Contact with Products of Conception, Urine, Blood, Saliva, and Feces

Bacteria	Viruses	Fungi	Helminths	Other
Bacillus anthracis *Brucella* species *Francisella tularensis* *Coxiella burnetii* *Pasteurella multocida* *Leptospira* species *Mycobacterium marinum* *Yersinia pestis*	Herpes B virus Vesicular stomatitis virus Orthopoxvirus (monkeypox) Parapoxvirus (orf) Marburg and Ebola viruses	*Microsporum canis* *Trichophyton mentagrophytes*	*Ancylostoma* species	*Sarcoptes scabei* var. *canis*

Prevention:
1. Reduce risk by prompt diagnosis, isolation, and treatment of infected animals.
2. With animal contact, use good hand washing, gloves, aprons, and protective clothing. Preferably, wash clothes at work.
3. Clean and disinfect fomites.
4. Use special care when assisting with animal deliveries, surgery, necropsy, and slaughterhouse work.

TABLE 159.3.   Fecal–Oral Transmission of Zoonoses

Bacteria	Helminths	Protozoa
Salmonella species *Shigella* species *Escherichia coli* O157:H7 *Campylobacter* species *Yersinia, pseudotuberculosis* *Yersinia enterocolitica*	*Toxocara canis, Toxocara cati* *Echinococcus* species	*Giardia lamblia* *Cryptosporidium* species *Toxoplasma gondii* *Baylisascaris procyonis* *Trichostrongylus* species

Prevention:
1. Reduce risk as for direct contact (see Table 159.2).
2. Use face mask when hosing cages.
3. Avoid eating, drinking, or smoking in potentially contaminated areas.
4. Culture or examine stools of potentially infectious animals, especially if they have diarrhea.

TABLE 159.4.   Zoonoses Transmitted by Consumption of Infected Meat, Poultry, Fish, and Dairy Products

Bacteria	Helminths	Protozoa
Salmonella species *Yersinia* species *Campylobacter* species *Shigella* species *Escherichia coli* O157:H7 *Brucella* species *Bacillus anthracis* *Vibrio parahaemolyticus* *Francisella tularensis* *Listeria monocytogenes* *Streptobacillus moniliformis*	*Taenia solium* *Trichinella spiralis* *Taenia saginata* *Diphyllobothrium latum* *Anisakis* species *Clonorchis sinensis* *Angiostrongylus cantonensis* *Opisthorchis* species *Paragonimus* species *Capillaria philippinensis*	*Toxoplasma gondii*

Prevention:
1. Use sanitary milking procedures, dairy inspection, mastitis control, brucellosis and tuberculosis testing of dairy animals, and pasteurization of milk.
2. Institute rodent control on farms (to reduce *Salmonella* and *Trichinella* in livestock), sanitary human sewage disposal (to reduce cysticercosis in cattle and swine), meat inspection, and proper refrigeration and freezing of meat.
3. Prevent salmonellosis by washing eggs and disposing of cracked eggs.
4. Instruct the public about the need for adequate cooking of all animal products.

TABLE 159.5.   Respiratory Transmission of Zoonoses

Bacteria	Viruses
Mycobacterium tuberculosis	Rabies virus
Bacillus anthracis	Influenza virus (swine, humans, chickens)
Coxiella burnetii	Lymphocytic choriomeningitis virus
Yersinia pestis	
Rhodococcus equi	Hantaan virus
Pseudomonas mallei	
Chlamydia psittaci	
Francisella tularensis	
Pasteurella multocida	
Brucella species	

Prevention:
1. Reduce risk with use of face masks and proper air circulation and filtration (e.g., in laboratories).
2. Test primates and cattle for tuberculosis. Tuberculin-positive animals are usually killed; rarely is any attempt made to treat them.

ZOONOTIC DISEASES IN IMMUNOCOMPROMISED PATIENTS

A number of diseases transmitted by pets are particularly serious in immunocompromised patients (15–17). The risks can be lowered as long as the pet owners use good hygiene after touching their pets, avoid handling the feces, and take the animal promptly to the veterinarian if it gets sick (46).

T. gondii oocysts can be shed in the feces of cats (usually kittens) and spread to those in contact with the cat litter or infected soil. Most human infections, however, are due to consumption of cysts in undercooked lamb or pork. Most infections in immunocompromised patients in the United States are a reactivation of a latent infection. It is prudent for patients at risk (including pregnant women) to know their *Toxoplasma* exposure history and, if susceptible, to use extreme caution when cleaning the litter box. The owner should attempt to limit the possibility of infection in the cat by keeping it inside and feeding it well-cooked food, or dry or canned food.

Bacillary angiomatosis is caused by *B. henselae* and *Bartonella quintana*. It is a rare disease even among immunocompromised patients. It can be transmitted by a cat scratch or possibly a bite from an infected flea. Cat owners should make sure that their cats are protected from fleas. Any scratches should be cleaned promptly with soap and water. Risk for *Bartonella* infection is diminished in cats older than 1 year of age. Immunocompromised cat owners must be aware that any unusual skin lesions should be examined promptly by a physician.

A number of zoonotic diarrheal illnesses are associated with significant morbidity in immunocompromised persons. The risk for transmission can be minimized by avoiding contact with animal feces.

Cryptosporidiosis is transmitted by infected farm animals and by contamination of drinking water. Dogs and cats have been shown to shed the organism occasionally, but there is no evidence that having these pets at home increases the likelihood of developing this illness. The younger the pet, the greater the potential for infection. Animals with diarrhea should be removed from the house. A pet owner purchasing a puppy or kitten may wish to have the animal's stool screened for *Cryptosporidium* species. Giardiasis may also be present in household pets, but it is unlikely that the pet owner is at a significantly increased risk for infection.

Campylobacter and *Salmonella* species are present in many animal species, any of which could potentially spread disease to immunocompromised patients. The most common route of infection is from contaminated and poorly cooked food. *Campylobacter* species infection in humans has also been associated with contact with infected dogs and cats, and *Salmonella* species infection in humans has been associated with infected pet birds,

TABLE 159.6.   Arthropod-borne Zoonoses

Bacteria	Viruses	Protozoa	Helminths
Tick-Borne			
Borrelia burgdorferi	Orbivirus (Colorado tick fever)	Babesia microti	
Borrelia species		Babesia divergens	
Ehrlichia chaffeensis			
Ehrlichia phagocytophilia			
Francisella tularensis			
Coxiella burnetii			
Rickettsia ricketsii			
Rickettsia species			
Mosquito-Borne			
	Flavivirus (yellow fever, St. Louis encephalitis, West Nile, Japanese encephalitis)		
	Bunyavirus (California and La Crosse encephalitis, Rift Valley fever)		Brugia species
	Alphavirus (eastern and Venezuelan equine encephalitis)		Dirofilaria immitis
Other Insect or Mite			
Rickettsia akari (mite)			
Yersinia pestis (flea)		Trypanosoma rhodesiense (tsetse fly)	
		Trypanosoma cruzi (reduviid bug)	
		Leishmania species (sandfly)	

Prevention:
1. The risk for transmission can be reduced by wearing protective clothing, using insect repellants, and using environmental insecticides in an appropriate way.
2. Mosquito bed netting should be used in some areas.
3. Ticks should be removed as soon as possible.
4. Pets should be protected from flea and tick infestations.

TABLE 159.7. Zoonotic Risks for Patients with Immunodeficiency

Bacteria	Protozoa	Fungi
Salmonella (dog, cat, bird)	*Toxoplasma* (cat)	*Cryptococcus*
Campylobacter (dog, cat)	*Cryptosporidium*	
Bartonella (cat)	(dog, cat)	
Rhodococcus (horse)[a]		
Mycobacterium avium (bird)[a]		
Mycobacterium marinum (fish)		

[a]More often from soil or other environmental sources.

turtles, lizards, dogs, and cats. Animals with diarrhea should be taken to the veterinarian. Puppies and kittens may be at higher risk for carrying these infections than older animals.

Inhalation has been considered the primary route of infection by *Cryptococcus* and *Rhodococcus*. *M. avium* complex infections are thought to enter the body through the gastrointestinal tract or the lungs. *Cryptococcus neoformans* is present in areas polluted with pigeon and other wild bird excrement. Patients who are immunocompromised should refrain from exposure to areas that may be contaminated with bird feces. *M. avium* complex infections occur in pet birds, but birds are rarely the source of infection in immunocompromised patients. *Rhodococcus equi* infection is rare, even in immunocompromised patients. The organism is probably transmitted from the soil more frequently than it is transmitted directly from farm animals.

Home aquariums have been documented as the source of infections by *Mycobacterium marinum* (47). In immunocompromised patients at risk for disseminated disease, use of gloves is recommended.

Arthropod-borne infections pose a risk to patients with immunodeficiency. Overwhelming parasitemia caused by *Babesia* species has been seen in asplenic patients and patients with HIV infection.

RESEARCH AREAS AND CONCLUSION

The emergence of many zoonotic pathogens during the past decade has made this one of the most active fields in infectious disease. Local and national public health organizations are needed to move rapidly into an area affected by a zoonotic outbreak, isolate the organism, and define the origin of infection. With this knowledge, interventions will be enacted and epidemics averted, if possible. We also need astute clinicians to be able to describe any illness that appears unusual. Asking about travel, pets, animal exposure, and insect bites should be routine when any infection is considered.

The need for, and benefit of, basic research is exemplified by work on the *Hantavirus* isolated in the southwestern United States in 1993 and West Nile virus in New York in 1998. Within weeks of their clinical appearance, these viruses were isolated and the environmental reservoir and mode of transmission defined.

Research is needed to develop vaccines to prevent or control zoonotic infections. Vaccines are already used for anthrax, Lyme disease, influenza, Japanese encephalitis, and rabies. Others are being developed. We also need to provide adequate water purification, rubbish removal, and rodent and mosquito control. Public health inspections of the food industry are important to keep standards high. Animals from other countries need to be examined and possibly quarantined. The best protection from zoonoses is to ensure good hand washing after handling animals, to clean and cook all food well, and to use insect repellant and protective clothing in mosquito- and tick-infested areas. Education, especially for travelers, farmers, pet owners, and people who are immunocompromised, is of great importance.

REFERENCES

1. Daszak P, Cunningham AA, Hyatt AD. Emerging infectious diseases of wildlife: threats of biodiversity and human health. *Science* 2000;287:443–449.
2. Petersen LR, Roehrig JT. West Nile virus: a reemerging global pathogen. *Emerg Infect Dis* 2001;7:4.
3. Rappole JH, Derrickson SR, Hubalek Z. Migratory birds and the spread of West Nile virus in the Western Hemisphere. *Emerg Infect Dis* 2001;6:319–328.
4. Ostrowski SR, Leslie MJ, Parrott T, et al. B-virus from pet macaque monkeys: an emerging threat in the United States? *Emerg Infect Dis* 1998;4:1.
5. Hummeler K, Davidson WL, Henle W, et al. Encephalomyelitis due to infection with *Herpesvirus simiae* (herpes B virus): report of two fatal laboratory acquired cases. *N Engl J Med* 1959;261:64–68.
6. Ohl ME, Spach DH. *Bartonella quintana* and urban trench fever. *Clin Infect Dis* 2000;31:131–135.
7. Schutze GE. Diagnosis and treatment of *Bartonella henselae* infections. *Pediatr Infect Dis J* 2000;19(12):1185–1187.
8. Koehler JE, Glaser CA, Tappero JW. *Rochalimaea henselae* infection: a new zoonosis with the domestic cat as reservoir. *JAMA* 1994;271:531–535.
9. Outbreak of *Escherichia coli* O157:H7 infections among children associated with farm visits: Pennsylvania and Washington, 2000. *MMWR Morb Mortal Wkly Rep* 2001;50(15):293–296.
10. Mead PS, Slutsker L, Dietz V, et al. Food-related illness and death in the United States. *Emerg Infect Dis* 1999;5:607–625.
11. Levy SB. Antibiotic resistance: an ecological imbalance. *Cibi Found Symp* 1997;207:1–9.
12. Angulo FJ, Johnson KR, Tauxe RV, et al. Origins and consequences of antimicrobial resistant nontyphoidal *Salmonella*: implications of the use of fluoroquinolones in animals. *Microb Drug Resist* 2000;6:77–83.
13. McDonald LC, Rossiter S, Mackinson C, et al. Quinupristin-dalfopristin-resistant *Enterococcus faecium* on chickens and in human stool specimens. *N Engl J Med* 2001;345:1155–1160.
14. White DG, Shao S, Sudler R, et al. The isolation of antibiotic resistant *Salmonella* from retail ground meats. *N Engl J Med* 2001;345:1147–1154.
15. Gorbach SL. Antimicrobial use in animal feed—time to stop [Editorial]. *N Engl J Med* 2001;345:1202–1203.
16. Prusiner SB. The prion diseases. *Sci Am* 1994;Jan:57.
17. Diringer H. Proposed link between transmissible spongiform encephalopathies of man and animals. *Lancet* 1995;346:1208–1210.
18. Brown P, Will RG, Bradley R, et al. Bovine spongiform encephalopathy and variant Creutzfeldt Jakob disease: background, evolution and current concerns. *Emerg Infect Dis* 2001;7:1.
18a. Ksiazek TG, Erdman D, Goldsmith CS, et al. A novel coronavirus associated with severe acute respiratory syndrome. *N Engl J Med* 2003;348:1953–1966.
19. Chua KB, Goh KJ, Wong KT, et al. Fatal encephalitis due to Nipah virus among pig-farmers in Malaysia. *Lancet* 1999;354:1257–1259.
20. Anonymous. Update: investigation of bioterrorism-related anthrax and interim guidelines for exposure management and antimicrobial therapy, October 2001. *MMWR Morb Mortal Wkly Rep* 2001;50(42);909–919.
21. Inglesby TV, Henderson DA, Bartlett JG, et al. Anthrax as a biological weapon: medical and public health management. *JAMA* 1999;281:1735–1963.
22. Dennis DT, Inglesby TV, Henderson DA, et al. Tularemia as a biological weapon: medical and public health management. *JAMA* 2001;285:2763–2773.
23. Inglesby TV, Dennis DT, Henderson DA, et al. Plague as a biological weapon: medical and public health management. *JAMA* 2000;283:2281–2290.
24. Radetsky M. Smallpox: a history of its rise and fall. *Pediatr Infect Dis J* 1999;18(2):85–93.
25. Ritchie SA, Rochester W. Wind-blown mosquitoes and introduction of Japanese encephalitis into Australia. *Emerg Infect Dis* 2001;7:5.
26. Bjoersdorff A, Bergstrom S, Massung RF, et al. *Ehrlichia*-infected ticks on migrating birds. *Emerg Infect Dis* 2001;7:5.
27. Hatta M, Gao P, Halfmann P, et al. Molecular basis for high virulence of Hong Kong H5N1 influenza A viruses. *Science* 2001;293(5536):1840–1842.
28. Claas ECJ, Osterhaus ADME, van Beek R, et al. Human influenza A H5N1 virus related to a highly pathogenic avian influenza virus. *Lancet* 1998;351:472–477.
29. Cyranoski D. Outbreak of chicken flu rattles Hong Kong. *Nature* 2001;412(6844):261.
30. Kilbourne ED. Epidemiology of influenza. In: Kilbourne ED, ed. *Influenza viruses and influenza.* New York: Academic Press, 1975:483–538.
31. CDC. 1999 USPHS/IDSA guidelines for the prevention of opportunistic infections in persons infected with human immunodeficiency virus. *MMWR Morb Mortal Wkly Rep* 1999;48(RR-10).
32. Potential risks: xenotransplantation. *MMWR Morb Mortal Wkly Rep* 2001;50(RR-15):1–46.

33. Hahn BH, Shaw GM, De Cock KM, et al. AIDS as a zoonosis: scientific and public health implications. *Science* 2000;287:607–614.
34. Anonymous. Anonymous survey for simian immunodeficiency virus (SIV) seropositivity in SIV-laboratory researchers—United States, 1992. *MMWR Morb Mortal Wkly Rep* 1992;41(43):814–815.
35. Khabbaz RF, Heneine W, George JR, et al. Brief report: infection of a laboratory worker with simian immunodeficiency virus. *N Engl J Med* 1994;330(3):172–177.
36. Glickman LT, Schantz PM. Epidemiology and pathogenesis of zoonotic toxocariasis. *Epidemiol Rev* 1981;3:230–250.
37. Saeed AM, Harris NV, DiGiacomo RF. The role of exposure to animals in the etiology of *Campylobacter jejuni/coli* enteritis. *Am J Epidemiol* 1993;137:108–114.
38. Croese J, Loukas A, Opdebeeck J, et al. Human enteric infection with canine hookworms. *Ann Intern Med* 1994;120:369–374.
39. Thompson C, Spielman A, Krause PJ. Coinfecting deer-associated zoonoses: Lyme disease, babesiosis and ehrlichiosis. *Clin Infect Dis* 2001;33:676–685.
40. Centers for Disease Control. Update: filovirus infection in animal handlers. *MMWR Morb Mortal Wkly Rep* 1990;39:221.
41. Peters CJ, Johnson ED, Jahrling PB. Filoviruses. In: Morse SS, ed. *Emerging viruses.* New York: Oxford University Press, 1993:159–175.
42. Gamble WG, Segal M, Schantz PM, et al. Alveolar hydatid disease in Minnesota: first human case acquired in the contiguous United States. *JAMA* 1979;241:904–907.
43. Mackenzie WR, Hoxie NJ, Proctor ME, et al. A massive outbreak in Milwaukee of *Cryptosporidium* infection transmitted through the public water supply. *N Engl J Med* 1994;331:161–167.
44. Duchin JS, Koster FT, Peters CJ, et al. Hantavirus pulmonary syndrome: a clinical description of 17 patients with a newly recognized disease. *N Engl J Med* 1994;330:949–955.
45. Nichol ST, Spiropoulou CF, Morzunov S, et al. Genetic identification of a hantavirus associated with an outbreak of acute respiratory illness. *Science* 1993;262:914–917.
46. Mayr B. Pets as permanent excretors of zoonoses pathogens. *Zentralbl Hyg Umweltmed* 1993;194:214–222.
47. Ries KM, White GL Jr, Murdock RT. Atypical mycobacterial infection caused by *Mycobacterium marinum* [Letter]. *N Engl J Med* 1990;322:633.

CHAPTER 160
Rabies

James E. Childs, Marta A. Guerra, and Charles E. Rupprecht

Rabies holds a special position in the universe of infectious diseases. The frightening circumstances leading to virus transmission, most often the bite from a "mad" dog, the fear of ensuing madness, and the nearly inevitable death that follows once clinical disease is apparent all contribute to the unique horror with which we regard rabies. It is a disease with one of the oldest pedigrees, recognizable as a malady of humans and animals from European, Middle Eastern, and Eastern texts dating from many centuries ago.

Rabies has been eliminated as a significant cause of human death in developed areas of the world. It is the only disease for which a vaccine is usually employed after the exposure, although preexposure prophylaxis is recommended for certain high-risk groups. Treatment with modern tissue culture vaccines, coupled with the appropriate use of immune globulin, is regarded as essentially 100% effective. Yet rabies remains a constant threat and the cause of more than 35,000 potentially preventable deaths per year in the developing world (1). Where human rabies has been eliminated or greatly reduced from historical levels, the economic costs of maintaining the programs that control and prevent the chain of events leading to human disease are formidable and beyond the grasp of many nations struggling with a host of other infectious diseases. Thus, human rabies is essentially a disease of poverty. The frustrations and conflict generated by the gap between scientific knowledge and product development and

their practical public health applications are nowhere more evident than with rabies. It is a preventable disease that has not been, and may not be for the foreseeable future, prevented over much of the globe. Rabies is an ancient disease that continues to challenge the way public health is practiced.

HISTORY

Early references to rabies can be found in ancient Babylonian, Greek, and Chinese texts. The genus to which the rabies virus now belongs, *Lyssavirus*, derives its name from the Greek word meaning "madness" (2). Observations found in these texts demonstrate that considerable knowledge of rabies was available in many cultures dating back thousands of years (3–5).

The history of rabies as a major cause of human disease is closely linked to the domestication of the dog. Although other carnivores, such as wolves, mongooses, and foxes, have played a role and continue to cause human exposures (6), no animal other than the dog has assumed this central role in maintaining and transmitting rabies virus to humans. It is now apparent that most of the dog rabies encountered by colonialists in the New World was initially imported from Europe with the transportation of domestic dogs incubating the infection. Comparisons of enzootic variants of dog rabies viruses collected from Asia, Africa, Europe, and the Americas by sequence analysis of the nucleocapsid (N) gene revealed that over broad geographic regions (including Europe, Africa, and the Americas), the limited variation of rabies virus strongly suggested a common European origin (7). Dogs have been imported into the New World since the sixteenth century (8), and most of the New World is still suffering the repercussions of this early transportation of animals.

The development of effective rabies vaccines for humans and domestic animals is one of the major success stories in infectious disease control and prevention. Louis Pasteur and his colleagues developed a "fixed" virus of high virulence and short incubation period (9). Through progressive attenuation of this virus, Pasteur produced, by a series of inoculations, a refractory state in dogs to subsequent intracerebral challenge with fully virulent rabies virus. Of additional major significance, Pasteur also demonstrated that his vaccine, consisting of progressively less attenuated preparations, was effective when used on dogs previously inoculated with rabies virus, demonstrating efficacy of the vaccine in postexposure treatment. This vaccine was first used successfully on a human, Joseph Meister, on July 6, 1885 (10), and similar treatments were subsequently used on thousands of exposed humans (11). Fermi and Semple introduced two improvements on the nervous tissue vaccines of Pasteur that allowed greater standardization of production. Phenol was used as a partial inactivating agent, and tissues used for vaccine were harvested at the same attenuation level and used for all injections in the series. The Fermi and Semple vaccines, made from sheep and goat brain, respectively, as well as the later Fuenzalida suckling mouse brain vaccine, have been used extensively in the past 80 years and still represent the most widely used rabies vaccines in Asia, Africa, and Latin America, which is about 90% of vaccine made and reported to the World Health Organization (WHO) (1). However, the high probability of adverse reactions associated with nervous tissue–derived vaccines, including neurologic complications such as meningitis and meningoencephalitis (12), gave added impetus to the development of highly immunogenic avian embryo– and cell culture–derived vaccines. Highly potent vaccines of tissue culture origin are now used to the exclusion of other rabies vaccines in developed nations, although the cost of these vaccines and the technology required

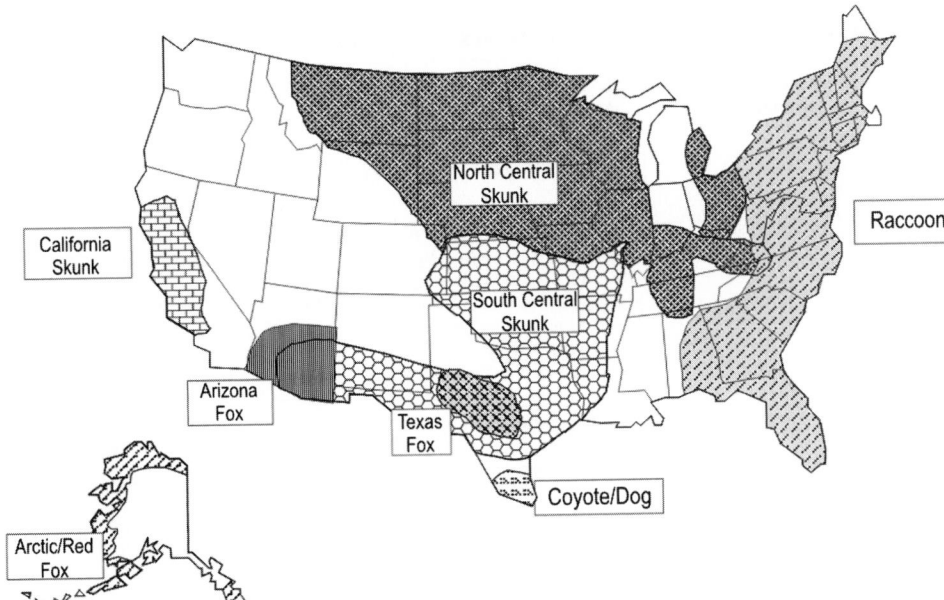

Figure 160.1. The approximate distributions of 8 genetically distinct rabies virus variants circulating in the United States, as of 2002, are indicated by shading patterns and labels. The virus variants depicted are maintained by terrestrial carnivore hosts (raccoon, skunk, fox, coyote) serving as reservoirs; rabies virus variants associated with various bat species (not shown) occur throughout the continental United States. The distribution of virus variants does not coincide with the geographic range of the host species, and a single species, such as the striped skunk, can act as a reservoir for multiple virus variants (see North Central Skunk and South Central Skunk in the figure). The rabies virus circulating in Puerto Rico (not shown) is a domestic dog variant.

to produce them have limited their availability in countries that require them most. The recommendation that immune globulin against rabies should be given in conjunction with vaccine (13) to ensure efficacy approaching 100% was a milestone in the evolution of effective treatment.

To date, the pathophysiology of rabies infection remains incompletely understood, although aspects of the molecular biology of viral replication and subsequent spread have been elucidated in detail. Some of the first observations of rabies at the cellular level were made in 1903 when Negri published his observations on pathology and described the cytoplasmic inclusion bodies that bear his name (14). Experiments involving amputations or neurectomies indicated that virus remained at local wound sites for prolonged periods (15) and spread as an ascending infection by retrograde axoplasmic flow (16) to the central nervous system, followed by centrifugal peripheral (anterograde) neural spread (17,18). The absolute neurotropism of rabies virus has been questioned because the initial site of replication may include myocytes (19). The long-term retention of virus within myocytes and the sequestering of virus in macrophages (20) have been proposed to explain the long incubation periods that occur with rabies (21). The virus has been found to spread to extraneural organs after infection of the central nervous system (22).

In the past two decades, a major leap in our understanding of the epidemiology of rabies has resulted from advances in the fields of immunology and molecular biology. In the late 1970s, monoclonal antibodies were used to demonstrate that antigenically unique variants of rabies virus circulate in different geographic areas and are usually associated with a primary reservoir species of carnivore or bat (23–25). Genetic analyses based on reverse transcription polymerase chain reaction (RT-PCR) and nucleic acid sequencing have permitted greater elucidation of the variability and specificity of rabies virus–host co-speciation and show promise in the area of disease diagnosis (7,26,27). These analyses have fundamentally changed the understanding of how different rabies viral variants are maintained and transmitted in distinct geographic regions (Fig. 160.1). Finally, only within the past few decades have methods been developed and adapted to the industrial scale, permitting public health officials to consider eliminating rabies within some terrestrial wildlife reservoirs. The rabies virus glycoprotein was one of the first genes to be incor-

porated into the vaccinia virus genome (28,29). These genetic constructs are now delivered in oral baits to wildlife in Europe (30,31) and the United States (32,33,34), an application of historical dimensions as the first use of a recombinant vaccine in the field. Research into rabies remains a dynamic field centuries after the disease was first described.

EPIDEMIOLOGY

Rabies is a zoonosis and is passed from human to human only under extraordinary circumstances (35). The epidemiology of human rabies is intimately linked to the cycles of virus maintenance in animals, and to understand the natural history of rabies that leads to human disease requires insight into wildlife ecology and animal behavior. Domestic and wild carnivores (e.g., foxes, skunks, raccoons) are the major reservoirs of terrestrial variants of the rabies virus (Table 160.1). Rabies in humans or animals is almost always the result of a bite containing rabies virus in the saliva. This tight linkage between animal rabies and human disease is best illustrated by the dramatic declines in human rabies that followed the initiation of effective animal control programs and the development of canine vaccines and vaccination campaigns (1,36). In the United States, the annual number of human rabies cases dropped from 100 per year during the early 1900s to 20 in 1951; during the past two decades, an average of less than two indigenously acquired cases have been reported annually. The cases of indigenously acquired rabies in the United States since 1980 have been caused primarily by virus variants maintained by insectivorous bats (26) (Fig. 160.2). In some cases of human rabies determined to be of canine origin, laboratory and epidemiologic data indicate that the exposures were received outside the United States (37,38). This decrease in the occurrence of human and domestic dog rabies has been accomplished at a time when wildlife rabies is at historically high levels, with 6,466 cases reported in 1999 (39). Thus, a central theme in the epidemiology of rabies has been established and used to guide our prevention strategies: effective control of dog-to-dog transmission, primarily through immunization, prevents human disease. This immune barrier in dogs also blocks the chain of events that could result in indirect transmission of wildlife variants of rabies virus to humans.

TABLE 160.1. Worldwide Distribution of Rabies and Rabies-related Viruses

Virus serotype/ genotype	Geographic region	Predominant animal cycle	Major animal affected	Comments
Rabies virus Serotype 1/genotype 1	North America	Wildlife	Raccoons, foxes, skunks, bats	Of 7,962 reported rabid animals in 1998, >92% wildlife in United States[a]
	Central America (including Mexico and the Caribbean islands)	Domestic	Dogs; cats and farm animals secondarily; vampire bat and mongoose rabies locally	Dog bite accounted for about 88% of reported human rabies
	South America	Domestic	Dogs; cats and farm animals secondarily; vampire bat rabies locally	Dog bite accounted for about 76% of reported human rabies
	Africa	Domestic	Dogs; cats and farm animals secondarily	Dog bite accounted for about 95% of reported human rabies
	Asia	Domestic	Dogs; cats and farm animals secondarily	Dog bite accounted for about 98% of reported human rabies
	Europe (Western)	Wildlife	Foxes, badgers, stone martens, bats	
	Europe (Eastern including Russian Federation)	Domestic	Dogs, cats, and farm animals	Dog bite accounted for about 29% of reported human rabies
	Oceania	Domestic	Dogs; cats and farm animals secondarily	
Lagos bat virus Serotype 2/genotype 2	Africa	Wildlife	Bats	Not identified as a human pathogen
Mokola virus Serotype 3/genotype 3	Africa	Wildlife	Bats	Not identified as a human pathogen
Duvenhage virus Serotype 4/genotype 4	South Africa	Wildlife	Bats	Caused rabies-like disease in humans
European bat lyssavirus 1 Genotype 5	Europe	Wildlife	Bats	Caused rabies-like disease in humans
European bat lyssavirus 2 Genotype 6	Europe	Wildlife	Bats	Caused rabies-like disease in humans
Australian bat lyssavirus Genotype 7	Australia[b]	Wildlife	Bats	Caused rabies-like disease in humans[b]

[a]Data from Krebs JW, et al. Rabies surveillance in the United States during 1998. *J Am Vet Med Assoc* 1999;215(12), with permission.
[b]Data from Scott JG. Australian bat lyssavirus: the public health response to an emerging infection. *Med J Aust*, 2000;172:573, with permission.
Except where noted, based on 1998 data of known animal exposures from World Health Organization. *World survey of rabies 34 for year 1998*. Geneva: World Health Organization, 2000:6, with permission.

In most areas of the world, accurate estimates of human rabies deaths or cases in animals are difficult to obtain because surveillance systems and regional diagnostic laboratories are inadequate or nonexistent. Annual reports of about 2,000 human deaths in Bangladesh and 30,000 deaths in India in 1998 convey a sense of the magnitude of the problem (1). In addition to deaths, 7.7 million persons received treatment for rabies exposure in the 60 of 92 rabies-endemic countries reporting to the WHO in 1998 (1). Most of these individuals received vaccines of nervous tissue origin, which translates into thousands of potentially serious adverse reactions. The incidence of rabies is highest among males and among individuals younger than 20 years old (40–43). Exposure to rabies has a seasonal and in some areas a cyclic component; cases of dog rabies occur most commonly in the spring or early summer (44,45). Bites to humans from dogs are also seasonal (46) and, like rabies, usually involve children (47). The risk for developing disease depends on the anatomic site and severity of the bite, the species inflicting the wound, and the virus variant (Fig. 160.2). However, in the United States, a clear history of animal bite has not been obtained in 24 of 32 cases that occurred between 1990 and 2000 (48,49). The indication that unnoticed exposure to bats may result in rabies transmission to humans has resulted in the additional recommendation to consider prophylaxis of individuals when bat bite cannot be ruled out (50) (Fig. 160.3).

Although animal bite remains the most important route of rabies virus transmission, cases of human rabies have been described after a variety of exposures. The best documented reports of human-to-human transmission involved eight recipients of transplanted corneas in France (51), the United States (52), Thailand (53), India (54), and Iran (55). Although human transplacental transmission of rabies virus has been reported in a single case (56), infants have survived delivery from mothers infected with rabies, when the child received postexposure treatment (57). Rabies infection presumably acquired by aerosol has been described in two persons visiting Frio cave in Texas, where millions of Mexican free-tailed bats congregate and where rabies virus is present in the bat population (58,59). Experimental studies with animals support the possibility of aerosol transmission under these exceptional circumstances (60). Laboratory exposure to aerosols has also resulted in infection (61). There is some documentation of natural rabies transmission by simple contact with virus-laden saliva or tissue (35,62), and isolated reports suggest infection after butchering of infected carcasses (63,64). Scratches from a rabid animal could potentially be contaminated with infectious saliva and, in the United States, are treated as an exposure, but documented cases of this injury leading to rabies are exceedingly rare (63,65,66).

In developing areas of the world, domestic dog rabies remains the most serious problem and results in tens of thousands of

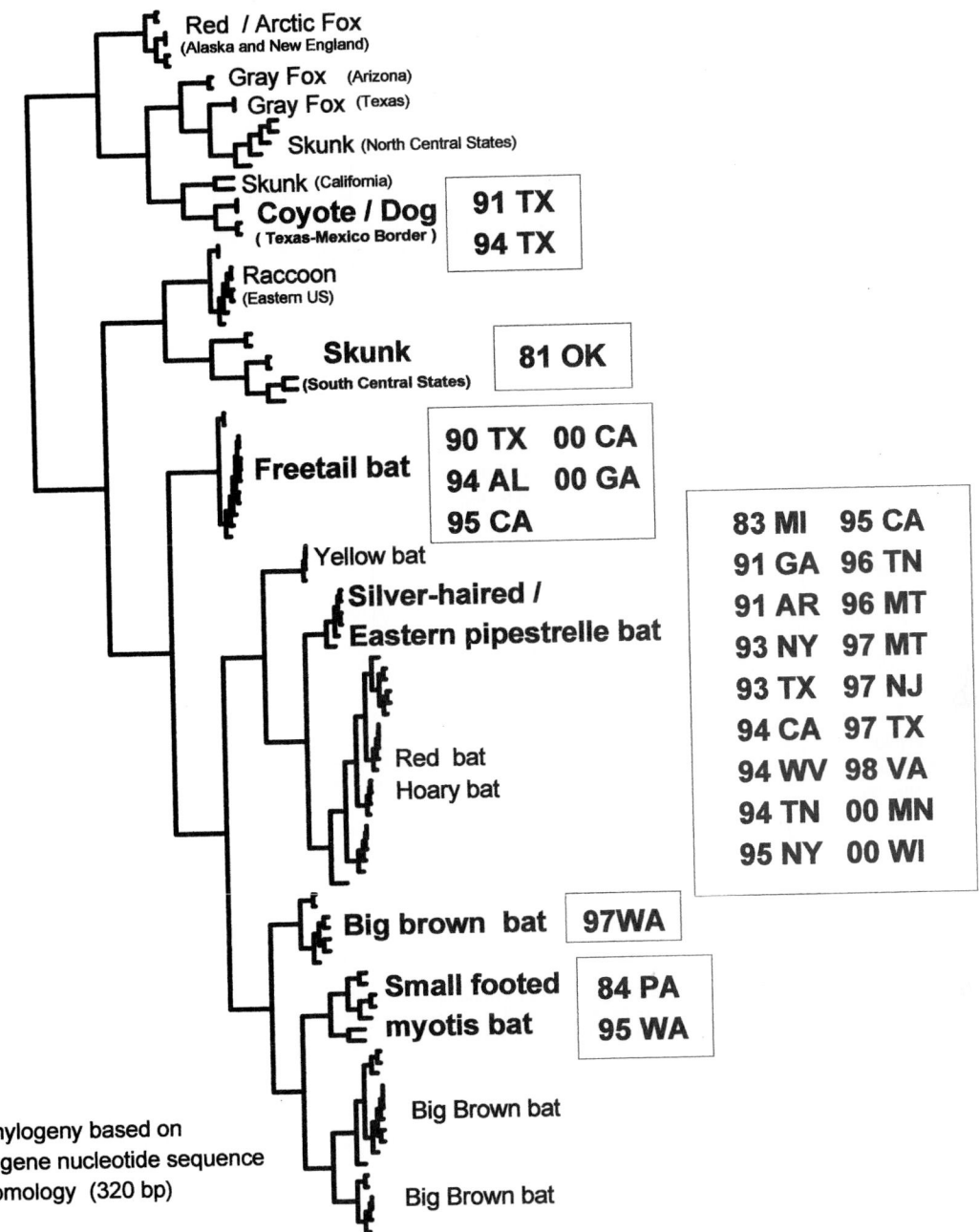

Within the figure:

Red / Arctic Fox (Alaska and New England)
Gray Fox (Arizona)
Gray Fox (Texas)
Skunk (North Central States)
Skunk (California)
Coyote / Dog (Texas-Mexico Border)

| 91 TX |
| 94 TX |

Raccoon (Eastern US)

Skunk (South Central States)

| 81 OK |

Freetail bat

90 TX	00 CA
94 AL	00 GA
95 CA	

Yellow bat
Silver-haired / Eastern pipestrelle bat
Red bat
Hoary bat

83 MI	95 CA
91 GA	96 TN
91 AR	96 MT
93 NY	97 MT
93 TX	97 NJ
94 CA	97 TX
94 WV	98 VA
94 TN	00 MN
95 NY	00 WI

Big brown bat

| 97WA |

Small footed myotis bat

| 84 PA |
| 95 WA |

Big Brown bat
Big Brown bat

Phylogeny based on N gene nucleotide sequence homology (320 bp)

Figure 160.2. Phylogeny of rabies virus variants in the United States and associated human deaths by state, 1981–2000. (From Smith JS: New aspects of rabies with emphasis on epidemiology, diagnosis, and prevention of the disease in the United States. *Clin Microbiol Rev* 1996;9:166–176, with permission.)

human deaths and millions of postexposure treatments each year (41,63). In some countries with enzootic canine rabies, past recommendations that advocated withholding postexposure treatment until a dog developed clinical rabies during a 10- to 14-day quarantine period have been reconsidered in favor of immediate treatment because of the high probability of rabies in dogs and short incubation after bites (67,68). Control of dog rabies in developing countries has been difficult to achieve for economic (69) as well as cultural (36) reasons. However, when large-scale canine vaccine campaigns are mounted in developing countries, they have the same dramatic effect on terminating epidemics of human and canine rabies (70,71). Vaccine coverage of 70% has been estimated to be sufficient to prevent at least 96.5% of po-

tential outbreaks of dog rabies (72). Vaccines designed for oral uptake and delivered in baits show promise for immunizing free-ranging dogs in developing countries (73–76).

Although dogs may in certain rare circumstances survive rabies infection and "carry" virus asymptomatically (77), this finding has not been shown to be epidemiologically important. Dogs can be naturally infected with other lyssaviruses, such as Mokola (78) and Lagos bat (79), but a significant role as reservoirs or vectors has not been suggested.

Wildlife species involved in rabies cycles vary with region. In North America, raccoons, skunks, foxes, and bats (several species) are the major wildlife reservoirs of rabies. Less is known about terrestrial wildlife reservoirs in Latin America,

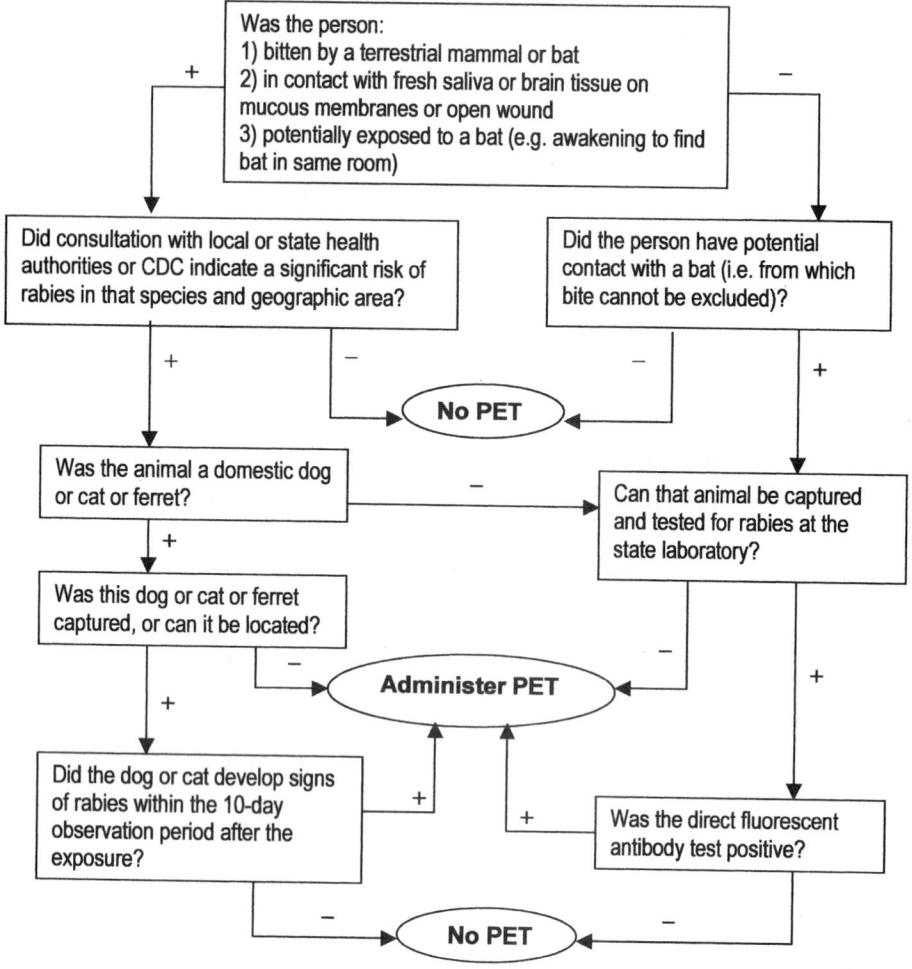

Figure 160.3. An algorithm for the administration of rabies postexposure prophylaxis. PET, postexposure treatment; CDC, Centers for Disease Control and Prevention; RVA, rabies vaccine absorbed; HDCV, human diploid cell vaccine; PCEC, purified chick embryo cell vaccine, IM, intramuscularly; HRIG, human rabies immune globulin. (Adapted with permission from Fishbein DB. Rabies in humans. In: Baer GM, ed. *The natural history of rabies*, 2nd ed. Boca Raton, FL: CRC Press, 1991:519–549, with permission. Copyright © 1991 CRC Press, Boca Raton, Florida.).

Notes:
1. Unless person previously received rabies immunoprophylaxis, PET consists of 5 doses (IM in the deltoid region) of HDCV, PCEC, or RVA on days 0, 3, 7, 14 and 28 and 1 dose of HRIG (divided between the bite site and IM in the gluteal region) on day 0.
2. This algorithm only addresses rabies prevention. Obviously, other treatments such as wound care and antibiotics may be indicated.
3. In the event that the biting animal is captured and tests negative after PET has begun, PET may be discontinued.

although vampire bat–transmitted rabies, which affects cattle and occasionally humans, is of special concern in some regions from northern Mexico to northern Argentina (80,81). Mongooses on some islands in the Caribbean (e.g., Puerto Rico), introduced to control rats and snakes in sugarcane fields, have provided a wildlife reservoir for rabies (82). Globally, rabies and other *Lyssavirus* infections of bats are widespread (83–84) and, although transmission cycles are distinct from those of terrestrial rabies, can occasionally spill over to terrestrial mammals (85).

Rabies in animals is considered a density-dependent disease. Population dynamics of reservoir hosts are regarded as critical to understanding the temporal and spatial patterns of wildlife rabies (86–88). Environmental factors, including habitat heterogeneity, play a major role in the rate of spread and persistence of the disease (89,90). Furthermore, multispecies interactions complicate the understanding of the ecology and epidemiology of rabies (91). Spillover of infection from the dominant reservoir of a region to other species is well documented (39), but the processes by which new epizootics and variants of ra-

bies virus emerge in different reservoir species are unknown. After epizootic rabies has abated, terrestrial reservoir populations are decreased. Reports of animal rabies in a given locale can decline precipitously, and rabies may disappear from regions for some time before reappearing (91). Some countries have eliminated or remain free of rabies for extended periods (1) (Table 160.2).

Rabies virus isolates from different geographic areas can be antigenically and genetically variable; at least five major antigenic variants from terrestrial carnivores (Fig. 160.1) are currently defined by monoclonal antibody analysis from 10 geographically overlapping areas of enzootic rabies in the United States (39,92). European isolates of rabies from terrestrial mammals are predominantly the red fox rabies virus variant (23).

Rabies virus variants circulating in bats are antigenically and genetically distinct from those associated with terrestrial carnivores and indicate largely independent transmission cycles of rabies (92–94). Rabies has been reported in more than 30 species of bats in the United States since the 1950s and occurs in each of the contiguous 48 states (95). Variants of rabies virus associated

TABLE 160.2. **Countries Not Reporting Animal or Human Rabies in 1998**[a]

Geographic region	Countries
Americas	Bahamas, Barbados, St. Kitts and Nevis, St. Vincent and the Grenadines, Uruguay
Africa	Cape Verde, Comoros, Libyan Arab Jamahiriya, Mauritius, Reunion, Seychelles
Asia	Bahrain, Brunei Darussalam, Cyprus, Hong Kong, Japan, Kuwait, Malaysia (Sabah), Malaysia (Sarawak), Qatar, Singapore
Europe	Albania, Andorra, Finland, Greece, Iceland, Ireland, Italy, Jersey Channel Islands, Luxembourg, Malta, Macedonia, Norway, Portugal, Sweden, Switzerland, United Kingdom of Great Britain
Oceania	Australia, Cook Islands, Fiji, French Polynesia, Guam, Kiribati, New Caledonia, New Zealand, Palau, Papua New Guinea, Samoa, Vanuatu

[a]Surveillance and reporting for rabies varies by country. Inclusion in this table does not necessarily indicate rabies-free status.
Based on 1998 data from World Health Organization. *World Survey of rabies 34 for year 1998*. Geneva: World Health Organization, 2001:15–24, with permission.

with bats have been responsible for 26 of 32 cases of human rabies reported from the United States from 1990 to 2000 (26,49) and 1 case in Canada (96). The rabies variant most commonly associated with human cases is recovered primarily from eastern pipistrelle and silver-haired bats (26), species rarely encountered or tested (97).

Two cases of human infection with rabies-related viruses have been reported from Europe (98). The viruses in European bats have been shown to be genetically unique and perhaps most similar to Duvenhage virus (98), and they may constitute two unique genotypes of *Lyssavirus* (99). There have been scattered reports of "rabid" bats from Asia, and bats infected with other lyssaviruses are found in Africa, but no isolates of rabies virus, serotype 1, have been collected from bats from either continent (100). Bats in Australia maintain a unique *Lyssavirus* that can cause a human disease clinically indistinguishable from rabies (83).

CLINICAL PRESENTATION

The clinical presentation of rabies is commonly reported as either "furious" and "paralytic" or "dumb"(101–105). Persons with rabies commonly present with a combination of symptoms, and attempts to distinguish between furious and paralytic forms may not serve to aid the diagnosis. Human disease resulting from exposures to the same animal species, and even the same animal, has resulted in cases with both clinical presentations (105). Human clinical presentation may be more dependent on inherent host factors than the exposing animal or virus virulence (103,106).

The course of human rabies infection generally progresses through five clinical phases: incubation, prodrome, neurologic phase, coma, and either death or recovery (107). The temporal lines separating phases are indistinct; however, each phase is marked by differing clinical presentations (Table 160.3).

Incubation

Although the usual period of incubation of rabies is 30 to 90 days, this phase is highly variable (41,104,107). In the extremes, incubation periods from 5 days to more than 19 years have been reported, but the chance of unknown or unreported exposures must be considered in these cases (20).

The period of incubation seems dependent on several factors. Bites on the head and neck or bites received in highly innervated areas, such as the face, hands, or genitalia (41,101,104,107), or higher titer of virus in the inoculum, shorten the incubation period. Children generally progress more quickly through the clinical stages (101,104,107). Finally, virus virulence and host immune status undoubtedly play important, although as yet undetermined, roles in disease progression. The administration of a full or partial course of postexposure treatment does not appear to alter the incubation period among those who subsequently develop rabies (41,106,108).

Prodrome

After the subclinical incubation period follows the prodromal phase of nonspecific symptoms. The local and systemic symptoms that last from several hours to several days are not

TABLE 160.3. **Hypothetical Human Rabies Clinical Phase Time Line**

	Exposure	First symptom	First neurologic sign	Coma onset	Death occurs or recovery begins
	Incubation	Prodrome	Neurologic phase	Coma	Recovery
Usual duration	30–80 days (variable)	Hours to days	2–7 days	0–14 days	Months
Main clinical signs	None	Fever	Hyperventilation	Pituitary dysfunction	
		Anorexia, nausea, vomiting	Hypoxia	Hypoventilation	
		Headache	Aphasia	Apnea	
		Malaise, lethargy	Incoordination	Hypotension	
		Pain or paresthesia at site	Paresis, paralysis	Cardiac arrhythmias	
		Anxiety, agitation	Pharyngeal spasms	Cardiac arrest	
		Depression	Hydrophobia	Coma	
			Marked hyperactivity	Pneumothorax	
			Confusion, delirium	Intravascular thrombosis	
			Hallucinations	Secondary infections	

Modified from Hattwick MAW. Human rabies. *Public Health Rev* 1994;3:229–274, with permission.

pathognomonic for rabies and may serve to direct the clinician's initial diagnostic efforts away from rabies. A common symptom is pain, numbness, or tingling at or near the inoculation site (101,102,104,106,l07). Additional manifestations may include vomiting, abdominal pain, muscle pain, weakness, and general malaise (fever, chills, headache) (101,102,104,105,107). Both local and systemic signs are probably due to the virus' replication in dorsal root ganglia and the central nervous system (107). The nonspecific nature of the initial presentation of the disease, coupled with the relative rarity of rabies in developed countries, helps to explain why many rabies diagnoses are made only post-mortem (26,38,109).

Neurologic Phase

The neurologic phase begins when central nervous system dysfunction dominates the clinical picture and generally lasts from 2 to 7 days. Hyperactivity and restlessness are common early features, which progress to marked agitation and nervousness. Hydrophobia presents in variable degrees and may not be initially obvious. Rather than a true fear of water, the response more probably represents a respiratory tract reflex resulting from central nervous system dysfunction. In addition to the mere proximity to water or liquid, reflex gagging and muscle fasciculations may be triggered by an attendant's touch or the anticipation of being touched, especially on the head or neck (101,103,106,107,110). Mental status continues to deteriorate until sudden death or coma results.

Ascending paralysis similar to that in Guillain-Barré syndrome is a less common manifestation of rabies in which mental status is preserved until much later in the clinical course. Average survival times are longer than in the more common hyperactive form (102,104,106). This clinical presentation occurs only rarely in the United States, and no clear molecular or epidemiologic explanation for this difference in presentation has been described. Finally, cardiac involvement with or without accompanying cardiovascular signs (111–114) and sexual manifestations, such as penile hyperexcitability and priapism, have been reported (115–117).

Tetanus, delirium tremens, poliomyelitis, Guillain-Barré syndrome, herpesvirus encephalitis, and arbovirus encephalitis should be differentiated from rabies early in the clinical course to focus treatment efforts and to minimize exposures among attending medical personnel.

Coma

Heralded by apneustic breathing patterns, this phase is reached when the central nervous system dysfunction results in generalized paralysis.

Death or Recovery

Death related to cerebral or cardiovascular dysfunction follows coma within hours or a few days unless intensive medical assistance is available. Among 25 human cases in the United States between 1980 and 1996, the average time from onset of clinical signs to death was 15.7 days (range, 6 to 32 days) (26).

There have been at least four reported instances of recovery from clinical rabies. A 6-year-old boy bitten by a bat developed clinical rabies after completing a 14-day course of duck embryo vaccine prophylaxis and experienced a complete recovery (118). A 45-year-old woman bitten by a rabid dog developed rabies (119) after receiving 12 daily doses of suckling mouse brain rabies vaccine and recovered over a 13-month period. Only partial

recovery occurred in the other two cases: a 32-year-old male laboratory technician who developed rabies about 45 days after exposure to modified live rabies vaccine (120) and a 9-year-old boy bitten by a rabid dog (121) and treated with rabies vaccine produced in Vero cells with a final dose of human diploid cell vaccine (HDCV).

TREATMENT OF CLINICAL RABIES

Intensive therapy for rabies patients is costly and nearly always futile, and some physicians have questioned its rationale (122). Nevertheless, such therapeutic efforts can delay the disease progression, and care providers continue to gain experience in preventing and controlling the many presenting complications.

Early consideration of rabies as a differential diagnosis is essential in anticipating these complications and instituting isolation procedures for the protection of attending medical personnel (105,123,124). These isolation precautions should be aimed at preventing contact with potentially infectious body fluids, including saliva, cerebrospinal fluid (CSF), and tears (107,123,125). Blood and feces are not considered infectious (50,123,125).

Once the neurologic phase is reached, intensive care and patient isolation become necessary (124). Because of the altered mentation and involuntary muscle activity associated with rabies, sedation and analgesia are important. Respiratory, cardiovascular, and neurologic complications require the most therapeutic attention. A common neurologic complication is increased intracranial pressure caused by cerebral edema resulting from hypoxia or inflammation of the brainstem resulting in localized swelling, occlusion of the cerebral aqueduct, and internal hydrocephalus (107). When hypoxia is successfully managed, complications due to cerebral edema occur less frequently (107).

Death most commonly results from the complications of hypoxemia, cardiac arrhythmias, cerebral edema, fluid imbalance, and hypotension (122). The concurrent presentation of multiple complications further frustrates therapy. Iatrogenic and nosocomial complications may appear at any time, although they are most common during the coma phase and probably correlated with the duration of hospitalization (107). These include thrombosis of the superior vena cava secondary to indwelling cardiac catheters, bilateral tension pneumothorax secondary to cardiac resuscitation, and opportunistic bacterial infections during prolonged disease progression (107).

Intravenous and intrathecal ribavirin therapy has not proved successful against human rabies infections (105,126). Similarly, vaccine and immune globulin administration, initiated after the onset of clinical signs, has not shown any positive effect and may quicken the disease progression (122,123,127). Finally, although high-dose interferon-α has not altered the eventual outcome (126), its use may delay the clinical progression, thus allowing more intensive and specific therapies (122,123).

LABORATORY DIAGNOSIS

In most countries of the world, the majority of human and animal rabies cases reported to the WHO are diagnosed solely on the basis of clinical presentation (1). This section deals with laboratory methods used to confirm a clinical diagnosis.

The diagnosis of human rabies depends on the isolation of virus; the demonstration of viral antigen or nucleic acid in saliva, corneal impressions, or tissue biopsy material; or the finding of specific antibody in serum (of previously unvaccinated persons) or CSF (128). Fluorescent antibody methods for antigen detection are the best available tests for the rapid diagnosis of rabies, and, since the 1980s, the use of monoclonal antibodies has allowed further epidemiologic typing of rabies viruses by their antigenic profiles (23,24,129,130). Virus isolation remains an important complement to direct fluorescent antibody (DFA) testing and provides material to further characterize the isolate. Nucleic acid–based detection systems using RT-PCR amplification are theoretically more sensitive than antigen-based detection and are being used by many laboratories as investigational new diagnostic tests (26,109,131). However, their cost, analysis time, and potential for contamination are drawbacks.

Virus isolation from infected tissues, saliva, throat swabs, and swabs of the nasal mucosa or eyes can be achieved by using a variety of cell lines or by direct intercerebral inoculation of laboratory rodents (132). Virus isolated in culture is identified in infected cells by the DFA test, but genetic assays may also be employed. Infected tissues may also be examined with hematoxylin-eosin or the Mann stain for the presence of pink-, lilac-, or red-staining cytoplasmic inclusions (Negri bodies) (14). Negri bodies are pathognomonic for rabies; however, in some cases, they may be absent, difficult to locate, or confused with other viral inclusions in some species (e.g., the Lentz bodies of canine distemper) (132). Intracerebral mouse inoculation using the specimens previously mentioned is a reliable method for isolating rabies virus and was the gold standard for rabies diagnosis to which DFA and cell culture isolation were compared. Suckling or weanling mice are preferred and should be checked at least daily until day 28 for paralysis, which typically occurs between days 5 and 12 (132,133). Confirmation of rabies in mice is usually performed with the DFA test on brain tissue.

The most widely used diagnostic test is the DFA test for detection of rabies antigen contained in intracytoplasmic inclusions, and the sensitivity and specificity approach 100% when guidelines for its use are followed (134,135). When it is applied antemortem, the materials most commonly tested are skin biopsy specimens (frequently obtained from the neck or scalp where the density of hair follicles is high) (136,137) and corneal impressions (1,138,139). A positive test result with these specimens is adequate to confirm a diagnosis of rabies, but a negative finding does not exclude the diagnosis (26). The sensitivity of all assays varies with the laboratory, the timing of specimen collection with regard to disease onset and viral dissemination, and the condition of the specimens when tested (26,140). For optimal postmortem diagnosis of rabies, samples of the hippocampus, cerebellum, and brainstem or spinal cord should be tested (134). Although usually fresh or frozen brain tissue has been used as the diagnostic tissue, formalin-fixed brain tissue may also be used in the DFA (41). Monoclonal antibodies applied to fresh frozen tissues can be used to characterize the antigenic variant responsible for infection and provide inferences about the animal species responsible for the exposure. Other labeled antibodies (e.g., horseradish peroxidase) have been applied to the diagnosis of rabies with good results (142,143); these methods have the advantage of employing conventional microscopy.

Serologic tests that measure antibody binding (e.g., indirect fluorescent antibody or enzyme immunoassay tests) or function (e.g., complement fixation or neutralization) can be useful in the diagnosis of human or animal rabies (26). Assays exist that readily distinguish between immunoglobulin G and immunoglobulin M (144). The finding of antibody in CSF can be an indication of intrathecal production and interpreted as indicating central nervous system infection. The finding of CSF antibody with oligoclonal bands has been used to support a documented human survival from rabies (121). Care must be taken in interpreting CSF results because of the risk for introducing serum antibody into the sample during the procedure and leakage across the blood–brain barrier (137). Binding assays, such as the indirect fluorescent antibody test or enzyme immunoassay, may be more sensitive than neutralizing assays in detecting early antibody (144,145). Serologic methods are also employed in documenting the immune response after rabies vaccination and in monitoring the immunologic status of individuals in high-risk professions to determine the necessity for boosters (50). In the United States, the test of choice is the rapid fluorescent focus inhibition test (146), a modified standard neutralization assay that replaced the *in vivo* mouse neutralization test; antibody titers can be converted to international units. Successful immunization is measured by the presence of a titer of 1:5 or greater (complete neutralization) with this fluorescent inhibition test, or about 0.5 IU, in sera collected 2 to 4 weeks after preexposure or postexposure prophylaxis (50).

Nucleic acid detection (based on RT-PCR) potentially offers considerable advantages in sensitivity over other assay systems and is the test of choice for slightly decomposed tissue (131). Single-step and nested RT-PCR methods have been developed (131,147). An added advantage of obtaining DNA fragments is that these can be sequenced and analyzed with existing databases of rabies virus variants to discriminate between virus variants that are identical by monoclonal antibody techniques (7,27,85,92). RT-PCR has already taken a place in many diagnostic laboratories as a complementary, but not a replacement, diagnostic and epidemiologic tool (26). The specialized equipment, expense of reagents, and potential for contamination of samples limit the widespread use of these methods in many laboratories without strong research missions.

PREVENTION

Prevention of rabies is best achieved by eliminating human exposure to rabid animals through both effective vaccination programs for domestic species and education of the public concerning the hazards of contact with certain wildlife. Mention has already been made of the effectiveness of rabies control efforts aimed at canine populations in both developed and developing nations. This section concentrates on preexposure and postexposure prophylaxis of individuals potentially exposed to the rabies virus and emerging methods for control of rabies in wildlife reservoirs.

Human-to-human transmission of rabies through the transplantation of corneas has been well documented, and recommendations for prevention exist (148). Rabies acquired by a physician during an autopsy has also been reported (149). Transmission through bites, saliva, or other contact with humans is rare, with two documented, but not laboratory-confirmed, cases in Ethiopia (35). The early consideration of rabies in any patient with clinical encephalitis and the initiation of contact isolation to exclude exposure to the patient's infectious tissues or fluids are the best methods of prevention (125). Laboratory transmission of rabies is preventable through preexposure prophylaxis and appropriate biosafety recommendations (150). The overwhelming majority of individuals who receive immunotherapy for prevention of rabies are vaccinated after the exposing event. Because the most important route of rabies transmission is through animal bite, essential preventative therapy begins with the careful cleansing of the wound with soap and water (or the cationic detergent benzalkonium chloride) (50,151,152).

The first problem facing the care provider is to assess the need for postexposure treatment (Table 160.4; Fig. 160.3) and whether treatment should be initiated immediately (e.g., is the biting animal a healthy dog, cat, or ferret available for 10-day quarantine or a wild animal unavailable for testing?). If treatment is

TABLE 160.4.   Postexposure Treatment (PET) Guide for the United States (ACIP) and Other Countries (WHO)

Guideline	ACIP	Expert committees WHO
Categories for assessing need for PET	Two categories considered, bite and nonbite. PET warranted if potential exposure to rabies virus by either route. Bite includes any penetration of skin. Nonbite exposures include scratches, abrasions, open wounds, or mucous membrane contaminated with saliva or other potentially infectious material (such as brain) from a rabid animal. Contact with a bat, where bite cannot be excluded, may also warrant PET.	Three categories of exposure (I–III). Category I (touching or feeding of rabid animal or licks on intact skin) does not warrant PET. Category II includes nibbling of uncovered skin, minor scratches or abrasions without bleeding, or licks on broken skin. Category III includes single or multiple transdermal bites or scratches or contamination of mucous membrane with saliva.
Recommended use of rabies immuneglobulin	Always given as part of PET, except when appropriate or proven effective preexposure prophylaxis has been previously given (see Table 160.5). Only products of human origin (HRIG; 20 IU/kg body weight) used in the United States.	Only given immediately with category III exposures. Both equine (40 IU/kg body weight) and human (20 IU/kg) products are recommended.
Use of rabies vaccine	Always part of PET and given intramuscularly. Can be halted if subsequent information indicates that animal is not rabid.[a]	Administered immediately with category II and III exposures. Can be given intradermally with rabies immune globulin. Can be halted if subsequent information indicates that animal is not rabid.[a]
Vaccine regimens	If previously vaccinated, then HRIG is not administered, and vaccine (HDVC, PCEC, or RVA) is given at 1.0 mL on days 0 and 3 (see Table 160.5). If not previously vaccinated, HRIG is administered, and vaccine is given at 1.0 mL on days 0, 3, 7, 14, and 28. Vaccine is never given intradermally.	Various tissue culture or purified duck or chick embryo vaccines are considered appropriate. A schedule similar to that of ACIP and an abbreviated schedule are recognized for 1.0-mL IM applications. An intradermal schedule using 0.1 mL of vaccine is also appropriate. For nervous tissue–derived vaccines, national authorities must be consulted.

ACIP, Advisory Committee on Immunization Practices; WHO, World Health Organization; HRIG, human rabies immune globulin; HDCV, human diploid cell vaccine; RVA, rabies vaccine adsorbed: PCEC, purified chick embryo cell vaccine.
[a]If a previously healthy dog or cat is involved in the biting incident, treatment can be delayed in some situations and in some countries during a 10-day observation period. If the dog or cat remains healthy during the 10-day incubation period, treatment can be stopped. If the animal is killed, tested for rabies, and found to be negative, treatment can be stopped.
Data from Centers for Disease Control and Prevention. Rabies prevention—United States, 1999. Recommendations of the Immunization Practices Advisory Committee (ACIP). *MMWR Morb Mortal Wkly Rep* 1999;48(RR-1):1–21, with permission; and World Health Organization: Expert Committee on Rabies. *Eighth report.* Geneva: World Health Organization, 1992:84, with permission.

required, human rabies immune globulin (HRIG) and the first of five vaccine doses are administered simultaneously (50). Equine immune globulin is less expensive than HRIG and is used in many parts of the world. Purified commercial equine immune globulin is considered a safe and effective product, although adverse reactions such as serum sickness are reported in 1% to 6% of recipients, depending on the product manufacturer (153,154). HRIG is administered at 20 IU/kg and equine immune globulin at 40 IU/kg, with the full dose infiltrated around the wound sites when anatomically feasible (50). HRIG should never be administered in the same syringe or at the same anatomic site as vaccine. If HRIG administration is delayed, it can be used through day 7 after the initial vaccine dose (50) but is not indicated after that because of the active induction of antibody and the potential interference with normal immune responses (155). Three vaccines, purified chick embryo cell (PCEC), HDCV, and rabies vaccine absorbed (RVA), are licensed for preexposure and postexposure treatment in the United States, and all can be used in the postexposure regimens described in Table 160.4 (50). Only intramuscular vaccines are available because the intradermal vaccine is no longer manufactured (156). It is important for physicians in the United States to recognize that the recommendations of the Advisory Committee on Immunization Practices for rabies postexposure treatment differ from those promulgated by the WHO (157). HRIG is used whenever vaccine is warranted according to Advisory Committee on Immunization Practices guidelines, but is restricted to category III exposures by the WHO.

Preexposure prophylaxis (Table 160.5) is offered only to individuals in high-risk occupational groups (veterinarians, animal handlers, and certain laboratory workers) and international travelers visiting locations considered to be high risk for exposure

and where access to medical care is limited (50). Preexposure vaccination does not eliminate the need for wound treatment and vaccination after exposure; however, the requirement for HRIG is obviated and the postexposure series is reduced to two 1.0-mL doses (Table 160.5). Booster doses of vaccine are recommended for some individuals who have received the preexposure series if their serum antibody titer falls to less than 1:5 (50) (Table 160.4). There is no requirement to test serum directly after the preexposure series because numerous studies have indicated nearly 100% immunologic response (50,158); immunity is long term, perhaps lifelong, in many recipients, and repeated boosters offer an additional measure of security (159).

Although not necessarily cost-effective (160), the preexposure prophylaxis of travelers is a luxury that many individuals choose. An important complication for preexposure vaccination that is most relevant to foreign travelers is the inhibitory effect of antimalarial drugs (e.g., chloroquine phosphate) on the development of the immune response (161,162). The 1.0-mL intramuscular route of vaccination should be employed, with individuals receiving concurrent chloroquine (50).

Postexposure protection achieved by proper wound treatment and use of modern tissue culture-derived vaccines with immune globulin is considered near 100% (158). However, postexposure vaccine failures have been reported when immune globulin has not been given (13) and in rare instances when appropriate postexposure treatment was given (163). Surgery under ketamine anesthesia, possibly resulting in depression of the immune response, has been suggested as a possible contribution to postexposure treatment failure (164). Strict adherence to recognized protocols for rabies management is critical (165,166). Elderly, obese, or immunocompromised individuals may not

TABLE 160.5.   Preexposure Prophylaxis Requirements and Schedules

Requirement for preexposure immunization	Route	Schedule
Preexposure vaccination should be given if exposure is continuous (e.g., rabies research laboratory workers, rabies biologicals production workers), frequent (rabies diagnostic laboratory workers, mammalogists, spelunkers, veterinarians and staff; animal control and wildlife workers in rabies epizootic areas; travelers visiting foreign areas of enzootic rabies for more than 30 d), or in some cases infrequent (veterinarians and animal control and wildlife workers in areas of low endemicity or veterinary students)	IM	HDCV, PCEC, or RVA, 1.0 mL in deltoid region on days 0, 7, and 21 or 28
Routine boosters after primary series[a]	IM	HDCV, PCEC, or RVA, 1.0 mL in deltoid area on day 0
Postexposure treatment for previously vaccinated persons	IM	HDCV, PCEC, or RVA, 1.0 mL in deltoid area on day 0 and 3; HRIG or other immune globulins not administered

IM, intramuscular; HRIG, human rabies immune globulin; HDCV, human diploid cell vaccine; RVA, rabies vaccine adsorbed; PCEC, purified chick embryo cell vaccine.
[a]For continuous exposures, booster is recommended if the antibody titer falls below 1:5 by rapid fluorescent focus inhibition testing done at 6-mo intervals. For frequent exposures, serologic testing and boosting, if necessary, are done at 2-y intervals.
Data from Centers for Disease Control and Prevention. Rabies prevention—United States, 1999. Recommendations of the Immunization Practices Advisory Committee (ACIP). *MMWR Morb Mortal Wkly Rep* 1999;48 (RR-1):1–21, with permission.

respond optimally to rabies preexposure (or postexposure) immunization, and a sixth dose of vaccine has been suggested by some for individuals older than 50 years, but the epidemiological data for this recommendation are not compelling (167). Very young age (50) and pregnancy (168) are not reasons to withhold treatment.

Both local and systemic adverse reactions are reported in preexposure and postexposure vaccinations. Local reactions among recipients of HDCV and HRIG include pain, redness, swelling, and itching; systemic reactions include fever, nausea, vomiting, lethargy, anorexia, general malaise, headache, immune complex–like disease, and rarely Guillain-Barré syndrome (169–173). Local reactions have been reported among 19% to 74% of recipients, whereas systemic reactions have been reported among 5% to 40% of recipients (50,170–172,174). Local reactions are usually manifested within a day or two, but the usual period between immunization and onset of systemic reactions is within 21 days, although longer periods have been reported (169,175). Reports of complications following PCEC are similarly rare (50,176).

Common local adverse reactions are treated symptomatically, if at all, and only rarely justify discontinuation of preventative immunotherapy (177). Systemic reactions appear to occur without relation to age, route, or timing of primary or booster vaccination, history of allergies, or history of immunization with products other than HDCV (178). As with local reactions, systemic reactions rarely preclude the necessity of continuing with a postexposure treatment regimen.

The ultimate prevention strategy for rabies is to eliminate the infection in animal reservoirs. Although control programs aimed at domestic animal populations dramatically reduce human deaths, they are expensive and must be maintained indefinitely in countries like the United States, where wildlife rabies is a constant threat. The successful use of modified live rabies vaccines designed for oral immunization and distributed in baits to immunize red foxes in Europe has demonstrated the potential to control terrestrial cycles of rabies (179,180). Efforts to control fox

and skunk rabies in Ontario, Canada, are promising and illustrate the difficulties in designing control programs when multiple species are involved (181). Recombinant rabies vaccines are now being used against red foxes in several countries in Europe (30,31,179,182), in raccoons in several states in the eastern United States (183), and in gray foxes and coyotes in Texas (184).

THE FUTURE

It has been more than 20 years since the advent of the HDCV, which revolutionized rabies vaccination, but most of the world continues to use multiple inoculations of neural tissue–based biologics (1,185). Although the HDCV and its modern progenitors from Vero cells and avian embryo-derived sources were important advances (186), issues of cost and availability are matters of major concern. Potent, safe, and inexpensive human rabies vaccines are still needed throughout the world. Less expensive but equally efficacious replacements for immune globulins of human or animal origin are also necessary, perhaps through murine, humanized, or human monoclonal antibodies (187). This development depends on identifying conserved *Lyssavirus* epitopes of immunologic relevance, to limit the number of hybridomas contained within any treatment "cocktail," without sacrificing efficacy or cost. The current Advisory Committee on Immunization Practices' five-dose cell culture vaccine treatment protocol is a major improvement over the required 14 to 28 doses of neural vaccines of the past century, but in the near future, it may be feasible to reconsider a further reduction in schedules and the potential elimination of immune globulin. If efficacious cytokine inducers or related immune mediators (188) are identified as the critical elements of human immunoprotection against rabies, a single inoculation with protection of lifetime duration may be within reach. Concomitant with a heightened focus on prevention of rabies among humans should be increased concentration on disease control in the animal reservoirs. Currently, wildlife rabies constitutes the ultimate source of most human and domestic exposures in the United States, Canada, and much of Europe. Research has progressed rapidly on the development of attenuated and genetically engineered vaccines for rabies in the past three decades. These products show great promise of being safe and effective oral vaccines for foxes, raccoons, and related wild carnivores, with more than 100 million doses delivered over 5 million km² in Europe to date (189). However, little attention has been paid to the feral dog in the same capacity, despite the paramount role of canine rabies in human mortality. In contrast to the more than half-dozen different vaccine types used in the field for wildlife, only two biologics have demonstrated preliminary oral efficacy in the dog under laboratory conditions (190). Given the close relationship between humans and domestic animals, additional safety considerations are inherent in the environmental release of organisms intended for canine use. Once this challenge is met, oral vaccination of the free-ranging dog may become a critical adjunct to traditional parenteral induction of herd immunity in the pariah animal.

REFERENCES

1. World Health Organization. *World survey of rabies no. 34 for year 1998.* Geneva: World Health Organization, 2000:1–31.
2. *Webster's ninth new collegiate dictionary.* Springfield, MA: Merriam-Webster, 1989.
3. Tierkel ES. Rabies. *Adv Vet Sci* 1959;5:183.
4. Steele JH, Fernandez PJ. History of rabies and global aspects. In: Baer GM, ed. *The natural history of rabies,* 2nd ed. Boca Raton, FL: CRC Press, 1991:24.
5. Yu WZ. Notes on Chinese medical history. *J Tradit Chin Med* 1985;5:232.
6. Fleming G. *Animal plagues.* London: Bailliere, 1882.
7. Smith JS, Orciari LA, Yager PA, et al. Epidemiologic and historical relationships among 87 rabies virus isolates as determined by limited sequence analysis. *J Infect Dis* 1992;166:296.
8. Varner JG, Varner JJ. *Dogs of conquest.* Norman, OK: University of Oklahoma Press, 1983:238.
9. Pasteur L. Nouvelle communication sur la rage. *C R Acad Sci* 1884;98:457.
10. Pasteur L. Méthode pour prévenir la rage après morsure. *C R Acad Sci* 1885;101:765.
11. Perrin P, Lafon M, Sureau P. Rabies vaccines from Pasteur's time up to experimental subunit vaccines today. *Adv Biotechnol Processes* 1990;14:325.
12. Hemachudha T, Phanuphak P, Johnson RT, et al. Neurologic complications of Semple-type rabies vaccine. *Neurology* 1987;37:550–556.
13. Devriendt J, Staroukine M, Costy F, et al. Fatal encephalitis apparently due to rabies. *JAMA* 1982;248:2304.
14. Negri A. Beitrag zum Studium der Aetiologie der Tollwurth. *Z Hyg Infektionskr* 1903;43:507.
15. Baer GM, Cleary WF. A model in mice for the pathogenesis and treatment of rabies. *J Infect Dis* 1972;125:520.
16. Tsiang H. Evidence for an intraaxonal transport of fixed and street rabies virus. *J Neuropathol Exp Neurol* 1979;38:286.
17. Murphy FA, Bauer SP, Harrison AK, et al. Comparative pathogenesis of rabies: viral infection and transit from inoculation site to the central nervous system. *Lab Invest* 1973;28:361.
18. Tsiang H, Lycke E, Ceccaldi PE, et al. The anterograde transport of rabies virus in rat sensory dorsal root ganglia neurons. *J Gen Virol* 1989;70:2075.
19. Shankar V, Dietzschold B, Koprowski H. Direct entry of rabies virus into the central nervous system without prior local replication. *J Virol* 1991;65:2736.
20. Charlton KM. The pathogenesis of rabies and other lyssaviral infections: recent studies. *Curr Top Microbiol Immunol* 1994;187:95.
21. Ray NB, Ewalt LC, Lodmell DL. Rabies virus replication in primary murine bone marrow macrophages and in human and murine macrophage-like cell lines: implications for viral persistence. *J Virol* 1995;69:764.
22. Jackson AC, Ye H, Phelan CC, et al. Extraneural involvement in human rabies. *Lab Invest* 1999;79(8):945–951.
23. Sureau P, Rollin P, Wiktor TJ. Epidemiologic analysis of antigenic variations of street rabies virus: detection by monoclonal antibodies. *Am J Epidemiol* 1983;117:605.
24. Rupprecht CE, Glickman LT, Spencer PA, et al. Epidemiology of rabies virus variants: differentiation using monoclonal antibodies and discriminant analysis. *Am J Epidemiol* 1987;126:298.
25. Smith JS, Reid Sanden FL, Roumillat LF, et al. Demonstration of antigenic variation among rabies virus isolates by using monoclonal antibodies to nucleocapsid proteins. *J Clin Microbiol* 1986;24:573.
26. Noah DL, Drenzek CL, Smith JS, et al. The epidemiology of human rabies in the United States, 1980 to 1996. *Ann Intern Med* 1998;128:922.
27. Smith JS, Orciari LA, Yager PA. Molecular epidemiology of rabies in the United States. *Semin Virol* 1995;6:387.
28. Wiktor TJ, Macfarlan RI, Reagan KJ, et al. Protection from rabies by a vaccinia virus recombinant containing the rabies virus glycoprotein gene. *Proc Natl Acad Sci USA* 1984;81:7194.
29. Kieny MP, Lathe R, Drillien R, et al. Expression of rabies virus glycoprotein from a recombinant vaccinia virus. *Nature* 1984;312:163.
30. Pastoret PP, Brochier B, Languet B, et al. First field trial of fox vaccination against rabies using a vaccinia-rabies recombinant virus. *Vet Rec* 1988;123:481.
31. Brochier B, Kieny MP, Costy F, et al. Large-scale eradication of rabies using recombinant vaccinia rabies vaccine. *Nature* 1991;354:520.
32. Rupprecht CE, Wiktor TJ, Johnston DH, et al. Oral immunization and protection of raccoons (*Procyon lotor*) with a vaccinia-rabies glycoprotein recombinant virus vaccine. *Proc Natl Acad Sci USA* 1986;83:7947.
33. Fearneyhough MG, Wilson PJ, Clark KA, et al. Results of an oral rabies vaccination program for coyotes. *J Am Vet Med Assoc* 1998;212:498.
34. Hanlon CA, Niezgoda M, Hamir AN, et al. First North American field release of a vaccinia-rabies glycoprotein recombinant virus. *J Wildl Dis* 1998;34:228.
35. Fekadu M, Endeshaw T, Alemu W, et al. Possible human-to-human transmission of rabies in Ethiopia. *Ethiopian Med J* 1996;34:123.
36. Beran GW, Frith M. Domestic animal rabies control: an overview. *Rev Infect Dis* 1988;10[Suppl 4]:S672.
37. Smith JS, Fishbein DB, Rupprecht CE, et al. Unexplained rabies in three immigrants in the United States: a virologic investigation. *N Engl J Med* 1991;324:205.
38. Centers for Disease Control and Prevention. Human rabies: New Hampshire, 1996. *MMWR Morbid Mortal Wkly Rep* 1997;46:267.
39. Krebs JW, Strine TW, Smith JS, et al. Rabies surveillance in the United States during 1999. *J Am Vet Med Assoc* 2000;205:1695.
40. Bhatia R, Bhardwaj M, Sehgal S. Canine rabies in and around Delhi: a 16 years study. *J Commun Dis* 1988;20:104.
41. Lakhanpal U, Sharma RC. An epidemiological study of 177 cases of human rabies. *Int J Epidemiol* 1985;14:614.
42. Eng TR, Fishbein DB, Talamante HE, et al. Urban epizootic of rabies in Mexico: epidemiology and impact of animal bite injuries. *Bull W H O* 1993;71:615.
43. Swaddiwudhipong W, Tiyacharoensri C, Singhachai C, et al. Epidemiology of human rabies post-exposure prophylaxis in Bangkok 1984–1986. *Southeast Asian J Trop Med Public Health* 1988;19:563.
44. Kappus KD. Canine rabies in the United States, 1971–1973: study of reported cases with reference to vaccination history. *Am J Epidemiol* 1976;103:242.
45. Ernst SN, Fabrega F. A time series analysis of the rabies control programme in Chile. *Epidemiol Infect* 1989;103:651.
46. Beck AM, Loring H, Lockwood R. The ecology of dog bite injury in St. Louis, Missouri. *Public Health Rep* 1975;90:262.
47. Bhanganada K, Wilde H, Sakolsataydorn P, et al. Dog-bite injuries at a Bangkok teaching hospital. *Acta Trop* (Basel) 1993;55:249.
48. Krebs JW, Smith JS, Rupprecht CS, et al. Mammalian reservoirs and epidemiology of rabies diagnosed in human beings in the United States, 1981–1998. *Ann N Y Acad Sci* 2000;916:345.
49. Centers for Disease Control and Prevention. Human rabies—California, Georgia, Minnesota, and Wisconsin, 2000. *MMWR Morb Mortal Wkly Rep* 2000;49:1111.
50. Centers for Disease Control. *Rabies prevention: United States, 1999.* Recommendations of the Immunization Practices Advisory Committee (ACIP). *MMWR Morb Mortal Wkly Rep* 1999;48(RR-1):1–21.
51. Centers for Disease Control and Prevention. Human-to-human transmission of rabies via a corneal transplant—France. *MMWR Morb Mortal Wkly Rep* 1980;29:25.
52. Houff SA, Burton RC, Wilson RW, et al. Human-to-human transmission of rabies virus by corneal transplant. *N Engl J Med* 1979;300:603.
53. Centers for Disease Control. Human-to-human transmission of rabies via corneal transplant—Thailand. *MMWR Morb Mortal Wkly Rep* 1981;30:473.
54. Gode GR, Bhide NK. Two rabies deaths after corneal grafts from one donor. *Lancet* 1988;2:791.
55. World Health Organization. Two rabies cases following corneal transplantation. *Wkly Epidemiol Rec* 1994;44:330.
56. Sipahioglu U, Alpaut S. Transplacental rabies in humans (in Turkish). *Mikrobiyol Bul* 1985;19:95.
57. Lumbiganon P, Wasi C. Survival after rabies immunisation in newborn infant of affected mother [Letter]. *Lancet* 1990;336:319.
58. Irons JV, Eads RB, Grimes JE, et al. The public health importance of bats. *Tex Rep Biol Med* 1957;15:292.
59. Humphrey GL, Kemp GE, Wood EG. A fatal case of rabies in a woman bitten by an insectivorous bat. *Public Health Rep* 1960;75:317.
60. Constantine DG. Rabies transmission by nonbite route. *Public Health Rep* 1962;77:287.
61. Winkler WG, Fashinell TR, Leffingwell L, et al. Airborne rabies transmission in a laboratory worker. *JAMA* 1973;226:1219.
62. Leach CN, Johnson HN. Human rabies with special reference to virus distribution and titer. *Am Soc Trop Med Hyg* 1940;20:335.
63. Kureishi A, Xu LZ, Wu H, et al. Rabies in China: recommendations for control. *Bull W H O* 1992;70:443.
64. Tariq WU, Shafi MS, Jamal S, et al. Rabies in man handling infected calf [Letter]. *Lancet* 1991;337:1224.
65. Tuncman ZM. A rare case of rabies without a bite. *Trop Dis Bull* 1949;46:139.
66. Babes V. *Traité de la Rage.* Paris: Bailliere, 1921:119.

67. Wilde H, Chutivongse S, Hemachudha T. Rabies and its prevention. *Med J Aust* 1994;160:83.
68. Wilde H, Choomkasien P, Hemachudha T, et al. Failure of rabies postexposure treatment in Thailand. *Vaccine* 1989;7:49.
69. Bogel K, Meslin FX. Economics of human and canine rabies elimination: guidelines for programme orientation. *Bull W H O* 1990;68:281.
70. Chomel B, Chappuis G, Bullon F, et al. Mass vaccination campaign against rabies: are dogs correctly protected? The Peruvian experience. *Rev Infect Dis* 1988;10[Suppl 4]:S697.
71. Belotto AJ. Organization of mass vaccination for dog rabies in Brazil. *Rev Infect Dis* 1988;10[Suppl 4]:S693.
72. Coleman PG, Dye C. Immunization coverage required to prevent outbreaks of dog rabies. *Vaccine* 1996;14:185–186.
73. Haddad N, Ben Khelifa R, Matter H, et al. Assay of oral vaccination of dogs against rabies in Tunisia with the vaccinal strain SADBern. *Vaccine* 1994;12:307.
74. Frontini MG, Fishbein DB, Garza Ramos J, et al. A field evaluation in Mexico of four baits for oral rabies vaccination of dogs. *Am J Trop Med Hyg* 1992;47:310.
75. Orciari LA, Niezgoda M, Hanlon CA, et al. Rapid clearance of SAG-2 rabies virus from dogs after oral vaccination. *Vaccine* 2001;19:4511.
76. Matter HC, Schumacher CL, Kharmachi H, et al. Field evaluation of two bait delivery systems for the oral immunization of dogs against rabies in Tunisia. *Vaccine* 1998;16:657.
77. Fekadu M, Shaddock JH, Chandler FW, et al. Rabies virus in the tonsils of a carrier dog. *Arch Virol* 1983;78:37.
78. Foggin CM. Mokola virus infection in cats and a dog in Zimbabwe. *Vet Rec* 1983;113:115.
79. Mebatsion T, Cox JH, Frost JW. Isolation and characterization of 115 street rabies isolates from Ethiopia by using monoclonal antibodies. *J Infect Dis* 1992;166:972.
80. Martinez-Burnes J, Lopez A, Medellin J, et al. An outbreak of vampire bat-transmitted rabies in cattle in northeastern Mexico. *Can Vet J* 1997;38:175–177.
81. Lopez A, Miranda P, Tejada E, et al. Outbreak of human rabies in the Peruvian jungle. *Lancet* 1992;339:408.
82. Everard CO, Everard JD. Mongoose rabies. *Rev Infect Dis* 1988;10[Suppl 4]:5610.
83. Scott JG. Australian bat lyssavirus: the public health response to an emerging infection. *Med J Aust* 2000;172:573.
84. de Mattos CA, Favi M, Yung V, et al. Bat rabies in urban centers in Chile. *J Wildl Dis* 2000;36:231.
85. McQuiston JH, Yager PA, Smith JS, et al. Epidemiologic characteristics of rabies virus variants in dogs and cats in the United States. *J Am Vet Med Assoc* 2001;218:1939–1942.
86. Bacon PJ. *Population dynamics of rabies in wildlife.* New York: Academic Press, 1985:358.
87. Thulke H, Tischendorf L, Staubach C, et al. The spatio-temporal dynamics of a post-vaccination resurgence of rabies in foxes and emergency vaccination planning. *Prev Vet Med* 2000;47:1–21.
88. Childs JE, Curns AT, Dey ME, et al. Predicting the local dynamics of epizootic rabies among raccoons in the United States. *Proc Natl Acad Sci USA* 2000;97:140.
89. Deal B, Farello C, Lancaster M, et al. A dynamic model of the spatial spread of an infectious disease: the case of fox rabies in Illinois. *Environ Modeling Assess* 2000;5:47.
90. Wandeler AI, Capt S, Gerber H, et al. Rabies epidemiology, natural barriers and fox vaccination. *Parassitologia* 1988;30:53.
91. Carey AB, McLean RG. The ecology of rabies: evidence of coadaptation. *J Appl Ecol* 1983;20:777.
92. Smith JS. New aspects of rabies with emphasis on epidemiology, diagnosis, and prevention of the disease in the United States. *Clin Microbiol Rev* 1996;9:166–176.
93. Smith JS. Monoclonal antibody studies of rabies in insectivorous bats of the United States. *Rev Infect Dis* 1988;10[Suppl 4]:S637.
94. Nadin-Davis SA, Huang W, Armstrong J, et al. Antigenic and genetic divergence of rabies viruses from bat species indigenous to Canada. *Virus Res* 2001;74:139–156.
95. Constantine DG. An updated list of rabies-infected bats in North America. *J Wildl Dis* 1979;15:347.
96. Turgeon N, Tucci M, Deshaies D, et al. Human rabies in Montreal, Quebec—October, 2000. *Can Commun Dis Rep* 2000;26(24):209.
97. Childs JE, Trimarchi CV, Krebs JW. The epidemiology of bat rabies in New York State, 1988–1992. *Epidemiol Infect* 1994;113:501.
98. Schneider LG, Cox JH. Bat lyssaviruses in Europe. *Curr Top Microbiol Immunol* 1994;187:207.
99. Bourhy H, Kissi B, Tordo N. Molecular diversity of the *Lyssavirus* genus. *Virology* 1993;194:70.
100. Pal SR, Arora B, Chuttani PN, et al. Rabies virus infection of a flying fox bat, *Pteropus poliocephalus* in Chandigarh, northern India. *Trop Geogr Med* 1980;32:265.
101. Toltzis P. Viral encephalitis. *Adv Pediatr Infect Dis* 1991;6:111.
102. Hatchett RP. Rabies: the disease and the value of intensive care treatment. *Intensive Care Nurs* 1991;7:53.
103. Tirawatnpong S, Hemachudha T, Manutsathit S, et al. Regional distribution of rabies viral antigen in central nervous system of human encephalitic and paralytic rabies. *J Neurol Sci* 1989;92:91.
104. Warrell DA. The clinical picture of rabies in man. *Trans R Soc Trop Med Hyg* 1976;70:188.
105. Hemachudha T. Human rabies: clinical aspects, pathogenesis, and potential therapy. *Curr Top Microbiol Immunol* 1994;187:121.
106. Chopra JS, Banerjee AK, Murthy JMK, et al. Paralytic rabies: a clinico-pathological study. *Brain* 1980;103:789.
107. Hattwick MAW. Human rabies. *Public Health Rev* 1974;3:229.
108. Held JR, Tierkel ES, Steele JH. Rabies in man and animals in the United States, 1946–1965. *Public Health Rep* 1967;82:1009.
109. Centers for Disease Control and Prevention. Human rabies—Montana and Washington, 1997. *MMWR Morb Mortal Wkly Rep* 1997;46:770–774.
110. Verma AK, Maheswari MC, Chawdhary C, et al. Acute ascending motor paralysis due to rabies: a clinicopathological report. *Eur Neurol* 1985;24:160.
111. Morais CF, Assis RVC. Cardiac involvement in human rabies: case report. *Rev Inst Med Trop Sao Paulo* 1985;27:145.
112. Araujo MF, Brito T, Machado CG. Myocarditis in human rabies. *Rev Inst Med Trop Sao Paulo* 1971;13:99.
113. Cheetham HD, Hart J, Coghill NF, et al. Rabies with myocarditis: two cases in England. *Lancet* 1970;1:921.
114. Raman GV, Prosser A, Spreadbury PL, et al. Rabies presenting with myocarditis and encephalitis. *J Infect* 1988;17:155.
115. Madhusadana SN. Rabies presenting with sexual manifestations. *J Indian Med Assoc* 1988;86:43.
116. Bhandari M, Kumar S. Penile hyperexcitability as the presenting symptom of rabies. *Br J Urol* 1986;58:224.
117. Udwadia ZF, Udwadia FE, Rao PP, et al. Penile hyperexcitability with recurrent ejaculations as the presenting manifestation of a case of rabies. *Postgrad Med J* 1988;64:85.
118. Hattwick MAW, Weiss TT, Stechsulte CJ, et al. Recovery from rabies: a case report. *Ann Intern Med* 1972;76:931.
119. Porras C, Barboza JJ, Fuenzalida E, et al. Recovery from rabies in man. *Ann Intern Med* 1976;85:44.
120. Centers for Disease Control. Rabies in a laboratory worker—New York. *MMWR Morb Mortal Wkly Rep* 1977;76:183.
121. Alvarez L, Fajardo R, Lopez E, et al. Partial recovery from rabies in a nine-year-old boy. *Pediatr Infect Dis J* 1994;13:1154.
122. Fishbein DB. Rabies in humans. In: Baer GM, ed. *The natural history of rabies,* 2nd ed. Boca Raton, FL: CRC Press, 1991:549.
123. Bernard KW. Clinical rabies in humans. In: Fishbein DB, Sawyer LA, Winkler WG, eds. *Rabies concepts for medical professionals,* 2nd ed. Miami: Mérieux Institute, 1986:48.
124. Ferguson CF. Human rabies. *Am J Nurs* 1981;81:1175.
125. Helmick CG, Tauxe RV, Vernon AA. Is there a risk to contacts of patients with rabies? *Rev Infect Dis* 1987;9:511.
126. Warrell MJ, White NJ, Looareesuwan S, et al. Failure of interferon alfa and tribavirin in rabies encephalitis. *BMJ* 1989;299:830.
127. Dutta JK, Dutta TK. Treatment of clinical rabies in man: drug therapy and other measures. *Int J Clin Pharmacol Ther* 1994;32:594.
128. Baer GM, ed. *The natural history of rabies,* 2nd ed. Boca Raton, FL: CRC Press, 1991.
129. Smith JS, Sumner JW, Roumillat LF, et al. Antigenic characteristics of isolates associated with a new epizootic of raccoon rabies in the United States. *J Infect Dis* 1984;149:769.
130. Rollin PE, Sureau P. Monoclonal antibodies as a tool for rabies epidemiological studies. *Dev Biol Stand* 1984;57:193.
131. Kamolvarin N, Tirawatnpong T, Rattanasiwanmoke R, et al. Diagnosis of rabies by polymerase chain reaction with nested primers. *J Infect Dis* 1993;167:207.
132. Sureau P, Ravisse P, Rollin PE. Rabies diagnosis by animal inoculation, identification of Negri bodies, or ELISA. In: Baer GM, ed. *The natural history of rabies,* 2nd ed. Boca Raton, FL: CRC Press, 1991:217.
133. Johnson HN, Emmons RW. Rabies virus. In: Lennette EH, ed. *Laboratory diagnosis of viral infections,* 2nd ed. New York: Marcel Dekker, 1992:684.
134. Trimarchi CV, Debbie JG. The fluorescent antibody in rabies. In: Baer GM, ed. *The natural history of rabies,* 2nd ed. Boca Raton, FL: CRC Press, 1991:233.
135. McQueen JL, Lewis AL, Schneider NJ. Rabies diagnosis by fluorescent antibody: its evaluation in a public health laboratory. *Am J Public Health* 1960;50:1743.
136. Blenden DC, Bell JF, Tsao AT, et al. Immunofluorescent examination of the skin of rabies-infected animals as a means of early detection of rabies virus antigen. *J Clin Microbiol* 18:631.
137. Warrell MJ, Looareesuwan S, Manatsathit S, et al. Rapid diagnosis of rabies and post-vaccinal encephalitides. *Clin Exp Immunol* 1988;71:229.
138. Schneider LG. The cornea test: a new method for the intravitam diagnosis of rabies. *Zentralbl Veterinarmed [B]* 1969;16:24.
139. Larghi OP, Gonzalez E, Held JR. Evaluation of the corneal test as a laboratory method for rabies diagnosis. *Appl Microbiol* 1973;25:187.
140. Lewis VJ, Thacker WL. Limitations of deteriorated tissue for rabies diagnosis. *Health Lab Sci* 1974;11:8.
141. Whitfield SG, Fekadu M, Shaddock JH, et al. A comparative study of the fluorescent antibody test for rabies diagnosis in fresh and formalin-fixed brain tissue specimens. *J Virol Methods* 2001;95:145–151.
142. Hamir AN, Moser G. Immunoperoxidase test for rabies: utility as a diagnostic test. *J Vet Diagn Invest* 1994;6:148.
143. Zimmer K, Wiegand D, Manz D, et al. Evaluation of five different methods for routine diagnosis of rabies. *Zentralbl Veterinarmed [B]* 1990;37:392.

144. Savy V, Atanasiu P. Rapid immunoenzymatic technique for titration of rabies antibodies IgG and IgM. *Dev Biol Stand* 1978;40:247.

145. Smith JS. Rabies serology. In: Baer GM, ed. *The natural history of rabies*, 2nd ed. Boca Raton, FL: CRC Press, 1991:252.

146. Smith JS, Yager PA, Baer GM. A rapid reproducible test for determining rabies neutralizing antibody. *Bull W H O* 1973;48:535.

147. Ermine A, Larzul D, Ceccaldi PE, et al. Polymerase chain reaction amplification of rabies virus nucleic acids from total mouse brain RNA. *Mol Cell Probes* 1990;4:189.

148. Gottesdiener KM. Transplanted infections: donor-to-host transmission with the allograft. *Ann Intern Med* 1989;110:1001.

149. Anonymous. Necrology (death from autopsical injury or infection). *JAMA* 1891;16:576.

150. Richardson JH, Barkeley WEE. *Biosafety in microbiological and biomedical laboratories*, 2nd ed. Department of Health and Human Services Publication (CDC) 88-8395. Washington, DC: U.S. Government Printing Office, 1988:100.

151. Dean DJ, Baer GM, Thompson WR. Studies on local treatment of rabies infected wounds. *Bull W H O* 1963;28:477.

152. Wiktor T, Koprowski H. Action locale de certains medicaments sur l'infection rabique de la souris. *Bull W H O* 1963;28:487.

153. Wilde H, Chomchey P, Prakongsri S, et al. Adverse effects of equine rabies immune globulin. *Vaccine* 1989;7:10.

154. Wilde H, Chutivongse S. Equine rabies immune globulin: a product with an undeserved poor reputation. *Am J Trop Med Hyg* 1990;42:175.

155. Glhck R, Wegmann A, Keller H, et al. Human rabies immunoglobulin assayed by the rapid fluorescent focus inhibition test suppresses active rabies immunization. *J Biol Stand* 1987;15:177.

156. Aventis Pasteur Inc. Letter addressing discontinuation of ID vaccine, March 12, 2001.

157. World Health Organization: Expert Committee on Rabies. *Eighth report*. Geneva: World Health Organization, 1992:84.

158. Thraenhart O, Marcus I, Kreuzfelder E. Current and future immunoprophylaxis against human rabies: reduction of treatment failures and errors. *Curr Top Microbiol Immunol* 1994;187:173.

159. Thraenhart O, Kreuzfelder E, Hillebrandt M, et al. Long-term humoral and cellular immunity after vaccination with cell culture rabies vaccines in man. *Clin Immunol Immunopathol* 1994;71:287.

160. Bernard KW, Fishbein DB. Pre-exposure rabies prophylaxis for travellers: are the benefits worth the cost? *Vaccine* 1991;9:833.

161. Bernard KW, Fishbein DB, Miller KD, et al. Pre-exposure rabies immunization with human diploid cell vaccine: decreased antibody responses in persons immunized in developing countries. *Am J Trop Med Hyg* 1985;34:633.

162. Pappaioanou M, Fishbein DB, Dreesen DW, et al. Antibody response to pre-exposure human diploid-cell rabies vaccine given concurrently with chloroquine. *N Engl J Med* 1986;314:280.

163. Raguin G, Nemeth J, Wassef M, et al. Additional reports of failure to respond to treatment after rabies exposure in Thailand. *Clin Infect Dis* 1999;28:143–144.

164. Fescharek R, Franke V, Samuel MR. Do anaesthetics and surgical stress increase the risk of post-exposure rabies treatment failure? *Vaccine* 1994;12:12.

165. Baer GM, Fishbein DB. Rabies post-exposure prophylaxis. *N Engl J Med* 1987;316:1270.

166. Fishbein DB, Arcangeli S. Rabies prevention in primary care: a four-step approach. *Postgrad Med* 1987;82:83.

167. Mastroeni I, Vescia N, Pompa MG, et al. Immune response of the elderly to rabies vaccines. *Vaccine* 1994;12:518.

168. Chutivongse S, Wilde H, Benjavongkulchai M, et al. Postexposure rabies vaccination during pregnancy: effect on 202 women and their infants. *J Infect Dis* 1995;20:818.

169. Dreesen DW, Bernard KW, Parker RA, et al. Immune complex-like disease in 23 persons following a booster dose of rabies human diploid cell vaccine. *Vaccine* 1986;4:45.

170. Anderson LJ, Winkler WG. The Centers for Disease Control's experience with a human diploid cell rabies vaccine. *Curr Chemother Infect Dis* 1980:1357.

171. Anderson LJ, Winkler WG, Hafkin B, et al. Clinical experience with a human diploid cell rabies vaccine. *JAMA* 1980;244:781.

172. Fishbein DB, Dreesen DW, Holmes DF, et al. Human diploid cell rabies vaccine purified by zonal centrifugation: a controlled study of antibody response and side effects following primary and booster pre-exposure immunizations. *Vaccine* 1989;7:437.

173. Bernard KW, Mallonee J, Wright JC, et al. Preexposure immunization with intradermal human diploid cell rabies vaccine: risks and benefits of primary and booster vaccination. *JAMA* 1987;257:1059.

174. Anderson LJ, Sikes RK, Langkop CW, et al. Postexposure trial of a human diploid cell strain rabies vaccine. *J Infect Dis* 1980;142:133.

175. Gamboa ET, Cowen D, Eggers A, et al. Delayed onset of postrabies vaccination encephalitis. *Ann Neurol* 1983;13:676.

176. Wasi C, Chaipraisithikul P, Thongcharoen P, et al. Progress and achievement of rabies control in Thailand. *Vaccine* 1997;15:7–11.

177. Nicholson KG, Turner GS, Aoki FY. Immunization with a human diploid cell strain of rabies virus vaccine: two year results. *J Infect Dis* 1978;137:783.

178. Nicholson KG. Rabies. *Lancet* 1990;335:1201.

179. Muller WW. Where do we stand with oral vaccination of foxes against rabies in Europe? *Arch Virol Suppl* 1997;13:83–94.

180. Aubert MF, Masson E, Artois M, et al. Oral wildlife rabies vaccination field trials in Europe, with recent emphasis on France. *Curr Top Microbiol Immunol* 1994;187:219.

181. Campbell JB. Oral rabies immunization of wildlife and dogs: challenges to the Americas. *Curr Top Microbiol Immunol* 1994;187:245.

182. Brochier B, Boulanger D, Costy F, et al. Towards rabies elimination in Belgium by fox vaccination using a vaccinia-rabies glycoprotein recombinant virus. *Vaccine* 1994;12:1368.

183. Rupprecht CE, Smith JS. Raccoon rabies: the re-emergence of an epizootic in a densely populated area. *Semin Virol* 1994;5:155.

184. Clark KA, Neill SU, Smith JS, et al. Epizootic canine rabies transmitted by coyotes in south Texas. *J Am Vet Med Assoc* 1994;204:536.

185. World Health Organization. *World survey of rabies no. 34 for the year 1998*. Geneva: World Health Organization, 1998:37.

186. Celis E, Rupprecht CE, Plotkin S. New and improved vaccines against rabies. In: Woodrow GC, Levine MM, eds. *New generation vaccines*. New York: Marcel Dekker, 1990:438.

187. Rupprecht CE, Shankar V, Hanlon CA, et al. Beyond Pasteur to 2001: future trends in lyssavirus research? *Curr Top Microbiol Immunol* 1994;187:325.

188. Baer GM. Animal models in the pathogenesis and treatment of rabies. *Rev Infect Dis* 1988;10[Suppl 4]:S739.

189. Stohr K, Meslin F-X. Progress and setbacks in oral immunization of foxes against rabies in Europe. *Vet Rec* 1996;139:32–35.

190. World Health Organization. *Report of the 5th Consultation on Oral Immunization of Dogs Against Rabies*. Geneva: World Health Organization, 1994:24.

CHAPTER 161
Bites

Fredrick M. Abrahamian and Ellie J. C. Goldstein

It is estimated that half of all Americans will be bitten by an animal or another human at some point in their lifetime (1). Dog, cat, and human bites account for the bulk of all mammalian bite injuries in the United States. Most animal bites result in minor injuries, and only about 15% to 20% of individuals bitten seek medical attention. Nevertheless, nearly 1% of all emergency department (ED) visits are related to animal and human bites (1). Because bites are common injuries for which patients seek medical attention, physicians' familiarity with this topic is essential. This chapter focuses on the epidemiology, microbiology, management, and complications of animal and human bites.

ANIMAL BITES

Epidemiology

Dog bites account for most mammalian bite injuries. More than 50 million dogs are kept as pets in about 35% of American families (2). Annually, more than 4 million and 200,000 individuals are bitten by dogs in the United States and United Kingdom, respectively (2,3). Each year, about 20 deaths are attributed to dog bites in the United States (2,4,5). It is estimated that for each U.S. dog bite fatality, there are about 670 hospitalizations, 16,000 ED visits, and 21,000 other medical visits (office and clinic) (4). Dog bite–related injuries constitute as many as 0.3% to 1.1% of all ED visits in the United States (4). Although these statistics are significant, it is believed that the true incidence of dog bite–related injuries is significantly underestimated (6,7). The accurate incidence of dog bites is difficult to quantify because there is no standardized national reporting system for nonfatal dog bite injuries, and not all patients injured by a dog seek medical attention.

Most dog bites occur in children and adult males (median age, 15 years) (4,6,8–10). A survey conducted among school-aged children in Pennsylvania found that 46% of children had been bitten by a dog by the time they reached twelfth grade (6). In comparison to older adults, children are more likely to sustain injuries that are fatal or require medical attention (2,5). Children are unable to defend themselves and, due to their short stature, are more vulnerable to head and neck injuries. They also have less muscle mass, which makes underlying organs and bony structures more vulnerable to injuries. In a U.S. survey of fatal dog attacks from 1989 to 1994, of the 109 dog bite–related fatalities, 57% were in children younger than 10 years of age. Similarly, in 1995 to 1996, of the 25 dog bite–related fatalities, 80% occurred among children younger than 12 years of age (11).

Most dog attacks occur during the summer, weekends, and afternoons and at or near the vicinity of the victim's home (4). The attacking dog is commonly known by the victim, and in most instances, the incident was provoked. In adults, the location of the bite is typically the upper (62%) and lower (20%) extremities (8,12). Bites to the hands make up the bulk of the injuries in the upper extremities. Head and neck injuries are more prevalent in children (7,9,10). The most commonly reported breeds implicated in dog bite–related injuries are medium to larger dogs such as pit bulls, German shepherds, rottweilers, and huskies (5,7–11). Although some dog breeds have received more media attention for their aggressive behavior than others, it is important to consider other factors, such as a dog's training, its quality of life and care, circumstances of the bite, and behavior of the victim, before blaming the incident entirely on the animal.

With more than 30% of American families owning cats, cat bites constitute the second most common type of mammalian bites in the United States (10). Unlike dog bites, cat bites occur more frequently among females, and the victims tend to be older (median age, 39 years) (1,8,10,12). Similar to dog bites, cat bites are often provoked, and typically the victim is the owner of the cat or knows the cat (10). The location of the bite typically is in the extremities, with most (86%) involving the upper extremities, especially the hands (63%) (8,10,12).

Infrequently, physicians encounter bites by other animals, such as snakes, monkeys, bears, lions, and sharks. Some of these animals are kept as pets. The annual incidence of snakebites in the United States is about 45,000, of which 10% to 18% are attributed to venomous snakes (e.g., rattlesnakes or coral snakes) (1,13). Each year, 5 to 10 deaths occur in the United States as a result of snakebites (14). The annual incidence of bites by the other exotic animals is sparse, and most reports come from anecdotal case reports.

Microbiology

Most of the bacteria isolated from bite wounds are related to organisms that colonize the oral cavity of the biting animal (1,15,16). The bacteriology of bite wounds most often reveals a microbiologic mix of aerobic and anaerobic organisms (12,15–19). Table 161.1 lists common organisms isolated from various animal bites (12,19–22).

In a prospective study of 107 infected dog and cat bite wounds, mixed aerobic and anaerobic bacteria were present in 56% of all wounds (dogs, 48%; cats, 63%). Thirty-six percent of the wounds demonstrated purely aerobic growth (dogs, 42%; cats, 32%). One dog bite had a growth of only two anaerobic organisms (*Bacteroides tectum* and *Porphyromonas gingivalis*), and the reminder 7% of cultures demonstrated no bacterial growth. The median number of isolates per culture was five, with approximately three aerobic and two anaerobic organisms. *Pasteurella* species was the most common pathogen isolated from both dog (50%) and cat (75%) bites. Classification beyond the genus and species level revealed that, of the *Pasteurella* species, *Pasteurella canis* dominated among dog bites (26%), whereas *Pasteurella multocida* subspecies *multocida* (54%) and subspecies *septica* (28%) were the most common isolates among cat bites. *Pasteurella* species were associated with shorter latency period and were more commonly isolated from abscesses and puncture wounds (12).

The next most frequently encountered aerobic organisms were streptococci (dogs and cats, 46%) and staphylococci (dogs, 46%; cats, 35%). Isolation of streptococci (59%) and staphylococci (52%) commonly occurred in wounds characterized as nonpurulent with cellulitis, lymphangitis, or both, in comparison to

TABLE 161.1.   Organisms Isolated from Various Animal Bites

Animal	Bacterial isolates from bite wounds
Dogs	*Pasteurella canis, P. multocida* subspecies *septica, P. stomatis; Streptococcus mitis, S. mutans; Staphylococcus aureus, S. epidermidis; Neisseria weaverii; Corynebacterium minutissimum; Moraxella* species; *Enterococcus faecalis; Bacillus firmus; Pseudomonas aeruginosa; Weeksella zoohelcum; Capnocytophaga* species; *Eikenella corrodens; Fusobacterium nucleatum; Bacteroides tectum; Porphyromonas macacae; Prevotella heparinolytica; Propionibacterium acnes; Peptostreptococcus anaerobius*
Cats	*Pasteurella multocida* subspecies *multocida, P. multocida* subspecies *septica; Streptococcus mitis, S. sanguis II; Staphylococcus epidermidis, S. warneri; Corynebacterium aquaticum, C. minutissimum; Moraxella* species; *Neisseria weaverii; Enterococcus durans; Capnocytophaga* species; *Acinetobacter baumannii; Erysipelothrix rhusiopathiae; Reimerella anatipestifer; Fusobacterium nucleatum, F. russii; Bacteroides tectum; Porphyromonas gingivalis; Prevotella heparinolytica; Propionibacterium acnes; Peptostreptococcus anaerobius; Filifactor villosus*
Primates	*Streptococcus* species; *Enterococcus* species; *Staphylococcus* species; *Eikenella corrodens; Neisseria* species; Enterobacteriaceae; *Bacteroides* species; *Prevotella* species; *Fusobacterium* species; B virus[a]
Pigs	*Staphylococcus* species; *Streptococcus sanguis, S. suis, S. milleri;* diphtheroids; *Pasteurella multocida; Actinobacillus suis; Bacteroides fragilis*
Horses	*Staphylococcus aureus; Streptococcus* species; *Neisseria* species; *Escherichia coli; Actinobacillus lignieresii; Pasteurella* species; *Bacteroides ureolyticus, B. fragilis; Prevotella melaninogenica, P. heparinolytica*
Snakes	*Pseudomonas aeruginosa; Proteus* species; *Staphylococcus* species; *Clostridium* species; *Bacteroides fragilis; Salmonella arizonae*
Marine animals	*Aeromonas hydrophila; Bacteroides fragilis; Chromobacterium violaceum; Clostridium perfringens; Erysipelothrix rhusiopathiae; Escherichia coli; Mycobacterium marinum; Pseudomonas aeruginosa; Salmonella enteritidis; Staphylococcus aureus; Streptococcus* species; *Vibrio* species

[a]Also known as cercopithecine herpesvirus type 1. Enzootic among monkeys of the genus *Macaca.* Most frequent among rhesus (*Macaca mulatta*) and cynomolgus (*Macaca fascicularis*) monkeys.

purulent wounds or abscesses. Of note was isolation of *Staphylococcus intermedius* from one dog and one cat bite (12). *S. intermedius* is a zoonotic pathogen often found in canine gingival flora (especially in dogs less than 40 pounds) (1). It is typically susceptible to penicillin and can be mistaken for *S. aureus* because it is coagulase positive about one fourth of the time (1). Other common organisms isolated belonged to *Neisseria* species (dogs, 16%; cats, 19%), *Corynebacterium* species (dogs, 12%; cats, 28%), and *Moraxella* species (dogs, 10%; cats, 35%) (12).

The most common anaerobic organisms isolated from infected dog and cat bites were *Fusobacterium nucleatum* (dogs, 16%; cats, 25%), *Bacteroides tectum* (dogs, 14%; cats, 28%), *Porphyromonas* species (dogs, 28%; cats, 30%), *Prevotella heparinolytica* (dogs, 14%; cats, 9%), and *Propionibacterium acnes* (dogs, 14%; cats, 16%). Anaerobes were usually present as mixed infections with aerobic organisms and were more prevalent in cat bites, abscesses, puncture wounds, and bites involving the upper extremities (12).

Management

A thorough history including information about the patient (e.g., drug allergies, history of tetanus and rabies immunizations, presence of comorbid conditions), and the animal (e.g., time and circumstances of the attack, behavior pattern and status of rabies immunization) should be obtained.

Essential elements of the physical examination include evaluation for signs of infection and injuries to deeper structures such as joints, tendons, and neurovascular structures. Animal bite injuries can range from insignificant wounds to wounds associated with fractures, amputations, and injuries to underlying organs (7,23). Some species of bats, due to their small, thin, sharp teeth, leave minimal signs of external injury (24). Wounds that appear to be "minor" may have underlying joint and other structural injuries. Cats, with their sharp, thin teeth, often produce small deep puncture wounds that seem to be trivial but that on further evaluation may include joint or cortical injuries. Joints should be taken through their full range of motion. Pain out of proportion to the wound and physical findings should raise suspicion for joint and bone injuries. For equivocal cases in which exclusion of injuries to deeper structures cannot be made by physical examination alone (e.g., wounds overlying the hands), open exploration by a trained specialist may be necessary.

Other important elements of the physical evaluation are best conveyed by a diagram of the bite wounds, including a description of the wound (e.g., abscess, purulent, nonpurulent, avulsion, puncture, laceration, crush); location and depth of the injury; existence of foreign materials; and presence and extent of edema, fluctuance, erythema, lymphadenopathy, or lymphangitis. Recognition of these elements is crucial because the presence of some of these factors places patients at a higher risk for wound infection (25) (Table 161.2). Demarcation of the fluctuant or erythematous areas with a pen will also aid in future wound assessments.

Ancillary studies helpful in further evaluation of animal bites may include wound cultures, Gram stain, and radiographic studies. Obtaining cultures in fresh or noninfected wounds routinely has not demonstrated a benefit in further care of the bite (17,26). Cultures (aerobic and anaerobic) are often reserved for infected wounds, deep wounds penetrating joint or bony structures, patients presenting with systemic signs of infection, and those not responding to conventional therapy. The potential benefit lies not only in the identification of the pathogenic organisms but also in determination of susceptibility of the recovered bacteria to antimicrobial agents. Bacterial cultures are best taken before any

---

TABLE 161.2.   Conditions Predisposing Patients to an Increased Risk for Wound Infection

Host factors
  Age <2 and >50 years
  Comorbidities (e.g., liver disease, splenectomy, diabetes mellitus, malignancy, human immunodeficiency virus)
  Preexisting edema in the area of bite
  Chronic alcohol consumption
  Use of immunosuppressive drugs (including chronic steroid use)
Wound type
  Cat and human bites
  Moderate to severe wounds
  Puncture wound, large avulsion, crush injury
  Presence of foreign material and/or heavily contaminated wounds
Wound location
  Hand, wrist, foot
  Scalp or face in infants and young children
  Associated injuries to bone, joint, tendon sheath, or neurovascular structures
  Adjacent to a prosthetic joint
Wound care
  Delay in care >24 hours
  Improper wound cleansing or débridement
  Noncompliance with prescribed antibiotics

Adapted from Abrahamian FM. Dog bites: bacteriology, management, and prevention. *Curr Infect Dis Rep* 2000;2:446–453, with permission.

---

wound manipulations. To decrease the possibility of contamination, it is best to cleanse the surrounding skin with alcohol or povidone-iodine solution.

For primate bites potentially inflicted with B virus, viral cultures or tissue biopsy specimen may be valuable for the diagnosis of B-virus infection. Viral cultures may be taken from the human wound, the monkey's buccal mucosa, and its cage. The cultures should be obtained after cleansing the wound. Scrubbing and irrigating the wound with a concentrated solution of soap or detergent for 15 minutes is the most important means of preventing B-virus infection. B-virus–specific antibody serology should also be obtained acutely and 3 weeks after exposure (20). The following reference laboratories perform B-virus identification and serologic testing: National B-virus Resource Center, Atlanta, Georgia, (404-651-0808); Esoterix Infectious Disease Center, San Antonio, Texas, (210-614-7350); Virus Reference Division, London, England (081-200-4400).

The Gram stain has somewhat limited clinical usefulness. It is specific but not sensitive due to the wide-ranging multiple flora of bite wounds (17). However, one exception might be in suspected cases of fulminant infection with *Capnocytophaga canimorsus* (formerly classified as dysgonic fermentor-2 [DF-2]). *C. canimorsus* commonly occurs in asplenic patients and those with liver disease. It is reported in variety of illnesses such as meningitis, endocarditis, and septicemia following dog bites. This organism grows slowly in blood cultures (mean, 6 days), and a rapid interim diagnosis can be made by Gram staining the buffy-coat preparations (27–30).

Plain radiographs are commonly used to identify fractures, cortical violations, foreign bodies (e.g., tooth), and subcutaneous air and serve as a baseline for the further evaluation of osteomyelitis. Cranial injuries are best evaluated by computed tomography scanning. Vascular pathologies (e.g., deep neck wounds) should be evaluated by Doppler or duplex ultrasonography, angiography, or both. Blood cultures and blood indices (e.g., white blood cell counts, hemoglobin and hematocrit levels, and platelet count) are not routinely performed unless clinically indicated.

The initial step in wound care is washing the wound under tap water or with a solution of soap and water. Debris and foreign bodies should be removed. Abscesses should be incised and drained. Necrotic and devitalized tissues should be cautiously débrided. Furthermore, the wound should be copiously irrigated under high-pressure (5 to 8 psi) with normal saline. This pressure can be achieved by attaching a 19-gauge needle or catheter tip to a 30- to 60-mL syringe. Concentrated forms of povidone-iodine, hydrogen peroxide, or ethyl alcohol should not be used as irrigating solutions because they can cause further tissue damage and toxicity (31). All of these steps in wound care help to prevent subsequent infections and are potential prophylaxis against the development of tetanus and rabies (26,32–35). It is also important to note that wound cleansing should not be significantly delayed for the purpose of obtaining wound cultures.

Primary wound closure is not typically performed on bite wounds. In general, bite wounds are left open, reevaluated within 2 to 3 days, and managed by secondary intention or delayed primary closure within 3 to 5 days of the injury. In selected cases, adhesive strips may be used for approximation of wound edges. Infected bite wounds should also be left open. Despite the absence of prospective studies, the accepted practice is to avoid closure of puncture wounds, crush injuries, wounds (including facial wounds) that are more than 24 hours old, extremity wounds more than 12 hours old, and wounds over the hands, wrists, feet, and joints (1,10,26,36,37). Noninfected facial wounds less than 24 hours old, because of a lower risk for infection, may be primarily repaired.

Antimicrobial therapy should be initiated for wounds with clinical evidence of infection. Antibiotic prophylaxis should also be considered for wounds with a higher risk for wound infection and for those undergoing primary closure (1,10,19,26,37,38) (Table 161.2). In comparison to dog bites, cat bites demonstrate a higher risk for wound infection; hence, prophylactic antibiotics are also recommended for noninfected cat bites (1,10,37). Prophylactic antibiotic use for wounds at low risk for infection or for noninfected dog bite wounds is somewhat controversial (38–40).

The choice of antimicrobial therapy is dependent on the oral flora of the biting animal (Table 161.1) and the skin flora of the victim. Antimicrobial susceptibilities of bacteria frequently isolated from animal and human bite wounds are presented in Table 161.3. For land-based animals, the initial empiric antibiotic therapy should demonstrate activity against the *Pasteurella* species, streptococci, staphylococci, and anaerobic organisms (12,18,19). Single antimicrobial therapy may include a combination of a β-lactam antibiotic and a β-lactamase inhibitor (e.g., amoxicillin-potassium clavulanate or ampicillin-sulbactam) or a second-generation cephalosporin with anaerobic activity (e.g., cefoxitin). Combination antimicrobial therapy may include penicillin with clindamycin. Other combinations with clindamycin can include a fluoroquinolone or trimethoprim-sulfamethoxazole. For monotherapy, first-generation cephalosporins, macrolides, clindamycin, and dicloxacillin should be avoided because many isolates from bite wounds demonstrate resistance to these agents (1,12,19).

For marine- and freshwater-acquired infection, the selected antimicrobial agent should cover *Vibrio* and *Aeromonas* species, respectively. Third-generation cephalosporins (e.g., cefotaxime) and fluoroquinolones cover both organisms (22). B-virus infection acquired from primate bites is treated with acyclovir. Routine prophylaxis of all primate bites for B virus with acyclovir is not recommended. The decision to initiate antiviral therapy is best made in conjunction with an infectious disease specialist familiar with B-virus infection (20).

In general, most infected wounds respond well to a course of therapy lasting about 10 to 14 days. Other factors, such as

TABLE 161.3. Antimicrobial Susceptibilities of Bacteria Frequently Isolated from Animal and Human Bite Wounds

Agent	Staphylococcus aureus	Streptococcus species	Pasteurella multocida	Fusobacterium species	Bacteroides species	Prevotella species	Porphyromonas species	Eikenella corrodens
Penicillins								
Penicillin	−	+	+	+/−*	+/−*	v	+	+
Ampicillin	−	+	+	+/−*	+/−*	v	+	+
Amoxicillin-clavulanate	+	+	+	+	+	+	+	+
Dicloxacillin	+	v	−	−	−	−	−	−
Cephalosporins								
Cephalexin	+	+	−	−	−	−	−	−
Cefoxitin	+	+	+	+	+	+	+	+
Cefuroxime	+	+	+	−	v	v	v	v
Tetracycline	v	−	+	v	v	+	+	+
Imipenem	+	+	+	+	+	+	+	+
PIP-TZ	+	+	+	+	+	+	+	+
Macrolides								
Erythromycin	v	+	−	−	v	v	+	−
Azithromycin	v	+	v	v	v	v	+	+
Clarithromycin	v	+	v	v	+	+	+	−
Clindamycin	+	+	+	−	−	−	−	+
TMP-SMX	+	−	+					
Fluoroquinolones								
Ciprofloxacin	v	v	+	−/+*	v	v	v	+
Levofloxacin	v	+	+	−/+*	v	+	+	+
Moxifloxacin	v	+	+	−/+*	v	v	+	v
Ketolides	v	+	v	+	+	+	+	−
Metronidazole	−	−	−	+	+	+	+	−

+, Usually susceptible; −, usually resistant; v, variable activity; TMP-SMX, trimethoprim-sulfamethoxazole; PIP-TZ, piperacillin-tazobactam;
*, animal/human bite susceptibilities.
Data compiled from various studies.

presence of complications (e.g., septic arthritis) and a slow rate of improvement, may extend this period. For patients undergoing prophylaxis, the course is typically 3 to 5 days (1,19,37).

The decision to hospitalize patients with bite injuries should be made on a case-by-case basis. The indications include multiple and severe injuries (especially head and hand wounds); spreading infection; systemic signs of infection (e.g., fever, hypotension); bites with injuries to bone, joints, and tendons; immunocompromised host; failure of outpatient therapy; and social reasons (1,25,37).

Other elements of animal bite wound management include attention to tetanus and rabies prophylaxis, elevation of the injured extremity for the first 2 to 3 days, and arrangement for close follow-up (36). Follow-up should take place within 24 to 48 hours of the initial visit. Patients should receive general wound care instructions and return earlier if signs and symptoms of developing or worsening infection appear. Physicians also need to be aware of their local and state animal bite reporting regulations.

Complications

Musculoskeletal, neurovascular, and infectious complications can accompany animal bite injuries. Potential musculoskeletal complications include fractures, cortical violations, osteomyelitis, septic arthritis, tenosynovitis, tendon disruption, and the development of compartment syndrome (7,23,41,42). Injuries to the skull, especially in children, may also lead to the formation of brain abscesses, cerebral contusions, and extracranial and intracranial hemorrhages (7,43). Neurovascular injuries may lead to loss of function, dissection, thrombosis, and embolism (44).

Infectious complications may include the development of necrotizing infection, sepsis, meningitis, and endocarditis. Clues to presence of necrotizing infections can include pain out of proportion to physical findings and subcutaneous emphysema. In addition to *Pasteurella* (especially *P. multocida* subspecies *multocida* and subspecies *septica*), *C. canimorsus* should be suspected as one of the potential etiologic agents in patients presenting with overwhelming systemic infection after dog and cat bites (15,27–30,45). Risk factors for this condition include splenectomy, liver dysfunction, and chronic steroid therapy, although cases among immunocompetent individuals have been reported (27–30). Clues to its diagnosis can include the presence of cutaneous gangrene at the site of the animal bite and purpura fulminans. *C. canimorsus* is usually susceptible to penicillins and fluoroquinolones and typically resistant to trimethoprim-sulfamethoxazole and aminoglycosides. The case fatality rate from 60 reported cases approached 30% (27).

Cat-scratch disease may also develop following a bite or a scratch from a cat or a dog due to *Bartonella henselae* or, in rare instances, *Afipia felis* (46,47). The disease is more prevalent in children and young adults during autumn and winter months. The typical clinical pattern is characterized by the presence of a papular or pustular cutaneous lesion followed by regional lymphadenopathy. The papular or pustular cutaneous lesion is often not observed by the physician because it typically resolves spontaneously within 3 to 5 days. Uncommon, atypical presentations can include encephalopathy, endocarditis, osteomyelitis, and granulomatous hepatitis (48,49). Because of the difficulty of growing *B. henselae* in culture mediums, the diagnosis is best made by serology or the polymerase chain reaction (47–49). Antimicrobial therapy is usually reserved for patients with severe disease or those with complications. Azithromycin, ciprofloxacin, and gentamicin demonstrate *in vitro* activity against *B. henselae* (48,49). In a prospective study of typical cat-scratch disease, a 5-day course of azithromycin re-

sulted in significant reduction of lymph node volume within the first month of treatment (50).

HUMAN BITES

Human bites account for the third most frequent type of mammalian bites encountered by physicians (1,37). The injury can be self-inflicted or acquired from another person either accidentally or unintentionally (e.g., in sports), or during an altercation. Self-inflected wounds typically occur in children around the nails (e.g., paronychia) and on the lips. Wounds inflicted by other humans are often associated with altercations, during sexual encounters ("love nips"), sex-assault crimes, and child abuse (51). In general, victims sustain multiple injuries. Male victims typically sustain injuries to the upper extremities and back, whereas female victims are frequently bitten on the breasts and the upper and lower extremities (52,53).

Similar to animal bites, the bacteriology of human bites is a mix of aerobic and anaerobic organisms. Typical organisms recovered from human bite wounds include α- and β-hemolytic streptococci, *S. aureus*, *Staphylococcus epidermidis*, *Corynebacterium* species, *Eikenella corrodens*, *Haemophilus influenza*, *H. parainfluenza*, *Klebsiella pneumoniae*, *Prevotella melaninogenica*, *Fusobacterium nucleatum*, *Peptostreptococcus* species; and *Prevotella* species (16,18,54). The anaerobic gram-negative bacilli recovered from human bites often produce β-lactamase (18). A synergistic relationship has been noted between *E. corrodens* and α-hemolytic streptococci (37). *E. corrodens* is more prevalent in injuries associated with direct contact with the gingival surface (e.g., clenched-fist injuries) (55).

As with animal bites, important elements of the history include time and circumstances of the injury, drug allergies, last tetanus immunization, hand dominance (e.g., for hand injuries), and recognition of comorbid conditions. In instances in which the offending individual is present or able to be located, a history of human immunodeficiency virus (HIV), hepatitis B and C, or herpesvirus infections should be elicited.

The physical examination should include assessment of the wound for signs and symptoms of infection and exclusion of injuries to deeper structures (e.g., tendon and joint capsule). Wounds overlying the third, fourth, or fifth metacarpal head are suggestive of a clenched-fist injury. In this type of the injury, the hand held in clenched-fist position strikes another person's mouth with resultant impalement of the tooth over the third, fourth, or fifth metacarpal head. Clenched-fist injuries may lead to extensor tendon tears, disruption of the joint capsule, and cortical and bony violations of the metacarpal head. For equivocal cases in which injuries to these underlying structures cannot be excluded by physical examination alone, it is best to consult a physician experienced in hand injuries to evaluate the wound by open exploration and direct inspection. Examination of the hand should be done both in open and clenched-fist positions (56). Tendon injury is best assessed by direct visualization while taking the hand through its full range of motion.

Common ancillary studies in the evaluation of human bite wounds include the Gram stain, cultures, and plain radiographs. Although there is no benefit from routine culture and Gram stain of noninfected wounds, aerobic and anaerobic cultures of infected human bite wounds are recommended. Cultures of infected wounds can aid in the identification of antimicrobial-resistant organisms. Plain radiographs are suggested for wounds with close proximity to bony structures. In addition to identifying fractures and cortical injuries, radiographs can serve as a baseline for future evaluation of osteomyelitis.

Wound care should begin by washing the wound with soap and water, followed by high-pressure (5 to 8 psi) irrigation with normal saline. Abscesses (e.g., paronychia) should undergo incision and drainage, and nonviable tissues should be débrided. Generally, because of the potential for subsequent infection, primary closure is avoided (26). Wounds are often repaired by delayed primary closure after 3 to 5 days or left to heal by secondary intention.

The initial empirical therapy should cover *S. aureus*, *H. influenza*, *E. corrodens*, and β-lactamase–producing oral anaerobic bacteria (1). As monotherapy, amoxicillin-clavulanic acid, ampicillin-sulbactam, cefoxitin, cefotetan, imipenem, meropenem, and piperacillin-tazobactam are appropriate choices. Combination therapy can include cefuroxime with clindamycin or metronidazole. For patients allergic to penicillins, a combination of clindamycin with either ciprofloxacin or trimethoprim-sulfamethoxazole is appropriate. Single use of first-generation cephalosporins (e.g., cephalexin), penicillinase-resistant penicillins (e.g., dicloxacillin), most aminoglycosides, clindamycin, erythromycin, and metronidazole should be avoided because of resistance of *E. corrodens* to these agents (37,56) (Table 161.3).

Indications for hospital admission and follow-up care are similar to those in animal bites. Human bite wounds also require tetanus prophylaxis. Wounds overlying the hand benefit from splinting and elevation. The appropriate authorities should be notified for cases involving child abuse or assault.

The approach to the management of paronychias is less complicated and dependent on the extent and severity of the infection. In cases with mild soft tissue swelling with no fluctuance and frank pus, remission may be achieved with frequent daily hot soaks and avoidance of activities that can exacerbate the condition (e.g., nail biting or finger sucking). If an abscess is present, drainage is the treatment of choice. This is most commonly achieved by elevating the eponychium (cuticle) at the site of its greatest fluctuance. More extensive drainage is required for cases involving a subungual abscess. Care should be taken not to confuse eponychium with herpetic whitlow because surgical intervention is contraindicated in the latter condition. In conjunction with the above measures, patients presenting with moderate to severe paronychias are also frequently treated with antimicrobials. A broad-spectrum antistaphylococcal antibiotic such as a first-generation cephalosporin (e.g., cephalexin) is proper empirical therapy. Mild paronychias without surrounding area of cellulitis often do well with drainage and hot soaks alone. Further care of the wound involves splinting the digit, elevation, and close follow-up.

Complications of human bite injuries may include arthritis, osteomyelitis, tenosynovitis, neurovascular injuries leading to loss of function, septicemia, toxic shock syndrome, and necrotizing fasciitis (57,58). Less frequent, but possible transmission of other infectious diseases (e.g., hepatitis B and C, HIV, herpes simplex virus) has also been reported (37,59–62). Postexposure prophylaxis and follow-up, as well as serologic assays for hepatitis B and HIV, should be considered for those at high risk for these infections (26,63,64).

REFERENCES

1. Goldstein EJC. Bite wounds and infection. *Clin Infect Dis* 1992;14:633–640.
2. Sacks JJ, Kresnow M, Houston B. Dog bites: how big a problem? *Injury Prev* 1996;2:52–54.
3. Moore F. "I've just been bitten by a dog." Surgical toilet, appropriate antibiotics, and device to come back if infection develops. *BMJ* 1997;314:88–90.
4. Weiss HB, Friedman DI, Coben JH. Incidence of dog bite injuries treated in emergency departments. *JAMA* 1998;279:51–53.
5. Sacks JJ, Lockwood R, Hornreich J, et al. Fatal dog attacks, 1989–1994. *Pediatrics* 1996;97:891–895.
6. Beck AM, Jones BA. Unreported dog bites in children. *Public Health Rep* 1985;100:315–321.
7. Brogan TV, Bratton SL, Dowd D, et al. Severe dog bites in children. *Pediatrics* 1995;96:947–950.
8. Patrick GR, O'Rourke KM. Dog and cat bites: epidemiologic analyses suggest different prevention strategies. *Public Health Rep* 1998;113:252–257.
9. Avner JR, Baker MD. Dog bites in urban children. *Pediatrics* 1991;88:55–57.
10. Garcia VF. Animal bites and *Pasteurella* infections. *Pediatr Rev* 1997;18:127–130.
11. Dog-bite–related fatalities—United States, 1995–1996. *MMWR Morb Mortal Wkly Rep* 1997;46:463–467.
12. Talan DA, Citron DM, Abrahamian FM, et al. Bacteriologic analysis of infected dog and cat bites. *N Engl J Med* 1999;340:85–92.
13. Snyder CC. Animal bite infections of the hand. *Hand Clin* 1998;14:691–711.
14. Langley RL, Morrow WE. Deaths resulting from animal attacks in the United States. *Wildl Environ Med* 1997;8:8–16.
15. Goldstein EJC. New horizons in the bacteriology, antimicrobial susceptibility and therapy of animal bite wounds. *J Med Microbiol* 1998;47:95–97.
16. Goldstein EJC, Citron DM, Wield B, et al. Bacteriology of human and animal bite wounds. *J Clin Microbiol* 1978;8:667–672.
17. Ordog GJ. The bacteriology of dog bite wounds on initial presentation. *Ann Emerg Med* 1986;15:1324–1329.
18. Brook I. Microbiology of human and animal bite wounds in children. *Pediatr Infect Dis J* 1987;6:29–32.
19. Goldstein EJC. Current concepts on animal bites: bacteriology and therapy. *Curr Clin Top Infect Dis* 1999;19:99–111.
20. Holmes GP, Chapman LE, Stewart J, et al. Guidelines for the prevention and treatment of B-virus infections in exposed persons. *Clin Infect Dis* 1995;20:421–439.
21. Goldstein EJC, Citron DM, Gonzalez H, et al. Bacteriology of rattlesnake venom and implications for therapy. *J Infect Dis* 1979;140:818–821.
22. Auerbach PS. Trauma and envenomations from marine fauna. In: Tintinalli JE, Kelen GD, Stapczynski JS, eds. *Emergency medicine: a comprehensive study guide*, 5th ed. New York: McGraw-Hill, 2000:1256–1261.
23. Huston HR, Anglin D, Pineda GV, et al. Law enforcement K-9 dog bites: injuries, complications, and trends. *Ann Emerg Med* 1997;29:637–642.
24. Feder HM, Nelson R, Reiher HW. Bat bite? *Lancet* 1997;350:1300.
25. Abrahamian FM. Dog bites: bacteriology, management, and prevention. *Curr Infect Dis Rep* 2000;2:446–453.
26. Fleisher GR. The management of bite wounds. *N Engl J Med* 1999;340:138–140.
27. Kullberg BJ, Westendorp RJ, van't Wout JW, et al. Purpura fulminans and symmetrical peripheral gangrene caused by *Capnocytophaga canimorsus* (formerly DF-2) septicemia: a complication of dog bite. *Medicine* 1991;70:287–292.
28. Mellor DJ, Bhandari S, Kerr K, et al. Man's best friend: life threatening sepsis after minor dog bite. *BMJ* 1997;314:129–130.
29. Pers C, Gahrn-Hansen B, Frederiksen W. *Capnocytophaga canimorsus* septicemia in Denmark, 1982–1995: review of 39 cases. *Clin Infect Dis* 1996;23:71–75.
30. Hovenga S, Tulleken JE, Möller LVM, et al. Dog-bite induced sepsis: a report of four cases. *Intensive Care Med* 1997;23:1179–1180.
31. Hollander JE, Singer AJ. Laceration management. *Ann Emerg Med* 1999;34:356–367.
32. Edlich RF, Rodeheaver GT, Morgan RF, et al. Principles of emergency wound management. *Ann Emerg Med* 1988;17:1284–1302.
33. Dean DJ, Baer GM, Thompson WR. Studies on the local treatment of rabies-infected wounds. *Bull W H O* 1963;28:477–486.
34. Human rabies prevention–United States, 1999. *MMWR Morb Mortal Wkly Rep* 1999;48(RR-1):1–21.
35. Abrahamian FM. Tetanus: an update on an ancient disease. *Infect Dis Clin Pract* 2000;9:228–235.
36. Wiggins ME, Akelman E, Weiss APC. The management of dog bites and dog bite infections to the hand. *Orthopedics* 1994;17:617–623.
37. Griego RD, Rosen T, Orengo IF, et al. Dog, cat, and human bites: a review. *J Am Acad Dermatol* 1995;33:1019–1029.
38. Cummings P. Antibiotics to prevent infection in patients with dog bite wounds: a meta-analysis of randomized trials. *Ann Emerg Med* 1994;23:535–540.
39. Dire DJ, Hogan DE, Walker JS. Prophylactic oral antibiotic for low-risk dog bite wounds. *Pediatr Emerg Care* 1992;8:194–199.
40. Callaham M. Prophylactic antibiotics in dog bite wounds: nipping at the heels of progress. *Ann Emerg Med* 1994;23:577–579.
41. Anderson PJ, Zafar I, Nizam M, et al. Compartment syndrome in victims of dog bites. *Injury* 1997;28:717.
42. Wass AR, Goodacre S. Dog bites causing upper-limb fractures in children. *Injury* 1996;27:433–435.
43. Jones N, Khoosal M. Infected dog and cat bites. *N Engl J Med* 1999;340:1841.
44. Meuli M, Glarner H. Delayed cerebral infarction after dog bites: case report. *J Trauma* 1994;37:848–849.
45. Rao N, Jain S. *Pasteurella multocida* meningitis from animal exposure. *Infect Dis Clin Pract* 1999;8:307–309.
46. Giladi M, Avidor B, Kletter Y, et al. Cat scratch disease: the rare role of *Afipia felis*. *J Clin Microbiol* 1998;36:2499–2502.
47. Del Prete R, Fumarola D, Fumarola L, et al. Detection of *Bartonella henselae* and *Afipia felis* DNA by polymerase chain reaction in specimens from patient with cat scratch disease. *Eur J Clin Microbiol Infect Dis* 2000;19:964–967.

48. Windsor JJ. Cat-scratch disease: epidemiology, aetiology, and treatment. *Br J Biomed Sci* 2001;58:101–110.
49. Maguina C, Gotuzzo E. Bartonellosis: new and old. *Infect Dis Clin North Am* 2000;14:1–22.
50. Bass JW, Freitas BC, Freitas AD, et al. Prospective randomized double blind placebo-controlled evaluation of azithromycin for treatment of cat-scratch disease. *Pediatr Infect Dis J* 1998;17:447–452.
51. Liston PN, Tong DC, Firth NA, et al. Bite injuries: pathophysiology, forensic analysis, and management. *N Z Dent J* 2001;97:58–63.
52. Vale GL, Noguchi TT. Anatomical distribution of human bite marks in a series of 67 cases. *J Forensic Sci* 1983;28:61–69.
53. Pretty IA, Sweet D. Anatomical location of bitemarks and associated findings in 101 cases from United States. *J Forensic Sci* 2000;45:812–814.
54. Brook I. Aerobic and anaerobic microbiology of paronychia. *Ann Emerg Med* 1990;19:994–996.
55. Goldstein EJ, Tarenzi LA, Agyare EO, et al. Prevalence of *Eikenella corrodens* in dental plaque. *J Clin Microbiol* 1983;17:636–639.
56. Faciszewski T, Coleman DA. Human bite infections of the hand. *Hand Clin* 1998;14:683–690.
57. Long WT, Filler BC, Cox E II, et al. Toxic shock syndrome after a human bite to the hand. *Am J Hand Surg* 1988;13:957–959.
58. Wienert P, Heiss J, Rinecker H, et al. A human bite. *Lancet* 1999;354:572.
59. Cancio-Bello TP, de Medina M, Shorey J, et al. An institutional outbreak of hepatitis B related to a human biting carrier. *J Infect Dis* 1982;146:652–656.
60. Dusheiko GM, Smith M, Scheuer PJ. Hepatitis C virus transmitted by human bite. *Lancet* 1990;336:503–504.
61. Vidmar L, Poljak M, Tomazic J, et al. Transmission of HIV-1 by human bite. *Lancet* 1996;347:1762.
62. Richman KM, Rickman LS. The potential for transmission of human immunodeficiency virus through human bites. *J Acquir Immune Defic Syndr Hum Retrovirol* 1993;6:402–406.
63. Moran GJ. Emergency department management of blood and body fluid exposures. *Ann Emerg Med* 2000;35:47–62.
64. Updated U.S. Public Health Service guidelines for the management of occupational exposures to HBV, HCV, and HIV and recommendations for postexposure prophylaxis. *MMWR Morb Mortal Wkly Rep* 2001;50(RR-11):1–52.

CHAPTER 162
Tularemia

David T. Dennis

Tularemia is an acute infectious disease caused by the aerobic gram-negative bacillus *Francisella tularensis*. It is a complex zoonosis, a disease of animals transmissible to humans, with a geographic range throughout much of the temperate northern hemisphere. Although *F. tularensis* is one of the most infectious agents known and is transmitted to humans from numerous environmental sources by various routes, it is not known to spread from person to person. The agent of tularemia has recently received renewed attention because of its potential use in bioterrorism.

HISTORY

In 1837, Homma Soken, a Japanese physician, described an unusual illness:

> Those who eat hare meat have often been found to suffer from poisoning . . . the symptoms appear on the day following, or even dozens of days after, eating the meat. At first the patient is attacked with chills and fever . . . then several glandular tumors will form on the neck, throat, arms, and armpits, resembling scrofula. For many days the tumors will not disappear nor suppurate . . . once the tumor suppurates and discharges, the symptoms will disappear and the tumors will cure (1).

This chapter was updated and modified from the chapter in the previous edition by Jay P. Sanford, deceased.

In the United States, in 1907, peculiar oculoglandular and ulceroglandular syndromes were reported in persons living in Arizona who had skinned and dressed wild rabbits. In 1911, McCoy and Chapin (2), investigating spread of sylvatic plague in California following epidemics of bubonic plague in San Francisco, discovered the causative bacterium of a "plague-like disease of rodents" prevalent among ground squirrels in Tulare county. They named the organism *Bacterium tularense*. Working with these squirrels, Chapin developed a febrile illness, and both he and his laboratory assistant were found to have serum antibodies against *B. tularense*. Thus, from the beginning, the tularemia agent was shown to be a laboratory hazard. In 1914, Wherry and Lamb isolated *B. tularense* from conjunctival scrapings of a "meat cutter in a cheap restaurant" in Cincinnati who had presented with an oculoglandular syndrome. At about this time, cases of an ulceroglandular illness were described in Utah in summer following deer fly bites. Two to 5 days after being bitten, patients became ill with fever and chills. Typically, they developed an erythematous lesion at the bite site that progressed to a punched-out, circular ulcer and that was accompanied by swelling and suppuration of afferent lymph nodes. Intrigued, the U.S. Public Health Service Surgeon Dr. Edward Francis went to Utah in 1919 to investigate the disease and its cause. He isolated *B. tularense* from patients' blood and published a report in 1921 entitled "The Occurrence of Tularemia in Nature as a Disease of Man" (3), naming the disease for the causative organism and its recovery from blood. In 1924, Parker and colleagues discovered the role of ticks in the transmission of tularemia (4). In a landmark paper in 1925, Francis described the principal microbiologic, clinical, and epidemiologic features of the disease (5). Concurrently, a Japanese physician, Ohara, described three patients who developed ulceroglandular disease after they had skinned, cooked, and eaten a dead hare (6). Ohara named the disease *yato-byo* (wild hare disease). Ohara and Francis soon recognized that *yato-byo* was tularemia, representing the first confirmation of the disease outside of North America. In the 1930s, Russian scientists recognized outbreaks of tularemia in rural agricultural areas, associated with epizootics in rodents and contaminated fields and watercourses. They also first described tularemia acquired by drinking contaminated water (7). A live attenuated vaccine was developed in the Soviet Union that was administered over the years to tens of millions of persons living in endemic areas, and this was the basis for a similar vaccine developed later in the United States.

ETIOLOGY

F. tularensis is a small (0.2 μm × 0.2 to 0.7 μm), pleomorphic, gram-negative coccobacillus. It is an intracellular pathogen. A strict aerobe, it grows optimally on media supplemented with sulfhydral compounds (cysteine, cystine, thiosulfate, isovitalex) and at 35° to 37°C. The medium most commonly used for growth is glucose-cysteine blood agar; thioglycolate broth or other sulfhydryl media will also support growth. Although it grows poorly or not at all on most ordinary media, it is occasionally isolated using automated blood culture systems (8). Selective media, such as those containing cycloheximide and penicillin, facilitate isolation from nonsterile specimens such as sputum or swabs of cutaneous ulcers or discharges.

F. tularensis comprises four subspecies (biovars) with differing clinical and epidemiologic features and biochemical reactions (9). *F. tularensis* subspecies *tularensis* (Jellison type A) is the predominate cause of tularemia in North America; it ferments glycerol to produce acid and contains the enzyme citrulline ureidase. *F. tularensis* subspecies *holarctica* (Jellison type B, formerly known as subspecies *palaearctica*) is found widely in North America, Europe, and northern Asia. Type B strains do not ferment glycerol and lack citrulline ureidase, and they have a unique 16S recombinant RNA (rRNA) signature sequence. Type A strains are more virulent in rabbits and collectively are associated with more severe disease in humans than type B strains. Other subspecies are *F. tularensis* subspecies *mediaasiatica*, which is found in nature in Central Asia but is not known to cause infections in humans, and *F. tularensis* subspecies *novicida*, isolated from a small number of patients with tularemia-like illness in the United States and Canada (10). A majority of strains of *F. tularensis* produce β-lactamase.

Human infections with *Francisella philomiragia*, a species related to *F. tularensis*, have been associated with saltwater exposures, including near-drownings, and with underlying diseases likely to impair host immunity, such as chronic granulomatous disease and myeloproliferative disorders (10). Small numbers of cases have been reported, mostly from the United States. Typically, they have presented as pneumonia and as undifferentiated bacteremia.

F. tularensis has multiple immunogenic antigens, including various outer membrane proteins and a lipopolysaccharide envelope. Patients with tularemia show variable reactivity to these antigens, and a formalin-killed whole-cell preparation with a broad reactivity is generally used for standard agglutination assays (11). Serologic cross-reactivity occurs between infections caused by *F. tularensis*, *Brucella abortus*, and *Yersinia enterocolitica*.

F. tularensis is a hardy non–spore-forming organism that may survive for weeks at low temperature in water, moist soil, hay, and decaying or frozen animal carcasses. However, it is sensitive to heat, and cooking at 56°C for 10 minutes renders meat of animals, such as rabbits, hares, and game birds, safe for eating. The organism does not survive in chlorinated water sources.

EPIDEMIOLOGY

Tularemia occurs worldwide in the Northern Hemisphere between latitudes 30 and 71 degrees North (12). Cases are reported from North America; throughout continental Europe, especially in Scandinavia and Finland; throughout the states of the former Soviet Union; and, in the Far East, in northern China, Korea, and Japan. Tularemia has not been described in sub-Saharan Africa, Central or South America, southern Asia, or Australia. In the

United States, tularemia has been reported from all states except Hawaii. There has been a marked decline in the number of cases reported in the United States since a peak of 2,900 cases in 1939; in recent decades, the number of annually reported cases has been between 100 and 200. During 1990 to 2000, a total of 1,368 cases were reported to the Centers for Disease Control and Prevention (CDC) from 44 states, averaging 124 cases (range, 86 to 193) per year (13). Four states accounted for 56% of all reported tularemia cases: Arkansas (315 cases, or 23%), Missouri (265 cases, or 19%), South Dakota (96 cases, or 7%), and Oklahoma (90 cases, or 7%) (Fig. 162.1). The age distribution was bimodal, with highest incidence rates in the age groups 5 to 9 years and 75 years of age or older. Males predominated in all age groups. Disease onsets peaked in the period from May to August (70% of all cases), but cases were reported from all months of the year. Although tularemia in the United States now mostly occurs as isolated cases or in small clusters of cases, several relatively large outbreaks were described in the past (14–16). Although the numbers of cases occurring worldwide is unknown, outbreaks involving thousands of persons occurred in the former Soviet Union in the 1930s and 1940s, and outbreaks affecting hundreds of persons have been described in recent decades from Sweden (17,18), Finland (19), and Yugoslavia (Kosovo) (20).

Evidence of infection with *F. tularensis* has been found in more than 100 species of wild mammals (rabbits, hares, squirrels, voles, muskrats, beavers) and in at least 9 species of domestic animals (sheep, cattle, dogs, cats). The organism has been isolated from 25 species of birds (grouse, pheasants, mallards, owls, crows, hawks), amphibians, fish, and more than 50 species of arthropods (ticks, deer flies, mosquitoes) as well as from mud and water (12).

The most common sources of infection in the United States are bites by ticks or deer flies and direct contact with carcasses of infected animals, especially rabbits, hares, and water rodents (12,21,22). In Scandinavia and Finland, the disease is associated in nature with hares and with voles, and mosquitoes are the most important arthropod vectors (18). Throughout the remainder of endemic Eurasia, hares, voles, water rodents and ticks are important sources of infection. In the United States, the summer peak of human cases reflects tick- and fly-borne disease (22). Although at least 13 species of ticks have been found to be naturally infected, the important species in transmitting infection to humans are the dog tick (*Dermacentor variabilis*), the lone star tick (*Amblyomma americanum*), and the Rocky Mountain wood

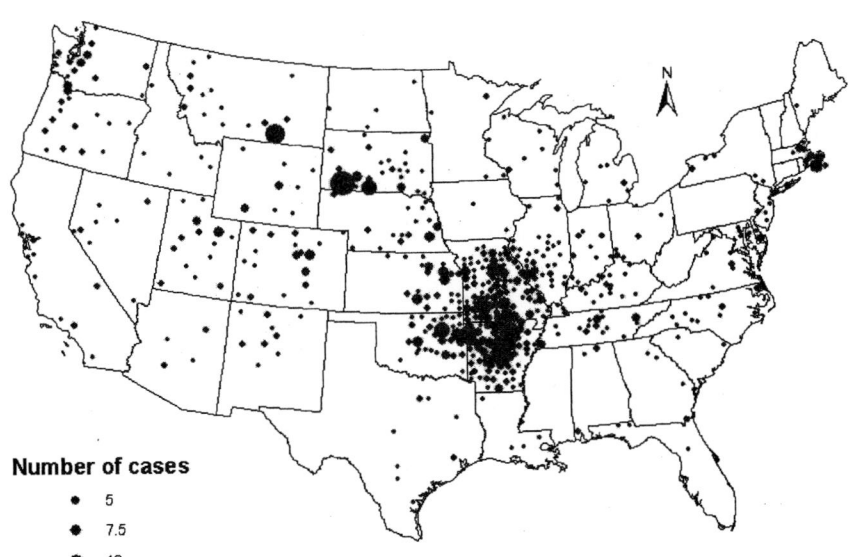

Number of cases

- •   5
- •   7.5
- ●   10

Figure 162.1. Reported cases of tularemia in the United States, 1990–2000. Based on 1347 cases reporting county of residence in the lower continental United States. Alaska reported 10 cases in 4 counties during 1990–2000. (From Centers for Disease Control and Prevention. Tularemia—United States, 1990–2000. *MMWR Morb Mortal Wkly Rep* 2002;51:181–184, with permission.)

tick (*Dermacentor andersoni*). Ticks are true biologic vectors because the organism is maintained within them and is transmitted from one tick stage to the next. Transmission by flies, especially deer flies and horse flies (tabanids), mostly occurs in arid environments of the western United States (16,21). Mosquitoes and biting flies are not biologic vectors, but mechanically transmit infection from contaminated mouthparts.

In the United States, most direct contact cases arise from handling cottontail rabbits (*Sylvilagus* species). The tularemia agent is transmitted between rabbits by the rabbit tick (*Haemaphysalis leporis-palustris*), which only rarely bites humans. Cottontail rabbits are extremely susceptible to infection, which usually results in their death. Jackrabbits (*Lepus* species) are also a source, whose importance was noted in early studies carried out in the western United States (21).

Less often, people acquire infection from the bite of an infected animal or the bite or scratch of one whose mouth or claws have become contaminated while preying on a diseased animal; this mode of transmission accounts for most instances of cat-associated tularemia (23) and has occasionally been associated with handling wild carnivores and raptors.

In both Europe and North America, outbreaks have been reported linked to trapping and skinning water rodents, such as muskrats and beavers (15). In Europe, large outbreaks have resulted from contamination of water or other environmental materials by voles, water rats, and field mice. Several recent outbreaks of ingestion tularemia in southern Europe have been associated with drinking contaminated water or eating contaminated food (20,24,25).

Infection may also occur through aerosolization of organisms. Aerosolized *F. tularensis* caused small summer outbreaks of pneumonic tularemia on Martha's Vineyard, Massachusetts in 1978 (26) and 2001 (27). The 2001 outbreak was epidemiologically associated with landscaping activities, such as mowing and brush cutting. Large outbreaks of inhalation and direct contact tularemia in Sweden and Finland have been linked to cutting fresh hay or handling stored hay contaminated with the carcasses and excrement of field voles (17,19). Exposure to water sprays in a beet processing plant caused an outbreak of inhalation tularemia in Austria. Aerosol transmission is also responsible for most laboratory-acquired cases (28). *F. tularensis* was weaponized for aerosol dispersal by the military establishments both in the United States and the Soviet Union during the Cold War, and the bacillus is considered by the CDC to be a category A critical biologic agent because it is easily disseminated as an aerosol, could cause high mortality with a major public health impact, might cause panic and social disruption, and requires special action for public health preparedness (29).

In the United States, the epidemiology of tularemia is changing. Before 1950, most cases were associated with hunting, skinning, and preparing wild rabbits for food (21), reflected in a large peak of cases in winter months corresponding to the rabbit hunting season. Spring and summer tick exposure has now become the most common mode of transmission, responsible for 71% of cases in one report (30), and the winter peak of cases has disappeared. These findings, as well as the steady decline of yearly reported cases, may be due to a number of factors, including a decline in hunting and eating of wild rabbits. Further, the expanding use of antimicrobials since 1950 may have led to early treatment of tularemia as an undifferentiated febrile illness, a modified clinical expression, and underrecognition of cases.

PATHOGENESIS AND PATHOLOGY

As with other infectious diseases, the host response reflects the balance of virulence, number of infecting organisms, the portal of entry, and immune status of the host. Systemic infection with the more severe disease-causing type A strains (subspecies *tularensis*) routinely follows intracutaneous inoculation of as few as 10 organisms, or inhalation of as few as 15 to 50 organisms (31,32). Following the entry of organisms through the skin, mucous membranes, or respiratory tract, they spread through blood and lymphatics. The incubation period is usually 3 to 6 days (range, 1 to 14 days) (33). Bacteremia has been detected as early as 3 days and as late as 12 days after onset of illness. After inoculation, organisms evoke a response by neutrophilic leukocytes, macrophages, and T lymphocytes. Neutrophils do not phagocytose wild strains of *F. tularensis* in the absence of antibody (34). Macrophages ingest the organisms, which multiply intracellularly and may kill the host cell. After about 2 weeks, T lymphocytes are activated; as expected, this response correlates with the development of reactivity to tularemia skin tests and blast transformation by T lymphocytes on exposure *in vitro* to tularemia antigens (34). Cell-mediated immunity persists for at least 25 years after natural infection; without reexposure, agglutinating antibody titers decline or become negative (34). Humoral antibodies appear between 12 days and 3 weeks after illness onset. In most cases, immunoglobulin G, M, and A antibodies appear simultaneously (34). Early lesions reveal areas of focal necrosis surrounded by neutrophilic leukocytes and a few macrophages. Later, the necrotic areas become surrounded by lymphocytes and epithelioid cells, finally resulting in caseating granulomata, with or without multinucleated giant cells (34). Viable *F. tularensis* organisms may persist in tissues for long periods.

CLINICAL MANIFESTATIONS

Tularemia has been classified into six primary clinical syndromes: ulceroglandular, glandular, oculoglandar, oropharyngeal, pneumonic, and typhoidal (5,35). Typhoidal tularemia is characterized by a lack of signs of a localized infection. The other primary syndromes reflect the portal of entry of infection, but there is often secondary spread. For example, any cutaneous or mucocutaneous exposure can result in secondary sepsis, pneumonia, or meningitis.

Regardless of primary syndrome, the general features of tularemia are similar. Onset of symptoms is abrupt. Symptoms consist of fever (85%), with the temperature usually higher than 38.3°C (101°F); chills (52%); headache (45%); cough (38%); generalized myalgia (31%); chest pain (20%); vomiting (17%); and pharyngitis (15% to 30%) (17,35,36). A pulse–temperature discrepancy was noted in up to 42% of evaluable patients in one series (35). Fever and generalized symptoms often subside after 24 to 96 hours, with a remission of 1 to 3 days, followed by a return of fever and other symptoms. Secondary skin lesions, such as papular or vesicular lesions, erythema nodosum, and erythema multiforme, may occur and have been reported to be common in some series. Untreated, illness typically continues for weeks, and sometimes for months. During this period, sweating, chills, progressive weakness, and weight loss are common. Before streptomycin was first used in 1947, the course of tularemia was described as "31 days of fever, 31 days in bed, and a total duration of disability of about 3½ months" (35).

ULCEROGLANDULAR DISEASE

In the United States, 45% to 85% of patients present with the ulceroglandular form of tularemia (22,35,36). Typically, 24 to 48 hours after the onset of fever and associated early generalized manifestations of infection, a painful red papule develops at the site of inoculation and over the next day or so develops into a vesicle that then ulcerates. The ulcer commonly expands to a size of 1 to 3 cm in diameter, having slightly raised, irregular borders and a flat, necrotic base. In the course of a week or so, an eschar may develop; the ulcer eventually heals, leaving a residual scar. In the first few days of illness, regional lymph nodes draining the site of inoculation become enlarged and painful. The nodes are firm and tender; the surrounding tissues are edematous, and the overlying skin is usually inflamed. The axillary, superficial femoral, and inguinal groups are most commonly involved, as would be expected from exposures related to handling infective carcasses and from tick or fly bite. Tick or mosquito bites on the head or neck, however, typically result in suboccipital or cervical lymphadenopathy. On the extremities, "sporotrichoid" nodules may appear along the ascending lymphatics. Adenopathy may persist for long periods, usually for several months. Half become fluctuant regardless of treatment and may develop fistulas. Patients undergoing incision and drainage should be treated with a bacteriocidal antibiotic to prevent possible hematogeneous spread of infection; excision of nodes should be avoided. Differential diagnostic possibilities include bubonic plague, streptococcal or staphylococcal lymphadenitis, sporotrichosis, chancroid, anthrax, and other causes of acute and subacute regional lymphadenitis having a primary skin lesion.

As well as the localized skin and glandular findings, patients commonly experience pharyngitis (up to one third of patients) and respiratory symptoms or signs (one half of patients) (17,35). Patients complaining of sore throat may have no observable signs of inflammation, but half have pharyngeal erythema, and some have an exudate. Chest radiographs may be abnormal, even in patients who have no symptoms or other signs of pleuropneumonic disease, and may disclose parenchymal infiltrates, usually in one lower lobe (two thirds of cases), pleural effusions, and hilar adenopathy; rarely, pericarditis has been reported (35).

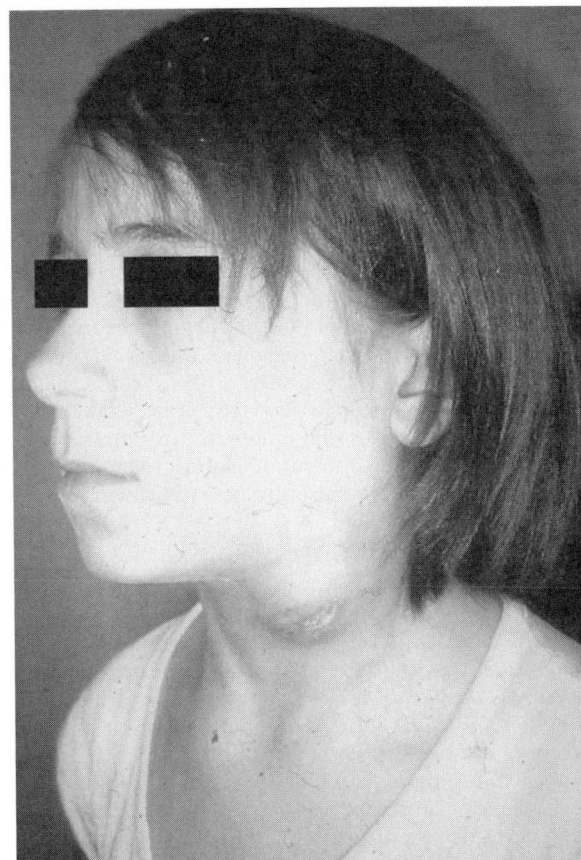

Figure 162.2. Girl with cervical adenitis and draining fistula—pharyngeal tularemia, Kosovo, 2000.

GLANDULAR DISEASE

The glandular form (8% to 25% of patients) is associated with a similar range of symptoms and signs as ulceroglandular disease, but without an ulcerative lesion. In addition to the causes listed previously for ulceroglandular tularemia, differential diagnostic possibilities include cat-scratch disease, tuberculosis, lymphogranuloma venereum, bubonic plague, and other causes of regional lymphadenitis without an accompanying skin lesion.

OCULOGLANDULAR DISEASE

Oculoglandular tularemia occurs in less than 5% of reported cases. The portal of entry is the conjunctival sac, most often self-inoculated by a person skinning or dressing an infected animal. Symptoms include marked conjunctivitis and inflamed, edematous eyelids. Small yellowish nodules and ulcers may be seen on the palpebral conjunctivae. Preauricular nodes are most commonly affected.

OROPHARYNGEAL DISEASE

In the United States, less than 5% of tularemia is oropharyngeal. This form follows the ingestion of contaminated water or food, or the eating of undercooked meat of an infected animal, most commonly a rabbit or hare. The usual features are pharyngitis and tonsillitis with cervical lymphadenopathy. Occasional patients present with stomatitis and submandibular lymphadenopathy (37). In the acute stage, tularemia may mimic β-hemolytic streptococcal infection, various viral causes of pharyngitis, and mumps. The nodes may suppurate and develop draining fistulae (Fig. 162.2). Disease seen in this latter stage may be confused with tuberculosis and various fungal conditions.

PNEUMONIC DISEASE

Pneumonic tularemia can arise directly from inhalation of organisms, or secondary to hematogeneous or lymphatic spread from another anatomic site. Aerosol exposures may result from disturbances of infected animal carcasses, breathing in contaminated water sprays, inhaling contaminated dusts from landscaping activities involving power tools (27), from agricultural activities involving contaminated hay and soil (17,19), and laboratory exposures (28). The usual incubation period for inhalation tularemia is 2 to 6 days, with onset of illness manifested as generalized flu-like symptoms, and further development of cough, retrosternal chest discomfort or pleuritic pains, and dyspnea. Radiographs or tomography scans of the chest show single or multiple-lobe infiltrates, often associated with pleural effusions and hilar adenopathy (38,39). In the laboratory-acquired cases reported by Overholt and colleagues (28), 15 of 17 patients with pneumonia had oval, 2- to 8-cm infiltrates (12 single, 3 multiple). Similar lesions have been reported by others, but not in more recent series. The largest outbreaks of inhalation tularemia, one in Sweden and one in Finland, affected farmers exposed to hay contaminated with dead voles and hay fields with many vole mounds (17,19). Half the patients experienced dry cough, retrosternal discomfort, pleuritic pain, or dyspnea. About 25% experienced sore throat. Some had conjunctivitis, suggesting direct ocular inoculation; many developed erythema multiforme or erythema nodosum skin lesions. The most common radiographic findings were hilar adenopathy (36%) and pulmonary infiltrates (14%). Many had typhoidal presentations without apparent pleuropneumonic disease. All patients were treated with streptomycin or tetracycline, there were no fatalities, and radiographic changes cleared within 3 months. The relatively benign course typifies infection with the type B biovar.

The pulmonary findings in tularemia are not specific, and tularemia needs to be distinguished from atypical and other community-acquired pneumonias of varying severity, such as those caused by *Mycoplasma pneumoniae*, *Chlamydia* species, respiratory viruses, *Legionella* species, *Streptococcus pneumoniae*, *Haemophilus influenzae*, *Histoplasma capsulatum*, *Coxiella burnetti*, and *Moraxella catarrhalis*, among others. In circumstances in which bioterrorism is a concern, inhalation tularemia needs to be distinguished from plague, anthrax, and Q fever.

TYPHOIDAL DISEASE

In the United States, typhoidal tularemia represents less than 5% of reported cases. Illness may present as sepsis, sometimes with serious complications, or as a less severe undifferentiated febrile illness. By definition, there is no apparent primary site of infection, although pulmonary infiltrates can be identified in many of these patients when appropriate examinations are made. Typhoidal presentations have been associated with underlying immune-compromising disorders. Typhoidal tularemia must be differentiated from a wide range of fevers of unknown etiology and, when severe, from other causes of life-threatening sepsis and septic complications. The diagnosis is often made fortuitously by blood culture.

UNUSUAL CLINICAL FORMS

Unusual clinical forms of tularemia include tularemia meningitis, pericarditis, endocarditis, and joint infections. An intestinal form of tularemia with enteritis, appendicitis, mesenteric adenitis, and ascites has been described in association with ingesting undercooked, contaminated game.

DIAGNOSIS

The diagnosis of tularemia should be made on clinical grounds, supported by laboratory findings. Clinical diagnostic specimens include acute and convalescent serum samples and blood for culture (all patients). Sputum, throat swabs, exudates from ulcers, and discharge from fistulas should be collected for Gram and direct fluorescence staining, as appropriate. Biopsy or necropsy specimens can be cultured and examined for *F. tularensis* by immunofluorescence or immunohistochemical staining. Physicians should inform the microbiology laboratory of a suspicion of tularemia because special enriched media need to be inoculated for culture and manipulation of cultures or other infective specimens might pose a biohazard unless performed with correct safety measures in place. At one time, tularemia was second only to viral hepatitis as a cause of laboratory-acquired infections in the United States (40). Procedures that pose a risk for aerosolization, including centrifugation and open-plate examination or manipulation of colonies, should be performed in a biosafety cabinet, preferably under BSL-3 conditions. *F. tularensis* grows slowly or not at all on routine media, blood cultures are often negative, and automated biochemical procedures may not code for *Francisella* species. Because of this, detecting a fourfold rise in serum antibodies is the most usual means of confirming infection. The microagglutination procedure is the most widely used serodiagnostic test method, although various enzyme-linked immunosorbent assay procedures are available and becoming more widely used. Antibodies usually do not appear before day 12 of illness, and sometimes not until the third week. Newer unstandardized diagnostic methods, such as polymerase chain reaction, antigen-capture assays (including handheld immunochromatographic assays), and immunohistochemical staining of tissues, are available in some specialized laboratories (41).

Routine nonspecific tests, such as differential counts of peripheral blood leukocytes (total count is usually 5,000 to 20,000 cells/mm^3) and measurements of various tissue enzymes, are not helpful in a differential diagnosis of tularemia. Nonspecific findings reported in severe cases, including sterile pyuria (one third of patients in one series), hyponatremia, and elevated serum levels of creatine kinase (with or without rhabdomyolysis) (42), may simply represent severe systemic infection.

TREATMENT AND PROGNOSIS

All *F. tularensis* strains are susceptible *in vitro* to several classes of antimicrobial agents (43,44). They are resistant to natural penicillins and first-generation cephalosporins. They are highly susceptible *in vitro* to the aminoglycosides (streptomycin, gentamicin, amikacin, tobramycin, netilmicin), tetracyclines (tetracycline, doxycycline), chloramphenicol, fluoroquinolones (ciprofloxacin, norfloxacin, pefloxacin, and ofloxacin), rifampin, and third-generation cephalosporins (cefotaxime, ceftriaxone). Streptomycin is the drug of choice, and the standard recommended dosing schedule for adults is 15 mg/kg given intramuscularly twice daily (not to exceed 2.0 gm per day) for 10 days. The response is prompt; in 80% of cases, fever drops within 48 hours, and patients have a slow but steady subjective improvement, although weakness and fatigue may persist for days or weeks. Streptomycin is often not readily available, and gentamicin is an acceptable alternative (45). The recommended dosage of gentamicin for adults is 3 to 5 mg/kg given intramuscularly or intravenously daily for 10 days; current evidence suggests that once-daily dosing of gentamicin is at least as effective as, and may be less toxic than, multiple-dose schedules (46). Tetracyclines are effective but require a longer course of treatment to prevent relapses, and primary treatment failures sometimes occur (45). Doxycycline is recommended because of its twice-daily dosing schedule and its rapid absorption when administered orally. The doxycycline dosage for adults is 100 mg given intravenously or orally twice daily for 14 to 21 days. Fluoroquinolones are increasingly used to treat tularemia, and ciprofloxacin has been found to be efficacious in doses of 500 or 750 mg given orally twice daily for 10 to 14 days (47,48). Ceftriaxone has not been shown to be clinically efficacious; eight of eight patients receiving 50 to 75 mg/kg daily for 4 to 7 days experienced clinical deterioration (49). Chloramphenicol is associated with a higher primary treatment failure and relapse rate than either the aminoglycosides or tetracyclines (45); it may, however, be useful in conjunction with one of these other drugs in treating the rare case of tularemia meningitis, because of its ability to cross the blood–brain barrier.

In the pre-antibiotic era, the overall mortality rate for untreated tularemia in the United States was 8%. For typhoidal or pneumonic tularemia, it was several times greater. Today, with early diagnosis and appropriate treatment, the mortality rate is less than 1%; it may be considerably higher in patients with underlying medical disorders and in those with a delayed diagnosis (42).

PREVENTION

To minimize the risk for tularemia, persons should avoid sick or dead animals and should wear impervious gloves to skin or dress wild rabbits, hares, water rodents, and other animals. Drinking unchlorinated water and eating undercooked game is ill advised for numerous reasons, including a risk for tularemia. When it is not possible to avoid tick- or biting fly–infested areas, protective clothing and use of repellents containing DEET or permethrin may reduce the risk for an infective bite. Persons who operate motorized landscaping equipment in areas where tularemia is a known risk should properly maintain and operate equipment to reduce dust exposures and consider the use of face masks designed to block fine particles. A live-attenuated tularemia vaccine was first made available in the United States in the 1960s. Although not fully protective, vaccine use was associated with a marked decline in laboratory-acquired tularemia in research laboratories and was recommended for use by laboratory workers routinely handling *F. tularensis* and for persons whose occupations involved direct contact with wildlife commonly associated with tularemia. The vaccine was, until recently, available through an Investigational New Drug (IND) protocol administered by the Department of Defense. It is currently under IND review by the Food and Drug Administration and is unavailable. In considering possible bioterrorist use of *F. tularensis*, protocols for antimicrobial treatment and for prophylaxis have been developed employing drugs that would be distributed from the National Pharmaceutical Stockpile. Guidelines for the medical and public health management of a bioterrorism event involving tularemia provide recommendations for both the contained and mass casualty situations (50). Standard precautions only are needed for hospital infection control because the disease is not contagious. Laboratory workers with a potentially infective exposure can be treated with 14 days of doxycycline if the risk is considered to be high (e.g., spill, centrifuge accident), or placed on a fever-watch for 14 days.

REFERENCES

1. Ohara S. Studies on Yato-byo (Ohara's disease, tularemia in Japan), report I. *Japan J Exp Med* 1954;24:69–79.
2. McCoy GW, Chapin CW. Further observations on a plague-like disease of rodents with a preliminary note on the causative agent, *Bacterium tularense*. *J Infect Dis* 1912;10:61–72.
3. Francis E. The occurrence of tularemia in nature as a disease of man. *Public Health Rep* 1921;36:1731–1738.
4. Parker RR, Spencer RR, Francis E. Tularaemia. XI. Tularaemia infection in ticks of the species *Dermacentor andersoni* Stiles in the Bitter Root Valley, Montana. *Public Health Rep* 1924;39:1052–1073.
5. Francis E. Tularemia. *JAMA* 1925;84:1243–1250.
6. Ohara H. On an acute febrile disease transmitted by wild rabbits. *Japan Med World* 1926;6:263–270.
7. Karpov SP, Antonoff NI. The spread of tularemia through water, as a new factor in its epidemiology. *J Bacteriol* 1936;32:243–258.
8. Provenza JM, Klotz SA, Penn RL. Isolation of *Francisella tularensis* from blood. *J Clin Microbiol* 1986;24:453–455.
9. Ellis J, Oyston PC, Green M, et al. Tularemia. *Clin Microbiol Rev* 2002;15:631–646.
10. Hollis DG, Weaver RE, Steigerwalt AG, et al. *Francisella philomiragia* comb. nov. (formerly *Yersinia philomiragia*) and *Francisella tularensis* biogroup Novicida (formerly *Francisella novicida*) associated with human disease. *J Clin Microbiol* 1989;27:1601–1608.
11. Bevanger L, MacLand JA, Naess AI. Agglutinins and antibodies to *Francisella tularensis* outer membranes antigens in early diagnosis of disease during an outbreak of tularemia. *J Clin Microbiol* 1988;26:433–437.
12. Bell JF. Tularemia. In: Steele JH, ed. *CRC handbook series in zoonoses*, Vol 2. Boca Raton, FL: CRC Press, 1980:161–193.
13. Centers for Disease Control and Prevention. Tularemia—United States, 1990–2000. *MMWR Morb Mortal Wkly Rep* 2002;51:181–184.
14. Warring WB, Ruffin JS. A tick-borne epidemic of tularemia. *N Engl J Med* 1946;234:137–140.
15. Young LS, Bicknell DS, Archer BG, et al. Tularemia epidemic, Vermont, 1968: forty-seven cases linked to contact with muskrats. *N Engl J Med* 1969;280:1253–1260.
16. Klock LE, Olsen PF, Fukushima T. Tularemia epidemic associated with the deerfly. *JAMA* 1973;226:149–152.
17. Dahlstrand S, Ringertz O, Zetterberg B. Airborne tularemia in Sweden. *Scand J Infect Dis* 1971;3:7–16.
18. Christensen B. An outbreak of tularemia in the northern part of Central Sweden. *Scand J Infect Dis* 1984;16:285–290.
19. Syrjälä H, Kujala P, Myllylä V, et al. Airborne transmission of tularemia in farmers. *Scand J Infect Dis* 1985;17:371–375.
20. Reintjes R, Dedushaj I, Gjini A, et al. Tularemia outbreak investigation in Kosovo: case control and environmental studies. *Emerg Infect Dis* 2002;8:69–73.
21. Jellison WL. *Tularemia in North America*. Missoula: University of Montana, 1974:1–276.
22. Boyce JM. Recent trends in the epidemiology of tularemia in the United States. *J Infect Dis* 1975;131:197–199.
23. Capellan J, Fong IW. Tularemia from a cat bite: case report and review of feline-associated tularemia. *Clin Infect Dis* 1993;16:472–475.
24. Greco D, Allegrino G, Tizzi T, et al. A waterborne tularemia outbreak. *Eur J Epidemiol* 1987;3:35–38.
25. Helvaci S, Gedikoglu S, Akalin H, et al. Tularemia in Bursa, Turkey: 205 cases in ten years. *Eur J Epidemiol* 2000;16:271–276.
26. Teutsch SM, Martone WJ, Brink EW, et al. Pneumonic tularemia on Martha's Vineyard. *N Engl J Med* 1979;301:826–828.
27. Feldman KA, Enscore R, Lathrop S, et al. Outbreak of primary pneumonic tularemia on Martha's Vineyard. *N Engl J Med* 2001;345:1601–1606.
28. Overholt EL, Tigertt WD, Kadull PJ, et al. An analysis of forty-two cases of laboratory-acquired tularemia: treatment with broad spectrum antibiotics. *Am J Med* 1961;30:785–806.
29. Khan AS, Morse S, Lillibridge S. Public health preparedness for biological terrorism in the USA. *Lancet* 2000;356:1179–1182.
30. Jacobs RF, Condrey YM, Yamaguchi T. Tularemia in adults and children: a changing presentation. *Pediatrics* 1985;76:818–822.
31. Saslaw S, Eigelsbach HT, Wilson HE, et al. Tularemia vaccine study. I. Intracutaneous challenge. *Arch Intern Med* 1961;107:121–133.
32. Saslaw S, Eigelsbach HT, Prior JA, et al. Tularemia vaccine study. II. Respiratory challenge. *Arch Intern Med* 1961;107:134–146.
33. Dienst FT. Tularemia: a perusal of three hundred thirty-nine cases. *J La State Med Soc* 1963;115:114–127.
34. Tärnvik A. Nature of protective immunity to *Francisella tularensis*. *Rev Infect Dis* 1989;11:440–451.
35. Evans ME, Gregory DW, Schaffner W, et al. Tularemia: a 30 year experience with 88 cases. *Medicine* (Baltimore) 1985;64:251–269.
36. Jacobs RF, Narain JP. Tularemia in children. *Pediatr Infect Dis J* 1983;2:487–491.
37. Luotonen J, Syrjälä H, Jokinen K, et al. Tularemia in otolaryngologic practice. *Arch Otolaryngol Head Neck Surg* 1986;112:77–79.
38. Stuart BM, Pullen RL. Tularemic pneumonia: review of American literature and report of 15 additional cases. *Am J Med Sci* 1945;210:223–236.
39. Dennis TM, Boudreau RP. Pleuropulmonary tularemia: its roentgen manifestations. *Radiology* 1957;68:25–30.
40. Pike RM. Laboratory-associated infections: Summary and analysis of 3921 cases. *Health Lab Sci* 1976;13:105–114.
41. Grunow R, Splettstoesser W, McDonald S, et al. Detection of *Francisella tularensis* in biological specimens using a capture enzyme-linked immunosorbent assay, an immunochromatographic handheld assay, and a PCR. *Clin Diagn Lab Immunol* 2000;7:86–90.
42. Penn RL, Kinasewitz GT. Factors associated with a poor outcome in tularemia. *Arch Intern Med* 1987;147:265–268.
43. Ikäheimo I, Syrjälä H, Karhukorpi J, et al. In vitro antibiotic susceptibility of *Francisella tularensis* isolated from humans and animals. *J Antimicrob Chemother* 2000;46:287–290.
44. Maurin M, Mersali NF, Raoult D. Bactericidal activities of antibiotics against intracellular *Francisella tularensis*. *Antimicrob Agents Chemother* 2000;44:3428–3431.
45. Enderlin G, Morales L, Jacobs RF, et al. Streptomycin and alternative agents for the treatment of tularemia: review of the literature. *Clin Infect Dis* 1994;19:42–47.
46. Ali MZ, Goetz MB. A meta-analysis of the relative efficacy and toxicity of single daily dosing vs. multiple daily dosing of aminoglycosides. *Clin Infect Dis* 1997;24:769–809.
47. Johansson A, Berglund L, Sjöstedt A, et al. Ciprofloxacin for treatment of tularemia. *Clin Infect Dis* 2001;33:267–268.
48. Johansson A, Berglund L, Gothefors L, et al. Ciprofloxacin for treatment of tularemia in children. *Pediatr Infect Dis J* 2000;19:449–453.
49. Cross JT, Jacobs RF. Tularemia: treatment failures with outpatient use of ceftriaxone. *Clin Infect Dis* 1993;17:976–980.
50. Dennis DT, Inglesby TV, Henderson DA, et al. Tularemia as a biological weapon: medical and public health management. *JAMA* 2001;285:2763–2773.

CHAPTER 163
Plague

Darwin L. Palmer

Plague, caused by the gram-negative bacillus *Yersinia pestis*, is marking the centennial of its discovery by Alexander Yersin in 1884 by its reemergence as a worldwide epidemic. Ominously, there has been an increase in the total world cases, outbreaks in several countries where it has been silent for many years, an increase in the foci in several areas including the United States, and the first evidence of major drug resistance (1). Originating in the Orient, the rat-borne plague epidemics of the Middle Ages caused such enormous population die-offs in Europe that their syndromic name, the Black Death, became synonymous with population decline. The epidemics killed 30% to 40% of the total population, a mortality not replicated by any other illness before or since. Subsequently established in enzootic rodent foci throughout the world, the prevalence of disease steadily declined in modern times as improved living conditions decreased rodent-flea human contact. Moreover, current early diagnosis and modern therapy has reduced the mortality from bubonic and pneumonic plague from 40% and 90%, respectively, to 5% and 10%. However, sporadic spread to humans as rodent populations wax and wane and as humankind increasingly encroaches on rural habitats and disrupts urban living conditions is a current problem in much of the world, including the western United States.

HISTORY

Biblical writings allude to a major pestilence with high mortality among the Philistines in 1320 BC. However, the description is so incomplete that one can only suspect plague as the source. The first pandemic clearly due to plague started in AD 542 during the reign of Justinian of the Ottoman empire (2,3). Imported from Asia Minor, as were subsequent pandemics, this lasted for about 100 years and devastated the Middle East and Mediterranean populations. The medieval European pandemic that later came to be called the Black Death was again imported from Asia in the fourteenth century, starting with the Ottoman invasion of the Genoese city of Caffa, where Mongol plague cadavers were hurled over the city walls as bacteriologic weapons. Subsequently spread by Genoese trading vessels to Messing, Genoa, and Marseilles, probably carrying the Asian black rat, which colonized the roofs and walls of human habitations, the disease rapidly spread throughout the rest of Europe between the years of 1347 and 1351. Killing an estimated 30% to 40% of the population, or 17 to 28 million persons, this decline has never subsequently been duplicated (Fig. 163.1). Known as the Black Death either because of popular dread or possibly a hemorrhagic diathesis in some victims, the disease became well established in and spread by urban rat populations. A recent study of dental pulp by polymerase chain reaction (PCR) from skeletons in a fourteenth century multiple-cadaver grave from Montpellier definitively identified *Y. pestis* as the cause of death (4). Periodic resurgence of human deaths were generally preceded by rat die-offs, and a major regional epidemic was often followed by local rodent decline. Thus, the Great Plague of London in 1665 was followed by a virtual absence of English cases until 1909. During the seventeenth century, the brown sewer rat (*Rattus norvegicus*) replaced the black house rat (*Rattus rattus*) in Europe. Because

the brown rat does not frequent house roofs and walls, and its fleas prefer it to humans, this change in rat ecology may have been instrumental in halting this second pandemic, which had lasted more than 130 years (5).

The third pandemic began in China in 1855; spread by war refugees to Hong Kong, its dissemination to the rest of the world was immensely enhanced by international shipping. Initially infecting waterfront areas of major port cities, *Y. pestis* was then spread inland by rats and other rodents. In Hong Kong, the hospital death rate was 95%, and the disease was rampant in neighboring Canton, where 30,000 people had died in 1 year. Alexander Yersin, a French ship's doctor who had worked previously on diphtheria toxin and trained with Pasteur, in June 1894 while visiting Hong Kong, cultured the organisms on peptone agar after detecting them microscopically as gram-negative bipolar bacilli from the buboes and blood of patients who had died of plague. He published his data on his return to Paris, naming the organism *Pasteurella pestis* in honor of his mentor. Returning to Vietnam, Yersin spent the rest of his life attempting to develop a plague vaccine. The genus was renamed *Yersinia* in the 1960s to honor its discoverer.

Rapidly spreading throughout the world, it ultimately killed more than 12 million people in India and China alone. Many nations, including the United States, sent plague commissions to India where the annual death rates were more than 1 million per year in 1903. The U.S. Surgeon General mailed a pamphlet to all his medical officers alerting them to its first appearance in the New World in Santos, Brazil in 1899; it was also found in the Philippines and Hawaii (6).

In 1900, bubonic plague was detected in the Chinatown slums of San Francisco, having been identified from the bubo of a dead Chinese worker (2). The case was astutely recognized and bacteriologically confirmed as *Y. pestis* by the chief quarantine officer, who recommended antipest serum, fumigation, and quarantine of Chinatown. In the next 5 days, two more plague deaths

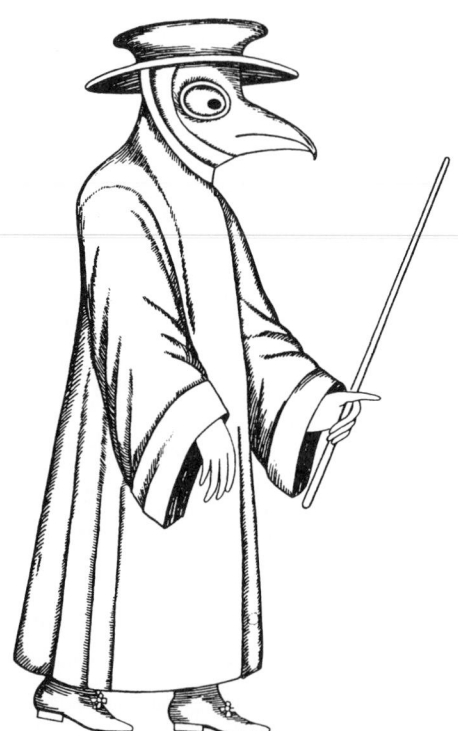

Figure 163.1. Antiplague costume of the sixteenth century. The nasal piece contained herbs to prevent inhaled contagion.

were detected in Chinese workers. However, the governor of California, fearing the effect of such adverse publicity on the tourist industry, initiated an investigation by the chamber of commerce, the railroad industry, and other business interests and concluded that plague "did not and never had existed." The control measures were halted by his mandate, and the warning concerning plague was officially scoffed at in the newspapers. By 1904, however, after 118 additional deaths due to plague, the new governor of California officially recognized the presence of the disease in San Francisco and the state of California. Rat-proofing of buildings and cleanup then commenced aggressively in the slums of San Francisco. By 1905, the local medical authorities had started rat eradication, and medical ecobiologists first recognized fleas as the vector between infected rats and humans. Despite the waning rat plague epidemic in the city, however, the lack of early disease containment may have assisted in transmitting plague to a focus of ground squirrels in the hills to the east of San Francisco. Detection of wild rodents as carriers (and transmitters) of plague bacillus led to the first understanding of sylvatic (rural) propagation of plague.

In 1919, a squirrel hunter in the Berkeley hills contracted bubonic, then secondary pneumonic, plague. He subsequently transmitted primary plague pneumonia to 13 others (including two nurses and two physicians), of whom 12 died. The transmission occurred sequentially over several weeks, especially among those not recognized or hospitalized. The epidemic was controlled by hospitalization and isolation of the patients. In 1924, a similar bubonic-pneumonic plague outbreak occurred in Los Angeles, again from sylvatic sources, but involving a total of 33 pneumonic cases. This time, a special isolation ward was established early, and a much larger outbreak was prevented. This was the last reported nosocomial cluster in the United States (7).

From this wild rodent population, it is suspected that the plague bacillus dispersed among other wild rodents, including ground squirrels, voles, chipmunks, and prairie dogs, gradually moving from California to the neighboring states (8,9). Initially causing only 5 to 10 cases per year, it gradually spread to the Pacific Northwest and inland to Nevada, Utah, Arizona, Colorado, and New Mexico. Now found as far east as western North Dakota, more than 14 states have had reported cases; however, more than 90% of the 362 cases reported in the past 50 years are from four western states with high concentrations of endemic disease (Arizona, California, Colorado, and New Mexico). The reason for this concentration west of the 100th meridian is unclear; possibly, the density of sylvatic rodents is sparse beyond this geographic boundary.

Transiently infecting the waterfront areas of New York City, New Orleans, and Galveston, plague did not cause major human outbreaks. The disease in the coastal cities was contained by rat-proofing buildings and rodent eradication. By not spreading to sylvatic rodents, plague eventually disappeared from these areas. Similar efforts to rat-proof ships halted dissemination to other cities in the United States.

EPIDEMIOLOGY

The plague bacillus exists on all continents of the world except for Australia and Antarctica. It is permanently established in more than 200 sylvatic rodent species in Eurasia, Africa, and North and South America. Whereas human cases must be reported to the World Health Organization, its presence among rodents often goes unrecognized because it circulates unobtrusively in discontinuous enzootic foci. The periodic increase and plague-associated die-off of rodent populations in the wild are the occasion for greater or lesser contact with rural-dwelling humans (10). This periodicity follows cooler, wetter seasons enhancing small-animal food resources, leading to an increase in the abundance of rodent hosts (11). The human cases rise and fall from year to year by 10-fold or more in New Mexico and are predictable on a local basis by the winter-spring precipitation.

Once established, sylvatic plague rarely completely disappears; an apparent exception may exist in Hawaii. There, 410 human cases were reported between 1899 and 1949. However, since 1957, continuous surveys of rats, other rodents, and carnivores (the mongoose) have failed to detect either plague bacilli or any serologic evidence of infection (6). Reports from other regions of the world, as in Russia or India, have shown reappearance of human plague after an apparent absence of 30 years, possibly resulting from inattention to sylvatic sources. Likewise, Africa has seen a recent resurgence, with outbreaks in 11 countries and Madagascar, and a high mortality because of poor health care.

Three separate biogroups of *Y. pestis*–*antigua*, *medievalis*, and *orientalis*–have distinct DNA homology, world localization, and sylvatic hosts, lending credence to the spread and establishment of plague bacilli in three pandemic waves (12). In Russia, tarbagans, marmots, and gerbils are infected; in Africa, spiny mice, giant grass rats, and insectivorous rodents are plague reservoirs. In the United States, prairie dogs, ground squirrels, and rock squirrels are the most commonly involved species, whereas voles, chipmunks, deer mice, and rabbits are less frequent hosts (8,10). More than 19 species of mammals have been found to be at least intermittent carriers. Rodents and their fleas vary in sensitivity to *Y. pestis*; thus, peridomestic rats, *R. rattus* and *R. norvegicus*, are readily killed, and their flea, *Xenopsylla cheopis*, carries and transmits plague bacillus well, both between rats and to humans. The bandicoot rat of India is relatively more resistant to lethal infection with *Y. pestis* and may serve as a permanent resident focus for infection. More susceptible species, such as ground squirrels of the western United States, may amplify the organism as the population of rodents increases. The prairie dog, if infected during the fall, may over-winter the organism in a dormant phase during hibernation, only to develop clinical disease and die with massive replication of *Y. pestis* during the spring. Rodent burrows are also able to maintain viable *Y. pestis* in cool, moist soil for many months. Dogs, both wild and domestic, are less susceptible to lethal infections and may serve as sentinel hosts to serologically document sylvatic infections; cats, on the other hand, sustain severe, oropharyngeal bacteremic infections, which they easily pass on to humans, before their own death. Since 1977, in excess of 15 peridomestic cases of plague, 5 of them pneumonic, have been acquired by owners from their cats.

Rodent fleas are partially specific for rodent species and have relative specificity for carriage of *Y. pestis*. Carriage of *Y. pestis* may persist for many weeks without death of the flea, and flea vector efficiency is variably dependent on environmental temperature and relative humidity (13). In addition, adverse conditions such as cold may enhance *Y. pestis* dormancy and maintenance in the flea; conversely, too much rainfall may promote growth of fungi that kill flea eggs and larvae. Fleas suck directly from venules, with the ingested blood going through the proventriculus to the stomach. Replication of *Y. pestis* in the proventriculus closes off this entranceway to the stomach. The flea, now unable to ingest a blood meal, will repeatedly attempt to feed and, because of the blocked proventriculus, will regurgitate infected material directly into the wound. Whereas *X. cheopis* is a good vector, other flea species, such as *Pulex irritans*, the human flea, carry and transmit *Y. pestis* less well.

Human plague has two epidemiologic forms (Fig. 163.2): the sporadic, acquired from endemic rural foci, and the epidemic, acquired from urban rat infestation. Sporadic human disease is

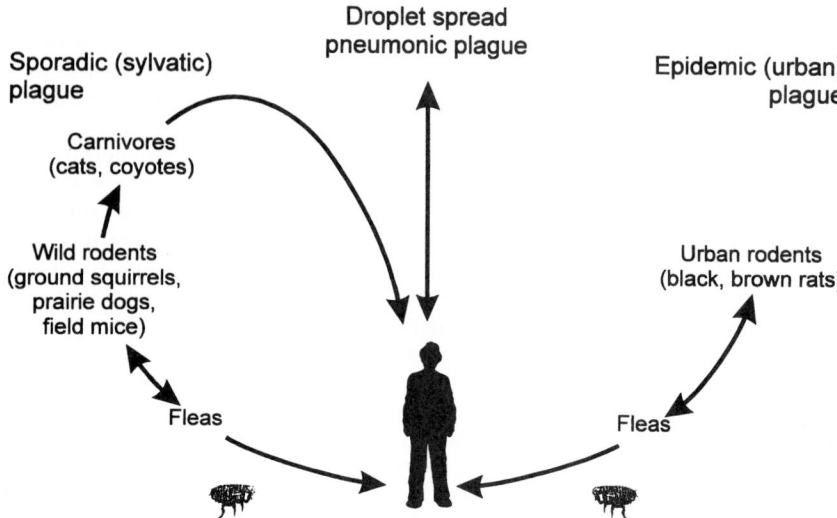

Figure 163.2. Human plague interaction with animal-flea sources. Sylvatic plague is ecologically distinct from urban plague.

probably underreported, especially in Africa, Asia, and Latin America. However, where epidemiologic tracking is precise, as in the southwestern United States, disease in humans closely follows that in wild rodent vectors (9,10). Thus, as rodent populations increase because of climatologic variation in foodstuffs, human disease will show resurgence (11). This has resulted in irregular periodicity in the southwestern United States, with cases in humans varying from 1 or 2 to 40 or 50 per year.

Epidemic disease in city-dwelling humans usually erupts after the infestation of large numbers of peridomestic urban rats. An often observed "rat fall" in which rats inhabiting the walls and ceilings of slum homes become infected, die, and drop to the ground, may precede the development of an urban outbreak in humans. This was noted before the 1994 epidemic of bubonic-pneumonic plague in south-central India (14). Human plague

occurs in settings of war and social disruption in cities; it almost always occurs among conditions of intense poverty, poor sanitation, and absence of control of rats and other vermin. Disease manifestations are identical in sylvatic and urban plague, that is, mostly bubonic disease with occasional (about 15%) secondary pneumonic illness. On occasion, urban population density may foster human-to-human spread of primary pneumonic plague from cough-generated aerosols of *Y. pestis*, with devastating consequences. Bubonic plague is essentially nontransmissible from person to person, whereas pneumonic plague is among the most contagious of all illnesses. With an accompanying mortality rate of almost 100% if untreated, pneumonic plague has been the apparent reason for extremely widespread die-offs of human populations in past pandemics, and the occasion for consideration as a bioterrorist weapon (7).

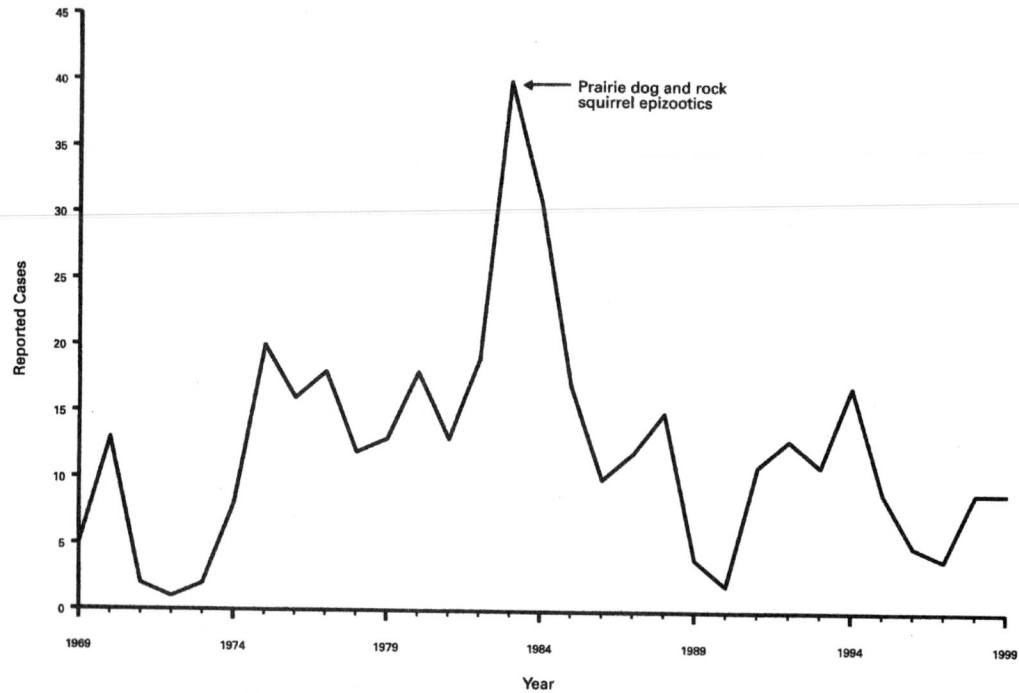

Figure 163.3. Human plague in the United States over 30 years. The rise and fall follows winter-spring moisture, subsequent plant growth and rodent increases. (From *MMWR Morb Mortal Wkly Rep* 2001;48:56, with permission.)

Plague occurs in zoonotic locations around the world; most cases are reported from the developing countries of Asia and Africa. In the past 15 years, more than 11 countries of Africa have reported outbreaks, with an overall case-fatality rate of 15% despite the availability of effective antibiotic treatment. Other sizable outbreaks have occurred in Brazil, Peru, Bolivia, Vietnam, Burma, and Madagascar, often after years of absence (7). From 1944 through 1993, 362 cases of human plague were reported in the United States; about 90% of these occurred in the four western states of Arizona, California, Colorado, and New Mexico, with more than 50% coming from New Mexico (15). Ranging from 1 to 40, these averaged 13 cases per year (Fig. 163.3). Rural homes and their surroundings accounted for 75% of the exposures. Mortality was greater in those in whom there was a delay in diagnosis, often occasioned by an atypical presentation or travel away from the endemic location during incubation of the illness. Males and females were affected about equally, with most cases occurring in those younger than 20 years (10,16), possible reflecting greater outdoor activity. Ground squirrels were the most frequently implicated source, but cases without known rodent or insect bite exposure were very common (17). Domestic cats have become recognized as increasingly important sources of exposure, causing no cases before 1977 but more than 15 human plague cases since then, including 4 in veterinarians (15,18). In addition, 4 of these 15 cases were primary pneumonic plague. Free-roaming cats catch wild rodents and either eat them or bring them back to the household, transmitting *Y. pestis* either by rodent fleas or, after developing illness, by direct contact (18). Because of similarities in clinical features and western state localization, Hantavirus pulmonary syndrome and plague may become diagnostically confused, especially in a patient with secondary plague pneumonia (15). Plague has also been acquired from rabbits during the winter months, usually by hunters (17). Native Americans have had an especially high attack rate (30% of all U.S. cases) because of their close contact with wild animals in a rural setting (19). In addition, the Navajos have used prairie dogs as a food source.

The continued residential expansion into high-risk areas of the rural environment has led to specific recommendations for control of human plague. These include increased surveillance of the rodent populations near human habitation; instruction concerning decrease in rodent harborage and food sources surrounding human households; control of wild rodents and their fleas by the use of appropriate insecticides and, occasionally, rodenticides; and care using gown, gloves, and masks when handling sick cats from endemic areas, especially if they have pharyngeal symptoms. Finally, advice should be given to avoid sick or dying rodents in the wild and warnings to health care providers about the signs, symptoms, and prevalence of plague in high-risk years and regions.

ETIOLOGIC AGENT

Y. pestis is a pleomorphic, gram-negative coccobacillus that is facultatively anaerobic and grows readily on most culture media (8). It is closely related to the pathogens *Yersinia enterocolitica* and *Yersinia pseudotuberculosis* but distinct from them in pathology, specific antigens, and certain culture characteristics (20). With Wayson or Giemsa stain, *Y. pestis* shows characteristic bipolar staining, giving it a characteristic "safety pin" appearance (Fig. 163.4).

Y. pestis tends to grow aerobically but slowly on blood agar and MacConkey agar, does not ferment lactose, and forms small colonies after 48 hours of incubation. Optimal temperature for growth is 28°C. Hence, prolonged incubation at temperatures below 37°C produces small, semitranslucent colonies that are gray and somewhat mucoid in appearance. The organism is nonmotile and urease negative and does not use citrate or indole. Automated laboratory diagnostic equipment may fail to identify *Yersinia* species or differentiate one *Yersinia* member from the other members of the genus. For definitive identification, the cultures should be forwarded to a reference laboratory, and a public health official should be notified about the possibility of a *Y. pestis* isolate.

The plague bacillus produces several virulence factors that correlate well with its antigenic, immunologic, and invasive characteristics. The organism has a temperature-dependent outer membrane capsule that contains an envelope antigen known as fraction one (F1). This is a protein–polysaccharide complex that is expressed at 37°C and appears to increase resistance to phagocytosis; V and W antigens are mediated by a

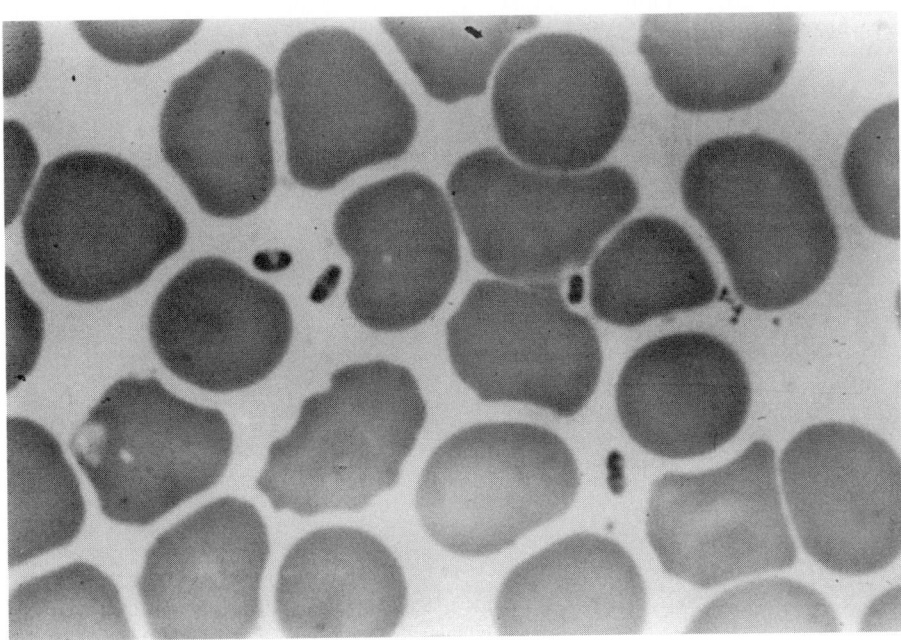

Figure 163.4. Peripheral blood smear in bacterium *Yersinia pestis,* showing characteristic bipolar ("safety pin") staining.

45-megadalton (MDa) plasmid and encode for dependence on calcium for growth of the bacterium at 37°C but not at lower temperatures. These V and W antigens confer virulence by enabling the organism to survive and grow intracellularly. Other virulence factors include a lipopolysaccharide endotoxin, the ability to absorb iron in the form of hemin from its surroundings, and the temperature-dependent enzymes coagulase and fibrinolysin. The last two characteristics are also plasmid mediated. Laboratory identification can be achieved by culture and by demonstration of a serologic response by using passive hemagglutination and enzyme-linked immunosorbent assay, both directed toward the F1 antigen of *Y. pestis*. A fourfold rise in titer from acute- to convalescent-phase serum or a presumptive titer of 1:16 is diagnostic of infection (8). For definitive identification, cultures can be sent to either one's own state laboratory or the Centers for Disease Control and Prevention, Plague Branch. Drug resistance has been detected only rarely in the United States, but recent isolates from South Africa and Madagascar have shown several resistant strains and multidrug resistance to the drugs currently recommended (chloramphenicol, streptomycin, and tetracycline). Susceptibility was retained to cephalosporins, other aminoglycosides, and quinolones (1).

PATHOGENESIS

Infection with *Y. pestis* is initiated when an infected flea attempts to feed on a human. Organisms are introduced when the flea regurgitates *Y. pestis* from the blocked proventriculus; or, if unblocked, the flea may contaminate the bite site by deposited fecal material, which is then scratched into the wound. On entering the vasculature, the organisms migrate to the nearest regional lymph node. Containing only small amounts of the F1 antigen because of their growth in the flea at temperatures of 30° to 35°C, the organisms are readily phagocytosed by polymorphonuclear or mononuclear cells. Because of contained V and W antigens, however, the *Y. pestis* organisms are able to grow and resist intracellular killing, with eventual destruction and lysis of the cell. At this point, at the end of a 3- to 6-day incubation period, organisms are released into surrounding tissue. With large amounts of F1 antigen now present because of growth in the mammalian host at 37°C, the organisms resist phagocytes. With continued rapid growth in a lymph node, the node becomes enlarged, inflamed, necrotic, and hemorrhagic. Vast numbers of these phagocytosis-resistant organisms are now released into the circulation, producing bacteremia in almost all infected humans. Clinical manifestations are those due to the typical gram-negative endotoxemia. These include fever, tachycardia, hypotension, leukocytosis, and laboratory evidence of disseminated intravascular coagulation. In the skin, purpura may be seen secondary to hemorrhage after disseminated intravascular coagulation. Splenic tissue may be engorged, inflamed, and hemorrhagic; the liver may show inflammation; and the kidneys often have glomerular fibrin thrombi as a manifestation of disseminated intravascular coagulation. If the host does not recover, organisms are found in most tissues but in highest concentrations in blood, lymph nodes, and splenic tissue.

CLINICAL FEATURES

Plague in humans generally presents as bubonic disease, in at least 75% of most sporadic presentations. The so-called septicemic form of plague is probably a variation with buboes located primarily intraabdominally or a more fulminant course (21). Pneumonic plague, developing in about 20% of humans, is secondary to dissemination to the lung (22). However, once established as secondary pneumonia, plague can be transmitted from person to person by cough-generated aerosols of *Y. pestis* causing primary plague pneumonia. Meningeal plague, like secondary pneumonia, is due to localization during bacteremia (23). Pharyngeal plague may be due to direct contact with infected tissues.

Bubonic plague occurs after an incubation period of 2 to 8 days, presenting with an abrupt onset of fever, chills, weakness, and headache. Although there is generally a history of possible animal exposure, more than 50% of patients do not remember or have evidence of an insect bite. Twelve to 24 hours after onset of fever, the patient will note painful adenopathy, the bubo. Found in a single anatomic area, the painful node is typically so tender that the patient avoids any movement that will provoke pain. Buboes are most commonly found in the groin (60%) (Fig. 163.5) but can be seen in the axilla (30%) or cervical area (10%) (8,17). The distribution of buboes is presumably due to the site of flea inoculation, and buboes at more than one anatomic site are unusual. When intraabdominal nodes are involved, which may either accompany or occur independently of an inguinal bubo, the patient may have severe abdominal pain, nausea, vomiting,

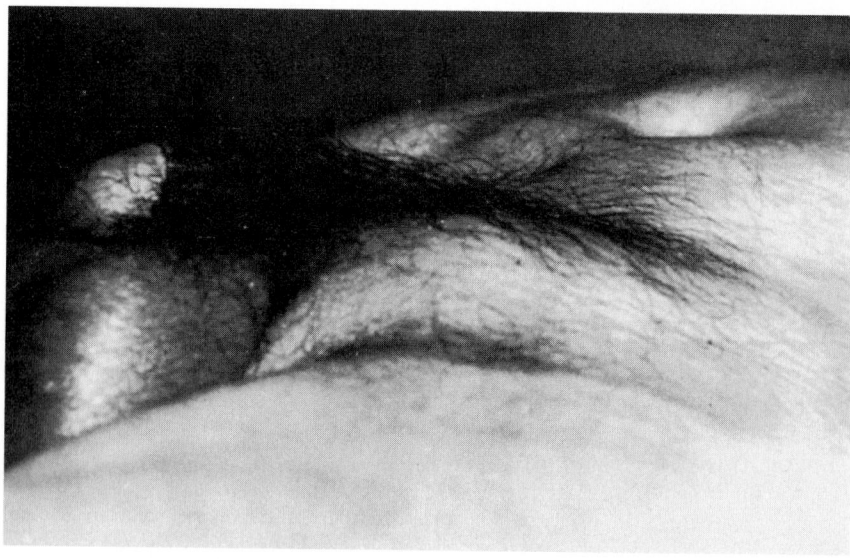

Figure 163.5. Inguinal bubo in a young man with bacteremic plague.

and diarrhea that may be so intense as to mimic an acute abdomen, or severe gastroenteritis (24). Buboes are swellings that vary from 1 to 10 cm in size and elevate the overlying skin, which is often red and stretched intensely. The surrounding tissue may be edematous, and there may be irregular smaller nodes surrounding the main nodular involvement. At presentation, the node is generally not fluctuant but can become secondarily infected with other bacteria, late in the course.

Depending on how early the patient has sought medical attention, the accompanying clinical manifestations may be severe and include modest hypotension, tachycardia, high fever, and shaking chills. As noted, more than 70% of patients with plague may have gastrointestinal complaints (24). Sometimes, neurologic symptoms may be overriding, with insomnia, mental confusion, stupor, weakness, staggering gait, and speech disorders. Most patients with bubonic plague do not have skin lesions, but about 25% of the patients in Vietnam presented with dermatologic findings, including pustules, vesicles, eschars, or papules, presumably at the site of the flea bite (25). These occasionally progress to cellulitis or abscesses. Less commonly, patients develop purpuric skin lesions that involve the extremities and can become necrotic, resulting in gangrene of the fingers, toes, nose, or penis. On abdominal examination, patients frequently show hepatic and splenic enlargement. Aside from tachycardia, the findings on cardiac examination are usually normal.

Laboratory findings are usually nondescript. Leukocytosis of 10,000 to 20,000 white cells/mm^3 is present, with an occasional leukemoid reaction with counts as high as 100,000 cells/mm^3. The peripheral smear will often reveal toxic granulations and Döhle's bodies. Platelet counts may be normal or low, depending on the presence of intravascular coagulopathy, which may also be manifested by fibrin degradation products. Abnormal liver enzyme activities, elevated bilirubin concentration, and hypoglycemia may be seen; with fever and dehydration, there may be a concentrated urine, elevation of the blood urea nitrogen, and some degree of proteinuria.

Although sometimes described as a separate syndrome, septicemia plague most probably represents a fulminant course with the sepsis and bacteremia often found in bubonic plague. Bacteremia is seen in at least 30% of all patients, and bacteremia without buboes is seen in about 10% of all patients. Bacteremia with sepsis is, like other gram-negative sepsis, manifested by hypotension, increased cardiac output, and depressed systemic vascular resistance. Multiorgan system failure results in an overall mortality rate of in excess of 50% despite therapy.

Pneumonic plague is one of the most feared complications of this disease and occurs in about 20% of all patients with *Y. pestis* infection (22). Plague pneumonia is generally a complication of bacteremia with secondary involvement of the lung. Some studies have suggested that in almost half of these, there is no evidence of an infection, and the pathologic process resembles that of classic endotoxin-associated adult respiratory distress syndrome. However, the clinical manifestations may initially be similar, with cough, shortness of breath, and thin, watery, blood-tinged sputum. The radiographic picture is that of a generalized, multilobed, patchy pneumonitis with consolidation in the case of secondary pneumonia and a generalized "white out" of the lung in adult respiratory distress syndrome. In plague pneumonia, the consolidation may occasionally progress to cavitation with air-fluid levels and involvement of the adjacent pleura with an exudative plural effusion (Fig. 163.6). In adult respiratory distress syndrome, frank respiratory failure requiring ventilatory support may supervene. The difference between the two is manifested by the presence of purulent sputum with white blood cells and *Y. pestis* in the case of secondary plague

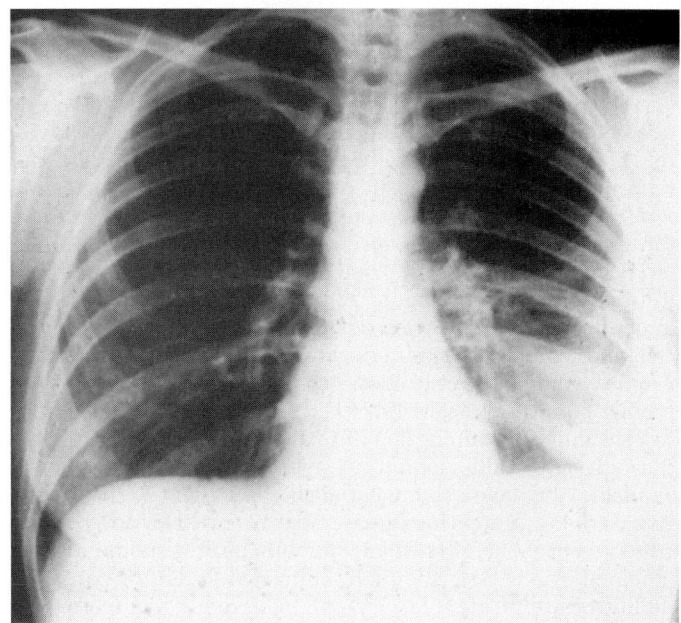

Figure 163.6. Chest radiograph of patient with secondary plague pneumonia, with cavitary changes.

pneumonia, and contagion due to cough-generated aerosols. Person-to-person transmission with the development of primary plague pneumonia may result in a major, rapidly spreading epidemic disease with a mortality rate in excess of 90%. Cases of primary plague pneumonia in the United States have been acquired from domestic cats with secondary pneumonia or pharyngeal infection. Many of these cat-acquired cases were fatal owing to lack of early detection and delay in initiating therapy. Feline plague has been detected in large numbers of cats in the hyperendemic region of New Mexico (more than 60 cases of cat plague) and presents a high risk to both pet owners and veterinarians (5,15,18).

Plague meningitis is an uncommon complication of bubonic plague, classically following an axillary bubo (23). It usually starts 1 week or more after the onset of disease, after antibiotic therapy has been started. Presumably, the plague bacillus, reaching the meninges during the early septicemia phase, is inadequately treated owing to the poor nervous system penetration of antibiotic. It may also appear without local adenitis, possibly more commonly in those handling infected animals. Patients typically have fever, headache, and a stiff neck.

DIAGNOSIS

The diagnosis of plague is critically dependent on obtaining a careful history to document the possibility of exposure to animals or their fleas in a plague endemic area. In a classic presentation with a bubo, fever, and appropriate travel or residence, the clinical diagnosis can be readily made and bacteriologically confirmed. However, not infrequently, patients have traveled to a nonplague location during the incubation period, an exposure history is not taken, and the connection with bubonic plague is not made. Such patients have had a 50% death rate, most commonly as a result of misdiagnosis and inappropriate therapy. Physical examination is usually dramatic and revealing in a patient presenting with an exquisitely painful, erythematous bubo, although the differential diagnosis can include incarcerated inguinal hernia, lymphogranuloma venereum, or localized lymphadenopathy due to regional infection. Finally, in the patient with prominent gastrointestinal symptoms and no bubo, the exposure history may be vital.

When a bubo is present, diagnostic confirmation is made by needle aspiration, using a 20-gauge needle while wearing gloves, mask, and goggles. Because the bubo does not contain liquid material, aspiration of diagnostic material is enhanced by injecting 1 ml of nonbacteriostatic saline and applying suction multiple times until a blood-tinged specimen is obtained. Aspirated material should be plated on blood and MacConkey agar and into infusion broth. Slides should be prepared, and microscopic examination should be carried out. Gram stain shows white blood cells and characteristic gram-negative bacilli. Wayson-stained (or Giemsa-stained) aspirate shows coccobacillary organisms with bipolar bodies characteristic of *Y. pestis* (Fig. 163.4). Direct fluorescent antibody staining is confirmatory and should be available through state health laboratories in endemic areas. If not locally available, the diagnostic material should be sent to the Plague Branch of the Centers for Disease Control and Prevention. Blood cultures and, when indicated, sputum cultures should also be obtained. All cultures should be cultivated at 28°C. Because the definitive culture identification of *Y. pestis* may be confused with that of *Y. pseudotuberculosis*, specific identification by bacteriophage and direct fluorescent antibody test of suspicious colonies is necessary. This may be conducted in special laboratories in states having endemic plague. If pneumonic plague is suspected, sputum should similarly be examined by Gram, Wayson, and fluorescent antibody staining.

Routine laboratory findings are nonspecific, with moderate leukocytosis present and evidence of organ system impairment and acidosis if sepsis has occurred. The peripheral blood smear may show bacteria in as many as 10% of patients. A serologic diagnosis is made by the passive hemagglutination test using the F1 antigen of *Y. pestis*, which demonstrates an antibody response in 2 weeks. A fourfold or greater increase in the titer of antibody is considered positive, as is a single titer of 1:16 or greater. When meningitic plague is suspected, lumbar puncture should be done and cerebrospinal fluid examined for cell count, glucose, protein, and Gram stain and culture. Cerebrospinal fluid should show moderate pleocytosis with polymorphonuclear cells, low glucose level, and modest elevation of protein.

TREATMENT

Untreated plague has a mortality rate of greater than 50%; when there is a high degree of clinical suspicion for this illness, treatment of patients should be started as soon as cultures have been obtained. With appropriate early antibiotic therapy, bubonic plague mortality may be reduced to about 5% to 10%. Most plague deaths in the United States are due to inappropriate delays in diagnosis or incorrect choice of antibiotic therapy. A delay in diagnosis is incurred because it is not recognized that plague may be indirectly transmitted to humans by pets; that plague can present without development of a bubo (septicemia plague); that plague can present with pulmonary symptoms; and that plague may present with severe gastrointestinal symptoms.

The drugs of choice for plague have classically been streptomycin for bubonic or septicemia disease, chloramphenicol for meningeal disease, and tetracycline for prophylaxis of contacts or exposed health care workers. Both streptomycin and chloramphenicol are very hard to find in most pharmacies because of very low usage and thus may not be readily available. Moreover, antibiotic resistance has arisen to these medications and to alternative therapies, such as ampicillin, kanamycin, and minocycline.

However, the organism appears to have retained sensitivity to other aminoglycosides, quinolones, cephalosporins, and doxycycline. The drug of first choice in bubonic, pneumonic, or septicemia plague should therefore be gentamicin, with doxycycline or trimethoprim-sulfamethoxazole for prophylaxis and a third-generation cephalosporin such as cefotaxime for the treatment of meningitis (1,26). The use of ciprofloxacin has been minimal, but it appears to be effective. All of these have been of proven effectiveness in small numbers of cases and are readily available. Gentamicin can be given once or twice daily and either intramuscularly or intravenously and should be continued for 10 days. The patient should become afebrile after 3 to 4 days, but the full 10 days should be given to prevent relapse because plague bacilli may remain viable in buboes for several days during therapy. If an oral drug is strongly preferred, a switch to doxycycline might be considered after 3 to 4 days of parenteral treatment to complete the 10-day course. For plague meningitis, or septic shock, intravenous therapy is necessary, and a combination of ciprofloxacin and gentamicin might be considered if chloramphenicol is not available. Neither the penicillins nor the first-generation cephalosporins have been proved to be effective in bubonic plague. Trimethoprim-sulfamethoxazole may be used in contacts of bubonic plague patients, but they should be asked to return for follow-up in 1 week or sooner if they become febrile. Because as many as 20% of patients with bubonic plague may develop pulmonary complications, it is probably wise to place all plague patients in isolation for observation for the first 48 hours of hospitalization and to get a chest radiograph in all.

Buboes generally resolve during the course of therapy. However, they may occasionally become secondarily infected, most commonly with *Staphylococcus aureus*. If a fluctuant bubo is noted during treatment, surgical drainage may be necessary.

PREVENTION

Other than respiratory isolation precautions in patients with pneumonic plague and the use of doxycycline or trimethoprim-sulfamethoxazole for case contacts of a pneumonic plague patient, no prophylaxis is generally necessary. Patients with bubonic plague are not contagious to health care workers or others around them (once pneumonia has been ruled out). A formalin-killed vaccine is available for laboratory workers who deal continuously with *Y. pestis* and for wildlife biologists working in plague endemic regions (27). The vaccine must be administered in two divided doses as a primary series 1 month apart and booster injections given at six month intervals thereafter to maintain immunity. Because the risk is low, travelers or tourists to plague endemic areas are generally not advised to use the vaccine. Individuals living in rural, plague endemic locations should reduce rodent harborage near their homes, keep pet foods stored in rodent-proof containers, and ensure that housing is rat-proof. Use of flea-directed insecticides (but not generally rodent poisons) may be warranted around houses and on pets.

REFERENCES

1. Galimand M, Guiyoule A, Gerbaud G, et al. Multidrug resistance in *Yersinia pestis* mediated by a transferable plasmid. *N Engl J Med* 1997;337:677–680.
2. Lipson LG. Plague in San Francisco in 1900. The United States Marine Hospital Service Commission to study the existence of plague in San Francisco. *Ann Intern Med* 1972;77:303–310.
3. Butler T. The black death past and present. I. Plague in the 1980s. *Trans R Soc Trop Med Hyg* 1989;83:458–460.

4. Raoult D, Aboudharam G, Crubezy E, et al. Molecular identification by "suicide PCR" of *Yersinia pestis* as the agent of Medieval Black Death. *Proc Natl Acad Sci U S A* 2000;97:12800–12803.
5. Christie AB. Plague: review of ecology. *Ecol Dis* 1982;1:111–115.
6. Tomich PQ, Barnes AM, Devick WS, et al. Evidence for the extinction of plague in Hawaii. *Am J Epidemiol* 1984;119:261–273.
7. Inglesby TA, Dennis DT, Henderson DA, et al. Plague as a biological weapon: medical and public health management. *JAMA* 2000;283:2281–2290.
8. Craven RB, Barnes AM. Plague and tularemia. *Infect Dis Clin North Am* 1991;5:165–175.
9. Kartman L. Historical and ecological observations on plague in the United States. *Trop Geogr Med* 1970;22:257–275.
10. Craven RB, Maupin GO, Beard ML, et al. Reported cases of plague infections in the United States, 1970–1991. *J Med Entomol* 1993;30:758–761.
11. Parmenter RR, Yadav EP, Parmenter CA, et al. Incidence of plague associated with increased winter-spring precipitation in New Mexico. *Am J Trop Med Hyg* 1999;615:814–821.
12. Guiyoule A, Grimont F, Iteman I, et al. Plague pandemics investigated by ribotyping of *Yersinia pestis* strains. *J Clin Microbiol* 1994;32:634–641.
13. Cavanaugh DC. Specific effect of temperature upon transmission of the plague bacillus by the oriental rat flea *Xenopsylla cheopis*. *Am J Trop Med Hyg* 1971;31:839–841.
14. Update: human plague–India, 1994. *MMWR Morbid Mortal Wkly Rep* 1994;43:722–723.
15. Emerging infectious diseases: human plague–United States, 1993–1994. *MMWR Morbid Mortal Wkly Rep* 1994;43:242–246.
16. Mann JM, Shandler L, Cushing AH. Pediatric plague. *Pediatrics* 1982;69:762–767.
17. Palmer DL, Kisch AL, Williams RI Jr, et al. Clinical features of plague in the United States: the 1969–70 epidemic. *J Infect Dis* 1971;124:367–371.
18. Eidson M, Tierney SL, Rollag OJ, et al. Feline plague in New Mexico: risk factors and transmission to humans. *Am J Public Health* 1988;78:1333–1335.
19. Crook LD, Tempest B. Plague: a clinical review of 27 cases. *Arch Intern Med* 1992;152:1253–1256.
20. Ferber DM, Brubaker RR. Plasmids in *Yersinia pestis*. *Infect Immun* 1981;31:839–841.
21. Lewieki EM. Primary plague septicemia. *Rocky Mt Med J* 1978;75:201–202.
22. Alsofrom DJ, Mettler FA, Mann JM. Radiographic manifestations of plague in New Mexico, 1975–1980. *Radiology* 1981;139:561–568.
23. Becker TM, Poland JD, Quan TJ, et al. Plague meningitis: a retrospective analysis of cases reported in the United States, 1970–1979. *Clin Med* 1987;147:554–557.
24. Hull BF, Montes JM, Mann JM. Plague masquerading as gastrointestinal illness. *West J Med* 1986;145:485–487.
25. Butler T, Bell WR, Link NM, et al. *Yersinia pestis* infection in Vietnam. I. Clinical and hematologic aspects. *J Infect Dis* 1974;129:s78–s83.
26. Frean JA, Arntzen L, Capper T, et al. In vitro activities of 14 antibiotics against 100 human isolates of *Yersinia pestis* from a southern African plague focus. *Antimicrob Agents Chemother* 1996;40:2646–2647.
27. *Plague: guide for adult immunizations*, 2nd ed. Philadelphia: American College of Physicians, 1989:89–91.

CHAPTER 164
Anthrax

Christopher C. Penn and Stephen A. Klotz

Anthrax is a disease of great antiquity and occupies an important place in the history of medicine because it was the first human disease to be attributed to a specific pathogen. The causative microorganism is *Bacillus anthracis*, an aerobic gram-positive rod measuring 3 to 8 μm by 1 to 1.5 μm that forms a large polypeptide capsule detectable in clinical specimens. Although the frequency of anthrax in industrialized nations has been reduced sharply in the twentieth and twenty-first centuries, terrorist activities in 2001 in the United States have thrust the disease into the limelight once again. Anthrax still remains an important disease of livestock in many arid and semiarid countries. It is especially prevalent in areas where poverty and nomadic grazing of unvaccinated livestock occur. Shipment of contaminated hides, hair, bone meal, and wool throughout the world gives rise to industry-related anthrax, often in industrialized, nonagrarian countries.

EPIDEMIOLOGY

Biologic Cycle of the Bacterium

It has been hypothesized that *B. anthracis* undergoes an independent propagation cycle in wet alkaline soils in North America followed by sporulation at the onset of dry weather (1). Notwithstanding, the persistence of anthrax in specific geographic regions is due to an environmental cycle that involves contaminated soil and susceptible wild animals and livestock (Fig. 164.1). Such a cycle, coupled with civil war, led to an epidemic in Zimbabwe from 1978 to 1982 with more than 10,000 human cases of anthrax (2). In southern Africa, spore counts in the soil can reach prodigious numbers. Disease is spread to animals and humans in these areas not only by contact with contaminated soil or infected carcasses but also by the bites of tabinid flies (deer flies and horseflies). After feeding on infected carcasses, tabinid flies deposit feces and vomitus containing spores on leaves that are subsequently ingested by browsing herbivores. Furthermore, vultures may spread disease from one location to another after feeding on infected carcasses. When spores are ingested by susceptible herbivores, these animals may die in epizootic proportions. Such has occurred in Africa with kudu and hippopotamuses and in west Texas with white-tailed deer. Cases of livestock anthrax occur regularly, if not yearly, on the Edwards plateau in West Texas and in South Dakota, indicating that the microorganism persists in these geographic regions. The spread of anthrax and endemicity of the disease in livestock in the United States may be due to the use in bygone centuries of popular and well-established cattle trails throughout the western states (3). Anthrax spores can survive for years in ecologically sparse xeric soils and also in workplaces.

Contact with carcasses of infected livestock leads to disease in animal husbandry workers and butchers. However, human cases in the United States, even among unvaccinated animal husbandry workers and veterinarians, are exceedingly uncommon, which may be a reflection of greater care surrounding dead livestock, the relative resistance of humans to anthrax, and diminishing contact with anthrax spores as urbanization continues.

Disease related to Industry

The industrial use of contaminated animal products such as hides, hair, and bone meal introduces a risk in persons who are far removed from the agrarian setting. Textile industries and tanneries are historically the principal sources of outbreaks in industrialized areas. The increasing use of synthetic fibers in the textile industry has contributed to the decline in the number of human cases of industrial anthrax.

In recent decades, disease has affected humans in Asia Minor, particularly Turkey and Iran; in southern Europe, principally Greece; and in Southern Africa as previously mentioned. Owing to inadequate reporting, the true worldwide frequency of disease in humans is unknown. In the twentieth century, most anthrax cases in the United States were industry related. The frequency has been declining in part as a result of preventive health measures such as dust control in the workplaces, import restrictions when deemed appropriate, and decontamination of raw materials.

Bioterrorism

Anthrax can also be spread by biologic weapons. The United States, Soviet Union, and Iraq have possessed weaponized anthrax. This form of warfare was a perceived threat in the Persian Gulf War that was not realized and a *casus belli* in the 2003 war

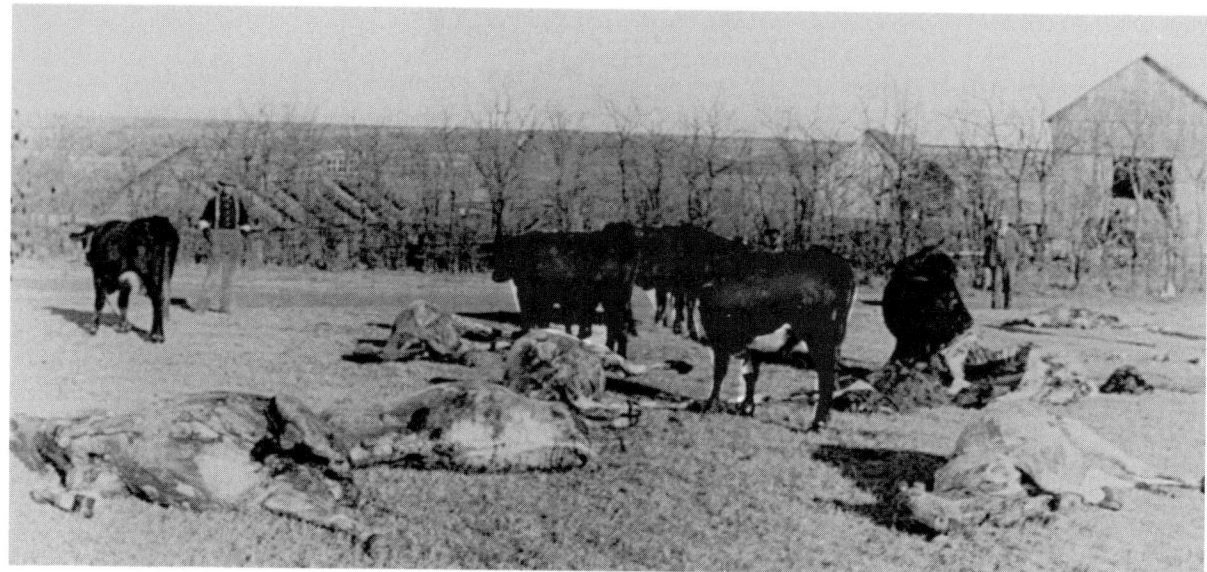

Figure 164.1. Headquarters area of a Smith Center, Kansas ranch in 1911 showing cattle dead from anthrax. Characteristic of this illness is the inability of the blood to clot, as demonstrated by the bloody fluids draining from the natural orifices and the where the hide has been removed. Hides will be contaminated. The same ranch experienced another outbreak of anthrax in cattle in 1990, likely due to the persisting spores. (Courtesy of M. W. Vorhees, DVM, Kansas State University, Manhattan, KS.)

in Iraq. The Aum Shinrikyo cult aerosolized *B. anthracis* Sterne (vaccine strain) over Kameido, Japan in 1993 (4). The accidental expulsion of spores from a biologic weapons plant in Sverdlovsk, now Ekaterinburg, in central Russia in 1979 resulted in significant mortality in livestock and humans (5). Recently, the United States postal system has been employed as a method of dispersing *B. anthracis* spores resulting in significant morbidity, mortality, and economic loss. Laboratorians are at risk for anthrax, as evidenced by a case of cutaneous anthrax in a laboratory technician handling specimens from a contaminated postal facility.

PATHOGENESIS

Inoculation of spores into the skin or contamination of preexisting abrasions leads to germination and vegetative reproduction. The capsule is antiphagocytic. The resulting skin lesion is known as a malignant pustule, although pus is not a hallmark of cutaneous anthrax unless there is secondary infection. Biopsy of cutaneous lesions reveals extensive tissue destruction with marked subepidermal edema, thrombosis of vessels, and hemorrhagic interstitium (6). Nonpitting edema around the lesion and a more generalized edema are thought to be due to toxin production. The draining lymph nodes of cutaneous lesions are avid scavengers of *B. anthracis*, but spread beyond this barrier may give rise to bacteremia.

Inhalation of spores leads to their phagocytosis by alveolar macrophages and transport to mediastinal lymph nodes, where the spores germinate, and hemorrhagic mediastinal lymphadenopathy follows. (It was formerly held that disease would follow only if 10^4 or more spores were inhaled in animal models. However, the nature of presumed contact with contaminated mail by several postal workers who subsequently contracted inhalational pneumonia would argue against the necessity for large numbers of spores.) Mediastinal widening then ensues, usually followed by bacteremia, which is massive and easily detectable in smears of blood. Death is likely due to toxin production. Autopsy specimens from inhalational anthrax victims in Sverdlovsk demonstrated that a primary pneumonia occurs in

the lung (7). Bacteria are not found in the sputum as a rule, but *B. anthracis* DNA is detectable in bronchial washings, pleural fluid, and blood by polymerase chain reaction (PCR) (8).

Gastrointestinal anthrax results from the ingestion of contaminated meat containing large numbers of bacilli or spores. Points of entry into the submucosa appear, particularly in the oropharynx and the ileocecal region. Ulceration develops at the point of inoculation, and hemorrhage occurs in the draining lymph nodes along with local edema. Disease in bowel segments can be accompanied by hemorrhagic ascites. Bacteremia is common in this form of the disease.

Meningitis, when it occurs, is hemorrhagic and secondary to bacteremia, which may arise in any form of the disease.

Immunity may develop from subclinical infection. Disease is thought to confer lasting protection, although reinfection with *B. anthracis* has been reported. Antibodies to toxin and capsule are measurable after infection. A skin test for delayed-type hypersensitivity, Anthraxin, developed in the former Soviet Union, has been reported to be useful in surveys of vaccinated humans and livestock.

CLINICAL MANIFESTATIONS

Anthrax in humans occurs in three principal forms: cutaneous, inhalational, and gastrointestinal. Most cases, 95% or more, are cutaneous disease. Inhalation anthrax comprises the remainder of cases in North America. An outbreak of gastrointestinal anthrax occurred in northern Thailand in 1982 (9) and in India in 1989. Anthrax meningitis, when it occurs, is always secondary to one of the three primary forms of disease and is hemorrhagic. Several cases of primary meningitis without pulmonary symptoms have been reported in recent years.

Cutaneous Anthrax

Cutaneous anthrax begins as a painless, pruritic papule that appears at the site of inoculation within 3 to 10 days. Lesions usually occur on the upper extremities, neck, and face. Several days

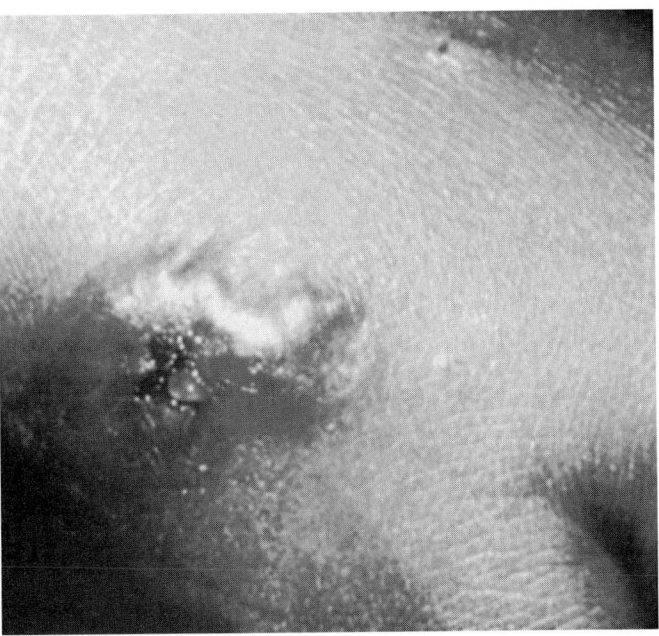

Figure 164.2. Early cutaneous lesion on the thumb of a 6-year old boy from Zimbabwe. (Courtesy of Wilhelm Kobuch, Toulouse, France.)

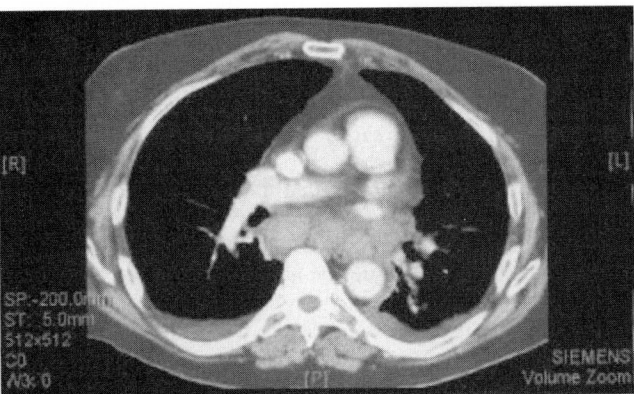

Figure 164.3. Computed tomography of the chest of a patient with inhalational anthrax. Note the mediastinal adenopathy and small pleural effusions. (Reproduced from Jernigan JA, Stephens DS, Ashford DA, et al. Bioterrorism-related inhalational anthrax: the first 10 cases reported in the United States. *Emerg Infect Dis* [serial online] 2001;7:933–944. Available at: http://www.cdc.gov/ncidod/EID.)

later, a vesicle or ring of vesicles develops, along with enlargement of the original lesion to 4 to 6 cm (Fig. 164.2). The base of the vesicle bleeds and may spontaneously discharge clear fluid, which on Gram stain demonstrates numerous microorganisms. The lesion ulcerates, and a central eschar is formed, which may remain *in situ* for up to 3 weeks. Healing usually results in scar formation, and reconstructive surgery may be required for lesions involving the face, particularly the eyelids. Painful regional adenopathy may persist long after successful treatment. Perilesional edema may be extensive, especially if the lesion is located on the face, neck, or upper chest. On occasion, edema may be so extensive as to embarrass respiratory function. Only about 50% of patients have fever, malaise, or leukocytosis. Untreated, cutaneous anthrax may have a mortality rate as high as 20%, probably related to the development of bacteremia. Rarely, multiple skin lesions occur. The evolution of the cutaneous lesion to an eschar is not interrupted by the use of antibiotics, although bacteremia is probably prevented. The appearance of the skin lesion of anthrax may vary, and this, combined with its rarity, may make diagnosis difficult in nonagricultural settings (10) (Table 164.1).

Inhalational Anthrax

Until recently, inhalational anthrax has remained peculiar to the textile industry (11) and is frequently biphasic in nature. After inhalation of spores, patients may complain of upper respiratory symptoms within 3 to 5 days. This viral illness–like prodrome is followed, often within hours, by dyspnea, diaphoresis, cyanosis, shock, and death. Analysis of recent cases confirms that the chest radiograph is helpful in initial evaluation, although findings may be subtle. Historical information regarding the use of computed tomography is lacking; however, information from the 11 victims of inhalational anthrax acquired by contact with contaminated mail in the United States in 2001 underscores the importance of this modality in making the diagnosis (12). Significant findings include hyperdense mediastinal adenopathy, pleural effusions, and occasionally, pericardial effusions (Fig. 164.3). Supraventricular arrhythmias are common. Bacteremia and occasionally splenomegaly accompany this form of the disease.

Before the anthrax outbreak in 2001 in the United States, the diagnosis of inhalational anthrax was usually confirmed at postmortem examination. However, heightened clinical suspicion, newer diagnostic modalities, sophisticated resuscitative efforts, and the use of combined antimicrobials have resulted in an apparent increase in survival from 5% to 60% of patients with inhalational anthrax.

Gastrointestinal Anthrax

Gastrointestinal anthrax may present as an acute abdomen, bloody diarrhea, or sometimes a cholera-like syndrome. A recent outbreak resembled a mild form of viral gastroenteritis, accompanied by high fever. Ascites may develop. Bacteremia usually accompanies this form of the disease. The oropharyngeal form often presents with a mucosal ulcer, regional lymphadenopathy, and accompanying neck edema.

TABLE 164.1.	Evolution of the Skin Lesions of Anthrax		
Features	**Papule**	**Papule with vesicles**	**Eschar**
Size (cm)	1	4–6	4–6
Characteristics	Pruritic, painless	Base of lesion becomes hemorrhagic	On occasion may be quite large
Duration of lesion (days)	2–3	3–5	7–21
Recovery of bacteria	?	Gram stain and culture of vesicular fluid are positive	Gram stain and culture may be positive if obtained from the base of the eschar
Can be confused with:	Orf	Staphylococcal skin lesions; bullous impetigo	Tularemia, plague, burn, cutaneous diphtheria

DIAGNOSIS

Knowledge of the geographic epidemiology of anthrax and clinical findings should suggest the diagnosis of cutaneous anthrax. A provisional diagnosis can be made by demonstrating large, encapsulated gram-positive bacilli, usually in short chains, obtained from a vesicle or the base of an ulcer. Culture will yield growth on most media, although prior antimicrobial treatment may inhibit growth, making isolation difficult. The clinical microbiology laboratory should be alerted to the fact that anthrax is suspected.

Although bacteremia is relatively uncommon in cutaneous anthrax, it occurs in most inhalational and gastrointestinal forms of disease. Microorganisms can be seen in blood smears (see Chapter 188). Gram stain of cerebrospinal fluid usually demonstrates the microorganism in cases of meningitis. Immunohistochemical studies for cell wall and capsule antigen may detect *B. anthracis* in pleural fluid. *B. anthracis* DNA can be detected by PCR in blood, bronchial washings, and pleural fluid (8). Serologic testing for antibody (immunoglobulin G) to *B. anthracis* is also available.

TREATMENT

Until recently, penicillin was recommended as the drug of choice for the treatment of anthrax, even though mean inhibitory concentrations for penicillin may be as high as 1 μg/mL. *In vitro*, *B. anthracis* is susceptible to many antimicrobials, including tetracyclines, chloramphenicol, imipenem, vancomycin, clarithromycin, cefazolin, and other first-generation cephalosporins as well as several quinolones (ciprofloxacin, ofloxacin, and gatifloxacin). It is resistant to cefuroxime, other extended spectrum cephalosporins, as well as trimethoprim-sulfamethoxazole. Inducible β-lactamase production has been reported.

Ciprofloxacin or doxycycline is recommended for empirical therapy of all forms of disease. For more severe cases, additional agents are recommended. Recent cases of inhalational anthrax were successfully treated with a combination of ciprofloxacin, rifampin, and clindamycin (12). The use of clindamycin is based on the theory that it may contribute to decreased toxin production. Hydrocortisone or other corticosteroids may be of benefit in cases of meningitis.

Knowledge about the optimal duration of therapy is expanding. It is thought that 7 to 10 days of oral ciprofloxacin, 500 mg twice a day, or doxycycline, 100 mg twice a day, is adequate treatment for cutaneous anthrax not related to aerosolized anthrax secondary to bioterrorism activity. Cutaneous anthrax in the setting of bioterrorism should be treated for 60 days as prophylaxis against an incubating form of inhalational anthrax. Inhalational anthrax should be treated with the same doses of ciprofloxacin or doxycycline combined with clindamycin and rifampin for a total of intravenous and oral drug for 60 days, or perhaps as long as 100 days (13). Additionally, patients and individuals exposed to aerosolized spores should receive the adsorbed vaccine, 3 injections over a 1-month period (see later) (14).

Extended prophylaxis for a 60-day period for postal workers potentially exposed to anthrax spores did not result in significant adverse events (15). The use of these same antibiotics over this time period, however, causes an increase in the minimal inhibitory concentration (MIC) of the respective drugs in *in vitro* experiments. In the case of quinolones, the rise in MIC may exceed resistant levels of the drug, whereas such is not the case with doxycycline (16). The clinical significance of such a phenomenon is unknown. Resources such as the Centers for Disease Control and Prevention (CDC) should be contacted for up-to-date recommendations (http://www.bt.cdc.gov/Agent/Anthrax/AnthraxGen.asp).

In addition to antimicrobial therapy, other supportive therapies are vital in treating inhalational anthrax. These include ventilatory support, fluid resuscitation, and thoracentesis. Future treatments are focusing on the use of combinations of antimicrobials and antitoxins, specifically targeting anthrax toxin receptors, which can be competitively inhibited by a soluble form of the protein (17).

PREVENTION

Vaccination of livestock is effective in eradicating disease in animals but must be repeated every year. Certain animal products, such as goat skin from Haiti and bristle brushes, are prohibited from entry into the United States or must be decontaminated before entry. However, goat hair, wool, and hides, even those from other known endemic regions, are not subject to import controls. The processing of these materials for use in clothing reduces spore counts to undetectable levels, and the finished products are not considered infectious.

The concept of postexposure prophylaxis relating to anthrax is relative new and continues to evolve. Generally, antimicrobial prophylaxis using either ciprofloxacin or doxycycline for 60 days is recommended. Pregnant women may be treated with penicillin or amoxicillin. Adverse reactions to these regimens were few in more than 8,000 postal employees treated prophylactically in New Jersey, New York City, and Washington, DC in 2001 (15). As with treatment recommendations, health care providers are directed to CDC information sources for up-to-date information (see above for web site).

Several vaccines are available worldwide. BioPort in Lansing, Michigan has now placed its product, an adsorbed vaccine from a formalin-killed avirulent strain of *B. anthracis*, back into production. Individuals who may be considered vaccine candidates include veterinarians, members of the armed forces, and individuals at risk for inhalational or gastrointestinal anthrax. Individuals exposed to aerosolized anthrax should receive vaccine in addition to a minimum of 40 days of antibiotics. Termination of antibiotics in vaccinated primates after 30 days resulted in appreciable mortality, likely from spores still resident in the lungs (18).

Technologic advances now allow for detection of *B. anthracis* in the environment by use of PCR and so-called smart tickets (handheld immunoassays for spores), whose efficacy has not yet been proved. Environmental surfaces can be decontaminated with 0.5% hypochlorite.

REFERENCES

1. Ness GBV. Ecology of anthrax. *Science* 1971;172:1303.
2. Davies JCA. A major epidemic of anthrax in Zimbabwe, part I. *Cent Afr J Med* 1982;28:291.
3. Coker PR, Smith KL, Hugh-Jones ME. Anthrax in the USA. Third International Conference on Anthrax, Plymouth, England, 1998.
4. Kiem P, Smith KL, Keys C, Takahashi H, et al. Molecular investigation of the Aum Shinrikyo anthrax release in Kameido, Japan. *J Clin Microbiol* 2001;39:4566–4567.
5. Meselson M, Guillemin J, Hugh-Jones M, et al. The Sverdlovsk anthrax outbreak of 1979. *Science* 1994;266:1202.
6. Dutz W, Kohout E. Anthrax. *Pathol Annu* 1971;6:209.
7. Abramova FA, Ginberg LM, Yampolskaya OV, et al. Pathology of inhalation anthrax in 42 cases from the Sverdlovsk outbreak of 1979. *Proc Natl Acad Sci U S A* 1993;90:2291.
8. Mina B, Dym JP, Kuepper F, et al. Fatal inhalational anthrax with unknown source of exposure in a 61-year-old woman in New York City. *JAMA* 2002;287:858–862.

9. Sirisanthana T, Navachareen N, Tharavichitkul P, et al. Outbreak of oral-oropharyngeal anthrax: an unusual manifestation of infection with *Bacillus anthracis*. *Am J Trop Med Hyg* 1984;33:144.
10. Gold H. Anthrax: a report of one hundred-seventeen cases. *Arch Intern Med* 1955;96:387.
11. Brachman PS. Inhalational anthrax. *N Y Acad Sci* 1980;353:83.
12. Jernigan JA, Stephens DS, Ashford DA, et al. Bioterrorism-related inhalational anthrax: the first 10 cases reported in the United States. *Emerg Infect Dis* 2001;7:933–944.
13. Anonymous. Update: investigation of bioterrorism-related anthrax and interim guidelines for exposure management and antimicrobial therapy, October 2001. *MMWR Morb Mortal Wkly Rep* 2001;50:909–919.
14. Anonymous. Notice to readers: additional options for preventive treatment for persons exposed to inhalational anthrax. *MMWR Morb Mortal Wkly Rep* 2001;50:1142.
15. Anonymous. Update: adverse events associated with anthrax prophylaxis among postal employees—New Jersey, New York City, and the District of Columbia metropolitan area, 2001. *MMWR Morb Mortal Wkly Rep* 2001;30:1051–1054.
16. Brook I, Elliott TB, Pryor HI, et al. In vitro resistance of *Bacillus anthracis* Sterne to doxycycline, macrolides, and quinolones. Forty-first Interscience Conference on Antimicrobial Agents and Chemotherapy. Chicago, IL: ASM Press, 2001.
17. Bradley KA, Mogridge J, Mourez M, et al. Identification of the cellular receptor for anthrax toxin. *Nature* 2001;414:225–229.
18. Friedlander AM, Welkos SL, Pitt MLM, et al. Postexposure prophylaxis against experimental inhalation anthrax. *J Infect Dis* 1993;167:1239–1242.

CHAPTER 165
Glanders

John G. Bartlett

Glanders is an infection with varied clinical features caused by *Burkholderia mallei*. The organism is usually acquired from equine sources, primarily horses. Glanders is found most often in Asia, Africa, and South America; there has been one reported case in the United States since 1944, and this was laboratory acquired (1).

CHARACTERISTICS OF THE PATHOGEN

B. mallei is a gram-negative aerobic bacterium that is related to *Burkholderia pseudomallei*, the agent of melioidosis. Like *Pseudomonas* species, *B. mallei* produces catalase and oxidase. *B. mallei* and *B. pseudomallei* are antigenically related, but differ in that *B. mallei* is nonmotile and grows poorly on ordinary laboratory media.

HISTORY

B. mallei was originally isolated by Loeffler and Schutz in 1882 from a horse that died with glanders (2). The name *Bacillus mallei* was applied by Zopf in 1885. A related organism was isolated from a man with a disease resembling glanders by Whitmore and Krishnaswami in 1912; that organism was designated *Bacillus pseudomallei* by Whitmore in 1913; Stanton and Fletcher subsequently applied the name *melioidosis* to the disease and *whitmori* to the agent. Both organisms were initially thought to be animal parasites, but it was subsequently found that *B. pseudomallei* was a natural inhabitant of soil in tropical areas. The close relationship of these two organisms was initially based on the fact that they were similar microbiologically and caused similar diseases, and it was subsequently shown that they are closely related biochemically with a guanine plus cytosine content of 68% to 69%. *B. mallei* infection differs in that it has always been a rare disease

in humans; it remains primarily a disease of horses, and infrequently, it is found in soil and other environmental sources. In 1906, Robins reported that only 156 cases of glanders in humans had been reported (3).

At one time, glanders was a severe and often lethal disease in horses throughout the world. It has been largely eliminated from the developed world through infection control measures as well as replacement of horse-drawn vehicles. Control of glanders in horses was achieved in England through the British Glanders or Farcy Order of 1907, which mandated that every animal with clinical evidence of these conditions was to be slaughtered and the carcass destroyed or buried. Mallein, a product of *B. mallei* grown in glycerol broth, was often used as an intradermal or conjunctival test for case detection in animals, and all positive reactors were also killed (4).

During World War I, Germany developed stocks of *B. mallei* and anthrax that were given to undercover agents to infect livestock shipped to allied countries (5). The goal was destruction of livestock and transmission to humans, but the plan failed to materialize. A current major interest in *B. mallei* is for developing an antibiotic-resistant form that could be aerosolized for germ warfare (6). The only case in the United States in 50 years was reported in a military microbiologist studying the organism for biodefense (1,7).

EPIDEMIOLOGY

Glanders is a serious infection of equine animals, principally horses but also mules and donkeys. The disease may occasionally affect goats, sheep, dogs, and cats.

The major diseases in horses are glanders and farcy. Glanders may be acute or chronic with primary involvement of the lung. There may also be nodular or ulcerative lesions of the nasal or tracheal mucosa. Many animals show subcutaneous abscesses, and there may be widespread dissemination with involvement of the spleen, liver, and other organs. With farcy, the typical lesions are found in the skin or subcutaneous tissue, primarily on the extremities and flanks, which appear as nodules that subsequently ulcerate. Involvement of lymphatic channels results in firm cords, sometimes referred to as *farcy pipes*, and large lymph nodes, referred to as *farcy buds*.

Glanders has largely been eliminated from the industrialized world. The major sources of infection in humans and animals at present are in Asia, Africa, and South America.

The disease is transmitted to humans by contact with infected animals, primarily horses. The disease may also be transmitted from person to person, emphasizing the importance of isolation. The animal source may have clinically silent infection. Infectious material includes nasal and pulmonary discharges and infected urine or stool from animals with glanders. Farcy is transmitted by subcutaneous inoculation. The organism also represents a laboratory hazard; several cases have been reported in laboratory workers.

CLINICAL FEATURES

Symptoms are varied and may be classified in four categories:

1. Localized infection reflects a cutaneous or mucosal site of inoculation that results in a nodule with lymphangitis. The usual incubation period is 1 to 5 days. The typical lesion is a nodule with cordlike induration of lymphatic channels, similar to farcy in animals. The nodules frequently break down and ulcerate.

2. Inoculation of the mucous membranes may cause localized infection of the eye, nose, or oral cavity, resulting in a similar type of ulcerating, granulomatous reaction, with or without a systemic response, including fever.

3. The septicemic form of the disease may occur 1 to 4 weeks after untreated infection in lymph nodes. This may cause widespread abscesses involving liver, spleen, and lung with signs of sepsis with or without a generalized papular rash that progresses to a pustular rash.

4. The pulmonary form shows an incubation period of 10 to 14 days, followed by fever, malaise, headache, and pleurisy. It is often uncertain whether the lung is involved through inhalation or by secondary invasion from other sites of involvement. The chest radiograph may show lobar pneumonia, bronchopneumonia, or nodular densities.

With all forms of glanders, the leukocyte count may show slight leukocytosis or leukopenia, there may be a relative lymphocytosis, or the peripheral leukocyte counts and differential may be entirely normal. The course of the disease is variable. Acute glanders with septicemia is usually fatal within 7 to 10 days. With chronic disease, there may be subcutaneous and muscle abscesses with lymphadenopathy and ulcerating lesions of mucosal surfaces. Abscesses should undergo surgical drainage. The disease may remain active for months or years. There may be apparent spontaneous recovery with subsequent relapse, and there may be latent periods for up to 10 years.

DIAGNOSIS

Gram stain examination of exudates may show typical small, gram-negative, slender bacilli, but the organisms are often present in small numbers and may be difficult to detect with direct stains. *B. mallei* and *B. pseudomallei* cannot be distinguished by Gram stain. *B. mallei* will grow slowly on most nutrient agar; growth is improved with media containing glycerol. Blood cultures usually fail to propagate the organism. Serologic tests include agglutination assays that demonstrate increased titers to at least 1:640 in the second week of infection. The complement fixation test is more specific but less sensitive. The mallein intradermal test has been primarily used for detecting the disease in animals.

TREATMENT

The only antimicrobial agent with established merit is sulfazine and trimethoprim plus sulfonamides, which have proved useful in experimentally infected hamsters and in a limited experience in patients with glanders (8,9). The organism is resistant to penicillin and can be grown selectively in media containing penicillin. It is sensitive *in vitro* to ceftazidime, gentamicin, imipenem, doxycycline, ciprofloxacin, and chloramphenicol. The use of these drugs in experimental animals has given variable results.

REFERENCES

1. Srinivasan A, Kraus CN, DeShazer D, et al. Glanders in a military research microbiologist. *N Engl J Med* 2001;345:256.
2. Wilson GS, Miles A. Diseases due to pseudomonads, including melioidosis and glanders. In: Wilson GS, ed. *Topley and Wilson's principles of bacteriology, virology and immunology*, Vol 2. Baltimore: Williams & Wilkins, 1975:18–43.
3. Robins GD. A study of chronic glanders in man with report of a case: analysis of 156 cases collected from the literature. *Stud R Victoria Hosp Montreal* 1906; 2:98.
4. McGilvray CD. The transmission of glanders from horse to man. *Can J Public Health* 1944;35:268.
5. Wheelis M. First shots fired in biological warfare. *Nature* 1998;395:213.
6. Centers for Disease Control and Prevention. Biological and chemical terrorism: strategic plan for preparedness and response. Recommendations of the CDC Strategic Planning Workshop. *MMWR Morb Mortal Wkly Rep* 2000;49(RR-4): 1–14.
7. Howe C, Miller WR. Human glanders: report of six cases. *Ann Intern Med* 1947; 26:93.
8. Miller WR, Pannell L, Ingalls MS. Experimental chemotherapy in glanders and melioidosis. *Am J Hyg* 1948;47:205.
9. Barmanov VP. Treatment of experimental glanders with combinations of sulfazine or sulfamonomethoxine with trimethoprim [in Russian]. *Antibiot Khimiter* 1993;38:18.

CHAPTER 166
Leptospirosis

Patrick W. Kelley

Leptospirosis is a spirochetal infection that is acquired by animals and humans, primarily through direct or indirect contact of skin or mucous membranes with the contaminated urine of infected wild and domestic mammals. It can develop clinically as an asymptomatic or influenza-like infection, or it may present with severe hemorrhagic manifestations and associated meningism, jaundice, myocarditis, and renal failure. The classic severe presentation that Adolph Weil described in 1886 became known as Weil's disease. As clinical understanding of leptospirosis has grown in the past 100 years, it has become clear that most human leptospiral infections represent the milder, self-limited end of the clinical spectrum. Transmission has been well documented in urban, suburban, and rural settings. Timely diagnosis is important because prompt initiation of antibiotic therapy is efficacious and potentially lifesaving in at least some situations. Efforts at prevention may include immunization of domestic animals, rodent control, antibiotic prophylaxis, surface decontamination, use of protective clothing, and education to reduce needless exposures.

HISTORY

Leptospirosis is considered one of the most widespread zoonoses, yet its recognition as a reported clinical entity dates only to the 1800s (1–3). In 1886, Weil lent his name to the most intense presentation of leptospirosis when he described four febrile men with a distinct syndrome characterized by "particularities of an acute infectious illness with spleen tumor, jaundice, and nephritis" (2). During the period 1914 to 1916, Inada and Ino concluded that the cause of leptospirosis was a spirochete; they found the organisms in the blood of jaundiced Japanese miners and in the liver of guinea pigs inoculated with blood from infected patients but not in the liver of guinea pigs inoculated with blood from control subjects (2). In 1916, Ido and co-workers reported that 40% of 86 house and ditch rats carried these spirochetes and thus implicated rats in the transmission cycle of leptospirosis (4).

In 1917 and 1918, Ido, Ito, and Wani concluded that a similar spirochete was associated with an anicteric illness called the *7-day fever* (2). This spirochete (then termed *Leptospira hebdomadis*) was serologically differentiated from the organism associated with Weil's syndrome (then termed *Leptospira icterohaemorrhagiae*); the field mouse (*Microtus montebelli*) was viewed as its animal host. The first U.S. case of leptospirosis was recognized in 1922. Although most then recognized U.S. cases were icteric, anicteric cases were occurring in the United States. This was documented in the 1950s by retrospective studies that proved that during the early 1940s at Fort Bragg, North Carolina, several summer outbreaks of a self-limited, anicteric, febrile illness accompanied by a pretibial rash were due to the *autumnalis* serovar (5). Numerous sporadic cases and other outbreaks have resulted in many colorful appellations, such as *sugarcane illness, swineherd's meningitis, rice-field fever, swamp fever, fish-handler disease, Japanese autumnal fever,* and *mouse fever* (6).

CHARACTERISTICS OF THE PATHOGEN

Taxonomy and Morphology

Pathogenic manifestations of leptospirosis can result from infection with any of more than 250 antigenically distinct serovars. At least 99 serovars have been isolated from humans, and at least 27 have been found in the United States (6). The family Leptospiraceae is divided into the pathogenic genus, *Leptospira*, and two nonpathogenic genera, *Leptonema* and *Turneria*. The traditional taxonomic classification of the Leptospiraceae based on serogroups and serovars has undergone considerable revision in recent years on the basis of genetic relatedness studies with the result that many new species classifications are being described that do not relate to the traditional serologic groupings based on the microagglutination test (MAT). Taxonomic divisions now include at least 12 species of *Leptospira*: *L. alexanderi, L. biflexa, L. borgpetersenii, L. fainei, L. inadai, L. interrogans, L. kirschneri, L. noguchii, L. santarosai, L. weilii, L. meyeri,* and *L. wolbachii*. These species have been classified as pathogen, intermediate, or saprophyte (3,7). The traditional serologically determined classifications into serogroups and serovars based on the MAT still remain common and useful but may be replaced by the molecular-based taxonomy. Strains that are serologically classified within a particular serovar have been assigned to more than one species based on molecular techniques. The molecular scheme may allow correlations between particular species and clinical manifestations that were not reliably detected with the serovar system. Further molecular studies may explain why, for example, a nonvirulent *hebdomadis* serovar in one part of the world might be serologically classified as identical to a virulent *hebdomadis* serovar from another region (6). Leptospires are obligate aerobes and appear as motile, flexible, tightly coiled, helicoid rods about 0.1 μm in diameter and 6 to 20 μm in length. One or both ends of the cells are usually hooked (8).

Laboratory Isolation

Media such as Fletcher semisolid or Tween 80-albumin (EMJH) allow leptospiral organisms to be isolated from blood and cerebrospinal fluid (CSF) during the first 7 to 10 days of illness and from urine after the first week of illness (8,9). Minimal inocula (1 mL of blood or urine in 10 mL of medium and diluted serially to produce three concentrations of 1:10, 1:100, and 1:1000) of blood, urine, or tissue are recommended to dilute out inhibitory substances. Multiple cultures should be made over time. In one study in which blood and urine cultures were obtained within 3 days of fever onset, more than 94% of the patients' cultures were positive (10). Because leptospires are slow growing, cultures should be incubated for 3 or 4 months in the dark at 28° to 30°C. If an appropriate medium is not readily available, blood may be collected before antibiotic therapy in a tube containing heparin or sodium oxalate as an anticoagulant. Viable leptospires may be recoverable from such specimens for more than a week after collection. Leptospires can also be isolated from contaminated specimens by passage through weanling hamsters or guinea pigs (11).

EPIDEMIOLOGY

Animals that survive the acute infection can harbor the spirochete in their renal tubules for months and even years. Chronic urinary shedding of leptospires can lead to further human or animal infections either through direct urinary contact or by contamination of soil and surface waters. Dogs immunized with canine bacterins to prevent clinical disease can still develop renal infections and leptospiruria (12). At least one outbreak of leptospirosis has been attributed to contact with the urine of immunized pet dogs (12). Mammals appear to be the only epidemiologically significant transmitters of leptospirosis, although the spirochetes have been isolated from birds, reptiles, amphibians, arthropods, mollusks, and helminths. In the United States from 1965 to 1974, dogs were implicated in transmission to humans about twice as often as rodents were. Cattle were also among the most important sources (13). The epidemiologic importance of any specific animal source at a given time is probably a function of the local ecology, the nature of human activities in that environment, and the dynamic shifts in the prevalence and virulence of different serovars. Although a particular host may harbor one or more serovars and a given serovar may occur in a variety of hosts, certain animals tend to serve as principal hosts for particular serovars.

Distribution

Leptospirosis has been reported in humans and animals in almost every country (6). Occurrence in a particular setting is a function of the presence of an appropriate animal host and local environmental conditions. In the United States, cases of leptospirosis have been reported from virtually all states, although most cases are recorded in Hawaii and in the less arid states in the southern half of the country (13). Significant U.S. outbreaks have been reported in recent years not only in rural settings but also in the inner city (14). A wet, alkaline environment favors survival of leptospires. Because the optimal temperature for survival is 28° to 32°C, tropical, unpolluted, nonsaline waters with a slightly alkaline pH provide a highly favorable situation. Pathogenic leptospires can survive a few hours in acid urine, but they survive much longer when the urine is diluted and less acid. Flooding after heavy tropical rains can facilitate saturation of the environment by subsurface leptospires, enhance the flushing of leptospires into surface waters, and draw rodents and other animals to swampy areas (8).

In the United States, leptospirosis cases occur year-round, but about half occur from July to October (13). Seasonality may be a function of agricultural cycles and increased levels of outdoor recreation in the warmer months; in some tropical countries, however, temporal increases in frequency coincide with the rainy season. Given the right association of animals and humans, even arid regions of the world can sustain significant levels of transmission. A drought may also create local conditions that can facilitate transmission (15).

Leptospirosis has traditionally been associated with occupations that bring people into direct or indirect contact with contaminated animal urine or infectious tissues. Leptospires enter through breaks in the skin or mucous membranes. Skin changes resulting from prolonged immersion in water may enhance the entrance of leptospires through otherwise intact skin. Occupational groups at particular risk for leptospirosis include persons employed in agriculture and aquaculture, sewer workers, construction workers, livestock handlers, abattoir workers, laboratory personnel, veterinarians, miners, and soldiers. Walking barefoot in places frequented by rodents or dogs would appear to be a risk factor in both rural and urban settings (14). In the past 20 years, avocational pursuits have been as epidemiologically important as occupational exposures and include the care of household pets, hunting, trapping, fishing, swimming in ponds or bodies of freshwater, rafting, and sports that result in contact with muddy fields (12,16,17). Contaminated well water, spring water, and food preparation surfaces have also been implicated in transmission to humans, as have animal bites and stagnant pools of water (1,4,8,18). Human-to-human transmission has been attributed to urine, breast milk, and sexual intercourse, but transmission by these routes is extremely rare (8,19).

Occurrence

During the mid-1980s, the number of cases of leptospirosis reported annually in the United States was in the range of 35 to 60 (20). Because the customary presentation of leptospirosis is fairly nonspecific and the index of suspicion is often low, this incidence should be regarded as a gross underestimate. Incidence rate estimates for various occupations can be high: 11,000 per 100,000 person-years for New Zealand dairy farmers; 3,700 per 100,000 person-years for Glasgow sewer workers; and 2,200 per 100,000 person-years for Hawaiian taro farmers (21). Between 1977 and 1982, surveillance of U.S. Army units undergoing a jungle warfare course in Panama during the fall rainy season yielded 91 confirmed and probable cases, for an annualized incidence estimate of 41,000 per 100,000 person-years (Takafuji E, unpublished data). This most likely underestimated the true risk because potential exposures did not occur every day.

PATHOGENESIS

The primary pathogenic manifestations of acute leptospirosis result from damage to the endothelial lining of capillaries coupled with renal tubular dysfunction and subcellular hepatic dysfunction (1,3). In many ways, it resembles other systemic infectious vasculitides. Among patients who die with severe leptospirosis, widespread hemorrhagic signs are evident and may include petechiae of skin, mucosal, and serosal surfaces. In some cases, gross visceral hemorrhage is also noted. One autopsy series found the cut surfaces of the lungs to be hemorrhagic in 60% of the cases (22). These hemorrhagic findings appear to reflect primarily endothelial damage rather than problems with blood clotting. In addition to hemorrhage, the endothelial changes in leptospirosis may facilitate fluid shifts from intravascular to extracellular spaces and thus contribute to hypovolemia (1). Cardiovascular abnormalities in addition to hemorrhage can include myocarditis, coronary arteritis, aortitis, pericarditis, and arrhythmias (23).

Historically, renal failure has been the cause of most leptospirosis-associated deaths, but the availability of dialysis has reduced the importance of this as a cause of death. The central pathogenic mechanism of renal failure in leptospirosis is probably ischemia, with consequent tissue hypoxia and renal tubule damage (1). Interstitial nephritis may follow this hypoxic effect and becomes most evident during the second week of illness. Proteinuria, pyuria, hematuria, hyaline and granular casts,

oliguria, and subsequent uremic manifestations clinically complement this picture.

Jaundice is common in fatal leptospirosis, although the overall architecture of the liver is fairly well preserved. When jaundice does occur, it appears related to hepatic cell dysfunction more than to hemolysis. Increased absorption of blood from tissue hemorrhage may contribute to the jaundice. Liver cell necrosis is uncommon, and liver transaminase values are increased only slightly. Deficiencies in serum prothrombin activity may be detected and can be corrected with vitamin K. Survivors of severe leptospirosis generally enjoy complete return of hepatic and renal function.

Myalgias may be prominent early in the clinical course of leptospirosis. Meningeal irritation is another hallmark of leptospirosis, although pathologic findings tend to be minimal (1). During the first week when spirochetes can be cultured from the CSF, the fluid is often normal otherwise. Meningismus tends to occur during the second week, coincident with the development of serum antibody and the disappearance of leptospires from the CSF. Similarly, leptospires may penetrate the anterior chamber of the eye and cause inflammation of the anterior uveal tract during the second week of the illness or as late as 1 year into the infection (3,8).

Antigen–antibody complexes or autoimmune responses may help explain effects observed in the eyes, nervous system, and kidney after the first week of illness (1). Immunity in leptospirosis is largely humoral, with circulating antibodies leading to opsonization of leptospires. Use of antibiotics may blunt the production of antibodies (1). Subsequent attacks with the same serovar do not seem to occur, but cross-immunity against other serovars is limited (4,24). Intrauterine infections can result in fetal death and abortion, stillbirth, premature labor, and signs of congenital leptospirosis soon after delivery (25). Lactating mothers may secrete leptospires in their milk during the septicemic phase.

CLINICAL MANIFESTATIONS

The incubation period of leptospirosis is 7 to 12 days (range, 2 to 26 days) (Table 166.1). Short incubation has been associated with laboratory and animal bite exposures (4). The variability in symptoms associated with infection is considerable, although few cases are thought to be entirely asymptomatic, as supported by the observation that in one prospective serosurvey, only 1 of 24 infected persons denied any symptoms (10). About 90% of cases present as a self-limited febrile illness that often escapes specific diagnosis because of a low index of suspicion or because the patient does not seek medical care. The other 10% of cases meet the description of Weil's disease and are often marked by fever, jaundice, hemorrhage, renal failure, and neurologic findings.

Patients with mild, anicteric leptospirosis often describe sudden onset of fever, mild to severe headache, profound myalgia, chills, back pain, joint pain, neck stiffness, and prostration. The fever may peak with temperature in the 38° to 40°C (100° to 105°F) range. The myalgias are often intense and most prominent in the lumbosacral spine, thighs, and calves. Merely lightly touching the skin over a muscle may cause pain. Conjunctival findings have been rarely noted in some series, yet other authors report them in virtually all cases (13,26). The most characteristic ocular finding during the first 3 days of the illness is conjunctival suffusion, a dilation of the conjunctival vessels without associated signs of inflammation. Generalized abdominal pain is not unusual and has led clinicians to suspect an acute abdomen or enteric fever. The pain may in fact be muscular, although

TABLE 166.1.   Clinical and Laboratory Manifestations of Leptospirosis in Six Published Series

Findings	Prevalence of findings (%) by investigators[a]					
	Berman et al. (31) n = 150, Vietnam	Heath et al. (27) n = 483, United States	Kaufmann (13) n = 368, United States	Alexander et al. (26) n = 106 (Anicteric), Puerto Rico	Alexander et al. (26) n = 107 (Icteric), Puerto Rico	Alston & Broom (4) n = 600 (Weil's), United Kingdom
Abrupt onset	—	78	—	—	—	62
Fever	97	100	62	100	99	—
Chills	78	66	16	84	90	—
Headache	98	77	50	82	95	87
Meningismus, stiff neck	12	37	40	12	5	34
Myalgias	79	68	29	97	97	—
Muscle tenderness	42	—	—	70	79	69
Nausea, vomiting	41/33	60	28	71/65	81/75	—
Diarrhea	29	15	5	25	30	—
Jaundice	2	43	33	0	100	74
Hepatomegaly	15	18	—	60	80	—
Splenomegaly	22	5	—	2	5	—
Abdominal tenderness	27	30	5	—	—	—
Conjunctival injection	42	33	8	100	98	72
Rash	7	9	9	—	—	—
Petechiae, ecchymoses	—	3	—	4	29	—
Anuria, oliguria	—	10	15	20	30	—
Azotemia	26	26	26	42	71	—
Albuminuria	≥67	19	21	64	79	75
Hematuria	5	27	22	9	13	—
Relapse (second pyrexia)	48	—	—	4	23	32
Case-fatality rate	0	7	8	0	13	—

[a] Number of subjects and location of the study are provided after the reference. Some reported percentages are based on a larger or smaller sample than that used to assess most manifestations.

gastrointestinal tract disease has been documented (1,26). Skin manifestations associated with mild leptospirosis can include a transient macular, maculopapular, erythematous, purpuric, or urticarial rash, the distribution of which is mainly truncal but can also include other areas of the body. Hepatomegaly may be noted in more than 50% of cases, though it is often less (26,27). Epistaxis and slightly bloody sputum may occur, but frank hemoptysis is uncommon. In 1995, however, a large outbreak of leptospirosis associated with pulmonary hemorrhage and without jaundice or renal manifestations was reported in Nicaragua (28). Cases and epidemics with pulmonary hemorrhage with few or no jaundiced patients have also been reported in Korea and China (29,30). Acute respiratory distress syndrome may also occur. Central nervous system effects may be reflected in meningeal irritation, photophobia, or mild to severe physiologic dysfunction. Variation in the clinical presentations reported by different authors may reflect differences in the prevalent serovars or in approaches to case identification (4,13,31,32).

Leptospirosis is classically described as a biphasic illness with an initial leptospiremic phase, a brief and fairly asymptomatic period, and then a secondary leptospiruric or "immune" phase (1–4). This classic course has been infrequently appreciated by some authors (26,31). In a review of 150 cases among U.S. soldiers in Vietnam by Berman and colleagues (31), only 48% of cases were marked by recurrence of fever, and that usually lasted only 1 day. The initial phase is notable for the presence of leptospires in the blood and CSF and typically lasts 4 to 7 days. The intervening asymptomatic period may last 1 to 5 days. Resolution of fever at the end of the initial phase has been noted to coincide with the appearance of agglutinating antibodies (31). The appearance of antibody also correlates with the disappearance of leptospiremia. The leptospiruric phase may begin with recurrence of fever and otherwise may be highly variable clinically. Headache and other signs of aseptic meningitis are frequent and prominent in the second phase. Meningeal symptoms can actu-

ally appear to be the initial manifestation of leptospirosis. The leptospiruric phase may last 4 to 30 days or longer.

In the minority of patients whose disease is at the most severe end of the clinical spectrum, the initial fever and generalized abnormalities can progress after several days to a life-threatening illness characterized by jaundice, azotemia, hemorrhage, anemia, shock, and severe mental status changes. The disease progresses during the second week, often without any significant interphase clinical improvement. Hemorrhagic signs may include petechiae, purpura, conjunctival hemorrhages, and bloody sputum. Clinical abnormalities peak in the second week, which is when fatally afflicted patients tend to expire (4). Renal failure may be accompanied by normal or reduced urine output or none. Low urine output may reflect volume depletion, hypotension, or acute tubular necrosis. In survivors, oliguria and anuria usually resolve during the second and third weeks, sometimes in association with notable diuresis. Before the availability of dialysis, the leading cause of death in many places was renal failure. Other potentially fatal complications include adult respiratory distress syndrome, congestive heart failure, and arrhythmias (32–34). Rarely, adrenal hemorrhage may result in sudden death. The severe hemorrhagic pneumonitis noted occasionally occurs usually during the second week. The liver derangements in leptospirosis are themselves rarely fatal. The liver, cardiac, and pulmonary abnormalities typically resolve completely in survivors, although the convalescent period may extend for several months.

The conjunctival suffusion associated with early leptospirosis is self-limited and usually resolves within a week without any specific intervention. A delayed ocular complication, however, is anterior uveal tract inflammation, which may become evident in up to 10% of patients during convalescence or as long as a year later. This may present clinically as iritis, iridocyclitis, and rarely chorioretinitis. Increased intraocular pressure secondary to the uveitis may be noted. The occurrence of cataracts and anterior chamber hypopyon may lead to blindness. Posterior ocular findings may also include retinal hemorrhage, vitreous membranes, and papilledema. Cotton-wool spots indicative of ischemic retinopathy have also been described (35). Some ophthalmic sequelae and headache may persist for decades (36).

Published figures for the duration of illness and case-fatality rates are confounded by the variable mix of mild and severe cases reported and by local medical practice. The case-fatality rate for U.S. cases reported in 1977 through 1983 ranged from 2.4% to 11.3% (37). In aggressive surveillance in which the proportion of mild cases reported is likely to be increased, the case-fatality rate is less than 1.0%. Reports from several tropical countries have noted case-fatality rates for severe leptospirosis of up to 18.8% (38).

Key laboratory abnormalities in leptospirosis include mild proteinuria (8,31). Pyuria, granular casts, and microscopic hematuria may be seen. Blood urea nitrogen levels vary with the severity of illness but are below 100 mg per 100 mL in most cases (39). Results of liver function tests are usually normal in anicteric illness. In jaundiced patients, transaminase and alkaline phosphatase levels may be increased twofold to threefold. The bilirubin level in icteric cases remains below 20 mg/dL in at least two thirds of cases and is predominantly conjugated (39). Although prothrombin levels are usually normal, vitamin K can correct the prothrombin deficiency that is sometimes seen. Creatine kinase (MM fraction) and amylase levels are commonly elevated (40,41). A complete blood count typically indicates a white cell count of 5,000 to 15,000 cells/mm^3, although it may be increased to more than 49,000 cells/mm^3 in severe disease. Neutrophilia is common. Anemia may be present, especially with more severe illness. Thrombocytopenia is common, although the platelet count is usually above 50,000 cells/mm^3; rarely, thrombocytopenia is severe (42,43). Examination of the CSF during the immune phase commonly shows pleocytosis, with generally less than 500 cells/mm^3. Early in the immune phase, the pleocytosis is mainly polymorphonuclear, but mononuclear cells subsequently predominate. The CSF glucose value is usually normal, and protein is not infrequently elevated (39).

Chest x-ray abnormalities have been noted in 23% to 67% of patients (44,45). Pulmonary abnormalities include nonsegmental opacities, basal linear opacities, and pleural effusions. Cardiac abnormalities may reflect myositis or a pericardial effusion. Electrocardiographic abnormalities are common in leptospirosis (46). These findings, which include tachycardia, small QRS complexes, an increase in the size of the S wave in leads I and V$_7$, and flat or inverted T waves, usually resolve within 10 days (46).

DIAGNOSIS

Early diagnosis of leptospirosis is important to maximize the benefits of antibiotic therapy, ensure intensive care monitoring when indicated, and institute warranted public health control measures. Because the clinical presentation is often nonspecific, a good epidemiologic history is useful in suggesting the diagnosis. Leptospirosis should be considered in the differential diagnosis of any febrile illness associated with an abrupt onset, myalgias, and severe headache. The initial diagnosis in most of these patients is variable and has often included dengue, meningitis, viral hepatitis, fever of unknown origin, influenza, nephritis, encephalitis, and viral illness (39). Other specific illnesses in the differential diagnosis can include heat injury, rickettsioses, typhoid fever, brucellosis, relapsing fever, toxoplasmosis, malaria, yellow fever, septicemia, Kawasaki syndrome, toxic

shock syndrome, Hantaan virus infection, human immunodeficiency virus seroconversion, and legionnaires' disease. Atypical pneumonia is a rare presentation (47). Leptospirosis can be differentiated from purulent bacterial meningitis by examination of the CSF and by the presence of severe myalgias, conjunctival suffusion, a suggestive epidemiologic history, and results of serologic tests. In contrast to viral hepatitis patients, those with leptospirosis are more likely to have prolonged fever, conjunctival suffusion, proteinuria, elevated creatine kinase levels, and only modest transaminase elevations. A particular challenge can be distinguishing between dengue and leptospirosis in the early stages of illness. Misdiagnosis of leptospirosis in the setting of dengue epidemics may lead to preventable mortality (48).

A specific diagnosis is usually based on demonstrating a fourfold rise in antibody titer. The MAT is the current reference standard; however, it is generally limited to reference institutions because it can require the maintenance in live culture of more than 15 different serovars representing the serogroups prevalent in the particular geographic region that generates patients for the laboratory (8). The importance of having local serovars in the MAT battery is emphasized by Gray's report, discussed by Thiermann (49), that 70% of U.S. soldiers' leptospirosis acquired in Panama could be diagnosed serologically only when Panamanian isolates were used in the MAT. The MAT often lacks sensitivity in early disease. Reflecting the limited availability of the MAT, a number of other methods have been studied in recent years (3). Immunoglobulin M enzyme-linked immunosorbent assays have been developed (50,51). A variety of other assays, including dipstick enzyme-linked immunosorbent assays, an immunohemagglutination assay, and a gold immunoblot technique, have been described (51–55). Assay performance may vary based on geographic setting. Polymerase chain reaction methods also hold promise for early diagnosis before a significant humoral response occurs (56,57). Blood, CSF, and urine cultures on specific media can be useful to confirm the diagnosis; however, it may take up to 4 months for leptospires to grow out. Demonstration of leptospira in a clinical specimen by immunofluorescence can also meet the criteria for diagnosis. Serologic studies of routine acute and convalescent specimens may fail to detect infection in up to 10% of culture-positive patients.

THERAPY

Recommendations concerning the antibiotic therapy for leptospirosis have historically been controversial owing to conflicting clinical studies (Table 166.2). On the basis of several published controlled trials, most consultants agree that antibiotic treatment of leptospirosis within the first 4 days of illness is beneficial (58–61). McClain and colleagues (58), for example, studied the effect of 100 mg doxycycline, taken orally twice a day for 7 days, in 29 U.S. soldiers with anicteric leptospirosis acquired in Panama. On average, therapy was initiated 45 hours after onset of illness. In comparison with the placebo group, the treated group received statistically significant benefits that included an overall 2.1-day reduction in illness, a 1.7-day reduction of fever, about 1 day less of headache and myalgia, and prevention of leptospiruria. No adverse effects of treatment were noted. Penicillin has also been used within the first week of illness (59). Erythromycin, some of the newer penicillins, and cephalosporins may also have a role (62).

Unfortunately, in clinical practice, the diagnosis of leptospirosis is often not made within the first 4 days of illness. To evaluate the benefits of therapy in severe and late leptospirosis, Watt

TABLE 166.2.   Duration of Fever in Seven Controlled Antibiotic Treatment Trials for Leptospirosis

Investigator	Drug and dosage regimen	Treated patients/ control subjects	Location	Day of illness when treated (mean)	Total mean duration of fever in days[a] (antibiotic vs. control)	Comments
Kocen (59)	Penicillin, 600,000 units q4h × 1 d, then q6h × 4 d	15/23	Malaya	≤4	3.7 vs. 8.1	Nonrandom
Kocen (59)	Penicillin, 600,000 units q4h × 1 d, then q6h × 4 d	13/10	Malaya	>4	6.4 vs. 8.6	Nonrandom
Edwards et al. (64)	Penicillin, 2 million units q6h × 5 d	38/41	Barbados	6.4	12.9 vs. 13.3	Randomized
Watt et al. (63)	Penicillin, 1.5 million units q6h × 7 d	23/19	Philippines	9	13.7 vs. 20.6	Randomized, blind
McClain et al. (58)	Doxycycline, 100 mg PO b.i.d. × 7 d	14/15	Panama	1.9	3.7 vs. 5.4	Randomized, blind
Russell (60)	Oxytetracycline, 1.5 mg PO, then 0.5 g q6h × 5+ d or until afebrile × 48 h (or similar IV regimen PRN)	27/25	Malaya	3.5	6.4 vs. 9.4	No effect on jaundice and renal failure
Hall et al. (61)	Penicillin, total of 1.5–16.9 million units in 5–20 d	5/12	Puerto Rico	4.2	7.9 vs. 8.6	Nonrandom, no placebo, control subjects' infections milder

IV, intravenously; PO, orally; b.i.d. twice daily; PRN, as required.
[a]For references 63 and 64, fever durations are approximate because either the overlap between the last day before treatment and the first day of treatment could not be determined or the mean pretreatment interval was not separately reported for antibiotic-treated and untreated groups.

and co-workers (63), in a double-blind study in the Philippines, randomized 42 patients (76% with severe disease) to receive a 7-day course of either intravenous penicillin (1.5 million units every 6 hours) or placebo. On average, the patients had been ill for 9 days before enrollment, and about half had received antibiotics. Treatment reduced the duration of fever from 11.6 to 4.7 days ($p < 0.005$). Creatinine elevations persisted more than three times longer in the placebo group (8.3 versus 2.7 days; $p < 0.01$), and penicillin markedly reduced the frequency of leptospiruria. By contrast, Edwards and colleagues (64) enrolled 79 icteric patients in Barbados in a randomized controlled trial of penicillin (2 million units every 6 hours for 5 days) or no antibiotic treatment. The mean duration of illness in both groups was 6 to 7 days. With the exception of eliminating leptospiruria, penicillin afforded these patients no measurable clinical benefit. Factors to explain the contrasting conclusions from different studies may include geographic differences in serovar virulence, differences in clinical status or prior antibiotic therapy at enrollment, dosage considerations, and random events. In a few reports, Jarisch-Herxheimer–type reactions (a sharp temperature rise, a marked drop in blood pressure, and precipitation or aggregation of symptoms and signs) have been reported to occur after antibiotic therapy for leptospirosis (65–67). This unusual phenomenon does not justify withholding antibiotics (67). Nonspecific therapy to manage pain, fever, vomiting, mental status changes, fluid and electrolyte imbalances, renal failure, hyperbilirubinemia, hypotension, and hemorrhage may be necessary. A course of steroids may be useful for bleeding associated with severe thrombocytopenia (42,43).

PREVENTION

Effective prevention of leptospirosis requires tailoring control measures to the particular situation. Efforts to control infection in domestic animal hosts can include isolation, chemotherapy, and selective slaughter of infected animals in addition to annual immunization. Immunization of animals, which may prevent disease but not chronic leptospiruria, requires use of biologicals that cover serovars endemic in the animal's locale. Physical barriers and various methods of habitat alteration or poisoning may help limit human exposure to free-living animal carriers such as rodents. Recognition of the hazards associated with certain swamps or bodies of water may necessitate putting those areas off-limits. Shoes and other forms of protective clothing (provided that it does not hold contaminated water near the skin or lead to skin conditions that would enhance penetration of leptospires), appropriate use of surface disinfectants, and other hygienic practices are useful in some settings. Chemoprophylaxis with 200 mg of doxycycline once a week has been effective in preventing leptospirosis among U.S. troops training in Panama during the rainy season; use of such a regimen should, however, be limited to prevention in the setting of short, high-risk exposures (10). At least one other study has also suggested prophylactic or postexposure benefits (68). No licensed human vaccine is available for use in the United States. Public and professional education is another important component of prevention.

REFERENCES

1. Feigin RD Anderson DC. Human leptospirosis. *Crit Rev Clin Lab Sci* 1975;5: 413.
2. Gsell O. The history of leptospirosis: 100 years. *Zentralbl Bakteriol Mikrobiol Hyg A* 1984;257:473.
3. Levett PN. Leptospirosis. *Clin Microbiol Rev* 2001;14:296–326.
4. Alston JM, Broom JC. *Leptospirosis in man and animals*. Edinburgh: E & S Livingstone, 1958.
5. Gochenour WS Jr, Smadel JE, Jackson EB, et al. Leptospiral etiology of Fort Bragg fever. *Public Health Rep* 1952;67:811.
6. Torten M. Leptospirosis. In: Steele JH, ed. *Handbook series in zoonoses*, Vol I. Boca Raton, FL: CRC Press, 1979:363–421.

7. Plank R, Dean D. Overview of the epidemiology, microbiology, and pathogenesis of *Leptospira* spp. in humans. *Microbes Infect* 2000;2:1265–1276.
8. Faine S, ed. *Guidelines for the control of leptospirosis.* Geneva: World Health Organization, 1982.
9. Ellinghausen HC, McCullough WG. Nutrition of *Leptospira pomona* and growth of 13 other serotypes: fractionation of oleic albumin complex and a medium of bovine albumin and polysorbate 80. *Am J Vet Res* 1965;26:45.
10. Takafuji ET, Kirkpatrick JW, Miller RN, et al. An efficacy trial of doxycycline chemoprophylaxis against leptospirosis. *N Engl J Med* 1984;310:497.
11. Johnson RC, Fame S. Family II. Leptospiraceae hovind-hougen. In: Krieg NR Holt JG, eds. *Bergeys manual of systematic bacteriology,* Vol 1. Baltimore: Williams & Wilkins, 1984:62–67.
12. Feigin RD, Lobes LA, Anderson D, et al. Human leptospirosis from immunized dogs. *Ann Intern Med* 1973;79:777.
13. Kaufmann AF. Epidemiologic trends of leptospirosis in the United States, 1965–1974. In: Johnson RC, eds. *The biology of parasitic spirochetes.* New York: Academic Press, 1976:177–190.
14. Vinetz JM, Glass GE, Flexner CE, et al. Sporadic urban leptospirosis. *Ann Intern Med* 1996;125:794–798.
15. Jackson LA, Kaufmann AF, Adams WG, et al. Outbreak of leptospirosis associated with swimming. *Pediatr Infect Dis* 1993;12:48.
16. Centers for Disease Control and Prevention. Update: leptospirosis and unexplained acute febrile illness among athletes participating in triathlons: Illinois and Wisconsin, 1998. *MMWR Morbid Mortal Wkly Rep* 1998;47:673–676.
17. Centers for Disease Control and Prevention. Public health dispatch: outbreak of acute febrile illness among participants in EcoChallenge Sabah 2000, Malaysia, 2000. *MMWR Morbid Mortal Wkly Rep* 2000;49:816–817.
18. Cacciapuoti B, Ciceroni L, Maffei C, et al. A waterborne outbreak of leptospirosis. *Am J Epidemiol* 1987;126:535.
19. Bolin CA, Koellner P. Human-to-human transmission of *Leptospira interrogans* by milk. *J Infect Dis* 1988;158:246.
20. Centers for Disease Control. Summary of notifiable diseases, United States, 1987. *MMWR Morbid Mortal Wkly Rep* 1987;36:1.
21. Gill ON, Coghlan JD, Calder IM. The risk of leptospirosis in United Kingdom fish farm workers. *J Hyg (Camb)* 1985;94:81.
22. Arean VM. The pathogenic anatomy and pathogenesis of fatal human leptospirosis (Weils disease). *Am J Pathol* 1962;40:393.
23. DeBrito T, Morais CF, Yasuda PH, et al. Cardiovascular involvement in human and experimental leptospirosis: pathologic findings and immunohistochemical detection of leptospiral antigen. *Ann Trop Med Parasitol* 1987;81:207.
24. Alexander AD. Immunity in leptospirosis. In: Johnson RC, ed. *The biology of parasitic spirochetes.* New York: Academic Press, 1976:339–349.
25. Shaked Y, Shpilberg O, Samra D, et al. Leptospirosis in pregnancy and its effect on the fetus: case report and review. *Clin Infect Dis* 1993;17:241.
26. Alexander A, Benenson A, Byrne R, et al. Leptospirosis in Puerto Rico. *Zoonoses Res* 1963;2:153.
27. Heath CW, Alexander AD, Galton MM. Leptospirosis in the United States: analysis of 483 cases in man, 1949–1961. *N Engl J Med* 1965;273:857.
28. Trevejo RT, Rigau-Perez JG, Ashford DA, et al. Epidemic leptospirosis associated with pulmonary hemorrhage—Nicaragua, 1995. *J Infect Dis* 1998;178:1457–1463.
29. Wang CN, Liu J, Chang TF, et al. Studies on anicteric leptospirosis: clinical manifestations and antibiotic therapy. *Chin Med J* 1965;84:283–291.
30. Park SK, Lee SH, Rhee YK, et al. Leptospirosis in Chonbuk Province of Korea in 1987: a study of 93 patients. *Am J Trop Med Hyg* 1989;41:345–351.
31. Berman SJ, Tsai C, Holmes K, et al. Sporadic anicteric leptospirosis in Viet Nam: a study in 150 patients. *Ann Intern Med* 1973;79:167.
32. Ramachandran S, Perera M. Cardiac and pulmonary involvement in leptospirosis. *Trans R Soc Trop Med Hyg* 1977;71:56.
33. Chee H, Ossenkoppele G, Bronsveld W, et al. Adult respiratory distress syndrome in *Leptospira icterohaemorrhagiae* infection. *Intensive Care Med* 1985;11:254.
34. ONeil KM, Rickman LS, Lazarus AA. Pulmonary manifestations of leptospirosis. *Rev Infect Dis* 1991;13:705.
35. Gutman I, Walsh JB, Knapp AB. Cotton-wool spots as a sign in leptospirosis (Weils disease). *Ophthalmologica* 1983;187:133.
36. Shpilberg O, Shaked Y, Maier MK, et al. Long-term follow-up after leptospirosis. *South Med J* 1990;83:405.
37. Centers for Disease Control. Annual summary 1984. Reported morbidity and mortality in the United States. *MMWR Morbid Mortal Wkly Rep* 1986;33:1.
38. Everard COR, Edwards CN, Webb GB, et al. The prevalence of severe leptospirosis among humans on Barbados. *Trans R Soc Trop Med Hyg* 1984;78:596.
39. Heath CW, Alexander AD, Galton MM. Leptospirosis in the United States (concluded): analysis of 483 cases in man, 1949–1961. *N Engl J Med* 1965;273:915.
40. Johnson WD, Coelho I, Rocha H. Serum creatinine phosphokinase in leptospirosis. *JAMA* 1975;233:981.
41. Kuriakose M, Eapen CK, Punnoose E, et al. Leptospirosis: clinical spectrum and correlation with seven simple laboratory tests for early diagnosis in the Third World. *Trans R Soc Trop Med Hyg* 1990;84:419.
42. Edwards CN, Nicholson GD, Hassell TA, et al. Thrombocytopenia in leptospirosis: the absence of evidence for disseminated intravascular coagulation. *Am J Trop Med Hyg* 1986;35:352.
43. Kahn JB. A case of Weil's disease requiring steroid therapy for thrombocytopenia and bleeding. *Am J Trop Med Hyg* 1982;31:1213.
44. Lee R, Terry S, Walter T, et al. The chest radiograph in leptospirosis in Jamaica. *Br J Radiol* 1981;54:939.
45. Wang C, Ch C, Lu F. Studies on anicteric leptospirosis. III. Radiographic observation of pulmonary changes. *Chin Med J (Engl)* 1965;84:298.
46. Parsons M. Electrocardiographic changes in leptospirosis. *Br Med J* 1965;2:201.
47. Alani FS, Mahoney MP, Ormerod LP, et al. Leptospirosis presenting as atypical pneumonia, respiratory failure and pyogenic meningitis. *J Infect* 1993;27:281.
48. Levett PN, Branch SL, Edwards CN. Detection of dengue infection in patients investigated for leptospirosis in Barbados. *Am J Trop Med Hyg* 2000;62:112–114.
49. Thiermann AB. Leptospirosis: current developments and trends. *J Am Vet Med Assoc* 1984;184:722.
50. Winslow WE, Merry DJ, Pirc ML, et al. Evaluation of a commercial enzyme-linked immunosorbent assay for detection of immunoglobulin M antibody in diagnosis of human leptospiral infection. *J Clin Microbiol* 1997;35:1938–1942.
51. Cumberland P, Everard COR, Levett PN. Assessment of the efficacy of an IgM-ELISA and microscopic agglutination test (MAT) in the diagnosis of acute leptospirosis. *Am J Trop Med Hyg* 1999;61:731–734.
52. Levett PN, Branch SL, Whittington CU, et al. Two methods for rapid serological diagnosis of acute leptospirosis. *Clin Diagn Lab Immunol* 2001;8:349–351.
53. Smits HL, Hartskeerl RA, Terpstra WJ. International multi-centre evaluation of a dipstick assay for human leptospirosis. *Trop Med Intl Health* 2000;5:124–128.
54. Levett PN, Whittington CU. Evaluation of the indirect hemagglutination assay for diagnosis of acute leptospirosis. *J Clin Microbiol* 1998;36:11–14.
55. Petchclai B, Hiranras S, Potha U. Gold immunoblot analysis of IgM-specific antibody in the diagnosis of human leptospirosis. *Am J Trop Med Hyg* 1991;45:672.
56. Merien F, Baranton G, Perolat P. Comparison of polymerase chain reaction with microagglutination test and culture for diagnosis of leptospirosis. *J Infect Dis* 1995;172:281–285.
57. Brown PD, Gravekamp C, Carrington DG, et al. Evaluation of polymerase chain reaction for early diagnosis of leptospirosis. *J Med Microbiol* 1995;43:110–114.
58. McClain JB, Ballou WR, Harrison SM, et al. Doxycycline therapy for leptospirosis. *Ann Intern Med* 1984;100:696.
59. Kocen RS. Leptospirosis: a comparison of symptomatic and penicillin therapy. *BMJ* 1962;1:1181.
60. Russell RW. Treatment of leptospires with oxytetracycline. *Lancet* 1958;2:1143.
61. Hall H, Hightower J, Diaz-Rivera R, et al. Evaluation of antibiotic therapy in human leptospirosis. *Ann Intern Med* 1951;35:981.
62. Alexander AD, Rule PL. Penicillins, cephalosporins, and tetracyclines in treatment of hamsters with fatal leptospirosis. *Antimicrob Agents Chemother* 1986;30:835.
63. Watt G, Padre LP, Tuazon ML, et al. Placebo-controlled trial of intravenous penicillin for severe and late leptospirosis. *Lancet* 1988;1:433.
64. Edwards CN, Nicholson GD, Hassell TA, et al. Penicillin therapy in icteric leptospirosis. *Am J Trop Med Hyg* 1988;39:388.
65. Mackay-Dick J, Robinson JF. Penicillin in the treatment of 84 cases of leptospirosis in Malaya. *J R Army Med Corps* 1957;103:186.
66. Friedland JS, Warrell DA. The Jarisch-Herxheimer reaction in leptospirosis: possible pathogenesis and review. *Rev Infect Dis* 1991;13:207.
67. Watt G, Padre LP, Tuazon M, et al. Limulus lysate positivity and Herxheimer-like reactions in leptospirosis: a placebo-controlled study. *J Infect Dis* 1990;1662:564.
68. Sehgal SC, Sugunan AP, Murhekar MV, et al. Randomized controlled trial of doxycycline prophylaxis against leptospirosis in an endemic area. *Int J Anti Agents* 2000;13:249–255.

CHAPTER 167

Relapsing Fever

Thomas Butler

HISTORY

The agent of relapsing fever was first established in Berlin in 1873 by Obermeier, who used a microscope to observe spirochetes in the blood of patients. Between 1910 and 1945, epidemics of louse-borne relapsing fever occurred in North Africa, Sudan, Ethiopia, West Africa, central Africa, eastern Europe, and Russia. In these epidemics, there were an estimated 15 million cases, more than 5 million deaths, and case-fatality rates as high as 73%.

CHARACTERISTICS OF THE PATHOGEN

Borrelia species spirochetes are spiral bacteria that measure 5 to 40 μm long and about 0.5 μm in diameter. They are too thin to be seen reliably by light microscopy of wet preparations, but they are easily visible when viewed by dark-field or phase-contrast microscopy. They are visible with aniline dyes, such as Wright and Giemsa stains, and stain well in tissue with silver stains, such as the Dieterle and Warthin-Starry stains.

Borrelia recurrentis is the cause of louse-borne relapsing fever. The species names of the tick-borne *Borrelia* are derived from the species names of *Ornithodorus* tick vectors that carry them, rather than from biochemical or antigenic characteristics. The more common ones are *Borrelia turicatae, Borrelia hermsii*, and *Borrelia parkeri* in North America and *Borrelia duttonii* in Africa. These spirochetes generate new serotypes based on variable major proteins that are responsible for relapses (1) (see Chapter 215).

EPIDEMIOLOGY

Louse-borne and tick-borne relapsing fevers differ so much in their epidemiology that they must be considered separately. *Epidemic relapsing fever* refers to the louse-borne kind and *endemic* or *sporadic relapsing fever* to the tick-borne variety.

The geographic distribution of the relapsing fevers remains widespread, occurring in most areas of the world. Louse-borne relapsing fever has disappeared from the United States but still occurs in parts of Latin America, such as the Guatemalan and Andean highlands. Ethiopia appears to be the country with the highest incidence, estimated at 10,000 or more cases per year.

Tick-borne relapsing fever occurs in endemic foci in southern British Columbia, the western United States, the plateau regions of Mexico, and Central and South America. This disease is present in most areas of Africa. It also occurs in Spain and Portugal. In Asia, tick-borne relapsing fever has been reported in Cyprus, Israel, Syria, Turkey, Iraq, Iran, southern Russia, China, Afghanistan, and India.

The persons at greatest risk for acquiring louse-borne relapsing fever are those living under crowded, unhygienic conditions that favor infestation with body lice. Migrant workers and soldiers in war are particularly susceptible to this infection. Males are at much greater risk than are females, presumably because their lives more often expose them to infected lice. A strain-specific and short-lived acquired immunity develops after infection. This immunity helps to explain why migrant workers coming into an endemic area are more susceptible to infection than are the permanent inhabitants. In some endemic areas, such as Addis Ababa, Ethiopia, there is an increase in frequency during the cool winter season, when people wear heavier clothing that becomes louse infested.

Persons at greatest risk for tick-borne infection are those who come into contact with infected ticks from wild rodents (2). In the United States, the largest outbreak of tick-borne relapsing fever occurred in 62 campers and employees in the national park at the northern rim of the Grand Canyon, Arizona, in 1973. In tropical countries, people who live in dwellings that are not rodent-proof are susceptible to infection.

PATHOGENESIS

After exposure to an infected louse or tick, spirochetes enter the skin and gain access to the blood and lymphatic circulations. The incubation period lasts 4 to 18 days after exposure, during which time the spirochetes divide in the blood plasma. After concentration has built up to 10^6 to 10^8 spirochetes per milliliter of blood, the illness begins. *Borrelia* spirochetes do not possess any known endotoxins or exotoxins. In general *Borrelia* spirochetes do not produce abscesses and are confined predominantly to the plasma space of their mammalian hosts (3). Symptoms are caused by elevated concentrations of tumor necrosis factor, interleukin-1, interleukin-6, and interleukin-8 (4).

CLINICAL MANIFESTATIONS

The typical patient suffers abrupt onset of shaking chills, fever, headache, and fatigue. Most patients have these symptoms almost continuously throughout the day, whereas some report the intermittent appearance of these symptoms several times a day. Patients complain frequently of myalgia, arthralgia, anorexia, dry cough, and abdominal pains. These symptoms are usually mild on the first day of illness and increase in intensity for a few days, leading to prostration. The nonspecific nature of these symptoms leads patients or their physicians to believe they have an influenza-like illness. In the differential diagnosis of relapsing fever in tropical regions, the most common diseases are malaria and typhoid fever.

The temperature is elevated in the range of 38.5° to 40°C, and the pulse rate increases to about 115 beats per minute. The blood pressure drops to about 105/70 mm Hg. Patients appear lethargic or may be delirious. Physical signs that are common but not necessarily present include conjunctival injection, petechial rash that is usually truncal in distribution, and hepatosplenomegaly with occasional jaundice (5–8). Disseminated intravascular coagulation also contributes to a decrease in platelets as well as producing prolonged prothrombin and partial thromboplastin times and elevated titers of fibrinogen-fibrin degradation products.

Untreated patients experience relapses after recovery. The first attack of louse-borne relapsing fever lasts about 6 days and is followed by an afebrile period of about 9 days. There is usually only one relapse, which characteristically lasts only 2 days. The first attack of tick-borne relapsing fever lasts about 3 days and is followed by an interval of about 7 days, after which an average of three relapses occur, each lasting about 2 days. Relapses are usually milder than the first attacks.

Autopsies performed in fatal cases of louse-borne relapsing fever showed that the spleen is enlarged to as much as 900 g, and the cut surface shows white microabscesses that consist of necrosis and hemorrhage in the white pulp. The liver is also enlarged, and the midzonal regions show scattered necrosis and hemorrhage. The heart is normal in size but frequently shows myocarditis consisting of interstitial edema and a cellular infiltrate of lymphocytes and plasma cells. The brain usually shows cerebral edema, and in some cases, there is hemorrhage into the subarachnoid space or cerebrum.

DIAGNOSIS

The diagnosis of relapsing fever depends on the demonstration of spirochetemia (Fig. 167.1). In most patients, this is readily accomplished by obtaining peripheral blood by either finger stick or venipuncture and preparing a thin film on a microscope slide. A routine blood smear stained with Wright or Giemsa stain is adequate, but blood smears prepared for examination for malaria parasites are also satisfactory. Smears from patients who are in the interval between relapses will not demonstrate the organism,

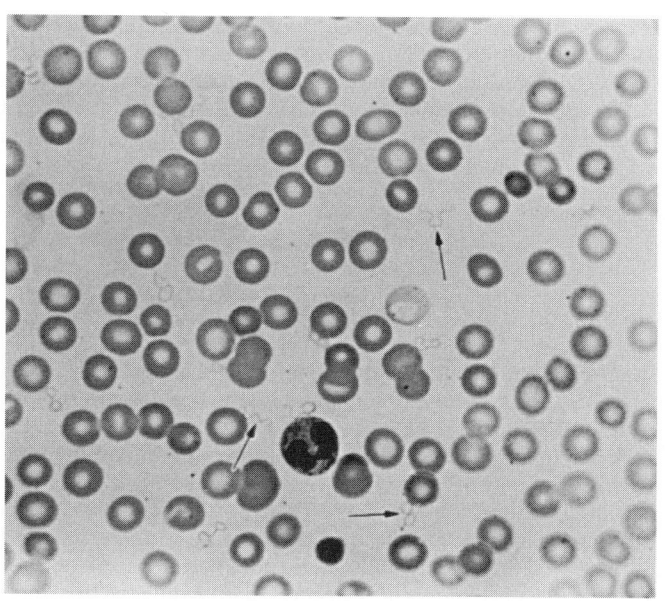

Figure 167.1. Blood smear from a patient with louse-borne relapsing fever shows spirochetes (*arrows*) (Wright stain, ×600).

and the examination should be repeated when the fever reappears.

Spirochetemia may be detected, alternatively, by dark-field or phase-contrast microscopy. A drop of fresh blood is diluted with a drop of 0.9% sodium chloride solution and overlaid with a coverslip. Spirochetes are readily identified by their characteristic rotational motility. Fluorescence microscopy of buffy coat has also been used (9).

Borrelia species can be cultivated in Kelly broth medium or inoculated intraperitoneally into laboratory mice or rats, whose blood is examined daily for 14 days for spirochetes. Louse-borne and tick-borne relapsing fevers are usually differentiated on epidemiologic grounds. If vectors can be collected from the patient or his or her household, they can be dissected and examined microscopically for the presence of spirochetes.

Serologic testing has been employed in endemic areas for purposes of seroepidemiology and examining convalescent patients. None of these tests, however, is standardized or available for general use.

TREATMENT

The relapsing fevers respond to tetracycline and erythromycin. Tetracycline is the treatment of choice except for children younger than 7 years and pregnant women. A single oral dose of tetracycline, 500 mg, is as effective in clearing spirochetemia and preventing relapse, as are longer courses. Erythromycin, 500 mg, given orally as a single dose, is a satisfactory alternative to tetracycline. For patients who are unable to take oral medication, intravenous injection of 250 mg of tetracycline or erythromycin is curative. For children smaller than 30 kg, the dose of tetracycline or erythromycin should be reduced to about 10 mg/kg. Penicillin G therapy results in slow clearance of spirochetes and frequent relapses.

In most patients with louse-borne relapsing fever and in some with tick-borne relapsing fever, antibiotic treatment provokes a distressing Jarisch-Herxheimer reaction. Rigor occurs 2 to 3 hours after treatment. Subsequently, the temperature rises sharply and the blood pressure drops while spirochetes are cleared from the blood. Patients may require intravenous infusions of 0.9% sodium chloride solution to maintain adequate blood pressure. During several hours, the temperature declines, and the patient feels better.

Attempts to ameliorate the severity of the reaction by giving antipyretic or antiinflammatory drugs have not been successful. The best approach is to anticipate the reaction and to provide intensive nursing care and intravenous fluid support during the first day of treatment. A low dose of procaine penicillin (100,000 units) causes less frequent reactions but results in more relapses than higher doses (10).

Complete recovery occurs in at least 95% of adequately treated cases of relapsing fever. The prognosis for untreated disease is variable, particularly for louse-borne relapsing fever, during epidemics of which mortality rates of 40% have been reported. The illness is usually fatal in neonates.

PREVENTION

Available approaches for control of the relapsing fevers include the detection and treatment of human cases, vector control, rodent control, and public health education. Vaccines are not available.

For louse-borne relapsing fever, the detection and treatment of cases have the effect of reducing the reservoir of infection and, consequently, reducing transmission. More important is the control of louse infestation. Instructing people to bathe and wash their clothes is the rational approach, but compliance is likely to be poor. Clothing and bodies can be deloused with insecticides or with insect repellents. In known epidemic situations, prophylactic antibiotics are a temporary measure to contain spread of infection to persons at high risk. The eventual control of this disease requires improvements in personal hygiene and housing conditions.

For tick-borne relapsing fever, the treatment of human cases has no impact on the animal reservoirs. Campers and hikers going into endemic areas should be advised to avoid staying in cabins that are inhabited by rodents and their ticks and to apply topical tick repellents to their skin. In endemic areas of Africa, people need to be assisted in building rodent-proof houses.

REFERENCES

1. Ras NM, Postic D, Ave P, et al. Antigenic variation of *Borrelia turicatae* Vsp surface lipoproteins occurs in vitro and generates novel serotypes. *Res Microbiol* 2000;151:5.
2. Trevejo RT, Schriefer ME, Gage KL, et al. An interstate outbreak of tick-borne relapsing fever among vacationers at a Rocky Mountain cabin. *Am J Trop Med Hyg* 1998;58:743.
3. Shamaei-Tousi A, Martin P, Bergh A, et al. Erythrocyte-aggregating relapsing fever spirochete *Borrelia crocidurae* induces formation of microemboli. *J Infect Dis* 1999;180:1929.
4. Fekade D, Knox K, Hussein K, et al. Prevention of Jarisch-Herxheimer reactions by treatment with antibodies against tumor necrosis factor α. *N Engl J Med* 1996;335:311.
5. Mekasha A. Louse-borne relapsing fever in children. *J Trop Med Hyg* 1992;95:206.
6. Barclay AJG, Coulter JBS. Tick-borne relapsing fever in central Tanzania. *Trans R Soc Trop Med Hyg* 1990;84:852.
7. Lovett MA, Goldstein EJC, Fleischmann J. Fever in a couple vacationing in the mountains of southern California. *Clin Infect Dis* 1992;14:1254.
8. Dupont HT, La Scola B, Williams R, et al. A focus of tick-borne relapsing fever in Southern Zaire. *Clin Infect Dis* 1997;25:239.
9. Van Dam AP, van Gool T, Wetsteyn JCFM, et al. Tick-borne relapsing fever imported from West Africa: diagnosis by quantitative buffy coat analysis and in vitro culture of *Borrelia crocidurae*. *J Clin Microbiol* 1999;37:2027.
10. Seboxa T, Rahlenbeck SI. Treatment of louse-borne relapsing fever with low dose penicillin or tetracycline: a clinical trial. *Scand J Infect Dis* 1995; 27:29.

CHAPTER 168
Rocky Mountain Spotted Fever

J. Stephen Dumler

Rocky Mountain spotted fever (RMSF) is a potentially severe, tick-borne, febrile illness caused by infection with *Rickettsia rickettsii*. Despite wide general awareness of the local prevalence, manifestations, and availability of highly effective therapeutic antimicrobial agents for RMSF, the disease is still frequently fatal (1,2). The reasons for this situation are incompletely understood but are partly explained by differences between the classic presentation and the actual situation in which the clinical diagnostic clues, such as rash, are often not present at the time of initial presentation (3,4). Regardless, RMSF can be severe and rapidly fatal if not recognized and treated early. It is the often undifferentiated presentation that can cause significant problems, and thus a complete understanding of the clinical manifestations, the appropriate historical and epidemiologic circumstances, appropriate use and interpretation of laboratory results, and pathophysiology of the infection provides the real key to early recognition and cure.

ECOLOGY AND TRANSMISSION OF *RICKETTSIA RICKETTSII*

RMSF is caused by *Rickettsia rickettsii*, a small, obligate intracellular bacterium that occupies part of its life cycle in tick tissues and in small animals. Historically, it is taught that *R. rickettsii* is maintained predominantly by vertical transmission in ticks (5); however, recent data suggest that the transient interval of rickettsemia in infected small mammal hosts that occurs before induction of immune clearance (horizontal transmission) is critical for propagating the agent into uninfected, cofeeding ticks (6). Progeny of infected female ticks are often nonviable or die, in part explaining the very low frequency with which *R. rickettsii* is detected in ticks. Small animal hosts include voles (*Microtus pennsylvanicus, Pitymys pinetorum*), white-footed mice (*Peromyscus leucopus*), cotton rats (*Sigmodon hispidus*), rabbits and hares (*Silvagus floridanus, Lepus americanus*), opossums (*Didelphis marsupialis virginia*), chipmunks (*Eutamius amoenus*), and squirrels (*Spermophilus lateralis tescorum*). Other wild and domestic animals such as dogs can be infected and sick. However, when infected, humans are dead-end hosts that offer no survival advantage for *R. rickettsii*.

Important tick species that are involved in the transmission of RMSF vary over geographic regions, including the American dog tick (*Dermacentor variabilis*) in much of the eastern and midwestern parts of the United States and the wood tick (*Dermacentor andersoni*) in the Rocky Mountain regions (5). Both the brown dog tick (*Rhipicephalus sanguineus*) and *Amblyomma cajennense* can transmit the rickettsia in parts of Mexico, Central America, and South America. Once acquired by blood meal, rickettsiae penetrate into midgut epithelial cells and disseminate to all tick tissues, including salivary glands. Infection of the latter tissue allows regurgitation of infectious salivary secretions into tick-bite wounds and the initiation of mammalian or human infection.

Prevalence of the agent and transmission by ticks are governed by several factors. Other spotted fever group rickettsiae in ticks preclude simultaneous infection with *R. rickettsii* (7). One explanation of the high seroprevalence of RMSF versus the low clinical prevalence of RMSF relates to infection by highly prevalent, presumed nonpathogenic spotted fever group rickettsiae that can induce *R. rickettsii* cross-reactive antibodies. *R. rickettsii* virulence for mammalian infection is minimal at the low ambient temperatures at which ticks live. After exposure to more elevated temperatures or exposure to blood for several hours, *R. rickettsii* becomes virulent (8). Thus, there is an interval ranging up to 48 hours or longer, before which rickettsiae are not reactivated. Thus, if attached ticks are removed when still flat, transmission of virulent *R. rickettsii* is unlikely.

Mammalian factors also influence transmission because immune animals will not support rickettsemia or horizontal amplification (5,9). Thus, risk for transmission is determined by (a) local prevalence of ticks that contain *R. rickettsii*, (b) local prevalence of ticks that contain nonpathogenic "interfering" rickettsiae, (c) the abundance, density, and immune status of susceptible small mammals for amplification of *R. rickettsii*, (d) large animals that support propagation of adult ticks, and (e) the probability that a human interrupts the ecological cycle (10).

DISTRIBUTION AND PREVALENCE

RMSF is the second most frequently diagnosed tick-borne disease next to Lyme disease in the United States, with 5,900 cases reported to the Centers for Disease Control and Prevention (CDC) between 1991 and 2000 (1). Between 1993 and 1996, the national rate of infections reported to the CDC was 2.2 cases per 1 million population. However, RMSF has undergone cyclical prevalence changes with a nadir in the early 1960s and a peak around 1980; yet another nadir appears to have occurred in 1993 to 1994, and the rate since has had an upward trend.

Most cases are recognized in the southeastern and central regions of the United States. For example, between 1993 and 1996, 1,208 (52%) cases occurred in the South Atlantic states, and North Carolina alone reported 57% of those (11). Other geographic regions with significant numbers of RMSF cases include the East and West South Central states (615 cases), especially Oklahoma, Arkansas, Mississippi, Tennessee, and Kentucky. Despite this geographic distribution, cases have been identified in nearly every state in the United States, including urban areas such as the Bronx, New York. Cases occur predominantly during summer months, with 92% of cases reported between April and September and 2.1% of cases reported in December through February (11).

RMSF has been considered chiefly a disease of children, with highest incidence in 5- to 9-year-old children (3.7 cases per million) and lowest incidence among individuals 70 years of age or older (1.4 cases per million). In general, most of the reported patients in the past have been male (56%) and white (88%) (11). RMSF in patients older than 70 years of age is particularly grave, with a case-fatality rate of 9% when recognized. Thus, a febrile illness in a child or adolescent or in a man older than 60 years of age that occurs during May through September with the potential for tick exposure should warrant the inclusion of RMSF in the differential diagnosis. Despite the availability of effective therapy, the case-fatality rate of RMSF is unacceptable and continues at levels as high as 8.5% (12).

PATHOGENESIS AND PATHOPHYSIOLOGY

After inoculation of *R. rickettsii* into the dermis, there is an incubation period that averages 7 days (range, 3 to 12 days) during which the initial proliferation and dissemination of the bacteria occurs. The rickettsiae that are inoculated into the dermal tick-bite wound apparently enter endothelial cells in the adjacent dermal capillaries, venules, or lymphatics. Dissemination from this site must occur rapidly because eschars and necrotic lesions at the tick-bite site are rare (13). Dissemination probably occurs through lymphatic or hematogenous spread, and the vascular beds of any or all tissues and organs can then become infected.

As the rickettsiae are spread, attachment to a surface receptor of vascular endothelium occurs. This process appears to be mediated through rickettsial outer membrane protein A (OmpA), a 190-kd protein of R. rickettsii (14). Once within the endothelial cell, the rickettsiae multiply and damage the cell by the accumulated effects of phospholipase A$_2$, phospholipase C (15), and free radical–mediated membrane damage (16). In vitro, infected endothelial cells are activated through NF-κB nuclear translocation to become proinflammatory and procoagulant; apoptosis is delayed (17,18). If analogous circumstances occur in vivo, these events lead to recruitment of inflammatory cells and deposition of fibrin and platelets on the surface of affected cells. In fact, the hallmark lesion of R. rickettsii infection is vasculitis characterized predominantly by an influx of lymphocytes and histiocytes, except where rickettsia-mediated necrosis has occurred that additionally elicits neutrophil influx and a pattern of leukocytoclastic vasculitis (19,20). Similarly, thrombosis is a relatively infrequent finding in most vasculitic lesions in vivo. The more frequent histopathologic lesion detected in patients with RMSF is a perivascular infiltrate of lymphohistiocytic inflammatory cells that may occur in almost any tissue. Regardless of whether vasculitis has compromised local perfusion, significant vascular injury can occur. The net result of this vascular injury is vascular leakage, leading to hypoperfusion, ischemia, and interstitial edema.

The septic shock–like course of RMSF might suggest a pathologic role for cytokines. However, experimental evidence now seems to indicate that the cytokines that are produced as an inflammatory and immune-initiating response to R. rickettsii are largely beneficial, decrease the rickettsial load, and eliminate rickettsia-infected cells (21,22). Animal models of spotted fever group rickettsiosis show that cytokines, including interferon-γ (IFN-γ), tumor necrosis factor-α (TNF-α), interleukin-1β (IL-1β), and IL-6, are an essential part of the protective immune and inflammatory responses and recovery from Rocky Mountain spotted fever early in the infectious process (21). In murine endothelial cells, the protective effects of IFN-γ and TNF-α are synergistic, apparently inducing endothelial nitric oxide synthase (22), resulting in nitric oxide production that leads to tryptophan sequestration and production of membrane-damaging hydrogen peroxide (23). An important role for CD8 cells and direct cell contact has been shown in perforin knockout mice (23). The net result is a reduction in rickettsial number and the number of rickettsia-infected cells.

Pathologic studies show a typical sequence of events that explain clinical and laboratory findings in RMSF (19,24). With rickettsial vasculitis and endothelial injury, increased vascular permeability yields edema, loss of plasma volume, hypoproteinemia, hypoalbuminemia, reduced serum oncotic pressure, and the hypovolemia and hypotension that are present in 17% of patients. The clinical manifestations depend on the degree of systemic vascular compromise and the specific organs damaged by hypoperfusion or direct rickettsia-mediated vascular damage. The frequent occurrence of acute renal insufficiency is best explained by this hypotension. As the rickettsial proliferation diminishes, either by specific antimicrobial therapy or by waxing immunity, microvascular integrity and tissue perfusion are reestablished, intravascular blood volume normalizes, and edema resolves.

The initial findings include fever, headache, malaise, and myalgias (3,25–27). After the initial signs and symptoms begin, some patients develop other findings, including chills or rigors, stiff neck, nausea, vomiting, diarrhea, abdominal pain and tenderness, conjunctival suffusion, photophobia, cough, facial or pedal edema, neurologic signs (meningismus, confusion, convulsions, coma), occasional cardiac abnormalities (arrhythmias, heart failure), hepatomegaly, splenomegaly, gangrene of digits or extremities, and hypotension (Table 168.1). RMSF is associated with a spectrum of clinical laboratory findings that suggest a systemic process (3,25,26). Clues to clinical suspicion of RMSF in a patient who appears infected, if not septic, include a normal leukocyte count or slight leukopenia with increased bands, thrombocytopenia, hyponatremia, mild to moderate elevations in serum aspartate and alanine aminotransferases, and acute elevations in serum urea nitrogen and creatinine levels (Table 168.2). Hypoproteinemia, hypoalbuminemia, and associated abnormalities in serum electrolyte concentrations (e.g., hypocalcemia) are often detected.

The involvement of the coagulation system in RMSF is greatly misunderstood. It is often assumed that much of the pathologic injury associated with the vasculitis results from thrombosis,

TABLE 168.1.   Frequent Clinical Features of Rocky Mountain Spotted Fever in Four Cases Series

History, signs, or symptoms	Helmick et al. (3) (n = 262)	Kaplowitz et al. (26) (n = 131)	Sexton & Burgdorfer (27) (n = 75)	Billings et al. (12) (n = 119)
Tick bite	60	NR	68	NR
Fever	99	100	100	NR
Rash	88	90	100	97
Rash on palms and soles	74	82	NR	84
Headache	91	79	92	NR
Myalgia	83	72	67	77
Nausea or vomiting	60	63	39	60
Abdominal pain	52	23	33	54
Conjunctivitis	30	30	15	NR
Edema	18	20	17	10
Pneumonitis	12	17	NR	NR
Any severe neurologic complication[a]	26	23	48	8
				6

NR, not reported. Data are expressed as a percentage of total cases in each series.
[a]Neurologic complications include stupor, delirium, seizures, ataxia, papilledema, focal neurologic deficits, and coma.

TABLE 168.2.   Selected Laboratory Abnormalities Reported in Patients with Rocky Mountain Spotted Fever, North Carolina Memorial Hospital, 1970 Through 1979

Laboratory finding	Patients tested (n)	Patients with finding	
		No.	Percentage
White blood cell count			
<10,000/μL	129	93	72
>10% bands	121	83	69
Platelet count/μL			
<150,000	117	61	52
<99,000	117	38	32
Serum sodium <132 mEq/L	131	72	56
AST ≥ twice normal value	71	44	62
ALT ≥ twice normal value	66	26	39
Bilirubin >1.4 mg/dL	53	16	30
Cerebrospinal fluid[a]			
Opening pressure ≤250 mm H₂O	35	5	14
Glucose ≤50 mg/dL	52	5	8
Protein ≥50 mg/dL	62	22	35
White blood cells ≥5/μL	63	24	48
Mononuclear cell predominance	24	11	46
Polymorphonuclear cell predominance	24	12	50

AST, aspartate transaminase; ALT, alanine aminotransferase.
[a]Lumbar puncture was performed in 63 of 131 patients before therapy was started.
Data from Kaplowitz LG, Fischer JJ, Sparling PF. Rocky Mountain spotted fever: a clinical dilemma. In: Remington JS, Swartz MN, eds. *Current clinical topics in infectious diseases*, Vol 2. New York: McGraw-Hill, 1981:89–108, with permission.

vascular occlusion, and tissue infarction; however, these situations are infrequent events that do not often influence the course of disease (13,28). Necrosis of the skin is seen in only 4% of patients and probably results from hypoperfusion rather than thrombosis in most patients (26). Overall, thrombosis is very infrequent, and nonocclusive vascular injury is the norm (19,20). The presence of small, nonocclusive thrombi that attach to sites of rickettsia-mediated vascular damage is more protec-

tive than damaging and precludes significant ischemic necrosis and hemorrhage by maintaining patency (13). True disseminated intravascular coagulation (DIC) due to systemic cytokine induction of leukocyte-endothelial adherence and damage is infrequent (3,26). Animal models do not demonstrate reductions in fibrinogen levels but have significant reductions in plasminogen activator and increases in plasminogen activator inhibitor with lethal infection (29). Most of the consumptive coagulopathy can be explained by the widespread rickettsia-mediated vasculitis and increased vascular permeability (3,13,26).

CLINICAL MANIFESTATIONS AND PATHOLOGY

Rash

Cutaneous manifestations occur in only 14% of patients on the first day of illness and in 49% during the first 3 days (3,26). In most patients, rash appears between days 3 and 5 of illness, and in 20% of patients, rash appears later than day 6; 9% to 34% of patients do not have a rash detected at any time (3,10,11,26). The absence of rash should not be taken as a sign of relatively mild illness because there is a clear association with an increased risk for severe or fatal outcome (3,4,30).

Rash often occurs in several stages, and an evolution toward petechiae and hemorrhagic lesions may be observed if not treated appropriately (3,13,31). Initially, the appearance is that of erythematous macules that occur first on the ankles or wrists in 70% of patients and subsequently on the trunk, palms, or soles (3,12,26). These lesions blanch with pressure and become papular as local edema and perivascular mononuclear inflammatory cell infiltrates accrue (19). As the rickettsiae proliferate, lymphohistiocytic or leukocytoclastic vasculitis with infiltration of the vascular wall and endothelial injury may be present (19,20) (Fig. 168.1). Irreversible endothelial cell injury results in extravasation of erythrocytes into the dermis and development of nonblanching petechiae, hemorrhagic lesions, or palpable purpura (Fig. 168.2). Petechiae are observed in 41% to 59% of patients and usually appear after the sixth day of illness (3,4,26). The petechial rash on the soles and palms that is often considered most typical of RMSF, in fact, only occurs in 43% of patients

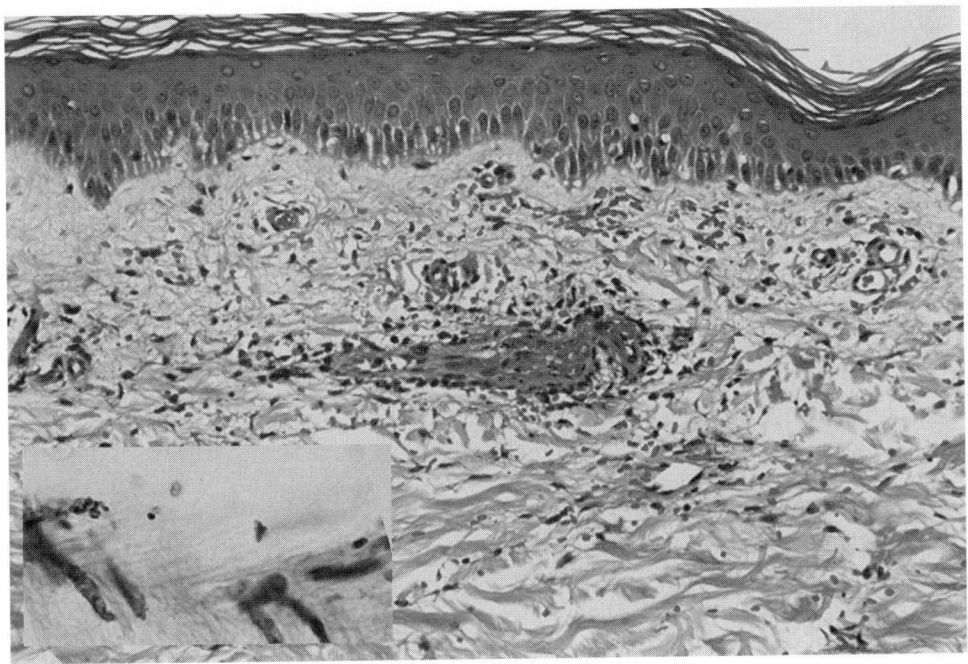

Figure 168.1. Rocky Mountain spotted fever. Skin biopsy of petechial lesion that shows moderate lymphohistiocytic perivascular infiltrate and lymphohistiocytic vasculitis. Note the endothelial cell necrosis, erythrocyte extravasation into the dermis, and minimal, nonocclusive thrombosis in this dermal venule (Hematoxylin & eosin, ×250). **Inset**: immunoalkaline phosphatase stain demonstrating *Rickettsia rickettsii* in endothelial cells (hematoxylin counterstain, ×1,000).

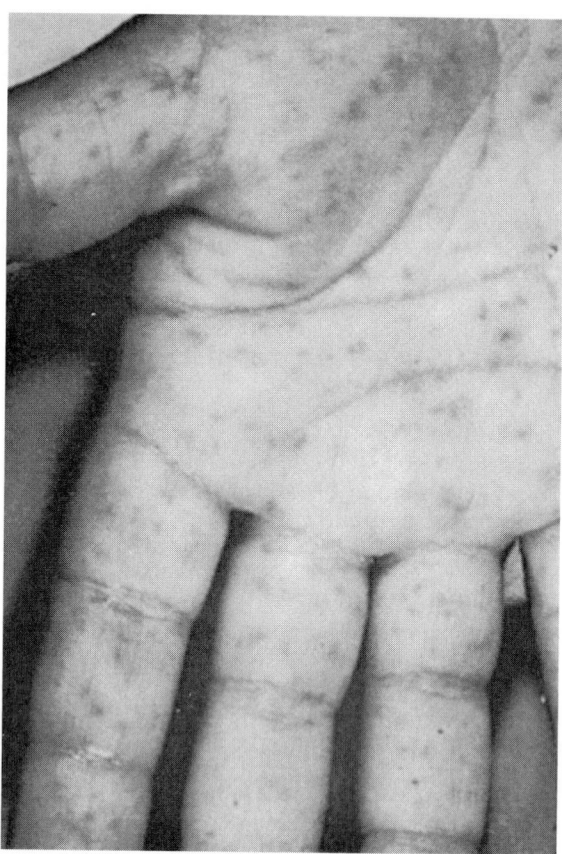

Figure 168.2. Petechial rash on the palm of a patient with Rocky Mountain spotted fever.

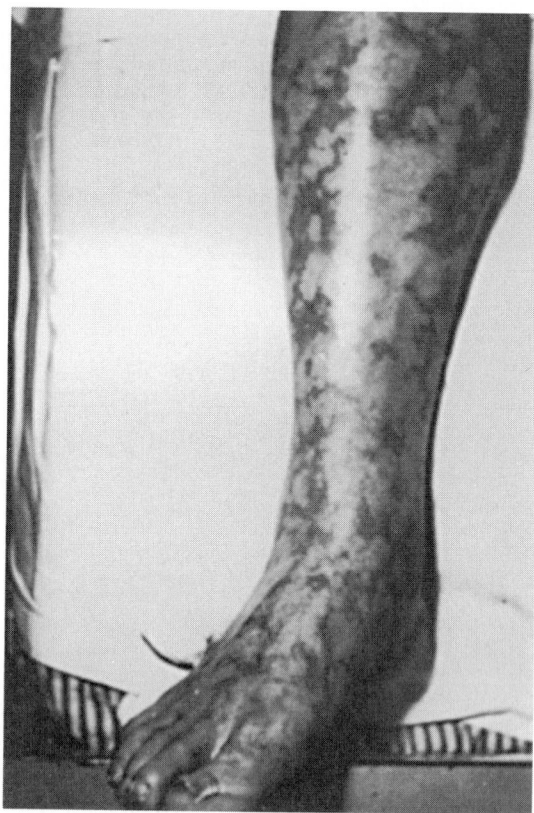

Figure 168.3. Purpuric rash in a patient with Rocky Mountain spotted fever complicated by widespread *Rickettsia rickettsii*–mediated vascular injury. (From Woodward TE. *Med Clin North Am* 1989;43:1516, with permission.)

with a rash and after day 5 of illness in between 36% and 82% of patients (3,4,12,26). Thus, at the typical time of presentation, about day 3 of illness, many patients lack the findings most often considered critical to render an accurate diagnosis of RMSF. In later disease, especially in severe cases with extensive vascular injury, many of the lesions may coalesce and become ecchymotic (Fig. 168.3).

Gastrointestinal System

Gastrointestinal abnormalities are frequent in RMSF and may lead to the erroneous diagnosis of an acute, surgical abdomen such as appendicitis, acute cholecystitis, or pancreatitis (3,26,32–34). These findings may present early and involve 39% to 63% of patients (3,35), and they result from vasculitis and rickettsia-mediated endothelial damage of the visceral wall and lamina propria (19,32). Liver involvement is very frequent with RMSF and is most often manifest by mild to moderate elevations in serum hepatic aminotransferase activities owing to infection of the endothelium in liver sinusoids and portal vascular structures but not hepatocytes (3,25,26,36). Jaundice is a risk factor for fatal disease (3), and severe liver injury is seen with fulminant RMSF in the absence of significant vasculitis (37).

Cardiopulmonary System

Among the most worrisome complications that occur with RMSF is the diffuse injury that occurs in the pulmonary vascular beds. The pathologic lesion is widespread interstitial pneumonitis with capillary endothelial injury (19). The resulting severe vascu-

lar permeability leads to noncardiogenic pulmonary edema and may be partly exacerbated by excessive intravenous fluid therapy for hypotension (13,24,38,39). Pulmonary involvement occurs in 17% to 30% of patients and is manifest by cough, rales, hypoxemia, or infiltrates on chest radiographs (26,40,41). Of these patients, 12% have severe respiratory dysfunction, and 8% require intubation and mechanical ventilation. Cardiopulmonary hemodynamic monitoring often shows relatively normal pulmonary capillary wedge pressures and left ventricular function, and careful monitoring will help effectively manage fluid volume, precluding worsening pulmonary function. When diffuse infiltrates are present, the mortality rate can be as high as 50% (40).

Cardiac involvement in RMSF is relatively infrequent and often clinically insignificant (38). Congestive heart failure in elderly patients may occur, particularly if volume overload occurs with therapy for hypotension. The principal evidence for myocardial involvement is the demonstration of arrhythmias, which occur in 7% to 16% of patients (3,26) and result from focal rickettsial nonnecrotizing lymphohistiocytic myocarditis near conduction tracts. Gallops, murmurs, cardiac enlargement, and electrocardiographic abnormalities (low voltage, ST-T changes, and atrioventricular conduction disturbances) have been reported (3,26,42). Significant clinical sequelae from these lesions are rare.

Renal System

Rickettsia-mediated interstitial nephritis is well documented (19,32), but the predominant renal abnormality in RMSF is prerenal azotemia that accounts for elevations in serum urea nitrogen and creatinine. However, continued hypoperfusion secondary to hypotensive shock can cause acute tubular necrosis and acute renal failure, a significant risk factor for severe or fatal infection (13,32,43). Glomerulonephritis is a very rare cause of renal dysfunction. Urinalysis may show proteinuria and hematuria, but an active urine sediment is very infrequent.

Neurologic System

Next to pulmonary involvement, central nervous system (CNS) infection is the most significant cause of severe and fatal outcome for RMSF (3,24,26,44–46). The *R. rickettsii* invade endothelial cells in the brain to cause focal vasculitis or perivascular infiltrates called *microglial* or *typhus nodules* (19). Encephalitis, manifest as confusion or lethargy, is present in 26% to 28% of patients, and more severe manifestations, such as stupor and delirium, occur in 21% to 26% of patients (3,26). Ataxia (18%), coma (9% to 10%), and convulsions (8%) are also frequent (3,46). Other neurologic involvement includes cranial nerve palsies, unilateral corticospinal signs, hearing loss, vertigo, dysarthria, aphasia, hemiplegia, paraplegia, paralysis, ankle clonus, nystagmus, hyperreflexia, spasticity, fasciculations, athetosis, and neurogenic bladder.

In the meninges, the presence of rickettsiae elicits a lymphohistiocytic meningitis. A cerebrospinal fluid (CSF) pleiocytosis and elevated CSF protein levels are present in about one third of patients (3,25,26). CSF examination usually reveals between 10 and 100 mononuclear cells/μL; however, patients with mostly polymorphonuclear cell pleiocytosis have been observed (25,26). CSF glucose values are usually normal. There is a strong association between severe CNS disease (coma and seizures) and fatality, presumably related to severe intracranial inflammation and edema. Thus, some have recommended the use of corticosteroids for rickettsial CNS infections, although no controlled trials have been performed.

Fulminant Disease

Fulminant RMSF is defined as illness that is unusually rapid (5 days or less from onset to death) (37). This form of the disease is characterized by early and rapid onset of clinical abnormalities, including neurologic signs and the absence or late appearance of rash. Host factors seem important for fulminant RMSF, and black male patients with glucose-6-phosphate dehydrogenase (G6PD) deficiency are prone to this form. The pathologic findings in this rare manifestation of RMSF include early and widespread vascular necrosis without significant accompanying inflammation.

Long-Term Sequelae

Nearly 50% of patients who recover from severe RMSF (hospitalized for more than 2 weeks) have long-term complications (30). Abnormalities that may persist for at least 1 year after the acute illness include paraparesis; hearing loss; peripheral neuropathy; bladder and bowel incontinence; cerebellar, vestibular, and motor dysfunction; language disorders; limb amputation; and scrotal pain following cutaneous necrosis.

LABORATORY FINDINGS

The results of clinical laboratory tests sometimes provide helpful clues for the diagnosis of RMSF. These findings vary depending on organ system involvement, severity of involvement, and duration of infection. Table 168.2 shows some of the frequent laboratory abnormalities associated with RMSF.

Hematologic Findings

One of the early (during the first week) findings is the occurrence of a normal leukocyte count or a slight leukopenia, accompanied by a high proportion of bands in the peripheral blood in a patient that appears seriously ill or septic (3,25,26,47). The mean high leukocyte count during the overall course of RMSF is 14,900 cells/μL, and the mean lowest value is 7,700 cells/μL, with a range from 3,800 to 16,800. An increased proportion of bands (more than 10%) is seen in nearly three fourths of patients, whereas thrombocytopenia (less than 150,000 platelets/μL), a sensitive early marker, is present in half. The mean platelet count is generally around the limits of low normal (143,000 platelets/μL), but profound thrombocytopenia may occasionally be present. After the first week of illness, leukocytosis and worsening thrombocytopenia occur more frequently.

Coagulation System

Evidence for activation of the coagulation system and other abnormalities of coagulation in RMSF is represented in several publications (25,48,49). About half of all patients have slight elevations in prothrombin time (PT) and activated partial thromboplastin times (aPTT), whereas hypofibrinogenemia and evidence for fibrin deposition (fibrin degradation products) may be detected in 36% to 67% of patients (25). These findings indicate that intravascular coagulation occurs at sites of rickettsia-infected endothelium, but not as a result of true DIC mediated by systemic release of proinflammatory cytokines and the induction of a generalized procoagulant state. Severe hemorrhage is very infrequent with RMSF (3,25,26).

Serum Electrolytes and Chemistry

Increased vascular permeability probably results in a net efflux of Na^+ ions from the serum and hyponatremia, which occurs in 56% to 91% of patients with RMSF (3,25,26). As the disease and accompanying hypotension progress, hyponatremia becomes more profound (10).

Liver function test abnormalities occur early and late in disease and are best reflected by elevations in serum aspartate transaminase (AST) or alanine aminotransferase (ALT) activities (3,25,26,35). These values are elevated more than twice the high-normal result in 40% to 80% of patients (3,25,26). Marked elevations, with levels above 1,000 IU/L, are sometimes identified in severely affected individuals (25,35). Similarly, bilirubin levels are elevated in 30% to 54% of patients at any time during the course of illness (3,25,26). With more severe illness and injury to other organs, aminotransferase and creatine phosphokinase isozyme activities may also be demonstrated in the serum (19,35). Serum urea nitrogen and serum creatinine levels may be elevated, usually secondary to prerenal mechanisms (13).

Cerebrospinal Fluid

With CNS involvement, a CSF pleiocytosis is sometimes identified. The opening pressure and glucose concentrations are usually within normal limits, whereas the protein concentration is slightly elevated in about half of all cases (25,26). When examined, the CSF may have a small number of cells (0 to 184 cells/μL), of which about 70% are mononuclear.

Electroencephalograms show diffusely slow cortical activity, and brain scans are normal (24,26). Neuroimaging studies may reveal a variety of findings, including infarcts, edema, and meningeal enhancement, and the identification of such abnormalities reveals an increased risk for severe and fatal disease (51).

DIAGNOSIS

Delay in recognition and treatment of RMSF is the most significant factor in severe morbidity, development of long-term sequelae, and fatality (3,4). The risk for death from RMSF is five times greater in patients treated after day 5 of illness, and most patients eventually diagnosed with RMSF are not treated with an antirickettsial antibiotic until after 5 days of illness, despite being examined by a physician before that time (4). Three major factors contribute to the ineffective diagnosis and delayed therapy: absence of rash, presentation during nonpeak season for tick activity, and presentation during the first 3 days of illness. Unfortunately, timely and highly sensitive laboratory-based diagnostic methods are not widely available, and serologic assays can be used safely only for retrospective diagnostic confirmation. Thus, all patients with a presumptive diagnosis of RMSF on the basis of clinical and epidemiologic history should be empirically treated.

The factors that are important to render an appropriate clinical diagnosis of RMSF are knowledge of the specific tick association and the presence of *D. variabilis* (American dog tick) or other appropriate vectors in the region, the seasonality of these tick vectors, human factors that predispose to tick exposure and tick bites, and the various clinical presentations, both typical and atypical (4,13). Tick vectors have specific seasons but may emerge and maintain activity for a longer season in warm climates or when local weather conditions are conducive. Although individual cases of RMSF have been acquired by aerosols and wound or conjunctival contamination, transmission must be assumed to be through a tick bite in all cases. Thus, exposure to ticks or tick bites during occupational or recreational activities are important clues. However, as few as 60% of patients report tick bites; thus, history of tick exposure should be sought, and its lack should not exclude the diagnosis in suspect cases.

Given that the epidemiologic hallmarks for RMSF are not always present, the diagnosis of RMSF should be considered in any patient who presents with an acute febrile illness with headache and myalgia, especially if presenting during a season with tick activity or with relevant tick exposure or bite (13). If a rash appears, RMSF must be considered in the differential diagnosis. Unfortunately, reliance on the clinical triad of fever, rash, and tick exposure is dangerous because it is identified in only 3% of patients during the first 3 days of illness (3), an interval within which 73% of patients will first seek medical attention (4), and in as few as 44% to 67% of patients with RMSF over the entire course of illness (3).

Differential Diagnosis

The differential diagnosis of RMSF is broad and modified by the presentation and degree of organ involvement. Within the first 3 days of illness, when rash is absent or inconspicuous, the list of potential diagnoses includes influenza, enteroviral infection, typhoid fever, leptospirosis, infectious mononucleosis, viral hepatitis, bacterial sepsis, and monocytic and granulocytic ehrlichiosis. Patients with RMSF often complain of very severe headache, a finding that might lead one to favor the diagnosis of RMSF. With manifestations that focus attention to a single organ system, such as nausea, vomiting, diarrhea, and abdominal pain, viral or bacterial gastroenteritis or perhaps a perforated viscus would be considered. Patients with a prominent cough and chest radiographic infiltrates or opacities might be considered to have an exacerbation of chronic bronchitis or acute bronchopneumonia.

When a rash develops, the differential list extends to include meningococcemia, disseminated gonococcal infection, secondary syphilis, bacterial endocarditis, toxic shock syndrome, scarlet fever, rheumatic fever, measles, rubella, murine typhus, rickettsialpox, recrudescent typhus, Lyme disease, drug hypersensitivity reactions, idiopathic thrombocytopenic purpura, thrombotic thrombocytopenic purpura, Kawasaki disease, immune complex vasculitis, or other connective tissue disorders.

Etiologic Laboratory Diagnosis

Unfortunately, most clinical laboratories have little to offer as timely, objective diagnostic assays for RMSF. There are several useful diagnostic methods, including serology, culture, demonstration of *R. rickettsii* antigens in skin biopsy or other tissue samples, and polymerase chain reaction (PCR) demonstration of *R. rickettsii* nucleic acids in blood (13,19,52–59). The standard confirmatory diagnostic measure is the demonstration of an increase in antibody titer to *R. rickettsii* during convalescence. Serologic reactivity is rarely present at the time of the acute infectious process; thus, withholding therapy while awaiting serologic confirmation is dangerous. A fourfold increase in antibody titer to *R. rickettsii* between acute and convalescent sera obtained 2 weeks apart confirms a clinical diagnosis.

Current serologic methods cannot distinguish *R. rickettsii* antibodies from those elicited by infection with other spotted fever group rickettsiae. Several highly sensitive and specific serologic assays have been developed: the indirect fluorescent antibody (IFA) test (52), enzyme-linked immunosorbent assay (ELISA), solid-phase enzyme immunoassays, and latex agglutination assays (53). Reliable serologic testing can usually be obtained by reference to state, federal, or territorial health laboratories. Reagents and kits for these assays may be purchased from commercial suppliers, or samples may be sent to commercial laboratories to have these tests performed. The standard serodiagnostic assay is IFA, in which a titer of at least 64 is generally first detected between days 7 and 10 of illness; confirmation requires a fourfold increase in titer. A single convalescent titer of at least 128 is considered as probable evidence of infection in the setting of a recent clinically compatible illness. This assay has been widely used and has a sensitivity that ranges between 94% and 100% with a specificity of nearly 100% (60,61). The latex agglutination test detects predominantly immunoglobulin M antibodies and is most useful after 7 to 9 days and within the first several weeks of RMSF (53). The sensitivity of the latex agglutination methods has been reported between 71% and 94% with a specificity of 96% to 99% (53). The archaic Weil-Felix reaction, a part of many laboratories' febrile agglutinins panel, is a relic of a previous serologic age and is based on cross-reactivity of *Proteus* species antigens with those of *Rickettsia* species. The sensitivity and specificity using the OX-19 agglutination test are 70% and 78%, respectively, and for the OX-2 antigen, the sensitivity is even lower, 47% (54).

Currently, the only test that may give a timely diagnosis during the acute phase of infection is the immunohistologic or immunfluorescent demonstration of *R. rickettsii* in tissue biopsy specimens of rash lesions (56,57,59). The test may be performed on either fresh tissue, on tissue stored in Michel's transport medium, or on formalin-fixed, paraffin-embedded tissues. The method is only useful for those patients with a rash or for postmortem examinations and thus is less useful during the first few days of illness. An appropriate rash lesion is selected, preferably a petechia. After preparation of the site, a 3- or 4-mm punch biopsy is performed, allowing that the lesion be centrally located within the biopsy. With frozen sections, *R. rickettsii* may be demonstrated as early as 3 hours after biopsy; if the tissue is fixed and paraffin embedded, a longer interval will be required. Unfortunately, this test and service are not widely available but may be obtained through public health or reference laboratories. Despite the consideration by many that this test is invasive, skin biopsy is a simple, relatively painless procedure that can provide reassuring diagnostic information.

Antigen demonstration of *R. rickettsii* in biopsy tissue specimens has a specificity of 100%; the sensitivity is 70% (26,57,62). A positive result is most useful and can allow a rapid focus of diagnostic considerations. However, the predictive values for negative *R. rickettsii* antigen tests on skin biopsy are 20%, 50%, and 80% for pretest probabilities of 80%, 50% and 20%, respectively and result in posttest probabilities of about 50%, 25%, and 7%, respectively. Thus, a negative result should not dissuade the physician from continuing the antirickettsial therapy. The skin biopsy should be obtained before initiation of therapy because sensitivity diminishes thereafter (56).

Other new diagnostic modalities have been developed but are incompletely evaluated and generally not available except in research laboratories. PCR amplification of *R. rickettsii* nucleic acids in acute-phase blood samples appears to lack sensitivity (58). Many consider rickettsial cultures to be hazardous, and this is generally not a diagnostic option; however, shell vial culture of blood is rapid and sensitive for diagnosis of boutonneuse fever (*R. conorii* infection) (55).

TREATMENT

Rocky Mountain spotted fever can be treated effectively with doxycycline or tetracycline, except in pregnant and allergic patients. Chloramphenicol has been extensively used in the treatment of RMSF, particularly in patients younger than 9 years of age, to preclude the potential for tooth staining observed with tetracyclines. However, recent epidemiologic data suggest that severity and fatality were more likely with chloramphenicol use when all other confounding factors were controlled (2). Although chloramphenicol would be considered an appropriate choice for therapy, especially in pregnant or allergic patients, most authorities now agree that doxycycline should be the drug of choice, even in young patients (2,63). No data currently support the use of macrolides or fluoroquinolones for treatment of RMSF, although *R. rickettsii* may be inhibited *in vitro* by achievable concentrations of levofloxacin (64).

Minimum inhibitory concentrations of antibiotics have been determined by several methods and have shown values of 0.06 to 0.1 μg/mL for doxycycline and 0.3 to 0.5 μg/mL for chloramphenicol (65). It must be noted that these antirickettsial drugs are bacteriostatic. Thus, recovery relies on effective induction of appropriate immunity. Moreover, prophylaxis should not be administered for tick bites because this would only delay the onset of illness and confound the epidemiologic history (66). Currently, the recommended dosages for the tetracyclines are (a) oral or intravenous doxycycline, 200 mg per day in two divided doses; (b) oral tetracycline, 25 to 50 mg/kg per day in four divided doses; or (c) chloramphenicol, 50 to 75 mg/kg per day in four divided doses. Therapy is continued for at least 2 days after defervescence.

Although effective for boutonneuse fever, evaluations of fluoroquinolone antibiotics for RMSF have not been performed. *In vitro* testing suggests that ciprofloxacin, ofloxacin, and lev-

ofloxacin may have activity against *R. rickettsii* (64,67), but lack of data prevents recommending these as therapy for RMSF. The use of sulfonamides is contraindicated in RMSF (24). The current recommendation for pregnant patients is therapy with chloramphenicol owing to the potential for adverse fetal and maternal reactions to tetracyclines; however, adverse fetal and maternal effects of doxycycline are not likely to be greater than with chloramphenicol, and a strong argument for its use in pregnant patients with RMSF can be made (68).

Response to therapy is usually prompt, within 48 to 72 hours. However, patients with severe complications may require a longer interval before recovery. On occasion, relapse may occur, especially in those treated very early in the course of disease before an effective immune response has occurred (66).

Mildly ill patients can often be managed effectively as outpatients. However, 52% to 78% of patients are moderately to severely ill enough to require hospitalization, potentially into an intensive care unit (11–13). Those patients with a particularly severe illness will require careful intravenous fluids management, preferably with hemodynamic monitoring to diminish the risk for noncardiogenic pulmonary edema, even if some degree of prerenal azotemia is present. Fluid replacement should not be restricted in patients with hyponatremia because it is usually not life threatening and responds to appropriate volume management (13,50).

Other therapies may be required, such as mechanical ventilation, hemodialysis, anticonvulsants, packed red blood cells, and platelet transfusions. Because the DIC-like appearance of RMSF is due to rickettsia-damaged endothelium, heparin therapy is contraindicated. Corticosteroids may be given to patients with rickettsial meningoencephalitis, but controlled trials to prove benefit have not been performed.

PREVENTION

There is currently no vaccine for RMSF. Prophylactic antirickettsial therapy for tick bites only delays the onset of disease. Thus, prevention of tick bites is the major preventive measure and may be achieved by avoidance of tick habitats with wooded or grassy terrains and the use of light-colored barrier clothing that helps identify ticks before reaching skin surfaces; tick repellents on clothing and skin may offer limited benefits. A careful search for ticks after potential exposure, including inspection of the scalp, axillae, and groin, will identify hidden sites of potential attachment. Similar inspection of pets will prevent animals from acting as vehicles that transport ticks into human environments.

Prompt removal of attached ticks often prevents infection even if the tick contains rickettsiae. Unengorged, flat ticks are unlikely to have activated rickettsiae or exchanged infectious salivary secretions. If attached, ticks are removed by gentle but firm retraction of the mouthparts from the skin with forceps. Generally, folklore remedies such as petroleum jelly or hot matches do little to encourage a tick to disattach and should be avoided. Although complete removal of the tick is encouraged, the additional trauma caused by removing remnant tick mouthparts probably does more harm than good. Crushing or handling of ticks that are potentially infectious should also be avoided to preclude mechanical transmission into conjunctivae or other mucous membranes.

REFERENCES

1. Centers for Disease Control. Summary of notifiable diseases, United States, 1999. *MMWR Morb Mortal Wkly Rep* 2001;48:1.

2. Dalton MJ, Clarke MJ, Holman RC, et al. National surveillance for Rocky Mountain spotted fever, 1981–1992: epidemiological summary and evaluation of risk factors for fatal outcome. *Am J Trop Med Hyg* 1995;52:405.

3. Helmick CG, Bernard KW, D'Angelo LJ. Rocky Mountain spotted fever: clinical, laboratory, and epidemiological features of 262 cases. *J Infect Dis* 1984;150:480.

4. Kirkland KB, Wilkinson WE, Sexton DJ. Therapeutic delay and mortality in cases of Rocky Mountain spotted fever. *Clin Infect Dis* 1995;20:1118.

5. McDade JE, Newhouse VF. Natural history of *Rickettsia rickettsii*. *Annu Rev Microbiol* 1986;40:287.

6. Niebylski ML, Peacock MG, Schwan TG. Lethal effect of *Rickettsia rickettsii* on its tick vector (*Dermacentor andersoni*). *Appl Environ Microbiol* 1999;65:773.

7. Burgdorfer W, Hayes SF, Mavros AJ. Nonpathogenic rickettsiae in *Dermacentor andersoni*: a limiting factor for the distribution of *Rickettsia rickettsii*. In: Burgdorfer W, Anacker RL, eds. *Rickettsiae and rickettsial diseases*. New York: Academic Press, 1981:585–594.

8. Hayes SF, Burgdorfer W. Reactivation of *Rickettsia rickettsii* in *Dermacentor andersoni* ticks: an ultrastructural analysis. *Infect Immun* 1982;37:779.

9. Gage KL, Burgdorfer W, Hopla CE. Hispid cotton rats (*Sigmodon hispidus*) as a source for infecting immature *Dermacentor variabilis* (Acari: Ixodidae) with *Rickettsia rickettsii*. *J Med Entomol* 1990;27:615.

10. Wilfert CM, MacCormack JN, Kleeman K, et al. Epidemiology of Rocky Mountain spotted fever as determined by active surveillance. *J Infect Dis* 1984;150: 469.

11. Treadwell TA, Holman RC, Clarke MJ, et al. Rocky Mountain spotted fever in the United States, 1993–1996. *Am J Trop Med Hyg* 2000;63:21.

12. Billings AN, Rawlings JA, Walker DH. Tick-borne disease in Texas: a 10-year retrospective examination of cases. *Texas Med* 1998;94:66.

13. Walker DH. Rocky Mountain spotted fever: a seasonal alert. *Clin Infect Dis* 1995;20:1111.

14. Li H, Walker DH. Characterization of rickettsial attachment to host cells by flow cytometry. *Infect Immun* 1992;60:2030.

15. Manor E, Carbonetti NH, Silverman DJ. *Rickettsia rickettsii* has proteins with cross-reacting epitopes to eukaryotic phospholipase A$_2$ and phospholipase C. *Microb Pathog* 1994;17:99.

16. Silverman DJ, Santucci L. Potential for free radical-induced lipid peroxidation as a cause of endothelial cell injury in Rocky Mountain spotted fever. *Infect Immun* 1988;56:3110.

17. Sporn LA, Marder VJ. Interleukin-1β production during *Rickettsia rickettsii* infection of cultured endothelial cells: potential role in autocrine cell stimulation. *Infect Immun* 1996;64:1609.

18. Clifton DR, Goss RA, Sahni SK, et al. NF-kappa B-dependent inhibition of apoptosis is essential for host cell survival during *Rickettsia rickettsii* infection. *Proc Natl Acad Sci U S A* 1998;95:4646.

19. Walker DH. Diagnosis of rickettsial diseases. *Pathol Annu* 1988;23:69.

20. Kao GF, Evancho CD, Ioffe O, et al. Cutaneous histopathology of Rocky Mountain spotted fever. *J Cutan Pathol* 1997;24:604.

21. Feng H-M, Wen J, Walker DH. *Rickettsia australis* infection: a murine model of a highly invasive vasculopathic rickettsiosis. *Am J Pathol* 1993;142:1471.

22. Feng H-M, Walker DH. Interferon-γ and tumor necrosis factor-α exert their antirickettsial effect via induction of synthesis of nitric oxide. *Am J Pathol* 1993;143:1016.

23. Walker DH, Olano JP, Feng HM. Critical role of cytotoxic T lymphocytes in immune clearance of rickettsial infection. *Infect Immun* 2001;69:1841.

24. Harrell GT. Rocky Mountain spotted fever. *Medicine* 1949;28:333.

25. Kirk JL, Fine DP, Sexton DJ, et al. Rocky Mountain spotted fever: a clinical review based on 48 confirmed cases, 1943–1986. *Medicine* 1990;69:35.

26. Kaplowitz LG, Fischer JJ, Sparling PF. Rocky Mountain spotted fever: a clinical dilemma. In: Remington JS, Swartz MN, eds. *Current clinical topics in infectious diseases*, Vol 2. New York: McGraw-Hill: 89–108.

27. Sexton DJ, Burgdorfer W. Clinical and epidemiological features of Rocky Mountain spotted fever in Mississippi, 1933–1973. *South Med J* 1975;68:1529.

28. Kirkland KB, Marcom PK, Sexton DJ, et al. Rocky Mountain spotted fever complicated by gangrene: report of six cases and review. *Clin Infect Dis* 1993;16: 629.

29. Schmaier AH, Srikanth S, Elghetany MT, et al. Hemostatic/fibrinolytic protein changes in C3H/HeN mice infected with *Rickettsia conorii*—a model for Rocky Mountain spotted fever. *Thromb Haemost* 2001;86:871.

30. Archibald LK, Sexton DJ. Long-term sequelae of Rocky Mountain spotted fever. *Clin Infect Dis* 1995;20:1122.

31. Hattwick MA, O'Brien RJ, Hanson BF. Rocky Mountain spotted fever: epidemiology of an increasing problem. *Ann Intern Med* 1976;84:732.

32. Walker DH, Mattern WD. Acute renal failure in Rocky Mountain spotted fever. *Arch Intern Med* 1979;139:443.

33. Davis AE, Bradford WD. Abdominal pain resembling acute appendicitis in Rocky Mountain spotted fever. *JAMA* 1982;247:2811.

34. Randall MB, Walker DH. Rocky Mountain spotted fever: gastrointestinal and pancreatic lesions and rickettsial infection. *Arch Pathol Lab Med* 1984;108: 963.

35. Middleton DB. Rocky Mountain spotted fever: gastrointestinal and laboratory manifestations. *South Med J* 1978;71:629.

36. Adams JS, Walker DH. The liver in Rocky Mountain spotted fever. *Am J Clin Pathol* 1981;75:156.

37. Walker DH, Hawkins HK, Hudson P. Fulminant Rocky Mountain spotted fever: its pathologic characteristics associated with glucose-6-dehydrogenase deficiency. *Arch Pathol Lab Med* 1983;107:121.

38. Walker DH, Mattern WD. Rickettsial vasculitis. *Am Heart J* 1980;100:896.

39. Donohue JF. Lower respiratory tract involvement in Rocky Mountain spotted fever. *Arch Intern Med* 1980;140:223.

40. Martin W, Choplin RH, Shertzer ME. The chest radiograph in Rocky Mountain spotted fever. *Am J Radiol* 1982;139:889.

41. Byrd RP, Vasquez J, Roy TM. Respiratory manifestations of tick-borne disease in the southeastern United States. *South Med J* 1997;90:1.

42. Marin GJ, Mirvis DM. Myocardial disease in Rocky Mountain spotted fever: clinical, functional, and pathologic findings. *Pediatr Cardiol* 1984;5:149.

43. Conlon PJ, Procop GW, Fowler V, et al. Predictors of prognosis and risk of acute renal failure in patients with Rocky Mountain spotted fever. *Am J Med* 1996;101:621.

44. Miller JQ, Price TR. The nervous system in Rocky Mountain spotted fever. *Neurology* 1972;22:561.

45. Massey EW, Thames T, Coffey CE, et al. Neurologic complications of Rocky Mountain spotted fever. *South Med J* 1985;78:1288.

46. Haynes RE, Sanders, Cramblett HG. Rocky Mountain spotted fever in children. *J Pediatr* 1970;76:685.

47. Hall GW, Schwartz RP. White blood cell count and differential in Rocky Mountain spotted fever. *N C Med J* 1971;40:212.

48. Rao AK, Shapira M, Clements ML, et al. A prospective study of platelets and plasma proteolytic systems during the early stages of Rocky Mountain spotted fever. *N Engl J Med* 1988;318:1021.

49. Yamada T, Harber P, Petit GW, et al. Activation of the kallikrein-kinin system in Rocky Mountain spotted fever. *Ann Intern Med* 1978;88:764.

50. Kaplowitz LG, Robertson GL. Hyponatremia in Rocky Mountain spotted fever: role of antidiuretic hormone. *Ann Intern Med* 1983;98:334.

51. Bonawitz C, Castillo M, Mukherji SK. Comparison of CT and MR features with clinical outcome in patients with Rocky Mountain spotted fever. *Am J Neuroradiol* 1997;18:459.

52. Philip RN, Casper EA, Ormsbee RA, et al. Microimmunofluorescence test for the serological study of Rocky Mountain spotted fever and typhus. *J Clin Microbiol* 1976;3:51.

53. Hechemy KE, Anacker RL, et al. Evaluation of latex *Rickettsia rickettsii* test for Rocky Mountain spotted fever in 11 laboratories. *J Clin Microbiol* 1983;18:938.

54. Hechemy KE, Stevens RW, Sasowski S, et al. Discrepancies in Weil-Felix and microimmunofluorescence test results for Rocky Mountain spotted fever. *J Clin Microbiol* 1979;9:292.

55. Marrero M, Raoult D. Centrifugation-shell vial technique for rapid detection of Mediterranean spotted fever rickettsiae in blood culture. *Am J Trop Med Hyg* 1989;40:197.

56. Walker DH, Cain BG, Olmstead PM. Laboratory diagnosis of Rocky Mountain spotted fever by immunofluorescent demonstration of *Rickettsia rickettsii* in cutaneous lesions. *Am J Clin Pathol* 1978;69:619.

57. Dumler JS, Gage WR, Pettis GL, et al. Rapid immunoperoxidase demonstration of *Rickettsia rickettsii* in fixed cutaneous specimens from patients with Rocky Mountain spotted fever. *Am J Clin Pathol* 1990;93:410.

58. Sexton DJ, Kanj SS, Wilson K, et al. The use of polymerase chain reaction as a diagnostic test for Rocky Mountain spotted fever. *Am J Trop Med Hyg* 1994; 50:59.

59. Procop GW, Burchette JL Jr, Howell DN, et al. Immunoperoxidase and immunofluorescent staining of *Rickettsia rickettsii* in skin biopsies: a comparative study. *Arch Pathol Lab Med* 1997;121:894.

60. Philip RN, Casper EA, MacCormack JN, et al. A comparison of serologic methods for diagnosis of Rocky Mountain spotted fever. *Am J Epidemiol* 1977;105:56.

61. Kaplan JE, Schonberger LB. The sensitivity of various serologic tests in the diagnosis of Rocky Mountain spotted fever. *Am J Trop Med Hyg* 1986;35:840.

62. Walker DH, Burday MS, Folds JD. Laboratory diagnosis of Rocky Mountain spotted fever. *South Med J* 1980;73:1443.

63. Abramson JS, Givner LB. Should tetracycline be contraindicated for therapy of presumed Rocky Mountain spotted fever in children less than 9 years of age? *Pediatrics* 1990;86:123.

64. Maurin M, Raoult D. Bacteriostatic and bactericidal activity of levofloxacin against *Rickettsia rickettsii*, *Rickettsia conorii*, 'Israeli spotted fever group rickettsia' and *Coxiella burnetii*. *J Antimicrob Chemother* 1997;39:725.

65. Wisseman CL Jr, Waddell A. In vitro sensitivity of *Rickettsia rickettsii* to doxycycline. *J Infect Dis* 1982;145:584.

66. DuPont HL, Hornick RB, Dawkins AT, et al. Rocky Mountain spotted fever: a comparative study of the active immunity induced by inactivated and viable pathogenic *Rickettsia rickettsii*. *J Infect Dis* 1973;128:340.

67. Jabarit-Aldighieri N, Torres H, Raoult D. Susceptibility of *Rickettsia conorii*, *R. rickettsii*, and *Coxiella burnetii* to PD 127,391, PD 131,628, pefloxacin, ofloxacin, and ciprofloxacin. *Antimicrob Agents Chemother* 1992;36:2529.

68. Stallings SP. Rocky Mountain spotted fever and pregnancy: a case report and review of the literature. *Obstet Gynecol Surv* 2001;56:37.

CHAPTER 169

The Human Ehrlichioses and Related Infections, Q Fever, Epidemic Typhus, Murine Typhus, Rickettsialpox, Scrub Typhus, and Other Rickettsioses

Jennifer H. McQuiston and James G. Olson

THE HUMAN EHRLICHIOSES AND RELATED INFECTIONS

Several members of the former genus *Ehrlichia* were recently recommended for reclassification as part of a taxonomic reorganization. *Ehrlichia chaffeensis* and *Ehrlichia ewingii* remained in the genus *Ehrlichia*. *Ehrlichia phagocytophilum* and related species were classified under the genus *Anaplasma* (i.e., *Anaplasma phagocytophilum*), and *Ehrlichia sennetsu* was classified under the genus *Neorickettsia* (i.e., *Neorickettsia sennetsu*). Thus, the term ehrlichiosis no longer accurately describes the nature of infections caused by these genetically distinct pathogens (1).

History of Disease

Current and former *Ehrlichia* species have long been recognized as animal pathogens and more recently have been recognized as an important cause of infection among humans. The first species reported to cause infections in humans was *Neorickettsia sennetsu* (formerly *Ehrlichia sennetsu*), the agent of Sennetsu fever. This agent, first described in a Japanese patient in 1954 (2), has rarely been diagnosed outside of Japan. Three additional forms of human ehrlichiosis have more recently been recognized in the United States. Human monocytic ehrlichiosis (HME), caused by *E. chaffeensis*, was described in 1986 (3). A second ehrlichial pathogen, *Anaplasma phagocytophilum* (formerly *Ehrlichia phagocytophilum*), was linked to human granulocytic ehrlichiosis (HGE) in 1994 (4). A third ehrlichial pathogen, *Ehrlichia ewingii*, was reported to cause human infection in 1999 (5). Although the epidemiology and pathogenicity of *E. chaffeensis* and *A. phagocytophilum* have been established, these characteristics are still being elucidated for *E. ewingii*.

Epidemiology

E. chaffeensis, *A. phagocytophilum*, and *E. ewingii* are transmitted to humans through the bite of infected ticks. Ticks typically acquire these pathogens by feeding on infected vertebrate hosts. The geographic distribution of these diseases, therefore, is similar to that of the specific tick vectors. *E. chaffeensis* and *E. ewingii* are transmitted by *Amblyomma americanum*, the Lone Star tick, which is commonly found throughout the southeastern and south-central United States (6). *A. phagocytophilum* is spread by *Ixodes scapularis* (the blacklegged tick) in the eastern and central United States and *Ixodes pacificus* (the western blacklegged tick) along the West

Coast (7). *I. scapularis* and *I. pacificus* are the same tick vectors responsible for transmission of *Borrelia burgdorferi* (Lyme disease) and *Babesia* species in the United States, and co-infection with *A. phagocytophilum* and these pathogens may be possible (8). The transmission cycle for *N. sennetsu* has not been well established but may involve exposure to water and a snail–fluke cycle, similar to that of the equine pathogen *Neorickettsia risticii* (9).

Data on the incidence of ehrlichiosis in the United States are incomplete because not all states consider it a reportable disease. Between 1986 and 1997, 742 cases of HME and 449 cases of HGE were reported to 30 state health departments in the United States; in addition, 32 cases were reported that were not ascribed to a particular agent (10). The highest average annual incidence rates of HME were reported from Arkansas, North Carolina, Missouri, and Oklahoma (10) (Fig. 169.1A). The highest average annual incidence rates for HGE were reported from Connecticut, Wisconsin, Minnesota, and New York (10) (Fig. 169.1B). Only four cases of *E. ewingii* infection have been described in the literature. These patients all resided in Missouri, and three of them were immunosuppressed at the time of diagnosis (5).

Ehrlichia species have been reported from many parts of the world. Although *N. sennetsu* has only been reported in western Japan and Malaysia (11), human infection with *A. phagocytophilum* has been confirmed in Slovenia and is suspected in other European countries (12). Although infections have not been confirmed, serologic evidence of human infections with *E. chaffeensis* or an antigenically related species have been reported from South America, Europe, and the Middle East as well as parts of Asia. Whether these represent endemic disease or were acquired through travel is not clear in all cases.

See Table 169.1 for the epidemiologic features of the rickettsial diseases discussed in this chapter.

Pathogenesis

N. sennetsu and *E. ewingii* have not been well studied to date, and most of our knowledge of disease pathogenesis comes from studies of *E. chaffeensis* and *A. phagocytophilum*. The incubation period for HME and HGE averages 1 week after a bite from an infected tick (range, 1 to 21 days) (13). *Ehrlichia* are obligate intracellular pathogens that infect circulating white blood cells, although they may also be found in platelets and tissue macrophages. *E. chaffeensis* and *N. sennetsu* predominantly infect monocytes, whereas *A. phagocytophilum* and *E. ewingii* predominantly infect granulocytes. The organisms cluster in intracytoplasmic membrane–lined vacuoles known as *morulae* that can sometimes be visualized on blood smears. Morulae can contain variable numbers of organisms and are more commonly seen in HGE than in HME.

Because these agents are intraleukocytic pathogens, there is a theoretical risk for transmission by blood transfusion, and at least one case of probable transfusion-transmission of HGE has been reported (14,15). Experimentally, both *E. chaffeensis* and *A. phagocytophilum* can survive in blood products stored under blood-banking conditions (16,17).

Clinical Manifestations

HME and HGE share clinical similarities and are typically characterized by acute onset of fever, headache, and malaise. Many patients report recent tick bites (68% for *E. chaffeensis*, 73% for *A. phagocytophilum*) (18,19). About one third of patients infected with *E. chaffeensis* may develop a generalized rash, although this percentage may be higher among children. A rash occurs only rarely among patients infected with *A. phagocytophilum*.

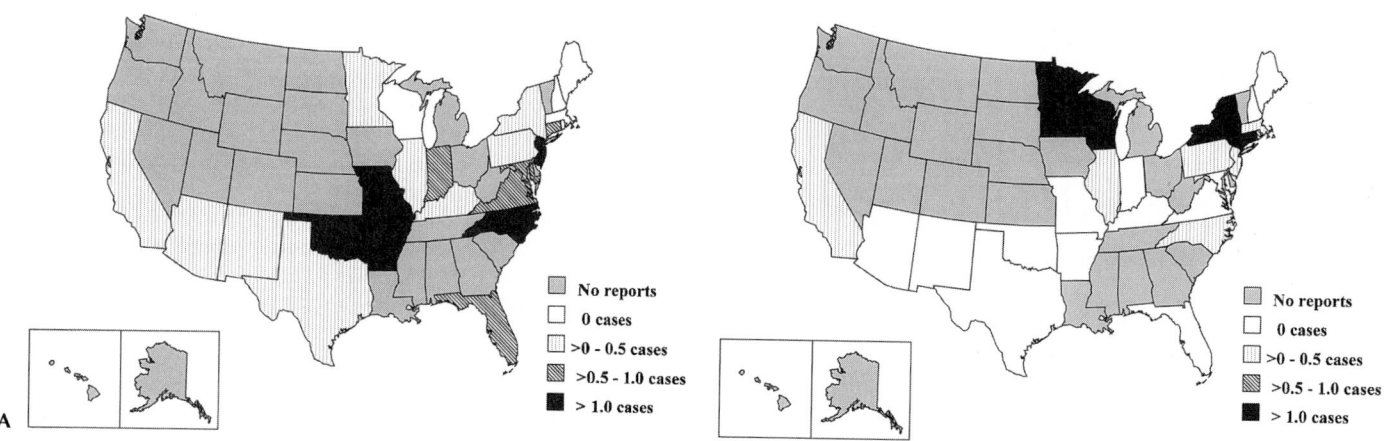

Figure 169.1. Average annual incidence of reported human monocytic ehrlichiosis (HME) (A) and human granulocytic ehrlichiosis (HGE) (B) by state in the United States, 1986–1997, per 1,000,000 population. Includes states that considered ehrlichiosis notifiable or routinely collected case information.

Ehrlichiosis and Rocky Mountain spotted fever (caused by *Rickettsia rickettsii*) may appear quite similar, and both diseases should be included in the diagnostic workup. Infected patients will typically develop thrombocytopenia, leukocytosis, and elevated hepatic transaminase levels (13,19). In some cases, infection may be severe, characterized by encephalitis or acute respiratory distress syndrome, or complicated by secondary infections (13,19). One case of perinatal transmission of HGE has been reported in the literature (20). Chronic ehrlichiosis has not been described. Asymptomatic ehrlichiosis infection may occur, and individuals may seroconvert without showing clinical signs of illness. However, it is sometimes unclear whether these are infections caused by *E. chaffeensis*, *A. phagocytophilum*, or an antigenically similar species.

HME and HGE are in most cases moderate illnesses, although severe disease and fatal infections have been reported. Case-fatality rates of 2% to 5% have been reported for HME and 0.7% to 10% for HGE (9,21), although some of these estimates may be inflated. Immunocompromised patients may be at higher risk for fatal infection (22).

Sennetsu fever is generally a mild to moderate illness that may resemble infectious mononucleosis, with characteristic signs of fever, lethargy, and lymphadenopathy (11). Hematologic changes may include lymphocytosis, whereas platelet counts are usually within normal limits (11). Fatal cases have not been reported.

Diagnosis

The indirect immunofluorescence assay (IFA) is most frequently used to diagnose acute ehrlichiosis. Because detectable antibody titers may not be present for as long as 10 to 14 days after the onset of clinical signs, the testing of both acute- and convalescent-phase serum specimens is important (23,24). Serologic confirmation of infection requires demonstration of a fourfold or greater change in antibody titers between paired sera (25). Because paired sera may not always be available for patients, physicians may interpret a high single titer or standing paired titers as a probable case (25). Because antibody titers may remain elevated for months to years after acute infection, serologic tests should always be interpreted within the epidemiologic and clinical context. Antibody cross-reactivity has been observed for *E. chaffeensis* and *A. phagocytophilum*. Therefore, in areas where the geographic ranges of responsible tick vectors overlap, physicians should request serologic tests for both agents.

Although frequently used, serologic tests are not very sensitive for testing sera acquired during early infection. Polymerase chain reaction (PCR) assays can provide earlier positive results than serology (24,26). Microscopic evaluation of peripheral blood smears for evidence of morulae may also be used for diagnosis, although this method is generally insensitive. Culture is not widely available.

Treatment

Because it can take several weeks to obtain paired serum specimens needed for laboratory confirmation, and because clinical signs may resemble those of the more severe disease Rocky Mountain spotted fever, physicians should always treat patients on the basis of clinical suspicion rather than awaiting laboratory confirmation. Tetracyclines are considered the treatment of choice, and patients should be given doxycycline, 100 mg twice daily, either orally or intravenously, for 7 to 10 days (27).

Prevention

Vaccines are not available for any of the human ehrlichioses. Tick-borne diseases are best prevented by avoiding tick bites and exposure to tick habitats. Persons can greatly decrease their risk for tick bites by wearing long sleeves and pants and by tucking pant legs into socks before entering tick habitats. Wearing light-colored clothing may make it easier to see ticks and remove them before they have a chance to attach. Use of permethrin-treated clothing and sprays may help decrease the chances of tick bites. Finally, persons should routinely perform body checks on themselves after visiting tick-infested areas because prompt removal of attached ticks may help reduce the risk for transmission of these pathogens.

Q FEVER

History of Disease

Q fever was first recognized as an outbreak of acute febrile illness among Australian slaughterhouse workers in 1935 (28). At that time, the etiology for the newly recognized disease was not known, and it was called *query (Q) fever*. Around the same time, researchers in the United States were investigating a rickettsial agent that had been isolated from ticks in Montana. The agent

TABLE 169.1. Epidemiologic Features of Selected Rickettsial Diseases

Features	Human monocytic ehrlichiosis	Human granulocytic ehrlichiosis	Q fever	Epidemic typhus	Murine typhus	Rickettsialpox	Scrub typhus	Other rickettsioses
Pathogen	*Ehrlichia chaffeensis*	*Ehrlichia phagocytophila*	*Coxiella burnetii*	*Rickettsia prowazekii*	*Rickettsia typhi*	*Rickettsia akari*	*Orientia tsutsugamushi*	*Rickettsia conorii, R. africae, R. australis*
Vector	Tick (*Amblyomma americanum*)	Tick (*Ixodes scapularis* or *I. pacificus*)	Infectious aerosols	Human body louse or fleas/lice associated with flying squirrels	Primarily rat flea; less often cat flea	Mouse mite	Chiggers	Exotic ticks
Animal reservoir	Wild rodents, other wild animals	Wild rodents, other wild animals	Parturient animals, especially sheep, cattle, goats	Worldwide: humans; flying squirrels in the U.S.	Rat; opossum in some parts of the U.S.	House mouse	Rats; unknown	Varies
Geographic distribution	Southeastern and south-central U.S.	Northeastern and upper midwestern U.S.	Worldwide	Developing countries; flying squirrel–associated typhus seen in eastern U.S.	Developing countries; U.S. border states, Hawaii	New York City	Asia, Pacific islands	Mediterranean, Africa (*R. conorii, R. africae*); Australia (*R. australis*)
Seasonality	Spring-fall	Spring-fall	Spring (livestock birthing season)	Winter	Summer-fall	Spring	Year-round	Varies
Severity of illness	Asymptomatic to severe	Asymptomatic to severe	Asymptomatic to severe	Moderate to severe	Mild to moderate	Mild	Moderate to severe	Mild (*R. australis*) to moderate (*R. conorii* and *R. africae*)
Case-fatality rate	2%–5%	1%–10%	<1%	15%–30% for untreated epidemic typhus; 0% for flying squirrel–associated typhus	<1%	0%	1%–10%	2.5% (*R. conorii*) 0%–2% for *R. africae* and *R. australis*
Patient characteristics	Exposure to tick habitats	Exposure to tick habitats	Farmers, slaughterhouse workers, researchers	War-torn location, famine; in U.S., history of exposure to flying squirrels	Geographic location, history of exposure to rats or oppossums	Urban residence (NYC), history of exposure to house mice	Travel to endemic area	Travel to endemic area

caused a febrile illness in guinea pigs and was called *nine-mile fever* (29). Subsequently, the agent was linked to human illness in a laboratory researcher. The two agents were eventually shown to be identical and were named *Coxiella burnetii* after two early researchers (Harold Cox and Frank Burnett).

Epidemiology

Q fever is a zoonotic disease that is most commonly transmitted to humans through contact with livestock, especially sheep, cattle, and goats. Although the agent can be shed in milk and urine, it is more commonly transmitted by products of parturition, such as placenta and amniotic fluid. Q fever has also been reported after contact with parturient cats and dogs and with wild rabbits (30–32). Humans typically acquire infection by inhalation of small-particle aerosols or dust contaminated with *C. burnetii*.

Q fever is considered endemic throughout most of the world. In the United States, human infections are often reported from rural areas owing to increased human–livestock contact. Outbreaks of disease have been associated with slaughterhouses, farms, and research institutions using parturient livestock in research projects. Between 1948 and 1979, 1,164 cases of Q fever were reported in the United States (mean, 39 cases per year) (33–35) (Fig. 169.2). However, human infection was just made nationally notifiable in 1999, and current national surveillance data for Q fever are still lacking.

Q fever is considered endemic in most European countries; at least 1,383 human cases were reported in France alone between 1985 and 1998 (36). It is also commonly reported in Australia, especially in Queensland and New South Wales; outbreaks are frequently linked to slaughterhouses, and national annual incidence rates range from 3 to 5 cases per 100,000 population (37). Human cases associated with parturient cats have been frequently reported from Nova Scotia and maritime Canada (31). Q fever has also been confirmed in children with pneumonia in Japan (38) and has been reported throughout Africa and South America. The only country where Q fever has not been documented is New Zealand, despite the presence of an intensive sheep farming industry in the country. A recent serologic survey of cattle and sheepdogs in New Zealand found no evidence of *C. burnetii* in those animal populations (39).

Pathogenesis

C. burnetii is an intracellular pathogen that replicates in the phagolysosomes of eukaryotic cells, usually macrophages (40). In the host, *C. burnetii* replicates to high numbers in the placenta of parturient animals and is shed in birthing materials, milk, and urine. The agent is highly resistant to desiccation, disinfectants, ultraviolet radiation, and pH changes and remains infectious for long periods in the environment (40). Humans are typically infected by inhalation of dust or droplets containing the agent, which can initiate infection with as little as a single organism. Although direct contact with parturient animals poses the highest risk for infection, contaminated dust can be dispersed over great distances by wind, and outbreaks have been associated with persons located downwind to infected animals (41,42).

Because *C. burnetii* can be shed in the milk, consumption of unpasteurized milk products may pose a risk for infection, although this route is not considered as likely for transmission as inhalation. *C. burnetii* has also been isolated from ticks; although tick bites may pose a risk for infection in animals, this means of transmission is not considered likely for human infections. Person-to-person transmission of *C. burnetii* is rare, although it has been reported between patients and obstetricians during delivery, and it may possibly be transmitted sexually (43,44).

Clinical Manifestations

There are two main recognized forms of Q fever: acute and chronic infection. The incubation period for acute Q fever averages 3 weeks (range, 14 to 39 days) after exposure and may depend on the inoculating dose or route of transmission. Many cases of acute Q fever are probably asymptomatic or mild enough to escape detection. In persons who become clinically ill, acute infection typically manifests as a nonspecific illness characterized by fever and malaise. Other clinical signs that may be observed are headache (especially retrobulbar), nonproductive cough, night sweats, and weight loss. Patients typically have elevated liver transaminase enzymes. Predominant features of illness may vary by strain and geographic area, but pneumonia and hepatitis are frequently reported. Encephalitis is an unusual but possible complication.

Most patients with acute Q fever recover within several weeks. However, *C. burnetii* may persist and result in chronic Q fever infection months to years after acute infection. Endocarditis is the most commonly reported chronic form of Q fever (45). Patients with a preexisting history of valvular disease or prosthetic valves are at higher risk for developing chronic Q fever endocarditis (45). Myocarditis and pericarditis have been associated with chronic Q fever infection as well, as has chronic granulomatous hepatitis. Recently, a chronic fatigue–like illness has been reported in some patients after acute Q fever infection, and there is some evidence of microbial persistence in these patients (46,47).

Diagnosis

As with other rickettsial diseases, diagnosis of acute Q fever usually depends on the documentation of changing antibody titers between acute- and convalescent-phase serum samples (48). A single high titer, or standing titer between paired samples, may be considered a probable case of Q fever if a clinically compatible illness is present (48). The IFA test is used most frequently in the United States, although enzyme immunoassay (EIA) and complement fixation may be used in some areas. The specific immune response may vary depending on the stage of infection and the predominant antigen-type. Acute infection typically shows an

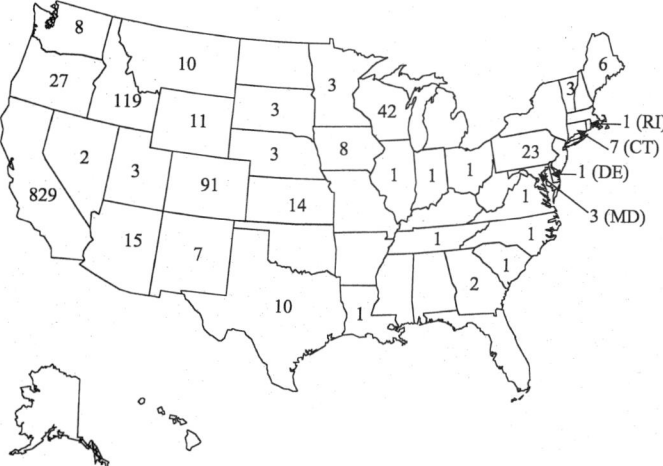

Figure 169.2. Reported cases of Q fever in the United States, 1948–1979. (Data from references 32 to 34.)

antibody response to phase II antigen; chronic infection usually demonstrates a phase I–to–phase II antibody response.

Culture of *C. burnetii* or demonstration of antigen in tissue samples by immunohistochemistry (IHC) may also be used for diagnosis, especially in cases of chronic Q fever endocarditis. Culture should be attempted only by laboratories with biosafety level 3 (BSL-3) capabilities because there is a high risk for laboratory-acquired infections. PCR can also be used to diagnose Q fever, using either whole blood or heart valve tissue (49).

Treatment

Patients with acute Q fever should be treated with tetracycline-class antibiotics. The standard treatment regimen is doxycycline, 100 mg by mouth twice a day (50). Children can receive 4.4 mg/kg per day, divided into two doses. Chronic Q fever endocarditis can be very difficult to treat. Affected patients may require several years of antibiotic therapy and may require surgical excision and replacement of affected heart valves. Currently, treatment with doxycycline and hydroxychloroquine for at least 18 months is recommended (51). Doxycycline is administered at 100 mg twice daily, and 300 mg hydroxychloroquine is given three times a day to start. Hydroxychloroquine levels in the blood should be monitored and regulated to maintain a plasma concentration between 0.8 and 1.2 $\mu g/mL$ (51). Treatment is generally continued until the phase I antibody titer declines and all clinical signs have resolved (50). Patients should be monitored periodically for relapse.

Prevention

An experimental vaccine is available in the United States for laboratory workers who may be at high risk for infection, but this vaccine is not available to the public. A vaccine is commercially available in Australia for slaughterhouse workers and others at high risk for infection.

Prevention of Q fever is not always possible, considering the role inhalation plays in transmission and the possibility of dissemination of *C. burnetii* by wind. However, the risk for infection can be decreased by maintaining good hygiene around birthing animals and products of parturition. Because consumption of unpasteurized dairy products may play a role in transmission of *C. burnetii*, persons should consume dairy products made only from pasteurized or boiled milk, both in the United States and when traveling in other countries. Finally, persons who have been previously diagnosed with acute Q fever and are diagnosed with endocarditis should inform their physician of their medical history.

EPIDEMIC TYPHUS

History of Disease

Epidemic (louse-borne) typhus is one of the oldest known diseases of humans. Although the first accurate clinical description of typhus can be traced back only to Hieronymus Fracastorius in 1546, brief references to a compatible illness can be found in the ancient writings of Greek and Arab physicians (52). Epidemic typhus has had a major effect on the history of civilization, periodically ravaging cities and decimating armies from antiquity to the present day (53). Before World War II, millions of cases were reported to the World Health Organization, especially from parts of Europe, Asia, and Africa (54).

The introduction of antibiotics and insecticides that were effective against lice vectors resulted in a dramatic decline in the numbers of epidemic typhus cases reported, from 18,359 in 1979 to 3,036 in 1982; in each of these years, more than 90% of the reported cases were from Ethiopia (55–57). However, typhus surveillance is limited, and the disease continues to occur in parts of Africa and Latin America (58). Outbreaks of epidemic typhus occurred in Burundi in 1997 during the civil war and in Russia following breakdown of the public health infrastructure (59,60). In the United States, the last outbreak of classic epidemic typhus occurred in 1922. Sporadic infections caused by *Rickettsia prowazekii* were reported in the United States in the 1970s and 1980s; these cases were subsequently linked to contact with the eastern flying squirrel (*Glaucomys volans*) or its ectoparasites (61–65).

Epidemiology

Epidemic typhus usually occurs in association with war, famine, and other factors that inflict poor living conditions on a given population. It is transmitted between humans by body lice (*Pediculus humanus corporis*), which shed the agent in their feces; humans become infected when contaminated louse feces are rubbed into abraded skin (66). Typhus rickettsiae have also been shown to be infectious for head lice (*Pediculus humanus capitis*), but head lice have not been proved to be a significant vector of disease. Body lice do not transmit infection to their progeny and die as a result of infection. They must feed on infected humans in order to transmit infection and thus are vectors but not reservoirs of typhus rickettsiae.

Humans are the principal interepidemic reservoir of *R. prowazekii*. Patients who recover from epidemic typhus develop a state of premunition, and viable typhus rickettsiae remain sequestered in their bodies. Recrudescent typhus, also known as Brill-Zinsser disease, may occur in patients years or even decades after initial infection (67–69). Recrudescent typhus is typically a milder disease, and patients usually lack the classic epidemiologic association with body lice. Depending on the prevalence of lice and immunity in the population, patients with Brill-Zinsser disease may be a source for continuing epidemics, thus repeating the infectious cycle.

In addition to primary louse-borne transmission cycles, the eastern flying squirrel (*G. volans*) has been determined to be a reservoir of *R. prowazekii* and a likely source of infection in humans (64,70,71). Sporadic cases of human *R. prowazekii* infection, which were clinically compatible with typhus and occurred after the patients had contact with flying squirrels, have been reported from various parts of the United States (61,62). Most infections were reported in winter months when flying squirrels may be more likely to enter homes. The mechanism by which disease is transmitted to humans is unclear, although squirrel fleas (*Orchopeas howardi*) have been found to be infected with *R. prowazekii* and occasionally bite humans (72). It is also possible that humans become infected by inhalation of contaminated feces from ectoparasites. It is not known whether humans who develop sporadic cases of flying squirrel–associated typhus could initiate an epidemic of human louse-borne typhus, although flying squirrel isolates of *R. prowazekii* have experimentally been shown to initiate infections in human body lice (65).

Pathogenesis

As with other rickettsial diseases, the basic underlying feature of typhus pathogenesis is damage to the endothelial cells lining the capillaries, arterioles, and venules. On entering the body, rickettsiae presumably infect cells at the bite site and replicate there for several days. Infected cells rupture and release rickettsiae into the lymphatic system, thus initiating systemic infection. Blood-borne dissemination of *R. prowazekii* causes the initial symptoms of chills and fever. Widespread infection of the endothelial cells of the capillaries and small blood vessels follows, producing the microvascular lesions that cause the characteristic rash and the many other features of the disease. Extensive damage to small vessels may in some instances restrict circulation to the point of skin necrosis, particularly at the extremities. Internal hemorrhage is frequently observed in the brain, heart, lungs, and kidneys. Characteristic typhus nodules are found in the brain and are marked by focal proliferation of glial cells and localized accumulation of mononuclear leukocytes (73). Both humoral and cellular immunity are important in the recovery from epidemic typhus, as demonstrated by studies with hyperimmune serum and activated T cells from typhus immune donors (74–76).

Clinical Manifestations

Primary louse-borne typhus is the most serious type of typhus infection, particularly when it occurs in epidemic form among malnourished populations. The onset of symptoms is usually abrupt and includes fever (a temperature higher than 39.5°C), chills, frontal headache, and myalgias; many patients report generalized weakness. Other symptoms include some that are constitutional (rigors, arthralgia, or generalized pain), whereas some symptoms are referable to the central nervous system (deafness, tinnitus, vertigo, drowsiness, disorientation, delirium) and the gastrointestinal system (anorexia, nausea, constipation, diarrhea, vomiting, abdominal pain). In 50% to 90% of patients, a generalized macular or maculopapular rash appears on the sides of the trunk between days 4 and 7, spreading centrifugally to the extremities (77). The face, the palms, and the soles are rarely involved. The white cell count is usually normal or mildly depressed, and thrombocytopenia is not uncommon. Abnormal results of liver function tests, microscopic hematuria, and proteinuria are common. Complications include hypotension, pneumonia, oliguria, azotemia, cerebral infarction, and gangrene. In the preantibiotic era, case-fatality rates of 10% to 50% were reported. More recent reports of case-fatality rates appear to be somewhat lower, both for treated (0.5%) and untreated (15%) cases (59).

In contrast to primary louse-borne typhus, recrudescent typhus (Brill-Zinsser disease) is a much milder disease. Initial symptoms of these patients include malaise, anorexia, nausea, headache, and myalgias. A febrile episode follows, accompanied by intensification of the headache and the appearance of a rash on the trunk, arms, and legs. Late in the second week of illness, the fever and headache subside abruptly, and patients generally convalesce uneventfully (58). The typical clinical presentation of patients with flying squirrel–associated typhus fever also appears to be milder than that observed in epidemic typhus, although the difference in clinical presentation may be related to the generally well-nourished status of squirrel-associated typhus patients when compared with populations classically at risk for louse-borne epidemic typhus (61,62).

Diagnosis

The diagnosis of any form of typhus must be prompted by the epidemiologic circumstances surrounding the development of disease. In developing countries, classic louse-borne typhus should be considered in persons who have been exposed to war, poverty, and famine and who are infested with lice and among dislocated persons who are arriving from areas where the disease is endemic. Recrudescent typhus should be suspected when refugees from countries with endemic typhus have unexplained febrile illnesses years after emigration. In the United States, flying squirrel–associated typhus should be suspected in the winter months in patients with a history of contact with flying squirrels.

Definitive diagnosis can be accomplished by visualizing rickettsiae in tissues, isolating rickettsiae, detecting rickettsiae by PCR, or testing paired acute- and convalescent-phase serum specimens (64,78,79). Serum can be tested for antibodies to typhus rickettsiae by any of several established procedures; the IFA technique is the method most commonly employed, but the enzyme-linked immunosorbent assay, microagglutination, latex agglutination, and other procedures have been used successfully. A positive result [a fourfold change in titer, a positive immunoglobulin M (IgM) titer, or a single high IgG titer in a clinically compatible case] indicates recent infection. Patients with Brill-Zinsser disease have IgG but not IgM antibodies to typhus rickettsiae.

Because *R. prowazekii* and *Rickettsia typhi* possess common antigens, serum specimens from epidemic or murine typhus patients may frequently exhibit cross-reactivity. Epidemiologic criteria can then be used to distinguish between epidemic and murine typhus infections, or antibody absorption or toxin neutralization tests can be employed to determine the specificity of serologic reactions (79). Such tests are usually available only from reference laboratories. Rickettsial isolation is hazardous and should be attempted only in a BSL-3 facility by experienced microbiologists.

Treatment

Because no rapid diagnostic test is readily available, treatment must be instituted before the diagnosis is confirmed. Doxycycline is considered the primary treatment of choice for *R. prowazekii* infection. Patients are normally given 200 mg of doxycycline per day in two divided doses. Single-dose (200 mg) doxycycline treatment has also been shown to be effective in treating patients with louse-borne typhus and may be the most practical approach in situations in which large numbers of patients must be managed (59,80). In some cases in which doxycycline is contraindicated, chloramphenicol may be administered. The temperature should begin to fall within 24 hours; patients should be treated until they remain afebrile for 48 to 72 hours. Other symptoms may persist for a week or more after treatment is begun (77,81).

Prevention

Typhus vaccines are not currently available in the United States. Cases of epidemic typhus can be reduced in disease-endemic areas by delousing campaigns and institution of hygienic measures that preclude reinfestation. Travelers to areas with endemic typhus are unlikely to contract epidemic typhus unless they are in constant, close association with louse-infested individuals. In the latter situation, maintenance of strict personal hygiene and frequent washing of clothing are recommended. Risk factors for contracting flying squirrel–associated typhus fever have not been firmly identified; hence, it is not possible to recommend prevention strategies for that particular illness.

MURINE TYPHUS

History of Disease

Originally known as Mexican typhus fever, or tabardillo, murine typhus was first reported in 1913 in patients in Atlanta, Georgia

(82). The disease was characterized by a milder form of illness than had been observed for classic louse-borne epidemic typhus. Early definitive identification of murine typhus as a distinct clinical entity was difficult because of its clinical similarity to Brill-Zinsser disease, and techniques for distinguishing the respective etiologic agents in the laboratory were not yet available. In 1929, a study of typhus patients in the southeastern United States reported that the disease had a different etiologic agent, the reservoir was probably rats or mice, and a bloodsucking ectoparasite was the likely vector (83). Shortly thereafter, *R. typhi* was isolated from rats and their fleas (84,85).

Epidemiology

R. typhi is a zoonosis, and rats of the genus *Rattus* are the primary reservoirs of *R. typhi*. The oriental rat flea, *Xenopsylla cheopis*, is the principal vector. Cats and peridomestic opossums infested with cat fleas (*Ctenocephalides felis*) have also been implicated in the transmission of murine typhus in the United States (86–89). There are no reliable data to implicate human lice, ticks, or mites as vectors of murine typhus (90). Fleas remain infected for life and transmit their infections to progeny (91); fleas themselves are apparently not harmed by the infection. Fleas shed organisms in their feces, which may cause infection in humans through contact with abraded skin or mucous membranes, or through the inhalation of infectious aerosols containing flea feces; laboratory studies have also indicated that fleas can transmit murine typhus directly during the feeding process (92).

Murine typhus exists on all continents, but its distribution is usually limited to areas where large numbers of *Rattus* are found. Typically, seaports, coastal areas, and the major commercial arteries are sites of endemic disease. Epidemiologic data suggest that murine typhus cases that occur in colder areas of the world are restricted to urban areas where *Rattus* species occupy warm indoor harborages. In contrast, murine typhus in southern areas occurs in both rural and urban areas, presumably because rodents and their fleas can thrive equally well indoors and outdoors in the relatively warm climate (90). The epidemiologic principles of cat- or opossum-associated murine typhus are not yet well defined.

Although sporadic cases may occur anywhere within an area in which the disease is endemic, murine typhus frequently occurs in small outbreaks. Murine typhus became a reportable disease in the United States in 1920, but surveillance did not really gain impetus until 1931. By World War II, more than 5,000 cases were documented annually, mostly from the southeastern and south-central United States, and the disease was believed to be underreported (93). Subsequent flea and rodent control programs caused a precipitous drop in the number of reported cases. Currently, fewer than 50 cases per year are reported, most frequently from Texas, California, and Hawaii (89,94–97). Murine typhus cases are no longer notifiable to the Centers for Disease Control and Prevention.

Pathogenesis and Clinical Manifestations

The pathogenesis and clinical presentation of murine typhus are similar to epidemic typhus and virtually identical to Brill-Zinsser disease. Murine typhus is usually much milder than epidemic typhus, but there are enough exceptions to the rule to confound the diagnosis of individual patients. Case-fatality rates of 0% to 4% have been reported (96–99).

Onset is usually abrupt, but occasionally a mild prodrome is present for a few days. Symptoms are usually severe enough to warrant hospitalization. Fever, usually a temperature higher than 39°C, is almost always present; headache, myalgia, and rash are noted in more than half of the cases, and chills, anorexia, nausea, and photophobia are usually reported less frequently (96–99). The rash, which appears an average of 5 to 6 days after symptoms begin, is usually macular (less often maculopapular or papular) and most often is found on the trunk, legs, or arms. Physical examination may reveal splenomegaly or hepatomegaly. Complications, including pneumonia and encephalitis, are occasionally reported. Most patients have mild thrombocytopenia and mildly elevated hepatic transaminase levels. Leukocytosis, mild leukopenia, and anemia have been reported (97). As with other rickettsial infections, humoral immunity and cellular immunity both contribute to recovery (100,101).

Diagnosis

The nonspecific clinical manifestations of murine typhus may make it difficult to diagnose without considering the patient's history and epidemiologic clues. In the United States, residence in a disease-endemic area and possible exposure to rodents provide important clues. A history of travel to a foreign country where the disease is endemic should also alert the physician to the possibility of murine typhus infection (102). Differentiation between louse-borne typhus and murine typhus is particularly difficult in areas of the world where both diseases are endemic. Each can occur sporadically and in small outbreaks. Moreover, in otherwise healthy individuals, the clinical presentations are similar. Disease confirmation follows the same guidelines that have been described for epidemic typhus. Serologic testing with typhus group antigens provides preliminary confirmation, although this will not differentiate *R. prowazekii* infections from *R. typhi* infections. If epidemiologic data are not helpful to distinguish infections, antibody absorption or toxin neutralization tests may provide additional information.

Treatment

The regimens for suspected *R. typhi* infections are the same as those for *R. prowazekii* infections, and prompt treatment shortens the duration of fever. Relapses have been reported in patients treated with chloramphenicol but not those treated with tetracycline, suggesting that tetracycline or tetracycline analogs may be preferable (98).

Prevention

Avoidance of rodent-infested areas is the best method of preventing murine typhus infection. Rodent and flea eradication programs are recommended for areas where harborages already exist. However, the latter programs should not be initiated until the relative potential environmental effect of poisons or insecticides has been considered. No vaccine is available. Risk factors for acquiring murine typhus from other sources (e.g., cats, opossums, and cat fleas) are not sufficiently defined to allow firm recommendations for prevention.

RICKETTSIALPOX

History

Rickettsia akari is the etiologic agent of rickettsialpox. It was first isolated in 1946 in association with an outbreak of rickettsialpox at a housing development in New York City. *R. akari* was isolated from the blood of two patients, from house mice (*Mus musculus*) trapped on the premises, and from rodent mites (*Liponyssoides sanguineus*) that were collected at the same site. The investigation also revealed a strong association between mite exposure and rickettsialpox, further incriminating mites as vectors of the disease (103–106).

Epidemiology

After the initial description of rickettsialpox in New York City, additional cases were reported in Massachusetts, Pennsylvania, Connecticut, and Ohio (107–110). *R. akari* was also isolated from a wild rodent (*Microtus fortis pelliceus*) in Korea (111) and is considered a worldwide disease. Rickettsialpox apparently occurs infrequently; however, human *R. akari* infections may be common among inner-city residents, and rickettsialpox cases may be misdiagnosed or go unreported (112,113).

R. akari is thought to exist in urban and sylvan cycles throughout the world; the rodent mite is the vector and principal reservoir. *R. akari* is maintained in successive generations of mites by transovarial transmission. Mice and other susceptible rodents become transient reservoirs of *R. akari* during periods of peak rickettsemia, and uninfected mites can become infected with *R. akari* if they imbibe infectious blood. However, it is uncertain whether infectious feeding contributes significantly to the establishment of new lines of persistently infected mites. Humans become infected when they intrude on these natural cycles of infection and are fed on aberrantly by these mites.

Clinical Manifestations

Compared with most rickettsioses, rickettsialpox is a relatively mild illness. Fatalities have not been reported. A clinical triad—an initial lesion (eschar), fever, and, usually 1 to 2 days later, a generalized rash—characterizes the disease (113–116). The eschar, which occurs in almost all patients, may be located anywhere on the body. It begins as an asymptomatic or pruritic erythematous papule 24 to 48 hours after the mite bite (117). A fluid-filled vesicle appears initially, and as it dries, it leaves a brown to black eschar surrounded by a 0.5- to 3-cm area of induration (114,117).

Chills, fever, sweats, and myalgia present acutely 7 to 14 days after the exposure, although incubation periods as long as 24 days have been reported. The peak temperature is usually 39° to 40°C; without treatment, fever persists for about 1 week. Other common symptoms include profuse diaphoresis, headache (usually frontal), and photophobia; occasionally, vertigo, rhinorrhea, cough, sore throat, nausea, and vomiting are present (114,115). Within 1 to 3 days after the onset of systemic symptoms, a sparse rash appears, with 5 to 100 discrete, firm erythematous papules on the face, trunk, and extremities. Less often, the lesions are maculopapular or are found on the palms and soles. In most cases, a vesicle develops at the summit of the papule, and the lesions then resolve by crusting. Except for toxicity, the rash, mild symptoms, and some regional lymphadenopathy, the findings of the physical examination are normal (115). Untreated, rickettsialpox usually resolves uneventfully in 2 to 3 weeks.

Differential diagnosis includes the other rickettsial diseases that may be accompanied by an eschar (scrub typhus and tick typhus), varicella, and infections caused by some coxsackieviruses. In contrast to rickettsialpox, the vesicles of varicella do not have a papular base or eschar (115).

Diagnosis

Diagnosis of rickettsialpox typically requires a combination of clinical and epidemiologic findings in conjunction with group-specific serologic tests. Patients with a compatible illness and known or possible mite exposure should be tested for antibodies to spotted fever group rickettsiae. *R. rickettsii* (the causative agent of Rocky Mountain spotted fever) is typically used as a surrogate antigen because it is antigenically related to *R. akari* and is more readily available. Seroconversion in a clinically compatible case would provide good evidence of rickettsialpox. Immunostaining of biopsy specimens taken from skin lesions has also been used to confirm the diagnosis (113).

Although the foregoing criteria are sufficient to diagnose probable cases of rickettsialpox, definitive confirmation requires the isolation of *R. akari* from the patient's blood. *R. akari* isolates can be propagated in any of a variety of cell cultures, provided that no antibiotics are added to supplement the medium. The identity of presumed isolates can be confirmed with monoclonal antibodies, with cross-neutralization tests, or by molecular methods (118).

Treatment

Although the disease eventually resolves without treatment, antibiotic therapy may hasten defervescence (119). Doxycycline should be administered at a dose of 100 mg twice daily for 2 to 5 days; chloramphenicol may be considered in situations in which doxycycline is contraindicated. As in other rickettsial infections, a response should occur within 48 hours; continued fever suggests another cause for the illness.

Prevention

Because rickettsialpox routinely occurs after exposure to mouse mites, the disease can best be prevented by enforcing sanitary measures that preclude the development of rodent harborages. Rodent eradication programs may be necessary to eliminate existing infestation problems.

SCRUB TYPHUS

History of Disease

Scrub typhus, caused by *Orientia tsutsugamushi*, gained prominence in World War II, when tens of thousands of soldiers in the Asiatic-Pacific theaters contracted the disease (120). Scrub typhus was also a serious problem in U.S. military personnel in Vietnam in the 1960s (121). Thousands of cases still occur each year in certain areas and may be important causes of fever among hospitalized patients and outpatients. The disease is endemic to an extremely large geographic area, ranging from the coastal portions of northern Australia to Asia and the Indian subcontinent and including, among others, Japan, Korea, southern China and Tibet, Indochina, the Philippines, New Guinea, Sri Lanka, and islands of the Chagos archipelago (Fig. 169.3). Proven habitats of *O. tsutsugamushi* range from sandy beaches and mountain deserts to equatorial rain forests. Thus, the term *scrub typhus* is a misnomer; *chigger-borne rickettsiosis* has been suggested as a more accurate term (122).

Epidemiology

Despite their apparent diversity, scrub typhus habitats do have one thing in common: they have experienced ecologic modifications by humans or nature that have resulted in transitional, nonclimactic vegetation (122). Such areas bring together the classic scrub typhus triad, *Rattus* rats, *Leptotrombidium* mites, and

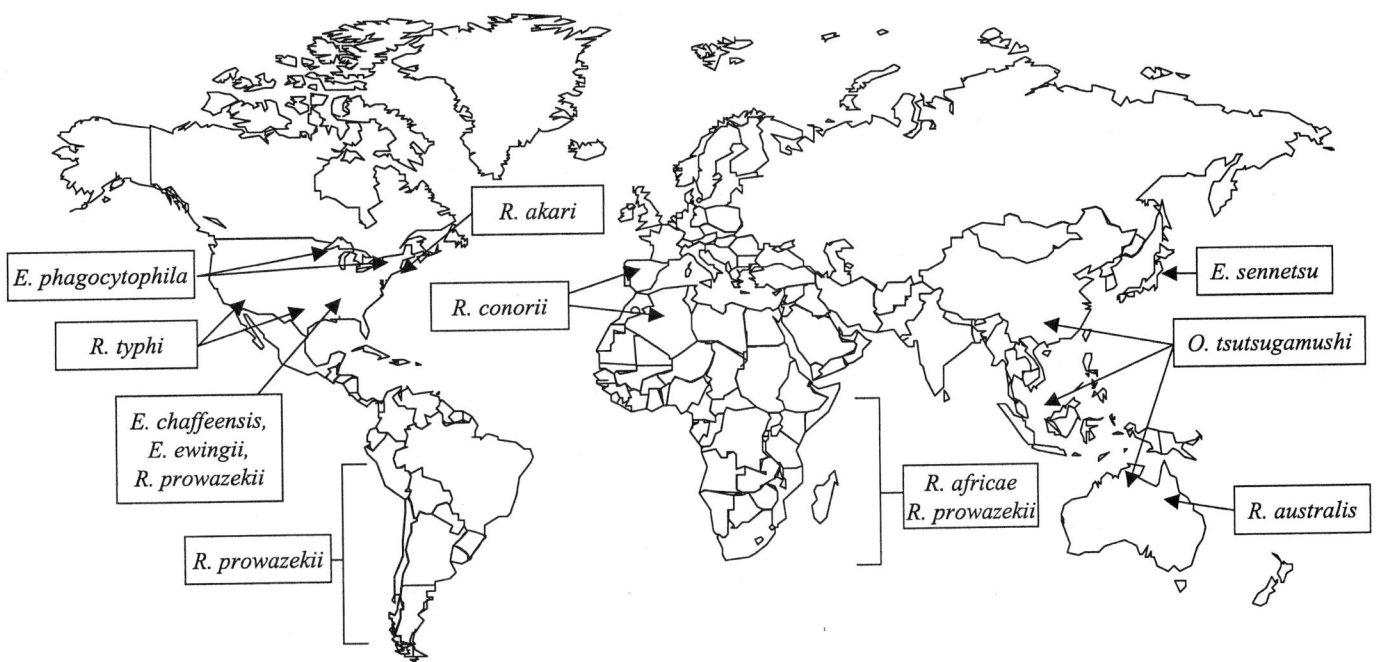

Figure 169.3. World map showing approximate distribution of selected rickettsial diseases. *C. burnetii* is reported from all over the world, except New Zealand. In addition to the areas specifically noted, *R. akari*, *R. typhi*, and *R. prowazekii* may be found worldwide where conditions are favorable for transmission.

O. tsutsugamushi. Chiggers (larval mites) of the *Leptotrombidium deliense* group are the principal vectors to humans, but other mite species are also vectors (122). *O. tsutsugamushi* is maintained in mites primarily by transovarial transmission. Although rats are hosts for the chiggers, they are not thought to contribute significantly to the maintenance of *O. tsutsugamushi*, except perhaps occasionally to infect a previously uninfected female mite that could pass the infection to its progeny.

Incidence figures for scrub typhus are generally unavailable because adequate surveillance systems are lacking. One study in a Malaysian community estimated the incidence there to be 3% to 4% per month (123). In a related study, 19.3% of all diagnosed febrile illnesses in a rural area of Malaysia were due to scrub typhus (124). Such a high incidence is not surprising because there are numerous strains of *O. tsutsugamushi*, and infection with one strain does not confer immunity to all infecting strains. Multiple scrub typhus infections are common among occupationally exposed persons.

Clinical Manifestations and Pathogenesis

The pathogenesis of *O. tsutsugamushi* resembles that of the spotted fever group rickettsiae, and pathologic changes usually result from the multiplication of rickettsiae within endothelial cells. Scrub typhus patients usually have nonspecific clinical manifestations (chills, fever, and headache). Other symptoms include cough, myalgias, arthralgias, retroorbital pain, and gastrointestinal abnormalities. Eschars are observed at the site of mite attachment in many patients. A macular rash frequently appears on the patient's trunk during the first week of illness and subsequently progresses to the face and extremities, sparing the palms and soles. Hepatomegaly and splenomegaly are common. Respiratory, neurologic, cardiovascular, and hematologic abnormalities may develop during the second week of illness, usually as a result of generalized vasculitis (125). Case-fatality rates of 0.5% to 10% have been reported (120,125). *O. tsutsugamushi* has been shown to survive in blood stored under blood-banking conditions (126), and at least one case of transfusion-transmitted illness has been reported.

Diagnosis

Scrub typhus is usually diagnosed by serologic tests, performed with the three prototype strains of *O. tsutsugamushi* (Karp, Gilliam, and Kato) as antigens. Currently, the IFA technique is the method of choice, but the immunoperoxidase test, EIAs, and passive hemagglutination assay have also been employed successfully (79,127–129). Minimal titers have not been established with certainty, and therefore tests of paired serum specimens are recommended, so that a rise in antibody titer can be demonstrated. PCR assays have confirmed *O. tsutsugamushi* infections in acute-phase blood of patients and may be of potential use as a diagnostic tool (130–132). Isolation attempts are performed only by referral laboratories.

Treatment

Doxycycline should be the primary therapy used to treat scrub typhus, at a dose of 100 mg twice daily. Chloramphenicol should be considered as an alternative treatment. Relapses are common with short therapeutic courses or when therapy is begun before 5 days after onset of symptoms (133). Documentation of scrub typhus resistant to doxycycline and chloramphenicol raises serious questions for appropriate treatment (134). *In vitro* data show that azithromycin is effective against scrub typhus rickettsiae that are resistant to doxycycline and chloramphenicol and may be an acceptable alternative for pregnant women, children, or patients in whom tetracyclines and chloramphenicol are contraindicated (135,136).

Prevention

Administration of chloramphenicol and tetracyclines (doxycycline 200 mg orally) has been investigated for chemoprophylaxis of scrub typhus (137,138). Although such treatment may delay onset of clinical signs, disease may occur after treatment is discontinued, and this means of prevention is not recommended (138). Additional prevention measures focus on avoidance of chigger-infested habitats and use of insecticides such as DEET (N,N-diethyl-meta-toluamide) on clothing to help prevent chigger bites. Currently, no vaccine is commercially available to protect against *O. tsutsugamushi* infection.

OTHER RICKETTSIOSES

History and Epidemiology

A variety of other rickettsial agents have been recognized as either confirmed or potential human pathogens throughout the world, including the following *Rickettsia* species: *R. conorii*, *R. africae*, *R. australis*, *R. honei*, *R. japonica*, *R. helvetica*, *R. slovaca*, *R. sibirica*, *R. mongolotimonae*, and *R. felis* (139,140). Most infections are geographically limited; however, physicians should be aware of these agents because they may be acquired during travel to endemic areas. A few of these agents that may be more commonly seen in travelers are discussed in further detail (Fig. 169.3).

R. conorii causes a tick-borne rickettsial disease known as boutonneuse fever or Mediterranean spotted fever. This disease is endemic in parts of France, Italy, and Spain and has also been reported from Africa (141,142). *R. conorii* is primarily transmitted by the common dog tick (*Rhipicephalus sanguineus*). In some disease-endemic areas, seroprevalence rates of 8% and 26% have been reported among humans and dogs, respectively (143). *R. africae* is a rickettsial agent transmitted by ticks in parts of Africa, causing a disease called *African tick-bite fever*; *Amblyomma* species of ticks are believed to be responsible for transmission (141,144). Queensland tick typhus is caused by the rickettsial agent *R. australis* and is transmitted by *Ixodes* species of ticks (141,145). These diseases may be diagnosed in persons residing in or traveling to disease-endemic areas (141,146).

Clinical Signs and Pathogenesis

R. conorii, *R. africae*, and *R. australis* belong to the spotted-fever rickettsiae group and are related to *R. rickettsii*, the causative agent of Rocky Mountain spotted fever. However, these agents typically cause disease that is less severe than Rocky Mountain spotted fever. During infection, rickettsiae invade the tissue surrounding the site of a tick bite and initiate infection in endothelial cells, causing vascular damage and resulting in characteristic clinical signs (141).

Onset of clinical signs occurs about 1 week following a tick bite, at which time a distinctive eschar is generally observed at the site of tick attachment. Fever, fatigue, and malaise are common (142,144,145). A maculopapular rash usually occurs after 3 to 5 days, first affecting the extremities and then the trunk. In some cases of *R. australis* infection, a vesicular rash has been reported (145,147). Unusual complications for *R. conorii* are similar to those seen for Rocky Mountain spotted fever and may include skin necrosis, bleeding disorders, and neuropathies. *R. africae* and *R. australis* are generally mild to moderate diseases, and unusual complications have not been frequently reported. Case-fatality rates of 2.5% have been reported for *R. conorii* (148); case-fatality rates for *R. africae* and *R. australis* are low (0% to 2%) (145).

Diagnosis

Diagnosis of these agents requires serologic confirmation by rising antibody titers in paired serum samples, as has been described for other the rickettsial pathogens. Physicians should request appropriate diagnostic tests on the basis of the patient's travel history. However, there is strong cross-reactivity between these agents and *R. rickettsia*; therefore, standard spotted fever rickettsial panels should be positive for these agents in infected patients. Confirmation of infecting species can be made through cross-adsorption, PCR, or culture (146).

Treatment and Prevention

Patients should be treated with doxycycline (100 mg twice daily) or chloramphenicol, as has been described for the other rickettsial agents. As with other tick-borne rickettsial disease, avoidance of tick habitats and exercising behaviors to prevent tick bites will help guard against infection.

REFERENCES

1. Dumler JS, Barbet AF, Bekker CP, et al. Reorganization of genera in the families Rickettsiaceae and Anaplasmataceae in the order Rickettsiales: unification of some species of *Ehrlichia* with *Anaplasma*, *Cowdria* with *Ehrlichia* and *Ehrlichia* with *Neorickettsia*, descriptions of six new species combinations and designation of *Ehrlichia equi* and 'HGE agent' as subjective synonyms of *Ehrlichia phagocytophila*. *Int J Syst Evol Microbiol* 2001;51:2145–2165.
2. Misao T, Kobayashi Y. Studies on infectious mononucleosis. I. Isolation of etiologic agent from blood, bone marrow, and lymph node of a patient with infectious mononucleosis by using mice. *Tokyo Iji Shinshi* 1954;71:683–686.
3. Anderson BE, Dawson JE, Jones DC, et al. *Ehrlichia chaffeensis*, a new species associated with human ehrlichiosis. *J Clin Microbiol* 1991;29:2838–2342.
4. Chen S, Dumler JS, Bakken JS, Walker DH. Identification of a granulocytotropic *Ehrlichia* species as the etiologic agent of human disease. *J Clin Microbiol* 1994;32:589–595.
5. Buller RS, Arens M, Hmiel SP, et al. *Ehrichia ewingii*, a newly recognized agent of human ehrlichiosis. *N Engl J Med* 1999;341:148–155.
6. Anderson BE, Sims KG, Olson JG, et al. *Amblyomma americanum*: a potential vector of human ehrlichiosis. *Am J Trop Med Hyg* 1993;49:239–244.
7. Telford SR3, Dawson JE, Katavolos P, et al. Perpetuation of the agent of human granulocytic ehrlichiosis in a deer tick-rodent cycle. *Proc Natl Acad Sci U S A* 1996;93:6209–6214.
8. Mitchell PD, Reed KD, Hofkes JM. Immunoserologic evidence of coinfection with *Borrelia burgdorferi*, *Babesia microti*, and human granulocytic *Ehrlichia* species in residents of Wisconsin and Minnesota. *J Clin Microbiol* 1996;34:724–727.
9. Reubel G, Barlough JE, Madigan JE. Production and characterization of *Ehrlichia risticii*, the agent of Potomac horse fever, from snails (*Pleuroceridae: Juga* spp.) in aquarium culture and genetic comparison to equine strains. *J Clin Microbiol* 1998;36:1501–1511.
10. McQuiston JH, Paddock CD, Holman RC, et al. Human ehrlichioses in the United States. *Emerg Infect Dis* 1999;5:635–642.
11. Rikihisa Y. The tribe *Ehrlichieae* and ehrlichial diseases. *Clin Microbiol Rev* 1991;4:286–308.
12. Lotric-Furlan S, Petrovec M, Avsic-Zupanc T, et al. Prospective assessment of the etiology of acute febrile illness after a tick bite in Slovenia. *Clin Infect Dis* 2001;33:503–510.
13. Eng TR, Harkess JR, Fishbein DB, et al. Epidemiologic, clinical, and laboratory findings of human ehrlichiosis in the United States, 1988. *JAMA* 1990;264:2251–2258.
14. McQuiston JH, Childs JE, Chamberland ME, et al. Transmission of tick-borne agents of disease by blood transfusion: a review of known and potential risks in the United States. *Transfusion* 2000;40:274–284.
15. Eastlund T, Persing D, Mathieson D, et al. Human granulocytic ehrlichiosis after red cell transfusion [Abstract S535-040N]. *Transfusion* 1999;39S:117S.
16. McKechnie DB, Slater KS, Childs JE, et al. Survival of *Ehrlichia chaffeensis* in refrigerated, ADSOL-treated RBCs. *Transfusion* 2000;40:1041–1047.
17. Kalantarpour F, Chowdhury I, Wormser GP, et al. Survival of the human granulocytic ehrlichiosis agent under refrigeration conditions. *J Clin Microbiol* 2000;38:2398–2399.
18. Fishbein DB, Dawson JE, Robinson LE. Human ehrlichiosis in the United States, 1985 to 1990. *Ann Intern Med* 1994;120:736–743.
19. Bakken JS, Krueth J, Wilson-Nordskog C, et al. Clinical and laboratory characteristics of human granulocytic ehrlichiosis. *JAMA* 1996;275:199–205.
20. Horowitz HW, Kilchevsky E, Haber S, et al. Perinatal transmission of the agent of human granulocytic ehrlichiosis. *N Engl J Med* 1998;339:375–378.
21. Dumler JS, Bakken JS. Ehrlichial diseases of humans: emerging tick-borne infections. *Clin Infect Dis* 1995;20:1102–1110.
22. Paddock CD, Sumner JW, Shore GM, et al. Isolation and characterization of *Ehrlichia chaffeensis* strains from patients with fatal ehrlichiosis. *J Clin Microbiol* 1997;35:2496–2502.

23. Horowitz HW, Aguero-Rosenfeld ME, McKenna DF, et al. Clinical and laboratory spectrum of culture-proven human granulocytic ehrlichiosis: comparison with culture-negative cases. *Clin Infect Dis* 1998;27:1314–1317.

24. Childs JE, Sumner JW, Nicholson WL, et al. Outcome of diagnostic tests using samples from culture-proven cases of human monocytic ehrlichiosis: implications for surveillance. *J Clin Microbiol* 1999;37:2997–3000.

25. Council of State and Territorial Epidemiologists. *Changes in the case definition for human ehrlichiosis, and addition of a new ehrlichiosis category as a condition placed under surveillance according to the National Public Health Surveillance System (NPHSS).* Position Statement 2000 ID-#3. Atlanta: Council of State and Territorial Epidemiologists, 2000. Available at: http://www.cste.org/ps/2000/2000-id-03.htm.

26. Comer JA, Nicholson WL, Sumner JW, et al. Diagnosis of human ehrlichiosis by PCR assay of acute-phase serum. *J Clin Microbiol* 1999;37:31–34.

27. Bakken JS, Dumler JS. *Ehrlichia* species. In: Yu VL, Merigan TCJ, Barriere SL, eds. *Antimicrobial therapy and vaccines.* Baltimore: Williams & Wilkins, 1999:546–550.

28. Derrick EH. "Q fever," new fever entity: clinical features, diagnosis, and laboratory investigation. *Med J Aust* 1937;2:281–299.

29. Davis GE, Cox HR. A filter-passing infectious agent isolated from ticks. I. Isolation from *Dermacentor andersoni,* reactions in animals, and filtration experiments. *Public Health Rep* 1938;53:2259–2261.

30. Marrie TJ, Williams JC. Q fever pneumonia associated with exposure to wild rabbits. *Lancet* 1986;1:427–429.

31. Marrie TJ, Durant H, Williams JC, et al. Exposure to parturient cats: A risk factor for acquisition of Q fever in maritime Canada. *J Infect Dis* 1988;158:101–108.

32. Buhariwalla F, Cann B, Marrie TJ. A dog-related outbreak of Q fever. *Clin Infect Dis* 1996;23:753–755.

33. D'Angelo LJ, Baker EF, Schlosser W. Q fever in the United States, 1948–1977. *J Infect Dis* 1979;139:613–615.

34. Centers for Disease Control. Summary: 1975–1978. *Rickettsial Disease Surveillance Report* 1979;1:1–15.

35. Centers for Disease Control. Summary: 1979. *Rickettsial Disease Surveillance Report* 1981;2:1–8.

36. Raoult D, Tissot-Dupont H, Foucault C, et al. Q fever 1985–1998: clinical and epidemiologic features of 1,383 infections. *Medicine* 2000;79:109–123.

37. Garner MG, Longbottom HM, Cannon RM, et al. A review of Q fever in Australia 1991–1994. *Aust N Z J Public Health* 1997;21:722–730.

38. Nagaoka H, Akiyama M, Sugieda M, et al. Isolation of *Coxiella burnetii* from children with influenza-like symptoms in Japan. *Microbiol Immunol* 1996;40:147–151.

39. Hilbink F, Penrose M, Kovacova E, et al. Q fever is absent from New Zealand. *Int J Epidemiol* 1993;5:945–949.

40. Maurin M, Raoult D. Q fever. *Clin Microbiol Rev* 1999;12:518–553.

41. Hawker JI, Ayres JG, Blair I, et al. A large outbreak of Q fever in the West Midlands: windborne spread into a metropolitan area? *Commun Dis Public Health* 1998;1:180–187.

42. Tissot-Dupont H, Torres S, Nezri M, et al. Hyperendemic focus of Q fever related to Sheep and Wind. *Am J Epidemiol* 1999;150:67–74.

43. Kruszewska D, Lembowicz K, Tylewska-Wierzbanowska S. Possible sexual transmission of Q fever among humans. *Clin Infect Dis* 1996;22:1087–1088.

44. Raoult D, Stein A. Q fever during pregnancy: a risk for women, fetuses, and obstetricians. *N Engl J Med* 1994;330:371.

45. Stein A, Raoult D. Q fever endocarditis. *Eur Heart J* 1995;16[Suppl B]:19–23.

46. Ayres JG, Flint N, Smith EG, et al. Post-infection fatigue syndrome following Q fever. *Q J Med* 1998;91:105–123.

47. Harris RJ, Storm PA, Lloyd A, et al. Long-term persistence of *Coxiella burnetii* in the host after primary Q fever. *Epidemiol Infect* 2000;124:543–549.

48. Council of State and Territorial Epidemiologists. *Placing Q fever* (Coxiella burnetii) *under national surveillance in the United States under the National Public Health Surveillance System (NPHSS).* ID-1. 1999. Available at: http://www.cste.org/ps/1999/1999-id-01.htm.

49. Stein A, Raoult D. Detection of *Coxiella burnetii* by DNA amplification using polymerase chain reaction. *J Clin Microbiol* 1992;30:2462–2466.

50. Marrie TJ. Part C. Rickettsia: *Coxiella burnetii.* In: Yu VL, Merigan TC, Barriere SL, eds. *Antimicrobial therapy and vaccines.* Baltimore: Williams & Wilkins, 1999:542–546.

51. Raoult D, Houpikian P, Tissot-Dupont H, et al. Treatment of Q fever endocarditis: comparisons of 2 regimens containing doxycycline and ofloxacin or hydroxychloroquine. *Arch Intern Med* 1999;159:167–173.

52. Hahon N. *Selected papers on the pathogenic rickettsiae.* Cambridge: Harvard University Press, 1968;369.

53. Woodward TE. A historical account of the rickettsial diseases with a discussion of unsolved problems. *J Infect Dis* 1973;127:583–594.

54. Weyer F. Progress in ecology and epidemiology of rickettsioses: a review. *Acta Trop* 1978;35:5–21.

55. World Health Organization. Louse-borne typhus in 1979. *Wkly Epidemiol Rec* 1981;56:129–131.

56. World Health Organization. Louse-borne typhus 1981–1982. *Wkly Epidemiol Rec* 1984;59:29–30.

57. Centers for Disease Control. Production of typhus vaccine discontinued in the United States. *MMWR Morb Mortal Wkly Rep* 1980;29:465.

58. Brill NE. An acute infectious disease of unknown origin: a clinical study based on 221 cases. *Am J Med Sci* 1910;139:484–501.

59. Raoult D, Ndihokubwayo JB, Tissot-Dupont H, et al. Outbreak of epidemic typhus associated with trench fever in Burundi. *Lancet* 1998;352:353–358.

60. Tarsevich I, Rydkina E, Raoult D. Epidemic typhus in Russia. *Lancet* 1998;352:1151.

61. McDade JE, Shepard CC, Redus MA, et al. Evidence of *Rickettsia prowazekii* infections in the United States. *Am J Trop Med Hyg* 1980;29:277–284.

62. Duma RJ, Sonenshine DE, Bozeman FM, et al. Epidemic typhus in the United States associated with flying squirrels. *JAMA* 1981;245:2318–2323.

63. Russo PK, Mendelson DC, Etkind PH, et al. Epidemic typhus (*Rickettsia prowazekii*) in Massachusetts: evidence of infection. *N Engl J Med* 1981;304:1166–1168.

64. Bozeman FM, Masiello SA, Williams MS, et al. Epidemic typhus rickettsiae isolated from flying squirrels. *Nature* 1975;255:545–547.

65. Bozeman FM, Sonenshine DE, Williams MS, et al. Experimental infection of ectoparasitic arthropods with *Rickettsia prowazekii* (GvF-16 strain) and transmission to flying squirrels. *Am J Trop Med Hyg* 1981;30:253–263.

66. Silverman DJ, Boese JL, Wisseman CL Jr. Ultrastructural studies of *Rickettsia prowazekii* from louse midgut cells to feces. *Infect Immun* 1974;10:257–263.

67. Murray ES, Baehr G, Schwartzman G, et al. Brill's disease. I. Clinical and laboratory diagnosis. *JAMA* 1950;142:1059–1066.

68. Murray ES, Snyder JC. Brill's disease. II. Etiology. *Am J Hyg* 1951;53:22–32.

69. Price WH. Studies on the interepidemic survival of louse-borne epidemic typhus fever. *J Bacteriol* 1955;69:105–106.

70. Woodman DR, Weiss E, Dasch GA, et al. Biological properties of *Rickettsia prowazekii* strains isolated from flying squirrels. *Infect Immun* 1977;16:853–860.

71. Dasch GA, Samms JR, Weiss E. Biochemical characteristics of typhus group rickettsiae with special attention to the *Rickettsia prowazekii* strains isolated from flying squirrels. *Infect Immun* 1978;19:676–685.

72. Sonenshine DE, Bozeman FM, Williams MS, et al. Epizootiology of epidemic typhus (*Rickettsia prowazekii*) in flying squirrels. *Am J Trop Med Hyg* 1978;27:339–349.

73. von Lichtenberg F. Rickettsial diseases. In: Cotran RS, Kumar V, Robbins SL, eds. *The pathologic basis of disease.* Philadelphia: WB Saunders, 1989:328–333.

74. Yeomans A, Snyder JC, Gilliam AG. The effects of concentrated hyperimmune rabbit serum in louse-borne typhus. *JAMA* 1945;129:19–24.

75. Beaman L, Wisseman CL Jr. Mechanisms of immunity in typhus infections. VI. Differential opsonizing and neutralizing action of human typhus rickettsia-specific cytophilic antibodies in cultures of human macrophages. *Infect Immun* 1976;14:1071–1076.

76. Carl M, Dasch GA. Characterization of human cytotoxic lymphocytes directed against cells infected with typhus group rickettsiae: evidence for lymphokine activation of effectors. *J Immunol* 1986;136:2654–2661.

77. Kamal AM, Messih GA. Typhus fever: Review of 11,410 cases. Symptomatology, laboratory investigations and treatment. *J Egyptian Public Health Assoc* 1943;1:125–213.

78. Carl M, Tibbs CW, Dobson ME, et al. Diagnosis of acute typhus infection using the polymerase chain reaction. *J Infect Dis* 1990;161:791–793.

79. Elisberg BL, Bozeman FM. The rickettsiae. In: Lennette EH, Schmidt NJ, eds. *Diagnostic procedures for viral, rickettsial, and chlamydial infections.* Washington, DC: American Public Health Association, 1979:1061–108.

80. Perine PL, Krause DW, Awoke S, et al. Single-dose doxycycline treatment of louse-borne relapsing fever and epidemic typhus. *Lancet* 1974;2:742–744.

81. Krause DW, Perine PL, McDade JE, et al. Treatment of louse-borne typhus fever with chloramphenicol, tetracycline or doxycycline. *East Afr Med J* 1975;52:421–427.

82. Paullin JE. Typhus fever with a report of cases. *Southern Med J* 1913;6:36–43.

83. Maxcy KF. Typhus fever in the United States. *Public Health Rep* 1929;44:1735–1742.

84. Mooser H, Castaneda MR, Zinsser H. Rats as carriers of Mexican typhus fever. *JAMA* 1931;97:231–232.

85. Dyer RE, Rumreich A, Badger LF. A virus of the typhus type derived from fleas collected from wild rats. *Public Health Rep* 1931;46:334–338.

86. Adams WJ, Emmons RW, Brooks JE. The changing ecology of murine (endemic) typhus in southern California. *Am J Trop Med Hyg* 1970;19:311–318.

87. Williams SG, Sacci JB, Schriefer ME, et al. Typhus and typhuslike rickettsiae associated with opossums and their fleas in Los Angeles County, California. *J Clin Microbiol* 1992;30:1758–1762.

88. Schriefer ME, Sacci JB Jr, Taylor JP, et al. Murine typhus: updated roles of multiple urban components and a second typhus-like rickettsia. *J Med Entomol* 1994;31:681–685.

89. Sorvillo FJ, Gondo B, Emmons R, et al. A suburban focus of endemic typhus in Los Angeles County: association with seropositive domestic cats and opossums. *Am J Trop Med Hyg* 1993;48:269–273.

90. Traub R, Wisseman CL Jr, Farhang-Azad A. The ecology of murine typhus—a critical review. *Trop Dis Bull* 1978;75:237–241.

91. Farhang-Azad A, Traub R, Baqar S. Transovarial transmission of murine typhus rickettsiae in xenopsylla chiopis fleas. *Science* 1985;227:543–545.

92. Farhang-Azad A, Traub R. Transmission of murine typhus rickettsiae by *Xenopsylla cheopis,* with notes on experimental infection and effects of temperature. *Am J Trop Med Hyg* 1985;34:555–563.

93. Pratt HD. The changing picture of murine typhus in the United States. *Ann N Y Acad Sci* 1958;130:516–527.

94. White PC Jr. Murine typhus in the United States. *Milit Med* 1965;130:469–473.
95. Manea SJ, Sasaki DM, Ikeda JK, et al. Clinical and epidemiological observations regarding the 1998 Kauai murine typhus outbreak. *Hawaii Med J* 2001;60:7–11.
96. Taylor JP, Betz TG, Rawlings JA. Epidemiology of murine typhus in Texas, 1980 through 1984. *JAMA* 1986;255:2173–2176.
97. Dumler JS, Taylor JP, Walker DH. Clinical and laboratory features of murine typhus in south Texas, 1980 through 1987. *JAMA* 1991;266:1365–1370.
98. Shaked Y, Samra Y, Maeir MK, et al. Murine typhus and spotted fever in Israel in the eighties: retrospective analysis. *Infection* 1988;16:283–287.
99. Whiteford SF, Taylor JP, Dumler JS. Clinical, laboratory, and epidemiologic features of murine typhus in 97 Texas children. *Arch Pediatr Adolesc Med* 2001;155:396–400.
100. Rollwagen FM, Dasch GA, Jerrells TR. Mechanisms of immunity to rickettsial infection: characterization of a cytotoxic effector cell. *J Immunol* 1986;136:1418–1421.
101. Rollwagen FM, Bakun AJ, Dorsey CH, et al. Mechanisms of immunity to infection with typhus rickettsiae: infected fibroblasts bear rickettsial antigens on their surfaces. *Infect Immun* 1985;50:911–916.
102. Stuart BM, Pullen PL. Endemic (murine) typhus fever: clinical observations of 180 cases. *Ann Intern Med* 1945;23:520–536.
103. Huebner RJ, Jellison WL, Armstrong C. Rickettsialpox: a newly recognized rickettsial disease. V. Recovery of *Rickettsia akari* from a house mouse (*Mus musculus*). *Public Health Rep* 1947;62:777–780.
104. Huebner RJ, Jellison WL, Pomerantz C. Rickettsialpox: a newly recognized rickettsial disease. IV. Isolation of a rickettsia apparently identical with the causative agent of rickettsialpox from *Allodermanyssus sanguineus*, a rodent mite. *Public Health Rep* 1946;61:1677–1682.
105. Huebner RJ, Stamps P, Armstrong C. Rickettsialpox: a newly recognized rickettsial disease. I. Isolation of the etiologic agent. *Public Health Rep* 1946;61:1605–1614.
106. Greenberg M, Pellitteri OJ, Jellison WL. Rickettsialpox: a newly recognized rickettsial disease. III. Epidemiology. *Am J Public Health* 1947;37:860–868.
107. Pike G, Cohen S, Murray ES. Rickettsialpox: report of a serologically proved case occurring in a resident of Boston. *N Engl J Med* 1950;243:913–915.
108. LaBoccetta AC, Israel HL, Perri AM, et al. Rickettsialpox: report of four apparent cases in Pennsylvania. *Am J Med* 1952;13:413–422.
109. Rindge ME. Connecticut has first rickettsialpox outbreak. *Conn Health Bull* 1952;66:73–75.
110. Hoeprich PD, Kent GT, Dingle JH. Rickettsialpox: report of a serologically proved case in Cleveland. *N Engl J Med* 1956;254:25–27.
111. Jackson EB, Danauskas JX, Coale MC, et al. Recovery of *Rickettsia akari* from the Korean vole *Microtus fortis pelliceus*. *Am J Hyg* 1957;66:301–308.
112. Comer JA, Tzianabos T, Flynn C, et al. Serologic evidence of rickettsialpox (*Rickettsia akari*) infection among intravenous drug users in inner-city Baltimore, Maryland. *Am J Trop Med Hyg* 1999;60:894–898.
113. Kass EM, Szaniawski WK, Levy H, et al. Rickettsialpox in a New York City hospital, 1980 to 1989. *N Engl J Med* 1994;331:1612–1617.
114. Greenberg M, Pellitteri O. Rickettsialpox. *Bull N Y Acad Med* 1947;23:338–351.
115. Barker LP. Rickettsialpox: clinical and laboratory study of twelve hospitalized cases. *JAMA* 1947;141:1119–1123.
116. Greenberg M, Pellitteri O, Klein IF, et al. Rickettsialpox: a newly recognized rickettsial disease. II. Clinical observations. *JAMA* 1947;133:901–906.
117. Brettman LR, Lewin S, Holzman RS, et al. Rickettsialpox: report of an outbreak and a contemporary review. *Medicine* (Baltimore) 1981;60:363–372.
118. Bell EJ, Stoenner HG. Immunologic relationships among the spotted fever group of rickettsiae determined by toxin neutralization tests in mice with convalescent animal serums. *J Immunol* 1960;84:171–182.
119. Rose HM. The treatment of rickettsialpox with antibiotics. *Ann N Y Acad Sci* 1952;55:1019–1026.
120. Farner DS, Katsampes CP. Tsutsugamushi disease. *U S Nav Med Bull* 1944;43:800.
121. Berman SJ, Kundin WD. Scrub typhus in South Vietnam: a study of 87 cases. *Ann Intern Med* 1973;79:26–30.
122. Traub R, Wisseman CL Jr. The ecology of chigger-borne rickettsioses (Scrub typhus). *J Med Entomol* 1974;11:237–303.
123. Brown GW, Robinson DM, Huxsoll DL. Serologic evidence for a high incidence of transmission of *Rickettsia tsutsugamushi* in two Orang Asli settlements in peninsular Malaysia. *Am J Trop Med Hyg* 1978;27:121–124.
124. Brown GW, Shirai A, Jegathesan M, et al. Febrile illness in Malaysia—an analysis of 1,629 hospitalized patients. *Am J Trop Med Hyg* 1984;33:311–315.
125. Sayen JJ, Pond HS, Forrester JS, et al. Scrub typhus in Assam and Burma: a clinical study of 616 cases. *Medicine* 1946;25:155–214.
126. Caselton BG, Salata K, Dasch GA, et al. Recovery and viability of *Orientia tsutsugamushi* from packed red blood cells and the danger of acquiring scrub typhus from blood transfusion. *Transfusion* 1998;38:680–689.
127. Suto T. A ten years experience on diagnosis of rickettsial diseases using the indirect immunoperoxidase methods. *Acta Virol* 1991;35:580–586.
128. Kim IK, Seong SY, Woo SG, et al. High-level expression of a 56-kilodalton protein gene (bor56) of *Rickettsia tsutsugamushi* Boryong and its application to enzyme-linked immunosorbent assays. *J Clin Microbiol* 1993;31:589–605.
129. Kim IK, Seong SY, Woo SG, et al. Rapid diagnosis of scrub typhus by passive hemagglutination assay using recombinant 56-kilodalton polypeptides. *J Clin Microbiol* 1993;31:2057–2060.
130. Kawamori F, Akiyama M, Sugieda M, et al. Two-step polymerase chain reaction for diagnosis of scrub typhus and identification of antigenic variants of *Rickettsia tsutsugamushi*. *J Vet Med Sci* 1993;55:749–755.
131. Murai K, Tachibana N, Okayama A, et al. Sensitivity of polymerase chain reaction assay for *Rickettsia tsutsugamushi* in patients' blood samples. *Microbiol Immunol* 1992;36:1145–1153.
132. Sugita Y, Yamakawa Y, Takahashi K, et al. A polymerase chain reaction system for rapid diagnosis of scrub typhus within six hours. *Am J Trop Med Hyg* 1993;49:636–640.
133. Olson JG, Bourgeois AL, Fang RC, et al. Prevention of scrub typhus: prophylactic administration of doxycycline in a randomized double blind trial. *Am J Trop Med Hyg* 1980;29:989–997.
134. Watt G, Chouriyagune C, Ruangweerayud R, et al. Scrub typhus infections poorly responsive to antibiotics in northern Thailand. *Lancet* 1996;348:86–89.
135. Choi EK, Pai H. Azithromycin therapy for scrub typhus during pregnancy. *Clin Infect Dis* 1998;27:1539–1540.
136. Strickman D, Sheer T, Salata K, et al. In vitro effectiveness of azithromycin against doxycycline-resistant and -susceptible strains of *Rickettsia tsutsugamushi*, etiologic agent of scrub typhus. *Antimicrob Agents Chemother* 1995;39:2406–2410.
137. Smadel JE, Traub R, Frick LP, et al. Chloramphenicol (chloromycetin) in the chemoprophylaxis of scrub typhus (Tsutsugamushi disease). III. Suppression of overt disease by prophylactic regimens of four-week duration. *Am J Hyg* 1950;51:216–228.
138. Twartz JC, Shirai A, Selvaraju G, et al. Doxycycline prophylaxis for human scrub typhus. *J Infect Dis* 1982;146:811–818.
139. Parola P, Raoult D. Ticks and tickborne bacterial diseases in humans: an emerging infectious threat. *Clin Infect Dis* 2001;32:897–928.
140. Bouyer DH, Stenos J, Crocquet-Valdes P, et al. *Rickettsia felis*: molecular characterization of a new member of the spotted fever group. *Int J Syst Evol Microbiol* 2001;51:339–347.
141. Gear JHS. Other spotted fever group rickettsioses: clinical signs, symptoms, and pathophysiology. In: Walker DH, ed. *Biology of rickettsial diseases*, Vol I. Boca Raton, FL: CRC Press, 1988:101–114.
142. Segura Porta F, Font-Creus B, Espejo-Arenas E, et al. New trends in Mediterranean spotted fever. *Eur J Epidemiol* 1989;5:438–443.
143. Segura Porta F, Diestre-Ortin G, Ortuno-Romero A, et al. Prevalence of antibodies to spotted fever group rickettsiae in human beings and dogs from an endemic area of Mediterranean spotted fever in Catalonia, Spain. *Eur J Epidemiol* 1998;14:395–398.
144. Brouqui P, Harle JR, Delmont J, et al. African tick-bite fever. *Arch Intern Med* 1997;157:119–124.
145. Sexton DJ, Dwyer B, Kemp R, et al. Spotted fever group rickettsial infections in Australia. *Rev Infect Dis* 1990;13:876–886.
146. Fournier PE, Roux V, Caumes E, et al. Outbreak of *Rickettsia africae* infections in participants of an adventure race in South Africa. *Clin Infect Dis* 1998;27:316–323.
147. Hudson BJ, McPetrie R, Kitchener-Smith J, et al. Vesicular rash associated with infection due to *Rickettsia australis*. *Clin Infect Dis* 1994;18:118–119.
148. Raoult D, Weiller PJ, Chagnon A, et al. Mediterranean spotted fever: clinical, laboratory and epidemiological features of 199 cases. *Am J Trop Med Hyg* 1986;35:845–850.

CHAPTER 170
Agents of Human Ehrlichiosis

John W. Sumner and Christopher D. Paddock

The genus *Ehrlichia* is composed of species of small, obligately intracellular bacteria that are gram-negative and have a coccobacillary morphology (1,2). They are included in the alpha subclass of the class *Proteobacteria* (3). Ehrlichiae reside and multiply within cytoplasmic vacuoles derived from the host cell membrane, where they characteristically form compact clusters of bacterial cells called *morulae*, a name derived from the mulberry-like appearance of these aggregates (1). Most species cause diseases of humans or wild or domesticated animals, and all are transmitted by invertebrate vectors (4). *Ehrlichia* species primarily infect white blood cells, and one disease classification scheme loosely divides pathogens on the basis of tropism for granulocytes or cells of monocytic lineage. Hence, the terms *granulocytic* (or granulocytotropic) and *monocytic* (or monocytotrpic) have been commonly used to describe different forms of ehrlichiosis and to characterize *Ehrlichia* species in the literature. However, in the context of taxonomic classification, the terms granulocytic and monocytic describe only cell tropism and do not accurately reflect phylogenetic relationships.

Recent studies involving analyses of gene sequences indicate that prior taxa designations involving the genera *Anaplasma*, *Cowdria*, *Ehrlichia*, *Neorickettsia*, and *Wolbachia* did not accurately reflect evolutionary relationships. Analyses of 16S ribosomal RNA (rRNA) gene (5–10) and *groESL* heat-shock operon (11–14) sequences showed that *Ehrlichia* species could be segregated into three distinct clades and that the individual clades were more closely related to species from the genera *Anaplasma*, *Cowdria*, or *Neorickettsia* than to each other. Using the more recent genetic information and other criteria, including antigenic relationships and natural histories, Dumler and colleagues proposed a reorganization of genera in the families Anaplasmataceae and Rickettsiaceae (15). The genus *Ehrlichia* was restructured so that *Ehrlichia* species in the clade represented by prototype species *Ehrlichia canis* form the emended genus *Ehrlichia* with the addition of *Ehrlichia* (formally *Cowdria*) *ruminantium*, the etiologic agent of the ruminant disease heartwater. *Ehrlichia* species in the clade represented by prototype species *Ehrlichia phagocytophila* were placed in the genus *Anaplasma*. The former *Ehrlichia sennetsu* and *Ehrlichia risticii* are now included in the genus *Neorickettsia*. This reorganization more accurately reflects phylogenetic relationships derived from genetic information. Here, we describe the agents of human ehrlichiosis in three separate sections corresponding to the emended classification of these bacteria.

EHRLICHIA CHAFFEENSIS (HUMAN MONOCYTIC EHRLICHIOSIS)

Characteristics of the Pathogen

Ehrlichia chaffeensis is one of three recognized species in the emended genus *Ehrlichia* that cause disease in humans. The other two pathogens, *Ehrlichia ewingii* and *E. canis*, have only recently been described as agents of human disease, predominantly in specialized patient cohorts (e.g., immunocompromised individuals) and as a single confirmed report, respectively (16,17), and are discussed in less detail.

E. chaffeensis is a small, nonmotile bacterium that resides and multiplies in cytoplasmic vacuoles of the host cell, where it forms morulae composed of a few to more than 40 individual bacteria that range from 1 to 6 μm in size and stain pale blue to dark violet by using various eosin-azure (Romanovsky)-type stains. Ultrastructural analyses of *E. chaffeensis* in cell culture reveals two morphologic types, namely coccobacillary forms that measure 0.4 to 0.6 μm by 0.7 to 1.9 μm and have ribosomes and nucleoid DNA fibrils uniformly dispersed throughout the cytoplasm (reticulate cells), and coccal forms that measure 0.4 to 0.6 μm and display centrally condensed nucleoid DNA and ribosomes (dense-cored cells). Both cell types replicate by binary fission (18,19). *E. chaffeensis* lacks pili or a capsule and may attach to host leukocytes by its outer membrane (20). An immunodominant 120-kd outer-membrane protein of *E. chaffeensis* may function as an adhesin that might also enhance internalization of ehrlichiae (21). Internalized ehrlichiae are contained within endosomes composed of the host cell membrane and maintain distinct cytoplasmic compartments that do not fuse with lysosomes (20).

In human hosts, *E. chaffeensis* infects predominantly monocytes and macrophages, but infection of other cell types has been described, including lymphocytes, promyelocytes, metamyelocytes, and band and segmented neutrophils (22,23). Infected cells typically contain only 1 or 2 morulae, although as many as 15 have been observed in leukocytes of immunosuppressed patients (24). Morulae can be visualized in smears of peripheral blood, buffy-coat preparations, cerebrospinal fluid (CSF), or bone marrow aspirates, but are infrequently identified in most infected patients. *E. chaffeensis* will grow in various cell lines; however, primary isolates from humans and animals have been obtained only in canine histiocytic cells (DH82 cells) and HEL 299 cells (23,25–32).

Nucleotide sequences identified for *E. chaffeensis* include the 16S rRNA gene (5), various genes coding for immunoreactive proteins, including the variable-length polymerase chain reaction (PCR) target (32), 120-kd, 106-kd, and 37-kd protein genes (33,34), the *groESL* heat-shock operon (35), a quinolate synthetase A (*nadA*) gene (36), and a locus that contains 22 homologous but not identical genes that code for immunodominant proteins (the *p28* multigene family) (37,38). Several of these sequences have been used as PCR targets, and some proteins expressed by these genes have been investigated as serodiagnostic reagents (34,39,40)

Relatively few genes of *E. chaffeensis* have been well characterized, but it is apparent that considerable genetic heterogeneity exists within this bacterium. The 120-kd protein gene contains a series of 2 to 4, 240–base pair (bp), serine-rich, tandem repeat units and encodes an extensively glycosylated, immunodominant surface protein that is preferentially expressed on dense-cored forms of *E. chaffeensis* (21,41). The *VLPT* gene exhibits isolate-dependent polymorphisms in the number (2 to 6), linear order, and nucleotide composition of the imperfect, 90-bp repeat units. The biologic function of the *VLPT* gene has not been determined; however, *VLPT* sequences code for immunoreactive proteins with apparent molecular masses of 30 to 60 kd (23,32). The greatest diversity among isolates of *E. chaffeensis* is created by a locus of 22 genes from 813 to 900 bp that encodes major outer membrane proteins, described as the *omp* cluster (37) or the *p28* multigene family (38). The *p28* genes code for mature proteins with predicted molecular sizes of about 26 to 32 kd; none of the proteins are identical, and the amino acid sequence identity varies from about 20% to 80% (38). Sequences of individual *p28* genes also vary among different isolates of *E. chaffeensis* (38,42).

Despite the identification of many genetically distinct isolates of *E. chaffeensis*, no molecular or antigenic markers have been linked with variations in disease severity or particular disease manifestations; however, most isolates have been obtained from patients with relatively severe or even fatal illnesses, and it is possible that intrinsic markers of disease will emerge as isolates are obtained from patients representing a range of clinical manifestations, including milder forms of the illness, and as knowledge of genetic composition of this pathogen increases (23,28). Because so few bacteria are generally detected in the blood or tissues of ill hosts, it has been proposed that disease manifestations result primarily from host immunity to the pathogen (19). As an example, the magnitude of multilineage cytopenias observed in most patients far exceeds the actual number of infected cells, implying nonspecific destruction of uninfected leukocytes and platelets during the host immune response.

Cellular and humoral processes also appear to play important and complementary roles in recovery following infection with *E. chaffeensis*. Immunologic models using mice deficient in toll-like receptor 4 or class II major histocompatibility complex alleles suggest that rapid and effective clearance of ehrlichiae from infected hosts requires macrophage activation and CD4[+] T-lymphocyte–mediated immunity (43). In a SCID mouse model, polyclonal anti–*E. chaffeensis* antibodies and monoclonal antibodies recognizing a P28 protein of *E. chaffeensis* effectively mediate clearance of ehrlichiae during active infection, even in the absence of T or B lymphocytes (44,45). Host humoral responses may also modulate the cellular response to infection with this agent and possibly stimulate immune responses that ultimately contribute to overt disease. Cell biology studies reveal that human monocytes infected with *E. chaffeensis* produce only two proinflammatory interleukins, interleukin-1β (IL-1β) and IL-8, and an immunosuppressive cytokine, IL-10. When infected cells are exposed to hyperimmune serum containing anti–*E. chaffeensis* immunoglobulin G (IgG) antibodies, additional proinflammatory cytokines, including tumor necrosis factor-α (TNF-α) and IL-6, are generated by the monocytes (46).

Little is known about long-term immunity to *E. chaffeensis* in persons infected with this pathogen. One case of sequential infection with two genetically distinct strains of *E. chaffeensis* has been described in an immunocompromised host (47); however, the susceptibility of previously infected, immune-intact persons to reinfection with different strains or the identical strain remains undetermined. Potential antigen diversity created by differential and sequential expression of *p28* genes to alter rapidly the composition of one or more immunodominant surface proteins has been proposed as a mechanism of immune evasion for *E. chaffeensis* (38,48,49).

Natural History and Ecology

E. chaffeensis is maintained in nature as part of a complex zoonosis involving perhaps several tick species as vectors and several vertebrate reservoir hosts. As with most vector-borne zoonoses, humans are only accidentally involved in the life cycle of this pathogen and represent dead-end hosts for this agent. *Amblyomma americanum* (the lone star tick) is the principal vector involved in the transmission of *E. chaffeensis* in the United States. In most regions throughout the southeastern United States, *A. americanum* represents a predominant tick species in terms of general distribution and absolute numbers. Lone star ticks are found from west-central Texas, north to Iowa and eastward in a broad swath that extends to the Atlantic coast. The range of this species also extends north through coastal areas of New England.

Larvae, nymphs, and adults feed from a wide host range that includes birds and medium and large mammals, and all stages readily bite humans; however, because *E. chaffeensis* appears to be transstadially but not transovarially passed in *A. americanum* (50), it is likely that only the nymph and adult transmit the infection to humans. These stages are most active during April through June and decline markedly in abundance and activity as summer progresses (51). In adult ticks tested individually using PCR, *E. chaffeensis* DNA has been reported from about 5% to 15% of specimens collected from areas where the disease is endemic (52–55); however, the stability of *E. chaffeensis* in defined tick populations is unknown, and prevalence rates of this agent among tick populations appear to vary considerably over time and space, even within a relatively circumscribed geographic region. DNA of *E. chaffeensis* has been detected in other tick species from the United States, including *Dermacentor variabilis* (54), and in *Amblyomma*, *Haemaphysalis*, and *Ixodes* species collected from Russia and China (56,57). However, the role of these or other tick species as significant vectors of *E. chaffeensis* has not been established.

Because *A. americanum* will feed readily from a wide variety of mammalian and avian hosts, it is possible that several vertebrate species serve as competent reservoirs for *E. chaffeensis*; however, the white-tailed deer (*Odocoileus virginianus*) currently represents the principal vertebrate host that maintains the transmission cycle of *E. chaffeensis*. Natural infections with *E. chaffeensis* have been identified in deer in the southeastern United States (30,53), and deer experimentally infected with *E. chaffeensis* maintain persistent viable bacteremia for at least several months (58). Serologic surveys have demonstrated seroprevalence rates of antibody reactive with *E. chaffeensis* antigens exceeding 50% among some white-tailed deer populations in regions where *E. chaffeensis* is endemic (53,59,60). DNA of *E. chaffeensis* has been detected in the blood of other wild and domesticated animals, including coyotes, dogs, and goats, but the role of these species in the life history of *E. chaffeensis* has not been definitively established (31,61,62). Similarly, antibodies reactive with *E. chaffeensis* have been detected in the blood of various animals, including raccoons (63) and opossums (53), although the significance of these observations is unknown.

EHRLICHIA CANIS AND *EHRLICHIA EWINGII*

E. canis and *E. ewingii* are zoonotic pathogens initially described as disease agents of dogs in 1935 and 1971, respectively. A definitive association with human disease was reported for *E. canis* in 1996 and for *E. ewingii* in 1999. Similar to *E. chaffeensis*, *E. canis* infects predominantly mononuclear leukocytes. Although considerable data exist on the microbial pathogenesis and immunology of *E. canis* infections in canines (64), almost nothing is known about the interaction of this bacterium with human hosts. *E. canis* is distributed widely throughout the world, but a case of human infection has been documented only in a single case in Venezuela (17). *Rhipicephalus sanguineus*, the brown dog tick, is the principal vector of *E. canis* (65). Populations of *R. sanguineus* in the United States seldom bite humans, which may explain the absence of documented human infections in this country. Nevertheless, *D. variabilis*, a human-biting tick distributed ubiquitously throughout many regions of the southeastern and western United States, is capable of transmitting *E. canis* (66), suggesting that human infections with this agent may not be restricted to South America.

E. ewingii has not been isolated in cell culture, and relatively few microbiologic data exist for this organism. In human hosts, *E. ewingii* infects predominantly mature neutrophils and occasionally eosinophils. In the few patients for whom morulae have been visualized in peripheral blood or CSF, as many as 50% of the granulocytes may be infected, although these observations have occurred largely for immunosuppressed patients (16,27). Various genetic sequences have been characterized, including the 16S rRNA gene, the *groESL* heat-shock operon, and a homolog of the *p28* gene of *E. chaffeensis* (6,12,67). The natural history of *E. ewingii* is also incompletely known. Natural infections have been reported from domestic dogs in the southeastern and midwestern United States (61,68); however, *A. americanum* is the probable vector of *E. ewingii* (69,70), and it is possible that reservoir species for this ehrlichia include one or several mammalian hosts also described for *E. chaffeensis*.

ANAPLASMA (FORMALLY *EHRLICHIA*) *PHAGOCYTOPHILA* (HUMAN GRANULOCYTIC EHRLICHIOSIS)

Characteristics of the Pathogen

In 1994, Johan Bakken described a cluster of human ehrlichiosis cases that occurred in Minnesota and Wisconsin (71). In these patients, morulae were observed primarily in neutrophils, which is not typical of ehrlichiosis caused by *E. chaffeensis*. A 16S rRNA gene sequence amplified from the blood of a patient was nearly identical to the sequences of two previously described veterinary pathogens that cause granulocytic ehrlichiosis, *Ehrlichia phagocytophila* and *Ehrlichia equi* (7). *E. phagocytophila* is the etiologic agent of tick-borne fever of ruminants, a disease described primarily in Europe (72). *E. equi* was first described in 1969 as an agent of granulocytic ehrlichiosis of horses in the United States (73). The newly discovered agent of human disease was called the *human granulocytic ehrlichiosis* (HGE) agent because its taxonomic position was uncertain. Over time, antigenic and genetic similarities among these three organisms became more apparent. Comparison of 16S rRNA gene and *groESL* operon sequences demonstrated a closer relationship to *Anaplasma* species than to *Ehrlichia* species aligned with *E. canis* or with the *Neorickettsia* species. Eventually, it became apparent that separate species designations were not justified, and taxonomic changes were proposed that included the consolidation of *E. phagocytophila*, *E. equi*, and the HGE agent into the single species *Anaplasma phagocytophila* (15).

After injection by tick bite, *A. phagocytophila* can cause a febrile illness that varies from a mild flu-like syndrome to severe disease that is occasionally fatal. The pathogenic mechanisms are not well understood. The organism likely infects a myeloid precursor in the bone marrow, and systemic disease may be initiated by adherence of infected neutrophils to endothelial tissues (74,75). Two cell types may be observed within the endosomes of infected neutrophils. They are described as reticulate cells and dense core bodies, and both cell types divide by binary fission, indicating they are not mandatory stages in a developmental cycle (76). The organs most often involved are the spleen, liver, lungs, bone marrow, and lymph nodes. *A. phagocytophila* does not appear to cause much tissue damage directly. Evidence indicates that lesions observed in these organs are the result of the accumulation of inflammatory cells, which initiate an immune response that results in local tissue damage (75). Pancytopenia usually occurs, and the cause is not completely understood. It has been suggested that cytokines produced by infected cells may exert a myelosuppressive effect (77). An interesting facet of the disease is the suppression of host immunity. Animals and humans infected with *A. phagocytophila* are predisposed to opportunistic fungal, viral, and bacterial infections, which have occasionally been associated with fatal outcomes in human cases (78).

A. phagocytophila has been propagated in undifferentiated HL-60 promyelocytic cells (79), HL-60 cells differentiated into neutrophil-like cells (80), and cell lines derived from *Ixodes scapularis* tick cells (81). HL-60 cells can be induced to differentiate to granulocytic or monocytic cell types, and it has been shown that with differentiation to the monocytic lineage, cells become refractory to infection by *A. phagocytophila* (82). The growth of the organism in cell culture has greatly facilitated the production of antigen for improved serologic testing methods, the isolation of *A. phagocytophila* DNA for construction of genomic libraries, and many other avenues of research (82–86). The mouse has also proved useful for isolation of the organism, for transmission studies, and as an animal model for studies on pathogenesis and immune response to infection (87,88).

The genome size of *A. phagocytophila* is estimated to be 1,494 kilobases (kb) (89). The nucleotide sequences of several *A. phagocytophila* genes have been determined. The 16S rRNA gene and *groESL* sequences have been used for phylogenetic studies and PCR detection. (12,90–93). More recently, the *gltA* (citrate synthase) gene has been sequenced for most of the species that were previously included in the genus *Ehrlichia*, and the relationships among these sequences correlate with those demonstrated for 16S rRNA gene and *groESL* sequences (94). One of

the more interesting genes is the 44-kd antigen gene, or *p44*. It represents a multigene family that encodes immunodominant outer-membrane proteins with an average molecular mass of 44 kd (95,96). Sequence similarities show that the *A. phagocytophila* *p44* is related to the *msp*-2 gene family of *Anaplasma marginale*, a polymorphic multigene family that contributes to antigenic variation and may have a role in immune evasion mechanisms. There is evidence that the P44 proteins induce proinflammatory cytokine gene expression, which may contribute to pathogenesis and immunomodulation (97). It has been shown that *p44* transcripts isolated from ticks and infected mammals are distinct, suggesting that the composition of surface proteins my change with environment (98). Recombinant P44 has been successfully used for enzyme-linked immunosorbent assay (ELISA) (99,100), and molecular typing methods based on the *p44* have been used to characterize genetic variation among PCR amplicons derived from samples collected in geographically disparate areas (101). A gene that contains ankyrin-like repeats has also been characterized (102,103). It has been used for PCR detection, and variant sequences have been shown to correlate with geographic origin (104).

Natural History and Ecology

The primary tick vectors of *A. phagocytophila* are *Ixodes* species. The organism has been detected in ticks by PCR amplification of *A. phagocytophila* DNA and by immunologic methods (105–108). Transmission studies have also been conducted to prove that specific tick species are capable of transmitting the organism to various animals, including rodents, horses, and sheep (72,109,110). It has been demonstrated that uninfected *I. scapularis* larval ticks acquired the organism from infected mice and that the molted nymphal ticks transmitted the infection to mice within 48 hours of attachment (111). In the United States, the principal tick vectors are *I. scapularis* (the deer tick, or black-legged tick) in the upper midwestern and northeastern states where most cases of HGE originate, and *Ixodes pacificus* in northern California. *I. spinipalpis* has been implicated in the transmission of *A. phagocytophila* to rodents in Colorado, but this species rarely feeds on humans (112).

A. phagocytophila DNA has been amplified from *I. ricinus* ticks collected in many European countries, suggesting that *I. ricinus* is the primary vector in Europe (93,113–120). *A. phagocytophila* DNA has also been detected in *I. persulcatus* ticks in Russia (121). Antibodies reactive with *A. phagocytophila* have been detected in sera collected from various animals and humans in most regions of Europe (83,91,117,122–127). There is also serologic evidence that HGE occurs in Israel (128), and recently, *A. phagocytophila* was detected by PCR in blood from HGE patients living in the Daxingan mountains in China (129).

To date, there is no evidence that transovarial transmission of *A. phagocytophila* occurs in ticks. If the organism is maintained in the tick population by transstadial transmission, maintenance in a reservoir host should be an essential part of the *A. phagocytophila* life cycle. Granulocytic ehrlichiosis caused by *A. phagocytophila* occurs in a variety of domestic animals, including cattle, sheep, goats, horses, llamas, and dogs (129–134), but it is likely that wildlife species constitute the primary reservoir hosts. Serologic methods have been used to demonstrate exposure to, and infection with, *A. phagocytophila* in various wild animals (91,135–138). *A. phagocytophila* has been detected by PCR in various wild animals in the United States and Europe, including pumas, foxes, coyotes, deer, and various rodents (137,139,140). The organism has also been detected in ticks removed from birds (141,142). To date, cervids and rodents have been studied most frequently. Infection with

A. phagocytophila occurs commonly among populations of white-tailed deer (*Odocoileus virginianus*) in some regions of the United States (138,143–145) and among roe deer (*Capreolus capreolus*), chamois (*Rupicapra rupicapra*), and red deer (*Cervus elaphus*) in Europe (91,146).

In a number of studies, *A. phagocytophila* DNA has been detected in questing nymphal-stage ticks, indicating the ticks acquired the organism while feeding as larvae (116). During their larval stage, ticks tend to feed on smaller animals, and therefore rodents may be important reservoir hosts (147). In the United States, *A. phagocytophila* has been detected by PCR in mice (*Peromyscus maniculatus* and *P. leucopus*) and in rats, including the dusky-footed wood rat (*Neotoma fuscipes*) and Mexican wood rat (*Neotoma mexicana*) (136,140,148–150). Nicholson and associates reported serologic evidence of infection for rodents trapped in Connecticut, California, Colorado, Florida, Maryland, New Jersey, and Wisconsin (135). Liz and colleagues have reported PCR detection of *A. phagocytophila* in tissue samples collected from voles (*Clethrionomys glareolus*) and mice (*Apodemus sylvaticus*) trapped in Switzerland (151). Wood rats (*Neotoma fuscipes*) have been shown to be seroreactive and PCR positive for *A. phagocytophila* for up to 14 months, providing a long period during which tick vectors might acquire the organism (148).

In summary, *A. phagocytophila* is maintained in nature in a life cycle involving tick vectors and various animal hosts. The relative importance of specific animal hosts is not clearly understood and may vary by geographic region. Humans are infected by the bite of tick vectors, and therefore, the likelihood of acquiring the disease increases with frequent tick exposure. The same tick vectors transmit *Borrelia burgdorferi*, the agent of Lyme disease, and dual infections with *A. phagocytophila* and *B. burgdorferi* have been described for several *Ixodes* species (152–154) and for human patients (155,156).

Anaplasma (formally *Ehrlichia*) *platys* and *Anaplasma* (formally *Ehrlichia*) *bovis* are veterinary pathogens closely related to *A. phagocytophila* (15). There is also a related organism commonly found in white-tailed deer, primarily in the southeastern region of the United States (157). This organism has not yet received a species designation and is called the *white-tailed deer agent*. These organisms have not been associated with human disease, but that was also the case for *A. phagocytophila* until 1994.

NEORICKETTSIA (FORMALLY EHRLICHIA) SENNETSU (SENNETSU FEVER)

Neorickettsia sennetsu causes sennetsu fever, a mononucleosis-like illness that has been described only in Japan and Malaysia (158). The organism was originally isolated by mouse inoculation of blood, bone marrow, and lymph node samples collected from a febrile Japanese man exhibiting lymphadenopathy and increased atypical lymphocytes (159). *N. sennetsu* exhibits a tropism for monocytes and macrophages and has been propagated in cell culture by using cells derived from canine monocytes (160). Epidemiologic studies indicate the disease is associated with the consumption of uncooked fish (1,161). It is likely, but not proven, that the disease is vectored by infected flukes that are parasites of fish. The organism was originally named *Rickettsia sennetsu* but was later included in the genus *Ehrlichia* after antigenic relatedness to the ehrlichiae was demonstrated and it was determined that development occurred in endosomes, not freely in the cytoplasm as is typical for *Rickettsia* species (162). Later studies revealed a close genetic and antigenic relationship to *Neorickettsia helminthoeca* (163). The taxonomic realignment proposed by Dumler and colleagues changed the genus designation of *Ehrlichia sennetsu* and *Ehrlichia risticii* to *Neorickettsia* (15). Relatively more is known about the life cycles of veterinary pathogens related to *N. sennetsu*. The prototype species of the genus, *N. helminthoeca*, is a parasite of the fluke *Nanophyetus helminthoeca*. Ingestion of fluke-infested fish causes salmon poisoning disease in dogs (1). A related organism, the SF agent, is found in the metacercarial stage of the fluke *Stellantchamus falcatus*, which also parasitizes fish (164). *Neorickettsia* (formally *Ehrlichia*) *risticii* causes an illness in horses that has been described regionally as *Potomac horse fever, equine monocytic ehrlichiosis*, or *Shasta river crud* (165). Recent studies suggest horses are infected by the ingestion of snails or aquatic insects parasitized by flukes (166). Exposure to these organisms is associated with aquatic habitats, and there is no evidence to indicate that ticks are involved in their life cycles. Only *N. sennetsu* has been associated with human disease.

REFERENCES

1. Rikihisa Y. The tribe *Ehrlichieae* and ehrlichial diseases. *Clin Microbiol Rev* 1991;4:286–308.
2. Ristic M, Holland CJ, Khondowe M. An overview of research on ehrlichiosis. *Eur J Epidemiol* 1991;7:246–252.
3. Weisburg WG, Dobson ME, Samuel JE, et al. Phylogenetic diversity of the *Rickettsiae*. *J Bacteriol* 1989;171:4202–4206.
4. Ogden NH, Woldehiwet Z, Hart CA. Granulocytic ehrlichiosis: an emerging or rediscovered tick-borne disease? *J Med Microbiol* 1998;47:475–482.
5. Anderson BE, Dawson JE, Jones DC, et al. *Ehrlichia chaffeensis*, a new species associated with human ehrlichiosis. *J Clin Microbiol* 1991;29:2838–2842.
6. Anderson BE, Greene CE, Jones DC, et al. *Ehrlichia ewingii* sp. nov., the etiologic agent of canine granulocytic ehrlichiosis. *Int J Syst Bacteriol* 1992;42:299–302.
7. Chen SM, Dumler JS, Bakken JS, et al. Identification of a granulocytotropic *Ehrlichia* species as the etiologic agent of human disease. *J Clin Microbiol* 1994;32:589–595.
8. van Vliet AH, Jongejan F, van der Zeijst BA. Phylogenetic position of *Cowdria ruminantium* (*Rickettsiales*) determined by analysis of amplified 16S ribosomal DNA sequences. *Int J Syst Bacteriol* 1992;42:494–498.
9. Wen B, Rikihisa Y, Mott J, et al. *Ehrlichia muris* sp. nov., identified on the basis of 16S rRNA base sequences and serological, morphological, and biological characteristics. *Int J Syst Bacteriol* 1995;45:250–254.
10. Wen B, Rikihisa Y, Yamamoto S, et al. Characterization of the SF agent, an *Ehrlichia* sp. isolated from the fluke *Stellantchasmus falcatus*, by 16S rRNA base sequence, serological, and morphological analyses. *Int J Syst Bacteriol* 1996;46:149–154.
11. Sumner JW, Nicholson WL, Massung RF. PCR amplification and comparison of nucleotide sequences from the *groESL* heat shock operon of *Ehrlichia* species. *J Clin Microbiol* 1997;35:2087–2092.
12. Sumner JW, Storch GA, Buller RS, et al. PCR amplification and phylogenetic analysis of *groESL* operon sequences from *Ehrlichia ewingii* and *Ehrlichia muris*. *J Clin Microbiol* 2000;38:2746–2749.
13. Yu XJ, Zhang XF, McBride JW, et al. Phylogenetic relationships of *Anaplasma marginale* and '*Ehrlichia platys*' to other *Ehrlichia* species determined by GroEL amino acid sequences. *Int J Syst Evolut Microbiol* 2001;51:1143–1146.
14. Zhang Y, Ohashi N, Lee EH, et al. *Ehrlichia sennetsu groE* operon and antigenic properties of the GroEL homolog. *FEMS Immunol Med Microbiol* 1997;18:39–46.
15. Dumler JS, Barbet AF, Bekker CP, et al. Reorganization of genera in the families *Rickettsiaceae* and *Anaplasmataceae* in the order Rickettsiales: unification of some species of *Ehrlichia* with *Anaplasma*, *Cowdria* with *Ehrlichia* and *Ehrlichia* with *Neorickettsia*, descriptions of six new species combinations and designation of *Ehrlichia equi* and 'HGE agent' as subjective synonyms of *Ehrlichia phagocytophila*. *Int J Syst Evolut Microbiol* 2001;51:2145–2165.
16. Buller RS, Arens M, Hmiel SP, et al. *Ehrlichia ewingii*, a newly recognized agent of human ehrlichiosis. *N Engl J Med* 1999;341:148–155.
17. Perez M, Rikihisa Y, Wen B. *Ehrlichia canis*-like agent isolated from a man in Venezuela: antigenic and genetic characterization. *J Clin Microbiol* 1996;34:2133–2139.
18. Popov VL, Chen SM, Feng HM, et al. Ultrastructural variation of cultured *Ehrlichia chaffeensis*. *J Med Microbiol* 1995;43:411–421.
19. Rikihisa Y. Clinical and biological aspects of infection caused by *Ehrlichia chaffeensis*. *Microbes Infect* 1999;1:367–376.
20. Rikihisa Y. Ehrlichial strategy for survival and proliferation in leukocytes. *Subcell Biochem* 2000;33:517–538.
21. Popov VL, Yu X, Walker DH. The 120 kDa outer membrane protein of *Ehrlichia chaffeensis*: preferential expression on dense-core cells and gene expression in *Escherichia coli* associated with attachment and entry. *Microb Pathog* 2000;28:71–80.

22. Maeda K, Markowitz N, Hawley RC, et al. Human infection with *Ehrlichia canis*, a leukocytic rickettsia. *N Engl J Med* 1987;316:853–856.

23. Paddock CD, Sumner JW, Shore GM, et al. Isolation and characterization of *Ehrlichia chaffeensis* strains from patients with fatal ehrlichiosis. *J Clin Microbiol* 1997;35:2496–2502.

24. Paddock CD, Suchard DP, Grumbach KL, et al. Brief report: fatal seronegative ehrlichiosis in a patient with HIV infection. *N Engl J Med* 1993;329:1164–1167.

25. Dawson JE, Anderson BE, Fishbein DB, et al. Isolation and characterization of an *Ehrlichia* sp. from a patient diagnosed with human ehrlichiosis. *J Clin Microbiol* 1991;29:2741–2745.

26. Standaert SM, Yu T, Scott MA, et al. Primary isolation of *Ehrlichia chaffeensis* from patients with febrile illnesses: clinical and molecular characteristics. *J Infect Dis* 2000;181:1082–1088.

27. Paddock CD, Folk SM, Shore GM, et al. Infections with *Ehrlichia chaffeensis* and *Ehrlichia ewingii* in persons coinfected with HIV. *Clin Infect Dis* 2001;33:1586–1594.

28. Dumler JS, Chen SM, Asanovich K, et al. Isolation and characterization of a new strain of *Ehrlichia chaffeensis* from a patient with nearly fatal monocytic ehrlichiosis. *J Clin Microbiol* 1995;33:1704–1711.

29. Chen SM, Yu XJ, Popov VL, et al. Genetic and antigenic diversity of *Ehrlichia chaffeensis*: comparative analysis of a novel human strain from Oklahoma and previously isolated strains. *J Infect Dis* 1997;175:856–863.

30. Lockhart JM, Davidson WR, Stallknecht DE, et al. Isolation of *Ehrlichia chaffeensis* from wild white-tailed deer (*Odocoileus virginianus*) confirms their role as natural reservoir hosts. *J Clin Microbiol* 1997;35:1681–1686.

31. Dugan VG, Little SE, Stallknecht DE, et al. Natural infection of domestic goats with *Ehrlichia chaffeensis*. *J Clin Microbiol* 2000;38:448–449.

32. Sumner JW, Childs JE, Paddock CD. Molecular cloning and characterization of the *Ehrlichia chaffeensis* variable-length PCR target: an antigen-expressing gene that exhibits interstrain variation. *J Clin Microbiol* 1999;37:1447–1453.

33. Yu XJ, Crocquet-Valdes P, Walker DH. Cloning and sequencing of the gene for a 120-kDa immunodominant protein of *Ehrlichia chaffeensis*. *Gene* 1997;184:149–154.

34. Yu XJ, Crocquet-Valdes PA, Cullman LC, et al. Comparison of *Ehrlichia chaffeensis* recombinant proteins for serologic diagnosis of human monocytotropic ehrlichiosis. *J Clin Microbiol* 1999;37:2568–2575.

35. Sumner JW, Sims KG, Jones DC, et al. *Ehrlichia chaffeensis* expresses an immunoreactive protein homologous to the *Escherichia coli* GroEL protein. *Infect Immun* 1993;61:3536–3539.

36. Yu XJ, Walker DH. Sequence and characterization of an *Ehrlichia chaffeensis* gene encoding 314 amino acids highly homologous to the NAD A enzyme. *FEMS Microbiol Lett* 1997;154:53–58.

37. Ohashi N, Rikihisa Y, Unver A. Analysis of transcriptionally active gene clusters of major outer membrane protein multigene family in *Ehrlichia canis* and *E. chaffeensis*. *Infect Immun* 2001;69:2083–2091.

38. Yu X, McBride JW, Zhang X, et al. Characterization of the complete transcriptionally active *Ehrlichia chaffeensis* 28 kDa outer membrane protein multigene family. *Gene* 2000;248:59–68.

39. Alleman AR, Barbet AF, Bowie MV, et al. Expression of a gene encoding the major antigenic protein 2 homolog of *Ehrlichia chaffeensis* and potential application for serodiagnosis. *J Clin Microbiol* 2000;38:3705–3709.

40. Unver A, Rikihisa Y, Ohashi N, et al. Western and dot blotting analyses of *Ehrlichia chaffeensis* indirect fluorescent-antibody assay-positive and -negative human sera by using native and recombinant *E. chaffeensis* and *E. canis* antigens. *J Clin Microbiol* 1999;37:3888–3895.

41. McBride JW, Yu XJ, Walker DH. Glycosylation of homologous immunodominant proteins of *Ehrlichia chaffeensis* and *Ehrlichia canis*. *Infect Immun* 2000;68:13–18.

42. Yu XJ, McBride JW, Walker DH. Genetic diversity of the 28-kilodalton outer membrane protein gene in human isolates of *Ehrlichia chaffeensis*. *J Clin Microbiol* 1999;37:1137–1143.

43. Ganta RR, Wilkerson MJ, Cheng C, et al. Persistent *Ehrlichia chaffeensis* infection occurs in the absence of functional major histocompatibility complex class II genes. *Infect Immun* 2002;70:380–388.

44. Winslow GM, Yager E, Shilo K, et al. Antibody-mediated elimination of the obligate intracellular bacterial pathogen *Ehrlichia chaffeensis* during active infection. *Infect Immun* 2000;68:2187–2195.

45. Li JS, Yager E, Reilly M, et al. Outer membrane protein-specific monoclonal antibodies protect SCID mice from fatal infection by the obligate intracellular bacterial pathogen *Ehrlichia chaffeensis*. *J Immunol* 2001;166:1855–1862.

46. Lee EH, Rikihisa Y. Absence of tumor necrosis factor alpha, interleukin-6 (IL-6), and granulocyte-macrophage colony-stimulating factor expression but presence of IL-1beta, IL-8, and IL-10 expression in human monocytes exposed to viable or killed *Ehrlichia chaffeensis*. *Infect Immun* 1996;64:4211–4219.

47. Liddell AM, Sumner JW, Paddock CD, et al. Reinfection with *Ehrlichia chaffeensis* in a liver transplant patient. *Clin Infect Dis* 2002;34:1644–1647.

48. Reddy GR, Streck CP. Variability in the 28-kDa surface antigen protein multigene locus of isolates of the emerging disease agent *Ehrlichia chaffeensis* suggests that it plays a role in immune evasion. *Mol Cell Biol Res Commun* 1999;1:167–175.

49. Reddy GR, Sulsona CR, Barbet AF, et al. Molecular characterization of a 28 kDa surface antigen gene family of the tribe Ehrlichiae. *Biochem Biophys Res Commun* 1998;247:636–643.

50. Ewing SA, Dawson JE, Kocan AA, et al. Experimental transmission of *Ehrlichia chaffeensis* (Rickettsiales: Ehrlichieae) among white-tailed deer by *Amblyomma americanum* (Acari: Ixodidae). *J Med Entomol* 1995;32:368–374.

51. Hair JA, Howell DE. *Lone star ticks: their biology and control in Ozark recreation areas.* Bulletin B-679. Oklahoma, Oklahoma State University, Agricultural Experiment Station, 1979:1–47.

52. IJdo JW, Wu C, Magnarelli LA, et al. Detection of *Ehrlichia chaffeensis* DNA in *Amblyomma americanum* ticks in Connecticut and Rhode Island. *J Clin Microbiol* 2000;38:4655–4656.

53. Lockhart JM, Davidson WR, Stallknecht DE, et al. Natural history of *Ehrlichia chaffeensis* (Rickettsiales: Ehrlichieae) in the piedmont physiographic province of Georgia. *J Parasitol* 1997;83:887–894.

54. Roland WE, Everett ED, Cyr TL, et al. *Ehrlichia chaffeensis* in Missouri ticks. *Am J Trop Med Hyg* 1998;59:641–643.

55. Whitlock JE, Fang QQ, Durden LA, et al. Prevalence of *Ehrlichia chaffeensis* (Rickettsiales: Rickettsiaceae) in *Amblyomma americanum* (Acari: Ixodidae) from the Georgia coast and Barrier Islands. *J Med Entomol* 2000;37:276–280.

56. Alekseev AN, Dubinina HV, Semenov AV, et al. Evidence of ehrlichiosis agents found in ticks (Acari: Ixodidae) collected from migratory birds. *J Med Entomol* 2001;38:471–474.

57. Cao WC, Gao YM, Zhang PH, et al. Identification of *Ehrlichia chaffeensis* by nested PCR in ticks from southern China. *J Clin Microbiol* 2000;38:2778–2780.

58. Davidson WR, Lockhart JM, Stallknecht DE, et al. Persistent *Ehrlichia chaffeensis* infection in white-tailed deer. *J Wildl Dis* 2001;37:538–546.

59. Irving RP, Pinger RR, Vann CN, et al. Distribution of *Ehrlichia chaffeensis* (Rickettsiales: Rickettsiaceae) in *Amblyomma americanum* in southern Indiana and prevalence of *E. chaffeensis*–reactive antibodies in white-tailed deer in Indiana and Ohio in 1998. *J Med Entomol* 2000;37:595–600.

60. Dawson JE, Childs JE, Biggie KL, et al. White-tailed deer as a potential reservoir of *Ehrlichia* spp. *J Wildl Dis* 1994;30:162–168.

61. Dawson JE, Biggie KL, Warner CK, et al. Polymerase chain reaction evidence of *Ehrlichia chaffeensis*, etiologic agent of human ehrlichiosis, in dogs from southeast Virginia. *Am J Vet Res* 1996;57:1175–1179.

62. Kocan AA, Levesque GC, Whitworth LC, et al. Naturally occurring *Ehrlichia chaffeensis* infection in coyotes from Oklahoma. *Emerg Infect Dis* 2000;6:477–480.

63. Comer JA, Nicholson WL, Paddock CD, et al. Detection of antibodies reactive with *Ehrlichia chaffeensis* in the raccoon. *J Wildl Dis* 2000;36:705–712.

64. Harrus S, Waner T, Bark H, et al. Recent advances in determining the pathogenesis of canine monocytic ehrlichiosis. *J Clin Microbiol* 1999;37:2745–2749.

65. Groves MG, Dennis GL, Amyx HL, et al. Transmission of *Ehrlichia canis* to dogs by ticks (*Rhipicephalus sanguineus*). *Am J Vet Res* 1975;36:937–940.

66. Johnson EM, Ewing SA, Barker RW, et al. Experimental transmission of *Ehrlichia canis* (Rickettsiales: Ehrlichieae) by *Dermacentor variabilis* (Acari: Ixodidae). *Vet Parasitol* 1998;74:277–288.

67. Gusa AA, Buller RS, Storch GA, et al. Identification of a p28 gene in *Ehrlichia ewingii*: evaluation of gene for use as a target for species-specific PCR diagnostic assay. *J Clin Microbiol* 2001;39:3871–3876.

68. Murphy GL, Ewing SA, Whitworth LC, et al. A molecular and serologic survey of *Ehrlichia canis*, *E. chaffeensis*, and *E. ewingii* in dogs and ticks from Oklahoma. *Vet Parasitol* 1998;79:325–339.

69. Anziani OS, Ewing SA, Barker RW. Experimental transmission of a granulocytic form of the tribe Ehrlichieae by *Dermacentor variabilis* and *Amblyomma americanum* to dogs. *Am J Vet Res* 1990;51:929–931.

70. Wolf L, McPherson T, Harrison B, et al. Prevalence of *Ehrlichia ewingii* in *Amblyomma americanum* in North Carolina. *J Clin Microbiol* 2000;38:2795.

71. Bakken JS, Dumler JS, Chen SM, et al. Human granulocytic ehrlichiosis in the upper Midwest United States: a new species emerging? *JAMA* 1994;272:212–218.

72. MacLeod J, Gordon WS. Studies in tick-borne fever in sheep. I. Transmission by the tick *Ixodes ricinus*, with a description of the disease produced. *Parasitology* 1933;25:273–283.

73. Gribble DH. Equine ehrlichiosis. *J Am Vet Med Assoc* 1969;155:462–469.

74. Walker DH, Dumler JS. Emergence of the ehrlichioses as human health problems. *Emerg Infect Dis* 1996;2:18–29.

75. Lepidi H, Bunnell JE, Martin ME, et al. Comparative pathology, and immunohistology associated with clinical illness after *Ehrlichia phagocytophila*–group infections. *Am J Trop Med Hyg* 2000;62:29–37.

76. Popov VL, Han V, Chen SM, et al. Ultrastructural differentiation of the genogroups in the genus Ehrlichia. *J Med Microbiol* 1998;47:235–251.

77. Klein MB, Hu S, Chao CC, et al. The agent of human granulocytic ehrlichiosis induces the production of myelosuppressing chemokines without induction of proinflammatory cytokines. *J Infect Dis* 2000;182:200–205.

78. Walker DH, Dumler JS. Human monocytic and granulocytic ehrlichioses: discovery and diagnosis of emerging tick-borne infections and the critical role of the pathologist. *Arch Pathol Lab Med* 1997;121:785–791.

79. Goodman JL, Nelson C, Vitale B, et al. Direct cultivation of the causative agent of human granulocytic ehrlichiosis. *N Engl J Med* 1996;334:209–215.

80. Heimer R, Van Andel A, Wormser GP, et al. Propagation of granulocytic *Ehrlichia* spp. from human and equine sources in HL-60 cells induced to differentiate into functional granulocytes. *J Clin Microbiol* 1997;35:923–927.

81. Munderloh UG, Madigan JE, Dumler JS, et al. Isolation of the equine granulocytic ehrlichiosis agent, *Ehrlichia equi*, in tick cell culture. *J Clin Microbiol* 1996;34:664–670.

82. Klein MB, Hayes SF, Goodman JL. Monocytic differentiation inhibits infection and granulocytic differentiation potentiates infection by the agent of human granulocytic ehrlichiosis. *Infect Immun* 1998;66:3410–3415.

83. Brouqui P, Salvo E, Dumler JS, et al. Diagnosis of granulocytic ehrlichiosis in humans by immunofluorescence assay. *Clin Diagn Lab Immunol* 2001;8:199–202.

84. Murphy CI, Storey JR, Recchia J, et al. Major antigenic proteins of the agent of human granulocytic ehrlichiosis are encoded by members of a multigene family. *Infect Immun* 1998;66:3711–3718.

85. Nicholson WL, Comer JA, Sumner JW, et al. An indirect immunofluorescence assay using a cell culture-derived antigen for detection of antibodies to the agent of human granulocytic ehrlichiosis. *J Clin Microbiol* 1997;35:1510–1516.

86. Ravyn MD, Goodman JL, Kodner CB, et al. Immunodiagnosis of human granulocytic ehrlichiosis by using culture-derived human isolates. *J Clin Microbiol* 1998;36:1480–1488.

87. Sun W, Ijdo JW, Telford SR III, et al. Immunization against the agent of human granulocytic ehrlichiosis in a murine model. *J Clin Invest* 1997;100:3014–3018.

88. Hodzic E, Ijdo JW, Feng S, et al. Granulocytic ehrlichiosis in the laboratory mouse. *J Infect Dis* 1998;177:737–745.

89. Rydkina E, Roux V, Raoult D. Determination of the genome size of *Ehrlichia* spp., using pulsed field gel electrophoresis. *FEMS Microbiol Lett* 1999;176:73–78.

90. Chae JS, Foley JE, Dumler JS, et al. Comparison of the nucleotide sequences of 16S rRNA, 444 Ep-ank, and *groESL* heat shock operon genes in naturally occurring *Ehrlichia equi* and human granulocytic ehrlichiosis agent isolates from Northern California. *J Clin Microbiol* 2000;38:1364–1369.

91. Liz JS, Sumner J, Pfister K, et al. PCR detection and serological evidence of granulocytic ehrlichial infection in roe deer (*Capreolus capreolus*) and chamois (*Rupicapra rupicapra*). *J Clin Microbiol* 2002;40:892–897.

92. Massung RF, Slater K, Owens JH, et al. Nested PCR assay for detection of granulocytic ehrlichiae. *J Clin Microbiol* 1998;36:1090–1095.

93. Petrovec M, Sumner JW, Nicholson WL, et al. Identity of ehrlichial DNA sequences derived from *Ixodes ricinus* ticks with those obtained from patients with human granulocytic ehrlichiosis in Slovenia. *J Clin Microbiol* 1999;37:209–210.

94. Inokuma H, Brouqui P, Drancourt M, et al. Citrate synthase gene sequence: a new tool for phylogenetic analysis and identification of *Ehrlichia*. *J Clin Microbiol* 2001;39:3031–3039.

95. Ijdo JW, Sun W, Zhang Y, et al. Cloning of the gene encoding the 44-kilodalton antigen of the agent of human granulocytic ehrlichiosis and characterization of the humoral response. *Infect Immun* 1998;66:3264–3269.

96. Zhi N, Ohashi N, Rikihisa Y, et al. Cloning and expression of the 44-kilodalton major outer membrane protein gene of the human granulocytic ehrlichiosis agent and application of the recombinant protein to serodiagnosis. *J Clin Microbiol* 1998;36:1666–1673.

97. Kim HY, Rikihisa Y. Expression of interleukin-1beta, tumor necrosis factor alpha, and interleukin-6 in human peripheral blood leukocytes exposed to human granulocytic ehrlichiosis agent or recombinant major surface protein P44. *Infect Immun* 2000;68:3394–3402.

98. Zhi N, Ohashi N, Tajima T, et al. Transcript heterogeneity of the p44 multigene family in a human granulocytic ehrlichiosis agent transmitted by ticks. *Infect Immun* 2002;70:1175–1184.

99. Magnarelli L, Ijdo J, Wu C, et al. Recombinant protein-44-based class-specific enzyme-linked immunosorbent assays for serologic diagnosis of human granulocytic ehrlichiosis. *Eur J Clin Microbiol Infect Dis* 2001;20:482–485.

100. Tajima T, Zhi N, Lin Q, et al. Comparison of two recombinant major outer membrane proteins of the human granulocytic ehrlichiosis agent for use in an enzyme-linked immunosorbent assay. *Clin Diagn Lab Immunol* 2000;7:652–657.

101. Carter SE, Ravyn MD, Xu Y, et al. Molecular typing of the etiologic agent of human granulocytic ehrlichiosis. *J Clin Microbiol* 2001;39:3398–3401.

102. Caturegli P, Asanovich KM, Walls JJ, et al. ankA: an *Ehrlichia phagocytophila* group gene encoding a cytoplasmic protein antigen with ankyrin repeats. *Infect Immun* 2000;68:5277–5283.

103. Storey JR, Doros-Richert LA, Gingrich-Baker C, et al. Molecular cloning and sequencing of three granulocytic *Ehrlichia* genes encoding high-molecular-weight immunoreactive proteins. *Infect Immun* 1998;66:1356–1363.

104. Massung RF, Owens JH, Ross D, et al. Sequence analysis of the *ank* gene of granulocytic ehrlichiae. *J Clin Microbiol* 2000;38:2917–2922.

105. Barlough JE, Madigan JE, Kramer VL, et al. *Ehrlichia phagocytophila* genogroup rickettsiae in ixodid ticks from California collected in 1995 and 1996. *J Clin Microbiol* 1997;35:2018–2021.

106. Fang QQ, Mixson TR, Hughes M, et al. Prevalence of the agent of human granulocytic ehrlichiosis in *Ixodes scapularis* (Acari: Ixodidae) in the coastal southeastern United States. *J Med Entomol* 2002;39:251–255.

107. Magnarelli LA, Stafford KC, III, Mather TN, et al. Hemocytic rickettsia-like organisms in ticks: serologic reactivity with antisera to Ehrlichiae and detection of DNA of agent of human granulocytic ehrlichiosis by PCR. *J Clin Microbiol* 1995;33:2710–2714.

108. Schwartz I, Fish D, Daniels TJ. Prevalence of the rickettsial agent of human granulocytic ehrlichiosis in ticks from a hyperendemic focus of Lyme disease. *N Engl J Med* 1997;337:49–50.

109. Des Vignes F, Fish D. Transmission of the agent of human granulocytic ehrli-

chiosis by host-seeking *Ixodes scapularis* (Acari: Ixodidae) in southern New York State. *J Med Entomol* 1997;34:379–382.

110. Reubel GH, Kimsey RB, Barlough JE, et al. Experimental transmission of *Ehrlichia equi* to horses through naturally infected ticks (*Ixodes pacificus*) from Northern California. *J Clin Microbiol* 1998;36:2131–2134.

111. Hodzic E, Fish D, Maretzki CM, et al. Acquisition and transmission of the agent of human granulocytic ehrlichiosis by *Ixodes scapularis* ticks. *J Clin Microbiol* 1998;36:3574–3578.

112. Zeidner NS, Burkot TR, Massung R, et al. Transmission of the agent of human granulocytic ehrlichiosis by *Ixodes spinipalpis* ticks: evidence of an enzootic cycle of dual infection with *Borrelia burgdorferi* in Northern Colorado. *J Infect Dis* 2000;182:616–619.

113. Alekseev AN, Dubinina HV, Van de Pol I, et al. Identification of *Ehrlichia* spp. and *Borrelia burgdorferi* in *Ixodes* ticks in the Baltic regions of Russia. *J Clin Microbiol* 2001;39:2237–2242.

114. Baumgarten BU, Rollinghoff M, Bogdan C. Prevalence of *Borrelia burgdorferi* and granulocytic and monocytic ehrlichiae in *Ixodes ricinus* ticks from southern Germany. *J Clin Microbiol* 1999;37:3448–3451.

115. Cinco M, Padovan D, Murgia R, et al. Detection of HGE agent-like *Ehrlichia* in *Ixodes ricinus* ticks in northern Italy by PCR. *Wien Klin Wochenschr* 1998;110:898–900.

116. Guy E, Tasker S, Joynson DH. Detection of the agent of human granulocytic ehrlichiosis (HGE) in UK ticks using polymerase chain reaction. *Epidemiol Infect* 1998;121:681–683.

117. Oteo JA, Gil H, Barral M, et al. Presence of granulocytic ehrlichia in ticks and serological evidence of human infection in La Rioja, Spain. *Epidemiol Infect* 2001;127:353–358.

118. Parola P, Beati L, Cambon M, et al. Ehrlichial DNA amplified from *Ixodes ricinus* (Acari: Ixodidae) in France. *J Med Entomol* 1998;35:180–183.

119. Pusterla N, Leutenegger CM, Huder JB, et al. Evidence of the human granulocytic ehrlichiosis agent in *Ixodes ricinus* ticks in Switzerland. *J Clin Microbiol* 1999;37:1332–1334.

120. Walker AR, Alberdi MP, Urquhart KA, et al. Risk factors in habitats of the tick *Ixodes ricinus* influencing human exposure to *Ehrlichia phagocytophila* bacteria. *Med Vet Entomol* 2001;15:40–49.

121. Semenov AV, Alekseev AN, Dubinina EV, et al. [Detection of the genotypic heterogeneity of *Ixodes persulcatus* Schulze (Acari: Ixodidae) of the North-West region of Russia and characteristics of distribution of tick-borne pathogens causing Lyme disease and Ehrlichia infections in various genotypes]. *Med Parazitol (Mosk)* 2001;11–15.

122. Bjoersdorff A, Berglund J, Kristiansen BE, et al. [Varying clinical picture and course of human granulocytic ehrlichiosis. Twelve Scandinavian cases of the new tick-borne zoonosis are presented]. *Lakartidningen* 1999;96:4200–4204.

123. Christova JS, Dumler JS. Human granulocytic ehrlichiosis in Bulgaria. *Am J Trop Med Hyg* 1999;60:58–61.

124. Cizman M, Avsic-Zupanc T, Petrovec M, et al. Seroprevalence of ehrlichiosis, Lyme borreliosis and tick-borne encephalitis infections in children and young adults in Slovenia. *Wien Klin Wochenschr* 2000;112:842–845.

125. Fingerle V, Goodman JL, Johnson RC, et al. Human granulocytic ehrlichiosis in southern Germany: increased seroprevalence in high-risk groups. *J Clin Microbiol* 1997;35:3244–3247.

126. Lotric-Furlan S, Avsic-Zupanc T, Petrovec M, et al. Clinical and serological follow-up of patients with human granulocytic ehrlichiosis in Slovenia. *Clin Diagn Lab Immunol* 2001;8:899–903.

127. Pusterla N, Weber R, Wolfensberger C, et al. Serological evidence of human granulocytic ehrlichiosis in Switzerland. *Eur J Clin Microbiol Infect Dis* 1998;17:207–209.

128. Keysary A, Amram L, Keren G, et al. Serologic evidence of human monocytic and granulocytic ehrlichiosis in Israel. *Emerg Infect Dis* 1999;5:775–778.

129. Gao D, Cao W, Zhang X, et al. [Investigations on human ehrlichia infectious people in Daxingan Mountains]. *Zhonghua Liu Xing Bing Xue Za Zhi* 2001;22:137–141.

130. Barlough JE, Madigan JE, Turoff DR, et al. An *Ehrlichia* strain from a llama (*Lama glama*) and llama-associated ticks (*Ixodes pacificus*). *J Clin Microbiol* 2002;35:1005–1007.

131. Engvall EO, Pettersson B, Persson M, et al. A 16S rRNA-based PCR assay for detection and identification of granulocytic *Ehrlichia* species in dogs, horses, and cattle. *J Clin Microbiol* 1996;34:2170–2174.

132. Greig B, Asanovich KM, Armstrong PJ, et al. Geographic, clinical, serologic, and molecular evidence of granulocytic ehrlichiosis, a likely zoonotic disease, in Minnesota and Wisconsin dogs. *J Clin Microbiol* 1996;34:44–48.

133. Madigan JE, Barlough JE, Dumler JS, et al. Equine granulocytic ehrlichiosis in Connecticut caused by an agent resembling the human granulocytotropic ehrlichia. *J Clin Microbiol* 1996;34:434–435.

134. Pusterla N, Anderson RJ, House JK, et al. Susceptibility of cattle to infection with *Ehrlichia equi* and the agent of human granulocytic ehrlichiosis. *J Am Vet Med Assoc* 2001;218:1160–1162.

135. Nicholson WL, Muir S, Sumner JW, et al. Serologic evidence of infection with *Ehrlichia* spp. in wild rodents (Muridae: Sigmodontinae) in the United States. *J Clin Microbiol* 1998;36:695–700.

136. Nicholson WL, Castro MB, Kramer VL, et al. Dusky-footed wood rats (*Neotoma fuscipes*) as reservoirs of granulocytic Ehrlichiae (Rickettsiales: Ehrlichieae) in northern California. *J Clin Microbiol* 1999;37:3323–3327.

137. Pusterla N, Chang CC, Chomel BB, et al. Serologic and molecular evidence of *Ehrlichia* spp. in coyotes in California. *J Wildl Dis* 2000;36:494–499.

138. Walls JJ, Asanovich KM, Bakken JS, et al. Serologic evidence of a natural infection of white-tailed deer with the agent of human granulocytic ehrlichiosis in Wisconsin and Maryland. *Clin Diagn Lab Immunol* 1998;5:762–765.

139. Foley JE, Foley P, Jecker M, et al. Granulocytic ehrlichiosis and tick infestation in mountain lions in California. *J Wildl Dis* 1999;35:703–709.

140. Stafford KC III, Massung RF, Magnarelli LA, et al. Infection with agents of human granulocytic ehrlichiosis, Lyme disease, and babesiosis in wild white-footed mice (*Peromyscus leucopus*) in Connecticut. *J Clin Microbiol* 1999;37:2887–2892.

141. Alekseev AN, Dubinina HV, Semenov AV, et al. Evidence of ehrlichiosis agents found in ticks (Acari: Ixodidae) collected from migratory birds. *J Med Entomol* 2001;38:471–474.

142. Bjoersdorff A, Bergstrom S, Massung RF, et al. *Ehrlichia*-infected ticks on migrating birds. *Emerg Infect Dis* 2001;7:877–879.

143. Belongia EA, Reed KD, Mitchell PD, et al. Prevalence of granulocytic *Ehrlichia* infection among white-tailed deer in Wisconsin. *J Clin Microbiol* 1997;35:1465–1468.

144. Foley JE, Barlough JE, Kimsey RB, et al. *Ehrlichia* spp. in cervids from California. *J Wildl Dis* 1998;34:731–737.

145. Magnarelli LA, Ijdo JW, Stafford KC III, et al. Infections of granulocytic ehrlichiae and *Borrelia burgdorferi* in white-tailed deer in Connecticut. *J Wildl Dis* 1999;35:266–274.

146. Stuen S, Engvall EO, van dP I, et al. Granulocytic ehrlichiosis in a roe deer calf in Norway. *J Wildl Dis* 2001;37:614–616.

147. Telford SR III, Dawson JE, Katavolos P, et al. Perpetuation of the agent of human granulocytic ehrlichiosis in a deer tick-rodent cycle. *Proc Natl Acad Sci U S A* 1996;93:6209–6214.

148. Castro MB, Nicholson WL, Kramer VL, et al. Persistent infection in *Neotoma fuscipes* (Muridae: Sigmodontinae) with *Ehrlichia phagocytophila sensu lato*. *Am J Trop Med Hyg* 2001;65:261–267.

149. Ravyn MD, Kodner CB, Carter SE, et al. Isolation of the etiologic agent of human granulocytic ehrlichiosis from the white-footed mouse (*Peromyscus leucopus*). *J Clin Microbiol* 2001;39:335–338.

150. Walls JJ, Greig B, Neitzel DF, et al. Natural infection of small mammal species in Minnesota with the agent of human granulocytic ehrlichiosis. *J Clin Microbiol* 1997;35:853–855.

151. Liz JS, Anderes L, Sumner JW, et al. PCR detection and serological evidence of granulocytic ehrlichiae in *Ixodes ricinus* ticks and wild small mammals in western Switzerland. *J Clin Microbiol* 2000;38:1002–1007.

152. Jenkins A, Kristiansen BE, Allum AG, et al. *Borrelia burgdorferi sensu lato* and *Ehrlichia* spp. in Ixodes ticks from southern Norway. *J Clin Microbiol* 2001;39:3666–3671.

153. Leutenegger CM, Pusterla N, Mislin CN, et al. Molecular evidence of coinfection of ticks with *Borrelia burgdorferi sensu lato* and the human granulocytic ehrlichiosis agent in Switzerland. *J Clin Microbiol* 1999;37:3390–3391.

154. Levin ML, Fish D. Acquisition of coinfection and simultaneous transmission of *Borrelia burgdorferi* and *Ehrlichia phagocytophila* by *Ixodes scapularis* ticks, *Infect Immun* 2000;68:2183–2186.

155. Duffy J, Pittlekow MR, Kolbert CP, et al. Coinfection with *Borrelia burgdorferi* and the agent of human granulocytic ehrlichiosis. *Lancet* 1997;349:399.

156. Nadelman RB, Horowitz HW, Hsieh TC, et al. Simultaneous human granulocytic ehrlichiosis and Lyme borreliosis. *N Engl J Med* 1997;337:27–30.

157. Dawson JE, Warner CK, Baker V, et al. *Ehrlichia*-like 16S rDNA sequence from wild white-tailed deer (*Odocoileus virginianus*). *J Parasitol* 1996;82:52–58.

158. Misao T, Katsuta K. Epidemiology of infectious mononucleosis. *Jpn J Clin Exp* 1956;33:73–82.

159. Misao T, Kobayashi Y. Studies on infectious mononucleosis. 1. Isolation of etiologic agent from blood, bone marrow and lymph nodes of a patient with infectious mononucleosis by using mice. *Tokyo Iji Shinshi* 1954;71:686.

160. Holland CJ, Ristic M, Huxsoll DL, et al. Adaptation of *Ehrlichia sennetsu* to canine blood monocytes: preliminary structural and serological studies with cell culture-derived *Ehrlichia sennetsu*. *Infect Immun* 1985;48:366–371.

161. Tachibana N. Sennetsu fever: the disease, diagnosis, and treatment. In: Microbiology—1986. American Society for Microbiology, 1986:205–208.

162. Ristic M, Huxsoll DL, Tachibana N, et al. Evidence of a serologic relationship between *Ehrlichia canis* and *Rickettsia sennetsu*. *Am J Trop Med Hyg* 1981;30:1324–1328.

163. Pretzman C, Ralph D, Stothard DR, et al. 16S rRNA gene sequence of *Neorickettsia helminthoeca* and its phylogenetic alignment with members of the genus *Ehrlichia*. *Int J Syst Bacteriol* 1995;45:207–211.

164. Wen B, Rikihisa Y, Yamamoto S, et al. Characterization of the SF agent, an *Ehrlichia* sp. isolated from the fluke *Stellantchasmus falcatus*, by 16S rRNA base sequence, serological, and morphological analyses. *Int J Syst Bacteriol* 1996;46:149–154.

165. Rikihisa Y, Perry BD. Causative ehrlichial organisms in Potomac horse fever. *Infect Immun* 1985;49:513–517.

166. Madigan JE, Pusterla N, Johnson E, et al. Transmission of *Ehrlichia risticii*, the agent of Potomac horse fever, using naturally infected aquatic insects and helminth vectors: preliminary report. *Equine Vet J* 2000;32:275–279.

CHAPTER 171
Cat-Scratch Disease

Jennifer S. Daly

HISTORY

Cat-scratch disease (CSD) was first diagnosed in 1931 by Debré and Semelaigne, and since that time this disorder has been a microbiologic, diagnostic, and therapeutic challenge to the medical community (Table 171.1). The first patient recognized with CSD was a 10-year-old boy with multiple cat scratches, epitrochlear lymphadenitis, and a draining fistula (1). Debré and Semelaigne at the University of Paris recognized the disease after the fistula and the adenitis resolved spontaneously, the skin test for tuberculosis was negative, and the patient's mother maintained that the disease was related to the boy's close contact with cats. Years later when Debré visited Cincinnati, he discussed his findings with Foshay, who had recognized the syndrome himself while studying patients thought to have tularemia. Foshay developed the first skin test antigen, and Rose and Hanger in New York used it. These U.S. physicians did not publish their work (1), but Debré and co-workers (2) published the first report on CSD in 1950, naming the syndrome "la maladie des griffes de chat."

Rapidly the literature expanded with case reports by Mollaret from the Institut Pasteur and Greer in the United States. By 1954, Daniels and MacMurray (3) had collected 160 cases from the Washington, DC area and published a review. Later, Margileth, Carithers, and their colleagues (4–7) independently published their findings on more than 1,000 cases collected by each author for decades and contributed extensively to the understanding and recognition of the disease. They have used the skin test extensively and have provided skin test material to other physicians. They have helped develop standard criteria for the diagnosis of CSD, but these criteria may now become less important as culture techniques and serologic testing become more reliable and available.

The infectious nature of the disorder was recognized soon after the disease was first seen, but the isolation of the etiologic agent or agents and pathogenesis of the disease continue to provoke controversy. In 1983, Wear and co-workers (8) related finding delicate pleomorphic gram-negative bacilli in 34 of 39 lymph nodes from patients with CSD. The organisms were best seen with the Warthin-Starry silver stain within the walls of capillaries and microabscesses and appeared as single organisms or in chains or clumps. Convalescent serum from patients who had reacted to the antigen skin test also reacted with the bacteria (using an immunoperoxidase stain) seen in the lymph nodes. The following year, Margileth and colleagues (9) reported finding the Warthin-Starry–staining bacteria at the primary inoculation site in three patients. The organisms were similar to those seen in 1913 when Verhoff first described a filamentous organism in the conjunctiva of patients with Parinaud's oculoglandular syndrome (10), a syndrome later recognized as a rare manifestation of CSD. These silver-staining organisms were found more consistently than the miscellaneous agents implicated in other studies that suggested a viral, mycobacterial, chlamydial, or bacterial etiology for CSD (10,11). Finally, in 1988, English and others (12), at the same institution (Armed Forces Institute of Pathology) as Wear, isolated and propagated a gram-negative bacterium from one patient with CSD. This isolate and three isolates from another patient were characterized more extensively and named *Afipia felis* by Brenner and colleagues (13). English and colleagues

TABLE 171.1. Cat-Scratch Disease History

Year	Event
1931	Debré and Semelaigne recognize the first case of cat-scratch disease (CSD).
1946	Foshay, Rose, and Hanger use cat-scratch antigen as a skin test.
1950	Debré and colleagues publish first report (in French) on CSD.
1954	Daniels and MacMurray report findings for 160 cases in the United States.
1983	Wear and colleagues discover bacilli using the Warthin-Starry stain.
1988	English and coworkers culture *Afipia felis*.
1990	Slater, Welch, and colleagues culture *Bartonella henselae* from the blood of immunocompromised patients with fever and bacteremia. Relman and others find *B. henselae* DNA in tissue specimens from patients with peliosis hepatis.
1992	Regnery and others find that patients with CSD have a serologic response to *B. henselae* and culture the organism from the blood of a cat.
1993	Dolan and colleagues recover *B. henselae* from lymph nodes of patients with CSD.
1995	Laboratories culture both *B. henselae* and *A. felis* from patients with CSD.
1997	*Bartonella clarridgeiae* recognized as a cause of CSD.

(12) described what they called "delicate pleomorphic forms" in nine other patients; the forms were reported to grow in culture in biphasic brain-heart infusion medium incubated at 30° to 32°C. Electron microscopy revealed that the delicate pleomorphic forms lacked a portion of their cell walls, which the authors thought helped explain the inability to subculture the unusual forms. The one patient whose lymph node grew *A. felis* had an antibody titer of 1:512 by immunofluorescence assay with antigen derived from the cultured organism. English and co-workers were able to produce lesions histologically similar to those of CSD by injecting the organism in the skin of an armadillo and, like others before them, thought they had isolated the etiologic agent of CSD. Several other laboratories have isolated *A. felis* from patients with CSD, and a few patients have developed a serologic reaction to *A. felis*, but most patients with CSD do not demonstrate a serologic reaction to this organism.

In the 1990s, several investigators brought a new pathogen, distinct from *A. felis*, to the attention of medical scientists. As the epidemic of acquired immunodeficiency syndrome (AIDS) progressed, patients with human immunodeficiency virus (HIV) infection were diagnosed with severe, disseminated CSD (14). About the same time, a new entity was recognized, bacillary angiomatosis, consisting of skin lesions similar histologically to those in CSD and containing organisms that stained with the Warthin-Starry silver stain preparation. Comparable organisms were found in the liver of patients with peliosis hepatis, and eventually the diseases bacillary angiomatosis and peliosis of the liver and spleen were linked. In 1990, Slater and colleagues (15) reported a new pathogen, later named *Bartonella henselae* (16,17), from the blood of immunocompromised individuals with fever and bacteremia, and Relman and co-workers (18) detected *B. henselae* in tissue from patients with AIDS who had bacillary angiomatosis or peliosis hepatis. Because of the similarities between CSD and bacillary angiomatosis, Regnery and colleagues (19) undertook a study using serum from patients with suspected CSD. By an indirect immunofluorescent antibody test, 88% of 41 patients with clinically suspected CSD had antibodies to *Bartonella* antigens (19). In the same year, they cultured

B. henselae from the blood of a domestic cat. In 1993, Zangwill and co-workers studied 60 persons with suspected CSD and found that 84% of cases had antibody to the *Bartonella* antigen versus 3.6% of healthy control subjects; 81% of the cats from households of patients with the disease also had antibody (20). Although these serologic studies showed that 84% to 96% of patients had antibody titers greater than or equal to 1:64 to *B. henselae*, these authors and other investigators have postulated that cross-reactions occur between some strains of *Bartonella quintana* (the agent of trench fever and some of the cases of bacillary angiomatosis) and *B. henselae* (21). Waldvogel and colleagues (22) have reported that the originally developed immunofluorescent antibody test should be regarded as genus rather than species specific. The relative importance of cross-reacting antibody has not been determined.

Bartonella species, most commonly *B. henselae* and sometimes *Bartonella clarridgeiae*, cause most cases of CSD. The evidence for the role of *B. henselae* in CSD goes beyond serologic studies. *B. henselae* DNA was detected in several preparations of CSD skin test antigen by using species-specific polymerase chain reaction (PCR) primers (23). In 1993, Dolan and colleagues (24) isolated *B. henselae* from the lymph nodes of two patients with CSD. Serology, direct detection, and culture techniques have confirmed a role for *B. henselae* in patients with typical and atypical manifestations of CSD. Evidence for the role of other *Bartonella* species is growing stronger as laboratories become more proficient at detecting or culturing members of this fastidious genus. French investigators cultured *B. quintana* from a cat owner with chronic lymphadenopathy (25) but not classic CSD, and Alkan and colleagues (26) have isolated both *B. henselae* and *A. felis* from the nodes of several patients with CSD. *B. henselae* and *B. clarridgeiae* have been isolated from the blood of cats (27–31). The extent of disease due to *B. clarridgeiae* has not been determined, but it is hoped that a specific antibody test using antigen from the polar flagella (not present in *B. henselae*) will produce more information (32). Neuroretinitis, one of the classic neurologic manifestations of CSD, has been described in a patient with serologic and molecular sequence evidence of infection with *B. vinsonii* subspecies *arupensis* (33,34) and in another patient with evidence of infection with *Bartonella grahamii*. The data suggest that *Bartonella* species other than *B. henselae* may produce similar syndromes to CSD (35,36), but further research is needed. In addition, there continues to be a small group of patients (5% to 15%) with negative skin tests, serology, and culture for any *Bartonella* species in whom CSD may be due to other pathogens, including *A. felis* (37–39). With careful study using molecular techniques, defined culture methods, and animal models, clinical syndromes and pathologic features of patients with CSD should become further defined.

CHARACTERISTICS OF THE PATHOGEN

Bartonella henselae

B. henselae was first cultured using a lysis-centrifugation blood culture system and was originally named *Rochalimaea henselae*, after Diane Hensel, a microbiologist who first isolated the organism from the blood of a patient at the University of Oklahoma (16,17). In 1993, the genera *Bartonella* and *Rochalimaea* were unified after DNA relatedness data, base content, and phenotypic similarities were recognized, with the result that the organism is now known as *B. henselae* (40). It is a member of the α-2 subgroup of the class Proteobacteria but is distinct from the branch that contains *A. felis*. *B. henselae* is a small, curved gram-negative bacillus that grows best on fresh chocolate agar plates or heart infusion agar with 5% rabbit blood, incubated at 35° to 37°C in 5% to 10% carbon dioxide with high humidity. Primary isolation usually requires 5 to 15 days from blood and 7 to 60 days from tissue. A chemically defined liquid medium containing hemin, developed by Wong and associates (41), allows recovery of *B. henselae* (and theoretically *A. felis*) from tissue after only 10 to 16 days of incubation. *B. henselae* has been cultured from cats (19,42), but a serologic response to *B. quintana* alone has been found in some cats (43). Other species of *Bartonella* may have a role in patients with findings similar to those of CSD (see Chapter 218).

Afipia felis

A. felis is a gram-negative, oxidase-positive rod in the α-2 subgroup of the class Proteobacteria. It was first cultured using brain-heart infusion biphasic medium incubated 1 to 6 days at 32°C aerobically. It is motile and grows on buffered charcoal-yeast extract agar and in nutrient broth. It grows best at 32°C and poorly at 35°C. The genus name is taken from the initials of the Armed Forces Institute of Pathology (AFIP), where it was first cultured, and the species designation after *felis* for cat (8).

EPIDEMIOLOGY

CSD occurs throughout the world where humans have contact with cats. It has been reported from many different countries and throughout the United States. Some authors have suggested that the disease is more common between August and December, and others have observed that the disease is seasonal only in temperate climates and occurs in the seasons when cats spend more time indoors, such as during the winter in the northern climates and during the summer and fall in the southern states (10,44,45). Prevalence of the *Bartonella* bacteremia in animals is most common in summer and early autumn when flea infestations are heaviest, and there seems to be a parallel seasonal increase in the incidence of CSD in humans. Seasonal patterns may reflect variations in the flea population parasitizing the cats, if transmission of the organism parallels transmission of other *Bartonella* species in small mammals. There do not appear to be epidemics of the disease, although there are periods during which physicians are more aware of the disease and thus report it more often. Accurate epidemiologic studies are difficult because the disease is not easily recognized or diagnosed definitively, and most patients with a diagnosis of CSD rarely require admission to the hospital. It has been estimated that 22,000 cases occur each year in the United States and that 2,000 patients are hospitalized (45). Thus, studies of hospital discharge data are not adequate to map the disease.

Traditionally, CSD is a disease of children who have had contact with a kitten. Studies by Margileth and Carithers suggest that about 80% of the cases occur in children, with the highest number occurring in children between 3 and 12 years old (5,6). The incidence of the disease is suspected to be between 6 and 9 cases per 100,000 people (45,46). It is slightly more common in boys than girls and is seen in households with kittens (a cat younger than 1 year) more often than households with older cats. In most series, 90% to 95% of the patients have a history of a contact with a cat; 75% report a scratch or a bite, and the disease may be transmitted by any close contact with a cat. It is thought that cases occurring after traumatic injury, such as a splinter of wood or an insect bite, are due to contact of the cat with the open wound, but proof is lacking. About 4% of the cases in one series occurred after contact with dogs (5), and a few cases

have no history of animal contact. When considering the diagnosis in patients without animal contact, the clinician should consider doing the skin test, serology, or a biopsy because these patients may have lymphadenopathy of another cause. Serologic reactivity or skin test reactivity is more likely to occur in cat owners, households of families of patients with CSD, and veterinary workers (5,10,44). In a case-control study in Connecticut, CSD was strongly associated with owning a kitten, owning a kitten with fleas, and being scratched or bitten by a kitten (20,47). The organism has been cultured from and can be transmitted by fleas (48).

B. henselae and *B. clarridgeiae* have been cultured from the blood of cats, who may remain bacteremic for long periods (months to years) without showing any ill effects or disease or may have pathologic findings similar to humans with CSD (46,49–52). Cats also mount an immune response to *B. henselae* that may protect cats against disease but not against bacteremia (52,53). In general, only one case occurs per family, yet studies using the skin test showed that 18% of family members were positive, with a difference between family members who liked cats (19% reacted) and those who disliked cats (1.5% reacted to the skin test).

PATHOGENESIS

The organism of CSD invades the human by way of a cat scratch, bite, or lick. Silver-staining organisms can be seen on biopsy of a primary papule that forms within 3 to 10 days at the inoculation site (9). Within about 2 to 3 weeks, patients develop regional lymphadenopathy involving one or multiple lymph nodes (5). The histology of the lesions reflects the host response to the organism. Initially, there is a neutrophilic response, and bacteria can be seen around vessels and in microabscesses. Later in the disease, as the node enlarges, lymphoid hyperplasia occurs with stellate necrotizing granulomata (5,8,54). Some lymph nodes have caseous necrosis. Few organisms are found with the silver stain in the tissue in the later stages. The pathologic findings are nonspecific, and without the finding of the organism on Warthin-Starry staining or probing of the tissue with a *Bartonella* species–specific primer, the diagnosis can only be suggested by the pathologist. About 10% of the nodes suppurate, and a fistulous tract may form. The disease usually remits spontaneously in normal hosts but may involve the central nervous system or other organs (6,7,55–58). In the immunocompromised patient, the clinical and pathologic manifestations of the disease are much different, and they are described in Chapter 218; in general, the organism density is greater, and the patients are frequently bacteremic.

CLINICAL MANIFESTATIONS

The most common presenting symptom of a patient with CSD is lymphadenopathy in the region draining the primary inoculation. Sites usually involved (in order of frequency) are the upper extremity, head and neck, and groin (5,20,44) (Table 171.2). The papule at the inoculation site is often unrecognized by physicians not used to dealing with the disease or may disappear by the time the lymphadenopathy is recognized. In a study from Connecticut, only 25% of patients' charts indicated the presence of a primary papule (20). This study was done using a survey mailed to physicians and may represent an atypical group of patients. In Carithers' study of 1,200 patients (including more than 250 he had seen as a primary care physician), 93% had a history of a lesion at the inoculation site (5). The lymphadenopathy

TABLE 171.2.   Presenting Features of Cat-Scratch Disease in Immunocompetent Patients

Feature	Frequency (%)
Adenopathy	95–100
Upper extremity	46–65
Head and neck	26–28
Groin	15–18
Other	8
Inoculation lesion	25–93
Fever	25–48
Malaise or fatigue	20–45
Headache	13
Anorexia	10–14
Splenomegaly	8–12
Parinaud's oculoglandular symptoms	3–6
Sore throat	3–9
Rash	3–4
Arthralgia	3
Conjunctivitis	2–7

Data compiled from references 4–6 and 24.

develops during 2 to 3 weeks but sometimes is not noticed for up to 8 weeks. About 30% to 50% of the patients have fever, and as many as 9% have temperatures as high as 102° to 105°F. In more than three fourths of the patients, the disease is mild, although these patients may have generalized aches, malaise, and anorexia. The lymphadenopathy usually disappears within 2 to 4 months. About 10% of the nodes suppurate and may require drainage or drain spontaneously. A few patients exhibit more unusual presentations, including Parinaud's oculoglandular fever, central nervous system manifestations, fever of unknown origin, granulomatous hepatitis, pulmonary symptoms, or persistent fatigue (7,55,59–63). The spectrum of neurologic symptoms and the list of unusual manifestations are given in Table 171.3. In some patients who present with meningoen-

TABLE 171.3.   Cat-Scratch Disease: Unusual Clinical Manifestations

Neurologic involvement
  Meningoencephalitis
  Combative behavior
  Seizures, including status epilepticus
  Coma
  Neuroretinitis
  Aseptic meningitis
  Facial nerve paralysis
  Myelopathy
  Radiculitis
  Cerebral arteritis
Other
  Granulomatous hepatitis
  Splenic granuloma or splenomegaly
  Fever of unknown origin
  Lytic bone lesions
  Prolonged or recurrent bacteremia
  Erythema nodosum
  Pleural effusion
  Atypical pneumonia
  Synovitis
  Pancytopenia
  Chronic malaise or fatigue
  Thrombocytopenic purpura

cephalitis, seizures (including status epilepticus) are the first recognized feature of CSD. Patients who are immunocompromised may develop widespread disease, including the skin lesions of bacillary angiomatosis, peliosis or microabscesses of the liver and spleen, lytic bone lesions, lymphadenopathy, or persistent bacteremia (46,63–65). A review of these infections is given in Chapter 218.

DIAGNOSIS

Diagnosis of CSD has traditionally relied on certain diagnostic criteria. These included (a) a history of animal contact with the presence of a scratch or primary skin or eye lesion, (b) regional lymphadenopathy developing about 2 weeks after contact, (c) negative studies for other causes, (d) a positive CSD skin test, and (e) a node biopsy revealing histopathologic features consistent with CSD (4). The difficulty with these criteria has been that only a few physicians use the cat-scratch antigen skin test, a serologic assay was not available until 1992, and most patients are not ill enough to warrant lymph node biopsy or require hospital admission.

In primary care practice today, the diagnosis of CSD is generally made clinically when a patient presents with lymphadenopathy after contact with a cat. The presence or history of a papule or pustule at the inoculation site in the absence of other causes of lymphadenopathy supports the diagnosis, and the clinician must rule out other causes. A complete blood count with differential, a rapid plasma reagin test for syphilis, a Monospot or heterophile test for mononucleosis, and a purified protein derivative skin test rule out some more common or treatable causes of lymphadenopathy. Often, physicians treat the patient with antibiotics active against usual suppurative bacteria, and in most series, 50% to 75% of patients have received antibiotics before their lymph node biopsy or referral to a specialist. The cat-scratch skin test is not available because it was never licensed by the U.S. Food and Drug Administration and was prepared using material from infected human lymph nodes. Serologic tests are available (37,39) and in many cases should be positive by the time a lymph node biopsy would be required, but the timing of the immunoglobulin M or immunoglobulin G antibody response varies. False-positive reactions to *Chlamydia* species occur in patients with *Bartonella* infections (66). Serologic responses to *B. henselae* vary from cat to cat and in people with different strain types (37,67,68).

One of the best clues to the diagnosis of CSD is the history of contact with cats. A careful history and consideration of the disease for every patient with chronic regional lymphadenopathy are required. If diagnostic needle aspiration is done, cultures for routine bacteria, mycobacteria, and fungi and cultures to detect *Bartonella* species should be performed. If the clinical course is atypical and the lymphadenopathy does not resolve, biopsy should be considered to rule out malignancy or infectious causes other than CSD. Details of the microbiology of these species may be found in Chapter 218.

TREATMENT

No treatment is required or has been proved effective in most of the cases of CSD in the normal host (57,69). In the normal host with suspected CSD, the most important aspect of treatment is careful follow-up to ensure that the disease resolves spontaneously in 2 to 4 months. If fatigue is present, bed rest may be required, and the patient should avoid trauma to the involved nodes and to the abdomen if the spleen is enlarged. Sometimes analgesics such as aspirin, acetaminophen, or ibuprofen may be used for relief of tender nodes. Warm compresses may provide local relief. Incision and drainage of nodes are not recommended because a chronic sinus tract may develop and persist for months. Needle aspiration of a markedly enlarged lymph node may relieve pain as well as provide material for culture. Biopsy may be indicated to rule out neoplasm.

Systemic antibiotics have not been uniformly successful in normal hosts with CSD (44,70,71). Although Collipp (72) reported oral trimethoprim-sulfamethoxazole effective, other investigators have found little improvement with this agent (70). One study suggests a decrease in volume of affected lymph nodes during therapy with azithromycin compared with controls receiving no treatment (73). Other agents have appeared to be successful, although oxacillin and first-generation cephalosporins appear to be the least active (69,74,75). Rifampin and ciprofloxacin have been reported to be effective (70). For immunocompromised patients, including those with HIV infection, erythromycin has been successful in clearing the bacteremia and skin lesions associated with bacillary angiomatosis (10,14,76) (see Chapter 218). *In vitro*, *B. henselae* is susceptible to many agents, including macrolides, tetracyclines, rifampin, amoxicillin, ceftriaxone, trimethoprim-sulfamethoxazole, and aminoglycosides (74,77). Only aminoglycosides have bactericidal activity (78). Experimental infections in cats have responded to antimicrobials, including doxycycline, ampicillin-clavulanic acid, and quinolones, but the infection is difficult to eradicate and *in vitro* minimal inhibitory concentrations did not parallel clinical response (79,80).

PREVENTION

The best way to prevent CSD is to avoid all contact with cats, especially kittens. Because there are more than 60 million cats in the United States, including 1 in up to 46% of American households (4), CSD is difficult to prevent. The disease seems to occur more often in young cats, and cats may be protected after experimental infection, suggesting that protective immunity may occur in felines (80). It is possible that a vaccine could be developed that could be given to cats at birth to prevent the prolonged bacteremia with *B. henselae*, but it appears that immunity to one serotype does not prevent infections with another strain or with other species of *Bartonella* (81). A vaccine for humans could also be feasible. If fleas or ticks are found on cats, ridding pets of these vectors may decrease the disease in the animals and decrease the transmission to humans. Treatment of pets with antibiotics is another option that has not yet been proved efficacious.

REFERENCES

1. Carithers HA. Cat-scratch disease: notes on its history. *Am J Dis Child* 1970; 119:200.
2. Debre R, Lany M, Jammet M-L, et al. La maladie des griffes de chat. *Bull Mem Soc Med Hop Paris* 1950;154:1247.
3. Daniels W, MacMurray F. Cat scratch disease: report of 160 cases. *JAMA* 1954;154:1247.
4. Margileth AM, Hayden GF. Cat scratch disease: from feline affection to human infection. *N Engl J Med* 1993;329:53.
5. Carithers HA. Cat-scratch disease: an overview based on a study of 1,200 patients. *Am J Dis Child* 1985;139:1124.
6. Margileth AM, Wear DJ, English CK. Systemic cat scratch disease: report of 23 patients with prolonged or recurrent severe bacterial infection. *J Infect Dis* 1987;155:390.
7. Carithers HA, Margileth AM. Cat-scratch disease: acute encephalopathy and other neurologic manifestations. *Am J Dis Child* 1991;145:98.
8. Wear DJ, Margileth AM, Hadfield TL, et al. Cat scratch disease: a bacterial infection. *Science* 1983;221:1403.
9. Margileth M, Wear D, Hadfield T, et al. Cat-scratch disease: bacteria in the skin at the primary inoculation site. *JAMA* 1984;252:928.
10. Adal KA, Cockerell CJ, Petri WA. Cat scratch disease, bacillary angiomatosis, and other infections due to Rochalimaea. *N Engl J Med* 1994;330:1509.
11. Gerber MA, Sedgwick AK, MacAlister TJ, et al. The aetiological agent of cat scratch disease. *Lancet* 1985;1:1236.
12. English CK, Wear DJ, Margileth AM, et al. Cat-scratch disease: isolation and culture of the bacterial agent. *JAMA* 1988;259:1347.
13. Brenner D, Hollis D, Moss C, et al. Proposal of *Afipia* gen. nov., with *Afipia felis* sp. nov. (formerly the cat scratch disease bacillus), *Afipia clevelandensis* sp. nov. (formerly the Cleveland Clinic Foundation strain), *Afipia broomeae* sp. nov., and three unnamed genospecies. *J Clin Microbiol* 1991;29:2450.
14. Koehler J, LeBoit P, Egbert B, et al. Cutaneous vascular lesions and disseminated cat-scratch disease in patients with the acquired immunodeficiency syndrome (AIDS) and AIDS-related complex. *Ann Intern Med* 1988;109:449.
15. Slater LN, Welch DF, Hensel D, et al. A newly recognized fastidious gram-negative pathogen as a cause of fever and bacteremia. *N Engl J Med* 1990;323:1587.
16. Regnery RL, Anderson BE, Clarridge JE 3rd, et al. Characterization of a novel *Rochalimaea* species, *R. henselae* sp. nov., isolated from blood of a febrile, human immunodeficiency virus–positive patient. *J Clin Microbiol* 1992;30:265.
17. Welch DF, Pickett DA, Slater LN, et al. *Rochalimaea henselae* sp. nov., a cause of septicemia, bacillary angiomatosis, and parenchymal bacillary peliosis. *J Clin Microbiol* 1992;30:275.
18. Relman DA, Loutit JS, Schmidt TM, et al. The agent of bacillary angiomatosis: an approach to the identification of uncultured pathogens. *N Engl J Med* 1990;323:1573.
19. Regnery RL, Olson JG, Perkins BA, et al. Serological response to "*Rochalimaea henselae*" antigen in suspected cat-scratch disease. *Lancet* 1992;339:1443.
20. Zangwill KM, Hamilton DH, Perkins BA, et al. Cat scratch disease in Connecticut: epidemiology, risk factors, and evaluation of a new diagnostic test. *N Engl J Med* 1993;329:8.
21. Drancourt M, Birtles R, Chaumentin G, et al. New serotype of *Bartonella henselae* in endocarditis and cat-scratch disease. *Lancet* 1996;347:441.
22. Waldvogel K, Regnery RL, Anderson BE, et al. Disseminated cat-scratch disease: detection of *Rochalimaea henselae* in affected tissue. *Eur J Pediatr* 1994;153:23.
23. Anderson B, Sims K, Regnery R, et al. Detection of *Rochalimaea henselae* DNA in specimens from cat scratch disease patients by PCR. *J Clin Microbiol* 1994;32:942.
24. Dolan MJ, Wong MT, Regnery RL, et al. Syndrome of *Rochalimaea henselae* adenitis suggesting cat scratch disease. *Ann Intern Med* 1993;118:331.
25. Raoult D, Drancourt M, Carta A, et al. *Bartonella* (*Rochalimaea*) *quintana* isolation in patient with chronic adenopathy, lymphopenia, and a cat. *Lancet* 1994;343:977.
26. Alkan S, Morgan MB, Sandin RL, et al. Dual role for *Afipia felis* and *Rochalimaea henselae* in cat-scratch disease [Letter]. *Lancet* 1995;345:385.
27. Kordick DL, Wilson KH, Sexton DJ, et al. Prolonged *Bartonella* bacteremia in cats associated with cat-scratch disease patients. *J Clin Microbiol* 1995;33:3245.
28. Bergmans AM, de Jong CM, van Amerongen G, et al. Prevalence of *Bartonella* species in domestic cats in the Netherlands. *J Clin Microbiol* 1997;35:2256.
29. Gurfield AN, Boulouis HJ, Chomel BB, et al. Coinfection with *Bartonella clarridgeiae* and *Bartonella henselae* and with different *Bartonella henselae* strains in domestic cats. *J Clin Microbiol* 1997;35:2120.
30. Gurfield AN, Boulouis HJ, Chomel BB, et al. Epidemiology of *Bartonella* infection in domestic cats in France. *Vet Microbiol* 2001;80:185.
31. Chomel BB, Carlos ET, Kasten RW, et al. *Bartonella henselae* and *Bartonella clarridgeiae* infection in domestic cats from the Philippines. *Am J Trop Med Hyg* 1999;60:593.
32. Sander A, Zagrosek A, Bredt W, et al. Characterization of *Bartonella clarridgeiae* flagellin (FlaA) and detection of antiflagellin antibodies in patients with lymphadenopathy. *J Clin Microbiol* 2000;38:2943.
33. Welch DF, Carroll KC, Hofmeister EK, et al. Isolation of a new subspecies, *Bartonella vinsonii* subsp. *arupensis*, from a cattle rancher: identity with isolates found in conjunction with *Borrelia burgdorferi* and *Babesia microti* among naturally infected mice. *J Clin Microbiol* 1999;37:2598.
34. Houpikian P, Fournier PE, Raoult D. Phylogenetic position of *Bartonella vinsonii* subsp. *arupensis* based on 16S rDNA and gltA gene sequences. *Int J Sys Evol Microbiol* 2001;51:179.
35. Anonymous. Case records of the Massachusetts General Hospital. Weekly clinicopathological exercises. Case 1-1998. An 11-year-old boy with a seizure [Clinical conference]. *N Engl J Med* 1998;338:112.
36. Kordick DL, Hilyard EJ, Hadfield TL, et al. *Bartonella clarridgeiae*, a newly recognized zoonotic pathogen causing inoculation papules, fever, and lymphadenopathy (cat scratch disease). *J Clin Microbiol* 1997;35:1813.
37. Bergmans AM, Peeters MF, Schellekens JF, et al. Pitfalls and fallacies of cat scratch disease serology: evaluation of *Bartonella henselae*–based indirect fluorescence assay and enzyme-linked immunoassay. *J Clin Microbiol* 1997;35:1931.
38. Del Prete R, Fumarola D, Fumarola L, et al. Detection of *Bartonella henselae* and *Afipia felis* DNA by polymerase chain reaction in specimens from patients with cat scratch disease. *Eur J Clin Microbiol Infect Dis* 2000;19:964.

39. Del Prete R, Fumarola D, Fumarola L, et al. Prevalence of antibodies to *Bartonella henselae* in patients with suspected cat scratch disease (CSD) in Italy. *Eur J Epidemiol* 1999;15:583.
40. Brenner DJ, SP OC, Winkler HH, et al. Proposals to unify the genera *Bartonella* and *Rochalimaea*, with descriptions of *Bartonella quintana* comb. nov., icomb. nov., *Bartonella henselae* comb. nov., and *Bartonella elizabethae* comb. nov., and to remove the family *Bartonellaceae* from the order *Rickettsiales*. *Int J Syst Bacteriol* 1993;43:777.
41. Wong MT, Thornton DC, Kennedy RC, et al. A chemically defined liquid medium that supports primary isolation of *Rochalimaea* (*Bartonella*) *henselae* from blood and tissue specimens. *J Clin Microbiol* 1995;33:742.
42. Olson PE, Wallace MR, Creek JG. Rochalimaea—a cosmopolitan zoonosis? *West J Med* 1994;161:428.
43. Childs JE, Olson JG, Wolf A, et al. Prevalence of antibodies to *Rochalimaea* species (cat-scratch disease agent) in cats. *Vet Rec* 1995;136:519.
44. Margileth A. Cat scratch disease: etiology, diagnosis, and therapy. *Infect Med* 1993;10:38.
45. Jackson L, Perkins B, Wenger J, et al. Cat scratch disease in the United States: an analysis of three national databases. *Am J Public Health* 1993;83:1707.
46. Koehler JE, Glaser CA, Tappero JW. *Rochalimaea henselae* infection: a new zoonosis with the domestic cat as reservoir. *JAMA* 1994;271:531.
47. Chomel BB, Abbott RC, Kasten RW, et al. *Bartonella henselae* prevalence in domestic cats in California: risk factors and association between bacteremia and antibody titers. *J Clin Microbiol* 1995;33:2445.
48. Higgins JA, Radulovic S, Jaworski DC, et al. Acquisition of the cat scratch disease agent *Bartonella henselae* by cat fleas (Siphonaptera: Pulicidae). *J Med Entomol* 1996;33:490.
49. Guptill L, Slater L, Wu CC, et al. Experimental infection of young specific pathogen-free cats with *Bartonella henselae*. *J Infect Dis* 1997;176:206.
50. Kordick DL, Brown TT, Shin K, et al. Clinical and pathologic evaluation of chronic *Bartonella henselae* or *Bartonella clarridgeiae* infection in cats. *J Clin Microbiol* 1999;37:1536.
51. Abbott RC, Chomel BB, Kasten RW, et al. Experimental and natural infection with *Bartonella henselae* in domestic cats. *Comp Immunol Microbiol Infect Dis* 1997;20:41.
52. Kordick DL, Breitschwerdt EB. Relapsing bacteremia after blood transmission of *Bartonella henselae* to cats. *Am J Vet Res* 1997;58:492.
53. O. Reilly K, Parr KA, Brown TP, et al. Passive antibody to *Bartonella henselae* protects against clinical disease following homologous challenge but does not prevent bacteremia in cats. *Infect Immun* 2001;69:1880.
54. Margileth AM. Dermatologic manifestations and update of cat scratch disease. *Pediatr Dermatol* 1988;5:1.
55. Wong MT, Dolan MJ, Lattuada CP Jr, et al. Neuroretinitis, aseptic meningitis, and lymphadenitis associated with *Bartonella* (*Rochalimaea*) *henselae* infection in immunocompetent patients and patients infected with human immunodeficiency virus type 1. *Clin Infect Dis* 1995;21:352.
56. Marra CM. Neurologic complications of *Bartonella henselae* infection. *Curr Opin Neurol* 1995;8:164.
57. Rosen BS, Barry CJ, Nicoll AM, et al. Conservative management of documented neuroretinitis in cat scratch disease associated with *Bartonella henselae* infection. *Aust N Z J Ophthalmol* 1999;27:153.
58. Suhler EB, Lauer AK, Rosenbaum JT. Prevalence of serologic evidence of cat scratch disease in patients with neuroretinitis. *Ophthalmology* 2000;107:871.
59. Dangman BC, Albanese BA, Kacica MA, et al. Cat scratch disease in two children presenting with fever of unknown origin: imaging features and association with a new causative agent, *Rochalimaea henselae*. *Pediatrics* 1995;95:767.
60. Carithers HA. Oculoglandular disease of Parinaud: a manifestation of cat-scratch disease. *Am J Dis Child* 1978;132:1195.
61. Lucey DDM, Moss CW, et al. Relapsing illness due to *Rochalimaea henselae* in immunocompetent hosts: implication for therapy and new epidemiological associations. *Clin Infect Dis* 1992;14:683.
62. Abbasi S, Chesney PJ. Pulmonary manifestations of cat-scratch disease: a case report and review of the literature. *Pediatr Infect Dis* 1995;14:547.
63. Caniza MA, Granger DL, Wilson KH, et al. *Bartonella henselae*: etiology of pulmonary nodules in a patient with depressed cell-mediated immunity. *Clin Infect Dis* 1995;20:1505.
64. Liston TE, Koehler JE. Granulomatous hepatitis and necrotizing splenitis due to *Bartonella henselae* in a patient with cancer: case report and review of hepatosplenic manifestations of *Bartonella* infection. *Clin Infect Dis* 1996;22:951.
65. Ahsan N, Holman MJ, Riley TR, et al. Peliosis hepatis due to *Bartonella henselae* in transplantation: a hemato-hepato-renal syndrome. *Transplantation* 1998;65:1000.
66. Maurin M, Eb F, Etienne J, et al. Serological cross-reactions between *Bartonella* and *Chlamydia* species: implications for diagnosis. *J Clin Microbiol* 1997;35:2283.
67. Pretorius AM, Kelly PJ, Birtles RJ, et al. Isolation of *Bartonella henselae* from a serologically negative cat in Bloemfontein, South Africa. *J S Afr Vet Assoc* 1999;70:154.
68. Guptill L, Slater L, Wu CC, et al. Immune response of neonatal specific pathogen-free cats to experimental infection with *Bartonella henselae*. *Vet Immunol Immunopathol* 1999;71:233.
69. Conrad DAMD. Treatment of cat-scratch disease. *Curr Opin Pediatr* 2001;13:56.
70. Margileth AM. Antibiotic therapy for cat-scratch disease: clinical study of therapeutic outcome in 268 patients and a review of the literature. *Pediatr Infect Dis* 1992;11:474.
71. Margileth AM. Cat scratch disease: a therapeutic dilemma. *Vet Clin North Am* 1987;17:91.
72. Collipp P. Cat-scratch disease therapy. *Am J Dis Child* 1989;143:1261.
73. Bass JW, Freitas BC, Freitas AD, et al. Prospective randomized double blind placebo-controlled evaluation of azithromycin for treatment of cat-scratch disease. *Pediatr Infect Dis* 1998;17:447.
74. Maurin M, Gasquet S, Ducco C, et al. MICs of 28 antibiotic compounds for 14 *Bartonella* (formerly *Rochalimaea*) isolates. *Antimicrob Agents Chemother* 1995;39:2387.
75. Rolain JM, Maurin M, Raoult D. Bactericidal effect of antibiotics on *Bartonella* and *Brucella* spp.: clinical implications. *J Antimicrob Chemother* 2000;46:811.
76. Spach DH, Koehler JE. *Bartonella*-associated infections. *Infect Dis Clin North Am* 1998;12:137.
77. Ives TJ, Manzewitsch P, Regnery RL, et al. In vitro susceptibilities of *Bartonella henselae*, *B. quintana*, *B. elizabethae*, *Rickettsia rickettsii*, *R. conorii*, *R. akari*, and *R. prowazekii* to macrolide antibiotics as determined by immunofluorescent-antibody analysis of infected Vero cell monolayers. *Antimicrob Agents Chemother* 1997;41:578.
78. Musso D, Drancourt M, Raoult D. Lack of bactericidal effect of antibiotics except aminoglycosides on *Bartonella* (*Rochalimaea*) *henselae*. *J Antimicrob Chemother* 1995;36:101.
79. Kordick DL, Papich MG, Breitschwerdt EB. Efficacy of enrofloxacin or doxycycline for treatment of *Bartonella henselae* or *Bartonella clarridgeiae* infection in cats. *Antimicrob Agents Chemother* 1997;41:2448.
80. Greene CE, McDermott M, Jameson PH, et al. *Bartonella henselae* infection in cats: evaluation during primary infection, treatment, and rechallenge infection. *J Clin Microbiol* 1996;34:1682.
81. Yamamoto K, Chomel BB, Kasten RW, et al. Homologous protection but lack of heterologous-protection by various species and types of Bartonella in specific pathogen-free cats. *Vet Immunol Immunopathol* 1998;65:191.

CHAPTER 172
Trichinellosis

Els Mathieu and Peter M. Schantz

HISTORY

Although the disease may date back to antiquity, *Trichinella* species cysts were first recognized in 1835 when, in the midst of an anatomic dissection, Paget noted distinct white flecks distributed throughout a muscle specimen (1). Microscopic examination of this material revealed what was to become recognized as the typical trichina cyst containing a single dormant larva. However, the association between the encysted organism and the ingestion of contaminated meat products was not realized until 1850, when Herbst demonstrated in Germany cysts in the musculature of dogs after they ate meat from an infected animal. In 1862, Friedreich diagnosed and described the first clinical case of acute trichinellosis (2). The first recognized fatality associated with this organism was documented by Zenker in 1860.

ETIOLOGY

Trichinellosis is caused by tissue-dwelling nematodes of *Trichinella* species. Formerly, the etiologic agent was considered a monotypic nematode species, *Trichinella spiralis*. However, there is accumulating evidence of species diversification that has led to taxonomic revision. Currently, seven genetically distinct species exist that vary according to major reservoir hosts and geographic distribution; three other forms exist whose classifications remain to be determined (3,4). *T. spiralis,* adapted to the domestic pig, is historically responsible for most of the infections in the United States and Europe and probably to other regions as well. *Trichinella nelsoni,* transmitted to humans through wild pigs, is found in Africa and southern Europe. *Trichinella murelli* is found in North America (5). *Trichinella nativa* is maintained in Arctic

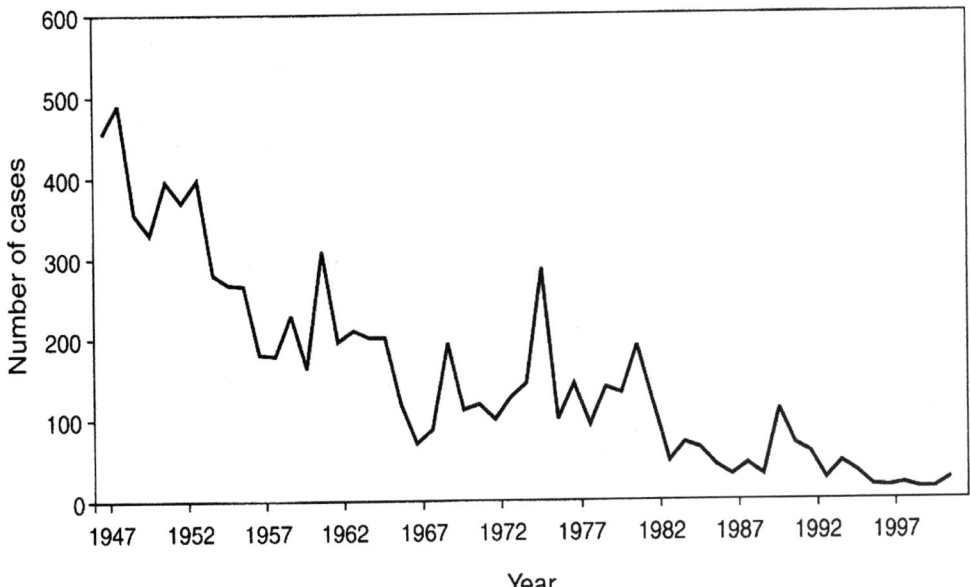

Figure 172.1. U.S. trichinellosis cases, by year, 1947 to 2001. Between 1997 and 2001, an average of 14 cases per year were reported, indicating continued decline. (Reproduced from *MMWR* July 25, 2003, 52:5.)

and sub-Arctic scavenging wildlife (e.g., polar and grizzly bears, arctic and red foxes). *Trichinella britovi* occurs in a variety of carnivores in northern Europe, Asia Minor, and India. *Trichinella pseudospiralis* infects small mammalian and marsupial predators, raptorial birds, and swine and has become increasingly recognized as a cause of human disease (6–8). *Trichinella papuae* was recently described in swine in Papua New Guinea (9). Most of the known variants are capable of infecting humans when ingested.

EPIDEMIOLOGY

Clinical trichinellosis was first reported in the United States in 1864. By the 1880s, this disease was recognized worldwide (2). In the United States, numerous outbreaks involving hundreds of cases were subsequently reported in the literature. Outbreaks occurring in the nineteenth century in Germany were associated with mortality rates between 17% and 30%. Surveys of human cadavers conducted between 1936 and 1941 revealed that one

of every six diaphragmatic muscle samples tested (16.7%) in the United States had *Trichinella* species organisms (10). National reporting of trichinellosis, however, did not begin until 1947, at which time 451 cases and 14 related deaths were documented (11). The incidence of this disease has declined (Fig. 172.1) as a result of legislation prohibiting the feeding of raw garbage to swine (Federal Swine Health Protection Act of 1980), improvements in management of swineherds, widespread commercial and home freezing of pork, and increased public awareness of the dangers of eating inadequately cooked pork products. From 1991 to 1996, an average of 38 cases were reported annually, including three associated fatalities, and during the period 1997 to 2001, the annual incidence of reported cases declined further, to an average of 14 per year with no fatalities (Table 172.1) (12,39). Due to specific food habits, immigrants from Southeast Asia and Europe (German, Italian Eastern European) have been at relatively high risk (13). The decline in human infection has been mainly accounted for by a decline in cases associated with the consumption of pork; however, cases caused by ingestion of meat from a variety of wild animals have continued to be

TABLE 172.1. Regional Cases of Trichinellosis in the United States, 1975–2001

Region	No. of cases (% of total) in indicated region				
	1975–1981	1982–1986	1987–1990	1991–1996	1997–2001
Northeast[a]	589 (55.3)	163 (56.8)	32 (15.5)	31 (13.5)	8 (11.1)
Midwest[b]	166 (15.6)	17 (5.9)	94 (45.6)	83 (36.1)	26 (36.1)
South[c]	131 (12.3)	47 (16.4)	21 (10.2)	23 (10.0)	4 (1.4)
Mountain west[d]	79 (7.4)	37 (12.9)	19 (9.2)	47 (20.4)	31 (43.0)
Alaska	101 (9.5)	23 (8.0)	38 (8.4)	45 (19.6)	6 (8.3)
TOTAL	1,066	287	206[e]	230[e]	72

[a]Includes Maine, New Hampshire, Vermont, Massachusetts, Rhode Island, Connecticut, New York, New Jersey, and Pennsylvania.
[b]Includes Ohio, Indiana, Illinois, Michigan, Wisconsin, Minnesota, Iowa, Missouri, North Dakota, South Dakota, Nebraska, and Kansas.
[c]Includes Delaware, Maryland, Washington DC, Virginia, West Virginia, North Carolina, South Carolina, Georgia, Florida, Kentucky, Tennessee, Alabama, Mississippi, Arkansas, Louisiana, Oklahoma, and Texas.
[d]Includes Montana, Idaho, Wyoming, Colorado, New Mexico, Arizona, Utah, Nevada, Washington, Oregon, California, and Hawaii.
[e]Cases from undefined States included.
Data from references 12, 14, 38, and 39.

TABLE 172.2.   Cases of Trichinellosis in the United States by Reported Food Source, 1975–2001

Food source	No. of cases (% of total) from indicated food source				
	1975–1981	1982–1986	1987–1990	1991–1996	1997–2001
Pork products	749 (70.3)	194 (67.6)	125 (60.7)	80 (59.7)	22 (31)
Domestic	740	172	123	78	21
Wild	9	22	2	2	1
Nonpork products	199 (18.7)	56 (19.5)	48 (23.3)	54 (40.3)	30 (42)
Bear meat	64	42	14	31	29
Other wild animal	68	2	36	23	1
Unknown	118 (11.1)	37 (12.9)	33 (16.0)	0 (0.0)	20 (28)
TOTAL	1,066	287	206	134	72

Data from references 12, 14, 38, and 39.

diagnosed at similar levels as in previous years. Meat from wild animals will probably continue to be an important source of infection (Table 172.2) (12,14).

PATHOGENESIS

Trichinellosis is acquired by eating raw or inadequately cooked meat products containing encysted larvae (Fig. 172.2). Larvae are released after gastric digestion of the cyst wall and invade the mucosa of the small bowel. Within 48 hours, female worms mature and are fertilized. Larval deposition begins within 5 to 6 days. Each female worm is capable of producing up to 1,500 larvae during its lifetime. Larval production generally continues for about 5 weeks before the adult worms are expelled from the intestine as a result of host immune responses (15). Newborn larvae penetrate the mucosa to enter the capillaries and lymphatics of the small intestine, from which they are distributed systemically. Immature larvae that reach striated muscle will enter and induce the myocyte to differentiate into a "nurse cell" unit, which subsequently contributes to and supports the process of encystation. These cystic structures may begin to calcify as early as 6 months after the initial infection; however, larvae may remain viable within cysts for several years. When infection occurs in wild game or animals destined for slaughter, the cycle may be reinitiated when a human eats the infected meat. Larvae that reach nonstriated muscles or other tissues do not encyst. These larvae continue to migrate within the tissues, resulting in marked inflammation and local tissue necrosis. Although this process is usually self-limited, severe multiorgan disease and chronic sequelae may develop.

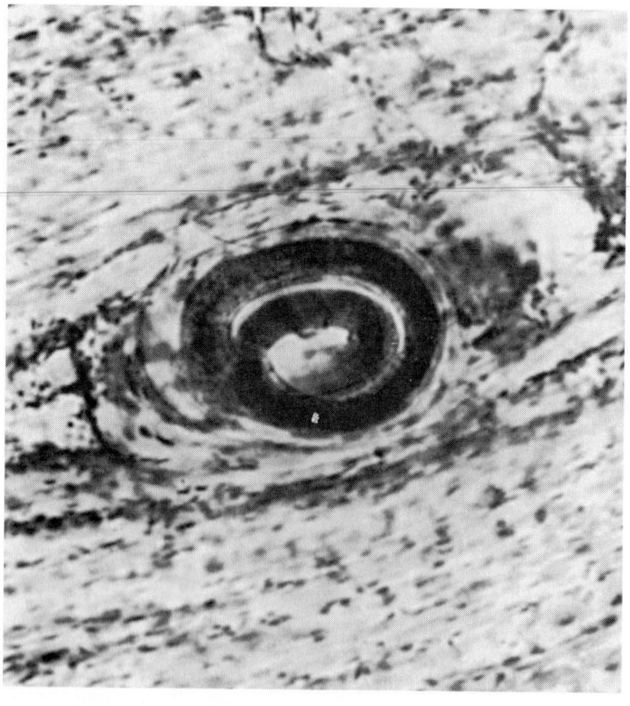

IMMUNOLOGY

Murine models of trichinellosis have provided an important model for the study of the complex mechanisms of host immune response to helminth parasites. Infection with *T. spiralis* elicits a strong immunologic response in the host that causes rapid expulsion of parasites, a reduction in reproductive capacity of the remaining parasites, a reduction in the number of larvae recovered from host muscles, and an impairment of the mobility of worms in the intestines (16–18). The worms are ejected from their niche in the mucosa of the intestine as a result of environmental changes, which makes the intestine inhospitable, and after having suffered damage. *Trichinella* species infections in most host species are characterized by strong protective immune responses against the worms to a primary infection and by high levels of resistance to reinfection.

CLINICAL MANIFESTATIONS

Trichinella species infections can range from asymptomatic or mildly symptomatic to severe life-threatening disease with neurologic and cardiac manifestations. The clinical symptoms and their severity are often correlated with the number and species of larvae ingested and with host factors (5,19). The clinical symptoms parallel the different development stages of the parasite and are frequently grouped into an enteric, a systemic or parenteral (muscular), and a convalescent phase. The incubation time of *T. spiralis*, responsible for most human infections, is generally 5 to 51 days and is inversely related to severity; that is, the shorter the incubation period, the more severe the disease.

Figure 172.2. Section of striated muscle demonstrating encysted *Trichinella* larva.

The intestinal phase is associated with larval penetration of intestinal mucosa. Symptoms during this phase include anorexia, nausea, malaise, upper abdominal pain, diarrhea or constipation, and afebrile state or low-grade fever. Diarrhea can range from mild to resembling severe cholera. Vomiting can persists up to 4 weeks. The enteric phase generally lasts 1 to 2 weeks but can be so mild that it is overlooked.

The parenteral phase begins 1 to 6 weeks after ingestion of larvae in meat. The symptoms are associated with the migration of the larva to striated musculature and other organs (20). A classic trichinellotic syndrome is described, consisting of fever, facial edema, myalgias, muscle swelling, and weakness. However, any organ can be involved, resulting in a wide range of symptoms. Ocular manifestations are common and very useful for diagnosis, especially periorbital edema that is highly suggestive of trichinellosis, especially when associated with peripheral eosinophilia. Edema begins 7 to 21 days after infection and usually lasts a week. Other eye symptoms are conjunctivitis, conjunctival and retinal hemorrhages, chemosis, and eye pain (19). Pneumonitis occurs in less than 5% of hospitalized patients and may be immunologically mediated (2,21). Chest radiographs may reveal pulmonary infiltrates, lesions characteristic of pulmonary vasculitis or disseminated emboli. Other pulmonary symptoms include dyspnea, bronchitis, pleuritis, and cough. Myocarditis and myocardial injury occurs in 20% of hospitalized patients. Symptoms include chest pain, shortness of breath, palpitations, and heart failure (19). Neurologic manifestations can occur in 10% to 24% of the infections and include headache, encephalitis, hemiplegia, convulsions, vertigo, tinnitus, deafness, loss of reflexes, neurologic sensations, paresthesias, focal motor deficits, insomnia, and incontinence (19,20). Mental changes have been reported, including psychosis and depression (22). Patients with neurologic manifestations should be evaluated for silent myocardial injury to exclude cardioneurologic syndrome of trichinellosis, which is characterized by encephalitis, hypereosinophilia (at least 4,000 cells/mm^3), and cardiovascular damage, including infarction (23). The various dermatologic symptoms include pruritus, urticaria, folliculitis, furunculosis, dermatographia, petechiae, and maculopapular skin rash resembling that of measles or rubella. Other symptoms include hot flashes, intermittent or remittent fever, chills, difficulty in speaking, diaphoresis, peripheral edema, diarrhea, constipation, hepatomegaly, splenomegaly, lymphadenopathy, and hoarseness (19,20). Myalgias are common and are characterized by continuous pain or contractions. The pain can be severe and can be accompanied by weakness and limited function and can have the appearance of paralysis (24). The mortality, usually related to congestive heart failure, is low (14).

The convalescent phase is heralded by lysis of fever and improvement in muscular symptoms, usually around week 5 to 6 after infection. Recovery is generally complete, although some patients demonstrate fatigue, weakness, and diarrhea for months after infection. Controversy exists regarding whether "chronic trichinellosis" is a real entity (24–26). Trichinellosis during pregnancy may result in spontaneous abortion, fetal death, placental parasitism, and passage to the fetus (21).

DIAGNOSIS

The diagnosis is based on clinical signs and laboratory findings (20). The classic symptoms of myalgias, periorbital edema, fever, and eosinophilia in a person who has recently eaten undercooked meat products suggests the diagnosis of trichinellosis. A variety of serologic tests have been developed to detect the human antibody response to antigens secreted by L1 (muscle-stage) larvae

(27). For most tests, seroconversion occurs by the third to fourth week after infection; however, antibodies can persist for months to years. Thus, serologic testing is most useful in conjunction with a thorough clinical evaluation. Most techniques, including enzyme-linked immunosorbent assay (ELISA) immunoglobulin G (IgG), indirect hemagglutination (IHA), and immunofluorescence (IF) IgG, have a high sensitivity. By day 14 after infection, clinically ill persons may be positive by ELISA for IgG, and the sensitivity of this assay may reach 100% after day 50 of infection (20). The IgG-ELISA test proved to be the most reliable test for detecting specific immunoglobulins in late (more than 1 year) infections (28). A commonly used test in the United States is the bentonite flocculation test, an IgM antibody test. False-negative and false-positive results are reported (19). The test cannot detect antibodies in the case of early or light infections. The diagnosis of trichinellosis can be made by muscle biopsy, although a negative biopsy does not rule out the disorder. Preferred sampling sites include the deltoid and gastrocnemius muscles. Ova and parasite examination of stool specimens is a low-yield procedure. Adult *Trichinella* species organisms do not produce eggs, newborn larvae are rapidly disseminated systemically from their submucosal location, and adult worms are rarely found in feces.

Differential Diagnosis

The nonspecificity of many of the symptoms associated with trichinellosis results in frequent misdiagnosis. This is particularly true during the intestinal phase, when the symptoms are often confused with those of viral syndrome or food poisoning (29). The parental phase should be distinguished from serum sickness, dermatomyositis, periarteritis nodosa, angioneurotic edema, periorbital edema, cavernous sinus thrombosis, typhoid fever, rheumatic fever, influenza, trypanosomiasis, hypothyroidism, and heart failure. Myositis associated with eosinophilia may occur in visceral larva migrans and, rarely, cysticercosis. Neurologic involvement may be confused with meningitis, encephalitis, cerebral infarct, or polyneuritis. Cardiac and pulmonary symptoms may be suggestive of myocarditis, endocarditis, or ischemic cardiomyopathy and pneumonia.

TREATMENT

The goal of the therapy is to alleviate symptoms and to eliminate the adult and larval-stage nematodes. The benzimidazole compounds are the most effective therapy against the larval stage nematode: mebendazole (200 mg per day for 5 days), albendazole (400 mg per day for 3 days for adults except pregnant women and 5 mg/kg per day for 4 days for children), or pyrantel pamoate (10 mg/kg per day for 5 days) (19,30). Prophylaxis with these agents may effectively prevent disease if they are taken within a few days of eating contaminated food (31). During the parenteral phase of infection, treatment is aimed at reducing muscle damage and eliminating encysted muscle larva and includes mebendazole, 5 mg/kg taken orally twice daily for 10 to 13 days, or albendazole (probably the more effective drug), 15 mg/kg taken orally for 10 to 15 days or until fever and allergic signs recede is indicated. Thiabendazole has also been used effectively, but adverse events are common and can be life threatening (32,33). Concurrent administration of corticosteroids (e.g., prednisone, 40 to 60 mg taken orally daily) is indicated in severe disease characterized by incapacitating symptoms such as prolonged fever or intense hypersensitivity reactions during the illness or associated with anthelminthic therapy (30). Use of the benzimidazole preparations during pregnancy can cause significant toxicity to the embryo and should be undertaken with caution.

PREVENTION

Reliable methods of killing *T. spiralis* larvae in meat include cooking to an internal temperature of 160°F (71°C), usually achieved if the meat is cooked until it is no longer pink inside. Pork cuts less than 6 inches thick can be rendered safe if frozen to 5°F (−17°C) for 20 days, −10°F (−23.3°C) for 10 days, or −20,°F (−28.9°C) for 6 days. Larger pieces require longer exposures or lower temperatures. The larvae of *T. nativa* and some other sylvatic variants are more resistant to freezing.

Curing (salting), drying, and smoking, except under rigidly defined conditions, may not be consistently effective in removing infective larvae. In addition, microwave cooking may not maintain meat at a sufficiently uniform temperature to guarantee elimination of all larvae (34). Low levels of ionizing radiation (0.15 kGy) are sufficient to kill larvae in infected meat (35). Although this process is now approved by the U.S. Food and Drug Administration and official authorities in many other countries, its application for control of trichinellosis requires acceptance by consumers and the industry. Many countries inspect every pig carcass for the presence of *Trichinella* species organisms (36,37).

REFERENCES

1. Kean B, Mott KE, Russel A. Trichinosis in tropical medicine and parasitology. In: Press CU, ed. *Classical investigations,* Vol II. Ithaca, NY: Cornell University Press, 1978.
2. Gould SE. *Trichinosis in man and animals.* Springfield, IL: Charles C Thomas, 1970.
3. Pozio E, Tamburrini A, Sacchi L, et al. Detection of *Trichinella spiralis* in a horse during routine examination in Italy. *Int J Parasitol* 1997;27:1613–1621.
4. Zarlenga DS, Chute MB, Martin A, et al. A multiplex PCR for unequivocal differentiation of all encapsulated and non-encapsulated genotypes of *Trichinella. Int J Parasitol* 1999;29:1859–1867.
5. Pozio E, La Rosa G. *Trichinella murrelli* n. sp: etiological agent of sylvatic trichinellosis in temperate areas of North America. *J Parasitol* 2000;86:134–139.
6. Andrews JR, Ainsworth R, Abernethy D. *Trichinella pseudospiralis* in humans: description of a case and its treatment. *Trans R Soc Trop Med Hyg* 1994;88:200–203.
7. Jongwutiwes S, Chantachum N, Kraivichian P, et al. First outbreak of human trichinellosis caused by *Trichinella pseudospiralis. Clin Infect Dis* 1998;26:111–115.
8. Ranque S, Faugere B, Pozio E, et al. *Trichinella pseudospiralis* outbreak in France. *Emerg Infect Dis* 2000;6:543–547.
9. Pozio E, Owen IL, La Rosa G, et al. *Trichinella papuae* n. sp. (Nematoda), a new non-encapsulated species from domestic and sylvatic swine of Papua New Guinea. *Int J Parasitol* 1999;29:1825–1839.
10. Wright WH, Kerr K, Jacobs L. Studies on trichinosis. XV. Summary of the findings of *Trichinella spiralis* in a random sampling and other samplings of the populations of the United States. *Public Health Rep* 1943;58:1293.
11. Schantz PM. Trichinosis in the United States, 1947–1981. *Food Technol* 1983;March:83.
12. Moorhead A, Grunenwald PE, Dietz VJ, et al. Trichinellosis in the United States, 1991–1996: declining but not gone. *Am J Trop Med Hyg* 1999;60:66–69.
13. Stehr-Green JK, Schantz PM. Trichinosis in Southeast Asian refugees in the United States. *Am J Public Health* 1986;76:1238–1239.
14. Bailey TM, Schantz PM. Trends in the incidence and transmission patterns of trichinosis in humans in the United States: comparisons of the periods 1975–1981 and 1982–1986. *Rev Infect Dis* 1990;12:5–11.
15. Despommier DD. *Immunodiagnosis of parasitic diseases in helminthic diseases,* Vol 1. Orlando, FL: Academic Press, 1986.
16. Wakelin D. *Immunity to parasites: how parasitic infections are controlled.* Cambridge, UK: Cambridge University Press, 1996.
17. Takahashi Y. Antigens of *Trichinella spiralis. Parasitol Today* 1997;:104–106.
18. Bell RG. The generation and expression of immunity to *Trichinella spiralis* in laboratory rodents. *Adv Parasitol* 19998;41:149–217.
19. Murrell KD, Bruschi F. Clinical trichinellosis. *Prog Clin Parasitol* 1994;4:117–150.

20. Capo V, Despommier DD. Clinical aspects of infection with *Trichinella* spp. *Clin Microbiol Rev* 1996;9:47–54.
21. Pawlowski ZS. Clinical aspects in man. In: Campbell WC, ed. *Trichinella and trichinosis.* New York: Plenum Publishing, 1983.
22. Simon JW, Riddell NJ, Wong WT, et al. Further observations on the first documented outbreak of trichinosis in Hong Kong. *Trans R Soc Trop Med Hyg* 1986;80:394–397.
23. Fourestie V, Douceron H, Brugieres P, et al. Neurotrichinosis: a cerebrovascular disease associated with myocardial injury and hypereosinophilia. *Brain* 1993;116:603–616.
24. Ferraccioli GF, Mercadanti M, Salaffi F, et al. [Clinico-biological aspects of myositis due to Trichinella T3 with special regard to a rheumatologic study]. *Ann Ist Super Sanita* 1989;25:641–647.
25. Cox PM, Schultz MG, Kagan IG, et al. Trichinosis: five-year serologic and clinical follow-up. *Am J Epidemiol* 1969;89:651–657.
26. Kassur B, Januszkiewicz J. On the inappropriateness of the idea of chronic trichinellosis. *Epidemiol Rev* 1970;24:68.
27. Gamble HR. Larval (L1) antigens for the serodiagnosis of trichinellosis in swine and other species. In: *Trichinellosis.* Proceedings of the 8th International Conference on Trichinellosis, Orvieto, Italy. Rome: 1st Sup Sanpress, 1994:323–325.
28. Bruschi F, Tassi C, Pozio E. Parasite-specific antibody response in Trichinella sp. 3 human infection: a one year follow-up. *Am J Trop Med Hyg* 1990;43:186–193.
29. Morse JW, Ridenour R, Unterseher P. Trichinosis: infrequent diagnosis or frequent misdiagnosis? *Ann Emerg Med* 1994;24:969–971.
30. Pozio E, Sacchini D, Sacchi L, et al. Failure of mebendazole in the treatment of humans with *Trichinella spiralis* infection at the stage of encapsulating larvae. *Clin Infect Dis* 2001;32:638–642.
31. Ozeretskovskaya N, Pereverzeva E, Tumolskaya N, et al. Benzimidazoles in the treatment and prophylaxis of synanthropic and sylvatic trichinellosis. In: Kim CW, Pawloski ZS, eds. *Trichinellosis.* Hanover, NH: England UPoN, 1978.
32. Cabie A, Bouchaud O, Houze S, et al. Albendazole versus thiabendazole as therapy for trichinosis: a retrospective study. *Clin Infect Dis* 1996;22:1033–1035.
33. Watt G, Saisorn S, Jongsakul K, et al. Blinded, placebo-controlled trial of antiparasitic drugs for trichinosis myositis. *J Infect Dis* 2000;182:371–374.
34. Murrell KD WG, Biehl LG. *Trichinellosis in pork industry handbook.* West Lafayette, IN: Service PUCE, 1991.
35. Loaharanu P, Murrell D. A role for irradiation in the control of foodborne parasites. *Trends Food Sci Technol* 1994;5:190–195.
36. Gamble HR. Detection of trichinellosis in pigs by artificial digestion and enzyme immunoassay. *J Food Prot* 1996;59:295–298.
37. Soule C, Guillou JP, Dupouy-Camet J, et al. Differentiation of *Trichinella* isolates by polymerase chain reaction. *Parasitol Res* 1993;79:461–465.
38. Centers for Disease Control and Prevention. Trichinosis surveillance, United States, 1987–1990. *MMWR Morb Mortal Wkly Rep* 1991;40(SS-3):35–42.
39. Centers for Disease Control and Prevention. Trichinellosis surveillance, United States, 1997–2001. *MMWR Morb Mortal Wkly Rep* 2002;52(SS-6):1–8.

CHAPTER 173
Toxoplasmosis

Rima McLeod and Jack S. Remington

The term *toxoplasmosis* has been used, imprecisely, to refer to both infection and disease caused by *Toxoplasma gondii*. The distinction between infection and disease caused by this organism is important, clinically and epidemiologically (1,2). *Toxoplasma* infection refers to the presence of the protozoan in persons regardless of whether they have clinical manifestations. Toxoplasmosis refers to the disease caused by the organism. *Toxoplasma* infection is usually asymptomatic in older children and adults, but when signs and symptoms are present, they are usually of short duration (acute) and self-limited. Chronic *Toxoplasma* infection describes persistence of the organism in the cyst form without clinical manifestations. The term *chronic toxoplasmosis* is best reserved to describe the disease in which active *Toxoplasma* infection is the proven cause of persistent or recrudescent clinical manifestations (e.g., encephalitis in infants, myocarditis, chorioretinitis, lymphadenopathy). Throughout the world, *Toxoplasma* infection occurs with significantly greater frequency than toxoplasmosis.

CHARACTERISTICS OF THE PATHOGEN

Classification of the Organism

T. gondii is an obligate intracellular protozoan. It has an enteroepithelial and extraintestinal cycle in members of the cat family and only an extraintestinal cycle in all other mammalian and avian hosts. The organism is classified among the Sporozoa and exists in three forms: tachyzoite, bradyzoites in cysts, and oocyst (3–7) (Fig. 173.1). The tachyzoite (Fig. 173.1A–C) is crescent or oval shaped, one end pointed and the other rounded. It measures about 3 by 7 μm. It stains well with either Wright or Giemsa stain. The nucleus is centrally located, and there are no flagella, cilia, or pseudopodia. Tachyzoites are found in tissues during the acute stage of infection and invade all mammalian cells except nonnucleated erythrocytes. Multiplication is by endodyogeny (i.e., two *Toxoplasma* organisms form within each parent cell). Division continues until the host cell ruptures or a tissue cyst forms. Desiccation, freezing and thawing, and gastric secretions kill tachyzoites.

Tachyzoites can be propagated in the peritoneum of mice, in tissue culture, and in eggs. Antigens of tachyzoites are used in complement fixation and hemagglutination tests for diagnosis of *Toxoplasma* infection, and whole tachyzoites are used in the Sabin-Feldman dye test, the agglutination test, and the fluorescent antibody method.

Bradyzoites in Cysts

The tissue cyst (Fig. 173.1D–F) develops within host cells and may contain thousands of organisms. Cysts range in size from 10 to 100 μm and stain well with periodic acid–Schiff stain. The cyst wall also stains with silver. Because cysts may be present in tissues ingested by carnivorous animals or humans, they are important in transmission. It seems probable that they are also the source of recrudescent disseminated infection in immunosuppressed persons and older children and adults who develop chorioretinitis. Cysts are demonstrable as early as the eighth day of infection in animals and may remain viable in multiple tissues throughout the life of the host. Skeletal and heart muscle and brain are the most common sites of chronic (latent) infection in humans, although cysts may exist in virtually every organ. Peptic and tryptic digestive fluids disrupt the cyst wall, thereby liberating viable *T. gondii* bradyzoites, which can survive several hours of exposure to these digestive enzymes. Freezing (20°C) and thawing, heating to 60°C, or desiccation destroys tissue cysts.

Oocysts

The oocyst (Fig. 173.1G–I) is ovoid and measures 10 to 12 μm in diameter. Only members of the cat family have been reported to excrete oocysts (Fig. 173.1H), and cats have systemic infection with *T. gondii* as well. After a cat eats food containing cysts or contaminated with oocysts, *T. gondii* organisms are released into the lumen of the stomach or small intestine. After invasion of the epithelial cells of the small intestine (Fig. 173.1G), the organism undergoes an asexual cycle (schizogony) and then a sexual cycle (gametogony), resulting in development of the noninfectious, unsporulated oocyst (Fig. 173.1H). A cat begins to excrete oocysts 3 to 24 days after the infection, depending on the form of the infecting organism. This excretion continues for 7 to 20 days, and as many as 10 million oocysts may be shed in the feces in a single day. Renewed oocyst excretion has been reported to occur when a cat becomes reinfected with *Toxoplasma* organisms or is acutely infected with *Isospora* species. Maturation (sporulation)

(Fig. 173.1I), which is required for the oocyst to become infectious, occurs only after the oocysts have been excreted. Sporulation occurs in 2 to 3 days at 24°C, in 5 to 8 days at 15°C, and in 14 to 21 days at 11°C. Oocysts do not sporulate in temperatures below 4°C or above 37°C. Under favorable conditions (e.g., warm, moist soil), oocysts remain infectious for several months to more than a year. Dry heat (above 66°C) or boiling water renders oocysts noninfectious. Ingestion of oocysts has been shown to cause infection.

Life Cycle and Modes of Transmission

T. gondii is ubiquitous and can infect herbivorous, omnivorous, and carnivorous animals, including all orders of mammals, some birds, and some reptiles. Most often, it infects humans or other animals when organisms are released from ingested cysts or oocysts. The tachyzoites invade intestinal epithelium and spread hematogenously or through lymphatics to tissues, where they form cysts. When humans or other animals (including the cat) eat infected tissues (from any animal) or mature oocysts (excreted only by members of the cat family), the life cycle is completed. Members of the family Felidae, including both domestic and feral cats, appear to be the definitive hosts in this life cycle because they are the only animals that are known to shed oocysts. Oocysts have been found in the feces of about 1% of cats in diverse areas of the world (including Costa Rica, Germany, Japan, and the United States).

Toxoplasma organisms are acquired mainly by ingestion and transplacental transmission, and less commonly through blood or leukocyte transfusion, organ transplantation (8), and laboratory accident (9) (Fig. 173.2). Reinfection from an exogenous source occurs but has not been recognized as a cause of clinical illness. *T. gondii* infection has occurred in family clusters (10).

INGESTION

T. gondii is acquired principally by eating food containing cysts or contaminated with oocysts. In most areas of the world, about 10% of lamb and 25% of pork contains cysts; the prevalence of cysts in beef is not known. Oocysts are ingested after direct contact with material contaminated by infected cat feces. Flies, cockroaches, and probably other insects can transport oocysts to food. Water, probably contaminated with oocysts, has been suggested to be the means of transmission in one outbreak of toxoplasmosis (11).

TRANSPLACENTAL TRANSMISSION

Toxoplasma may be transmitted transplacentally to the fetus *in utero* or at vaginal delivery. This transmission occurs if infection is acquired by the mother during pregnancy. Infection acquired by the mother during pregnancy most often results in birth of an uninfected infant but may also result in spontaneous abortion, stillbirth, or birth of a premature or full-term infected infant.

About one third of infants born to mothers who acquire infection during pregnancy are infected. Congenital infection is least common in infants born to mothers infected during the first trimester (about 17%), but disease is most severe; congenital infection is most common in infants born to mothers infected during the third trimester (about 65%) but is usually asymptomatic.

Toxoplasma infection that is acquired by the mother during pregnancy is symptomatic in only about 10% to 20% cases, but whether or not the infection is symptomatic, the fetus is still at risk.

The following are guidelines for ascertaining the risk to the fetus of a woman who has been infected before the pregnancy in

TACHYZOITE (acute, active infection)

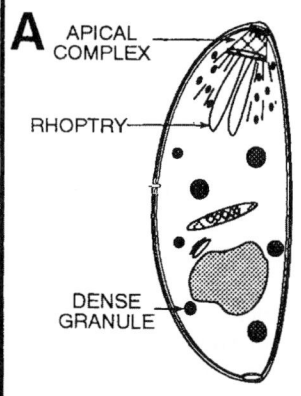

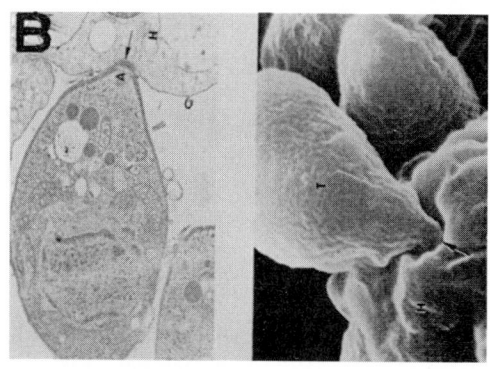

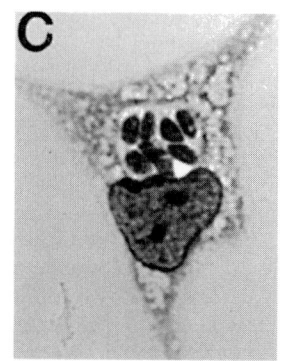

BRADYZOITE IN CYST (latent infection)

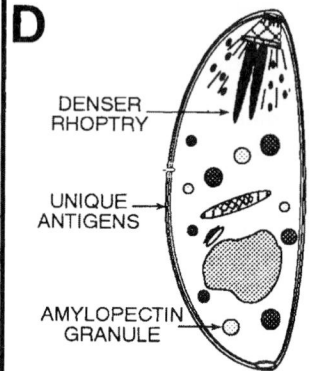

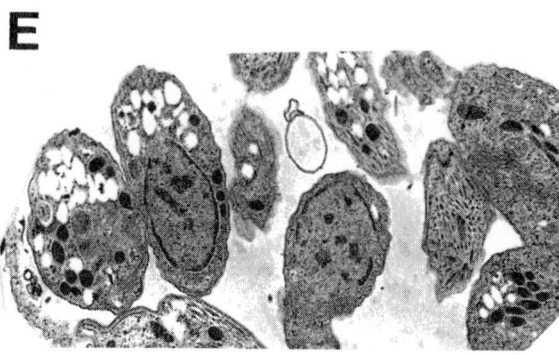

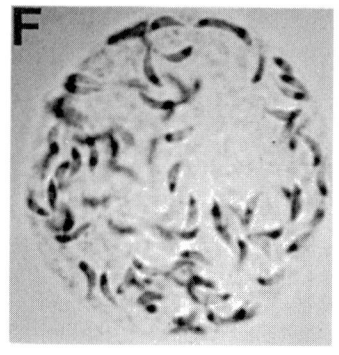

SPOROZOITE IN OOCYST (feline intestine and soil)

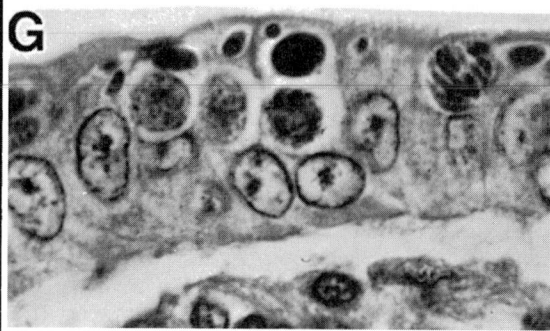

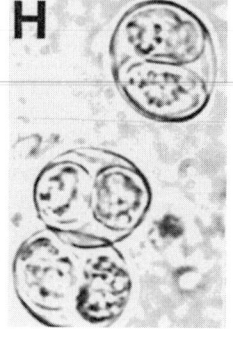

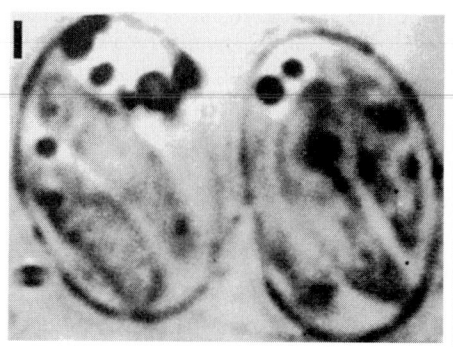

Figure 173.1. Stages of *Toxoplasma gondii*. Tachyzoites: **A:** Schematic diagram. **B:** Transmission and scanning electron micrographs of tachyzoite invading a host cell. **C:** Light micrograph of tachyzoites replicating within a parasitophorous vacuole in the host cell cytoplasm. Bradyzoites: **D:** Schematic diagram. **E:** Transmission electron micrograph of cyst containing bradyzoites, with the arrow indicating amylopectin granules. **F:** Light micrograph of cyst containing bradyzoites. Sporozoites: **G:** Development of oocysts in cat intestine. **H:** Oocysts in lumen of cat intestine. **I:** Sporulating oocysts that contain sporozoites. [From Boyer K, McLeod R. *Toxoplasma gondii* (toxoplasmosis). In: Long SS, Proeber GC, Pickering LK, eds. *Principles and practice of pediatric infectious diseases.* New York: Churchill Livingstone, 1996:645–672.

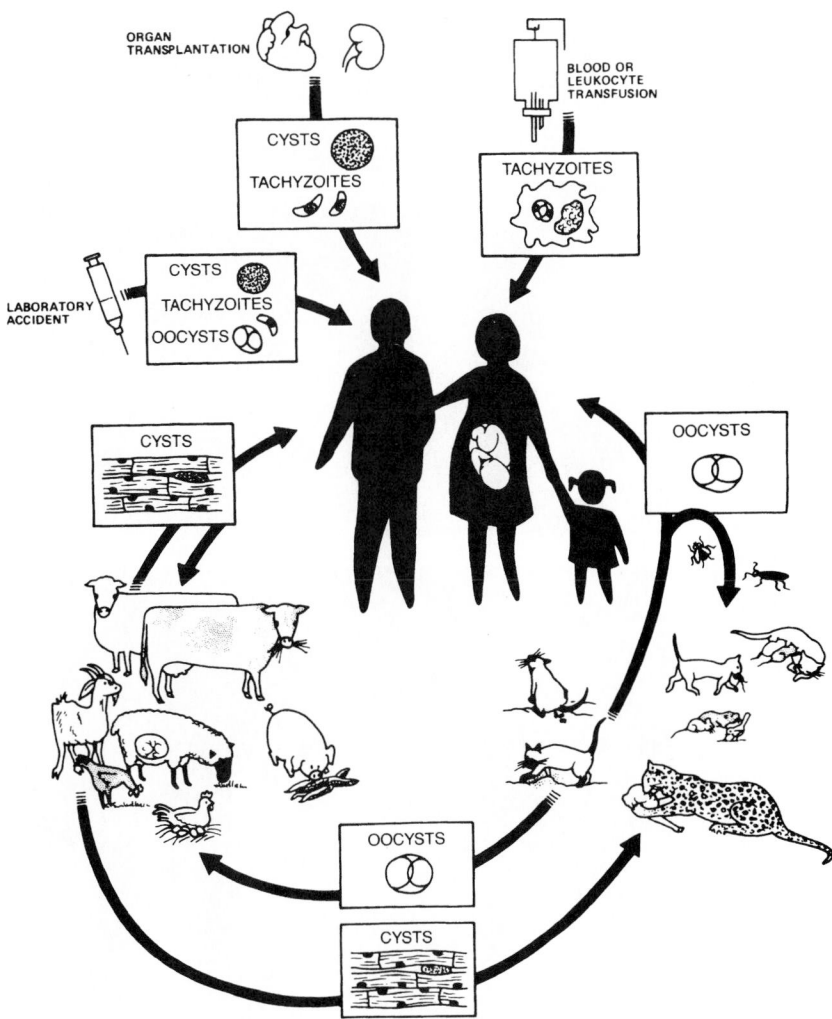

Figure 173.2. Life cycle and modes of transmission of *Toxoplasma gondii*. Infection in humans and other animals occurs primarily after ingestion of either the cyst or the oocyst. Released organisms invade the intestinal epithelium, spread to tissues (either hematogenously or through lymphatics), and form cysts. When humans or other animals (including the cat) eat infected tissues (from any animal) or mature oocysts (excreted only by members of the cat family), the life cycle is completed. Laboratory accidents, organ transplantation, and blood and white blood cell transfusion have also been implicated in transmission of the organism. (From Remington JS, McLeod R. Toxoplasmosis. In Braude AI, ed. *International textbook of medicine*, Vol II. *Medical microbiology and infectious diseases*. Philadelphia: WB Saunders, 1981:1816–1832, with permission.)

question:

- An immunocompetent woman who acquired *Toxoplasma* infection more than 6 months before gestation does not deliver an infected infant.
- When conception occurs less than 6 months after acquisition of the infection, the risk to the fetus is exceedingly low, but transplacental transmission has been documented in this setting.
- *Toxoplasma* organisms have been isolated on rare occasions from abortuses of women with chronic (latent) infection. The frequency of *Toxoplasma* infection as a cause of abortion is unknown and is a controversial subject.

TRANSMISSION THROUGH BREAST-FEEDING

Transmission by human milk has not been demonstrated. It might occur if infection were acquired in the last weeks of gestation; however, the incidence of transplacental transmission approaches 100% if infection is acquired at this time, so the possible additional risk associated with breast-feeding would be insignificant.

TRANSMISSION BY BLOOD OR LEUKOCYTE TRANSFUSION OR ORGAN TRANSPLANTATION

Parasitemia has been reported to persist in otherwise normal persons for up to 1 year after acquisition of infection, and *Toxoplasma* organisms have been recovered from leukocytes of persons who have no recognized clinical evidence of *Toxoplasma* infection. The organism can survive for up to 50 days in whole citrated blood stored at 4°C. This poses a particular threat to immunodeficient patients who require multiple blood transfusions. *Toxoplasma* has been transmitted by heart, bone marrow, liver, and kidney transplantation from acutely infected donors to recipients who were not previously infected with *Toxoplasma* and has caused morbidity and death.

Figure 173.1. (*continued*) **A** from McLeod R, Mack D, Brown C. New advances in cellular and molecular biology of *Toxoplasma gondii*. *Exp Parasitol* 1991;72:109–121; **B** and **C** from Aikawa M, Komata Y, Asai T, et al. Transmission and scanning electron microscopy of host cell entry by *Toxoplasma gondii*. *Am J Pathol* 1977;87:285–296; **F** from Weiss L, LaPlace D. Bradyzoite development in vitro. *J Eukaryot Microbiol* 1995;42:150–157; **G** from Remington JS. In discussion, Lainson R. Observations on the nature and transmission of *Toxoplasma gondii* in light of its wide host and geographical range. Toxoplasmosis. *Surv Ophthalmol* 1961;6:721–758; **H** from Dubey JP, Miller NL, Frenkel JK. The *Toxoplasma gondii* oocyst from cat feces. *J Exp Med* 1970;132:636–662; **I** from Dubey JP, unpublished, with permission.]

PATHOGENESIS

After their release from cysts or oocysts, the organisms enter gastrointestinal cells, where they multiply, disrupt cells, and infect contiguous cells. Extracellular organisms or organisms within leukocytes may be transported through the lymphatics and bloodstream to every organ and tissue. Proliferating tachyzoites usually produce necrotic foci of invaded cells surrounded by an intense cellular reaction. The outcome of the acute process depends on both humoral and cell-mediated immunity. In some apparently normal people, and especially in immunodeficient persons, the acute infection may progress and cause potentially lethal lesions, such as acute necrotizing encephalitis, pneumonitis, or myocarditis. With development of the normal immune response, tachyzoites disappear from the tissues.

A unique aspect of the infection is that organisms persist as cysts in multiple organs for the life span of the host. The tissue cysts, which are characteristic of chronic infection, provoke little or no inflammatory response. Either rupture of cysts or persistence of viable tachyzoites within monocytes and macrophages may be the source of recurrent parasitemia in some asymptomatic persons who have chronic infection. Cysts are the likely source of organisms that cause recrudescent disease in immunocompromised patients or chorioretinitis in older children and adults with congenital toxoplasmosis.

PATHOLOGY

The meager information on the pathologic changes of toxoplasmosis in immunologically normal persons is derived largely from lymph node biopsy because most of these infections are asymptomatic and self-limited. Limited information is available concerning changes in other organs. Pathology has been defined most clearly in congenitally infected infants and in immunosuppressed patients with disseminated infection.

The degree of organ and tissue involvement of infants with congenital infection varies considerably. In some, autopsy reveals only central nervous system (CNS) and eye involvement, whereas in others, there is wide dissemination of lesions and organisms. The CNS is never spared. In extraneural organs, whose tissues can regenerate, residual lesions may be so slight that they are easily overlooked. In the CNS and eye, on the other hand, the inability of nerve cells to regenerate leads to more severe, permanent damage.

The pathologic changes described in the following are the same in adults and in congenitally infected infants unless otherwise specified.

Lymph Node

In older children and adults, the histopathologic changes in toxoplasmic lymphadenitis are distinctive (12) (Fig. 173.3). The characteristic lesion is a reactive follicular hyperplasia, with irregular clusters of epithelioid histiocytes that encroach on and blur the margins of germinal centers. There is also an associated focal distention of sinuses with monocytoid cells. Giant cells are absent, and *T. gondii* can be demonstrated only rarely.

Eye

The earliest changes in the eye are single or multiple foci of necrosis. The infiltrate consists largely of lymphocytes, plasma cells, and mononuclear phagocytes (13). Intracellular and extracellular tachyzoites and numerous cysts may be found in the retinal

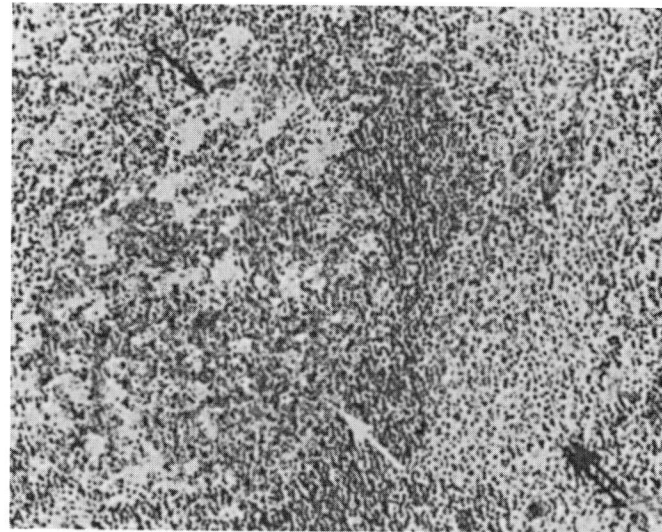

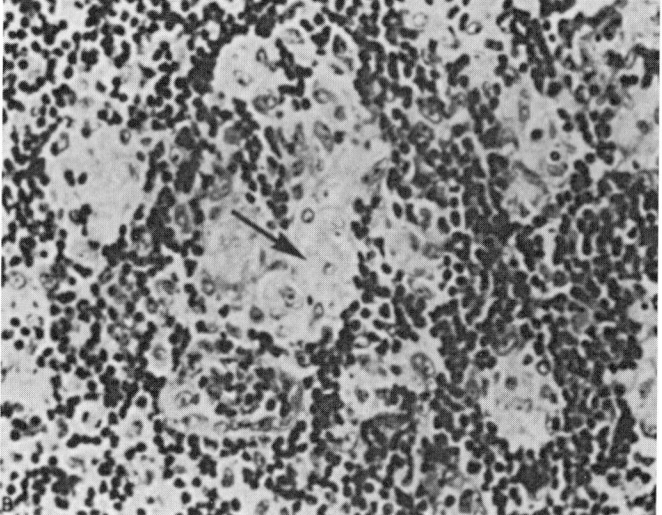

Figure 173.3. Characteristic lymph node pathology in lymphadenitis caused by *Toxoplasma* species. **A:** Epithelioid cells (*black arrow*) encroach on and blur margins of germinal center (*white arrow*), and there is focal distention of subcapsular and trabecular sinuses by monocytoid cells (*double black arrows*). **B:** Irregular clusters of epithelioid cells (*arrow*) scattered throughout paracortical lymphoid stroma. (**A** and **B** from Dorfman RF, Remington JS. Value of lymph-node biopsy in the diagnosis of acute acquired toxoplasmosis. *N Engl J Med* 1973;289:878–881, with permission.)

lesions. It has been suggested that the retinitis originates from cyst rupture. Granulomatous inflammation of the choroid is secondary to the necrotizing retinitis. Iridocyclitis, glaucoma, and cataracts may occur as complications of the chorioretinitis.

Central Nervous System

In acute infection, there is a focal or diffuse meningoencephalitis, with necrosis and microglial nodules. Multinucleated giant cells are not a characteristic feature. Perivascular mononuclear inflammation is frequent and is contiguous to areas of necrosis. Occasionally, there is necrosis of vessel walls. Areas of necrosis may mimic mass lesions, and intracellular and extracellular tachyzoites are usually found at the periphery of areas of necrosis. Cysts in the brain may occur during acute infection or reflect infection of long duration (Fig. 173.4). The extent and location of CNS involvement, as well as the size of lesions, vary

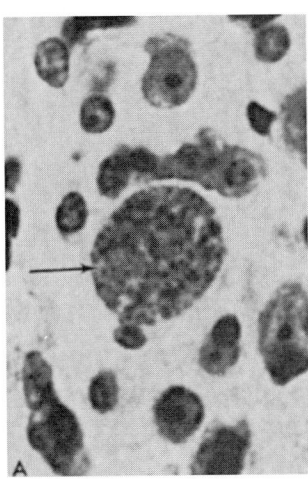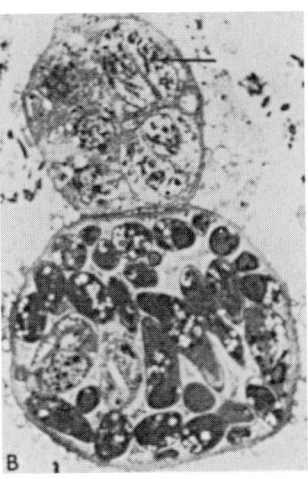

Figure 173.4. Infection of the central nervous system (CNS) with *Toxoplasma* species. **A:** Cyst in brain (*arrow*) is seen in acute infection as early as 8 days, or in chronic (latent) infection. **B:** Electron micrograph of CNS *Toxoplasma* species infection. The diagnosis may be established by electron microscopic identification of the organism (*arrow*) when light microscopic examination is not definitive. (**A** and **B** from Ghatak NR, Poon TP, Zimmerman HM. Toxoplasmosis of the central nervous system in the adult: a light and electron microscopic study of three cases. *Arch Pathol* 1970;89:337–348, with permission.)

considerably. The lesions in the CNS in adults and congenitally infected infants are similar. Periaqueductal or periventricular vasculitis with necrosis is a unique aspect of severe congenital infection. Necrotic tissue sloughs into the ventricles, obstructing the aqueduct of Sylvius or the foramen of Monro and causing hydrocephalus. Obstruction of the aqueduct of Sylvius in congenitally infected persons may also occur later in life. The pathogenesis of this lesion has not been delineated. Calcification of necrotic areas is especially prominent in congenital infection but rarely may also occur in older children or adults.

Lung

Pulmonary infection may cause clinically significant interstitial pneumonitis in congenitally infected infants, in immunocompromised patients, and sometimes, in persons who have no apparent underlying disease. In each of these settings, there are thickened and edematous alveolar septa that, along with peribronchial areas, may be infiltrated with mononuclear cells, occasional plasma cells, and rare eosinophils. The walls of small blood vessels may also be infiltrated with lymphocytes and mononuclear cells, and *Toxoplasma* may be present in endothelial cells. Both tachyzoites and cysts have been seen within alveolar lining cells. Necrosis within granulomatous foci is prominent in some patients with disseminated toxoplasmosis and malignancy but is rarely seen in infants or in patients without malignancy. In many cases, there is some bronchopneumonia, often caused by superimposed infection with other organisms.

Heart

Myocarditis is associated with congenital infection, infection of immunocompromised persons, and, rarely, severe acute infection of apparently otherwise healthy persons. In patients with acquired immunodeficiency syndrome (AIDS) who die with toxoplasmosis, autopsies have revealed involvement of the heart and lung in 40% to 70% of cases. Cysts and large aggregates of tachyzoites occur within muscle fibers (Fig. 173.1C). Single organisms

are found adjacent to and within areas of necrotic tissue. Foci of inflammatory cells (lymphocytes, plasma cells, mononuclear cells, and occasionally eosinophils) are associated with hyaline necrosis and fragmentation of myocardial cells, usually without organisms. Hemorrhagic pericarditis has also been reported in some patients with toxoplasmosis.

Kidney

In congenital toxoplasmosis and disseminated infection in older children and adults, the pathologic changes in the kidney resemble those in other organs (i.e., necrosis and the presence of cysts, tachyzoites, and inflammatory cells). Necrosis may occur in both glomeruli and tubules. In addition, glomerulonephritis with deposits of immunoglobulin M (IgM), fibrinogen, and *Toxoplasma* antigen and antibody has been reported.

Other Sites

The organisms and foci of necrosis have been found in the adrenal cortex, testes, and ovaries of infected infants; and *Toxoplasma* organisms, usually without inflammation, have been found in the pituitary. In infected infants and adults, cysts or tachyzoites, with or without inflammation, have been reported in multiple organs, including liver, spleen, bone marrow, thyroid, pancreas, adipose tissue, and skin. Involvement of pancreas, stomach, and intestine in patients with AIDS and toxoplasmosis is striking. Involvement of skeletal muscles varies from parasitized fibers without pathologic changes to focal areas of infiltration or widespread myositis with necrosis.

Immunologic Abnormalities

Monoclonal gammopathy of the IgG class has been described in infants with congenital toxoplasmosis. IgM levels may be elevated in newborns with congenital toxoplasmosis. Circulating immune complexes have been detected by C1q-binding assay in sera from adults with the systemic, febrile, and lymphadenopathic forms of toxoplasmosis and in an infant with congenital toxoplasmosis but not after signs and symptoms resolved. Reversible IgA deficiency has been reported in infants with congenital toxoplasmosis.

Marked and prolonged alterations in T-lymphocyte subpopulations are associated with *T. gondii* infection, which can be correlated with disease syndromes but not necessarily with disease outcome. Some patients with prolonged fever and malaise exhibit lymphocytosis, increased numbers of suppressor T cells, and a depressed helper-to-suppressor T-cell ratio. Some patients have fewer helper cells even when they are asymptomatic. Sometimes, with lymphadenopathy, the number of helper cells diminishes for longer than 6 months after onset of infection. Asymptomatic patients have abnormal T-cell subpopulations. Some patients with disseminated disease have a markedly reduced number of T cells and a markedly depressed ratio of helper-to-suppressor lymphocytes.

CLINICAL MANIFESTATIONS

Lymphadenopathy and Other Manifestations

The most commonly recognized clinical manifestation of acute acquired toxoplasmosis is lymphadenopathy (14). The cervical nodes (either a single posterior one or multiple nodes) are involved most frequently, and discovery of their involvement is often incidental. Asymptomatic lymphadenopathy may mimic lymphoma. Involvement of a pectoral node may be mistaken for carcinoma of the breast in females. Suboccipital, supraclavicular, axillary, and inguinal nodes are involved frequently. It is important to recognize that mediastinal, mesenteric, and retroperitoneal nodes may also be involved. With infection of the mesenteric or retroperitoneal nodes there may be abdominal pain and fever, with a temperature to 40°C. Involved lymph nodes are usually discrete and vary in firmness; they may be tender but do not suppurate. Confusion, malaise, fever, stiff neck, myalgias, arthralgias, headache, sore throat, maculopapular rash (which spares the palms and soles), urticaria, hepatosplenomegaly, hepatitis, or reactive lymphocytes may occur. In one epidemic, 35 of 37 persons who had serologic evidence of acute acquired *Toxoplasma* infection had signs or symptoms of infection. Although 25 persons consulted physicians, toxoplasmosis was correctly diagnosed in only three. The lymphadenopathic form of toxoplasmosis is self-limited, but lymphadenopathy or malaise may persist or recur for months. If toxoplasmosis is in the differential diagnosis in a patient with lymphadenopathy, serologic studies to exclude acute *T. gondii* infection should be performed before lymph node biopsy to exclude lymphoma.

Rarely, someone whose immune system seems to be normal may develop any of the following, alone or in combination: myocarditis, pericarditis, pericardial effusion, polymyositis, hepatitis, pneumonitis, encephalitis, or meningoencephalitis. None of the signs or symptoms resulting from involvement of these organs is specific for infection with *T. gondii*. Some of these patients have died.

Ocular Involvement

Toxoplasma has been estimated to cause about 35% of the cases of chorioretinitis in the United States and in Central and Western Europe. In older children and adults, ocular disease is most frequently a consequence of congenital *Toxoplasma* infection, but chorioretinitis does occur in patients with acute acquired *Toxoplasma* infection. In Erecim, Brazil, toxoplasmic chorioretinitis occurs in about 18% of the 80% of adults who acquire *T. gondii* (15). Severe ocular disease may be associated with the more virulent type I strain parasites or recombinant parasites (16).

The frequency of *Toxoplasma* chorioretinitis is lower than that of cytomegalovirus retinitis in patients with AIDS, but it does occur, usually in conjunction with CNS or systemic infection. Active chorioretinitis may produce blurred vision, scotomata, pain, photophobia, or epiphora. Central vision may be impaired or lost if the macula is involved. Strabismus may be an early sign of chorioretinitis in children. In congenital toxoplasmosis, microophthalmia, small cornea, posterior cortical cataract, anisometropia, strabismus, nystagmus, and leukocoria also occur. Nystagmus may result either from poor fixation related to the chorioretinitis or from involvement of the CNS. Convergent or divergent strabismus may be caused by involvement of extraocular muscles or the brain. Associated systemic signs of infection are uncommon. Because ocular involvement may cause the only clinical sign of infection in newborns, newborn infants suspected to have congenital toxoplasmosis require ophthalmologic examination to exclude toxoplasmosis. As inflammation subsides, vision improves but often incompletely. Episodic flares of chorioretinitis are common and destroy retinal tissue. Such multiple recurrences may result in glaucoma.

On ophthalmoscopic examination, the acute lesions appear as yellowish white, cottony patches that have elevated, indistinct margins surrounded by a zone of hyperemia. The inflammatory exudate in the vitreous may obscure the fundus. Older lesions are atrophic, whitish gray plaques with distinct borders

and black spots of choroidal pigment. The lesions may be single or, more commonly, multiple and are usually located near the posterior pole of the retina, although they may be peripheral. Lesions of varying age may be seen simultaneously (Fig. 173.5A). Less common are panuveitis and papillitis with optic atrophy. Isolated anterior uveitis related to toxoplasmosis has never been proved. Infants with congenital toxoplasmosis may have (a) unilateral or bilateral macular involvement, (b) other unilateral or bilateral lesions, (c) peripheral involvement in one or more quadrants of the retina and choroid, (d) punched-out lesions in the late phase, (e) massive chorioretinal degeneration,

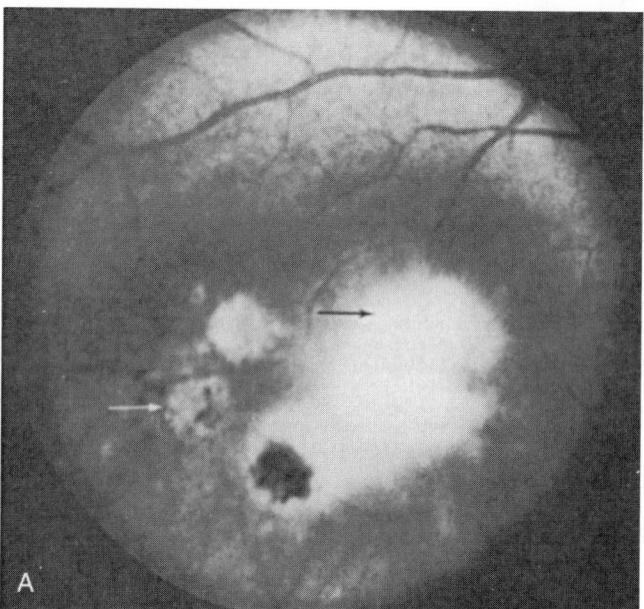

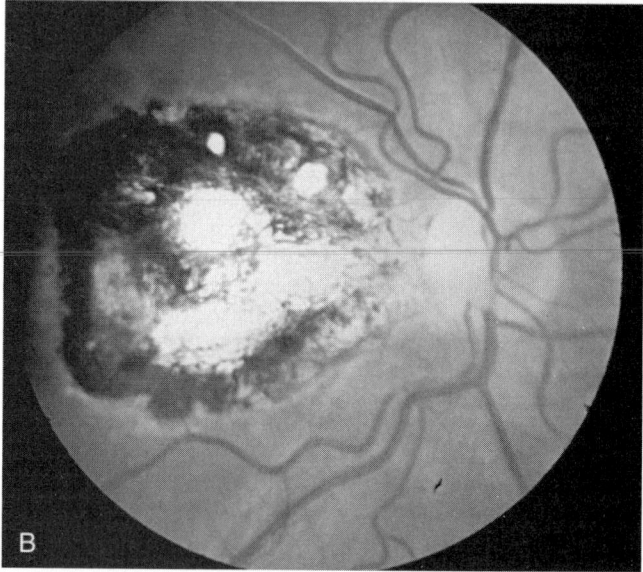

Figure 173.5. A: Chorioretinitis caused by *Toxoplasma* species. The characteristic lesion is a focal necrotizing retinitis with cotton-like patches in the fundus. Note that the acute lesions (*black arrow*) have indistinct borders and appear soft and white, whereas older lesions (*white arrow*) are whitish gray, sharply outlined, and spotted by accumulations of choroidal pigment. **B:** Toxoplasmic chorioretinitis in a patient with AIDS. (**A** from O'Connor GR. Ocular toxoplasmosis. In: Locatcher-Khorazo D, Seegal BC, eds. *Microbiology of the eye.* St. Louis: CV Mosby, 1972:199; **B** from Polis MA. Differential diagnosis of retinal lesions in persons with HIV infection. *Opportunistic Infect Interaction* 1994;3:1, with permission.)

(f) extensive fibrosis and heavy pigmentation (in contrast to the dissociation of these changes in other chorioretinal lesions), (g) normal retina and vasculature surrounding the lesions throughout the infection, (h) rapid development of sequential optic nerve atrophy, and (i) clarity of the media despite severe chorioretinitis. In patients with AIDS, *Toxoplasma* retinal lesions are often large, and there is diffuse necrosis of the retina with substantial numbers of encysted organisms and free tachyzoites. They usually do not have well-developed granulomatous chorioiditis, significant inflammatory, cell infiltrate, or preexisting chorioretinal scar formation (Fig. 173.5B).

Toxoplasmosis in Immunocompromised Patients

All forms of toxoplasmosis that occur in normal persons also occur in those whose immune system is compromised (17–19). Acute toxoplasmosis in an immunocompromised patient may be due to reactivation of latent infection or to acquisition of infection from exogenous sources, including organ transplants and blood or leukocyte transfusion (20). Immunosuppressed patients with the greatest predilection for life-threatening toxoplasmosis are those with AIDS and those receiving immunosuppressive therapy for lymphoproliferative disorders (especially Hodgkin's disease), hematologic malignancy, or prevention of organ graft rejection. Although not frequent, toxoplasmosis in bone marrow recipients is often severe and lethal and, because the manifestations are protean, not diagnosed during life (21). Disease is often fulminant and rapidly fatal in immunocompromised patients, and because effective therapy is available, it is incumbent on clinicians to be aware of the clinical presentation in this type of patient. An emerging problem is infants born with both human immunodeficiency virus (HIV) and *T. gondii* infection. This results from reactivation of toxoplasmosis in the HIV-infected mother. CNS toxoplasmosis is among the 10 most commonly occurring opportunistic infections and malignancies in patients with AIDS and a significant cause of mortality and morbidity, even in the era of highly active antiretroviral therapy (HAART) and trimethoprim-sulfamethoxazole (TMP-SMX) prophylaxis. Toxoplasmic encephalitis remains one of the major CNS presentations of AIDS, even in the era of HAART. Reported lifetime risk for developing CNS toxoplasmosis for seropositive AIDS in the era of HAART patients is 6% to 12%, with a mortality rate of more than 50%. *T. gondii* causes 20% of intracerebral infections of AIDS patients, often undiagnosed until autopsy.

The most characteristic clinical manifestations of toxoplasmosis in immunocompromised patients result from brain involvement, which is present in more than 50% of documented cases. The symptoms and signs are manifestations of diffuse encephalopathy, meningoencephalitis, or cerebral mass lesions and include changes in mental status, headache, seizures, and focal neurologic deficits. In AIDS patients, *Toxoplasma* encephalitis is fatal without treatment. It is the major cause of focal intracerebral lesions in AIDS. At least 30% of persons who have HIV infection and antibodies to *T. gondii* will develop *Toxoplasma* encephalitis if they are not receiving prophylaxis. It may be the presenting manifestation of AIDS. Geographic origin (e.g., residence in Germany and France, where meat is consumed raw or undercooked), proximity to cats that may be excreting oocysts, and dietary habits (e.g., exposure to undercooked meat) may suggest that *T. gondii* infection is likely. Typical findings include fever (in 10% to 74% of patients), headache (56%), altered mental status, psychosis, cognitive impairment, seizures (33%), and focal neurologic defects (60%), including hemiparesis, aphasia, ataxia, visual field loss, cranial nerve palsies, dysmetria, or movement disorders. Uncommon findings include meningismus; involve-

ment of heart, abdomen, or testes; panhypopituitarism; and the syndrome of inappropriate secretion of antidiuretic hormone. Between 97% and 99% of patients with AIDS and *Toxoplasma* encephalitis have IgG antibody to *T. gondii* in serum; however, *Toxoplasma* IgM antibodies are usually not demonstrable. Intrathecal antibody production may be present. A therapeutic trial of antitoxoplasma medications in AIDS patients who have characteristic findings on neuroradiologic imaging studies is often used to help establish this diagnosis. Alternative causes are sought by brain biopsy if the patient fails to respond clinically or "radiographically." Time to resolution at computed tomography (CT) usually varies between 20 days and 6 months. Positron emission tomographic scans appear to be useful in differentiating toxoplasmic encephalitis (hypometabolic lesions) and lymphoma (hypermetabolic lesions).

Areas of predilection for CNS toxoplasmosis in patients with AIDS are the basal ganglia and corticomedullary junction. Lesions may occur anywhere and are generally enhanced when contrast is administered. Magnetic resonance imaging is significantly more sensitive than CT and frequently reveals multiple focal lesions in patients with toxoplasmic encephalitis who have only a single lesion at CT.

Persons who have not been infected previously with *Toxoplasma* and receive a heart transplant from an infected person often develop signs and symptoms of toxoplasmosis. The diagnosis of brain involvement can be made by finding tachyzoites in a biopsy specimen or in material aspirated from mass lesions that resemble a brain abscess at CT. The cerebrospinal fluid (CSF) typically shows mononuclear pleocytosis, a moderate elevation in protein concentration, and a normal glucose level. In any immunosuppressed patient with symptoms or signs of brain involvement, the diagnosis of toxoplasmosis must be excluded. Other manifestations of the disease in immunocompromised patients may be nonspecific or reflect inflammation and necrosis of the organs involved, particularly the heart and lungs.

T. gondii infection has also been transmitted by liver transplantation and resulted in multiorgan failure in the early period after liver transplantation. We recommend serologic testing to detect acute acquired *T. gondii* infection in the evaluations of all organ donors and recipients because, in a number of instances, disseminated infection has resulted from transplantation of an organ from an individual with acute acquired infection into a seronegative recipient.

Toxoplasmosis and *Toxoplasma* Infection in Pregnant Women

Toxoplasma infection acquired in pregnancy causes symptoms in only about 10% to 20% of mothers, but the fetus is at risk whether symptoms are present or not. Guidelines on toxoplasmosis and *Toxoplasma* infection in pregnant women were offered earlier (in the section "Transplacental Transmission").

Congenital Toxoplasmosis

Most infected newborns have no symptoms at birth and may suffer untoward sequelae of the infection: without treatment most develop chorioretinitis, about half with impairment of vision, by the time they reach adolescence (22–24). Less frequent manifestations of infection include strabismus, blindness, epilepsy, and psychomotor or mental retardation, which may occur weeks, months, or even years later. Those with clinically apparent infection at birth may have all or any combination of the following signs: mild nonspecific illness, fever, hypothermia, vomiting, diarrhea, jaundice, rash (most commonly petechiae caused by thrombocytopenia), hydrocephalus, microcephaly, cerebral calcifications, microphthalmia, strabismus, cataracts, glaucoma, chorioretinitis, optic atrophy, deafness, lymphadenopathy, pneumonitis, myocarditis, hepatosplenomegaly, convulsions, psychomotor retardation, other CNS signs, anemia, abnormal bleeding, thrombocytopenia, eosinophilia, monocytosis, and abnormal CSF with xanthochromia, mononuclear pleocytosis, and high protein value (grams per deciliter). Although they are not specific for toxoplasmosis in infants, these CSF changes should prompt consideration of toxoplasmosis even in subclinical cases. *Toxoplasma* infection does not cause fetal malformation.

COMPLICATIONS AND SEQUELAE

The lymphadenopathic form of acquired toxoplasmosis is usually self-limited but may persist or recur for months, in the presence or absence of constitutional symptoms.

When clinical signs of infection are present at birth, mental retardation, epilepsy, spasticity, palsies, and severe vision impairment sometimes develop in children who are treated, and they are common sequelae for untreated children. Prompt treatment induces resolution of signs of active infection, and many treated children function normally. Deafness has been reported in untreated children. Microcephaly has been reported in about 13% and hydrocephalus in about 28% of untreated infants with signs or symptoms of toxoplasmosis involving the CNS. These serious sequelae are a threat to all congenitally infected infants, whether or not they exhibit signs in the perinatal period.

Ocular toxoplasmosis is characterized by frequent relapses. It may result in glaucoma or loss of vision and ultimately may necessitate enucleation.

Acute infection is extremely serious in immunodeficient patients. Although the mortality rate is high, the actual death rate is not known. Relapse is frequent in patients with AIDS who do not receive chronic suppressive therapy.

GEOGRAPHIC VARIATIONS IN DISEASE AND INFECTION

There are considerable geographic variations in prevalence of infection with *Toxoplasma* (Fig. 173.6). In all areas surveyed, the prevalence of positive serologic reactions increases with age. Generally, there are fewer human infections in cold regions, in hot and arid areas, and at high elevations. Exceptions do exist: Eskimos, once thought to be free of this infection, have been found to have prevalence rates of 13% to 46%, whereas some isolated tropical communities have little or no *Toxoplasma* infection. It is interesting that these tropical communities have no known exposure to domestic or feral cats. However, there are also populations who are infected with *T. gondii* and who have no known exposure to cats. Most of the variations in prevalence and incidence of infections from area to area have not been explained, but personal habits and exposure to cat feces are important in transmission. For example, in the United States and Europe, ingestion of undercooked meat is common and is probably important in transmission. In Costa Rica, proximity of the area where cats defecate to human habitation is important in transmission. In Erecim, Brazil, retinal disease is frequent in acute acquired infection (15). There have been recent outbreaks in Victoria (25) and Brazil (15).

The actual incidence of congenital toxoplasmosis is unknown. Approximations, per 1,000 live births, are as follows: Vienna, 6 to 7; Paris, 3; New York City, 1.3; and Mexico City, 2.

Association of certain major histocompatibility complex haplotypes and susceptibility has been documented for humans (both congenitally infected infants with hydrocephalus and patients with AIDS and toxoplasmic encephalitis). Epidemics of toxoplasmosis have been documented in humans and in domestic animals in several countries, including the United States,

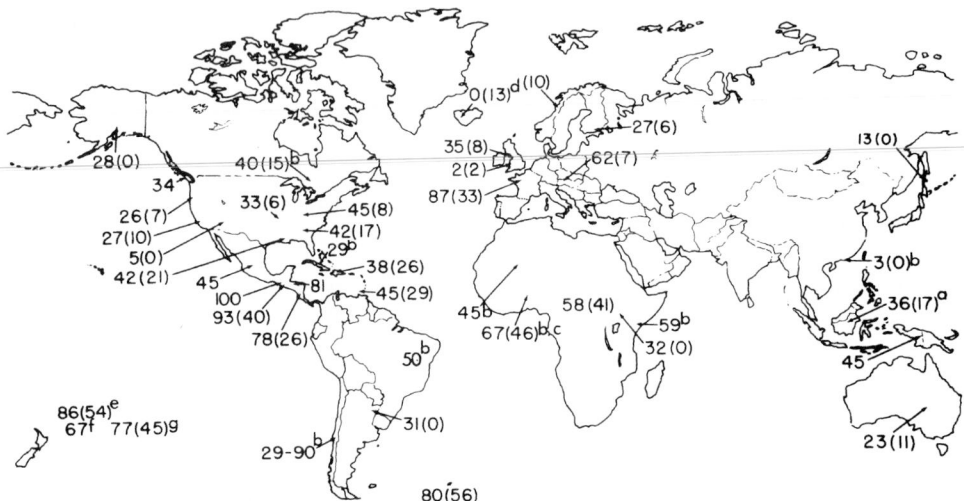

Figure 173.6. Prevalence of antibodies against *Toxoplasma gondii* in persons in selected locales. Unless otherwise specified, figures outside parentheses represent the percentage of seropositive adults about 30 to 40 years of age; figures inside parentheses are the percentage of seropositive children younger than 10 years of age. Notes: *a*, IHA antibodies; others were IFA or dye test. *b*, Adults with either age range not clearly specified or wider age range than about 30 to 40 years. *c*, "Juveniles." *d*, Although 14 individuals 30 to 39 years old had no *Toxoplasma* species antibody, 29% of 14 individuals 40 to 49 years old did have *Toxoplasma* species antibody. *e*, Society Island. *f*, American Samoa. *g*, Tahiti. (From Remington JS, McLeod R. Toxoplasmosis. In: Braude AL, ed. *International textbook of medicine*, Vol II. *Medical microbiology and infectious diseases*. Philadelphia: WB Saunders, 1981:1816–1832, with permission.)

Canada, Brazil, and Spain. Simultaneous infections in multiple members of the same family who cohabit have been reported.

DIAGNOSIS

The diagnosis of acute infection with *Toxoplasma* is made by isolation of *T. gondii* from blood or body fluids. It is also made by demonstration of tachyzoites in sections or preparations of tissues and body fluids; of cysts in the placenta or tissues of a fetus or newborn; and of characteristic lymph node histology. Serologic tests are also useful for diagnosis.

The organism can be isolated by inoculation of body fluids, leukocytes, or tissue specimens into the peritoneal cavity of mice or into tissue cultures. Body fluids should be processed and inoculated immediately; tissues and blood may be stored overnight at 4°C. Freezing or treating specimens with formalin kills the organism.

Mice should be examined for *Toxoplasma* in their peritoneal fluid 6 to 10 days after inoculation or earlier if they die. Mice that survive 6 weeks should be tested for *Toxoplasma* antibody in serum. If antibody is present, definitive diagnosis is made by visualization of *Toxoplasma* cysts in the mouse's brain. If no cysts are seen in mice with *Toxoplasma* antibody, portions of brain, liver, and spleen from the mice should be inoculated into other mice. *T. gondii* organisms can be isolated using tissue cultures by diagnostic microbiology or virology laboratories. When examined microscopically, plaques stained with Wright or Giemsa stain show necrotic, heavily infected cells with numerous extracellular tachyzoites. They may form as early as in 4 days (Fig. 173.7).

Isolation of *T. gondii* from body fluids reflects acute infection, as does isolation from the blood in most patients. Persistent parasitemia in asymptomatic people with latent infection appears to be rare, except perhaps in chronic myelogenous leukemia. Isolation from tissues (e.g., skeletal muscle, lung, brain, eye) obtained by biopsy or at autopsy may reflect the presence of tissue cysts and thus is not proof of acute infection.

Histologic Diagnosis

Demonstration of tachyzoites in tissue sections (e.g., endomyocardial biopsy in heart transplant recipients), smears (e.g., brain biopsy, bone marrow aspirate, bronchoalveolar lavage), or in body fluids (e.g., CSF, amniotic fluid) establishes the diagnosis of acute toxoplasmosis. Although it is difficult to see the tachyzoite with ordinary stains, immunofluorescent antibody techniques and a peroxidase-antiperoxidase immunohistochemical staining technique have been successful (26). Demonstration of the tissue cyst is diagnostic of *Toxoplasma* infection but does not differentiate between acute and chronic infection. Numerous cysts in any organ usually indicate recent acute infection. The presence of cysts in the placenta or tissues of the newborn infant establishes the diagnosis of congenital infection. The characteristic histologic criteria are sufficient to establish the diagnosis of *Toxoplasma* lymphadenitis (12) (Fig. 173.3).

Serologic Tests

It is important to understand that the diagnosis of toxoplasmosis usually requires results from more than one serologic test. The titers in such tests may vary when performed by different laboratories or with different commercial test kits. Thus, it is the responsibility of each laboratory to provide adequate standardization and interpretation with its test results. Results that affect therapy should be confirmed in a reference laboratory.

The Sabin-Feldman dye, indirect fluorescent antibody (IFA), and indirect hemagglutination (IHA) tests are the methods most widely used for diagnosis of acute toxoplasmosis. Tests to detect parasite DNA by polymerase chain reaction (PCR) are particularly promising for diagnosis in newborns and in immunocompromised persons. Immunosorbent assays and radioimmunoassay are potentially valuable because they allow automation.

The dye test is sensitive and specific and measures principally IgG antibodies (27). The World Health Organization has recommended that dye test titers be expressed in international units per milliliter. An international standard reference serum for this purpose is available on request from the World Health Organization.

The IFA test appears to measure the same antibodies as the dye test. In both tests, the titers tend to be parallel. Dye test and IFA test antibodies usually appear 1 to 2 weeks after infection, reach high titers in 6 to 8 weeks, and then gradually decline over months to years; low titers (1:4 to 1:64) commonly persist for life. Magnitude of antibody titer does not correlate with severity of illness. Commercially available kits produce significant numbers of false-positive or false-negative results.

The agglutination test (28) is available commercially (BioMerieux, Lyon, France). It employs formalin-preserved whole parasites and detects IgG. This method should not be used to measure IgM antibodies. It is accurate, simple to perform, and inexpensive. The agglutination test has special usefulness for serologic screening to diagnose acute infection in pregnant women. Because it takes 2 to 6 months for IgG antibodies detected with the whole-cell agglutination test to reach a steady high titer (28), the existence of a steady high titer signifies that the infection was acquired more than 2 months earlier. As a

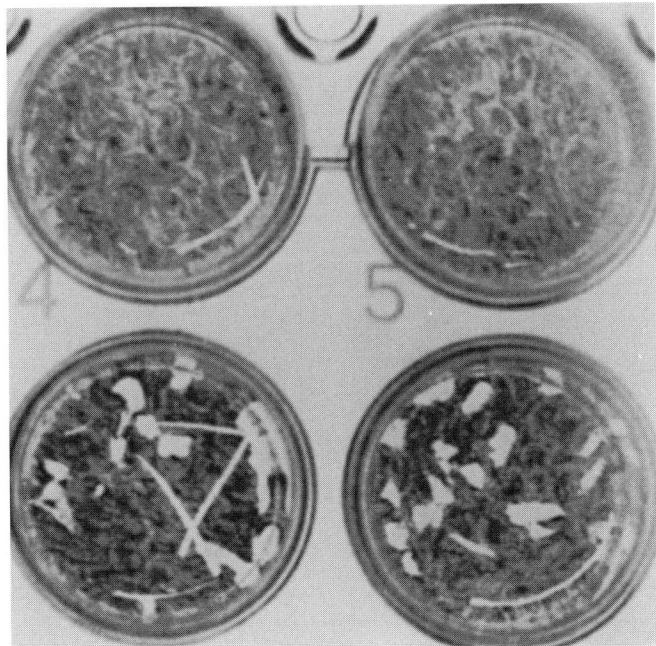

Figure 173.7. Plaque formation by *Toxoplasma gondii:* 100 RH strain *Toxoplasma* tachyzoites were inoculated onto semiconfluent monolayers of human foreskin fibroblasts. Plaques (*bottom row*) were observed at 96 hours. *Top row:* Uninfected (control) monolayers. (Adapted from Israelski DM, Remington JS. Toxoplasmic encephalitis in patients with AIDS. In: Sande MA, Volberding PA, eds. *The medical management of AIDS.* Philadelphia: WB Saunders, 1988:193, with permission.)

TABLE 173.1.   Criteria Used for Interpretation of AC/HS Test Results[a]

HS test result (IU/mL)	Interpretation with the following AC test result (IU/mL)							
	<50	50	100	200	400	800	1,600	>1,600
<100	NA[b]	NA[b]	A	A	A[c]	A[c]	A[c]	A[c]
100	NA	NA	A	A	A	A	A[c]	A[c]
200	NA	NA	A	A	A	A	A	A[c]
400	NA	NA	A	A	A	A	A	A
800	NA	NA	NA	A	A	A	A	A
1,600	NA	NA	NA	NA	A	A	A	A
3,200	NA	NA	NA	NA	NA	A	A	A
>3,200	NA	NA	NA	NA	NA	NA	A	A

A, acute pattern; NA, not acute pattern.
[a]The AC/HS test was performed as described in reference 29.
[b]HS titer of >0 but <100; this pattern may be seen in the earliest stages of infection. Follow-up serum samples are necessary to clarify whether the infection is acute.
[c]Results were not observed in routine use of the test.
From Dannemann BR, Vaughn WC, Thulliez P, et al. Differential agglutination test for diagnosis of recently acquired infection with *Toxoplasma gondii*. *J Clin Microbiol* 1990;28:1928–1933, with permission.

consequence, if the first sample of serum has been obtained during the first 2 months of pregnancy, a stable agglutination test titer demonstrates that the infection occurred before the time of conception and that there is little risk to the baby for congenital infection.

The differential agglutination test [AC/HS (acetone-fixed parasites/formalin-fixed parasites)] has proved useful in the differentiation of recent infection in contrast to more distant infection (27,29,30) (Table 173.1).

The IgM fluorescent antibody (IgM-IFA) test is useful for the diagnosis of acute infection with *T. gondii* because IgM antibodies appear faster (as early as 5 days after infection) and disappear sooner than IgG antibodies. In most cases, IgM-IFA test antibody levels rise rapidly (to levels of 1:80 to 1:1,000) and fall to low titers (1:10 or 1:20) or disappear within a few weeks or months (31) (Fig. 173.8). In some patients, they remain positive at low titers for as long as several years. IgM antibodies in neonates represent synthesis *in utero* by the infected fetus because IgM does not normally pass the placental barrier. IgM *Toxoplasma* antibodies may not be demonstrable in some immunodeficient patients with acute toxoplasmosis and in most patients with active toxo-

plasmosis limited to the eye and are demonstrable in only about 25% of newborns with congenital toxoplasmosis. Antinuclear antibodies may cause false-positive reactions in both the IFA and IgM-IFA tests; rheumatoid factor may cause false-positive reactions in the IgM-IFA test.

Detection of IgM antibodies by the double-sandwich IgM enzyme-linked immunosorbent assay (32) (DS-IgM-ELISA) is more sensitive and specific than the IgM-IFA test. Rheumatoid factor and antinuclear antibodies do not cause false-positive test results. The DS-IgM-ELISA detects about 75% of infants with proven congenital infection, whereas the IgM-IFA detects only 25% of such cases. The DS-IgM-ELISA avoids false-positive results associated with rheumatoid factor, which the infant can produce *in utero*, and false-negative results related to competition from high levels of maternal IgG antibody, which occur in the IgM-IFA test. IgM antibodies are detected by the IgM-IFA test for a shorter time than by the DS-IgM-ELISA. The IgM immunosorbent agglutination assay (IgM-ISAGA) is more sensitive than the IgM-ELISA and may detect specific IgM antibodies before and for a longer time than the IgM-ELISA.

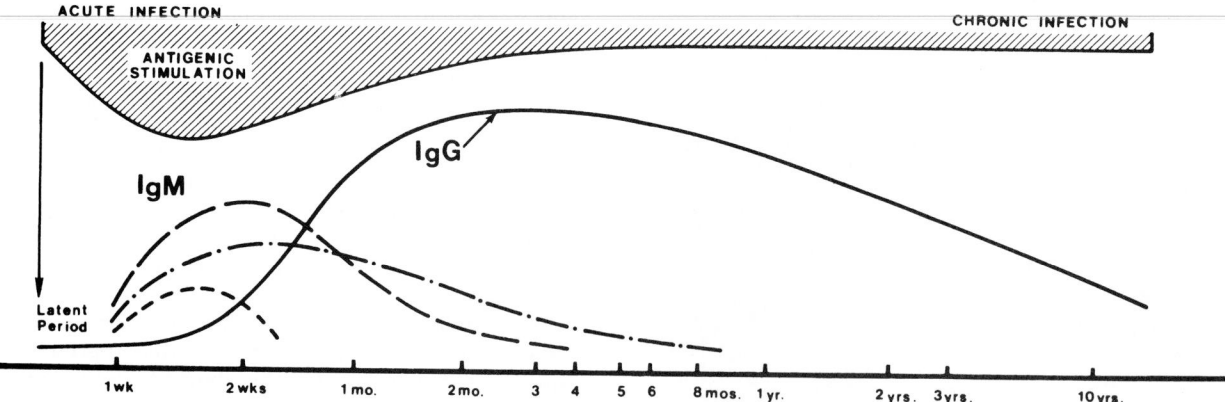

Figure 173.8. Antibody response of humans to *Toxoplasma* species infection. Immunoglobulin M (IgM) antibodies (the three broken curves), detectable by the IgM indirect fluorescent antibody (IFA) test, reach their maximal titer within the first weeks after infection and may decline within a few weeks or persist for months. IgG antibodies (the continuous curve), detectable by either the Sabin-Feldman dye test or the conventional IFA test, reach their maximal titer within 2 months, maintain a plateau for months or years, and then decline, but usually persist at a low titer for life. (Data from Desmonts G. Sérodiagnostic de la toxoplasmose. *Feuill Biol* 1975;16:61, with permission.)

The IgM-ISAGA, which combines trapping of a patient's IgM to a solid surface and formalin-fixed organisms or antigen-coated latex particles to detect the IgM antibodies, is specific and sensitive. The test is read as an agglutination test. It avoids false-positive results caused by rheumatoid factor or antinuclear antibodies and is more sensitive and specific than the IgM-IFA test. We use it routinely in newborns. The IgA and IgE-ELISA and IgE-ISAGA are also useful tests in establishing the diagnosis of newly acquired or congenital toxoplasmosis (33).

The antibodies measured in the IHA test are different from those measured in the IFA and dye tests and may persist for years. Because IHA titers rise later than IFA or dye test titers, the IHA test may be helpful when these titers have stabilized. The IHA test should not be used for infants with suspected congenital infection or to screen for infection acquired during pregnancy because the result may be negative for too long a period early in the infection. There is a great need for proper standardization of methodology for this and all other serologic tests and particularly for quality control of commercial kits that are often used by laboratories inexperienced in performing these serologic tests.

The level of *Toxoplasma* antibody in CSF or aqueous humor may be used to demonstrate local production of antibody in active ocular or CNS toxoplasmosis. Local antibody production is assessed by application of the following equation:

$$c = \text{antibody titer in body fluid} / \text{antibody titer in serum}$$
$$\times \text{concentration of } \gamma\text{-globulin in serum} / \text{concentration of}$$
$$\gamma\text{-globulin in body fluid}$$

A significant correlation coefficient (*c*) is 8 and reflects local antibody production related to active infection of the CNS or eye. If the dye test serum titer is 1:1,000 or more, it is usually not possible to demonstrate significant local antibody production by application of this formula. The formula has been applied by using dye test titers and IgM-IFA test titers.

Toxoplasma antigen has been detected in serum of adults with the lymphadenopathic form of toxoplasmosis or with other acute *Toxoplasma* infection but not in serum of uninfected or chronically infected persons. It was detected in serum, amniotic fluid, and CSF from the few congenitally infected infants tested.

More avid *T. gondii*–specific IgG antibody (using an avidity ELISA) has been described in association with more remotely but not recently acquired chronic infection. This test is clinically very useful in differentiating recently (within the preceding 12 to 16 weeks) and more remotely acquired infection (high avidity) (34).

Comparative Western blots of serum samples from a mother and her baby demonstrating that both contain antibodies that react with different antigens have been reported as a means of diagnosing congenital toxoplasmosis.

Enzyme-linked immunofiltration assay is carried out on a micropore membrane and permits simultaneous study of antibody specificity by immunoprecipitation and characterization of antibody isotypes by immunofiltration with enzyme-labeled antibodies. The authors reported that this method detects 85% of cases of congenital infection in the first few days of life. Although the method has not been used in sufficient numbers of laboratories to define its usefulness, it appears promising. It is interesting that by this method, IgE may by found at birth in the infant's CSF or serum. IgA antibodies were present in 5% of cases of congenital infection after the fifth month of life and were found in the CSF.

PCR can be used to amplify DNA of *T. gondii*, which can then be detected using a DNA probe (35). This is a useful technique for detecting *T. gondii* DNA in CSF and amniotic fluid.

The lymphocyte blastogenic response to *Toxoplasma* antigens has also been useful in the diagnosis of congenital toxoplasmosis.

ACUTE ACQUIRED *TOXOPLASMA* INFECTION IN THE IMMUNOCOMPETENT PERSON

In settings in which acute acquired *Toxoplasma* infection is suspected in an immunocompetent person, a negative dye test or IFA test virtually excludes the diagnosis. The diagnosis of recent acute acquired infection is confirmed if there is seroconversion from a negative to a positive titer (in the absence of transfer of antibody by transfusion) or if there is a serial two-tube rise in titer when serum samples drawn at 3-week intervals are run in parallel. Although suggestive of active infection, one high titer in any test is not diagnostic.

Titers obtained using each kit and results as performed by each laboratory may vary. It is the responsibility of each laboratory to provide reliable information concerning results they consider indicative of recently or remotely acquired infection for each clinical illness. Some representative guidelines are based on results from the laboratory of one of the authors (JSR). Tables 173.2 and 173.3 (and review Table 173.1) are helpful in interpreting test results, but exceptions may occur (36,37). A dye test or IFA test titer of 1:1,000 or greater in the presence of a high IgM-IFA test titer (1:80 or greater) or DS-IgM-ELISA or IgM-ISAGA titer is probably diagnostic of recent acute infection, with or without symptoms. In immunologically normal people with positive titers in the dye test or IFA test, the absence of IgM-IFA test or DS-IgM-ELISA or IgM-ISAGA antibodies almost always excludes the diagnosis of acute infection.

OCULAR TOXOPLASMOSIS

The diagnosis of ocular toxoplasmosis in older children and adults is difficult because the titer of antibody in the serum does not necessarily correlate with presence of active lesions in the fundus. Indeed, low serologic test titers (1:4 to 1:64) are usual in older children and adults with active *Toxoplasma* chorioretinitis. For practical purposes, *Toxoplasma* chorioretinitis is probably excluded if results of serologic tests are negative when performed on undiluted serum. If retinal lesions are characteristic and serologic test results are positive, the diagnosis can be made with a high degree of confidence. If the retinal lesion is atypical and the result is positive, the diagnosis of toxoplasmosis is only presumptive; a high prevalence of antibodies in the normal population precludes the assumption of a causal relationship in this situation.

ACTIVE INFECTION IN THE IMMUNOCOMPROMISED INDIVIDUAL

The available diagnostic techniques, including the IgM-EFA test, DS-IgM-ELISA, and IgM-ISAGA, are at times insufficient for detection of active infection in immunocompromised patients because antibody responses may be abnormal. Serologic tests in immunocompromised persons can identify those at risk for primary infection or reactivation of latent infection (see the later section "Prevention").

Kinetics of serologic responses in heart transplant recipients who receive a heart donated by a seropositive person are variable. Seronegative patients who received hearts donated by seropositive persons exhibited seroconversion 4 to 7 weeks later and severe illness 1 week to 9 months after transplantation. About 50% of patients who were seropositive before transplantation demonstrated a significant rise in IgG and IgM antibodies, although all remained asymptomatic.

Detection of *Toxoplasma* DNA in blood and CSF or vitreous, by PCR (35), seems promising for identifying disseminated *Toxoplasma* infection in immunocompromised persons.

TABLE 173.2. Approach to Serologic Diagnosis of Toxoplasmosis

Patient and specimen	Toxoplasma gondii–specific IgG[a]				T. gondii–specific IgM[b]				T. gondii–specific IgA	T. gondii–specific IgE	T. gondii–specific IgE	Other tests			
	Dye test	IFA	IgG-ELISA	Direct agglutination	DS-IgM-ELISA	IgM-ISAGA	ELISA for IgM to P30	IFA	IgA-ELISA	IgE-ELISA	IgE-ISAGA	PCR	Isolation	AC/HS	Avidity
Newborn congenital toxoplasmosis															
Serum	C	C	C	C	C	C	C	Do not use	C	C	C		C		C
CSF	C	C		C	C	C	C						C		
Peripheral blood clot or peripheral blood cells												R	C		
Placenta												R	C		
Pregnant woman															
Maternal serum	C	C	C	C	C	C	C	C	C	C	C			C	C
Amniotic fluid									C			C	C		
Immunologically normal patient															
Serum	C	C	C	C	C	C	C	C						C	C
CSF	C	C			C	C	C	C				C			
Immunologically deficient patient															
Serum, or peripheral blood	C	C	C	C	C[c]	C[c]	C[c]	C[c]				C	C		
CSF	C	C	C	C	C[c]	C[c]	C[c]	C[c]				C	C		

IFA, indirect fluorescent antibody; Ig, immunoglobulin; ELISA, enzyme-linked immunosorbent assay; IgM-ISAGA, immunosorbent test for IgM; PCR, polymerase chain reaction; AC/HS, differential agglutination test; CSF, cerebrospinal fluid; C, commercially available; R, research test at present in reference laboratories.

[a]When properly standardized, any one of these tests is useful for demonstration of IgG antibody.

[b]ISAGA is usually most sensitive; IFA is least sensitive (do not use for congenital infection).

[c]Rarely positive.

Source: Adapted from Roberts F, Boyer KM, McLeod R. Toxoplasmosis. In: Krugman S, Gershon AA, Katz SL, et al., eds. Infectious Diseases of Children, ed 10. St. Louis: Mosby–Year Book, 1997, with permission.

TABLE 173.3.   Guidelines for Interpretation of Serologic Tests for Toxoplasmosis

Test	Positive titer	Titer in congenital infection (infant) or acute infection (older child, adult)	Titer in chronic infection	Duration of elevation of titer
IgG				
Sabin-Feldman dye test	Undiluted	NC: S OCA: 1:4 to ≥1:1,000 (usual)	1:4 to 1:2,000	Years
Direct agglutination test	≥1:20	NC:S OCA: Rises slowly from negative to low to high titer (1:512)	Stable (≥1:1,000) or slowly decreasing titer	≥1 yr
Indirect fluorescent IgG antibody	≥1:10	NC: S OCA: ≥1:1,000	1:8 to 1:2,000	Years
Indirect hemagglutination test	≥1:16	NC: S OCA: ≥1:1,000	1:16 to 1:256	Years
Complement fixation	≥1:4	NC: S OCA: varies among laboratories	Negative to 1:8	Years
IgM				
Indirect fluorescent for IgM	≥1:10, adults	OCA: ≥1:80 (use only for OCA, not NC)	Negative to 1:20	Weeks to months, occasionally years
Double-sandwich IgM-ELISA	≥0.2, newborn fetus; ≥1.7, older children, adults	NC: ≥0.2 OCA: ≥1.7	Negative to 1.7 (OCA)	Can be ≥1 yr
Immunosorbent test for IgM	≥3, infant; 8, adult	NC: ≥3 OCA: >8	Negative to 1	Unknown, can be ≥1 yr
IgA				
IgA, ELISA	≥1.0, infants; ≥2.1, adults	NC: ≥1.0 OCA: >2.1	Negative to <1.0 Negative to ≤2.1	Weeks to months, occasionally longer
IgE				
IgE, ELISA	≥1.9, infants and adults	NC and OCA: ≥1.9	Negative	Weeks to months, occasionally longer
Immunosorbent test for IgE	≥4, infants and adults	NC and OCA: ≥4	Negative	Weeks to months, occasionally longer
AC/HS	See Table 173.1	See Table 173.1	See Table 173.1	Usually <9 mo
PCR (amniotic fluid; CSF)	Positive	Positive	Negative	Only when *Toxoplasma* DNA present during active infection
IgG avidity	Not applicable	Not applicable, low or high	High	High avidity, infection not likely acquired in preceding 12 to 16 wk

Ig, Immunoglobulin; NC, titer in newborn with congenital infection; OCA, titer in older child or adult with acute, acquired infection; S, usually the same as the mother; ELISA; enzyme-linked immunosorbent assay; AC/HS, differential agglutination test; PCR, polymerase chain reaction; CSF, cerebrospinal fluid. *Note:* values are those of one reference laboratory; each laboratory must provide its own standards and interpretation of results in each clinical setting.
Adapted from McLeod R, Remington JS. Toxoplasmosis. In: Braunwald E, Isselbacher K, Petersdorf R, et al., eds. *Harrison's principles of internal Medicine,* 11th ed. New York: McGraw-Hill, 1987:791–797. Reproduced by permission of The McGraw-Hill Companies.

TOXOPLASMOSIS AND *TOXOPLASMA* INFECTION IN PREGNANT WOMEN

Any woman who is considering becoming pregnant should have a *Toxoplasma* serologic test to determine whether she has *Toxoplasma* infection before pregnancy. (See the section "Transplacental Transmission" for a complete discussion of risks to the fetus in relation to *Toxoplasma* infection acquired by the mother before pregnancy versus during pregnancy.)

In systematic monthly screening of pregnant women, serum IgM antibodies usually appear first, but low titers of IgG antibodies as measured in the dye test also appear early. Sera in which only IgM antibodies are detectable are uncommon. Because IgM antibodies measured by ELISA or ISAGA can persist for many months or even years, their greatest value is for determining that a pregnant woman has not recently been infected. A negative result virtually rules out recently acquired infection, unless serum samples are tested so early after acute infection that the antibody response has not yet occurred. In this case, acute infection would be identified in a screening program in which follow-up serology is performed in seronegative pregnant women. IgM antibodies that are measured by the IFA test may disappear earlier than those measured by IgM-ELISA or ISAGA. Thus, a negative IgM-IFA test late in gestation may not necessarily exclude recent acute infection. A positive IgM test is more difficult to evaluate unless it is possible to demonstrate a significant rise in IgG or IgM titer when serum samples are run in parallel or when other tests (e.g., tests for IgA and IgE antibody and the AC/HS test) suggest recent infection. A high IgM titer is more likely to reflect recent infection, but such high titers may persist for months. Such positive serum samples should be tested with additional methods, such as the AC/HS test and tests that detect IgE antibodies. Usually, this requires use of and consultation with a reference laboratory. A rise in IgM antibody titer is infrequent, suggesting that the rise was steep and reached its peak in 1 or 2 weeks. In contrast, the rise in IgG antibody is initially slow. The dye test titer usually remains relatively low (2 to 50 IU/mL or 1:10 to 1:200) for 3 to 6 weeks. Thus, acute infection cannot be ruled out when two samples collected 2 or even 3 weeks apart show no significant rise in titer, especially if the dye test is performed with fourfold dilutions of the sera, which would require an eightfold (two-tube) rise in titer to be considered significant. For this reason, twofold dilutions are imperative. A fourfold rise is often difficult to detect in the IgG-IFA test. After the initial 3 to 6 weeks, the rise in IgG antibody becomes steeper, and high titers (400 IU/mL or 1:1,000) are usually reached within an additional 3 weeks. Thereafter, the rise is slower but still detectable over an additional 3 to 6 weeks by careful methodology, avoiding fourfold dilutions of serum. Thus, although the rise in IgG antibody in the dye test differs from case to case, it lasts more than 2 months and sometimes 3 months. In the agglutination test with 2-mercaptoethanol, the IgG antibody value may parallel exactly the dye test response or may rise more slowly, reaching the peak no earlier than 6 months after infection. By 6 months, the IgM-IFA test result is negative in most cases, whereas the DS-IgM-ELISA and the IgM-ISAGA results usually remain positive; in women who become infected during pregnancy, the latter two tests are usually positive at the time of parturition.

When *Toxoplasma* infection is treated during the initial antibody response (when the IgG titer is low), the rise in IgG antibody titer slows and the titer (e.g., in the dye test or conventional IFA test) may remain low as long as treatment is continued. A late (delayed) rise often occurs after cessation of treatment.

In the absence of a routine screening program in which *Toxoplasma* serologic tests are performed each month in pregnant women, an IgM-IFA or DS-IgM-ELISA or IgM-ISAGA test should be performed if any other serologic test result is positive at any titer. If the IgM-IFA or DS-IgM-ELISA or IgM-ISAGA test is unavailable, the serologic test should be repeated in 3 or 4 weeks with serial twofold dilutions, to determine whether the titer is stable or rising. If the IgM-IFA test or DS-IgM-ELISA or IgM-ISAGA is negative and an IFA or dye test titer is stable and less than 1:1,000 (300 IU), no further evaluation is necessary. Because titers in the dye test or IFA test usually stabilize at high levels

[1:1,000 6 to 8 weeks after acquisition of infection or longer, if the dye test or IFA test titer is 1:1,000 (300 IU) and stable regardless of titer in the IgM-IFA test or DS-IgM-ELISA or IgM-ISAGA], the infection was acquired at least 4 weeks earlier and probably more than 8 weeks before the serum was obtained. Thus, for practical purposes, if the dye test or IFA test titer is 1:1,000 and stable when measured in the first 2 months of pregnancy, risk to the fetus is low.

Whereas titers in the dye test or IFA test may have stabilized and peaked by 8 weeks after onset of infection, titers in the complement fixation or IHA test may continue to rise for 4 to 6 months or longer after acquisition of infection. Therefore, rises in the last two test results may not be helpful in defining when the infection occurred relative to conception. The AC/HS test is also useful in determining that an infection was recently acquired. If the AC/HS test has an acute pattern (Table 173.1), infection has usually been acquired in the preceding 9 months.

A common problem is the interpretation of serologic test results in an asymptomatic woman who is tested for *Toxoplasma* antibody late in the first trimester or in the second trimester of pregnancy. If her IFA or dye test titer is found to be in the range of 1:2,000, her IgM-IFA test titer or DS-IgM-ELISA or IgM-ISAGA test is negative, and no significant rise in titer in any test is demonstrable, it is impossible to determine whether her infection occurred before, at, or after conception.

Detection of the *Toxoplasma B1* gene in amniotic fluid (35) is useful in establishing the diagnosis of congenital toxoplasmosis in the fetus.

CONGENITAL TOXOPLASMOSIS

Guidelines for evaluation of a neonate when serology of the mother or illness in the neonate indicates that the diagnosis of congenital toxoplasmosis is suspected or likely are presented in Table 173.4. When the diagnosis of toxoplasmosis is suspected in a neonate, evaluation should proceed as outlined in Table 173.4.

TABLE 173.4.   Evaluation of Neonate When Serology of Mother or Illness of Neonate Indicates that Diagnosis of Congenital Toxoplasmosis Is Suspected or Likely

In addition to a careful examination, the infant is examined by the following:
Clinical Evaluation and Nonspecific Tests
  A pediatric ophthalmologist
  A pediatric neurologist
  Brain computed tomography
  Blood tests
    Complete blood count with differential and platelet counts
    Serum total IgM, IgG, IgA, and albumin
    Serum alanine aminotransferase, total and direct bilirubin
    CSF cell count, glucose, protein, and total IgG
***Toxoplasma gondii*–specific Tests**
  Newborn serum analyzed for antibody detected by the Sabin-Feldman dye test, IgM-ISAGA, IgA-ELISA, IgE-ELISA/ISAGA (0.5 mL of serum to *Toxoplasma* Serology Laboratory, Palo Alto Medical Foundation, 795 El Camino Real, Ames Building Palo Alto, CA 94301, 650-326-8120); if value for IgA-ELISA measured in the first day of life is borderline, another sample on day 7 to 10 of life may be useful in establishment of the diagnosis
  Newborn blood for inoculation into mice (1–2 mL of clotted whole blood in red-topped tube to *Toxoplasma* Serology Laboratory, address above)
  Lumbar puncture: CSF dye test and IGM-ELISA (0.5 mL of CSF to *Toxoplasma* Serology Laboratory, address above); consider PCR (1 mL of frozen CSF to *Toxoplasma* Serology Laboratory, address above) (PCR with peripheral blood WBCs and urine may also be useful)
  Sterile placental tissue (100 g in saline, from fetal side near insertion of cord, no formalin) to *Toxoplasma* Serology Laboratory for subinoculation
  Maternal serum analyzed for antibody detected by dye test, IgM-ELISA, IgA-ELISA, IgE-ELISA/ISAGA, and AC/HS

Ig, immunoglobulin; CSF, cerebrospinal fluid; ISAGA, immunosorbent agglutination assay; ELISA, enzyme-linked immunosorbent assay; PCR, polymerase chain reaction; WBCs, white blood cells; AC/HS, differential agglutination test. Adapted from Roberts F, Boyer KM, McLeod R. Toxoplasmosis. In: Krugman S, Gershon AA, Katz SL, et al., eds. *Infectious diseases of children*, 11th ed. St. Louis: Mosby–Year Book, 2003, with permission.

Representative results of specific serologic tests indicative of congenital infection are shown in Table 173.2. Persistent or rising titers in the dye test or a positive IgM, IgA, or IgE test specific for *T. gondii* in the absence of placental leak indicates infection. Repeating these tests on the seventh to tenth day of life may help to establish the significance of a borderline or indeterminate value obtained initially at birth. It may be necessary to utilize multiple diagnostic tests because none is positive in all infected infants. Because rheumatoid factor may be present in a newborn with congenital infection, it is important to exclude the presence of this antibody in an infant with a positive IgM-IFA test. If a placental leak of maternal blood has occurred, an elevated level of human chorionic gonadotropin-β may be present in the infant's serum, and the IgM test titer in the neonate drops significantly within a week because the half-life of IgM is about 3 to 5 days. IgM synthesis by the infant could also have stopped at this time, resulting in the fall in titer, however. Passively transferred maternal antibodies may require 6 to 12 months or longer to disappear from the infant's serum, depending on the original titer. The serum half-life of IgG is about 1 month. Synthesis of *Toxoplasma* antibody by the infected infant is usually demonstrable by the third month of life if the infant is not treated, but it may be delayed until the sixth or ninth month if the infant is treated. Infrequently, it may not occur at all. Thus, at the time the infant begins to synthesize antibody, infection may be documented serologically, even when IgM antibodies are not demonstrable. This may be accomplished by computation of the specific antibody "load" (i.e., the ratio of specific serum antibody titer to the level of serum IgG in mother and infant). For example, in an uninfected infant with only maternal antibody, there is no change in antibody load because, as the titer of antibody decreases in the infant's serum, total IgG decreases in a similar manner. During the second and third months, the amount of IgG synthesized by the infant increases. Because this newly synthesized IgG does not contain *Toxoplasma* antibodies, the antibody load decreases and continues to decrease as IgG synthesis in the child progresses. In congenitally infected infants, the production of antibody may vary considerably from one case to another. Early and delayed antibody production can be demonstrated by increases in antibody load. The diagnosis of congenital toxoplasmosis has also been established as follows: demonstration of *Toxoplasma* DNA in the infant's blood or CSF; demonstration of antibodies to unique *T. gondii* epitopes in the infant's serum not present in the mother's serum; lymphocyte blastogenic response of the infant to lymphocyte *T. gondii* antigens; and isolation of *T. gondii* from placenta, blood, or CSF of the infant. The approach to serologic diagnosis of toxoplasmosis in each of these clinical settings is summarized in Table 173.2.

TREATMENT

Treatment in Specific Clinical Settings

The need for and duration of therapy are determined by the clinical severity of the illness and by the person who is infected.

Immunologically normal patients with the lymphadenopathic form of acute toxoplasmosis do not require specific treatment unless there are severe and persistent symptoms or evidence of damage to vital organs (38). Infections acquired in laboratory accidents or through transfusions may be more severe than naturally acquired infections and probably should be treated.

Patients with active chorioretinitis should be treated with specific drug therapy (39–41). Patients with active ocular toxoplasmosis should receive pyrimethamine and sulfadiazine 7 days beyond the time that active lesions resolve. Within 10 days

of initiation of treatment, the borders of retinal lesions should sharpen, and the vitreous haze (caused by inflammatory cells) should disappear. A favorable clinical response is seen in most cases; if unfavorable, the courses of pyrimethamine and sulfadiazine are repeated. Systemic corticosteroids are administered if vision is endangered by lesions involving the macula, optic nerve head, or papillomacular bundle. Occasionally, vitrectomy and removal of the lens may be necessary to restore visual acuity.

Toxoplasmosis should be treated in a patient whose resistance to infection is compromised by an underlying disease or by therapy (e.g., corticosteroids or cytotoxic drugs) (18,20,41,42). Either serologic evidence of acute infection in an immunocompromised patient, whether or not signs and symptoms of infection are present, or the demonstration of tachyzoites in tissue, regardless of serologic test titers, is an indication for therapy. In 80% of immunocompromised patients in whom the diagnosis was established ante mortem, improvement occurred when specific therapy was administered. The major problem lies in making the diagnosis early enough to institute treatment. This is especially the case in bone marrow transplant recipients, for whom fever, pneumonia, or diffuse encephalitis may be nonspecific, presenting manifestations.

Concerning the treatment of toxoplasmosis in patients with AIDS (43,44), at present the dosage of pyrimethamine used is 75 to 100 mg per day after a 100- to 200-mg loading dose. This is given with 4 to 6 g of sulfadiazine or triple sulfonamides. Ten to 15 mg of leucovorin daily is also administered. Alternative treatment regimens are listed in Table 173.5 (45). Treatment with pyrimethamine plus clindamycin was found to have comparable initial efficacy to treatment with pyrimethamine and sulfadiazine. AIDS patients are treated with pyrimethamine (25 to 50 mg) and sulfadiazine (2 to 4 g) each day for maintenance therapy. Other potentially effective regimens are listed in Table 173.6. Patients whose lesions completely resolve and have CD4 counts higher than 200 cells/mm³ for 4 to 6 months may discontinue maintenance therapy. TMP-SMX or other prophylaxis is recommended for seropositive patients without toxoplasmic encephalitis with less than 200 CD4 lymphocytes/mm³. Flares of infection may occur with initiation of HAART.

If a woman who acquires infection at any time during pregnancy is treated, the chance of congenital infection in her infant is decreased but not eliminated. In one series, the incidence of infection was decreased from 17% to 5%, and in another series, it was decreased from 60% to 23%. The drugs effective in the only two reported studies were spiramycin in France (46) and pyrimethamine plus sulfonamide in Germany (47). Because of the potential teratogenicity of pyrimethamine, sulfadiazine (which is highly effective in animal models when used alone) should be used alone if treatment is to be given in the first trimester of pregnancy. Spiramycin [available in the United States through the U.S. Food and Drug Administration (telephone 302-443-7580)] has also been used safely for prevention during the first trimester of pregnancy.

An approach, with apparent good outcome, for prevention, diagnosis, and treatment of congenital toxoplasmosis during a fetus' gestation is used in France and in part has been described by Hohlfeld and coworkers as outlined in Table 173.7 (34,47–49). In France, the methods for prevention include education about methods to avoid acquisition of *T. gondii* (Table 173.8). In one study, in one hospital, little or no information was given to pregnant women about how they might avoid acquisition of infection. The observed incidence of 59 per 1,000 per year remained essentially identical to the incidence observed before the mode of transmission of the infection was discovered. In another hospital, the observed incidence was 37 per 1,000 per year in 1973, when verbal instructions about hygienic measures

TABLE 173.5. Guidelines for Acute or Primary Therapy of Toxoplasmic Encephalitis in Patients with Acquired Immunodeficiency Syndrome

Drug	Dosage schedule
Standard regimens	
Pyrimethamine	Oral 200 mg loading dose, then 50 to 75 mg/d
Folinic acid (leucovorin)[a]	Oral, intravenous, or intramuscular 10–20 mg/d (up to 50 mg/d)
plus	
Sulfadiazine	Oral 1–1.5 g q6h
or	
Clindamycin	Oral or intravenous 600 mg q6h (up to intravenous 1,200 mg q6h)
Possible alternative regimens[b]	
Trimethoprim-sulfamethoxazole[c]	Oral or intravenous 5 mg (trimethoprim component) per kg q6h
Pyrimethamine and folinic acid	As in standard regimens plus one of the following:
Clarithromycin	Oral 1 g q12h
Azithromycin	Oral 1,200–1,500 mg/d
Atovaquone	Oral 750 mg q6h
Dapsone	Oral 100 mg/d

Note: This table is intended as a guide only, and readers are referred to detailed reviews for individual regimens (57–72).
[a] The dose of folinic acid can be titrated on the basis of the hemogram to reduce pyrimethamine-associated myelotoxicity. Up to 50 mg/d has been used.
[b] These agents have been used in clinical studies with small numbers of patients and have response rates lower than those of the standard regimens. They should be used only in patients who are intolerant of the standard regimens. Alternative agents must be used in combination with another antimicrobial agent (most frequently, pyrimethamine with folinic acid) that has proven clinical activity against *Toxoplasma gondii*.
[c] In a small study, trimethoprim-sulfamethoxazole at a dose of 6.6 mg (trimethoprim component) per kg per day has been reported to have similar efficacy to 20 mg of trimethoprim per kg per day. Further studies are required to determine the optimal dosage schedule (see text).
[d] The optimal dose of azithromycin for the treatment of toxoplasmic encephalitis is being investigated in a dose escalation trial conducted by the AIDS Clinical Trials Group. The dosages given here are those that appear to have been effective in a small number of patients.
Adapted from Wong SY, Remington JS. Toxoplasmosis in the setting of AIDS. In: Broder S, Merigan TC Jr, Bolognesi D, eds. *Textbook of AIDS medicine.* Baltimore: Williams & Wilkins, 1994:223–257, with permission. © by Samuel Broder, MD.

were given to seronegative women, and 11 per 1,000 per year in 1974, when explanatory drawings were given to patients. From these results, health education appears to be moderately effective in reducing incidence rates, and pictures and graphics appear to be more effective than the written word for such education.

In addition, acquisition of *T. gondii* by mothers during gestation is detected in a systematic serologic screening program (46,48,50) (Table 173.7). An acutely infected woman receives oral spiramycin (1 g three times a day), which reduces the incidence of transmission to the fetus. Fetal ultrasonography is performed every 2 weeks, with special attention to whether there are cerebral calcifications, hydrocephalus, hepatic calcification, hepatomegaly, or ascites. Amniocentesis is performed at about 18 weeks' gestation or later until term, as described before, and PCR is performed to determine whether DNA of *T. gondii* is present. Diagnostic amniocentesis should not be limited to 17- to 18-week-gestation pregnancies when it is likely that the fetus may be infected. Overall sensitivity of PCR using amniotic fluid is 85%: sensitivity of PCR using amniotic fluid is less earlier and later in gestation than in the middle of gestation (49). The cell pellet from a separate aliquot of amniotic fluid is inoculated into mice. If an infant is found to be infected using these tests, the well-informed pregnant patient can choose either to treat the fetus *in utero* with pyrimethamine, sulfadiazine, and leucovorin

TABLE 173.6. Primary Prophylaxis and Suppressive Treatment

Medications with documented efficacy for primary prophylaxis for seropositive patients with $CD4^+$ cell counts <200 cells/mm^3
  Trimethoprim-sulfamethoxazole [same as doses for *Pneumocystis carinii* pneumonia (PCP)]
  Pyrimethamine-dapsone (same as doses for PCP)
  Sulfadoxine-pyrimethamine (Fansidar)
Suppressive regimens
  Pyrimethamine (25 mg/d) plus sulfadiazine (500 mg q.i.d.)—lowest relapse rate
  Pyrimethamine (25 mg/d) plus clindamycin (1,200 mg/d); often unacceptable gastrointestinal toxicity
  Pyrimethamine-dapsone two or three times per week
  Fansidar

TABLE 173.7. French Approach to Prenatal Prevention, Diagnosis, and Treatment

Diagnosis of mother: systematic serologic screening, before conception and intrapartum
Treatment of mother: if acute serology, spiramycin reduces transmission. Untreated 94 (60%) of 154 versus treated 91 (23%) of 388 (46)
Diagnosis of fetus: ultrasound examinations; amniocentesis, PCR at ≥17 wk of gestation. Sensitivity 37 (97%) of 38; specificity 301 of 301 (48,49)
Treatment of fetus: pyrimethamine, sulfadiazine, or termination. n = 54 live births; 34 terminations (74)
Outcome: all 54 had normal development; 10 (19%) subtle findings; 7 (13%) intracranial calcifications; 3 (6%) chorioretinal scars (50)

TABLE 173.8. Effect of Attempts at Health Education on the Incidence Rate of *Toxoplasma* Infection in Selected Populations of Pregnant Women in the Paris Area

Hospital	Period	Instruction	Seroconversion	Incidence per 1,000 per year
Hospitals Pinard and Baudelocque	Pre-1960	None	11 of 356	60
Centres Medico-Sociaux CPCAM	1961–1970	None	73 of 2496	64
Hospital X	1973–1975	None	18 of 710	59
Saint Antoine	1973	Verbal drawings	7 of 463	37
	1974		3 of 658	11
Longjumeau	1974–1981	Verbal	20 of 1938	22

Adapted from Remington JS, McLeod R, Desmonts G. Toxoplasmosis. In: Remington JS, Klein JO, eds. *Infectious diseases of the fetus and newborn infant,* 4th ed. Philadelphia: WB Saunders, 1995:140–263, with permission.

or to terminate the pregnancy. In the description of this method by Daffos and colleagues, 28 such pregnancies were terminated, and 15 infants of women who acquired *T. gondii* between the 16th and 25th weeks of gestation were treated *in utero* (i.e., their mothers received 3-week courses of spiramycin alternating with 3-week courses of 50 mg of pyrimethamine daily and 3 g of sulfadiazine daily until term) and then during their first year of life, beginning at birth. All the children are functioning normally at 2 years of age. Four had cerebral calcifications demonstrated during the first year of life, and two had peripheral retinal lesions.

Hohlfeld and colleagues (50) described their experience in detail. They presented results of treatment of 54 infants, 43 of whom were treated *in utero* with a mean follow-up of 19 months. Forty-one infants had subclinical infection, 12 had isolated asymptomatic signs (intracerebral calcifications and normal neurologic status, chorioretinal scar without visual impairment), and l had severe congenital toxoplasmosis. This outcome is considerably better than that found for historical controls without treatment *in utero*.

Recent studies (2) demonstrate that there is less brain and eye disease in the fetus or infant when there is a shorter interval between diagnosis and treatment of the fetus *in utero*. In Austria, Aspock and coworkers (47) treated all pregnant women with evidence of acquisition of *T. gondii* during their gestation with spiramycin until the 17 weeks' gestation and then with pyrimethamine and sulfonamide until the infant was born. Studies are needed to determine the best approach. There are no carefully controlled studies to support the contention that a pregnant woman who has *Toxoplasma* antibody and a history of habitual abortion benefits from treatment.

We suggest that pregnant women who have depressed cell-mediated immunity (e.g., a pregnant woman with systemic lupus erythematosus who is receiving corticosteroids) and with serologic or other clinical evidence of *Toxoplasma* infection receive antitoxoplasma therapy in an attempt to prevent transmission to the fetus, whether the infection is newly acquired or chronic.

Both symptomatic and asymptomatic infants with congenital toxoplasmosis should be treated in an effort to prevent further destruction of vital organs (40,51–54). Guidelines for treatment of congenitally infected infants in whom the diagnosis is strongly suspected are outlined in Table 173.9 (36). Data from Europe and the United States suggest that early institution of specific treatment in these infants may prevent some sequelae and that it corrects manifestations of this infection, such as active chorioretinitis, meningitis, encephalitis, hepatitis, splenomegaly, and thrombocytopenia. Hydrocephalus caused by aqueductal obstruction may develop or worsen during therapy. Such treatment also may reduce the incidence of some sequelae, such as chorioretinitis. Children with extensive involvement at birth may function normally later in life. Treatment does not eradicate the parasite in most children (51).

Therapeutic Agents

PYRIMETHAMINE PLUS SULFADIAZINE OR TRISULFAPYRIMIDINES

Pyrimethamine and sulfadiazine act synergistically against *Toxoplasma in vivo* with a combined activity that is eight times the amount expected if their effects were merely additive. Clinical experience confirms their efficacy. There is evidence that treatment of an acutely infected pregnant woman may prevent infection of her fetus (see the earlier section "Treatment in Specific Clinical Settings"). The simultaneous use of both drugs is indicated except during the first trimester of pregnancy. Comparative tests have shown that sulfapyrazine, sulfamethazine, and sulfamerazine are about as effective as sulfadiazine. All the other sulfonamides tested (sulfathiazole, sulfapyridine, sulfadimetine, and sulfisoxazole) are much less effective.

PYRIMETHAMINE

For adults, a loading dose of 100 to 200 mg of pyrimethamine should be given orally in two divided doses on the first day of treatment. For young children, a loading dose of 1 mg/kg b.i.d. should be given for the first 2 days of treatment. Infants are given 1 mg/kg b.i.d. for the first 2 days of treatment as a loading dose. Thereafter, a usual dosage for an immunologically normal adult is 25 mg per day in one dose. Higher dosages (e.g., 50 to 70 mg day) have been used in adults with AIDS to treat toxoplasmosis (44,55). Doses in young children should not exceed 1 mg/kg to a maximum of 25 mg per day. Because there are no data on absorption of the drug in patients who are quite ill, daily administration is recommended. Daily therapy is recommended for active ocular infection. Pyrimethamine is available only in tablet form. For infants, it may be crushed and administered with food or fluid (51).

Pyrimethamine is a folic acid antagonist and therefore produces a dose-related, reversible, and usually gradual depression of the bone marrow. Thrombocytopenia, leukopenia, and anemia may occur. All patients treated with pyrimethamine should have platelet and peripheral blood cell counts twice weekly.

TABLE 173.9.   Treatment of Toxoplasmosis

Manifestation of infection	Medication	Dosage	Duration of therapy
Pregnant women with acute toxoplasmosis First 18 wk of gestation or until term if fetus not infected.	Spiramycin[a]	1 g q8h without food	Until fetal infection is documented or excluded at 18–20 wk; if documented, has been used in France in alternate months with pyrimethamine, sulfadiazine, and leucovorin until term[b]
Fetal infection confirmed after 17th wk of gestation or if maternal infection acquired in last few weeks of gestation (after amniocentesis and PCR to determine whether there is *Toxoplasma* infection in the fetus)	Pyrimethamine	Loading dose: 100 mg/d in two divided doses for 2 d, then 50 mg/d	Until term (leucovorin is continued 1 wk after pyrimethamine is discontinued)
	Sulfadiazine	Loading dose: 75 mg/kg/d in two divided doses (maximum 4 g/d) for 2 d, then 100 mg/kg/d in two or four divided doses (maximum 4 g/d)	
	Leucovorin (folinic acid)	5–20 mg/d[c]	
Congenital *Toxoplasma* infection in infants	Pyrimethamine[d]	Loading dose: 1 mg/kg b.i.d. for 2 d, then 1 mg/kg/d for 2 or 6 mo,[e] then this dose every Monday, Wednesday, and Friday	1y[f] (leucovorin is continued 1 wk after pyrimethamine is discontinued)
	Sulfadiazine[d]	100 mg/kg/d in two divided doses	
	Leucovorin[d]	5–10 mg three times weekly[c]	
CSF protein value ≥1 g/dL or active chorioretinitis that threatens vision	Corticosteroids (prednisone)	1 mg/kg/d in two divided doses[g]	Until resolution of elevated CSF protein level or active chorioretinitis
Active chorioretinitis in older children	Pyrimethamine	Loading dose: 1 mg/kg b.i.d. (maximum 50 mg) for 2 d, then maintenance, 1 mg/kg/d (maximum 25 mg)	Usually 1–2 wk beyond resolution of signs and symptoms (leucovorin is continued 1 wk after pyrimethamine is discontinued)
	Sulfadiazine	Loading dose: 75 mg/kg, then maintenance, 50 mg/kg every 12 h or 6 h	
	Leucovorin	5–20 mg three times weekly[c]	
	Corticosteroids	1 mg/kg/d of prednisone in two divided doses[g]	Until resolution[g]
Immunologically normal children Lymphadenopathy Significant organ damage that is life threatening	No therapy Pyrimethamine, sulfadiazine, leucovorin	Same as above for active chorioretinitis in older children; no corticosteroids	Usually 4–6 wk or 2 wk beyond resolution of signs and symptoms
Immunocompromised children Non-AIDS	Pyrimethamine, sulfadiazine, leucovorin	Same as above for active chorioretinitis in older children; no corticosteroids	Usually 4–6 wk beyond complete resolution of signs and symptoms
AIDS	Pyrimethamine, sulfadiazine, leucovorin	Same as above for active chorioretinitis in older children; no corticosteroids	Lifetime
	Clindamycin in place of sulfadiazine	Reported trials for adults, but not infants and children	

PCR, polymerase chain reaction; CSF, cerebrospinal fluid; AIDS, acquired immunodeficiency syndrome.

[a]Available only on request from the U.S. Food and Drug Administration; telephone 301-443-5680.

[b]The only studies are those of Hohlfeld et al. (48). However, because Hohlfeld and colleagues found pyrimethamine-sulfadiazine therapy to be superior to spiramycin for treatment of the fetus, continuous therapy with pyrimethamine, sulfadiazine, and leucovorin should be considered in the third trimester.

[c]Adjusted for megaloblastic anemia, granulocytopenia, or thrombocytopenia; blood counts, including platelets, should be monitored as described in text.

[d]Optimal dosage, feasibility, and toxicity are currently being evaluated or planned in ongoing Chicago-based National Collaborative Treatment Trial; telephone 312-791-4152.

[e]These two regimens are currently being compared in a randomized National Collaborative Treatment Trial. Data are not yet available to determine which, if either, is superior. Both regimens appear to be feasible and relatively safe.

[f]In infants with AIDS. The duration of therapy is unknown. Please see discussion in section on congenital toxoplasmosis and AIDS.

[g]Corticosteroids should be continued until signs of inflammation (high CSF protein value ≥1 g/dL) or active chorioretinitis that threatens vision have subsided; dosage can then be tapered and discontinued; use only with pyrimethamine, sulfadiazine, and leucovorin.

From Roberts F, Boyer KM, McLeod R. Toxoplasmosis. In: Krugman S, Gershon AA, Katz SL, et al., eds. *Infectious diseases of children*, 10th ed. St. Louis: Mosby–Year Book, 1997, with permission.

Leucovorin calcium (folinic acid) should be administered with pyrimethamine to prevent suppression of the bone marrow. The optimal frequency for administration of folinic acid is unknown. An oral dose of 10 mg or more is recommended daily for older children and adults, or 10 mg three times weekly or more frequently for infants.

SULFADIAZINE OR TRISULFAPYRIMIDINE

Sulfadiazine or trisulfapyrimidine is administered to older children and adults in a dose of 100 mg/kg (maximum 4–6 g total daily). This dose is administered daily in two doses 12 hours apart or four doses 6 hours apart. In infants, a total daily dose of 100 mg/kg is administered in two doses every 12 hours. Only a tablet form is available.

The potential toxic effects of sulfonamides (e.g., crystalluria, hematuria, rash) must be carefully monitored. Hypersensitivity reactions to sulfonamides may be a particular problem for patients with AIDS (56).

OTHER DRUGS

Treatment of pregnant women with spiramycin to reduce transplacental transmission of *T. gondii* has been with 3 g daily (i.e., 1.0 g morning, noon, and evening). Food impairs absorption of spiramycin. Toxicity is infrequent and has included paresthesia, allergic rash, nausea, vomiting, and diarrhea.

In a small number of patients with AIDS, high doses of pyrimethamine and large doses of clindamycin appeared as efficient as sulfonamides and high doses of pyrimethamine (44). Azithromycin or clarithromycin and pyrimethamine have also been used in this setting (57).

Other agents that have had some success when used in combination with pyrimethamine for treatment of toxoplasmosis in immunocompromised patients are azithromycin, clarithromycin, atovaquone, and interferon-γ. Because of potential interactions between zidovudine and pyrimethamine and possible additive bone marrow toxicity, when possible zidovudine therapy should be discontinued during treatment with pyrimethamine. Concomitant therapy with phenobarbital may reduce the half-life of pyrimethamine by induction of hepatic enzymes that degrade pyrimethamine (58). Usual therapeutic doses of sulfadiazine interfere with metabolism of other agents such as phenytoin and warfarin by hepatic microsomal enzymes.

Duration of Therapy

The optimal duration of specific therapy of toxoplasmosis is not known. Patients who appear to be immunologically normal but have severe and persistent symptoms or damage to vital organs (e.g., chorioretinitis, myocarditis) require specific therapy until these specific symptoms resolve, followed by therapy for an additional 2 weeks. This is usually for at least 4 to 6 weeks and sometimes longer.

For immunocompromised patients, therapy should continue for at least 4 to 6 weeks beyond complete resolution of all signs and symptoms of active disease. Careful follow-up of these patients is imperative because relapse requires prompt reinstitution of therapy.

Relapse is frequent in patients with AIDS. Prolonged prophylaxis should be given (41,43,59–70). Although therapy may be effective against *T. gondii* tachyzoites and may induce a beneficial response clinically, it does not eradicate the cyst from the CNS and perhaps not from other tissues. Patients infected with HIV who have neurologic signs or symptoms, CD4+ cell counts less than 100 cells/mm³, and radiographic scans consistent with toxoplasmic encephalitis are treated empirically with pyrimethamine plus either clindamycin or sulfadiazine. Clinical

response to treatment is noted in 1 to 2 weeks and radiographic resolution in 3 to 6 weeks. Relapse occurs after this treatment in more than 50% of such individuals if treatment is discontinued. Daily pyrimethamine (25 mg) and sulfadiazine (2 g) prophylaxis reduced the relapse rate to 6% in one study, and tolerance of this regimen was reasonable. In this study, twice-weekly prophylaxis with the same dosages of medications resulted in a 30% relapse rate. Other suppressive regimens for individuals who cannot tolerate sulfadiazine, the efficacy of which has not been proved are listed in Table 173.6. For seropositive individuals with HIV infection who have not had toxoplasmic encephalitis, TMP-SMX prophylaxis can be discontinued when CD4 counts are higher than 200 cells/mm³ for more than 4 to 6 months.

Desmonts and Couvreur (46) treated acutely infected pregnant women with 3 g of spiramycin daily, administered orally in three doses, from the time of diagnosis until term. Aspock (47) in Germany gave a course of sulfonamide and pyrimethamine followed by one to two courses of sulfonamide administered alone or in combination with pyrimethamine. Each course was given for about 2 weeks. The courses of treatment were separated by 3- to 4-week intervals of no treatment. Pyrimethamine was not given in the first trimester of pregnancy.

Infants with congenital toxoplasmosis should be treated as outlined in Table 173.9.

PREVENTION

Prophylaxis against *Toxoplasma* involves intervention in the cycle of transmission (71,72) (Table 173.10). Prevention of infection by *T. gondii* is most important in immunodeficient patients and seronegative pregnant women (71–73).

Meat and eggs should be heated to 60°C to kill cysts. Freezing to −20°C kills cysts in meat, but commercial freezers in most areas of the world do not reach or maintain this

---

TABLE 173.10. Methods for Preventing Congenital Toxoplasmosis

Prevention of infection in adults
Cook meat to 66°C (well done), smoke it, or cure it in brine.
Cook eggs and do not drink unpasteurized milk.
Avoid touching mucous membranes of mouth and eyes while handling raw meat.
Wash hands thoroughly after handling raw meat.
Wash kitchen surfaces that come into contact with raw meat.
Wash fruits and vegetables before consumption.
Prevent access of flies, cockroaches, and so on to fruits and vegetables.
Avoid contact with materials that are potentially contaminated with cat feces (e.g., cat litter boxes) or wear gloves when handling such materials or when gardening or playing with children in a sandbox.
Disinfect cat litter box for 5 min with nearly boiling water.

Prevention of infection in fetus
Identify women at risk by serologic testing.
Treatment during pregnancy results in about a 50% reduction in infected infants and can treat manifestations of infection in the fetus.
Therapeutic abortion prevents birth of infected infant; used only when women acquire infection in first or second trimester (50% of cases).

Adapted from Wilson CB, Remington JS. What can be done to prevent congenital toxoplasmosis? *Am J Obstet Gynecol* 1980;138:357–363, with permission.

temperature reliably. Hands should be washed after touching uncooked meat. Fruits and vegetables may be contaminated with oocysts and should be washed. Contact with cat feces should be avoided.

Although there are no definitive data on the risks of using seropositive donors, the following are our recommendations: blood or blood products donated by people with *Toxoplasma* antibody should not be given to immunosuppressed recipients, and organs of those with *Toxoplasma* antibody should not be given to seronegative recipients. If organs (especially heart transplants) from seropositive individuals are given to seronegative recipients, prophylactic antimicrobial treatment is recommended. Prophylaxis with TMP-SMX for AIDS patients with serum antibodies to *T. gondii* may be discontinued when CD4 counts are more than 200 cells/mm^3.

A nontoxic drug that eliminates the organism in the tissue cyst form as well as in the tachyzoite form is needed to prevent the devastating complications of recrudescent infection in immunocompromised patients.

For prevention of transmission of *Toxoplasma* to the fetus, see the section "Treatment in Specific Clinical Settings." There is no effective vaccine to prevent *Toxoplasma* infection. Because maternal immunity appears to prevent congenital transmission of *T. gondii*, development of a vaccine should be explored. Vaccines that prevent oocyst development in household cats could interrupt the life cycle of *T. gondii*.

REFERENCES

1. Boyer K, McLeod R. *Toxoplasma gondii* (toxoplasmosis). In: Long SS, Prober CG, Pickering LK, eds. *Principles and practice of pediatric infectious diseases.* New York: Churchill Livingstone, 2002:1303–1322.
2. Remington JS, McLeod R, Thulliez P, et al. Toxoplasmosis. In: Remington JS, Klein JO, eds. *Infectious diseases of the fetus and newborn infant,* 5th ed. Philadelphia: WB Saunders, 2001:205–346.
3. McLeod R, Mack D, Brown C. New advances in cellular and molecular biology of *Toxoplasma gondii. Exp Parasitol* 1991;72:109.
4. Aikawa M, Komata Y, Asai T, et al. Transmission and scanning electron microscopy of host cell entry by *Toxoplasma gondii. Am J Pathol* 1977;87:285.
5. Weiss LM, Laplace D, Takvorian PM, et al. Development of bradyzoites of *Toxoplasma gondii* in vitro. *J Eukaryol Microbiol* 1994;41:185.
6. Remington JS. In Lainson R. Observations on the nature and transmission of *Toxoplasma gondii* in light of its wide host and geographical range: toxoplasmosis [Discussion]. *Surv Ophthalmol* 1961;6:721.
7. Dubey JP, Miller NL, Frenkel JK. The *Toxoplasma gondii* oocyst from cat feces. *J Exp Med* 1970;132:636.
8. Mayes JT, O'Connor BJ, Avery R, et al. Transmission of *Toxoplasma gondii* infection by liver transplantation. *Clin Infect Dis* 1995;21:511.
9. Remington JS, McLeod R. Toxoplasmosis. In: Braude AL, ed. *International textbook of medicine,* Vol II. Medical microbiology and infectious diseases. Philadelphia: WB Saunders, 1981:1816–1832.
10. Luft BJ, Remington JS. Acute *Toxoplasma* infection among family members of patients with acute lymphadenopathic toxoplasmosis. *Arch Intern Med* 1984; 144:53.
11. Bennenson MW, Takafuji ET, Lemon SM, et al. Oocyst-transmitted toxoplasmosis associated with ingestion of contaminated water. *N Engl J Med* 1982; 307:666.
12. Dorfman RF, Remington JS. Value of lymph-node biopsy in the diagnosis of acute acquired toxoplasmosis. *N Engl J Med* 1973;289:878.
13. Roberts F, McLeod R. Pathogenesis of toxoplasmic retinochoroiditis. *Parasitol Today* 1999;15:51.
14. McCabe RE, Brooks RG, Dorfman RF, et al. Clinical spectrum in 107 cases of toxoplasmic lymphadenopathy. *Rev Infect Dis* 1987;9:754.
15. Glasner PD, et al. An unusually high prevalence of ocular toxoplasmosis in southern Brazil. *Am J Ophthalmol* 1992;1(4):136–144.
16. Grigg M, Bonnefoy S, Hehl AB, et al. Success and virulence in *Toxoplasma* as the result of sexual recombination between two distinct ancestries. *Science* 2001;294:161–165.
17. Polis MA. Differential diagnosis of retinal lesions in persons with HIV infection. *Opportunistic Infect Interaction* 1994;3:1.
18. Ruskin J, Remington JS. Toxoplasmosis in the compromised host. *Ann Intern Med* 1976;84:193.
19. Israelski DM, Remington JS. Toxoplasmic encephalitis in patients with AIDS. In: Sande MA, Volberding PA, eds. *The medical management of AIDS.* Philadelphia: WB Saunders, 1988:193–211.
20. Luft BJ, Naot Y, Araujo FG, et al. Primary and reactivated toxoplasma infection in patients with cardiac transplants: clinical spectrum and problems in diagnosis in a defined population. *Ann Intern Med* 1983;99:27.
21. Deroin F, Devergie A, Auber P. Toxoplasmosis in bone marrow-transplant recipients: report of seven cases and review. *Clin Infect Dis* 1992;15:267–270.
22. Desmonts G, Couvreur J. Natural history of congenital toxoplasmosis. *Ann Pediatr* 1984;31:799.
23. Koppe JG, Loewer-Sieger DH, De Roever-Bonnet H. Results of 20-year follow-up of congenital toxoplasmosis. *Lancet* 1986;1:254.
24. Wilson CB, Remington JS, Stagno S, et al. Development of adverse sequelae in children born with subclinical congenital *Toxoplasma* infection. *Pediatrics* 1980;66:767.
25. Burnett AJ, Shortt SG, et al. Multiple cases of acquired toxoplasmosis retinitis presenting in an outbreak. *Ophthalmology* 1998;105(6):1032–1037.
26. Conley FK, Remington JS. *Toxoplasma gondii* infection of the central nervous system: use of the PAP method to demonstrate *Toxoplasma* in formalin-fixed paraffin-embedded tissue sections. *Hum Pathol* 1981;12:690.
27. Montoya JG, Remington J. Studies on the serodiagnosis of toxoplasmic lymphadenopathy. *Clin Infect Dis* 1995;20:781.
28. Desmonts G, Remington JS. Direct agglutination test for diagnosis of *Toxoplasma* infection: method for increasing sensitivity and specificity. *J Clin Microbiol* 1980;11:562.
29. Dannemann BR, Vaughan WC, Thulliez P, et al. The differential agglutination test for diagnosis of recently acquired infection with *Toxoplasma gondii. J Clin Microbiol* 1990;28:1928.
30. Thulliez P, Remington JS, Santoro F, et al. Une nouvelle réaction d'agglutination pour le diagnostic du stade évolutif de la toxoplasmose acquise. *Pathol Blot* 1986;34:173.
31. Desmonts G. Sérodiagnostic de la toxoplasmose. *Feuill Blot* 1975;16:61.
32. Naot Y, Remington JS. An enzyme-linked immunosorbent assay for detection of IgM antibodies to *Toxoplasma gondii:* use for diagnosis of acute acquired toxoplasmosis. *J Infect Dis* 1980;142:757.
33. Stepick-Biek P, Thulliez P, Araujo FG, et al. IgA antibodies for diagnosis of acute congenital and acquired toxoplasmosis. *J Infect Dis* 1990;162:270.
34. Liesenfeld 0, Montoya J, Kinney S, et al. Effect of testing for IgG avidity in the diagnosis of toxoplasmosis in pregnant women: experience in a US reference laboratory. *J Infect Dis* 2001;183:1248–1253.
35. Grover CM, Thulliez P, Remington JS, et al. Rapid prenatal diagnosis of congenital *Toxoplasma* infection by using polymerase chain reaction and amniotic fluid. *J Clin Microbiol* 1990;28:2297.
36. Roberts F, Boyer KM, McLeod R. Toxoplasmosis. In: Krugman S, Gershon AA, Katz SL, et al., eds. *Infectious diseases of children,* 11th ed. St. Louis: Mosby–Year Book, 2003.
37. McLeod R, Remington JS. Toxoplasmosis. In: Braunwald E, Isselbacher K, Petersdorf R, et al., eds. *Harrison's principles of internal medicine,* 11th ed. New York: McGraw-Hill, 1987:791–797.
38. Townsend JJ, Wolinsky JS, Baringer JR, et al. Acquired toxoplasmosis. *Arch Neurol* 1975;32:335.
39. Montoya JG, Remington JS. Toxoplasmic chorioretinitis in the setting of acute acquired toxoplasmosis. *Clin Infect Dis* 1996;23:277–282.
40. Mets M, Holfels E, Boyer KM, et al. Eye manifestations of congenital toxoplasmosis. *Am J Ophthalmol* 1996;122:309.
41. Couvreur J, Thulliez P. Toxoplasma acquise or localization oculaire ou neurologiqne. *Press Med* 1996;25:438–442.
42. Luft BJ, Hafner R, Korzun AH, et al. Toxoplasmic encephalitis in patients with the acquired immunodeficiency syndrome. Members of the ACTG 077p/ANRS 009 Study Team. *N Engl J Med* 1993;329:995.
43. Consensus recommendations: disease-specific recommendations; toxoplasmic encephalitis. *Clin Infect Dis* 1995;21[Suppl 1].
44. Dannemann BR, McCutchan JA, Israelski D, et al. Treatment of toxoplasmic encephalitis in patients with AIDS: a randomized trial comparing pyrimethamine plus clindamycin to pyrimethamine plus sulfadiazine. *Ann Intern Med* 1992;116:33.
45. Liesenfeld O, Wong SY, Remington JS. Toxoplasmosis in the setting of AIDS. In: Bartlett JG, Merigan TC, Bolognesi D, eds. *Textbook of AIRD medicine.* Baltimore: Williams & Wilkins, 1999.
46. Desmonts G, Couvreur J. Congenital toxoplasmosis: a prospective study of 378 pregnancies. *N Engl J Med* 1974;290:1110.
47. Aspock H. Prevention of congenital toxoplasmosis by serological surveillance during pregnancy: current strategies and future perspectives. In: Marget W, Lang W, Gabler-Sandberger E, eds. *Parasitic infections, immunology, mycotic infections, general topics,* Vol 3. Munich: MMV Medizin Verlag, 1986:69–72.
48. Hohlfeld P, Daffos F, Costa JM, et al. Prenatal diagnosis of congenital toxoplasmosis with a polymerase-chain-reaction test on amniotic fluid. *N Engl J Med* 1994;331:695.
49. Romand S, Wallon J, Franck J, et al. Prenatal diagnosis using polymerase chain reaction on amniotic fluid for congenital toxoplasmosis. *Obstet Gynecol* 2001;97:296–300.
50. Hohlfeld P, Daffos F, Thulliez P, et al. Fetal toxoplasmosis outcome of pregnancy and infant follow-up after in utero treatment. *J Pediatr* 1989;115:765.
51. McAuley J, Boyer K, Patel D, et al. Early and longitudinal evaluations of treated infants and children and untreated historical patients with congenital toxoplasmosis: the Chicago Collaborative Treatment Trial. *Clin Infect Dis* 1994; 18:38.

52. McLeod R, Boyer K, Roizen N, et al. The child with congenital toxoplasmosis. *Curr Clin Top Infect Dis* 2000;20:189–208.
53. Roizen N, Swisher C, Stein M, et al. Developmental and neurologic outcome in treated congenital toxoplasmosis. *Pediatrics* 1995;95:11.
54. Patel D, Holfels EM, Vogel NP, et al. Resolution of intracerebral calcifications in children with treated congenital toxoplasmosis. *Radiology* 1996;199:433.
55. Weiss LM, Harris C, Berger M, et al. Pyrimethamine concentrations in serum and cerebrospinal fluid during treatment of acute *Toxoplasma* encephalitis in patients with AIDS. *J Infect Dis* 1988;157:580.
56. Moreno JN, Poblete RB, Maggio C, et al. Rapid oral desensitization for sulfonamides in patients with the acquired immunodeficiency syndrome. *Ann Allergy Asthma Immunol* 1995;74:140.
57. Fernandez-Martin J, Leport C, Morlat P, et al. Pyrimethamine-clarithromycin combination for therapy of acute *Toxoplasma* encephalitis in patients with AIDS. *Antimicrob Agents Chemother* 1991;35:2049.
58. McLeod R, Mack D, Foss R, et al. Levels of pyrimethamine in sera and cerebrospinal and ventricular fluids from infants treated for congenital toxoplasmosis. *Antimicrob Agents Chemother* 1992;36:1040.
59. de Gans J, Portegies P, Reiss P, et al. Pyrimethamine alone as maintenance therapy for central nervous system toxoplasmosis in 38 patients with AIDS. *J Acquir Immune Defic Syndr* 1992;5:137.
60. Kovacs JA. Toxoplasmosis in AIDS: keeping the lid on. *Ann Intern Med* 1995;123:230.
61. Leport C, Cherie G, Morlat P, et al. Pyrimethamine for primary prophylaxis of toxoplasmic encephalitis in patients with human immunodeficiency virus infection: a double-blind, randomized trial. *J Infect Dis* 1996;173:91.
62. Katlama C, De Wit S, O'Doherty E, et al. Pyrimethamine-clindamycin vs. pyrimethamine-sulfadiazine as acute and long-term therapy for toxoplasmic encephalitis in patients with AIDS. *Clin Infect Dis* 1996;22:268.
63. Heald A, Flepp M, Chave JP, et al. Treatment for cerebral toxoplasmosis protects against *Pneumocystis carinii* pneumonia in patients with AIDS. The Swiss HIV Cohort Study. *Ann Intern Med* 1991;155:760.
64. Pedrol E, Gonzalez-Clemente JM, Gatell JM, et al. Central nervous system toxoplasmosis in AIDS patients: efficacy of an intermittent maintenance therapy. *AIDS* 1990;4:511.
65. Podzamczer D, Salazar A, Jimenez J, et al. Intermittent trimethoprim-sulfamethoxazole compared with dapsone-pyrimethamine for the simultaneous primary prophylaxis of *Pneumocystis pneumonia* and toxoplasmosis in patients infected with HIV. *Ann Intern Med* 1995;122:755.
66. Podzamczer D, Miro JM, Bolao F, et al. Twice weekly maintenance therapy with sulfadiazine-pyrimethamine to prevent recurrent toxoplasmic encephalitis in patients with AIDS. *Ann Intern Med* 1995;123:175.
67. Porter SB, Sande MA. Toxoplasmosis of the central nervous system in the acquired immunodeficiency syndrome. *N Engl J Med* 1992;327:1643.
68. Richards F Jr, Kovacs J, Luft B. Preventing toxoplasmic encephalitis in persons infected with human immunodeficiency virus. *Clin Infect Dis* 1995;21[Suppl 1]:S49.
69. Ruf B, Schurmann D, Bergmann F, et al. Efficacy of pyrimethamine/sulfadoxine in the prevention of toxoplasmic encephalitis relapses and *Pneumocystis carinii* pneumonia in HIV infected patients. *Eur J Clin Microbiol Infect Dis* 1993;12:325.
70. Saba J, Morlat P, Raffi F, et al. Pyrimethamine plus azithromycin for treatment of acute toxoplasmic encephalitis in patients with AIDS. *Eur J Clin Microbiol Infect Dis* 1993;12:853.
71. McCabe R, Remington JS. Toxoplasmosis: the time has come. *N Engl J Med* 1988;318:313.
72. Wilson CB, Remington JS. What can be done to prevent congenital toxoplasmosis? *Am J Obstet Gynecol* 1980;138:357.
73. Wong SY, Remington JS. State of the art clinical article: Toxoplasmosis in pregnancy. *Clin Infect Dis* 1994;18:853.
74. Daffos F, Forestier F, Capella-Pavlovsky M, et al. Prenatal management of 746 pregnancies at risk for congenital toxoplasmosis. *N Engl J Med* 1988;318:271–275.

CHAPTER 174
Larva Migrans Syndromes Caused by Toxocara Species and Other Helminths

Peter M. Schantz

HISTORY

Certain parasitic helminths of lower animals can infect a variety of mammals that are not their definitive hosts. Under such conditions, the invading larvae usually do not develop further but survive indefinitely in the tissues. If these animals, called paratenic or transport hosts, form part of the food chain of the definitive host, the parasite's life cycle is eventually completed. In the first half of this century, several parasitologists speculated that such animal parasites might cause disease in human beings. In 1952, Beaver and colleagues (1) described larvae of *Toxocara canis*, an intestinal roundworm of dogs, in the tissues of children with eosinophilia and hepatomegaly, a common clinical syndrome of previously unknown cause. The authors proposed the term visceral larva migrans (VLM) to describe the syndrome. Wilder (2) observed nematode larvae in 24 of 46 eyes that had been enucleated, in most instances after a clinical diagnosis of retinoblastoma. She identified the worms as third-stage hookworm larvae, but Nichols (3) reexamined the specimens and identified the larvae as *T. canis*. The concept of larva migrans was redefined by Beaver (4) to describe the prolonged migration and long persistence of larvae whose behavior reflects the behavior of larvae in paratenic hosts. Subsequently, Sprent (5) described the complex life cycles of *Toxocara* spp. The development of a sensitive and specific serologic test greatly stimulated clinical and epidemiologic research (6). Toxocaral larva migrans syndromes are now recognized as common zoonotic infections in all countries (7). In developed countries, toxocariasis ranks as the most frequent human helminth infection (8).

Other species of helminth larvae have been reported to infect human beings and cause larva migrans syndromes (Table 174.1). The clinical manifestations of the larva migrans syndromes vary according to the helminth species, number of infective larvae, mode of transmission, migration of larvae to critical locations, and other factors.

TOXOCARA SPECIES

Characteristics of the Pathogen

Toxocara species (family Ascaridae) are large (8 to 18 cm long), heavy-bodied nematodes, the adult stages of which reside in the small intestine of their final host. Two species infect dogs and cats: *T. canis* of dogs and other canids, and *T. cati* of cats and other felines (9). Clinical and epidemiologic evidence indicates that the majority of human infections are caused by *T. canis*. The infective stage for humans is the egg (75 to 90 × 65 to 75 μm) containing the third-stage larva. When released by hatching, the larva measures 350 to 450 × 16 to 20 μm and is capable of migrating extensively in tissues (Fig. 174.1).

Epidemiology

Toxocara species are well adapted for transmission and survival. Dogs can become infected with *T. canis* by ingestion of infective

TABLE 174.1.   Some Helminth Agents of Larva Migrans Syndromes, Their Natural Hosts, and Modes of Transmission to Humans

Helminth agent	Natural definitive hosts	Source and mode of transmission to humans
Toxocara canis	Dogs, other canids	Ingestion of infective eggs
Toxocara cati	Cats, other felids	Ingestion of infective eggs
Ancylostoma spp.	Dogs, cats	Direct skin penetration by larvae or ingestion of larvae
Baylisascaris spp.	Raccoons and other wild mammals	Ingestion of infective eggs
Gnathostoma spp.	Cats, other carnivores	Ingestion of larvae in uncooked flesh of fish, amphibian, avian, or mammalian transport hosts
Spirometra spp.	Cats	Ingestion of larvae in aquatic crustaceans or vertebrate transport hosts

eggs, ingestion of larvae in tissues of paratenic hosts (mice, birds, pigs, earthworms), transplacental migration of larvae from a pregnant bitch to her developing pups, transmammary passage of larvae in milk from a lactating bitch to nursing pups, and ingestion of late-stage larvae or immature adults in the vomitus or feces of infected pups (9). By the fourth postpartum week, these larvae have matured in the pups' intestines and are producing eggs. The life cycle of *T. cati* in cats is similar to that of *T. canis* in dogs, except that there is no placental transfer of larvae. The life span of adult *Toxocara* organisms averages 4 months. Individual female *T. canis* organisms can produce 200,000 eggs per day; because intestinal worm burdens range from one to several hundred worms, infected animals can contaminate the environment daily with millions of eggs. Fertilized eggs passed in dog or cat feces require a minimum of 14 to 21 days in optimal temperature and humidity to molt and develop to the infective larval stage. Direct sunlight and desiccation are rapidly lethal to eggs; in humid soil, however, they may survive for months or even years.

The immense popularity of pets (nearly 60% of U.S. households have dogs or cats), the high prevalence of toxocariasis in puppies and kittens, and the intimate association of dogs and children favor widespread environmental contamination and transmission to children (7). Almost all cases of severe VLM are diagnosed in children 18 months to 3 years old. In the United States, studies have implicated household dogs, particularly puppies, in combination with pica as the principal risk factors for infection (7). Children with geophagic pica (compulsion to eat dirt), a behavior disorder noted in 2% to 10% of children 1 to 6 years old (10), are extremely vulnerable to infection

if they are in a contaminated environment. Older children and adults exposed to the same environments may avoid infection altogether or ingest fewer eggs. Ocular larva migrans (OLM) and milder signs and symptoms of VLM are seen more frequently in older children and adults than in extremely young children (7). Most children with toxocariasis have kept a dog in the house or yard within 1 year of onset of symptoms. However, numerous surveys have verified that soil in parks and other public places is frequently contaminated by *Toxocara* eggs (11).

Although under-recognized and under-reported, *Toxocara* larva migrans is a relatively common infection. Serosurveys in the United States suggest that many thousands of persons are infected every year (7); the great majority of new infections are apparently asymptomatic. One indication of the number of clinical cases is the number of serum specimens submitted every year to state health laboratories for serodiagnosis of toxocariasis. From 1978 through 1987, this number varied from 2,500 to 3,500 samples, 25% to 30% of which tested positive (8).

Pathogenesis

Toxocariasis in humans is acquired by ingestion of the eggs of *Toxocara* spp. that contain the infective-stage larvae. The eggs hatch in the proximal small intestine, and the released larvae penetrate the mucosa, migrate to the liver via the portal circulation, follow vascular channels to the lungs, and then enter the systemic circulation. When the size of the larvae exceeds the diameter of the blood vessel, they are impeded and actively bore through the vessel wall and migrate in the surrounding tissue. Larvae migrate extensively through the body and have been found in every tissue and organ system, including liver, lungs, heart, and brain (1). The distribution and survival of larvae are determined by the size of the inoculum and the frequency of reinfection. In *Toxocara*-naive animals, the total number of recoverable larvae, especially in the liver and lungs, is reduced markedly after the first week after infection (12). Thereafter, however, most larvae survive for many months or even years, although the distribution in the host's tissues may continue to shift. Larvae accumulate progressively in the brain while disappearing from other tissues (13). Larvae in the brain may be relatively free from the harmful effects of the host immunologic response. The number of larvae retained in the liver is greater with superinfection and reinfection than with lower doses or single infections. The migrating larvae leave tracks of hemorrhage, necrosis, and inflammatory cells. The earliest response, for example, 2 weeks, is an acute inflammatory reaction consisting of aggregates of eosinophils, neutrophils, and some monocytes (12). As a result of rapid migration, most larvae visualized at this time in

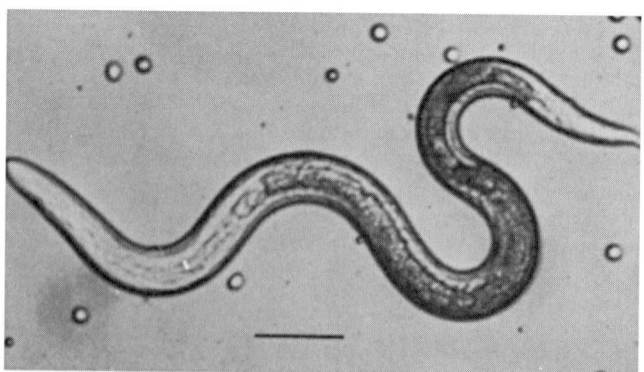

Figure 174.1. Infective-stage larva of *Toxocara canis* after artificial hatching from egg. Bar = 50 μm.

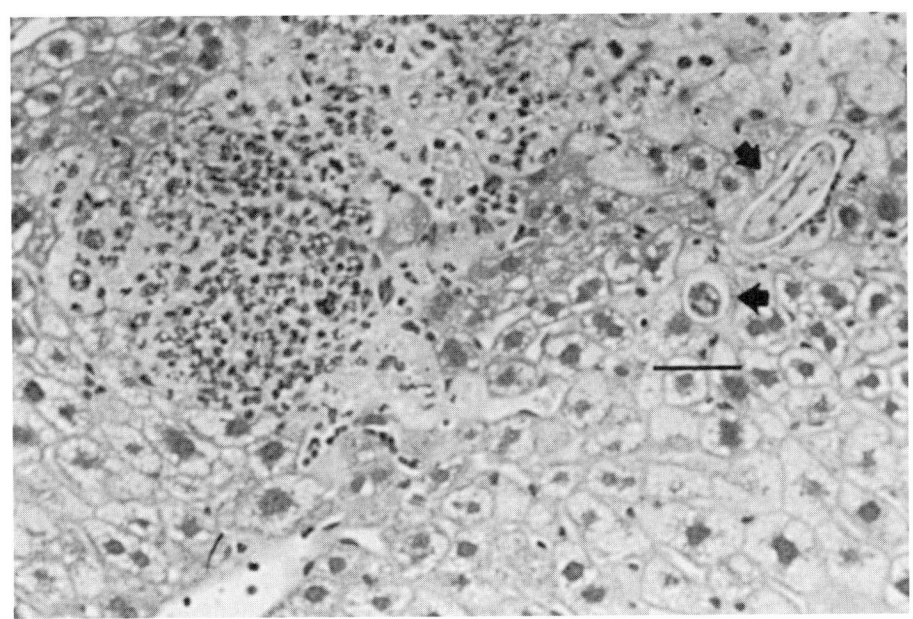

Figure 174.2. Section of mouse liver 2 days after experimental infection with 5,000 eggs of *T. canis*. Areas of hepatocellular necrosis and infiltration of neutrophils associated with a *T. canis* larva (*arrows*). Note that larva is free of inflammatory cells. Hematoxylin-eosin; bar = 50 μm. (Courtesy of Dr. Jim C. Parsons, Victorian Institute of Animal Sciences, Victoria, Australia.)

tissues are not associated with inflammatory cells (Fig. 174.2). By 1 month, larvae and larval tracks are surrounded by rudimentary collagenous capsules. In chronic infections, most larvae are encapsulated by mature granulomata composed of a central core of multinucleated cells and leukocytes. A narrow zone of fibroblastic tissue may delineate the granuloma from the adjacent hepatic parenchyma (Fig. 174.3). Although larvae are not seen in most granulomata, those that are seen usually appear intact and are presumably viable. The remarkable capacity of *Toxocara* larvae to survive and continue migrating in host tissues despite vigorous immunologic responses seems to be associated with the larvae's capacity to shield themselves from host antibody and cells by producing and shedding substances from the larval surface (14,15).

Clinical Manifestations

Overt clinical disease does not develop in most people with *Toxocara* infection. The spectrum of clinical manifestations reflects the numbers of larvae ingested, the frequency of reinfection, the distribution of larvae in the tissues, and the intensity of the inflammatory response.

Two syndromes caused by *Toxocara* infection, VLM and OLM, are well defined (7,16). VLM, usually diagnosed in quite young children (average age 2 years), is a marked inflammatory immune response to numerous larvae migrating in the liver and other tissues. VLM is characterized by persistent eosinophilia, leukocytosis, fever, hepatomegaly, hypergammaglobulinemia, and elevated titers of blood group isohemagglutinins. Clinical signs often include wheezing or coughing, and pulmonary infiltration is evident in one third of patients (16,17). Toxocara has been suggested as possible etiologic agent of asthma (18); however, a recent study found no significant association between the two conditions (19). Neurologic manifestations, including focal or generalized seizures and behavior disorders, have been reported in as many as 28% of patients with VLM (16). The term covert toxocariasis has been suggested to describe the signs and symptoms of patients with clinical features that singly are

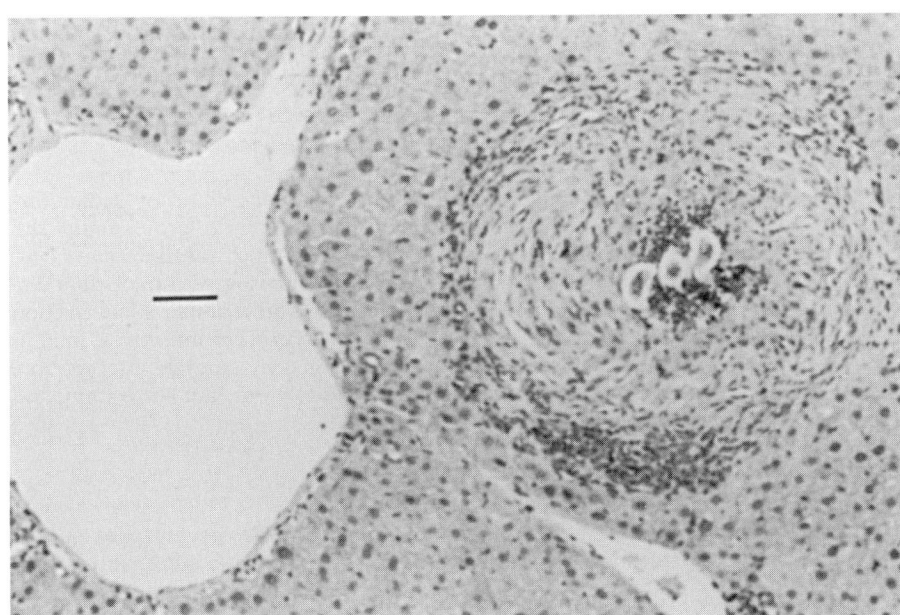

Figure 174.3. Section of mouse liver 5 months after experimental infection with 500 eggs of *T. canis*. Note granuloma containing a coiled larva within a central core of eosinophils surrounded by epithelioid cells and a collagenous capsule. Hematoxylin-eosin; bar = 100 μm. (Courtesy of Dr. Jim C. Parsons, Victorian Institute of Animal Sciences, Victoria, Australia.)

nonspecific but together form a recognizable symptom complex (20). Such signs include abdominal pain, anorexia, sleep and behavior disturbances, cervical adenitis, wheezing, limb pains, and fever. VLM is ordinarily self-resolving once patients are prevented from reinfecting themselves. Rare fatal cases have resulted from larval migration through the myocardium or the central nervous system.

Larval invasion of the eye, typically unilateral, is not uncommon. Common complaints include visual loss, strabismus, and more rarely, eye pain. On funduscopic examination, the lesion may range from a solitary posterior pole or peripheral granuloma in a "quiet" eye to severe exudative endophthalmitis with retinal detachment. In addition, *Toxocara* infection may cause posterior and peripheral retinochoroiditis, optic papillitis, uveitis, and other lesions (21). The average age of patients with OLM is approximately 8 years, but the condition is often diagnosed in adults as well (16).

Clinical and epidemiologic differences between VLM and OLM suggest distinct pathogenetic mechanisms (7,16). These differences seem to be related to the number of infective larvae ingested (7). Lower doses of *Toxocara* are associated with a higher probability of OLM than VLM. As the number of ingested larvae increases, the probability of OLM decreases and the chance of VLM increases. As the parasite load increases further, the likelihood of OLM (concurrent with VLM) once again increases as does the severity of systemic signs. This may explain why most children with VLM have a history of pica and recent exposure to puppies, both of which indicate exposure to large numbers of *Toxocara* eggs. In contrast, patients with OLM are usually older, lack systemic signs, and do not have pica. In these persons, infection with only a small number of eggs is more likely. This may explain why *Toxocara* serum antibody titers are generally lower in persons with OLM than in those with VLM.

Diagnosis

The diagnosis of *Toxocara* infection should be considered in any person with persistent hypereosinophilia. A history of geophagia and association with dogs or cats is helpful. The clinical and laboratory findings (other than specific serologic tests) are nondiagnostic and do not help to differentiate toxocaral LM from other conditions associated with eosinophilia. As the parasite does not mature beyond the larval stage in human tissues, adult worms do not develop in the intestine and diagnosis by egg detection in feces is not possible. Medical imaging methods (ultrasound, computed tomography, magnetic resonance imaging) are useful for detecting the migratory tracks or granulomas induced by tissue-migrating *Toxocara* larvae in many tissues (11).

OLM should be considered in any patients who have raised, unilateral, whitish or gray lesions in the fundus.

Identification of larvae in biopsy tissue permits the definitive diagnosis of *Toxocara* infection; other larval nematodes can be differentiated on the basis of characteristic morphologic features (3). Biopsy is often unrewarding, however. Even in the liver, biopsy specimens may not yield larvae unless the infection is massive.

The enzyme-linked immunosorbent assay (ELISA), using excretory-secretory antigens from infective-stage larvae, is the most useful diagnostic test for toxocaral VLM and OLM (6). In the patient whose clinical signs and history suggest VLM, a positive toxocaral ELISA titer supports the diagnosis. A significantly rising titer in a recently ill patient is consistent with VLM infection. Because toxocaral antibody titers may remain elevated for years after infection, a measurable titer is not proof of a causative relationship between *T. canis* and the current illness.

Surveys have shown that as many as 1% to 10% of asymptomatic children have positive ELISA titers (8). In patients with ocular lesions compatible with OLM, positive serum ELISA titers support the diagnosis but do not rule out retinoblastoma or other ocular pathology. Demonstration of specific toxocaral antibody reactivity in aqueous or vitreous fluid strongly supports the diagnosis.

Toxocaral VLM must be differentiated from signs and symptoms caused by other tissue-migrating helminths (ascarids, hookworm, *Gnathostoma*, *Strongyloides stercoralis*, and *Trichinella spiralis*) and hypereosinophilic syndromes. Ocular disease may be confused with retinoblastoma, ocular tumors, developmental anomalies, exudative retinitis (Coats disease), trauma, and other childhood uveitides (21).

Treatment

Asymptomatic toxocariasis does not require the institution of anthelmintic therapy. Although there are isolated reports of ocular disease occurring years after an episode of VLM, available data suggest that asymptomatic individuals have spontaneous resolution of their eosinophilia and seroreactivity without adverse sequelae (22).

Treatment of patients with symptoms of toxocaral VLM is primarily supportive. Severe pulmonary, myocardial, or central nervous system involvement may warrant corticosteroid therapy. The efficacy and indications for specific anthelmintic treatment remain unclear because of the complexity of the clinical picture and occult localization of the infecting larval parasites (23). Diethylcarbamazine, 50 to 150 mg by mouth (PO) three times a day for 1 to 3 weeks, and thiabendazole, 25 to 50 mg/kg per day PO for 1 to 3 weeks, have been used in the management of VLM but have not been consistently effective. The newer benzimidazole compounds, mebendazole (20 to 25 mg/kg per day PO for 21 days) and albendazole (10 to 15 mg/kg per day PO for 5-15 days), are preferable to other anthelmintics because of their greater safety (23). Ivermectin is not recommended for larval toxocariasis.

Treatment of acute ocular toxocariasis is directed toward suppressing the inflammatory response associated with larval migration or worm death (21). Systemic and intraocular corticosteroids (prednisone, 30 to 60 mg PO each day for 2 to 4 weeks; triamcinolone acetonide, 40 mg sub-Tenon weekly for 2 weeks; or topical prednisolone acetate) are the most consistently effective form of intervention if instituted within the first 4 weeks of illness. The concurrent use of anthelmintic drugs has not been shown to be of any additive benefit in managing OLM. If visualization of the nematode is made possible by clearing of the vitreal inflammatory reaction, laser photocoagulation becomes an effective means of destroying the migrating larva.

The management of patients with long-standing ocular *Toxocara* infection (longer than 8 weeks) is more problematic (23). Corticosteroids may be effective in treating exacerbations of ocular inflammation; however, relapse and progression of ocular disease are common. Intraocular fibrous adhesions, retinal traction and detachment, retrolental plaques, and chronic vitreal inflammation are most effectively managed by surgical intervention. Commonly used procedures include pars plana vitrectomy and scleral buckling (24).

Prevention

Most cases of human toxocariasis can be prevented by simple measures, such as careful personal hygiene, elimination of intestinal parasites from pets, and not allowing children to play in potentially contaminated environments. Unfortunately, few people are aware of the health hazards associated with pets and therefore lack motivation to inquire about or to take the necessary precautions. Efforts must be directed at increasing awareness, especially among pet owners, about potential zoonotic hazards and how to minimize them. Veterinarians are uniquely suited to provide pet owners with sound advice: they have the knowledge, they have established rapport with clients, and a high proportion of pet owners use veterinary services (8).

All pet dogs and cats should receive anthelmintics periodically to prevent the dissemination of infectious eggs. It is particularly important to treat puppies and bitches shortly after whelping and several times during the first year to prevent passage of infectious eggs (25). Laws prohibiting puppies and dogs from running free and defecating in public areas, particularly areas used by children, are neither strictly followed nor strictly enforced. Therefore, parents should not allow children, especially those with pica, to play unattended outdoors where they are likely to have access to infectious eggs.

ANCYLOSTOMA SPECIES

Characteristics of the Pathogen

Ancylostoma braziliense, a hookworm of dogs and cats, and *Ancylostoma caninum*, a common hookworm of dogs, are found throughout North, Central, and South America, most commonly in tropical and subtropical areas. Other *Ancylostoma* spp. are found in animal hosts in other parts of the world. Some species of animal *Strongyloides* can cause cutaneous larva migrans syndromes.

Epidemiology

Cutaneous larva migrans is a disease of utility workers, gardeners, children, sea bathers, and others who come in contact with damp sandy soil that has been contaminated with feces of cats or dogs infected with hookworms. Humans become infected, usually manifest by cutaneous migration when the infective larvae enter the skin by direct penetration (26). *A. caninum* can also reach the human intestine; the enteric form of infection by *A. caninum* is seen relatively commonly in northern Australia (27) and has been diagnosed in the United States (28).

Pathogenesis and Disease

In humans, these animal-hookworm larvae cause a dermatitis called creeping eruption. The larvae, which enter the skin, migrate intracutaneously for long periods but eventually may penetrate to deeper tissues (26). Each larva causes a serpiginous tract, advancing 1 mm to a few centimeters a day, with intense itching that becomes more marked at night. The disease is self-limited; cure is spontaneous after several weeks or months. *A. caninum* may occasionally enter and partially mature in the small intestine and has been causally associated with eosinophilic enteritis (27). Enteric infection may occur most commonly when infection results from ingestion of hookworm larvae rather than by skin penetration.

Diagnosis

Cutaneous larva migrans is diagnosed from the clinical appearance and history of possible exposure (25). Eosinophilic enteritis caused by *A. caninum* is diagnosed on the basis of obscure abdominal pain and blood eosinophilia. Serologic tests, not widely available, do not distinguish infection by *A. caninum* from that caused by human-adapted forms of hookworm.

Treatment

Albendazole (200 mg PO twice a day for 1 to 3 days) (28) and ivermectin (200 μg/kg PO for 1 day) (29) are effective in eliminating signs and symptoms of cutaneous larval migration. These same anthelmintic drugs or mebendazole (100 mg twice a day PO for 3 days) are effective for eliminating hookworms that reach the intestinal lumen.

BAYLISASCARIS SPECIES

Characteristics of the Pathogen

Baylisascaris procyonis, an intestinal ascarid of raccoons, is prevalent throughout North America, usually at rates greater than 50% (31). Other species of *Baylisascaris*, which are found in skunks, bears, and other hosts, may also be capable of infecting human beings.

Epidemiology

Humans are infected when they ingest infective eggs in soil or other contaminated materials; pica and geophagia are behaviors documented in most patients that were conducive to accidental ingestion of infectious eggs. Fewer than 20 clinical cases in humans have been documented through 2001 (32); however, infections resulting in less severe disease may go undiagnosed. The potential for exposure is widespread and growing as the numbers of raccoons in suburban and urban areas increase.

Pathogenesis and Disease

Ingested eggs hatch in the intestine, released larvae penetrate the gut wall, and are carried throughout the body by the circulatory system. Pathogenesis is similar to that of *Toxocara* infection; however, the disease is usually more severe because the larvae increase in size by several factors and have a predilection for the heart and central nervous system (31). Severe neurologic illness results from traumatic damage caused by migrating larvae and release of eosinophil-derived neurotoxin from associated eosinophilic inflammation (33). Consequently, the disease is a severe or fatal cerebrospinal nematodiasis (32). Ocular invasion may occur, causing an OLM syndrome (34,35).

Diagnosis

A diagnosis of baylisascariasis should be considered in patients with progressive neurologic disease and elevated eosinophilia; in several human cases the specific cause was not suspected before the patients died and the *Baylisascaris* larvae were identified at autopsy. Specific serologic tests have been described but are not yet widely available (32).

Treatment

High-dose albendazole (25 to 50 mg/kg per day) given early in the course of infection has the potential to prevent or halt progression of central nervous system (CNS) disease; however, in most reported cases the specific diagnosis was made after extensive damage had already occurred (33).

GNATHOSTOMA SPECIES

Characteristics of the Pathogen

Gnathostoma spp. are spiruroid nematodes parasitic in the intestines of wild and domestic carnivores. The life cycles of these nematodes include successive parasitic stages first in aquatic invertebrates; second in vertebrates including fish, amphibians, and reptiles; and finally in carnivorous mammals, including human beings. *G. spinigerum*, the most common agent of human zoonotic gnathostomiasis, is a parasite of cats and dogs (36).

Epidemiology

Humans become infected when they ingest raw or undercooked dishes prepared from second intermediate hosts (fish, frogs, snakes) containing third-stage *Gnathostoma* spp. larvae. Human infection is common in Southeast Asia, Japan, Ecuador, and Mexico (36).

Pathogenesis and Disease

After ingestion the larval parasite migrates through the tissues, forming transient inflammatory lesions or abscesses in various parts of the body. The disease is characterized systemically by eosinophilia and locally by localized or migratory ("creeping eruption") swelling of the skin and various visceral organs (36). Larvae may invade the brain, producing focal cerebral lesions associated with eosinophilic pleocytosis; ocular invasion may also occur (37).

Diagnosis

Diagnosis is usually by biopsy of lesions. Serologic tests available in Asia are reportedly specific (38).

Treatment

Ivermectin (0.2 mg/kg single dose) and albendazole (400 mg twice a day for 28 days) were comparably effective (greater than 93%) in cases involving dermal and subcutaneous localization (39); in cases involving the CNS helminthicidal medical treatment may not resolve all symptoms due to residual damage (40). Surgical removal of the worm was recommended for larvae localized in the eye or brain (37).

SPIROMETRA SPECIES (SPARGANOSIS)

Characteristics of the Pathogen

Sparganosis is infection by the second-stage larva (plerocercoid or sparganum) of pseudophyllidean cestodes, usually assumed to be of the genus *Spirometra*. The sparganum is a fleshy, motile, ribbon-shaped elongated larva (3 to 40 cm in length) that is flattened dorsoventrally and has a broad evaginated anterior end, which is the future scolex.

Epidemiology

The adult tapeworms are parasitic in the intestines of domestic and wild carnivores. Intermediate hosts for the larval stages include aquatic crustaceans and a variety of amphibians, reptiles, birds, and mammals. People become infected by (a) drinking water containing infected copepods; (b) ingesting tissues of an amphibian, reptilian, mammalian, or avian host of second-stage larvae; or (c) applying the flesh of an infected intermediate host as a poultice to the eye or an open wound. Human sparganosis has been reported worldwide but is more common in Japan, China, Korea, and Southeast Asia. In the United States, approximately 60 cases have been confirmed, but many more cases go undescribed (41).

Pathogenesis and Disease

Larvae migrate from the human intestine to peripheral tissues, where they coil or remain elongated. Sparganosis most commonly presents as a palpable firm mass or nodule (2 to 3 cm), which may be inflamed, tender, painful, or pruritic. Spargana are most commonly localized in subcutaneous connective tissue and in superficial muscles, but infection can develop anywhere on the body. Spargana can migrate to internal organs, eyes or brain, giving rise to the rare visceral, ocular and cerebral forms of the disease (42,43). A rare but serious form is proliferative sparganosis, in which spargana proliferate throughout the body and is ultimately fatal (44).

Diagnosis

The diagnosis may be suggested by the clinical manifestations (migrating nodule) or serpiginous tubular tracts in imaging studies (45), but is usually not confirmed until sparganum tissue is identified in a biopsy specimen.

Treatment

Preferred treatment is surgical removal of the nodules. When the nodules are inaccessible treatment with praziquantel (50 mg/kg per day for 14 days) may be effective (42); however, chemotherapy of the proliferative form has not been successful (46).

REFERENCES

1. Beaver PC, Snyder MD, Carrera GM, et al. Chronic eosinophilia due to visceral larva migrans. *Pediatrics* 1952;9:7.
2. Wilder HC. Nematode endophthalmitis. *Trans Am Acad Ophthalmol* 1951;55:99.
3. Nichols RL. The etiology of visceral larva migrans. 1. The diagnostic morphology of infective second-stage *Toxocara* larvae. *J Parasitol* 1956;42:349.
4. Beaver PC. The nature of visceral larval migrans. *J Parasitol* 1969;55:3.
5. Sprent JFA. Observations on the development of *Toxocara canis* (Werner, 1782) in the dog. *Parasitology* 1958;48:184.
6. Glickman LT, Schantz PM, Grieve RB. Toxocariasis. In: Walls KW, Schantz PM, eds. *Immunodiagnosis of parasitic diseases*, vol 1, *Helminthic diseases*. New York: Academic Press, 1986:201–231.
7. Glickman LT, Schantz PM. Epidemiology and pathogenesis of zoonotic toxocariasis. *Epidemiol Rev* 1981;3:230.
8. Schantz PM. Toxocaral larva migrans now. *Am J Trop Med Hyg* 1989;41[Suppl]:21.
9. Parsons JC. Ascarid infections of cats and dogs. *Vet Clin North Am Small Anim Pract* 1987;17:1307.
10. Bicknell J. *Pica: a childhood symptom*. London: Butterworth, 1975:4–25.
11. Magnaval J-F, Glickman LT, Dorchies P, Morassin B. Highlights of human toxocariasis. *Kor J Parasitol* 2001;39:1–11.
12. Kayes SG, Oaks JA. Effect of inoculum size and length of infection on the distribution of *Toxocara canis* larvae in the mouse. *Am J Trop Med Hyg* 1976;25:573.
13. Dunsmore JD, Thompson RCA, Bates IA. The accumulation of *Toxocara canis* larvae in the brains of mice. *Int J Parasitol* 1983;13:517.
14. Parsons JC, Bowman DD, Grieve RB. Tissue localization of excretory-secretory antigens of larval *Toxocara canis* in acute and chronic murine toxocariasis. *Am J Trop Med Hyg* 1986;35:974.
15. Maizels RM, de Savigny D, Ogilvie BM. Characterization of surface and excretory-secretory antigens of *Toxocara canis* infective larvae. *Parasite Immunol* 1984;6:23.
16. Zinkham WH. Visceral larva migrans. A review and reassessment indicating two forms of clinical expression: visceral and ocular. *Am J Dis Child* 1978;132:627.
17. Huntley CC, Costas MC, Lyerly A. Visceral larval migrans syndrome: clinical characteristics and immunologic studies in 51 patients. *Pediatrics* 1965;36:523.

18. Buijs J, Borsboom G, van Gemond JJ, et al. *Toxocara* seroprevalence in 5-year-old elementary school children: relation with allergic asthma. *Am J Epidemiol* 1994;140:839.

19. Sharghi N, Schantz PM, Caramico L, et al. Environmental exposure to *Toxocara* as a possible risk factor for asthma: a clinic-based case-control study. *Clin Inf Dis* 2001;32:e111–e116.

20. Taylor MRH, Keane CT, O'Connor P, et al. The expanded spectrum of toxocaral disease. *Lancet* 1988;1:692.

21. Shields JA. Ocular toxocariasis: a review. *Surv Ophthalmol* 1984;28:361.

22. Bass JL, Mehta KA, Glickman LT, et al. Asymptomatic toxocariasis in children. *Clin Pediatr* 1987;26:441.

23. Magnaval J-F, Dorchies P, Glickman LT. *Toxocara* species. In: Liu VL, Raoult D, Weber R, eds. *Antimicrobial therapy and vaccines.* New York: Lippincott, Williams and Wilkins, 2003 (*in press*).

24. Hagler WS, Pollard ZF, Jarrett WH, Donnelly EH. Results of surgery for ocular *Toxocara canis.* *Ophthalmology* 1981;88:1081.

25. Centers for Disease Control/American Association of Veterinary Parasitologists. Recommendations for veterinarians. How to prevent transmission of intestinal roundworms from pets to people. 1995. Available at: www.cdc.gov/ncidod/diseases/roundwrm/roundwrm.htm.

26. Enander MW Adam RC. Cutaneous larva migrans: a literature review and case report. *J Am Podiatr Assoc* 1988;79:83.

27. Croese J, Lookas A, Opdebeeck J, Prociv P. Occult enteric infection by *Ancylostoma caninum*: a previously unrecognized zoonosis. *Gastroenterology* 1994;106:3.

28. Khoshoo V, Schantz P, Craver R et al. Dog hookworm: a cause of eosinophilic enterocolitis in humans. *J Pediatr Gastroenterol Nutr* 1994;19:448.

29. Orihuela AR, Torres JR. Single dose of albendazole in the treatment of cutaneous larva migrans. *Arch Dermatol* 1990;126:396.

30. Caumes E, Datry A, Paris L, et al. Efficacy of ivermectin in the therapy of cutaneous larva migrans. *Arch Dermatol* 1992;128:994.

31. Kazacos KR. Neurology chapter. *Baylisascaris procyonis* and related species. In: Samuel WM, Pybus MJ, Kocan AA, eds. *Parasitic diseases of wild mammals,* 2nd ed. Ames, IA: Iowa State University Press, 2001:301–341.

32. Kazacos KR, Gavin PJ, Shulman ST, et al. Raccoon roundworm (*Baylisascaris procyonis*) encephalitis—Chicago and Los Angeles 2000. *MMWR* 2002;50(51):1153–1155.

33. Moertel CL, Kazacos KR, Butterfield JH, et al. Eosinophil-derived inflammation and elaboration of eosinophil-derived proteins in two children with raccoon roundworm (*Baylisascaris procyonis*) encephalitis. *Pediatrics* 2001;108:E93.

34. Kazacos KR, Raymond LA, Kazacos EA, Vestre WA. The raccoon ascarid: a probable cause of human ocular larva migrans. *Ophthalmology* 1985;92:1735.

35. Goldberg MA, Kazacos KR, Boyce WM, et al. Diffuse unilateral subacute neuroretinitis. *Ophthalmology* 1993;100:1695.

36. Rosnak JM, Lucey DR. Clinical gnathostomiasis: case report and review of the English-language literature. *Clin Infect Dis* 1993;16:33.

37. Qahtani F, Deschenes J, Ali-Khan Z, et al. Intraocular gnathostomiasis: a rare Canadian case. *Can J Ophthalmol* 2000;35:35–39.

38. Tapchaisri P, Nopparatana C, Chaicumpa W, et al. Specific antigen of *Gnathostoma spinigerum* for immunodiagnosis of human gnathostomiasis. *Int J Parasitol* 1991;21:315–319.

39. Nontasut P, Bussaratid V, Chullawichit S, et al. Comparison of ivermectin and albendazole treatment for gnathostomiasis. *SE Asian J Trop Med Pub Health* 2000;31:374–377.

40. Chandenier J, Husson J, Canaple S, et al. Medullary gnathostomiasis in a white patient: use of immunodiagnosis and magnetic resonance imaging. *Clin Infect Dis* 2001;32:e154–157.

41. Norman SH, Kreutner A Jr. Sparganosis: clinical and pathologic observations in ten cases. *South Med J* 1980;73:297.

42. Munckhof WJ, Grayson ML, Susil BJ, et al. Cerebral sparganosis in an East Timorese refugee. *Med J Aust* 1994;161:263–264.

43. Kim CY, Cho BK, Kim IO, et al. Cerebral sparganosis in a child. *Pediatr Neurosurg* 1997;26:103–106.

44. Beaver PC, Rolon FA. Proliferating larval cestodes in a man in Paraguay: a case report and review. *Am J Trop Med Hyg* 1981;30:625.

45. Cho J-H, Lee K-B, Yong TS, et al. Subcutaneous and musculoskeletal sparganosis: imaging characteristics and pathologic correlation. *Skel Radiol* 2000;29:402–408.

46. Torres J, Noya OO, Noya BA, et al. Treatment of proliferative sparganosis with mebendazole and praziquantel. *Trans Roy Soc Trop Med Hyg* 1981;75:846–847.

Lymph Node Syndromes

CHAPTER 175
Epstein-Barr Virus Infection and Infectious Mononucleosis

Elliott Kieff

HISTORY

The initial descriptions of infectious mononucleosis (IM) are attributed to Filatov and Pfeiffer, who independently described clinical syndromes of lymphadenopathy with fever in 1885 (1,2). Sprunt and Evans first used the term "infectious mononucleosis" in 1921 when they described six cases of fever, lymphadenopathy and atypical lymphocytosis in healthy adults (3). In 1932, Paul and Bunnell described the association of heterophile antibodies with IM (4). Davidsohn devised a more specific heterophile test using differential absorption of patient serum with guinea pig kidney and beef erythrocytes (5). After the description by Dennis Burkitt of an endemic lymphoma in African children, Epstein and associates discovered the herpesvirus that is now called Epstein-Barr virus (EBV) in electron micrographs of Burkitt tumor cell lines (6,7). Gertrude and Werner Henle developed an indirect immunofluorescent assay for EBV and found that 90% of U.S. adults had antibody directed against EBV (8). The Henles discovered seroconversion to EBV positivity in a laboratory technician with acute IM, generated an EBV-infected lymphoblastoid cell line from the patient, and recognized that EBV was a suitable candidate etiologic agent for IM (9). Subsequent epidemiologic studies confirmed that EBV is the usual cause of heterophile-positive IM (10–13).

This chapter describes the epidemiology, pathogenesis, clinical manifestations, diagnosis, and treatment of EBV-induced IM.

EPIDEMIOLOGY

EBV infection is usually transmitted through contact of saliva from an infected person with the oropharyngeal epithelium of an uninfected individual. Primary EBV infection in children often occurs by sharing food with infected family members. Adolescents or adults usually are infected by salivary transfer during kissing; IM is called the "kissing disease" (14–17). Transmission among children in nurseries or during play has not been investigated. EBV most likely does not survive very long on fomites. Infection is not readily spreads among roommates (12).

After exposure to infected saliva, EBV replicates in epithelial cells of the oropharynx. EBV is shed most consistently into saliva during primary infection. Virus shedding into saliva continues intermittently throughout life. Immunocompromised individuals have higher rates of oropharyngeal shedding of EBV as compared to immunocompetent individuals (18–21). After infecting oropharyngeal epithelium, EBV infects B-lymphocytes. Virus persists indefinitely in a small fraction of circulating B-lymphocytes and in lymph nodes. Transfusion of blood products that contain white blood cells to susceptible (nonimmune) persons can result in primary infection (22). In patients who have undergone allogeneic bone marrow or solid organ transplantation, EBV shed from the oropharynx can frequently be traced to the donor, indicating that infected B-cells may serve as a source of EBV, which can infect pharyngeal epithelium. EBV may also be shed in salivary gland secretions and secretions from the cervix (23), indicating that epithelial tissues other than that of the oropharynx may serve as sources of EBV infection.

In less industrialized societies or among lower socioeconomic groups in industrialized societies, children are usually infected with EBV in the first decade of life (24,25), while it is more common for those in higher socioeconomic groups to remain uninfected until adolescence or adulthood. Primary EBV infection during adolescence or adulthood often causes the syndrome of IM (26). IM accounts for approximately 5% of hospitalizations in the university setting (27,28). More than 90% of adults worldwide have serologic evidence of EBV infection and latent infection with EBV (24,29).

PATHOGENESIS

Because primary EBV infection usually occurs during the first 3 years of life and is usually asymptomatic in this age group, little is known about the pathogenesis of infection in this population (24,25). EBV pathogenesis is best studied in the less common circumstance where infection occurs during adolescence or adulthood because these patients often have symptomatic disease, which can be readily identified (26). EBV initially infects oropharyngeal epithelial cells and most likely subsequently infects circulating B-lymphocytes as they pass near the infected oropharyngeal cells. In two studies (30,31), EBV-infected lymphoblastoid cell lines were established from the blood of patients during the incubation period of IM, before the onset of symptoms and before the onset of an EBV-specific immune response. Therefore, EBV infection of B cells precedes the symptoms of IM. Immunofluorescent staining of circulating B cells from patients with IM has shown 0.1% to 1% of these cells are usually EBV-infected, although more than 10% of cells may be EBV-infected in some cases (31–34). The numbers of EBV-infected cells decrease rapidly with disease progression and mounting of an immune response. Histologic analysis of lymphoid tissue from patients in the acute phase of IM reveal considerable numbers of EBV infected B cells in extrafollicular areas (35).

The most commonly used serologic tests of EBV infection measure antibody responses to: EBV nuclear antigen (EBNA) expressed in latently infected cells (36); early antigen (EA), which is divisible into diffuse (EA-D, methanol-resistant) and restricted (EA-R, methanol-sensitive) components that are expressed in early lytic infection (37); and virus capsid antigen (VCA), which is expressed in late lytic infection (8). Typically, such tests are done using indirect immunofluorescence microscopy or enzyme-linked immunoassay (ELISA). Each of these "antigens" is actually a composite of several viral proteins. Attempts to replace these older assays with more specific tests have been partially successful. Most clinical testing is still done with the original assays (38–41).

At the onset of IM symptoms, IgM antibodies to EA and VCA are usually present and IgG titers to both VCA and EA (most frequently to the D component) are rising. IgM antibodies to

VCA are diagnostic of IM and disappear within several months of illness in most patients (42–46). Patients in the recovery phase of IM have low EBNA titers that then rise and persist for years. Documentation of EBNA seroconversion is also diagnostic of IM. IgG anti-VCA titers reach a peak after illness and then slowly fall over several months to a steady-state level. IgG anti-EA titers fall faster and further than IgG anti-VCA, and become undetectable or stabilize at low levels (47). Low titer virus neutralizing antibodies directed at the gp350 antigen are present in acute IM and persist at relatively stable levels (48). This antibody response is summarized in Fig. 175.1.

There is usually a polyclonal increase in total immune globulin in IM, which is most likely related to EBV activation of B cells (47). As part of this nonspecific antibody response, heterophile antibodies appear in 90% of patients with IM (49). The Paul-Bunnell-Davidsohn test for heterophile antibodies is positive when antibodies are present that agglutinate sheep or horse erythrocytes. However, serum must first be absorbed with guinea pig kidney to remove antibodies of serum sickness or naturally occurring Forssman antibodies (4). The Monospot test assays for the ability of serum to agglutinate horse red blood cells after absorption with guinea pig kidney. A further control may include absorption of serum with beef red blood cells, which reduces or eliminates agglutination of horse erythrocytes when heterophile antibodies are present. Horse erythrocyte agglutination tends to be somewhat more sensitive and specific than sheep erythrocyte agglutination ($\cong$7% versus $\cong$12% false-positive results, respectively). Horse erythrocyte agglutinins also persist longer than sheep erythrocyte agglutinins (75% versus 30%, respectively, present one year after infection) (42). In young children, particularly those younger than 4 years of age, the heterophile test result is often negative in primary EBV infection (50). When IM is suspected and the heterophile test result is negative, specific EBV antibody titers can distinguish EBV induced IM from other causes of IM-like illness (i.e., cytomegalovirus or *Toxoplasma*) (47).

In addition to specific and nonspecific antibody responses, IM is associated with a strong cell-mediated immune response. The "atypical" lymphocytes seen in IM are predominantly CD8 but also CD4 T cells and not the EBV-infected B lymphocytes (51,52). During IM, there is suppression of delayed type hypersensitivity responses (53).

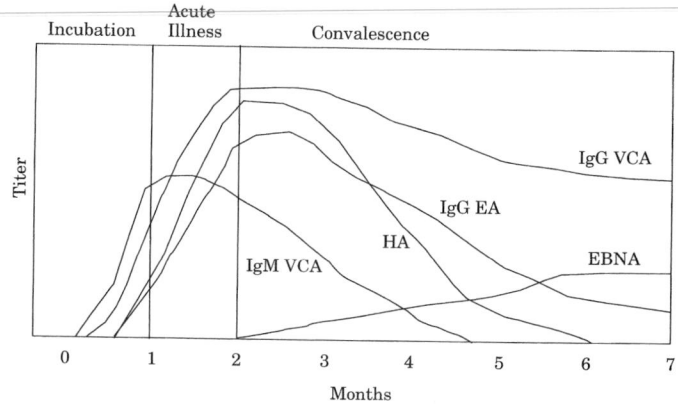

Figure 175.1. Antibody response to acute infection with EBV. VCA, virus capsid antigen; HA, heterophile antibody; EA, early antigen; EBNA, EBV nuclear antigen. (Adapted from Henle W, Henle G. Seroepidemiology of the virus. In: Epstein M, Achong B, eds. *The Epstein-Barr virus*. Berlin: Springer-Verlag, 1979:61–78; and Tomkinson B, Sullivan J. Epstein-Barr virus Infection and mononucleosis. In: Gorbach S, Bartlett J, Blacklow N, eds. *Infectious diseases*. Philadelphia, WB Saunders, 1991:1348–1356.)

CLINICAL MANIFESTATIONS

After exposure to EBV, there is a 2- to 5-week incubation period before the onset of IM. Symptoms include pharyngitis, lymphadenopathy, fever, headache, and malaise, which may last from 1 to several weeks. The presenting complaint of IM is often pharyngitis, which is exudative in approximately 50% of patients. Cervical lymph nodes (posterior more often than anterior) may be significantly enlarged and are usually moderately tender. The range of fever is generally between 38°C and 40°C (54,55). Tonsils may enlarge dramatically and may meet at the midline of the oropharynx. Other findings may include splenomegaly (50%), hepatitis (20% to 90%), palatal petechiae (11% to 33%), periorbital or facial edema (33%), vomiting (5% to 20%), and jaundice (5% to 9%) (54–58). Rash occurs in approximately 10% of IM cases and may be maculopapular, urticarial, petechial, or erythema multiforme-like. If ampicillin or amoxicillin is administered, a distinctive, diffuse maculopapular rash may develop (58). Intermittent malaise or weakness may persist for several months after IM.

Complications occur in IM and occasionally result in fatal outcomes. An infrequent complication of IM may present as the predominant or only clinical finding and may occur without atypical lymphocytosis or heterophile antibodies. Neurologic complications include encephalitis (cerebellar dysfunction often predominates), aseptic meningitis, mono- or polyneuritis, transverse myelitis, Guillain-Barré syndrome, uveitis, optic neuritis, seizures, or cranial nerve palsies (59–68). Hematologic complications include autoimmune hemolytic anemia due to anti-i antibodies (69), thrombocytopenia likely due to anti-platelet antibodies (70), neutropenia, pancytopenia, or a hemophagocytic syndrome (71). Splenic rupture can occur in IM even without clinical evidence of splenomegaly or significant trauma. Splenic rupture occurs most commonly at the height of illness or early in the convalescent stage of IM. Signs of splenic rupture include abdominal pain, pain referred to the left shoulder, and signs of hypovolemia. Due to the possibility of splenic rupture, contact sports should be avoided during IM (72,73). Cardiac complications of IM include myocarditis, pericarditis and conduction abnormalities. Renal complications of IM include nephrotic syndrome and renal dysfunction. Interstitial pneumonia or pleuritis also occur in IM (74,75).

In X-linked lymphoproliferative disease (Duncan's syndrome), progressive, severe, primary EBV infections may occur. Children with this syndrome have no obvious manifestation of immune deficiency until they become infected with EBV, which then leads to severe disease during primary infection. In these patients, there is early polyclonal proliferation of EBV-infected B cells. Fulminant hepatic failure frequently occurs and can be fatal. When patients do recover, long-term complications may occur such as anemia, pancytopenia or hypogammaglobulinemia. EBV-associated lymphoproliferative disease can occur during the initial illness or after recovery (76–78). The underlying genetic defect in x-linked lymphoproliferative disease has been traced to the gene, *SH2D1A*, which encodes a small SH2 binding domain protein. *SD2D1A* likely affects the immune response to EBV-infected lymphocytes (79).

Rarely, severe, chronic EBV infection occurs in previously well individuals without X-linked lymphoproliferative disease. Clinical findings may include lymphadenopathy, uveitis, hepatosplenomegaly and polyneuropathy (80,81). These patients usually have antibody titers directed against EBV replicative proteins that are ten- to 100-fold higher than titers typically found in IM.

Patients infected with human immunodeficiency virus (HIV) may manifest oral hairy leukoplakia, which causes white, corrugated lesions on the inferolateral surfaces of the tongue and typically occurs once the CD4 count drops below $150,000/mm^3$. The lesions of oral hairy leukoplakia contain foci of EBV replication in squamous epithelial cells (82–84).

Chronic fatigue syndrome is characterized by recurrent malaise, weakness, myalgias, arthralgias, pharyngitis, lymphadenitis, and self-reports of low-grade fever. Initially, EBV was thought to be the etiologic agent of the chronic fatigue syndrome. However, after extensive study, this hypothesis has been disproved because it has been found that titers of antibodies directed against EBV and objective findings of EBV infection in patients with the chronic fatigue syndrome are not significantly different from controls (85,86).

DIAGNOSIS

Laboratory findings in IM include a relative or absolute lymphocytosis and lymphocytes may account for more than 50% of the total leukocyte count. Atypical lymphocytes often comprise over 10% of the total white blood cell count. Atypical lymphocytes are large cells with abundant, basophilic, vacuolated cytoplasm. Relatively mild neutropenia with an absolute neutrophil count less than 2000 may occur during the second week of illness. Mild thrombocytopenia with platelet counts 100,000 to $140,000/mm^3$ occur in approximately 50% of patients. Hepatic transaminases, alkaline phosphatase and bilirubin are elevated two- to threefold in up to 90% of IM patients and levels usually peak in the second or third week of illness (54,87–91).

Typically, the diagnosis of IM is made when patients present with fever, pharyngitis, lymphadenopathy, atypical lymphocytosis, and a positive heterophile titer. Specific serology for EBV (see Fig. 175.1) is helpful diagnostically in cases with negative heterophile tests. Direct culturing of EBV involves infecting and immortalizing primary human B lymphocytes with EBV and is not available commercially.

The differential diagnosis of EBV-induced IM includes other diseases that can cause pharyngitis or atypical lymphocytosis. Group A streptococcal pharyngitis presents with an exudative pharyngitis, cervical lymphadenopathy and fever and can be diagnosed with a throat culture or rapid streptococcal antigen test. Because 3% to 30% of IM patients are throat culture positive for group A streptococcus, these patients should be given penicillin or erythromycin to avoid amoxicillin- or ampicillin-induced rash (55). Cytomegalovirus-induced IM can present similarly to EBV-induced IM with fever and lymphocytosis with atypical lymphocytes. Pharyngitis and cervical lymphadenopathy are usually absent. The heterophile test result is negative. Acute viral hepatitis caused by hepatitis A, B, or C can also cause an atypical lymphocytosis but the level is usually less than 10% of the total white blood cell count. More significantly, transaminases rise substantially higher in acute viral hepatitis than the mild two- to threefold elevation seen in IM. Acute toxoplasmosis can cause a mononucleosis syndrome with cervical lymphadenopathy and fever but the atypical lymphocytosis is usually less than 10% and the heterophile test result is negative. Other causes of atypical lymphocytosis include rubella, acute HIV infection, mumps, other herpesvirus infections, rickettsial infections, and drug hypersensitivity reactions (92–96).

TREATMENT

Therapy of IM is primarily supportive and aspirin or acetaminophen may help alleviate fever and symptoms of pharyngitis. It is generally recommended that patients rest during the initial phase of disease and then to slowly resume normal activities but firm data are lacking. Due to the risk of splenic rupture, sports (especially contact) or strenuous activity such as heavy lifting should be avoided for at least 1 month and patients with enlarged or tender spleens should avoid such activity until splenomegaly and tenderness have resolved. Ultrasound can be used to ensure normal spleen size before resuming strenuous activity (54,55)

The therapeutic use of corticosteroids for IM is controversial. Although corticosteroids enhance the rapidity of resolution of pharyngitis and fever in uncomplicated IM, their routine use is not recommended. It is possible corticosteroids might enhance EBV infection due to immune suppression and there have been rare reports of an association between corticosteroids and encephalitis or myocarditis in IM (55). The least controversial role for corticosteroids is for impending airway obstruction due to enlarged tonsils meeting at the midline. Short courses of corticosteroids (i.e., 60 mg prednisone per day for approximately 4 days followed by a rapid taper) usually result in significant improvement in the obstruction with shrinkage of the tonsils within 24 hours (54,55,97). Corticosteroids may be beneficial in cases of severe hemolytic anemia or thrombocytopenia (98–101). The efficacy of corticosteroids for other complications of IM is less clear.

Acyclovir has activity against EBV *in vitro* and *in vivo* but is not approved for use in EBV infection and has not been shown to alter the course of IM (55,102–104). Acyclovir can be effective for oral hairy leukoplakia because EBV replication appears to be the cause of this illness. Neither acyclovir nor corticosteroids are effective in treating EBV infection in X-linked lymphoproliferative disease. Instead, these patients may partially respond to gamma interferon or alpha interferon plus immune globulin (55,105,106). Patients with well-documented severe, progressive EBV infection may respond to acyclovir. Corticosteroids plus a cytotoxic agent induced responses in three of five patients with progressive EBV infection (55,80). Acyclovir does not improve outcome in EBV-associated lymphoproliferative syndromes. Partial restoration of immune function by decreasing immune suppression when possible has been beneficial in treating EBV-associated lymphoproliferative disease. There have been reports of responses of EBV-associated lymphoproliferative disease to alpha interferon plus immune globulin or to the use of monoclonal antibodies directed against B cells (55). In bone narrow transplant recipients donor T lymphocytes sometimes specifically expanded, in vitro, have been beneficial in achieving regression of EBV-induced lymphoproliferation disease (109,110)

REFERENCES

1. Filatov N. Lektuse ob ostrikh infektsion Nikj Lolieznyak (Lectures on acute infectious diseases of children). Moscow: U Deitel, 1885.
2. Pfeiffer E. Drusenfieber. *Jahrb f Kinderheilk* 1889;29:257.
3. Sprunt T, Evans F. Mononuclear leukocytosis in reaction to acute infections ("infectious mononucleosis"). *Johns Hopkins Hosp Bull* 1923;374:410.
4. Paul J, Bunnell W. The presence of heterophile antibodies in infectious mononucleosis. *Am J Med Sci* 1932;183:91.
5. Davidsohn I, Walker P. The nature of the heterophilic antibodies in infectious mononucleosis. *Am J Clin Pathol* 1935;5:455.
6. Epstein MA, Achong BG. Discovery and general biology of the virus. In: Epstein M, Achong B, eds. *The Epstein-Barr virus.* Heidelberg: Springer-Verlag, 1979:1–22.
7. Rickinson AB, Kieff E. Epstein-Barr virus. In: Fields B, Knipe D, Howley P, et al., eds. *Virology.* New York: Raven Press, 1996:2397–2446.
8. Henle G, Henle W. Immunofluorescence in cells derived from Burkitt lymphoma. *J Bacteriol* 1966;91:1248–1256.
9. Henle G, Henle W, Diehl F. Relation of Burkitt's tumor-associated herpes-type virus to infectious mononucleosis. *Proc Natl Acad Sci USA* 1968;59:94.
10. Niederman J, McCollum R, Henle G, et al. Infectious mononucleosis: clinical manifestations in relation to EB virus antibodies. *JAMA* 1968;203:205–209.
11. Evans A, Niderman J, McCollum R. Seroepidemiologic studies of infectious mononucleosis with EB virus. *N Engl J Med* 1968;279:1121–1127.
12. Sawyer R, Evans A, Niederman J, et al. Prospective studies of a group of Yale University freshmen. I. Occurrence of infectious mononucleosis. *J Infect Dis* 1971;123:263–279.
13. Laboratories UHPaP. A joint investigation of infectious mononucleosis and its relation ship to EB virus antibody. *BMJ* 1971;4:643.
14. Lipman M, Andrews L, Niederman J, Miller G. Direct visualization of enveloped Epstein-Barr herpesvirus in throat washing with leukocyte-transforming activity. *J Infect Dis* 1975;132(5):520–523.
15. Hoagland R. The transmission of infectious mononucleosis. *Am J Med Sci* 1955;229:262–272.
16. Fleisher GR, Pasquariello PS, Warren WS, et al. Intrafamilial transmission of Epstein-Barr virus infections. *J Pediatr* 1981;98(1):16–19.
17. Larsson BO, Linde A. Intrafamilial transmission of symptomatic Epstein-Barr virus infection among six adult members of one family. *Scand J Infect Dis* 1990;22(3):363–366.
18. Miller G, Niederman JC, Andrews LL. Prolonged oropharyngeal excretion of Epstein-Barr virus after infectious mononucleosis. *N Engl J Med* 1973;288(5):229–232.
19. Strauch B, Andrews LL, Siegel N, Miller G. Oropharyngeal excretion of Epstein-Barr virus by renal transplant recipients and other patients treated with immunosuppressive drugs. *Lancet* 1974;1(851):234–237.
20. Chang RS, Lewis JP, Reynolds RD, Sullivan MJ, Neuman J. Oropharyngeal excretion of Epstein-Barr virus by patients with lymphoproliferative disorders and by recipients of renal homografts. *Ann Intern Med* 1978;88(1):34–40.
21. Chang R, Lewis J, Abildgaard C. Prevalence of oropharyngeal excreters of leukocyte transforming agents among a human population. *N Engl J Med* 1973;289:1325–1329.
22. Gerber P, Walsh J, Rosenblum E, et al. Association of EB virus infection with the post perfusion syndrome. *Lancet* 1969;1:593–595.
23. Sixbey JW, Lemon SM, Pagano JS. A second site for Epstein-Barr virus shedding: the uterine cervix. *Lancet* 1986;2(8516):1122–1124.
24. Henle G, Henle W, Clifford P, et al. Antibodies to Epstein-Barr virus in Burkitt's lymphoma and control groups. *J Natl Cancer Inst* 1969;43(5):1147–1157.
25. Lang DJ, Garruto RM, Gajdusek DC. Early acquisition of cytomegalovirus and Epstein-Barr virus antibody in several isolated Melanesian populations. *Am J Epidemiol* 1977;105(5):480–487.
26. Henle G, Henle W. Observations on childhood infections with the Epstein-Barr virus. *J Infect Dis* 1970;121(3):303–310.
27. Evans A. Infectious mononucleosis in University of Wisconsin students. Report of a 5 year investigation. *Am J Hyg* 1960;71:342–362.
28. Evans A. Epidemiology and pathogenesis of infectious mononucleosis. International Infectious Mononucleosis Symposium, Evanston, IL, 1967.
29. Pereira M, Blake J, Macrae A. EB virus antibody at different ages. *BMJ* 1969;4:526–527.
30. Diehl V, Henle G, Henle W, Kohn G. Demonstration of a herpes group virus in cultures of peripheral leukocytes from patients with infectious mononucleosis. *J Virol* 1968;2:663–669.
31. Svedmyr E, Ernberg I, Seeley J, et al. Virologic, immunologic, and clinical observations on a patient during the incubation, acute, and convalescent phases of infectious mononucleosis. *Clin Immunol Immunopathol* 1984;30:437–450.
32. Robinson JE, Smith D, Niederman J. Plasmacytic differentiation of circulating Epstein-Barr virus-infected B lymphocytes during acute infectious mononucleosis. *J Exp Med* 1981;153(2):235–244.
33. Katsuki T, Hinuma Y, Saito T, et al. Simultaneous presence of EBNA positive and colony-forming cells in peripheral blood of patients with infectious mononucleosis. *Int J Cancer* 1979;23:746–750.
34. Klein G, Svedmyr E, Jondal M, Persson PO. EBV-determined nuclear antigen (EBNA)-positive cells in the peripheral blood of infectious mononucleosis patients. *Int J Cancer* 1976;17(1):21–26.
35. Niedobitek G, Herbst H, Young LS, et al. Patterns of Epstein-Barr virus infection in non-neoplastic lymphoid tissue. *Blood* 1992;79(10):2520–2526.
36. Reedman BM, Klein G. Cellular localization of an Epstein-Barr virus (EBV)-associated complement-fixing antigen in producer and non-producer lymphoblastoid cell lines. *Int J Cancer* 1973;11(3):499–520.
37. Henle W, Henle G, Zajac BA, Pearson G, Waubke R, Scriba M. Differential reactivity of human serums with early antigens induced by Epstein-Barr virus. *Science* 1970;169(941):188–190.
38. Henle W, Henle G, Andersson J, et al. Antibody responses to Epstein-Barr virus-determined nuclear antigen (EBNA)-1 and EBNA-2 in acute and chronic Epstein-Barr virus infection. *Proc Natl Acad Sci USA* 1987;84(2):570–574.
39. Hille A, Klein K, Baumler S, Grasser FA, Mueller-Lantzsch N. Expression of Epstein-Barr virus nuclear antigen 1,2A and 2B in the baculovirus expression system: serological evaluation of human antibodies to these proteins. *J Med Virol* 1993;39(3):233–241.
40. Pearson G, Luka J. Characterisation of the virus-determined antigens. In: Epstein M, Achong B, eds. *The Epstein-Barr virus: recent advances.* London: Heinemann, 1986:47–73.
41. van Grunsven WM, Spaan WJ, Middeldorp JM. Localization and diagnostic application of immunodominant domains of the BFRF3-encoded Epstein-Barr virus capsid protein. *J Infect Dis* 1994;170(1):13–19.

42. Evans AS, Niederman JC, Cenabre LC, West B, Richards VA. A prospective evaluation of heterophile and Epstein-Barr virus- specific IgM antibody tests in clinical and subclinical infectious mononucleosis: specificity and sensitivity of the tests and persistence of antibody. *J Infect Dis* 1975;132(5):546–554.

43. Schimitz H, Scherer M. IgM antibodies to Epstein-Barr virus in infectious mononucleosis. *Arch Gesamte Virusforsch* 1972;37:332–339.

44. Henle W, Henle GE, Horwitz CA. Epstein-Barr virus specific diagnostic tests in infectious mononucleosis. *Hum Pathol* 1974;5(5):551–565.

45. Horwitz CA, Henle W, Henle G, et al. Clinical and laboratory evaluation of infants and children with Epstein-Barr virus-induced infectious mononucleosis: report of 32 patients (aged 10-48 months). *Blood* 1981;57(5):933–938.

46. Wahren B. Diagnosis of infectious mononucleosis by the Monospot test. *Am J Clin Pathol* 1968;52:303.

47. Henle G, Henle W. The virus as the etiologic agent of infectious mononucleosis. In: Epstein M, Achong B, eds. *The Epstein-Barr virus.* Berlin: Springer-Verlag, 1979:279–320.

48. Pearson GR, Qualtiere LF, Klein G, Norin T, Bal IS. Epstein-Barr virus-specific antibody-dependent cellular cytotoxicity in patients with Burkitt's lymphoma. *Int J Cancer* 1979;24(4):402–406.

49. Garzelli C, Taub FE, Scharff JE, Prabhakar BS, Ginsberg-Fellner F, Notkins AL. Epstein-Barr virus-transformed lymphocytes produce monoclonal autoantibodies that react with antigens in multiple organs. *J Virol* 1984;52(2):722–725.

50. Sumaya CV, Ench Y. Epstein-Barr virus infectious mononucleosis in children. II. Heterophil antibody and viral-specific responses. *Pediatrics* 1985;75(6):1011–1019.

51. Reinherz EL, O'Brien C, Rosenthal P, Schlossman SF. The cellular basis for viral-induced immunodeficiency: analysis by monoclonal antibodies. *J Immunol* 1980;125(3):1269–1274.

52. Sheldon P, Papamichael M, Hemsted E, et al. Thymic origin of atypical lymphoid cells in infectious mononucleosis. *Lancet* 1973;1:1153–1155.

53. Mangi R, Niederman J, Kelleher J, et al. Depression of cell-mediated immunity during acute infectious mononucleosis. *N Engl J Med* 1974;291:1149–1153.

54. Chetham M, Roberts K. Infectious mononucleosis in adolescents. *Pediatr Ann* 1991;20(4):206–213.

55. Straus SE, Cohen JI, Tosato G, Meier J. NIH conference. Epstein-Barr virus infections: biology, pathogenesis, and management. *Ann Intern Med* 1993;118(1):45–58.

56. Decker GR, Berberian BJ, Sulica VI. Periorbital and eyelid edema: the initial manifestation of acute infectious mononucleosis. *Cutis* 1991;47(5):323–324.

57. Halevy J. Clinical presentation and course of infectious mononucleosis in older patients. *Int Med* 1989;10(10):48–57.

58. Finkel M, Parker G, Fanselau H. The hepatitis of infectious mononucleosis: experience with 235 cases. *Milit Med* 1964;129:533–538.

59. Silverstein A, Steinberg G, Nathanson M. Nervous system involvement in infectious mononucleosis. The heralding and-or major manifestation. *Arch Neurol* 1972;26(4):353–358.

60. Bennett D, Peter H. Acute cerebellar syndrome secondary to infectious mononucleosis in a 52 year old man. *Ann Intern Med* 1961;55:147–149.

61. Gilbert JW, Culebras A. Cerebellitis in infectious mononucleosis. *JAMA* 1972;220(5):727.

62. Bejada S. Cerebellitis in glandular fever. *Med J Aust* 1976;1:153–156.

63. Joncas JH, Chicoine L, Thivierge F, Bertrand M. Epstein-Barr virus antibodies in the cerebrospinal fluid. A case of infectious mononucleosis with encephalitis. *Am J Dis Child* 1974;127(2):282–285.

64. Grose C, Henle W, Henle G, Feorino PM. Primary Epstein-Barr-virus infections in acute neurologic diseases. *N Engl J Med* 1975;292(8):392–395.

65. Tanner O. Ocular manifestations of infectious mononucleosis. *Arch Ophthalmol* 1954;51:229–241.

66. Schechter F, Lipsius E, Rasansky H. Retrobulbar neuritis. *Am J Dis Child* 1955;89:58–61.

67. Gautier-Smith PC. Neurological complications of glandular fever (infectious mononucleosis). *Brain* 1965;88(2):323–334.

68. Cotton PB, Webb-Peploe MM. Acute transverse myelitis as a complication of glandular fever. *BMJ* 1966;5488:654–655.

69. Capra JD, Dowling P, Cook S, Kunkel HG. An incomplete cold-reactive gamma G antibody with i specificity in infectious mononucleosis. *Vox Sang* 1969;16(1):10–17.

70. Ellman L, Carvalho A, Jacobson BM, Colman RW. Platelet autoantibody in a case of infectious mononucleosis presenting as thrombocytopenic purpura. *Am J Med* 1973;55(5):723–726.

71. Mroczek E, Weisenburger D, Grierson H, et al. Fatal infectious mononucleosis and virus-associated hemophagocytic syndrome. *Arch Pathol Lab Med* 1987;111:530–535.

72. Farley D, Zietlow S, Bannon M, et al. Spontaneous rupture of the spleen due to infectious mononucleosis. *Mayo Clin Proc* 1992;67:846–853.

73. Aldrete J. Spontaneous rupture of the spleen in patients with infectious mononucleosis (editorial). *Mayo Clin Proc* 1992;67:910–912.

74. Mundy GR. Infectious mononucleosis with pulmonary parenchymal involvement. *BMJ* 1972;1(794):219–220.

75. Offit PA, Fleisher GR, Koven NL, Plotkin SA. Severe Epstein-Barr virus pulmonary involvement. *J Adolesc Health Care* 1981;2(2):121–125.

76. Purtilo DT, Szymanski I, Bhawan J, et al. Epstein-Barr virus infections in the X-linked recessive lymphoproliferative syndrome. *Lancet* 1978;1(8068):798–801.

77. Purtilo DT, Cassel CK, Yang JP, Harper R. X-linked recessive progressive combined variable immunodeficiency (Duncan's disease). *Lancet* 1975;1(7913):935–940.

78. Purtilo DT, Cassel C, Yang JP. Fatal infectious mononucleosis in familial lymphohistiocytosis [Letter]. *N Engl J Med* 1974;291(14):736.

79. Hwang PM, Li C, Morra M, et al. A "three-pronged" binding mechanism for the SAP/SH2D1A SH2 domain: structural basis and relevance to the XLP syndrome. *EMBO J* 2002;21:314–312.

80. Schooley RT, Carey RW, Miller G, et al. Chronic Epstein-Barr virus infection associated with fever and interstitial pneumonitis. Clinical and serologic features and response to antiviral chemotherapy. *Ann Intern Med* 1986;104(5):636–643.

81. Straus S. The chronic mononucleosis syndrome. *J Infect Dis* 1988;157:405–412.

82. Resnick L, Herbst JS, Raab-Traub N. Oral hairy leukoplakia. *J Am Acad Dermatol* 1990;22(6 Pt 2):1278–1282.

83. Greenspan D, Greenspan JS, Hearst NG, et al. Relation of oral hairy leukoplakia to infection with the human immunodeficiency virus and the risk of developing AIDS. *J Infect Dis* 1987;155(3):475–481.

84. Greenspan JS, Greenspan D. Oral hairy leukoplakia: diagnosis and management. *Oral Surg Oral Med Oral Pathol* 1989;67(4):396–403.

85. Holmes G, Kaplan J, Gantz N, et al. Chronic fatigue syndrome: a working case definition. *Ann Intern Med* 1988;108:387–389.

86. Holmes G. Defining the chronic fatigue syndrome. *Rev Infect Dis* 1991;13:S53–S55.

87. Hoagland R. Infectious mononucleosis. *Am J Med* 1952;13:158–171.

88. Mason WJ, Adams E. Infectious mononucleosis. An analysis of 100 cases with particular attention to diagnosis, liver function tests, and treatment of selected cases with prednisone. *Am J Med Sci* 1958;236:447–459.

89. Carter R. Granulocyte changes in infectious mononucleosis. *J Clin Pathol* 1966;19:279–283.

90. Cantow E, Kostinas J. Studies on infectious mononucleosis. IV. Changes in the granulocytic series. *Am J Clin Pathol* 1966;46:43–47.

91. Walter RB, Hong TC, Balchli EB. Life-threatening thrombocytopenia associated with acute Epstein-Barr virus infection in an older adult. *Ann Hematol* 2002;81:672–675.

92. Wood TA, Frenkel EP. The atypical lymphocyte. *Am J Med* 1967;42(6):923–936.

93. Chin TD. Diagnosis of infectious mononucleosis. *South Med J* 1976;69(5):654–658.

94. Horwitz CA, Henle W, Henle G, et al. Heterophile negative infectious mononucleosis and mononucleosis-like illnesses. Laboratory confirmation of 43 cases. *Am J Med* 1977;63(6):947–957.

95. Cooper DA, Gold J, Maclean P, et al. Acute AIDS retrovirus infection. Definition of a clinical illness associated with seroconversion. *Lancet* 1985;1(8428):537–540.

96. Goudsmit J, de Wolf F, Paul DA, et al. Expression of human immunodeficiency virus antigen (HIV-Ag) in serum and cerebrospinal fluid during acute and chronic infection. *Lancet* 1986;2(8500):177–180.

97. Bender CE. The value of corticosteroids in the treatment of infectious mononucleosis. *JAMA* 1967;199(8):529–531.

98. Clark B, Davies S. Severe thrombocytopenia in infectious mononucleosis. *Am J Med Sci* 1964;248:703–708.

99. Radel E, Schorr J. Thrombocytopenic purpura with infectious mononucleosis. *J Pediatr* 1963;63:46–60.

100. Goldstein E, Porter DY. Fatal thrombocytopenia with cerebral hemorrhage in mononucleosis. *Arch Neurol* 1969;20(5):533–535.

101. Grossman L, Wolff S. Acute thrombocytopenic purpura in infectious mononucleosis. *JAMA* 1959;171:2208–2210.

102. van der Horst C, Joncas J, Ahronheim G, et al. Lack of effect of peroral acyclovir for the treatment of acute infectious mononucleosis. *J Infect Dis* 1991;164(4):788–792.

103. Andersson J, Britton S, Ernberg I, et al. Effect of acyclovir on infectious mononucleosis: a double-blind, placebo-controlled study. *J Infect Dis* 1986;153(2):283–290.

104. Andersson J, Skoldenberg B, Henle W, et al. Acyclovir treatment in infectious mononucleosis: a clinical and virological study. *Infection* 1987;15(Suppl 1):S14–S20.

105. Okana M, Pirruccelo S, Grierson H, et al. Immunovirological studies of fatal infectious mononucleosis in a patient with X-linked lymphoproliferative syndrome treated with intravenous immunoglobulin and interferon-alpha. *Clin Immun Immunopathol* 1990;54:410–418.

106. Okana M, Thiele G, Kobayashi R, et al. Interferon-gamma in a family with X-linked lymphoproliferative syndrome with acute Epstein-Barr virus infection. *J Clin Immunol* 1989;9:48–54.

107. Henle W, Henle G. Seroepidemiology of the virus. In: Epstein M, Achong B, eds. *The Epstein-Barr virus.* Berlin: Springer-Verlag, 1979:61–78.

108. Tomkinson B, Sullivan J. Epstein-Barr virus Infection and mononucleosis. In: Gorbach S, Bartlett J, Blacklow N, eds. *Infectious diseases.* Philadelphia, WB Saunders, 1991:1348–1356.

109. Savoldo B, Cubbage ML, Durett AG, et al. Generation of EBV-specific CD4+ cytotoxic T cells from virus naive individuals. *J Immunol* 2002;168(2):909–918.

110. Koehne G, Smith KM, Ferguson TL, et al. Quantitation, selection, and functional characterization of Epstein-Barr virus-specific and alloreactive T cells detected by intracellular interferon-gamma production and growth of cytotoxic precursors. *Blood* 2002;99(5):1730–1740.

CHAPTER 176
Chronic Fatigue Syndrome

Stephen E. Straus

HISTORY

The chronic fatigue syndrome is a new name for what is, in all likelihood, an ancient condition. As currently defined, it comprises a subset of heterogeneous disorders of uncertain pathogenesis that are associated with chronic fatigue and a variety of other physical, constitutional, and neuropsychological symptoms (1–3) (Fig. 176.1).

An early, clear reference to chronic fatigue was made with the description in 1750 of febricula as an illness exhibiting "low, continued fever ... transient chilliness ... listlessness with great lassitude and weariness ... and little flying pains" (4).

In 1869, Beard (5) postulated that an acquired weakness of the nerves, or neurasthenia, causes severe exhaustion. Examinations of battle-worn veterans of the U.S. Civil War led his contemporary DaCosta to conclude, however, that the chronic fatigue resulted from an irritable heart (6). Beard's concept of neurasthenia was widely acknowledged; the term persisted in the psychiatric lexicon for over a century. Among cardiologists, DaCosta's hypothesis was well entrenched until World War II, when detailed investigations failed to confirm defects in cardiac physiology (7).

Discussion of chronic fatigue syndrome in this book is warranted because of its alleged causal relationship, in many instances, with infections. In the 1930s, Evans (8) argued that chronic brucellosis includes not only osteomyelitis and endocarditis, but also a syndrome with chronic fatigue with other subjective complaints. Spink, Cluff, and their colleagues, however, could not verify persistent infection in patients whose brucellosis devolved solely into the fatiguing form of illness. They reported, instead, that such patients manifested features of psychoneurosis (9,10).

From 1960 to 1970, these findings induced Cluff's group and several others to explore reasons for delayed convalescence from a variety of infections. The most careful work involved influenza and infectious mononucleosis (11–13). The cumulative evidence indicated that patients who experienced subjective symptoms long after the acute illness tended to differ in premorbid personality from patients who recovered promptly.

Against this historical backdrop, in the early 1980s Epstein-Barr virus was postulated to cause chronic fatigue (14–17). The hypothesis rested on three observations: that the virus persists for life and reactivates frequently, affording a biologic potential for chronic infection; that patients often possess abnormal titers of antibodies to Epstein-Barr virus antigens in patterns suggesting recent or active infection; and that prolonged fatigue developed in some patients in the wake of a mononucleosis-like illness.

Critical studies verified that chronic Epstein-Barr virus infection can persist as a rare, severe illness of the compromised host, but it is not the cause of chronic fatigue syndrome. The abnormal serologic profiles of patients with chronic fatigue syndrome proved to be nonspecific (17,18).

In 1988, the Centers for Disease Control recommended that the name chronic fatigue syndrome be used for such patients, rather than chronic Epstein-Barr virus infection or other terms then in vogue, and to move beyond the idea of a unitary infectious cause (19). Tentative criteria for the syndrome were field-tested for several years and then revised, because several of its elements proved vague, redundant and unnecessarily exclusionary. The criteria formulated in 1994 are now preferred (3) (Table 176.1).

EPIDEMIOLOGY

Chronic fatigue is a remarkably common complaint. One study of patients in a primary care setting reported 24% to have fatigue for longer than 1 month (20,21), but a far smaller proportion appears to have chronic fatigue syndrome. Estimates based on the original CDC definition ranged from two to seven cases per 100,000 people (22). The revised case definition is far more inclusive and yields estimates ranging up to 250 cases or more per 100,000 (21,23).

Chronic fatigue syndrome is primarily a disorder of young to middle-aged adults, but cases in children have been recognized. It appears to also occur in the elderly, but coexisting medical conditions usually preclude its consideration. Virtually all studies show that chronic fatigue syndrome is more common in women than in men by a ratio of at least 2:1 (14–17,21–23). The facts that the prevalence in African-American and Hispanic populations in the United States is at least as great as that among whites, and rates are relatively greater in lower rather than upper income strata reveal that the sobriquet, the "Yuppie Flu" is incorrect (21).

Chronic fatigue syndrome usually arises sporadically, but closely related, if not identical, illnesses have occurred in outbreaks. One early such outbreak led to temporary closure of the Los Angeles County Hospital in 1934; more than 1,000 people, including many staff members, fell ill. Other well-known outbreaks occurred in Iceland in 1948, in the Royal Free Hospital of London in 1955, and in Lake Tahoe, Nevada, in 1985 (18,24–27). The name epidemic neuromyasthenia is often attached to these outbreaks (26). Myalgic encephalomyelitis is another term for epidemic illnesses such as these, particularly when neurologic features are prominent (27).

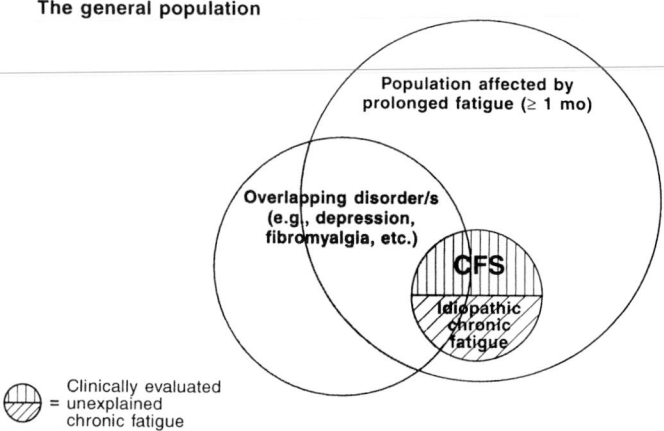

The general population

Population affected by prolonged fatigue (≥ 1 mo)

Overlapping disorder/s (e.g., depression, fibromyalgia, etc.)

CFS

Idiopathic chronic fatigue

Clinically evaluated = unexplained chronic fatigue

Figure 176.1. A schematic depiction of how chronic fatigue syndrome (CFS) relates to other sets of diagnoses associated with fatigue. Idiopathic chronic fatigue is the term proposed for cases that resemble—but do not fully conform to the definition of—chronic fatigue syndrome. (From Fukuda K, Straus SE, Hickie I, et al. The chronic fatigue syndrome: a comprehensive approach to its definition and study. *Ann Intern Med* 1994;121:953–959, with permission.)

TABLE 176.1. Revised Centers for Disease Control and Prevention Criteria for Chronic Fatigue Syndrome

A case of chronic fatigue syndrome is defined by the presence of
1. Clinically evaluated, unexplained, persistent, or relapsing fatigue that is of new or definite onset; is not the result of ongoing exertion; is not alleviated by rest; and results in substantial reduction in previous levels of occupational, educational, social, or personal activities
2. Four or more of the following symptoms that persist or recur during 6 or more consecutive months of illness and that do not predate the fatigue:
   - Self-reported impairment in short-term memory or concentration
   - Sore throat
   - Tender cervical or axillary nodes
   - Muscle pain
   - Multijoint pain without redness or swelling
   - Headaches of a new pattern or severity
   - Unrefreshing sleep
   - Postexertional malaise lasting $\geq$24 h

From Fukuda K, Straus SE, Hickie I, et al. The chronic fatigue syndrome: A comprehensive approach to its definition and study. *Ann Intern Med* 1994;121:953–959, with permission.

PATHOGENESIS

The genesis of chronic fatigue syndrome remains unsettled. While chronic fatigue syndrome often has its onset in the context of an acute infection, no known agent can be reliably credited with being a primary contributor to it. Besides the *Brucella* species and Epstein-Barr virus mentioned previously, there have been attempts to implicate human herpesvirus type 6, retroviruses, enteroviruses, *Mycoplasma*, and *Candida*. Antibodies to some of these agents have been reported to be more prevalent in patients with chronic fatigue syndrome than in control subjects. Subsequent studies could never confirm these findings or establish their specificity (18,28). Various reports of microbial antigens or nucleic acids in patients specimens could also never be confirmed (28–32).

Because there is no compelling evidence of infection or contagion as consistent features of chronic fatigue syndrome, research on pathogenesis has shifted. Several studies have shown immunologic abnormalities in chronic fatigue syndrome (17,33–36). There are a few reports of modest reductions in the number and activity of a subset of natural killer cells and increases in the proportion of circulating lymphocytes displaying activation or adhesion markers. These findings led to the speculation that many of the disease symptoms are caused by dysregulation of lymphokines or interleukins, substances that induce fever, myalgias, and fatigue (17). Unfortunately, the degree of immune abnormalities has not correlated consistently with the severity of complaints, nor do these abnormalities appear to be specific for chronic fatigue syndrome. Patients with depression, for example, also possess natural killer cell deficiencies and other abnormalities similar to those reported in chronic fatigue syndrome.

Depression is a theme that has pervaded chronic fatigue syndrome literature for years. It is a charged issue that patients prefer to dismiss because of the personal and societal stigma attached to psychiatric diagnoses. Small studies verified that two thirds or more of patients with chronic fatigue syndrome meet existing psychiatric criteria for anxiety disorders, dysthymia, or depression (37–39). Some interpret these findings as implying that the fatigue results from a psychiatric disorder; others argue that the psychiatric problems arise from the chronic fatigue and disability.

A prospective study of patients with an acute viral-type illness found that psychiatric morbidity, the patient's belief about viruses as the cause of his or her complaints, and how the physician reinforced those beliefs conspire to predict chronic fatigue. The infective symptoms predicted fatigue initially, but not 6 months later (40).

Regarding the premorbid profile of patients, a recent study in the United Kingdom showed that those in whom chronic fatigue syndrome develops had been consulting their general practitioners significantly more frequently than did control subjects in the 15 years before chronic fatigue syndrome developed (41).

Several other contributors to the etiology and persistence of chronic fatigue have also been investigated in recent years. Dysfunction of hypothalamic-pituitary-adrenal axis regulation has been documented in chronic fatigue syndrome (42–44). Patients with chronic fatigue syndrome have reduced exercise tolerance and perceive greater effort during exercise even than sedentary controls (45). Finally, patients with chronic fatigue syndrome can have impaired autonomic responses to sustained upright tilting, leading to paradoxical bradycardia and syncope (46–48). It is unclear whether these diverse physiologic differences in chronic fatigue syndrome are of primary importance to the development of the disorder, or secondary to prolonged illness.

CLINICAL MANIFESTATIONS

Besides fatigue, there are numerous other subjective features of chronic fatigue syndrome that fluctuate with time but do not appear to progress (Table 176.2). Once the inciting illness, if any, is resolved, the physical examination is typically normal. Although patients commonly feel febrile, few ever demonstrate elevated temperatures. Joints ache, but there is no erythema, effusion, or limitation of motion. Although the muscles are easily

TABLE 176.2. Patients with Chronic Fatigue Syndrome Reporting the Indicated Symptoms

Symptom	Percentage[a]
Easy fatigability	100
Difficulty concentrating	90
Headache	90
Sore throat	85
Tender lymph nodes	80
Muscle aches	80
Joint aches	75
Feverishness	75
Difficulty sleeping	70
Psychiatric problems	65
Allergies	55
Abdominal cramps	40
Weight loss	20
Rash	10
Rapid pulse	10
Weight gain	5
Chest pain	5
Night sweats	5

[a]Percentages are approximate.
From Straus SE. The chronic mononucleosis syndrome. *J Infect Dis* 1988;157:405–412, by The University of Chicago, with permission.

fatigued, strength is normal, as are biopsy results and electromyograms. Mild lymphadenitis is occasionally noted but not true lymphadenopathy. Biopsy specimens of lymph nodes show only reactive hyperplasia.

Routine hematologic and chemical tests are typically normal. Patients may have intermittent low positive titers of antinuclear antibodies, slightly elevated levels of circulating immune complexes, or partial hypogammaglobulinemia (15,16).

Many patients with chronic fatigue syndrome are partially or totally disabled by its manifestations. Their outward, healthy appearance belies the internal sense of ill health. It is common for relatives and colleagues to accuse them of malingering. A vicious circle of frustration, anger, and depression commonly ensues.

Chronic fatigue syndrome does not progress, but it does lead to prolonged debility. The likelihood of sustained remissions is greatest in adolescents and younger adults (49,50). In contrast, remissions are least likely in people over age 38, with less total years of education, with more somatic complaints, and a lifetime history of dysthymia (50).

DIAGNOSIS

Chronic fatigue syndrome remains a diagnosis of exclusion (3). As such, there is a temptation to conduct an exhaustive laboratory evaluation. Such a workup is expensive and does not add measurably to management. Although the chronic fatigue syndrome may have numerous somatic and psychosomatic causes, it is useful for family practitioners, pediatricians, and internists to recognize its common features and its prognosis, which are distinct from those of many other chronic conditions.

TREATMENT

While there are no specific treatments for chronic fatigue syndrome, it can be treated successfully. Commonsense recommendations to patients include a balanced diet, reduction in stress, attention to sleep habits, and regular exercise below the threshold at which further exhaustion is induced. Symptomatic therapies help reduce pain and feverishness.

Claims for other treatments abound. Few have been seriously tested. Anecdotes regarding amantadine, doxycycline, magnesium, evening primrose oil, vitamin B_{12}, and cimetidine are but a few that do not hold up in clinical studies (51). Systematic reviews of the better designed studies of treatments for chronic fatigue syndrome concluded that only two approaches can be said to afford positive outcomes—cognitive behavioral therapy and graded exercise (52–55). Data regarding immunoglobulin therapy and low dose hydrocortisone were considered equivocal (47,56–58). While antidepressants are widely prescribed, the studies to date have been too small to permit conclusions as to their efficacy, but they are effective in fibromyalgia, which is a closely related somatic disorder that is present in many patients with chronic fatigue syndrome (60,61).

REFERENCES

1. Bock GR Whelan J (eds). *Chronic fatigue syndrome.* Ciba Foundation Symposium 173. West Sussex, England: John Wiley & Sons, 1993.
2. Straus SE (ed). *Chronic fatigue syndrome.* New York: Marcel Dekker, 1994.
3. Fukuda K, Straus SE, Hickie I, et al. The chronic fatigue syndrome: a comprehensive approach to its definition and study. *Ann Intern Med* 1994;121:953.
4. Manningham R. *The symptoms, nature, causes and cure of the febricula or little fever: commonly called the nervous or hysteric fever; the fever on the spirits; vapours, hypo, or spleen,* 2nd ed. London: J Robinson, 1750.
5. Beard G. Neurasthenia or nervous exhaustion. *Boston Med Surg J* 1869; 3 (new series):217.
6. DaCosta JM. On irritable heart: a clinical study of a form of functional cardiac disorder and its consequences. *Am J Med Sci* 1871;121:17.
7. Wood P. DaCosta's syndrome (or effort syndrome). *BMJ* 1941;1:767, 805.
8. Evans AC. Brucellosis in the United States. *Am J Public Health* 1947;37:139.
9. Spink WW. What is chronic brucellosis? *Ann Intern Med* 1951;35:358.
10. Imboden JB, Canter A, Cluff LE, Trever RW. Brucellosis. III. Psychologic aspects of delayed convalescence. *Arch Intern Med* 1959;103:406.
11. Imboden JB, Canter A, Cluff LE. Convalescence from influenza: a study of the psychological and clinical determinants. *Arch Intern Med* 1961;108: 393.
12. Greenfield NS Roessler R, Crosley AP. Ego strength and length of recovery from infectious mononucleosis. *J Nerv Ment Dis* 1959;128:125.
13. Kasl SV, Evans AS, Niederman JC. Psychological risk factors in the development of infectious mononucleosis. *Psychosom Med* 1979;41:445.
14. DuBois RE, Seeley JK Brus L, et al. Chronic mononucleosis syndrome. *South Med J* 1984;77:1376.
15. Jones JF, Ray CF, Minnich LL, et al. Evidence for active Epstein-Barr virus infection in patients with persistent, unexplained illnesses: elevated anti-early antigen antibodies. *Ann Intern Med* 1985;102:1.
16. Straus SE, Tosato G, Armstrong G, et al. Persisting illness and fatigue in adults and evidence of Epstein-Barr virus infection. *Ann Intern Med* 1985;102:7.
17. Straus SE. The chronic mononucleosis syndrome. *J Infect Dis* 1988;157: 405.
18. Holmes GP, Kaplan JE, Steward JA, et al. A cluster of patients with a chronic mononucleosis-like syndrome: is Epstein-Barr virus the cause? *JAMA* 1987;257:2297.
19. Holmes GP, Kaplan JE, Gantz NM, et al. Chronic fatigue syndrome: a working case definition. *Ann Intern Med* 1988;108:387.
20. Kroenke K, Wood DR, Mangelsdorf AD, et al. Chronic fatigue is primary care. Prevalence, patient characteristics, and outcome. *JAMA* 1988;206:929.
21. Steele L, Dobbins JG, Fukuda K, et al. The epidemiology of chronic fatigue syndrome in San Francisco. *Am J Med* 1998;105:83S–90S.
22. Gunn WJ, Connell DB, Randall B. Epidemiology of chronic fatigue syndrome: the Centers for Disease Control study. In: Bock GR Whelan J, eds. *Chronic fatigue syndrome.* Ciba Foundation Symposium 173. West Sussex, England: John Wiley & Sons, 1993:83–93.
23. Jason LA, Richman JA, Rademaker AW, et al. A community-based study of chronic fatigue syndrome. *Arch Intern Med* 1999;159:2129.
24. Gilliam AG. Epidemiologic study of an epidemic diagnosed as poliomyelitis, occurring among personnel of Los Angeles County General Hospital during the summer of 1934. Washington, DC: US Public Health Service, Division of Infectious Diseases, Institute of Health, 1938, bulletin 240.
25. Acheson ED. The clinical syndrome variously called benign myalgic encephalomyelitis, Iceland disease and epidemic neuromyasthenia. *Am J Med* 1959;26:569.
26. Henderson DA Shelokov A. Epidemic neuromyasthenia: clinical syndrome? *N Engl J Med* 1959;260:757.
27. Medical Staff of the Royal Free Hospital. An outbreak of encephalomyelitis in the Royal Free Hospital Group, London, in 1955. *BMJ* 1957;3:895.
28. Ablashi DV, Josephs SF, Buchbinder A, et al. Human B-lymphotropic virus (human herpesvirus-6). *J Virol Methods* 1988;21:29.
29. Archard LC, Bowles NE, Behan PO, et al. Postviral fatigue syndrome: persistence of enterovirus RNA in muscle and elevated creatine kinase. *J R Soc Med* 1988;81:326.
30. DeFreitas E Hilliard B, Cheney PR, et al. Retroviral sequences related to human T-lymphotropic virus type II in patients with chronic fatigue immune dysfunction syndrome. *Proc Natl Acad Sci USA* 1991;88:2922.
31. Khan AS, Heneine WM, Chapman LE, et al. Assessment of a retrovirus sequence and other possible risk factors for the chronic fatigue syndrome in adults. *Ann Intern Med* 1993;118:241.
32. Reeves WC, Stamey FR, Black JB, et al. Human herpesviruses 6 and 7 in chronic fatigue syndrome: a case control study. *Clin Infect Dis* 2000;31:48.
33. Borysiewicz LK, Haworth SJ, Cohen J, et al. Epstein-Barr virus-specific immune defects in patients with persistent symptoms following infectious mononucleosis. *Q J Med* 1986;58:111.
34. Caliguiri M, Murray C, Buchwald D, et al. Phenotypic and functional deficiency of natural killer cells in patients with chronic fatigue syndrome. *J Immunol* 1987;139:3306.
35. Lloyd A, Wakefield D, Boughton C, Dwyer J. Immunological abnormalities in the chronic fatigue syndrome. *Med J Aust* 1989;151:122.
36. Strober W. Immunological function in chronic fatigue syndrome In: Straus SE, ed. *Chronic fatigue syndrome.* New York: Marcel Dekker, 1994:207–237.
37. Taerk GS, Toner BB, Salit IE, et al. Depression in patients with neuromyasthenia (benign myalgic encephalomyelitis). *Int J Psychiatry Med* 1987;17:49.
38. Kruesi MJP, Dale JK, Straus SE. Psychiatric diagnoses in patients who have the chronic fatigue syndrome. *J Clin Psychiatry* 1989;50:53.
39. Manu P, Lane TJ, Matthews DA. The frequency of the chronic fatigue syndrome in patients with symptoms of persistent fatigue. *Ann Intern Med* 1988; 109:554.
40. Cope H, David A, Pelosi A Mann A. Predictors of chronic "postviral" fatigue. *Lancet* 1994;344:864.
41. Hamilton WT, Hall GH, Round AP. Frequency of attendance in general practice and symptoms before development of chronic fatigue syndrome: a case-control study. *Br J Gen Pract* 2001;51:553.

42. Demitrack MA, Dale J, Straus SE, et al. Evidence for impaired activation of the hypothalamic-pituitary-adrenal axis in patients with chronic fatigue syndrome. *J Clin Endocrinol Metab* 1991;73:1224.

43. Ehlert U, Gaab J, Heinrichs M. Psychoneuroendocrinological contributions to the etiology of depression, posttraumatic stress disorder, and stress-related bodily disorders: the role of the hypothalamic-pituitary-adrenal axis. *Biol Psych* 2001;57:141.

44. Cleare AJ, Miell J, Heap E, et al. Hypothalamo-pituitary-adrenal axis dysfunction in chronic fatigue syndrome, and effects of low-dose hydrocortisone therapy. *J Clin Endocrinol Metab* 2001;86:3545.

45. Fulcher KY, White PD. Strength and physiological response to exercise in patients with chronic fatigue syndrome. *J Neurol Neurosurg Psychiatry* 2000; 69:302.

46. Bou-Holaigah I, Rowe P, Kan J, Calkins H. the relationship between neurally mediated hypotension and the chronic fatigue syndrome. *JAMA* 1995;274: 961.

47. Rowe PC, Calkins H, DeBusk K, et al. Fludrocortisone actetate to treat neurally mediated hypotension in chronic fatigue syndrome: a randomized controlled trial. *JAMA* 2001;285:52.

48. Streeten DH, Thomas D, Bell DS. The roles of orthostatic hypotension, orthostatic tachycardia, and subnormal erythrocyte volume in the pathogenesis of chronic fatigue syndrome. *Am J Med Sci* 2000;320:1.

49. Bell DS, Jordan K, Robinson M. Thirteen-year follow-up of children and adolescents with chronic fatigue syndrome. *Pediatrics* 2001;107:994.

50. Clark MR, Katon W, Russo J, et al. Chronic fatigue: risk factors for symptom persistence in a 2 1/2-year follow-up study. *Am J Med* 1995;98:187.

51. McCluskey DR. Pharmacological approaches to the therapy of chronic fatigue syndrome. In: Bock GR Whelan J, eds. *Chronic fatigue syndrome.* Ciba Foundation Symposium 173. West Sussex, England: John Wiley & Sons, 1993:280–287.

52. Reid S, Chalder T, Cleare A, et al. Extracts from "clinical evidence": chronic fatigue syndrome. *BMJ* 2000;320:292.

53. Whiting P, Bagnall AM, Sowden AJ, et al. Interventions for the treatment and management of chronic fatigue syndrome: a systematic review *JAMA* 2001;286:1360.

54. Deale A, Chalder T, Marks J et al. Cognitive behavioral therapy for chronic fatigue syndrome: a randomized controlled trial. *Am J Psychiatry* 1997;154: 408.

55. Fulcher KY, White PD. A randomized controlled trial of graded exercise therapy in patients with chronic fatigue syndrome. *BMJ* 1997;314:1647.

56. DuBois RE. Gamma globulin therapy for chronic mononucleosis syndrome. *AIDS Res* 1986;2(Suppl 1):S191.

57. Peterson PK, Shepard J, Macres M, et al. A controlled trial of intravenous immunoglobulin G in chronic fatigue syndrome. *Am J Med* 1990;89:554.

58. Cleare A, Heap E, Mahli G et al. Low-dose hydrocortisone in chronic fatigue syndrome: a randomized controlled trial. *Lancet* 1999;353:455.

59. Yunus MB. Diagnosis, etiology, and management of fibromyalgia syndrome: An update. *Compr Ther* 1988;14:8.

60. Aaron LA, Burke MM, Buchwald D. Overlapping conditions among patients with chronic fatigue syndrome, fibromyalgia, and temporomandibular disorder. *Arch Intern Med* 2000;160:221.

CHAPTER 177
Cytomegalovirus Infections

Sarah H. Cheeseman and Laura L. Gibson

HISTORY

The clinical importance of cytomegalovirus (CMV) was first recognized in infants with cytomegalic inclusion disease. Transplant and postperfusion syndromes were defined in the 1960s. CMV was one of the candidate viruses considered as a cause of acquired immunodeficiency syndrome (AIDS) when the disease appeared in the early 1980s. Its current clinical prominence, and perhaps some progress in therapy, reflect its frequent and severe manifestations in patients with AIDS, as well as the increasing frequency of organ transplantation.

CHARACTERISTICS OF THE PATHOGEN

See Chapter 235.

EPIDEMIOLOGY

Approximately 1% of mothers infected with CMV before conception transmit virus to their children in utero. For primary maternal infection during pregnancy, the transmission rate is nearly 50% (1–3). In studies prior to 1990, virtually all of the severe disease and major neurologic sequelae occurred in infants infected as a result of maternal primary infection (1,4–7), although there were isolated case reports of mothers who had more than one child with cytomegalic inclusion disease (8,9). More recent series have found that as many as 17% of infants with symptomatic congenital CMV infection are born to mothers with preconceptional antibody to CMV (10). Many, if not most, of these women have acquired infection with a new strain of CMV (11). Polymerase chain reaction demonstrates viremia more often in women with recently acquired CMV infection and among those who subsequently give birth to congenitally infected infants (12). CMV can replicate in cytotrophoblasts, placental cells directly exposed to maternal blood (13), and this may well be the route of transmission to the fetus.

Postnatal CMV may be derived from maternal cervical secretions (14), but the most common source is breast milk (15–17). Young children appear to be effective vectors of CMV transmission, both in daycare and at home. In families with young children, the introduction of CMV results in infection of 50% of the remaining susceptible family members within 6 months. (18). This is probably the result of close contact with virus-containing urine and saliva characteristic of this age group, as occurs with diaper changing and sharing of toys that have been mouthed (19). By contrast, health care workers, even in pediatric and transplantation settings, have not generally been found to have higher seroconversion rates than the general population (1% to 2% per year) (20–26), nor have they been shown by genomic analysis to have the same virus as their patients (25,27–29). This suggests that the norms of professional hygiene are sufficient to protect against what might seem to be equally close contact with urine and other infected secretions (24,30).

Sexual transmission is the other major route of spread of CMV (31). Twelve of 34 seronegative homosexual men in San Francisco in the early 1980s became infected during an average follow-up period of 13.6 months (32). All women older than 30 years seen in a sexually transmitted disease clinic in Kansas City, Missouri, in 1970 were seropositive, compared with only 45% of 30-year-old nuns working as nurses or school teachers (33).

Transfusion-transmitted CMV disease occurs in both seronegative and seropositive adults (34) and in preterm infants who require transfusion as part of neonatal intensive care (35). In the case of newborns, molecular methods have confirmed transfusion as the source of infection (36,37) and demonstrated the absence of nosocomial transmission by other routes (37). The risk of infection is related both to total number of units transfused and to the number of units from seropositive donors (38–40). Overall, the risk has been estimated at 2.5 to 7.0 cases per 100 units transfused (32) and may be as high as 25% for seronegative persons receiving 30 or more units (41). The rate of CMV infection can be reduced to zero by the use of seronegative blood products for seronegative recipients or by filtration to remove contaminating white blood cells (42).

The serologic status of the blood product donor, organ donor, and recipient all contribute to the risk of CMV infection after transplantation. In kidney transplantation, which does not require massive blood product support, the kidney plays the dominant role, with organs from seropositive donors conferring a high rate of CMV infection (43,44). A seropositive donor organ is also the major risk for CMV infection in liver transplantation (45,46). In heart transplantation, the donor heart can be shown to transmit virus, but its effect is overwhelmed by that of transfusion unless CMV-seronegative blood is used for seronegative recipients (47).

In all three types of solid organ transplantation, the highest risk of CMV disease occurs in the recipient who acquires a primary infection (45–53). However, severe, even fatal, CMV disease is occasionally seen in patients with pretransplant antibody. A study that distinguished between reinfection and reactivation in kidney transplantation identified the same spectrum of illness in reinfection as in primary infection, albeit at a somewhat lower rate of occurrence, whereas reactivation appeared clinically benign (54).

By contrast, in bone marrow transplantation the major risk for CMV infection derives from the recipient's seropositivity before transplantation (55). In a few instances, the identity of a patient's pretransplant and posttransplant CMV isolates has been confirmed by genomic analysis (56). However, if the recipient is seronegative, the infection rate is the same for recipients of either seropositive marrow or seropositive granulocyte transfusions (55). Although these patients are at lower risk of overt CMV disease than seropositive recipients, their post-transplant mortality is higher (57).

IMMUNITY AND PATHOGENESIS

See Chapter 235.

Severe CMV infection has not been reported among persons with isolated immunoglobulin deficiency. However, it is common in patients with cell-mediated immunodeficiency associated with transplantation or human immunodeficiency virus infection, indicating the importance of cell-mediated response in controlling this infection.

Our understanding of the mechanisms responsible for the clinical manifestations of CMV infection is fragmentary. The atypical lymphocyte in CMV mononucleosis has been identified as a killer cell (58), as in classic infectious mononucleosis induced by Epstein-Barr virus. Also like Epstein-Barr virus, CMV induces broad-spectrum helper cell activity (59), but CMV infection of a monocyte may render it capable of suppressing natural killer cell activity (60). An explanation for the frequent association of leukopenia with CMV infection may lie in the capability of even abortive infection of bone marrow monocytes to suppress both granulocyte-macrophage and erythroid colony-forming activity (61). Vasculitis, perhaps due to CMV infection of endothelial cells, may underlie ulcerative and necrotizing lesions (62).

CLINICAL MANIFESTATIONS

More than 90% of congenitally infected infants appear normal at birth (63, 64). CMV syndromes are rarely recognized in early childhood. Even in prospectively followed adults, only about 10% of seroconverters have any clinical syndrome (7). The most common feature of CMV disease at any age is a nonspecific illness. The signs and symptoms seen in infants with symptomatic congenital CMV infection do not differ greatly from those of other congenital infections.

Cytomegalic Inclusion Disease of the Newborn

Infants with cytomegalic inclusion disease are recognizably ill within the first few days of birth. Hepatosplenomegaly is nearly universal, petechiae and thrombocytopenia are quite common,

and there may be a "blueberry muffin" appearance due to cutaneous islands of extramedullary erythropoiesis. Although congenital anomalies have been reported in association with congenital CMV infection, none are particularly characteristic and causation has not been established (63). Intrauterine growth retardation and postnatal failure to thrive may occur. Encephalitis is a frequent part of this process and is of a progressive and ongoing nature, because the active phase of the infection does not cease until some time after birth. In fact, these infants are quite slow to mount a cell-mediated immune response to the infection (64) and continue to shed large quantities of virus in urine for up to 8 years (65). Thus, microcephaly may not be present at birth, but it is found in a majority of surviving children by the end of the first year, often in association with periventricular calcifications (66–71). The neurologic outcome of this form of CMV infection is usually devastating. Severe mental and motor retardation may occur in up to 90% of patients (63–71), although one report suggests a slightly better prognosis (72). This form of CMV disease affects approximately 3,000 to 4,000 infants in the United States each year (73).

Subclinical Congenital Infection

The dire outcome of overt congenital CMV infection has led to long-term scrutiny of congenitally infected infants without severe symptoms at birth. Instances of severe mental retardation and motor impairment have been reported in children of mothers with recurrent as well as primary infection during pregnancy (74). The most consistent finding in children asymptomatic at birth has been an 11% to 25% risk of profound sensorineural hearing loss (75–77). A battery of neuropsychologic tests predicted school failure in asymptomatic congenitally-infected children 2.8 times more often than in control subjects in lower socioeconomic groups, but this effect was not seen in the higher socioeconomic stratum, suggesting that these deficits can be overcome (76).

Acquired Cytomegalovirus in Neonates

Preterm infants who acquire CMV often have an episode of "gray baby" syndrome, with pallor and hypotension, and may have renewed respiratory distress requiring reintubation and ventilatory support (38). This infection may be the direct cause of death in very small infants (those weighing less than 1,200 g) (78). The frequency of this complication has declined, probably because of screening for other bloodborne pathogens, but significant CMV disease has also been recognized among premature infants of seropositive as well as seronegative mothers (79).

Cytomegalovirus Mononucleosis

CMV mononucleosis is the disease resulting from acute primary CMV infection. Perhaps the most famous case is that of Pope John Paul II, who acquired CMV infection from blood transfusion after an assassination attempt (80). Burn victims, who may be slightly immunocompromised by their injury, have the same clinical manifestations (81,82). Heterophile-negative mononucleosis and postperfusion syndrome, the latter named for its occurrence after heart-lung bypass for cardiac surgery, are other terms for the same illness, which may be due to either primary acquisition of CMV or recurrence (whether reinfection or reactivation is not yet established).

Table 177.1 compares the frequency of signs and symptoms of this condition in two series (83,84) with summary data for primary infection in kidney (85) and heart transplant recipients

TABLE 177.1. Symptoms of Primary Cytomegalovirus Infection

Symptom	Normal hosts[a]		Transplant recipients[b]		
				Heart or lung	
	Literature review (N = 62) [83]	Consecutive cases (N = 82) [84]	Renal (N = 31–51) [85]	(N = 12) [52]	(N = 16) [53]
Fever	98	94	84	90	69
Leukopenia	0		57	50	
Pneumonia			25	44	31
Pharyngitis	38	31			
Atypical lymphocytes	88	100[c]	70	67	
Elevated liver function tests	91	92	46	75	

[a]Percentage of reported or recognized patients (all symptomatic).
[b]Percentage of all pretransplant seronegative patients with cytomegalovirus infection documented after transplantation.
[c]Required for inclusion in series.

(52,53) to demonstrate the common features. The most frequent finding is fever, usually accompanied by profound fatigue and malaise. In classic (Epstein-Barr virus) infectious mononucleosis, sore throat and lymphadenopathy are the next most common symptoms, but they occur in a much smaller proportion of patients with CMV disease: pharyngitis in 30% to 40% and lymphadenopathy in 17% to 27%. The laboratory features of the two forms of mononucleosis are nearly identical: atypical lymphocytosis and mild elevation of serum transaminase values are seen in the vast majority of patients. Leukopenia is a frequent part of the CMV syndrome in transplant recipients and may be seen in normal hosts as well. One series reported leukocytosis in most patients (83), but another recorded it in only 3.8% (84). Approximately 15% to 20% of these patients have more severe abnormalities of liver enzyme tests, and a hepatitis-like presentation of CMV can certainly occur in the normal host. In summary, in a patient who "feels ill" and has fever but no real localizing signs by history and physical examination, the finding of abnormal liver chemistries or atypical lymphocytosis points in the direction of CMV or Epstein-Barr virus mononucleosis.

Infrequent but recurrently reported sequelae of CMV mononucleosis are Guillain-Barré syndrome and Bell palsy (83,86,89). Other specific organ syndromes are rare but reported in the normal host, including interstitial pneumonia, colitis, and even encephalitis. Many of these cases rest primarily on serologic evidence and have not been confirmed histologically. Nonetheless, the fact that the same syndromes are well-established expressions of CMV in the immunosuppressed patient lends credence to their relation to the virus in the ostensibly normal host.

Transplant Syndromes

The CMV syndrome after kidney transplantation was once called 40-day fever (87). The time of onset and the nature of CMV disease after liver and heart transplantation are similar (52,88). There may be transient and benign fever without localizing signs, or the patient may become progressively more ill with hepatitis, leukopenia, and pneumonitis constituting a "deadly triad" (89). Significant superinfection, either bacterial or opportunistic, is common in these latter patients, particularly in the lung. Although viral damage to the lung, as in influenza, and low numbers of circulating granulocytes may both predispose to bacterial infection, the reason for the high attack rate of *Pneumocystis carinii* and fungi in these patients appears to be a decline in CD4+ cells and increase in CD8+ cells attributable to the CMV infec-

tion (90). Thus, the finding of CMV makes it more imperative to exclude other pathogens in this setting. However, in some patients CMV infection is the only demonstrable pathologic process. More rarely seen is a progressive wasting syndrome associated with failure to mount a complement-fixing antibody response to the CMV infection (91). This illness progresses inexorably to death over several weeks, and disseminated CMV is found at autopsy.

Isolated involvement of specific organs may also occur. CMV is the most common cause of esophagitis in bone marrow transplant recipients (92). CMV chorioretinitis can be a late complication, occurring as a result of prolonged viremia (93,94).

CMV tends to affect the transplanted organ disproportionately. In kidney transplant recipients, renal dysfunction during active CMV infection seems to be due to glomerulitis rather than rejection (95). CMV hepatitis is most prominent in liver transplantation, and accelerated atherosclerosis is associated with CMV infection in heart transplantation (96–98). CMV infection also increases the risk of rejection (48,96,99–106) and rejection increases the risk for late-onset CMV disease in patients who receive chemoprophylaxis against CMV in the early post-transplant period (104). Decreased rejection and improved graft survival were the most striking results of the use of a candidate CMV vaccine in patients awaiting kidney transplantation (107).

The interaction between CMV infection and the allogeneic response comes to the fore in bone marrow transplantation. In this setting, the disease has its onset at 50 to 70 days after grafting (55,92,108). CMV and graft-versus-host disease contribute jointly to the pathogenesis of a devastating form of interstitial pneumonitis (55,109,110). This complication affects 15% to 20% of patients and had an 87% mortality until reports of successful treatment with the combination of ganciclovir and CMV hyperimmune globulin (111,112). The failure of antiviral therapy alone to affect clinical outcome despite 1,000-fold reduction in lung viral titers (113) demonstrates the important role of the allogeneic reaction in this syndrome; the contribution of the immune globulin may well be to the immunopathologic part of the process rather than its anti-CMV properties.

CMV infection is a major risk factor for invasive bacterial and fungal infections in both hematopoietic and solid organ transplant recipients. Leukopenia due to the virus or to its treatment, organ and mucosal damage due to viral replication, and immune perturbations all probably contribute. In fact, the increased mortality associated with stem cell transplantation from a CMV-seropositive donor to a CMV-seronegative recipient is due to excess bacterial and fungal infection even in the absence of demonstrable CMV disease (57).

Cytomegalovirus Syndromes in Acquired Immunodeficiency Syndrome

Although a large majority of persons infected with the human immunodeficiency virus type 1 are coinfected with CMV, disease attributable to CMV is usually restricted to those with the most severe levels of immunodeficiency. In fact, most studies of CMV syndromes in AIDS report median CD4+ cell counts of 25/mm^3 or less at diagnosis (114–116). Preservation of CD4+ cell counts above this level by highly active antiretroviral therapy has dramatically reduced the frequency of CMV disease in HIV-infected persons, although an occasional patient may present with CMV disease with a higher number of CD4+ cells. When this occurs shortly after the initiation of potent antiretroviral therapy, immune reconstitution of host response may be contributing to the pathogenesis.

The most frequent form of CMV disease in AIDS is retinitis, with characteristic funduscopic findings of yellow-white exudate, often accompanied by hemorrhage. Alternatively, a white granular lesion may occur (117). CMV retinitis is painless; the symptoms are floaters, blurring of vision, and loss of portions of the visual field, sometimes described as though a veil were covering the area. These symptoms in a person at risk demand prompt ophthalmologic evaluation, even if recent routine ophthalmologic examination showed no evidence of disease. In the absence of treatment, CMV retinitis progresses rapidly (118) and eventually leads to blindness. In the pre-HAART era, monocular CMV retinitis treated intravitreally but not systemically carried a 50% risk of CMV retinitis in the other eye within 6 months and a considerable risk of other organ involvement (115). A distinct syndrome of vitreous inflammation and cystoid macular edema, termed "immune recovery vitreitis," occurs in some patients with inactive CMV retinitis when CD4+ cell counts rise following initiation of highly active antiretroviral therapy (119,120). Retinal detachment may also cause sudden visual loss in the course of CMV retinitis.

The gastrointestinal tract is the next most frequently recognized site of CMV involvement in AIDS. Colitis, characterized by diarrhea, bleeding, and abdominal pain, may progress to perforation. Some patients have macroscopically normal colonic mucosa with typical cytomegalic inclusions on biopsy, but patchy erythematous lesions are more common; ulcers may also occur (121). CMV esophagitis typically presents with odynophagia; endoscopy demonstrates large, usually solitary, ulcers. Biopsy specimens taken at the edge of the lesions show CMV inclusions in endothelial cells (122).

In the past, it was difficult to attribute specific neurologic syndromes in AIDS to CMV because of a lack of diagnostic tools, although response to ganciclovir therapy strongly suggested a role for CMV in some patients with encephalitis who had not improved with zidovudine (123). Several distinct clinical entities have now been described, and the development of polymerase chain reaction for CMV DNA in cerebrospinal fluid offers a firm basis for diagnosis in the future (124). A polyradiculopathy or cauda equina syndrome associated with CMV causes lower extremity weakness associated with bowel and bladder dysfunction, most commonly urinary retention (125,126). Cerebrospinal fluid of persons with this syndrome shows a predominantly polymorphonuclear pleocytosis (124,127), somewhat surprising for a viral etiology, and hypoglycorrhachia may occur relatively frequently (128). Another syndrome that may coexist with polyradiculopathy or occur independently has been recognized by a pattern of periventricular enhancement at magnetic resonance imaging of the brain corresponding to necrotizing ependymitis (129). Interestingly, this is the same anatomic distribution as the intracranial calcification that occurs in infants with severe congenital cytomegalic inclusion disease. Oculomotor and other cranial nerve palsies and nystagmus are frequent clues to this syndrome, as are elevated cerebrospinal fluid protein level and depressed glucose values (124,129). Progression from lethargy and confusion to coma and death is rapid, usually within 1 to 2 months.

In the absence of these relatively characteristic features, CMV encephalitis is difficult to distinguish clinically from that caused by human immunodeficiency virus. One third to one half of patients with CMV retinitis may have coexisting CMV encephalitis, and half of those ultimately diagnosed with CMV encephalitis at autopsy had CMV retinitis during life (124). A necropsy-verified series also demonstrated associations with quasi-psychiatric symptoms, such as delirium, confusion, apathy, and withdrawal, and electrolyte abnormalities (130). Coexisting CMV adrenalitis was found in nearly all cases in this autopsy series, but the electrolyte abnormalities at the time of presentation were not always related to adrenal insufficiency.

CMV adrenalitis may be the cause of postural hypotension in some patients with AIDS (131–133), and biliary tract disease may be related to the virus as well (134). CMV pneumonia is believed to be much less common than isolation of virus from bronchoalveolar lavage specimens (135, 136) and probably constitutes only about 4% of pneumonias in patients with AIDS (133).

DIAGNOSIS

The presence of the typical enlarged cell with "owl's eye" basophilic nuclear inclusion in affected tissue is the gold standard proving CMV as the etiology of disease involving that tissue. Mere detection of CMV is not sufficient evidence of a causative role in the syndrome in question. For example, CMV is frequently isolated from bronchoalveolar lavage specimens in patients with AIDS who have other diagnosed pulmonary infections (usually *Pneumocystis carinii* pneumonia) and respond to treatment directed solely at the other pathogen (135). Formal criteria incorporating clinical findings, CMV detection at the site in question, and often, exclusion of other pathogens, have been developed for the definition of specific CMV syndromes in transplant recipients (136).

Virus Detection

Isolation of CMV from urine of a newborn within the first 3 weeks of life unequivocally establishes congenital infection (virus acquired postnatally is not shed until after that time) but does not distinguish symptomatic from asymptomatic infants. Virus shedding can persist for up to 8 years from congenitally infected children (65) and last for an average of 18 months when children are infected in daycare (137). One fourth of patients studied 2 to 14 years after kidney transplantation excreted CMV in urine (94).

The isolation of virus from buffy coat leukocytes has a high correlation with the presence of disease but is not highly sensitive (138,139). Detection of pp65 in circulating leukocytes by fluorescent antibody or immunoperoxidase staining has improved sensitivity without loss of specificity, but performance characteristics of this test differ among centers (140–145). Detection of CMV DNA by polymerase chain reaction is more sensitive and should be more reproducible (see Chapter 235 for a more detailed discussion of this technique). Although there are reports of high predictive value (128,146–148), a clinical trial based on this assay for CMV DNA in leukocytes of liver transplant recipients found the positive predictive value to be only 36% and the negative predictive value 90% (149). Polymerase chain reaction identifies CMV DNA in the cerebrospinal fluid of both AIDS patients and congenitally infected infants with central nervous system disease (150–152).

Serology

In adults, the presence of serum antibody establishes a diagnosis of CMV infection but not disease. Conversion from seronegative to seropositive status defines the time of acquisition and could confirm CMV as the cause of an episode of heterophile-negative mononucleosis. However, most patients will already have detectable or peak antibody levels by the time they are investigated for this possibility. A fourfold rise in antibody titer is accepted as evidence of active infection, although it may occur in the absence of symptoms—and presumably in the presence of symptoms of other causes. Theoretically, a test for serum immunoglobulin M antibody should solve these problems, but the difficulties with CMV specific immunoglobulin M assays are numerous, as discussed in Chapter 235. Centers that specialize in the evaluation of pregnancies at risk for symptomatic congenital infection confirm primary CMV infection in only one fourth of women referred for the finding of CMV IgM by routine laboratory testing (153). In the presence of a compatible clinical syndrome such as CMV mononucleosis, the IgM test may be useful supporting evidence because it does not require collection of a second serum sample after adequate time for further antibody rise. Clearly, this test should not be used as the sole means of identifying primary infection in a pregnant woman.

Assay for CMV antibody of the immunoglobulin G class can be extremely useful in excluding the diagnosis. Absence of antibody in a newborn excludes congenital infection except in rare circumstances, because maternal antibody should be present even if the child has failed to make any response. In a patient with a puzzling febrile illness of several weeks' duration, absence of CMV antibody would exclude the diagnosis. If a serum sample obtained early in illness is negative or has a low antibody titer or an indeterminate reaction, that serum sample should be saved to be retested at the same time as subsequent specimens.

Prenatal Diagnosis

Detection of CMV in amniotic fluid by culture or PCR is highly predictive of congenital infection but does not identify which infants will be seriously affected (154–156). Quantitative polymerase chain reaction showing $>10^5$ CMV genome copies/mL of amniotic fluid (154) or CMV-specific IgM in fetal blood (156) strongly predict symptomatic disease at birth. The occasional instance of positive amniotic fluid PCR or culture followed by birth of a baby without congenital infection seems to be explained by very low copy numbers of CMV genome in the amniotic fluid (154) and may represent prenatal clearance of the infection. False-negative results may occur when amniocentesis is performed before 22 weeks of gestation or too early after maternal acquisition of infection (155,156) (at least 9 weeks after seroconversion is recommended) (154).

TREATMENT

Antiviral treatment is warranted for established CMV disease in AIDS and transplant settings. In the past, the choice of agent

has usually been based on the toxicity profiles of the three parenteral drugs active against CMV, ganciclovir, foscarnet and cidofovir. Ganciclovir's primary toxicity is bone marrow suppression, while foscarnet is nephrotoxic and can produce electrolyte disturbances such as hypocalcemia even in the absence of impairment of renal function. Cidofovir requires administration with probenecid and normal saline to protect renal tubular cells from drug accumulation, but even with these precautions, nephrotoxicity can be dose-limiting. The recent demonstration of efficacy of the oral prodrug valganciclovir for CMV retinitis in AIDS (157) has opened the possibility of oral therapy for other serious CMV infections.

The major reason to select an agent other than ganciclovir for initial treatment is suspicion of ganciclovir resistance. The majority of ganciclovir-resistant CMV isolates have mutations in *UL97*, which do not affect susceptibility to foscarnet and cidofovir. However, exposure to ganciclovir alone can also select for mutations in *UL54*, the viral DNA polymerase, and the target of all three drugs. The most frequent pattern associated with single mutations in *UL54* is resistance to both ganciclovir and cidofovir. Foscarnet resistance may occur in isolation or combined with resistance to either of the other two drugs. Viral isolates resistant to all three compounds have multiple mutations in *UL54* (158).

Therapy customarily involves an induction period, followed by maintenance at a lower dose. In transplant recipients, plasma CMV DNAemia is commonly used as the indicator of response to therapy, with reduction to maintenance dose when plasma DNA has been undetectable for at least a week and discontinuation after undetectable DNA for several more weeks at the lower dose. In CMV retinitis, induction lasts 2 to 3 weeks and until there is definite response of the lesion; some prefer to continue induction-level dosing until there is complete healing. Before highly active antiretroviral therapy, patients with AIDS required lifelong therapy for CMV and progression of retinitis occurred despite continued drug therapy. The median duration to clinical progression after first induction was about 60 days with ganciclovir or foscarnet (159). Patients whose retinitis progressed responded equally well to re-induction with the same drug they had initially received or to a switch from ganciclovir to foscarnet or vice versa (in fact, clinical assessment of duration of response favored ganciclovir, even though it was the first agent used in nearly 75%), but duration of control was improved for those who continued their original maintenance therapy and added the alternate drug at induction doses (median time to progression 4.3 mos, or about 130 days) (160). Cidofovir, given as two once-weekly doses followed by infusions every other week, delayed progression 120 days or more (161-163). Intravitreal implants that release ganciclovir over 4 to 8 months provide the longest duration of local control of CMV retinitis (164).

A trial to evaluate the best approach to protecting the contralateral eye and other organs demonstrated dramatic reduction in these events resulting from the introduction of protease inhibitors for the treatment of HIV (165). Clinical experience found that maintenance therapy for CMV could be safely discontinued in patients with a good response to highly active antiretroviral therapy (166). Current guidelines recommend discontinuation when the CD4$^+$ cell count has been above 100 to 150 cells/mm^3 for more than 6 months and when reactivation of disease would not lead quickly to blindness; ophthalmologic monitoring should continue (167). Treatment of other types of CMV disease in AIDS follows the experience in CMV retinitis, with some authors advocating combined foscarnet and ganciclovir for CNS disease.

Early results of treatment of infants with symptomatic congenital CMV infection with daily intravenous ganciclovir for

6 weeks include improvement or stabilization of hearing in five (16%) of 30 children at 6 months (168). Ganciclovir therapy alone is inadequate for the treatment of interstitial pneumonitis in bone marrow transplant recipients, but ganciclovir combined with immune globulin has reduced mortality to 30% to 48% (111,112,169).

PREVENTION

Immunoprophylaxis

Intravenous CMV immune globulin does not prevent CMV infection but does modify disease in seronegative recipients of seropositive kidneys (170). In liver transplantation, seronegative recipients with seropositive donors did not benefit from this therapy, but there was a modest overall reduction in serious CMV-related disease, including fungal superinfection (171). Hyperimmune globulin did not protect premature infants of seronegative mothers from either CMV infection or disease (79). No effective vaccine for CMV is currently available; see Chapter 235 for a review of vaccine development.

Chemoprophylaxis

A number of studies have demonstrated prophylactic efficacy for intravenous ganciclovir, oral ganciclovir, and the oral prodrug of acyclovir, valacyclovir, in various transplant settings (153,172–178). The high cost of these agents, their toxicity, and concern about selecting for ganciclovir resistance have led some transplant centers to prefer a strategy of preemptive therapy, triggered by detection of CMV by culture, antigenemia, or polymerase chain reaction (179–182). Some patients may already have disease by the time the indicator for initiation of preemptive therapy turns positive (148,183). Patients who receive either prophylaxis or preemptive therapy may have CMV disease deferred rather than prevented, but the hope is that they will be better able to handle the infection later after transplant. Late-onset disease appears to correlate with high viral load in stem cell transplant recipients and also in solid organ transplants, where it occurs in seronegative patients whose graft comes from a seropositive donor (148,183, 184). These patients may have low-level viral replication in the presence of the drug. Clinically-significant ganciclovir resistance has been documented in this setting even in patients who received only preemptive therapy (183,184). At the time of this writing, the outcomes of clinical trials of valganciclovir for transplant prophylaxis have not yet been reported, nor has a reliable and reproducible level of CMV DNA determined by a commercially-available test been validated as the trigger for initiation of preemptive therapy.

REFERENCES

1. Stagno S, Pass RE, Dworsky ME, et al. The relative importance of primary and recurrent maternal infection. *N Engl J Med* 1982;306:945.
2. Kumar ML, Gold E, Jacobs IB, et al. Primary cytomegalovirus infection in adolescent pregnancy. *Pediatrics* 1984;74:493.
3. Stagno S, Pass RF, Cloud G, et al. Primary cytomegalovirus infection in pregnancy. *JAMA* 1986;256:1904.
4. Monif GRG, Egan EA, Held B, Eitzman DV. The correlation of maternal cytomegalovirus infection during varying stages in gestation with neonatal involvement. *J Pediatr* 1972;80:17.
5. Stern H, Tucker SM. Prospective study of cytomegalovirus infection in pregnancy. *BMJ* 1973;2:268.
6. Griffiths PD, Campbell-Benzie A, Heath RB. A prospective study of primary cytomegalovirus infection in pregnant women. *Br J Obstet Gynaecol* 1980;87:308.
7. Ahlfors K, Forsgen M, Ivarsson S, et al. Congenital cytomegalovirus infection: on the relation between type and time of maternal infection and infant's symptoms. *Scand J Infect Dis* 1983;15:129.
8. Embil JA, Ozere RL, Haldane EV. Congenital cytomegalovirus infection in two siblings from consecutive pregnancies. *J Pediatr* 1970;77:417.
9. Ahlfors K Harris S, Ivarsson S, Svanberg L. Secondary maternal cytomegalovirus infection causing symptomatic congenital infection. *N Engl J Med* 1981;305:284.
10. Boppana SB, Fowler KB, Britt WJ, et al. Symptomatic congenital cytomegalovirus infection in infants born to mothers with preexisting immunity to cytomegalovirus. *Pediatrics* 1999;104:55–60.
11. Boppana SB, Rivera LB, Fowler KB, et al. Intrauterine transmission of ytomegalovirus to infants of women with preconceptional immunity. *N Engl J Med* 2001;344:1366–1371.
12. Balcarek KB, Oh MK, Pass RF. Maternal viremia and congenital CMV infection. In: Michelson S, Plotkin SA, eds. *Multidisciplinary approach to understanding cytomegalovirus disease.* Amsterdam: Elsevier, 1993:169–173.
13. Fisher S, Genbacev O, Maidji E, Pereira L. Human cytomegalovirus infection of placental cytotrophoblasts in vitro and in utero: implications for transmission and pathogenesis. *J Virol* 2000;74:6808–6820.
14. Reynolds DW, Stagno S, Hosty TS, et al. Maternal cytomegalovirus excretion and perinatal infection. *N Engl J Med* 1973;289:1.
15. Hayes K, Danks DM, Gibas H, Jack I. Cytomegalovirus in human milk. *N Engl J Med* 1972;287:177.
16. Cheeseman SH, McGraw BR. Studies on cytomegalovirus in human milk. *J Infect Dis* 1983;148:615.
17. Dworsky M, Yow M, Stagno S, et al. Cytomegalovirus infection of breast milk and transmission in infancy. *Pediatrics* 1983;72:295.
18. Taber LH, Frank AL, Yow MD, Bagley A. Acquisition of cytomegaloviral infections in families with young children: a serological study. *J Infect Dis* 1985;151:948.
19. Hutto C, Little EA, Ricks R, et al. Isolation of cytomegalovirus from toys and hands in a day care center. *J Infect Dis* 1986;154:527.
20. Tolkoff-Rubin NE, Rubin RH, Keller EE, et al. Cytomegalovirus infection in dialysis patients and personnel. *Ann Intern Med* 1978;89:625.
21. Betts RF, Cestero RVM, Freeman RB, Douglas RG. Epidemiology of cytomegalovirus infection in end stage renal disease. *J Med Virol* 1979;4:89.
22. Dworsky ME, Welch K, Cassady G, Stagno S. Occupational risk for primary cytomegalovirus infection among pediatric healthcare workers. *N Engl J Med* 1983;390:950.
23. Hatherley LI. Is primary cytomegalovirus infection an occupational hazard for obstetrics nurses? *Infect Control* 1986;7:452.
24. Balfour CL, Balfour HH Jr. Cytomegalovirus is not an occupational risk for nurses in renal transplant and neonatal units. *JAMA* 1986;256:1909.
25. Demmler GJ, Yow MD, Spector SA, et al. Nosocomial cytomegalovirus infections within two hospitals caring for infants and children. *J Infect Dis* 1987;156:9.
26. Gerberding JL. Incidence and prevalence of human immunodeficiency virus, hepatitis B virus, hepatitis C virus, and cytomegalovirus among health care personnel at risk for blood exposure: final report from a longitudinal study. *J Infect Dis* 1994;170:1410.
27. Yow MD, Lakeman AD, Stagno S, et al. Use of restriction enzymes to investigate the source of a primary cytomegalovirus infection in a pregnant nurse. *Pediatrics* 1982;70:713.
28. Wilfert CM, Eng-Shang H, Stagno S. Restriction endonuclease analysis of cytomegalovirus deoxyribonucleic acid as an epidemiologic tool. *Pediatrics* 1982;70:717.
29. Dworsky ME, Lakeman A, Stagno S. Cytomegalovirus transmission within a family. *Pediatr Infect Dis* 1984;3:286.
30. Haneberg B, Bertnes, E, Haukenes G. Antibodies to cytomegalovirus among personnel at a children's hospital. *Acta Paediatr Scand* 1980;69:407.
31. Forbes BA. Acquisition of cytomegalovirus infection: an update. *Clin Microbiol Rev* 1989;2:204.
32. Drew WL, Mills J, Levy J, et al. Cytomegalovirus infection and abnormal T-lymphocyte subset ratios in homosexual men. *Ann Intern Med* 1985;103:61.
33. Davis LE, Stewart JA, Garvin S. Cytomegalovirus infection: a seroepidemiologic comparison of nuns and women from a venereal disease clinic. *Am J Epidemiol* 1975;102:327.
34. Adler SP. Transfusion-associated cytomegalovirus infections. *Rev Infect Dis* 1983;5:977.
35. Yeager AS. Transfusion-acquired cytomegalovirus infection in newborn infants. *Am J Dis Child* 1974;128:478.
36. Tolpin MD, Stewart JA, Warren D, et al. Transfusion transmission of cytomegalovirus confirmed by restriction endonuclease analysis. *J Pediatr* 1985;107:953.
37. Adler SP, Baggett J, Wilson M, et al. Molecular epidemiology of cytomegalovirus in a nursery: lack of evidence for nosocomial transmission. *J Pediatr* 1986;108:117.
38. Ballard RA, Drew WL, Hufnagle KG, Riedel PA. Acquired cytomegalovirus infection in preterm infants. *Am J Dis Child* 1979;133:482.
39. Spector SA, Schmidt K, Ticknor W, Grossman M. Cytomegalovirus in older infants in intensive care nurseries. *J Pediatr* 1979;95:444.
40. Beneke JS, Tegtmeier GE, Alter HJ, et al. Relation of titers of antibodies to CMV in blood donors to the transmission of cytomegalovirus infection. *J Infect Dis* 1984;150:883.

41. Preiksaitis JK, Brown L, McKenzie M. The risk of cytomegalovirus infection in seronegative transfusion recipients not receiving exogenous immunosuppression. *J Infect Dis* 1988;157:523.

42. Hillyer CD, Emmens RK, Zago-Novaretti M, Berkman EM. Methods for the reduction of transfusion-transmitted cytomegalovirus infection: filtration versus the use of seronegative donor units. *Transfusion* 1994;34:929.

43. Ho M, Suwansirikul S, Dowling JN, et al. The transplanted kidney as a source of cytomegalovirus infection. *N Engl J Med* 1975;293:1109.

44. Betts RF, Freeman RB, Douglas RG Jr, et al. Transmission of cytomegalovirus infection with renal allograft. *Kidney Int* 1975;8:385.

45. Rakela J, Wiesner RH, Taswell HF, et al. Incidence of cytomegalovirus infection and its relationship to donor-recipient serologic status in liver transplantation. *Transplant Proc* 1987;19:2399.

46. Gorensek MJ, Carey WD, Vogt D, Goormastic M. A multivariate analysis of risk factors for cytomegalovirus infection in liver transplant recipients. *Gastroenterology* 1990;98:1326.

47. Preiksaitis JK, Rosno S, Grumet C, Merigan TC. Infections due to herpesviruses in cardiac transplant recipients: role of the donor heart and immunosuppressive therapy. *J Infect Dis* 1983;147:974.

48. Betts RF, Freeman RB, Douglas RJ Jr, Talley TE. Clinical manifestations of renal allograft derived primary cytomegalovirus infection. *Am J Dis Child* 1977;131:759.

49. Naraqi S, Jackson GG, Jonasson O, Yamashiroya HM. Prospective study of prevalence, incidence, and source of herpes-virus infections in patients with renal allografts. *J Infect Dis* 1977;136:531.

50. Pass RF, Long WK, Whitley RJ, et al. Productive infection with cytomegalovirus and herpes simplex virus in renal transplant recipients: role of source of kidney. *J Infect Dis* 1978;137:556.

51. Suwansirikul S, Rao N, Dowling JN, Ho M. Primary and secondary cytomegalovirus infection. *Arch Intern Med* 1977;137:1026.

52. Pollard RB, Rand KH, Arvin AM, Merigan TC. Cell-mediated immunity to cytomegalovirus infection in normal subjects and cardiac transplant recipients. *J Infect Dis* 1978;137:541.

53. Dummer JS, White LT, Ho M, et al. Morbidity of cytomegalovirus infection in recipients of heart or heart-lung transplants who received cyclosporine. *J Infect Dis* 1985;152:1182.

54. Grundy JE, Super M, Sweny P, et al. Symptomatic cytomegalovirus infection in seropositive kidney recipient: reinfection with donor virus rather than reactivation of recipients virus. *Lancet* 1988;2:132.

55. Meyers JD, Fluornoy N, Thomas ED. Risk factors for cytomegalovirus infection after human marrow transplantation. *J Infect Dis* 1986;153:478.

56. Winston DJ, Huang ES, Miller MJ, et al. Molecular epidemiology of cytomegalovirus infections associated with bone marrow transplantation. *Ann Intern Med* 1985;102:16.

57. Nichols WG, Corey L, Gooley T, et al. High risk of death due to bacterial and fungal infection among cytomegalovirus (CMV)-seronegative recipients of stem cell transplants from seropositive donors: evidence for indirect effects of primary CMV infection. *J Infect Dis* 2002;185:273–282.

58. Lemon SM, Hutt LM, Huang YT. Cytotoxicity of circulating leukocytes in cytomegalovirus mononucleosis. *Clin Microbiol Immunopathol* 1977;8:513.

59. Yachie A, Tosato G, Straus SE, Blaese RM. Immunostimulation by cytomegalovirus: helper T cell-dependent activation of immunoglobulin production in vitro by lymphocytes from CMV-immune donors. *J Immunol* 1985;135:1305.

60. Kapasi K, Rice GPA. Role of the monocyte in cytomegalovirus-mediated immunosuppression in vitro. *J Infect Dis* 1986;154:881.

61. Rakusan TA, Juneja HS, Fleischmann WR. Inhibition of hemopoietic colony formation by human cytomegalovirus in vitro. *J Infect Dis* 1989;159:127.

62. Golden MP, Hammer SM, Wanke CA, Albrecht MA. Cytomegalovirus vasculitis. *Medicine (Baltimore)* 1994;73:246.

63. Hanshaw JB, Dudgeon JA, Marshall WC. *Viral diseases of the fetus and newborn,* 2nd ed. Philadelphia: WB Saunders, 1985:92–131.

64. Stagno S, Whitley RJ. Herpesvirus infections of pregnancy. Part I. Cytomegalovirus and Epstein-Barr virus infection. *N Engl J Med* 1985;313:1270.

65. Hanshaw JB. Congenital cytomegalovirus infection: a fifteen year perspective. *J Infect Dis* 1971;123:555.

66. Weller TH, Hanshaw JB. Virological and clinical observations on cytomegalic inclusion disease. *N Engl J Med* 1964;266:1233.

67. Medearis DN Jr. Observation concerning human cytomegalovirus infection and disease. *Bull Johns Hopkins Hosp* 1964;114:181.

68. McCracken GH Jr, Shinefleld HR, Cobb K, et al. Congenital cytomegalic inclusion disease a longitudinal study of 20 patients. *Am J Dis Child* 1969;117:522.

69. Berenberg W, Nankervis G. Long-term follow-up of cytomegalic inclusion disease of infancy. *Pediatrics* 1970;46:403.

70. Pass RF, Stagno S, Meyers GJ, Alford CA. Outcome of symptomatic congenital cytomegalovirus infection: results of long-term longitudinal follow-up. *Pediatrics* 1980;66:758.

71. Williamson WD, Desmond MM, LaFevers N, et al. Symptomatic congenital cytomegalovirus: disorders of language, learning and hearing. *Am J Dis Child* 1982;136:902.

72. Conboy TJ, Pass RF, Stagno S, et al. Early clinical manifestations and intellectual outcome in children with symptomatic congenital cytomegalovirus infection. *J Pediatr* 1987;111:343.

73. Yow MD. Congenital cytomegalovirus disease: a NOW problem. *J Infect Dis* 1989;159:163.

74. Ahlfors K, Ivarsson SA, Harris S. Report on a long-term study of maternal and congenital cytomegalovirus infection in Sweden: review of prospective studies available in the literature. *Scand J Infect Dis* 1999;31:443–457.

75. Reynolds DW, Stagno S, Stubbs KG, et al. Inapparent congenital cytomegalovirus infection with elevated cord IgM levels: causal relation with auditory and mental deficiency. *N Engl J Med* 1974;2290:291.

76. Hanshaw JB, Scheiner AP, Moxley AW, et al. School failure and deafness after "silent" congenital cytomegalovirus infection. *N Engl J Med* 1976;295:468.

77. Saigal S, Lunyk O, Larke RPB, Chernesky MA. The outcome in children with congenital cytomegalovirus infection: a longitudinal follow-up study. *Am J Dis Child* 1982;136:896.

78. Yeager AS, Grumet FC, Hafleigh EB, et al. Prevention of transfusion-acquired cytomegalovirus infections in newborn infants. *J Pediatr* 1981;98:281.

79. Snydman DR, Werner BG, Meissner HC, et al. Use of cytomegalovirus immunoglobulin in multiply transfused premature neonates. *Pediatr Infect Dis J* 1995;14:34.

80. CMV: Pathogenesis and prevention of human infection. *Birth Defects Original Article Series* 1984;20:1.

81. Linnemann CC, MacMillan BG. Viral infections in pediatric burn patients. *Am J Dis Child* 1981;135:750.

82. Deepe G, MacMillan BG, Linnemann CC. Unexplained fever in burn patients due to cytomegalovirus infection. *JAMA* 1982;248:2299.

83. Cohen JI, Corey GRE. Cytomegalovirus infection in the normal host. *Medicine (Baltimore)* 1985;64:100.

84. Horwitz CA, Henle W, Henle G, et al. Clinical and laboratory evaluation of cytomegalovirus-induced mononucleosis in previously healthy individuals: report of 82 cases. *Medicine (Baltimore)* 1986;65:124.

85. Hirsch MS, Cheeseman SH, Hammer SM. Human herpesvirus infections: Pathogenesis and clinical implications. In: Weinstein L, Fields BN, eds. *Seminars in infectious diseases.* New York: Stratton Intercontinental Medical Book, 1979:217–264.

86. Kaplan JE, Greenspan JR, Bomgarrs M, et al. Simultaneous outbreaks of Guillain-Barré syndrome and Bell's palsy in Hawaii in 1981. *JAMA* 1983;250:2635.

87. Coulson AS, Lucas ZJ, Condy M, Cohn R. Forty-day fever: an epidemic of cytomegalovirus disease in a renal transplant population. *West J Med* 1974;120:1.

88. Gorensek MJ, Stewart RW, Keys TF, et al. A multivariate analysis of the risk of cytomegalovirus infection in heart transplant recipients. *J Infect Dis* 1988;157:515.

89. Rubin RH, Cosimi AB, Tolkoff-Rubin NE, et al. Infectious disease syndromes attributable to cytomegalovirus and their significance among renal transplant recipients. *Transplantation* 1977;24:458.

90. Schooley RT, Hirsch MS, Colvin RB, et al. Association of herpesvirus infections with T-lymphocyte subset alterations, glomerulopathy, and opportunistic infections after renal transplantation. *N Engl J Med* 1983;308:307.

91. Simmons RL, Matas AJ, Rattazzi LC, et al. Clinical characteristics of the lethal cytomegalovirus infection following renal transplantation. *Surgery* 1977;82:537.

92. McDonald GB, Sharma PJ, Hackman RC, et al. Esophageal infections in immunosuppressed patients after marrow transplantation. *Gastroenterology* 1985;88:1111.

93. Fiala M, Payne JE, Berne TV, et al. Epidemiology of cytomegalovirus after transplantation and immunosuppression. *J Infect Dis* 1975;132:421.

94. Cheeseman SH, Stewart JA, Winkle S, et al. Cytomegalovirus excretion 2-14 years after renal transplantation. *Transplant Proc* 1979;11:71.

95. Richardson WP, Colvin RB, Cheeseman SH, et al. Glomerulopathy associated with cytomegalovirus viremia in renal allografts. *N Engl J Med* 1981;305:57.

96. Grattan MT, Moreno-Cabral CE, Starnes VA, et al. Cytomegalovirus infection is associated with cardiac allograft rejection and atherosclerosis. *JAMA* 1989;261:3561.

97. Speir E, Modali R, Huang E, et al. Potential role of human cytomegalovirus and p53 interaction in coronary restenosis. *Science* 1994;265:391.

98. Valentine HA, Gao SZ, Menon SG, et al. Impact of prophylactic immediate posttransplant ganciclovir on development of transplant atherosclerosis: a post hoc analysis of a randomized, placebo-controlled study. *Circulation* 1999;100:61–66.

99. David DS, Millian SJ, Whitsell JC, et al. Viral syndromes and renal homograft rejection. *Ann Surg* 1972;175:257.

100. Lopez C, Simmons RL, Mauer SM, et al. Association of renal allograft rejection with virus infections. *Am J Med* 1974;56:280.

101. Simmons RL, Lopez C, Balfour HH, et al. Cytomegalovirus: clinical virological correlations in renal transplant recipients. *Ann Surg* 1974;180:623.

102. May AG, Betts RF, Freeman RB, Andrus CH. An analysis of cytomegalovirus infection and HLA antigen matching on the outcome of renal transplantation. *Ann Surg* 1978;187:110.

103. Rubin RH, Tolkoff-Rubin NE, Oliver D, et al. Multicenter seroepidemiologic study of the impact of cytomegalovirus infection on renal transplantation. *Transplantation* 1985;40:243.

104. Razonable RR, Rivero A, Rodriguez A, et al. Allograft rejection predicts the occurrence of late-onset cytomegalovirus (CMV) disease among CMV-mismatched solid organ transplant patients receiving prophylaxis with oral ganciclovir. *J Infect Dis* 2001;184:1461.

105. Humar A, Gregson D, Caliendo AM, et al. Clinical utility of quantitative

cytomegalovirus load determination for predicting cytomegalovirus disease in liver transplant recipients. *Transplantation* 1999;68:1305–1311.

106. Evans PC, Soin A, Wreghitt TG, et al. An association between cytomegalovirus infection and chronic rejection after liver transplantation. *Transplantation* 2000;69:30–35.

107. Brayman KL, Dafoe DC, Smythe WR, et al. Prophylaxis of serious cytomegalovirus infection in renal transplant candidates using live human cytomegalovirus vaccine: interim results of a randomized controlled trial. *Arch Surg* 1988;123:1502.

108. Miller W, Flynn P, McCullough J, et al. Cytomegalovirus infection after bone marrow transplantation: an association with acute graft-v-host disease. *Blood* 1986;4:1162.

109. Meyers JD, Spencer HC, Watts JC, et al. Cytomegalovirus pneumonia after human marrow transplantation. *Ann Intern Med* 1975;82:181.

110. Thomas ED, Buckner CD, Banaji M, et al. One hundred patients with acute leukemia treated by chemotherapy, total body irradiation, and allogeneic marrow transplantation. *Blood* 1977;49:511.

111. Emanuel D, Cunningham I, Jules-Elysee K, et al. Cytomegalovirus pneumonia after bone marrow transplantation successfully treated with the combination of ganciclovir and high-dose intravenous immune globulin. *Ann Intern Med* 1988;109:777.

112. Reed EC, Bowden RA, Dandliker PS, et al. Treatment of cytomegalovirus pneumonia with ganciclovir and intravenous cytomegalovirus immunoglobulin in patients with bone marrow transplants. *Ann Intern Med* 1988;109:783.

113. Shepp DH, Dandliker PS, de Miranda P, et al. Activity of 9-(2-hydroxy-l-hydroxymethylethoxymethyl)guanine in the treatment of cytomegalovirus pneumonia. *Ann Intern Med* 1985;103:368.

114. Studies of Ocular Complications of AIDS Research Group in Collaboration with the AIDS Clinical Studies Group. Mortality in patients with the acquired immunodeficiency syndrome treated with either foscarnet or ganciclovir for cytomegalovirus retinitis. *N Engl J Med* 1992;326:213.

115. Martin DF, Parks DJ, Mellow SD, et al. Treatment of cytomegalovirus retinitis with an intraocular sustained-release ganciclovir implant. *Arch Ophthalmol* 1994;112:1531.

116. Wilcox CM, Straub RF, Schwartz DA. Cytomegalovirus esophagitis in AIDS: A prospective evaluation of clinical responses to ganciclovir therapy, relapse rate, and long-term outcome. *Am J Med* 1995;98:169.

117. Bloom JN, Palestine AG. The diagnosis of cytomegalovirus retinitis. *Ann Intern Med* 1988;109:963.

118. Spector SA, Weingeist T, Pollard RB, et al. A randomized, controlled study of intravenous ganciclovir therapy for cytomegalovirus peripheral retinitis in patients with AIDS. AIDS Clinical Trials Group and Cytomegalovirus Cooperative Study Group. *J Infect Dis* 1993;168:557.

119. Karavellas MP, Lowder CY, Macdonald JC, Avila CP Jr, Freeman WR: Immune recovery vitritis associated with inactive cytomegalovirus retinitis: a new syndrome. *Arch Ophthalmol* 1998;116:169–175.

120. Zegans ME, Walton RC, Holland GN, O'Donnell JJ, Jacobson MA, Margolis TP. Transient vitreous inflammatory reactions associated with combination antiretroviral therapy in patients with AIDS and cytomegalovirus retinitis. *Am J Ophthalmol* 1998;125:292–300.

121. Dieterich DT, Rahmin M. Cytomegalovirus colitis in AIDS: Presentation in 44 patients and a review of the literature. *J AIDS Hum Retrovirol* 1991; 4(Suppl 1):S29.

122. Wilcox CM, Diehl DL, Cello JP, et al. Cytomegalovirus esophagitis in patients with AIDS. A clinical, endoscopic, and pathologic correlation. *Ann Intern Med* 1990;113:589.

123. Fiala M, Cone LA, Cohen N, et al. Responses of neurologic complications of AIDS to 3'-azido-3'-deoxythymidine and 9-(1,3-dihydroxy-2-propoxymethyl) guanine. 1. Clinical features. *Rev Infect Dis* 1988;10:250.

124. McCutchan JA. Cytomegalovirus infections of the nervous system in patients with AIDS. *Clin Infect Dis* 1995;30:747.

125. Behar R, Wiley C, McCutchan A. Cytomegalovirus polyradiculoneuropathy in acquired immune deficiency syndrome. *Neurology* 1987;37:557.

126. Kim YS, Hollander H. Polyradiculopathy due to cytomegalovirus: report of two cases in which improvement occurred after prolonged therapy and review of the literature. *Clin Infect Dis* 1993;17:32.

127. de Gans J, Tiessens G, Portegies P, et al. Predominance of polymorphonuclear leukocytes in cerebrospinal fluid of AIDS patients with cytomegalovirus polyradiculomyelitis. *J AIDS* 1990;3:1155.

128. Wolf DG, Spector SA. Early diagnosis of human cytomegalovirus disease in transplant recipients by DNA amplification in plasma. *Transplantation* 1993;56:330.

129. Kalayjian RC, Cohen ML, Bonomo RA, Flanigan TP. Cytomegalovirus ventriculoencephalitis in AIDS. *Medicine (Baltimore)* 1993;72:67.

130. Holland N, Power C, Mathews V, et al. Cytomegalovirus encephalitis in acquired immunodeficiency syndrome (AIDS). *Neurology* 1994;44:507.

131. Tapper ML, Rotterdam HZ, Lerner CW, et al. Adrenal necrosis in the acquired immunodeficiency syndrome. *Ann Intern Med* 1984;100:239.

132. Greene LW, Cole W Greene LB, et al. Adrenal insufficiency as a complication of the acquired immunodeficiency syndrome. *Ann Intern Med* 1984;101:497.

133. Jacobson MA, Mills J. Serious cytomegalovirus disease in the acquired immunodeficiency syndrome (AIDS): clinical findings, diagnosis and treatment. *Ann Intern Med* 1988;108:585.

134. Schneiderman DJ, Cello JP, Laing FC. Papillary stenosis and sclerosing cholangitis in patients with the acquired immunodeficiency syndrome. *Ann Intern Med* 1987;106:546.

135. Bozzette SA, Arcia J, Bartok AE, et al. Impact of *Pneumocystis carinii* and cytomegalovirus on the course and outcome of atypical pneumonia in advanced human immunodeficiency virus disease. *J Infect Dis* 1992;165:93.

136. Ljungman P, Griffiths P, Paya C. Definitions of cytomegalovirus infection and disease in transplant recipients. *Clin Infect Dis* 2002;34:1094–1097.

137. Adler SP, Starr SF, Plotkin SA, et al. Immunity induced by primary cytomegalovirus infection protects against secondary infection in women of childbearing age. *J Infect Dis* 1995;171:26.

138. Cheeseman SH, Rubin RH, Stewart JA, et al. Controlled clinical trial of prophylactic human-leukocyte interferon in renal transplantation: effects on cytomegalovirus and herpes simplex virus infection. *N Engl J Med* 1979;300: 1345.

139. Meyers JD, Ljungman P, Fisher LD. Cytomegalovirus excretion as a predictor of cytomegalovirus disease after marrow transplantation: importance of cytomegalovirus viremia. *J Infect Dis* 1990;162:373.

140. van der Bij W, Torensma R, van Son W, et al. Rapid immunodiagnosis of active cytomegalovirus infection by monoclonal antibody staining of blood leukocytes. *J Med Virol* 1988;25:179.

141. Erice A, Holm MA, Gill PC, et al. Cytomegalovirus (CMV) antigenemia assay is more sensitive than shell vial cultures for rapid detection of CMV in polymorphonuclear blood leukocytes. *J Clin Microbiol* 1992;30:2822.

142. Mazzulli T, Rubin RH, Ferraro MJ, et al. Cytomegalovirus antigenemia: clinical correlations in transplant recipients and in persons with AIDS. *J Clin Microbiol* 1993;31:2824.

143. Landry ML, Ferguson D. Comparison of quantitative cytomegalovirus antigenemia assay with culture methods and correlation with clinical disease. *J Clin Microbiol* 1993;31:2851.

144. Storch GA, Buller RS, Bailey TC, et al. Comparison of PCR and pp65 antigenemia assay with quantitative shell vial culture for detection of cytomegalovirus in blood leukocytes from solid organ transplant recipients. *J Clin Microbiol* 1994;32:997.

145. Singh N, Paterson DL, Gayowski T, Wagener MM, Marino IR. Cytomegalovirus antigenemia directed pre-emptive prophylaxis with oral versus iv ganciclovir for the prevention of cytomegalovirus disease in liver transplant recipients: a randomized, controlled trial. *Transplantation* 2000;70:717–722.

146. Spector SA, Wolf D, Salunga K. Human cytomegalovirus (HCMV) DNA detected in plasma by PCR predicts development of HCMV disease in patients with AIDS or following transplantation. In: Michelson S, Plotkin SA, eds. Multidisciplinary approach to understanding cytomegalovirus disease. Amsterdam: Elsevier Science, 1993:225–230.

147. Rasmussen S, Morris S, Zipeto D, et al. Quantitation of human cytomegalovirus DNA from peripheral blood cells of human immunodeficiency virus-infected patients could predict cytomegalovirus retinitis. *J Infect Dis* 1995;171:177.

148. Limaye AP, Corey L, Koelle DM, et al. Emergence of ganciclovir-resistant cytomegalovirus disease among recipients of solid-organ transplants. *Lancet* 2000;356:645–649.

149. Paya CV, Wilson JA, Espy MJ, et al. Preemptive use of oral ganciclovir to prevent cytomegalovirus infection in liver transplant patients: a randomized, placebo-controlled trial. *J Infect Dis* 2002;185:854–860.

150. Wolf DG, Spector SA. Diagnosis of human cytomegalovirus central nervous system disease in AIDS patients by DNA amplification from cerebrospinal fluid. *J Infect Dis* 1992;166:1412.

151. Anque P, Vago L, Brytting M, et al. Cytomegalovirus infection of the central nervous system in patients with AIDS: diagnosis by DNA amplification from cerebrospinal fluid. *J Infect Dis* 1992;166:1408.

152. Atkins J, Demmler GJ, Williamson WD, et al. Polymerase chain reaction to detect cytomegalovirus DNA in the cerebrospinal fluid of neonates with congenital infection. *J Infect Dis* 1994;169:1334.

153. Mullen GM, Silver MA, Malinowska K, et al. Effective oral ganciclovir prophylaxis against cytomegalovirus disease in heart transplant recipients. *Transplant Proc* 1998;30:4110–4112.

154. Lazzarotto T, Varani S, Guerra B, et al. Prenatal indicators of congenital cytomegalovirus infection. *J Pediatr* 2000;137:90–95.

155. Gouarin S, Palmer P, Cointe D, et al. Congenital HCMV infection: a collaborative and comparative study of virus detection in amniotic fluid by culture and by PCR. *J Clin Virol* 2001;21:47–55.

156. Enders G, Bäder U, Lindemann L, et al. A Prenatal diagnosis of congenital cytomegalovirus infection in 189 pregnancies with known outcome. *Prenatal Diagn* 2001;21:362–377.

157. Martin DF, Sierra-Madero J, Walmsley S, et al. A controlled trial of valganciclovir as induction therapy for cytomegalovirus retinitis. *N Engl J Med* 2002; 346:1119–1126.

158. Erice A. Resistance of human cytomegalovirus to antiviral drugs. *Clin Microbiol Rev* 1999;12:286–297.

159. Studies of Ocular Complications of AIDS Research Group in Collaboration with the AIDS Clinical Study Group. Foscarnet-ganciclovir cytomegalovirus retinitis trial: 4. Visual outcomes. *Ophthalmology* 1994;101:1250.

160. The Studies of Ocular Complications of AIDS Research Group in Collaboration with the AIDS Clinical Trials Group. Combination foscarnet and ganciclovir therapy vs monotherapy for the treatment of relapsed cytomegalovirus retinitis in patients with AIDS: the cytomegalovirus retreatment trial. *Arch Ophthalmol* 1996;114:23–33.

161. Lalezari JP, Stagg RJ, Kupperman BD, et al. Intravenous cidofovir for peripheral cytomegalovirus retinitis in patients with AIDS: a randomized, controlled trial. *Ann Intern Med* 1997;126:257–263.

162. Studies of Ocular Complications of AIDS Research Group in Collaboration with the AIDS Clinical Trials Group. Parenteral cidofovir for cytomegalovirus retinitis in patients with AIDS: the HPMPC peripheral cytomegalovirus retinitis trial. *Ann Intern Med* 1997;126:264–274.

163. Lalezari JP, Holland GN, Kramer F, et al. Randomized, controlled study of the safety and efficacy of intravenous cidofovir for the treatment of relapsing cytomegalovirus retinitis in patients with AIDS. *J AIDS Hum Retrovirol* 1998;17:339–344.

164. Musch DC, Martin DF, Gordon JF, et al. Treatment of cytomegalovirus retinitis with a sustained-release ganciclovir implant. *N Engl J Med* 1997;337:83–90.

165. Martin DF, Kuppermann BD, Wolitz RA, et al. Oral ganciclovir for patients with cytomegalovirus retinitis treated with a ganciclovir implant. *N Engl J Med* 1999;340:1063–1070.

166. Whitcup SM, Fortin E, Lindblad AS, et al. Discontinuation of anticytomegalovirus therapy in patients with HIV infection and cytomegalovirus retinitis. *JAMA* 1999;282:1633–1637.

167. Centers for Disease Control and Prevention. Guidelines for Preventing Opportunistic Infections Among HIV-Infected Persons, 2002 Recommendations of the U.S. Public Health Service and the Infectious Diseases Society of America. *MMWR* 2002;51(RR–8):1–52. Updates available at http://aidsinfo.nih.gov/guidelines/

168. Whitley RJ, Cloud G, Gruber W, et al. Ganciclovir treatment of symptomatic congenital cytomegalovirus infections: results of a phase II study. *J Infect Dis* 1997;175:1080–1086.

169. Schmidt GM, Kovacs A, Zaia JA, et al. Ganciclovir/immunoglobulin combination therapy for the treatment of human cytomegalovirus-associated interstitial pneumonia in bone marrow allograft recipients. *Transplantation* 1988;46:905.

170. Snydman DR, Werner BG Heinze-Lacey B, et al. Use of cytomegalovirus immune globulin to prevent cytomegalovirus disease in renal-transplant recipients. *N Engl J Med* 1987;317:1049.

171. Snydman DR, Werner BG, Dougherty NN, et al. Cytomegalovirus immune globulin prophylaxis in liver transplantation. *Ann Intern Med* 1993;119:984.

172. Winston DJ, Ho WG, Bartoni K, et al. Ganciclovir prophylaxis of cytomegalovirus infection and disease in allogeneic bone marrow transplant recipients. *Ann Intern Med* 1993;118:179.

173. Goodrich JM, Bowden RA, Fisher L, et al. Ganciclovir prophylaxis to prevent cytomegalovirus disease after allogeneic marrow transplant. *Ann Intern Med* 1993;118:173.

174. Merigan TC, Renlund DG, Keay S, et al. A controlled trial of ganciclovir to prevent cytomegalovirus disease after heart transplantation. *N Engl J Med* 1992;326:1182.

175. Gane E, Saliba F, Valdecasas GJC, et al. Randomized trial of efficacy and safety of oral ganciclovir in the prevention of cytomegalovirus disease in liver-transplant recipients. *Lancet* 1997;350:1729–1733.

176. Lowance D, Neumayer H-H, Legendre CM, et al. Valacyclovir for the prevention of cytomegalovirus disease after renal transplantation. *N Engl J Med* 1999;340:1462–1470.

177. Wreghitt TG, Abel SJC, McNeil K, et al. Intravenous ganciclovir prophylaxis for cytomegalovirus in heart, heart-lung, and lung transplant recipients. *Transpl Int* 1999;12:254–270.

178. Winston DJ, Wirin D, Shaked A, Busuttil RW. Randomized comparison of ganciclovir and high-dose acyclovir for long-term cytomegalovirus prophylaxis in liver-transplant recipients. *Lancet* 1995;346:69–74.

179. Schmidt GM, Horak DA, Niland JC, et al. A randomized controlled trial of prophylactic ganciclovir for cytomegalovirus pulmonary infection in recipients of allogeneic bone marrow transplants. *N Engl J Med* 1991;324:1005.

180. Goodrich JM, Mori M, Gleaves CA, et al. Early treatment with ganciclovir to prevent cytomegalovirus disease after bone marrow transplantation. *N Engl J Med* 1991;325:1601.

181. Singh N, Yu UL, Mieles L, et al. High-dose acyclovir compared with short-course preemptive ganciclovir to prevent cytomegalovirus disease in liver transplant recipients: a randomized trial. *Ann Intern Med* 1994;120:375.

182. Singh N. Preemptive therapy versus universal prophylaxis with ganciclovir for cytomegalovirus in solid organ transplant recipients. *Clin Infect Dis* 2001;32:742–751.

183. Zaia JA, Gallez-Hawkins GM, Tegtmeier BR, et al. Late cytomegalovirus disease in marrow transplantation is predicted by virus load in plasma. *J Infect Dis* 1997;176:782–785.

184. Limaye AJ, Raghu G, Koelle DM, et al. High incidence of ganciclovir-resistant cytomegalovirus infection among lung transplant recipients receiving preemptive therapy. *J Infect Dis* 2002;185:20–27.

CHAPTER 178
Kawasaki Syndrome

H. Cody Meissner and Donald Y. M. Leung

INTRODUCTION

Kawasaki syndrome is an acute vasculitis that primarily affects infants and young children. The illness was first described by Tomisaku Kawasaki in 1967 in Japanese in the *Journal of Allergology* (1). Although Kawasaki syndrome was originally described as a benign illness of early childhood, it is now recognized that this disease is a leading cause of acquired heart disease in children in the United States and Western Europe (2,3). Children with Kawasaki syndrome who do not receive treatment with intravenous immune globulin (IVIG) and aspirin within the first 10 days of onset of fever have a 20% to 25% risk of coronary artery abnormalities. Early recognition and prompt treatment reduces the prevalence of coronary artery abnormalities to less than 5%, placing emphasis on the need for early diagnosis and treatment (4–7). A diagnosis of Kawasaki syndrome is based on the presence of fever plus at least four of five criteria, just as a diagnosis of rheumatic fever is based on the Jones criteria. While the etiology of Kawasaki syndrome is not fully defined, features of this syndrome are similar to those found in certain illnesses which are known to be caused by toxin producing bacteria, including toxic shock syndrome and scarlet fever.

EPIDEMIOLOGY

Kawasaki syndrome has been reported from countries throughout the world although the highest rates of disease are found in Japan and children of Japanese ancestry living outside of Japan. In the United States, the prevalence of Kawasaki syndrome is highest in Asians, intermediate in African Americans, and lowest in whites. The hospitalization rate for Kawasaki syndrome among American Indians and Alaskan natives appears to be lower than among whites (8). Disease occurs in males about 1.5 times more often than in females (2). The peak age at which disease occurs is 12 to 24 months. More than 80% of cases occur in patients before 5 years of age and most cases occur before 2 years. The onset of disease after 8 years is rare, representing less than 10% of cases reported to the CDC. Recurrent disease develops in fewer than 2% of patients. Some reports suggest that cardiac sequelae may be more common in children who are 8 or older (9,10). It is not clear whether older patients are predisposed to more severe disease or whether older patients are more likely to have a delay in diagnosis and initiation of treatment later in the course of their illness with correspondingly greater morbidity. Infants less than 12 months of age and particularly those less than 6 months appear to be at increased risk of coronary artery abnormalities (11).

Person-to-person transmission of Kawasaki syndrome is uncommon, although one Japanese study suggested a second case in a family may be higher than in the general population. Three national epidemics have occurred in Japan in 1979, 1987, and in 1985 to 1986 (2). One well-documented epidemiologic study demonstrated spread of disease outward from Tokyo during an epidemic period in a manner clearly suggesting transmission of an infectious agent. Endemic Kawasaki syndrome occurs in Japan with an incidence rate of 110 cases/100,000 children younger than 5 years of age per year. In industrialized countries, there is a seasonality of disease with a peak in activity in late winter and spring.

CLINICAL DISEASE

The possibility of Kawasaki syndrome should be considered in any patient with a fever lasting 5 or more days without an alternative explanation and the presence of at least four of the five clinical criteria listed in Table 178.1 (12). Kawasaki syndrome typically begins with an acute onset with daily fevers to 40°C or greater in a toxic-appearing child. Fever may last 2 weeks or longer without treatment. It is important to consider Kawasaki syndrome in the differential diagnosis of a child who presents with fever of unknown origin.

The mucocutaneous manifestations of Kawasaki syndrome are varied and not all patients will exhibit each feature. In the first days of acute febrile illness, a polymorphous exanthem that may demonstrate a variety of forms develops in approximately 90% of children with Kawasaki syndrome. The eruption tends to be most prominent on the trunk and extremities. The rash is rarely vesicular, pustular, or bullous. One early sign may be accentuation of a perineal rash (13). This may occur before the rash appears on the trunk or extremities.

In most patients a nonexudative, bilateral conjunctival injection begins shortly after the onset of fever and generally involves the bulbar conjunctiva to a greater extent than the palpebral conjunctiva. Conjunctival vessels become engorged and dilated. Purulent discharge is generally not present. Conjunctival injection is associated with anterior uveitis in approximately 80% of patients (14).

Oral mucosal findings occur in almost all typical cases. The lips become red, dry, and often cracked, producing small hemorrhagic fissures. There are no punctate ulcerations such as those seen in herpes gingivostomatitis and no erosions suggestive of Stevens-Johnson syndrome. The tongue is often "strawberry" in appearance with hypertrophied papillae and hyperemia, similar to that seen with streptococcal infections. A generalized erythema of the oropharynx is common although ulceration of the mucosal surface is not characteristic.

Changes in the extremities may be the most distinctive finding among the five criteria. Erythema and edema of the hands and feet with fusiform swelling of the fingers and toes are often observed. Swelling usually begins within a few days of the onset of illness. The hyperemic areas desquamate during the second or third week. The desquamation characteristically begins at the tips of the fingers and toes (the periungual region) and may extend to involve the palms and soles in a manner similar to that seen in scarlet fever. Lymphadenopathy is the least frequent find-

TABLE 178.2.   Associated Features of Kawasaki Syndrome

Cardiovascular abnormalities including myocarditis, arterial aneurysms, pericarditis, aortic or mitral regurgitation, ventricular arrhythmias
Arthralgia and arthritis
Hepatic dysfunction
Urethritis with sterile pyuria
Aseptic meningitis
Hydrops of the gallbladder
Diarrhea, vomiting or abdominal pain
Peripheral gangrene
Uveitis
Sensorineural hearing loss

ing and is seen in only 50% to 75% of patients. It is most often unilateral and the nodes are firm and nontender.

Other associated clinical features of Kawasaki syndrome are listed in Table 178.2. Polyarticular arthralgia and arthritis may occur soon after onset of fever and involve the small joints (15). Pauciarticular arthritis involving the large weight-bearing joints (hips, knees, and ankles) may occur in the second or third week of illness. Urethritis associated with sterile pyuria is common. A mononuclear cell pleocytosis of the cerebrospinal fluid with normal glucose and protein levels occur in approximately one third of patients who undergo lumbar puncture (16). It should be remembered that aseptic meningitis will develop in a small number of patients (fever, headache, vomiting, nuchal rigidity) within 48 following IVIG infusion (17). Hydrops of the gallbladder may be present with or without obstructive jaundice. Diarrhea, vomiting, abdominal pain, cranial nerve palsies, tympanitis, and infarction of organs whose vascular supply are compromised by thrombosis may also be presenting symptoms.

CARDIAC INVOLVEMENT

Cardiac abnormalities are the major complication of Kawasaki syndrome and constitute the most serious complication of this disease (18). Myocarditis may develop during the first few days following onset of fever and is manifest by tachycardia out of proportion to fever elevation, conduction irregularities, a gallop rhythm, or electrocardiogram changes (19). Pericardial effusion may develop as a manifestation of carditis. Congestive heart failure may develop as a complication of myocardial dysfunction secondary to ischemia or infarct.

Coronary artery abnormalities occur in 20% to 25% of untreated patients. Dilatation of the coronary arteries can be detected by echocardiography soon after the onset of fever. Aneurysms of the coronary arteries may be demonstrable by echocardiography as soon as a few days after onset of illness, but more typically occur between 1 and 4 weeks of illness. Rarely patients experience aortic regurgitation or mitral regurgitation due to valvulitis, transient papillary muscle dysfunction, or myocardial infarction. Occasionally, aneurysm of the brachial, renal, or iliac arteries develops (20). This usually occurs in association with coronary artery abnormalities.

Factors associated with an increased risk for coronary artery involvement include male sex, age younger than 12 months, and prolonged signs of inflammation, such as fever lasting longer than 10 days. The major complication of aneurysms includes thrombosis and stenosis leading to myocardial infarction. Aneurysms greater than 8 mm in diameter (giant aneurysms) pose the greatest risk for myocardial infarction and sudden

TABLE 178.1.   Diagnostic Criteria for Kawasaki Syndrome

Fever for ≥5 days without other explanation, and at least four of the following five criteria:
  Non-exudative bulbar conjunctival injection
  Oropharyngeal changes, including injected or fissured lips, injected pharynx or strawberry tongue
  Extremity changes, including erythema of the palms or soles, edema of the hands or feet, or periungal desquamation
  Polymorphous rash
  Acute non-suppurative cervical lymphadenopathy
A diagnosis of atypical Kawasaki syndrome can be made when
  <4 criteria are present when coronary artery aneurysms are present.

death. Infarction most commonly occurs within 1 year after onset of disease. Approximately 50% of aneurysms regress within 1 year because of intimal proliferation as assessed by angiography. In those children with aneurysms that do not regress, long-term studies suggest that most will continue to show normal blood flow and normal myocardial function during stress testing.

During the acute stage, two-dimensional echocardiography should be performed as soon as possible in an appropriately sedated child to assess ventricular function, coronary artery structure, valvular function, and the presence of pericardial effusion. Follow-up echocardiography is generally performed 6 to 8 weeks later if the initial study shows no aneurysm formation and inflammation promptly subsides with treatment. The next echocardiogram should be performed 12 months later if the earlier studies remain normal. If the initial echocardiogram is abnormal, management involves therapy to reduce the risk for thrombosis, restrictions on physical activity, and consideration of cardiac catheterization. Such management should be conducted by a physician experienced in pediatric cardiology.

DIFFERENTIAL DIAGNOSIS

The clinical manifestations of Kawasaki syndrome are not specific for this disease and occur in a number of other infectious and rheumatologic diseases. Other diseases that may resemble Kawasaki syndrome (KS) are shown in Table 178.3.

A firm diagnosis of KS is often difficult because the symptoms of KS are not unique to this disease and because not all symptoms are seen in all patients. Because therapy within the first 10 days of onset of fever is clearly desirable in terms of reducing the risk for cardiac complications, rapid diagnosis and treatment are important. In many patients, differentiation of KS from other illnesses that resemble this syndrome may be difficult. When measles is common in the community, this diagnosis may be among the most difficult to exclude. Considerations that may eliminate measles from the differential diagnosis include local epidemiology, vaccination history, and culture results. Other viral illnesses that may enter the differential diagnosis include Epstein-Barr virus, adenovirus, and influenza virus infections. Nasal secretions should be cultured in a patient whose symptoms include evidence of an upper respiratory tract infection, especially to rule out adenovirus infection. Group A β-hemolytic streptococcus and *Staphylococcus aureus* infections may also mimic KS. Noninfectious diseases that frequently appear in the differential diagnosis include drug reactions and juvenile rheumatoid arthritis. Findings at physi-

cal examination that are not typical of KS include discrete intraoral ulcerations, exudative conjunctivitis, and generalized lymphadenopathy.

LABORATORY FINDINGS

Leukocytosis with a predominance of neutrophils and an increase in band counts develop in the first week of illness. A normocytic, normochromic anemia may also be present. Thrombocytosis is generally present by the end of the first week of illness. A mild elevation of liver transaminase levels is common usually with elevated bilirubin and alkaline phosphatase. Sterile pyuria due to urethritis occurs in approximately 75% of patients during the first week of illness. Early in the disease, acute phase reactants are elevated and remain high for 1 to 2 months.

Electrocardiographic changes include prolonged PR or QT intervals, ST segment depression, T wave changes, evidence of left ventricular hypertrophy, and ventricular arrhythmias. A baseline two-dimensional echocardiogram should be obtained at diagnosis. If the results are abnormal, a pediatric cardiology consultation and serial echocardiograms are indicated.

ATYPICAL KAWASAKI SYNDROME

KS is based on diagnostic criteria that use clinical signs and symptoms that overlap with other illnesses. This can result in diagnostic dilemmas, particularly in atypical cases that do not completely fulfill the diagnostic criteria but are associated with the development of coronary artery abnormalities. Reports of atypical KS have increased in recent years (21). In certain cases, the decision to treat with IVIG and aspirin can be a difficult diagnostic dilemma. The risk of coronary artery abnormalities increases in direct proportion to the interval between the onset of fever and administration of IVIG. Instances of atypical KS are most common in infants, the age group that is at greatest risk of coronary artery abnormalities. The decision to initiate therapy in children who do not satisfy the American Heart Association criteria can be supported by laboratory results showing acute phase reactants (elevated white blood cell count, elevated sedimentation rate), an ultrasound showing a pericardial effusion, or a slit lamp examination showing anterior uveitis.

ETIOLOGY

A number of epidemiologic and clinical observations suggest that KS is caused by an infectious agent. These include the geographic clustering of outbreaks often with a seasonal predominance and the acute self-limited nature of the illness. The fever and clinical findings (as defined by the six diagnostic criteria) overlap with well-defined bacterial toxin–mediated illnesses, including toxic shock syndrome and scarlet fever. The unique susceptibility of infants and young children to develop KS is consistent with the theory that illness is caused by a common, widely circulating infectious agent that induces immunity in most individuals before the beginning of the second decade of life. While the lack of demonstrable person to person transmission of KS is not typical of many infectious diseases, it may be that infection leads to an immune-mediated syndrome only in an immunologically susceptible host. The increased prevalence of KS in children of Japanese and Korean descent suggests that a genetic

---

TABLE 178.3. Differential Diagnosis of Kawasaki Syndrome

Measles
Scarlet fever
Drug reactions
Toxic shock syndrome
Staphylococcal scalded skin syndrome
Stevens-Johnson syndrome
Rocky Mountain spotted fever
Viral exanthems
Leptospirosis
Juvenile rheumatoid arthritis
Adenovirus infection
Epstein-Barr virus infection

TABLE 178.4. Immunologic Abnormalities Reported in Patients with Kawasaki Syndrome

Increase in acute phase reactants
Complement activation
Circulating immune complexes
Endothelial cell activation
    Expression of class II HLA proteins
    Expression of adhesion molecules
Endothelial tissue infiltration
    Activated CD4+ T cells
    Macrophages
    B cells
    IgA-producing B cells
T lymphocytes
    Depressed circulating CD8+ T cells
    Activated circulating CD4 cells
    Expansion/deletion V β2-restricted CD8+ T cells
    Increased CD45RO expression in CD8+ T cells
B lymphocytes
    Polyclonal activation
Increased cytokine production
    IFN-gamma, TNF-alpha
    IL-1, IL-2, IL-4, IL-6, IL-10
    Increased neopterin levels
    Increased soluble TNF receptor levels
Autoantibodies
    Antibody to cytokine-induced neoantigens on endothelial cells
    Anti-neutrophil cytoplasmic antibody
    Anticardiolipin
    IgM antibody to cardiac myosin

predisposition will be found, even though no consistent HLA association has been identified.

Despite more than 25 years of effort to identify an etiologic agent using serologic as well as standard and advanced culture techniques, no microbe has been consistently associated with this syndrome. In contrast to the difficulty in identifying an infectious agent, investigation into the immune status of children with KS has consistently revealed a profound degree of immunoregulatory abnormalities that are not characteristic of most other febrile exanthems of childhood (Table 178.4). This unusual degree of immune activation in patients with KS is a feature of disease caused by bacterial and viral protein toxins that act as superantigens, such as staphylococcal enterotoxins (toxic shock syndrome toxin, exfoliative toxin) and streptococcal pyrogenic exotoxins B and C (22).

Superantigens differ from conventional antigens in a number of important ways (23). Characteristics of an immune response induced by a superantigen include polyclonal B cell activation (in contrast to monoclonal activation), extensive proinflammatory cytokine production and changes in the number of circulating T lymphocytes which bear a specific surface receptor (specifically, Vβ-restricted T cells). Superantigens cause extensive T-cell proliferation and cytokine secretion after direct binding to major histocompatability complex (MHC) class II proteins that reside on the surface of an antigen-presenting cell. A traditional protein antigen elicits an immune response only after ingestion by an antigen-presenting cell. Peptides from that antigen are expressed on the surface of the cell within a specific antigen-binding groove formed by MHC class II molecules. Only a limited number of lymphocytes respond to a conventional, processed antigen, typically less than one cell per 10,000 lymphocytes. In contrast, superantigens bind to MHC class II molecules on the surface of the antigen presenting cell without ingestion and at a site outside the classical binding groove. The MHC-bound superantigen interacts with a T-cell receptor (TCR) by means of a variable

portion of the β chain. All T cells possessing a specific sequence on the TCR receptor (Vβ2+ T cells) will be activated by the MHC-superantigen complex and this may represent as many as 20% of circulating lymphocytes. The result is a release of unusually large amounts of cytokines from activated T cells (hence, the name superantigen). Cytokines then mediate the disease process.

One recognized hallmark of T-cell activation due to a toxin with superantigenic activity is an increase in the number of T cells expressing a specific T-cell receptor (TCR Vβ) region. The first of two early reports on TCR Vβ skewing in patients with KS was published in 1992 (24,25). Subsequently, three other laboratories reported similar findings (26–28), although some investigators have failed to detect these abnormalities (29,30).

Other observations support a toxin-mediated disease. The clinical features of KS are similar to those seen in patients with staphylococcal and streptococcal toxin (TSST)–mediated disease. Case reports describe children who were initially diagnosed with toxic shock syndrome and whose illness progressed to satisfy the clinical criteria of KS, including the development of coronary artery disease (31,32). These observations suggest a common pathophysiology for these two diseases and that TSST has the ability to cause both hypotension, and vasculitis and coronary artery aneurysms, depending on the clinical setting.

There is evidence that the effect of TSST on the immune response may be a function of toxin concentration (33). This provides one explanation why different clinical syndromes may be caused by the same toxin. Other factors may play a role in determining host response to TSST including: (a) location of site of infection by toxin-producing bacteria, which may influence the amount of toxin secreted based on pH, oxygen, and glucose concentration in the local environment; and (b) the age of the host.

In a controlled trial conducted in 1993, cultures from several anatomic sites were analyzed in a blinded fashion from 16 consecutive patients with Kawasaki syndrome and from 15 age matched febrile control patients (33). Superantigen producing bacteria were present in 13 of 16 patients with KS and only one of 15 febrile control patients ($P<.001$). Eleven of 13 superantigen positive culture results from patients with KS contained TSST-secreting *S. aureus* and two of 13 cultures contained streptococci producing streptococcal pyrogenic exotoxin B or C.

The following hypothesis has been proposed to explain the pathogenesis of this illness (34): a genetically susceptible host becomes colonized on the mucous membranes of the gastrointestinal tract by an organism which produces a toxin that behaves as a superantigen. Toxin is absorbed through the inflamed mucosal surface and stimulates local or circulating mononuclear cells to produce proinflammatory cytokines that in turn result in fever and the clinical picture of KS. In response to cytokine-induced stimulation, antigens are expressed on the surface of vascular endothelial cells, rendering them susceptible to attack by cytotoxic antibodies and activated T cells. Neoantigens on endothelial cells render the vessels more thrombogenic.

TREATMENT

Treatment of patients with KS is directed at reducing inflammation in the myocardium and coronary artery wall during the acute phase (12). Once the acute stage has passed, therapy is directed at prevention of coronary artery thrombosis. Aspirin (ASA) in combination with high dose IVIG forms the basis of current therapy (Table 178.5). ASA is used for both anti-inflammatory and antithrombotic actions, although convincing

TABLE 178.5.   Treatment of Kawasaki Syndrome

Acute phase
  IVIG 2 g/kg over 10–12 h
  Aspirin, 80–100 mg/kg/day in 4 divided doses until afebrile
Convalescent phase in patients with uncomplicated Kawasaki
    syndrome
  Aspirin 3–5 mg/kg/day once daily for 6–8 weeks
For patients with coronary artery disease
  Aspirin 3–5 mg/kg/day once daily
  Dipyridamole 1 mg/kg/day in selected patients
  Anticoagulant therapy as needed in patients with arterial thrombosis

data that ASA reduces coronary artery abnormalities are not available. ASA is administered at a dose of 80 to 100 mg/kg per day in four divided doses to achieve a serum salicylate level of 20-25 mg/dl during the acute phase of the illness (4–7). This is the only dose of ASA that has been carefully studied in the United States. Lower doses of ASA may have equal efficacy, but a minimum of 30 to 50 mg/kg per day in combination with IVIG should be used (36,37). Efficacy from IVIG therapy has only been demonstrated when administered within the first 10 days of illness. Patients who present beyond the 10th day of fever should still be treated with IVIG and ASA, although supporting data is not available. It is not clear whether different preparations of IVIG have similar efficacy in the prevention of coronary artery abnormalities. In afebrile children, the ASA dose is reduced to 3 to 5 mg/kg per day to continue antithrombosis activity. ASA is discontinued if no coronary abnormalities have been detected by 6 to 8 weeks after onset of the illness. ASA therapy is continued indefinitely if coronary artery aneurysms develop.

Several studies have demonstrated high-dose IVIG in combination with ASA therapy is safe and effective in reducing the prevalence of coronary artery abnormalities in KS (5,6). Rowley and associates demonstrated that IVIG and ASA not only reduce the overall prevalence of coronary artery abnormalities but also prevent the formation of giant aneurysms, the most serious form of coronary abnormality caused by KS (7). Newburger and associates have also found that abnormalities of left ventricular systolic function and contractility improve more rapidly in children treated in the acute phase with high dose IVIG together with ASA as compared with those treated with ASA alone (38).

At present, the treatment of choice for acute KS is a single dose of IVIG at 2 gm/kg administered over 10-12 hours in combination with ASA. Using this regimen, the prevalence of coronary artery abnormalities falls to less than 5%. Compared with multiple-dose regimens of approximately equivalent total dose, this single high dose of IVIG has been associates with a lower incidence of coronary abnormalities, more rapid resolution of fever and laboratory indices of acute inflammation, reduced duration of hospitalization and higher peak serum IgG levels. Peak adjusted serum globulin levels are lower among patients who subsequently develop coronary artery abnormalities and are inversely related to fever duration and laboratory indices of acute inflammation.

Other symptoms are treated symptomatically. Digitalis and diuretics are used as needed in the patient with congestive heart failure. In patients at risk of cardiovascular complications, some physicians add dipyridamole, 1 mg/kg of body weight per day to further inhibit platelet aggregation. Therapy of the mucocutaneous manifestations of the disease includes emollients for desquamation and antihistamines for pruritus.

All children diagnosed with KS should undergo two-dimensional echocardiography at the time of diagnosis. Repeat studies are recommended at 4 to 6 weeks and again at 6 to 12 months (12).

RETREATMENT

Approximately 5% to 10% of patients who receive IVIG have persistent fever 48 hours after completion of the infusion. Other patients may demonstrate initial defervescence but then experience recurrence of fever after being afebrile for 24 hours or more. Due to concern that persistent fever correlates with elevated levels of proinflammatory cytokines, which are associated with increased risk for the development of coronary artery abnormalities, retreatment with 2 g/kg of IVIG is often provided for both types of patients.

CORTICOSTEROID THERAPY

At present, the use of systemic steroids in the treatment of KS is controversial (39). Several studies from Japan have reported that patients treated with steroids alone or in combination with ASA have a higher frequency of coronary artery aneurysms and of subsequent myocardial infarction and death. Therefore, despite the use of corticosteroids in other forms of vasculitis, there has been a reluctance to use steroids in children with KS. A more recent uncontrolled study of 4 patients with KS resistant to repeat doses of IVIG suggested a response to high-dose pulse methylprednisolone (30 mg/kg per day for 1 to 3 days) therapy (40). In 1999, Shinohara reviewed the experience with prednisolone in children with KS (41). The authors concluded that prednisolone resulted in a shorter duration of fever and a lower prevalence of coronary artery aneurysms. However, this study was a retrospective review of patients who received different doses and different schedules of IVIG than what is currently used in the United States. Case reports of either oral or intravenous corticosteroid use in patients with unresponsive disease despite at least two adequate doses of IVIG suggest a possible role in the reduction in the acute inflammatory phase as well as control of the vasculitis (42). Before steroid use can be recommended for treatment of KS, both the efficacy and safety of steroid therapy should be evaluated in randomized, controlled trials.

MECHANISM OF ACTION OF INTRAVENOUS IMMUNE GLOBULIN

The mechanism by which high-dose IVIG works to reduce the vasculitis associated with KS is unknown. The observation that IVIG works rapidly in reducing the laboratory parameters of the acute phase response associated with KS suggests a generalized anti-inflammatory effect. In this regard, it has been reported that prior to IVIG therapy, peripheral blood mononuclear cells from patients with acute KS secrete high levels of IL-1, an endogenous pyrogen and tissue vascular endothelial cells express IL-1 inducible endothelial activation antigens. IL-1 secretion remained elevated in IVIG-treated patients in whom coronary artery abnormalities developed. However, IL-1 secretion levels fell to normal in-patients who responded to IVIG therapy. These data support the notion that IVIG may work in KS by reducing cytokine inducible endothelial activation.

Takei and associates have demonstrated that IVIG contains high concentrations of neutralizing antibodies that inhibit the

T cell response to staphylococcal superantigens (43). Using affinity absorption techniques, it was shown that this T-cell inhibiting effect was mediated by antitoxin-specific antibodies in IVIG. Thus, the beneficial effect of IVIG may be partially due to antibodies that inhibit bacterial toxin-induced stimulation of the immune response.

LONG-TERM MANAGEMENT

Patients in whom cardiovascular disease develops must be monitored closely (44). Stress echocardiography and coronary angiography may be indicated for patients with evidence of myocardial ischemia. For patients with obstructive changes in their coronary arteries, anticoagulation therapy may be required. For more severe cardiovascular symptoms, the options include intravenous streptokinase when a thrombus is present, balloon angioplasty, or coronary artery bypass grafting. Long-term patency of saphenous vein grafts has been a problem, but the use of internal mammary artery grafts has been reported to give improved results.

The major long-term morbidity in KS is related to cardiovascular complications. Approximately 50% of children with arterial aneurysms will show angiographic regression within 6 months to 2 years after onset of their disease. The likelihood of resolution of the aneurysm is determined by the initial size of the aneurysm, with smaller aneurysms having a greater likelihood of regression. Patients with giant aneurysms (diameter greater than 8 mm) have the worst prognosis. Nakano and associates have reported that 71% of patients with giant aneurysms progress to stenosis or obstruction over an 11-month follow-up period. Thirty percent of giant aneurysms develop obstruction at a mean follow-up of 32 months. Nearly all late deaths from KS occur in patients with this complication. Cardiac transplantation for patients with severe ischemic heart disease has been completed in a small number of patients.

Understanding the etiology of KS remains a major unresolved issue of pediatrics. It is important that the etiology of this illness be resolved so that a definitive test can be developed to identify children with typical KS as well as those who present with atypical disease and who do not satisfy the diagnostic criteria but are still at risk for coronary artery disease. In addition, it is unlikely that a more specific form of therapy than intravenous immune globulin will be found without understanding the etiology.

REFERENCES

1. Kawasaki T. Acute febrile mucocutaneous syndrome with lymphoid involvement with specific desquamation of the fingers and toes in children: clinical observations of 50 cases. *Jpn J Allergol* 1967;16:178–222.
2. Yanagawa H, Nakamura Y, Yashiro M, et al. A nationwide incidence survey of Kawasaki disease in 1985 1986 in Japan. *J Infect Dis* 1988;158:1296–1301.
3. Taubert K, Rowely A, Shulman S. A nationwide survey of Kawasaki disease and acute rheumatic fever. *J Pediatr* 1991;119:279–282.
4. Furusho K, Kamiya T, Nakano H, et al. High dose intravenous gammaglobulin for Kawasaki disease. *Lancet* 1984;2:1055–1058.
5. Newburger JW, Takahashi M, Burns JC, et al. The treatment of Kawasaki syndrome with intravenous gammaglobulin. *N Engl J Med* 1986:315:341–347.
6. Newburger JW, Takahashi M, Beiser AS, et al. A single intravenous infusion of gamma globulin as compared with four infusions in the treatment of acute Kawasaki syndrome. *N Engl J Med* 1991;324:1633–1639.
7. Rowley AH, Duffy CE, Shulman ST. Prevention of giant coronary artery aneurysms in Kawasaki disease by intravenous gamma globulin therapy. *J Pediatr* 1989;114:1065–1066.
8. Holman RC, Belay ED, Clarke MJ, Kaufman SF, Schonberger LB. Kawasaki syndrome among American Indian and Alaska native children, 1980 through 1995. *Pediatr Infect Dis J* 1999;18:451–455.
9. Stockbeim JA, Innocentini N, Shulman ST. Kawasaki disease in older children and adolescents. *J Pediatr* 2000;137:250–252.
10. Momenah T, Sanatani S, Potts J, Sandor GS, Human DG, Paterson MWH. Kawasaki disease in the older child. *Pediatrics* 1998;102:e7.
11. Rosenfield EA, Corydon KE, Shulman ST. Kawasaki disease in infants less than one year of age. *J Pediatr* 1995;126:524–529.
12. Dajani AS, Taubert KA, Gerber MA, et al. Diagnosis and therapy of Kawasaki disease in children. *Circulation* 1993;87:1776–1780.
13. Friter BS, Lucky AW. The perineal eruption of Kawasaki syndrome. *Arch Dermatol* 1988;124:1805–1810.
14. Burns JC, Joffe L, Sargent RA, Glode MP. Anterior uveitis associated with Kawasaki syndrome. *Pediatr Infect Dis* 1985;4:258–261.
15. Hicks RV, Melish ME. Kawasaki disease. *Pediatr Clin North Am* 1986;33:1151–1175.
16. Dengler LD, Capparelli EV, Bastian JF, et al. CSF profile in Kawasaki disease. *Pediatr Infect Dis J* 1998;17:478–481.
17. Boyce TG, Spearman P. Acute aseptic meningitis in a patient with Kawasaki syndrome. *Pediatr Infect Dis J* 1998;17:1054–1056.
18. Kato H, Ichinose E, Kawasaki Y. Myocardial infarction in Kawasaki disease: clinical analyses in 195 cases. *J Pediatr* 1986;108:923–927.
19. Yutani C, Okano K, Kamiya T, et al. Histopathological study on right endomyocardial biopsy of Kawasaki disease. *Br Heart J* 1980;43:589–592.
20. Fukushige J, Nihill MR, McNamara DG. Spectrum of cardiovascular lesions in mucocutaneous lymph node syndrome: analysis of eight cases. *Am J Cardiol* 1980;45:98–107.
21. Witt MD, Minich L, Bohnsack JF, Young PC. Kawasaki disease: more patients are being diagnosed who do not meet America Heart Association criteria. *Pediatrics* 1999;104:e10.
22. Meissner HC, Leung DYM. Superantigen, conventional antigens and the etiology of Kawasaki syndrome. *Pediatr Infect Dis J* 2000;19:91–94.
23. Kotb M. Bacterial pynogenic exotoxins as superantigens. *Clin Microbiol Rev* 1995;8:411–426.
24. Abe J, Kotzin BL, Jujo K, et al. Selective expansion of T cells expressing T-cell receptor variable regions VB2 and VB8 in Kawasaki disease. *Proc Natl Acad Sci* 1992;89:4066–4070.
25. Abe J, Kotzin BL, Meissner C, et al. Characterization of T cell repertoire changes in acute Kawasaki disease. *J Exp Med* 1993;177:791–796.
26. Curtis N, Zheng R, Lamb JR, Levin M. Evidence for a superantigen mediated process in Kawasaki disease. *Arch Dis Child* 1995;72:308–311.
27. Yamashiro Y, Nagata S, Oguchi S, Shimizu T. Selective increase of VB2 T cells in the small intestine mucosa in Kawasaki disease. *Pediatr Res* 1996;39:264–266.
28. Yoshioka T, Matsutani T, Iwagami S, et al. Polyclinic expansion of TCRBV2- and TCRBV6- bearing T cells in patients with Kawasaki disease. *Immunology* 1999;96;465–472.
29. Pietra BA, De Inocencio J, Giannini EH, Hirsch R. T cell receptor VB family repertoire and T cell activation markers in Kawasaki disease. *J Immunol* 1994;153;1881–1888.
30. Barron KS, Shulman ST, Rowley A, et al. Report of the National Institute of Health on Kawasaki disease. *J Rheumatol* 1999;26:170–190.
31. Wiesenthal AM, Todd JK. Toxic shock syndrome in children aged 10 years or less. *Pediatrics* 1984;74:112–117.
32. Davies HD, Kirk V, Jadavji T, Kotzin BL. Simultaneous presentation of Kawasaki disease and toxic syndrome in an adolescent male. *Pediatr Infect Dis J* 1996;155:1136–1137.
33. Hofer MF, Newell K, Duke RC, Schlievert PM, Freed JH, Leung DY. Differential effects of staphylococcal toxic syndrome toxin-1 on B cell apoptosis. *Proc Nat Acad Sci* 1996;93:5425–5430.
34. Leung DYM, Meissner HC, Fulton DR, Murray DL, Kotzin BL, Schlievert PM. Toxic shock syndrome toxin-secreting *Staphylococcus aureus* in Kawasaki syndrome. *Lancet* 1993;342:1385–1387.
35. Meissner HC, Schlievert PM, Leung DYM. Mechanisms of immunoglobulin action: observation on Kawasaki syndrome and RSV prophylaxis. *Immun Rev* 1994;139:109–123.
36. Terai M, Shulman ST. Prevalence of coronary artery abnormalities in Kawasaki disease is highly dependent on gamma globulin dose but independent of salicylate dose. *J Pediatr* 1997;131:888–893.
37. Durongpisitkul K, Gururaj VJ, Park JM, Martin CF. Prevention of coronary artery aneurysms in Kawasaki disease: a meta-analysis on the efficacy of aspirin and immunoglobulin treatment. *Pediatrics* 1995;96:1057–1061.
38. Newbuger JW, Sanders SP, Burns JC, Parness IA, Beiser AS, Colan SD. Left ventricular and function in Kawasaki syndrome: effect of intravenous gamma-globulin. *Circulation* 1989;79:1237–1246.
39. Newburger JW. Treatment of Kawasaki disease: corticosteroids revisited. *J Pediatr* 1999;135:411–413.
40. Wright DA, Newburger JW, Baker A, Sundel RP. Treatment of immune globulin-resistant Kawasaki disease with pulsed doses of corticosteroids. *J Pediatr* 1996;128:146–149.
41. Shinohara M, Sone K Tomomasa T, Morikawa A, Corticosteroids in the treatment of the acute phase of Kawasaki disease. *J Pediatr* 1999;135:465–469.
42. Dale R, Saleem MA, Daw S, Dillon MJ. Treatment of severe complicated Kawasaki disease with oral prednisolone and aspirin. *J Pediatr* 2000;137:723–726.
43. Takei S, Arora YK, Walker SM. Intravenous immunoglobulin contains specific antibodies inhibitory to activation of T cells by staphylococcal toxin superantigens. *J Clin Invest* 1993;91:602–607.
44. Dajani AS, Taubert KA, Takahashi M, et al. Guidelines for long-term management of patients with Kawasaki disease. *Circulation* 1994;89:916–922.

Other Infections

CHAPTER 179
Infections in a Prosthetic Device

Adolf W. Karchmer

Insertion of prosthetic devices to provide relief for an increasing array of symptoms is a major advance in medical therapeutics, but this treatment has created diseases of medical progress—infections of prosthetic devices (Table 179.1). Although infection is a rare complication with devices that are completely implanted, it is not unusual for those devices that traverse a cutaneous or mucosal surface. Nevertheless, infections of both partially and fully implanted devices produce major morbidity, mortality, and expense.

Prosthetic devices are always vulnerable to infection. Whenever a patient with a prosthesis presents with systemic symptoms or signs of infection, evidence of prosthesis dysfunction, or periprosthesis inflammation, the possibility of an infected device must be entertained. When a prosthesis is found to be infected, the clinical importance of both the infection and the device must be considered. The patient's life may be threatened acutely by systemic infection or prosthesis dysfunction or conversely merely inconvenienced by the potential loss of a cosmetic device or the need for antimicrobial therapy. Formulating a diagnostic and therapeutic plan for an infected prosthesis requires an understanding of the pathogenesis of infection of the specific device and of foreign bodies in general, as well as the pathologic physiology that arises with a dysfunctional device. The infecting organism must be recovered so that appropriate antimicrobial therapy can be selected. The limitations of host defenses and antimicrobial therapy in eradicating infection associated with foreign material must be understood. In addition, detailed knowledge of prior experience treating infections of the device must be considered, particularly those caused by the specific pathogen. In selecting therapy, the morbidity and mortality risks of the treatment required to eradicate infection, to salvage or replace the device, and to correct infection-induced pathologic physiology must be balanced against the hazards of the infection itself, the role of the device, and the alternatives to the device. The device may be essential for life (prosthetic heart valve), essential for life but with convenient alternatives (hemodialysis shunt), necessary for important activities (prosthetic hip joint), an aid in performing nonessential activities (penile prosthesis), or primarily cosmetic (breast prosthesis). Thus, salvaging, replacing, and eliminating the device are fundamental considerations in designing therapy.

PATHOGENESIS

The introduction of foreign material into the complex interaction between a microorganism and the host and its defenses increases the likelihood of infection. Elek and Conen (1) demonstrated that the minimal number of staphylococci required to induce infection could be reduced from 10^6 to 10^2 by the presence of a braided silk suture. Foreign material not only enhances the pathogenic-

ity of known virulent microorganisms by reducing the inoculum necessary to initiate infection but also allows organisms that are typically not pathogenic to establish infection. The latter is illustrated by the striking frequency with which usually avirulent *Staphylococcus epidermidis* cause prosthetic device infection. Foreign material was required in order for subcutaneously injected *S. epidermidis* or *Staphylococcus aureus* Wood 46 strain to cause infection in mice and guinea pigs (2,3). The pathogenetic interactions between host, organism and foreign material that culminate in an infection uniquely resistant to treatment will be considered briefly; detailed reviews can be found elsewhere (4–8).

Adherence of an organism to a device and its proliferation to a microcolony is the initial step in establishing an infection. Physiochemical interactions between the device and the microorganism promote adherence, but studies suggest that species-specific selective binding also occurs. These specific mechanisms have been best elucidated for *S. aureus* and *S. epidermidis*, the dominant pathogens in foreign device infection (4,6,8). Host proteins, including fibrinogen, its derivative fibrin, and fibronectin, promptly and progressively coat implanted foreign materials. Complex dynamic interactions occur between specific bacterial surface adhesins and foreign body–bound receptors derived from host proteins, glycoproteins, and cellular elements (6,8).

The adhesins expressed on the surface of *S. aureus*, given the acronym MSCRAMMs (microbial surface components recognizing adhesive matrix molecules), the genes encoding them, and the molecular basis of adherence to host proteins coating foreign bodies have been studied extensively (5,6). The major surface exposed adhesins, which are covalently linked to cell wall peptidoglycan, include two fibrinogen-binding proteins called ClFA (called clumping factor) and ClFB, fibronectin binding proteins A (FnbA) and B (FnbB), and a collagen adhensin (Cna) (5). *In vitro* exposure of various foreign materials to plasma, serum, or albumin inhibits the binding of staphylococci. This inhibition is overcome by *in vivo* exposure of devices to host proteins and cellular elements. Studies of polymethylmethacrylate (PMMA) and titanium plates implanted subcutaneously or fixed to iliac bone, respectively, for 4 to 6 weeks demonstrate progressive coating with cellular and connective tissue components, including fibronectin, and that fibronectin-binding adhesins of *S. aureus* specifically mediate the adherence of the organism to these explanted plates even in the presence of serum or albumin (6). The fibrinogen-binding protein (clumping factor) mediates the attachment *ex vivo* of *S. aureus* to polyvinyl chloride tubing exposed briefly to blood, indicating the major role of fibrinogen, and platelet-fibrin aggregates in promoting organism adhesion to foreign material after initial interaction with blood (9). In contrast, studies of long-term intravenous catheters removed from patients reveal that, over time, fibrinogen-fibrin on catheters are degraded by plasmin and no longer facilitate the adherence of *S. aureus* but that residual fibronectin determines adhesion (10). Thus, different MSCRAMMs interacting with specific but variable and time-dependent host proteins adherent to foreign devices facilitate *S. aureus* attachment and thereby device infection.

S. epidermidis and other coagulase-negative staphylococci express a more limited array of surface adhesins and react with host proteins less avidly than do *S. aureus* (4). Coagulase negative staphylococci adhere to fibronectin, but not fibrinogen, bound *in vitro* to PMMA or *in vivo* to chronic intravenous catheters removed from patients (6). An autolysin designated ahe, encoded by *ahe* gene, facilitates adherence to vitronectin-coated polystyrene (4). However, it appears that *S.epidermidis* initial adherence to polymers depends on a hydrophobic interaction with the surface and is impaired by plasma proteins which render surfaces hydrophilic (4,8). The extracellular substance associated

TABLE 179.1.   Infections of Prosthetic Devices

Device	Prevalence of infection	Common pathogens	Major syndromes
Heart valve	3% at 1 y 4%–6% at 4–5 y	*Staphylococcus epidermidis* *Staphylococcus aureus* Streptococci	Endocarditis
Joints	Hip 0.5%–1.3% Knee 1.3%–2.9%	*S. aureus* *S. epidermidis*	Indolent, progressively painful joint; acute septic arthritis
Transvenous permanent Pacemaker	Pocket sepsis 1%–7% Lead only <1%	*S. aureus* *S. epidermidis*	Localized pocket infection, bacteremia (infected intravascular wire)
Arterial graft	Aortoiliac <1%–1.5% Femoropopliteal 2%–7%	*S. aureus* *S. epidermidis*	Bacteremia, false aneurysm, occlusion, anastomotic rupture
Intraocular lens	<1%	*S. epidermidis* *S. aureus*	Endophthalmitis
CSF shunt	1.5%–15%	*S. epidermidis* *S. aureus*	Ventriculitis, meningitis, hydrocephalus, bacteremia
CAPD catheter	60% first year; 0.5–1.0 episodes/patient/y	*S. epidermidis* *S. aureus* Streptococci	Mild peritonitis; catheter track wound infection
Breast implant	Augmentation 2%–3% Reconstruction >3%	*S. aureus* *S. epidermidis*	Wound infection
Penile prosthesis	1%–5%	*S. epidermidis* Enterobacteriaceae	Indolent or purulent wound infection

CSF, cerebrospinal fluid; CAPD, continuous ambulatory peritoneal dialysis.

with *S. epidermidis*, called glycocalyx or slime, does not appear to be associated with initial adherence and forms only after attachment (4,8).

The chemical composition of slime is not fully established. A variety of substances have been identified in slime from *S. epidermidis*; these include slime-associated antigen (SAA), capsular polysaccharide adhesin (PS/A), and most recently a polysaccharide involved in intercellular adhesion, termed polysaccharide intercellular adhesin (PIA). It is likely that these are the same or closely related and under the control of *ica* operon (*icaR* [regulatory gene] and *ica ADBC* [biosynthesis] genes). PIA appears important in the colonization of foreign devices by coagulase-negative staphylococci and necessary to develop the multilayer, organism-embedded slime matrix or biofilm (4,8). In addition to being essential in the biofilm, slime has been found to decrease phagocytic activity of macrophages and to prompt degranulation and impair intracellular killing by polymorphonuclear neutrophils (PMN) (8). It thus facilitates foreign body infection. Accordingly, slime or glycocalyx has been significantly associated with those coagulase-negative staphylococci, particularly *S. epidermidis*, that infect foreign bodies (11–16).

Foreign body infection is difficult to eradicate without removing the foreign material. This difficulty results, in part, from impairment of host defenses in the immediate environment of the foreign body. The opsonizing capability of fluid surrounding foreign materials is reduced relative to that of serum and deteriorates further during local infection as the C3 component of complement is degraded by PMN elaborated elastase. Nevertheless, preopsonizing *S. aureus* organisms before inoculating them into an implanted foreign body fails to prevent infection. Thus, although reduced opsonization may contribute to the pathogenesis of foreign body infection, the opsonization defect is not the dominant abnormality (6).

The bactericidal capacity of PMNs that have been in contact with foreign materials is significantly weaker than that of PMNs from acute and chronic inflammatory exudates and from peripheral blood (6). This abnormality is associated with defective oxygen-dependent PMN killing mechanisms, deficient PMN superoxide production, and evidence of prior degranulation by the defective PMNs (17). Defective PMNs appear to play an im-

portant role in the initiation of foreign body infection by small inocula of bacteria and also likely contribute to the persistence of these infections. Functional PMNs infused locally before or shortly after a bacterial challenge prevent infection of a subcutaneously implanted foreign body (17).

Other host-parasite-foreign body interactions also make eradication of these infections difficult. For example, the ability of fully effective PMNs to phagocytose and kill *S. aureus* organisms that are adherent to polymethylmethacrylate is reduced (18). Alterations in the production of cytokines, for example, tumor necrosis factor, in the immediate vicinity of foreign devices may impair PMN bactericidal activity (19). Resistance to the bactericidal action of many antibiotics by organisms adherent to foreign devices reduces the efficacy of therapy. Bacteria recovered from infected foreign bodies and from glycocalyx biofilms and those adherent to foreign materials are less susceptible to killing by selected antibiotics when studied immediately after recovery from the foreign material than are the same strains grown in a planktonic fashion (20–22). This resistance to killing, a phenotypic tolerance, is demonstrable *in vivo* and *in vitro* and differs from *in vitro* antibiotic resistance or tolerance, which are constant inherited properties. This tolerance correlates with slow-growth or stationary-growth phase, is unstable, and is reversible after incubation as planktonic organisms in antibiotic-free growth medium (4,6,7).

The clinical events that lead to infection of a prosthesis are powerful determinants of the time of clinical onset and microbial etiology of infection. Intraoperative or perioperative contamination, which accounts for a large portion of infections involving fully implanted devices, results in infections clustered in the initial months after surgery. Often these are indolent infections caused by coagulase-negative staphylococci or other components of normal skin flora. Foreign body infections that present within the early weeks after surgery as typical wound infections are caused by more virulent bacteria. In a review of 205 vascular graft infections, early infections were often caused by *S. aureus* and occurred in association with inguinal wound infection (23).

Small epidemics result from contamination of the devices or materials used during surgery. In these epidemics, the infections share clinical and epidemiologic features, a pathogen, and cluster in time according to the virulence of the contaminating microorganism. Occasionally, an infection resulting from perioperative contamination of a prosthesis by avirulent organisms remains asymptomatic for many months. This sequence has been postulated for coagulase-negative staphylococcal and other bacterial infections of prosthetic heart valves (24,25), joint replacements (26–28), and synthetic vascular grafts (29). Usually, infection beginning 1 year or more after surgery results from proximate seeding of a device. This seeding may occur hematogenously, by extension of adjacent infection to the device, or by erosion of the device into a contaminated area as seen with the development of an aortoenteric fistula or erosion of a pacemaker generator through the skin. The virulence of the causative organism determines the toxicity associated with these late-onset infections. Toxicity can range from the subacute presentations of viridans streptococcal prosthetic valve endocarditis (PVE) (30) to highly febrile presentations of acute septic arthritis involving a joint prosthesis (26,31). Devices placed transcutaneously and manipulated regularly (e.g., Tenckhoff peritoneal dialysis catheters) are infected repeatedly by organisms that are part of the patient's flora (32). In addition, contamination of medical materials or machines used with a device can lead to epidemic infection.

CLINICAL MANIFESTATIONS

The diversity of clinical presentations among patients with infected prosthetic devices exceeds that attributable to the spectrum of devices in use. Typical clinical syndromes seen in the absence of implanted devices are associated with infection involving some prostheses (e.g., acute or subacute endocarditis with prosthetic valve infection (30,33), and endophthalmitis with infection of an intraocular lens implant (34). Infections in a given prosthesis may present variably. Signs and symptoms may be localized, systemic, or both and may range in severity from dramatic to minimal. These extremes are contingent in part on the location of the device—depth of implantation, surrounding tissue or space, intravascular position—and on the pathogen. For example, infection involving a total hip prosthesis may manifest as an early postoperative wound infection with local and systemic symptoms, postoperative pain on weight bearing without local or systemic signs of infection beginning months after surgery, or an acute septic arthritis with marked systemic toxicity and local pain. Infection of cerebrospinal fluid (CSF) shunts developing shortly after surgery may present as fever and inflammation along the subcutaneous path of the shunt (35). Less than one third of patients with CSF shunt infections have clinical features characteristic of meningitis (35). Patients with infected ventriculoperitoneal CSF shunts may present primarily with abdominal pain, tenderness, peritonitis, or occasionally a loculated collection of infected cerebrospinal fluid that is palpable and detectable by ultrasound (35).

The predominant signs provoked by prosthesis infection are not always those of inflammation. Instead, they may reflect physiologic alterations caused by prosthesis dysfunction or the immune consequences of chronic infection. These symptoms can be dramatic, masking those of inflammation, or can be subtle and indolent. Patients with PVE with minimal symptoms of infection may present with severe congestive heart failure caused by acute aortic valve regurgitation or with neurologic symptoms resulting from a massive cerebrovascular event.

Symptoms and signs of increased intracranial pressure may indicate CSF shunt dysfunction due to infection (35). With infection of a ventriculoatrial CSF shunt with immune complex–induced vasculitis and glomerulonephritis, presenting manifestations may be palpable purpuric skin lesions and azotemia with proteinuria and hematuria (36–38). Infection involving a synthetic vascular graft may present with signs of local incisional infection or septicemia, or with graft dysfunction, including occlusion, hemorrhage, or formation of a false aneurysm. Infection of the artery-graft anastomosis eventually produces suture line breakdown. When this occurs at the aorta-graft anastomosis, the presentations include a painful abdominal mass, hydronephrosis due to ureteral compression, or low-grade fever and intermittent gastrointestinal tract bleeding due to an aortoenteric fistula (29,39). If the diagnosis of aortoenteric fistula is not made promptly, there may be brisk gastrointestinal bleeding as the false aneurysm ruptures into the bowel lumen (29,39).

MICROBIOLOGY

An awareness of the unusually broad array and variable virulence of microorganisms that infect prosthetic devices is important in approaching the patient with a possibly infected prosthesis. It is crucial, however, to realize that staphylococci are the predominant cause of these infections (see Table 179.1). The microbiology of device infections is the consequence of interrelated circumstances: (a) the presence of the foreign body; (b) the placement of the device entirely within the body or across a skin or mucosal surface; (c) the anatomic location of the prosthesis; and (d) the clinical events leading to contamination. The clinical circumstances that lead to an infection are often a strong predictor of the infecting microorganism. Placement of a foreign body across an external surface affords microorganisms continuous access along the insertion route to the implanted portion. Similarly, repeated manipulation of a totally implanted device affords increased opportunity for direct seeding. Until it is covered with a pseudoendothelium, a prosthesis implanted in the circulatory system is vulnerable to organisms in the blood. Unless there is a major break in sterile technique, perioperative contamination of a prosthesis favors infection with skin flora, particularly *S. aureus* and coagulase-negative staphylococci, and occasionally streptococci and diphtheroids. The prominent role of *S. aureus* and coagulase-negative staphylococci, which are usually *S. epidermidis*, is more than a chance occurrence; it reflects, in addition to the likelihood that these organisms contaminate wounds by virtue of their presence on the skin, biologic properties that facilitate their adherence to and proliferation on foreign materials. The result of perioperative contamination is reflected in the microbiology of PVE that occurs within the year after valve surgery (30,33), in early and delayed-onset prosthetic joint infections (26), in CSF shunt infections (35), and in infections of intraocular lenses (34) and prosthetic arterial grafts (23,29). Transient bacteremia is the predominant clinical event that leads to both non-nosocomial, non-addict associated native valve endocarditis and to PVE with onset 1 year or more after surgery; consequently, the microbiology of these two forms of endocarditis is similar (30,33). The location of a prosthesis renders it vulnerable to invasion by microorganisms that are normally resident in the contiguous areas. Thus, transmural spread of enteric bacteria from the bowel causes peritoneal dialysis–associated peritonitis (32), and gram-negative bacteria, as part of perineal skin flora are important causes of infection of penile prostheses (40,41). Peripheral infections give rise to bacteremia that seeds prosthetic devices; thus, the presence of a distant infection provides an important clue to the organism causing device infection. *S. aureus*, β-hemolytic streptococci, or enteric gram-negative bacilli have spread via the blood from skin or urinary tract infection to well-established, functioning prosthetic joints (26,42). In contrast, the unanticipated discovery of bacteremia due to an avirulent organism (e.g., *S. epidermidis*, diphtheroids) should prompt consideration of infection of an intravascular device such as a prosthetic valve, vascular graft, ventriculoatrial CSF shunt, or transvenous pacemaker (25,33,36–38).

DIAGNOSIS

A prosthesis exposed in the base of an unhealed surgical wound or at the end of a sinus track is obviously infected. Typically, however, the impetus to pursue potential device infection hinges on recognizing subtle findings. Prosthesis dysfunction, particularly as a new development or one that progresses over a brief interval, may be an important clue to infection. Occasionally the inflammatory process is subclinical or minimal and the dysfunction itself is the major manifestation of infection. Mild local inflammation adjacent to a device, although appearing more consistent with a sterile reaction to the foreign body, may be indicative of infection.

Ultimately, the diagnosis of device infection hinges on demonstrating microorganisms on the prosthesis or in the area immediately surrounding it. Documentation of local inflammation and infection is difficult. Leukocytosis and an accelerated erythrocyte sedimentation rate are rarely noted, but even when they are, at best they are nonspecific. The discriminatory capacity of radiography, nuclear imaging, and sonography is often reduced by the presence of implanted devices. Frequently these modalities cannot distinguish between changes produced by infection and those induced by the disease that necessitated placement of the prosthesis, by local tissue reaction to the prosthesis itself, or by the implant insertion procedure. For example, when persistent hip pain develops 6 months after insertion of a joint prosthesis, none of these signs—lucency at the bone-cement interface, periosteal reaction on radiographs, uptake of technetium-99m diphosphonate–labeled or gallium-111–labeled PMNs—is specific enough to distinguish between changes related to recent surgery, infection, or aseptic loosening (the major alternative diagnosis to low-grade infection) (26,31). The capability of other modalities may also be limited; device-induced artifacts in computed tomography and magnetic resonance imaging and prominent reflective properties in sonography compromise their utility, although with careful interpretation of results in the context of the clinical problem, selected noninvasive studies can provide important information even if they are not diagnostic. Echocardiography, with Doppler, particularly using a transesophageal approach, may detect perivalvular abscess formation, fistulae, or transvalvular pressure gradients indicative of prosthetic valve dysfunction, which in the context of fever, bacteremia, or clinical signs of endocarditis is highly suggestive of PVE (43). Similarly, even if ultrasonography, computed tomography, magnetic resonance imaging, and arteriography cannot provide direct evidence of inflammation or infection, they may disclose a false aneurysm arising at the artery-graft anastomosis, perigraft air or fluid collection, or graft occlusion (29). Negative findings may be of importance also; no increase in uptake of technetium-99m around a joint prosthesis argues against local infection. Failure to demonstrate dysfunction or local inflammation of a prosthesis does not always rule out infection. For example, radionuclide scans are not sufficiently sensitive to eliminate the possible diagnosis of vascular graft infection (29).

If infection is suspected, it is necessary to attempt to recover microorganisms from the device or adjacent tissues before initiating antibiotic therapy, even if treatment is delayed briefly. Empirical antimicrobial therapy is rarely justifiable before optimal cultures are obtained. With devices that are intravascular (at least in part), such as prosthetic heart valves, transvenous

cardiac pacers, synthetic arterial grafts, and ventriculoatrial CSF shunts, repeated isolation of an organism from blood establishes the pathogen. If blood cultures fail to demonstrate the organism and an extravascular or partially extravascular device is in place, material for culture must be obtained, where feasible, by direct aspiration of fluid in or adjacent to the device. For example, aspiration of the intraarticular space, the pacemaker generator pocket, the subcutaneous space adjacent to a CSF shunt, or the CSF shunt valve reservoir may be necessary. Scrupulous sterile technique must be used to avoid contaminating the device and the aspirated material.

Even with diligent efforts it may be difficult to recover organisms from an infected device or to conclude that an isolated organism is responsible for an infection. The density of organisms at the site of infection may be low, which would reduce the sensitivity of cultures, especially when the inoculum is small. In addition, organisms infecting prosthetic devices may be fastidious and difficult to recover. Anticipating these problems and using generous inocula, multiple media, and in selected situations, special culture techniques to recover anaerobic bacteria, fungi, mycobacteria, *Legionella* species, or mycoplasmas enhance the yield of cultures. Foreign body infection characterized by organisms embedded in surface biofilms may be difficult to document microbiologically. The recovery of organisms in cultures, especially coagulase-negative staphylococci, is increased by culturing a fragment of the device and its attached biofilm. Similarly, organisms can be recovered from surface biofilms that have been mechanically disrupted by ultrasonic oscillations or grinding tissue (29).

Concluding that an isolate is the cause of infection and not a contaminant can be challenging. This quandary arises because organisms that are usually dismissed as contaminants, such as coagulase-negative staphylococci, a-hemolytic streptococci, and diphtheroids, often cause these infections. Such organisms are implicated when they are present in large numbers. If material is cultured promptly, recovering the organism in at least moderate amounts on one or more solid media, rather than only in broth media, indicates that large numbers of organisms are present. In addition, when inflammatory cells and the organism are seen at microscopic examination of the specimen, or when identical organisms are recovered from, multiple independently obtained specimens, from sequential aspirates or from preoperative and intraoperative specimens, it is likely that the organism is the pathogen (31,44). Organisms commonly viewed as contaminants must not be disregarded when they are recovered from a prosthetic device. When the significance of an organism is not clear, efforts to recover it from additional specimens are warranted. Determining that coagulase-negative staphylococci isolated sporadically from a device are identical increases the likelihood that the unique organism is causing the infection.

Because most coagulase-negative staphylococci isolated are *S. epidermidis* and possess similar antibiotic susceptibility profiles, special tests such as molecular finger printing with pulse field gel electrophoresis are required to establish the uniqueness of isolates from sequential cultures (24,45). Thus, determining that an organism isolated from a foreign body is causing infection may require semiquantitative assessment of specimens, repeated cultures, or special tests to establish the uniqueness of a sporadically isolated organism.

DIFFERENTIAL DIAGNOSIS

The presence of fever or of signs and symptoms of inflammation in the patient with an indwelling medical device invariably raises the possibility that the device is infected. In seeking an explanation for these signs and symptoms, the temporal relationship of the febrile episode to the insertion of the device helps to focus the investigation, as do symptoms suggestive of a remote infection. Shortly after surgery, the usual causes of early postoperative fever, including infections and noninfectious entities, are sought. In addition, during the early postoperative period, causes of fever that are peculiar to the specific device must be considered. For example, fever after prosthetic valve placement may be due to the postpericardiotomy syndrome, and that after neurosurgery that included placement of a CSF shunt may be due to surgically induced aseptic meningitis. When surgical placement of the prosthesis is more distant, the number of possible explanations is greatly increased; in the evaluation of fever of unclear origin a device infection is simply one consideration. If there is inflammation around a recently inserted device but no fever, infection must still be excluded; however, alternative causes, including reactions to the trauma of surgery, to the device itself, and materials used in the insertion, and hematoma must be considered also. Inflammation of the eye after cataract extraction and intraocular lens implantation results from infection, surgical trauma, toxicity due to residual polishing compounds or sterilizing agents on the lens implant, or allergic reactions to crystalline lens cortical remnants (34).

Prosthesis dysfunction, a possible clue to infection, may also result from noninfectious problems. Technical problems can account for persistently elevated intracranial pressure after placement of a CSF shunt or a murmur of valvular incompetence after insertion of a prosthetic heart valve. Interactions between the device and surrounding tissues can result in the late appearance of prosthesis dysfunction. For example, aseptic loosening of the femoral component of a total hip replacement causes late onset of pain on weight bearing. Inflammatory signs and symptoms in the area of the prosthesis can be caused by unrelated diseases that coincidentally involve that anatomic region. Distinguishing a ventriculoperitoneal CSF shunt infection from acute appendicitis may be difficult. Similarly, diverticulitis, cholecystitis, and the many other causes of abdominal pain must be considered in the differential diagnosis of abdominal pain or peritonitis in patients undergoing continuous ambulatory peritoneal dialysis (CAPD).

TREATMENT

Effective treatment of an infected prosthesis must achieve two objectives: eradication of the infection and maintenance of a functioning device or provision of a functional alternative. Failure to achieve both objectives is less than optimal. The clinical dictum that an infected device must be removed to eliminate infection is inaccurate and oversimplified. Some foreign body infections can be eradicated with aggressive antimicrobial therapy. Furthermore, the ultimate goal of eradicating infection and maintaining function, while limiting the risks of therapy itself, is not always best served by removing the prosthesis.

The fundamentals of effective antimicrobial therapy include identifying the infecting organism or organisms and their antimicrobial susceptibility profiles, designing a bactericidal antimicrobial regimen with minimal toxicity, and administering the antimicrobial so as to produce an adequate concentration at the site of infection. The bactericidal activity of antibiotics against stationary-phase organisms and those that are adherent to foreign material correlates directly with the eradication of infection involving foreign bodies (46). Rifampin possesses this type of bactericidal activity against susceptible staphylococci. Furthermore, when used in combination with one or two additional antibiotics to prevent the emergence of rifampin resistance

during therapy, treatment with rifampin-containing regimens eradicated infections caused by *S. epidermidis* and *S. aureus* in animal models without removing the foreign body (46–48). These studies suggest a specific important role for rifampin in combination therapy for foreign body infection. Also, combination antibiotic therapy may be necessary to achieve bactericidal activity, to provide a synergistic or enhanced bactericidal effect, or to broaden the spectrum of antimicrobial activity when treating a polymicrobial infection. The duration and route of antibiotic administration are based on experience with analogous infections. Prolonged courses of intravenous antibiotics are used for PVE and infected orthopedic devices; more abbreviated courses are used for peritonitis complicating CAPD and soft tissue infections that persist after a device has been removed. Direct instillation of antibiotics at the infection site is used to treat selected infections, e.g. CAPD-associated peritonitis. Because systemically administered antibiotics penetrate the anterior and posterior chambers of the eye poorly, infected intraocular lens replacements are treated by local injections of antibiotics (34). Although the benefit has not been clearly documented, local treatment with antibiotic-impregnated cement has been used in conjunction with systemic antibiotics in the replacement of an infected orthopedic prosthesis with a new device (26,49). Occasionally, device-related infection that is totally confined to a closed body space (e.g., peritonitis associated with CAPD) can be treated solely by instillation of antimicrobials directly into the infected area (32).

The essential considerations in deciding whether an infection can be successfully treated without removing the device are the initial and continued functional status of the prosthesis, prior experience in treating the specific infection, and the infecting organism. PVE occurring 1 year or more after valve placement and caused by avirulent, antibiotic-susceptible organisms, such as viridans streptococci or fastidious gram-negative coccobacilli, can usually be cured by intensive antibiotic therapy; however, if valve dysfunction and congestive heart failure develop, cardiac surgery is necessary to remove the infected valve and to restore valve function (30,50,51). Often, removal of the prosthesis is necessary to eradicate infection by highly virulent, destructive, antibiotic-resistant organisms, such as *S. aureus*, enteric and nonenteric gram-negative bacilli, and fungi. Intraperitoneal antibiotic treatment without removing a functioning Tenckhoff catheter often eradicates CAPD-associated peritonitis caused by coagulase-negative staphylococci or enteric gram-negative bacilli, but peritonitis due to *S. aureus*, *Pseudomonas aeruginosa*, or fungi, particularly if there is tunnel infection or dialysis catheter dysfunction, usually requires catheter removal (32). In selected clinical settings, the device and the associated function are most likely to be salvaged with aggressive antibiotic treatment. Because of the hazards of hemorrhage and retinal tears when operating on an inflamed eye, eradication of infection with maintenance of visual function is best achieved by antibiotic treatment of infected intraocular lens implants without lens removal (34).

Although marked virulence or antibiotic resistance of an infecting organism suggests the need to remove a device to eliminate infection, the clinical setting and other characteristics of the infecting agent are important considerations. Infection of a prosthetic joint by a highly virulent organism can be cured by surgical débridement and intensive antibiotic therapy without removal of the prosthesis, if the infection is recognized early, before the bone-cement-prosthesis interface is involved and the prosthesis becomes loosened, painful, and dysfunctional (26,31,52). In contrast, successful treatment of smoldering infection of a painful, loosened, joint prosthesis, although the infection is caused by an avirulent organism, requires removal of the device (26,31,53,54).

Slime or glycocalyx formation by avirulent coagulase-negative staphylococci has been associated with a decreased likelihood of eradicating infection from CSF shunts (16,55) and other devices (15) without removing the infected foreign material.

In planning therapy, the role of a prosthetic device in sustaining a patient's well-being must be considered as well as the patient's general health and prognosis. Attempting to salvage a device by antibiotic therapy must be weighed against the consequences of further injury to periprosthetic tissue if the infection does not respond. If additional damage during attempted salvage would compromise survival or functional outcome, optimal therapy includes early prosthesis removal and either reinsertion of another device or provision of a functional alternative. For example, in patients with PVE, prolonged antibiotic therapy and delay of surgery in spite of persistent fever, progressive destruction of the valve annulus, or worsening congestive heart failure results in higher mortality rates than prompt valve replacement (30,33,56). Infection involving synthetic arterial grafts in the lower extremity, wherein the anastomoses are intact and the grafts are fully functional, may be treated effectively without graft removal. Treatment includes not only intensive antibiotic therapy but also aggressive wound drainage and débridement and often rotational muscle flaps to cover the exposed synthetic graft (53,57–59). In contrast, attempted cure with antibiotic therapy of an infected dysfunctional synthetic arterial graft (leaking anastomosis, partial occlusion), particularly one in a body cavity where further deterioration in function cannot be continuously monitored, is likely to be associated with increased morbidity and mortality due to graft occlusion or rupture of the anastomosis (29,39). In this latter setting, better results are obtained with antibiotic therapy in combination with graft resection and vascular reconstruction through an uninfected extraanatomic route (29,59). Failure to eradicate infection involving a breast implant and the need to subsequently remove the device are unlikely to jeopardize the patient's life or the potential for reconstructive surgery (60). Finally, aggressive surgical intervention may not be feasible because of the patients poor general health or refusal to allow removal of the infected prosthesis. In this setting, attempted medical therapy, including long-term antibiotic suppression, may be the sole option. To be successful or at least to temporize using this approach, the prosthesis must function adequately and the infecting organism must be highly susceptible to antibiotics.

SPECIFIC PROSTHETIC DEVICE INFECTIONS

Prostheses and medical devices can be categorized by their position: (a) intravascular (prosthetic valve); (b) partially intravascular (transvenous pacemaker or cardioverter-defibrillator, synthetic vascular graft); (c) extravascular (prosthetic joint, ventriculoperitoneal shunt); and (d) partially implanted (Tenckhoff catheter, implanted central nervous system catheters). An examination of infections involving a prosthesis from several of these categories illustrates features that are common to device-related infections as well as some that are unique to the category and the prosthesis. In addition, the principles that guide the evaluation and treatment of patients with device-related infection are demonstrated. Other specific device related infections are reviewed in detail elsewhere (4).

Prosthetic Valve Endocarditis

The risk of prosthetic valve infection, while it continues indefinitely, is greatest in the first year after surgery. The cumulative rate of PVE is 1.5% to 3.0% 1 year after valve surgery and increases to 3.2% to 5.7% after 4 to 5 years (25,30,33). Thus, PVE must be considered when any valve recipient has unexplained fever. The microbiology of PVE at various times after surgery is relatively predictable (Table 179.2). Coagulase-negative staphylococci, which are almost exclusively methicillin-resistant *S. epidermidis*, are the predominant agent of PVE during the initial year after surgery (25,30,61). Thereafter, although they are still an important cause of PVE, organisms that are commonly associated with native valve endocarditis become prominent: viridans streptococci, enterococci, *S. aureus*, and fastidious gram-negative coccobacilli (25,30,33). The coagulase-negative staphylococci that cause these later onset cases are often species other than *S. epidermidis*, and less than 30% of the isolates are resistant to methicillin (25,30,33). Despite the relative predictability of the microbiology of PVE a vast array of organisms including unusual bacteria, fungi, mycobacteria, rickettsia, and mycoplasma have caused sporadic cases (30,33).

PVE is a highly invasive disease. Annulus invasion and myocardial abscess occur in at least 40% and 14% of patients with mechanical valve infection, respectively (62–65). Partial dehiscence of the prosthesis from the infected annulus results in paravalvular regurgitation. Vegetations on the mitral valve

TABLE 179.2. Microbiology of Prosthetic Valve Endocarditis

Organism	No. of cases (%) at time of onset after cardiac surgery		
	<2 mo N = 161	2–12 mo N = 53	>12 mo N = 194
Coagulase-negative staphylococci	51 (32)	24 (45)	22 (11)
Staphylococcus aureus	36 (22)	6 (11)	34 (18)
Gram-negative bacilli	19 (11)	2 (4)	11 (6)
Streptococci	5 (3)	4 (8)	61 (31)
Enterococci	13 (8)	5 (9)	22 (11)
Diphtheroids	9 (5)	1 (2)	5 (3)
Fastidious gram-negative coccobacilli (HACEK)	0	1 (2)	11 (6)
Fungi	12 (7)	4 (8)	3 (2)
Miscellaneous/polymicrobial	4 (2)	2 (4)	9 (5)
Culture-negative	7 (4)	4 (8)	16 (8)

Data from references 75,111–115.
HACEK indicates *Hemophilus* sp., *Actinobacillus actinomycetemcomitans*, *Cardiobacterium hominis*, *Eikenella* sp., *Kingella* sp.

occasionally encroach on the valve orifice and cause functional stenosis (63,65).

Infection involving bioprosthetic valves is highly invasive during the first year after surgery and thereafter is more frequently confined to the leaflets (30,33,66). Infection may destroy tissue leaflets resulting in regurgitation or cause valve stenosis by rendering the leaflet stiff and immobile (30,67).

The diagnosis of PVE requires a high index of suspicion. The clinical features of PVE resemble those of acute or subacute native valve endocarditis, except that new murmurs indicative of valve dysfunction are more frequent among patients with infected prosthetic valves. Although complications of recent surgery, hemodynamic instability, or neurologic complications may obscure the clinical features, the diagnosis is suggested by the endocarditis syndrome, unexplained fever, persistent bacteremia especially with endocarditis-associated organisms or evidence of new prosthesis dysfunction. Patients in whom PVE is suspected can be systemically evaluated by applying the highly sensitive, modified Duke criteria for the diagnosis of endocarditis (68). When these criteria were used retrospectively to assess patients with PVE that had been confirmed by pathology, 76% to 79% of cases were classified as definite and 21% to 24% as possible endocarditis (69–71). Even though these patients were not uniformly evaluated by transesophageal echocardiography (TEE), in only 1% of cases was the diagnosis rejected erroneously. TEE, as contrasted with transthoracic echocardiography, has been repetitively demonstrated to be the optimal imaging technique for anatomic confirmation of PVE regardless of prosthesis type or valve setting (30,33,43). TEE is also superior for detecting intracardiac complications, i.e. paravalvular abscesses, fistulae, valve dehiscence and paravalvular leaks, which are major considerations in defining management strategy (33).

Treatment of PVE uses principles evolved from treating native valve endocarditis. If an optimal antimicrobial regimen is to be selected, the specific cause of PVE must be identified. This may necessitate blood cultures in special media, serologic testing, microbiologic and histologic examination of embolic vegetations, or judicious delay of antimicrobial therapy for patients who recently received inadequate antibiotic therapy. Antibiotic therapy for patients with PVE, although more prolonged in duration, is similar to that used for patients with native valve endocarditis caused by the analogous organism (72). One difference, however, is the recommended treatment of patients with staphylococcal PVE. In this instance, a multi-drug regimen is recommended. Treatment includes vancomycin or a penicillinase-resistant penicillin, depending upon the susceptibility of the isolate to methicillin, combined with rifampin and either gentamicin or a fluoroquinolone, again depending upon the susceptibility of the causative staphylococcus (30,33,46–48,72).

Valve replacement surgery will be necessary to eliminate infection and maintain effective valve function for 50% to 65% of patients with PVE (30,33,73). This requirement is the consequence of invasive disease causing valve dysfunction or infection by destructive antibiotic-resistant organisms. Surgical intervention is necessary for patients with valve dysfunction (with or without congestive heart failure), fever unresponsive to appropriate antibiotic therapy, evidence of invasive perivalvular disease by echocardiogram or new-onset electrocardiographic conduction abnormalities, infection that has relapsed after appropriate therapy, or fungal PVE (30,33,74,75). Valve replacement is usually indicated for patients with PVE caused by S. aureus, and antibiotic-resistant gram-negative bacilli, especially Pseudomonas aeruginosa (30,33,69,73,75). Aggressive surgical treatment of patients with PVE, including surgery early during antibiotic therapy, extensive reconstruction using pros-

thetic devices, and reconstruction of the aortic outflow tract using cryopreserved allografts, combined with appropriate antibiotic therapy yields survival rates of 70% to 90% in patients with PVE complicated by perivalvular invasion and valve dysfunction (30,33,51,76–82).

Infected Electrophysiologic Cardiac Devices (Pacemakers and Cardioverter-Defibrillator)

The frequency of infections complicating electrophysiologic cardiac devices has decreased in recent years coincident with improved surgical techniques and with the nearly universal use of transvenous devices. Nevertheless, these devices become infected in 1% to 7% of recipients (33,83–85). Infection can involve one or more sites along the device: the generator or defibrillator pocket, the subcutaneous tissue or venous intravascular space along the electrode, or the endocardium of the right atrium, tricuspid valve, or right ventricle in contact with the lead or its tip. Occasionally devices use epicardial leads which can also become infected.

Several mechanisms result in infection. Infection within the month after device placement or generator exchange commonly involve the pocket and may extend along the electrode to the intravascular space, occasionally causing lead-associated right sided endocarditis. Usually these infections arise as a consequence of intraoperative contamination (33,86–89). Later onset pocket infections result from mechanical erosion of the generator through the skin or low-grade smoldering infection in the pocket that necessitates. Hematogenous seeding of the intravascular component from infection at a remote site occurs infrequently, except in the setting of S. aureus bacteremia wherein 30% of episodes result in device infection (89,90).

Although a variety of organisms have caused electrophysiologic device infections, including gram-negative bacilli, viridans streptococci, Corynebacterium species, and Candida species, staphylococci are the most common cause (33,85,87–89). S. aureus is the predominant cause of bacteremia and generator site infections that occur within weeks of surgery (88,89). Polybacterial infections are generally confined to the generator site (87). In a recent larger series, the most common organisms causing these infections were coagulase-negative staphylococci (68%), S aureus (24%), and gram-negative bacilli (17%). Polymicrobial infection occurred in 13% of cases. The causes of infection of pacemakers and cardioverter-defibrillators were similar (84).

The clinical manifestations of electrophysiologic device infection, which are contingent on the site of infection, are highly variable, not surprising because infection ranges from erosion of the generator through overlying skin to S. aureus right sided endocarditis (Table 179.3). In a recent report examining all device infections, the majority of patients (69%) presented with findings localized to the device pocket, 20% experienced local pocket and systemic symptoms, and 11% had only systemic symptoms (84). Fever was reported in only 29% and bacteremia detected in 33%. In other reports limited to pacemaker-associated endocarditis, fever (86% to 100%) and chills (75% to 84%) are common and bacteremia is universal (88,91,92). In these patients, pulmonary findings, including pneumonia, abscesses or embolism occur in 20% to 45%.

Infection is documented by recovery of organisms from an inflamed area or sinus tracks associated with the pacer or from blood cultures. In the absence of infection at a remote site, sustained staphylococcal bacteremia strongly suggests infection involving the intravascular electrode (89,90). In contrast, gram-negative bacillus bacteremia, particularly if remote sites

TABLE 179.3. Signs and Symptoms of Electrophysiologic Device Infection at Presentation[a]

Sign or symptom	Number (%) N = 123
Generator pocket pain	68 (55)
Generator pocket erythema	67 (55)
Generator pocket erosion/drainage	52 (42)
Fever (history)	35 (29)
Fever (detected)	23 (19)
Chills	27 (22)
Malaise	26 (21)
Anorexia	14 (11)
Nausea	10 (8)

[a]Includes infection localized to the generator pocket and device related endocarditis.
Data from Chua JD, Wilkoff BL, Lee I, Juralti N, Longworth DL, Gordon SM: Diagnosis and management of infections involving implantable electrophysiologic cardiac devices. *Ann Intern Med* 2000;133:604–608.

of infection are noted, does not necessarily indicate infection of the intravascular lead (89).

Echocardiography demonstrating vegetations on the pacing leads or the right side of the heart helps to confirm infection of the intravascular electrode. For this purpose, TEE, which detects vegetations in 91% to 96% of patients with proven pacemaker endocarditis, is more sensitive than transthoracic evaluation, which demonstrates vegetations in only 23% to 54% of cases (88,91–93).

Optimal management of infected electrophysiologic devices, especially the requirement for device removal, has not been studied prospectively and remains debated. Fundamental to management is establishing the extent of infection, otherwise the entire device should be assumed to be infected. Conservative therapy—débridement, local irrigation, and systemic antibiotics for generator pocket infection and intensive intravenous antibiotic therapy for intravascular electrode infection—has occasionally eradicated these infections (33). Failure of conservative therapy, however, hazards septicemia that may be life threatening. When infection is limited to the subcutaneous tissue surrounding the generator pocket partial device removal (the generator and adjacent electrode) plus antibiotic therapy may be successful (94–96). Prompt eradication of subcutaneous or intravascular infection is almost universal when the entire pacing unit is removed in conjunction with intravenous antimicrobial therapy; hence, this approach is preferred (33,84,87–89,91,92). Mortality rates among patients with pacemaker endocarditis were 41% (12 of 29) when treated with antibiotics alone versus 19% (30 of 161) when antibiotic therapy was combined with removal of the entire device (92). Patients with bacteremia or electrode-related endocarditis are generally treated with parenteral therapy as recommended for endocarditis; whereas those with infection limited to the generator pocket can be treated with abbreviated parenteral therapy followed by oral therapy plus wound care for residual infected pocket (33,84). If bacteremia and infection is suppressed by antibiotic therapy, insertion of a replacement pacemaker at a new site when the infected unit is removed does not increase the risk of recurrent infection (33). If infection cannot be controlled before the infected device is removed, placement of a new permanent unit should be delayed. A temporary pacer is used until the infection is controlled. Technical considerations and the degree to which an infection is under control determine whether a new transvenous or epicardial electrode is used. After reassessment of their cardiac disease, some patients will not require another electrophysiologic device (84).

Although recently placed generators and electrodes are easily removed, electrodes that have been in place for an extended period, particularly those with tines and wire mesh tips, are often bound by fibrous tissue to the venous and intracardiac endothelium and difficult to remove by traction without disrupting endothelial and intracardiac structures. Use of the Excimer laser sheath to extract pacing leads allows non-thoracotomy removal of the vast majority of leads, including most that failed attempted removal by traction (97). Transvenous electrodes that cannot be removed transcutaneously and infected older epicardial leads should be removed surgically with cardiopulmonary bypass support if necessary (33). If surgical removal entails unacceptable risks, prolonged intravenous antibiotic therapy followed by long term oral suppressive therapy is occasionally successful (87,88,92).

A meta-analysis suggests that infectious complications of electrophysiologic device implantation can be reduced by using prophylactic antibiotics at the time of placement (98).

Prosthetic Joint Infection

The cumulative rate (hazard) of infection involving total hip and knee arthroplasty is greatest during the initial 6 months after surgery and declines thereafter. During the initial 2 years after hip and knee arthroplasty surgery, 5.9 infections per 1,000 joint-years were noted whereas during years 3 through 10, 2.3 infections per 1,000 joint-years were seen (26). Infection rates for other replaced joints are not available. Perioperative wound infection that extends to the device and intraoperative contamination of the prosthesis with delay in onset and diagnosis of infection result in the high rate noted during the initial 2 years after hip and knee replacement. Late hematogenous seeding and extension from adjacent soft tissue infection are the mechanisms whereby joint prostheses become infected in year 3 and thereafter. Rheumatoid arthritis, prior joint surgery, perioperative wound complications, malignancy noted within previous 5 years, increased National Nosocomial Infection Surveillance System score, and metal-on-metal prostheses are factors associated with increased risk for arthroplasty infection (26,99).

The presentation of a patient with an infected arthroplasty is highly variable and depends on the time and route of infection and the virulence of the pathogen. From 35% to 50% of patients with an infected prosthesis present within 3 months of surgery with joint pain and clinical evidence of wound infection, although systemic toxicity often is absent. The challenge for the physician, particularly if the treatment goal is salvage of the implant, is to distinguish mechanical complications and superficial infections from infections that involve the prosthesis. In some patients these questions can be answered only by aspirating or re-exploring the wound in the operating room (31). Another 30% to 45% of patients with infected arthroplasties present from 3 to 24 months postoperatively with joint pain as the predominant symptom (26,31). Signs of local inflammation, fever, and sinus tracks are uncommon and clinical differentiation from aseptic loosening is not feasible (26,31,54). Approximately 6% to 15% of patients with infected prostheses present with acute septic arthritis due to hematogenous seeding from a remote infection (26,31). These infections, which may present within 2 years of implant surgery but typically present later, are characterized by systemic toxicity, local inflammation, and signs of acute septic arthritis. These infections usually develop in patients whose prosthesis has been functioning normally (26,31,100). The diagnosis is established by examination of periprosthetic fluid.

The diagnosis of late onset chronic infection in a joint replacement (or other orthopedic implant) is challenging. While blood cell counts, erythrocyte sedimentation rate, C-reactive protein, radiographs, radionuclide scans, and arthrographs often fail to distinguish low-grade infection from aseptic loosening of the prosthesis, and, most important, they do not identify the infecting organism (26,31,54). To diagnose infection, antibiotics are omitted for at least 2 weeks and fluid is aspirated with sterile technique from the joint for microscopic examination and culture anaerobically and aerobically using multiple media. Although the fluid Gram stain is unreliable, the sensitivity and specificity of the culture result for the diagnosis of infection is 86% (95% CI, 63% to 96%) and 94% (95% CI, 89% to 97%) (101). Three specimens should be sent because recovery of the same organism from multiple specimens increases diagnostic accuracy (44,100). It may be beneficial to repeat the aspiration and reconfirm the presence of the organism, using careful speciation or molecular techniques in the case of organisms such as coagulase-negative staphylococci, which could be a contaminant or pathogen. If further confirmation of infection is needed, histologic examination and multiple cultures of periprosthetic tissue obtained at surgery (before antibiotic administration) are useful. Finding 10 or more neutrophils per high-power field on frozen section has an 89% positive predictive value for infection and recovering the same organism from three or more of six intraoperative specimens has a post test probability of 96% for infection (26,44). If only one specimen yields an organism, the probability of infection is markedly reduced unless the same organism has been recovered on aspiration preoperatively or the prosthesis is failing within 2 years of implantation.

Staphylococci are isolated from 55% of the infected arthroplasties (Table 179.4). Gram-negative bacilli are involved when arthroplasty infection results from acute wound complications or late hematogenous seeding. Indolent infections presenting 3 to 24 months after surgery are caused by avirulent organisms such as coagulase-negative staphylococci, viridans streptococci, anaerobic gram-positive cocci, and corynebacteria. *Candida* organisms that contaminate the wound perioperatively cause rare episodes of indolent prosthetic joint infection (102). Hematogenous infections of arthroplasties are caused by virulent organisms such as *S. aureus*, β-hemolytic streptococci, and gram-negative bacilli.

Multiple factors effect the surgical management and antibiotic treatment of an infected joint prosthesis: acute versus chronic infection, the virulence and antibiotic susceptibility of the pathogen, the degree of loosening (and associated pain) of the device, the general health of the patient and local health of the bone stock, and the anticipated compliance of the patient. In patients with chronic infection and a painful loosened prosthesis, eradication of infection and achieving a pain-free, fully functional joint requires removal of the prosthesis, meticulous débridement of all infected bone and cement, intensive antimicrobial therapy targeted to the specific pathogen, and subsequent reinsertion of a prosthesis. In nonpurulent arthroplasty infections caused by highly antibiotic susceptible, avirulent organisms, satisfactory results can be achieved with removal of the infected device, débridement, and immediate reinsertion of a new prosthesis (generally using antibiotic-impregnated cement) followed by prolonged antibiotic therapy (26,31,49,54). More often, a two-stage procedure is used whereby the new prosthesis is implanted after 4 to 6 weeks of intensive organism-specific antibiotic therapy (26,31,49,54,103).

Although impacted by significant selection bias, one stage and two-stage reimplantations for infected hip and knee prostheses are associated with cure rates ranging from 80% to 83% and 88% to 92%, respectively (26). When a hip arthroplasty is infected by virulent, antibiotic-resistant organisms, some authors advise a delay of 6 to 12 months after completion of antibiotic therapy before implanting a new prosthesis. If a knee prosthesis is to be reimplanted, technical considerations prohibit delays significantly longer than 6 weeks after device removal (26).

Discontinuation of antibiotics and delaying perioperative prophylaxis to allow optimal microbiologic assessment of the bone at the time of the second stage reimplantation is recommended and allows optimal postoperative antimicrobial management.

In approximately 20% of patients, the original prosthesis can be salvaged by débridement and intensive antibiotic therapy.

TABLE 179.4. Microbiology of Infected Hip, Knee, or Elbow Prostheses

Organism	All infections (314 joints)	Hematogenous infections (54 joints)
Staphylococcus aureus	109	20
Coagulase-negative staphylococci	79	4
Enterococci	17	5
β-Hemolytic streptococci	12	4
Group B streptococci	5	1
Other streptococci	15	5
Corynebacteria	9	1
Other gram-positive bacteria	8	1[a]
Escherichia coli	13	5
Klebsiella spp.	4	—
Enterobacter spp.	7	1
Pseudomonas spp.	20	3
Proteus spp.	9	2
Other gram-negative bacilli	10	6[b]
Peptostreptococci	3	—
Peptococci	9	—
Bacteroides spp.	6	2
Propionibacterium acnes	2	—
Clostridium spp.	1	—
Mycobacterium fortuitum	1	—

[a] *Listeria monocytogenes.*
[b] *Pasteurella multocida* (two infections).

This approach is likely to be successful only when infection is diagnosed early (less than 14 to 28 days of symptoms), the prosthesis remains securely fixed and the bone-cement interface is not disrupted by infection, there is a clear single implicated pathogen susceptible to oral antimicrobial agents of proven efficacy, and the patient is willing to undergo long-term antimicrobial therapy (26,31,52,104–106). Using regimens that included rifampin and a second antimicrobial, this strategy has allowed salvage of prostheses and internal fixation devices infected by staphylococci. Therapy has been initiated intravenously for 2 to 6 weeks and thereafter given orally for 3 months to patients with infected hip prostheses or internal fixation devices or for 6 months for infected knee prostheses (31,107–109). Ciprofloxacin alone and in combination with ceftazidime (initial 6 weeks only) have been effective for treatment of orthopedic device infection caused by *Salmonella* and *P. aeruginosa* (31,105). Decision analysis modeling suggests that in elderly patients with non-loosened infected prostheses, debridement and prosthesis retention is cost-effective and associated with increased life expectancy (110). When removal or debridement of an infected prosthesis is not possible, chronic suppressive oral antibiotic therapy has permitted satisfactory retention of the arthroplasty if the pathogen is avirulent and exquisitely susceptible to the antibiotic and the prosthesis is not loose or painful (26).

In patients who are unable or unwilling to undergo extensive surgery, who are nonambulatory (if infection involves the knee or hip), when debridement will be incomplete, who have failed multiple treatments for an infected device, who lack sufficient bone stock or have other technical limitations, resection arthroplasty, including arthrodesis when the knee is involved, may be recommended. This approach while yielding major functional limitations is effective treatment for infection and associated pain (26).

REFERENCES

1. Elek SD, Conen PE: Virulence of *Staphylococcus pyogenes* for man: a study of the problems of wound infection. *Br J Exp Pathol* 1957;38:573.
2. Christensen GD, Simpson WA, Bisno AL. Experimental foreign body infections in mice challenged with slime-producing *Staphylococcus epidermidis*. *Infect Immun* 1983;40:407.
3. Zimmerli W, Waldvogel F, Vaudaux P. Pathogenesis of foreign body infection: Description and characteristics of an animal model. *J Infect Dis* 1982;146:487.
4. Gotz F, Peters G. Colonization of medical devices by coagulase-negative staphylococci. In: Waldvogel F, Bisno AL, eds. *Infections associated with indwelling medical devices*. Washington, DC: ASM Press, 2000:55–88.
5. Foster TJ, Hook M. Molecular basis of adherence to *Staphylococcus aureus* to biomaterials. In: Waldvogel F, Bisno AL, eds. *Infections associated with indwelling medical devices*. Washington, DC: ASM Press, 2000:27–39.
6. Vaudaux P, Francois P, Lew DP, Waldvogel FA. Host factors predisposing to and influencing therapy of foreign body infections. In: Waldvogel F, Bisno AL, eds. *Infections associated with indwelling medical devices*. Washington, DC: ASM Press, 2000:1–26.
7. Stewart PS. Mechanisms of antibiotic resistance in bacterial biofilms. *Int J Med Microbiol* 2002;292:107–113.
8. von Eiff C, Peters G, Heilmann C. Pathogenesis of infections due to coagulase-negative staphylococci. *Lancet* 2002;2:677–685.
9. Vaudaux PE, Francois P, Proctor RA, et al. Use of adhesion-defective mutants of *Staphylococcus aureus* to define the role of specific plasma proteins in promoting bacterial adhesion to canine arteriovenous shunts. *Infect Immun* 1995;63:585–590.
10. Vaudaux P, Pittet D, Hacberli A, et al. Fibronectin is more active than fibrin or fibrinogen in promoting *Staphylococcus aureus* adherence to inserted intravascular catheters. *J Infect Dis* 1993;167:633–641.
11. Bayston R, Penny SR. Excessive production of mucoid substance in staphylococcus SIIA: a possible factor in colonization of Holter shunts. *Dev Med Child Neurol* 1972;14(Suppl 27):25.
12. Christensen GD, Parisi JT, Bisno AL. Characterization of clinically significant strains of coagulase-negative staphylococci. *J Clin Microbiol* 1983;18:258.
13. Christensen GD, Bisno AL, Parisi JT. Nosocomial septicemia due to multiply antibiotic-resistant *Staphylococcus epidermidis*. *Ann Intern Med* 1982;96:1.
14. Ishak MA, Groschel DHM, Mandell GL. Association of slime with pathogenicity of coagulase-negative staphylococci causing nosocomial septicemia. *J Clin Microbiol* 1985;22:1025.
15. Davenport DS, Massanari RM, Pfaller MA. Usefulness of a test for slime production as a marker for clinically significant infections with coagulase-negative staphylococci. *J Infect Dis* 1986;153:332.
16. Diaz-Mitoma F, Harding GKM, Hoban DJ. Clinical significance of a test for slime production in ventriculoperitoneal shunt infections caused by coagulase-negative staphylococci. *J Infect Dis* 1987;156:555.
17. Zimmerli W, Lew DP, Waldvogel FA. Pathogenesis of foreign body infection. Evidence for a local granulocyte defect. *J Clin Invest* 1984;73:1191.
18. Vaudaux PE, Zulian G, Huggler E. Attachment of *Staphylococcus aureus* to polymethylmethacrylate increases its resistance to phagocytosis in foreign body infection. *Infect Immun* 1985;50:472.
19. Vaudaux P, Grau GE, Huggler E, et al. Contribution of tumor necrosis factor to host defense against staphylococci in a guinea pig model of foreign body infections. *J Infect Dis* 1992;166:58–64.
20. Chuard C, Vaudaux P, Waldvogel FA, Lew DP. Susceptibility of *Staphylococcus aureus* growing on fibronectin-coated surfaces to bactericidal antibiotics. *Antimicrob Agents Chemother* 1993;37:625–632.
21. Chuard C, Lucet JC, Rohner P, et al. Resistance of *Staphylococcus aureus* recovered from infected foreign body in vivo to killing by antimicrobials. *J Infect Dis* 1991;163:1369–1373.
22. Gilbert P, Collier PJ, Brown MRW. Influence of growth rate on susceptibility to antimicrobial agents: biofilms, cell cycle, dormancy, and stringent response. *Antimicrob Agents Chemother* 2990;34:1865–1868.
23. Bunt TJ. Synthetic vascular graft infections. I. Graft infections. *Surgery* 1983;93:733.
24. Archer GL, Vishniavsky N, Stiver HG. Plasmid pattern analysis of *Staphylococcus epidermidis* isolates from patients with prosthetic valve endocarditis. *Infect Immun* 1982;35:627–632.
25. Calderwood SB, Swinski LA, Waternaux CM, Karchmer AW, Buckley MJ. Risk factors for the development of prosthetic valve endocarditis. *Circulation* 1985;72:31–37.
26. Steckelberg JM, Osmon DR. Prosthetic joint infections. In: Waldvogel FA, Bisno AL, eds. *Infections associated with indwelling medical devices*. Washington, DC: ASM Press, 2000:173–209.
27. Lidwell OM, Lowbury EJL, Whyte W. Effect of ultraclean air in operating rooms on deep sepsis in the joint after total hip or knee replacement: a randomized study. *BMJ* 1982;285:10.
28. Glynn MK, Sheehan JM. An analysis of causes of deep infection after hip and knee arthroplasties. *Clin Orthop* 1983;178:202.
29. Bandyk DF. Diagnosis and treatment of biomaterial-associated vascular infections. *Infect Dis Clin North Am* 1992;6:719–729.
30. Karchmer AW. Infections of prosthetic heart valves. In: Waldvogel FA, Bisno AL, eds. *Infections associated with indwelling medical devices*. Washington, DC: ASM Press, 2000:145–172.
31. Widmer AF. New developments in diagnosis and treatment of infection in orthopedic implants. *Clin Infect Dis* 2001;33(Suppl 2):S94–S106.
32. Oliver MJ, Schwab SJ. Infections related to hemodialysis and peritoneal dialysis. In: Waldvogel FA, Bisno AL, eds. *Infections associated with indwelling medical devices*. Washington, DC: ASM Press, 2000:345–372.
33. Karchmer AW, Longworth DL. Infections of intracardiac devices. *Infect Dis Clin North Am* 2002;16:477–505.
34. Barequet IS, Baker AS, Schein OD. Ocular infections. In: Waldvogel FA, Bisno AL, eds. *Infections associated with indwelling medical devices*. Washington, DC: ASM Press, 2000:287–306.
35. Yogev R, Bisno AL. Infections of central nervous system shunts. In: Waldvogel FA, Bisno AL, eds. *Infections associated with indwelling medical devices*. Washington, DC: ASM Press, 2000:231–246.
36. Rames L, Wise B, Goodman JR. Renal disease with *Staphylococcus albus* bacteremia. *JAMA* 1970;8:1671.
37. Becker BA, Crowder JG, Smith JW. *Propionibacterium acnes*: pathogen in central nervous system infection. Report of three cases including immune complex glomerulonephritis. *Am J Med* 1976;61:935.
38. Bolton WK, Sande MA, Normansell DE. Ventriculojugular shunt nephritis with *Corynebacterium bovis*. *Am J Med* 1975;59:417.
39. Champion MC, Sullivan SN, Coles JC. Aortoenteric fistula. Incidence, presentation, recognition, and management. *Ann Surg* 1982;195:314.
40. Blum MD: Infections in genitourinary prostheses. *Infect Dis Clin North Am* 1989;3:259.
41. Montague DK, Angermeier KW, Lakin MM. Penile prosthesis infection. *Int J Impot Res* 2001;13:326–328.
42. Murdoch DR, Roberts SA, Fowler VG Jr, et al. Infection of orthopedic prostheses after *Staphylococcus aureus* bacteremia. *Clin Infect Dis* 2001;32:647–649.
43. Daniel WG, Mugge A, Grote J, et al. Comparison of transthoracic and transesophageal echocardiography for detection of abnormalities of prosthetic and bioprosthetic valves in the mitral and aortic positions. *Am J Cardiol* 1993;71:210–215.
44. Atkins BL, Athanasou N, Deeks JJ, et al, The OSIRIS Collaborative Study Group. Prospective evaluation of criteria for microbiological diagnosis of prosthetic-joint infection at revision arthroplasty. *J Clin Microbiol* 1998;36:2932.
45. Archer GL, Karchmer AW, Vishniavsky N, Johnston JL. Plasmid-pattern analysis for the differentiation of infecting from noninfecting *Staphylococcus epidermidis*. *J Infect Dis* 1984;149:913–920.

46. Widmer AF, Frei R, Rajacic Z, Zimmerli W. Correlation between in vivo and in vitro efficacy of antimicrobial agents against foreign body infections. *J Infect Dis* 1990;162:96–102.

47. Lucet JC, Herrmann M, Rohner P, Auckenthaler R, Waldvogel FA, Lew DP. Treatment of experimental foreign body infection caused by methicillin-resistant *Staphylococcus aureus*. *Antimicrob Agents Chemother* 1990;34:2312–2317.

48. Chuard C, Herrmann M, Vaudaux P, Waldvogel FA, Lew DP. Successful therapy of experimental chronic foreign-body infection due to methicillin-resistant *Staphylococcus aureus* by antimicrobial combinations. *Antimicrob Agents Chemother* 1991;35:2611–2616.

49. Hanssen AD, Rand JA, Osmon DR. Treatment of the infected total knee arthroplasty with insertion of another prosthesis: the effect of antibiotic-impregnated bone cement. *Clin Orthop Relat Res* 1994;309:44–55.

50. Meyer DJ, Gerding DN. Favorable prognosis of patients with prosthetic valve endocarditis caused by gram-negative bacilli of the HACEK group. *Am J Med* 1988;85:104–107.

51. Lytle BW, Priest BP, Taylor PC, et al. Surgery for acquired heart disease: surgical treatment of prosthetic valve endocarditis. *J Thorac Cardiovasc Surg* 1996;111:198–210.

52. Tattevin P, Cremieux AC, Pottier P, Huten D, Carbon C. Prosthetic joint infection: when can prosthesis salvage be considered? *Clin Infect Dis* 1999;29:292–295.

53. Cherry JJ Jr, Roland CF, Pairolero PC, et al. Infected femorodistal bypass: is graft removal mandatory? *J Vasc Surg* 1992;15:295–305.

54. Gillespie WJ. Prevention and management of infection after total joint replacement. *Clin Infect Dis* 1997;25:1310–1317.

55. Jounger JJ, Christensen GD, Bartley DL. Coagulase-negative staphylococci isolated from cerebrospinal fluid shunts: importance of slime production, species identification, and shunt removal to clinical outcome. *J Infect Dis* 1987;156:548.

56. Boyd AD, Spencer FC, Isom OW, et al. Infective endocarditis: an analysis of 54 surgically treated patients. *J Thorac Cardiovasc Surg* 1977;73:23–30.

57. Perler BA, Vander Kolk CA, Manson PM, Williams GM. Rotational muscle flaps to treat localized prosthetic graft infection: long-term follow-up. *J Vasc Surg* 1993;18:358–364.

58. Calligaro KD, Veith FJ, Sales CM, Dougherty MJ, Savarese RP, DeLaurentis DA. Comparison of muscle flaps and delayed secondary intention wound healing for infected lower extremity arterial grafts. *Ann Vasc Surg* 1994;8:32–37.

59. Calligaro KD, Veith FJ, Schwartz ML, et al. Selective preservation of infected prosthetic arterial grafts: analysis of a 20-year experience with 120 extracavitary-infected grafts. *Ann Surg* 1994;220:461–471.

60. Freedman AM, Jackson IT. Infections of breast implants. *Infect Dis Clin North Am* 1989;3:275.

61. Karchmer AW, Archer GL, Dismukes WE. *Staphylococcus epidermidis* causing prosthetic valve endocarditis: microbiologic and clinical observations as guides to therapy. *Ann Intern Med* 1983;98:447–455.

62. Richardson JV, Karp RB, Kirklin JW, Dismukes WE. Treatment of infective endocarditis: a 10-year comparative analysis. *Circulation* 1978;58:589–597.

63. Anderson DJ, Bulkley BH, Hutchins GM. A clinicopathologic study of prosthetic valve endocarditis in 22 patients: morphologic basis for diagnosis and therapy. *Am Heart J* 1977;94:325–332.

64. Dismukes WE, Karchmer AW, Buckley MJ, Austen WG, Swartz MN. Prosthetic valve endocarditis: analysis of 38 cases. *Circulation* 1973;XLVIII:365–377.

65. Arnett EN, Roberts WC. Prosthetic valve endocarditis: clinicopathologic analysis of 22 necropsy patients with comparison of observations in 74 necropsy patients with active infective endocarditis involving natural left-sided cardiac valves. *Am J Cardiol* 1976;38:281–291.

66. Fernicola DJ, Roberts WC. Frequency of ring abscess and cuspal infection in active infective endocarditis involving bioprosthetic valves. *Am J Cardiol* 1993;72:314–323.

67. Magilligan DJ Jr. Bioprosthetic valve endocarditis. In: Magilligan DJ Jr, Quinn EL, eds. *Endocarditis—medical and surgical management.* New York: Marcel Decker, 1986:253–263.

68. Li JS, Sexton DJ, Mick N, Nettles R, et al. Proposed modifications to the Duke criteria for the diagnosis of infective endocarditis. *Clin Infect Dis* 2000;30:633–638.

69. John MVD, Hibberd PL, Karchmer AW, Sleeper LA, Calderwood SB. *Staphylococcus aureus* prosthetic valve endocarditis: optimal management and risk factors for death. *Clin Infect Dis* 1998;26:1302–1309.

70. Nettles RE, McCarty DE, Corey RG, Li J, Sexton DJ. An evaluation of the Duke criteria in 25 pathologically confirmed cases of prosthetic valve endocarditis. *Clin Infect Dis* 1997;25:1401–1403.

71. Perez-Vazquez A, Farinas MC, Garcia-Palomo JD, Bernal JM, Revuelta JM, Gonzalez-Macias J. Evaluation of the Duke criteria in 93 episodes of prosthetic valve endocarditis: could sensitivity be improved? *Arch Intern Med* 2000;160:1185–1191.

72. Wilson WR, Karchmer AW, Bisno AL, et al. Antibiotic treatment of adults with infective endocarditis due to viridans streptococci, enterococci, other streptococci, staphylococci, and HACEK microorganisms. *JAMA* 1995;274:1706–1713.

73. Calderwood SB, Swinski LA, Karchmer AW, Waternaux CM, Buckley MJ. Prosthetic valve endocarditis: analysis of factors affecting outcome of therapy. *J Thorac Cardiovasc Surg* 1986;92:776–783.

74. Karalis DG, Blumberg EA, Vilaro JF, et al. Prognostic significance of valvular regurgitation in patients with infective endocarditis. *Am J Med* 1991;90:193–197.

75. Wolff M, Witchitz S, Chastang C, Regnier B, Vachon F. Prosthetic valve endocarditis in the ICU: prognosis factors of overall survival in a series of 122 cases and consequences for treatment decision. *Chest* 1995;108:688–694.

76. Pansini S, di Summa M, Patane F, Forsennati PG, Serra M, Del Ponte S. Risk of recurrence after reoperation for prosthetic valve endocarditis. *J Heart Valve Dis* 1997;6:84–87.

77. d'Udekem Y, David TE, Feindel CM, Armstrong S, Sun Z. Long-term results of operation for paravalvular abscess. *Ann Thorac Surg* 1996;62:48–53.

78. David TE. The surgical treatment of patients with prosthetic valve endocarditis. *Sem Thorac Cardiovasc Surg* 1995;7:47–53.

79. Glazier JJ, Verwilghen J, Donaldson RM, Ross DN. Treatment of complicated prosthetic aortic valve endocarditis with annular abscess formation by homograft aortic root replacement. *J Am Coll Cardiol* 1991;17:1177–1182.

80. Dossche KM, Defauw JJ, Ernst SM, Craenen TW, DeJongh BM, de la Riviere AB. Allograft aortic root replacement in prosthetic aortic valve endocarditis: a review of 32 patients. *Ann Thorac Surg* 1997;63:1644–1649.

81. Jault F, Gandjbakheh I, Chastre JC, et al. Prosthetic valve endocarditis with ring abscesses: Surgical management and long-term results. *J Thorac Cardiovasc Surg* 1993;105:1106–1113.

82. Nataf P, Jault F, Dorent R, et al. Extra-annular procedures in the surgical management of prosthetic valve endocarditis. *Eur Heart J* 1995;16(Suppl B):99–102.

83. Lai KK, Fontecchio SA. Infections associated with implantable cardioverter-defibrillators placed transvenously and via thoracotomies: epidemiology, infection control, and management. *Clin Infect Dis* 1998;27:265–269.

84. Chua JD, Wilkoff BL, Lee I, Juratli N, Longworth DL, Gordon SM. Diagnosis and management of infections involving implantable electrophysiologic cardiac devices. *Ann Intern Med* 2000;133:604–608.

85. Kearney RA, Eisen HJ, Wolf JE. Nonvalvular infections of the cardiovascular system. *Ann Intern Med* 1994;121:219–230.

86. DaCosta A, Lelievre H, Kirkorian G, et al. Role of the preaxillary flora in pacemaker infections: a prospective study. *Circulation* 1998;97:1791–1795.

87. Lewis AB, Hayes DL, Holmes DR, Jr., Vliestra RE, Pluth JR, Osborn MJ. Update on infections involving permanent pacemakers: characterization and management. *J Thorac Cardiovasc Surg* 1985;89:758–763.

88. Arber N, Pras E, Copperman Y, et al. Pacemaker endocarditis: report of 44 cases and review of the literature. *Medicine* 1994;73:299–305.

89. Camus C, Leport C, Raffi F, Michelet C, Cartier F, Vilde JL. Sustained bacteremia in 26 patients with a permanent endocardial pacemaker: assessment of wire removal. *Clin Infect Dis* 1993;17:46–55.

90. Chamis AL, Peterson GE, Cabell CH, et al. *Staphylococcus aureus* bacteremia in patients with permanent pacemakers or implantable cardioverter-defibrillators. *Circulation* 2001;104:1029–1033.

91. Klug D, Lacroix D, Savoye C, et al. Systemic infection related to endocarditis on pacemaker leads: clinical presentation and management. *Circulation* 1997;95:2098–2107.

92. Cacoub P, Leprince P, Nataf P, et al. Pacemaker infective endocarditis. *Am J Cardiol* 1998;82:480–484.

93. Victor F, DePlace C, Camus C, et al. Pacemaker lead infection: echocardiographic features, management and outcome. *Heart* 1999;81:82–87.

94. Trappe HJ, Pfitzner P, Klein H. Infections after cardioverter-defibrillator implantation: observations in 335 patients over 10 years. *Br Heart J* 1995;73:20–24.

95. Molina JE. Undertreatment and overtreatment of patients with infected antiarrhythmic implantable devices. *Ann Thorac Surg* 1997;63:504–509.

96. Samuels LE, Samuels FL, Kaufman MS, Morris RJ, Brockman SK. Management of infected implantable cardiac defibrillators. *Ann Thorac Surg* 1997;64:1702–1706.

97. Wilkoff BL, Byrd CL, Love CJ, et al. Pacemaker lead extraction with the laser sheath: results of the pacing lead extraction with the excimer sheath (PLEXES) trial. *J Am Coll Cardiol* 1999;33:1671–1676.

98. DaCosta A, Kirkorian G, Cucherat M, et al. Antibiotic prophylaxis for permanent pacemaker implantation: a meta-analysis. *Circulation* 1998;97:1796–1801.

99. Berbari EF, Hanssen AD, Duffy MC, et al. Risk factors for prosthetic joint infection: case-control study. *Clin Infect Dis* 1998;27:1247–1254.

100. Spangehl MJ, Younger ASE, Masri BA, Duncan CP. Diagnosis of infection following total hip arthroplasty. *J Bone Joint Surg Am* 1997;97:1578–1588.

101. Spangehl M, Masri B, O'Connell J, Duncan C. Prospective analysis of preoperative and intraoperative investigations for the diagnosis of infection at the sites of 202 revision total hip arthroplasties. *J Bone Joint Surg Am* 1999;81:672–683.

102. Phelan DM, Osmon DR, Keating MR, Hanssen AD. Delayed reimplantation arthroplasty for candidal prosthetic joint infection: a report of 4 cases and review of the literature. *Clin Infect Dis* 2002;34:930–938.

103. Lieberman JR, Callaway GH, Salvati EA, Pellicci PM, Brause BD. Treatment of the infected total hip arthroplasty with a two-stage reimplantation protocol. *Clin Orthoped Relat Res* 1994;301:205–212.

104. Brandt CM, Sistrunk WW, Duffy MC, et al. *Staphylococcus aureus* prosthetic joint infection treated with debridement and prosthesis retention. *Clin Infect Dis* 1997;24:914–919.

105. Brouqui P, Rousseau MC, Stein A, Drancourt M, Raoult D. Treatment of *Pseudomonas aeruginosa*–infected orthopedic prostheses with ceftazidime-ciprofloxacin antibiotic combination. *Antimicrob Agents Chemother* 1995;39: 2423–2425.

106. Karchmer AW. Salvage of infected orthopedic devices [Editorial response]. *Clin Infect Dis* 1998;27:714–716.

107. Widmer AF, Gaechter A, Ochsner PE, Zimmerli W. Antimicrobial treatment of orthopedic implant-related infections with rifampin combinations. *Clin Infect Dis* 1992;14:1251–1253.

108. Zimmerli W, Widmer AF, Blatter M, Frei R, Ochsner PE, the Foreign-Body Infection Study Group. Role of rifampin for treatment of orthopedic implant-related staphylococcal infections: a randomized controlled trial. *JAMA* 1998;279:1537–1541.

109. Drancourt M, Stein A, Argenson JN, Zannier A, Curvale G, Raoult D. Oral rifampin plus ofloxacin for treatment of *Staphylococcus*-infected orthopedic implants. *Antimicrob Agents Chemother* 1993;37:1214–1218.

110. Fisman DN, Reilly DT, Karchmer AW, Goldie SJ. Clinical effectiveness and cost-effectiveness of 2 management strategies for infected total hip arthroplasty in the elderly. *Clin Infect Dis* 2001;32:419–430.

111. Arvay A, Lengyel M. Incidence and risk factors of prosthetic valve endocarditis. *Eur J Cardio-thorac Surg* 1988;2:340–346.

112. Chen SC, Sorrell TC, Dwyer DE, Collignon PJ, Wright EJ. Endocarditis associated with prosthetic cardiac valves. *Med J Aust* 1990;152:458–463.

113. Keys TF. Early-onset prosthetic valve endocarditis. *Clev Clin J Med* 1993;60: 455–459.

114. Sett SS, Hudon MPJ, Jamieson WRE, Chow AW. Prosthetic valve endocarditis: experience with porcine bioprostheses. *J Thorac Cardiovasc Surg* 1993;105:428–434.

115. Tornos P, Sanz E, Permanyer-Miralda G, Almirante B, Planes AM, Soler-Soler J. Late prosthetic valve endocarditis: immediate and long-term prognosis. *Chest* 1992;101:37–41.

CHAPTER 180
Fever of Unknown Origin

Burke A. Cunha

The term fever of unknown origin (FUO) should be applied to prolonged fevers the cause of which are not readily apparent after routine physical examination, laboratory, and roentgenographic studies. In 1961, Petersdorf and Beeson coined the term "FUO." They defined FUO as a prolonged febrile disorder lasting 3 weeks or longer, with a temperature of 101°F or higher, that remained undiagnosed after 1 week of in-hospital testing. The original definition has been termed the "classical FUO." The original intent of describing patients with undiagnosed febrile disorders of long duration was to separate these patients from those with undiagnosed acute febrile illnesses. The term FUO should not be applied to patients who have acute, otherwise unexplained fevers, who have not undergone complete investigation, or whose diagnostic test results are pending (1–10) (Table 180.1).

There are also special populations who have FUOs. It is appropriate to use the term FUO in conjunction with patients and children who are infected by human immunodeficiency virus (HIV) and fit the definition of classical FUO (Tables 180.2 and 180.3). There is little rationale for using the term FUO in conjunction with neutropenic patients or with nosocomial infections. Elderly patients with FUO should not be a separate category because most medical patients with FUO are elderly. These special populations are best considered as having prolonged undiagnosed fevers rather than as FUOs. Some have changed the definition of FUO to include these special population groups as separate categories by changing the definition to three days of undiagnosed fever. In the clinical context there are so many reasons why test results are not back within 3 days, and labeling such patients, even as a separate category of FUO, is clinically unhelpful; these patients should be considered as having acute fevers, (see Chapter 5 on Clinical Approach to Fever). What has changed in defining classical FUOs is that this term may also be applied to ambulatory patients who remain undiagnosed after three ambulatory visits (11–25) (Tables 180.4 and 180.5).

The classic FUO as initially described, was due primarily to infectious diseases and to a lesser extent, malignancies and collagen vascular diseases. Currently, malignancies and infectious etiologies constitute the majority of patients with classic FUO. Collagen vascular diseases, excluding polymyalgia/temporal arteritis, or adult Still disease (a type of juvenile rheumatoid arthritis [JRA]) are currently relatively uncommon causes of FUO (13–15). Subacute bacterial endocarditis and intra-abdominal/pelvic abscesses, and extrapulmonary tuberculosis are still important causes of classic FUO. Unusual causes of FUO continue to be described in the literature. Malignancy, among the noninfectious disorders, continues to be an important cause of FUO.

In spite of the best diagnostic efforts, there are a small but definite group of patients who remain undiagnosed. There is a subgroup of FUO patients who continue to have fevers for periods of longer than 6 months. Such prolonged FUOs are nearly always due to noninfectious or neoplastic causes (26,28) (Table 180.6).

THE DIAGNOSTIC APPROACH

The diagnostic approach to FUO depends on pursuing historical, physical, or laboratory clues that suggests a pattern of organ involvement. The pattern of organ involvement, in turn, defines diagnostic possibilities. The clinician approaching the patient with FUO, should attempt to arrive at a working diagnosis based on a clinical syndrome presentation. Both infectious and noninfectious disorders usually present with a characteristic pattern of organ involvement, which is an important diagnostic clue. The majority of patients with classic FUO have some etiologic clue in the history, physical, or routine laboratory tests that should suggest specific diagnostic possibilities. It is important that the clinician approaching the patient with an FUO not order tests in a shotgun fashion, but rather the workup should be based on clues from the history, physical examination, or routine laboratory tests (4–10) (Tables 180.7 to 180.10).

FEVER OF UNKNOWN ORIGIN WITHOUT LOCALIZING SIGNS

In patients without localizing findings, the diagnostic workup is guided by an analysis of fever patterns and subtle abnormalities on routine laboratory testing. The fever pattern has diagnostic importance. The relationship of the pulse to the temperature also has diagnostic importance, i.e., the presence or absence of relative bradycardia. Relative bradycardia may suggest lymphoma, drug fever, psittacosis, typhoid fever, etc. Other fever patterns that may be of diagnostic importance include the double quotidian fever, e.g., two fever spikes within a 24-hour period. Double quotidian fever may suggest the diagnosis of miliary tuberculosis, malaria, visceral leishmaniasis, or adult Still disease. Fevers with a periodic or relapsing pattern might suggest lymphoma, malaria, or cyclic neutropenia. Intermittent fevers with a hectic septic pattern should suggest an occult abscess, miliary tuberculosis, or lymphoma. Most patients with FUOs, excluding abscesses, lymphomas and drug fevers, have temperatures of 102°F or less. Low-grade fevers of 102°F or less may be on an infectious or noninfectious basis, but temperatures 102°F or greater usually are a clue to an infectious etiology, lymphoma, or vasculitis (4,5,10).

TABLE 180.1. Diseases Causing Classical Fever of Unknown Origin

Type of disorder	Common	Uncommon	Rare
Malignancy	Lymphoma Metastases to liver/CNS Hypernephromas	Hepatomas Pancreatic carcinoma Pre-leukemias Colon carcinoma	Atrial myxomas CNS tumors Myelodysplastic diseases

Infections	Extrapulmonary TB
	Renal TB
	TB meningitis
	Miliary TB
	Intra-abdominal abscesses
	Subdiaphragmatic abscesses
	    peri-appendiceal
	    peri-colonic
	    hepatic
	Pelvic abscesses
		SBE
		CMV
		Toxoplasmosis
		Salmonella enteric fevers
		Intra/perinephric abscess
		Splenic abscess
			Periapical dental abscesses
			Small brain abscesses
			Chronic sinusitis
			Subacute vertebral osteomyelitis
			Chronic meningitis/encephalitis
			Listeria
			Yersinia
			Brucellosis
			Relapsing fever
			Rat-bite fever
			Chronic Q fever
			Cat-scratch Fever
			HIV
			EBV mononucleosis (elderly)
			Malaria
			Leptospirosis
			Blastomycosis
			Histoplasmosis
			Coccidioidomycosis
			Cryptococcosis
			Infected aortic aneurysm
			Infected vascular grafts
			RMSF
			Lyme disease
			Leischmaniasis
			Trypanosomiasis
			LGV
			Permanently placed central IV-line infection
			Trichinosis
			Prosthetic device infections
			Relapsing mastoiditis
			Septic jugular phlebitis

Rheumatologic	Adult Still disease Temporal arteritis (elderly)	PAN Rheumatoid arthritis (elderly)	SLE Vasculitis (e.g., Takayasu's arteritis hypersensitivity vasculitis) Felty's syndrome Pseudo gout Acute rheumatic fever Sjogren's syndrome Behcet's disease FMF
Miscellaneous Causes	Drug fever Cirrhosis Alcoholic hepatitis	Granulomatous hepatitis	Regional enteritis Whipple's disease Fabray's disease Hyperthyroidism Hyperparathyroidism Pheochromocytomas Addison's disease Subacute thyroiditis Cyclic neutropenia Polymyositis Wegener's granulomatosis Occult hematomas Subacute aortic dissecting aneurysm Weber-Christian disease Sarcoidosis (e.g., basilar meningitis, hepatic granulomas Pulmonary emboli (multiple, recurrent) Hypothalamic dysfunction Habitual hyperthermia Factitious fever Giant hepatic hemangiomas Mesenteric fibromatosis Pseudolymphomas Idiopathic granulomatosis Kikuchi's disease Malakoplakia Hyper IgD syndrome

CMV; cytomegalovirus; CNS, central nervous system; EBV, Epstein-Barr virus; FMF, familial Mediterranean fever; HIV, human immunodeficiency virus; LGV, lymphogranuloma venereum; RMSF, Rocky Mountain spotted fever; SBE, subacute bacterial endocarditis; SLE, systemic lupus erythematosus.

TABLE 180.2.   Fever of Unknown Origin in HIV Infection

Infectious causes	Noninfectious causes
Common	Common
Mycobacterium tuberculosis	Drug fever
Mycobacterium avium-intracellulare	Thrombophlebitis
Visceral leishmaniasis	
Histoplasmosis	
Uncommon	Uncommon
Mycobacteria other than *M. tuberculosis*	Non-Hodgkins
or *M. avium intracellulare*	lymphomas
Pneumocystis carinii pneumonia	
Toxoplasmosis	
C. neoformans	

TABLE 180.3.   Fever of Unknown Origin in Children

Infectious causes	Noninfectious causes
Common	Common
Mastoiditis (chronic)	Leukemia
Salmonellosis	Lymphoma
Sinusitis	Juvenile rheumatoid arthritis
Subdiaphragmatic abscess	Systemic lupus erythematosus
Cytomegalovirus	Periodic fever
Hepatitis viruses	
Epstein-Barr virus	
Rocky Mountain spotted fever	
Malaria	
Visceral larva migrans	
Uncommon	Uncommon
Perinephric abscess	Polyarteritis nodosa
Pyelonephritis	Neuroblastomas
Psittacosis	Serum sickness
Rare	Rare
Histoplasmosis (disseminated)	Pancreatitis
Toxoplasmosis	Drug fever
Subacute bacterial endocarditis	
Brucella	
Leptospirosis	

TABLE 180.4.   Prolonged Nosocomial Fevers

Infectious causes	Noninfectious causes
Common	Common
Abdominal abscess	Drug fever
Pelvic abscess	GI bleed
Sinusitis (secondary to	Pancreatitis
prolonged nasotracheal	Adrenal insufficiency
intubation)	Acute MI (silent)
Central IV-line infection	Pulmonary emboli
Nosocomial procedure-related	Retroperitoneal hematomas
endocarditis	Septic thrombophlebitis
C. difficile diarrhea/colitis	Central fevers
	Cardiovascular accident/
	irritable colon hemorrhage
	Dressler's syndrome
Uncommon	Uncommon
HSV pneumonia	Ischemic colitis
CNS shunt infection	Cholesterol emboli syndrome
Suppurative parotitis	Gout (flare)
	SLE (flare)

CNS, central nervous system; GI, gastrointestinal; HSV, herpes simplex virus; MI, myocardial infarction; SLE, systemic lupus erythematosus.

TABLE 180.5.   Prolonged Neutropenic Fevers

Infectious causes	Noninfectious causes
Common	Common
Primary bacteremias	Drug fever
Semi-permanent central IV-lines	Central nervous system
Hepato-splenic candidiasis	metastases
Perirectal/ischiorectal abscess	Liver metastases
Uncommon	Uncommon
Bacteremia (rare organism)	"Tumor fever"
Fungemia (rare organism)	

FEVER OF UNKNOWN ORIGIN WITH LOCALIZING SIGNS

In patients with localizing signs, the diagnostic workup should be directed according to the pattern of organ involvement. In addition, appropriate serological tests should be ordered only if a specific etiological agent is suggested by the history or findings on physical diagnosis. In the diagnostic workup in FUO, the history often suggests the diagnosis. Clinicians should carefully interrogate the patient regarding previous medical illnesses, travel exposure, zoonotic exposures, a careful medication history, and contact with potentially toxic fumes. During the history, the patient should also be queried, in the review of systems, regarding nonspecific findings that, together with physical or laboratory findings, may suggest the diagnosis. Particular attention should be paid to eliciting a history of myalgias, fatigue, and localized pain, such as eye pain, back pain, neck pain, or abdominal pain. Mental confusion or headache also provide additional useful historical information. Prolonged fatigue and loss of appetite should also be specifically inquired for (8–10).

CAUSES OF FEVER OF UNKNOWN ORIGIN

Neoplastic Neoplasms

LYMPHOMAS

Occult lymphomas located in the retroperitoneal area are a common cause of neoplastic FUO. Retroperitoneal lymphomas are common in the elderly and present with few symptoms or clinical clues. Occasionally, lymphomas will present with a Pell-Epstein type of intermittent fever, or a hectic-septic fever curve that suggests an infection or abscess (17). Retroperitoneal lymphomas may be associated with systemic symptoms, such as weight loss,

TABLE 180.6.   Prolonged Fevers of Unknown Origin[a]

Common
Resolved without definitive diagnosis
Granulomatous hepatitis
Adult Still disease
Uncommon
SLE
Familial Mediterranean fever
Factitious fever
Rare
Malignancy infections

[a]Fever for ≥6 months.

TABLE 180.7.   Historic Clues to Classical Fever of Unknown Origin

Medication or toxic substances	Mental confusion	Fatigue
Drug fever	Sarcoid meningitis	Carcinomas
Fume fever	TB meningitis	Lymphomas
Tick exposure	Cryptococcal meningitis	CMV, EBV
Relapsing fever	Carcinomatous meningitis	Typhoid fever
RMSF	CNS neoplasms	SLE
Lyme disease	Brucellosis	Rheumatoid arthritis
Animal contact	Typhoid fever	Toxoplasmosis
Psittacosis	HIV	Abdominal pain
Leptospirosis	Cardiovascular accident	PAN
Brucellosis	SBE	FMF
Toxoplasmosis	Takayasu's arteritis	Relapsing fever
Cat-scratch fever	PAN	Back pain
Q fever	RMSF	Brucellosis
Rat-bite fever	Nonproductive cough	SBE
Myalgias	TB	Neck pain
Trichinosis	Q fever	Subacute thyroiditis
SBE	Psittacosis	Adult Still disease
PAN	Typhoid fever	Temporal arteritis
Rheumatoid arthritis	Pulmonary neoplasms	(angle of jaw)
FMF	RMSF	Relapsing mastoiditis
Polymyositis	Acute rheumatic fever	Septic jugular phlebitis
Headache	Vision disorders or eye pain	
Relapsing fever	Temporal arteritis (emboli)	
Rat-bite fever	SBE	
Chronic meningitis/encephalitis	Relapsing fever	
Malaria	Brain abscess	
Brucellosis	Takayasu's arteritis	
CNS neoplasms		
RMSF		

CMV, cytomegalovirus; CNS, central nervous system; FMF, familial Mediterranean fever; HIV, human immunodeficiency virus; PAN, periarteritis nodosa; RMSF, Rocky Mountain spotted fever; SBE, subacute bacterial endocarditis; SLE, systemic lupus erythematosus.

decreased appetite, malaise, etc. suggesting disseminated tuberculosis. Abdominal hepatosplenomegaly is not present with these lymphomas, and the only clue may be an unexpectedly elevated erythrocyte sedimentation rate (ESR), eosinophilia, or basophilia. The presumptive diagnosis is suggested by finding retroperitoneal node involvement by computed tomography (CT) or magnetic resonance imaging (MRI), and definitive diagnosis is by node biopsy (1,3–7).

HYPERNEPHROMAS

Another common malignancy that presents as an FUO is renal cell carcinoma, e.g., hypernephroma. Fever is an important feature of both the primary tumor and its metastases. Metastatic hypernephromas with multisystem involvement is a difficult diagnostic challenge, since most patients with hypernephroma will not have hematuria. A left varicocele, thrombocytosis, elevated alkaline phosphatase, and eosinophilia are diagnostic clues. Diagnosis is by tissue biopsy (2–5,10).

METASTATIC NEOPLASMS

Fever may be the sole presenting sign of early metastatic disease to the liver or central nervous system (CNS) in elderly patients. Small metastatic infiltrations in the liver are frequently clinically silent and present only with low-grade fevers. Physical findings are usually absent early and an unexplained elevation of the alkaline phosphatase, especially if accompanied by an increase in the ESR, should suggest the hepatic involvement. Metastatic disease to the CNS resulting in meningeal carcinomatosis or basilar infiltration of the brain, with or without hypothalamic involvement, occurs secondary to neoplasms that frequently metastasize to the brain, i.e., primary brain tumors, either in children or

those infected by HIV. These may be difficult to diagnose in the early stage in the absence of definite neurologic abnormalities (3,4,10).

HEPATIC AND PANCREATIC CARCINOMAS

Pancreatic carcinoma remains a difficult diagnosis and may be suggested by vague changes in mental status, hyperglycemia, vague abdominal discomfort, or abnormalities on gallium/indium scanning or CT or MRI (1–6).

Hepatomas often manifest wit hepatomegaly, hepatic bruit or rub, and the diagnosis is usually made by liver biopsy. Hepatomas are indistinguishable from metastatic liver disease with current imaging techniques. Laboratory clues include an elevated alkaline phosphatase, ESR, or alpha fetoprotein (AFP), and definitive diagnosis is by liver biopsy (31–33).

PRE-LEUKEMIAS

Pre-leukemic monocytic leukemia is the most frequent cause of FUO among the acute and chronic leukemias. Patients usually have vague and nonspecific symptoms in addition to prolonged fevers. On physical examination, sternal tenderness may be the only positive finding. Blast cells are not present in the peripheral blood smear, and diagnosis is by bone marrow aspirate (4–8,10).

ATRIAL MYXOMAS

Atrial myxomas may present with low-grade fevers, embolic phenomena, or heart murmur that may or may not be influenced by changes in position. Atrial myxomas mimic and are most frequently confused with subacute bacterial endocarditis (SBE). Although renal involvement is not a feature of atrial myxomas, the clinical presentation closely resembles SBE in many respects.

TABLE 180.8.   Physical Clues to Classical Fever of Unknown Origin

Skin hyperpigmentation	Sternal tenderness	Splenic abscess
Whipple disease	Metastatic carcinoma	SBE
Hypersensitivity vasculitis	Pre-leukemias	Brucellosis
Band keratopathy	Heart murmur	Salmonella
Adult Still disease	SBE	Epididymo-orchitis
Dry eyes	Atrial myxoma	Tuberculosis
Rheumatoid arthritis	Hepatomegaly	Lymphoma
SLE	Hepatoma	Brucellosis
Sjogren's syndrome	Relapsing fever	Leptospirosis
Watery eyes	Lymphomas	PAN
PAN	Metastatic carcinoma	EBV
Epistaxis	Alcoholic liver disease	Spinal tenderness
Relapsing fever	Granulomatous hepatitis	Subacute vertebral osteomyelitis
Psittacosis	Q fever	SBE
Conjunctivitis	Typhoid fever	Brucellosis
TB	Splenomegaly	Typhoid fever
Cat-scratch fever	Leukemia	Arthritis/joint pain
SLE	Lymphomas	FMF
Conjunctival suffusion	TB	Pseudo-gout
Leptospirosis	Brucellosis	Rat-bite fever
Relapsing fever	SBE	Rheumatoid arthritis
RMSF	CMV	SLE
Subconjunctival hemorrhage	EBV	Lyme disease
SBE	Rheumatoid arthritis	LGV
Trichinosis	Sarcoidosis	Whipple's disease
Uveitis	Psittacosis	Brucellosis
TB	Relapsing fever	Hyper IgD syndrome
Adult Still disease	Alcoholic liver disease	Calf tenderness
Sarcoidosis	Typhoid fever	RMSF
SLE	RMSF	Polymyositis
Lymphadenopathy	Kikuchi's disease	Tongue tenderness
Lymphomas	Trapezius tenderness	Relapsing fever
Cat-scratch fever	Subdiaphragmatic abscess	Thrombophlebitis
TB	Thigh tenderness	Psittacosis
LGV	Brucellosis	
EBV	Polymyositis	
CMV	Relative bradycardia	
Toxoplasmosis	Typhoid fever	
HIV	Malaria	
Adult Still disease	Leptospirosis	
Brucellosis	Psittacosis	
Whipple's disease	Central fever	
Pseudo-lymphoma	Drug fever	
Kikuchi's disease		

CMV, cytomegalovirus; EBV, Epstein-Barr virus; FMF, familial Mediterranean fever; LGV, lymphogranuloma venereum; PAN, periarteritis nodosa; RMSF, Rocky Mountain spotted fever; SBE, subacute bacterial endocarditis; SLE, systemic lupus erythematosus; TB, tuberculosis.

Polyclonal gammopathy on serum protein electrophoresis suggests atrial myxoma versus SBE, and an intracardiac mass is diagnostic by echocardiography (5,7,10).

Infectious Diseases

SUBACUTE BACTERIAL ENDOCARDITIS

SBE is less common as a cause of FUO because of the widespread practice of obtaining blood cultures in patients with prolonged fevers. Fastidious or unculturable organisms produce prolonged unexplained fevers, and brucellosis or Q fever are the commonest causes of culture-negative endocarditis presenting as FUO (1,3–10).

INTRAABDOMINAL AND PELVIC ABSCESSES

Perforation of the pelvic or gastrointestinal organs by procedures, surgery, or disease may result in abscess formation in various parts of the pelvis or abdomen. Location of the abscess depends upon the degree of intra-abdominal spillage and the location of the patient following organ perforation. Most commonly, periappendiceal or pericolonic collections are responsible for prolonged fevers. Subdiaphragmatic collections and intrahepatic abscesses are also responsible for prolonged fevers. The majority of these patients will have some, albeit subtle, physical findings suggesting intra-abdominal or pelvic pathology. Trapezius tenderness may be the only manifestation of a sub-diaphragmatic abscess. With CT or MRI, pelvic and intra-abdominal abscesses are less common causes of obscure and prolonged fevers. Splenic abscesses associated with endocarditis, typhoid fever or brucellosis are invariably part of multisystem infection. Perinephric abscesses may result from hematogenous dissemination from a distant source or from previous pyelonephritis. If there is not communication between the collecting system, urine may show only sterile pyuria. Intrarenal abscesses associated with medullary sponge kidney, medullary polycystic kidneys or stone disease, rarely cause diagnostic confusion as renal causes of FUO (2–4,15,30–33).

TABLE 180.9.   Laboratory Clues to Classical Fever of Unknown Origin

Monocytosis	Atypical lymphocytosis	Increased serum transaminases
TB	EBV mononucleosis	EBV mononucleosis
PAN	CMV	CMV
Temporal arteritis	Brucellosis	Q fever
CMV	Toxoplasmosis	Psittacosis
Sarcoidosis	Drug fever	Drug fever
Brucellosis	Thrombocytosis	Leptospirosis
SBE	Myeloproliferative diseases	Toxoplasmosis
SLE	TB	Brucellosis
Lymphomas	Carcinomas	Relapsing fever
Carcinomas	Lymphomas	Kikuchi's disease
Regional enteritis	Sarcoidosis	SPEP (Polyclonal gammopathy)
Myeloproliferative diseases	Vasculitis	Atrial myxoma
Eosinophilia	Temporal arteritis	Alcoholic cirrhosis
Trichinosis	Subacute osteomyelitis	Sarcoidosis
Lymphomas	Hypernephroma	Lymphomas
Drug fever	Rheumatoid factor	PAN
Addison's disease	SBE	HIV
PAN	Chronic active hepatitis	Takayasu's arteritis
Hypersensitivity vasculitis	Rheumatoid arthritis	Idiopathic granulomatosis
Hypernephroma	Malaria	Abnormal renal tests
Myeloproliferative diseases	Hypersensitivity vasculitis	SBE
Leukopenia	ESR (>100 mm/hr)	Renal TB
Miliary TB	Adult Still disease	PAN
Brucellosis	Temporal arteritis	Fabray's disease
SLE	Hypernephroma	Leptospirosis
Lymphomas	SBE	Brucellosis
Pre-leukemias	Drug fever	Lymphomas
Typhoid fever	Carcinomas	SLE
Kikuchi's disease	Lymphomas	Hypernephroma
Basophilia	Myeloproliferative diseases	HIV
Carcinomas	Abscesses	Malakoplakia
Lymphomas	Subacute osteomyelitis	Quantitative immunoglobulins
Pre-leukemias	Polymyositis	Hyper IgD syndrome
Myeloproliferative diseases	Hyper IgD syndrome	Thrombocytopenia
Lymphocytosis	Alkaline phosphatase	Leukemias
TB	Hepatoma	Lymphomas
EBV mononucleosis	Miliary TB	Myeloproliferative diseases
CMV	Lymphomas	Relapsing fever
Toxoplasmosis	EBV mononucleosis	EBV
Non-Hodgkins lymphoma	CMV	Drug fever
Lymphocytopenia	Adult Still disease	Vasculitis
HIV	Subacute thyroiditis	SLE
Whipple's disease	Temporal arteritis	HIV
Miliary TB	Hypernephroma	
SLE	PAN	
Sarcoidosis	Liver metastases	
	Granulomatous hepatitis	

CMV, cytomegalovirus; EBV, Epstein-Barr virus; ESR, erythrocyte sedimentation rate; HIV, human immunodeficiency virus; PAN, periarteritis nodosa; SBE, subacute bacterial endocarditis; SLE, systemic lupus erythematosus; TB, tuberculosis.

EXTRAPULMONARY TUBERCULOSIS

Disseminated tuberculosis is a less common cause of FUO than was seen previously, but tuberculous meningitis and miliary tuberculosis are not uncommon and remain difficult diagnostic problems. Renal tuberculosis may present with sterile pyuria, microscopic hematuria, or clinically with slowly progressive renal failure or epididymal orchitis in males. Diagnosis is suggested by microscopic hematuria/sterile pyuria in patients with simultaneous upper and lower tract involvement by IVP or CT or MRI. Renal tuberculosis is one of the few diseases that simultaneously affects the upper and lower urinary tracts. The upper tract changes resemble chronic pyelonephritis and the ureters are frequently scalloped, kinked, or have a corkscrew configuration. Diagnosis is by recovery of the organism in the urine (8,10).

Early tuberculous meningitis presents with subtle neurologic abnormalities, i.e., cognitive difficulties, mild headaches, difficulties in concentration, etc. with intermittent low-grade fevers. Cranial nerve abnormalities, unilateal or bilateral abducens nerve palsies are late findings in basilar meningitis due to tuberculosis. CT or MRI early is frequently unremarkable and cerebrospinal fluid (CSF) abnormalities may not be present. As tuberculous meningitis progresses without treatment, the CSF glucose will fall in concert with a rise in the CSF protein. The need for serial lumbar punctures cannot be underestimated in making the diagnosis of tuberculous meningitis to detect the protein glucose dissociation. Definitive diagnosis is by culture of the organism from the CSF. Not infrequently, the chest radiography is unremarkable in patients with CNS tuberculosis (1,8,10).

Miliary tuberculosis remains an important cause of FUO. Elderly patients and those on corticosteroids may silently disseminate previously quiescent disease and slowly become chronically ill with disseminated tuberculosis. Miliary tuberculosis has no

TABLE 180.10. Organ System Involvement in Classical Fever of Unknown Origin

CNS
  TB meningitis
  Sarcoid meningitis
  Tumors/hemorrhage
  Chronic encephalitis
  Brain abscess
  SBE
  Takayasu's arteritis
Neck
  Subacute thyroiditis
  Adult Still disease
  Dental abscess
  Relapsing mastoiditis
  Septic jugular phlebitis
  Kikuchi's disease
Lymph nodes
  Lymphomas
  Cat-scratch fever
  TB
  LGV
  EBV
  CMV
  Toxoplasmosis
  HIV
  Adult Still disease
  Brucellosis
  Whipple's disease
  Kikuchi's disease
Joints
  Whipple's disease
  Rat bite fever
  Brucellosis
  FMF
  Acute rheumatic fever
  LGV
  Hyper IgD syndrome
Small intestine
  FMF
  Lymphomas
  Regional enteritis
  Whipple's disease

Pelvis
  Pelvic abscess
  Pelvic tumors
No localizing signs
  Infected aortic aneurysm
  Dissecting aortic aneurysm
  SBE
  Miliary TB
  Brucellosis
  Q fever
  Colon cancer
  HIV
  Lymphomas
  Typhoid fever
  Drug fever
  Factitious fever
  Pre-leukemias
  Myeloproliferative diseases
Heart
  SBE
  Atrial myxomas
  Takayasu's arteritis
Kidneys
  Subacute endocarditis
  Hypernephroma
  Intra/perinephric abscess
  PAN
  Renal TB
  HIV
  Fabray's disease
  Lymphomas
  SLE
  Leptospirosis
  Brucellosis
  Malakoplakia
Spleen
  SBE
  Splenic abscess
  Lymphomas
  CMV
  HIV

Liver
  Metastatic carcinoma
  Hepatoma
  Cirrhosis
  Alcoholic hepatitis
  Liver abscess
  Miliary TB
  Sarcoidosis
  Giant hemangioma
  Granulomatous hepatitis
  Brucellosis
  Q fever
  EBV
  CMV
  Rat-bite fever
  Adult Still disease
  Drug fever
  Kikuchi's disease
  Idiopathic granulomatosis
Biliary tract
  Subacute cholangitis
  PAN
  Gallbladder wall abscess
Bone marrow
  Lymphomas
  Carcinomas
  Miliary TB
  Histoplasmosis
  Brucellosis
  Typhoid fever

CMV, cytomegalovirus; EBV, Epstein-Barr virus; FMF, familial Mediterranean fever; HIV, human immunodeficiency virus; LGV, lymphogranuloma venereum; PAN, periarteritis nodosa; SBE, subacute bacterial endocarditis; SLE, systemic lupus erythematosus; TB, tuberculosis.

localizing signs and the diagnosis may be made retrospectively by analysis of serial chest radiographs appreciating the gradual appearance of miliary infiltrates. Since miliary tuberculosis involves the reticular endothelial system, the diagnosis may be made by biopsy of the liver or bone marrow. Not infrequently, the only way to make a definite diagnosis is by empiric trial of antituberculous agents in a rapidly deteriorating patient with presumed miliary tuberculosis (34–37).

EPSTEIN-BARR VIRUS

Epstein-Barr virus (EBV), except in elderly patients, is a rare cause of FUO. Elderly patients with EBV usually present without prominent posterior cervical adenopathy or pharyngitis. Such patients may have hepatic tenderness or enlargement, but usually have mildly abnormal liver function tests. The combination of mild "hepatitis" in an elderly patient with atypical lymphocytosis should suggest EBV, and positive EBV serology is diagnostic (1,8,10).

TOXOPLASMOSIS

Toxoplasmosis in the immunocompetent adult with an FUO may present with a prolonged mono-like illness, or isolated lymphadenopathy. Except for adenopathy, there is a paucity of

physical findings sometimes with atypical lymphocytosis and mild liver abnormalities. Biopsy of the affected node is characteristic and a serologic diagnosis is by demonstrating increased IgM IFA anti-toxoplasmosis titers (1–6).

ENTERIC FEVERS

Enteric fever due to *Salmonella typhi* or other invasive *Salmonella* strains are associated with infection of the reticuloendothelial system and multisystem involvement.

Established typhoid fever may present with splenomegaly or spinal tenderness, but frequently there are no localizing signs with typhoid fever. The white blood cell count is normally decreased, the ESR is minimally, if at all, elevated, and the only clue may be a sustained fever with a pulse-temperature deficit. Eosinophilia is not a feature of the *Salmonella* enteric fevers. Febrile agglutinins to *Salmonella* may suggest the diagnosis, which may be confirmed by recovery of the organism from body fluids or bone marrow aspiration (10,37,38).

Other Infectious Causes

Any chronic infectious disease is capable of presenting as an FUO. Certain diseases such as malaria, Rocky Mountain spotted fever, Q fever, visceral leishmaniasis or histoplasmosis may present as FUOs in nonendemic areas where clinicians are not familiar with their protean manifestations. CMV mononucleosis may be a difficult diagnosis months after disease onset, when atypical lymphocytes are no longer present and the only diagnostic clue is a mild serum transaminase elevation. HIV may present with prolonged fevers, but with improved serological tests and increased index of suspicion, HIV should be considered as an important cause of prolonged fevers, even without opportunistic infections or neoplasms. Cat-scratch fever primarily occurs in children but may occur in adults. Tissue biopsy may be needed to rule out other causes of infectious or neoplastic node enlargement. Disseminated histoplasmosis, and to a lesser extent disseminated cryptococcosis, may mimic miliary tuberculosis. Parasitic diseases, fungi and rickettsia are rare causes of FUO. Subacute vertebral osteomyelitis in males is a difficult diagnosis to make if the preceding history of urinary tract infection is not appreciated. The organisms ascend from the urinary tract via Batson's plexus to the spine. Such patients may have fever, nonspecific low back pain, or complain of symptoms of disk disease or sciatica. Other infections including chronic sinusitis, brain abscesses or periapical dental abscesses, have infrequently been associated with FUO. Periapical dental abscesses are particularly difficult to diagnose since there is no local tenderness or pyorrhea, and the jaws appear normal on panoramic film of the jaw. Diagnosis may be made by doing a local gallium scan of the jaws, which may reveal the periapical collection. Dental abscesses may metastasize to the brain, presenting as a brain tumor that at craniotomy proves to be a brain abscess (1,10,39,40).

Rheumatologic Causes

PERIARTERITIS NODOSA
Periarteritis nodosa is a mid-size vasculitis characterized by multisystem involvement. Abdominal pain, headache, or arthritic complaints are common. The constellation of hypertension, peripheral eosinophilia, with a history of acalculous cholecystitis, or epididymo-orchitis, should suggest the diagnosis. Renal insufficiency, heart failure or stroke in someone with hepatitis B surface antigenemia should suggest periarteritis nodosa (1,10).

Granulomatous arteritis of the temporal arteries is a common cause of FUO in the elderly. Patients often complain of visual disturbances, vague headache or stiffness/myalgias. Tenderness over the temporal arteries is not unusual, but complaints of pain over the angle of the jaw, when present, may provide a clue to the diagnosis, and characteristically the ESR is very rapid, i.e., 100 mm/hour or less. Definitive diagnosis is by temporal artery biopsy of the involved segments (41,45).

VASCULITIS
Many vasculitides produce intermittent or prolonged fevers. Hypersensitivity vasculitis and Takayasu's arteritis are infrequent but important causes of FUO. Multisystem organ involvement is characteristic and diagnosis is made by tissue biopsy.

Kikuchi disease is necrotizing adenitis with fever and leukopenia that usually occurs in young women. Necrotizing mediastinal and retroperitoneal adenopathy has been reported, as has splenomegaly in Kikuchi disease presenting as an FUO (46–48).

RHEUMATOID ARTHRITIS
Rheumatoid arthritis presenting as an FUO in the elderly can be a difficult diagnosis because of the absence of joint involvement or elevated rheumatoid factors. Prolonged fevers and rheumatic complaints may be the only manifestation of late onset rheumatoid arthritis in aged individuals. SLE is only a rare cause of FUO today (3,10).

ADULT STILL DISEASE
Still disease is one type of juvenile rheumatoid arthritis (JRA). Adult Still disease remains an important cause of FUO in adults. Patients usually present with hepatosplenomegaly and evanescent truncal "salmon colored" rash, with or without the Koebner phenomenon, and minimal joint or eye findings. Rheumatoid factors are negative and the only clue to the diagnosis may be double quotidian fever (1,49,50).

Other Causes

A variety of other diseases rarely present as FUOs, including dissecting aortic aneurysms, occult hematomas, subacute thyroiditis, hyperthyroidism, hyperparathyroidism, Fabry's disease, cyclic neutropenia. In addition, multiple recurrent pulmonary emboli may present a difficult diagnostic problem in the patient with prolonged obscure fevers. The diagnosis is suggested by the appropriate setting, such as an immobilized patient who may or may not have wheezing. The diagnosis may be suspected by vague chest discomfort or shortness of breath, and the only laboratory clues may be an increase in the ESR or fibrin split products (3,10).

ALCOHOLIC LIVER DISEASE
Alcoholic liver disease is a common cause of prolonged fevers. Cirrhosis and particularly alcoholic hepatitis are frequently missed causes of prolonged fevers in the patient with alcoholic liver disease. Alcoholic hepatitis is suggested by mildly abnormal liver function tests and a white count of greater than 10,000 cu mm^3. Definitive diagnosis is by liver biopsy (10,31,51).

GRANULOMATOUS HEPATITIS
Granulomatous hepatitis is a diagnosis of exclusion and is characterized by normochromic-normocytic anemia, occasional liver enlargement, and mildly abnormal liver function tests. Liver biopsy shows granuloma formation which also occurs with regional enteritis, sarcoidosis, lymphoma, histoplasmosis or tuberculosis in the FUO differential (1,10).

SARCOIDOSIS
Sarcoidosis is a disease not characterized by fever. However, sarcoidosis may be associated with fever if there is bilateral hilar adenopathy with or without erythema nodosum, uveal tract-parotid involvement (Heerfordt syndrome), or hepatic granuloma infiltration. On liver biopsy specimens, sarcoid granulomata are numerous and accompanied by many giant cells. This is in contrast to tuberculosis where giant cells and granulomata are few. If sarcoidosis is accompanied by fevers in the absence of these clinical conditions, co-existing tuberculosis should be suspected (3–6,10).

FAMILIAL MEDITERRANEAN FEVER
Familial Mediterranean fever is characterized by intermittent pleuritic or abdominal pain, with or without join pain or headache. Unexplained persistent chest pain or abdominal pain with fever in individuals of western European Mediterranean ancestry should suggest the diagnosis (5,6,10).

REGIONAL ENTERITIS
Vague abdominal pain and persistent low-grade fevers are the usual presentations of FUO in patients with regional enteritis. Malabsorption or a right lower quadrant mass are late features. Fever may precede gastrointestinal symptoms and the ESR is usually elevated (2–5).

WHIPPLE'S DISEASE

Patients with Whipple's disease usually have knee or ankle joint symptoms and changes in mentation are also common. Skin hyperpigmentation and adenopathy are variably present. The majority of patients have low carotene serum levels and diagnosis is by periodic acid-Schiff-positive material on small intestine biopsy (1–10).

HYPERGAMMAGLOBULINEMIA D PERIODIC FEVER SYNDROME

Hypergammaglobulinemia D syndrome presents as periodic prolonged febrile episodes with abdominal pain, arthralgias, cervical adenopathy and splenomegaly (children). Large joints are usually affected and some patients have an erythematous extremity rash. The ESR and white cell count are elevated in addition to serum immunoglobulin D and A levels. Serum immunoglobulin D levels are elevated in sarcoidosis, Hodgkin's lymphoma, HIV infection, and tuberculosis, but are very highly elevated in the hyperimmunoglobulinemia D syndrome (100 units/mL, and greater). This syndrome is benign and is a problem of clinical recognition, since it may be confused with many diseases.

FACTITIOUS FEVER

Patients with factitious fever may present as FUO, but with the advent of electronic thermometers, factitious temperature elevations are less common. Patients with factitious fevers are usually young women in the medical field. Factitious fevers are usually high and are not accompanied by an appropriate pulse response. The single best way to determine the true temperature of a patient with a suspected factitious fever is to measure the temperature of a recently voided urine, which closely approximates core temperature. Some individuals have higher core temperatures that are 1°F to 2°F above normal, without any physical or laboratory abnormalities, just as some individuals have lower than normal temperatures. Individuals with higher than normal temperatures should not be regarded as abnormal. Such individuals should be reassured because they are usually preoccupied with their apparent fevers (28,52–55).

DRUG FEVERS

An important cause of FUO is drug fever. Most drugs are potentially sensitizing and therefore may cause fever as the sole manifestation of their hypersensitivity reaction. It is a popular misconception that antibiotics are primarily responsible for drug fevers. Although antibiotics, particularly sulfonamides and the β-lactam antibiotics remain important causes of drug fever, antiarrythmics, pain medications, diuretics, sulfa-containing stool softeners, sleep medications, antiseizure medications, antithyroid medications, and tranquilizers are more frequent causes of drug fever. The temperature range with a drug fever is variable, but if the temperature is greater than 102°F, a pulse-temperature deficit is usually apparent. Patients with drug fever often have low-grade eosinophilia, usually within the normal ranges. Eosinophils are commonly present, but infrequently present above normal elevations of serum transaminases or alkaline phosphatase. The diagnosis of drug fever is made on the basis of excluding other causes of fever and withdrawing the potentially offending drug. The patient with drug fever does not necessarily give a history of allergic reactions to medications, and appears to be surprisingly well. Patients may be on medications for many years without developing hypersensitivity reactions to their medications. It should never be assumed that because the patient has been on a particular medication for an extended time, that it is not the cause of the drug fever. Patients occasionally develop hypersensitivity reactions to fumes or toxin exposures. Fume fevers are exceedingly rare, but have been reported to cause FUO (10,56,57).

LABORATORY TESTS

The history and physical examination should suggest the appropriate diagnostic direction of laboratory testing. Routine laboratory tests may provide important clues and should be obtained on all patients with FUO. The hemogram should include a complete white cell count with differential and platelet count. Leukopenia may suggest miliary tuberculosis, brucellosis, lupus, or lymphoma. A monocytosis may be the initial clue to cytomegalovirus infection, tuberculosis, brucellosis, lymphoma, regional arteritis, or carcinoma. Eosinophilia in a patient with FUO suggests lymphoma, trichinosis, drug fever, or periarteritis nodosa; basophilia almost invariably points to carcinoma or lymphoma in patients with prolonged fevers. Chronic lymphocytosis suggests cytomegalovirus or EBV mononucleosis, tuberculosis, or toxoplasmosis.

The ESR is a sensitive although nonspecific test, but is diagnostically useful in combination with other clinical or laboratory abnormalities. In a patient with FUO and eosinophilia, an ESR of 2 mm/hour would immediately suggest the possibility of trichinosis. A rapid ESR (i.e., 100 mm/hour or greater) in a patient with FUO suggests drug fever, adult Still disease, giant cell arteritis, subacute endocarditis, abscess, osteomyelitis, carcinoma, lymphoma, or hyperimmunoglobulinemia D syndrome. Moderate elevations of ESR are seen with most disease entities causing FUO. The absence of an elevated ESR does not rule out the presence of infectious, rheumatic, or neoplastic disease as a cause of prolonged fever.

Liver function tests are particularly important as part of the workup in a patient with FUO because so many of the diseases causing FUO are characterized by hepatic involvement. Elevation of the alkaline phosphatase out of proportion to serum transaminases suggests an infiltrative or obstructive process, and may be the only clue to adult Still disease, subacute thyroiditis, giant cell arteritis, or periarteritis nodosa. An isolated, modest elevation of the alkaline phosphatase is a normal finding in healthy elderly adults. Elevations of the serum transaminases, with minimal or no elevations of the serum alkaline phosphatase suggests infectious disease of the liver, particularly CMV or EBV mononucleosis, Q fever, or psittacosis, but is also common with drug fever. The serum protein electrophoresis may provide a clue to lymphoma with an isolated elevation of the α_2-globulin fraction. A diffuse polyclonal gammopathy in a patient with an FUO would suggest atrial myxoma, sarcoidosis, lymphoma, or HIV infection. Fibrin split products may be the only clue to multiple recurrent pulmonary emboli, not detectable by scanning methods or angiography (1–10).

OTHER DIAGNOSTIC MODALITIES

The naproxen (Naprosyn) test has been used to differentiate malignant from benign fevers. This simple and safe, noninvasive test differentiates neoplastic from infectious fever. Therapeutic agents can be used diagnostically in selected cases to support or confirm the diagnosis, when diagnosis is not possible by other means. Patients with drug fevers can only be diagnosed with certainty by discontinuation of the drug. Temperature elevations due to drug fever will return to nearly normal within 72 hours if the sensitizing medication is discontinued (58–60) (Fig. 180.1).

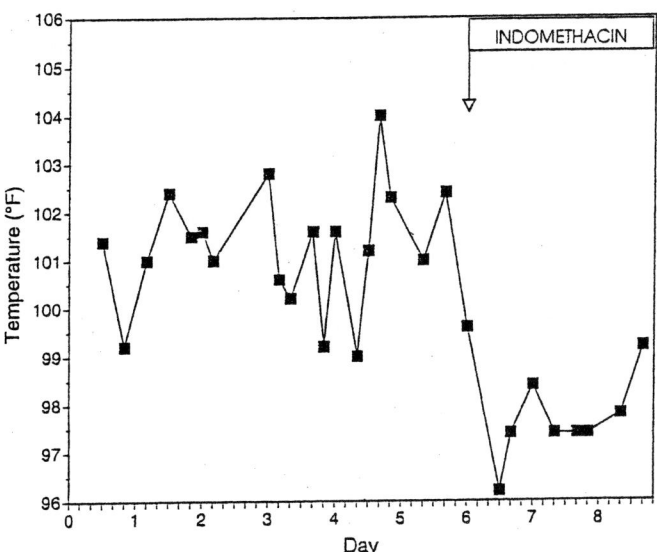

Figure 180.1. Defervescence of fever with Indocin in an 81-year-old man with a FUO due to metastatic colon cancer. (From Reme P, Cunha BA. Indocin and the naprosyn test in fever of unknown origin (FUO). *Infect Dis Pract* 2000;24:32, with permission.)

RADIOGRAPHIC IMAGING TESTS

Noninvasive imaging techniques have made the diagnosis of many cryptic processes presenting with prolonged fevers possible. Abdominal ultrasonography has been useful in detecting intrahepatic, intrasplenic, and intra-perinephric mass lesions. Percutaneous or transesophageal echocardiography has been useful in detecting vegetations and intracardiac myxomas. CT and MRI have been most sensitive in detecting intracranial, intraabdominal and pelvic pathology. CT and MRI are the best way to detect retroperitoneal lymphomas or subacute vertebral osteomyelitis. The diagnosis of intraabdominal/pelvic abscesses has been greatly improved by CT and MRI and fewer of these diseases present now as FUOs. Gallium and indium scans are useful in detecting abscesses or malignancies, but these scans are associated with problems of false-positive and false-negative findings and should be interpreted with caution. Gallium scans should be used early in the diagnostic workup, and abnormal findings should be confirmed by CT and MRI. Steroids and a variety of antibiotics may result in false-negative results of gallium scans (31,32,39,40,61,62).

TISSUE BIOPSY

Invasive techniques usually provide the definitive diagnosis in many patients with FUO. Because most of the neoplastic and infectious diseases that result in FUO invade the reticuloendothelial system, liver biopsy, and bone marrow biopsy are important diagnostic procedures in patients with clinical or laboratory involvement of these organ systems. Liver biopsy may be the only way to make a diagnosis of miliary tuberculosis, or metastatic carcinoma, if the deposits are small and below the resolution of liver or spleen on gallium and indium scanning. Bone marrow biopsy may provide the diagnosis in patients with lymphoma, miliary tuberculosis, or typhoid fever. Small bowel biopsy is indicated in patients with the possibility of intestinal lymphoma or Whipple's disease. Patients with findings suggesting a CNS source should have a lumbar puncture, which may

provide clues to the presence of meningeal carcinomatosis, HIV infection, CNS lymphoma, or basilar meningitis due to tuberculosis or sarcoidosis. If temporal arteritis is a reasonable diagnostic possibility, biopsy of the affected segments of the artery is usually diagnostic. A trial of low-dose steroids would support the diagnosis of giant cell arteritis where there is shoulder stiffness and rapid ESR, when temporal biopsy is not possible (10,12,63–67).

THERAPY FOR FEVERS OF UNKNOWN ORIGIN

Therapeutic trials of antibiotics for FUOs are to be discouraged. True culture-negative endocarditis is uncommon, and an empirical trial of antimicrobial therapy should not be given to patients with a fever and heart murmur. Extrapulmonary tuberculosis may be difficult to diagnose, and clinically silent dissemination may occur in patients taking steroids or in elderly patients. Therefore, because miliary tuberculosis and CNS tuberculosis are frequently difficult to diagnose, an empirical trial of antituberculous therapy may be lifesaving (68,69).

REFERENCES

1. Petersdorf RG, Beeson PB. Fever of unexplained origin: report on 100 cases. *Medicine (Baltimore)* 1961;40:1–30.
2. Louria DB. Fever of unknown etiology. *Del Med J* 1971;43:343–348.
3. Keefer CS, Leard SE. *Prolonged and perplexing fevers.* Boston, Little Brown, 1955:1–248.
4. Larson EB, Featherstone HJ, Petersdorf RG. Fever of undetermined origin. Diagnosis and follow-up of 105 cases, 1970–1980. *Medicine* 1982;61:269–292.
5. Brusch JL, Weinstein L. Fever of unknown origin. *Med Clin North Am* 1988;72:1247–1261.
6. Wolf SM, Fauci SS, Dale DC. Unusual etiologies of fever and their evaluation. *Annu Rev Med* 1975;26:277–279.
7. Knockaert DC, Vanneste LJ, Vanneste SB, Bobbaers HJ. Fever of unknown origin in the 1980s: an update of the diagnostic spectrum. *Arch Intern Med* 1992;152:51–55.
8. Kazanjian PH. Fever of unknown origin. Review of 86 patients treated in community hospitals. *Clin Infect Dis* 1992;15:968–973.
9. DiNubile MJ. Acute fevers of unknown origin. A plea for restraint. *Arch Intern Med* 1993;153:2525–2526.
10. Cunha BA. Fever of unknown origin. *Infect Dis Clin North Am* 1996;10:111–128.
11. Bissuel F, Leport C, Perrone C, et al. Fever of unknown origin in HIV-infected patients: a critical analysis of a retrospective series of 57 cases. *J Intern Med* 1994;236:529–535.
12. Engels E, Marks PW, Kazanjian P. Usefulness of bone marrow evaluation of unexplained fever in patients infected with human immunodeficiency virus. *Clin Infect Dis* 1995;21:427–428.
13. Lambertucci JR, Rayes AA, Nunes F, et al. Fever of undetermined origin in patients with acquired immunodeficiency syndrome in Brazil: report on 55 cases. *Rev Inst Med Trop Sao Paulo* 1999;41:27–32.
14. Cunha BA. Fever of unknown origin in HIV/AIDS patients. *Drugs Today* 1999;35:429–434.
15. Pizzo PA, Lovejoy FH, Smith DH. Prolonged fever in children: review of 100 cases. *Pediatrics* 1975;55:468–473.
16. Lohr JA, Hendley JO. Prolonged fever of unknown origin: a record of experiences with 54 childhood patients. *Clin Pediatr* 1977;16:768–773.
17. Gartner JC Jr. Fever of unknown origin. *Adv Pediatr Infect Dis* 1992;7:1–24.
18. Majeed HA. Differential diagnosis of fever of unknown origin in children. *Curr Opin Rheumatol* 2000;12:439–444.
19. Akpede GO, Akenzua GI. Aetiology and management of children with acute fever of unknown origin. *Paediatr Drugs* 2001;3:169–193.
20. Akpede GO, Akenzua GI. Management of children with prolonged fever of unknown origin and difficulties in the management of fever of unknown origin in children in developing countries. *Paediatr Drugs* 2001;3:247–262.
21. Esposito AL, Gleckman R. Fever of unknown origin in the elderly. *J Am Geriatr Soc* 1978;26:498–505.
22. Cunha BA. Fever of unknown origin in the elderly. *Geriatrics* 1982;37:27–44.
23. Kauffman CA, Jones PG. Diagnosing fever of unknown origin in older patients. *Geriatrics* 1984;39:46–51.
24. Knockaert DC, Vanneste LJ, Bobbears HJ. Fever of unknown origin in elderly patients. *J Am Geriatr Soc* 1993;41:1187–1192.
25. Cunha BA. Commentary: FUO in the elderly. *Infect Dis Clin Pract* 1993;2:380–383.

26. Sharma BK, Kumari S, Varma SC. Prolonged undiagnosed fever in Northern India. *Trop Geogr Med* 1992;44:32–36.
27. Knockaert DC, Vanneste LJ, Bobbaers HJ. Recurrent or episodic fever of unknown origin: review of 45 cases and survey of the literature. *Medicine* 1993; 72:184–196.
28. Weinstein L. Clinically benign fever of unknown origin: a personal retrospective. *Rev Infect Dis* 1985;7:692–699.
29. Sen P, Louria DB. Noninvasive and diagnostic procedures and laboratory methods. In: Murray HW (eds). *FUO: fever of undetermined origin.* Mount Kisco, NY: Futura Publishing, 1983:159–190.
30. Mitchell DP, Hanes TE, Hoyumpa AM Jr, Shenker S. Fever of unknown origin: assessment of the value of percutaneous liver biopsy. *Arch Intern Med* 1977;137(8):1001–1004.
31. Quinn MJ, Sheedy PF II, Stephen DH, Hattery RR. Computed tomography of the abdomen in evaluation of patients with fever of unknown origin. *Radiology* 1980;136:407–411.
32. Rowland MD, Del Bene VE. Use of body computed tomography to evaluate fever of unknown origin. *J Infect Dis* 1987;156:408–409.
33. Blockmans D, Knockaert D, Maes A, et al. Clinical value of [(18)F] fluoro-deoxyglucose positron emission tomography for patients with fever of unknown origin. *Clin Infect Dis* 2001;32:191–196.
34. Harris HW, Menitove S. Miliary tuberculosis. In: Schlossberg D (ed). *Tuberculosis*, ed 3. New York: Springer-Verlag 1994:233–245.
35. Zedtwitz-Liebenstein K, Podesser B, Peck-Radosavljevic M, et al. Intestinal tuberculosis presenting as fever of unknown origin in a heart transplant patient. *Infection* 1999;27:289–290.
36. Collazos J, Guerra E, Mayo J, Martinez E. Tuberculosis as a cause of recurrent fever of unknown origin. *J Infect* 2000;41:269–272.
37. Volk EE, Miller ML, Kirkley BA, Washington JA. The diagnostic usefulness of bone marrow cultures in patients with fever of unknown origin. *Am J Clin Pathol* 1998;110:150–153.
38. Rubin RH, Weinstein L. *Salmonellosis: microbiologic, pathologic, and clinical features.* New York: Stratton International Medical Book, 1977.
39. Knockaert DC, Mortelmans LA, De Roo MC, Bobbaers HJ. Clinical value of gallium-67 scintigraphy in evaluation of fever of unknown origin. *Clin Infect Dis* 1994;18:601–605.
40. Peters AM. Nuclear medicine imaging in fever of unknown origin. *Q J Nucl Med* 1999;43:61–73.
41. Goodman BW. Temporal arteritis. *Am J Med* 1979;67:839–852.
42. Wu YJJ, Martin BR, Ong K, et al. Takayasu's arteritis presenting as a cause of fever of unknown origin. *Am J Med* 1989;87:476–477.
43. Ghose MK, Shensa S, Lerner PI. Arteritis of the aged (giant cell arteritis) and fever of unexplained origin. *Am J Med* 1976;60:429–436.
44. Fauchald P, Rygvold O, Oipstese B. Temporal arteritis and polymyalgia rheumatica. *Ann Intern Med* 1972;77:845–852.
45. Uthman IW, Bizri AR, Hajj Ali RA. et al. Takayasu's arteritis presenting as fever of unknown origin: report of two cases and literature review. *Semin Arthritis Rheum* 1999;28:280–285.
46. Bailey EM, Klein NC, Cunha BA. Kikuchi's disease with liver dysfunction presenting as fever of unknown origin. *Lancet* 1989;2:986.
47. Norris AH, Krasinskas AM, Salhany KE, Glickman SJ. Kikuchi-Fujimoto disease: a benign cause of fever and lymphadenopathy. *Am J Med* 1996;101:401–405.
48. Pearl D, Strauchen JA. Kikuchi's disease as a cause of fever of unknown origin. *N Engl J Med* 1989;320:1147–1148.
49. Pouchot J, Sampalis JS, Beaudet F, et al. Adult Still's disease: manifestations, disease course, and outcome in 62 patients. *Medicine* 1991;70:118–136.
50. Calabro JJ, Marchesano JM. Juvenile rheumatoid arthritis. *N Engl J Med* 1967;277:746–749.
51. Anceno-Reyes RI. Acute fevers of unknown origin. *Arch Intern Med* 1994;154: 2253–2254.
52. Murray HW. Factitious or fraudulent fever. In: Murray HW (ed). *FUO: fever of undetermined origin.* Mount Kisco, NY: Futura Publishing, 1983:87–108.
53. Petersdorf RG, Bennett IL. Factitious fever. *Ann Intern Med* 1957;46:1039–1062.
54. Rumans LW, Vosti KL. Factitious and fraudulent fever. *Am J Med* 1978;65:745–755.
55. Sawari AR, Mackowiak PA. Factitious fever. *Curr Clin Topics Infect Dis* 1997; 17:88–94.
56. Cunha BA. Drug fever. *Postgrad Med* 1986;80:123–129.
57. Johnson DH, Cunha BA. Drug fever. *Infect Dis Clin North Am* 1996;10:85–91.
58. Chang JC, Gross HM. Utility of naproxen in the differential diagnosis of fever of undetermined origin in patients with cancer. *Am J Med* 1984;76:597–603.
59. Reme P, Cunha BA. Indocin and the naprosyn test in fever of unknown origin (FUO). *Infect Dis Pract* 2000;24:32.
60. Chang JC, Hawley BH. Neutropenic fever of undetermined origin (N-FUO): why not use the naproxen test? *Cancer Invest* 1995;13:448–450.
61. Hilson AJW, Maisey MN. Gallium-67 scanning in pyrexia of unknown origin. *BMJ* 1979;II:1330–1331.
62. Datz FL, Anderson CE, Ahluwalia R, et al. The efficacy of indium-111 polyclonal IgG for the detection of infection and inflammation. *J Nucl Med* 1994;35: 74–83.
63. Mitchell DP, Hanes TE, Hoyumpa AM Jr, Schenker S. Fever of unknown origin: assessment of the value of percutaneous liver biopsy. *Arch Intern Med* 1977;137:1001–1004.
64. Kilby JM, Margues MB, Jaye DL, et al. The yield of bone marrow biopsy and culture compared with blood culture in the evaluation of HIV-infected patients for mycobacterial and fungal infections. *Am J Med* 1998;104:123–128.
65. Garcia-Ordonez MA, Colmenero JD, Jimenez-Onate F, et al. Diagnostic usefulness of percutaneous liver biopsy in HIV-infected patients with fever of unknown origin. *J Infect* 1999;38:94–98.
66. Benito N, Nunez A. de Gorgolas M, et al. Bone marrow biopsy in the diagnosis of fever of unknown origin in patients with acquired immunodeficiency syndrome. *Arch Intern Med* 1997;157:1577–1580.
67. Rajwanshi A, Gupta D, Kapoor S, et al. Fine needle aspiration biopsy of the spleen in pyrexia of unknown origin. *Cytopathology* 1999;10:195–200.
68. Cunha BA. Antipyretic therapy in infectious disease. *Antibiotics Clinicians* 2000;4:60–62.
69. Cunha BA. Fever of unknown origin. In: Schlossberg D (Ed). *Current therapy of infectious disease*, 2nd ed. Philadelphia: Elsevier Science, 2000.

CHAPTER 181
Toxic Shock Syndrome

Patrick M. Schlievert and Aristides P. Assimacopoulos

HISTORY

Staphylococcal toxic shock syndrome (TSS) is an acute multisystem illness characterized by fever, hypotension, erythematous rash, desquamation of the skin on recovery, and a variable multiorgan component. The illness has been reported in the literature sporadically since 1927, principally as staphylococcal scarlet fever, but it was brought to the attention of the medical community as a major entity in 1978 by Todd and coworkers (1), who also named the illness. A TSS-like illness has also been described that is associated with group A streptococcal infection (2,3). Since these articles were published, a large number of articles have provided additional clinical information, epidemiologic risk factors, and determinants of pathogenicity in a relatively short time. Both staphylococcal TSS and streptococcal TSS are discussed in this chapter.

CHARACTERISTICS OF THE PATHOGENS

Staphylococcus aureus is a gram-positive, coagulase-positive coccus that grows in clusters and causes numerous infections, ranging from mild to life threatening. The organisms are facultative anaerobes. It is now generally accepted that staphylococcal TSS is caused by certain strains of *S. aureus*; coagulase-negative strains do not cause TSS. Numerous studies indicate that the superantigen (SAg) TSS toxin-1 (TSST-1) is the cause of all or nearly all menstrual cases and approximately half of nonmenstrual cases (4,5). The toxin, which was formerly known as pyrogenic exotoxin type C and enterotoxin F, is capable of inducing TSS symptoms in experimental animals, notably rabbits (4–7). It has been shown that the SAgs enterotoxins B and C are the causes of nearly 50% of nonmenstrual cases (6). Other enterotoxins, of which there are now A to Q serotypes, may also rarely cause the illness. *S. aureus* strains that make TSST-1 do not make enterotoxin B (SEB) but may simultaneously express SEA or C. The mechanism for this toxin exclusion is not known.

The majority of streptococcal TSS is caused by group A streptococcal strains, but groups B, C, F, and G occasionally cause the illness. Most of the group A streptococcal strains associated with TSS belong to M protein types 1 and 3, but other M types may also be associated (8,9). Group A streptococci (*Streptococcus pyogenes*) are β-hemolytic, catalase-negative, gram-positive cocci that grow in chains and cause large numbers of mucous membrane (pharyngitis) and skin (impetigo) acute inflammatory infections. The organisms also cause invasive infections (including streptococcal TSS) and delayed sequelae, including rheumatic fever, acute glomerulonephritis, and erythema nodosum. Group A streptococci are aerotolerant anaerobes and are serotyped on the basis of cell surface, antiphagocytic M proteins, of which 80 types have been identified. Large numbers of nontypeable organisms also occur; these organisms presumably have M proteins, but they have not yet been characterized. Immunity against group A streptococcus depends on development of opsonic antibodies against M protein.

Group A streptococci that cause TSS have been associated with production of the SAgs streptococcal pyrogenic exotoxins (SPEs, scarlet fever toxins), notably types A and C but also type B (which has been characterized as a cysteine protease, and whose superantigenicity is debatable) and type F (mitogenic factor, which has been characterized as a DNase and whose superantigenicity is debatable), streptococcal superantigen, and streptococcal mitogenic exotoxin Z (8–12).

SAgs are a large family of proteins, secreted by both *S. aureus* (also *S. intermedius*) and group A streptococci (also other groups of β-hemolytic streptococci), that share biologic activity and in many instances amino acid sequence similarity (13–15). All these toxins (TSST-1; SEs serotypes A, B, Cn, D-Q; and the SPE serotypes A, B, C, F, G-M, streptococcal superantigen, and streptococcal mitogenic exotoxin Z) are relatively low molecular weight (20,000 to 30,000 kD), simple proteins that are secreted into the culture medium either in exponential (such as SEA, K, and Q) or in the late logarithmic (such as TSST-1, SEB, SEC, SPE A, and SPE C) phase of growth, though SPE B is primarily made during late stationary phase, consistent with it being a cysteine protease). The toxins induce fever, enhance host susceptibility to lethal endotoxin shock, nonspecifically stimulate T lymphocyte proliferation (superantigenicity) (16), and induce sustained release of cytokines from both macrophages and T lymphocytes as a consequence of superantigenicity. The T lymphocyte proliferation results in sufficient interferon γ release to suppress immunoglobulin synthesis in experimental animals and amplify delayed hypersensitivity, which may explain the erythematous rash, erythrophagocytosis, and failure to develop neutralizing antibodies seen in TSS illnesses. The shared properties of the toxins are summarized in Table 181.1. The staphylococcal enterotoxins have the additional capacity, not shared with other SAgs, to induce vomiting and diarrhea by an unknown mechanism after oral administration. The scarlet fever toxins are also more capable than other SAgs of inducing myocardial damage. Finally, TSST-1 has the unique property of being able both to cross mucosal surfaces more efficiently than other SAgs, which may explain its menstrual association, and reactivate arthritis in experimental animals (17,18).

Because the SAgs have in common many biologic activities, it may be expected that they share structural similarities. The crystal structures of all known SAgs thus far evaluated (TSST-1, SEA-E, and numerous streptococcal SAgs) indicate the three dimensional structures of the toxins are highly similar (13,14). The prototype SAg structure is illustrated by that of TSST-1 (19) shown in Fig. 181.1. The toxins have a short N-terminal α-helix of amino acids followed by a barrel of β strands that compose domain B. Domain B is connected to a wall of β strands in domain A by a central diagonal α-helix. The enterotoxins have a loop of amino acids (referred to as a cystine loop) that is not present in TSST-1 and appears to participate in emetic activity. Minor other differences in structure are seen in some of the toxins.

TABLE 181.1. Shared Properties of Toxic Shock Syndrome-Associated Superantigens
Biochemical
Relatively low molecular weight (20,000–30,000), simple proteins, secreted mainly in logarithmic or late logarithmic phase of growth.
Relatively resistant to heat, protease, and desiccation treatment
Biologic
Pyrogenicity (interleukin 1 and tumor necrosis factor α)
Enhancement of susceptibility to endotoxin shock (interferon γ and tumor necrosis factor α) and cellular killing (contribute to hypotension?)
T lymphocyte mitogenicity (superantigenicity) which results in: B cell immunosuppression
Rash
Erythrophagocytosis
Lymphokine release (tumor necrosis factor β, interferon γ, interleukin 2) (contribute to hypotension)
Induction of monokine release from macrophages (tumor necrosis factor α, interleukin 1) (contribute to hypotension)
Alteration of liver clearance function

All of the toxins have been cloned and sequenced (13,14). With two exceptions (SPE G and streptococcal mitogenic exotoxin Z), the SAg genes are variable traits, being present in some strains and not in others. Many of the streptococcal SAgs, including SPEs A and C, and SEA and E are phage-encoded, SED is plasmid-encoded, and the remainder of the toxins, including TSST-1, SEB, and SEC, are present in the bacterial genome on mobile elements referred to as pathogenicity islands (20).

Several animal models for the study of TSS have been developed, mostly in rabbits, and observations indicate that SAgs have the ability to induce TSS illness (7,21–23). In one type of experiment, isogenic pairs of *S. aureus* strains that differ only in ability to express SAgs were used to examine toxin role in TSS (21). Only the toxin positive organism was capable of inducing TSS symptoms. In another set of experiments, several members of the SAg family were implanted subcutaneously in miniosmotic pumps designed to release toxin during a 7-day period (7,22,23). On administration of approximately 100 to 200 ug of toxin to a 1- to 2-kg rabbit, typical TSS symptoms were seen that culminated in

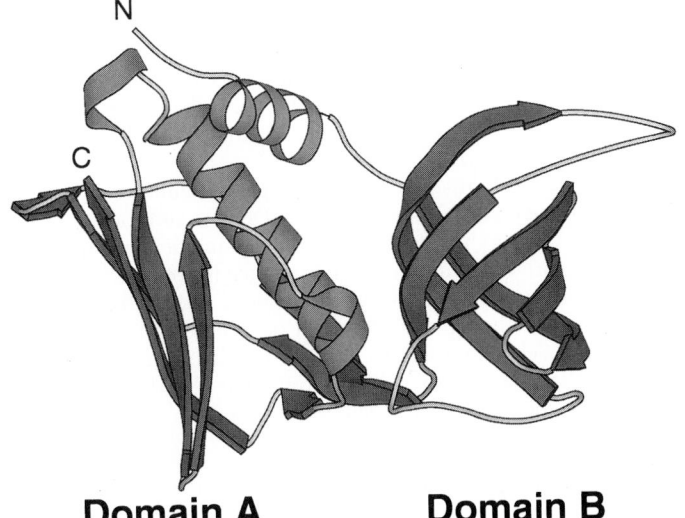

Domain A   **Domain B**

Figure 181.1. Ribbon diagram of the three dimensional structure of toxic shock syndrome toxin-1. The α carbon backbone is shown.

death. It appeared that continuous exposure to the toxins for a period of days was necessary for the development of TSS symptoms, because single injections of up to 1.5 mg per animal often did not produce TSS manifestations. The need for continuous exposure to toxin is consistent with the observation menstrual TSS most often begins on the third or fourth day of menstruation, despite the fact that numbers of *S. aureus* increase vaginally early in menstruation. Finally, studies with viable group A streptococci administered to rabbits indicate that immunity against SPE A can protect the animals from both streptococcal TSS and necrotizing fasciitis due to M1 and M3 organisms (23). However, SPE A alone did not have the ability to cause necrotizing fasciitis despite having the capacity to cause TSS. It appeared that other streptococcal factors were required to induce soft tissue necrosis.

EPIDEMIOLOGY

The epidemiology of TSS has been thoroughly examined and will be addressed by reviewing available studies of *S. aureus* and *Streptococcus pyogenes* separately. Nearly all of the epidemiologic studies of staphylococcal TSS were conducted in the 1980s. Cases of staphylococcal TSS can be categorized as menstruation-associated cases and nonmenstrual cases. A large proportion of cases recognized in the early 1980s were menstruation associated and related to use of high absorbency tampons. With changes in the tampon industry and the recognition of more subsets of nonmenstrual TSS, menstrual cases have both declined significantly in numbers and in proportion to nonmenstrual. Today staphylococcal TSS is split approximately 50:50 between menstrual and nonmenstrual cases. It is also important to mention that many staphylococcal cases are being recognized, that are not severe enough to meet the case definition criteria, and it has been proposed that such cases be referred to as toxin mediated disease rather than TSS. Cases of TSS associated with *Streptococcus pyogenes* first received a high level of attention after a report in 1987, continuing up to the present.

TRENDS IN OCCURRENCE OF STAPHYLOCOCCAL TOXIC SHOCK SYNDROME

In the early 1980s, the incidence of staphylococcal TSS was six to 12 cases per 100,000 women (24–27). In 1986, the Centers for Disease Control (CDC) conducted an active surveillance project for TSS in Los Angeles County and in the states of Missouri, New Jersey, Oklahoma, Tennessee, and Washington (28). The overall incidence of TSS detected in this surveillance project was 0.53 case per 100,000 persons with an incidence of 1.05 cases per 100,000 women aged 15 to 44 years.

Another mechanism for obtaining surveillance data is through passive surveillance, which CDC has conducted since 1980. Their data demonstrated a peak in the incidence of cases in mid-1980, with a decline in incidence since that time. The peak in 1980 was in part due to publicity about the syndrome and enhanced surveillance activities that occurred at that time. Although the decline may in part reflect a decrease in reporting, it is consistent with active surveillance data that also demonstrated a decline in incidence from 1980 to 1986 (29,30).

MENSTRUATION-ASSOCIATED STAPHYLOCOCCAL TOXIC SHOCK SYNDROME

When TSS was first widely recognized in 1980, multiple studies demonstrated the association between tampon use and on-

set of TSS in menstruating women (25–27,31,32). In addition, early studies demonstrated elevated odds ratios with use of tampons of very high absorbency; as a result of these studies, Rely tampons [Procter & Gamble, Cincinnati, Ohio] were taken off the market in September 1980 (32). For example, the tri-state (Minnesota, Wisconsin, and Iowa) TSS study demonstrated clearly an increased risk related to use of any tampons with high absorbency and not just Rely (25). Subsequent studies confirmed these findings and demonstrated that the risk for TSS increased proportionately to the absorbency of tampon brand used (33,34). In 1985, polyacrylate was removed from tampons, and because tampons containing polyacrylate were generally of high absorbency, this led to a decrease in TSS cases (29,30). Although the number of reported menstrual cases has declined since the peak was identified in the early 1980s, cases still occur.

NONMENSTRUAL STAPHYLOCOCCAL TOXIC SHOCK SYNDROME

Nonmenstrual cases of TSS caused by *S. aureus* have been reported in a variety of clinical settings, including nearly any type of mucous membrane, skin, or soft tissue infection. For example TSS has been associated with a variety of respiratory tract infections, including sinusitis, pharyngitis, tracheitis, rhinoplasty with nasal packing, and post viral (35–47). Postpartum cases of TSS have been recognized after both vaginal and cesarean deliveries. Use of barrier contraceptives has also been demonstrated to be a risk factor for nonmenstrual TSS with a reported incidence of approximately one per 100,000 women (48,49). A recalcitrant erythematous desquamating syndrome has been described associated with acquired immunodeficiency syndrome in which patients experience 70 or more days of illness (50). TSS associated with pneumonia and community-acquired methicillin-resistant *S. aureus* has recently been recognized. This illness poses a serious treatment challenge because of the high levels of SEs B or C made by the strains. Most importantly, it is necessary to recognize that TSST-1, SEB, and SEC producing *S. aureus* strains are very common today, and any individual with skin or mucous membrane damage, either acute or chronic, is susceptible to infection by such a strain. In the absence of neutralizing antibodies to the toxins, TSS is likely to occur.

TOXIC SHOCK SYNDROME CAUSED BY *STREPTOCOCCUS PYOGENES*

TSS caused by *Streptococcus pyogenes* was first described by Cone and coworkers in 1987 (2). Subsequently, a larger report of 20 patients identified in the Rocky Mountain region was published (3). Of the patients described in that latter study, 19 had shock and most had associated soft-tissue infections. Less than half had underlying risk factors for disease, including diabetes, obesity, alcoholism, cerebella ataxia, or intravenous drug use. The median age of patients was 35 years, and 16 of the patients were younger than 60 years.

Studies have assessed incidence rates for invasive group A streptococcal disease. The first incidence study was a retrospective medical record review of cases of invasive group A streptococcal disease occurring between April 1985 and March 1990 in hospitals located in Pima county, Arizona (51). In that study, the overall incidence rate of invasive group A streptococcal disease was 4.3 per 100,000 population. On the basis of this finding, the authors concluded that the incidence of streptococcal TSS had increased in Pima County during the 5 years of observation. A prospective, population-based study on the incidence of invasive group A streptococcal infections has also been published. During

1992 and 1993, investigators conducted active surveillance of invasive disease in Ontario, Canada (52). Three hundred twenty-three patients were identified, for an annual incidence rate of 1.5 cases per 100,000 population; 42 (13%) of these patients were classified as having streptococcal TSS. The overall case:fatality rate for patients with streptococcal TSS was 81% compared with 5% of invasive group A streptococcal cases without TSS. Streptococcal TSS occurred in 11 (55%) of 20 patients with necrotizing fasciitis compared with 31 (10%) of 303 patients who had invasive group A streptococcal disease with a diagnosis other than necrotizing fasciitis.

Community-based outbreaks of invasive group A streptococcal infection, including TSS, have been reported. One outbreak involved seven cases of severe invasive group A streptococcal disease, including four with TSS (53). All cases occurred in three adjacent southeastern Minnesota counties in a 3-month period. Epidemiologic investigation demonstrated a high rate of carriage (approximately 35%) of the outbreak clone of group A streptococcus among children attending an elementary school in the outbreak area. Another outbreak involved 13 cases, 5 with streptococcal TSS, in the Shenandoah Valley of Virginia between December 1, 1994, and the end of February 1995 (54).

PATHOGENESIS

A model for the production of TSS symptoms by pyrogenic toxins is presented in Fig. 181.2 (13,14). The model depends primarily on the toxins' ability to alter immune system function, causing sustained release of monokines, tumor necrosis factor-α, and interleukin 1 from macrophages. The effect of these two endogenous pyrogens, or in some cases the direct action of the toxins on the hypothalamus, probably explains the production of fever (13–15). In addition, monokine release explains many of the other TSS symptoms, most notably hypotension.

All of the SAgs are potent T lymphocyte mitogens (16). This activity depends on two properties of the toxins: (a) the ability of the toxins to interact directly with class II major histocompatibility complex products (without the need for processing) on the surface of antigen presenting cells, such as macrophages, and to be presented to T lymphocytes; and (b) the toxins' ability to bind the subsets of the variable part of the β chain of the T cell receptor complex. Because the toxins stimulate only a subset, although without regard for antigen specificity, they have been referred to as SAgs. Primarily CD4$^+$ but also CD8$^+$ cells are induced to proliferate.

Toxin stimulation of CD4$^+$ cells leads to production of high levels of interferon γ, which activates macrophages and thus has been proposed to explain the TSS-associated rash as a manifestation of amplified delayed hypersensitivity (13–15). This activity many also result from release of high levels of interleukin 2. Macrophage activation also explains the erythrophagocytosis seen on autopsy in staphylococcal TSS. The high levels of interferon γ released have been shown in experimental animals to lead to suppression of B cell function and may, therefore, explain the failure of approximately 85% of patients to develop neutralizing antibody against TSST-1 in TSST-1 associated illness. Thus, most TSS patients remain susceptible to the illness on recovery. Indeed, large numbers of recurrences have been reported, particularly in menstrual cases (55).

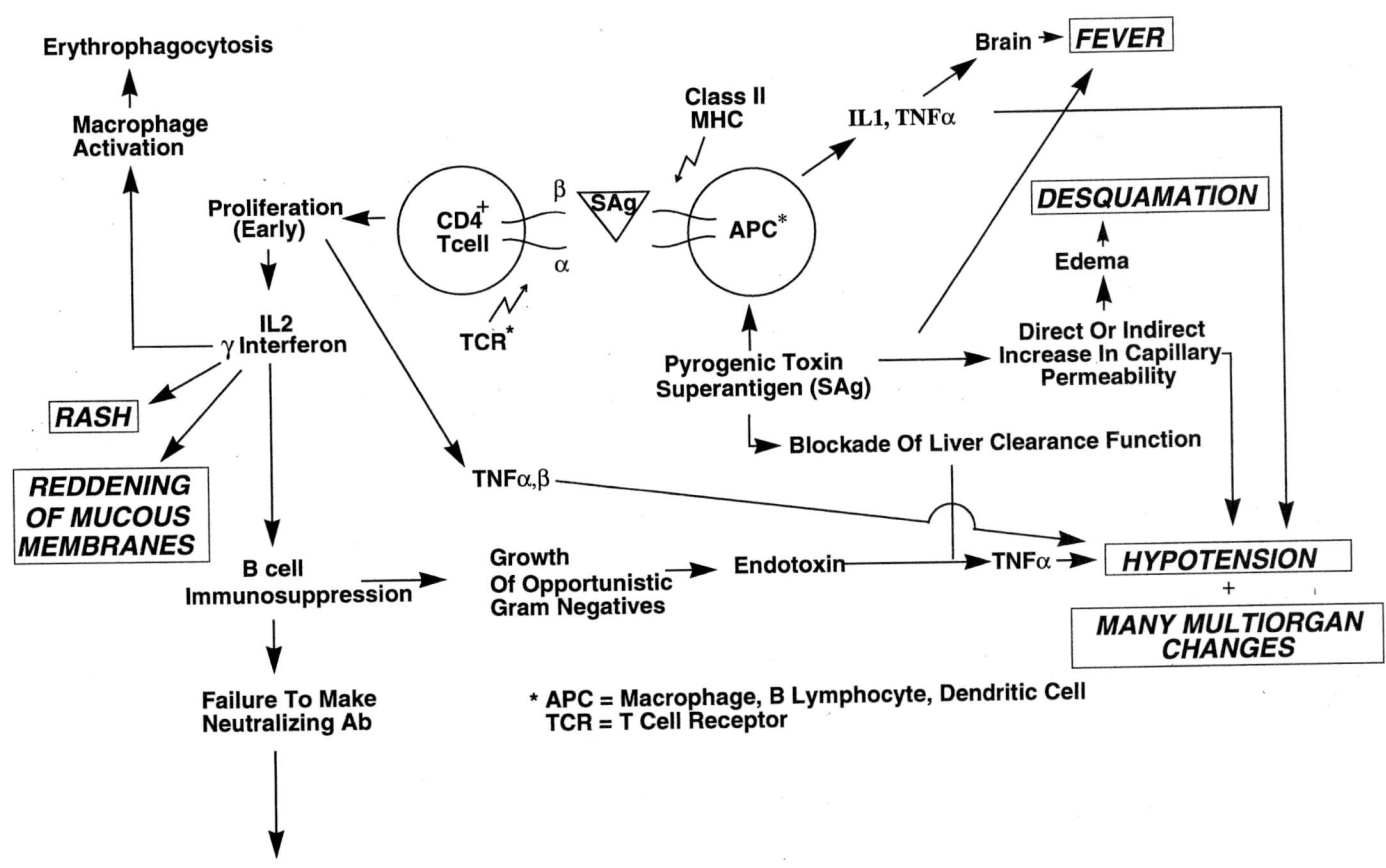

Figure 181.2. Model for the development of toxic shock syndrome and related illnesses. Ab, Antibody; IL1, interleukin 1; IL2, interleukin 2; MHC, major histocompatibility complex; SAg, superantigen; TNF, tumor necrosis factor.

A dramatic and potentially important biologic property of SAgs is their capacity to enhance host susceptibility to lethal endotoxin shock (13–15). Thus, an animal may show up to 100,000-fold enhanced susceptibility to the lethal effects of endotoxin, and this may represent picogram amounts in humans. Although it is still controversial, there is evidence to suggest that this activity plays a role in the most severe manifestations of TSS or at least increases the severity of illness.

A major difference between staphylococcal and streptococcal TSS is the association of streptococcal TSS with necrotizing fasciitis, whereas soft tissue necrosis is not often associated with staphylococcal TSS. Studies in experimental animals suggest that induction of necrotizing fasciitis depends on production of high levels of tumor necrosis factor-α, which appears have the opposite effect of its expected pro-inflammatory property, thus downregulating chemotactic receptors on polymorphonuclear leukocytes and delaying phagocytosis (23). The consequence of this delay is growth of the streptococci and production of virulence factors such as streptolysins, nucleases, and proteases (notably SPE B) that are likely to cause the soft tissue necrosis. The reason that staphylococcal TSS is not associated with necrotizing fasciitis is unclear.

One of the most controversial and publicized aspects of staphylococcal TSS is the role of certain tampons in the illness. Several theories have been put forward, but only two remain as viable possibilities. Investigators have identified the physicochemical factors necessary to promote TSST-1 production (56). Toxin production occurs in protein (or amino acid)-containing media, at 37°C to 40°C, in a pH range of 6.5 to 8, and in the presence of oxygen and carbon dioxide; the toxin is susceptible to catabolite repression by glucose. With the exception of oxygen, these conditions are present in the human vagina at times of menstruation or of trauma that causes bleeding. It has been shown that tampons increase the oxygen content of the vagina to an extent that toxin can be induced (57). These data, combined with the observation that nearly 3% to 5% of menstruating women have TSST-1 positive *S. aureus* in the vagina, have given rise to the oxygen theory for the role of tampons in TSS. Interestingly, data obtained by Todd and colleagues showed that the oxygen content of staphylococcal abscesses is sufficient to permit TSST-1 production, which is contrary to the usual thinking that abscesses are anaerobic environments (58).

The second theory is that the TSS association with Rely tampon is in part explained by the amplification of TSST-1 production by the surfactant Pluronic L-92 contained in the tampon. In vitro studies have shown the surfactant increases toxin production.

Postsurgical staphylococcal TSS represents an important subset of TSS in that the causative bacterium is typically nonpyogenic. Thus, in many cases of postsurgical TSS, the infected incision site may heal and show only minimal signs of inflammation or none. This may allow the illness to progress to severe disease before the cause is recognized. The mechanism underlying the lack of pyogenic response in postsurgical cases, as well as in other cases, may be twofold: (a) the organism does not express many inflammation-inducing factors; and (b) TSST-1 induces overproduction of tumor necrosis factor-α from macrophages, which in turn inhibits polymorphonuclear leukocyte chemotaxis (59).

The physicochemical factors that influence production of the streptococcal pyrogenic toxin superantigens are similar to those required for production of staphylococcal toxins except that SPE production is independent of oxygen levels (as would be expected because streptococci are aerotolerant anaerobes) and is not as susceptible to catabolite repression by glucose (again as expected because streptococci are fermentative).

CLINICAL FEATURES

The CDC has developed case definitions for TSS caused by both *S. aureus* and *S. pyogenes* (Tables 181.2 and 181.3) (13,14,24,51,60). Both case definitions include hypotension (systolic blood pressure less than or equal to 90 mm Hg in adults or less than the fifth percentile by age for children). The case definition for TSS caused by *S. aureus* also requires fever, presence of a diffuse macular rash, and desquamation (particularly of palms and soles) 1 to 2 weeks after onset of illness. Whereas a generalized erythematous rash followed by desquamation can occur with streptococcal TSS, it is less common than with staphylococcal TSS and not an essential feature of the case definition. Conversely, soft tissue necrosis, including necrotizing fasciitis or myositis, tends to occur relatively frequently with streptococcal TSS. TSS caused by both organisms tends to involve multiple organ systems, including renal impairment, hepatic involvement, adult respiratory distress syndrome, and disseminated intravascular coagulation or thrombocytopenia. Central nervous system involvement with disorientation or alteration in consciousness can also occur. With staphylococcal TSS, mucous membrane changes have often been noted. The most common of these include erythema of conjunctivae and mucous membranes of mouth, tongue, vagina, and tympanic membranes; strawberry tongue; subconjunctival hemorrhages; and ulcerations of the mouth, vagina, and esophagus. Telogen effluvium can also occur after staphylococcal TSS; hair and nail loss occurs 1 to 2 months after onset of illness, with regrowth approximately 6 months later.

The hypotension present in TSS is clinically similar to that seen in septic shock. Hypotension in the setting of TSS is most commonly caused by a decrease in systemic vascular resistance and hypovolemia secondary to capillary leakage into the interstitial space. With hemodynamic monitoring, patients typically have a low central venous pressure, low pulmonary artery wedge pressure, low intravascular volume, low systemic vascular resistance, and increased cardiac index. However, these parameters may vary in individual patients. A report of clinical characteristics associated with streptococcal TSS noted a greater degree of decreased cardiac output with diminished ventricular

---

TABLE 181.2. Diagnostic Criteria for Staphylococcal Toxic Shock Syndrome

1. Temperature >38.9°C
2. Systolic blood pressure <90 mm Hg for adults, less than the fifth percentile for children, or greater than 15 mm Hg orthostatic drop in diastolic blood pressure or orthostatic dizziness/syncope.
3. Diffuse macular rash with subsequent desquamation
4. Three involved organ systems:
   Liver: bilirubin, ALT, AST > twice the upper normal limit
   Blood: platelets <100,000/mm³
   Renal: BUN or creatinine > twice the upper normal limit or pyuria without urinary tract infection.
   Mucous membranes: Hyperemia of the vagina, oropharynx, or conjunctivae
   Gastrointestinal: Diarrhea or vomiting
   Muscular: Myalgias or CPK > twice the normal upper limit
   Central nervous system: Disorientation or lowered level of consciousness in the absence of hypotension, fever or focal neurologic deficits.
5. Negative serologic studies for measles, leptospirosis, and Rocky Mountain spotted fever. Blood or CSF culture results negative for organisms other than *Staphylococcus aureus*.

AST, aspartate transaminase; ALT, alanine aminotransferase; BUN, blood urea nitrogen; CPK, creatine phosphokinase.

TABLE 181.3. Diagnostic Criteria for Streptococcal Toxic Shock Syndrome

1. Isolation of group A streptococci:
   From a sterile site for a *definite* case
   From a non-sterile site for a *probable* case
2. Two clinical criteria:
   Hypotension
   and two of the following:
   Renal dysfunction
   Liver involvement
   Erythematous macular rash
   Coagulopathy
   Adult respiratory distress syndrome
   Soft-tissue necrosis

performance and less significant decreases in systemic vascular resistance (61). In that report, primary myocardial depression appeared to be the major determinant of refractory shock. Because cardiomyopathy can also occur with staphylococcal TSS, hemodynamic monitoring of patients with TSS due to either *S. aureus* or *Streptococcus pyogenes* is particularly important to ensure that therapy is appropriate.

DIAGNOSIS

A patient who presents with fever, rash, and hypotension represents little diagnostic challenge, especially if she is menstruating or has an obvious focus of invasive infection. The diagnosis of necrotizing fasciitis is likewise little challenge once tissue death has begun. The greater difficulty lies in making an early diagnosis, when the patient presents to the physician with non-specific flu-like symptoms. In many cases this may be impossible. However, if clinicians maintain a high degree of suspicion, they may be able to identify cases prior to the development of critical illness. The prodrome of staphylococcal TSS may include nausea, vomiting and diarrhea and thus mimic gastroenteritis. Clinical gastroenteritis in association with a menstrual period should raise the question of TSS. The presenting rash may be so subtle that it can be seen only with close examination in a brightly-lit room. Orthostatic symptoms or orthostatic hypotension may be the precursor of frank sepsis. The initial presentation of necrotizing fasciitis (NF) may be quite subtle. Re-development of pain in an area of previous trauma, no matter how minor, should bring the diagnosis to mind. Ironically, development of pain out of proportion to physical findings in an area without previous trauma should also suggest the diagnosis. Although nonsteroidal anti-inflammatory drugs (NSAIDs) have not definitively been shown to increase the risk of NF, they may be a marker to identify those patients who are experiencing the severe, localized pain that may first bring them to medical attention. NSAIDS, however, do have effects on immune modulators such as tumor necrosis factor and it is conceivable that there may be some interaction that will increase the risk of necrotizing fasciitis. With close examination, there may be early subtle changes in the overlying tissue with NF, such as blanching or edema. If the diagnosis is suspected, orthostatic changes in blood pressure and pulse should be measured and laboratory investigation initiated. Though the white blood cell count is likely to be normal, or even low, a differential may show a profound bandemia of 20% to 30% or greater. The serum creatinine may be mildly or markedly elevated as well as the total creatine kinase. In the patient with the right clinical picture, who has already been hospitalized, isolation of *S. aureus* of *Streptococcus pyogenes* from a sterile site is definitive evidence of TSS and isolation from a non-sterile site such as the throat, sputum, vagina, skin lesions, or wound is supportive of the diagnosis. *S. aureus* isolates may be assayed for toxin production and, in staphylococcal TSS, the patient's serum may be assayed for anti-TSST-antibody to demonstrate the absence of immunity.

There are cases that do not fit neatly into classic definitions of TSS. These patients tend to have low-grade fever, a subtle rash, a left shift with a bandemia and staphylococcal or streptococcal isolate from vagina, wound, or other suspect site. They may have little or no hypotension, negligible desquamation and no signs of systemic involvement. Predictably, these patients do very well with appropriate medical management. Though they do not fit the classic definition, they clearly have a superantigen-mediated process. Further, some patients may have a streptococcal fasciitis which is not necrotizing or a "myositis," which does not lead to acute and extensive tissue death.

THERAPY

In both staphylococcal and streptococcal TSS, appropriate antibiotic therapy should be given and any necessary supportive therapies such as intravenous fluids, plasma expanders, inotropic agents and vasopressors, which may be required. Large volumes of intravenous fluids are often necessary because of the profound capillary leak and subsequent third spacing of intravascular fluids. For staphylococcal TSS, cefazolin would be one appropriate choice, or vancomycin for the allergic patient. For streptococcal infections, penicillin, ampicillin or ceftriaxone would be appropriate choices with vancomycin or clindamycin for the allergic patient. Some authors have also recommended the addition of clindamycin to a beta-lactam antibiotic, because of its ability to inhibit toxin production even at antibiotic doses that do not inhibit bacterial growth. In light of the high morbidity and mortality of streptococcal TSS/NF it seems prudent to utilize both agents unless the patient is quite stable. Urgent surgical debridement of any infected or traumatic wound or areas of necrosis with removal of any suspected foreign bodies is advisable.

Intravenous immunoglobulin (IVIG) and steroids have been suggested as possible adjunctive therapies for patients with TSS. IVIG may inhibit the activation of T cells or bind SAgs and may be of value. Various studies have shown that some preparations of IVIG inhibit the activity of certain staphylococcal and streptococcal toxins (62–64). A murine model of necrotizing fasciitis did not show any benefit (65). However, some case reports and one human observational study with historical controls suggests that IVIG has a positive effect on survival in streptococcal TSS (66–69). Steroids are not routinely administered, but may have a role, especially in severe cases. Each case must be judged individually. IVIG and possibly steroids should be given to the critically ill patient that either fails to respond, or responds only poorly, to initial attempts at stabilization with fluids, pressors, monitoring, etc. and thus is feared to be at significant risk of death or sustaining severe morbidity from uncontrolled hypotension or rapidly progressive tissue loss. Regardless of the presence of sepsis, IVIG should be seriously considered for the patient with necrotizing fasciitis, unless the extent of disease is small and responds well to antibiotics and limited surgical debridement.

REFERENCES

1. Todd J, Fishaut M, Kapral F, Welch T. Toxic shock syndrome associated with phage group I staphylococci. *Lancet* 1978;2:1116.
2. Cone LA, Woodard DR, Schlievert PM, Tomory GS. Clinical and bacteriologic observations of a toxic shock-like syndrome due to *Streptococcus pyogenes*. *N Engl J Med* 1987;317:146.

3. Stevens DL, Tanner MH, Winship J, et al. Severe group A streptococcal infections associated with a toxic shock-like syndrome and scarlet fever toxin A. *N Engl J Med* 1989;321:1.

4. Schlievert PM, Shands KN, Dan BB, et al. Identification and characterization of an exotoxin from *Staphylococcus aureus* associated with toxic-shock syndrome. *J Infect Dis* 1981;143:509.

5. Bergdoll MS, Crass B, Reiser RF, et al. A new staphylococcal enterotoxin, enterotoxin F, associated with toxic shock syndrome *Staphylococcus aureus* isolates. *Lancet* 1981;1:1017.

6. Schlievert PM. Staphylococcal enterotoxin B and toxic-shock syndrome toxin-1 are significantly associated with nonmenstrual TSS. *Lancet* 1986;1:1149.

7. Parsonnet J, Gillis ZA, Richter AG, Pier GB. A rabbit model of toxic shock syndrome that uses a constant, subcutaneous infusion of toxic shock syndrome toxin-l. *Infect Immun* 1987;55:1070.

8. Hauser AR, Stevens DL, Kaplan EL, Schlievert PM. Molecular analysis of pyrogenic exotoxins from *Streptococcus pyogenes* isolates associated with toxic shock-like syndrome. *J Clin Microbiol* 1991;29:1562.

9. Musser JM, Hauser AR, Kim M, et al. *Streptococcus pyogenes* causing toxic shock-like syndrome and other invasive diseases: clonal diversity, and pyrogenic exotoxin expression. *Proc Natl Acad Sci USA* 1991;88:2668.

10. Reda KB, Kapur V, Mollick JA, et al. Molecular characterization and phylogenetic distribution of the streptococcal superantigen gene (SSA) from *Streptococcus pyogenes*. *Infect Immun* 1994;62:1867.

11. Wheeler MC, Roe MH, Kaplan EL, et al. Clinical, epidemiological, and microbiological correlates of an outbreak of group A streptococcal septicemia in children. *JAMA* 1991;266:533.

12. Iwasaki M, Igarashi H, Hinuma Y, Yutsudo T. Cloning, characterization and overexpression of a *Streptococcus pyogenes* gene encoding a new type of mitogenic factor. *FEBS Lett* 1993;331:187.

13. Dinges MM, Orwin PM, Schlievert PM: Exotoxins of *Staphylococcus aureus*. *Clin Microbiol Rev* 2000;13:16.

14. McCormick JK, Yarwood JM, Schlievert PM. Toxic shock syndrome and bacterial superantigens: an update. *Annu Rev Microbiol* 2001;55:77.

15. Bohach GA, Fast DJ, Nelson RD, Schlievert PM. Staphylococcal and streptococcal pyrogenic toxins involved in toxic shock syndrome and related illnesses. *Crit Rev Microbiol* 1989;17:251.

16. Marrack P, Kappler J. The staphylococcal enterotoxins and their relatives. *Science* 1990;248:705.

17. Schlievert PM, Joblonski LM, Roggiani M, et al. Pyrogenic toxin site specificity in toxic shock syndrome and food poisoning in animals. *Infect Immun* 2000;68:3630.

18. Schwab JH, Brown RR, Anderle SK, Schlievert PM. Superantigen can reactivate bacterial cell wall-induced arthritis. *J Immunol* 1993;150:4151.

19. Prasad GS, Earhart CA, Murray DL, et al. Structure of toxic shock syndrome toxin-1. *Biochemistry* 1993;32:13761.

20. Novick RP, Schlievert P, Ruzin A. Pathogenicity and resistance islands of staphylococci. *Microbes Infect* 2001;3:585.

21. de Azavedo JCS, Foster TJ, Hartigan PJ, et al. Expression of the cloned toxic shock syndrome toxin-1 gene (*tst*) in vivo with a rabbit uterine model. *Infect Immun* 1985;50:304.

22. Lee PK, Schlievert PM. Group A streptococcal pyrogenic exotoxins: quantification and toxicity in an animal model of toxic shock syndrome-like illness. *J Clin Microbiol* 1989;27:1890.

23. Schlievert PM, Assimacopoulos AP, Cleary PP. Severe invasive group A streptococcal disease: clinical description and mechanisms of pathogenesis. *J Lab Clin Med* 1996;127:13.

24. Centers for Disease Control. Toxic-shock syndrome: United States. *MMWR* 1980;29:229.

25. Osterholm MT, Davis JP, Gibson RW, et al. Tri-state toxic-shock syndrome study. 1. Epidemiologic findings. *J Infect Dis* 1982;145:431.

26. Latham RH, Kehrberg MW, Jacobson JA, Smith CB. Toxic shock syndrome in Utah: a case-control and surveillance study. *Ann Intern Med* 1982;96:906.

27. Davis JP, Chesney PJ, Wand PJ, La Venture M, the Investigation and Laboratory Team. Toxic shock syndrome: epidemiologic features, recurrence, risk factors, and prevention. *N Engl J Med* 1980;303:1429.

28. Gaventa S, Reingold AL, Hightower AW, et al. Active surveillance for toxic shock syndrome in the United States, 1986. *Rev Infect Dis* 1989;2(Suppl 1):S28.

29. Schuchat A, Broome CV. Toxic shock syndrome and tampons. *Epidemiol Rev* 1991;13:99.

30. Broome CV. Epidemiology of toxic shock syndrome in the United States: overview. *Rev Infect Dis* 1989;2(Suppl 1):S14.

31. Shands KN, Schmid GP, Dan BB, et al. Toxic shock syndrome in menstruating women. *N Engl J Med* 1980;303:1436.

32. Schlech WF, Shands KN, Reingold AL, et al. Risk factors for development of toxic shock syndrome: association with a tampon brand. *JAMA* 1982;248:835.

33. Berkley SF, Hightower AW, Broome CV, Reingold, AL. The relationship of tampon characteristics to menstrual toxic shock syndrome. *JAMA* 1987;258:917.

34. Reingold AL, Broome CV, Gaventa S, Hightower AW, the Toxic Shock Syndrome Study Group. Risk factors for menstrual toxic shock syndrome: results of a multistate case-control study. *Rev Infect Dis* 1989;2(Suppl 1):S35.

35. Reingold AL, Hargrett NT, Dan BB, et al. Nonmenstrual toxic shock syndrome: a review of 130 cases. *Ann Intern Med* 1982;96(pt 2):871.

36. Parsonnet J. Nonmenstrual toxic shock syndrome: new insights into diagnosis, pathogenesis, and treatment. *Curr Clin Top Infect Dis* 1996;16:1.

37. Navazesh M, Mulligan R, Sobel S. Toxic shock and Down syndromes in a dental patient: a case report and review of the literature. *Spec Care Dent* 1994;14:246.

38. Bartlett P, Reingold AL, Graham DR, et al. Toxic shock syndrome associated with surgical wound infections. *JAMA* 1982;247:1448.

39. Solomon R, Truman T, Murray DL. Toxic shock syndrome as a complication of bacterial tracheitis. *Pediatr Infect Dis* 1985;4:298.

40. Surh L, Read SE. Staphylococcal tracheitis and toxic shock syndrome in a young child. *J Pediatr* 1984;105:585.

41. Hirsch B, Stair T, Horowitz Z, et al. Toxic shock syndrome from staphylococcal pharyngitis. *Ear Nose Throat J* 1984;63:494.

42. Wilkins EGL, Nye F, Roberts C, et al. Case report: probable toxic shock syndrome with primary staphylococcal pneumonia. *J Infect* 1985;11:231.

43. Barbour SD, Shlaes DM, Guertin SR. Toxic shock syndrome associated with nasal packing: analogy to tampon-associated illness. *Pediatrics* 1984;73:163.

44. Hull HF, Mann IM, Sands CH, et al. Toxic shock syndrome related to nasal packing. *Arch Otolaryngol Head Neck Surg* 1983;109:624.

45. MacDonald KL, Osterholm MT, Hedberg CW, et al. Toxic shock syndrome: a newly recognized complication of influenza and influenza-like illness. *JAMA* 1987;257:1053.

46. Sperber SJ, Francis JB. Toxic shock syndrome during an influenza outbreak. *JAMA* 1987;257:1086.

47. Tolan RW Jr. Toxic shock syndrome complicating influenza A in a child: case report and review. *Clin Infect Dis* 1993;17:43.

48. Faich G, Pearson K, Fleming D, et al. Toxic shock syndrome and the vaginal contraceptive sponge. *JAMA* 1986;255:216.

49. Schwartz B, Gaventa S, Broome CV, et al. Nonmenstrual toxic shock syndrome associated with barrier contraceptives: report of a case-control study. *Rev Infect Dis* 1989;2[Suppl 1]:S43.

50. Cone LA, Woodard DR, Byrd RG, Schulz K, Kopp SM, Schlievert PM. A recalcitrant, erythematous, desquamating disorder associated with toxin-producing staphylococci in patients with AIDS. *J Infect Dis* 1992;165:638.

51. Hoge CW, Schwartz B, Talkington DF, et al. The changing epidemiology of invasive group A streptococcal toxic shock-like syndrome. *JAMA* 1993;269:384.

52. Davis HD, McGeer A, Schwartz B, et al. Invasive group A streptococcal infections in Ontario, Canada. *N Engl J Med* 1996;335:547.

53. Cockerill FR, MacDonald KL, Thompson RL, et al. An outbreak of invasive group A streptococcal disease associated with high carriage rates of the invasive clone among school-age children. *JAMA* 1997;277:38.

54. Levine OS, Turf E, Ginsberg R, et al. An outbreak of invasive group A streptococcal (GAS) disease in the Shenandoah Valley of Virginia (Abstr K134). Presented at the 35th Interscience Conference on Antimicrobial Agents and Chemotherapy; September 17–20, 1995; San Francisco, CA; p 312.

55. Davis JP, Osterholm MT, Helms CM, et al. Tri-state toxic shock syndrome study, II. Clinical and laboratory findings. *J Infect Dis* 1982;145:441.

56. Schlievert PM, Blomster DA. Production of staphylococcal pyrogenic exotoxin type C: influence of physical and chemical factors. *J Infect Dis* 1983;146:236.

57. Wagner G Bohr L, Wagner P. Tampon-induced changes in vaginal oxygen and carbon dioxide tension. *Am J Obstet Gynecol* 1984;148:147.

58. Todd JK, Todd BH, Franco-Fuff A, et al. Influence of focal growth conditions on the pathogenesis of toxic shock syndrome. *J Infect Dis* 1987;155:673.

59. Fast DJ, Schlievert PM, Nelson RD. Nonpurulent response to toxic shock syndrome toxin-1 producing *Staphylococcus aureus*: Relationship to toxin-stimulated production of tumor necrosis factor. *J Immunol* 1988;140:949.

60. The Working Group on Severe Streptococcal Infections. Defining the group A streptococcal toxic shock syndrome. *JAMA* 1993;269:390.

61. Forni AL, Kaplan EL, Schlievert PM, Roberts RB. Clinical and microbiological characteristics of group A streptococcus infections and streptococcal toxic shock syndrome. *Clin Infect Dis* 1995;21:333.

62. Basma H, Norrby-Teglund A, McGeer A, et al. Opsonic antibodies to the surface M protein of group A streptococci in pooled normal immunoglobulins (IVIG): potential impact on the clinical efficacy of IVIG therapy for severe invasive group A streptococcal infections. *Infect Immun* 1998;66:2279.

63. Norrby-Teglund A, Low DE, McGeer A, Kotb M. Superantigenic activity produced by group A streptococcal isolates is neutralized by plasma from IVIG-treated streptococcal toxic shock syndrome patients. *Adv Exp Med Biol* 1997;418:563.

64. Norrby-Teglund A, Ihendyane N, Kansal R, et al. Relative neutralizing activity in polyspecific IgM, IgA, and IgG preparations against group A streptococcal superantigens. *Clin Infect Dis* 2000;31:1175.

65. Patel R, Rouse MS, Florez MV, et al. Lack of benefit of intravenous immune globulin in a murine model of group A streptococcal necrotizing fasciitis. *J Infect Dis* 2000;181:230.

66. Kaul R, McGeer A, Norrby-Teglund A, et al. Intravenous immunoglobulin therapy for streptococcal toxic shock syndrome-a comparative observational study. The Canadian Streptococcal Study Group. *Clin Infect Dis* 1999;28:800.

67. Perez CM, Kubak BM, Cryer HG, et al. Adjunctive treatment of streptococcal toxic shock syndrome using intravenous immunoglobulin: case report and review. *Am J Med* 1997;102:111.

68. Lamothe F, D'Amico P, Ghosn P, et al. Clinical usefulness of intravenous human immunoglobulins in invasive group A streptococcal infections: case report and review. *Clin Infect Dis* 1995;21:1469.

69. Barry W, Hudgins L, Donta ST, Pesanti EL. Intravenous immunoglobulin therapy for toxic shock syndrome. *JAMA* 1992;267:3315.

Gram-Positive Cocci

CHAPTER 182
Staphylococci

John N. Sheagren and Dennis R. Schaberg

HISTORY

A summary of the history of staphylococci was provided by A. C. Baird-Parker (1). Briefly, cocci were first associated with human diseases when they were observed in purulent material obtained from human abscesses. The Scottish surgeon Sir Alexander Ogston demonstrated conclusively in 1880 that "cluster-forming coccus was the cause of certain pyogenous abscesses in man." Louis Pasteur had reached a similar conclusion in Paris. Ogston named the cluster-forming coccus "staphylococcus" in 1882, deriving the name from the Greek nouns *staphyle* ("a bunch of grapes") and *kokkus* ("berry"). Ogston also showed that injection of pus containing staphylococci into mice produced the same symptoms seen in humans and observed that heat treatment of the pus prevented infection.

CHARACTERISTICS OF THE PATHOGEN

The two genera in the Micrococcaceae family are *Staphylococcus* and *Micrococcus* (Table 182.1). The genus *Staphylococcus* contains at least 13 species, several of which have been classified into subspecies or biotypes (1). Three species, however, are responsible for almost all human infections: *Staphylococcus aureus*, the agent of most acute pyogenic and toxin-related staphylococcal infections in humans; *Staphylococcus epidermidis*, a major component of the normal flora of the skin and mucous membranes but increasingly a pathogen of infections of skin and skin structures, of foreign bodies, and of deep infections in immunocompromised patients; and *Staphylococcus saprophyticus*, which produces lower urinary tract infections in young women.

Structure

The staphylococci are gram-positive organisms with a diameter between 0.7 and 1.2 μm. The organisms divide randomly

in three planes, and because the daughter cells do not separate completely, they form grapelike clusters (Fig. 182.1) which, when viable, are densely stained by Gram stain. In electron micrographs of thin sections, the cell wall of staphylococci usually consists of a thick (up to 80 nm) layer that is more or less homogeneous. The cell envelope is surrounded by a unit membrane (cytoplasmic membrane), and the cell wall outside the plasma membrane is thick, rather homogeneous, and less electron dense. Some strains also have a capsule surrounding the cell wall.

Biologic and Biochemical Properties

S. aureus isolates growing on blood agar typically produce opaque, golden-yellow (*aureus* is Latin for "golden") colonies, approximately 2 to 3 mm in diameter, that usually produce beta hemolysis on blood agar plates. When encapsulated, *S. aureus* colonies may appear mucoid and sticky. Small-colony variants of *S. aureus* produce small, nonpigmented, nonhemolytic colonies, which can be misidentified in the microbiology laboratory (2,3). These organisms revert to normal growth in the presence of menadione, hemin, or carbon dioxide supplementation. They are usually resistant to aminoglycosides. Their importance lies in the fact that they may play a role in chronic relapsing infections characterized by long periods of quiescence, especially osteomyelitis. In contrast to *S. aureus*, coagulase-negative colonies (e.g., *S. epidermidis*, *S. saprophyticus*) are usually white and nonhemolytic.

The pathogenic genus *Staphylococcus*, with its three species of major significance, *S. aureus*, *S. epidermidis*, and *S. saprophyticus*, is differentiated in the standard laboratory by a number of tests. The most important is that for coagulase, which distinguishes *S. aureus* from all the other species which are designated as coagulase-negative. Other tests that differentiate *S. aureus* from the coagulase-negative species include mannitol fermentation (positive in *S. aureus* and only rarely positive in coagulase-negative strains) and the deoxyribonuclease test (also positive only in *S. aureus*). An additional test, usually performed only on urine isolates of staphylococci, is the ability to grow in the presence of concentrations of 1.6 μg/mL or more of novobiocin. Staphylococci that are found to be both novobiocin resistant and coagulase-negative can be identified presumptively as *S. saprophyticus*. Rapid screening tests that identify *S. aureus* are becoming more readily available. These tests identify organisms as *S. aureus* if protein A is detected on the surface.

The Cell Wall

The cell wall structure of staphylococci is important because the actions of many of the effective classes of antibiotics involve

TABLE 182.1. Microbiologic Characteristics of Staphylococci and Micrococci

Characteristic	*Staphylococcus* species	*Micrococcus* species
Anaerobic acid production from glucose	+	−
Anaerobic acid production from glycerol (in presence of erythromycin, 0.4 mg/mL)	+	−
Selective media		
SK medium	+	−
FTO medium	−	+
Modified oxidase and benzidine tests (to identify presence of cytochrome *c*)	− (most)	+
Sensitivity to lysostaphin, 200 mg or less	+	−

inhibition of cell wall synthesis and because a number of diagnostic tests that are potentially useful in the management of staphylococcal disease depend on cell wall characteristics (4). The Gram stain examination depends on the ability of the bacterial cell when washed with ethanol to retain the basic dye crystal violet. Gram-positive bacteria retain the stain principally because their cell walls contain large quantities of peptidoglycan. Surrounding the entire cell is a huge macromolecule consisting of glycan chains composed of alternating β-1,4-linked units of the amino sugars N-acetylglucosamine and N-acetylmuramic acid, all of which are cross-linked through short peptide chains (usually tetrapeptides of L-alanine, D-isoglutamine, L-lysine, and D-alanine). These tetrapeptides are further cross-linked (in a second dimension) by interpeptide bridges usually consisting of pentaglycine or hexaglycine peptides which extend from the C-terminal D-alanine in position 4 of one peptide to the amino group of L-lysine in position 3 of an adjacent peptide. In the coagulase-negative species of staphylococci, the peptidoglycan differs mainly in the interpeptide bridges (some of the glycines are replaced by L-serines).

The other major cell wall component of staphylococci is teichoic acid. Teichoic acids are water-soluble polymers of glycerol or ribitol phosphate, sugars, and sometimes D-alanine. They are linked covalently to the peptidoglycan backbone. *S. aureus* contains predominantly ribitol teichoic acid, whereas most of the other coagulase-negative staphylococci contain glycerol teichoic acid. Antibodies are generated against ribitol teichoic acid in many patients with deep invasive *S. aureus* infections, and the presence of such antibodies may be helpful in diagnosing and guiding the duration of therapy for patients who have suffered *S. aureus* bacteremia (5,6).

Capsule formation is variable among staphylococci may be important pathogenically. For example, strains of *S. epidermidis* that produce a slimelike glycocalyx adhere much more avidly to foreign bodies and so are more import pathogens in infections of prosthetic implants of all types (7). The few strains of *S. aureus* that are encapsulated in vitro seem to be more pathogenic in animal models; however, role of the capsule in *S. aureus* foreign body infections, for example, is not clear.

The adherence of *S. aureus* to heart valves and foreign bodies appears to be mediated in part by receptors for fibronectin on the surface of *S. aureus*. Fibronectin is a large glycoprotein important in various adhesive functions, including clot stabilization. *S. aureus* strains that express large numbers of receptors for fibronectin appear to be more invasive and better able to adhere (8). The role of surface-associated proteins of *S. aureus* and their possible roles in virulence have been reviewed (9). These substances include not only fibronectin binding proteins but protein A, collagen, and fibrinogen binding proteins as well (10).

ENZYMES AND TOXINS

Enzymes and toxins (11,12) have been strongly implicated as potential pathogenic factors in diseases produced by *S. aureus*. Among the more important enzymes is catalase, which can inactivate potentially bactericidal hydrogen peroxide. Other enzymes that may be important in the pathogenicity of *S. aureus*, by permitting the organism to spread through tissues, include hyaluronidase (which hydrolyzes hyaluronic acids, part of the

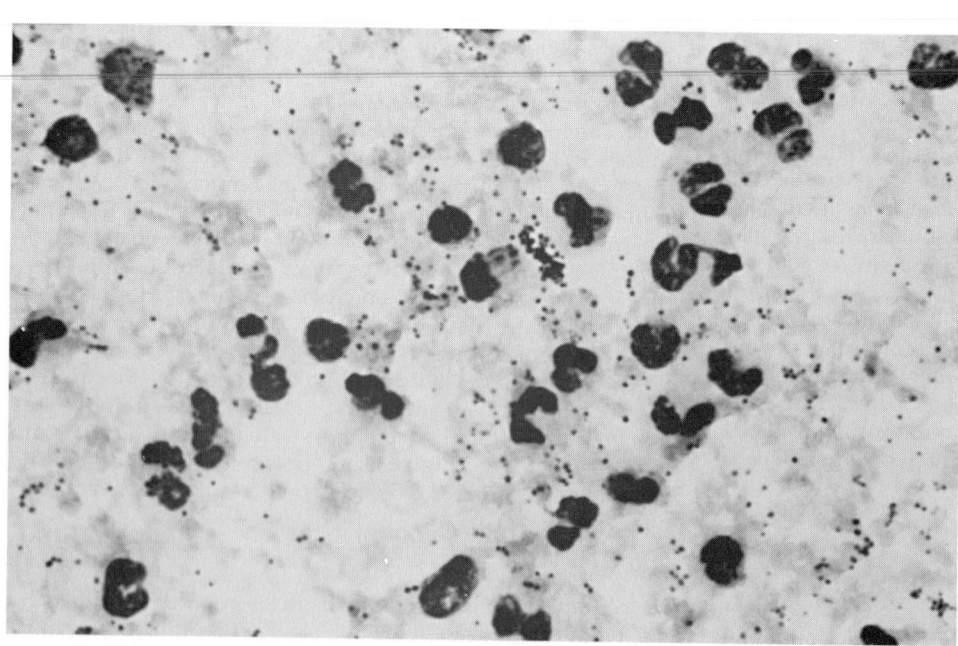

Figure 182.1. Gram stain of pus from typical abscess caused by *Staphylococcus aureus*.

connective tissue matrix) and lipase (which breaks down tissue lipid components).

In addition to the extracellular enzymes, a number of extracellular protein products of *S. aureus* have been identified. These have been called toxins because either of adverse effects on cell function or the production of cell lysis. The α-toxin is a protein that acts on a wide variety of cell membranes and, when injected parenterally, rapidly produces an area of necrosis. Most pathogenic strains of *S. aureus* elaborate α-toxin. The β-toxin is another enzyme-like protein, which breaks down sphingomyelin. The γ- and δ-toxins may also lyse cells or stimulate intestinal secretion. Leukocidin has a dramatic effect on granulocytes, resulting in degranulation and lysis. Finally, three toxins are related specifically to human diseases caused by *S. aureus*: exfoliatin (responsible for the staphylococcal scalded skin syndrome), enterotoxin (an important cause of food poisoning), and the toxic shock syndrome toxin-1 (the agent of a potentially lethal multisystem disorder that mimics bacteremic septic shock). The most important new concept with regard to toxin-associated diseases is that these protein toxins (especially toxic shock syndrome toxin 1) function as "superantigens" (13). Superantigens interact simultaneously with immune receptors on macrophages and lymphocytes, resulting in release of large amounts of inflammatory cytokines.

Strain Characterization

Serotyping of staphylococci has not been successful. Strains of staphylococci within individual species have been best delineated by their biochemical characteristics (biotyping), by phage typing, or by various genomic DNA "fingerprinting" methods (see later). Clinically, antibiotic sensitivity patterns can occasionally help identify an epidemic strain of *Staphylococcus* involved in a hospital outbreak.

EPIDEMIOLOGY

Transmission

The central event in diseases caused by all types of staphylococci seems to be the carrier state. Coagulase-negative staphylococci are important components of the normal flora of the body, and it is presumed that virtually all humans carry *S. epidermidis* on the skin and in and around body orifices. Contamination by coagulase-negative staphylococci carried by the patient is believed to be the most important event in infections associated with foreign bodies (intravascular devices, heart valves, prosthetic joints), although some studies have demonstrated hospital acquisition of strains that are resistant to several antibiotics (14).

Human carriers of *S. aureus* are at risk not only of transmitting the organism to others but of inoculating their own portals of entry, which could result in self-infection (15). Approximately 25% of adults are asymptomatic carriers of *S. aureus* in the anterior nares or intertriginous regions (axillae, groin, perineum). *S. aureus* carriers may experience recurrent staphylococcal infections of the skin and mucous membranes and are at substantially higher risk than noncarriers of developing more serious, deep *S. aureus* infections (e.g., intravenous line infections, wound infections, pneumonias and bacteremias) (15,16). This concept is now coming to clinical fruition in that pretreatment of *S. aureus* carriers can help prevent nosocomial infections (17–19).

Certain subgroups of patients are more likely to be *S. aureus* carriers (15): patients with chronic dermatologic conditions (up to 100% are carriers); patients who regularly undergo hemodialysis (approximately 75%); diabetic patients who take insulin (approximately 50%); patients receiving allergy shots (up to 50%); and intravenous drug abusers (approximately 40%). Such persons may also have other immune deficits that predispose them to more frequent and more serious infections with *S. aureus*. Another group of patients at extremely high risk are those receiving interleukin-2 (20).

Human immunodeficiency virus-infected patients have a significantly increased carriage rate of *S. aureus*, which increases as patients progress to full-blown acquired immunodeficiency syndrome (21,22). Such patients are at particularly high risk for symptomatic infections, especially if neutropenic and/or require an indwelling line (22). Colonization of patients who have acquired immunodeficiency syndrome with strains of *S. aureus* that produce toxic shock syndrome toxin-1 may result in what has been described as a recalcitrant, erythematous desquamating disorder (23), thought to be due to low-grade, toxic shock syndrome toxin-1 induced systemic inflammatory cytokine activation (24,25).

Distribution and Prevalence

S. aureus is now the single most frequently identified isolate from true-positive blood cultures in the hospital setting (26). It is the most common cause of postsurgical wound infections and of other traumatic infections of the skin and skin structures. It is the leading cause of both soft tissue and bone and joint infections. *S. epidermidis* is a frequent (25% to 50%) cause of infections of foreign bodies such as prosthetic heart valves and prosthetic joints of all types; like *S. aureus*, it may infect intravascular lines, becoming increasingly important in infections of indwelling central lines such as those used for chemotherapy of patients with neoplastic disease, for parenteral hyperalimentation, or for vascular monitoring devices and pacemakers. *S. saprophyticus* accounts for approximately 10% of urinary tract infections in otherwise healthy young women (27).

Typing systems for studying the epidemiology of staphylococcal infections have been investigated intensively. Phage typing of *S. aureus* has been in use since the 1940s, and it has been quite valuable in investigating the epidemiology of staphylococcal infections (28). Because of problems with the interpretation of phage-typing data, such information is far more useful in *excluding* possible epidemiologic relationships than it is in defining groups of related staphylococcal strains in an epidemic situation.

Because as many as 50% of strains have not been phage-typeable, continued attempts to identify relationships between isolated organisms have been undertaken. Plasmid profile analysis has been used to identify the reservoir and mode of transmission of *S. aureus* infections, especially in hospitals (29). The technique of the arbitrarily primed polymerase chain reaction combined with plasmid profile analysis has provided complementary epidemiologic information in several nosocomial *S. aureus* outbreaks (30).

PATHOGENESIS

Staphylococci produce disease in two ways: directly, by invasion and subsequent tissue destruction, whether locally or after having spread via the blood stream, (15) and through the effects of toxins (11,15) Table 182.2 lists the types of infections produced by *S. aureus*; Table 182.3, the various virulence factors the organisms produce; and Table 182.4, the sequence of pathogenic events associated with serious infections.

**TABLE 182.2.   Infections Produced by
*Staphylococcus aureus***

Direct invasion
  Superficial
    Pyodermas, including impetigo, paronychia
    Skin and soft tissue infections—boils, furuncles, carbuncles,
      cellulitis, lymphangitis, lymphadenitis
  Deep
    Septic arthritis
    Osteomyelitis
    Pyomyositis
Dissemination via the bloodstream
    Bacteremia (sometimes accompanied by bacterial vasculitis), with
      or without septic shock or multiple organ system failure
    Metastatic abscess formation (brain, lung, liver, spleen,
      retroperitoneum, kidney, genital tract)
Toxin-mediated
    Skin disease: staphylococcal scalded skin syndrome
    Gastrointestinal disease: gastroenteritis (staphylococcal food
      poisoning)
    Multisystem disease: toxic shock syndrome

**TABLE 182.4.   Sequence of Pathogenic Events in Serious
Staphylococcus aureus Infections**

Colonization → carriage → toxin production
Barrier breach or break
Invasion (all are enhanced by the presence of a foreign body)
    Cellulitis, lymphangitis
    Abscess formation
    Bloodstream invasion
Bacteremia or septicemia
Syndrome of severe sepsis
    Cell wall components
    Toxic shock syndrome toxin 1
    Role of triggered mediators
Complications
    Suppurative: metastatic abscesses, endocarditis, and others
    Inflammatory: septic shock or multiple organ system failure
      syndromes
Death

Invasive Staphylococcal Infections

In invasive infections, the primary event is the presence of staphylococci as colonizing organisms, which then invade, usually through breaches in the barrier systems of the skin and mucous membranes. The *sine qua non* of staphylococcal infections is the abscess, presenting on the skin as a boil or furuncle. This lesion is an exquisitely tender, erythematous warm lesion that, during the course of 24 to 48 hours, develops a central white pustule. The purulent material is creamy, yellowish, and often contains a "core" (the follicle and its debris) at the site where the infection was initiated. Around foreign bodies, the inoculum of staphylococci necessary to produce disease is quite small and antibiotic therapy is much less successful. *S. aureus* bacteremia develops "spontaneously" in some people (i.e., no identifiable primary focus of infection), and it is assumed either that the patient had subclinical infection of the skin and skin structures or that the organism invaded from a nasopharyngeal—or even, possibly, a gastrointestinal—source.

Once through barrier systems and into the subcutaneous or submucous tissues, *S. aureus* organisms spread quickly, forming abscesses and seeking deep, chronically inflamed or avascular areas. Once in and around bones and other support structures or sequestered in blood clots, the organisms become resistant to attack and eradication by host defenses, the most important host defense cell being the polymorphonuclear leukocyte. The bacteria frequently enter the blood stream, through which they can

spread around the body, sometimes forming multiple metastatic abscesses. From venous foci (e.g., septic thrombophlebitis), they can seed the lungs, causing bacteremic pneumonia with or without the presence of septic thrombi. Once into the arterial circulation, they can adhere directly to damaged endothelial surfaces (deformed valves, arterial aneurysms) and can seed to the major organ systems served by the arterial circulation. In the course of an overwhelming infection, bacterial vasculitis may develop. In such cases, the patient often develops coagulopathy, and the combined vasculitis and a coagulopathy produce a petechial rash that is difficult to distinguish from those of meningococcemia, Rocky Mountain spotted fever, and other septicemic, coagulopathic states (31,32).

The sequence of events during fulminant *S. aureus* bacteremia is still not entirely clear, but it probably duplicates that which has been studied more extensively in gram-negative bacteremic infections. Specifically, in the latter situation, endotoxin from the gram-negative cell wall triggers a series of "mediators," which together produce the manifestations of both hemodynamic instability (septic shock) and end organ failure. We assume that the same sequence is occurring in gram-positive infections (see Table 182.4). In the case of gram-positive microbes, especially staphylococci, it is the cell wall peptidoglycan and/or the teichoic acid complex that trigger(s) the release of mediators (33). Clinically, septic shock or multiple organ system failure is more common with gram-negative infections, but the same sequence can transpire in gram-positive bacteremia. On the other hand, peripheral seeding of the microbe itself (e.g., into organs and tissues to cause metastatic abscesses, endocarditis) is much more common with gram-positive infections, especially staphylococcal infections, than with gram-negative ones (15). The probable reason for this phenomenon is that gram-positive microbes have receptors (surface-associated proteins) (9) on their cell walls for subendothelial vascular components (fibronectin, laminin) and for components of clots, whereas gram-negative microbes have none (or have fewer or less avid ones) and so are much less likely to seed around the body. Bacterial seeding and a propensity to cause secondary abscess formation are hallmarks of *S. aureus* bacteremia. All such specific infections are discussed at length in other chapters of this book.

S. epidermidis, even though it is frequently a cause of low-grade bacteremia (usually from intravenous lines or infected prostheses), rarely produces a septic shock-like picture and does not secondarily seed as frequently as *S. aureus* to deep organs and tissues. Immunocompromised hosts with high-grade

**TABLE 182.3.   Virulence Factors of Coagulase-Producing
Staphylococcus aureus Species**

Enzymes	Catalase, hyaluronidase, lipase
Toxins	α-, β-, γ-, δ-toxins, leukocidin, exfoliatin, enterotoxin, toxic shock syndrome toxin 1
Immune system factors	Antigen-antibody complexes, pseudoimmune complexes, superantigens
Cell wall components	Activated complement, tumor necrosis factor, interleukin-1, and other cytokines and mediator systems

S. epidermidis bacteremia, however, can took quite septic and develop secondary foci of infection. *S. saprophyticus* seems quite specifically to affect only the urinary tract, usually of young women (27), and it seems to have an unusual propensity to adhere to uroepithelial cells. It hardly ever causes urinary tract infection in men (34).

Toxigenic Staphylococcus Infections

The classic syndromes associated with toxin-producing strains of *S. aureus* are the staphylococcal scalded skin syndrome (see Chapter 132), gastroenteritis (see Chapter 77), and the toxic shock syndrome (see Chapter 181). None of the coagulase-negative strains of staphylococci produce clinically significant toxins.

CLINICAL MANIFESTATIONS

Invasive Infections

While patients with peripheral, localized infections caused by staphylococci (and especially those who develop bacteremia) may exhibit the usual manifestations of sepsis, initially, such patients are usually afebrile. Later, fever may develop; some patients experience a chill; and confusion, tachypnea, tachycardia, and ultimately signs of peripheral organ hyperperfusion develop in a few patients. Some patients with septicemia may develop a vasculitic rash consisting of palpable purpuric lesions, which eventually develop small pustules (31,32). These small pustules are the key to differentiating the petechial rash of *S. aureus* bacteremia from that of meningococcal infection, Rocky Mountain spotted fever, and idiopathic thrombocytopenic purpura, among others. Patients with severe but localized organ infections—for example, pneumonia, urinary tract infection, septic arthritis, or osteomyelitis—usually present as does any such patient, with symptoms and signs relevant to the involved organ.

Toxigenic *Staphylococcus aureus* Infections

See Chapters 77, 132, and 181.

DIAGNOSIS

Specific Laboratory Diagnostic Procedures

On Gram stain examination, purulent material from staphylococcal infections exhibits clusters of large gram-positive cocci (see Fig. 182.1). Interpretation of results of cultures is complicated by the need to discriminate colonization from infection. Careful specimen collection and communication between clinician and laboratory personnel are vital for accurate assessment. Initially, the laboratory will report from blood cultures only the presence of "gram-positive cocci," and empirical therapy to cover staphylococci usually will already have been initiated. Later, the laboratory will be able to determine whether the organism produces coagulase and so differentiate *S. aureus* from coagulase-negative staphylococci. At that point, *S. aureus* is generally considered to be a true pathogen until proved otherwise; *S. epidermidis* is rarely (15% or less) a true bacteremic pathogen and is usually a skin contaminant from the site where blood was taken for culture. True *S. epidermidis* bacteremia is identified by the findings of multiple positive blood cultures over a brief time in the presence of an appropriate clinical syndrome and epidemiologic setting (35).

TREATMENT

Specific treatment of all staphylococcal infections is one or more antibiotics. *S. saprophyticus* continues to be sensitive to all the β-lactam antibiotics, including penicillin. A brief course of large doses of penicillin (or for penicillin-allergic patients, a cephalosporin or trimethoprim-sulfamethoxazole) suffices to treat most *S. saprophyticus* urinary tract infections in young women.

Treatment of *S. aureus* and *S. epidermidis* infections is now becoming much more difficult because an increasingly large percentage of strains, both nosocomial *and* community acquired, have become resistant to all of the β-lactam antibiotics (36–38). Detection of β-lactam antibiotic-resistant staphylococci is a complicated procedure, often requiring special testing conditions to ensure that resistance is not overlooked (39–41). Thus, whenever the clinical setting is such that a resistant strain cannot be ruled out, vancomycin must be added to the initial antibiotic regimen. The quinolone group of antibiotics has been effective initially against many resistant strains of *S. aureus* and *S. epidermidis*; however, with increasing use, resistance is a significant problem. More recently, two new agents, quiniquistin/dalfopristin and linezolid have been approved for use by the U.S. Food and Drug Administration and show promise for the treatment of infections due to *S. aureus*, including the β-lactam antibiotic resistant strains. Data have been presented suggesting that the glycopeptide antibiotics (e.g., vancomycin and teicoplanin) are not as effective in controlling complicated *S. aureus* infections as are the β-lactam antibiotics, especially the penicillinase-resistant penicillins (e.g., nafcillin or oxacillin) (42,43). These data have been well summarized by Mortara and Bayer (44). Thus, whenever a β-lactam antibiotic-susceptible strain of staphylococcus is found to be the cause of an infection, nafcillin or oxacillin should be used long term. Note that every effort should be made to reduce vancomycin usage, as continued use is a major factor in selecting for vancomycin-resistant enterococci, which *in vitro* can transmit vancomycin resistance to other gram-positive microbes. Although not based on this transfer mechanism, the report of *S. aureus* isolates with markedly increased minimal inhibitory concentrations for vancomycin from both Japan and the United States reinforce the careful use of vancomycin for therapy (45), and readiness to implement stringent infection control (46).

PREVENTION

Immunization

Despite the multiple immune sequelae of staphylococcal infections and exerted attempts to develop vaccines, no type of immunization has been shown to be effective in ameliorating *S. aureus* infections in humans.

Treatment of the *Staphylococcus aureus* Carrier State

In day-to-day practice, patients with recurrent staphylococcal infections of the skin (e.g., boils, furuncles) benefit from having the strain of *S. aureus* they harbor eliminated from the nose. Oral therapy with rifampin or topical mupirocin nasal ointment have been used to eradicate the carrier state (47,48). Repeated treatment is sometimes necessary anywhere from 6 to 12 weeks later, and individual patients have different cycles of recurrence.

General Preventive Measures

Because the agent of most staphylococcal infections is on, the patient's own colonizing organisms, eradication of carried microbe may be prophylactic. The colonization rate of hemodialysis patients is approximately 75% for *S. aureus* (49,50); prospective treatment of colonized patients with rifampin has been shown to reduce the number of subsequent infections (49). As anticipated, nasal carriage of *S. aureus* has been shown to be a major risk factor for post-cardiac sugery sternotomy wound infections. (19,51) Thus, it seems reasonable to recommend identification of patients at high risk of being nasal *S. aureus* carriers before major surgical procedures wherein postoperative *S. aureus* wound and prosthesis infections are known to be common (e.g., cardiac, orthopedic, neurosurgical, ear-nose-throat). Treatment of potential carriers would permit the operation to occur during the subsequent carriage-free period. This approach, by Cimochowski and associates (19), resulted in a 67% reduction in sternal wound infections after open heart surgery both in diabetic and nondiabetic patients.

Identification and treatment of carriers among hospital personnel has occasionally been found to be helpful during outbreaks of staphylococcal infections. In day-to-day medical practice, simply washing the hands *before and after* interacting with each patient essentially *stops* the spread of organisms. Strict adherence to standard protocols for the placement and maintenance of intravascular lines can substantially reduce rate of line infections. Mupirocin applied intranasally eliminates *S. aureus* nasal carriage in healthy persons for up to 3 months and appears to decrease hand carriage at 72 hours after therapy. Thus, mupirocin may have a role in decreasing hand carriage of colonized medical personnel (52,53).

REFERENCES

1. Baird-Parker AC. Classification of staphylococci and their resistance to physical agents. In: Cohen JO, ed. *The staphylococci.* New York: Wiley, 1972: 1–20.
2. Oeding P. Taxonomy and identification. In: Easmon CSF, Adlam C, eds. *Staphylococci and staphylococcal infections.* New York: Academic Press, 1983: 1–31.
3. Proctor RA, van Langeveld P, Kristjansson M, et al. Persistent and relapsing infections associated with small-colony variants of *Staphylococcus aureus. Clin Infect Dis* 1995;20:95.
4. Schleifer KH. The cell envelope. In: Easmon CSF, Adlam C, eds. *Staphylococci and staphylococcal infections.* New York: Academic Press, 1983:385–428.
5. Tuazon CU, Sheagren JN, Choa MS, et al. *Staphylococcus aureus* bacteremia: relationship between teichoic acid antibody formation and the development of metastatic abscesses. *J Infect Dis* 1978;131:57.
6. Sheagren JN. Guidelines for the use of the teichoic acid antibody assay. *Arch Intern Med* 1984;144:250.
7. Christensen GD, Simpson WA, Bisno AL, et al. Experimental foreign body infections in mice challenged with slime-producing *Staphylococcus epidermidis. Infect Immun* 1983;40:407.
8. Proctor RA. The staphylococcal fibronectin receptor: evidence for its importance in invasive infections. *Rev Infect Dis* 1987;9[Suppl]:S317.
9. Foster TJ, McDevitt D. Surface-associated proteins of *Staphylococcus aureus*: their possible roles in virulence. *FEMS Microbiol Lett* 1994;118:199.
10. Arvidson SO. Extracellular enzymes from *Staphylococcus aureus.* In: Easmon CSF, Adlam C, eds. *Staphylococci and staphylococcal infections.* New York: Academic Press, 1983:745–808.
11. Lowy FD. *Staphylococcus aureus* infections. *N Engl J Med* 1998;339:520.
12. Wadstrom T. Biological effects of cell-damaging toxins. In: Easmon CSF, Adlam C, eds. *Staphylococci and staphylococcal infections.* New York: Academic Press, 1983:671–704.
13. Kotb M. Bacterial pyrogenic exotoxins as superantigens. *Clin Microbiol Rev* 1995;8:411.
14. Archer GL, Tenenbaum MJ. Antibiotic-resistant *S. epidermidis* in patients undergoing cardiac surgery. *Antimicrob Agents Chemother* 1980;17:269.
15. Sheagren JN. *Staphylococcus aureus*: the persistent pathogen. *N Engl J Med* 1984;310:1368, 1437.
16. Weinstein HJ. The relation between the nasal staphylococcal carrier state and the incidence of postoperative complications. *N Engl J Med* 1959;260: 1303.
17. Wenzel RP, Perl TM. The significance of nasal carriage of *Staphylococcus aureus* and the incidence of post operative wound infection. *J Hosp Infect* 1995;31:13.
18. von Eiff C, Becker K, Machka K, et al. Nasal carriage as a source of *Staphylococcus aureus* bacteremia. *N Engl J Med* 2001;344:11.
19. Cimochowski GE, Harostock MD, Brown R, et al. Intranasal mupirocin reduces sternal wound infection after open heart surgery in diabetics and nondiabetics. *Ann Thorac Surg* 2001;71:1572.
20. Pockaj BA, Topalian SL, Steinberg SM, et al. Infectious complications associated with interleukin 2 administration: a retrospective review of 935 treatment courses. *J Clin Oncol* 1993;11:136.
21. Raviglione MC, Mariuz P, Pablos-Mendez A, et al. High *Staphylococcus aureus* nasal carriage rate in patients with acquired immunodeficiency syndrome of AIDS-related complex. *Am J Infect Control* 1990;18:64.
22. Senthilkumar A, Kumar S, Sheagren JN. Increased incidence of *Staphylococcus aureus* bacteremia in hospitalized patients with acquired immunodeficiency syndrome. *Clin Infect Dis* 2001;33:1412.
23. Cone LA, Woodward DR, Byrd RG, et al. A recalcitrant erythematous desquamating disorder associated with toxin-producing staphylococci in patients with AIDS. *J Infect Dis* 1992;165:638.
24. Dondorp AM, Veenstra J, van der Poll T, et al. Activation of the cytokine network in a patient with AIDS and the recalcitrant erythematous desquamating disorder. *Clin Infect Dis* 1994;18:942.
25. Fast DJ, Schlievert PM, Nelson RD. Toxic shock syndrome-associated staphylococcal and streptococcal pyrogenic toxins are potent inducers of tumor necrosis factor production. *Infect Immun* 1989;57:291.
26. National Nosocomial Infection Surveillance (NNIS) System. Data Summary from October 1986 – April 1998. Atlanta: Hospital Infections Program, National Center for Infectious Diseases, Centers for Disease Control and Prevention. Public Health Service, U.S. Department of Health and Human Services, 1998.
27. Hovelius B, Mardh PA, Bygren P. Urinary tract infections caused by *Staphylococcus saprophyticus. J Urol* 1979;122:645.
28. Parker MT. The significance of phage-typing patterns in *Staphylococcus aureus.* In: Easmon CSF, Adlam C, eds. *Staphylococci and staphylococcal infections.* New York: Academic Press, 1983:33–62.
29. Cohen ML, Wong ES, Falkow S. Common R plasmids in *Staphylococcus aureus* in a nosocomial *Staphylococcus aureus* outbreak. *Antimicrob Agents Chemother* 1982;21:210.
30. Fang FC, McClelland M, Guiney DG, et al. Value of molecular epidemiologic analysis in a nosocomial methicillin resistant *Staphylococcus aureus* outbreak. *JAMA* 1993;270:1323.
31. Murray HW, Tuazon CU, Sheagren JN. Staphylococcal septicemia and disseminated intravascular coagulation: *S. aureus* endocarditis mimicking meningococcemia. *Arch Intern Med* 1977;137:844.
32. Mitunski MR, Gallis HA, Fuekerson WJ. *Staphylococcus aureus* septicemia mimicking fulminant Rocky Mountain spotted fever. *Am J Med* 1987;83:801.
33. Sheagren JN. Inflammation induced by *Staphylococcus aureus.* In: Gallin JI, Goldstein IM, Synderman R, eds. *Inflammation: basic principles and clinical correlates.* New York: Raven Press, 1988:829–840.
34. Kauffman CA, Hertz CS, Sheagren JN. *Staphylococcus saprophyticus*: role in urinary tract infections in men. *J Urol* 1983;130:493.
35. Kirchhoff LV, Sheagren JN. Epidemiology and clinical significance of blood cultures positive for coagulase-negative *Staphylococcus. Infect Control* 1985;6: 479.
36. Brumfitt W Hamilton-Miller J. Methicillin-resistant *Staphylococcus aureus. N Engl J Med* 1989;320:1188.
37. Mulligan ME, Murray-Leisure KA, Ribner BS, et al. Methicillin resistant *Staphylococcus aureus*: a consensus review of the microbiology, pathogenesis and epidemiology with implications for prevention and management. *Am J Med* 1993;94:313.
38. Shopsin B, Mathema B, Martinez J, et al. Prevalence of methicillin-resistant and methicillin-susceptible *Staphylococcus aureus* in the community. *J Infect Dis* 2000;182:359.
39. McDougal LK, Thornsberry C. The role of β-lactamase in staphylococcal resistance to penicillinase penicillins and cephalosporins. *J Clin Microbiol* 1986; 23:832.
40. Hackbarth CJ, Chambers HF. Methicillin-resistant staphylococci: genetics and mechanisms of resistance. *Antimicrob Agents Chemother* 1989;33:991.
41. Kloos WE, Jorgensen JH. Staphylococci. In: Lennette EM, ed. *Manual of clinical microbiology.* Washington, DC: American Society for Microbiology, 1985:143–153.
42. Small PM, Chambers HF. Vancomycin for *Staphylococcus aureus* endocarditis in intravenous drug users. *Antimicrob Agents Chemother* 1990;34:1917.
43. Levine DP, Fromm BS, Reddy BR. Slow response to vancomycin or vancomycin plus rifampin in methicillin resistant *Staphylococcus aureus* endocarditis. *Ann Intern Med* 1991;115:674.
44. Mortara LA, Bayer AS. *Staphylococcus aureus* bacteremia and endocarditis: new diagnostic and therapeutic concepts. *Infect Dis Clin North Am* 1993; 7:53.
45. Tenover FC, Lancaster MV, Hill BC, et al. Characterization of staphylococci with reduced susceptibilities to vancomycin and other glycopeptides. *J Clin Microbiol* 1998;36:1020.
46. Wenzel RP, Edmond MB. Vancomycin-resistant *Staphylococcus aureus*: infection control considerations. *Clin Infect Dis* 1998;27:245.
47. Wheat LJ, Kohler RB, Shite AL, et al. Effect of rifampin on nasal carriers of coagulase-positive staphylococci. *J Infect Dis* 1984;144:177.

48. Parenti MA, Hatfield SM, Leyden JJ. Mupirocin: a topical antibiotic with a unique structure and mechanism of action. *Clin Pharmacol* 1987;6:761.
49. Yu VL, Goetz A, Wagener M, et al. *Staphylococcus aureus* nasal carriage and infection in patients on hemodialysis: efficacy of antibiotic prophylaxis. *N Engl J Med* 1986;315:91.
50. Kirmani N, Tuazon CU, Murray HW, et al. *Staphylococcus aureus* carriage rate among patients on chronic hemodialysis. *Arch Intern Med* 1978;138:1657.
51. Kluytmans JAJW, Mouton JW, Pljzerman EPF, et al. Nasal carriage of *Staphylococcus aureus* as a major risk factor for wound infections after cardiac surgery. *J Infect Dis* 1995;171:216.
52. Reagan DR, Doebbeling BN, Pfaller MA, et al. Elimination of coincident *Staphylococcus aureus* nasal and hand carriage with intranasal application of mupirocin calcium ointment. *Ann Intern Med* 1991;114:101.
53. Doebling BN, Breneman DL, Neu HC, et al. Elimination of *Staphylococcus aureus* nasal carriage in health care workers: analysis of six clinical trials with calcium mupirocin ointment. *Clin Infect Dis* 1993;17:466.

CHAPTER 183
Streptococcus pyogenes
(*Group A Streptococci*)

Gene H. Stollerman

INTRODUCTION

As a result of the great variety of clinical syndromes it causes, *Streptococcus pyogenes* (group A streptococcus) is one of the most extensively studied human pathogens. *S. pyogenes* owes its species name to its role in causing pyogenic infections, either as an invader of the throat (pharyngitis) and lower respiratory tract (pneumonia) or of the skin (impetigo, erysipelas), of the endometrium (puerperal sepsis), or of traumatic or surgical wounds (cellulitis, lymphangitis, and necrotizing fasciitis). Certain of its strains may cause scarlet fever, toxic shock, or post-infectious non-suppurative sequels, such as acute rheumatic fever (ARF) and acute glomerulonephritis (AGN). Poststreptococcal reactive arthritis (PSRA) and postinfectious autoimmune neurologic diseases (PANDAS) are other syndromes with a more recently recognized relationship to antecedent group A streptococcal infection.

CLINICAL MICROBIOLOGY

The diversity of these clinical syndromes, their geographic variation, and the secular changes in their epidemiology within the relatively short history of their discovery speak for the diversity of the strains of this single species classified among the 30 or more of the genus *Streptococcus*. It has been classified on the basis of hemolysis observed on blood agar plates, antigenic composition, growth characteristics, biochemical reactions, and currently by genetic analysis. It is likely that rapid current progress in the latter will lead to better future strain characterization.

Microscopic Appearance

Streptococci are spherical or ovoid gram-positive organisms, no larger than 2 μm in diameter. Cell division occurs in one plane by the formation of an equatorial plate, which results in the formation of chains of varied length, usually 6 to 12 cocci. Electron microscopy reveals fine hair-like fimbriae by which the organism apparently adheres to cell surfaces (1) (Fig. 183.1).

Colonial Morphology

On blood agar plates, the great majority of group A streptococci colonies have a clear zone around them resulting from complete lysis of red blood cells referred to as β-hemolysis. In contrast, α-hemolysis differentiates colonies of *Streptococcus viridans* that incompletely lyse red blood cells in the surrounding medium and convert hemoglobin to a greenish pigment. γ-Hemolysis refers to colonies that are nonhemolytic. Sheep blood is ideal for primary isolation of cultures on blood agar. Strains of group A streptococci that are well-encapsulated form large mucoid colonies, which on fresh isolation have the appearance of a drop of oil. With dehydration, the colony surface becomes roughened (matte) (2) (Fig 183.2). Nonencapsulated or slightly encapsulated colonies have an opaque, pearly appearance. Freshly isolated, virulent strains dissociate rapidly on artificial media. Passage of selected mucoid colonies through mice or fresh human blood is necessary to preserve cultures in the virulent phase. Virulence is also well preserved by freeze-drying.

Cultural Characteristics

Group A streptococci are facultative anaerobes. They do not produce catalase or oxidase and do not contain heme compounds. They are sensitive to heat, requiring only 30 minutes at 60°C for sterilization. The cultures are optimally made in blood-enriched media at pH 7.4 to 7.6 incubated at 37°C under reduced oxygen tension and a 10% carbon dioxide atmosphere. Under anaerobic conditions, hemolysis is enhanced. Reducing substances such as thioglycollate shorten the lag period of growth.

CELL STRUCTURE AND COMPONENTS

The Cell Wall

MURAMYL PEPTIDOGLYCANS
These basic cell wall structures are mucopeptides (peptidoglycans) consisting of repeating subunits of *N*-acetyl-D-glucosamine and *N*-acetyl-D-muramic acid, connected to a tripeptide, D-glutamic acid, L-lysine, and D- and L-alanine. They are potent immunologic adjuvants.

GROUP A CARBOHYDRATE
Linked to the peptidoglycan is the group A carbohydrate, a branched polymer composed of dimers of L-rhamnose, *N*-acetyl-D-glucosamine in a 2:1 ratio, the latter comprising the antigenic determinant. Classically, it is identified by precipitin tests made with specific antiserum.

M PROTEINS
Hemolytic streptococci were first serotyped in agglutinin tests by Griffith (3). Later, Lancefield found the organisms that she classified by their carbohydrate as group A to contain three heterotypic surface protein antigens, M, T, and R (4). More than 100 M serotypes have been identified to date. Strains that have dissociated and lost M protein still may be identified serologically by their T antigens. More than 90% of strains may be classified serotypically by using M and T antigens. Genes encoding many M proteins (*emm*) have been identified and are being used increasingly to better identify group A strains (5,6,6a).

Molecular Structure and Biological Properties of M Protein
Strains expressing M protein resist phagocytosis when incubated in nonimmune blood, whereas M-negative strains are readily phagocytosed and killed. Homologous type M antibodies are

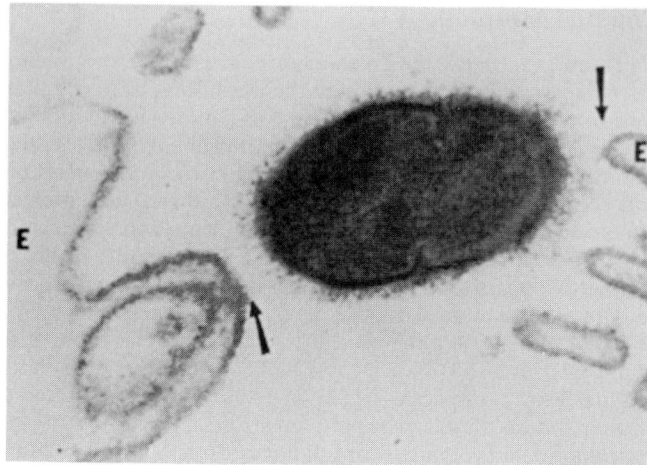

Figure 183.1. Electron micrograph of group A streptococci adhering to the surface of a buccal mucosal cell. Prominent surface projections (fimbriae) contain both M protein and lipoteichoic acid. E = buccal mucosal cell. (From Beachey EH, Ofek L. Epithelial cell binding of group A streptococci by lipoteichoic acid on fimbriae denuded of M protein. Reproduced with permission from *The Journal of Experimental Medicine*, 1976;143:759–771.)

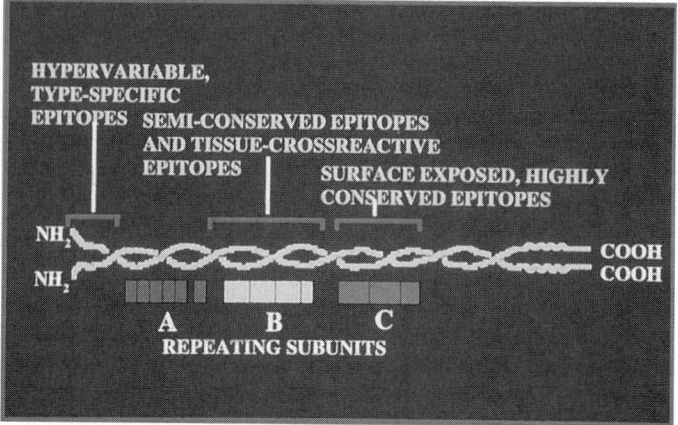

Figure 183.3. Functional domains of M protein: Schema depicting the location on the M protein molecule of the epitopes cross-reactive with myocardium, synovia, and brain. They are shown located within and flanking the repeats of the M5 molecule, well proximal to the type-specific epitopes within the N-terminal. (Courtesy of Dr. James B. Dale.)

type-specifically protective, and therefore M protein contains the immunologic potential for a streptococcal vaccine (see section "Prospects for a Vaccine Against Rheumatic Fever"). Gentle treatment of the organism with dilute pepsin removes the terminal piece of the M protein molecule from surface fimbriae (5). The extracted "Pep M" is a filamentous macromolecule with a spring-like, α-helical coiled-coil structure (6). The N-acetyl terminus of pep M contains the peptide's type-specific epitope (5). It can be separated from the proximal portion of the Pep M molecule that contains epitopes cross-reactive with host tissues, heart, skin, synovia, and brain (7,8) (Fig 183.3) (see section "Prospects for a Vaccine Against Rheumatic Fever").

The molecular structure of M protein differs in strains that cause pharyngitis ("throat strains") from that of the "skin strains" associated with pyoderma (see later). Nucleotide sequences of M protein genes (*emms*) form five distinctive chromosomal patterns, labeled A to E. Skin strains are virtually all of the D,E pattern, whereas throat strains (including those associated with rheumatic fever) are almost all of the A,B,C pattern. Some throat strains appear to be distributed between both of these groupings (9,10).

OTHER SURFACE PROTEINS

Streptococcal protective antigen (Spa) contains newly identified epitopes that are clearly separable from M protein but that also evoke protective homologous type antibodies in humans (11). Expression of both Spa and M protein is apparently required for optimal virulence of the strains in which it has been found. The distribution of Spa in various M serotypes is under investigation.

Serum opacity factor (OF), also closely associated with M protein, is an α-lipoproteinase that opacifies serum. Strains of at least 29 known M types elaborate this type-specific antigen (12). It is a useful epidemiologic marker, and a common component of skin strains. OF positive strains produce weaker anti-M immune responses than those of OF negative strains and are apparently not rheumatogenic.

CELL ADHERENCE FACTORS

In addition to M proteins, adherence of group A streptococci to host mucosal cells is mediated by other ligands binding to fibronectin. These include lipoteichoic acid and the F proteins (F1 and Sfb1) (13,14). These promote internalization of the organism by mucosal epithelial cells. F1 also has been associated with strains stubbornly carried in the throat asymptomatically following penicillin therapy (15).

The hyaluronate capsule has a major anti-phagocytic effect and therefore is an important virulence factor (16,17). It is responsible for the "mucoid" appearance of colonies on blood agar (see Fig 183.2) and is well demonstrated by India ink preparations or polychrome staining of liquid cultures. Streptococcal hyaluronate is chemically identical to that of the human host. Highly polymerized, intact hyaluronate was not found to be immunogenic until sensitive immunologic methods (enzyme-linked immunosorbent assay) revealed that antibodies can be raised against streptococcal hyaluronate that has been partially denatured (18). New insights into the control of genetic

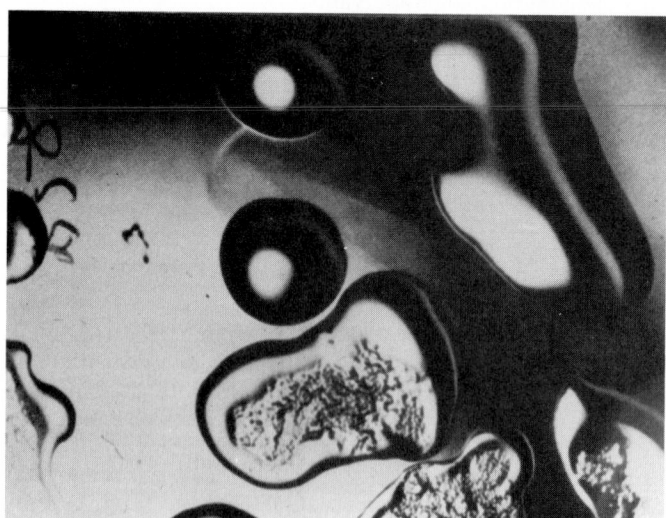

Figure 183.2. "Mucoid" colonies of highly encapsulated group A streptococci growing on the surface of blood agar. Some of the colonies have begun to dry to form a "matte" surface. (From Wilson AT. The relative importance of the capsule and the M antigen in determining colony form of group A streptococci. *J Exp Med* 1959;109:257, with permission from The Rockefeller University Press.)

repression and expression of the capsule along with other important virulence factors are discussed below.

Extracellular Products

S. pyogenes releases a great variety of biologically active products into the culture medium during growth The β-hemolysins, streptolysin O (SLO) and streptolysin S (SLS), are both produced by most group A strains and by streptococci belonging to groups C and G as well (19). SLO is so named because of its sensitivity to oxygen by which it is reversibly inactivated. SLO is cytotoxic to a variety of cells and is a potent cardiac toxin. Antistreptolysin O antibodies are clinically useful indicators of antecedent group A streptococcal infection (see later).

SLS is related to the bacteriocin family of microbial toxins. By weight, it is one of the most potent cytotoxins known, destroying cell membranes and organelles. It is oxygen-stable, of low molecular weight and exists in intracellular, cell-surface-bound and extracellular forms. It is readily extracted from the group A streptococcal (GAS) surface by serum (hence its name "serum streptolysin") or by media containing other high-molecular-weight carriers such as albumin, ribonucleic acid (RNA), and polysorbate detergents (Tween 80). Such carriers stabilize its potent hemolytic activity. Unlike SLO, SLS is non-antigenic. Its hemolytic activity is inhibited by serum lipoproteins and other phospholipids (20). The genetic determinants involved in SLS production (*sag*, for SLS-associated genes) have been identified in a nine-gene locus (21). Its expression, along with other virulence factors will be discussed.

PYROGENIC EXOTOXINS (ERYTHROGENIC EXOTOXINS)

Streptococcal pyrogenic exotoxins (A, B, C mitogenic factor, and streptococcal superantigen) are responsible for the rash of scarlet fever and have been implicated in the pathogenesis of toxic shock syndrome (22). Like diphtheria toxin, they appear to be synthesized as the consequence of infection with temperate bacteriophages, probably accounting for the striking strain variation in the capacity of group A streptococci to cause scarlet fever, toxic shock, or both. As with streptolysin S, the biologic effects of these toxins can be seen in the intense hypersensitivity and characteristic erythema they evoke in the skin of susceptible subjects. These reactions were the historical basis of positive Dick tests (23). Persons with adequate immunity to erythrogenic toxins do not react (negative Dick test). Antitoxin injected into the skin of a patient with scarlet fever causes localized blanching because of neutralization of the erythrogenic toxin (Schultz-Charlton reaction).

DEOXYRIBONUCLEASES A, B, C, AND D

Four deoxyribonucleases (DNases) have been purified and serologically distinguished. They account for the breakdown of nucleoproteins and thus for the thin pus of group A streptococcal infections. Anti-Dnase B is a serum antibody useful, such as antistreptolysin O to detect recent group A streptococcal infection (25).

STREPTOKINASE

Two different streptokinases are produced by group A streptococci. These enzymes are antigenically distinct from group C streptokinase, the source of the commercial streptokinase used in therapeutic thrombolysis. Streptokinase forms complexes with plasminogen activator and catalyzes the conversion of plasminogen to plasmin. Plasmin in turn digests fibrinogen and fibrin. Thus, streptokinase also contributes to the thinning of streptococcal pus. With hyaluronidase it may facilitate the rapid spread of streptococci through the skin and lymphatics that is seen in cellulitis. Streptokinase antibodies are raised after most streptococcal infections, and these can be measured by the antistreptokinase serologic test (26,27).

Streptococcal hyaluronidase hydrolyzes hyaluronic acid, present in the streptococcal capsule, and also that found in the matrix of animal connective tissues. Known as a "spreading factor" in the skin, this enzyme is also produced readily in the infected host, eliciting antibodies with approximately the same frequency as SLO and DNase B and streptokinase (28). Other extracellular enzymes produced by many GAS strains include proteinases, NADase, adenosinetriphosphatase, phosphatases, esterases, amylase, and neuraminidase.

STREPTOCOCCAL INFECTIONS

Virulence Properties of Infecting Strains

Streptococci can divide every 20 minutes in the log phase of growth, but when phagocytosed are rapidly killed because they are highly susceptible to the antibacterial action of oxygen radicals and other antibacterial substances within phagosomes. Streptococcal infection, therefore, is principally extracellular, and virulence is related primarily to resistance to phagocytosis and toxin production. Strains that lack M protein and capsules are easily recognized and killed by phagocytes (16). They readily interact with receptors on phagocytes and activate complement components through the alternative and classical complement pathways (29). Encapsulated strains that are rich in M protein strikingly resist phagocytosis and grow rapidly in fresh human blood unless recognized by M-type-specific antibodies. Resistance to phagocytosis is enhanced by M protein's precipitation of fibrinogen, further blocking surface interactions with complement components and phagocyte receptors (30). In addition, a cell-surface-bound C5a peptidase cleaves human C5, inactivating this potent chemoattractant (31). Highly encapsulated mutants apparently are less readily internalized by epithelial cells (32) or skin keratinocytes (33–35) than less or non-encapsulated strains so that the latter less virulent strains may be more likely to be carried asymptomatically.

Genetic Control of Virulence

Genes of many GAS virulence factors have been identified and cloned. Control of their expression at various stages of infection and growth underlies their capacity for variation of strain virulence. GAS can apparently sense environmental changes through a two-component response regulator (CsrRS or CovRS, for "control of virulence genes") that represses transcription of several virulence operons (36) (Table 183.1). One of these, a two-component regulatory system originally designated CsrR/CsrS (capsule synthesis regulation) (37,38) represses genes that encode the synthesis of the hyaluronate capsule (*hasA*), streptolysin S (*saga*), pyrogenic exotoxin B (*speB*), and streptokinase (*ska*). CsrS is a membrane-spanning sensor kinase, and CsrR is a DNA-binding cytoplasmic protein. Mutations that affect expression of CsrR result in enhanced expression of the regulated genes. Such CsrR mutants are highly mucoid and produce increased SLS activity and SpeB protein (39).

An independent multiple gene regulator (Mga) (40–42) that is autoregulated (no negative regulator has been yet identified), activates transcription of several other virulence genes including those encoding M protein (*emm*), C5a peptidase (*scpA*), itself (*mga*) and other factors. Some genes such as *emm*, *scpA*, *mga*, and *hasA* are expressed during exponential growth but

TABLE 183.1. Group A Streptococcal Virulence Genes

Gene	Gene product
mga[a]	Multiple gene regulator for
emm[a]	M protein
scpA[a]	C5a peptidase
covR[b]	CovR (control of virulence genes)
hasA[a]	capsule synthesis
sagA[c]	streptolysin S
ska	streptokinase
speMF#[c]	mitogenic factor
slo	streptolysin O
speA, speB, speC	pyrogenic exotoxins A, B, C

[a]Maximal expression during growth phase.
[b]Originally named *csrRS* gene for two-component negative control of capsule synthesis.
[c]Maximal expression during stationary phase.
Based on data from references 36–40.

not in the stationary growth phase (36,40). These genetic insights promise to explain changes in strain virulence among group A streptococci that by environmental signals or mutation, or both, lead to the emergence of clones that may produce either severe or mild infections or relatively harmless mucosal or skin carriage (40a,42).

SPECIFIC INFECTIONS: CLINICAL SYNDROMES AND INFECTING STRAINS

Group A streptococci may be classified clinically as the agents of pharyngitis (throat strains), pyoderma (skin strains), rheumatic fever (throat only), glomerulonephritis (skin or throat), and scarlet fever and toxic shock (throat or skin strains). Invasive infections of skin and soft tissues may be produced by any of these strains that contain the relevant virulence factors. As noted earlier, the M protein gene emm patterns on chromosomes are distinctive for either impetigo strains (pattern D,E) or rheumatogenic throat strains (A,B,C), whereas nonrheumatogenic strains isolated from the throat may belong to either or both patterns (9,10). Some of the strains isolated from the throat may have spread there secondarily from skin lesions. Of special interest is the difference between rheumatogenic and nonrheumatogenic strains of the A,B,C pattern (see later).

Streptococcal Pharyngitis

EPIDEMIOLOGY

Group A streptococcal pharyngitis is one of the most common bacterial human infections. It differs much in frequency, severity, and clinical characteristics, depending on the patient's age, the character of the infecting strains, and the epidemiologic circumstances that affect their transmission. The high attack rate in families, institutions and military recruits is the result of contact among susceptible persons that is close enough to ensure droplet spread of infection. Explosive food-borne or waterborne outbreaks are also well documented. Less virulent strains of group A streptococci cause asymptomatic colonization but are readily transmitted. During convalescence from pharyngitis, GAS strains lose M protein and capsules. Yet, such attenuated strains may be carried stubbornly, making throat carriage among school children very common (43). Although much lower in adults, throat carriage rates of 15% to 20% have been reported

in school-age children. Streptococci that contaminate fomites and dust rapidly lose virulence and infectivity (44).

Host susceptibility to streptococcal pharyngitis does not appear to be influenced by race, ethnic group, climate, geography, or nutrition alone. Age is important in that infants may express only mild rhinorrhea rather than acute local symptoms and signs of pharyngitis but they are prone to develop secondary suppurative complications of otitis media, sinusitis, cervical adenitis, and even bacteremia. By childhood, however, increased nonspecific immunity develops and pharyngeal infection becomes explosive, with intense local and systemic responses. Peak rates of streptococcal pharyngitis and throat carriage occur between 5 and 15 years. In temperate climates during winter months, approximately 25% of all children complaining of sore throat may have a positive culture result for GAS. Of these mild, sporadic infections, less than half can be demonstrated to have immunologically significant infections (45), whereas in outbreaks the percentage may reach 85% or greater (46). In the absence of M-type–specific immunity, adults acquire infection at a rate similar to that for children.

CLINICAL FEATURES

The incubation period of GAS pharyngitis is brief, 2 to 4 days. Onset of sore throat and fever is sudden. Pain on swallowing may be severe. Coryza, rhinitis, laryngitis, cough and bronchitis, and hoarseness are not associated symptoms as they frequently are in viral respiratory infections. Systemic symptoms include fever, headache, malaise, anorexia, and, especially in younger children, abdominal pain and vomiting. Chilliness is common but not rigors. Examination of the pharynx reveals diffuse erythema, edema, patchy or confluent tonsillar exudates, and hypertrophy of the lymphoid tissues of the posterior pharynx. The anterior cervical nodes are typically enlarged and tender. The course of the infection is relatively brief. Fever abates within several days, and sore throat and constitutional symptoms rarely last more than 1 week. Indeed, in controlled studies in military recruits, significant differences in duration of fever were not observed in patients treated with penicillin compared with those treated symptomatically. Milder infections often do not express these classic findings and are not clearly diagnosed by clinical manifestations alone. Indeed, even the proposed criteria for a presumptive clinical diagnosis of GAS pharyngitis, fever, exudative pharyngitis., tender, enlarged cervical lymph nodes, and absence of cough, have a positive predictive value of less than 70% (47).

DIAGNOSIS

Group A streptococcal pharyngitis must be differentiated from sore throat produced by other bacterial and viral agents. Of the former, group C and G streptococcal infections may be most confusing, but these are milder, do not often cause suppurative complications, and do not cause rheumatic fever. Gonococcal pharyngitis must be considered in populations in which fellatio is practiced, and its clinical appearance may be readily confused with that of group A streptococcal infection. Although diphtheria is now rare, it should be considered in vulnerable, nonimmunized populations. *Mycoplasma pneumoniae* may cause sore throat, but the infection usually involves some other part of the respiratory tract as well, usually the bronchi. *Arcanobacterium* (formerly *Corynebacterium haemolyticum*) is a rare cause of pharyngitis. It usually affects teenagers and adults and may produce exudative pharyngitis and a scarlatiniform rash, thus closely mimicking *S. pyogenes* pharyngitis.

The major confusion in differential diagnosis stems from common viral nasopharyngeal infections (47) (see Chapter 46), some of which cause pharyngeal and tonsillar exudate, particularly those due to adenovirus infections and infectious mononucleosis. Failure to respond to a trial of penicillin therapy should alert the clinician to a cause other than GAS and to the fact that in such cases culture isolation of streptococci from throat secretions represents throat carriage from an earlier infection. Experienced clinicians using clinical impressions alone might fail to treat one quarter to one half of the patients with positive throat cultures and might needlessly treat one in four patients who are neither infected or colonized by group A streptococci. Laboratory confirmation is therefore particularly helpful when epidemiologic conditions require precise diagnosis.

LABORATORY DIAGNOSIS

The white blood cell count is usually greater than 12,000/mm^3 and the serum level of C-reactive protein increased. Confirmation of the presence of pharyngeal GAS is achievable by the following methods.

Culture of Throat Secretions

If specimens are properly taken the throat culture propagates large numbers of group A β-hemolytic streptococci in 90% to 95% of patients with characteristic clinical symptoms and signs. To obtain culture material from the throat, swabs should be passed under direct vision over the pharyngeal tonsils and posterior pharynx. The swab should then be streaked directly, as soon as possible, on a sheep's blood agar plate of low dextrose content. Stabbing through the agar with the inoculating loop is recommended to grow some colonies below the surface at low oxygen tension to encourage hemolysis from streptolysin O production. Colonies should be noted for mucoid characteristics (see earlier). For definitive epidemiologic studies, serologic grouping and typing or strain identification by genetic markers should be made by reference laboratories.

Rapid Antigen Detection Tests

Rapid antigen (group A) detection tests (RADTs) made from throat swabs are currently popular with clinicians because they can be processed and reported within hours and are available in commercial kits (48,49). Whereas the specificity of some RADTs has been reported as 95% or greater, their sensitivity may be considerably less. A negative throat culture or RADT reported in a patient with pharyngitis has great negative predictive value, sparing overuse of ineffective antibiotic therapy.

However, in sporadic infections, previously acquired throat carriage lowers the positive predictive value for throat cultures or RADTs to approximately 75%. The practical value of throat cultures for adults in current clinical practice in the United States and the United Kingdom is controversial. Guidelines by expert committees of the American Academy of Pediatrics (49), the Infectious Disease Society of America (48), and the American Heart Association (50) favor greater precision in diagnosis by the use of throat cultures. American College of Physicians' guidelines for diagnosis in adults (51,52), however, eschews throat cultures in favor of RADTs, and suggests that even the latter are unnecessary criteria for antibiotic therapy in the presence of typical clinical manifestations of GAS pharyngitis (see Treatment).

Streptococcal Antibodies

Although not relevant to the prompt diagnosis of acute GAS infection, a significant increase in the convalescent titer of streptococcal antibodies is the gold standard for establishing antecedent streptococcal infection (53,54). Extensive studies have established the behavior and usefulness of antibodies to streptococcal extracellular products such as SLO, DNase B, hyaluronidase, streptokinase, and NADase, among others. Antistreptolysin O and anti-Dnase B have become the most commonly available tests commercially. Repeated streptococcal infections set the expected mean level of "normalcy" of antibody titers in a given population, and such values therefore relate to both the age groups studied and the epidemiologic setting. The curve of the rate of decline of elevated streptococcal antibody titers has been established in patients with ARF who received monthly injections of benzathine penicillin G to prevent intercurrent streptococcal infection (53). When such patients receive continuous penicillin prophylaxis, the decline in titer is rapid for the first 2 to 3 months. Anti-SLO titers, for example, fall much more slowly when levels decline to approximately 200 units/mL. After streptococcal pharyngitis (except in quite young children) the increase in titer is rapid, consistent with secondary antigenic stimulation, and peak titers are usually observed within a few weeks. When titers are initially increased above 300 units/mL in serum samples obtained during the acute phase of infection, further increases may be more difficult to demonstrate. Given an initial titer of less than 200 units/mL, approximately 80% of patients demonstrate a twofold or greater increase between acute- and convalescent-phase values. When two different antibodies are tested with the same serum, a boost in titer is observed in one or the other in at least 90% of patients who have streptococcal pharyngitis. Type-specific antibodies to M protein can be detected by several methods (55,56), but the methods are technically complex and are used principally for investigative and epidemiologic purposes. Prompt and effective antibiotic therapy suppresses anti-M immune responses that are primary. In contrast, other streptococcal antibodies commonly measured, such as anti-SLO, are usually secondary immune responses and are therefore less readily suppressed by antibacterial therapy.

TREATMENT OF GROUP A STREPTOCOCCAL PHARYNGITIS

Group A streptococci are uniformly highly sensitive to the action of penicillin. For multiplying organisms, penicillin G is rapidly bactericidal in a concentration of 0.01 to 0.04 units/mL in a standard broth culture. No penicillin-resistant strains have emerged despite almost half a century of intense clinical use. Sustained bactericidal blood levels, however low, eradicate proliferating group A streptococci. Since World War II, the treatment of GAS pharyngitis has been strongly directed toward the primary prevention of rheumatic fever and suppurative complications. Where rheumatic fever persists in the world, and particularly in undeveloped countries, primary rheumatic fever prevention is still the major aim of the treatment of group A streptococcal pharyngitis. Such treatment should ensure effective penicillin levels for at least 10 days (57). Because this can be achieved by a single intramuscular injection of 1.2 million units of benzathine penicillin G, or 600,000 units for children who weigh less than 27 kg or 60 pounds, this regimen is a favored one. Intramuscular injections of repository penicillins, however, produce some local pain and discomfort, and they must be administered by physicians or nurses. Injectable benzathine penicillin G for pharyngitis, therefore, has declined in popularity in developed countries in which the fear of ARF has virtually disappeared, and it has been replaced by oral penicillin, usually penicillin V (48–50). Treatment of GAS sore throat should be started promptly, although a delay of a few days while awaiting culture results does not seem to interfere with prevention of attacks of ARF (60).

Oral penicillin regimens appear to be adequate, however, to provide rapid symptomatic relief and to prevent suppurative complication of pharyngitis. Penicillin V, the current preferred oral penicillin, may be given twice daily in 1.0-g doses and has been shown to be at least as effective as 0.5 g administered four times daily, with greater compliance seen with a twice-daily regimen (61). Oral cephalosporins are also highly effective in the treatment of streptococcal pharyngitis, and some reports show even a slightly higher rate of clinical cure and eradication of convalescent carriage than that achieved with penicillin therapy (62). Despite these observations, penicillin remains the drug of choice because of its proven efficacy in preventing rheumatic attacks, its low cost, and its relatively narrow spectrum. In non-epidemic settings in which rheumatic fever is rare or nonexistent, shorter coursers of oral penicillin may be clinically effective.

If penicillin allergy is suspected or known to exist, erythromycin has been the drug of choice, in doses of 20 mg/pound per day (not to exceed 1 g/day) for a period of 10 days. Although erythromycin resistance is not a serious problem in the United States, the drug has caused resistance with striking frequency in some countries when it is used as the first-line drug for treatment of sore throat. Newer macrolides, azithromycin, clarithromycin are also effective but more expensive. Treating streptococcal pharyngitis with sulfonamides does not prevent rheumatic fever. Sulfonamides are quite effective, however, as secondary prophylactic agents for rheumatic fever recurrences (see later). Tetracycline-resistant group A streptococci are prevalent in many areas; therefore, this drug is not recommended.

SCARLET FEVER

Epidemiology of scarlet fever (23) is closely related to that of streptococcal pharyngitis and also to that of streptococcal pyoderma because it depends on the capability of any strain to produce one or more of the pyrogenic exotoxins (see previous section). Scarlet fever may be produced by rheumatogenic strains as well, and the epidemiology of the two diseases was often superimposed in the pre-antibiotic era. In the 19th century, the severe toxicity of scarlet fever in industrializing nations made it a dreaded, and sometimes fatal, disease. By the 1920s, however, its severity and frequency waned, and by the 1950s the prevalence of scarlet fever dramatically declined. Pyrogenic exotoxin-producing strains have been reappearing in the United States, principally as a result of soft tissue infections. Most of these infections are relatively mild but some may result in severe systemic symptoms, frequently associated with fatal shock or severe multiorgan damage. Streptococcal strains, therefore, can produce any of the erythrogenic toxins in any kind of streptococcal disease, and the independent expression of the pyrogenic toxins may account for the vagaries of scarlatina throughout modern medical history (63).

Clinical manifestations of scarlet fever, in addition to pharyngitis, may include the classic enanthema, strawberry tongue (one that is coated with red, protruding papillae) or raspberry tongue (bright red with large papillae). Within a day or 2 of the sore throat, the scarlatinal rash appears on the face, sparing the area around the lips (circumoral pallor) and spreading to the neck, chest, back, and remainder of the trunk and extremities. The rash is a diffuse erythema, blanching on pressure, and may have punctate elevations that roughen the skin. The inner aspects of the trunk, arms, and thighs are most intensely affected. Pastia lines are linear striations of confluent petechiae related to capillary fragility induced by the erythrogenic toxin, which may be demonstrated by an applied tourniquet (the Rumpel-Leede sign). The erythema abates in 6 to 9 days, followed by a characteristic desquamation of the skin during the second week, most often affecting the palms and soles. Striking eosinophilia often occurs during this stage of desquamation. The scarlatinal rash must be differentiated from the rashes of viral exanthems, Kawasaki disease, staphylococcal TSS, and drug eruptions.

COMPLICATIONS

Suppurative complications of pharyngitis most frequently affect contiguous pharyngeal cavities, such as the middle ear and paranasal sinuses. Mastoiditis and meningitis caused by *S. pyogenes* are now quite rare. Bacteremia leading to metastatic involvement of joints, bones, and other sites and group A streptococcal pneumonia also now occur mostly in epidemics caused by highly virulent strains, as has been observed in military recruit camps (64,65). Streptococcal pneumonia also occurs in economically depressed populations where medical care is inadequate and living conditions are crowded.

Peritonsillar abscess, or quinsy, is not usually caused by group A streptococcal infection alone but is due, rather, to the formation of a polymicrobial abscess in which anaerobic throat flora predominate. Aerobic cultures of aspirate from such abscesses therefore may not isolate a pathogen, but the infecting anaerobic throat flora is exquisitely sensitive to penicillin treatment, which, with adequate drainage, produces a dramatic response. Peritonsillar abscess must be suspected when an abrupt increase in pain and dysphagia, swelling of the neck, and fever arise after a primary pharyngitis. Displacement of the tonsil can be seen on the affected side, and a fluctuant mass can be readily palpated with a gloved finger. Early diagnosis and prompt penicillin therapy are essential to prevent the development of necrotizing fasciitis of the neck, which can be a fatal complication (Ludwig angina) (66).

Patients with more severe suppurative complications may require larger doses of penicillin administered parenterally.

Streptococcal Skin Infections

Pyoderma is a term used to denote localized purulent streptococcal infections of the skin. Skin wounds or burns can be secondarily infected by any virulent group A streptococcus, but certain streptococcal strains have particular tropism for the skin causing common superficial pyodermas usually referred to as streptococcal impetigo or impetigo contagiosa (see Chapter 132 on skin infection) (67). In temperate climates, impetigo is most common during summer months, when children frequently sustain insect bites and trauma to exposed skin, particularly in populations whose poor hygiene and sanitation promote transmission. Streptococci responsible for pyoderma can adhere to and colonize intact skin, so insect bites and minor abrasions and trauma can initiate the superficial lesions. Washing and proper hygiene are therefore major preventive measures. Skin strains find their way within a few weeks from skin to the mucosa of the nose and throat, where they may cause pharyngitis and acute glomerulonephritis but not rheumatic fever.

Skin strains of streptococci are distinguished by certain features. In general, they belong to certain M and T types. Their chromosomal arrangement of M proteins genes are distinctive (see above). Such strains rarely form highly mucoid colonies and have relatively low virulence for mice. They do not resist phagocytosis in human blood as strikingly as heavily encapsulated, M-rich throat strains. The skin infections they cause are associated with blunted anti-SLO but brisk anti-DNase B responses (68). Type-specific anti-M responses are also relatively weak (69). Skin strains usually produce the serum opacity factor SOR (see earlier). Pyoderma is not associated with rheumatic fever (67).

The lesions of pyoderma begin as papules, usually on an exposed area of the body that is traumatized by an abrasion or an insect bite. They are often multiple, and within a few days form thick crusts that heal slowly and leave depigmented areas. Systemic symptoms are absent but regional lymphadenitis may occur. Culture of material from the surface of these lesions usually yields staphylococci (aerobic) much more often than group A streptococci (facultatively anaerobic). The latter are easily overgrown by the former on surfaces exposed to air. When crusts and scabs are removed, however, and the deeper exudate is propagated in culture, virtually pure isolates of group A streptococci result. Staphylococcal infection, however, may coexist.

The association of certain pyoderma-producing strains with epidemic acute glomerulonephritis is well recognized (see later). A more serious form of pyoderma is the deeper ulcerated lesion known as ecthyma. These lesions may be caused by skin irritation and maceration by footwear (especially in tropical climates). They are often located on the ankle or dorsum of the foot and may be complicated by cellulitis and lymphangitis.

Impetigo is readily prevented with good personal hygiene and adequate cleansing of the skin. It usually responds well to penicillin therapy except in the presence of coinfection with a penicillinase-producing strain of *S. aureus*. It then may require treatment with cloxacillin, or a cephalosporin such as cephalexin, cefadroxil, or cefaclor given orally for 10 days (70). Erythromycin's effectiveness is limited in areas in which erythromycin-resistant strains are prevalent. Mupirocin ointment is an effective but expensive alternative therapy for stubborn cases (71).

ERYSIPELAS

The features of erysipelas make it unique clinically because of its explosive onset. Unlike the indolent pyoderma lesions described earlier, this infection spreads rapidly through skin lymphatics from a small abrasion, particularly around the nares. Erysipelas often erupts across the cheeks and nose and affects the eyelids, which may become edematous or shut, so that the presentation may resemble angioneurotic edema (Fig.183.4). The lesion is intensely painful and erythematous, has a characteristic elevated advancing margin, and may vesiculate and even form bullae that rupture and crust. Erysipelas can lead to bacteremia and death, particularly in infants and in frail elders. Attempts at culture isolation of material from the lesions are usually frustrated because bacteria are not numerous locally, suggesting hypersensitivity or toxin-producing features. Management, therefore, depends on prompt clinical recognition and penicillin therapy, which is curative.

Perianal, vulvovaginal and penile infections due to group A streptococci may be a relatively common diagnosis in a pediatric

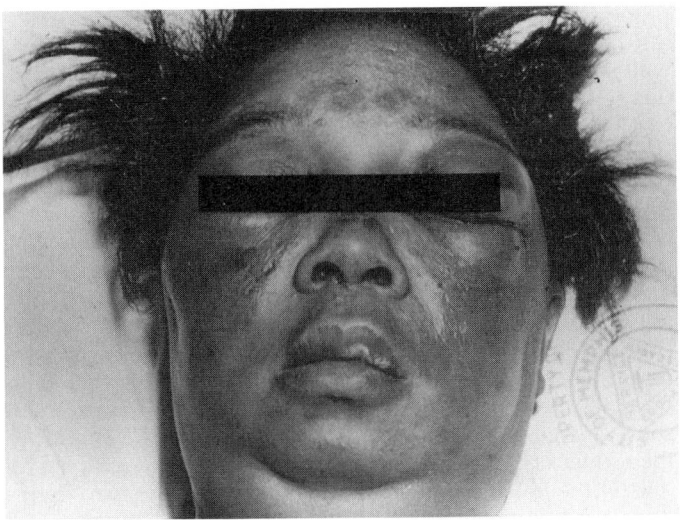

Figure 183.4. Erysipelas due to an M56 group A streptococcal strain in a patient who subsequently developed acute glomerulonephritis.

or family practice setting. Mostly affected are children with an average age of 5 years, often in day care and preschool settings, where they are associated with a range of perineal, gastrointestinal and urinary tract symptoms (72).

Invasive Streptococcal Infections

CELLULITIS

Rapid spread of group A streptococci through the skin and subcutaneous tissues with lymphangitis and bacteremia is a distinctive feature of wound infection with virulent group A streptococci. It may occur as a complication of burns and traumatic and surgical wounds but may also follow mild trauma and other skin lesions. It is differentiated from erysipelas in that the lesion is not raised; the demarcation between involved and uninvolved skin is indistinct (long red streaks rather than an advancing border of intradermal swelling). A strong predisposing factor is impaired lymphatic drainage such as that seen after radical mastectomy, saphenous vein removal for coronary bypass grafting (73), intravenous drug abuse (74), and recurrent lymphangitis secondary to chronic tinea pedis and other skin lesions (75).

Streptococcal cellulitis responds brilliantly to intravenous or repository intramuscular penicillin G therapy. Semisynthetic penicillinase-resistant penicillin may be used when staphylococcal infection cannot be excluded on initial presentation. In the absence of a positive blood culture, a clear distinction between streptococcal and staphylococcal infection may not be made because aspirate or biopsy results are often negative or because surface skin contamination by staphylococci is quite common and may confuse the diagnosis.

RECENT INCREASE AND SPREAD OF SEVERE INFECTIONS BY INVASIVE STRAINS

After a dramatic decline in the 1970s, focal outbreaks of acute rheumatic fever appeared in military and civilian populations in the United States. These were associated with the reappearance of highly virulent, encapsulated ("mucoid") rheumatogenic, M protein serotypes (see acute rheumatic fever). Shortly thereafter, unusually severe invasive streptococcal infections were reported in the United States, Europe, Australia, Japan and elsewhere (76). Many of these life-threatening infections were caused by M types 1 and 3. The portal of entry for these infections was usually the skin and soft tissues. Some of these infections gave rise to shock and multiorgan failure, with manifestations similar to those of the staphylococcal toxic shock syndrome (77).

Streptococcal toxic shock syndrome (TSS) is characterized as the sudden onset of shock and multiple organ failure and may be associated with any streptococcal infection by pyrogenic toxin-producing strains (see above). Most cases of streptococcal TSS have occurred in healthy patients with an initial focal infection of the skin and soft tissue. Severe puerperal infections associated with disseminated intravascular coagulation are also well documented (78). TSS occurs only rarely in association with pharyngeal infection alone. Secondary cases of TSS are very uncommon, although streptococcal strains causing TSS may be readily transmitted from person to person and may initiate invasive disease in susceptible contacts (79). Treatment of contacts is advised by some authorities but deemed unnecessary by others (80). The clinical features and management of toxic shock is discussed in more detail elsewhere (81) (see Chapter 181).

NECROTIZING FASCIITIS (STREPTOCOCCAL GANGRENE)

This terrifying and often fatal fulminating infection has received much media publicity as due to a "flesh-eating organism" because of its involvement of the deeper subcutaneous tissues and fascia, characterized by rapidly spreading necrosis and gangrene of the skin and underlying structures. The infection may be polymicrobial with both aerobic and anaerobic microorganisms. Originally called "streptococcal gangrene" by Meleney (82), it characteristically begins at the site of a trivial or inapparent trauma as a mild erythema progressing rapidly to an extensive, dusky bluish swelling. Bullae containing yellowish or hemorrhagic fluid may appear. Bacteremia and frank gangrene follow within a few days. Mortality is high even with appropriate medical and surgical intervention. To aid in diagnosis, a biopsy with frozen sections should be made as soon as the diagnosis is suspected (83). In addition to intravenous penicillin therapy, prompt surgical intervention with extensive debridement of dead and devitalized tissues is necessary as soon as the diagnosis is confirmed (66,84).

OTHER INVASIVE GROUP A STREPTOCOCCUS INFECTIONS

Streptococcal bacteremia, pneumonia, infective endocarditis, and puerperal sepsis may complicate deep streptococcal infections and their current incidence morbidity and mortality have been recently reviewed (84). Most suppurative streptococcal infections respond well to intramuscular injections of procaine penicillin G, 600,000 units once or twice daily. For life-threatening infections in hospitalized patients, intravenous penicillin may be employed and is recommended in larger doses. Although secondary cases are rare, family member and health care workers are most likely to acquire and carry these strains asymptomatically and transmit such dangerous clones (85,86). Decisions for antimicrobial prophylaxis should be individualized.

POSTINFECTIOUS SEQUELAE

Acute Rheumatic Fever

ARF is a post-streptococcal systemic inflammation characterized predominantly by polyarthritis and pancarditis. Sydenham's chorea is a less common, but no less clinically characteristic manifestation. Though relatively uncommon, erythema marginatum and subcutaneous nodules, the other two major manifestations, are important only because they improve diagnostic accuracy. The lesions of rheumatic fever are sterile, so that it has been called a nonsuppurative sequela. ARF appears after a latent period of 10 to 30 days when residual symptoms and signs of the pharyngeal infection are gone. In fact, approximately 30% of patients may not recall it at all. The history, pathology, detailed clinical manifestations and global significance are described extensively elsewhere (87–89). In this chapter I am concerned mainly with the diagnosis and management of ARF as an infectious disease, because the group A streptococcus has been established as the sole agent of ARF and the prevention of rheumatic heart disease, its most important complication, depends on the proper treatment and prevention of group A streptococcal pharyngitis.

ETIOLOGY

To initiate ARF, the site of group A streptococcal infection must be pharyngeal (90). The characteristics of the strains clearly responsible for the great ARF epidemics of World War II are well known (91). They are very rich in M-protein, heavily encapsulated by hyaluronic acid, and highly mouse virulent (Fig 183.5). They produce striking "mucoid" colonies on blood agar plates. They are tropic primarily for the throat rather than the skin, infecting the latter secondarily through wounds. They evoke strong type-specific immune responses. They do not seem to contain lipoproteinase (the serum opacity factor) that is usually found in skin

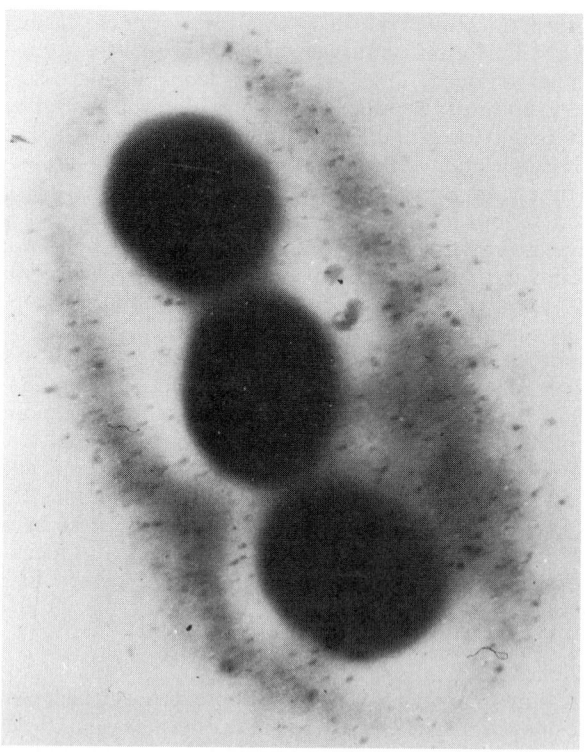

Figure 183.5. Electron microphotograph of a chain of group A streptococci (type M24) isolated during a rheumatic fever epidemic in a military population. The cocci are enclosed by a large hyaluronic acid capsule shadowed by M24 antibody precipitated on its surface. (Reprinted with permission from Stollerman GH. The return of rheumatic fever. *Hosp Pract* 1988;23:100–106.)

strains. Streptococci that are clearly rheumatogenic have been found so far among but a limited number of M serotypes, notably 1,3,5,6,18, 19, and 24, and some others. They possess "class I" rather than "class II" epitopes (92) and their M proteins have the characteristic chromosomal patterns of throat strains (9,10) (see above). In addition, they contain epitopes cross-reactive with host tissues (94) and their M-associated proteins have potent superantigenic properties (95) (see the section on M protein). It should be noted, however, that none of these characteristics are specific for rheumatogenic strains alone so that no one virulence property has been identified as uniquely rheumatogenic.

The attack rate of streptococcal pharyngitis among healthy, well-nourished military recruits in controlled studies of previous epidemics was approximately 3% (46), varying with the intensity of the immune response evoked. In civilian populations, however, not all strains identified within the above M serotypes have retained a high degree of virulence (96), a fact that caused much confusion about the notion of the rheumatogenic potential of specific M proteins (97). ARF has not been observed following pharyngeal infection with strains belonging to some other common pharyngeal serotypes, notably types 2, 4, and 28 (98,99), nor to strains causing sporadic mild pharyngitis in U.S. school children (100) (Table 183.2). The M types associated with pyoderma (see above) are not associated with ARF, even when these infect the throat. For example, in the southern United States, seasonal changes virtually completely dissociated ARF and AGN, the former occurring following group A streptococcal pharyngitis in the fall and winter, and the latter following pyoderma during the summer (101).

Recurrences of rheumatic fever (secondary attacks) are also caused solely by group A streptococcal pharyngitis, but occur at

TABLE 183.2.   Virulence Studies of Strains Obtained from Throat Cultures of 1,000 Children with Untreated Nonexudative Pharyngitis

No. β-hemolytic: 292
No. group A: 233   No. patients who developed rheumatic fever: 0
　Group A, M typable: 95/233
　　Amount of M protein:[a] Low 86, Moderate 9, High 0
　　Colony morphology: Mucoid 1, Glossy 94
　　Mouse virulence:[b] None 74 Slight 16 Moderate 5 High 0
　　Growth in fresh human blood[c] 20
　Group A with capsules[a] (India ink): Large 1, Small 31, None 2

Virulence studies of strains of group A streptococci obtained from throat cultures made in Chicago school children with untreated mild (nonexudative) pharyngitis. In the 95 M typable strains, virulence was determined by: amount of extractable M protein, degree of encapsulation, mouse virulence, and growth in fresh human blood, all compared with a virulent M19 strain that caused an epidemic of rheumatic fever.
[a]Compared with standard epidemic strain M19, high in extractable M protein.
[b]High = LD_{50} 1000; Low = LD_{50} <100.
[c]Ability to increase inoculum 2× or > in 3 hr.
Based on data from Stollerman GH, Siegel AC, Johnson EE. Variable epidemiology of streptococcal disease and the changing pattern of rheumatic fever. *Mod Concepts Cardiovasc Dis* 1965;34:45–48.

much higher attack rates after such infection than those of primary attacks. The most important variables determining the secondary attack rate are: the presence or absence of heart disease, the number of previous attacks, the duration since the last attack, and the intensity of the immune response to the antecedent infection (102) (Table 183.3). Recurrences tend to be mimetic, that is, similar in manifestations to the original attack (103).

CHANGING EPIDEMIOLOGY OF ACUTE RHEUMATIC FEVER

Rheumatic heart disease (RHD) was once the major cardiac disease of children and young adults, and before World War II ARF was a greater cause of death in school-age children than all other diseases combined (87). In the industrialized nations of the world, however, the prevalence of ARF and RHD declined dramatically after World War II, and precipitously in the 1970s (104) along with the disappearance of the strains once known to be rheumatogenic (97). Yet, ARF and RHD has remained widespread in many developing countries of the world (105) where in-depth coordinated clinical and microbiological studies of the causative group A streptococcal strains remain to be made.

TABLE 183.3.   Ratio of Rheumatic Recurrences to Streptococcal Infections in Patients Stratified for Heart Disease and for Anti-Streptolysin O Rise

Anti-SLO (Tube dilutions)	Heart disease		No heart disease	
	Ratio	%	Ratio	%
0–1	3/24	13	1/72	1
2	10/36	28	2/46	4
3	6/16	37	4/32	13
4	9/14	65	9/25	36

From Taranta A, Wood HF, Feinstein AR, et al. Rheumatic fever in children and adolescents. A long-term epidemiologic study of subsequent prophylaxis, strepococcal infections, and clinical sequelae. IV. Relation of the rheumatic fever recurrence rate per streptococcal antibodies to the titers of streptococcal antibodies. *Ann Intern Med* 1964;60[Suppl 5]:47–57, with permission.

—Fort Leonard Wood, Missouri, 1987 and 1988

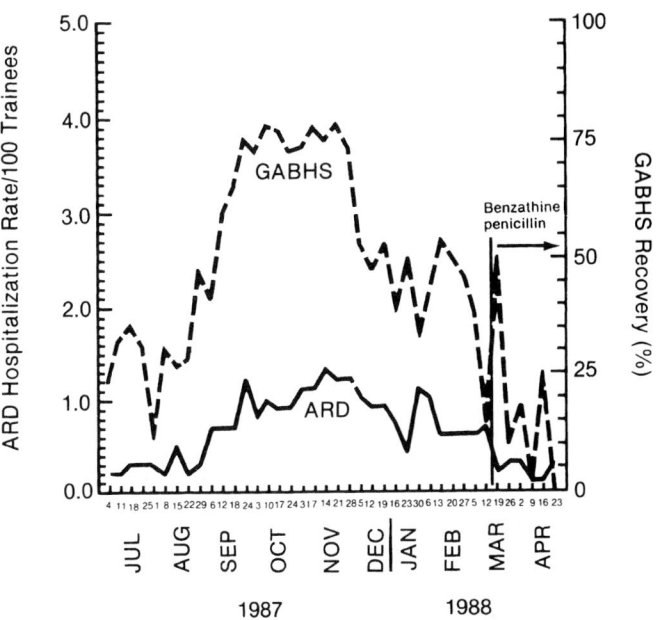

Figure 183.6. **A:** Patient with group A streptococcal pharyngitis. **B:** Throat culture from patient in **A** showing colonies of β-hemolytic streptococci growing on sheep's blood agar. Bacitracin disks marked **A** show zone of inhibition of growth.

In the 1980s, focal outbreaks of rheumatic fever reappeared in the United States among military recruits (106,107) and among schoolchildren in many civilian communities belonging to middle-class populations with relatively high health care standards (108–110) (Fig. 183.6). Among contacts of these cohorts were found "mucoid" strains of GAS belonged to some of the same M serotypes that caused the great World War II military epidemics of ARF (97,109,110). This resurgence of rheumatic fever in the 1980s was followed later in the decade by the reappearance in North America, Europe and Japan of invasive streptococcal infections of unusual virulence (97) (see above). These invasive infections, however, were not associated with ARF, although rheumatogenic strains may produce pyrogenic toxins (e.g., as in scarlet fever).

DECLINING RECURRENCES OF RHEUMATIC FEVER

In the late 1970s, streptococcal infections that were detected retrospectively by streptococcal immune responses in rheumatic subjects failed to reactivate the disease (111). Such studies supported the concept of disappearing rheumatogenic strains. In a local Santiago, Chile cohort of rheumatic subjects (112) penicillin prophylaxis was safely discontinued after several years when rheumatic recurrences virtually disappeared along with the prevalent M typable strains of streptococci (only 7% recognizable by M typing, compared with the initial rate of 52%). Still, rheumatic fever persisted in high incidence among cohorts in other sections of the city. Such a situation resembles that of other places in the world where focal populations are heavily affected by ARF, while nearby populations are almost completely spared.

HOST FACTORS

The predisposition of rheumatic hosts to recurrences may be genetic or acquired, or both. ARF is rare in very young children, and reaches its peak incidence between 6 to 15 years of age after repeated group A streptococcal pharyngeal infections. Streptococcal antibody responses in ARF patients are exaggerated compared with cohorts in whom acute streptococcal pharyngitis is uncomplicated by rheumatic fever (113). This observation is consistent with strain virulence of the antecedent pharyngitis since rheumatic hosts do not produce exaggerated responses to nonstreptococal antigens (114). Both the observed hyperimmunity and the intensity of antigenic stimulation by the initiating infection have been considered relevant to the pathogenesis of rheumatic fever (46).

The role of genetic predisposition is less clear. ARF is far less concordant in identical twins (about 20%) than it is in twins with other immunologic diseases such as atopic allergy and hyperthyroidism, or in infections such as tuberculosis or poliomyelitis (115). No clear association of class I human leukocyte antigens (HLAs) with rheumatic fever has been found. The trend toward an association of HLA-B5 may be related to an increased response to streptococcal antigens produced by these persons. HLA-DR2, -3, and -4 have been detected with increased frequency in black, white, and Indian patients, respectively, principally those with rheumatic heart disease. HLA-DR1 and -DRw6 were observed with increased frequency in South African black persons (116,117). Recent analyses indicate that certain class II alleles/haplotypes are associated with risk or protection from rheumatic heart disease and that these associations are stronger and more consistent when analyzed in patients with relatively more homogeneous clinical manifestations (118).

In contrast to the lack of a definitive association with specific HLA-DR antigens, a strong relationship has been detected with a non-HLA B-cell antigen designated 883 and detected in widely distributed populations from New York to Bogota, Colombia, and New Mexico to India (119). Studies with a series of monoclonal antibodies directed against B cells from rheumatic fever patients have identified another B-cell alloantigen labeled D8/17 (117). It is present in a relatively large percentage of the total B cells of rheumatic fever probands: 33.5% compared with 14.6% and 13%, respectively, of the B cells of unaffected siblings and parents. Two sets of identical twins were included in these studies. The proband with rheumatic fever had 43% positive B cells, whereas the unaffected twin had only 15%. In the other set of unaffected twins, 20% and 10%, respectively, had D8/17 B cells. Thus, this B-cell alloantigen is not unique to rheumatic hosts but is expressed more vigorously in those who have had rheumatic fever. Perhaps a predisposing host factor, present to some degree in all persons, is more expressible in rheumatic hosts who are stimulated by antigens, and perhaps superantigens contained in virulent pharyngeal strains of group A streptococci (see below).

PATHOGENESIS

Autoimmunity is often hypothesized to cause inflammation of the heart and its valves (94). Purified synthetic peptides of M protein isolated from rheumatogenic strains contain epitopes cross-reactive with cardiac tissues. Some of these react with myosin and keratin, coiled proteins of primary and secondary (and perhaps tertiary) molecular structure similar to that of M protein (120). Other streptococcal antigens cross-react with heart valve glycoproteins and fibroblasts, synovia and articular cartilage, brain tissues and skeletal muscles, smooth muscle, liver, lymphocytes, thymus, skin, and kidney (121). Large amounts of group A streptococcal antigens swallowed in the course of GAS pharyngitis may result in the production of protective type-specific IgE (122). In susceptible hosts, such an immunologic stress may break immune tolerance. Resulting autoimmune complexes may produce the non-destructive synovitis of ARF, the non-destructive reversible reactions in the basal ganglia observed in Sydenham's chorea, and autoimmune, cell-mediated cytotoxic reactions may destroy heart valves (123).

CLINICAL FEATURES OF ACUTE RHEUMATIC FEVER

ARF is remarkable for the unity and diversity of the syndrome. The major manifestations of rheumatic fever may sometimes appear as isolated findings, but more impressive is the relative consistency of their association. For example, in the outbreak of ARF in Utah (108), polyarthritis, carditis, and chorea occurred with the same frequency as they did many years ago in the cities of the temperate zone of the United States, before the great decline of ARF began. Moreover, when careful prospective observations were made in a pediatric population served by a general medical clinic in New Delhi, India, the relative respective frequencies of these manifestations were similar to those reported in the Western world (87).

Polyarthritis

Migratory polyarthritis of rheumatic fever is its least specific but most common major manifestation. Because of its dramatic onset 10 to 30 days from the antecedent streptococcal pharyngitis streptococcal antibodies are at or near their peak. These high titers help to support the diagnosis of rheumatic fever. Because polyarthritis due to causes other than rheumatic fever may also occur coincidentally following streptococcal pharyngitis, increased streptococcal antibody titers may be a false-positive finding. However, negative streptococcal antibody titers virtually exclude the diagnosis of rheumatic polyarthritis (27). Rheumatic polyarthritis does not respond to penicillin or other antibiotics. A therapeutic trial of penicillin may be useful, therefore, to rule out a highly responsive pyogenic polyarthritis, such as acute gonococcal polyarthritis. A fuller discussion of rheumatic polyarthritis appears elsewhere (87,88) and its relation to poststreptococcal reactive arthritis is discussed below.

Carditis

The pancarditis of ARF is symptomatic only when cardiac insufficiency is expressed as fatigue or shortness of breath or when pericarditis (usually "silent") is painful. Most cases of carditis are not severe enough to produce such symptoms and therefore carditis is usually diagnosed by detection of the murmurs produced by its invariable valvulitis (124) or by Doppler echocardiography (125,126). These facts account for the frequency of the discovery of rheumatic valvular disease in patients who do not recall having ARF, particularly in populations who do not receive adequate medical attention. Mild, sporadic bouts of ARF can therefore lead to a confusing global epidemiologic pattern of rheumatic heart disease in populations wherein overt ARF is claimed to be rare despite the high prevalence of rheumatic heart disease.

The mildest cases of apparent rheumatic carditis, so-called "silent" (subauscultatory) episodes of valvular regurgitation, have been identified by Doppler echocardiography in 15–20% of cases. Whether or not subauscultatory mitral regurgitation will be generally accepted as the sole diagnostic criterion of acute rheumatic carditis RF is at issue. That diagnosis depends on the experience of the examining cardiologist, not only with the technique of echocardiography but with the diagnostic criteria of rheumatic valvulitis. A more detailed discussion of the clinical features of acute rheumatic carditis can be found elsewhere (87,89,91).

Sydenham's Chorea

In its florid form, chorea is easily recognized by the patient's erratic, jerky, purposeless movements, stumbling gait (St. Vitus' dance), fleeting local muscular weakness, emotional lability, and personality changes. In its mildest form it is often overlooked or misdiagnosed. Like polyarthritis, it is most often evanescent, over in a few weeks, but occasionally it may be stubborn, persisting for many months. The sex distribution of chorea is noteworthy. Before puberty, it is equally common in both sexes. Thereafter, chorea disappears in mature men, accounting for its absence in military epidemics. On the other hand, pregnancy aggravates and exacerbates chorea (chorea gravidarum). The latent period between streptococcal pharyngitis and chorea is prolonged, often to 2 to 3 months or more, by which time evidence of antecedent streptococcal infection may be absent if streptococcal antibody titers have returned to relatively low levels by the time they are measured (127). At such time, all evidence of rheumatic inflammation, including C-reactive protein and erythrocyte sedimentation rate elevation, may also have abated. If polyarthritis was not noted in the initial phase of the disease and carditis was also either transient or absent, the syndrome of "pure" chorea may emerge. Like other chorea patients, they suffer similarly frequent recurrences of this manifestation following intercurrent streptococcal pharyngitis (129).

Erythema Marginatum

Erythema marginatum is a vasohumoral, focal, evanescent erythema localized mostly to parts of the body usually covered by clothes (trunk and proximal extremities). Its pink color is not readily seen except on fair skin and with the aid of natural light. Although it is less frequently expressed as part of the rheumatic syndrome and is often difficult to recognize, it is a characteristic, if nonspecific, manifestation of ARF.

Subcutaneous Nodules

These are also easily overlooked because they are pea sized, painless, and movable and appear evanescently over bony prominences. They are most often associated with rheumatic carditis.

Minor manifestations that are entirely non-specific but constant include fever (almost invariable), arthralgias (common), abdominal pain (more often in younger patients), and epistaxis (occasional). All are regularly associated with an increase in serum acute phase reactants (e.g., C-reactive protein) and erythrocyte sedimentation rate, and commonly with electrocardiographic changes, most often prolongation of the PR-interval.

DIAGNOSIS

The modified Jones criteria (124,126) continue to be a useful guideline for the diagnosis of ARF. They require the presence of either one major and two minor or two major manifestations supported by evidence of antecedent streptococcal infection. The latter relies heavily on evidence of increased levels of streptococcal antibodies, but an understanding of the rise and fall of such antibodies after streptococcal infection is necessary to appreciate their advantages and limitations (87–89) (see previous section).

Two syndromes may occur as complications of GAS pharyngitis and may or may not be considered part of the rheumatic fever syndrome (91):

Poststreptococcal Reactive Arthritis

The characteristics of poststreptococcal reactive arthritis (PSRA) that are not typical of ARF are: persistence of arthritis for several months, non-migratory polyarthritis, poor response to nonsteroidal antiinflammatory drugs and, in adults, an apparent predilection for females. Thus, some authors claim that PSRA does not meet the characteristic description of polyarthritis presented in the Jones criteria and should therefore be excluded (130). Although a different etiology of polyarthritis may be inadvertently included in this type of reactive arthritis, some authorities prefer to retain so-called PSRA patients on antibiotic prophylaxis, but for a modified duration, the exact time dependent on other variables, particularly the age of the patient and the prevalence of ARF in the community (see secondary prophylaxis). Moreover, some PSRA patients have developed rheumatic valvular disease after several years of follow-up, in-

deed, in some reports as high as 7% of PSRA in children (130). Although the numbers of the reported cases of so-called PSRA are still rather few, and not always similarly defined, they deserve further study.

Post-Infectious Autoimmune Neurologic Diseases

These include tics, Tourette's syndrome, and obsessive-compulsive behavior, all of which have been observed in some patients during or after an attack of rheumatic chorea (131). PANDAS that did not express choreiform movement usually were not previously referred to rheumatic fever investigators (132). Antibasal ganglia antibodies, however, are now well-known for their association with both Sydenham's chorea and with PANDAS (134), the latter of which are recognized as possible sequelae to group A streptococcal infection (132–136). If studies that are in progress reveal them to be totally or partially preventable by antistreptococcal prophylaxis, they might well be included, like PSRA, as variable features of the syndrome of ARF.

TREATMENT OF ACUTE RHEUMATIC FEVER

Once ARF has appeared treatment with penicillin does not alter the course of the disease. Neither is antiinflammatory therapy curative nor does it shorten the attack. Both salicylates and corticosteroids are highly effective, however, in suppressing inflammation but do not prevent ultimate cardiac valvular damage (137). The prognosis of rheumatic valvular damage depends on the severity of initial rheumatic carditis (138,139). Recommended anti-inflammatory therapy and general management is considered more fully elsewhere (87,88).

PREVENTION OF ACUTE RHEUMATIC FEVER: PROPHYLAXIS OF STREPTOCOCCAL INFECTIONS

Mass Prophylaxis

Prophylactic treatment of an entire population may be required when rheumatic sequelae are associated with a focal epidemic of streptococcal pharyngitis. Such events are rare now except in military populations or in closed institutions. A single injection of 1.2 million units of benzathine penicillin G to each person in the population affected has promptly terminated such epidemics (107,140,141) (see Fig. 183.6).

Primary Prophylaxis

Primary rheumatic fever prophylaxis consists of prompt and effective treatment of GAS pharyngitis (48,50,91) (see above). For patients who have had a previous bout of rheumatic fever, primary prophylaxis is inadequate and secondary (continuous) prophylaxis is mandatory.

Secondary Prophylaxis

Secondary attacks prophylaxis begins as soon as the diagnosis of ARF is made. Continuous prophylaxis is initiated with either a single intramuscular injection of 1.2 million units of benzathine penicillin G, or a 10 day course of penicillin V orally (50). Prevention of recurrences of ARF is most effective by monthly injections of 1.2 million units of intramuscular benzathine penicillin G. (58,142,143). Oral prophylactic regimens are also effective but less reliable (50). They are recommended when the risk of rheumatic recurrences is low. Penicillin V orally is recommended in doses of 250 mg twice daily. The recommended dose of oral sulfadiazine is 0.5 g once daily for patients who weigh less than 27 kg (60 pounds) and 1 g daily for heavier persons. For the rare patient who is sensitive to both penicillin and sulfonamides, erythromycin may be substituted in a dose of 250 mg twice daily.

The duration of continuous prophylaxis for rheumatic subjects cannot be stated arbitrarily because of the number of variables influencing the rate of recurrences (128). Such variables include the presence or absence of rheumatic heart disease, the duration from the previous attack, the number of previous attacks, and the severity of the antecedent infection. To these should now be added variation in the local prevalence of rheumatogenic streptococci (111,112).

Prospects for a Vaccine Against Rheumatic Fever

Pep M (see previous section) is immunogenic in animals and humans (4,5). An effective vaccine against rheumatic fever may not require the inclusion of all known M protein serotypes, but rather those identified most clearly as containing rheumatogenic strains. The *N*-acetyl-terminal type–specific epitope of pep M protein can be separated from the proximal, toxic parts of the molecule and from the epitopes cross-reactive with host tissues (8) (see Fig. 183.3). By recombinant DNA techniques, numerous M serotype epitopes now have been linked to form a multivalent polypeptide vaccine that is protective in animal studies (8,144–146). The potential of such preparations for oral human immunization for the production of IgA antibodies to M proteins is also suggested by recent studies (8,144a,146).

Poststreptococcal Acute Glomerulonephritis

ETIOLOGY

Acute glomerulonephritis (AGN) may follow infection with specific nephritogenic strains of group A streptococci. These may be either pharyngeal or skin strains (67). Nephritogenic strains have been associated with strains within a well-defined group of M serotypes: 1, 2, 3, 4, 12, 15, 49, 55, 56, 59, 60, 61 and probably others (147,148). Type 12 is most frequent among the pharyngeal strains that have caused AGN (149), but most M12 strains are not nephritogenic. Thus, M serotype alone is not an adequate marker for nephrogenicity (150). Seasonal peaks of AGN have been clearly dissociated from those of ARF in climates and populations in which both diseases are endemic, such as the southern United States (101). In the Caribbean island of Trinidad, the epidemiologic patterns of AGN and ARF are also distinct—ARF is present year-round and AGN occurs in approximately 6-year cycles and the streptococcal strains that cause each sequela appear to be distinct as well (151). Unlike rheumatic fever, however, the clinical syndrome of AGN is not specific for *S. pyogenes* alone. There have been well-documented outbreaks due to strains of group C streptococci from other host species (152).

The attack rate of AGN after throat or skin infection with a nephritogenic strain may be high (10% to 15%). Unlike ARF, however, AGN recurrences are quite rare. Progression of poststreptococcal AGN to chronic glomerulonephritis has been documented in very few patients, so that the opportunity to study the effect of recurrent streptococcal infection on its course has been quite limited. Reports from areas as distant from each other as Memphis, Tennessee (153) and Singapore (154) indicate a marked decline in the disease during the past two decades.

PATHOGENESIS

The latent period between streptococcal infection and the appearance of AGN is 1 to 2 weeks after pharyngitis and perhaps 2 to 3 weeks after skin infection, although the exact onset of the latter is more difficult to establish. The pathogenesis of most cases of PSAGN like those of other causes of acute proliferative glomerulonephritis is thought to be related to the deposition of circulating insoluble antigen-antibody complexes in the glomeruli (155) and possibly as well to autoimmunity resulting from shared components among glomerular and streptococcal membranes (156). When made early in the course of the disease, renal biopsies reveal a typical picture of diffuse proliferative glomerulonephritis without significant vasculitis. Immunofluorescence studies reveal complement components and/or immunoglobulins (immunoglobulin G and C3) deposited in a granular pattern. Such deposits can be shown by electron microscopy to be subepithelial on the glomerular basement membrane. The binding of complement by such complexes may explain the low serum complement levels associated with the acute stage of proliferative AGN. The putative nephritogenic factor in certain strains of *S. pyogenes*, however, has not been identified. Renal glomerular autoimmune epitopes have been identified in a variety of M-associated proteins (156,157). The gene of an M-like protein (Szp5058) has been found to be identical in several independent isolates from PSAGN patients and in other hypervariable regions of *szp* genes from various human and animal hosts (152).

PREVENTION

The prevention of AGN by the treatment of streptococcal pharyngitis or pyoderma caused by a nephritogenic strain has not been systematically studied, but isolated reports of failure of such treatment suggest that treating the antecedent infection prevents AGN far less often than it does ARF (158). In outbreaks of poststreptococcal AGN, however, treatment of GAS pharyngitis or skin infections with intramuscular benzathine penicillin G or oral penicillin V prevents spread of nephritogenic strains throughout the family and community and may terminate AGN epidemics if used appropriately in the affected population (159). As in the case of ARF, the incidence of AGN has declined greatly where cleanliness and good hygiene prevail and adequate medical facilities exist.

REFERENCES

1. Beachey EH, Ofek I. Epithelial cell binding of group A streptococci by lipoteichoic acid on fimbriae denuded of M protein. *J Exp Med* 1976;143:759–771.
2. Wilson AT. The relative importance of the capsule and the M antigen in determining colony form of group A streptococci. *J Exp Med* 1959;109:257.
3. Griffith F. Types of haemolytic streptococci in relation to scarlet fever. *J Hyg* 1926;25:385–397.
4. Lancefield RC. Specific relationship of cell composition to biological activity of hemolytic streptococci. *Harvey Lect* 1941;35:251.
5. Beachey EH, Stollerman GH, Johnson RH, et al. Human immune response to immunization with a structurally defined polypeptide fragment of streptococcal M protein. *J Exp Med* 1979;150:862–877.
6. Fischetti VA, Jones KF, Hollingshead SK, Scott JR. Structure, function and genetics of streptococcal M protein. *Rev Infect Dis* 1988;10[Suppl 2]:S356–S359.
6a. Facklam RF, Martin DR, Lovgren M, et al. Extension of the Lancefield classification for group A streptococci by addition of 22 new M protein gene sequence types from clinical isolates: emm103 to emm124. *Clin Infect Dis* 2002;34:28–38.
7. Bronze MS, Dale JB. Epitopes of streptococcal M proteins that evoke antibodies that cross-react with human brain. *J Immunol* 1993;151:2820–2828.
8. Dale JB, Group A streptococcal vaccines. *Infect Dis Clinics North Am* 1999;13:227–234.
9. Bessen DE, Sotir CM, Readdy TL, Hollingshead SK. Genetic correlates of throat and skin isolates of group A streptococci. *J Infect Dis* 1996;173:896–900.
10. Bessen DE, Carapetis JR, Beall B, et al. Contrasting molecular epidemiology of group A streptococci causing tropical and nontropical infections of skin and throat. *J Infect Dis* 2000;182:1109–1116.
11. McLellan DGJ, Chiang EY, Courtney HS, et al. Spa contributes to the virulence of type 18 group A streptococci. *Infect Immun* 2001;69:2943–2949.
12. Widdowson JP, Maxted WR, Grant DL, et al. The relationship between M antigen and opacity factor in group A streptococci. *J Gen Microbiol* 1971;65:69–80.
13. Courtney HS, Hasty DL, Dale JB. Molecular mechanisms of adhesion, colonization and invasion of group A streptococci. *Ann Med* 2002;34:77–87.
14. Ozeri V, Rosenshine I, Mosher DF, Fassler R, Hanski E. Roles of integrins and fibronectin in the entry of *Streptococcus pyogenes* into cells via protein F1. *Mol Microbiol* 1998;30:625–637.
15. Neeman R, Keller N, Barzalai A, Korenman Z, Sela S. Prevalence of internalization-associated gene, prtF1, among persisting group-A streptococcus strains isolated from asymptomatic carriers. *Lancet* 1998;352:1974–1977.
16. Stollerman GH, Ekstedt RD, Cohen IR. Natural resistance of germ-free mice and colostrum-deprived piglets to group A streptococci. *J Immunol* 1965;95:131–140.

17. Moses AE, Wessels MR, Zalcman K, et al. Relative contributions of hyaluronic acid capsule and M protein to virulence in a mucoid strain of the group A streptococcus. *Infect Immun* 1997;65:64–71.
18. Fillit HM, Blake M, MacDonald C, McCarty M. Immunogenicity of liposome-bound hyaluronate in mice. *J Exp Med* 1988;168:971–982.
19. Todd EW. The differentiation of two distinct serological varieties of streptolysin, streptolysin O and streptolysin S. *J Pathol Bacteriol* 1938;47:423–445.
20. Stollerman GH, Bernheimer AW, MacLeod CM. The association of lipoproteins with the inhibition of streptolysin S by serum. *J Clin Invest* 1950;29:1636–1645.
21. Nizet V, Beall B, Bast DJ, et al: Genetic locus for streptolysin S production by group A streptococcus. *Infect Immun* 2000;68:4245–4254.
22. Stevens DL, Tanner MH, Winship J, et al: Severe group A streptococcal infections associated with toxic shock-like syndrome and scarlet fever toxin A. *N Engl J Med* 1989;321:1–7.
23. Stollerman GH. The historical role of the Dick test. *JAMA* 1983;250:3097–3099.
25. Ayoub EM, Wannamaker LW. Evaluation of the streptococcal DNase B and DPNase antibody in acute rheumatic fever and acute glomerulonephritis. *Pediatrics* 1962;29:527–538.
26. Christensen LR. Methods for measuring the activity of components of the streptococcal fibrinolytic system and streptococcal deoxyribonuclease. *J Clin Invest* 1949;28:163–172.
27. Stollerman GH, Lewis AJ, Schultz I, et al. Relationship of the immune response to group A streptococci to the course of acute, chronic and recurrent rheumatic fever. *Am J Med* 1956;20:163–169.
28. Whitnack E, Stollerman GH. Antistreptococcal antibodies in the diagnosis of rheumatic fever. In: Cohen AS, ed. *Laboratory diagnostic procedures in rheumatic diseases,* 3rd ed. Boston: Little, Brown, 1985:273–292.
29. Bisno AL. Alternate complement pathway activation by group A streptococci: role of M-protein. *Infect Immun* 1979;26:1172–1176.
30. Whitnack E, Beachey EH. Inhibition of complement mediated opsonization and phagocytosis of *Streptococcus pyogenes* by D fragments of fibrinogen and fibrin bound to cell surface M protein. *J Exp Med* 1985;162:1983–1997.
31. O'Connor SP, Cleary PD. Localization of the streptococcal C_{5a} peptidase to the surface of the group A streptococci. *Infect Immun* 1986;53:432–434.
32. Jadoun J, Sela S. Mutation in *csr* R global regulator reduces *Streptococcus pyogenes* internalization. *Microb Pathogenesis* 2000;29:1–7.
33. Schrager HM, Rheinwald JG, Wessels MR. Hyaluronic acid capsule and the role of streptococcal entry into keratinocytes in invasive skin infection. *J Clin Invest* 1996;98:1954–1958.
34. Ashbaugh CD, Warren HB, Carey VJ, Wessels MR. Molecular analysis of the role of the group A streptococcal cysteine proteinase, hyaluronic acid, capsule and M protein in a murine model of human invasive soft-tissue infections. *J Clin Invest* 1998;102:550–560.
35. Ravins MR, Jaffe J, Hanski E, et al. Characterization of a mouse-passaged, highly encapsulated variant of group A streptococcus in in vitro and in vivo studies. *J Infect Dis* 2000;182;1702–1711.
36. Federle MJ, McIver KS, Scott JR. A response regulator that represses transcription of several virulence operons in the group A streptococcus. *J Bacteriol* 1999;181:3649–3657.
37. Dougherty BA, van de Rijn. Molecular characterization of *hasA* from an operon required for hyaluronic acid synthesis in group A streptococci. *J Biol Chem* 1994;2:69–75.
38. Levin JC, Wessels MR. Identification of *csr R/csrS,* a genetic locus that regulates hyaluronic acid capsule synthesis in group A streptococcus. *Mol Microbiol* 1998;30:209–219.
39. Engelberg NC, Heath A, Miller A, et al. Spontaneous mutations in the CsRS two-component regulatory system of *Streptococcus pyogenes* result in enhanced virulence in a murine model of skin and soft tissue infection. *J Infect Dis* 2001;1043–1054.
40. Scott JR, Fischetti VA. Expression of streptococcal M protein in *Escherichia coli. Science* 1983;221:758–760.
40a. Chaussee MS, Sylva GL, Sturdevant DE, et al. Rgg influences the expression of multiple regulatory loci to coregulate virulence factor expression in Streptococcus pyogenes. *Infect Immun* 2002;70(2):762–770.
41. Chen C, Bormann N, Cleary PP. VirR and Mry are homologous trans-acting regulators of M protein and C5a peptidase expression in group A streptococci. *Mol Gen Genet* 1993;241:685–693.
42. Bisno AL, Brito MO, Collins CM. Molecular basis of group A streptococcal virulence. *Lancet Infect Dis* 2003;3:191–198.
43. Kaplan EL, Top FH, Dudding BA, Wannamaker LW. Diagnosis of streptococcal pharyngitis: Differentiation of active infection from the carrier state in the symptomatic child. *J Infect Dis* 1971;123:490–501.
44. Perry WD, Siegel AC, Rammelkamp CH Jr. Transmission of group A streptococci. II The role of contaminated dust. *Am J Hyg* 1957;66:96–101.
45. Siegel AC, Johnson EE, Stollerman GH. Controlled studies of streptococcal pharyangitis in a pediatric population. 1. Factors related to the attack rate. *N Engl J Med* 1961;265:559–566.
46. Rammelkamp CH, Denny FW, Wannamaker LW. Studies on the epidemiology of rheumatic fever in the armed services. In: Thomas L, ed. *Rheumatic fever.* Minneapolis, MN: University of Minnesota Press, 1952:72–89.
47. Bisno AL. Acute pharyngitis. *N Eng J Med* 2001;344:205–211.
48. Bisno AL, Gerber MA, Gwaltney JM Jr, et al. Diagnosis and management of group A streptococcal pharyngitis: a practice guideline. Infectious Diseases Society of America. *Clin Infect Dis* 1997;25:574–583.
49. American Academy of Pediatrics. Group A streptococcal infections. In:
50. Dajani A, Taubert K, Ferreri P, et al. Treatment of acute streptococcal pharyngitis and prevention of rheumatic fever: a statement for health professionals. Committee on Rheumatic Fever, Endocarditis, and Kawasaki Disease of the Council on Cardiovascular Disease in the Young, the American Heart Association. *Pediatrics* 1995;96:758–764.
51. Cooper RJ, Hoffman JR, Bartlertt JG, et al. Principles of appropriate antibiotic use for pharyngitis in adults: background. *Ann Intern Med* 2001;134:506–508.
52. Snow S, Mottur-Pilson C, Cooper RI, Hoffman JR. Principles of appropriate use for acute pharyngitis in adults. *Ann Intern Med* 2001;134:506–508.
53. Stollerman GH, Lewis AJ, Schultz I, et al. Relationship of the immune response to group A streptococci to the course of acute, chronic and recurrent rheumatic fever. *Am J Med* 1956;20:163.
54. Whitnack E, Stollerman GH. Antistreptococcal antibodies in the diagnosis of rheumatic fever. In: Cohen AS, ed. *Laboratory diagnostic procedures in rheumatic diseases,* 3rd ed. Boston: Little, Brown, 1985:273–292.
55. Lancefield RC. Persistence of type specific antibodies in man following infection with group A streptococci. *J Exp Med* 1959;110:271–292.
56. Stollerman GH, Siegel AC, Johnson EE. Evaluation of the "long chain reaction" as a means for detecting type specific antibody to group A streptococci in human sera. *J Exp Med* 1959;110:887–897.
57. Denny FW Jr, Wannamaker LW, Brink WR, et al. Prevention of rheumatic fever. Treatment of the preceding streptococcal infection. *JAMA* 1950;143:151–153.
58. Stollerman GH, Rusoff JR. Prophylaxis against group A streptococcal infections in rheumatic fever patients. Use of a new repository penicillin. *JAMA* 1952;150:1571–1575.
59. Stollerman GH, Rusoff JH, Hirshfield I. Prophylaxis against group A streptococci in rheumatic fever. The use of single monthly injections of benzathine penicillin G. *N Engl J Med* 1955;252:787–792.
60. Catanzaro FJ, Stetson CA, Morris AJ, et al. The role of the streptococcus in the pathogenesis of rheumatic fever. *Am J Med* 1954;17:749–756.
61. Stollerman GH. Penicillin for streptococcal pharyngitis: has anything changed? *Hosp Pract* 1995;30:80–83.
62. Picherero ME. Cephalosporins are superior to penicillin for the treatment of tonsillopharyngitis: is the difference worth it? *Pediatr Infect Dis J* 1993;123:268–274.
63. Dochez AR. Etiology of scarlet fever. *Harvey Lect* 1926;20:131–155.
64. Centers for Disease Control. Acute rheumatic fever at a Navy training center—San Diego, California. *JAMA* 1988;259(12):1782, 1787.
65. Leads from the MMWR. Acute rheumatic fever among army trainees—Fort Leonard Wood, Missouri, 1987–1988. *JAMA* 1988;260:2185–2188.
66. Steinberg DG, Stollerman GH. Dangerous pyogenic skin infections. *Hosp Pract* 1989;24:101–103.
67. Wannamaker LW. Differences between streptococcal infections of the throat and of the skin. I. *N Engl J Med* 1970;282:23–31.
68. Kaplan EL, Anthony BF, Chapman SS, et al. The influence of the site of infection on the immune response to group A streptococci. *J Clin Invest* 1970;49:1405–1414.
69. Bisno AL, Nelson KE, Waytz P, et al. Factors influencing serum antibody responses in streptococcal pyoderma. *J Lab Clin Med* 1973;81:410–420.
70. Demidovich CW, Wittler RR, Ruff ME, et al. Impetigo. Current etiology and comparison of penicillin, erythromycin and cephalexin therapies. *Am J Dis Child* 1990;144:1313–1315.
71. Rice TD, Duggan AK, DeAngelis C. Cost-effectiveness of erythromycin versus mupirocin for treatment of impetigo in children. *Pediatrics* 1992;89:210–214.
72. Mogielnicki NP, Schwartzman JD, Elliott JA. Perineal group A streptococcal disease in a pediatric practice. *Pediatrics* 2001;106:276–281.
73. Greenberg J, DeSanctis RW, Mills RM Jr. Vein-door-leg cellulitis after coronary by-pass surgery. *Ann Intern Med* 1982;97;565–566.
74. Barg NL, Kish MA, Kauffman CA, et al. Group A streptococcal bacteremia in intravenous drug abusers. *Am J Med* 1985;78:569–574.
75. Hook EWI, Hooten TM, Horton CA, et al. Microbiologic evaluation of cutaneous cellulitis in adults. *Arch Intern Med* 1986;146:295–297.
76. Stevens DL, Tanner MH, Winship J, et al. Severe group A streptococcal infections associated with a toxic shock-like syndrome and scarlet fever toxin A. *N Engl J Med* 1989;321:1–7.
77. Bartter T, Doscal A, Carroll K, et al. "Toxic strep syndrome:" manifestation of group A streptococcal infection. *Arch Intern Med* 1988;148:1421–1424.
78. Silver RM, Heddleston LN, McGregor JA, et al. Life-threatening puerperal infection due to group A streptococci. *Obstet Gynecol* 1992;79:894–896.
79. Cockerill FR 3rd, MacDonald KL, Thompson RL, et al. An outbreak of invasive group A streptococcal disease associated with high carriage rates of the invasive clone among school-aged children. *JAMA* 1997;277:38–43.
80. Carapetis JR, Currie BJ, Kaplan EL. Epidemiology and prevention of group A streptococcal infections: acute respiratory tract infections, skin infections, and their sequelae at the close of the twentieth century. *Clin Infect Dis* 1999;28:205–210.
81. Freedman JD, Beer DJ. Expanding perspectives on the toxic shock syndrome. *Adv Intern Med* 1991;96:363–425.
82. Meleney FL. Hemolytic streptococcus gangrene. *Arch Surg* 1924;9:317–364.
83. Stamenkovic I, Lew PD. Early recognition of potentially fatal necrotizing fasciitis: the use of frozen-section biopsy. *N Engl J Med* 1984;312:1689–1693.
49. (cont.) Pickering LK, ed. *Red book: report of the committee on infectious diseases,* 25th ed. Elk Grove Village, IL: American Academy of Pediatrics, 2000:526–536.

84. Bisno AL, Stevens DL. Streptococcal infections of skin and soft tissues. *N Engl J Med* 1996;334:240–244.

85. DiPersio JR, File TM Jr, Stevens DL, Gardner WG, Petropoulos G, Dinsa K. Spread of serious disease-producing M3 clones of group A streptococcus among family members and health care workers. *Clin Infect Dis* 1996;22:490–495.

86. Weiss K, Laverdiere M, Lovgren M, Delorme J, Poirier L, Beliveau C. Group A Streptococcus carriage among close contacts of patients with invasive infections. *Am J Epidemiol* 1999;149:863–868.

87. Stollerman GH. *Rheumatic fever and streptococcal infection.* New York: Grune & Stratton, 1975.

88. Bisno AL. *Textbook of rheumatology,* 5th ed. Philadelphia: WB Saunders, 1997.

89. Narula J, Virmani R, Reddy KS, Tandon R, eds. *Rheumatic fever.* Washington, DC: American Registry of Pathology, 1999.

90. Wannamaker LW. The chain that links the heart to the throat. *Circulation* 1973;48:9–18.

91. Stollerman GH. Rheumatic fever in the 21st century. *Clin Infect Dis* 2001;33:806–814.

92. Bessen D, Jones KF and Fischetti VA. Evidence for two distinct classes of streptococcal M-protein and their relationship to rheumatic fever. *J Exp Med* 1989;169:269–283.

93. Bessen DE, Veasy LG, Hill HR, Augustine NH, Fischetti VA. Serologic evidence for a class I group A streptococcal infection among rheumatic fever patients. *J Infect Dis* 1995;172:1608–1611.

94. Cunningham MW. Pathogenesis of group A streptococcal infections. *Clin Microbiol Rev* 2000;13:470–511.

95. Watanabe-Ohnishi R, Aelion J, LeGros L, et al. Characterization of unique human TCR V-beta specificities for a family of streptococcal superantigens represented by rheumatogenic serotypes of M protein. *J Immunol* 1994;152:2066–2073.

96. Maxted WR, Valkenburg HA. Variation in the M-antigen of group A streptococci. *J Med Microbiol* 1969;2:199–210.

97. Kaplan EL. Global assessment of rheumatic fever and rheumatic heart disease at the close of the century. *Circulation* 1993;88:1964–1972.

98. Coburn AF, Pauli RH. Studies on the immune response of the rheumatic subject and its relationship to activity of the rheumatic process. IV. Characteristics of strains of hemolytic streptococcus, effective and noneffective in initiating rheumatic activity. *J Clin Invest* 1935;14:755–762.

99. Kuttner AG, Krumwiede E. Observations on the effect of streptococcal upper respiratory infections on rheumatic children. A three-year study. *J Clin Invest* 1941;20:273–287.

100. Stollerman GH, Siegel AC, Johnson EE. Variable epidemiology of streptococcal disease and the changing pattern of rheumatic fever. *Mod Concepts Cardiovasc Dis* 1965;34:45–48.

101. Bisno AL, Pearce IA, Wall HP, et al. Contrasting epidemiology of acute rheumatic fever and acute glomerulonephritis. Nature of the antecedent streptococcal infection. *N Engl J Med* 1970;283:561–565.

102. Taranta A, Wood HF, Feinstein AR, et al. Rheumatic fever in children and adolescents. IV. Relation of the rheumatic fever recurrence rate per streptococcal antibodies. *Ann Intern Med* 1964;[Suppl 5] 60:47–57.

103. Feinstein AR, Spagnuolo M. Mimetic features of of rheumatic recurrences. *N Engl J Med* 1960;262:533–540.

104. Schwartz B, Facklam RR, Breiman RF. Changing epidemiology of group A streptococcal infection in the USA. *Lancet* 1990;336:1167–1171.

105. McLaren MJ, Markowitz MM. Rheumatic heart disease in developing countries: the consequences of inadequate protection. *Ann Intern Med* 1994;120:243–245.

106. Centers for Disease Control. Acute rheumatic fever at a navy training center—San Diego, California. *MMWR* 1988;37:101.

107. Centers for Disease Control. Acute rheumatic fever among army trainees—Ft. Leonard Wood, Missouri, 1987–1988. *MMWR* 1988;37:519–521.

108. Veasy LG, Wiedmeier SE, Garth SO, et al. Resurgence of acute rheumatic fever in the intermountain area of the United States. *N Engl J Med* 1987;316:421–427.

109. Centers for Disease Control. Acute rheumatic fever—Utah. *MMWR* 1987;36:108–110.

110. Smoot JC, Korgenski EK, Daly JA. Molecular analysis of group A streptococcus type emm 18 isolates temporally associated with acute rheumatic fever outbreaks in Salt Lake City, Utah. *J Clin Microbiol* 2002;40:1805–1810.

111. Bisno AL, Pearce IA, Stollerman GH. Streptococcal infections that fail to cause recurrences of rheumatic fever. *J Infect Dis* 1977;136:278–285.

112. Berrios X, del Campo E, Guzman B, Bisno AL Discontinuing rheumatic fever prophylaxis in selected adolescents and young adults. A prospective study. *Ann Intern Med* 1993;118:401–406.

113. Bernhard GC, Stollerman GH. Serum inhibition of streptococcal diphosphopyridine nucleotidase in uncomplicated streptococcal pharyngitis and in rheumatic fever. *J Clin Invest* 1959;38:1942–1949.

114. Kuhns WJ, McCarty M. Studies of diphtheria toxin in rheumatic fever subjects. Analysis of reactions to the Schick test and of antitoxin responses following hyperimmunization with diphtheria toxoid. *J Clin Invest* 1954;33:759–767.

115. Taranta A, Torosdag S, Metrakos JD, et al. Rheumatic fever in monozygotic and dizygotic twins. *Circulation* 1959;20:778.

116. Ayoub EM. Susceptibility to rheumatic fever: host factors. In: Narula J et al, eds. *Rheumatic fever.* Washington, DC: Armed Forces Institute of Pathology, American Registry of Pathology, 1999:181–194.

117. Carreno-Manjarrez R, Visvanathan K, Zibriskie JB. Immunogenic and genetic factors in rheumatic fever. *Curr Infect Dis Rep* 1998;2:302–307.

118. Guedez Y, Kotby A, El-Demellawry M, et al. HLA class II associations with rheumatic heart disease are more evident and consistent among clinically homogeneous patients. *Circulation* 1999;99:2784–2790.

119. Khanna AK, et al. Presence of a non-HLA B cell antigen in rheumatic fever patients and their families as defined by a monoclonal antibody. *J Clin Invest* 1989;83:1710–1716.

120. Quinn A, Kosanke S, Fischetti VA, et al. Induction of autoimmune valvular heart disease by recombinant streptococcal m protein. *Infect Immun* 2001;69:4072–4078.

121. Roberts S, Kosanke S, Terrence Dunn S, et al. Pathogenic mechanisms in rheumatic carditis: focus on valvular endothelium. *J Infect Dis* 2001;183:507–511.

122. Dale JB, Chiang EC. Intranasal immunization with recombinant group A streptococcal M protein fragment fused to the B subunit of *Escherichia coli* labile toxin protects mice against systemic challenge infections. *J Infect Dis* 1995;171:1038–1041.

123. Galvin JE, Hemric ME, Ward K, Cunningham MW. Cytotoxic mAb from rheumatic carditis recognizes heart valves and laminin. *J Clin Invest* 2000;106:217–224.

124. Dajani AS, et al. Guidelines for the diagnosis of rheumatic fever (Jones Criteria, update). *JAMA* 1992;268:2069–2073.

125. Veasy LG. Echocardiography for diagnosis and management of rheumatic fever. *JAMA* 1993;269:2084.

126. Narula J, Chandrasekhar Y, Rahimtoola S. Diagnosis of active carditis. The echos of change. *Circulation* 1999;100:1576–1581.

127. Taranta A, Stollerman GH. The relationship of Sydenham's chorea to infection with group A streptococci. *Am J Med* 1956;20:170–175.

128. Taranta A, Wood HF, Feinstein AR, et al. Rheumatic fever in children and adolescents. IV. Relation of the rheumatic fever recurrence rate per streptococcal antibodies. *Ann Intern Med* 1964;[Suppl 5]60:47–57.

129. Taranta A. Relation of isolated recurrences of Sydenham's chorea to infection with group A streptococci. *N Engl J Med* 1959;260:1204–1210.

130. Ayoub EM, Ahmed S. Update on complications of group A streptococcal infections. *Curr Probl Pediatr* 1997;27:90–101.

131. Swedo SE. Sydenham's chorea. A model for childhood autoimmune neuropsychiatric disorders. *JAMA* 1994;72:1788–1791.

132. Swedo SE. Pediatric autoimmune neuropsychiatric disorders associated with streptococcal infections (PANDAS). *Mol Psychiatry* 2002;7-Suppl 2:S24–S25.

133. Garvey MA, Perlmutter SJ, Allen AJ, et al. A pilot study of penicillin prophylaxis for neuropsychiatric exacerbations triggered by streptococcal infections. *Biol Psychiatry* 1999;45:1564–1571.

134. Morshed SA, Parveen S, Leckman JF, et al. Antibodies against neural, nuclear, cytoskeletal and streptococcal epitopes in children and adults with Tourette's syndrome, Sydenham's chorea, and autoimmune disorders. *Biol Psychiatry* 2001;50:566–578.

135. Leckman JF. Tourette's syndrome *Lancet* 2002;360:1577–1586.

136. Arnold PD, Richter MA. Is obsessive-compulsive disorder an autoimmune disease? *CMAJ* 2001;165:1353–1358.

137. Albert DA, Harel L, Karrison T. The treatment of rheumatic carditis: a review and metanalysis. *Medicine* 1995;74:1–12.

138. Feinstein AR, DiMassa R. Prognostic significance of valvular involvement in acute rheumatic fever. *N Engl J Med* 1959;260:1001–1007.

139. United Kingdom and United States Joint Report: The natural history of rheumatic fever and rheumatic heart disease: ten-year report of a cooperative clinical trial of ACTH, cortisone and aspirin. *Circulation* 1965;32:457–476.

140. Frank PF, Stollerman GH, Miller LF. Protection of a military population from rheumatic fever. *JAMA* 1965;193:775–783.

141. Brundage JF, Gunzenhauser JD, Longfield JN, et al. Epidemiology and control of acute respiratory diseases with emphasis on group A beta-hemolytic streptococcus: a decade of U.S. Army experience. *Pediatrics* 1996;97:964–970.

142. Wood HF, Stollerman GH, Feinstein AR, et al. A controlled study of three methods of prophylaxis against streptococcal infection in a population of rheumatic children. *N Engl J Med* 1957;106:345–356.

143. Feinstein AR, Spagnuolo M, Jonas S, et al. Prophylaxis of recurrent rheumatic fever. Therapeutic-continuous oral penicillin vs. monthly injections. *JAMA* 1968;206:565–568.

144. Dale JB. Multivalent group A streptococcal vaccine designed to optimize the immunogenicity of six tandem M protein fragments. *Vaccine* 1999;17:193–200.

144a. Fischetti VA. Vaccine approaches to protect against group A streptococcal pharyngitis. In: Fischetti VA, Novick RP, Ferretti JJ, et al, eds. *Gram-positive pathogens.* Washington, DC: American Society for Microbiology 2000:96–104.

145. Brandt ER, Teh T, Relf WA, et al. Protective and nonprotective epitopes from amino termini of M proteins from Australian aboriginal isolates and reference strains of group A streptococci. *Infect Immun* 2000;68:6587–6594.

146. Brandt ER, Hayman WA, Currie B, et al. Functional analysis of IgA antibodies specific for a conserved epitope within the M protein of group A streptococci from Australian aboriginal endemic communities. *Int Immunol* 1999;11:569–576.

147. Potter EV, Ortiz JS, Sharrett R, et al. Changing types of nephritogenic streptococci in Trinidad. *J Clin Invest* 1971;150:1197–1205.

148. Dillon HC, Derrick CW. Dillon MS. M-antigens common to pyoderma and acute glomerulonephritis. *J Infect Dis* 1974;130:257–267.

149. Rammelkamp CH, Jr., Weaver RS. Acute glomerulonephritis. The significance of the varuiations in the incidence of the disease. *J Clin Invest* 1953;32:345–358.
150. Stollerman GH. Rheumatogenic and nephritogenic streptococci. *Circulation* 1971;43:915–921.
151. Potter EV, Svartman M, Mohammed I, et al. Tropical acute rheumatic fever and associated streptococcal infections compared with concurrent acute glomerulonephritis. *J Pediatr* 1978;92:325–333.
152. Nicholson ML, Ferdinand L, Sampson JS, et al. Analysis of immunoreactivity to a *Streptococcus equi* subsp. *zooepidemicus* M-like protein to confirm an outbreak of poststreptococcal glomerulitis, and sequences of M-like proteins from isolates obtained from different host species. *J Clin Microbiol* 2000;38:4126–4130.
153. Roy S, Stapleton FB. Changing perspectives in children hospitalized with post-streptococcal glomerulonephritis. *Pediatr Nephrol* 1990;4:585–588.
154. Yap HK, Chia KS, Murugasu B, et al. Acute glomerulonephritis—changing patterns in Singapore children. *Pediatr Nephrol* 1990;4:482–484.
155. Van de Rijn I, Fillit HM, Brandeis WE, et al. Serial studies on circulating immune complexes in post-streptococcal sequelae. *Clin Exp Immunol* 1978; 34:318–325.
156. Johnson KJ, Zabriskie JB. Purification and partial characterization of the nephritis strain-associated protein from *Streptococcus pyogenes*, group A. *J Exp Med* 1986;163:697–712.
157. Yashizawa N, Oshima S, Sagel I, et al. Role of a post-streptococcal antigen in the pathogenesis of acute poststreptococcal glomerulonephritis. *J Immunol* 1992;148:3110–3116.
158. Weinstein L, Le Frock J. Does antimicrobial therapy of streptococcal pharyngitis or pyoderma alter the risk of glomerulonephritis? *J Infect Dis* 1971;124:229–231.
159. Johnston F, Carapetis J, Patel M, et al. Evaluating the use of penicillin to control outbreaks of acute poststreptococcal glomerulonephritis. *Pediatr Infect Dis J* 1999;18:327–332.

CHAPTER 184
Streptococcus pneumoniae

Robert Austrian

HISTORY

The pneumococcus, *Streptococcus pneumoniae*, was isolated first in 1880 from carriers of the organism by Sternberg and by Pasteur. Its role as the principal cause of community-acquired bacterial pneumonia was established by Fraenkel and by Weichselbum in the 1880s (1), as was its ability to cause otitis media, meningitis, and arthritis.

CHARACTERISTICS OF THE PATHOGEN

The pneumococcus is a member of the genus *Streptococcus*, bacteria characterized by a lack of cytochromes and catalase (2). Absence of catalase prevents degradation of hydrogen peroxide formed by the cells and necessitates an exogenous source of the enzyme, such as intact erythrocytes, to prevent the death of cultures. Pneumococci are gram-positive and grow as single cells, diplococci, and in chains of variable length. They are α-hemolytic. Their nutritional requirements are complex and include choline, which is incorporated into the teichoic acid of the cell wall. Pneumococci produce an autolytic enzyme, L-alaninemuramyl amidase (Lyt A), which hydrolyzes the cell wall and is activated by detergents, including bile, resulting in lysis of the cell wall (3). It is one of a group of choline-binding proteins (4). The growth of most strains of pneumococci is inhibited by ethylhydrocupreine hydrochloride (Optochin), although resistant strains occur (5).

Several well-characterized surface antigens of *S. pneumoniae* are known. They are the choline-containing teichoic acid (C polysaccharide) of the cell wall, Psp A and Psp C choline-binding proteins (6,7) and type-specific capsular polysaccharides. Ninety distinct capsular polysaccharides have been identified (8). These polymers, though nontoxic, exert an antiphagocytic effect; and their presence is essential to the virulence of the organism and its ability to cause infection (9,10).

Pneumococci grown on transparent solid media have been recognized to undergo phase variation giving rise to opaque and transparent colonies (11). Transparent variants of a given capsular type producing larger amounts of C polysaccharide and lesser amounts of capsular polysaccharide appear better adapted to colonization of the upper respiratory tract than are opaque variants producing lesser amounts of C polysaccharide and larger amounts of capsular polysaccharide, the latter form being recovered most often from sites of systemic infection (12).

EPIDEMIOLOGY

S. pneumoniae is an obligate parasite of humans, although occasionally it may be isolated from other mammalian species. Colonization of the human upper respiratory tract may occur on the first day of life (13). As many as four distinct capsular types may be carried simultaneously, although colonization with one or two capsular types is more usual. Children are more likely to be carriers of pneumococci than are adults, but the latter are colonized frequently. Antibodies to pneumococcal capsular polysaccharides do not eliminate established carriage of organisms of the homologous type but do reduce by half or more, both in adults (14) and in children (15), the likelihood of becoming colonized with the same organism. Pneumococci are spread from person to person by direct contact with secretions bearing the organism. Infection is thought to result most frequently after acquisition of a previously unencountered capsular type.

Not all pneumococcal types are equally invasive. In childhood, capsular types 4, 6A, 6B, 9V, 12F, 14, 18C, 19F, 19A, and 23F account for 82% of invasive pneumococcal infections (16). In adults, capsular types 1, 3, 4, 6A, 6B, 7F, 8, 9N, 9V, 10A, 11A, 12F, 14, 15B, 17F, 18C, 19F, 19A, 20, 22F, 23F, and 33F cause approximately 90% of bacteremic pneumococcal infections in the United States.

At present, *S. pneumoniae* causes approximately 500,000 cases of otitis media in the United States annually (17). The minimum annual attack rate of pneumococcal bacteremia, determined retrospectively, is 30 per 100,000 (18); that of pneumococcal pneumonia is one to two per 1,000 and that of pneumococcal meningitis, one to 1.5 per 100,000 (19).

PATHOGENESIS

Pneumococci are a component of the normal bacterial flora of the human nasopharynx and, in the absence of injury to the epithelial lining of the upper and lower respiratory tract, live in a commensal state with humans. Anatomic alterations in the cells lining the respiratory tract, be they viral, mechanical, or chemical, predispose to bacterial infection of the affected region (20). Viral infections of the upper respiratory tract causing edema of the eustachian tube and negative pressure in the middle ear predispose to bacterial otitis media, of which pneumococci are the most common cause (21,22). Any disturbance of the complex and coordinated neuromuscular reflexes protecting the lower respiratory tract from aspiration of foreign material may be followed by infection of the lungs. Bacteria reaching the alveoli of the normal lung are usually cleared rapidly. Injury to the alveolar lining cells by viral infection such as that caused by influenza virus or rhinoviruses or by chemical agents, trauma, or aspirated material delays clearance of bacteria and allows the establishment of progressive infection furthered by the inflammatory properties of fragments of the pneumococcal cell wall (23) and the oxygen-labile intracellular hemolysin, pneumolysin (24). Pharmacologically active substances retarding the migration of polymorphonuclear leukocytes, including alcohol, anesthetics, and corticosteroids, facilitate the establishment and spread of pneumonia. Failure of the host's defensive mechanisms to limit infection to the lung results in extension of bacteria to hilar lymph nodes and, in cases developing bacteremia, from the latter site to the systemic circulation via the thoracic duct. Pneumococci in infants, and less commonly in adults, like meningococci and *Haemophilus influenzae*, appear capable of penetrating the nasopharyngeal mucosa and gaining access to the systemic circulation via the cervical lymphatic vessels in the absence of a demonstrable focus of infection (25). Bacteremia, once established, may be followed by metastatic foci of infection, notably of serous cavities such as the meninges, joints, and peritoneum. Meningitis may also arise by extension of infection from the middle ear or paranasal sinuses and pleural empyema or pericarditis by direct extension from the lung. Pneumococcal endocarditis, a complication of bacteremic infection, occurs most commonly in persons older than 40 years.

Spontaneous recovery from pneumococcal infection is mediated by the development of type-specific anticapsular antibodies that, acting with complement (26), combine with the polysaccharide capsule surrounding the infecting pneumococci, causing them to adhere to one another and to alveolar walls and to be phagocytosed with increased efficiency. Antibodies of both the immunoglobulin M and immunoglobulin G classes are formed. Reinfection with the same pneumococcal capsular type is rare in the absence of agammaglobulinemia or dysgammaglobulinemia, and immunity to reinfection with a given pneumococcal type is usually lifelong. Congential or acquired deficiency of the early components of complement also predisposes to pneumococcal bacteremia (27) and to infection of soft tissues (28).

CLINICAL MANIFESTATIONS

The prototypic clinical picture of lobar pneumonia in the adult is characterized by an antecedent history of a common cold or influenza marked by a sudden worsening of the patient's condition manifested by a shaking chill and rise in body temperature, development of cough productive of rusty sputum, pleural pain, dyspnea, anorexia, and prostration (29). With the illness unmodified by therapy, signs of segmental or lobar pulmonary consolidation evolve in the next 24 to 48 hours. Elevation of temperature persists for 5 to 10 days and may fall abruptly in one third of patients ("crisis") or by lysis. Defervescence frequently coincides with the demonstrable presence of circulating anticapsular antibody. In infants and the elderly, the clinical picture may deviate significantly from that described and mimic that of pneumonia of any cause. The clinical manifestations of otitis media, meningitis, arthritis, pleural empyema, pericarditis, peritonitis, and endocarditis caused by *S. pneumoniae* do not differ significantly from those of infections of these sites with other pyogenic bacteria, and diagnosis rests on isolation and identification of the infecting organism. Patients who have anatomic or functional asplenia are at risk of fulminant pneumococcal sepsis manifesting itself not infrequently with a clinical picture resembling that of the Waterhouse-Friderichsen syndrome and running its course from onset to death in 24 to 48 hours. The incidence of bacteremic

pneumococcal infection in children and in adults infected with human immunodeficiency virus is greatly increased both before and after the development of the acquired immunodeficiency syndrome, approximating ten times that in the uninfected population, and results apparently from multiple disturbances of host defenses (30). In other respects, pneumococcal infection in persons infected with human immunodeficiency virus resembles clinically that seen in immunocompetent hosts.

Laboratory investigations should include determination of the concentration of hemoglobin and of polymorphonuclear leukocytes in the blood, measurement of arterial blood gas levels in the more seriously ill, and both posteroanterior and lateral radiographs of the chest.

DIAGNOSIS

Although differences exist among the historical and clinical manifestations of pneumonias caused by different infectious agents, identification of the cause of a given illness rests on the proper use and interpretation of the appropriate microbiologic and immunologic tests in relation to that illness.

Diagnosis of pneumococcal infection with certainty rests on isolation of the organism from a normally sterile body site such as the blood, middle ear, subarachnoid space, or other serous cavity. A strongly presumptive diagnosis of pneumococcal pneumonia can be made from microscopic and cultural examination of expectorated respiratory secretions (sputum), but because pneumococci are normal inhabitants of the upper respiratory tract, isolation of the organism from material passing through it does not establish absolutely its role in infection of the lung. In the absence of bacteremia, the causal role of pneumococci in pneumonia can be demonstrated by recovery of the organism from material obtained by transtracheal or transthoracic lung puncture; however, because both procedures are accompanied by small but finite morbidity, their use should be limited to situations in which they are deemed necessary for the patient's welfare.

Because pneumococci may be highly sensitive to most antimicrobial drugs, it is essential that material for culture be obtained before their administration. Sputum should be collected in a sterile container by the physician to ensure that it is expectorated from the lung. After microscopic examination, sputum should be plated on nutrient blood agar and incubated in an atmospheric concentration of 5% carbon dioxide (candle jar). Characteristic colonies of pneumococci are depicted in Figures 184.1 and 184.2.

Most strains of pneumococci lyse in the presence of bile, bile salts, or other detergents and their growth is inhibited by ethylhydrocupreine hydrochloride (Optochin). The most useful test for identification of pneumococci in the diagnostic laboratory is the quellung or capsular precipitin reaction (31). The test can be carried out either directly with sputum or other body fluids such as cerebrospinal fluid or with organisms isolated from cultures. When type-specific anticapsular antibodies combine with capsular polysaccharide of the same type surrounding the pneumococcal cell, a refractile gel is formed that can be seen readily in the light microscope (Fig. 184.3). Visualization of the reaction is facilitated by the use of a substage concave mirror and oblique illumination. The test is performed by allowing a loopful of suspension of the material to be examined to dry on a glass slide. A loopful of 1% methylene blue is deposited on a coverslip, and a loopful of anticapsular antiserum is placed on the dried suspension on the slide. The residual serum in the loop is then mixed sequentially with the methylene blue on the coverslip

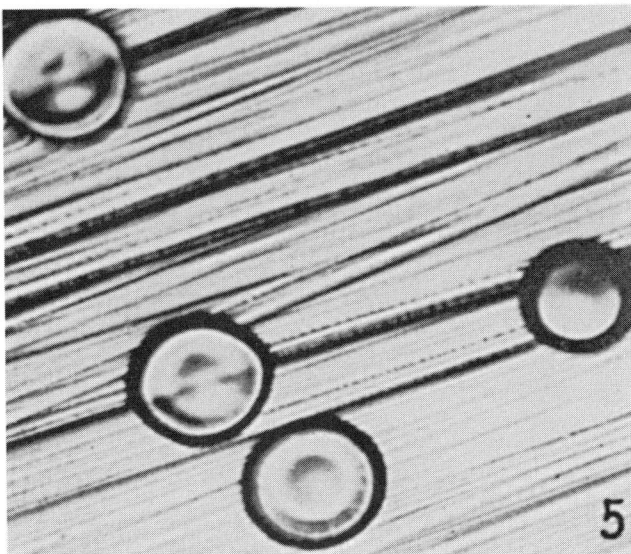

Figure 184.1. Typical colonies of *Streptococcus pneumoniae* on the surface of a blood agar plate. Central autolysis gives the colony the appearance of a checker (X18). (Reproduced from *The Journal of Experimental Medicine*, 1953;98:21–34, by copyright permission of The Rockefeller University Press.)

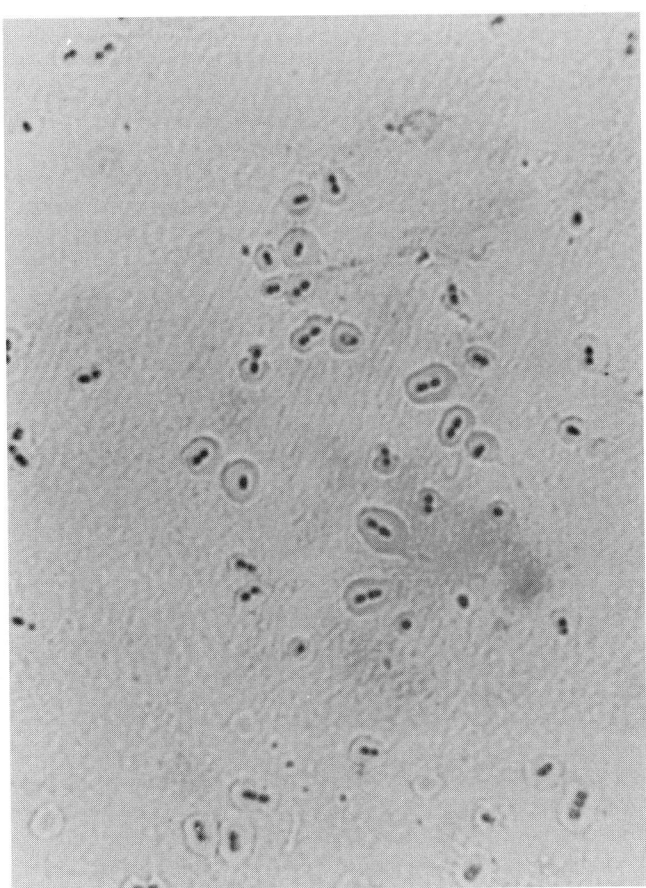

Figure 184.3. Quellung preparation of pneumococcal cells showing the refractile halo surrounding the bacterial cell (X1,100). (Reproduced from *The Journal of Experimental Medicine*, 1953;98:21–34, by copyright permission of The Rockefeller University Press.)

and then with the serum on the slide. The coverslip is placed over the suspension, and the preparation is examined under the oil immersion lens of the microscope. To avoid interference by excess antigen (prozone), no more than 50 to 100 pneumococci should be present in a single microscopic field. Sera for identifying all the pneumococcal types known currently are available commercially from the Danish Statens Seruminstitut, including a reagent designated Omniserum, which contains antibodies to 90 pneumococcal capsular polysaccharides and is an invaluable reagent for the rapid presumptive identification of pneumococcal infection.

Methods for identifying pneumococci by examination of bacterial nucleic acids remain essentially investigational (32) and have not yet found significant applicability in diagnostic laboratories.

TREATMENT

Since recognition of *S. pneumoniae* as a pathogen of humans, treatment of pneumococcal infections has undergone continual change, the result of better understanding of the biology of such infection and of pharmacologic advances. The case-fatality rate of pneumococcal pneumonia of 30% to 35%, affected little if at all by symptomatic therapy, fell to 20% to 25% among the infections for which serum therapy became available after recognition of the diversity of pneumococcal types in 1910. A further

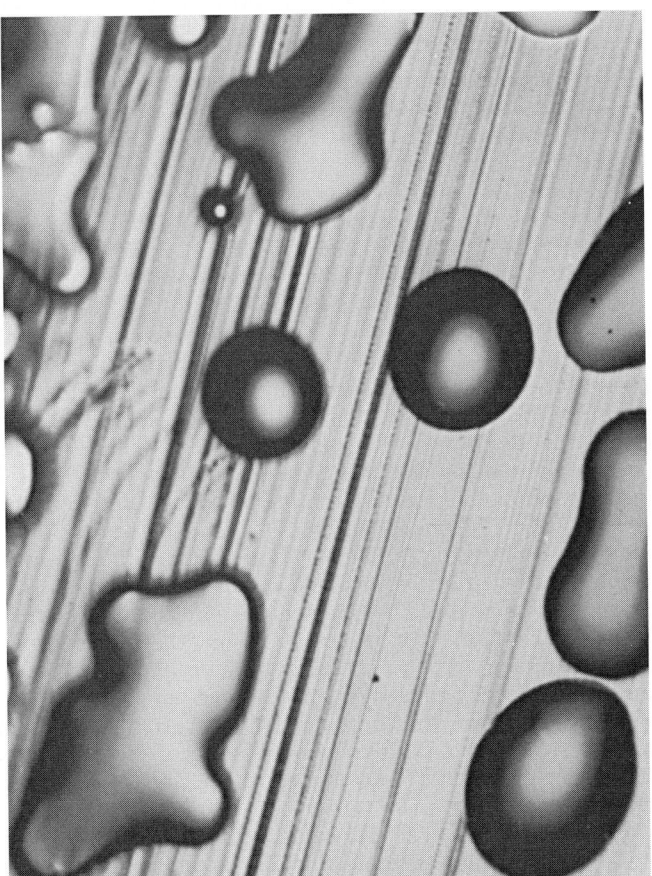

Figure 184.2. Typical mucoid colonies of *S. pneumoniae* type 3 (X21). (Reproduced from *The Journal of Experimental Medicine*, 1953;98:21–34, by copyright permission of The Rockefeller University Press.)

decline in case-fatality rate to 12% to 15% followed the introduction of sulfapyridine and its congeners, and the case-fatality rate reached its present nadir of 5% to 8% when penicillin and other comparably effective antibiotics became the accepted therapeutic agents (33).

Although mutants of pneumococci resistant to penicillin G (benzylpenicillin) were recovered from experimentally infected animals treated with the drug a year before the report in 1944 of its efficacy in the management of both nonbacteremic and bacteremic pneumococcal pneumonia in humans, penicillin G became the unquestioned drug of first choice in the management of such infections in those not hypersensitive to it. Two decades were to elapse before resistant mutants similar to those described earlier were isolated from humans; since their initial recovery, both their frequency and the degree of resistance manifested by them have increased steadily. In addition, strains of pneumococci resistant to cephalosporins (ceftriaxone, cefotaxime), macrolides (erythromycin, azithromycin, clarithromycin), clindamycin, fluoroquinolones, (levofloxacin, grepafloxacin, trovafloxacin), tetracylines, chloramphenicol, cotrimoxazole, and aminoglycosides have been recognized, posing potential problems for the treatment of pneumococcal infection. Although no strain of pneumococcus resistant to vanomycin has been identified, strains tolerant of the drug; i.e., ones the growth of which is inhibited by vancomycin but are not killed by it, have been recovered, posing an additional potential problem in the management of pneumococcal meningitis (34). Whatever the choice of therapy, it is now mandatory that the susceptibilities of the infecting strain to the drug (s) to be employed be determined promptly. For such determinations, the standards recommended by the NCCLS should be followed (35).

Resistance of pneumococci to penicillin is the result of mutations in one or more of the penicillin binding proteins concerned with the synthesis of the pneumococcal cell wall (36). Strains sensitive to 0.1 μg/mL or less are classified as sensitive, those inhibited by concentrations between 0.1 and 2 μg/mL are said to manifest intermediate resistance, and those inhibited only by concentrations greater than 2 μg/mL are considered to be fully resistant (37). Resistance of any degree to penicillin is independent of capsular type but is observed most frequently among the types that most often affect children, types 6A, 6B, 9V, 14, 18C, 19F, 19A, and 23F. The proportion of penicillin-resistant pneumococcal strains varies with time and place, and knowledge of its extent may play an ancillary role in the choice of therapy. In some geographic areas pneumococcal strains defined as fully resistant to penicillin constitute more that 25% of the total isolated from blood cultures (39) and strains resistant to 16 μg/mL have been recovered from man (40).

For the treatment of pneumococcal pneumonia caused by normally sensitive organisms, conventional doses of penicillin G of 300,000 to 600,000 units administered parenterally every 6 hours are adequate. For those gravely ill or with complications, especially where strains manifesting increased resistance to penicillin are known to exist, penicillin G in parenteral doses of 1,200,000 units every two hours (14,400,000 units per day) results in serum levels of penicillin of approximately 5 μg/ml (41), a level sufficiently high to inhibit the growth of 98% of 4148 isolates recovered in world-wide surveillance in 2000 (Jacobs, MR, personal communication). This regimen, however, is not adequate for the treatment of pneumococcal meningitis caused by strains of the organism that manifest increased resistance to penicillin. Because strains of pneumococci with increased resistance to ceftriaxone and cefotaxime, alternatives to penicillin G, have also been observed, vancomycin should be included in the initial treatment of all cases of pneumococcal meningitis until the sensitivity of the infecting strain to antimicrobials has been

determined (42). Its administration may be discontinued if the isolate is sensitive to a β-lactam drug.

Several new agents of potential utility in the treatment of infections caused by pneumococci resistant to one or more of the drugs currently employed are under investigation, (43) but additional clinical experience is required before the role of any can be determined.

Symptomatic treatment of pneumococcal infections entails bed rest, a liquid or light diet, adequate hydration, analgesics for pleural pain, and oxygen when cyanosis is present in pneumonia. During the acute phase of illness, vital signs should be recorded no less often than every 4 hours, and temperature should be measured rectally or by thermocouple in the auditory canal.

PROPHYLAXIS

Because the case-fatality rate of uncomplicated bacteremic pneumococcal pneumonia in adults treated optimally is 17% (44) and that of pneumococcal meningitis in person older than 40 years treated in similar fashion exceeds 40%, polyvalent vaccines of pneumococcal capsular polysaccharides have been developed for the prevention of such infections. A second reason for their availability is the slow but steady increase of the number of pneumococcal strains manifesting resistance to one or more antimicrobial drugs. The currently available 23-valent vaccine, containing 25 μg each of the capsular polysaccharides of pneumococcal types 1, 2, 3, 4, 5, 6B, 7F, 8, 9N, 9V, 10A, 11A, 12F, 14, 15B, 17F, 18C, 19F, 19A, 20, 22F, 23F, and 33F, has been shown to be safe, immunogenic, and effective. It has an aggregate efficacy of 60% to 70% in both young and elderly adults in preventing infection with any of the 23 immunologically distinct capsular types represented in it. (45–47) It is recommended by the Advisory Committee on Immunization Practices of the Centers for Disease Control (48) and by the American College of Physicians (49) that the vaccine be administered to all persons 65 years of age or older and to any immunocompetent adult with chronic underlying systemic illness. Among the latter are those infected with HIV. Studies of the efficacy of pneumococcal vaccine in persons infected with HIV have given rise to discrepant results, in part because of the heterogenicity of the populations under scrutiny. There is evidence, nonetheless, of its efficacy in some cohorts (50); and, because of the heightened vulnerability of those infected with this virus, the vaccine should be administered to such persons as early in the course of their infection as possible. Although agammaglobulinemic and dysgammaglobulinemic individuals and those with other forms of compromised immunity resulting from illness or treatment manifest heightened susceptibility to pneumococcal infection and may be vaccinated without risk, the likelihood of their being protected against such infection is, in most instances, reduced. All individuals with anatomic or functional asplenia, however, regardless of age, should receive the 23-valent pneumococcal vaccine. In light of the increasing frequency of infection caused by pneumococci resistant to one or more antimicrobial drugs, modification of current recommendations to include immunocompetent adults of all ages as candidates for the receipt of pneumococcal vaccine is now highly desirable.

Pneumococcal infections are most frequent in the first 2 years of life and include bacteremia, pneumonia, meningitis, and otitis media. They impose, in addition, a significant financial burden. Although the human infant is immunologically immature in the first years of life and unresponsive to bacterial polysaccharides, when the latter are coupled chemically to a protein and injected, antibodies of both the immunoglobulin M and immunoglobulin G classes develop together with immunologic memory. A heptavalent vaccine containing the polysaccharide-protein conjugates of pneumococcal types 4, 6B, 9V, 14, 18C, 19F, and 23F, which account for 82% of systemic pediatric infections in the United States (16), has been shown to be highly effective in preventing bacteremia caused by organisms of those capsular types and, to a lesser degree, in preventing otitis media (50). The Advisory Committee on Immunization Practices recommends that the conjugate vaccine be given to all children aged 2 to 23 months and to those aged 24 to 59 months at increased risk of pneumococcal infection (51). The conjugate vaccine should be given to be followed by the 23-valent polysaccharide vaccine after an interval of 2 or more months to all children 5 years of age and older to whom the 23-valent polysaccharide vaccine was recommended because of their increased vulnerability. An 11-valent conjugate vaccine including the additional polysaccharides of types 1, 3, 5, and 7F is currently under development (52).

REFERENCES

1. Austrian R. The gram stain and the etiology of lobar pneumonia, an historical note. *Bacteriol Rev* 1960;24:261–265.
2. Austrian R. Pneumococci. In: Davis BD, Dulbecco R, Eisen HN, Ginsberg HS (eds): *Microbiology*, ed 4. Philadelphia: JB Lippincott, 1990:515–524.
3. Mosser JL, Tomasz A. Choline-containing teichoic acid as a structural component of pneumococcal cell wall and its role in sensitivity to lysis by an autolytic enzyme. *J Biol Chem* 1970;245:287–298.
4. Rosenow C, Ryan P, Weiser JN, et al. Contributions of novel choline–binding proteins to adherence, colonization, and immunogenicity of *Streptococcus pneumoniae. Mol Microbiol* 1997;25:819–829.
5. Ragsdale AR, Sanford JP. Interfering effect of incubation in carbon dioxide on the identification of pneumococci by optochin discs. *Appl Microbiol* 1971;22:854–855.
6. Briles DE, Creech Tart R, Swiatlo E, et al. Pneumococcal diversity: considerations for new vaccine strategies with emphasis on pneumococcal surface protein A (Psp A). *Clin Microbiol Rev* 1998;11:645–657.
7. Boulnois GJ. Pneumococcal proteins and pathogenesis of disease caused by *Streptococcus pneumoniae. J Gen Microbiol* 1992;138:249–259.
8. Henrichsen J. Six newly recognized types of *Streptococcus pneumoniae. J Clin Microbiol* 1995;33:2759–2762.
9. Avery OT, Dubos R. Protective action of a specific enzyme against type III pneumococcus in mice. *J Exp Med* 1931;54:73–89.
10. Rich AR, McKee CM. The pathogenicity of avirulent pneumococci for animals deprived of leukocytes. *Bull Johns Hopkins Hosp* 1939;64:434–446.
11. Weiser JN, Austrian R, Sreenivasan PK, et al. Phase variation in pneumococcal opacity; relationship between colonial morphology and nasal colonization. *Infect Immun* 1994;62:2582–2589.
12. Kim JO, Weiser JN. Association of intrastrain phase variation in quantity of capsular polysaccharide and teichoic acid with virulence of *Streptococcus pneumoniae. J Infect Dis* 1998;177:368–377.
13. Austrian R. Some aspects of the pneumococcal carrier state. *J Antimicrob Chemother* 1986;18[Suppl A]:35–45.
14. MacLeod CM, Hodges RG, Heidelberger M, et al. Prevention of pneumococcal pneumonia by vaccination. *J Exp Med* 1945;82:445–465.
15. Dagan R, Melamed R, Muallem M, et al. Reduction of nasopharyngeal carriage during the second year of life by a heptavalent conjugate vaccine. *J Infect Dis* 1996;174:1271–1278.
16. Robinson KA, Baughman W, Rothrock G et al. Epidemiology of invasive *Streptococcus pneumoniae* infections in the United States, 1995–1998. Opportunities for prevention in the conjugate vaccine era. *JAMA* 2001;285:1729–1735.
17. Austrian R, Howie VM, Ploussard JH. The bacteriology of pneumococcal otitis media. *Johns Hopkins Med J* 1977;141:104–111.
18. Austrian R. Pneumococcal pneumonia. Diagnostic, epidemiologic, therapeutic and prophylactic considerations. *Chest* 1986;90:738–743.
19. Fraser DW, Geil CC, Feldman RA. Bacterial meningitis in Bernalillo County, New Mexico. A comparison with three other American populations. *Am J Epidemiol* 1974;100:29–34.
20. Harford CG, Hara M. Pulmonary edema in influenzal pneumonia of the mouse and the relation of fluid in the lung to the inception of pneumococcal pneumonia. *J Exp Med* 1950;91:245–260.
21. Giebink GS. The pathogenesis of pneumococcal otitis media in chinchillas and the efficacy of vaccination in prophylaxis. *Rev Infect Dis* 1981;3:342–353.
22. Klein JO. Otitis media. *Clin Infect Dis* 1994;19:823–832.
23. Tuomanen EI, Austrian R, Masure HR. Pathogensis of pneumococcal infection. *N Engl J Med* 1995;332:1280–1284.
24. Boulnois GJ, Paton JC, Mitchell TJ, et al. Structure and function of pneumolysin, multifunctional, thiol-activated toxin of *Streptococcus pneumoniae, Mol Microbiol* 1991;5:2611–2616.
25. Austrian R. Untreated pneumococcal bacteremia of cryptic origin in the human adult with spontaneous recovery. *S Afr Med J* 1986;70[Suppl]:46–49.
26. Hosea SW, Brown EJ, Frank MM. The critical role of complement in experimental pneumococcal sepsis. *J Clin Invest* 1980;142:903–909.
27. Ross SC, Densen P. Complement deficiency states and infection: Epidemiology, pathogenesis and consequences of neisserial and other infections in an immune deficiency. *Medicine (Baltimore)* 1984;63:243–273.
28. Taylor SN, Sanders CV. Unusual manifestations of invasive pneumococcal infection. *Am J Med* 1999;107(1A):12S–27S.
29. Heffron R. *Pneumonia with special reference to pneumococcus lobar pneumonia*, 2nd printing. Boston: Harvard University Press, 1979.
30. Janoff EN, Breiman RF, Daley CL, et al. Pneumococcal disease during HIV infection. Epidemiologic, clinical, and immunologic perspectives. *Ann Intern Med* 1992;117:314–324.
31. Austrian R. The Quellung reaction, a neglected microbiologic technique. *Mt Sinai J Med* 1976;43:699–709.
32. Garcia A, Roson B. Pérez JL, et al. Usefulness of PCR and latex agglutination test with samples obtained by transthoracic needle aspiration for diagnosis of pneumococcal pneumonia. *J Clin Microbiol* 2000;37:709–714.
33. Austrian R. Confronting drug-resistant pneumococci [Editorial]. *Ann Intern Med* 1994;121:807–809.
34. Wormark BH, Novak R, Ortquist A, et al. Clinical isolates of *Streptococcus pneumoniae* that exhibit tolerance of vancomycin. *Clin Infect Dis* 2001;32:552–558.
35. *NCCLS Performance Standards for Antimicrobial Sensitivity Testing.* 11th Informational Supplement. NCCLS document M100-S11. Wayne, PA, 2001.
36. Zighelboim S, Tomasz A. Penicillin-binding proteins of multiply-resistant South African strains of *Streptococcus pneumoniae. Antimicrob Agents Chemother* 1980;17:434–442.
37. Klugman KP. Pneumococcal resistance to antibiotics. *Clin Microbiol Rev* 1990; 3:171–196.
38. Hoban DJ, Doern GV, Fluit AC, et al. Worldwide prevalence of antimicrobial resistance in *Streptococcus pneumoniae, Haemophilus influenzae* and *Moraxella catarrhalis* in the SENTRY antimicrobial surveillance program, 1997–1999. *Clin Infect Dis* 2001;32[Suppl 2]:S81–S83.
39. Lee HJ, Park J-Y, Jang S-H, et al. High incidence of resistance to multiple antimicrobials in clinical isolates of *Streptococcus pneumoniae* from a university hospital in Korea. *Clin Infect Dis* 1995;20:826–833.
40. Corso A, Severina EP, Petruk VF, et al. Molecular characterization of penicillin-resistant *Streptococcus pneumoniae* isolates causing respiratory disease in the United States. *Microb Drug Resist* 1998;4:325–337.
41. Tucker HA, Eagle H. Serum concentrations of penicillin G in man following intramuscular injections in aqueous solution and in peanut oil-beeswax. *Am J Med* 1948;4:343–354.
42. Viladrich PF, Gudiol F, Liñares J, et al. Evaluation of vancomycin for therapy of adult pneumococcal meningitis. *Antimicrob Agents Chemother* 1991;35:2467–2472.
43. Livermore DM. Quinupristin/dolfopristin and linezolid: where, when, which and whether to use? *J Antimicrob Chemother* 2000;46:347–350.
44. Austrian R, Gold J. Pneumococcal bacteremia with especial reference to bacteremic pneumococcal pneumonia. *Ann Intern Med* 1964;60:759–776.
45. Shapiro ED, Clemens JD. A controlled evaluation of the protective efficacy of pneumococcal vaccine for patients at high risk of serious pneumococcal infections. *Ann Intern Med* 1986;101:325–330.
46. Bolan G, Broome CV, Facklam RR, et al. Pneumococcal vaccine efficacy in selected populations in the United States. *Ann Intern Med* 1986;104:1–6.
47. Shapiro ED, Berg AT, Austrian R, et al. The protective effect of polyvalent pneumococcal polysaccharide vaccine. *N Engl J Med* 1991;325:1453–1460.
48. Recommendations of the Advisory Committee on Immunization Practices (ACIP). Prevention of pneumococcal disease. *MMWR* 1997;46(RR-08):1–24.
49. American College of Physicians. *Guide for adult immunization*, 3rd ed. Philadelphia: American College of Physicians, 1994:108–114.
50. Black S, Shinefeld S, Fireman B, et al. Efficacy, safety and immunogenicity of heptavalent pneumococcal conjugate vaccine in children. *Pediatr Infect Dis J* 2000;19:187–195.
51. Recommendations of the Advisory Committee on Immunization Practices (ACIP). Preventing pneumococcal disease among infants and young children. *MMWR* 2000;49(RR-9):1–35.
52. Puumalainen T, Ekström N, Zeta-Capeding R, et al. Functional antibodies elicited by an 11-valent diphtheria-tetanus toxoid-conjugated pneumococcal vaccine. *J Infect Dis* 2003;187:1704–1708.

CHAPTER 185
Enterococci

Barbara E. Murray and John G. Bartlett

The name enterococcus derives from a paper in France published in 1899 that described an "entérocoque," a new gram-positive coccus of intestinal origin (1). The name *Streptococcus faecalis* (faecalis, related to feces) was given in 1906 to an organism isolated from the blood of a patient with endocarditis (2). Probably the first description of *Streptococcus faecium* was in 1919, but this organism was not formally recognized as a separate species for several decades (3). Through the years, a number of other types of enterococci were recognized, including *Streptococcus durans* and *Streptococcus avium*; motile enterococci, which were also known as *S. faecium* var. *mobilis*; and organisms producing a yellow pigment, referred to as *S. faecium* var. *casseliflavus*.

Two decades ago, deoxyribonucleic acid (DNA)-DNA and DNA-ribosomal ribonucleic acid hybridization studies showed that enterococci, contrary to their long-standing classification, are not actually members of the genus *Streptococcus* 4, 5 and the common name enterococcus became the new genus. In addition to *Enterococcus faecalis, Enterococcus faecium, Enterococcus durans*, and *Enterococcus avium*, a number of other organisms have been classified in this genus (6,7), an updated list of which is shown in Table 185.1.

IDENTIFICATION

For a number of years, enterococci have been presumptively identified by their morphologic appearance in culture and on Gram stain together with their ability to hydrolyze esculin in the presence of bile and to grow in the presence of 6.5% NaCl. Many laboratories also test organisms with group D antiserum. It is now clear that a number of other, less often encountered organisms may have these characteristics including most pediococci and a number of *Leuconostoc* that test positive with group D antiserum. Lactococci, pediococci, and *Leuconostoc* are often bile esculin–positive and able to grow in high salt concentrations (8,9). *Leuconostoc* and pediococci are characteristically resistant to vancomycin, which formerly was useful for distinguishing these organisms from enterococci (9). Other helpful tests include the demonstration of pyrrolidyl arylamidase (the PYRase test), growth at 45°C, and leucine aminopeptidase, which are characteristic of enterococci but not *Leuconostoc*, and the production of gas from glucose, which is characteristic of *Leuconostoc* but not enterococci (8,9). This topic has been reviewed, and the reader is referred to these articles for more details (6,10). It is important to note that some of the rapid kit identification systems for species identification of enterococci were evaluated before some of the newer species were recognized and may not be accurate, particularly for species other than *E. faecalis*.

HABITAT AND TYPING SCHEMES

As the names of the two most common species suggest, *E. faecalis* and *E. faecium* are commonly found in the feces of normal individuals. In most studies, *E. faecalis* has been more com-

mon than other enterococcal species and is usually present in higher numbers, often 10^5 to 10^7 colony-forming units per gram of stool (3,9,11,12). Enterococci are also found at other sites, although much less frequently than in fecal contents (13,14).

Epidemiologic studies of enterococcal infections have been difficult in the past because of the lack of convenient and reliable subspecies typing schemes. Although phage and bacteriocin typing have been described for enterococci for at least two decades, this system has not gained widespread use (15). Total plasmid content analysis, a technique used with a variety of other organisms, has also been used to compare strains of enterococci (16), although plasmid analysis has not been as convenient or reproducible, at least in our hands, with enterococci as with other organisms. Pulsed-field gel electrophoresis of enterococcal chromosomal DNA has shown that enterococci, like other nosocomial pathogens, can be spread within and even between hospitals (17–19).

CLINICAL INFECTIONS

Endocarditis

It is estimated that enterococci cause between 5% and 15% of cases of bacterial endocarditis (Table 185.2) (20–22). The first report of this disease was probably in 1899; although the organism was called *Micrococcus zymogenes*, it was probably a β-hemolytic enterococcus (3). The authors who first coined the name *S. faecalis* in 1906 isolated the organism from a patient with endocarditis (2). Although most enterococcal endocarditis isolates are *E. faecalis, E. faecium* is also seen and, with the emergence of vancomycin resistance, may be increasing. Enterococcal endocarditis occurs rarely in infants, occasionally in children, and more often in older individuals. Risk factors include genitourinary and biliary tract infections; in one study, 50% of men had had genitourinary instrumentation or urinary tract infection and 38% of women had a genitourinary source, including instrumentation or abortion (20–22). The disease can occur on valves that are apparently normal as well as on those with underlying disease. In drug addicts, enterococci are estimated to cause between 5% and 10% of cases, although in one study 53% of 20 cases of endocarditis were caused by enterococci (3,23). The valves

TABLE 185.1.   List of Generally Recognized *Enterococcus* Species

Predominant human isolates	No known reports of human infections
E. faecalis[a]	*E. malodoratus*
E. faecium[a]	*E. pseudoavium*
Occasional human isolates	*E. sulfureus*
E. casseliflavus[b]	*E. cecorum*[d]
E. gallinarumt[b]	*E. columbae*[d]
E. flavescens[b,c]	*E. saccharolyticus*[d]
E. avium	
E. raffinosus	
E. mundtii	
E. durans	
E. hirae	

[a]The ratio of *E. faecalis* to *E. faecium* among clinical specimens is typically 8:1 to 9:1, unless organisms are vancomycin-resistant.
[b]May express vancomycin resistance because of VanC phenotype.
[c]Some evidence suggests that this species is the same as *E. casseliflavus* (90).
[d]These species have less genetic similarity to other enterococcal species (91).

TABLE 185.2.   Clinical Infections Caused by Enterococci

Type of infection	% of cases caused by enterococci
Endocarditis	5–15
Urinary tract infections	<5 in young otherwise healthy women; ~15 of nosocomial infections
Intraabdominal pelvic and wound infections	15; frequently isolated, but other organisms are more important
Spontaneous peritonitis (cirrhosis)	5–10
Nosocomial bacteremia	10–15
Neonatal sepsis	Unusual
Central nervous system infections	Rare
Osteomyelitis	Rare
Pneumonia	Rare

most often involved in drug addicts are the mitral and aortic valves.

Bacteremia

Bacteremia caused by enterococci is increasing in frequency (3,24–26), possibly due to antimicrobial pressure. In most series, the enterococcus ranks in the top four organisms to cause bacteremia, accounting for 10% to 20% of cases (20). In most cases, it is a true pathogen rather than a contaminant. The most likely portals of entry are the urinary tract, intra-abdominal sepsis, and vascular catheters (20–23).

Urinary Tract Infections

Enterococci are also a common cause of urinary tract infections (UTIs). Perinephric abscesses and prostatitis are occasionally seen. Enterococcal urinary tract infections are more common among hospitalized individuals, those who have had instrumentation, those who have structural abnormalities or recurrent urinary tract infections, and those who have received antibiotics (3). In one study from a Veterans Administration hospital, for example, enterococci were found in 21% of urinary tract infections (26). A multicenter study in the United States showed the enterococcus accounted for 13% of UTIs in 1,510 hospitalized patients in 1998 (27). In contrast, enterococci cause less than 5% of urinary tract infections in young, healthy women with cystitis who do not have structural abnormalities and have not had instrumentation or recurrent infections.

Intraabdominal and Pelvic Infections

Enterococci are found in the feces of most normal adults and in approximately 17% of routine vaginal cultures (13). Enterococci are common components of mixed infections involving the female genital tract and in intra-abdominal sepsis (28,29). It has been difficult to know the importance of these organisms because they are generally part of a complex mixed flora. Suggesting that they are not usually pathogenic are the observations that other bacteria are usually predominant by quantitative analysis, treatment directed against other components of the mixed flora (anaerobes and coliforms) is usually effective (29–32) and studies in an animal model suggest enterococci have no pathogenic potential (33). Nevertheless, there are clinical settings in which enterococci play a more convincing role in the pathogenic process

as suggested by positive blood cultures (34,35) in cases where they are the dominant pathogens on Gram stain or culture, and with superinfections (36,37).

Miscellaneous Infections

Enterococci can also cause primary peritonitis in adults and children, although less frequently than coliforms and pneumococci (38,39). With neonates, a study of more than 30,000 live births at Parkland Memorial Hospital in Dallas in the 1970s showed enterococci caused between 0.6 and 2.0 infections per 1,000 live births in a 4-year period, compared with the rates for *E. coli* of 0.4 to 1.4 infections per 1,000 live births (40). Infection can occur in apparently normal infants, but those with severe underlying disease, intravascular devices, nasogastric endotracheal intubation, and prematurity appear to be more susceptible (41,42). Some of these risk factors are also thought to predispose adults to enterococcal infection.

Enterococcal infections of the central nervous system are uncommon but have been described in all age groups. The predisposing factors are thought to be underlying long-term primary disease, invasive procedures of the central nervous system, and prior therapy with antimicrobial agents. For example, case reports have included the development of enterococcal meningitis in patients with underlying meningeal leukemia while receiving intrathecal chemotherapy; after basilar skull fracture; and after intracranial surgery. Enterococcal meningitis has also occurred in patients with central nervous system shunts, particularly ventriculoperitoneal and lumbo-ureteral shunts (3,43,44).

Nosocomial Infections and Superinfections, Including Those with Vancomycin-Resistant Enterococci

The Centers for Disease Control and Prevention's National Nosocomial Infection Surveillance survey listed the enterococcus as one of the three most common organisms recovered from nosocomial infections beginning in the early 1990s. At that time, enterococci were found in about 10% of all nosocomial infections, 9% of bacteremias, and approximately 16% of urinary tract infections (45). In the past, it was assumed that nosocomial enterococcal disease resulted from the endogenous flora with which the patient was admitted, but it is now clear that nosocomial spread of these organisms can occur (16–19,41). Several factors appear to be involved in the emergence of enterococci as important nosocomial pathogens, including the multiple resistances characteristic of these organisms, heavy use of cephalosporins and other antimicrobial agents to which these organisms are resistant, use of mechanically compromising devices such as intravascular lines and urinary catheters, and increasing numbers of seriously ill and debilitated patients in hospitals.

Enterococci have now become far more important in the hospital setting because of the emergence of strains resistant to vancomycin. In the United States, vancomycin-resistant enterococci (VRE) were first a problem in intensive care units the northeastern part of the country but have now spread to all states, are found throughout the hospital, and are common in long-term care facilities (42,43). A survey of 4,998 strains of enterococci from throughout the world collected from 1997–99 showed the overall rate of vancomycin resistance in the United States was 17%, far higher than in other countries (44,45). Some published outbreaks of VRE from the United States have reported a predominant strain or "clone," and one report found the same strain in three hospitals in two states, indicating spread of specific organisms between patients. Most of these reports have also identified some distinctly different strains, indicating that horizontal spread of the vancomycin resistance gene cluster(s) has also occurred. Of interest, although *E. faecalis* has traditionally outnumbered *E. faecium* among clinical isolates of enterococci by about 10:1, among VRE, isolates of *E. faecium* outnumber those of *E. faecalis* by 10:1.

A number of risk factors have been identified for VRE colonization and infection, and many of these are the same risks that drive high rates of nosocomial infections involving methicillin-resistant *S. aureus*, extended spectrum β-lactam–resistant *Enterobacteriaceae*, *C. difficile*, and *Candida* (46). They include exposure to antimicrobial agents (especially cephalosporins, vancomycin, and anti-anaerobic antibiotics), age, length of stay, and severe underlying disease (46–48).

To control transmission of VRE within the hospital, the Hospital Infection Control Practices Advisory Committee of the CDC recommends identification of those infected or colonized (rectal swabs) for high-risk patients. Those who are VRE-infected or VRE-colonized should be placed in a private room or with other culture-positive patients, gloves should be worn when entering a room with a VRE-positive patient, and gowns are to be worn if contact with environmental surfaces (which have frequently been contaminated with VRE) is anticipated. Gowns and gloves should be removed before exiting the room, and hands should be washed with an antiseptic soap (e.g., chlorhexidine) (49–51). The effectiveness of these methods to contain VRE has been documented (41).

An unexpected and interesting twist in the epidemiology of VRE is that in Europe, but apparently not in the United States, VRE have been found as part of the normal flora of animals and normal community volunteers. This is due to the previous practice of using glycopeptides for growth promotion in agriculture with gastrointestinal colonization following consumption (52–54).

RESISTANCE

With the emergence of resistance to vancomycin, enterococci have displayed resistance to essentially every antimicrobial agent used to treat them except linezolid and quinupristin-dalfopristin (55–57). Rare strains of VRE are resistant to linezolid; quinupristin-dalfopristin is inactive against all *E. faecalis* and occasional *E. faecium* (44,58). Resistance to antimicrobial agents can be divided into that which is an intrinsic or natural property of the species and that which is acquired (Table 185.3).

Intrinsic Resistance

Enterococci are intrinsically resistant or at least relatively resistant to β-lactams. The most effective agents in this group include penicillin, ampicillin, ureidopenicillins, and imipenem. Minimal inhibitory concentrations (MICs) of these agents typically range between 0.5 and 8 μg/mL for *E. faecalis* but are higher for *E. faecium* (3,59); occasional strains of *E. faecium* have quite high MICs (3). Enterococci are less susceptible to ticarcillin and carbenicillin and are more resistant to the penicillinase-resistant semisynthetic penicillins, such as methicillin, and the cephalosporins, including the third-generation compounds (3,60,61). In addition to the high MICs of β-lactams displayed by enterococci, these organisms often have high minimal bactericidal concentrations, greater than 100 μg/mL for β-lactams, and are thus a natural example of β-lactam-"tolerant" organisms (3). As discussed later, the high minimal bactericidal concentrations pre-

TABLE 185.3. Resistances Found in Enterococci

Intrinsic (naturally occurring) resistances
  Aminoglycosides (low level)
  β-Lactams, particularly semisynthetic penicillinase-resistant penicillins, cephalosporins, and aztreonam
  Clindamycin (low level)
Acquired resistances
  Aminoglycosides (high level; minimal inhibitory concentration usually greater than 2,000 μg/mL)
  Chloramphenicol
  Erythromycin and high levels of clindamycin
  Fluoroquinolones
  Penicillins via penicillinase or low-affinity penicillin binding proteins
  Rifampin
  Tetracycline
  Trimethoprim
  Vancomycin

sumably explain why endocarditis (a disease for which bactericidal activity is required for optimal results) caused by enterococci has an unacceptably low cure rate when treated with β-lactams alone.

Enterococci frequently show intrinsic low-level resistance to clindamycin and aminoglycosides (3,59,60,62). However, when strains with low-level aminoglycoside resistance (typically MICs of 8 to 250 μg/mL) are treated with penicillin or ampicillin plus the aminoglycoside, there is markedly enhanced killing or synergism (which is described in more detail later). *E. faecium* has an additional problem not seen with *E. faecalis*. For these organisms, MICs of certain aminoglycosides, namely tobramycin, kanamycin, netilmicin, and sisomicin are higher than for *E. faecalis*, although still less than 2,000 μg/mL, and combinations of penicillin or ampicillin plus these aminoglycosides fail to show synergism against *E. faecium*; this appears to be true of all members of this species (59). These organisms normally produce an aminoglycoside-modifying enzyme (a 6′-acetyltransferase) that is an inherent species characteristic (63).

Problems are also seen with enterococci and other antimicrobial agents. Currently available fluoroquinolones are only moderately active against enterococci, and true resistance has emerged in isolates apparently as a result of mutations (64). The value of trimethoprim-sulfamethoxazole for enterococcal infections is also debatable. This is related partially to the ability of enterococci to use both thymidine and thymine (unlike most other bacteria) and to use preformed dihydrofolate and tetrahydrofolate (60,65,66). The MICs of trimethoprim-sulfamethoxazole are increased in media containing these compounds and in urine, which raises the question of *in vivo* efficacy (67). Unless clinical data are published to indicate *in vivo* efficacy, this compound should be considered for therapy only as a last possible resort. The potential problem is illustrated by a report of two patients in whom enterococcal bacteremia developed during or shortly after therapy with trimethoprim-sulfamethoxazole for enterococcal urinary tract infections and by poor results in some animal models (68–70).

Acquired Resistance

In addition to the intrinsic resistance just described, enterococci may acquire resistance to antimicrobial agents. This can occur either by mutation in existing DNA or by the acquisition of new DNA, such as a plasmid or a transposon. Resistance to chloramphenicol, erythromycin, high levels of clindamycin, tetracycline, high levels of aminoglycosides, and vancomycin is common and often plasmid- and/or transposon-mediated (63), whereas resistance to rifampin and fluoroquinolones arises via mutations.

Resistance to Aminoglycosides and β-Lactams

Enterococci with low-level aminoglycoside resistance are usually killed by the combination of an agent that inhibits cell wall synthesis, such as vancomycin or penicillin, with an aminoglycoside. There is characteristically a greater than or equal to 2 $\log_{10}$ increase in killing versus the effect of the cell wall-active agent alone, even when the aminoglycoside is used in a subinhibitory concentration (71). The first description of high-level resistance (MIC of 2,000 μg/mL or greater) to aminoglycosides involved streptomycin. High-level resistance to streptomycin can occur because of a mutation leading to ribosomal resistance or via the acquisition of new DNA, which encodes an enzyme that adenylates streptomycin (72). High-level resistance to kanamycin has also been recognized for some years; when not accompanied by high-level gentamicin resistance, this trait is due to the production of a 3'-phosphotransferase (73). Although high-level resistance to kanamycin is per se of little clinical significance, the 3'-phosphotransferase also modifies amikacin. The MICs for amikacin may not be elevated (i.e., no high-level resistance), but the 3'-phosphotransferase eliminates the synergistic effect that would otherwise be seen with a cell wall-active agent plus amikacin (73). High-level resistance to gentamicin is due to the presence of a bifunctional fusion protein that has both acetyltransferase and phosphotransferase activities (16,58,74,75). This enzyme confers high-level resistance or resistance to synergism for all commercially available aminoglycosides (gentamicin, sisomicin, netilmicin, tobramycin, kanamycin, and amikacin) except streptomycin. Some strains have acquired high-level resistance to all aminoglycosides by a combination of mechanisms; for such strains, there is no synergism with any aminoglycoside and thus no value in adding an aminoglycoside to a therapeutic regimen (62,75).

A β-lactamase-producing strain of E. faecalis was first reported in the early 1980s (76). Currently, such strains are still apparently rare but have been reported from a variety of locations (77,78). The structural gene for the enterococcal β-lactamase enzyme is the same as the gene for the common β-lactamase of staphylococci, strongly suggesting spread from these organisms (79); as expected, the enzyme is highly active against penicillin, ampicillin, and the ureidopenicillins. It is important to note that the amount of β-lactamase produced by enterococci is low, and thus the resistance of strains may not be detected by routine susceptibility testing (77). At higher inocula and in animal model studies, the resistance of β-lactamase-producing strains to penicillin and ampicillin is obvious (80). Although the enzyme is not active against the semisynthetic penicillinase-resistant penicillins or cephalosporins, these agents have little intrinsic activity against enterococci and are not useful for such strains. Imipenem and vancomycin remain active against β-lactamase-producing E. faecalis, but, as with other cell wall-active agents, are not bactericidal (77,81).

In addition to β-lactamase production as a mechanism of penicillin resistance, many enterococci, particularly E. faecium, are resistant to penicillin by a nonpenicillinase mechanism. E. faecium are typically more resistant than E. faecalis to penicillins, and this appears to be related to the fact that their cell wall synthesis enzymes are less inhibitable by (i.e., have lower affinity for) penicillin. Higher levels of penicillin resistance have been reported to arise from either increased production of these low-affinity cell wall synthesis enzymes (referred to as penicillin binding proteins) or a further reduction in the affinity of these penicillin binding proteins for penicillin.

Resistance to Vancomycin

The latest and most disturbing resistance to appear in enterococci is resistance to vancomycin, which was first reported in 1988 (82,83). In at least some instances, the resistance has been found to be plasmid and transposon mediated and has been transferable by conjugation to other species, including Staphylococcus aureus (84). This highly feared potential resistance to create VRSA was first reported in the lab in 1992 and first reported in a patient in 2002. 85 The mechanism of vancomycin resistance has been best defined for the VanA phenotype, which is associated with the vanA gene cluster. This cluster has been shown to be part of a transposon named Tn1546. On the basis of polymerase chain reaction and hybridization data, this transposon or related elements have a wide geographic distribution and appear to account for much of the VanA type resistance. Two genes on this transposon encode proteins associated with transposition function, and at least six of the other seven genes (vanS, vanR, vanA, vanH, vanX, vanY, and vanZ) encode proteins involved with the vancomycin resistance phenotype. The genes vanR and vans encode two proteins that function as part of a two-component regulatory system that somehow senses (VanS, the sensor) the presence (or the effect) of vancomycin and then regulates (VanR, the response regulator) the response of other genes of this cluster. Vanes (encoded by vanH) is a dehydrogenase that generates D-lactate; VanA (encoded by vanA) is a ligase that ligates D-alanine with D-lactate to form the depsipeptide, D-alanine-D-lactate; VanX is a dipeptidase that cleaves the dipeptide D-alanine-D-alanine; VanY is a carboxypeptidase that can cleave the terminal unit (e.g., D-alanine or D-lactate) from the pentapeptide part of cell wall precursors; and VanZ is of unknown function.

To understand the mechanism of resistance to vancomycin, it is necessary to understand how vancomycin inhibits cell wall synthesis. It does this by binding to the terminal two amino acids (D-alanine-D-alanine) of N-acetylmuramyl-N-acetylglucosamine pentapeptide, which is a precursor unit for cell wall peptidoglycan synthesis. Once vancomycin binds to this pentapeptide-containing precursor, it blocks the rest of cell wall peptidoglycan synthesis and thus leads to inhibition of cell growth. Resistance to vancomycin associated with the VanA phenotype and, by analogy, the VanB phenotype occurs when the cell wall pentapeptide precursor ends in something to which vancomycin cannot bind. This is accomplished through a complex system of steps that involves the generation of a new peptidoglycan pentadepsipeptide precursor, as well as the destruction of the cell's normal pentapeptide-containing precursor. Vancomycin resistance is normally inducible; that is, the presence of vancomycin leads to the synthesis of the resistance-associated proteins. As just mentioned, Vanes generates D-lactate, which is the substrate for the ligase, VanA. After generation, by VanA, of D-alanine-D-lactate, the cells own enzymes apparently add D-alanine-D-lactate to the peptidoglycan precursor tripeptide, resulting in the pentadepsipeptide precursor containing a terminal D-alanine-D-lactate. The action of VanX, the dipeptidase, results in cleavage of the normally present D-alanine-D-alanine, thus preventing the formation of normal, vancomycin-susceptible pentapeptide precursor. Should any D-alanine-D-alanine escape cleavage and end up in cell wall subunits, the carboxypeptidase VanY can cleave the terminal D-alanine, resulting in a tetrapeptide chain to which vancomycin does not bind. The purpose of the remaining gene, vanZ, in the van cluster is unknown.

The VanB phenotype shows the homologs of each of the genes of the *vanA* cluster and the mechanism of resistance is similar. Cell wall precursor units of strains expressing the VanB phenotype also end in D-alanine-D-lactate. The VanC phenotype is a naturally occurring trait of *Enterococcus gallinarum* and *Enterococcus casseliflavus* and confers low-to-moderate levels of resistance (MICs of 32 μg/mL or less), although most strains have MICs of 8 μg/mL or less. Two genes, *vanC-1* and *vanC-2*, are found in *E. gallinarum* and *E. casseliflavus*, respectively. Cell wall peptidoglycan of *E. gallinarum* has been shown to end in D-alanine-D-serine, which appears to have lower affinity for vancomycin than does D-alanine-D-alanine.

In addition to the remarkable complexity of the vancomycin resistance mechanism, two additional interesting phenomena related to this resistance are vancomycin dependence and penicillin-vancomycin synergy. Enterococci dependent on vancomycin for growth have been isolated from patients who have been treated with vancomycin. In cases described, cultures were negative but patients were strongly suspected of being infected. Organisms were eventually recovered either by using vancomycin-containing media or by noting growth around vancomycin disks. It appears that these vancomycin-dependent cells turned off their normal production of D-alanine-D-alanine, which, in the presence of vancomycin, was being destroyed by VanX or VanY. In the presence of vancomycin, the cells make D-alanine-D-lactate, and D-alanine-D-alanine is unnecessary for survival. However, when cells are removed from vancomycin, no VanA or VanB ligase is made, so no D-alanine-D-lactate is made. If neither D-alanine-D-alanine nor D-alanine-D-lactate is made, the cell cannot survive. Revertants can survive independent of vancomycin by either turning back on the production of its normal D-alanine-D-alanine ligase (to make once again the dipeptide D-alanine-D-alanine) or by mutating to constitutive production of the VanA or VanB ligase, to make D-alanine-D-lactate independent of the presence of vancomycin.

The phenomenon of penicillin-vancomycin synergy refers to the fact that some strains of VRE, in the presence of vancomycin, have a lower MIC of penicillin. The proposed mechanism for this enhanced activity is that not all of the cell wall synthesis enzymes are able to use D-alanine-D-lactate pentadepsipeptide precursor to make cell wall and that when this precursor is present and D-alanine-D-alanine-ending pentapeptide is not, the cell must shift to enzymes that can use D-alanine-D-lactate-containing precursor to survive. If these enzymes are more susceptible to inhibition by penicillin, the MIC of penicillin is decreased in the presence of vancomycin. Unfortunately, many VRE do not display this phenomenon and even for those that do, mutants arise frequently, in vitro as well as in animal models that no longer show this beneficial interaction, so the clinical usefulness of this phenomenon appears to be limited.

Susceptibility Testing

In most instances, susceptibility of enterococci to penicillin, ampicillin, and vancomycin should be determined; for urinary isolates, a fluoroquinolone and/or nitrofurantoin may be considered. Because routine testing may not detect β-lactamase-producing strains, the possible presence of this enzyme should be determined with nitrocefin for isolates from patients with serious enterococcal infections; nitrocefin is a chromogenic cephalosporin that changes color when hydrolyzed by penicillinase (72,85,86). Isolates from patients with endocarditis and possibly those with other serious infections, including meningitis, should also be tested for the presence of high-level aminoglycoside resistance. This resistance can be detected by several methods, including a plate screening method with plates containing streptomycin at 2,000 μg/mL or gentamicin at 500 μg/mL, a single-concentration broth test with 1,000 μg/mL streptomycin or 500 μg/mL gentamicin (it should be noted that discrepancies have arisen with some commercial microdilution susceptibility methods), or use of disks impregnated with a high concentration of aminoglycosides (120 mg of gentamicin and 300 mg of streptomycin) (85,86).

MANAGEMENT OF ENTEROCOCCAL INFECTION

Formerly, most enterococcal soft tissue and urinary tract infections could be treated with single-drug therapy such as penicillin, ampicillin, or vancomycin. Although the MICs of penicillin are approximately twice those of ampicillin, adequate concentrations are normally achieved. Ureidopenicillins such as piperacillin and mezlocillin also appear adequate, but these drugs have a broader spectrum of activity than is needed, unless mixed infection is suspected. Ticarcillin and carbenicillin are only moderately active in vitro and probably have little role in therapy for enterococcal infections. For the occasional isolates of *E. faecalis* that produce penicillinase, vancomycin, imipenem, ampicillin-sulbactam, and amoxicillin-clavulanate all appear active (76,81). The fluoroquinolones have been successful in enterococcal urinary tract infections, but susceptibility is marginal. Rifampin, like other agents, lacks bactericidal activity against enterococci, does not appear to enhance the efficacy of other agents, and is associated with rapid emergence of resistant strains (88).

Enterococcal endocarditis, and probably meningitis and other serious enterococcal infections, should be treated with a combination of a cell wall-active agent such as penicillin or vancomycin plus an aminoglycoside to which the strain is not highly resistant (21). The rationale for this therapy dates back to the early antibacterial chemotherapeutic era, when it was observed that therapy with penicillin alone was associated with an unacceptably high relapse rate and that the empirical combination of streptomycin with penicillin was much more likely to produce cure. 3 Unfortunately, high-level resistance to streptomycin has become quite common, and high-level resistance to gentamicin (and all other aminoglycosides) is increasing (16,45,62). Optimal therapy for patients with serious infections caused by strains with high-level resistance to all aminoglycosides is unknown, but adding an aminoglycoside to the cell wall-active agent adds nothing to the therapy except for toxicity (62,89). No current clinical data suggest that any single-drug regimen reliably produces cure. However, animal model studies with one strain showed that continuous infusion ampicillin was more effective than intermittent ampicillin in therapy for enterococcal endocarditis caused by a single strain that was highly resistant to gentamicin (89).

For infections caused by VRE, there are some strains that are sensitive to ampicillin, tetracycline, chloramphenicol, or a fluoroquinolone; nitrofurantoin may be used for urinary tract infections with normal renal function. The usual drugs for most cases are linezolid or, less commonly, quinupristin-dalfopristin (55–57). Other treatment barriers to address are resolution of neutropenia, reduction in antibiotic pressure, drained closed space infection, and removal of foreign bodies.

CONCLUSION

The enterococcus is an old pathogen with a newly recognized role as a nosocomially transmitted pathogen. Although the organism is normally of relatively low virulence, its remarkable native antibiotic resistance has always made it difficult to treat.

However, the addition of high-level aminoglycoside resistance, β-lactamase, and vancomycin resistance to the enterococcal armamentarium makes it one of our greatest challenges to both contain it with infection control and cure it with new and novel therapeutic strategies.

REFERENCES

1. Thiercelin ME. Sur un diplocoque saprophyte de l'intestin susceptible de devenir pathogène. *C R Seances Soc Biol Paris* 1899;5:269.
2. Andrewes FW, Horder TJ. A study of the streptococci pathogenic for man. *Lancet* 1906;2:708.
3. Murray BE. The life and times of the enterococcus. *Clin Microbiol Rev* 1990;3:46.
4. Farrow JAE, Jones D, Phillips BA, Collins MD. Taxonomic studies on some group D streptococci. *J Gen Microbiol* 1983;129:1423.
5. Schleifer KH, Kilpper-Balz R. Transfer of *Streptococcus faecalis* and *Streptococcus faecium* to the genus *Enterococcus* nom. rev. as *Enterococcus faecalis* comb. nov. and *Enterococcus faecium* comb. nov. *Int J Syst Bacteriol* 1984;34:31.
6. Facklam RR, Hollis D, Collins MD. Identification of gram-positive coccal and coccobacillary vancomycin-resistant bacteria. *J Clin Microbiol* 1989;27:724.
7. Collins MD, Facklam RR, Farrow JAE, Williamson R. *Enterococcus raffinosus* sp. nov, *Enterococcus solitarius* sp. nov. and *Enterococcus pseudoavium* sp. nov. *FEMS Microbiol Lett* 1989;57:283.
8. Facklam RR, Collins MD. Identification of *Enterococcus* species isolated from human infections by a conventional test scheme. *J Clin Microbiol* 1989;27:731.
9. Benno Y, Suzuki K, Suzuki K, et al. Comparison of the fecal microflora in rural Japanese and urban Canadians. *Microbiol Immunol* 1986;30:521.
10. Facklam RR, Sahm DA. *Enterococcus*. In: Murray PR. Baron EJ, Pfaller MA, et al, eds. *Manual of clinical microbiology*, 6th ed. Washington, DC: American Society for Microbiology, 1995:308–314.
11. Mead GC. Streptococci in the intestinal flora of man and other non-ruminant animals. In: Skinner FA, Quesnel LB, eds. *Streptococci*. London: Academic Press, 1978:245–261.
12. Noble CJ. Carriage of group D streptococci in the human bowel. *J Clin Pathol* 1978;31:1182.
13. Beargie R, Lynd P, Tucker E, Duhring J. Perinatal infection and vaginal flora. *Am J Obstet Gynecol* 1975;122:31.
14. Kurrie E, Bhaduri S, Krieger D, et al. Risk factors for infections of the oropharynx and the respiratory tract in patients with acute leukemia. *J Infect Dis* 1981;144:128.
15. Kuhnen E, Richter F, Richter K, Andries L. Establishment of a typing system for group D streptococci. *Zentralbl Bakteriol Mikrobiol Hyg A* 1988;267:322.
16. Zervos MJ, Kauffman CA, Therasse PM, et al. Nosocomial infection by gentamicin-resistant *Streptococcus faecalis*: an epidemiologic study. *Ann Intern Med* 1987;106:687.
17. Chow JW, Kuritza A, Shlaes DM, et al. Clonal spread of vancomycin-resistant *Enterococcus faecium* between patients in three hospitals in two states. *J Clin Microbiol* 1993;31:1609.
18. Handwerger S, Raucher B, Altarac D, et al. Nosocomial outbreak due to *Enterococcus faecium* highly resistant to vancomycin, penicillin and gentamicin. *Clin Infect Dis* 1993;16:750.
19. Murray BE, Singh KV, Markowitz SM, et al. Evidence for clonal spread of a single strain of β-lactamase-producing *Enterococcus faecalis* to six hospitals in five states. *J Infect Dis* 1991;163:780.
20. Hoen B, Alla F, Selton-Suty C, et al. Changing profile of infective endocarditis: results of a one year survey in France. *JAMA* 2002;288:75.
21. Mylonakis E, Calderwood SB. Infective endocarditis in adults. *N Engl J Med* 2001;345:1318.
22. Wilson WR, Wilkowske CJ, Wright AJ, et al. Treatment of streptomycin-susceptible and streptomycin-resistant enterococcal endocarditis. *Ann Intern Med* 1984;100:816.
23. Maki DG, Agger WA. Enterococcal bacteremia: clinical features, the risk of endocarditis, and management. *Medicine (Baltimore)* 1988;67:248.
24. Edmond MB, Wallace SE, McClish DK, et al. Nosocomial bloodstream infections in United States hospitals: a three year analysis. *Clin Infect Dis* 1999;29:239.
25. Raad II, Hanna HA. Intravascular catheter-related infections. *Arch Intern Med* 2002;162:871.
26. Mermel LA, Farr BM, Sherertz RJ, et al. Guidelines for the management of intravascular catheter-related infection. *Clin Infect Dis* 2001;32:1249.
27. Mathai D, Jones RN, Pfaller MA. Epidemiology and frequency of resistance among pathogens causing urinary tract infections in 1,510 hospitalized patients: a report from the SENTRY Antimicrobial Surveillance Program. *Diag Microbiol Infect Diag* 2001;40:129.
28. Pitkin D, Sheikh W, Wilson S, et al. Comparison of the activity of meropenem with that of other agents in the treatment of intraabdominal, obstetric/gynecologic and soft tissue. *Clin Infect Dis* 1995;[Suppl 2]:S372.
29. Patterson JH, Sweeney AH, Simms M, et al. An analysis of 100 serious enterococcal infections. *Medicine* 1995;74:191.
30. Canadian Metronidazole Study Group. Prospective, randomized comparison of metronidazole and clindamycin, each with gentamicin, for the treatment of serious intraabdominal infection. *Surgery* 1983;93:221.
31. Hemsell DW, Wendel GD, Gall SA, et al. Multicenter comparison of cefotetan and cefoxitin in the treatment of acute obstetric and gynecologic infections. *Am J Obstet Gynecol* 1988;158:722.
32. Stone HH, Morris ES, Geheber CE, et al. Clinical comparison of cefotaxime with gentamicin plus clindamycin in the treatment of peritonitis and other soft tissue infections. *Rev Infect Dis* 1982;4[Suppl]:439.
33. Bartlett JG, Onderdonk AB, Louis T, et al. A review: lessons from an animal model of intra-abdominal sepsis. *Arch Surg* 1978;113:850.
34. Dougherty SH, Flahr AB, Simmons RL. Breakthrough enterococcal septicemia in surgical patients. Nineteen cases and a review of the literature. *Arch Surg* 1983;118:232.
35. Garrison RN, Fry DE, Berberich S, Polk HC. Enterococcal bacteremia: clinical implications and determinants of death. *Ann Surg* 1982;196:43.
36. Zervos MJ, Bacon AE, Patterson JE, et al. Enterococcal superinfection in patients treated with ciprofloxacin. *J Antimicrob Chemother* 1988;21:113.
37. Dougherty SH. Role of enterococcus in intraabdominal sepsis. *Am J Surg* 1984;148:308.
38. Gorensek MJ, Lebel MH, Nelson JD. Peritonitis in children with nephrotic syndrome. *Pediatrics* 1988;81:849.
39. Leigh DA. Peritoneal infections in patients on long-term peritoneal dialysis before and after human cadaveric renal transplantation. *J Clin Pathol* 1969;22:539.
40. Siegel JD, McCracken GH Jr. Group D streptococcal infections. *J Pediatr* 1978;93:542.
41. Ostrowsky BE, Trick WE, Sohn AH, et al. Control of vancomycin-resistant enterococcus and health care facilities in a region. *N Engl J Med* 2001;344:1427.
42. Vergis EN, Hayden MK, Chow JW, et al. Determinants of vancomycin resistance and mortality rates in enterococcal bacteremia: a prospective multicenter study. *Ann Intern Med* 2001;135:484.
43. Elizaga ML, Weinstein RA, Hayden MK. Patients in long-term care facilities: a reservoir for vancomycin-resistant enterococci. *Clin Infect Dis* 2002;34:441.
44. Low DE, Keller N, Barth A, Jones RN. Clinical prevalence, antimicrobial susceptibility and geographic resistance patterns of enterococci: results from the SENTRY Antimicrobial Surveillance Program 1997–1999. *Clin Infect Dis* 2001;32[Suppl 2]:S133.
45. Shouten MA, Voss A, Hoogkamp-Korstanje JA. Antimicrobial susceptibility patterns of enterococci causing infections in Europe. *Antimicrob Agents Chemother* 1999;43:2542.
46. Safdar N, Maki DG. The commonality of risk factors for nosocomial colonization and infection with antimicrobial-resistant *Staphylococcus aureus*, enterococcus, gram-negative bacilli, *Clostridium difficile* and Candida. *Ann Intern Med* 2002;136:834.
47. Donskey CJ, Chowdhry TK, Hecker MT, et al. Effect of antibiotic therapy on the density of vancomycin-resistant enterococci in the stool of colonized patients. *N Engl J Med* 2000;343:1925.
48. Fridkin SK, Edwards JR, Courval JM, et al. The effect of vancomycin and third generation cephalosporins on prevalence of vancomycin-resistant enterococci in 126 U.S. adult intensive care units. *Ann Intern Med* 2001;135:175.
49. Jones RN, Sader HS, Erwin ME, et al. Emerging multiply resistant enterococci among clinical isolates. I. Prevalence data from 97 medical center surveillance study in the United States. *Diagn Microbiol Infect Dis* 1995;21:85.
50. Centers for Disease Control and Prevention. Preventing the spread of vancomycin resistance-Report from the Hospital Infection Control Practices Advisory Committee. *Fed Regist* 1994;59:25757.
51. Centers for Disease Control and Prevention. Recommendations for preventing the spread of vancomycin resistance. *Infect Control Hosp Epidemiol* 1995;16:105.
52. Murray BE. Editorial response: what can we do about vancomycin-resistant enterococci? *Clin Infect Dis* 1995;20:1134.
53. Aarestrup FM, Seyfarth AM, Emborg HD, et al. Effect of abolishment of the use of antimicrobial agents for growth promotion on occurrence of antimicrobial resistance in fecal enterococci from food animals in Denmark. *Antimicrob Agents Chemother* 2001;45:2054.
54. Sorensen TL, Blom M, Monnet DL, et al. Transient intestinal carriage after ingestion of antibiotic-resistant *Enterococcus faecium* from chicken and pork. *N Engl J Med* 2001;345:1161.
55. Linden PK, Moellering RC Jr, Wood CA, et al. Treatment of vancomycin-resistant *Enterococcus faecium* infections with quinupristin/dalfopristin. *Clin Infect Dis* 2001;33:1816.
56. McNeil SA, Clark NM, Chandrasekar PH, Kaufman CA: Successful treatment of vancomycin-resistant *Enterococcus faecium* bacteremia with linezolid after failure of treatment with synercid (quinupristin/dalfopristin) *Clin Infect Dis* 2000;30:403.
57. Rybak MJ, Hershberger E, Moldovan T, Grucz RG. In vitro activities of daptomycin, vancomycin, linezolid and quinupristin-dalfopristin against Staphylococci and Enterococci including vancomycin intermediate and resistant strains. *Antimicrob Agents Chemother* 2000;44:1062.
58. Gonzales RD, Schreckenberger PC, Graham MB, et al. Infections due to vancomycin-resistant *Enterococcus faecium* resistant to linezolid. *Lancet* 2001;357:1179.
59. Moellering RC Jr, Korzeniowski OM, Sande MA, Wennersten CB. Species-specific resistance to antimicrobial synergism in *Streptococcus faecium* and *Streptococcus faecalis*. *J Infect Dis* 1979;140:203.

60. Tofte RW, Solliday J, Crossley KB. Susceptibilities of enterococci to twelve antibiotics. *Antimicrob Agents Chemother* 1984;25:532.

61. Fass RJ. In vitro activities of β-lactam and aminoglycoside antibiotics: a comparative study of 20 parenterally administered drugs. *Arch Intern Med* 1988;140:766.

62. Mederski-Samoraj BD, Murray BE. High-level resistance to gentamicin in clinical isolates of enterococci. *J Infect Dis* 1983;147:751.

63. Costa Y, Galimand M, Leclercq R, et al. Characterization of the chromosomal *aac(6')-Ii* gene specific for *Enterococcus faecium*. *Antimicrob Agents Chemother* 1993;37:1896.

64. Korten V, Huang WM, Murray BE. Analysis by PCR and direct DNA sequencing of *gyrA* mutations associated with fluoroquinolone resistance in *Enterococcus faecalis*. *Antimicrob Agents Chemother* 1994;38:2091.

65. Hamilton-Miller JMT. Reversal of activity of trimethoprim against gram-positive cocci by thymidine, thymine and "folates." *J Antimicrob Chemother* 1988;22:35.

66. Crider SR, Colby SD. Susceptibility of enterococci to trimethoprim and trimethoprim-sulfamethoxazole. *Antimicrob Agents Chemother* 1985;27:71.

67. Zervos MJ, Schaberg DS. Reversal of the in vitro susceptibility of enterococci to trimethoprim-sulfamethoxazole by folinic acid. *Antimicrob Agents Chemother* 1985;28:446.

68. Chenoweth CE, Robinson KA, Schaberg DR. Efficacy of ampicillin versus trimethoprim-sulfamethoxazole in a mouse model of lethal enterococcal peritonitis. *Antimicrob Agents Chemother* 1990;34:1800.

69. Goodhart GL. In vivo v in vitro susceptibility of enterococcus to trimethoprim-sulfamethoxazole. A pitfall. *JAMA* 1984;252:2748.

70. Grayson ML, Thauvin-Eliopoulos C, Eliopoulos GM, et al. Failure of trimethoprim-sulfamethoxazole therapy in experimental enterococcal endocarditis. *Antimicrob Agents Chemother* 1990;34:1792.

71. Calderwood SA, Wennersten C, Moellering RC Jr, et al. Resistance to six aminoglycoside aminocyclitol antibiotics among enterococci: prevalence, evolution, and relationship to synergism with penicillin. *Antimicrob Agents Chemother* 1977;12:401.

72. Eliopoulos GM, Farber BF, Murray BE, et al. Ribosomal resistance of clinical enterococcal isolates to streptomycin. *Antimicrob Agents Chemother* 1984;25:398.

73. Krogstad DJ, Korfhagen TR, Moellering RC Jr, et al. Aminoglycoside-inactivating enzymes in clinical isolates of *Streptococcus faecalis*: an explanation for antibiotic synergism. *J Clin Invest* 1978;62:480.

74. Horodniceanu T, Bougueleret T, El-Solh N, et al. High-level, plasmid-borne resistance to gentamicin in *Streptococcus faecalis* subsp. *zymogenes*. *Antimicrob Agents Chemother* 1979;16:686.

75. Murray BE, Tsao J, Panida J. Enterococci from Bangkok, Thailand, with high-level resistance to currently available aminoglycosides. *Antimicrob Agents Chemother* 1983;23:799.

76. Murray BE, Mederski-Samoraj B. Transferable β-lactamase: a new mechanism for in vitro penicillin resistance in *Streptococcus faecalis*. *J Clin Invest* 1983;72:1168.

77. Murray BE, Church DA, Wanger A, et al. Comparison of two β-lactamase-producing strains of *Streptococcus faecalis*. *Antimicrob Agents Chemother* 1986;30:861.

78. Rhinehart E, Smith NE, Wennersten C, et al. Rapid dissemination of β-lactamase-producing, aminoglycoside-resistant *Enterococcus faecalis* among patients and staff on an infant-toddler surgical ward. *N Engl J Med* 1990;323:1814.

79. Zscheck K, Murray BE. Nucleotide sequence of the β-lactamase gene from *Enterococcus faecalis* HH22 and its similarity to staphylococcal β-lactamase genes. *Antimicrob Agents Chemother* 1991;35:1736.

80. Ingerman M, Pitsakis PG, Rosenberg A, et al. β-Lactamase production in experimental endocarditis due to aminoglycoside-resistant *Streptococcus faecalis*. *J Infect Dis* 1987;155:1226.

81. Scheld WM, Keeley JM. Imipenem therapy of experimental *Staphylococcus aureus* and *Streptococcus faecalis* endocarditis. *J Antimicrob Chemother* 1983;12[Suppl D]:65.

82. Leclercq R, Deriot E, Duval J, Courvalin P. Plasmid-mediated resistance to vancomycin and teicoplanin in *Enterococcus faecium*. *N Engl J Med* 1988;319:157.

83. Uttley AHC, Collins CH, Naidoo J, George RC. Vancomycin-resistant enterococci. *Lancet* 1988;1:57.

84. Noble WD, Virani Z, Cree RGA. Co-transfer of vancomycin and other resistance genes from *Enterococcus faecalis* NCTC 12201 to *Staphylococcus aureus*. *FEMS Microbiol Lett* 1992;93:195.

85. Center for Disease Control and Prevention. *Staphylococcus aureus* resistant to vancomycin–United States, 2002. *MMWR* 2002;51:565.

86. National Committee for Clinical Laboratory Standards. *Methods for dilution antimicrobial susceptibility tests for bacteria that grow aerobically*, 3rd ed. Approved Standard. Villanova, PA: National Committee for Clinical Laboratory Standards, 1993; NCCLS document M7-A3.

87. Murray BE, Mederski-Samoraj B, Foster SK, et al. In vitro studies of plasmid-mediated penicillinase from *Streptococcus faecalis* suggest a staphylococcal origin. *J Clin Invest* 1986;77:289.

88. Moellering RC Jr, Wennersten CB. Therapeutic potential of rifampin in enterococcal infections. *Rev Infect Dis* 1983;5[Suppl]:528.

89. Thauvin C, Eliopoulos GM, Willey S, et al. Continuous-infusion ampicillin therapy of enterococcal endocardidtis in rats. *Antimicrob Agents Chemother* 1987;31:139.

CHAPTER 186
Group B Streptococcus

Michael R. Wessels and Dennis L. Kasper

HISTORY

The bacterial species now known as *Streptococcus agalactiae*, or group B *Streptococcus*, was recognized in the dairy industry for many years as an important cause of mastitis in cows. Definition of the organism as distinct from other hemolytic streptococci, however, did not come until the 1930s, when Rebecca Lancefield developed a classification scheme for streptococci based on serologic reactions of specific antisera with hot hydrochloric acid extracts of the organisms. On the basis of antigenic differences among strains, Lancefield distinguished several groups of streptococci as distinct from *Streptococcus pyogenes* (group A *Streptococcus*) (1). The strains she classified as belonging to group B came from bovine sources, though within a few years group B streptococci also were isolated from the vaginas of postpartum women (2). While vaginal colonization appeared, in most women, not to be associated with clinical disease, occasional cases of postpartum fever were noted, and in 1938, Fry reported 3 cases of fatal postpartum sepsis due to group B *Streptococcus* (3), demonstrating the potential of the organism to cause invasive disease in humans. Multiple subsequent reports documented the role of group B streptococci as occasional causes of serious infections in adults, most commonly postpartum sepsis, and also as a cause of neonatal bacteremia and meningitis. Beginning in the early 1960s, reports appeared implicating group B *Streptococcus* as a more important cause of neonatal septicemia than had been appreciated previously (4,5). By the early 1970s, group B *Streptococcus* had been clearly established as a major cause of neonatal sepsis and meningitis; it continues to be the leading cause of serious bacterial infection among neonates in the United States.

CHARACTERISTICS OF THE PATHOGEN

When cultured on sheep blood agar, group B streptococci form glistening gray-white colonies surrounded by a narrow zone of β-hemolysis. The colonies of group B *Streptococcus* are usually somewhat larger, more definitely gray, and surrounded by a narrower hemolytic zone than those of group A *Streptococcus*. Although definitive identification of a strain as group B *Streptococcus* is based on serologic reaction with specific antiserum, clinical laboratory identification can be done quite reliably on the basis of biochemical reactions. Helpful tests for presumptive identification of group B *Streptococcus* include hydrolysis of sodium hippurate (99% of strains are positive) (6), bile-esculin hydrolysis (99% to 100% of strains are negative) (6), bacitracin sensitivity (greater than 90% of strains are resistant) (6,7), and production of CAMP factor (greater than 98% of strains are positive). CAMP factor, named after the authors of its description (8) is a product produced by group B *Streptococcus*, which produces synergistic hemolysis on blood agar with the β-lysin of *Staphylococcus aureus*. A reasonable combination of tests for presumptive identification of streptococci as belonging to group B includes bacitracin sensitivity, CAMP factor production, and bile-esculin hydrolysis (9). Definitive identification of a strain as group B *Streptococcus* is made serologically, using group specific antiserum. Commercially available kits utilizing latex agglutination or staphylococcal coagglutination compare favorably with the standard Lancefield microprecipitin method for identification of the organisms in culture.

Surface Antigens

In Lancefield's early studies, the acid-extractable antigen which gave a positive precipitin reaction with group B–specific antiserum was found to be a complex carbohydrate associated with the cell wall of the organisms (1). Subsequent studies have shown the common group B antigen to be a complex polysaccharide of rhamnose, *N*-acetylglucosamine, galactose, and glycerol phosphate (10–12). The group B carbohydrate molecule appears to be anchored in the cell wall, with a tetra-antennary branching structure extending outward from the cell surface, each branch terminating in an α(1,2)-linked rhamnose trisaccharide (13). Lancefield also found that strains of group B *Streptococcus* could be divided into serotypes based on antigenic differences in a carbohydrate antigen distinct from the group B carbohydrate, the type-specific antigen (14,15). The type-specific antigen has been shown to represent the polysaccharide capsule of the organisms (Fig. 186.1) (16). The capsular polysaccharides from the four serotypes described by Lancefield (Ia, Ib, II, and III) have been isolated and their structures determined (17–19). Additional capsular types IV, V, VI, VII, and VIII (also called JM9) have been identified, subsequently. Each of the group B *Streptococcus* capsular polysaccharides is a high molecular weight

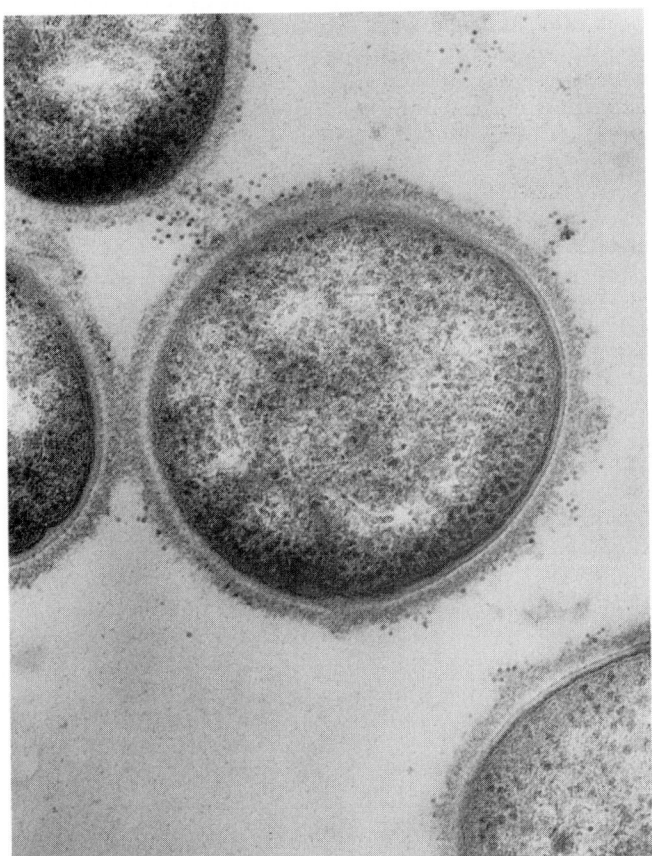

Figure 186.1. Transmission electron micrograph of group B *Streptococcus*. Organisms of group B *Streptococcus* were incubated with type-specific antiserum followed by ferritin-labeled anti-IgG. An irregular layer of capsular polysaccharide is visible exterior to the cell wall, decorated by ferritin particles (original magnification, X55,000).

(100,000 to 500,000) polymer made up of a linear backbone with short side chains. The types Ia, Ib, II, III, IV, V, and VII polysaccharides contain galactose, glucose, *N*-acetylglucosamine, and *N*-acetylneuraminic acid (sialic acid) as exclusive sugars. The component sugars of some of the more recently described capsular polysaccharides are similar, with minor variations: types VI and VIII lack *N*-acetylglucosamine and type VIII contains rhamnose (20–27).

Group B streptococci also express cell surface protein antigens. A serologically defined protein antigen, originally called the Ibc antigen, is present on all strains of capsular type Ib, many strains of capsular type Ia (greater than 90%), type II (50%), type IV (greater than 90%), and infrequently on type III strains (less than 5%) (28–30). According to a proposed convention for classification of group B *Streptococcus* strains, the presence of the Ibc antigen (now, termed C protein) is indicated by /C, following the capsular type designation, e.g., Ia/C (formerly termed Ic) (31). At least two distinct types of C proteins have been defined, the alpha- and beta-C proteins, one or both of which may be present on an individual strain. The beta-C protein appears to be relatively invariant in structure, and it is found on approximately 10% of GBS isolates, primarily those of capsular type Ib. The alpha-C protein is variable in size depending on the number of identical 82 amino acid repeat sequences that comprise the majority of the protein (32,33). It has become apparent that the alpha-C protein is one of a family of closely related, repeat-containing GBS surface proteins. Other members of this protein family include Rib, Rib-like or Alp2, and Alp3, only one of which is expressed on an individual strain (34–36). Evidence has been presented that the C proteins (alpha and beta) and Rib can elicit protective antibodies in animals, suggesting that one or more of these proteins might be useful as a component of a vaccine against group B streptococci (28,29,34,37,38). Surface proteins that appear to be conserved among most or all GBS clinical isolates include Sip and C5a-peptidase, both of which have been shown to evoke protective or opsonic antibodies as experimental vaccines in mice (39,40).

EPIDEMIOLOGY

Neonatal infections with group B *Streptococcus* (GBS) have been divided into two clinical syndromes based on time of onset after delivery: early onset, occurring within the first 5 to 7 days of life, and usually within the first 24 hours; and late onset, occurring after the first week, but rarely after 3 months. The attack rate for early onset disease was estimated to be 1.4 per 1,000 live births, based on 1990 incidence data from a multistate active surveillance system (41); the same study estimated the incidence of late onset disease at 0.3 to 0.4 per 1,000 live births. A population-based study of metropolitan Atlanta, as well as several smaller hospital-based surveys from the 1980s, reported similar or slightly higher rates of neonatal group B streptococcal disease (42–44). There was a striking decline in the incidence of early onset GBS infection during the mid-1990s, coincident with the dissemination of prevention guidelines and the wider use of intrapartum chemoprophylaxis (see section on Prevention). Surveys during the late 1990s documented substantially lower rates of early onset neonatal infection (0.5 to 0.6 cases per 1,000 live births) in the United States and Australia, countries in which selective intrapartum antibiotic prophylaxis has been used extensively (45,46). In contrast, the incidence of late-onset disease in the same populations has not changed significantly since the 1980s.

While the rate of GBS infection is lower in adults than in neonates, infections in adults now account for more than one-half of all invasive group B streptococcal infections. GBS disease in adults occurs primarily in the peripartum period or among individuals with underlying chronic conditions, particularly diabetes mellitus or a malignancy (41,47,48).

The GBS serotypes most commonly associated with invasive neonatal disease are types Ia, III, and V, and, less commonly, types II and Ib (49–51). The same serotypes are associated with GBS infection in non-pregnant adults, but type V is the most frequent cause of infection in this population (52). Although types IV, VI, VII, and VIII appear to be uncommon among human disease isolates in the United States, type VI and VIII strains predominated in a series of vaginal colonizing isolates in Japanese women (53).

Asymptomatic colonization of the vagina and lower gastrointestinal tract occurs commonly, and of the upper respiratory tract, occasionally. Surveys of pregnant and nonpregnant women have indicated carriage rates of 10% to 35% in both groups, with higher rates in sexually active women and African American women (54). Vertical transmission of GBS from mother to infant at the time of vaginal delivery occurs with a frequency of approximately 60% (43,55); of infants who are colonized at birth, symptomatic infection develops in only 1% to 3%. Neonatal acquisition of the organism at or shortly before birth has been shown to be the source of infection in early onset neonatal disease; in late-onset infection, the organism may be acquired in this manner, or may be transmitted to the infant after birth from the mother, from nursery personnel, or from other contacts. Risk factors for neonatal GBS infection include maternal GBS bacteriuria during pregnancy, GBS rectovaginal colonization at delivery, a sibling with a history of invasive GBS infection, black race, maternal age of less than 20, and obstetric complications including prematurity, birth weight of 2,500 g, prolonged rupture of membranes, peripartum fever, and chorioamnionitis (42,44,56).

PATHOGENESIS

In vitro studies have demonstrated marked stimulation of tumor necrosis factor-α (TNF-α) release from human cord blood monocytes in response to GBS, and TNF-α is thought to play an important role in the pathogenesis of GBS septic shock in neonates (57). The observation that colonization of both women and neonates with GBS is common while clinical infection is relatively uncommon indicates that particular strain characteristics of the organisms and/or differences in host susceptibility must play a role in the development of invasive disease. Studies by Baker and Kasper and coworkers in the 1970s and a multicenter study in the 1990s demonstrated that the presence of antibodies directed against the capsular polysaccharide was a key factor in neonatal immunity to GBS (58,59). Cord blood of infants with type III GBS bacteremia and meningitis invariably contained low or undetectable levels of specific antibody against the type III capsule (58). Whether capsule-specific antibodies are protective against infection in adults has not been determined (60). *In vitro* studies have shown that virulent strains of GBS require serum complement for opsonophagocytic killing by peripheral blood leukocytes, and opsonophagocytosis is more efficient in the presence of specific antibody (61,62). The importance of the capsule in pathogenesis has been born out by studies of genetically manipulated strains of type III GBS. Unencapsulated mutants derived from type III strains by transposon mutagenesis had reduced virulence in a neonatal rat model of lethal GBS infection (63,64). Resistance to opsonophagocytosis appears to be conferred by the capsular polysaccharide, with more highly encapsulated strains being more resistant than those with only a thin capsular layer (65). The presence of capsular sialic acid residues may play a

role in pathogenesis by inhibiting complement activation, as has been suggested for the sialic acid-containing capsules of *Neisseria meningitidis* groups B and C, and for *Escherichia coli* K1 (66,67). The importance of capsular sialic acid was supported by studies showing reduced virulence of type III GBS mutants that elaborated a sialic acid-deficient capsular polysaccharide (68,69).

Group B streptococci elaborate a variety of other potential virulence factors including hemolysin, CAMP factor, C5a peptidase, and an enzyme, previously called neuraminidase, but subsequently shown to be a hyaluronidase (70,71). While each of these products might play a role in pathogenesis, none has been clearly shown to be a virulence factor during infection.

CLINICAL MANIFESTATIONS

Early onset neonatal sepsis with GBS typically presents with the same manifestations characteristic of other types of bacterial sepsis in the newborn: respiratory distress, apnea, hypothermia or fever, lethargy, hypotension. The risk of early onset disease is increased in premature infants, and in those born after prolonged rupture of membranes or maternal peripartum fever (44). Premature rupture of membranes with infection of the infant *in utero* probably accounts for the fact that approximately half of infants with early onset infection are symptomatic at birth. Respiratory symptoms are very common, and often constitute the initial clinical indication of infection. Surfactant deficiency may contribute to susceptibility to pulmonary GBS infection, and treatment with surfactant appeared beneficial in a nonrandomized clinical trial (72,73). Radiographic evidence of pneumonia, often indistinguishable from hyaline membrane disease, is present in 40% of cases. Autopsies of infants dying of early onset disease have shown pathologic findings in the lungs resembling hyaline membrane disease in patients with GBS pneumonia (74). Meningitis is present in approximately 5% to 10% of early onset cases. Since there are rarely distinctive clinical features to suggest the presence of meningitis, all patients with suspected sepsis should undergo lumbar puncture, ideally before initiation of antibiotic therapy.

The mean age of presentation of infants with late onset infection is 24 days, with a range of 7 days to 3 months, and rarely, later (58). Usual manifestations are nonspecific and include fever, poor feeding, lethargy or irritability, and respiratory distress. Approximately two thirds of late-onset infections are caused by type III strains (43,75). Type III strains appear to have a predilection for meningeal invasion, and meningitis is more common in late onset disease, occurring in about one third of cases. While bacteremia and meningitis are the usual manifestations of late onset infection, a variety of other sites of infection have been described, including septic arthritis, osteomyelitis, endocarditis, cellulitis, sinusitis, pyelonephritis. Except for bone and joint infections, focal infections are uncommon. Osteomyelitis due to group B *Streptococcus* generally has an indolent onset, and most often occurs in the proximal humerus, or less commonly, in other long bones. Septic arthritis may occur in association with osteomyelitis, or as an isolated entity, usually in the lower extremity (Table 186.1).

GBS infections in adults may be divided into two groups: those that occur in peripartum women, and those that occur in patients with underlying predisposing conditions. Peripartum infections are often manifested by fever and bacteremia. While these infections typically produce only mild symptoms, occasional patients have severe and sometimes rapidly fatal sepsis. Symptoms and signs of chorioamnionitis or endometritis are often, but not always, present. Less common manifestations include meningitis and endocarditis. Outside the peripartum

TABLE 186.1. Characteristics of Early and Late-onset Neonatal Infection due to Group B *Streptococcus*

Characteristic	Early onset	Late-onset
Mean age (range)	20 h (0–7 d)	24 d (7–90 d)
Signs	Respiratory distress	Fever
	Apnea	Lethargy
	Fever or hypothermia	Irritability
	Hypotension	
Affected sites	Bacteremia	Bacteremia
	Pneumonia (40%)	Meningitis (30%)
	Meningitis (5–10%)	Focal infections (esp. bone and joint)
Serotypes	All types (Ia, III, and V most common)	Type III (60%–70%)

period, GBS infections in otherwise healthy adults are unusual. Most adult patients with GBS have some underlying condition such as diabetes mellitus, liver disease, malignancy, stroke, decubitus ulcer, or neurogenic bladder (76). Skin and soft tissue are the most frequent sites of infection, particularly in association with diabetic foot ulcers (47). A wide variety of other infections in adults have been described including endocarditis, pneumonia, pyelonephritis, osteomyelitis, and septic arthritis (77–79). GBS endocarditis often has an acute presentation, and is frequently associated with embolization and metastatic infection (77,79). Recurrent infection can occur weeks to months after an episode of invasive GBS infection and is usually due to the same GBS strain (80).

DIAGNOSIS

The clinical manifestations of neonatal sepsis due to GBS are non-specific and do not distinguish GBS from sepsis caused by other agents. Suggestive findings include respiratory distress, apnea, lethargy, disturbed thermoregulation, and hypotension. Laboratory findings also are nonspecific; the presence of metabolic acidosis and leukopenia are poor prognostic signs. Diagnosis generally depends on identification of the organism in blood cultures (positive results in essentially all cases of untreated neonatal GBS sepsis), in cultures of cerebrospinal fluid (positive in 5% to 10% of early onset cases and in 30% of late onset disease) or in cultures of other normally sterile sites. Rapid diagnostic tests are available for detection of group B antigen in cerebrospinal fluid and urine; these assays use antibodies against the group B carbohydrate to detect antigen shed from the organisms during bacteremic infections. The latex agglutination assays currently available have a sensitivity of approximately 90% in cases of neonatal sepsis, when both cerebrospinal fluid and concentrated urine samples are tested. The occasional false negative results of the antigen detection tests means that empiric therapy must often be initiated on the basis of clinical suspicion of infection while awaiting culture results. While rapid antigen detection tests are useful for detecting GBS antigen in body fluids of infected neonates, these tests lack sufficient sensitivity to be reliable for detection of the organism in maternal vaginal or anorectal swab specimens.

TREATMENT

Penicillin is the drug of choice for treatment of all forms of GBS infection. All strains are sensitive, although the minimal inhibitory concentrations are higher than for group A *Streptococcus*, ranging from 0.01 to 0.4 μg/mL (5). Although *in vitro* synergy with aminoglycosides has been demonstrated, no adequate data exist to evaluate the role of combination therapy in human infection. However, it is common practice to initiate therapy for suspected neonatal sepsis and meningitis (in infants less than 7 days of age) with ampicillin (200 to 300 mg/kg per day) and gentamicin (5 mg/kg per day), changing to high-dose penicillin (150,000 units/kg per day for bacteremia, 300,000 units/kg per day for meningitis) alone after culture results are back and clinical improvement is evident. Infants older than 7 days of age should receive penicillin at 200,000 units/kg per day for group B streptococcal bacteremia or 450,000 units/kg per day for meningitis. Adults should receive penicillin G 12 to 18 million units per day in divided doses for bacteremia or serious local infection, 24 million units per day for meningitis or endocarditis. For patients allergic to penicillin, vancomycin may be used. Clindamycin is another alternative but should only be used if susceptibility results are known, because 8% of clinical isolates are resistant (81,82).

PREVENTION

With advances in intensive care, mortality from neonatal GBS infection has fallen to approximately 5% (41,83). However, substantial morbidity in the form of persistent neurologic sequelae occurs in approximately 30% of survivors of group B streptococcal meningitis. Therefore, considerable attention has been focused on strategies to prevent neonatal infection. Attempts to eradicate maternal carriage by antibiotic treatment during pregnancy have had an unacceptably high failure rate; 30% or more of women treated during pregnancy had positive culture results at the time of delivery. Presumptive antibiotic treatment of high risk infants also was unsuccessful, with no effect on mortality. Therefore, recent approaches to prevention have focused on three strategies: (a) prophylactic antibiotic treatment of colonized pregnant women during delivery; (b) passive immunization of mother (with transplacental transfer of antibody to the infant *in utero*) or of the infant after delivery, using immune globulin; (c) active immunization of women with a GBS vaccine containing purified components of one or more antigens, to elicit maternal antibodies that would cross the placenta and persist in the neonate through the first several weeks of life. While each of these approaches has its theoretical advantages and disadvantages, only the first (antibiotic prophylaxis) has had sufficient clinical testing to permit evaluation of efficacy. Several trials have shown that intrapartum administration of antibiotics reduces transmission of GBS to the infants, and prevents GBS disease (44,84–86). In a well-designed, randomized trial, Boyer and Gotoff administered ampicillin intrapartum to 83 prenatally colonized women with risk factors for early onset GBS disease (premature labor or prolonged rupture of membranes). No cases of group B *Streptococcus* disease occurred in the infants of these women, while five cases of early onset sepsis occurred among infants of 76 untreated control women (P = .02) (84). In this study, ampicillin was given to the infants in the treatment group for 36 hours following delivery.

On the basis of these studies, consensus guidelines for intrapartum prevention of GBS infection were developed in 1996 by the Centers for Disease Control and Prevention (87), the American Academy of Pediatrics (88), and the American College of Obstetrics and Gynecology (89). Two alternative approaches were endorsed: (a) screening all women for vaginal and anorectal carriage of GBS at 35 to 37 weeks' gestation and offering intrapartum chemoprophylaxis to all carriers, or (b) a risk-based strategy in which intrapartum chemoprophylaxis is offered to all women who have risk factors at the time of labor (temperature 38°C, rupture of membranes at 18 hours, or delivery at less than 37 weeks' gestation). For both approaches, prophylaxis is offered to women who deliver at less than 37 weeks' gestation unless a screening culture is known to be negative, to women who have had GBS bacteriuria during pregnancy, and to those who previously have delivered an infant with GBS disease. Studies of the impact of the two strategies have concluded that while institution of either approach reduces the incidence of early onset infection, the use of screening cultures appears to be somewhat more effective than the risk-based strategy, since approximately 25% to 40% of early onset cases occur in infants of women without risk factors (90,91). This topic has recently been reviewed by a working group of experts in the field, and updated recommendations on prevention strategies will be available from the Centers for Disease Control and Prevention at *www.cdc.gov/mmwr* (MMWR Recommendations and Reports).

The recommended regimen for intrapartum chemoprophylaxis is penicillin G, 5 million units initially, then 2.5 million units every 4 hours until delivery. Clindamycin or erythromycin may be substituted in women allergic to penicillin. There has been concern that widespread use of intrapartum prophylaxis might mask early signs of illness in neonates with GBS sepsis; however, in a large retrospective study that included 172 term infants with culture-positive GBS infection, all GBS-infected term infants exposed to intrapartum antibiotics exhibited clinical signs of infection within 24 hours of delivery (92). Therefore, a 48-hour hospital stay may not be required for routine monitoring of asymptomatic term infants exposed to intrapartum chemoprophylaxis.

The observations that antibodies directed against the capsular polysaccharide of group B *Streptococcus* are protective in animal models and that maternal antibody levels appear to correlate with immunity in the neonate have led to efforts to prevent neonatal GBS disease by passive or active immunization. Administration of intravenous immunoglobulin (IVIG) has been shown to protect neonatal rats against experimental GBS infection (93,94). However, no adequate clinical trials in human neonates have shown IVIG to be effective in preventing GBS neonatal sepsis. Because individual lots of IVIG vary considerably in specific antibody levels, standard IVIG preparations may not contain sufficient quantities of antibodies to GBS. Until data from larger randomized trials are available, routine use of IVIG for prevention or treatment of neonatal GBS disease is not recommended.

Another strategy for prevention of neonatal GBS disease is the immunization of pregnant women with a vaccine based on the purified GBS capsular polysaccharide(s). Purified capsular polysaccharides from three of the major serotypes (Ia, II, and III) have been tested in human subjects; immunogenicity rates in nonimmune volunteers range from 40% for type Ia to 88% for type II (95–99). Baker and associates showed that the type III polysaccharide vaccine elicited levels of antibody thought to be sufficient for protection in 57% of pregnant women and that comparable levels of antibody were detectable in the infants' sera after delivery, establishing the feasibility of this approach for preventing neonatal GBS infection (97). Because the purified polysaccharides are not immunogenic in all recipients, efforts are underway currently to develop a polysaccharide or oligosaccharide-protein conjugate vaccine to increase the immunogenicity of these antigens. Conjugate vaccines based on the type Ia, Ib, II, III, and V GBS capsular polysaccharides have been synthesized by coupling the polysaccharide to tetanus toxoid (100–105). These polysaccharide-protein conjugate vaccines have been highly immunogenic in experimental animals and

vaccines of similar design are currently being tested in volunteers. Phase I clinical testing of vaccines comprised of GBS type III, Ia, Ib, or II polysaccharide coupled to tetanus toxoid indicated the vaccines were safe, well-tolerated, and highly immunogenic (106,107,108). Encouraging results have been obtained also in animal testing of a vaccine consisting of type III polysaccharide coupled to the group B streptococcal beta-C protein (109). A vaccine for clinical use will probably consist of several group B streptococcal polysaccharides, representing the prevalent serotypes, coupled to carrier protein(s), one or more of which also may be derived from group B streptococci. If fully protective, a vaccine that included polysaccharide conjugates of the five prevalent serotypes (Ia, Ib, II, III, and V) could theoretically confer immunity to more than 95% of the group B streptococcal isolates associated with neonatal infection in the United States (49,50,51). Although still in the investigational stage, active immunization of childbearing women ultimately may prove an effective approach for prevention of neonatal GBS infection.

REFERENCES

1. Lancefield RC. A serological differentiation of human and other groups of hemolytic streptococci. *J Exp Med* 1933;57:571.
2. Lancefield RC. The serological differentiation of pathogenic and non-pathogenic strains of hemolytic streptococci from parturient women. *J Exp Med* 1935;61:335.
3. Fry RM. Fatal infection by haemolytic streptococcus group B. *Lancet* 1938;1:199.
4. Hood M, Janney A, Dameron G. Beta hemolytic streptococcus group B associated with problems of perinatal period. *Am J Obstet Gynecol* 1961;82:809.
5. Eickhoff TC, Klein JO, Daly AK, et al. Neonatal sepsis and other infections due to group B beta-hemolytic streptococci. *N Engl J Med* 1964;271:1221.
6. Facklam RR, Padula JR, Thacker LG, et al. Presumptive identification of group A, B, and D streptococci. *Appl Microbiol* 1974;27:107.
7. Pollack HM, Dahlgren BJ. Distribution of streptococcal groups in clinical specimens with evaluation of bacitracin screening. *Appl Microbiol* 1974;27:141.
8. Christie R, Atkins NE, Munch-Petersen E. A note on a lytic phenomenon shown by group B streptococci. *Aust J Exp Biol Med Sci* 1944;22:197.
9. Facklam RR, Padula JR, Wortham EC, et al. Presumptive identification of group A, B and D streptococci on agar plate medium. *J Clin Microbiol* 1979;9:665.
10. Kane JA, Karakawa WW. Multiple polysaccharide antigens of group B *Streptococcus*, type Ia: emphasis on a sialic acid type-specific polysaccharide. *J Immunol* 1977;118:2155.
11. Carey RB, Eisenstein TK, Shockman GD, et al. Soluble group- and type-specific antigens from type III group B *Streptococcus*. *Infect Immun* 1980;28:195.
12. Pritchard DG. Characterization of the group-specific polysaccharide of group B *Streptococcus*. *Arch Biochem Biophys* 1984;235:385.
13. Michon F, Brisson JR, Dell A, et al. Multiantennary group-specific polysaccharide of group B *Streptococcus*. *Biochemistry* 1988;27:5341.
14. Lancefield RC. A serological differentiation of specific types of bovine hemolytic streptococci (group B). *J Exp Med* 1934;59:441.
15. Lancefield RC. Two serological types of group B hemolytic streptococci with related, but not identical, type-specific substances. *J Exp Med* 1938;67:25.
16. Kasper DL, Baker CJ. Electron microscopic definition of surface antigens of group B *Streptococcus*. *J Infect Dis* 1979;139:147.
17. Jennings HJ, Rosell K-G, Katzenellenbogen E, Kasper DL. Structural determination of the capsular polysaccharide antigen of type II group B streptococci. *J Biol Chem* 1983;258:1793.
18. Jennings HJ, Katzenellenbogen E, Lugowski C, Kasper DL. Structure of the native polysaccharide antigens of type Ia and type Ib group B *Streptococcus*. *Biochemistry* 1983;22:1258.
19. Wessels MR, Pozsgay V, Kasper DL, Jennings HJ. Structure and immunochemistry of an oligosaccharide repeating unit of the capsular polysaccharide of type III group B *Streptococcus*. *J Biol Chem* 1987;262:8262.
20. Jelinkova J, Motlova J. Worldwide distribution of two new serotypes of group B streptococci: type IV and provisional type V. *J Clin Microbiol* 1985;21:361.
21. Wessels MR, Benedi V-J, Jennings HJ, et al. Isolation and characterization of type IV group B *Streptococcus* capsular polysaccharide. *Infect Immun* 1989;57:1089.
22. DiFabio JL, Michon F, Brisson J-R, et al. Structure of the capsular polysaccharide antigen of type IV group B *Streptococcus*. *Can J Chem* 1989;67:877.
23. Wessels MR, DiFabio JL, Benedi V-J, et al. Structural determination and immunochemical characterization of the type V group B *Streptococcus* capsular polysaccharide. *J Biol Chem* 1991;266:6714.

24. von Hunolstein C, d'Ascenzi S, Wagner B, et al. Immunochemistry of capsular type polysaccharide and virulence properties of type VI *Streptococcus agalactiae* (group B streptococci). *Infect Immun* 1993;61:1272.

25. Kogan G, Uhrin D, Brisson J-R, et al. Structure of the type VI group B *Streptococcus* capsular polysaccharide determined by high resolution NMR spectroscopy. *J Carbohydrate Chem* 1994;13:1071.

26. Kogan G, Brisson J-R, Kasper DL, et al. Structure of the novel type VII group B *Streptococcus* capsular polysaccharide by high resolution NMR spectroscopy. *Carbohydrate Res* 1995;277:1.

27. Kogan G, Uhrin D, Brisson J-R, et al. Structural and immunochemical characterization of the type VIII group B *Streptococcus* capsular polysaccharide. *J Biol Chem* 1996;271:8786.

28. Wilkinson HW, Eagon RG. Type-specific antigens of group B type Ic streptococci. *Infect Immun* 1971;4:596.

29. Lancefield RC, McCarty M, Everly WN. Multiple mouse-protective antibodies directed against group B streptococci. Special reference to antibodies effective against protein antigens. *J Exp Med* 1975;142:165.

30. Johnson DR, Ferrieri P. Group B streptococcal Ibc protein antigen: distribution of two determinants in wild-type strains of common serotypes. *J Clin Microbiol* 1984;19:506.

31. Henrichsen J, Ferrieri P, Jelinkova J, et al. Nomenclature of antigens of group B streptococci. *Int J Syst Bacteriol* 1984;34:500.

32. Madoff LC, Hori S, Michel JL, et al. Phenotypic diversity in the alpha C protein of group B *Streptococcus. Infect Immun* 1991;59:2638.

33. Michel JL, Madoff LC, Olson K, et al. Large, identical, tandem repeating units in the C protein alpha antigen gene, *bca*, of group B streptococci. *Proc Natl Acad Sci USA* 1992;89:10060.

34. Stalhammer-Carlemalm M, Stenberg L, Lindahl G. Protein Rib: a novel group B streptococcal cell surface protein that confers protective immunity and is expressed by most strains causing invasive infections. *J Exp Med* 1993;177:1593.

35. Areschoug T, Stalhammar-Carlemalm M, Larsson C, Lindahl G. Group B streptococcal surface proteins as targets for protective antibodies: identification of two novel proteins in strains of serotype V. *Infect Immun* 1999;67:6350.

36. Lachenauer CS, Creti R, Michel JL, Madoff LC. Mosaicism in the alpha-like protein genes of group B streptococci. *Proc Natl Acad Sci USA* 2000;97:9630.

37. Michel JL, Madoff LC, Kling DE, et al. Cloned alpha and beta c-protein antigens of group B streptococci elicit protective immunity. *Infect Immun* 1991;59:2023.

38. Madoff LC, Michel JL, Gong EW, et al. Protection of neonatal mice from group B streptococcal infection by maternal immunization with beta C protein. *Infect Immun* 1992;60:4989.

39. Cheng Q, Carlson B, Pillai S, et al. Antibody against surface-bound C5a peptidase is opsonic and initiates macrophage killing of group B streptococci. *Infect Immun* 2001;69:2302.

40. Brodeur BR, Boyer M, Charlebois I, et al. Identification of group B streptococcal Sip protein, which elicits cross-protective immunity. *Infect Immun* 2000;68:5610.

41. Zangwill KM, Schuchat A, Wenger JD. Group B streptococcal disease in the United States, 1990: report from a multistate active surveillance system. *MMWR* 1992;41:25.

42. Schuchat A, Oxtoby M, Cochi S, et al. Population-based risk factors for neonatal group B streptococcal disease: results of a cohort study in metropolitan Atlanta. *J Infect Dis* 1990;162:672.

43. Dillon HC Jr, Khare S, Gray BM. Group B streptococcal carriage and disease: a 6-year prospective study. *J Pediatr* 1987;110:31.

44. Boyer KM, Gadzala CA, Burd LI, et al. Selective intrapartum chemoprophylaxis of neonatal group B streptococcal early-onset disease. I. Epidemiologic rationale. *J Infect Dis* 1983;148:795.

45. Isaacs D, Royle JA. Intrapartum antibiotics and early onset neonatal sepsis caused by group B *Streptococcus* and by other organisms in Australia. Australasian Study Group for Neonatal Infections. *Pediatr Infect Dis J* 1999;18:524.

46. Schrag SJ, Zywicki S, Farley MM, et al. Group B streptococcal disease in the era of intrapartum antibiotic prophylaxis. *N Engl J Med* 2000;342:15.

47. Schwartz B, Schuchat A, Oxtoby MJ, et al. Invasive group B streptococcal disease in adults, a population-based study in metropolitan Atlanta. *JAMA* 1991;266:1112.

48. Farley MM, Harvey RC, Stull T, et al. A population-based assessment of invasive disease due to group B *Streptococcus* in nonpregnant adults. *N Engl J Med* 1993;328:1807.

49. Lin FY, Clemens JD, Azimi PH, et al. Capsular polysaccharide types of group B streptococcal isolates from neonates with early-onset systemic infection. *J Infect Dis* 1998;177:790.

50. Harrison LH, Elliott JA, Dwyer DM, et al. Serotype distribution of invasive group B streptococcal isolates in Maryland: implications for vaccine development. *J Infect Dis* 1998;177:998.

51. Zaleznik DF, Rench MA, Hillier S, et al. Invasive disease due to group B streptococcus in pregnant women and neonates from diverse population groups. *Clin Infect Dis* 2000;30:276.

52. Tyrrell GJ, Senzilet LD, Spika JS, et al. Invasive disease due to group B streptococcal infection in adults: results from a Canadian, population-based, active laboratory surveillance study—1996. Sentinel Health Unit Surveillance System Site Coordinators. *J Infect Dis* 2000;182:168.

53. Lachenauer CS, Kasper DL, Shimada J, et al. Serotypes VI and VIII predominate among group B streptococci isolated from pregnant Japanese women. *J Infect Dis* 1999;179:1030.

54. Campbell JR, Hillier SL, Krohn MA, et al. Group B streptococcal colonization and serotype-specific immunity in pregnant women at delivery. *Obstet Gynecol* 2000;96:498.

55. Hoogkamp-Korstanje JAA, Gerards LJ, Cats BP. Maternal carriage and neonatal acquisition of group B streptococci. *J Infect Dis* 1982;145:800.

56. Benitz WE, Gould JB, Druzin ML. Risk factors for early-onset group B streptococcal sepsis: estimation of odds ratios by critical literature review. *Pediatrics* 1999;103:e77.

57. Vallejo JG, Knuefermann P, Mann DL, Sivasubramanian N. Group B Streptococcus induces TNF-alpha gene expression and activation of the transcription factors NF-kappa B and activator protein-1 in human cord blood monocytes. *J Immunol* 2000;165:419.

58. Baker CJ, Kasper DL. Correlation of maternal antibody deficiency with susceptibility to neonatal group B streptococcal infection. *N Engl J Med* 1976;294:753.

59. Lin FY, Philips IJ, Azimi PH, et al. Level of maternal antibody required to protect neonates against early-onset disease caused by group B streptococcus type ia: a multicenter, seroepidemiology study. *J Infect Dis* 2001;184:1022.

60. Wessels MR, Kasper DL, Johnson KD, Harrison LH. Antibody responses in invasive group B streptococcal infection in adults. *J Infect Dis* 1998;178:569.

61. Shigeoka AO, Hall RT, Hemming VG, et al. Role of antibody and complement in opsonization of group B streptococci. *Infect Immun* 1978;21:34.

62. Baltimore RS, Kasper DL, Baker CJ, Goroff DK. Antigenic specificity of opsonophagocytic antibodies in rabbit anti-sera to group B streptococci. *J Immunol* 1977;118:673.

63. Rubens CE, Wessels MR, Heggen LM, Kasper DL. Transposon mutagenesis of group B streptococcal type III capsular polysaccharide: correlation of capsule expression with virulence. *Proc Natl Acad Sci USA* 1987;84:7208.

64. Rubens CE, Heggen LM, Haft RF, Wessels MR. Identification of cpsD, a gene essential for type III capsule expression in group B streptococci. *Mol Microbiol* 1993;8:843.

65. Marques MB, Kasper DL, Pangburn MK, Wessels MR. Prevention of C3 deposition is a virulence mechanism of type III group B *Streptococcus* capsular polysaccharide. *Infect Immun* 1992;60:3986.

66. Edwards MS, Nicholson-Weller A, Baker CJ, Kasper DL. The role of specific antibody in alternative pathway-mediated opsonophagocytosis of type III, group B *Streptococcus. J Exp Med* 1980;151:1275.

67. Edwards MS, Kasper DL, Jennings HJ, et al. Capsular sialic acid prevents activation of the alternative complement pathway by type III, group B streptococci. *J Immunol* 1982;128:1278.

68. Wessels MR, Rubens CE, Benedi V-J, Kasper DL. Definition of a bacterial virulence factor: sialylation of the group B streptococcal capsule. *Proc Natl Acad Sci USA* 1989;86:8983.

69. Wessels MR, Haft RF, Heggen LM, Rubens CE. Identification of a genetic locus essential for capsule sialylation in type III group B streptococci. *Infect Immun* 1992;60:392.

70. Bohnsack JF, Mollison KW, Buko AM, et al. Group B streptococci inactivate complement component C5a by enzymic cleavage at the C-terminus. *Biochem J* 1991;273:635.

71. Pritchard DG, Lin B. Group B streptococcal neuraminidase is actually a hyaluronidase. *Infect Immun* 1993;61.

72. LeVine AM, Bruno MD, Huelsman KM, et al. Surfactant protein A-deficient mice are susceptible to group B streptococcal infection. *J Immunol* 1997;158:4336.

73. Herting E, Gefeller O, Land M, et al. Surfactant treatment of neonates with respiratory failure and group B streptococcal infection. Members of the Collaborative European Multicenter Study Group. *Pediatrics* 2000;106:957.

74. Katzenstein A, Davis C, Braude A. Pulmonary changes in neonatal sepsis due to group B beta-hemolytic streptococcus: relation to hyaline membrane disease. *J Infect Dis* 1976;133:430.

75. Wenger JD, Hightower AW, Facklam RR, et al. Bacterial meningitis in the United States, 1986: report of a multistate surveillance study. *J Infect Dis* 1990;162:1316.

76. Jackson LA, Hilsdon R, Farley MM, et al. Risk factors for group B streptococcal disease in adults. *Ann Intern Med* 1995;123:415.

77. Lerner PI, Gopalakrishna KV, Wolinsky E, et al. Group B streptococcus (*S. agalactiae*) bacteremia in adults: analysis of 32 cases and review of the literature. *Medicine* 1977;56:457.

78. Verghese A, Mireault K, Arbeit R. Group B streptococcal bacteremia in men. *Rev Infect Dis* 1986;8:912.

79. Gallagher PG, Watanakunakorn C. Group B streptococcal endocarditis: report of seven cases and review of the literature. *Rev Infect Dis* 1986;8:175.

80. Harrison LH, Ali A, Dwyer DM, et al. Relapsing invasive group B streptococcal infection in adults. *Ann Intern Med* 1995;123:421.

81. Lin FY, Azimi PH, Weisman LE, et al. Antibiotic susceptibility profiles for group B streptococci isolated from neonates, 1995–1998. *Clin Infect Dis* 2000;31:76.

82. Bland ML, Vermillion ST, Soper DE, Austin M. Antibiotic resistance patterns of group B streptococci in late third-trimester rectovaginal cultures. *Am J Obstet Gynecol* 2001;184:1125.

83. CDC. Decreasing incidence of perinatal group B streptococcal disease—United States, 1993–95. *MMWR* 1997;46:473.

84. Boyer KM, Gotoff SP. Prevention of early-onset neonatal group B streptococcal disease with selective intrapartum chemoprophylaxis. *N Engl J Med* 1986;314:1665.

85. Easmon CSF, Hastings MJG, Deeley J, et al. The effect of intrapartum chemoprophylaxis on the vertical transmission of group B streptococci. *Br J Obstet Gynecol* 1983;90:633.

86. Morales WJ, Lim DV, Walsh AF. Prevention of neonatal group B streptococcal sepsis by the use of a rapid screening test and selective intrapartum chemoprophylaxis. *Am J Obstet Gynecol* 1986;155:979.

87. CDC. Prevention of perinatal group B streptococcal disease: a public health perspective. *MMWR* 1996;45(RR-7):1.

88. American Academy of Pediatrics Committee on Infectious Diseases and Committee on Fetus and Newborn. Revised guidelines for prevention of early-onset group B streptococcal (GBS) infection. *Pediatrics* 1997;99:489.

89. American College of Obstetricians and Gynecologists, Committee on Obstetric Practice. Prevention of early-onset group B Streptococcal disease in newborns [Opinion 173]. *Int J Gynaecol Obstet* 1996;54:197.

90. Gilson GJ, Christensen F, Romero H, et al. Prevention of group B streptococcus early-onset neonatal sepsis: comparison of the Center for Disease Control and prevention screening- based protocol to a risk-based protocol in infants at greater than 37 weeks' gestation. *J Perinatol* 2000;20:491.

91. Main EK, Slagle T. Prevention of early-onset invasive neonatal group B streptococcal disease in a private hospital setting: the superiority of culture-based protocols. *Am J Obstet Gynecol* 2000;182:1344.

92. Bromberger P, Lawrence JM, Braun D, et al. The influence of intrapartum antibiotics on the clinical spectrum of early-onset group B streptococcal infection in term infants. *Pediatrics* 2000;106:244.

93. Fischer GW, Hunter KW, Wilson SR. Modified human immune serum globulin for intravenous administration: *in vitro* protection against group B streptococcal disease in suckling rats. *Acta Paediatr Scand* 1982;71:639.

94. Santos JI, Shigeoka AO, Hill HR. Protective efficacy of a modified immune serum globulin in experimental group B streptococcal infection. *J Pediatr* 1981;99.

95. Baker CJ, Edwards MS, Kasper DL. Immunogenicity of polysaccharides from type III, group B *Streptococcus. J Clin Invest* 1978;61:1107.

96. Baker CJ, Kasper DL. Group B streptococcal vaccines. *Rev Infect Dis* 1985; 7:458.

97. Baker CJ, Rench MA, Edwards MS, et al. Immunization of pregnant women with a polysaccharide vaccine of group B *Streptococcus. N Engl J Med* 1988;319:1180.

98. Eisenstein TK, De Cueninck BJ, Resavy D, et al. Quantitative determination in human sera of vaccine-induced antibody to type-specific polysaccharides of group B streptococci using an enzyme-linked immunosorbent assay. *J Infect Dis* 1983;147:847.

99. Kasper DL, Baker CJ, Galdes B, et al. Immunochemical analysis and immunogenicity of the type II group B streptococcal capsular polysaccharide. *J Clin Invest* 1983;72:260.

100. Wessels MR, Paoletti LC, Rodewald AK, et al. Stimulation of protective antibodies against type Ia and Ib group B streptococci by a type Ia polysaccharide-tetanus toxoid conjugate vaccine. *Infect Immun* 1993;61:4760.

101. Paoletti LC, Wessels MR, Michon F, et al. Group B *Streptococcus* type II polysaccharide-tetanus toxoid conjugate vaccine. *Infect Immun* 1992;60:4009.

102. Wessels MR, Paoletti LC, Kasper DL, et al. Immunogenicity in animals of a polysaccharide-protein conjugate vaccine against type III group B *Streptococcus. J Clin Invest* 1990;86:1428.

103. Lagergard T, Shiloach J, Robbins JB, Schneerson R. Synthesis and immunological properties of conjugates composed of group B streptococcus type III capsular polysaccharide covalently bound to tetanus toxoid. *Infect Immun* 1990;58:687.

104. Paoletti LC, Wessels MR, Rodewald AK, et al. Neonatal mouse protection against infection with multiple group B streptococcal serotypes by maternal immunization with a tetravalent GBS polysaccharide-tetanus toxoid conjugate vaccine. *Infect Immun* 1994;62:3236.

105. Wessels MR, Paoletti LC, Pinel J, Kasper DL. Immunogenicity and protective activity in animals of a group B *Streptococcus* type V polysaccharide-tetanus toxoid conjugate vaccine. *J Infect Dis* 1995;171:879.

106. Kasper DL, Paoletti LC, Wessels MR, et al. Immune response to type III group B streptococcal polysaccharide- tetanus toxoid conjugate vaccine. *J Clin Invest* 1996;98:2308.

107. Baker CJ, Paoletti LC, Wessels MR, et al. Safety and immunogenicity of capsular polysaccharide-tetanus toxoid conjugate vaccines for group B streptococcal types Ia and Ib. *J Infect Dis* 1999;179:142.

108. Baker CJ, Paoletti LC, Rench MA, et al. Use of capsular polysaccharide-tetanus toxoid conjugate vaccine for type II group B streptococcus in healthy women. *J Infect Dis* 2000;182:1129.

109. Madoff LC, Paoletti LC, Tai JY, Kasper DL. Maternal immunization of mice with group B streptococcal type III polysaccharide-beta C protein conjugate elicits protective antibody to multiple serotypes. *J Clin Invest* 1994;94:286.

Gram-Positive Bacilli

CHAPTER 187
Corynebacteria

Neal Halsey and John G. Bartlett

CHARACTERISTICS OF THE PATHOGEN

The genus *Corynebacterium* contains one important pathogen of normal hosts, *Corynebacterium diphtheriae*, and nondiphtheria corynebacteria, often referred to as diphtheroids, which cause disease principally in persons whose host defenses are altered, occasional cases of endocarditis (the "C" of HACEK), and infections associated with catheters and devices (1,2). The genus has been substantially revised in more recent years, with many species reclassified on the basis of ribosomal RNA sequencing (2,3). Some organisms such as *Corynebacterium* Centers for Disease Control and Prevention (CDC) group JK have been reclassified as *C. jeikeium* (2). Some organisms formerly classified as corynebacteria have been reclassified as belonging in the *Arcanobacterium*, *Actinomyces*, and *Rhodococcus* genera. Other species are under consideration for reclassification.

Corynebacteria are nonmotile unencapsulated bacilli. The organisms stain gram positive, but decolorization occurs readily, and they are tapered or slightly curved. Methylene blue stains are particularly useful and bring out the characteristic purple-red metachromatic granules of *C. diphtheriae*. On Gram stains of colonies, many corynebacteria are club shaped, owing to a weakness in one side of the cell wall. The organisms frequently remain attached after division and form sharp angles, resulting in a "Chinese letter" configuration. Biochemical testing is essential for proper identification of individual species. Corynebacteria are generally catalase positive and do not hydrolyze esculin or gelatin; clinically relevant strains are negative for lactose, xylose, and mannitol utilization (2).

C. diphtheriae strains are divided into three biotypes (*mitis*, *gravis*, *intermedius*) on the basis of colony morphology and biochemical characteristics. Tentative differentiation may be made by colony morphology and the formulation of starch and glycogen in heart infusion broth (3). The use of antibiotic susceptibility patterns and phage typing has largely been replaced by phage-DNA restriction enzyme patterns, bacterial polypeptide analysis, and DNA probes as epidemiologic markers (4–8). Although *C. diphtheriae* is not a spore-forming organism, it survives drying and can be transported in silica gel packs at room temperature (9).

Diphtheria toxin is produced by lysogenized strains of *C. diphtheriae, Corynebacterium ulcerans,* and occasionally other strains; however, toxin-mediated disease is caused primarily by *C. diphtheriae*. The gene sequence of this 62,000-dalton protein has been identified, and the receptor site on the organism for the phage can be identified with molecular techniques (10,11).

EPIDEMIOLOGY

Corynebacteria have been identified in all climates and regions of the world. Nondiphtheria corynebacteria, normal inhabitants of the skin and respiratory tract, often produce disease by entering the bloodstream through breaks in the skin and seeding of foreign material such as valves, patches, and catheters in the vascular tree or central nervous system (2). Other specific disease entities are described later. Disease caused by *C. diphtheriae* has been identified in all countries where laboratory facilities are available. *C. diphtheriae* is transmitted from person to person by respiratory secretions or droplets, by direct skin-to-skin contact, and from skin to respiratory tract via hands. Silent carriers of the organisms on skin and in the pharynx are common sources of transmission in outbreaks. In crowded impoverished urban settings and in tropical climates, skin diphtheria has been more common than have respiratory infections (12–16). Contaminated cow's milk has been identified as a source of *C. diphtheriae* infections and has been a common mode of transmission for *Corynebacterium pseudotuberculosis*. The latter organism has also been acquired by humans in close contact with animals, especially livestock (17–19). *Corynebacterium aquaticum* is found in freshwater and has been recovered from distilled water (1,20,21).

Diphtheria has occurred principally during the winter months in temperate zones (22). In tropical climates, infections occur throughout the year, but peaks in disease have been observed in some but not all countries during the rainy season (23,24). Cutaneous disease is also less frequent during summer in temperate climates, presumably owing to decreased contact among impoverished persons (12).

Infants born to immune mothers are protected against toxin-mediated disease for several months by passively acquired maternal immunoglobulin G antibodies (25). Before routine immunization with diphtheria toxoid, the peak incidence of respiratory disease was in school-aged children. After widespread immunization of young children became a reality, the peak incidence shifted to older persons (26,28). In most tropical countries, persons often acquire antibodies to toxin through repeated low-grade skin infections (29). In the United States, the peak incidence of skin infections has been in persons older than 30 years, and the highest incidence of skin disease has been in coastal regions (12,17,28). Outbreaks have occurred among the homeless populations in urban centers, especially Seattle (12).

Higher attack rates of both skin and respiratory disease have occurred in populations of lower socioeconomic status in all areas of the world. Contributing factors probably include crowding, skin abrasions, use of less clothing in warm climates, decreased availability of water for hand washing, and lower immunization rates. In the United States and Canada, the incidence of diphtheria has been higher among the native populations (12,17,28). However, the case-fatality rate has been lower in these populations, presumably owing to a high incidence of skin disease. The incidence of the nasopharyngeal carrier state of toxigenic *C. diphtheriae* strains has been similar for males and females, but the incidence of respiratory disease and case-fatality rates have been higher for males. The occurrence of skin infections in persons over 19 years of age has been eight times higher for men than for women, presumably because of the larger numbers of homeless men in the population.

The incidence of diphtheria in the United States has diminished to only a few cases per year during the past 25 years (Fig. 187.1); however, many persons have suboptimal immunity and additional outbreaks could occur, especially among homeless persons in coastal cities (12) (see the later prevention section). An epidemic of diphtheria affecting primarily adults involving more than 125,000 cases and 4,000 deaths took place in the Newly Independent States of the former Soviet Union from 1990 to 1995 and then decreased from 16.7 cases per 100,000 population per year to 2.7 cases per 100,000 population per year in 1997 (29–31) (Fig. 187.2). Factors contributing to this epidemic have included decreased immunization rates in children, the use of adult tetanus and diphtheria toxoid preparations for primary immunization in children in place of full-strength diphtheria-tetanus-pertussis vaccine in some areas, waning immunity among adults who did not receive booster doses, and increased movement of the population after the break-up of the Soviet Union (31). The epidemic appears to have peaked in 1995 in response to intensive efforts to improve immunization of children and adults.

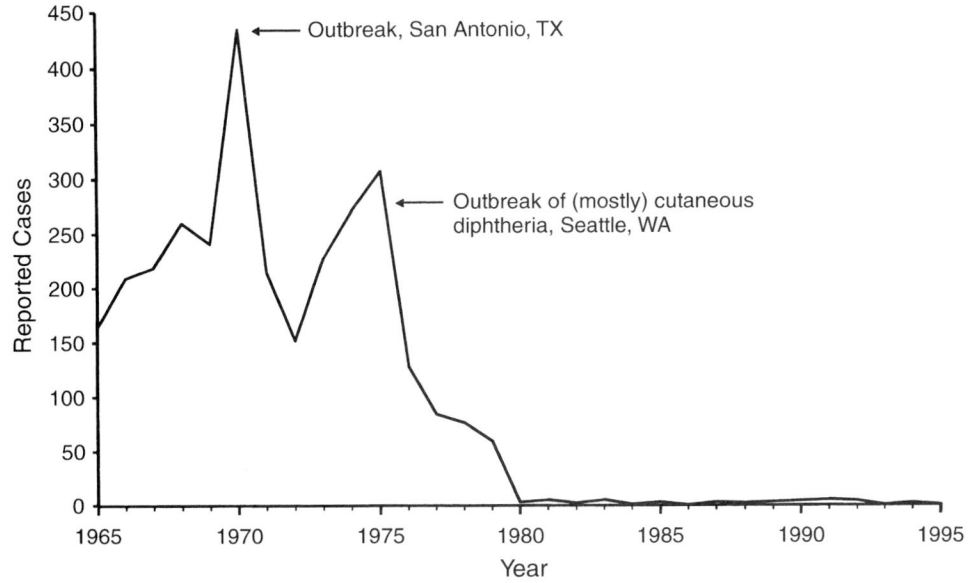

Figure 187.1. Diphtheria by year in the United States, 1965 to 1995. (From Centers for Disease Control and Prevention. Summary of notifiable diseases, United States 1995. *MMWR* 1995;44:1–87, with permission.)

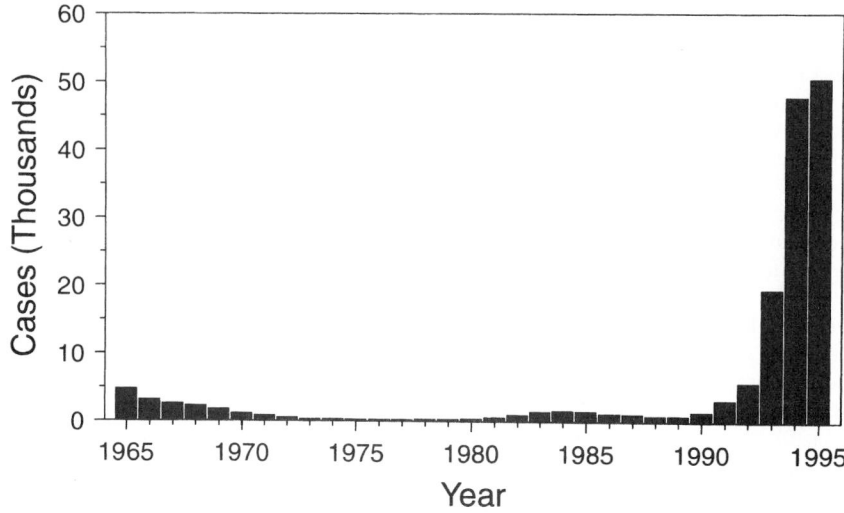

Figure 187.2. Number of reported cases of diphtheria in the former Soviet Union, 1965 to 1995. (From Centers for Disease Control and Prevention. Update: diphtheria epidemic—New Independent States of the Former Soviet Union, January 1995–March 1996. *MMWR* 1996;45:693–697, with permission.)

PATHOGENESIS

Nondiphtheria corynebacteria produce disease principally by colonizing foreign bodies introduced into host tissue (catheters, shunts, prosthetic valves), by attaching to damaged cardiac valves, or by producing systemic infections (e.g., sepsis, abscess, meningitis) in immunocompromised hosts after disruption of the skin (1,2,32–36). Several nondiphtheria corynebacteria cause skin and soft tissue infections and lymphadenitis by direct extension from local breaks in the skin (see the later section on clinical manifestations).

Most disease caused by *C. diphtheriae* is related to toxin production and excretion. Diphtheria toxin is a 62,000-dalton protein produced by strains that have been lysogenized by phages containing the genetic material for toxin production (11,37). *C. diphtheriae* replicates on the mucous membrane of the respiratory tract or in superficial skin infections and the toxin is disseminated via the bloodstream. Toxin induces local cell death, producing more favorable growth conditions for the organism and increased toxin production (11). The toxin is composed of two fragments. Attachment to specific receptors on host cells is via the B fragment. All cells of the body are susceptible to the action of the active A fragment, but differential effects are noted in tissues, depending on the availability of specific receptor sites (37). Proteolytic cleavage, usually by trypsin, results in the breaking of two disulfide bonds and release of the A fragment, which enters the host cell by endocytosis. The A fragment catalyzes an enzymatic reaction, binding elongation factor 2 to adenosine diphosphate, and the product becomes irreversibly bound to the surface of ribosomes. Bacteria do not have elongation factor 2 and therefore are not affected by the toxin. The production of protein is stopped by preventing the addition of further amino acids into polypeptide chains. Chang and co-workers (38) found evidence for nuclease activity as an alternative mechanism of cell killing by diphtheria toxin. However, several investigators questioned those findings and presented evidence that the nuclease activity was a contaminant in the studies of Chang and colleagues. One molecule of fragment A can produce cell death within a few hours. The fatal dose for humans has been estimated to be 13 μg/kg (10,37).

Local tissue necrosis in the respiratory tract results in the formation of a thin gray membrane composed of necrotic cell material, exudative fluid, bacteria, and red and white blood cells. The surrounding tissues become edematous, and local and regional lymph nodes are usually enlarged. Circulating toxin affects all tissues, but the tissues and organs most affected are heart muscle, kidneys, and the peripheral nervous system. Pathologic changes in muscle tissue include lipid accumulation, hyaline degeneration, edema, and mononuclear cell infiltration (39–43). Muscle regeneration is observed in survivors, but fibrosis is evident in biopsy specimens. Neuronal changes consist primarily of demyelination and tubular necrosis and are found in kidneys (44). The A subunit of diphtheria toxin has been purified, placed inside microcarriers, and selectively targeted to cancer cells, resulting in clinical responses in animals (45,46).

CLINICAL MANIFESTATIONS

Disease Caused by Nondiphtheria Corynebacteria

Because nondiphtheria corynebacteria colonize the skin, they are frequently found as contaminants in blood cultures, but septicemia, endocarditis, and other serious diseases are being seen with increasing frequency owing to the growing population of immunocompromised patients and large numbers of patients with catheters and prosthetic devices in vessels and the central nervous system. Neutropenia appears to be the most important predisposing factor for severe systemic diseases, but patients with breaks in the skin who have received prolonged courses of antibiotics are at increased risk for disease.

Species identified lately have been assigned to groups rather than being given specific names. Some organisms have been associated with specific disease entities. Erythrasma, caused by *Corynebacterium minutissimum*, is a commonly diagnosed skin infection (1). Pruritic reddish brown macular lesions that fluoresce coral-red under a Wood lamp occur in intertriginous areas.

C. ulcerans, formerly thought to be a separate species, is now considered to be a variant of *C. diphtheriae* and causes clinical disease indistinguishable from diphtheria including cardiac and nervous system involvement (3,47–50). With toxigenic cases, diphtheria antitoxin should be given. Erythromycin is the preferred antibiotic.

C. pseudotuberculosis produces a dermonecrotic toxin and has been identified as the agent of suppurative granulomatous lymphadenitis in several patients, primarily those from Australia (3,18,19,51,52). The organism is a common cause of infections in farm animals, and most affected humans have been persons exposed to cattle or horses or who are consumers of raw milk (51,52). Therapy requires a several weeks' course of erythromycin or tetracycline.

Corynebacterium jeikeium (formerly *Corynebacterium* CDC group JK) has been recognized as an important cause of sepsis, primarily in cancer patients. Common features of these cases are neutropenia, skin disruption, exposure to multiple antibiotics, and prolonged hospitalization (53,54). These organisms are components of the normal skin flora of the inguinal, axillary, and perirectal areas, especially in hospitalized patients (55). Vancomycin is the preferred antibiotic.

Corynebacterium pseudodiphtheriticum has most commonly been reported as a cause of endocarditis involving both natural and prosthetic valves (56,57). It has also been reported to cause a diverse array of pulmonary infections, including tracheitis, bronchitis, pneumonia, and lung abscess (58,59). Supporting evidence is based on large concentrations in sputum, within neutrophils, and response to antibiotic therapy.

Many nondiphtheria corynebacteria species have been shown to cause endocarditis or intravenous line sepsis (1,3,60,61). *C. diphtheriae* can also cause endocarditis, septic arthritis, and septicemia (3,62–64). Patients with artificial cardiac valves or indwelling vascular catheters are at particular risk. Intraocular lenses have been contaminated, leading to endophthalmitis (65).

Diphtheria

The incubation period for respiratory tract disease is usually less than 1 week. Although the onset is insidious in most patients, severe cases involving the posterior pharynx may present as acute disease. Fever is usually low grade, and the initial findings include erythema of the posterior pharynx, followed by white or gray spots that subsequently coalesce to form a thin veil-like membrane, which thickens and becomes gray. The membrane is usually asymmetric and extends beyond the usual tonsillar borders to involve the soft palate and uvula. The advancing border of the membrane is deep red. Clinical severity is correlated with the size of the membrane. The membrane is adherent, and bleeding occurs readily after attempts to remove it. Mildly affected patients have been mistakenly diagnosed as having acute streptococcal pharyngitis, and simultaneous infections with group A streptococci do occur. The submandibular and anterior cervical lymph nodes are usually enlarged, and soft tissue edema may be present. Severely affected persons have a bull-necked appearance and are at high risk for airway obstruction and sudden death. Severe cases may be complicated by bleeding secondary to thrombocytopenia or disseminated intravascular coagulation (43,66). Laryngeal and tracheal involvement may occur primarily or by extension from the pharynx. Hoarseness, respiratory stridor, and dyspnea develop and progress to respiratory obstruction and death in young children unless an artificial airway is provided. Older children and adults are less likely to have complete obstruction because of the larger size of the airway. The membrane may form a cast of the trachea and upper bronchi in severe cases. Nasal diphtheria presents with purulent and often serosanguineous discharge. Nasal diphtheria can be chronic, and patients are efficient transmitters during outbreaks. Otitis media can occur primarily or by extension from the pharynx, and conjunctivitis has been reported. Corneal involvement can be severe, resulting in severe scarring, blindness, and loss of the eye. Cutaneous lesions may resemble a variety of dermatologic conditions, including impetigo, pyoderma, ecthyma, insect bites, and deep, punched-out lesions with a leathery eschar (12,67,68). Underlying conditions that predispose to skin lesions include eczema, psoriasis, scabies, insect bites, human bites, trauma, and surgical wounds (12). Coinfection with β-hemolytic streptococci and staphylococci is common. Most lesions occur on the extremities, but the trunk and genitals are also affected. Endocarditis has

been reported, but bacteremia is exceedingly rare, and almost all systemic complications are due to circulating toxin. Myocarditis and neuropathies are much more common in patients with symptomatic nasopharyngeal diphtheria than in patients with only cutaneous infections; however, the rate of systemic complications from cutaneous infections with toxigenic strains of *C. diphtheriae* is sufficient to warrant antitoxin therapy in most instances (12).

Myocarditis presents during the second week of clinical symptoms in 20% to 65% of patients. The presentation may be insidious, with progressive weakness and dyspnea, but acute congestive heart failure and circulatory collapse do occur. Physical examination reveals muffled heart sounds and loss of the difference in the first and second heart sounds with progression to cardiac dilatation and a gallop rhythm. Endocardial thrombi may be dislodged, with resultant embolic phenomena. Conduction disturbances are common, ranging from prolongation of the PR interval to bundle branch blocks or complete atrioventricular block. High mortality rates occur in patients with atrioventricular conduction disturbances, and many are left with permanent damage. Although patients often recover completely, cardiac arrest, apparently caused by conduction disturbances, has occurred 4 to 8 weeks after onset. In cutaneous diphtheria the incidence of myocarditis is lower, the onset is usually later (between the third and eighth week of illness), and the disease is usually milder than in pharyngeal diphtheria (12). A late form of myocarditis with onset in the fourth to sixth week and milder clinical findings is less common.

The incidence of neurologic complications is related directly to the severity of respiratory symptoms. Approximately 20% of all symptomatic respiratory infections are followed by polyneuritis, but 75% of patients with severe disease develop some form of neuropathy. In patients with faucial diphtheria the initial finding is usually palatal paralysis beginning 1 to 2 weeks after onset of symptoms. Paralysis of swallowing and involvement of other cranial nerves follow. Peripheral polyneuritis, with a glove-and-stocking distribution of motor and sensory loss, may resemble Guillain-Barré syndrome. The neuropathy can progress for 1 to 3 months and may take up to 6 months for complete recovery. Residual pharyngeal paralysis occurred in approximately 3% of patients in the preantibiotic era, and rare cases of partial paralysis may present with swallowing disorders (43,69,70).

DIAGNOSIS

In severe cases of pharyngeal diphtheria the clinical diagnosis is not difficult. The presence of an asymmetric gray, adherent membrane with lymph node enlargement and soft tissue swelling in a toxic-looking person should be easily identified as diphtheria. The presence of hoarseness and stridor helps to suggest laryngeal disease. Unilateral palatal paralysis with an exudate is most likely diphtheria.

Laboratory confirmation should be sought for all cases, especially mild ones. Interpretation of Gram stains of scabs from lesions has been discouraged, but some institutions with extensive clinical and laboratory experience have found methylene blue stains of pharyngeal and skin lesions to be sensitive and specific (12). These stains have allowed rapid decision making in suspect cases. Cultures should be obtained from under the membrane if possible or by rubbing the surface of the membrane. Because the nasopharynx is usually colonized, culture material should be collected from every patient's nose. In cutaneous disease, cultures should be obtained from more than one skin lesion and from the nasopharynx. Selective media should be utilized to avoid overgrowth by normal respiratory and skin flora.

Corynebacteria grow on the media routinely used to culture organisms from skin, wounds, and throats, but the colonies resemble the abundant normal flora and selective media are needed to distinguish *C. diphtheriae* from other organisms. Suspect infections should be cultured on tellurite-containing agar. Because cystine-tellurite agar may inhibit some *C. diphtheriae* strains, blood agar cultures should also be propagated and colonies should be examined as possible *C. diphtheriae* in suspect cases when no characteristic colonies grow on selective media. Tinsdale medium has been useful in outbreak situations, but its short shelf life precludes routine use. Also, some commercial preparations have been too inhibitory. If selective media are not available, blood agar with a fosfomycin disk can be inoculated (3). Coryneforms growing in the zone of inhibition should be selected for identification.

Presumptive identification can be made rapidly by examining immunofluorescent-stained specimens from 4- to 8-hour cultures. Classification is based on colony morphology and biochemical profiles, but definitive identification can be difficult (3,71).

Toxin production can be demonstrated *in vivo* by the guinea pig lethality test, and some laboratories use the more rapid Elek test *in vitro* (3). Filter paper strips or circles soaked in diphtheria antitoxin (100 units/mL) are allowed to dry on supplemental Elek agar containing 2% sterile rabbit serum and 0.3% potassium tellurite. Suspect colonies are streaked up to the filter paper with appropriate known toxigenic and nontoxigenic control strains on the same plate. Toxigenic strains produce an arrow-shaped line of precipitation pointing toward the filter paper. Polymerase chain reaction, Vero cell cytotoxicity test, and a reversed passive latex agglutination assay are also available (72).

Polymerase chain reaction methods have allowed rapid probing of suspect isolates for genetic sequences responsible for producing the B subunit of diphtheria toxin (73,74). Commercial application of these methods would simplify laboratory procedures. Other causes of pharyngeal disease that could cause confusion include group A β-hemolytic streptococcal infections. Although group A streptococci are found in up to one third of pharyngeal diphtheria cases, the appearance of the diphtheria membrane is not changed. The asymmetric appearance of the membrane and involvement of the soft palate and uvula are helpful diagnostic signs. Other causes of exudative lesions include Vincent angina, Epstein-Barr virus, adenovirus, and herpes simplex virus or *Candida* (severe infections) in immunocompromised hosts. A foreign body in the nose of a child results in profuse, foul-smelling nasal discharge. Epiglottitis caused by *Haemophilus influenzae* type b can present in a similar manner, and Ludwig angina, with severe soft tissue infection of the neck, can be caused by mixed mouth flora. The clinical manifestations of retropharyngeal and peritonsillar abscesses can resemble those of diphtheria, and the presence of exudative streptococcal pharyngitis could be confusing. Ulcerative lesions have been seen with chemical or thermal burns of the posterior pharynx.

TREATMENT

Nondiphtheria Corynebacteria

Treatment of nondiphtheria corynebacteria depends on susceptibility testing. Although some species are highly susceptible to penicillins, many corynebacteria are resistant to multiple antibiotics. Many of these strains are resistant to macrolides and tetracycline (75). Initial therapy with vancomycin is encouraged for serious systemic infections, and combination therapy may be necessary (2,53,54). Some strains are resistant to vancomycin (76). Removal of devices associated with these infections is often necessary.

Diphtheria

For patients with moderate to severe respiratory disease, initial management must be based on the clinical impression, because delays in therapy can increase the rates of complications and mortality. When antitoxin was administered on the first day of illness, mortality was less than 1%, as compared with 30% when treatment was initiated after 6 days' illness (43). Diphtheria antitoxin neutralizes circulating toxin but is ineffective against intracellular toxin and toxin that has been bound to cells for more than a short time. There is no effective specific therapy to reverse toxin-mediated neurologic or cardiac disease. Only horse serum antitoxin is available commercially and approved for treatment of diphtheria. Patients should be tested for hypersensitivity before the full dose is administered.

The conjunctival test involves administering one drop of antitoxin diluted 1:10 in one eye. Saline is placed in the other eye. Skin testing with a 1:1,000 dilution of antitoxin in normal saline can be used for uncooperative infants or adults. If the result is negative after 20 minutes, the full dose of antitoxin is administered intravenously. Desensitization is required for allergic patients. Antitoxin should be diluted 1:20 in physiologic saline and administered at a rate not to exceed 1 mL/min. The dose is dependent on the location and severity of disease and the duration of disease before therapy rather than on the age or weight of the patient. For pharyngeal or laryngeal disease of less than 48 hours' duration, the dose is 20,000 to 40,000 units; nasopharyngeal disease, 40,000 to 60,000 units; extensive disease of 3 or more days' duration, 80,000 to 100,000 units (77).

Antitoxin has no proven value in cutaneous disease, but toxin-mediated illness occurs, and some experts advise administering 20,000 to 40,000 units of antitoxin. Serum sickness occurs in 5% to 20% of patients who receive antitoxin. Intravenous preparations of human immune globulin contain diphtheria antitoxin, but the products have not been evaluated or approved for use in clinical diphtheria.

Antibiotics are administered to prevent further toxin formation, to treat local infection, and to prevent transmission of *C. diphtheriae* to contacts (78). Treated patients are usually infectious for less than 4 days, although some remain carriers. Erythromycin, 40 to 50 mg/kg per day (maximum, 2 g per day), is the drug of choice unless large proportions of resistant organisms have been identified in the area (12). Procaine penicillin G, 600,000 units per day for patients who weigh more than 10 kg, is an acceptable alternative. Severely affected patients should be treated with intravenous penicillin initially. Treatment should continue for 14 days, and elimination of the organism should be confirmed by three consecutive negative cultures after completion of therapy. Rifampin, 600 mg per day for 7 days, has been used successfully to eliminate the carrier state of erythromycin-resistant strains (12). Recurrent infections have been reported to be associated with erythromycin resistance and chronic dermatoses (12). It is not known whether these patients had experienced a relapse because of inadequate therapy or repeated infection. Material for respiratory tract cultures should be collected 7 days after completion of erythromycin therapy, as up to 20% of patients are colonized at this time (79). There is a need for clinical trials to determine whether rifampin is more effective than erythromycin for eliminating the carrier state.

Supportive care and management of complications, especially maintenance of an airway, are essential to minimize mortality. Tracheostomy or intubation should be undertaken early in moderate to severe laryngeal disease, and equipment for suction must be available at all times. Sudden obstruction of the respiratory tract by sloughing of tracheal membranes may occur with little notice 48 to 96 hours after initiation of therapy.

Strict bed rest is recommended during the acute phase of pharyngeal diphtheria, to minimize the risks of arrhythmias and exacerbation of myocarditis. Severe cardiac failure can develop rapidly. Digitalis and monitoring for cardiac arrhythmias are indicated for patients with myocarditis. Cardiac pacing may be necessary. Steroids are not effective for the prevention of neuropathy or carditis (80). Patients with neuropathies require intensive nursing care similar to that provided for quadriplegic patients. Pharyngeal paralysis can lead to difficulty in swallowing. Elevation of the foot of the bed and keeping the patient on his or her side should minimize the risk for aspiration. Because clinical diphtheria does not reliably induce an antitoxin immune response adequate to prevent recurrent disease, all patients should be immunized with diphtheria toxoid.

PREVENTION

Three doses of diphtheria toxoid are recommended in infancy as part of routine childhood immunization. Diphtheria and tetanus toxoid combined with pertussis vaccine contains 5 to 25 limit flocculation units (Lf) per dose. The vaccine is available in whole-cell (DPT) or acellular (DTaP) forms. The acellular vaccine is preferred in children because the incidence of adverse events is significantly less. Efficacy is reported at 70% to 89% for three doses (81). The risk of encephalitis with the whole-cell vaccine is estimated at 0 to 10.5 per million (82). Three doses are given in the first year of life 4 to 8 weeks apart (usually at 2, 4, and 6 months), a fourth dose is given 6 to 12 months later, and a booster is given at 4 to 6 years. Immunity wanes with age, and 10% to 60% of persons over 30 years of age have antitoxin levels below the protective level (0.01 IU/mL) (29,83–89). Booster doses of tetanus-diphtheria toxoid contain only 1 to 2 Lf diphtheria toxoid and should be administered every 10 years. Unfortunately, many practitioners administer tetanus toxoid alone, contributing to the high rates of inadequate protection in older individuals. Preparations containing 5 Lf diphtheria toxoid induce higher antitoxin levels and are used in some Scandinavian countries. Preparations containing less than 6 Lf diphtheria toxoid are less effective for primary immunization of persons who did not receive diphtheria-tetanus-pertussis vaccine during infancy. Immunization does not protect against becoming a carrier during outbreaks, but immune persons do not become ill and harbor small numbers of organisms. In populations with high rates of immunization coverage, reduced rates of carriage are seen and shifts toward nontoxigenic strains have occurred (90).

Contacts of patients with diphtheria should be observed closely for 7 days, and they should receive erythromycin, 40 to 50 mg/kg per day (maximum 2 g) for 7 days, or benzathine penicillin intramuscularly, 600,000 units if they weigh less than 30 kg and 1.2 million units for larger patients. Benzathine penicillin is preferred for patients who cannot be depended on for close surveillance. Antitoxin is not indicated for contacts because of the risk for serum sickness. Individuals with inadequate or uncertain immunization status should receive a dose of diphtheria toxoid at the first visit and complete the immunization series with the appropriate product (diphtheria-tetanus-pertussis or tetanus and diphtheria toxoid).

REFERENCES

1. Lipsky BA, Goldberger AC, Tompkins LS, et al. Infections caused by nondiphtheria corynebacteria. *Rev Infect Dis* 1982;4:1220.
2. Janda WJ. *Corynebacterium* species and the coryneform bacteria. *Clin Microbiol News* 1998;20:41–66.
3. Colins MD, Jones D, Scholfield GM. Reclassification of *Corynebacterium haemolyticum* (MacLean, Liebow & Rosenberg) in the genus *Arcanobacterium* gen. nov. as *Arcanobacterium haemolyticum* nom. rev., comb. nov. *J Gen Microbiol* 1982;128:1279.
4. Clarridge JE, Spiegel CA. *Corynebacterium* and miscellaneous irregular gram-positive rods, *Erysipelothrix*, and *Gardnerella*. In: Murray PR, Baron EJ, Pfaller MA, et al., eds. *Manual of clinical microbiology*, 6th ed. Washington, DC: ASM Press, 1995:357–378.
5. Rappuoli R, Perugini M, Falsen E. Molecular epidemiology of the 1984–1986 outbreak of diphtheria in Sweden. *N Engl J Med* 1988;318:12.
6. Gruner E, Opravil M, Altwegg M, et al. Nontoxigenic *Corynebacterium diphtheriae* isolated from intravenous drug users. *Clin Infect Dis* 1994;18:94.
7. De Zoysa A, Efstratiou A, George RC, et al. Molecular epidemiology of *Corynebacterium diphtheriae* from northwestern Russia and surrounding countries studied by using ribotyping and pulsed-field gel electrophoresis. *J Clin Microbiol* 1995;33:1080.
8. Coyle MB, Groman NB, Russell JQ, et al. The molecular epidemiology of three biotypes of *Corynebacterium diphtheriae* in the Seattle outbreak, 1972–1982. *J Infect Dis* 1989;159:670.
9. Sacchi CT, de Lemos AP, Casagrande ST, et al. Genetic relationships of *Corynebacterium diphtheriae* strains isolated from a diphtheria case and carriers by restriction fragment length polymorphism of rRNA genes. *Rev Inst Med Trop Sao Paulo* 1995;37:291.
10. Kim-Farley RJ, Soewarso TI, Rejeki S, et al. Silica gel as transport medium for *Corynebacterium diphtheriae* under tropical conditions (Indonesia). *J Clin Microbiol* 1987;25:964.
11. Uchida T. Diphtheria toxin. *Pharmacol Ther* 1983;19:107.
12. Pappenheimer A. The diphtheria bacillus and its toxin: a model system. *J Hyg (Lond)* 1984;93:397.
13. Harnisch JP, Tronca E, Nolan CM, et al: Diphtheria among alcoholic urban adults: a decade of experience in Seattle. Clinical review. *Ann Intern Med* 1989;111:71.
14. Liebow AA, MacLean PD, Bumstead JH, et al. Tropical ulcers and cutaneous diphtheria. *Arch Intern Med* 1946;78:225.
15. Bacon DF, Marples MJ. Researches in western Samoa. II. Lesions of the skin and their bacteriology. *Trans R Soc Trop Med Hyg* 1955;49:76.
16. Galazka AM, Robertson SE. Diphtheria: changing patterns in the developing world and the industrialized world. *Eur J Epidemiol* 1995;11:107–117.
17. Bray JP, Burt EG, Potter EV, et al. Epidemic diphtheria and skin infections in Trinidad. *J Infect Dis* 1972;126:34.
18. Dixon JMS. Diphtheria in North America. *J Hyg (Lond)* 1984;93:419.
19. Richards M, Hurse A. *Corynebacterium pseudotuberculosis* abscesses in a young butcher. *Aust N Z J Med* 1985;15:85.
20. House RW, Schousboe M, Allen JP, et al. *Corynebacterium bovis* (pseudotuberculosis) lymphadenitis in a sheep farmer: a new occupational disease in New Zealand. *N Z Med J* 1986;99:659.
21. Casella P, Bosoni MA, Tommasi A. Recurrent *Corynebacterium aquaticum* peritonitis in a patient undergoing continuous ambulatory peritoneal dialysis. *Clin Microbiol Newslett* 1988;10:62.
22. Moore C, Norton R. *Corynebacterium aquaticum* septicaemia in a neutropenic patient. *J Clin Pathol* 1995;48:971.
23. Brooks GF, Bennett JV, Feldman RA. Diphtheria in the United States, 1959–1970. *J Infect Dis* 1974;129:172.
24. Chakraborty SM. The incidence and treatment of faucial diphtheria in a rural West Bengal population. *J Ind Med Assoc* 1970;55:371.
25. Bennett SW. Investigation of tropical pattern of diphtheria in Buenaventura, Colombia. In: *Proceedings of the International Symposium of Tropical Dermatoses in the Pacific Region*, Tokyo, 1966:38.
26. Halsey N, Galazka A. The efficacy of DPT and oral poliomyelitis immunization schedules initiated from birth to 12 weeks of age. *Bull WHO* 1985;63:1151.
27. Khuri-Bulos N, Hamzah Y, Sammerrai SM, et al. The changing epidemiology of diphtheria in Jordan. *Bull WHO* 1988;66:65.
28. Centers for Disease Control and Prevention. *Diphtheria surveillance.* Report No. 12. Atlanta: Centers for Disease Control and Prevention, July 1978.
29. Centers for Disease Control and Prevention. Update: diphtheria epidemic—new independent states of the former Soviet Union, January 1995–March 1996. *MMWR* 1996;45:693.
30. Dittmann S. Epidemic diphtheria in the newly independent states of the former USSR—situation and lessons learned. *Biologicals* 1997;25:179–186.
31. Galazka AM, Robertson SE, Oblapenko GP. Resurgence of diphtheria. *Fur J Epidemiol* 1995;11:95.
32. Murray BA, Karchmer AW, Moellering RC. Diphtheroid prosthetic valve endocarditis. *Am J Med* 1980;69:838.
33. Johnson WD, Kaye D. Serious infections caused by diphtheroids. *Ann N Y Acad Sci* 1970;174:568.
34. Kaplan K, Weinstein L. Diphtheroid infections of man. *Ann Intern Med* 1969;70:919.

35. Washington JA II. Bacteriology, clinical spectrum of disease, and therapeutic aspects in coryneform bacterial infection. *Curr Clin Top Infect Dis* 1981; 2:68.

36. Hoy CM, Kerr K, Livingston JH. Cerebrospinal fluid-shunt infection due to *Corynebacterium striatum. Clin Infect Dis* 1997;25:1486–1487.

37. Pappenheimer AM, Harper AA, Moynihan M, et al. Diphtheria toxin and related proteins: effect of route of injection of toxicity and the determination of cytotoxicity for various cultured cells. *J Infect Dis* 1982;145:94.

38. Chang MP, Baldwin RL, Bruce C, et al. Second cytotoxic pathway of diphtheria toxin suggested by nuclease activity. *Science* 1989;246:1165.

39. Bodley JW. Does diphtheria toxin have nuclease activity? *Science* 1990;250:832.

40. Johnson VG. Does diphtheria toxin have nuclease activity? *Science* 1990; 250:834.

41. Wilson BA, Blanke SR, Murphy JR, et al. Does diphtheria toxin have nuclease activity? *Science* 1990;250:835.

42. Boyer NH, Weinstein L. Diphtheritic myocarditis. *N Engl J Med* 1948;239:913.

43. Naiditch MJ, Bower AG. Diphtheria: a study of 1,433 cases observed during a ten year period at the Los Angeles County Hospital. *Am J Med* 1954;17:229.

44. Solders G, Nennesmo I, Persson A. Diphtheritic neuropathy, an analysis based on muscle and nerve biopsy and repeated neurophysiological and autonomic function tests. *J Neurol Neurosurg Psychiatry* 1989;52:876.

45. Carroll SF, Barbieri JT, Collier RJ. Diphtheria toxin: purification and properties. *Methods Enzymol* 1988;165:68.

46. Maxwell IH, Maxwell F, Glode LM. Regulated expression of a diphtheria toxin A-chain gene transfected into human cells: possible strategy for inducing cancer cells suicide. *Cancer Res* 1986;46:4660.

47. Meers PD. A case of classical diphtheria and other infections due to *Corynebacterium ulcerans. J Infect* 1979;1:139.

48. Hadfield TL, Monson MH. *Corynebacterium ulcerans* infection. *Clin Microbiol Newslett* 1983;5:104.

49. Centers for Disease Control and Prevention. Respiratory diphtheria caused by *Corynebacterium ulcerans*—Terre Haute, Indiana. *MMWR* 1996;46:330–332.

50. Siegel SM, Haile CA. *Corynebacterium ulcerans* pneumonia. *South Med J* 1985;78:1267.

51. Augustine JL, Renshaw HW. Survival of *Corynebacterium pseudotuberculosis* in axenic purulent exudate on common barnyard fomites. *Am J Vet Res* 1986;47:713.

52. Peel MM, Palmer GG, Stacpoole AM, et al. Human lymphadenitis due to *Corynebacterium pseudotuberculosis*: report of ten cases from Australia and review. *Clin Infect Dis* 1996;24:185–191.

53. Young VM, Meyers WF, Moody MR, et al. The emergence of coryneform bacteria as a cause of nosocomial infection in compromised hosts. *Am J Med* 1981;70:646–650.

54. Stamm WE, Tompkins LS, Wagner KF, et al. Infection due to *Corynebacterium* species in marrow transplant patients. *Ann Intern Med* 1979;91:167–173.

55. McGinley KJ, Labows JN, Zeckman JM, et al. Pathogenic JK group corynebacteria and their similarity to human cutaneous lipophilic diphtheroids. *J Infect Dis* 1985;152:801–806.

56. Morris A, Guild I. Endocarditis due to *Corynebacterium pseudodiphtheriticum*: five case reports, review and antibiotic susceptibilities of nine strains. *Rev Infect Dis* 1991;13:887–892.

57. Wilson ME, Shapiro DS. Native valve endocarditis due to *Corynebacterium pseudodiphtheriticum. Clin Infect Dis* 1992;15:1059–1060.

58. Ahmed K, Kawakami K, Watanabe K, et al. *Corynebacterium pseudodiphtheriticum*: a respiratory tract pathogen. *Clin Infect Dis* 1995;20:41–46.

59. Manzella JP, Kellogg JA, Parsey KS. *Corynebacterium pseudodiphtheriticum*: a respiratory tract pathogen in adults. *Clin Infect Dis* 1995;20:37–40.

60. Wilson AP. The return of *Corynebacterium diphtheriae*: the rise of non-toxigenic strains. *J Hosp Infect* 1995;30(suppl):306.

61. Claeys G, Vanhouteghem H, Riegel P, et al. Endocarditis of native aortic and mitral valves due to *Corynebacterium accolens*: report of a case and application of phenotypic and genotypic techniques for identification. *J Clin Microbiol* 1996;34:1290.

62. Pennie RA, Malik AS, Wilcox L. Misidentification of toxigenic *Corynebacterium diphtheriae* as a *Corynebacterium* species with low virulence in a child with endocarditis. *J Clin Microbiol* 1996;34:1275.

63. Tiley SM, Kociuba KR, Heron LG, et al. Infective endocarditis due to non-toxigenic *Corynebacterium diphtheriae*: report of seven cases and review [see comments]. *Clin Infect Dis* 1993;16:271.

64. Damade R, Pouchot J, Delacroix I, et al. Septic arthritis due to *Corynebacterium diphtheriae. Clin Infect Dis* 1993;16:446.

65. Doyle A, Beigi B, Early A, et al. Adherence of bacteria to intraocular lenses: a prospective study. *Br J Ophthalmol* 1995;79:347.

66. Wesley AG, Father M, Chrystol V. The haemorrhagic diathesis in diphtheria with special reference to disseminated intravascular coagulation. *Ann Trop Pediatr* 1981;1:51.

67. Betsey MA, Sinclair M, Roder MR, et al. *Corynebacterium diphtheriae* skin infections in Alabama and Louisiana. A factor in the epidemiology of diphtheria. *N Engl J Med* 1969;176:273.

68. Liebow AA, MacLean PD, Bumstead JH, et al. Tropical ulcers and cutaneous diphtheria. *Arch Intern Med* 1946;78:255.

69. Scheid W. Diphtheria paralysis: an analysis of 2292 cases of diphtheria which include 174 cases of polyneuritis. *J Nerv Ment Dis* 1952;116:1095.

70. Obana KK, Fee WE. Unusual pharyngeal lesion causing dysphagia. *Ann Otol Rhinol Laryngol* 1987;96:527.

71. Efstratiou A, George RC. Laboratory guidelines for the diagnosis of infections caused by *Corynebacterium diphtheriae* and *C. ulcerans*. World Health Organization. *Commun Dis Public Health* 1999;2:250–257.

72. Toma C, Sisavatu L, Iwanaga M. Reversed passive agglutination assay for detection of toxigenic *Corynebacterium diphtheriae. J Clin Microbiol* 1997;35:3147–3149.

73. Aravena-Roman M, Bowman R, O'Neill G. Polymerase chain reaction for the detection of toxigenic *Corynebacterium diphtheriae. Pathology* 1995;27:71.

74. Mikhailovich VM, Melnikov VG, Mazurova IK, et al. Application of PCR for detection of toxigenic *Corynebacterium diphtheriae* strains isolated during the Russian diphtheria epidemic, 1990 through 1994. *J Clin Microbiol* 1995;33:3061.

75. Eady EA, Coates P, Ross JI, et al. Antibiotic resistance patterns of aerobic coryneforms and furazolidone-resistant gram-positive cocci from the skin surface of the human axilla and fourth toe cleft. *J Antimicrob Chemother* 2000;46:205–13.

76. Kremery V, Sefton A. Vancomycin resistance in gram-positive bacteria other than *Enterococcus* spp. *Int J Antimicrob Agents* 2000;14:99–105.

77. Wilson AP. Treatment of infection caused by toxigenic and non-toxigenic strains of *Corynebacterium diphtheriae. J Antimicrob Chemother* 1995;35:717.

78. Farizo KM, Strebel PM, Chen RT, et al. Fatal respiratory disease due to *Corynebacterium diphtheriae*: case report and review of guidelines for management, investigation, and control. *Clin Infect Dis* 1993;16:59.

79. Miller LW, Bickham S, Jones WL, et al. Diphtheria carriers and the effect of erythromycin therapy. *Antimicrob Agents Chemother* 1974;6:166.

80. Thisyakorn USA, Wongvanich J, Kumpeng V. Failure of corticosteroid therapy to prevent diphtheritic myocarditis or neuritis. *Pediatr Infect Dis* 1984;3:126.

81. Centers for Disease Control and Prevention. Pertussis vaccination. Use of acellular pertussis vaccines among infants and young children. *MMWR* 1997;46:1–25.

82. Miller D, Wadsworth J, Diamond J, et al. Pertussis vaccine and whooping cough as risk factors in acute neurologic illness and death in young children. *Der Biol Stand* 1985;61:389–394.

83. Koblin BA, Townsend TR. Immunity to diphtheria and tetanus in inner-city women of childbearing age. *Am J Public Health* 1989;79:1297.

84. Bjorkholm B, Wahl M, Granstrom M, et al. Immune status and booster effects of low doses of diphtheria toxoid in Swedish medical personnel. *Scand J Infect Dis* 1989;21:429.

85. Simonsen O, Kjeldsen K, Vendborg HA, et al. Revaccination of adults against diphtheria. I: Responses and reactions to different doses of diphtheria toxoid in 30 to 70 year old persons with low serum antitoxin levels. *Acta Pathol Microbiol Immunol Scand [C]* 1986;94:213.

86. Simonsen O, Klaerke M, Klaerke A, et al. Revaccination of adults against diphtheria. II: Combined diphtheria and tetanus revaccination with different doses of diphtheria toxoid 20 years after primary vaccination. *Acta Pathol Microbiol Immunol Scand [C]* 1986;94:219.

87. Jones AE, Johns A, Magrath DI, et al. Durability of immunity to diphtheria, tetanus and poliomyelitis after a three dose immunization schedule completed in the first eight months of life. *Vaccine* 1989;7:300.

88. Cellesi C, Zanchi A, Michelangeli C, et al. Immunity to diphtheria in a sample of adult population from central Italy. *Vaccine* 1989;7:417.

89. Kjeldsen K, Simonsen O, Heron I. Immunity against diphtheria and tetanus in the age group 30–70 years. *Scand J Infect Dis* 1988;20:177.

90. Pappenheimer AM Jr. Diphtheria: studies on the biology of an infectious disease. *Harvey Lect* 1982;76:45.

CHAPTER 188

Bacillus anthracis *and Other Aerobic Gram-Positive Spore Forming Bacilli*

Christopher C. Penn and Stephen A. Klotz

Bacillus anthracis, the agent of anthrax, has long been recognized as a pathogen since the early work by Davaine, Koch, and Pasteur in the 19th century. The pathogenic role of the other species of *Bacillus* has only become appreciated in the last several decades and disease caused by these bacteria is often an accompaniment of advances in medical technology. *Bacillus* is a genus in the family, Bacillaceae, microorganisms that are aerobic and facultatively anaerobic bacilli. They are motile by means of peritrichous flagella with the notable exception on *B. anthrax*, which

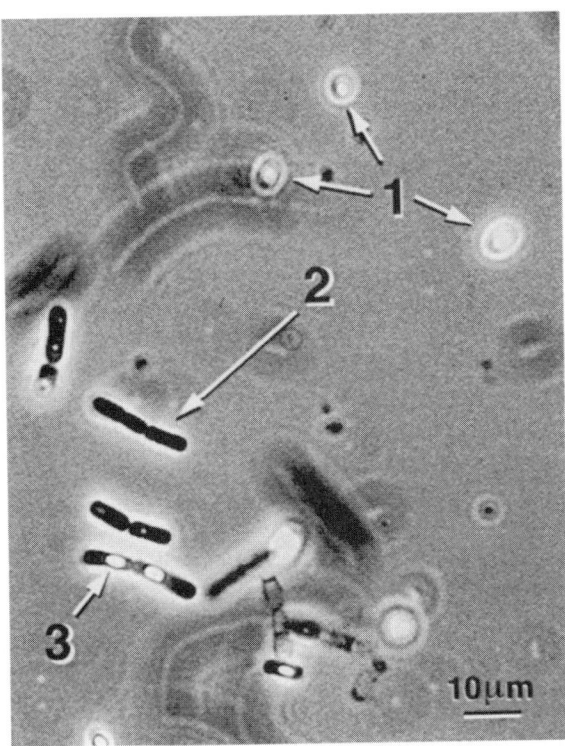

Figure 188.1. Morphologic forms of *Bacillus anthracis. Arrow 1*, spores; *arrow 2*, vegetative forms; *arrow 3*, spores forming subterminally. (Sterne strain, isolate courtesy of Dr. Max Glass, Bayer, Lenexa, KS.)

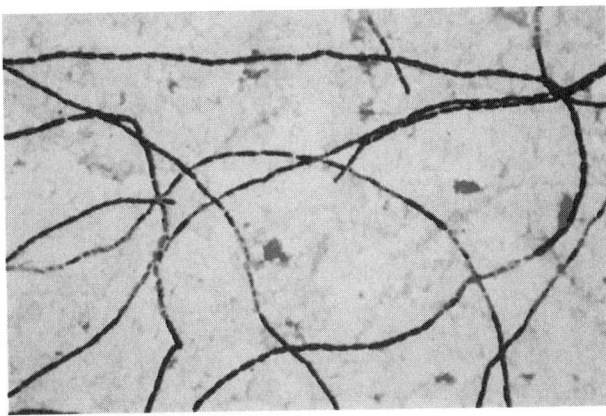

Figure 188.2. Gram stain of *Bacillus anthracis* in blood culture of patient with inhalational anthrax. (Reproduced from Quintiliani R Jr, Mahajan A, Quintiliani R. Fatal case of inhalational anthrax mimicking intra-abdominal sepsis. *Clin Infect Dis* 2001;33, with permission.)

is non-motile. The major characteristic of the genus is the ability to form spores (Fig. 188.1). The spores are central, subterminal, or terminal and are oval or round. They may cause swelling of the cell in some species but not in *B. anthracis*. The size of the vegetative cells varies from a width of 0.4 μm and length of 3 μm in the small species to a width of 2.0 μm and length of 9.0 μm in the large species. The majority of species are gram positive, although some species stain gram variable.

BACILLUS ANTHRACIS

Characteristics of the Pathogen

B. anthracis can be provisionally identified by finding large gram-positive rods in material swabbed from cutaneous lesions, blood, or the cerebrospinal fluid (Fig. 188.2). Capsules are always present in tissue specimens. Giemsa, polychrome methylene blue, and India ink stains demonstrate the presence of the capsule. The production of the capsule is mediated by the presence of a 60-kDa plasmid. *B. anthracis* grows in extended chains on solid medium, giving rise to the formation of a Medusa head recognized by finger-like projections from the edge of the colonies. It is not encapsulated on a solid medium unless it is grown in the presence of 0.7% sodium bicarbonate or in the presence of carbon dioxide. Under these growth conditions, it exhibits exuberant capsule formation. Furthermore, in the presence of increased carbon dioxide and bicarbonate, colonies are smooth and mucoid, but in their absence colonies are rough. If grown in a liquid medium containing bicarbonate *B. anthracis* produces an aromatic acid that colors the medium from brown to red.

The spore of *B. anthracis* is central to terminal in location and does not swell the vegetative cell. Some strains are asporoge-

nous, but the ability to form spores is independent of virulence. The bacterium is non-motile, unlike the majority of members of the *Bacillus* genus. It is catalase positive and almost never causes hemolysis on blood agar. The bacterium does not grow on MacConkey's agar. *B. anthracis* grows well on PLET agar (polymyxin, B-lysozyme ethylenediamine tetraacetic acid [EDTA]–thallous acetate), which is selective for the species (1) and a rapid selective medium has recently been described (2). Typical virulent strains of *B. anthracis* can be differentiated from other *Bacillus* species with accuracy by determining the reaction pattern to a battery of preformed substrates, the API 50CHB strip (Analytab Products, Plainview, New York) in conjunction with the API 20E strip (Anyltab Products) (3). Due to changes in the taxonomy of the genus, as discussed below, some of the criteria in these tests have changed. Additionally, *B. anthracis* can be identified by serologic means, polymerase chain reaction and strains (arising in different geographic locales) can be differentiated by comparison of specific tandem repeats occurring within fragment length polymorphism analysis (4).

Virulence and Immunity

Several virulence factors are produced by *B. anthracis* and are encoded on two plasmids: capsule formation on one plasmid and production of protective antigen, edema factor and lethal factor on another plasmid. The capsule is composed of a poly-γ-D-glutamic acid, is antigenic but not protective, and can be visualized when stained with polychrome methylene blue (M'Fadyean reaction). *Bacillus subtilis, B. lichenformis*, and *B. megaterium* can also produce capsule in the presence of bicarbonate.

B. anthracis produces an antigenic exotoxin that is responsible for many of the clinical symptoms in anthrax. The toxin is tripartite, consisting of protective antigen, edema factor, and lethal factor. Toxin production is mediated by a 110-kDa plasmid and occurs in response to the presence of bicarbonate and temperature (5).

Protective antigen (PA) is a protein that binds a cell surface receptor (anthrax toxin receptor, ATR). ATR is a membrane protein that possesses an extracellular von Willebrand factor A domain and binds directly to PA (6). After binding to ATR, the shape of PA is modified by enzymatic cleavage with seven cleaved moieties joining together to form a heptamer. This heptamer facilitates movement of the edema and lethal factors into the cytosol. Without PA, edema factor and lethal factor are biologically inactive. PA does not appear to have any specific toxic effects.

Edema factor is a secreted adenylyl cyclase of about 92 kDa that is activated by host cell calmodulin (7). This toxin is distinct from, but closely related to *Bordetella pertussis* toxin (8). Edema toxin is the combination of edema factor and PA, and is responsible for prominent edema at the site of infection, impaired neutrophil function and the interruption of tumor necrosis factor and interleukin-6 production.

Lethal factor is a zinc metalloproteinase (approximately 90 kDa) that deactivates mitogen-activated protein kinase and whose crystal structure is known (9). The combination of lethal factor with PA to form lethal toxin results in impaired intracellular signaling and release of tumor necrosis factor-α and interleukin-1-β, both of which may contribute to cell death.

After infection, antibodies are detectable to all four virulence factors: capsule, protective antigen, edema factor, and lethal factor.

Prevention

Greenfield in London, England (10) and later, Pasteur in Pouilly-leFort, France demonstrated that anthrax could be prevented in livestock by the use of a vaccine containing *B. anthracis* attenuated through *in vitro* cultivation (11). The highly effective animal vaccine (Sterne vaccine) is a live spore vaccine derived from an isolate cured of the plasmid required for capsule formation (pX02-strain). The human vaccines used in the Western Hemisphere are cell-free filtrate vaccines composed principally of PA. Annual booster injections of both vaccines are required. The present supplier in the United States is BioPort (Lansing, Mich), which has recently recommenced its production of anthrax vaccine absorbed for the U.S. Department of Defense. At present, the vaccine is in short supply and is not recommended for the general public, including health care workers. A live spore vaccine (pXO2-strain) has been developed and used extensively in the former Soviet Union. This vaccine has been shown to be effective in challenge experiments with humans in large field trials but has not found favor in the Western world.

Infected animals should be quarantined and carcasses burned or buried after being covered with quicklime (calcium oxide). Given recent anthrax threats, specific guidelines have been issued by the Centers for Disease Control (CDC). Buildings, equipment, and mail suspected of being contaminated with anthrax should be reported to local authorities at which time quarantine and rapid testing for the presence of anthrax may be used. These methods include nucleic acid signatures and antigen detection by enzyme-linked immunosorbent assay. Decontamination of such environments has been achieved with chlorine dioxide. Formaldehyde has been employed as an agent of decontamination as well.

Obviously, care should be taken in handling specimens thought to be *B. anthracis*. Such specimens should be referred to a level B laboratory of the Laboratory Response Network for Bioterrorism. The organism and contaminated containers should be autoclaved or treated with dilute hypochlorite (Clorox) solution. Laboratory personnel should be alerted by clinicians to the possibility of isolating this microorganism.

Treatment

While penicillin has been the drug of choice for many years, current recommendations include the use of either ciprofloxacin or doxycycline (either orally or intravenously, depending on the site and severity of infection) plus one or two additional antimicrobial agents. Recent reports on the treatment of inhalational anthrax have demonstrated improvement over expected mortality with the use of ciprofloxacin, rifampin, and clindamycin. The possibility of an inducible β-lactamase in the microorganism raises concern over the use of penicillins and cephalosporins. The duration of treatment depends on the route of exposure, the severity of disease, and the site of infection. Treatment and prophylaxis regimes may include vaccination. The CDC should be consulted in any case of suspected exposure or infection (*www.bt.cdc.gov/Agent/Anthrax/AnthraxGen.asp*).

In addition to traditional antimicrobial therapy, there is significant interest in "anti-toxin" therapy against *B. anthracis*. Proposed targets of such therapies include the prevention of protective antigen attaching to the ATR as well as the disabling of the protective antigen heptamer itself.

OTHER *BACILLUS* SPECIES

The taxonomy of the genus, *Bacillus*, underwent extensive revision in the 1990s. It has been subdivided into 5 new genera. Most of the medically important species remain within the genus *Bacillus*, although the former *B. alvei* has been renamed *Paenobacillus alvei*. Other new genera include: *Alicyclobacillus, Brevibacillus, Aneurinibacillus*, and *Virgibacillus*. It is likely that several more new genera will be forthcoming (1). The vast majority of the 50 species of *Bacillus* are presumed to be saprophytes, with the major exception of *B. anthracis*. In common with *B. anthracis*, and indeed the entire family of *Bacillaceae*, these bacteria form endospores, likely as a maneuver to survive unfavorable environmental conditions. All of these microorganisms are believed to be important in the recycling of carbon and nitrogen on the earth's crust. Five *Bacillus* species are known insect pathogens, yet two of these species have caused disease in man.

The genus is gram positive and most species hemolyze blood agar. A combination of morphology and special tests is usually sufficient to allow speciation of an isolate. Morphologic features important in speciation are size of vegetative cells, the location of spores, and whether or not the spores swell the vegetative cells. Special biochemical tests useful in identification are casein hydrolysis, sugar fermentation reactions, production of lecithinase (phospholipase), nitrate reduction, and the Voges-Proskauer reaction. Further information regarding identification to the species level can be found elsewhere (1).

The *Bacillus* species, in particular *B. cereus*, possess the ability to elaborate a number of extracellular products such as collagenase, phospholipase C, an hemolysin, and a soluble toxin that is lethal for mice. Some authorities believe *B. cereus* and *B. anthracis* to be the same species, the latter, a variant of *B. cereus*. In any case, *B. anthracis* is closely related to *B. cereus, B. mycoides,* and *B. thuringiensis*, which may pose problems in identification.

REFERENCES

1. Logan NA, Turnbull PCB. *Bacillus* and recently derived genera. In: Murray PR, Barron EJ, Pfaller MA, Tenover FC, Yolken RH, eds. *Manual of clinical microbiology.* Washington, DC: ASM Press, 1999:357–369.
2. Kiel JL, Parker JE, Alls JL, et al. Rapid recovery and identification of anthrax bacteria from the environment. *Ann NY Acad Sci* 2000;916:240–252.
3. Logan NA, Berkeley RCW. Identification of *Bacillus* strains using the API system. *Gen J Microbiol* 1984;130:1871–1872.
4. Keim P, Klevytska AM, Price LB, et al. Molecular diversity in *Bacillus anthracis*. *J Appl Microbiol* 1999;87:215.
5. Sirard JC, Mock M, Fouet A. The three *Bacillus anthracis* toxin genes are coordinately regulated by bicarbonate and temperature. *J Bacteriol* 1994;176:5188.
6. Bradley KA, Mogridge J, Mourez M, Collier RJ, Young JA. Identification of the cellular receptor for anthrax toxin. *Nature* 2001;414:225–229.
7. Drum CL, Yan SZ, Bard J, et al. Structural basis of the activation of anthrax adenylyl cyclase exotoxin by calmodulin. *Nature* 2002;415:396–402.

8. Masure HR, Shattuck RL, Storm DR. Mechanisms of bacterial pathogenicity that involve production of calmodulin-sensitive adenylate cyclases. *Microbiol Rev* 1994;51:60.
9. Pannifer AD, Wong TY, Schwarzenbacher R, et al. Crystal structure of anthrax lethal factor. *Nature* 2001;414:229–233.
10. Tigertt WD. Anthrax. William Smith Greenfield, M.D., F.R.C.P., Professor Superintendent, the Brown Animal Sanatory Institution (1878–1881). Concerning the priority due to him for the production of the first vaccine against anthrax. *J Hyg* 1980;85:415.
11. Turnbull PCB. Anthrax vaccines: past, present and future. *Vaccine* 1991;9:533.

CHAPTER 189
Bacillus *Species Infections*

Christopher C. Penn and Stephen A. Klotz

The history of a patient's illness, to include exposure to bioterrorism activities, should alert the clinician to the possibility of isolating *B. anthracis*. The isolation of the other *Bacillus* species is almost always unexpected, and one must determine whether or not the isolate is playing a pathogenic role or is a contaminant. The taxonomy of the genus *Bacillus* underwent extensive revision in the 1990s. It has been subdivided into five new genera. Most of the medically important species remain within the genus *Bacillus*, although the former *B. alvei* has been renamed *Paenobacillus alvei*. Other new genera include *Alicyclobacillus*, *Brevibacillus*, *Aneurinibacillus*, and *Virgibacillus*. It is likely that several new genera will be forthcoming (1). The vast majority of the 50 species of *Bacillus* are presumed to be saprophytes, with the major exception of *B. anthracis*. *Bacillus* species have been described as pathogenic in infections involving all sites of the body. Two excellent reviews provide the reader a flavor for the spectrum of illness caused by these microorganisms (2,3). Clinical experience over the past several decades has demonstrated that much the same as with *Candida* species and coagulase-negative staphylococci, *Bacillus* isolates must be considered pathogenic until proven otherwise. Reasonable criteria to establish whether or not an isolate of *Bacillus* is truly implicated in a significant infection are (a) at least two positive blood cultures for *Bacillus* drawn on different occasions; (b) an isolate from a normally sterile body site along with at least one positive blood culture; or (c) isolation of *Bacillus* species from a surgical specimen (sometimes in conjunction with another bacterium particularly in posttraumatic wounds) obtained during an open surgical procedure, with clinical evidence of infection at that site (i.e., local tenderness or swelling on examination or obvious purulence noted at surgery) (3). More than a single isolation of the bacterium is important before assigning a causative role for disease with the *Bacillus* species when the isolate is from the blood, trauma is involved, or the patient is an intravenous drug abuser.

There have now been numerous reports of bacteremia with these microorganisms in neutropenic hosts; therefore, the isolation of *Bacillus* species in immunosuppressed patients warrants prompt empiric coverage with appropriate antibiotics. Table 189.1 provides a list of some of the most frequently encountered clinical infections caused by *Bacillus* species and some recent reports of new associations. It includes comments on how to support the diagnosis, other gram-positive bacilli that may present differential diagnostic problems, and empiric therapy. *Bacillus* species are also capable of causing prosthetic device–associated infections in the hip, knee, eye, peritoneum, soft tissue, and heart valves. Many other clinical presentations with these microorganisms have been described (for a review, see references 4 and 5).

PSEUDOINFECTIONS

The clinician should appreciate that the ability of *Bacillus* species to form spores explains the uncanny habit of these bacteria to appear in unusual circumstances, often where one would anticipate sterility. For example, *Bacillus* species have been responsible for outbreaks of pseudomeningitis (6) and pseudobacteremia (7); the former, by contamination of sterile broth used in the culture of cerebral spinal fluid and the latter by contamination of gloves worn by phlebotomists (8). *Bacillus* species have been implicated in other pseudobacteremias through the use of contaminated cotton alcohol swabs (9) and contamination of the rubber stoppers of blood culture bottles (7). Contamination of the rubber stoppers of blood culture bottles occurred following environmental disturbance caused by hospital construction (7).

INFECTIONS ASSOCIATED WITH ADVANCED MEDICAL PRACTICE

Infections have been associated with the advanced technology of medicine. For example, *B. cirulans* contaminating lens implants was responsible for an outbreak of postoperative endophthalmitis (10,11). *Bacillus* species have been responsible for line sepsis due to contamination of intravenous coupling devices (12), cross-contamination of hemodialysis tubing (13), and contaminated solutions infused into patients (14). "Sterile" loofah sponges used in cosmetics may harbor a number of microorganisms, including *Bacillus* species, and have been associated with infections (15).

TREATMENT

Effective antibiotic treatment schemes have been reported for infections caused by a wide range of *Bacillus* species. Theoretically, the choice of an appropriate antibiotic is complicated by the fact that there exist no standards for testing antibiotic susceptibility for the *Bacillus* species (16). Furthermore, the recent change in taxonomy of the genus has invalidated the previous identification schemata used in automated identification systems. In practice, however, there are adequate reported patient cases that one can with confidence treat the majority of *Bacillus* species infections. As a "rule of thumb" most isolates of *B. cereus* and *Bacillus* species are highly susceptible (>95% of strains) to imipenem, vancomycin, ciprofloxacin, and chloramphenicol, and moderately susceptible (70%–95% of strains) to clindamycin and gentamicin (4).

Some disease presentations and effective regimens can be found in Table 189.1. The treatment of *B. anthracis* is discussed in Chapter 164. *B. cereus* and *B. thuringiensis* are predictably resistant to the use of penicillin and the cephalosporins due to the production of β-lactamase. Clindamycin, vancomycin, and gentamicin have had the widest clinical use and the most apparent success for the treatment of *Bacillus* species infections; therefore, one or more of these drugs should be incorporated in any empiric regimen. In serious infections it may be prudent to administer gentamicin in addition to vancomycin or clindamycin. Combination regimens may be synergistic against *B. cereus* ocular isolates (17). Clindamycin penetrates the vitreous and is probably the drug of choice for treating endophthalmitis due to *B. cereus*. Imipenem penetrates the vitreous and aqueous humors to high levels and may be useful in disease of the eye. Similarly, ciprofloxacin, intravenously, may be useful in *Bacillus* species eye infections.

TABLE 189.1. *Bacillus* Species Infections: Associated Conditions, Detection, Differential Diagnoses, and Empiric Therapy

Clinical presentation	Associated problems	Gram stain results	Likely gram-positive bacterium	Empiric therapy (reference)
Meningitis	Ventricular shunt		Coagulase-negative staphylococci; *Proprionibacterium acnes*	Removal of shunt plus vancomycin (18)
Endophthalmitis Endogenous	Intravenous drug use (often with positive blood culture)	Smears of vitreous are positive	*B. cereus; B. subtilis;* intravenous drug use with positive blood culture	Intensive systemic, topical, intravitreal vancomycin, clindamycin, gentamicin with vitrectomy (19,20) (11)
Exogenous	Following trauma or postoperative	Smears of the vitreous and some aqueous humor are positive	*P. acnes* or *Corynebacterium* species; *B. circulans* associated with contaminated lens implants; (smears from chronic infection with *B. circulans* show coccobacillary elements)	
Keratitis	Trauma from foreign object with soil; contact lens	Scrapings of the cornea are positive	*B. cereus*	Topical vancomycin or clindamycin with gentamicin (21)
Pneumonia	Occupational hazard of welding?	Blood culture and Gram stain of sputum show gram-positive rods	*B. cereus* (syndrome may cause confusion with *B. anthracis*)	(22)
Pneumonia associated with ventilator		Gram stain of aspirated material may be positive	*Bacillus* species; must now include *B. anthracis*	(23)
Bacteremia	Intravenous drug abuse; neutropenia	May be associated with endophthalmitis	*B. cereus*	Clindamycin (24)
Bacteremia with central venous catheter	Usually catheter indwelling for a long period; cancer therapy	Blood cultures are positive	*B. licheniformis; B. cereus*	Remove catheter (25–28)
Osteomyelitis	Motor vehicle trauma	Culture of involved tissue with heavy growth of *Bacillus*	*B. cereus; Clostridium* species	Flucloxacillin (29); vancomycin, gentamicin (30); vancomycin, clindamycin (31)

REFERENCES

1. Logan NA, Turnbull PCB. *Bacillus* and recently derived genera. In: Murray PR, Barron EJ, Pfaller MA, et al., eds. *Manual of clinical microbiology.* Washington, DC: ASM Press, 1999:357–369.
2. Tuazon CU, Murray HW, Levy C, et al. Serious infections from *Bacillus* sp. *JAMA* 1979;241:1137–1140.
3. Sliman R, Rehm S, Shlaes DM. Serious infections caused by *Bacillus* species. *Medicine* 1987;66:218–223.
4. Weber DJ, Rutala WA. *Bacillus* species. *Infect Control Hosp Epidemiol* 1988;9:368–373.
5. Weber DJ, Saviteer SM, Rutala WA, et al. Clinical significance of *Bacillus* species isolated from blood cultures. *South Med J* 1989;82:705–709.
6. Lettau LA, Benjamin D, Cantrell HF, et al. *Bacillus* species pseudomeningitis. *Infect Control Hosp Epidemiol* 1988;9:394–397.
7. Loeb M, Wilcox L, Thornley D, et al. *Bacillus* species pseudobacteremia following hospital construction. *Can J Infect Control* 1995;10:37–40.
8. York MK. *Bacillus* species pseudobacteremia traced to contaminated gloves used in collection of blood from patients with acquired immunodeficiency syndrome. *J Clin Microbiol* 1990;28:2114–2116.
9. Berger SA. Pseudobacteremia due to contaminated alcohol swabs. *J Clin Microbiol* 1983;18:974–975.
10. Roy M, Chen JC, Miller M, et al. Epidemic *Bacillus* endophthalmitis after cataract surgery. I. Acute presentation and outcome. *Ophthalmology* 1997;104:1768–1772.
11. Chen JC, Roy M. Epidemic *Bacillus* endophthalmitis after cataract surgery. II. Chronic and recurrent presentation and outcome. *Ophthalmology* 2000;107:1038–1041.
12. Matsumoto S, Suenaga H, Naito K, et al. Management of suspected nosocomial infection: an audit of 19 hospitalized patients with septicemia caused by *Bacillus* species. *Jpn J Infect Dis* 2000;53:196–202.
13. Longfield RN, Wortham WG, Fletcher LL, et al. Clustered bacteremias in a hemodialysis unit: cross-contamination of blood tubing from ultrafiltrate waste. *Infect Control Hosp Epidemiol* 1992;13:160–164.
14. Thuler LCS, Velasco EA. An outbreak of *Bacillus* species in a cancer hospital. *Infect Control Hosp Epidemiol* 1998;19:856–858.
15. Bottone EJ, Perez AA II, Oeser JL. Loofah sponges as reservoirs and vehicles in the transmission of potentially pathogenic bacterial species to human skin. *J Clin Microbiol* 1994;32:469–472.
16. National Committee for Clinical Laboratory Standards. *Performance standards for antimicrobial susceptibility testing: twelfth informational supplement.* Vol. 21, No. 1. National Committee for Clinical Laboratory Standards. January 2002.
17. Gigantelli JW, Gomez JT, Osato MS. *In vitro* susceptibilities of ocular *Bacillus cereus* isolates to clindamycin, gentamicin, and vancomycin alone or in combination. *Antimicrob Agents Chemother* 1991;35:201.
18. Berner R, Heinen F, Pelz K, et al. Ventricular shunt infection and meningitis due to *Bacillus cereus*. *Neuropediatrics* 1997;28:333–334.
19. Davey RTJ, Tauber WB. Posttraumatic endophthalmitis: the emerging role of *Bacillus cereus* infection. *Rev Infect Dis* 1987;9:110.
20. Donahue SP, O'Day DM. *Bacillus cereus* endophthalmitis. In: Fraunfelder FT, Roy FH, Randall J, eds. *Current ocular therapy.* Philadelphia: WB Saunders, 2000:11–12.
21. Suh DW, Pulido JS. *Bacillus* species infections. In: Fraunfelder FT, Roy FH, Randall J, eds. *Current ocular therapy.* Philadelphia: WB Saunders, 2000:12–14.
22. Miller JM, Hair JG, Hebert M, et al. Fulminating bacteremia and pneumonia due to *Bacillus cereus*. *J Clin Microbiol* 1997;35:504–507.
23. Bryce EA, Smith JA, Tweeddale M, et al. Dissemination of *Bacillus cereus* in an intensive care unit. *Infect Control Hosp Epidemiol* 1993;14:459.
24. Weller PF, Nicholson A, Braslow N. The spectrum of *Bacillus* bacteremias in heroin addicts. *Arch Intern Med* 1979;139:293–294.
25. Blue SR, Singh VR, Saubolle MA. *Bacillus licheniformis* bacteremia: five cases associated with indwelling catheters. *Clin Infect Dis* 1995;20:629–633.
26. Cotton DJ, Gill VJ, Marshall DJ, et al. Clinical features and therapeutic interventions in 17 cases of *Bacillus* bacteremia in an immunosuppressed patient population. *J Clin Microbiol* 1987;25:672.
27. Banerjee C, Bustamante CI, Wharton R, et al. *Bacillus* infections in patients with cancer. *Arch Intern Med* 1988;148:1769.
28. Zinner SH. Changing epidemiology of infections in patients with neutropenia and cancer: emphasis on gram-positive and resistant bacteria. *Clin Infect Dis* 1999;29:490–494.

29. Akesson A, Hedstrom SA, Ripa T. *Bacillus cereus*: a significant pathogen in postoperative and post-traumatic wounds on orthopaedic wards. *Scand J Infect Dis* 1991;23:71–77.
30. Wong MT, Dolan MJ. Significant infections due to *Bacillus* species following abrasions associated with vehicle-related trauma. *Clin Infect Dis* 1992;15:855–857.
31. Schricker ME, Thompson GH, Schreiber JR. Osteomyelitis due to *Bacillus cereus* in an adolescent: case report and review. *Clin Infect Dis* 1994;18:863–867.

CHAPTER 190

Listeria monocytogenes

Claire Broome, Robert Pinner, Anne Schuchat, and John G. Bartlett

Listeria monocytogenes has been recognized as a human pathogen since 1929, but food-borne outbreaks and ensuing concern about food safety have brought this bacterium into the spotlight. An intracellular pathogen, *L. monocytogenes* has provided a classic model for investigating cell-mediated immunity. Comprehensive reviews of the epidemiology (1) and pathogenesis (2) of listeriosis have been published.

CHARACTERISTICS OF THE PATHOGEN

Taxonomic work has demonstrated that the genus *Listeria* is located in the *Clostridium* sub-branch, which also includes the genera *Staphylococcus*, *Streptococcus*, and *Lactobacillus* (3). The genus *Listeria* comprises six species: *L. monocytogenes*, *Listeria innocua*, *Listeria ivanovii* (subspecies *ivanovii* and *londoniensis*), *Listeria welshimeri*, and *Listeria seeligeri* are genetically closely related to one another, whereas *Listeria grayii* stands apart. Virtually all human disease is caused by *L. monocytogenes*; rare cases of human disease caused by *L. ivanovii*, *L. seeligeri*, and *L. welshimeri* have been reported.

Listeria organisms are gram-positive, non–spore-forming rods that are aerobic and facultatively anaerobic. The organisms are 0.4 to 0.5 μm in diameter and 0.5 to 2.0 μm long. In older cultures, filaments up to 20 μm or more may develop; some cells in older cultures may lose the ability to retain the Gram stain. *Listeria* organisms have one to five peritrichous flagella, which produce a "tumbling" motility in cultures grown at 20° to 25°C and a characteristic "umbrella" below the surface of motility medium. The organisms grow readily on the usual bacteriologic media for isolations from sterile sites, although they do not grow on selective media typically used to isolate agents causing diarrhea from stool cultures, which inhibit growth of gram-positive bacteria such as *Listeria*. They grow best at neutral to slightly alkaline pH but die at pH below 5.5. *Listeria* species grow optimally between 30° and 37°C but are capable of growth at the wide range of 1° to 45°C. The ability of these bacteria to grow better than other bacteria at low temperatures formed the basis for cold enrichment, a method now mainly of historic interest for isolating *Listeria* from nonsterile sites, foods, or environmental specimens. A variety of selective media and techniques have been developed and are currently used to enhance the yield of *Listeria* from nonsterile sites (3).

Colonies of *L. monocytogenes* on blood-free agar have a characteristic blue-green sheen when viewed in obliquely transmitted light. On blood agar, *L. monocytogenes*, as well as *L. ivanovii* and *L. seeligeri*, shows β-hemolysis.

Biochemical features of *L. monocytogenes* include catalase positivity, oxidase negativity, fermentative metabolism, methyl red positivity, and Voges-Proskauer reaction positivity. The CAMP test (named after the original investigators who described the test: Christie, Atkins, and Munch-Petersen) can be used to distinguish among the hemolysis patterns produced by the various species of *Listeria* (4). Table 190.1 lists biochemical characteristics of the species of *Listeria* (3).

Strains of *L. monocytogenes* can be classified by several methods. A serotyping scheme based on both cellular O and flagellar H antigens defines 13 different serotypes; however, because only three of these (1/2a, 1/2b, and 4b) account for about 95% of all human cases of listeriosis, serotyping is of limited value for epidemiologic studies. Other, more discriminating methods have been devised to further classify *Listeria*, including phage typing, multilocus enzyme electrophoretic analysis, subtyping based on patterns of endonuclease restriction of chromosomal or ribosomal DNA, and polymerase chain reaction–based typing. Because many *L. monocytogenes* isolates were not typeable, phage typing has been of limited utility for epidemiologic studies. Several studies that illuminated the role of foods in outbreaks and sporadic cases of listeriosis have used multilocus enzyme electrophoretic analysis to compare clinical and food isolates of *L. monocytogenes* (1,5).

ECOLOGY

L. monocytogenes is distributed widely in the environment. It is a well-known cause of disease among sheep and cattle, in which it causes septic abortion and "circling" disease (basilar meningoencephalitis). Many mammalian and avian species can harbor the organism, and it has been recovered from dust, soil, water, sewage, animal feed, and silage. *L. monocytogenes* has been isolated from many different foods, including meats, vegetables, seafood, and dairy products. In addition, the organism inhabits the gastrointestinal tract of 1% to 5% or more of asymptomatic humans (6,7). The organism contains a surface protein, internalin, that binds to E-cadherin of enterocytes. This interaction appears necessary for translocation from the gut and may be important in penetration of the blood-brain barrier and the fetoplacental barrier (8). Exposure appears to be extensive, but disease is largely dependent on the integrity of the immune system and possibly on inoculum size (9).

EPIDEMIOLOGY

Listeriosis tends to occur in well-defined risk groups—pregnant women, neonates, and immunocompromised adults—but the disease also occasionally occurs in persons who have no predisposing underlying condition.

A multistate active surveillance project conducted by the Centers for Disease Control and Prevention has provided information on trends in listeriosis in the United States (10). Through regular contact with all acute care hospital laboratories in an aggregate population of 19 million to 34 million to identify bacteriologically confirmed cases, this investigation estimated that the annual incidence of listeriosis in the United States declined from 7.9 cases per million in 1989 (or 1,965 cases and 481 deaths) to 4.4 cases per million in 1993 (or 1,092 cases and 248 deaths). Of more than 600 invasive listeriosis cases identified through this surveillance system, 32% occurred in association with pregnancy, affecting pregnant women, newborns, or both. No pregnant women died from listeriosis, but 22% of pregnancy-associated

TABLE 190.1. Characteristics of *Listeria* Species

Characteristic	*L. grayi*	*L. innocua*	*L. ivanovii* subspecies *ivanovii*	*L. ivanovii* subspecies *londoniensis*	*L. monocytogenes*	*L. seeligeri*	*L. welshimeri*
β-hemolysis	−	−	++	++	+	+	−
AMP test reaction							
Staphylococcus aureus	−	−	−	−	+	+	−
Rhodococcus equi	−	−	+	+	−	−	−
Acid production from							
Mannitol	+	−	−	−	−	−	−
α-Methyl-D-mannoside	+	+	−	−	+	−	+
L-rhaxnnose	V	V	−	−	+	−	V
Soluble starch	+	−	−	−	−	−	−
D-xylose	−	−	+	+	−	ND	ND
Ribose	V	−	+	+	−	+	+
N-acetyl-β-D-mannosamine			−	+			
Hippurate hydrolysis	−	+	+	+	+	ND	ND
Reduction of nitrate	−	−	−	−	−	ND	ND
Pathogenicity for mice	−	−	+	?	+	−	−
Serotype	S	4ab, US, 6a, 6b	5	5	1/2a, 1/2b, 1/2c, 3a, 3b, 3c, 4a, 4ab, 4b, 4c, 4d, 4e, 7	1/2a, 1/2b, 1/2c, US, 4b, 4d, 6b	1/2b, 4c, 6a, bb, US

+, ≥90% of strains are positive; −, ≥90% of strains are negative; ND, not determined; V, variable; US, undesignated serotype; S, specific. Usually a wide zone or multiple zones.

Adapted from Swaminathan B, Rocourt J, Bille J. *Listeria*. In: Murray PR, Baron EJ, Pfaller MA, et al., eds. *Manual of clinical microbiology*, 6th ed. Washington, DC: ASM Press, 1995:344, with permission.

cases resulted in either fetal loss or neonatal death. Among nonperinatal cases, 28% were fatal.

Large studies in the United States, Europe, and Australia demonstrated that the vast majority of patients with nonperinatal listeriosis have immunosuppressive conditions (9,11–13). A summary of 1,808 reported cases from 1967 to 1999 showed that 74% of the patients were immunosuppressed (9). The most common predisposing conditions include immunosuppressive therapy, malignancy, diabetes mellitus, organ transplantation, and in some populations acquired immunodeficiency syndrome. Although listeriosis is not common among patients with acquired immunodeficiency syndrome, such persons had approximately 280 times the risk for listeriosis of the general population in the era before highly active antiretroviral therapy (HAART) (11).

Geographic differences have been observed in the incidence of perinatal listeriosis within the United States (10,11). The rate of perinatal listeriosis in Los Angeles County has been consistently higher than the rate in other surveillance areas. This geographic variation may reflect differences in dietary habits, host susceptibility, or enhanced diagnosis by obstetric providers in Los Angeles. The Centers for Disease Control and Prevention surveillance project did not find clear evidence of a seasonal pattern, although other reports have observed a peak of listeriosis during the summer months.

Investigations of several outbreaks of listeriosis have enhanced understanding of the epidemiology of this disease (Table 190.2). In 1981, an outbreak in Nova Scotia, Canada, was caused by locally produced coleslaw. Investigation of this outbreak first established listeriosis as a food-borne illness (14). The epidemiologic investigation of a 1983 outbreak of listeriosis in Massachusetts implicated a particular brand of pasteurized milk (15). This controversial finding prompted several studies that concluded that properly performed pasteurization is adequate to kill *L. monocytogenes*, but products can be contaminated after pasteurization or if pasteurization is not done properly. The largest outbreak in the United States involved 142 cases in Los Angeles in 1985, the result of consumption of Mexican-style cheese made from contaminated milk that was not adequately pasteurized. Recall of the implicated product ended the epidemic (16). Several large outbreaks in Europe were associated with ready-to-eat foods: soft cheese, paté, and pork tongue in jelly (17–19). One outbreak in Italy resulted in gastroenteritis in 1,566 of 2,189 (72%) exposed by consumption of a contaminated corn salad; 292 (19%) were hospitalized (20).

TABLE 190.2. Major Food-Borne Outbreaks of Invasive Listeriosis

Date	Place	No. of cases (deaths)[a]	Implicated vehicle	Reference
1981	Nova Scotia, Canada	41 (18)	Coleslaw	14
1983	Massachusetts, United States	49 (14)	Pasteurized milk	15
1985	Los Angeles, California, United States	142 (48)	Soft Mexican-style cheese	16
1983–1987	Switzerland	122 (34)	Soft cheese	17
1988–1989	United Kingdom	NA	Paté	18
1992	France	279 (86)	Pork tongue in jelly	19

[a]Total number of listeriosis deaths includes stillbirths and spontaneous abortions. NA, not available.

These investigations confirmed that *L. monocytogenes* organisms can cause epidemic food-borne disease, but the role of foods in sporadic listeriosis has been of considerable interest. Epidemiologic and microbiologic studies implicated uncooked hot dogs, undercooked chicken, soft cheeses, and food purchased from delicatessen counters as causes of sporadic listeriosis (5,11,21). Further evidence was provided by a report documenting the isolation of the same rare enzyme type of *L. monocytogenes* from the blood of a patient, an opened package of turkey franks in her refrigerator, and an unopened package of the same brand of turkey franks purchased at a local store (22). Evaluation of foods collected from patients with listeriosis suggested that foods that are ready to eat, heavily contaminated, or contaminated with serotype 4b are more often associated with cases than are other contaminated foods (5).

On the basis of well-documented cases of food-borne listeriosis, the incubation period between ingestion of contaminated food and bacteremia may be much longer than that for other food-borne illnesses (median of 3 weeks, range of 11–70 days) (13,23), although some outbreaks indicate an incubation period of only about 24 hours (20). The long incubation period sometimes encountered may make it difficult to identify specific food vehicles responsible for sporadic cases. The infectious dose for this organism is not known, and host susceptibility probably alters the number of organisms necessary to produce symptoms. Human feeding experiments are not appropriate for *L. monocytogenes*, given the high mortality associated with infection.

A substantial proportion of listeriosis is due to food-borne transmission, but other modes of transmission occur. Newborns can acquire the organism transplacentally from bacteremic mothers or during passage through an infected birth canal. Some reports have suggested cross-infection in neonatal nurseries (24), and one common-source nosocomial outbreak was caused by contaminated mineral oil used for infant baths (25). Cutaneous, nonsystemic infections have occurred in veterinarians and ranchers who have delivered infected and aborted calves and in workers who have handled infected poultry.

PATHOGENESIS

The pathogenesis of listeriosis involves a complex interaction of host immunologic response, organism factors, and dose. The association of listeriosis with underlying malignancies and immunosuppressive therapy such as corticosteroids implies that cell-mediated immune function plays a key role in the immune response to *L. monocytogenes*. Mackaness (26) used a mouse model of listeriosis in an early demonstration of the phenomenon of cell-mediated immunity to this intracellular pathogen, and later experiments suggested that helper T cells, suppressor cells, and macrophages all figure in the cell-mediated immune response to *Listeria*. Other murine experiments have shown that genetically determined characteristics, age, nutritional status, and pregnancy all affect susceptibility to *L. monocytogenes*.

Listeriosis is one of several diseases that are more common or more severe during pregnancy. The phenomenon may represent an immune compromise that permits tolerance of the fetus and diminishes cell-mediated resistance to certain infections. Whether this immunologic alteration is systemic, local, or both remains uncertain.

Humoral immunity plays a limited role in establishing immunity to *Listeria*. Both immunoglobulin M (absent in newborns) and classical complement activity (low in newborns) appear to be necessary for efficient opsonization of *L. monocytogenes*, suggesting possible mechanisms for the susceptibility of newborns to this infection (27).

Experimental evidence supports the epidemiologic conclusion that *Listeria* organisms are transmitted by the food-borne route. Listeriosis can be induced in laboratory animals by oral feeding of pathogenic *L. monocytogenes* (28). Experiments using a rat model of food-borne *Listeria* infection found that cimetidine significantly lowered the infective dose of *L. monocytogenes*, supporting an association found in a few epidemiologic studies of listeriosis and decreased gastric acidity (29). *Listeria* has also been shown to invade and even multiply in enterocytes, supporting its role as an enteroinvasive pathogen.

Applications of newer technology, particularly transposon mutagenesis and tissue culture models of infection, have enhanced understanding of the cell biology of *Listeria* infections and identified several potential virulence factors (2). After entry into host cells, *Listeria* organisms escape from host cell vacuoles and multiply in the cytoplasm. Listeriolysin O, the best characterized of the molecular virulence determinants of *L. monocytogenes*, appears to participate in the dissolution of host vacuoles. Once free in the cell cytoplasm, the bacteria are soon surrounded by actin filaments, which mediate intracytoplasmic movement and propel them toward the cell surface, where they protrude in pseudopod-like structures. These structures are apparently recognized and phagocytosed by a neighboring cell; this direct cell-to-cell spread reflects at the cellular level the limited role humoral factors play in immunity to *Listeria* infection.

CLINICAL MANIFESTATIONS

Listeriosis During Pregnancy

Pregnant women generally have mild clinical illness, but maternal infection can result in intrauterine infection, spontaneous abortion, and neonatal infection (Table 190.3). The most common clinical picture in pregnant women is an influenza-like illness with fever and myalgias, sometimes accompanied by gastrointestinal symptoms. The organism may grow in blood cultures. Listeriosis during pregnancy can cause amnionitis, premature labor, premature rupture of membranes, and stillbirth. Infants with no clinical infection have been born to women treated for listeriosis during pregnancy, suggesting that listeriosis does not invariably affect the fetus and that treatment of maternal cases may prevent adverse pregnancy outcomes.

Listeriosis in Neonates

In contrast to the mild clinical syndrome that usually occurs in pregnant women, in neonates listeriosis can be a serious and often fatal illness (9). As with disease caused by group B streptococci, two clinical forms of neonatal listeriosis are recognized: early-onset and late-onset disease. Early-onset disease generally occurs in infants infected *in utero* from bacteremic mothers, whereas infection in late-onset disease may result from passage through an infected birth canal or nosocomial transmission. Early-onset disease usually presents as sepsis rather than meningitis. It often occurs in preterm infants, perhaps causing prematurity. Classically, widely disseminated microabscesses are noted, to which the term *granulomatosis infantisepticum* has been applied. No findings are specific for neonatal sepsis caused by *Listeria*, but papular skin lesions may occur. Late-onset disease tends to occur in full-term infants of uncomplicated pregnancies. These infants are usually healthy at birth, and symptoms develop several days to weeks after birth. In late neonatal listeriosis, the clinical syndrome is more likely to be meningitis than sepsis. The mortality rate is lower than for early-onset disease.

TABLE 190.3.   Syndromes Associated with Infection with *Listeria monocytogenes*

Population	Clinical presentation	Diagnosis	Predisposing conditions or circumstances
Pregnant women	Fever, ± myalgias ± diarrhea Preterm delivery Abortion/stillbirth	Blood culture ± amniotic fluid culture	
Newborns			
<7 days old	Sepsis, pneumonia	Blood, cerebrospinal fluid cultures	Prematurity
≥7 days old	Meningitis, sepsis		
Nonpregnant adults	Sepsis, meningitis, encephalitis, focal infections	Culture of blood, cerebrospinal fluid, or other normally sterile site	Immunosuppressed, elderly
Healthy adults	? Diarrhea and fever	Stool culture in selective enrichment broth	? High inoculum ? Unusual strains

Nonperinatal Listeriosis

Nonperinatal listeriosis is generally an infection of patients immunocompromised by underlying illness or immunosuppressive therapy, accounting for 74% of reported cases (9), but some patients who develop listeriosis have no apparent immunocompromising conditions. Sepsis and meningitis are the usual clinical presentations of nonperinatal listeriosis (9). Although meningitis has been reported to be the most common form of listeriosis in adults, bacteremia without meningitis was more common in the Centers for Disease Control and Prevention active surveillance project (30). Patients with bacteremia generally have fever but may have a variety of symptoms, including myalgias and gastrointestinal complaints. No symptoms or findings are specific for *L. monocytogenes* bacteremia. Central nervous system findings such as tremors, seizures, ataxia, and fluctuating consciousness seem to be characteristic of *Listeria* meningitis, however. Unlike other common bacterial pathogens that cause pyogenic meningitis, *Listeria* more commonly causes brain abscess, especially subcortical brain abscess with bacteremia (31). In *Listeria* meningitis, the cerebrospinal fluid is abnormal, but a wide range of values may occur for the cerebrospinal fluid white cell count and differential, glucose value, and protein level. Gram stain is positive in only about 40% and may be misinterpreted as *S. pneumoniae*, so the cerebrospinal fluid profile cannot be easily used to distinguish *Listeria* meningitis from meningitis caused by other bacteria. Monocytosis is not a characteristic feature of listeriosis. As noted, *Listeria* causes other infections of the central nervous system, such as meningoencephalitis, cerebritis, brainstem abscesses, and spinal cord abscesses. Brainstem encephalitis (rhombencephalitis) is characterized by asymmetric cranial nerve palsies, cerebellar signs, motor or sensory loss, and impaired consciousness (31,32). *Listeria* endocarditis resembles other forms of subacute endocarditis; it usually occurs in patients who previously had valvular disease. A variety of focal infections with *L. monocytogenes* have been reported, including endophthalmitis, septic arthritis, osteomyelitis, liver abscesses, cholecystitis, hepatitis, peritonitis, pleuropulmonary infection, and arterial infections. These collectively account for only about 4% of reported cases (9).

Mild Gastrointestinal Illness

L. monocytogenes may cause, like other food-borne pathogens, a gastrointestinal syndrome characterized by fever, nausea, diarrhea, and abdominal pain (20). However, the role of *L. monocytogenes* in acute gastrointestinal illness is difficult to prove because the routine stool cultures, which use *selective media* that inhibit the growth of gram-positive organisms such as *Listeria*, are not adequate for isolation of the organism. In addition, asymptomatic gastrointestinal carriage is well described (6,7). Diarrheal illness that occurs in healthy adults within 2 days of exposure to heavily contaminated foods, and the same strain of *L. monocytogenes*, confirms this association (20).

DIAGNOSIS

The diagnosis of listeriosis should be suspected with (a) neonatal sepsis or meningitis; (b) meningitis or parenchymal brain infection in patients with compromised cell-mediated immunity or over 50 years of age; (c) subcortical brain abscess; (d) fever during pregnancy; (e) blood or spinal fluid with diphtheroids or gram-positive bacilli; or (f) food-borne outbreak with negative routine cultures. A confirmed diagnosis depends on isolation of the organism from a normally sterile site such as blood or cerebrospinal fluid. Because *L. monocytogenes* may be mistaken for diphtheroid contaminants with Gram stain, complete bacteriologic evaluation is important. From specimens collected from normally sterile sites, *Listeria* grows readily in routine media, and culture results are usually positive within 36 hours. Isolation of *L. monocytogenes* from sites containing other flora may pose problems, however. Selective enrichment media permit isolation of *L. monocytogenes* from stool cultures. Methods using fluorescent antibody reagents and DNA probes coupled with polymerase chain reaction technology may prove useful in identifying *L. monocytogenes* in some specimens. Serologic tests have been neither sufficiently sensitive nor specific to be useful for routine diagnosis in clinical practice. However, serologic assays for antibody to listeriolysin O (33) may be useful in some epidemiologic investigations and have been used to suggest the diagnosis in culture-negative central nervous system infection (34).

TREATMENT

The optimal antibiotic therapy of human listeriosis has not been defined by controlled clinical trials. The most commonly recommended therapy is ampicillin; some evidence suggests synergy with the addition of an aminoglycoside, and this combination is often used. Penicillin may be comparably effective (3,31,35,36). Treatment failures are common with cephalosporins, which should not be used to treat listeriosis. *Listeria* organisms are susceptible *in vitro* to a number of commonly available antibiotics, except cephalosporins, but clinical experience is limited (37). For penicillin-allergic patients, trimethoprim-sulfamethoxazole may be useful; this combination demonstrates bactericidal activity against *Listeria*, and there have been reports of its effectiveness. Other drugs, including erythromycin, tetracycline, and rifampin, have been suggested. Information is inadequate to judge the use of the newer macrolide antibiotics in listeriosis. Case reports on the use of vancomycin in listeriosis have included both treatment successes and failures. The outcome of antibiotic therapy depends on the severity of the infection; therapy is made difficult because listeriosis often occurs in immunocompromised hosts and because, as an intracellular pathogen, the organism may be relatively inaccessible to antibiotics. The mortality is high for listeriosis in its two common forms: neonatal infection and CNS infection in the compromised host. Among all food-borne illnesses, *Listeria* is one of the least frequently identified pathogens, accounting for less than 0.1% of cases, but second only to *Salmonella* in causing 27% of all food-borne–related deaths (38).

Optimal duration of therapy also remains uncertain. A prudent treatment course is 2 weeks for listeriosis in pregnancy; 2 to 3 weeks for neonatal listeriosis; 2 to 4 weeks for adults with bacteremia; and longer for complicated infections such as meningitis, parenchymal central nervous system infections, or endocarditis.

PREVENTION

Because *L. monocytogenes* is commonly found in the environment, avoiding exposure to the organism is difficult. For persons at increased risk, however (including those who are pregnant or immunocompromised), several dietary measures can be taken to minimize risk. Such measures include thorough cooking of foods of animal origin, avoiding foods made from unpasteurized milk, and avoiding cross-contamination when handling raw foods of animal origin and foods that are ready to eat without further cooking. Pregnant women and immunosuppressed persons may also choose to avoid soft cheeses, paté, and other foods that have been epidemiologically linked with listeriosis, such as ready-to-eat processed meats with long shelf lives. Currently, U.S. regulatory agencies recommend recalls when *L. monocytogenes* is detected in processed foods that are available for consumption without further cooking. Food industry approaches to minimizing the risk for food-borne listeriosis, introduced in response to regulatory policy, are temporally related to a decline in the incidence of listeriosis in the United States (10).

REFERENCES

1. Schuchat A, Swaminathan B, Broome CV. Epidemiology of human listeriosis. *Clin Microbiol Rev* 1991;4:169–183.
2. Portnoy DA, Chakraborty T, Goebel W, et al. Molecular determinants of *Listeria monocytogenes* pathogenesis. *Infect Immun* 1992;60:1263–1267.
3. Lorber B. Listeriosis. *Clin Infect Dis* 1997;24:1–11.
4. Seeliger HPR, Jones D. Genus *Listeria* Pirie 1940, 383. In: Sneath PHA, Mair NS, Sharpe ME, et al., eds. *Bergey's manual of systematic bacteriology*, Vol. 2. Baltimore: Williams & Wilkins, 1986:1235–1245.
5. Pinner RW, Schuchat A, Swaminathan B, et al. Role of foods in sporadic listeriosis. II: Microbiologic and epidemiologic investigation. *JAMA* 1992;267:2046–2050.
6. Kampelmacher EH, van Noorle Jansen LM. Isolation of *Listeria monocytogenes* from feces of clinically healthy humans and animals. *Zentralbl Bakteriol* 1969;211:353–359.
7. Schuchat A, Deaver KA, Hayes PS, et al. Gastrointestinal carriage of *Listeria monocytogenes* in household contacts of patients with listeriosis. *J Infect Dis* 1993;167:1261–1262.
8. Lecuit M, Vandomael-Poumin S, Lefort J, et al. A transgenic model for listeriosis: role of internalin in crossing the intestinal barrier. *Science* 2001;292:1722–1725.
9. Siegman-Igra Y, Levin R, Weinberger M, et al. *Listeria monocytogenes* infection in Israel and review of cases worldwide. *Emerg Infect Dis* 2002;8:305–310.
10. Tappero JW, Schuchat A, Deaver KA, et al. Reduction in the incidence of human listeriosis in the United States: effectiveness of prevention efforts. *JAMA* 1995;273:1118–1122.
11. Schuchat A, Deaver K, Wenger JD, et al. Role of foods in sporadic listeriosis. I: Case-control study of dietary risk factors. *JAMA* 1992;267:2041–2045.
12. Skogberg K, Syrjanen J, Jahkola M, et al. Clinical presentation and outcome of listeriosis in patients with and without immunosuppressive therapy. *Clin Infect Dis* 1992;14:815–821.
13. Paul ML, Dwyer DE, Chow C, et al. Listeriosis—a review of eighty-four cases. *Med J Aust* 1994;160:489–493.
14. Schlech WF, Lavigne PM, Bortolussi RA, et al. Epidemic listeriosis—evidence for transmission by food. *N Engl J Med* 1983;308:203–206.
15. Fleming DW, Cochi SL, MacDonald KL, et al. Pasteurized milk as a vehicle of infection in an outbreak of listeriosis. *N Engl J Med* 1985;312:404–407.
16. Linnan MJ, Mascola L, Lou XD, et al. Epidemic listeriosis associated with Mexican-style cheese. *N Engl J Med* 1988;319:823–828.
17. Bille J. Epidemiology of human listeriosis in Europe, with special reference to the Swiss outbreak. In: Miller AJ, Smith JL, Somkuti GA, eds. *Foodborne listeriosis*. Amsterdam: Elsevier Science, 1990:71–74.
18. McLauchlin J, Hall SM, Velani SK, et al. Human listeriosis and paté: a possible association. *BMJ* 1991;303:773–775.
19. Goulet V, Lepoutre A, Rocourt J, et al.: Épidémie de listeriose en France: Bilan final et résultats de l'enquête épidémiologique. *Bull Epidemiol Hebd* 1993;39:13–14.
20. Aureli P, Fiorucci Gc, Caroli D, et al. An outbreak of febrile gastroenteritis associated with corn contaminated by *Listeria monocytogenes*. *N Engl J Med* 2000;342:1236–1241.
21. Schwartz B, Ciesielski CA, Broome CV, et al. Association of sporadic listeriosis with consumption of uncooked hotdogs and undercooked chicken. *Lancet* 1988;2:779–782.
22. Centers for Disease Control and Prevention. Listeriosis associated with consumption of turkey franks. *MMWR* 1989;38:267–268.
23. Riedo FX, Pinner RW, Tosca ML, et al. A point-source foodborne listeriosis outbreak: documented incubation period and possible mild illness. *J Infect Dis* 1994;170:693–696.
24. McLauchlin J, Audurier A, Taylor AG. Aspects of the epidemiology of human *Listeria monocytogenes* infections in Britain 1967–1984; the use of serotyping and phage typing. *J Med Microbiol* 1986;22:367–377.
25. Schuchat A, Lizano C, Broome CV, et al. Outbreak of neonatal listeriosis associated with mineral oil. *Pediatr Infect Dis J* 1991;10:183–189.
26. Mackaness GB. Cellular resistance to infection. *J Exp Med* 1962;116:381–406.
27. Bortolussi R, Issekutz A, Faulkner G. Opsonization of *Listeria monocytogenes* type 4b by human adult and newborn sera. *Infect Immun* 1986;52:493–498.
28. Schlech WF 3d. New perspectives on the gastrointestinal mode of transmission in invasive *Listeria monocytogenes* infection. *Clin Invest Med* 1984;7:321–324.
29. Schlech WF III, Chase DP, Badley A. A model of food-borne *Listeria monocytogenes* infection in the Sprague-Dawley rat using gastric inoculation: development and effect of gastric acidity on infective dose. *Int J Food Microbiol* 1993;18:15–24.
30. Gellin BG, Broome CV, Bibb WF, et al. The epidemiology of listeriosis in the United States—1986. *Am J Epidemiol* 1991;133:392–401.
31. Mylonakis E, Hohmann EL, Calderwood SB. Central nervous system infection with *Listeria monocytogenes*: 33 years' experience at a general hospital and review of 776 episodes from the literature. *Medicine* 1998;77:313–336.
32. Armstrong RW, Fung PC. Brainstem encephalitis (rhombencephalitis) due to *Listeria monocytogenes*: case report and review. *Clin Infect Dis* 1993;16:689–702.
33. Berche P, Reich KA, Bonnichon M, et al. Detection of antilisteriolysin O for serodiagnosis of human listeriosis. *Lancet* 1990;335:624–627.
34. Gaillard JL, Beretti JL, Boulot-Tolle M, et al. Serological evidence for culture-negative listeriosis of central nervous system [Letter]. *Lancet* 1992;340:560.
35. McLauchlin J, Audurier A, Taylor AG. Treatment failure and recurrent human listeriosis. *J Antimicrob Chemother* 1991;27:851–857.
36. Cherubin CE, Appleman MD, Heseltine PNR, et al. Epidemiological spectrum and current treatment of listeriosis. *Rev Infect Dis* 1991;13:1108–1114.
37. Hof H. Therapeutic activities of antibiotics in listeriosis. *Infection* 1991;19:229–233.
38. Mead PS, Slutsker L, Dietz V, et al. Food-related illness and death in the United States. *Emerg Infect Dis* 1999;5:607–625.

CHAPTER 191
Erysipelothrix rhusiopathiae

Judith L. Nerad

Erysipelothrix rhusiopathiae is a Gram-positive bacillus that causes occupationally related skin infections (erysipeloid) and, rarely, septicemia in humans. It is a significant cause of swine morbidity (swine erysipelas). The disease was first clinically described in butchers by Fox and Baker (in 1873), who named it erythema serpens (1). Koch (in 1880) first isolated the organism from infected mouse blood and named it *Erysipelothrix muriseptica*. Pasteur and Thullier (in 1883) demonstrated that swine could be immunized with a strain of *E. muriseptica,* which would prevent erysipelas in swine. Löffler (in 1886) definitively identified *Erysipelothrix* as the causative agent of erysipelas in swine. Rosenbach (in 1909) was the first to identify *E. muriseptica* as the pathogen responsible for the human skin disease and named it erysipeloid. He made the association among the human, swine, and mouse diseases, stating, however, that the organisms were different strains. Rickman (in 1909) did not concur but thought that the strains were not sufficiently different on morphologic, cultural, or serologic grounds. This was later confirmed by Kohl (in 1940) (2).

CHARACTERISTICS OF THE PATHOGEN

E. rhusiopathiae is a gram-positive, non–spore-forming bacillus that is nonmotile, is facultatively anaerobic, and has no capsule (3,4). However, evidence in mice suggests that a capsule may play a role in virulence (5). It is easily decolorized with Gram stain and may appear gram negative with gram-positive granules or beads. Rods are usually 0.2 to 0.4 μm in diameter and 0.8 to 2.5 μm long. They can occur singly or in short chains and may form filaments up to 60 μm long. Colonies grow on sheep blood agar (not human blood agar) and form small, non-pigmented, transparent colonies that may be smooth or rough. Smooth colonies are often more coccobacillary or coryneform, whereas rough colonies are often larger, more beaded, and associated with long filaments. *E. rhusiopathiae* causes narrow zones of α-hemolysis on blood agar. Optimal growth temperature is 30° to 37°C. The organisms are killed by heating for 15 minutes at 60°C but tolerate cold (35 days at 3°C). The organisms prefer alkaline pH; are able to be grown aerobically or anaerobically; and grow better in 5% serum, low oxygen tension, and enhanced carbon dioxide environments. *E. rhusiopathiae* tolerates a high-salt environment and can survive in seawater. Specific nutrients (riboflavin and oleic acid, several amino acids, and glucose) are necessary for growth. On gelatin stab culture at 22° to 28°C, *E. rhusiopathiae* forms a characteristic "pipe cleaner" or "test-tube brush" growth pattern.

E. rhusiopathiae is catalase negative, oxidase negative, and weakly fermentative (Table 191.1). The organisms produce acid from glucose and lactose within 48 hours, but not galactose and fructose. Most strains produce hydrogen sulfide on triple sugar iron agar, a differentiating characteristic from other gram-positive rods. Serologically, there are heat- and acid-stable type-specific antigens and heat-labile antigens. Twenty-three serotypes are described, types 1 and 2 being most common in swine erysipelas (6). These antigens are thought to be peptidoglycans (7).

There are two species in the genus, *E. rhusiopathiae* and *Erysipelothrix tonsillarum,* and strains can be heterogeneous (6,8–11). Thus far, only *E. rhusiopathiae* has been reported as a pathogen in humans. *E. rhusiopathiae* can easily be confused with other gram-positive bacilli (3,12). Major differentiating factors can be found in Table 191.1.

EPIDEMIOLOGY

E. rhusiopathiae is ubiquitous in nature (1,2,13). It is associated with many types of animals (mammals, birds, fish, insects), organic matter, and water. It causes disease most commonly in pigs, and its prevention and treatment have a major economic impact on industry relevant to hog marketing (7). In humans, the major manifestation of *E. rhusiopathiae* infection is erysipeloid; however, septicemia and endocarditis are also seen. More common names for erysipeloid include whale finger, seal finger (14), speck finger, blubber finger, and fish handler's disease (15). The general route of transmission in humans is thought to be by direct contact with contaminated animals, animal products including leather (16), or soil with a break in the skin. Veterinarians, abattoir workers, fish handlers, farmers, butchers, poultry workers, and housewives handling infected meat or fish are most commonly exposed, but cases have been described in people without known exposures; males predominate over females, probably because of the occupational exposure. Reports of two patients suggest oral transmission: (a) a woman with *E. rhusiopathiae* endocarditis whose consumption of infected pork was her only exposure risk (2), and (b) a woman with a history of ethanol abuse and subsequent pancreatitis with persistent *E. rhusiopathiae* bacteremia whose consumption of shellfish was her only exposure risk (17). In humans, the incubation period is 1 to 4 days, rarely up to 1 week (18). The organism can persist in the environment (3,19), remaining viable for 5 to 15 days in water and for weeks to 3 months in salted or pickled bacon or smoked ham; it has been grown after 9 months in a buried carcass. One study from Lund, Sweden, reported isolation of *E. rhusiopathiae* from 30% to 60% of retail samples of pork, cod, and herring (20).

CLINICAL MANIFESTATIONS

In humans, *E. rhusiopathiae* manifests itself primarily as a skin disease. However, systemic disease has also been reported (1,2,13,14,21).

Erysipeloid of Rosenbach

These skin lesions are the most common clinical presentation of *E. rhusiopathiae* infection (22). They are characterized by a purplish red, indurated lesion, usually on the hands or fingers, that probably represents the site of inoculation 1 to 3 days prior. The margins are slightly raised and sharp and spread peripherally with central clearing. The area can be swollen, and contiguous lesions may occur despite improvement in the initial area. Hemorrhagic vesicles may be present. Pitting edema and suppuration are rare, and their presence serves to differentiate *E. rhusiopathiae* infection from other cutaneous lesions (cellulitis, erythema multiforme, diphtheria, and anthrax). Lesions may be pruritic or burning and painful. Arthralgia in the area of the lesion occurs. Arthritis may occur concomitantly. Systemic symptoms, diffuse arthralgias, fever, lymphangitis, and regional lymphadenopathy are seen approximately 10% of the time.

TABLE 191.1. Major Morphologic and Biochemical Differentiating Factors Among Gram-Positive Rods

Factor	*Bacillus*	*Corynebacterium*	*Erysipelothrix*	*Lactobacillus*	*Listeria*
Quality					
Gram stain	Large rods, square ends with sports	Pleomorphic	Slender with filaments	Straight rods, few coccobacilli	Short rods with short chains
Rod diameter	$1–1.3 \times 3–10\ \mu m$	$0.5–1 \times 2–3\ \mu m$ in palisades	$0.2–0.5 \times 0.5–2.5\ \mu m$	$0.5–1.1 \times 2–3\ \mu m$	$0.4–0.5 \times 1–2\ \mu m$
Colony size	2 mm to several	0.5–1 mm	Rough >1 mm, or smooth 0.5–1 mm	<0.5 mm	0.5–1 mm
Spores	Yes	No	No	No	No
Motility	Usually	Usually	No	No	Yes (20°–25°C)
Hemolysis	Large zone of beta	Variable	Alpha	Usually alpha	Beta
Atmosphere requirement	Aerobic	Usually aerobic	Facultatively aerobic	Microaerophilic	Aerobic
Biochemistry					
Catalase	Positive	Variable	Negative	Negative	Positive
Oxidase	Positive	Negative	Negative	Negative	Negative
Hydrogen sulfide from triple sugar iron agar	Negative (usually)	Negative	Positive	Negative	Negative
Nitrate reduction	Variable	Variable	Negative	Negative	Positive
Neomycin	Resistant	Variable	Resistant	Resistant	Sensitive
Vancomycin	Sensitive	Sensitive (JK diphtheroids)	Resistant	Variable	Sensitive

A severe, diffuse cutaneous form occurs rarely. This is manifested by similar spreading violaceous lesions with central pallor. Diffuse vesicobullous lesions have also occurred. Patients have systemic symptoms (e.g., fever and lymphadenopathy); however, blood cultures are negative.

Septicemia and Endocarditis

Most cases of endocarditis have a documented history of appropriate contact with an infected animal (89%) or an erysipeloid lesion (36%) (14,21,23–25). Bacteremia and septic shock without endocarditis have also been reported (17,26–30).

In more than 75% of septicemic cases, acute or subacute bacterial endocarditis develops. Factors predisposing to this condition include a chronic debilitating disease, ethanol abuse (33%), an immunocompromised state (17%) (21), or intravenous drug abuse (31). The presence of valvular heart disease is less commonly a predisposing factor. Only 40% of *E. rhusiopathiae* endocarditis cases have preexisting valvular disease compared with 60% to 80% of all cases of endocarditis. The aortic valve is affected in about 60% of cases of *E. rhusiopathiae* endocarditis. The disease tends to be virulent, with complications such as aortic valve perforation, myocardial abscess, and heart failure. It is not uncommon for patients with *E. rhusiopathiae* endocarditis to require valve replacement. *E. rhusiopathiae* is the most common cause of native valve endocarditis caused by gram-positive bacilli. Prosthetic valve endocarditis with *E. rhusiopathiae* has also been reported (32,33).

Rare Complications

There are rare complications of *E. rhusiopathiae* infection that occur less than 1% of the time. These include diffuse cerebral involvement (34), intracranial brain abscess (35), optic neuritis (22), pulmonary infarction, probably from an infected intravascular source (36), pericarditis (37), valvular and myocardial abscesses (38), renal failure (39), septic bursitis (40), osseous necrosis (41), and chronic arthritis (18,22) and osteomyelitis (22).

DIAGNOSIS

Most cases of *E. rhusiopathiae* are diagnosed on the basis of clinical presentation and a history of exposure. Gram stain and culture of skin biopsy specimens yield a definitive diagnosis. Gram-positive rods growing in blood cultures may not be diphtheroids and should be further identified. Small α-hemolytic colonies growing on blood agar may be confused with *Streptococcus viridans*. Besides culturing techniques, identification of *E. rhusiopathiae* DNA by polymerase chain reaction techniques has allowed rapid detection of the organism, especially in commercial slaughterhouses (42).

TREATMENT AND PROPHYLAXIS

Penicillin is the drug of choice for treating *E. rhusiopathiae* infections (1,13,21). Minimum inhibitory concentrations and minimum bactericidal concentrations to penicillin are in the range of 0.0025 to 0.75 μg/mL. *E. rhusiopathiae* is generally susceptible to all classes of the penicillin family, cephalosporins, and clindamycin. It has variable sensitivity to erythromycin, chloramphenicol, and tetracycline (43). A new ketolide, telithromycin, may be an effective alternate therapy (44). It is notably resistant to vancomycin (minimum inhibitory concentration >25 μg/mL), aminoglycosides, sulfa derivatives, neomycin, and polymyxin (21,43). The minimum inhibitory concentrations of teicoplanin and daptomycin are better than that of vancomycin; however, the activity *in vitro* is poor (43). Although clinical data on the quinolones and *E. rhusiopathiae* infections are minimal, ofloxacin (200 mg orally twice daily) was successful in eradicating soft tissue infections (45), and ciprofloxacin has successfully been used to treat tricuspid valve endocarditis and pneumonia (23). Studies of *in vitro* susceptibility of veterinary strains have shown ciprofloxacin to have more activity than norfloxacin (46) and sensitivity to levofloxacin (44).

Uncomplicated skin infections may be treated with either oral penicillin (1 g per day for 5–10 days) or intramuscular procaine or benzathine penicillin. The disease is usually self-limited.

However, treatment decreases the duration of symptoms and potentially reduces the development of complications.

The recommended antibiotic therapy for endocarditis is 12 to 20 million units of penicillin per day in divided doses for 4 to 6 weeks. Synergy with streptomycin has not been demonstrated. Shorter courses of intravenous penicillin (2 weeks) followed by 2 to 4 weeks of oral penicillin therapy have been reported to be successful. Surgery has been necessary in 36% of cases with *E. rhusiopathiae* endocarditis (21) and should be determined on the basis of general criteria for valve replacement in endocarditis. Despite seemingly appropriate antibiotic therapy, the mortality rate for treated *E. rhusiopathiae* endocarditis is 38%.

In patients who are allergic to penicillin, clindamycin or erythromycin plus rifampin may be the drugs of choice. Two cases of septicemia in penicillin-allergic immunocompromised hosts have been successfully treated with either clindamycin alone for 2 weeks (47) or erythromycin (6 weeks) and rifampin (3 weeks) (40).

At present, there is no effective vaccine against *E. rhusiopathiae* in humans. Protective clothing (gloves, aprons, boots) is helpful in preventing occupational exposure.

REFERENCES

1. Freland C: Erysipeloid. In: Braude AI, Davis CE, Fierer J, eds. *Infectious diseases and medical microbiology*, 2nd ed. Philadelphia: WB Saunders, 1986:1512–1514.
2. Woodbine M. *Erysipelothrix rhusiopathiae*. Bacteriology and chemotherapy. *Bacteriol Rev* 1950–1951;14–15:161.–178
3. Jones D. Genus *Erysipelothrix* Rosenbach 1909, 367. In: Sneath PHA, Mair NS, Sharpe ME, et al., eds. *Bergey's manual of systematic bacteriology*, Vol. 2. Baltimore: Williams & Wilkins, 1986:1245–1249.
4. Bille J, Doyle MP. *Listeria* and *Erysipelothrix*. In: Balows A, Hausler WJ Jr, Herrmann KL, et al., eds. *Manual of clinical microbiology*, 5th ed. Washington, DC: American Society for Microbiology, 1991:287–295.
5. Shimoji Y, Yokomizo Y, Sekizaki T, et al. Presence of a capsule in *Erysipelothrix rhusiopathiae* and its relationship to virulence for mice. *Infect Immun* 1994;62:2806–2810.
6. Takahashi T, Fujisawa T, Tamura Y, et al. DNA relatedness among *Erysipelothrix rhusiopathiae* strains representing all twenty-three serovars and *Erysipelothrix tonsillarum*. *Int J Syst Bacteriol* 1992;42:469–473.
7. Wood RL. Swine erysipelas—a review of prevalence and research. *J Am Vet Med Assoc* 1984;184:944–949.
8. Feresu SB, Jones D. Taxonomic studies on *Brochothrix*, *Erysipelothrix*, *Listeria* and atypical lactobacilli. *J Gen Microbiol* 1988;134:1165–1183.
9. Takahashi T, Fujisawa T, Benno Y, et al. *Erysipelothrix tonsillarum* sp. nov. isolated from tonsils of apparently healthy pigs. *Int J Syst Bacteriol* 1987;37:166–168.
10. Ahrne S, Inga-Maj S, Jensen NE, et al. Classification of *Erysipelothrix* strains on the basis of restriction fragment length polymorphisms. *Int J Syst Bacteriol* 1995;45:382–385.
11. Okatani AT, Hatashidani H, Takahashi T, et al. Randomly amplified polymorphic DNA analysis of *Erysipelothrix* spp. *J Clin Microbiol* 2000;38:4332–4336.
12. Yu PKW, Washington JA II. Identification of aerobic and facultatively anaerobic bacteria. In: Washington JA II, ed. *Laboratory procedures in clinical microbiology*. New York: Springer-Verlag, 1985:164–179.
13. Grieco MH, Sheldon C. *Erysipelothrix rhusiopathiae*. *Ann NY Acad Sci* 1970; 174:523–532.
14. Proctor WI. Subacute bacterial endocarditis due to *Erysipelothrix rhusiopathiae*. *Am J Med* 1965;38:820–824.
15. Auerbach PS. Natural microbiologic hazards of the aquatic environment. *Clin Dermatol* 1987;5:52–61.
16. Popugailo VM, Podkin IUA, Gurvich VB, et al. Erysipeloid as an occupational disease of workers in shoe enterprises [in Russian]. *Zh Microbiol Epidemiol Immunobiol* 1983;10:46–49.
17. Shuster M, Brennan P, Edelstein P. Persistent bacteremia with *Erysipelothrix rhusiopathiae* in a hospitalized patient. *Clin Infect Dis* 1993;17:783–784.
18. Klauder JV. Erysipeloid as an occupational disease. *JAMA* 1938;111:1345–1348.
19. David CE. *Erysipelothrix rhusiopathiae*. In: Braude AI, Davis CE, Fierer J, eds. *Infectious diseases and medical microbiology*, 2nd ed. Philadelphia: WB Saunders, 1986:310–315.
20. Stenstrom I, Norrung V, Ternstrom A, et al. Occurrence of different serotypes of *Erysipelothrix rhusiopathiae* in retail pork and fish. *Acta Vet Scand* 1992;33:169–173.
21. Gorby GL, Peacock JE Jr. *Erysipelothrix rhusiopathiae* endocarditis: microbiologic, epidemiologic, and clinical features of an occupational disease. *Rev Infect Dis* 1988;10:317–325.
22. Ehrlich JC. *Erysipelothrix rhusiopathiae* infection in man. *Arch Intern Med* 1946;78:565–577.
23. MacGowan A, Reeves D, Wright C, et al. Tricuspid valve infective endocarditis and pulmonary sepsis due to *Erysipelothrix rhusiopathiae* fully treated with high doses of ciprofloxacin but complicated by gynaecomastia [Letter]. *J Infect* 1991;22:100–101.
24. Venditti M, Gelfusa V, Castelli F, et al. *Erysipelothrix rhusiopathiae* endocarditis. *Eur J Clin Microbiol Infect Dis* 1990;9:50–52.
25. Bibler M. *Erysipelothrix rhusiopathiae* endocarditis [Letter]. *Rev Infect Dis* 1988;10:1062–1063.
26. Ognibene FP, Cunnion RE, Gill V, et al. *Erysipelothrix rhusiopathiae* bacteremia presenting as septic shock. *Am J Med* 1985;78:861–864.
27. Fakoya A, Bendall R, Churchill D, et al. *Erysipelothrix rhusiopathiae* bacteraemia in a patient without endocarditis. *J Infect* 1995;30:180–181.
28. Asnis D, Bresciani A. Bacteremia due to *Erysipelothrix rhusiopathiae* [Letter]. *South Med J* 1992;85:332–333.
29. Callon R Jr, Brady P. Toothpick perforation of the sigmoid colon: an unusual case associated with *Erysipelothrix rhusiopathiae* septicemia. *Gastrointest Endosc* 1990;36:141–143.
30. Garcia-Restoy E, Espejo E, Bella F, et al. Bacteremia due to *Erysipelothrix rhusiopathiae* in immunocompromised hosts without endocarditis [Letter]. *Rev Infect Dis* 1991;13:1252–1253.
31. Kramer Mr, Gombert ME, Corrado ML, et al. *Erysipelothrix rhusiopathiae* endocarditis. *South Med J* 1982;75:892.
32. Gransden WR, Eykyn SJ. *Erysipelothrix rhusiopathiae* endocarditis [Letter]. *Rev Infect Dis* 1988;10:1228.
33. Hayek LF. *Erysipelothrix rhusiopathiae* endocarditis affecting a porcine xenograft heart valve [Letter]. *J Infect* 1993;27:203–204.
34. Silberstein EB. *Erysipelothrix* endocarditis. *JAMA* 1965;191:862–864.
35. Torkildsen A. Intracranial erysipeloid (swine-erysipelas) abscess: a variety of abscess not hitherto observed. *Bull Hyg* 1943;18:1013.
36. Townshend RH, Jephcott AE, Yekta MH. *Erysipelothrix* septicaemia without endocarditis. *BMJ* 1973;1:464.
37. Quabeck K, Muller J, Wendt F, et al. Pericarditis in *Erysipelothrix rhusiopathiae* septicemia [Letter]. *Infection* 1986;14:301.
38. Nandish S, Khardori N. Valvular and myocardial abscesses due to *Erysipelothrix rhusiopathiae*. *Clin Infect Dis* 1999;29:1351–1352.
39. Gimenez M, Fernandez P, Padilla E, et al. Endocarditis and acute renal failure due to *Erysipelothrix rhusiopathiae*. *Eur J Clin Microbiol Infect Dis* 1996;15:347–348.
40. Shumack SL, McDonald S, Baer P, et al. *Erysipelothrix* septicemia in an immunocompromised host. *Can Med Assoc J* 1987;136:273–274.
41. Klauder JV, Kramer DW, Nicholas L. *Erysipelothrix rhusiopathiae* septicemia: diagnosis and treatment. *JAMA* 1943;122:938–943.
42. Takeshi K, Makino S, Ikeda T, et al. Direct and rapid detection by PCR of *Erysipelothrix* sp. DNAs prepared from bacterial strains and animal tissues. *J Clin Microbiol* 1999;37:4093–4098.
43. Venditti M, Gelfusa V, Tarasi A, et al. Antimicrobial susceptibilities of *Erysipelothrix rhusiopathiae*. *Antimicrob Agents Chemother* 1990;34:2038–2040.
44. Soriano F, Fernandez-Roblas R, Calvo R, et al. *In vitro* susceptibilities of aerobic and facultative non–spore-forming Gram-positive bacilli to HMR 3647 (RU 55547) and 14 other antimicrobials. *Antimicrob Agents Chemother* 1998;42:1028–1033.
45. Fritzen T, Marx E, Uy J. Treatment of surgical infections with a modern quinolone: therapy of soft tissue infections and pneumonia with ofloxacin. *Infection* 1996;14(suppl 4):S293–S296.
46. Prescott J, Yielding K. *In vitro* susceptibility of selected veterinary bacterial pathogens to ciprofloxacin, enrofloxacin and norfloxacin. *Can J Vet Res* 1990;54:195–197.
47. Berg RA. *Erysipelothrix rhusiopathiae* [Letter]. *South Med J* 1984;77:1614.

Gram-Negative Cocci

CHAPTER 192
Neisseria gonorrhoeae

Khalil Ghanem and Jonathan Zenilman

HISTORY

Urethritis and its association with copulation was known to biblical authors, thus suggesting that gonorrhea is one of the oldest diseases known. The word *gonorrhea* comes from the Greek words *gene* ("seed") and *rhoia* ("flow"). *Neisseria gonorrhoeae* was first described in urethral pus by Albert Neisser in 1879. It was soon thereafter isolated on artificial culture media and definitively recognized as the agent causing the clinical disease gonorrhea.

In the preantibiotic era, treatment modalities were rather disparate and included such drastic measures as intraurethral inoculation of heavy metals and other disinfectants. Successful therapy was introduced with the advent of the sulfa drugs during the 1930s, but widespread resistance developed in less than 6 years. Subsequently, penicillin afforded single-dose outpatient therapy. On introduction in 1944, as little as 50,000 units of penicillin cured gonorrhea (1). Although the required dose increased over the next 30 years, high-level resistance did not emerge until 1976.

In 1976, plasmid-mediated penicillinase-producing *N. gonorrhoeae* (PPNG) emerged in Southeast Asia and Africa and quickly spread. This was followed by chromosomally mediated penicillin resistance in 1983 and plasmid-mediated tetracycline resistance in 1985 (2). More recently, increasing resistance to the quinolones, one of the most frequently used drug classes for the treatment of gonorrhea, has been rapidly increasing throughout many parts of the world, including the United States (especially Hawaii and California) (3).

CHARACTERISTICS OF THE PATHOGEN

N. gonorrhoeae belongs to the family Neisseriaceae, which includes, *Neisseria meningitidis* (see Chapter 193) and many nonpathogenic species such as *Neisseria sicca*, *Neisseria subflava*, and *Neisseria flava* (4).

On Gram stain, *N. gonorrhoeae* characteristically appears as a gram-negative diplococcus (Fig. 192.1). It is a fastidious organism with complex growth requirements that include enriched media, a 3% to 5% carbon dioxide atmosphere (candle jar), and an incubation temperature of 35°C to 37°C. It can be maintained for 5 to 7 days in special transport media (5). Gonococci grow *in vivo* under relatively anaerobic conditions and are capable of growing anaerobically *in vitro*. As with other bacteria, the growth conditions alter the antigenic makeup of the microorganism.

N. gonorrhoeae produces unusually high levels of catalase, an enzyme that converts hydrogen peroxide into oxygen and water. Hydrogen peroxide is produced by most lactobacilli, which are part of the normal flora of the vagina, and catalase production is likely an important survival mechanism for gonococci (6).

N. gonorrhoeae also produces an oxidase. Because this characteristic can be easily and quickly identified in the laboratory, gram-negative diplococci obtained from appropriate clinical specimens (e.g., urethral exudate) that are "oxidase-positive" and grow on selective media (supplemented with antimicrobials such as vancomycin, colistin, and nystatin to suppress commensal organisms) are presumed to be *N. gonorrhoeae* by the vast majority of clinical laboratories. For example, the predictive value of oxidase-positive isolates obtained from genital sites is high, especially in a sexually transmitted disease (STD) clinic setting. Species verification is usually reserved for problem cases (e.g., blood isolates), antibiotic sensitivity testing, and research endeavors.

The gold standard for distinguishing *N. gonorrhoeae* from other *Neisseria* species is sugar fermentation patterns (Table 192.1). *N. gonorrhoeae* organisms utilize only glucose, pyruvate, and lactate as carbon sources. Newer and more rapid techniques have occasionally resulted in misdiagnosis, a potential problem because of the social and medicolegal consequences of infections that are sexually transmitted. Besides other *Neisseria* species, other gram-negative cocci such as *Kingella denitrificans*, *Moraxella* species, and *Branhamella* (*Moraxella*) *catarrhalis* may be mistaken for *N. gonorrhoeae*.

Colonies examined from cultures of fresh clinical specimens within 16 to 20 hours contain organisms that are piliated and are designated P^+, P^{++} or T_1, T_2. As colonies incubate longer *in vitro* or are passed blindly on artificial media, there is a loss of pilus expression and these organisms and colonies are labeled P^- or T_3, T_4. Any colonial type (P^+, P^{++}, or P^-) may also differ in opacity (O^-, O^+, O^{++}, O^{+++}, O^{++++}) owing to the presence of an outer membrane protein termed Opa protein or protein II. Both pilin and Opa are related to pathogenicity.

The organism cell wall (Fig. 192.2) consists of pili, a putative capsule, a number of distinctive outer membrane proteins known as protein I, Opa protein (protein II), protein III (Rmp), iron-regulating proteins, lipooligosaccharide (LOS), and H.8 (Lip), as well as a series of other unnamed proteins induced by varying growth or stress conditions such as reduced or increased oxygen tension (7) and heat (8). As such, *N. gonorrhoeae* can undergo both phase variation (control of expression of a certain protein is either on or off) and antigenic variation (protein changes in its primary sequence). This latter aspect has significant implications on the ability of the gonococcus to evade the host's immune response, its antigenicity, hydrophobicity, agglutination, drug resistance, and nutritional requirements (9). The genome sequence for *N. gonorrhoeae* strain FA-1090 can be located on the World Wide Web at: *www.genome.ou.edu/gono.html*.

Pili and Pilin

The pili of *N. gonorrhoeae* are hairlike filamentous appendages about 7 nm in diameter and up to 2.5 μm in length that extend from the cell surface as individual fibrils or fibrillar aggregates. They consist of protein subunits of approximately 160 amino acids (10), called pilin, which are encoded by the chromosomal gene *pilE* (11). Pili are an important virulence factor and appear to mediate adherence to host epithelial cells (115). In human challenge studies in men, piliated organisms produced classic gonococcal urethritis, but nonpiliated organisms did not (12,13). A multitude of pilin structural variants can arise owing to recombinant events between silent (*pilS*) and expressed (*pilE*) pilin gene sequences (14). Their primary function is mediating adherence of the gonococcus to the host cell, especially to microvilli of

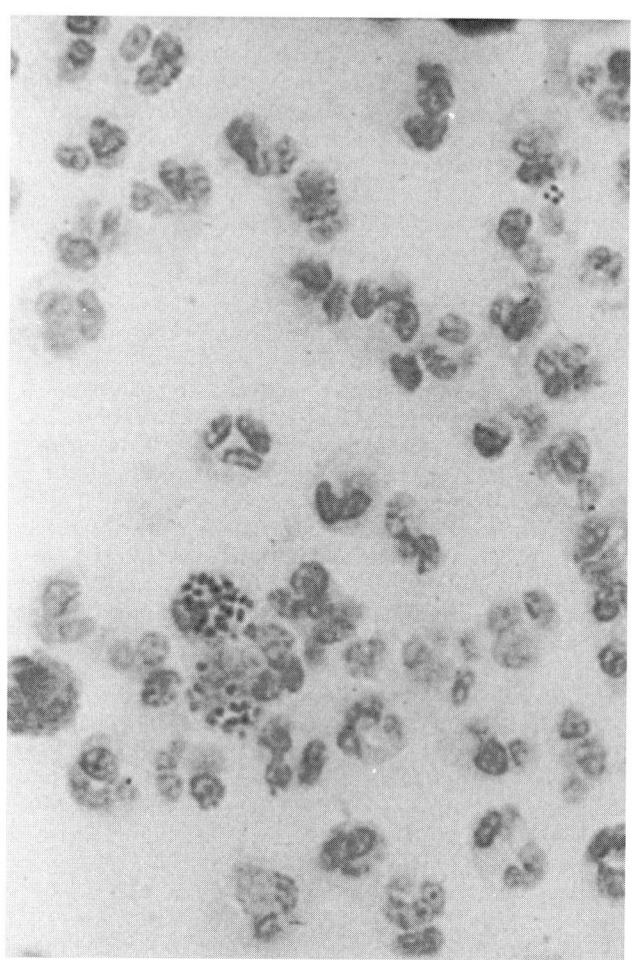

Figure 192.1. Urethral exudate with gram-negative diplococci.

(15). It is thought that attachment to this receptor allows the organism to manipulate the host's cell-mediated immune response.

The gonococcus can switch between a piliated and a nonpiliated state (phase variation), depending on whether pilin genes are being expressed. Obviously, when pilin genes are deleted (a common consequence of prolonged blind passage *in vitro*) the organism cannot revert to a piliated state.

In addition to this phase variation, there is extensive antigenic interstrain and intrastrain variation in pilin (116), predominantly in the C-terminal portion of the pilin, which can be mediated by many mechanisms. The genes responsible for these tremendous antigenic variations appear to be distributed in a random fashion along the gonococcal chromosome. Antigenic variation may be mediated by insertions and deletions of one to four amino acid residues (16), or conversion of pilin gene copies into an expression site may give rise to expressed pilin of different antigenic types (11,17–21). Furthermore, this variable portion is immunodominant with regard to the primary humoral immune response. As with other organisms, DNA transformation of pilin genes between organisms may also occur (22). Thus, the gonococcal pilus is engineered for altering the antigenic nature of this important virulence factor and likely represents a major escape mechanism of the organism for evading immune-mediated control by the host. It also appears to be important for selective individual strain tropisms necessary to colonize different hosts and host cells (23).

In contrast to the C-terminal, the N-terminal region is highly conserved and is homologous to pilin of many other species, including *N. meningitidis, Pseudomonas aeruginosa, Vibrio cholerae,* enteropathogenic *Escherichia coli,* and *Moraxella* and *Bacteroides* species. Expression of these proteinaceous appendages is also associated with a phenomenon known as twitching motility (modes of migration along liquid-solid or liquid-air interfaces). This property is due to a protein located in the cytoplasmic membrane encoded by the gene *pilT* (24).

Because of the demonstrated pivotal role of gonococcal pili in the pathogenesis of clinical gonorrhea, pili were one of the approaches initially investigated as vaccine candidates. However, despite the limited success of a pilus vaccine in a human challenge study (25) and the demonstration of an immune response that blocked pilus function (26), a phase II field trial failed to

nonciliate columnar cells. This is thought to be the result of PilC protein, an adhesin component that mediates pilus binding. The gonococcal pilus has been shown to interact with CD46 (a member of the superfamily of complement resistance proteins, and the receptor for measles and HHV-6)

TABLE 192.1. Differentiation of *Neisseria gonorrhoeae* from Related Species That May Be Isolated on Gonococcal Selective Media

Species	Produces acid from				Superoxol	Hydroxyprolyl aminopeptidase	γ-Glutamyl-aminopeptidase	Nitrate reduction
	Glucose	Maltose	Lactose	Sucrose				
Neisseria gonorrhoeae	+	−	−	−	+	+	−	−
Neisseria meningitidis[a]	+	+	−	−	−	NA	+	−
Neisseria cinerea[b]	+[c]	−	−	−	−	+	−	−
Branhamella (Moraxella) catarrhalis	−	−	−	−	−	−	−	+[d]
Kingella denitrificans	+	−	−	−	−	+	−	+
Neisseria lactamica	+	+	+	−	−	NA	−	−
Neisseria polysaccharea	+	+	−	+	−	+	−	−
Neisseria kochii[e]	+	−	−	−	+	NA	−	−
Neisseria flavescens	−	−	−	−	−	+	−	−

[a]Maltose-negative strains.
[b]Some strains grow on selective media that do not contain colistin.
[c]Some strains produce weak acid reactions that are not delayed and are not glucose-positive in all test systems.
[d]Reaction is weak or delayed; cannot be performed reliably as a rapid test (unpublished observations).
[e]*N. kochii* grows without CO_2 and at 35°C.
NA, not available.
Adapted from Knapp JS. Historical perspectives and identification of *Neisseria* and related species. *Clin Microbiol Rev* 1988;1:415, with permission.

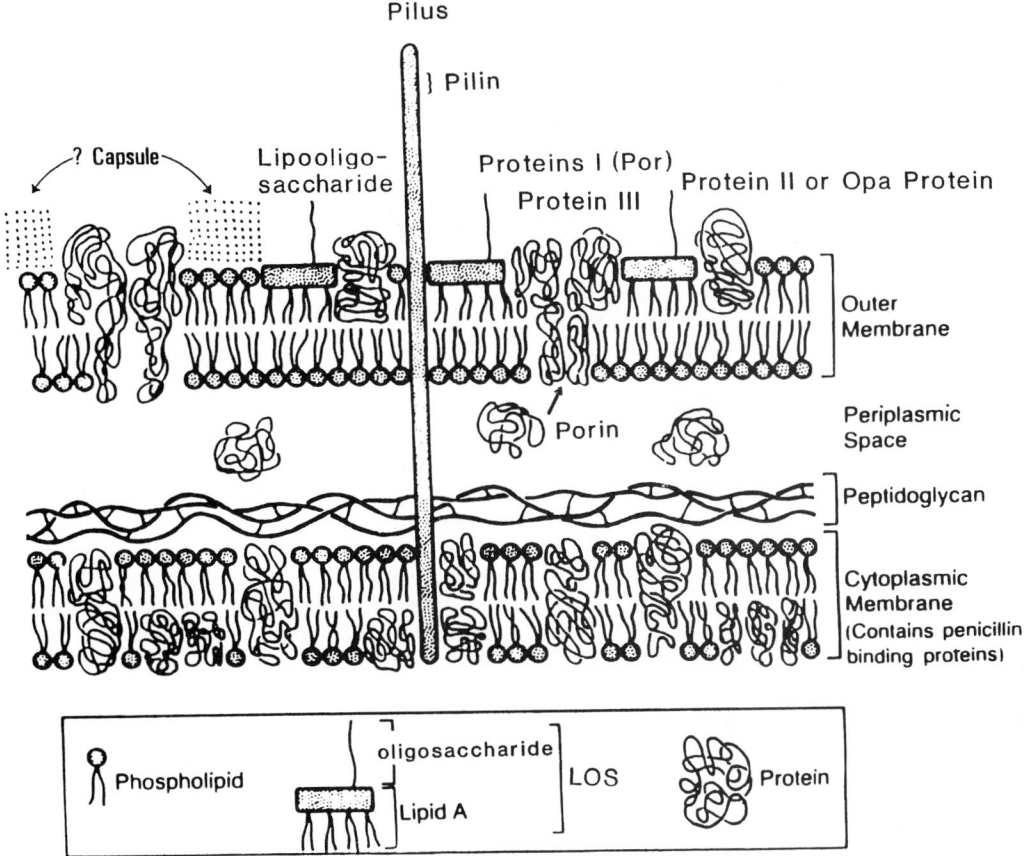

Figure 192.2. Cell wall of *Neisseria gonorrhoeae*. (Adapted from Hook EW III, Holmes KK. Gonococcal infections. *Ann Intern Med* 1985;102:229–243, with permission.)

demonstrate broad protection (27), probably because of the extreme degree of pilin antigenic diversity.

Protein I

The *porB* locus codes for protein I, the most prominent outer membrane protein of *N. gonorrhoeae*. It ranges in molecular mass from 32 to 37 kd (25). It functions as a porin, forming a hydrophilic channel through the outer membrane. Protein I appears to trigger endocytosis of the organism by the host mucosal cell (28,29), it may disrupt neutrophil degranulation (30,31) and phagosome maturation (32), and it appears to mediate apoptosis of phagocytes and epithelial cells (33). It is located on the cell wall proximate to LOS and protein III, thus making up a unique antigenic constellation.

Unlike most other proteins in the outer membrane surface, protein I is always expressed, and because a single strain produces only one antigenically stable protein I, it has proved to be a useful tool for classifying gonococci. Recently, however, gonococci with IA/IB hybrid porins have been described (34). There are two principal subclasses of protein I, known as protein IA and protein IB, that respectively represent a family of structurally related proteins (30). The most commonly used coagglutination assay uses six protein IA monoclonal antibodies and six protein IB monoclonal antibodies. On the basis of a reaction pattern to a panel of these antibodies, a given strain can be classified into a serovar (4,28). At least 24 protein IA and 32 protein IB serovars have been recognized. In any given geographic region, the vast majority of strains belong to a small number of serovars.

Antibodies to protein I develop in both serum and genital secretions (35–37). Serum antibodies exhibit both bactericidal and opsonic properties (38,39). Furthermore, in women this antibody appears to be protective against infection of the same protein I type (40) and serovar (41).

In addition, organisms with protein IA are more often associated with disseminated gonococcal infection and resistance to the bactericidal action of normal (uninfected) human serum (42). Conversely, protein IB organisms are more closely associated with urethritis, cervicitis, and increased antibiotic resistance (43).

Opa Protein, or Protein II

Opa protein, or protein II, is a family of 24- to 30-kd heat-modifiable outer membrane proteins that manifest extensive intrastrain and interstrain antigenic and phase variation analogous to pilus variation. Opa protein is not always expressed. It imparts to an organism the capability of forming opaque colonies *in vitro*, a property associated with isolates obtained from the male urethra (44) and from the cervix about midway in the menstrual cycle (day 15). Functionally, Opa protein allows greater gonococcal cell-to-cell adhesion (45), thus encouraging the formation of an infectious unit, which is possibly an important virulence factor (46). It appears to enhance adhesion to human conjunctival cells, epithelial cells, and, in particular, neutrophils (47,48). When Opa protein is not expressed, the organism forms "transparent" colonies, a characteristic more often found in isolates obtained from asymptomatic and disseminated gonococcal infections (49), and is associated with increased resistance to killing by normal (uninfected) human serum as well as trypsin. It predominates in cervical cultures obtained at times other than midcycle and in isolates from blood, synovial fluid, and fallopian tubes. Expression is clearly related to environmental growth conditions. Two classes of cellular receptors for Opa protein are known: heparan-sulfate-proteoglycan present on epithelial cells, and CD66 (a member of the carcinoembryonic antigen family) present on epithelial cells and neutrophils (50).

Protein III (Rmp)

In sharp contrast to other outer membrane proteins of gonococci, protein III (Rmp) is antigenically stable and invariant among gonococcal strains (51). An analogous protein exists on *N. meningitidis*, and it is structurally similar to the OmpA proteins of *E. coli* and other Enterobacteriaceae, and protein F of *P. aeruginosa*. It is poorly immunogenic in humans, but protein III antibody appears to possess the capacity to block bactericidal antibodies directed at other surface antigens (LOS, protein I) to which it is closely aligned on the cell surface. Its role in pathogenesis is not known, although antibodies to Rmp have been associated with an increased susceptibility to infection (52). Finally, it has been shown recently that acidic conditions reduced the expression of Rmp (53).

Nonpilin Protein Adhesins

Proteins that copurify with gonococcal pilin have been described (54,55). They mediate the binding of gonococci to host cells by incorporation onto the tip of the pilus in a manner similar to the protein adhesins that mediate the binding of uropathogenic *E. coli*. They may also mediate binding of nonpiliate strains to eukaryotic cells.

Environmentally Induced, or Stress, Proteins

A variety of environmental stress conditions such as reduced carbon dioxide or oxygen tension, iron-poor conditions, or temperature variations can result in the expression of a variety of other surface and cytoplasmic proteins (7,56,57). Their significance in the pathogenesis of gonococcal infection is still unclear, although antibodies to them have been demonstrated in women with pelvic inflammatory disease (58).

Major Iron-Regulated Proteins

Most bacteria, especially those that reside on mucous membranes, must acquire iron from their environment. Hence, iron-scavenging systems are essential for survival. The ferric uptake regulator protein (Fur) has been described in many gram-negative organisms, including *N. gonorrhoeae* (59). This protein is a global gene regulator, controlling not only iron-scavenging functions, but possibly virulence factors as well. It has been shown that Fur binds to the *opa* promoters, and thus may have direct influence on the virulence of the organism (60). For the most part, bacteria synthesize proteins called siderophores that perform iron-scavenging functions. Rather than producing siderophores, *N. gonorrhoeae* uses outer membrane proteins that bind to host iron sources such as transferrin and lactoferrin. The transferrin receptor is made up of two proteins: an outer membrane receptor (TbpA) and a surface exposed lipoprotein (TbpB). These proteins bind transferrin, removing its iron, and internalizing it in an energy-dependent fashion (61–63).

Immunoglobulin A Protease

Many bacteria that normally reside on a mucosal surface, such as the *Neisseria* species, *Haemophilus influenzae*, or *Streptococcus pneumoniae*, produce a protease that cleaves human immunoglobulin A1 (IgA1) at the hinge region (64). Secretory IgA, significant for its predominance in local mucosal secretions, can thus be rendered inactive. IgA1 prevents microbial adherence, neutralizes toxins, and promotes phagocytosis. Recent studies have implicated IgA1 protease as an inducer of proinflammatory cytokines, especially tumor necrosis factor (TNF)-α (65), and as a proinflammatory T-cell antigen (66). Moreover, IgA1 protease has been shown to cleave human chorionic gonadotropin, which could have serious implications on the fetus in pregnant women (67).

H.8 Outer Membrane Protein

H.8 (Lip) refers to a conserved and stable epitope contained on two different lipoproteins. H.8 outer membrane protein is present on *N. gonorrhoeae*, *N. meningitidis*, *Neisseria lactamica*, and *Neisseria cinerea*, but not on other nonpathogenic *Neisseria* species (68). The protein consists of a repeating heptapeptide of 22 to 30 kd. Its exact function is not known. The presence of serum antibody to the H.8 epitope does not protect against a subsequent infection (69). Recently, Lip has been used as an adjunct for the subtyping of *N. gonorrhoeae* strains (70).

A second lipoprotein that contains the H.8 epitope is lipid-modified azurin (Laz). It is present on all *Neisseria* species and is believed to function in electron transport during bacterial respiration.

Lipooligosaccharide (Lipopolysaccharide)

Like all gram-negative organisms, lipopolysaccharide makes up part of the gonococcal cell wall. Because it lacks long, hydrophilic, and neutral polysaccharides that are found in Enterobacteriaceae, it is referred to as LOS (71). Gonococcal LOS has been shown to mediate most of the toxic damage that occurs to human oviduct mucosa in organ culture. It is the principal target of bactericidal antibodies, regulates complement activation on the bacterial cell surface, and thus appears to be the principal determinant of serum-sensitive and serum-resistant phenotypes (72).

Like pili, gonococcal LOS exhibits both intra- and interstrain antigenic variability. Some LOS moieties have carbohydrate structures that are analogous to mammalian glycosphingolipids, especially human erythrocyte glycosphingolipids (73). There is growing evidence in human challenge studies that LOS plays a key role in the pathogenesis of gonococcal infection (74–76) and may be responsible for the gonococcus' ability to escape an effective immune response through molecular mimicry (77,78). In vitro, LOS has been recently shown to be involved in promoting cellular invasion by *N. gonorrhoeae* organisms independent of Opa (79).

Capsule

A gonococcal capsule has been described by two different laboratories (80), but it has never been isolated or purified. Its role in pathogenesis is not known.

Plasmids

Most gonococci possess a 2.6-megadalton (MDa) cryptic plasmid (81). A number of β-lactamase plasmids have been described that independently result in PPNG strains: 4.2 to 4.4 MDa (Asia), 3.2 MDa (Africa), 2.9 MDa (Rio de Janeiro), 3.05 MDa (Toronto), 3.8 MDa (Nîmes, France), and 6.5 MDa (New Zealand). These six plasmid types are genetically related. Gonococci may also possess a 24.5-MDa plasmid that mediates conjugation and transfer of genetic material. Organisms with high-level plasmid-mediated tetracycline resistance have a 25.2-MDa plasmid, representing recombination of the conjugative plasmid with the *tetM* tetracycline resistance determinant found in group B streptococci. New plasmids carrying antibiotic resistance determinants are also being found with increased frequency among commensal *Neisseria* species, a precursor of their eventual appearance in pathogenic species.

MOLECULAR EPIDEMIOLOGY

The epidemiology of *N. gonorrhoeae* is discussed in detail in Chapter 103. Here we will review certain aspects of its molecular epidemiology.

Gonorrhea is a sexually transmitted disease and remains a frequently reported infectious disease in the United States (361,705 cases reported in 2001). In some developing countries, the morbidity caused by gonorrhea rivals that of the more traditional tropical diseases. As with all sexually transmitted diseases, the principal risk factor is unprotected sex with multiple sexual partners.

The need to (a) characterize gonococcal isolates to gain a greater understanding of the spread of disease; (b) devise and evaluate strategies to control outbreaks caused by a single strain or a limited number of strains; (c) determine epidemiologic and molecular correlates of pathogenicity; and (d) study reinfection versus treatment failure, coinfection, and forensics has resulted in numerous classification strategies (Table 192.2). Antibiograms, the characterization of gonococcal strains by susceptibility to various antibodies and plasmid profiles, are not discriminating enough for most epidemiologic studies. Auxotyping, the characterization of gonococcal strains according to nutritional requirements, also has limited discriminatory utility but has offered some interesting insights. For example, arginine-dependent isolates are rare in the Far East; isolates that require arginine, hypoxanthine, and uracil (AXU), rare before 1950, appear to cause asymptomatic urethral infections in men and disseminated gonococcal infection in both sexes. They are suscepti-

ble to lower doses of penicillin G, produce type 1 IgA1 protease and *dam* methylase (DNA adenine methyltransferase, EC 2.1.1), grow atypically as small colonies, are normally serum bactericidal resistant, and because they are sensitive to vancomycin at 4 μg/mL they may not grow on selective culture media. Isolates that require proline, citrulline, and uracil (PCU) do not contain the 2.6-MDa plasmid found in most other gonococci.

Pulsed field gel electrophoresis, utilizing enzymes that cleave the chromosome at rare restriction sites, has been shown to be stable, reproducible, and sensitive (82). Other DNA-based techniques have recently been devised, such as sequence analysis of the *porB* gene (83), amplification and restriction fragment length polymorphism analysis of the *por* gene (84), and typing of the *opa* gene (85).

As noted earlier, protein I (Por) serotyping, utilizing a standard panel of protein IA–specific and protein IB–specific monoclonal antibody reagents, has been widely used. The auxotype/serotype (A/S) classification utilizes auxotypes and Por serotyping. The most useful serologic typing system at present utilizes a standard panel of protein IA–specific and protein IB–specific monoclonal antibody reagents (86), alone or in conjunction with other tests (82). Because no single antigen has yet to be correlated with protective immunity, new, more sophisticated typing systems are continuously being devised (70,87). Although sensitive systems have been devised, practical issues remain that have hindered broad field implementation.

PATHOGENESIS

N. gonorrhoeae is uniquely a human pathogen. It is spread from person to person by contact with infected secretions, most often through sexual contact. Once the pathogen is deposited on a mucosal surface, a complex series of molecular interactions ensue that result in invasion of mucosal columnar cells (88). The steps include, first, distant attachment mediated by pili (PilC) likely attaching to CD46, leading to host cell calcium release from intracellular stores (89) and the induction of cortical plaques (90). Second, close attachment is most likely mediated by protein I and Opa protein (protein II) via CD66 or heparansulfate-proteoglycan receptors located on epithelial cells. Third, ingestion by the host mucosal cell is likely also mediated by Opa through stimulation of lipid hydrolysis enzymes, leading to endocytosis (91). However, Opa binding to vitronectin, leading to aggregation and uptake of the bacterium into the host cell, has also been shown as a potential mechanism for invasion (92). Fourth, there is transportation through the cell in phagosomes and possible egestion into the submucosa; and, on rare occasions, bloodstream invasion (Fig. 192.3). In organ culture models, the integrity of the epithelial lining is markedly affected, with loss of ciliary motility (mediated by LOS) and extrusion of ciliated cells.

Attachment is the critical first step in establishing infection. Human challenge studies have clearly established the importance of pili and Opa proteins (protein II) in this event (12,45), and the rapid selection *in vivo* of new types of these proteins (13,45). It is speculated that these latter events are an adaptation by the gonococcus to selective pressures mediated by diverse host cell tropisms (26,93,94) or immune pressures, or both (93,94). Pili may also interfere with phagocytosis. Once colonization is established, the gonococcus is well armed to evade mucosal defenses. For example, IgA protease may degrade secretory IgA (64), the gonococcus can utilize the iron-binding proteins transferrin and lactoferrin as an iron source, and bactericidal antibody, the critical protective host immune response to *N. meningitidis*, a close relative of gonococci, can be overcome by blocking antibodies to protein III (Rmp) (51) or sialylation of LOS (72).

TABLE 192.2. Characterization of *Neisseria gonorrhoeae* for Epidemiologic Purposes

Test	Comment
Antimicrobial susceptibility patterns (antibiograms)	Quick, easy, broad categories; limited utility, with resistant strains
Auxotyping (nutritional requirements)	Broad categories; certain auxotypes more often associated with certain clinical states; cluster in certain geographic areas
Serologic tests Polyclonal antibody Monoclonal antibody (utilizes protein I; stable, flexible, destined to be continuously refined and expanded)	Historical interest only
Combined auxotyping plus serotyping (A/S) antibiograms plus auxotyping, or any combination thereof	Provides greater discrimination of gonococcal isolates; can be specifically tailored (e.g., to monitor antimicrobial resistance patterns); method most likely to be used in future
Pulsed field gel electrophoresis	Stable, reproducible, sensitive

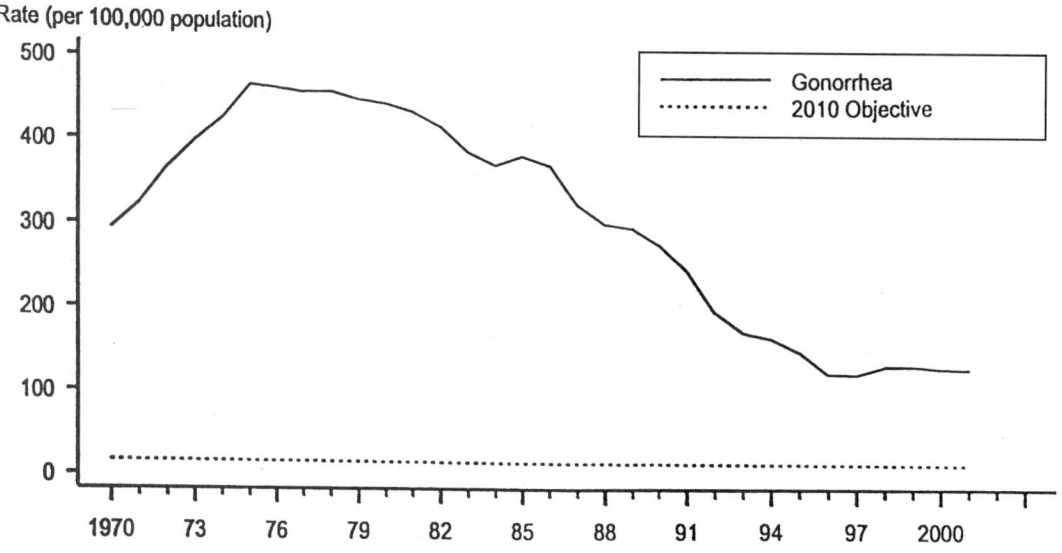

Rate (per 100,000 population)

Figure 192.3. Gonorrhea. Reported rates: United States, 1970 to 2000 and the year 2010 objective. (Data from STD Surveillance, 2002. Atlanta Centers for Disease Control and Prevention.)

Protein I, and especially protein III, may interfere with bactericidal activity. Serum-resistant isolates and variants generate chemotaxins at a slower rate and at a quantitatively smaller concentration than do serum-sensitive isolates and variants. The former is more common in symptomatic (brisk inflammatory) disease, and the latter is more common in asymptomatic urethral infections (73). LOS may be directly cytotoxic to some host cells.

It is highly likely that the tissue damage resulting from a gonococcal infection is related to the degree of inflammation (leukorrhea), making this interaction critical in the pathogenesis. *In vitro* studies have shown that epithelial cells are a major source of proinflammatory cytokine release (95). The induction of leukorrhea correlates well with the expression of LOS, which closely mimics mammalian cell glycosphingolipid (78). Also, sialylation of the LOS, which can occur during active infection (72), renders the organism resistant to bactericidal activity. Finally, it has been shown that the interaction of Opa and pili proteins may facilitate phagocytosis of the organism by monocytes (96) and that PorB is responsible for the arrest of phagosome maturation within the monocytes (32). This allows the organism to survive within these cells, thereby making these cells partially responsible for further transmission of the organism.

The host's response is usually inflammatory and brisk, producing the classic exudate that contains host inflammatory cells [principally polymorphonuclear leukocytes (PMNs)], epithelial cells, and gonococci, most of which have been ingested by PMNs (Fig. 192.1). However, a mild or even quiescent infection may ensue. The reasons for the modulation of the host response are only partially known and include both host and microbial factors. For example, gonococcal strains isolated from patients with a milder inflammatory response are quite sensitive to antibiotics, have unique nutritional requirements, are more resistant to bactericidal activity, or have limited ability to generate neutrophil chemotactic activity (93). IgA protease may inactivate secretory IgA, which can block attachment of gonococci to host mucosal cells (97).

The anti-gonococcal T-cell response has not been as extensively investigated as the humoral one. A recent study has shown a Th2-type immune response against the Por protein manifested by an increase in interleukin-4 production by CD4 T-helper lymphocytes (98). On the other hand, IgA1 protease elicited CD4 T-helper lymphocyte activation, and production of interferon-γ suggesting a Th1-type immune response (99).

Because repeated gonococcal infections are not unusual, it has been suggested that humans do not develop immunity to gonorrhea. However, a relative resistance to infection has been correlated with a history of previous infection (40,41) and protein I (37). Serovar-specific protection has been described (41), suggesting that at least some modulation of the infection does occur.

CLINICAL MANIFESTATIONS

A complete discussion of the clinical manifestations of gonorrhea is presented in Chapter 103. In brief, the spectrum of disease ranges from local infection (urethritis, cervicitis, oropharyngitis) to invasion restricted to sex organs (pelvic inflammatory disease, epididymitis), to invasion of the bloodstream, with or without dissemination to distant organs (e.g., joints, heart valves, pericardium). Like other organisms that may colonize the oropharynx, gonococci have a tropism for serous membranes such as the synovial membrane, pericardium, aortic valve, and conjunctiva. When the peritoneum is invaded, the gonococcus can cause perihepatitis (Fitz-Hugh-Curtis syndrome). Systemic invasion is usually characterized by a subacute course and a relatively small antigen load, attested to by the difficulty often experienced in attempts to isolate the causative organism from blood or synovial fluid. Gonococcal endocarditis is an exception and usually presents with florid symptoms because there is a predilection to involve the aortic valve. Premature and low birth rates are associated in particular with genital gonococcal infection (100).

Asymptomatic carriage is most common in women (at least 50% of cases). It occurs in approximately 15% of men with gonorrhea. Asymptomatic carriage has been associated more often with transparent colony types and certain auxotypes, and serovars, but these same "types" have often been associated with pelvic inflammatory disease. Thus, they are an important reservoir for the most common significant sequelae of gonococcal infections, namely salpingitis, sterility, and ectopic pregnancy (101). Whether this reflects a predisposition of the infecting organism to involve the fallopian tubes or the reluctance of asymptomatic men to seek medical consultation is not known. Disseminated gonococcal infection occurs most frequently in women, especially during menses. It also occurs more frequently during the later stages of pregnancy. Whether this increased virulence is innately due to the increased utilization of iron or to an increased antigen load is not known.

Tenosynovitis and septic arthritis are the most common complications of disseminated gonococcal infection. The usual course is manifested by fever, asymmetric arthralgias, and "migrating" tenosynovitis that later "settles" in one joint, usually the knee, elbow, ankle, wrist, or small joints of the hands and feet, in that order. Skin lesions secondary to a microscopic septic arteritis often develop, usually on the extremities. They range from macular lesions to discrete pustules, which may become hemorrhagic and necrotic. Endocarditis, meningitis, and pericarditis are unusual complications. The diagnosis is made by isolation of *N. gonorrhoeae* from blood, synovial fluid, the urogenital tract, oropharynx, or rectum or from a sexual partner of a patient who has typical joint and cutaneous manifestations. Isolation from blood and joint fluid is often difficult and may require culturing relatively large amounts of blood, synovial fluid, and cerebrospinal fluid, and using osmotically stabilized (hypertonic) media. Disseminated gonococcal infection occurs most frequently in persons with a concomitant asymptomatic genital infection.

TREATMENT

Antibiotic Resistance

Penicillin remained the drug of choice for more than 40 years (1945–1988). Nevertheless, slowly increasing resistance to penicillin steadily progressed over time, as did resistance to the macrolides and tetracyclines. In recent years, there has been increasing resistance to the fluoroquinolones.

Resistance to penicillin and tetracycline can be either plasmid mediated, or chromosomally mediated. For penicillin resistance, the former is due to the production of TEM-1–like β lactamases. Those strains are called penicillinase-producing *Neisseria gonorrhoeae*. PPNG strains have a minimum inhibitory concentration (MIC) of at least 16 μg/mL to penicillin, in contrast to susceptible strains whose MIC is no more than 1 μg/mL. PPNG strains are characterized by a sudden increase in MIC to penicillin. This is in contradistinction to chromosomally mediated resistance, which tends to be gradual and stepwise. Chromosomal resistance results from the acquisition of multiple resistance genes that affect the penicillin-binding proteins or the outer membrane permeability. This results in strains whose MIC to penicillin is greater than 1 μg/mL but not as high as the ones due to plasmid resistance. Thus far, some of the loci identified have been designated *penA, penB, penC, mtr, tem, pem, ampA, ampB, ampC, ampD, ponA* and *mom*. Because the effects are additive, resistance at 2 μg/mL, the level associated with an unacceptable failure rate in patients treated with a standard course of penicillin, has increased in prevalence to the point at which penicillin is no longer the antibiotic of choice. Resistance is conferred by decreasing the affinity of penicillin-binding proteins for β-lactam antibiotics, decreasing the permeability of the gonococcal outer membrane, and altering the concentration of penicillin-binding proteins (102–104).

As previously mentioned, resistance to tetracycline can also be mediated via plasmids or chromosomally (117). Similar to penicillin resistance, the MIC to tetracycline of plasmid-mediated resistant strains ($\geq$16 μg/mL) are much higher than the chromosomal ones (>0.25 μg/mL).

Chromosomal resistance is also the mechanism of resistance to spectinomycin, the aminoglycosides, erythromycin, trimethoprim-sulfamethoxizole, and most recently the fluoroquinolones.

Fluoroquinolone-resistant *Neisseria gonorrhoeae* has become a serious threat in many parts of the world, including the Far East and certain parts of the United States (Hawaii and California)

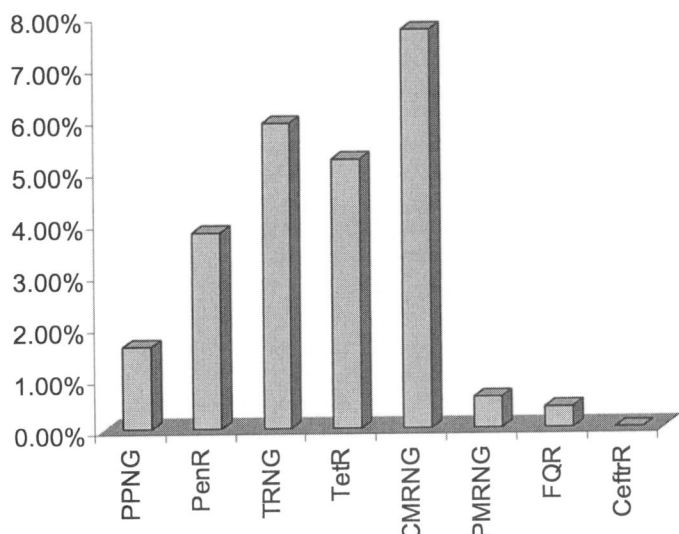

Figure 192.4. Antibiotic resistance in the 2000 Gonococcal Isolate Surveillance Project isolates. PPNG, plasmid-mediated penicillin resistance; PenR, chromosomal penicillin resistance; TRNG, plasmid-mediated tetracycline resistance; TetR, chromosomal tetracycline resistance; CMRNG, chromosomal tetracycline and penicillin resistance; PMRNG, plasmid-mediated tetracycline and penicillin resistance; FQR, fluoroquinolone resistance; CeftrR, ceftriaxone resistance. (Adapted from the Centers for Disease Control and Prevention. *Sexually transmitted diseases surveillance 2000 supplement: gonococcal isolate surveillance program annual report—2000.* Atlanta: U.S. Department of Health and Human Services, October 2001.)

(105). The use of fluoroquinolones in those areas has been all but abandoned. It is only a matter of time before widespread quinolone resistance renders these drugs as useless as penicillin. Quinolone resistance can be the result of mutations in the *gyrA* subunit of DNA gyrase or mutations in the *parC* subunit of topoisomerase IV. When both mutations are present, a concomitant decrease in susceptibility to cephalosporins has been observed in some strains (106). Figure 192.4 summarizes the distribution of antibiotic resistance of the gonococcal isolates from the Gonococcal Isolate Surveillance Project (GISP) in the year 2000 (107). The percentage of PPNG has decreased from a peak of 11% in 1995 to 1.6% in 2000. The number of penicillin and tetracycline coresistant isolates was 8.3% of the total number of isolates. There has been no documented resistance to ceftriaxone or any other cephalosporin in the United States. However, several isolates with decreased susceptibility to ceftriaxone have been seen.

PREVENTION

Immunization

The quest for a gonococcal vaccine has been ongoing for many years. Unfortunately, none has so far proved efficacious (108,118). Attempts have included whole-cell vaccines (109), autolyzed gonococcal piliate vaccines (110), and purified pili vaccines (27). Other vaccine candidates include the porin proteins, antiidiotypic antibodies that mimic regions in the lipopolysaccharide (LPS), and some of the iron-regulated proteins (111). One of the issues with regard to gonococcal vaccines is philosophical: should the aim be to protect against the local infection (e.g., urethritis or cervicitis) or is it sufficient to protect only against the systemic complications associated with greater morbidity, such as pelvic inflammatory disease? Would a vaccine result in more asymptomatic disease and thus a broader epidemic?

General Measures

As with any sexually transmitted disease, abstinence and preexposure and postexposure antibiotic prophylaxis have been used successfully (98,112,113). Most spermicides are toxic to gonococci, and some findings have suggested that they reduce the incidence of infection. However, in a recently published metaanalysis of randomized controlled trials comparing Nonoxynol-9 to placebo for prevention of STDs, there was no benefit in STD or human immunodeficiency virus risk reduction (114). The effectiveness of a number of home remedies, such as washing the genitals or urinating after sexual intercourse, has been asserted to be effective anecdotally through the years, but none has been evaluated clinically. Epidemiologic treatment refers to the treatment of sexual partners after high-risk exposure and before culture verification. Its effectiveness has been proved, and it is recommended because of the great probability of acquired secondary infections.

REFERENCES

1. Sternberg TH, Howard EB, Dewey LA, et al. Venereal disease. In: *Preventive medicine in World War II*, Vol. V. Washington, DC: U.S. Government Printing Office, 1961:139–332.
2. Boslego JW, Tramont EC, Takafuji ET, et al. Effect of spectinomycin on the prevalence of spectinomycin-resistant and penicillinase-producing *Neisseria gonorrhoeae*. *N Engl J Med* 1987;517:27.
3. Division of STD Prevention. *Sexually transmitted disease surveillance 2001*. U.S. Department of Health and Human Services, Public Health Service. Atlanta: Centers for Disease Control and Prevention, 2002.
4. Knapp JS. Historical perspectives and identification of *Neisseria* and related species. *Clin Microbiol Rev* 1988;1:415.
5. Carlson BL, Haley MS, Tisei NA, et al. Evaluation of four methods for isolation of *Neisseria gonorrhoeae*. *J Clin Microbiol* 1980;12:301.
6. Zheng H, Alcor TM, Cohen MS. Effects of H_2O_2-producing lactobacilli or *Neisseria gonorrhoeae* growth and catalase activity. *J Infect Dis* 1994;170:1209.
7. Clark VL, Campbell LA, Palmero DA, et al. Induction and repression of outer membrane proteins by anaerobic growth of *Neisseria gonorrhoeae*. *Infect Immun* 1987;55:1359.
8. Woods ML, Bonfigholi, McGee ZA, et al. Synthesis of a select group of proteins by *Neisseria gonorrhoeae* in response to thermal stress. *Infect Immun* 1990;58:719.
9. Merz A, Magdalene S. Interactions of pathogenic neisseriae with epithelial cell membranes. *Annu Rev Cell Dev Biol* 2000;16:423.
10. Schoolnik GK, Fernandez R, Tay JY, et al. Gonococcal pili: primary structure and receptor binding domain. *J Exp Med* 1984;159:1351.
11. Meyer TF, Billyard E, Haas R, et al. Pilus gene of *Neisseria gonorrhoeae*: chromosomal organization and DNA sequence. *Proc Natl Acad Sci USA* 1984;81:6110.
12. Kellogg DS, Cohen IR, Norins LC, et al. *Neisseria gonorrhoeae*. II. Colonial variation and pathogenicity during 35 months *in vitro*. *J Bacteriol* 1968;96:596.
13. Swanson J, Robbins K, Barrera O, et al. Gonococcal pilin variants in experimental gonorrhea. *J Exp Med* 1987;165:1344.
14. Rytkonen A, Johansson L, Asp V, et al. Soluble pilin of *Neisseria gonorrhoeae* interacts with human target cells and tissue. *Infect Immun* 2001;69:6419.
15. Kallstrom H, Liszewski MK, Atkinson JP, et al. Membrane cofactor protein (MCP or CD46) is a cellular pilus receptor for pathogenic *Neisseria*. *Mol Microbiol* 1997;25:639.
16. Taha M, Marchal C. Conservation of *Neisseria gonorrhoeae* pilus expression regulatory genes *pilA* and *pilB* in the genus *Neisseria*. *Infect Immun* 1990;58:4145.
17. Meyer TF, Mlawer N, So M. Pilus expression in *Neisseria gonorrhoeae* involves chromosomal rearrangement. *Cell* 1982;30:45.
18. Potts WJ, Saunders JR. Nucleotide sequence of the structural gene for class I pilin from *Neisseria meningitidis*. *Mol Microbiol* 1988;2:647.
19. Bergström S, Robbins K, Koomey JM, et al. Filiation control mechanisms in *Neisseria gonorrhoeae*. *Proc Natl Acad Sci USA* 1986;83:3890.
20. Haas R, Meyer TF. The repertoire of silent pilus genes in *Neisseria gonorrhoeae*: evidence for gene conversion. *Cell* 1986;44:107.
21. Meyer TF, Haas R. Phase and antigenic variation by DNA rearrangements in procaryotes. *Symp Soc Gen Microbiol* 1988;43:193.
22. Seifert HS, Ajioka R, So M. Alternative model for *Neisseria gonorrhoeae* pilin variation. *Vaccine* 1988;6:107.
23. Tramont EC, Hodge WC, Gilbreath MJ, et al. Differences in attached antigens of gonococci in reinfection. *J Lab Clin Med* 1979;93:730.
24. Brossay L, Paradis G, Fox R, et al. Identification, localization, and distribution of the NIT protein in *Neisseria gonorrhoeae*. *Infect Immun* 1994;62:2302.
25. Brinton CC, Wood SW, Brown A, et al. The development of a neisserial pilus vaccine for gonorrhea and meningococcal meningitis. In: Robbins JB, Hill JC, Sadoff JC, eds. *Seminars in infectious diseases*, Vol. IV. Bacterial vaccines. New York: Thieme-Stratton, 1982:140–159.
26. Tramont EC, Boslego JW, Chung R, et al. Parenteral gonococcal pilus vaccine. In: Schoolnik GK Brooks GF, Falkow S, et al., eds. *The pathogenic neisseriae*. Washington, DC: American Society for Microbiology, 1985:316–322.
27. Boslego JW, Tramont EC, Chung R, et al. Efficacy trial of a parenteral gonococcal pilus vaccine. *Vaccine* 1991;9:154.
28. Judd RC. Protein I: structure, function, and genetics. *Clin Microbiol Rev* 1989;2:541.
29. Bjerknes R, Guttormsen HK, Solberg CO, et al. Neisserial porins inhibit human neutrophil actin polymerization, degranulation, opsonin receptor expression, and phagocytosis but prime the neutrophils to increase their oxidative burst. *Infect Immun* 1995;63:160.
30. Carbonetti NH, Simnad VI, Seifert HS, et al. Genetics of protein I of *Neisseria gonorrhoeae*: construction of hybrid porins. *Proc Natl Acad Sci USA* 1988;85:6841.
31. Haines KA, Reibman J, Tang XY, et al. Effects of protein I of *Neisseria gonorrhoeae* on neutrophils activation: generation of diacylglycerol from phosphatidylcholine via a specific phospholipase C is associated with exocytosis. *J Cell Biol* 1991;114:433.
32. Mosleh IM, Huber LA, Steinlein P, et al. *Neisseria gonorrhoeae* porin modulates phagosome maturation. *J Biol Chem* 1998;273:35332.
33. Muller A, Gunther D, Dux F, et al. Neisserial porin (PorB) causes rapid calcium influx in target cells and induces apoptosis by the activation of cysteine proteases. *EMBO J* 1999;18:339.
34. Gill MJ, Jayamohan J, Lessing MPA, et al. Naturally occurring PIA/PIB hybrids of *Neisseria gonorrhoeae*. *FEMS Microbiol Lett* 1994;119:161.
35. Hicks CB, Boslego JW, Brandt B. Evidence of serum antibodies to *Neisseria gonorrhoeae* before gonococcal infection. *J Infect Dis* 1987;155:1276.
36. Hook EW III, Olsen DA, Buchanan TM. Analysis of antigen specificity of the human sera immunoglobulin G immune response to complicated gonococcal infection. *Infect Immun* 1984;43:706.
37. Ison CA, Hadfield SG, Bellinger CM, et al. The specificity of serum and local antibodies in female gonorrhea. *Clin Exp Immunol* 1986;65:198.
38. Sarafian SK, Tam MR, Morse SA. Gonococcal protein I–specific opsonic IgG in normal human serum. *J Infect Dis* 1983;148:1025.
39. Heckels JE, Virji M, Zak K, et al. Immunobiology of gonococcal outer membrane protein I. *Antonie Van Leeuwenhoek* 1987;53:461.
40. Buchanan T, Eschenbach D, Knapp J, et al. Gonococcal salpingitis is less likely to recur with *Neisseria gonorrhoeae* of the same principal outer membrane protein antigenic type. *Am J Obstet Gynecol* 1981;138:978.
41. Plummer FA, Simonsen JN, Chubb H, et al. Epidemiologic evidence for the development of serovar-specific immunity after gonococcal infection. *J Clin Invest* 1989;83:1472.
42. Brunham RC, Plummer F, Slaney L, et al. Correlation of auxotype and protein I type with expression of disease due to *Neisseria gonorrhoeae*. *J Infect Dis* 1985;152:339.
43. Rice RJ, Biddle JW, JeanLouise YA, et al. Chromosomally mediated resistance in *Neisseria gonorrhoeae* in the United States: results of surveillance and reporting, 1983–1984. *J Infect Dis* 1986;153:340.
44. Swanson J, Barrera O, Sela J, et al. Expression of outer membrane protein II by gonococci in experimental gonorrhea. *J Exp Med* 1988;168:221.
45. Blake MS, Blake CM, Apicella MA, et al. Gonococcal opacity: lectin-like interactions between Opa proteins and lipooligosaccharide. *Infect Immun* 1995;63:1434.
46. Novotry P, Caronley K. Immunological anatomy of *Neisseria gonorrhoeae*. In: Brooks GE, Gotschlich EC, Holmes KK, et al., eds. Immunobiology of *Neisseria gonorrhoeae*. Washington, DC: American Society for Microbiology, 1978:263–271.
47. Naids FL, Belisle B, Lee N, et al. Interactions of *Neisseria gonorrhoeae* with human neutrophils: studies with purified PII (Opa) outer membrane proteins and synthetic Opa peptides. *Infect Immun* 1991;59:4628.
48. Elkins C, Rest RF. Monoclonal antibodies to outer membranes protein PII block interactions of *Neisseria gonorrhoeae* with human neutrophils. *Infect Immun* 1990;58:1078.
49. James JF, Swanson J. Studies on gonococcus infection. XIII. Occurrence of color/opacity colonial variants in clinical cultures. *Infect Immun* 1978;19:332.
50. Dehio C, Gray-Owen SD, Meyer TF. The role of neisserial Opa proteins in interactions with host cells. *Trends Microbiol* 1998;6:489–495.
51. Blake MS, Wetzler LM, Gotschlich C, et al. Protein III: structure, function and genetics. *Clin Microbiol Rev* 1989;2(suppl):60.
52. Plummer FA, Chubb H, Simonsen JN, et al. Antibody to Rmp (outer membrane protein 3) increases susceptibility to gonococcal infection. *J Clin Invest* 1993;91:339.
53. Pettit RK, McAllister SC, Hamer TA. Response of gonococcal clinical isolates to acidic conditions. *J Med Microbiol* 1999;48:149.
54. Muir LL, Strugnell RA, Davies JK. Proteins that appear to be associated with pili in *Neisseria gonorrhoeae*. *Infect Immun* 1988;56:1743.
55. Rudel T, Scheuerpflug 1, Meyer TF. *Neisseria PilC* protein identified as type-4 pilus tip-located adhesin. *Nature* 1995;373:357.
56. Frangipane JV, Rest R. Anaerobic growth and cytidine 5'-mono-phospho-N-acetylneuraminic acid act synergistically to induce high-level serum resistance in *Neisseria gonorrhoeae*. *Infect Immun* 1993;61:1657.

57. Hoehn GT, Clark VL. Distribution of a protein antigenically related to the major anaerobically induced gonococcal outer membrane protein among other *Neisseria* species. *Infect Immun* 1990;38:3929.

58. Clark VL, Knapp JS, Thompson S, et al. Presence of antibodies to the major anaerobically induced gonococcal outer membrane protein in sera from patients with gonococcal infections. *Microb Pathog* 1988;5:381.

59. Berish SA, Subbarao S, Chen CY, et al. Identification and cloning of a *fur* homolog from *Neisseria gonorrhoeae*. *Infect Immun* 1993;61:4599.

60. Shite S, Agarwal S, Murphy J, et al. The gonococcal fur regulation: identification of additional genes involved in major catabolic, recombination and secretory pathways. *J Bacteriol* 2002;184:3965.

61. Cornelissen CN, Anderson JE, Sparling PF. Energy-dependent changes in the gonococcal transferrin receptor. *Mol Microbiol* 1997;26:25.

62. Cornelissen CN, Biswas GD, Tsai J, et al. Gonococcal transferrin-binding protein 1 is required for transferrin utilization and is homologous to TonB-dependent outer membrane receptors. *J Bacteriol* 1992;174:5788.

63. Kenney CD, Cornelissen CN. Demonstration and characterization of a specific interaction between gonococcal transferrin binding protein A and TonB. *J Bacteriol* 2002;184:6138.

64. Lomholt H, Mogens K. Antigenic relationships among immunoglobulin AI proteases from *Haemophilus, Neisseria,* and *Streptococcus* species. *Infect Immun* 1994;62:3178.

65. Lorenzen DR, Dux F, Wolk U. Immunoglobulin A1 protease, an exoenzyme of pathogenic neisseriae, is a potent inducer of proinflammatory cytokines. *J Exp Med* 1999;190:1049.

66. Tsirpouchtsidis A, Hurwitz R, Brinkmann V, et al. Neisserial immunoglobulin A1 protease induces specific T-cell responses in humans. *Infect Immun* 2002;70:335.

67. Senior BW, Stewart WW, Galloway C, et al. Cleavage of the hormone human chorionic gonadotropin by the type 1 IgA1 protease of *Neisseria gonorrhoeae,* and its implications. *J Infect Dis* 2001;184:922.

68. Cannon JG, Black W, Nachamkin I, et al. Monoclonal antibody that recognizes an outer membrane antigen common to pathogenic *Neisseria* species but not to most nonpathogenic *Neisseria* species. *Infect Immun* 1985;43:994.

69. Chow AW, Malkasian KL, Marshall JR, et al. The bacteriology of acute pelvic inflammatory disease. *Am J Obstet Gynecol* 1975;122:876.

70. Trees DL, Schultz AJ, Knapp JS. Use of the neisserial lipoprotein (Lip) for subtyping *Neisseria gonorrhoeae*. *J Clin Microbiol* 2000;38:2914.

71. Griffiss JM, Schneider H, Mandrell RE, et al. Lipooligosaccharides: the principal glycolipids of the neisserial outer membrane. *Rev Infect Dis* 1988;10(suppl):287.

72. Mandrell RE, Lesse AJ, Sugai JV, et al. *In vitro* and *in vivo* modification of *Neisseria gonorrhoeae* lipooligosaccharide epitope structure by sialylation. *J Exp Med* 1990;171:1649.

73. Mandrell RE, Griffiss JM, Macher BA. Lipooligosaccharides (LOS) of *Neisseria gonorrhoeae* and *Neisseria meningitidis* have components that are immunochemically similar to precursors of human blood group antigens: carbohydrate sequence specificity of the mouse monoclonal antibodies that recognize cross-reacting antigens on LOS and human erythrocytes. *J Exp Med* 1988;168:107.

74. Schneider H, Griffiss JM, Boslego JW, et al. Expression of paragloboside-like lipooligosaccharides may be a necessary component of gonococcal pathogenesis in men. *J Exp Med* 1991;174:1601.

75. Schneider H, Schmidt KA, Skillman D, et al. Sialylation lessens the infectivity of *Neisseria gonorrhoeae* MS11mkC. *J Infect Dis* 1996;173:1422.

76. Smith H, Parsons NJ, Cole JA. Sialylation of neisserial lipopolysaccharide: a major influence on pathogenicity. *Microb Pathog* 1995;19:365.

77. Mandrell RE. Further antigenic similarities of *Neisseria gonorrhoeae* lipooligosaccharides and human glycosphingolipids. *Infect Immun* 1992;60:3017.

78. Ramsey KH, Schneider H, Cross AS, et al. Inflammatory cytokines produced in response to experimental human gonorrhea. *J Infect Dis* 1995;172:186.

79. Song W, Ma L, Chen R, et al. Role of lipooligosaccharide in Opa-independent invasion of *Neisseria gonorrhoeae* into human epithelial cells. *J Exp Med* 2000;191:949.

80. Richardson WP, Sadoff JC. Production of a capsule by *Neisseria gonorrhoeae*. *Infect Immun* 1977;15:663.

81. Roberts MC. Plasmids of *Neisseria gonorrhoeae* and other *Neisseria* species. *Clin Microbiol Rev* 1989;2(suppl):18.

82. Xia M, Whittinghan WL, Holmes KK, et al. Pulsed-field gel electrophoresis for genomic analysis of *Neisseria gonorrhoeae*. *J Infect Dis* 1995;17:455.

83. Unemo M, Olcen P, Berglund T, et al. Molecular epidemiology of *Neisseria gonorrhoeae*: sequence analysis of the *porB* gene confirms presence of two circulating strains. *J Clin Microbiol* 2002;40:3741.

84. Lau QC, Chow VTK, Poh CL. Differentiation of *Neisseria gonorrhoeae* strains by polymerase chain reaction and restriction fragment length polymorphism of outer membrane protein IB genes. *Genitourin Med* 1995;71:363.

85. Cooke SJ, de la Paz H, Poh CL, et al. Variation within serovars of *Neisseria gonorrhoeae* detected by structural analysis of outer membrane protein PIB and by pulsed-field gel electrophoresis. *Microbiology* 1997;143:1415.

86. Gill MJ. Serotyping *Neisseria gonorrhoeae,* a report of the Fourth International Workshop. *Genitourin Med* 1991;67:53.

87. O'Rourke M, Ison CA, Renton AM, et al. Opa-typing: a high-resolution tool for studying the epidemiology of gonorrhoea. *Mol Microbiol* 1995;17:865.

88. Apicella MA, Ketterer M, Lee FKN, et al. The pathogenesis of gonococcal urethritis in men: confocal and immunoelectron microscopic analysis of urethral exudates from men infected with *Neisseria gonorrhoeae*. *J Infect Dis* 1996;173:636.

89. Kallstrom H, Islam MS, Berggren PO, et al. Cell signaling by the type IV pili of pathogenic *Neisseria*. *J Biol Chem* 1998;273:21777.

90. Merz AJ, Enns CA, So M. Type IV pili of pathogenic neisseriae elicit cortical plaque formation in epithelial cells. *Mol Microbiol* 1999;32:1316.

91. Grassme H, Gulbins E, Brenner B, et al. Acidic sphingomyelinase mediates entry of *N. gonorrhoeae* into nonphagocytic cells. *Cell* 1997;91:605.

92. Dehio M, Gomez-Duarte OG, Dehio C, et al. Vitronectin-dependent invasion of epithelial cells by *Neisseria gonorrhoeae* involves αv integrin receptors. *FEBS Lett* 1998;424:84.

93. Cohen MS, Sparling PF. Mucosal infection with *Neisseria gonorrhoeae*. Bacterial adaption and mucosal defenses. *J Clin Invest* 1992;89:1699.

94. Britigan BE, Cohen MS, Sparling PF. Gonococcal infection: a model of molecular pathogenesis. *N Engl J Med* 1985;312:1683.

95. Fichorova RN, Desai PJ, Gibson FC III, et al. Distinct proinflammatory host responses to *Neisseria gonorrhoeae* infection in immortalized human cervical and vaginal epithelial cells. *Infect Immun* 2001;69:5840.

96. Knepper B, Heuer I, Meyer TF, et al. Differential response of human monocytes to *Neisseria gonorrhoeae* variants expressing pili and opacity proteins. *Infect Immun* 1997;65:4122.

97. Tramont EC. Inhibition of adherence of *Neisseria gonorrhoeae* by genital secretions. *J Clin Invest* 1977;59:117.

98. Simpson SD, Ho Y, Rice PA, et al. T lymphocyte response to *Neisseria gonorrhoeae* porin in individuals with mucosal gonococcal infections. *J Infect Dis* 1999;180:762.

99. Tsirpouchtsidis A, Hurwitz R, Brinkmann V, et al. Neisserial immunoglobulin A1 protease induces specific T-cell responses in humans. *Infect Immun* 2001;70:335.

100. Elliott B, Brunham RC, Laga M, et al. Maternal gonococcal infection as a preventable risk factor for low birth weight. *J Infect Dis* 1990;161:531.

101. Sarafian SK, Knapp JC. Molecular epidemiology of gonorrhea. *Clin Microbiol Rev* 1989;2(suppl):49.

102. Dougherty TJ. Peptidoglycan biosynthesis in *Neisseria gonorrhoeae* strains sensitive and intrinsically resistant to β-lactam antibiotics. *J Bacteriol* 1983;153:429.

103. Dillon JR, Yeung K. β-lactamase plasmids and chromosomally mediated antibiotic resistance in pathogenic *Neisseria* species. *Clin Microbiol Rev* 1989;2(suppl):125.

104. Dougherty TJ, Koller AE, Tomasz A. Competition of β-lactam antibiotics for the penicillin-binding proteins of *Neisseria gonorrhoeae*. *Antimicrob Agents Chemother* 1981;20:109.

105. Division of STD Prevention. Sexually transmitted disease surveillance 2001. U.S. Department of Health and Human Services, Public Health Service. Atlanta: Centers for Disease Control and Prevention, 2002.

106. Acar JF, Goldstein FW. Trends in bacterial resistance to fluoroquinolones. *Clin Infect Dis* 1997;24:67.

107. Centers for Disease Control and Prevention. *Sexually transmitted diseases surveillance 2000 supplement: gonococcal isolate surveillance program annual report—2000.* Atlanta: U.S. Department of Health and Human Services, October 2001.

108. Tramont EC. Gonococcal vaccines. *Clin Microbiol Rev* 1989;2(uppl):74.

109. Greenberg L, Diena FA, Ashton FA, et al. Gonococcal vaccine studies in Inuvik. *Can J Public Health* 1974;65:29.

110. Johnson S, Chung RCY, Deal CD, et al. Human immunization with Pgh 3-2 gonococcal pilus results in cross-reactive antibody to the cyanogen bromide fragment-2 of pilin. *J Infect Dis* 1991;163:128.

111. Darrow WW, Weisner PJ. Personal prophylaxis for venereal disease. *JAMA* 1975;233:444.

112. Harrison WO, Hooper RR, Weisner PJ, et al. A trial of microcycline given after exposure to prevent gonorrhea. *N Engl J Med* 1979;300:1074.

113. Jick H, Hannan MT, Stergachis A, et al. Vaginal spermicides and gonorrhea. *JAMA* 1982;248:1619.

114. Wilkinson D, Tholandi M, Ramjee G, et al. Nonoxynol-9 spermicide for prevention of vaginally acquired HIV and other sexually transmitted infections: systematic review and meta-analysis of randomized controlled trials including more than 5000 women. *Lancet Infect Dis* 2002;2:613.

115. Heckels JE. Structure and function of pili of *Neisseria* species. *Clin Microbiol Rev* 1989;2:566.

116. Hagblom P, Segal E, Billyard E, et al. Intragenic recombination leads to pilus antigenic variation in *Neisseria gonorrhoeae*. *Nature* 1985;315:156.

117. Morse SA, Johnson SR, Biddle JW, et al. High level tetracycline resistance in *Neisseria gonorrhoeae* is result of acquisition of streptococcal TetM determinant. *Antimicrob Agents Chemother* 1986;30:664.

118. Blake MS, Wetzler LM. Vaccines for gonorrhea: where are we on the curve? *Trends Microbiol* 1995;3:469.

CHAPTER 193
Neisseria meningitidis

John W. Boslego, Edmund C. Tramont,
and John G. Bartlett

HISTORY

The history of meningococcal disease is both fascinating and humbling—fascinating when one reflects on what we have learned over the years about the epidemiology, pathogenesis, pathophysiology, and the principal determinant of host susceptibility (the lack of bactericidal antibody) (1), but humbling from the standpoint of how little we understand about the virulence properties of the organism or the dynamics involved in epidemic disease.

From 1805 to 1810, *Neisseria meningitidis* was the likely cause of a series of epidemics of meningitis that ravaged the Napoleonic and Persian armies (*meningitic de congélation*) as well as an epidemic in New England known as "spotted fever." The next 150 years were marked by a peculiar pattern of periodic outbreaks occurring every 8 to 15 years interspersed with sporadic cases. At first, high rates of meningococcal disease predominated in Europe and North America, but over time the disease spread throughout the world, especially to sub-Saharan Africa, leaving in its wake milder and less explosive outbreaks with each successive epidemic wave.

The first description of the etiologic agent appeared in 1886 when Anton Weichselbaum demonstrated gram-negative diplococci in the cerebrospinal fluid (CSF) of a young Viennese patient who had died of purulent meningitis. Five years later, Quincke introduced the lumbar puncture as a therapeutic measure to reduce the increased pressure associated with meningitis. But its major impact was diagnostic: the isolation of *N. meningitidis* (and other bacteria) in pure culture. Armed with the knowledge of the etiologic agent of epidemic "cerebrospinal meningitis," numerous investigative studies quickly elucidated basic information concerning (a) epidemiology, that is, the episodic nature of epidemics interspersed with sporadic cases, the difficulty in linking cases with one another, the propensity for higher attack rates during the winter months, the predilection to occur in young children and young adults, and the asymptomatic carrier state; (b) bacteriology, that is, serogrouping and characterization of strains; (c) clinical aspects, that is, a bacterium that is usually a normal saprophyte but that can become one of the quickest killers of humans; and (d) immunology, that is, the lack of serum bactericidal activity predisposing to invasive disease. Such studies set the stage for attempts at innovative treatments such as passive immunotherapy and eventually vaccine development.

Meningococcal Disease and the Military

Meningococcal disease has had a long and special relationship with the military (2). The collection of a large number of young adults from disparate localities who train, eat, and sleep in proximity creates an ecologic setting highly favorable for the spread of meningococci. Indeed, some of the most dramatic outbreaks of meningococcal meningitis have occurred in military training camps.

The introduction of sulfa drugs successfully controlled such outbreaks when it became routine practice to give prophylaxis to entire units after the occurrence of a single case. This approach was highly effective until sulfadiazine-resistant strains emerged in the early 1960s.

Against this backdrop, the classic studies of Goldschneider and co-workers (3) on the natural history of meningococcal infections firmly established that the absence of bactericidal antibody against the infecting strain predisposed an individual to develop invasive meningococcal disease soon after colonization of the oropharynx. They further demonstrated that bactericidal antibody could be elicited by purified, high-molecular-weight meningococcal capsular polysaccharides. Their studies quickly led to the development of the highly effective group C meningococcal vaccine (4).

Antimicrobial Therapy and Prophylaxis

The introduction of antimicrobial agents dramatically transformed this highly fatal disease into a usually curable one, particularly when the diagnosis is made early.

Antimicrobial prophylaxis continues to play a role in the management of meningococcal outbreaks. With the inevitable advent of antimicrobial resistance, however, the effectiveness of routine prophylaxis of contacts has become less predictable (5).

CHARACTERISTICS OF THE PATHOGEN

The genus *Neisseria* is a member of the family Neisseriaceae, which also includes *Moraxella, Acinetobacter,* and *Kingella* (6) (Table 193.1). Although 12 species of *Neisseria* have been isolated from humans, only *N. meningitidis* and *Neisseria gonorrhoeae* are regularly pathogenic. The other species are usually part of the normal flora and only rarely cause disease.

TABLE 193.1. Taxonomy of Neisseriaceae

Genus: *Neisseria*
  N. meningitidis[a]
  N. gonorrhoeae[a] (includes subspecies *kochii*[a])
  N. subflava[a] (includes biovars *perflava*[a] *flava*[a])
  N. flavescens[a]
  N. caviae
  N. mucosa[a]
  N. canis
  N. cinerea[a]
  N. cuniculi
  N. denitrificans
  N. elongata
  N. lactamica[a]
  N. ovis
  N. polysaccharea[a]
Genus: *Acinetobacter*
  A. calcoaceticus
Genus: *Kingella*
  K. kingae
  K. indologenes
  K. denitrificans
Genus: *Moraxella*
  M. lacunata
  M. bovis
  M. nonliquefaciens
  M. phenylpyruvica
  M. osloensis
  Branhamella (Moraxella) catarrhalis

[a] *Neisseria* strains that have been isolated from humans.

N. meningitidis is an aerobic, oxidase-positive, gram-negative diplococcus. Under culture conditions, it grows best at 35° to 37°C in a moist 5% to 7% CO_2 environment (candle jar).

The optimal isolation medium depends on the source of the specimen. Antibiotic-containing medium (such as modified Thayer-Martin or New York City medium) is necessary when the culture specimen is obtained from a nonsterile site such as the oropharynx. When a normally sterile site such as blood or CSF is cultured, nonselective chocolate agar is preferable.

Oxidative metabolism of specific carbohydrates with resultant acid production is the major means for differentiating *Neisseria* species (Table 193.1). *N. meningitidis* produces acid from glucose and maltose but not sucrose, lactose, or fructose. A pure subculture of the organism is required for proper evaluation.

A wide array of tests has been developed to provide a more rapid, specific identification of *N. meningitidis*. Such tests utilize acid production, enzyme elaboration, and serologic specificity (6). These tests have greatly aided quick and accurate diagnosis in the laboratory but can occasionally result in misidentification. Acid fermentation reactions by an occasional strain may not be easily interpreted. Likewise, enzyme identification may sometimes be difficult to interpret. For example, *N. meningitidis* produces γ-glutamylaminopeptidase, but so does an occasional nonpathogenic *Neisseria* species. Therefore, the combined use of biochemical and enzyme tests is necessary to obtain the greatest diagnostic precision.

Structurally, the meningococcus resembles other gram-negative bacteria. The organism is surrounded by a polysaccharide capsule. Beneath it, the cell envelope consists of a lipid bilayer, outer-membrane proteins (OMPs), lipooligosaccharide (LOS), pili (filamentous projections that extend through the capsule), and a dense peptidoglycan layer. A cytoplasmic membrane encloses the cytoplasm and nucleus.

The capsule is composed of an anionic polysaccharide. This serves as the basis for categorizing the organism into serogroups. To date, 13 serogroups have been identified: A, B, C, D 29E, H, I, K, L, W135, X, Y, and Z. Serogroups A, B, C, W135, and Y are the serogroups responsible for the overwhelming majority of cases of invasive disease. All serogroups except D have been chemically and structurally defined (7–11). The presence of a capsule is associated with virulence. Invasive meningococci are almost always encapsulated, whereas meningococci colonizing mucous membranes frequently are not.

Subcapsular antigens are used to classify meningococci further into serotypes, subtypes, and immunotypes (12). There are five classes of major OMPs, designated class 1 to class 5 and differentiated on the basis of molecular weight, peptide maps, and electrophoretic behavior (13). The serotype is based on serologic (monoclonal antibody) reactivity to the class 2 or 3 OMP (a strain has either a class 2 or a class 3 OMP but not both). The subtype is based on serologic reactivity to the class 1 OMP The LOS immunotype is based on serologic reactivity to LOS. Each serogroup contains strains with a variety of types, subtypes, and LOS immunotypes, and each type is not restricted to a given serogroup. For example, approximately 15 serotypes, 13 subtypes, and 13 LOS immunotypes have been identified among group B strains, but many strains remain nontypable. According to convention, a strain can be designated as B:15:P1.3:L3,8, which means serogroup B, serotype 15, subtype 3, immunotypes 3 and 8.

These grouping and typing schemes have been quite useful for epidemiologic studies and for vaccine development, but continued studies are required to develop a more complete, standardized, and universally accepted set of typing reagents.

Another method of classifying meningococci is based on the electrophoretic mobilities of metabolic enzymes produced by *N. meningitidis* (14). Multilocus enzyme electrophoresis provides a mechanism for characterizing the chromosomal genome and grouping strains by their genetic relatedness. Analysis of hundreds of isolates from around the world has yielded 78 electrophoretic types representing multilocus genotypes. Only a small number of electrophoretic types are responsible for most of the invasive disease cases. Preliminary studies indicate that strains that colonize the throat are usually from clones different from those that cause invasive disease (15). With continued experience, this enzyme typing system should provide a better understanding of the virulence determinants of meningococci.

EPIDEMIOLOGY

Meningococcal infections are a worldwide health problem. The vast majority of cases occur in childhood. Attack rates are highest in infants 6 months to 1 year of age and then decrease over time. A minor secondary peak occurs in the late teens and early twenties and reflects outbreaks in military recruits and college populations (16). In temperate climates, disease rates peak during the winter months. Even with the introduction of effective antibiotics, the fatality rate remains high at 5% to 15%. In the United States, *N. meningitidis* causes approximately 3,000 cases a year and has replaced *Haemophilus influenzae* type b as the most frequent cause of bacterial meningitis in children. This is the result of a substantial reduction in the incidence of *H. influenzae* type b infections because of the high effectiveness and widespread use of protein-polysaccharide conjugate vaccines in infants.

The sub-Saharan "meningitis belt" in Africa is one of the areas most severely affected. Major epidemics have occurred in that region every 8 to 12 years during the past century, resulting in an estimated 500,000 deaths in the past 50 years. One of the largest more recent epidemics occurred in China between 1963 and 1970 (17). The peak year was 1967, when there was an attack rate of 400 cases per 100,000 persons per year, resulting in more than 3 million cases and 166,000 deaths.

N. meningitidis is a uniquely human pathogen. Humans are the only reservoir, and the organism is carried on the nasopharyngeal mucosa. Transmission occurs from person to person, presumably through passage of respiratory secretions or aerosolized droplets.

Carrier rates of meningococci among cohorts vary tremendously. The bacteria serogroup and strain, age and socioeconomic status of the person, prevalence of disease activity, and crowded living conditions are all factors (18,19). However, there is no critical "carrier rate" that accurately predicts an epidemic or outbreak.

In an individual person, the virulence of a particular strain, host susceptibility (immunity), and environmental influences all play a role in the development of invasive disease. These interrelationships have not yet been fully defined. Often, a preceding respiratory infection such as influenza occurs and may facilitate entry of meningococci through respiratory mucosa. Additional precipitating factors are probably needed for an epidemic to occur, such as exceptional climatic conditions, an infectious cofactor, or the introduction of a new virulent strain to which many individuals lack immunity.

Epidemics of meningococcal disease normally result from a single dominant strain or clone. Specific combinations of serotype and subtype have been found to be associated with epidemic group B, group C, and W135 disease (18,20). Conversely, endemic disease is caused by diverse serogroups, serotypes, and subtypes.

Serogroups A, B, and C have been responsible for practically all known epidemics. Serogroup A has been most often associated with explosive widespread epidemics. In sub-Saharan Africa, outbreaks generally occur during the dry season, terminate at the onset of the rainy season, and generally occur in cycles with an interval of 8 to 12 years. The large epidemics in China have been due exclusively to group A as well and have also followed an 8- to 10-year cyclic pattern. Group A outbreaks in industrialized countries are now rare and, when they occur, are generally small and affect those of the lowest socioeconomic status.

Although serogroup C can cause large outbreaks, it is more often associated with smaller outbreaks and endemic disease. Sao Paulo, Brazil, experienced a large group C outbreak in the early 1970s, but the responsible serogroup later shifted to group A (18). Subsequently, Los Angeles, California, experienced clusters of group C cases (19,21).

Serogroup B does not generally cause the extraordinarily high attack rates of meningitis common with group A or C disease. However, this serogroup is now the major cause of endemic disease and small outbreaks in industrialized countries (19,22). During the 1970s, group B disease emerged in northwest Europe and caused sustained outbreaks in Norway Iceland, the Faeroe Islands, Great Britain, Denmark, and the Netherlands. Clonally related group B strains [electrophoretic type 5 (ET5) complex] have also spread to the Western Hemisphere, causing outbreaks in Cuba, Chile, and Brazil (19).

As noted earlier, the diverse patterns of disease imply differences in virulence determinants, host immunity, and efficiency of transmission. Unfortunately, little is understood about these differences.

PATHOGENESIS

Although the organism may cause an oropharyngitis, it is primarily a saprophyte that asymptomatically colonizes the majority of human beings sometime during their lives. As with other neisserial species, it can sometimes colonize the genital tract or conjunctiva. Rarely, the organism escapes from its customarily benign ecologic niche and invades the bloodstream. The frequency of this event or the reasons why it occurs are poorly understood. On the basis of studies in military recruits, invasion probably takes place within hours or days after colonization. Once the organism has disseminated, an overlapping array of clinical outcomes may ensue (Fig. 193.1). The host's immune status plays a critical role in the ultimate course (3,23).

Host Immunity

Serum bactericidal antibody is the cornerstone of an effective host defense against meningococcal disease (1,3). Protective antibody may be acquired transplacentally or actively, as a result of colonization or infection with meningococci or other organisms possessing cross-reactive antigens (i.e., other neisserial species or commensal organisms in the oropharynx or gut) or by vaccination. Transplacental (maternal) antibodies protect newborn infants up to 6 months of age, after which susceptibility increases until age 2. It then wanes over time as the child's immune experience broadens, reflected by the acquisition of serum bactericidal activity against *N. meningitidis* species. Apparently, the development of antibody protective against invasion by colonizing strains of *N. meningitidis* is commonplace because in military recruits the oropharyngeal carriage rate can be as high as

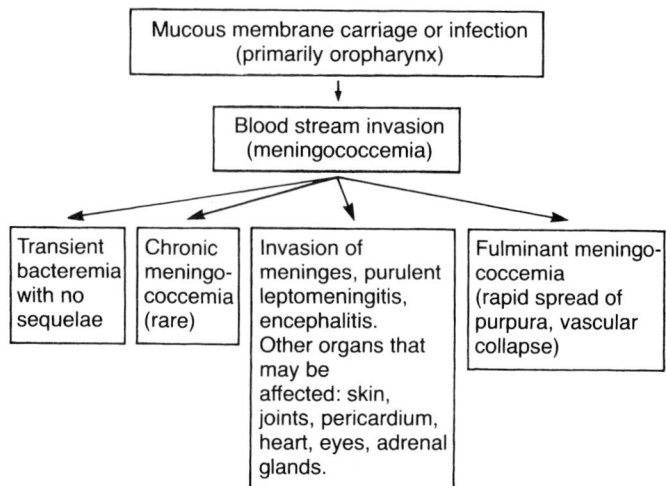

Figure 193.1. Pathogenesis of meningococcal disease.

95%, yet the incidence of systemic disease remains well under 1% (3).

Meningococcal Disease

When bactericidal antibody is present in the serum, the meningococcus appears to be rapidly destroyed on entry into the bloodstream. If bactericidal antibody is absent, the organism multiplies and disseminates. If inadequate amounts or low-affinity antibody is present, the disease process may be modulated, but the factors that determine the clinical presentation (transient bacteremia, chronic meningococcemia, meningococcal meningitis, fulminant meningococcemia, or any combination thereof) are unknown (Fig. 193.1).

At least three host factors can influence the efficiency of bactericidal antibody: complement deficiency, blocking immunoglobulin A (IgA) antibody, and IgM deficiency. Meningococcal disease is a common infection experienced by complement-deficient individuals. Inherited deficiencies of properdin, early complement components (C1, C4, C2), or late complement components (C6, C7, C8) all predispose to invasive meningococcal disease (24). Specific antibody can partially overcome deficiencies of properdin and early complement components. But patients with late component complement deficiencies exhibit a striking susceptibility to initial and recurrent infections, emphasizing the importance of serum bactericidal activity in the control of this infection. Some persons may also develop transient blocking IgA antibody. Because IgA does not effectively bind complement, the organisms are not killed (25). Removing the IgA experimentally restores the serum's ability to lyse the bacterium. Because the IgM class of antibody readily binds complement, persons with an IgM deficiency lyse meningococci less efficiently (26).

Like many other encapsulated organisms, *N. meningitidis* has a predilection to invade the meninges (pia and arachnoid) and cause a leptomeningitis. In most instances, acute infection is common and is probably the result of rapid multiplication of meningococci and the release of endotoxin (LOS), which in turn invokes an intense, acute inflammatory response characterized by an exudate consisting primarily of polymorphonuclear cells. Direct invasion of brain parenchyma is rare, but encephalitis commonly results from swelling secondary to impeded venous drainage. However, the ultimate outcome in appropriately treated patients is not related to the intensity of the inflammatory response.

In the bloodstream, endotoxin from propagating organisms reacts with macrophages to release cytokines (e.g., tumor necrosis factor), prostaglandins, and free radicals. Disruption of activated endothelial protein C complex results in the early development of widespread thrombosis (27). The result is petechiae, ecchymoses, and disseminated intravascular coagulation, sometimes with shock and multiorgan system failure (28,29).

CLINICAL MANIFESTATIONS

The clinical manifestations of meningococcal disease have already been alluded to. An oropharyngitis may occur. Rarely, a pneumonia may develop, usually with serogroup Y or B strains (30). The cultural diagnosis of these infections is often missed unless the clinical microbiology laboratory has been alerted to use selective media. Occasionally, a person can develop a meningococcal genital tract infection, proctitis, or conjunctivitis.

Once the bloodstream is invaded, a spectrum of clinical manifestations may ensue (Fig. 193.1). The mildest form is a transient bacteremia that usually begins insidiously with fever and malaise. Only a few, if any, petechial skin lesions occur. No meningeal signs develop. The symptoms spontaneously resolve in 24 to 48 hours. Blood cultures subsequently grow *N. meningitidis.*

In rare instances, a chronic meningococcemia develops. This curious clinical entity is similar to the gonococcal dermatitis-arthritis syndrome and consists of intermittent febrile episodes lasting 2 to 10 days associated with a variety of skin lesions (macular, maculopapular, pustular) and migratory arthralgias and myalgias. Blood cultures may be continuously or intermittently positive. Sometimes multiple blood cultures are required to isolate the organism. The infection may last months and may resolve spontaneously; the effect of appropriate antibiotic treatment is dramatic (31).

Acute meningococcemia occurs most often after several days of upper respiratory symptoms. The patient's temperature increases abruptly followed by chills and malaise. Weakness, myalgias, arthralgias, nausea, vomiting, and headache usually develop quickly, but the most remarkable manifestation is the development of characteristic petechial skin lesions. They are the most common type of skin lesion occurring with meningococcal disease, usually appearing in crops on the ankles, wrists, and armpits, but may progress to involve any part of the body. The palms, soles, and head are usually spared. The number of lesions can advance rapidly within a few hours, and new lesions may continue to develop for up to 24 hours after appropriate treatment. Other skin manifestations include macular and maculopapular lesions. The patients tend to have only a moderate fever (39.5°C) but a marked leukocytosis. Signs of vascular collapse are infrequent.

Fulminant meningococcemia, also referred to as Waterhouse-Friderichsen syndrome or purpura fulminans, is the toxic extension of acute meningococcemia. It occurs in 5% to 15% of cases and is characterized by apprehension, restlessness, and delirium developing in a few hours. The skin lesions rapidly become widespread, purpuric, and ecchymotic. Vascular collapse eventually ensues (27,32). Acute renal failure, pulmonary insufficiency, and cardiac insufficiency, the most frequently reported autopsy finding (33), are secondary complications. High fever is usually present, but sometimes a febrile response fails to develop, which represents a poor prognostic sign. The white cell

count can be high, normal, or low (neutropenia), and thrombocytopenia is frequent. Evidence of intravascular coagulation is common. Mortality rates remain high despite appropriate antibiotic treatment.

With the exception of mild transient bacteremia, all of the foregoing syndromes can be associated with acute meningitis (see Chapter 148). Clinically, meningococcal meningitis resembles acute bacterial meningitis of any cause.

DIAGNOSIS

Clinical diagnosis rests on a high index of suspicion and, in a patient presenting with a febrile illness, a rapid and thorough search for petechiae and purpura. Evidence of meningeal irritation is helpful but may be absent early in the disease course. Diagnostic specimens should be collected as rapidly as possible but should not delay initiation of treatment.

The laboratory diagnosis of meningococcal disease is based on the isolation of the organism from blood, CSF, or skin lesions. Blood cultures are positive in up to 75% of patients with proven meningococcal disease (34). They may be positive when CSF cultures are not, even in the setting of inflamed meninges.

An abnormal CSF demonstrating an elevated white cell count consisting of predominantly polymorphonuclear cells, associated with a low glucose level, is highly suggestive of bacterial meningitis. A CSF Gram stain is positive in about 70% of cases, but meningococci may sometimes be confused with pneumococci or *H. influenzae*, particularly when few organisms are seen. Culture of the CSF is the most reliable diagnostic test and is positive in about 70% of cases. Because of the organism's fragility, efforts must be made to plate the CSF on chocolate agar as soon as possible (within minutes) and place it in a 5% to 7% carbon dioxide environment (candle jar). This usually allows the culture to remain viable for up to 8 hours before incubation at 35° to 37°C. Rarely, the culture of an otherwise normal CSF specimen may yield *N. meningitidis* (35).

Petechial skin lesions also represent a potential diagnostic specimen. Meningococci are often present in petechiae, and Gram-stained smears of needle aspirates or punch biopsies from skin lesions are positive in up to 75% of cases (34). This can be particularly useful when antibiotics were started before cultures were obtained.

Nasopharyngeal cultures for *N. meningitidis* must be interpreted with caution. A positive throat culture may reveal serogroupable *N. meningitidis* in patients with invasive disease. However, a positive throat culture alone should not be considered proof of meningococcal infection because patients with other forms of meningitis may be coincident carriers of *N. meningitidis.*

Newer techniques for the rapid identification of *N. meningitidis* capsular polysaccharide in blood and CSF are available. Countercurrent immunoelectrophoresis, latex particle agglutination, and coagglutination techniques have been developed (36). CSF is the optimal specimen for analysis by these techniques. Although antigen can be detected in serum, urine, and other body fluids, the sensitivity is lower than with CSF. The main advantage of these tests is to provide a rapid identification (minutes to hours) of the specific bacterium responsible for infection. These tests should not replace the Gram stain. Their most appropriate use is in cases in which the Gram stain is negative or confusing, such as early in the course of infection or when prior antibiotics have been administered. The sensitivity of these tests is lower than that of a positive Gram stain (approximately

10^5 organisms per milliliter). Group B polysaccharide antigen is generally the most difficult to detect, and sensitivity is lowest for this serogroup.

Commercial countercurrent immunoelectrophoresis kits are available for serogroups A, B, and C and can detect as little as 50 ng of purified polysaccharide per milliliter. Only rarely is an organism misidentified.

Latex particle agglutination is simpler, faster, and probably more sensitive than countercurrent immunoelectrophoresis. Commercial kits for detection of serogroups A, C, Y, W135, and B are available. Most of the published data reflect antigen detection in serogroup A and C disease with a sensitivity of about 80%. Data on detection of antigen in serogroup B, Y, and W135 disease are limited.

Coagglutination tests for *N. meningitidis* have been evaluated in research settings (36). This technique appears less sensitive than countercurrent immunoelectrophoresis or latex particle agglutination.

Preliminary data on the use of the polymerase chain reaction for the diagnosis of meningococcal meningitis are promising. In one study, the sensitivity and specificity of this technique were both 91% (37). Moreover, sensitivity was not affected by prior antibiotic treatment. As the polymerase chain reaction technology becomes more widely available in clinical laboratories, additional studies will be needed to define its utility in various demographic populations.

TREATMENT

Few infections progress with the rapidity of those caused by *N. meningitidis,* and a successful outcome is highly dependent on early, appropriate antibiotic administration.

Penicillin G has remained the treatment of choice for more than 50 years, although it is used somewhat less frequently now (38,39). In infants and children, 300,000 units/kg per day (in divided doses every 4 hours) should be given intravenously for at least 7 days, longer in more serious cases. In adults, 24 million units per day intravenously (in divided doses every 2–4 hours) should be given initially; the dose can be reduced after a few days depending on the clinical status of the patient. Treatment duration is usually 10 to 14 days, depending on the clinical response.

The antibiotic armamentarium for bacterial meningitis has greatly expanded. Unlike the first-generation cephalosporins (e.g., cephalothin), the third-generation cephalosporins exhibit excellent CSF penetration (40). This feature, combined with their excellent *in vitro* activity against common meningeal pathogens, makes them an attractive selection in cases in which the etiologic diagnosis is uncertain or for patients with a nonanaphylactic history of penicillin intolerance. Clinical experience with cefotaxime and ceftriaxone has verified the pharmacologic data. Chloramphenicol [75–100 mg/kg per day (up to 4 g per day) intravenously in divided doses every 6 hours] also remains an alternative regimen. Fluoroquinolones have good *in vitro* activity against *N. meningitidis* and reasonable CSF penetration, and their role in the treatment of meningococcal meningitis must await the results of clinical trials.

Occasional isolates of *N. meningitidis* from clinical cases have demonstrated a relative resistance to penicillin (39,41,42). These isolates are termed penRR and are defined by a minimum inhibitory concentration of penicillin of 0.1 to 1.0 mg/L. These isolates do not produce β-lactamase, and the mechanism of resistance is related to a decreased affinity of one of the organism's penicillin-binding proteins to penicillin. The penRR isolates have

been reported from Spain, South Africa, the United Kingdom, Canada, Greece, Switzerland, Romania, Belgium, and the United States. In Spain, penRR *N. meningitidis* strains account for up to 50% of isolates, but the incidence is much lower in other regions.

The clinical significance of this relative resistance is not established. Patients infected with penRR strains recover when treated with penicillin or ampicillin, although there are suggestions of a higher rate of complications or a slightly prolonged clinical course.

Third-generation cephalosporins continue to demonstrate low minimum inhibitory concentrations for penRR strains. Until more information is available, clinical cases caused by penRR meningococci should be treated with a third-generation cephalosporin. In addition, continued surveillance for penRR isolates and β-lactamase–producing isolates is warranted.

As in other patients with vascular collapse, supportive therapy is vitally important for a successful outcome (see Chapter 61). Monitoring of fluid replacement and renal and cardiovascular function is essential. The value of steroid therapy in meningococcal infections is still unknown. Short-term administration of high-dose dexamethasone decreased the likelihood of moderate to severe hearing loss in infants and children with bacterial meningitis primarily caused by *H. influenzae.* Although an effect is probable, there were too few cases of meningococcal meningitis in the study to document a beneficial effect for this subgroup (43,44). Obviously, steroid replacement is essential in patients with acute adrenal insufficiency secondary to adrenal gland infarction. Heparin therapy for an accompanying intravascular coagulopathy has not proved beneficial.

PREVENTION

Immunoprophylaxis

Currently licensed meningococcal vaccines consist of mixtures of purified, high-molecular-weight capsular polysaccharides from serogroups A, C, Y, and W135. Serogroup A and C vaccines were developed in the late 1960s and were shown to be remarkably safe and highly effective (4,45–47). In 1982, serogroups Y and W135 were added to serogroup A and C polysaccharides to form a single tetravalent vaccine. Use of this vaccine in all U.S. military recruits has virtually eliminated meningococcal disease except for serogroup B in this cohort (2,48).

The tetravalent vaccine is indicated for all intimate contacts of meningococcal cases, except for those known to be caused by group B organisms. The vaccine can also be used in institutional settings when one or more cases occur (49). Travelers to regions experiencing epidemics or high rates of endemic disease should be immunized before departure (50). All patients with meningococcal disease should be evaluated for inherited complement deficiencies after their recovery from acute infection. Patients and their family members with properdin and early component deficiencies respond well to vaccination and should be immunized (51). Patients with late complement component deficiencies respond less well, but periodic immunization should be considered as part of their management strategy.

Despite their safety and effectiveness, there remain several important limitations of the current meningococcal vaccines. In addition to cost and distribution difficulties similar to those for other vaccines in worldwide use, the duration of immunity of capsular polysaccharide vaccines is unknown but estimated to be 2 to 3 years. Consequently, disease unpredictability, logistic difficulties, and cost considerations often delay the initiation of immunization until the onset of an outbreak or epidemic. More important, these vaccines, particularly the group C component, are poorly immunogenic in children younger than 2 years, the age group at highest risk for infection. Lastly, no licensed vaccine is currently available for serogroup B.

Efforts to improve the immunogenicity of capsular polysaccharide vaccines in infants and young children have focused on the conjugation of polysaccharides to carrier proteins. This approach has been used successfully with *H. influenzae* polysaccharide vaccine, with resultant improved immunogenicity and protection in children under 1 year of age (52). Improvements in the immunogenicity of meningococcal polysaccharides conjugated to proteins bode well for an effective vaccine for infants (46,53).

Unlike those of the other major serogroups, purified group B meningococcal capsular polysaccharide is not immunogenic in humans (54). Efforts to enhance its immunogenicity have been generally unsuccessful. These results, coupled with the shared antigenicity of B polysaccharide and determinants on gangliosides of animal and human cells, have dampened enthusiasm for purified B polysaccharide as a vaccine component (55).

Chemoprophylaxis

Antibiotic administration for the prevention of invasive meningococcal disease is based on the premise that close contacts (e.g., defined as living and sleeping in the same household, dormitory, or barracks) of meningococcal disease cases are at a considerably higher risk than the normal population for development of disease. Although close contacts are at a 500- to 1,000-fold higher risk than are control subjects, the risk of invasive disease in an individual contact is still quite low (34). Nonetheless, the standard practice is to prescribe an antibiotic course designed to eradicate meningococcal throat carriage in all close contacts. Nonimmunized contacts should also receive the tetravalent meningococcal vaccine in all situations except group B outbreaks because protective antibody develops quickly after immunization. Time does not permit bacteriologic screening to determine an individual's carrier status, because those who develop invasive disease usually do so within a few days of exposure to the index case.

Because chemoprophylaxis is not uniformly successful or sufficient for treatment of invasive disease, patients must be advised to seek prompt evaluation in the event of symptoms even remotely suggestive of meningococcal infection.

Sulfadiazine was employed as chemoprophylaxis with great success in the 1940s and 1950s. But the emergence and high prevalence of sulfadiazine-resistant meningococci in the 1960s rendered it inadequate. Although the prevalence of sulfadiazine resistance has waned, sulfadiazine prophylaxis is rarely practical because of the time involved in determining sulfadiazine susceptibility.

Despite their efficacy in the treatment of invasive disease, penicillins do not predictably eradicate carriage and consequently are not used (34).

Rifampin and ciprofloxacin are the mainstays of chemoprophylaxis (56). Rifampin, given twice daily for 2 days in a dose of 10 mg/kg (up to 600 mg per dose), eradicates meningococci from 75% to 98% of carriers. Side effects are few, but treatment failure has been associated with rifampin resistance (57). Ciprofloxacin (500 mg orally one time) appears more effective (58) and is often preferred for adults, although failures have been reported (59). Other options are ceftriaxone (250 mg intramuscularly one time for adults), which is sometimes preferred for pregnant women, or minocycline (100 mg orally twice daily for 5 days), which can be used in persons over 8 years of age (60,61).

REFERENCES

1. Heist GD, Solis-Cohen S, Solis-Cohen M: A study of the virulence of meningococci for man and of human susceptibility of meningococcic infection. *J Immunol* 1922;7:1.
2. Brundage JF, Zollinger WD. Evolution of meningococcal disease epidemiology in the US Army. In: Vedros NA, ed. *Evolution of meningococcal disease*, Vol. 1. Boca Raton, FL: CRC Press, 1987:6–25.
3. Goldschneider 1, Gotschlich EC, Artenstein MS. Human immunity to the meningococcus. I. The role of humoral antibodies. *J Exp Med* 1969;129:1307.
4. Artenstein MS, Gold R, Zimmerly JG, et al. Prevention of meningococcal disease by group C polysaccharide vaccine. *N Engl J Med* 1970;282:417.
5. Artenstein MS. Chemoprophylaxis of meningococcal carriers. *N Engl J Med* 1969;281:678.
6. Knapp JS. Historical perspectives and identification of *Neisseria* and related species. *Clin Microbiol Rev* 1988;1:415.
7. Jenning HJ. Capsular polysaccharides as human vaccines. *Adv Carbohydr Chem Biochem* 1983;41:155.
8. Michon F, Roy R, Jennings HJ, et al. Structural elucidation of the capsular polysaccharide of *Neisseria meningitidis* group H. *Can J Chem* 1984;62:1519.
9. Michon F, Brisson JR, Roy R, et al. Structural determination of the capsular polysaccharide of *Neisseria meningitidis* group I: a two-dimensional NMR analysis. *Biochemistry* 1985;24:5592.
10. Michon F, Brisson JR, Roy R, et al. Structural determination of the group K capsular polysaccharide of *Neisseria meningitidis*: a 2D-NMR analysis. *Can J Chem* 1985;63:2781.
11. Jenning HJ. The structure of the capsular polysaccharide obtained from a new serogroup (L) of *Neisseria meningitidis*. *Carbohydr Res* 1983;112:105.
12. Frasch CE, Zollinger WD, Footman JT. A proposed nomenclature for designation of serotypes within *Neisseria meningitidis*. *Rev Infect Dis* 1985;7:504.
13. Tsai CM, Frasch CE, Mocca LF. Five structural classes of major outer membrane proteins in *Neisseria meningitidis*. *J Bacteriol* 1981;146:69.
14. Caugant DA, Froholm LO, Borre K, et al. Intercontinental spread of a genetically distinctive complex of clones of *Neisseria meningitidis* causing epidemic disease. *Proc Natl Acad Sci USA* 1986;83:4927.
15. Caugant DA, Kristiansen BE, Froholm LO, et al. Clonal diversity of *Neisseria meningitidis* from a population of asymptomatic carriers. *Infect Immun* 1988;56:2060.
16. Harrison LH, Pass MA, Mendelsohn AB, et al. Invasive meningococcal disease in adolescents and young adults. *JAMA* 2001;286:694.
17. Zhen H. Epidemiology of meningococcal disease in China. In: Vedros NA, ed. *Evolution of meningococcal disease*, Vol. II. Boca Raton, FL: CRC Press, 1987:19–32.
18. Mastrantonio P, Stefanelli P, Fazio C, et al. Serotype distribution, antibiotic susceptibility, and genetic relatedness of *Neisseria meningitides* strains recently isolated in Italy. *Clin Infect Dis* 2003;36:422.
19. Schwartz B, Moore PS, Broome CV. Global epidemiology of meningococcal disease. *Clin Microbiol Rev* 1989;2(suppl):118.
20. Mayer LW, Reeves MW, Al-Hamdan N, et al. Outbreak of W135 meningococcal disease in 2000: not emergence of a new W135 strain but clonal expansion within the electrophoretic type-37 complex. *J Infect Dis* 2002;185:1596.
21. Tappero JW, Reporter R, Wenger JD, et al. Meningococcal disease in Los Angeles County, California, and among men in the county jails. *N Engl J Med* 1996;335:833.
22. Peltola H. Meningococcal disease: still with us. *Rev Infect Dis* 1983;5:71.
23. DeVoe IW. The meningococcus and mechanisms of pathogenicity. *Microbiol Rev* 1982;46:162.
24. Densen P. Interaction of complement with *Neisseria meningitidis* and *Neisseria gonorrhoeae*. *Clin Microbiol Rev* 1989;2(suppl):11.
25. Griffiss JM, Bertram MA. Immuno-epidemiology of meningococcal disease in military recruits. II. Blocking of serum bactericidal activity by circulating IgA early in the course of invasive disease. *J Infect Dis* 1977;136:733.
26. Hobbs JR, Milner RDG, Watt PJ. Gamma M deficiency predisposing to meningococcal septicaemia. *BMJ* 1967;4:583.
27. Faust SN, Levin M, Harrison OB, et al. Dysfunction of endothelial protein C activation in severe meningococcal sepsis. *N Engl J Med* 2001;345:408.
28. Brandtzaeg P, Ovstebo R, Kierrulf P. Compartmentalization of lipopolysaccharide production correlates with clinical presentation in meningococcal disease. *J Infect Dis* 1992;166:650.
29. Brandtzaeg P, van Deuren M. Current concepts in the role of the host response in *Neisseria meningitides* septic shock. *Curr Opin Infect Dis* 2002;15:247.
30. Irwin RS, Woelk WK, Condon WL. Primary meningococcal pneumonia. *Ann Intern Med* 1975;82:493.
31. Benoit FL. Chronic meningococcemia. *Am J Med* 1963;35:103.
32. Waage A, Brandizag P, Holstensen A, et al. The complex pattern of cytokines in serum from patients with meningococcal septic shock. *J Exp Med* 1989;169:333.
33. Hardman JM. Fatal meningococcal infections: the changing pathologic picture in the '60's. *Milit Med* 1968;12:951.
34. Gold R. Clinical aspects of meningococcal disease. In: Vedros NA, ed. *Evolution of meningococcal disease*, Vol. II. Boca Raton, FL: CRC Press, 1987:69–97.
35. Rosenthal J, Golan A, Dagan R. Bacterial meningitis with initial normal cerebrospinal fluid findings. *Isr J Med Sci* 1989;25:186.

36. Wilson CB, Smith AL. Rapid tests for the diagnosis of bacterial meningitis. In: Remington J, Swartz MN, eds. *Current clinical topics in infectious diseases,* Vol. XII. New York: McGraw-Hill, 1986:134–156.

37. Ni H, Knight AI, Cartwright K, et al. Polymerase chain reaction for diagnosis of meningococcal meningitis. *Lancet* 1992;340:1432.

38. Cherubin CE, Eng RHK, Norrby R, et al. Penetration of newer cephalosporins into cerebrospinal fluid. *Rev Infect Dis* 1989;11:526.

39. Richter SS, Gordon KA, Rhomberg PR, et al. *Neisseria meningitides* with decreased susceptibility to penicillin: report from the SENTRY antimicrobial surveillance program, North America, 1998–99. *Diagn Microbiol Infect Dis* 2001;41:83.

40. Scheld NM. Quinolone therapy for infections of the central nervous system. *Rev Infect Dis* 1989;11(suppl):1194.

41. Jackson LA, Tenover FC, Baker C, et al. Prevalence of *Neisseria meningitidis* relatively resistant to penicillin in the United States, 1991. *J Infect Dis* 1994;169: 438.

42. Woods CR, Smith AL, Wasilauskas BL, et al. Invasive disease caused by *Neisseria meningitides* relatively resistant to penicillin in North Carolina. *J Infect Dis* 1994;170:453.

43. Molyneux EM, Walsh AL, Forsyth H, et al. Dexamethasone treatment in childhood bacterial meningitis in Malawi: a randomized controlled trial. *Lancet* 2002;360:211.

44. Lebel MH, Freig BJ, Syrogiannopoulos A, et al. Dexamethasone therapy for bacterial meningitis: results of two double-blind, placebo-controlled trials. *N Engl J Med* 1988;319:964.

45. Wahdan MH, Rizk F, El-Addad AM, et al. A controlled field trial of a serogroup A meningococcal polysaccharide vaccine. *Bull WHO* 1973;48:667.

46. Wildes SS, Tunkel AR. Meningococcal vaccines: a progress report. *BioDrugs* 2002;16:321.

47. Jodar L, Feavers JL, Salisbury D, et al. Development of vaccines against meningococcal disease. *Lancet* 2002;359:1499.

48. Campbell JD, Edelman R, King JC Jr, et al. Safety, reactogenicity, and immunogenicity of a tetravalent meningococcal polysaccharide-diphtheria toxoid conjugate vaccine given to healthy adults. *J Infect Dis* 2002;186:1848.

49. Lingappa JR, Rosenstein N, Zell ER, et al. Surveillance for meningococcal disease and strategies for use of conjugate meningococcal vaccines in the United States. *Vaccine* 2001;19:4566.

50. Memish ZA. Meningococcal disease and travel. *Clin Infect Dis* 2002;34:84.

51. Wilder-Smith A, Barkham TM, Ravindran S, et al. Persistence of W135 *Neisseria meningitides* carriage in returning Hajj pilgrims: risk for early and late transmission to household contacts. *Emerg Infect Dis* 2003;9:123.

52. Eskola J, Peltola H, Takala AK, et al. Efficacy of *Haemophilus influenzae* type b polysaccharide-diphtheria toxoid conjugate vaccine in infancy. *N Engl J Med* 1987;317:717.

53. Twumasi PA Jr, Kumah S, Leach A, et al. A trial of a group A plus group C meningococcal polysaccharide-protein conjugate vaccine in African infants. *J Infect Dis* 1995;171:632.

54. Wyle FA, Artenstein MS, Brandt BL, et al. Immunologic response of man to group B meningococcal polysaccharide vaccines. *J Infect Dis* 1972;126: 514.

55. Finne J, Leinonen M, Makela PH. Antigenic similarities between brain components and bacteria causing meningitis: implications for vaccine development and pathogenesis. *Lancet* 1983;2:355.

56. Centers for Disease Control and Prevention. Control and prevention of meningococcal disease. *MMWR* 1997;46(RR-5):1.

57. Cooper ER, Ellison RT, Smith GS, et al. Rifampin-resistant meningococcal disease in a contact patient given prophylactic rifampin. *J Pediatr* 1986;108:93.

58. Cuevas LE, Kazembe P, Mughogho GK, et al. Eradication of nasopharyngeal carriage of *Neisseria meningitidis* in children and adults in rural Africa: a comparison of ciprofloxacin and rifampin. *J Infect Dis* 1995;171:728.

59. Shehab S, Keller N, Barkay A, et al. Failure of mass antibiotic prophylaxis to control a prolonged outbreak of meningococcal disease in an Israeli village. *Eur J Clin Microbiol Infect Dis* 1998;17:749.

60. Guttler RB, Beaty HN. Minocycline in the chemoprophylaxis of meningococcal disease. *Antimicrob Agents Chemother* 1972;1:397.

61. Schwartz B, Al-Tobaiqi A, Al-Ruwais A, et al. Comparative efficacy of ceftriaxone and rifampicin in eradicating pharyngeal carriage of group A *Neisseria meningitidis.* *Lancet* 1988;1:1239.

CHAPTER 194
Miscellaneous Gram-Negative Cocci: Other Neisseria, Moraxella, and Kingella Species

Timothy F. Murphy

The family Neisseriaceae is composed of five genera. These include *Neisseria, Moraxella, Acinetobacter, Kingella,* and *Oligella.* Table 194.1 lists some of the characteristics that are used to differentiate genera of the family.

In this chapter, *Neisseria* strains other than *N. gonorrhoeae* and *N. meningitidis* will be discussed. *N. gonorrhoeae* and *N. meningitidis* are discussed in Chapters 192 and 193, respectively. *Acinetobacter* is discussed in Chapter 207.

OTHER *NEISSERIA* SPECIES

N. meningitidis and *N. gonorrhoeae* have long been recognized as the pathogenic *Neisseria,* while other *Neisseria* species have been regarded as the nonpathogenic or commensal *Neisseria.* These other *Neisseria* species, listed in Table 194.2, are unusual causes of disease in humans. DNA hybridization studies have demonstrated that these other *Neisseria* species lack several markers associated with virulence in the meningococcus and gonococcus. These include pili, the protein II outer membrane protein and the H8 antigen (1).

Neisseria species can be distinguished from one another by a variety of methods, which are based on carbohydrate utilization, colorimetry involving chromogenic substrates, monoclonal antibody reactivity, and isoenzyme electrophoresis. Several kits are commercially available.

Other *Neisseria* species are common inhabitants of the normal upper respiratory tract (2–4). Asymptomatic carriage of *Neisseria lactamica* induces antibody that cross-reacts with lipooligosaccharide (LOS) of *N. meningitidis;* this antibody may be important in protection from meningococcal infection (5). *N. lactamica* has rarely been recovered from the female genital tract (6).

Other *Neisseria* species are unusual causes of human disease. Infections that are caused by these organisms are documented primarily by small series and case reports. These infections include meningitis (7–9), endocarditis (10–13), bacteremia (14–16), ocular infections (17–19), pericarditis (20), empyema (21), septic arthritis (22,23), bursitis (24,25), osteomyelitis (16,26), otitis media (27), peritonitis (28,29), soft tissue infections associated with dog and cat bites (30), and Bartholin gland abscess (31). The former Centers for Disease Control and Prevention (CDC) group M5 strains have been characterized as the *Neisseria* species *N. weaveri* (32). These strains are strongly associated with dog bite wounds in humans (32,33).

Many of these infections have been treated successfully with penicillin or ampicillin. However, isolates of *Neisseria* species showing increased resistance to penicillin have emerged in recent years (34,35). One mechanism of resistance in *Neisseria* species is an alteration of penicillin-binding protein 2 genes (*penA*) (36). Interspecies transfer of *penA* genes by genetic transformation from commensal *Neisseria* species to pathogenic *Neisseria* is an important mechanism of acquisition of penicillin

TABLE 194.1. Differential Characteristics of the Genera of the Family Neisseriaceae

Characteristics	Neisseria	Moraxella species	Moraxella catarrhalis	Acinetobacter	Kingella	Oligella (146)
Cell morphology						
Cocci	+	−	+	−	+	−
Rods	+	+	−	+	−	+
Oxidase test	+	+	+	−	+	+
Catalase test	+	+	+	+	−	+
Presence of carbonic anhydrase	+	−	−			
Acid from glucose	[+]	−	−	D	+	−
Nitrite reduction	+	−	D	−	+	+
Mol% G + C of DNA	46.5–53.5	40–47.5	40–47.5	38–47	47–55	46–47.5

Symbols: +, positive for the majority of strains and some strains of each species; [+], positive for all strains of the majority of species (only one species uniformly negative); D, positive and negative species (or strains of *Acinetobacter*) about equally represented; −, all strains negative; G, guanine; C, cytosine.
Adapted from *Bergey's manual of systematic bacteriology*. Baltimore: Williams & Wilkins, 1984, with permission.

resistance of *N. gonorrhoeae* and *N. meningitidis* (36–40). Susceptibility testing should be performed on all isolates associated with invasive infections.

Moraxella catarrhalis

Moraxella (Branhamella) catarrhalis was previously known as *Neisseria catarrhalis* and had been regarded as a harmless saprophyte of the upper respiratory tract. Over the past 20 years, *M. catarrhalis* has emerged as an important human respiratory tract pathogen.

The taxonomic relationship of *M. catarrhalis* to other *Moraxella* and related genera continues to be confusing. Originally called *Micrococcus catarrhalis*, the bacterium was renamed *Neisseria catarrhalis* in the 1960s based on phenotypic similarities with *Neisseria* species. In 1970, the organism was transferred to the new genus *Branhamella* on the basis of differences in fatty acid content and DNA hybridization studies compared to other Neisseriaceae (41). An alternative scheme had *Branhamella* as a subgenus of *Moraxella* (42). The organism was subsequently placed into the genus *Moraxella*, and it is now most widely referred to as *Moraxella catarrhalis*.

TABLE 194.2. Bacteria of the Family Neisseriaceae

Family: Neisseriaceae	*Moraxella*
Genus	*M. catarrhalis*
Neisseria	*M. lacunata*
N. gonorrhoeae	*M. liquefaciens*
N. meningitidis	*M. nonliquefaciens*
Other *Neisseria*	*M. osloensis*
N. lactamica	*M. phenylpyruvica*
N. sicca	*M. atlantae*
N. subflava	*M. bovus*
N. mucosa	*M. lincolnii*
N. flavescens	*Kingella*
N. cinerea	*K. kingae*
N. perflava	*K. indologenes*
N. flava	*K. dentrificans*
N. weaveri	*K. oralis*
N. elongata	*Acinetobacter*
Branhamella	*A. calcoaceticus (anitratus)*
B. caviae	*A. lwoffi*
B. ovis	*Oligella*
B. cuniculi	*O. urethralis*
	O. urealytica

M. catarrhalis is predominantly a mucosal pathogen. It is a common cause of otitis media in children, sinusitis in children and adults, and lower respiratory tract infection in the elderly and in the setting of chronic bronchitis (43–48).

Characteristics of the Pathogen

GROWTH AND IDENTIFICATION

M. catarrhalis grows well on blood agar, chocolate agar, and a variety of media. Its colony morphology is difficult to distinguish from *Neisseria* species. *M. catarrhalis* is a gram-negative diplococcus with kidney-shaped cells. Isolates of *M. catarrhalis* produce cytochrome oxidase, catalase, and DNAse. They are unable to utilize maltose, glucose, lactose, and sucrose as carbohydrate sources. Several kits to speciate strains of *M. catarrhalis* are commercially available.

SURFACE ANTIGENS

The surface of *M. catarrhalis* is composed of outer membrane proteins, LOS, and pili. Analysis of strains of *M. catarrhalis* from diverse clinical and geographic sources reveals that the molecular weights of eight major outer membrane proteins are nearly identical from strain to strain (49). This contrasts with other species of nonenteric gram-negative bacteria, where differences in outer membrane protein patterns among isolates are generally observed. Table 194.3 summarizes information on outer membrane proteins of *M. catarrhalis*. Current lines of investigation are evaluating several of these proteins as potential virulence factors for the organism and as potential vaccine antigens (50).

The LOS of *M. catarrhalis* consists of a lipid A core coupled to oligosaccharides. The molecule lacks the long O-polysaccharide side chains observed in enteric gram-negative bacteria. The molecular mass is approximately 5,500 daltons and the molecule shares many structural features with the LOS of other nonenteric gram-negative bacteria that colonize mucosal surfaces (51,52). A serotyping system based on antigenic differences in the LOS molecule has been developed. Three antigenic types have been identified by using adsorbed antisera in an inhibition enzyme-linked immunosorbent assay (53). The LOS of *M. catarrhalis* exhibits biologic activity that is characteristic of endotoxin (54). Although specific studies have not yet been performed, LOS is likely an important virulence factor in *M. catarrhalis* infections.

Clinical isolates of *M. catarrhalis* express pili that are lost with progressive passage *in vitro* (55). Preliminary studies suggest a

TABLE 194.3. Outer Membrane Proteins of _Moraxella catarrhalis_

Outer-membrane protein	Molecular mass (kd)	Function
UspA1	88 (oligomer)[a]	Adhesin
UspA2	62 (oligomer)[a]	Involved in serum resistance
200-kd protein	200	? Hemagglutination
OMP CD	46[b]	Porin
OMP E	50	Unknown
MID	200	Binds IgD
Proteins involved in iron uptake		
TbpA	115–120	Transferrin transport
TbpB (OMP B1)	80–84	Binds transferrin
CopB (OMP B2)	80	Under study
LbpA	110	Binds lactoferrin
LbpB	98	Binds lactoferrin

[a]Molecular mass varies among strains.
[b]OMP CD runs aberrantly (apparent molecular mass, ~60 kd) in sodium dodecyl sulfate polyacrylamide gel electrophoresis.

role for pili in adherence (56,57), but elucidation of the precise role of pili in adherence will await the development of appropriate model systems for the study of _M. catarrhalis_ adherence.

TYPING SYSTEMS

A variety of approaches have been used to develop methods for typing strains of _M. catarrhalis_. Table 194.4 lists seven systems that have been used to help elucidate the epidemiology of colonization and infection. Each system has advantages and limitations. An ideal serotyping system for _M. catarrhalis_ has not yet been developed. This system would divide strains into several groups based on antigenic differences in important surface antigens, be convenient and reproducible, and be capable of placing all strains into a serotype. Such a system would be a powerful tool in understanding the epidemiology, pathogenesis, and protection from infection by _M. catarrhalis_.

Epidemiology

M. catarrhalis colonizes primarily the upper respiratory tract, although it has occasionally been recovered from genital mucosa. Nasopharyngeal colonization with _M. catarrhalis_ is common throughout infancy (58–61). A prospective study in which nasopharyngeal cultures were obtained monthly showed that 66% of infants were colonized at some time during the first year of life, and 78% were colonized by the age of 2 years (59). A high rate of colonization with _M. catarrhalis_ is associated with an increased incidence of otitis media (59). Healthy adults have a low rate of respiratory tract colonization by _M. catarrhalis_ (60). A subset of patients with bronchiectasis is colonized with _M. catarrhalis_ (62). Analysis of prospectively collected strains from the sputum of patients with bronchiectasis has shown that one strain colo-

TABLE 194.4. Typing Systems for _Moraxella catarrhalis_

Sodium dodecyl sulfate polyacrylamide gel electrophoresis and immunoblot assays
Esterase electrophoretic polymorphism
Lipooligosaccharide serotyping
Restriction enzyme analysis of genomic DNA
Southern blot assays with DNA probes
Ribotyping
Pulsed field gel electrophoresis of genomic DNA

nizes for a mean duration of 2.3 months (62). These observations indicate that colonization by _M. catarrhalis_ is a dynamic process.

M. catarrhalis is an important cause of otitis media. Studies from several centers in the 1990s have established that _M. catarrhalis_ is the third most common cause of otitis media (Table 194.5). In all of the series in Table 194.5, cultures of middle ear aspirates were performed; this is the most reliable method to establish the cause of otitis media. As strategies for preventing otitis media caused by pneumococcus and nontypable _Haemophilus influenzae_ are developed, the relative importance of _M. catarrhalis_ as a cause of otitis media will increase in the next decade.

M. catarrhalis causes sinusitis in adults and children (63–65). The organism can be recovered alone or in combination with other bacteria from direct sinus aspirates from patients with clinical and radiographic evidence of acute bacterial sinusitis.

M. catarrhalis causes lower respiratory tract infections, particularly in the setting of chronic bronchitis and chronic obstructive pulmonary disease (COPD) (45,46). Four sets of observations indicate that _M. catarrhalis_ is a lower respiratory tract pathogen:

1. Some patients with COPD have exacerbations in which a sputum Gram stain shows a predominance of intracellular and extracellular gram-negative diplococci and culture reveals _M. catarrhalis_.
2. _M. catarrhalis_ can be obtained in pure culture from transtracheal aspirates and from samples obtained by the protected specimen brush from patients with clinical evidence of respiratory infection (66–70).
3. Administration of specific antimicrobial therapy directed at β-lactamase–producing _M. catarrhalis_ results in clinical improvement in these patients after failure of therapy with β-lactams.
4. Patients with clinical, Gram stain, and culture evidence of respiratory infection with _M. catarrhalis_ develop bactericidal antibodies specific for their own isolate (71).

In addition to causing purulent exacerbations of COPD, which are generally not associated with infiltrates on chest films, _M. catarrhalis_ also causes pneumonia, particularly in the elderly (72–75). A highly characteristic feature is a predominance of Gram-negative diplococci on sputum Gram stain. When _M. catarrhalis_ is the etiologic agent of pneumonia or an exacerbation of COPD, the organism is usually present in large numbers in the sputum.

Nosocomial outbreaks of lower respiratory tract infections caused by _M. catarrhalis_ have been recognized since the

TABLE 194.5. Causes of Otitis Media: Results of Tympanocentesis

			Percentage of cases caused by		
Reference	Year	Location	*Streptococcus pneumoniae*	*Haemophilus influenzae*	*Moraxella catarrhalis*
147	1990	Norway and Finland	28	16	16
148	1991	Dallas, Texas	29	30	15
149	1991	Cleveland, Ohio	25	27	11
150	1992	Buffalo, New York	19	35	18
151	1992	Philadelphia, Pennsylvania	48	20	23
152	1992	Galveston, Texas	39	34	18
153	1993	Galveston, Texas	29	37	15
154	1994	United States (five centers)	39	27	14
155	1996	France	28	43	10
156	1998	Israel	28	45	7
157	2000	United States (several centers)	52	33	11
158	2000	United States (several centers)	39	39	12
159	2001	Finland	26	23	23

mid-1980s. Reports from several centers indicate that clusters of *M. catarrhalis* infections occur in hospitals. The reservoir of infection and the mode of transmission are largely unknown. Several of these outbreaks have occurred in respiratory units, suggesting that the presence of a susceptible population contributed to the clusters.

In addition to the relatively common clinical manifestations noted above, *M. catarrhalis* is also a rare cause of invasive infection. These are documented predominantly by case reports. Invasive infections rarely caused by *M. catarrhalis* include meningitis (76), endocarditis (77), bacteremia (78,79), septic arthritis (80,81), osteomyelitis (82), epiglottitis (83), cellulitis (84), shunt-associated ventriculitis (85), peritonitis (86), pericarditis (87), and wound infection (88), among others. In addition, *M. catarrhalis* is an unusual cause of acute urethritis (89,90) and can cause conjunctivitis (91,92).

Clinical Manifestations and Diagnosis

The clinical manifestations of otitis media and sinusitis caused by *M. catarrhalis* are indistinguishable from those of infection by other organisms. Otitis and sinusitis caused by *M. catarrhalis* may be associated with less fever and fewer constitutional symptoms of infection compared with pneumococcus and nontypable *H. influenzae*, but substantial overlap exists. The diagnosis of otitis media is best made by pneumatic otoscopy. A compatible clinical picture and radiograph suggest a diagnosis of sinusitis. Tympanocentesis is required to establish an etiologic diagnosis of otitis media, and sinus aspiration is necessary to establish the etiology of sinusitis, but these are not routinely performed. Nasopharyngeal and throat cultures are not helpful in establishing an etiology of either otitis media or sinusitis because bacteria colonize the nasopharynx and throat in the absence of infection.

The clinical manifestations of lower respiratory tract infection caused by *M. catarrhalis* are similar to those of infection by other bacteria such as nontypable *H. influenzae*. Exacerbations of COPD are characterized by increased sputum production, increased purulence of sputum, and increased shortness of breath compared with baseline. When fever is present, it is usually low grade. Pneumonia due to *M. catarrhalis* occurs almost exclusively in the elderly and in patients with COPD. It is characterized by fever as high as 103°F, cough, purulent sputum, and shortness of breath. Auscultation sometimes reveals signs of consolidation. The chest film shows either patchy or lobar alveolar infiltrates.

Pleural effusion and empyema are uncommon. The most practical method for making a diagnosis is a sputum Gram stain. A Gram-stained sputum that shows a predominance of intracellular and extracellular gram-negative diplococci is a rapid, simple, and reliable indicator for making a diagnosis (71).

Treatment

Approximately 90% of strains of *M. catarrhalis* produce β-lactamase (93). Two major β-lactamase forms, BRO-1 and BRO-2, are produced, with BRO-1–producing strains predominating (93–97). The β-lactamases of *M. catarrhalis* are inducible, cell-associated, more active against penicillins than against cephalosporins, and inhibited by β-lactamase inhibitors such as clavulanic acid and sulbactam. β-lactamase–producing strains show an inoculum-dependent susceptibility to ampicillin. Therefore, ampicillin should not be used for β-lactamase–producing strains, regardless of the results of susceptibility testing. One study showed persistently positive middle ear cultures during ampicillin therapy for *M. catarrhalis* otitis media caused by a β-lactamase producing strain (58). Most *M. catarrhalis* infections can be treated with orally administered antimicrobial agents. Oral agents active against *M. catarrhalis* include the combination of amoxicillin and clavulanic acid, macrolides, extended-spectrum cephalosporins, fluoroquinolones, trimethoprim-sulfamethoxazole, and tetracycline (98,99). *M. catarrhalis* is also uniformly susceptible to ticarcillin, piperacillin, mezlocillin, azlocillin, chloramphenicol and aminoglycosides. *M. catarrhalis* is resistant to penicillin, ampicillin, vancomycin, clindamycin, and methicillin.

Other *Moraxella* Species

Moraxella are normal inhabitants of the upper respiratory tract and occasionally can be recovered from the skin and genital tract. Species can be differentiated biochemically, but genetic transformation assays are useful for identification of some species (100–102). The taxonomy of *Moraxella* species is an active area of research and is constantly changing as more is learned about these bacteria (103–106). Indeed, the classification of some of these bacteria is controversial (107–109). Some species of *Moraxella* are listed in Table 194.2.

M. bovis causes bovine keratoconjunctivitis, the most common ocular disease of cattle throughout the world. *Moraxella* species are unusual pathogens in humans, although recent studies have emphasized the role of these bacteria as ocular pathogens (110–114). *Moraxella* is often overlooked as a causative agent of conjunctival infection; *M. nonliquefaciens* is the most common *Moraxella* species associated with eye infection, and in one study represented the fourth most common cause of corneal infection after pneumococcus, *Staphylococcus,* and *Pseudomonas* species (112). *Moraxella* are susceptible to all conventional topical ocular antibiotics. Topical treatment of these infections should continue for 7 to 10 days.

Moraxella species are uncommon causes of invasive infection in humans, including endocarditis (115,116), bacteremia (117–119), septic arthritis (120,121), pneumonia (122), lymphadenitis (123), soft tissue infection (124), purulent pericarditis (125), and meningitis (33,126). A high frequency of inherited or acquired complement deficiency exists in patients with meningitis due to *Moraxella* species; therefore, such patients should be studied for complement deficiency (126). *Moraxella* species are generally susceptible to penicillins and cephalosporins.

Kingella

In 1976, *Moraxella kingae* was transferred to the new genus *Kingella* (127,128). *Kingella* has four species: *K. kingae, K. indologenes, K. dinitrificans,* and *K. oralis* (129). *Kingella* is recovered from the human upper respiratory tract. *K. kingae* has recently emerged as an important invasive pathogen in children (33,130,131). The organism has a propensity to cause skeletal infections, including septic arthritis and osteomyelitis (132,133). In some regions, *K. kingae* is the most common cause of septic arthritis in children under 2 years of age. Inoculation of joint fluid into blood culture bottles increases the yield in recovering *K. kingae* from joint fluid (130,134). In addition to skeletal infections, *Kingella* species are unusual causes of other invasive infections, including endocarditis (135–138), epiglottitis (139), bacteremia (140), intervertebral diskitis (141), soft tissue infection (142), and meningitis (136,143). *Kingella* are generally susceptible to a wide variety of antimicrobial agents, including penicillins and cephalosporins (144,145).

REFERENCES

1. Aho EL, Murphy GL, Cannon JG. Distribution of specific DNA sequences among pathogenic and commensal *Neisseria* species. *Infect Immun* 1987;55:1009–1013.
2. Saez Nieto JA, Marcos C, Vindel A. Multicolonization of human nasopharynx due to *Neisseria* spp. *Int Microbiol* 1998;1:59–63.
3. Knapp JS, Hook EWI. Prevalence and persistence of *Neisseria cinerea* and other *Neisseria* spp. in adults. *J Clin Microbiol* 1988;26:896–900.
4. Gold R, Goldschneider I, Lepow ML, et al. Carriage of *Neisseria meningitidis* and *Neisseria lactamica* in infants and children. *J Infect Dis* 1978;137:112–121.
5. Kim JJ, Mandrell RE, Griffiss JM. *Neisseria lactamica* and *Neisseria meningitidis* share lipooligosaccharide epitopes but lack common capsular and class 1, 2, and 3 protein epitopes. *Infect Immun* 1989;57:602–608.
6. Brunton WAT, Young H, Fraser DRK. Isolation of *Neisseria lactamica* from the female genital tract. *Br J Vener Dis* 1980;56:325–326.
7. Baraldes MA, Domingo P, Barrio JL, et al. Meningitis due to *Neisseria subflava*: case report and review. *Clin Infect Dis* 2000;30:615–617.
8. Sartin JS. *Neisseria sicca* meningitis in a woman with nascent pernicious anemia. *Am J Med* 2000;109:175–176.
9. Stotka JL, Rupp ME, Meier FA, et al. Meningitis due to *Neisseria mucosa*: case report and review. *Rev Infect Dis* 1991;13:837–841.
10. Dominguez EA, Smith TL. Endocarditis due to *Neisseria elongata* subspecies nitroreducens: case report and review. *Clin Infect Dis* 1998;26:1471–1473.
11. Apisarnthanarak A, Dunagan WC, Dunne WM. *Neisseria elongata* subsp. elongata, as a cause of human endocarditis. *Diagn Microbiol Infect Dis* 2001;39:265–266.
12. Lopez-Velez R, Fortun J, de Pablo C, et al. Native-valve endocarditis due to *Neisseria sicca*. *Clin Infect Dis*. 1994;18:660–661.
13. Heiddal S, Sverrisson JT, Yngvason FE, et al. Native-valve endocarditis due to *Neisseria sicca*: case report and review. *Clin Infect Dis* 1993;16:667–670.
14. Carlson P, Kontiainen S, Anttila P, et al. Septicemia caused by *Neisseria weaveri*. *Clin Infect Dis* 1997;24:739.
15. Hofstad T, Hope O, Falsen E. Septicaemia with *Neisseria elongata* ssp. nitroreducens in a patient with hypertrophic obstructive cardiomyopathia. *Scand J Infect Dis* 1998;30:200–201.
16. Wong JD, Janda JM. Association of an important *Neisseria* species, *Neisseria elongata* subsp. nitroreducens, with bacteremia, endocarditis, and osteomyelitis. *J Clin Microbiol* 1992;30:719–720.
17. Gini GA. Ocular infection in a newborn caused by *Neisseria mucosa*. *J Clin Microbiol* 1987;25:1574–1575.
18. Au Y-K, Reynolds MD, Rambin ED, et al. *Neisseria cinerea* acute purulent conjunctivitis. *Am J Opthalmol* 1990;109:96–97.
19. Bourbeau P, Holla V, Piemontese S. Ophthalmia neonatorum caused by *Neisseria cinerea*. *J Clin Microbiol* 1990;28:1640–1641.
20. Fainstein V, Musher DM, Young EJ. Purulent pericarditis due to *Neisseria mucosa*. *Chest* 1978;74:476–477.
21. Thorsteinsson SB, Minuth JN, Musher DM. Postpneumonectomy empyema due to *Neisseria mucosa*. *Am J Clin Pathol* 1975;64:534–536.
22. Geisler WM, Markovitz DM. Septic arthritis caused by *Neisseria sicca*. *J Rheumatol* 1998;25:826–828.
23. Obeid EMH. *Neisseria subflava* causing septic arthritis of the ankle in a child. *J Infect* 1993;27:100–101.
24. Linquist PR, Linquist JA. *Neisseria mucosa* bursitis. A rare cause of gas in soft tissue. *Clin Orthop* 1988;231:222–224.
25. Halla JT. Septic olecranon bursitis caused by *Neisseria sicca*. *J Rheumatol* 1990;17:1240–1241.
26. Doern GV, Blacklow NR, Gantz NM, et al. *Neisseria sicca* osteomyelitis. *J Clin Microbiol* 1982;16:595–597.
27. Orden B, Amerigo MA. Acute otitis media caused by *Neisseria lactamica*. *Eur J Clin Microbiol Infect Dis* 1991;10:986–987.
28. Vermeij CG, van Dam DW, Oosterkamp HM, et al. *Neisseria subflava* biovar perflava peritonitis in a continuous cyclic peritoneal dialysis patient. *Nephrol Dial Transplant* 1999;14:1608.
29. George MJ, DeBin JA, Preston KE, et al. Recurrent bacterial peritonitis caused by *Neisseria cinerea* in a chronic ambulatory peritoneal dialysis (CAPD) patients. *Diagn Microbiol Infect Dis* 1996;26:91–93.
30. Talan DA, Citron DM, Abrahamian FM, et al. Bacteriologic analysis of infected dog and cat bites. Emergency Medicine Animal Bite Infection Study Group. *N Engl J Med* 1999;340:85–92.
31. Berger SA, Gorea A, Peyser MR, et al. Bartholin's gland abscess caused by *Neisseria sicca*. *J Clin Microbiol* 1988;26:1589.
32. Holmes B, Costas M, On SLW, et al. *Neisseria weaveri* sp. nov. (formerly CDC group M-5), from dog bite wounds of humans. *Int J Syst Bacteriol* 1993;43:687–693.
33. Graham DR, Band JD, Thornsberry C, et al. Infections caused by *Moraxella, Moraxella urethralis, Moraxella*-like groups M-5 and M-6, and *Kingella kingae* in the United States, 1953–1980. *Rev Infect Dis* 1990;12:423–431.
34. Roberts MC, Moncla BJ. Tetracycline resistance and TetM in oral anaerobic bacteria and *Neisseria perflava-N. sicca*. *Antimicrob Agents Chemother* 1988;32:1271–1273.
35. Piot P, Roberts M, Ninane G. Beta-lactamase production in commensal *Neisseriaceae*. *Lancet* 1979;1:619.
36. Lujan R, Zhang Q-Y, Saez-Nieto JA, et al. Penicillin-resistant isolates of *Neisseria lactamica* produce altered forms of penicillin-binding protein 2 that arose by interspecies horizontal gene transfer. *Antimicrob Agents Chemother* 1991;35:300–304.
37. Orus P, Vinas M. Transfer of penicillin resistance between neisseriae in microcosm. *Microb Drug Resist* 2000;6:99–104.
38. Frosch M, Meyer TF. Transformation-mediated exchange of virulence determinants by co-cultivation of pathogenic *Neisseria*. *FEMS Microbiol Lett* 1992;100:345–350.
39. Spratt BG, Bowler LD, Zhang Q-Y, et al. Role of interspecies transfer of chromosomal genes in the evolution of penicillin resistance in pathogenic and commensal *Neisseria* species. *J Mol Evol* 1992;34:115–125.
40. Bowler LD, Zhang Q-Y, Riou J-Y, et al. Interspecies recombination between the *penA* genes of *Neisseria meningitidis* and commensal *Neisseria* species during the emergence of penicillin resistance of *N. meningitidis*: natural events and laboratory simulation. *J Bacteriol* 1994;176:333–337.
41. Catlin BW. Transfer of the organism named *Neisseria catarrhalis* to *Branhamella* genus. *Int J Syst Bacteriol* 1970;20:155–159.
42. Bovre K. Proposal to divide the genus *Moraxella* into two subgenera, subgenus *Moraxella* and subgenus *Branhamella*. *Int J Syst Bacteriol* 1979;29:403–406.
43. Murphy TF. *Branhamella catarrhalis*: epidemiology, surface antigenic structure, and immune response. *Microbiol Rev* 1996;60:267–279.
44. Karalus R, Campagnari A. *Moraxella catarrhalis*: a review of an important human mucosal pathogen. *Microbes Infect* 2000;2:547–559.
45. Sethi S, Murphy TF. Bacterial infection in chronic obstructive pulmonary disease in 2000. A state of the art review. *Clin Microbiol Rev* 2001;14:336–363.
46. Murphy TF. *Branhamella catarrhalis*: epidemiological and clinical aspects of a human respiratory tract pathogen. *Thorax* 1998;53:124–128.
47. Christensen JJ. *Moraxella (Branhamella) catarrhalis*: clinical, microbiological and immunological features in lower respiratory tract infections. *APMIS* 1999;107(suppl):1–36.
48. Enright MC, McKenzie H. *Moraxella (Branhamella) catarrhalis*—clinical and molecular aspects of a rediscovered pathogen. *J Med Microbiol* 1997;46:360–371.

49. Bartos LC, Murphy TF. Comparison of the outer membrane proteins of 50 strains of *Branhamella catarrhalis*. *J Infect Dis* 1988;158:761–765.

50. McMichael JC. Vaccines for *Moraxella catarrhalis*. *Vaccine* 2000;19(suppl):101–108.

51. Edebrink P, Jansson P-E, Rahman MM, et al. Structural studies of the O-polysaccharide from the lipopolysaccharide of *Moraxella (Branhamella) catarrhalis* serotype A (strain ATCC 25238). *Carbohydrate Res* 1994;257:269–284.

52. Masoud H, Perry MB, Richards JC. Characterization of the lipopolysaccharide of *Moraxella catarrhalis*. Structural analysis of the lipid A from *M. catarrhalis* serotype A lipopolysaccharide. *Eur J Biochem* 1994;220:209–216.

53. Vaneechoutte M, Verschraegen G, Claeys G, et al. Serological typing of *Branhamella catarrhalis* strains on the basis of lipopolysaccharide antigens. *J Clin Microbiol* 1990;28:182–187.

54. Fomsgaard JS, Fomsgaard A, Hoiby N, et al. Comparative immunochemistry of lipopolysaccharides from *Branhamella catarrhalis* strains. *Infect Immun* 1991;59:3346–3349.

55. Ahmed K, Rikitomi N, Matsumoto K. Fimbriation, hemagglutination and adherence properties of fresh clinical isolates of *Branhamella catarrhalis*. *Microbiol Immunol* 1992;36:1009–1017.

56. Rikitomi N, Andersson B, Matsumoto K, et al. Mechanism of adherence of *Moraxella (Branhamella) catarrhalis*. *Scand J Infect Dis* 1991;23:559–567.

57. Ahmed K. Fimbriae of *Branhamella catarrhalis* as possible mediators of adherence to pharyngeal epithelial cells. *APMIS* 1992;100:1066–1072.

58. Van Hare GF, Shurin PA, Marchant CD, et al. Acute otitis media caused by *Branhamella catarrhalis*: biology and therapy. *Rev Infect Dis* 1987;9:16–27.

59. Faden H, Harabuchi Y, Hong JJ, Tonawanda/Williamsville Pediatrics. Epidemiology of *Moraxella catarrhalis* in children during the first 2 years of life: relationship to otitis media. *J Infect Dis* 1994;169:1312–1317.

60. Vaneechoutte M, Verschraegen G, Claeys G, et al. Respiratory tract carrier rates of *Moraxella (Branhamella) catarrhalis* in adults and children and interpretation of the isolation of *M. catarrhalis* from sputum. *J Clin Microbiol*. 1990;28:2674–2680.

61. Aniansson G, Alm B, Andersson B, et al. Nasopharyngeal colonization during the first year of life. *J Infect Dis* 1992;165(suppl):38–42.

62. Klingman KL, Pye A, Murphy TF, et al. Dynamics of respiratory tract colonization by *Moraxella (Branhamella) catarrhalis* in bronchiectasis. *Am J Respir Crit Care Med* 1995;152:1072–1078.

63. Penttila M, Savolainen S, Kiukaanniemi H, et al. Bacterial findings in acute maxillary sinusitis—European study. *Acta Otolaryngol Suppl* 1997;529:165–169.

64. Brorson J-E, Axelsson A, Holm SE. Studies on *Branhamella catarrhalis (Neisseria catarrhalis)* with special reference to maxillary sinusitis. *Scand J Infect Dis* 1976;8:151–155.

65. Wald ER, Reilly JS, Casselbrant M, et al. Treatment of acute maxillary sinusitis in childhood: a comparative study of amoxicillin and cefaclor. *J Pediatr* 1984;104:297–302.

66. Ninane G, Joly J, Kraytman M. Bronchopulmonary infection due to *Branhamella catarrhalis*: 11 cases assessed by transtracheal puncture. *BMJ* 1978;1:276–278.

67. Fagon J-Y, Chastre J, Trouillet J-L, et al. Characterization of distal bronchial microflora during acute exacerbation of chronic bronchitis. *Am Rev Respir Dis* 1990;142:1004–1008.

68. Soler N, Torres A, Ewig S, et al. Bronchial microbial patterns in severe exacerbations of chronic obstructive pulmonary disease (COPD) requiring mechanical ventilation. *Am J Respir Crit Care Med* 1998;157:1498–1505.

69. Monso E, Ruiz J, Rosell A, et al. Bacterial infection in chronic obstructive pulmonary disease. A study of stable and exacerbated outpatients using the protected specimen brush. *Am J Respir Crit Care Med* 1995;152:1316–1320.

70. Pela R, Marchesani F, Agostinelli C, et al. Airways microbial flora in COPD patients in stable clinical conditions and during exacerbations: a bronchoscopic investigation. *Monaldi Arch Chest Dis* 1998;53:3–262.

71. Chapman AJ, Musher DM, Jonsson S, et al. Development of bactericidal antibody during *Branhamella catarrhalis* infection. *J Infect Dis* 1985;151:878–882.

72. Carr B, Walsh JB, Coakley D, et al. Prospective hospital study of community acquired lower respiratory tract infection in the elderly. *Respir Med* 1991;85:185–187.

73. Barreiro B, Esteban L, Prats E, et al. *Branhamella catarrhalis* respiratory infections. *Eur Respir J* 1992;5:675–679.

74. Choo PW, Gantz NM. *Branhamella catarrhalis* pneumonia with bacteremia. *South Med J* 1989;82:1317–1318.

75. Verghese A, Berk SL. *Moraxella (Branhamella) catarrhalis*. *Infect Dis Clin North Am* 1991;5:523–38.

76. Newing WJ, Christie R. Meningitis: isolation of an organism resembling *Neisseria catarrhalis* from cerebrospinal fluid; report of a case. *Med J Aust* 1947;1:306.

77. Stefanou J, Agelopoulou AV, Sipsas NV, et al. *Moraxella catarrhalis* endocarditis: case report and review of the literature. *Scand J Infect Dis* 2000;32:217–218.

78. Wallace MR, Oldfield ECI. *Moraxella (Branhamella) catarrhalis* bacteremia. *Arch Intern Med* 1990;150:1332–1334.

79. Cimolai N, Adderley RJ. *Branhamella catarrhalis* bacteremia in children. *Acta Paediatr Scand* 1989;78:465–468.

80. Craig DB, Wehrle PA. *Branhamella catarrhalis* septic arthritis. *J Rheumatol* 1983;10:985–986.

81. Melendez PR, Johnson RH. Bacteremia and septic arthritis caused by *Moraxella catarrhalis*. *Rev Infect Dis* 1991;13:428–429.

82. Prallet B, Lucht F, Alexandre C. Vertebral osteomyelitis due to *Branhamella catarrhalis*. *Rev Infect Dis* 1991;13:769.

83. Vernham GA, Crowther JA. Acute myeloid leukaemia presenting with acute *Branhamella catarrhalis* epiglottitis. *J Infect* 1993;26:93–95.

84. Rotta AT, Asmar BI. *Moraxella catarrhalis* bacteremia and preseptal cellulitis. *South Med J* 1994;87:541–542.

85. Cooke RPD, Williams R, Bannister CM. Shunt-associated ventriculitis caused by *Branhamella catarrhalis*. *J Hosp Infect* 1990;15:197–198.

86. Contreras MR, Ash SR, Swick SD, et al. Peritonitis due to *Moraxella (Branhamella) catarrhalis* in a diabetic patient receiving peritoneal dialysis. *South Med J* 1993;86:589–590.

87. Kostiala AAI, Honkanen T. *Branhamella catarrhalis* as a cause of acute purulent pericarditis. *J Infect* 1989;19(3):291–292.

88. Gray LD, Van Scoy RE, Anhalt JP, et al. Wound infection caused by *Branhamella catarrhalis*. *J Clin Microbiol* 1989;27:818–820.

89. Smith GL. *Branhamella catarrhalis* infection imitating gonorrhea in a man. *N Engl J Med* 1987;316:1277.

90. Doern GV, Gantz NM. Isolation of *Branhamella (Neisseria) catarrhalis* from men with urethritis. *Sex Transm Dis* 1982;9:202–204.

91. Lue YA, Simms DH, Ubriani R, et al. Ophthalmia neonatorum caused by penicillin-resistant *Branhamella catarrhalis*. *NY State J Med* 1981;81:1775–1776.

92. Kawakami Y, Segawa K, Kandi M. A case of acute catarrhal conjunctivitis due to *Branhamella catarrhalis*. *Microbiol Immunol* 1983;27:641–642.

93. McGregor K, Chang BJ, Mee BJ, et al. *Moraxella catarrhalis*: clinical significance, antimicrobial susceptibility and BRO beta-lactamases. *Eur J Clin Microbiol Infect Dis* 1998;17:234.

94. Bootsma HJ, van Dijk H, Vauterin P, et al. Genesis of β-lactamase–producing *Moraxella catarrhalis*: evidence for transformation-mediated horizontal transfer. *Mol Microbiol* 2000;36:93–104.

95. Bootsma HJ, van Dijk H, Verhoef J, et al. Molecular characterization of the BRO β-lactamase of *Moraxella (Branhamella) catarrhalis*. *Antimicrob Agents Chemother* 1996;40:966–972.

96. Bootsma HJ, Aerts PC, Posthuma G, et al. *Moraxella (Branhamella) catarrhalis* BRO β-lactamase: a lipoprotein of gram-positive origin? *J Bacteriol* 1999;181:5090–5093.

97. Richter SS, Winokur PL, Brueggemann AB, et al. Molecular characterization of the β-lactamases from clinical isolates of *Moraxella (Branhamella) catarrhalis* obtained from 24 U.S. medical centers during 1994–1995 and 1997–1998. *Antimicrob Agents Chemother* 2000;44:444–446.

98. Barry AL, Pfaller MA, Fuchs PC, et al. In vitro activities of 12 orally administered antimicrobial agents against four species of bacterial respiratory pathogens from U.S. medical centers in 1992 and 1993. *Antimicrob Agents Chemother* 1994;38:2419–2425.

99. Fung CP, Powell M, Seymour A, et al. The antimicrobial susceptibility of *Moraxella catarrhalis* isolated in England and Scotland in 1991. *J Antimicrob Chemother* 1992;30:47–55.

100. Juni E, Heym GA, Maurer MJ, et al. Combined genetic transformation and nutritional assay for identification of *Moraxella nonliquefaciens*. *J Clin Microbiol* 1987;25:1691–1694.

101. Henriksen SD. *Moraxella, Neisseria, Branhamella*, and *Acinetobacter*. *Ann Rev Microbiol* 1976;30:63–83.

102. Henriksen SD. *Moraxella, Acinetobacter*, and the *Mimeae*. *Bacteriol Rev* 1973;37:522–61.

103. Tonjum T, Caugant DA, Bovre K. Differentiation of *Moraxella nonliquefaciens*, *M. lacunata*, and *M. bovis* by using multilocus enzyme electrophoresis and hybridization with pilin-specific DNA probes. *J Clin Microbiol* 1992;30:3099–3107.

104. Veron M, Lenvoise-Furet A, Coustere C, et al. Relatedness of three species of "false Neisseria," *Neisseria caviae*, *Neisseria cuniculi*, and *Neisseria ovis*, by DNA-DNA hybridizations and fatty acid analysis. *Int J Syst Bacteriol* 1993;43:210–220.

105. Jannes G, Vaneechoutte M, Lannoo M, et al. Polyphasic taxonomy leading to the proposal of *Moraxella canis* sp. nov. for *Moraxella catarrhalis*-like strains. *Int J Syst Bacteriol* 1993;43:438–449.

106. Vandamme P, Gillis M, Vancanneyt M, et al. *Moraxella lincolnii* sp. nov., isolated from the human respiratory tract, and reevaluation of the taxonomic position of *Moraxella osloensis*. *Int J Syst Bacteriol* 1993;43:474–481.

107. Catlin BW. Branhamaceae fam. nov., a proposed family to accommodate the genera *Branhamella* and *Moraxella*. *Int J Syst Bacteriol* 1991;41:320–323.

108. Rossau R, Van Landschoot A, Gillis M, et al. Taxonomy of Moraxellaceae fam. nov., a new bacterial family to accommodate the genera *Moraxella, Acinetobacter*, and *Psychrobacter* and related organisms. *Int J Syst Bacteriol* 1991;41:310–319.

109. Catlin BW. *Branhamella catarrhalis*: an organism gaining respect as a pathogen. *Clin Microbiol Rev* 1990;3:293–320.

110. Garg P, Mathur U, Athmanathan S, et al. Treatment outcome of *Moraxella keratitis*: our experience with 18 cases—a retrospective review. *Cornea* 1999;18:176–181.

111. Schaefer F, Bruttin O, Zografos L, et al. Bacterial keratitis: a prospective clinical and microbiological study. *Br J Ophthalmol* 2001;85:842–847.

112. Cobo LM, Coster DJ, Peacock J. *Moraxella* keratitis in a nonalcoholic population. *Br J Opthalmol* 1981;65:683–686.

113. Schmidt ME, Smith MA, Levy CS. Endophthalmitis caused by unusual gram-negative bacilli: three case reports and review. *Clin Infect Dis* 1993;17:686–690.

114. Sherman MD, York M, Irvine AR, et al. Endophthalmitis caused by β-lactamase–positive *Moraxella nonliquefaciens. Am J Opthalmol* 1993;115:674–676.

115. Silberfarb PM, Lawe JE. Endocarditis due to *Moraxella liquefaciens. Arch Intern Med* 1968;122:512–513.

116. Sanyal SK, Wilson N, Twum-Danso K, et al. *Moraxella* endocarditis following balloon angioplasty of aortic coarctation. *Am Heart J* 1990;119:1421–1423.

117. Shah SS, Ruth A, Coffin SE. Infection due to *Moraxella osloensis*: case report and review of the literature. *Clin Infect Dis* 2000;30:179–181.

118. Guttigoli A, Zaman MM. Bacteremia and possible endocarditis caused by *Moraxella phenylpyruvica. South Med J* 2000;93:708–709.

119. Buchman AL, Pickett MJ. *Moraxella atlantae* bacteraemia in a patient with systemic lupus erythematosis. *J Infect* 1991;23:197–199.

120. Johnson DW, Lum G, Nimmo G, et al. *Moraxella nonliquefaciens* septic arthritis in a patient undergoing hemodialysis. *Clin Infect Dis* 1995;21:1039–1040.

121. Juvin Ph, Boulot-Telle M, Triller R, et al. *Moraxella lacunata* infectious arthritis. *J R Soc Med* 1991;84:629–630.

122. Goetz MB, Jones J. Pneumonia and bacteremia caused by a previously undescribed Moraxella-like bacterium. *J Clin Microbiol* 1982;15:720–722.

123. Vaneechoutte M, Claeys G, Steyaert S, et al. Isolation of *Moraxella canis* from an ulcerated metastatic lymph node. *J Clin Microbiol* 2000;38:3870–3871.

124. Christensen JJ, Fabrin J, Fussing V, et al. A case of *Moraxella canis*–associated wound infection. *Scand J Infect Dis* 2001;33:155–156.

125. Appelbaum A, Giladi A, Borman JB. *Moraxella* purulent pericarditis. *J Cardiovasc Surg* 1974;15:479–481.

126. Fijen CAP, Kuijper EJ, Tjia HG, et al. Complement deficiency predisposes for meningitis due to nongroupable meningococci and *Neisseria*-related bacteria. *Clin Infect Dis* 1994;18:780–784.

127. Snell JJS, Lapage SP. Transfer of some saccharolytic *Moraxella* species to *Kingella* Henriksen and Bovre 1976, with descriptions of *Kingella indologenes* sp. nov. and *Kingella dentrificans* sp. nov. *Int J Syst Bacteriol* 1976;26:451–458.

128. Henriksen SD, Bovre K. Transfer of *Moraxella kingae* Henriksen and Bovre to the genus *Kingella* gen. nov. in the family *Neisseriaceae. Int J System Bacteriol* 1976;26:447–450.

129. Chen C. Distribution of a newly described species, *Kingella oralis*, in the human oral cavity. *Oral Microbiol Immunol* 1996;11:425–427.

130. Yagupsky P, Dagan R. *Kingella kingae*: an emerging cause of invasive infections in young children. *Clin Infect Dis* 1997;24:860–866.

131. Yagupsky P, Dagan R, Howard CB, et al. Clinical features and epidemiology of invasive *Kingella kingae* infections in southern Israel. *Pediatrics* 1993;92:800–804.

132. Esteve V, Porcheret H, Clerc D, et al. Septic arthritis due to *Kingella kingae* in an adult. *Joint Bone Spine* 2001;68:85–86.

133. La Scola B, Lorgulescu I, Bollini G. Five cases of *Kingella kingae* skeletal infection in a French hospital. *Eur J Clin Microbiol Infect Dis* 1998;17:512–515.

134. Host B, Schumacher H, Prag J, et al. Isolation of *Kingella kingae* from synovial fluids using four commercial blood culture bottles. *Eur J Clin Microbiol Infect Dis* 2000;19:608–611.

135. Chakraborty RN, Meigh RE, Kaye GC. *Kingella kingae* prosthetic valve endocarditis. *Indian Heart J* 1999;51:438-39.

136. Wolak T, Abu-Shakra M, Flusser D, et al. *Kingella* endocarditis and meningitis in a patient with SLE and associated antiphospholipid syndrome. *Lupus* 2000;9:393.

137. Lewis MB, Bamford JM. Global aphasia without hemiparesis secondary to *Kingella kingae* endocarditis. *Arch Neurol* 2000;5":1774–1775.

138. Wells L, Rutter N, Donald F. *Kingella kingae* endocarditis in a sixteen-month-old-child. *Pediatr Infect Dis J* 2001;20:454–455.

139. Kennedy CA, Rosen H. *Kingella kingae* bacteremia and adult epiglottitis in a granulocytopenic host. *Am J Med* 1988;85:701–702.

140. Redfield DC, Overturf GD, Ewing N, et al. Bacteria, arthritis, and skin lesions due to *Kingella kingae. Arch Dis Child* 1980;55:411–414.

141. Amir J, Schockelford PG. *Kingella kingae* intervertebral disk infection. *J Clin Microbiol* 1991;29:1083–1086.

142. Rolle U, Schille R, Hormann D, et al. Soft tissue infection caused by *Kingella kingae* in a child. *J Pediatr Surg* 2001;36:946–947.

143. Reekmans A, Noppen M, Naessens A, et al. A rare manifestation of *Kingella kingae* infection. *Eur J Intern Med* 2000;11:343–344.

144. Yagupsky P, Katz O, Peled N. Antibiotic susceptibility of *Kingella kingae* isolates from respiratory carriers and patients with invasive infections. *J Antimicrob Chemother* 2001;47:191–193.

145. Jensen KT, Schonheyder H, Thomsen VF. *In-vitro* activity of β-lactam and other antimicrobial agents against *Kingella kingae. J Antimicrob Chemother* 1994;33:635–640.

146. Rossau R, Kersters K, Falsen E, et al. *Oligella*, a new genus including *Oligella urethralis* comb. nov. (formerly *Moraxella urethralis*) and *Oligella ureolytica* sp. nov. (formerly CDC group IVe): relationship to *Taylorella equigenitalis* and related taxa. *Int J Syst Bacteriol* 1987;37:198–210.

147. Stenfors L-E, Raisanen S. Quantitative analysis of the bacterial findings in otitis media. *J Laryngol Otol* 1990;104:749–757.

148. Gan VN, Kusmiesz H, Shelton S, Nelson JD. Comparative evaluation of loracarbef and amoxicillin-clavulanate for acute otitis media. *Antimicrob Agents Chemother* 1991;35:967–971.

149. Johnson CE, Carlin SA, Super DM, et al. Cefixime compared with amoxicillin for treatment of acute otitis media. *J Pediatr* 1991;119:117–122.

150. Faden H, Bernstein J, Stanievich J, et al. Effect of prior antibiotic treatment on middle ear disease in children. *Ann Otol Rhinol Laryngol* 1992;101:87–91.

151. DelBeccaro MA, Mendelman PM, Inglis AF, et al. Bacteriology of acute otitis media: A new perspective. *J Pediatr* 1992;120:81–84.

152. Chonmaitree T, Owen MJ, Patel JA, et al. Effect of viral respiratory tract infection on outcome of acute otitis media. *J Pediatr* 1992;120:856–862.

153. Owen MJ, Anwar R, Nguyen HK, et al. Efficacy of cefixime in the treatment of acute otitis media in children. *AJDC* 1993;147:81–86.

154. Aspin MM, Hoberman A, McCarty J, et al. Comparative study of the safety and efficacy of clarithromycin and amoxicillin-clavulanate in the treatment of acute otitis media in children. *J Pediatr* 1994;125:135–141.

155. Gehanno P, Lenoir G, Barry B, et al. Evaluation of nasopharyngeal cultures for bacteriologic assessment of acute otitis media in children. *Pediatr Infect Dis J* 1996;15:329–332.

156. Dagan R, Leibovitz E, Greenberg D, et al. Early eradication of pathogens from middle ear fluid during antibiotic treatment of acute otitis media is associated with improved clinical outcome. *Pediatr Infect Dis J* 1998;17:776–782.

157. Block SL, Hedrick JA, Kratzer J, et al. Five-day twice daily cefdinir therapy for acute otitis media: microbiologic and clinical efficacy. *Pediatr Infect Dis J* 2000;19(suppl):153–158.

158. Block SL, McCarty JM, Hedrick JA, et al. Comparative safety and efficacy of cefdinir vs amoxicillin/clavulanate for treatment of suppurative acute otitis media in children. *Pediatr Infect Dis J* 2000;19(suppl):159–165.

159. Kilpi T, Herva E, Kaijalainen T, et al. Bacteriology of acute otitis media in a cohort of Finnish children followed for the first two years of life. *Pediatr Infect Dis J* 2001;20:654–662.

Gram-Negative Bacilli

CHAPTER 195
Enterobacteriaceae

Henry D. Isenberg and Richard F. D'Amato

The family of Enterobacteriaceae—obviously mislabeled in view of its numerous, diverse, extraintestinal habitats—is a fitting example of the mastery exerted by the microbial world over all living forms. Their very ubiquity and the beneficial and harmful effects of these bacteria have contributed to their role as favorite test objects. The haploid nature of the prokaryotic chromosome has complicated the application of Linnaean taxonomy to all "primitive" organisms, requiring special definitions of species and genera, based lately on the degree of DNA homology achieved under the most stringent environmental conditions and the determination of bacterial relationships based on recombinant RNA genes. Fortunately, many of the accepted classifications within the family, based on biochemical and immunologic characteristics, have been confirmed by this approach. Still, new genera and species have emerged: in 1972, 11 genera and 26 species made up the family; in 1995, there were 28 genera, 115 species, and 7 enteric groups (1).

This expansion, based on ongoing analyses, continues unabated, and it is complicated further by the discovery that variants within a species represent a spectrum of interactions, some of which are injurious to the host, others of which are beneficial, and some of which have no effect, all depending on the individual host (2–8). (The reader is referred to references 4–8 for detailed scientific treatments of this significant family.) Thus, the oxidase-positive *Plesiononas shigelloides* has been tentatively based in the family Enterobacteriaceae (J.J. Farmer III, personal communication).

All members of Enterobacteriaceae are straight gram-negative rods. When motile, they possess peritrichous flagella. The cellular organization of these bacteria is typical of gram-negative organisms: an outer membrane overlies the murein sacculus, and there is a periplasmic space between the peptidoglycan cell wall and the cytoplasmic membrane. The outer membrane, in contact with the environment, displays protective properties such as hydrophilic, mostly negatively charged carbohydrate chains and acidic proteins to prevent phagocytosis. Enterobacteriaceae organisms display in their somatic (O) and capsular (K) polysaccharides incredible structural variations that may prevent interactions with preexisting host antibodies or enzymes. This outer membrane (9) contains lipids, proteins, and various polysaccharides arranged in concert with the peptidoglycan layer in a hexagonal lattice that ionically links the outer membrane and cell wall. In addition, a small lipoprotein in the outer membrane anchors to the C-terminal of the several diaminopimelic acid constituents of the peptidoglycan.

The Enterobacteriaceae lipopolysaccharides that are so fascinating to investigators are composed of three distinct regions: lipid A, closest to the cell wall; core antigen; and the polysaccharide chains responsible for the O or somatic antigenicity of species and subspecies variants (Fig. 195.1). Lipid A consists of a phosphorylated glucosamine sequence linked by β-glycosidic bonds. Generally, the amino group of the glucosamine is substituted by D-3-hydroxy fatty acids; the hydroxyl groups of the molecule are esterified with various long-chain saturated fatty acids. The core polysaccharide unites the outer O polysaccharide with the lipid A moiety. This core is usually composed of glucosamine, heptose, 3-deoxy-D-manooctulosonic acid (also known as 2-keto-3-deoxyoctonate), galactose, and other hexoses and pentoses. It is attached through a ketocytic link of 2-keto-3-deoxyoctonate to glucosamines of lipid A. The complex somatic antigens consist of various polysaccharides, many of them peculiar to Enterobacteriaceae, in addition to a "common" antigen, an acidic polysaccharide composed of

N-acetyl-D-glucosamine, N-acetylmannosaminuronic acid, and 4-acetamido-4,6-dideoxygalactose. The presence, absence, linkage types, and sequences of glucose, galactose, acetylglucosamine, 3-deoxy-D-manooctulosonic acid, mannose, ribose, xylose, rhamnose, fucose, and 2,6-dideoxyhexoses such as abequose, colitose, and tyvelose account for the display of antigenic diversity observed in the outermost hydrophilic polysaccharide chains.

Several members of the family express additional antigenic polysaccharides in the form of capsules or envelopes (K antigens) as well as fimbriae, structures useful for adhesion of bacteria to environmental surfaces, including mammalian cells. The K antigens are specific polysaccharides that are found in *Escherichia coli*; specific polysaccharides are also found as Vi and M antigens among *Salmonella* species and as capsular antigens of *Klebsiella* species. These polysaccharides are acidic, always containing different uronic acids in addition to hexoses, deoxyhexoses, and hexosamines. Considerable variation in the expressions of all antigens must be expected. Although the antigenicity of various outer membrane proteins and polypeptides has not been exploited for laboratory recognition of these bacteria, more than 20 different representatives have been recognized, including matrix proteins, proteins in combination with lipid moieties, and the proteins of the porin channels. The explanation of the significance of these molecules in the reaction of bacteria to antibiotics and other environmental challenges is in its infancy; the molecules may function as receptors for bacteriophage attachments, transporters of selected nutrients, and barriers to hydrophobic substances such as dyes or detergents.

Bacterial survival depends on the organism's ability to adhere to surfaces and to form microcolonies on them. The latter is accomplished by exopolysaccharide production that forms a protective cement that is rarely penetrated by host immune

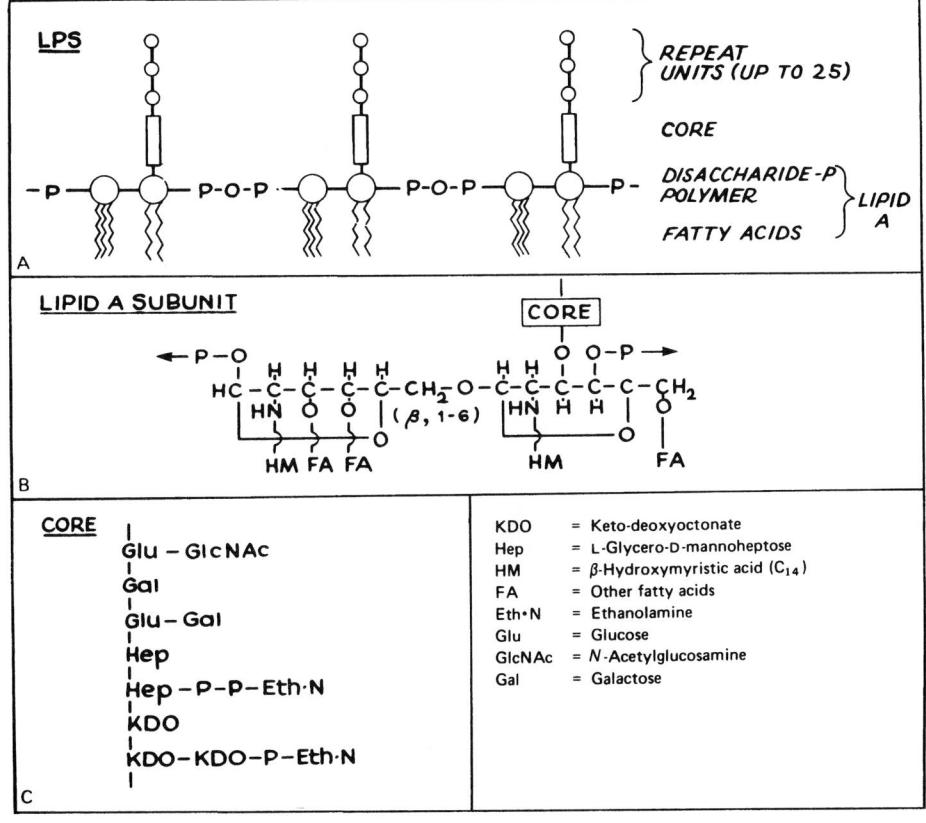

Figure 195.1. The outer membrane of Enterobacteriaceae. *LPS*, lipopolysaccharide.

TABLE 195.1.   Environmental Sources of Enterobacteriaceae

Genus	Animals	Water	Soil	Environment (not specified)	Food	Unknown[a]	Human
Budvicia		+					+
Cedecea							+
Citrobacter	+	+	+		+	+	+
Edwardsiella	+	+			+	+	+
Enterobacter	+	+		+	+	+	+
Escherichia	+	+	+	+	+	+	+
Ewingella					+	+	+
Hafnia						+	+
Klebsiella	+	+		+		+	+
Kluyvera	+	+	+	+	+	+	+
Leclercia	+	+		+	+		+
Leminorella	+						+
Moellerella		+					+
Morganella							+
Pragia		+					+
Proteus	+						+
Providencia						+	+
Rhanella		+				+	+
Salmonella	+	+	+	+	+	+	+
Serratia	+	+	+	+	+	+	+
Shigella	Primates						+
Tatumella							+
Trabulsiella						+	+
Yersinia	+	+	+	+	+	+	+
Yokenella						+	+
Xenorhabdus	+						+

Different species of each genus are recovered from different environmental sources.
[a] The exact source of all species has not been determined.

defenses or antibiotics. These exopolysaccharides probably also serve as reservoirs for nutrients required by the constituents of the microbial mats that are not necessarily monomicrobial (10). Adherence mechanisms determined by fimbriae and other structures are described and discussed in other chapters of this book, as are the mechanisms of bacterial responses to environmental and host challenges resulting from conjugation and extrachromosomal DNA in the form of plasmids.

The widespread distribution of the family in nature complicates the interpretation of laboratory results with respect to significance of an isolate. The sources listed in Table 195.1 do not necessarily constitute permanent habitats; they may reflect contamination of these environments by animals or humans. Traditionally, the major diseases attributed to the members of the family are intestinal disorders, ranging from diarrhea and food poisoning to dysentery and typhoid-like fever. The inclusion of *Yersinia* in the family now warrants consideration of plague and other yersinioses.

In addition to urinary tract infections, the major role of Enterobacteriaceae representatives in developed countries is in extraintestinal infections as agents of enteric bacterioses, which are acquired through colonization of prostheses or lesions in patients whose immunity is impaired (11). Enteric bacteriosis manifests as bacteremia; pneumonia; urinary tract, wound, or central nervous system infections; abscess formation; and colonization of implants, prostheses, and catheters, these last-named devices serving as niches for the spread of infection. The various clinical consequences of these bacteria are described in the relevant chapters of this book. Still, it is worth remembering the assertion of Farmer and colleagues (12) that in the United States as many as 90% of Enterobacteriaceae isolates from clinical specimens are composed of three species: *E. coli*, *Klebsiella pneumoniae*, and *Proteus mirabilis* (12).

SPECIMEN COLLECTION

Appropriate specimens for laboratory analysis should be collected in suitable transport media that ensure the preservation of the organisms and, for polymicrobial infections, that preserve the proportions of representative bacteria. Special neutralizing buffers are recommended when salmonellae, and especially shigellae, are sought in stool specimens, because room temperature lowers the pH to levels that most of these bacteria cannot tolerate (13).

ISOLATION AND IDENTIFICATION

All Enterobacteriaceae species grow readily on nutrient media. In most instances laboratorians use, besides general media, selective agars that allow presumptive identification of the organisms in the specimen after 18 to 24 hours' incubation. Media such as MacConkey, deoxycholate, and eosinmethylene blue agar are used (13–16) for their isolation in general. Only *Yersinia pestis* and *Yersinia pseudotuberculosis* may not grow on selective media. The isolation and separation of the so-called enteric pathogens, *Salmonella* and *Shigella* organisms, are aided by the use of an entire array of selective agars supplemented by enrichment broths that enhance the detection of these organisms in the presence of many other bacteria. For this purpose, *Salmonella-Shigella* agar, bismuth sulfite agar (for the isolation of *Salmonella*), brilliant green agar (for the isolation of *Salmonella*), Hektoen enteric agar, lysine-deoxycholate agar, and many others are used widely (14–16). Separation on the basis of lactose fermentation is still a widely accepted tool for sequestering the diarrheogenic salmonellae and shigellae; however, not all of the genera designated as lactose fermenters do so invariably. The next level of identification tests usually involves soliciting fermentation reactions on various carbohydrate substrates and the detection of enzymes. Many commercial systems are available and have been incorporated into automated devices linked to computers (17). Identification on the basis of 12 to more than 30 substrates can be provided in this manner. Most such methods require that a lack of oxidase be demonstrated. These biochemical examinations usually allow identification of the species. For certain isolates, further identifications are required; usually they involve serologic classifications. Although molecular tools are useful taxonomically and epidemiologically and for the recognition of plasmid-associated so-called virulence factors, routine applications of these markers are not yet practical.

SEPARATION OF ENTEROBACTERIACEAE INTO GENERA AND SPECIES

Taxonomists and clinical microbiologists, aware that they always deal with enormous populations of organisms, prefer to score bacterial action on individual substrates in percentages.

Once the genus has been designated, identification at the species level may be indicated, but this step may be expensive and not clinically warranted. Laboratorians must decide whether more information will affect the choice of therapy as well as determine the epidemiologic implications of the isolate. Antibiotic profiles, the patient's history, the anatomic source of the clinical specimen, and the desires of the responsible clinician are factors in the decision.

ESCHERICHIA

E. coli, the best-known and most common member of Enterobacteriaceae, shares with other members of the family the characteristic shape and tinctorial properties, and when motile, peritrichous flagella. *Escherichia* organisms may have capsules or extracellular slime. These chemoorganotrophic bacteria can attack carbohydrates fermentatively or oxidatively, producing pyruvate that may lead to lactic, acetic, and formic acids. These acids can be attacked by a complex hydrogenlyase enzyme system, leading to the liberation of carbon dioxide and hydrogen, one of the earliest clues used to detect *E. coli* in water and clinical specimens. *E. coli* is a common inhabitant of the human and animal large intestine. It is easily recognized by a few salient tests: indole production, a positive result on methyl red tests, negative Voges-Proskauer reaction, and inability to utilize citrate.

The serologic analysis of *E. coli* has established the antigens previously discussed. At present, there are 171 O antigens, approximately 80 K antigens, and 56 H antigens of *E. coli*. The outermost border of *E. coli* displays fimbriae, fibrils, or colonizing factors now classified as F antigens. The more recently recognized members of the genus *Escherichia* are rarely encountered in clinical specimens. *Escherichia blattae,* a cockroach resident, has not as yet been discovered in the intimate human biosphere. *Escherichia fergusonii* and *Escherichia hermannii* have been isolated from stool and extraintestinal sources, whereas *Escherichia vulneris* has been recovered from extraintestinal specimens, mostly wounds. The differences between the various *Escherichia* and *Shigella* species are shown in Table 195.2. *E. coli,* always suspect when encountered in appropriate quantity extraintestinally, has now been recognized for the diarrheogenic potential of certain variants. Those capable of producing intestinal disease are much more prevalent in developing countries; extraintestinal involvement of *E. coli* in disease complications is more common in developed areas. One group of *E. coli* serotypes, the enterotoxigenic *E. coli,* associated with traveler's diarrhea in developing countries, are characterized by the production of enterotoxins, a thermolabile (LT) and two thermostable (STa and STb) toxins. The former resembles cholera toxin in action and attachment sites in the small intestine. These toxins can be recognized by specialized tests, but these tests are not yet available in most laboratories. The following serotypes have been involved in the production of these toxins, which lead to cholera-like diarrhea: O6, O8, O15, O20, O25, O27, O63, O78, O80, O85, O114, O115, O128ac, O148, O153, O159, and O167. However, the genetic determinants for the production of enterotoxins reside on transmissible plasmids that can be lost. Thus, typing of isolates by biochemical or serologic methods may be unreliable for detecting enterotoxigenic *E. coli.*

Another group of *E. coli* strains, the enteropathogenic group, were prominent causes of neonatal diarrhea in Europe and the United States during the 1950s and 1960s. For unknown reasons their pathogenicity seems to have declined in developed countries, but they are still a major problem in the developing world. The serotypes implicated in this group of diseases are O18, O26, O44, O55, O86, O111, O114, O119, O125, O126, O127, O128ab, O142, and O158. The enteroinvasive *E. coli* strains cause

TABLE 195.2. Differentiation of *Escherichia* and *Shigella* Species

Organism	Indole	Decarboxylases Lysine	Decarboxylases Ornithine	Growth in potassium cyanide	Fermentation Lactose	Adonitol	Sorbitol	Cellobiose	Mucate	Acetate
Escherichia										
E. coli	+	+	d	0	+	0	+	0	+	+
E. coli (inactive)[a]	d	d	d	0	d	0	d	0	d	d
E. fergusonii	+	+	+	0	0	+	0	+	0	+
E. hermannii	+	0	+	+	d	0	0	+	+	d
E. vulneris	0	d	0	d	d	0	0	+	d	d
E. blattae[b]	0	+	+	0	0	0	0	0	d	0
Shigella										
S. sonnei[a]	0	0	+	0	0	0	0	0	0	0
Serogroups A, B, C	d	0	0	0	0	0	d	0	0	0

[a]Immotile at 36°C; no gas from glucose.
[b]Not found in clinical specimens.
+, ≥90% positive; 0, ≤10% positive; d, 11%–89% positive.

illness similar to that caused by *Shigella*. Serogroups O28, O29, O112, O124, O136, O143, O144, O152, O164, and O167 can cause ulceration of the intestine and symptoms resembling those of bacterial dysentery. The enterohemorrhagic *E. coli* O157:H7 causes a range of illnesses, from mild diarrhea to hemorrhagic colitis and hemolytic-uremic syndrome. Asymptomatic colonization may also occur. A cardinal feature of *E. coli* O157:H7 is its inability to ferment sorbitol in 24 hours, which allows it to be detected in the stool microbiota through the use of a selective medium, a modified MacConkey agar, that demonstrates the absence of sorbitol fermentation and is specific for this pathogen. The ability to produce hemorrhagic colitis is associated with *E. coli* strains other than O157:H7, which produce a Shiga-like toxin or verotoxin, both terms describing the identical toxic moiety. The common occurrence of *E. coli*, especially in stool specimens, makes it difficult for the laboratory to readily recognize these potentially harmful members of the species. Usually, it is the absence of any other causative microorganisms or virus that prompts a search for these strains. Often, especially in developed countries, such a search is fruitless, because most of the disease manifestations of diarrheogenic *E. coli* are self-limiting. Specimens from travelers to areas where diarrheogenic species are endemic should be submitted with appropriate encouragement to search for representatives of these groups.

Certain serogroups of *E. coli* occur with greater frequency in extraintestinal infections as well. Many share somatic antigens. Urinary tract infections are most often caused by representatives of serogroups O1, O2, O4, O6, O7, O8, O9, O11, O18, O22, O25, O62, and O75, and the selfsame representatives (except O62) produce bacteremia. *E. coli* meningitis seems to involve fewer serogroups: O1, O6, O7, O16, O18, and O83. In the neonatal period, *E. coli* K1 is the principal agent of *E. coli* meningitis and bacteremia. Unfortunately, specialty laboratories or reference laboratories must identify these variants. The role of the somatic antigens in the pathogenesis of extraintestinal *E. coli* infections has not been established. The numerous plasmids carried by *E. coli* explain the spectrum of antibiotic susceptibility displayed by clinical isolates, even in a single geographic area. Communication with genera within the family and even extrafamilial exchanges account for this resistance. We can only hope that advances in molecular epidemiology provide appropriate tools for understanding the mechanisms through which these organisms disseminate in hospitals and communities (4,8,18).

SHIGELLA

Genetically, shigellae are *E. coli*. They may be separated from classically reacting *E. coli* by a variety of tests (Table 195.2). Inability to grow on acetate is the most useful characteristic of *Shigella* species, which separates them from the nonmotile, nonaerogenic groups of *E. coli*, especially the alkalescens-dispar group. For convenience, the genus *Shigella* is divided into four "species" with 32 serotypes and more subserotypes. Biochemical reactions are not helpful or conclusive in separating the four species. Inability to ferment mannitol separates the *Shigella dysenteriae* group from the remainder of the genus, but this distinction is best made by serologic tests. For epidemiologic purposes, biotyping and pulsed field gel electrophoresis (PFGE) can be performed (7).

The shigellae are pathogenic for only humans and primates. On rare occasions they have been isolated from domestic dogs. Disease in humans is usually limited to the colon and rectum (see Chapter 66). In severe cases the terminal ileum may also be involved. The organisms cause an acute inflammatory reaction and ulceration of the epithelium, especially when *S. dysenteriae* and *Shigella flexneri* are involved. Usually the organisms do not spread beyond the lamina propria, and bacteremic phases are uncommon. There is still some hesitation by investigators to declare certain aspects of *S. dysenteriae* toxin as being truly related to the labile enterotoxin of *E. coli* and the enterotoxin of *Vibrio cholerae*. It has now been shown that under stringent conditions the Shiga toxin does behave similarly (19).

SALMONELLA

All salmonellae possess the potential to cause disease in humans and animals and to engender disagreements among bacterial taxonomists (Table 195.3). The mosaic of somatic antigens displayed by the genus, coupled with numerous flagellar antigens capable of phase variations due to two chromosomal genes, have led microbiologists to recognize more than 2,000 different variants, regarded as species by some and as subspecies by others. Some agreement is now emerging based on molecular analyses that indicate that the genus contains but one species, *Salmonella choleraesuis*. It has been proposed that all salmonellae, including the *Salmonella arizonae* strains, be considered variants of the newly created species *Salmonella enterica*, to avoid confusion with the serotype (serovar) *S. choleraesuis* (7). The various earlier

---

TABLE 195.3.   Differences Between the Major Subgroups of *Salmonella* Organisms

Property or test	DNA subgroup						
	1	2	3a	3b	4	5	6
DNA hybridization group	1	2	3	4	5	?	?
Fermentation							
Dulcitol	+	+	0	0	0	+	d
Lactose	0	0	d	d	0	0	d
Mucate	+	+	+	d	0	+	d
o-Nitrophenyl-β-galactoside	0	d	+	+	0	+	d
Malonate utilization	0	+	+	+	0	0	0
Growth in potassium cyanide	0	0	0	0	+	+	0
Gelatin hydrolysis	0	+	0	+	+	+	0

+, ≥90% positive; 0, ≤10% positive; d, 11%–89% positive.
Modified from Farmer JJ III. Enterobacteriaceae. Introduction and identification. In: Murray PR, Baron EJ, Pfaller MA, et al., eds. *Manual of clinical microbiology*, 6th ed. Washington, DC: ASM Press, 1995:438–449.

divisions are regarded as subspecies, and a second species, *Salmonella bongor,* has been proposed for those errant salmonellae that may occasionally display confusing biochemical reactions.

Salmonellae have selected the intestinal tract of humans and warm- and cold-blooded wild and domestic animals as their habitat. They may be present as colonizers, but all can cause infections in humans, usually after ingestion of food or water. Two major disease manifestations characterize *Salmonella* infections: enteric fever and food poisoning. The former is characterized by headache, malaise, anorexia, and symptoms not referable to the gastrointestinal tract, as well as fever. Food poisoning presents with diarrhea, abdominal cramps, and vomiting, often accompanied by fever. The salmonellae invade the small bowel lumen, penetrate the ileum (more rarely the colonic epithelium), and induce an inflammatory reaction. After the bacteria reach the lymph nodes, the follicles enlarge and many ulcerate. The bacteria finally enter the bloodstream and produce enteric fever, of which typhoid fever is the classic example. In food poisoning, *Salmonella* organisms remain confined to the intestine (see Chapter 68).

The isolation of salmonellae from clinical specimens can be accomplished with differential media grouped on the basis of their selectivity for the genus (14,16). Salmonellae grow readily on all routine media, including those selected for members of the Enterobacteriaceae. Moderately selective media, such as *Salmonella-Shigella* agar, Hektoen enteric agar, and xylosedeoxycholate agar, are also helpful in their isolation and produce a high degree of suspicion for the presence of the genus. Highly selective media, such as bismuth sulfite and brilliant green agar, should be used when salmonellae are suspected on clinical grounds. Enrichment broths are helpful, especially for investigating food-borne outbreaks or ruling out the carrier state (14–16). Members of the genus *Salmonella* are usually recognized by their biochemical reactions. Simple media may be used, such as triple sugar iron agar supplemented with lysine-iron agar and certain other reactions (7). Commercial, manual, and automated systems approaches have gained favor in most clinical laboratories to achieve this level of identification. Commercially available antisera permit the clinical laboratory to group isolates. The capability to type to the serotype (serovar) level is the province of specialty or reference laboratories. *Salmonella typhi* can be recognized by biochemical reactions producing minimal amounts of hydrogen sulfide and fermenting glucose without producing gas. Such isolates may not group readily with group D antisera until the blocking Vi antigen has been removed by boiling for 30 minutes. Vi antiserum is part of the commercially available battery.

Recognition of a serogroup is based on the presence of shared somatic antigens. More than 90% of clinically encountered salmonellae belong to DNA group 1. Serotypes of group B share O antigen 4; group C1, 7; C2, 6 and 8; C3, 8; D, 9; E1, 10; E2, 15; E3, 34; E4, 19; F, 11; and G, 13. The somatic antigens can occur among other bacteria, but the flagellar antigens are highly specific for the individual salmonellae. Fimbriae, other antigens such as M and the aforementioned Vi antigens, antigenic polysaccharide changes induced by bacteriophages, and other findings may confound identification of an isolate (7). Bacteriophage typing has helped epidemiologic analyses, now largely supplanted by PFGE and other molecular tools (20).

The salmonellae and shigellae are the traditional enteric pathogens of the Enterobacteriaceae. *K. pneumoniae* and *P. mirabilis* are second only to *E. coli* in the frequency with which they are isolated from clinical specimens. Both organisms may be involved in community-acquired urinary tract infections, and *K. pneumoniae* can be found in lower respiratory tract specimens of older persons who have a history of ethanol abuse or chronic obstructive pulmonary disease. *Klebsiella* and *Proteus* species and most other members of the family have attained significance as agents of nosocomial infections called enteric bacterioses (11). The ability of Enterobacteriaceae to meet environmental challenges has brought into the intimate human biosphere genera and species that were unknown there only a few years ago. The introduction of these organisms reflects the selective pressures in communities and medical facilities. Most of the genera and species were considered commensal organisms in the past but have now been shown to participate in complicating the recovery of patients in medical facilities (3). The one characteristic that these diverse species share is their almost exclusive involvement with immunocompromised patients. Rarely are these bacteria isolated from patients in the community, and when they are it is often from persons who have an underlying disease that is in remission. In the hospital setting, where many procedures, therapies, and devices permit colonization of patients with microorganisms residing in the institution, the Enterobacteriaceae bacteria behave as infectious agents. Antimicrobial agents may well have been the most influential factor leading to their ubiquitous presence in hospitals, where their inherent and plasmid-mediated antibiotic resistance capabilities allow them to replace susceptible members of the institutional microbiota and to complicate patients' recovery. They may enter the intimate human biosphere from the sources listed in Table 195.1 (to which plants should be added for *Klebsiella, Enterobacter,* and *Serratia* species). Practically all clinical specimens may harbor these organisms. It bears repeating that these bacteria are involved in all types of infections that plague patients whose immunity is compromised by disease or therapy or who may require a prosthesis. All these bacteria grow well on ordinary laboratory media, including those designed specifically to isolate all Enterobacteriaceae, such as MacConkey and eosin-methylene blue agars.

KLEBSIELLA

Klebsiella species are characteristically nonmotile; attack most carbohydrates; do not, except for *Klebsiella ornithinolytica,* produce ornithine decarboxylase; and display few somatic antigens but numerous capsular ones. Most representatives produce acetylmethylcarbinol, utilize citrate, grow on potassium cyanide medium, and utilize malonate. *Klebsiella oxytoca* is isolated with increasing frequency from blood, urine, and respiratory tract specimens, but stool remains its principal source. *Klebsiella planticola* is a plant organism that has intruded into drinking water and into occasional clinical specimens; *Klebsiella terrigena* has not yet been found in clinical specimens. *K. pneumoniae* is now divided into three subspecies, which are differentiated by certain tests (Table 195.4). *Klebsiella ozaenae* and *Klebsiella rhinoscleromatis* are inactive variants of *K. pneumoniae* that have adapted to specific disease manifestations (21) rarely encountered in the United States.

THE TRIBE PROTEAE

Members of the tribe Proteae are distinguished by their ability to elaborate phenylalanine deaminase; they may be separated from one another by DNase production (some *Proteus* species), swarming, and xylose fermentation by DNase-negative *Proteus* species that separates them from *Morganella* and *Providencia,* members of Ewing's tribe Proteae (7). The species of *Proteus* are separated by reactions given in Table 195.5. Clinical laboratories have no difficulty in recognizing *P. mirabilis* and *Proteus vulgaris* organisms. Certain variants of the latter display variation, especially in esculin hydrolysis and salicin fermentation (1); this

TABLE 195.4.   Differentiation of *Klebsiella pneumoniae* Subspecies

Test	Subspecies *pneumoniae*	Subspecies *ozaenae*	Subspecies *rhinoscleromatis*
Acid from lactose	+	+	0
Acid from dulcitol	d	0	0
Voges-Proskauer	+	0	0
Urease	+	d	0
Mucate	+	d	0
Lysine decarboxylase	+	d	0

+, ≥90% positive; 0, ≤10% positive; d, 11%–89% positive.

suggests a need for taxonomic investigation but is of no consequence in the clinical setting. The epidemiology of cluster outbreaks may require that these variations be used and may lead to the establishment of new species, as was the case for *Proteus penneri* (22), a bacterium of increasing significance in infections of agranulocytic patients. Another species, *Proteus myxofaciens* (1), has not yet been observed in clinical specimens. *Providencia rettgeri* and *Providencia stuartii* have caused an appreciable number of nosocomial urinary tract infections. The natural habitat and means by which these organisms gain access to patients are not known. *Providencia rustigianii* and *Providencia alcalifaciens* have been isolated occasionally from diarrheal stools of infants and children, but their role in producing disease has not been clearly defined (Table 195.6). A newly described species, *Providencia heimbachae*, has not yet been isolated from humans.

Morganella morganii may be distinguished from *Proteus* organisms by an absence of swarming; hydrogen sulfide production; absence of gelatinase, lipase, and citrate utilization; but production of acid from mannose. *Morganella* species differ from *Providencia* species by producing ornithine decarboxylase and by their inability to produce acid from inositol, D-mannitol, adonitol, D-arabitol, and erythritol. *M. morganii* is suspected to be the agent of summer diarrhea (23), and it is isolated with considerable frequency from wounds, urine, and respiratory tract specimens of hospitalized patients.

SERRATIA

The several *Serratia* species (Table 195.1) are widely distributed in nature—in freshwater and saltwater, and on leaves, shrubs, fruits, vegetables, herbs, mushrooms, and mosses. They are also recovered from a considerable number of insects, and some may be pathogenic for the insect species from which they have been

TABLE 195.5.   Differentiation of *Proteus* Species

Test	*P. mirabilis*	*P. vulgaris*	*P. penneri*
Indole	0	+	+
Ornithine decarboxylase	+	0	0
Acid from maltose	0	+	+
Esculin hydrolysis	0	d	0
Chloramphenicol susceptibility[a]	+	d	0

+, ≥90% positive; 0, ≤10% positive; d, 11%–89% positive.
[a]Usual clinical isolates; exceptions can be encountered.

isolated. Several of the *Serratia* species have become established in hospitals, where they complicate the recovery of immunocompromised patients. The frequency with which these bacteria are involved in nosocomial disease varies from hospital to hospital in a given geographic area and may reflect the antibiotic use patterns of the institution. Ingestion of raw vegetables and salads by patients and flowers in patients' rooms may play a role in colonization of patients who subsequently develop disease manifestations caused by *Serratia* species.

Serratia species (Table 195.7) produce extracellular DNase at 25°C and gelatinase at 22°C. They also elaborate lipase and are resistant to colistin and cephalothin. The combination of these biochemical activities and the responses to the two antimicrobial agents do not characterize any other Enterobacteriaceae.

The only *Serratia* species isolated frequently is *Serratia marcescens*. The inability to ferment L-arabinose is an important biochemical feature, because not all *S. marcescens* organisms produce the typical red pigment prodigiosin (2-methyl-3-amyl-6-methoxyprodigiosene), elaborated also by *Serratia rubidaea* and *Serratia plymuthica* (1). Serologic identification of *S. marcescens* is difficult, because the 20 somatic and 20 flagellar antigens recognized to date cross-react. In the hospital setting, *S. marcescens* is characterized by its ability to resist antimicrobial challenges (24).

Serratia liquefaciens, a common inhabitant of water, plants, insects, and foods, is encountered less frequently in human specimens than is *S. marcescens*, but it can become established as a nosocomial bacterium with antimicrobial resistance patterns similar to those of *S. marcescens*.

S. rubidaea and *S. plymuthica* are rarely isolated from hospitalized patients. *Serratia odorifera* and *Serratia ficaria* are even rarer. All the *Serratia* species may display susceptibility to cephalosporins and aminocyclitols initially but manifest resistance during therapy.

CITROBACTER

Citrobacter organisms, comprising 11 different species, are easily differentiated from other members of the family by their ability to utilize citrate as the sole carbon source, by not producing acetylmethylcarbinol, and especially by their inability to produce lysine decarboxylase (1). These bacteria are considered normal inhabitants of the intestinal tract of humans and animals, including mammals, birds, reptiles, and some insects. They are also encountered in soil, water, sewage, food, and industrial wastewater. Disease production is once again opportunistic, as the bacteria take advantage of the underlying disease of hospitalized patients. Organisms are recovered from clinical specimens such as urine, sputum, blood, cerebrospinal fluid, and otitis media exudates, and from surgical and traumatic wounds, abscesses, and postmortem specimens. *Citrobacter freundii* is by far the most common isolate, but the others have been isolated from nosocomial infections, at times from cluster epidemics. *C. freundii* representatives possess 42 somatic antigens and more than 70 flagellar ones. These antigens are closely related to those of *Salmonella* and *Escherichia*. *Citrobacter diversus* has displayed some 6 to 17 O antigens and at least 7 flagellar antigens. Investigations of *Citrobacter amalonaticus* reveal to date 13 somatic antigens, some of which seem to be related to those of *Shigella boydii* and *S. dysenteriae*.

ENTEROBACTER AND HAFNIA

These two genera are considered together because the similarity of *Hafnia alvei* to *Enterobacter* organisms is considerable.

TABLE 195.6. Differentiation of *Providencia* Species

Test	*P. alcalifaciens*	*P. rettgert*	*P. rustigianii*	*P. stuartii*	*P. heimbachae*
Urease	0	+	0	d	0
Produces acid from					
myo-inositol	0	+	0	+	d
Adonitol	+	+	0	0	+
Arabitol	0	+	0	0	+
Trehalose	0	0	0	+	0
Indole	+	+	+	+	0

+, >90% positive; 0, <10% positive; d, 11%–89% positive.

The former designation of the organism was *Enterobacter hafnia*. The organisms share many biochemical characteristics (Table 195.8). These bacteria are widely distributed in nature. They are found in human and animal feces, quite probably as transients. They are encountered in soil, sewage, milk and dairy products, animal hides, meat, and fish from contaminated waters, and on grasses, feed, corn, sugar cane, and bananas. *Enterobacter sakazakii* and *Enterobacter gergoviae* have been encountered only in clinical specimens; their natural habitats are not known. In addition, *Enterobacter intermedium*, *Enterobacter cancerogenus*, *Enterobacter dissolvens*, biogroup 1 of *H. alvei*, and *Enterobacter nimipressuralis* have not yet been isolated from human specimens.

These organisms represent typical examples of opportunistic enteric bacteriosis. They constitute approximately 5% of nosocomial infections and have been isolated from blood, urinary tract, surgical wound infections, lungs, and burn wounds. The frequency with which they are encountered reflects their ability to resist an appreciable number of antibiotic agents. The resistance mechanisms involve constitutive and inducible chromosomal mechanisms as well as plasmid-mediated ones. They are thought to contribute to the resistance plasmid pools in institutions by their ability to transfer extrachromosomal resistance factors to susceptible bacteria.

Although they can be recognized fairly readily on routine media in the microbiology laboratory, the biochemical activities of *Enterobacter agglomerans* are a challenge to clinical microbiologists. This bacterium, recognized by agricultural microbiologists as *Erwinia herbicola*, may be divided into two major groups that are distinguished by their ability to form gas from glucose. This bacterium is readily confused with other Enterobacteriaceae; several tests are required to identify *E. agglomerans* with some degree of certainty.

The somatic and capsular antigens of the genus are presently under intensive investigation for epidemiologic purposes, as are bacteriocins, plasmids, and bacteriophages. Molecular and immunochemical probes may aid in the detection of *Enterobacter* species in clinical specimens.

The versatility of *Enterobacter* and *Hafnia* in their response to antimicrobial agents requires the caveat that each clinically significant isolate be tested for its antibiotic susceptibility. Whereas laboratory tests may indicate susceptibility to ampicillin and the first-generation cephalosporins, clinical experience has not supported the use of these agents in the treatment of patients. The problem of inducible β-lactamase resistance of many *Enterobacter* species must be kept in mind when their laboratory response is evaluated, especially because second- and third-generation cephalosporins and the broad-spectrum penicillins are powerful β-lactamase inducers.

H. alvei, separated from *Enterobacter* species on the basis of DNA evaluations, has been implicated as a possible agent of diarrhea and gastroenteritis; it has been recovered from normal stool. As an opportunistic pathogen, it has been found in feces, sputum, urine, wounds, abscesses, peritonitis, and upper respiratory tract infections. Rarely has it been isolated in pure culture from these patients, except from ones who had severe underlying disease. The cardinal laboratory characteristic that separates it from *Enterobacter* species is the inability of *Hafnia* to ferment melibiose and cellobiose.

TABLE 195.7. Differentiation of *Serratia* Species

Test	*S. marcescens*	*S. liquefaciens*	*S. rubidaea*	*S. plymuthica*	*S. odorifera*	*S. ficari*
DNase 25°C	+	+	+	+	+	+
Lipase	+	+	+	d	d	+
Gelatinase 22°C	+	+	+	d	+	+
Lysine decarboxylase	+	+	d	0	+	0
Ornithine decarboxylase	+	+	0	0	d	0
Distinct odor	0	0	0	0	+	+
Prodigiosin production	d	0	0	0	0	0
Fermentation						
L-Arabinose	0	+	+	+	+	+
D-Arabitol	0	0	+	0	0	+
D-Sorbitol	+	+	0	d	+	+
Adonitol	d	0	+	0	d	0

+, ≥90% positive; 0, ≤10% positive; d, 11%–89% positive.

TABLE 195.8. Differentiation of *Enterobacter* and *Hafnia* Species

Test	*E. aerogenes*	*E. cloacae*	*E. agglomerans*	*E. gergoviae*	*E. sakazakii*	*E. taylorae*	*E. amnigenus*	*E. asburiae*	*E. hormaechei*	*Hafnia alvei*
Indole	0	0	d	0	0	0	0	0	0	0
Methyl red	0	0	d	0	0	0	0	+	d	d
Urease	0	d	d	+	0	0	0	d	d	0
Lysine decarboxylase	+	0	0	+	0	0	0	0	0	+
Ornithine decarboxylase	+	+	0	+	+	+	d	+	+	+
Arginine dihydrolase	0	+	0	+	0	0	0	d	d	0
Growth in potassium cyanide	+	+	d	0	+	+	+	+	+	+
Gas from glucose	+	+	d	+	+	+	+	+	d	+
Fermentation										
Lactose	+	+	d	d	+	0	d	d	0	0
Sucrose	+	+	d	+	+	0	+	+	+	0
Dulcitol	0	d	0	+	0	0	+	+	d	0
Adonitol	+	d	0	0	0	0	0	0	0	0
D-arabitol	+	d	d	+	0	0	0	0	0	0

+, ≥90% positive; 0, <10% positive; d, 11%–89% positive.

EDWARDSIELLA

Edwardsiella tarda organisms have been isolated from a wide variety of animals. They have been recovered on occasion in stool specimens of healthy persons. They are regarded as opportunistic pathogens that have been involved in wound infections and implicated in some cases of diarrhea. Of the two remaining species in the genus, *Edwardsiella ictaluri* has not yet intruded into the human environment, whereas *Edwardsiella hoshinae* has been isolated from normal human feces. To date, *E. ictaluri* has been recognized only as a pathogen of catfish (25). The members of the genus grow more slowly than do other Enterobacteriaceae on ordinary media. *E. tarda* may be differentiated by its motility, inability to produce DNase and urease, production of hydrogen sulfide and indole, and inability to ferment lactose or utilize citrate.

EWINGELLA

Ewingella americana is the only species in this genus (1). Little is known about its normal habitat; to date it has been isolated only from food. The organism has been recovered from various clinical specimens, including blood, wounds, respiratory tract specimens, and stools. The bacterium is a nonmotile member of Enterobacteriaceae that does not ferment adonitol and has a positive Voges-Proskauer reaction. It may thus present problems of separation from *Yersinia* species.

KLUYVERA

Kluyvera ascorbata is distinguished from *Kluyvera cryocrescens* by the fact that it uses D-ascorbate and by the ability of *K. cryocrescens* to ferment glucose at 5°C after 21 days. The precise habitat of these organisms has not been established; they have been found in water, sewage, soil, and food. These bacteria have complicated the recovery of hospitalized patients and have been isolated from blood, urine, wounds, respiratory tract, and feces. Both rapidly acquire resistance to antimicrobial agents. The bacteria are motile and do not produce DNase, urease, hydrogen sulfide, or acetylmethylcarbinol. Both may or may not produce lysine decarboxylase–negative variants and attack esculin, which helps to distinguish them from *Citrobacter*. A significant isolation of the organisms should lead to a reexamination of their antibiotic profile during therapy to detect the emergence of resistant variants.

CEDECEA

The five species of the genus *Cedecea* can be differentiated by their reaction with ornithine decarboxylase; malonate utilization; and fermentation of sucrose, D-sorbitol, raffinose, D-xylose, and melibiose (1). The natural habitat of the members of the genus has not been discovered. They were identified as isolates from blood, urine, wound, respiratory tract, and stool specimens. *Cedecea* organisms produce lipase and are resistant to colistin and cephalothin, properties they share with *Serratia*. *Cedecea davisae* has been isolated principally from the respiratory tract. *Cedecea lapagei* was derived from sputum and the throat, but no real clinical significance has been attributed to it. *Cedecea neteri* may have been involved in complicating the recovery of a few patients, but it has not been encountered with any frequency in the clin-

ical setting to date. The two unnamed species, *Cedecea* species 3 and 5, are rarely isolated in the clinical setting. Their significance in nosocomial infections depends on the ability of clinical laboratories to identify them.

YERSINIA

The genus *Yersinia* has been included in the family of Enterobacteriaceae as the result of DNA hybridization findings, the presence of common enterobacterial antigens in all representatives, its biochemical activities, and its antibiotic susceptibility profiles (see Chapter 200). With the exception of *Yersinia ruckeri*, DNA hybridization studies indicate a close relationship between the remaining members of the genus. Molecular analysis of *Y. pestis* and *Y. pseudotuberculosis* indicates that they are so closely related as to probably constitute two subspecies of one species (26). *Yersinia* is nonmotile at 37°C, but all species except *Y. pestis* move with peritrichous flagella when grown at temperatures below 30°C. The organisms are widely distributed in nature. All members of the genus grow on the usual laboratory media, although they form smaller colonies and often require a longer period of incubation, especially at temperatures above 30°C. Their slow growth is not accelerated by the incorporation of enrichments such as serum, blood, or yeast extracts. These observations are especially true for *Y. pestis*. The organisms also grow more slowly in broth. The following four species have been added to the genus: *Yersinia aldovae*, *Yersinia bercovieri*, *Yersinia mollaretii*, and *Yersinia rohdei*; all except *Y. aldovae* have been recovered from clinical material.

Plasmids in *Yersinia* species may be rare, but metabolic plasmids that enable the organisms to ferment lactose and raffinose have been observed in *Yersinia enterocolitica* and appear to be the result of 40- to 48-kd DNA. The antigens of *Yersinia* represent a complex group of carbohydrate and protein moieties. Their use in classification has not been studied sufficiently. Epidemiologically significant serogrouping of *Y. enterocolitica* depends on 34 different O antigens and 20 different H antigens.

Yersinia species are susceptible *in vitro* to drugs such as tetracycline, chloramphenicol, streptomycin, gentamicin, kanamycin, neomycin, sulfonamides, and nalidixic acid. They are not susceptible to β-lactam antibiotics, and the more modern agents have not been studied.

Six different factors are involved in the ability of *Y. pestis* to produce disease, of which the production of V and W antigens is probably the most significant. *Y. pestis* causes disease in rodents. The disease is transmitted when fleas regurgitate bacteria while taking a blood meal from animals—or from humans when no other hosts are readily available. Bubonic, septicemic, or pneumonic plague follow. The organisms are phagocytosed and killed in polymorphonuclear neutrophils, but those ingested by macrophages survive and multiply, acquiring resistance to further phagocytosis. Invasion of other organs leads to the usual presentation of the disease. Plague is enzootic in North and South America, Africa, the Middle East, and Asia. In the United States, wild rodents and similar animals are the reservoir. Several methods are available for testing the virulence of a *Y. pestis* strain (see Chapter 200).

Y. pseudotuberculosis causes epizootics in many animal species, especially rodents. It involves primarily the lymphatic system. On occasion, humans acquire *Y. pseudotuberculosis* infection and may develop mesenteric adenitis that mimics acute appendicitis; immunocompromised patients can develop severe septicemia. *Y. enterocolitica*, on the other hand, is pathogenic for hares, monkeys, and humans. In animals, the disease caused by this organism resembles *Y. pseudotuberculosis* infection. In children, *Y. enterocolitica* is introduced via the oral route and the bacteria gain access to and multiply in Peyer's patches. The serogroup and the presence of certain virulence-associated plasmids determine the subsequent manifestations of human disease. *Yersinia* organisms may remain localized and cause ileitis, or they may invade the lymphatics, producing mysenteric adenitis. When they reach the circulation, septicemia ensues. *Yersinia* arthritis is caused by *Y. enterocolitica* serogroup O9, organisms that share an antigen with *Brucella*. Patients who have human leukocyte antigen type 27 seem especially prone to this type of infection. The role in human disease of the remaining *Yersinia* species has not been clearly established. Many behave as opportunistic pathogens (27). *Y. ruckeri*, an organism suspected of belonging to a different group of bacteria, is the agent of red-mouth disease of fish; it is a rare cause of human disease (1).

NEW ENTEROBACTERIACEAE GENERA

Rhanella aquatalis has been isolated principally from water and rarely from human sources. It is difficult to distinguish from other Enterobacteriaceae, especially *E. agglomerans* (1).

Tatumella ptyseos has occasionally been isolated from clinical specimens (blood, urine, stool) and mostly respiratory tract specimens. Its habitat is not known.

Xenorhabdus is divided into two species, *Xenorhabdus nematophilus* and *Xenorhabdus luminescens*, which are pathogenic for nematodes and were believed to be incapable of intruding into the human biosphere because they do not grow at 35°C. They have been isolated from clinical specimens, however, and eventually they may become occasional nosocomial bacteria.

A number of other genera have been added to Enterobacteriaceae. *Budvicia*, *Leclercia*, *Leminorella*, and *Yokenella* have been recovered from clinical material. *Trabulsiella* and *Pragia* are genera as yet unknown in the human biosphere.

Obviously, the family Enterobacteriaceae continues to grow. The various enteric groups will eventually receive genus and species designations. In addition, the application of molecular biology methods to understanding relationships among microorganisms may lead to the creation of more genera. The continued advances in medicine may also make it possible for organisms hitherto unknown in the intimate human biosphere to gain access and to complicate the recovery of patients receiving therapy. That some of these organisms may be members of the family Enterobacteriaceae is not unlikely, although there seems to be little chance that the predominance of *E. coli*, *K. pneumoniae*, and *P. mirabilis* will be challenged by newcomers to the human environment. However, these bacteria are significant for the care of hospitalized—and especially of immunocompromised—patients. We need to recognize them to control cluster epidemics. The Enterobacteriaceae that are established, albeit not necessarily autochthonous residents, will continue to dominate in the economy of human health and disease.

REFERENCES

1. Farmer JJ III. Enterobacteriaceae: introduction and identification. In: Murray PR, Baron EJ, Pfaller MA, et al., eds. *Manual of clinical microbiology*, 6th ed. Washington, DC: ASM Press, 1995:438–449.
2. Isenberg HD, Balows A. Bacterial pathogenicity in man and animals. In: Starr MP, Stolp H, Truper HG, et al., eds. *The prokaryotes—a handbook on habitats, isolation and identification of bacteria*. Berlin: Springer-Verlag, 1981: 83–122.
3. Isenberg HD. Pathogenicity and virulence: another view. *Clin Microbiol Rev* 1988;1:40.
4. Brenner DJ. Family Enterobacteriaceae. In: Krieg NR, Holt JG, eds. *Bergey's manual of systematic bacteriology*, Vol. 1. Baltimore: Williams & Wilkins, 1984:408–420.
5. Krieg NR, Holt JG, eds. *Bergey's manual of systemic bacteriology*, Vol. 1. Baltimore: Williams & Wilkins, 1984.
6. Kauffman F. *The bacteriology of Enterobacteriaceae*. Baltimore: Williams & Wilkins, 1966.
7. Ewing WH. *Edwards and Ewing's identification of Enterobacteriaceae*. New York: Elsevier Science, 1986.
8. Neidhardt FC, Ingraham JL, Low KB, et al., eds. *Escherichia coli* and *Salmonella typhimurium: cellular and molecular biology*. Washington, DC: American Society for Microbiology, 1987.
9. Nikaido H, Vaara M. Outer membrane. In: Neidhardt FC, Ingraham JL, Low KB, et al., eds. *Escherichia coli* and *Salmonella typhimurium: cellular and molecular biology*, Vol. 1. Washington, DC: American Society for Microbiology, 1987: 7–22.
10. Costerton JW, Cheng KJ, Geesay GG, et al. Bacterial biofilms in nature and disease. *Annu Rev Microbiol* 1987;41:435.
11. D'Amato RF, Isenberg HD. Enteric bacteriosis. In: Balows A, Hausler WJ Jr, Ohashi M, et al., eds. *Laboratory diagnosis of infectious disease: principles and practice*, Vol. 1. New York: Springer-Verlag, 1988:217–231.
12. Farmer JJ II, Davis BR, Hickman-Brenner FW, et al. Biochemical identification of new species and biogroups of Enterobacteriaceae isolated from clinical specimens. *J Clin Microbiol* 1985;21:46.
13. Miller JM, Holmes HT. Specimen collection, transport and storage. In: Murray PR, Baron EJ, Pfaller MA, et al., eds. *Manual of clinical microbiology*, 6th ed. Washington, DC: ASM Press, 1995:19–32.
14. Isenberg HD. *Clinical microbiology procedures handbook*. Washington, DC: American Society for Microbiology, 1992.
15. McFaddin JF. *Media for isolation, cultivation, identification, maintenance of medical bacteria*. Baltimore: Williams & Wilkins, 1985.
16. Baron EJ, Peterson LIZ, Finegold SM. *Bailey and Scott's diagnostic microbiology*, ed 9. St. Louis: Mosby-Year Book, 1994.
17. Isenberg HD, MacLowry JC. Automated methods and data handling in bacteriology. *Annu Rev Microbiol* 1976;30:483.
18. Smith GR, ed. Topley and Wilson's principles of bacteriology virology and immunity, 7th ed. Baltimore: Williams & Wilkins, 1984.
19. Rowe B, Gross RJ. *Shigella*. In: Krieg NR, Holt JG, eds. *Bergey's manual of systematic bacteriology*, Vol. 1. Baltimore: Williams & Wilkins, 1984: 423–427.
20. Parker MT. *Salmonella*. In: Smith GR, ed. *Topley and Wilson's principles of bacteriology, virology and immunity*, 7th ed, Vol. 2. Baltimore: Williams & Wilkins, 1984:337–355.
21. Orskov I. *Klebsiella*. In: Krieg NR, Holt JG, eds. *Bergey's manual of systematic bacteriology*, Vol. 1. Baltimore: Williams & Wilkins, 1984:461–465.
22. Hickman FW, Steigerwalt AG, Farmer JJ III, et al. Identification of *Proteus penneri*, sp. nov., formerly known as *Proteus vulgaris* indole negative or as *Proteus vulgaris* biogroup 1. *J Clin Microbiol* 1982;15:1097.
23. Penner JL. The tribe Proteae. In: Starr MP, Stolp H, Truper HG, et al., eds. *The prokaryotes—a handbook on habitats, isolation and identification of bacteria*. Berlin: Springer-Verlag, 1981:1204–1244.
24. Grimont PAD, Grimont F. *Serratia*. In: Krieg NR, Holt JG, eds. *Bergey's manual of systematic bacteriology*, Vol. 1. Baltimore: Williams & Wilkins, 1984:477–484.
25. Farmer JJ III, McWhorter AC. *Edwardsiella*. In: Krieg NR, Holt JG, eds. *Bergey's manual of systematic bacteriology*, Vol. 1. Baltimore: Williams & Wilkins, 1984:486–491.
26. Bercovier H, Mollaret HH. *Yersinia*. In: Krieg NR, Holt JG, eds. *Bergey's manual of systematic bacteriology*, Vol. 1. Baltimore: Williams & Wilkins, 1984:498–506.
27. Bottone EJ. *Yersinia enterocolitica*: a panoramic view of a charismatic microorganism. *Crit Rev Microbiol* 1977;5:211.

CHAPTER 196
Salmonella: *Pathogenesis and Vaccines*

Arthur Y. Kim, Robert H. Rubin, and
Marcia B. Goldberg

Salmonella serotypes are distributed worldwide and are adapted to a wide spectrum of ecologic niches. They are found throughout the animal kingdom and cause a broad spectrum of diseases in their various hosts. Certain pathogenic characteristics, such as the ability to enter into mammalian cells, are shared by all virulent salmonellae, whereas other characteristics, such as factors that determine host or organ specificity, are probably more variable.

SEROTYPING AND BACTERIOLOGY

More than 2,500 serotypes of salmonellae are found in nature. They can be categorized simply according to their habitats: *Salmonella typhi* and *S. paratyphi* are highly adapted to human hosts, other serotypes are highly adapted to nonhuman hosts, and others are not adapted to any specific host. Serotypes in the first category cause a large number of infections in developing countries. Serotypes in the second category rarely produce disease in humans with the exception of the equine pathogen *S. dublin* and the swine pathogen *S. choleraesuis*. In the third category are more than 1,800 serotypes, which cause more than 80% of *Salmonella* infections in the United States and Europe (1).

Salmonellae are aerobic or facultatively anaerobic, usually flagellated and thereby motile, non–spore-forming, gram-negative bacilli. They grow well on rich media, such as blood agar, chocolate agar, and nutrient broth. These nonselective media are appropriate for culture of normally sterile body fluids.

Growth of salmonellae and shigellae is less inhibited by citrate than is growth of the coliform organisms that are part of the normal fecal flora. As a consequence, *Salmonella-Shigella* agar, which contains citrate and bile salts, selects for growth of either *Salmonella* or *Shigella*. Normally nonsterile body fluids (e.g., stool), should be plated on such selective media. If *S. typhi* is suspected, the specimen should also be plated on bismuth sulfite agar, which is the most efficient medium for its isolation and on which *S. typhi* forms characteristic black colonies.

In the laboratory, *Salmonella* species are distinguished from other Enterobacteriaceae by biochemical reactions (Table 196.1). Like *Shigella, Proteus,* and *Yersinia* species, they are unable to ferment lactose and thus give rise to white colonies on solid media containing lactose and the color indicator neutral red (e.g., MacConkey or *Salmonella-Shigella* agar). Most salmonellae produce abundant hydrogen sulfide, form gas in glucose media, decarboxylate lysine and ornithine, and do not ferment sucrose. Hydrogen sulfide production gives a green color to colonies grown on blood agar. *Salmonella* species are distinguished from several *Proteus* species by their inability to metabolize urea. An important exception to these biochemical rules is *S. typhi*, which produces little or no hydrogen sulfide, does not form gas in glucose media, and does not decarboxylate ornithine. Lactose-fermenting strains of *S. typhi* have also been reported rarely.

Salmonella serotypes are traditionally classified on the basis of two surface antigens, somatic O antigens and flagellar H antigens (Fig. 196.1), which represent specific structures on the bacterial surface that vary in their protein or chemical composition among various serotypes. Lipopolysaccharide, a major component of the cell wall of gram-negative bacteria, consists of a long chain of sugar units that are called O antigens, covalently linked to a basal core polysaccharide, which in turn is covalently linked to an outer membrane–anchored lipid moiety designated lipid A. The core polysaccharide is structurally similar among all salmonellae. The O antigens are linear polymers of repeating oligosaccharide units that vary biochemically and structurally among salmonellae; the structural differences among the oligosaccharides of different *Salmonella* serotypes form the primary basis of serotype classification. H antigens are the proteins that constitute the bacterial flagellar filaments. These also vary structurally among *Salmonella* serotypes and form the secondary basis of serotype classification. In a process that is known as phase variation, an individual bacterium can switch back and forth between two different flagellar filament proteins. As a result, a *Salmonella* isolate may carry two types of H antigen, referred to as phase 1 and phase 2 antigens.

The traditional Kauffmann-White classification system of salmonellae is based on O and H antigens (Table 196.2). Nine serogroups (A through I) are defined by O antigens. All members of a serogroup carry the same major O antigen, but individual members of a serogroup may carry different minor O antigens. Serotypes within the serogroups are defined by H antigens. Ninety percent of human isolates are from serogroups A through E, which collectively contain fewer than 40 serotypes.

Certain serotypes are linked with particular clinical syndromes. For example, within serogroup D, *S. typhi* isolates commonly cause enteric fever, *S. enteritidis* isolates result in gastroenteritides, and *S. dublin* isolates often result in bacteremias (2). In addition to being useful for the prediction of the clinical course, the serotyping of clinical isolates is important in the characterization and control of epidemics.

Only a few highly specialized laboratories maintain collections of specific antisera that are adequate to type strains precisely. Most clinical laboratories group their *Salmonella* isolates both by agglutination reactions using group-specific antisera and by biochemical tests. In the United States, all *Salmonella* isolates confirmed by appropriate biochemical tests should be forwarded to reference laboratories in state health departments for more exhaustive serotyping as part of the national *Salmonella* surveillance system (3).

The Widal agglutination test for the detection of serum antibodies against the O and H antigens is in common use but lacks adequate sensitivity and specificity in most clinical settings. For a nonimmune person, a positive test is one in which either the anti-O antibody rises fourfold or a titer of greater than 1:50 or 1:100 is present in a single sample drawn during the initial 2 to 3 weeks of disease (4). Because the antibody response to gastroenteritis and to the chronic carrier state is minimal, the test is potentially useful only in typhoid fever and some chronic infections, such as osteomyelitis. Nevertheless, not all cases of typhoid fever, treated or untreated, produce diagnostic titers. Moreover, the specificity of the test is low, because both anti-O and anti-H antibodies are acute-phase reactants, often increasing in response to nonspecific inflammatory processes. After immunization, the anti-O antibody titer may remain elevated for months, and that of anti-H antibody for years, making interpretation of the test difficult. Finally, some cross-reactivity occurs with non-typhi salmonellae (5).

A third type of antigen, the virulence or Vi antigen, is present on *S. typhi* and occasionally on *S. paratyphi* C. The Vi antigen is a capsular polysaccharide (a polymer of *N*-acetylgalactosaminic acid, Fig. 196.1) that appears to protect the organisms from the

TABLE 196.1.   Useful Biochemical Reactions for Distinguishing *Salmonella* from Other Enterobacteriaceae and *Aeromonas* and *Vibrio* Organisms

REACTION	ESCHERICHIA SPP.	SHIGELLA SPP.	EDWARDSIELLA SPP.	SALMONELLA SPP.	ARIZONA SPP.	CITROBACTER FREUNDII	CITROBACTER DIVERSUS	KLEBSIELLA PNEUMONIAE	ENTEROBACTER CLOACAE	ENTEROBACTER AEROGENES	ENTEROBACTER HAFNIAE	ENTEROBACTER AGGLOMERANS
Hydrogen sulfide	−	−	+	+	+	+/−	−	−	−	−	−	−
Urease	−	−	−	−	−	a	a	−	−	−	−	−
Motility	+/−	−	+	+	+	+	+	+	+/−	−	−	a
Lysine decarboxylase	a	−	+	+	+	−	−	+	+	+	+	+/−
Ornithine decarboxylase	a	a	+	+	+	a	+	−	+	+	+	−
Gas production from glucose	+	−	+	+	+	a	+	−	+	+	+	−/+
Lactose	+	−	−	−	a	c	a	+	c	+	a	a
Sucrose	a	−	−	−	−	a	−/+	+	+	+	a	a

+, 90% or more are positive in 1 to 2 days; −, 90% or more are negative; +/−, majority are positive; −/+, majority are negative; a, different biochemical types are found; b, positive between 22° and 37°C; c, positive or delayed positive; d, positive reaction delayed.
Modified from Holt JG, Krieg NR, Sneath PHA, et al. *Bergey's manual of determinative bacteriology,* 9th ed. Baltimore: Williams & Wilkins, 1994:203–222, with permission.

actions of complement and can be detected during serotyping (Table 196.2).

In the epidemiologic characterization of outbreaks, the definition of *Salmonella* strains or subtypes within a single serotype is informative and aides in outbreak management. Several techniques are useful in this process, including phage typing, plasmid profile analysis, restriction endonuclease digestion of chromosomal DNA, and nucleic acid hybridization (6,7).

MOLECULAR PATHOGENESIS OF *SALMONELLA* INFECTION

Disease caused by *Salmonella* serotypes can be loosely divided into two categories: gastroenteritis and enteric (typhoid) fever. *Salmonella* serotypes in both categories gain access to the host via the digestive tract. Gastric acid is an important barrier to infection; treatments that reduce gastric acid lead to a decrease in the infectious dose of *Salmonella* (8,9). On the other hand, upon exposure to low pH, *Salmonella* demonstrates an adaptive response that leads to enhancement of its survival in low-pH environments (10). After passage into the small intestine, *Salmonella* crosses the mucus layer and adheres to intestinal epithelial cells via several surface adhesive structures called fimbriae (11).

Salmonella Entry into Mammalian Cells

Salmonella has the remarkable capacity to induce uptake or entry into mammalian cells, which leads to its placement in a cellular vacuole or phagosome. Entry into mammalian cells presumably aids in *Salmonella*'s avoidance of the host humoral immune response, permits bacterial access to deeper tissues, and places the bacterium in an intracellular niche in which it is equipped to survive. The molecular mechanism of induced uptake will be described in detail below. *Salmonella* serotypes that cause gastroenteritis are likely limited to those that adhere to and enter into cells of the intestinal mucosa, whereas *Salmonella* serotypes that cause enteric fever infect and induce hypertrophy of the reticuloendothelial system, including intestinal Peyer's patches, mesenteric lymph nodes, the liver, the spleen, and the bone marrow. Evidence suggests that enteric fever–causing *Salmonella* serotypes gain access to these sites by traversing the intestinal mucosa and invading and surviving within macrophages (12).

The intestinal mucosa is lined with enterocytes and patches of microfold (M) cells. Data from murine models suggest that *Salmonella* preferentially adheres to and is taken up by M cells (13), although some is taken up into enterocytes as well. Enteric fever–causing *Salmonella* serotypes are able to traverse the intestinal mucosa by transcytosis (i.e., by transport within a vacuolar compartment from the apical to the basal side of a mucosal cell). After traversing the intestinal mucosa, these salmonellae enter into macrophages present in the intestinal submucosa and are transported within migrating macrophages throughout the reticuloendothelial system. Organisms may also be phagocytosed in the intestinal lumen by migrating CD18-positive phagocytes and then be transported across the intestinal mucosa and enter the

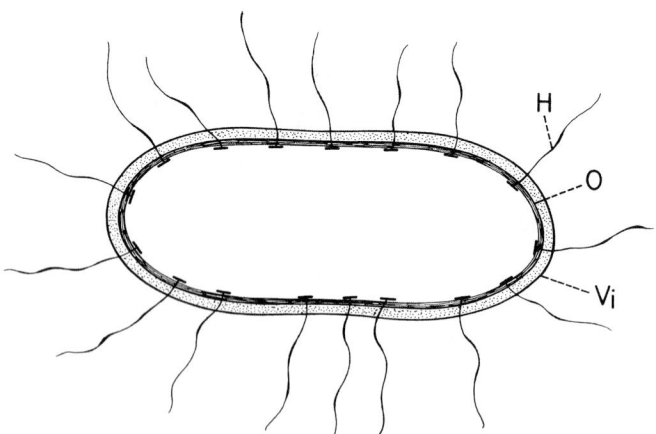

Figure 196.1. Schematic representation of the *Salmonella* bacterium. Surface antigens are indicated as follows: *O*, somatic O-specific chains; *H*, flagellar H antigens; *Vi*, virulence antigen.

TABLE 196.1. (*continued*)

SERRATIA MARCESCENS	SERRATIA LIQUEFACIENS	SERRATIA RUBIDAEA	PROTEUS VULGARIS	PROTEUS MIRABILIS	PROTEUS MORGANII	PROTEUS RETTGERI	PROVIDENCIA ALCALIFACIENS	PROVIDENCIA STUARTII	YERSINIA ENTEROCOLITICA	YERSINIA PSEUDOTUBERCULOSIS	YERSINIA PESTIS	AEROMONAS HYDROPHILA	VIBRIO CHOLERAE
−	−	−	+	+							−	−	−
a	a	a	+	+	+	+	−	−	+	+	−/a	−	−
+	+	+/−	+	+	+/−	+	+	+	b	b	b	+	+
+	c	c	−	−	−	+	−	+	−	−	−	−	++
+	+	−	−	+	+	−	−	−	+	−	−	−	++
+/−	+/−	a	+/−	+	+/−	−/+	+/−	−	−	−	−	+/−	−
−	a	+	−	−	−	−	−	−	−	−	−	−/+	d
+	+	+	+	a	−	a	a	c	+	−	−	+	+

systemic lymphatics within these phagocytes (14). As will be described below, *Salmonella* have evolved mechanisms for prolonged survival within macrophages.

Salmonella induction of its own uptake into mammalian host cells involves a highly coordinated series of molecular interactions between proteins released by *Salmonella* and proteins of the host cell. Upon contact with mammalian cells, secreted *Salmonella* proteins induce a dramatic reorganization of the mammalian cell cytoskeleton (15). As a result, the cell forms large "ruffles" with its plasma membrane that engulf the bacterium (Fig. 196.2), leading to its uptake into a cellular vacuole or phagosome. Rapidly thereafter, the cellular cytoskeleton returns to its normal architecture, despite the presence of intracellular

Salmonella (16). The net effect of this *Salmonella*-induced process is the entry of the bacterium into the mammalian host cell with relatively minor permanent alteration of the host cell cytoskeleton (17).

The highly specialized mechanism by which *Salmonella* delivers the proteins that induce these cytoskeletal changes is known as type III secretion (18–20). The genes that encode the type III secretion machinery that is involved in membrane ruffle formation are encoded in a region of the genome called *Salmonella* pathogenicity island 1 (21). The bacterial organelle that mediates delivery of these proteins looks remarkably like a needle and syringe (22,23) (Fig. 196.3). The base of the organelle, which is shaped like a syringe, spans the two bacterial membranes.

TABLE 196.2. Kauffmann-White Classification of Common *Salmonella* Serotypes

Serotype	Group	O antigens	H antigens Phase 1	H antigens Phase 2
S. paratyphi A	A	1,2,12	a	(1),(5)
S. paratyphi B[a]	B	1,4,(5),12	b	1,2
S. typhimurium	B	1,4,(5),12	i	1,2
S. heidelberg	B	1,4,(5),12	r	1,2
S. canada	B	4,12	b	1,6
S. saintpaul	B	1,4,(5),12	e,h	1,2
S. paratyphi C[b]	C1	6,7,(Vi)	a	1,5
S. bareilly	C1	6,7	y	1,5
S. choleraesuis	C1	6,7	(c)	1,5
S. montevideo	C1	6,7	g,m,(p),s	(1),(2),(7)
S. oranienburg	C1	6,7	m,t	—
S. newport	C2	6,8	e,h	1,2
S. typhi	D1	9,12,(Vi)	d	—
S. enteritidis	D1	1,9,12	g,m	(1),(7)
S. gallinarum-pullorum	D1	1,9,12	—	—
S. anatum	E1	3,10	e,h	1,6
S. vancouver	1	16	c	1,5

Parentheses indicate that the antigenic determinant may be absent or difficult to detect.
[a]Also designated *S. schottmülleri.*
[b]Also designated *S. hirschfeldii.*
Adapted from Le Minor L. Genus III. *Salmonella* lignières 1900, 389. In: Krieg NR, Holt JG, eds. *Bergey's manual of systematic bacteriology,* Vol 1. Baltimore: Williams & Wilkins, 1984:427–458, with permission.

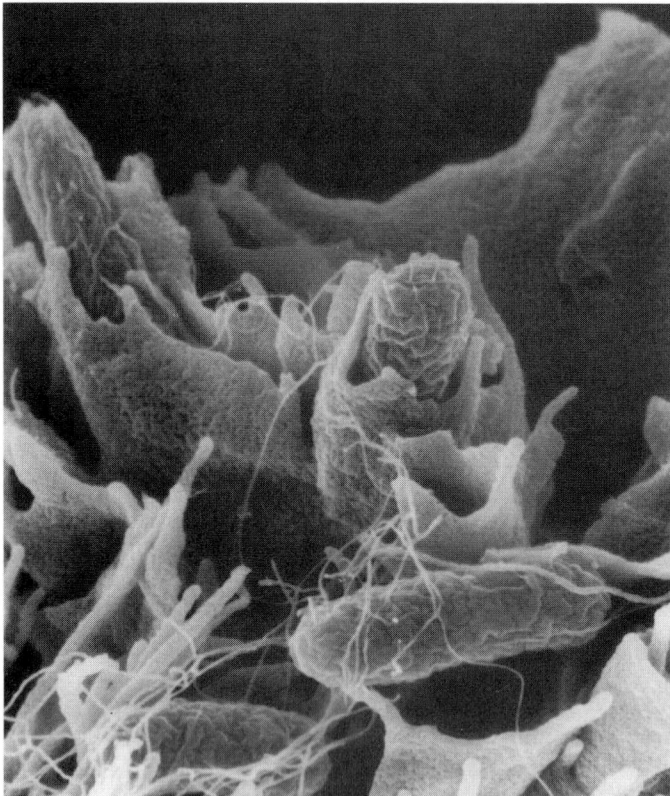

Figure 196.2. *Salmonella* entering into a mammalian cell. Scanning electron micrograph of bacteria being engulfed by cellular membranes during *Salmonella*-induced uptake (118).

Attached to it and protruding from the bacterial surface is a long needle-like structure. The bacterial proteins that mediate mammalian cytoskeletal changes (the type III "effector" proteins) are secreted from the bacterial cytoplasm through the syringe and needle (Fig. 196.3B). Among the secreted effectors are proteins that are thought to form a pore in the cellular plasma membrane, through which additional effector proteins appear to be translocated from the tip of the needle across the plasma membrane and into the host cell cytosol. The timing of secretion of all the effector proteins is precisely regulated, such that full activation of their release occurs in an orderly temporally-regulated fashion following bacterial contact with mammalian cells (22,24). *Salmonella* encodes a second type III secretion system (described

below), and type III secretion systems are present and function similarly in several other gram negative pathogens as well, including *Shigella*, *Yersinia*, and pathogenic *E. coli*.

In the initial step of *Salmonella* entry, *Salmonella* effector proteins activate mammalian signal transduction pathways that regulate the actin cytoskeleton. Two Rho-family guanosine triphosphatases (GTPases), Cdc42 and Rac1, are activated at the mammalian cell membrane in proximity to the site of bacterial contact (25). Rho-family GTPases are active when bound to GTP and inactive when bound to guanosine diphosphate. Activated (GTP-bound) Cdc42 and Rac1 activate downstream effector molecules. The activation of these pathways causes rearrangements in the actin cytoskeleton that lead to membrane ruffle formation at the site of bacterial contact. Each of three *Salmonella* proteins, SopE, SopE2, and SopB, is able to induce these changes in the host cell actin cytoskeleton (26–29); this functional redundancy suggests the evolutionary importance of this process for *Salmonella* pathogenesis. Additional *Salmonella* effector proteins contribute to the cytoskeletal rearrangements by binding cellular actin and modulating actin dynamics (30–33).

The actin cytoskeletal rearrangements induced by *Salmonella* are reversible, and reversal of these rearrangements is directly aided by *Salmonella* effector proteins. The *Salmonella* protein SptP catalyzes the conversion of Cdc42 and Rac1 to their inactive states by enhancing their intrinsic nucleotide hydrolyzing activities (16). SptP also possesses tyrosine phosphatase activity, which appears to contribute to the reversal process (28a,34). Other *Salmonella* effectors secreted by *Salmonella* pathogenicity island 1 induce proinflammatory cytokine production, stimulate the migration of polymorphonuclear leukocytes into the intestinal lumen, and modulate chloride secretion (25,26,35–45). The outcome of effector protein interaction with host cells is *Salmonella* entry into host cells, diarrhea, and an intense inflammatory response.

Salmonella Survival Within Macrophages

To survive within macrophages, *Salmonella* must resist several macrophage microbicidal mechanisms. Most important in macrophage killing of *Salmonella* are the phagocyte NADPH oxidase (*phox*) and inducible nitric oxide synthase (*iNOS*) systems (46). The *phox* system produces superoxide, hydrogen peroxide, and peroxynitrite (47), and the *iNOS* system produces nitric oxide (48). Each of these reactive oxygen and nitrogen compounds is toxic to microbes. The importance of the NADPH oxidase system is demonstrated by the observation that *Salmonella* is the second most common infection in chronic granulomatous

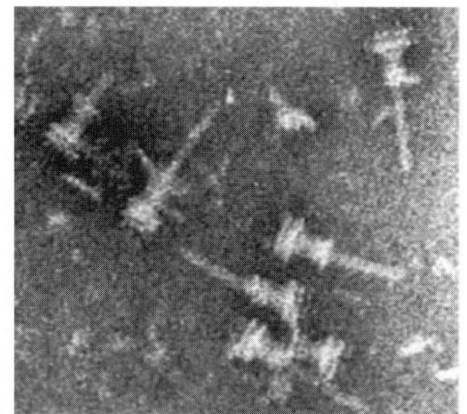

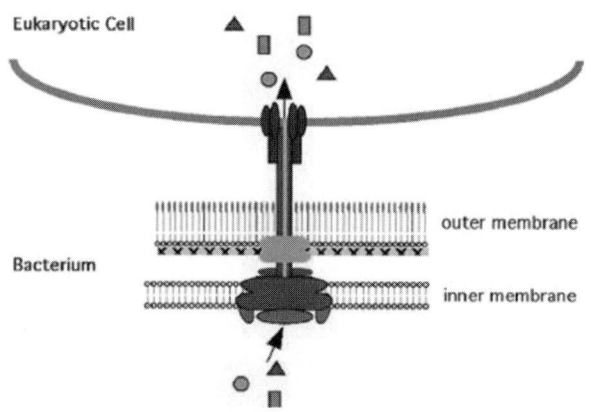

Figure 196.3. Type III secretion apparatus of *Salmonella*. **A:** Electron micrograph of isolated type III secretion organelle, demonstrating its resemblance to a syringe and needle. **B:** Model of the orientation of the type III secretion organelle in the bacterial cell wall, extending through the mammalian cell membrane, thereby allowing secretion of bacterial effector proteins directly into the mammalian cytoplasm (118).

disease (49), a syndrome in which the phagocyte oxidase system is defective due to either a recessive X-linked *gp91-* or autosomal *p22-, p47-,* or *p67-phox* mutation. Mutations in the *iNOS* system have not been described in humans.

Killing by the *phox* system appears to be most important in the first several hours after *Salmonella* uptake into macrophages, whereas killing by the *iNOS* system appears to be most important several days later. Mice that carry a mutation in the *phox* system are extraordinarily susceptible to systemic *Salmonella* infection, dying early in the course of disease (50–52). Mice that carry a mutation in *iNOS* are also markedly susceptible to *Salmonella* infection, but these mice are able to control the infection during the first several days, developing progressive infection only in the second and third weeks (50,51).

Salmonella serotypes that cause enteric fever must be able to survive within macrophages (53). To do so, the bacteria must both acquire nutrients in the nutrient-poor environment of the phagosome and resist the reactive oxygen and nitrogen compounds produced by the macrophage. *Salmonella* has evolved several mechanisms for each. *Salmonella* produces antagonists to both reactive oxygen and reactive nitrogen compounds (54,55). *Salmonella* senses the phagosome environment and, in response, induces the expression of virulence factors that enhance its survival in that environment. Included among these factors is the response regulator PhoP/PhoQ (56), which regulates the expression of over 40 genes, including some that lead to alterations in the *Salmonella* cell wall that make it more resistant to host antimicrobial peptides (57). Also included among the virulence factors that are induced in the phagosome is a second type III secretion system, called *Salmonella* pathogenicity island 2, that translocates bacterial effector proteins from the phagosome into the macrophage cytosol. Some of the bacterial effectors secreted by this type III secretion system exclude a component of the NADPH oxidase from *Salmonella*-containing phagosomes, thereby protecting the bacteria from its toxic effects (58,59). The precise role of others of these bacterial effector proteins remains uncertain, but it appears that some interfere with the normal maturation of the phagosome (60). It is interesting to speculate whether others of these effectors will be involved in the acquisition of essential nutrients from the cytosol or in modifying macrophage gene expression.

Immune Response to *Salmonella*

The host immune response to *Salmonella* infection is largely specific to the serotype that causes the infection (61–70). *Salmonella* serotypes are determined by the O antigen of the lipopolysaccharide in the bacterial cell wall. The O antigen is a carbohydrate constituent, and the immune response induced by this, and by most other carbohydrate constituents, is a humoral or antibody response. Thus, following human infection with *Salmonella*, significant elevations occur in antilipopolysaccharide and anti-O antigen antibody titers. Elevation of these titers is correlated with protection against subsequent infection of the same serotype, but such protection is at best only partial.

S. typhi infection can result in protective immunity against subsequent infection with *S. typhi* (71). Evidence suggests that this protective immunity is dependent on both humoral and cellular immune responses (71,72). Recurrence of enteric fever is unusual; it has been reported only in the setting of prior immunization or antibiotic administration shortly after the onset of clinical illness, either of which may attenuate the natural immune response (73).

VACCINES

An ideal *Salmonella* vaccine should fulfill five criteria. First, the vaccine should induce lasting and protective immune responses both locally, that is, in the intestinal tract, and systemically. Vaccines prepared from live attenuated strains are more apt to meet this requirement than are vaccines prepared from killed or inactivated organisms, as has been demonstrated in a comparison of immune responses to various oral formulations of the *S. typhi* Ty21a vaccine (74). Second, an ideal vaccine should induce protective immunity with only a single dose. Third, the vaccine should be administered orally. Fourth, vaccine preparations should be stable under field conditions; for example, they should not require refrigeration. Finally, an ideal vaccine strain should have an extremely low rate of reversion to a virulent strain.

To date, the *Salmonella* vaccines that have been developed provide protection against single serotypes only. Two vaccines for *S. typhi* are currently approved for use in the United States (Table 196.3). A third vaccine, the heat-phenol-killed parenteral vaccine (75–77), has recently been discontinued for use by the general public in the United States. An acetone-inactivated derivative continues to be available to the military (78).

The first *S. typhi* vaccine available in the United States is a live attenuated form of strain Ty21a. The primary immunization series consists of ingestion of an enteric-coated capsule containing 2 to 6×10^9 viable and 5 to 50×10^9 nonviable *S. typhi* Ty21a organisms every other day for a total of four doses. Multiple field trials conducted using various preparations and dosing schemes have yielded a wide range of levels of protection. Field trials conducted among schoolchildren in Chile that involved administration of an enteric-coated capsule in three doses during a 1-week period demonstrated 66% protection during a 5-year period (79), but only 33% protection during a 3-year period (80). In a follow-up trial, also in Chile, designed to test the protective effect of one or two doses of the enteric-coated formulation among school-aged children, efficacies of 29% and 59% were obtained in the first 2 years after vaccination with one or two doses, respectively; ominously, no protective efficacy was demonstrable with either dosing regimen 3 to 5 years after vaccination (81). An earlier clinical trial conducted in Egypt among children who received a liquid formulation of the oral Ty21a vaccine reported an efficacy of 96% during a 3-year period (82). Direct comparison of the oral formulations in two trials demonstrated higher efficacy for the liquid versus the enteric-coated preparation: 77% versus 33% efficacy during a 3-year period for the Chilean study and

TABLE 196.3. Currently Available *Salmonella typhi* Vaccines

Vaccine	Efficacy	Administration	Adverse reactions
Live attenuated, oral Ty21a	29%–96% for 2 yr or longer (79–83)	Four doses of capsule	None
Vi capsular polysaccharide, parenteral[a]	65%–75% for 17 mo or longer (86, 87)	One 0.5-mL intramuscular dose; booster every 2 yr	Fever, headache, and erythema or induration at injection site (87–89)

[a]Not approved for children younger than 2 yr.

53% versus 42% efficacy for an Indonesian study, respectively (80,83). Long-term follow-up of the Chilean study revealed continued protection for up to 7 years (84). This vaccine is unable to elicit immune responses in infants (85) and in the United States is not recommended for children under 6 years of age. In addition, the vaccine is contraindicated in immunocompromised persons or those receiving antimicrobial agents (78). This vaccine produces no significant adverse reactions. If exposure continues, booster doses may be required every 5 years.

The second typhoid vaccine available in the United States is a parenteral vaccine that consists of the Vi capsular polysaccharide of *S. typhi*. The vaccine is administered in the primary series as a single intramuscular injection of 25 μg of antigen in 0.5 mL. The efficacy of this antigen has been evaluated in two field trials: one large clinical trial in Nepal demonstrated 75% protection for 17 months or longer (86), and a trial in South Africa reported 65% protection during a 2-year period (87). The Vi capsular polysaccharide vaccine is not approved for children under 2 years of age. Adverse reactions included fever, headache, and erythema or induration at the site of injection (87–89). Advantages of this vaccine include the single-dose administration schedule and stability at ambient temperature, precluding the need for refrigeration.

In the United States, vaccination is recommended for travel to regions where there is a recognized risk of exposure to *S. typhi*, especially to developing countries in Latin America, Asia, and Africa. The recommendations apply to persons who expect to be exposed to potentially contaminated food or water for prolonged periods. For less prolonged or less significant exposure, as might apply to tourists lodging in international hotels in these countries, many physicians advocate dietary precautions rather than vaccination. Vaccination is also recommended for persons with intimate exposure to documented carriers of *S. typhi* and for laboratory personnel who work with virulent strains of *S. typhi* (78).

Newer and potentially more effective vaccines for *S. typhi* are on the horizon. One promising vaccine is a conjugate polysaccharide vaccine that consists of Vi antigen covalently linked to a nontoxic recombinant protein derivative of *Pseudomonas aeruginosa* exotoxin A (Vi-rEPA) (90). Preliminary trials revealed increased immunogenicity as compared with the traditional Vi-conjugate vaccine (91). A double-blind randomized trial among 5,525 two-to five-year-olds in Vietnam revealed that two doses of Vi-rEPA administered 6 weeks apart yielded an efficacy of 91.5% when compared with placebo, the highest reported efficacy of any vaccine against *S. typhi*. Among children in the vaccine group, levels of immunoglobulin G antibodies to Vi increased by a factor of more than 575. Adverse reactions largely consisted of local reactions and fever following administration of vaccine (92). As of this writing, the Vi-rEPA vaccine is not yet licensed for use in the United States.

Several *Salmonella* strains containing genetically defined mutations are currently under study. These include strains that are auxotrophic for chorismic acid biosynthesis (the *aro* mutants) (93–99), which have deletions in genes encoding adenylate cyclase (*cya*) or cyclic 3′,5′-adenosine monophosphate receptor protein (*crp*) (100), which carry mutations in the regulatory locus involved in the protection of *Salmonella* from microbicidal host proteins (56), and which harbor mutations in the gene encoding the regulatory histidine kinase inner membrane protein, *ompR* (101). More recent candidates for potential vaccine strains include *hemA* (deficient in functional transfer RNA reductase), *htrA* (deficient in a serine protease that degrades aberrant periplasmic proteins), *guaBA* (deletion of an operon critical for guanine nucleotide synthesis) (102–104), and the double auxotroph *his pur* strains 1771 and 3334 (105). Modifying certain bacterial virulence genes in *Salmonella* results in alteration of murine immune responses; a *phoP* mutant promoted potent and protective innate immune responses, while an *aro* mutant elicited strong and spe-

cific antibody and T-helper cell responses (106). All of these mutants are attenuated, yet highly immunogenic in murine models, and several show promise or are under study in human volunteers (107–111).

Live attenuated strains of *Salmonella* have the exciting ability to serve as carriers of heterologous antigens of other human pathogens (112). Genes encoding such antigens can be introduced into the vaccine strain (113). Hosts challenged with these recombinant strains can be expected to manifest an immune response to both the foreign antigen and antigens of the vaccine strain. Several experimental difficulties must be overcome before widespread use of such antigen delivery systems is feasible. Specifically, the foreign antigens must be expressed at levels that simultaneously have negligible effects on carrier strain physiology but are sufficient to elicit the desired immune response. In addition, if the heterologous gene is carried on a plasmid, to be maintained in the bacterial population, this plasmid must segregate equally among progeny bacteria during division. In routine molecular biology work, plasmids are most commonly maintained among progeny by placement of antibiotic resistance–encoding genes onto the plasmid and propagation of the plasmid-carrying strains in the presence of the antibiotic in question, thereby allowing survival only of organisms that maintain the plasmid. As the use of antibiotic resistance genes is obviously precluded in candidate vaccine strains, investigators have either placed foreign genes on plasmids that complement auxotrophic mutations in recipient strains, and hence must be carried by the bacteria to allow their survival in the host, or have stably integrated the heterologous genes into the chromosome of the carrier strain.

Of particular interest is the use of attenuated *Salmonella* to deliver antigens of human immunodeficiency virus type 1 (HIV-1) to the human immune system (114). Studies in murine models have demonstrated that such vectors successfully induce both mucosal and systemic cytotoxic T-lymphocyte–mediated immunity against HIV-1 antigens (115–117). Although still in the early stages of development, this vaccine approach shows scientific promise. In addition, these vaccines are of relatively low cost, are administered orally, and are stable under field conditions.

REFERENCES

1. Goldberg MB, Rubin RH. The spectrum of *Salmonella* infection. *Infect Dis Clin North Am* 1988;2:571.
2. Rubin RH, Weinstein L. *Salmonellosis: microbiologic, pathologic and clinical features.* New York: Stratton Intercontinental, 1977.
3. Farmer JJ, Kelly MT. Enterobacteriaceae. In: *Manual of clinical microbiology.* Washington, DC: American Society for Microbiology, 1991:371.
4. Schroeder SA. Interpretation of serologic tests for typhoid fever. *JAMA* 1968;206:839.
5. Reynolds DW, Carpenter RL, Simon WH. Diagnostic specificity of Widal's reaction for typhoid fever. *JAMA* 1970;214:2192.
6. O'Brien TF, Hopkins JD, Gilleece ES, et al. Molecular epidemiology of antibiotic resistance in *Salmonella* from animals and human beings in the United States. *N Engl J Med* 1982;307:1.
7. Bender JB, Hedberg CW, Boxrud DJ, et al. Use of molecular subtyping in surveillance for *Salmonella enterica* serotype typhimurium. *N Engl J Med* 2001;344:189.
8. Giannella RA, Broitman SA, Zamcheck N. Gastric acid barrier to ingested microorganisms in man: studies *in vivo* and *in vitro*. *Gut* 1972;13:251.
9. Takeuchi A. Electron microscopic studies of experimental *Salmonella* infection. 1. Penetration into the intestinal epithelium by *Salmonella typhimurium*. *Am J Pathol* 1967;50:109.
10. Garcia del Portillo F, Foster JW, Finlay BB. Role of acid tolerance response genes in *Salmonella typhimurium* virulence. *Infect Immun* 1993;61:4489.
11. Baumler AJ, Tsolis RM, Heffron F. Contribution of fimbrial operons to attachment to and invasion of epithelial cell lines by *Salmonella typhimurium*. *Infect Immun* 1996;64:1862.
12. Alpuche-Aranda CM, Racoosin EL, Swanson JA, et al. Salmonellae stimulate macrophage macropinocytosis and persist within spacious phagosomes. *J Exp Med* 1994;179:601.
13. Jones BD, Ghori N, Falkow S. *Salmonella typhimurium* initiates murine infection

by penetrating and destroying the specialized epithelial M cells of the Peyer's patches. *J Exp Med* 1994;180:15.

14. Vazquez-Torres A, Jones-Carson J, Baumler AJ, et al. Extraintestinal dissemination of *Salmonella* by CD18-expressing phagocytes. *Nature* 1999;401:804.

15. Francis CL, Ryan TA, Jones BD, et al. Ruffles induced by *Salmonella* and other stimuli direct macropinocytosis of bacteria. *Nature* 1993;364:639.

16. Fu Y, Galan JE. A salmonella protein antagonizes Rac-1 and Cdc42 to mediate host-cell recovery after bacterial invasion. *Nature* 1999;401:293.

17. Galan JE. Molecular and cellular bases of *Salmonella* entry into host cells. *Curr Top Microbiol Immunol* 1996;209:43.

18. Cornelis GR, Van Gijsegem F. Assembly and function of type III secretory systems. *Annu Rev Microbiol* 2000;54:735.

19. Galan JE, Collmer A. Type III secretion machines: bacterial devices for protein delivery into host cells. *Science* 1999;284:1322.

20. Hueck CJ. Type III protein secretion systems in bacterial pathogens of animals and plants. *Microbiol Mol Biol Rev* 1998;62:379.

21. Galan JE. Interaction of *Salmonella* with host cells through the centisome 63 type III secretion system. *Curr Opin Microbiol* 1999;2:46.

22. Kubori T, Sukhan A, Aizawa SI, et al. Molecular characterization and assembly of the needle complex of the *Salmonella typhimurium* type III protein secretion system. *Proc Natl Acad Sci USA* 2000;97:10225.

23. Kubori T, Matsushima Y, Nakamura D, et al. Supramolecular structure of the *Salmonella typhimurium* type III protein secretion system. *Science* 1998;280:602.

24. Lucas RL, Lee CA. Unravelling the mysteries of virulence gene regulation in *Salmonella typhimurium*. *Mol Microbiol* 2000;36:1024.

25. Chen LM, Hobbie S, Galan JE. Requirement of CDC42 for *Salmonella*-induced cytoskeletal and nuclear responses. *Science* 1996;274:2115.

26. Zhou D, Chen LM, Hernandez L, et al. A *Salmonella* inositol polyphosphatase acts in conjunction with other bacterial effectors to promote host cell actin cytoskeleton rearrangements and bacterial internalization. *Mol Microbiol* 2001;39:248.

27. Hardt WD, Chen LM, Schuebel KE, et al. *S. typhimurium* encodes an activator of Rho GTPases that induces membrane ruffling and nuclear responses in host cells. *Cell* 1998;93:815.

28. Bakshi CS, Singh VP, Wood MW, et al. Identification of SopE2, a *Salmonella* secreted protein which is highly homologous to SopE and involved in bacterial invasion of epithelial cells. *J Bacteriol* 2000;182:2341.

28a. Murli S, Watson RO, Galan JE. Role of tyrosine kinases and the tyrosine phosphatase SptP in the interaction of Salmonella with host cells. *Cell Microbiol* 2001;3:795.

29. Stender S, Friebel A, Linder S, et al. Identification of SopE2 from *Salmonella typhimurium*, a conserved guanine nucleotide exchange factor for Cdc42 of the host cell. *Mol Microbiol* 2000;36:1206.

30. Zhou D, Mooseker MS, Galan JE. An invasion-associated *Salmonella* protein modulates the actin-bundling activity of plastin. *Proc Natl Acad Sci USA* 1999;96:10176.

31. Zhou D, Mooseker MS, Galan JE. Role of the *S. typhimurium* actin-binding protein SipA in bacterial internalization. *Science* 1999;283:2092.

32. Mitra K, Zhou D, Galan JE. Biophysical characterization of SipA, an actin-binding protein from *Salmonella enterica*. *FEBS Lett* 2000;482:81.

33. Hayward RD, Koronakis V. Direct nucleation and bundling of actin by the SipC protein of invasive *Salmonella*. *EMBO J* 1999;18:4926.

34. Kaniga K, Uralil J, Bliska JB, et al. A secreted protein tyrosine phosphatase with modular effector domains in the bacterial pathogen *Salmonella typhimurium*. *Mol Microbiol* 1996;21:633.

35. Arnold JW, Niesel DW, Annable CR, et al. Tumor necrosis factor-alpha mediates the early pathology in *Salmonella* infection of the gastrointestinal tract. *Microb Pathog* 1993;14:217.

36. Eckmann L, Kagnoff MF, Fierer J. Epithelial cells secrete the chemokine interleukin-8 in response to bacterial entry. *Infect Immun* 1993;61:4569.

37. Hess CB, Niesel DW, Klimpel GR. The induction of interferon production in fibroblasts by invasive bacteria: a comparison of *Salmonella* and *Shigella* species. *Microb Pathog* 1989;7:111.

38. Jung HC, Eckmann L, Yang SK, et al. A distinct array of proinflammatory cytokines is expressed in human colon epithelial cells in response to bacterial invasion. *J Clin Invest* 1995;95:55.

39. McCormick BA, Colgan SP, Delp-Archer C, et al. *Salmonella typhimurium* attachment to human intestinal epithelial monolayers: transcellular signalling to subepithelial neutrophils. *J Cell Biol* 1993;123:895.

40. Pace J, Hayman MJ, Galan JE. Signal transduction and invasion of epithelial cells by *S. typhimurium*. *Cell* 1993;72:505.

41. Hobbie S, Chen LM, Davis RJ, et al. Involvement of mitogen-activated protein kinase pathways in the nuclear responses and cytokine production induced by *Salmonella typhimurium* in cultured intestinal epithelial cells. *J Immunol* 1997;159:5550.

42. Lee CA, Silva M, Siber AM, et al. A secreted *Salmonella* protein induces a proinflammatory response in epithelial cells, which promotes neutrophil migration. *Proc Natl Acad Sci USA* 2000;97:12283.

43. Wood MW, Jones MA, Watson PR, et al. The secreted effector protein of *Salmonella dublin*, SopA, is translocated into eukaryotic cells and influences the induction of enteritis. *Cell Microbiol* 2000;2:293.

44. Eckmann L, Rudolf MT, Ptasznik A, et al. D-*myo*-inositol 1,4,5,6-tetrakisphosphate produced in human intestinal epithelial cells in response to *Salmonella* invasion inhibits phosphoinositide 3-kinase signaling pathways. *Proc Natl Acad Sci USA* 1997;94:14456.

45. Norris FA, Wilson MP, Wallis TS, et al. SopB, a protein required for virulence of *Salmonella dublin*, is an inositol phosphate phosphatase. *Proc Natl Acad Sci USA* 1998;95:14057.

46. Vazquez-Torres A, Fang F. Oxygen-dependent anti-*Salmonella* activity of macrophages. *Trends Microbiol* 2001;9:29.

47. Vazquez-Torres A, Jones-Carson J, Mastroeni P, et al. Antimicrobial actions of NADPH phagocyte oxidase and inducible nitric oxide synthase in experimental salmonellosis. I. Effects on microbial killing by activated peritoneal macrophages. *J Exp Med* 2000;192:227.

48. Nathan C, Xie QW. Nitric oxide synthases: roles, tolls and controls. *Cell* 1994;78:915.

49. Mouy R, Fischer A, Vilmer E, et al. Incidence, severity, and prevention of infections in chronic granulomatous disease. *J Pediatr* 1989;114:555.

50. Mastroeni P, Vazquez-Torres A, Fang F, et al. Antimicrobial action of the NADPH oxidase and inducible nitric oxide synthase in experimental salmonellosis. II. Effects on microbial proliferation and host survival *in vivo*. *J Exp Med* 2000;192:237.

51. Shiloh MU, MacMicking JD, Nicholson S, et al. Phenotype of mice and macrophages deficient in both phagocyte oxidase and inducible nitroc oxide synthase. *Immunity* 1999;10:29.

52. De Groote MA, Ochsner UA, Shiloh MU, et al. Periplasmic superoxide dismutase protects *Salmonella* from products of phagocyte NADPH-oxidase and nitric oxide synthase. *Proc Natl Acad Sci USA* 1997;94:13997.

53. Fields PI, Swanson JV, Haidaris CG, et al. Mutants of *Salmonella typhimurium* that cannot survive within the macrophage are avirulent. *Proc Natl Acad Sci USA* 1986;83:5189.

54. DeGroote MA, Testerman T, Xu Y, et al. Homocysteine antagonism of nitric oxide–related cytostasis in *Salmonella typhimurium*. *Science* 1996;272:414.

55. Fang FC, DeGroote MA, Foster JW, et al. Virulent *Salmonella typhimurium* has two periplasmic Cu, Zn-superoxide dismutases. *Proc Natl Acad Sci USA* 1999;96:7502.

56. Miller SI, Kukral AM, Mekalanos JJ. A two-component regulatory system (*phoP phoQ*) controls *Salmonella typhimurium* virulence. *Proc Natl Acad Sci USA* 1989;86:5054.

57. Guo L, Lim KB, Poduje CM, et al. Lipid A acylation and bacterial resistance against vertebrate antimicrobial peptides. *Cell* 1998;95:189.

58. Vazquez-Torres A, Xu Y, Jones-Carson J, et al. *Salmonella* pathogenicity island 2–dependent evasion of the phagocyte NADPH oxidase. *Science* 2000;287:1655.

59. Gallois A, Klein JR, Allen LA, et al. *Salmonella* pathogenicity island 2–encoded type III secretion system mediates exclusion of NADPH oxidase assembly from the phagosomal membrane. *J Immunol* 2001;166:5741.

60. Uchiya K, Barbieri MA, Funato K, et al. A *Salmonella* virulence protein that inhibits cellular trafficking. *EMBO J* 1999;18:3924.

61. Hsu HS. Pathogenesis and immunity in murine salmonellosis. *Microbiol Rev* 1989;53:390.

62. Ding HF, Nakoneczna I, Hsu HS. Protective immunity induced in mice by detoxified *Salmonella* lipopolysaccharide. *J Med Microbiol* 1990;31:95.

63. Hormaeche CE, Joysey HS, Desilva L, et al. Immunity conferred by Aro-*Salmonella* live vaccines. *Microb Pathog* 1991;10:149.

64. O'Callaghan D, Maskell D, Tite J, et al. Immune responses in BALB/c mice following immunization with aromatic compound or purine-dependent *Salmonella typhimurium* strains. *Immunology* 1990;69:184.

65. Mastroeni P, Villarreal-Ramos B, Hormaeche CE. Role of T cells, TNF alpha and IFN gamma in recall of immunity to oral challenge with virulent salmonellae in mice vaccinated with live attenuated aro-*Salmonella* vaccines. *Microb Pathog* 1992;13:477.

66. Mastroeni P, Villarreal-Ramos B, Hormaeche CE. Adoptive transfer of immunity to oral challenge with virulent salmonellae in innately susceptible BALB/c mice requires both immune serum and T cells. *Infect Immun* 1993;61:3981.

67. Villarreal B, Mastroeni P, de Hormaeche RD, et al. Proliferative and T-cell specific interleukin (IL-2/IL-4) production responses in spleen cells from mice vaccinated with aroA live attenuated *Salmonella* vaccines. *Microb Pathog* 1992;13:305.

68. Muotiala A, Makela PH. Role of gamma interferon in late stages of murine salmonellosis. *Infect Immun* 1993;61:4248.

69. Blanden RV, Mackaness GB, Collins FM. Mechanisms of acquired resistance in mouse typhoid. *J Exp Med* 1966;124:585.

70. Udhayakumar V, Muthukkaruppan VR. Protective immunity induced by outer membrane proteins of *Salmonella typhimurium* in mice. *Infect Immun* 1987;55:816.

71. Levine MM, Ferreccio C, Black RE, et al. Progress in vaccines against typhoid fever. *Rev Infect Dis* 1989;11(suppl 3):552.

72. Nencioni L, Villa L, De Magistris MT, et al. Cellular immunity against *Salmonella typhi* after live oral vaccine. *Adv Exp Med Biol* 1987;75:1669.

73. Marmion DE, Naylor GRE, Stewart IO. Second attacks of typhoid fever. *J Hygiene* 1953;51:260.

74. Kantele A, Arvilommi H, Kantele JM, et al. Comparison of the human immune response to live oral, killed oral or killed parenteral *Salmonella typhi* TY21A vaccines. *Microb Pathog* 1991;10:117.

75. Ashcroft MT, Singh B, Nicholson CC, et al. A seven-year field trial of two typhoid vaccines in Guyana. *Lancet* 1967;2:1056.

76. Hejfec LB, Salmin LV, Lejtman MZ, et al. A controlled field trial and laboratory study of five typhoid vaccines in the USSR. *Bull WHO* 1966;34:321.

77. Yugoslav TC. A controlled trial of the effectiveness of acetone-dried and inactivated and heat-phenol-inactivated typhoid vaccines in Yugoslavia. *Bull WHO* 1964;30:623.

78. Typhoid immunization: recommendations of the Advisory Committee on Immunization Practices (ACIP). *MMWR* 1994;43:1.

79. Levine MM, Ferreccio C, Black RE, et al. Large-scale field trial of Ty21a live oral typhoid vaccine in enteric-coated capsule formulation. *Lancet* 1987;1:1049.

80. Levine MM, Ferreccio C, Cryz S, et al. Comparison of enteric-coated capsules and liquid formulation of Ty21a typhoid vaccine in randomised controlled field trial. *Lancet* 1990;336:891.

81. Black RE, Levine MM, Ferreccio C, et al. Efficacy of one or two doses of Ty21a *Salmonella typhi* vaccine in enteric-coated capsules in a controlled field trial. Chilean Typhoid Committee. *Vaccine* 1990;8:81.

82. Wahdan MH, Serie C, Cerisier Y, et al. A controlled field trial of live *Salmonella typhi* strain Ty 21a oral vaccine against typhoid: three-year results. *J Infect Dis* 1982;145:292.

83. Simanjuntak CH, Paleologo FP, Punjabi NH, et al. Oral immunisation against typhoid fever in Indonesia with Ty21a vaccine. *Lancet* 1991;338:1055.

84. Levine MM, Ferreccio C, Abrego P, et al. Duration of efficacy of Ty21a, attenuated *Salmonella typhi* live oral vaccine. *Vaccine* 1999;17(suppl 2):22.

85. Murphy JR, Grez L, Schlesinger L, et al. Immunogenicity of *Salmonella typhi* Ty21a vaccine for young children. *Infect Immun* 1991;59:4291.

86. Acharya IL, Lowe CU, Thapa R, et al. Prevention of typhoid fever in Nepal with the Vi capsular polysaccharide of *Salmonella typhi*. A preliminary report. *N Engl J Med* 1987;317:1101.

87. Klugman KP, Gilbertson IT, Koornhof HJ, et al. Protective activity of Vi capsular polysaccharide vaccine against typhoid fever. *Lancet* 1987;2:1165.

88. Keitel WA, Bond NL, Zahradnik JM, et al. Clinical and serological responses following primary and booster immunization with *Salmonella typhi* Vi capsular polysaccharide vaccines. *Vaccine* 1994;12:195.

89. Cumberland NS, St Clair Roberts J, Arnold WS, et al. Typhoid Vi: a less reactogenic vaccine. *J Int Med Res* 1992;20:247.

90. Szu SC, Stone AL, Robbins JD, et al. Vi capsular polysaccharide-protein conjugates for prevention of typhoid fever. Preparation, characterization, and immunogenicity in laboratory animals. *J Exp Med* 1987;166:1510.

91. Kossaczka Z, Lin FY, Ho VA, et al. Safety and immunogenicity of Vi conjugate vaccines for typhoid fever in adults, teenagers, and 2- to 4-year-old children in Vietnam. *Infect Immun* 1999;67:5806.

92. Lin FY, Ho VA, Khiem HB, et al. The efficacy of a *Salmonella typhi* Vi conjugate vaccine in two-to-five-year-old children. *N Engl J Med* 2001;344:1263.

93. Hoiseth SK, Stocker BA. Aromatic-dependent *Salmonella typhimurium* are nonvirulent and effective as live vaccines. *Nature* 1981;291:238.

94. Dougan G, Maskell D, Pickard D, et al. Isolation of stable aroA mutants of *Salmonella typhi* Ty2: properties and preliminary characterisation in mice. *Mol Gen Genet* 1987;207:402.

95. Dougan G, Chatfield S, Pickard D, et al. Construction and characterization of vaccine strains of *Salmonella* harboring mutations in two different aro genes. *J Infect Dis* 1988;158:1329.

96. Miller IA, Chatfield S, Dougan G, et al. Bacteriophage P22 as a vehicle for transducing cosmid gene banks between smooth strains of *Salmonella typhimurium*: use in identifying a role for aroD in attenuating virulent *Salmonella* strains. *Mol Gen Genet* 1989;215:312.

97. Jones PW, Dougan G, Hayward C, et al. Oral vaccination of calves against experimental salmonellosis using a double aro mutant of *Salmonella typhimurium*. *Vaccine* 1991;9:29.

98. Chatfield SN, Fairweather N, Charles I, et al. Construction of a genetically defined *Salmonella typhi* Ty2 aroA, aroC mutant for the engineering of a candidate oral typhoid-tetanus vaccine. *Vaccine* 1992;10:53.

99. Hone DM, Harris AM, Chatfield S, et al. Construction of genetically defined double aro mutants of *Salmonella typhi*. *Vaccine* 1991;9:810.

100. Curtiss R 3rd, Kelly SM. *Salmonella typhimurium* deletion mutants lacking adenylate cyclase and cyclic AMP receptor protein are avirulent and immunogenic. *Infect Immun* 1987;55:3035.

101. Dorman CJ, Chatfield S, Higgins CF, et al. Characterization of porin and ompR mutants of a virulent strain of *Salmonella typhimurium*: ompR mutants are attenuated *in vivo*. *Infect Immun* 1989;57:2136.

102. Benjamin WH Jr, Hall P, Briles DE. A hemA mutation renders *Salmonella typhimurium* avirulent in mice, yet capable of eliciting protection against intravenous infection with *S. typhimurium*. *Microb Pathog* 1991;11:289.

103. Chatfield SN, Strahan K, Pickard D, et al. Evaluation of *Salmonella typhimurium* strains harbouring defined mutations in htrA and aroA in the murine salmonellosis model. *Microb Pathog* 1992;12:145.

104. Wang JY, Pasetti MF, Noriega FR, et al. Construction, genotypic and phenotypic characterization, and immunogenicity of attenuated DeltaguaBA *Salmonella enterica* serovar typhi strain CVD 915. *Infect Immun* 2001;69:4734.

105. Mitov I, Denchev V, Linde K. Humoral and cell-mediated immunity in mice after immunization with live oral vaccines of *Salmonella typhimurium*: auxotrophic mutants with two attenuating markers. *Vaccine* 1992;10:61.

106. VanCott JL, Chatfield SN, Roberts M, et al. Regulation of host immune responses by modification of *Salmonella* virulence genes. *Nat Med* 1998;4:1247.

107. Tacket CO, Hone DM, Losonsky GA, et al. Clinical acceptability and immunogenicity of CVD 908 *Salmonella typhi* vaccine strain. *Vaccine* 1992;10:443.

108. Sztein MB, Tanner MK, Polotsky Y, et al. Cytotoxic T lymphocytes after oral immunization with attenuated vaccine strains of *Salmonella typhi* in humans. *J Immunol* 1995;155:3987.

109. Hohmann EL, Oletta CA, Killeen KP, et al. phoP/phoQ-deleted *Salmonella typhi* (Ty800) is a safe and immunogenic single-dose typhoid fever vaccine in volunteers. *J Infect Dis* 1996;173:1408.

110. Tacket CO, Sztein MB, Losonsky GA, et al. Safety of live oral *Salmonella typhi* vaccine strains with deletions in htrA and aroC aroD and immune response in humans. *Infect Immun* 1997;65:452.

111. Eisenstein TK, Meissler JJ Jr, Miller SI, et al: Immunosuppression and nitric oxide production induced by parenteral live *Salmonella* vaccines do not correlate with protective capacity: a phoP:Tn10 mutant does not suppress but does protect. *Vaccine* 1998;16:24.

112. Chatfield SN, Strugnell RA, Dougan G. Live *Salmonella* as vaccines and carriers of foreign antigenic determinants. *Vaccine* 1989;7:495.

113. Darji A, Guzman CA, Gerstel B, et al. Oral somatic transgene vaccination using attenuated *S. typhimurium*. *Cell* 1997;91:765.

114. Fouts TR, Lewis GK, Hone DM. Construction and characterization of a *Salmonella typhi*–based human immunodeficiency virus type 1 vector vaccine. *Vaccine* 1995;13:561.

115. Berggren RE, Wunderlich A, Ziegler E, et al. HIV gp120-specific cell-mediated immune responses in mice after oral immunization with recombinant *Salmonella*. *J Acquir Immune Defic Syndr Hum Retrovirol* 1995;10:489.

116. Wu S, Pascual DW, Lewis GK, et al. Induction of mucosal and systemic responses against human immunodeficiency virus type 1 glycoprotein 120 in mice after oral immunization with a single dose of a *Salmonella*-HIV vector. *AIDS Res Hum Retrovir* 1997;13:1187.

117. Shata MT, Reitz MS Jr, DeVico AL, et al. Mucosal and systemic HIV-1 Env-specific CD8(+) T-cells develop after intragastric vaccination with a *Salmonella* Env DNA vaccine vector. *Vaccine* 2001;20:623.

118. Ohl ME, Miller SI. *Salmonella*: a model for bacterial pathogenesis. *Annu Rev Med* 2001;52:259.

CHAPTER 197
Shigella

Gerald T. Keusch

The genus *Shigella* is probably best considered as an end stage of differentiation of *Escherichia coli*, achieved by acquisition of virulence attributes to the point where *Shigella* species are almost always pathogens rather than usually being a commensal in the normal gut flora. It is because the genus *Shigella* is so closely related to *E. coli* that the two actually cannot be distinguished by DNA hybridization methods (1). It is not surprising that the majority of microbiologic properties of the four *Shigella* species are also identical to those of *E. coli*. Like *E. coli*, they are also classified in the family Enterobacteriaceae and belong to the tribe Escherichieae. Their common evolutionary path is further suggested by the striking frequency with which they share surface carbohydrate antigens (2) and specific virulence factors, including plasmid-mediated invasion determinants (3) and cytotoxins closely related to Shiga toxin (4). Nonetheless, *Shigella* species are highly host adapted to humans, whereas *E. coli* strains are widely distributed among animals.

The genus *Shigella* was discovered because of its association with the clinical picture of epidemic dysentery (5), resulting in a severe, febrile, inflammatory colitis characterized by a triad of clinical findings, including (a) a characteristic small volume of stool composed primarily of blood, mucus, and inflammatory cells; (b) abdominal cramps and pain; and (c) tenesmus (painful straining to pass stool) (6). The discovery of *Entamoeba histolytica* in 1875 and the description of histologic criteria for its diagnosis in humans in 1891 set the stage for the subsequent identification of *Shigella* (7). Although the first isolation can probably be attributed to Chantemesse and Widal in 1888, a much more complete description was provided by Kiyoshi Shiga during an epidemic of dysentery in Japan in the late 1890s (5). Not only did Shiga isolate a distinct non–lactose-fermenting organism from the stool of patients that was not present in healthy subjects or in patients with other clinical entities, but he also proved its importance by demonstrating the development of agglutinating antibodies during the course of the infection. For this classic work, Shiga's name ultimately was honored in the genus designation, *Shigella*, and the organism he reported and called *Bacillus dysenteriae* is now known as *Shigella dysenteriae* type 1.

Three years after Shiga's report on *B. dysenteriae*, Kruse isolated a similar organism from dysenteric cases except that it was mannitol fermenting (in contrast to the mannitol-negative *B. dysenteriae*) and serologically distinct, that is, it would not agglutinate in convalescent serum from patients with *B. dysenteriae* (7). This bacterium was designated *Bacillus pseudodysenteriae* and was quickly confirmed by Flexner and by Castellani in Ceylon. Others referred to these isolates as *B. dysenteriae* Flexner, and when the genus name was formally established, these organisms were designated *Shigella flexneri*. Boyd, working somewhat later in Bangalore, India, identified a common isolate biochemically resembling *S. flexneri* except for its inability to agglutinate in group- or type-specific antiserum to *S. flexneri*. The nonagglutinable organisms could of course, be agglutinated by homologous antiserum (7). These strains were ultimately defined as a third *Shigella* species, *Shigella boydii*. The fourth species was described by Kruse, Castellani, and Duval as a late lactose-fermenting variant that was serologically distinct from the other known dysentery bacilli (7). Kruse first called this organism *B. pseudodysenteriae* type E, but because of the extensive work on these organisms carried out by Sonne, it became known as *B. pseudodysenteriae* Sonne, and ultimately as *Shigella sonnei*.

Thus, during the 40 years from 1898 to 1938, the four clinically virulent species of *Shigella* were biochemically and serologically distinguished by group- and type-specific antigens. These include *S. dysenteriae* (serogroup A, 12 serotypes), *S. flexneri* (serogroup B, 14 serotypes), *S. boydii* (serogroup C, 15 serotypes), and *S. sonnei* (serogroup D, 1 serotype, but multiple colicin types).

CHARACTERISTICS OF THE PATHOGEN

Shigella organisms are gram-negative, facultatively anaerobic rod-shaped bacilli that are devoid of flagella. Although they share major biochemical properties with *E. coli* (Table 197.1), *Shigella* species can be distinguished from nearly all *E. coli* species by their failure to ferment lactose within 24 hours, their inability to produce gas from glucose (with rare exceptions), and, of course, their lack of motility. In fact, diagnostic microbiology schemata utilize these characteristics to quickly separate putative *Shigella* species from *E. coli* within the first 24 hours of culture. *S. sonnei*, which is positive for *o*-nitrophenyl-*β*-D-galactopyranoside, can utilize lactose, but only after a delay of

TABLE 197.1. Shared Biochemical Characteristics of *Shigella* and *Escherichia coli*

Test or substrate used	Result
Adonitol	Negative
DNase	Negative
Hydrogen sulfide on triple sugar iron agar	Negative
Inositol	Negative
Potassium cyanide	Negative
Malonate	Negative
Mannitol	Positive (except *S. dysenteriae*)
Methyl red	Positive
Mucate	Variable
Phenylalanine deaminase	Negative
Urease	Negative
Voges-Proskauer	Negative

TABLE 197.2. Differentiation of *Shigella* and *Escherichia coli*

Test or substrate	*Shigella* (%)[a]	*E. coli* (%)[a]
Acetate	Negative (0)	Positive (84)
Arginine decarboxylase	Negative (8)	Variable (17)
Citrate	Negative (0)	Variable (24)
Esculin	Negative (0)	Variable (31)
Gas from glucose[b]	Negative (<2)	Positive (91)
Indole	Variable (38)	Positive (99)
Lactose fermentation[c]	Negative (<1)	Positive (91)
Lysine decarboxylase	Negative (0)	Positive (90)
Motility	Negative (0)	Positive (80)
Mucate	Negative (0)	Positive (92)
Ornithine decarboxylase[d]	Variable (20)	Positive (63)
Salicin	Negative (0)	Positive (40)
Sucrose	Negative (<1)	Positive (50)
Xylose	Negative (2–5)	Positive (95)

[a]Percentage positive are in parentheses.
[b]Some *S. flexneri* type 6 organisms produce gas from glucose.
[c]*S. sonnei* usually ferments lactose or sucrose after several days in culture.
[d]Some *S. sonnei* organisms decarboxylate ornithine.

several days. Biochemical characteristics that differentiate *E. coli* and *Shigella* are shown in Table 197.2. It should be noted that *Shigella* is one of the least biochemically active members of the Enterobacteriaceae family.

The four *Shigella* species are also biochemically similar to one another, except for the inability of *S. dysenteriae* to ferment mannitol, positive ornithine utilization by *S. sonnei*, and the ability of most *S. sonnei* strains to ferment lactose after several days in culture. In practice, differentiation among species is usually accomplished by serologic methods, and group- and type-specific antisera can be used to identify the four serogroups and different serotypes.

Virulence Attributes

LIPOPOLYSACCHARIDE O ANTIGENS

Considerable information has been obtained about the specific structures of the O antigens of the most clinically relevant *Shigella* species and the structural basis for the known serologic cross-reactivity with certain *E. coli* (8). For example, *S. dysenteriae* type 1 has a unique repeating unit (→3α-D-GlcNAc1→3-α-L-Rha1→3-α-L-Rha1→2-α-D-Gal1→), which is shared only with *E. coli* O1 and O120 and not with other species of *Shigella*. The somatic antigens of two other group A serotypes, *S. dysenteriae* types 2 and 3, are also known to be identical to the O antigens of *E. coli* O112 and O124, respectively, but distinct from that of *S. dysenteriae* type 1.

All *S. flexneri* serotypes except *S. flexneri* type 6 have a common repeating unit of four sugars (→2α-L-Rha1→2-α-L-Rha1→3-α-L-Rha1→3-β-D-GlcNac→), which constitutes the serologic specificity termed group Y (8). The more frequently found 1a-5b seroreactivities of *S. flexneri* result from the attachment of a-D-glucopyranosyl and O-acetyl groups to various sites on the basic repeat unit. These sorts of antigens are relatively common among Enterobacteriaceae; as a result, there are many cross-reactions between *S. flexneri* and *E. coli* (8). In addition to possessing unique sequences, *S. flexneri* type 6 shares the α-L-Rha1→2-α-L-Rha1→ disaccharide with *S. flexneri* 1–5, so that it is recognized by convalescent sera from patients with the latter infections.

S. sonnei has a disaccharide of unusual nature in common with *Plesiomonas shigelloides,* consisting of 2-acetamido-2-deoxy-L-altruronic acid-$\alpha 1 \rightarrow 4$-2-acetamido-4-amino-2,4,6-trideoxy-D-Gal, linked to one another in a $\beta 1 \rightarrow 6$ linkage (8).

The rest of the lipopolysaccharide molecule is similar among all gram-negative organisms (9). The 2-keto-3-deoxyoctonate inner core region of the *Shigella* lipopolysaccharide resembles that of *Salmonella* or *E. coli,* whereas the short outer core region is markedly similar in all *Shigella* species. There is no evidence of significant variation in lipid A structure or biologic activity from *Shigella* to *E. coli* (10).

Although it is known that rough mutants are avirulent, the actual role of lipopolysaccharide in virulence of *Shigella* is unclear. Evidence suggests that this may be related to a requirement for O antigens in the transport and insertion of IcsA, a critical virulence determinant involved in intra- and intercellular spread of an organism, within the outer membrane of the organism (11). Further evidence of the role of lipopolysaccharide comes from Tn5 mutagenesis experiments in which insertional inactivation of the *rfa* locus involved in the synthesis of lipopolysaccharide basal core structures results in inefficient cell-to-cell spread in *in vitro* models and reduced inflammatory lesions in *in vivo* models (12). Previous speculations that O antigens were helpful to the organisms by blocking the complement-dependent serum bacteriolytic system appear to be incorrect. The invasive strains most frequently causing shigellemia, *S. dysenteriae* type 1 and *S. flexneri,* are sensitive to complement-mediated lysis; rather, it is a host serum bactericidal activity that is lacking (13). This explains why patients with bacteremic shigellosis are usually under 1 year of age and are significantly malnourished (14). Endotoxemia has been described in patients with hemolytic-uremic syndrome due to *S. dysenteriae* type 1, and, as described later, circulating endotoxin may play a role in pathogenesis (15).

CELL INVASION

There is little doubt that the ability to invade epithelial cells is central to the virulence of *Shigella* species (16). Creation of noninvasive *Shigella* variants renders those organisms avirulent (17). Invasiveness is now known to be a complex process dependent on gene products and regulatory elements present on both chromosomal and plasmid DNA (Fig. 197.1). *In vivo,* invasion occurs predominantly in the human colon; however, most of our information comes from either animal models or *in vitro* studies of HeLa or other extraenteric cells in tissue culture. Early studies using conjugal transfer or transduction of *E. coli* chromosomal DNA from the *xyl-rha, his,* or *purE* loci to virulent *Shigella flexneri* type 2a recipients resulted in hybrids that were able to invade but not survive within cells (18). The *xyl-rha* region of *S. flexneri* codes for iron-binding hydroxymate proteins and several iron-regulated outer membrane proteins (19), which may directly affect intracellular survival of the organisms, although no effect on survival in HeLa cells of a Tn10-induced aerobactin mutation has been detected (20). The *his* region controls synthesis of somatic antigen side chains (14), but it is not at all clear how this might condition intracellular survival. Selection of spontaneously appearing opaque *S. flexneri* colonial mutants or rough phase II *S. sonnei* also results in noninvasive avirulent isolates (17).

The clue to the extensive unraveling of the puzzle was the demonstration that noninvasive organisms have invariably lost a large 140- to 160-megadalton (MDa) plasmid present in all virulent *Shigella* strains and enteroinvasive *E. coli* (21–23). These plasmids contain certain highly conserved regions common to all, constituting an operon that encodes a group of outer membrane proteins termed invasion plasmid antigens (Ipas) (24,25). Of the multiple Ipas, IpaA to IpaD (polypeptides of 78, 62, 43, and

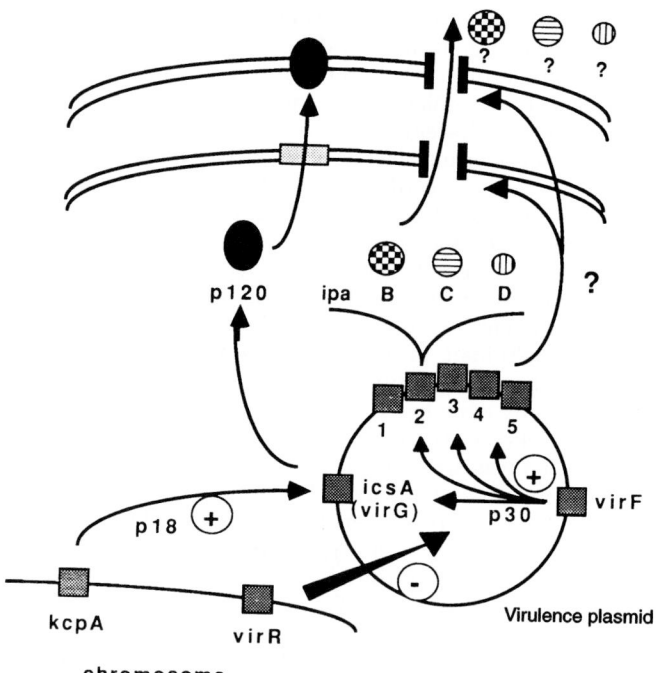

Figure 197.1. Location of some virulence determinant genes and regulatory elements in *Shigella flexneri.* Structural genes for the invasion plasmid antigens (*Ipas*) are present on the large 140-kd *S. flexneri* plasmid and are positively regulated by the nearby *virF* locus at the transcriptional level. *virF* encodes a 30-kd protein, which also positively regulates the *icsA* gene (formerly known as *virG*), along with the chromosomal locus *kcpA.* The *icsA* product, a 120-kd protein, which is inserted in the outer membrane of the organism, is necessary for intracellular spread of the organism. *virR* is a chromosomal negative regulator of the *ipa* genes. [From Sansonetti PJ. Genetic and molecular basis of epithelial cell invasion by *Shigella* spp. *Rev Infect Dis* 1991;13(suppl 4):285–291, with permission.]

38 kDa, respectively) are usually recognized by convalescent human serum (25). Tn5 insertions in the genes for IpaB, IpaC, and IpaD, but not IpaA, have been found to impair *Shigella* invasiveness, indicating their importance in the process (24). These essential virulence factors are transported and inserted in the bacterial surface membrane under the control of two regulatory gene sets known as mxi (membrane export of Ipa) (26) and spa (surface presentation of Ipas) (27). Growth of *Shigella* on cultured epithelial cells leads to release of Ipa proteins (28). In response, host cells respond with complex changes in the cytoskeleton that result in formation of phagocytic vesicles and bacterial uptake (29).

Significant insights into invasion have resulted from the realization that it is essentially analogous to phagocytosis of bacteria by neutrophils or macrophages (30) (Fig. 197.2). This followed from observations that internalization of *Shigella* by tissue culture or intestinal cells occurs within membrane-bounded vesicles and that the process requires polymerization of actin filaments (31–33). Sansonetti and colleagues (33) have effectively used transposon mutagenesis to define the further functions and antigens of importance to virulence. Electron microscopy has demonstrated that virulent *Shigella* organisms are able to lyse the phagocytic vacuole within a few minutes and gain rapid entry to the cytoplasm (Fig. 197.3). This has been correlated with a plasmid-mediated acid-activated contact hemolysin, activated at a pH known to occur in phagocytic vesicles. Hemolysin-negative isolates are invasive but avirulent. Tn5 mutants, which delete the hemolysin function, also eliminate the ability to invade cells and escape from vesicles. Ipa proteins are also required for vesicle

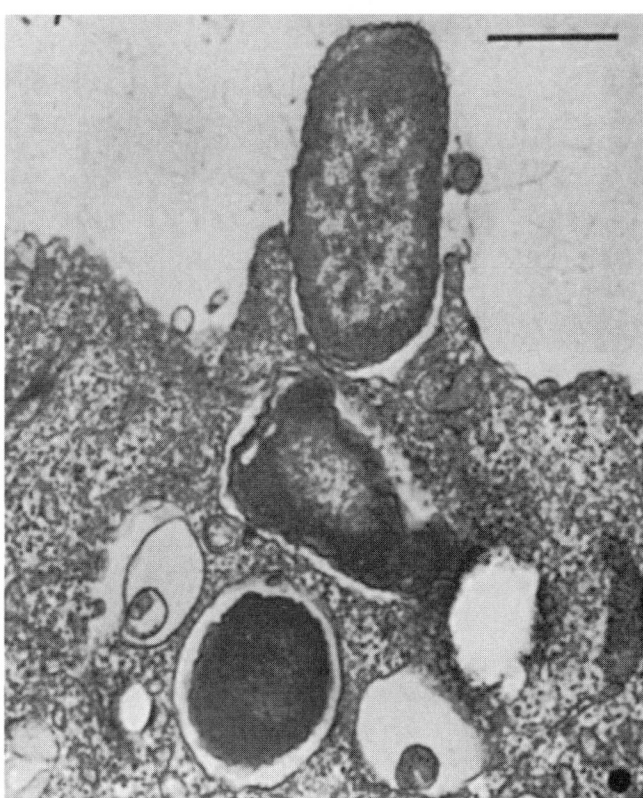

Figure 197.2. Entry of *S. flexneri* into a HeLa cell. Pseudopods extend from the surface of the nonprofessional phagocytic HeLa cell and ultimately engulf the organism, which comes to lie within the cytoplasm in a vacuole analogous to a phagosome. [From Sansonetti PJ. Genetic and molecular basis of epithelial cell invasion by *Shigella* spp. *Rev Infect Dis* 1991;13(suppl 4):285–291, with permission.]

lysis, because nonpolar inactivation mutants of IpaB, IpaC, or IpaD are inhibited in both entry and vesicle lysis (34).

Another characteristic of intracellular *Shigella* organisms is their impressive ability to multiply (33). However, the basis for this is uncertain. Intracellular multiplication is necessary for virulence, because mutants defective in folic acid synthesis via the aromatic pathway, or bearing mutations of the porins OmpC and OmpF, or their regulatory gene, ompB (35,36), are unable to do

so and are avirulent as well. The reason may be related to events during cell division that assist the organism in spreading from cell to cell.

An avirulent Tn*phoA* mutant, SC557, has helped delineate the mechanism of intracellular spread, the next step in pathogenesis (37). This strain invades cells and rapidly lyses the vacuole but it fails to spread within the cytoplasm or to spread from cell to cell, forming plaques in HeLa cell monolayers. This strain fails to synthesize an immunogenic 120-kd outer membrane protein named IcsA and coded for by a plasmid gene, *icsA* (intraintercellular spread). This same gene locus was previously identified as *virG* and defined as a plasmid gene needed for continuing reinfection of adjacent cells in culture (38). It turns out that expression of IcsA occurs during bacterial division at the back pole of the organism (which is defined with respect to the direction of subsequent motion of the bacterial cell) (39). Expression of IcsA is associated with actin polymerization at the site, forming an actin tail just behind the organism. An actin-binding host protein, plastin, is present in the same location, and actin crosslinking causes a sphincter-like contraction and generation of a forward propulsive force. This is referred to as the actin "motor," which apparently uses energy derived from adenosine triphosphate by the adenosine triphosphatase activity of IcsA itself (40). By this means, the organisms create and utilize an intracellular network of polymerized actin to spread throughout the cell interior to reach the plasma membrane (41), where they use the propulsive force of the actin motor to protrude beyond the plane of the host cell and extend into the adjacent cell, still within the plasma membrane of the first host cell (Fig. 197.4). Addition of cytochalasins after initial invasion to block the polymerization of actin filaments also inhibits spread of the organism within the cell (37). IcsA functions are regulated via phosphorylation mediated by cyclic nucleotide–dependent host cell protein kinases (42). Because phosphorylation mutations lead to enhanced microbial spread, it is possible that the host cell modulates bacterial virulence through its own protein kinases.

Shigella organisms also move to the cell periphery along actin stress fibers, following the architecture of the cytoskeleton. This has been termed organelle-like movement (Olm) (43). Although Olm is distinct from IcsA-mediated propulsion, the former could act together with the latter in a complementary manner (44). Once at the host cell surface, membrane-bounded organisms spread to the adjacent cell by fusion of the two host cell membranes, permitting the bacterium to enter the second cell within a vesicle to begin the process again. An important host target for

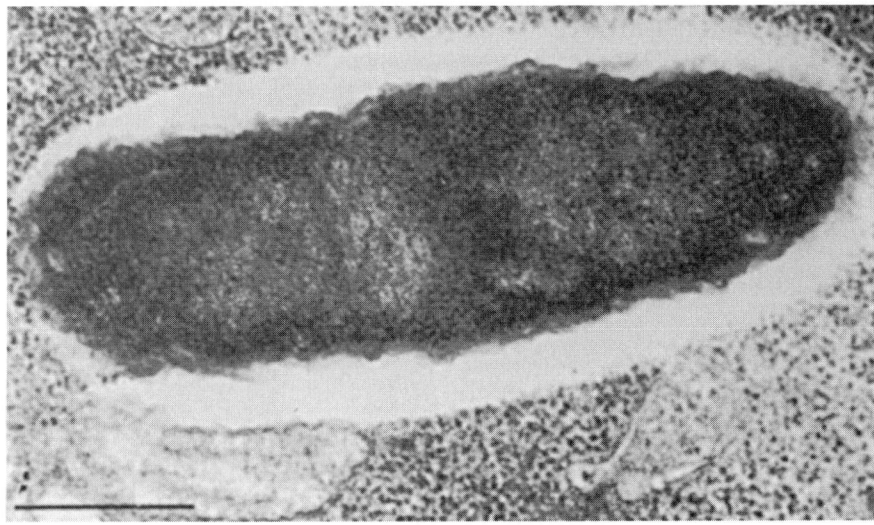

Figure 197.3. Shortly after invasion of a HeLa cell, *S. flexneri* lyses the phagosomal membrane and lies freely within the cytoplasm of the cell. Note the lack of host cell membrane surrounding the bacterium. [From Sansonetti PJ. Genetic and molecular basis of epithelial cell invasion by *Shigella* spp. *Rev Infect Dis* 1991;13(suppl 4):285–291, with permission.]

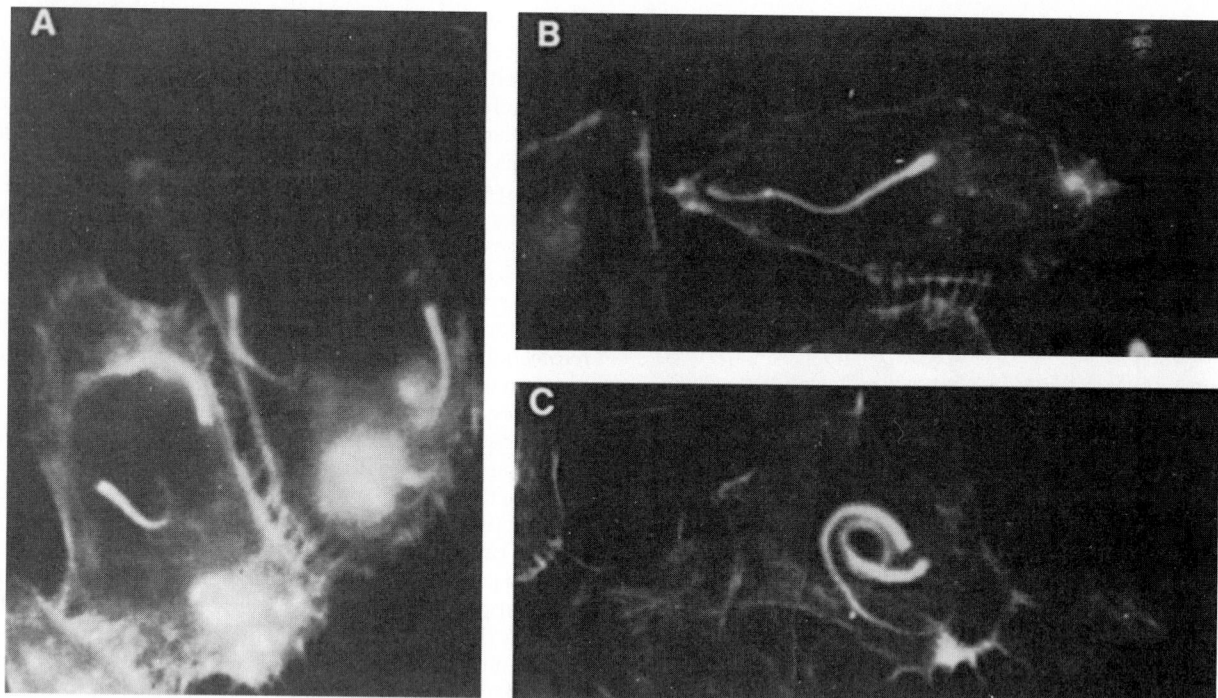

Figure 197.4. Intracellular spread of *S. flexneri* within HeLa cells is detected by the trail of polymerized F-actin it produces. Three views of actin trails are shown in an experimental tissue culture system. F-actin is brightly stained with fluorescein-tagged NBD-phallacidin, a fungal product that reacts specifically with F-actin. [From Sansonetti PJ. Genetic and molecular basis of epithelial cell invasion by *Shigella* spp. *Rev Infect Dis* 1991;13(suppl 4):285–291, with permission.]

this membrane fusion event appears to be a calcium-dependent adhesin, L-CAM (45). When L-CAM is altered, bacteria containing protrusions fail to complete the intercellular microbial transfer process. A second gene within the ics operon, *icsB,* is required for this final stage of microbial spread (41). If *icsB* is mutationally inactivated, the double host membrane-bounded vesicle cannot lyse and the organism cannot spread. Such mutants are also avirulent.

Both *in vitro* and *in vivo,* invasion and cell-to-cell spread of *Shigella* are accompanied by host cell death by an as yet unknown mechanism. Some evidence suggests that apoptosis is involved, at least when macrophages are used as targets for invasion by *Shigella flexneri* (46). Ipa proteins may be required as well, because when these are mutationally inactivated in a strain engineered to still express low levels of a cloned *E. coli* hemolysin to allow lysis of the phagocytic vesicle, apoptosis is not observed (47).

Just as there are several genes involved in invasion, there are also several levels of regulation of these genes (Fig. 197.1). One such locus, termed *virF,* is located on the invasion plasmid and acts in trans as a positive inducer (48). It codes for a 30-kd protein that up-regulates production of Ipas and also of the *icsA* gene product. A second locus, termed *virR,* is located on the chromosome at 27 minutes between *trp* and galU (49). It is a temperature-dependent repressor of the plasmid invasion genes, and it acts in trans at 30°C but not at 37°C. Another chromosomal gene, *kcpA,* located at 12 minutes near the *purE* gene, originally defined as a necessary locus for induction of keratoconjunctivitis in guinea pigs (50), has been shown to positively regulate expression of *icsA* (51).

TOXINS

S. dysenteriae type 1 was first shown in 1903 to produce a lethal toxin that became known as Shiga neurotoxin because it resulted first in limb paralysis in animals (52). Since then, this toxin has been found to cause fluid accumulation in rabbit gut and to be cytotoxic for cells in culture (53,54). Shiga toxin is the prototype of a family of enzymatically and structurally similar toxins, known as Shiga-like toxins, that are produced by other members of the genus and by certain *E. coli* serotypes (4). On the basis of these common features, the toxin nomenclature has changed (Table 197.3). Although the *E. coli* –produced Shiga toxins Stx-1 and Stx-2 are encoded by genes present in transforming phage, the Shiga toxin gene in *Shigella, stx,* is uniquely present on the chromosome of *S. dysenteriae* type 1, near the *pyrF* locus (55).

The toxin is composed of two different peptide subunits, an enzymatically active 32-kd A subunit and a complex of five identical 7.8-kd B subunits responsible for binding to the host cell receptor (56), a glycolipid containing a terminal disaccharide composed of galactose-linked $\alpha 1 \rightarrow 4$ to galactose (57). The A subunit is an *N*-glycosidase identical in action to the plant toxin ricin, which cleaves a specific adenine base in the 28S ribosomal RNA of the 60S ribosomal subunit and permanently inactivates the ribosome in protein synthesis (58). The active site of the A

TABLE 197.3.   Nomenclature for Shiga Family Toxins

New name (old name)	Nomenclature	
	Gene	Gene product
Shiga toxin (Shiga toxin)	*stx*	Stx
Shiga toxin type 1 (SLT-1, VT-1)	*stx1*	Stx-1
Shiga toxin type 2[a] (SLT-2, VT-2)	*stx2*	Stx-2

[a]Variant Stx-2 toxins, such as the toxin associated with porcine edema disease, are designated Stx-2e (formerly SLT-2e or VT-2e).

subunit has not been fully characterized; however, glutamic acid 167 appears to be a critical residue, and even a conservative change to aspartic acid reduces the A subunit enzymatic activity by more than 1,000-fold (59). The x-ray crystallographic structure of the B subunit of *E. coli* Stx-1, which is identical to Shiga toxin itself, has been solved (60). The three-dimensional view suggests that a conserved carbohydrate binding site is formed by β-sheet interactions between adjacent B monomers, which are arranged in a pentameric structure, producing five potential binding sites per holo-B subunit. Site-directed mutagenesis of aspartate residues at positions 16 and 17, which are within the potential binding cleft noted in the crystal structure (60), alters the toxin's binding capability (61).

The structural genes for the A and B subunits form an operon that is organized in tandem and translated in-frame, with the open reading frame for *stxA* 5′ to *stxB* and separated from one another by 12 nucleotides (55). Shiga toxin production is regulated by iron concentration through the *fur* locus (62), an iron-dependent negative regulator of a number of iron-regulated genes, including those controlling the synthesis of iron-binding siderophores and inner and outer membrane proteins involved in the uptake of the iron-siderophore complex. The *fur* gene also appears to control the *E. coli* Stx-1 gene but not the Stx-2 gene (63). A binding site for the *fur* gene product has been found 5′ to *stxA* in *S. dysenteriae* type 1 and in a region of dyad symmetry within the *stx* promoter (64). When iron is present in sufficient quantities, it complexes with the Fur protein, enabling Fur to bind to sites near or within the promoters of iron-regulated genes, which serves to down-regulate these genes at the transcriptional level.

Two new *Shigella* toxins have been reported, called ShET1 and ShET2 (for *Shigella* enterotoxin) because they increase net electrolyte transport by rabbit small bowel tissue *in vitro* and cause net fluid secretion *in vivo* in ligated rabbit ileal loops (65,66). These toxins are much less active on a weight basis than is Shiga toxin, which causes the same physiologic response by intestinal tissue. Humans infected with *Shigella* develop neutralizing antibody to ShET1 and ShET2, indicating that they are produced *in vivo*. The former is encoded by a chromosomal gene, whereas the latter is controlled by an iron-regulated plasmid gene and is homologous with a previously described enteroinvasive *E. coli* enterotoxin (67). Although the role of the ShET toxins in disease pathogenesis remains uncertain, the potential importance of ShET1 is limited by the observation that the gene is found predominantly in *S. flexneri* type 2 and not other *S. flexneri* serotypes or *Shigella* species (68).

DIAGNOSTIC MICROBIOLOGY

Diagnostic microbiology depends first on screening agar plates inoculated with stool samples for the presence of lactose-negative bacterial colonies. For this purpose, stool is streaked onto selective media such as MacConkey, Hektoen enteric, *Shigella-Salmonella*, or other agars that contain inhibitors of the growth of gram-positive organisms and a dye indicator to show acid production resulting from lactose fermentation. Lactose-negative colonies are then picked and streaked onto the slant of triple sugar iron agar or Kligler iron agar and stabbed into the butt to create anaerobic conditions. These media are designed to show several typical features of the genus, the failure of *Shigella* to ferment lactose aerobically on the slant and its ability to anaerobically utilize glucose in the butt, which results in a decrease in pH and a local color change of the pH dye indicator from red to yellow. *Salmonella* species also produce a red slant and yellow butt but can be distinguished from *Shigella* because the organisms characteristically produce hydrogen sulfide, which forms

an easily detected black reaction product, and their motility can often be seen on the slant. In the clinical laboratory, rapid presumptive identification can be made by agglutination of suspect colonies in group-specific antisera, which are available commercially. Further tests can be performed to distinguish the presumptive *Shigella* from other organisms, but this is rarely necessary in the clinical laboratory.

Modern molecular and immunologic diagnosis is also possible with the use of gene probes and polymerase chain reaction primers to identify virulence genes of *Shigella* or virulence gene products such as Ipa proteins or Shiga toxin. Some of these assays can be carried out directly on clinical samples such as stool or may serve a useful purpose after the initial isolation of organisms by more conventional bacteriologic methods. However, except for experimental studies of pathogenesis and molecular epidemiology, DNA-based tests and immunoassays are not in clinical use, and it is unlikely that they will displace the time-honored traditional culture and identification methods in the near future.

REFERENCES

1. Brenner DJ. Characterization and clinical identification of Enterobacteriaceae by DNA-hybridization. *Prog Clin Pathol* 1978;7:71–117.
2. Cheasty T, Rowe B. Antigenic relationships between the enteroinvasive *Escherichia coli* O-antigen O28ac, O112ac, O124, O136, O143, O144, O152, and O164 and *Shigella* O-antigens. *J Clin Microbiol* 1983;17:681–684.
3. Sansonetti PJ, d'Hauteville H, Ecobichon C, et al. Molecular expression of virulence plasmids in *Shigella* and enteroinvasive *E. coli*. *Ann Microbiol (Paris)* 1983;134A:295–318.
4. Acheson DWK, Donohue Rolfe A, Keusch GT. The family of Shiga and Shiga-like toxins. In: Alouf JE, Freer JH, eds. *Sourcebook of bacterial protein toxins.* London: Academic, 1991:415–433.
5. Shiga K. Ueber den Dysenterie-bacillus (*Bacillus dysenteriae*). *Zentralbl Bakteriol Orig* 1898;24:913–918.
6. Keusch GT. *Shigella* infections. *Clin Gastroenterol* 1979;8:645–662.
7. Keusch GT, Bennish ML. Shigellosis. In: Evans AE, Brachman P, eds. *Bacterial infections of humans,* 3rd ed. New York: Plenum, 1998.
8. Ewing WH, Lindberg AA. Serology of *Shigella*. In: Bergan T, ed. *Methods in microbiology,* Vol. 14. London: Academic, 1984:113–142.
9. Galanos C, Luderitz O, Rietschel ET, et al. Newer aspects on the chemistry and biology of bacterial lipopolysaccharides with special reference to the lipid A component. In: Goodwin KW, ed. *International review of biochemistry.* Vol. 2. Biochemistry of lipids. Baltimore: University Park Press, 1977:239–335.
10. Hase S, Rietschel ET. Isolation and analysis of the lipid A backbone. Lipid A structure of lipopolysaccharides from various bacterial groups. *Eur J Biochem* 1976;63:101–107.
11. Sandlin RC, Lampel KA, Keasler SP, et al. Avirulence of rough mutants of *Shigella flexneri*: Requirement of O antigen for correct unipolar localization of IcsA in the bacterial outer membrane. *Infect Immun* 1995;63:229–237.
12. Okada N, Sasakawa C, Tobe T, et al. Virulence-associated chromosomal loci of *Shigella flexneri* identified by random Tn5 insertion mutagenesis. *Mol Microbiol* 1991;5:187–195.
13. Struelens MJ, Mondal G, Roberts M, et al. Role of bacterial and host factors in the pathogenesis of *Shigella* septicemia. *Eur J Clin Microbiol Infect Dis* 1990;9:337–344.
14. Struelens MJ, Patte D, Kabir I, et al. *Shigella* septicemia: prevalence, presentation, risk factors and outcome. *J Infect Dis* 1985;152:784–790.
15. Koster F, Levin J, Walker L, et al. Hemolytic-uremic syndrome after shigellosis: relation to endotoxin and circulating immune complexes. *N Engl J Med* 1978;298:927–933.
16. LaBrec EH, Schneider H, Magnani TJ, et al. Epithelial cell penetration is an essential step in the pathogenesis of bacillary dysentery. *J Bacteriol* 1964;88:1503–1518.
17. Formal SB, Hale TL, Sansonetti PJ. Invasive enteric pathogens. *Rev Infect Dis* 1983;5(suppl):702–707.
18. Formal SB, LaBrec EH, Kent TH, et al. Abortive intestinal infection with an *Escherichia coli–Shigella flexneri* hybrid strain. *J Bacteriol* 1965;89:1374–1382.
19. Griffiths E, Stevenson P, Hale TL, et al. Synthesis of aerobactin and a 76,000 dalton iron-regulated outer membrane protein by *Escherichia coli* K-12–*Shigella flexneri* hybrids and by enteroinvasive strains of *Escherichia coli*. *Infect Immun* 1985;49:67–71.
20. Nassif X, Mazert M-C, Mounier J, et al. Evaluation with an iuc:Tn10 mutant of the role of aerobactin production in the virulence of *Shigella flexneri*. *Infect Immun* 1987;55:1963–1969.
21. Kopecko DJ, Washington O, Formal SB. Genetic and physical evidence for plasmid control of *Shigella sonnei* form I cell surface antigen. *Infect Immun* 1980;29:207–214.

22. Sansonetti PJ, Kopecko DJ, Formal SB. *Shigella sonnei* plasmids: evidence that a large plasmid is necessary for virulence. *Infect Immun* 1981;34:75–83.

23. Sansonetti PJ, Kopecko DJ, Formal SB. Involvement of a plasmid in the invasive ability of *Shigella flexneri*. *Infect Immun* 1982;35:852–860.

24. Baudry B, Maurelli AT, Clerc P, et al. Localization of plasmid loci necessary for the entry of *Shigella flexneri* into HeLa cells, and characterization of one locus encoding four immunogenic polypeptides. *J Gen Microbiol* 1987;133:3409–3413.

25. Hale TL, Oaks EV, Formal SB. Identification and antigenic characterization of virulence-associated, plasmid-coded proteins of *Shigella* spp. and enteroinvasive *Escherichia coli*. *Infect Immun* 1985;50:620–629.

26. Andrews GP, Hromockyj AE, Coker C, et al. Two novel virulence loci, *mxiA* and *mxiB*, in *Shigella flexneri* 2a facilitate excretion of invasion plasmid antigens. *Infect Immun* 1991;59:1997–2005.

27. Venkatesan MM, Buysse JM, Oaks EV. Surface presentation of *Shigella flexneri* invasion plasmid antigens requires the products of the *spa* locus. *J Bacteriol* 1992;174:1990–2001.

28. Menard R, Sansonetti P, Parsot C. The secretion of the *Shigella flexneri* Ipa invasins is activated by epithelial cells and controlled by IpaB and IpaD. *EMBO J* 1994;13:5293–5302.

29. Goldberg MB, Sansonetti PJ. *Shigella* subversion of the cellular cytoskeleton: a strategy for epithelial colonization. *Infect Immun* 1993;61:4941–4946.

30. Clerc P, Sansonetti PJ. Entry of *Shigella flexneri* into HeLa cells: evidence for directed phagocytosis involving actin polymerization and myosin accumulation. *Infect Immun* 1987;55:2681–2688.

31. Hale TL, Bonventre PF. *Shigella* infection of Henle intestinal epithelial cells: role of the bacteria. *Infect Immun* 1979;24:879–886.

32. Hale TL, Morris RE, Bonventre PF. *Shigella* infection of Henle intestinal epithelial cells: role of the host cell. *Infect Immun* 1979;24:887–894.

33. Sansonetti PJ, Ryter A, Clerc P, et al. Multiplication of *Shigella flexneri* within HeLa cells: lysis of the phagocytic vacuole and plasmid mediated contact hemolysis. *Infect Immun* 1986;55:521–527.

34. Menard R, Sansonetti PJ, Parsot C. Nonpolar mutagenesis of the ipa genes defines IpaB, IpaC, and IpaD as effectors of *Shigella flexneri* entry into epithelial cells. *J Bacteriol* 1993;175:5899–5906.

35. Sansonetti PJ, Arondel J, Fontaine A, et al. OmpB (osmo-regulation) and *icsA* mutants of *Shigella flexneri*: Vaccine candidates and probes to study the pathogenesis of shigellosis. *Vaccine* 1991;9:416–422.

36. Bernardini ML, Sanna MG, Fontaine A, et al. OmpC is involved in invasion of epithelial cells by *Shigella flexneri*. *Infect Immun* 1993;61:3625–3635.

37. Bernardini ML, Mounier J, d'Hauteville H, et al. Identification of *icsA*, a plasmid locus of *Shigella flexneri* that governs bacterial intra- and intercellular spread through interactions with F-actin. *Proc Natl Acad Sci USA* 1989;86:3867–3871.

38. Makino S, Sasakawa C, Kamata K, et al. A genetic determinant required for continuous reinfection of adjacent cells on a large plasmid in *Shigella flexneri* 2a. *Cell* 1986;46:551–555.

39. Goldberg MB, Theriot JA, Sansonetti PJ. Regulation of surface presentation of IcsA, a *Shigella* protein essential to intracellular movement and spread, is growth phase dependent. *Infect Immun* 1994;62:5664–5668.

40. Goldberg MB, Barzu O, Parsot C, et al. Unipolar localization and ATPase activity of IcsA, a *Shigella flexneri* protein involved in intracellular movement. *J Bacteriol* 1993;175:2189–2196.

41. Allaoui A, Mounier J, Prevost MC, et al. icsB: a *Shigella flexneri* virulence gene necessary for the lysis of protrusions during intercellular spread. *Mol Microbiol* 1992;6:1605–1616.

42. d'Hauteville H, Sansonetti PJ. Phosphorylation of IcsA by cAMP-dependent protein kinase and its effect on intercellular spread of *Shigella flexneri*. *Mol Microbiol* 1992;6:833–841.

43. Vasselon T, Mounier J, Prevost MC, et al. A stress fiber-based movement of *Shigella flexneri* within cells. *Infect Immun* 1991;59:1723–1732.

44. Vasselon T, Mounier J, Hellio R, et al. Movement along actin filaments of the perijunctional area and *de novo* polymerization of cellular actin are required for *Shigella flexneri* colonization of epithelial Caco-2 cell monolayers. *Infect Immun* 1992;60:1031–1040.

45. Sansonetti PJ, Mounier J, Prevost MC, et al. Cadherin expression required for formation and internalization of *Shigella flexneri*–induced intercellular protrusions involved in spread between epithelial cells. *Cell* 1994;76:829–839.

46. Zychlinsky A, Prevost MC, Sansonetti PJ. *Shigella flexneri* induces apoptosis in infected macrophages. *Nature* 1992;358:167–169.

47. Zychlinsky A, Kenny B, Menard R, et al. IpaB mediates macrophage apoptosis induced by *Shigella flexneri*. *Mol Microbiol* 1994;11:619–627.

48. Sakai T, Sasakawa C, Makino S, et al. DNA sequence and product analysis of the *virF* locus responsible for Congo red binding and cell invasion in *Shigella flexneri* 2a. *Infect Immun* 1986;54:395–402.

49. Maurelli AT, Sansonetti PJ. Identification of a chromosomal gene controlling temperature regulated expression of *Shigella* virulence. *Proc Natl Acad Sci USA* 1988;85:2820–2824.

50. Formal SB, Gemski P Jr, Baron LS, et al. A chromosomal locus which controls the ability of *Shigella flexneri* to evoke keratoconjunctivitis. *Infect Immun* 1971;3:73–79.

51. Pal TL, Newland JW, Tall BD, et al. Intracellular spread of *Shigella flexneri* associated with the *kcpA* locus and a 140-kilodalton protein. *Infect Immun* 1989;57:477–486.

52. Conradi H. Ueber lösliche durch aseptische Autolyse erhalten Giftstoffe von Ruhr und Typhusbazillen. *Dtsch Med Wochenschr* 1902;29:26–28.

53. Keusch GT, Grady GF, Mata LJ, et al. The pathogenesis of *Shigella* diarrhea. 1. Enterotoxin production by *Shigella dysenteriae* 1. *J Clin Invest* 1972;51:1212–1218.

54. Vicari G, Olitzki AL, Olitzki Z. The action of the thermolabile toxin of *Shigella dysenteriae* on cells cultivated *in vitro*. *Br J Exp Pathol* 1960;41:179–189.

55. Strockbine NA, Jackson MP, Sung LM, et al. Cloning and sequencing of the genes for Shiga toxin from *Shigella dysenteriae* type 1. *J Bacteriol* 1988;170:1116–1122.

56. Donohue-Rolfe A, Jacewicz M, Keusch GT. Isolation and characterization of functional Shiga toxin subunits and renatured holotoxin. *Mol Microbiol* 1989;3:1231–1236.

57. Jacewicz M, Clausen H, Nudelman E, et al. Pathogenesis of *Shigella* diarrhea. XI. Isolation of a shigella toxin-binding glycolipid from rabbit jejunum and HeLa cells and its identification as globotriaosylceramide. *J Exp Med* 1986;163:1391–1404.

58. Endo Y, Tsurugi K, Yutsudo T, et al. Site of action of a Vero toxin (VT2) from *Escherichia coli* O157:H7 and of Shiga toxin on eukaryotic ribosomes. *Eur J Biochem* 1988;171:45–50.

59. Hovde CJ, Calderwood SB, Mekalanos JJ, et al. Evidence that glutamic acid 167 is an active-site residue of Shiga-like toxin I. *Proc Natl Acad Sci USA* 1988;85:2568–2572.

60. Stein PE, Boodhoo A, Tyrrell GJ, et al. Crystal structure of the cell-binding B oligomer of verotoxin-1 from *E. coli*. *Nature* 1992;355:748–750.

61. Jackson MP, Wadolkowski EA, Weinstein DL, et al. Functional analysis of the Shiga toxin and Shiga-like toxin type II variant binding subunits by using site-directed mutagenesis. *J Bacteriol* 1990;172:653–658.

62. Calderwood SB, Mekalanos JJ. Iron regulation of Shiga-like toxin expression is *Escherichia coli* is mediated by the *fur* locus. *J Bacteriol* 1987;169:4759–4764.

63. Weinstein DL, Jackson MP, Samuel JE, et al. Cloning and sequencing of a Shiga-like toxin type II variant from an *Escherichia coli* strain responsible for edema disease of swine. *J Bacteriol* 1988;170:4223–4230.

64. de Lorenzo V, Wee S, Herrero M, et al. Operator sequences of the aerobactin operon of plasmid Co1V-K30 binding site of the ferric uptake regulation (*fur*) repressor. *J Bacteriol* 1987;169:2624–2630.

65. Fasano A, Noriega FR, Maneval DR Jr, et al. *Shigella* enterotoxin 1: an enterotoxin of *Shigella flexneri* 2a active in rabbit small intestine *in vivo* and *in vitro*. *J Clin Invest* 1995;95:2853–2861.

66. Nataro JP, Seriwatana J, Fasano A, et al. Cloning a sequencing of a new plasmid-encoded enterotoxin in enteroinvasive *E. coli* and *Shigella*. In: *Program and Abstracts of the 29th Joint Conference on Cholera and Related Diseases*. Bethesda, MD: National Institutes of Health, 1993:144–147.

67. Fasano A, Kay BA, Russell RG, et al. Enterotoxin and cytotoxin production by enteroinvasive *Escherichia coli*. *Infect Immun* 1990;58:3717–3723.

68. Noriega FR, Liao FM, Formal SB, et al. Prevalence of *Shigella* enterotoxin 1 (ShET1) among *Shigella* clinical isolates of diverse serotypes. *J Infect Dis* 1995;172:1408–1411.

CHAPTER 198
Campylobacters

Ban Mishu Allos

Campylobacters were recognized as a cause of human diarrheal illness in the 1970s and 1980s. Soon after, studies showed that these organisms are not only capable of causing gastrointestinal illness, they are among the most common causes of diarrhea worldwide. In addition, *Campylobacter jejuni* and *Campylobacter coli* are the most common causes of food-borne bacterial illness in the United States and other industrialized nations. *C. jejuni* and *C. coli* are very closely related species; *C. jejuni*, however, is predominant and the name is commonly used to refer to both organisms (1). In this chapter, *C. jejuni* shall refer to both species unless otherwise indicated. Other *Campylobacter* species are discussed in Chapter 71.

MICROBIOLOGY AND ISOLATION

Campylobacters are slender, curved or spiral gram-negative rods. Recently, the complete genome sequence of *Campylobacter* was characterized. Of note was the finding of hypervariable regions that might be important in the survival of the organism

(2). Campylobacters are motile via a single polar flagellum at one or both ends (3). They are microaerophilic, requiring 3% to 15% oxygen for growth. *C. jejuni* grows best at 42°C, unlike other *Campylobacter* species, which grow best at 37°C. *C. jejuni* grows slowly, up to 2 weeks may be required for primary isolation from blood (4). The organism may be isolated from stools within 72 hours (1). If more than 2 hours is anticipated before arrival of the specimen to the laboratory, a transport medium such as Cary Blair should be used (5). Because most *C. jejuni* strains are resistant to cephalothin, they may be isolated from stools using a medium that contains cephalothin or another antibiotic to which the organism is resistant. These *Campylobacter*-selective media will inhibit the growth of more rapidly growing components of the enteric flora. However, some *Campylobacter* species are susceptible to cephalothin; culture techniques using antibiotic-free media are needed to isolate these organisms (see Chapter 71).

When using *Campylobacter*-selective media, colonies that appear after 24 to 48 hours and that are gray, mucoid, or wet appearing should be suspected of being *Campylobacter*. The organism may be identified using standard biochemical tests (6). A rapid presumptive identification can be made by the following characteristics: (a) typical colonial morphology, (b) Gram stain showing gram-negative curved rods, (c) oxidase and catalase positivity, and (d) motility.

The two most widely used serotyping systems for *C. jejuni* and *C. coli* are the Penner system, which identifies heat-stable (somatic, O) antigens, and the Lior system, which measures heat-labile (flagellar, H) antigens (7). There are over 90 reference serotypes defined by the Penner system and 112 by the Lior system. Both systems identify over 90% of *Campylobacter* isolated from human and nonhuman sources (8,9). The Lior system is quicker and easier to use and consequently more applicable for use outside reference laboratories (10).

EPIDEMIOLOGY

Incidence and Seasonality

Campylobacter infections occur everywhere in the world. Isolations have been made in tropical, temperate, and arctic climates (11). The incidence of *C. jejuni* infections in the United States peaks in the late summer and early fall (12). Infants have the highest rate of infections, but a second surge occurs in young adulthood. Not surprisingly, *C. jejuni* infections are the most common cause of diarrheal disease at U.S. universities (13,14). In developing countries too, the highest isolation rate occurs in young children; however, no second peak occurs in the early adult years (10). Isolation rates for *C. jejuni* in males are higher than in females from infancy through age 40 years; no explanation for this phenomenon is available.

The incidence of *Campylobacter* infections in developed countries is difficult to estimate. *Campylobacter* infections became reportable illnesses in many states in the United States in the early 1980s; from the outset, however, the reporting systems routinely underestimated the impact of these infections. In the early years of *Campylobacter* surveillance, many hospital microbiology laboratories did not culture stools for *Campylobacter* when they were searching for other enteric pathogens. Later studies confirmed that when diarrheal stools were cultured for *Campylobacter* every time they cultured for *Salmonella* or *Shigella*, *Campylobacter* was identified between two and seven times more frequently than *Salmonella* or *Shigella*. Even currently, estimates have shown that only 1 in 38 cases of detected *Campylobacter* infection are ever reported (15).

Accurate estimates of the true incidence of *Campylobacter* infections in the United States and other industrialized nations depend on many data sources. In 1996, the U.S. Centers for Disease Control and Prevention (CDC) Emerging Infections Program Foodborne Diseases Active Surveillance Network (Foodnet) began collecting data on nine food-borne illnesses in selected U.S. cities. In the first year, *Campylobacter* infections were detected more frequently than any other pathogen, more frequently than *Salmonella* and *Shigella* combined. However, from 1996 to 1999, the incidence of *Campylobacter* infection declined 26%, although it remained the most commonly identified enteric pathogen (16). The decreased rates were attributed to disease prevention efforts that had been implemented in food service establishments, meat and poultry processing plants, and egg production farms (16). Currently, the CDC estimates that 2.4 million cases of *Campylobacter* infection occur in the United States each year—almost 1% of the entire population (17). Similarly, in England studies at the level of community-based physicians show that the true annual incidence is 1,100 per 100,000 population (18).

In developing countries, campylobacters are ubiquitous in the environment and infection is hyperendemic among young children. Breast-fed children have a lower risk for infection, but once weaned, a high proportion develop symptomatic infection. *Campylobacter* infection is an important cause of morbidity from watery diarrhea in this age group. In adults and children over 3 years of age, infections are usually asymptomatic (19,20), suggesting that acquired immunity is protective.

Sources and Mechanisms of Infection

The principal route of infection with *C. jejuni* in developed countries is through preparation and consumption of chicken. Indeed, case-control studies of sporadic cases of *C. jejuni* infection show that more than 70% are associated with eating chicken (21–24). Perhaps this should not be surprising when one considers the frequency with which poultry products are consumed and the nearly universal contamination of chicken carcasses with *Campylobacter* (25). Recent studies suggest that the greatest risk comes from eating chicken prepared outside the home (26). Other foods of animal origin (e.g., beef, pork) may occasionally be related to *C. jejuni* infection (27). In contrast to sporadic cases, outbreaks of *C. jejuni* infection are associated most commonly not with eating chicken but with drinking raw milk (12). From 1981 to 1990, 20 raw milk–associated outbreaks of *C. jejuni* occurred in the United States involving 458 teenagers and children (28). In the United Kingdom, pasteurized, bottled milk may be a source of *Campylobacter* infections because of the contamination of milk by birds pecking the bottle tops (29,30).

Waterborne outbreaks of *C. jejuni* infection have been reported in the United States, Europe, and Israel (31–33). Contamination of drinking water with feces from birds or animals is usually the cause. In Colorado, ingestion of untreated water from rivers or streams is an important cause of *C. jejuni* infections (34). Indeed, in the Rocky Mountain states, diarrhea occurring after drinking untreated surface water is more often caused by *C. jejuni* than by *Giardia* (35).

C. jejuni infections have been associated with foreign travel and with exposure to dogs and cats (22,36–39). Person-to-person transmission of *C. jejuni* infection has been reported (40,41) but is rare. Likewise, transmission via infected food handlers or health care workers has been described but is rare (42). Unlike *Shigella*, *Giardia*, or hepatitis A infections, there have been no outbreaks of *C. jejuni* infection reported in day care centers or institutions for the mentally retarded.

CLINICAL FEATURES

The consequences of *C. jejuni* infection vary from complete absence of symptoms to fulminant sepsis and death (Table 198.1). The proportion of asymptomatic infected persons depends on the population studied. For example, in developing countries where *Campylobacter* is endemic, many infected persons may be asymptomatic (43,44). Alternatively, a high proportion of infected persons may become severely ill and require hospitalization (45,46). The case-fatality rate for *Campylobacter* infections is 0.05 per 1,000 infections (47).

Signs and Symptoms of Gastrointestinal Illness

The typical infection with *C. jejuni* is characterized by an acute diarrheal illness which is indistinguishable from gastroenteritis caused by *Salmonella*, *Shigella*, or other enteric bacterial pathogens. Usually the illness has an abrupt onset with abdominal cramps and diarrhea. Some patients, however, have a flu-like prodrome consisting of fever, headache, myalgias, and dizziness. Nevertheless, the most common symptom experienced by most patients with *C. jejuni* infection is diarrhea. The diarrhea may be severe, and many patients have at least 1 day with eight or more stools; 20% report more than 15 stools on at least 1 day (48). Almost half describe grossly bloody diarrhea. Occasionally the diarrhea is minimal or absent and the abdominal pain (which can be intense) may be mistakenly attributed to appendicitis. Exploratory laparotomy and appendectomy is not unusual in *C. jejuni*–infected persons whose infections have not yet been diagnosed (46,49–51). Although nausea is frequently reported, vomiting is uncommon. Subjective fever is reported by more than 90% of infected persons. Resolution of symptoms in most patients occurs within 1 week; however, 20% experience more prolonged or relapsing illness lasting several weeks (46,52). Rarely, *C. jejuni* infection may cause mild, chronic diarrhea lasting many months (53–55).

The signs and laboratory findings associated with *C. jejuni* infection are also not distinguishable from those produced by other enteric bacterial pathogens. Almost two thirds of persons with documented infection have fever greater than 37.5°C (56), however, temperatures of over 40°C are unusual. Fecal leukocytes are found in 75% of cases; gross or occult blood is seen in 50%. Sigmoidoscopic examination reveals diffuse colonic inflammation; *Campylobacter* enteritis may be confused with early inflammatory bowel disease. Although the peripheral white blood cell count may be mildly elevated, other laboratory findings, including liver function tests, serum electrolytes, and hematocrit are normal.

Local and Systemic Complications

Gastrointestinal complications of *C. jejuni* infection are relatively rare and are the result of local invasion. Massive gastrointestinal hemorrhage may occur. Infection of the biliary tract may lead to cholecystitis, pancreatitis, or obstructive hepatitis (51,57,58). Eleven (6%) of 188 patients hospitalized with *C. jejuni* enteritis developed pancreatitis—a far higher rate than that seen with *Salmonella* or *Shigella* infections (51). In patients on peritoneal dialysis, *C. jejuni* infection may cause peritonitis (59). Spontaneous bacterial peritonitis due to *C. jejuni* infection may occur in patients with cirrhosis. *C. jejuni* infection has been reported to cause splenic rupture (60). *Campylobacter* infections may exacerbate inflammatory colitis, but there are no data to suggest it causes the disease. Infections in pregnant women are likely to be mild and self-limited, but neonatal sepsis and death can occur if the woman is infected during her third trimester (61).

Extraintestinal complications of *C. jejuni* infection such as bacteremia, meningitis, and purulent arthritis usually are the result of systemic spread. *C. jejuni* bacteremia occurs in approximately 1.5 per 1,000 intestinal infections (62). The rate is higher in the elderly and in immunodeficient persons (63). It is possible that transient bacteremia occurs in many cases of *C. jejuni* enteritis but is not detected because blood cultures are not routinely performed in healthy persons with uncomplicated diarrheal illness. Clinically significant bacteremia is infrequently observed because most *C. jejuni* strains are susceptible to killing by normal human serum. In contrast, *Campylobacter fetus* is intrinsically serum resistant, and infection is less likely to be contained within the gastrointestinal tract. Although a far higher proportion of *C. fetus* infections are bacteremias, *C. jejuni* still accounts for most (89%) *Campylobacter* isolates from blood (62). One minor extraintestinal manifestation of infection is urticaria (64,65). *C. jejuni* has occasionally been isolated from the urinary tract in women.

Postinfectious Complications

The most important and recently recognized postinfectious complication of *C. jejuni* infection is the Guillain-Barré syndrome (GBS). GBS is an infrequent complication of *C. jejuni* infection; approximately 1 in 2,000 to 5,000 infections is followed by GBS. However, because these infections are common, they account for 30% of cases of GBS occurring in the United States each year (66). Furthermore, GBS occurring after *C. jejuni* infection may be more severe, with a greater likelihood of irreversible neurologic damage. The likelihood of developing GBS after *C. jejuni* infection does not appear to be related to the severity of gastroenteritis. Indeed GBS may occur following asymptomatic infections. In the United States, GBS is more likely to occur following infection with *C. jejuni* Penner serotype O:19 (67); in South Africa, the most common serotype associated with GBS is O:41 (68).

The pathogenic mechanism of *C. jejuni*–associated GBS is not known precisely. However, because neurologic symptoms usually begin 1 to 3 weeks after onset of diarrhea (69,70), a humoral immunopathogenic mechanism is likely. Recent studies suggest possible antibody cross-reactivity between structures on the cell surface of *Campylobacter* and peripheral nerve glycolipids or myelin proteins (71).

TABLE 198.1. Consequences of Infection with *Campylobacter jejuni*

Asymptomatic	Systemic complications
Gastrointestinal symptoms	Bacteremia
Diarrhea	Meningitis
Fever	Purulent arthritis
Abdominal cramps	Osteomyelitis
Nausea	Neonatal sepsis
Vomiting	Death
Malaise	Post-infectious
Myalgias	complications
Local complications	Guillain-Barre syndrome
Cholecystitis	Reactive arthritis
Pancreatitis	Uveitis
Peritonitis	Encephalopathy
Gastrointestinal	Hemolytic-uremic
hemorrhage	syndrome
"Pseudo"-appendicitis	Hemolytic anemia
Toxic megacolon	Carditis

Another postinfectious complication of *C. jejuni* infection, reactive arthritis, is most likely in persons who carry the HLA-B27 phenotype. Like GBS, it may follow symptomatic or asymptomatic *C. jejuni* infection (72,73). Reactive arthritis also occurs following *Salmonella*, *Shigella*, and *Yersinia* infections. The rate of this postinfectious complication of *C. jejuni* infection is not known but is likely low. In Scandinavia, 1% to 2% of patients with *Campylobacter* enteritis develop arthritis 4 days to 4 weeks after onset of diarrhea (74). Interestingly, in another Scandinavian study, 32 patients in a hospital for rheumatic diseases developed culture-confirmed *C. jejuni* infection during a hospital outbreak; none of these patients had exacerbations of their existing conditions (75).

Uveitis without arthritis has been reported in two patients with *Campylobacter* enteritis (76,77); erythema nodosum has been reported in five (78–82). Nine cases of hemolytic uremic syndrome developing during the course of *C. jejuni* enteritis have been reported (83–90); however, the presence of *E. coli O:157, H7* was not excluded in these patients. Other reported but rare postinfectious complications of *C. jejuni* infection include nephritis, carditis, hemolytic anemia, and encephalopathy.

C. jejuni Infections in Immunodeficient Persons

Among persons with acquired immunodeficiency syndrome (AIDS), *C. jejuni* infections are detected almost 40 times as frequently as in the general population (91). This excess of infections impacts on patients with the lowest CD4 cell counts; patients with early human immunodeficiency virus (HIV) infection are not especially likely to develop *C. jejuni* infections (92). *C. jejuni* infections in AIDS patients are generally more persistent and more severe (92–97). Hypogammaglobulinemic patients develop severe persistent and relapsing infections due to *C. jejuni* (98,99). Asplenic patients or others who lack opsonizing activity are predisposed to extraintestinal spread of infection, including meningitis, osteomyelitis, and cellulitis (100–102). Immunodeficient persons with even mild *C. jejuni* infections should receive prompt antibiotic treatment.

Campylobacter jejuni Infections in Developing Countries

The epidemiology of *Campylobacter* infections is quite different in developing countries than in the industrialized world. In tropical developing countries, *Campylobacter* infections are hyperendemic among young children, especially those under 2 years of age. Asymptomatic infections occur commonly in both children and adults, whereas in developed countries, asymptomatic *Campylobacter* infections are unusual. Additionally, in developing countries, outbreaks of infection are uncommon and the illness lacks the marked seasonal nature observed in industrialized nations. Nevertheless, in both developed and developing countries, *Campylobacter* remains one of the most common bacterial causes of diarrhea.

PATHOGENESIS AND IMMUNITY

Despite the ubiquity of *C. jejuni* and the frequency of both symptomatic and asymptomatic infections, the pathogenesis of *C. jejuni* enteritis remains poorly understood. The organism's motility, conferred by its flagella, enables it to directly invade and proliferate within the intestinal epithelium. The virulence of individual strains may depend on the activity of their flagella (103,104) as well as on their ability to adhere to intestinal cells (105,106).

The incubation period depends on the number of organisms ingested but can range from 1 day to 1 week (107). The attack rate is also dose dependent; infection may be induced with as few as 500 organisms (107,108). Serum and mucosal serum responses are elicited in both natural and experimental infections (109). Serum IgA, IgG, and IgM responses peak within 2 to 4 weeks then decline rapidly (110,111). The increased frequency and severity of *C. jejuni* infections in HIV-infected persons suggest that cellular immunity also plays a protective role.

Enterotoxins are unlikely to play a role in the pathogenesis of *C. jejuni* infections. Toxins were once thought to play an important role because some isolates were reported to be enterotoxigenic (112,113) and because infection frequently produces watery diarrhea. It appears clear now that enterotoxins are not involved in *C. jejuni* pathogenesis. First of all, enterotoxin production by *C. jejuni* cannot be demonstrated *in vivo*. Secondly, infected patients do not form antibodies against toxin (114). Finally, the clinical picture of *C. jejuni* enteritis (fever, bloody stools, fecal leukocytes) is not consistent with illness produced by enterotoxins.

The ability of *C. jejuni* to adhere to and colonize epithelial cells may be an important virulence factor (115). A superficial antigen, PEB$_1$, may be the major adhesin (116); it is a target of the immune response and is considered a potential vaccine candidate (117,118).

Infection with *C. jejuni* produces an acute inflammatory enteritis affecting the small intestine and the colon. Acute exudative and hemorrhagic inflammation may be seen; the appendix, mesenteric lymph nodes, and gall bladder may also be affected (50,119). Histopathologically, epithelial cell injury, edema, and infiltration of the lamina propria by mononuclear cells and neutrophils may be seen; eosinophils also may be present (120). In general, the findings of *C. jejuni* enteritis are nonspecific; there are no pathognomatic features (120). A trained pathologist will recognize that *C. jejuni* enteritis may produce crypt abscesses (which can look similar to ulcerative colitis) and granulomas (which can look like Crohn's disease) (120–122).

DIAGNOSIS

Because the signs, symptoms, and laboratory findings associated with *C. jejuni* infection are not distinctive from other bacterial enteric pathogens, diagnosis depends on the isolation of the organism from stool or other infected site (Table 198.2). Cultures for *Campylobacter* are indicated in nonhospitalized patients with acute onset of fever and diarrhea. The suspicion of *C. jejuni* gastroenteritis is even higher if the stools contain blood or fecal leukocytes. Stool cultures should not be routinely ordered on patients who develop fever and diarrhea after being hospitalized longer than 3 days. However, hospitalized patients with appendicitis should be cultured for *C. jejuni* because infection may mimic appendicitis. Identification of *C. jejuni* in stools could eliminate the need for surgery, although culture results may not be available in time to prevent many laparotomies. Some

---

TABLE 198.2. Groups of Patients in whom Diagnosis of *Campylobacter* Infection should be Considered

Nonhospitalized persons with acute onset of fever and diarrhea
Persons with symptoms of appendicitis
Persons being worked up for inflammatory bowel disease
Immunocompromised patients with chronic diarrhea
Travelers to developing countries who develop diarrhea

laboratories have begun performing the polymerase chain reaction (PCR) of stools for *Campylobacter,* but this is not yet a standard practice. Species-specific assays using PCR enzyme-linked immunosorbent assays to detect *Campylobacter* antigens in stools have been developed and also may become useful in the diagnosis of *Campylobacter* infections (123). Persons suspected of having inflammatory bowel disease should have cultures for *C. jejuni* and other campylobacters and related organisms as part of their diagnostic workup. Other persons who are at high risk for *C. jejuni* infection include travelers to developing countries and persons with possible occupational or recreational exposure to campylobacters in whom an acute diarrheal illness develops. Immunocompromised persons should have stool cultures for *Campylobacter* even if their diarrhea is chronic.

TREATMENT

The most important tenet of treatment of patients with acute gastroenteritis due to *C. jejuni* or any other organism is maintenance of proper hydration and electrolyte balance. In almost all cases, this can be accomplished by encouraging proper oral intake of liquids; occasionally, intravenous fluids are required, especially in the very young and very old.

C. jejuni is susceptible to a number of antimicrobial agents, but not all infected patients require such treatment. Many infections result in mild illness, and only rest and rehydration are required. Some studies show shortened duration of symptoms and *Campylobacter* excretion in patients who receive antibiotics at the onset of their illness (124,125). However, most healthy persons do not seek medical care until they have been ill a few days and, therefore, would not benefit from antibiotics. Patients in whom antimicrobial therapy is indicated include those with persistent or severe illness, fever above 38.5°C, or bloody diarrhea. Because immunocompromised persons, the elderly, and pregnant women may have more dire consequences of infection, these people also should receive prompt antibiotic therapy.

Until a few years ago, if antimicrobial therapy was indicated to treat a *Campylobacter* infection, fluoroquinolones were considered the treatment of choice. This approach was the simplest for physicians and patients alike because the symptoms of *Campylobacter* enteritis (fever, abdominal cramps, and diarrhea) are clinically indistinguishable from bacterial gastroenteritis due to other organisms such as *Salmonella* or *Shigella*. Because these other pathogens were also generally susceptible to fluoroquinolones, empiric treatment with these drugs could be used without waiting for the results of stool cultures. Fluoroquinolones were especially apt to be used for the treatment of traveler's diarrhea. However, in the past few years, a rapidly increasing proportion of *Campylobacter* strains from all over the world have been found to be fluoroquinolone resistant (126–134). Primary quinolone resistance in humans was first noted in the early 1990s in Asia and in European countries such as Sweden, the Netherlands, Finland, and Spain. Not surprisingly, this coincided with the introduction of the fluoroquinolone enrofloxacin into food animals in those countries (135). A similar increase in fluoroquinolone resistance rates among human *Campylobacter* isolates was observed in the United Kingdom following the approval of the use of fluoroquinolones in veterinary animals there as well (126). In the United States, the licensure of sarafloxacin in 1995 and enrofloxacin in 1996 for use in poultry flocks contributed to an increase in the number of domestically acquired fluoroquinolone-resistant *Campylobacter* infections in Minnesota (127). In that state, fluoroquinolone resistance among human *Campylobacter* isolates increased from 1.3% in 1992 to 10.2% in 1998. The impact of fluoroquinolone use in food animals upon human health was the subject of a recent World Health Organization (WHO) Meeting (136). In addition to more prudent use of these agents in people, international controls on the use of antibiotics in food animals may become necessary to curtail the development of additional resistance among food-borne bacterial pathogens.

Most *C. jejuni* infections are still susceptible to erythromycin. Because this drug is safe, inexpensive, easy to administer, and has less of an inhibitory effect on fecal flora than do other antibiotics, it remains the treatment of choice for *C. jejuni* infections (Table 198.3). The newer macrolides (azithromycin, clarithromycin) are also effective in the treatment of *C. jejuni* infections,

---

TABLE 198.3. Oral Antimicrobial Agents Effective for Treatment of *Campylobacter* Infections

Agent	Doses	
	Adults	**Children**
Macrolides		
Erythromycin stearate[a]	250 mg p.o. q.i.d. for 5 days	10–15 mg/kg p.o. t.i.d. for 5 days
Azithromycin	500 mg p.o. on day 1; 250 mg/day on days 2–5	Not recommended for children <16 years old
Clarithromycin	250 mg p.o. every 12 h for 5 days	Safe doses not established
Quinolones		
Ciprofloxacin	500 mg p.o. b.i.d. for 5 days	Safe doses not established
Ofloxacin	200–400 mg p.o. b.i.d. for 5 days	Safe doses not established
Levofloxacin	500 mg p.o. daily for 5 days	Safe doses not established
Nitrofurans		
Furazolidone	100 mg p.o. q.i.d. for 5 days	1.25 mg/kg p.o. q.i.d. for 5 days
Alternatives		
Clindamycin	150–300 mg p.o. every 6 h for 5 days	2–4 mg/kg every 6 h for 5 days
Tetracycline	250–500 mg p.o. q.i.d.	6–12 mg/kg p.o. q.i.d. for children >8 years old

[a] Treatment of choice.
p.o., orally; b.i.d., twice daily; t.i.d., three times daily; q.i.d., four times daily.

but they are more expensive and have no proven advantage over erythromycin. For persons who reside in areas where fluoroquinolone resistance rates remain low, these agents have retained the advantage of being effective against a wide range of enteric pathogens. Because *Campylobacter* infections are clinically indistinguishable from infections caused by other bacterial enteric pathogens, fluoroquinolones may still be a good choice where rates of fluoroquinolone resistant *Campylobacter* are known to be low and when a bacterial gastroenteritis is suspected but no organisms have yet been isolated.

C. jejuni strains are almost universally resistant to cephalosporins, vancomycin, and rifampin; 25% are resistant to tetracycline. Susceptibility to ampicillin and trimethoprimsulfamethoxazole is variable. Fewer than 1% of *C. jejuni* strains are resistant to aminoglycosides and imipenem. Aminoglycosides may be used in extraintestinal *C. jejuni* infections, but oral therapy must also be given because they are ineffective against gut infections.

PREVENTION

Because most *C. jejuni* infections are transmitted via eating chicken, ultimately, the most effective way to control *C. jejuni* enteritis is to control infections in broiler flocks. *Campylobacter* infection of chickens is nearly universal. One raw chicken carcass may contain 10^6 *Campylobacter* organisms (110). Current mass processing and distribution of chicken may amplify the bacterial load; perhaps future work will devise a system that will produce chickens that are free of or only lightly colonized with campylobacters. Observing careful food preparation habits in the kitchen is also important in preventing infections. Chicken should be adequately cooked—not charred on the outside and left pink near the bone. Cutting boards and utensils used in handling uncooked poultry or other meats should be washed with hot soapy water before being used for preparation of salads or other foods eaten raw.

Although person-to-person transmission of *C. jejuni* infection is unusual, persons with any acute diarrheal illness should avoid preparation and handling of food until their illness resolves. Of course, as part of good general hygiene, all persons should wash their hands after using the bathroom, especially if they have diarrhea. Similarly, all people, but especially those who handle pets or other animals, should wash their hands before eating. Prevention of many outbreaks of *C. jejuni* infection could be accomplished by avoiding consumption of unpasteurized milk; this should be emphasized to pregnant women, the elderly, immunocompromised persons, or other persons in whom *C. jejuni* infection may have serious consequences. Travelers to developing countries and campers should be cautioned against drinking untreated water. Routine use of antibiotic prophylaxis to prevent *Campylobacter* infections is not recommended.

REFERENCES

1. Nachamkin I. *Campylobacter* and *Arcobacter*. In: Murray PR, Baron EJ, Pfaller MA, et al., eds. *Manual of clinical microbiology*, 6th ed. Washington, DC: American Society for Microbiology 1995:483–491.
2. Parkhill J, Wren BW, Mungall K, et al. The genome sequence of the foodborne pathogen *Campylobacter jejuni* reveals hypervariable sequences. *Nature* 2000;403:667–668.
3. Vandamme P, De Ley J. Proposal for a new family, Campylobacteraceae. *Int J Syst Bacteriol* 1991;41:451–455.
4. Wang WL, Blaser MJ. Detection of pathogenic *Campylobacter* species in blood culture systems. *J Clin Microbiol* 1986;23:709–714.
5. Wang WL, Reller LB, Smallwood B, et al. Evaluation of transport media and filtration for the isolation of *Campylobacter* in human fecal specimens. *J Clin Microbiol* 1983;18:803–807.
6. Smibert RM. Genus *Campylobacter* Sebald and Véon 1963, 907. In: Krieg NR, Holt JG, eds. *Bergey's manual of systematic bacteriology*, Vol. 1. Baltimore: Williams & Wilkins, 1984:111–118.
7. Lior H, Woodward DL, Edgar JA, et al. Serotyping of *Campylobacter jejuni* by slide agglutination based on heat-labile antigenic factors. *J Clin Microbiol* 1982;15:761–768.
8. Jones DM, Sutcliffe EM, Abbott JD. Serotyping of *Campylobacter* species by combined use of two methods. *Eur J Clin Microbiol* 1985;4:562–565.
9. Patton CM, Barrett TJ, Morris GK. Comparison of the Penner and Lior methods of serotyping *Campylobacter* spp. *J Clin Microbiol* 1985;22:558–565.
10. Nicholson MA, Patton CM. Application of Lior biotyping by use of genetically identified *Campylobacter* strains. *J Clin Microbiol* 1993;31:3348–3350.
11. Taylor DN, Blaser MJ. *Campylobacter* infections. In: Evans A, Brachman P, eds. *Bacterial infections of humans*. New York: Plenum, 1991:151–172.
12. Tauxe RV, Hargrett-Bean N, Patton CM, et al. *Campylobacter* isolates in the United States, 1982–1986. *MMWR* 1988;37:1–14.
13. Murray BJ. *Campylobacter* enteritis. A college campus average incidence and a prospective study of the risk factors for exposure. *West J Med* 1986;145:341–342.
14. Tauxe RV, Deming MS, Blake PA. *Campylobacter jejuni* infections on college campuses: a national survey. *Am J Public Health* 1985;75:659–660.
15. Mead PS, Slutsker L, Dietz V, et al. Food-related illness and death in the United States. *Emerg Infect Dis* 1999;5:607–625.
16. Preliminary FoodNet data on the incidence of foodborne illness—selected sites, United States, 1999. *MMWR* 2000;45(10):201–205.
17. Friedman CR, Neimann J, Wegener HC, et al. Epidemiology of *Campylobacter jejuni* infections in the United States and other industrialized nations. In: Nachamkin I, Blaser MJ, eds. *Campylobacter*, 2nd ed. Washington, DC: ASM Press, 2000:121–138.
18. Kendall EJ, Tanner El. *Campylobacter* enteritis in general practice. *J Hyg* 1982;88:155–163.
19. Taylor DN, Echeverria P, Pitarangsi C, et al. The influence of strain characteristics and immunity on the epidemiology of *Campylobacter* infections in Thailand. *J Clin Microbiol* 1988;26:863–868.
20. Glass RI, Stoll BJ, Huq MI, et al. Epidemiology and clinical features of endemic *Campylobacter jejuni* infection in Bangladesh. *J Infect Dis* 1983;148:292–296.
21. Seattle-King County Department of Public Health. Surveillance of the flow of *Salmonella* and *Campylobacter* in a community. Seattle, Communicable Disease Control Section, Seattle-King County Department of Public Health, 1984.
22. Deming MS, Tauxe RV, Blake PA, et al. *Campylobacter* enteritis at a university: transmission from eating chicken and from cats. *Am J Epidemiol* 1984:126:526–534.
23. Studahl A, Andersson Y. Risk factors for indigenous *Campylobacter* infection: a Swedish case-control study. *Epidemiol Infect* 2000;125(2):269–275.
24. Neal KR, Slack RC. The autumn peak in campylobacter gastro-enteritis. Are the risk factors the same for travel- and UK-acquired *Campylobacter* infections? *J Pub Health Med* 1995;17(1):98–102.
25. Food Safety and Inspection Service. Nationwide broiler chicken microbiologic baseline data collection program, 1994–1995. Washington, DC: U.S. Department of Agriculture, 1996.
26. Effler P, Ieong MC, Kimura A, et al. Sporadic *Campylobacter jejuni* infections in Hawaii: associations with prior antibiotic use and commercially prepared chicken. *J Infect Dis* 2001;183(7):1152–1155.
27. Harris NV, Thomson D, Martin DC, et al. A survey of *Campylobacter* and other bacterial contaminants of pre-market chicken and retail poultry and meats, King County, Washington. *Am J Public Health* 1986;76:401–406.
28. Wood RC, MacDonald KL, Osterholm MT. *Campylobacter* enteritis outbreaks associated with drinking raw milk during youth activities. *JAMA* 1992;268:3228–3230.
29. Palmer SR, McGuirk SM. Bird attacks on milk bottles and *Campylobacter* infections [Letter]. *Lancet* 1994;35:326–327.
30. Lighton LL, Kaczmarski EB, Jones DM. A study of risk factors for *Campylobacter* infections in late spring. *Public Health* 1991;105:199–203.
31. Mentzing LO. Waterborne outbreaks of *Campylobacter* enteritis associated with contaminated water. *Ann Intern Med* 1982;96:292–296.
32. Vogt RL, Sours HE, Barrett T, et al. *Campylobacter* enteritis associated with contaminated water. *Ann Intern Med* 1982;96:292–296.
33. Melby K, Dahl OP, Crisp L, Penner JL. Clinical and serological manifestations in patients during a waterborne epidemic due to *Campylobacter jejuni*. *J Infect* 1990;21:309–316.
34. Hopkins RS, Olmsted R, Istre GR. Endemic *Campylobacter jejuni* infection in Colorado: identified risk factors. *Am J Public Health* 1984;74:249–250.
35. Taylor DN, McDermott KT, Little JR, et al. *Campylobacter* enteritis from untreated water in the Rocky Mountains. *Ann Intern Med* 1983;99:38–40.
36. Kapperud G, Skjerve E, Bean NH, et al. Risk factors for sporadic *Campylobacter* infections: results of a case-control study in southeastern Norway. *J Clin Microbiol* 1992;30:3117–3121.
37. Wolfs TF, Duim B, Geelen SP, et al. Neonatal sepsis by *Campylobacter jejuni*: genetically proven transmission from a household puppy. *Clin Infect Dis* 2001;32(5):E97–E99.
38. Neimann J, Engberg J, Moelbak K, et al. Foodborne risk factors associated with sporadic campylobacteriosis in Denmark. *Dansk Veterinaertidsskrift* 1998;81:702–705.
39. Schorr D, Schmid H, Rieder HL, et al. Risk factors for *Campylobacter* enteritis in Switzerland. *Zentbl Hyg Umweltmed* 1994;196:327–337.

40. Blaser MJ, Waldman RJ, Barrett T, et al. Outbreaks of *Campylobacter* enteritis in two extended families: evidence for person-to-person transmission. *J Pediatr* 1981;98:254–257.

41. Oosterom J, den Uyl CH, Banffer JR, et al. Epidemiological investigations on *Campylobacter jejuni* in households with a primary infection. *J Hyg* 1984;93:325–332.

42. Olsen SJ, Hansen GR, Bartlett L, et at. An outbreak of *Campylobacter jejuni* infections associated with food handler contamination: the use of pulsed-field gel electrophoresis. *J Infect Dis* 2001;183(1):164–67.

43. Riordan T. Intestinal infection with *Campylobacter* in children [Letter]. *Lancet* 1988;1:992.

44. Calva JJ, Ruiz-Palacioz GM, Lopez-Vidal AB, et al. Cohort study of intestinal infection with *Campylobacter* in Mexican children. *Lancet* 1988;1:992.

45. Walder M. Epidemiology of *Campylobacter* enteritis. *Scand J Infect Dis* 1982; 14:27–33.

46. Kapperud G, Lassen J, Ostroff SM, et al. Clinical features of sporadic *Campylobacter* infections in Norway. *Scand J Infect Dis* 1992;24:741–749.

47. Smith GS, Blaser MJ. Fatalities associated with *Campylobacter jejuni* infections. *JAMA* 1985;253:2873–2875.

48. Blaser MJ, Wells JG, Feldman RA, et al. *Campylobacter* enteritis in the United States: a multicenter study. *Ann Intern Med* 1983;98:360–365.

49. Ponka A, Pitkanen T, Kosunen TU. *Campylobacter* enteritis mimicking acute abdominal emergency. *Acta Chir Scand* 1981;147:663–666.

50. Skirrow MB. *Campylobacter* enteritis: a "new" disease. *BMJ* 1977;2:9–11.

51. Pitkanen T, Ponka A, Pettersson T, et al. *Campylobacter* enteritis in 188 hospitalized patients. *Arch Intern Med* 1983;143:215–219.

52. Blaser MJ, Reller LB, Leuchtefeld NW, et al. *Campylobacter* enteritis in Denver. *West J Med* 1982;136:287–290.

53. Paulet P, Coffernils M. Very long-term diarrhea due to *Campylobacter jejuni*. *Postgrad Med J* 1990;66:410–411.

54. Richardson NJ, Koornhof HJ, Bokkenheuser VD. Long-term infections with *Campylobacter fetus subsp.* jejuni. *J Clin Biol* 1981;13:846–849.

55. Berezin S, Newman LJ. Prolonged mild diarrhea caused by *Campylobacter* [Letter]. *NY State J Med* 1986;86:29.

56. Blaser MJ, Berkowitz ID, LaForce M, et al. *Campylobacter* enteritis: clinical and epidemiologic features. *Ann Intern Med* 1979;91:179–185.

57. Van der Hoop AG, Veringa EM. Cholecystitis caused by *Campylobacter jejuni*. *Clin Infect Dis* 1993;17:133.

58. Ezpeleta C, de Ursa PR, Obregon F, et al. Acute pancreatitis associated with *Campylobacter jejuni* bacteremia. *Clin Infect Dis* 1992;15:1050.

59. Wood CJ, Fleming V, Turridge J, et al. *Campylobacter* peritonitis in continuous ambulatory peritoneal dialysis: report of eight cases and a review of the literature. *Am J Kidney Dis* 1992;19:257–263.

60. Frizelle FA, Rietveld JA. Spontaneous splenic rupture associated with *Campylobacter jejuni* infection. *Br J Surg* 1994;81:718.

61. Simor AE, Ferro S. *Campylobacter jejuni* infection occurring during pregnancy. *Eur J Clin Microbiol Infect Dis* 1990;9:142–144.

62. Skirrow MB, Jones DM, Sutcliffe E, et al. *Campylobacter* bacteremia in England and Wales, 1981–91. *Epidemiol Infect* 1993;110:567–573.

63. de Guevara CL, Gonzalez J, Pena P. Bacteraemia caused by *Campylobacter* spp. *J Clin Pathol* 1994;47:174–175.

64. Bretag AH, Archer RS, Atkinson HM, et al. Circadian urticara: another *Campylobacter* association [Letter]. *Lancet* 1984;1:954.

65. Lopez-Brea M, Fontelos PM, Baquero M, et al. Urticaria associated with *Campylobacter* enteritis [Letter]. *Lancet* 1984;1:954.

66. Mishu B, Blaser MJ. Role of infection due to *Campylobacter jejuni* in the initiation of Guillain-Barré syndrome. *Clin Infect Dis* 1993;17:104–108.

67. Allos BM, Lippy FE, Carlsen AR, et al. Serotype, serum resistance and ^{125}I-C3 binding among *C. jejuni* strains from patients with Guillain-Barré syndrome or with uncomplicated enteritis. *Emerg Infect Dis* 1998;4:263–268.

68. Wassenaar TM, Fry BN, Lastovica AJ. Genetic characterization of *Campylobacter jejuni* O:41 isolates in relation with Guillain-Barré syndrome. *J Clin Microbiol* 2000;38:874–876.

69. Mishu B, Amjad AA, Koski CL, et al. Serologic evidence of previous *Campylobacter jejuni* infection in patients with the Guillain-Barré syndrome. *Ann Intern Med* 1993;188:947–953.

70. Kuroki S, Saida T, Nukina M, et al. *Campylobacter jejuni* strains from patients with Guillain-Barré syndrome belong mostly to Penner serogroup 19 and contain β-N-acetylglucosamine. *Ann Neurol* 1993;22:243–247.

71. Yuki N, Taki T, Inagaki F, et al. A bacterium lipopolysaccharide that elicits Guillain-Barré syndrome has a GM1 ganglioside-like structure. *J Exp Med* 1993;178:1771–1775.

72. Gumpel JM, Martin C, Sanderson PJ. Reactive arthritis associated with *Campylobacter* enteritis. *Ann Rheum Dis* 1981;40:64–65.

73. Bremell T, Bjelle A, Svedhem A. Rheumatic symptoms following an outbreak of *Campylobacter* enteritis: a five year follow up. *Ann Rheum Dis* 1991;50:934–938.

74. Eastmond CJ, Rennie JA, Reid TM. An outbreak of *Campylobacter* enteritis: a rheumatological follow-up survey. *J Rheumatol* 1983;10:107–108.

75. Rautelin H, Koota K, von Essen R, et al. Waterborne *Campylobacter jejuni* epidemic in a Finnish hospital for rheumatic diseases. *Scand J Infect Dis* 1990;22:321–326.

76. Lever AML, Dolby JM, Webster ADB, et al. Chronic campylobacter colitis and uveitis in patient with hypogammaglobulinaemia. *BMJ* 1984;288:531.

77. Howard RS, Sarkies NJC, Sanders MD. Anterior uveitis associated with *Campylobacter jejuni* infection. *J Infect* 1987;14:186–187.

78. Wilson PG, Davies JR, Hoskins TW, et al. Epidemiology of an outbreak of milkborne enteritis in a residential school. In: Pearson AD, Skirrow MB, Rowe B, et al., eds. Campylobacter *II: Proceedings of the Second International Workshop on* Campylobacter *Infections*. London: Public Health Laboratory Service, 1983:143.

79. Lambert M, Marion E, Coche E, et al. *Campylobacter* enteritis and erythema nodosum. *Lancet* 1982;1:1409.

80. Ellis ME, Pope J, Mokashi A, et al. *Campylobacter* colitis associated with erythema nodosum. *BMJ* 1982;285:937.

81. Eastmond CJ, Reid TMS. *Campylobacter* enteritis and erythema nodosum. *BMJ* 1982;285:1421–1422.

82. Ashworth J, English JSC. Recurrent erythema nodosum and prolonged *Campylobacter jejuni* excretion. *BMJ* 1984;288:830.

83. Denneberg T, Freidberg M, Holmberg L, et al. Combined plasmapheresis and hemodialysis treatment for severe hemolticuremic syndrome following *Campylobacter* colitis. *Acta Paediatr Scand* 1982;71:243–245.

84. Chamovitz BN, Hartstein Al, Alexander SR, et al. *Campylobacter jejuni*–associated hemolytic-uremic syndrome in a mother and daughter. *Pediatrics* 1983;71:253–256.

85. Shulman ST, Moel D. *Campylobacter* infection [Letter]. *Pediatrics* 1983;72:437.

86. Dickgiesser A. Campylobakterinfektion und hämolytisch-uramisches Syndrom. *Immun Infect* 1983;11:71–74.

87. Delans RJ, Biuso JD, Saba SR, et al. Hemolytic uremic syndrome after *Campylobacter*-induced diarrhea in an adult. *Arch Intern Med* 1984;144:1074–1076.

88. Haq JA, Rahman KM, Akbar MS. Haemolytic-uraemic syndrome and *Campylobacter*. *Med J Aust* 1985;142:662–663.

89. Morton AR, Yu R, Waldek S, et al. *Campylobacter*-induced syndrome and *Campylobacter*. *Med J Aust* 1985;142:662–663.

90. May TH, Gerard A, Voiriot P, et al. Entéite á *Campylobacter jejuni* associée á un syndrome hémolytique et urémique. *Presse Med* 1986;15:803–804.

91. Sorvillo FJ, Lieb LE, Waterman SH. Incidence of campylobacteriosis among patients with AIDS in Los Angeles County. *J AIDS* 1991;4:598–602.

92. Nelson MR, Shanson DC, Hawkins DA, et al. *Salmonella, Campylobacter* and *Shigella* on HIV-seropositive patients. *AIDS* 1992;6:1495–1498.

93. Johnson RJ, Nolan C, Wang SP, et al. Persistent *Campylobacter jejuni* infection in an immunocompromised patient. *Ann Intern Med* 1984;100:832–834.

94. Wheeler AP, Gregg CR. *Campylobacter* bacteremia, cholecystitis, and the acquired immunodeficiency syndrome [Letter]. *Ann Intern Med* 1986;105:804.

95. Bernard E, Roger PM, Bonaldi CV, et al. Diarrhea and *Campylobacter* infections in patients infected with human immunodeficiency virus. *J Infect Dis* 1989;159:143–144.

96. Peterson MC, Farr RW, Castiglia M. Prosthetic hip infections and bacteremia due to *Campylobacter jejuni* in a patient with AIDS. *Clin Infect Dis* 1993;16:439–440.

97. Perlman DM, Ampel NM, Schifman RB, et al. Persistent *Campylobacter jejuni* infections in patients infected with human immunodeficiency virus (HIV). *Ann Intern Med* 1988;108:540–546.

98. Melamed I, Bujanover Y, Igra YS, et al. *Campylobacter* enteritis in normal and immunodeficient children. *Am J Dis Child* 1983;137:752–753.

99. Van der Meer JWM, Mouton RP, Daha MR, et al. *Campylobacter jejuni* bacteraemia as a cause of recurrent fever in a patient with hypogammaglobulinaemia. *J Infect* 1986;12:235–239.

100. Melamed A, Zakuth V, Schwartz D, et al. The immune system response to *Campylobacter* infection. *Microbiol Immunol* 1988;32:75–82.

101. Kerstens PJSM, Endtz HP, Meis JFGM, et al. Erysipelas-like skin lesions associated with *Campylobacter jejuni* septicemia in patients with hypogammaglobulinemia. *Eur J Clin Microbiol Infect Dis* 1992;11:842–847.

102. Hammarstrom V, Smith CIE, Hammarstrom L. Oral immunoglobulin treatment in *Campylobacter jejuni* enteritis [Letter]. *Lancet* 1993;341:1036.

103. Guerry P, Logan SM, Thornton S, et al. Genomic organization and expression of *Campylobacter* flagellin genes. *J Bacteriol* 1990;172:1853–1860.

104. Alm RA, Guerry P, Trust TJ. Distribution and polymorphism of the flagellin genes from isolates of *Campylobacter coli* and *Campylobacter jejuni*. *J Bacteriol* 1993;175:3051–3057.

105. McSweegan E, Walker RI. Identification and characterization of two *Campylobacter jejuni* adhesins for cellular and mucous substrates. *Infect Immun* 1986;53:141–148.

106. Lindblom GB, Cervantes LE, Sjogren E, et al. Adherence, enterotoxigenicity, invasiveness, and serogroups in *Campylobacter jejuni* and *Campylobacter coli* strains from adult humans with acute enterocolitis. *APMIS* 1990;98:179–184.

107. Black RE, Levine MM, Clements ML, et al. Experimental *Campylobacter jejuni* infection in humans. *J Infect Dis* 1988;157:472–479.

108. Robinson DA. Infective dose of *Campylobacter jejuni* in milk. *BMJ* 1981;282:1584.

109. Black RE, Perlman D, Clements ML, et al. Human volunteer studies with *Campylobacter jejuni*. In: Nachamkin I, Blaser MJ, Tompkins LS, eds. Campylobacter jejuni—current strategy and future trends. Washington, DC: American Society for Microbiology, 1992:207–215.

110. Hood AM, Pearson AD, Shahamat M. The extent of surface contamination of retailed chickens with *Campylobacter jejuni* serogroups. *Epidemiol Infect* 1988;100:17–25.

111. Blaser MJ, Duncan D. Human serum antibody response to *Campylobacter jejuni* infection as measured in an enzyme-linked immunosorbent assay. *Infect Immun* 1984;44:292–298.

112. Goossens H, Butzler JP, Takeda Y. Demonstration of cholera-like enterotoxin production by *Campylobacter jejuni*. *FEMS Microbiol Lett* 1985;29:73–76.

113. Lindblom GB, Johny M, Khalil K, et al. Enterotoxigenicity and frequency of *Campylobacter jejuni*, *C. coli*, and *C. laridis* in human and animal stool isolates from different countries. FEMS *Microbiol Lett* 1990;54:163–168.

114. Pérez-Pérez GI, Taylor DN, Echeverria PD, et al. Lack of evidence of enterotoxin involvement in pathogenesis of *Campylobacter* diarrhea. In: Nachamkin I, Blaser MJ, Tompkins LS, eds. *Campylobacter jejuni—current strategy and future trends*. Washington, DC: American Society for Microbiology, 1992:184–192.

115. Fauchere JL, Rosenau A, Veron M, et al. Association with HeLa cells of *Campylobacter jejuni* and *Campylobacter coli* isolated from human feces. *Infect Immun* 1986;54:283–287.

116. Kervella M, Pages J-M, Pei Z, et al. Isolation and characterization of two *Campylobacter* glycine-extracted proteins that bind to HeLa cell membranes. *Infect Immun* 1993;61:3440–448.

117. Pei Z, Blaser MJ. PEB1, the major cell-binding factor of *Campylobacter jejuni* is a homolog of the binding component in gram negative nutrient transport systems. *J Biol Chem* 1993;267:18717–18725.

118. Pei Z, Burucoa C, Grignon B, et al. Mutation in the *peb1A* locus of *Campylobacter jejuni* reduces interactions with epithelial cells and intestinal colonization of mice. *Infect Immun* 1998;66:935–943.

119. Bayerdorffer E, Hochter W, Schwarzkopf-Steinhauser G, et al. Bioptic microbiology in the differential diagnosis of enterocolitis. *Endoscopy* 1986;18:177–181.

120. Blaser MJ, Parsons RB, Wang WLL. Acute colitis caused by *Campylobacter fetus* ssp. *jejuni*. *Gastroenterology* 1980;78:448–453.

121. Surawicz CM, Belic L. Rectal biopsy helps to distinguish acute self-limited colitis from idiopathic inflammatory bowel disease. *Gastroenterology* 1984;86:104–113.

122. Price AB, Jewkes J, Sanderson PJ. Acute diarrhoea: *Campylobacter* colitis and the role of rectal biopsy. *J Clin Pathol* 1979;32:990–997.

123. Lawson AJ, Logan JM, O'Neill GL, et al. Large-scale survey of *Campylobacter* species in human gastroenteritis by PCR and PCR-enzyme-linked immunosorbent assay. *J Clin Microbiol* 1999;37:3860–3864.

124. Goodman LJ, Trenholme GM, Kaplan RL, et al. Empiric antimicrobial therapy of domestically acquired acute diarrhea in urban adults. *Arch Intern Med* 1990;150:541–546.

125. Petruccelli BP, Murphy GS, Sanchez JL, et al. Treatment of traveler's diarrhea with ciprofloxacin and loperamide. *J Infect Dis* 1992;165:557–560.

126. Sam WIC, Lyons MM, Waghorn DJ. Increasing rates of ciprofloxacin resistant *Campylobacter*. *J Clin Pathol* 1999;52:709–710.

127. Smith KE, Besser JM, Hedberg CW, et al. Quinolone-resistant *Campylobacter jejuni* infections in Minnesota, 1992–1998. *N Engl J Med* 1999;340:1525–1532.

128. Sjogren E, Lindblom G-B, Kaijser B. Norfloxacin resistance in *Campylobacter jejuni* and *Campylobacter coil* isolates from Swedish patients. *J Antimicrob Chemother* 1997;40:257–261.

129. Prasad KN, Mathur SK, Dhole TN, et al. Antimicrobial susceptibility and plasmid analysis of *Campylobacter jejuni* isolated from diarrhoeal patients and healthy-chickens in northern India. *J Diarrhoeal Dis Res* 1994;12(4):270–273.

130. Hoge CW, Gambel JM, Srijan A, et al. Trends in antibiotic resistance among diarrheal pathogens isolated in Thailand over 15 years. *Clin Infect Dis* 1999;1998;26:341–345.

131. Saenz Y, Zarazaga M, Lantero M, et al. Antibiotic resistance in *Campylobacter* strains isolated from animals, foods, and humans in Spain in 1997–1998. *Antimicrob Agent Chemother* 2000;44:267–271.

132. Engberg J, Aarestrup FM, Taylor DE, et al. Quinolone and macrolide resistance in *Campylobacter jejuni* and *C. coli*: resistance mechanisms and trends in human isolates. *Emerg Infect Dis* 2001;7(1):24–34.

133. Wistrom J, Jertborn M, Ekwall E, et al. Empiric treatment of acute diarrheal disease with norfloxacin. *Ann Intern Med* 1992;117:202–208.

134. Rautelin H, Renkonen OV, Kosunen TU. Emergence of fluoroquinolone resistance in *Campylobacter jejuni* and *Campylobacter coil* in subjects from Finland. *Antimicrob Agents Chemother* 1991;35:2065–2069.

135. Endtz HP, Ruijs GJ, van Klingeren B, et al. Quinolone resistance in *Campylobacter* isolated from man and poultry following the introduction of fluoroquinolones in veterinary medicine. *J Antimicrob Chemother* 1991;27:199–208.

136. *Use of quinolones in food animals and potential impact on human health. Report and proceedings of a WHO meeting, Geneva, Switzerland, June 2–June 5, 1998.* Geneva, Switzerland: World Health Organization, 1998.

CHAPTER 199
Vibrios

G. Balakrish Nair and David A. Sack

In the recent issue of the *Bergey's Manual of Systematic Bacteriology*, the family Vibrionaceae is classified into six genera, namely *Vibrio*, *Allomonas*, *Enhydrobacter*, *Listonella*, *Photobacterium* and *Salinivibrio* (1). The vibrios are a group of gram-negative, curved or straight motile rods that normally inhabit the aquatic environments. Currently, the genus consists of 51 species, of which at least 12 are known to be associated with human disease. Six of the *Vibrio* species (*V. cholerae*, *V. parahaemolyticus*, *V. fluvialis*, *V. furnissii*, *V. hollisae* and *V. mimicus*) are primarily associated with diarrheal disease, two generally cause wound infections (*V. alginolyticus* and *V. damsela*), *V. vulnificus* is an important cause of septicemia in alcoholics and immunosuppressed hosts, while the significance of isolation of three species (*V. cincinnatiensis*, *V. carchariae* and *V. metschnikovii*) from humans remains to be determined. Many of the strains have specific virulence factors, such as toxins, capsules, or colonization factors that increase virulence or explain the mechanism of the symptoms that the organisms produce. Also, certain host factors, especially hypochlorhydria, immunodeficiency, cirrhosis, hemochromatosis, and diabetes, increase susceptibility to or severity of the infection. The natural habitat of vibrios is the aquatic ecosystem, where they can be found as free-living bacterium or in association with phytoplankton and crustaceans. All *Vibrio* species are common to marine and estuarine environments and exhibit dramatic increases in cell densities in warmer months (particularly in temperate climates), correlating with corresponding increases in disease prevalence. The biochemical characteristics of the clinically important vibrios that are useful for their laboratory identification are shown in Table 199.1.

VIBRIO CHOLERAE O1 AND O139

V. cholerae is of special interest because it includes the serogroups that cause epidemic and pandemic cholera, serogroups O1 and O139. The current serotyping scheme of *V. cholerae* recognizes 206 serogroups. Strains belonging to other serogroups (e.g., serogroups O2 to O138 or O140 to O206; collectively known as non-O1 non-O139 serogroups or also as nonepidemic *V. cholerae*) and strains that are not toxin producing (even if they are serogroup O1 or O139) may cause sporadic illnesses, but they have never caused widespread epidemics and thus are of less public health importance. Epidemic strains of O1 and O139 are also distinguished from most others by their production of cholera toxin (CT) and a toxin-coregulated pilus (TCP).

Cholera is an illness characterized by severe watery diarrhea. In suspected cases of cholera, fecal specimens should be cultured for vibrios. Cholera is more likely in patients who live in cholera-endemic areas or have recently (within the preceding week) traveled to a cholera area or eaten seafood from a cholera area (including the Gulf Coast of the United States) during the warm months. *V. cholerae* survives well in fecal specimens en route to the laboratory if kept moist, but if there is a delay of more than a few hours, Cary-Blair transport medium should be used. The feces (either fresh or in the transport medium) should then be plated onto thiosulfate citrate bile salts sucrose (TCBS) agar, a medium that inhibits most normal flora but supports the growth of the vibrios. In addition, the specimen should be

TABLE 199.1.   Key Differential Tests for Clinically Important *Vibrio* Species

Species	Growth in nutrient broth 0% NaCl	1% NaCl	Oxidase	Nitrate to nitrite	Myoinositol fermentation	Arginine dihydrolase	Lysine decarboxylase	Ornithine decarboxylase
V. cholerae	+	+	+	+	−	−	+	+
V. mimicus	+	+	+	+	−	−	+	+
V. metschnikovii	−	+	−	−	V	V	V	+
V. cincinnatiensis	−	+	+	+	+	V	V	−
V. hollisae	−	+	+	+	+	−	−	−
V. damsela	−	+	+	+	−	+	V	−
V. fluvialas	−	+	+	+	−	+	−	−
V. furnissii	−	+	+	+	−	+	−	−
V. alginolyticus	−	+	+	+	−	−	−	−
V. parahaemolyticus	−	+	+	+	−	−	+	V
V. vulnificus	−	+	+	+	+	−	+	V

+, more than 90% positive; −, less than 10% positive; V, 10%–90% positive.
Adapted from Bopp CA, Kay BA, Wells JG. *Laboratory methods for the diagnosis of Vibrio cholerae.* Atlanta: National Center for Infectious Diseases, Centers for Disease Control and Prevention, 1994.

inoculated into alkaline peptone water, a high-pH enrichment broth, which preferentially supports the growth of vibrios. After 6 to 18 hours of incubation at 37°C, a second TCBS plate is inoculated. The TCBS plates are incubated for 18 to 24 hours at 37°C. *V. cholerae* colonies appear as smooth yellow colonies. Presumptive identification of *V. cholerae* O1 can be made on the basis of typical colonies, which are oxidase positive and agglutinate with O1 or O139 antiserum. Agglutination should be carried out after subculture onto a nonselective agar (e.g., nutrient or trypticase soy agar) because colonies from TCBS may give atypical agglutination results. If such colonies are recovered, they should be reported immediately to the state health department and sent to the appropriate referral laboratory for confirmation.

V. cholerae organisms are short, curved rods (hence their historic name, the comma bacillus). They are oxidase positive; have a single polar flagellum; ferment glucose, sucrose, and mannitol; and produce lysine and ornithine decarboxylase. Strains associated with epidemics produce a potent enterotoxin, but not all strains of *V. cholerae* O1 produce the toxin. Isolates, especially from surface waters, may be serogroup O1 but do not produce the toxin, and these nontoxigenic strains do not represent a cholera threat.

V. cholerae serogroup O1 is classified into two serotypes (Ogawa and Inaba) and two biotypes (classical and *eltor*). Classical strains predominated until they were replaced by the *eltor* strains during the seventh pandemic, which began in the 1960s. Until 1995, classical strains could be isolated only in southern Bangladesh but it has now completely disappeared. *Eltor* strains are found throughout Asia, Africa, and South America. The *eltor* strains appear better suited to the environmental waters and persist there once established. Fewer of those infected with *eltor* strains develop severe cholera, and there are more asymptomatic infections. Among patients with severe cholera, however, the clinical illness is identical regardless of biotype. The *eltor* strains are distinguished from classical strains by agglutination with chicken red blood cells, their resistance to polymyxin B and resistance to specific lytic phages.

The serotype, defined by agglutination with monovalent antiserum, is a useful marker for strains, but the clinical illness of Ogawa and Inaba strains is identical. Also, strains occasionally switch between the two serotypes during an epidemic season, so this marker is not altogether stable. A few unusual strains agglutinate with both Inaba and Ogawa monospecific antiserum and are designated Hikojima strains.

The major virulence factor for *V. cholerae* O1 and O139 is cholera toxin (CT), but additional properties include the colonization pili (mannose-sensitive hemagglutinin and toxin-coregulated pilus). The flagellum can also be considered a virulence factor because motility increases virulence. The cholera toxin genes are within the genome of a filamentous M-13–related phage designated CTXφ (2). Although a CTXφ prophage can be carried as a plasmid, it is usually found integrated into the chromosome, often in a multicopy tandem array, and controlled by a prophage repressor. The genes for TCP form part of a 40-kb segment that is absent from nonepidemic strains that has been designated as pathogenicity island (3) and that might also correspond to a temperate filamentous phage (4). As remarkable examples of evolutionary coadaptation, the CTXφ virion uses TCP as receptor during infection (2). The entire genome sequence of *V. cholerae* O1 (biotype eltor) was recently completed, which showed that the genome consists of two circular chromosomes (5). The large chromosome contains most of the genes that are required for growth and pathogenicity while some of the components of several essential metabolic and regulatory pathways reside on the small chromosome. Unlike *V. cholerae* O1, serogroup O139 possesses a capsule distinct from the lipopolysaccharide antigens and has 3,6-dideoxyhexose (abequose or colitose), quinovosamine and glucosamine, and traces of tetradecanoic and hexadecanoic fatty acids (6).

The nature of the persistence of *V. cholerae* between epidemic seasons has been of great interest because, in many locations, cases completely disappear and the bacterium cannot be cultured from surface waters. It now appears that *V. cholerae* (and other vibrios) may enter a viable but nonculturable survival form— a form in which the bacterium metabolizes slowly but is not detectable with use of usual culture media (7). Under certain conditions, it can then revert to the normal form.

Molecular methods (e.g., plasmid profiles, ribotyping, restriction fragment length polymorphisms, multilocus enzyme electrophoresis, DNA sequencing of selected genes, and others) have become useful in characterizing strains of *V. cholerae* and have revealed a great diversity of subtypes. By use of these molecular techniques, strains can be characterized as belonging to clusters associated with certain geographic regions (8). Furthermore, by using polymerase chain reaction techniques, specimens can be screened for both culturable and nonculturable forms. These methods provide a greatly improved understanding of the molecular epidemiology of the organism and improve the sensitivity of detecting the bacterium.

Clinically useful rapid methods are now also available to detect cases of cholera. The most practical of the rapid tests include dark-field examination of stool specimens; coagglutination tests using antibody-coated *Staphylococcus aureus* cells (Cowan 1 strain); and the sensitive membrane antigen rapid test (9), a membrane-bound monoclonal antibody-based test that uses a gold label to detect the O antigen in the specimen in about 5 minutes. If the case is the first in a geographic area, the results of the rapid test must be confirmed with culture.

In the past, most strains of *V. cholerae* were sensitive to the clinically useful antibiotics, but in recent years, reports of toxigenic *V. cholerae* strains resistant to the antibiotics commonly used for treatment are appearing with increasing frequency. Many recent epidemics have been due to plasmid-containing strains, which render them resistant to multiple antibiotics including tetracycline (which was the drug of choice), ampicillin, chloramphenicol, trimethoprim, and others. Thus, antibiotic sensitivity patterns of local strains must be determined to establish optimal antibiotic therapy.

OTHER VIBRIOS

Vibrio cholerae non-O1, non-O139

Strains of *V. cholerae* that do not agglutinate with O1 or O139 antiserum are known as non-O1, non-O139 *V. cholerae* (formerly called nonagglutinating vibrios). The non-O1, non-O139 serogroups comprise a heterogeneous group, which give the same reactions in microbiologic tests as that of the O1 and O139 serogroups. Few laboratories perform serotyping for these strains, and from a clinical perspective, knowing the specific serogroup is not important; hence, except in unusual outbreaks, sending these strains to a reference laboratory for serotyping is not needed. These bacteria most often cause watery diarrhea, but they may rarely cause systemic infections (bacteremia or meningitis) and wound infections, especially in patients with increased susceptibility due to immunodeficiency, cirrhosis, or hemochromatosis.

Although cholera toxin (CT) and nonagglutinable vibrio heat-stable enterotoxin (NAG-ST) have been described as important virulence factors for non-O1 *V. cholerae*, these toxins are relatively rare among clinical isolates. A wide range of other determinants, including cytotoxins, hemolysins, colonization factors, and a CT-like toxin, have been described as virulence factors for non-O1 non-O139 *V. cholerae* (10). Although not associated with epidemics, there has been an increasing tendency to isolate these organisms from hospitalized patients, in recent years. At least three localized outbreaks of diarrhea caused by non-O1 non-O139 have been described in the recent past. These include an outbreak caused by *V. cholerae* O10 and O12 in February 1994 in Lima, Peru (11), another caused by O10 in East Delhi, India (12), and an epidemic caused by non-O1 *V. cholerae* that produced ST among Khmers in a camp in Thailand (13). Other nonepidemic serogroups of *V. cholerae* have been associated primarily with sporadic cases (10,14).

Vibrio mimicus

The species *V. mimicus* was first proposed to encompass biochemically atypical non-O1 *V. cholerae* isolates. *V. mimicus* can be readily differentiated from *V. cholerae* on the basis of

negative reactions in sucrose, Voger-Proskauer, corn oil, and Jordan tartarate reactions (15). Some strains of *V. mimicus* produce a heat-labile enterotoxin similar to CT as well as other toxins and toxic substances that might contribute to its pathogenesis. CT, however, is the main factor responsible for the severity of the diarrhea (16). It differs from *V. cholerae* epidemiologically in not being associated with epidemics. Cases occur mostly in patients in the Indian subcontinent but are occasionally seen in other areas. Consumption of *V. mimicus*–contaminated shellfish has been linked to the development of gastroenteritis. Turtle eggs serve as potential sources of *V. mimicus* diarrhea in tropical countries where turtle eggs are used for human consumption (17).

Vibrio parahaemolyticus

V. parahaemolyticus is a halophilic (salt-loving) marine *Vibrio* that causes gastroenteritis in humans by consumption of contaminated seafoods and is especially common among people who eat raw or undercooked seafood. Unlike *V. cholerae*, where only two serogroups (O1 and O139) are involved in causing epidemic and pandemic disease, *V. parahaemolyticus* gastroenteritis is a multiserogroup affliction, and as many as 76 different combinations of O and K serotypes are currently recognized and known to be associated with gastroenteritis. *V. parahaemolyticus* was commonly isolated in Japan, but is now recognized as a pathogen in all parts of the world, including both industrialized and developing countries. Outbreaks do occur and are nearly always due to consumption of seafood.

V. parahaemolyticus diarrheal disease is toxin mediated, and at least two toxins have been identified as potential virulence factors that include the thermostable direct hemolysin (TDH) and the TDH-related hemolysin (TRH) (18). The TDH strains are β-hemolytic on Wagatsuma agar and are known as Kanagawa-positive strains, but those that produce TDH-related hemolysin may be Kanagawa negative. The presence of either one or both of the virulence genes, namely *tdh* or *trh,* differentiates the pathogenic strains from the nonpathogenic strains. The exact mechanism by which TDH or TRH causes gastroenteritis is still not clearly known. However, these factors can now best be detected with use of gene probe techniques. *V. parahaemolyticus* produces a capsular polysaccharide whose role in pathogenesis is unknown but whose antigenic properties have been used for serotyping. Because most environmental strains, as well as other vibrios, are negative for both TDH and TDH-related hemolysin, detection of these markers helps in differentiating pathogenic from nonpathogenic strains. Most patients with *V. parahaemolyticus* infection have acute watery diarrhea, but occasionally systemic infections (e.g., sepsis and wound infections) may occur (19), especially in patients at increased risk because of immunodeficiency or liver cirrhosis.

Before 1996, *V. parahaemolyticus* was sporadically isolated with diverse serogroups being involved in disease in different geographic areas. Beginning in February 1996, a new clone of *tdh*- positive and *trh*-negative *V. parahaemolyticus* belonging to the O3:K6 serotype was responsible for a dramatic increase in the number of cases of diarrhea in Calcutta, India (20). An increase in incidence of *V. parahaemolyticus* food poisoning observed during 1997 and 1998 was also ascribed to increased incidence of O3:K6 food poisoning in Japan (21). Evidence supporting the hypothesis that the O3:K6 clone emerged recently and had pandemic potential was recently presented (22). The *V. parahaemolyticus* pandemic has presently spread into at least eight countries, and the emergence of two other serotypes (O4:K68 and O1:KUT) possessing the pandemic potential has been documented (23,24). Three large outbreaks caused by this serogroup have also been reported in the United States on the Gulf, Atlantic, and Pacific coasts (24). Molecular analysis of these additional serotypes indicates that they may have diverged from the pandemic O3:K6 strains by alteration of the O:K antigens (21,23). Thus, *V. parahaemolyticus* is an emerging pathogen and the second *Vibrio* that has acquired the potential of causing pandemics.

Fecal specimens of patients with a suspected *Vibrio* infection should be cultured with use of TCBS agar because these organisms may not be recognized on the routine media used for isolation of *Salmonella* and *Shigella*, unless oxidase-positive colonies are identified. On TCBS agar, green, sucrose-negative colonies are seen. Once isolated, the colonies can be identified by use of biochemical tests. *V. parahaemolyticus* is a halophilic vibrio (e.g., the organisms grow in nutrient broth containing 1% sodium chloride, but not in the same broth without salt). Other biochemical tests useful in differentiating this from other vibrios are shown in Table 199.1. If there is a delay in transporting the specimen to the laboratory, Cary-Blair transport medium should be used to preserve the strains en route.

Vibrio vulnificus

V. vulnificus has become the most common *Vibrio* causing serious morbidity and mortality in the United States (25,26) and is associated primarily with systemic infections. Rarely, it causes diarrhea. When persons with an underlying illness (e.g., immunodeficiency, cirrhosis, hemochromatosis, diabetes) ingest foods contaminated with the bacteria, the bacteria can invade and cause severe sepsis associated with high case-fatality rates (about 50%). The organism may also infect wounds, leading to severe necrotic wound infections and sepsis, also associated with high case-fatality rates (about 25%). The wound infections frequently have bullous lesions, which provide a clue to the cause, and the organism can often be identified in the bullous fluid. Among the survivors of the wound infection, disability is common because the infections are so destructive to the tissue.

A hemolytic toxin, encoded by the *vvh* gene, has been identified, but mutants that do not express the toxin remain virulent in animal models (27). Capsular polysaccharide is clearly required for virulence of this organism (28) and may play a direct role in the disease lethality by mediating host cytokine responses (29). *V. vulnificus* produces several enzymes (e.g., lipase, hyaluronidase, mucinase, DNase) (30). Encapsulated strains predominate among clinical isolates but are unusual in environmental specimens. Encapsulated strains of *V. vulnificus* also persist longer in oyster tissues than unencapsulated isolates, either by evading phagocytic hemocytes of oysters or by surviving within the hemocytes (31).

In the United States, there is a marked seasonality of *V. vulnificus* infections, with most occurring during the warm months of the year. Persons with a predisposing risk factor should be warned against consumption of raw or undercooked seafood (especially raw oysters), especially during the summer.

OTHER HALOPHILIC VIBRIOS

Vibrio fluvialis is closely related to *Aeromonas* and is commonly found in brackish waters. It can cause severe diarrhea (31). *Vibrio hollisae* and *Vibrio furnissii* similarly are causes of diarrhea. Like *V. vulnificus*, *V. hollisae* may rarely cause sepsis in susceptible hosts. Unlike other vibrios, *V. hollisae* does not grow well on TCBS agar.

Vibrio alginolyticus and *Vibrio damsela* are rare causes of sepsis or wound infections and are associated with exposure to seawater or seafood. The other vibrios of medical importance listed in Table 199.1 (*V. metschnikovii, V. cincinnatiensis, V. carchariae*) are extremely rare causes of systemic illness in humans, and descriptions of infection caused by these organisms have been restricted to case reports.

REFERENCES

1. Garrity GM, Winters M, Searies DB. Taxonomic outline of the Procaryotes. *Bergey's manual of systematic bacteriology,* 2nd ed. (Release 1.0, April 2001). New York: Springer-Verlag, 2001.
2. Waldor MK, Mekalanos JJ. Lysogenic conversion by a filamentous phage encoding cholera toxin. *Science* 1996;272:1910–1914.
3. Karaolis DKR, Johnson JA, Bailey CC, et al. A *Vibrio cholerae* pathogenicity island associated with epidemic and pandemic strains. *Proc Natl Acad Sci USA* 1998;95:3134–3139.
4. Karaolis DKR, Somara S, Maneval DR, et al. A bacteriophage encoding a pathogenicity island, a type IV pilus and a phage receptor in cholera bacteria. *Nature* 1999;399:375–379.
5. Heidelberg JF, Eisen JA, Nelson WC, et al. DNA sequence of both chromosomes of the cholera pathogen *Vibrio cholerae*. *Nature* 2000;406:477–483.
6. Colwell RR, Huq A. Vibrios in the environment: viable but nonculturable *Vibrio cholerae*. *Vibrio cholerae* and cholera. Washington, DC: American Society for Microbiology, 1994:117–133.
7. Johnson JA, Salles CA, Panigrahi P, et al. *Vibrio cholerae* O139 synonym Bengal is closely related to *Vibrio cholerae* O1 ElTor, but has important differences. *Infect Immun* 1994;62:2108–2110.
8. Wachsmuth IK, Evins GM, Fields PI, et al. The molecular epidemiology of cholera in Latin America. *J Infect Dis* 1993;167:621–626.
9. Hasan JA, Huq A, Tamplin ML, et al. A novel kit for rapid detection of *Vibrio cholerae* O1. *J Clin Microbiol* 1994;32:249–252.
10. Morris JG Jr. Non-O group 1 *Vibrio cholerae*: a look at the epidemiology of an occasional pathogen. *Epidemiol Rev* 1990;12:179–191.
11. Dalsgaard A, Albert MJ, Taylor DN, et al. Characterization of *Vibrio cholerae* non-O1 serogroup obtained from an outbreak of diarrhea in Lima, Peru. *J Clin Microbiol* 1995;33:2715–2722.
12. Rudra S, Mahajan R, Mathur M, et al. Cluster of cases of clinical cholera due to *Vibrio cholerae* O10 in east Delhi. *Ind J Med Res* 1996;103:71–73.
13. Bagchi K, Echeverria P, Authur JD, et al. Epidemic diarrhea caused by *Vibrio cholerae* non-O1 that produced heat-stable toxin among Khmers in a camp in Thailand. *J Clin Microbiol* 1993;31:1315–1317.
14. Ramamurthy T, Bag PK, Pal A, et al. Virulence patterns of *Vibrio cholerae* non-O1 strains isolated from hospitalized patients with acute diarrhea in Calcutta, India. *J Med Microbiol* 1993;39:310–317.
15. Davis BR, Fanning GR, Madden JM, et al. Characterization of biochemically atypical *Vibrio cholerae* strains and designation of a new pathogenic species, *Vibrio mimicus*. *J Clin Microbiol* 1976;14:631–639.
16. Chowdhury MA, Aziz KM, Kay BA, et al. Toxin production by *Vibrio mimicus* strains isolated from human and environmental sources in Bangladesh. *J Clin Microbiol* 1987;25:2200–2203.
17. Campos E, Bolanos H, Teresa M, et al. *Vibrio mimicus* diarrhea following ingestion of raw turtle eggs. *Appl Environ Microbiol* 1996;62:1141–1144.
18. Shirai H, Ito H, Hirayama T, et al. Molecular epidemiologic evidence for association of thermostable direct hemolysin (TDH) and TDH-related hemolysin of *Vibrio parahaemolyticus* with gastroenteritis. *Infect Immun* 1990;58:3568–3573.
19. Klontz KC. Fatalities associated with *Vibrio parahaemolyticus* and *Vibrio cholerae* non-O1 infections in Florida (1981 to 1988). *South Med J* 1990;83:500–502.
20. Okuda J, Ishibashi M, Hayakawa E, et al. Emergence of a unique O3:K6 clone of *Vibrio parahaemolyticus* in Calcutta, India, and isolation of strains from the same clonal group from southeast Asian travellers arriving in Japan. *J Clin Microbiol* 1997;35:3150–3155.
21. World Health Organization. *Vibrio parahaemolyticus*, Japan, 1996–1998. *Weekly Epidemiol Rec* 1999;74:357–364.
22. Matsumoto C, Okuda J, Ishibashi M, et al. Pandemic spread of an O3:K6 clone of *Vibrio parahaemolyticus* and emergence of related strains evidenced by arbitrarily primed PCR and *toxRS* sequence analyses. *J Clin Microbiol* 2000;38:578–585.
23. Chowdhury NR, Chakraborty S, Ramamurthy T, et al. Molecular evidence of clonal *Vibrio parahaemolyticus* pandemic strains. *Emerg Infect Dis* 2000;6:631–636.
24. Centers for Disease Control and Prevention. Vibrio *surveillance system, summary data, 1997–1998*. Atlanta, GA: Centers for Disease Control and Prevention, 1999.
25. Hlady WG, Mullen RC, Hopkin RS: *Vibrio vulnificus* from raw oysters. Leading cause of reported deaths from foodborne illness in Florida. *J Fla Med Assoc* 1993;80:536–538.
26. Morris JG Jr. *Vibrio vulnificus*—a new monster of the deep? *Ann Intern Med* 1988;109:261–263.
27. Wright AC, Morris JG Jr, Maneval DR Jr, et al. Cloning of the cytotoxin-hemolysin gene of *Vibrio vulnificus*. *Infect Immun* 1985;50:922–924.

28. Wright AC, Powell JL, Tanner MK, et al. Differential expression of *Vibrio vulnificus* capsular polysaccharide capsular polysaccharide. *Infect Immun* 1999;67:717–724.
29. Powell JL, Wright AC, Wasserman SS, et al. Release of tumor necrosis factor alpha in response to *Vibrio vulnificus* capsular polysaccharide in *in vivo* and *in vitro* models. *Infect Immun* 1997;65:3713–3718.
30. Hayat U, Reddy GP, Bush CA, et al. Capsular types of *Vibrio vulnificus*: an analysis of strains from clinical and environmental sources. *J Infect Dis* 1993;168:758–762.
31. Klontz KC, Desenclos JC. Clinical and epidemiological features of sporadic infections with *Vibrio fluvialis* in Florida, USA. *J Diarrhoeal Dis Res* 1990;8:24–26.

CHAPTER 200
Francisella tularensis, Pasteurella, *and* Yersinia pestis

Shirish S. Huprikar and Edward J. Bottone

FRANCISELLA TULARENSIS

The species *Francisella tularensis* consists of several subspecies that differ in their virulence and epidemiology. *F. tularensis* biovar tularensis (type A) is the most virulent subspecies and is predominantly isolated in North America. *F. tularensis* biovar palaearctica (type B) is less virulent and predominantly isolated in Asia and Europe, and to a lesser extent in North America.

Types A and B are the causative agents of tularemia, a human zoonosis affecting skin and internal organs. *F. tularensis* biovar novicida (type C) is less virulent in humans and is primarily an animal pathogen (1). *F. philomiragia* (formerly *Yersinia philomiragia*) represents another species within the genus *Francisella* that rarely causes disease in humans (1).

F. tularensis is maintained in nature through an enzootic cycle involving rodents, lagomorphs (rabbits, hares, and pikas), ticks, mosquitoes, and other blood-sucking arthropods (2) and has been isolated from approximately 250 wildlife species. *F. tularensis* is widely distributed geographically with cases of tularemia reported in North America, Scandinavia, Russia, Japan, and the Middle East (3,4). In 1997, an outbreak of tularemia associated with hare hunting affected 585 patients in Spain (5). One year later, another outbreak of ulceroglandular tularemia associated with crayfish in a contaminated freshwater stream, geographically distant from the prior outbreak, affected 19 patients in Spain (6). Most of the infections occurred following crayfish-related injuries while fishing or cleaning. In the United States, the disease occurs in the central, southern, and southwestern parts of the country, but the incidence of reported cases has steadily declined since 1950 (7). A tick-borne outbreak involving 50 soldiers occurred in Tennessee in 1943 (8). Although the disease is rare in New England states (9), 47 cases linked to contact with muskrats occurred in Vermont (10).

F. tularensis is a minute, nonmotile, non–spore-forming and faintly staining gram-negative coccobacillus. Capsules may be discerned in clinical material. Although uniform morphologic features are observed *in vivo* and in young cultures, marked pleomorphism, manifested by swollen oval bodies and teardrop-shaped bacillary forms, may prevail in older cultures. Bipolar morphology is particularly evident with Giemsa stain.

Growth occurs optimally under aerobic conditions at 37°C in media supplemented with cystine or cysteine and defibrinated rabbit blood or human packed red blood cells (3,11). Cysteine heart agar (CHA) supplemented with 9% chocolatized sheep red blood cells is the preferred medium for isolation of *F. tularensis* (7). Colonies typically develop within 3 to 5 days of incubation but may take as long as 3 weeks. For contaminated clinical specimens (e.g., skin, sputum, gastric lavage fluid), antibiotic-containing media such as Thayer-Martin chocolate agar, which is also supplemented with cysteine-containing Isovitalex, may also be used for isolation (12). *F. tularensis* also grows on buffered charcoal yeast extract (BCYE) media, typically used for *Legionella* isolation. Inoculation of thioglycollate broth, which contains cysteine, is also recommended (7). Due to the highly infectious nature of *F. tularensis*, it is stressed that attempts at cultivation be undertaken only under aseptic technique with meticulous laboratory conditions (class I or III exhaust cabinet) (11). Once isolated, *F. tularensis* may be confirmed serologically through agglutination with specific antisera. Rapid techniques such as immunofluorescence and enyme-linked immunosorbent assays (ELISA) have been developed to detect *F. tularensis* antigens in clinical specimens. The polymerase chain reaction (PCR) has been used to detect *F. tularensis* DNA in wound specimens in 30 of 40 patients with serologically confirmed ulceroglandular tularemia. Positive cultures were achieved in only 10 of the 40 patients (13). Differentiation of the virulent *F. tularensis* biovar tularensis from the serologically identical but less virulent *F. tularensis* biovar palaearctica (14) and the virulent animal pathogen *F. tularensis* biovar novicida may be achieved through comparison of biochemical characteristics (15). PCR has also been used to discriminate between the human pathogens (16).

The clinical manifestations of tularemia and their categorization into glandular, ulceroglandular, oculoglandular, oropharyngeal, typhoidal, and pneumonic depend on the route of acquisition or portal of entry of the organism (Table 200.1). Infection is initiated by as few as 25 aerosolized cells or 10 subcutaneously inoculated biovar tularensis organisms (17,18). General symptoms accompanying infection include fever, chills, headache, cough, and myalgias (3). Infection with *F. tularensis* induces serum agglutinin titers of 1:160 or greater, which usually develop during the second week of infection (19). Natural infection confers lifelong immunity.

Virulence of *F. tularensis* is associated with the presence of a capsule composed of lipid, protein, and carbohydrate (20). In contrast to the attenuated live vaccine strain, which is poorly encapsulated, or a capsule-deficient mutant of the live vaccine strain that shows decreased virulence (21), wild-type encapsulated strains are slowly phagocytosed (22) and are able to withstand the lethal effects of polymorphonuclear lysosomal oxidants, including hypochlorous acid (23). Although the capsules of wild-type *F. tularensis* may protect against hypochlorous acid, the exact mechanism underscoring resistance to polymorphonuclear oxidants by wild-type *F. tularensis* is unknown. The capsule also seems to protect *F. tularensis* against complement-mediated serum bactericidal activity (24).

F. tularensis is a facultative intracellular pathogen that survives and grows in macrophages (25). Host defense against this species therefore depends on cell-mediated immunity propelled by cytokines (especially interferon-γ) produced by antigen-specific T-lymphocytes to enhance the microbicidal activity of inflammatory macrophages. Toxic levels of nitric oxide, generated by activated macrophages, have been identified as the effector molecule that inhibits intracellular growth of *F. tularensis* (26). T-cell (CD4$^+$, CD8$^+$)–independent host defense mechanisms may also be operative in resolving *F. tularensis* infection (27).

The recommended antimicrobial treatment for *F. tularensis* infection has traditionally been streptomycin (3). Cure rates of 97% without relapse have been achieved with streptomycin (28),

TABLE 200.1.   Clinical Presentation and Route of Acquisition of *Francisella tularensis* Infection

Clinical form	Route of acquisition	Clinical signs and symptoms
Ulceroglandular-glandular	Direct contact by skinning and dressing infected animals (rabbits, squirrels, muskrats) Animal bites, scratches Bites of ticks, deerflies, mosquitoes	Cutaneous ulcers Predominantly on hands Lymphadenopathy Autoinoculation to other sites possible Ulcers: head, neck, back
Oculoglandular	Rubbing of eyes after handling infected animals	Absence of primary lesion at site of inoculation Regional lymphadenopathy Conjunctivitis with discrete ulcers Periauricular, parotid, submaxillary lymphadenopathy Erythema and edema of eyelids
Oropharyngeal	Inhalation of large infected droplets Ingestion of contaminated food or water	Exudative pharyngitis Anterior-posterior cervical lymphadenopathy Enteritis, peritonitis, and appendicitis rare complications
Typhoidal	Unclear	Local signs possibly absent Fever, shaking chills; meningitis rare
Pneumonic	Inhalation of contaminated aerosols, dust Hematogenous spread Pulmonary involvement possible regardless of route of transmission	Bronchopneumonia Pleural effusion Hilar lymphadenopathy

but alternative therapies are needed given the unavailability of streptomycin. A review of the literature demonstrated that gentamicin is an acceptable alternative to streptomycin based on cure rates of 86% and relapse rates of 6% (28). The tetracyclines and fluoroquinolones may also be reasonable alternatives (28–30). Although relapse has been reported with ciprofloxacin (31), significantly better results were reported with ciprofloxacin compared with other therapies during the tularemia epidemic associated with hare hunting in Spain (5). A live attenuated vaccine derived from the avirulent live vaccine strain is currently under review by the U.S. Food and Drug Administration (32). Doxycycline and ciprofloxacin have been proposed as prophylactic agents in the early postexposure period if *F. tularensis* were to be used as a biological weapon (32).

PASTEURELLA

Members of the genus *Pasteurella* within the family Pasteurellaceae share their small coccobacillary morphology with *Actinobacillus* and *Haemophilus* species (11).

Pasteurellae, especially *Pasteurella multocida*, are considered zoonotic agents and colonize the mucous membranes of the upper respiratory tract of a wide variety of wild and domesticated animals including livestock, poultry, and especially dogs and cats (11). Most human infections with *P. multocida* result from direct contact (bites and scratches) with dogs and cats. Some cases may occur as a result of indirect cat contact with catheters used for peritoneal dialysis (33,34) or chemotherapy (35). An association with animal exposure cannot be established in all cases of *P. multocida* infection (36). For example, a nosocomial outbreak of *P. multocida* infection occurred among seven patients in a chronic care facility in which epidemiologic investigation failed to identify the source for these infections (37).

Pasteurella species are gram-negative, non–spore-forming minute coccobacilli with a tendency toward pleomorphism. Bipolar staining may be observed and heightened with Wright, Giemsa, or Wayson stains. *P. multocida* is an encapsulated organism, a feature best recognized directly in purulent exudates (11).

When grown on 5% sheep blood agar, *Pasteurella* species produce small convex colonies with a glistening consistency. Isolates of *P. multocida* derived from respiratory secretions of patients with underlying chronic pulmonary diseases, such as bronchitis, emphysema, or bronchiectasis, are often mucoid and watery (11). *Pasteurella* species are nonhemolytic with the exception of *Pasteurella haemolytica*, which produces β-hemolytic colonies. Growth of *P. multocida* on blood agar is accompanied by a distinct musty odor, possibly due to indole production from tryptone in the blood agar.

Pasteurellae are fermentative and, with the exception of *P. aerogenes*, anaerogenic (Table 200.2). All species are oxidase, catalase, and nitrate reductase positive. Several species are urease positive (Table 200.2). Biotyping of *P. multocida* may be achieved through assessment of sugar fermentation reactions (11).

Virulence factors of *P. multocida* include an antiphagocytic capsule (38) that allows classification into six serotypes (39) and confers resistance to complement-mediated lysis (38,40); an outer membrane protein also with antiphagocytic activity (41); and iron-scavenging capacity (42).

P. multocida is the most common *Pasteurella* species involved in human infections. Table 200.3 summarizes the clinical manifestations of *P. multocida* infections. Skin and soft tissue infections via traumatic introduction of *P. multocida* after a dog or cat bite represent the vast majority of cases. Complications of skin and soft tissue infections may include abscesses, tenosynovitis, septic arthritis, and osteomyelitis. Infections at other sites are rarely reported in the literature, but *P. multocida* can mimic infections caused by *Haemophilus influenzae*. After skin and soft tissue infections, the respiratory tract represents the next most common site of isolation of *P. multocida* (43). Asymptomatic colonization of devitalized lung tissue in patients with chronic lung disease can occur, and pneumonia may ensue in some patients. Bacteremia and shock are rare but have been noted, especially in patients with severe underlying medical conditions. Neonatal meningitis is the most commonly reported central nervous system infection. Spontaneous bacterial peritonitis in patients with liver cirrhosis and appendicitis represent the most common intraabdominal infections. *P. multocida* peritonitis associated with peritoneal dialysis has been reported in nine cases in which *P. multocida* was introduced into the peritoneal cavity through a bite or scratch to the dialysis tubing (44). Patients were usually

TABLE 200.2. Salient Characteristics Differentiating *Pasteurella* Species

	Pasteurella species					
Characteristic	*multocida*	*haemolytica*	*pneumotropica*	*ureae*	*dagmatis*	*aerogenes*
Fermentation						
Glucose	+	+	+	+	+ (gas)	+ (gas)
Xylose	V	V	(+)	0	0	V
Lactose	V	V	V	0	0	V
Production of						
Urease	0	0	+	+	V	+
Indole	+	0	+	0	+	0
Ornithine decarboxylase	+	0	+	0	0	V
Growth						
MacConkey agar	0	V	V	0	0	+
Beta hemolysis	0	+	0	0	0	0

All species are oxidase and catalase positive, reduce nitrates, and are nonmotile.
+, positive; 0, negative; V, variable; (+), delayed positive.

symptomatic within 24 hours, suggesting that the rich dialysate enhances the growth of *P. multocida*, even if the inoculum density is small, as might be expected with a scratch to the tubing. Because of the large numbers of patients undergoing peritoneal dialysis in households with pet cats, one can anticipate a continuing incidence of cat bite/scratch peritonitis (45). A case of *P. pneumotropica* peritonitis developed in a patient undergoing peritoneal dialysis as a result of contamination of the dialysis tubing by a pet hamster (46). Infections caused by *Pasteurella* species other than *P. multocida* are listed in Table 200.4.

Penicillin remains the drug of choice for treating *Pasteurella* infections. Penicillin G, penicillin VK, ampicillin, and amoxicillin demonstrate good *in vitro* activity. Later-generation cephalosporins also demonstrate good *in vitro* activity and are considered reasonable alternatives. Other antibiotics with good activity include tetracyclines, quinolones, and chloramphenicol, but clinical data are limited with these agents. β-lactamase producing strains of *P. multocida* have been isolated from humans

(47,48). The use of β-lactamase inhibitor antibiotic combinations may be necessary in the future if these strains are increasingly isolated from humans.

YERSINIA PESTIS

Within the family Enterobacteriacae, the genus *Yersinia* is composed of 11 species. *Y. pestis, Y. enterocolitica,* and *Y. pseudotuberculosis* are the major human pathogens. The latter two species predominantly cause gastrointestinal tract disease and are discussed separately from *Y. pestis,* which mainly causes a systemic disease.

Y. pestis, the causative agent of human plague, is primarily an infectious agent of rodents transmitted to humans by the bite of a flea carrying *Y. pestis* or through the handling of *Y. pestis*–infected carcasses of rodents and rabbits or other infected animals, including dogs and cats (65–68). The bacterium multiplies in the flea's esophagus and is transmitted by the flea during the course of a blood meal. *Y. pestis* may also be transmitted by aerosols generated by humans or animals with pneumonic plague. Interestingly, both forms of plague, bubonic (65,66) and pneumonic (67,68), have been transmitted to humans by the

TABLE 200.3. Spectrum of Human *Pasteurella multocida* Infections

Local	Respiratory
Skin and bone infections	Pneumonia
Cellulitis	Empyema
Subcutaneous abscesses	Epiglottitis
Osteomyelitis	Pharyngitis
Septic arthritis	Sinusitis
Wound infection	Chronic otitis
Systemic	Lung abscess
Blood and vascular	Rare
Septicemia	Abdominal
Endocarditis-native and	Spontaneous bacterial
prosthetic	peritonitis
Mycotic aneurysm	Peritonitis related to cat
Infected vascular graft	bite/scratch
Pericarditis/tamponade	Appendicitis
Central nervous system	Hepatosplenic abscesses
Meningitis	Renal abscess
Cerebral abscesses	Genitourinary tract
	Ocular
	Corneal ulcer
	Conjunctivitis
	Endophthalmitis

TABLE 200.4. Human Infections Associated with *Pasteurella* Species Other Than *Pasteurella multocida*

Species	Infection	Reference
Pasteurella aerogones	Vertebral osteomyelitis	49
Pasteurella haemolytica	Cutaneous infection	50
	Endocarditis	51
	Septicemia, shock	52
Pasteurella dagmatis	Endocarditis	53
	Wound infection	11
	Septicemia	54
Pasteurella pneumotropica	Wound infection	55–57
	Bone and joint infection	58
	Septicemia	59
	Peritonitis (CAPD)	46
Pasteurella ureae	Meningitis	60,61
	Peritonitis	62
	Septicemia	63
	Pneumonia	64

domestic cat in plague endemic areas of the southwestern United States—the bubonic form through a scratch and bite from an infected cat; the pneumonic form through face-to-face exposure to a cat with pneumonic plague. Twenty-three cases were reported between 1977 and 1998 following exposure to domestic cats (69).

Y. pestis is a gram-negative encapsulated coccobacillus with distinct bipolar ("safety pin") staining when it is viewed directly in clinical material after Wright, Wayson, or Giemsa staining (70). Like other pathogenic *Yersinia* species, *Y. pestis* grows slowly and produces pinpoint colonies on most bacteriologic media including MacConkey agar within 24 hours of incubation. Optimal growth occurs at 28° to 30°C rather than 37°C. Hemolysis is absent on blood agar, but colonies of fully virulent *Y. pestis* have a "hammered copper" or "fried egg" appearance after 48 hours of incubation at 37°C (71). On nutrient agar, colonies may become mucoid and glistening, an attribute associated with the proteinaceous capsular material (F1). In liquid media, *Y. pestis*, in contrast to *Y. enterocolitica* and *Y. pseudotuberculosis*, produces granular growth at the bottom of the tube with streaking of growth upward along the inner aspect of the tube (71). Smears of such cultures show chains of bacilli.

Like other yersiniae, *Y. pestis* is oxidase negative and fermentative, producing acid without gas from a variety of carbohydrates (Table 200.5). Unlike *Y. pseudotuberculosis*, with which it may easily be confused (68), *Y. pestis* is nonmotile regardless of incubation temperature (28° or 37°C), does not produce urease, and fails to ferment melibiose and rhamnose (Table 200.5). Many microbiology laboratories use automated or semiautomated identification systems that may misidentify *Y. pestis* as *Y. pseudotuberculosis* (72,73). Care in choosing the rapid biochemical identification system, especially in plague endemic areas, is critical. Suspected *Y. pestis* isolates can be confirmed at plague reference laboratories by bacteriophage sensitivity testing at 20° to 22°C and agglutination with *Y. pestis*–specific antisera (71). The development of a 41.7 kb *Y. pestis*—specific primer has been used in PCR amplification to distinguish *Y. pestis* from *Y. pseudotuberculosis* (74).

Fully virulent wild-type *Y. pestis* possesses several plasmid species, ranging from 70 to 75 kb, that it shares with *Y. enterocolitica* and *Y. pseudotuberculosis* and that encode a number of virulence determinants (75). Interestingly, *Y. pestis* is considered to be a recently emerged clone that arose from *Y. pseudotuberculosis* 1,500 to 20,000 years ago (76). Furthermore, *Y. pseudotuberculosis* shows greater than 90% DNA-DNA homology with *Y. pestis* (77).

Y. pestis has two distinct plasmids, a 110-kb plasmid and a 9.5-kb plasmid, that encode virulence determinants. Expression of the 70- to 75-kb plasmid-encoded virulence attributes is under exquisite control of temperature and calcium concentration (75). In the absence of Ca^{2+} at 37°C, several virulence determinants (e.g., V and W antigens, outer-membrane proteins) are produced. In the presence of millimolar concentrations of Ca^{2+} at 37°C, plasmid function is down-regulated but still higher than at 25°C. The 70- to 75-kb (45-MDa) plasmid encodes a series of outer membrane proteins (Yops) involved in adherence, invasion, and antiphagocytic activity and a set of Ca^{2+}+ and temperature-sensitive regulatory genes (*lcr*) that control synthesis of other plasmid genes. The 110-kb plasmid encodes an antiphagocytic protein capsule termed fraction 1 (Fra). The 9.5-kb plasmid encodes an outer membrane protease (Pla) that activates plasminogen, which aids in systemic spread of *Y. pestis* (Table 200.6). This plasmid also encodes coagulase activity and pesticin synthesis. *Y. pestis* also contains a chromosomally encoded surface antigen, termed pH6 antigen, that is expressed at 37°C and acidic pH (78). This outer-membrane protein may serve as an epithelial cell adhesin and function maximally in the acid environment induced by an inflammatory response. This antigen is also produced intracellularly in macrophage phagolysosomes and may aid intracellular survival (79). Chromosomally controlled virulence factors also include purine synthesis (Pur⁺) and production of surface structures involved in absorption and storage of hemin (71).

Virulent plague strains produce two phage-encoded toxins: a soluble heat-labile exotoxin that is highly toxic for rats and mice (murine toxin), and a lipopolysaccharide endotoxin that is lethal for guinea pigs and rabbits. The role of these toxins in human plague is still uncertain (80), although endotoxin-mediated shock and disseminated intravascular coagulation (DIC) can occur in plague.

Plague ensues clinically after the bite of a flea or infected animal or by inhalation of *Y. pestis*–infected aerosols from individuals with pneumonic plague. After being introduced into the victim's skin by a fleabite, *Y. pestis* migrates via the lymphatic system to the nearest lymph node, where the bacterium is sequestered. *Y. pestis* is subsequently phagocytosed by local macrophages but survives intracellular killing and multiplies in the regional lymph node, which ultimately necroses. Proliferation produces swelling of the lymph node (bubo), and organisms gain access to the bloodstream after 5 to 10 days, which may result in septicemia, endotoxemia, and potentially DIC. In a

TABLE 200.5. Differential Characteristics of Pathogenic *Yersinia* Species

Characteristic	*Yersinia* species		
	pestis	*pseudotuberculosis*	*enterocolitica*
Motility (25°C)	0	+	+
Urease production	0	+	+
Ornithine decarboxylase production	0	0	+
Voges-Proskauer test	0	0	+ (25°C)
Indole production	0	0	V
Fermentation			
Glucose	+	+	+
Rhamnose	0	V	0
Melibiose	V	V	0
Sucrose	0	0	+

+, positive; 0, negative; V, variable.

TABLE 200.6. Virulence Factors of *Yersinia pestis*

Factor	Determinant	Role in pathogenesis
Serum resistance	Chromosome	Resistance to complement-mediated lysis
Fraction 1 (Fra) (protein capsule)	110-kb plasmid	Antiphagocytic
V antigen (LcrV) (protein)	72-kb plasmid	Unknown; essential for virulence; neutralized by antibody; intracellular survival and multiplication
W antigen (envelope lipoprotein)	72-kb plasmid	Unknown; essential for virulence; intracellular survival and multiplication
pH6 antigen	Chromosome	Epithelial cell adherence; intracellular survival?
Plasminogen activator	9.5-kb plasmid	Dissolves fibrin clots; enhances systemic spread; degrades Cab, C5a
Coagulase	9.5-kb plasmid	Dissolves fibrin clots
Hemin absorption	Chromosome	Iron source masks bacterial surface
Pesticin	9.5-kb plasmid	Unknown

minority of patients, lung involvement may result in pneumonic plague. Aerosols from such individuals are highly infectious and lead to a form of plague more rapidly progressive than that initiated by a fleabite. This may be attributed to the release of fully virulent bacilli expressing all virulence factors, subsequent to host passage.

Plague is linked epidemiologically to rodent (rats, ground squirrels, prairie dogs) and flea populations in warmer geographic regions such as the southwestern states of New Mexico, Arizona, Colorado, and California. Plague-endemic areas also include Southeast Asia (Myanmar, China), South America (Bolivia, Brazil, Ecuador, Peru), Africa, and the Middle East (Saudi Arabia, Afghanistan) but not Australia (81,82). Reemergence of plague has been observed in Madagascar (83).

Interestingly, a warm climate may actually favor the development of *Y. pestis* virulence factors in an infected flea such as plasminogen activator, which would enhance spread of the bacillus subsequent to a fleabite. *Y. pestis* infection in the flea results in blockage of the flea digestive track by massive bacterial multiplication in the proventriculus, a valve-like chamber situated between the esophagus and midgut that is lined with spikes. Infected fleas with blocked digestive tracts are unable to pump blood into their stomachs. As the starving flea attempts to feed, *Y. pestis* is released or regurgitated from the proventriculus into the bite wound. In the cold-blooded flea the heme storage (*hms*) genes, essential for *Y. pestis* colonization of the proventriculus and flea blockage, are activated. Infected fleas with blocked digestive tracts ultimately starve to death (84).

Plague is treated with antibiotics such as streptomycin, tetracycline, and chloramphenicol (85). *Y. pestis* isolates remain highly susceptible to these and newer antibiotics (i.e., broad-spectrum cephalosporins and quinolones) (86), despite reports of multidrug resistance in human isolates (87). Control and prevention are achieved through a formalin-inactivated vaccine, control of wild rodent and flea populations, and quarantine measures.

REFERENCES

1. Hollis DG, Weaver RE, Steigerwalt AG, et al. *Francisella philomiragia* comb. nov. (formerly *Yersinia philomiragia*) and *Francisella tularensis* biogroup novicida (formerly *Francisella novicida*) associated with human disease. *J Clin Microbiol* 1989;27:1601–1608.
2. Leighton FA, Artsob HA, Chu MC, et al. A serological survey of rural dogs and cats on the southwestern Canadian prairie for zoonotic pathogens. *Can J Public Health* 2001;92:67–71.
3. Evans ME, Gregory DW, Schaffner W, et al. Tularemia: a 30-year experience with 88 cases. *Medicine (Baltimore)* 1985;64:251–269.
4. Ohara Y, Sato T, Fugita H, et al. Clinical manifestations of tularemia in Japan—analysis of 1,355 cases observed between 1924 and 1987. *Infection* 1991;19:14–17.
5. Perez-Castrillon JL, Bachiller-Luque P, Martin-Luquero M, et al. Tularemia epidemic in northwestern Spain: clinical description and therapeutic response. *Clin Infect Dis* 2001;33:573–576.
6. Anda P, Segura Del Pozo J, Diaz Garcia JM, et al. Waterborne outbreak of tularemia associated with crayfish fishing. *Emerg Infect Dis* 2001;7(3 suppl):575–582.
7. Centers for Disease Control and Prevention. *Basic laboratory protocols for the presumptive identification of* Francisella tularensis. Bethesda, MD: Centers for Disease Control and Prevention, April 18, 2001 (*www.bt.cdc.gov/Agent/Tularemia/tularemia20010417.pdf*).
8. Warring WB, Ruffin JS Jr. A tick-borne epidemic of tularemia. *N Engl J Med* 1946;234:137.
9. Francis E. A summary of present knowledge of tularemia. *Medicine (Baltimore)* 1928;7:411.
10. Young LS Bickwell DS, Archer BG, et al. Tularemia epidemic: Vermont, 1968. Forty-seven cases linked to contact with muskrats. *N Engl J Med* 1969;280:1253–1260.
11. Weaver RE, Hollis DG, Bottone EJ. Gram-negative fermentative bacteria and *Francisella tularensis*. In: Lennette E, Balows A, Hausler WJ Jr, et al., eds. *Manual of clinical microbiology*, 4th ed. Washington, DC: American Society for Microbiology, 1985:305–329.
12. Berdal BP, Soderlund E. Cultivation and isolation of *Francisella tularensis* on selective chocolate agar as used routinely for the isolation of gonococci. *Acta Pathol Microbiol Scand B* 1977;85:108–109.
13. Johansson A, Berglund L, Eriksson U, et al. Comparative analysis of PCR versus culture for diagnosis of ulceroglandular tularemia. *J Clin Microbiol* 2000;38(1):22–26.
14. Schmid GP, Komblatt AN, Connors CA, et al. Clinically mild tularemia associated with tick-borne *Francisella tularensis*. *J Infect Dis* 1983;148:63–67.
15. Holt JG, Krieg NR, Sneath PHA, et al. Gram-negative aerobic microaerophilic rods and cells. In: Holt JG, Krieg NR, Sneath PHA, et al., eds. *Bergey's manual of determinative bacteriology*, 9th ed. Baltimore: Williams & Wilkins, 1994:83, 141.
16. Johansson A, Ibrahim A, Goransson I, et al. Evaluation of PCR-based methods for discrimination of *Francisella* species and subspecies and development of a specific PCR that distinguishes the two major subspecies of *Francisella tularensis*. *J Clin Microbiol* 2000;38(11):4180–4185.
17. Saslaw S, Eigelsbach HT, Wilson HE, et al. Tularemia vaccine study. I. Intracutaneous challenge. *Arch Intern Med* 1961;107:689.
18. Saslaw S, Eigelsbach HT, Prior JA, et al. Tularemia vaccine study. II. Respiratory challenge. *Arch Intern Med* 1961;107:702.
19. Tärnvik A. Nature of protective immunity to *Francisella tularensis*. *Rev Infect Dis* 1989;11:440–451.
20. Hood AM. Virulence factors of *Francisella tularensis*. *J Hyg* 1977;79:47–60.
21. Cherwonogrodzky JW, Knodel MH, Spence MR. Increased encapsulation and virulence of *Francisella tularensis* live vaccine strain (LVS) by subculturing on synthetic medium. *Vaccine* 1994;12:773–775.
22. Lofgren S, Tärnvik A, Blood GD, et al. Phagocytosis and killing of *Francisella tularensis* by human polymorphonuclear leukocytes. *Infect Immun* 1983;39:715–720.
23. Lofgren S, Tärnvik A, Thore M, et al. A wild and an attenuated strain of *Francisella tularensis* differ in susceptibility to hypochlorous acid: a possible explanation to their different handling by polymorphonuclear leukocytes. *Infect Immun* 1984;43:730–734.
24. Sandstrom G, Lofgren S, Tärnvik A. A capsule-deficient mutant of *Francisella tularensis* LVS exhibits enhanced sensitivity to killing by serum but diminished sensitivity to killing by polymorphonuclear leukocytes. *Infect Immun* 1988;56:1194–1202.

25. Anthony LSD, Burke RD, Nano FE. Growth of *Francisella* spp. *in rodent macrophages*. *Infect Immun* 1991;59:3291–3296.

26. Fortier AH, Polsinelli T, Green SJ, et al. Activation of macrophages for destruction of *Francisella tularensis*: identification of cytokines, effector cells, and effector molecules. *Infect Immun* 1992;60:817–825.

27. Conlan JW, Sjöstedt A, North RJ. CD4+ and CD8+ T-cell–dependent and – independent host defense mechanisms can operate to control and resolve primary and secondary *Francisella tularensis* LVS infection in mice. *Infect Immun* 1994;62:5603–5607.

28. Enderlin G, Morales L, Jacobs RF, et al. Streptomycin and alternative agents for the treatment of tularemia: review of the literature. *Clin Infect Dis* 1994;19:42–47.

29. Syrjala H, Schildt R, Raisainen S. *In vitro* susceptibility of *Francisella tularensis* to fluoroquinolones and treatment of tularemia with norfloxacin and ciprofloxacin. *Eur J Clin Microbiol Infect Dis* 1991;10:68–70.

30. Limaye AP, Hooper CJ. Treatment of tularemia with fluoroquinolones: two cases and review. *Clin Infect Dis* 1999;29:9224.

31. Chocarro A, Gonzales A, Garcia I. Treatment of tularemia with ciprofloxacin. *Clin Infect Dis* 2000;31:623.

32. Dennis DT, Inglesby TV, Henderson DA, et al. Tularemia as a biological weapon: medical and public health management. *JAMA* 2001;285:2763–2773.

33. Paul RV, Rostand SG. Cat-bite peritonitis: *Pasteurella multocida* peritonitis following feline contamination of peritoneal dialysis tubing. *Am J Kidney Dis* 1987;10:318–319.

34. London RD, Bottone EJ. *Pasteurella multocida*: zoonotic cause of peritonitis in a patient undergoing peritoneal dialysis. *Am J Med* 1991;91:202–204.

35. Majeed H, Verghese A, Rivera RR. The cat and the catheter [Letter]. *N Engl J Med* 1995;332:338.

36. Hubbert WT, Rosen MN. *Pasteurella multocida* infection in man unrelated to animal bites. *Am J Public Health* 1970;60:1109–1117.

37. Itoh M, Tierno PM, Milstoc M, et al. A unique outbreak of *Pasteurella multocida* in a chronic disease hospital. *Am J Public Health* 1983;70:1170–1173.

38. Boyce JD, Adler B. The capsule is a virulence determinant in the pathogenesis of *Pasteurella multocida* M1404(B:2). *Infect Immun* 2000;68:3463–3468.

39. Rimler RB, Rhoades KR. Serogroup F, a new capsule serogroup of *Pasteurella multocida*. *J Clin Microbiol* 1987;25:615–618.

40. Snipes KP, Hirsch DC. Association of complement sensitivity with virulence of *Pasteurella multocida* isolated from turkeys. *Avian Dis* 1986;30:500–504.

41. Truscott WM, Hirsch DC. Demonstration of an outer membrane protein with antiphagocytic activity from *Pasteurella multocida* of avian origin. *Infect Immun* 1988;56:1538–1544.

42. Snipes KP, Hansen LM, Hirsch DC. Plasma and iron-regulated expression of high molecular weight outer membrane proteins by *Pasteurella multocida*. *Am J Vet Res* 1988;49:1336–1338.

43. Weber DJ, Wolfson JS, Swartz MN, et al. *Pasteurella multocida* infections. Report of 34 cases and review of the literature. *Medicine (Baltimore)* 1984;63:133–154.

44. Van Langenhove G, Daelemans R, Zachee P, et al. *Pasteurella multocida* as a rare cause of peritonitis in peritoneal dialysis. *Nephron* 2000;85:283–284.

45. Uribarri J, Bottone EJ, London RD. *Pasteurella multocida* peritonitis: are peritoneal dialysis patients on cyclers at increased risk? *Perit Dial Int* 1996;16:648–649.

46. Campos A, Taylor JH, Campbell M. Hamster bite peritonitis: *Pasteurella pneumotropica* peritonitis in a dialysis patient. *Pediatr Nephrol* 2000;15:31–32.

47. Rosenau A, Labigne A, Escande F, et al. Plasmid-mediated ROB-1 beta-lactamase in *Pasteurella multocida* from a human specimen. *Antimicrob Agents Chemother* 1991;35:2419–2422.

48. Naas T, Benaoudia F, Lebrun L, et al. Molecular identification of TEM-1 beta-lactamase in a *Pasteurella multocida* isolate of human origin. *Eur J Clin Microbiol Infect Dis* 2001;20:210–213.

49. Quiles I, Blazquez JC, De Teresa L, et al. Vertebral osteomyelitis due to *Pasteurella aerogenes*. *Scand J Infect Dis* 2000;32:566–567.

50. Muraski TF, Smith CK, Miller JK. Primary cutaneous (ulceroglandular) infection due to *Pasteurella* hemolytica. *N Y State J Med* 1962;62:3137.

51. Doty GL, Loomus GN, Wolf PL. *Pasteurella* endocarditis. *N Engl J Med* 1963;268:830.

52. Bitterman H, Shmilovitz M, Rotfeld M, et al. Septic shock due to *Pasteurella hemolytica*. *Isr J Med Sci* 1985;21:397–398.

53. Gump DW, Holden RA. Endocarditis caused by a new species of *Pasteurella*. *Ann Intern Med* 1972;76:275–278.

54. Deschilder I, Gordts B, Van Landuyt H et al. *Pasteurella dagmatis* septicaemia in an immunocompromised patient without a history of dog or cat bites. *Acta Clin Belg* 2000;55:225–226.

55. Olson JR, Meadows TR. *Pasteurella pneumotropica* infection resulting from a cat bite. *Am J Clin Pathol* 1969;51:709–710.

56. Medley S. A dog bite wound infected with *Pasteurella pneumotropica*. *Med J Aust* 1977;2:224–225.

57. Winton FW, Mair NS. *Pasteurella pneumotropica* isolated from a dog bite wound. *Microbios* 1969;2:155.

58. Gadberry JL, Zipper R, Taylor JA, et al. *Pasteurella pneumotropica* isolated from bone and joint infections. *J Clin Microbiol* 1984;19:926–927.

59. Rogers BT, Anderson JC, Palmer A, et al. Septicemia due to *Pasteurella pneumotropica*. *J Clin Pathol* 1973;26:396–398.

60. Wang WLL, Haiby G. Meningitis caused by *Pasteurella ureae*. *Am J Clin Pathol* 1966;45:562–565.

61. Brass EP, Wray LM, McDuff T. *Pasteurella ureae* meningitis associated with endocarditis. Report of a case and review of the literature. *Eur Neurol* 1983;22:138–141.

62. Noble RC, Marek BJ, Overman SB. Spontaneous bacterial peritonitis caused by *Pasteurella ureae*. *J Clin Microbiol* 1987;25:442–444.

63. Gatti F, Seynhaeve V, Weaver R. First description of a case of human septicemia due to *Pasteurella ureae*. *Ann Soc Belg Med Trop* 1968;48:463–468.

64. Starkebaum GA, Plorde JJ. *Pasteurella* pneumonia: report of a case and review of the literature. *J Clin Microbiol* 1977;5:332–335.

65. Weniger BG, Warren AJ, Forseth V, et al. Human bubonic plague transmitted by a domestic scratch. *JAMA* 1984;251:927–928.

66. Thornton DJ, Tustin RC, Pienaar BJ, et al. Cat bite transmission of *Yersinia pestis* infection to man. *J S Afr Vet Assoc* 1975;46:165–169.

67. Werner SB, Weidmer CE, Nelson BC, et al. Primary plague pneumonia contracted from a domestic cat at South Lake Tahoe, CA. *JAMA* 1984;251:929–931.

68. Doll JM, Zeitz DS, Ettestad P, et al. Cat-transmitted fatal pneumonic plague in a person who traveled from Colorado to Arizona. *Am J Trop Med Hyg* 1994;51:109–114.

69. Gage KL, Dennis DT, Orloski KA, et al. Cases of cat-associated human plague in the Western US, 1977–1998. *Clin Infect Dis* 2000;30:893–900.

70. Mann JD, Hull HF, Schmid GP, et al. Plague and the peripheral smear. *JAMA* 1984;251:953.

71. Quan TJ. Yersinia pestis. In: Balows A, ed. *The prokaryotes: a handbook on the biology of bacteria: ecophysiology, isolation, identification, applications*, 2nd ed. New York: Springer-Verlag, 1992:2888–2898.

72. Centers for Disease Control and Prevention. Fatal human plague—Arizona and Colorado, 1996. *MMWR* 1997;46:617.

73. Wilmoth BA, Chu MC, Quan TJ. Identification of *Yersinia pestis* by BBL Crystal Enteric/Nonfermenter Identification System. *J Clin Microbiol* 1996;34:2829–2830.

74. Radnedge L, Gamez-Chin S, McCready PM, et al. Identification of nucleotide sequences for the specific and rapid detection of *Yersinia pestis*. *Appl Environ Microbiol* 2001;67:3759–3762.

75. Straley SS, Skrzypek E, Plano GV, et al. Yops of *Yersinia* species pathogenic for humans. *Infect Immun* 61:3105-10, 1993.

76. Achtman M, Zurth K, Morelli G et al. *Yersinia pestis*, the cause of plague, is a recently emerged clone of *Yersinia pseudotuberculosis*. *Proc Natl Acad Sci USA* 1999;96:14043–14048.

77. Bercovier H, Mollaret HH, Alonso JM, et al. Intra- and interspecies relatedness of *Yersinia pestis* by DNA hybridization and its relationship to *Y. pseudotuberculosis*. *Curr Microbiol* 1980;4:225.

78. Ben-Efrain S, Aronson M, Bichowsky-Slomnicki L. New antigen component of *Pasteurella pestis* formed under specific conditions of pH and temperature. *J Bacteriol* 1961;81:704.

79. Linder LE, Tall B. *Y. pestis* pH6 antigen forms fimbriae and is induced by intracellular association with macrophages. *Mol Microbiol* 1993;8:311.

80. Ferber DM, Brubaker JR. Plasmids in *Yersinia pestis*. *Infect Immun* 1981;31:839.

81. World Health Organization. *Weekly Epidemiol Rec 1974–1987*. Plague in 1973, 49:253; plague in 1974, 59:317; plague in 1975, 51:237; plague in 1976, 53:229; human plague in 1986, 40:299.

82. Perry RD, Fetherston JD. *Yersinia pestis*—etiologic agent of plague. *Clin Microbiol Rev* 1997;10:35–66.

83. Ratsitorahina M, Chanteau S, Rahalison L et al. Epidemiological and diagnostic aspects of the outbreak of pneumonic plague in Madagascar. *Lancet* 2000;355:111–113.

84. Hinnebusch BJ. Bubonic plague: a molecular genetic case history of the emergence of an infectious disease. *J Mol Med* 1997;75:645–652.

85. Barnes AM, Quan TJ. Plague. In: Gorbach SL, Bartlett JG, Blacklow NR, eds. *Infectious diseases*. Philadelphia: WB Saunders, 1992:1285–1291.

86. Wong JD, Barash JR, Sandfort RF, et al. Susceptibilities of *Yersinia pestis* strains to 12 antimicrobial agents. *Antimicrob Agents Chemother* 2000;44:1995–1996.

87. Galimand M, Guiyoule A, Gerbaud G, et al. Multidrug resistance in *Yersinia pestis* mediated by a transferable plasmid. *N Engl J Med* 1997;337:677–680.

CHAPTER 201
Pseudomonas aeruginosa *and Related Bacteria*

Christopher A. Ohl and Matthew Pollack

Pseudomonas aeruginosa and other *Pseudomonas* species, *Burkholderia* (formerly *Pseudomonas*) *cepacia,* and *Stenotrophomonas* (formerly *Xanthomonas*) *maltophilia* are aerobic, nonfermentative, nonenterobacterial gram-negative bacilli (1). These bacteria are cosmopolitan in their distribution, inhabiting soil, water, plants, and animals. Their medical importance derives principally from their being opportunistic pathogens, and the clinical diseases they cause are usually nosocomial in origin. Approximately 15% of all gram-negative clinical isolates are non–glucose-fermenting gram-negative rods; of these, more than two thirds are *P. aeruginosa.*

P. aeruginosa and related bacteria share many epidemiologic and clinical characteristics. They are hearty, free-living organisms with minimal nutritional requirements and a predilection for wet environments. They are widely distributed in nature, despite the absence of a discrete natural reservoir, and they abound in hospitals. They rarely infect normal persons but are capable of producing serious, sometimes life-threatening disease in immunocompromised persons, particularly those with persistent neutropenia. They exhibit innate resistance to many commonly used antibiotics and are capable of developing new resistance on exposure to antimicrobial agents. They are found in the inanimate hospital environment and may be spread from patient to patient on the hands of hospital personnel or by other fomites.

PSEUDOMONAS AERUGINOSA

Microbiologic Characteristics of the Pathogen

P. aeruginosa is isolated from clinical sources more often than all other *Pseudomonas* species combined and is more often associated with clinical disease. Most *P. aeruginosa* strains are identifiable on the basis of their colony morphology, grape-like odor, and production of pyocyanin, a blue-green, nonfluorescent pigment. Apyocyanogenic strains are identified on the basis of their polar monotrichous flagella, motility, acid production from glucose but not lactose or sucrose on open oxidation fermentation medium, positive indophenol oxidase and L-arginine dihydrolase reactions, and growth at 42°C (2). *P. aeruginosa* is usually identifiable by computer-based, automated gram-negative identification systems.

Epidemiology

P. aeruginosa frequents moist microenvironments in hospitals, such as sinks, water faucets, disinfectant solutions, inhalation equipment medicines, and food. Although not usually part of normal human bacterial flora, *P. aeruginosa* does colonize hospitalized patients. The frequency of colonization and subsequent infection is increased by underlying disease or injury, immunosuppression, prior antimicrobial therapy, and by invasive procedures that breach, circumvent, or impair normal physical barriers to bacterial invasion or other host defense mechanisms. Although discrete sources for these infections are

rarely identified, occasional epidemics are traced to a single source, such as an operating room suction apparatus, respiratory equipment, sink or faucet, endoscope, or physiotherapy pool (3–8).

P. aeruginosa is an important hospital-acquired pathogen, particularly in critical care settings. According to data from the Centers for Disease Control and Prevention, National Nosocomial Infections Surveillance (NNIS) system covering the period 1990 to 1999 (9), *P. aeruginosa* was the second most common cause of hospital-acquired pneumonia (17% of isolates), the third most common urinary tract isolate (11%), and the sixth most common cause of bacteremia (4%). It is particularly problematic in units caring for patients with cystic fibrosis, burns, and cancer. Horizontal transmission of a single strain or genotype of *P. aeruginosa* is frequently documented during patient-unit outbreaks, presumably due to health care worker–mediated cross-contamination (10,11). Outbreaks of *P. aeruginosa* nosocomial infection have been traced to health care workers' hands and fingernails (natural or artifical) that became colonized through patient contact or contaminated hand lotions and creams (12–15).

Community-acquired infection due to *P. aeruginosa* has been increasingly recognized. These infections include folliculitis, otitis externa and malignant external otitis, contiguous focus osteomyelitis following trauma, endocarditis in injection drug users, and bacteremia and pneumonia in patients with human immunodeficiency virus infection.

Pathogenesis

The pathogenesis of *Pseudomonas* infections is complex. A classic opportunistic pathogen, *P. aeruginosa* is a rare cause of disease in normal persons but is highly virulent in patients with impaired host defense mechanisms. The broad spectrum of disease produced by *Pseudomonas* suggests pathogenic versatility based on use of multiple virulence factors. The opportunistic virulence of *P. aeruginosa* is related to its ability to colonize a variety of anatomic sites (owing to effective adherence mechanisms, minimal nutritional requirements, and antibiotic resistance), its capacity for local tissue invasion and damage, and its propensity for bloodstream invasion with resulting systemic disease. Insight into these versatile properties of *P. aeruginosa* was recently gained when the organism's entire genome was successfully sequenced (16). Contained within the large, 6.3 million–base pair genome is a considerable number of genes involved in regulatory functions, catabolism, and organic compound transport and efflux. These elements presumably allow the organism to thrive in diverse environments and contribute to its intrinsic resistance to antimicrobials.

The colonization by *Pseudomonas* of mucosal surfaces such as respiratory epithelium is facilitated by its attachment to epithelial cells by means of pili or fimbriae and is enhanced by prior tissue injury. So-called mucoid exopolysaccharide (MEP) elaborated by mucoid strains of *P. aeruginosa* isolated from the respiratory secretions of cystic fibrosis (CF) patients also acts as an adhesin for tracheal epithelial cells and for tracheobronchial mucin. The MEP produced by mucoid *Pseudomonas* contains a polymer of mannuronic and guluronic acid called alginate. MEP serves a virulence function by protecting mucoid CF respiratory isolates from mucociliary and opsonophagocytic clearance mechanisms. In addition, it is important in the formation of biofilms within which sessile microcolonies of *Pseudomonas* are protected from host defenses and antimicrobial agents. The genetic regulation of MEP production in *P. aeruginosa* has been elucidated and found to be encoded by the *algD* gene, the first gene of the alginate biosynthetic operon (17).

The locally invasive and destructive properties of *Pseudomonas* appear to be interrelated. *P. aeruginosa* elaborates a number of extracellular enzymes or toxins that act selectively on various host tissues. Alkaline protease and elastase, for example, produce necrosis in lung, cornea, and skin (18). Proteases potentiate the invasive properties of *Pseudomonas* through tissue breakdown and the proteolysis of immunoglobulins and complement. Elastase dissolves the internal elastic lamina of blood vessels and is in part responsible for the hemorrhage and necrosis observed in certain locally invasive *Pseudomonas* infections. These enzymes are not cytotoxic but disrupt connective tissue architecture and connections between cells, thus facilitating bacterial invasion. *P. aeruginosa* produces heat-labile and heat-stable hemolysins; the heat-labile hemolysin is referred to as phospholipase C, which breaks down lipids and lecithin (19,20). Like protease, these enzymes produce tissue necrosis and contribute to the invasive properties of the organism.

Pseudomonas lipopolysaccharide (endotoxin) and exotoxin A appear to be responsible for many of the systemic manifestations of *Pseudomonas* disease. Endotoxin causes fever, leukocytosis or leukopenia, hypotension, and oliguria and is a direct participant in events leading to disseminated intravascular coagulation, adult respiratory distress syndrome, and the systemic inflammatory response. Exotoxin A, a single polypeptide chain of 613 amino acids, is a potent inhibitor of protein synthesis by a mechanism involving adenosine diphosphate ribosylation of elongation factor-2, which is inactivated by this reaction and is no longer capable of catalyzing polypeptide biosynthesis (21,22). Exotoxin A has direct cytopathic effects on a wide variety of mammalian cells and additionally appears to mediate systemic toxic effects. It is lethal in exceedingly small quantities for animals, including subhuman primates. Data suggest a lethal pathogenic role for toxin A in septicemic *Pseudomonas* infections and a protective role for toxin A–specific antibodies (23).

Four other extracellular cytotoxins of *P. aeruginosa*—ExoS, ExoT, ExoU, and ExoY—are deleterious to host cells due to their ability to disrupt host cell actin cytoskeletons (ExoS, ExoT), cause acute cytotoxicity (ExoU), and increase intracellular cyclic adenosine monophosphate levels (ExoY) (24–26). These cytotoxins are directly introduced into the cytosol of the host cell using a type III secretion apparatus, a complex array of transmembrane proteins that are under the control of genes located on discrete plasmid or chromosomal pathogenicity islands (27). Expression of type III secretion systems by *P. aeruginosa* is associated with increased bacterial virulence and pathogenicity in infections of tissue cultures, animals, and patients (28).

The production and secretion of many of the extracellular virulence factors of *P. aeruginosa*, as well as the assembly and maturation of its biofilm, are ultimately under the regulatory control of a complex cell-to-cell signaling system called quorum sensing (29–32). Quorum sensing is the process in which the entire population of *Pseudomonas* organisms that inhabit a biofilm, colonized mucosa, or infected tissue is able to sense its environment, discern its own cell density, and communicate as a community. It is mediated through two distinct homoserine lactone signal molecules that are secreted and sensed by each *Pseudomonas* organism in the community. This system presumably allows *P. aeruginosa* to produce virulence factors and extracellular matrix in a coordinated fashion only when conditions are optimal for it to overcome the host's defenses. Supporting this concept are data indicating that *P. aeruginosa* strains, which are incapable of quorum sensing because of mutation of the system's regulatory genes, are incapable of forming a competent biofilm, secreting virulence factors, or establishing a pronounced inflammatory response in infected tissues (33,34).

Clinical Manifestations and Treatment

GENERAL PRINCIPLES

P. aeruginosa is responsible for a broad spectrum of disease in a variety of clinical settings (Table 201.1). Some *P. aeruginosa* infections are acute, even fulminant; others are subacute or chronic in their presentation. The varying levels of severity and acuteness of *Pseudomonas* disease, the anatomic location of infection, and the nature and severity of a patient's underlying disease and immune status dictate different therapies and signal different prognoses. Because *P. aeruginosa* is a common human saprophyte and is ubiquitous in the hospital environment, it may be difficult to distinguish infection from colonization, particularly in the case of specimens obtained from superficial sites such as wounds,

TABLE 201.1. Infections Caused by *Pseudomonas aeruginosa*

Acquired immunodeficiency syndrome–related infections	Eye infections
	Keratitis (corneal ulcer)
Bacteremia	Endophthalmitis
Primary	Gastrointestinal infections
Secondary	Necrotizing enterocolitis
Bone and joint infections	Shanghai fever
Sternoarticular pyarthrosis	Respiratory infections
Vertebral osteomyelitis	Pneumonia
Symphysis pubis infection	Nonbacteremic
Osteochondritis of the foot	Bacteremic
Chronic contiguous osteomyelitis	Lower respiratory tract infection in cystic fibrosis
Central nervous system infections	Skin and soft tissue infections
Meningitis	Ecthyma gangrenosum
Brain abscess	Pyoderma
Ear infections	Wound infection
Otitis externa	Dermatitis
Malignant external otitis	Burn wound sepsis
Chronic suppurative otitis media	Urinary tract infections
Endocarditis	Acute
Native heart valve infection in intravenous drug users	Chronic (frequently with sites of persistence or obstruction)
Prosthetic heart valve infection	

TABLE 201.2. Antimicrobials with Activity Against *Pseudomonas aeruginosa*

Antimicrobial	Dose[a]	Antimicrobial	Dose[a]
Antipseudomonal penicillins		**Aminoglycosides**	
Piperacillin	3–4 g every 4–6 h i.v.	Tobramycin	MDD: 2 mg/kg load then 1.7 mg/kg every 8 h i.v.
Piperacillin/Tazobactam[b]	3.375 g every 4 h i.v.		ODD: 5–7 mg/kg every 24 h i.v.
Ticarcillin	3 g every 3–6 h i.v.	Gentamicin	MDD: Same as tobramycin
Ticarcillin/clavulanate[b]	3.1 g every 4–6 h i.v.		ODD: Same as tobramycin
Antipseudomonal cephalosporins		Amikacin	MDD: 7.5 mg/kg every 12 h i.v.
Ceftazadime	2 g every 8 h i.v.		ODD: 15 mg/kg every 24 h i.v.
Cefoperazone	2 g every 6 h i.v.	**Antipseudomonal fluoroquinolones**	
Cefepime	2 g every 8–12 h i.v.	Ciprofloxacin	400 mg every 8–12 h i.v. or 750 mg every 12 h p.o.
Carbapenems[c]		Levofloxacin	750 mg every 24 h i.v. or 750 mg every 24 h p.o.
Imipenem	0.5 g every 6 h i.v.	**Other Antimicrobials**	
Meropenem	1 g every 8 h i.v.	Polymyxin B	0.75–1.25 mg/kg every 12 h i.v.
Monobactams		Colistin	1.7 mg/kg every 8 h i.v.
Aztreonam	2 g every 6–8 h i.v.		

[a]Use higher indicated doses for neutropenic or severely immunocompromised patients. Doses shown for patients with normal renal function.
[b]Piperacillin/tazobactam or ticarcillin/clavulanate have little added activity over piperacillin or ticarcillin against *P. aeruginosa.*
[c]Ertapenem, a third drug in this class, has less activity against *P. aeruginosa* than imipenem or meropenem and has no clinical utility for therapy of this organism.
[d]Trovafloxacin, an additional fluoroquinolone with antipseudomonal activity, has limited usefulness due to hepatotoxicity. Gatifloxacin and moxifloxacin have less *in vitro* activity against *P. aeruginosa* than ciprofloxacin or levofloxacin and there are few clinical studies to support their use in *Pseudomonas* or nosocomial infections.
i.v., intravenously; MDD, multiple-daily dosing; ODD, once-daily dosing; p.o., orally.

sinus drainage, or respiratory secretions. Clinical evidence of infection must therefore accompany simple demonstration of the organism at a potential infection site. *P. aeruginosa* exhibits innate or acquired resistance to many commonly used antibiotics, thus complicating therapy. This and other mechanisms of bacterial persistence at sites of infection, such as biofilm formation, make *P. aeruginosa* infections difficult to treat and the organism difficult to eradicate. These factors often necessitate aggressive therapy using maximal safe antibiotic doses, synergistic antimicrobial combinations, and prolonged treatment.

Table 201.2 lists antimicrobials available in the United States that have intrinsic activity against *P. aeruginosa*. These include selected β-lactam antibiotics in the extended-spectrum penicillin, third- and fourth-generation cephalosporin, carbapenem, and monobactam classes. Other effective antibiotics include aminoglycosides and the fluoroquinolones (particularly ciprofloxacin and levofloxacin). Initial, empiric antibiotic selection should be based on the local institutional antimicrobial susceptibility profile for *Pseudomonas* and the subsequent, definitive therapy on the susceptibilities of the specific culture isolate. One of the more controversial aspects of antimicrobial therapy for *P. aeruginosa* has been the relative merits of two-agent combination therapy as opposed to that of single agent monotherapy. The putative benefits of combination therapy include synergistic killing (seen best *in vitro* between the β-lactams and aminoglycosides or to a lesser extent ciprofloxacin), diminished potential for acquired resistance while on therapy, and superior efficacy as shown in early clinical studies (35–37). However, more recently these benefits have been questioned, and advocates for monotherapy have emerged (38). Specifically, advocates of monotherapy correctly point out that there are few data that support the assertion that synergy has clinical significance, or that combination therapy prevents the emergence of acquired resistance. Regarding the later concept, while there is evidence that acquired resistance not uncommonly arises during imipenem monotherapy of *Pseudomonas* pneumonia, it has been shown that adding a second antibiotic agent to imipenem does not prevent or influence the emergence of resistance to this drug (40,41). To further complicate the debate, there are conflicting data from

clinical trials that were designed to either support or oppose the superiority of combination therapy. In fact, several trials have shown it to be equivalent to monotherapy for the treatment of *Pseudomonas* infections of various sites and severity (41–45). It should be noted, however, that any one of these studies lacks the statistical power to show a significant outcome difference between double- and single-agent therapies. Thus, until a large randomized study is designed to answer the question, this conundrum will continue to exist, and most clinicians will advocate combination therapy (excluding a combination of two β-lactam drugs) for serious or life-threatening *P. aeruginosa* infections.

ANTIMICROBIAL RESISTANCE

Antimicrobial resistance in *P. aeruginosa* is both intrinsic and acquired. Acquired resistance may occur through chromosomal- or plasmid-mediated β-lactamases (e.g., penicillins and cephalosporins; occasionally carbapenems and aztreonam), decreased outer-membrane permeability through porin loss (e.g., carbapenems), DNA gyrase mutation (e.g., fluoroquinolones), and aminoglycoside-inactivating enzymes. High-level, multidrug-resistant *Pseudomonas* isolates often express energy-dependent efflux pumps in addition to one or more of the resistance determinants described above (46–49). These transmembrane proteins actively transport selected antimicrobials from the intracellular to extracellular space, which effectively increases the minimum inhibitory concentration (MIC) for those antimicrobials over and above that attributed to another discrete mechanism of resistance.

Acquired antimicrobial resistance in *P. aeruginosa* is rapidly increasing, particularly in isolates from CF patients, or those associated with burn or intensive care units (ICUs). According to data from the NNIS and the Intensive Care Antimicrobial Resistance Epidemiology (ICARE) projects between 1998 and 2002, for *P. aeruginosa* the pooled mean rate of resistance in all types of ICUs to piperacillin, ceftazidime, imipenem, and ciprofloxacin was 14.3%, 10.5%, 13.7%, and 28.9%, respectively (50). Resistant organisms may be transmitted to patients from hospital staff, other patients, or the environment, or they may appear *de novo* in an individual during antimicrobial therapy or prophylaxis with any given agent (3,40,51–55). Patient unit specific outbreaks of drug-resistant *Pseudomonas* occur, and city-wide clonal outbreaks have been described (56). The emergence of antibiotic resistance in *Pseudomonas* has been associated with increased rates of secondary bacteremia, higher patient mortality, and greater hospitalization stays and costs (57).

Antimicrobial therapy for patients with resistant *P. aeruginosa* infections should be directed by extended antimicrobial susceptibility testing. For organisms that are resistant to all traditional antimicrobials, there may be a role for systemic or inhaled therapy with either polymyxin B or colistin (58–63). Unfortunately, both of these older antibiotics may exhibit significant renal and neurotoxicity and variable clinical responses.

BACTEREMIA

P. aeruginosa is reported to be the sixth leading cause of hospital-acquired bacteremia in intensive care units in the United States (9) and the fourth most common bloodstream isolate in Europe (64,65). The mortality attributed to *P. aeruginosa* bacteremia is high, with rates ranging from approximately 15% to 55%, depending on the source of infection, underlying disease, and presence or absence of septic shock (45,66–68). *Pseudomonas* bacteremia may result from identifiable focal infections but is described as primary when no other infection site is discernible. Primary *Pseudomonas* bacteremia is particularly common in patients with hematologic malignant neoplasms who suffer from chemotherapy-induced neutropenia and have undergone an invasive procedure. Secondary bacteremias are most commonly associated with respiratory, gastrointestinal, pancreatobiliary, urinary tract, or skin and soft tissue infections. Indwelling intravenous catheter infections are also common sources of *Pseudomonas* bacteremia.

Most of the clinical signs and symptoms of *Pseudomonas* bacteremia are indistinguishable from those associated with gram-negative sepsis caused by other bacteria. Exceptions are the greater likelihood of respiratory failure associated with bacteremic *Pseudomonas* pneumonia; more frequent jaundice; and ecthyma gangrenosum skin lesions, which, although found in a minority of bacteremic patients, are virtually pathognomonic when they are present (69). Other types of skin lesions have also been reported in association with *Pseudomonas* bacteremia, including small painful vesicles; flat, sharply demarcated areas of cellulitis, which may expand rapidly, becoming hemorrhagic and necrotic; diffuse maculopapular eruptions concentrated on the trunk; and metastatic abscesses on the extremities (70).

Empiric, and in most cases, directed therapy of *P. aeruginosa* bacteremia should be with an antibiotic combination, such as a β-lactam agent with antipseudomonal activity and an aminoglycoside or fluoroquinolone antibiotic. Monotherapy of *P. aeruginosa* bacteremia with a single β-lactam or fluoroquinolone antimicrobial, but not an aminoglycoside agent, has been shown to be equivalent to combination therapy in a number of investigations (42–45,71). However, until more clinical data and experience are available, monotherapy of bacteremia should be limited to treatment of patients with *P. aeruginosa* isolates of known susceptibility that do not have neutropenia, septic shock, concomitant *P. aeruginosa* pneumonia, or a life-threatening comorbidity. The initial choice of antibiotics should be governed by local antibiotic susceptibility patterns, and maximum safe doses of both agents should be used. Indwelling intravenous catheters or other devices suspected of being infected and the source of the bacteremia should be removed if possible. In those patients with an indwelling catheter that cannot be removed and who are hemodynamically stable without hypoperfusion or organ system dysfunction, a combination of systemic and catheter antibiotic lock therapy can be attempted (72). The optimal duration of therapy is dictated by the severity of the infection, therapeutic response, and presence or persistence of neutropenia.

BONE AND JOINT INFECTIONS

Pseudomonas infections of the bones and joints result from direct inoculation, contiguous spread, or hematogenous dissemination from distant sites. They often occur in the face of underlying diseases such as diabetes mellitus or other predisposing factors such as chronic debilitation, intravenous drug abuse, and penetrating trauma. *Pseudomonas* has a particular affinity for fibrocartilaginous joints of the axial skeleton, involving cartilage, synovium, joint space, and contiguous bone. *Pseudomonas* osteomyelitis tends to be more indolent and less destructive than bone infections caused by *Staphylococcus aureus* (73).

Pseudomonas pyarthrosis of the sternoclavicular or sternochondral joints occurs principally in intravenous drug users (74). The most common symptoms, which may begin months before diagnosis, are anterior chest pain at the site of involvement and restriction of movement of the ipsilateral shoulder. Swelling, erythema, and tenderness occur over the affected joint; range of motion of the shoulder may be limited on the affected side; and fever is usually present. There is typically an accompanying leukocytosis, and the erythrocyte sedimentation rate is almost always elevated. Aspiration of synovial fluid reveals characteristics of a pyogenic infection, and cultures yield *Pseudomonas* despite the frequent difficulty in identifying organisms on Gram stain of joint fluid. Radiographs reveal soft tissue swelling; demineralization or lytic lesions of adjacent bone; and periosteal elevation of the sternum, rib, or clavicular head. Arthrotomy may be required to débride contiguous areas of involved bone, and perisynovial or retrosternal abscesses may necessitate surgical drainage. A β-lactam or fluoroquinolone antibiotic with activity against *P. aeruginosa* should be administered for a minimum of 6 weeks. Immunosuppressed patients and those with concomitant bacteremia should receive combination therapy with a β-lactam plus aminoglycoside or fluoroquinolone antibiotic. For adherent patients with a functioning gut, a fluoroquinolone agent can be given orally.

P. aeruginosa produces vertebral osteomyelitis in elderly patients in association with complicated urinary tract infections and genitourinary instrumentation or surgery (75). The lumbosacral spine is most commonly involved. *Pseudomonas* vertebral osteomyelitis also occurs in intravenous drug users where it predominately involves the cervical spine (76). Symptoms, including neck or back pain, may last weeks or months. Local tenderness and decreased range of motion of the spine are found on physical examination, whereas neurologic signs are observed in approximately 15% of patients. Fever, when present, is usually low grade. Leukocytosis is variable, and the erythrocyte sedimentation rate is almost always elevated. Radiographs of the affected spine may demonstrate loss of bone density, lytic lesions of vertebral bodies, sclerosis, a narrowed interspace, destruction of adjacent vertebral end plates, and osteophyte formation. Computed tomography (CT) or magnetic resonance imaging (MRI) reveals changes in bone density or adjacent soft tissue densities and may be the most sensitive and specific means for defining the extent of disease. Technetium- and gallium-enhanced scans are also useful for this purpose, although they have lower specificity. *Pseudomonas* may be established as the cause of vertebral osteomyelitis by culture and histologic examination of specimens obtained by needle biopsy or aspiration under fluoroscopic guidance. Surgery is sometimes necessary for adequate exploration and bone biopsy or for decompression of a rare associated epidural or paravertebral abscess.

The choice and length of antimicrobial therapy is similar to that described for pyarthrosis above. A longer course of therapy may be advisable if the area of involvement is extensive, the erythrocyte sedimentation rate remains elevated, or a single antibiotic is used.

Pseudomonas infections of the symphysis pubis are associated with pelvic surgery and intravenous drug abuse (77). Symptoms include groin, thigh, hip, and lower abdominal pain, which is made worse by walking. There is typically exquisite tenderness over the symphysis pubis, and the patient may be febrile. Symptoms may be present for weeks or months before the patient seeks medical attention. Leukocytosis is variable, whereas an elevated erythrocyte sedimentation rate is common. Radiography shows irregularity of the pubic margins, separation of the symphysis pubis, and involvement of the pubic rami, in most cases. Findings of bone scans are usually abnormal. Biopsy or needle aspiration of the symphysis pubis is necessary to make the diagnosis and to distinguish osteomyelitis from osteitis pubis, a presumably noninfectious disease. Most *Pseudomonas* infections of the symphysis pubis are curable with 4 to 6 weeks of antibiotics alone and do not require surgical débridement.

P. aeruginosa is the most common cause of osteochondritis after puncture wounds of the foot by a nail or other sharp object (78). This infection is seen primarily in children but also occurs occasionally in adults. In many cases the infection is acquired via direct inoculation of the foot by *P. aeruginosa* that resides in the moist environment that exists in the soles of shoes. It involves cartilage and bone surrounding small joints and bones of the foot, reflecting the peculiar predilection of *Pseudomonas* for fibrocartilaginous joints. Pain and swelling may develop a number of days after a puncture wound of the foot, and weeks may pass before the patient seeks medical attention. Fever and other systemic signs are usually absent. Tenderness or frank cellulitis is discernible over the affected joint. Possible areas of involvement include the proximal phalanges, metatarsals, metatarsophalangeal joints, tarsal bones, and calcaneus. Radiography and bone scan findings are usually abnormal, and aspiration of the infected joint may yield a small amount of purulent, culture-positive fluid. Treatment consists of extensive surgical débridement and antipseudomonal antibiotics, which are continued for 2 to 4 weeks. One study successfully used oral ciprofloxacin (750 mg twice daily for 7–14 days) after surgical débridement (79).

Chronic contiguous osteomyelitis arises by direct extension from infected overlying soft tissue or direct inoculation rather than by hematogenous spread. *P. aeruginosa* is frequently implicated in this type of infection, which may follow a compound fracture, penetrating trauma, or surgery involving bone. These infections may also complicate peripheral neuropathy or peripheral vascular disease associated with pressure necrosis of skin and soft tissue or decubitus ulcers overlying bone. The heterogeneity of these infections makes it difficult to establish general therapeutic guidelines. Adequate debridement of necrotic bone and tissues along with hardware removal is usually necessary. Antimicrobial therapy is administered parenterally for 4 to 6 weeks; complicated infections may require longer treatment. While combination therapy with a β-lactam and aminoglycoside or fluoroquinolone antibiotic is often employed initially, single agents such as ceftazidime, imipenem, and intravenous or oral ciprofloxacin have been used successfully in all or part of the treatment duration of chronic *Pseudomonas* osteomyelitis (80–82).

CENTRAL NERVOUS SYSTEM INFECTIONS

P. aeruginosa central nervous system infections (meningitis or brain abscess) may result from (a) direct inoculation of the subarachnoid space or brain secondary to penetrating head trauma or surgery; (b) extension from a contiguous focus, such as infected paranasal sinus or mastoid; or (c) bloodstream infection. Other predisposing factors or conditions include previous lumbar puncture, spinal anesthesia, intraventricular shunt or reservoir, cerebrospinal fluid (CSF) leak, and cancer involving the head or subarachnoid space. In one study of postneurosurgical meningitis *Pseudomonas* represented 21% of gram negative meningitis with a mortality of 36% (83).

Pseudomonas meningitis presents, as do other forms of meningitis, with fever, headache, irritability, and obtundation. The onset of meningitis symptoms may be acute, or even fulminant, particularly in association with bacteremia. The clinical course may be compressed into several hours or days and may be accompanied by septic shock. In contrast, *Pseudomonas* meningitis may sometimes develop insidiously, especially when it is associated with a contiguous site of infection or cancer involving the subarachnoid space.

Appropriate antibiotic therapy for *Pseudomonas* meningitis is dictated by the relative bactericidal activity of various agents and their ability to penetrate into the subarachnoid space (84). Ceftazidime has generally been dependable *in vitro* and *in vivo* against *Pseudomonas* and achieves CSF concentrations well in excess of the mean inhibitory concentration for most strains. Ceftazidime may therefore be considered the drug of first choice for the treatment of *Pseudomonas* meningitis (85–87). The need for combination therapy with a second agent such as an aminoglycoside or ciprofloxacin is unclear. Although neither of these second agents achieves useful CSF levels when given systemically, they would generally be advised for those patients who are suspected to have concomitant *Pseudomonas* pneumonia or bacteremia, particularly if the infection is rapidly progressive or life threatening. Because ceftazidime crosses the blood-brain barrier efficiently, there is ordinarily no need for intrathecal administration of either it or an accompanying aminoglycoside. When there is obstruction of the subarachnoid space or ventriculitis is present, an aminoglycoside may have to be instilled directly into the ventricular system through a catheter or reservoir (88,89). Ciprofloxacin has been used successfully in high-dose (400 mg every 8 hours) monotherapy according to anecdotal reports (90,91); however, given its poor penetration into the CSF compared with β-lactam antibiotics, its use as a single drug for these infections should be reserved for therapy of highly resistant *Pseudomonas* or for patients with severe β-lactam allergies. Carbapenems such as imipenem and meropenem, and the monobactam aztreonam, achieve reasonable levels in the CSF and have also been successfully used in the treatment of *Pseudomonas* meningitis (92,93). There is not as much published experience, however, with these agents as with ceftazidime or other β-lactam antibiotics. There are no data on the efficacy of the fourth-generation cephalosporin cefepime in this infection. The proper duration of antibiotic treatment of *Pseudomonas* meningitis is determined by the extent of disease, structural integrity of the involved central nervous system, and initial response to therapy. A minimum of 2 weeks' treatment is usually appropriate. Relapses are common and must be managed aggressively.

Pseudomonas brain abscess is treated with surgical drainage and prolonged antibiotic therapy. The choice of antimicrobial agents should be determined as it is for meningitis. Abscess size is monitored by CT or MRI, and antibiotic therapy is continued until a marked diminution in abscess size or closure is achieved. Failure of initial therapy may necessitate surgical reexploration and drainage, with additional antibiotic treatment.

EAR INFECTIONS

P. aeruginosa is isolated from the external auditory canal of most patients with external otitis (sometimes called "swimmer's ear"), a superficial, self-limited infection that usually resolves spontaneously or responds to local measures (94). On occasion, however, *Pseudomonas* penetrates the epithelium at the junction between cartilage and bone in the floor of the lateral portion of the external auditory canal and invades underlying soft tissue, cartilage, and bone. This invasive, necrotizing process is commonly referred to as malignant external otitis (95,96).

Malignant external otitis is principally a disease of elderly diabetic patients but occasionally affects young infants with serious underlying diseases (95–97). Antecedent ear irrigation and aural water exposure have been found to be risk factors for its development (98,99). Once the infection enters the parotid space or retromandibular area, bypassing the tympanic membrane and middle ear, it enters the mastoid airspaces and temporal bone. It may spread through the temporal bone and the base of the skull, involving the seventh cranial nerve at the stylomastoid foramen; the ninth, tenth, and eleventh cranial nerves at the jugular foramen; and the twelfth cranial nerve at the hypoglossal canal. The lateral and sigmoid sinuses may also become involved, with further extension through vascular channels across the base of the skull. Meningitis and brain abscess are infrequent complications.

The most common symptoms of malignant external otitis are severe otalgia and otorrhea. Facial nerve paralysis occurs early, and other nerve palsies are observed later in the disease. The pinna of the involved ear may be tender; trismus may be present; and diminished hearing is sometimes reported. Fever is uncommon. Physical examination reveals a swollen, erythematous external auditory canal with purulent discharge. The tympanic membrane is intact in some patients, perforated in others, or hidden from view by edema, granulation tissue, and debris. Pain and tenderness are often noted in the pinna and soft tissue adjacent to the ear.

Leukocytosis and CSF pleocytosis are occasional laboratory findings in malignant external otitis. A marked elevation in the erythrocyte sedimentation rate is almost always observed. CT may reveal bony erosions and new bone formation in the mastoid and temporal bone. Soft tissue densities are associated with areas of cellulitis involving the floor of the skull. MRI is superior to CT in defining the extent of disease and soft tissue involvement (100). Technetium 99m–enhanced bone scans may document early bone involvement, whereas gallium 67 scans help distinguish infection from neoplastic disease. *P. aeruginosa* is isolated from the external auditory canal or from surgical specimens in virtually all cases of malignant external otitis. Although other bacteria may also be present, *P. aeruginosa* should be considered the primary agent of this disease.

Malignant external otitis is treated with antipseudomonal antibiotics, occasionally in conjunction with surgical débridement of accessible tissue. Therapy with fluoroquinolone antibiotics, particularly ciprofloxacin, has been shown to have high clinical cure rates and few adverse effects (101–106). Initial intravenous therapy with ciprofloxacin may be switched to oral therapy with this drug (750 mg twice a day) once the patient begins to show a clinical response. Fluoroquinolone susceptibility of clinical isolates of *Pseudomonas* should be ensured when this approach is used, because ciprofloxacin-resistant *Pseudomonas* infections have become increasingly more common. Alternatives to ciprofloxacin include intravenous ceftazidime, cefepime, or other antipseudomonal β-lactams with or without an aminoglycoside.

The duration of therapy should be a minimum of 4 weeks in the case of relatively limited disease and 6 to 8 weeks when the infection is more extensive or oral fluoroquinolone therapy is used. Long-term follow-up, necessitated by the risk for relapse, should include the monitoring of pain, erythrocyte sedimentation rate, and serial CT or MRI studies. There is some evidence for the use

of single-photon emission computed tomography (SPECT) for following the response to therapy (107).

Chronic suppurative otitis media is most often caused by *P. aeruginosa*, sometimes in combination with other organisms. Tympanomastoid surgery is frequently used when medical treatment alone is unsuccessful; however, evidence suggests that aggressive antibiotic therapy, in conjunction with daily otic toilet, may be curative, precluding surgery in cases in which cholesteatoma is not present (108,109).

ENDOCARDITIS

P. aeruginosa causes infections of native heart valves in intravenous drug abusers as well as infections of prosthetic heart valves (110–112). The tricuspid valve is most frequently involved in drug addicts, but the pulmonic, aortic, or mitral valve and mural endocardium of either atrium may also be affected. Right-sided involvement is often subacute in onset, whereas left-sided disease tends to be more acute. Septic pulmonary emboli occur in tricuspid valve endocarditis and may be associated with productive cough, pleuritic chest pain, and pulmonary infiltrates. Left-sided disease, on the other hand, is particularly fulminant and may be accompanied by large systemic arterial embolization and intractable congestive heart failure. Cardiac murmurs are usual. Diagnosis is based on positive blood cultures and appropriate clinical signs. Abnormal transthoracic or transesophageal echocardiographic findings are often confirmatory.

Medical therapy for tricuspid endocarditis should include the higher indicated doses of an antipseudomonal β-lactam antibiotic plus an aminoglycoside. If bacteremia persists beyond 2 weeks' therapy or recurs after 6 weeks' therapy, tricuspid valvulectomy should be undertaken, without valve replacement (110–112). The pulmonic valve should be inspected at the time of surgery and also removed if it is involved. Left-sided *Pseudomonas* endocarditis represents a medical and surgical emergency. Antibiotic therapy, as described for right-sided disease, should be started and the involved aortic or mitral valve replaced immediately. CT should be performed before surgery, and if splenic abscesses are found, splenectomy should be accomplished before cardiac surgery. Antibiotic therapy should be continued for at least 6 weeks, with peak gentamicin or tobramycin serum levels maintained at 12 to 20 μg/mL or at least 10 times the mean bactericidal concentration. Limited animal data may indicate a role for therapy with ciprofloxacin, but clinical data are lacking (113). The prognosis for cure of tricuspid endocarditis, with valvulectomy if necessary, is approximately 80%. Mortality from left-sided infection remains high despite prompt antibiotic therapy and surgery.

EYE INFECTIONS

P. aeruginosa causes keratitis (corneal ulcer) and endophthalmitis. When introduced by direct inoculation or hematogenous spread into the avascular, immunologically sequestered environment of the eye, *P. aeruginosa* can produce rapidly destructive and sometimes sight-threatening disease. Treatment is complicated by the existence of the so-called blood-eye barrier, which limits the delivery of antibiotics to infected intraocular structures.

Eye trauma, sometimes extremely minor, predisposes to *P. aeruginosa* corneal infections by causing a break in the epithelial surface and allowing access of bacteria to the underlying stroma. *Pseudomonas* keratitis appears to be more common in warm, humid environments and is associated with contact lens use, particularly the soft extended-wear type (114). There also is a higher frequency of *Pseudomonas* keratitis in patients with underlying ocular conditions and in those treated with topical steroids or contaminated eye medications (115). Other predisposing conditions include coma, tracheostomy or endotracheal intubation, extensive burns, intensive care, and ocular irradiation (116–118).

Pseudomonas keratitis often starts as a small central ulcer that spreads centrifugally to involve the entire cornea and portions of the surrounding sclera. The infection may also penetrate more deeply into underlying stroma, causing corneal perforation in some instances. Typical clinical signs of *Pseudomonas* keratitis include a rapidly evolving grayish, necrotic stromal infiltrate in the bed of an epithelial injury; tenacious mucopurulent discharge; surrounding epithelial edema; and severe anterior chamber reaction. The lesion may spread rapidly in 24 to 48 hours to involve the entire cornea, leading in some cases to perforation.

Pseudomonas corneal ulcer should be considered a medical emergency because of the chance of perforation into the anterior chamber, leading to a rapidly destructive intraocular infection and possible blindness. Scrapings from the floor of the ulcer are examined by Gram stain and cultured. Susceptibility testing of all culture isolates is indicated due to increasing antimicrobial resistance in *Pseudomonas* corneal infections (119–121). Treatment entails the use of combined topical and subconjunctival or subtenon therapy with an aminoglycoside and β-lactam antibiotic. A fortified antibiotic ophthalmic solution (e.g., gentamicin/tobramycin at 14 mg/mL; piperacillin/ticarcillin at 6–12 mg/mL) should be instilled every 15 to 60 minutes in the affected eye. A fortified ophthalmic solution containing a quinolone antibiotic such as ciprofloxacin, ofloxacin, or lomefloxacin may also be effective for topical therapy. Although small ulcers can often be treated effectively with topical therapy alone, more advanced lesions require simultaneous treatment with subconjunctival or subtenon injections of an aminoglycoside (122). This is particularly critical if perforation into the anterior chamber appears imminent. Gentamicin can be used at a dose of 20 mg, administered once or twice daily for 3 days or until cultures are negative. Subconjunctival ceftazidime may represent an effective alternative to gentamicin.

Pseudomonas endophthalmitis may occur as a complication of perforating corneal ulcer, penetrating injuries, intraocular surgery, or bacteremia originating outside the eye (123–125). It is an acute, fulminant disease that can lead rapidly to the loss of sight. This characteristic of *Pseudomonas* endophthalmitis distinguishes it from other less severe forms of endophthalmitis caused by less virulent bacteria such as *Staphylococcus epidermitis*. Clinical features include pain, decreased visual acuity, conjunctival chemosis and hyperemia, lid edema, hypopyon, and anterior uveitis. These are followed by involvement of the vitreous and panophthalmitis. Proper management of *Pseudomonas* endophthalmitis begins with aspiration of the anterior chamber or vitreous cavity to obtain material for Gram stain and culture. Wound drainage after intraocular surgery may be cultured in lieu of aspirated material from the eye, although superficial conjunctival cultures are undependable. Appropriate antibiotic therapy includes the intravitreal administration of ceftazidime (2.25 mg) or aminoglycosides (e.g., amikacin, 0.4 mg) in addition to their topical or subconjunctival (or subtenon) administration. Concomitant systemic therapy with ceftazidime or antipseudomonal penicillin with or without ciprofloxacin or an aminoglycoside is often instituted. Meropenem or cefepime may provide effective alternative systemic therapy, although there is limited published experience with these agents in this infection. Vitrectomy is frequently useful to clear areas of loculated infection, dispose of necrotic material, and enhance antibiotic penetration into the eye. Antibiotic therapy should be continued until clinical improvement occurs and signs of infection in the eye have subsided. The prognosis for *Pseudomonas* endophthalmitis diagnosed early and treated aggressively has improved markedly compared with that in the past.

GASTROINTESTINAL INFECTIONS

The gastrointestinal tract represents a common portal of entry for *Pseudomonas* bloodstream infections as well as a frequent site of primary infection. *Pseudomonas* is a common cause of necrotizing enterocolitis in young infants (126,127), in which affected patients present with irritability, vomiting, diarrhea, and dehydration. Physical findings include fever, abdominal distention, and signs of peritonitis. A similar disease, known as "typhlitis," occurs in neutropenic cancer patients where *Pseudomonas* is one of the most important isolates in this polymicrobial infection (128–130). The most common sites of involvement are the distal ileum, cecum, and proximal ascending colon. Necrosis and gangrene, sometimes leading to perforation with resultant peritonitis, are most often seen in patients with acute leukemia. CT and ultrasonography are useful for establishing the diagnosis. Necrotizing enterocolitis is best treated with a broad-spectrum β-lactam antibiotic that has antipseudomonal as well as anaerobic activity (e.g., piperacillin/tazobactam, ticarcillin/clavulanate, or a carbapenem) with or without an aminoglycoside or fluoroquinolone antibiotic. Surgical intervention may be necessary in the event of bowel gangrene or perforation. Death is common despite aggressive therapy.

P. aeruginosa has also been associated historically with a syndrome that resembles enteric fever. So-called Shanghai fever (131,132) presents with constipation or diarrhea, rash, and fever lasting 1 to 2 weeks. *Pseudomonas* is isolated from stool, but its causal role is unclear, and the curative action of antibiotics is not known.

RESPIRATORY INFECTIONS

P. aeruginosa causes acute, life-threatening, bacteremic (133–135) or nonbacteremic pneumonia (136) in immunocompromised patients, including those with acquired immunodeficiency syndrome (AIDS) (137). In addition, it can cause a chronic lower respiratory tract infection in patients with CF or bronchiectasis. Patients exposed to the hospital environment, particularly in an intensive care setting, are subject to upper respiratory tract colonization by *P. aeruginosa*. Previous antibiotic administration and ventilator or respiratory inhalation therapy, as well as underlying chronic lung disease and congestive heart failure, predispose colonized patients to lower respiratory tract infection through aspiration of upper respiratory secretions. Thus, it is not surprising that this organism has been found to be one of the leading causes of pneumonia in the intensive care unit (9). Unfortunately, because airway colonization with *P. aeruginosa* is common in critically ill patients, it is often difficult to determine the significance of a respiratory culture yielding this organism. Occasionally, epidemics of *Pseudomonas* pneumonia due to a unique strain of the organism are identified in intensive care and other closed units. Sources of these outbreaks have included respiratory devices, unit water sources, drains, and contaminated bronchoscopes (3,6,7). Although community-acquired pneumonia due to *P. aeruginosa* has been described in normal hosts, it is distinctly uncommon (138).

Pseudomonas pneumonia may present as a fulminant infection accompanied by chills, fever, dyspnea, productive cough, cyanosis, and signs of severe systemic toxic effects (136). Chest radiographs may show a diffuse bronchopneumonia, often bilateral, with distinctive nodular infiltrates, sometimes associated with areas of radiolucency. Lobar consolidation is sometimes seen, pleural effusions are common, but empyema is rare. Microabscesses occur in *Pseudomonas* pneumonia, and necrosis of alveolar septa is observed, but blood vessels are not involved in nonbacteremic infections.

Bacteremic *Pseudomonas* pneumonia occurs principally in neutropenic patients (133–135). It begins in the lower respiratory tract, is accompanied by bloodstream invasion, and often spreads to metastatic sites of infection. Small, nodular, hemorrhagic (and sometimes necrotic) lesions form diffusely in both lung fields. On microscopic examination, these lesions involve small blood vessels and contain many bacteria but lack a leukocytic reaction. They represent the pulmonary counterpart of ecthyma gangrenosum involving the skin. The radiographic picture of bacteremic *Pseudomonas* pneumonia is typified by rapid progression from pulmonary vascular congestion to pulmonary edema to necrotizing bronchopneumonia (133). The course of this disease is usually fulminant and ends fatally, particularly in neutropenic patients.

Most patients with CF suffer from chronic lower respiratory tract infection by mucoid strains of *P. aeruginosa* beginning between the ages of 3 and 18 years (139). Once established, these infections usually persist for life and follow a progressive waxing and waning course punctuated by frequent acute exacerbations. Lower respiratory tract infection by *Pseudomonas* contributes substantially to acute exacerbations and chronic progression of CF lung disease. The clinical signs and symptoms of *Pseudomonas* pulmonary infection in CF patients vary considerably as a function of the extent of underlying lung disease and the frequency and severity of acute exacerbations (140). Patients develop a chronic productive cough, decreased appetite, weight loss, and diminished activity, particularly during acute episodes. Wheezing and tachypnea may be present, and low-grade fever is usually documented during acute exacerbations. Physical signs include evidence of undernutrition, clubbing, increased anteroposterior diameter, retractions, cyanosis, wheezing, moist rales and rhonchi, and abdominal distention. Leukocytosis with a leftward shift is usual. Blood gas values demonstrate hypoxemia with or without hypercapnia. Results of pulmonary function tests indicate an obstructive defect and restriction in the presence of chronic fibrosis. Radiographs of the chest show overaeration, peribronchial thickening, patchy atelectasis, and pneumonia.

The treatment of life-threatening *Pseudomonas* lower respiratory tract infections requires the early, aggressive use of antibiotics. Because of the increasing problem with antimicrobial resistance in the organism, the initial empiric choice of antimicrobials should be made based on the local antimicrobial susceptibility patterns of *Pseudomonas* that are endemic to the institution. Continuing therapy should be guided by specific susceptibility testing of any respiratory or blood culture isolates. Initially, an antipseudomonal β-lactam agent in combination with an aminoglycoside or ciprofloxacin should be combined in maximum tolerated doses to attain optimal bactericidal activity in lung tissue, pulmonary secretions, and blood. Such combination therapy is meant to achieve synergistic killing or to maximize coverage of potentially resistant strains prior to the results of susceptibility testing. Although combination therapy has traditionally been advocated for the duration of therapy, some researchers have recently suggested that treatment may be streamlined to a single agent once culture results are available and the patient shows a favorable clinical response (38). The duration of therapy, dictated by the severity of disease and clinical response, should be no less than 10 days in most cases. As an alternative to or in conjunction with intravenous therapy, there may be a role for inhalational antibiotic therapy in selected non-CF patients with acute *Pseudomonas* pneumonia, as well as in patients with bronchiectasis and chronic pseudomonas lung infection (138,141). Ceftazidime and aminoglycosides have both been administered via this route.

The treatment of acute exacerbations of *Pseudomonas* lower respiratory tract infections in CF follows the same principles as those just outlined (139,142–148). Antibiotics may be expected to produce temporary improvement in both respiratory symptoms and pulmonary function. *P. aeruginosa* may disappear temporarily from the patient's sputum or persist, sometimes developing resistance to the antibiotic used (144,149). After cessation of treatment, however, *P. aeruginosa* often returns to the sputum or reverts to its original antibiotic susceptibility pattern. Moreover, the clinical improvement associated with antibiotic treatment appears to bear little relation to the microbiology of sputum. Acute exacerbations of *Pseudomonas* lung disease are treated with antibiotics until clinical improvement is noted, customarily within 1 to 2 weeks. Larger than usual doses of aminoglycosides, β-lactam agents, and fluoroquinolones are frequently required by CF patients because of altered antibiotic pharmacokinetics (150). Because of the emergence of respiratory infections in patients with CF due to *P. aeruginosa* that is resistant to all available conventional drugs, therapy with aerosolized and intravenous colistin is sometimes necessary and has been used with some success (58).

Another treatment strategy entails intermittent antibiotic therapy for chronic *Pseudomonas* lung disease aimed at preventing acute exacerbations. This approach, employed in Denmark using quinolone antibiotics, may be responsible in part for improvements in mortality rates (151,152). In addition, intermittent aerosolization of antibiotics including tobramycin or colistin into the lower respiratory tract of CF patients has also been shown to result in symptomatic improvement, improved pulmonary function, and a reduced number of hospitalizations (153–156). Finally, lung transplantation has been used successfully in CF patients with end-stage *P. aeruginosa*–associated lower respiratory tract disease (157–159).

SKIN AND SOFT TISSUE INFECTIONS

Ecthyma gangrenosum is a focal skin lesion characterized by hemorrhage, necrosis, surrounding erythema, and vascular invasion by bacteria (69,160). Ecthyma lesions are usually associated with *Pseudomonas* bacteremia, although they occur in a minority of such cases. Whereas it is sometimes claimed that ecthyma gangrenosum is pathognomonic for *P. aeruginosa* infections, it has been reported, albeit rarely, in association with *S. maltophilia* sepsis (161,162) and other forms of gram-negative sepsis (163). *P. aeruginosa* septicemia, on the other hand, has also been associated with vesicular or pustular skin lesions, subcutaneous nodules, deep abscesses, cellulitis, and bullae (164,165). Large, destructive lesions of the skin or mucous membranes can complicate *Pseudomonas* sepsis, particularly in neutropenic patients (166–168). These lesions may produce frank gangrene involving the face, oropharynx, perineum, or extremities.

Primary *Pseudomonas* skin lesions may be focal or diffuse. Predisposition to such infections results from skin breakdown secondary to severe burns, trauma, dermatitis, or local ulcerations; moisture involving the perineum, diaper area of small infants, swimmers' ears, soldiers' feet in the tropics; and neutropenia secondary to cancer chemotherapy. Primary *Pseudomonas* pyoderma looks much like ecthyma lesions associated with *Pseudomonas* bacteremia. Both lesions appear hemorrhagic and necrotic, and both are likely to demonstrate vascular invasion by bacteria.

Pseudomonas wound infections usually do not have a characteristic appearance that distinguishes them from those caused by other bacteria. However, *Pseudomonas* wound infections or pyoderma may occasionally give rise to a blue-green exudate resulting from the production by *P. aeruginosa* of pyocyanin pigment (169), and a characteristic fruity odor may be noted. The pyocyanin pigment produced by *Pseudomonas* may be seen more readily on wound dressings or bandages than within the wound itself. Virtually any nonoperative or postoperative wound infection may be caused by *P. aeruginosa*, but the organism should be seriously considered in any wound, such as a compound fracture, that is contaminated with soil, water, or plant material.

Nosocomial, common source outbreaks of *Pseudomonas* surgical wound infections occasionally occur. One such outbreak of sternal wound infections following median sternotomy operations was traced to a surgical scrub nurse afflicted with onychomycosis colonized by *P. aeruginosa* (14).

In contrast to the severe manifestations of skin and soft tissue discussed above, *P. aeruginosa* is also capable of causing self-limited, diffuse, pruritic, maculopapular, or vesiculopustular rashes in association with exposure to contaminated hot tubs, spas, or whirlpools (170–172). Many cases are reported as a part of a common-source outbreak. Rashes tend to be more pronounced in the area covered by the bathing suit but can be diffuse. Systemic symptoms rarely include fever but may involve headache, dizziness, sore eyes, earache, sore nose, sore throat, breast tenderness, and abdominal pain. *Pseudomonas* rashes occurring in this setting usually require no specific therapy. Possible exceptions are immunocompromised patients, including those with neutropenia and AIDS, whose skin involvement may be more extensive and require systemic antimicrobial therapy (173,174). The source of exposure should be identified, if possible, and reexposure prevented. A similar condition, termed *Pseudomonas* hot foot syndrome, was reported in a group of children exposed to a wading pool containing high concentrations of *P. aeruginosa*. This infection was characterized by the acute onset of exquisitely painful plantar nodules that followed a benign, self-limited course (175).

P. aeruginosa is a common cause of hospital-acquired burn wound infection with a high mortality rate. *Pseudomonas* burn wound infections typically occur at least 1 to 2 weeks after severe thermal injury. During the lag period, the patient's normal skin flora may be replaced by hospital flora, including *Pseudomonas*, particularly under the selective pressure of antibiotics. Sepsis results from colonization of the burn eschar, invasion of the subeschar space, and bloodstream invasion. Clinical manifestations include multifocal discoloration of the burn eschar, degeneration of underlying granulation tissue leading to premature eschar separation and hemorrhage, edema or hemorrhagic necrosis of tissue adjacent to the infected burn site, and brown or black neoeschar formation. Systemic symptoms may include fever or hypothermia, disorientation, hypotension, oliguria, and abdominal distention. Ecthyma gangrenosum lesions may appear at sites distant from the infected burn wound, and pneumonia may be present, especially if inhalation injury has occurred.

Early recognition of *Pseudomonas* burn wound sepsis is essential for successful treatment. Daily surveillance of burn sites should focus on signs of inflammation or fresh tissue damage, and systemic symptoms should be closely monitored. There may be a role for biopsy of suspicious skin sites that includes quantitative culture of the specimen. Diagnostic features include greater than 10^5 organisms per gram of tissue, bacteria in unburned tissue, masses of organisms in the subeschar space, perivascular inflammation, hemorrhage, and an inflammatory reaction at the burn wound margin (176,177). If *Pseudomonas* burn wound sepsis is suspected, it should be treated presumptively and immediately with maximum doses of at least two antibiotics to which the infecting strain is likely to be susceptible. The specific choice of antibiotics is dictated by local susceptibility patterns and complicated by the fact that burn centers tend to harbor highly resistant strains of *P. aeruginosa* (178,179). Single-agent antimicrobial therapy should not ordinarily be used for *Pseudomonas* burn wound sepsis because of the huge populations of bacteria present in burned tissues and the limited access of antibiotics to poorly perfused burn sites. An absorbable topical agent such as mafenide acetate (Sulfamylon, Bertek Pharmaceuticals, Morgantown, WV, U.S.A.) should be applied to burn sites colonized or infected by *Pseudomonas* organisms to reduce the population of bacteria present. In addition, subeschar antibiotic injections have been advocated in the case of infections that do not extend beneath the investing fascia (180). Finally, surgical débridement of necrotic tissue, eschar removal, or even amputation may be necessary in addition to systemic and local antibiotic therapy.

URINARY TRACT INFECTIONS

Many *Pseudomonas* urinary tract infections are hospital acquired, and some are iatrogenic. Common predisposing factors are urinary tract catheterization, instrumentation, and surgery, including renal transplantation (181–183). Outbreaks of invasive *Pseudomonas* urinary tract infections related to contaminated urodynamic devices have been described (5). *Pseudomonas* urinary tract infections are frequently associated with persistent sites of infection (such as chronic prostatitis or stones), obstruction, or previous antibiotic therapy. Recurrences are common, and chronic *Pseudomonas* urinary tract infections are often seen. Multidrug-resistant *Pseudomonas* often complicates recurrent or chronic infection. Clinical symptoms and signs of uncomplicated *Pseudomonas* urinary tract infection are similar to those due to other bacteria.

Proper therapy for *Pseudomonas* urinary tract infections is governed by the area of involvement, extent of infection, association with bacteremia, chronicity, presence of a persistent focus or obstruction, and antibiotic susceptibility of the infecting strain. Most symptomatic *Pseudomonas* urinary tract infections should be treated. Sites of persistence (such as an indwelling Foley catheter or stone) should be removed if possible, obstructions relieved, or abscesses drained. Due to the achievable concentrations in urine, aminoglycosides are the first-line drugs for single-agent treatment of *Pseudomonas* urinary tract infection that is not complicated by bacteremia. Antipseudomonal penicillins, extended-spectrum cephalosporins, carbapenems, aztreonam, and the oral fluoroquinolones are all possible alternatives.

Ciprofloxacin has been widely employed for the treatment of *Pseudomonas* urinary tract infections because of its superior activity against *P. aeruginosa* and good systemic distribution following oral dosing (184–186). Oral ciprofloxacin has been used effectively in acute, complicated, and chronic *Pseudomonas* urinary tract infections, even in the presence of a persistent focus. Unfortunately, treatment failure and relapse rates are generally high in complicated *Pseudomonas* urinary tract infections, and ciprofloxacin-resistant strains have been become increasingly common in these settings. Parenteral therapy for *Pseudomonas* urinary tract infections limited to the bladder should be administered for 3 to 5 days; urosepsis should be treated for at least 10 days; and documented or suspected upper tract involvement associated with obstruction or abscess formation is best treated for 2 to 3 weeks. Although optimal dosing schedules for oral quinolones have not been firmly established, ciprofloxacin may be administered at a dose of 250 to 500 mg twice daily for 5 to 14 days, depending on the extent and severity of a particular infection. Longer courses of treatment using ciprofloxacin have been employed for certain chronic *Pseudomonas* urinary tract infections, especially those associated with a persistent focus, and chronic suppression has been attempted in some instances, with varying success.

PSEUDOMONAS AERUGINOSA INFECTIONS IN PATIENTS WITH ACQUIRED IMMUNODEFICIENCY SYNDROME

P. aeruginosa infections have been reported in patients with advanced stages of AIDS (137,139,187,188). These infections have been documented in the presence or absence of traditional risk factors for the development of *Pseudomonas* disease, such as hospitalization, previous antibiotic therapy, neutropenia, indwelling vascular catheters, or other factors associated with the interruption of normal anatomic barriers to infection. The majority of such infections occur in human immunodeficiency virus (HIV)-infected individuals with profoundly low CD4+ T-cell counts (<50 cells/mL) and a history of opportunistic infections. Although earlier reports suggested that *P. aeruginosa* infections in AIDS patients were primarily nosocomial, later studies documented that the majority of such infections are actually community acquired, albeit associated, in some instances, with previous hospitalization or antibiotic therapy. Morbidity and mortality are high, and relapse or recurrence is common.

The immunologic factors in AIDS that predispose patients to *Pseudomonas* disease have not been specifically identified or prioritized. It has been speculated, nonetheless, that impaired host defense mechanisms, including loss of mucosal integrity, defects in humoral and cellular immunity, and leukocyte abnormalities, may render HIV-infected patients more susceptible to life-threatening *P. aeruginosa* infections (188).

P. aeruginosa bronchopulmonary infections account for a substantial proportion of *Pseudomonas* disease observed in patients with late-stage HIV infections (168,189–194). Most of these infections are community acquired, many are recurrent or chronic despite appropriate antibiotic therapy, and a substantial proportion are associated with cavitary pulmonary lesions. This pattern of recurrent or chronic *Pseudomonas* lower respiratory tract infection has been compared with that observed in patients with CF (191). AIDS-related *P. aeruginosa* lung infections have been reported to produce bronchopneumonia (191), lobar pneumonia (189), diffuse interstitial involvement (190), cavitary lesions (192,195), empyema (188), acute and chronic bronchitis, and bronchiectasis (194).

P. aeruginosa bacteremia occurs in children (196,197) as well as in adults (198) with AIDS. It can be either community or hospital acquired and may be associated with a primary site of infection involving the lungs, upper respiratory tract, ear, or indwelling vascular catheter (198). Bacteremic infections are often fulminant, particularly in children, and may be associated with signs of sepsis as well as with skin manifestations. Mortality rates are high, and relapse is common, although complications can be lessened by early and appropriate antimicrobial therapy (197,198).

Bacterial infections of the paranasal sinuses are a common complication of advanced HIV disease (199,200), and *P. aeruginosa* is a frequent cause of these infections (199–201). Like AIDS-associated *Pseudomonas* infections at other sites, *P. aeruginosa* sinus infections are usually community acquired, although sometimes associated with previous hospitalization or antibiotic therapy. Multiple sinuses are typically involved, and infections tend to be recurrent or chronic. Therapy includes antibiotics with antipseudomonal activity and appropriate irrigation or drainage procedures. Repeated courses of treatment or chronic suppressive therapy are often indicated.

Other AIDS-associated *Pseudomonas* infections may involve the skin (including ecthyma gangrenosum) (173,202), soft tissues (203,204), bone (205), and urinary tract (206). In addition, malignant external otitis unassociated with diabetes mellitus has been reported (207–209).

The treatment of *P. aeruginosa* infections in AIDS patients relies on antimicrobial agents and ancillary measures similar to those employed in treating *Pseudomonas* infections in other immunocompromised patients. The widespread use of trimethoprim-sulfamethoxazole and dapsone for prophylaxis against opportunistic infections has not been found to be protective against *Pseudomonas* infections in AIDS patients and in fact, in some studies, has been shown to increase their risk for infection (210–212). Since the late 1990s the incidence of *P. aerug-*

inosa infections in patients with AIDS appears to be declining, possibly due to widespread use of highly active antiretroviral therapy and the consequent increase in CD4 cell counts (213,214). In addition, a few patients with recalcitrant, relapsing *P. aeruginosa* bronchopulmonary infections have experienced resolution of infection after the initiation of intense antiretroviral therapy (215). Unfortunately, advanced HIV patients whose virus has developed antiretroviral resistance continue to be at risk for *Pseudomonas* infection (215,216).

STENOTROPHOMONAS MALTOPHILIA

S. maltophilia, like *P. aeruginosa*, is a ubiquitous free-living organism. It colonizes various body sites of hospitalized patients and has emerged as an important opportunistic pathogen. Factors that lead to colonization and infection with this organism include prolonged hospitalization, malignancy, catheterization (urinary, peritoneal, and central venous), and prior administration of broad-spectrum antibiotics (217). Among the documented infections caused by this organism are bacteremia, pneumonia, endocarditis, urinary tract infection, meningitis, wound infection, peritonitis, and cholangitis (162,218–222). A salient characteristic of *S. maltophilia* is its resistance to antibiotics, including agents such as the aminoglycosides and carbapenems, which are active against *P. aeruginosa*. *S. maltophilia* is resistant, or develops resistance, to many β-lactam agents because of low outer-membrane permeability and at least two inducible broad-spectrum β-lactamases (223). The antibiotic resistance of *S. maltophilia* has contributed to its emergence as a nosocomial pathogen in areas, such as the intensive care unit, where patients are severely ill and broad-spectrum antibiotic use is commonplace.

S. maltophilia is sometimes associated with pseudoinfection, particularly pseudobacteremia, as a result of contamination of blood-drawing materials. Authentic intravenous line–related sepsis due to this organism is well recognized, as are bacteremias associated with a number of different primary sites of infection. *S. maltophilia* urosepsis occurs in the setting of chronic indwelling urinary catheterization or urologic procedures. It is generally indistinguishable from urinary tract sepsis caused by other organisms. *S. maltophilia* peritonitis has been reported in patients undergoing chronic ambulatory peritoneal dialysis. Pneumonia, although relatively uncommon, is seen increasingly among critically ill or debilitated intensive care unit patients; positive blood cultures may accompany as many as 75% of such cases (220). *S. maltophilia* has been reported as a cause of native valve endocarditis among intravenous drug abusers (162) and of prosthetic valve infections (219). *S. maltophilia* endocarditis is usually subacute, although extensive abscess and fistula formation has been reported. Ecthyma gangrenosum skin lesions, apparently identical to those associated with *P. aeruginosa* infections, have been observed in two leukemia patients with *S. maltophilia* bacteremia (161,162). Postoperative *S. maltophilia* meningitis has also been reported (162).

S. maltophilia infections have been treated successfully with trimethoprim-sulfamethoxazole, to which the organism is usually sensitive. Other effective antibiotics may include ticarcillin-clavulanate and third-generation cephalosporins such as cefoperazone or ceftazidime, although susceptibility must be documented initially and monitored during therapy. Long-acting tetracyclines such as doxycycline also have activity against most *S. maltophilia* strains. Limited *in vitro* and clinical data suggest a possible future role for aztreonam plus clavulanate for treatment of multidrug-resistant *S. maltophilia* infections (141,161,162,224).

BURKHOLDERIA CEPACIA

B. cepacia has been identified as both an endemic and an epidemic nosocomial pathogen (225–227). Hospital outbreaks are often traced to a contaminated liquid reservoir or moist environmental surface. It is often difficult to distinguish between *B. cepacia* colonization and infection, and pseudoinfections are common because of the capacity of the organism to contaminate liquids of all kinds, including antiseptics and disinfectants (228). At least two outbreaks of *B. cepacia* pseudobacteremia (and bacteremia) have been traced to contaminated blood gas analyzers (229). *B. cepacia* colonization of various body sites is relatively common in the hospital setting and often precedes serious infections, including surgical and burn wound infections, bacteremia, urinary tract infections, pneumonia, meningitis, and peritonitis. In addition, *B. cepacia* endocarditis has been reported as a complication of intravenous drug abuse (230).

The increasing frequency of *B. cepacia* lower respiratory tract infections in CF patients is a trend of growing concern (227,231,232). *B. cepacia* is being isolated, alone or in combination with *P. aeruginosa,* from respiratory secretions of patients from many CF centers. Isolation of *B. cepacia* correlates, in a general way, with clinical deterioration. Of special concern is a subgroup of such patients who, when colonized with *B. cepacia,* exhibit a fulminant downhill disease course. These patients suffer extensive necrotizing pneumonia, sometimes accompanied by *B. cepacia* bacteremia (233). Some, but not all, cystic fibrosis centers segregate patients infected or colonized with *B. cepacia* in an attempt to reduce horizontal transmission of this organism to uninfected patients.

Therapy for *B. cepacia* infections is complicated by intrinsic resistance of the organism to many β-lactam agents as well as to the aminoglycosides (234). Although they are traditionally susceptible to trimethoprim-sulfamethoxazole, chloramphenicol, and minocycline, some *B. cepacia* strains have developed resistance to these agents as well. Carbapenems and third-generation cephalosporins and fluoroquinolones have variable activity against *B. cepacia.* The aminoglycosides and colistin are generally inactive against *B. cepacia.* Synergy against *B. cepacia in vitro* has been demonstrated for various antibiotic combinations such as tobramycin or gentamicin and aztreonam (142) or ciprofloxacin, imipenem, and rifampin (235). The clinical significance of these interactions *in vitro* is unknown. Unfortunately, cystic fibrosis patients with *B. cepacia* infection have a high mortality rate following lung transplantation, which limits the potential for this procedure in many medical centers.

OTHER RELATED BACTERIA

Pseudomonas fluorescens, together with *P. aeruginosa* and *Pseudomonas putida,* composes the so-called fluorescent group of pseudomonads; it is a rare cause of iatrogenic human infections. Although it has been implicated in bacteremia, pneumonia, urinary tract infections, and soft tissue infections, its best known association is with blood transfusion-induced bacteremia (236,237). The ability of psychrophilic *P. fluorescens* to grow, multiply, and survive in blood at 4°C is the primary basis for its causative role in bacteremia associated with the administration of contaminated blood products. Transfusion-associated *P. fluorescens* bacteremia can be fatal, even when it is suspected and treated promptly. *P. fluorescens* pseudobacteremia has also been reported, after inoculation of contaminated blood culture collection tubes (238,239).

Rare infections have been associated with *P. mosselli, P. putida, Pseudomonas stutzeri, Pseudomonas alcaligenes,* and *Pseu-* *domonas pseudoalcaligenes; Burkholderia pickettii; Comomonas acidovorans* and *Comomonas testosteroni; Brevundimonas diminuta* and *Brevundimonas vesicularis;* and other related species (2). Although unusual human pathogens, the aforementioned species share common features with *P. aeruginosa*: wide distribution in nature, primarily saprophytic or commensal relationship to humans, and occasional emergence as opportunistic pathogens in the face of impaired host defenses.

REFERENCES

1. Bruckner DA, Colonna P. Nomenclature for aerobic and facultative bacteria. *Clin Infect Dis* 1995;21:263–272.
2. Kiska D, Gilligan P. *Pseudomonas.* In: Murray P, Baron E, Pfaller M, et al., eds. *Manual of clinical microbiology.* Washington, DC: American Society for Microbiology, 1999:517–525.
3. Bukholm G, Tannaes T, Kjelsberg AB, et al. An outbreak of multidrug-resistant *Pseudomonas aeruginosa* associated with increased risk of patient death in an intensive care unit. *Infect Control Hosp Epidemiol* 2002;23:441–446.
4. Cortes P, Mariscal D, Valles J, et al. Presence of polyclonal *Pseudomonas aeruginosa* in an intensive care unit: a 27-month prospective study on molecular epidemiology. *Infect Control Hosp Epidemiol* 2001;22:720–723.
5. Yardy GW, Cox RA. An outbreak of *Pseudomonas aeruginosa* infection associated with contaminated urodynamic equipment. *J Hosp Infect* 2001;47:60–63.
6. Srinivasan A, Wolfenden LL, Song X, et al. An outbreak of *Pseudomonas aeruginosa* infections associated with flexible bronchoscopes. *N Engl J Med* 2003;348:221–227.
7. Berrouane YF, McNutt LA, Buschelman BJ, et al. Outbreak of severe *Pseudomonas aeruginosa* infections caused by a contaminated drain in a whirlpool bathtub. *Clin Infect Dis* 2000;31:1331–1337.
8. Schlech WF III, Simonsen N, Sumarah R, et al. Nosocomial outbreak of *Pseudomonas aeruginosa* folliculitis associated with a physiotherapy pool. *CMAJ* 1986;134:909–913.
9. National Nosocomial Infections Surveillance (NNIS) System report, data summary from January 1990–May 1999, issued June 1999. *Am J Infect Control* 1999;27:520–532.
10. Miranda G, Leanos B, Marquez L, et al. Molecular epidemiology of a multiresistant *Pseudomonas aeruginosa* outbreak in a paediatric intensive care unit. *Scand J Infect Dis* 2001;33:738–743.
11. Bertrand X, Thouverez M, Talon D, et al. Endemicity, molecular diversity and colonisation routes of *Pseudomonas aeruginosa* in intensive care units. *Intens Care Med* 2001;27:1263–1268.
12. Becks VE, Lorenzoni NM. *Pseudomonas aeruginosa* outbreak in a neonatal intensive care unit: a possible link to contaminated hand lotion. *Am J Infect Control* 1995;23:396–398.
13. Foca M, Jakob K, Whittier S, et al. Endemic *Pseudomonas aeruginosa* infection in a neonatal intensive care unit. *N Engl J Med* 2000;343:695–700.
14. McNeil SA, Nordstrom-Lerner L, Malani PN, et al. Outbreak of sternal surgical site infections due to *Pseudomonas aeruginosa* traced to a scrub nurse with onychomycosis. *Clin Infect Dis* 2001;33:317–323.
15. Moolenaar RL, Crutcher JM, San Joaquin VH, et al. A prolonged outbreak of *Pseudomonas aeruginosa* in a neonatal intensive care unit: did staff fingernails play a role in disease transmission? *Infect Control Hosp Epidemiol* 2000;21:80–85.
16. Stover CK, Pham XQ, Erwin AL, et al. Complete genome sequence of *Pseudomonas aeruginosa* PA01, an opportunistic pathogen. *Nature* 2000;406:959–964.
17. Chitnis CE, Ohman DE. Genetic analysis of the alginate biosynthetic gene cluster of *Pseudomonas aeruginosa* shows evidence of an operonic structure. *Mol Microbiol* 1993;8:583–593.
18. Morihara K. Production of elastase and proteinase by *Pseudomonas aeruginosa.* *J Bacteriol* 1964;88:745–749.
19. Berka RM, Vasil ML. Phospholipase C (heat-labile hemolysin) of *Pseudomonas aeruginosa*: purification and preliminary characterization. *J Bacteriol* 1982;152:239–245.
20. Johnson MK, Boese-Marrazzo D. Production and properties of heat-stable extracellular hemolysin from *Pseudomonas aeruginosa. Infect Immun* 1980;29:1028–1033.
21. Allured VS, Collier RJ, Carroll SF, et al. Structure of exotoxin A of *Pseudomonas aeruginosa* at 3.0-Angstrom resolution. *Proc Natl Acad Sci USA* 1986;83:1320–1324.
22. Iglewski BH, Kabat D. NAD-dependent inhibition of protein synthesis by *Pseudomonas aeruginosa* toxin. *Proc Natl Acad Sci USA* 1975;72:2284–2288.
23. Pollack M, Young LS. Protective activity of antibodies to exotoxin A and lipopolysaccharide at the onset of *Pseudomonas aeruginosa* septicemia in man. *J Clin Invest* 1979;63:276–286.
24. Finck-Barbancon V, Goranson J, Zhu L, et al. ExoU expression by *Pseudomonas aeruginosa* correlates with acute cytotoxicity and epithelial injury. *Mol Microbiol* 1997;25:547–557.
25. Kulich SM, Yahr TL, Mende-Mueller LM, et al. Cloning the structural gene for the 49-kDa form of exoenzyme S (exoS) from *Pseudomonas aeruginosa* strain 388. *J Biol Chem* 1994;269:10431–10437.

26. Yahr TL, Vallis AJ, Hancock MK, et al. ExoY, an adenylate cyclase secreted by the *Pseudomonas aeruginosa* type III system. *Proc Natl Acad Sci USA* 1998; 95:13899–13904.

27. Winstanley C, Hart CA. Type III secretion systems and pathogenicity islands. *J Med Microbiol* 2001;50:116–126.

28. Hauser AR, Cobb E, Bodi M, et al. Type III protein secretion is associated with poor clinical outcomes in patients with ventilator-associated pneumonia caused by *Pseudomonas aeruginosa*. *Crit Care Med* 2002;30:521–528.

29. Davies DG, Parsek MR, Pearson JP, et al. The involvement of cell-to-cell signals in the development of a bacterial biofilm. *Science* 1998;280:295–298.

30. Parsek MR, Greenberg EP. Acyl-homoserine lactone quorum sensing in gram-negative bacteria: a signaling mechanism involved in associations with higher organisms. *Proc Natl Acad Sci USA* 2000;97:8789–8793.

31. Pesci EC, Iglewski BH. The chain of command in *Pseudomonas* quorum sensing. *Trends Microbiol* 1997;5:132–134.

32. Rumbaugh KP, Griswold JA, Hamood AN. The role of quorum sensing in the *in vivo* virulence of *Pseudomonas aeruginosa*. *Microbes Infect* 2000;2:1721–1731.

33. Lesprit P, Faurisson F, Join-Lambert O, et al. Role of the quorum-sensing system in experimental pneumonia due to *Pseudomonas aeruginosa* in rats. *Am J Respir Crit Care Med* 2003;167:1478–1482.

34. Pearson JP, Feldman M, Iglewski BH, et al. *Pseudomonas aeruginosa* cell-to-cell signaling is required for virulence in a model of acute pulmonary infection. *Infect Immun* 2000;68:4331–4334.

35. Hilf M, Yu VL, Sharp J, et al. Antibiotic therapy for *Pseudomonas aeruginosa* bacteremia: outcome correlations in a prospective study of 200 patients. *Am J Med* 1989;87:540–546.

36. Bodey GP, Jadeja L, Elting L. *Pseudomonas* bacteremia. Retrospective analysis of 410 episodes. *Arch Intern Med* 1985;145:1621–1629.

37. Craig W, Ebert S. Antimicrobial therapy in *Pseudomonas aeruginosa* infections. In: Baltch A, Smith R, eds. Pseudomonas aeruginosa *infections and treatment*. New York: Marcel Dekker, 1994:441–518.

38. Acharya A, Paterson D. *Pseudomonas aeruginosa*. In: Yu VL, Weber R, Raoult D, eds. *Antimicrobial therapy and vaccines*. New York: Apple Trees Productions 2002:549–562.

39. Kanj SS, Sexton DJ. *Pseudomonas aeruginosa*: bacteremia and endocarditis: clinical manifestations, diagnosis, and treatment. In: Rose BD, Rush JM, eds. *UpToDate* (CD-ROM or online at *www.uptodate.com*). Wellesley, MA: UpToDate, 2002.

40. Carmeli Y, Troillet N, Eliopoulos GM, et al. Emergence of antibiotic-resistant *Pseudomonas aeruginosa*: comparison of risks associated with different antipseudomonal agents. *Antimicrob Agents Chemother* 1999;43:1379–1382.

41. Cometta A, Baumgartner JD, Lew D, et al. Prospective randomized comparison of imipenem monotherapy with imipenem plus netilmicin for treatment of severe infections in nonneutropenic patients. *Antimicrob Agents Chemother* 1994;38:1309–1313.

42. Chow JW, Yu VL. Combination antibiotic therapy versus monotherapy for gram-negative bacteraemia: a commentary. *Int J Antimicrob Agents* 1999;11:7–12.

43. Leibovici L, Paul M, Poznanski O, et al. Monotherapy versus beta-lactam-aminoglycoside combination treatment for gram-negative bacteremia: a prospective, observational study. *Antimicrob Agents Chemother* 1997;41:1127–1133.

44. Siegman-Igra Y, Ravona R, Primerman H, et al. *Pseudomonas aeruginosa* bacteremia: an analysis of 123 episodes, with particular emphasis on the effect of antibiotic therapy. *Int J Infect Dis* 1998;2:211–215.

45. Vidal F, Mensa J, Almela M, et al. Epidemiology and outcome of *Pseudomonas aeruginosa* bacteremia, with special emphasis on the influence of antibiotic treatment. Analysis of 189 episodes. *Arch Intern Med* 1996;156:2121–2126.

46. Poole K. Bacterial multidrug resistance—emphasis on efflux mechanisms and *Pseudomonas aeruginosa*. *J Antimicrob Chemother* 1994;34:453–456.

47. Li XZ, Zhang L, Poole K. Interplay between the MexA-MexB-OprM multidrug efflux system and the outer membrane barrier in the multiple antibiotic resistance of *Pseudomonas aeruginosa*. *J Antimicrob Chemother* 2000;45:433–436.

48. Nakae T. Multiantibiotic resistance caused by active drug extrusion in *Pseudomonas aeruginosa* and other gram-negative bacteria. *Microbiologia* 1997; 13:273–284.

49. Poole K. Multidrug efflux pumps and antimicrobial resistance in *Pseudomonas aeruginosa* and related organisms. *J Mol Microbiol Biotechnol* 2001;3:255–264.

50. National Nosocomial Infections Surveillance (NNIS) System Report, data summary from January 1992 to June 2002, issued August 2002. *Am J Infect Control* 2002;30:458–475.

51. Bertrand X, Thouverez M, Talon D, et al. Endemicity, molecular diversity and colonisation routes of *Pseudomonas aeruginosa* in intensive care units. *Intens Care Med* 2001;27:1263–1268.

52. Douglas MW, Mulholland K, Denyer V, et al. Multi-drug resistant *Pseudomonas aeruginosa* outbreak in a burns unit—an infection control study. *Burns* 2001;27:131–135.

53. Gillespie TA, Johnson PR, Notman AW, et al. Eradication of a resistant *Pseudomonas aeruginosa* strain after a cluster of infections in a hematology/oncology unit. *Clin Microbiol Infect* 2000;6:125–130.

54. Gulay Z, Atay T, Amyes SG. Clonal spread of imipenem-resistant *Pseudomonas aeruginosa* in the intensive care unit of a Turkish hospital. *J Chemother* 2001;13:546–554.

55. Galanakis N, Giamarellou H, Moussas T, et al. Chronic osteomyelitis caused by multi-resistant gram-negative bacteria: evaluation of treatment with newer quinolones after prolonged follow-up. *J Antimicrob Chemother* 1997;39:241–246.

56. Landman D, Quale JM, Mayorga D, et al. Citywide clonal outbreak of multiresistant *Acinetobacter baumannii* and *Pseudomonas aeruginosa* in Brooklyn, NY: the preantibiotic era has returned. *Arch Intern Med* 2002;162:1515–1520.

57. Carmeli Y, Troillet N, Karchmer AW, et al. Health and economic outcomes of antibiotic resistance in *Pseudomonas aeruginosa*. *Arch Intern Med* 1999;159:1127–1132.

58. Beringer P. The clinical use of colistin in patients with cystic fibrosis. *Curr Opin Pulmon Med* 2001;7:434–440.

59. Denton M, Kerr K, Mooney L, et al. Transmission of colistin-resistant *Pseudomonas aeruginosa* between patients attending a pediatric cystic fibrosis center. *Pediatr Pulmonol* 2002;34:257–261.

60. Gales AC, Reis AO, Jones RN. Contemporary assessment of antimicrobial susceptibility testing methods for polymyxin B and colistin: review of available interpretative criteria and quality control guidelines. *J Clin Microbiol* 2001;39:183–190.

61. Hamer DH. Treatment of nosocomial pneumonia and tracheobronchitis caused by multidrug-resistant *Pseudomonas aeruginosa* with aerosolized colistin. *Am J Respir Crit Care Med* 2000;162:328–330.

62. Levin AS, Barone AA, Penco J, et al. Intravenous colistin as therapy for nosocomial infections caused by multidrug-resistant *Pseudomonas aeruginosa* and *Acinetobacter baumannii*. *Clin Infect Dis* 1999;28:1008–1011.

63. Stein A, Raoult D. Colistin: an antimicrobial for the 21st century? *Clin Infect Dis* 2002;35:901–902.

64. Luzzaro F, Vigano EF, Fossati D, et al. Prevalence and drug susceptibility of pathogens causing bloodstream infections in northern Italy: a two-year study in 16 hospitals. *Eur J Clin Microbiol Infect Dis* 2002;21:849–855.

65. Fluit AC, Jones ME, Schmitz FJ, et al. Antimicrobial susceptibility and frequency of occurrence of clinical blood isolates in Europe from the SENTRY antimicrobial surveillance program, 1997 and 1998. *Clin Infect Dis* 2000;30:454–460.

66. Maschmeyer G, Braveny I. Review of the incidence and prognosis of *Pseudomonas aeruginosa* infections in cancer patients in the 1990s. *Eur J Clin Microbiol Infect Dis* 2000;19:915–925.

67. Carratala J, Roson B, Fernandez-Sevilla A, et al. Bacteremic pneumonia in neutropenic patients with cancer: causes, empirical antibiotic therapy, and outcome. *Arch Intern Med* 1998;158:868–872.

68. Sifuentes-Osornio J, Gonzalez R, Ponce-de-Leon A, et al. Epidemiology and prognosis of *Pseudomonas aeruginosa* bacteremia in a tertiary care center. *Rev Invest Clin* 1998;50:383–388.

69. Dorff GJ, Geimer NF, Rosenthal DR, et al. *Pseudomonas* septicemia. Illustrated evolution of its skin lesion. *Arch Intern Med* 1971;128:591–595.

70. Forkner C, Frei E, Edgcomb J. *Pseudomonas* septicemia. Observations on twenty-three cases. *Am J Med* 1958;25:877–884.

71. Kuikka A, Valtonen VV. Factors associated with improved outcome of *Pseudomonas aeruginosa* bacteremia in a Finnish university hospital. *Eur J Clin Microbiol Infect Dis* 1998;17:701–708.

72. Mermel LA, Farr BM, Sherertz RJ, et al. Guidelines for the management of intravascular catheter-related infections. *Clin Infect Dis* 2001;32:1249–1272.

73. Norden CW, Myerowitz RL, Keleti E. Experimental osteomyelitis due to *Staphylococcus aureus* or *Pseudomonas aeruginosa*: a radiographic-pathological correlative analysis. *Br J Exp Pathol* 1980;61:451–460.

74. Bayer AS, Chow AW, Louie JS, et al. Sternoarticualr pyoarthrosis due to gram-negative bacilli. Report of eight cases. *Arch Intern Med* 1977;137:1036–1040.

75. Forkner C. Pseudomonas aeruginosa *infections*. New York: Grune & Stratton, 1960.

76. Sapico FL, Montgomerie JZ. Vertebral osteomyelitis in intravenous drug abusers: report of three cases and review of the literature. *Rev Infect Dis* 1980; 2:196–206.

77. Sequeira W, Jones E, Siegel ME, et al. Pyogenic infections of the pubic symphysis. *Ann Intern Med* 1982;96:604–606.

78. Jacobs RF, McCarthy RE, Elser JM. *Pseudomonas* osteochondritis complicating puncture wounds of the foot in children: a 10-year evaluation. *J Infect Dis* 1989;160:657–661.

79. Raz R, Miron D. Oral ciprofloxacin for treatment of infection following nail puncture wounds of the foot. *Clin Infect Dis* 1995;21:194–195.

80. Bach MC, Cocchetto DM. Ceftazidime as single-agent therapy for gram-negative aerobic bacillary osteomyelitis. *Antimicrob Agents Chemother* 1987;31:1605–1608.

81. Gilbert DN, Tice AD, Marsh PK, et al. Oral ciprofloxacin therapy for chronic contiguous osteomyelitis caused by aerobic gram-negative bacilli. *Am J Med* 1987;82:254–258.

82. Greenberg RN, Tice AD, Marsh PK, et al. Randomized trial of ciprofloxacin compared with other antimicrobial therapy in the treatment of osteomyelitis. *Am J Med* 1987;82:266–269.

83. Lu CH, Chang WN, Chuang YC, et al. Gram-negative bacillary meningitis in adult post-neurosurgical patients. *Surg Neurol* 1999;52:438–443.

84. Rahal JJ, Simberkoff MS. Host defense and antimicrobial therapy in adult gram-negative bacillary meningitis. *Ann Intern Med* 1982;96:468–474.

85. Fong IW, Tomkins KB. Review of *Pseudomonas aeruginosa* meningitis with special emphasis on treatment with ceftazidime. *Rev Infect Dis* 1985;7:604–612.

86. Marone P, Concia E, Maserati R, et al. Ceftazidime in the therapy of pseudomonal meningitis. *Chemioterapia* 1985;4:289–292.

87. Norrby SR. Role of cephalosporins in the treatment of bacterial meningitis in adults. Overview with special emphasis on ceftazidime. *Am J Med* 1985;79:56–61.

88. Swartz MN. Intraventricular use of aminoglycosides in the treatment of gram-negative bacillary meningitis: conflicting views. *J Infect Dis* 1981;143:293–296.

89. Wright PF, Kaiser AB, Bowman CM, et al. The pharmacokinetics and efficacy of an aminoglycoside administered into the cerebral ventricles in neonates: implications for further evaluation of this route of therapy in meningitis. *J Infect Dis* 1981;143:141–147.

90. Lipman J, Allworth A, Wallis SC. Cerebrospinal fluid penetration of high doses of intravenous ciprofloxacin in meningitis. *Clin Infect Dis* 2000;31:1131–1133.

91. Wong-Beringer A, Beringer P, Lovett MA. Successful treatment of multidrug-resistant *Pseudomonas aeruginosa* meningitis with high-dose ciprofloxacin. *Clin Infect Dis* 1997;25:936–937.

92. Chmelik M, Gutvirth J. Meropenem treatment of post-traumatic meningitis due to *Pseudomonas aeruginosa*. *J Antimicrob Chemother* 1993;32:922–923.

93. Kilpatrick M, Girgis N, Farid Z, Bishay E. Aztreonam for treating meningitis caused by gram-negative rods. *Scand J Infect Dis* 1991;23:125–126.

94. Feinmesser R, Wiesel YM, Argaman M, et al. Otitis externa—bacteriological survey. *J Otorhinolaryngol Relat Spec* 1982;44:121–125.

95. Rubin J, Yu VL. Malignant external otitis: insights into pathogenesis, clinical manifestations, diagnosis, and therapy. *Am J Med* 1988;85:391–398.

96. Zaky DA, Bentley DW, Lowy K, et al. Malignant external otitis: a severe form of otitis in diabetic patients. *Am J Med* 1976;61:298–302.

97. Sherman P, Black S, Grossman M. Malignant external otitis due to *Pseudomonas aeruginosa* in childhood. *Pediatrics* 1980;66:782–783.

98. Rubin J, Yu VL, Kamerer DB, et al. Aural irrigation with water: a potential pathogenic mechanism for inducing malignant external otitis? *Ann Otol Rhinol Laryngol* 1990;99:117–119.

99. Zikk D, Rapoport Y, Himelfarb MZ. Invasive external otitis after removal of impacted cerumen by irrigation. *N Engl J Med* 1991;325:969–970.

100. Grandis JR, Curtin HD, Yu VL. Necrotizing (malignant) external otitis: prospective comparison of CT and MR imaging in diagnosis and follow-up. *Radiology* 1995;196:499–504.

101. Levenson MJ, Parisier SC, Dolitsky J, et al. Ciprofloxacin: drug of choice in the treatment of malignant external otitis (MEO). *Laryngoscope* 1991;101:821–824.

102. Leggett JM, Prendergast K. Malignant external otitis: the use of oral ciprofloxacin. *J Laryngol Otol* 1988;102:53–54.

103. Sade J, Lang R, Goshen S, et al. Ciprofloxacin treatment of malignant external otitis. *Am J Med* 1989;87(suppl):138–141.

104. Morrison GA, Bailey CM. Relapsing malignant otitis externa successfully treated with ciprofloxacin. *J Laryngol Otol* 1988;102:872–876.

105. Hickey SA, Ford GR, O'Connor AF, et al. Treating malignant otitis with oral ciprofloxacin. *BMJ* 1989;299:550–551.

106. Lang R, Goshen S, Kitzes-Cohen R, et al. Successful treatment of malignant external otitis with oral ciprofloxacin: report of experience with 23 patients. *J Infect Dis* 1990;161:537–540.

107. Stokkel MP, Boot CN, Eck-Smit BL. SPECT gallium scintigraphy in malignant external otitis: initial staging and follow-up. Case reports. *Laryngoscope* 1996;106:338–340.

108. Kenna MA, Bluestone CD, Reilly JS, et al. Medical management of chronic suppurative otitis media without cholesteatoma in children. *Laryngoscope* 1986;96:146–151.

109. Lang R, Goshen S, Raas-Rothschild A, et al. Oral ciprofloxacin in the management of chronic suppurative otitis media without cholesteatoma in children: preliminary experience in 21 children. *Pediatr Infect Dis J* 1992;11:925–929.

110. Levine DP, Crane LR, Zervos MJ. Bacteremia in narcotic addicts at the Detroit Medical Center. II. Infectious endocarditis: a prospective comparative study. *Rev Infect Dis* 1986;8:374–396.

111. Reyes MP, Brown WJ, Lerner AM. Treatment of patients with pseudomonas endocarditis with high dose aminoglycoside and carbenicillin therapy. *Medicine (Baltimore)* 1978;57:57–67.

112. Reyes MP, Lerner AM. Current problems in the treatment of infective endocarditis due to *Pseudomonas aeruginosa*. *Rev Infect Dis* 1983;5:314–321.

113. Papadakis JA, Samonis G, Maraki S, et al. Efficacy of amikacin, ofloxacin, pefloxacin, ciprofloxacin, enoxacin and fleroxacin in experimental left-sided *Pseudomonas aeruginosa* endocarditis. *Chemotherapy* 2000;46:116–121.

114. Butrus SI, Klotz SA, Misra RP. The adherence of *Pseudomonas aeruginosa* to soft contact lenses. *Ophthalmology* 1987;94:1310–1314.

115. Schein OD, Wasson PJ, Boruchoff SA, Kenyon KR: Microbial keratitis associated with contaminated ocular medications. *Am J Ophthalmol* 1988;105:361–365.

116. Hansen KD, Meyer RF. Amikacin treatment of *Pseudomonas*-caused corneal ulcer. *Arch Ophthalmol* 1980;98:1991–1992.

117. Hutton WL, Sexton RR. Atypical *Pseudomonas* corneal ulcers in semicomatose patients. *Am J Ophthalmol* 1972;73:37–39.

118. Tarr KH, Constable IJ. *Pseudomonas* endophthalmitis associated with scleral necrosis. *Br J Ophthalmol* 1980;64:676–679.

119. Alexandrakis G, Alfonso EC, Miller D. Shifting trends in bacterial keratitis in south Florida and emerging resistance to fluoroquinolones. *Ophthalmology* 2000;107:1497–1502.

120. Schaefer F, Bruttin O, Zografos L, et al. Bacterial keratitis: a prospective clinical and microbiological study. *Br J Ophthalmol* 2001;85:842–847.

121. Garg P, Sharma S, Rao GN. Ciprofloxacin-resistant *Pseudomonas* keratitis. *Ophthalmology* 1999;106:1319–1323.

122. Golden B. Subtenon injection of gentamicin for bacterial infections of the eye. *J Infect Dis* 1971;124(suppl):271–281.

123. Ayliffe GA, Barry DR, Lowbury EJ, et al. Postoperative infection with *Pseudomonas aeruginosa* in an eye hospital. *Lancet* 1966;1:1113–1117.

124. Forster R. Endophthalmitis: In: Duane T, ed. *Clinical ophthalmology*. New York: Harper and Row, 1978:1–20.

125. Yannis RA, Rissing JP, Buxton TB, et al. Multistrain comparison of three antimicrobial prophylaxis regimens in experimental postoperative *Pseudomonas* endophthalmitis. *Am J Ophthalmol* 1985;100:404–407.

126. Leigh L, Stoll BJ, Rahman M, et al. *Pseudomonas aeruginosa* infection in very low birth weight infants: a case-control study. *Pediatr Infect Dis J* 1995;14:367–371.

127. Rowe MI, Reblock KK, Kurkchubasche AG, et al. Necrotizing enterocolitis in the extremely low birth weight infant. *J Pediatr Surg* 1994;29:987–990.

128. Otaibi AA, Barker C, Anderson R, et al. Neutropenic enterocolitis (typhlitis) after pediatric bone marrow transplant. *J Pediatr Surg* 2002;37:770–772.

129. Pastore D, Specchia G, Mele G, et al. Typhlitis complicating induction therapy in adult acute myeloid leukemia. *Leuk Lymphoma* 2002;43:911–914.

130. Sherman NJ, Woolley MM. The ileocecal syndrome in acute childhood leukemia. *Arch Surg* 1973;107:39–42.

131. Chakravarti D, Tyagi N. Pyrexia simulating that of enteric fever by *Pseudomonas pyocyaneus* in children. *Ind Med Gaz* 1937;72:367–372.

132. Dold H. On *pyocyaneus* sepsis and intestinal infections in Shanghai due to *Bacillus pyocyaneus*. *Chin Med J* 1918;32:435–444.

133. Iannini PB, Claffey T, Quintiliani R. Bacteremic *Pseudomonas* pneumonia. *JAMA* 1974;230:558–561.

134. Pennington JE, Reynolds HY, Carbone PP. *Pseudomonas* pneumonia. A retrospective study of 36 cases. *Am J Med* 1973;55:155–160.

135. Rose HD, Heckman MG, Unger JD. *Pseudomonas aeruginosa* pneumonia in adults. *Am Rev Respir Dis* 1973;107:416–422.

136. Tillotson JR, Lerner AM. Characteristics of nonbacteremic *Pseudomonas* pneumonia. *Ann Intern Med* 1968;68:295–307.

137. Dropulic LK, Leslie JM, Eldred LJ, et al. Clinical manifestations and risk factors of *Pseudomonas aeruginosa* infection in patients with AIDS. *J Infect Dis* 1995;171:930–937.

138. Hatchette TF, Gupta R, Marrie TJ. *Pseudomonas aeruginosa* community-acquired pneumonia in previously healthy adults: case report and review of the literature. *Clin Infect Dis* 2000;31:1349–1356.

139. Shepp DH, Tang IT, Ramundo MB, et al. Serious *Pseudomonas aeruginosa* infection in AIDS. *J AIDS* 1994;7:823–831.

140. Reynolds H, Fick R. *Pseudomonas aeruginosa* pulmonary infections (emphasizing nosocomial pneumonia and respiratory infections in cystic fibrosis). In: Sabath L, ed. Pseudomonas aeruginosa: *the organism, diseases it causes, and their treatment*. Bern, Switzerland: Hans Huber, 1980:71–98.

141. Downhour NP, Petersen EA, Krueger TS, et al. Severe cellulitis/myositis caused by *Stenotrophomonas maltophilia*. *Ann Pharmacother* 2002;36:63–66.

142. Bosso JA, Saxon BA, Matsen JM. *In vitro* activity of aztreonam combined with tobramycin and gentamicin against clinical isolates of *Pseudomonas aeruginosa* and *Pseudomonas cepacia* from patients with cystic fibrosis. *Antimicrob Agents Chemother* 1987;31:1403–1405.

143. Gold R, Overmeyer A, Knie B, et al. Controlled trial of ceftazidime vs. ticarcillin and tobramycin in the treatment of acute respiratory exacerbations in patients with cystic fibrosis. *Pediatr Infect Dis* 1985;4:172–177.

144. Hyatt AC, Chipps BE, Kumor KM, et al. A double-blind controlled trial of anti-*Pseudomonas* chemotherapy of acute respiratory exacerbations in patients with cystic fibrosis. *J Pediatr* 1981;99:307–314.

145. Jackson MA, Kusmiesz H, Shelton S, et al. Comparison of piperacillin vs. ticarcillin plus tobramycin in the treatment of acute pulmonary exacerbations of cystic fibrosis. *Pediatr Infect Dis* 1986;5:440–443.

146. Webb AK. The treatment of pulmonary infection in cystic fibrosis. *Scand J Infect Dis Suppl* 1995;96:24–27.

147. Wientzen R, Prestidge CB, Kramer RI, et al. Acute pulmonary exacerbations in cystic fibrosis. A double-blind trial of tobramycin and placebo therapy. *Am J Dis Child* 1980;134:1134–1138.

148. Banerjee D, Stableforth D. The treatment of respiratory *Pseudomonas* infection in cystic fibrosis: what drug and which way? *Drugs* 2000;60:1053–1064.

149. Moller NE, Hoiby N. Antibiotic treatment of chronic *Pseudomonas aeruginosa* infection in cystic fibrosis patients. *Scand J Infect Dis Suppl* 1981;29:87–91.

150. Lindsay CA, Bosso JA. Optimisation of antibiotic therapy in cystic fibrosis patients. Pharmacokinetic considerations. *Clin Pharmacokinet* 1993;24:496–506.

151. Jensen T, Pedersen SS, Nielsen CH, et al. The efficacy and safety of ciprofloxacin and ofloxacin in chronic *Pseudomonas aeruginosa* infection in cystic fibrosis. *J Antimicrob Chemother* 1987;20:585–594.

152. Pedersen SS, Jensen T, Hoiby N, et al. Management of *Pseudomonas aeruginosa* lung infection in Danish cystic fibrosis patients. *Acta Paediatr Scand* 1987;76:955–961.

153. Hodson ME, Gallagher CG, Govan JR. A randomised clinical trial of nebulised tobramycin or colistin in cystic fibrosis. *Eur Respir J* 2002;20:658–664.

154. Moss RB. Long-term benefits of inhaled tobramycin in adolescent patients with cystic fibrosis. *Chest* 2002;121:55–63.

155. Mukhopadhyay S, Singh M, Cater JI, et al. Nebulised antipseudomonal antibiotic therapy in cystic fibrosis: a meta-analysis of benefits and risks. *Thorax* 1996;51:364–368.

156. Ratjen F, Doring G, Nikolaizik WH. Effect of inhaled tobramycin on early *Pseudomonas aeruginosa* colonisation in patients with cystic fibrosis. *Lancet* 2001;358:983–984.

157. Massard G, Shennib H, Metras D, et al. Double-lung transplantation in mechanically ventilated patients with cystic fibrosis. *Ann Thorac Surg* 1993;55:1087–1091.

158. Ramirez JC, Patterson GA, Winton TL, et al. Bilateral lung transplantation for cystic fibrosis. The Toronto Lung Transplant Group. *J Thorac Cardiovasc Surg* 1992;103:287–293.

159. Whitehead B, Helms P, Goodwin M, et al. Heart-lung transplantation for cystic fibrosis. 2: Outcome. *Arch Dis Child* 1991;66:1022–1026.

160. Greene SL, Su WP, Muller SA. Ecthyma gangrenosum: report of clinical, histopathologic, and bacteriologic aspects of eight cases. *J Am Acad Dermatol* 1984;11:781–787.

161. Bottone EJ, Reitano M, Janda JM, et al. *Pseudomonas maltophilia* exoenzyme activity as correlate in pathogenesis of ecthyma gangrenosum. *J Clin Microbiol* 1986;24:995–997.

162. Muder RR, Yu VL, Dummer JS, et al. Infections caused by *Pseudomonas maltophilia*. Expanding clinical spectrum. *Arch Intern Med* 1987;147:1672–1674.

163. Rajan RK. Spontaneous bacterial peritonitis with ecthyma gangrenosum due to *Escherichia coli*. *J Clin Gastroenterol* 1982;4:145–148.

164. Fleming MG, Milburn PB, Prose NS. *Pseudomonas* septicemia with nodules and bullae. *Pediatr Dermatol* 1987;4:18–20.

165. Roberts R, Tarpay MM, Marks MI, et al. Erysipelaslike lesions and hyperesthesia as manifestations of *Pseudomonas aeruginosa* sepsis. *JAMA* 1982;248:2156–2157.

166. Berg A, Armitage JO, Burns CP. Fournier's gangrene complicating aggressive therapy for hematologic malignancy. *Cancer* 1986;57:2291–2294.

167. Koopmann CF Jr, Coulthard SW. Infectious facial and nasal cutaneous necrosis: evaluation and diagnosis. *Laryngoscope* 1982;92:1130–1134.

168. Schuster DI. Palatopharyngeal and lower extremity soft tissue loss in an infant secondary to *Pseudomonas* gangrenous cellulitis. *Ann Plast Surg* 1981;6:138–141.

169. Hall JH, Callaway JL, Tindall JP, et al. *Pseudomonas aeruginosa* in dermatology. *Arch Dermatol* 1968;97:312–324.

170. Pseudomonas dermatitis/folliculitis associated with pools and hot tubs—Colorado and Maine, 1999–2000. *MMWR* 2000;49:1087–1091.

171. Thomas P, Moore M, Bell E, et al. *Pseudomonas* dermatitis associated with a swimming pool. *JAMA* 1985;253:1156–1159.

172. Washburn J, Jacobson JA, Marston E, et al. *Pseudomonas aeruginosa* rash associated with a whirlpool. *JAMA* 1976;235:2205–2207.

173. Berger TG, Kaveh S, Becker D, et al. Cutaneous manifestations of *Pseudomonas* infections in AIDS. *J Am Acad Dermatol* 1995;32:279–280.

174. El Baze P, Thyss A, Caldani C, et al. Pseudomonas aeruginosa O-11 folliculitis. Development into ecthyma gangrenosum in immunosuppressed patients. *Arch Dermatol* 1985;121:873–876.

175. Fiorillo L, Zucker M, Sawyer D, et al. The pseudomonas hot-foot syndrome. *N Engl J Med* 2001;345:335–338.

176. Pruitt BA Jr, Foley FD. The use of biopsies in burn patient care. *Surgery* 1973;73:887–897.

177. Williams HB, Breidenbach WC, Callaghan WB, et al. Are burn wound biopsies obsolete? A comparative study of bacterial quantitation in burn patients using the absorbent disc and biopsy techniques. *Ann Plast Surg* 1984;13:388–395.

178. Hansbrough JF, Carroll WB, Zapata-Sirvent RL, et al. Identification and antibiotic susceptibility of bacterial isolates from burned patients. *Burns Incl Therm Inj* 1985;11:393–403.

179. Estahbanati HK, Kashani PP, Ghanaatpisheh F. Frequency of *Pseudomonas aeruginosa* serotypes in burn wound infections and their resistance to antibiotics. *Burns* 2002;28:340–348.

180. McManus WF, Goodwin CW Jr, Pruitt BA Jr. Subeschar treatment of burn-wound infection. *Arch Surg* 1983;118:291–294.

181. Anderson RJ, Schafer LA, Olin DB, et al. Septicemia in renal transplant recipients. *Arch Surg* 1973;106:692–694.

182. Marrie TJ, Major H, Gurwith M, et al. Prolonged outbreak of nosocomial urinary tract infection with a single strain of *Pseudomonas aeruginosa*. *Can Med Assoc J* 1978;119:593–596.

183. Moore B. An outbreak of urinary *Pseudomonas aeruginosa* infection acquired during urological operations. *Lancet* 1966;2:929–931.

184. Brown EM, Morris R, Stephenson TP. The efficacy and safety of ciprofloxacin in the treatment of chronic *Pseudomonas aeruginosa* urinary tract infection. *J Antimicrob Chemother* 1986;18(suppl D):123–127.

185. Leigh DA, Emmanuel FX, Petch VJ. Ciprofloxacin therapy in complicated urinary tract infections caused by *Pseudomonas aeruginosa* and other resistant bacteria. *J Antimicrob Chemother* 1986;18(suppl D):117–121.

186. Malinverni R, Glauser MP. Comparative studies of fluoroquinolones in the treatment of urinary tract infections. *Rev Infect Dis* 1988;10(suppl 1):153–163.

187. Fichtenbaum CJ, Woeltje KF, Powderly WG. Serious *Pseudomonas aeruginosa* infections in patients infected with human immunodeficiency virus: a case-control study. *Clin Infect Dis* 1994;19:417–422.

188. Kielhofner M, Atmar RL, Hamill RJ, et al. Life-threatening *Pseudomonas aeruginosa* infections in patients with human immunodeficiency virus infection. *Clin Infect Dis* 1992;14:403–411.

189. Ainsworth JG, Mitchell D, Harris JR. Successful prevention of recurrent pneumonia caused by *Pseudomonas aeruginosa* in a patient with AIDS. *Int J STD AIDS* 1995;6:123–124.

190. Ali NJ, Kessel D, Miller RF. Bronchopulmonary infection with *Pseudomonas aeruginosa* in patients infected with human immunodeficiency virus. *Genitourin Med* 1995;71:73–77.

191. Baron AD, Hollander H. *Pseudomonas aeruginosa* bronchopulmonary infection in late human immunodeficiency virus disease. *Am Rev Respir Dis* 1993;148:992–996.

192. Gallant JE, Ko AH. Cavitary pulmonary lesions in patients infected with human immunodeficiency virus. *Clin Infect Dis* 1996;22:671–682.

193. Miller RF, Foley NM, Kessel D, et al. Community acquired lobar pneumonia in patients with HIV infection and AIDS. *Thorax* 1994;49:367–368.

194. Verghese A, al Samman M, Nabhan D, et al. Bacterial bronchitis and bronchiectasis in human immunodeficiency virus infection. *Arch Intern Med* 1994;154:2086–2091.

195. Schuster MG, Norris AH. Community-acquired *Pseudomonas aeruginosa* pneumonia in patients with HIV infection. *AIDS* 1994;8:1437–1441.

196. Flores G, Stavola JJ, Noel GJ. Bacteremia due to *Pseudomonas aeruginosa* in children with AIDS. *Clin Infect Dis* 1993;16:706–708.

197. Roilides E, Butler KM, Husson RN, et al. *Pseudomonas* infections in children with human immunodeficiency virus infection. *Pediatr Infect Dis J* 1992;11:547–553.

198. Mendelson MH, Gurtman A, Szabo S, et al. *Pseudomonas aeruginosa* bacteremia in patients with AIDS. *Clin Infect Dis* 1994;18:886–895.

199. Godofsky EW, Zinreich J, Armstrong M, et al. Sinusitis in HIV-infected patients: a clinical and radiographic review. *Am J Med* 1992;93:163–170.

200. Tami TA. The management of sinusitis in patients infected with the human immunodeficiency virus (HIV). *Ear Nose Throat J* 1995;74:360–363.

201. O'Donnell JG, Sorbello AF, Condoluci DV, et al. Sinusitis due to *Pseudomonas aeruginosa* in patients with human immunodeficiency virus infection. *Clin Infect Dis* 1993;16:404–406.

202. Khan MO, Montecalvo MA, Davis I, et al. Ecthyma gangrenosum in patients with acquired immunodeficiency syndrome. *Cutis* 2000;66:121–123.

203. Higgins SP, Stedman YF, Bundred NJ, et al. Periareolar breast abscess due to *Pseudomonas aeruginosa* in an HIV antibody positive male. *Genitourin Med* 1994;70:147–148.

204. Roca B, Vilar C, Perez EV, et al. Breast abscess with lethal septicemia due to *Pseudomonas aeruginosa* in a patient with AIDS. *Presse Med* 1996;25:803–804.

205. McNaghten AD, Adams MR, Dworkin MS. Case 23-2000: osteomyelitis in HIV-infected patients. *N Engl J Med* 2001;344:66–67.

206. Manfredi R, Nanetti A, Ferri M, et al. *Pseudomonas* spp. complications in patients with HIV disease: an eight-year clinical and microbiological survey. *Eur J Epidemiol* 2000;16:111–118.

207. Daniels DG, Nelson MR, Barton SE, et al. Malignant otitis externa in a patient with AIDS. *Int J STD AIDS* 1992;3:214.

208. Hern JD, Almeyda J, Thomas DM, et al. Malignant otitis externa in HIV and AIDS. *J Laryngol Otol* 1996;110:770–775.

209. Weinroth SE, Schessel D, Tuazon CU. Malignant otitis externa in AIDS patients: case report and review of the literature. *Ear Nose Throat J* 1994;73:772–778.

210. Dworkin MS, Williamson J, Jones JL, et al. Prophylaxis with trimethoprim-sulfamethoxazole for human immunodeficiency virus–infected patients: impact on risk for infectious diseases. *Clin Infect Dis* 2001;33:393–398.

211. Meynard JL, Barbut F, Guiguet M, et al. *Pseudomonas aeruginosa* infection in human immunodeficiency virus infected patients. *J Infect* 1999;38:176–181.

212. Sorvillo F, Beall G, Turner PA, et al. Incidence and determinants of *Pseudomonas aeruginosa* infection among persons with HIV: association with hospital exposure. *Am J Infect Control* 2001;29:79–84.

213. Mayaud C, Parrot A, Cadranel J. Pyogenic bacterial lower respiratory tract infection in human immunodeficiency virus–infected patients. *Eur Respir J Suppl* 2002;36(suppl):28–39.

214. Pedro-Botet ML, Modol JM, Valles X, et al. Changes in bloodstream infections in HIV-positive patients in a university hospital in Spain (1995–1997). *Int J Infect Dis* 2002;6:17–22.

215. Domingo P, Ferre A, Baraldes MA, et al. *Pseudomonas aeruginosa* bronchopulmonary infection in patients with AIDS, with emphasis on relapsing infection. *Eur Respir J* 1998;12:107–112.

216. Rosenberg AL, Seneff MG, Atiyeh L, et al. The importance of bacterial sepsis in intensive care unit patients with acquired immunodeficiency syndrome: implications for future care in the age of increasing antiretroviral resistance. *Crit Care Med* 2001;29:548–556.

217. Sattler CA, Mason EO Jr, Kaplan SL. Nonrespiratory *Stenotrophomonas maltophilia* infection at a children's hospital. *Clin Infect Dis* 2000;31:1321–1330.

218. Elting LS, Bodey GP. Septicemia due to *Xanthomonas* species and non-aeruginosa *Pseudomonas* species: increasing incidence of catheter-related infections. *Medicine (Baltimore)* 1990;69:296–306.

219. Gutierrez RF, Masia MM, Cortes J, et al. Endocarditis caused by *Stenotrophomonas maltophilia*: case report and review. *Clin Infect Dis* 1996;23:1261–1265.

220. Morrison AJ Jr, Hoffmann KK, Wenzel RP. Associated mortality and clinical characteristics of nosocomial *Pseudomonas maltophilia* in a university hospital. *J Clin Microbiol* 1986;24:52–55.

221. Schoch PE, Cunha BA. *Pseudomonas maltophilia*. *Infect Control* 1987;8:169–172.

222. Szeto CC, Li PK, Leung CB, et al. *Xanthomonas maltophilia* peritonitis in uremic patients receiving continuous ambulatory peritoneal dialysis. *Am J Kidney Dis* 1997;29:91–95.

223. Mett H, Rosta S, Schacher B, et al. Outer membrane permeability and beta-lactamase content in *Pseudomonas maltophilia* clinical isolates and laboratory mutants. *Rev Infect Dis* 1988;10:765–769.

224. Krueger TS, Clark EA, Nix DE. In vitro susceptibility of *Stenotrophomonas maltophilia* to various antimicrobial combinations. *Diagn Microbiol Infect Dis* 2001;41:71–78.

225. Yamagishi Y, Fujita J, Takigawa K, et al. Clinical features of *Pseudomonas cepacia* pneumonia in an epidemic among immunocompromised patients. *Chest* 1993;103:1706–1709.

226. Martone WJ, Tablan OC, Jarvis WR. The epidemiology of nosocomial epidemic *Pseudomonas cepacia* infections. *Eur J Epidemiol* 1987;3:222–232.

227. Pitt TL, Kaufmann ME, Patel PS, et al. Type characterisation and antibiotic susceptibility of *Burkholderia* (*Pseudomonas*) *cepacia* isolates from patients with cystic fibrosis in the United Kingdom and the Republic of Ireland. *J Med Microbiol* 1996;44:203–210.

228. Goldmann DA, Klinger JD. *Pseudomonas cepacia*: biology, mechanisms of virulence, epidemiology. *J Pediatr* 1986;108:806–812.

229. Henderson DK, Baptiste R, Parrillo J, et al. Indolent epidemic of *Pseudomonas cepacia* bacteremia and pseudobacteremia in an intensive care unit traced to a contaminated blood gas analyzer. *Am J Med* 1988;84:75–81.

230. Mandell IN, Feiner HD, Price NM, et al. Pseudomonas cepacia endocarditis and ecthyma gangrenosum. *Arch Dermatol* 1977;113:199–202.

231. Tablan OC, Martone WJ, Jarvis WR. The epidemiology of *Pseudomonas cepacia* in patients with cystic fibrosis. *Eur J Epidemiol* 1987;3:336–342.

232. Taylor RF, Gaya H, Hodson ME. *Pseudomonas cepacia*: pulmonary infection in patients with cystic fibrosis. *Respir Med* 1993;87:187–192.

233. Tomashefski JF, Thomassen MJ, Bruce MC, et al. *Pseudomonas cepacia*–associated pneumonia in cystic fibrosis. Relation of clinical features to histopathologic patterns of pneumonia. *Arch Pathol Lab Med* 1988;112:166–172.

234. Aronoff SC. Outer membrane permeability in *Pseudomonas cepacia*: diminished porin content in a beta-lactam-resistant mutant and in resistant cystic fibrosis isolates. *Antimicrob Agents Chemother* 1988;32:1636–1639.

235. Kumar A, Wofford-McQueen R, Gordon RC. Ciprofloxacin, imipenem and rifampicin: *in-vitro* synergy of two and three drug combinations against *Pseudomonas cepacia*. *J Antimicrob Chemother* 1989;23:831–835.

236. Murray AE, Bartzokas CA, Shepherd AJ, et al. Blood transfusion–associated *Pseudomonas fluorescens* septicaemia: is this an increasing problem? *J Hosp Infect* 1987;9:243–248.

237. Scott J, Boulton FE, Govan JR, et al. A fatal transfusion reaction associated with blood contaminated with *Pseudomonas fluorescens*. *Vox Sang* 1988;54:201–204.

238. Simor AE, Ricci J, Lau A, et al. Pseudobacteremia due to *Pseudomonas fluorescens*. *Pediatr Infect Dis* 1985;4:508–512.

239. Smith J, Ashhurst-Smith C, Norton R. *Pseudomonas fluorescens* pseudobacteraemia: a cautionary lesson. *J Paediatr Child Health* 2002;38:63–65.

CHAPTER 202
Brucella

Eduardo Gotuzzo and Carlos Carrillo

Brucellosis is an anthropozoonosis and an important cause of morbidity in humans and animals, with an estimated half a million new cases every year (1). Some nations such as Peru and Mexico in Latin America, Spain and Greece in Europe, and Iraq, Iran, Jordan, and Kuwait in the Middle East (2) are defined as hyperendemic areas with more than 4,000 cases per year, caused mainly by *Brucella melitensis*. In the United States, with the implementation of bovine brucellosis eradication programs and the pasteurization of milk, the number of cases dropped to only 172 in 1978; these were found mainly in Iowa, California, and Texas (3). Because the incidence is small (0.1 case per 100,000 inhabitants per year in 1985), the Centers for Disease Control and Prevention has listed brucellosis as a notifiable disease of low frequency (4). In the past 10 years, fewer than 100 cases a year have been reported, usually associated with dairy products from endemic areas.

HISTORICAL ASPECTS

In 1885, Sir David Bruce (5) described "a disease of long duration, clinically characterized by fever, profuse perspiration, splenomegaly, frequent relapses, rheumatoid or neuralgic pain, swelling of the joints and orchitis." He isolated the pathogen from the spleen of soldiers who died as a consequence of "Malta disease."

In 1905, Zammit (6) discovered that the goat was the reservoir of *B. melitensis* and produced an immediate decrease in deaths and infection in members of the army by prohibiting the use of untreated goat milk.

Brucella abortus was isolated in Denmark by Bang (7) from intrauterine membranes of aborting cows. *Brucella suis* is a cause of enzootic disease in swine. Carmichael (7a) described *Brucella canis* as an epidemic in beagle dogs and their trainers.

BACTERIOLOGIC ASPECTS

Brucellae are small coccoid or rodlike aerobic, gram-negative bacteria 0.5 to 1.5 μm in length. The genus *Brucella* comprises six species that can be distinguished by their oxidative utilization and by their sensitivity to bacteriophages. *B. melitensis* has three biotypes, *B. abortus* has nine, *B. suis* has four, and other species have one (8). Brucellae are parasites of mammalian cells and have a facultative intracellular reproduction.

Brucella organisms can survive in soil for up to 10 weeks, in liquid manure for up to 2 years, in goat cheese for up to 180 days at 4°C to 8°C, and in tap water for up to 60 days (9,10). They are quite sensitive to heat, to ionizing radiation, and to the most commonly used disinfectants, and they are killed by pasteurization.

EPIDEMIOLOGY

Brucellosis is a disease affecting various domesticated animals, including cattle (*B. abortus*), goats (*B. melitensis*), swine (*B. suis*), and dogs (*B. canis*). The disease incidence worldwide is estimated at 500,000 cases per year. In developed countries, brucellosis is considered an occupational hazard, especially among farmers, veterinarians, and butchers, who may become infected through the skin or conjunctiva (11–14). Ingestion of unpasteurized dairy products is another common mechanism, especially in Texas and Florida, which account for 50% of reported cases in the United States. *Brucella* is also one of the most infectious bacteria to laboratory personnel, probably by means of aerosols (15,16). Human-to-human transmission of brucellosis does not exist (Table 202.1).

Internationally, the most important mechanism of transmission is the consumption of fresh, unpasteurized goat cheese and untreated milk (1,17,18). *B. melitensis* produces a more severe disease, and the attack rate is high, especially in family infections (19). *B. abortus* has been the most frequent cause of brucellosis in the United States and produces a mild clinical disease. It has a low rate of clinical disease, with more subclinical infections; there are only rare family outbreaks (20).

CLINICAL MANIFESTATIONS

Brucellosis has been recognized as a disease of great clinical polymorphism (21). In our experience, which includes observation of nearly 2,000 patients with brucellosis caused by *B. melitensis*, we have classified the disease as acute, subacute or undulant, and chronic (Table 202.2).

Acute Form

The acute form of brucellosis is the typical form, with a temperature of 100°F to 104°F, especially in the evenings. It is accompanied by general discomfort, weakness, headache, and profuse diaphoresis, arthralgias, and myalgias. Back pain is frequent. Anorexia, constipation, and weight loss in the first 3 to 4 weeks are commonly seen. Physical examination shows fever and hepatomegaly (two thirds of cases) and splenomegaly (50%

TABLE 202.1.   Species of *Brucella* and Animal Reservoirs

Species	Reservoir	Other hosts	Human cases (worldwide)
Brucella melitensis	Goat, sheep	Cattle or antelope	+++++ (70% of cases)
Brucella abortus	Cattle, water buffalo, jackal, and hyena	Horse	+++ (25% of cases)
Brucella suis	Pig, wolf, and fox	Cattle or caribou	++ (5% of cases)
Brucella ovis	Sheep	—	No
Brucella canis	Dog	—	Few
Brucella neotomae	Desert wood rat	—	No

in children and young adults). In other types of *Brucella* infection, hepatomegaly is uncommon.

Subacute (Undulant) Form

At present, we recognize patients who have relapsed because of incomplete or partial antibiotic treatment and patients who have received incorrect antibiotic treatment because of erroneous diagnoses. The clinical pattern is more protean and may be an important cause of fever of unknown origin (22). The symptoms are milder; arthritis is more common (23) and orchiepididymitis is more common among young male patients.

Chronic Form

The chronic form of brucellosis includes patients who have had the disease for more than 1 year. It is extremely rare in children but common in older people, with a cyclic course of depressive episodes and a reappearance of sweating. Fever is rare. Chronic brucellosis is similar to chronic fatigue syndrome. Hepatic and hematologic complications are rare; however, ocular damage, such as cyclic episcleritis and uveitis (24), is common. Spondylitis can be present in this form (23).

COMPLICATIONS

Liver

The most common manifestation is granulomatous hepatitis. Authors from Mediterranean countries and Latin America highlight the frequency of granulomatous hepatitis (25–27). In our group, a review of 59 liver biopsies showed that more than 95% had granulomata and the liver function tests showed a mild increase of aminotransferase and a substantial increase in alkaline phosphatase. With electron microscopy (28), we observed a cell-mediated immune response with epithelioid histiocytes and typical granulomata. Other more severe hepatic lesions were described in 1951 by Arias Stellar (29), who showed sub-

acute atrophy of the liver in six patients who had died from brucellosis.

Arthritis

Huddleson (30), in his classic book, indicated a low frequency of articular involvement related to *B. abortus*, but Debono (31) showed a high frequency with brucellosis caused by *B. melitensis* in Malta. In an extensive retrospective revision (32), we pointed out sacroiliitis, the most common articular lesion, as shown by Debono (31). This complication appears in 33.6% of our patients, and the published range of articular involvement is between 9% and 57% (14,33–36). Most cases are unilateral and are usually accompanied by a positive Lasègue sign and night pain. Radiographs in a Ferguson view showed blurring with erosions; a bone scan may be helpful for early detection (37).

In our prospective series, peripheral arthritis was the most common finding, present in 40% to 45% of those with the articular form (32). It primarily affects young adults and children, especially during relapse, and is rare in persons older than 55 years. Most cases are monarticular, involving a large lower extremity joint such as the knee, hip, or ankle, but one fourth of patients have polyarthritis with pauciarticular involvement, some of them having a rheumatoid-like syndrome.

We propose two pathogenic patterns: The first is infectious arthritis with monarticular involvement and isolation of *Brucella* organisms in synovial fluid using a Ruiz-Castañeda medium modified by Gotuzzo et al. (38). The second form is reactive arthritis with polyarticular involvement and failure to isolate *Brucella* organisms from the joint. This type affects the ankles, wrists, elbows, and both knees. Joint fluid analysis does not distinguish between the groups; the white blood cell count is usually 300 to 10,000 cells/mm³ and protein level exceeds 3 g/dL (23). Low levels of lactate in joint fluid have been reported in infectious arthritis (39) when the biopsy does not show the difference between these two forms. In our hospital, the main cause of sternoclavicular arthritis is brucellosis and not *Staphylococcus aureus*, as has been reported in intravenous drug abusers (40).

TABLE 202.2.   Clinical Differences between Various Forms of Brucellosis

Observation	Acute form (bacteremia, <8 wk)	Undulant form (<52 wk)	Chronic form (>52 wk)
Age	Young adults, children	Young adults	Adults older than 40 yr
Arthralgia	Common, ++	Common, +++	Quite common, +++
High fever	95%	50%–70%	No
Hepatomegaly	66%	50%	Only occasional
Splenomegaly	50%–70%	<40%	Rare
Hematologic involvement	Occasional	Common	Rare
Psychiatric disorders	No	Occasional	Frequent depression, neurasthenia
Ocular damage (uveitis)	No	Rare, 1%–2%	Common, 5%–10%

Extraarticular rheumatism is seen in about 10% to 15% of our patients, mainly in women between 30 and 55 years of age. Tendinitis, bursitis, and fibrositis are common.

Spondylitis occurs in 3% to 15% of cases, is age dependent, and usually involves the lumbar spine. About 20% of the spondylitis cases show involvement of two or more vertebrae. The narrowing of the disk space and epiphysitis are the earliest signs, but the erosions of the anterosuperior margin of the vertebral body (pons sign), with rounding off of the corner and narrowing of the intervertebral disk the most characteristic radiographic manifestations. The distinction from Pott's disease (or spinal tuberculosis) is early bone repair with dense sclerosis and syndesmophytes resulting in "parrot peak" (41). The combination of lytic and blastic lesions is rare in tuberculosis but common in *Brucella* infections (Fig. 202.1).

Spondylitis may occur in the course of systemic brucellosis with fever, sweating, and back pain (42) but may also occur without systemic symptoms (32,43), as in chronic brucellosis. High suspicion based on clinical, radiologic, and epidemiologic clues may enable the diagnosis to be made. Computed tomography has been shown to be effective in the detection of paravertebral abscess and in guided needle aspiration of abscess or vertebral bone. Between 10% and 20% of patients with spondylitis have paravertebral abscess (42,44). In summary, brucellar arthritis is common, but the different clinical patterns are primarily associated with age (Fig. 202.2).

Hematologic Involvement

Anemia, leukopenia, and thrombocytopenia were frequently found. Bleeding complications were significantly associated with clotting abnormalities, and lymphopenia was significantly correlated with the severity of clinical manifestations (45). In our study of 60 patients, the evaluation of bone marrow aspirate showed iron deficiency in 34.5% of the patients (46). Pancytopenia has been described, caused by granulomata in the bone marrow (47,48), although cytophagocytosis is an important mechanism in the pathogenesis of these abnormalities (46,49) and sometimes suggests the diagnosis of medullary malignant histiocytosis (Robb-Smith syndrome) (50).

Thrombocytopenic purpura has been described in 1% of adults and 4% of children with brucellosis. Thrombocytopenia can be severe and some patients need steroids or splenectomy (51). In our series, we detected 2.5% of patients with severe

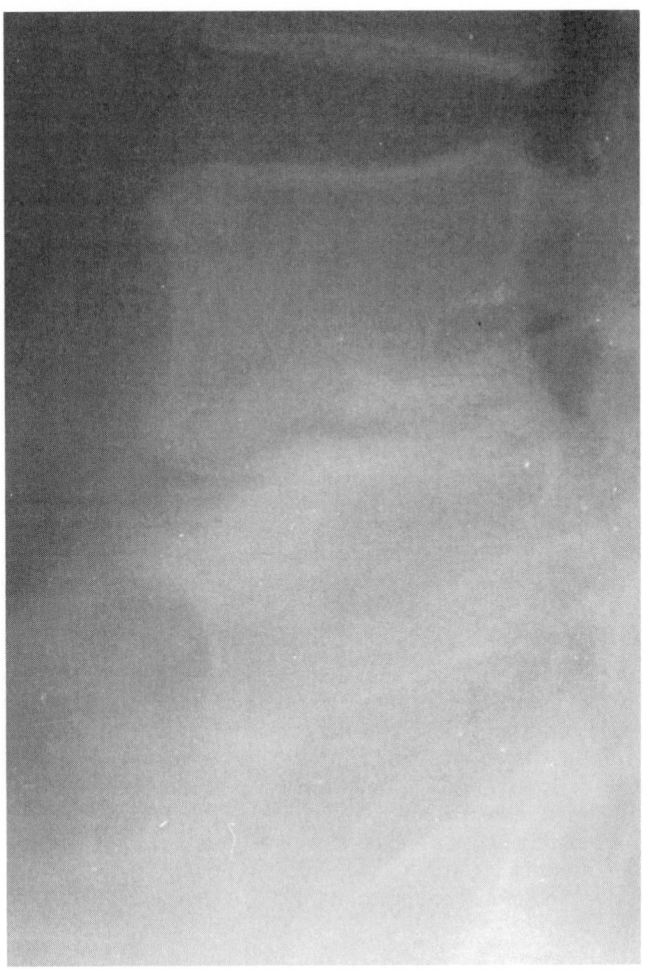

Figure 202.1. Narrowing of the disk space, epiphysitis, and erosion of the anterosuperior margin of the vertebrae with blastic reaction.

thrombocytopenia; 6 of 485 were men and 21 of 606 women ($p < 0.05$). In these cases, bone marrow showed absence of iron in 59.1%, and 12 of 13 of the patients with iron absence were women.

In most infectious diseases, thrombocytopenia is transitory and disappears when the infection is under control. In

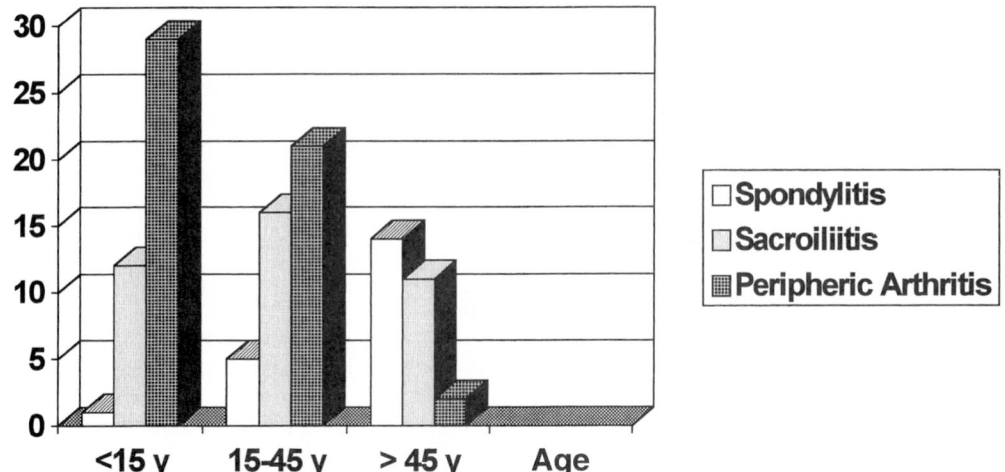

Figure 202.2. Brucellosis: arthritis by age. Variances among brucellar arthritis patterns according to age-groups, showing important differences.

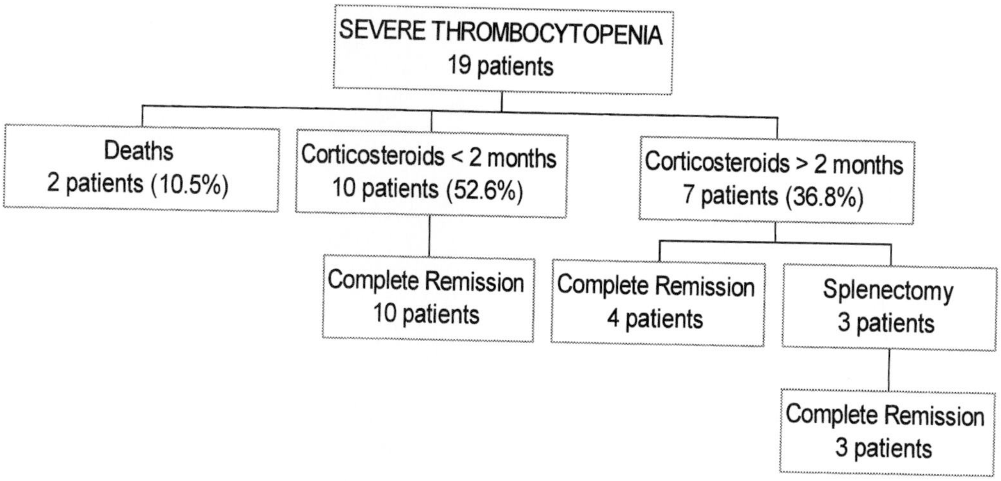

Figure 202.3. Severe thrombocytopenia complicating brucellosis: treatment and evolution. Evolution of severe thrombocytopenia purpura (less than 50,000 platelets/mm^3) after patients received standard anti-*Brucella* treatment. (From Ulloa V, Rojas J, Gotuzzo E. Púrpura thrombocitopénica asociada a brucelosis. *Rev Med Hered* 1992;3:87–93, with permission.)

brucellosis, an important number of cases have severe thrombocytopenia persisting for several weeks despite administration of corticosteroid and having the infection controlled with appropriate antibiotics. As shown in Figure 202.3, it is an important cause of death (rarely observed in brucellosis). An adequate response is obtained in 52.6%, but 37% require prolongation of corticosteroid treatment for more than 2 months, and in some cases after 4 to 6 months, if thrombocytopenia was not controlled, we had to use splenectomy to control it (52).

Neurologic Involvement

The incidence of neurobrucellosis is reported to be 3% to 5% (53,54), although Spink (14) estimated that 10% of patients suffered neuropsychiatric complications. In children, neurobrucellosis has been reported as a rare complication (55). Lubani et al. (56) reported nine children with neurobrucellosis: six with meningitis, one with encephalitis, one with meningoencephalitis, and one with meningomyeloencephalitis. *B. melitensis* was recovered from the cerebrospinal fluid (CSF) in three patients. Mousa et al. (57) described acute *Brucella* meningitis characterized by fever, headache, nuchal rigidity, and altered consciousness. We have sometimes seen Guillain-Barré syndrome, as has been reported by Bashir et al. (58).

The CSF analysis in *Brucella* meningitis is similar to that for other chronic meningitides, with lymphocytic pleocytosis, an increase in protein content, and a slight decrease in glucose level; the CSF culture may also be useful (but the organism has been isolated in only a few cases), as may the finding of *Brucella* antibodies in CSF (59). In chronic brucellosis, psychiatric disorders are common, including depression, chronic fatigue, amnesia, and even suicide (21).

Eye Involvement

Uveitis, optic neuritis, papilledema, and corneal involvement have been reported (60–63). Woods (64) reinforced the role of *Brucella* as an etiologic agent of uveitis; in Peru, it is one of the most common causes of uveitis (65).

Circulating immune complexes in brucellosis may have a role in the physiopathology of the uveal damage, as in reactive arthritis of brucellosis (66,67). Uveitis was present in 14 (20%) of 71 patients with chronic brucellosis. All these cases showed circulating immune complexes by the Raji cell assay and solid-phase C1q assay (68,69). In our series, the uveal syndrome occurred as follows: anterior uveitis, six; posterior uveitis, nine; and total uveitis, eight. The evolution showed the following complications: cataract, detachment of the macula, phthisis bulbi, and secondary glaucoma. The prognosis was poor for those with total uveitis compared with those with posterior or anterior involvement, who had a good visual prognosis (70). A rare case of retinal detachment in chronic brucellosis has been reported (68,69).

Other Complications

Unilateral epididymoorchitis occurs in approximately 10% of men and is rare in children. With treatment, most patients recover without sequelae. *Brucella* endocarditis occurs mainly on the aortic valve; 50% of the patients have had preexisting valvular abnormalities. In some series, 85% of the deaths occur as a consequence of infective endocarditis (21), and most patients require valve replacement with 8 to 12 weeks of systemic antibiotic therapy (70a).

BRUCELLOSIS IN CHILDHOOD

In endemic *B. melitensis* areas, children represent 20% to 25% of cases (71). Reports of sporadic outbreaks (72) and some *reviews* of brucellosis in children have been published (73–78). The infection occurs more frequently in school-aged children and in familial outbreaks; the attack rate in children younger than 5 years is significantly less ($p < 0.05$) than that in older children and adults (19).

The clinical disease in children is usually mild and moderate (progression to the chronic form is rare), and it is sometimes described as a self-limiting infection (79). In our hospital, cases are moderate and articular involvement is common. A monarticular arthritis of the knee is the most commonly reported form (23,32,80). Spondylitis is rare. Liver involvement and hematologic changes are common in this age-group.

BRUCELLOSIS AND PREGNANCY

Spink (14) claimed that there was "no definitive evidence that *Brucella* produces human abortions any more often than other species of bacteria" because erythritol does not exist in the human placenta. However, we consider this to be true only of *B. abortus* infections (81). Abortion is a common feature in animals with brucellosis and appears to be related to high concentrations of erythritol in placental tissues (81,82). Nevertheless, in areas where brucellosis (*B. melitensis*) is endemic, there is an increased rate of abortion in asymptomatic women with serologic evidence of brucellosis (83). Asymptomatic women with agglutination titers greater than 1:160 had significantly more frequent abortions than women with low or negative titers.

In our series, among 75 pregnant women with clinical evidence of brucellosis, we observed increased rates of abortion, premature delivery, miscarriage, and intrauterine infection with fetal death. These complications were especially common in patients with several weeks of untreated disease. Women with early diagnosis and adequate treatment had a good maternal and fetal outcome.

Tetracyclines, the drug of choice for the treatment of brucellosis, should not be administered during pregnancy; for this reason, the tendency of pregnant women is to have relapses 2 to 4 months after having completed treatment.

FAMILY STUDIES IN BRUCELLOSIS

Several outbreaks of brucellosis have been reported in individuals infected through contaminated edible products (84–87), but brucellosis occurring within family groups has been reported only rarely (88,89). Spink (89a) studied several family groups over 16 years in an endemic area for *B. abortus* and emphasized the relatively low rate of symptomatic infection in family members. In our study of 39 families with a family member infected with *B. melitensis,* 19 with a follow-up period of 6 months, half of those affected became symptomatic, confirming the high degree of infectivity of *B. melitensis* (90). The attack rate was lowest in children younger than 10 years. The clinical manifestations were more severe in women. Articular involvement was also more common in women—34.5% versus only 8.1% in men (*p* < 0.01) (87). Genetically determined susceptibility factors may also play a role in this arthritis; however, immunogenetic studies have not shown any association between a given human leukocyte antigen (HLA) type and osteoarticular involvement (91,92) even in Peruvian family studies (93). Only Hodinka et al. (94) in Hungary have published a relationship between HLA-B27 and brucellar spondylitis.

DIAGNOSIS

Worldwide, the diagnosis of brucellosis is usually made by serology (95,96), with the agglutination assay, rose bengal test, immunofluorescence, enzyme-linked immunosorbent assay, or counterimmunoelectrophoresis (97–99).

In Spain, the rose bengal test is extensively used, especially in acute brucellosis; it is easily and rapidly performed, with a low rate of false-positive results (97,98). A titer of 1:160 or more in any of the agglutination tests could be interpreted as positive. False-positive results may be caused by *Francisella tularensis* infection, *Yersinia enterocolitica* infection, and *Vibrio cholerae* vaccine (100) and in our experience rare cases of lymphoma and tuberculosis (101).

With the cholera pandemic in Latin America, where brucellosis is endemic, there was a restriction caused by the cross-reaction detected in patients with cholera. We studied 44 patients with cholera, and of those, 7 had titers greater than 1:80, which decreased at the fourth week (102). Another Peruvian publication also indicated this cross-reaction (103).

In patients with relapses, in this clinical situation we prefer the addition of 2-mercaptoethanol, permitting detection of immunoglobulin G. Any titer higher than 1:40 with 2-mercaptoethanol indicates active infection. The main problem in chronic brucellosis is its diagnosis. In this case, we recommend the Coombs test (97,104) and/or blocking antibodies (101,105), and we recommend, in addition, bone marrow culture as routine.

BACTERIOLOGIC DIAGNOSIS

The diagnosis of brucellosis is established with certainty by the isolation of *Brucella.* Blood culture in 10% carbon dioxide is the simplest and most frequently used method, and the yield is 50% to 80%, even in afebrile patients (105a).

The original medium of Ruiz-Castañeda (106) was useful; however, a modification by Gotuzzo et al. (38), with the addition of 0.025% sodium polyethylene sulfonate and 0.05% cysteine, increased the yield of organisms, especially in patients with the acute form of disease (38). The yield with blood cultures decreases significantly with chronic and subacute forms of brucellosis.

Bone marrow aspirates from the iliac crest (0.5 to 1.0 mL) showed a yield of 92% in comparison with a 70% yield for two blood cultures (*p* < 0.001). Bacteria multiplied significantly faster in bone marrow culture.

We recommend the bone marrow culture for patients for whom there is clinical and/or epidemiologic suspicion of brucellosis but whose serologic test results are negative in the diagnostic evaluation of fever of unknown origin, unexplained arthritis, unexplained hematologic abnormalities, and relapsing or severe uveitis, and suspicion of chronic brucellosis.

IMMUNE RESPONSE AND PHYSIOPATHOLOGY

The immune response induced by *Brucella* is complex and results are sometimes contradictory. The response involves humoral and cellular immunity. In the humoral response, antibodies appear early in the infection and may persist for months, especially immunoglobulin M (104,107).

Some clinical manifestations such as glomerulonephritis, uveitis, arthritis, and hepatitis are highly suggestive of immune complex disease (circulating immune complexes). We showed high levels of circulating immune complexes by Raji cell C1q assay in a group of patients with acute brucellosis (67); the level was decreased several months after therapy. Also, 25% of patients had antinuclear antibodies and 37.5% had rheumatoid factors positive during the acute phase. Impaired cell-mediated immune response was studied extensively by Spink et al. (108). The classic pathologic response is the granuloma.

Brucella infection has some analogies to infections with other intracellular pathogens such as *Listeria.* The role of macrophages in resistance to these intracellular pathogens was described by Mackaness (see reference 109). A genetic susceptibility to brucellosis was described by Serre et al. (109a), although the influencing factors appear to be more complex than those described in the

Listeria model. A Hungarian group suggested that brucellosis, like yersiniosis and salmonellosis, can be associated with HLA-B27 with spondyloarthritis (94). However, in our studies with arthritis, spondylitis, and familial infection, we found no relation between HLA haplotypes and *Brucella*-induced arthritis in Peruvians (8,90–92).

TREATMENT

Antibiotics should have *in vitro* activity and adequate intracellular concentrations. Tetracyclines are drugs that have shown excellent *in vitro* activity against *Brucella* (110–112). In our experience, tetracyclines, mainly doxycycline, had excellent activity, and during the past 25 years, the pattern has not changed. The minimum inhibitory concentration for 90% of the strains (MIC_{90}) is 0.125 μg/mL for doxycycline and 2.0 μg/mL for tetracyclines. The MIC and the minimal bactericidal concentration are 1 μg/mL; this means that tetracyclines are bactericidal to *Brucella* (113). These features and the worldwide experience indicate that tetracyclines are the "gold standard" drug (Table 202.3). Another therapeutic aspect in brucellosis is the necessity to combine antibiotics to reduce relapse rates and chronicity of the disease (114,115).

Other drugs for which there is substantial experience in the treatment of brucellosis are aminoglycosides, which maintain excellent *in vitro* activity. The MIC_{90} for streptomycin was 8.0 μg/mL but for gentamicin, netilmicin, and amikacin was less than 4.0 μg/mL, in our strains. The largest experience was with streptomycin; sometimes other intravenous aminoglycosides are required because of the presence of purpura. Aminoglycosides have moderate activity against *Brucella* (11–13,111,116). With streptomycin, there is more clinical experience, especially in synergic activity (117); most authors use 1 g per day intramuscularly for 2 weeks (14,18,21,115,118). Prolonging treatment with streptomycin for more than 2 weeks has not proved more effective (38). Other aminoglycosides have documented activity *in vitro*, especially gentamicin (116,119), but there is limited clinical information (120). We showed good *in vitro* activity for netilmicin, gentamicin, spectinomycin, and amikacin (113). In a prospective study of 64 patients with the administration of doxycycline, 100 mg twice a day for 45 days, plus netilmicin, 300 mg intramuscularly once a day for 7 days, Solera et al. (121) showed a cure rate of 92.3%; the relapse rate was 12.5% (confidence interval 5.6% to 23.2%). For children, Lubani et al. (80) recommended therapy for 5 to 10 days with gentamicin in association with co-trimoxazole for 4 weeks.

Rifampin is also considered one of the first-line drugs because of its excellent *in vitro* activity and good intracellular penetration.

In Peruvian strains, it has maintained an MIC_{90} of 4.0 μg/mL in the past 15 years; however, lately an MIC_{90} of 16.0 μg/mL has been found (113). The World Health Organization recommendation is for doxycycline, 200 mg per day, combined with rifampin, 600 to 900 mg per day for 6 weeks. In a metaanalysis of five comparative studies done in Spain with doxycycline plus rifampin versus doxycycline plus streptomycin, both schedules showed high cure rates, but doxycycline plus rifampin was associated with a significantly higher relapse rate ($p < 0.01$) (121).

Colmenero et al. (122) in Spain presented an interaction between doxycycline and rifampin. Results were found in rapid acetylators with high clearance of doxycycline. In addition, the area under the curve and half-life of doxycycline were significantly lower with the use of rifampin compared with the doxycycline-streptomycin association. They assumed that this interaction would explain the high rate of relapses, nearly 40%, in Spain; however, the results of this experience are not the same as those in other countries, where the relapse rate with this combination is between 5% and 15%.

In spondylitis, some authors prolong therapy for several months. We recommend standard treatment during 6 weeks, followed by low-dose oxytetracyclines for 2 to 4 months (e.g., 100 mg of doxycycline daily) to reduce relapse.

Doxycycline is preferred because it is used twice a day and is little affected when administered with meals. There is high gastrointestinal tract intolerance for tetracyclines, because four to eight capsules are required daily, resulting in an important interaction with meals and antacids. Our standard treatment in adults is doxycycline (or minocycline), 100 mg twice a day, plus aminoglycoside for 10 to 14 days, or rifampin for 6 weeks could be used.

In children 7 years of age or younger, tetracyclines are contraindicated because these agents are deposited in bones and on teeth enamel. The treatment is only for 4 weeks because the relapse rate is low and the chronic form is rare in children.

Rifampin for 4 weeks plus 10 days of aminoglycosides is highly effective in this age-group. In a large series in Kuwait, Lubani et al. (122a) used co-trimoxazole for 4 weeks plus 5 to 10 days of gentamicin and obtained excellent results.

Different antibiotics, such as chloramphenicol, ampicillin, erythromycin, and cephalosporins, show moderate *in vitro* activity, but despite the decrease in fever with most of the antibiotics, the rate of cure is low and the relapse rate is high.

In some studies, including our *in vitro* study (113), good *in vitro* activity was found for ciprofloxacin, lomefloxacin, and fleroxacin and only mild susceptibility for norfloxacin. The clinical response in a few patients with norfloxacin or ciprofloxacin was poor; however, fluoroquinolones have good intracellular penetration. In Ankara, Akova et al. (123) published a

---

TABLE 202.3. Brucellosis: Treatment

Patients	Treatment		
Adults	Doxycycline, 100 mg twice a day for 6 wk	plus	Rifampin, 600–900 mg/d (in 2 doses) for 6 wk *or* Streptomycin or netilmicin, once a day for 14 d
Children older than 7 yr	Same treatment as adults for 4 wk		
Children younger than 7 yr	Rifampin, 10 mg/kg/d (in 2 doses) for 4 wk	plus	Streptomycin, once a day for 14 d *or* Co-trimoxazole for 4 wk
Pregnancy	Rifampin, 600 mg/d for 4 wk	plus	Streptomycin, once a day for 14 d *or* Co-trimoxazole for 4 wk

comparative trial of ofloxacin, 400 mg per day, plus rifampin, 600 mg per day, for 6 weeks in comparison with doxycycline, 200 mg per day, plus rifampin for 6 weeks; both regimens resulted in a greater than 95% cure, but gastric discomfort or intolerance was more common with doxycycline (43.3%), whereas only 6.5% of patients were affected with ofloxacin (see Table 202.3).

Garcia-Rodriguez et al. (124) in Spain studied the lack of bactericidal activity of fluoroquinolones against *Brucella* (123), and in experimental murine brucellosis, fluoroquinolones yielded poor therapeutic results (125).

A special problem is brucellosis in pregnant women, because the best treatment, tetracyclines or doxycycline, is contraindicated. In these cases, we recommend rifampin for 4 weeks plus streptomycin for 2 weeks, or 4 weeks of rifampin plus trimethoprim-sulfamethoxazole for 4 weeks with close follow-up.

Rifampin is safe in leprosy and in tubercular pregnant women without fetal problems associated with the drug. Short treatments with aminoglycosides—14 days or less—are safe. The information about co-trimoxazole is still controversial because of trimethoprim restriction; however, worldwide experience with trimethoprim-sulfamethoxazole in pregnant women with urinary tract infection shows no side effects.

Early diagnosis and proper treatment can improve maternal and fetal prognosis. Women who had the disease for less than 3 weeks and who had proper treatment had newborns at term, healthy, with normal weight.

REFERENCES

1. Thimm BM. *Brucellosis: distribution in man, domestic and wild animals.* Berlin: Springer-Verlag, 1982.
2. Lulu AR, Braj GF, Khateeb MI, et al. Human brucellosis in Kuwait: a prospective study of 400 cases. *Q J Med* 1988;66:39.
3. Centers for Disease Control and Prevention. *Brucellosis surveillance annual summary 1978.* Atlanta: Centers for Disease Control and Prevention, 1979.
4. Centers for Disease Control and Prevention. Annual summary 1984. *MMWR Morb Mortal Wkly Rep* 1986;32:54.
5. Bruce D. Note on discovery of a micrococcus in Malta fever. *Practitioner* 1887;39:161.
6. Zammit T. A preliminary note of examination of the blood of goats suffering from Mediterranean fever. In: *Reports of the Royal Society of London. Mediterranean Fever Commission,* part III. London: Harrison Sons, 1905:83.
7. Bang BF. Die actiologie des Sevchenhattern (infectiosen). *Verwerfens Z Tiormed* 1897;1:241.
7a. Carmichael LE. Canine brucellosis: isolation diagnosis, transmission. *Proc U S Livestock Sanit Assoc* 1967;71:517.
8. Alton GG, Elberg SS. *Brucella melitensis* vaccine: a review of ten years of study. *Vet Bull* 1967;37:793.
9. Corbel MJ. Microbiology of the genus *Brucella.* In: Young EJ, Corbel MJ, eds. *Brucellosis: clinical and laboratory aspects.* Boca Raton, FL: CRC Press, 1989:53–72.
10. Daminova LF. Survival of brucella in soil, water and animal buildings. *Vetemeriya (Moscow)* 1967;44:103.
11. Buchanan TM, Feber LC, Feldman RA. Brucellosis in the United States, 1960–1972, an abattoir-associated disease. Part I. Clinical features and therapy. *Medicine (Baltimore)* 1974;53:402.
12. Buchanan TM, Hendricks ST, Patton DM, et al. Brucellosis in the United States 1960–1972, an abattoir-associated disease. Part III. Epidemiology and evidence for acquired immunity. *Medicine (Baltimore)* 1974;53:427.
13. Buchanan TM, Sulzeir CR, Frix MK, et al. Brucellosis in the United States, 1960–1972, an abattoir-associated disease. Part II. Diagnostic aspects. *Medicine (Baltimore)* 1974;53:415.
14. Spink WW. *The nature of brucellosis.* Minneapolis: University of Minnesota Press, 1956:207–208.
15. Pike RM. Laboratory associated infections. Incidence, fatalities, causes and prevention. *Annu Rev Microbiol* 1979;33:41.
16. Pike RM. Laboratory associated infections. Summary and analysis of 3921 cases. *Health Lab Sci* 1976;13:105–114.
17. Roux J. Epidémiologie et prevention de la brucellose. *Bull WHO* 1979;57:179.
18. Elberg SS, ed. *A guide to the diagnosis, treatment and prevention of human brucellosis.* Geneva: World Health Organization, 1981.
19. Gotuzzo E, Carrillo C, Seas C, et al. Características epidemiológicas y clínicas de la brucelosis en 39 grupos familiares. *Rev Esp Enferm Infecc Microbiol Clin* 1989;7:519.
20. Jordan CF, Borths IH. Brucellosis and infections caused by three species of *Brucella:* clinical, laboratory and epidemiological observations. *Am J Med* 1947;2:156.
21. Pacheco G, Thiago de Mello M. *Brucellose monograph del Instituto Brasileiro de Geografia y Estadfsticas.* Rio de Janeiro: Instituto Oswaldo Cruz, 1956.
22. Farid Z, Trabolsi B, Yassin W, et al. Acute brucellosis presenting as fever of unknown origin (FUO). *Trans R Soc Trop Med Hyg* 1980;74:402.
23. Gotuzzo E, Alarcón G, Bocanegra T, et al. Articular involvement in human brucellosis. A retrospective analysis of 304 cases. *Semin Arthritis Rheum* 1982;12:245.
24. Carbone A, Rolando I, Gotuzzo E, et al. La brucelosis lesiones oftalmológicas. *Diagnostico* 1983;12:196.
25. Fernández-Guerrero ML, Días-Curiel, Cortez-Cansino JM. Hepatic granulomas in brucellosis [Letter]. *Ann Intern Med* 1980;92:572.
26. Jordans HGM, De Bruin KD. Granulomas in *Brucella melitensis* infection [Letter]. *Ann Intern Med* 1980;92:264.
27. Lang R, Raz R, Sacks T, et al. Failure of prolonged treatment with ciprofloxacin in acute brucellosis. In: Program and abstracts of the 28th Interscience Conference on Antimicrobial Agents and Chemotherapy; Washington, DC; American Society for Microbiology; 1988. Abstract no. 386.
28. Recavarren S, Gotuzzo E. Patogenesis de la hepatitis granulomatosa por *Brucella;* estudios ultraestructurales. *Acta Med Peru* 1975;4:39.
29. Arias Stella J. Brucellosis. Contribución al conocimiento patológico. *Ann Fac Med (Peru)* 1951;34:429.
30. Huddleson IF. *Brucellosis in man and animals.* New York: The Commonwealth Fund, 1943.
31. Debono JE. Brucellosis in Malta. In: Huddleson IF, ed. *Brucellosis in man and animals.* New York: The Commonwealth Fund, 1943:115–143.
32. Gotuzzo E, Carrillo C. *Brucella* arthritis. In: Espinoza L, Goldberg D, Arnett F, et al, eds. *Infections in the rheumatic disease.* Orlando, FL: Grune & Stratton, 1988.
33. Brito M, Gonzales-Díaz J, Marques J, et al. Brucelosis osteoarticular. Revision de 20 casos observados recientemente. *Rev Esp Reum Enferm Osteoartic* 1972;15:219.
34. Feldman JL, Menkes GJ, Weil B, et al: Les sacro-ileites infectieuses.Étude multicentrique sur 214 observations. *Rev Rheum Mal Osteartic* 1981;48:83.
35. Norton WL. Brucellosis and rheumatic syndromes in Saudi Arabia. *J Rheumatol* 1984;43:810.
36. Porat S, Shapiro M. *Brucella* arthritis of the sacro-iliac joint. *Infection* 1984;12:205.
37. Cano R, Falcon S, Gotuzzo E, et al. La gamagrafta ósea: un procedimiento diagnóstico de valor en la artritis brucelar. Paper presented at IV Jornadas Científicas; September 1986; Universidad Peruana Cayetano Heredia; Lima, Peru. Abstract.
38. Gotuzzo E, Carrillo C, Guerra J, et al. Evaluation of diagnostic methods in brucellosis. Value of bone marrow culture. *J Infect Dis* 1986;153:122.
39. Mavidris AK, Drossos AA, Tsolas O, et al. Lactate levels in *Brucella* arthritis. *Rheumatol Int* 1984;4:169.
40. Berrocal A, Gotuzzo E, Calvo A, et al. Sternoclavicular brucellar arthritis: a report of seven cases and a review of the literature. *J Rheumatol* 1993;20:1184.
41. Pons P. Le spondylitis melitoccocita. *Ann Med* 1929;5:227.
42. Ariza J, Gudiol F, Valverde J, et al. Brucellar spondylitis: a detailed analysis based on current findings. *Rev Infect Dis* 1985;7:656.
43. Martin WJ, Nichols DR, Beahrs OH. Chronic localized brucellosis. *Arch Intern Med* 1961;107:143.
44. Rotes-Querol J. Osteo-articular sites of brucellosis. *Ann Rheum Dis* 1957;16:63.
45. Crosby E, Llosa L, Miroquesada M, et al. Hematologic changes in human brucellosis. *J Infect Dis* 1984;150:419.
46. Garcia P, Yrivarren JL, Argumans C, et al. Evaluación de la médula ósea en pacientes con brucelosis. Correlación clinicopatoldgica. *Rev Esp Enferm Infecc Microbiol Clin* 1990;8:37.
47. Lynch EC, McKechnie JC, Alfrey CP Jr. Brucellosis with pancytopenia. *Ann Intern Med* 1968;69:319.
48. Stoll DB, Blum S, Pasquale D, et al. Thrombocytopenia with decreased megakaryocytes. *Ann Intern Med* 1981;94:170.
49. Martin-Moreno S, Soto-Guzmán O, Bernardo-de-Quiros J, et al. Pancytopenia due to hemophagocytosis in patients with brucellosis; a report of four cases. *J Infect Dis* 1983;147:445.
50. Zuazu J, Duran J, Julia A. Hemofagocitosis en brucelosis aguda. *Rev Clin Esp* 1981;152:231.
51. McGaraty WC, Serafin D. Brucellosis, indications for splenectomy. *Am J Surg* 1968;115:355.
52. Ulloa V, Rojas J, Gotuzzo E. Púrpura trombocitopúnica asociada a brucelosis. *Rev Med Hered* 1992;3(3):87.
53. Bouza E, Garcia de la Torre M, Parras F, et al. Brucellar meningitis. *Rev Infect Dis* 1987;9:810.
54. Shakir RA, Al-Din ASN, Araj GF, et al. Clinical categories of neurobrucellosis. A report on 19 cases. *Brain* 1987;110:213.
55. Swick HM. *Brucella* meningoencephalitis in childhood. *Neuropediatrics* 1981;12:330.

56. Lubani MM, Dudin KI, Araj GF, et al. Neurobrucellosis in children. *Pediatr Infect Dis* 1989;8:779.
57. Mousa AR, Koshy TS, Araj GF, et al. *Brucella* meningitis: presentation, diagnosis and treatment, a prospective study of ten cases. *Q J Med* 1986;60:873.
58. Bashir R, Al-Kawl Z, Harder EJ, et al. Nervous system brucellosis: diagnosis and treatment. *Neurology* 1985;35:1576.
59. Bouza E. Brucellosis crónica. In: Baquero F, Buzon L, eds. *Encuentro Internacional sobre Brucellosis*. Madrid, 1985:57–60.
60. Corrado A, Toselli C. Contributo clinico alto studio delle complicanze ocularinella brucellosi. *Rass Ital Oftalmol* 1979;18:163.
61. Lyall M. Ocular brucellosis. *Trans Ophthalmol Soc U K* 1973;93:689.
62. Oppermann A, Royer I, Joubert L, et al. La brucellose oculaire. *Ann Anat Pathol* 1969;3:499.
63. Pichon A. L'Uvéite brucelliene [Thesis]. Tours, Faculté de Médecine de Tours, 1976.
64. Woods A. *Endogenous uveitis*. Baltimore: Williams & Wilkins, 1960.
65. Tobaru L. Uveitis: aspectos clinicos y etiologicos. Estudio prospectivo [Thesis Especialidad]. Lima Universidad Peruona Cayetano Heredia, 1983.
66. Bocanegra T, Gotuzzo E, Alarcón G, et al. Circulating immune complexes in acute fever and brucellosis. *Clin Res* 1981;29:381.
67. Gotuzzo E, Bocanegra T, Carrillo C, et al. Immunological abnormalities in human brucellosis. *Allergol Immunopathol (Madr)* 1985;13:417.
68. Rolando I, Carbone O, Gotuzzo E, et al. Circulating immune complexes in the pathogenesis of human brucellar uveitis. *Chibret Int J Ophthalmol* 1985;3:30.
69. Rolando I, Carbone O, Haro D, et al. Retinal detachment in chronic brucellosis. *Am J Ophthalmol* 1985;99:733.
70. Rolando I, Tobaru L, Hinostroza S, et al. Clinical manifestations of 25 *Brucella* uveitis. *Ophthalmic Pract* 1987;5:12.
70a. Jacobs F, Abramowicz D, Vereerstraeten P, et al. *Brucella* endocarditis: the role of combined medical and surgical treatment. *Rev Infect Dis* 1990;12:740.
71. Burgio R. Brucellosis. In: Sala Ginebra JD, ed. *Tratado de las enfermedades infecciosas en la infancia*, Barcelona: Editorial Cientifico-Medico, 1962:vol 2.873–900.
72. Chattas A, Ramaccio HF, Zamar R, et al. Brucelosis en el niño. *Gaceta Sanit (Argent)* 1963;6:69.
73. Gorbar JP. Brucelosis en el niño. *El Dia Mex* 1961;3(2):21.
74. Llorens-Terol J, Busquets RM. Brucellosis treated with rifampicin. *Arch Dis Child* 1980;55:486.
75. Martín-Fontelos P, Barreiro Casal B, Pérez Jurado M, et al. Brucelosis en la infancia. Paper presented at II Congreso Sociedad Española de Enfermedad Infecciosas y Microbiologia Clinico (SEIMC); May 1986; Palma de Mallorca, Spain. Abstract no. 12/4.
76. McCullough NB. Brucellosis in children. Symposium of unusual infections in childhood. *Pediatr Clin North Am* 1955;2:73.
77. Sattarov AI, Ambeev SA. Characteristics of brucellosis epidemiology in children in the Kasakh SSR. *Zh Microbiol Epidemiol Immunobiol* 1979;9:92.
78. Shan PM, Joshi VG. Brucellosis in children. *Indian Pediatr* 1967;4:226.
79. Hagebusch OE, Frei CF. Undulant fever in children. *Am J Clin Pathol* 1947;11:497.
80. Lubani MM, Dudin KI, Sharda DC, et al. A multicenter therapeutic study of 1100 children with brucellosis. *Pediatr Infect Dis J* 1989;8:75.
81. Keppie J, Williams AE, Witt K, et al. The role of erythritol in the tissue localization of the brucellae. *Br J Exp Pathol* 1965;46:104.
82. Smith H, Williams AE, Pearce JH, et al. Fetal erythritol: a cause of the localization of *Brucella abortus* in bovine contagious abortion. *Nature* 1962;193:47.
83. Criscuolo E, DiCarlo FB. El aborto y otras manifestaciones ginecobstétricas en el curso de la brucelosis humana. *Rev Fac Cienc Min Educ Univ Cordoba* 1954;12:321.
84. Arnow PM, Smaron M, Ormiste V. Brucellosis in a group of travelers to Spain. *JAMA* 1984;251:505.
85. Eckman MR. Brucellosis linked to Mexican cheese. *JAMA* 1975;232:636.
86. Galbraith NS, Ross MS, De Mowbray RR, et al. Outbreak of *Brucella melitensis* type 2 infection in London. *Br Med J* 1969;1:612.
87. Gotuzzo E, Seas C, Guerra J, et al. Brucellar arthritis—study of 39 Peruvian families. *Ann Rheum Dis* 1987;46:506.
88. Dalrymple-Champneys W. Undulant fever, a neglected problem. *Lancet* 1950;1:429.
89. Damdhere M, Bhagwat R, Sainini G. Outbreak of brucellosis in family. *Indian J Med Sci* 1964;18:145.
89a. Spink WW. Family studies in brucellosis. *Am J Med Sci* 1954;227:128.
90. Williams E. Brucellosis. *Practitioner* 1982;226:1507.
91. Alarcón GS, Bocanegra T, Gotuzzo E, et al. Reactive arthritis associated with brucellosis: HLA studies. *J Rheumatol* 1981;8:621.
92. Alarcón GS, Gotuzzo E, Hinostroza SA, et al. HLA studies in brucellar spondylitis. *Clin Rheumatol* 1985;4:312.
93. Alarcón GS, Gotuzzo E, Hinostroza TS, et al. Familial studies in human brucellosis. *Tissue Antigens* 1985;26:77.
94. Hodinka L, Gomor B, Meretey K, et al. HLA-B27 associated spondyloarthritis in chronic brucellosis. *Lancet* 1978;1:499.
95. Elberg SS. *Brucella melitensis*. Part II 1968–1980. *Vet Bull* 1981;51:67.
96. Spink WW, Cullough NB, Hutchings LM, et al. Diagnostic criteria for human brucellosis: report no. 2 of the National Research Council, Committee of Public Health Aspects of Brucellosis. *JAMA* 1952;149:805.
97. Díaz R, Moriyón I. Laboratory techniques in the diagnosis of human brucellosis. In: Young EJ, Corbel MI, eds. *Brucellosis: clinical and laboratory aspects.* Boca Raton, FL: CRC Press, 1989:73–83.
98. Díaz RE, Maraví-Poma E, Rivero A. Comparison of counterimmunoelectrophoresis with other serological tests in the diagnosis of human brucellosis. *Bull WHO* 1976;53:417.
99. Sippel JE, El-Masry NA, Farid Z. Diagnosis of human brucellosis with ELISA. *Lancet* 1982;2:19.
100. Ahvonen P, Sievers K. *Yersinia enterocolitica* infection associated with brucella agglutinins. Clinical features of 24 patients. *Acta Med Scand* 1969;185:121.
101. Carrillo C, Sanchez-Griñan E, Guerra J, et al. Evaluación de las metodologías diagnósticas en brucellosis, según las diferentes formas clínicas. In: *Libro de Resúmenes del 3rd Congreso Peruano de Medicina Interna.* Lima: Peruvian Society of Internal Medicine, 1984:102.
102. Goicochea C, Gotuzzo E, Carrillo C. Cholera-*Brucella* cross-reaction: a new potential diagnostic problem for travelers to Latin America. *J Travel Med* 1996;3:37.
103. Begue R, Guillen A, Meza R. *Brucella* antibodies and oral cholera vaccination [Letter]. *Lancet* 1995;346:115.
104. Foz A, Garriga S. Relation entre la fixation de complément et les anticorps incomplets (test de Coombs) dans la brucellose humaine. *Rev Immunol* 1954;18:288.
105. Ruiz-Castañeda M, Tovar R, Velez R. Studies on brucellosis in Mexico. Comparative study of various diagnostic tests and classification of the isolated bacteria. *J Infect Dis* 1942;70:97.
105a. Rodriguez-Torres A, Fermoso J, Landinez A. Brucellosis. *Medicina* 1983;48:3126.
106. Ruiz-Castañeda MA. Equipo perfeccionado para el aislamiento de *Brucella, Salmonella*, etc, por hemocultivo. *Bol Sanit Panam* 1957;42:564.
107. Bradstreet PCM, Tannahill AJ, Pollack TM, et al. Intradermal test and serological tests in suspected brucella infection in man. *Lancet* 1970;26:653.
108. Spink WW, Hoffbauer FW, Walker WW, et al. Histopathology of the liver in human brucellosis. *J Lab Clin* 1949;34:40.
109. Young EJ. Clinical manifestations of human brucellosis. In: Young EJ, Corbel MI, eds. *Brucellosis. Clinical and laboratory aspects.* Boca Raton, FL: CRC Press, 1989:97–126.
109a. Serre H, Kalfa G, Brousson A, et al. Manifestations osteoarticulaires de la brucellose. Aspects actuels. *Rev Rheum Mal Osteoartic* 1981;48:143.
110. Bertrand A, Roux J, Jonquet O. Place de la rifampicine dans le traitement de la brucellose. In: Baquero F, ed. *Proceedings of the first Mediterranean Congress of Chemotherapy.* Madrid, 1978:785–791.
111. Hall WH, Mannion RE. *In vitro* susceptibility of brucella to various antibiotics. *Appl Microbiol* 1970;20:600.
112. Spink WW, Braude AI, Castañeda MR, Goytia RS. Aureomycin therapy in human brucellosis due to *Brucella melitensis*. *JAMA* 1948;138:1145.
113. Carrillo C, Gotuzzo E, Adachi J, et al. Sensibilidad antimicrobiana in vitro de cepas de *Brucella* melitensis aisladas en un area endémica (Lima, Peru). *Rev Esp Quimioter* 1993;6:309.
114. Al-Majed SA, Al-Aska AK, Al-Mitwalli A, et al. Use of antibiotics in the treatment of human brucellosis. *Curr Ther Res* 1986;57:175.
115. Young EJ. Human brucellosis. *Rev Infect Dis* 1983;15:821.
116. Robertson L, Farell ID, Hinchliffe PM. The sensitivity of *Br. abortus* to chemotherapeutic agents. *J Med Microbiol* 1973;6:549.
117. Richardson M, Holt JN. Synergist action of streptomycin with other antibiotics on intracellular *Br. abortus in vitro. J Bacteriol* 1962;84:638.
118. Schirger A, Nichols DR, Martin WJ, et al. Brucellosis, experiences with 224 patients. *Ann Intern Med* 1960;52:827.
119. Waitz JA, Weinstein MJ. Recent microbiological studies with gentamicin. *J Infect Dis* 1969;119:355.
120. Novotny A, Moeschlin S. Klinische Erfahrung mit dem Breitspektrumantibisti kum Gentamizin. *Schweiz Med Wochenschr* 1972;102:24.
121. Solera J, Martínez-Alfaro E, Saez L. Meta-análisis sobre la eficacia de la combinación de rifampicina y doxiciclina en el tratamiento de la brucelosis humana. *Med Clin (Barc)* 1994;102:731.
122. Colmenero JD, Ferández-Gallardo LC, Agundez JAG, et al. Possible implication of doxycycline-rifampicin interaction for treatment of brucelosis. *Antimicrob Agents Chemother* 1994;38:2798.
122a. Lubani MM, Dudin KI, Sharda DC, et al. A multicenter therapeutic study of 1100 children with brucellosis. *Pediatr Infect Dis* 1989;8:75.
123. Akova M, Uzun O, Akalin HE, et al. Quinolones in treatment of human brucellosis: comparative trial of ofloxacin-rifampicin versus doxycycline-rifampicin. *Antimicrob Agents Chemother* 1993;37:1831.
124. García-Rodríguez JA, García-Sánchez JE, Trujillano I. Lack of bactericidal activity of new quinolones against *Brucella* spp. *Antimicrob Agents Chemother* 1991;35:756.
125. Shasha B, Lang R, Rubinstein E. Therapy of experimental murine brucellosis with streptomycin, co-trimoxazole, ciprofloxacin, ofloxacin, pefloxacin, doxycyclines, and rifampicin. *Antimicrob Agents Chemother* 1992;36:973.

CHAPTER 203

Haemophilus

Timothy F. Murphy

HAEMOPHILUS INFLUENZAE

Characteristics of the Pathogen

Haemophilus influenzae is a small nonmotile, non–spore-forming gram-negative bacterium. The bacterium was first recognized in 1892 by Pfeiffer, who erroneously concluded that the bacterium was the cause of influenza. On microscopic examination, *H. influenzae* is a small about 1.0- by 0.3-μm) gram-negative organism whose shape is variable; hence, it is often described as a pleomorphic coccobacillary form. In clinical specimens such as cerebrospinal fluid (CSF) and sputum, it often stains faintly with safranin dye and therefore can easily be overlooked.

H. influenzae is capable of both aerobic and anaerobic growth. Aerobic growth requires two factors: hemin (X factor) and nicotinamide adenine dinucleotide (V factor). The growth requirement for these two factors is used in the clinical laboratory to identify the bacterium.

CAPSULAR SEROTYPES

Six major serotypes of *H. influenzae* have been identified (1). These serotypes, designated A through F, are based on antigenically distinct polysaccharide capsules. In addition, some strains lack a polysaccharide capsule and these strains are referred to as nontypeable strains. Type B and nontypeable strains are the clinically relevant strains of *H. influenzae*.

Slide agglutination using serotype-specific antiserum has been the most widely used method to determine the serotype of a strain of *H. influenzae*. The accuracy of this method is variable, and the results must be interpreted cautiously. The most common error is that a nontypeable strain is misidentified as a typeable strain (2). Counterimmunoelectrophoresis using serotype-specific antiserum is a more accurate and reproducible method for determining the capsular serotype of a strain of *H. influenzae* (2).

H. influenzae: *Type B and Nontypeable Strains.* Type B strains are distinguished by their antigenically distinct capsule consisting of a linear polymer of ribosyl ribitol phosphate [polyribosyl ribitol phosphate (PRP)]. *H. influenzae* type B strains cause disease primarily in infants and children younger than 6 years. These strains are an important cause of meningitis in children and cause a variety of other serious invasive infections, including epiglottitis, pneumonia, septic arthritis, cellulitis, and others.

As a result of difficulty in defining disease caused by nontypeable *H. influenzae*, these unencapsulated organisms have been overlooked. However, nontypeable strains have gained increasing attention in the past two decades (2–5). These strains are important human pathogens but differ from type B strains in several respects. Nontypeable strains lack a polysaccharide capsule. They are primarily mucosal pathogens, although they occasionally cause invasive disease; indeed the incidence of invasive disease caused by nontypeable strains may be increasing (4,6,7). The most common clinical manifestations of infection with nontypeable *H. influenzae* are otitis media in children and respiratory tract infections in adults with chronic bronchitis and in children in developing countries. Therefore, clear distinctions exist between type B and nontypeable strains. These organisms affect different patient populations, cause different infections, and present different surface antigens to the host. In addition, type B and nontypeable strains are genetically different. Type B strains represent a restricted subset of genotypes of the species as a whole, suggesting a clonal origin for type B strains (8). By contrast, nontypeable strains are genetically diverse (9,10). Table 203.1 summarizes these differences.

Typing Systems. In addition to determining the capsular serotypes of strains of *H. influenzae*, it is now possible to subtype strains by various methods. These typing methods make it possible to discriminate among strains of the same capsular serotype, allowing for studies of pathogenesis and epidemiology of infections by both type B and nontypeable strains. Table 203.2 lists the typing systems that have been developed and the basis of strain differentiation for each system. Studies in which epidemiologically well-characterized strains have been subjected to molecular typing have revealed important new information regarding the dynamics of colonization of the human respiratory tract, the pathogenesis of otitis media, the role of nontypeable *H. influenzae* infections in adults with chronic lung disease, and mechanisms of immune evasion by *H. influenzae*.

Epidemiology and Transmission

H. influenzae is an exclusively human pathogen. The bacterium resides on the upper respiratory mucosa of adults and children. Nontypeable strains are common inhabitants of the normal human upper respiratory tract, being present in up to three fourths of healthy adults. Colonization with nontypeable *H. influenzae* is a dynamic process, with new strains being acquired and replacing old strains periodically (11). Children colonized with nontypeable *H. influenzae* in the first year of life are at increased risk of otitis media compared with children who remained free of nontypeable *H. influenzae* (12). Otitis media occurs earlier in colonized children and is directly related to age at the initial time of colonization. A direct relationship exists between the number of times a child is colonized with nontypeable *H. influenzae* and the number of episodes of otitis media (12).

Type B strains colonized the nasopharynx of children at a rate of 3% to 5% before the widespread use of conjugate vaccines, with higher rates seen in settings such as day care centers. The rate of nasopharyngeal colonization by type B strains has decreased with the widespread use of conjugate vaccines to prevent invasive infections caused by *H. influenzae* type B (13–17).

H. influenzae is spread by airborne droplets or by direct contact with secretions or fomites. Young children in the same household as a child with *H. influenzae* meningitis are at an increased risk of secondary disease; this risk is estimated at 2% to 4% (18–20). Controversy exists regarding the secondary attack rate in nonhousehold settings such as day care centers (21–24).

Studies of siblings with otitis media caused by nontypeable *H. influenzae* indicate that person-to-person transmission of nontypeable strains occurs among children in the same household (25). The epidemiology and transmission of nontypeable strains in patients with chronic bronchitis is yet to be defined.

Certain populations have a higher incidence of invasive type B disease than the general population. African American children have a three to four times higher incidence of meningitis caused by *H. influenzae* type B infection than white children in several studies (26,27). This might be related to the effect of different immunoglobulin allotypes in the populations on susceptibility to infection by encapsulated bacteria (28,29). Certain Native American groups have a markedly increased incidence of invasive type B disease. These include Apache (30) and Navajo (31), and Alaskan Eskimos (32,33), who have a rate that is

TABLE 203.1. Characteristics of *Haemophilus influenzae* Type B Versus Nontypeable Strains

	Type B	Nontypeable
Capsule	Ribosyl ribitol Phosphate polysaccharide capsule	Unencapsulated
Pathogenesis	Invasive infections	Mucosal infections
Clinical manifestations	Meningitis in infants; invasive disease in infants and children	Otitis media in infants and children; respiratory tract infection in adults with chronic obstructive pulmonary disease
Immunity	Primarily antibody to capsule	Antibody to noncapsular somatic antigens
Evolutionary history	Basically clonal	Genetically diverse

10 times higher than that of the general population. Although the precise explanation for this increased incidence is not yet defined, several factors might explain the observation. These include early age at exposure to the bacterium and genetic differences in the populations with regard to ability to mount an immune response.

Pathogenesis

COLONIZATION AND INVASION

H. influenzae resides predominantly on the human upper respiratory mucosal surface. Many strains that are recovered from the mucosal surface are piliated, including both type B and nontypeable strains. Pili likely play an important role in colonization of the upper respiratory mucosa by *H. influenzae*. Other surface molecules in addition to pili are involved in adherence to human respiratory epithelial cells and likely play a role in the ability of *H. influenzae* to colonize the human respiratory tract (34).

Type B strains cause systemic disease after invasion and hematogenous spread to distant sites such as meninges and epiglottis. The type B polysaccharide capsule is an important virulence factor in the bacterium's ability to invade and cause systemic disease. Isolates recovered from blood and CSF are invariably nonpiliated, indicating that the bacterium turns off expression of these structures after invasion.

Nontypeable strains cause disease by local invasion of mucosal surfaces. Otitis media results when bacteria migrate from the nasopharynx to the middle ear by way of the eustachian tube (25). Adults with chronic bronchitis experience recurrent lower respiratory tract infection resulting from nontypeable strains (35). Nontypeable strains cause invasive disease infrequently, although the incidence appears to be increasing (4,6,7).

ANIMAL MODELS OF INFECTIONS

An infant rat model of meningitis and bacteremia due to *H. influenzae* type B strains has provided useful information regarding pathogenesis of infection and preliminary identification of potentially protective antigenic determinants. Bacteria are inoculated intraperitoneally into infant rats and blood is obtained for quantitative culture 24 hours later (36). *H. influenzae* type B causes bacteremia in most infant rats thus inoculated. In a somewhat different version of the model, infant rats are infected in their nasopharynx and the bacteria disseminate from there (37). This model has allowed for the study of virulence factors and the investigation of the potential protective effect of antibodies to specific bacterial antigens.

An experimental model of otitis media caused by nontypeable *H. influenzae* has been developed in chinchillas (38,39). Bacteria are directly inoculated into the middle ear of the animal. This model has provided insight into the pathogenesis and immune response to infection and evaluation of potential vaccine

TABLE 203.2. Typing Systems for *Haemophilus influenzae*

Typing system	Assay	Basis of strain differentiation
Capsular serotype	Counterimmunoelectrophoresis with type-specific antiserum (1,2)	Antigenically distinct polysaccharide capsule
OMP subtype	SDS-PAGE of outer membranes (50)	Molecular weights of major OMPs
LOS serotype	Western blot assay of LOS with adsorbed antisera (61)	Antigenic heterogeneity of LOS
OMP serotype	Kinetic ELISA of OMPs with polyclonal antiserum (196)	Antigenic heterogeneity of OMPs
Biotype	Tests for ornithine, indole, and urease (197,198)	Biochemical differences among strains
Electrophoretic type	Starch gel electrophoresis and selective enzyme stains (8,199)	Genetic diversity among strains
Pulsed field gel electrophoresis	Pulsed field gel electrophoresis of restriction enzyme digested genomic DNA (200,201)	Genetic diversity among strains
Restriction endonuclease analysis of genomic DNA	Agarose gel electrophoresis of restriction enzyme digested genomic DNA (202–204)	Genetic diversity among strains
PCR	PCR using primers with common sequences (205,206)	Genetic diversity among strains
PCR ribotyping	Agarose gel electrophoresis of restriction enzyme digested ribosomal DNA (207,208)	Genetic diversity among strains

ELISA, enzyme-linked immunosorbent assay; LOS, lipooligosaccharide; OMP, outer-membrane protein; PCR, polymerase chain reaction; SDS-PAGE, sodium dodecyl sulfate polyacrylamide gel electrophoresis.

antigens. In a modification of this model, intranasal inoculation of nontypeable *H. influenzae* causes otitis media in animals that have been previously infected with adenovirus type 1 (40,41). This model offers the advantage studying pathogenesis of mucosal infection and avoids direct inoculation of bacteria into the middle ear.

A pulmonary challenge model in which nontypeable *H. influenzae* are inoculated directly into the trachea of rodents has been useful in studying potential vaccine antigens and in elucidating mechanisms of pulmonary clearance (42–45).

One must be cautious in extrapolating results in animal models to humans in view of the observation that *H. influenzae* is an exclusively human pathogen. Furthermore, differences in the immune responses between animals and humans have been demonstrated.

SURFACE ANTIGENS

Type B strains express on their surface a polysaccharide capsule that is a linear polymer of ribose, ribitol, and phosphate. Serum antibody to type B capsule is bactericidal *in vitro* (46), confers protection from bacteremia in experimental animals (47), and protects against disease in humans (48,49). The capsule is an important virulence factor in the ability of type B strains to cause invasive disease.

The outer-membrane protein (OMP) composition of *H. influenzae* is typical for that of nonenteric gram-negative bacteria in that approximately 20 proteins are present, with 4 to 6 proteins predominating. The sodium dodecyl sulfate polyacrylamide patterns of OMPs are the basis of subtyping systems for both type B and nontypeable strains (25,50,51). In general, OMPs are similar for type B and nontypeable strains except that those of nontypeable *H. influenzae* show more diversity from strain to strain.

The outer membrane of *H. influenzae* has a single major porin protein called *P2* or *b/c:* Its molecular mass varies among strains from 36,000 to 42,000 daltons (52–55). P2 exists as a trimer in the outer membrane and its molecular weight exclusion limit is approximately 1,400 daltons (56,57). OMP P6 (g) is a peptidoglycan-associated lipoprotein that has a molecular weight of 16,000 daltons. Antigenic and molecular studies show that P6 is highly conserved among strains (58,59). *H. influenzae* expresses several adhesins on its surface and these molecules mediate adherence to host tissue (34). Several other OMPs are the focus of antigenic and molecular studies in an effort to identify virulence factors and mediators of the human immune response to infection (45).

The outer membrane of *H. influenzae* contains lipooligosaccharide (LOS). It is similar to that of other nonenteric gram-negative bacteria in that it lacks the repeating polysaccharide side chains and demonstrates all the biologic activity characteristic of endotoxins (60). The LOS of *H. influenzae* demonstrates marked antigenic heterogeneity and undergoes phase variation (61–63). Approximately half of strains of *H. influenzae* have sialylated LOS (64). Sialylation of LOS may represent a form of molecular mimicry because its structure mimics host cell membrane glycosphingolipids (64,65). The precise role of LOS in pathogenesis is an area of active investigation.

IMMUNE RESPONSE

Antibody to capsule is important in protection from infection. The age-related susceptibility to *H. influenzae* type B disease is inversely related to the presence of serum bactericidal antibody (66). Much of this serum bactericidal antibody is directed at capsular polysaccharide (46). After the level of serum antibody to PRP declines from birth to 6 months of age (maternal antibody), the titer stays low until around 2 to 3 years of age in the absence of vaccination. The antibody nadir correlates with the peak age incidence of type B disease. Antibody to PRP then appears partly as

a result of exposure to *H. influenzae* type B or other cross-reacting antigens and partly as a result of the ability of older children to respond to polysaccharide antigens. Systemic type B disease is unusual after the age of 6 years because of the presence of protective antibody. Vaccines in which PRP is conjugated to diphtheria toxoid, tetanus toxoid, and meningococcal OMP complex have been developed in an effort to stimulate an antibody response to the polysaccharide antigen in young infants. These vaccines generate an antibody response to PRP in infants and are effective in preventing invasive infections in infants and children (67–74).

Noncapsular antigens of *H. influenzae* have generated considerable interest as targets of the human immune response and as potential vaccine components. Nontypeable strains lack a capsule so the immune response to infection is to noncapsular antigens. Characterization of molecular mechanisms of pathogenesis, structural analysis of surface antigens, elucidation of the human immune response to infection, and the search for potential vaccine antigens are areas of exciting and active investigation (34,35,45,75).

Clinical Manifestations

H. INFLUENZAE TYPE B

The most serious manifestation of infection with *H. influenzae* type B is meningitis. The peak age incidence of disease varies somewhat among populations, but this is primarily an infection of infants younger than 2 years. There is little distinction about the clinical manifestations of meningitis caused by *H. influenzae* type B compared with meningitis caused by other bacterial pathogens. Fever and altered central nervous system function are the most common presentation. Nuchal rigidity may or may not be present. Subdural effusion is the most common complication. One suspects this complication when the infant has seizures, hemiparesis, or continued obtundation in spite of 2 or 3 days of appropriate antibiotic therapy. The overall mortality of meningitis caused by *H. influenzae* type B is approximately 5% and the rate of morbidity is high. Six percent of survivors have permanent sensorineural hearing loss and about one fourth of survivors have significant handicap. If more subtle handicaps are sought, up to half of survivors have some neurologic sequelae such as partial hearing loss and delay in language development (76–78).

Epiglottitis is a life-threatening infection involving cellulitis of the epiglottis and supraglottic tissues (79,80). It can lead to acute upper airway obstruction. Unique epidemiologic features are that it occurs in an older age-group (2 to 7 years old) compared with other *H. influenzae* type B infections, and it is not seen in Navajo Indians and Alaskan Eskimos. Sore throat and fever rapidly progress to dysphagia, drooling, and airway obstruction.

Cellulitis caused by *H. influenzae* type B infection occurs in young children. The most common location is on the face or neck and the involved area sometimes has a characteristic bluish-red color. Bacteremia is usually present and 10% will have an additional focus of infection (81).

H. influenzae type B infection causes pneumonia in infants with a similar age distribution compared with meningitis. The infection is clinically indistinguishable from other bacterial pneumonias such as pneumococcal pneumonia except that *H. influenzae* is more likely to involve the pleura. Children with human immunodeficiency virus (HIV) infection have a higher incidence of *H. influenzae* type B pneumonia compared with healthy children (82).

Several less common invasive infections are seen as important clinical manifestations of *H. influenzae* type B infection in children. These include osteomyelitis, septic arthritis, pericarditis, orbital cellulitis, endophthalmitis, urinary tract infection, abscesses, and bacteremia without an identifiable focus (83–89). Invasive infections caused by *H. influenzae* type B have become rare in countries in which *H. influenzae* type B conjugate vaccines are widely used (13,90–97).

NONTYPEABLE *H. INFLUENZAE*

Nontypeable *H. influenzae* infection is an important cause of community-acquired bacterial pneumonia in adults (98). It is especially common in the setting of chronic obstructive pulmonary disorder (COPD) and in patients with acquired immunodeficiency syndrome (AIDS) (99–101). The clinical features of pneumonia caused by *H. influenzae* infection are indistinguishable from those of other bacterial pneumonias including pneumococcal pneumonia. Patients present with fever, cough, and purulent sputum, usually of several days' duration. The chest radiograph shows alveolar infiltrates in a patchy or lobar distribution. The sputum Gram stain shows a predominance of small, pleomorphic, coccobacillary gram-negative bacteria.

Exacerbations of COPD caused by nontypeable *H. influenzae* infection are characterized by increased cough, sputum production, and shortness of breath. Fever is low grade or absent and infiltrates are not present on the chest film. It is often difficult to establish the specific microbial cause of exacerbations of COPD in individual patients (35).

Nontypeable *H. influenzae* is one of the three most common causes of childhood otitis media, along with *Streptococcus pneumoniae* and *Moraxella catarrhalis* (102). There is nothing distinctive about the clinical presentation of otitis media caused by nontypeable *H. influenzae* infection compared with other middle ear pathogens such as *S. pneumoniae* and *M. catarrhalis*. Infants present with fever and irritability, whereas older children complain of ear pain. Symptoms of viral upper respiratory tract infection often precede otitis media. The diagnosis is established by pneumatic otoscopy. An etiologic diagnosis can be established by tympanocentesis and culture of middle ear fluid, but this is not routinely done.

Nontypeable *H. influenzae* is also an obstetric pathogen. It causes puerperal sepsis and is now an important cause of neonatal bacteremia. These strains tend to be biotype IV and cause invasive disease after colonizing the female genital tract (103,104).

Nontypeable *H. influenzae* infection causes sinusitis in adults and children (105,106). In addition, the bacterium is a less common cause of a variety of invasive infections that are documented primarily by small series and case reports. These include empyema, adult epiglottitis, pericarditis, cellulitis, septic arthritis, osteomyelitis, endocarditis, cholecystitis, intraabdominal infections, urinary tract infections, mastoiditis, aortic graft infection, scleritis, and bacteremia without a detectable focus of infection (97,107–121). In studies performed before the early 1980s, nontypeable strains were often misidentified as type B strains.

Diagnosis

The most reliable method for establishing a diagnosis of *H. influenzae* type B infection depends on recovery of the organism in culture. The CSF of a patient with suspected meningitis should be subjected to Gram stain and culture. The presence of gram-negative coccobacilli in Gram-stained CSF is strong evidence for *H. influenzae* type B meningitis. Recovery of the organism from CSF confirms the diagnosis. Cultures of other normally sterile body fluids such as blood, joint fluid, pleural fluid, pericardial fluid, and subdural effusion are confirmatory in other infections.

Detection of capsular antigen (PRP) is an important adjunct to culture in reaching a diagnosis. Several methods have been effective and these include immunoelectrophoresis, latex agglutination, coagglutination, and enzyme-linked immunosorbent assay. PRP can be detected in CSF, serum, and sterile body fluids of patients and this is quite specific for *H. influenzae* type B infection. Antigen detection can provide a rapid diagnosis before culture results are available. In addition, these assays are particularly helpful in patients who have received prior antimicrobial therapy and are, therefore, more likely to have negative cultures.

Because nontypeable *H. influenzae* is primarily a mucosal pathogen, the organism is present as part of a mixed flora, making it challenging to establish an etiologic diagnosis. A Gram-stained sputum specimen from a patient suspected of pneumonia or tracheobronchitis is highly suggestive of nontypeable *H. influenzae* infection when a predominance of gram-negative coccobacilli are seen among abundant polymorphonuclear leukocytes (122). A sputum culture is helpful when interpreted along with results of the Gram stain.

A diagnosis of otitis media is made by demonstrating the presence of fluid in the middle ear by pneumatic otoscopy. An etiologic diagnosis requires a tympanocentesis, but this is not routinely performed. Treatment is generally empirical, based on the pathogens known to be the most likely to cause otitis media. These include *S. pneumoniae*, nontypeable *H. influenzae*, and *M. catarrhalis*. As is the case with otitis media, it is necessary to perform an invasive procedure to determine the etiology of sinusitis, so treatment is often empirical once a diagnosis is suspected from clinical symptoms and sinus radiographs.

Treatment

Initial therapy for meningitis caused by *H. influenzae* type B infection should be ceftriaxone or cefotaxime (123). An alternative regimen for initial therapy is ampicillin plus chloramphenicol (123). When ampicillin is administered, it should be given initially in combination with chloramphenicol. If the isolate is ampicillin sensitive on susceptibility testing, chloramphenicol can be discontinued. If the isolate is ampicillin resistant, the patient should receive chloramphenicol alone. Chloramphenicol resistance is rare. Because chloramphenicol levels are unpredictable, serum levels should be determined and doses adjusted accordingly. Therapy should continue for 1 to 2 weeks.

Administration of corticosteroids to patients with meningitis caused by *H. influenzae* infection is beneficial with regard to reducing the incidence of subsequent neurologic sequelae. The presumed mechanism is that steroids reduce the inflammation induced by bacterial cell wall mediators of inflammation when cells are killed by antimicrobial agents. Dexamethasone therapy is recommended for infants and children 2 months and older with *H. influenzae* type B meningitis (123).

Invasive infections other than meningitis are treated with the same antimicrobial agents. Epiglottitis is a medical emergency and maintenance of an airway is critical. Duration of therapy is determined by the clinical response. One to two weeks of therapy is usually appropriate.

Many infections caused by nontypeable strains of *H. influenzae* can be treated with oral antimicrobial agents. These include otitis media, sinusitis, and exacerbations of COPD. Approximately 25% of nontypeable strains produce β-lactamase and are resistant to ampicillin. Infections caused by ampicillin-resistant strains can be treated with a variety of agents, including sulfonamides, trimethoprim-sulfamethoxazole, erythromycin-sulfasoxazole, extended-spectrum cephalosporins, amoxicillin–clavulanic acid, and newer macrolides (124–126). Fluoroquinolones are active against *H. influenzae* infection but are generally contraindicated in children younger than 18 years because of cartilage damage observed in juvenile animal models (123).

TABLE 203.3. Conjugate Vaccines for *Haemophilus influenzae* Type B

Vaccine	Carrier	PRP	Trade Name
PRP-T	Tetanus toxoid	Polysaccharide	ActHIB
HbOC	CRM_{197}, a mutant diphtheria toxin	Oligosaccharide	HibTITER
PRP-OMP	Group B *Neisseria meningitidis* outer-membrane complex	Polysaccharide	PedvaxHIB

Prevention

VACCINES

The development of conjugate vaccines to prevent invasive infections by *H. influenzae* type B in infants and children represents a dramatic success in the prevention of an infectious disease. Conjugating the PRP capsular polysaccharide to protein carriers has resulted in vaccine formulations that effectively induce protection from invasive *H. influenzae* type B infections in infants. Three such vaccines are licensed and are available in the United States (Table 203.3). Studies from several centers in the United States and Europe have established that conjugate vaccines are highly effective in preventing disease (70–74,127). One mechanism by which these vaccines prevent disease is by reducing pharyngeal colonization by *H. influenzae* type B (15,128–132). The reduction of pharyngeal colonization in infants may delay the age at initial acquisition of *H. influenzae* type B in a population (133,134). It will be important to monitor colonization patterns and disease incidence now that conjugate vaccines are in widespread use in many countries (6,7,135,136).

All children should be immunized with an *H. influenzae* type B conjugate vaccine beginning at approximately 2 months of age. Infants should receive a primary series of immunizations between 2 and 6 months of age and a booster vaccination at 12 to 15 months of age. Specific recommendations vary for the different conjugate vaccines. The reader is referred to the recommendations by the American Academy of Pediatrics for specific details (123).

No vaccines are available for prevention of disease caused by nontypeable *H. influenzae*. The PRP conjugates will not elicit antibody that is protective against nontypeable strains, because none of the conjugate vaccines contain noncapsular antigens of *H. influenzae*. Work is underway to identify somatic antigens that will elicit protective antibodies (45). Such a vaccine would be useful in preventing otitis media caused by nontypeable *H. influenzae*.

CHEMOPROPHYLAXIS

An increased risk of secondary disease is seen in household contacts of patients with *H. influenzae* type B disease (18–20). The attack rate can be as high as 4% of susceptible infants. Therefore, in households where there are contacts younger than 4 years, rifampin prophylaxis should be administered (123). All members (children and adults) of a household with a child in the susceptible age-group should receive oral rifampin. Based on the high rate of efficacy of conjugate vaccines, rifampin prophylaxis is not required when all of the household contacts younger than 4 years have completed their immunization. Children younger than 12 years should receive 20 mg/kg once daily for 4 days and adults should receive 600 mg daily for 4 days. The index case should receive rifampin before or at the time of discharge from the hospital because antimicrobial agents used to treat meningitis do not reliably eradicate the organism from the nasopharynx.

When two or more cases of invasive disease caused by *H. influenzae* type B have occurred within 60 days and unimmunized or incompletely immunized children attend the child care facility, rifampin should be administered to all children and personnel at the facility (123). When a single case has occurred, the question of rifampin prophylaxis is controversial, but many authorities recommend no prophylaxis. The decision should be individualized based on the size of the center, extent of contact, and other factors. In addition, a dose of conjugate vaccine should be administered to contacts younger than 4 years who are unvaccinated or incompletely vaccinated.

H. influenzae Biogroup *aegyptius*

H. influenzae biogroup *aegyptius* was formerly called *Haemophilus aegyptius* because of phenotypic characteristics distinct from *H. influenzae*. These include a distinct rod shape, susceptibility to troleandomycin, inability to grow on tryptic soy agar with added hemin and nicotinamide adenine dinucleotide, agglutination of human erythrocytes, and inability to ferment xylose. However, studies involving deoxyribonucleic acid (DNA) hybridization and DNA transformation studies have demonstrated that *H. aegyptius* and *H. influenzae* are members of the same species (137,138). Therefore, strains that were previously called *H. aegyptius* are now referred to as *H. influenzae* biogroup *aegyptius*.

H. influenzae biogroup *aegyptius* has long been associated with conjunctivitis. This strain is now also known to be the cause of Brazilian purpuric fever (BPF), first recognized in 1984, in the rural Brazilian town of Promissao (139). The peak age incidence of BPF is 1 to 4 years, with a range of 3 months to 8 years. The illness can occur sporadically or in outbreaks. Typically, following an episode of purulent conjunctivitis, high fever is seen initially in association with vomiting and abdominal pain. Within 12 to 48 hours from onset, the patient experiences petechiae, purpura, peripheral necrosis, and vascular collapse. The laboratory features of the illness are characterized by thrombocytopenia, prolonged prothrombin time, a uniformly unrevealing CSF, and positive blood cultures for *H. influenzae* biogroup *aegyptius* (139,140). The mortality in initial reports was high (about 70%), but subsequent studies have indicated that milder forms of the illness exist. Most patients have resolved or resolving purulent conjunctivitis and culture of the conjunctiva is positive in approximately one third of patients with BPF. The illness has been seen in several towns in Brazil and on two occasions in Australia (141,142).

Strains of *H. influenzae* biogroup *aegyptius* that cause BPF are of a clonal origin (143). Case clone strains share the following characteristics: (a) a 24-MDa plasmid that has a characteristic restriction digest pattern, (b) a typical banding pattern in sodium dodecyl sulfate polyacrylamide gel electrophoresis of whole organism lysates, (c) identical electrophoretic type in multilocus enzyme typing, (d) typical ribosomal DNA restriction patterns, (e) trimethoprim-sulfamethoxazole resistance, (f) a highly conserved surface epitope on the P1 OMP (144), and (g) a unique immunoglobulin A1 protease (145). Of interest, the Australian strains do not share these characteristics and represent a second clone (146). More recently, strains recovered from Valparaiso, Brazil, lack the 24-MDa plasmid typical of case clone strains yet are capable of causing BPF (147).

Several potentially useful model systems have been developed to study the pathogenesis of BPF. Case clone strains (a) are relatively serum resistant in spite of the absence of capsular genes (148,149), (b) show increased virulence in an infant rat model of bacteremia (150,151), and (c) are cytotoxic in an *in vitro* model using a human microvascular endothelial cell line (152). These models distinguish strains of *H. influenzae* biogroup *aegyptius* capable of causing BPF from strains not associated with the fulminant syndrome. They hold promise in facilitating the identification of virulence factors that enable these strains to cause invasive disease.

Several surface structures on BPF case clone strains have been identified and characterized. A unique surface-exposed epitope on the P1 OMP is highly predictive of disease-causing strains (144). The pilus gene has been sequenced and shares extensive homology with pili of other strains of *H. influenzae* (153,154). A phase-variable 145-kd surface protein is present in case clone strains (155). LOS phenotype is related to virulence in the infant rat model (156). Identifying the virulence factors expressed by case clone strains is important in understanding BPF. In addition, the identification and characterization of factors that enable a clone of an otherwise noninvasive bacterium (nontypeable *H. influenzae*) to become invasive is of general importance in understanding the pathogenesis of invasive bacterial infections.

HAEMOPHILUS DUCREYI (CHANCROID)

Haemophilus ducreyi is the etiologic agent of chancroid, a sexually transmitted disease characterized by genital ulceration and inguinal adenitis. *H. ducreyi* is a major health problem in developing countries. In the United States, the incidence of reported cases of chancroid peaked in 1987 with 4,986 cases reported. In 1999, 143 cases of chancroid were reported in the United States. However, the incidence of disease is undoubtedly higher because chancroid is underdiagnosed and underreported (157). In addition to morbidity associated with chancroid itself, it is associated with HIV infection by virtue of the role of genital ulceration in transmission of the virus (158–160).

Characteristics of the Pathogen

H. ducreyi is a coccobacillary gram-negative bacterium that has a growth requirement for X factor (hemin). Therefore, the bacterium is placed within the genus *Haemophilus*. However, studies of DNA homology (161) and chemotaxonomic studies established major differences between *H. ducreyi* and other *Haemophilus* species. Transfer in taxonomic assignment of the organism is likely in the future, but this awaits further study (162).

H. ducreyi is highly fastidious in its growth requirements. It is inert to most standard biochemical tests. There is not yet an established method for typing strains. Several methods have been studied. These include sodium dodecyl sulfate polyacrylamide gel electrophoresis of OMPs (163), indirect immunofluorescence using absorbed polyclonal antiserum (164), and specific

aminopeptidase activities (165). More recently, plasmid analysis and restriction fragment length polymorphism of genomic DNA have provided information on the epidemiology of *H. ducreyi* infection (166).

The classic test for virulence of *H. ducreyi* strains was the rabbit intradermal test (167,168). More recent work has resulted in the development of better model systems to study pathogenesis (169). A temperature-dependent rabbit model of experimental chancroid has been developed. Lesion development requires both a viable inoculum of *H. ducreyi* and housing of animals at reduced ambient temperatures (15° to 17°C) (170). Immunization with killed whole bacteria induces protection upon rechallenge (171). Experimental infections that produce lesions similar to those in humans have been established in macaques (172). A human model involving dermal challenge with live *H. ducreyi* is providing important insight into the pathogenesis of infection and the human immune response to the organism (173–175). In addition to these *in vivo* systems, several *in vitro*–cultured cells are being used to study adherence, invasion and cytopathic effect of *H. ducreyi* (176–178).

H. ducreyi expresses hemolysins and these are likely involved in pathogenesis. Several surface structures, including LOS, pili, OMPs, have been identified and their role in pathogenesis is being investigated.

Epidemiology and Prevalence

The epidemiology of *H. ducreyi* infections is not well defined because of difficulty in reliable cultures of chancroid lesions. Most studies have relied on the clinical picture to establish a diagnosis. A clinical diagnosis based on the appearance of the ulcer is often inaccurate, particularly in areas where the incidence of chancroid is low. Chancroid is a common cause of genital ulcers in developing countries. Several large outbreaks of chancroid have been identified in the United States since 1981 (166,179). In addition, when newer diagnostic methods including polymerase chain reaction (PCR) and serologic tests are used to evaluate patients with genital ulcers, *H. ducreyi* is found to be a more common cause of ulcers than when culture alone is used (157,160,180,181). Recurring epidemiologic themes in outbreaks in the United States are apparent: (a) Affected patients were primarily black and Hispanic, (b) transmission was predominantly heterosexual, (c) men outnumbered women by 3:1 to 25:1, and (d) prostitutes were important in transmission of the infection.

Clinical Manifestations

Infection occurs as a result of a break in the epithelium during sexual contact with an infected individual. After an incubation period of 4 to 7 days, the initial lesion is a papule with surrounding erythema. In 2 to 3 days, the papule evolves into a pustule, which spontaneously ruptures and forms a sharply circumscribed ulcer that is generally not indurated. The ulcers are painful and bleed easily and little or no inflammation of the surrounding skin is seen. Approximately half of the patients develop enlarged tender inguinal lymph nodes, which frequently become fluctuant and spontaneously rupture.

Chancroid does not usually present with all of the typical clinical features and sometimes manifests atypically. Multiple ulcers can coalesce to form giant ulcers. Ulcers can appear and then resolve, followed by inguinal adenitis with suppuration 1 to 3 weeks later. This can be confused with lymphogranuloma venereum. Multiple small ulcers can look like folliculitis.

Other differential diagnostic considerations include the causes of genital ulceration such as primary syphilis, condyloma latum of secondary syphilis, genital herpes, and donovanosis. Rarely, chancroid lesions can become secondarily infected with bacteria leading to extensive inflammation.

Diagnosis

Clinical diagnosis is often inaccurate, and laboratory confirmation should be attempted in suspected cases (162). Gram stain of a swab of the lesion can show a predominance of characteristic gram-negative coccobacilli, but the presence of other bacteria can often confuse the interpretation. PCR-based and serologic tests are under development but are not yet widely available. An accurate diagnosis of chancroid relies on cultures of *H. ducreyi* from the lesion. The organism can be difficult to grow, and the use of selective and supplemented media is necessary. The highest rate of recovery from clinical samples has been obtained with GC agar base containing 1% to 2% of hemoglobin, 5% fetal bovine serum, and 3 μg/mL of vancomycin. Media containing a variety of other supplements have been used. The use of more than one media will enhance the likelihood of obtaining a positive culture because of differing growth requirements of strains of *H. ducreyi* (182). Colonies are pinpoint at 24 hours and grow to 1 to 2 mm in diameter at 48 hours. Laboratory strains tend to grow more readily than clinical strains.

Treatment

Clinical isolates often have plasmid-mediated resistance to ampicillin, chloramphenicol, tetracyclines, and sulfonamides. *H. ducreyi* can acquire resistance determinants and can exchange plasmids with other human pathogens such as *H. influenzae* and *Neisseria gonorrhoeae*. Chancroid can be treated effectively with several regimens (183,184). These include (a) ceftriaxone, 250 mg intramuscularly as a single dose; (b) azithromycin, 1 gram orally as a single dose; (c) ciprofloxacin, 500 mg orally twice daily for 3 days; and (d) erythromycin, 500 mg orally four times daily for 7 days. Patients with HIV infection do not respond as well as otherwise healthy hosts. Susceptibility testing of isolates for patients who do not respond promptly to treatment should be performed.

OTHER *HAEMOPHILUS* SPECIES

Haemophilus species are often recovered as part of the normal upper respiratory tract flora in humans. However, these bacteria are uncommon causes of infection because of their low pathogenic potential. *Haemophilus* species have fastidious growth requirements and generally grow slowly. The species implicated in human infections are noted in Table 203.4. *Haemophilus* species are differentiated by several characteristics. Requirements for factor X and factor V are the primary means. Species designated "para" require factor V only for growth, whereas others require either factors X and V or factor X only. Other tests to differentiate species include hemolysis, the porphyrin test, nitrate reduction, lysine decarboxylase activity, and acid production from glucose, sucrose, lactose, and xylose (185).

Haemophilus species, particularly *Haemophilus parainfluenzae*, are an increasingly recognized cause of infective endocarditis (186–194). Several recent series indicate that *H. parainfluenzae* must be considered as a cause of endocarditis, especially when initial blood cultures are negative but when the clinical suspicion

TABLE 203.4. Other *Haemophilus* species[a] Associated with Human Disease

Haemophilus parainfluenzae
Haemophilus aphrophilus
Haemophilus paraphrophilus
Haemophilus parahemolyticus
Haemophilus hemolyticus
Haemophilus segnis

[a]Not including *H. influenzae* and *H. ducreyi*.

of endocarditis is present. It is likely that some cases of what has been called "culture-negative endocarditis" are actually caused by fastidious slow-growing bacteria such as *H. parainfluenzae* and *Haemophilus paraphrophilus*. To increase the chances of recovering the organisms, blood cultures should be subcultured onto chocolate agar and incubated in 5% carbon dioxide.

Endocarditis caused by *Haemophilus* species usually presents with a subacute course, but variability in the presentation is seen. The diagnosis is often delayed because of the difficulty in recovering the organism from blood cultures, which is a result of fastidious growth requirements and the intermittent nature of the bacteremia seen with these organisms. Preexisting valvular heart disease and other underlying conditions can be seen, but these are not constant features. Several series have noted a propensity for large-vessel embolization; this might be a result of large vegetations seen in the face of a frequently delayed diagnosis.

A variety of other infections in addition to endocarditis can be caused by *Haemophilus* species and these are listed in Table 203.5. It should be noted that these are unusual manifestations of infection with these bacteria and most are documented by case reports and small series.

The antimicrobial susceptibility characteristics of *Haemophilus* species are similar to those of *H. influenzae*. Some strains produce β-lactamase and these are resistant to ampicillin (195). Other strains are sensitive to ampicillin, which has been used successfully to treat many of these infections. Alternative agents with

TABLE 203.5. Human Infections Caused by Other *Haemophilus* Species[a]

Infection	Reference
Endocarditis	(187,209–212)
	(188–194,213–220)
Pulmonary infection	(187,209,212,221,222)
Epiglottitis	(209,223,224)
Meningitis	(209,225)
Bacteremia without an identifiable focus	(187,212,217)
Intraabdominal infection	(187,222,226,227)
Septic arthritis, osteomyelitis	(209,228–231)
Soft tissue infection or abscess	(187,212)
Neonatal sepsis	(232)
Otitis media	(216)
Brain abscess	(187)
Sinusitis	(187)
Necrotizing fasciitis	(233)
Urinary tract infection	(234)
Biliary tract infection	(235–238)

[a]Not including *H. influenzae* and *H. ducreyi*.

good activity against most *Haemophilus* species include chloramphenicol, trimethoprim-sulfamethoxazole, third-generation cephalosporins, tetracycline, and aminoglycosides and fluoroquinolones. Endocarditis caused by ampicillin-sensitive strains should be treated with ampicillin plus aminoglycoside. In addition, careful observation is required because surgical intervention is sometimes required because of the large size of vegetations and their propensity for embolization

REFERENCES

1. Pittman M. Variation and type specificity in the bacterial species *Haemophilus influenzae*. *J Exp Med* 1931;53:471–492.
2. Wallace RJ Jr, Musher DM, Septimus EJ, et al. *Haemophilus influenzae* infections in adults: characterization of strains by serotypes, biotypes, and beta-lactamase production. *J Infect Dis* 1981;144:101–106.
3. Murphy TF, Apicella MA. Nontypable *Haemophilus influenzae*: a review of clinical aspects, surface antigens, and the human immune response to infection. *Rev Infect Dis* 1987;9:1–15.
4. Farley MM, Stephens DS, Brachman PS Jr, et al. Invasive *Haemophilus influenzae* disease in adults. *Ann Intern Med* 1992;116:806–812.
5. Falla TJ, Dobson SRM, Crook DWM, et al. Population-based study of nontypable *Haemophilus influenzae* invasive disease in children and neonates. *Lancet* 1993;341:851–854.
6. Sarangi J, Cartwright K, Stuart J, et al. Invasive *Haemophilus influenzae* disease in adults. *Epidemiol Infect* 2000;124:441–447.
7. Hargreaves RM, Slack MPE, Howard AJ, et al. Changing patterns of invasive *Haemophilus influenzae* disease in England and Wales after introduction of the Hib vaccination programme. *BMJ* 1996;312:160–161.
8. Musser JM, Granoff DM, Pattison PE, et al. A population genetic framework for the study of invasive diseases caused by serotype b strains of *Haemophilus influenzae*. *Proc Natl Acad Sci USA* 1985;82:5078–5082.
9. Musser JM, Barenkamp SJ, Granoff DM, et al. Genetic relationships of serologically nontypable and serotype b strains of *Haemophilus influenzae*. *Infect Immun* 1986;52:183–191.
10. Porras O, Caugant DA, Gray B, et al. Difference in structure between type b and nontypable *Haemophilus influenzae* populations. *Infect Immun* 1986;53:79–89.
11. Spinola SM, Peacock J, Denny FW, et al. Epidemiology of colonization of nontypable *Haemophilus influenzae* in children: a longitudinal study. *J Infect Dis* 1986;154:100–109.
12. Harabuchi Y, Faden H, Yamanaka N, et al. Nasopharyngeal colonization with nontypeable *Haemophilus influenzae* and recurrent otitis media. *J Infect Dis* 1994;170:862–866.
13. Madore DV. Impact of immunization on *Haemophilus influenzae* type b disease. *Infect Agents Dis* 1996;5:8–20.
14. Barbour ML. Conjugate vaccines and the carriage of *Haemophilus influenzae* type b. *Emerg Infect Dis* 1996;2:176–182.
15. Barbour ML, Mayon-White RT, Coles C, et al. The impact of conjugate vaccine on carriage of *Haemophilus influenzae* type b. *J Infect Dis* 1995;171:93–98.
16. Forleo-Neto E, de Oliveira CF, Maluf EM, et al. Decreased point prevalence of *Haemophilus influenzae* type b (Hib) oropharyngeal colonization by mass immunization of Brazilian children less than 5 years old with Hib polyribosylribitol phosphate polysaccharide-tetanus toxoid conjugate vaccine in combination with diphtheria-tetanus toxoids-pertussis vaccine. *J Infect Dis* 1999;180:1153–1158.
17. Fernandez J, Levine OS, Sanchez J, et al. Prevention of *Haemophilus influenzae* type b colonization by vaccination: correlation with serum anti-capsular IgG concentration. *J Infect Dis* 2000;182:1553–1556.
18. Ward JI, Fraser DW, Baraff LJ, et al. *Haemophilus influenzae* meningitis: a national study of secondary spread in household contacts. *N Engl J Med* 1979;301:122–126.
19. Filice GA, Andrews JS Jr, Hudgins MP, et al. Spread of *Haemophilus influenzae*: secondary illness in household contacts of patients with *H. influenzae* meningitis. *Am J Dis Child* 1978;132:757–759.
20. Campbell LR, Zedd AJ, Michaels RH. Household spread of infection due to *Haemophilus influenzae* type b. *Pediatrics* 1980;66:115–117.
21. Makintubee S, Istre GR, Ward JI. Transmission of invasive *Haemophilus influenzae* type b disease in day care settings. *J Pediatr* 1987;111:180–186.
22. Osterholm MT, Pierson LM, White KE, et al. The risk of subsequent transmission of *Haemophilus influenzae* type b disease among children in day care. *N Engl J Med* 1987;316:1–5.
23. Murphy TV, Clements JF, Breedlove JA, et al. Risk of subsequent disease among day-care contacts of patients with systemic *Haemophilus influenzae* type b disease. *N Engl J Med* 1987;316:5–10.
24. Broome CV, Mortimer EA, Katz SL, et al. Use of chemoprophylaxis to prevent the spread of *Haemophilus influenzae* b in day-care facilities. *N Engl J Med* 1987;316:1226–1228.
25. Murphy TF, Bernstein JM, Dryja DD, et al. Outer membrane protein and lipooligosaccharide analysis of paired nasopharyngeal and middle ear isolates in otitis media due to nontypable *Haemophilus influenzae*: pathogenetic and epidemiological observations. *J Infect Dis* 1987;156:723–731.
26. Granoff DM, Basden M. *Haemophilus influenzae* infections in Fresno County, California: a prospective study of the effects of age, race, and contact with a case on incidence of disease. *J Infect Dis* 1980;141:40–46.
27. Parke JC, Schneerson R, Robbins JB. The attack rate, age, incidence, social distribution, and case fatality rate of *Haemophilus influenzae* type b meningitis in Mecklenburg County, North Carolina. *J Pediatr* 1972;81:765–769.
28. Ambrosino DM, Schiffman G, Gotschlich EC, et al. Correlation between G2m(n) immunoglobulin allotype and human antibody response and susceptibility to polysaccharide encapsulated bacteria. *J Clin Invest* 1985;75:1935–1942.
29. Granoff DM, Pandey JP, Boies E, et al. Response to immunization with *Haemophilus influenzae* type b polysaccharide-pertussis vaccine and risk of *Haemophilus influenzae* meningitis in children with Km(1) immunoglobulin allotype. *J Clin Invest* 1984;74:1708–1714.
30. Santosham M, Reid R, Ambrosino DM, et al. Prevention of *Haemophilus influenzae* type b infections in high-risk infants treated with bacterial polysaccharide immune globulin. *N Engl J Med* 1987;317:923–929.
31. Coulehan JL, Michaels RH, Williams KE, et al. Bacterial meningitis in Navajo Indians. *Public Health Rep* 1976;91:464–468.
32. Ward JI, Lum MKW, Bender TR. *Haemophilus influenzae* disease in Alaska: Epidemiologic, clinical and serologic studies of a population at high risk of invasive disease. In: Sell SH, Wright PF, eds. Haemophilus influenzae: *epidemiology, immunology and prevention of disease.* New York: Elsevier Science, 1982:23–34.
33. Ward JI, Margolis HS, Lum MKW, et al. *Haemophilus influenzae* disease in Alaskan Eskimos: characteristics of a population with an unusual incidence of invasive disease. *Lancet* 1981;1:1281–1285.
34. Rao VK, Krasan GP, Hendrixson DR, et al. Molecular determinants of the pathogenesis of disease due to non-typable *Haemophilus influenzae*. *FEMS Microbiol Rev* 1999;23:99–129.
35. Sethi S, Murphy TF. Bacterial infection in chronic obstructive pulmonary disease in 2000. A state of the art review. *Clin Microbiol Rev* 2001;14:336–363.
36. Granoff DM, Rockwell R. Experimental *Haemophilus influenzae* type b meningitis: immunological investigation of the infant rat model. *Infect Immun* 1978;20:705–713.
37. Moxon ER, Smith AL, Averill DR, et al. *Haemophilus influenzae* meningitis in infant rats after intranasal inoculation. *J Infect Dis* 1974;129:154–162.
38. Giebink GS. Experimental otitis media due to *Haemophilus influenzae* in the chinchilla. In: Sell SH, Wright PF, eds. Haemophilus influenzae: *epidemiology, immunology and prevention of disease.* New York: Elsevier Science, 1982:73–80.
39. Doyle WJ, Supance JS, Marshack G, et al. An animal model of acute otitis media consequent to beta lactamase–producing nontypable *Haemophilus influenzae*. *Otolaryngol Head Neck Surg* 1982;90:831–836.
40. Suzuki K, Bakaletz LO. Synergistic effect of adenovirus type 1 and nontypeable *Haemophilus influenzae* in a chinchilla model of experimental otitis media. *Infect Immun* 1994;62:1710–1718.
41. Bakaletz LO, Kennedy B-J, Novotny LA, et al. Protection against development of otitis media induced by nontypeable *Haemophilus influenzae* by both active and passive immunization in a chinchilla model of virus-bacterium superinfection. *Infect Immun* 1999;67:2746–2762.
42. Kyd JM, Cripps AW. Potential of a novel protein, OMP26, from nontypeable *Haemophilus influenzae* to enhance pulmonary clearance in a rat model. *Infect Immun* 1998;66:2272–2278.
43. Foxwell AR, Kyd JM, Cripps AW. Characteristics of the immunological response in the clearance of non-typeable *Haemophilus influenzae* from the lung. *Immunol Cell Biol* 1998;76:323–331.
44. Kyd JM, Dunkley ML, Cripps AW. Enhanced respiratory clearance of nontypeable *Haemophilus influenzae* following mucosal immunization with P6 in a rat model. *Infect Immun* 1995;63:2931–2940.
45. Foxwell AR, Kyd JM, Cripps AW. Nontypeable *Haemophilus influenzae*: pathogenesis and prevention. *Microbiol Mol Biol Rev* 1998;62:294–308.
46. Anderson P, Johnston RB, Smith DH. Human serum activities against *Haemophilus influenzae* type b. *J Clin Invest* 1972;51:31–38.
47. Gigliotti F, Insall RA. Protection from infection with *Haemophilus influenzae* type b by monoclonal antibody to the capsule. *J Infect Dis* 1983;146:249–254.
48. Peltola H, Kayhty H, Sivonen A, et al. *Haemophilus influenzae* type b capsular polysaccharide vaccine in children: a double-blind field study of 100,000 vaccinees 3 months to 5 years of age in Finland. *Pediatrics* 1977;60:730–737.
49. Peltola H, Kayhty H, Virtanen M, et al. Prevention of *Haemophilus influenzae* type b bacteremic infections with the capsular polysaccharide vaccine. *N Engl J Med* 1984;310:1561–1566.
50. Murphy TF, Dudas KC, Mylotte JM, et al. A subtyping system for nontypable *Haemophilus influenzae* based on outer-membrane proteins. *J Infect Dis* 1983;147:838–846.
51. Barenkamp SJ, Munson RS Jr, Granoff DM. Subtyping isolates of *Haemophilus influenzae* type b by outer-membrane protein profiles. *J Infect Dis* 1981;143:668–676.

52. Vachon V, Lyew DJ, Coulton JW. Transmembrane permeability channels across the outer membrane of *Haemophilus influenzae* type b. *J Bacteriol* 1985;162:918–924.

53. Munson RS Jr, Shenep JL, Barenkamp SJ, et al. Purification and comparison of outer membrane protein P2 from *Haemophilus influenzae* type b isolates. *J Clin Invest* 1983;72:677–684.

54. Murphy TF, Bartos LC. Purification and analysis with monoclonal antibodies of P2, the major outer membrane protein of nontypable *Haemophilus influenzae*. *Infect Immun* 1988;56:1084–1089.

55. Munson R Jr, Tolan RW Jr. Molecular cloning, expression, and primary sequence of outer membrane protein P2 of *Haemophilus influenzae* type b. *Infect Immun* 1989;57:88–94.

56. Klingman KL, Jansen EM, Murphy TF. Nearest neighbor analysis of outer membrane proteins of nontypeable *Haemophilus influenzae*. *Infect Immun* 1988;56:3058–3063.

57. Vachon V, Kristjanson DN, Coulton JW. Outer membrane porin protein of *Haemophilus influenzae* type b pore size and subunit structure. *Can J Microbiol* 1988;34:134–140.

58. Deich RA, Metcalf BJ, Finn CW, et al. Cloning of genes encoding a 15,000-dalton peptidoglycan-associated outer membrane lipoprotein and an antigenically related 15,000-dalton protein from *Haemophilus influenzae*. *J Bacteriol* 1988;170:489–498.

59. Nelson MB, Munson RS Jr, Apicella MA, et al. Molecular conservation of the P6 outer membrane protein among strains of *Haemophilus influenzae*: analysis of antigenic determinants, gene sequences, and restriction fragment length polymorphisms. *Infect Immun* 1991;59:2658–2663.

60. Flesher AR, Insel RA. Characterization of lipopolysaccharide of *Haemophilus influenzae*. *J Infect Dis* 1978;138:719–730.

61. Campagnari AA, Gupta MR, Dudas KC, et al. Antigenic diversity of lipooligosaccharides of nontypable *Haemophilus influenzae*. *Infect Immun* 1987;55:882–887.

62. Weiser JN. Relationship between colony morphology and the life cycle of *Haemophilus influenzae*: the contribution of lipopolysaccharide phase variation to pathogenesis. *J Infect Dis* 1993;168:672–680.

63. Weiser JN. The oligosaccharide of *Haemophilus influenzae*. *Microb Pathogen* 1992;13:335–342.

64. Mandrell RE, McLaughlin R, Abu Kwaik Y, et al. Lipooligosaccharides (LOS) of some *Haemophilus* species mimic human glycosphingolipids, and some LOS are sialylated. *Infect Immun* 1992;60:1322–1328.

65. Phillips NJ, Apicella MA, Griffis JM, et al. Structural characterization of the cell surface lipooligosaccharides from a nontypable strain of *Haemophilus influenzae*. *Biochemistry* 1992;31:4515–4526.

66. Fothergill LD, Wright J. Influenzal meningitis: the relation of age incidence to the bactericidal power of blood against the causal organism. *J Immunol* 1933;24:273–284.

67. Eskola J, Peltola H, Takala AK, et al. Efficacy of *Haemophilus influenzae* type b polysaccharide-diphtheria toxoid conjugate vaccine in infancy. *N Engl J Med* 1987;317:717–722.

68. Centers for Disease Control and Prevention. FDA approval of use of a new *Haemophilus* b conjugate vaccine and a combined diphtheria-tetanus-pertussis and *Haemophilus* b conjugate vaccine for infants and children. *JAMA* 1993;269:2359.

69. Eskola J, Peltola H, Kayhty H, et al. Finnish efficacy trials with *Haemophilus influenzae* type b vaccines. *J Infect Dis* 1992;165(S1):S137–S138.

70. Vadheim CM, Greenberg DP, Eriksen E, et al. Eradication of *Haemophilus influenzae* type b disease in Southern California. *Arch Pediatr Adolesc Med* 1994;148:51–56.

71. Peltola H, Kilpi T, Anttila M. Rapid disappearance of *Haemophilus influenzae* type b meningitis after routine childhood immunisation with conjugate vaccines. *Lancet* 1992;340:592–594.

72. Singleton RJ, Davidson NM, Desmet IJ, et al. Decline of *Haemophilus influenzae* type b disease in a region of high risk: impact of passive and active immunization. *Pediatr Infect Dis J* 1994;13:362–367.

73. Murphy TV, White KE, Pastor P, et al. Declining incidence of *Haemophilus influenzae* type b disease since introduction of vaccination. *JAMA* 1993;269:246–248.

74. Santosham M, Wolff M, Reid R, et al. The efficacy in Navajo infants of a conjugate vaccine consisting of *Haemophilus influenzae* type b polysaccharide and *Neisseria meningitidis* outer membrane protein complex. *N Engl J Med* 1991;324:1767–1772.

75. Murphy TF. Bacterial otitis media: pathogenetic considerations. *Pediatr Infect Dis J* 2000;19:S9–S16.

76. Sell SH, Merrill RE, Doyne EO. Long term sequelae of *Haemophilus influenzae* meningitis. *Pediatrics* 1972;49:206–211.

77. Feigin RD, Stechenberg BW, Chaig MJ. Prospective evaluation of treatment of *Haemophilus influenzae* meningitis. *J Pediatr* 1976;88:542–548.

78. Ferry PC, Culbertson JL, Cooper JA, et al. Sequelae of *Haemophilus influenzae* meningitis: preliminary report of a long-term follow-up study. In: Sell SH, Wright PF, eds. Haemophilus influenzae: *epidemiology, immunology and prevention of disease*. New York: Elsevier Science, 1982:111–117.

79. Bottenfield GW, Arcinue EL, Sarnaik A. Diagnosis and management of acute epiglottitis. Report of 90 consecutive cases. *Laryngoscope* 1980;90:822–825.

80. Trollfors B, Nylen O, Carenfelt C, et al. Aetiology of acute epiglottitis in adults. *Scand J Infect Dis* 1998;30:49–51.

81. Fleisher G, Ludwig S, Campos J. Cellulitis: bacterial etiology, clinical features, and laboratory findings. *J Pediatr* 1980;97:591–592.

82. Madhi SA, Petersen K, Madhi A, et al. Increased disease burden and antibiotic resistance of bacteria causing severe community-acquired lower respiratory tract infections in human immunodeficiency virus type 1-infected children. *Clin Infect Dis* 2000;31:170–176.

83. Ricketts RR, Ilbawi MN, Idriss FS. Management of *Haemophilus influenzae* pericarditis. *J Pediatr Surg* 1982;17:285–289.

84. Cheatham JE Jr, Grantham RN, Peyton MD. *Haemophilus influenzae* purulent pericarditis in children. *J Thorac Cardiovasc Surg* 1980;79:933–936.

85. Boomla K, Quilliam RP. *Haemophilus influenzae* endophthalmitis. *Br Med J* 1981;2828:989–990.

86. Liechty E, Kleiman MB, Ballantine TVN. Primary *Haemophilus influenzae* lung abscesses with bronchial obstruction. *J Pediatr Surg* 1982;17:281–284.

87. McCarthy LG. *Haemophilus influenzae* associated with periappendiceal abscess. *Am J Gastroenterol* 1981;76:157–159.

88. Broughton RA, Edwards MS, Taber LH. Systemic *Haemophilus influenzae* type b infection presenting as fever of unknown origin. *J Pediatr* 1981;98:925–928.

89. Marshall R, Teele DW, Klein JO. Unsuspected bacteremia due to *Haemophilus influenzae*: Outcome in children not initially admitted to hospital. *J Pediatr* 1979;95:690–695.

90. Herrera GA, Smith P, Daniels D, et al. National, state, and urban area vaccination coverage levels among children aged 19–35 months—United States, 1998. *Morb Mortal Wkly Rep CDC Surveill* 2000;49:1–26.

91. Dagan R, Fraser D, Greif Z, Keller N, et al. A nationwide prospective surveillance study in Israel to document pediatric invasive infections, with an emphasis on *Haemophilus influenzae* type b infections. Israeli Pediatric Bacteremia and Meningitis Group. *Pediatr Infect Dis J* 1998;17:S198–S203.

92. Barone SR, Aiuto LT. Periorbital and orbital cellulitis in the *Haemophilus influenzae* vaccine era. *J Pediatr Ophthalmol Strabismus* 1997;34:293–296.

93. Luhmann JD, Luhmann SJ. Etiology of septic arthritis in children: an update for the 1990s. *Pediatr Emerg Care* 1999;15:40–42.

94. Howard AW, Viskontas D, Sabbagh C. Reduction in osteomyelitis and septic arthritis related to *Haemophilus influenzae* type b vaccination. *J Pediatr Orthop* 1999;19:705–709.

95. Garpenholt O, Hugosson S, Fredlund H, et al. Epiglottitis in Sweden before and after introduction of vaccination against *Haemophilus influenzae* type b. *Pediatr Infect Dis J* 1999;18:490–493.

96. Midwinter KI, Hodgson D, Yardley M. Paediatric epiglottitis: the influence of the *Haemophilus influenzae* b vaccine, a ten-year review in the Sheffield region. *Clin Otolaryngol* 1999;24:447–448.

97. Sarria JC, Vidal AM, Kimbrough RCI. *Haemophilus influenzae* osteomyelitis in adults: a report of 4 frontal bone infections and a review of the literature. *Scand J Infect Dis* 2001;33:263–265.

98. Bartlett JG, Dowell SF, Mandell LA, et al. Practice guidelines for the management of community-acquired pneumonia in adults. *Clin Infect Dis* 2000;31:347–382.

99. Steinhart R, Reingold AL, Taylor F, et al. Invasive *Haemophilus influenzae* infections in men with HIV infection. *JAMA* 1992;268:3350–3352.

100. Schlamm HT, Yancovitz SR. *Haemophilus influenzae* pneumonia in young adults with AIDS, ARC, or risk of AIDS. *Am J Med* 1989;86:11–14.

101. Afessa B, Green B. Bacterial pneumonia in hospitalized patients with HIV infection. *Chest* 2000;117.

102. Klein JO. Otitis media. *Clin Infect Dis* 1994;19:823–833.

103. Wallace RJ Jr, Baker CJ, Quinones FJ, et al. Nontypable *Haemophilus influenzae* (biotype 4) as a neonatal, maternal, and genital pathogen. *Rev Infect Dis* 1983;5:123–135.

104. Quentin R, Goudeau A, Wallace RJ Jr, et al. Urogenital, maternal and neonatal isolates of *Haemophilus influenzae*: identification of unusually virulent serologically non-typeable clone families and evidence for a new *Haemophilus* species. *J Gen Microbiol* 1990;136:1203–1209.

105. Wald ER, Milmoe GJ, Bowen A, et al. Acute maxillary sinusitis in children. *N Engl J Med* 1981;304:749–754.

106. Evans FO Jr, Sydnor JB, Moore WEC, et al. Sinusitis of the maxillary antrum. *N Engl J Med* 1975;293:735–739.

107. Spagnuolo PJ, Ellner JJ, Lerner PI, et al. *Haemophilus influenzae* meningitis: the spectrum of disease in adults. *Medicine* 1982;61:74–85.

108. Snyder SN, Brunjes S. *Haemophilus influenzae* meningitis in adults. Review of the literature and report of 18 cases. *Am J Med Sci* 1965;250:658–667.

109. Eykyn SJ, Thomas RD, Phillips I. *Haemophilus influenzae* meningitis in adults. *Br Med J* 1974;2:463–465.

110. Addy MG, Ellis PDM, Turk DC. *Haemophilus* epiglottitis: nine recent cases in Oxford. *Br Med J* 1972;1:40–42.

111. Black MJ, Harbour J, Remsen KA, et al. Acute epiglottitis in adults. *J Otolaryngol* 1981;10:23–27.

112. Ossoff RH, Wolff AP, Ballenger JJ. Acute epiglottitis in adults: experience with fifteen cases. *Laryngoscope* 1980;90:1155–1161.

113. Alsever RN, Stiver HG, Dinerman N, et al. *Haemophilus influenzae* pericarditis and empyema and thyroiditis in an adult. *JAMA* 1974;230:1426–1427.

114. Lev EI, Onn A, Levo OY, et al. *Haemophilus influenzae* biotype III cellulitis in an adult. *Infection* 1999;27:42–43.

115. Ligtenberg JJ, van der Werf TS, Zijlstra JG, et al. Non-surgical treatment of purulent pericarditis, due to non-encapsulated *Haemophilus influenzae*, in an immunocompromised patient. *Neth J Med* 1999;55:151–154.

116. Personius CD, Camp CJ. Vertebral osteomyelitis: nontypeable beta-lactamase–negative *Haemophilus influenzae* in an adult: case report. *Diagn Microbiol Infect Dis* 1997;28:205–208.

117. Lesage V, Van Pee D, Luyx C, et al. Septic arthritis caused by *Haemophilus influenzae* associated with endocarditis. *Clin Rheumatol* 1998;17:340–342.

118. Melhus A, Svernell O. Polyarticular septic arthritis caused by non-encapsulated *Haemophilus influenzae* biotype I in a rheumatic adult. *Scand J Infect Dis* 1998;30:630–631.

119. Sykes SO, Riemann C, Santos CI, et al. *Haemophilus influenzae* associated scleritis. *Br J Ophthalmol* 1999;83:410–413.

120. McDonald CL, Crafton EM, Covin FA, et al. Pericarditis: a probable complication of endocarditis due to *Haemophilus influenzae*. *Clin Infect Dis* 1994;18:648–649.

121. Rolle U. *Haemophilus influenzae* cellulitis after bite injuries in children. *J Pediatr Surg* 2000;35:1408–1409.

122. Musher DM, Kubitschek KR, Crennan J, et al. Pneumonia and acute febrile tracheobronchitis due to *Haemophilus influenzae*. *Ann Intern Med* 1983;99:444–450.

123. Pickering LK, ed. *The red book: report of the Committee on Infectious Diseases*, 25th ed. Elk Grove, IL: American Academy of Pediatrics, 2000.

124. Bandak SI, Turnak MR, Allen BS, et al. Antibiotic susceptibilities among recent clinical isolates of *Haemophilus influenzae* and *Moraxella catarrhalis* from fifteen countries. *Eur J Clin Microbiol Infect Dis* 2001;20:55–60.

125. Mathai D, Lewis T, Kugler KC, et al, for the SENTRY Participants Group (North America). Antibacterial activity of 41 antimicrobials tested against over 2773 bacterial isolates from hospitalized patients with pneumonia: I—results from the SENTRY Antimicrobial Surveillance Program (North America, 1998). *Diagn Microbiol Infect Dis* 2001;39:105–116.

126. Hoban DJ, Doern GV, Fluit AC, et al. Worldwide prevalence of antimicrobial resistance in *Streptococcus pneumoniae*, *Haemophilus influenzae*, and *Moraxella catarrhalis* in the SENTRY Antimicrobial Surveillance Program, 1997–1999. *Clin Infect Dis* 2001;32(S2):S81–S93.

127. Shapiro ED. Infections caused by *Haemophilus influenzae* type b. The beginning of the end? *JAMA* 1993;269:264–266.

128. Takala AK, Eskola J, Leinonen M, et al. Reduction of oropharyngeal carriage of *Haemophilus influenzae* type b (Hib) in children immunized with an Hib conjugate vaccine. *J Infect Dis* 1991;164:982–986.

129. Kauppi M, Saarinen L, Kayhty H. Anti-capsular polysaccharide antibodies reduce nasopharyngeal colonization by *Haemophilus influenzae* type b in infant rats. *J Infect Dis* 1993;167:365–371.

130. Takala AK, Santosham M, Almeido-Hill J, et al. Vaccination with *Haemophilus influenzae* type b meningococcal protein conjugate vaccine reduces oropharyngeal carriage of *Haemophilus influenzae* type b among American Indian children. *Pediatr Infect Dis J* 1993;12:593–599.

131. Murphy TV, Pastor P, Medley F, et al. Decreased *Haemophilus* colonization in children vaccinated with *Haemophilus influenzae* type b conjugate vaccine. *J Pediatr* 1993;122:517–523.

132. Mohle-Boetani JC, Ajello G, Breneman E, et al. Carriage of *Haemophilus influenzae* type b in children after widespread vaccination with conjugate *Haemophilus influenzae* type b vaccines. *Pediatr Infect Dis J* 1993;12:589–593.

133. Barbour ML, Mayon-White RT, Coles C, et al. The impact of conjugate vaccine on carriage of *Haemophilus influenzae* type b. *J Infect Dis* 1995;171:93–98.

134. Singleton R, Bulkow LR, Levine OS, et al. Experience with the prevention of invasive *Haemophilus influenzae* type b disease by vaccination in Alaska: the impact of persistent oropharyngeal carriage. *J Pediatr* 2000;137:313–320.

135. Olowokure B, Hawker J, Blair I, et al. Decrease in effectiveness of routine surveillance of *Haemophilus influenzae* disease after introduction of conjugate vaccine: comparison of routine reporting with active surveillance system. *BMJ* 2000;321:731–732.

136. Heath PT, Booy R, Azzopardi HJ, et al. Non–type b *Haemophilus influenzae* disease: clinical and epidemiologic characteristics in the *Haemophilus influenzae* type b vaccine era. *Pediatr Infect Dis J* 2001;20:300–305.

137. Albritton WL, Setlow JK, Thomas M, et al. Heterospecific transformation in the genus *Haemophilus*. *Mol Gen Genet* 1984;193:358–363.

138. Leidy G, Jaffee I, Alexander HE. Further evidence of a high degree of genetic homology between *H. influenzae* and *H. aegyptius*. *Proc Soc Exp Biol Med* 1965;118:671–679.

139. Brazilian Purpuric Fever Study Group. Brazilian purpuric fever: epidemic purpura fulminans associated with antecedent purulent conjunctivitis. *Lancet* 1987;2:757–761.

140. Brazilian Purpuric Fever Study Group. *Haemophilus aegyptius* bacteremia in Brazilian purpuric fever. *Lancet* 1987;2:761–763.

141. McIntyre P, Wheaton G, Erlich J, et al. Brasilian purpuric fever in central Australia. *Lancet* 1987;2:112.

142. Wild BE, Pearman JW, Campbell PB, et al. Brazilian purpuric fever in Western Australia [Letter]. *Med J Aust* 1989;150:344, 346.

143. Brenner DJ, Mayer LW, Carlone GM, et al. Biochemical, genetic, and epidemiologic characterization of *Haemophilus influenzae* biogroup aegyptius (*Haemophilus aegyptius*) strains associated with Brazilian purpuric fever. *J Clin Microbiol* 1988;26:1524–1534.

144. Lesse AJ, Gheesling LL, Bittner WE, et al. Stable, conserved outer membrane epitope of strains of *Haemophilus influenzae* biogroup aegyptius associated with Brazilian Purpuric Fever. *Infect Immun* 1992;60:1351–1357.

145. Carlone GM, Gorelkin L, Gheesling LL, et al. Potential virulence factors of *Haemophilus influenzae* biogroup aegyptius in Brazilian purpuric fever. *Pediatr Infect Dis J* 1989;8:245–247.

146. Mayer LW, Bibb WF, Birkness KA, et al. Distinguishing clonal characteristics of the Brazilian purpuric fever–producing strain. *Pediatr Infect Dis J* 1989;8:241–243.

147. Tondella MLC, Quinn FD, Perkins BA. Brazilian purpuric fever caused by *Haemophilus influenzae* biogroup *aegyptius* strains lacking the 3031 plasmid. *J Infect Dis* 1995;171:209–212.

148. Porto MH, Noel GJ, Edelson PJ, for the Brazilian Purpuric Fever Study Group. Resistance to serum bactericidal activity distinguishes Brazilian purpuric fever (BPF) case strains of *Haemophilus influenzae* biogroup *aegyptius* (*H. aegyptius*) from non-BPF strains. *J Clin Microbiol* 1989;27:792–794.

149. Dobson SRM, Kroll JS, Moxon ER. Insertion sequence IS1016 and absence of *Haemophilus* capsulation genes in the Brazilian purpuric fever clone of *Haemophilus influenzae* biogroup aegyptius. *Infect Immun* 1992;60:618–622.

150. Rubin LG, Gloster ES, Carlone GM, for the Brazilian Purpuric Fever Study Group. An infant rat model of bacteremia with Brazilian purpuric fever isolates of *Haemophilus influenzae* biogroup *aegyptius*. *J Infect Dis* 1989;160:476–482.

151. Rubin LG, Carlone GM, for the Brazilian Purpuric Fever Study Group. An infant rat model of bacteremia with Brazilian purpuric fever isolates of *Haemophilus influenzae* biogroup *aegyptius* (*Haemophilus aegyptius*). *Pediatr Infect Dis J* 1989;8:247–248.

152. Weyant RS, Quinn FD, Utt EA, et al. Human microvascular endothelial cell toxicity caused by Brazilian purpuric fever–associated strains of *Haemophilus influenzae* biogroup aegyptius. *J Infect Dis* 1994;169:430–433.

153. Whitney AM, Farley MM. Cloning and sequence analysis of the structural pilin gene of Brazilian purpuric fever–associated *Haemophilus influenzae* biogroup *aegyptius*. *Infect Immun* 1993;61:1559–1562.

154. St. Geme JW III, Falkow S. Isolation, expression, and nucleotide sequencing of the pilin structural gene of the Brazilian purpuric fever clone of *Haemophilus influenzae* biogroup *aegyptius*. *Infect Immun* 1993;61:2233–2237.

155. Rubin LG. Phase-variable expression of the 145-kDa surface protein of Brazilian purpuric fever case-clone strains of *Haemophilus influenzae* biogroup *aegyptius*. *J Infect Dis* 1995;171:713–717.

156. Rubin LG, St. Geme JW III. Role of lipooligosaccharide in virulence of the Brazilian purpuric fever clone of *Haemophilus influenzae* biogroup *aegyptius* in infant rats. *Infect Immun* 1993;61:650–655.

157. Mertz KJ, Trees D, Levine WC, et al. Etiology of genital ulcers and prevalence of human immunodeficiency virus coinfection in 10 US cities. *J Infect Dis* 1998;178:1795–1798.

158. Kreiss JK, Koech D, Plummer FA, et al. AIDS virus infection in Nairobi prostitutes. Spread of the epidemic to East Africa. *N Engl J Med* 1986;314:414–418.

159. Quinn TC, Mann JM, Curran JW, et al. AIDS in Africa: an epidemiologic paradigm. *Science* 1986;234:955–963.

160. Mertz KH, Weiss JB, Webb RM, et al. An investigation of genital ulcers in Jackson, Mississippi, with use of a multiplex polymerase chain reaction assay: high prevalence of chancroid and human immunodeficiency virus infection. *J Infect Dis* 1998;178:1060–1066.

161. Casin I, Grimont F, Grimont PAD, et al. Lack of deoxyribonucleic acid relatedness between *Haemophilus ducreyi* and other *Haemophilus* species. *Int J Syst Bacteriol* 1985;35:23–25.

162. Morse SA. Chancroid and *Haemophilus ducreyi*. *Clin Microbiol Rev* 1989;2:137–157.

163. Odumeru JA, Ronald AR, Albritton WL. Characterization of cell proteins of *Haemophilus ducreyi* by polyacrylamide gel electrophoresis. *J Infect Dis* 1983;148:710–714.

164. Slootmans L, Vanden Berghe DA, Piot P. Typing *Haemophilus ducreyi* by indirect immunofluorescence assay. *Genitourin Med* 1985;61:123–126.

165. Van Dyck E, Piot P. Enzyme profile of *Haemophilus ducreyi* strains isolated on different continents. *Eur J Clin Microbiol* 1987;6:40–43.

166. Flood JM, Sarafian SK, Bolan GA, et al. Multistrain outbreak of chancroid in San Francisco, 1989–91. *J Infect Dis* 1993;167:1106–1111.

167. Dienst RB. Virulence and antigenicity of *Haemophilus ducreyi*. *Am J Syph Gonorrhea Vener Dis* 1948;32:289–291.

168. Feiner RR, Mortara F. Infectivity of *Haemophilus ducreyi* for the rabbit and the development of skin hypersensitivity. *Am J Syph Gonorrhea Vener Dis* 1945;29:71–79.

169. Lagergard T. *Haemophilus ducreyi*: pathogenesis and protective immunity. *Trends Microbiol* 1995;3:87–92.

170. Purcell BK, Richardson JA, Radolf JD, et al. A temperature-dependent rabbit model for production of dermal lesions by *Haemophilus ducreyi*. *J Infect Dis* 1991;164:359–367.

171. Hansen EJ, Lumbley SR, Richardson JA, et al. Induction of protective immunity to *Haemophilus ducreyi* in the temperature-dependent rabbit model of experimental chancroid. *J Immunol* 1994;152:184–192.

172. Totten PA, Morton WR, Knitter GH, et al. A primate model for chancroid. *J Infect Dis* 1994;169:1284–1290.

173. Spinola SM, Wild LM, Apicella MA, et al. Experimental human infection with *Haemophilus ducreyi*. *J Infect Dis* 1994;169:1146–1150.

174. Gelfanova V, Humphreys TL, Spinola SM. Characterization of *Haemophilus ducreyi*-specific T-cell lines from lesions of experimentally infected human subjects. *Infect Immun* 2001;69:4224–4231.

175. Bauer ME, Goheen MP, Townsent CA, et al. *Haemophilus ducreyi* associates with phagocytes, collagen, and fibrin and remains extracellular throughout infection of human volunteers. *Infect Immun* 2001;69:2549–2557.

176. Alfa MJ. Cytopathic effect of *Haemophilus ducreyi* for human foreskin cell culture. *J Med Microbiol* 1992;37:43–50.

177. Lammel CJ, Dekker NP, Palefsky J, et al. *In vitro* model of *Haemophilus ducreyi* adherence to and entry into eukaryotic cells of genital origin. *J Infect Dis* 1993;167:642–650.

178. Brentjens RJ, Spinola SM, Campagnari AA. *Haemophilus ducreyi* adheres to human keratinocytes. *Microb Pathogen* 1994;16:243–247.

179. Schmid GP, Sanders LL Jr, Blount JH, et al. Chancroid in the United States. Reestablishment of an old disease. *JAMA* 1987;258:3265–3268.

180. Elkins C, Yi K, Olsen B, et al. Development of a serological test for *Haemophilus ducreyi* for seroprevalence studies. *J Clin Microbiol* 2000;38:1520–1526.

181. Totten PA, Kuypers JM, Chen C-Y, et al. Etiology of genital ulcer disease in Dakar, Senegal, and comparison of PCR and serologic assays for detection of *Haemophilus ducreyi*. *J Clin Microbiol* 2000;38:268–273.

182. Pillay A, Hoosen AA, Loykissoonlal D, et al. Comparison of culture media for the laboratory diagnosis of chancroid. *J Med Microbiol* 1998;47:1023–1026.

183. Aldridge KE, Cammarata C, Martin DH. Comparison of the in vitro activities of various parenteral and oral antimicrobial agents against endemic *Haemophilus ducreyi*. *Antimicrob Agents Chemother* 1993;37:1986–1988.

184. Schmid GP. Treatment of chancroid, 1997. *Clin Infect Dis* 1999;28(S1):S14–S20.

185. Albritton WL. Species identification in *Haemophilus* infection. *Rev Infect Dis* 1988;6:1226.

186. Lynn DJ, Kane JG, Parker RH. *Haemophilus parainfluenzae* and *influenzae* endocarditis: a review of forty cases. *Medicine* 1977;56:115–128.

187. Bieger RC, Brewer NS, Washington JAI. *Haemophilus aphrophilus*: a microbiologic and clinical review and report of 42 cases. *Medicine* 1978;57:345–355.

188. Elster SK, Mattes LM, Meyers BR, et al. *Haemophilus aphrophilus* endocarditis: review of 23 cases. *Am J Cardiol* 1975;35:72–79.

189. Bangsborg JM, Tvede M, Skinhoj P. *Haemophilus segnis* endocarditis. *J Infect* 1988;16:81–85.

190. Raucher B, Dobkin J, Mandel L, et al. Occult polymicrobial endocarditis with *Haemophilus parainfluenzae* in intravenous drug abusers. *Am J Med* 1989;86:169–172.

191. Darras-Joly C, Lortholary O, Mainardi J-L, et al. *Haemophilus* endocarditis: report of 42 cases in adults and review. *Clin Infect Dis* 1997;24:1087–1094.

192. Coll-Vinent B, Suris X, Lopez-Soto A, et al. *Haemophilus paraphrophilus* endocarditis: case report and review. *Clin Infect Dis* 1995;20:1381–1383.

193. Berbara EF, Cockerill FR III, Steckelberg JM. Infective endocarditis due to unusual or fastidious microorganisms. *Mayo Clin Proc* 1997;72:532–542.

194. Patel A, Asirvatham S, Sebastian C, et al. Polymicrobial endocarditis with *Haemophilus parainfluenzae* in an intravenous drug user whose transesophageal echocardiogram appeared normal. *Clin Infect Dis* 1998;26:1245–1246.

195. Brunton J, Clare D, Meier MA. Molecular epidemiology of antibiotic resistance plasmids of *Haemophilus* species and *Neisseria gonorrhoeae*. *Rev Infect Dis* 1986;8:713–724.

196. Murphy TF, Apicella MA. Antigenic heterogeneity of outer membrane proteins of nontypable *Haemophilus influenzae* is a basis for a serotyping system. *Infect Immun* 1985;50:15–21.

197. Kilian M. A rapid method for the differentiation of *Haemophilus* strains: the porphyrin test. *Acta Pathol Microbiol Scand B* 1974;82:835–842.

198. Oberhofer TR, Back AE. Biotypes of *Haemophilus* encountered in clinical laboratories. *J Clin Microbiol* 1979;10:168–174.

199. Porras O, Caugant DA, Lagergard T, et al. Application of multilocus enzyme gel electrophoresis to *Haemophilus influenzae*. *Infect Immun* 1986;53:71–78.

200. Saito M, Umeda A, Yoshida S-I. Subtyping of *Haemophilus influenzae* strains by pulsed-field gel electrophoresis. *J Clin Microbiol* 1999;2142:2147.

201. Yano H, Suetake M, Kuga A, et al. Pulsed-field gel electrophoresis analysis of nasopharyngeal flora in children attending a day care center. *J Clin Microbiol* 1999;38:625–629.

202. Groeneveld K, van Alphen L, Eijk PP, et al. Changes in outer membrane proteins of nontypable *Haemophilus influenzae* in patients with chronic obstructive pulmonary disease. *J Infect Dis* 1988;158:360–365.

203. Loos BG, Bernstein JM, Dryja DM, et al. Determination of the epidemiology and transmission of nontypeable *Haemophilus influenzae* in children with otitis media by comparison of total genomic DNA restriction fingerprints. *Infect Immun* 1989;57:2751–2757.

204. Bruce KD, Jordens JZ. Characterization of noncapsulate *Haemophilus influenzae* by whole-cell polypeptide profiles, restriction endonuclease analysis, and rRNA gene restriction patterns. *J Clin Microbiol* 1991;29:291–296.

205. Jordens JZ, Leaves NI, Anderson EC, et al. Polymerase chain reaction–based strain characterization of noncapsulate *Haemophilus influenzae*. *J Clin Microbiol* 1993;31:2981–2987.

206. Van Belkum A, Duim B, Regelink A, et al. Genomic DNA fingerprinting of clinical *Haemophilus influenzae* isolates by polymerase chain reaction amplification: comparison with major outer-membrane protein and restriction fragment length polymorphism. *J Med Microbiol* 1994;41:63–68.

207. Smith-Vaughan HC, Sriprakash KS, Mathews JD, et al. Long PCR-ribotyping of nontypeable *Haemophilus influenzae*. *J Clin Microbiol* 1995;33:1192–1195.

208. Smith-Vaughan HC, Leach AJ, Shelby-James TM, et al. Carriage of multiple ribotypes of non-encapsulated *Haemophilus influenzae* in Aboriginal infants with otitis media. *Epidemiol Infect* 1996;116:177–183.

209. Oill PA, Chow AW, Guze LB. Adult bacteremic *Haemophilus parainfluenzae* infections. *Arch Intern Med* 1979;139:985–988.

210. Jemsek JG, Greenberg SB, Gentry LO, et al. *Haemophilus parainfluenzae* endocarditis. Two cases and review of the literature in the past decade. *Am J Med* 1979;66:51–57.

211. Blair DC, Weiner LB. Prosthetic valve endocarditis due to *Haemophilus parainfluenzae* biotype II. *Am J Dis Child* 1979;133:617–618.

212. Hable KA, Logan GB, Washington JAI. Three *Haemophilus* species. *Am J Dis Child* 1971;121:35–37.

213. Parker SW, Apicella MA, Fuller CM. *Haemophilus* endocarditis. Two patients with complications. *Arch Intern Med* 1983;143:48–51.

214. Geraci JE, Wilkowske CJ, Wilson WR, et al. *Haemophilus* endocarditis. Report of 14 patients. *Mayo Clin Proc* 1977;52:209–215.

215. Geraci JE, Wilson WR. Endocarditis due to gram-negative bacteria. Report of 56 cases. *Mayo Clin Proc* 1982;57:145–148.

216. Sutter VL, Finegold SM. *Haemophilus aphrophilus* infections: clinical and bacteriologic studies. *Ann N Y Acad Sci* 1970;174:468–487.

217. Julander I, Lindberg AA, Svanbon M. *Haemophilus parainfluenzae*—an uncommon cause of septicemia and endocarditis. *Scand J Infect Dis* 1980;12:85–89.

218. Coll-Vinent B, Suris X, Lopez-Soto A, et al. *Haemophilus paraphrophilus* endocarditis: case report and review. *Clin Infect Dis* 1995;20:1381–1383.

219. Hamed KA, Dormitzer PR, Su CK, et al. *Haemophilus parainfluenzae* endocarditis: application of a molecular approach for identification of pathogenic bacterial species. *Clin Infect Dis* 1994;19:677–683.

220. Hricak V, Kovacik J, Marx P, et al. Etiology and risk factors of 180 cases of native valve endocarditis. Report from a 5-year national prospective survey in Slovak Republic. *Diagn Microbiol Infect Dis* 1998;31:431–435.

221. Cooney TG, Harwood BR, Meisner DJ. *Haemophilus parainfluenzae* thoracic empyema. *Arch Intern Med* 1981;141:940–941.

222. Kiddy K, Webberley J. *Haemophilus aphrophilus* as a cause of chronic suppurative pulmonary infection and intra-abdominal abscesses. *J Infect* 1987;15:161–163.

223. Jones RN, Slepack J, Bigelow J. Ampicillin-resistant *Haemophilus paraphrophilus* laryngo-epiglottitis. *J Clin Microbiol* 1976;4:405–407.

224. Dudley JP. Supraglottitis and *Haemophilus parainfluenzae*: pathogenic potential of the organism. *Ann Otol Rhinol Laryngol* 1987;96:400–402.

225. Bachman DS. *Haemophilus* meningitis: comparison of *H. influenzae* and *H. parainfluenzae*. *Pediatrics* 1975;55:526–530.

226. Welch WD, Southern PM Jr, Schneider NR. Five cases of *Haemophilus segnis* appendicitis. *J Clin Microbiol* 1986;24:851–852.

227. Gallant TE, Malinak LR, Gump DW, et al. *Haemophilus parainfluenzae* peritonitis associated with an intrauterine contraceptive device. *Am J Obstet Gynecol* 1977;129:702–703.

228. Warman ST, Reinitz E, Klein RS. *Haemophilus parainfluenzae* septic arthritis in an adult. *JAMA* 1981;246:868–869.

229. von Essen R, Kostiala AA, Anttolainen I, et al. Arthritis caused by *Haemophilus paraphrophilus* and isolation of the organism by using an improved culture protocol. *J Clin Microbiol* 1987;25:2447–2448.

230. Merino D, Saavedra J, Pujol E, et al. *Haemophilus aphrophilus* as a rare cause of arthritis. *Clin Infect Dis* 1994;19:320–322.

231. Hung CC, Hsueh PR, Chen YC, et al. *Haemophilus aphrophilus* bacteremia complicated with vertebral osteomyelitis and spinal epidural abscess in a patient with liver cirrhosis. *J Infect* 1997;35:304–308.

232. Milne LM, Isaacs D, Crook PJ. Neonatal infections with *Haemophilus* species. *Arch Dis Child* 1988;63:83–85.

233. Crawford SA, Evans JA, Crawford GE. Necrotizing fasciitis associated with *Haemophilus aphrophilus*. *Arch Intern Med* 1978;138:1714–1715.

234. Blaylock BL, Baber S. Urinary tract infection caused by *Haemophilus parainfluenzae*. *Am J Clin Pathol* 1980;73:285–287.

235. Carson HJ, Rezmer S, Belli J. *Haemophilus segnis* cholecystitis: a case report and literature review. *J Infect* 1997;35:85–86.

236. Black CT, Kupferschmid JP, West KW, et al. *Haemophilus parainfluenzae* infections in children, with the report of a unique case. *Rev Infect Dis* 1988;10:342–346.

237. Bottone EJ, Zhang DY. *Haemophilus parainfluenzae* biliary tract infection: rationale for an ascending route of infection from the gastrointestinal tract. *J Clin Microbiol* 1995;33:3042–3043.

238. Alvarez M, Potel C, Rey L, et al. Biliary tract infection caused by *Haemophilus influenzae*. *Scand J Infect Dis* 1999;31:212–213.

CHAPTER 204
Streptobacillus moniliformis

Gary Doern

MICROBIOLOGY

Streptobacillus moniliformis, one of the causative agents of rat-bite fever, is a facultatively anaerobic, pleomorphic, nonmotile, gram-negative bacillus. Its general dimensions are approximately 0.3 by 3.0 μm; however, one of the principal distinguishing attributes of this organism is its morphologic variability. Depending on age, condition of culture, and composition of growth media, single bacillary forms, many with central round enlargements, may be observed or chains of bacilli may be seen. The filamentous forms, when found to possess the central swellings, resemble a string of beads. In addition, stable cell wall–defective L-phase variants often arise both *in vivo* and *in vitro*.

S. *moniliformis* may be visualized with Gram, Wayson, Giemsa, or acridine orange stain; Gram stain yields the least consistent results. The organism is readily propagated on or within standard microbiologic agar and broth media, assuming the media are supplemented with blood, serum, or ascites fluid from practically any animal source (1,2). Indeed, the patient's blood will act as a satisfactory supplement, which perhaps explains the relatively frequent isolation of *S. moniliformis* from broth-based blood cultures. One concern with respect to detecting *S. moniliformis* bacteremia is the relative sensitivity of this organism to sodium polyanetholesulfonate (Liquoid). Sodium polyanetholesulfonate is an anticoagulant that is added to most broth-based blood culture bottles at a concentration of 0.025%, a concentration inhibitory to many strains of *S. moniliformis* (3). Therefore, sodium polyanetholesulfonate should probably be eliminated from broth blood culture media or neutralized by the addition of 1.5% sterile gelatin when an effort is made to document *S. moniliformis* bacteremia. Finally, supplementation of blood culture broth with papain digest of ox liver (Panmede) has been shown to yield early growth of small inocula of *S. moniliformis* (4).

Cultures should be incubated at 35°C to 37°C in an atmosphere of 5% to 8% carbon dioxide. In broth, *S. moniliformis* forms characteristic puffball aggregates. On solid media, 1- to 2-mm grayish, round, glistening colonies appear after 2 to 6 days of incubation. L-phase variants pit the agar and resemble a fried egg. Positive biochemical reactions useful in the identification of *S. moniliformis* include starch and esculin hydrolysis; production of oxidase, catalase, and alkaline phosphatase; reduction of 2,3,5-triphenyltetrazolium chloride, potassium tellurite, and nitrate; and use of glucose, maltose, fructose, galactose, mannose, dextrin, and glycogen. Gas is not produced from carbohydrate fermentation (5,6). Last, gas-liquid chromatography has been used to achieve rapid identification of *S. moniliformis*. The characteristic fatty acid profile of this organism includes palmitic, linoleic, oleic, and stearic acids (7).

EPIDEMIOLOGY AND PATHOGENESIS

The primary reservoir of *S. moniliformis* is the respiratory tract of rodents. More than 50% of wild and laboratory rats harbor this organism in the nasopharynx or oral cavity (8). The organism has also been isolated from various respiratory tract sources from wild and laboratory mice (9), turkeys, and guinea pigs (10,11). Furthermore, rat-bite fever is reported to have occurred after close contact with cats, dogs, pigs, and squirrels (3,12).

Human infections usually arise after one of two distinct modes of transmission: traumatic implantation of the organism through the skin or ingestion of contaminated food with subsequent penetration of the organism through the mucosal epithelium of the gastrointestinal (GI) tract. In the first case, the most common trauma is the bite of a rat or another rodent. However, handling a colonized animal without incurring a bite also can lead to infection. In the second case, the most common vehicle has been raw milk, presumably contaminated by rodents harboring *S. moniliformis* (13–15). Water has also been incriminated (16). *S. moniliformis* infection that occurs as a consequence of ingesting contaminated food or water has been termed *Haverhill fever*; it typically arises in the setting of a common-source outbreak.

After the organism penetrates the skin or the GI tract mucosa, it presumably multiplies locally and then is disseminated throughout the host by the bloodstream. Hematogenous seeding of any organ may result; however, joints are most often involved.

Infection caused by *S. moniliformis* is relatively uncommon. Thirteen cases were reported between 1958 and 1983 in the United States (17). Approximately half of cases occur in laboratory workers who have extensive contact with laboratory rats and mice (18). Most cases among persons who do not work in laboratories occur in children, presumably because they suffer more rodent bites (12).

CLINICAL MANIFESTATIONS

Infection caused by *S. moniliformis* characteristically manifests with fever, rash, and constitutional symptoms (19). Patients usually experience abrupt onset of fever and shaking chills. The incubation period is extremely variable (1 day to 3 weeks, mean of 10 days). Constitutional symptoms (headache, malaise, myalgias) are prominent. A characteristic rash occurs in 90% of cases within 1 week of the onset of symptoms, usually an erythematous macular eruption that is widely distributed but most prominent on the soles and palms (20). Skin lesions may be discrete or confluent, petechial or purpuric. In cases in which infection arises after a rodent bite, the bite wound is often initially conspicuous; however, it heals rapidly and is inapparent by the time the rash appears. Half of all patients suffer arthralgias (12,20). Knees, wrists, and elbows are most often affected. Joint involvement may be monarticular or polyarticular and may progress to frank arthritis with purulent effusion. Abscess formation in the female genital tract and endocarditis in human immunodeficiency virus (HIV)–infected individuals have also been described (21,22). Excepting these two conditions, the symptoms of *S. moniliformis* infection, without treatment, usually abate within 2 weeks; however, episodic relapses have been described at intervals of weeks to months.

Rat-bite fever can also be due to infection with another commensal organism of the respiratory tract of rodents, *Spirillum minus*. *S. minus* infection, also referred to as *sodoku*, differs clinically from that caused by *S. moniliformis* insofar as the disease usually has a more insidious onset, there is rarely any evidence of the bite entry wound, and joints are not involved. Only a single case of *S. minus* infection has been reported in the United States in the past 31 years. Most infections due to this bacterium occur in Asia (10).

TREATMENT

When a patient is seen soon after a rodent bite, the lesion should be cleaned thoroughly and tetanus immunization administered. There is no proven benefit of antimicrobial prophylaxis for rat-bite fever.

Recommended therapy of uncomplicated rat-bite fever and Haverhill fever for penicillin-tolerant patients consists of intravenous procaine penicillin G, 600,000 U every 12 hours (12). Therapy should be continued for 10 to 14 days. It is possible to switch to oral therapy (penicillin, 2 g per day) after 1 week of parenteral therapy if a favorable clinical response is achieved. Systemic focal infections such as endocarditis require larger doses of antimicrobial agent administered for a longer period (23). For penicillin-allergic patients, tetracycline, 500 mg orally every 6 hours, is the therapy of choice (11).

PREVENTION

The only measure effective in preventing rat-bite fever and Haverhill fever in the general public is the elimination of rodent reservoirs (i.e., rats and mice) from environments in which humans live, work, and play. Disease among laboratory workers can be prevented by exercising care in handling laboratory animals, especially mice, rats, and guinea pigs, so the risk for bites and scratches is minimized.

REFERENCES

1. Faro S, Walker C, Pierson RL. Amnionitis with intact amniotic membranes involving. *Streptobacillus moniliformis. Obstet Gynecol* 1980;55:9S.
2. Portnoy BL, Satterwhite TK, Dyckman JD. Rat-bite fever misdiagnosed as Rocky Mountain spotted fever. *South Med J* 1979;72:607.
3. Lambe DW, McPhedran AM, Mertz JA, et al. *Streptobacillus moniliformis* from a case of Haverhill fever. *Am J Clin Pathol* 1973;60:854.
4. Shanson DC, Pratt J, Greene P. Comparison of media with and without Panmede for the isolation of *Streptobacillus moniliformis* from blood cultures and observations on the inhibitory effect of sodium polyanethol sulphonate. *J Med Microbiol* 1985;19:181.
5. Rogesa M. *Streptobacillus moniliformis* and *Spirillum minor.* In: Linnete EH, Balows A, Hausler WJ, et al, eds. *Manual of clinical microbiology,* 4th ed. Washington, DC: American Society for Microbiology, 1985:400–406.
6. Edwards R, Finch RG. Characterization and antibiotic susceptibility of *Streptobacillus moniliformis. J Med Microbiol* 1986;21:39.
7. Rowbotham TJ. Rapid identification of *Streptobacillus moniliformis. Lancet* 1983;2:567.
8. Strangeways WI. Rats as carriers of *Streptobacillus moniliformis. J Pathol Bacteriol* 1933;37:45.
9. Glastonbury JR, Morton JG, Matthews LM. *Streptobacillus moniliformis* infection in Swiss white mice. *J Vet Diagn Invest* 1996;8:202.
10. Josephson SL. Rat-bite fever. In: Balows A, Hausler WJ, Lennette EH, eds. *Laboratory diagnosis of infectious disease: principles and practices,* vol 1. New York: Springer-Verlag, 1988:443–447.
11. Murray HW. *Streptobacillus moniliformis* (rat-bite fever). In: Mandell GL, Douglas RG, Bennett JE, eds. *Principles and practice of infectious diseases,* 2nd ed. New York: John Wiley & Sons, 1985:1305–1306.
12. Roughgarden JW. Antimicrobial therapy of rat-bite fever. *Arch Intern Med* 1965;116:39.
13. Parker F, Hudson NP. The etiology of Haverhill fever. *Am J Pathol* 1926;2:357.
14. Place EH, Sutton LE. Erythema arthriticum epidemicum (Haverhill fever). *Arch Intern Med* 1934;54:659.
15. Shanson DC, Midgley J, Gazzard BG, et al. *Streptobacillus moniliformis* isolated from blood in four cases of Haverhill fever. *Lancet* 1983;1:92.
16. McEvoy MB, Noak ND, Pilsworth R. Outbreak of fever caused by *Streptobacillus moniliformis. Lancet* 1987;2:1361.
17. Hadfield TL. Bartonellosis, cat-scratch disease and rat-bite fever. In: Wentworth BB, ed. *Diagnostic procedures for bacterial infections,* 7th ed. Washington, DC: American Public Health Association, 1987:147–154.
18. Anderson LC, Leary SL, Manning PJ. Rat-bite fever in animal research laboratory personnel. *Lab Anim Sci* 1983;33:292.
19. Hagelskjaer L, Sorensen I, Randers E. *Streptobacillus moniliformis* infection: 2 cases and a literature review. *Scand J Infect Dis* 1998;30:309.
20. Raffin BJ, Freemark M. Streptobacillary rat-bite fever: a pediatric problem. *Pediatrics* 1979;64:214.
21. Rordorf T, Zuger C, Zbinden R, et al. *Streptobacillus moniliformis* endocarditis in an HIV-positive patient. *Infection* 2000;28:393.
22. Pin MR, Holden JM, Yang JM, et al. Isolation of presumptive *Streptobacillus moniliformis* from abscesses associated with the female genital tract. *Clin Infect Dis* 1996;22:471.
23. McCormack RC, Kaye D, Hook EW. Endocarditis due to *Streptobacillus moniliformis. JAMA* 1967;200:77.

CHAPTER 205
Legionella

Sue M. Mietzner and Janet E. Stout

In the United States, approximately 600,000 adults are diagnosed each year with community-acquired pneumonia that is severe enough to require hospitalization (1). Approximately 2% to 5% of these cases are caused by a bacterium that was unrecognized before 1977 (2,3). The dramatic outbreak of pneumonia at an American Legion Convention in Philadelphia, Pennsylvania, in 1976 resulted in the isolation of a new disease-causing agent. The newly discovered bacterium was isolated by investigators at the Centers for Disease Control and Prevention in Atlanta, Georgia, and assigned to the family Legionellaceae, the genus *Legionella,* and the species *pneumophila.* Now more than 60 serogroups are among the more than 40 *Legionella* species (4), however, most cases of legionellosis are caused by *Legionella pneumophila,* serogroups 1, 3, 4, and 6 (3,5). The other *Legionella* species most commonly associated with illness are *Legionella micdadei, Legionella longbeachae, Legionella dumoffii,* and *Legionella bozemanii* (6,7). Among the more than 40 named species, at least 20 have been implicated in human disease (Table 205.1); the remaining species have been isolated from environmental water sources (4,8,9).

CLASSIFICATION

Early classification of the family Legionellaceae included *L. pneumophila* as the only genus and species (10). Subsequent recognition of other *Legionella*-like bacteria and analysis of deoxyribonucleic acid (DNA) relatedness led to a proposed separation of the family into three genera: *Legionella, Tatlockia,* and *Fluoribacter* (11). Further analysis by DNA–DNA hybridization, guanine-plus-cytosine content, and 16S ribosomal ribonucleic acid (rRNA)–encoding sequencing supports the delineation of the phylogeny within the Legionellaceae as one monophyletic family belonging to the gamma subdivision of the Proteobacteria (4,12–14). Some of the species within this family have been isolated from co-cultivation with amebae. These bacteria have been designated *Legionella*-like amebal pathogens (LLAPs) (15,16). One such organism, *Sarcobium lyticum,* was transferred to the genus *Legionella* as *Legionella lytica* comb. nova (13).

Physiologically defined as obligate aerobic slow-growing nonfermenters, Legionellaceae are distinguished from other saccharolytic bacteria by their requirement for L-cysteine and iron salts for primary isolation, as well as by their unique cellular fatty acids and ubiquinones. Gas-liquid chromatography demonstrates unusually large amounts of cellular branched-chain fatty acids and respiratory ubiquinones with 10 or more isoprene units (17). Differences among the *Legionella* species have

TABLE 205.1. Biochemical and Phenotypic Differentiation of *Legionella* Species Implicated in Infections

Species	Browning on tyrosine-supplemented agar	Gelatinase production	Hippurate hydrolysis	Oxidase	β-Lactamase production	Autofluorescence (365-nm UV light)	Flagella
Legionella pneumophila	+	+	+	+/−	+	−	+
Legionella micdadei	−	−	−	+	−	−	+
Legionella bozemanii	+	+	−	+/−	+/−	+(BW)	+
Legionella dumoffii	+	+	−	−	+	+(BW)	+
Legionella longbeachae	+	+	−	+	+/−	−	+
Legionella jordanis	+	+	−	+	+	−	+
Legionella feeleii	+	−	+/−	−	+	−	+
Legionella gormanii	+	+	−	−	+	+(BW)	+
Legionella wadsworthii	−	+	−	−	+	+(YG)	+
Legionella hackeliae	+	+	−	+	+	−	+
Legionella maceachernii	+/−	+/−	−	+	+	−	+
Legionella oakridgensis	+	+	−	−	+(W)	−	−
Legionella birminghamensis	+/−	+	−	+/−	+	+(YG)	+
Legionella cherrii	+	+	−	−	+	+(BW)	+
Legionella sainthelensi	+	+	−	+	+	−	+
Legionella cincinnatiensis	+	+	−	−	+	−	+
Legionella tucsonensis	−	+	−	−	+	+(BW)	+
Legionella anisa	+	+	−	+	+	+(BW)	+
Legionella lansingensis	−	−	−	+	−	−	+
Legionella parisiensis	+	+	−	+	+	+(BW)	+

+, positive; −, negative; +/−, variable reaction; W, weak reaction; BW, blue-white autofluorescence; YG, yellow-green autofluorescence.
Source: references 13, 43, and 165. Reprinted with permission from the American Society for Microbiology, ASM Press.

been assessed by phenotypic and chemotaxonomic tests. Phenotypic tests include composition of lipopolysaccharide (LPS) (18,19), electrophoretic protein profiles (20), monoclonal antibodies (21), fatty acid composition (22), and cellular carbohydrates (23). Genotypic tests include randomly amplified polymorphic DNA profiles (24,25), heteroduplex analysis of 5S rRNA gene sequences (26), and computer-assisted matching of tDNA-intergenic length polymorphism patterns (27).

LABORATORY DIAGNOSIS AND IDENTIFICATION

Legionella species are small (0.3 to 0.9 μm in width and approximately 2 μm in length), faintly staining gram-negative rods with polar flagella (except *Legionella oakridgensis*) (28). They generally appear as small coccobacilli in infected tissue or secretions, whereas long filamentous forms (up to 20 μm in length) can be seen when they are grown in culture media.

Morphologically, *Legionella* organisms are similar to other oropharyngeal flora; therefore, Gram stain is of little diagnostic use with respiratory tract specimens. Suggested alternative staining methods include carbol fuchsin (without heating and acid–alcohol decolorizing) and crystal violet with or without Lugol's iodine (the half–Gram stain) (29). Silver impregnation stains, including the Dieterle stain and Warthin-Starry stain, allow visualization in paraffin-fixed tissue sections. *Legionella micdadei* can stain weakly acid fast in tissue with the Kinyoun and Fite stains, and in smears with the modified Ziehl-Neelsen stain from tissue or sputum specimens (30). Interestingly, the acid fastness is rarely seen in *L. micdadei* grown from culture.

Direct fluorescent antibody (DFA) stain is most commonly used to visualize *Legionella* in respiratory tract specimens. However, with 25% to 75% sensitivity, DFA should not be performed as the only diagnostic test (31). If the direct culture of the specimen is overgrown by competing microflora, the specimen undergoes acid pretreatment and DFA staining can be performed in lieu of pending culture results. In our experience, the mono-

clonal antibody DFA reagent (MONOFLUO, Bio-Rad Laboratories, Redmond, Washington) is superior to polyclonal reagents because background fluorescence is reduced and cross-reactivity with non-*Legionella* bacteria has not occurred.

Culture remains the definitive method for diagnosis. *Legionella* are primary pathogens of the lower respiratory tract and can be isolated from expectorated sputum, tracheal aspirate, bronchoscopy specimens, pleural fluid, and lung tissue. Although not routinely tested, *Legionella* has been detected in the following specimens/sites: blood, pleural, pericardial, and peritoneal fluids, prosthetic valves, and sternal wounds (32,33). A single colony isolated in culture will confirm the diagnosis of Legionnaires' disease.

Buffered charcoal yeast extract (BCYE) agar, buffered with ACES [N-(2-acetamido)-2-aminoethane sulfonic acid] and supplemented with α-ketoglutarate, L-cysteine, and ferric pyrophosphate (pH = 6.9) is the primary medium for isolation of *Legionella* by culture. Both α-ketoglutarate and charcoal stimulate *Legionella* growth by decreasing production of toxic peroxides: α-ketoglutarate indirectly by inhibiting cysteine oxidation (34) and charcoal directly by promoting decomposition of peroxides (35). Yeast extract, L-cysteine, and ferric pyrophosphate supply vitamins, minerals, and other specific nutrients essential for growth, whereas the ACES buffer maintains a critical pH level of 6.85 to 6.95. Addition of albumin, which blocks the toxic effects of starch products, also increases the yield of *L. micdadei*, *L. bozemanii*, and *Legionella anisa* in culture (36). Optimal recovery of legionellae from respiratory tract specimens requires the use of dye and antibiotic containing selective media with acid (pH = 2.2 HCL–KCL buffer) or heat pretreatment of the specimen to minimize overgrowth of competing microorganisms (37). For maximal sensitivity, three media are generally used: BCYE; BCYE with polymyxin, anisomycin, and cefamandole (PAC); BCYE with polymyxin, anisomycin, vancomycin (PAV) and dyes. *Legionella* characteristically demonstrates a speckled green, blue, or pinkish-purple iridescence on BCYE and BCYE-selective media (Fig. 205.1). This iridescence can be seen easily through the

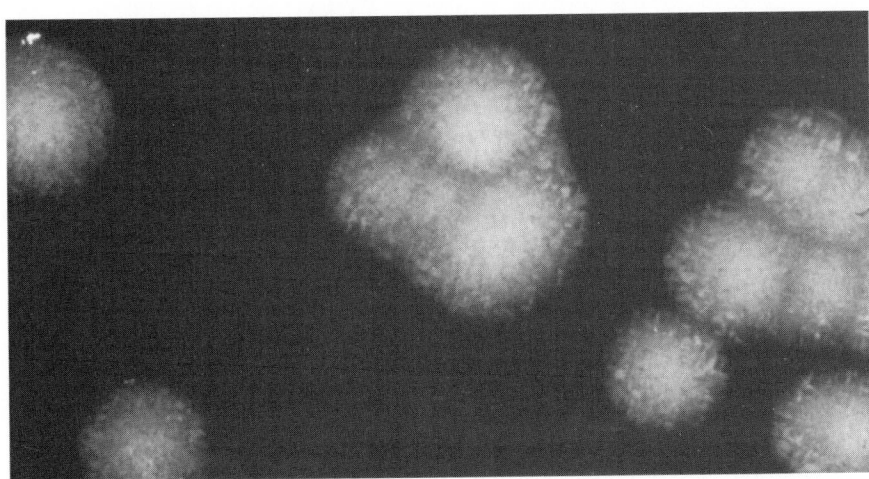

Figure 205.1. Colonies of *Legionella pneumophila* with characteristic ground glass surface texture (magnification approximately ×10).

dissecting stereomicroscope if a light source is directed toward the plates at a slight angle. Colonies mature in 3 or 4 days and are 3 to 4 mm in diameter, entire, and convex and have a frosted-glass internal appearance. When exposed to long-wave ultraviolet light (365 nm), certain species of *Legionella* (*L. bozemanii, L. dumoffii, Legionella cherrii, Legionella gormanii, Legionella tucsonensis, L. anisa, Legionella parisiensis*) demonstrate a blue-white autofluorescence. Other species, *Legionella rubrilucens* and *Legionella erythra,* demonstrate a red autofluorescence; and *Legionella wadsworthii* and *Legionella birminghamensis,* a yellow-green autofluorescence (Table 205.1). Colonies demonstrating characteristic morphology are tested to determine whether L-cysteine is essential for growth by subculturing the isolate in parallel to BCYE agar and 5% sheep blood agar. Those isolates found only to grow on BCYE, with typical colony morphology and staining characteristics, can be presumptively identified as *Legionella.*

The urinary antigen test for the detection of *L. pneumophila* serogroup 1 is a practical alternative to culture in diagnosing pneumonia caused by this species and serogroup. The antigen test has several advantages over culture. Obtaining an adequate sputum specimen from patients with Legionnaires' disease is difficult if not impossible; urine, on the other hand, is easily obtained. In addition, the results of urinary antigen testing can be available within hours, whereas culture results require 3 to 5 days. The disadvantage of the urinary antigen test is that it detects only *L. pneumophila* serogroup 1. Because the vast majority of cases of Legionnaires' disease are caused by this species and serogroup (5), this limitation has not been considered a major disadvantage of the test.

The primary format for the urinary antigen test has been an enzyme immunoassay (EIA), which is available commercially from two U.S. suppliers (Wampole Laboratories, a division of Carter-Wallace Inc., New Jersey; and Bartels, Issaquash, Washington). A new, rapid immunochromatographic (ICT) assay that yields results in less than 15 minutes is performed using a swab dipped in urine, which is inserted into a card-type test device (Binax NOW *Legionella* Urinary Antigen Test, Portland, Maine). The ICT format of the urinary antigen test seems to be less prone to false-positive reactions.

Other diagnostic tests include serologic testing by the indirect fluorescent antibody (IFA) stain or the enzyme-linked immunosorbent assay and the polymerase chain reaction (PCR). Serologic tests are most useful for epidemiologic studies but less helpful in making an immediate diagnosis of Legionnaires' disease for an individual patient. Diagnosis is based on a fourfold rise in antibody titer to more than 1:128; therefore, both acute-and convalescent-phase sera are required. Although PCR-based assays for the detection of *Legionella* in clinical samples have been shown to be highly specific, they have not been shown to be more sensitive than culture (38,39). It is for this reason that the Centers for Disease Control and Prevention does not recommend the routine use of PCR or genetic probes for the detection of *Legionella* in clinical samples (40). The primary advantage of PCR is the ability to detect *Legionella* rapidly and to detect species other than *L. pneumophila.*

The Legionellaceae share a number of phenotypic characteristics (Table 205.1); however, these characteristics are of limited value in species identification (13). With variable degrees of accuracy, the combinations of culture characteristics (requirement for cysteine), nonfermentative metabolism, and serotyping (either by slide agglutination or DFA staining) are more appropriately used in distinguishing the numerous *Legionella* species (41–43).

Testing to confirm the identification of *Legionella* includes fluorescent antibody (FA) staining (direct and indirect), crossed immunoelectrophoresis (44), slide agglutination (45), and immunodiffusion (46). FA reagents are available as monoclonal and polyclonal, monovalent and polyvalent reagents. One reagent is a polyclonal-polyvalent reagent capable of reacting with 22 species and 31 serogroups of *Legionella* (REMEL, Lenexa, Kansas). A latex agglutination test is now available that allows presumptive identification of *L. pneumophila* serogroup 1 or serogroups 2 to 14 and detection of seven other *Legionella* species (Oxoid Limited, Hampshire, England).

To link patient isolates of *L. pneumophila* to an environmental reservoir in epidemiologic investigations, phenotypic, and genotypic methods are used (47,48). These methods include serotyping (49), monoclonal antibody subtyping, isoenzyme analysis, protein and carbohydrate profiling, plasmid analysis, restriction endonuclease analysis, restriction fragment length polymorphism of rRNA (ribotyping) (48,50) or chromosomal DNA, amplified fragment length polymorphism (AFLP) (51), repetitive element PCR (53), restriction endonuclease analysis of whole-cell DNA with or without pulsed-field gel electrophoresis (PFGE) (52,54), arbitrarily primed PCR (48,52,55,56), and 16S–23S spacer analysis (48). It has been recommended that both a phenotypic method (monoclonal subtyping) and a genotypic method (e.g., PFGE) be used for optimal discrimination (57) because there may be limited genetic heterogeneity among subtypes of *L. pneumophila* (57–59).

Among the available techniques for molecular subtyping of *Legionella* isolates, PFGE, AFLP, or arbitrarily primed PCR are used for epidemiologic investigations (52,56,60,61).

ANTIGENIC PROPERTIES

L. pneumophila is a gram-negative bacterium with LPS as a major constituent of the outer membrane. *Legionella* species possess various antigens in addition to LPS, including heat-shock proteins (Hsps), outer-membrane proteins, and flagella (62). LPS is the predominant antigen recognized by human antisera and is the serogroup-specific antigen (63,64). *L. pneumophila* LPS also stimulates macrophages to produce the cytokine tumor necrosis factor, which has been shown to augment the bactericidal activity of polymorphonuclear leukocytes (65,66). An LPS antigenic determinant in the outer membrane that is recognized by a monoclonal antibody is used in the preliminary identification of *L. pneumophila* (67,68).

Protein profiles of *L. pneumophila* serogroup 1 show two major immunoreactive proteins (24-kd and 38-kd) (69,70). The 24-kd macrophage infectivity potentiator (Mip) is a peptidyl-prolyl, *cis-trans* isomerase that is exported to the cell surface (71) and is involved in establishing intracellular infection (62). A 38-kd exoprotease termed the *zinc metalloprotease* or major secretory protein (Msp) has been shown to induce cell-mediated immune responses and protective immunity against lethal aerosol challenge with *L. pneumophila* in a guinea-pig model (72,73). A 60-kd Hsp (Hsp60) is the genus common antigen of the Legionellaceae. It is the immunodominant major cytoplasmic membrane protein (74–76). Anti-Hsp60 antibodies have been demonstrated in convalescent sera of culture-confirmed cases (77). This protein has been implicated in attachment and entry of *L. pneumophila* into host cells, and has been shown to induce protective immunity in a guinea pig model (62,78).

PATHOGENESIS AND VIRULENCE FACTORS

Cell-mediated immunity is the primary host defense against *Legionella*. Human mononuclear, polymorphonuclear, and alveolar macrophages readily phagocytize *Legionella*. Phagocytosis occurs by a coiling mechanism mediated by complement receptors, which bind to the outer-membrane protein of *Legionella* (79). Interferon-γ (IFN-γ) activation of macrophages limits internalization of the bacterium and intracellular multiplication by restricting complement receptors and limiting the availability of iron. Polymorphonuclear leukocytes are the predominant cells seen on histologic smears from the lungs of infected patients; however, these cells do not support intracellular replication of *Legionella*.

L. pneumophila is a facultative intracellular bacterial pathogen that causes disease via perturbation of normal intracellular killing mechanisms (62,71,80). *Legionella* are internalized most efficiently (but not exclusively) by opsonin-dependent CR3-mediated phagocytosis (81). Attachment of *Legionella* to host cells has been shown to be mediated by type IV pili (82), Hsp60 (83), and the major-outer membrane protein. The bacteria bind to complement CR1 and CR3 integrin receptors on the surface of the host cell (62,84,85).

After entry into a host macrophage or monocyte, *Legionella* evades intracellular destruction by inhibiting phagosome–lysosome fusion. Replication occurs within the phagosome, which has an uncharacteristically neutral pH level. This specialized compartment will traffic through the cell until it becomes associated with the rough endoplasmic reticulum. The *dot* (defective organelle trafficking) and *icm* (intracellular multiplication) gene products redirect phagosome trafficking, establish the intracellular compartment for growth, and are involved in the formation of a transmembrane transport channel (pore) (71). Altered endocytic trafficking, cytotoxicity, and pore formation by *L. pneumophila* appear to be mediated by a variety of proteins encoded by the *pmi, mil, dot, icm,* and the *enh* loci (71,86–90). The ability of *L. pneumophila* to enter host cells may be regulated by one of the genes of the *enh1* locus, the *rtxA* gene. The *rtxA* gene appears to be involved in adherence, cytotoxicity, and pore formation (90).

The susceptibility of macrophages to *L. pneumophila* is also related to the intracellular availability of iron (91). For example, IFN-γ inhibits the growth of *L. pneumophila* within human monocytes by reducing intracellular iron (91–93). *Legionella* has been shown to produce iron-binding siderophores, called *legiobactin*, which transports iron to the bacterium (94).

Epidemiologic and genetic studies have revealed a number of factors that affect the virulence of *Legionella* (95,96). Multiple strains of *L. pneumophila* may colonize a water system, but only a few strains will cause disease in patients exposed to the water. Although more than 40 *Legionella* species have been identified, less than half of these have been linked to disease in humans. *L. pneumophila* is the most pathogenic, accounting for 90% of the cases of legionellosis, followed by *L. micdadei* and *L. longbeachae* (3,5). Although more than 15 serogroups of *L. pneumophila* have been identified, serogroup 1 accounts for more than 80% of the reported cases of legionellosis caused by *L. pneumophila*. A surface antigen of *L. pneumophila* serogroup 1 that is recognized by one particular monoclonal antibody (MAB-2) may be associated with virulence (97–99).

The presence of flagella is one phenotypic difference between virulent and avirulent *L. pneumophila*; isogeneic avirulent strains obtained by laboratory passage lose their flagella (100–102). It has also been suggested that the virulence of *Legionella* may be increased by replication in amebae (103–106). Avirulent strains of *Legionella* were unable to multiply intracellularly in a ciliated protozoan (107).

ENVIRONMENTAL ECOLOGY

Legionella organisms are natural inhabitants of aquatic bodies and some species have been recovered from soil (108,109). The organisms have been detected in a wide range of conditions, including temperatures of 0°C to 63°C, pH level of 5.0 to 8.5, and dissolved oxygen concentrations of 0.2 to 15 parts per million in water (110). *Legionella* and other microorganisms attach to submerged surfaces and form a biofilm. *Legionella* has been shown to attach to and colonize various materials found in water systems including plastics, rubber, and wood (111,112). *Legionella* has been shown to form microcolonies in biofilms on these surfaces (112). Commensal organisms such as bacteria and blue-green algae (Cyanobacteria) can stimulate the growth of *Legionella* in the aquatic environment (113–116).

L. pneumophila can also infect and multiply within soil and aquatic species of amebae (*Hartmannella, Naegleria, Acanthamoeba*) and the ciliated protozoa (*Tetrahymena*), including the amebae isolated from hot-water tanks, spas, and hot springs (109,117). This intracellular parasitism parallels that seen in humans, except that mononuclear cells are the targets in humans. These protozoan hosts appear to play a pivotal role in the growth and transmission of *Legionella* from the environment to humans. Intracellular growth in amebae enhances virulence of *L. pneumophila* for replication in human cells (62,105,106,109,118). When the protozoan host ruptures, large numbers of motile *Legionella* are freed (119). It has been suggested that *Legionella* could be transmitted to humans via inhalation of the amebic vesicles (120–122); however, there has been no clinical evidence to support this theory. A/J mice developed more severe disease when infected with a mixture of *L. pneumophila* and amebae, suggesting that amebae exacerbate *Legionella* lung infections (123). Growth within amebae may also protect *Legionella* from harsh environmental conditions by survival within amebae cysts (124).

Legionella survive the water treatment process because of relative resistance to low levels of chlorine (125) and pass into water distribution systems. *Legionella* are present in all segments of municipal water supplies, including water treatment facilities (126–129). As a result, *Legionella* are found in human-made habitats such as cooling towers, evaporative condensers, whirlpool spas, decorative fountains, and potable water distribution systems (130,131). Hot-water distribution systems are the primary source for nosocomial infections and a significant source for sporadic community-acquired cases (131–137). In fact, the water distribution systems of hospitals have been the source of the majority of nosocomial cases in the United States and Europe (7,138,139). Legionnaires' disease has been linked to exposure to contaminated water supplies in residences, rehabilitation centers, nursing homes, and industrial water supplies (140).

Environmental and clinical surveillance for *Legionella* in hospitals is recommended as a proactive approach to prevention (141–143). *Legionella* environmental culture is performed using acid-buffer pretreatment and glycine-containing selective media (144). A potentially sensitive method for the detection of *Legionella* in water samples is the PCR (145). A *Legionella* PCR kit has been developed for detection of *Legionella* in water samples (Perkin-Elmer EnviroAmp). Two primers are used to detect and amplify gene sequences of legionellae: One is genus specific and detects the 5S rRNA and the other is species specific and detects the *mip* gene sequence of *L. pneumophila*. PCR does not appear to be more sensitive than culture, particularly with respect to detecting *L. pneumophila*.

Ultimately, control of nosocomial Legionnaires' disease has been achieved via disinfection of the hospital water system (137). Three primary disinfection methods have been used with variable success, superheat and flush, hyperchlorination, and copper-silver ionization (Liqui-Tech, Bolingbrook, Illinois). Comparison of the efficacy of thermal eradication and copper-silver ionization has shown ionization to be superior (146,147).

ANTIBIOTIC SUSCEPTIBILITY

As facultative intracellular pathogens, *Legionella* species can avoid the effects of antimicrobial agents that cannot penetrate the host cell membranes. Agents that cannot penetrate macrophages, such as penicillins and cephalosporins, demonstrate activity in minimum inhibitory concentration (MIC) assays but are clinically ineffective (148). Because of the lack of standardized methodology, *in vitro* antibiotic susceptibility studies have been problematic. Three methods are generally used for susceptibility testing, extracellular testing in broth or agar, intracellular testing in tissue culture, and studies using infected guinea pigs (148).

In vitro and *in vivo* results have shown the following agents to be highly active: azithromycin, clarithromycin, ciprofloxacin, pefloxacin, levofloxacin, moxifloxacin, fleroxacin, trovafloxacin, minocycline, doxycycline, and the ketolides (149–156). Synergy *in vitro* has also been shown for trimethoprim-sulfamethoxazole, erythromycin-rifampin, and macrolide-quinolone combinations (157,158). Variable results (including antagonism) have been reported for quinolones and rifampin (157,159).

Erythromycin, rifampin, tetracycline, fluoroquinolones, and newer macrolide-azolide antimicrobial agents are considered effective agents in the treatment of Legionnaires' disease (160). However, with the availability of intravenous formulations of the newer macrolides, the newer quinolones and macrolides have displaced erythromycin as the drug of choice (161,162).

Resistance to antimicrobial therapy has been suspected because of persistent recovery of *Legionella* from respiratory tract cultures despite macrolide therapy (163,164). When the MICs of isolates recovered from specimens taken early and late in the course of therapy were compared, no difference in MIC was observed (163).

REFERENCES

1. File TM, Bartlett JG, Bernstein A, et al. Management of community-acquired pneumonia: an appropriate-use tool. *Infect Med* 2001;18:462–472.
2. Marston BJ, Plouffe JF, File TM, et al. Incidence of community-acquired pneumonia requiring hospitalization; results of a population based active surveillance study in Ohio. *Arch Intern Med* 1997;157:1709–1718.
3. Marston BJ, Lipman HB, Breiman RF. Surveillance for Legionnaires' disease. Risk factors for morbidity and mortality. *Arch Intern Med* 1994;154:2417–2422.
4. Benson RF, Fields BS. Classification of the genus *Legionella*. *Semin Respir Infect* 1998;13:90–99.
5. Yu VL, Plouffe JF, Pastoris MC, et al. Distribution of *Legionella* species and serogroups isolated by culture in consecutive patients with community acquired pneumonia: an international collaborative survey. *J Infect Dis* 2002;186:127–128.
6. Fang GD, Yu VL, Vickers RM. Disease due to *Legionellaceae* (other than *Legionella pneumophila*): historical, microbiological, clinical and epidemiological review. *Medicine* 1989;68:116–139.
7. Butler JC, Fields BS, Breiman RF. Prevention and control of legionellosis. *Infect Dis Clin Pract* 1997;6:458–464.
8. Harrison TG, Saunders NA. Taxonomy and typing of legionellae. *Rev Med Microbiol* 1994;5:79–90.
9. Thacker WL, Dyke JW, Benson RF, et al. Legionella lansingensis sp. nov. isolated from a patient with pneumonia and underlying chronic lymphocytic leukemia. *J Clin Microbiol* 1992;30:2398–2401.
10. Brenner DJ, Steigerwalt AG, McDade JE. Classification of the Legionnaires' disease bacterium: *Legionella pneumophila* genus novum, species nova, of the family Legionellaceae. *Ann Intern Med* 1979;90:656–658.
11. Garrity GM, Brown A, Vickers RM. *Tatlockia* and *Fluoribacter*: two new genera of organisms resembling *Legionella pneumophila*. *Int J Syst Bacteriol* 1980;30:609–614.
12. Heuner K, Steinert M, Marre R, et al. Genomic structure and evolution of *Legionella* species. *Curr Topics Microbiol Epidemiol* 2002;264:61–78.
13. Hookey JV, Saunders NA, Fry NK, et al. Phylogeny of *Legionellaceae* based on small-subunit ribosomal DNA sequences and proposal of *Legionella lytica* comb. nov. for *Legionella*-like amoebal pathogens. *Int J Syst Bacteriol* 1996;46:526–531.
14. Fry NK, Warwick S, Saunders NA, et al. The use of 16S ribosomal RNA analysis to investigate the phylogeny of the family Legionellaceae. *J Gen Microbiol* 1991;137:1215–1222.
15. Adeleke A, Pruckler J, Benson R, et al. *Legionella*-like amebal pathogens—phylogenetic status and possible role in respiratory diseases. *Emerg Infect Dis* 1996;2:225–230.
16. Newsome AL, Scott TM, Benson RF, et al. Isolation of an amoeba naturally harboring a distinctive *Legionella* species. *Appl Environ Microbiol* 1998;64:1688–1693.
17. Waite R. Confirmation of identity of legionellae by whole cell fatty-acid and isoprenoid quinone profiles. In: Harrison TG, Taylor AG, eds. *A laboratory manual for* Legionella. Chichester, UK: John Wiley, 1988:69–101.
18. Sonesson A, Jantzen E, Bryn K, et al. Composition of 2, 3-dihydroxy fatty acid-containing lipopolysaccharides from *Legionella israelensis*, *Legionella maceachernii*, and *Legionella micdadei*. *Microbiology* 1994;140:1261–1271.
19. Sonesson A, Jantzen D, Bryn K, et al. Chemical composition of lipopolysaccharide from *Legionella pneumophila*. *Arch Microbiol* 1989;153:72.
20. Lema M, Brown A. Electrophoretic characterization of soluble protein extracts of *Legionella pneumophila* and other members of the family Legionellaceae. *J Clin Microbiol* 1983;17:1132–1140.
21. Brindle RJ, Bryant TN, Draper PW. Taxonomic investigation of *Legionella pneumophila* using monoclonal antibodies. *J Clin Microbiol* 1989;27:536–539.
22. Diogo A, Verissimo A, Nobre MF, et al. Usefulness of fatty acid composition for differentiation of *Legionella* species. *J Clin Microbiol* 1999;37:2248–2254.
23. Fox A, Lau PY, Brown A, et al. Capillary gas chromatographic analysis of carbohydrates of *Legionella pneumophila* and other members of the family Legionellaceae. *J Clin Microbiol* 1984;19:326–332.
24. Lo Presti F, Riffard S, Vandenesch F, et al. Identification of *Legionella* species by random amplified polymorphic DNA profiles. *J Clin Microbiol* 1998;36:3193–3197.
25. Bansal NS, McDonell F. Identification and DNA fingerprinting of *Legionella* strains by randomly amplified polymorphic DNA analysis. *J Clin Microbiol* 1997;35:2310–2314.
26. Pinar A, Ahkee S, Miller RD, et al. Use of heteroduplex analysis to classify legionellae on the basis of 5S rRNA gene sequences. *J Clin Microbiol* 1997;35:1609–1611.

27. Gheldre YD, Maes N, Lo Presti F, et al. Rapid identification of clinically relevant *Legionella* spp. by analysis of transfer DNA intergenic spacer length polymorphism. *J Clin Microbiol* 2001;39:162–169.

28. Brenner DJ. Classification of legionellae. *Semin Respir Infect* 1987;2:90–205.

29. Winn WC Jr, Pasculle AW. Laboratory diagnosis of infections caused by *Legionella* species. *Clin Lab Med* 1982;2:343–369.

30. Hilton E, Freedman RA, Cintron F, et al. Acid-fast bacilli in sputum: a case of *Legionella micdadei* pneumonia. *J Clin Microbiol* 1986;24:1102–1103.

31. Edelstein PH. Legionnaires' disease. *Clin Infect Dis* 1993;16:741–749.

32. Lowry PW, Tompkins LS. Nosocomial legionellosis: a review of pulmonary and extrapulmonary syndromes. *Am J Infect Cont* 1993;21:21–27.

33. Pasculle AW. Update on *Legionella*. *Clin Microbiol Newsletter* 2000;22:97–101.

34. Pine L, Hoffman PS, Malcolm GB, et al. Role of keto acids and reduced oxygen-scavenging enzymes in the growth of *Legionella* species. *J Clin Microbiol* 1986;23:33–42.

35. Hoffman PS, Pine L, Bell S. Production of superoxide and hydrogen peroxide in medium used to culture *L. pneumophila*: catalytic decomposition by charcoal. *Appl Environ Microbiol* 1983;45:784–791.

36. Morrill WE, Barbaree JM, Fields BS, et al. Increased recovery of *Legionella micdadei* and *Legionella bozemanii* on buffered charcoal yeast extract agar supplemented with albumin. *J Clin Microbiol* 1990;28:616–618.

37. Vickers RM, Stout JE, Yu VL, et al. Culture methodology for the isolation of *Legionella pneumophila* and other *Legionellaceae* from clinical and environmental specimens. *Semin Respir Infect* 1987;2:274–279.

38. Kessler HH, Reinthaler FF, Pschaid A, et al. Rapid detection of *Legionella* species in bronchoalveolar lavage fluids with the EnviroAmp *Legionella* PCR amplification and detection kit. *J Clin Microbiol* 1993;31:3325–3328.

39. Matsiota-Bernard P, Pitsouni E, Legakis N, et al. Evaluation of commercial amplification kit for detection of *Legionella pneumophila* in clinical samples. *J Clin Microbiol* 1994;32:1503–1505.

40. Centers for Disease Control and Prevention. Guidelines for prevention of nosocomial pneumonia. *MMWR Morb Mortal Wkly Rep* 1997;46(RR-1)3:1–79.

41. Vickers RM, Yu VL. Clinical laboratory differentiation of Legionellaceae family members with pigment production and fluorescence on media supplemented with aromatic substrates. *J Clin Microbiol* 1984;19:583–587.

42. Fox KF, Brown A. Application of numerical systematics to the phenotypic differentiation of legionellae. *J Clin Microbiol* 1989;27:1952–1955.

43. Vesey G, Dennis PJ, Lee J, et al. Further development of simple tests to differentiate the *Legionella*. *J Appl Bacteriol* 1988;65:339–345.

44. Bangsborg JM, Shand G, Pearlman E, et al. Cross-reactive *Legionella* antigens and the antibody response during infection. *APMIS* 1991;99:854–865.

45. Wilkinson HW, Fikes BJ. Slide agglutination tests for serogrouping *Legionella pneumophila* and atypical *Legionella*-like organisms. *J Clin Microbiol* 1980;11:99–101.

46. Orrison LH, Bibb WF, Cherry WB, et al. Determination of antigenic relationships among legionellae and non-legionellae by direct fluorescent-antibody and immunodiffusion tests. *J Clin Microbiol* 1983;17:332–337.

47. Barbaree JM. Selecting a subtyping technique for use in investigations of legionellosis epidemics. In: Barbaree JM, Brieman RF, Dufour AP, eds. *Legionella: current status and emerging perspectives*. Washington, DC: American Society for Microbiology, 1993:169–172.

48. van Belkum A, Mass H, Verbrugh H, et al. Serotyping, ribotyping, PCR-mediated ribosomal 16S-23S spacer analysis, and arbitrarily primed PCR for epidemiological studies on *Legionella pneumophila*. *Res Microbiol* 1996;147:405–413.

49. Venezia RA, Agresta MD, Hanley EM, et al. Nosocomial legionellosis associated with aspiration of nasogastric feedings diluted in tap water. *Infect Cont Hosp Epidemiol* 1994;15:529–533.

50. Bangsborg JM, Gerner-Smidt P, Colding H, et al. Restriction fragment length polymorphism of rRNA genes for molecular typing of members of the family Legionellaceae. *J Clin Microbiol* 1995;33:402–406.

51. Valsangiacomo C, Baggi F, Gaia V, et al. Use of amplified fragment length polymorphisms in molecular typing of *Legionella pneumophila* and application to epidemiological studies. *J Clin Microbiol* 1995;33:1716–1719.

52. Lawrence C, Ronco E, Dubrou S, et al. Molecular typing of *L. pneumophila* serogroup 1 isolates from patients and the nosocomial environment by arbitrarily primed PCR and pulsed-field gel electrophoresis. *J Med Microbiol* 1999;48:327–333.

53. Georghiou PR, Doggett AM, Kielhofner MA, et al. Molecular fingerprinting of *Legionella* species by repetitive element PCR. *J Clin Microbiol* 1994;32:2989–2994.

54. Schoonmaker D, Heimberger T, Birkhead G. Comparison of ribotyping and restriction enzyme analysis using pulsed-field gel electrophoresis for distinguishing *Legionella pneumophila* isolates obtained during a nosocomial outbreak. *J Clin Microbiol* 1992;30:1491–1498.

55. Jonas D, Heinz-Georg WM, Matthes F, et al. Comparative evaluation of three different genotyping methods for investigation of nosocomial outbreaks of Legionnaires' disease in hospitals. *J Clin Microbiol* 2000;38:2284–2291.

56. Pruckler JM, Mermel LA, Benson RF. Comparison of *Legionella pneumophila* isolates by arbitrarily primed PCR and pulsed-field gel electrophoresis: Analysis from seven epidemic investigations. *J Clin Microbiol* 1995;33:2872–2875.

57. Drenning SD, Stout JE, Joly JR, et al. Unexpected similarity of pulsed-field gel electrophoresis patterns of unrelated clinical isolates of *Legionella pneumophila* serogroup 1. *J Infect Dis* 2001;183:628–632.

58. Struelens MJ, Maes N, Rost F, et al. Genotypic and phenotypic methods for the investigation of a hospital-acquired *Legionella pneumophila* outbreak and efficacy of control measures. *J Infect Dis* 1992;166:22–30.

59. Lawrence C, Reyrolle M, Dubrou S, et al. Single clonal origin of a high proportion of *Legionella pneumophila* serogroup 1 isolates from patients and the environment in the area of Paris, France, over a 10-year period. *J Clin Microbiol* 1999;37:2652–2655.

60. Saunders NA, Harrison TG, Haththotuwa A, et al. A method for typing strains of *Legionella pneumophila* serogroup 1 by analysis of restriction fragment length polymorphisms. *J Med Microbiol* 1990;31:45–55.

61. Fry NK, Bangsborg JM, Bernander S, et al. Assessment of intercenter reproducibility and epidemiological concordance of *Legionella pneumophila* serogroup 1 genotyping by amplified fragment length polymorphism analysis. *Eur J Clin Microbiol Infect Dis* 2000;19:773–780.

62. Swanson MS, Hammer BK. *Legionella pneumophila* pathogenesis: a fateful journey from amoebae to macrophages. *Annu Rev Microbiol* 2000;54:567–613.

63. Ciesielski CA, Blaser MJ, Wang WLL. Serogroup specificity of *Legionella pneumophila* is related to lipopolysaccharide characteristics. *Infect Immun* 1986;51:397–404.

64. Gabay J, Blake M, Niles W, et al. Purification of *Legionella pneumophila* major outer membrane protein and demonstration that it is a porin. *J Bacteriol* 1985;162:85–91.

65. Blanchard DI, Friedman H, Klein TW, et al. Induction of interferon-gamma and tumor necrosis factor by *Legionella pneumophila*—augmentation of human neutrophil bactericidal activity. *J Leukocyte Biol* 1989;45:538–545.

66. Arata S, Newton C, Klein TW, et al. *Legionella pneumophila* induced tumor necrosis factor production in permissive versus nonpermissive macrophages. *Proc Soc Exp Biol Med* 1993;203:26–29.

67. Barthe C, Joly JR, Ramsay D, et al. Common epitope on the lipopolysaccharide of *Legionella pneumophila* recognized by monoclonal antibody. *J Clin Microbiol* 1988;26:1016–1023.

68. Helbig JH, Kurtz JB, Pastoris MC, et al. Antigenic lipopolysaccharide components of *Legionella pneumophila* recognized by monoclonal antibodies: possibilities and limitations for division of the species into serogroups. *Journal of Clinical Microbiology* 1997;35:2841–2845.

69. Pearlman E, Engleberg NC, Eisenstein BI. Identification of protein antigens of *Legionella pneumophila* serogroup 1. *Infect Immun* 1985;47:74–79.

70. Engleberg NC, Drutz DJ, Eisenstein BI. Cloning and expression of *Legionella pneumophila* antigens in *Escherichia coli*. *Infect Immun* 1984;44:222–227.

71. Roy CR. Trafficking of the *Legionella pneumophila* phagosome. *ASM News* 1999;65:416–421.

72. Szeto L, Shuman HA. The *Legionella pneumophila* major secretory protein, a protease, is not required for intracellular growth or cell killing. *Infect Immun* 1990;58:2585–2592.

73. Blander SJ, Breiman R, Horwitz MA. A live avirulent mutant *L. pneumophila* vaccine induces protective immunity against lethal aerosol challenge. *J Clin Invest* 1989;83:810–815.

74. Lema MW, Brown A, Butler CA, et al. Heat-shock response in *Legionella pneumophila*. *Can J Microbiol* 1988;34:1148–1153.

75. Hoffman PS, Butler CA, Quinn FC. Cloning and temperature-dependent expression in *Escherichia coli* of a *Legionella pneumophila* gene coding for a genus-common 60-Kilodalton antigen. *Infect Immun* 1989;57:1731–1739.

76. Sampson JS, Plikaytis BB, Wilkinson HW. Immunologic response of patients with legionellosis against major protein-containing antigens of *Legionella pneumophila* serogroup 1 as shown by immunoblot analysis. *J Clin Microbiol* 1986;23:92–99.

77. Hoffman PS, Houston L, Butler CA. *Legionella* pneumophila htpAb heat shock operon: nucleotide sequence and expression of the 60-kilodalton antigen in *L. pneumophila*–infected HeLa cells. *Infect Immun* 1990;58:3380–3387.

78. Blander SJ, Horwitz MA. Major cytoplasmic membrane protein of *L. pneumophila*, a genus common antigen and member of hsp 60 family of heat shock proteins induces protective immunity in a guinea pig model of Legionnaires' disease. *J Clin Invest* 1993;91:717–723.

79. Horwitz MA. Toward an understanding of host and bacterial molecules mediating *L. pneumophila* pathogenesis. In: Barbaree JM, Breiman RF, Dufour AP, eds. *Legionella: current status and emerging perspectives*. Washington, DC: American Society of Microbiology, 1993:55–62.

80. Abu Kwaik Y. Fatal attraction of mammalian cells to *Legionella pneumophila*. *Mol Microbiol* 1998;30:689–696.

81. Payne NR, Horwitz MA. Phagocytosis of *Legionella pneumophila* is mediated by human monocyte complement receptors. *J Exp Med* 1987;166:1377–1389.

82. Stone BJ, Kwaik YA. Expression of multiple pili by *Legionella pneumophila*: identification and characterization of a type IV pilin gene and its role in adherence to mammalian and protozoan cells. *Infect Immun* 1998;66:1768–1775.

83. Garduno RA, Garduno E, Hoffman PS. Surface-associated hsp60 chaperonin of *Legionella pneumophila* mediates invasion in a HeLa cell model. *Infect Immun* 1998;66:4602–4610.

84. Zuckman DM, Hung JB, Roy CR. Pore-forming activity is not sufficient for *Legionella pneumophila* phagosome trafficking and intracellular replication. *Mol Microbiol* 1999;32:990–1001.

85. Gao L-Y, Abu Kwaik Y. Activation ov caspase 3 during *Legionella pneumophila*–induced apoptosis. *Infect Immun* 1999;67:4886–4894.

86. Berger KH, Isberg RR. Two distinct defects in intracellular growth complemented by a single genetic locus in *Legionella pneumophila*. *Mol Microbiol* 1993;7:7–19.

87. Marra A, Shuman HA. Genetics of *Legionella pneumophila* virulence. *Annu Rev Genet* 1992;26:51–69.

88. Engleberg CN. Genetic studies of Legionella pathogenesis. In: Barbaree JM, Breiman RF, Dufour AP, eds. *Legionella—current Status and Emerging Perspectives*. Washington, DC: American Society of Microbiology, 1993: 63–68.

89. Segal G, Shuman HA. How is the intracellular fate of the *Legionella pneumophila* phagosome determined. *Trends Microbiol* 1998;6:253–255.

90. Crillo SL, Bermudez LE, El-Etr SH, et al. *Legionella pneumophila* entry gene rtxA is involved in virulence. *Infect Immun* 2001;69:508–517.

91. Viswanathan VK, Cianciotto NP. Role of iron acquisition in *Legionella pneumophila* virulence. *ASM News* 2001;67:253–258.

92. Gebran SJ, Newton C, Yamamoto Y, et al. Macrophage permissiveness for *L. pneumophila* growth modulated by iron. *Infec Immun* 1994;62:564–568.

93. Aberrantly low transferrin receptor expression on human monocytes is associated with nonpermissiveness for *Legionella pneumophila* growth. *J Infect Dis* 2000;181:1394–4000.

94. Viswanathan VK, Edelstein PH, Pope CD, et al. The *Legionella pneumophila* iraAB locus is required for iron assimilation, intracellular infection, and virulence. *Infect Immun* 2000;68:1069–1079.

95. Dowling JN, Saha AK, Glew RH. Virulence factors of the family Legionellaceae. *Microbiol Rev* 1992;56:32–60.

96. Shuman HA, Purcell M, Segal G, et al. Intracellular multiplication of *Legionella pneumophila*: human pathogen or accidental tourist? *Curr Topics Microbiol Immunol* 1998;225:99–112.

97. Stout JE, Joly J, Para M, et al. Comparison of molecular methods for subtyping patients and epidemiologically-linked environmental isolates of *L. pneumophila*. *J Infect Dis* 1988;157:486–494.

98. Dournon E, Bibb WF, Rajagopalan P, et al. Monoclonal antibody reactivity as a virulence marker for *Legionella pneumophila* serogroup 1 strains. *J Infect Dis* 1988;157:496–501.

99. Joly JR, McKinney RM, Tobin J, et al. Development of a standardized subtyping scheme for *L. pneumophila* serogroup 1, using monoclonal antibodies. *J Clin Microbiol* 1986;23:768–771.

100. Pruckler J, Benson R, Martin W, et al. Association of flagella and intracellular growth of *L. pneumophila*. *Annual Meeting of the American Society of Microbiology*. Washington, DC: American Society of Microbiology. 1995;B-391 (Abstract).

101. Dietrich CK, Heuner K, Brand BC, et al. Flagellum of *Legionella pneumophila* positively affects the early phase of infection of eukaryotic host cells. *Infect Immun* 2001;2001:2116–2122.

102. Bryne B, Swanson MS. Expression of *Legionella pneumophila* virulence traits in response to growth conditions. *Infect Immun* 1998;66:3029–3034.

103. Cirillo JD, Falkow S, Tompkins LS. *Legionella pneumophila* in *Acanthamoeba castellanii* enhances invasion. *Infect Immun* 1994;62:3254–3261.

104. Moffat JF, Tompkins LS. A quantitative model of intracellular growth of *Legionella pneumophila* in *Acanthamoeba castellanii*. *Infect Immun* 1992;60:296–301.

105. Cirillo JD, Cirillo SLG, Yan L, et al. Intracellular growth in *Acanthamoeba castellanii* affects monocyte entry mechanisms and enhances virulence of *Legionella pneumophila*. *Infect Immun* 1999;67:4427–4434.

106. Harb OS, Gao LY, Kwaik YA. From protozoa to mammalian cells: a new paradigm in the life cycle of intracellular bacterial pathogens. *Environ Microbiol* 2000;2:251–265.

107. Fields BS, Barbaree JM, Shotts EB, et al. Comparison of guinea pig and protozoan models for determining virulence of *Legionella* species. *Infect Immun* 1986;53:553–559.

108. Steele TW, Moore CY, Sangster N. Distribution of *Legionella longbeachae* serogroup 1 and other legionellae in potting soil in Australia. *Appl Environ Microbiol* 1990;56:2984–2988.

109. Atlas RM. *Legionella:* from environmental habitats to disease pathology, detection and control. *Environ Microbiol* 1999;1:283–293.

110. Fliermans CB. Philosophical ecology: *Legionella* in historical perspective. In: Thornsberry C, Ballows A, Feeley JC, eds. *Legionella—proceedings of the 2nd International Symposium*. Washington, DC: American Society of Microbiology, 1984:285–289.

111. Wright JB, Ruseska I, Athar M, et al. *Legionella pneumophila* grows adherent to surfaces in vitro and in situ. *Infect Control Hosp Epidemiol* 1989;10:408–415.

112. Rogers J, Dowsett AB, Dennis PJ, et al. Influence of temperature and plumbing material selection on biofilm formation and growth of *Legionella pneumophila* in a model potable water system containing complex microbial flora. *Appl Environ Microbiol* 1994;60:1585–1592.

113. Wadowsky RM, Yee RB. Effect of non-Legionellaceae bacteria on the multiplication of *Legionella pneumophila* in potable water. *Appl Environ Microbiol* 1985;49:1206–1210.

114. Wadowsky RM, Yee RB. Satellite growth of *Legionella pneumophila* with an environmental isolate of *Flavobacterium breve*. *Appl Environ Microbiol* 1983;46:1147–1149.

115. Stout JE, Yu VL, Best M. Ecology of *Legionella pneumophila* within water distribution systems. *Appl Environ Microbiol* 1985;49:221–228.

116. Tison DL, Pope DH, Cherry WB, et al. Growth of *Legionella pneumophila* in association with blue-green algae (Cyanobacteria). *Appl Env Microbiol* 1980;39:456–459.

117. Fields BS. *Legionella* and protozoa: interaction of a pathogen and its natural host. In: Barbaree JM, Breiman RF, Dufour AP, eds. *Legionella: current status and emerging perspectives*. Washington, DC: American Society of Microbiology, 1993:129–136.

118. Abu Kwaik Y, Gao L-Y, Stone BJ, et al. Invasion of protozoa by *Legionella pneumophila* and its role in bacterial ecology and pathogenesis. *Appl Environ Microbiol* 1998;64:3127–3133.

119. Berk S, Ting R, Turner G, et al. Production of respirable vesicles containing live *Legionella pneumophila* cells by two *Acanthamoeba* spp. *Appl Environ Microbiol* 1999;64:279–286.

120. Rowbotham TJ. Current views on the relationships between amoebae legionellae, and man. *Isr J Med Sci* 1986;22:678–689.

121. Rowbotham TJ. *Legionella*-like amoebal pathogens. In: Barbaree JM, Brieman RF, Dufour AP, eds. *Legionella: current status and emerging perspectives*. Washington, DC: American Society of Microbiology, 1993:139–140.

122. Barker J, Brown MRW. Trojan horses of the microbial world: protozoa and the survival of bacterial pathogens in the environment. *Microbiology* 1994;140:1253–1259.

123. Brieland JK, et al. Coinoculation with *Hartmannella vermiformis* enhances replicative *Legionella pneumophila* lung infection in a murine model of Legionnaires' disease. *Infect Immun* 1996;64:2449–2456.

124. Kilvington S, Price J. Survival of *Legionella pneumophila* within cysts of *Acanthamoeba polyphaga* following chlorine exposure. *J Appl Bacteriol* 1990;68:519–525.

125. Kuchta JM, States SJ, McGlaughlin JE, et al. Enhanced chlorine resistance of tap water—adapted *Legionella pneumophila* as compared with agar medium-passage strains. *J Appl Microbiol* 1985;50:21–26.

126. Colbourne JS, Dennis PJ. The ecology and survival of *Legionella pneumophila*. *Thames Water Authority Journal of the Institution of Water and Environmental Management* 1989;3:345–350.

127. Palmer C, Tsai Y-L, Paszko-Kolva C, et al. Detection of *Legionella* species in sewage and ocean water by polymerase chain reaction, direct fluorescent antibody, and plate culture methods. *App Environ Microbiol* 1993;59:3618–3624.

128. States SJ, Conley L, Kuchta JM, et al. Survival and multiplication of *Legionella pneumophila* in municipal drinking water systems. *Appl Environ Microbiol* 1987;53:979–986.

129. Voss L, Button KS, Lorenz RC, et al. *Legionella* contamination of a preoperational treatment plant. *J Am Water Works Assoc* 1986;78:70–75.

130. Muraca PW, Stout JE, Yu VL. Environmental aspects of Legionnaires' disease. *J Am Water Works Assoc* 1988;80:78–86.

131. Lin YE, Stout JE, Yu VL. Disinfection of water distribution systems for *Legionella*. *Semin Respir Infect* 1998;13:147–159.

132. Yu VL. Nosocomial legionellosis. *Curr Opin Infect Dis* 2000;13:385–388.

133. Yu VL. *Legionella* surveillance: political and social implications—a little knowledge is a dangerous thing. *J Infect Dis* 2002;185:259–261.

134. Stout JE, Yu VL, Muraca P, et al. Potable water as the cause of sporadic cases of community-acquired Legionnaires' disease. *New Engl J Med* 1992;326:151–154.

135. Best M, Yu VL, Stout J, et al. *Legionellaceae* in the hospital water supply—epidemiological link with disease and evaluation of a method of control of nosocomial Legionnaires' disease and Pittsburgh pneumonia. *Lancet* 1983;2:307–310.

136. Straus WL, Plouffe JF, File TM Jr, et al. Risk factors for domestic acquisition of Legionnaires' disease. *Arch Intern Med* 1996;156:1685–1692.

137. Lin YE, Vidic RD, Stout JE, et al. *Legionella* in water distribution systems. *J Am Water Works Assoc* 1998;90:112–121.

138. Butler JC, Fields BS, Breiman RF. Issues in the control of nosocomial Legionellosis. *Infect Dis Clin Pract* 1997;7:117–118.

139. Joseph C. Surveillance of Legionnaires' disease in Europe. In: Marre R, et al., ed. *Legionella*. Washington, DC: ASM Press, 2002:311–317.

140. Stout JE, Yu VL. Current concepts: legionellosis. *N Engl J Med* 1997;337:682–687.

141. Allegheny County Health Department. *Approaches to prevention and control of Legionella infection in Allegheny County Health Care Facilities*, 2nd ed. Pittsburgh, PA: Allegheny County Health Department, 1997:1–15. Available at: www.legionella.org.

142. State of Maryland Department of Health & Mental Hygiene. Report of the Maryland Scientific Working Group to Study *Legionella* in Water Systems in Healthcare Institutions, June, 2000.

143. Stout JE, Yu VL. *Legionella* in the hospital water supply: a plea for decision making based on evidence-based medicine. *Infect Control Hosp Epidemiol* 2001;22:670–672.

144. Mietzner SM, Stout JE. Laboratory detection of Legionella in environmental samples. *Clin Microbiol Newsletter* 2002;24:81–85.

145. Bej AK, Mahbubani MD, Atlas RM. Detection of viable *Legionella pneumophila* in water by polymerase chain reaction and gene probe methods. *Appl Environ Microbiol* 1991;57:597–600.

146. Mietzner S, Schwille RC, Farley A, et al. Efficacy of thermal treatment and copper-silver ionization for controlling *Legionella pneumophila* in high volume hot water plumbing systems in hospitals. *Am J Infect Control* 1998;25:452–457.

147. Stout JE, Lin YSE, Goetz AM, et al. Controlling *Legionella* in hospital water systems: experience with the superheat-and-flush method and copper-silver ionization. *Infect Control Hosp Epidemiol* 1998;19:911–914.

148. Edelstein PH. Antimicrobial chemotherapy for Legionnaires' disease: a review. *Clin Infect Dis* 1995;21[Suppl 3]:S265–S276.

149. Sens K, Mietzner S, Sagnimeni A, et al. Activity of new quinolones, macrolides, and ketolide against 100 strains of *Legionella* species using broth dilution and intracellular susceptibility testing methods. *Intersci Conf Antimicrob Agents Chemother* 2000(abstr). No 2159.
150. Baltch A, Smith RP, Franke WJ, et al. Antibacterial effect of telithromycin (HMR 3647) and comparative antibiotics against intracellular *Legionella pneumophila*. *J Antimicrob Chemother* 2000;46:51–55.
151. Edelstein PH, Edelstein MAC. In vitro activity of the ketolide HMR 3647 (RU 6647) for *Legionella* spp., its pharmacokinetics in guinea pigs and use of the drugs to treat guinea pigs with *Legionella pneumophila* pneumonia. *Antimicrob Agents Chemother* 1999;43:90–95.
152. Jung R, Danziger LH, Pendlard SL. Intracellular activity of ABT-773 and other antimicrobial agents against *Legionella pneumophila*. *J Antimicrob Chemother* 2002;49:857–861.
153. Walz A, Nichterlein T, Hof H. Excellent activity of newer quinolones on *Legionella pneumophila* in J774 macrophages. *Zbl Bakt* 1997;285:431–439.
154. Edelstein PH, Shinzato T, Doyle E, et al. In vitro activity of gemifloxacin (SB-265805, LB20304a) against *Legionella pneumophila* and its pharmacokinetics in guinea pigs with *L. pneumophila* pneumonia. *Antimicrob Agents Chemother* 2001;45:2204–2209.
155. Edelstein PH, Edelstein MAC, Lehr KH, et al. In-vitro activity of levofloxacin against clinical isolates of *Legionella* spp., its pharmacokinetics in guinea pigs, and use in experimental *Legionella pneumophila* pneumonia. *J Antimicrob Chemother* 1996;37:117–126.
156. Edelstein PH, Edelstein MAC, Ren J, et al. Activity of trovafloxacin (CP-99, 219) against *Legionella* isolates: in vitro activity, intracellular accumulation and killing in macrophages, and pharmacokinetics and treatment of guinea pigs with *L. pneumophila* pneumonia. *Antimicrob Agents Chemother* 1996;40:314–331.
157. Moffie BG, Mouton RP. Sensitivity and resistance of *Legionella pneumophila* to some antibiotics and combination of antibiotics. *J Antimicrob Chemother* 1988;22:457–462.
158. Martin SJ, Pendland SL, Chen C, et al. In vitro synergy testing of macrolide-quinolone combinations against 41 clinical isolates of *Legionella*. *Antimicrob Agents Chemother* 1996;40:1419–1421.
159. Havlichek D, Saravolatz L, Pohlod D. Effect of quinolones and other antimicrobial agents on cell-associated *Legionella pneumophila*. *Antimicrob Agents Chemother* 1987;31:1529–1534.
160. Yu VL. *Legionella* infections. In: Neu HD, Young LS, Zinner SH, eds. *The new macrolides, azolides, and streptogramins*. New York: Marcel Dekker, 1993:141–146.
161. Vergis EN, Yu VL. Macrolides are ideal for empiric therapy of community-acquired pneumonia in the immunocompetent host. *Semin Respir Infect* 1998;12:327–328.
162. Edelstein PH. Antimicrobial chemotherapy for Legionnaires' disease: time for a change. *Ann Intern Med* 1998;129:328–330.
163. Tan JS, File TM Jr, DiPersio LP, et al. Persistently positive culture results in a patient with community-acquired pneumonia due to *Legionella pneumophila*. *Clin Infect Dis* 2001;32:1562–1566.
164. Ko Y-Y, Chen C-H, Lai C-L, et al. Recurrent infection of *Legionella* pneumonia: a case report. *Chin Med J* 1996;57:365–369.
165. Wilkinson HW. *Hospital laboratory diagnosis of* Legionella *infections*. Atlanta, GA: Centers for Disease Control and Prevention, 1988.

CHAPTER 206
Bordetella

William Jerry Durbin

HISTORY

Pertussis (literally, *intensive cough*) is a highly contagious disease caused by organisms of the genus *Bordetella*, which have a highly selective tropism for the ciliated epithelium of the respiratory tract. The name is more appropriate than the familiar term *whooping cough* because coughing paroxysms in small infants and older people with pertussis are often not associated with a whoop. Despite its distinctive clinical presentation, this illness was not described until 1578 when an epidemic occurred in Paris (1). The term *pertussis* was introduced a century later. As recently as the 1940s in the United States, pertussis accounted for more deaths in infants younger than 1 year than meningitis, measles, diphtheria, poliomyelitis, and scarlet fever combined (2). Even now, on a worldwide basis, pertussis ranks in the top ten of fatal infections and is estimated to cause more than 40,000,000 cases and 360,000 deaths each year, mostly in unimmunized infants (3).

CHARACTERISTICS OF THE PATHOGEN

Bordetella species are small (0.2 to 1.0 μm) gram-negative coccobacilli that are catalase-positive obligate aerobes with many nutritional requirements that grow slowly *in vitro*, even on enriched media (4). Seven species are recognized. *Bordetella pertussis* is the agent responsible for most cases of human pertussis and is difficult to recover in the microbiology laboratory. Less fastidious than *B. pertussis* are *Bordetella parapertussis*, associated with a pertussis-like illness in humans (5), and *Bordetella bronchiseptica*, an agent associated with respiratory illness in horses, rabbits (snuffles), dogs (kennel cough), and pigs (atrophic rhinitis) that may rarely cause respiratory disease in immunocompetent humans (6) and systemic disease in immunosuppressed individuals (7). A fourth species, *Bordetella avium*, which may grow on MacConkey's agar, causes turkey coryza (8) and has been associated with human disease (chronic otitis) (9). Newly recognized species are *Bordetella hinzii* [associated with sepsis (10) and with pulmonary infections in cystic fibrosis (11)]; *Bordetella trematum* [associated with wound and ear infections (12)]; and *Bordetella holmesii* [associated with a severe systemic illness (13) and with respiratory tract illness including a pertussis-like illness (14)].

B. pertussis was first cultured by Bordet and Gengou in 1906, in a medium of potato starch infusion, glycerol, and defibrinated blood. This medium, freshly made up or frozen and thawed, is still used today. Regan-Lowe agar (a more stable medium consisting of charcoal, horse blood, and cephalexin) may be used for transport and culture. CHB agar, consisting of charcoal and horse blood supplemented with cephalexin, is associated with the highest recovery rate (15). All *Bordetella* species require organic sulfur, organic nitrogen, and either niacin or nicotinamide for growth; unsaturated fatty acids (such as those potentially found on glassware or on cotton swabs) inhibit their growth. On Bordet-Gengou medium, *B. pertussis* forms tiny, glistening, translucent colonies with a hazy zone of hemolysis; on CHB agar, colonies are small, shiny, round, and mercury-silver. Growth generally takes at least 3 days to appear. Other *Bordetella* species have fewer growth requirements, are generally recovered more quickly, and are distinguished from *B. pertussis* by colonial morphology, biochemical testing, and agglutination reactions. In general, plates should be held at least 7 days, and holding for a second week may even further enhance recovery rates (16).

A number of biologically active virulence components of *B. pertussis* have been identified that appear to contribute to pathogenicity (17,18). Unlike diphtheria, tetanus, and botulism, pertussis is not a single-toxin disease (19). Filamentous hemagglutinin (FHA) is a surface protein of *B. pertussis* that is an important mediator of attachment of the organism to ciliated epithelial cells. Pertussis agglutinogens also are protein surface antigens that may play a role in bacterial attachment; agglutinating antibodies have provided serologic markers for epidemiologic studies and may contribute to protection. Pertussis toxin (PT), the best-studied virulence factor, is composed of a hemagglutinin envelope protein and has many important biologic functions, including mediation of attachment, toxin production, and the induction of leukocytosis. Other recognized antigenic components of *B. pertussis* for which potential biologic roles have been described include adenylate cyclase, pertactin, fimbria-3, dermonecrotic toxin, *Bordetella* lipopolysaccharide, tracheal cytotoxin, tracheal colonization factor, serum resistance factor, and type III secretion (20,21).

Of interest, *Bordetella* species can alternate between two phenotypic phases: the Bvg-positive or virulent phase and the Bvg-negative or avirulent phase (22). It appears that regulation of expression of virulence factors is in response to environmental changes. In the Bvg-positive phase, the organism makes adhesins and toxins critical to gaining colonization and infection, whereas in the Bvg-negative phase, the organism may evade host defenses by living intracellularly (23).

The pathogenesis of pertussis has been divided arbitrarily into several steps: attachment, evasion of host defenses, production of local tissue damage, and production of systemic disease (24). *B. pertussis* has a striking tropism in humans for ciliated cells of the respiratory epithelium. Attachment by *B. pertussis* to the cilia of epithelial cells is mediated by FHA, PT, and pertactin. Once attachment occurs, adenylate-cyclase toxin and PT impair phagocytic function, whereas tracheal cytotoxin disturbs mucociliary clearance. Subsequent local tissue damage, with sloughing of the respiratory mucosal surface, is mediated by tracheal cytotoxin, adenylate-cyclase toxin, and dermonecrotic toxin. Systemic manifestations of pertussis are caused by PT; however, PT is not solely responsible for disease manifestations, and a similar illness caused by *B. parapertussis* occurs in the absence of PT. The mechanism of the most important systemic complication of pertussis, encephalopathy, is not known; anoxia related to coughing paroxysms with obstructive apnea probably accounts for most of the central nervous system insult. Whether metabolic disturbances, hypoglycemia, hemorrhage, or toxins play a role is unclear (25,26).

EPIDEMIOLOGY

Pertussis demonstrates a number of striking epidemiologic features. *B. pertussis* and *B. parapertussis* are strictly human pathogens that have no animal reservoir. Pertussis occurs in all parts of the world with no clearcut yearly pattern, although some regions have a higher seasonal attack rate. Both endemic disease and epidemic disease can occur, the latter every 2 to 5 years even in highly immunized populations (27–29), suggesting that immunization may protect individuals but not prevent spread (30). Unlike most other infections, pertussis is more common in females (2). Attack rates do not vary appreciably by race.

Pertussis is highly contagious. Person-to-person transmission occurs through aerosolized large respiratory droplets. Transmission occurs during the catarrhal stage and during the first 2 to 3 weeks of the paroxysmal phase. The attack rate ranges from 70% to 100% in susceptible household contacts, and from 25% to 50% in schools (17). Hospital outbreaks have been reported (31–34), as have outbreaks in schools and day care centers (35,36), even in communities with high immunization rates. In urban areas, pertussis infection clusters in areas of poverty (37). Asymptomatic carriage is not well documented and is not felt to represent a source of spread (38). Disease transmission usually occurs in settings in which symptomatic coughing adults with unrecognized infection (39) spread disease to inadequately immunized infants, who in turn become more dramatically ill, ultimately prompting recognition of the correct diagnosis of pertussis. Immunity after natural infection is thought to be lifelong, with second symptomatic episodes being uncommon (2). On the other hand, vaccine-induced immunity is not durable; by 5 to 10 years after immunization, most individuals are susceptible to infection (40–42). Serologic surveys demonstrate a high frequency of undiagnosed infection in young men (43) and studies of young adults with cough lasting more than 1 to 2 weeks demonstrate evidence of recent pertussis infection in more than 20% (44–47).

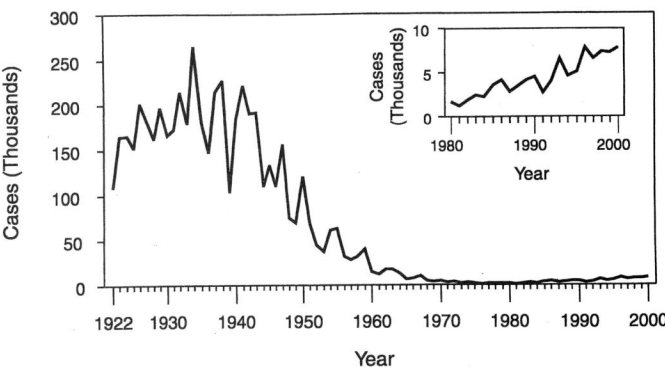

Figure 206.1. Reported cases of pertussis in the United States, from 1922 to 2000. (From Centers for Disease Control and Prevention. Pertussis—United States, 1997–2000. *MMWR Morb Mortal Wkly Rep* 2002;51:73–76, with permission.)

Practice guidelines for managing cough and bronchitis emphasize the importance of pertussis (48,49).

Before a vaccine was introduced, more than 90% of persons in the United States developed clinical pertussis, with young children (ages 1 to 5 years) being most frequently infected (2). Attack rates started to decline in the early 1900s, and a more precipitous decrease followed introduction of vaccine in the 1940s (50,51). Before routine vaccination was implemented, there were approximately 150 cases per 100,000 population in the United States, with 115,000 to 270,000 cases per year and 5,000 to 10,000 deaths. By the mid-1970s, the incidence decreased to its lowest point, about 1 case per 100,000 per year with 5 to 10 deaths reported annually (28). However, since the late 1970s and 1980s, more pertussis cases have been reported, with one third occurring in young infants (52–56) (Fig. 206.1). [It is estimated that only about 10% of cases are formally reported in the United States (56).] The highest incidence of severe disease is in infants younger than 6 months, who represent 80% of hospital days and virtually all the mortality (an average of 15 deaths per year in the late 1990s) (56). Newborns do not necessarily gain transplacental protection even when mothers are immune because of natural infection. Currently, children between ages 1 and 9 years (the population with the highest vaccination rate) represent just 20% of reported pertussis cases, much lower than in prevaccination days (56) (Table 206.1).

The population of pertussis-susceptible teenagers and young adults is increasing because of waning vaccine protection, whereas the population of older persons who have lifelong immunity as a consequence of natural disease is declining (59) (Fig. 206.2). The increase in reported incidence of pertussis recently is mainly due to increased disease in adolescents and young adults, and it is likely that most patients now infected with *B. pertussis* are adults (46). This trend is worrisome, because young susceptible infants are inevitably exposed to young adult parents and caretakers and will increasingly have exposure to pertussis. Thus, even with widespread use of an effective childhood vaccine, pertussis outbreaks will continue to occur unless adolescents and young adults receive booster immunizations.

CLINICAL MANIFESTATIONS

Traditionally, pertussis has been arbitrarily divided into catarrhal, paroxysmal, and convalescent stages, the entire duration of illness usually being 6 to 12 weeks (thus the Chinese term "the 100-day cough"). Illness is most severe in young infants, in

TABLE 206.1. Pertussis-Related Hospitalizations and Deaths, by Age-Group—United States, 1997–2000

Age-group	No. with pertussis		Hospitalized		Deaths	
	No.	(%)	No.	(%)	No.	(%)
<6 mo	7,203	(25.6)	4,543	(63.1)	56	(0.8)
6–11 mo	1,073	(3.8)	301	(28.1)	1	(0.1)
1–4 yr	3,137	(11.1)	324	(10.3)	1	(<0.1)
5–9 yr	2,756	(9.8)	86	(3.1)	2	(0.1)
10–19 yr	8,273	(29.4)	174	(2.1)	0	—
≥20 yr	5,745	(20.4)	202	(3.5)	2	(<0.1)
Total	28,187[a]		5,630	(20.0)	62	(0.2)

[a]Excludes 92 (0.3%) persons of unknown age with pertussis.
Source: From centers for Disease Control and Prevention. Pertussis—United States. 1997–2000. *MMWR Morb Mortal Wkly Rep* 2002;51:73–76, with permission.

those who were either remotely or never immunized (60) and in persons with *B. pertussis* (as opposed to *B. parapertussis*) infection. After an average incubation period of 7 days (range, 6 to 20 days), the patient develops mild upper respiratory tract symptoms with coryza, conjunctival injection, tearing, and sneezing. After the first week, a cough develops; usually dry and hacking, it becomes more intense and frequent and may be triggered by such stimuli as exercise, eating, or drinking. Fever is usually low grade or absent, and patients generally feel systemically well. Except in outbreak situations, the disease generally goes unrecognized during this catarrhal stage; unfortunately, this is also the period of greatest contagiousness.

After the first week, the illness enters the paroxysmal stage, which generally lasts 2 to 4 weeks. The cough becomes more pronounced, with increasingly severe attacks that often are debilitating. A paroxysm consists of a long series of forceful, staccato coughs during a single expiration. During these attacks, there may be protruding of the tongue and drooling, tearing, bulging of the eyes, facial cyanosis, and bulging of the head and neck veins. At the end of the violent expiration, during which the patient is reflexly trying to clear the tenacious secretions from the upper airway, there is a sudden inspiratory gasp as air is forcefully inhaled through the glottic opening, producing the characteristic stridulous "whoop" (61).

A whoop is usually heard in young preschool children, but not in infants in the first months of life, and it is usually absent or less pronounced in adolescents and adults. Paroxysms may be triggered by a number of events, including eating, drinking, yawning, sneezing, or being examined, and even by suggestion. Vomiting or coughing of clear fluid often follows the attacks, and patients may become transiently exhausted. Between paroxysms, however, patients generally appear well and are comfortable with no fever and a normal respiratory rate. The physical examination may be entirely normal between attacks, or it may reveal some manifestations of the increased pressure generated during the violent cough and vomiting, such as facial or eyelid edema, petechiae, subconjunctival hemorrhages, or erosion of the lingual frenulum. The chest examination is usually normal or may reveal scattered rhonchi; wheezing and signs of consolidation are generally absent.

During the convalescent stage (usually lasting 2 weeks to 3 months), the coughing spells gradually decrease in number and severity. Mild cough may persist for several months, and coughing paroxysms may be triggered by subsequent respiratory tract infections in the absence of new pertussis infection.

Pertussis-related morbidity and mortality are greatest for small infants (62–64). For children younger than 3 to 6 months, in whom whoop is usually absent, *B. pertussis* sometimes may not be considered among the numerous respiratory tract pathogens that commonly cause illness in this age-group (65). In *B. pertussis*–infected infants, feeding difficulties, choking spells, and apnea may be seen, with or without apparent coughing paroxysms. Because the less effective cough mechanism of small infants leads to inability to clear upper airway secretions, respiratory tract obstruction with apnea, hypoxemia, and resultant asphyxia may occur (66). Infants presenting with an apparent life-threatening event may have pertussis (67), but sudden infant death syndrome *per se* is not associated with this infection (68). Older children and adults tend to have milder disease, especially those who have been immunized. Adults with pertussis are typically only mildly ill, with a cough that lasts several weeks (69). Occasionally the coughing spells may be paroxysmal and incapacitating, with affected individuals gasping, choking, and even collapsing because of difficulty getting their breath, despite feeling well between attacks. Complications such as sinusitis, sleep

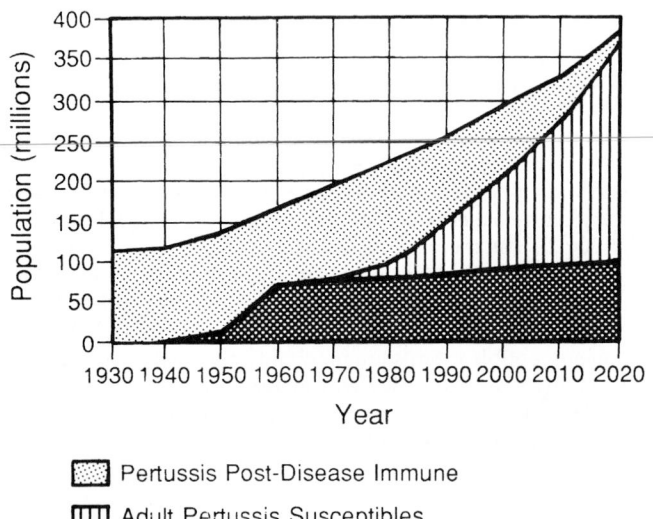

Pertussis Post-Disease Immune

Adult Pertussis Susceptibles

Pertussis Vaccine Immune (1 to 20 years old)

Figure 206.2. Projected pertussis epidemiology in the United States through the year 2020 with continued use of childhood pertussis vaccines. (Adapted from Bass JW, Stephenson SR. The return of pertussis. *Pediatr Infect Dis J* 1987;6:141–144, with permission.)

disturbance, and incontinence are described (70). Unfortunately, however, unless there are unusual epidemiologic circumstances, the possibility of pertussis is unlikely to be considered in adults (71,72).

Complications of pertussis are usually confined to the respiratory tract and central nervous system or are related to the intense mechanical forces generated during coughing paroxysms. Otitis media is a common complication. In addition, pneumonia, usually secondary to bacterial superinfection or to aspiration (rather than to primary infection caused by *Bordetella*) may result, in part due to the damaged respiratory tract epithelium. Such patients usually develop fever, tachypnea, and focal infiltrates, features that distinguish their condition from those with uncomplicated pertussis. In addition, patients with pertussis may develop atelectasis, particularly of the right upper lobe, which may persist for months. Longitudinal studies are inconclusive about whether there is detectable long-term impairment of pulmonary function in children who have recovered from pertussis (73,74).

Central nervous system dysfunction is unusual during pertussis but can be severe and rarely can even occur in adults (75,76). It may be manifested by seizures; by encephalopathy with development of gradual coma (with or without seizures); or by specific abnormalities such as hemiplegia, paraplegia, blindness, or deafness. In some cases, the manifestations are thought to be secondary to anoxia; in others, there is evidence of cerebral hemorrhage and thrombosis (77). In addition, toxins may play a role in some cases (25). The cerebrospinal fluid is usually normal; mild pleocytosis (less than 100 cells/mm^3) and protein elevation (less than 100 mg/dL) are occasionally seen. Long-term follow-up of children with pertussis suggests that those with uncomplicated disease have normal intelligence and reading performance (78), whereas those with apnea or seizures may sustain long-term intellectual and school impairment (79).

The high pressures generated by the explosive cough of pertussis have resulted in a number of hemorrhagic events ranging from subconjunctival hemorrhages, petechiae, and epistaxis to melena and subdural and spinal epidural hematomas. Other mechanical consequences of the violent cough and vomiting include ulceration of the frenulum, umbilical and inguinal hernias, rectal prolapse, herniated disc, pneumothorax, mediastinal and subcutaneous emphysema, and diaphragmatic rupture.

DIAGNOSIS

The diagnosis of pertussis can often be made readily on clinical grounds, especially during outbreaks, because of the distinctive findings during the paroxysmal stage and the protracted nature of the cough. Laboratory tests may be helpful. During the late catarrhal and paroxysmal stages, the white blood cell (WBC) count is typically elevated, often in the range of 20,000 to 30,000 cells/mm^3, with a predominance of small, mature lymphocytes. Hyperleukocytosis (WBC count more than 100,000) is occasionally encountered in infants and is associated with respiratory failure and death (80). However, the WBC count may be normal, especially in small infants and in older persons. The erythrocyte sedimentation rate is generally normal or even low (81). The chest radiograph is usually normal; on occasion, it may demonstrate dense markings that fan out from the heart borders, the so-called *shaggy heart sign* (82). These densities reflect peribronchial thickening rather than pneumonic infiltrates.

The differential diagnosis of severe paroxysmal coughing includes infection by other agents that may be associated with a severe coughing illness. *B. parapertussis* and *B. bronchiseptica*

cause a similar illness that is generally milder than that caused by *B. pertussis*. A number of adenovirus serotypes have been recovered from patients with clinical pertussis, but usually from those who have concurrent *B. pertussis* infection; an independent role for adenoviruses in causing a pertussis syndrome has not been conclusively established (83). Respiratory syncytial virus may also be isolated from patients with proven *B. pertussis* infection, but it does not appear to cause the pertussis syndrome by itself (84). *Chlamydia trachomatis* respiratory tract infection in infants, which generally occurs between 4 and 8 weeks of life, is also associated with a prominent cough, but that of chlamydial disease is described as a series of staccato expirations, each followed by an inspiration (as opposed to pertussis, in which the inspiration comes only at the end of the paroxysm) (85). In addition, infants with chlamydial respiratory tract disease, unlike those with pertussis, usually have resting tachypnea and hypoxemia, with rales on auscultation and infiltrates on chest radiography; laboratory studies may demonstrate peripheral eosinophilia and hypergammaglobulinemia. Noninfectious diseases to be considered with pertussis include conditions associated with severe coughing such as cystic fibrosis, foreign body aspiration, tracheoesophageal fistula, gastroesophageal reflux, and mass lesions compressing the trachea.

Diagnosis of pertussis requires recovery of the organism in culture; demonstration of its presence by deoxyribonucleic acid (DNA) detection techniques, direct fluorescein-labeled immunofluorescence antibody (DFA) stains, or other immunohistochemical technique; or the development of specific antibody responses. The most definitive means for making a diagnosis of pertussis is recovery of the organism from nasopharyngeal specimens, but *B. pertussis* is fastidious and grows slowly, and attempts to isolate it may fail up to 50% of the time (compared with seroconversion) (4). Highest rates of recovery are achieved by collecting nasopharyngeal secretions with calcium alginate swabs on a flexible wire and inoculating them immediately onto suitable selective media at the patient's bedside. Use of cotton-tipped swabs or delayed inoculation of media decreases the likelihood of successful isolation. Recovery rates may also be increased by obtaining both a nasopharyngeal swab and a nasal suction aspirate (86). The recovery rate for *B. pertussis* is highest during the first 2 to 3 weeks of illness and declines thereafter, even in the absence of antibiotic administration. Specimens from patients who have received antimicrobial therapy or who were previously immunized are less likely to yield the organism.

A DFA staining technique has been used in an attempt to circumvent some of the difficulties of culture. Although attractive because of the ability to obtain rapid results, sensitivity and specificity are suboptimal (87,88). The DFA test is less sensitive than culture early in the illness and more sensitive in later stages. Quality-control issues and technical experience affect the results. Unfortunately, culture is an insensitive "gold standard" for comparison. In experienced hands, a positive DFA test determination is useful in making a presumptive diagnosis of pertussis, but such results should be confirmed by culture, DNA detection, or serologic studies.

The use of polymerase chain reaction (PCR) to diagnose pertussis has evolved over the past decade (89–91) and may supplant culture and DFA techniques where available. PCR results in general correlate with culture, with PCR-negative culture-positive results generally only seen in patients with very low colony counts. On the other hand, PCR-positive culture-negative results occur more often, reflecting the fastidious microbiologic nature of the organism and the high sensitivity of PCR assays, which can detect low numbers and even dead organisms (90,91). PCR is more sensitive than culture, and aside from its expense and unavailability in all clinical settings, appears to be the diagnostic procedure of choice (92).

Several antibody responses to *B. pertussis* have been described. A frequently used and well-studied response in the past has been the agglutination reaction; however, because of the absence of a standardized method, the test's poor sensitivity, and the lack of commercially available test reagents, it has a limited role in the diagnosis of pertussis. Currently the most useful tests for diagnosing pertussis are assessment of immunoglobulin A (IgA) and immunoglobulin G (IgG) antibodies to PT and FHA with an enzyme-linked immunosorbent assay (4,92). IgA develops after infection but not after immunization and generally declines to low levels after a few months in the absence of exposure. Immunoglobulin M assays have not been consistently reliable. Clinical case definitions that do not depend on laboratory confirmation (e.g., cough longer than 2 weeks or paroxysmal cough longer than 1 week) have been used in monitoring community outbreaks (56,93).

TREATMENT

The most important aspect of treatment of patients with pertussis is the provision of general supportive care. Infants younger than 3 to 6 months are at greatest risk for serious complications and generally should be hospitalized, monitored closely, and supported until coughing paroxysms, apnea, cyanosis, and feeding problems have resolved or have diminished to the point that they can be managed safely at home. Such support includes the use of oxygen and judicious suctioning, avoidance of unnecessary stimuli, and fluid and nutritional support. In terms of pharmacologic support, the few data available on corticosteroids suggest that these drugs are safe in small children and may ultimately reduce the number of coughing paroxysms if administered for more than a few days (94,95). Similarly, inhaled β-adrenergic agents are safe and may reduce coughing (96,97). Administration of specific antipertussis immunoglobulin is under study and may prove beneficial in reducing cough frequency and duration (98,99).

Because of the contagiousness of *B. pertussis*, droplet (mask) precautions are recommended until the index case has received antibiotic therapy for 5 days (100) to prevent transmission and hospital outbreaks. *In vitro* and *in vivo*, erythromycin has been demonstrated to be the most efficacious antimicrobial agent (101,102), although resistance has been reported (103,104). The most important role of antibiotic therapy is to reduce contagiousness by eliminating the organism from the nasopharyngeal secretions of the index patient. If erythromycin is given during the incubation period or early catarrhal stage, it may also prevent or ameliorate clinical disease (105). Therapy not begun until the paroxysmal stage generally has no immediate discernible impact on the clinical course, but in fact, whoop frequency may ultimately be reduced in such patients (106,107). Erythromycin therapy for 2 weeks has been recommended to avoid bacterial relapse (100), but 1 week of therapy appears to be equally effective (108). Erythromycin estolate may be the preferred form of the drug, especially for children (104). In small infants, erythromycin administration for pertussis has been associated with pyloric stenosis (109). Shorter course treatment with azithromycin or clarithromycin also appears to be sufficient (110,111). Trimethoprim-sulfamethoxazole is generally considered to be the second drug of choice for persons who are allergic to or intolerant of erythromycin, but efficacy data are much more limited. The fluoroquinolones also demonstrate *in vitro* activity, but clinical data are lacking.

Intimate contacts of pertussis-infected persons, including household, day care, and classroom contacts, and health care providers who did not adhere to droplet precautions, should also receive a full prophylactic course of erythromycin or equivalently effective agent, regardless of their immunization status. Contacts younger than 7 years should also generally receive diphtheria and tetanus toxoids and acellular pertussis vaccine if they are not fully immunized, as outlined in official guidelines (100).

PREVENTION

Vaccines for pertussis were first studied in the 1920s and came into widespread use in the late 1940s and early 1950s. The whole-cell vaccine developed in the United States was composed of a suspension of inactivated *B. pertussis* combined with diphtheria and tetanus toxoids (DTP) and adsorbed onto an aluminum salt adjuvant. The protective efficacy in fully immunized children was 80% to 90%. Durability of humoral protection, however, is limited to about a decade, as previously discussed. Five doses of vaccine are recommended (100). The primary series consists of a dose administered at 2 months of age; two additional doses given at intervals of 2 months; a fourth dose given at 12 to 18 months of age, and a fifth and last dose given as a kindergarten booster at age 4 to 6 years. In outbreak situations, immunizations may be started as early as 2 weeks of age, and doses may be scheduled at intervals as short as 1 month. Minor adverse reactions to vaccine are common: erythema, swelling, or pain at the injection site and fever, drowsiness, fretfulness, and anorexia. These reactions generally occur on the day of administration and subside uneventfully.

Less common but more severe sequelae of whole-cell pertussis immunization include convulsions (usually associated with fever); persistent uncontrollable screaming or an unusual, high-pitched cry; collapse or shocklike state (hypotonic-hyporesponsive episode); and temperature greater than 40.5°C. Anaphylaxis has been exceedingly rare. No causal relationship between pertussis immunization and sudden infant death syndrome or infantile spasms is recognized (17), and a family history of seizures does not constitute a contraindication to pertussis immunization.

Complacency about the seriousness of pertussis combined with concerns about whole-cell pertussis vaccine toxicity led to a marked decline in use of the vaccine in many countries during the 1970s and, subsequently, a large increase in the number of reported cases of pertussis in England, Japan, and Sweden. Careful analysis of the available data suggests that neurologic illness associated with DTP whole-cell vaccine was not actually caused by the vaccine. Rather, DTP immunization may have unmasked (i.e., accelerated the onset of) a neurologic disorder that would have eventually become manifest anyway. Results of numerous careful risk/benefit analyses indicate that the benefits of vaccination far outweigh the risk (17), and most experts including the American Academy of Pediatrics have concluded that pertussis vaccine has not been proven to cause brain damage (100).

In the past decade, acellular pertussis vaccines, which have been used in Japan for more than two decades, have come into use in the United States (112,113). These vaccines, extensively studied in the United States and Europe, consist of at least one of the components of the organism. All contain inactivated PT; other components include FHA, pertactin and types 2 and 3 fimbriae. Studies searching for a serologic marker of protection have shown that high antibody levels against pertactin, PT, and fimbriae (but not FHA) correlated with lower rates of pertussis (115,116). In general, vaccines with three or more antigens have been found to be more immunogenic than those containing one or two components (114). Although serum antibodies decline after immunization, cellular responses are more sustained (117,118). Duration of immunity is not known. Acellular vaccines are less reactigenic, with fewer local, systemic, and neurologic reactions than with whole-cell vaccines. As with DTP, reactions may become more pronounced over time; for example, the fourth and fifth dose may rarely be associated with swelling of the entire limb (119). Overall, the acellular vaccines appear to be as efficacious as whole-cell vaccines. Several acellular vaccines have been licensed and approved for use in the United States, and whole-cell vaccine is no longer used.

Acellular vaccines have been studied in adolescents and adults (120), and data supporting immunogenicity and efficacy are encouraging (121). It is clear that overall reduction of pertussis and elimination of disease in infants will require administration of vaccine to adolescents and perhaps young adults (122,123). If booster doses are administered beyond age 6 years, it is possible that pertussis could join diphtheria and tetanus as diseases for which serial immunizations could reduce disease incidence to very low levels (124).

REFERENCES

1. Cone TE. Whooping cough is first described as a disease *sui generis* by Baillou in 1640. *Pediatrics* 1970;46:522.
2. Gordon JE, Hood RL. Whooping cough and its epidemiological anomalies. *Am J Med Sci* 1951;222:333–361.
3. Ivanoff B, Robertson SE. Pertussis: a worldwide problem [Review]. *Dev Biol Stand* 1997;89:3–13.
4. Hoppe JE. *Bordetella*. In: Murray PR, ed. *Manual of clinical microbiology*, 7th ed. Washington, DC: American Society for Microbiology, 1999:614–624.
5. He Q, Viljanen MK, Arvilommi H, et al. Whooping cough caused by *Bordetella pertussis* and *Bordetella parapertussis* in an immunized population. *JAMA* 1998;280:635–637.
6. Stefanelli P, Mastrontonio P, Hausman SZ, et al. Molecular characterization of two *Bordetella bronchiseptica* strains isolated from children with coughs. *J Clin Microbiol* 1997;35:1550–1555.
7. Woolfrey BF, Moody JA. Human infections associated with *Bordetella bronchiseptica*. *Clin Microbiol Rev* 1991;4:243–255.
8. Kersters K, Hinz KH, Hertle A. *Bordetella avium* sp. nov. isolated from the respiratory tracts of turkeys and other birds. *Int J Syst Bacteriol* 1984;34:56–58.
9. Vandamme P, Hinz KH, Schemken-Birk EM, et al. Isolations of a *Bordetella avium*–like organism from a human specimen. *Eur J Clin Microbiol Infect Dis* 1995;14:451–454.
10. Kattar MM, Chavez JF, Limaye AP, et al. Applications of 16S rRNA gene sequencing to identify *Bordetella hinzii* as the causative agent of fatal septicemia. *J Clin Microbiol* 2000;38:789–794.
11. Furke G, Hess T, Vandamme P. Characteristics of *Bordetella hinzii* strains isolated from a cystic fibrosis patient over a 3-year period. *J Clin Microbiol* 1996;34:966–969.
12. Vandamme P, Heyndrickx M, Vancanneyt M, et al. *Bordetella trematum* sp. nov., isolated from wounds and ear infections in humans. *Infect J Syst Bacteriol* 1996;46:849–858.
13. Russell FM, Davis JM, Whipp MJ, et al. Severe *Bordetella holmesii* infection in a previously healthy adolescent confirmed by gene sequence analysis. *Clin Infect Dis* 2001;33:129–130.
14. Mazenqiu E, Silva EA, Peppe JA, et al. Recovery of *Bordetella holmesii* from patients with pertussis-like symptoms. *J Clin Microbiol* 2000;38:2330–2333.
15. Hoppe JE, Vogel R. Comparison of three media for culture of *Bordetella Pertussis* spp. *Eur J Clin Microbiol* 1986;5:361–362.
16. Katzko GM, Hofmeister M, Church D. Extended incubation of culture plates improves recovery of *Bordetella* spp. *J Clin Microbiol* 1996;34:1563–1564.
17. Cherry JD, Brunnel PA, Golden GJ, et al. Report of the task force on pertussis and pertussis immunization—1988. *Pediatrics* 1988;81[Suppl]:939–984.
18. Cattaneo L, Edwards K. *Bordetella pertussis* (whooping cough). *Semin Pediatr Infect Dis* 1995;6:107–117.
19. Pittman M. The concept of pertussis as a toxin-mediated disease. *Pediatr Infect Dis* 1984;3:467–486.
20. Smith AM, Guzman CA, Walker MJ. The virulence factors of *Bordetella pertussis*: a matter of control. *FEMS Microbiol Rev* 2001;25:309–333.
21. Kerr JR, Mathews RC. *Bordetella pertussis* infection: pathogenesis, diagnosis, management, and the role of protective immunity. *Eur J Clin Microbiol Infect Dis* 2000;19:77–88.
22. Weiss AA, Hewlett EL, Myers GA, et al. Tn S-induced mutations affecting virulence factors of *Bordetella pertussis*. *Infect Immun* 1983;42:33–41.
23. Friedman RL, Nordensson K, Wilson C, et al. Uptake and intracellular survival of *Bordetella pertussis* in human macrophages. *Infect Immun* 1992;60:4578–4585.
24. Hewlett EL. Pertussis: current concepts of pathogenesis and prevention. *Pediatr Infect Dis J* 1997;16:578–584.
25. Davis LE, Burstyn DG, Manclark CR. Pertussis encephalopathy with a normal brain biopsy and elevated lymphocytosis-promoting factor antibodies. *Pediatr Infect Dis* 1984;3:448–451.
26. Halperin SA, Marrie TJ. Pertussis encephalopathy in an adult: case report and review. *Rev Infect Dis* 1991;13:1043–1047.
27. Thomas M. Epidemiology of pertussis. *Rev Infect Dis* 1989;11:255–262.
28. Farizo KM, Cochi SL, Zell ER, et al. Epidemiologic features of pertussis in the United States, 1980–1989. *Clin Infect Dis* 1992;14:708–719.
29. Wright PF. Pertussis in developing countries: definition of the problem and prospects for control. *Rev Infect Dis* 1991;13[Suppl 6]:S528–S534.
30. Fine PEM, Clarkson SA. The recurrence of whooping cough: possible implications for assessment of vaccine efficacy. *Lancet* 1982;1:666–669.
31. Kurt TL, Yeager AS, Guenette S, et al. Spread of pertussis by hospital staff. *JAMA* 1972;221:264–267.
32. Shefer A, Dales L, Nelson M, et al. Use and safety of acellular pertussis vaccine among adult hospital staff during an outbreak of pertussis. *J Infect Dis* 1995;171:1053–1057.
33. Haiduven DJ, Hench CP, Simpkins SM, et al. Standardized management of patients and employees exposed to pertussis. *Infect Control Hosp Epidemiol* 1998;19:861–864.
34. Sherertz RJ, Bassetti S, Bassetti-Wyss B. "Cloud" health-care workers. *Emerg Infect Dis* 2001;7:241–244.
35. Brennan M, Strebel P, George H, et al. Evidence for transmission of pertussis in schools, Massachusetts, 1996. *J Infect Dis* 2000;18:210–215.
36. Christie CD, Marx ML, Daniels JA, et al. Pertussis containment in schools and day care centers during the Cincinnati epidemic of 1993. *Am J Public Health* 1997;87:460–462.
37. Siegol C, Davidson A, Kafadar K, et al. Geographic analysis of pertussis infection in an urban area: a tool for health services planning. *Am J Public Health* 1997;87:2022–2026.
38. Bass JW. Is there a carrier state in pertussis? *Lancet* 1987;1:96–98.
39. Deville JG, Cherry JD, Christenson PD. Frequency of unrecognized *Bordetella pertussis* infections in adults. *Clin Infect Dis* 1995;21:639–642.
40. Lambert H. Epidemiology of a small pertussis outbreak in Kent County Michigan. *Public Health Rep* 1965;80:365–369.
41. Jenkinson D. Duration of effectiveness of pertussis vaccine: evidence from a 10 year community study. *Br Med J* 1988;296:612–614.
42. Mink CM, Sirota NM, Nugent S. Outbreak of pertussis in a fully immunized adolescent and adult population. *Arch Pediatr Adolesc Med* 1994;148:153–157.
43. Cherry J, Beer T, Chartrand S, et al. Comparison of values of antibody to *Bordetella pertussis* antigens in young German and American men. *Clin Infect Dis* 1995;20:1271.
44. Mink CM, Cherry JD, Christenson P, et al. A search for *Bordetella pertussis* in university students. *Clin Infect Dis* 1992;14:464–471.
45. Wright SW, Edwards KM, Decker MD, et al. Pertussis infection in adults with persistent cough. *JAMA* 1995;273:1044–1046.
46. Black S. Epidemiology of pertussis. *Pediatr Infect Dis J* 1997;16:585–589.
47. Miller E, Fleming DM, Ashworth LA, et al. Serological evidence of pertussis in patients presenting with cough in general pediatric in Birmingham. *Commun Dis Public Health* 2000;3:132–134.
48. Irwin RJ, Madison JM. Primary care: the diagnosis and treatment of cough. *N Engl J Med* 2000;343:1715–1721.
49. Gonzales R, Sande MA. Uncomplicated acute bronchitis. *Ann Intern Med* 2000;133:981–991.
50. Cherry JD. The epidemiology of pertussis and pertussis immunization in the United Kingdom and the United States: a comparative study. *Curr Probl Pediatr* 1984;14:1–77.
51. Hodder S, Mortimer E. Epidemiology of pertussis and reactions to pertussis vaccine. *Epidemiol Rev* 1992;14:243–267.
52. Centers for Disease Control and Prevention. Resurgence of pertussis—United States, 1993. *MMWR Morb Mortal Wkly Rep* 1993;42:952–956.
53. Bass J, Wittler R. Return of epidemic pertussis in the United States. *Pediatr Infect Dis J* 1994;13:343–345.
54. Guris D, Strebel P, Bardenheier B, et al. Changing epidemiology of pertussis in the United States: increasing reported incidence among adolescents and adults, 1990–96. *Clin Infect Dis* 1999;28:1230–1237.
55. Sutter RW, Cochi SL. Pertussis hospitalizations and mortality in the United States, 1985–1988: evaluation of the completeness of national reporting. *JAMA* 1992;267:386–391.
56. Centers for Disease Control and Prevention. Pertussis—United States, 1997–2000. *MMWR Morb Mortal Wkly Rep* 2002;51:73–76.
57. Marchant C, Loughlin A, Lett S, et al. Pertussis in Massachusetts, 1981–1991: incidence, serologic diagnosis, and vaccine effectiveness. *J Infect Dis* 1994;169:1297–1305.

58. Gordon M, David HD, Gold R. Clinical and microbiologic features of children presenting with pertussis to a Canadian pediatric hospital during an eleven-year period. *Pediatr Infect Dis J* 1994;13:617.

59. Bass JW, Stephenson SR. The return of pertussis. *Pediatr Infect Dis J* 1987;6:141–144.

60. Stojunov S, Liese J, Belohradsky BH. Hospitalization and complications in children under two years of age with *Bordetella pertussis* infection. *Infection* 2000;28:106–110.

61. Olson LC. Pertussis. *Medicine (Baltimore)* 1975;54:427–465.

62. Runganattan S, Tasker R, Booy R, et al. Pertussis is increasing in unim-munized infants: is a change in policy needed? *Arch Dis Child* 1999;80:297–299.

63. Hoppe JE. Neonatal pertussis. *Pediatr Infec Dis J* 2000;19:244–247.

64. Smith C, Vyas H. Early infantile pertussis; increasingly prevalent and poten-tially fatal. *Eur J Pediatr* 2000;159:898–900.

65. Sotomayor J, Wiener LB, McMillan JA. Inaccurate diagnosis in infants with pertussis: an 8 year experience. *Am J Dis Child* 1985;139:724–727.

66. Southall DP, Thomas MG, Lambert HP. Severe hypoxemia in pertussis. *Arch Dis Child* 1988;163:598–605.

67. Davies F, Gupta R. Apparent life-threatening events in infants presenting to an emergency department. *Emerg Med J* 2002;19:11–16.

68. Jan MSJ, Halperin S. Pertussis epidemic and sudden infant death syndrome. *Clin Pediatr* 1998;37:449–452.

69. Jenkinson D. Natural course of 500 consecutive cases of whooping cough: a general practice population study. *BMJ* 1995;310:299–302.

70. De Serres G, Shadmani R, Duval B, et al. Morbidity of pertussis in adolescents and adults. *J Infect Dis* 2000;182:174–179.

71. Deeks S, De Serres G, Boulianne N. Failure of physicians to consider the di-agnosis of pertussis. *Clin Infect Dis* 1999;28:840–846.

72. Cherry JD. Pertussis in adults. *Ann Intern Med* 1998;128:64–66.

73. Johnston IDA, Bland JM, Ingram D, et al. Effect of whooping cough in infancy on subsequent lung infection. *Am Rev Respir Dis* 1986;134:270–275.

74. Howenstine M, Eigen H, Tepper R. Pulmonary function in infants after per-tussis. *J Pediatr* 1991;118:563–566.

75. Hewlett EL. *Bordetella pertussis* and the central nervous system. In: Scheid WM, ed. *Infections of the central nervous system.* New York: Raven Press, 1991:625–635.

76. Halperin SA, Morrie TJ. Pertussis encephalopathy in an adult: case report and review. *Rev Infect Dis* 1991;13:1043–1047.

77. Zellweger H. Pertussis encephalopathy. *Arch Pediatr* 1959;76:381–382.

78. Johnston IDA. Reading attainment and physical development after whooping cough. *J Epidemiol Commun Health* 1985;39:314.

79. Swansea Research Unit of the Royal College of General Practitioners. Study of intellectual performance of children in ordinary school after certain serious complications of whooping cough. *Br Med J* 1987;295:1044–1047.

80. Pierie C, Klein N, Peters M. Is leukocytosis a predictor of mortality in severe pertussis? *Intensive Care Med* 2000;26:1512–1514.

81. Lagergren G. The white blood cell count and the erythrocyte sedimentation rate in pertussis. *Acta Paediatr* 1963;52:405–409.

82. Barnhard HJ, Kniker WT. Roentgenologic findings in pertussis with partic-ular emphasis on the "shaggy heart" sign. *AJR Am J Roentgenol* 1960;84:445–447.

83. Keller MA, Affandelians R, Connor JD. Etiology of pertussis syndrome. *Pedi-atrics* 1980;66:50–55.

84. Nelson WL, Hopkins RS, Roe MH, et al. Simultaneous infection with *Bordetella pertussis* and respiratory syncytial virus in hospitalized children. *Pediatr Infect Dis* 1986;5:540–544.

85. Beem MO, Saxon EM. Respiratory-tract colonization and a distinctive pneu-monia syndrome in infants infected with *Chlamydia trachomatis.* *N Engl J Med* 1977;296:306–310.

86. Bejuk D, Beguvac J, Buce A, et al. Culture of *Bordetella pertussis* from three upper respiratory tract specimens. *Pediatr Infect Dis J* 1995;14:64–65.

87. Evanowich CA, Chai LWL, Paranchuych MG, et al. Major outbreak of per-tussis in northern Alberta, Canada: analysis of discrepant direct fluorescent-antibody and culture results by using polymerase chain reaction methodology. *J Clin Microbiol* 1993;31:1715–25.

88. Halperin SA, Bartolussi R, Wert JR. Evaluation of culture, immunofluores-cence, and serology for the diagnosis of pertussis. *J Clin Microbiol* 1989;27:752–757.

89. Farrell DJ, McKeon M, Duggard G, et al. Rapid-cycle PCR method to detect *Bordetella pertussis* that fulfills all consensus recommendations for use of PCR in diagnosis of pertussis. *J Clin Microbiol* 2000;38:4499–4502.

90. Heininges U, Schmidt-Schläpfer G, Cherry J, et al. Clinical validation of a polymerase chain reaction assay for the diagnosis of pertussis by comparison with serology, culture and symptoms during a large pertussis vaccine efficacy trial. *Pediatrics* 2000;105:E31.

91. He Q, Schmidt-Schläpfer G, Just M, et al. Impact of polymerase chain reac-tion on clinical pertussis research: Finnish and Swiss experiences. *J Infect Dis* 1996;174:1288–1295.

92. Müller FM, Hoppe JE, Wirsing VM, et al. Laboratory diagnosis of pertussis: state of the art in 1997. *J Clin Microbiol* 1997;35:2435–2443.

93. Strebel PM, Cochi SL, Farizo KM, et al. Pertussis in Missouri: evaluation of nasopharyngeal culture, direct fluorescent antibody testing, and clinical case definitions in the diagnosis of pertussis. *Clin Infect Dis* 1993;16:276–285.

94. Torre D, Tambini R, Ferrario G, et al. Treatment with steroids in children with pertussis. *Pediatr Infect Dis J* 1993;2:419–420.

95. Roberts I, Gavin R, Lennon D. Randomized controlled trial of steroids in pertussis. *Pediatr Infect Dis J* 1992;11:982–983.

96. Krantz I, Norrby JR, Trollfors B. Salbutamol vs. placebo for treatment of per-tussis. *Pediatr Infect Dis J* 1985;4:638–640.

97. Mertsula J, Viljaned MK, Ruuskanen O. Salbutamol in the treatment of whoop-ing cough. *J Infect Dis* 1986;18:593–594.

98. Granstrom M, Olinder-Nielsen, Holmblad P. Specific immunoglobulin for treatment of whooping cough. *Lancet* 1991;338:1230–1232.

99. Bruss JB, Malley R, Halperin S, et al. Treatment of severe pertussis: a study of the safety and pharmacology of intravenous pertussis immunoglobulin. *Pediatr Infect Dis J* 1999;18:505–511.

100. American Academy of Pediatrics. Pertussis. In: Pickering LK, ed. *Red Book Report of the Committee on Infectious Diseases,* 26th ed. Elk Grove Village, IL: American Academy of Pediatrics, 2003:472–486.

101. Bass JW. Erythromycin for treatment and prevention of pertussis. *Pediatr Infect Dis* 1986;5:154–157.

102. Hoppe JE. State of art in antibacterial susceptibility of *Bordetella pertussis* and antibiotic treatment of pertussis. *Infection* 1998;26:242–246.

103. Lewis K, Soubolle MA, Tenover FC, et al. Pertussis caused by an erythromycin-resistant strain of *Bordetella pertussis.* *Pediatr Infect Dis J* 1995;14:388–391.

104. Korgenski EK, Daly JA. Surveillance and detection of erythromycin resistance in *Bordetella pertussis* isolates recovered from a pediatric population in the Intermountain West region of the United States. *J Clin Microbiol* 1997;35:2989–2991.

105. Bergquist S-O, Bernander S, Dahnsjo H, et al. Erythromycin in the treatment of pertussis: a study of bacteriologic and clinical effects. *Pediatr Infect Dis J* 1987;6:458–461.

106. Hoppe R. Comparison of erythromycin estolate and erythromycin ethylsuc-cinate for treatment of pertussis. *Pediatr Infect Dis J* 1991;11:189–193.

107. Hoppe JE, Haug A. Treatment and prevention of pertussis by antimicrobial agents (Part II). *Infection* 1988;16:148–152.

108. Halperin SA, Bartolussi R, Langley JM, et al. Seven days of erythromycin estolate is as effective as fourteen days for the treatment of *Bordetella pertussis* infections. *Pediatrics* 1997;100:65–71.

109. Anon. Hypertrophic pyloric stenosis in infants following pertussis prophy-laxis with erythromycin—Knoxville, Tennessee, 1999. *MMWR Morb Mortal Wkly Rep* 1999;48:1117–1120.

110. Bace A, Zrnic T, Begovac J, et al. Short-term treatment of pertussis with azithromycin in infants and young children. *Eur J Clin Microbiol Infect Dis* 1999;18:296–298.

111. Aoyama T, Sunakawa K, Iwata S, et al. Efficacy of short-term treatment of pertussis with clarithromycin and azithromycin. *J Pediatr* 1996;129:761–764.

112. Deiker MD, Edwards KM. Acellular pertussis vaccines. *Pediatr Clin North Am* 2000;47:309–335.

113. Schleiss MR, Dahl K. Acellular pertussis vaccines. *Curr Probl Pediatr* 2000;30:185–201.

114. Cherry JD. Comparative efficacy of acellular pertussis vaccines: an analysis of recent trials. *Pediatr Infect Dis J* 1997;165:590–596.

115. Cherry JD, Gornbein J, Heininger, et al. A search for serologic correlates of immunity to *Bordetella pertussis. Vaccine* 1998;16:1901–1906.

116. Stursaeter J, Hallender HO, Gustafsson L, et al. Levels of anti-pertussis anti-bodies related to protection after household exposure to *Bordetella pertussis. Vaccine* 1998;16:1907–1914.

117. Tran Minh NN, He Q, Edelman K, et al. Cell-mediated immune responses to antigens of *Bordetella pertussis* and protection against pertussis in school children. *Pediatr Infect Dis J* 1999;18:366–370.

118. Mills KH. Immunity to *Bordetella pertussis* [Review]. *Microbes Infect* 2001;3:655–677.

119. Use of diphtheria-tetanus toxoid-acellular pertussis vaccine as a five-dose series: supplemental recommendations of the Advisory Committee on Im-munization Practices (ACIP). *MMWR Morb Mortal Wkly Rep* 2000;49(RR-13): 1–16.

120. Keitel WA, Edwards KM. Acellular pertussis vaccines in adults. *Infect Dis Clin North Am* 1999;13:83–94.

121. Halperin S. Should all adolescents and adults be vaccinated against pertussis? *Infect Med* 2001;18:473–475.

122. Gardner P. Issues related to the decennial tetanus-diphtheria toxoid booster recommendations in adults. *Infect Dis Clin North Am* 2001;15:143–153.

123. Edwards KM. Is pertussis a frequent cause of cough in adolescents and adults? Should routine pertussis immunization be recommended? *CID* 2001;32:1698–1699.

124. Centers for Disease Control and Prevention. *Guidelines for the control of pertus-sis outbreaks.* Atlanta, GA: Centers for Disease Control and Prevention, 2000. Available at: *www.cdc.gov/nip/publications.* Accessed March 2002.

CHAPTER 207
Miscellaneous Gram-Negative Bacilli: Acinetobacter, Cardiobacterium, Actinobacillus, Chromobacterium, Capnocytophaga, *and Others*

Judith L. Nerad and Stephanie Black

Although most gram-negative infections that are clinically significant are caused by members of the Enterobacteriaceae and Pseudomonadaceae, a small percentage of infections are caused by various uncommon gram-negative organisms.

These are usually identified by Gram stain and growth characteristics, biochemical reactions, and appropriate epidemiologic circumstances. Patients infected with these more unusual gram-negative organisms may present with both localized and systemic infections, be normal or immunocompromised hosts, and present with acute or chronic disease. These infections arise from endogenous or environmental exposures.

These heterogeneous organisms are often grouped according to their ability to ferment glucose (produce acid from carbohydrate in the absence of oxygen). Therefore, they are considered here as such and are discussed in the groupings glucose fermenters and nonfermenters (Table 207.1). See subsequent tables for other general characteristics regarding natural reservoirs (Table 207.2), clinical manifestations of infection (Table 207.3), antimicrobial susceptibilities (Table 207.4), and host immune defects (Table 207.5).

GLUCOSE FERMENTERS

Actinobacillus

The genus *Actinobacillus* consists of several species: *Actinobacillus lignieresii* (type species), *Actinobacillus equuli*, *Actinobacillus suis*, *Actinobacillus hominis*, *Actinobacillus pleuropneumoniae*, and *Actinobacillus actinomycetemcomitans* (1). The last affects only humans; the others have rarely been associated with disease in humans and more often infect domestic animals. *A. pleuropneumoniae* (2) is a significant pathogen in pigs. *A. actinomycetemcomitans* was initially described in 1912. For 50 years, the organism was thought to be a contaminant and not a pathogen because of the frequency with which it was isolated in infections with *Actinomyces israelii* (1). There is some debate whether *A. actinomycetemcomitans* should be classified in the genus *Haemophilus* (2).

A. actinomycetemcomitans refers to a bacillus in ray form that accompanies an actinomycete. It is a gram-negative bacillus predominantly but is found in both coccobacillary and filamentous forms. Biochemically, it is oxidase variable and catalase positive, does not hydrolyze urea or form indole, and does reduce ni-

trates. It is nonmotile and does not grow on MacConkey's agar. It ferments glucose, not lactose or sucrose. Growth in blood culture media may not be seen until 3 to 6 days of incubation, and cultures should be held for 2 to 3 weeks. Early growth is manifested by discrete floccules in sedimented blood or adherence to the wall of the bottle. *A. actinomycetemcomitans* organisms are facultatively anaerobic or aerobic and require carbon dioxide for growth. Colonies are smooth, translucent, and slightly domed with a corrugated surface. They are quite "sticky" and, with further incubation, about 3 to 5 days, a four- to six-pointed star shape forms with the colony or "crossed cigars" form. *A. actinomycetemcomitans* has eight biotypes depending on sugar fermentation and serotype, although these are not clinically relevant. Local and serum antibodies develop to *A. actinomycetemcomitans*, but it has not been established that they are protective (1,3–5). *A. actinomycetemcomitans* are easily confused with *Pasteurella*, *Haemophilus*, and *Yersinia*. None of these forms sticky colonies, however.

Virulence properties possessed by actinobacilli include endotoxin (6) and leukotoxin (7,8), which may be significant in the development of periodontal disease (9). Endotoxin may indirectly enhance collagen breakdown (via prostaglandin E_2 or interleukin-1 involvement) and interfere with monocyte defenses recruited against the bacteria. Leukotoxin may lyse polymorphonuclear cells and inhibit chemotaxis and is variably produced depending on genotype (10). Interference with lymphocyte function either directly or indirectly, via altered monocyte integrity, occurs. There is no evidence that *A. actinomycetemcomitans* degrades fibronectin (11). Because it grows in environments with low oxygen tension (e.g., tissues), neutrophil myeloperoxidase systems may not be effective in killing *A. actinomycetemcomitans*.

A. actinomycetemcomitans has been isolated from oral flora of about 20% of healthy adults and children (5,12). It has been found in food, dental plaque, buccal mucosa, tonsils, and the gastrointestinal and genital tracts of humans and animals (1,5). Clinical isolates include oral pharynx (especially in young adults with localized juvenile periodontitis), abscesses, sinus tracts, and pleural fluid. Sites distant from the oral cavity are thought to be infected through hematogenous spread. Common clinical syndromes include endocarditis, periodontal disease, and soft tissue abscesses either alone or in association with *Actinomyces*.

ENDOCARDITIS
Endocarditis is the most common serious infection associated with *A. actinomycetemcomitans*. In a review by Kaplan et al. (12), 60% of patients had underlying valvular heart disease and 46% of patients had periodontal disease or recent dental manipulation. Of those with valvular heart disease, roughly 40% had prosthetic valves. Most of the patients were men, presenting with subacute disease (after 1 to 16 weeks). One third had presenting manifestations of classic endocarditis (hepatosplenomegaly, peripheral manifestations). Anemia and elevated erythrocyte sedimentation rate were seen in 90% or more of patients. Emboli occurred in 39% of patients and were associated with a poor prognosis. Similar findings were reported by Chen et al. (13) in a much smaller series.

The presentation of symptoms can occur during a prolonged time. In patients with prosthetic valve endocarditis caused by *A. actinomycetemcomitans*, presentation generally occurred more than 1 year after surgery. Of 13 patients reviewed, all but 1 were treated medically and only 1 died (12,14). There is one reported case of pulmonary valve endocarditis related to *A. actinomycetemcomitans* with a presenting course after 18 months (15). Additionally, persistent bacteremia (more than 1 year in duration) with an infected pacemaker and positive dental cultures (16),

TABLE 207.1.   Growth and Biochemical Characteristics of Selected Gram-negative Organisms

Organism	Growth characteristics				Biochemical characteristics			
	Gram stain morphology	CO$_2$ requirement	Growth on MacConkey agar	Growth on blood agar	Oxidase	Catalase	Indole	Reduce nitrates
Glucose fermenters								
Actinobacillus	Coccobacilli	↑ CO$_2$	−	Slow (3–6 days)	Weak +	+	−	+
Capnocytophaga	Long, thin rods (fusiform)	↑ CO$_2$	−	Slow (2–4 days), gliding	−	−	−	+
Capnocytophaga canimorsus	Long, thin rods (curved)	↑ CO$_2$	−	Slow (2–3 days), gliding	+	+	−	+
Dysgonomonas	Coccobacilli	Facultative anaerobe	−	Slow (2–3 days), fruity odor	−	−	+	−
Cardiobacterium	Pleomorphic rods, small to medium	↑ CO$_2$	−	Slow (>2 days)	+	−	+	−
Chromobacterium	Long curved rod	Facultative anaerobe	+	Violet pigment	+	+	−	+
Glucose non-fermenters								
Acinetobacter	Diplococci-coccobacilli	Aerobe	+	Within 1 day	−	+	−	−
Achromobacter	Medium straight rods	Aerobe	+	Within 1 day	+	+	−	+
Alcaligenes	Medium straight rods	Obligate aerobe	+	Within 1 day	+	+	−	(+)[a]
Eikenella	Coccobacilli	Facultative anaerobe and hemin required with ↑ CO$_2$	−	Pitting (2–3 days)	+	−	−	+
Ochrobactrum	Rods	Aerobe	+	Within 1 day	+	+	−	+
Flavobacterium	Long, thin rods, occasionally filamentous	Aerobe	+	Within 1 day, yellow pigment	+	+	+/−[a]	−

[a]Species dependent.

endarteritis with aortic coarctation (17), endocarditis with vasculitis and glomerulonephritis (18,19), and endocarditis with left atrial myxoma (20) have all been reported. One case of endocarditis caused by *A. suis* infection (21) has recently been documented.

Most patients were treated with penicillin or ampicillin and an aminoglycoside. The overall mortality rate was about 23% and was the same for native valve versus prosthetic valve involvement. Valve replacement was generally required in about 25%. Patients with prosthetic valve endocarditis caused by gram-negative bacilli of the HACEK group (*Haemophilus aphrophilus, A. actinomycetemcomitans, Cardiobacterium hominis, Eikenella corrodens,* and *Kingella kingae*) generally have a more favorable outcome than patients with a non-HACEK gram-negative bacilli in-

fection on a prosthetic or native valve. Specifically, they have less mortality and do not require valve replacement as often (22).

LOCALIZED JUVENILE PERIODONTITIS OR ACUTE NECROTIZING ULCERATIVE GINGIVITIS

A. actinomycetemcomitans is thought to be involved in the pathogenesis of localized juvenile periodontitis or acute necrotizing ulcerative gingivitis. Predisposing factors include a neutrophil chemotactic defect that is either familial or acquired, perhaps

TABLE 207.2.   Natural Reservoirs of Selected Gram-negative Organisms

Environmental sources	Endogenous sources
Soil, water	Normal oral flora
Achromobacter	*Acinetobacter*
Acinetobacter	*Actinobacillus*
Alcaligenes	*Capnocytophaga*
Chromobacterium	*Cardiobacterium*
Flavobacterium	*Eikenella*
Hospital equipment	Skin
Achromobacter	*Acinetobacter*
Acinetobacter	*Alcaligenes*
Alcaligenes	Stool
Flavobacterium	*Achromobacter*
Ochrobactrum	*Alcaligenes*
	Chromobacterium
	Eikenella
	Dysgonomonas
	Ochrobactrum

TABLE 207.3.   Common Clinical Syndromes Associated with Selected Gram-negative Bacteria

Sepsis	Endocarditis
Achromobacter	*Actinobacillus*
Acinetobacter	*Alcaligenes*
Capnocytophaga	*Cardiobacterium*
Chromobacterium	*Eikenella*
Dysgonomonas	Meningitis
Ochrobactrum	*Achromobacter*
Flavobacterium	*Acinetobacter*
Associated with bites (human or animal)	*Capnocytophaga*
Acinetobacter	*Flavobacterium*
Actinobacillus	Abscess formation
Capnocytophaga	*Acinetobacter*
Eikenella	*Actinobacillus*
Soft tissue infection	*Capnocytophaga*
Acinetobacter	*Chromobacterium*
Achromobacter	*Eikenella*
Actinobacillus	Chronic diarrhea
Alcaligenes	*Dysgonomonas*
Chromobacterium	
Eikenella (often mixed infections)	

TABLE 207.4. Antibiotic Sensitivities of Miscellaneous Gram-negative Bacilli

Organism	Penicillins	Expanded-spectrum penicillins	Cephalosporins 1°, 2°, 3°	Vancomycin	Erythromycin	Tetracycline	Clindamycin	Aminoglycosides
Glucose fermenters								
Actinobacillus	R, V	S	V S	R	R	S	R	S
Capnocytophaga	V	S	V S	R		S	S	R
Capnocytophaga canimorsus	S	S	S	S	S		S	S[a]
Dysgonomonas	R		R	R	V	S	S	R
Cardiobacterium	V	S	S S	V	V	S		S
Chromobacterium	R	R, V	R R		R	S		S
Glucose nonfermenters								
Acinetobacter	R	V +	R S			V		V
Achromobacter	R	V +	R V			V		R
Alcaligenes	V	V	V V					V
Eikenella	S	S	V S	R		V	R	R
Ochrobactrum	R	R	R R			V		S
Flavobacterium	R	R	R R	S	V		S	

Organism	Chloramphenicol	T-S	Metronidazole	Rifampin	Aztreonam	Quinolones	Imipenem
Glucose fermenters							
Actinobacillus	S				S	S	
Capnocytophaga	S	R	S		R	V	S
Capnocytophaga canimorsus	S	S		S	R	S	S
Dysgonomonas	R	S			R	R	S
Cardiobacterium	S					S	
Chromobacterium	S	S				S	
Glucose nonfermenters							
Acinetobacter	R	S			V		S
Achromobacter	V	S					S
Alcaligenes	S	S					
Eikenella	S		R	V			
Ochrobactrum	R	S				R	S
Flavobacterium	V	S		S		R	R

R, most strains are resistant *in vitro*; V, variable resistance; S, most strains are sensitive; S[a], not sensitive in older literature because of different techniques of evaluation; +, imipenem is a consistently effective agent against these organisms; 1°, 2°, first- and second-generation cephalosporins; 3°, third-generation cephalosporins; T-S, trimethoprim-sulfamethoxazole.

from infection with *A. actinomycetemcomitans* (23,24). More than 90% of patients with localized juvenile periodontitis have had *A. actinomycetemcomitans* identified from plaque samples or gingival tissue. Most cases are successfully treated with penicillin. Pavicic et al. (25) reported success in treating patients with chronic periodontitis with mechanical débridement and oral amoxicillin and metronidazole.

OTHER CLINICAL PRESENTATIONS

A. actinomycetemcomitans infections have included pericarditis (26), parotitis, endophthalmitis (27,28), tenosynovitis (29), arthritis (30,31), osteomyelitis (vertebral), urinary tract infections, pneumonia (32–34), empyema, synovitis, mycetoma (35), lymphadenitis (36), and abscess formation (12,37). Abscesses in the brain, thyroid gland, chest wall, hand, and head and neck have all been described (12), including co-infection with *Actinomyces* (38–40). *A. lignieresii, A. suis,* and *A. equuli*–like bacteria have been isolated from infected horse, sheep, and pig bite wounds in humans (41–43).

On the basis of data from the review by Kaplan et al. (12), *A. actinomycetemcomitans* is generally susceptible to chloramphenicol, tetracycline, streptomycin, aminoglycosides, and cephalosporins. More than 90% of isolates are also susceptible to mezlocillin and carbenicillin. About 80% of isolates are susceptible to ampicillin and penicillin (12). *Actinobacillus* is generally resistant (less than 30% of isolates sensitive) to erythromycin, clindamycin, vancomycin (44), and methicillin. Excellent *in vitro* activity has been demonstrated by quinolones (45,46), azithromycin, and amoxicillin-clavulanate on clinical isolates from bite wounds (45).

Topical potassium iodide may be beneficial in chronic periodontal infections. Reviews studying *in vitro* susceptibilities of periodontal isolates have found 100% susceptibility to cefaclor, cefuroxime, cefixime (47), tetracycline, doxycycline, trimethoprim-sulfamethoxazole, and ciprofloxacin (47,48).

TABLE 207.5. Host Immune Status Related to Infecting Organisms

Organism	Host immune defect
Acinetobacter	Debilitation, prolonged hospital stay, after surgery, trauma
Achromobacter	As for *Acinetobacter*
Actinobacillus	Neutrophil chemotactic defect
Alcaligenes	Neutrophil chemotactic defect and IVDU
Eikenella	IVDU
Capnocytophaga	Neutropenia, periodontal disease
Capnocytophaga canimorsus	Splenectomy, alcohol abuse
Chromobacterium	Chronic granulomatous disease
Dysgonomonas	Malignancy, human immunodeficiency virus infection, common variable hypogammaglobulinemia, chronic illness
Ochrobactrum	Immunosuppressive therapy
Flavobacterium	Premature and small-for-gestational-age infants, immunocompromised status, debilitation

IVDU, intravenous drug user.

Amoxicillin or ciprofloxacin synergy with metronidazole has been demonstrated and has been successfully used in combination with mechanical débridement for therapy of periodontitis (47). Photodynamic therapy is effective *in vitro* and may be a promising adjunctive treatment for periodontitis (49).

Conservative therapy for endocarditis would dictate 4 to 6 weeks of therapy with a cephalosporin and aminoglycoside. However, one case of prosthetic valve endocarditis treated with oral ciprofloxacin for 8 weeks has been reported (50). Reports show that penicillin, erythromycin, and vancomycin have all failed as prophylaxis against endocarditis with *A. actinomycetemcomitans* infection after dental procedures (12). It has been suggested that patients with valvular disease and severe periodontitis who are undergoing dental work have prophylaxis 14 days before the procedure with tetracycline.

Capnocytophaga

Capnocytophaga species were first described in the 1950s and were known as a variant of *Fusobacterium nucleatum* or *Bacteroides oralis*. King named the strain DF-1 (dysgonic fermenter-1) in the 1960s. In 1972, the earlier strains of capnophilic, fastidious gram-negative bacteria were recognized as the same organism and named *Bacteroides ochraceus*. In 1979, the genus *Capnocytophaga* was described to include the DF-1 and *Bacteroides* species (51,52).

There are seven species: *Capnocytophaga ochracea, Capnocytophaga sputigena, Capnocytophaga gingivalis* (53), *Capnocytophaga granulosa, Capnocytophaga haemolytica* (54,55) (all DF-1–like), *Capnocytophaga canimorsus* [formerly dysgonic fermenter-2 (DF-2)], and *Capnocytophaga cynodegmi* (DF-2–like organisms) (56). *C. canimorsus* and *C. cynodegmi* were established later as *Capnocytophaga* species and are discussed separately. *C. granulosa* and *C. haemolytica* have recently been described in dental plaque (54,55) and like the other DF-1 organisms are part of normal human oral flora, whereas the DF-2 organisms are found as part of normal animal (dog, cat) oral flora.

Capnocytophaga organisms are gram-negative long, thin rods, often fusiform that are "gliding" or spreading on agar. They grow slowly, during at least 2 to 4 days, require carbon dioxide under either aerobic or anaerobic growth conditions, and have the capacity to ferment glucose. Colonies leave a yellow pigment on the agar. Special selective media (57,58) are required for optimal growth because the organisms do not grow on MacConkey's agar. Biochemically, they are oxidase, catalase, and indole negative, and reduction of nitrates is variable between species. Each species also ferments a different profile of carbohydrates (53). Of note, *C. ochracea* has been reported to cause a false-positive *Legionella* latex agglutination test (59).

Virulence factors are important regarding pathogenesis (53). Endotoxin is biologically active and contains a unique C15 branched-chain fatty acid. Endotoxin, a peptidoglycan, and a slime layer may be immunomodulators. Patients with neutrophil dysfunction or deficiency are predisposed to developing periodontitis (60) and septicemia in granulocytopenic hosts caused by *Capnocytophaga* (61). *Capnocytophaga* infection may induce a chemotactic defect in polymorphonuclear leukocytes by elaborating a dialyzable substance that interferes with neutrophil migration. Other *Capnocytophaga* species have been shown to enhance (B-cell activation, lymphocyte, and macrophage proliferation) or inhibit (fibroblast proliferation) various immunologic functions that may interfere with optimal host response to infection. *Capnocytophaga* species also synthesize trypsin and an immunoglobulin A (IgA) protease. β-Lactamase production has been described (62). A review of clinical isolates from oral and nonoral lesions demonstrated a reduced ability to activate complement by nonoral isolates and hence reduced serum bactericidal capacity (63).

The major site of *Capnocytophaga* colonization is the oral cavity; however, organisms have been isolated from the vagina and upper and lower respiratory tract sources (nose and throat, sputum, trachea, bronchial specimens, pleural fluid) (64,65). Clinical isolates have been obtained from blood, cerebrospinal fluid (CSF), wounds (especially bite wounds), eyes (both the corneal ulcers and vitreous fluid), vagina (66), and amniotic fluids (65).

Clinically important infections are most commonly seen with cases of juvenile periodontitis (67) or systemic disease in patients with granulocytopenic cancer who have oral lesions. A variety of infections have been reported in nonimmunocompromised hosts as well. The cases of juvenile periodontitis are thought to be related to an acquired neutrophil defect secondary to *Capnocytophaga* infection (60); the defect resolves as the infection is treated. Other local immunosuppressive actions may occur, including IgA protease activity. Immunocompromised patients with *Capnocytophaga* infection tend to be young, mostly children with malignancies, have low neutrophil counts (e.g., chemotherapy-induced granulocytopenia), and have significant oral diseases (65) [oral ulcers (64) or glossitis (68)]. Clinical presentations include bacteremia and septicemia (64,65,69). One case of *C. gingivalis* meningitis has been reported, which is unusual because most cases of *Capnocytophaga* meningitis are due to *C. canimorsus* (70).

Nonimmunocompromised patients have had a variety of clinically significant infections with *Capnocytophaga* species. These include ocular infections (65,71) [keratitis (72,73), conjunctivitis, endophthalmitis (74), corneal ulcer (75)], cardiothoracic infections [endocarditis (76), pericardial abscess (77), mediastinitis (78), lung and subphrenic abscess, empyema (65)], septic arthritis (79), cervical (80) and inguinal (81) lymphadenitis, sinusitis (82), thyroiditis (83), osteomyelitis (84,85), peritonitis (86), liver abscess (87), abdominal abscess, and traumatic hand wounds (65). Cases of peripartum infections (88) including amniotic fluid infection associated with premature delivery (89,90) and congenital bacteremia (91,92) have been described. Endometritis secondary to an intrauterine device has also been reported (93). Like *Actinobacillus* infection, *Capnocytophaga* infection has been reported in association with *A. israelii* infection (94). Most infections reported to be caused by *Capnocytophaga* are of the species *C. ochracea, C. sputigena*, or *C. gingivalis* or are listed as *Capnocytophaga* species. However, a lumbosacral abscess in a 14-year-old immunocompetent boy has recently been reported, which grew *Staphylococcus aureus* and *C. granulosa* (95).

Capnocytophaga species are sensitive to clindamycin, third-generation cephalosporins, newer penicillins, imipenem, and the quinolones (ciprofloxacin, ofloxacin) (96–100). Although in a recent series of 28 patients with *Capnocytophaga* bacteremia, 9 of 16 isolates tested were resistant to ciprofloxacin (101). Chloramphenicol, tetracycline, and metronidazole also have activity against *Capnocytophaga*. Penicillin, ampicillin, amoxicillin, and first- and second-generation cephalosporins have variable activity against these organisms. β-Lactamase production has been reported in as many as 32% to 79% of strains and may be overcome clinically with the addition of β-lactamase inhibitors (102,103). In general, *Capnocytophaga* organisms are resistant to aztreonam, aminoglycosides, vancomycin, trimethoprim, and polymyxin B. Resistance may be plasmid mediated. Special media are usually required to assess *in vitro* susceptibility. Susceptibility testing by E-tests correlated well with results using agar dilution (104) and may provide an easier method for testing antimicrobial susceptibility of *Capnocytophaga* strains.

CAPNOCYTOPHAGA CANIMORSUS (FORMERLY CDC GROUP DF-2) AND CAPNOCYTOPHAGA CYNODEGMI (FORMERLY GROUP DF-2–LIKE)

In 1976, the first case report of a "previously undescribed gram-negative bacillus causing septicemia and meningitis" was published. This was followed by further reports and reviews of similar cases, and the gram-negative bacilli were classified as Centers for Disease Control and Prevention (CDC) group DF-2. Later, on the basis of deoxyribonucleic acid (DNA) hybridization studies, DF-2 was classified as a new species, *C. canimorsus*, and DF-2–like organisms as *C. cynodegmi* (56).

Both species are long filamentous gram-negative rods, often curved, that grow slowly on blood or chocolate agar and not on MacConkey's agar. Optimal growth is on brain-heart infusion agar supplemented with 5% rabbit or sheep blood incubated at 37°C in a candle extinction jar (carbon dioxide present). Neither species has flagella, but both exhibit gliding motility. As opposed to the other *Capnocytophaga* species, *C. canimorsus* and *C. cynodegmi* are oxidase and catalase positive. Both species are indole negative and reduce nitrates and show variable reduction of nitrites. They all differ from each other in the pattern of sugar fermentation; however, they all ferment glucose (4,56).

Virulence factors are not well defined. *C. canimorsus* is thought to have low virulence because it has been demonstrated to be serum sensitive and immunocompromised hosts are more commonly affected. Studies evaluating the humoral aspects of DF-2 infection suggested that the early response may be immunoglobulin G (IgG) mediated as the immunoglobulin M (IgM) response does not occur or thus far has not been observed (105).

Sources of *C. canimorsus* in nature include oral flora of dogs and cats (106). Clinical isolates have included blood and CSF most frequently, but also wounds from dog bites and cat scratches, heart valve, petechiae, adrenal gland, and cornea (DF-2–like organism) (56). Of note is that a false-positive cryptococcal latex agglutination result was obtained from the CSF of an immunocompetent patient with septicemia caused by DF-2. Blood and CSF cultures were positive and the CSF Gram stain, white cell differential, and biochemistry values were negative (107).

Infection with *C. cynodegmi* has been reported only in wound infections after dog bites or cat scratches; however, *C. canimorsus* has been reported with similar exposure or as a severe systemic infection, without known exposure, particularly in splenectomized individuals (56). In 1977, Butler et al. (108) described 17 patients with systemic infection, 13 with bacteremia, 3 with meningitis, and 1 with both. Hicklin, Verghese, and Alvarez (105) reviewed 41 cases reported in the English literature by 1987 (including cases studied by Butler et al.). Of these 41 cases, 34 had either septicemia or bacteremia, 4 had meningitis, and 3 had both presentations. Predisposing factors to infection include splenectomy for any reason (35%), alcohol abuse (35%), and evidence for immune dysfunction (steroids, hematologic malignancies, autoimmune disease) (17%). Four patients had no known predisposing factors for infection. More than 75% of cases involved previous exposure to a dog either through ownership or direct bite. In 50% of splenectomized patients, the clinical course was fulminant, that is, hypotension, renal failure, disseminated intravascular coagulation, gangrene, pulmonary infiltrates, and death. Gram stain of the buffy coat demonstrated the organism in all splenectomized patients examined and may prove helpful in early diagnosis. The overall mortality rate was 27% to 31% (105,109). A recent review of *C. canimorsus* sepsis in Denmark corroborates these findings (109).

Other clinical presentations include endocarditis, renal failure, disseminated intravascular coagulation, adrenal hemorrhage [Waterhouse-Friderichsen syndrome (110)], rash (107) (urticarial, petechial, macular), joint effusion and arthritis, cellulitis,

pneumonia, empyema (111), and mononeuropathy (112). *C. canimorsus* keratitis (113) and endophthalmitis (114) have also been reported, both related to cat exposure.

Antimicrobial susceptibility studies *in vitro* must use appropriate techniques for fastidious organisms. For *Capnocytophaga* isolates, longer incubation times and carbon dioxide are required for optimal growth. Broth dilution techniques in a carbon dioxide–enriched atmosphere are desirable. On this basis, Verghese et al. (115) examined eight clinical isolates. With the exception of aztreonam, all eight isolates were sensitive to penicillin, piperacillin, imipenem, erythromycin, vancomycin, clindamycin, third-generation cephalosporins, gentamicin, amikacin, chloramphenicol, rifampin, trimethoprim-sulfamethoxazole, and ciprofloxacin. Previous studies (100,107) using disk diffusion or agar dilution assays have demonstrated resistance to aminoglycosides.

DYSGONOMONAS CAPNOCYTOPHAGOIDES (FORMERLY CDC GROUP DF-3)

An organism thought to be closely related to *Capnocytophaga* is *Dysgonomonas capnocytophagoides* (formerly CDC DF-3) (116). It is a facultatively anaerobic gram-negative coccobacillus that does not grow on MacConkey's, *Salmonella-Shigella*, or xylose-lysine-deoxycholate agars or most *Campylobacter* media incubated at 42°C (117) and thus is not detected on routine stool culture. It grows well on blood agar, chocolate agar, and cefoperazone-vancomycin-amphotericin B agar incubated at 35°C within 48 to 72 hours. Colonies are usually nonhemolytic and have a unique fruity odor. This organism is catalase and oxidase negative, like the DF-1 organisms, but can be distinguished by being indole positive and fermenting different sugars. The presence of 12-methyltetradecanoate in cell wall fatty acid analysis assists in identification (118).

DF-3 has been isolated from multiple sites (119), the most frequent being stools, blood, and wounds. It has been isolated from asymptomatic persons and is rarely pathogenic. The most common clinical presentation is chronic diarrhea (120), which is usually not bloody and not accompanied by fever. It has also been reported to cause bacteremia with sepsis (121), urinary tract infection (122), and abscess (123). The majority of those infected are immunocompromised [malignancy, human immunodeficiency virus infection (HIV), common variable hypogammaglobulinemia, corticosteroid therapy] or have chronic illness (diabetes mellitus, cirrhosis).

Most strains of DF-3 are susceptible to clindamycin, trimethoprim-sulfamethoxazole, tetracycline, and chloramphenicol. They are variably susceptible to erythromycin and imipenem but are generally resistant to penicillin, ampicillin, cephalosporins, aminoglycosides, ciprofloxacin, aztreonam, and vancomycin. Patients with diarrhea usually show clinical improvement within a few days to a week into a 2-week course of antibiotics. Of note, in HIV-infected patients with diarrhea believed to be due to DF-3, therapy has been associated with clinical improvement and clearance of infection was maintained for months after therapy was discontinued.

Cardiobacterium

The only species in the genus *Cardiobacterium* is *C. hominis*. It is a gram-negative rod occurring in pleomorphic form including rosette clusters, teardrops, and enlargement of one or both ends. Retention of crystal violet may occur, resulting in a gram-positive appearance. Biochemically, *C. hominis* is oxidase positive, catalase negative, and nitrate-reduction negative. It forms indole in small amounts, a major identifying characteristic, but usually after 24 to 48 hours and extraction with xylene. *C. hominis* ferments glucose to lactic acid. It is nonmotile and requires 5% to 10% carbon dioxide for growth. On blood agar after 48 hours, colonies are 1 to 2 mm, circular, convex, smooth, and moist without hemolysis. It does not grow well aerobically, unless air is humidified, or anaerobically, accounting for its fastidious nature. Cultures must be held for 2 to 3 weeks (5,124).

Virulence properties of *C. hominis* have not been documented. The organisms do not produce exotoxins or cause disease in laboratory animals (5). *C. hominis* has been isolated from normal nasal and pharyngeal flora of 68% of humans as well as cervical and vaginal cultures. *C. hominis* has *not* been isolated from animals, soil, water, or hospital equipment (3–5).

Clinical isolates have been obtained from blood, CSF, and valve tissue (125). The major clinical syndromes are subacute endocarditis and late prosthetic valve endocarditis, including endocarditis after endoscopic procedures (126,127). The best estimate of prevalence of *C. hominis* infective endocarditis is 0.1% of all cases of endocarditis (128). To date, approximately 50 cases of *C. hominis* endocarditis have been reported in the literature (125,129–132). The course is generally insidious (mean duration of symptoms is 169 days), with many of the classic features of subacute bacterial endocarditis (fever, splenomegaly, petechiae, anemia, elevated erythrocyte sedimentation rate, hematuria) occurring in more than 40% of the cases. Large vegetations and emboli are not uncommon. Seventy-five percent of the cases occur in patients with abnormal valves. Emboli and congestive heart failure occur in 44% of cases. The mitral and aortic valves most often are affected. A high proportion (87%) of patients can be cured, most (70%) with antimicrobial therapy alone (130,133,134). Aortic homograft valve endocarditis (135) and mycotic aneurysm (136,137), probably secondary to endocarditis, have been described. Other reported clinical infections include bacteremia without endocarditis in a patient with an abdominal abscess caused by *C. hominis* and *Clostridium bifermentans* (138), pacemaker lead infection with vertebral osteomyelitis (139), and meningitis (140).

C. hominis is generally quite sensitive to penicillin and ampicillin, as well as cephalothin, chloramphenicol, tetracycline, and aminoglycosides. However, recent reports document β-lactamase production and high-level penicillin resistance (with reduced sensitivity to vancomycin) (141,142). Susceptibility to vancomycin and erythromycin is variable. Results of tests *in vitro* are difficult to interpret, given the slow-growing nature of the organism. Most cases have been treated with either penicillin or ampicillin, with or without an aminoglycoside for bacteriologic and clinical cure. Second- and third-generation cephalosporins also have excellent activity *in vitro* and have been used clinically (143). Endocarditis successfully treated with ciprofloxacin has been reported (144).

Chromobacterium

Chromobacterium violaceum is the type species for the genus *Chromobacterium*. It is the only known pathogenic member of the genus and the only violet pathogenic bacterium (145). Other names have included *Bacillus violaceous* and *Chromobacterium janthinum*. *Chromobacterium lividum* is a nonpathogenic species that can be differentiated by its lack of violet color and growth at 4°C but not at 37°C (3,4,146).

C. violaceum is a gram-negative, sometimes slightly curved rod, facultatively anaerobic, that produces a violet tryptophan metabolite (violacein) that is insoluble in water. The pigment is not produced when the organism is grown anaerobically, and not all strains produce the pigment. The organisms grow within 24 hours on conventional media (blood and MacConkey's agar)

and media containing tryptophan. *C. violaceum* organisms are motile with both polar and lateral flagella (antigenically distinct). They are usually oxidase positive, but the pigment may interfere with the reading and they can be confused with *Aeromonas* species. They are catalase positive, are generally indole negative, and reduce nitrates and nitrites. They ferment glucose to acid, sometimes produce gas (20%), and produce hydrogen cyanide. *C. violaceum* organisms also produce substances that are inhibitory to gram-positive and some gram-negative bacteria. Two such agents with antibacterial properties, aerocavin (147) and aerocyanidin (148), have been described. *C. violaceum* may be confused with *B. pseudomallei* using biochemical test panels only (149).

Virulence properties include production of a biologically active endotoxin, chromosomally mediated β-lactamase (145), and possibly an extracellular slime layer. A report comparing a virulent clinical isolate and an avirulent soil isolate demonstrated greater superoxide dismutase and catalase production from the virulent isolate (150). There is evidence that humans with neutrophil defects may be more susceptible to infections with *C. violaceum*.

Chromobacterium is generally found in the environment; sources include soil, freshwater, stagnant water, and food (refrigerated food grows only *C. lividum*) (151,152). It has recently been reported as a colonizer in the stools of infants and toddlers in Atlanta, Georgia (153). Because *C. violaceum* grows optimally at 20°C to 37°C, most infections have been documented in tropical or subtropical climates between the latitudes 35 degrees north and 35 degrees south. In the United States, most infections are reported from Florida and Louisiana between the months of June and September (154), although one case has been reported from Ohio (after exposure in New England) (155) and one case in Florida (156) during January. Recently the first case was reported from Japan (157).

C. violaceum is an uncommon to rare cause of infection in that fewer than 40 cases have been reported in the world literature (158). Clinical isolates have included visceral and skin abscesses, blood, CSF, brain, eye and ear specimens, urine, feces, sputum, throat, bone, and joint fluid (145,153,154). Clinically, the portal of entry of *C. violaceum* is thought to be a break in the skin, although ingestion of contaminated food or water may also play a role because it has been isolated from feces when near drowning (159) has been the only source of exposure.

Typically, the infection begins around a break in the skin followed by local cellulitis, regional or diffuse lymphadenitis, and then hematologic dissemination. Septicemia, acute respiratory distress syndrome, disseminated intravascular coagulation, and multiple organ system failure subsequently occur. Multiple liver abscesses develop and can be seen by hepatic imaging. The mortality rate is 60% to 70% and is probably related to underlying disease (e.g., neutrophil defects), appropriateness of antibiotic therapy, and accuracy of diagnosis. Autopsy specimens have frequently demonstrated multiple liver, lung, and spleen abscesses. Other clinical presentations besides septicemia include fever, cutaneous (160,161) lesions (minor abrasions, rashes, cellulitis), lymphadenitis, deep neck tissue infection (162), abdominal pain, osteomyelitis, arthritis, meningitis (163,164), hemophagocytic syndrome (157), ocular infections (165,166) (necrotizing conjunctivitis, periorbital cellulitis), and pneumonia (154,156,158,159).

Multiple reports suggest an association with chronic granulomatous disease and *C. violaceum* infection (154,155,160,165,167). Most patients with overwhelming infection are younger than 28 years. *C. violaceum* infection in patients with other neutrophil defects such as glucose-6-phosphate dehydrogenase deficiency (168) of the polymorphonuclear leukocyte (and red blood cell) and leukemia (161,169) has been described. Normal hosts with overwhelming exposure (near drowning) and minimal exposure (barefoot in mud) have been described; however, formal leukocyte testing has not been performed in these cases (159).

C. violaceum is generally quite susceptible to ciprofloxacin, chloramphenicol, gentamicin, and tetracycline. It is uniformly resistant to cephalosporins and is generally resistant to most penicillins. It has variable sensitivity to some of the carboxy penicillins and ureidopenicillins (145,153,154,169,170). Treatment failure and relapse have occurred with the use of erythromycin (155). Trimethoprim-sulfamethoxazole has been used successfully as outpatient therapy after prolonged (4-week) intravenous therapy with other agents (145,156,170).

GLUCOSE NONFERMENTERS

Acinetobacter

The first descriptions of Acinetobacter species were made by DeBord in 1939 when he isolated gram-negative coccobacilli from urethral specimens (171). The classification has changed frequently during the past 50 years. Acinetobacter is a member of the family Neisseriaceae and according to Bergey's Manual of Systematic Bacteriology (172) has only one species, Acinetobacter calcoaceticus. Acinetobacter derives from the Greek for nonmotile rod and calcoaceticus (from Latin) for its ability to use calcium acetate as a carbon source. Previously, the most common isolates involved in human disease included A. calcoaceticus var. anitratus (formerly Herellea vaginicola, Bacterium anitratum, Achromobacter anitratum, Micrococcus calcoaceticus), which oxidizes carbohydrates to acid, and A. calcoaceticus var. lwoffii (formerly Mima polymorpha var. nonoxidans, Moraxella lwoffii, B5W organism), which does not form acid. Subsequently, four major biotypes of Acinetobacter were described: A. calcoaceticus var. anitratus and var. haemolyticus both oxidize glucose to acid, whereas var. lwoffii and var. alcaligenes do not. A. calcoaceticus var. anitratus and var. lwoffii are not hemolytic, whereas var. haemolyticus and var. alcaligenes are.

The taxonomy of Acinetobacter has been evolving during the past several years; it was redefined by Bouvet and Grimont (173) in 1986 on the basis of DNA hybridization techniques with which they identified 17 genospecies of Acinetobacter, including A. calcoaceticus, Acinetobacter baumannii, A. haemolyticus, Acinetobacter junii, Acinetobacter johnsonii, A. lwoffii, Acinetobacter radioresistens, and 10 undesignated species (3,174–176). These genospecies are the currently accepted taxonomic definitions. Because A. calcoaceticus, A. baumannii, and DNA groups 3 and 13 are genotypically and phenotypically similar, they are often referred to as A. calcoaceticus-baumannii complex (175,176). Speciation versus subspeciation may not be clinically relevant to the individual patient; however, it may be useful in epidemiologic investigations of outbreaks.

Acinetobacter is a gram-negative rod, predominantly coccobacillary or diplococcoid (172,177,178). Acinetobacter may be difficult to decolorize on Gram stain, hence appearing gram positive. It is nonmotile but may exhibit twitching motility as a result of polar fimbriae. Acinetobacter organisms are oxidase negative, catalase positive, and indole negative and do not reduce nitrates. Some strains may be encapsulated. Capsules consist of a polysaccharide and, at least from one strain, have cross-reacted with antisera made to group B and G streptococci and pneumococci. Some strains cross-react with antichlamydial antibodies (179,180). More than 28 serotypes of the acid-forming strains have been described.

Acinetobacter organisms grow well on complex media and selective media including MacConkey's agar. They grow aerobically and produce gray-white colonies 2 to 3 mm in diameter after 18 to 24 hours at 33°C to 35°C (177). Acinetobacter species differ from Enterobacteriaceae in that they cannot grow anaerobically or reduce nitrates. They are distinguished from Neisseria and Moraxella in their reaction to the oxidase test (172).

Acinetobacter has a low potential for virulence. Most infections are nosocomial and occur in severely ill patients who have had previous antibiotics, surgery, trauma, or instrumentation. Potential virulence factors include a polysaccharide capsule, which may prevent phagocytosis, fimbriae that potentiate adherence to epithelial cells, and a lipopolysaccharide known to be biologically active (178). In addition, human serum resistance is more common among A. anitratus than A. lwoffii strains (181).

Acinetobacter is widely distributed in the environment. It is found in soil, food (182), water (154), and sewage (172) and has been transmitted by contact with these sources. Infections in foundry workers (183) and others (184,185) have suggested airborne transmission. Chickens (186), septic hens (187,188), rubber and stainless steel milk pipelines (189), and bottled uncarbonated mineral drinking water (190) have also been sources in nature. Typically, moist environments including hospital equipment such as ventilator tubing and resuscitation bags (191), peak flowmeters (192), humidifiers (193), sinks (194), mist tents (195), dialysis baths (196) and dialysis hardware (0 rings) (197), duodenoscopes (198), angiography catheters (199), intravenous catheters (200), pressure transducers (201), caloric testing water tanks (202), and latex gloves (203) or pharmacologic solutions such as plasma protein solutions (204), intravenous anesthetics (205), and enteral feeding solutions (206) contain this organism or have been associated with outbreaks. Acinetobacter is known to survive up to 16 weeks on dry surfaces (207). Several outbreaks have been linked to dry sources such as mattresses (208) and pillows (209). It is found on the skin of many animal species and humans, usually as a commensal organism. From 2% to 25% of humans carry it on their skin (210,211) including the hands of hospital personnel (212). It is also found as part of normal oral flora (up to 7% of healthy people are colonized) (210) and in the upper respiratory tract, genitourinary tract, and lower gastrointestinal tract. Acinetobacter has been isolated from tracheostomy sites in adults, sputum, urine, feces (213), vaginal secretions, saliva, conjunctiva (210), frozen human milk (214), wound sites, and blood (215–217). It has been identified as one of the five most common gram-negative rods isolated from the pharyngeal flora of normal healthy infants older than 1 week (218).

Factors predisposing to infection include debilitating conditions (e.g., alcoholism, advanced age, chronic disease, acute and severe illness), major surgery, major trauma, and burn injury, previous antibiotic therapy, intensive care unit stay, and prior instrumentation in the hospital (171). These procedures include endotracheal tube intubation, tracheostomy, urinary tract catheterization, peripheral and central intravenous catheter placement, and chest tube insertion.

Acinetobacter infections have been reported for almost all organ systems. It is usually an opportunistic pathogen as evidenced by the fact that 14% to 62% of infections are mixed infections (171,212,219). The most common sites involved are the respiratory and urinary tracts. The mortality rate can be up to 36% depending on the site and the presence of factors indicating poor prognosis such as polymicrobial sepsis and shock.

Acinetobacter species accounted for 1% of all nosocomial infections reported to the CDC by 1990 to 1996 National Nosocomial Infections Surveillance (NNIS) participating hospitals (2% of bloodstream infections and 4% of pneumonias) (220). A seasonal peak incidence in the late summer has also been noted (221). One hypothesis explaining this seasonality is that summer weather increases the number of Acinetobacter species in the natural environment, leading to increased number in the hospital environment, promoting nosocomial transmission (221).

Nosocomial infections include septicemia in adults (171,212,222,223) and neonates (224), which can be associated with vascular catheters (225), oral or nasopharyngeal intubation (226), or transhepatic cholangiography (227), and endocarditis, including prosthetic valve endocarditis (228). Meningitis, often associated with neurosurgical procedures, and brain abscesses have been reported (229–232). Respiratory tract infections include pneumonia, usually multilobar, occasionally with associated pleural effusion, cavity formation, and rarely bronchopulmonary fistula (171) and are associated with increased morbidity and mortality rates compared with those for other gram-negative organisms (233). Pneumonia may be chronic (234). Empyema, lung abscess, and tracheobronchitis have also been reported. Upper and lower urinary tract infections occur, with upper tract infections being associated with renal calculi. Wound infections, cellulitis, skin abscess, phlebitis, an infected abdominal aortic aneurysm (235), intraabdominal abscess, and suppurative thyroiditis associated with *Acinetobacter* bacteremic pneumonia (236) have been described. Peritonitis associated with continuous ambulatory peritoneal dialysis has also been reported and can be successfully treated with intraperitoneal, intravenous, or oral antibiotics often without removal of the catheter (237–240). Musculoskeletal infections including pyarthrosis and osteomyelitis (241) may occur. Conjunctivitis, exposure keratitis (242), endophthalmitis (243) and corneal ulcer (244) secondary to trauma, and blepharitis (245) have been reported.

Community-acquired infections with *Acinetobacter* are not uncommon. Pneumonia has been reported infrequently in the United States (Texas) (211), foundry workers in Connecticut (183), Chicago (246), Papua, New Guinea (247), and Australia (248). Compared with nosocomially acquired pneumonia, community-acquired pneumonia tends to be more fulminant, is associated with bacteremia, and has a higher mortality rate (43%) (211). Predisposing factors in patients include chronic pulmonary disease, cigarette smoking, alcohol abuse, diabetes mellitus, and non-Hodgkin's lymphoma. Community-acquired meningitis (249) is rarely reported. Native valve endocarditis (250) can be more aggressive than prosthetic valve endocarditis in this setting. Long-term indwelling tunneled catheters used for home intravenous therapy have also been associated with *Acinetobacter* infections (251). *Acinetobacter* infection has been reported after a dog bite (252).

Acinetobacter organisms are commonly multidrug resistant (253,254), and isolated pathogens must be evaluated for specific sensitivity patterns within each hospital. Antibacterial resistance is greater among *A. baumannii* strains than among other *Acinetobacter* species. Nosocomial strains are more resistant to β-lactams than community-acquired strains. They are generally resistant to penicillin, ampicillin, most first- and second-generation cephalosporins, gentamicin, chloramphenicol, and nalidixic acid (178,255,256). They are variably resistant to tetracycline, tobramycin, kanamycin, ureidopenicillins, and aztreonam. Most strains are still sensitive to imipenem, ceftazidime, cefotaxime, amikacin, trimethoprim-sulfamethoxazole (257), and minocycline. Imipenem is the most reliable agent against *Acinetobacter*; however, imipenem-resistant strains have been reported. SENTRY investigators examined 1,078 *Acinetobacter* isolates from 1997 to 1999 from five countries (including the United States) and found that 8% of 150 nosocomial isolates from the United States and Canada were resistant to imipenem compared with 3% in all 552 reported isolates. Seventy-four percent of imipenem-resistant isolates were nosocomial (258). However, carbapenems and aminoglycosides continue to be the most active agents

against this organism (259). In cases of carbapenem resistance, the addition of sulbactam *in vitro* killed the *Acinetobacter* and treating the patients with ampicillin-sulbactam resulted in clinical improvement in 9 of 10 cases (260).

Recent studies have demonstrated *in vitro* susceptibility of clinical isolates of *Acinetobacter* species to fluoroquinolones such as ciprofloxacin and Levaquin (259,261), although resistance (up to 50%) has been reported. Clinical multidrug-resistant *Acinetobacter* isolates have been tested *in vitro* against nontraditional antimicrobials including cefepime, meropenem, netilmicin, azithromycin, doxycycline, and rifampin. Minimum inhibitory concentration (MIC_{90}) for each antimicrobial against multidrug-resistant *Acinetobacter* were as follows: doxycycline (1 μg/mL), azithromycin (4 mg/mL), rifampin (8 μg/mL), and netilmicin (1 μg/mL). However, these drugs have not been tested *in vivo* (262).

Many mechanisms of resistance to antibiotics have been reported for *Acinetobacter*. Resistance to β-lactam antibiotics (including resistance to imipenem) is mediated by altered penicillin-binding proteins (263,264), reduced outer-membrane permeability (263,265), and both constitutive and plasmid-mediated β-lactamases (266,267). *Acinetobacter* exhibits high-level resistance to aminoglycosides by producing acetylating and phosphorylating enzymes to inactivate these agents (266,267). The particular chromosomal resistance gene against amikacin may be species specific (268,269).

Depending on the severity of infection and the sensitivities of the clinical isolate, conservative therapy dictates individualized, combination therapy for *Acinetobacter* infections—for example, imipenem or a third-generation cephalosporin with or without amikacin. For imipenem-resistant strains, ampicillin-sulbactam and piperacillin-tazobactam may be better alternatives. The ability of *Acinetobacter* to remain viable on inanimate surfaces, combined with the organism's intrinsic resistance mechanisms, require rigorous infection-control practices and tailored antimicrobial therapy.

Alcaligenes and *Achromobacter*

The taxonomy of the *Alcaligenes* and *Achromobacter* genera is controversial. Both genera are in the family Alcaligenaceae and species names are often interchanged. The clinically relevant species include *Alcaligenes faecalis* (inclusive of the strain formerly known as *A. odorans*) (270), *Achromobacter xylosoxidans* (subspecies *denitrificans* and subspecies *xylosoxidans*), and *Achromobacter piechaudii*. In 1998, Yabuuchi, et al. proposed a revision of the genus *Achromobacter* based on RNA analysis. *Alcaligenes piechaudii* was transferred to the genus *Achromobacter*, creating the species *Achromobacter piechaudii*. *Alcaligenes denitrificans* was also transferred to the genus *Achromobacter* and renamed *A. xylosoxidans*. Two subspecies names were created: *A. xylosoxidans* subspecies *denitrificans* and *A. xylosoxidans* subspecies *xylosoxidans* (271). *Achromobacter xylosoxidans* subspecies *denitrificans* was formerly identified as CDC group Vc or *Alcaligenes xylosoxidans* subspecies *dentrificans*. *A. xylosoxidans* subspecies *xylosoxidans* was formerly known as CDC groups IIIa and IIIb or *Alcaligenes xylosoxidans* subspecies *xylosoxidans* or *Alcaligenes denitrificans* subspecies *xylosoxidans* (272). Species differentiation occurs on the basis of ability to grow with 6% NaCl, reduce nitrates, and use carbohydrates.

The name *Alcaligenes* means alkali-producing bacteria. Organisms are gram-negative rods or cocci on Gram stain and are motile with peritrichous flagella, and most are obligately aerobic (e.g., *A. faecalis*). Some strains grow anaerobically, reducing nitrate or nitrite to nitrogen gas (e.g., *A. denitrificans*). *Alcaligenes* are oxidase and catalase positive and indole negative. They grow using a variety of organic acids, including amino acids, but generally not carbohydrates, for energy. Strains grow on blood and selective media (MacConkey). Virulence factors include production of bacteriocins and resistance via β-lactamase production (177,270).

Sources of *Alcaligenes* include soil and water (154), as well as part of normal human flora, especially the skin and gastrointestinal tract. Dairy products and rotten eggs have been sources for *Alcaligenes* infection. Clinical isolates include blood, sputum, urine, feces, chronic ear discharge, material from wounds, CSF, pleural fluid, eye and throat swabs, and bronchial washings. Isolation is not always associated with infections, especially respiratory and urinary tract isolates. *Alcaligenes* have been isolated from hospital equipment including respirators, hemodialysis systems, intravenous solution, and disinfectants (273).

Clinically important infections are found in patients with severe underlying illnesses. *A. faecalis* isolated from the urine is often considered a contaminant. Blood isolates from patients with septicemia are thought to be associated with contaminated hospital equipment, although blood isolates have also been obtained from patients without clinical evidence of sepsis. Clinical syndromes are varied (273), including endocarditis [late prosthetic valve endocarditis (133) and native valve endocarditis (274)], meningitis (275), chronic purulent otitis (276), meibomianitis (277), corneal ulcer (278), pyelonephritis, hepatitis, appendicitis, and diarrhea. Many infections are mixed with other flora.

Alcaligenes organisms are generally susceptible to trimethoprim-sulfamethoxazole and chloramphenicol. Sensitivity to β-lactams and aminoglycosides is variable; however, *A. faecalis* is more likely to be sensitive to these than the other species. Greater resistance is seen in the hospital setting, especially with *A. xylosoxidans* subspecies *denitrificans* and *A. xylosoxidans* subspecies *xylosoxidans*. Piperacillin and ciprofloxacin may be reasonable therapeutic alternatives (279–281).

Achromobacter differs from *Alcaligenes* by its ability to reduce nitrate to nitrite and grow anaerobically in the presence of nitrate. *Achromobacter* organisms are gram-negative rods that are oxidase and catalase positive, exhibit motility related to peritrichous flagella, and do not produce indole. They can be easily confused with *Pseudomonas* species unless a stain for flagella is done. They can grow in the presence of various sugars including glucose, xylose, and gluconate, whereas other *Alcaligenes* do not. Colonies grow well on blood and MacConkey's agar.

Achromobacter is found widely distributed in nature, including soil and water (swimming pools, well water) (154,282). It may be part of the normal flora of the lower gastrointestinal tract. *Achromobacter* has been isolated from pharyngeal swabs, sputum, skin, feces, and vaginal secretions. Clinical isolates include blood, urine, wounds, abscesses, orbital swabs, purulent ear discharge, CSF and brain tissue, and pleural and peritoneal fluids (172,270,283,284). The organisms have been found as contaminants in disinfectants (chlorhexidine) (284), diagnostic tracer solution (285) (presumably in nonbacteriostatic saline), intravenous computed tomography contrast solution (286), and hemodialysis solutions. *Achromobacter* has been isolated from hospital equipment (284) including ventilators, humidifiers, pressure transducers (287), and hand-washing machines (288).

Yabuuchi and Oyama (289) first described *A. xylosoxidans* in 1971 from the purulent discharge from the ears of seven patients with chronic otitis media. Subsequently, it has been reported as an uncommon causative agent in a variety of nosocomial and community-acquired infections. Community-acquired infections include a case of bacteremia in a 79-year-old woman with metastatic breast cancer in whom the only identifiable source was well water that she had ingested (282). A second case resulted in meningitis in a young man after a gunshot wound to the chest (290), presumably the source of contamination. This patient underwent spinal surgery within 24 hours of hospital admission and did not develop meningitis until 2 weeks into the hospital course, however. In other reports of *Achromobacter* meningitis, almost all cases were related to previous neurosurgical manipulation (291,292). Maternal–fetal transmission has been reported in a case of a mother with chorioamnionitis and neonate with fatal meningitis caused by *A. xylosoxidans* (293).

Achromobacter has been described in nosocomial outbreaks (284,294). Clinical presentations include meningitis (295,296), ventriculitis (related to neurosurgical procedures), septicemia and bacteremia (297–300) (including prosthetic valve endocarditis and catheter-associated infections), bacteremia in HIV-positive patients (301), pseudobacteremia (302), otitis, endophthalmitis (303), corneal ulcer (304), keratitis (305), pharyngitis, pneumonia (283), wounds (skin, burns, ulcers), peritonitis, urinary tract infection, arthritis [native (306,307) and prosthetic (308) joints], osteomyelitis (309–311), and abscesses [lung (312)]. Mandell, Garvey, and Neu (283) have reviewed cases of bacteremia with *A. xylosoxidans* and described the major predisposing factor as severe underlying disease. The mortality rate was approximately 52% in the seven well-documented cases of bacteremia. A subsequent review of 77 cases of *A. xylosoxidans* bacteremias demonstrated a mortality of 30%. The majority (70%) of bacteremias were nosocomial, including 36% associated with a common source (313). The first episode of clinically significant bacteremia due to *A. piechaudii* was reported in an elderly man with large-cell lymphoma receiving chemotherapy via a Hickman catheter. Treatment required removal of the catheter and responded to cefepime (314).

A. xylosoxidans is generally resistant to penicillin, ampicillin, first- and second-generation cephalosporins, and aminoglycosides. Resistance may occur via β-lactamases and either plasmid-mediated (294) or constitutively expressed cephalosporinases or penicillinases (279,296,315). Trimethoprim-sulfamethoxazole, chloramphenicol, tetracycline, and the quinolones exhibit variable activity (279); however, trimethoprim-sulfamethoxazole is active for most strains (279,281,315,313). Imipenem was the most consistently active agent *in vitro* against 37 clinical isolates (316). Piperacillin, carbenicillin, ticarcillin-clavulanate, and ceftazidime were active against at least 50% of strains. Clinical isolates should be tested for their sensitivity to these antibiotics. For severe infections, more than one drug may be necessary; however, synergistic combination therapy has not been established.

Ochrobactrum anthropi

Ochrobactrum anthropi (formerly CDC group Vd) is another organism previously included under the genus *Achromobacter* (317). In contrast to *A. xylosoxidans*, *O. anthropi* is urease positive, does not use the same carbon sources, and does not grow on cetrimide agar (154,270,318). *O. anthropi* is also oxidase positive, non–lactose fermenting, and motile by peritrichous flagella. *Ochrobactrum* is gram negative, although it can stain gram positive even after the agar or broth is boiled (319).

Ochrobactrum has been isolated from blood, wounds, stool, urine, throat, and vaginal secretions. It has also been isolated from the hospital environment. In general, infections are rare; however, the most common clinical presentation is bacteremia associated with a central venous catheter (320–326). It has caused an outbreak of bacteremia in organ transplant recipients associated with contaminated vials of rabbit antithymocyte globulin (327). Another outbreak of meningitis was reported in children receiving pericardial allograft transplant tissue for dural defect repair (328). Other reported cases include pancreatic abscess (329), osteochondritis of the foot secondary to a puncture wound (330), wound infection and cellulitis (331), empyema (331), necrotizing fasciitis in which the tissue grew group G streptococci but blood cultures grew *Ochrobactrum* (332), endogenous endophthalmitis in a patient receiving hyperalimentation via a central line (333), and pyogenic infections related to foreign bodies [retained pacemaker leads (334), a draining T tube, and a chest tube (335,336)]. Most of the patients are immunocompromised (resulting from malignancy) or receiving immunosuppressive therapy. The first cases of *O. anthropi* bacteremia in HIV-infected patients have been described. Both patients had acquired immunodeficiency syndrome (AIDS) (CD4$^+$ counts of 95 cells/μL and 8 cells/μL, respectively). Although the bacteremias in both patients were hospital acquired, no obvious source of bacteremia was identified (337).

Ochrobactrum is typically resistant to the penicillins, cephalosporins, aztreonam, and chloramphenicol. The drugs most frequently active are ciprofloxacin, trimethoprim-sulfamethoxazole, imipenem, and amikacin (320–326). Therapy should be guided by *in vitro* susceptibility testing, although there have been reports of treatment failure using drugs active *in vitro* (320) and likewise, clinical response with inactive drugs based on susceptibility tests (321). The recommendations are contradictory regarding the removal of central venous catheters. Catheter removal may be necessary only for patients not responding to antimicrobial therapy alone.

Eikenella

Eikenella corrodens is a gram-negative, pleomorphic coccobacillus that after 48 to 72 hours has the characteristic colonial morphology of "corroding" or pitting the agar surface on which it is grown. It was formerly known as bacillus HB-1 of King and *Bacteroides corrodens*. The genus was established in 1972 by Jackson and Goodman (338), who differentiated the genus from *Bacteroides ureolyticus* by genetic analysis and growth characteristics. *E. corrodens* is a facultative anaerobe, whereas *B. ureolyticus* is an obligate anaerobe. *Eikenella* is nonmotile but exhibits twitching motility on agar. About half of the strains corrode; those that do not corrode also do not exhibit twitching motility. There is a characteristic musty odor on agar similar to "hypochlorite bleach, crackers, or musty mouse cages" (339). It is often grown from mixed cultures but can easily be overgrown. Clindamycin disks on media can be used to select for *E. corrodens* because it is resistant to this drug. Aerobic, but not anaerobic, growth requires the presence of hemin (blood or chocolate agar); 3% to 10% carbon dioxide also enhances growth. It does not grow on MacConkey's agar. It is oxidase positive and catalase, indole, and urease negative. It reduces nitrate to nitrite and does not use carbohydrate as a carbon source (172,338,339). A species-specific DNA probe has been used to detect *E. corrodens* in advanced periodontitis (340) and may provide an alternative means of diagnosis.

Virulence properties include a slime layer that may be immunosuppressive and a biologically active lipopolysaccharide. A number of hydrolytic enzymes, particularly proline aminopeptidase and a thiol-dependent hemolysin, may also be important virulence factors (341). Isolation of *E. corrodens* has been associated with mixed infections with α-hemolytic or nonhemolytic streptococci and Enterobacteriaceae, as well as *Actinomyces* infection, although pure cultures have been obtained. These other organisms may enhance the virulence of *E. corrodens* (172,338,339).

E. corrodens is found in normal human oral flora, dental plaques, and gastrointestinal and genitourinary tract flora. It may behave as an opportunistic pathogen when breaks in the mucosal surface or trauma contaminated by oral flora lead to

hematogenous dissemination. Treatment with inappropriate antibiotics may select for *E. corrodens* growth. It is well documented that drug abusers who use methylphenidate have subcutaneous abscesses with *E. corrodens* near the site of injection, probably from chewing the tablets before injection (342). In a series of 43 cases of invasive *E. corrodens* infections, malignancy of the head and neck was the most common underlying disease (35%) (343).

Clinical manifestations are varied but most often are associated with a history of abnormal exposure to oral flora contamination, for example, human bites, dental extractions, or trauma. In a review by Stoloff and Gillies (344), 22 of 33 infections with *E. corrodens* occurring in an 18-month period were related to human bites, fistfights, or trauma. These included face or hand abscesses, septic arthritis, and osteomyelitis. Other infections, either pure or mixed, involving *E. corrodens* include cellulitis (345) or abscess formation [tooth, wound (346), brain (347,348), liver, spleen (349), appendix (344), intraabdominal (350,351), Brodie abscess (352), or intervertebral diskitis (353)]. *Eikenella* has been associated with a suppurative mediastinal lymphadenitis leading to a benign superior vena cava syndrome (354) and intrathoracic infections (355) [empyema (356,357), pneumonia (358–360), lung abscess (361), mediastinitis, and pericarditis (362)]. Head and neck infections including calvarial osteomyelitis (363), dacryocystitis, conjunctivitis, keratitis (364), orbital cellulitis (365), canaliculitis (366), otitis externa, gingivitis (67,367), parotitis (368), thyroiditis (369), and thyroid abscess (370,371), meningitis and subdural empyema (342), and obstetric and gynecologic infections [chorioamnionitis (372), endometritis associated with an intrauterine device (373), and Bartholin's abscess (374)] have been reported. Cardiovascular involvement has been described including endocarditis (22,133,274,375,376) (native and prosthetic valve), mycotic aneurysm (377), intravascular space infections (376), and septic pulmonary emboli from internal jugular vein phlebitis (378).

E. corrodens is generally susceptible to penicillin, ampicillin, carbenicillin, ticarcillin, piperacillin, mezlocillin, second- and third-generation cephalosporins, chloramphenicol, and the quinolones (379–381). *E. corrodens* is variably sensitive to tetracycline and rifampin (382) and uniformly resistant to clindamycin and metronidazole (344). Aminoglycosides and vancomycin are relatively inactive, as are first-generation cephalosporins and isoxazolyl penicillins (379–381). β-Lactamase production (350) and tetracycline resistance (166) have been reported. A review of *Eikenella* infections in children and adolescents stresses the importance of adjunctive surgical débridement in addition to appropriate antimicrobial therapy; 16 of 20 patients for whom outcome information was available underwent at least one surgical procedure for resolution of infection (383).

In the review by Stoloff and Gillies (344), 25 of 32 strains were resistant to penicillin as tested by the disk-diffusion method. This is quite misleading, because the only reliable way to evaluate *in vitro* sensitivity of *E. corrodens* is by agar dilution techniques. This is because of the slow rate of growth of *E. corrodens* and the higher MIC (1 to 4 μg/mL) needed to be effective (380).

Flavobacterium

Organisms belonging to the genus *Flavobacterium* are common inhabitants of soil and water that occasionally cause human disease. *Flavobacterium meningosepticum* is the species most commonly isolated, but *Flavobacterium odoratum*, *Flavobacterium balustinum*, and other *Flavobacterium* species have been reported to cause human infections.

Flavobacterium organisms are long, thin, slightly curved, occasionally filamentous gram-negative rods. They are nonmotile and are catalase, oxidase, gelatinase, and phosphatase positive

(384). They are weakly fermentative but are usually strongly proteolytic, with diffuse β-hemolysis on blood agar plates (3). They grow on blood agar and MacConkey's agar under aerobic conditions, and colonies are visible in 1 to 2 days. Colonies are translucent, circular, convex, smooth, and typically pigmented (yellow to orange), although nonpigmented strains occur. DNA amplification using universal polymerase chain reaction primers along with a specific *Bacteroides-Flavobacterium* probe was used to identify *F. meningosepticum;* this may provide an alternative to culture for diagnosis of *Flavobacterium* infections (385).

The pathogenicity of *Flavobacterium* may be derived from production of an elastase. This elastase is structurally similar to that produced by *Pseudomonas* species; however, it has been shown to be less proteolytic than the latter in animal studies (386). *Flavobacterium* species are generally of low virulence. They are uncommon pathogens in adults, rarely causing infections beyond the newborn period. In neonates, infections present as sepsis and meningitis. Premature and small-for-gestational-age infants seem to be at particular risk. The development of meningitis may be insidious. The prognosis is extremely poor, with mortality rates of more than 60%. Half of the survivors develop significant neurologic complications, often with hydrocephalus.

In adults, infections with *Flavobacterium* are seen among immunocompromised or debilitated patients. Meningitis has been reported in adults. Other clinical presentations include bacteremia, endocarditis (387,388), pneumonia (389), sinusitis (390), peritonitis (391), keratitis (392), cellulitis (389,393), prostatitis (394), and pyomyositis in an intravenous drug user (395). Bacteremia caused by *F. indologenes* was reported in 12 patients in southern Taiwan (eight of whom had polymicrobial bacteremia). Six patients had ventilator-associated pneumonia, two had primary bacteremia, and the remaining four patients had pyonephrosis, peritonitis, biliary tract disease, and surgical wound infection (396). Most of the described cases were nosocomial, and some were associated with prolonged antibiotic use.

In hospitals, *Flavobacterium* organisms have been isolated from ice machines (397), sinks, humidifiers, drinking fountain bubblers (398), nebulizers, and contaminated disinfectants (399). They have also been isolated from tap water, sink traps, tube feedings (400), the hands of hospital personnel, the air in the operating room (401), and pasteurization tanks (402). There is evidence to suggest that *Flavobacterium* organisms enter the hospital through the municipal water supply (400). These organisms have been shown to survive chlorination, resisting levels of chlorine as high as 100 parts per million (398). It has been suggested that susceptible patients acquire *Flavobacterium* through contaminated water or ice. Colonized patients could then serve as secondary reservoirs, with bacterial transmission to noncolonized patients occurring through hand carriage by contaminated hospital personnel.

Flavobacterium species have an unusual antimicrobial susceptibility pattern in that they are resistant to most drugs but are usually susceptible to antibiotics used for gram-positive bacteria. Antimicrobial susceptibilities vary depending on the method used, with dilution methods being more reliable than the agar disk-diffusion method (403,404). Most *Flavobacterium* species produce β-lactamases and carbapenemases and are thus resistant to β-lactam drugs, including aztreonam (391) and imipenem (391,405). Clindamycin, trimethoprim-sulfamethoxazole, rifampin, and ciprofloxacin are active *in vitro* against most strains. Other drugs that have been used alone or in combination with some success include erythromycin, chloramphenicol, and vancomycin. Erythromycin and rifampin have both been given concurrently intravenously and intrathecally with some success. In a study of *in vitro* antibiotic synergy, four isolates of *F. meningosepticum* from neonates with sepsis

and meningitis showed synergy between rifampin and vancomycin against three isolates, whereas combinations of vancomycin, ciprofloxacin, and linezolid showed additive effect. Vancomycin and meropenem were antagonistic (406). Development of resistance during therapy has been documented with erythromycin, rifampin, trimethoprim-sulfamethoxazole, and ciprofloxacin; this should be considered in case of persistence of infection.

Recovery is the rule in immunocompetent older patients infected with contaminated materials. There have been reports of patients with bacteremia that resolved spontaneously without sequelae (407). In immunocompromised patients and neonates, however, prognosis is poor, with mortality rates up to 75% and development of neurologic sequelae.

REFERENCES

Actinobacillus

1. Phillips JE. Genus III. *Actinobacillus* Brumpt 1910, 849. In: Krieg NR, Holt JG, eds. *Bergey's manual of systematic bacteriology*, vol. 1. Baltimore: Williams & Wilkins, 1984:570–575.
2. Negrete-Abascal E, Tenorio V, Garcia C, et al. *Actinobacillus pleuropneumoniae:* virulence and gene cloning. *Arch Med Res* 1994;25:229–233.
3. Pickett M, Hollis D, Bottone E. Miscellaneous gram-negative bacteria. In: Balows A, Hausler W Jr, Herrmann K, et al, eds. *Manual of clinical microbiology.* Washington, DC: American Society for Microbiology, 1991:410–428.
4. Weaver RE, Hollis DG, Bottone EJ. Gram-negative fermentative bacteria and *Francisella tularensis.* In: Lennette EH, Balows A, Hausler WJ Jr, et al, eds. *Manual of clinical microbiology.* Washington, DC: American Society for Microbiology, 1985:309–329.
5. Slotnick IJ. *Actinobacillus* and *Cardiobacterium.* In: Braude AI, ed. *Infectious diseases and medical microbiology,* 2nd ed. Philadelphia: WB Saunders, 1986:348–352.
6. Heath JK, Atkinson SJ, Hembry RM, et al. Bacterial antigens induce collagenase and prostaglandin E_2 synthesis in human gingival fibroblasts through a primary effect on circulating mononuclear cells. *Infect Immun* 1987;55:2148–2154.
7. Rabie G, Lally ET, Shenker BJ. Immunosuppressive properties of *Actinobacillus actinomycetemcomitans* leukotoxin. *Infect Immun* 1988;56:122–127.
8. Simpson DL, Berthold P, Taichman NS. Killing of human myelomonocytic leukemia and lymphocytic cell lines by *Actinobacillus actinomycetemcomitans* leukotoxin. *Infect Immun* 1988;56:1162–1166.
9. Loesche W. Bacterial mediators in periodontal disease. *Clin Infect Dis* 1993;16[Suppl 4]:S203–S210.
10. Saarela M, Saxen L, Slots J. Clonal specificity of *Actinobacillus actinomycetemcomitans* in destructive periodontal disease. *Clin Infect Dis* 1997;25[Suppl 2]:S227–S229.
11. Wikstrom M, Linde A. Ability of oral bacteria to degrade fibronectin. *Infect Immun* 1986;51:707–711.
12. Kaplan AH, Weber DJ, Oddone EZ, et al. Infection due to *Actinobacillus actinomycetemcomitans:* 15 cases and review. *Rev Infect Dis* 1989;11:46–63.
13. Chen Y, Chang S, Luh K, et al. *Actinobacillus actinomycetemcomitans* endocarditis: a report of four cases and review of the literature. *Q J Med* 1991;81:871–878.
14. Grace CJ, Levitz RE, Katz-Pollak H, et al. *Actinobacillus actinomycetemcomitans* prosthetic valve endocarditis. *Rev Infect Dis* 1988;10:922–929.
15. Collazos J, Diaz F, Ayarza R, et al. *Actinobacillus actinomycetemcomitans:* a cause of pulmonary-valve endocarditis of 18 months duration with unusual manifestations [Letter]. *Clin Infect Dis* 1994;18:115–116.
16. van Winkelhoff A, Overbeek B, Pavicic M, et al. Long-standing bacteremia caused by oral *Actinobacillus actinomycetemcomitans* in a patient with a pacemaker. *Clin Infect Dis* 1993;16:216–218.
17. Idir M, Denisi R, Parrens M, et al. Endarteritis and false aneurysm complicating aortic coarctation. *Ann Thorac Surg* 2000;70:966–969.
18. Collazos J, Diaz F, Mayo J, et al. Infectious endocarditis, vasculitis, and glomerulonephritis. *Clin Infect Dis* 1999;28:1342–1343.
19. Steitz A, Orth T, Feddersen A, et al. A case of endocarditis with vasculitis due to *Actinobacillus actinomycetemcomitans:* a 16S rDNA signature for distinction from related organisms. *Clin Infect Dis* 1998;27:224–225.
20. Marshall C, McDonald M. Recurrent subacute bacterial endocarditis as a presentation of left atrial myxoma. *Austr N Z J Med* 1998;28:350.
21. Arana-Domondon LC, Chen S, Mann L, et al. Boar hunter's endocarditis. *JAMA* 1998;279:198.
22. Meyer DJ, Gerding DN. Favorable prognosis of patients with prosthetic valve endocarditis caused by gram-negative bacilli of the HACEK group. *Am J Med* 1988;85:104–107.

23. Wilson ME, Genco RJ. The role of antibody, complement and neutrophils in host defense against *Actinobacillus actinomycetemcomitans*. *Immunol Invest* 1989;18:187–209.

24. Genco RJ, Van-Dyke TE, Levine MJ, et al. 1985 Kreshover Lecture. Molecular factors influencing neutrophil defects in periodontal disease. *J Dent Res* 1986;65:1379–1391.

25. Pavicic M, van Winkelhoff A, Douque N, et al. Microbiological and clinical effects of metronidazole and amoxicillin in *Actinobacillus actinomycetemcomitans*–associated periodontitis. A 2-year evaluation. *J Clin Periodontol* 1994;21:107–112.

26. Horowitz EA, Pugsley MP, Turbes PG, et al. Pericarditis caused by *Actinobacillus actinomycetemcomitans*. *J Infect Dis* 1987;155:152–153.

27. Ishak MA, Zablit KV, Duman J. Endogenous endophthalmitis caused by *Actinobacillus actinomycetemcomitans*. *Can J Ophthalmol* 1986;21:284–286.

28. Schmidt M, Smith M, Levy C. Endophthalmitis caused by unusual gram-negative bacilli: three case reports and review. *Clin Infect Dis* 1993;17:686–690.

29. Burgess RC. Chronic tenosynovitis caused by *Actinobacillus actinomycetemcomitans*. *J Hand Surg* 1987;12:294–295.

30. Molina F, Echaniz A, Duran M, et al. Infectious arthritis of the knee due to *Actinobacillus actinomycetemcomitans* [Letter]. *Eur J Clin Microbiol Infect Dis* 1994;13:687–689.

31. Cuende E, de Pablos M, Gomez M, et al. Coexistence of pseudogout and arthritis due to *Actinobacillus actinomycetemcomitans*. *Clin Infect Dis* 1996;23:657–658.

32. Morris J, Sewell D. Necrotizing pneumonia caused by mixed infection with *Actinobacillus actinomycetemcomitans* and *Actinomyces israelii*: case report and review. *Clin Infect Dis* 1994;18:450–452.

33. Yuan P, Yand P, Lee L, et al. *Actinobacillus actinomycetemcomitans* pneumonia with chest wall involvement and rib destruction. *Chest* 1992;101:1450–1452.

34. Chen A, Liu C, Yao W, et al. *Actinobacillus actinomycetemcomitans* pneumonia with chest wall and subphrenic abscess. *Scand J Infect Dis* 1995;27:289–290.

35. Dommann S, Widmer M, Dommann-Scherrer C, et al. *Actinobacillus actinomycetemcomitans* isolated from a mycetoma (of the forearm) [in German]. *Hautarzt* 1994;45:402–405.

36. Hammerberg O, Gregson D, Gopaul D, et al. Recurrent cervical and submandibular lymphadenitis due to *Actinobacillus actinomycetemcomitans* [Letter]. *Clin Infect Dis* 1993;7:1077–1078.

37. Page MI, King EO. Infection due to *Actinobacillus actinomycetemcomitans* and *Haemophilus aphrophilus*. *N Engl J Med* 1966;275:181–188.

38. Kuijper E, Wiggerts H, Jonker G, et al. Disseminated actinomycosis due to *Actinomyces meyeri* and *Actinobacillus actinomycetemcomitans*. *Scand J Infect Dis* 1992;24:667–672.

39. Tyrrell J, Noone P, Prichard J. Thoracic actinomycosis complicated by *Actinobacillus actinomycetemcomitans*: case report and review of literature. *Respir Med* 1992;86:341–343.

40. Zijlstra E, Swart G, Godfroy F, et al. Pericarditis, pneumonia and brain abscess due to a combined *Actinomyces-Actinobacillus actinomycetemcomitans* infection. *J Infect* 1992;25:83–87.

41. Benaoudia F, Escande F, Simonet M. Infection due to *Actinobacillus lignieresii* after a horse bite [Letter]. *Eur J Clin Microbiol Infect Dis* 1994;13:439–440.

42. Peel M, Hornidge K, Luppino M, et al. *Actinobacillus* spp. and related bacteria in infected wounds of humans bitten by horses and sheep. *J Clin Microbiol* 1991;29:2535–2538.

43. Escande F, Bailly A, Bone S, et al. *Actinobacillus suis* infection after a pig bite. *Lancet* 1996;348:888.

44. Baker PJ, Wilson ME. Effect of clindamycin on neutrophil killing of gram-negative periodontal bacteria. *Antimicrob Agents Chemother* 1988;32:1521–1527.

45. Goldstein EJC, Citron DM. Comparative activities of cefuroxime, amoxicillin-clavulanic acid, ciprofloxacin, enoxacin, and ofloxacin against aerobic and anaerobic bacteria isolated from bite wounds. *Antimicrob Agents Chemother* 1988;32:1143–1148.

46. Goldstein EJC, Citron DM, Merriam CV, et al. Activity of gatifloxacin compared to those of five other quinolones versus aerobic and anaerobic isolates from skin and soft tissue samples of human and animal bite wound infections. *Antimicrob Agents Chemother* 1999;43:1475–1479.

47. Pavicic M, van Winkelhoff A, de Graaf J. *In vitro* susceptibilities of *Actinobacillus actinomycetemcomitans* to a number of antimicrobial combinations. *Antimicrob Agents Chemother* 1992;36:2634–2638.

48. Pajukanta R, Asikainen S, Saarela M, et al. *In vitro* antimicrobial susceptibility of different serotypes of *Actinobacillus actinomycetemcomitans*. *Scand J Dent Res* 1993;101:299–303.

49. Rovaldi CR, Pievsky A, Sole NA, et al. Photoactive porphyrin derivative with broad-spectrum activity against oral pathogens in vitro. *Antimicrob Agents Chemother* 2000;44:3364–3367.

50. Babinchak TJ. Oral ciprofloxacin therapy for prosthetic valve endocarditis due to *Actinobacillus actinomycetemcomitans*. *Clin Infect Dis* 1995;21:1517.

Capnocytophaga

51. Williams BL, Hollis D, Holdeman IV. Synonymy of strains of Centers for Disease Control group DF-1 with species of *Capnocytophaga*. *J Clin Microbiol* 1979;10:550–556.

52. Newman MG, Suffer VL, Pickett MJ, et al. Detection, identification, and comparison of *Capnocytophaga, Bacteroides ochraceus*, and DF-1. *J Clin Microbiol* 1979;10:557–562.

53. Davis CE. *Capnocytophaga*. In: Braude AI, ed. *Infectious diseases and medical microbiology*, 2nd ed. Philadelphia: WB Saunders, 1986:361–364.

54. Yamamoto T, Kajiura S, Hirai Y, et al. *Capnocytophaga haemolytica* sp. nov. and *Capnocytophaga granulosa* sp. nov., from human dental plaque. *Int J Syst Bacteriol* 1994;44:324–329.

55. Ciantar M, Spratt DA, Newman DA, et al. *Capnocytophaga granulosa* and *Capnocytophaga haemolytica*: a novel species in subgingival plaques. *J Clin Periodontol* 2001;28:701–705.

56. Brenner DJ, Hollis DG, Fanning R, et al. *Capnocytophaga canimor sus* sp. nov. (formerly CDC group DF-2), a cause of septicemia following dog bite, and *C. cynodegmi* sp. nov., a cause of localized wound infection following dog bite. *J Clin Microbiol* 1989;27:231–235.

57. Rummens JL, Fossepre JM, De Gruyter M, et al. Isolation of *Capnocytophaga* species with a new selective medium. *J Clin Microbiol* 1985;22:375–378.

58. Mashimo PA, Yamamoto Y, Nakamura M, et al. Selective recovery of oral *Capnocytophaga* spp. with sheep blood agar containing bacitracin and polymyxin B. *J Clin Microbiol* 1983;17:187–191.

59. Chen S, Hicks L, Mitchell D, et al. Serological cross-reaction between *Legionella* spp. and *Capnocytophaga ochracea* by using latex agglutination test. *J Clin Microbiol* 1994;32:3054–3055.

60. Shurin SB, Socransky SS, Sweeney E, et al. A neutrophil disorder induced by *Capnocytophaga*, a dental micro-organism. *N Engl J Med* 1979;301:849–854.

61. Forlenza SW, Newman MG, Lipsey AI, et al. *Capnocytophaga* sepsis: a newly recognised clinical entity in granulocytopenic patients. *Lancet* 1980;1:567–568.

62. Arlet G, Sanson-Le Pors MJ, Castaigne S, et al. Isolation of a strain of β-lactamase–producing *Capnocytophaga ochracea* [Letter]. *J Infect Dis* 1987;155:1346.

63. Wilson ME, Jonak-Urbanczyk JT, Bronson PM, et al. *Capnocytophaga* species: increased resistance of clinical isolates to serum bactericidal action. *J Infect Dis* 1987;156:99–106.

64. Warren JS, Allen SD. Clinical, pathogenetic, and laboratory features of *Capnocytophaga* infections. *Am J Clin Pathol* 1986;86:513–518.

65. Parenti DM, Snydman DR. *Capnocytophaga* species: infections in nonimmunocompromised and immunocompromised hosts. *J Infect Dis* 1985;151:140–147.

66. Miller K, Hansen W, Labbe M, et al. Isolation of *Neisseria elongata* and of *Capnocytophaga ochracea* from vaginal specimens [Letter]. *J Infect* 1985;10:174–175.

67. Newman MG, Socransky SS, Savitt ED, et al. Studies of the microbiology of periodontosis. *J Periodontol* 1976;47:373–379.

68. Gandola C, Butler T, Badger S, et al. Septicemia caused by *Capnocytophaga* in a granulocytopenic patient with glossitis. *Arch Intern Med* 1980;140:851–852.

69. Applebaum PC, Ballard JO, Eyster ME. Septicemia due to *Capnocytophaga* (*Bacteroides ochraceus*) in Hodgkin's disease. *Ann Intern Med* 1979;90:716–717.

70. Kim JO, Ginsberg J, McGowan KL. *Capnocytophaga* meningitis in a cancer patient. *Pediatr Infect Dis J* 1996;15:636–637.

71. Ormerod LD, Foster CS, Paton BG, et al. Ocular *Capnocytophaga* infection in an edentulous, immunocompetent host. *Cornea* 1988;7:218–222.

72. Roussel TJ, Osato MS, Wilhelmus KR. *Capnocytophaga* keratitis. *Br J Ophthalmol* 1985;69:187–188.

73. Heidemann DG, Pflugfelder SC, Kronish J, et al. Necrotizing keratitis caused by *Capnocytophaga ochracea*. *Am J Ophthalmol* 1988;105:655–660.

74. Rubsamen PE, McLeish WM, Pflugfelder S, et al. *Capnocytophaga* endophthalmitis. *Ophthalmology* 1993;100:456–459.

75. Eiferman RA, Levartovsky S, Box JD. Anaerobic *Capnocytophaga* corneal ulcer. *Am J Ophthalmol* 1988;105:427.

76. Buu-Hoi AY, Joundy S, Acar JF. Endocarditis caused by *Capnocytophaga ochracea*. *J Clin Microbiol* 1988;26:1061–1062.

77. Matlow A, Vellend H. *Capnocytophaga*: a pathogen in immunocompetent hosts. *J Infect Dis* 1985;152:233–234.

78. Mosher CB, Corp R. Mediastinal abscess with *Capnocytophaga* spp. in a competent host. *J Clin Microbiol* 1986;24:161–162.

79. Winn RE, Chase WF, Lauderdale PW, et al. Septic arthritis involving *Capnocytophaga ochracea*. *J Clin Microbiol* 1984;19:538–540.

80. Seger R, Kloeti J, Von Graevenitz A, et al. Cervical abscess due to *Capnocytophaga ochracea*. *Pediatr Infect Dis* 1982;1:170–172.

81. Johnson CC, Poupard J. Inguinal lymphadenitis associated with *Capnocytophaga* bacilli. *J Clin Microbiol* 1991;29:832–833.

82. Brown R, McCann MP. *Capnocytophaga* bacteremia in a neutropenic patient with sinusitis. *Ala Med* 1985;54:33–35.

83. Goudreau E, Comtois R, Bayardelle P, et al. *Capnocytophaga ochracea* and group F beta-hemolytic *Streptococcus* suppurative thyroiditis. *J Otolaryngol* 1986;15:59–61.

84. Elster AD, Macone AB, Kasser JR. Osteomyelitis caused by *Capnocytophaga ochracea*. *J Pediatr Orthop* 1983;3:613–615.

85. Duong M, Besancenot JF, Neuwirth C, et al. Vertebral osteomyelitis due to *Capnocytophaga* species in immunocompetent patients: report of two cases and review. *Clin Infect Dis* 1996;22:1099–1101.

86. Tarrero MT, Baranda MM, Arizaga JI, et al. Peritonitis involving *Capnocytophaga ochracea*. *Am J Gastroenterol* 1989;84:206–207.

87. Weber G, Abu-Shakra M, Hertzanu Y, et al. Liver abscess caused by *Capnocytophaga* species. *Clin Infect Dis* 1997;25:152–153.

88. Hager H, DeLasho G, Zenn R. Peripartum infections with *Capnocytophaga*. A case report. *J Reprod Med* 1988;33:657–660.

89. Ernest JM, Wasilauskas B. *Capnocytophaga* in the amniotic fluid of a woman in preterm labor with intact membranes. *Am J Obstet Gynecol* 1985;153:648–649.

90. McDonald H, Gordon DL. *Capnocytophaga* species: a cause of amniotic fluid infection and preterm labour. *Pathology* 1988;20:74–76.

91. Mercer LJ. *Capnocytophaga* isolated from the endometrium as a cause of neonatal sepsis: a case report. *J Reprod Med* 1985;30:67–68.

92. Feldman JD, Kontaxis EN, Sherman MP. Congenital bacteremia due to *Capnocytophaga*. *Pediatr Infect Dis* 1985;4:415–416.

93. Arlet G, Sanson-Le-Pors MJ, Ortenberg M, et al. Infections a *Capnocytophaga*. A propos de huit observations. *Ann Biol Clin (Paris)* 1986;44:373–379.

94. Juhl G, Brzezinski WA. Disseminated actinomycosis associated with infection by *Capnocytophaga* species. *J Infect Dis* 1984;149:654.

95. Ebinger M, Nichterlein T, Schumacher UK, et al. Isolation of *Capnocytophaga granulosa* from an abscess in an immunocompetent adolescent. *Clin Infect Dis* 2000;30:606–607.

96. Forlenza SW, Newman MG, Horikoshi AL, et al. Antimicrobial susceptibility of *Capnocytophaga*. *Antimicrob Agents Chemother* 1981;19:144–146.

97. Sutter VL, Pyeatt D, Kwok YY. In vitro susceptibility *Capnocytophaga* strains of to 18 antimicrobial agents. *Antimicrob Agents Chemother* 1981;20:270–271.

98. Rummens JL, Gordts B, Van Landuyt HW. *In vitro* susceptibility of *Capnocytophaga* species to 29 antimicrobial agents. *Antimicrob Agents Chemother* 1986;30:739–742.

99. Hawkey PM, Smith SD, Haynes J, et al. *In vitro* susceptibility of *Capnocytophaga* species to antimicrobial agents. *Antimicrob Agents Chemother* 1987;31:331–332.

100. Fuchs PC. *In vitro* antimicrobial activity and susceptibility testing of ofloxacin. *Am J Med* 1989;87[Suppl 6C]:10S–13S.

101. Martino R, Ramila E, Cap de Vila JA, et al. Bacteremia caused by *Capnocytophaga* species in patients with neutropenia and cancer: results of a multicenter study. *Clin Infect Dis* 2001;33:E20–E22.

102. Roscoe DL, Zemcov SJV, Thornber D, et al. Antimicrobial susceptibilities and β-lactamase characterization of *Capnocytophaga* species. *Antimicrob Agents Chemother* 1992;36:2197–2200.

103. Jolivet-Gougron A, Buffet A, Dupuy C, et al. *In vitro* susceptibilities of *Capnocytophaga* isolates to β-lactam antibiotics and β-lactamase inhibitors. *Antimicrob Agents Chemother* 2000;44:3186–3188.

104. Nachnani S, Scuteri A, Newman MG, et al. E-test: a new technique for antimicrobial susceptibility testing for periodontal microorganisms. *J Periodontol* 1992;63:576–583.

105. Hicklin H, Verghese A, Alvarez S. Dysgonic fermenter 2 septicemia. *Rev Infect Dis* 1987;9:884–890.

106. Bailie WE, Stowe EC, Schmitt AM. Aerobic bacterial flora of oral and nasal fluids of canines with reference to bacteria associated with bites. *J Clin Microbiol* 1978;7:223–234.

107. Westerink MAJ, Amsterdam D, Petell RJ, et al. Septicemia due to DF-2. *Am J Med* 1987;83:155–158.

108. Butler T, Weaver RE, Ramani TKV, et al. Unidentified gram-negative rod infection: a new disease of man. *Ann Intern Med* 1977;86:1–5.

109. Pers C, Gahrn-Hansen B, Frederiksen W. *Capnocytophaga canimorsus* septicemia in Denmark, 1982–1995: review of 39 cases. *Clin Infect Dis* 1996;23:71–75.

110. Mirza I, Wolk J, Toth L, et al. Waterhouse-Friderichsen syndrome secondary to *Capnocytophaga canimorsus* septicemia and demonstration of bacteremia by peripheral blood smear. *Arch Pathol Lab Med* 2000;124:859–863.

111. Chambers GW, Westblom TU. Pleural infection caused by *Capnocytophaga canimorsus*, formerly CDC group DF-2. *Clin Infect Dis* 1992;15:325–326.

112. Banerjee TK, Grubb W, Otero C, et al. Musculocutaneous mononeuropathy complicating *Capnocytophaga canimorsus* infection. *Neurology* 1993;343:2411–2412.

113. Chadosh I. Cat's tooth keratitis: human corneal infection with *Capnocytophaga canimorsus*. *Cornea* 2001;20:661–663.

114. Zimmer-Galler IE, Pach JM. *Capnocytophaga canimorsus* endophthalmitis. *Retina* 1996;16:163–164.

115. Verghese A, Fawwaz H, Berk S, et al. Susceptibility of dysgonic fermenter 2 to antimicrobial agents *in vitro*. *Antimicrob Agents Chemother* 1988;32:78–80.

Dysgonomonas capnocytophagoides (Formerly CDC Group DF-3)

116. Hofstad T, Olsen I, Eribe ER, et al. *Dysgonomonas* gen. nov. to accommodate *Dysgonomonas gadei* sp. nov., an organism isolated from a human gall bladder, and *Dysgonomonas capnocytophagoides* (formerly CDC Group DF-3). *Int J Syst Eval Microbiol* 2000;50:2189–2195.

117. Blum RN, Berry CD, Phillips MG. Clinical illnesses associated with isolation of dysgonic fermenter 3 from stool samples. *J Clin Microbiol* 1992;30:396–400.

118. Gill VJ, Travis LB, Williams DY. Clinical and microbiological observations on CDC group DF-3, a gram-negative coccobacillus. *J Clin Microbiol* 1991;29:1589–1592.

119. Wagner DK, Wright JJ, Ansher AF, et al. Dysgonic fermenter 3-associated gastrointestinal disease in a patient with common variable hypogammaglobulinemia. *Am J Med* 1988;84:315–318.

120. Melhus A. Isolation of dysgonic fermenter 3, a rare isolate associated with diarrhoea in immunocompromised patients. *Scand J Infect Dis* 1997;29:195–196.

121. Aronson NE, Zbick CJ. Dysgonic fermenter 3 bacteremia in a neutropenic patient with acute lymphocytic leukemia. *J Clin Microbiol* 1988;26:2213–2215.

122. Schonheyder H, Ejlertsen T, Frederiksen W. Isolation of a dysgonic fermenter (DF-3) from urine of a patient. *Eur J Clin Microbiol Infect Dis* 1991;10:530–531.

123. Bangsborg JM, Frederiksen W, Bruun B. Dysgonic fermenter 3-associated abscess in a diabetic patient. *J Infect* 1990;20:237–240.

Cardiobacterium

124. Weaver RE. Genus *Cardiobacterium* Slotnick and Dougherty 1964, 271. In: Krieg NR, Holt JG, eds. *Bergey's manual of systematic bacteriology*, vol. 1. Baltimore: Williams & Wilkins, 1984:583–585.

125. Taveras J III, Campo R, Segal N, et al. Apparent culture-negative endocarditis of the prosthetic valve caused by *Cardiobacterium hominis*. *South Med J* 1993;86:1439–1440.

126. Pritchard T, Foust R, Cantely J, et al. Prosthetic valve endocarditis due to *Cardiobacterium hominis* occurring after upper gastrointestinal endoscopy. *Am J Med* 1991;90:516–518.

127. Schlaeffer F, Riesenberg K, Mikolich D, et al. Serious bacterial infections after endoscopic procedures. *Arch Intern Med* 1996;156:572–574.

128. Ben-Chetrit E, Nashif M, Levo Y. Infective endocarditis caused by uncommon bacteria. *Scand J Infect Dis* 1983;15:179–183.

129. Kiwan Y, Shuhaiber H, Chungh T. *Cardiobacterium hominis* endocarditis. *J Cardiovasc Surg* 1989;39:281–283.

130. Wormser GP, Bottone EJ. *Cardiobacterium hominis*: review of microbiologic and clinical features. *Rev Infect Dis* 1983;5:680–691.

131. Zehnter E, Seifert H, Petit M, et al. A protracted course in *Cardiobacterium hominis* endocarditis [in German]. *Dtsch Med Wochenschr* 1991;116:768–771.

132. Lecluse E, Scanu P, Saloux E, et al. Endocarditis caused by *Cardiobacterium hominis* [in French]. *Presse Med* 1994;23:325–328.

133. Geraci JE, Wilson WR. Endocarditis due to gram-negative bacteria: report of 56 cases. *Mayo Clin Proc* 1982;57:145–148.

134. Ellner JJ, Rosenthal MS, Lerner PI, et al. Infective endocarditis caused by slow-growing, fastidious, gram-negative bacteria. *Medicine (Baltimore)* 1979;58:145–158.

135. Currie PF, Codispoti M, Mankad PS, et al. Late aortic homograft valve endocarditis caused by *Cardiobacterium hominis*: a case report and review of the literature. *Heart* 2000;83:579–581.

136. Lin B, Vieco P. Intracranial mycotic aneurysm in a patient with endocarditis caused by *Cardiobacterium hominis*. *Can Assoc Radiol J* 1995;46:40–42.

137. Silver SE. Ruptured mycotic aneurysm of the superior mesenteric artery that was due to *Cardiobacterium* endocarditis. *Clin Infect Dis* 1999;29:1573–1574.

138. Rechtman D, Nadler J. Abdominal abscess due to *Cardiobacterium hominis* and *Clostridium bifermentans*. *Rev Infect Dis* 1991;13:418–419.

139. Nurnberger M, Treadwell T, Lin B, et al. Pacemaker lead infection and vertebral osteomyelitis presumed due to *Cardiobacterium hominis*. *Clin Infect Dis* 1998;27:890–891.

140. Francioli PB, Roussianos D, Glauser MP. *Cardiobacterium hominis* endocarditis manifesting as bacterial meningitis. *Arch Intern Med* 1983;143:1483–1484.

141. Le Quellec A, Bessis D, Perez C, et al. endocarditis due to beta-lactamase–producing *Cardiobacterium hominis*. *Clin Infect Dis* 1994;19:994–995.

142. Lu P, Hsueh P, Hung C, et al. Infective endocarditis complicated with progressive heart failure due to β-lactamase–producing *Cardiobacterium hominis*. *J Clin Microbiol* 2000;38:2015–2017.

143. Watanakunakorn C. The use of beta-lactam antibiotics in the treatment of septicaemia and endocarditis. *Scand J Infect Dis Suppl* 1984;42:110–116.

144. Vogt K, Klefisch F, Hahn H, et al. Antibacterial efficacy of ciprofloxacin in a case of endocarditis due to *Cardiobacterium hominis*. *Int J Med Microbiol Virol Parasitol Infect Dis* 1994;28:80–84.

Chromobacterium

145. Davis CE. *Chromobacterium*. In: Braude AI, ed. *Infectious diseases and medical microbiology*, 2nd ed. Philadelphia: WB Saunders, 1986:358–361.

146. Peter HAS. Genus *Chromobacterium* Bergonzini 1881, 153. In: Krieg NR, Holt JG, eds. *Bergey's manual of systematic bacteriology*, vol 1. Baltimore: Williams & Wilkins, 1984:580–582.

147. Singh PD, Liu WC, Gougoutas JZ, et al. Aerocavin, a new antibiotic produced by *Chromobacterium violaceum*. *J Antibiot (Tokyo)* 1988;41:446–453.

148. Parker WL, Rathnum ML, Johnson JH, et al. Aerocyanidin, a new antibiotic produced by *Chromobacterium violaceum*. *J Antibiot (Tokyo)* 1988;41:454–463.

149. Inglis TJJ, Chiang D, Lee GSH, et al. Potential misidentification of *Burkholderia pseudomallei* by API 2ONE. *Pathology* 1998;30:62–64.

150. Miller DP, Blevins WT, Steele DB, et al. A comparative study of virulent and avirulent strains of *Chromobacterium violaceum*. *Can J Microbiol* 1988;34:249–255.

151. Ponte R, Jenkins S: Fatal *Chromobacterium violaceum* infections associated with exposure to stagnant waters. *Pediatric Infect Dis J* 1992;11:583–586.

152. Koburger JA, May SO. Isolation of *Chromobacterium* spp. from foods, soil, and water. *Appl Environ Microbiol* 1982;44:1463–1465.

153. Berkowitz FE, Metchock B. Third generation cephalosporin-resistant Gram-negative bacilli in the feces of hospitalized children. *Pediatr Infect Dis J* 1995;14:97–100.

154. Auerbach PS. Natural microbiologic hazards of the aquatic environment. *Clin Dermatol* 1987;5:52–61.

155. Macher AM, Casale TB, Fauci AS. Chronic granulomatous disease in childhood and *Chromobacterium violaceum* infections in the southeastern United States. *Ann Intern Med* 1982;97:51–55.

156. Sorensen RU, Jacobs MR, Shurin SB. *Chromobacterium violaceum* adenitis acquired in the northern United States as a complication of chronic granulomatous disease. *Pediatr Infect Dis* 1985;4:701–702.

157. Hiraoka N, Yoshioka K, Inoue K, et al. *Chromobacterium violaceum* sepsis accompanied by bacteria-associated hemophagocytic syndrome in a Japanese man. *Arch Intern Med* 1999;159:1623–1624.

158. Suarez AE, Wenokur B, Johnson JM, et al. Nonfatal chromobacterial sepsis. *South Med J* 1986;79:1146–1148.

159. Kaufman SC, Ceraso D, Schugurensky A. First case report from Argentina of fatal septicemia caused by *Chromobacterium violaceum*. *J Clin Microbiol* 1986;23:956–958.

160. Centers for Disease Control and Prevention. Chromobacteriosis—Florida. *MMWR Mortal Wkly Rep* 1991;29:613–615.

161. Ti T, Tan W, Chong A, et al. Nonfatal and fatal infections caused by *Chromobacterium violaceum*. *Clin Infect Dis* 1993;17:505–507.

162. Roberts SA, Morris AJ, McIvor N, et al. *Chromobacterium violaceum* infection of the deep neck tissues in a traveler to Thailand. *Clin Infect Dis* 1997;25:334–335.

163. Hassan H, Suntharalingam S, Dhillon K. Fatal *Chromobacterium violaceum* septicaemia. *Singapore Med J* 1993;34:456–458.

164. Shetty M, Venkatesh A, Shenoy S, et al. *Chromobacterium violaceum* meningitis—a case report. *Indian J Med Sci* 1987;41:275–276.

165. Martin J, Brimacombe J. *Chromobacterium violaceum* septicaemia: the intensive care management of two cases. *Anaesth Intensive Care* 1992;20:88–90.

166. Feldman RB, Stern GA, Hood CI. *Chromobacterium violaceum* infection of the eye. A report of two cases. *Arch Ophthalmol* 1984;102:711–713.

167. Macher AM, Casale TB, Gallin JI, et al. *Chromobacterium violaceum* infections and chronic granulomatous disease [Letter]. *Ann Intern Med* 1983;98:259.

168. Mamlok RJ, Mamlok V, Mills GC, et al. Glucose-6-phosphate dehydrogenase deficiency, neutrophil dysfunction and *Chromobacterium violaceum* sepsis. *J Pediatr* 1987;111:852–854.

169. Dreizen S, McCredie KB, Bodey GP, et al. Unusual mucocutaneous infections in immunosuppressed patients with leukemia—expansion of an earlier study. *Postgrad Med* 1986;79:287–294.

170. Aldridge KE, Valainis GT, Sanders CV: Comparison of the in vitro activity of ciprofloxacin and 24 other antimicrobial agents against clinical strains of *Chromobacterium violaceum*. *Diagn Microbiol Infect Dis* 1988;10:31–39.

Acinetobacter

171. Glew RH, Moellering RC, Kunz LJ. Infections with *Acinetobacter calcoaceticus* (*Herellea vaginicola*): clinical and laboratory studies. *Medicine (Baltimore)* 1977;56:79–97.

172. Juni E. Genus III. *Acinetobacter* Brisou and Prevot 1954, 727. In: Krieg NR, Holt JG, eds. *Bergey's manual of systematic bacteriology*, vol 1. Baltimore: Williams & Wilkins, 1984:303–307.

173. Bouvet PJM, Grimont PAO. Taxonomy of the genus Acinetobacter with the recognition of *Acinetobacter baumannii* sp. nov., *Acinetobacter haemolyticus* sp. nov., *Acinetobacter johnsonii* sp. nov., and *Acinetobacter junii* sp. nov. and extended descriptions of *Acinetobacter calcoaceticus* and *Acinetobacter lwoffii*. *Int J Syst Bacteriol* 1986;36:228–240.

174. Traub WH. *Acinetobacter baumannii* serotyping for delineation of outbreaks of nosocomial cross-infection. *J Clin Microbiol* 1989;27:2713–2716.

175. Gerner-Smidt P, Frederiksen W. *Acinetobacter* in Denmark: I. Taxonomy, antibiotic susceptibility, and pathogenicity of 112 clinical strains. *APMIS* 1993;101:815–825.

176. Dijkshoom L, van der Toorn J. *Acinetobacter* species: which do we mean [Letter]? *Clin Infect Dis* 1992;15:748–749.

177. Rubin SJ, Granato PA, Wasilauskas BL. Glucose-nonfermenting gram-negative bacteria. In: Lennette EH, Balows A, Housler NJ, eds. *Manual of clinical microbiology*. Washington, DC: American Society for Microbiology, 1985:330–349.

178. Davis CE, Baer H. *Moraxella, Kingella* and *Acinetobacter*. In: Braude AI, ed. *Infectious diseases and medical microbiology*, 2nd ed. Philadelphia: WB Saunders, 1986:287–292.

179. Saikku P, Puolakkainen M, Leiononen M, et al. Cross-reactivity between Chlamydiazyme and *Acinetobacter* strains [Letter]. *N Engl J Med* 1986;314:922–923.

180. Brade H, Brunner H. Serological cross-reactions between *Acinetobacter calcoaceticus* and chlamydiae. *J Clin Microbiol* 1979;10:819–822.

181. Jankowski S, Grzybek-Hryncewicz K, Fleischer M, et al. Susceptibility of isolates of *Acinetobacter anitratus* and *Acinetobacter lwoffii* to the bactericidal activity of normal human serum. *FEMS Microbiol Immunol* 1992;4:255–260.

182. Gennari M, Lombardi P. Comparative characterization of *Acinetobacter* strains isolated from different foods and clinical sources. *Int J Med Microbiol Virol Parasitol Infect Dis* 1993;279:553–564.

183. Cordes LG, Brink EW, Checko PJ, et al. A cluster of *Acinetobacter* pneumonia in foundry workers. *Ann Intern Med* 1981;95:688–693.

184. Allen KD, Green HT. Hospital outbreak of multi-resistant *Acinetobacter anitratus*: an airborne mode of spread? *J Hosp Infect* 1987;9:110–119.

185. Daschner FD, Habel H. Hospital outbreak of multi-resistant *Acinetobacter anitratus*: an airborne mode of spread? *J Hosp Infect* 1987;10:211–212.

186. Vivian A, Hinchliffe E, Fewson CA. *Acinetobacter calcoaceticus*: some approaches to a problem. *J Hosp Infect* 1981;2:199–203.

187. Erganis O, Corlu M, Kaya O, et al. Isolation of *Acinetobacter calcoaceticus* from septicaemic hens. *Vet Rec* 1988;123:374.

188. Kaya O, Ates M, Erganis O, et al. Isolation of *Acinetobacter lwoffii* from hens with septicemia. *Zentralbl Veterinarmed B* 1989;36:157–158.

189. Lewis SJ, Gilmour A. Microflora associated with the internal surfaces of rubber and stainless steel milk transfer pipeline. *J Appl Bacteriol* 1987;62:327–333.

190. Gonzalez C, Gutierrez C, Grande T. Bacterial flora in bottled uncarbonated mineral drinking water. *Can J Microbiol* 1987;33:1120–1125.

191. Hartstein AI, Rashad AL, Liebler JM, et al. Multiple intensive care unit outbreak of *Acinetobacter calcoaceticus* subspecies *anitratus* respiratory infection and colonization associated with contaminated, reusable ventilator circuits and resuscitation bags. *Am J Med* 1988;85:624–631.

192. Ahmed J, Brutus A, D'Amato R, et al. *Acinetobacter calcoaceticus anitratus* outbreak in the intensive care unit traced to a peak flow meter. *Am J Infect Control* 194;22:319–321.

193. Smith RW, Masanari M. Room humidifiers as the source of *Acinetobacter* infection. *JAMA* 1977;237:795–797.

194. Van-Saene HK, Van-Putte JC, Van-Saene JJ, et al. Sink flora in a long-stay hospital is determined by the patients' oral and rectal flora. *Epidemiol Infect* 1989;102:231–238.

195. Snydman DR, Mallow MF, Brock SM, et al. Pseudobacteremia: false-positive blood cultures from mist tent contamination. *Am J Epidemiol* 1977;106:154–159.

196. Abrutyn E, Goodhard GL, Roos K, et al. *Acinetobacter calcoaceticus* outbreak associated with peritoneal dialysis. *Am J Epidemiol* 1978;107:328–335.

197. Flaherty J, Garcia-Houchins S, Chudy R, et al. An outbreak of gram-negative bacteremia traced to contaminated O-rings in reprocessed dialyzers. *Ann Intern Med* 1993;119:1072–1078.

198. Alfa M, Sitter D. In-hospital evaluation of contamination of duodenoscopes: a quantitative assessment of the effect of drying. *J Hosp Infect* 1991;19:89–98.

199. Shawker TH, Kluge RM, Ayella RJ. Bacteremia associated with angiography. *JAMA* 1974;229:1090–1092.

200. Haslett TM, Isenberg HD, Hilton E, et al. Microbiology of indwelling central intravascular catheters. *J Clin Microbiol* 1988;26:696–701.

201. Beck-Sague CM, Jarvis WR. Epidemic bloodstream infections associated with pressure transducers: a persistent problem. *Infect Control Hosp Epidemiol* 1989;10:54–59.

202. Baguley D, Whipp J, Farrington M. A microbiological hazard in caloric testing. *Br J Audiol* 1991;25:427–428.

203. Patterson J, Vecchio J, Pantelick E, et al. Association of contaminated gloves with transmission of *Acinetobacter calcoaceticus* var. *anitratus* in an intensive care unit. *Am J Med* 1991;91:479–483.

204. Matsen JM. The source of hospital infection. *Medicine (Baltimore)* 1973;52:271–277.

205. Arduino M, Bland L, McAllister S, et al. Microbial growth and endotoxin production in the intravenous anesthetic propofol. *Infect Control Hosp Epidemiol* 1991;12:535–539.

206. Oie S, Kamiya A, Hironaga K, et al. Microbial contamination of enteral feeding solution and its prevention. *Am J Infect Control* 1993;21:34–38.

207. Wendt C, Dietze B, Dietz, E, et al. Survival of *Acinetobacter baumannii* on dry surfaces. *J Clin Microbiol* 1997;35:1394–1397.

208. Sherertz R, Sullivan M. An outbreak of infections with *Acinetobacter calcoaceticus* in burn patients: contamination of patients' mattresses. *J Infect Dis* 1985;151:252–258.

209. Weernink A, Severin WP, Tjernberg I, et al. Pillows, an unexpected source of *Acinetobacter*. *J Hosp Infect* 1995;29:189–199.

210. Rosenthal SL. Sources of *Pseudomonas* and *Acinetobacter* species found in human culture materials. *Am J Clin Pathol* 1974;62:807–811.

211. Rudin ML, Michael JR, Huxley EJ. Community-acquired *Acinetobacter* pneumonia. *Am J Med* 1979;67:39–43.

212. Smego RA. Endemic nosocomial *Acinetobacter calcoaceticus* bacteremia: clinical significance, treatment, and prognosis. *Arch Intern Med* 1985;145:2174–2179.

213. Timsit J, Garrait V, Misset B, et al. The digestive tract is a major site for *Acinetobacter baumannii* colonization in intensive care unit patients [Letter]. *J Infect Dis* 1993;168:1336–1337.

214. el-Mohandes A, Schatz V, Keiser J, et al. Bacterial contaminants of collected and frozen human milk used in an intensive care nursery. *Am J Infect Control* 1993;21:226–230.

215. Henriksen SD. *Moraxella, Acinetobacter* and the Mimeae. *Bacteriol Rev* 1973;37:522–561.

216. Weinstein MP, Reller LB, Murphy JR, et al. The clinical significance of positive blood cultures: a comprehensive analysis of 500 episodes of bacteremia and fungemia in adults. I. Laboratory and epidemiologic observations. *Rev Infect Dis* 1983;5:35–53.

217. Seifert H, Baginski R, Schulze A, et al. The distribution of *Acinetobacter* species in clinical culture materials. *Int J Med Microbiol Virol Parasitol Infect Dis* 1993;279:544–552.

218. Baltimore RS, Duncan RL, Shapiro ED, et al. Epidemiology of pharyngeal colonization of infants with aerobic gram-negative rod bacteria. *J Clin Microbiol* 1989;27:91–95.

219. Horan TC, White JW, Jarvis WR, et al. Nosocomial infection surveillance, 1984. *MMWR CDC Surveill Summ* 1986;35:17SS–29SS.

220. Centers for Disease Control and Prevention. National Nosocomial Infections Study Report, data summary from October 1986–April 1996, issued May 1996. *Am J Infect Control* 1996;24:380–388.

221. McDonald LC, Banerjee SN, Jarvis WR. Seasonal variation of *Acinetobacter* infections: 1987–1996. *Clin Infect Dis* 1999;29:1133–1137.

222. Tilley P, Roberts F. Bacteremia with *Acinetobacter* species: risk factors and prognosis in different clinical settings. *Clin Infect Dis* 1994;18:896–900.

223. Chen Y, Chang S, Hsieh W, et al. *Acinetobacter calcoaceticus* bacteremia: analysis of 48 cases. *J Formos Med Assoc* 1991;90:958–963.

224. Regev R, Dolfin T, Zelig I, et al. *Acinetobacter* septicemia: a threat to neonates? Special aspects in a neonatal intensive care unit. *Infection* 1993;21:394–396.

225. Seifert H, Strate A, Schulze A, et al. Vascular catheter-related bloodstream infection due to *Acinetobacter johnsonii* (formerly *Acinetobacter calcoaceticus* var.*lwoffii*): report of 13 cases. *Clin Infect Dis* 1993;17:632–636.

226. Ali M, Tremewen D, Hay A, et al. The occurrence of bacteremia associated with the use of oral and nasopharyngeal airways. *Anaesthesia* 1992;47:153–155.

227. Sacks-Berg A, Calubiran O, Epstein H, et al. Sepsis associated with transhepatic cholangiography. *J Hosp Infect* 1992;20:43–50.

228. Weinberger I, Davidson E, Rotenberg Z, et al. Prosthetic valve endocarditis caused by *Acinetobacter calcoaceticus* subsp. *lwoffii*. *J Clin Microbiol* 1987;25:955–957.

229. Nguyen M, Harris S, Muder R, et al. Antibiotic-resistant *Acinetobacter* meningitis in neurosurgical patients. *Neurosurgery* 1994;35:851–855.

230. Seigman-Igra Y, Bar-Yosef S, Gorea A, et al. Nosocomial *Acinetobacter* meningitis secondary to invasive procedures: report of 25 cases and review. *Clin Infect Dis* 1993;17:843–849.

231. Baltas I, Tsoulfa S, Sakellariou P, et al. Posttraumatic meningitis: bacteriology, hydrocephalus, and outcome. *Neurosurgery* 1994;35:422–426.

232. Lu C-H, Chang W-N, Chuang Y-C, et al. Gram-negative bacillary meningitis in adult post-neurosurgical patients. *Surg Neurol* 1999;52:438–444.

233. Fagon J, Chastre J, Hance A, et al. Nosocomial pneumonia in ventilated patients: a cohort study evaluating attributable mortality and hospital stay. *Am J Med* 1993;94:281–288.

234. Suchyta MR, Peters JI, Black RD. Chronic *Acinetobacter calcoaceticus* var *anitratus* pneumonia. *Am J Med Sci* 1987;294:117–119.

235. Ishihara H, Yamamori Y, Ihaya A, et al. Successful management of abdominal aortic aneurysm due to bacterial infection: report of a case. *Nippon Geka Gakkai Zasshi* 1987;88:907–911.

236. Yu EH, Ko W-C, Chuang Y-C, et al. Suppurative *Acinetobacter baumannii* thyroiditis with bacteremic pneumonia: case report and review. *Clin Infect Dis* 1998;27:1286–1290.

237. Galvao C, Swartz R, Rocher L, et al. *Acinetobacter* peritonitis during chronic peritoneal dialysis. *Am J Kidney Dis* 1989;14:101–104.

238. Benzakour M, Lagarde C, Benevent D, et al. Peritonitis during continuous ambulatory peritoneal dialysis. *Nephron* 1988;50:175–176.

239. Lye W, Lee E, Ang K. *Acinetobacter* peritonitis in patients on CAPD: characteristics and outcome. *Adv Perit Dial* 1991;7:176–179.

240. Valdez J, Asperilla M, Smego R Jr. *Acinetobacter* peritonitis in patients receiving continuous ambulatory peritoneal dialysis. *South Med J* 1991;84:607–610.

241. Volpin G, Krivoy N, Stein H. *Acinetobacter* sp. osteomyelitis of the femur: a late sequel of unrecognized foreign body implantation. *Injury* 1993;24:345–346.

242. Marcovoch A, Levartovsky S. *Acinetobacter* exposure keratitis. *Br J Ophthalmol* 1994;78:489–490.

243. Melki T, Sramek S. Trauma-induced *Acinetobacter lwoffii* endophthalmitis [Letter]. *Am J Ophthalmol* 1992;113:598–599.

244. Zabel RW, Winegarden T, Holland EJ, et al. *Acinetobacter* corneal ulcer after penetrating keratoplasty. *Am J Ophthalmol* 1989;107:677–678.

245. Groden J, Murphy B, Rodnite J, et al. Lid flora in blepharitis. *Cornea* 1991;10:50–53.

246. Bick J, Semel J. Fulminant community-acquired *Acinetobacter* pneumonia in a healthy woman. *Clin Infect Dis* 1993;17:820–821.

247. Barnes DJ, Naraqi S, Igo JD. Community-acquired *Acinetobacter* pneumonia in adults in Papua New Guinea. *Rev Infect Dis* 1988;10:636–639.

248. Anstey N, Currie B, Withnall K. Community-acquired *Acinetobacter* pneumonia in the Northern Territory of Australia. *Clin Infect Dis* 1992;14:83–91.

249. Reindersma P, Nohlmans L, Korten J. *Acinetobacter*, an infrequent cause of community acquired bacterial meningitis. *Clin Neurol Neurosurg* 1993;95:71–73.

250. Gradon J, Chapnick E, Lutwick L, et al. Infective endocarditis of a native valve due to *Acinetobacter*: case report and review. *Clin Infect Dis* 1992;14:1145–1148.

251. Brown R, Cipriani D, Schulte M, et al. Community-acquired bacteremias from tunneled central intravenous lines: results from studies of a single vendor. *Am J Infect Control* 1994;22:149–151.

252. Auerbach PS, Morris JA Jr. *Acinetobacter calcoaceticus* infection following a dog bite. *J Emerg Med* 1987;5:363–366.

253. Vila J, Almela M, Jimenez de Anta T. Laboratory investigation of hospital outbreak caused by two different multi-resistant *Acinetobacter calcoaceticus* subsp.*anitratus* strains. *J Clin Microbiol* 1989;27:1086–1089.

254. Muller-Serieys C, Lesquoy JB, Perez E, et al. Nosocomial infections caused by *Acinetobacter*. Epidemiology and therapeutic difficulties. *Presse Med* 1989;18:107–110.

255. Rolston KVI, Bodey GP. *In vitro* susceptibility of *Acinetobacter* species to various antimicrobial agents. *Antimicrob Agents Chemother* 1986;30:769–770.

256. Bergogne-Berezin E, Joly-Guillou ML. Comparative activity of imipenem, ceftazidime and cefotaxime against *Acinetobacter calcoaceticus*. *J Antimicrob Chemother* 1986;18[Suppl E]:35–39.

257. Overturf GD. Use of trimethoprim-sulfamethoxazole in pediatric infections: relative merits of intravenous administration. *Rev Infect Dis* 1987;9[Suppl 2]:S168–S176.

258. Gales AC, Jones RN, Forward KR, et al. Emerging importance of multidrug-resistant *Acinetobacter* species and *Stenotrophomonas maltophilia* as pathogens in seriously ill patients: geographic patterns, epidemiological features, and trends in the SENTRY antimicrobial surveillance program (1997–1999). *Clin Infect Dis* 2001;32[Suppl 2]:104–113.

259. Heinemann B, Wisplinghoff H, Edmond M, et al. Comparative activities of ciprofloxacin, clinafloxacin, gatifloxacin, gemifloxacin, levofloxacin, moxifloxacin, and trovafloxacin against epidemiologically defined *Acinetobacter baumannii* strains. *Antimicrob Agents Chemother* 2000;44:221–2213.

260. Urban C, Go E, Mariano N, et al. Effect of sulbactam on infections caused by imipenem-resistant *Acinetobacter calcoaceticus* biotype *anitratus*. *J Infect Dis* 1993;167:448–451,1993.

261. Sahm DF, Critchley IA, Kelly LJ, et al. Evaluation of current activities of fluoroquinolones against gram-negative bacilli using centralized *in vitro* testing and electron surveillance. *Antimicrob Agents Chemother* 2001;45:267–274.

262. Appleman MD, Belzberg H, Citron DM, et al. *In vitro* activities of nontraditional antimicrobials against multiresistant *Acinetobacter baumannii* strains isolated in an intensive care unit outbreak. *Antimicrob Agents Chemother* 2000;44:1035–1040.

263. Obaraa M, Nakae T. Mechanisms of resistance to beta-lactam antibiotics in *Acinetobacter calcoaceticus*. *J Antimicrob Chemother* 1991;28:791–800.

264. Gehrlein M, Leying H, Cullmann W et al. Imipenem resistance in *Acinetobacter baumannii* is due to altered penicillin-binding proteins. *Chemotherapy* 1991;37:405–412.

265. Sato K, Nakae T. Outer membrane permeability of *Acinetobacter calcoaceticus* and its implication in antibiotic resistance. *J Antimicrob Chemother* 1991;28:35–45.

266. Joly-Guillou ML, Bergogne-Berezin E, Moreau N. Enzymatic resistance to beta-lactams and aminoglycosides in *Acinetobacter calcoaceticus*. *J Antimicrob Chemother* 1987;20:773–776.

267. Vila J, Marcos A, Marco F, et al. *In vitro* antimicrobial production of beta-lactamases, aminoglycoside-modifying enzymes, and chloramphenicol acetyltransferase by and susceptibility of clinical isolates of *Acinetobacter baumannii*. *Antimicrob Agents Chemother* 1993;37:138–141.

268. Lambert T, Gerbaud G, Courvalin P. Characterization of the chromosomal *AAC (6′)-IJ* gene of *Acinetobacter* sp 13 and the *AAC (6′)-IH* plasmid gene of *Acinetobacter baumannii*. *Antimicrob Agents Chemother* 1994;38:1883–1889.

269. Lambert T, Gerbaud G, Galimand M, et al. Characterization of *Acinetobacter haemolyticus AAC (6′)-IG* gene encoding an aminoglycoside 6′-*N*-acetyltransferase which modifies amikacin. *Antimicrob Agents Chemother* 1993;37:2093–2100.

Alcaligenes and *Achromobacter*

270. Kersters K, De Ley J. Genus *Alcaligenes* Castellani and Chalmece 1919, 936. In: Krieg NR, Holt JG, eds. *Bergey's manual of systematic bacteriology*, vol. 1. Baltimore: Williams & Wilkins, 1984:361–373.

271. Yabuuchi E, Kawamura Y, Kosako Y, et al. Emendation of genus *Achromobacter* and *Achromobacter xylosoxidans* (Yabuuchi and Yano) and proposal of *Achromobacter ruhlandii* (Packer and Vishniac) comb. nov., *Achromobacter piechaudii* (Kiredjian et al.) comb. nov., and *Achromobacter xylosoxidans* subsp. *denitrificans* (Ruger and Tan) comb. nov. *Microbiol Immunol* 1998;42:429–438.

272. Bruckner DA, Colonna P, Bearson BL. Nomenclature for aerobic and facultative bacteria. *Clin Infect Dis* 1999;29:713–723.

273. Gardner P, Griffin WB, Swartz MN, et al. Nonfermentative gram-negative bacilli of nosocomial interest. *Am J Med* 1970;48:735–749.

274. Cohen PS, Maguire JH, Weinstein L. Infective endocarditis caused by gram-negative bacteria: a review of the literature, 1945–1977. *Frog Cardiovasc Dis* 1980;22:205–242.

275. Kishan J, Elzouki AY, Mir NA. Bacillus *Alcaligenes faecalis* septicemia and meningitis in the newborn. *Indian J Pediatr* 1988;55:443–444.

276. Peel MM, Hibberd AJ, King BM, et al. *Alcaligenes piechaudii* from chronic ear discharge. *J Clin Microbiol* 1988;26:1580–1581.

277. Ooishi M, Miyao M. A clinical evaluation of sultamicillin fine granules in the treatment of meibomianitis. *Jpn J Antibiot* 1988;41:2059–2064.

278. Tayeri T, Kelly L. *Alcaligenes faecalis* corneal ulcer in a patient with cicatricial pemphigoid [Letter]. *Am J Ophthalmol* 1993;115:255–256.

279. Auckenthaler R, Michea-Hamzehpour M, Pechere JC. *In-vitro* activity of newer quinolones against aerobic bacteria. *J Antimicrob Chemother* 1986;17[Suppl B]:29–39.

280. Schell RF, Francisco M, Bihl JA, et al. The activity of ceftazidime compared with those of aztreonam, newer cephalosporins, and Sch 29482 against nonfermentative gram-negative bacilli. *Chemotherapy* 1985;31:181–190.

281. Bizet C, Tekaia F, Philippon A. *In-vitro* susceptibility of *Alcaligenes faecalis* compared with those of other *Alcaligenes* spp. to antimicrobial agents including seven beta-lactams [Letter]. *J Antimicrob Chemother* 1993;32:907–910.

282. Spear JB, Fuhrer J, Kirby BD. *Achromobacter xylosoxidans* (*Alcaligenes xylosoxidans* subsp. *xylosoxidans*) bacteremia associated with a well-water source: case report and review of the literature. *J Clin Microbiol* 1988;26:598–599.

283. Mandell WF, Garvey GJ, Neu HC. *Achromobacter xylosoxidans* bacteremia. *Rev Infect Dis* 1987;9:1001–1005.

284. Reverdy ME, Freney J, Fleurette J, et al. Nosocomial colonization and infection by *Achromobacter xylosoxidans*. *J Clin Microbiol* 1984;19:140–143.

285. McGuckin MB, Thorpe RJ, Koch KM, et al. An outbreak of *Achromobacter xylosoxidans* related to diagnostic tracer procedures. *Am J Epidemiol* 1982;115:785–793.

286. Reina J, Antich M, Siquier B, et al. Nosocomial outbreak of *Achromobacter xylosoxidans* associated with a diagnostic contrast solution. *J Clin Pathol* 1988;41:920–921.

287. Gahm-Hansen B, Alstrup P, Dessau R, et al. Outbreak of infection with *Achromobacter xylosoxidans* from contaminated intravascular pressure transducers. *J Hosp Infect* 1988;12:1–6.

288. Wurtz R, Moye G, Jovanovic B. Handwashing machines, handwashing compliance, and potential for cross-contamination. *Am J Infect Control* 1994;22:228–230.

289. Yabuuchi E, Oyama A. *Achromobacter xylosoxidans* n. sp. from human ear discharge. *Jpn J Microbiol* 1971;15:477–481.

290. D'Amato RF, Salemi M, Mathews A, et al. *Achromobacter xylosoxidans* (*Alcaligenes xylosoxidans* subsp. *xylosoxidans*) meningitis associated with a gunshot wound. *J Clin Microbiol* 1988;26:2425–2426.

291. Sepkowitz DV, Bostic DE, Maslow MJ. *Achromobacter xylosoxidans* meningitis: case report and review of the literature. *Clin Pediatr* 1987;26:483–485.

292. Namnyak SS, Holmes B, Fathalla SE. Neonatal meningitis caused by *Achromobacter xylosoxidans*. *J Clin Microbiol* 1985;22:470–471.

293. Hearn Y, Gander R. *Achromobacter xylosoxidans*. An unusual neonatal pathogen. *Am J Clin Pathol* 1991;96:211–214.

294. Arroyo JC, Jordan W, Lema MW, et al. Diversity of plasmids in *Achromobacter xylosoxidans* isolates responsible for a seemingly common-source nosocomial outbreak. *J Clin Microbiol* 1987;25:1952–1955.

295. Boukadida J, Monastiri K, Snoussi N, et al. Nosocomial neonatal meningitis by *Alcaligenes xylosoxidans* transmitted by aqueous eosin. *Pediatr Infect Dis J* 1993;12:696–697.

296. Decre D, Arlet G, Danglot C, et al. A beta-lactamase–overproducing strain of *Alcaligenes dentrificans* subsp. *xylosoxidans* isolated from a case of meningitis. *J Antimicrob Chemother* 1992;30:769–779.

297. Legrand C, Anaissie E. Bacteremia due to *Achromobacter xylosoxidans* in patients with cancer. *Clin Infect Dis* 1992;14:479–484.

298. Dupon M, Winnock S, Rogues A, et al. *Achromobacter xylosoxidans* (*Alcaligenes xylosoxidans* subsp. *xylosoxidans*) bacteremia after liver transplantation [Letter]. *Intensive Care Med* 1993;19:480.

299. Cieslak T, Robb M, Drabick, et al. Catheter-associated sepsis caused by *Ochrobactrum anthropi*: report of a case and review of related nonfermentative bacteria. *Clin Infect Dis* 1992;14:902–907.

300. Cieslak T, Raszka W. Catheter-associated sepsis due to *Alcaligenes xylosoxidans* in a child with AIDS [Letter]. *Clin Infect Dis* 1993;16:592–593.

301. Manfredi R, Nanetti A, Ferri M, et al. Bacteremia and respiratory involvement by *Alcaligenes xylosoxidans* in patients with the human immunodeficiency virus. *Eur J Clin Microbiol Infect Dis* 1997;16:933–938.

302. Kerr J, Webb C. Five cases of *Alcaligenes* pseudobacteraemia. *Ulster Med J* 1992;61:163–165.

303. Ficker L, Meredith, TA, Wilson LA, et al. Chronic bacterial endophthalmitis. *Am J Ophthalmol* 1987;103:745–748.

304. Newman PE, Hider P, Waring GO, et al. Corneal ulcer due to *Achromobacter xylosoxidans*. *Br J Ophthalmol* 1984;68:472–474.

305. Siganos D, Tselentis I, Papatzanaki M, et al. *Achromobacter xylosoxidans* keratitis following penetrating keratoplasty. *Refractive Corneal Surg* 1993;9:71–73.

306. San Miguel V, Lavery J, York J, et al. *Achromobacter xylosoxidans* septic arthritis in a patient with systemic lupus erythematosus. *Arthritis Rheum* 1991;34:1484–1485.

307. Taylor P, Fischbein L. Septic arthritis in Waldenström's macroglobulinemia [Letter]. *J Rheumatol* 1994;21:776–777.

308. Taylor P, Fischbein L. Prosthetic knee infection due to *Achromobacter xylosoxidans*. *J Rheumatol* 1992;19:992–993.

309. Barton LL, Hoddy DM. Osteomyelitis due to *Achromobacter xylosoxidans* [Letter]. *Clin Infect Dis* 1993;17:296–297.

310. Hoddy D, Barton L. Puncture wound-induced *Achromobacter xylosoxidans* osteomyelitis of the foot [Letter]. *Am J Dis Child* 1991;145:599–600.

311. Walsh R, Klein N, Cunha B. *Achromobacter xylosoxidans* osteomyelitis [Letter]. *Clin Infect Dis* 1993;16:176–178.

312. Gradon J, Mayrer A, Hayes J. Pulmonary abscess associated with *Alcaligenes xylosoxidans* in a patient with AIDS [Letter]. *Clin Infect Dis* 1993;17:1071–1072.

313. Duggan JM, Goldstein SJ, Chenoweth CE, et al. *Achromobacter xylosoxidans* bacteremia: report of four cases and review of the literature. *Clin Infect Dis* 1996;23:569–576.

314. Kay SE, Clark RA, White KL, et al. Recurrent *Achromobacter piechaudii* bacteremia in a patient with hematological malignancy. *J Clin Microb* 2001;39:808–810.

315. Rolston K, Messer M. The *in-vitro* susceptibility of *Alcaligenes dentrificans* subsp. *xylosoxidans* to 40 antimicrobial agents. *J Antimicrob Chemother* 1990;26:857–859.

316. Glupczynski Y, Hansen W, Freney J, et al. *In vitro* susceptibility of *Alcaligenes denitrificans* subsp. *xylosoxidans* to 24 antimicrobial agents. *Antimicrob Agents Chemother* 1988;32:276–278.

Ochrobactrum anthropi

317. Holmes B, Popoff M, Kiredjian M, et al. *Ochrobactrum anthropi* gen. nov., sp. nov. from human clinical specimens and previously known as group Vd. *Int J Syst Bacteriol* 1988;38:406–416.

318. Chester B, Cooper LH. *Achromobacter species* (CDC group Vd): Morphological and biochemical characterization. *J Clin Microbiol* 1979;9:425–436.

319. Van Horn KG, Gedris CA, Ahmed T, et al. Bacteremia and urinary tract infection associated with CDC group Vd biovar 2. *J Clin Microbiol* 1989;27:201–202.

320. Kern WV, Oethinger M, Kaufhold A, et al. *Ochrobactrum anthropi* bacteremia: report of four cases and short review. *Infection* 1993;21:306–310.

321. Haditsch M, Binder L, Tschurtschenthaler G, et al. Bacteremia caused by *Ochrobactrum anthropi* in an immunocompromised child. *Infection* 1994;22:291–292.

322. Klein JD, Eppes SC. *Ochrobactrum anthropi* bacteremia in a child. *Del Med J* 1993;65:493–495.

323. Kish MA, Buggy BP, Forbes BA. Bacteremia caused by *Achromobacter* species in an immunocompromised host. *J Clin Microbiol* 1984;19:947–948.

324. Cieslak TJ, Robb ML, Drabick CJ, et al. Catheter-associated sepsis caused by *Ochrobactrum anthropi*: report of a case and review of related nonfermentative bacteria. *Clin Infect Dis* 1992;14:902–907.

325. Gransden WR, Eykyn SJ. Seven cases of bacteremia due to *Ochrobactrum anthropi* [Letter]. *Clin Infect Dis* 1992;15:1068–1069.

326. Alnor D, Frimodt-Moller N, Espersen F, et al. Infections with the unusual human pathogens *Agrobacterium* species and *Ochrobactrum anthropi*. *Clin Infect Dis* 1994;18:914–920.

327. Ezzedine H, Mourad M, Van Ossel C, et al. An outbreak of *Ochrobactrum anthropi* bacteraemia in five organ transplant patients. *J Hosp Infect* 1994;27:35–42.

328. Chang HJ, Christenson JC, Pavia AT, et al. *Ochrobactrum anthropi* meningitis in pediatric pericardial allograft transplant recipients. *J Infect Dis* 1996;173:656–669.

329. Applebaum PC, Campbell DB. Pancreatic abscess associated with *Achromobacter* group Vd biovar 1. *J Clin Microbiol* 1980;12:282–283.

330. Barson WJ, Cromer BA, Marcon MJ. Puncture wound osteochondritis of the foot caused by CDC group Vd. *J Clin Microbiol* 1987;25:2014–2016.

331. Cieslak TJ, Drabick CJ, Robb ML. Pyogenic infections due to *Ochrobactrum anthropi*. *Clin Infect Dis* 1996;22:845–847.

332. Brivet F, Guibert M, Kiredjian M, et al. Necrotizing fasciitis, bacteremia, and multiorgan failure caused by *Ochrobactrum anthropi*. *Clin Infect Dis* 1993;17:516–518.

333. Berman AJ, Del Priore LV, Fischer CK. Endogenous *Ochrobactrum anthropi* endophthalmitis. *Am J Ophthalmol* 1997;123:560–562.

334. Earhart KC, Boyce K, Bone WD, et al. *Ochrobactrum anthropi* infection of retained pacemaker leads. *Clin Infect Dis* 1997;24:281–282.

335. Cieslak TJ, Drabnick CJ, Robb ML. Pyogenic infections due to *Ochrobactrum anthropi*. *Clin Infect Dis* 1996;22:845–847.

336. Alnor D, Frimodt-Moller N, Espersen F, et al. Infections with the unusual human pathogens *Agrobacterium* species and *Ochrobactrum anthropi*. *Clin Infect Dis* 1994;18:914–920.

337. Manfredi R, Nanetti A, Ferri M, et al. *Ochrobactrum anthropi* as an agent of nosocomial septicemia in the setting of AIDS. *Clin Infect Dis* 1999;28:692–694.

Eikenella

338. Jackson FL, Goodman Y. Genus *Eikenella* Jackson and Goodman 1972, 74. In: Krieg NR, Holt JG, eds. *Bergey's manual of systematic bacteriology*, vol. 1. Baltimore: Williams & Wilkins, 1984:591–597.
339. Brooks GF. *Eikenella corrodens*. In: Braude AI, ed. *Infectious diseases and medical microbiology*, 2nd ed. Philadelphia: WB Saunders, 1986:346–348.
340. Soder P-O, Jin LJ, Soder B. DNA probe detection of periodontopathogens in advanced periodontitis. *Scand J Dent Res* 1993;101:363–370.
341. Alkaler RP, Young KA, Hardie JM. Production of hydrolytic enzymes by oral isolates of *Eikenella corrodens*. *FEMS Microbiol Lett* 1994;123:69–74.
342. Brooks GF, O'Donoghue JM, Rissing JP, et al. *Eikenella corrodens*, a recently recognized pathogen: infections in medical-surgical patients and in association with methylphenidate abuse. *Medicine (Baltimore)* 1974;53:325–342.
343. Sheng W-S, Hsueh P-R, Hung C-C, et al. Clinical features of patients with invasive *Eikenella corrodens* infections and microbiological characteristics of the causative isolates. *Eur J Clin Microbiol Infect Dis* 2001;20:231–236.
344. Stoloff AL, Gillies ML. Infections with *Eikenella corrodens* in a general hospital: a report of 33 cases. *Rev Infect Dis* 1986;8:50–53.
345. Datar SD, Shafran SD. Cellulitis of the foot due to *Eikenella corrodens* [Letter]. *Arch Dermatol* 1989;125:849–850.
346. Rayan GM, Putnam JL, Cahill SL, et al. *Eikenella corrodens* in human mouth flora. *J Hand Surg* 1988;13:953–956.
347. Cheng AF, South JR, French GL. *Eikenella corrodens* as a cause of brain abscess. *Scand J Infect Dis* 1988;20:667–671.
348. Burdick CO, Erasmus D, Jayaram A, et al. *Eikenella* brain abscess [Letter]. *JAMA* 1982;248:1972–1973.
349. Ramos JM, Pacho E, Garcia-Valle B, et al. Splenic abscess due to *Eikenella corrodens*. *Postgrad Med J* 1994;70:848–849.
350. Perez Trallero E, Garcia Arenzana JM, Cilla Eguiluz G, et al. β-Lactamase–producing *Eikenella corrodens* in an intraabdominal abscess [Letter]. *J Infect Dis* 1986;153:379–380.
351. Danziger LH, Schoonover LL, Kale P, et al. *Eikenella corrodens* as an intraabdominal pathogen. *Am Surg* 1994;60:296–299.
352. Kyi MS, Al Wali W, Gillespie SH, et al. Brodie's abscess caused by *Eikenella corrodens*. *J Infect* 1991;23:213–214.
353. Noordeen MHH, Godfrey LW. Case report of an unusual cause of low back pain: intervertebral diskitis caused by *Eikenella corrodens*. *Clin Orthop* 1992;280:175–178.
354. Roy D, Thompson KC, Price JP. Benign superior vena cava syndrome due to suppurative mediastinal lymphadenitis: anterior mediastinoscopic management. *Mayo Clin Proc* 1998;73:1185–1187.
355. Allen MB. Intrathoracic infections due to *Eikenella corrodens* [Letter]. *Thorax* 1988;43:344.
356. Harcombe A, Allen M. Empyema due to *Eikenella corrodens* [Letter]. *J Infect* 1988;17:86–87.
357. St. John MA, Belda AA, Matlow A, et al. *Eikenella corrodens* empyema in children. *Am J Dis Child* 1981;135:415–417.
358. Goldstein EJ, Kirby BD, Finegold SM. *Eikenella corrodens* and pulmonary infections [Letter]. *Am Rev Respir Dis* 1979;120:217.
359. Goldstein EJ, Kirby BD, Finegold SM. Isolation of *Eikenella corrodens* from pulmonary infections. *Am Rev Respir Dis* 1979;119:55–58.
360. Green SL, Oster SE, Tillman TJ. Pneumonia due to *Eikenella corrodens*: case report. *VA Med* 1983;110:257–259.
361. Kentos A, De Vuyst P, Struelens MJ, et al. Lung abscess due to *Eikenella corrodens*: three cases and review. *Eur J Clin Microbiol Infect Dis* 1995;14:146–148.
362. Hardy CC, Roza SN, Isalska B, et al. A traumatic suppurative mediastinitis and pericarditis due to *Eikenella corrodens*. *Thorax* 1988;43:494–495.
363. Arana E, Vallcanera A, Santamaria JA, et al. *Eikenella corrodens* skull infection: a case report with review of the literature. *Surg Neurol* 1997;47:389–391.
364. Kelly L, Eliason J. *Eikenella corrodens* keratitis: case report. *Br J Ophthalmol* 1989;73:22–24.
365. Hemady R, Zimmerman A, Katzen BW, et al. Orbital cellulitis caused by *Eikenella corrodens*. *Am J Ophthalmol* 1992;114:584–588.
366. Jordan DR, Agapitos RJ, McCunn PD. *Eikenella corrodens* canaliculitis. *Am J Ophthalmol* 1993;115:823–824.
367. Page RC. Gingivitis. *J Clin Periodontol* 1986;13:345–359.
368. Bissell P, Glew RH, Liland JB. Parotitis associated with *Eikenella corrodens* in a healthy adult. *Arch Otolaryngol* 1983;109:772–773.
369. Queen JS, Clegg HW, Council JC, et al. Acute suppurative thyroiditis caused by *Eikenella corrodens*. *J Pediatr Surg* 1988;23:359–361.
370. Cheng AF, Man DW, French GL. Thyroid abscess caused by *Eikenella corrodens*. *J Infect* 1988;16:181–185.
371. Vichyanond P, Howard CP, Olson LC. *Eikenella corrodens* as a cause of thyroid abscess. *Am J Dis Child* 1983;137:971–973.
372. Jeppson KG, Reimer LG. *Eikenella corrodens* chorioamnionitis. *Obstet Gynecol* 1991;78:503–505.
373. Drouet E, De Montclos H, Boude M, et al. *Eikenella corrodens* and intrauterine contraceptive device [Letter]. *Lancet* 1987;2:1089.
374. Riche O, Vernet V, Megier P. Bartholin's abscess associated with *Eikenella corrodens* [Letter]. *Lancet* 1987;2:1089.
375. Landis SJ, Korver J. *Eikenella corrodens* endocarditis: case report and review of the literature. *Can Med Assoc J* 1983;128:822–824.
376. Decker MD, Graham BS, Hunter EB, et al. Endocarditis and infections of intravascular devices due to *Eikenella corrodens*. *Am J Med Sci* 1986;292:209–212.
377. Burger AJ, Messineo FC, Schulman P, et al. Mycotic aneurysm of the sinus of Valsalva due to *Eikenella corrodens* bacterial endocarditis. *Cardiology* 1984;71:220–228.
378. Celikel TH, Muthuswamy PP. Septic pulmonary emboli secondary to internal jugular vein phlebitis (postanginal sepsis) caused by *Eikenella corrodens*. *Am Rev Respir Dis* 1984;130:510–513.
379. Goldstein EJ, Cherubin CE, Corrado ML, et al. Comparative susceptibility of *Yersinia enterocolitica*, *Eikenella corrodens*, and penicillin-resistant and penicillin-susceptible *Streptococcus pneumoniae* to beta-lactam and alternative antimicrobial agents. *Rev Infect Dis* 1982;4[Sept-Oct Suppl]:S406–S410.
380. Goldstein EJC, Citron DM. Susceptibility of *Eikenella corrodens* to penicillin, apalcillin, and twelve new cephalosporins. *Antimicrob Agents Chemother* 1984;26:947–948.
381. Goldstein EJC, Citron DM, Vagvolgyi AE, et al. Susceptibility of *Eikenella corrodens* to newer and older quinolones. *Antimicrob Agents Chemother* 1986;30:172–173.
382. Knapp JS, Johnson SR, Zenilman JM, et al. High-level tetracycline resistance resulting from TetM in strains of *Neisseria* spp. *Kingella denitrificans*, and *Eikenella corrodens*. *Antimicrob Agents Chemother* 1988;32:765–767.
383. Paul K, Patel SS. *Eikenella corrodens* infections in children and adolescents: case reports and review of the literature. *Clin Infect Dis* 2001;33:54–61.

Flavobacterium

384. Holmes B, Owen RJ, McMeekin TA. Genus *Flavobacterium* Bergey, Harrison, Breed, Hammer and Huntoon 1923, 97. In: Krieg NR, Holt JG, eds. *Bergey's manual of systematic bacteriology*, vol. 1. Baltimore:, Williams & Wilkins, 1984:353–360.
385. Greisen K, Loeffelholz M, Purohit A, et al. PCR primers and probes for the 16S rRNA gene of most species of pathogenic bacteria, including bacteria found in cerebrospinal fluid. *J Clin Microbiol* 1994;32:335–351.
386. Miyazaki S. Biological activities of partially purified elastase produced by *Flavobacterium meningosepticum*. *Microbiol Immunol* 1984;28:1083–1092.
387. Schiff J, Suter LS, Gourley RD, et al. *Flavobacterium* infection as a cause of bacterial endocarditis. *Ann Intern Med* 1961;55:499–506.
388. Ferrer C, Jakob E, Pastorino G, et al. Right-sided bacterial endocarditis due to *Flavobacterium odoratum* in a patient on chronic hemodialysis. *Am J Nephrol* 1995;15:82–84.
389. Ashdown LR, Previtera S. Community-acquired *Flavobacterium meningosepticum* pneumonia and septicemia. *Med J Aust* 1992;156:69–70.
390. Skapek SX, Jones WS, Hoffman KM, et al. Sinusitis and bacteremia caused by *Flavobacterium meningosepticum* in a sixteen-year-old with Shwachman Diamond syndrome. *Pediatr Infect Dis* 1992;11:411–413.
391. Marnejon T, Watanakunakorn C. *Flavobacterium meningosepticum* septicemia and peritonitis complicating CAPD. *Clin Nephrol* 1992;38:176–177.
392. Bucci FA, Holland EJ. *Flavobacterium meningosepticum* keratitis successfully treated with topical trimethoprim/sulfamethoxazole. *Am J Ophthalmol* 1991;111:116–118.
393. Abter EIM, Lutwick LI, Torrey MJ, et al. Cellulitis associated with bacteremia due to *Flavobacterium meningosepticum*. *Clin Infect Dis* 1993;17:929–930.
394. Riley DE, Berger RE, Miner DC, et al. Diverse and related 16s rRNA-encoding DNA sequences in prostate tissues of men with chronic prostatitis. *J Clin Microbiol* 1998;36:1646–1652.
395. Hsueh P-R, Hsiue T-R, Hsieh W-C. Pyomyositis in intravenous drug abusers: report of a unique case and review of the literature. *Clin Infect Dis* 1996;22:858–860.
396. Hsueh P-R, Hsiue T-R, Wu J-J, et al. *Flavobacterium indologenes* bacteremia: clinical and microbiological characteristics. *Clin Infect Dis* 1996;23:550–555.
397. Stamm WE, Colella JJ, Anderson LL, et al. Indwelling arterial catheters as a source of nosocomial bacteremia: an outbreak caused by *Flavobacterium* species. *N Engl J Med* 1975;292:1099–1102.
398. Herman LG, Himmelsbach CK. Detection and control of hospital sources of flavobacteria. *Hospitals* 1965;39:72–76.
399. Coyle-Gilchrist MM, Crewe P, Roberts G. *Flavobacterium meningosepticum* in the hospital environment. *J Clin Pathol* 1976;29:824–826.
400. du Moulin GC. Airway colonization by *Flavobacterium* in an intensive care unit. *J Clin Microbiol* 1979;10:155–160.
401. Olsen H. An epidemiological study of hospital infection with *Flavobacterium meningosepticum*. *Dan Med Bull* 1967;14:6–9.
402. Pokrywka M, Viazanko K, Medvick J, et al. A *Flavobacterium meningosepticum* outbreak among intensive care patients. *Am J Infect Control* 1993;21:139–145.
403. Aber RC, Wennersten C, Moellering RC. Antimicrobial susceptibility of flavobacteria. *Antimicrob Agents Chemother* 1978;14:483–487.
404. Von Graevenitz A, Grehn M. Susceptibility studies on *Flavobacterium* II-b. *FEMS Microbiol Lett* 1977;2:289–292.
405. Blahova J, Hupkova M, Krcmery V, et al. Resistance to and hydrolysis of imipenem in nosocomial strains of *Flavobacterium meningosepticum* [Letter]. *Eur J Clin Microbiol Infect Dis* 1994;13:833.
406. DiPentima MC, Mason EO Jr, Kaplan SL. *In vitro* antibiotic synergy against *Flavobacterium meningosepticum*: implications for therapeutic options. *Clin Infect Dis* 1998;26:1169–1176.
407. Olsen H. *Flavobacterium meningosepticum*: a bacteriological, epidemiological and clinical study. *Dan Med Bull* 1970;17:171–172.

Anaerobic Bacteria

CHAPTER 208
Anaerobic Bacteria

John G. Bartlett

Anaerobic bacteria are the predominant components of the abundant microbial flora of the human body. The role of these microbes as pathogens was well established at the turn of the century, but fastidious growth requirements often limit recovery, and ubiquity on mucocutaneous surfaces often raised doubts about pathogenic potential. During the past three decades, there has been renewed interest in anaerobic infections, particularly with regard to the definition of virulence factors and response to antimicrobial therapy.

DEFINITION OF ANAEROBES

Anaerobic bacteria are defined as bacteria that grow in the absence of oxygen and fail to show surface growth in 10% carbon dioxide in air. Anaerobes may be further classified by aerotolerance: Strict anaerobes cannot tolerate 0.5% oxygen; most clinically important anaerobes [*Bacteroides fragilis, Prevotella melaninogenica* (formerly classified as *Bacteroides melaninogenicus*), and *Fusobacterium nucleatum*] are moderate anaerobes that tolerate 2% to 8% oxygen.

HISTORICAL PERSPECTIVE

Louis Pasteur is credited with the discovery of anaerobes with the successful cultivation of *Clostridium butyricum* in the absence of atmospheric oxygen (1). Veillon, and subsequently Veillon and Zuber, from the Faculty of Medicine of Paris, published a series of important contributions in the 1890s concerning the role of anaerobic bacteria as the cause of putrid discharge and of infections at multiple anatomic sites, including pelvic infections, purulent arthritis, brain abscess, lung gangrene, and appendicitis (2).

The classic histotoxic clostridial syndromes, botulism and tetanus, were also well recognized by the end of the nineteenth century. In fact, by 1890, *Clostridium tetani* organisms were recovered in pure culture, and studies of immunization had begun (1).

Around the turn of the twentieth century, numerous papers in the French and German literature reviewed the role of anaerobic bacteria in diverse types of infections. Many were described as "fusospirochetal infections" characterized by the appearance of fusiform gram-negative rods (presumably *F. nucleatum*) and anaerobic spirochetes. In retrospect, it seems that these infections were probably analogous to those encountered in present-day practice, but the organisms identified generated considerable interest owing to the unique morphologic character of *F. nucleatum* and to the special interest in spirochetes because of the importance at that time of syphilis.

Among the major contributions was the observation by Schottmueller (3) that anaerobic streptococci, rather than group A β-hemolytic streptococci, were actually the predominant pathogens in puerperal sepsis. He postulated that the infection was acquired endogenously from the normal genital flora; this suggested an unconventional pathophysiologic mechanism at a time when contagion was a dominant thesis in the field of infectious diseases.

Contributions by British and American investigators in the early 1900s were modest, but hallmark studies were provided by David Smith (4,5) from Duke, who studied the bacteriology and pathophysiology of lung abscess in the late 1920s. Smith noted that the organisms in the abscess walls obtained at autopsy resembled the organisms seen in the gingival crevice, leading to the postulate that aspiration was the mechanism of infection. He subsequently supported this notion by intratracheal inoculation of pyorrhea pus into experimental animals to demonstrate the sequential progression from pneumonitis ("aspiration pneumonia") to lung abscess. In a tedious series of subsequent experiments, he isolated 17 different organisms from the inoculum; he challenged animals with each component alone and then with various microbes in combination. Eventually he showed that four microbial species were required to reproduce lung abscess: anaerobic streptococci, an anaerobic spirochete, an anaerobic *Vibrio,* and the fusiform *Bacillus*. This was one of the first studies of synergy, the demonstration that two or more organisms could produce a pathologic event that could not be reproduced with a simpler inoculum.

Additional important contributions were noted by two American surgeons—Meleney and subsequently Altemeier. Meleney made many important observations about anaerobic bacteria and their role in soft tissue infections and surgical infections. Especially noteworthy is his work with the condition subsequently known as Meleney's synergistic gangrene. Altemeier (6) examined the bacteriology of appendicitis in the late 1930s and was able to isolate anaerobic bacteria from 96 of 100 patients. He also noted that putrid discharge was found exclusively in the presence of infections involving anaerobic bacteria and that these were also the only organisms to produce the characteristic odor *in vitro* (7).

Interest in anaerobic infections seemed to subside during the first two decades of the antibiotic era. This was the period when there were relatively few clinical reports; most important, clinical laboratories either made no attempt to recover anaerobes or used only a broth culture, which was a problem because anaerobic bacteria were readily overgrown by aerobic bacteria that were also present. When anaerobes were recovered, there was often confusion about their role because of the multiplicity of bacterial species at the infection site, the failure to use standard methods of identification and classification, and the lack of demonstrable benefit from antimicrobial treatment directed against anaerobes.

Renewed interest in anaerobic infections in the middle and late 1960s reflected three simultaneous developments. First, and most important, was the availability of the GasPak system, in which anaerobiosis could be easily produced with a sealed jar and a commercial packet to which one simply added water. This made isolation of anaerobes relatively easy for most microbiology laboratories. The second important development was that the taxonomic classification of anaerobic bacteria was finally put in order by the outstanding work of many contributors but especially workers from the Virginia Polytechnic Institute. Third, the therapeutic implication of infections involving anaerobes was the subject of many studies *in vitro* and clinical trials by Sydney Finegold and others; this work initially highlighted the potential role of lincomycin, and subsequent reports dealt with clindamycin, metronidazole, cefoxitin, and then a host of others (8).

Later work has shown that anaerobic bacteria account for a relatively large number of infections, although the frequency is profoundly influenced by the anatomic site of infection, the mechanism of disease acquisition (exogenous versus endogenous), and clinical features. Detection of anaerobes in the laboratory is also highly variable, depending on the methods used to collect, transport, and process specimens. A review of the experience at the Mayo Clinic in the early 1970s found that *B. fragilis* was second only to *Escherichia coli* as a cause of gram-negative bacillary bacteremia (9). Brook (10) reported that anaerobes accounted for 28% of positive blood cultures in two military hospitals from 1973 to 1985. These results have been translated into practical application by the use of drugs directed specifically at anaerobic bacteria. Among the most commonly used drugs in hospital practice are three whose raison d'être is largely anaerobic infections: clindamycin, metronidazole, and cefoxitin. The extensive publicity accorded anaerobic bacteria and anaerobic infections in the 1960s and 1970s resulted in widespread acceptance of these organisms as major pathogens in selected types of infections. This was accompanied by widespread use of appropriate antimicrobials. Anaerobes are neither gone nor forgotten, but their role as major agents of mortality and morbidity is notably reduced by what must be viewed as one of the most successful education campaigns in the history of modern medicine. The result is a virtual disappearance of bacteremia to the extent that some authorities have proposed a discontinuation of routine anaerobe blood cultures (11).

NORMAL FLORA

Most mucocutaneous surfaces of humans harbor a rich indigenous flora composed of aerobic and anaerobic bacteria, the microbial species and concentrations of which vary at different anatomic sites (Table 208.1). Anaerobic bacteria are the dominant forms, often accounting for 99% to 99.9% of the culturable flora (12). The total number of bacterial species in a single individual probably exceeds 500.

The upper airways, including the oral cavity, nasal passages, oropharynx, and nasopharynx, harbor a complex flora that differs at various sites known as *ecologic niches* (12). Concentrations of bacteria in saliva are approximately 10^8/mL, of which approximately 90% are anaerobic bacteria, the predominant organism being *Veillonella parvula*. Dental plaque includes a complicated matrix of bacteria, including *Streptococcus mutans*, the principal organism implicated in dental caries, but also anaerobic bacteria that have been similarly implicated. The gingival crevice may be likened to the colon in that the oxidation-reduction potential is as low as −300 mV, concentrations of bacteria reach 10^{12}/mL

(the geometric limits with which bacteria may occupy space), and anaerobic bacteria account for 99% of the culturable flora. In healthy persons, the sinuses, eustachian tubes, and respiratory passages below the level of the glottis are generally sterile.

The most important anaerobic potential pathogens found in the upper airways include *Fusobacterium* species, especially *Fusobacterium nucleatum*; *P. melaninogenica*; the *Prevotella oralis* group; the *Bacteroides ureolyticus* group; and *Peptostreptococcus* species. These are the predominant organisms in anaerobic infections of the oral cavity and anaerobic pleuropulmonary infections.

The gastrointestinal (GI) tract shows marked variations in bacteriologic patterns in concentrations at different levels (13–16). The stomach is protected by gastric acidity (the "gastric barrier") and consequently harbors relatively small numbers of bacteria derived from swallowed salivary bacteria that are predominately gram positive. The number and types of bacteria increase with loss of gastric acidity (histamine H_2 blockers, antacids, aging), gastric bleeding, gastric obstruction, or gastric carcinoma. In the small bowel, the major mechanism of population control is intestinal motility, so the organisms commonly found are simply passing through. Interruption of this flow, as with a stagnant segment (stricture, obstruction, diverticulum, blind loop), may result in high concentrations of bacteria with a predominance of anaerobes, similar to the flora of the colon (13). This bacterial overgrowth pattern may be responsible for malabsorption and is best treated with antibiotics directed against anaerobes.

The largest concentrations of anaerobic bacteria are found in the relatively stagnant terminal ileum and colon, where concentrations reach $10^{11.7}$/g and anaerobic bacteria account for approximately 99.9% (14,15). The total number of microbial species is estimated at 300 to 400, but the most important anaerobic bacteria with respect to frequency of isolation from infected sites of intraabdominal sepsis are *Bacteroides* species (principally members of the *B. fragilis* group), *Prevotella* species, *Clostridium* species, and *Peptostreptococcus* species.

The colon flora becomes established after weaning and is thought to remain relatively stable throughout life unless it is disrupted by antibiotic treatment. The role of the flora in health is debated, but many believe that it is important in maintaining an ecologic balance by preventing colonization with exogenous organisms. This protection, known as *colonization resistance*, is compromised with antibiotic treatment, which presumably enhances the potential for infection with enteric pathogens and colonization by gram-negative bacilli that eventually are the agents of many or most nosocomial infections and bacteremia complicating neutropenia. A logical extension of this thesis is "selective modulation of the fecal flora" by use of antibiotics that are directed against aerobic gram-negative bacilli but preserve the anaerobic component of the flora in an effort to prevent colonization by resistant strains (17). Antibiotics may have a major impact in the normal colonic flora on the basis of multiple contributing factors, including activity versus components of the flora, concentrations (reflecting enterohepatic circulation or failed absorption), susceptibility to inactivating enzymes such as β-lactamases, and activity in the environmental conditions of the gut.

The flora of the female genital tract is far less stable than that of the GI tract. Concentrations of bacteria in the vagina or cervix average approximately 10^8/mL during reproductive years (18–20). There is considerable variation (10^5 to 10^{11}/mL), simultaneous cultures of material from the cervix and vagina show unique bacteriologic patterns, and sequential cultures show considerable shifts at various stages of the menstrual cycle that may be hormonally influenced (18–21). Approximately 50% are anaerobic

TABLE 208.1. Bacteriology of the Normal Flora

Anatomic site	Total bacteria (per mL or g)	Anaerobe/aerobe ratio
Upper airways		
Nasal washings	10^3–10^4	3–5:1
Saliva	10^8–10^9	1:1
Tooth surface	10^{10}–10^{11}	1:1
Gingival crevice	10^{11}–10^{12}	1,000:1
Gastrointestinal tract		
Stomach	0–10^5	1:1
Small bowel	10^2–10^4	1:1
Ileum	10^4–10^7	1:1
Colon	10^{11}–10^{12}	1,000:1
Female genital tract		
Endocervix	10^7–10^9	1–5:1
Vagina	10^7–10^9	1–5:1

bacteria, but there is considerable variation, and approximately 20% of women have no detectable anaerobes or at least low concentrations. The dominant organisms are aerobic, microaerobic, and anaerobic lactobacilli; the dominant anaerobes are *Lactobacillus*, *Peptostreptococcus*, and *Bacteroides* species, including *Prevotella bivia*(formerly *Bacteroides bivius*). *B. fragilis* is found in only 2% to 10%. Studies of premenarchal or postmenopausal genital tract flora show a substantial difference in the flora, with an especially high yield of coliforms (22). Other factors that appear to influence the bacteriologic findings in the genital tract include pregnancy, antibiotic therapy, and gynecologic surgery (23–26). The role of the genital tract flora in maintaining homeostasis is not well studied, although antibiotic treatment clearly predisposes to vaginal candidiasis; bacterial vaginosis (*Gardnerella vaginitis* or nonspecific vaginitis) appears to reflect dysbiosis of the genital tract flora in which concentrations of lactobacilli are notably reduced, the dominant organisms are anaerobic bacteria, vaginal effluent contains a predominance of the short-chain volatile fatty acids produced by anaerobes, and current therapeutic recommendations are restricted to drugs directed against anaerobes (metronidazole and clindamycin) (19,27).

The skin flora contains large numbers of anaerobic bacteria, the predominant organisms being *Propionibacterium acnes* and to a lesser extent other species of *Propionibacterium* and *Peptostreptococcus* species (27). The skin flora of the perineum, and to some extent of the lower extremities, often contains the usual components of the colon flora. *P. acnes* and *Propionibacterium granulosum* colonize hair follicles and sebaceous glands, where concentrations correlate with sebum content.

PATHOPHYSIOLOGY

Anaerobic infections are usually endogenous, meaning that they originate from the host's own flora. The only important exceptions are some of the histotoxic clostridial syndromes, such as botulism, *Clostridium perfringens* food poisoning, enteritis necroticans, tetanus, and gas gangrene. Even this tabulation is somewhat deceptive, because many or most cases of *Clostridium difficile*–associated diarrhea or colitis, most cases of gas gangrene, and some cases of tetanus appear to involve clostridia that are residents of the host's normal colonic flora.

The usual pathophysiologic mechanism for anaerobic infection is a breach in the mucocutaneous defense barrier resulting in displacement of the normal flora. This simplistic mechanism applies to most of the anaerobic infections encountered in clinical practice. Host defense mechanisms are obviously important, but patients with neutropenia, defective complement systems, previous splenectomy, congenital or acquired defects in humoral immunity, defective cell-mediated immunity, advanced human immunodeficiency virus infection, cancer chemotherapy, or corticosteroid treatment infrequently acquire infections involving anaerobic bacteria. The exception is infections associated with defects of mucocutaneous barriers, such as carcinoma with obstruction, mucositis, perirectal lesions, or compromised consciousness with aspiration.

VIRULENCE FACTORS

One of the most important observations to lend credibility to microbes as pathogens is the identification of specific mechanisms or virulence factors that account for pathologic events. Such studies have been applied to anaerobes with use of traditional methods to detect capsules, toxins, and other virulence factors *in vitro* and *in vivo*.

One of the more common approaches to the study of anaerobes has been investigation of the concept of synergy, reflecting the fact that most such infections are polymicrobial. The work of David Smith was alluded to earlier; this showed that four anaerobic species were necessary to produce lung abscess in experimental animals (4,5). Meleney's studies of synergistic gangrene are other good examples of the interaction between microbial species, in this case *Staphylococcus aureus* and an anaerobic or microaerophilic streptococcus (28). These organisms were frequently found at the infection site, but inoculation of either in pure culture failed to reproduce typical lesions; the disease known as Meleney's synergistic gangrene could be reproduced only when both microbes were injected. Subsequent studies showed that *S. aureus* produced a collagenase that permitted the anaerobic streptococcus to invade tissue as an explanation of *in vivo* observations. Altemeier (29) also demonstrated that multiple microbial species produced more extensive disease with intraabdominal challenge. Despite these studies suggesting synergy, results of other investigations in experimental animals have not always supported the concept. More important, the identification of specific virulence factors has increased interest in these organisms as legitimate pathogens without the necessity for multiple bacterial species.

The most clearly identified virulence factors for anaerobic bacteria are the exotoxins produced by clostridial species: that of *Clostridium botulinum* and *C. tetani*, the most potent microbial toxin known; toxins A and B of *C. difficile* that are only about 100 times less active according to mouse lethality tests; and the 11 toxins produced by *C. perfringens* (as well as many other clostridial species), including 5 that are lethal to experimental animals. Clinical expression of these histotoxic clostridial syndromes depends on the site of toxin production and the physiologic effects of the toxin.

Anaerobic gram-negative bacteria, like all gram-negative bacteria, contain lipopolysaccharide that can be extracted from the envelope, but the biologic activity of this endotoxin (mouse lethality assays, the chick embryo death test, and the Shwartzman reaction) is 100 to 1,000 times less than that of lipopolysaccharide from Enterobacteriaceae (30). The lipopolysaccharide of *B. fragilis* is structurally similar to the lipid A of *E. coli* but lacks a phosphate group on the C4 of the nonreducing amino sugar and has a limited number of monosaccharides. These structural differences appear to explain the weak endotoxicity (30). Other anaerobic gram-negative bacteria, such as fusobacteria, are thought to contain endotoxin with more biologic activity.

One of the most extensively studied virulence properties of *B. fragilis* is the capsular polysaccharide that promotes abscess formation by resistance to opsonophagocytosis. This polysaccharide is capable of inducing abscesses in the absence of viable bacteria (31–33). There are actually a family of *B. fragilis* polysaccharides composed of oligosaccharide repeating units possessing sugars with positively charged free amino groups and negatively charged carboxyl or phosphonate groups. These positively and negatively charged groups mediate the capacity to induce abscess formation (34). The capsule also serves as an immunogen that confers protection to experimental animals on repeated challenge, a protective effect that appears to rely on cellular rather than humoral mechanisms (33,35).

Another virulence factor of *B. fragilis* that is shared by many other anaerobic bacteria is the production of short-chain fatty acids that inhibit phagocytic killing at low pH values (36,37). Short-chain volatile fatty acids are metabolic products of anaerobic bacteria that are used to classify these organisms, and some, such as butyric or succinic acid, are probably responsible for the putrid odor noted at the bedside and in the laboratory with growth of anaerobic bacteria. The best studied as a possible virulence factor is succinic acid, which inhibits phagocytic killing, an effect that is pH dependent (increased inhibition in acid conditions as found in abscesses) and nonselective in the sense that all microbial species are protected (36,37).

Host Defenses

Studies of host resistance to *B. fragilis* began in the mid-1970s with the observation that fecal isolates were susceptible to killing by serum. Subsequent work indicated that clinical isolates of *B. fragilis* were substantially more resistant, and heat inactivation suggested that this effect was mediated by complement (38,39). Of the various species of the *B. fragilis* group, *B. fragilis* is the most resistant to the bactericidal action of serum (39,40). Clinical isolates require opsonization with serum before ingestion and killing by neutrophils (41); the alternative pathway is the major complement mechanism for opsonization by all species of the *B. fragilis* group (42). Natural antibodies in serum directed against these bacteria belong primarily to the immunoglobulin M class (43) and are directed against strain-specific antigenic determinants in the outer-membrane complex (44). The polysaccharide capsule, as expected, influences opsonization and phagocytosis, so natural variants lacking capsules are more susceptible (45).

Biphasic Disease Model

Numerous animal models have been used to examine the pathophysiologic mechanism of anaerobic infections, but one of the most extensively studied during the past three decades has been the rat model of intraabdominal sepsis (31,46). Rats are challenged with an intraperitoneal implant of fecal contents with an adjuvant in an effort to simulate the septic complications of colonic perforation. The initial phase of the infection is characterized by generalized peritonitis, followed by the second phase characterized by abscess formation. Initial work showed a 43% mortality rate, with all deaths occurring during the first 4 days after challenge. Abscesses were defined as loculated collections with the characteristic outer collagen wall, an interface of polymorphonuclear cells, and a central area of necrotic debris and bacteria. Lesions satisfying this definition were initially detected 5 days after challenge, and all animals sacrificed 7 days or more after challenge had typical abscesses; follow-up evaluations of untreated animals at 3 months showed that some developed large abscesses and others had spontaneous resolution.

Studies of this animal model were designed to distinguish the role of various bacteria by use of quantitative cultures, antimicrobial probes (such as gentamicin for its selective activity against coliforms and clindamycin for its selective activity against anaerobes), and monomicrobial challenge with the organisms recovered from infected sites. This work supported the role of *E. coli* as the major pathogen in the initial phase of infection characterized by generalized peritonitis, bacteremia, and death. Supporting evidence was the presence of *E. coli* in 95% of blood cultures obtained during the first 5 days after challenge; this organism was the numerically dominant one in peritoneal exudate; gentamicin prevented the early mortality; and this was the only isolate that reproduced acute mortality with monomicrobial challenge. *B. fragilis* assumed unique importance in the second phase of the infection characterized by abscess formation. The role of this microbe in abscess formation was supported by evidence that it was the numerically dominant microbe in abscesses, clindamycin prevented this complication, and it was the only organism that caused abscesses with monomicrobial challenge. Further testimony to the "abscessogenic potential" of *B. fragilis* was the demonstration of typical abscesses after challenge with the capsular polysaccharide of *B. fragilis* (31–33).

The conclusion is that both coliforms and anaerobic bacteria represent pathogens in this model of intraabdominal sepsis, although they appear to be responsible for different biologic events as the infection evolves through its two stages. Although *E. coli* was the principal coliform in the inoculum in this work, other coliforms could be equally devastating—effects that may well reflect the biologic activity of endotoxin shared by these organisms. Similarly, it is now known that many members of the *B. fragilis* group, as well as some in the *P. melaninogenica* group, also possess polysaccharide capsules and produce short-chain fatty acids. The practical application of these data is that antimicrobial therapy should be directed against both coliforms and anaerobes, a thesis that is well supported in clinical studies (47,48).

CLUES TO ANAEROBIC INFECTIONS

Clinical clues to the probable presence of anaerobic bacteria at infected sites are summarized in Table 208.2. Infections that occur in continuity with mucosal surfaces where anaerobic bacteria compose the normal flora often involve these microbes. In most cases, an associated condition—oral or dental infection, intraabdominal sepsis, infections of the female genital tract—has caused a breach in the barrier defense mechanisms.

Infections associated with tissue necrosis and abscess formation are often due to anaerobic bacteria. The specific role of virulence factors such as capsular polysaccharide and short-chain fatty acids to possibly account for this association is summarized previously. Thus, anaerobic bacteria are reported as the dominant isolates in abscesses at virtually all anatomic sites, including cerebral, dental, peritonsillar, lung, intraabdominal, tuboovarian, prostatic, and cutaneous abscess.

The putrid odor of infections or discharges is considered diagnostic of anaerobic infection. This tends to be a relatively late feature of most anaerobic infections and is seen in approximately one third to half of patients. The chemical basis for the odor is not well established, but it presumably reflects the metabolic products of anaerobic bacteria, including volatile fatty acids such as succinic and butyric acid, as well as methylmercaptan. As noted, these short-chain fatty acids are used to identify anaerobic bacteria; they may represent virulence factors, and direct detection of these acids in exudate by gas-liquid chromatography may be used as an early clue to the presence of anaerobes (49).

TABLE 208.2. Clues to Probability of Anaerobic Bacteria at Infection Site

Infection adjacent to surfaces that harbor anaerobes as normal flora

Infections characterized by abscess formation or tissue necrosis

Infections associated with putrid odor

Infections characterized by gas formation

Gram stain or exudate showing polymicrobial flora or organisms with morphological features of anaerobes

Failure to cultivate likely pathogens from infected site, possibly because of failure to perform anaerobic cultures, suboptimal anaerobic microbiologic technique, or prior use of antimicrobial agents active against anaerobes

Classic features of toxins produced by histotoxic clostridia: tetanus, botulism, *Clostridium perfringens* food poisoning, gas gangrene, *Clostridium difficile*-induced diarrhea or colitis, enteritis necroticans

Infections that by prior experience usually involve anaerobic bacteria

Gas in the tissue is another clue to the presence of anaerobic bacteria, but it is not considered diagnostic because occasional aerobic bacteria produce gas (50). Gas may be detected by palpation, radiography, or scanning techniques. This may reflect not only gas production by microbes but also air introduced during irrigations or other manipulations such as the release of carbon dioxide with hydrogen peroxide.

Infections involving a polymicrobial flora are often anaerobic or represent mixtures of both obligate and facultative anaerobic bacteria. This may be easily suspected when Gram stain examination of exudate shows multiple different morphotypes at infected sites. This examination may also indicate the unique morphologic features of many anaerobes, especially *Bacteroides* species, *Fusobacterium* species, and clostridia; by contrast, *Peptostreptococcus,* the other major genus of clinically significant anaerobes, cannot be distinguished from aerobic or microaerophilic gram-positive cocci on the basis of Gram stain appearance.

The failure to grow likely pathogens in the laboratory often serves as a clue to the presence of relatively fastidious bacteria, including anaerobes. This may reflect failure to obtain an appropriate specimen for anaerobic culture, failure of the laboratory to use appropriate microbiologic techniques, or the impact of prior antimicrobial therapy. With regard to the last, it is well established that treatment with clindamycin, metronidazole, and possibly other antimicrobial agents rapidly modifies the cultur-able flora from infection sites. Perhaps the best clue to the presence of anaerobic bacteria is simply the clinical features of the infection based on a century of published data to document microbial associations.

MICROBIOLOGIC METHODS

Microbiologist and clinician must work together to achieve optimal recovery of anaerobic bacteria, giving proper attention to collection, transport, and processing of specimens (51). Anaerobic bacteriology is relatively expensive because of the often tedious and technically demanding additional laboratory work required and the multiplicity of bacteria found at infected sites. In an era of cost restraint, it is likely that emphasis on anaerobic bacteriology will be reduced, technical expertise will decrease, and management strategies ("clinical pathways") including antibiotic decisions will be increasingly empirical.

Specimen Selection

Specimens appropriate for anaerobic culture must be devoid of the normal flora. Optimal specimens are normally sterile body fluids and aspirates or biopsy material from normally sterile sites (Table 208.3). On occasion, the problem of contamination may be obviated by quantitative cultures, although most

TABLE 208.3. Specimens Appropriate for Anaerobic Culture

Specimen and collection method	Comment
Normally sterile body fluids	Includes blood, pleural fluid, peritoneal fluid, bile, cerebrospinal fluid.
Abscess contents	Needle aspirates are preferred.
Wound[a]	Exudate, preferably collected by syringe aspiration using care to decontaminate surface areas.
Pulmonary	
Pleural fluid	Results of growth in broth cultures only are difficult to interpret.
Transtracheal aspirate[a]	
Transthoracic needle aspirate	
Thoracotomy specimen	
Bronchoscopic aspirate[a]	Requires double-lumen catheter brush with distal occluding plug or bronchoalveolar lavage, each combined with quantitative culture.
Tracheostomy aspirate[a]	Validity is not well established; one third of patients without evidence of infection yield anaerobes, and quantitative cultures may be required.
Urinary tract	Rare source of anaerobic infections.
Suprapubic aspirate	
Female genital tract	
Culdocentesis	Experience is varied, seldom done.
Specimens obtained above pelvic reflection at surgery or laparoscopy	
Transabdominal needle aspirates of uterus	
Intrauterine brush using double catheter with a distal occluding plug[a]	Requires quantitative culture.
Intraabdominal	
Aspirates, biopsy specimens	Specimen must be devoid of the gastrointestinal flora.
Small bowel aspirate	Quantitative culture is necessary to detect overgrowth syndromes.
Oral dental	
Aspirate of closed spaces	Collected from endodontal canal and preferably transported in conditions that preserve hydration and anaerobiosis.
Paper point specimen	
Paranasal sinuses	
Aspirate using catheter or syringe[a]	Plastic catheter inserted into depths of sinus tract is preferred.
Middle ear aspirate	Optimal specimens are obtained with intact tympanic membrane.
Soft tissue	
Aspirate of closed spaces, e.g., abscesses	
Biopsies using 3-mm dermal punch[a]	

[a]Because contamination with normal flora is common, broth cultures are inappropriate and interpretation is facilitated with quantitative or semiquantitative culture.

laboratories do not provide this service. As a general rule, liquid or tissue specimens are preferred; swab specimens should be avoided.

Specimen Transport

The optimal way to transport specimens is immediate delivery to permit prompt microbiologic processing. A variety of specialized transport devices are available that provide an atmosphere of oxygen-free gas, such as a mixture of carbon dioxide, hydrogen, and nitrogen; also included in most is an indicator such as resazurin, to document anaerobic conditions, and a reducing agent, such as cysteine, to eliminate small amounts of oxygen that are inadvertently introduced. Tissue specimens may be placed in a sterile tube flushed with carbon dioxide; if the tube is held upright with the stopper removed, the heavier carbon dioxide will exclude oxygen until the stopper is replaced. Although they are theoretically attractive, there is little evidence that such techniques are actually necessary. A study of survival of anaerobic bacteria in clinical specimens using quantitated culture techniques of exudate left for various periods showed nearly complete qualitative and quantitative recovery of anaerobic bacteria with exposure to room air for periods of up to 48 to 72 hours (52). Swabs are different due to drying rather than oxygen sensitivity. When swab specimens are necessary, the best transport medium is a specially prepared, prereduced, and anaerobically sterilized semisolid medium such as Cary-Blair medium.

Laboratory Processing

Direct microscopic examination is an important clue to the probable presence of anaerobic bacteria and an important method of quality assurance of microbiology culture technique. Three systems are generally advocated for anaerobic culture: the anaerobic jar (GasPak, evacuation replacement, and Bio-bags); the anaerobic glove box; and prereduced, anaerobically sterilized roll tubes (the Virginia Polytechnic Institute system). Several studies indicate comparable results in the yield of anaerobes from clinical specimens with these various systems (51). Consequently, the decision of which system to use depends on previous training of personnel, the volume of specimens, and the resources of the laboratory. Many clinical laboratories have found the GasPak jar method particularly convenient, although the jar should remain inviolate for at least 48 hours after the GasPak has been generated. An alternative, more convenient method for one or two plates is Bio-bags. Anaerobic chambers may be preferred when a large number of specimens are processed. Quality assurance with anaerobic technology indicates that the major discrepancies in most clinical laboratories are (a) failure to use the initial Gram-stained specimen to ensure that culture results account for all recognized morphotypes, (b) improper use of anaerobic jars, especially by opening before 48 hours has elapsed, (c) failure to use plate media that have not been maintained in a reduced environment, (d) premature discarding of plates, (e) inadequate picking of colonies from primary isolation plates, and (f) inadequate selective and nonselective plate media or excessive dependence on broth cultures.

Identification

The major clinically significant anaerobes are summarized in Table 208.4 according to prior taxonomic classification. Most clinical laboratories should be able to identify most of these organisms; however, peptostreptococci, which account for approximately 25% of all anaerobic isolates in most microbiology laboratories, rarely merit speciation, except for research studies, because these organisms lack distinctive virulence properties and appear to be susceptible to the same antimicrobial agents. The non–spore-forming gram-positive bacilli require chromatographic analysis for genus designation and extensive biochemical testing for speciation. With the exception of *Actinomyces*, these organisms have minimal documented pathogenic potential, and cursory identification is generally adequate. A rational approach is to separate *Propionibacterium*, a common contaminant, from the others simply by a catalase test and indole reaction. Clostridia are identified by spores seen on Gram stain examination or by survival with exposure to ethanol for

---

TABLE 208.4.   Clinically Important Anaerobes Seen with Greatest Frequency

Gram-negative bacteria
  Bacteroides fragilis group: *B. fragilis, Bacteroides thetaiotaomicron, Bacteroides distasonis, Bacteroides ovatus, Bacteroides vulgatus*
  Pigmented *Prevotella* (formerly *Bacteroides*): *Prevotella intermedia, Prevotella melaninogenica, Prevotella corporis, Prevotella denticola, Prevotella loescheii, Prevotella nigrescens*
  Prevotella (other): *Prevotella bivia* (formerly *Bacteroides bivius*), *Prevotella disiens* (formerly *Bacteroides disiens*), *Prevotella oralis* (formerly *Bacteroides oralis*)
  Porphyromonas asaccharolytica (formerly *Bacteroides asaccharolyticus*)
  Fusobacterium: Fusobacterium nucleatum, Fusobacterium necrophorum, Fusobacterium varium
  Bilophila: B. wadsworthia
Gram-positive cocci
  Peptostreptococcus: Peptostreptococcus intermedius, Peptostreptococcus micros, Peptostreptococcus anaerobius, Peptostreptococcus magnus, Peptostreptococcus asaccharolyticus, Peptostreptococcus prevotii
Gram-positive spore-forming bacilli
  Clostridium: Clostridium perfringens, Clostridium difficile, Clostridium sporogenes, Clostridium sordellii, Clostridium septicum, Clostridium tertium, Clostridium ramosum, Clostridium novyi, Clostridium histolyticum, Clostridium bifermentans, Clostridium innocuum, Clostridium tetani, Clostridium botulinum
Gram-positive non–spore-forming bacilli
  Propionibacterium: Propionibacterium acnes
  Eubacterium: Eubacterium lentum
  Bifidobacterium: Bifidobacterium dentium
  Actinomyces: Actinomyces israelii, Actinomyces naeslundii, Actinomyces odontolyticus, Actinomyces viscosus

30 minutes or to 80°C for 10 minutes. Extensive biochemical testing is required for speciation, which generally is unnecessary but desirable in selected cases and for detection of the most clinically significant and common isolates, *C. perfringens*, *Clostridium ramosum*, and occasionally others such as *C. difficile*. The *B. fragilis* group (*B. fragilis*, *Bacteroides thetaiotaomicron*, *Bacteroides distasonis*, *Bacteroides ovatus*, and *Bacteroides vulgatus*) is distinguished by the ability to grow in the presence of 20% bile, and most are catalase positive. Pigmented *Prevotella* species (*P. melaninogenica*, *Prevotella corporis*, *Prevotella denticola*, *Prevotella intermedia*, *Prevotella loescheii*, and *Prevotella nigrescens*) are distinguished by the production of brown or black pigment, although this may take a week or more and may require rabbit blood agar medium; this is a clinically important group of anaerobes that are relatively fastidious, and frequency of recovery provides testimony to anaerobic expertise. Fusobacteria are also relatively fastidious, are distinguished from *Bacteroides* species by susceptibility to the 1,000-μg kanamycin disk, are indole positive, are nonmotile, produce butyric acid, and show distinctive morphologic features on Gram stain. The major anaerobic gram-positive cocci of clinical importance are peptostreptococci.

ANAEROBIC BACTERIA AT INFECTION SITES

Anaerobes have been encountered in infections at virtually all anatomic sites, although the frequency of recovery is highly variable and the bacteriologic patterns depend largely on the flora at adjacent mucocutaneous sites (Table 208.5).

Central Nervous System Infections

Pyogenic intracranial infections that commonly involve anaerobic bacteria include cerebral and epidural abscess and subdural empyema. Meningitis rarely involves these bacteria.

The most extensively studied is cerebral abscess, which is usually a polymicrobial infection with some variation in bacteriologic patterns, depending on the associated condition. One of the first careful bacteriologic studies of nontraumatic brain abscesses in which anaerobic cultures were performed systematically showed anaerobes in 16 of 18 cases (53). *B. fragilis* is usually present when the associated condition is a middle ear or mastoid infection with local extension, usually to the temporal lobe; coliforms, *Pseudomonas aeruginosa*, various streptococci, and other anaerobic bacteria are often present as well (101). When sinusitis is the source of the infection, the usual bacteriologic pattern includes a variety of anaerobic bacteria other than *B. fragilis* and streptococci, especially *Streptococcus milleri*. Metastatic abscesses tend to involve polymicrobial flora like that at the site of origin, most often a pulmonary infection and less frequently intraabdominal sepsis. The exception is cerebral abscess associated with endocarditis or cyanotic heart disease, in which there is usually a single microbe, either *Staphylococcus* or an anaerobic or microaerophilic *Streptococcus*. Occasional cerebral abscesses involve *Actinomyces* species. Brain abscess associated with neurosurgery or head trauma is usually due to a diverse array of predominantly aerobic bacteria. Other central nervous system infections likely to involve anaerobes are subdural empyema and epidural empyema (54).

Antibiotic recommendations reflect these bacteriologic patterns. In cases in which anaerobes are suspected or established pathogens, good results have been achieved with metronidazole, which produces demonstrably high levels within the cerebral abscess, and clinical outcome is good (101). However, metronidazole is ill advised as a single agent because of its inactivity against aerobic streptococci, especially *S. milleri*, gram-negative aerobes, and *Actinomyces* species. For this reason, metronidazole is often combined with penicillin or a third-generation cephalosporin. Neurosurgical drainage, once the mainstay of treatment for cerebral abscess, has now been largely supplanted by medical management because of improved evaluation techniques using computed tomography and magnetic resonance imaging and by more appropriate selection of antimicrobial agents (102).

Infections of the Upper Airways

Anaerobic bacteria are involved in various infections of the oral cavity and adjacent structures. Bacteriologic patterns reflect the flora at these sites, with the dominant isolates being the *Bacteroides oralis* group, the pigmented *Prevotella* (formerly *B. melaninogenicus* group), *Porphyromonas asaccharolytica*, *Fusobacterium* species, *Peptostreptococcus*, microaerophilic streptococci, and aerobic streptococci.

Nearly all clinically important dental infections are likely to involve anaerobes, including pulpitis (endodontal infection) (103,104), periapical or dental abscess, and perimandibular space infections (57,58). These three infections usually represent a continuum. The initial lesion is endodontal; the infection progresses to the periapical region, and then it may extend through the mandible to involve the potential spaces created by insertions of fascia along the mandible. The perimandibular spaces are contiguous, although infections are usually localized to specific anatomic sites adjacent to the portal of entry. The usual presentation is pain and swelling, and the mainstay of therapy is surgical drainage. Life-threatening forms of perimandibular infections that are important to recognize clinically include Ludwig's angina (105) and Lemierre's syndrome (106–108). Ludwig's angina is an infection characterized by bilateral involvement of the sublingual and submandibular spaces that causes swelling of the base of the tongue and potential airway compromise. Lemierre's syndrome is an infection involving the posterior compartment of the lateral pharyngeal space complicated by suppurative thrombophlebitis of the jugular vein with *Fusobacterium* bacteremia and metastatic abscesses, primarily to the lung (106–108).

Infections of the gingival crevice and gums, including gingivitis, periodontitis, and pyorrhea, usually involve anaerobic bacteria (109). An uncommon but distinct form is necrotizing ulcerative gingivitis, sometimes known as *Vincent's angina* or *trench mouth*. This is a relatively fulminant infection associated with severe pain, tissue destruction, pseudomembrane formation, and putrid discharge. The bacterial agent is not well established, although anaerobic spirochetes have been detected within tissue at the advanced edge of inflammation, and antibiotic treatment directed against anaerobes is necessary. A possibly related necrotizing infection of the oral mucous membranes is cancrum oris, or noma, characterized by destruction of soft tissue and bone. It occurs most often in children with malnutrition or systemic disease; this is usually fatal in the absence of intensive antibiotic therapy.

Anaerobic bacteria are also frequently implicated in chronic sinusitis (55), chronic otitis media (56), and mastoiditis but play a minimal role in acute otitis media or acute sinusitis. Peritonsillar abscesses are frequently caused by anaerobic bacteria, especially *Peptostreptococcus* species, which appear to be more common than *Streptococcus pyogenes* (59,60). Human bites—and to a lesser extent animal bites—often involve anaerobic bacteria (97,110). These include the clenched-fist injury that is the equivalent of a human bite. Also important are *Eikenella*

TABLE 208.5. Recovery Rates of Anaerobic Bacteria in Infectious Disease

Disease category: reference no.	Cases studied (no.)	Anaerobes recovered	
		No.	%
Head and neck			
Nontraumatic brain abscess: 53	18	16	89
Subdural empyema: 54	84	24	29
Chronic sinusitis: 55	83	44	53
Chronic otitis: 56	68	35	51
Perimandibular space infection: 57	31	29	94
58	21	21	100
Peritonsillar abscess: 59	30	23	76
60	45	38	84
Dental abscess: 61	10	9	90
Chest infections			
Aspiration pneumonia: 62	70	61	87
63	47	29	62
Lung abscess: 64	57	53	93
65	26	22	85
Empyema: 66	83	63	76
67	37	23	62
Bronchiectasis: 68	18	17	94
Unselected patients: 69	89	29	33
70	74	16	22
Hospital-acquired pneumonia: 71	159	56	35
Intraabdominal sepsis: 72	759	627	83
Abscess or peritonitis: 73	72	68	94
74	110	98	89
75	64	52	81
Appendiceal abscess: 76	100	96	96
Liver abscess: 77	40	21	52
Female genital tract			
Miscellaneous types: 78	33	33	100
79	91	67	74
80	50	36	72
Pelvic abscess: 81	25	22	88
Pelvic inflammatory disease: 82	54	13	25
83	74	57	77
84	70	53	78
Septic abortion: 85	29	20	69
Postpartum endometritis: 86	128	49	38
Soft tissue			
Wound infection after elective colon surgery: 87	19	18	95
Postappendectomy wound: 88	65	15	79
Cutaneous abscess: 89	135	81	60
Pilonidal abscess: 9	41	36	88
Perirectal abscess: 90	74	57	77
Diabetic foot ulcer: 91	19	12	63
Pilonidal sinus: 92	45	33	73
Breast abscess: 93	52	41	79
Necrotizing synergistic cellulitis: 94	57	51	89
Necrotizing soft tissue: 95	182	85	47
Paronychia: 96	32	23	72
Bite wound infections: 97	34	18	53
Bacteremia			
All blood cultures: 10	4,659	296	6
98	2,025	81	4
Intraabdominal sepsis: 87	8	7	88
Septic abortion: 99	76	48	63
Decubitus ulcers: 100	62	10	16
Endometritis: 86	28	15	54

corrodens and aerobic and microaerophilic streptococci from the oral flora; *S. aureus* from the recipient's skin may also be involved.

Penicillin was previously regarded as the drug of choice for oral and dental infections involving anaerobic bacteria; however, increasing resistance has been noted among these organisms, principally with β-lactamase production by *Bacteroides,* *Prevotella,* and *Fusobacterium* species (110,111). For infections that are serious, the preferred drugs for oral use are clindamycin, metronidazole, metronidazole plus penicillin, gatifloxacin, moxifloxacin, and amoxicillin-clavulanate. Macrolides and ketolides are usually active *in vitro* with the exception of *Fusobacterium,* which is usually resistant (112). Ciprofloxacin, trimethoprim-sulfamethoxazole, tetracyclines, oral cephalosporins, and

TABLE 208.6. Bacteriology of Anaerobic Infections of the Lung

Measure	Bartlett (113)	Marina et al. (114)
Period reviewed	1968–1975	1976–1991
Cases	193	110
Total anaerobic isolates	461	404
Average anaerobic isolates per case	2.4	3.5
Former *Bacteroides* species		
Bacteroides fragilis group	38[a]	18
Pigmented *Prevotella*	76[a]	63
Nonpigmented *Prevotella*	—	40
Bacteroides ureolyticus	—	23
Other	37	38
Fusobacterium nucleatum	56	34
Peptostreptococci	87	39
Peptococci	39[a]	—
Gram-positive bacilli		
Clostridium species	18	12
Eubacterium species	18	22
Actinomyces	5	19
Lactobacillus species	8	22
Propionibacterium species	10	9
Bifidobacterium species	9	4
Veillonella	23	18

[a]Numbers refer to the number of isolates. Differences in the two series reflect, in part, taxonomic changes and variations in microbiologic methods. In the earlier series (113), the "black-pigmented *Bacteroides* species" were reported as *Bacteroides melaninogenicus,* whereas the later series reported these according to reclassification as *B. melaninogenicus, Bacteroides intermedius,* and *Bacteroides asaccharolyticus.* These organisms are now classified as pigmented *Prevotella,* including *Prevotella nelaninogenica* and *Prevotella intermedia.* For gram-positive cocci, the clinically important organisms formerly classified as *Peptococcus* have been reclassified as *Peptostreptococcus.*

antistaphylococcal penicillins are not active or are less predictably active.

Pleuropulmonary Infections

Anaerobic bacteria are relatively common and often overlooked pathogens in the lower airways. The usual mechanism is aspiration of oral and dental secretions, which results in aspiration pneumonitis, which may be an indolent form of pneumonia but may also simulate other forms of acute bacterial pneumonia, including pneumococcal pneumonia (113). Patients seen at this early or pneumonitis stage of infection rarely have putrid sputum and may well be classified as having atypical pneumonia, because no likely pathogen is recovered with routine aerobic culture of the expectorated specimen. The usual clues to the likelihood of anaerobes are the features seen in the later stages of disease, when there is likely to be putrid discharge and necrosis of tissue with abscess formation or empyema. Another clue to anaerobic involvement with chronic infections is the indolent course of many of these infections. Patients often present with weight loss, anemia, and chronic pulmonary complaints, all features that are relatively uncommon in pneumonia due to most aerobic bacteria other than mycobacteria (113).

The frequency of anaerobic pulmonary infections was studied most extensively from 1970 through the early 1980s, when transtracheal aspiration was a common method of obtaining uncontaminated specimens from the lower airways. This work showed that 60% to 90% of cases of aspiration pneumonia, lung abscess, and empyema involved anaerobic bacteria (62–67,113). Studies of nosocomial pneumonia also showed a 35% frequency of anaerobes, although in contrast to community-acquired cases, these tended to be mixed infections involving aerobic gram-negative bacilli or *S. aureus* as well (71). Two studies attempted to define the role of anaerobes in unselected patients with community-acquired pneumonia; one used transtracheal

aspiration with a yield of 33% (69) and the other used fiberoptic bronchoscopy with quantitative cultures and showed a yield of 22% (70). These studies suggest that anaerobic pulmonary infections are substantially more common than is generally appreciated.

Bacteriologic patterns in anaerobic pulmonary infection are similar to those described for oral and dental infections (Table 208.6). Many reports from the 1970s showed that *B. fragilis* was recovered in 15% to 20% of cases (62–67,113). This finding was somewhat surprising, because studies of the oral flora, the presumed source of the inoculum, have not observed *B. fragilis.* More recent findings suggest that *B. fragilis* was identified erroneously and that other penicillin-resistant *Bacteroides* species presumably account for the discrepancies (113–115).

With regard to therapeutic recommendations, clinicians from the 1950s and 1960s often did not know what pathogen was involved in aspiration pneumonia or lung abscess, but penicillin became widely recognized as the drug of choice for both conditions (116–119). Somewhat paradoxically, when the pathogens were identified by the combination of transtracheal aspiration and meticulous anaerobic bacteriologic tests, considerable controversy developed about the preferred treatment, because 20% to 25% of patients harbored penicillin-resistant anaerobes. Two comparative trials of large doses of intravenous penicillin versus clindamycin for patients with anaerobic lung abscesses have subsequently shown clear superiority for clindamycin in terms of clinical response rates, time to defervescence, and time to elimination of putrid sputum (118,119). Clindamycin is often considered the drug of choice for lung abscess and aspiration pneumonia. Other options include any combination of a β-lactam–β-lactamase inhibitor or metronidazole and penicillin. It is possible that cephalosporins, macrolides, gatifloxacin, or moxifloxacin would be effective, but experience is limited. Metronidazole should not be used alone because of the importance of aerobic and microaerophilic strep infection (121).

Intraabdominal Sepsis

Infections within the abdominal cavity may be classified as monomicrobial or polymicrobial, depending on the number of bacterial species at the infection site. Infections likely to be monomicrobial include biliary tract infections, primary or "spontaneous" peritonitis, and pancreatic infections (pancreatic abscess, infected pseudocyst). In each instance, the dominant organism is a coliform, especially *E. coli*. Polymicrobial infections include peritonitis, which may be generalized or localized (phlegmon), and intraabdominal abscess. The predominant bacteria in these cases are combinations of coliforms and anaerobic bacteria. There is an average of four to six microbial species per specimen, and the dominant isolates in most series are *B. fragilis* and *E. coli* (72,73,75) (Table 208.7).

The usual pathophysiologic mechanism is a breach in the mucosal defense barrier that affords entry for an inoculum composed of the normal intestinal flora. Colonic flora is especially common, reflecting the frequency of associated diseases at this anatomic site, including appendicitis, diverticulitis, carcinoma of the colon, inflammatory bowel disease, and previous colon surgery. In such cases, the inoculum of bacteria presumably involves the approximately 400 species that compose the normal flora. Thus, the pathogens at the infection site, an average of four to six species, represent a distillate of the inoculum in which the organisms presumably survive because of virulence factors and their ability to accommodate to the new environmental conditions. Perforation of the proximal bowel, as with perforated peptic ulcer, results in an infection that is microbiologically distinct, reflecting the flora of the upper GI tract; the predominant microbial species in such cases often include aerobic and anaerobic gram-positive bacteria or *Candida* species.

The outcome of intraabdominal sepsis is highly variable, depending largely on the Acute Physiology and Chronic Health Evaluation (APACHE) score. The most important facet of treatment is usually surgical intervention or percutaneous drainage. With regard to antibiotic decisions, most patients are treated empirically without benefit of bacteriologic studies using drugs directed against both coliforms and anaerobes. Single agents that can serve this role are imipenem, meropenem, or a combination of a β-lactam–β-lactamase inhibitor (120,122,123). The alternative is a two-drug regimen using one agent for coliforms (such as a third-generation cephalosporin or an aminoglycoside) and a second for anaerobes (such as clindamycin, cefoxitin, or metronidazole) (124–126).

TREATMENT OF ENTEROCOCCAL INFECTION

Enterococcus is encountered in 15% to 20% of cases, and some of these, primarily in nosocomial cases, may be vancomycin-resistant *Enterococcus faecium.* (127,128). Prior studies suggested that *Enterococcus* species in mixed infections were of doubtful clinical significance. The animal model failed to show virulence of *Enterococcus* with intraperitoneal challenge, 46 clinical studies showed that use of antibiotics active against enterococci did not improve outcome (120–123), and enterococci were rarely recovered in blood cultures (129). The issue, once seemingly resolved, is increasingly controversial because of increased rates of enterococcal bacteremia and concern for vancomycin-resistant enterococci (127,128). Some authorities advocate adding a third drug (ampicillin or vancomycin) to counter the enterococci, although clinical and experimental animal studies do not support this tactic.

BOWEL PREPARATION FOR COLON SURGERY

All patients undergoing elective colon surgery should receive prophylactic antibiotics directed against coliforms and anaerobes. Many authorities prefer the erythromycin plus neomycin oral preparation because of its extensive track record of excellent results, relatively low cost, ease of administration, and lack of impact on the therapeutic options for postoperative infections in the event that resistance emerges (130). Others prefer a parenteral preparation such as cefoxitin or metronidazole plus tobramycin (131).

Infections of the Female Genital Tract

Nearly all infections of the female genital tract that are not caused by sexually transmitted pathogens are likely to involve anaerobic bacteria. Early investigators emphasized the role of *Peptostreptococcus* species in these infections (7,81). Later work suggested that anaerobic gram-negative bacilli are common and often dominant. Reports during the 1970s emphasized the frequency of *B. fragilis,* coliforms, and *Enterococcus* organisms, drawing an analogy to the bacteriologic patterns of intraabdominal sepsis (78–80). The recovery of *B. fragilis* in these infections was mysterious. Studies of genital tract flora identify this organism in less than 2% of women. Subsequent work showed that *B. fragilis* was probably erroneously identified in the earlier studies and that far more common were other penicillin-resistant anaerobes, especially *P. bivia* and to a lesser extent *Prevotella disiens* (formerly *Bacteroides disiens*) (83–86,132) (Table 208.8).

Infections likely to involve anaerobic bacteria include Bartholin's gland abscess, tuboovarian abscess, pyometra, endometritis, adnexal abscess, salpingitis, pelvic cellulitis, amnionitis, septic thrombophlebitis of the pelvic veins, and wound infections after gynecologic surgery or obstetric procedures. Bacterial vaginosis is now added to this tabulation of anaerobic infections, although the pathophysiology is poorly understood except for dysbiosis of the genital flora with reduced lactobacilli and increased anaerobes (133). One of the great difficulties encountered in many of these infections is obtaining appropriate material for meaningful anaerobic culture. The problem of contamination by the normal genital tract flora may be obviated by using culdocentesis, laparoscopy, or quantitative cultures with

---

TABLE 208.7. Bacteriology of Intraabdominal Sepsis
(72,73,75)

Cases studied	759
Bacteriology	
Aerobes only	132 (17%)
Anaerobes only	7 (1%)
Anaerobes and aerobes	620 (82%)
Bacterial isolates	
Aerobes	1,256
Escherichia coli	306
Pseudomonas aeruginosa	121
Klebsiella	119
Other gram-negative bacilli	270
Enterococcus	277
Staphylococcus aureus	111
Other gram-positive cocci	62
Anaerobes	1,187
Bacteroides species	443
Bacteroides fragilis	133
Clostridium species	306
Peptostreptococcus	220
Fusobacterium	35
Miscellaneous	116

Source: Adapted from Stone HH, Strom PR, Fabian TC, et al. Third-generation cephalosporins for polymicrobial surgical sepsis. *Arch Surg* 1983;118:193–200, with permission.

TABLE 208.8. Bacteria Recovered from the Upper Genital Tract of 188 Women Hospitalized with Acute Pelvic Inflammatory Disease

Bacteria	No. of isolates
Anaerobes	
Prevotella species	88
Prevotella bivia	72
Prevotella disiens	25
Bacteroides species	99
Peptostreptococcus asaccharolyticus	93
Peptostreptococcus anaerobius	72
Facultative bacteria	
Gardnerella vaginalis	121
Escherichia coli	25
Group B streptococci	29
α-Hemolytic streptococci	45
Nonhemolytic streptococci	49
Coagulase-negative staphylococci	72

Source: From Sweet RL. Role of bacterial vaginosis in pelvic inflammatory disease. _Clin Infect Dis_ 1995;20[Suppl 2]:S271–S275, with permission.

telescoping catheters for transcervical sampling of the endometrium (82–86).

Choosing antimicrobial agents for mixed aerobic-anaerobic infections of the pelvis follows many of the principles noted for intraabdominal sepsis (134,135). Recommendations for patients with pelvic inflammatory disease require regimens active against the usual aerobic and anaerobic flora, _Chlamydia trachomatis,_ and _Neisseria gonorrhoeae_; these include doxycycline combined with cefoxitin, cefotetan, clindamycin, or ampicillin-sulbactam. Clinical trials indicate that these regimens are equally effective (83,135). Infections of the female pelvis that do not represent sexually transmitted diseases are usually complications of pregnancy or gynecologic surgery. The major anaerobic pathogens are _P. bivia, P. disiens,_ and _Peptostreptococcus._

Infections of Soft Tissue

Anaerobic bacteria are common pathogens in a diverse array of skin and soft tissue infections. Most involve the cutaneous flora, especially _Peptostreptococcus,_ or the flora of adjacent mucosal surfaces.

S. aureus and _S. pyogenes_ are commonly viewed as the dominant pathogens in soft tissue infections, although anaerobic bacteria account for a major portion. With regard to superficial soft tissue infections, cutaneous abscesses above the waist usually involve _S. aureus_ or _Peptostreptococcus_ species; abscesses below the waist are more likely to involve anaerobic bacteria and often reflect the organisms in the colon (89). Similarly, anaerobes are the predominant isolates in breast abscesses (93), infected sebaceous cysts, infected pilonidal cysts, and paronychia (92,96). Other soft tissue infections that show a high yield of anaerobes are wound infections after surgery, bite wounds, diabetic foot ulcers, and decubitus ulcers (87,88,91,97,100). Quantitative cultures of diabetic foot ulcers show anaerobes to be the numerically dominant microbes (136), and osteomyelitis secondary to decubitus ulcers or diabetic foot ulcer is also likely to involve anaerobes (137).

Deep soft tissue infections likely to involve anaerobic bacteria include necrotizing fasciitis, necrotizing synergistic cellulitis, crepitant cellulitis, and gas gangrene (94,95). These infections involve the fascia, the muscle compartment formed by the enveloping fascia, or both. Major pathogens in these deep infections are group A β-hemolytic streptococci, clostridia, and combina-

tions of aerobic and anaerobic bacteria. The most common is synergistic necrotizing cellulitis, a deep soft tissue infection involving both the fascial plane and muscle compartment caused by a mixed aerobic-anaerobic flora. Clinical features are severe pain, gas in the soft tissue, and surgical drainage yielding putrid "dishwater" pus (thin, grayish discharge) (94). Clinical clues in these and other deep soft tissue infections that specifically suggest anaerobic bacteria include the putrid discharge; Gram stains showing a mixed factor; and gas in the soft tissue as detected by palpation, radiography, or scans.

Bacteremia

Anaerobes account for 2% to 5% of blood culture isolates from patients with clinically significant bacteremia (10,98,139). This excludes _Propionibacterium,_ which almost invariably represents a skin contaminant. The yield of anaerobes was substantially higher 20 to 30 years ago when recognition was less, and commonly used antibiotics in hospital practice showed poor activity against anaerobes. The use of metronidazole, imipenem, clindamycin, cefoxitin, cefotetan, and β-lactam–β-lactamase inhibitors for infections involving anaerobes is largely based on studies done in the 1970s and 1980s. The most common blood culture isolates among anaerobes are the _B. fragilis_ group, which account for 60% to 80% (139). A review of the suspected portal of entry for 855 episodes of bacteremia involving anaerobes indicated an intraabdominal source in 52%, the female genital tract in 20%, the lower respiratory tract in 6%, the upper respiratory tract in 5%, and soft tissue infections in 8% (139). Anaerobes previously accounted for most of the blood culture isolates in patients with bacteremia complicating infections of the female genital tract (86,99), intraabdominal sepsis (87), decubitus ulcers (100), and synergistic necrotizing cellulitis (94). The mortality rate is reported to be 15% to 35%; as expected, it is lower when appropriate antimicrobial agents are used (140).

ANTIBIOTIC SELECTION

A unique feature of anaerobic infections is that the decision regarding antimicrobial agents is usually made empirically, without the benefit of _in vitro_ susceptibility tests. This reflects the difficulties in obtaining test results within a useful time frame, with interpretation of culture results, and of performing sensitivity tests. In fact, it is difficult to justify the cost of such testing when considering that the results take a long time to deliver, the infections are polymicrobial, which multiplies the work, the testing is technically demanding, and the results are largely predictable (Table 208.9). Consequently, the National Committee for Clinical Laboratory Standards Working Group on Anaerobic Susceptibility Testing has recommended this type of testing for four settings: (a) to monitor susceptibility patterns in various geographic areas to determine changing sensitivity profiles, (b) to determine the activity of newly introduced antibiotics, (c) to monitor sensitivity patterns in local hospitals as a reflection of local antimicrobial pressure, and (d) to assist in the management of infections in selected patients (141). The last recommendation applies to infections in which intensive and often prolonged pathogen-directed treatment is generally required. Specific examples are cerebral abscess, joint infections, osteomyelitis, endocarditis, infections associated with prosthetic devices, and refractory or recurrent bacteremia. Most clinical laboratories will not do susceptibility tests unless they are specifically requested; many hospitals do not offer this service, and those that do often use techniques that are not considered reliable. Despite this deemphasis on _in vitro_ testing, it should be noted that the _in vitro–in vivo_ correlation

TABLE 208.9.   Activity of Antimicrobial Agents Versus Anaerobes

Agents	Comments
Nearly always active	
Metronidazole	Inactive versus microaerophilic strep (strep milleri, etc.), *Propionibacterium*, and *Actinomyces* species; bactericidal versus most true anaerobe strains (110,121,143–151)
Chloramphenicol	Good activity versus virtually all clinically significant anaerobes (110,143–151)
Imipenem	Resistant to most *Bacteroides* β-lactamases (110,120,143–151), although a novel β-lactamase that inhibits imipenem was found in rare *B. fragilis* strains (148)
β-Lactam plus β-lactamase inhibitor	Only carbapenems (imipenem) and cefamycins (cefoxitin) are β-lactams resistant to hydrolysis by the β-lactams produced by most *B. fragilis* strains. The addition of a β-lactamase inhibitor dramatically increases activity *in vitro* (110,120,143–152)
Usually active	
Clindamycin	*B. fragilis* group: 10%–20% of strains resistant; some clostridia other than *C. perfringens* are resistant (104,110,118,119,143–152)
Cefoxitin	*B. fragilis* group: 5%–15% of strains resistant with considerable institutional variation at least partly reflecting use patterns (143–151); poor activity versus clostridia
Antipseudomonad penicillins	Relatively resistant to β-lactamases of *Bacteroides* species; large doses usually employed (143–151)
Variable activity	
Penicillin	Inactive versus some or most penicillinase-producing anaerobes, including most of the *B. fragilis* group and many strains of *Prevotella melaninogenica*, *Prevotella intermedia*, *Prevotella bivia*, *Prevotella distens*, and some clostridia (110,143–152)
Cephalosporins other than cefotetan, cefoxitin, and cefmetazole	Less activity *in vitro* than penicillin G versus most anaerobes and limited published clinical experience to document efficacy (143–151)
Tetracycline	Inactive versus many anaerobes and most strains of *B. fragilis*; doxycycline and minocycline are somewhat more active than tetracycline
Vancomycin	Active against gram-positive anaerobes; inactive versus gram-negative anaerobes
Macrolides	Inactive versus many *Fusobacterium* species and some *B. fragilis* species (112,119); ketolides also show reduced activity versus fusobacteria (145,152)
Fluoroquinolones	Third generation (trovafloxacin, gatifloxacin, moxifloxacin, and gemifloxacin) show good *in vitro* activity; limited published data (150,151)
Poor activity	
Aminoglycosides	
Trimethoprim-sulfamethoxazole	
Monobactams (aztreonam)	

between activity in the test tube and survival with anaerobic bacteremia is impressive (142).

REFERENCES

1. Finegold SM, George WL, Mulligan ME. Anaerobic infections, part 1. *Dis Mon* 1985;31:1.
2. Veillon A, Zuber A. Sur quelques microbes strictment anaerobies et leur role clans la pathologie humaine. *C R Soc Biol (Paris)* 1897;49:253.
3. Schottmueller H. Allgemeinen krankenhaus hamburg-eppendorf. *Mitt Grenzt Med Chir* 1910;21:450.
4. Smith DT. Fusospirochetal disease of the lungs, its bacteriology, pathology and experimental reproduction. *Am Rev Tuberc* 1927;16:584.
5. Smith DT. Fusospirochetal disease of the lungs produced with cultures from Vincent's angina. *J Infect Dis* 1930;46:303.
6. Altemeier WA. Bacterial flora of acute perforated appendicitis with peritonitis: bacteriologic study based upon 100 cases. *Ann Surg* 1938;107:517.
7. Altemeier WA. The cause of the putrid odor of perforated appendicitis with peritonitis. *Ann Surg* 1938;107:634.
8. Gorbach SL, Bartlett JG. Anaerobic infections. *N Engl J Med* 1974;290:1177.
9. Wilson WR, Martin WJ, Wilkowske CJ, et al. Anaerobic bacteremia. *Mayo Clin Proc* 1972;47:639.
10. Brook I. Recovery of anaerobic bacteria from clinical specimens in 12 years at two military hospitals. *J Clin Microbiol* 1988;26:1181.
11. James PA, al-Shafi KM. Clinical value of anaerobic blood culture: a retrospective analysis of positive patient episodes. *J Clin Pathol* 2000;53:231.
12. Sutter VL. Anaerobes as normal oral flora. *Rev Infect Dis* 1984;6[Suppl]:S62.
13. Broido PW, Gorbach SL, Condon RE, et al. Upper intestinal microflora control. *Arch Surg* 1973;106:90.
14. Finegold SM, Attebery HR, Sutter V. Effect of diet on human fecal flora. *Am J Clin Nutr* 1974;27:1456.
15. Moore WEC, Holdeman LV. Human fecal flora: the normal flora of 20 Japanese-Hawaiians. *Appl Microbiol* 1974;27:961.
16. Mackowiak PA. The normal microbial flora. *N Engl J Med* 1982;307:83.
17. Van der Waaij D. Colonization resistance of the digestive tract: clinical consequences and implications. *J Antimicrob Chemother* 1982;10:263.
18. Bartlett JG, Polk BF. Bacterial flora of the vagina: quantitative study. *Rev Infect Dis* 1984;6[Suppl 1]:567.
19. Rendondo-Lopez V, Cook R, Sobel JD. Emerging role of lactobacilli in the control and maintenance of the vaginal bacterial microflora. *Rev Infect Dis* 1990;12:856.
20. Hillier S, Krohn MA, Klebanoff SJ, et al. The relationship of hydrogen peroxide-producing lactobacilli to bacterial vaginosis and genital microflora in pregnant women. *Obstet Gynecol* 1992;79:369.
21. Sautter RL, Brown WJ. Sequential vaginal cultures from normal young women. *J Clin Microbiol* 1980;11:479.
22. Hammerschlag MR, Alpert S, Rosner I, et al. Microbiology of the vagina in children: normal and potentially pathogenic organisms. *Pediatrics* 1978;62:57.
23. Goplerud CP, Ohm MJ, Galask RP. Aerobic and anaerobic flora of the cervix during pregnancy and the puerperium. *Am J Obstet Gynecol* 1976;126:858.
24. Ohm MJ, Galask RP. Bacterial flora of the cervix from 100 prehysterectomy patients. *Am J Obstet Gynecol* 1975;122:683.
25. Ohm MJ, Galask RP. The effect of antibiotic prophylaxis on patients undergoing vaginal operations. *Am J Obstet Gynecol* 1975;123:597.
26. Spiegel CA. Bacterial vaginosis. *Clin Microbial Rev* 1991;4:485.
27. Nielsen ML, Raahave D, Stage JG, et al. Anaerobic and aerobic skin bacteria before and after skin disinfection with chlorhexidine: an experimental study in volunteers. *J Clin Pathol* 1975;28:793.
28. Meleney FL. *Clinical aspects and treatment of surgical infections.* Philadelphia: WB Saunders, 1949.
29. Altemeier WA. The pathogenicity of the bacteria of appendicitis peritonitis. *Surgery* 1942;11:374.
30. Lindberg AA, Weintraub A, Zahringer U, et al. Structure-activity relationships in lipopolysaccharides of *Bacteroides fragilis*. *Rev Infect Dis* 1990;12:5133.
31. Onderdonk AB, Cisneros RL, Finberg R, et al. Animal model system for studying virulence of and host response to *Bacteroides fragilis*. *Rev Infect Dis* 1990;12:5169.
32. Pantosti A, Tzianabos AO, Onderdonk AB, et al. Immunochemical characterization of two surface polysaccharides of *Bacteroides fragilis*. *Infect Immun* 1991;59:2075.
33. Pantosti A, Tzianabos AO, Reinap BG, et al. *Bacteroides fragilis* strains express multiple capsular polysaccharides. *J Clin Microbiol* 1993;31:1850.
34. Tzianabos AO, Onderdonk AB, Zaleznik DF, et al. Structural characteristics of polysaccharides that induce protection against intra-abdominal abscess formation. *Infect Immun* 1994;62:4881.

35. Tzianabos AO, Kasper DL, Cisneros RL, et al. Polysaccharide-mediated protection against abscess formation in experimental intra-abdominal sepsis. *J Clin Invest* 1995;96:2727.

36. Rotstein OD, Nasmith PE, Grinstein S. The *Bacteroides* by-product succinic acid inhibits neutrophil respiratory burst by reducing intracellular pH. *Infect Immun* 1987;55:864.

37. Rotstein OD, Vittorini T, Kao J, et al. A soluble *Bacteroides* byproduct impairs phagocytic killing of *Escherichia coli* by neutrophils. *Infect Immun* 1989;57:745.

38. Casciato DA, Rosenblatt JE, Goldberg LS, et al. *In vitro* interaction of *Bacteroides fragilis* with polymorphonuclear leukocytes and serum factors. *Infect Immun* 1975;11:337.

39. Casciato DA, Rosenblatt JE, Bluestone R, et al. Susceptibility of isolates of *Bacteroides* to the bactericidal activity of normal human sera. *J Infect Dis* 1979;140:109.

40. Rotimi VO, Eke PI. The bactericidal action of human serum on *Bacteroides* species. *J Med Microbiol* 1984;18:355.

41. Bjornson AB, Bjornson HS. Participation of immunoglobulin and alternative complement pathway in opsonization of *Bacteroides fragilis* and *Bacteroides thetaiotaomicron*. *J Infect Dis* 1978;138:351.

42. Dahlen G, Nygren H. An electron microscopic study of surface polysaccharides in *Bacteroides*. *Microbios* 1982;35:119.

43. Sonnenwirth AC. Antibody response to anaerobic bacteria. *Rev Infect Dis* 1979;1:337.

44. Bjornson AB, Bjornson HS, Kitko BP. Specificity of immunoglobulin M antibodies in normal human serum that participate in opsonophagocytosis and intracellular killing of *Bacteroides fragilis* and *Bacteroides thetaiotaomicron* by human polymorphonuclear leukocytes. *Infect Immun* 1980;30:263.

45. Reid JH, Patrick S. Phagocytic and serum killing of capsulate and noncapsulate *Bacteroides fragilis*. *J Med Microbiol* 1984;17:247.

46. Bartlett JG, Onderdonk AB, Louie T, et al. A review: lessons from an animal model of intra-abdominal sepsis. *Arch Surg* 1978;113:853.

47. Thadepalli H, Gorbach SL, Broido PW, et al. Abdominal trauma, anaerobes and antibiotics. *Surg Gynecol Obstet* 1973;137:270.

48. diZerega GS, Yonekura ML, Roy S, et al. A comparison of clindamycin-gentamicin and penicillin-gentamicin in the treatment of postcesarean endomyometritis. *Am J Obstet Gynecol* 1979;134:238.

49. Gorbach SL, Mayhew JW, Bartlett JG, et al. Rapid diagnosis of anaerobic infections by direct gas-liquid chromatography of clinical specimens. *J Clin Invest* 1976;57:478.

50. Gorbach SL, Proppe KH. Fulminant illness with subcutaneous crepitance: case records of the Massachusetts General Hospital. *N Engl J Med* 1979;301:1276.

51. Citron DM. Specimen collection and transport, anaerobic culture techniques and identification of anaerobes. *Rev Infect Dis* 1984;6:551.

52. Bartlett JG, Sullivan-Sigler N, Louie TJ, et al. Anaerobes survive in clinical specimens despite delayed processing. *J Clin Microbiol* 1976;3:133.

53. Heineman HS, Braude AL. Anaerobic infection of the brain: observations on eighteen consecutive cases of brain abscess. *Am J Med* 1963;35:682.

54. Swartz MN. Central nervous infections. In: Finegold SM, George WL, eds. *Anaerobic infections in humans.* San Diego: Academic Press, 1989:156–232.

55. Frederick J, Braude AL. Anaerobic infection of the paranasal sinuses. *N Engl J Med* 1974;290:135.

56. Brook I. The role of anaerobic bacteria in otitis media: microbiology, pathogenesis, and implications on therapy. *Am J Otolaryngol* 1987;8:109.

57. Bartlett JG, O'Keefe P. The bacteriology of perimandibular space infections. *J Oral Surg* 1979;37:407.

58. Chow AW, Roser AM, Brady FA. Orofacial odontogenic infections. *Ann Intern Med* 1978;88:392.

59. Flodstrom A, Hallander HO. Microbiological aspects on peritonsillar abscesses. *Scand J Infect Dis* 1976;8:157.

60. Mitchelmore IJ, Prior AJ, Montgomery PQ, et al. Microbiological features and pathogenesis of peritonsillar abscesses. *Eur J Clin Microbiol Infect Dis* 1995;14:870.

61. Williams BL, McCann GF, Schoenknecht FD. Bacteriology of dental abscesses of endodontic origin. *J Clin Microbiol* 1983;18:770.

62. Bartlett JG, Finegold SM. Anaerobic infections of the lung and pleural space. *Am Rev Respir Dis* 1974;110:56.

63. Lorber B, Swenson RM. Bacteriology of aspiration pneumonia: a prospective study of community and hospital acquired cases. *Ann Intern Med* 1974;81:329.

64. Bartlett JG, Gorbach SL, Tally FP, et al. Bacteriology and treatment of primary lung abscess. *Am Rev Respir Dis* 1974;109:510.

65. Beerens H, Tahon-Castel M. *Infections humaines à bactéries Anaérobies non-toxigènes.* Bruxelles: Presses Académiques Européenes, 1965:91114.

66. Bartlett JG, Gorbach SL, Thadepalli H, et al. The bacteriology of empyema. *Lancet* 1974;1:338.

67. Varkey B, Rose H, Kutty K, et al. Empyema thoracis during a ten-year period. *Arch Intern Med* 1981;141:1771.

68. Greey PH. The bacteriology of bronchiectasis: an analysis based on nine cases in which lobectomy was done. *J Infect Dis* 1932;50:203.

69. Ries K, Levison ME, Kaye D. Transtracheal aspiration in pulmonary infection. *Arch Intern Med* 1974;133:453.

70. Pollack HM, Hawkins EL, Bonner JR, et al. Diagnosis of bacterial pulmonary infections and quantitative protected catheter cultures obtained during bronchoscopy. *J Clin Microbiol* 1983;17:255.

71. Bartlett JG, O'Keere P, Tally FP, et al. The bacteriology of hospital-acquired pneumonia. *Arch Intern Med* 1986;146:868.

72. Stone HH, Strom PR, Fabian TC, et al. Third-generation cephalosporins for polymicrobial surgical sepsis. *Arch Surg* 1983;118:193.

73. Gorbach SL. Management of anaerobic infections: intra-abdominal sepsis. *Ann Intern Med* 1975;83:377.

74. Brook I, Frazier EH. Aerobic and anaerobic microbiology in intra-abdominal infections associated with diverticulitis. *J Med Microbiol* 2000;49:827.

75. Swenson RM, Lorber B, Michaelson TC, et al. The bacteriology of intra-abdominal infections. *Arch Surg* 1974;109:398.

76. Brook I. Microbiology of subphrenic abscesses: a 14-year experience. *Am Surg* 1999;65:1049.

77. Sabbaj J, Sutter VL, Finegold SM. Anaerobic pyogenic liver abscess. *Ann Intern Med* 1972;77:629.

78. Thadepalli H, Gorbach SL, Keith L. Anaerobic infections of the female genital tract: bacteriologic and therapeutic aspects. *Am J Obstet Gynecol* 1973;117:1034.

79. Swenson RM, Michaelson TC, Daly MJ, et al. Anaerobic bacterial infections of the female genital tract. *Obstet Gynecol* 1973;42:538.

80. Ledger WJ, Gee CL, Pollin P, et al. The use of prereduced media and a portable jar for the collection of anaerobic organisms from clinical sites of infection. *Am J Obstet Gynecol* 1976;125:677.

81. Altemeier WA. The anaerobic streptococci in tuboovarian abscess. *Am J Obstet Gynecol* 1940;39:1038.

82. Eschenbach DA, Buchanan TM, Pollock HM. Polymicrobial etiology of acute pelvic inflammatory disease. *N Engl J Med* 1975;193:166.

83. Sweet RL. Role of bacterial vaginosis in pelvic inflammatory disease. *Clin Infect Dis* 1995;20[Suppl 2]:S271.

84. Sweet RL, Schachter J, Landers DV, et al. Treatment of hospitalized patients with acute pelvic inflammatory disease: comparison of cefotetan plus doxycycline and cefoxitin plus doxycycline. *Am J Obstet Gynecol* 1988;158:736.

85. Chow AW, Marshall JR, Guze LB. A double-blind comparison of clindamycin with penicillin plus chloramphenicol in treatment of septic abortion. *J Infect Dis* 1977;135:535.

86. Rosene K, Eschenbach DA, Tompkins LS, et al. Polymicrobial early postpartum endometritis with facultative and anaerobic bacteria, genital mycoplasmas, and *Chlamydia trachomatis:* treatment with piperacillin or cefoxitin. *J Infect Dis* 1986;153:1028.

87. Bartlett JG, Condon RE, Gorbach SL, et al. Veterans Administration Cooperative study on bowel preparation for elective colon surgery. *Ann Surg* 1978;188:126.

88. Sanderson Pi, Wren MWD, Baldwin AWF. Anaerobic organisms in postoperative wounds. *J Clin Pathol* 1979;32:143.

89. Meislin HW, Lerner SA, Graves MH, et al. Cutaneous abscesses. *Ann Intern Med* 1977;87:145.

90. Whitehead SM, Leach RD, Eykyn SJ, et al. The aetiology of perirectal sepsis. *Br J Surg* 1982;69:166.

91. Louie TJ, Bartlett JG, Tally FP, et al. The microbiology of diabetic foot ulcers. *Ann Intern Med* 1976;85:461.

92. Pearson HE, Smiley DF. *Bacteroides* in pilonidal sinuses. *Am J Surg* 1968;115:336.

93. Edmiston CE Jr, Walker AP, Krepel CJ, et al. The nonpuerperal breast infection: aerobic and anaerobic microbial recovery from acute and chronic disease. *J Infect Dis* 1990;162:695.

94. Stone HH, Martin JD Jr. Synergistic necrotizing cellulitis. *Ann Surg* 1972;175:702.

95. Elliott D, Kufera JA, Myers RA. The microbiology of necrotizing soft tissue infections. *Am J Surg* 2000;179:361.

96. Brook I. Bacteriologic study of paronychia in children. *Am J Surg* 1981;141:703.

97. Goldstein EJC, Citron DM, Finegold SM. Role of anaerobic bacteria in bite-wound infections. *Rev Infect Dis* 1984;6:S177.

98. Salonen JH, Eerola E, Meurman O. Clinical significance and outcome of anaerobic bacteremia. *Clin Infect Dis* 1998;26:1413.

99. Smith JW, Southern PM Jr, Lehmann JD. Bacteremia in septic abortion: complications and treatment. *Obstet Gynecol* 1970;35:404.

100. Bryan CS, Dew CE, Reynolds KL. Bacteremia associated with decubitus ulcers. *Arch Intern Med* 1983;143:2093.

101. Ingham HR, Selkon JB, Roxby CM. Bacteriological study of otogenic cerebral abscesses: chemotherapeutic role of metronidazole. *Br Med J* 1977;2:991.

102. Boom WH, Tuazon CU. Successful treatment of multiple brain abscesses with antibiotics alone. *Rev Infect Dis* 1985;7:189.

103. Zavistoski J, Dzink JA, Onderdonk AB, et al. Quantitative bacteriology of endodontic infections. *Oral Surg Oral Med Oral Pathol* 1980;1:46.

104. Kuriyana T, Karasawa T, Nakagawa K, et al. Bacteriologic features and antimicrobial susceptibility in isolates from orofacial odogenic infections. *Oral Surg Oral Med Oral Pathol Oral Radiol Endod* 2000;90:600.

105. Ferra PC, Busino LJ, Snyder H. Uncommon complications of odontogenic infections. *Am J Emerg Med* 1996;14:317.

106. Lemierre A. On certain septicaemias. *Lancet* 1936;1:701.

107. Hagelskjaer KL, Prag J. Human necrobacillosis with emphasis on Lemierre's syndrome. *Clin Infect Dis* 2000;31:524.

108. Sinave CP, Hardy GJ, Fardy PW. The Lemierre syndrome: suppurative thrombophlebitis of the internal jugular vein secondary to oropharyngeal infection. *Medicine (Baltimore)* 1989;68:85.

109. Loesche WJ, Syed SA, Laughon BE, et al. The bacteriology of acute necrotizing ulcerative gingivitis. *J Periodontol* 1982;53:223.

110. Appelbaum PC, Spangler SK, Jacobs MR. β-Lactamase production and susceptibilities to amoxicillin, amoxicillin-clavulanate, ticarcillin, ticarcillin-clavulanate, cefoxitin, imipenem, and metronidazole of 320 non–*Bacteroides fragilis Bacteroides* isolates and 129 fusobacteria from 28 U.S. centers. *Antimicrob Agents Chemother* 1990;34:1546.

111. Fosse T, Madinier I, Hitzig C, et al. Prevalence of beta-lactamase–producing strains among 149 anaerobic gram-negative rods isolated from periodontal pockets. *Oral Microbiol Immunol* 1999;14:352.

112. Goldstein EJ, Citron DM, Merriam CV, et al. Activities of telithromycin (HMR 3647, RU66647) compared to erythromycin, azithromycin, clarithromycin, roxithromycin, and other antimicrobial agents against unusual anaerobes. *Antimicrob Agents Chemother* 1999;43:2801.

113. Bartlett JG. Anaerobic bacterial infections of the lung and pleural space. *Clin Infect Dis* 1993;16[Suppl 4]:S248.

114. Marina M, Strong CA, Civen R, et al. Bacteriology of anaerobic pleuropulmonary infections: preliminary report. *Clin Infect Dis* 1993;16[Suppl 4]: S256.

115. Levinson M. Anaerobic pleuropulmonary infection. *Curr Opin Infect Dis* 2001;14:187.

116. Bartlett JG. Treatment of anaerobic pleuropulmonary infections. *Ann Intern Med* 1975;83:376.

117. Weiss W. Oral antibiotic therapy of acute primary lung abscess: comparison of penicillin and tetracycline. *Curr Ther Res* 1970;12:154.

118. Levison ME, Mangura CT, Lorber B, et al. Clindamycin compared with penicillin for the treatment of anaerobic lung abscess. *Ann Intern Med* 1983;98: 466.

119. Gudiol F, Manresa F, Pallares R, et al. Clindamycin vs. penicillin for anaerobic lung infections: high rate of penicillin failures associated with penicillin-resistant *Bacteroides melaninogenicus*. *Arch Intern Med* 1990;150:2525.

120. Medical Letter Consultants. The choice of antibiobacterial drugs. *Med Lett* 2001;43:69.

121. Sanders CV, Hanna BJ, Lewis AC. Metronidazole in the treatment of anaerobic infections. *Am Rev Respir Dis* 1979;120:337.

122. Barie PS, Vogel SB, Dellinger EP, et al. A randomized, double-blind clinical trial comparing cefepime plus metronidazole with imipenem-cilastatin in the treatment of complicated intra-abdominal infections. *Arch Surg* 1997;132:1294.

123. Younes Z, Johnson DA. New developments and concepts in antimicrobial therapy for intra-abdominal infections. *Curr Gastroenterol Rep* 2000;2:277.

124. Malangoni MA, Condon RE, Spiegel CA. Treatment of intraabdominal infections is appropriate with single-agent or combination antibiotic therapy. *Surgery* 1985;98:648.

125. Harding GKM, Buckwold FJ, Ronald AR, et al. Prospective, randomized comparative study of clindamycin, chloramphenicol, and ticarcillin, each in combination with gentamicin, in therapy for intraabdominal and female genital tract sepsis. *J Infect Dis* 1980;142:384.

126. Smith JA, Skidmore AG, Forward AD, et al. Prospective, randomized, double-blind comparison of metronidazole and tobramycin with clindamycin and tobramycin in the treatment of intraabdominal sepsis. *Ann Surg* 1980;192:213.

127. Centers for Disease Control and Prevention. Recommendation for preventing the spread of vancomycin resistance. *MMWR Morb Mortal Wkly Rep* 1995;44(RR-12):1.

128. Gold HS. Vancomycin-resistant enterococci: mechanisms and clinical observations. *Clin Infect Dis* 2001;33:210.

129. Barie PS, Christou NV, Dellinger EP, et al. Pathogenicity of the enterococcus in surgical infections. *Ann Surg* 1990;212:155.

130. Condon RE, Bartlett JG, Greenlee H, et al. Efficacy of oral and systemic antibiotic prophylaxis in colorectal operations. *Arch Surg* 1983;118:496.

131. Solla JA, Rothenberger DA. Preoperative bowel preparation: a survey of colon and rectal surgeons. *Dis Colon Rectum* 1990;33:154.

132. Walker CK, Workowski KA, Washington AE, et al. Anaerobes in pelvic inflammatory disease: implications for the Centers for Disease Control and Prevention's treatment guidelines for sexually transmitted diseases. *Clin Infect Dis* 1999;28[Suppl 1]:S29.

133. Spiegel CA, Eschenbach DA, Amsel R, et al. Curved anaerobic bacteria in bacterial (nonspecific) vaginosis and their response to antimicrobial therapy. *J Infect Dis* 1983;148:817.

134. Ledger WJ. Selection of antimicrobial agents for treatment of infections of the female genital tract. *Rev Infect Dis* 1983;5:598.

135. Hemsell DL, Little BB, Faro S, et al. Comparison of three regimens recommended by the Centers for Disease Control and Prevention for the treatment of women hospitalized with acute pelvic inflammatory disease. *Clin Infect Dis* 1994;19:720.

136. Sapico FL, Canawati HN, Witte JL, et al. Quantitative aerobic and anaerobic bacteriology of infected diabetic feet. *J Clin Microbiol* 1980;12:413.

137. Templeton WC III, Wawrukiewicz A, Melo JC, et al. Anaerobic osteomyelitis of long bones. *Rev Infect Dis* 1983;5:692.

138. Nakata MM, Lewis RP. Anaerobic bacteria in bone and joint infections. *Rev Infect Dis* 1984;6[Suppl]:S165.

139. Finegold SM, George WL, Mulligan ME. Anaerobic infections. *Dis Mon* 1988;31:4.

140. Condo RE. *Bacteroides* bacteremia. *Arch Surg* 1984;119:897.

141. Finegold SM. Perspective on susceptibility testing of anaerobic bacteremia. *Clin Infect Dis* 1997;25[Suppl 2]:S251.

142. Nguyen MH, Yu VL, Morris AJ, et al. Antimicrobial resistance and clinical outcome of *Bacteroides* bacteremia: findings of a multicenter prospective observational trial. *Clin Infect Dis* 2000;30:870.

143. Cuchural GJ, Tally FP, Jacobus NV, et al. Comparative activities of newer β-lactam agents against members of the *Bacteroides fragilis* group. *Antimicrob Agents Chemother* 1990;34:479.

144. Grollier G, Mory F, Quentin C, et al. Susceptibility of strict anaerobic bacteria to antibiotics in France: a multicenter study. *Pathol Biol* 1994;42:498.

145. Wexler HM, Molitoris E, Molitoris D, et al. *In vitro* activity of telithromycin (HMR 3647) against 502 strains of anaerobic bacteria. *J Antimicrob Chemother* 2001;47:467.

146. Hoellman DB, Kelly LM, Jacobs MR, et al. Comparative antianaerobic activity of BMS 284756. *Antimicrob Agents Chemother* 2001;45:589.

147. Aldridge KE, Ashcraft D, Cambre K, et al. Multicenter survey of the changing in vitro antimicrobial susceptibilities of clinical isolates of *Bacteroides fragilis* group, *Prevotella*, *Fusobacteria*, *Porphyromonas*, and *Peptostreptococcus* species. *Antimicrob Agents Chemother* 2001;45:1238.

148. Pfaller MA, Jones RN. A review of the *in vitro* activity of meropenem and comparative antimicrobial agents tested against 30,254 aerobic and anaerobic pathogens isolated world wide. *Diagn Microbiol Infect Dis* 1997;28:157.

149. Jung R, Messick CR, Pendland SL, et al. Postantibiotic effects and bactericidal activities of clarithromycin, hydroxy-clarithromycin, versus those of amoxicillin-clavulanate against anaerobes. *Antimicrob Agents Chemother* 2000;44:778.

150. Ackermann G, Schaumann R, Pless B, et al. Comparative activity of moxifloxacin *in vitro* against obligately anaerobic bacteria. *Eur J Clin Microbiol Infect Dis* 2000;19:228.

151. Rotimi VO, Mokaddas EM, Jamal WY, et al. Susceptibility of 497 clinical isolates of gram negative anaerobes to trovafloxacin and eight other antibiotics. *J Chemother* 1999;11:349.

152. Goldstein EJ, Citron DM, Merriam CV. Comparative *in vitro* activities of ABT-773 against aerobic and anaerobic pathogens isolated from skin and soft tissue animal and human bite infections. *Antimicrob Agents Chemother* 2000;44:2525.

CHAPTER 209
Anaerobic Cocci

John G. Bartlett

Anaerobic cocci are prominent components of the normal flora on virtually all mucocutaneous surfaces in humans, and they are common clinical isolates in endogenous infections, usually as components of a polymicrobial flora. The organisms most frequently isolated and considered clinically important are in the genus *Peptostreptococcus*.

TAXONOMY

Anaerobic gram-positive cocci include the genera *Peptostreptococcus*, *Streptococcus*, and *Gemella* (previously *Streptococcus morbillorum*). Other anaerobic cocci that are less important clinically include *Coprococcus*, *Peptococcus*, *Ruminococcus*, *Sarcina*, and *Staphylococcus saccharolyticus*. Older studies showed high yields of *Peptococcus* in various types of specimens, but most of the former species in the genus have now been transferred to *Peptostreptococcus* on the basis of deoxyribonucleic acid (DNA) content of guanine plus cytosine (1,2). *Peptococcus niger* is retained in the *Peptococcus* genus but is an infrequent clinical isolate. Another taxonomic change has been gram-positive cocci that produce abundant lactic acid and were formerly considered anaerobic but are now classified as *Streptococcus* on the basis of aerotolerance. These include *Streptococcus intermedius*, *Streptococcus constellatus*, and *Gemella morbillorum*. These organisms produce lactic acid as the sole major end product and show morphologic characteristics of variable size and form in chains and pairs. *S. intermedius* and *S. constellatus* usually grow initially on anaerobic plate media but become aerotolerant after subculturing. *S. intermedius*, *S. constellatus*, and *Streptococcus anginosus* were formerly classified as *S. anginosus* or *Streptococcus milleri*. They are common isolates in infectious diseases and abscesses, and they are often found in polymicrobial infections that include anaerobic bacteria (3,4). Unlike true anaerobes, these species of *Streptococcus* are resistant to metronidazole (5).

Of the peptostreptococci, the most common isolates are *Peptostreptococcus magnus* and *Peptostreptococcus asaccharolyticus*; less common are *Peptostreptococcus micros* and *Peptostreptococcus anaerobius* (6–8). More recently described species are *Peptostreptococcus vaginalis*, *Peptostreptococcus lactolyticus*, and *Peptostreptococcus pydrogenalis*. With regard to anatomic site, *P. magnus* is usually associated with skin and soft tissue infections and is commonly found with other anaerobes. *P. asaccharolyticus* is found at widely distributed sites, and *P. anaerobius* is usually found in subdiaphragmatic locations (6).

The anaerobic gram-negative cocci include *Veillonella*, *Acidaminococcus*, and *Megasphaera*. *Veillonella* is virtually always found as indigenous flora of the mouth and is common in the gastrointestinal (GI) tract and vaginal flora. *Megasphaera* and *Acidaminococcus* are common components of the intestinal flora. The pathogenic role of these organisms is unclear, but they are usually considered nonpathogens or contaminants.

MICROBIOLOGIC CHARACTERISTICS

The anaerobic cocci grow well on nonselective plate and broth media that are commonly recommended for recovering anaerobic bacteria (9) These include Schaedler agar, *Brucella* agar, brain-heart infusion agar, and Centers for Disease Control and Prevention (CDC) anaerobic blood agar. Selective media include blood agar plates containing phenylethyl alcohol or neomycin. Growth is generally slow, usually requiring 48 hours or longer. Gram stain does not distinguish among anaerobic, microaerophilic, and aerotolerant gram-positive cocci. Exposure of strict anaerobes to oxygen may result in loss of integrity of cell walls, causing Gram stain variability (10). Sensitivity to vancomycin with use of a 5-μg disk on *Brucella* blood agar will confirm Gram stain results. *Peptostreptococcus productus* and *P. anaerobius* may appear as coccobacilli. Identification at the genus and species levels is based on fermentation reaction and product of metabolism detected by gas-liquid chromatography; rapid tests such as RapID ANA 11 and ID32A have been useful for rapid identification of *P. micros*, *P. anaerobius*, and *P. asaccharolyticus* but are unreliable for other species such as *Peptostreptococcus prevotii* (11). Nevertheless, the utility of speciation is often questioned on the basis of the time and resources required. Differences between these organisms based on virulence and *in vitro* sensitivity test results are minimal.

NORMAL FLORA

Anaerobic cocci are found at virtually all mucocutaneous surfaces that harbor a normal flora. *Veillonella* species, primarily *Veillonella parvula*, are universally present in saliva and may be used as a marker of salivary contamination of respiratory specimens (12). In addition, numerous anaerobic gram-positive cocci are found in the normal flora of the upper airways (13). Concentrations are often on the order of 10^7 to 10^9 bacteria/mL of saliva (12). Quantitative studies of the vaginal and cervical flora indicate anaerobic gram-positive cocci in 60% to 80% of women of childbearing age in mean concentrations of 10^{10}/g of secretions (14,15). The dominant species are *P. anaerobius*, *P. asaccharolyticus*, *P. magnus*, and *P. micros* (11). The fecal flora show anaerobic gram-positive cocci usually present in mean concentrations of approximately 10^{10}/g (16,17). The most common species are *P. productus*, *P. magnus*, *P. prevotii*, *P. micros*, and *P. asaccharolyticus*. This flora also commonly includes *Veillonella*, *Ruminococcus*, *Acidaminococcus fermentans*, and *Megasphaera elsdenii*. Anaerobic gram-positive cocci are also constituents of the normal flora of skin, urethra, stomach, and small bowel.

CLINICAL INFECTIONS

Anaerobic gram-positive cocci are often found in clinical specimens with appropriate culture techniques (Table 209.1). They are usually found as components of mixed infections. Experience at the Mayo Clinic indicates that these bacteria are present in 17% to 31% of all specimens that yield anaerobic bacteria (9,18,19); the experience at St. Bartholomew's Hospital is that these bacteria account for about 27% of all clinical anaerobic isolates (20).

BACTEREMIA

Peptostreptococci account for 4% to 7% of blood culture isolates involving anaerobic bacteria (9,18–21). Transient bacteremia is common with dental procedures (22). Anaerobic or microaerophilic streptococci account for 5% to 10% of endocarditis cases, but a relatively small portion of these organisms are now classified as *Peptostreptococcus* (23). These organisms constitute normal skin flora, and their appearance in blood may often represent contaminants.

Respiratory Tract Infections

Peptostreptococci constitute a major component of the flora of upper airways (24,25) and are commonly noted in dental infections, perimandibular space infections, chronic sinusitis, and chronic otitis (26–30). They are the most common isolates in peritonsillar abscesses (31). These organisms are found in 10% to 20% of anaerobic infections of the lung (21,32,33).

Genital Tract Infections

Peptostreptococci have been reported in 25% to 40% of infections of the female pelvis, including pelvic abscess, Bartholin's gland abscess, endometritis, puerperal sepsis, infections after gynecologic surgery, and pelvic inflammatory disease (34–40).

TABLE 209.1. Recovery of *Peptostreptococcus* from Clinical Specimens

Clinical setting	Reference	No. of patients	Total number of anaerobic isolates	Total number of peptostreptococcal isolates
Anaerobic infections of the lung	32	193	461	136 (29.5%)
Intraabdominal sepsis	41	759	1,187	220 (18.5%)
Infections of the female genital tract	38	188	449	165 (36.7%)

Intraabdominal Sepsis

Peptostreptococci account for 10% to 30% of bacteria recovered in intraabdominal sepsis (21,41–45). These organisms, including microaerophilic streptococci, are common and are considered clinically important in pyogenic liver abscess and ascending cholangitis (42).

Skin and Soft Tissue Infections

Peptostreptococci are common isolates in infections of skin and soft tissue, including cutaneous abscesses below the waist, diabetic foot ulcers, infected decubitus ulcers, necrotizing fasciitis, necrotizing synergistic gangrene, and infected sebaceous cysts. They are also common in wound infections after intestinal or gynecologic surgery (46–49). Infections involving human bites and animal bites often involve these organisms (21). Streptococcal myositis is often attributed to *Streptococcus pyogenes*, but *Peptostreptococcus* species appear to cause the same syndrome.

Osteomyelitis

P. magnus appears to play a prominent role in septic arthritis and osteomyelitis among patients who have orthopedic surgical implants (19). The clinical course in these cases is typically chronic and indolent; removal of the prosthesis is eventually necessary in most.

TREATMENT

Peptostreptococci are usually recovered as part of a mixed flora, so a pathogenic role is difficult to determine. Many of these organisms are relatively fastidious, and they may be readily apparent on Gram stain but difficult to recover in culture. They usually have predictable sensitivity patterns, making empirical treatment relatively easy. For these reasons, most authorities do not recommend routine sensitivity testing except in selected clinical settings such as endocarditis, cerebral abscess, osteomyelitis, and septic arthritis (50).

Penicillin G is usually considered the preferred agent for infections involving peptostreptococci. Because these organisms are usually present in polymicrobial infections, therapeutic decisions are often dictated by other components that may be more resistant. Other drugs that are usually effective *in vitro* are other penicillins (except nafcillin or oxacillin), vancomycin, linezolid, telithromycin, gatifloxacin, moxifloxacin, imipenem, chloramphenicol, macrolides, many cephalosporins (other than ceftazidime), and any combination of a β-lactam–β-lactamase inhibitor (51–61). Drugs that are not active include aztreonam, aminoglycosides, and early generation fluoroquinolones (53). Metronidazole and clindamycin are somewhat unpredictable because 12% to 15% of peptostreptococci are resistant. Some strains that are initially clindamycin sensitive but erythromycin resistant often have inducible clindamycin resistance (62). Strains belonging to the *Streptococcus milleri* group show occasional resistance to penicillin (63) and consistent resistance to metronidazole.

VEILLONELLA

Veillonella is generally regarded as a nonpathogen and is a frequent contaminant reflecting near-universal presence in the normal oral flora. There have been rare cases of infection including endocarditis (64,65), meningitis (66), prosthetic joint infection (67), and bacteremia with no identified source (68,69). Penicillin is generally regarded as the preferred drug.

REFERENCES

1. Ezaki T, Yamamoto N, Ninomiya K, et al. Transfer of *Peptococcus indolicus, Peptococcus asaccharolyticus, Peptococcus prevotii,* and *Peptococcus magnus* to the genus *Peptostreptococcus* and proposal of *Peptostreptococcus tetradius* sp. nov. *Int J Syst Bacteriol* 1983;33:683.
2. Huss VAR, Festl H, Schleifer KH. Nucleic acid hybridization studies and deoxyribonucleic acid base compositions of anaerobic gram-positive cocci. *Int J Syst Bacteriol* 1984;34:95.
3. Cato EP. Transfer of *Peptostreptococcus parvulus* (Weinberg, Nativelle, and Prevot 1937) Smith 1957 to the genus *Streptococcus: Streptococcus parvulus* (Weinberg, Nativelle, and Prevot 1937) comb. nov., rev., emend. *Int J Syst Bacteriol* 1983;33:82.
4. Gossling J. Occurrence and pathogenicity of the *Streptococcus milleri* group. *Rev Infect Dis* 1988;10:257.
5. Madinger NE, McGregor JA, McKinney PJ, et al. Comparative antibiotic susceptibilities of anaerobes associated with infection of the female reproductive tract. *Clin Infect Dis* 1993;16[Suppl 4]:S349.
6. Murdoch DA, Mitchelmore IJ, Tabaqchali S. The clinical importance of gram-positive anaerobic cocci isolated at St. Bartholomew's Hospital, London, in 1987. *J Med Microbiol* 1994;41:36.
7. Murdoch DA, Magee T. A numerical taxonomic study of the gram-positive anaerobic cocci. *J Med Microbiol* 1995;43:148.
8. Brook I. Peptostreptococcal infection in children [Review]. *Scand J Infect Dis* 1994;26:503.
9. Rosenblatt J. Anaerobic cocci. In: Lennette EH, ed. *Manual of clinical microbiology,* 4th ed. Washington, DC: American Society for Microbiology, 1985:445–449.
10. Johnson MJ, Thatcher E, Cox ME. Techniques for controlling variability in Gram staining of obligate anaerobes. *J Clin Microbiol* 1995;33:755.
11. Ng J, Ng LK, Chow AW, et al. Identification of five *Peptostreptococcus* species isolated predominantly from the female genital tract by using the rapid ID32A system. *J Clin Microbiol* 1994;32:1302.
12. Bartlett JG, Finegold SM. Bacteriology of expectorated sputum with quantitative culture and wash technique compared to transtracheal aspiration. *Am Rev Respir Dis* 1978;117:1010.
13. Socransky SS, Manganiello SD. The oral microbiota of man from birth to senility. *J Periodontol* 1971;42:485.
14. Bartlett JG, Onderdonk AB, Drude E, et al. Quantitative bacteriology of the vaginal flora. *J Infect Dis* 1977;136:271.
15. Ohm MJ, Galask RP. Bacterial flora of the cervix from 100 prehysterectomy patients. *Am J Obstet Gynecol* 1975;122:683.
16. Finegold SM, Attebery HR, Sutter VL. Effect of diet on human fecal flora: comparison of Japanese and American diets. *Am J Clin Nutr* 1974;27:1456.
17. Hentges DJ. The anaerobic microflora on the human body. *Clin Infect Dis* 1993;16[Suppl 4]:S175.
18. Martin WJ. Isolation and identification of anaerobic bacteria in the clinical laboratory: a 2-year experience. *Mayo Clin Proc* 1974;49:300.
19. Bourgault A-M, Rosenblatt JE, Fitzgerald RH. *Peptococcus magnus:* a significant human pathogen. *Ann Intern Med* 1980;93:244.
20. Murdoch DA, Mitchelmore LJ, Tabaqchali S. The clinical importance of gram-positive anaerobic cocci isolated at St. Bartholomew's Hospital, London in 1987. *J Med Microbiol* 1994;41:36.
21. Finegold SM, George WL, Mulligan ME. Anaerobic infections. *Dis Mon* 1985;31:8.
22. Montejo M, Ruiz-Irastorza G, Aguirrebengoa K, et al. Prosthetic valve endocarditis caused by *Peptostreptococcus anaerobius* [Letter]. *Clin Infect Dis* 1995;20:1431.
23. van der Vorm ER, Dondorp AM, van Ketel RJ, et al. Apparent culture-negative prosthetic valve endocarditis caused by *Peptostreptococcus magnus. J Clin Microbiol* 2000;38:4640.
24. von Troil-Linden B, Torkko H, Alaluusua S, et al. Salivary levels of suspected periodontal pathogens in relation to periodontal status and treatment. *J Dent Res* 1995;74:1789.
25. Gomes BP, Lilley JD, Drucker DB. Clinical significance of dental root canal microflora. *J Dent* 1996;24:47.
26. Bartlett JG, O'Keefe P. The bacteriology of perimandibular space infections. *J Oral Surg* 1979;37:407.
27. Frederick J, Braude AI. Anaerobic infection of the paranasal sinuses. *N Engl J Med* 1974;290:135.
28. Brook I. The role of anaerobic bacteria in otitis media: microbiology, pathogenesis, and implications on therapy. *Am J Otolaryngol* 1987;8:109.
29. Ito K, Ito Y, Mizuta K, et al. Bacteriology of chronic otitis media, chronic sinusitis, and paranasal mucopyocele in Japan. *Clin Infect Dis* 1995;20[Suppl 2]:S214.
30. Brook I, Frazier EH. Correlation between microbiology and previous sinus surgery in patients with chronic maxillary sinusitis. *Ann Otol Rhinol Laryngol* 2001;110:148.
31. Mitchelmore IJ, Prior AJ, Montgomery PQ, et al. Microbiological features and pathogenesis of peritonsillar abscesses. *Eur J Clin Microbiol Infect Dis* 1995;14:870.

32. Bartlett JG. Systemic infection involving anaerobes: anaerobic bacterial infections of the lung and pleural space. *Clin Infect Dis* 1993;16[Suppl 4]:S248.

33. Civen R, Jousimies-Somer H, Marina M, et al. A retrospective review of cases of anaerobic empyema and update of bacteriology. *Clin Infect Dis* 1995;20[Suppl 2]:S224.

34. Rotheram EB Jr, Schick SF. Nonclostridial anaerobic bacteria in septic abortion. *Am J Med* 1969;46:80.

35. Smith JW, Southern PM Jr, Lehmann JD. Bacteremia in septic abortion: complications and treatment. *Obstet Gynecol* 1970;35:704.

36. Chow AW, Malkasian KL, Marshall JR, et al. The bacteriology of acute pelvic inflammatory disease. *Am J Obstet Gynecol* 1975;122:876.

37. Eschenbach DA, Buchanan TM, Pollock HM, et al. Polymicrobial etiology of acute pelvic inflammatory disease. *N Engl J Med* 1975;293:166.

38. Sweet R, Schachter J, Landers DV, et al. Treatment of hospitalized patients with acute pelvic inflammatory disease: comparison of cefotetan plus doxycycline and cefoxitin plus doxycycline. *Am J Obstet Gynecol* 1988;158:736.

39. Sweet R. Role of bacterial vaginosis in pelvic inflammatory disease. *Clin Infect Dis* 1995;20[Suppl 2]:S271.

40. Smayevsky J, Canigia LF, Lanza A, et al. Vaginal microflora associated with bacterial vaginosis in non-pregnant women: reliability of sialidase detection. *Infect Dis Obstet Gynecol* 2001;9:17.

41. Stone HH, Strom PR, Fabian TC, et al. Third-generation cephalosporins for polymicrobial surgical sepsis. *Arch Surg* 1983;118:193.

42. Sabbaj J, Sutter VL, Finegold SM. Anaerobic pyogenic liver abscess. *Ann Intern Med* 1972;77:629.

43. Gorbach SL. Management of anaerobic infections: intra-abdominal sepsis. *Ann Intern Med* 1975;83:377.

44. Moore WEC, Cato EP, Holdeman LV. Anaerobic bacteria of the gastrointestinal flora and their occurrence in clinical infections. *J Infect Dis* 1969;119:641.

45. Swenson RM, Lorber B, Michaelson TC, et al. The bacteriology of infraabdominal infections. *Arch Surg* 1974;109:398.

46. Gerding DN. Foot infections in diabetic patients: the role of anaerobes [Review]. *Clin Infect Dis* 1995;20[Suppl 2]:S283.

47. MacLennan JD. The histotoxic clostridial infections of man. *Bacteriol Rev* 1962;26:232.

48. Summanen PH, Talan DA, Strong C, et al. Bacteriology of skin and soft-tissue infections: comparison of infections in intravenous drug users and individuals with no history of intravenous drug use. *Clin Infect Dis* 1995;20[Suppl 2]:S279.

49. Brook I, Frazier EH. Clinical and microbiological features of necrotizing fasciitis. *J Clin Microbiol* 1995;33:2382.

50. Finegold SM, and the National Committee for Clinical Laboratory Standards Working Group on Anaerobic Susceptibility Testing. Susceptibility testing of anaerobic bacteria. *J Clin Microbiol* 1988;26:1253.

51. Edson RS, Rosenblatt JE, Lee DT, et al. Recent experience with antimicrobial susceptibility of anaerobic bacteria. *Mayo Clin Proc* 1982;57:737.

52. Bourgault A-M, Harding GK, Smith JA, et al. Survey of anaerobic susceptibility patterns in Canada. *Antimicrob Agents Chemother* 1986;30:798.

53. Garcia-Rodriguez JA, Garcia-Sanchez JE, Trujillano-Martin I, et al. *In vitro* activity of BAY y3118 and nine other antimicrobial agents against anaerobic bacteria. *J Chemother* 1995;7:189.

54. Krepel CJ, Gohr CM, Edmiston CE, et al. Surgical sepsis: constancy of antibiotic susceptibility of causative organisms. *Surgery* 1995;117:505.

55. Aldridge KE, Morice N, Schiro DD. Increased *in vitro* activity of ceftriaxone by addition of tazobactam against clinical isolates of anaerobes. *Diagn Microbiol Infect Dis* 1994;19:227.

56. Goldstein EJ, Citron DM, Merriam CV, et al. Activities of telithromycin compared to erythromycin, azithromycin, clarithromycin, roxithromycin, and other antimicrobials against unusual anaerobes. *Antimicrob Agents Chemother* 1999;43:2801.

57. Ackermann G, Schaumann R, Pless B, et al. Comparative activity of moxifloxacin in vitro against obligately anaerobic bacteria. *Eur J Clin Microbiol Infect Dis* 2000;19:228.

58. Clemett D, Markham A. Linezolid. *Drugs* 2000;59:815.

59. Aldridge KE, Ashcraft D, Cambre K, et al. Multicenter survey of the changing *in vitro* antimicrobial susceptibilities of clinical isolates of *Bacteroides fragilis* group, *Prevotella, Fusobacterium, Porphyromonas,* and *Peptostreptococcus* species. *Antimicrob Agents Chemother* 2001;45:1238.

60. Winkel EG, Winkelhoff AJ, Timmerman MF, et al. Ampicillin plus metronidazole in the treatment of adult periodontitis patients. *J Clin Periodontol* 2001;28:296.

61. Wexler HM, Molitoris E, Molitoris D, et al. *In vitro* activity of levofloxacin against a selected group of anaerobic bacteria isolated from skin and soft tissue infections. *Antimicrob Agents Chemother* 1998;42:984.

62. Reig M, Moreno A, Baquero F. Resistance of *Peptostreptococcus* spp to macrolides and lincosamides: inducible and constitutive phenotypes. *Antimicrob Agents Chemother* 1992;36:662.

63. Bantar C, Canigia LF, Relloso S, et al. Species belonging to the *Streptococcus milleri* group: antimicrobial susceptibility and comparative prevalence in significant clinical specimens. *J Clin Microbiol* 1996;34:2020.

64. Houston S, Taylor D, Rennie R. Prosthetic valve endocarditis due to *Veillonella dispar*: successful medical treatment following penicillin desensitization. *Clin Infect Dis* 1997;24:1013.

65. Prpic-Mehicic G, Marsan T, Miletic I, et al. Infective endocarditis caused by *Veillonella* of dental origin. *Coll Antropol* 1998;22:39.

66. Bhatti MA, Frank MO. *Veillonella parvula* meningitis: case report and review of *Veillonella* infections. *Clin Infect Dis* 2000;31:839.

67. Marchandin H, Jean-Pierre H, Carriere C, et al. Prosthetic joint infection due to *Veillonella dispar*. *Eur J Clin Microbiol Infect Dis* 2001;20:340.

68. Fisher RG, Denison MR. *Veillonella parvula* bacteremia without an underlying source. *J Clin Microbiol* 1996;34:3235.

69. Liu JW, Wu JJ, Want LR, et al. Two fatal cases of *Veillonella* bacteremia. *Eur J Clin Microbiol Infect Dis* 1999;17:62.

CHAPTER 210

Anaerobic Gram-negative Rods: Bacteroides, Prevotella, Porphyromonas, Fusobacterium, Bilophila, Sutterella, Tannerella

Sydney M. Finegold

In this chapter, I describe members of the genera *Anaerobiospirillum, Anaerorhabdus, Anaerovibrio, Bacteroides, Bilophila, Butyrivibrio, Campylobacter, Catonella, Centipeda, Desulfomonas, Desulfovibrio, Dialister, Dichelobacter, Fibrobacter, Fusobacterium, Johnsonella, Leptotrichia, Megamonas, Mitsuokella, Porphyromonas, Prevotella, Rikenella, Ruminobacter, Sebaldella, Selenomonas, Succinimonas, Succinivibrio, Sutterella,* and *Tannerella*. These organisms are part of the normal flora of the mouth and upper respiratory, intestinal, and urogenital tracts of humans and animals.

CHARACTERISTICS OF THE PATHOGENS

The initial differentiation of these genera is based on motility, flagellar arrangement, cellular morphology, and gas-liquid chromatography (GLC) analysis of cellular fatty acids and metabolic end products (1–41) (Table 210.1). Species definition is based on 16S ribosomal ribonucleic acid (rRNA) sequencing comparisons and deoxyribonucleic acid (DNA)–DNA hybridization (25–27). For most clinical specimens, only the genera *Bacteroides, Prevotella, Porphyromonas,* and *Fusobacterium* need to be considered. However, *Bilophila* and *Sutterella* do occur fairly commonly in intraabdominal and other infections (6,14). The taxonomy of anaerobic gram-negative bacilli has been in a state of great change recently, and the trend will continue. It has been proposed that only the present *Bacteroides fragilis* group should be included in the genus *Bacteroides* and that other species that have not yet been reclassified should be (29). Actually, *Bacteroides distasonis* and *Bacteroides merdae* will be taken out of the *B. fragilis* group also. *Prevotella* includes the moderately saccharolytic organisms previously in the genus *Bacteroides* (7). This includes the species *Prevotella oris, Prevotella buccae,* the *Prevotella oralis* group, *Prevotella melaninogenica, Prevotella denticola, Prevotella loescheii, Prevotella intermedia, Prevotella nigrescens* (30), *Prevotella corporis, Prevotella bivius,* and *Prevotella disiens*. Nonsaccharolytic pigmented rods are in the genus *Porphyromonas* (8). This includes

TABLE 210.1. Differentiation of Genera of Gram-negative Anaerobic Bacilli

Characteristic	Genus
Nonmotile or peritrichous flagella	
Produce butyric acid (without isobutyric and isovaleric acid)	*Fusobacterium*
Produce major lactic acid	*Leptotrichia*
Produce acetic acid and hydrogen sulfide; reduce sulfate	*Desulfomonas*
Not as above	*Anaerorhabdus*
	Bacteroides
	Bilophila
	Fibrobacter
	Megamonas
	Mitsuokella
	Porphyromonas
	Prevotella
	Rikenella
	Ruminobacter
	Sebaldella
	Sutterella
Polar flagella	
Fermentative	
Produce butyric acid	*Butyrivibrio*
Produce succinic acid	
Spiral-shaped cells	*Succinivibrio*
Ovoid cells	*Succinimonas*
Produce propionic and acetic acids	*Anaerovibrio*
Nonfermentative, produce succinic acid from fumarate	*Campylobacter*
Tufts of flagella on concave side of curved cells, fermentative	*Selenomonas*
	Centipeda
Bipolar tufts of flagella	*Anaerobiospirillum*

the species *Porphyromonas asaccharolytica, Porphyromonas gingivalis, Porphyromonas endodontalis,* and *Porphyromonas macacae.* For recent taxonomic changes see Table 210.2. The most commonly encountered gram-negative anaerobic rods are listed in Table 210.3.

B. fragilis (Fig. 210.1), one of the most important of all anaerobes because of its frequent occurrence in clinical infection and its resistance to antimicrobial agents, is a gram-negative bacillus with rounded ends 0.5 to 0.8 μm in diameter and 1.5 to 4.5 μm long with rounded ends. Most strains are encapsulated. Vacuolization, irregular staining, and pleomorphism are common, particularly in broth media. The ultrastructure of *B. fragilis* is similar to that of other gram-negative bacteria. The guanine plus cytosine (G+C) content is 42%. *Bacteroides thetaiotaomicron* is even more resistant to antimicrobials than *B. fragilis* and is involved in infections with some frequency. *P. melaninogenica* and *P. asaccharolytica* are short to coccoid gram-negative rods that produce a distinctive brown to black pigment, which is a heme derivative (Figs. 210.2 and 210.3). *P. asaccharolytica* is encapsulated. Many strains of *P. melaninogenica* require vitamin K or similar compounds as well as heme. Other anaerobic gram-negative rods are much less common.

Numerous studies of the endotoxin of gram-negative anaerobic bacilli have determined that in *B. fragilis* the endotoxin contains little or no lipid A, 2-ketodeoxyoctonate, or heptose. It also lacks β-hydroxymyristic acid. This endotoxin exhibits little biologic activity (42). Poor biologic activity of endotoxin also has been demonstrated for the other *B. fragilis* group members, and for *P. melaninogenica* and *P. asaccharolytica.*

Members of the genus *Fusobacterium* (Fig. 210.4) may be spindle shaped or may have parallel sides and rounded ends. G+C ratios range from 26% to 34%. Cells of *Fusobacterium mortiferum* (and sometimes *Fusobacterium necrophorum*) often are elongated or filamentous and curved and possess spherical enlargements and large, free, round bodies. *Fusobacterium nucleatum,* usually does not produce infections as serious as those caused by *F. necrophorum,* but it is certainly a virulent organism and is encountered clinically much more often. The cells of this species are usually spindle shaped, 5 to 10 μm long, and are often seen in pairs, end to end.

The 2-ketodeoxyoctonate and sugar content of the lipopolysaccharide of *F. necrophorum* vary from strain to strain. Although biologic activity varies, many or most strains do show strong biologic activity, comparable to that of *Salmonella enteritidis* (42). The biologic activity of the endotoxin of *F. nucleatum* is also variable but often strong.

Bilophila wadsworthia (Fig. 210.5) is a very large, pale-staining, gram-negative bacillus with some pleomorphism and irregular staining. Its G+C ratio is 33% to 34%. It is commonly encountered in intraabdominal infection and has been involved in such serious infections as bacteremia and brain abscess.

Plasmids have been found in about half of the *Bacteroides* strains studied. For the most part, their biologic and clinical significance are not known; however, some have been found to code for resistance to antimicrobial agents.

Most strains of the *B. fragilis* group can deconjugate bile acids (43). *P. melaninogenica, P. oralis,* and *F. nucleatum* are inhibited by bile. *Bilophila* and *Sutterella,* as well as the *B. fragilis* group, are resistant to bile (4,10). *F. necrophorum* deconjugates bile acids, primarily taurine conjugates (43). Some *Bacteroides* species can convert primary bile acids to secondary ones. Glucuronidase produced by anaerobic gram-negative bacilli may be of special significance in deconjugating compounds that previously had been detoxified in the liver by combination with glucuronide.

Certain *Bacteroides* species possess distinguishing enzymes. Superoxide dismutase has been found in *B. fragilis, B. thetaiotaomicron, Bacteroides vulgatus,* and *Bacteroides ovatus* (44). In general, a good correlation exists between superoxide dismutase activity and oxygen tolerance. β-Lactamase activity has been demonstrated in several species of anaerobic gram-negative rods; it accounts for most of the resistance to various β-lactam antibiotics, such as certain penicillins and cephalosporins, although occasionally other mechanisms are responsible (45,46). Urease is produced by *B. wadsworthia* (6) and by *Bacteroides ureolyticus. B. ureolyticus* also produces an agarase, which leads to pitting of the agar by the colonies. A related pitting organism *Sutterella wadsworthensis* (14) is more pathogenic and relatively resistant to antimicrobial drugs.

EPIDEMIOLOGY

All anaerobic, gram-negative bacillary infections arise when mucosal damage related to surgery, trauma, or disease permits indigenous flora to penetrate tissue. Knowledge of the indigenous flora at various sites under different circumstances permits the clinician to anticipate the likely infecting flora in acute infections. The pathogenicity of various species also must be considered. Ecologic determinants include oxygen sensitivity, ability of organisms to adhere, and microbial interrelationships.

At birth, an infant's oral cavity usually is sterile, but by age 12 months, *Fusobacterium* species can be cultured from 50% of infants and *Bacteroides* from a smaller percentage. In the human gingival crevice area, gram-negative anaerobic rods account for 16% to 20% of the total cultivatable flora. *P. melaninogenica* is seldom isolated before age 6 years, but by the early teens, this organism can be isolated from the gingival crevice area of most

TABLE 210.2.   Recent Taxonomic Changes and Trends Among Anaerobic Gram-negative Rods

Current nomenclature	Synonym/taxonomic position
Anaerobiospirillum thomasii	New species
Bacteroides distasonis/merdae	Related to *Porphyromonas* cluster
Bacteroides furcosus	Related to *Porphyromonas* cluster
Bacteroides putredinis	Possibly related to *Rikenella*
Bacteroides pyogenes[a]	*Bacteroides tectum* homology group II (some strains)
Bacteroides splanchnicus	Possibly represents a new genus
Bacteroides tectus	*Bacteroides tectum*, related to *Bacteroides fragilis*
Butyrivibrio species	Related to *Clostridium* subphylum, cluster XIVa
Campylobacter gracilis	*Bacteroides gracilis* (some strains)
Campylobacter hominis	New species
Campylobacter showae	New species
Capnocytophaga granulosa	New species
Capnocytophaga haemolytica	New species
Catonella morbi	Related to *Clostridium* subphylum, cluster XIVa
Centipeda periodontii	Related to *Selenomonas* species
Desulfomicrobium orale	New species
Desulfovibrio piger	*Desulfovibrio pigra*
Dialister pneumosintes	Related to *Sporomusa* branch of *Clostridium* subphylum, cluster IX
Dysgonomonas	CDC group DF-3, related organisms
Fusobacterium varium	*Fusobacterium pseudonecrophorum*
Johnsonella ignava	Related to *Clostridium* subphylum, cluster XIVa
Leptotrichia sanguinegens	New species
Mitsuokella multacida	Related to *Sporomusa* branch of *Clostridium* subphylum, cluster IX
Porphyromonas cangingivalis[a]	New species
Porphyromonas canoris[a]	New species
Porphyromonas cansulci[a]	New species
Porphyromonas catoniae	*Oribaculum catoniae*
Porphyromonas crevioricanis	New species
Porphyromonas gingivicanis[a]	New species
Porphyromonas gulae[a]	Animal version of *P. gingivalis*
Porphyromonas levii[a]	*Bacteroides levii*
Porphyromonas macacae[a]	*Bacteroides macacae, Porphyromonas salivosa*
Prevotella albensis[a]	*Bacteroides ruminicola* subsp. *ruminicola* biovar 7, *Prevotella ruminicola* (some strains)
Prevotella brevis[a]	*Bacteroides ruminicola* subsp. *brevis* biovars 1,2, *Prevotella ruminicola* (some strains)
Prevotella bryantii[a]	*B. ruminicola* subsp. *brevis* biovar 3, *Prevotella ruminicola* (some strains)
Prevotella dentalis	*Mitsuokella dentalis, Hallella seregans*
Prevotella enoeca	New species
Prevotella heparinolytica	Related to *Bacteroides fragilis* group
Prevotella nigrescens	New species; *Prevotella intermedia* (some strains)
Prevotella pallens	New species
Prevotella ruminicola	*B. ruminicola* subsp. *ruminicola* biovar 1
Prevotella tannerae	New species
Prevotella zoogleoformans	Related to *Bacteroides fragilis* group
Selenomonas species	Related to *Sporomusa* branch of *Clostridium* subphylum, cluster IX
Sutterella wadsworthensis	New genus and species, *Campylobacter (Bacteroides) gracilis* (some strains)
Tannerella forsythensis	*Bacteroides forsythus*
Tissierella praeacuta	Related to *Clostridium* subphylum, cluster XII

[a]Of animal origin; many found in infections secondary to animal bites.

humans. In the presence of acute ulcerative gingivitis or advanced chronic periodontal disease, *Fusobacterium* counts in saliva are higher than the usual 10^4 to 10^6/mL. Gram-negative anaerobic rods usually constitute 8% to 17% of the cultivatable flora of human dental plaque. Selective localization is illustrated by the fact that *P. melaninogenica* is routinely found in the gingival crevice but only rarely on the tongue, cheek, or coronal tooth surface (47,48).

The normal stomach has few organisms and, as a rule, no anaerobic bacteria; however, in the presence of pathologic con-

ditions such as duodenal ulcer with bleeding or obstruction, abnormal colonization with *B. fragilis* can occur in the stomach (49). The terminal ileum has approximately equal numbers of facultative aerobes and anaerobes, *Bacteroides* being one of the major anaerobes. Almost invariably, *Bacteroides* organisms are found in the feces of adult subjects; the mean count is 10^{11}/g. *Fusobacterium* species are found in 18% of adults (mean 10^8/g). *B. thetaiotaomicron* and *B. vulgatus* are the dominant species of *Bacteroides* in feces, followed by *B. distasonis, B. ovatus*, and *B. fragilis*. It has been found in animal studies that *Bacteroides*

TABLE 210.3. **Commonly Encountered Gram-Negative Anaerobic Rods**

Bacteroides fragilis group	Nonpigmented bile-sensitive
B. fragilis	*Prevotella and Bacteroides*
B. thetaiotaomicron	*Prevotella*
B. distasonis	P. oris
B. ovatus	P. buccae
B. vulgatus	P. oralis
B. uniformis	P. buccalis
B. caccae	P. veroralis
B. merdae	P. oulora
B. stercoris	P. disiens
B. eggerthii	P. heparinolytica
Bacteroides splanchnicus	P. zoogleoformans
Pigmented *Porphyromonas*	*Bacteroides*
and *Prevotella*	B. capillosus
Porphyromonas	B. putredinis
P. asaccharolytica	*Tannerella forsythensis*
P. gingivalis	*Fusobacterium* species
P. endodontalis	F. nucleatum
P. macacae	F. necrophorum
Prevotella	F. gonidiaformans
P. intermedia	F. naviforme
P. nigrescens	F. necrogenes
P. corporis	F. varium
P. melaninogenica	F. mortiferum
P. denticola	F. russii
P. loescheii	F. periodonticum
P. bivia	Miscellaneous bile-resistant
P. tannerae	anaerobes
	Bilophila wadsworthia
	Sutterella wadsworthensis

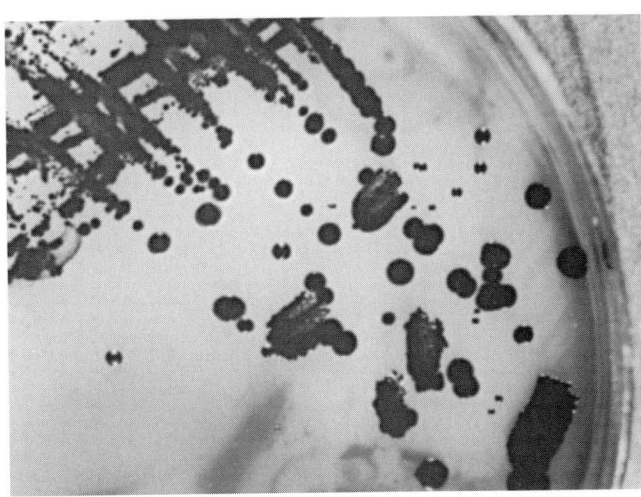

Figure 210.2. Colony morphology of pigmented *Prevotella*. Pigment varies from brown to black.

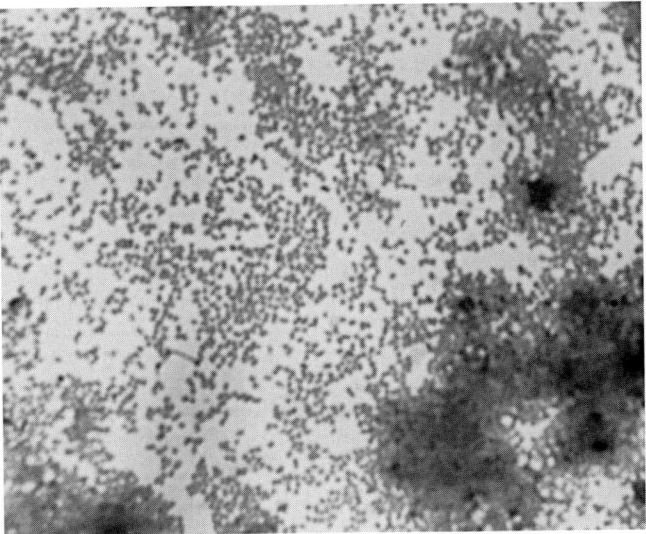

Figure 210.3. Microscopic morphology of pigmented *Prevotella*. Organisms are coccobacilli.

protect against intestinal infections due to *Salmonella* and *Shigella* organisms (47).

Bacteroides, *Prevotella*, and *Fusobacterium* organisms have often been found in the vaginal flora. Vaginal and cervical flora studies show that *Bacteroides* species are recovered from half of patients; mean concentrations are 10^6/g. Species of *Bacteroides* and *Prevotella* recovered from the normal cervical flora of healthy women include *P. oralis*, *B. fragilis*, *B. capillosus*, *P. bivia*, *P. disiens*, *P. oris*, *P. buccae*, and *B. ureolyticus* (47,50).

Studies of normal urethral flora are relatively limited, but various *Fusobacterium* and *Bacteroides* species have been isolated.

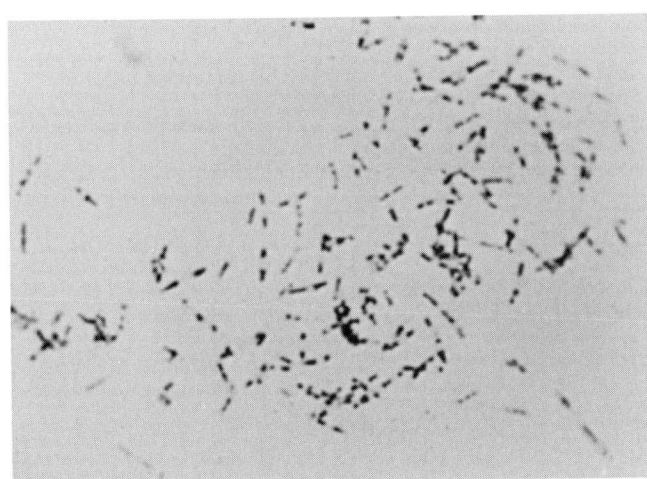

Figure 210.1. Microscopic morphology of *Bacteroides fragilis*. Note irregularity of staining.

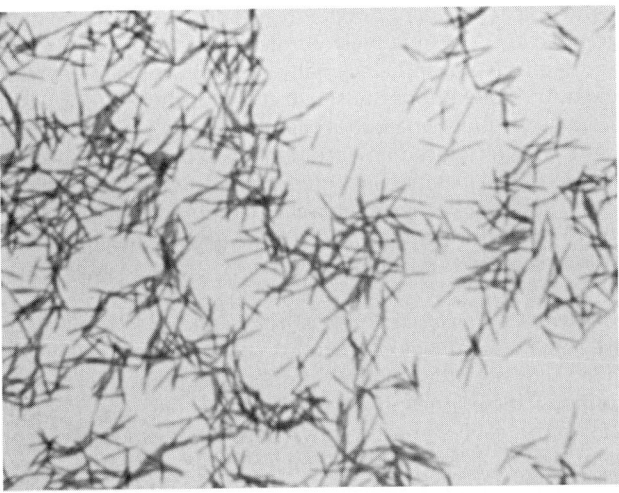

Figure 210.4. Microscopic morphology of *Fusobacterium nucleatum*. Note delicate rods with tapered ends.

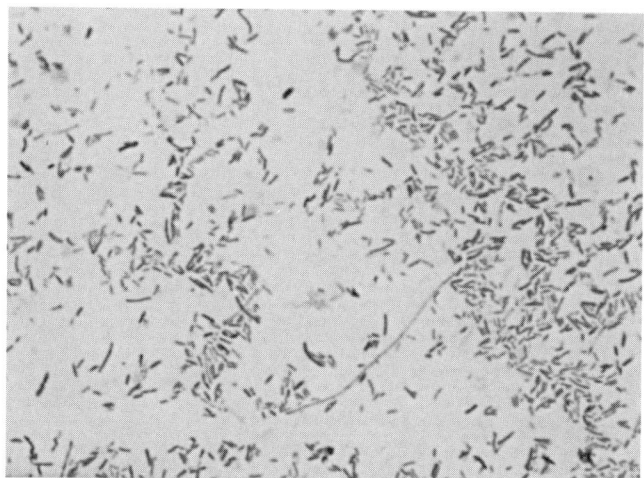

Figure 210.5. Microscopic morphology of *Bilophila wadsworthia*. Organism is very large and shows some pleomorphism.

Fusiform bacilli and *P. melaninogenica* are found regularly on the external genitalia.

Bilophila organisms are found in about half of normal stool specimens, usually in counts of 10^5 to 10^6/g of dry feces. They are part of the normal oral or vaginal flora in 2% of subjects.

PATHOGENESIS

Bacteroides, Prevotella, Porphyromonas, and *Fusobacterium* organisms are prevalent as indigenous flora on all mucosal surfaces. Under circumstances such as surgical or other trauma or when tumors arise or other diseases occur at the mucosal surface, they may penetrate tissues and set up an infection. In certain cases, for example, aspiration pneumonia, anaerobic bacteria from a site of normal carriage may move into another site that is normally free of bacteria and infect that site. Tissue necrosis and poor blood supply lower the oxidation-reduction potential, favoring the growth of anaerobes; accordingly, vascular disease, cold, shock, trauma, surgery, foreign bodies, malignancy, edema, and gas production by bacteria may significantly predispose tissue to infection with anaerobes, as may prior infection with aerobic or facultative bacteria. Antimicrobial agents, such as aminoglycosides, trimethoprim-sulfamethoxazole, or the earlier quinolones, to which anaerobes are notably resistant, may facilitate anaerobic infection. The relatively aerotolerant anaerobes are more likely to survive after the normally protective mucosal barrier is broken until conditions are satisfactory for their multiplication and invasion. Once anaerobes begin to multiply, they can maintain their own reduced environment by excreting end products of fermentative metabolism. Infections involving gram-negative anaerobic bacilli often are characterized by abscess formation and tissue destruction, as are most anaerobic infections. Table 210.4 lists common infections that involve gram-negative anaerobic bacilli.

Bacteroides, Prevotella, Porphyromonas, and *Fusobacterium* produce enzymes that may play a role in pathogenesis: collagenase, trypsin-like enzymes, various proteinases, neuraminidase, deoxyribonuclease, phosphatase, heparinase, and phospholipase (42). Fibrinolysin is produced by many *P. melaninogenica*–group strains and by a few of the *B. fragilis* group strains. Strains of *Bacteroides, Prevotella,* and *Porphyromonas* have been shown to degrade complement factors and immunoglobulin G and immunoglobulin M. The lipopolysaccharides of *B. fragilis, B. vul-*

gatus, and *F. mortiferum* activate Hageman's factor and thereby initiate the intrinsic pathway of coagulation. *F. necrophorum* produces a leukocidin, hemolysin, and a hemagglutinin. *B. fragilis* produces an enterotoxin.

Other factors may be involved in pathogenicity of certain anaerobes (Table 210.5). *P. melaninogenica* may inhibit phagocytosis and killing of other organisms in mixed infections. Constituents of the cell envelope and cell surface may contribute to pathogenicity. The capsule of organisms such as *B. fragilis* is an important virulence factor, as fimbriae, pili, and lectin-like adhesions may be. Butyrate and succinate produced by *Bacteroides* are cytotoxic.

TABLE 210.4. Common Syndromes of Gram-negative Anaerobic Rod Infection

Bite infection
Oral or dental infection
Aspiration pneumonia, lung abscess, empyema
Postabortion and puerperal infections
Infection following bowel, gallbladder, or gynecologic surgery
Appendicitis, diverticulitis
Septicemia with malignant neoplasm, diabetes, corticosteroid therapy, negative blood cultures
Septic thrombophlebitis
Gas-forming infection
Putrid infection

TABLE 210.5. Potential Virulence Factors of Gram-negative Anaerobic Bacilli

Putative virulence factor or property	Possible significance
Adherence to peritoneal mesothelium	Factor in development of peritonitis
Adherence to gingival crevicular epithelium	Factor in development of periodontal disease
Polysaccharides of capsule	Inhibit macrophage migration, antiphagocytic for aerobes and anaerobes, promote abscess formation
Superoxide dismutase and catalase	Confer oxygen tolerance
Immunoglobulin proteases	Resist host defenses
Hyaluronidase, collagenase, chondroitin sulfatase, neuraminidase, fibrinolysin	Tissue digestion or dissolution (i.e., "spreading factors")
Heparinase and other coagulation-promoting factors	Impair blood supply to infected area
Lipopolysaccharide	Causes inflammation and bone resorption in periodontal disease
"Leukotoxin"	Cytopathic for a variety of mammalian cell types
Butyrate	Cytotoxic substance
Soluble inhibitors of chemotaxis	Blunting of inflammatory response
Enterotoxin (fragilysin)	Diarrhea secondary to cleavage of E-cadherin, which appears to lead to stimulation of intestinal secretion and changes in the tight junctional complex
Modulation of surface antigens	Escape host immune response

Polymorphonuclear leukocytes have oxygen-dependent and oxygen-independent microbicidal systems. Polymorphonuclear leukocytes normally kill *B. fragilis* under anaerobic and aerobic conditions. In response to factors generated by bacteria in plasma, however, chemotaxis is depressed markedly under anaerobic conditions, and products of *Bacteroides* may suppress neutrophil chemotaxis and phagocytic killing (51,52).

Studies of host defenses indicate that various other interactions may occur between the bacteria and the host cells. *B. fragilis* is more resistant to the normal bactericidal activity of serum than other members of the *B. fragilis* group.

Immunoglobulin and components of the classical and alternate complement pathways participate in chemotaxis, bacteriolysis, and opsonophagocytic killing of various gram-negative anaerobic bacilli. Antibody to the capsular polysaccharide of *B. fragilis* confers significant protection against subsequent abscess development from *B. fragilis* strains (42); furthermore, a study of women with acute pelvic inflammatory disease whose infecting flora contained *B. fragilis* demonstrated antibody to its capsular antigen (53).

F. necrophorum has been demonstrated to persist for an extended period in the liver, where its proliferation in Kupffer's cells impairs macrophage function. T cells are involved in immunity to *B. fragilis*, specifically linked to early stages of abscess formation (42,54–57). Enterotoxin-producing *B. fragilis* strains may play a role in diarrhea in children and older adults (58,59).

CLINICAL MANIFESTATIONS

The clinical characteristics of infection with gram-negative anaerobic rods are primarily those of anaerobic infections in general: foul-smelling discharge, location of infection in proximity to mucosal surfaces, tissue necrosis, gas in tissues or discharge fluid, association of infection with malignancy, infection related to the use of aminoglycosides or other antimicrobials with poor activity against anaerobes, septic thrombophlebitis, infection following human or animal bites, and certain distinctive clinical features. The clinical presentation of *F. necrophorum* sepsis may be distinctive in that onset is characterized by sore throat and fever, often accompanied by chills. Membranous tonsillitis with foul-smelling breath may be noted, and in the absence of effective therapy, bacteremia and widespread metastatic infection may occur (61,62). Black discoloration of bloody exudates or red fluorescence of such exudates under ultraviolet light indicates infection with a pigmented anaerobic gram-negative rod.

Table 210.4 lists common syndromes of infection involving gram-negative anaerobic rods; in addition, infections such as brain abscess are uncommon but usually involve anaerobic gram-negative rods and other anaerobes. The incidence of specific gram-negative anaerobic rods in various infections is noted in Table 210.6.

Gram-negative anaerobic bacilli, the most common anaerobes in clinical infections, are found in more than half of specimens yielding anaerobes (63–65). *B. fragilis* and *B. thetaiotaomicron* are the members of the *B. fragilis* group that have the greatest clinical significance. They are recovered from most intraabdominal infections and may be found in infections of all types at other sites. *B. fragilis* is the most common anaerobic isolate from clinical specimens overall and from bacteremia. Enterotoxigenic *B. fragilis* strains are disproportionately represented in bacteremia (59) and are found in diarrheal disease in children 1 year or older and in adults 60 years or older, both in developing countries and in industrialized countries (59). They may also be found in stools of healthy children and adults.

The pigmenting anaerobic gram-negative bacilli are composed of saccharolytic and asaccharolytic species of the genera *Prevotella* and *Porphyromonas*. At least 10 species of these genera are found in human clinical material (66). *P. corporis, P. denticola, P. intermedia, P. nigrescens P. loescheii, P. melaninogenica, P. endodontalis, P. asaccharolytica,* and *P. gingivalis* are found in the human oral cavity. Some are important pathogens in oral, dental, and bite wound infections and may produce infections of the head, neck, and lower respiratory tract. *P. asaccharolytica* and some of the pigmenting organisms already mentioned are also prevalent in the urogenital and intestinal tract and are important in various infections. Other pigmenting species—*Porphyromonas levii, P. macacae,* and others—are of animal origin and may be found in humans with infected animal bite wounds.

The bile-sensitive, saccharolytic, nonpigmented gram-negative bacilli are found in the same setting as the pigmenting gram-negative rods (67). *Prevotella bivia* and *P. disiens*, particularly, are found in female genital tract infections and less frequently in oral infections. It is important that they be recognized because these strains are often resistant to the β-lactam antibiotics, including penicillin, aminopenicillins, and most cephalosporins. *P. oris* and *P. buccae* are found in a variety of oral (39) and other infections. The *P. oralis* group is represented by *P. oralis, P. veroralis, Prevotella buccalis,* and *P. oulora* (1,2,32,33). *P. gingivalis* and *P. endodontalis* are the key pathogens in adult periodontitis and endodontic infections, respectively. *P. catoniae* organisms are occasionally involved in oral infections and may produce β-lactamase.

Strains that produce a viscous material in broth are represented by (indole-negative) *Prevotella zoogleoformans* and (indole-positive) *Prevotella heparinolytica* (40,41); they are found in the oral cavity and in related infections. Phylogenetically, they cluster with the *B. fragilis* group. *Prevotella dentalis* has been isolated from infected dental root canals and other oral infections (13,68).

The bile-sensitive asaccharolytic species, *Bacteroides capillosus* and *putredinis*, inhabit the intestinal tract and occasionally have been recovered from various infections (67). *Tannerella forsythensis* (24,34), a fusiform, gram-negative rod, has been recovered from subgingival sites in patients with periodontitis.

The asaccharolytic, formate- and fumarate-requiring, nitrate- or nitrite-reducing gram-negative rods include *B. ureolyticus, Campylobacter gracilis* (formerly *Bacteroides gracilis*), *Campylobacter curvus* (formerly *Wolinella curva*), *Campylobacter rectus* (formerly *Wolinella recta*), and *Wolinella succinogenes*. *Campylobacter showae* is found in the oral cavity and *Campylobacter hominis* in the intestinal tract. *S. wadsworthensis* has been recovered from a variety of infections including infections of the lungs, head and neck, abdomen, urogenital tract, bone, and soft tissue and others. Almost half of *Sutterella* strains produce β-lactamase and *Sutterella* is resistant to metronidazole about one third of the time (14). *W. succinogenes* is also an oral isolate found primarily in periodontitis and periodontosis (10). *B. wadsworthia* resembles *B. ureolyticus* and *Desulfomonas* species but is stimulated by bile, is strongly catalase positive, and does not reduce sulfate. *Bilophila* is present in normal bowel flora in low numbers yet is the third most common anaerobe recovered from gangrenous or perforated appendices and is found in a variety of significant infections, including bacteremia, brain abscess, and liver abscess (69). About 95% of *Bilophila* strains are resistant to penicillin by virtue of β-lactamase production (8).

F. nucleatum is often found in clinical infections. The organism is found in the mouth and in the genital, gastrointestinal, and upper respiratory tracts. It is often involved in the same types of infection as the pigmented *Prevotella* species and *Porphyromonas* species (70). *F. nucleatum* was isolated more often in pure culture from cases of pleural empyema than any other organism, an

TABLE 210.6. Incidence of Specific Anaerobes in Various Infections (Wadsworth VA Medical Center Experience 1991–1997)

									Miscellaneous skin soft tissue and bone infections[a]					
	Blood	Central nervous system	Head and neck	Dental	TTA and pleural	Lung	Perirectal abscess	Decubitus ulcer	Below the waist	Above the waist	Appendiceal tissue or abscess	Peritoneal fluid	Gall bladder	Abdominal, other
No. of specimens	[b]	103	225	8	651	128	17	22	777	327	183	170	155	165
No. of specimens yielding anaerobes	83	16	123	8	48	28	15	16	241	98	133	61	17	46
Bacteroides fragilis	26				1	3	5	9	33	6	70	23	2	18
B. thetaiotaomicron	4						2		9		41		1	12
Other, B. fragilis group	12	1	2		1	3	7	6	31	4	177	140	3	44
Bilophila species						1		6	2	1	49	32	6	
Campylobacter gracilis			4		1	2				3	1	1		
Campylobacter/B. ureolyticus		4	5	9	2	1	2		16	4	7	2	1	
Fusobacterium nucleatum	3		23		10	5	1		18	26	23	24	7	
F. necrophorum			2					3	3		13	9		
F. mortiferum/varium	1							1	3					
Other Fusobacterium species	2		3				1			5	8		1	5
Porphyromonas asaccharolytica		1	2				2	2	3		1	3	1	2
P. gingivalis			2	3					12		2	5	1	
P. levii			2		1				12	2	14	10	1	
Porphyromonas species			1					2	6	2		1		
Prevotella melaninogenica/denticola	1	1	7	1	3	2			12	10	9	3		
P. intermedia-nigrescens-pallens	1	1	23	5	9	3			9	9				
P. loeschii (P. corporis)			7	1	3	1	1		7	10	15	8		
P. bivia/disiens			5		2		1		15	3	2	1	1	
P. oralis group			2		2	1			3	3	3	2		
P. oris/buccae		1	29		5	1	1		10	7	2	3		
Prevotella species	1		9	5	1	2	4		22	8		6	2	2
Desulfomonas/Desulfovibrio	1							1			7	6	3	
Sutterella wadsworthensis							1		2	1	17	19	2	

[a]Includes foot ulcer and osteomyelitis specimens.
[b]Total number of specimens was not available.
Source: From Jousimies-Somer H, Summanen P, Citron DM, et al. Wadsworth—KTL anaerobic bacteriology manual, 6th ed. Belmont, CA: Star Publishing, 2002, with permission.

indication of its virulence (71). *Fusobacterium periodonticum* is primarily isolated from subgingival sites in gingivitis and periodontitis. *F. necrophorum* is a very virulent anaerobe that may cause severe infection originating from pharyngotonsillitis, usually in children or young adults. Local complications include peritonsillar abscess and jugular vein septic thrombophlebitis. There may also be multiple metastatic abscesses (most commonly in the lungs, pleural space, liver, soft tissue, bone, and large joints) related to bacteremia (postanginal sepsis syndrome or Lemierre's disease) (62,70). *F. necrophorum* is found less often now than in the era before antimicrobial agents. *F. ulcerans* is found in tropical ulcer (35).

Leptotrichia buccalis is a common mouth organism that may also be found in the vagina and intestinal tract. It has caused septicemia in immunocompromised patients with oral mucosal infections (72), as has *Capnocytophaga* species. *Dysgonomonas* species, formerly CDC DF-3, and related organisms have been involved in various infections including bacteremia and may be resistant to certain cephalosporins, fluoroquinolones, and macrolides (22).

Selenomonas sputigena, *Selenomonas artemidis*, *Selenomonas dianae*, *Selenomonas flueggei*, *Selenomonas infelix*, and *Selenomonas noxia* (36) are all oral organisms, as is *Centipeda periodontii* (1,2), which is found in subgingival sites in patients with periodontitis.

Desulfomonas piger (formerly *Desulfomonas pigra*), *Desulfovibrio* species, *Succinimonas amylolytica*, *Succinivibrio dextrinosolvens*, and *Butyrivibrio fibrisolvens*, all normal colon flora, may occasionally be encountered in clinical infections as well (73). The normal sites of carriage of *Anaerobiospirillum succiniciproducens* in humans are not known at present, but *Anaerobiospirillum* species are common in the fecal flora of cats and dogs (23,74). Strains of *A. succiniciproducens* have been isolated from blood cultures of immunocompromised patients (73,75). *Anaerobiospirillum thomasii* organisms have been recovered from feces of patients with diarrhea (23).

Specific clinical entities involving anaerobic gram-negative rods are discussed elsewhere in this text and are described in numerous reports (45,63,64,71,76–85). Most gram-negative bacillary anaerobic infections are characterized by a prolonged course, significant tissue destruction, and abscess formation. Virtually all of these infections are mixed, containing other anaerobes and aerobic and facultative organisms as well.

DIAGNOSIS

Anaerobic culture is the major method for specific laboratory diagnosis. Relatively good educated guesses about the involvement of certain specific anaerobic gram-negative rods can be made from examination of Gram stain of clinical specimens; however, different species can resemble one another. A limited number of fluorescent antibody reagents are available commercially, but they are not as specific as one might wish. Although gas chromatographic analysis of clinical specimens (or blood cultures) may provide definitive identification of an anaerobe, principally at the genus level (e.g., fusobacteria produce large amounts of butyric acid without isoacids), there are many potential pitfalls. DNA probes have been developed for a few gram-negative anaerobic rods, but none is yet available commercially except for diagnosis of periodontal disease.

Optimum culture requires pre-reduced or fresh media. It is probably desirable to use an anaerobic chamber for at least the initial culture; obviously, it is critical that optimum specimen collection and transport techniques be used. Collection must avoid sources of indigenous flora; tissue and pus collected in a syringe

TABLE 210.7. Mechanisms of Resistance in Anaerobes

Mechanisms
  Drug inactivation (e.g., beta-lactamases)
  Failure of drug to get into bacterial cells (e.g., porin channel changes)
  Pumping drug out of bacterial cells (efflux pumps)
  Changes in targets for drugs
  Failure to reduce drug to active form (e.g., metronidazole)
Facilitators
  Inducibility
  Conjugation
  Plasmid transfer

are the best specimens. A variety of good transport setups are available commercially.

Species are identified presumptively based on a few observations: colonial and cellular morphology, pigment production, fluorescence under long-wave ultraviolet light, susceptibility to special-potency antibiotic disks, and certain rapidly determined biochemical characteristics (2). Definitive identification requires the determination of multiple characteristics with a battery of biochemical tests (1–4,21,28). Cellular fatty acid determination is particularly helpful (26). Definitive identification is not feasible for all anaerobic isolates because of financial constraints and is not ordinarily important for clinical purposes. Such detailed bacteriologic tests should be available in certain teaching centers or reference laboratories for special circumstances, such as unusual clinical cases, organisms never before encountered, and publication and teaching purposes. For clinical purposes, it is commonly sufficient to know the broad groupings of isolates, whether they produce β-lactamase or not, and their usual patterns of susceptibility to antimicrobial agents. Details on definitive identification may be found in anaerobic laboratory manuals (1–3).

TREATMENT

Surgical or percutaneous computed tomography- or ultrasonography-guided drainage of abscesses and surgical débridement or excision of necrotic tissue are crucial to successful treatment. Hyperbaric oxygen is of doubtful value in non–spore-forming anaerobic infections.

Mixed infections involving anaerobic and aerobic or facultative bacteria typically involve a complex flora, so results of cultures do not become available for some time; accordingly, initial therapy for such infections must be empirical, although information such as that derived from examination of a Gram-stained specimen may be used effectively to assist in the choice of drug. The physician should base the initial choice of therapeutic

TABLE 210.8. β-Lactamase–producing Gram-negative Anaerobic Rods

Bacteroides fragilis group	*Prevotella buccae*
Bacteroides splanchnicus	*Fusobacterium nucleatum*
Bacteroides coagulans	*Fusobacterium mortiferum*
Pigmented *Prevotella* and	*Fusobacterium varium*
Porphyromonas	*Bilophila wadsworthia*
Porphyromonas catoniae	*Sutterella wadsworthensis*
Prevotella oralis group	*Megamonas hypermegas*
Prevotella disiens	
Prevotella oris	

TABLE 210.9. Activity of Various Drugs Against Anaerobic Gram-negative Bacteria (Wadsworth Agar Dilution Procedure)[a]

Drug	NCCLS breakpoint (µg/mL)		Percent susceptible[b]							
	Susceptible	Intermediate	B. fragilis	B. fragilis group[c]	Prevotella species	Porphyromonas species	Fusobacterium species	C. gracilis[d]	Sutterella species[d]	Bilophila species[e]
Cefotaxime	16	32	50–69	<50	>95	>95	85–95			70–84
Cefotetan	16	32	85–95	50–69			85–95			>95
Cefoxitin	16	32	>95	85–95	>95	>95	>95	>95	>95	>95
Ceftizoxime	32	64	85–95	85–95	>95	>95	>85–95	>95	85–95	>95
Ceftriaxone	16	32	70–84	<50	85–95	>95	>85–95	>95	>95	
Chloramphenicol	8	16	>95	>95	>95	>95	>95	>95	>95	>95
Clindamycin	2	4	85–95	70–84	>95	>95	70–95	>95	50–69	85–95
Imipenem	4	8	>95	>95	>95	>95	>95	>95	>95	>95
Meropenem	4	8	>95	>95	>95	>95	>95	>95	>95	>95
Metronidazole	8	16	>95	>95	>95	>95	>95	>95	70–84	>95
Penicillin G[f]	0.5	1	<50	<50	<50	85–95	70–95	>95	>95	<50
Amoxicillin-clavulanate	4/2	8/4	>95	85–95	>95	>95	85–95	>95	85–95	>95
Piperacillin	32	64	>95	85–95	>95	>95	85–95	>95	85–95	>95
Piperacillin-tazobactam	32/4	64/4	>95	>95	>95	>95	>95	>95	85–95	>95
Ticarcillin	32	64			>95	>95				>95
Ticarcillin-clavulanate	32/2	64/2	>95	>95	>95	>95	85–95	>95	>95	>95
Newer fluoroquinolones[g]	2	4	85–95	70–95	50–95	>95	70–95	>95	85–95	>95

[a]National Committee for Clinical Laboratory Standards (NCCLS M11-A5) approved method; data from Wadsworth Anaerobic Bacteriology Laboratory.

[b]According to the NCCLS-approved breakpoints (M11-A5), using the intermediate category as susceptible.

[c]Includes the species B. fragilis.

[d]The use of formate-fumarate additive is presently recommended.

[e]Addition of 1% pyruvate in the test medium recommended.

[f]Strains producing β-lactamase should be considered resistant.

[g]Includes clinafloxacin, gatifloxacin, gemifloxacin, levofloxacin, moxifloxacin, sitafloxacin, and trovafloxacin.

TABLE 210.10.   Antimicrobial Susceptibility of Motile, Anaerobic Gram-negative Bacilli *in vitro*

Organism[b]	Drugs eliciting indicated result in susceptibility tests[a]		
	Susceptible	Variable	Resistant
Butyrivibrio (1)	Penicillin G, choloramphenicol, erythromycin, tetracyclines		Bacitracin, streptomycin, kanamycin, lincomycin, sulfonomides
Succinimonas (1)[c]	Bacitracin, oxytetracycline, penicillin G		Kanamycin, streptomycin, erythromycin
Succinivibrio (2)	Penicillin G, tetracycline, erythromycin, chloramphenicol	Clindamycin	
Wolinella (19)[d]	Metronidazole, clindamycin, chloramphenicol, tetracycline, erythromycin, imipenem, ciprofloxacin	Penicillin G, piperacillin, cephalosporins, gentamicin, rifampin, polymyxins	Vancomycin, bacitracin, nalidixic acid
Campylobacter (7)	Clindamycin, chloramphenicol, metronidazole, penicillin G, tetracycline, erythromycin		Vancomycin, bacitracin, rifampin
Desulfovibrio (1)	Penicillin G, clindamycin, chloramphenicol, tetracycline, erythromycin		Vancomycin, colistin
Selenomonas (32)	Clindamycin, chloramphenicol, metronidazole	Penicillin G, ampicillin, erythromycin, tetracycline	Vancomycin, colistin
Anaerobiospirillum (17)	Cephalothin, chloramphenicol, tetracycline, rifampin	Ampicillin, erythromycin, metronidazole, nalidixic acid	Vancomycin, trimethoprim, penicillin G

[a]Strains are reported as susceptible if more than 90% of tested isolates were susceptible, as variable if 50% to 90% of tested isolates were susceptible, and as resistant if less than 50% of tested isolates were susceptible. The susceptibility of all isolates was not reported for all antimicrobial agents.
[b]Approximate number of isolates is given in parentheses.
[c]Susceptibility data are for a strain isolated from an animal rumen. (From Johnson CC, Finegold SM. Uncommonly encountered, motile, anaerobic gram-negative bacilli associated with infection. *Rev Infect Dis* 1987;9:1150, with permission.)
[d]Now reclassified as *Campylobacter;* various species are involved.
Source: From Finegold SM. Therapy of anaerobic infections. In: Finegold SM, George WL, eds. *Anaerobic infections in humans.* San Diego, CA: Academic Press, 1989:793–818, with permission.

agents on the nature and location of the infection, the usual flora anticipated in infections of the type being treated, factors that might have modified such flora, Gram stain results, and severity of the infection.

It must be remembered that most anaerobic infections are mixed: If the agent chosen for the anaerobes does not provide adequate coverage for the nonanaerobes, an additional agent may be needed. Other factors to be considered in certain circumstances include central nervous system penetration and bactericidal effect. Clearly, the toxicity of various agents under consideration for therapy is important, as is their impact on the normal flora. Agents that produce relatively little disturbance of indigenous flora are less likely to lead to significant superinfection. One major superinfection to be kept in mind is pseudomembranous colitis, which is usually caused by *Clostridium difficile,* although other clostridia and *Staphylococcus aureus* may cause it on occasion. Agents that suppress normal colon flora significantly and have relatively poor activity against *C. difficile,* of course, are more likely to lead to this complication. The cost of the various antimicrobial agents that may be suitable in terms of activity is certainly an important consideration, and pharmacokinetic characteristics that may permit less frequent dosing must be factored into the decision.

The breakpoint is the concentration of drug in the body at or below which infection with the organism in question will generally respond to therapy; this is usually equivalent to peak levels achievable in serum with the maximum approved dosage in the case of anaerobes.

Finally, the severity of infection should be considered. The most potent agents should not be used for relatively mild infections. This practice is likely to lead eventually to the development of resistance and to the consequent loss of important agents for treating serious infections. Less powerful agents may be perfectly adequate for milder infections in patients with good host defense mechanisms; indeed, it may be impossible to demonstrate any advantage for a more potent agent in such a setting. Young, otherwise healthy patients with a community-acquired infection (such as appendicitis without generalized peritonitis or with pelvic inflammatory disease) will usually respond well to less potent agents if needed surgical management is provided. If the less effective agents have other advantages (e.g., low toxicity, low cost), it makes good sense to use them. On the other hand, an elderly diabetic patient in an intensive care unit with a hospital-acquired intraabdominal infection needs the best antimicrobial agents available.

TABLE 210.11. Anaerobic Bacteria Isolated from Infected Human, Dog and Cat Bite Wounds

| | % of patient specimens positive | | | |
| | | | Human | |
Isolate	Dog bite	Cat bite	CFI	Bite
Fusobacterium species	32	33	19	6
F. nucleatum	16	25	19	6
F. russi	2	14		
Other species	16	9		
Prevotella species	28	19		
P. melaninogenica	2	2	13	17
P. intermedia	8	0	31	22
P. buccae			19	17
P. heparinolytica	14	9		
P. zoogleoformans	4	2		
Other species	2	7	32	33
Porphyromonas species	28	30		
P. macacae	6	7		
P. cansulci	6	2		
P. gingivalis	4	11		
P. canoris	4	9		
P. cangingivalis	4	4		
P. circumdentaria	2	5		
P. levii–like	2	0		
Other species	4	0		
Bacteroides species	30	28		
B. tectum	16	32		
B. forsythus[a]	4	0		
B. ureolyticus	4		6	
Campylobacter gracilis	4			

[a] Now *Tannerella forsythensis*.
CFI, clenched first injury
Source: From Jousimies-Somer H, Summanen P, Citron DM, et al. *Wadsworth—KTL anaerobic bacteriology manual,* 6th ed. Belmont, CA: Star Publishing, 2002, with permission.

Antimicrobial resistance is as much a problem with anaerobic gram-negative rods as with most other bacteria. (Various major mechanisms of resistance are noted in Table 210.7, and gram-negative anaerobic rods known to produce β-lactamases are listed in Table 210.8.) Susceptibility data for various anaerobic gram-negative rods isolated at the Wadsworth Veterans Hospital are given in Table 210.9; for motile, anaerobic, gram-negative rods in Table 210.10 (mostly from reports in the literature); and for isolates from bite wounds in Table 210.11. Details of therapy for anaerobic infections are found in specific chapters.

SUSCEPTIBILITY TESTING

A number of problems are encountered in susceptibility testing of anaerobic bacteria: lack of standardized techniques, failure to use recent clinical isolates, testing too few strains, use of nonrepresentative species, clustering at the breakpoint, difficulty in reading end points, poor growth of certain anaerobes, and the need for clinical correlation. Interlaboratory variations in testing procedures have produced confusion about the extent of resistance among anaerobes. The current National Committee for Clinical Laboratory Standards (NCCLS) reference method is unsatisfactory because the medium does not support the growth of a number of strains of clinically important anaerobes, such as pigmented anaerobic bacilli, *F. nucleatum,* and anaerobic cocci. The phenomenon of clustering of end points within one dilution of the breakpoint is relatively common with certain β-lactam agents, clindamycin, and chloramphenicol (39). Because the error factor common to most of the procedures used is one twofold dilution, this clustering effect may lead to significant variability, even within one laboratory. The broth disk elution procedure, a simple test preferred by many clinical laboratories, has given undependable results with a number of antimicrobial agents and is no longer approved by the NCCLS. However, gradient end-point procedures such as the E-test are easy to use and useful.

Susceptibility testing of anaerobes should be done to determine the activity of new agents, to monitor susceptibility patterns periodically in various centers, to monitor susceptibility patterns in a particular hospital or community, and to guide the management of infections in individual patients. In the last case, indications would include failure, relapse, persistence of infection despite empiric therapy, and serious illness (e.g., brain abscess, endocarditis, osteomyelitis, and infected prosthetic device or vascular graft) requiring prolonged therapy.

These problems notwithstanding, a great deal of valuable information has been accumulated on the activity of various drugs against different anaerobic pathogens. There are no simple answers, unfortunately, as to the "best" or "correct" test *in vitro* for susceptibility. The most practical tests available for studying small numbers of isolates in clinical laboratories are the broth microdilution test (available commercially in frozen or lyophilized form in trays already containing serial twofold dilutions of various antimicrobial agents) and the E-test strips containing gradients of antibiotic concentrations. Agar plate dilution procedures and the spiral gradient agar procedure are preferred for larger numbers of strains.

The information gleaned from susceptibility studies provides us with good guidance for empiric therapy. There is a considerable mass of clinical data that show a good correlation with data from *in vitro* tests, although more correlative studies are clearly needed, particularly with certain newer agents and with older agents to which significant resistance has developed.

REFERENCES

1. Holdeman LV, Cato EP, Moore WEC, eds. *Anaerobe laboratory manual*, 4th ed. Blacksburg, VA: Virginia Polytechnic Institute and State University, 1977:1–156.
2. Moore LVH, Cato EP, Moore WEC. *Anaerobe laboratory manual update. Published as a supplement to the VPI anaerobe laboratory manual*, 4th ed. Blacksburg, VA: Virginia Polytechnic Institute and State University, 1987.
3. Jousimies-Somer H, Summanen P, Citron DM, et al. *Wadsworth—KTL anaerobic bacteriology manual*, 6th ed. Belmont, CA: Star Publishing, 2002.
4. Jousimies-Somer H, Summanen P. Recent taxonomic changes and terminology update of clinically significant anaerobic gram-negative bacteria (excluding spirochetes). *Clin Infect Dis* 2002;35(Suppl 1):S17.
5. Shah HN, Collins MD. Reclassification of *Bacteroides furcosus* Veillon and Zuber (Hauduroy, Ehringer, Urbain, Guillot and Magrou) in a new genus *Anaerorhabdus*, as *Anaerorhabdus furcosus* comb. nov. *Syst Appl Microbiol* 1986;8:86.
6. Baron EJ, Summanen P, Downes J, et al. *Bilophila wadsworthia*, a unique gram-negative anaerobic rod recovered from appendicitis specimens and human feces. *J Gen Microbiol* 1989;135:3405.
7. Shah HN, Collins MD. *Prevotella*, a new genus to include *Bacteroides melaninogenica* and related species formerly classified in the genus *Bacteroides*. *Int J Syst Bacteriol* 1989;40:205.
8. Shah HN, Collins MD. Proposal for reclassification of *Bacteroides asaccharolyticus*, *Bacteroides gingivalis*, and *Bacteroides endodontalis* in a new genus, *Porphyromonas*. *Int J Syst Bacteriol* 1988;38:128.
9. Hudspeth MK, Hunt Gerardo S, Citron DM, et al. Growth characteristics and a novel method for identification (the WEE-TAB System) of *Porphyromonas* species isolated from infected dog and cat bite wounds in humans. *J Clin Microbiol* 1997;35:2450.
10. Tanner ACR, Badger S, Lai C-H, et al. *Wolinella* gen. nov., *Wolinella succinogenes* (*Vibrio succinogenes* Wolin et al.) comb. nov., and description of *Bacteroides gracilis* sp. nov., *Wolinella recta* sp. nov., *Campylobacter concisus* sp. nov., and *Eikenella corrodens* from humans with periodontal disease. *Int J Syst Bacteriol* 1981;31:432.
11. Gharbia SE, Shah HN. Characteristics of glutamate dehydrogenase, a new diagnostic marker for the genus *Fusobacterium*. *J Gen Microbiol* 1988;134:327.
12. Conrads G, Claros MC, Citron DM, et al. 16S-23S rDNA internal transcribed spacer sequences for analysis of the phylogenetic relationships among species of the genus *Fusobacterium*. *Int J Syst Evol Microbiol* 2002;52:493.
13. Willems A, Collins MD. 16S rRNA gene similarities indicate that *Hallella seregens* (Moore and Moore) and *Mitsuokella dentalis* (Haapasalo et al.) are genealogically highly related and are members of the genus *Prevotella*: emended description of the genus *Prevotella* (Shah and Collins) and description of *Prevotella dentalis* comb. nov. *Int J Syst Bacteriol* 1995;45:832.
14. Wexler HM, Reeves D, Summanen PH, et al. *Sutterella wadsworthensis* gen. nov., sp.nov., bile-resistant microaerophilic *Campylobacter gracilis*–like clinical isolates. *Int J Syst Bacteriol* 1996;46:252.
15. Vandamme P, Daneshvar MI, Dewhirst FE, et al. Chemotaxonomic analyses of *Bacteroides gracilis* and *Bacteroides ureolyticus* and reclassification of *B. gracilis* as *Campylobacter gracilis* comb. nov. *Int J Syst Bacteriol* 1995;45:145.
16. Vandamme P, Falsen E, Rossau R, et al. Revision of *Campylobacter*, *Helicobacter*, and *Wolinella* taxonomy: emendation of generic descriptions and proposal of *Arcobacter* gen. nov. *Int J Syst Bacteriol* 1991;41:88.
17. Willems A, Collins MD. Reclassification of *Oribaculum catoniae* (Moore and Moore 1994) as *Porphyromonas catoniae* comb. nov. and emendation of the genus *Porphyromonas*. *Int J Syst Bacteriol* 1995;45:578.
18. Kononen E, Vaisanen M-L, Finegold SM, et al. Cellular fatty acid analysis and enzyme profiles of *Porphyromonas catoniae*—a frequent colonizer of the oral cavity in children. *Anaerobe* 1996;2:329.
19. Love D. *Porphyromonas macacae* comb. nov., a consequence of *Bacteroides macacae* being a senior synonym of *Porphyromonas salivosa*. *Int J Syst Bacteriol* 1995;45:90.
20. Love DN, Bailey GD, Collings S, et al. Description of *Porphyromonas circumdentaria* sp. nov. and reassignment of *Bacteroides salivosus* (Love, Johnson, Jones, and Calverley 1987) as *Porphyromonas* (Shah and Collins 1988) *salivosa* comb. nov. *Int J Syst Bacteriol* 1992;42:434.
21. Fournier D, Mouton C, Lapierre P. *Porphyromonas gulae* sp. nov., an anaerobic gram-negative coccobacillus from the gingival sulcus of various animal hosts. *Int J Syst Evol Microbiol* 2001;51:1179.
22. Hofstad T, Olsen I, Eribe ER, et al. *Dysgonomonas* gen. nov. to accommodate *Dysgonomonas gadei* sp. nov., an organism isolated from a human gall bladder, and *Dysgonomonas capnocytophagoides* (formerly CDC group DF-3). *Int J Syst Evol Microbiol* 2000;50;2189.
23. Malnick H. *Anaerobiospirillum thomasii* sp. nov., an anaerobic spiral bacterium isolated from the feces of cats and dogs and from diarrheal feces of humans, and emendation of the genus *Anaerobiospirillum*. *Int J Syst Bacteriol* 1997;47:381.
24. Sakamoto M, Suzuki M, Umeda M, et al. Reclassification of *Bacteroides forsythus* (Tanner et al 1986) as *Tannerella forsythensis* corrig., gen. nov., comb. nov. *Int J Syst Evol Microbiol* 2002;52:841.
25. Tanner A, Maiden MFJ, Paster BJ, et al. The impact of 16S ribosomal RNA-based phylogeny on the taxonomy of oral bacteria. *Periodontology 2000* 1994;5:26.
26. Moore LVH, Bourne DM, Moore WEC. Comparative distribution and taxonomic value of cellular fatty acids in thirty-three genera of anaerobic gram-negative bacilli. *Int J Syst Bacteriol* 1994;44:338.
27. Wayne LG, Brenner DJ, Colwell RR, et al. Report of the ad hoc committee on reconciliation of approaches to bacterial systematics. *Int J Syst Bacteriol* 1987;37:463.
28. Jousimies-Somer HR, Summanen PH, Finegold SM. *Bacteroides, Porphyromonas, Prevotella, Fusobacterium*, and other anaerobic gram-negative bacteria. In: Baron EJ, Pfaller MA, Tenover FC, et al., eds. *Manual of clinical microbiology*. Washington, DC: ASM Press, 1995:603.
29. Shah HN, Collins MD. Proposal to restrict the genus *Bacteroides* (Castellani and Chalmers) to *Bacteroides fragilis* and closely related species. *Int J Syst Bacteriol* 1989;39:85.
30. Shah HN, Gharbia SE. Biochemical and chemical studies on strains designated *Prevotella intermedia* and proposal of a new pigmented species, *Prevotella nigrescens* sp. nov. *Int J Syst Bacteriol* 1992;42:542.
31. Haapasalo M. *Bacteroides buccae* and related taxa in necrotic root canal infections. *J Clin Microbiol* 1986;24:940.
32. Shah HN, Collins MD, Watabe J, et al. *Bacteroides oulorum* sp. nov., a nonpigmented saccharolytic species from the oral cavity. *Int J Syst Bacteriol* 1985;35:193.
33. Watabe J, Benno Y, Mitsuoka T. Taxonomic study of *Bacteroides oralis* and related organisms and proposal of *Bacteroides veroralis* sp. nov. *Int J Syst Bacteriol* 1983;33:57.
34. Tanner ACR, Listgarten MA, Ebersole JL, et al. *Bacteroides forsythus* sp. nov., a slow-growing, fusiform *Bacteroides* sp. from the human oral cavity. *Int J Syst Bacteriol* 1986;36:213.
35. Adriaans B, Shah H. *Fusobacterium ulcerans* sp. nov. from tropical ulcers. *Int J Syst Bacteriol* 1988;38:447.
36. Moore LVH, Johnson JL, Moore WEC. *Selenomonas noxia* sp.nov., *Selenomonas flueggei* sp. nov., *Selenomonas infelix* sp. nov., *Selenomonas dianae* sp. nov., and *Selenomonas artemidis* sp. nov., from the human gingival crevice. *Int J Syst Bacteriol* 1987;36:271.
37. Love DN, Bailey GD. Chromosomal DNA probes for the identification of *Bacteroides tectum* and *Bacteroides fragilis* from the oral cavity of cats. *Vet Microbiol* 1993;34:89.
38. Moore LV, Johnson JL, Moore WE. Descriptions of *Prevotella tannerae* sp. nov. and *Prevotella enoeca* sp. nov. from the human gingival crevice and emendation of the description of *Prevotella zoogleoformans*. *Int J Syst Bacteriol* 1994;44:599.
39. Bolstad AI, Jensen HB. Polymerase chain reaction-amplified nonradioactive probes for identification of *Fusobacterium nucleatum*. *J Clin Microbiol* 1993;31:528.
40. Bailey GD, Moore LVH, Love DN, et al. *Bacteroides heparinolyticus*: deoxyribonucleic acid relatedness of strains from the oral cavity and oral-associated disease conditions of horses, cats, and humans. *Int J Syst Bacteriol* 1988;38:42.
41. Okuda K, Kato T, Shiozu J, et al. *Bacteroides heparinolyticus* sp. nov. isolated from humans with periodontitis. *Int J Syst Bacteriol* 1985;35:438.
42. Zaleznik DF, Kasper DL. Role of bacterial virulence factors in pathogenesis of anaerobic infections. In: Finegold SM, George WL, eds. *Anaerobic infections in humans*. San Diego: Academic Press, 1989:81–95.
43. Shimada K, Sutter VL, Finegold SM. Effect of bile and desoxycholate on gram-negative anaerobic bacteria. *Appl Microbiol* 1970;20:737.
44. Goldin BR, Gorbach SL. Impact of anaerobic bowel flora on metabolism of endogenous and exogenous compounds. In: Finegold SM, George WL, eds. *Anaerobic infections in humans*. San Diego: Academic Press, 1989:691–714.
45. Nord CE. The role of anaerobic bacteria in recurrent episodes of sinusitis and tonsillitis. *Clin Infect Dis* 1995;20:1512.
46. Wexler HM, Finegold SM. Antimicrobial resistance in *Bacteroides*. Leading article. *J Antimicrob Chemother* 1987;19:143.
47. Hentges DJ. Anaerobes as normal flora. In: Finegold SM, George WL, eds. *Anaerobic infections in humans*. San Diego: Academic Press, 1989:37–53.
48. Hentges DJ. The anaerobic microflora of the human body. *Clin Infect Dis* 1993;16[Suppl 4]:S175.
49. Nichols RL, Smith JW. Intragastric microbial colonization in common disease states of the stomach and duodenum. *Ann Surg* 1975;182:557.
50. Hillier SL, Krohn MA, Rabe LK, et al. The normal vaginal flora, H_2O_2-producing lactobacilli, and bacterial vaginosis in pregnant women. *Clin Infect Dis* 1993;16[Suppl 4]:S273.
51. Rotstein OD. Interactions between leukocytes and anaerobic bacteria in polymicrobial surgical infections. *Clin Infect Dis* 1993;16[Suppl 4]:S190.
52. Bjornson AB. Host defense mechanisms against non–spore-forming anaerobic bacteria.In: Finegold SM, George WL, eds. *Anaerobic infections in humans*. San Diego: Academic Press, 1989:97–110.
53. Eschenbach DA, Holmes KK. The etiology of acute pelvic inflammatory disease. *Sex Transm Dis* 1979;6:224.
54. Tzianabos AO, Kasper DL, Onderdonk AB. Structure and function of *Bacteroides fragilis* capsular polysaccharides: relationship to induction and prevention of abscesses. *Clin Infect Dis* 1995;20[Suppl 2]:S132.
55. Kalka-Moll WM, Wang Y, Comstock LE, et al. Immunochemical and biological characterization of three capsular polysaccharides from a single *Bacteroides fragilis* strain. *Infect Immun* 2001;69:2339.

56. Coyne MJ, Tzianabos AO, Mallory BC, et al. Polysaccharide biosynthesis locus required for virulence of *Bacteroids fragilis. Infect Immun* 2001;69:4342.

57. Tzianabos AO, Kasper DL. Role of T cells in abscess formation. *Curr Opin Microbiol* 2002;5:92.

58. Sears CL, Myers LL, Lazenby A, et al. Enterotoxigenic *Bacteroides fragilis. Clin Infect Dis* 1995;20[Suppl 2]:S142.

59. Sears CL. The toxins of *Bacteroides fragilis. Toxicon* 2001;39:1737.

60. Krinos CM, Coyne MJ, Weinacht KG, et al. Extensive surface diversity of a commensal microorganism by multiple DNA inversins. *Nature* 2001;414:555.

61. Mulligan ME. Ear, nose, throat, and head and neck infections. In: Finegold SM, George WL, eds. *Anaerobic infections in humans.* San Diego: Academic Press, 1989:263–288.

62. Moreno S, Altozano JG, Pinilla B, et al. Lemierre's disease: postanginal bacteremia and pulmonary involvement caused by *Fusobacterium necrophorum. Rev Infect Dis* 1989;11:319.

63. Finegold SM. *Anaerobic bacteria in human disease.* New York: Academic Press, 1977:1–710.

64. Finegold SM, George WL, eds. *Anaerobic infections in humans.* San Diego: Academic Press, 1989.

65. Finegold SM. Overview of clinically important anaerobes. *Clin Infect Dis* 1995;20[Suppl 2]:S205.

66. Finegold SM, Strong CA, McTeague M, et al. The importance of black-pigmented gram-negative anaerobes in human infections. *FEMS Immunol Med Microbiol* 1993;6:77.

67. Kirby BD, George WL, Sutter VL, et al. Gram-negative anaerobic bacilli: their role in infection and patterns of susceptibility to antimicrobial agents, I: little-known *Bacteroides* species. *Rev Infect Dis* 1980;2:914.

68. Haapasalo M, Ranta H, Shah H, et al. *Mitsuokella dentalis* sp. nov. from dental root canals. *Int J Syst Bacteriol* 1986;36:566.

69. Summanen PH, Jousimies-Somer H, Manley S, et al. *Bilophila wadsworthia* isolates from clinical specimens. *Clin Infect Dis* 1995;20[Suppl 2]:S210.

70. Bennett KW, Eley A. Fusobacteria: new taxonomy and related diseases. *J Med Microbiol* 1993;39:246.

71. Civen R, Jousimies-Somer H, Marina M, et al. A retrospective review of cases of anaerobic empyema and update of bacteriology. *Clin Infect Dis* 1995;20[Suppl 2]:S224.

72. Baquero F, Fernández J, Dronda F, et al. Capnophilic and anaerobic bacteremia in neutropenic patients: an oral source. *Rev Infect Dis* 1990;12[Suppl 2]:S157.

73. Johnson CC, Finegold SM. Uncommonly encountered, motile, anaerobic gram-negative bacilli associated with infection. *Rev Infect Dis* 1987;9:1150.

74. Malnick H. *Anaerobiospirillum thomasii* sp. nov., an anaerobic *spiral* bacterium from the feces of cats and dogs and from diarrheal feces of humans, and emendation of the genus *Anaerobiospirillum. Int J Syst Bacteriol* 1997;47:381.

75. McNeil MM, Martone WJ, Dowell VR Jr. Bacteremia with *Anaerobiospirillum succiniciproducens. Rev Infect Dis* 1987;9:737.

76. Tanner A, Stillman N. Oral and dental infections with anaerobic bacteria: clinical features, predominant pathogens, and treatment. *Clin Infect Dis* 1993;16[Suppl 4]:S304.

77. Gharbia SE, Haapasalo M, Shah HN, et al. Characterization of *Prevotella intermedia* and *Prevotella nigrescens* isolates from periodontic and endodontic infections. *J Periodontol* 1994;65:56.

78. Tabaqchali S. Anaerobic infections in the head and neck region. *Scand J Infect Dis* 1988;Suppl 57:24.

79. Jousimies-Somer H, Savolainen S, Makitie A, et al. Bacteriologic findings in peritonsillar abscess in young adults. *Clin Infect Dis* 1993;16[Suppl 4]:S292.

80. Bennion RS, Baron EJ, Thompson JE Jr. et al. The bacteriology of gangrenous and perforated appendicitis—revisited. *Ann Surg* 1990;211:165.

81. Vandamme P, Falsen E, Pot B, et al. Identification of EF group 22 campylobacters from gastroenteritis cases as *Campylobacter concisus. J Clin Microbiol* 1989;27:1775.

82. Germain M, Krohn MA, Hillier SL, et al. Genital flora in pregnancy and its association with intrauterine growth retardation. *J Clin Microbiol* 1994;32:2162.

83. Hillier SL, Krohn MA, Cassen E, et al. The role of bacterial vaginosis and vaginal bacteria in amniotic fluid infection in women in preterm labor with intact fetal membranes. *Clin Infect Dis* 1995;20[Suppl 2]:S276.

84. McGregor JA, French JI, Bloom BS, et al. Bacterial vaginosis and preterm birth [Letter]. *N Engl J Med* 1996;334:1337.

85. Summanen PH, Talan DA, Strong C, et al. Bacteriology of skin and soft-tissue infections: comparison of infections in intravenous drug users and individuals with no history of intravenous drug use. *Clin Infect Dis* 1995;20[Suppl 2]:S279.

CHAPTER 211
Clostridium tetani

John G. Bartlett

Tetanus (lockjaw) is a neurologic syndrome caused by a neurotoxin elaborated by *Clostridium tetani* at a site of injury. This disease is relatively uncommon in the United States and the developed world, but the estimated worldwide annual mortality exceeds 1 million, largely because of the failure of immunization programs in developing countries.

PATHOGENESIS

C. tetani is an anaerobic, gram-positive, slender, motile bacillus. The spore form has a characteristic drumstick or tennis-racket shape (Fig. 211.1). Vegetative forms of *C. tetani* are highly susceptible to heat and disinfectants, but the spores are highly resistant, and killing them requires boiling for at least 4 hours or autoclaving for 12 minutes at 121°C.

Tetanospasmin is the neurotoxin responsible for tetanus. This is a protein with a molecular mass of about 150 kd that may be proteolytically cleaved to a light chain and a heavy chain linked by a disulfide bond (1). The heavy chain (100 kd) is responsible for binding to eukaryotic cells, and the light chain (50 kd) is responsible for blocking the release of neurotransmitters. The entire amino acid sequence has been defined (2) and shows considerable homology with *botulinum* toxin (3). Tetanospasmin ranks with *botulinum* toxin as the most potent known microbial toxins. One milligram is capable of killing 50 million to 70 million mice.

The clinical syndrome requires a source of the organism, local tissue conditions that promote production by vegetative forms, and immune system naïveteé. The organism is introduced at the site of injury. The prevalence of *C. tetani* spores in soil samples is 2% to 23% (4). Local factors that are important at the site of injury in promoting toxin elaboration by vegetative forms are necrotic tissue, suppuration, and the presence of a foreign body. The toxin is produced as a protoplasmic protein and is released with lysis of bacilli. Tetanospasmin is taken up by peripheral nerve terminals and then transported intraaxonally within membrane-bound vesicles to spinal neurons at a transport rate of 75 to

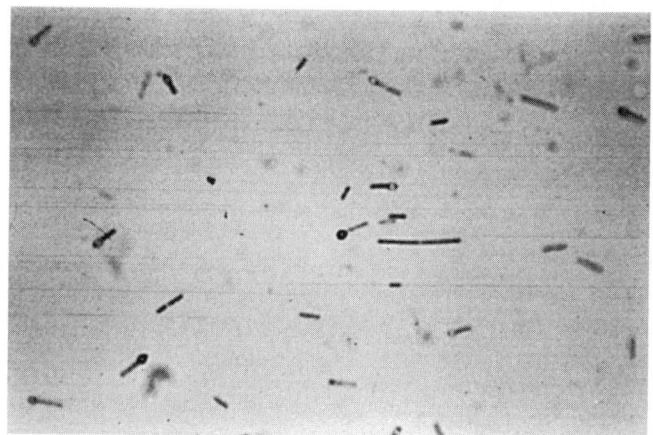

Figure 211.1. Gram stain of *Clostridium tetani* showing typical "drumstick" forms.

250 mm per day (5). Large amounts of the toxin may spread by blood and lymphatics to myoneural junctions throughout the body. After retrograde transport the neurotoxin reaches the perikarya of the motor neuron and passes to the presynaptic terminals, where it blocks release of neurotransmitters, including glycine and γ-aminobutyric acid (GABA), the neurotransmitters used by group 1A inhibitory afferent motor neurons (6). The absence of inhibition results in unrestrained firing with sustained muscle contraction of both agonist and antagonist muscles. Toxin binding is irreversible, so recovery requires the generation of new axonal terminals. In severe cases, there is also involvement of the sympathetic chain, resulting in autonomic dysfunction.

EPIDEMIOLOGY

Tetanus is most common in warm climates and heavily cultivated rural areas (6–9). The greatest problem is in economically deprived countries, reflecting poor immunization standards and poor hygiene (8,10,11). The greatest toll is in neonates, reflecting the prevalent practices of dressing the umbilical wound with animal dung and performing circumcision without aseptic technique on children born to unimmunized mothers. Neonatal tetanus accounts for about 400,000 deaths annually in resource-limited areas but has been rare in the developed world for the last 50 years (8–10).

The rate of tetanus in the United States decreased approximately 20-fold since immunization became generally available in the early 1940s. The tetanus rate was 0.39 per 100,000 population when reporting began in 1947 and is now 0.02 per 100,000

(9,10). About 50 cases of tetanus are reported annually in the United States; reporting efficiency is estimated at 40%. The reported experience with tetanus for the United States is summarized in Table 211.1, which shows that most patients are older than 60 years, reflecting declining immunity that is observed in patients older than 40 years (13). Most of the patients had puncture wounds with sharp objects, most did not seek medical attention, and none received prophylaxis with tetanus immune globulin (TIG).

CLINICAL FEATURES

The forms of tetanus are generalized, localized, cephalic, and neonatal. Generalized tetanus is most common (14–22). The usual incubation period from the time of injury is 4 to 14 days, depending to some extent on the distance of the site of injury from the central nervous system. The onset period refers to the interval between the first symptoms of tetanus and the first generalized spasm. An incubation period of less than 9 days and an onset period of less than 48 hours are associated with more severe disease.

The initial symptoms of tetanus may include localized or generalized weakness and difficulty in swallowing or chewing. Muscles served by nerves with the shortest neural pathways are usually the first to be affected, including cervical, facial, and masticatory muscles. Trismus, the presenting complaint in about 75% of patients, reflects increased tone in the masseter muscle, accounting for the term *lockjaw*. Muscle rigidity then increases progressively, in a descending or ascending pattern. Other early features include irritability, diaphoresis, listlessness, dysphagia, and drooling. Sustained contracture of the orbicularis oris may result in a characteristic sardonic smile, risus sardonicus; persistent spasm of the back musculature may result in opisthotonos. Reflex spasms are a common feature of the disease, with waves of tonic contractions of various muscle groups that are often triggered by sensory stimuli. The spasms may cause waves of opisthotonos, flexion and adduction of the arms with clenched fists over the lower part of the chest, and extension of the legs resulting in a characteristic posturing. The autonomic nervous system is often involved with arrhythmias, extreme oscillation in blood pressure, diaphoresis, rhabdomyolysis, laryngeal spasms, hyperthermia, and urinary retention (16). The patient generally remains lucid and suffers intense pain with the spasms, which may be precipitated by noise, light, or touch. Generalized tetanus often progresses over 2 weeks, representing the time required for completion of toxin transport, which is intraaxonal when antitoxin is given. Complications include fractures resulting from the sustained contractions and convulsions, aspiration, pulmonary emboli, bacterial superinfections, dehydration, respiratory failure, and cardiac arrest.

Localized tetanus refers to involvement of an extremity with a contaminated wound (5,12,14,15). There is considerable variation in severity. There may be muscle weakness and diminished tone that resolves spontaneously or may persist in a chronic form. More severe cases are characterized by intense, painful spasms, and most cases progress to generalized tetanus. This is a relatively unusual form of tetanus, and the prognosis for survival is excellent.

Cephalic tetanus usually occurs in association with a head injury or with *C. tetani* infection of the middle ear (14,15,21,22). Clinical features consist of an isolated or combined cranial motor nerve dysfunction, most often the seventh cranial nerve. This also may remain localized or progress to generalized tetanus. Cephalic tetanus is an unusual form of the disease; the incubation period is only 1 or 2 days and the prognosis variable (21,22).

TABLE 211.1. Experience with Tetanus in the United States for 1989 and 1990

Reported cases (1989, 1990): 110
Demographic data
  Female: 57 (52%)
  Age older than 60 yr: 63 (58%)
  Age younger than 20 yr: 7 (6%)
Portal of entry
  Acute injury: 86 (78%)
    Puncture wound: 45 (52%)
    Lacerations: 20 (23%)
    Abrasion: 15 (17%)
  Chronic wound: 14[a] (9%)
  Intravenous drug abuse: 5 (5%)
Neonatal tetanus: 1 (1%)
No portal of entry or associated condition: 10 (9%)
Persons who sought medical care for initial injury: 27/86 (32%)
Persons treated with tetanus toxoid: 15 (58%)
Persons treated with tetanus immunoglobulin (TIG): 0[b]
Persons who had received primary immunization: 12/57 (21%)[c]
Type of tetanus (90 patients)
  Generalized: 79 (88%)
  Localized: 8 (9%)
  Cephalic: 3 (3%)
Outcome of tetanus
  Length of hospitalization (median): 17 d
  No. requiring assisted ventilation: 55/94 (58%)
  TIG dosage (median): 3,000 IU
  Mortality rate: 24%

---

[a]Skin ulcers, abscesses, or gangrene (three diabetic patients).
[b]Seven were considered candidates for tetanus and diphtheria toxoids absorbed for adult use (Td) and TIG, of whom four received Td and none received TIG.
[c]Vaccination status was unknown for 53 patients.
Source: From Prevots R, Sutter RW, Strebel PM, et al. Tetanus surveillance—United States, 1989–1990. *MMWR CDC Surveill Summ* 1992;41(8):1–9, with permission.

Tetanus neonatorum is generalized tetanus in neonates that occurs almost exclusively in underdeveloped countries (8,11,23,24). The incubation period after birth is 3 to 10 days, and it is sometimes referred to as the "disease of the seventh day." The child typically shows facial grimacing, irritability, and severe spasms in response to being touched. The mortality rate is about 90%, and this disease accounted for an estimated 400,000 neonatal deaths annually and is widely viewed as one of the world's major health problems that could be easily eliminated with maternal vaccines and simple hygienic measures (10,11,24).

DIAGNOSIS

The diagnosis is usually established by clinical observation. The organism is rarely recovered from cultures of wound material. A confirmed history of immunization or a serum antitoxin level of 0.01 U/mL or higher makes tetanus unlikely but does not exclude the diagnosis. Cerebrospinal fluid analysis findings are normal, imaging studies of the brain are normal, and the electroencephalogram usually shows a sleep pattern. Electrophysiologic studies of the masseter muscle show a characteristic absence or shortening of the silent period ascribed to the failure of Renshaw cell inhibition (25). This may also show exaggerated F responses, indicating hyperexcitability. The differential diagnosis depends to some extent on the dominant clinical features and includes dental infection with trismus, seizure disorder, oculogyric crisis secondary to phenothiazine toxicity, subarachnoid hemorrhage, meningitis, hypocalcemic or alkalotic tetany, alcohol withdrawal, stiff man syndrome (26), and strychnine poisoning. The last produces similar symptoms, but patients usually recover rapidly with supportive care. Strychnine poisoning can be excluded with toxicologic studies of serum and urine.

TREATMENT

Generalized tetanus requires an intensive care unit setting with an aggressive, multidisciplinary coordinated effort to avoid noxious stimuli, direct primary attention to ventilatory support, liberal use of benzodiazepines, an attack on *C. tetanus* and its toxin, attention to defects in the autonomic nervous system, and supportive care (15–17,27–31).

Most important is the effort to secure the airway. This may be done by orotracheal or nasotracheal intubation, or it may require a tracheostomy. Patients with severe muscle spasms may require therapeutic paralysis with mechanical ventilation.

Treatment directed against *C. tetanus* toxin should include passive immunoglobulin as TIG, 500 mg intramuscularly (31), or pooled intravenous immune globulin, which should be as effective (32). Active immunization should be initiated as well using 0.5 mL of tetanus toxoid, often as diphtheria-tetanus absorbed. This should be given at a site distant from TIG. With regard to *C. tetani*, local wounds should be treated and the putative agent should be treated with metronidazole based on a therapeutic trial showing metronidazole to be superior to penicillin (33). Penicillin has the additional theoretical disadvantage that like tetanus toxin, it is a GABA antagonist. Alternative antibiotics include erythromycin, tetracycline, and chloramphenicol.

Benzodiazepines have become standards for management because of established merit, enhancement of GABA-mediated central inhibition, and utility in controlling spasms, reducing anxiety, promoting muscle relaxation, and preventing seizures (15,16,17,27–30). The most extensively studied is diazepam, usually in doses of 10 to 30 mg every 1 to 8 hours, but doses up to 40 mg per hour may be required. A possible complication is lactic acidosis from the propylene glycol vehicle (20). Midazolam, lorazepam, or propofol are alternatives that are probably equally effective (30,34,35). If muscle spasms are severe or interfere with ventilation, therapeutic paralysis may be required using pancuronium bromide or metocurine. Dantrolene has been used for peripheral muscle relaxation, but prolonged use of large doses risks hepatic dysfunction.

Supportive care is critical and includes nasogastric feedings and intravenous fluids with careful attention to fluid balance, because there may be large losses resulting from profuse sweating. Other supportive measures to consider are anticoagulation to prevent pulmonary emboli, sucralfate for gastrointestinal bleeding, a cooling blanket for hyperthermia, antibiotics for established infections, and dialysis for renal failure secondary to rhabdomyolysis with myoglobinuria.

Autonomic nervous system involvement may cause hypertension and tachycardia, increased cardiac output, and arrhythmias. With the ventilatory support that is currently available in intensive care units, autonomic instability now represents the major cause of lethality. This may be treated with combined α- and β-adrenergic blocking agents using intravenous labetalol. Additional therapeutic modalities include morphine sulfate, esmolol, epidural blockage, and infusions of magnesium sulfate (30,36–39).

PROGNOSIS

The overall mortality rate for generalized tetanus in industrialized countries is 20% to 25% (9,14–16,20,30,40,41). Prognostic indicators are the form of tetanus, the incubation period, the onset period, and the patient's age (41). Some patients have only trismus with minor muscle spasms and do quite well. Moderately severe disease is often characterized by trismus, dysphagia, rigidity, and intermittent muscle spasms. Severe tetanus is associated with generalized convulsions and respiratory failure. Patients with moderate or severe generalized tetanus usually require 3 to 6 weeks to recover, and most of this time is usually spent in the intensive care unit. The most common causes of death are pneumonia and autonomic instability (42).

PREVENTION

Tetanus is a preventable disease: Virtually all victims are not immunized or are inadequately immunized. The Immunization Practices Advisory Committee recommends active immunization for infants and children with diphtheria and tetanus toxoids and pertussis absorbed at ages 2 months, 4 months, 6 months, 15 months, and 4 to 6 years (13,43). Tetanus toxoid is an excellent antigen, and protective levels among persons who complete the primary series persist for a minimum of 10 years. Tetanus and diphtheria toxoids absorbed for adult use (Td) are recommended every 10 years at mid decade (ages 15 years, 25 years, and so on).

Nearly all states now require diphtheria, pertussis, and tetanus immunization for school enrollment, but booster vaccinations after the primary series are often neglected. Serosurveys indicate that 31% of persons older than 70 years in the United States lack protective levels of 0.15 IU/mL (enzyme immunoassay) or higher (3). These observations account for the frequency of tetanus in older persons in the United States. Some authorities advocate hospital-based Td immunization programs for adults unless there is proof of immunization within 10 years or a convincing history of a severe reaction to the toxoid (44). On a global

TABLE 211.2. Recommendations of Advisory Committee on Immunization Practices for Tetanus Prophylaxis in Routine Wound Management

History of tetanus toxoid immunization	Clean minor wounds		Other wounds[a]	
	Td[b]	TIG	Td[b]	TIG
Unknown or <3 doses	Yes	No	Yes	Yes
At least 3 doses[c]	No unless >10 yr since last dose	No	No unless >5 yr since last dose	No

[a]Including wounds contaminated with dirt, soil, feces, or saliva; puncture wounds; avulsions; and wounds resulting from missiles, crushing, burns, or frostbite.
[b]Td, tetanus toxoid ± diphtheria toxoid; TIG, tetanus immune globulin; children younger than 7 years should receive diphtheria and tetanus toxoids and pertussis absorbed; persons 7 years or older should receive Td.
[c]If only three doses of fluid toxoid were given, the fourth dose of toxoid, preferably an absorbed toxoid, should be given.
Source: From Advisory Committee on Immunization Practices. Adult immunization. *MMWR Morb Mortal Wkly Rep* 1991;40(RR-12):1, with permission.

scale, the World Health Organization has adopted a resolution for worldwide elimination of neonatal tetanus. To achieve this goal, we will need to protect 80% or more of infants through maternal vaccination with at least two doses of toxoid or through clean delivery and cord care practices.

Also important for preventing tetanus is appropriate management of patients with wounds, especially in emergency departments, where mistakes are common (9,45–47). The goal is to provide adequate wound management, ensure adequate immunity, and consider antibiotic prophylaxis. The goal of surgery is to remove necrotic tissue, drain purulent collections, and remove foreign bodies that promote the environmental conditions necessary for the germination of spores.

Guidelines for immunoprophylaxis are based on the immunization status and characteristics of the wound (Table 211.2). Passive immunization with TIG is recommended for wounds described as tetanus prone if the patient has not been immunized. *Tetanus prone* is defined as having wounds contaminated with dirt, soil, stool, or saliva; puncture wounds; avulsions; and wounds resulting from missiles, crush injuries, burns, or frostbite. The definition of a tetanus-prone wound also depends on the interval between injury and treatment, the severity of contamination, the extent of devitalized tissue or foreign bodies at the site of the wounding, and the depth of the injury. The usual dose of TIG is 250 U intramuscularly, but up to 500 U is given for highly tetanus prone wounds. Active immunization is done simultaneously using separate syringes for TIG and tetanus toxoid. Simultaneous administration does not appear to blunt the immune response to the toxoid.

Antimicrobial agents, including penicillin, erythromycin, and metronidazole, may be given to prevent replication of vegetative forms of *C. tetani*; however, the local management of the wound and immunoprophylaxis are considered much more important.

REFERENCES

1. Habermann E, Dreyer F. Clostridial neurotoxins: handling and action at the cellular and molecular level. *Curr Top Microbiol Immunol* 1986;129:93.
2. Fairweather NF, Lyness VA. The complete amino acid sequence of tetanus toxin. *Nucleic Acids Res* 1986;14:7809.
3. Halpern JL, Smith LA, Seamon KB, et al. Sequence homology between tetanus and *botulinum* toxins detected by an antipeptide antibody. *Infect Immun* 1989;57:18.
4. Boyd JSK, MacLennan JD. Tetanus in the Middle East: effect of active immunization. *Lancet* 1942;2:745.
5. Griffin JW. Local tetanus. *Johns Hopkins Med J* 1981;149:84.
6. Dowell VR Jr. Botulism and tetanus: selected epidemiologic and microbiologic aspects. *Rev Infect Dis* 1984;6[Suppl 1]:202.
7. Schiavo G, Benfenati B, Poulain B, et al. Tetanus and *botulinum*-B neurotoxins block neurotransmitter release by proteolytic cleavage of synaptobrevin. *Nature* 1992;359:832.
8. Schofield F. Selective primary health care: strategies for control of disease in the developing world. XXII. Tetanus: a preventable problem. *Rev Infect Dis* 1986;8:144.
9. Prevots R, Sutter RW, Strebel PM, et al. Tetanus surveillance—United States, 1989–1990. *MMWR CDC Surveill Summ* 1992;41(8):1.
10. Maple PA, al-Wali W. The prevention of tetanus in England and Wales. *Comm Dis Public Health* 2001;4:106.
11. Meegan ME, Conroy RM, Lengensy SO, et al. Effect neonatal tetanus mortality after a culturally-based health promotion programme. *Lancet* 2002;359:262.
12. Centers for Disease Control and Prevention. Tetanus surveillance—United States, 1995–97. *MMWR Morb Mortal Wkly Rep* 1998;47(SS-2):1.
13. McQuillan GM, Kruszon-Moran D, Deforest A, et al. Serologic immunity to diphtheria and tetanus in the United States. *Ann Intern Med* 2002;136:660.
14. Weinstein L. Tetanus. *N Engl J Med* 1973;289:1293.
15. Bleck TP. Tetanus: dealing with the continuing clinical challenge. *J Crit Illness* 1987;2:41.
16. Al-Kaabi JM, Scrimgeour EM, Louon A, et al. Tetanus: a clinical review. *Saudi Med J* 2001;22:606.
17. Kanchanapongkul J. Tetanus in adults: a review of 85 cases at Chon Buri Hospital. *J Med Assoc Thai* 2001;84:494.
18. Kerr JH, Corbett JL, Prys-Roberts C, et al. Involvement of the sympathetic nervous system in tetanus: studies on 82 cases. *Lancet* 1968;2:236.
19. LaForce FM, Young LS Bennett JV. Tetanus in the United States (1965–1966): epidemiologic and clinical features. *N Engl J Med* 1969;280:569.
20. Sanford JP. Tetanus—forgotten but not gone. *N Engl J Med* 1995;332:812.
21. Abde VW, Dekate MP. Cephalic tetanus. *J Indian Med Assoc* 1980;74:111.
22. Mayo J, Berciano J. Cephalic tetanus presenting with Bell's palsy. *J Neurol Neurosurg Psychiatry* 1985;48:290.
23. Salimpour R. Cause of death in tetanus neonatorum: study of 233 cases with 54 necropsies. *Arch Dis Child* 1977;52:587.
24. Progress towards the global elimination of neonatal tetanus, 1989–1993. *MMWR Morb Mortal Wkly Rep* 1994;43:885.
25. Risk WS, Bosch EP, Kimura J, et al. Chronic tetanus: clinical report and histochemistry of muscle. *Muscle Nerve* 1981;4:363.
26. Solimena M, Folli F, Denis-Donini S, et al. Autoantibodies to glutamic acid decarboxylase in a patient with stiff-man syndrome, epilepsy, and type I diabetes mellitus. *N Engl J Med* 1988;318:1012.
27. Olsen KM, Hiller FC. Management of tetanus. *Clin Pharm* 1987;6:570.
28. Trujillo MH, Castillo A, Espana J, et al. Impact of intensive care management on the prognosis of tetanus: analysis of 641 cases. *Chest* 1987;92:63.
29. Bleck TP. Tetanus. *Dis Mon* 1991;37:547.
30. Bleck TP. *Clostridium tetani.* In: Mandell GL, Bennett JE, Dolin R, eds. *Principles and practice of infectious diseases*, 5th ed, vol 2. New York, Churchill Livingstone, 2000:2537.
31. Blake PA, Feldman RA, Buchanan TM, et al. Serologic therapy of tetanus in the United States. *JAMA* 1976;236:42.
32. Lee DC, Lederman HM. Anti-tetanus toxoid antibodies in intravenous gammaglobulum: an alternative to tetanus immune globulin. *J Infect Dis* 1992;166:642.
33. Ahmadsyah I, Salim A. Treatment of tetanus: an open study to compare the efficacy of procaine penicillin and metronidazole. *Br Med J* 1985;291:648.
34. Orko R, Rosenberg PH, Himberg JJ. Intravenous infusion of midazolam, propofol and vecuronium in a patient with severe tetanus. *Acta Anaesthesiol Scand* 1988;32:590.
35. Borgeat A, Dessibourg C, Rochani M, et al. Sedation by propofol in tetanus—is it a muscular relaxant? *Intensive Care Med* 1991;17:427.
36. King WW, Cave DR. Use of esmolol to control autonomic instability of tetanus. *Am J Med* 1991;91:425.

37. Rocke DA, Wasley AG, Father M, et al. Morphine in tetanus: the management of sympathetic nervous system overactivity. *S Afr Med J* 1986;70:666.
38. Lipman J, James MFM, Erskine J, et al. Autonomic dysfunction in severe tetanus: magnesium sulfate as an adjunct to deep sedation. *Crit Care Med* 1987;15:987.
39. Southorn PA, Blaise GA. Treatment of tetanus-induced autonomic dysfunction with continuous epidural blockade. *Crit Care Med* 1986;14:251.
40. Armitage P, Clifford R. Prognosis in tetanus: use of data from therapeutic trials. *J Infect Dis* 1978;138:1.
41. Nolla-Salas M, Garces-Bruses J. Severity of tetanus in patients older than 80 years: comparative study with younger patients. *Clin Infect Dis* 1993;16:591.
42. Edmondson RS, Flowers MWW. Intensive care in tetanus: management, complications and mortality in 100 patients. *Br Med J* 1979;1:1401.
43. Advisory Committee on Immunization Practices. General recommendations on immunization. *MMWR Morb Mortal Wkly Rep* 2002;51(RR-2):1.
44. Thorley JD, Holmes RK, Sanford JP. Tetanus and diphtheria antitoxin levels following a hospital-based adult immunization program. *Am J Epidemiol* 1975;101:438.
45. Brand DA, Acampora D, Gotlieb LD, et al. Adequacy of antitetanus prophylaxis in six hospital emergency rooms. *N Engl J Med* 1983;309:636.
46. Giangrosso J, Smith RK. Misuse of tetanus immunoprophylaxis in wound care. *Ann Emerg Med* 1985;14:573.
47. Hsu SS, Groleau G. Tetanus in the emergency department: a current review. *J Emerg Med* 2001;20:357.

CHAPTER 212
Clostridium botulinum

Charles L. Hatheway and John G. Bartlett

HISTORY

Botulism has long been recognized as a food-borne illness. The name is derived from the Latin word *botulus,* which means "sausage," because of the association of the illness with the consumption of sausages and other preserved meat products over the centuries in Europe (1). The bacterial etiology and toxicologic mechanism of the illness were elucidated by van Ermengem (2) in 1895 in the investigation of a large outbreak in Belgium. The name *Bacillus botulinus* was given to the toxigenic organism that was responsible for the outbreak. Investigations of subsequent incidents repeatedly confirmed van Ermengem's findings, but they also revealed that the toxins in different outbreaks might have different serologic specificities and that the implicated toxigenic organisms could have various physiologic and cultural characteristics. Foods other than meat products were encountered as vehicles. Botulism was seen to occur also in cattle (3) and chickens (4), as well as in other mammalian and avian species (1). A second form of human botulism (wound botulism) was found on rare occasions to result from growth of toxigenic organisms in infected wounds (5,6). A third form, resulting from colonization of the intestinal tract of infants (infant botulism) was recognized in 1976 (7–9). In 1978, a fourth category of human botulism was established by the Centers for Disease Control and Prevention (CDC) for single-case incidents involving adults and noninfant children for whom there was no apparent food vehicle (10); this provided a classification for cases that might actually have been due to intestinal colonization. The most recent form is botulism toxin as a mechanism of biological warfare, either by the standard mechanism via contaminated food or by aerosolization with inhalation of botulinum toxin (11).

Because the organisms that cause botulism are anaerobic spore formers, they were placed in the genus *Clostridium* on the recommendation of the Committee on Classification of the Society of American Bacteriologists (12). The name *Clostridium botulinum* is applied to four diverse groups of organisms that produce potent neurotoxins that can cause botulism.

CHARACTERISTICS OF THE PATHOGEN

C. botulinum spores are found in soil samples throughout the world. The most distinguishing characteristic of the organisms is their ability to produce botulism neurotoxin. All the organisms noted to date clearly fit into the genus *Clostridium.* They are all anaerobic spore-forming bacilli that are usually referred to as *gram positive,* although the Gram reaction is variable, often appearing as positive in young cultures but changing to negative in cultures after 18 hours. A single strain always produces only a single toxin type.

Toxin Types

The first differential characteristic among the toxin-producing organisms is the serologic specificity of the neurotoxins. There are seven toxin types, each designated by a letter of the alphabet, A through G (1). The biologic activity of each type of toxin is specifically neutralized by its corresponding antitoxin. There is no cross-neutralization except for a low-level reciprocal cross-reactivity between types E and F (13).

The toxin is a binary polypeptide with a 105-kd chain linked by a disulfide bond to a 50-kd chain. Biologic activity resides with the light chain, which contains a Zn^{2+}-containing endopeptidase that blocks fusion of acetylcholine-containing vesicles with motor neuron membrane terminals (14,15). The result is a flaccid paralysis. The estimated lethal dose for a 70-kg man is 0.09 to 0.15 μg by intravenous administration, 0.7 to 0.9 μg by inhalation, and 70 μg by mouth (11).

Types C and D neurotoxins are phage mediated, that is, the genes that code for them are carried by bacteriophages with which the toxigenic organisms are infected (16,17). Studies with toxigenic (type E) *C. botulinum* have provided evidence that the toxin gene in that organism is phage associated (18). There is evidence that the gene for type G toxin is present on a plasmid (19,20). Because all attempts so far have failed to show evidence of phage or plasmid association with toxigenicity of types A, B, or F, the genes for those types are presumed to be present on the chromosome.

Physiologic Groups

C. botulinum is divided into four groups (17,21) on the basis of different metabolic characteristics. The differences are sufficient to designate a separate species name for each group. Group I consists of "proteolytic" organisms, that is, those that can digest complex proteins such as casein or coagulated serum or egg albumin (12). All organisms that produce type A toxin and certain strains that produce type B or type F toxin belong in this group. Group II includes all type E strains, some type B strains (notably those implicated in botulism outbreaks associated with meat products in Europe), and some type F strains. These organisms have a notably lower optimal growth temperature (25°C to 30°C) and are nonproteolytic. Group III consists of the organisms that produce type C or type D toxin and have shown cultural and metabolic characteristics, for example, production of propionic acid, that distinguish them from both group I and group II (22). All three of these groups are saccharolytic and produce lipase (18). Group IV was established to classify the organism isolated from soil in Argentina that produces type G toxin (23) and is proteolytic, asaccharolytic, and lipase negative.

The four groups are clearly distinguishable by deoxyribonucleic acid (DNA) relatedness studies (24–27). Analysis of the phylogeny of the clostridia by 16S ribosomal ribonucleic acid (RNA) gene sequences has reinforced these groupings (28).

TABLE 212.1. Groups of *Clostridium botulinum* and Other Species Capable of Producing Botulism Neurotoxin: Differential Characteristics and Related Nontoxigenic Species

| Group or species | Type of toxin | Ferment glucose | Digest casein | Liquefy gelatin | Reactions on egg yolk agar | | Metabolic acids[a] | Related species |
					Lipase	Lecithinase		
I	A, B, F	+	+	+	+	−	A, iB, B, iV	*Clostridium sporogenes*
II	B, E, F	+	−	+	+	−	A, B	—
III	C, D	+	±	+	+	±	A, P, B	*Clostridium novyi*
Clostridium argentinense[b]	G	−	+	+	−	−	A, iB, B, iV	—
Clostridium barati	F	+	−	−	−	+	A, B	—
Clostridium butyricum	E	+	−	−	−	−	A, B	—

[a]Volatile metabolic acids produced in peptone–yeast extract glucose, analyzed by gas-liquid chromatography.
[b]Also commonly known as *C. botulinum* type G.
A, acetic; iB, isobutyric; B, butyric; iV, isovaleric.

Some nonneurotoxigenic organisms known by other clostridial species names are phenotypically and genetically related to group I *(Clostridium sporogenes)* and group III *(Clostridium novyi).* Thus, in essence, there are toxigenic and nontoxigenic members of the same "species." Because neurotoxigenic organisms identifiable as *Clostridium barati* and *Clostridium butyricum* (29) have been implicated in human botulism, it is difficult to insist that all organisms that produce the neurotoxin be called *C. botulinum.* The groups of organisms identified to date that produce botulism neurotoxin and their characteristics are listed in Table 212.1.

TOXIN TYPES IN HUMAN BOTULISM

Human botulism is essentially restricted to toxin types A, B, and E (1). The occurrence of botulism in the United States since 1950 is summarized in Table 212.2 by disease form and toxin type. Of the more than 2,000 cases whose types are known, all are type A, B, or E, except for nine cases identified as type F.

Type F botulism was first recognized in a food-borne outbreak in Denmark in 1958 (30). It has since been recognized in the United States in eight instances involving nine patients (31–35). Although toxin type C is often associated with botulism in birds

and in domestic and wild mammals (1), only one poorly confirmed type C human food-borne outbreak has been reported. One type D outbreak was reported by Demarchi et al. (37). The occurrence of type G botulism is controversial. Although one laboratory has reported isolating type G organisms from autopsy specimens (38), there was no convincing evidence that botulism had occurred in those cases.

EPIDEMIOLOGY

Food-borne Botulism

Food-borne botulism remains the most common form of botulism worldwide, although in the United States infant cases have become the most common. Hauschild (35) reviewed the incidence of food-borne botulism in 1993. Poland, China, the United States, and France lead in the number of reported food-borne cases. The foods are largely home processed. In Europe, they are most often meat products, and the toxin is largely type B. In China, the vehicle is more commonly a vegetable (or cereal grain) product and type A toxin predominates (1,35).

Food-borne botulism in the continental United States is typically due to inadequately processed home-preserved vegetables.

TABLE 212.2. Incidence of Food-borne, Wound, and Infant Botulism in the United States Since 1950[a]

| Disease form | Years | Toxin type | | | | Unknown | Total | Case-fatality rate (%) |
		A	B	E	F			
Food-borne	1950–1993	436	183	196	3	303[b]	1,126	17.9
Wound	1950–1993	37	15	0	0	6[c]	58	10.3
Infant	1975–1993	575	603	0	2	10[d]	1,190	1.1
Other	1978–1993	17	6	0	4	4	31	29.0

[a]Number of cases of botulism (Centers for Disease Control and Prevention, unpublished data).
[b]Toxin type not determined.
[c]Botulism diagnosed on clinical evidence; no confirmatory laboratory evidence.
[d]Three cases without report of toxin type, two due to single organism producing two types of toxin (B, F), and one due to colonization by two organisms (A, B).

In these cases, the causative organism is almost always type A or B (group I), and the incidence of each type correlates with the toxin type distribution in the soil of the region of origin of the food. Type A predominates in the western part of the country and type B in the eastern part (39). Type E food-borne botulism, associated with fish and other marine foods, is common in Alaska and is enhanced by fish and marine animals prepared by nontraditional fermentation methods used by the Alaska Native populations (40–44). Type E *C. botulinum* is well represented in the soil and beach flora in areas where those foods are obtained, processed, and consumed. The average number of food-borne cases reported in the United States from 1951 to 1998 was 24 per year (45).

Wound Botulism

The first case of wound botulism was documented in 1943 (46). Weber et al. (6) reviewed 47 cases of laboratory-confirmed wound botulism that occurred between 1943 and 1990 in the United States. Through 1993, 58 cases were reported to the CDC (see Table 212.2); the toxin types have been either A or B, and the causative organisms, when identified, are always group I strains. Of the known types of associated wounds listed by Weber et al., 30 were traumatic, 5 were surgical, and 9 were associated with illicit drug abuse. The case-fatality rate for wound botulism is about 10%. In 1994, there was a sudden increase in cases attributed to the use of black-tar heroin in California (45).

Infant Botulism

Infant botulism (caused by colonization of infants younger than 1 year) was first recognized in 1976 as distinct from food-borne botulism (7,8). It has been documented in at least 14 countries (47) and since 1980 has become the most frequently recognized form of botulism in the United States with an average of 71 cases per year (45) (see Table 212.2). Approximately 50% of the U.S. cases are found in California. The usual source of the organisms is most likely the soil, but honey has been implicated in 26 instances (45). The case-fatality rate for infant botulism is about 1%.

The organisms that cause infant botulism are almost exclusively group I strains of *C. botulinum* of toxin type A or B. One case in Japan was identified by Oguma et al. (48) as type C, two type F cases in the United States were caused by *C. barati* (32), and two type E cases in Italy were caused by *C. butyricum* (49).

Biological Warfare

There has been an attempt to use botulinum toxin for bioterrorism with an aerosol dispersed over Tokyo at least three times by the Japanese cult Aum Shinrikyo (11). Not surprisingly, all were unsuccessful. Botulinum toxin was also tested by the Soviet bioweapons site, Aralsk-7, on Vozrozhdeniye Island in the Aral Sea (11,50). More recently, there is suspicion that at least four nations (Iraq, Iran, North Korea, and Syria) are stockpiling botulism for potential use in bioterrorism (11). The mechanism of dispersal would be by aerosol of toxin from missiles for inhalation. It is estimated that a point-source release of 50 kg of botulinum toxin would incapacitate or kill 10% of persons within 0.5 km downstream (11). The CDC maintains a surveillance system to facilitate detection of such outbreaks (51).

Undetermined Classification

Single cases of botulism for which there are neither plausible food sources for botulinum toxin nor any wound site for possible infection with *C. botulinum* are sometimes confirmed on the basis of detection of toxin in serum or feces or both and isolation of the organism from the feces. This suggests the possibility of botulism due to intestinal colonization, which though quite rare, has been documented (52). Several cases of botulism were confirmed among patients who had surgical alteration of the bowel (53–55). The altered environment of the intestinal lumen appears to be conducive to germination and outgrowth of spores of toxigenic organisms. The occurrence of botulism immediately after surgery (56) might be due to infection of the surgical wound rather than colonization of the lumen. One case of botulism associated with Crohn's disease has been documented (57); whether this was due to colonization or to infection of the lesions associated with the disease is not clear.

PATHOGENESIS

Botulism is a neuroparalytic disease caused by blockage of acetylcholine release by the nerves that activate skeletal muscles (14,15,58). Botulinum neurotoxin may also interfere with certain autonomic nervous system functions, as has been evidenced by abnormal heart rate and blood pressure responses to cardiovascular reflex tests (59). Botulism neurotoxins, regardless of toxin type, consist of a dichain peptide molecule with a molecular mass of about 150,000. They exist in the native state as complexes with nontoxic proteins, which greatly enhance their stability. All forms of botulism result from absorption of the toxin into the systemic circulation via the intestine, lung, or wound. The toxin molecules bind to specific receptors on the nerve endings, and a portion of the molecule gains entrance into the nerve cell (58). The light-chain fragment has endopeptidase activity and cleaves membrane proteins essential for exocytosis of the neurotransmitter. The paralytic signs of the disease reflect the specific nerve fibers to which the toxin binds. Death from botulism in the absence of intensive supportive care is usually due to respiratory failure.

CLINICAL MANIFESTATIONS

Botulism is characterized by a descending paralysis of the muscles of the limbs and trunk that is symmetric and always begins with the bulbar musculature (Table 212.3). This is recognized as the "4 *D*s": diplopia, dysarthria, dysphonia, and dysphagia (11). The course is a descending flaccid paralysis. Parasympathetic involvement may cause a dry mouth and red throat. Deep tendon reflexes decrease and then disappear. The loss of a gag reflex may predispose to aspiration. Sensation is intact. The patient is afebrile and remains alert. The major cause of death is respiratory failure that often requires ventilatory support. The frequency of mechanical ventilation is usually 40% to 60% for hospitalized adults with food-borne disease and 60% for infant botulism. Some patients may have mild forms of disease that is detected only because they are part of an outbreak investigation (43). The classic triad is (a) a symmetric descending paralysis with prominent bulbar palsies, (b) afebrile patient, and (c) clear sensorium (11). The reported mortality in U.S. cases from 1976 to 1995 was 6.6%. Recovery is usually slow over weeks or months because of the necessity to regenerate new axons (59).

The neurologic symptoms of botulism are similar regardless of toxin type or route of entry (60). The infant form may be somewhat different, reflecting the age of the host (Table 212.4), and the mortality rate is only about 1% (61). The pathophysiology of the four forms of botulism is also distinctive. Infant and wound

TABLE 212.3. **Symptoms and Signs of Illness Observed in Food-borne Botulism Outbreaks Occurring 1953 to 1973 Expressed as Number of Outbreaks in Which One or More Patients Experienced Symptoms or Exhibited Signs**

Symptoms and signs	Type A: 34 outbreaks, 97 cases	Type B: 15 outbreaks, 46 cases	Type E: 10 outbreaks, 36 cases	Type F: 1 outbreak, 3 cases	Undetermined[a]: 44 outbreaks, 90 cases	Total: 104 outbreaks, 272 cases	With signs and symptoms (%)
Symptoms							
Blurred vision, diplopia, photophobia	31	13	9	1	40	94	90.4
Dysphagia	27	14	3	—	35	79	76.0
Generalized weakness	22	12	4	—	22	60	57.7
Nausea and/or vomiting	15	13	10	1	19	58	55.8
Dysphonia	25	8	5	—	19	57	54.8
Dizziness or vertigo	8	4	5	—	15	32	30.8
Abdominal pain, cramps, fullness	5	6	3	—	7	21	20.2
Diarrhea	5	6	—	—	5	16	15.4
Urinary retention or incontinence	2	2	1	—	2	7	6.7
Sore throat	4	2	1	—	—	7	6.7
Constipation	2	2	—	1	3	6	5.8
Paresthesias	1	—	—	—	—	1	1.0
Signs							
Respiratory impairment	32	7	7	—	30	76	73.1
Specific muscle weakness or paralysis	23	9	3	—	13	48	46.2
Eye muscle involvement	16	9	3	1	17	46	44.2
Dry mouth, throat, or tongue	7	6	2	—	7	22	21.2
Dilated, fixed pupils	3	4	2	—	8	16	15.4
Ataxia	3	1	—	1	4	9	8.7
Postural hypotension	—	—	1	—	2	3	2.9
Nystagmus	1	—	1	—	1	3	2.9
Somnolence	—	—	1	—	—	1	1.0

[a]Toxin type undetermined or unspecified.
Source: From Centers for Disease Control and Prevention. Botulism in the United States, 1899–1977. Handbook for epidemiologic, clinicians, and laboratory workers. Public Health Service. Atlanta: US Department of Health, Education, and Welfare, 1979, with permission.

botulism are associated with *in vivo* production of *C. botulinum.* By contrast, inhalation and food-borne forms involve exposure only to preformed toxin; there is speculation that food-borne botulism may actually include *C. botulinum* ingestion with *in vivo* production in a fashion analogous to the infant form.

The incubation period usually ranges from 6 hours to as late as 10 days after exposure; the incubation period varies inversely with the amount of toxin consumed. The incubation period is shortest for type E botulism, but type A botulism is more severe, as indicated by a greater number of patients requiring intubation (67%, 52%, and 39% for types A, B, and E, respectively) (60).

TABLE 212.4. **Physical Findings in 44 Cases of Infant Botulism in Pennsylvania**

Finding[a]	% of infants
Weakness	100
Hypotonia	95
Constipation	95
Failure of oral feeding	93
Diminished gagging or sucking reflex	91
Respiratory failure	89
Facial diparsis or ptosis	84
Decreased spontaneous movement	82
Decreased deep tendon reflexes	57

[a]Findings in more than 50% of cases.
Source: From Long SS, Gajewski JL, Brown LW, et al. Clinical, laboratory, and environmental features of infant botulism in southeastern Pennsylvania. *Pediatrics* 1985;75:935–941, with permission.

Patients with wound botulism show the same paralytic signs as those with food-borne disease, but the initial gastrointestinal tract features are absent.

DIAGNOSIS

Botulism is first recognized or suspected on the basis of the clinical signs and symptoms. Epidemiologic evidence in multipatient outbreaks can make the diagnosis rather easy. In single-case noninfant incidents, recognition may be difficult when there is no obvious suggestive food history. Diseases sometimes confused with botulism are Guillain-Barré syndrome, myasthenia gravis, stroke, and chemical poisoning. Confirmation of botulism requires detection of toxin in the patient's serum or stool or in the suspected food vehicle (62). Finding *C. botulinum* in the stool of a patient exhibiting signs consistent with botulism is fairly good confirmatory evidence because it is rarely ever recovered in the absence of botulism (63,64). Wound botulism is confirmed by detecting toxin in the serum or by culturing *C. botulinum* from the wound. Failure to find toxin or the organism in a noninfant patient does not rule out the diagnosis. In infants, however, botulism can generally be ruled out if two or more stools obtained during the acute phase of the illness are toxin and culture negative. Serum is usually negative in infant botulism (65). Antitoxin has not been detected in postrecovery serum, except in the unusual case associated with Crohn's disease mentioned earlier (57). Rubin, Dezfulian, and Yolkin (66) reported that convalescent serum from two infants gave positive reactions in enzyme-linked immunosorbent assays against botulism toxin.

At present, the only reliable diagnostic test for identifying the toxin is the mouse bioassay. Many *in vitro* tests have been proposed, but none has been adequately evaluated (67). Because botulism is so rare, and because even a single case may represent a public health emergency, emergency diagnostic services should be obtained through state public health departments or the CDC. Consultation on the diagnosis and arranging for therapeutic antitoxin laboratory testing may be obtained through one of these facilities. Outside the United States, appropriate local and national health departments should be consulted. Detailed laboratory procedures for toxin testing and culturing for *C. botulinum* are described elsewhere (62,68).

Electrophysiologic studies are sometimes used in the diagnosis of botulism using repetitive stimuli at 20 to 50 Hz to distinguish causes of flaccid paralysis (69–72). They may be more successful for diagnosis of infant botulism (72), but for this form of the disease, fecal analysis is reliable and virtually conclusive (65).

TREATMENT

Intensive supportive care is most important in treating persons with botulism. Improvements in mechanical ventilatory support have been the most important factor in lowering the case-fatality rate for food-borne botulism from about 70% in 1910 to about 6% more recently (44,73). Therapeutic antitoxin (trivalent, types A, B, and E) is available for specific treatment of adult (but not infant) botulism in the United States through the CDC. The standard dose is one vial (5,500 to 8,500 IU) delivered by slow intravenous infusion. There is an experimental pentavalent vaccine (types A through G) held by the U.S. Army that could be used for unusual types (11). An analysis of 132 cases of type A food-borne botulism in which 115 of the patients received standard equine antitoxin therapy supports efficacy (74), but animal studies show that unless antitoxin is given early, usually before the onset of signs of illness, the protective effect is questionable (75). Antitoxin will not reverse paralysis or the binding of toxin to nerve endings but will neutralize any unbound toxin in the circulation and prevent further paralysis. Because the antitoxin is of equine origin, hypersensitive reactions occur in about 9% of treated patients, including anaphylaxis in 2% (76). Standard treatment can provide serum antitoxin levels more than sufficient to neutralize unbound toxin, and residual circulating antitoxins have half-lives of up to 1 week (77). Paralysis may progress for a while after antitoxin administration because of the effects of the bound toxin. If one or two vials fail to stabilize the patient's condition, the failure is unlikely to be due to insufficient antitoxin (77).

Other facets of care are supportive: ventilatory support for respiratory failure, tube feedings, intravenous hydration, and antibiotics for secondary infections. Antibiotics directed against *C. botulinum* are indicated in wound botulism, but not other forms. With infants, the concern is lysis of the organism with toxin release in a subset that shows a 99% recovery rate with supportive care alone. This also accounts for the lack of antitoxin use in this group.

PREVENTION

Food-borne botulism is prevented by careful food preservation and handling practices. Specific recommendations are (a) spore destruction with heating to 120°C for 30 minutes (pressure cooker); (b) prevention of germination by reducing pH level, refrigeration, freezing, drying, or adding inhibitory substances— salt, sugar, or sodium nitrate; and (c) inactivation of preformed toxin with heating at 80°C for 20 minutes or 90°C for 10 min-

utes. Careful surveillance, immediate reporting, and swift public health investigation of suspected incidents to determine the source can prevent further cases in an outbreak. If commercial food products or food sources are involved, a single case may herald the beginning of a large outbreak. Therefore, close coordination with local and state public health epidemiologists is critical to management of even apparently isolated cases of botulism. Good sterile practice in surgery and wound management may lessen the rare incidence of wound botulism. Because honey has been implicated as a vehicle for spores in infant botulism, it should not be fed to infants younger than 1 year (78). Pentavalent (A, B, C, D, and E) botulism toxoid (79) may be available from the CDC for immunization of laboratory workers who work with the neurotoxins or neurotoxigenic organisms and pentavalent antitoxin may be available from the U.S. Army if there is reason to suspect an unusual toxin type (11).

REFERENCES

1. Smith LDS, Sugiyama H. *Botulism: the organism, its toxins, the disease,* 2nd ed. Springfield, IL: Charles C Thomas, 1988.
2. Van Ermengem E. Ueber einen neuen anaeroben bacillus und seine beziehungen zum botulismus. *Z Hyg Infektionskr* 1897;26:1.
3. Seddon HR. Bulbar paralysis in cattle due to the action of a toxicogenic bacillus with a discussion of the relationship of the condition to forage poisoning (botulism). *J Comp Pathol Ther* 1922;35:147.
4. Bengtson IA. Preliminary note on a toxin-producing anaerobe isolated from the larvae of *Lucilia Caesar. Public Health Rep* 1922;37:164.
5. Merson MH, Dowell VR Jr. Epidemiologic, clinical, and laboratory aspects of wound botulism. *N Engl J Med* 1973;289:1105.
6. Weber JT, Goodpasture HC, Alexander H, et al. Wound botulism in a patient with a tooth abscess: case report and review. *Clin Infect Dis* 1993;16:635.
7. Pickett J, Berg B, Chaplin E, et al. Syndrome of botulism in infancy: clinical and electrophysiologic study. *N Engl J Med* 1976;295:770.
8. Midura TF, Amon SS. Infant botulism: identification of *Clostridium botulinum* and its toxin in faeces. *Lancet* 1976;2:934.
9. Amon SS: Infant botulism. In: Borriello SP, ed. *Clostridia in gastrointestinal disease.* Boca Raton, FL: CRC Press, 1985:39–57.
10. Centers for Disease Control and Prevention. Botulism—United States, 1978. *MMWR Morb Mortal Wkly Rep* 1979;28:73.
11. Arnon SS, Schechter R, Inglesby TV, et al. Botulinum toxin as a biological weapon. *JAMA* 2001;285:1059.
12. Bengtson IA. Studies on organisms concerned as causative factors in botulism. *Hyg Lab Bull* 1924;136:101.
13. Yang KH, Sugiyama H. Purification and properties of *Clostridium botulinum* type F toxin. *Appl Microbiol* 1975;29:598.
14. Hatheway CL. Toxigenic clostridia. *Clin Microbiol Rev* 1990;3:67.
15. Montecucco C, Schiavo G. Mechanism of action of tetanus and botulinum neurotoxins. *Mol Microbiol* 1994;13:1.
16. Jansen BC. *Clostridium botulinum* type C, its isolation and taxonomic position. In: Eklund MW, Dowell VR Jr, eds. *Avian botulism.* Springfield, IL: Charles C Thomas, 1987:123–132.
17. Cato EP, George WL, Finegold SM. Genus *Clostridium* Prazmuwski 1880, 23. In: Sneath PHA, Mair NS, Sharpe ME, et al, eds. *Bergey's manual of systematic bacteriology,* vol 2. Baltimore: Williams & Wilkins, 1986:1141–1200.
18. Zhou Y, Sugiyama H, Johnson EA. Transfer of neurotoxigenicity from *Clostridium butyricum* to a nontoxigenic *Clostridium botulinum* type E-like strain. *Appl Environ Microbiol* 1993;59:3825.
19. Eklund MW, Poysky FT, Mseitif LM, et al. Evidence for plasmid mediated toxin and bacteriocin production in *Clostridium botulinum* type G. *Appl Environ Microbiol* 1988;54:1405.
20. Zhou Y, Sugiyama H, Nakano H, et al. The genes for the *Clostridium botulinum* type G toxin complex are on a plasmid. *Infect Immun* 1995;63:2087.
21. Bleck TP. *Clostridium botulinum.* In: Mandell GL, Bennett JE, Dolin R, eds. *Principles and practice of infectious diseases,* 5th ed. Philadelphia: Churchill Livingstone, 2000:2543.
22. Eklund MW, Poysky F, Oguma K, et al. Relationship of bacteriophages to toxin and hemagglutinin production and its significance in avian botulism outbreaks. In: Eklund MW, Dowell VR Jr, eds. *Avian botulism.* Springfield, IL: Charles C Thomas, 1987:191–222.
23. Holdeman LV, Cato EP, Moore WEC. *Anaerobe laboratory manual,* 4th ed. Blacksburg, VA: Department of Anaerobic Microbiology, Virginia Polytechnic Institute and State University, 1977.
24. Giménez DF, Ciccarelli AS. Another type of *Clostridium botulinum. Zentralbl Bakteriol Orig A* 1970;215:221.
25. Schroeder K, Tollefsrud A. Botulism fra rekorret. *Tidsskr Nors Laegeforen* 1962;82:1084.
26. Lee WH, Riemann H. The genetic relatedness of proteolytic *Clostridium botulinum* strains. *J Gen Microbiol* 1970;64:85.

27. Nakamura S, Okado I, Nakashio S, et al. *Clostridium sporogenes* isolates and their relationship to *C. botulinum* based on deoxyribonucleic acid reassociation. *J Gen Microbiol* 1977;100:395.

28. Collins MD, Lawson PA, Willems A, et al. The phylogeny of the genus *Clostridium*: proposal of five new genera and eleven new species combinations. *Int J Syst Bacteriol* 1994;44:812.

29. Hatheway CL, McCroskey LM. Unusual neurotoxigenic clostridia recovered from human fecal specimens in the investigation of botulism. In: Hattori T, Ishida Y, Maruyama Y, et al, eds. *Recent advances in microbial ecology.* Tokyo: Japan Scientific Societies Press, 1989:477–481.

30. Moller V, Scheibel I. Preliminary report on the isolation of an apparently new type of *C. botulinum. Acta Pathol Microbiol Scand* 1960;48:80.

31. Midura TF, Nygaard GS, Wood RM, et al. *Clostridium botulinum* type F: isolation from venison jerky. *Appl Microbiol* 1972;24:165.

32. Hall JD, McCroskey LM, Pincomb BJ, et al. Isolation of an organism resembling *Clostridium barati* which produces type F botulinal toxin from an infant with botulism. *J Clin Microbiol* 1985;21:654.

33. McCroskey LM, Hatheway CL, Woodruff BA, et al. Type F botulism due to neurotoxigenic *Clostridium barati* from an unknown source in an adult. *J Clin Microbiol* 1991;29:2618.

34. Green J, Spear H, Brinson RR. Human botulism type F—a rare type. *Am J Med* 1983;75:893.

35. Hauschild AHW. Epidemiology of human foodborne botulism. In: Hauschild AHW, Dodds KL, eds. Clostridium botulinum: *ecology and control in foods.* New York: Marcel Dekker, 1993:69–104.

36. Prevot AR, Terrasse J, Daumail J, et al. Existence en France du botulisme humain de type C. *Bull Acad Natl Med Paris* 1955;139:355.

37. Demarchi J, Mourgues C, Orio J, et al. Existence du botulisme humain de type D. *Bull Acad Natl Med Paris* 1958;142:580.

38. Sonnabend OA, Sonnabend WF, Krech U, et al. Continuous microbiological study of 70 sudden and unexpected infant deaths: toxigenic intestinal *Clostridium botulinum* infection in nine cases of sudden infant death syndrome. *Lancet* 1985;2:237.

39. Smith LDS. The occurrence of *Clostridium botulinum* and *Clostridium tetani* in the soil of the United States. *Health Lab Sci* 1978;15:74.

40. Wainwright RB, Heyward WL, Middaugh JP, et al. Food-borne botulism in Alaska, 1947–1985: epidemiology and clinical findings. *J Infect Dis* 1988;157:1158.

41. Shaffer N, Wainwright RB, Middaugh JP, et al. Botulism among Alaskan Natives. The role of changing food preparation and consumption practices. *West J Med* 1990;153:390.

42. Miller LG, Clark PS, Kunkle GA. Possible origin of *Clostridium botulinum* contamination of Eskimo foods in northwestern Alaska. *Appl Microbiol* 1972;23:427.

43. Centers for Disease Control and Prevention. Botulism outbreak associated with eating fermented food—Alaska 2001. *MMWR Morb Mortal Wkly Rep* 2001;50:680.

44. Centers for Disease Control and Prevention. *Botulism in the United States 1899–1996: handbook for epidemiologists, clinicians, and laboratory workers.* Atlanta: Centers for Disease Control and Prevention, 1998. Available at: www.cdc.gov/ncidod/dbmd/diseaseinfo/botulism.pdf. Accessed September 1, 2001.

45. Shapiro RL, Hatheway C, Swerdlow DL. Botulism in the United States. *Ann Intern Med* 1998;129:221.

46. Davis JB, Mattman LH, Wiley M. *Clostridium botulinum* in a fatal wound infection. *JAMA* 1951;146:646.

47. Dodds KL. Worldwide incidence and ecology of infant botulism. In: Hauschild AHW, Dodds KL, eds. Clostridium botulinum: *ecology and control in foods.* New York: Marcel Dekker, 1993:105–117.

48. Oguma K, Yokota K, Hayashi S, et al. Infant botulism due to *Clostridium botulinum* type C toxin. *Lancet* 1990;336:1449.

49. Aureli P, Fenicia L, Pasolini B, et al. Two cases of type E infant botulism caused by neurotoxigenic *Clostridium butyricum* in Italy. *J Infect Dis* 1986;154:201.

50. Alibek K, Handleman S. *Biohazard.* New York: Random House, 1999.

51. Shapiro RL, Hatheway C, Becher J, et al. Botulism surveillance and emergency response: a public health strategy for a global challenge. *JAMA* 1997;278:433.

52. McCroskey LM, Hatheway CL. Laboratory findings in four cases of adult botulism suggest colonization of the intestinal tract. *J Clin Microbiol* 1988;26:1052.

53. English WL, Williams LP, Bryant RE, et al. Case 48-1980: botulism [Letter]. *N Engl J Med* 1981;304:789.

54. Freedman M, Armstrong RM, Killian JM, et al. Botulism in a patient with jejunoileal bypass. *Ann Neurol* 1986;20:641.

55. Chia JK, Clark JB, Ryan CA, et al. Botulism in an adult associated with food-borne intestinal infection with *Clostridium botulinum. N Engl J Med* 1986;315:239.

56. Isacsohn M, Cohen A, Steiner A, et al. Botulism intoxication after surgery in the gut. *Isr J Med Sci* 1985;21:150.

57. Griffin PM, Hatheway CL, Rosenbaum RB, et al. Endogenous antibody production to *botulinum* toxin in an adult with intestinal colonization botulism and underlying Crohn's disease. *J Infect Dis* 1997;175:633.

58. Simpson LL. Peripheral actions of the *botulinum* toxins. In: Simpson LL, ed. *Botulinum neurotoxin and tetanus toxin.* San Diego, CA: Academic Press, 1989:153–178.

59. Vita G Girlanda P, Puglisi RM, et al. Cardiovascular-reflex testing and single-fiber electromyography in botulism. *Arch Neurol* 1987;44:202.

60. Woodruff BA, Griffin PM, McCroskey LM, et al. Clinical and laboratory comparison of botulism from toxin types A, B, and E in the United States, 1975–1988. *J Infect Dis* 1992;166:1281.

61. Long SS, Gajewski JL, Brown LW, et al. Clinical, laboratory, and environmental features of infant botulism in southeastern Pennsylvania. *Pediatrics* 1985;75:935.

62. Hatheway CL. Botulism. In: Balows A, Hausler WH Jr, Ohashi M, et al, eds. *Laboratory diagnosis of infectious diseases: principles and practice,* vol 1. New York: Springer-Verlag, 1988:111–133.

63. Dowell VR Jr, McCroskey LM, Hatheway CL, et al. Coproexamination for botulinal toxin and *Clostridium botulinum.* A new procedure for laboratory diagnosis of botulism. *JAMA* 1977;238:1829.

64. Easton EJ, Meyer KF. Occurrence of *Bacillus botulinus* in human and animal excreta. *J Infect Dis* 1924;35:207.

65. Hatheway CL, McCroskey LM. Examination of feces and serum for diagnosis of infant botulism in 336 patients. *J Clin Microbiol* 1987;25:2334.

66. Rubin LG, Dezfulian M, Yolkin RH. Serum antibody response to *Clostridium botulinum* toxin in infant botulism. *J Clin Microbiol* 1982;16:770.

67. Hatheway CL, Ferreira JL. Detection and identification of *Clostridium botulinum* neurotoxins. *Adv Exp Med Biol* 1996;391:481.

68. Centers for Disease Control and Prevention. *Botulism in the United States, 1899–1977. Handbook for epidemiologists, clinicians, and laboratory workers.* Public Health Service. Atlanta: US Department of Health, Education, and Welfare, 1979.

69. Cherrington M. Electrophysiologic methods as an aid in diagnosis of botulism: a review. *Muscle Nerve* 1982;5:S28.

70. Masilli RA, Bakshi N. American Association of electrodiagnostic medicine case report 16: botulism. *Muscle Nerve* 2000;23:1137.

71. Cherington M. Clinical spectrum of botulism. *Muscle Nerve* 1998;21:701.

72. Cornblath DR, Sladky JT, Sumner AJ. Clinical electrophysiology of infantile botulism. *Muscle Nerve* 1983;6:448.

73. Morris JG. Current trends in therapy of botulism in the United States. In: Lewis GE Jr, ed. *Biomedical aspects of botulism.* New York: Academic Press, 1981:317–326.

74. Tacket CO, Shandera WX, Mann JM, et al. Equine antitoxin use and other factors that predict outcome in type A food-borne botulism. *Am J Med* 1984;76:794.

75. Lewis GE Jr, Metzger JF. Studies on the prophylaxis and treatment of botulism. In: Eaker D, Wadström T, eds. *Natural toxins.* Oxford, UK: Pergamon Press, 1980:601–606.

76. Black RE, Gunn RA. Hypersensitivity reactions associated with botulinal antitoxin. *Am J Med* 1980;69:567.

77. Hatheway CL, Snyder JD, Seals JE, et al. Antitoxin levels in botulism patients treated with trivalent equine botulism antitoxin to toxin types A, B, and E. *J Infect Dis* 1984;150:407.

78. Amon SS, Midura TF, Damus K, et al. Honey and other environmental risk factors for infant botulism. *J Pediatr* 1979;94:331.

79. Cardella MA. Botulinum toxoids. In: Lewis KH, Cassel K Jr, eds. *Botulism: proceedings of a symposium.* Cincinnati, OH: US Department of Health, Education, and Welfare, 1964:113–130. Public Health Service publication no. 999 FP-1.

CHAPTER 213
Clostridium perfringens *and Other Clostridia*

Sherwood L. Gorbach

The genus *Clostridium* is composed of gram-positive, spore-forming, anaerobic rods that live in soil and in animals. To date, more than 80 species have been defined biochemically and metabolically, and numerous others await characterization (1,2). Usually, these organisms reside in peaceful coexistence with their human or animal host, but given the proper circumstances, their pathogenic potential can be realized. Various clostridia are capable of endogenous and exogenous infection, producing disease that is either toxin mediated or suppurative (3–5).

CHARACTERISTICS OF THE PATHOGEN

Clostridia are ubiquitous throughout nature in animals and soil. All species grow better under anaerobic conditions, but some—*Clostridium perfringens, Clostridium septicum, Clostridium histolyticum,* and *Clostridium tertium*—are remarkably aerotolerant. Clostridia can be distinguished from *Bacillus* species by the absence of catalase, peroxidase, and cytochrome oxidase.

TABLE 213.1. *Clostridium* Species Isolated from Clinical Specimens

Species	Blood cultures	Soft tissue infections	Intraabdominal sepsis	Total
C. perfringens	37	20	4	61
C. ramosum	3	15	5	23
C. bifermentans	2	5	4	11
C. sphenoides	2	4	1	7
C. sporogenes	—	3	3	6
C. innocuum	1	3	2	6
C. difficile	1	3	1	5
C. butyricum	—	3	2	5
C. septicum	2	2	—	4
C. tertium	2	1	—	3
C. sordellii	—	3	—	3
C. limosum	2	—	1	3
C. baratii	1	1	1	3
C. pseudotetanicum	1	1	—	2
C. beijerinckii	—	1	—	2
C. fallax	—	1	1	2
C. ghoni	—	1	1	2
C. carnis	—	1	1	2
C. subterminale	—	2	—	2
C. novyi	—	2	—	1
C. putrificum	1	—	—	1
C. hastiforme	1	—	—	1
C. cadaveris	—	1	1	1
C. paraputrificum	—	—	1	1
Clostridium (unclassified)	11	12	13	36
Total	65	87	43	195

Data from Gorbach SL, Thadepalli H. Isolation of *Clostridium* in human infections: evaluation of 114 cases. *J Infect Dis* 1975;131:581–S85, and Gorbach SL, Thadepalli H, Norsen J. Anaerobic microorganisms in intraabdominal infections. In: Balows A, DeHann RM, Dowell VR Jr, et al., eds. *Anaerobic bacteria: role in disease.* Springfield, IL: Charles C Thomas, 1974:399–407, with permission.

Spore formation, a trait that is useful in species identification, may be either terminal or subterminal, but it is not noted in all clinical isolates, particularly *C. perfringens* and *Clostridium ramosum*, and it may be necessary to use ethanol or heat shock to induce sporulation. By electron microscopy, most clostridia appear as fat, boxcar-shaped rods with a typical gram-positive cell wall. Because many species appear to be gram-negative in clinical material or in late cultures, the tinctorial characteristics should not be an absolute criterion for classification.

About 30 of the 83 clostridial strains described in *Bergey's Manual of Systematic Bacteriology* (6) are involved in infection in humans (Table 213.1). Production of protein toxins has been noted in 14 species, and these species have been associated with certain classic infections such as botulism, tetanus, gas gangrene, pseudomembranous colitis, and food poisoning (Table 213.2).

Normal Flora

Clostridia are present in the normal intestinal flora of humans and of many animal species (1,7–9). The organisms can be isolated from the feces of 70% of humans, at a concentration of 10^8 to 10^9 per gram (9,10). Clostridia are cultured from the vagina of 4% to 10% of healthy women (11–13) and from 19% to 29% after unsanitary abortion (14). A variety of *Clostridium* species are present in the fecal flora, *C. ramosum* being the most common, followed by *C. perfringens* and, in smaller numbers, 30 or more other species. Occasionally, the organisms can be isolated from the skin of the perineum and other cutaneous sites.

Clostridium perfringens

C. perfringens is the species most frequently isolated from clinical material. It has been recovered from virtually every organ site, including infections in the abdomen, female pelvis, skin and soft tissues, and bloodstream (3,15,16). The organism is relatively aerotolerant and exhibits "stormy fermentation" when cultured in milk. It is the fastest growing clostridial species: generation time is 8 minutes under ideal conditions (6). *C. perfringens* can be recognized by its gray, spreading colonies, which often produce a double zone of hemolysis on blood agar, depending on the isolate and culture medium. The organism is known to produce 12 toxins: four major toxins (α, β, ϵ, and ι) and eight minor toxins, including the enterotoxin (1,2) (Table 213.2). On the basis of the distribution of the four major toxins, the species has been divided into five types, A through E (Table 213.3). The α toxin has phospholipase C (lecithinase, PLC) and sphingomyelinase activities, which interact with eukaryotic cell membranes and hydrolyze phosphatidylcholine and sphingomyelin, leading to cell death (17). Its activity, as measured in medium containing egg yoke (Nagler), can be inhibited by specific antitoxin. The α toxin has been purified and crystallized, and its C-terminal domain has been expressed in *Escherichia coli* (18,19). This toxin plays an essential role in the causation of gas gangrene; α toxin causes muscle inflammation and necrosis, platelet aggregation, hemolysis, lethality in animals, vasodilation, and increased vascular permeability (17,20,21). The α toxin directly suppresses myocardial contractility and is associated with reductions in cardiac output and hypotension (22). A hemolysin, θ toxin (perfingolysin O, PFO) is also lethal to mice, and it causes a fall in peripheral vascular resistance,

TABLE 213.2. Toxigenic *Clostridium* Species and Their Toxins

Species	Toxins		Size of molecule (kd)	Activity or disease
C. botulinum	Neurotoxin		150	Botulism
	C_2 (binary)			Permease
		Component I	50	ADP-ribosylation
		Component II	105	Binding
	C_3		25	ADP-ribosylation
C. argentinense (C. botulinum type G)	Neurotoxin		ND[a]	Botulism (experimental)
C. tetani	Neurotoxin		150	Tetanus
	Tetanolysin		48	Oxygen-labile hemolysin
C. perfringens	Major			
	α		43	Phospholipase C/myonecrosis
	β		40	Lethal, necrotic/enterotoxemia
	ε		34	Lethal, permease/enterotoxemia
	ι (binary)			Enterotoxemia
		Component a	48	ADP-ribosylation
		Component b	72	Binding
	Other			
	Enterotoxin		35	Food-borne diarrhea
	δ		42	Hemolysin
	θ		51	Oxygen-labile hemolysin
	κ		80	Collagenase
	λ		ND	Protease
	μ		ND	Hyaluronidase
	ν		ND	DNase
	Neuraminidase		43, 64, 105, 310	N-acetylneuraminic acid glycohydrolase
C. difficile	Toxin A		400–500	Enterotoxin/AAPMC
	Toxin B		360–470	Cytotoxin/AAPMC
	CDT		43	ADP-ribosylation
C. sordellii (C. bifermentans)	α		43	Phospholipase C
	β			Lethal
		HT	525	Equivalent to C. difficile toxin A
		LT	250	Equivalent to C. difficile toxin B
	Hemolysin		43	Oxygen-labile hemolysin
C. novyi, C. haemolyticum	α		260–280	Lethal
	β		32	Phospholipase C
	γ		30	Phospholipase C
	δ		ND	Oxygen-labile hemolysin
	ε		ND	Lipase
C. chauvoei, C. septicum	α		27	Lethal, necrotizing
	β		45	DNase
	γ		ND	Hyaluronidase
	δ		ND	Oxygen-labile hemolysin
C. histolyticum	α		ND	Necrotizing
	β			Collagenases
		Class I	68, 115, 79, 130	
		Class II	100, 110, 125	
	γ		>10, <50	Proteinase, thiol activated
	δ		ND	Proteinase
	ε			Oxygen-labile hemolysin
C. spiroforme	ι (binary)			Diarrhea in rabbits
		Component a	43–47	ADP-ribosylation
		Component b	ND	Binding
C. butyricum	Neurotoxin		145	Botulism, type E
C. baratii	Neurotoxin		ND	Botulism, type F

ND, not determined; AAPMC, antibiotic-associated pseudomembranous colitis; ADP, adenosine diphosphate.
[a]For neurotoxin of *C. argentinense,* a 16S complex of 500 kd has been purified, but the size of its toxic subcomponent has not been determined.
From Hatheway CL. Toxigenic clostridia. *Clin Microbiol Rev* 1990;3:66–98, with permission.

resulting in "warm shock" (22,23). PLC and PLO appear to act synergistically to produce hypotension, hypoxia, and reduced cardiac output, which are the systemic hallmarks of gas gangrene.

C. perfringens type A is responsible for virtually all the infections of humans caused by this species. Types B, D, and E cannot be isolated from soil samples and only rarely are associated with human disease. *C. perfringens* type C is found in pigs. It causes enteritis necroticans (EN), also known as *Darmbrand* (24) and pigbel (25) (see later).

Clostridium septicum

C. septicum distinguished itself in early reports by causing generalized edema and bacteremia in animals (1), and it was the second or third most common cause of gas gangrene in wartime (26).

TABLE 213.3. Distribution of the Major Lethal Toxins Among the Types of *Clostridium perfringens*

Type	TOXIN			
	α	β	ϵ	ι
A	+	−	−	−
B	+	+	+	−
C	+	+	−	−
D	+	−	+	−
E	+	−	−	+

From Smith L, Williams BL. *The pathogenic anaerobic bacteria,* 3rd ed. Springfield, IL: Charles C Thomas, 1984, with permission.

More recently, it has been associated with bacteremia and neutropenic enterocolitis seen in conjunction with malignancy (see later). *C. septicum* is unusually aerotolerant, perhaps accounting for its ability to survive in the bloodstream. Four major toxins and neuraminidase are produced by *C. septicum*; the lethal, necrotizing α toxin and the hemolysin (δ toxin) appear to be responsible for pathogenicity (27,28).

CLINICAL CONDITIONS

A wide range of clostridial species can be isolated from soft tissues (Table 213.1). *C. perfringens* is the most common, although it represents only one fourth of all isolates. *C. ramosum* is nearly as common in soft tissues, and a host of other species are seen with regularity. Clostridia can be recovered from suppurative processes without local or systemic signs of toxin activity. Indeed, it is often impossible to separate the role of clostridia from the roles of multiple other organisms at the same site. In one study, 84% of soft tissue infections that harbored clostridia also contained other bacteria, often as many as 5 to 10 different types (3).

Simple contamination by clostridia, without clinical signs or symptoms, is by all accounts the most frequent setting for isolating clostridial species from clinical material (5). Before antibiotics came into widespread use, clostridia could be isolated from 10% to 30% of wounds in civilians and from up to 80% of war wounds. Even with antibiotic treatment, such as with cephalothin and kanamycin, clostridia were isolated from 16% of penetrating abdominal wounds (29). Clostridia are isolated with similar frequency from suppurating wounds and from well-healing wounds. Indeed, recovery of clostridia from a wound does not determine its clinical status, nor does it dictate specific therapeutic decisions. Clostridial infections (as opposed to contamination) are clinical entities, not bacteriologic diagnoses.

Gas production, detected by palpation or radiologic studies, has been noted in infections caused by clostridia such as gas gangrene, crepitant cellulitis (30), emphysematous cholecystitis (31,32), emphysematous gastritis (33), and emphysematous cystitis. (34–36). Yet, gas production is not unique to clostridial infections: it can be associated with infections by coliforms, streptococci, staphylococci, and *Bacteroides* species (30,37), and even in noninfectious settings such as trauma (air hose injuries, penetrating wounds of the airway or thorax), benzine injection, wound irrigation with hydrogen peroxide, and tracking along an intravascular catheter.

The histotoxic clostridial syndromes include neurologic diseases, botulism (Chapter 212), and tetanus (Chapter 211); enteric diseases such as food poisoning (Chapter 77), EN, and

pseudomembranous colitis (Chapter 74); and soft tissue infections, such as gas gangrene and spontaneous (nontraumatic) myonecrosis (Chapter 95).

Intraabdominal infections, especially those caused by bowel perforation, are associated with clostridia in 30% to 50% of cases (38–41). In a study of 67 patients with intraabdominal infection (29,45), clostridial strains were isolated, including 16 known species and a number of nontypeable ones. *C. ramosum* was the most common isolate, followed by *C. perfringens* and *Clostridium bifermentans*. None of these patients had gas gangrene, and it was impossible to differentiate on clinical grounds those whose specimens yielded *Clostridium* organisms in culture.

The diseased gallbladder is contaminated by clostridia in 10% to 20% of cases sampled at surgery (42–45). Gas gangrene of the abdominal wall can follow cholecystectomy and even laparoscopic cholecystectomy (46). A particularly virulent form of cholangitis, termed *emphysematous cholecystitis* because of gas formation in the biliary tract radicles and the wall of the gallbladder, is caused in at least 50% of cases by clostridial species (31,47–50). More common in male diabetic patients, this complication has a higher mortality rate than other biliary tract infections. There is, however, no evidence of muscle invasion or systemic signs of clostridial toxin; rather, patients succumb to severe sepsis.

Female pelvic infections are associated with clostridia in 4% to 20% of cases, and they are particularly common in patients with tuboovarian or pelvic abscess (51–55). In the era before antibiotic therapy, clostridia were often isolated from discharge of women with septic abortions, indeed, with such frequency in women with mild infection that Ramsey (56) referred to *Clostridium welchii* (*perfringens*) as a harmless saprophyte. Nevertheless, this organism continues to cause severe postpartum infection in the modern era, even in uncomplicated deliveries (57). (For discussion of uterine gas gangrene, see Chapter 102).

Pulmonary infections can be caused by clostridia, but usually they are mixed infections. Clostridia have been isolated from about 10% of patients with various aspiration syndromes, either from empyema fluid or from transtracheal aspirates, and *C. perfringens* is the most frequent isolate (58). There are scattered reports in the older literature of pure *C. perfringens* pulmonary infections (59–66). Clostridia have also been associated with infection after chest injury or thoracotomy (67,68). Like other suppurative clostridial infections, these typically show no signs of local or systemic toxin production; they are indistinguishable from pulmonary infections that do not involve clostridia, notwithstanding the rare case of myonecrosis with gas formation (61,64).

Central nervous system infections involving clostridia are relatively rare, consisting mostly of case reports of penetrating head wounds (69), brain abscess (70–73), or purulent meningitis (74,75). Seventeen cases of clostridial bacterial endocarditis have been reported, including the case of an intravenous drug user who was infected with *C. bifermentans* (76) and a patient with colon cancer who developed endocarditis caused by *C. septicum* (77). When clostridia cause suppurative arthritis, the isolate is usually *C. perfringens*, and the setting is penetrating trauma to the joint, an immunocompromised host, or knee arthroplasty (78–80). A miscellany of chronic wound infections have been associated with clostridia as part of a mixed flora, including diabetic foot ulcers, stump infections, decubitus ulcers, and perirectal infections (4,81).

Intestinal Disorders

Clostridia are known to cause three types of intestinal illness: food poisoning, related to *C. perfringens* type A; EN, caused by

C. perfringens type C; and pseudomembranous colitis (PMC) and its milder form, antibiotic-associated diarrhea, caused by *Clostridium difficile*. These toxin diseases are entirely distinct, and each has its own epidemiology and pathogenesis. (*C. difficile* is discussed in Chapter 74; the epidemiology of food poisoning, in Chapter 77).

EN is a severe, necrotizing disease of the small intestine caused by β-toxin–producing strains of *C. perfringens* type C (82). Known originally by its German name, *Darmbrand*, EN was described in malnourished people in Germany and Norway after World War II (24). Subsequently, the same condition, with the name *pigbel*, was recognized in the highlands of Papua New Guinea (25,83). Scattered reports of EN have come from Africa, Southeast Asia, Nepal, China, and most recently Thailand (83,84). In New Guinea, pigbel accounts for 10% of deaths of children between the ages of 1 and 15 years. It is the most common cause of death in children 6 to 10 years of age, the mortality rate being as high as 30 in 10,000 in some districts (85). Pork consumption is the mode of transmission, either in ritual pig feasting or in a family setting (now the more common venue) (86).

The major pathologic focus of EN is the small intestine, particularly the jejunum, where a spotty coagulative necrosis causes transmural destruction of the intestinal wall (87). The result is a friable mucosa, which often sloughs, leaving deep ulcers that are liable to perforate.

In Papua New Guinea, the disease is said to occur when a specific set of cultural and epidemiologic circumstances coincide (83). The organism, usually acquired by eating undercooked pork, colonizes the host's intestine (88). The basic requirement for disease is a disturbance of the fine balance in the intestinal lumen between toxin production by the organism and toxin destruction by intestinal proteases such as trypsin. Because the unfortunate hosts habitually consume a low-protein diet, the concentration of trypsin in their intestine is low. Trypsin activity is further reduced during the pork meal by simultaneous consumption of sweet potatoes, which contain trypsin inhibitors. In addition, many people are infected with *Ascaris* worms, which produce protein inhibitors. The result is low proteolytic activity in the intestine, with failure to degrade the toxin elaborated by the clostridia that are now attached to the intestinal surface (89). This hypothesis is supported by experiments in which pigbel developed in guinea pigs given *C. perfringens* type C only when sweet potatoes were fed concomitantly (90).

In view of the high mortality rate and the frequent need for surgery (pigbel is the most common indication for laparotomy in the highland hospitals of Papua New Guinea), it is most encouraging to learn of the successful development of a vaccine based on the β toxin. In a field trial, the vaccine conferred significant protection, and subsequent studies in Papua New Guinea have shown a marked reduction in pigbel incidence and mortality (83,91).

Clostridial food poisoning, caused by enterotoxin-producing strains of *C. perfringens* type A, ranks second or third on the list of types of food poisoning in the United States (92,93) (see Chapter 77). Such strains are responsible for about 10% of the diagnosed outbreaks; about 25 epidemics are reported each year, each involving an average of 24 persons (94,95). Hospital outbreaks of clostridial food poisoning have also been reported (96). The usual vehicle is meat or meat products, and there is a high attack rate, often greater than 50%. The organisms are more likely to be heat resistant in outbreaks reported in England, but they tend to be heat sensitive in the United States (2,97). The optimal temperature for *C. perfringens* is 43° to 47°C (98). Although it was originally thought that the toxin was ingested preformed in food, it is now believed that the organism is ingested in its vegetative state and that the toxin is elaborated in the intestinal tract. About 10^8 colony-forming units are required to initiate infection in volunteers; the viable forms cause disease, but spores and cell-free fluid cannot induce clinical symptoms (99,100). The toxin was believed to be related to sporulation, but subsequently it has been shown that nonsporulating cultures can elaborate toxin (101). Enterotoxin-producing strains are isolated from most ill patients; when sensitive methods are employed they can also be recovered from the stools of about 30% of healthy persons (102).

The clinical illness is caused by a heat-labile protein, *C. perfringens* enterotoxin (cpe) with a molecular mass of about 35,000 (103). It is encoded by the *cpe* gene, which is either chromosomal or plasma borne (104). Clostridial enterotoxin induces fluid production in the rabbit ileal loop model (105). It also causes vomiting in monkeys, death in mice, and cytotoxicity in Vero cells (106–108). The toxin differs from cholera toxin in the following respects: clostridial toxin has its maximal activity in the ileum and minimal activity in the duodenum, just the opposite of cholera toxin. Clostridial enterotoxin inhibits glucose transport, damages the intestinal epithelium, and causes protein loss into the intestinal lumen, none of which are observed with cholera toxin (105). It does not affect cyclic adenosine monophosphate (cAMP) levels. *C. perfringens* enterotoxin has a unique mechanism for disturbing cell membrane permeability of eukaryotic cells (109). It binds to a protein receptor on the plasma membrane and inserts into the membrane. The plasma membrane becomes freely permeable to small molecules such as ions and amino acids. The toxin causes cytoskeleton collapse and inhibition of cell metabolism, with resulting cell death and loss of the ability of the intestinal cell to secrete fluid and electrolytes (108,110–112).

The most prominent symptoms of clostridial food poisoning are diarrhea (90% of cases) and moderate to severe midepigastric pain (80%); additional findings include nausea (25%), vomiting (9%), and fever (24%), but the entire illness generally lasts less than 24 hours (95,113,114).

An outbreak of clostridial food poisoning should be suspected when the incubation period is short (8 to 12 hours), a meat product is incriminated, the attack rate is 50% or greater, and the illness lasts less than 24 hours.

Three criteria are used to establish the diagnosis of *C. perfringens* food poisoning: more than 10^5 *C. perfringens* organisms per gram of incriminated food; a median spore count of more than 10^6 *C. perfringens* organisms per gram of stool from ill persons; or isolation of the same serotype of *C. perfringens* from stools and suspected food (115,116).

For *C. perfringens* type A, serotyping has limited value in the United States because only 40% of strains can be typed (94); nevertheless, this method may be useful in some epidemics, especially when tests of food items fail to demonstrate clostridia (117). Plasmid profiles can be a helpful typing system, but their role is limited because not all enterotoxin strains have detectable plasmids (118). The fecal spore count can also be unreliable because in an outbreak, ill and healthy people can have the same count. Alternative methods of enterotoxin detection in stool are enzyme-linked assay (119), Vero cell assay (120), and the preferred test, reverse passive latex agglutination assay (121).

Bacteremia

In a large general hospital, in which good anaerobic technique was used, clostridia were found in 0.3% of all blood cultures and represented 2.6% of the positive isolates (3). *C. perfringens* accounts for 60% of the blood cultures that grow clostridia;

the prevalence of *C. perfringens* in soft tissues is about 25% of all clostridia isolated in culture (Table 213.1). Yet, clostridia bacteremia often represents an intriguing paradox, in that a "positive" blood culture is not necessarily associated with serious illness—and in some cases cannot be correlated with the patient's clinical condition. Of patients who had a septic abortion, for example, positive clostridial blood cultures were noted in 18% to 27%, most of whom had a benign disease course, even without antibiotics, and none of whom had evidence of gas gangrene (56,122–124). In another series of 29 patients with clostridial bacteremia, only 12 had a concurrent infection involving clostridia, whereas the others had "spontaneous" clostridial bacteremia documented at the time of admission to the hospital for a variety of unrelated medical conditions (3). These patients recovered from their primary illness, and the source of the *Clostridium* in the bloodstream was never uncovered. On the other hand, three studies reported that more than 95% of cases of clostridial bacteremia were clinically significant. These patients' mortality rate was 43% to 48%, nearly all attributable to the clostridial infection (125–127). Two thirds of these infections were related to intraabdominal sources; half were associated with malignancy, mostly colon cancer. Several studies have shown that anaerobic bacteremia has decreased, probably as a result of early and appropriate use of antimicrobial drugs in suspected cases. Nevertheless, clostridia accounted for 31% of significant anaerobic bacteremias in one series, with an attributable mortality rate of 45%. *C. perfringens* and *C. septicum* were present in equal frequencies, 38% each (128). Thus, clostridial bacteremia must be treated with respect, and colon cancer should be suspected, but the experience in at least some hospitals is that many such cases are in fact benign or spontaneous.

Several clostridial species have been associated with malignancy, including *C. perfringens* (1,129,130), *C. ramosum* (3), *C. difficile* (3), *Clostridium sordellii* (131), *C. histolyticum* (132), *C. tertium* (133), and *Clostridium sporogenes* (134). Yet, when cases of clostridial bacteremia were reviewed in a general hospital, only 3% to 4% were, in fact, associated with malignancy (3,135).

C. septicum bacteremia represents a special case. Under healthy conditions, *C. septicum* is a rather rare inhabitant of the normal intestinal flora (9,129,136–138), although it has been isolated from the ileum and appendix, especially from patients with leukemia (139). In a review of 162 bacteremia cases in the world literature, 89% were related to malignancy (140); this percentage is nearly identical to that cited in the initial review of *C. septicum* bacteremia published some 20 years earlier (141). About half of the patients with bacteremia had colon cancer, whereas most of the others had hematologic malignancies, and a few had some other tumor. Nearly 20% of the subjects had diabetes. Remarkably, 37% of patients presenting with *C. septicum* bacteremia were found at a later examination to have an occult malignancy, of which 84% were located in the large bowel.

Besides the usual signs of sepsis, *C. septicum* bacteremia often has findings related to the abdomen, including abdominal pain, tenderness, vomiting, and diarrhea. About one fourth of patients have metastatic infection and myonecrosis at a distant site (see Chapter 95). Although the clinical picture is often dramatic, such cases are relatively rare, and *C. septicum* is responsible for only 1% to 3% of all clostridial bacteremias (3,142,143).

Neutropenia, associated with leukemia or lymphoproliferative disorders or with cyclic neutropenia, has also been correlated with *C. septicum* bacteremia (3,135,144–146). The intestinal mucosa of the terminal ileum and cecum in such patients is often involved with neutropenic enterocolitis, a condition characterized by mucosal infiltrates of leukemic deposits and necrosis (147). *C. septicum* can be seen penetrating the bowel wall at sites of

mucosal damage. Many patients with leukemia, especially those with neutropenia secondary to disease or to chemotherapy, have inflamed, necrotic areas in the ileum and colon, even without evidence of infection (148–151). It is likely that *C. septicum* makes its way through an intestinal mucosa damaged by the underlying disease, aided and abetted by toxin production and its relative aerotolerance (140,149); the absence of neutrophils, which is almost universal in leukemia patients with clostridial bacteremia, facilitates dissemination of the organism into the bloodstream and to other parts of the body (152).

About 20% of patients with *C. septicum* bacteremia have diabetes (140,153). Complications of diabetes, such as foot ulcers and amputation stumps, may be contaminated with this species and other clostridia (81,154).

C. tertium bacteremia is also associated with neutropenia (155–157). This species is somewhat unusual in that it is resistant to β-lactam antibiotics as well as to clindamycin and metronidazole, but it is sensitive to vancomycin, trimethoprim-sulfamethoxazole, and ciprofloxacin. Presenting symptoms are often related to the abdomen or perirectal area. In contrast to *C. septicum* bacteremia, the outcome with *C. tertium* bacteremia is often favorable when appropriate antibiotics are employed.

TREATMENT

The therapeutic approach, whether medical or surgical, must be tailored to the specific clinical condition and the incriminated *Clostridium* strain. Simple contamination of open wounds by clostridia is managed with good wound care and calculated avoidance of antibiotics. Judicious surgical débridement may be necessary, depending on clinical circumstances. Suppurative infections that involve clostridia—for example, in the abdomen or female pelvis—should be treated with broad-spectrum antibiotics to suppress the aerobic and anaerobic bacteria that are invariable components of this infection. Patients with benign clostridial bacteremia generally should not be treated with antibiotics, although the incriminated pathogen may dictate otherwise (e.g., patients with *C. septicum* or *C. tertium* bacteremia require early and aggressive treatment). Obviously, when bacteremia is associated with organ site involvement or soft tissue infection, therapy is indicated. Clostridial infections that are related to toxin production may, in some circumstances, be treated with immunotherapy. Tetanus and botulism should be managed with passive antibodies in the form of specific immunoglobulin. Vaccines can be used for tetanus and EN. On the other hand, immunotherapy is not indicated for *C. difficile* diarrhea, *C. perfringens* food poisoning, or gas gangrene (see Chapter 95).

Antibiotic therapy should be used in clinically significant clostridial infections (with the notable exception of *C. perfringens* food poisoning). Antimicrobial susceptibility tests *in vitro* have shown a somewhat variable pattern (158–165) (Table 213.4). Most strains of *C. perfringens* are sensitive to β-lactam antibiotics, although some resistance to penicillin at low concentrations has been encountered. Clindamycin is also active against this species, but resistance has been noted in *C. ramosum* and *C. tertium*. In general, antibiotic resistance has been seen most often in strains of *C. ramosum*, *C. sporogenes*, and *C. tertium* (which is resistant to β-lactam antibiotics, clindamycin, and metronidazole) (155–157).

Resistance of clostridia to β-lactam antibiotics can be explained by β-lactamase production or decreased affinity of penicillin-binding proteins (PBPs) (166). Three species, *Clostridium butyricum*, *Clostridium clostridioforme*, and *C. ramosum*, produce β-lactamase (166–170); the enzymes are usually inducible,

TABLE 213.4. Susceptibility (%) of *Clostridium* Species to Antimicrobial Agents

Antimicrobial drug (μg/mL)	C. perfringens	C. difficile	C. septicum	C. botulinum	C. ramosum	C. bifermentans
Penicillin (1)	93	92	100	95	49	100
Metronidazole (4)	73	99	100	100	50	—
Clindamycin (4)	99	77	100	94	30	100
Cephalothin (16)	100	49	100	98	—	—
Cefoxitin (16)	100	15	100	99	—	—
Cefotaxime (16)	—	—	100	—	—	—
Inipenem (4)	100	0	—	—	—	—
Vancomycin (4)	—	99	100	88	49	—
Chloramphenicol (16)	99	93	100	100	100	100

Data from references 156–163.

and some of the strains can be inhibited by cefoxitin and sulbactam. Plasmid-mediated β-lactamase has been found only in *C. ramosum* (171), and most of the other enzyme-producing strains are thought to be chromosomally mediated. PBPs have been found in *C. perfringens*: β-lactam affinity is greatest for PBP 3 and PBP 4 (172). Reduced affinity to PBP 1 of *C. perfringens* has been associated with increased resistance to penicillin (173).

Animal models of clostridial infections, mostly *C. perfringens*, have shown that antibiotics that inhibit protein synthesis (clindamycin, tetracycline, chloramphenicol) produce higher survival rates than cell wall drugs such as penicillin, and this may be related to inhibition of toxin production (174,175). Metronidazole and rifampin are also superior to penicillin in animal models (174,176,177). Yet, animal models are artificial, especially because surgery and adjunctive therapy are not used. Furthermore, penicillin can be given in large doses to humans because it is not toxic, whereas most other drugs have a limited safe dose range.

Penicillin therapy for *C. perfringens* infections has enjoyed a long and largely untarnished record (4,165–182), although it must be conceded that this experience is based on anecdotal observation rather than controlled trials. With regard to *C. septicum*, data from studies *in vitro* (165,182) and clinical experience establish its extreme sensitivity to penicillin as well as to other antibiotics. Resistance to penicillin may be encountered with *C. tertium*, *C. ramosum*, and *C. sporogenes*, and infections with these organisms should be treated with other antibiotics, according to their sensitivity.

REFERENCES

1. Smith LD, Williams BL. *The pathogenic anaerobic bacteria*. Springfield, IL: Charles C Thomas, 1984.
2. Hatheway CL. Toxigenic clostridia. *Clin Microbiol Rev* 1990;3:66.
3. Gorbach SL, Thadepalli H. Isolation of *Clostridium* in human infections: evaluation of 114 cases. *J Infect Dis* 1975;131:S81.
4. Finegold SM. *Anaerobic bacteria in human disease*. New York: Academic Press, 1977.
5. MacLennan JD. The histotoxic clostridial infections of man. *Bacteriol Rev* 1962;26:177.
6. Cato EP, George WL, Finegold SM. Genus *Clostridium* Prazmowski 1880, 23. In Sneath PHA, Mair NS, Sharpe ME, et al., eds. *Bergey's manual of systematic bacteriology*, Vol 2. Baltimore: Williams & Wilkins, 1986:1141–1200.
7. Smith LDS, Gardner VM. Vegetative cells of *Clostridium perfringens* in soil. *J Bacteriol* 1949;58:407.
8. Beerens H, Delcourte F. Caractère différential entre *Clostridium perfringens* fécal et tellurique. *Ann Inst Pasteur* 1958;195:739, 1958.
9. Finegold SM, Attebery HR, Sutter VL. Effect of diet on human fecal flora: comparison of Japanese and American diets. *Am J Clin Nutr* 1974;27:1456.
10. Stringer MF, Watson GN, Gilbert RJ, et al. Fecal carriage of *Clostridium perfringens*. *J Hyg* 1985;95:277.
11. Gorbach SL, Menda KB, Thadepalli H, et al. Anaerobic microflora of the cervix in healthy women. *Am J Obstet Gynecol* 1973;117:1053.
12. Ohm MJ, Galask RP. The effect of antibiotic prophylaxis on patients undergoing vaginal operations. *Am J Obstet Gynecol* 1975;123:597.
13. Bartlett JG, Onderdonk AB, Drude E, et al. Quantitative bacteriology of the vaginal flora. *J Infect Dis* 1977;136:271.
14. Holtz F, Mauch EW. Gas gangrene of uterus: survival following hysterectomy. *Obstet Gynecol* 1962;19:545.
15. Martin WJ. Isolation and identification of anaerobic bacteria in the clinical laboratory: a 2-year experience. *Mayo Clin Proc* 1974;49:300.
16. Finegold SM, George WL, Mulligan ME. Anaerobic infections. *Dis Mon* 1985;31:10.
17. Titball RW. Bacterial phospholipases C. *Microbiol Rev* 1993;57:347.
18. Basak AK, Stuart DI, Nikura T, et al. Purification, crystallization and preliminary X-ray diffraction studies of alpha-toxin of *Clostridium perfringens*. *J Mol Biol* 1994;244:648.
19. Titball RW Fearn AM, Williamson ED. Biochemical and immunological properties of the C-terminal domain of the alpha-toxin of *Clostridium perfringens*. *FEMS Microbiol Lett* 1993;110:45.
20. Williamson ED, Titball RW. A genetically engineered vaccine against the alpha-toxin of *Clostridium perfringens* protects mice against experimental gas gangrene. *Vaccine* 1993;11:1253.
21. Awad MM, Bryant AE, Stevens DL, et al. Virulence studies on chromosomal alpha-toxin and theta-toxin mutants constructed by allelic exchange provide genetic evidence for the essential role of alpha-toxin in *Clostridium perfringens*–mediated gas gangrene. *Mol Microbiol* 1995;15:191.
22. Stevens DL, Bryant AE. The role of clostridial toxins in the pathogenesis of gas gangrene. *Clin Infect Dis* 2002;35:S93–S100.
23. Awad MM, Ellemor DM, Boyd RL, et al. Synergistic effects of alpha-toxin and perfringolysin O in *Clostridium perfringens*–mediated gas gangrene. *Infect Immun* 2001;69(12):7904–7910.
24. Zeissler J, Rassfeld-Sternberg L. Enteritis necroticans due to *Clostridium welchii* type F. *Br Med J* 1949;1:267.
25. Murrell TCG, Egerton JR, Rampling A, et al. The ecology and epidemiology of the pig bel syndrome in New Guinea. *J Hyg* 1966;64:375.
26. MacLennan JD. Anaerobic infections of war wounds in the Middle East. *Lancet* 1943;2:94.
27. Bernheimer AW. Parallelism in the lethal and hemolytic activity of the toxin of *Cl. septicum*. *J Exp Med* 1944;80:309.
28. Moussa RS. Complexity of toxins from *Clostridium septicum* and *Clostridium chauvoei*. *J Bacteriol* 1958;76:538.
29. Thadepalli H, Gorbach SL, Broido PW, et al. Abdominal trauma, anaerobes, and antibiotics. *Surg Gynecol Obstet* 1973;137:270.
30. Nichols RL, Smith JW. Gas in the wound: What does it mean? *Surg Clin North Am* 1975;55:1289.
31. Ram MD, Ghavari MA. Biliary infections and the choice of antibiotics. *Am J Gastroenterol* 1974;62:134.
32. Mentzer RM Jr, Golden GT, Chandler JG, et al. Emphysematous cholecystitis: an important clinical variant of acute cholecystitis. *Rev Surg* 1974;31:454.
33. Stephenson SE Jr, Yasrebi H, Rhatigan R, et al. Acute phlegmasia of the stomach. *Am Surg* 1970;36:225.
34. Lazurus JA. *Bacillus welchii* infections complicating surgical procedures upon the upper urinary tract. *J Urol* 1944;51:315.
35. Greene MH. Emphysematous cystitis due to *Clostridium perfringens* and *Candida albicans* in two patients with hematologic malignant conditions. *Cancer* 1992;70:2658.
36. Katz DS, Aksoy E, Cunha BA. *Clostridium perfringens* emphysematous cystitis. *Urology* 1993;41:458.
37. Bessman AN, Wagner W. Nonclostridial gas gangrene: report of 48 cases and review of the literature. *JAMA* 1962;182:23.
38. Gorbach SL, Thadepalli H, Norsen J. Anaerobic microorganisms in intraabdominal infections. In: Balows A, DeHann RM, Dowell VR Jr, et al., eds.

Anaerobic bacteria: role in disease. Springfield, IL: Charles C Thomas, 1974: 399–407.

39. Dunn DL, Simmons RL. The role of anaerobic bacteria in intra-abdominal infections. *Rev Infect Dis* 1984;6:5139.

40. Moore WEC, Cato EP, Holdeman LV. Anaerobic bacteria of the gastrointestinal flora and their occurrence in clinical infections. *J Infect Dis* 1969;119:641.

41. Stone HH, Kolb LD, Geheber CE. Incidence and significance of intraperitoneal anaerobic bacteria. *Ann Surg* 1975;181:705.

42. Gordon-Taylor G, Whitby LEK. The incidence of anaerobic infections in the gallbladder. *Br J Surg* 1932;19:619.

43. England DM, Rosenblatt JE. Anaerobes in human biliary tract. *J Clin Microbiol* 1977;6:494.

44. Lykkegaard NM, Justesen T. Anaerobic and aerobic bacteriological studies in biliary tract disease. *Scand J Gastroenterol* 1976;11:437.

45. Shimada K, Inamatsu R, Yamashiro M. Anaerobic bacteria in biliary disease in elderly patients. *J Infect Dis* 1977;135:850.

46. Samel S, Post S, Martell J, et al. Clostridial gas gangrene of the abdominal wall after laparoscopic cholecystectomy. *J Laparoendosc Adv Surg Tech* 1997;7:245–247.

47. Sarmiento RV. Emphysematous cholecystitis: report of four cases and review of the literature. *Arch Surg* 1966;93:1099.

48. Edinburgh A, Geffen A. Acute emphysematous cholecystitis. *Am J Surg* 1958;96:66.

49. Mentzer RM Jr, Golden GT, Chandler JG, et al. A comparative appraisal of emphysematous cholecystitis. *Am J Surg* 1975;129:11.

50. Hegner CF. Gaseous pericholecystitis with cholecystitis and cholelithiasis. *Arch Surg* 1931;22:993.

51. Thadepalli H, Gorbach SL, Keith L. Anaerobic infections of the female genital tract: bacteriologic and therapeutic aspects. *Am J Obstet Gynecol* 1973;117:103.

52. Swenson RM, Michaelson TC, Daly MJ, et al. Anaerobic bacterial infections of the female genital tract. *Obstet Gynecol* 1973;42:538.

53. DiZerega GS, Yonekura ML, Keegan K, et al. Bacteremia in postcesarean section endomyometritis: differential response to therapy. *Obstet Gynecol* 1980;55:587.

54. Sweet RL. Anaerobic infections of the female genital tract. *Am J Obstet Gynecol* 1975;122:891.

55. Ledger WJ, Norman M, Gee C, et al. Bacteremia on an obstetric-gynecologic service. *Am J Obstet Gynecol* 1975;121:205.

56. Ramsay AM. The significance of *Clostridium welchii* in the cervical swab and blood stream in postpartum and postabortum sepsis. *J Obstet Gynaecol Br Commonw* 1949;56:247.

57. Dylewski J, Wiesenfeld H, Latour A. Postpartum uterine infection with *Clostridium perfringens*. *Rev Infect Dis* 1989;11:470.

58. Bartlett JG. Anaerobic bacterial infections of the lung. *Chest* 1987;91:901.

59. Bayer AS, Nelson SC, Galpin JE, et al. Necrotizing pneumonia and empyema due to *Clostridium perfringens*. *Am J Med* 1975;59:851.

60. O'Donnell AE. Primary clostridial pneumonia: report of a case. *Lancet* 1952;2:367.

61. Sweeting J, Rosenberg L. Primary clostridial pneumonia. *Ann Intern Med* 1959;151:805.

62. Jacox R. A case report of an unusual lung abscess due to *Clostridium perfringens* (B. welchii). *Ann Intern Med* 1951;34:479.

63. Glaser LF, Glynn R, Ernest HB. Gas bacillus gangrene of lung. *JAMA* 1941;116:827.

64. Goldberg NM, Rifkind D. Clostridial empyema. *Arch Intern Med* 1941;116:421.

65. Mamborg AS, Rylander M, Selander H. Primary thoracic empyema caused by *Clostridium sporogenes*. *Scand J Infect Dis* 1970;2:155.

66. Hardison JE. Primary clostridial pneumonia and empyema. *Chest* 1970;57:390.

67. Elliot TR, Henry H. Infections of hemothorax by anaerobic gas producing bacilli. *Br Med J* 1917;1:413.

68. Lynch JF, Strieder J. Hemothorax complicated by infection with *Clostridium welchii*. *N Engl J Med* 1942;226:685.

69. Cairns H, Calbert CA, Daniel P, et al. Complications of head wounds with special reference to infection. *Br J Surg* 1947;(War Surg Suppl):198.

70. Keogh AJ. Clostridial brain abscess and hyperbaric oxygen. *Postgrad Med J* 1973;49:64.

71. Russell JA, Taylor JC. Circumscribed gas gangrene abscess of the brain: case report together with an account of the literature. *Br J Surg* 1963;50:434.

72. Clark PR. Gas gangrene abscess of the brain. *J Neurol Neurosurg Psychiatry* 1958;31:391.

73. Gilbert AI, Tolmach RS, Farrell JJ. Gas gangrene of the brain. *Am J Surg* 1961;101:366.

74. Colwell FG, Sullivan J, Shuman HH, et al. Acute purulent meningitis due to *Clostridium perfringens*. *N Engl J Med* 1960;262:618.

75. Heidemann SM, Meert KL, Perrin E, et al. Primary clostridial meningitis in infancy. *Pediatr Infect Dis J* 1989;8:126.

76. Kolander SA, Cosgrove EM, Molavi A. Clostridial endocarditis: report of a case caused by *Clostridium bifermentans* and review of the literature. *Arch Intern Med* 1989;149:455.

77. Ridgway EJ, Grech ED. Clostridial endocarditis: report of a case caused by *Clostridium septicum* and review of the literature. *J Infect* 1993;26:309.

78. Fauser DJ, Zuckerman JD. Clostridial septic arthritis: case report and review of the literature. *Arthritis Rheum* 1988;31:295.

79. Wilde AH, Sweeney RS, Borden LS. Hematogenously acquired infection of a total knee arthroplasty by *Clostridium perfringens*. *Clin Orthop* 1988;229:228.

80. Stern SH, Sculco TP. *Clostridium perfringens* infection in a total knee arthroplasty: A case report. *J Arthroplasty* 1988;3(Suppl):S37.

81. George WL. Other infections of skin, soft tissue, and muscle. In: Finegold SM, George WL, eds. *Anaerobic infections in humans.* San Diego: Academic Press, 1989:485–506.

82. Rood JI. Virulence genes of clostridium perfringens. *Annu Rev Microbiol* 1998;52:333–360.

83. Murrell TGC. Enteritis necroticans. In: Finegold SM, George LW, eds. *Anaerobic infections in humans.* San Diego: Academic Press, 1989:639–659.

84. Johnson S, Escheverria P, Taylor DN, et al. Enteritis necroticans among Khmer children at an evacuation site in Thailand. *Lancet* 1987;2:496.

85. Smith D. Mortality from pig-bel (enteritis necroticans) in children in Tari 1971 to 1976. *Papua New Guinea Med J* 1979;22:24.

86. Millar JS, Smellie S. Antecedent nutritional status of children with enteritis necroticans. In: Davis MW, ed. *Pig bel: necrotizing enteritis in Papua New Guinea.* Goroka: Papua New Guinea Institute of Medical Research, 1984:47–49.

87. Cooke R. The pathology of pig bel. *Papua New Guinea Med J* 1979;22:35.

88. Murrell TGC, Walker PD. Pig bel: a zoonosis? *J Trop Med Hyg* 1978;81:231.

89. Lawrence G. Necrotizing enteritis and *Clostridium perfringens*. *J Infect Dis* 1986;153:803.

90. Lawrence G, Cooke R. Experimental pigbel: the production and pathology of necrotizing enteritis due to *Clostridium welchii* type C in the guinea pig. *Br J Exp Pathol* 1980;61:261.

91. Lawrence G, Shann F, Freestone DS, et al. Prevention of necrotising enteritis in Papua New Guinea by active immunisation. *Lancet* 1979;1:227.

92. MacDonald KL, Griffin PM. Foodborne disease outbreaks, annual summary, 1982. *MMWR Morb Mortal Wkly Rep* 1985;35:7SS.

93. Johnson CC. *Clostridium perfringens* food poisoning. In: Finegold SM, George WL, eds. *Anaerobic infections in humans.* San Diego: Academic Press, 1989:629–638.

94. Hatheway CL, Whaley DN, Dowell VR Jr. Epidemiological aspects of *Clostridium perfringens* foodborne illness. *Food Technol* 1980;34:77, 90.

95. Shandera WX, Tacker CO, Blake PA. Food poisoning due to *Clostridium perfringens* in the United States. *J Infect Dis* 1983;147:167.

96. Regan CM, Syed Q, Tunstall PJ. A hospital outbreak of *Clostridium perfringens* food poisoning: implications for food hygiene review in hospitals. *J Hosp Infect* 1995;29:69.

97. Hall HE, Angelotti R. *Clostridium perfringens* in meat and meat products. *Appl Microbiol* 1965;13:353.

98. Hobbs BC. *Clostridium welchii* and *Bacillus cereus* infection and intoxication. *Postgrad Med J* 1974;50:597.

99. Dische FE, Elek SD. Experimental food poisoning by *Clostridium welchii*. *Lancet* 1957;2:71.

100. Hauschild AHW, Thatcher FS. Experimental food poisoning with heat-susceptible *Clostridium perfringens* type A. *J Food Sci* 1967;32:467.

101. Goldner SB, Solberg M, Jones S, et al. Enterotoxin synthesis by nonsporulating cultures of *Clostridium perfringens*. *Appl Environ Microbiol* 1986;52:407.

102. Uemura T. Incidence of enterogenic *Clostridium perfringens* in healthy humans in relation to the enhancement of enterotoxin production by heat treatment. *J Appl Bacteriol* 1978;44:411.

103. Stark RL, Duncan CL. Biological characteristics of *Clostridium perfringens* type A enterotoxin. *Infect Immun* 1971;4:89.

104. Brynestad S, Granum PE. Clostridium perfringens and foodborne infections. *Int J Food Microbiol* 2002;74(3):195–202.

105. McDonel JL, Duncan CL. Regional localization of activity of *Clostridium perfringens* type A enterotoxin in the rabbit ileum, jejunum and duodenum. *J Infect Dis* 1977;136:661.

106. Niilo L. Measurement of biological activities of purified and crude enterotoxin of *Clostridium perfringens*. *Infect Immun* 1975;12:440.

107. Granum PE, Skjelkvale R. Chemical modification and characterization of enterotoxin from *Clostridium perfringens* type A. *Acta Pathol Microbiol Scand* 1977;95:89.

108. McDonel JL, McClane BA. Binding versus biologic activity of *Clostridium perfringens* enterotoxin in Vero cells. *Biochem Biophys Res Commun* 1979;87:497.

109. McClane BA. *Clostridium perfringens* enterotoxin acts by producing small molecule permeability alterations in plasma membranes. *Toxicology* 1994;87:43.

110. McDonel JL. Binding of *Clostridium perfringens* enterotoxin to rabbit intestinal cells. *Biochemistry* 1980;21:4801.

111. McClane BA, McDonel JL. The effects of *Clostridium perfringens* enterotoxin on morphology, viability and macromolecular synthesis in Vero cells. *J Cell Physiol* 1979;99:191.

112. McClane BA, Hanna PC, Wnek AP. *Clostridium perfringens* enterotoxin. *Microb Pathog* 1988;5:317.

113. Finegold SM. *Anaerobic bacteria in human disease.* New York: Academic Press, 1977:511–512.

114. Skjelkvale R, Uemura R. Experimental diarrhoea in human volunteers following oral administration of *Clostridium perfringens* enterotoxin. *J Appl Bacteriol* 1977;43:281.
115. Hauschild AHW. Criteria and procedures for implicating *Clostridium perfringens* in foodborne outbreaks. *Can J Public Health* 1975;66:388.
116. Birkhead G, Vogt RL, Heum EM, et al. Characterization of an outbreak of *Clostridium perfringens* food poisoning by quantitative fecal culture and fecal enterotoxin measurement. *J Clin Microbiol* 1988;26:471.
117. Gross TP, Kamara LB, Hathaway CL, et al. *Clostridium perfringens* food poisoning: use of serotyping in an outbreak setting. *J Clin Microbiol* 1989;4:660.
118. Eisgruber H, Wiedmann M, Stolle A. Use of plasmid profiling as a typing method for epidemiologically related *Clostridium perfringens* isolates from food poisoning cases and outbreaks. *Lett Appl Microbiol* 1995;20:290.
119. McClane BA, Strouse RJ. Rapid detection of *Clostridium perfringens* type A enterotoxin by enzyme-linked immunosorbent assay. *J Clin Microbiol* 1984;19:112.
120. Larson HE, Borriello SP. Infectious diarrhea due to *Clostridium perfringens*. *J Infect Dis* 1988;157:390.
121. Harmon SM, Kautter DA. Evaluation of a reverse passive latex agglutination test kit for *Clostridium perfringens* enterotoxin. *J Food Prot* 1986;49:523.
122. Decker WH, Hall W. Treatment of abortion infected with *Clostridium welchii*. *Am J Obstet Gynecol* 1966;95:394.
123. Smith LP, McLean AP, Maughan GB. *Clostridium welchii* septicotoxemia. *Am J Obstet Gynecol* 1971;110:135.
124. Pritchard JA, Whalley PJ. Abortion complicated by *Clostridium perfringens* infection. *Am J Obstet Gynecol* 1971;111:484.
125. Chu DZ, Fainstein V, Bodey GP, et al. Necrotizing gas-forming infections in cancer patients. *South Med J* 1989;82:860.
126. Tanable KK, Jones WG, Barie PS. Clostridial sepsis and malignant disease. *Surg Gynecol Obstet* 1989;169:423.
127. Rechner PM, Agger WA, Mruz K, et al. Clinical features of clostridial bacteremia: a review from a rural area. *Clin Infect Dis* 2001;33(3):349–353.
128. Lombardi DP, Engleberg NC. Anaerobic bacteremia: incidence, patient characteristics, and clinical significance [see Comments]. *Am J Med* 1992;92:53.
129. Cabrera A, Tsukada Y, Pickren JW. Clostridial gas gangrene and septicemia in malignant disease. *Cancer* 1965;18:800.
130. Burrell MI, Hyson EA, Walker-Smith GI. Spontaneous clostridial infection and malignancy. *AJR Am J Roentgenol* 1980;134:1153.
131. Thys JP, Ectors P, Noel P. Nontraumatic clostridial myositis: an unusual feature of brain death. *Postgrad Med J* 1980;56:501.
132. Kaiser CW, Milgrom ML, Lynch JA. Distant nontraumatic clostridial myonecrosis and malignancy. *Cancer* 1986;57:885.
133. Mzabi R, Himal HS, MacLean LD. Gas gangrene of the extremity: the presenting clinical picture in perforating carcinoma of the caecum. *Br J Surg* 1975;62:373.
134. Jones LE, Wirth WA, Farrow CC. Clostridial gas gangrene and septicemia complicating leukemia. *South Med J* 1960;53:863.
135. Epidemiological Research Laboratory of the Public Health Service. *Clostridium welchii* from blood culture. *Br Med J* 1976;1:845.
136. Draser BS, Goddard P, Heaton S, et al. Clostridia isolated from faeces. *J Med Microbiol* 1976;9:63.
137. Moore WEC, Holdeman IV. Human fecal flora: the normal flora of 20 Japanese-Hawaiians. *Appl Microbiol* 1974;27:961.
138. Holdeman LV, Good IJ, Moore WEC. Human fecal flora: variations in bacterial composition with individuals and a possible effect of emotional stress. *Appl Environ Microbiol* 1974;31:359.
139. Borriello SP. Newly described clostridial diseases of the gastrointestinal tract: *Clostridium perfringens* enterotoxin-associated diarrhea and neutropenic enterocolitis due to *Clostridium septicum*. In: Borriello SP, ed. *Clostridia in gastrointestinal disease*. Boca Raton, FL: CRC Press, 1985:223–229.
140. Kornbluth AA, Danzig JB, Bernstein LH. *Clostridium septicum* infection and associated malignancy. *Medicine* (Baltimore) 1989;68:30.
141. Alpern RJ, Dowell VR. *Clostridium septicum* infections and malignancy. *JAMA* 1969;209:385.
142. Wilson WR, Martin WJ, Wilkowske CJ, et al. Anaerobic bacteremia. *Mayo Clin Proc* 1972;47:639.
143. Lewis JF, Mullins N, Johnson P. Isolation and evaluation of clostridia from clinical sources. *South Med J* 1980;73:427.
144. Gazzaniga AB. Nontraumatic, clostridial gas gangrene of the right arm and adenocarcinoma of the cecum: report of a case. *Dis Colon Rectum* 1967;10:298.
145. Graham BS, Johnson AC, Sawyers JL. Clostridial infection of renal cell carcinoma. *J Urol* 1986;135:354.
146. Bretzke ML, Bubrick MP, Hitchcock CR. Diffuse spreading *Clostridium septicum* infections, malignant disease and immune suppression. *Surg Gynecol Obstet* 1988;166:197.
147. Lev R, Sweeney KG. Neutropenic enterocolitis: two unusual cases with review of the literature. *Arch Pathol Lab Med* 1993;117:524.
148. Amromin GD, Solomon RD. Necrotizing enteropathy: a complication of treated leukemia or lymphoma patients. *JAMA* 1962;182:23.
149. Prolla JC, Kirsner JB. The gastrointestinal lesion and complication of the leukemias. *Ann Intern Med* 1964;61:1084.
150. Moir DH, Bale PM. Necropsy findings in childhood leukemia emphasizing neutropenic colitis and cerebral calcification. *Pathology* 1976;8:247.
151. Dosik GM, Luna M, Valdivieso M, et al. Necrotizing colitis in patients with cancer. *Am J Med* 1979;67:646.
152. Caya JG, Farmer SG, Ritch PS, et al. *Clostridial septicemia* complicating the course of leukemia. *Cancer* 1986;57:2045.
153. Koransky JR, Stargel MD, Dowell VR. *Clostridium septicum* bacteremia: its clinical significance. *Am J Med* 1979;66:63.
154. Louie TJ, Bartlett JG, Tally FB, et al. Aerobic and anaerobic bacteria in diabetic foot ulcers. *Ann Intern Med* 1976;85:461.
155. Thaler M, Gill V, Pizzo PA. Emergence of *Clostridium tertium* as a pathogen in neutropenic patients. *Am J Med* 1986;81:596.
156. Spiers G, Warren RE, Rampling A. *Clostridium tertium* septicemia in patients with neutropenia. *J Infect Dis* 1988;158:1336.
157. Valtonen M, Sivonen A, Elonen E. A cluster of seven cases of *Clostridium tertium* septicemia in neutropenic patients. *Eur J Clin Microbiol Infect Dis* 1990;9:40.
158. Tally FP, Armfield AY, Dowell VR, et al. Susceptibility of *Clostridium ramosum* to antimicrobial agents. *Antimicrob Agents Chemother* 1975;5:589.
159. Sutter VL, Finegold SM. Susceptibility of anaerobic bacteria to 23 antimicrobial agents. *Antimicrob Agents Chemother* 1976;10:736.
160. Scheartzman JD, Reller LB, Wang WL. Susceptibility of *Clostridium perfringens* isolated from human infections to twenty antibiotics. *Antimicrob Agents Chemother* 1977;11:695.
161. Applebaum PC, Chatterton SA. Susceptibility of anaerobic bacteria to ten antimicrobial agents. *Antimicrob Agents Chemother* 1978;14:271.
162. Brown WJ, Waatti PE. Susceptibility testing of clinically isolated anaerobic bacteria by an agar dilution technique. *Antimicrob Agents Chemother* 1980;17:629.
163. Dzink J, Bartlett JG. In vitro susceptibility of *Clostridium difficile* isolates from patients with antibiotic-associated diarrhea or colitis. *Antimicrob Agents Chemother* 1980;17:695.
164. Swenson JM, Thornsberry C, McCroskey LM, et al. Susceptibility of *Clostridium botulinum* to thirteen antimicrobial agents. *Antimicrob Agents Chemother* 1980;18:13.
165. Gabey EL, Rolfe RD, Finegold SM. Susceptibility of *Clostridium septicum* to 23 antimicrobial agents. *Antimicrob Agents Chemother* 1981;20:852.
166. Nord CE, Hedberg M. Clinical infections and treatment: resistance to β-lactam antibiotics in anaerobic bacteria. *Rev Infect Dis* 1990;12[Suppl 2]:S231.
167. Blandino G, Olsson-Liljequist B, Nord CE. Characterization of β-lactamase from *Clostridium butyricum*. *Chemioterapia* 1983;2:95.
168. Hart CA, Barr K, Makin T, et al. Characteristics of a β-lactamase produced by *Clostridium butyricum*. *J Antimicrob Chemother* 1982;10:31.
169. Magot M. Some properties of the *Clostridium butyricum* group β-lactamase. *J Gen Microbiol* 1981;127:113.
170. Weinrich AE, Del Bene VE. β-Lactamase activity in anaerobic bacteria. *Antimicrob Agents Chemother* 1976;10:106.
171. Matthew M. Plasmid-mediated β-lactamases of gram-negative bacteria: properties and distribution. *J Antimicrob Chemother* 1979;5:349.
172. Murphy IF, Barza M, Park JT. Penicillin-binding proteins in *Clostridium perfringens*. *Antimicrob Agents Chemother* 1981;20:809.
173. Williamson R. Resistance of *Clostridium perfringens* to β-lactam antibiotics mediated by a decreased affinity of a single essential penicillin-binding protein. *J Gen Microbiol* 1983;129:2339.
174. Stevens DL, Maier KA, Laine BM, et al. Comparison of clindamycin, rifampin, tetracycline, metronidazole, and penicillin for efficacy in prevention of experimental gas gangrene due to *Clostridium perfringens*. *J Infect Dis* 1987;155:220.
175. Stevens DL, Maier KA, Mitten JE. Effect of antibiotics on toxin production and viability of *Clostridium perfringens*. *Antimicrob Agents Chemother* 1987;31:213.
176. Altemeier WA, Furste WL. Gas gangrene. *Surg Gynecol Obstet* 1947;84:507.
177. Altemeier WA, McMurrin JA, Alt AP. Chloromycetin and aureomycin in experimental gas gangrene. *Surgery* 1950;28:621.
178. Altemeier WA, Fullen WD. Prevention and treatment of gas gangrene. *JAMA* 1971;217:806.
179. Knight RJ. Reception and resuscitation of casualties in South Vietnam: experience at the first Australian Field Hospital. *Lancet* 1972;2:29.
180. Darke SG, King AM, Slack WK. Gas gangrene and related infection: classification, clinical features and aetiology, management and mortality. A report of 88 cases. *Br J Surg* 1977;64:104.
181. Weinstein L, Barza MA. Gas gangrene. *N Engl J Med* 1973;289:1129.
182. Brazier JS, Levett PN, Stannard AJ, et al. Antibiotic susceptibility of clinical isolates of clostridia. *J Antimicrob Chemother* 1985;15:181.

Spirochetes

CHAPTER 214
Lyme Disease

Raymond J. Dattwyler and Gary P. Wormser

HISTORY

In 1982, Willy Burgdorfer and his colleagues isolated a new *Borrelia* species from ixodid ticks (1). This discovery directly led to the establishment of this new species as the etiologic agent of Lyme disease when two separate groups, Benach and colleagues (2) and Steere and associates (3), subsequently isolated this newly described spirochete from patients with Lyme disease. The newly defined pathogen was named *Borrelia burgdorferi* in honor of Willy Burgdorfer.

As a result of that finding, it was subsequently established that an array of clinical syndromes described in the European medical literature since the early twentieth century were due to infection with pathogens of this species complex. For example, erythema migrans (EM), the earliest sign of Lyme borreliosis, was first appreciated by Afzelius, a Swedish dermatologist, in 1909 (4). Afzelius hypothesized that this cutaneous lesion was the result of a tick bite from which the causative agent could be transmitted to humans from an animal source. Subsequently, in 1921, Lipshitz identified *Ixodes ricinus* as the vector for this disease (5). By the 1940s, European investigators had demonstrated that EM could be associated with the subsequent development of several neurologic syndromes, including acute meningitis, meningopolyneuritis, meningoencephalitis, and chronic lymphocytic meningitis, as well as other types of illnesses, such as musculoskeletal complaints and a number of dermatologic conditions, including acrodermatitis chronicum atrophicans (ACA) and lymphadenosis benigna cutis (lymphocytoma) (6–12), Lenhoff, a Swedish pathologist, in 1948 observed spirochete-like structures in skin biopsies from EM lesions (5). By 1950, European investigators had demonstrated the efficacy of penicillin for EM (13,14).

The first well-documented case of EM acquired in the United States was reported in 1970 by Scrimenti, a Wisconsin dermatologist (15). Mast and Burrows reported a cluster of cases of EM in Southeastern Connecticut in 1976 (16). Subsequently, Steere and colleagues reported an association between EM and arthritis in a small group of patients living around the town of Old Lyme, Connecticut (17). They coined the name *Lyme arthritis* for this entity. Once it was realized that organs such as the heart and nervous system could also be involved, the name was changed to *Lyme disease*.

PATHOGEN

Organisms of the *Borrelia burgdorferi sensu lato* group belong to the family Spirochaetaceae, genus *Borrelia* (18). These loosely coiled spirochetes are motile with a flexible helix structure, measuring about 10 to 30 μm in length and 0.18 to 0.25 μm in width. Like most spirochetes, *B. burgdorferi* is difficult to visualize under bright-field conditions but is readily visible in phase-contrast or dark-field conditions. It can be identified with acridine orange,

Giemsa, or silver stains, such as the Dieterle or Warthin-Starry stains, and by immunohistochemical techniques (19). Demonstration of the spirochete in tissue sections is difficult, especially in late disease; therefore, histopathologic identification of the organism cannot be used routinely to diagnose this infection. The organism is microaerophilic and can be grown in a modified Kelly medium (Barbour-Stoener-Kelly) at 33°C (20,21). *B. burgdorferi* is easily isolated from the tick vector. However, culture from the human host has proved to be more difficult, and culture is not a routine diagnostic tool at this time. Although yields as high as 80% or more have been reported from cultures of skin biopsies of EM lesions, and up to nearly 50% from plasma samples of patients with EM (22), the culture yield from whole blood, cerebrospinal fluid (CSF), or synovial tissue is much lower (23).

There are at least 11 species in the *B. burgdorferi* complex (24–26) and an unknown but large number of substrains (25–27). Of this group of spirochetes, three species, *B. burgdorferi sensu stricto*, *Borrelia garinii*, and *Borrelia afzelii* are known to be human pathogens (24–28) (Fig. 214.1). All three pathogenic genospecies are found in Europe, but only *B. burgdorferi sensu stricto* is found in North America. Because of the greater diversity in Europe, European studies of this disease cannot be expected to apply precisely to North American patients. Although there is overlap in the clinical manifestations, the particular genospecies of *Borrelia* causing infection will affect clinical presentation (28–31). For example, two dermatologic manifestations of Lyme disease, borrelial lymphocytoma and ACA, are rarely if ever seen in the United States because the genospecies that cause these clinical manifestations are found exclusively in Eurasia (31,32).

The *B. burgdorferi* species complex evolved by differentiation of lineages (asexually) and is consequently composed of an array of clones (27). Sequence analysis of chromosomal genes and *OspA* genes from a number of variant strains shows that there has been no horizontal transfer of chromosomal genes and very little plasmid transfer within or between species (27). The diversity of this species complex has been defined by analyzing organisms isolated from patients, ticks, and reservoir animals. In Europe, all three known pathogenic genospecies and at least two other genospecies have been isolated. By contrast,

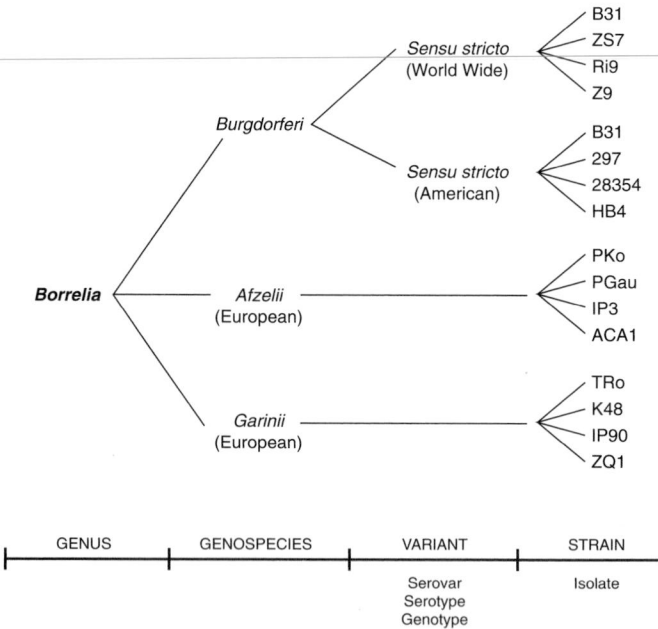

Figure 214.1. Taxonomy of *Borrelia* species.

TABLE 214.1. *Borrelia burgdorferi* Major antigens

Bb protein	Molecular weight (kd)	Function
p93 or p80/100	93	Good serodiagnostic antigen
p73	73	Common bacterial antigen HSP 70 family
p66	66	Common bacterial antigen, HSP 60 family; its possible contact with OspA may hinder the effectiveness of anti-OspA antibodies
p58	58	Serodiagnostic antigen
BBK32	47	Fibronectin binding protein, serodiagnosic antigen—early and late LD
Fla or p41	41	Flagellar antigen; immunodominant; highly cross-reactive with other bacterial flagellins
p39 (BmpA)	39	Serodiagnostic antigen for early LD
p35	35	Adds to diagnostic sensitivity, role in protective immunity, indicator of natural infections in dogs
VlsE	34	Invariable region peptide (VlsE-IR6) is a good diagnostic antigen, C-terminal invariable domain does not induce protective response
OspB	34	Induces strain-specific immunity, bactericidal antibodies have been generated
OspA	30	Immunogenic, has been used as a human vaccine
OspD	28	Expressed only by some *Borrelia* strains, not immunogenic, not a good serodiagnostic antigen
OspF	26	Induces partial protection in mouse models, indicator of natural infection in dogs
pG	22	Induces T-cell proliferation in patients with LD, could be used as diagnostic marker other than serodiagnosis
OspC	21	Induces strain-specific immunity, possible vaccine alternative being tested in humans, good for serodiagnosis
DbpA	20	Decorin-binding protein, good serodiagnostic antigen for Lyme arthritis and neuroborreliosis but not for EM, role in protective immunity
OspE	19	Induces partial protection in mouse models

HSP, heat-shock protein; LD, Lyme disease; Em, erythema migrans.

in the United States, only one of the pathogenic genospecies, *B. burgdorferi sensu stricto*, exists along with *Borrelia andersonii*, *Borrelia bissettii* and two unnamed nonpathogenic genospecies (33,34). Two other species, *Borrelia japonica*, and *Borrelia sinica*, have been found in Japan and China, respectively (33). European studies have demonstrated that humans can be multiply infected with spirochetes representing each of the three pathogenic genospecies of *B. burgdorferi sensu lato* (32). Using polymerase chain reaction (PCR) with primers specific for the *OspA* gene from each of the three genospecies, it was possible to detect multiple species in clinical specimens obtained from selected patients exhibiting neurologic Lyme disease. The results were corroborated by immunoblot analyses, which showed a pattern of activity that could differentiate among the three phylogenetic groups. It is not known whether pluri-infection is the result of consecutive infections or simultaneous infection from a single tick. *I. ricinus* ticks can carry more than genospecies of *B. burgdorferi sensu lato*.

Ixodes scapularis ticks from North America can harbor more than one variant of *B. burgdorferi sensu stricto* (35). We have found that multiple strains can also be found in the skin of patients with erythema migrans (35). Taken together, these data are consistent with the hypothesis that the multisystem nature of Lyme disease may in part be the result of infection with multiple strains of *B. burgdorferi sensu lato*, which vary in their antigenic properties, tropisms, and types of clinical symptoms they elicit (36).

The genome of *B. burgdorferi sensu stricto* has been sequenced and many of its key antigens have been characterized (37) (Table 214.1). Two major outer surface proteins OspA and OspB are encoded on a 54-kilobase linear plasmid (38); the plasmid is present in nearly all strains. Although quantitatively OspA is the major surface protein expressed in cultured organisms and in the midgut of the tick, an immune response to OspA develops in only a minority of infected patients and then only late in the course of infection (39). Recent evidence has shown that OspA expression is down-regulated and that in some spirochetes, OspC is expressed as the spirochetes migrate from the tick gut into the tick's salivary glands during the course of tick feeding (40,41).

OspC is highly polymorphic (42–45). The alleles of OspC *sensu stricto* can be grouped into at least 21 major OspC groups based on sequence divergence. By comparing the OspC alleles in 162 human *B. burgdorferi sensu stricto* isolates, Seinost found that disseminated infection was limited to just 4 of the 21 OspC groups (46). Among the three pathogenic genospecies of *B. burgdorferi*, a total of 58 OspC groups have been described. Of these, only 10 groups are associated with invasive disease in humans (47).

Additional outer-surface lipoproteins have been identified (OspD, E, and F). Although it had previously been proposed as a virulence factor (48–50), OspD is not present in all *B. burgdorferi sensu stricto* isolates. Using the classification system devised by Liveris and associates (50a), all RFLP-2 strains are OspD deficient, even those isolated from humans (Gui-qing Wang, personal communication with the authors, 2003). Thus, OspD is not essential for infectivity. OspE and F form a plasmid-encoded operon. As with OspC, OspF can induce a protective immune response in rodents; however, it is less pronounced than the response to OspC.

Structurally, these spirochetes possess outer cell and cytoplasmic membranes. Between these membranes are 7 to 11 flagella inserted at the ends of the spirochete (51). In contrast to the outer surface proteins, the structure of the 41-kd flagellar antigen is consistent among strains. Immune responses to this latter antigen are elicited early in the course of infection. This 41-kd protein is highly cross-reactive with similar flagella antigens of both other *Borrelia* and *Treponema* species. The 60-kd protein is a common heat-shock antigen found in a variety of bacteria (52).

EPIDEMIOLOGY

Lyme disease is the most common vector-borne infectious disease in North America. It has a limited geographic distribution. Within the United States, cases occur primarily in specific areas of the Northeast, Mid Atlantic, Midwest, and Far West. Just nine states, New York, Connecticut, Rhode Island, Pennsylvania, Delaware, New Jersey, Maryland, Massachusetts, and Wisconsin, account for more than 90% percent of the Lyme disease cases reported each year. Even in New York, the state with the largest number of cases, more than 80% of cases are reported from just 5 of 62 counties (53).

In the United States, Lyme disease occurs in all age groups and is found almost equally in males and females (53). There is a bimodal age distribution, with the highest rates of infection in 5- to 9-year-old children and in 45- to 54-year-old adults (53).

Although there are reported cases of EM-like skin lesions associated with tick bites in the Southeastern and South Central United States, human *B. burgdorferi* infection has not been documented. Also, the illness in these areas appears to be associated with the bite of a different tick species (*Amblyomma americanum*) (54–56).

Lyme disease is transmitted exclusively by hard ticks of the genus *Ixodes* (57), and throughout the world, cases are limited to areas where this genus is endemic (58–60).

Unlike the distantly related soft ticks, hard ticks differ in that feeding occurs only once during each developmental stage. In addition, in contrast to soft ticks, *Ixodes* ticks seek hosts widely in the environment rather than confining their search for hosts to burrows or nests (61). Although many *Ixodes* species transmit *B. burgdorferi* in natural enzootic cycles, only those species belonging to the *Ixodes persulcatus* complex of ixodid ticks transmit *B. burgdorferi sensu lato* to humans (62–64). *I. persulcatus* in Eurasia, *I. ricinus* in Europe, *Ixodes pacificus* in the western United States, and *I. scapularis* in the middle and eastern United States (65) are included in this group. These ixodid ticks require high surface humidity to survive and thus are more common along river valleys, lake shores, and coastal areas (66,67). Because they have a broad host range for all feeding stages (68), they are efficient vectors of zoonotic pathogens forming a transmission bridge from wildlife reservoir hosts to humans. Studies suggest that migrating birds may have a role in the spread of ticks and *B. burgdorferi* to new locations (69). Lyme disease–like illnesses are reported in Australia, Africa, and South America, but *B. burgdorferi* has not been isolated from patients there, and these locations should not be considered endemic for this infection (70).

In the United States, *I. scapularis*, the black-legged or deer tick, is responsible for more than 95% of Lyme disease cases (71). These ixodid ticks, like all ixodid ticks, have a three-stage life cycle with larval, nymphal, and adult stages. Larval ticks can be distinguished from nymphs by their smaller size and the presence of only six legs, which is characteristic of insects (*Hexapoda*). In contrast to true insects, both nymphal and adult ticks have eight legs.

Larval-stage ticks are born uninfected and only become infected with *B. burgdorferi* after feeding on an infected animal.

Depending on the vertebrate host species composition in a given area, infection prevalence in host-seeking nymphs can reach as high as 30% (72,73). Although all tick stages can be found on various animal species, not all animals are equally favored as hosts (67). *Peromyscus leucopus*, the white-footed mouse, is the primary source of infection for *I. scapularis*. These mice are ubiquitous in forested environments and can remain infected with *B. burgdorferi* for life (74,75). However, other mammals, such as chipmunks, and some bird species, such as robins, may also serve as sources of infection (76–80).

After 2 to 3 days of feeding, engorged larvae drop to the ground, molt into the nymphal stage and overwinter until the following spring when they are ready to feed again (81). The peak season for *B. burgdorferi* transmission to both wildlife and humans is June and July when nymphal *I. scapularis* seek a blood meal (82). The enzootic cycle is completed as reservoir hosts become infected just before peak larval feeding in August.

By the time they have reached the adult stage, *I. scapularis* have had two opportunities to acquire *B. burgdorferi* infection, first as a larva and second as a nymph. Thus, infection prevalence in adults commonly exceeds 50% (72,83). Transmission by adult ticks is an ecological dead end because white-tailed deer, the preferred host for adults, are incapable of maintaining *B. burgdorferi* infection (84).

In contrast to *I. scapularis*, the larvae of *I. pacificus* tend to feed on reptiles. Reptiles do not harbor *B. burgdorferi*, and this may be one of the reasons why the prevalence of this pathogen in adult *I. pacificus* (about 5%) is so much less than that observed in adult *I. scapularis* (30% to 70% in highly endemic areas) (85).

Within the tick, spirochetes can be found in the midgut and, to a lesser extent, systemically. As the tick begins to feed, spirochetes multiply and migrate from the midgut into the tick's salivary glands and are eventually carried along with saliva into the skin. The gene encoding OspA is down-regulated, and OspC expression is up-regulated, causing a change in the major outer surface protein from OspA to OspC. From experimental animal studies, it has been estimated that it requires at least 48 or more hours of feeding for the tick to be able to transmit *B. burgdorferi* to its host (62). Human studies by Sood and colleagues (86), Berger and associates (87), and Nadelman and co-workers (88) support these animal findings.

Ixodid ticks can carry other infectious agents in addition to *B. burgdorferi*. These other pathogens vary by geographic location. In the United States, ixodid ticks are competent vectors for the agent *Anaplasma phagocytophilum*, the agent of human granulocytic ehrlichiosis (HGE), and *Babesia microti*, whereas in Europe, possible co-infecting agents include *A. phagocytophilum*, *Babesia divergens*, and the tick-borne encephalitis virus. Co-infections with one or more of these agents may influence disease manifestation and severity (89,90).

CLINICAL MANIFESTATIONS

The frequency and type of clinical manifestations observed in this infectious disease have changed because of the greater recognition of early infection, more attention paid to the accuracy of diagnosis, and the prompt use of effective antibiotic regimens. Lyme arthritis, once considered by many to be the most important aspect of Lyme disease in North America, has become very rare. Overemphasis of the rheumatologic aspects of Lyme disease has skewed the view of this infectious disease. Some have divided this disease into three distinct stages: stage 1, EM; stage 2, neurologic or cardiac involvement; and stage 3, arthritis (91). This staging scheme implies that the clinical manifestations proceed from one discrete entity to the next in an orderly fashion.

It has become apparent that this staging scheme is intrinsically flawed, in that *B. burgdorferi* infection is a progressive infectious disease that may disseminate early in its course. Between the time of acute dissemination to the onset of the manifestations of late disease, there is usually a disease-free interval in which the infection remains latent. The earliest and most easily recognized manifestation of *B. burgdorferi* infection is EM, a characteristic skin lesion observed in 90% or more of patients with objective manifestations (92,93). EM usually develops 7 to 10 days after a painless and often unnoticed tick bite. In some patients, there may be a nonspecific viral-like illness with no obvious skin lesions, but diagnosis in these patients is less certain, and most patients presenting in this manner do not have *B. burgdorferi* infection. One or more systemic signs or symptoms, such as low-grade fever, malaise, headache, stiff neck, or mild fatigue, may occur concurrently with EM in most North American patients (94,95). Although the development of these systemic signs and symptoms may herald the systemic spread of this spirochete, the presence of multiple EM lesions is a more reliable indicator of early disseminated infection. Most recent series report an 8% to 15% incidence of multiple lesions, although rates as high as 50% were reported in earlier studies (95).

Other clinical manifestations, including acute meningitis, cranial nerve palsy, myocarditis with or without conduction block abnormalities, anicteric hepatitis, and less commonly, frank arthritis, can be observed during the acute disseminated phase of infection (96).

Localized inflammatory processes tend to predominate in the late phase of the illness, although multiple organ systems may also be involved. There tend to be few constitutional signs and symptoms. Three organ systems (skin, nervous system, and musculoskeletal system) are predominantly involved during this phase. Fatigue, malaise, or nonspecific musculoskeletal complaints in the absence of clear objective abnormalities are not compatible with a diagnosis of late *B. burgdorferi* infection.

In assessing the clinical manifestations of Lyme disease, it is important to remember the possibility of co-infection with babesia, *A. phagocytophilum*, or tick-borne encephalitis virus (89,90,97), Signs and symptoms may be more severe and longer lasting in patients co-infected with one of these agents. Previously, Russian investigators noticed a relationship between tick-borne encephalitis due to flavivirus and EM (98,99). Because Lyme borreliosis itself can be associated with meningitis, meningoencephalitis, or encephalitis, it is not clear whether these particular cases of tick-borne encephalitis associated with EM were due to flavivirus infection or not. Lyme disease should be considered in all patients suspected of arbovirus encephalitis in regions where the ixodid tick is endemic.

DERMATOLOGIC MANIFESTATIONS

EM is most often characterized as an expanding annular erythematous skin lesion that clears centrally. However, variations, including vesicular, purpuric, and homogeneously erythematous lesions, are common. The lesion is usually sharply demarcated. Scaling, commonly associated with fungal dermatitis, is not observed with EM (100) (Fig. 214.2).

Primary EM develops at the site of the tick bite. The tick bite is painless, and after 72 hours or more of the tick taking its blood meal, the tick generally falls off spontaneously. In more than half the cases in the United States, the patient is totally unaware of the tick bite. Lesions are usually asymptomatic but can occasionally be associated with mild, local pruritus or dysesthesia but are rarely very painful. EM can be located anywhere but in adults is more commonly found below the waist. Regional lymphadenopathy may occur. Associated constitutional symptoms can vary from none to mild and transitory, including malaise, fatigue, headache, low-grade fever, and chills (95,101). Secondary lesions tend to be smaller and lack an indurated center. In untreated patients, EM will often clear spontaneously within weeks to months after onset. If inadequately treated, EM can very rarely relapse. Patients with a prior history of EM are still susceptible to reinfection and therefore to recurrent episodes.

Borrelial lymphocytoma is not associated with *B. burgdorferi sensu stricto* infection and therefore is not observed in patients acquiring Lyme disease in North America (101,102). This dermatologic manifestation has only been reported in Europe. It may occur concurrently with the acute infection or may occur months later (101). These solitary, bluish red nodules have a predilection for occurring on the ear lobes of children and on the nipple areas of adults. Other manifestations of infection, such as meningitis, arthritis, and ACA, can be present along with the lymphocytoma. The clinical appearance of this lesion may be confused with breast malignancy. Histopathologically, borrelial lymphocytoma is characterized by a dense lymphocytic infiltrate in the dermis or subcutaneous tissue, and at times, it can be difficult to differentiate lymphocytoma from lymphoma. *B. burgdorferi sensu lato* has rarely been isolated from lymphocytoma (101).

ACA is a chronic and insidious skin infection occurring predominantly in elderly women (103). It is well described throughout Northern, Central, and Eastern Europe but is rarely reported

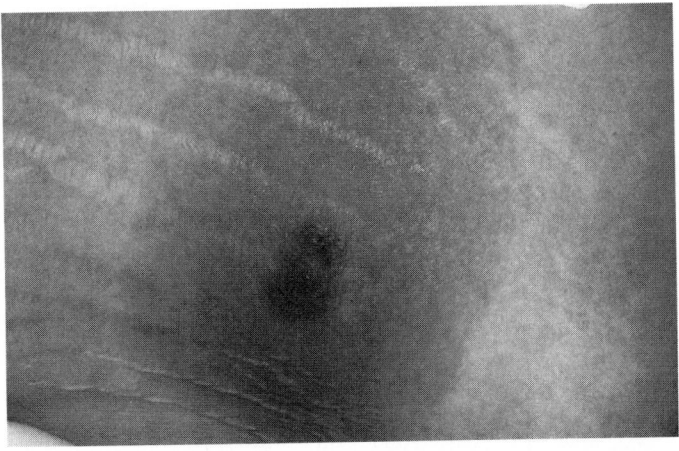
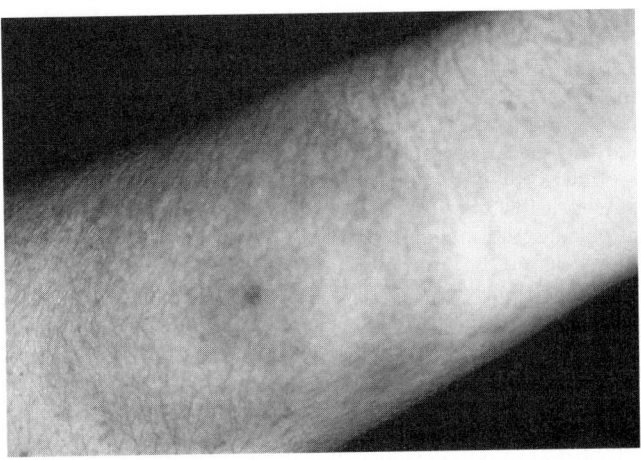

Figure 214.2. Examples of erythema migrans skin lesions.

in the United States. Generally, ACA develops 10 years after the onset of infection. Characteristically, the skin lesions are described as violet to bluish discolored areas with a doughy consistency. The erythematous component may be variable, and swelling of soft tissue with relatively normal-appearing skin may be present. The lesions eventually become atrophic or sclerotic. Most commonly, these lesions are found on the distal extremities, typically sparing the face, palms, and soles. The trunk, however, may also be the initial site. Concomitant with ACA, neurologic and rheumatologic evidence of *B. burgdorferi* infection may be present (103,104). Polyneuropathy, small joint arthritis with subluxation, arthritis of the large joints, and periosteal thickening of the bones frequently occur in the same extremity as ACA.

MUSCULOSKELETAL MANIFESTATIONS

Arthralgias are the most common musculoskeletal manifestation associated with EM. Rarely, some patients with EM develop acute arthritis, usually involving the knee, while the EM is still present. However, musculoskeletal involvement in early infection is most frequently manifested as pain in joints, tendons, bursae, muscle, or bones. Usually, there is no joint swelling or other signs of active inflammation. One or two sites at a time are affected, and symptoms last from a few hours to several days.

If untreated, about one half of patients with EM in North America develop arthritis a mean of about 6 months after onset of EM (105). Bursitis, epicondylitis, and tendonitis have also been reported. Lyme arthritis is primarily a monoarticular or oligoarticular large-joint arthritis, which is characteristically episodic in nature. Episodes last a few days to a few months before spontaneously resolving. Patients may have just one or multiple episodes of arthritis. In most, the interval between episodes gradually increases, and the arthritis spontaneously remits. Only 10% of those who develop arthritis have a more chronic course, a year or more of continuous joint swelling. Even those who develop this complication tend to remit spontaneously. In more than 90% of Lyme arthritis patients, the knee is the affected joint, but other large joints can be affected. Although it was once thought that arthritis was not associated with this infection in Europe, it may occur in European patients, especially those infected with the genospecies *B. burgdorferi sensu stricto* (106,107).

Lyme arthritis has become uncommon and chronic Lyme arthritis extremely rare. This is undoubtedly due to the prompt treatment of patients with EM with highly effective antibiotic regimens. Because the overall incidence of frank arthritis has dramatically decreased, one should be cautious in making a diagnosis of Lyme arthritis. In patients with symmetric polyarthritis, especially if there is small-joint involvement, alternate diagnoses besides Lyme disease should be considered, even in patients with serologic evidence of exposure to *B. burgdorferi*.

PCR studies have demonstrated that appropriate antibiotic regimens are highly effective in eradicating *B. burgdorferi* from the joint (108). Yet, there are very rare individuals who have ongoing arthritis with no evidence of continued infection. At the present, the major interest in Lyme arthritis is as a model to help define the immunopathology of postinfectious illness. Much attention has been placed on the few patients with antibiotic refractory arthritis. In part, this is to explain why some individuals continue to experience ongoing signs or symptoms after they have had Lyme disease. Animal and human studies have demonstrated that helper T-cell subtype 1 (T_H1) responses mediate refractory disease (109–112).

Early reports attempting to link the development of refractory Lyme arthritis with certain HLA haplotypes were not consistent (113–115). More recent studies have associated chronic or antibiotic refractory arthritis both with certain HLA-DR4 genotypes, HLA-DRB1*0401, and HLA-DRB1*0101, (112,115), and with the development of immune reactivity to OspA (114). These findings raised the possibility of a link between the two. Of note, both of these genotypes are also more common in patients with rheumatoid arthritis (114).

The 60 COOH-terminal amino acids of OspA contain epitopes recognized by antibodies and T cells from patients with Lyme disease (116,117), and immunoglobulin G (IgG) antibodies to the COOH-terminus of OspA are linked with arthritis (118). In individuals with Lyme arthritis and the HLA DR4 genotype HLA-DRB1, T-cell reactivity to OspA epitopes (amino acids 154 to 173 and 214 to 233) has been associated with antibiotic refractory disease (119).

A 9–amino acid peptide from the OspA *B. burgdorferi sensu stricto*, strain B31, was predicted by Hammer (120) to bind effectively to HLA-DRB1*0401. The amino acid sequence of this peptide is similar to a sequence contained in human leukocyte function-associated antigen-1 (hLFA-1). T_H1 cells from a patient with refractory Lyme arthritis were found to react to this OspA peptide and to the analogous hLFA-1 peptide. Thus, it was hypothesized that the OspA helper T-cell epitope YVLEGTLTA in OspA B31 (amino acids 165 to 173) is cross-reactive with the similar sequence YVIEGTSKQ in hLFA-1 (amino acids 332 to 340) (112) and that this peptide within hLFA-1 is a candidate autoantigen in HLA-DRB1*0401–positive individuals with treatment-resistant Lyme arthritis.

Gross and co-workers proposed a model to describe how priming by *B. burgdorferi* infection or at least by OspA may be required for development of an autoimmune response to hLFA-1 in the joint (112). They proposed that because of the cross-reactivity between the two similar epitopes in OspA (*B. burgdorferi sensu stricto* strain B31) and hLFA-1, even after elimination of the spirochetes by antibiotic therapy, the OspA-primed T cells recruited in the joint remain activated by stimulation of the previously interferon-γ (IFN-γ)–recruited LFA-1–expressing T cells.

The hypothesis that the rare antibiotic-refractory patients have infection-induced autoimmune-mediated joint inflammation that continues despite eradication of the spirochete remains unproved. Benoist and Mathis pointed out that the finding of T_H1 cells reactive to LFA-1 may merely reflect the promiscuous nature of the T-cell receptor (121). Our findings support this possibility. We found T_H1 reactivity to hLFA-1 (amino acids 326 to 345) in the peripheral blood of both patients with Lyme disease and healthy individuals. Thus, these results suggest that the ability of the average T cell to recognize 105 to 106 different peptides is responsible for the finding that T cells can recognize epitopes in both OspA and hLFA-1. Other investigators, Hammer and associates (122) and Maier and colleagues (123), have found additional epitopes in OspA that are predicted to be cross-reactive and are candidates for autoimmune reactions in susceptible individuals.

NERVOUS SYSTEM MANIFESTATIONS

Clinical data support but do not necessarily prove the hypothesis that *B. burgdorferi* can invade the central nervous system (CNS) early in the course of infection. The most compelling evidence is the frequency of complaints referable to the nervous system in patients with EM. In one U.S. study, 64% of patients with EM had headaches, and 48% had neck stiffness (124). The possibility of early invasion of the CNS was confirmed anecdotally by PCR detection of borrelial DNA in the CSF of two thirds of patients with acute disseminated infection (125).

About 15% of untreated patients with EM will develop one or more of three acute disorders—meningitis, cranial neuritis, or painful radiculitis—in the first 3 months after infection. CSF abnormalities in patients with meningitis include pleocytosis, moderate elevations of CSF protein, and a normal CSF glucose (126). Cranial neuropathies are commonly associated with acute disseminated infection. These may occur with or without meningitis, which may be asymptomatic. Seventh-nerve palsy, both unilateral and bilateral, is by far the most common cranial nerve abnormality. Also reported is involvement of the optic, third, fourth, fifth, sixth, and eighth cranial nerves along with the recurrent laryngeal nerves (127). These cranial nerve abnormalities can occur alone or with other evidence of polyneuritis. Very rarely, optic disc edema can occur because of optic neuritis or increased intracranial pressure.

Although late disseminated *B. burgdorferi* infection may also be associated with symptoms of nervous system dysfunction, proving that any symptom is directly related to active *B. burgdorferi* infection is difficult. At present, the most commonly used test for making the initial diagnosis of nervous system infection is the measurement of intrathecal *B. burgdorferi* antibody production in CSF (128,129). The role of PCR in demonstrating borrelial DNA in CSF and in establishing a diagnosis of CNS infection remains to be defined.

B. burgdorferi can cause unifocal or multifocal areas of inflammation in the brain and spinal cord. Whether this is due to vasculitis, direct infection, or immune-mediated mechanisms has yet to be determined. The clinical manifestations of this process range from prominent focal CNS abnormalities to more subtle alterations of cognitive function (130–132). Although some reports have confused the more dramatic focal form of this disorder with multiple sclerosis, these two disorders can usually be easily differentiated. Neuroborreliosis is less likely to follow a relapsing–remitting course, does not cause abnormal evoked responses, and is associated with intrathecal production of specific antibody against *B. burgdorferi*. Other patients with apparent *B. burgdorferi* infection have alteration of cognitive function but lack clinical or laboratory evidence of CNS infection. Whether these patients represent the coincidental occurrence of other disorders in patients with anti–*B. burgdorferi* immunoreactivity or whether this represents a remote noninfectious CNS manifestation of this disorder remains to be clarified. There is no clear evidence that infection directly causes any specific psychiatric disorder. Patients with well-documented Lyme borreliosis given the Beck Depression Inventory did not demonstrate significant levels of depression (130).

The peripheral nervous system can also be involved in patients with *B. burgdorferi* infection (130,133–135). The type and frequency of neurologic involvement differ in Europe and North America. A spectrum of disease severity has been noted, ranging from the severe, painful, debilitating meningopolyneuritis (Garin-Bujadoux-Bannwarth syndrome) to a milder axonal neuropathy in patients with late infection. Meningopolyneuritis, the most dramatic of the peripheral nervous system abnormalities, is much more common in Europe than in the United States. Occurring early in the course of the infection, this syndrome is characterized by intense radicular pain, paresthesias, and hyperesthesias (136–139). CSF examination may reveal lymphocytic pleocytosis (137). Concomitant encephalitis and myelitis occur in more than 20% of the patients. In these patients, long-term sequelae such as spastic paraparesis and neurogenic bladder may persist even after appropriate therapy (137–138).

Peripheral neuropathies may be distributed symmetrically or asymmetrically and can resemble polyneuritis multiplex. Some patients with late infection complain of paresthesia and hyperesthesia (130,133–135). Nerve conduction studies can reveal abnor-malities due to an axonopathy of the peripheral nerves in such patients.

Although the literature has repeatedly emphasized the rather protean neurologic manifestations of this disorder, it appears that it is now becoming possible to be more restrictive in the disorders considered causally linked to *B. burgdorferi* infection. As the common threads unifying these different disorders are elucidated, it should become possible to design more specific studies to clarify the pathogenetic mechanisms underlying them. Differences in the infecting strain or substrain of the infecting organism may play a significant role in the clinical manifestations observed. It is clear that *B. burgdorferi sensu stricto* causes less acute neurologic disease than *B. garinii*.

CARDIAC MANIFESTATIONS

Acute cardiac involvement has been reported in up to 8% of adult patients (140), although in our experience, it occurs in only 1% or 2% of patients with acute disseminated infection. About 90% of patients with cardiac involvement develop varying degrees of atrioventricular block, including complete heart block. However, heart block is virtually always reversible, even in patients with third-degree block (141). Atrioventricular block can fluctuate rapidly. In most cases, the block is proximal to the bundle of His, and only rarely is it diffuse. Syncope can occur in patients with third-degree block. Myocarditis or pericarditis is observed in about 65% of patients with cardiac involvement. Although left ventricular dysfunction can be documented in almost half of these patients, it is usually not severe and does not significantly compromise cardiac function (140,142–145). Congestive heart failure should lead to an evaluation for underlying cardiac disease. Myopericarditis can be associated with chest pain or mild shortness of breath. Late cardiac manifestations associated with *B. burgdorferi* infection have not been well defined. Stanek reported in European patients that chronic infection can be associated with a chronic carditis and the development of cardiomyopathy (146,147). Similar cases have not been well documented in the United States.

OTHER ORGANS

B. burgdorferi has been associated with abnormalities of other organs and systems during acute infection. Hepatitis with mild elevation of transaminases has been reported in early Lyme disease (93). Some question of this finding is warranted in view of the fact that in many areas of North America where *B. burgdorferi* is endemic, ixodid ticks are frequently co-infected with *A. phagocytophilum*, the agent of HGE. HGE is frequently associated with hepatic dysfunction.

DIAGNOSIS

EM is the classic marker for this infection, and in endemic areas, its presence is virtually diagnostic. This characteristic skin lesion is recognized in more than 90% of patients with objective clinical manifestations of this spirochetosis (148,149). Unfortunately, it is typically only seen early in the course of infection. In the absence of EM, definitively diagnosing Lyme borreliosis cannot be done on the clinical presentation alone.

PCR, although widely available, has a limited role in the diagnosis of this illness owing to lack of standardization among clinical laboratories and problems with both sensitivity and specificity in some laboratories. Therefore, unlike most bacterial diseases, which can be defined microbiologically by direct observation or culture of the pathogen, Lyme disease is defined indirectly. In the absence of EM, the basis for diagnosis is the demonstration of an immune response against *B. burgdorferi*, in an appropriate clinical setting. This is not optimum, especially in view of the widespread myth that Lyme disease is responsible for a wide array of vague nonspecific symptoms and the substantial frequency of background seropositivity in endemic areas (4% in highly endemic areas of North America and 8% in Europe) (150–151). Lack of agreement on a precise clinical definition for this illness and lack of standardization of serologic assays with a high rate of false-positive results in some laboratories have led to confusion.

Antibody responses to *B. burgdorferi* in the infected host follow the usual pattern: IgM antibody appears first, followed by IgG and IgA responses (150). Within 2 to 3 weeks after the onset of infection, a rise in antibody against two or more spirochetal antigens can be detected in virtually all infected individuals. During the second and third months of infection, specific IgG and IgA responses gradually increase and, once established, may remain detectable for years, even with curative treatment. In most humans, the earliest immune response to *B. burgdorferi* is directed to the protein antigens, flagellin (p41) and OspC (25-kd), with 37-kd and 39-kd protein antigens also eliciting an early response in many individuals (152). Sensitive techniques can detect a response to OspA in early infection in some individuals, but large amounts of antibodies to the major outer-surface lipoproteins OspA and OspB generally appear only much later in the course of infection, if at all. The delayed immune response to OspA with respect to OspC may be the result of host-dependent differential expression of these surface proteins by the spirochete (153). OspA expression is adapted to spirochetes present in the tick gut, whereas OspC is expressed only by spirochetes in a feeding tick and in the mammal during the earliest phase of infection.

In the clinical laboratory, antibodies against *B. burgdorferi* are usually detected by either indirect immunofluorescence assay (IFA) or enzyme-linked immunosorbent assay (ELISA). Whole *B. burgdorferi* preparations are generally used for these assays. For the IFA, fixed *B. burgdorferi* is used as the antigen substrate, and for most ELISAs, crude fractions of sonicated organisms are used. None of these assays is standardized. Consequently, there is wide variability between laboratories regarding how assays are performed and reported. The sensitivity, specificity, and normal values are not comparable between laboratories. The positive predictive value of current IFA and ELISA assays is poor (150). Spirochetes make up part of the normal human flora, and most individuals have circulating antibodies that are cross-reactive with one or more *B. burgdorferi* antigens. This is especially true for the 41-kd flagellin antigen and some of the common bacterial antigens expressed by this pathogen (150). Further complicating the assessment of the humoral response is that, like syphilis, prompt antimicrobial therapy can abort the development of a mature humoral response, and patients treated before they develop a mature humoral response may lack diagnostic levels of *Borrelia*-specific antibodies (150,154).

Using highly sensitive immunoblots, we have found that greater than half of normal healthy adults with no history *B. burgdorferi* infection had circulating anti–41-kd IgG antibody. Many also had antibodies against other spirochetal antigens, most commonly, the 60-kd common bacterial antigen and the 66-kd antigen. This high level of cross-reactive antibodies is why most laboratories performing the IFA have established negative cutoffs between 1:64 and 1:256. ELISA can be more easily used to screen large numbers of serum samples and do not have the problem of observer error intrinsic to the IFA. Most laboratories using ELISA have established their norms and negative cutoffs statistically. Absorbency of 3 standard deviations or more above the mean of healthy controls is the value that most laboratories use to establish their cutoff. Although IFA can be as useful as ELISA for detection of antibodies against *B. burgdorferi* in the peripheral blood, to measure antibody concentrations in CSF, the superior sensitivity of ELISA offers a marked advantage. With the exception of demonstrating intrathecal antibody production in CSF, the positive predictive value of a positive assay by itself is low, no matter which test is used, IFA or ELISA.

To improve the specificity of serologies, the Centers for Disease Control and Prevention (CDC) recommend that all positive ELISAs and IFAs be followed by Western blot analysis (150). Only if both the first-tier assay and the Western blot are positive should the patient be considered seropositive. The IgM blot is thought to be helpful only early in the course of infection, that is, infection of less than 4 weeks' duration, whereas the IgG Western blot is useful at any point. IgM Western blots should not be done on patients with late disease. IgM assays have a higher rate of false-positive results and can lead to inappropriate diagnoses. To be considered positive, there should be IgM reactivity against any two of the following proteins: the 23-kd (OspC), 39-kd, or 41-kd protein. The criteria proposed by Dressler are recommended for IgG blot interpretation (155). It is recognized that the apparent molecular weight of individual proteins can vary among strains or under different growth conditions.

Recently, new recombinant-based assays and peptide-based assays have been developed. A peptide-based ELISA using a 26–amino acid peptide from the conserved region of the VLS protein is highly promising (156). This assay has become available for routine clinical use. It is highly specific and in early disease is highly sensitive (157). A sensitive and specific rapid recombinant-based assay using portions of key borrelial antigens is approved for doctors' office use and yields results in 20 minutes or less (158,159). Both of these new assays still require that Western blot analysis be performed on all positive patients.

It should be remembered that the finding that an individual has significant amounts of antibody reactive to *B. burgdorferi* can only be interpreted in the context of the clinical setting. Simply demonstrating that someone has an immune response against this organism does not mean that person is actively infected or that any symptoms have anything to do with *B. burgdorferi* infection. A diagnosis of Lyme borreliosis requires that objective clinical abnormalities be documented. Likewise, if an individual has objective neurologic abnormalities clinically compatible with Lyme borreliosis, examination of CSF should be considered, even if the peripheral antibody studies are negative. Very rarely, individuals with negative peripheral serologies have evidence of local antibody production in the CNS. Individuals without diagnostic levels of antibody in either their serum or CSF are highly unlikely to have active *B. burgdorferi* infection, and other reasons for their signs and symptoms should be sought. Seronegative extracutaneous Lyme disease is extremely rare (160). Earlier reports of this entity all occurred in patients treated with antibiotic regimens that are no longer recommended.

PREVENTION

Risk Assessment

Assessing the risk for Lyme disease is essential for planning effective prevention measures. The seasonal nature of Lyme disease risk is determined by the onset and duration of host-seeking activity by nymphal *I. scapularis* (161,162). This is quite predictable because onset is controlled by the duration of sunlight. In the

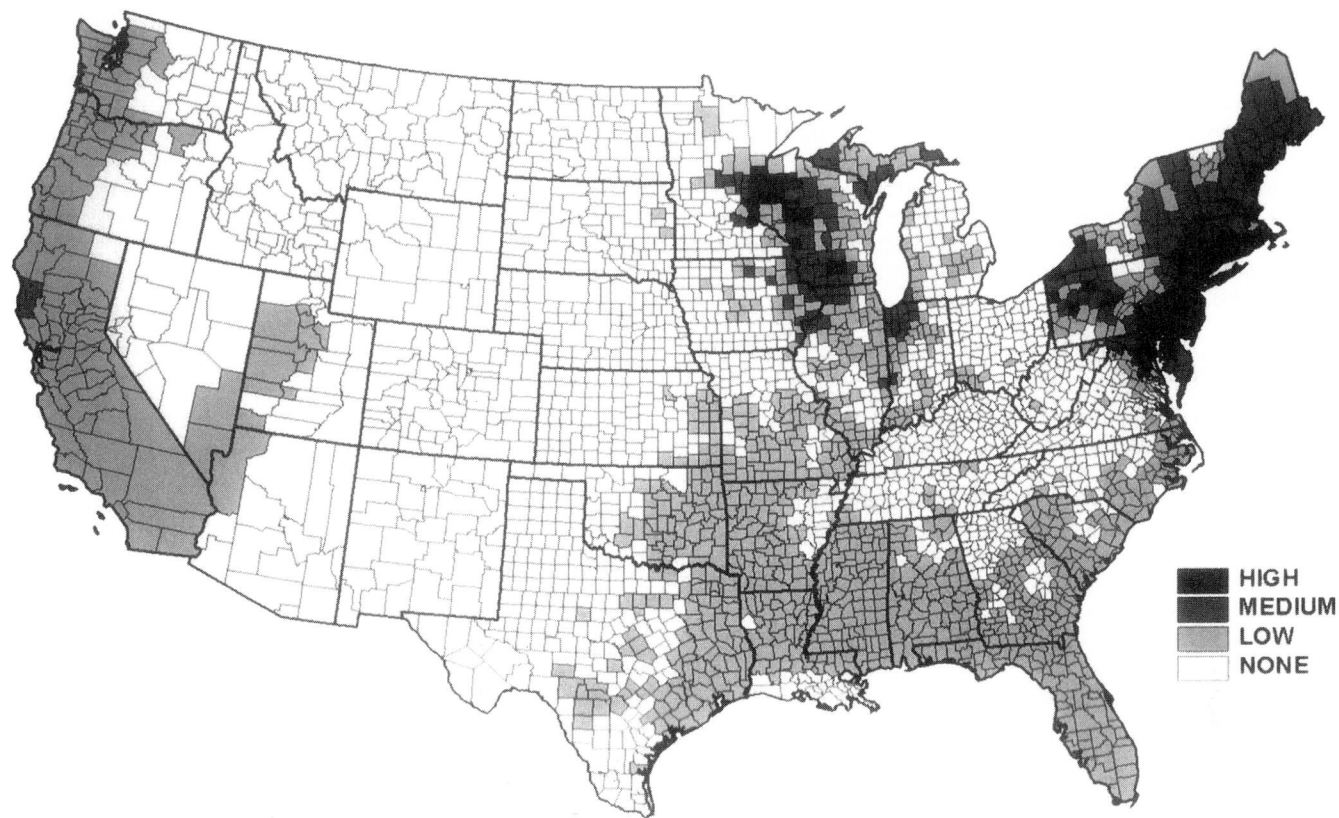

Figure 214.3. National Lyme disease risk map differentiated into counties with high, moderate, low, or minimal to no risk.

northeastern United States, nymphal tick feeding starts in late May, and duration, although dependent on local climate, rarely lasts until September (161). Thus, the seasonal period of risk is roughly equivalent each year.

In the United States, the geographic distribution of infected *I. scapularis* in the upper Midwest and Northeast is expanding, suggesting that risk is not geographically stable (163,164). The geographic incidence of human Lyme disease follows the geographic distribution of *B. burgdorferi*–infected ixodid ticks, with more than 90% of cases reported from the Northeast and upper Midwest (165). The National Lyme Disease Risk Map produced for the CDC (166) provides information on geographic Lyme disease risk Fig. 214.3. All counties within the contiguous United States are placed within one of four risk categories ranging from high to low or none. Even within high-risk counties, risk at the local scale is dependent on habitat suitability for the establishment and maintenance of vector ticks and human activities that result in exposure (167,168). In the Northeast, the risk is primarily from peridomestic exposure due to the expansion of suburban developments into forested areas and an overabundance of deer, which contribute to high densities of *I. scapularis* ticks (169–171). However, in the upper Midwest, exposure to infected ticks from recreational activities appears to be the predominant mode of acquiring Lyme disease (172). Information on the local distribution of *I. scapularis* and delineation of areas of high human risk for exposure can frequently be obtained from local or state departments of public health.

Vector Control

Reduction or elimination of the vector species is a key measure in the control of vector-borne disease. For controlling ticks, three approaches have been found to be effective: area application of insecticides, wildlife host management, and environmental alteration. Several studies have demonstrated the efficacy of applying insecticides to tick-infested areas to reduce Lyme disease risk (173–177). A single application in early spring targeted against nymphal ticks is effective. New nymphs will not appear until later in the summer when larvae develop into nymphal ticks, and these nymphs will not feed until the following year (176). Nymphs attached to animals will complete feeding and molt into adults. There is no mechanism for recruitment of new nymphs until the following year, once they are eradicated from an area. Thus, short-acting insecticides are effective and long-acting ones are not necessary. Although adult ticks pose little risk for Lyme disease, a second application of insecticide during September will reduce the densities of both fall and spring adults.

Studies have shown that almost any insecticide registered for lawn insect control will also control ticks (177). Management of wildlife hosts is less practical. Deer are the preferred host of *I. scapularis* adults, and eliminating deer is a potential means of controlling tick populations (178). Although eliminating deer totally is impractical, they can be excluded from high-risk residential or recreational areas by fencing. Studies of fencing to exclude deer from individual residential properties in New York and Connecticut reduced nymphal *I. scapularis* by 47% to 83% (179,180). Because a single deer can support more than 100 female ticks, each of which can produce 3,000 larvae, exclusion must be total. Fencing may be limited to October to April to coincide with the activity period of adult *I. scapularis* (161).

Pyrethin-treated cotton made available for mice to use as nesting material, and bait-boxes that attract and directly treat small mammals with insecticide have had limited success in independent studies (181–184). These products only reduce the prevalence of *B. burgdorferi* infection in nymphal ticks and do not reduce or eliminate the tick population.

Creating habitats less suitable for wildlife attraction and tick survival by altering residential or recreational environments is another option. Clearing leaf litter and providing an inhospitable barrier for mammals and ticks by surrounding the property with a narrow strip of wood chips has been found to reduce nymphal abundance by more than 70% in residential properties (185–187). Thinning canopy trees and shrubs and removing leaf litter lowers surface humidity levels, reducing the survival of overwintering ticks (187,188).

Personal Protection

Ticks are attracted by heat and carbon dioxide. They seek passing animals by ascending blades of grass or leaves and waiting for an animal to brush against the vegetation. Larval and nymphal-stage ticks usually ascend less than 0.5 m (20 inches) and adults from 0.5 to 1.0 m (20 to 40 inches). Because host-seeking ticks are close to the ground, restriction of tick access below the knees is important for preventing nymphs from contacting skin. In addition, wearing light-colored clothing makes crawling ticks more visible, providing greater opportunity to remove ticks before they bite.

DEET (N-N-diethyl-meta toluamide) can be used on skin or on clothing to prevent ticks from crawling on skin or clothing (189–192). Application should be limited to exposed skin, and not skin underneath clothing. Clothing can be treated with 1% permethrin, but permethrin should not be applied to skin (190). Permethrin-treated clothes can be used along with DEET skin application for protection. However, no combination of protective clothing and repellants is 100% effective in preventing tick bites.

Prompt removal of ticks is the best defense against infection, even when all other preventive measures are followed. Using a fine-tipped forceps to grab the tick as close to the skin as possible and pulling the tick away from the attachment site at an angle perpendicular to the skin is one of the best ways to remove a tick (193). Complete removal of tick mouthparts (hypostome) is frequently impossible because of associated barbs (denticles). There is no need to remove retained mouthparts surgically. Warm soaks can be used to facilitate their expulsion.

If identification is in doubt, ticks may be sent to a local health department, cooperative extension service, or academic ento-

mology department. Testing ticks for the presence of pathogens is not warranted or practical because blood accumulated in the gut of feeding ticks even after 24 hours of feeding can compromise both immunofluorescent and molecular-based pathogen detection methods (194,195). Outdoor clothing and pets can transport nymphal *I. scapularis* inside a home (196). Placing clothing in a clothes dryer for 30 minutes kills any ticks on the clothes. Flea and tick products are effective in protecting pets from ticks (197). The low humidity in most homes prevents the survival of *I. scapularis* within houses.

Chemoprophylaxis

Four prospective, randomized, placebo-controlled studies of antibiotic prophylaxis have been conducted to assess the efficacy of antibiotics in preventing Lyme disease in patients with recent *I. scapularis* tick bites (198–201). Antibiotic efficacy varied from 87% to 100% in preventing EM at the tick bite site (the most reliable indicator of transmission of *B. burgdorferi* by a specific tick bite). Although three of the studies had an antibiotic efficacy rate of 100%, antibiotics were not significantly more effective than placebo (198–200). This is mainly attributable to the low risk for transmission of *B. burgdorferi* from tick bites in the United States that are recognized and removed (1.1% to 3.2%) and to the relatively small number of subjects enrolled. Transmission of *B. burgdorferi* is slow, and removing the tick during the feeding process interrupts transmission (202–204). In animal experiments using *I. scapularis* ticks, transmission rarely occurs before 48 hours of feeding (205). However, transmission of spirochetes within 24 hours to laboratory animals is well documented in experiments in Europe using *I. ricinus* ticks. In addition, two United States studies have demonstrated that the frequency of transmission to humans is significantly greater after tick bites in which the ticks were estimated to have fed for at least 72 hours. Studies in two of the most highly endemic areas of the Northeast found that the risk for Lyme disease after 72 hours of *I. scapularis* tick feeding was 20% among patients bitten on Eastern Long Island, NY (206) and 25% among patients bitten in Westchester County, NY (201). In a United States study using an experimentally validated estimate of the duration of *I. scapularis* tick feeding based on the degree of blood engorgement of the tick, 63% of the ticks were removed before 24 hours, 9% between 24 and 48 hours, 15% between 48 and 72 hours, and only 13% after 72 hours of feeding (207) (Fig. 214.4). The high incidence of

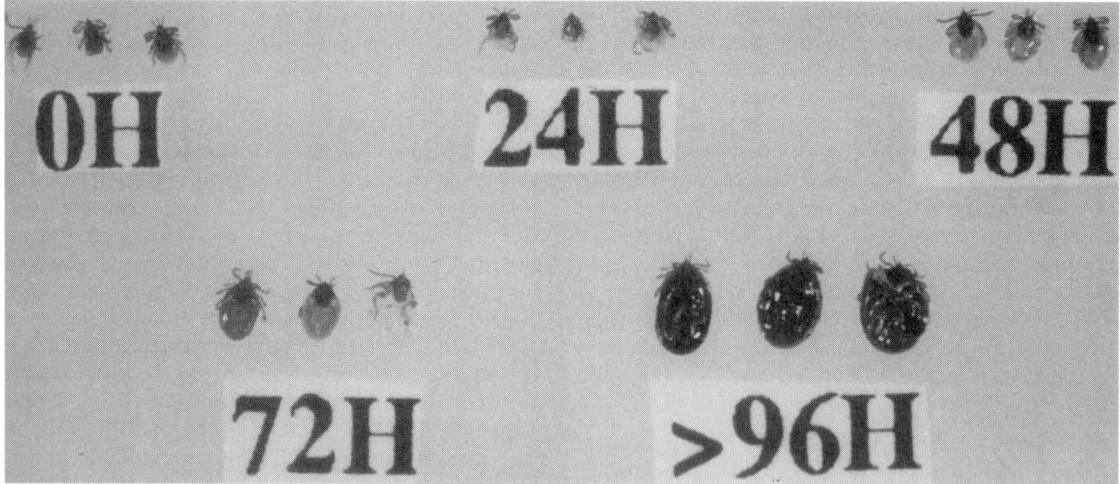

Figure 214.4. Nymphal *Ixodes scapularis* ticks demonstrating changes in blood engorgement after various durations of attachment to an animal host. (Photograph is a generous gift from Dr. Richard Falco.)

feeding durations of less than 72 hours is probably responsible for the minimal risk of Lyme disease observed among placebo recipients in the chemoprophylaxis trials.

Although adult *I. scapularis* ticks have a higher *B. burgdorferi* infection rate than nymphal-stage ticks, human infection associated with adult tick bites is infrequent. This is presumably because adult ticks are larger and therefore more readily observed and more quickly removed. In one study, the estimated median duration of attachment was 10 hours for 76 adult ticks compared with 30 hours for 115 nymphal-stage ticks ($p < 0.001$) (201). Infection is also more likely to result from nymphal-stage tick bites because bites from nymphs are more common. The latter is true for several reasons, including the greater number of nymphal-stage ticks in the environment (more than 10-fold higher than adult-stage ticks) (29) and seasonal differences in the abundance of nymphal- versus adult-stage ticks pertinent to human exposure (208).

Most of the studies on antibiotic prophylaxis of tick bites (198–200), as well as a cost-effectiveness analysis of antibiotic treatment (209), used a 10- to 14-day course of antibiotics, a course similar to that used to treat EM (210,211). Because a single dose of antibiotic therapy had previously been established as successful in preventing syphilis (212) or leptospirosis (213), Nadelman and colleagues tried a similar approach in a randomized study of 482 patients with an *I. scapularis* tick bite (201). Using a single 200-mg dose of doxycycline as the treatment arm, only one doxycycline-treated patient developed EM at the tick bite site (this patient was bitten by a nymphal-stage tick), whereas 3.2% of placebo recipients, including 5.6% of 142 patients bitten by nymphal-stage ticks and 0% of 97 patients bitten by adult-stage ticks, developed EM at the tick bite site. The efficacy rate for doxycycline was 87% (95% confidence interval, 25% to 98%; $p < 0.04$). The single dose of doxycycline effectively prevented EM (201).

Before publication of the single-dose doxycycline study, our practice had been not to offer antibiotic prophylaxis for tick bites. We would instead monitor patients with tick bites for signs and symptoms of tick-borne illness for up to 30 days after the bite. We have reevaluated this approach and now recommend in highly endemic areas 200 mg of doxycycline as prophylaxis for adult patients who have removed an engorged nymphal-stage *I. scapularis* tick and who have no contraindications to receipt of tetracycline antibiotics. Children younger than 8 years of age and pregnant or lactating women should not receive tetracyclines. Although it has never been systematically studied, based on a crude extrapolation from the single-dose doxycycline study, a 72-hour course of amoxicillin may be offered to individuals who are unable to take tetracyclines. There is less of a rationale for antibiotic prophylaxis of *I. pacificus* tick bites because their infection rate with *B. burgdorferi* is considerably lower (214–217). Because all genospecies of *B. burgdorferi* are highly susceptible to doxycycline *in vitro* (218), a single prophylactic dose of doxycycline should be effective for *I. ricinus* or *I. persulcatus* tick bites (the vectors of Lyme borreliosis in Eurasia), but no data are available to substantiate this hypothesis. Larval-stage ixodid ticks are virtually always uninfected with *B. burgdorferi* because of the rarity of transovarian transmission of the spirochete; therefore, prophylaxis is unnecessary (219).

Tick bite chemoprophylaxis has a number of limitations. The primary limitation is that about 75% of patients with Lyme disease in the United States do not recognize the tick bite in the first place (220). Single-dose therapy is not 100% effective, and there is no evidence that such treatment would prevent transmission of other potential tick-borne pathogens. In addition, even single-dose antibiotic treatment can cause an array of potential adverse effects, including, but not limited to, allergic reactions, nausea,

and vomiting (201). Insects and scabs may be confused with ticks, and vector-tick species may not be distinguished from nonvector species, leading to unwarranted use of antibiotic prophylaxis (206,221). Also, many practitioners and patients cannot reliably differentiate an engorged from an unengorged nymphal-stage tick.

Immunoprophylaxis

Immunoprophylaxis is a potential option to prevent Lyme disease. In experimental animals, humoral immunity can provide protection against *B. burgdorferi* infection (222–224), and in some model systems, passive immunization may also ameliorate or eliminate preexistent infection (225–228).

An efficacy study of 10,936 subjects aged 15 to 70 years who received either three doses of a recombinant OspA vaccine or placebo (93) demonstrated a reduction of Lyme disease in the vaccine group of 76%. In December 1998, the U.S. Food and Drug Administration (FDA) approved an aluminum hydroxide adjuvanted lipidated recombinant OspA vaccine known as LYMErix (229). This vaccine was withdrawn from the market in 2002 because of poor sales.

TREATMENT

Although *in vitro* susceptibility testing has not been standardized, available studies suggest that *B. burgdorferi* is highly susceptible to a number of antimicrobial drug classes, including tetracyclines, penicillins, second- and third-generation cephalosporins, and macrolides (210,230). These microorganisms are resistant to fluoroquinolones, rifampin, and first-generation cephalosporins (210,231,232). Published randomized controlled antibiotic studies have demonstrated that a number of regimens are highly efficacious. With very rare exceptions, courses of antibiotics of 10 to 28 days' duration are successful for treatment of patients with Lyme disease (210). Considering the risk-to-benefit ratio, there is no justification for extended courses of antibiotics in this infectious disease. Even without treatment, most manifestations of Lyme disease resolve spontaneously. Antibiotics hasten the resolution of symptoms and prevent disease progression. When treated appropriately, less than 5% of infected individuals fail to respond to antibiotic therapy as evidenced by objective manifestations, and repeat treatment with antimicrobials is rarely required (210) (Tables 214.2 and 214.3).

Erythema Migrans

EM is the best-studied manifestation of Lyme disease with regard to antibiotic therapy. At least eight randomized prospective trials have addressed the treatment of individuals with EM in the United States, and many other studies on this topic have been conducted in Europe (96,154,210,232–236). It is clear from these studies that doxycycline, amoxicillin, and cefuroxime axetil, when given orally for time periods ranging from 10 to 21 days, are highly effective (210), with most patients responding promptly and completely. Ceftriaxone was compared with oral doxycycline in patients with multiple EM lesions without active signs of CNS infection (237). Both antibiotics were equally effective; there was no additional benefit in using parenteral ceftriaxone. Macrolides are highly active against *B. burgdorferi in vitro* (238), yet in treatment trials of erythromycin and azithromycin in the United States (154,232) and in a roxithromycin study performed in Europe (239), these macrolides were significantly less effective than the comparator antibiotics used. In several small European

TABLE 214.2. Recommended Antimicrobial Regimens for Treatment of Patients with Lyme Disease

Recommended drug	Dosage for adults	Dosage for children
Preferred oral		
Amoxicillin	500 mg t.i.d.	50 mg/kg/d divided into 3 doses (maximum, 500 mg/dose)
Doxycycline	100 mg b.i.d.[a]	Age < 8 y: not recommended; age ≥ 8 y: 1–2 mg/kg b.i.d. (maximum, 100 mg/dose)
Alternative oral		
Cefuroxime axetil	500 mg b.i.d.	30 mg/kg/d divided into 2 doses (maximum, 500 mg/dose)
Preferred parenteral		
Ceftriaxone	2 g i.v. once daily	75–100 mg/kg iv per day in a single dose (maximum, 2 g)
Alternative parenteral		
Cefotaxime	2 g i.v. t.i.d.	150–200 mg/kg/d i.v. divided into 3 or 4 doses (maximum, 6 g/d)
Penicillin G	18–24 million units i.v./d divided into doses given q4h[b]	200,000–400,000 units/kg/d, divided into doses given q4h[b] (maximum, 18–24 million units/d)

[a]Tetracyclines are relatively contraindicated for pregnant or lactating women.
[b]The penicillin dosage should be reduced for patients with impaired renal function.
From Wormser GP, Nadelman RB, Dattwyler RJ, et al. Practice guidelines for the treatment of Lyme disease. *Clin Infect Dis* 2000;31[Suppl 1]:S1–14, with permission.

trials, azithromycin was not significantly different in efficacy compared with comparators (240–244). It is unclear whether the different genospecies of *Borrelia* in Europe or methodologic limitations in study design, such as small sample size, account for the observed greater effectiveness of azithromycin in Europe.

No controlled comparative studies of clarithromycin have been carried out (245).

Patients with multiple EM lesions and those with numerous and more severe systemic manifestations at the time of diagnosis are more likely to have persistent or intermittent subjective

TABLE 214.3. Treatment of Lyme Disease

Indication	Treatment	Duration (d)
Cutaneous lesions		
Erythema migrans	Oral regimen[a,b]	10–21
Lymphocytoma	Oral regimen[a,b]	14–21
Acrodermatitis chronica atrophicans[a]	Oral regimen[a]	28
Acute neurologic disease		
Meningitis or radiculopathy	Parenteral regimen[a,c]	14–28
Cranial nerve palsy	Oral regimen[a]	14–21
Cardiac disease		
First- or second-degree heart block	Oral regimen[a]	14–21
Third-degree heart block	Parenteral regimen[a,d]	14–21
Late disease		
Arthritis without neurologic disease	Oral regimen[a]	28
Recurrent arthritis after oral regimen	Oral regimen[a] or parenteral regimen[a]	28 / 14–28
Persistent arthritis after 2 courses of oral antibiotics or 1 course of a parenteral antibiotic	Symptomatic therapy	
Central or peripheral nervous system disease	Parenteral regimen	14–28
Post–Lyme disease syndrome	Symptomatic therapy	

[a]See Table 214.2.
[b]For adult patients who are intolerant of amoxicillin, doxycycline, and cefuroxime axetil, alternatives are azithromycin (500 mg orally daily for 7–10 d), erythromycin (500 mg orally 4 times per day for 14–21 d), or clarithromycin (500 mg orally twice daily for 14–21 days, except during pregnancy). The recommended dosages of these agents for children are as follows: azithromycin, 10 mg/kg daily (maximum, 500 mg/d); erythromycin 12.5 mg/kg 4 times daily (maximum, 500 mg/dose); clarithromycin 7.5 mg/kg twice daily (maximum, 500 mg/dose). Patients treated with macrolides should be closely followed.
[c]For nonpregnant adult patients intolerant of both penicillin and cephalosporins, doxycycline (200–400 mg/d orally, or i.v. if oral medications cannot be taken, divided into 2 doses) may be adequate.
[d]A temporary pacemaker may be required.

complaints following treatment (246). Unrecognized CNS infection or co-infection with other tick-borne infections may be responsible for treatment failures in a minority of cases (247,248).

Rarely, within 24 hours of initiating appropriate antibiotic therapy for patients with EM, patients experience arthralgias, an increase in temperature, or malaise (210). This Jarisch-Herxheimer–like reaction is not observed in patients treated for later manifestations of Lyme disease. Classical Jarisch-Herxheimer–like reactions are not observed in Lyme disease. All antimicrobials can cause side effects. Both amoxicillin and cefuroxime axetil can cause drug-induced rashes, and doxycycline is also associated with photosensitivity and photodermatitis. Fortunately, doxycycline, amoxicillin, and cefuroxime axetil, which are recommended for the treatment of patients with EM, have a low frequency of serious adverse effects (210). A limitation of doxycycline therapy is that EM is most common in the late spring and summer when the chance for photosensitivity reactions is greatest. Individuals treated with doxycycline should be advised to avoid sun exposure while receiving therapy. Tetracyclines have the advantage over β-lactams in that they are also effective therapy for HGE, which can occur simultaneously with Lyme disease (249).

Cefuroxime axetil is the only FDA-approved drug for the treatment of EM. However, it is not an attractive first-line agent because it is much more expensive than either doxycycline or amoxicillin (210). Although cefuroxime axetil has been proved effective in the treatment of Lyme disease, no other oral cephalosporin antibiotic has proven efficacy, and no others should be used. First-generation cephalosporins such as cephalexin have been demonstrated to be ineffective clinically (231).

There are no prospective treatment trials of pregnant patients. Nevertheless, other than avoiding tetracyclines, there are no data to suggest, and little rationale to believe, that pregnant patients should be treated differently from other patients with Lyme disease (210,250–252). Amoxicillin is the most commonly recommended antibiotic for the treatment of pregnant patients with EM.

Early Neuroborreliosis

No randomized antibiotic treatment trial in North America has specifically addressed early neuroborreliosis. The relatively few studies on therapy of early neurologic Lyme disease have mainly been carried out in Europe (210). Ceftriaxone is the most commonly studied antibiotic in neurologic infection, and it has efficacy in patients with Lyme meningitis or acute radiculopathy. Oral doxycycline has also been used successfully in Europe, but experience with this agent for treatment of patients with Lyme meningitis in the United States is limited (210).

No placebo-controlled studies on patients with active neurologic disease have been (nor will be) done in North American Lyme disease. Comparing antibiotic treatment, mainly with penicillin, to historical series of untreated patients or of patients treated with only corticosteroids, the data are conflicting as to whether there is an advantage favoring antibiotics (253–258). Nonetheless, the accepted standard of care for patients with neurologic Lyme disease is antimicrobial treatment (210,259).

The natural history of untreated patients is slow resolution of clinical and CSF abnormalities over the course of 2 to 6 months or longer (254,256,260). Clinical findings typically fluctuate in intensity over this period.

Radiculoneuritis with severe pain is a prominent symptom among some European patients with early neuroborreliosis. In the United States, seventh-nerve palsy and meningitis are the two most common acute neurologic manifestations of Lyme disease, whereas radiculoneuritis is extremely rare. In one report on the treatment of North American Lyme meningitis, 12 patients treated with parenteral penicillin were compared retrospectively with 15 patients previously treated only with corticosteroids (254). The patients treated with penicillin responded significantly faster, with resolution of headache and stiff neck beginning by the second day of antibiotic therapy. In another study, clinical improvement was noted in most patients by the third to fifth day of antimicrobial therapy (261).

Ceftriaxone, given once daily intravenously, has become standard practice for both adults and children with early neuroborreliosis. It is the most convenient regimen (because of the drug's long serum half-life) (210). An exception to this is that oral antibiotic therapy may be sufficient in patients with uncomplicated seventh-nerve palsy (210). Any patient with seventh-nerve palsy for whom there is a strong clinical suspicion of CNS involvement (i.e., those with severe headache or meningismus) should undergo a lumbar puncture before a treatment decision is made. If CSF pleocytosis is found, the patient should be treated with parenteral antibiotics. It is not clear that antibiotics affect the rate or frequency of recovery of seventh-nerve palsy. The principal goal of therapy may be to prevent development of later clinical manifestations. One study has addressed neuroborreliosis that remained untreated for more than 10 years (262). The most common complaint in the 11 patients in that study was arthralgia. The treatment of patients with peripheral nervous system manifestations is likewise ill defined. Parenteral antibiotic therapy (i.e., ceftriaxone) is often used for these patients, but given the absence of data or clear rationale to justify parenteral therapy, comparative studies with oral regimens appear warranted (210,259).

Lyme Carditis

Controlled studies on the treatment of cardiac manifestations of Lyme disease and acute Lyme carditis with heart block are lacking. Lyme carditis will usually remit spontaneously, even without treatment, but the standard of care is to give antibiotics. An expert panel has recommended that patients with first- or second-degree heart block resulting from Lyme disease may be treated with oral antibiotic therapy (210). Patients with third-degree heart block should be closely monitored, preferably in a hospital setting (263). These latter patients are usually treated at least initially with parenteral antibiotic therapy; insertion of a temporary pacemaker also may be necessary (210).

Lyme Arthritis

About 90% of patients with Lyme arthritis can be expected to respond to antibiotics or spontaneously remit (264) even without treatment. Both oral and intravenous antibiotic regimens shorten the course of arthritis and eradicate DNA evidence of *B. burgdorferi* from the joint (210,264–270). In the absence of concurrent neurologic involvement, oral therapy is more cost effective than intravenous therapy for Lyme arthritis. Although a few patients may develop nervous system manifestations after oral treatment, oral therapy is safer and substantially less costly (271). An expert panel concluded that oral antibiotics are preferred in the initial treatment of Lyme arthritis (210). There are rare individuals with Lyme arthritis who do not respond to antibiotics but continue to have joint swelling. In one treatment trial, 16 patients with unremitting Lyme arthritis despite prior treatment with parenteral or oral antibiotic regimens were treated with ceftriaxone, and all continued to have arthritis during the 3-month posttherapy observation period (272). These 16 patients were also found to have distinctive immunogenetic and immune markers, including a high frequency of HLA-DR4 specificity and of antibody reactivity with OspA (115).

For patients who have persistent or recurrent joint swelling for 3 months after a 28-day course of oral antibiotic therapy, an expert panel recommended repeat treatment with another 28-day course of oral antibiotics or with a 14- to 28-day course of ceftriaxone (210). A 3-month observation period after the initial course of therapy is recommended because of the anticipated slow resolution of inflammation. If joint inflammation persists, no further antibiotic therapy is recommended. A trial of symptomatic therapy is warranted.

For patients with persistent arthritis, arthroscopic synovectomy may be effective. In a study of 20 patients who underwent this procedure for refractory chronic Lyme arthritis of the knee, 16 (80%) had resolution of joint inflammation during the first month following surgery or soon thereafter (273). The remaining 4 patients (20%) had persistent or recurrent synovitis.

Late Neuroborreliosis

The natural history of untreated late peripheral neuropathy and encephalopathy is not well defined. However, these manifestations appear to progress very slowly and to develop in only a small fraction of untreated patients (130–132). Whether spontaneous resolution occurs or not is also unclear. It is clear that most of these patients, as well as those with encephalomyelitis, improve coincident with antibiotic therapy, although often without complete resolution of signs and symptoms (132,274). Analysis of two comparative studies of the treatment of late Lyme disease including patients who had rheumatologic or neurologic manifestations suggests that the third-generation cephalosporins, ceftriaxone and cefotaxime, are more efficacious than parenteral penicillin (275,276). Whether penicillin is truly less effective than third-generation cephalosporins is not important because the convenience of once-daily dosing makes ceftriaxone the preferred agent (210). After antibiotic therapy, rapid recovery should not be expected. Patients with late neuroborreliosis improve slowly over the course of months (132–135). The role of systemic corticosteroids has never been systematically evaluated.

In a trial of 27 adult patients with Lyme encephalopathy, polyneuropathy, or both treated with intravenous ceftriaxone for 2 weeks, response to therapy was usually gradual and did not begin until several months after treatment (132). Outcome measures included CSF analyses and neuropsychological tests of memory, in addition to assessment of clinical signs and symptoms. Measuring the response 6 months after treatment, 17 patients (63%) had uncomplicated improvement, 6 (22%) had improvement but then relapsed, and 4 (15%) were unchanged. In a subsequent study, 18 adult patients with Lyme encephalopathy were treated with a 30-day course of intravenous ceftriaxone (274). The same outcome measures were used. Six months after treatment, 14 (93%) of the 15 evaluable patients reported diminished symptoms, and verbal memory scores for the 15 patients were significantly improved ($p < 0.01$). For the 10 patients who had follow-up analyses, CSF protein values were significantly reduced ($p < 0.05$). One patient was retreated at 8 months. All evaluable patients had returned to normal or had improved by 12 to 24 months after treatment. The authors concluded that Lyme encephalopathy can be treated successfully with a 30-day course of intravenous ceftriaxone, suggesting that this entity may be associated with active infection of the nervous system. No trial has compared length of treatment; thus, whether a 30-day course is superior to 14 days of treatment remains to be defined (210). It is clear, however, that these studies do not support the need for treatment for more than 30 days. Children with neurocognitive abnormalities attributed to Lyme disease have not been well studied but also appear to improve after 2 to 4 weeks of intravenous ceftriaxone (277).

Post–Lyme Disease Syndrome

Regardless of the manifestation of Lyme disease being treated, a small proportion of patients may experience either constantly or intermittently a variety of subjective complaints after treatment, including myalgia, arthralgia, or fatigue. Some have labeled this phenomenon *post–Lyme disease syndrome* or *chronic Lyme disease*. A strict case definition for this entity does not exist, nor have its underlying mechanisms been defined (210). The frequency and type of complaints reported are indistinguishable from those that occur in otherwise healthy matched controls without Lyme borreliosis (278). To determine whether post–Lyme disease syndrome is antibiotic responsive, two treatment trials of patients with at least 6 months of post–Lyme disease symptoms were carried out (279). Identical treatments were used in the two trials: patients were randomized to receive either 1 month of intravenous ceftriaxone followed by 2 months of oral doxycycline or identical-appearing placebo therapies. Both of these antimicrobials are active against *B. burgdorferi in vitro*, have the ability to cross the blood–brain barrier, and have been proved efficacious in prospective trials. In the first trial, patients were required to have serologic evidence of exposure to *B. burgdorferi*, and in the second, serologic evidence was not required. The primary outcome measure in both studies was symptom improvement based on patient responses to a health-related quality-of-life questionnaire given 90 days after they completed the course of antibiotic treatment or placebo. Both studies were terminated early by a data and safety monitoring board because of lack of efficacy of the antibiotic therapy. There was no evidence that antibiotics were more effective than placebo. In both studies, regardless of whether antibiotic or placebo was administered, about one third of patients improved, one third remained unchanged, and one third worsened. In both trials, there was systematic testing by use of culture and PCR techniques of CSF and blood samples for evidence of active infection. None of the 129 patients had evidence of persistent *B. burgdorferi* infection. The investigators concluded that the patients' subjective complaints were not due to active *B. burgdorferi* infection and that it would be highly unlikely that different antibiotic regimens involving either alternative antimicrobial agents or longer durations of therapy would be beneficial. To our knowledge, *B. burgdorferi* has not been recovered from any patient in the United States following a recommended course of antibiotic treatment (280,281), although this phenomenon has rarely been reported in Europe (282). In light of current knowledge, antibiotics are not indicated for the treatment of ongoing symptoms after Lyme disease. These patients should receive only symptomatic therapy (210).

REFERENCES

1. Burgdorfer W, Hayes SF, Benach JL, et al. Lyme disease: a tick-borne spirochetosis? *Science* 1982;216:1317–1319.
2. Benach JL, Bosler EM, Hanrahan JP, et al. Spirochetes isolated from the blood of two patients with Lyme disease. *N Engl J Med* 1983;308:740–742.
3. Steere AC, Grodzicki RL, Kornblatt AN, et al. The spirochetal etiology of Lyme disease. *N Engl J Med* 1983;308:733–740.
4. Afzelius A. Verhandlungen der dermatologischen Gesellschaft zu Stockholm. *Arch Dermatol Syphilol* 1910;101:405–406.
5. Burgdorfer W. Discovery of the Lyme disease spirochete: a historical review. *Zentralbl Bakteriol Mikrobiol Hyg* 1986;263:7–10.

6. Garin C, Bujadoux C. Paralysie par les tiques. *J Med Lyon* 1922;3:765–767.
7. Hellerstrom S. Erythema chronicum migrans Afzelii. *Acta Derm Venereol (Stockh)* 1930;11:315–321.
8. Bannwarth A. Chronische Lymphocytare Meningitis entzudliche Polypeuritis and Rheumatismus. *Arch Psychiatr Nervenkr* 1941;113:284–376.
9. Bannwarth A. Zur Klinik and Pathogenese der "chronischen lymphocytaren Meningitis." *Arch Psychiatr Nervenkr* 1944;117:161–185.
10. Herxheimer K, Hartmann K. Uber Acrodermatitis chronica atrophicans. *Arch Dermatol Syphilis* 1902;61:57–76, 255—300.
11. Buchwald A. Ein Fall vor diffuser idiopathischer Haut-Atrophie. *Arch Dermatol Syphilis* 1883;15:553–556.
12. Bafverstedt B. Uber Lymphadenosis benigna cutis. *Acta Derm Venereol* 1943;24: 1–202.
13. Bianchi GE. Penicillinbehandlung der Lymphozytome. *Dermatologia* 1950;100: 270–273.
14. Hollstrom E. Successful treatment of erythema migrans Afzelius. *Acta Derm Venereol(Stockh)* 1951;31:325–332.
15. Scrimenti RJ. Erythema chronicum migrans. *Arch Dermatol* 1970;236:859–860.
16. Mast WE, Burrows WM. Erthema chronicum migrans in the United States. *JAMA* 1976;236:859–860.
17. Steere AC, Malawista SE, Snydman DR, et al. Lyme arthritis: an epidemic of oligoarticular arthritis in children and adults in three Connecticut communities. *Arthritis Rheum* 1977;20:7–17.
18. Wang G, Van Dam AP, Schwartz I, et al. Molecular typing of *Borrelia burgdorferi sensu lato*: taxonomic, epidemiologic, and clinical implications. *Clin Microbiol Rev* 1999;12:633–653.
19. De Koning J, Bosma RB, Hoogkamp-Korstanje JA. Demonstration of spirochaetes in patients with Lyme disease with a modified silver stain. *J Med Microbiol* 1987;23:261–267.
20. Barbour AG. Isolation and cultivation of Lyme disease spirochetes. *Yale J Biol Med* 1984;57:521–525.
21. Asbrink E, Hovmark A. Successful cultivation of spirochetes from skin lesions of patients with erythema chronicum migrans Afzelius and acrodermatitis chronica atrophicans. *Acta Path Microbiol Immunol* 1985;93B:161–163.
22. Wormser GP, Bittker S, Cooper D, et al. Comparison of the yields of blood cultures using serum or plasma from patients with early Lyme disease. *J Clin Microbiol* 2000;38(4):1648–1650.
23. Nadelman RB, Nowakowski J, Forseter G, et al. The clinical spectrum of early Lyme borreliosis in patients with culture-confirmed erythema migrans. *Am J Med* 1996;100:502–508.
24. Wang G, Van Dam AP, Schwartz I, et al. Molecular typing of *Borrelia burgdorferi sensu lato*: taxonomic, epidemiologic, and clinical implications. *Clin Microbiol Rev* 1999;12:633–653.
25. Rauter C, Oehme R, Diterich I, et al. Distribution of clinically relevant *Borrelia* genospecies in ticks assessed by a novel, single-run, real-time PCR. *J Clin Microbiol* 2002;40(1):36–43.
26. Wilske B, Barbour AG, Bergstrom S, et al. Antigenic variation and strain heterogeneity in *Borrelia* spp. *Res Microbiol* 1992;143:583–596.
27. Dykhuizen DE, Polin DS, Dunn JJ, et al. *Borrelia burgdorferi* is clonal: implications for taxonomy and vaccine development. *Proc Natl Acad Sci U S A* 1993;90:10163–10167.
28. O'Connell S, Granstrom M, Gray JS, et al. Epidemiology of European Lyme borreliosis. *Zentbl Bakteriol* 1998;287:229–240.
29. Strle F, Nadelman RB, Cimperman J, et al. Comparison of culture-confirmed erythema migrans caused by *Borrelia burgdorferi sensu stricto* in New York State and by *Borrelia afzelii* in Slovenia. *Ann Intern Med* 1999;130:32–36.
30. Lunemann JD, Zarmas S, Priem S, et al. Rapid typing of *Borrelia burgdorferi sensu lato* species in specimens from patients with different manifestations of Lyme borreliosis. *J Clin Microbiol* 2001;39(3):1130–1133.
31. Van Dam AP, Kuiper H, Vos K, et al. Different genospecies of *Borrelia burgdorferi* are associated with distinct clinical manifestations of Lyme borreliosis. *Clin Infect Dis* 1993;17:708–717.
32. Tazelaar DJ, Molkenboer MJ, Noordhoek GT, et al. Detection of *Borrelia afzelii*, *Borrelia burgdorferi sensu stricto*, *Borrelia garinii* and group VS 116 by PCR in skin biopsies of patients with erythema migrans and acrodermatitis chronica atrophicans. *Clin Microbiol Infect* 1997;3(1):109–116.
33. Wang G, van Dam AP, Schwartz I, et al. Molecular typing of *Borrelia burgdorferi sensu lato*: taxonomic, epidemiological, and clinical implications. *Clin Microbiol Rev* 1999;12(4):633–653.
34. Lin T, Oliver JH Jr, Gao L, et al. Genetic heterogeneity of *Borrelia burgdorferi sensu lato* in the southern United States based on restriction fragment length polymorphism and sequence analysis. *J Clin Microbiol* 2001;39(7):2500–2507.
35. Seinost G, Golde WT, Berger BW, et al. Infection with multiple strains of *Borrelia burgdorferi sensu stricto* in patients with Lyme disease. *Arch Dermatol* 1999;135(11):1329–1333.
36. Baranton G, Seinost G, Theodore G, et al. Distinct levels of genetic diversity of *Borrelia burgdorferi* are associated with different aspects of pathogenicity. *Res Microbiol* 2001;152(2):149–156.
37. Fraser CM, Casjens S, Huang WM, et al. Genomic sequence of a Lyme disease spirochete, *Borrelia burgdorferi*. *Nature* 1997;390:580–586.
38. Howe TR, LaQuier FW, Barbour AG. Organization of genes encoding two outer membrane proteins of the Lyme disease agent *Borrelia burgdorferi* within a single transcriptional unit. *Infect Immun* 1986;54:207–212.
39. Craft JE, Fischer D, Shimamoto GT, et al. Antigens of *Borrelia burgdorferi* recognized during Lyme disease: appearance of a new immunoglobulin in response and expansion of the immunoglobulin G response late in the illness. *J Clin Invest* 1986;78:934–939.
40. Schwan TG, Piesman J, Golde WT, et al. Induction of an outer surface protein on *Borrelia burgdorferi* during tick feeding. *Proc Natl Acad Sci U S A* 1995;92:2909–2913.
41. Gilmore RD Jr, Mbow ML, Stevenson B. Analysis of *Borrelia burgdorferi* gene expression during life cycle phases of the tick vector *Ixodes scapularis*. *Microbes Infect* 2001;3(10):799–808.
42. Theisen M, Frederiksen B, Lebech AM, et al. Polymorphism in OspC gene of *Borrelia burgdorferi* and immunoreactivity of OspC protein: implications for taxonomy and for use of OspC protein as a diagnostic antigen. *J Clin Microbiol* 1993;31:2570–2576.
43. Wilske B, Preac-Mursic V, Jauris S, et al. Immunological and molecular polymorphisms of OspC, an immunodominant major outer surface protein of *Borrelia burgdorferi*. *Infect Immun* 1993;61:2182–2191.
44. Livey I, Gibbs CP, Schuster R, et al. Evidence for lateral transfer and recombination in OspC variation in Lyme disease *Borrelia*. *Mol Microbiol* 1995;18:257–269.
45. Theisen M, Borre M, Mathiesen MJ, et al. Evolution of the *Borrelia burgdorferi* outer surface protein OspC. *J Bacteriol* 1995;177:3036–3044.
46. Seinost G, et al. Four clones of *Borrelia burgdorferi sensu stricto* cause invasive infection in humans. *Infect Immun* 1999;67(7):3518–3524.
47. Bunikis J, Mirian H, Bunikiene E, et al. Non-heritable change of a spirochaete's phenotype by decoration of the cell surface with exogenous lipoproteins. *Mol Microbiol* 2001;40(2):387–396.
48. Bunikis J, Barbour AG. Access of antibody or trypsin to an integral outer membrane protein (P66) of *Borrelia burgdorferi* is hindered by Osp lipoproteins. *Infect Immun* 1999;67(6):2874–2883.
49. Akins DR, Bourell KW, Caimano MJ, et al. A new animal model for studying Lyme disease spirochetes in a mammalian host-adapted state. *J Clin Invest* 1998;101(10):2240–2250.
50. Hovind-Hougen K, Asbrink E, Stiernstedt G, et al. Ultrastructural differences among spirochetes isolated from patients with Lyme disease and related disorders, and from *Ixodes ricinus*. *Zentralbl Bakteriol Mikrobiol Hyg [A]* 1986; 263(1–2):103–111.
50a. Liveris D, Wormser GP, Nowakowski J, et al. Molecular typing of *Borrelia burgdorferi* from Lyme disease patients by PCR-restriction fragment length polymorphism analysis. *J Clin Microbiol* 1996;34:1306–1309.
51. Wilske B, Preac-Mursic V, Schierz G, et al. Antigenic variability of *Borrelia burgdorferi*. *Ann N Y Acad Sci* 1988;539:126–143.
52. Hansen K, Bangsborg JM, Fjordvang H, et al. Immunochemical characterization of and isolation of the gene for a *Borrelia burgdorferi* immunodominant 60-kilodalton antigen common to a wide range of bacteria. *Infect Immun* 1988;56:2047–2053.
53. Orloski KA, Hayes EB, Campbell GL, et al. Surveillance for Lyme disease-United States, 1992–1998. *MMWR Morb Mortal Wkly Rep* 2000;49(SS-3):1–12.
54. James AM, Liveris D, Wormser GP, et al. *Borrelia lonestari* infection after a bite by an *Amblyomma americanum* tick. *J Infect Dis* 2001;183:1810–1814.
55. Felz MW, Chandler FW Jr, Oliver JH Jr, et al. Solitary erythema migrans in Georgia and South Carolina. *Arch Dermatol* 1999;135:1317–1326.
56. Masters E, Granter S, Duray P, et al. Physician-diagnosed erythema migrans and erythema migrans-like rashes following lone star tick bites. *Arch Dermatol* 1998;134:955–960.
57. Barbour AG, Fish D. The biological and social phenomenon of Lyme disease. *Science* 1993;260:1610–1616.
58. Benach JL, Coleman JL, Skinner RA, et al. Adult *Ixodes dammini* on rabbits: a hypothesis for the development and transmission of *Borrelia burgdorferi*. *J Infect Dis* 1987;155:1300–1306.
59. Kawabata M, Baba S, Iguchi K, et al. Lyme disease in Japan and its possible incriminated tick vector, *Ixodes persulcatus*. *J Infect Dis* 1987;156:854–860.
60. Lane RS, Burgdorfer W. Transovarial and transstadial passage of *Borrelia burgdorferi* in the Western black-legged tick, *Ixodes pacificus*. *Am J Trop Med Hyg* 1987;37:188–192.
61. Sonenshine DE. *Biology of ticks*, Vol 1. New York: Oxford University Press, 1991.
62. Benach JL, Coleman JL, Skinner RA, et al. Adult *Ixodes dammini* on rabbits: a hypothesis for the development and transmission of *Borrelia burgdorferi*. *J Infect Dis* 1987;155:1300–1306.
63. Telford SR 3rd, Spielman A. Enzootic transmission of the agent of Lyme disease in rabbits. *Am J Trop Med Hyg* 1989;41:482–490.
64. Maupin GO, Gage KL, Piesman J. Discovery of an enzootic cycle of *Borrelia burgdorferi* in *Neotoma mexicana* and *Ixodes spinipalpis* from northern Colorado, an area where Lyme disease is nonendemic. *J Infect Dis* 1994;170:636–643.
65. Barbour AG, Fish D. The biological and social phenomenon of Lyme disease. *Science* 1993;260:1610–1616.
66. Bosler EM, Coleman J, Benach JL, et al. Natural distribution of the Ixodes dammini spirochete. *Science* 1983;220:321–322.
67. Stafford KC 3rd. Survival of immature *Ixodes scapularis* (*Acari: Ixodidae*) at different relative humidities. *J Med Entomol* 1994;31:310–314.
68. Fish D. Population ecology of Ixodes dammini In: Ginsberg H, ed. *Ecology and environmental management of Lyme disease*. New Brunswick, NJ: Rutgers University Press, 1993:25–42.
69. Smith RP, Rand PW, Lacombe EH, et al. Role of bird migration in the long-distance dispersal of *Ixodes dammini*, the vector of Lyme disease. *J Infect Dis* 1996;174:221–224.
70. Nadelman RB, Wormser GP. Lyme borreliosis. *Lancet* 1998;352:557–565.

71. Dennis DT, Nekomoto TS, Victor JC, et al. Reported distribution of *Ixodes scapularis* and *Ixodes pacificus* (Acari: Ixodidae) in the United States. *J Med Entomol* 1998;35:629–638.

72. Fish D. Environmental risk and prevention of Lyme disease. *Am J Med* 1995;98:2S–7S.

73. Schwartz I, Fish D, Daniels TJ. Prevalence of the rickettsial agent of human granulocytic ehrlichiosis in ticks from a hyperendemic focus of Lyme disease. *N Engl J Med* 1997;337:49–50.

74. Donahue JG, Piesman J, Spielman A. Reservoir competence of white-footed mice for Lyme disease spirochetes. *Am J Trop Med Hyg* 1987;36:92–96.

75. Levine JF, Wilson ML, Spielman A. Mice as reservoirs of the Lyme disease spirochete. *Am J Trop Med Hyg* 1985;34:355–360.

76. Mannelli A, Kitron U, Jones CJ, et al. Role of the eastern chipmunk as a host for immature Ixodes dammini (Acari: Ixodidae) in northwestern Illinois. *J Med Entomol* 1993;30:87–93.

77. Slajchert T, Kitron UD, Jones CJ, et al. Role of the eastern chipmunk (*Tamias striatus*) in the epizootiology of Lyme borreliosis in northwestern Illinois, USA. *J Wildl Dis* 1997;33:40–46.

78. Falco RC, Fish D. Prevalence of *Ixodes dammini* near the homes of Lyme disease patients in Westchester County, New York. *Am J Epidemiol* 1988;127:826–830.

79. Richter DS, Komar A, Matuschka N. Competence of American robins as reservoir hosts for Lyme disease spirochetes. *Emerg Infect Dis* 2000;6:133–138.

80. Smith RP, Rand PW, Lacombe EH, et al. Role of bird migration in the long-distance dispersal of *Ixodes dammini*, the vector of Lyme disease. *J Infect Dis* 1996;174:221–224, 1996.

81. Fish D. Population ecology of *Ixodes dammini*. In: Ginsberg H, ed. *Ecology and environmental management of Lyme disease.* New Brunswick, NJ: Rutgers University Press, 1993:25–42.

82. Falco RC, McKenna DF, Daniels TJ, et al. Temporal relation between *Ixodes scapularis* abundance and risk for Lyme disease associated with erythema migrans. *Am J Epidemiol* 1999;149:771–776.

83. Schwartz I, Fish D, Daniels TJ. Prevalence of the rickettsial agent of human granulocytic ehrlichiosis in ticks from a hyperendemic focus of Lyme disease. *N Engl J Med* 1997;337:49–50.

84. Telford SR 3rd, Mather TN, Moore SI, et al. Incompetence of deer as reservoirs of the Lyme disease spirochete. *Am J Trop Med Hyg* 1988;39:105–109.

85. Piesman J, Clark KL, Dolan MC, et al. Geographic survey of vector ticks (*Ixodes scapularis* and *Ixodes pacificus*) for infection with the Lyme disease spirochete, *Borrelia burgdorferi.* *J Vector Ecol* 1999;24:91–98.

86. Sood SK, Salzman MB, Johnson BJB, et al. Duration of tick attachment as a predictor of the risk of Lyme disease in an area in which Lyme disease is endemic. *J Infect Dis* 1997;175:996–999.

87. Berger BW, Johnson RC, Kodner C, et al. Cultivation of *Borrelia burgdorferi* from human tick bite sites: a guide to the risk of infection. *J Am Acad Dermatol* 1995;32(2 Pt 1):184–187.

88. Nadelman RB, Nowakowski J, Fish D, et al. Prophylaxis with single-dose doxycycline for the prevention of Lyme disease after an Ixodes scapularis tick bite. *N Engl J Med* 2001;345:79–86.

89. Krause PJ, Telford SR III, Spielman A, et al. Concurrent Lyme disease and babesiosis: evidence for increased severity and duration of illness. *JAMA* 1996;275:1657–1660.

90. Nadelman RB, Horowitz HW, Hsieh T-C, et al. Simultaneous human ehrlichiosis and Lyme borreliosis. *N Engl J Med* 1997;337:27–30.

91. Steere AC, Schoen RT, Taylor E. The clinical evolution of Lyme arthritis. *Ann Intern Med* 1987;107:725–731.

92. Wormser GP, Nowakowski J, Nadelman RB, et al. Efficacy of an OspA vaccine preparation for prevention of Lyme disease in New York State. *Infection* 1998;26:208–212.

93. Steere AC, Sikand VK, Meurice F, et al. Vaccination against Lyme disease with recombinant *Borrelia burgdorferi* outer-surface lipoprotein A with adjuvant. *N Engl J Med* 1998;339:209–215.

94. Steere AC, Hutchinson GJ, Rahn DW, et al. Treatment of the early manifestations of Lyme disease. *Ann Intern Med* 1983;99:22–28.

95. Steere AC, Hutchinson GJ, Craft JE, et al. The early clinical manifestations of Lyme disease. *Ann Intern Med* 1983;99:76–82.

96. Dattwyler RJ, Luft BJ, Kunkel M, et al. Ceftriaxone compared with doxycycline for the treatment of acute disseminated Lyme disease. *N Engl J Med* 1997;337:289–2894.

97. Piesman J, Hicks T, Sinsky RJ, et al. Simultaneous transmission of *Borrelia burgdorferi* and *Babesia microti* by individual nymphal Ixodes dammini ticks. *J Clin Microbiol* 1987;25:2012–2013.

98. Edlinger E, Rodhain F, Perez C. Lyme disease in patients previously suspected of arbovirus infection [Letter]. *Lancet* 1985;2:93.

99. Rodhain F, Edlinger E. Serodiagnostic of erythema chronicum migrans (Lyme disease) in cases initially suspected as caused by arboviruses. *Zentralbl Bakteriol Mikrobiol Hyg [A]* 1987;263:425–426.

100. Berger BW. Erythema migrans. *Clin Dermatol* 1993;11(3):359–362.

101. Asbrink E, Hovmark A. Early and late cutaneous manifestations in Ixodes-borne borreliosis (erythema migrans borreliosis, Lyme borreliosis). *Ann N Y Acad Sci* 1988;539:4–15.

102. Hovmark A, Asbrink E Olsson I. The spirochetal etiology of *Lymphadenosis benigna cutis solitaria. Acta Derm Venereol(Stockh)* 1986;66:479–484.

103. Asbrink E, Brehmer-Andersson E, Hovmark A. *Acrodermatitis chronica atrophicans-A* spirochetosis, clinical and histopathological picture based on 32 patients: course and relationship to erythema chronicum migrans afzelius. *Am J Dermatopathol* 1986;8:209–219.

104. Kristoferitsch W, Sluga E, Graf M, et al. Neuropathy associated with *Acrodermatitis chronica atrophicans*: clinical and morphological features. *Ann N Y Acad Sci* 1988;539:35–45.

105. Steere AC, Schoen RT, Taylor E. The clinical evolution of Lyme arthritis. *Ann Intern Med* 1987;107(5):725–731.

106. Steere AC. Lyme disease. *N Engl J Med* 2001;345(2):115–125.

107. Herzer P. Joint manifestations of Lyme borreliosis. *Acta Dermatovenerologica Alpina, Panonica et Adriatica.* 1996;5(3–4):143–146.

108. Nocton JJ, Dressler F, Rutledge BJ, et al. Detection of *Borrelia burgdorferi* by polymerase chain reaction in synovial fluid from patients with Lyme arthritis. *N Engl J Med* 1994;330:229–234.

109. Dong Z, Edelstein MD, Glickstein LG. CD8+ T cells are activated during the early Th l and Th2 immune responses in a murine Lyme disease model. *Infect Immun* 1997;65(12):5334–5337.

110. Kang I, et al. T-helper-cell cytokines in the early evolution of murine Lyme arthritis. *Infect Immun* 1997;65(8):3107–3111.

111. Gross DM, Steere AC, Huber BT. T helper 1 response is dominant and localized to the synovial fluid in patients with Lyme arthritis. *J Immunol* 1998;160(2):1022–1028.

112. Gross DM, et al. Identification of LFA-1 as a candidate autoantigen in treatment-resistant Lyme arthritis. *Science* 1998;281(5377):703–706.

113. Steere AC, Gibofsky A, Patarroyo ME, et al. Chronic Lyme arthritis: clinical and immunogenetic differentiation from rheumatoid arthritis. *Ann Intern Med* 1979;90(6):896–901.

114. Steere AC, Feld J, Winchester RJ. Association of chronic Lyme arthritis with increased frequencies of DR4 and DR3 [Abstract]. *Arthritis Rheum* 1988;31:S98.

115. Kalish RA, Leong JM, Steere AC. Association of treatment-resistant chronic Lyme arthritis with HLA-DR4 and antibody reactivity to OspA and OspB of *Borrelia burgdorferi. Infect Immun* 1993;61:2774–2779.

116. Shanafelt MC, Anzola J, Soderberg C, et al. Epitopes on the outer surface protein A of *Borrelia burgdorferi* recognized by antibodies and T cells of patients with Lyme disease. *J Immunol* 1992;148(l):218–224.

117. Lahesmaa R, Shanafelt MC, Allsup A, et al. Preferential usage of T cell antigen receptor V region gene segment V beta 5.1 by *Borrelia burgdorferi* antigen-reactive T cell clones isolated from a patient with Lyme disease. *J Immunol* 1993;150(9):4125–4135.

118. Akin E, McHugh GL, Flavell RA, et al. The immunoglobulin (IgG) antibody response to OspA and OspB correlates with severe and prolonged Lyme arthritis and the IgG response to P35 correlates with mild and brief arthritis. *Infect Immun* 1999;67(1):173–181.

119. Chen J, Field JA, Glickstein L, et al. Association of antibiotic treatment-resistant Lyme arthritis with T cell responses to dominant epitopes of outer surface protein A of *Borrelia burgdorferi. Arthritis Rheum* 1999;42(9):1813–1822.

120. Hammer J, Bono E, Gallazzi F, et al. Precise prediction of major histocompatibility complex class II–peptide interaction based on peptide side chain scanning. *J Exp Med* 1994;180(6):2353–2358.

121. Benoist C, Mathis D. Autoimmunity provoked by infection: how good is the case for T cell epitope mimicry? *Nat Immunol* 2001;2(9):797–801.

122. Hemmer B, Gran B, Zhao Y, et al. Identification of candidate T-cell epitopes and molecular mimics in chronic Lyme disease. *Nat Med* 1999;5(12):1375–1382.

123. Maier B, et al. Multiple cross-reactive self-ligands for *Borrelia burgdorferi-specific* HLA-DR4-restricted T cells. *Eur J Immunol* 2000;30(2):448–457.

124. Steere AC, Hutchinson GJ, Craft JE, et al. The early clinical manifestations of Lyme disease. *Ann Intern Med* 1983;99:76–82.

125. Luft BJ, Steinman CR, Shubach WH, et al. Invasion of the central nervous system by *Borrelia burgdorferi* in acute disseminate infection. *JAMA* 1992;267(10):1364–1367.

126. Halperin JJ, Luft BJ, Anand AK, et al. Lyme neuroborreliosis: central nervous system manifestations. *Neurology* 1989;39:753–759.

127. Schmutzhard E, Stanek G, Pohl P. Polyneuritis cranialis associated with *Borrelia burgdorferi. J Neurol Neurosurg Psychiatry* 1985;48:1182–1184.

128. Kaiser R, Lucking CH. Intrathecal synthesis of specific antibodies in neuroborreliosis: comparison of different ELISA techniques and calculation methods. *J Neurol Sci* 1993;118(1):64–72.

129. Stanek G. Laboratory diagnosis and seroepidemiology of Lyme borreliosis. *Infection* 1991;19(4):263–267.

130. Halperin JJ, Pass HL, Anand AK, et al. Nervous system abnormalities in Lyme disease. *Ann N Y Acad Sci* 1988;539:24–34.

131. Halperin JJ, Luft BJ, Anand AK, et al. Lyme neuroborreliosis: central nervous system manifestations. *Neurology* 1989;39:753–759.

132. Logigian EL, Kaplan RF, Steere AC. Chronic neurologic manifestations of Lyme disease. *N Engl J Med* 1990;323:1438–1444.

133. Halperin JJ, Coyle PK, Little BV, et al. Lyme disease: a treatable cause of peripheral neuropathy. *Neurology* 1987;37:1700–1706.

134. Halperin JJ, Luft BJ, Volkman DJ, et al. Lyme neuroborreliosis: peripheral nervous system manifestations. *Brain* 1990;113:1207–1221.

135. Logigian EL, Steere AC. Clinical and electrophysiologic findings in chronic neuropathy of Lyme disease. *Neurology* 1992;42:303–311.

136. Kristoferitsch W, Baumhackl U, Sluga E, et al. High-dose penicillin therapy in meningopolyradiculitis Garin-Bujadoux-Bannwarth: clinical and cerebrospinal fluid data. *Zentralbl Bakteriol Mikrobiol Hyg [A]* 1987;263:357–364.

137. Kampner AL, Andersen J. Reversible bladder denervation in acute polyradiculitis. *Scand J Urol Nephrol* 1982;16:291–293.

138. Maida E, Kristoferitsch W, Spiel G. Cerebrospinal fluid changes in Garin-Bujadoux-Bannwarth meningoradiculitis. *Nervenarzt* 1986;57:149–152.

139. Stiernstedt G, Gustafsson R, Karlsson M, et al. Clinical manifestations and diagnosis of neuroborreliosis. *Ann N Y Acad Sci* 1988;539:46–55.

140. Steere AC, Batsford WP, Weinberg M, et al. Lyme carditis: cardiac abnormalities of Lyme disease. *Ann Intern Med* 1980;93:8–16.

141. McAlister HF, Klementowicz PT, Andrews C, et al. Lyme carditis: an important cause of reversible heart block. *Ann Intern Med* 1989;110:339–345.

142. Reznick JW, Braunstein D, Walsh RL, et al. Lyme carditis: electrophysiologic and histopathologic study. *Am J Med* 1986;81:923–927.

143. Ponsonnaille J, Citron B, Karsenty B, et al. Acute myocarditis in Lyme's syndrome: value of myocardial scintigraphy with gallium. *Arch Mal Coeur* 1986;79:1946–1950.

144. Rienzo RJ, Morel DE, Prager D, et al. Gallium avid Lyme myocarditis. *Clin Nucl Med* 1987;12:475–476.

145. Lorcerie B, Boutron M, Portier H, et al. Pericardial manifestations of Lyme disease. *Ann Med Interne* (Paris) 1987;138:601–603.

146. Klein J, Stanek G, Bittner R, et al. Lyme borreliosis as a cause of myocarditis and heart muscle disease. *Eur Heart J* 1991;12[Suppl D]:73–75.

147. Bergler-Klein J, Stanek G. Myocarditis. *N Engl J Med* 2001;15;344(11):857.

148. Steere AC, Sikand VK, Meurice F, et al. Vaccination against Lyme disease with recombinant *Borrelia burgdorferi* outer-surface lipoprotein A with adjuvant. Lyme Disease Vaccine Study Group. *N Engl J Med* 1998;339:209–215.

149. Sigal LH, Zahradnik JM, Lavin P, et al. A vaccine consisting of recombinant *Borrelia burgdorferi* outer-surface protein A to prevent Lyme disease. Recombinant Outer-Surface Protein A Lyme Disease Vaccine Study Consortium. *N Engl J Med* 1998;339:216–222.

150. Centers for Disease Control and Prevention. Recommendations for test performance and interpretation from the Second National Conference on Serologic Diagnosis of Lyme Disease. *MMWR Morb Mortal Wkly Rep* 1995;44:590–591.

151. Gutierrez J, Guerrero M, Nunez F, et al. Antibodies to *Borrelia burgdorferi* in European populations. *J Clin Lab Anal* 2000;14(1):20–26.

152. Engstrom SM, Shoop E, Johnson RC. Immunoblot interpretation criteria for serodiagnosis of early Lyme disease. *J Clin Microbiol* 1995;33(2):419–427.

153. de Silva AM, Fikrig E. Arthropod- and host-specific gene expression by *Borrelia burgdorferi*. *J Clin Invest* 1997;99(3):377–379.

154. Luft BJ, Dattwyler RJ, Johnson RC, et al. Azithromycin compared with amoxicillin in the treatment of erythema migrans: a double-blind, randomized, controlled trial. *Ann Intern Med* 1996;124:785–791.

155. Dressler F, Whalen JA, Reinhardt BN, et al. Western blotting in the serodiagnosis of Lyme disease. *J Infect Dis* 1993;167(2):392–400.

156. Liang FT, Philipp MT. Epitope mapping of the immunodominant invariable region of *Borrelia burgdorferi* V1sE in three host species. *Infect Immun* 2000;68(4):2349–2352.

157. Liang FT, Steere AC, Marques AR, et al. Sensitive and specific serodiagnosis of Lyme disease by enzyme-linked immunosorbent assay with a peptide based on an immunodominant conserved region of *Borrelia burgdorferi* vlsE. *J Clin Microbiol* 1999;37(12):3990–3996.

158. Gomes-Solecki MJ, Dunn JJ, Luft BJ, et al. Recombinant chimeric *Borrelia* proteins for diagnosis of Lyme disease. *J Clin Microbiol* 2000;38(7):2530–2535.

159. Gomes-Solecki MJ, Wormser GP, Persing DH, et al. A first-tier rapid assay for the serodiagnosis of *Borrelia burgdorferi* infection. *Arch Intern Med* 2001;10;161(16):2015–2020.

160. Dattwyler RJ, Volkman DJ, Luft BJ, et al. Seronegative Lyme disease: dissociation of specific T- and B-lymphocyte responses to *Borrelia burgdorferi*. *N Engl J Med* 1988;1;319(22):1441–1446.

161. Fish D. Population ecology of *Ixodes dammini*. In: Ginsberg H, ed. *Ecology and environmental management of Lyme Disease*. New Brunswick, NJ: Rutgers University Press, 1993:25–42.

162. Falco RC, McKenna DF, Daniels TJ, et al. Temporal relation between *Ixodes scapularis* abundance and risk for Lyme disease associated with erythema migrans. *Am J Epidemiol* 1999;149:771–776.

163. Bouseman JK, Kitron U, Kirkpatrick CE, et al. Status of *Ixodes dammini* (Acari: Ixodidae) in Illinois. *J Med Entomol* 1990;27:556–560.

164. White DJ, Chang HG, Benach JL, et al. The geographic spread and temporal increase of the Lyme disease epidemic. *JAMA* 1991;266:1230–1236.

165. Orloski KA, Hayes EB, Campbell GL, et al. Surveillance for Lyme disease-United States, 1992–1998. *MMWR Morb Mortal Wkly Rep* 2000;49(SS-3):1–12.

166. Fish D, Howard C. Methods used for creating a national Lyme disease risk map. *MMWR Morb Mortal Wkly Rep* 1999;48(RR07):21–24.

167. Fish D. Environmental risk and prevention of Lyme disease. *Am J Med* 1995;98:2S–7S.

168. Mount G, Haile DG, Daniels E. Simulation of backlegged tick (Acari: Ixodidae) population dynamics and transmission of *Borrelia burgdorferi*. *J Med Entomol* 1997;34:461–484.

169. Falco RC, Fish D. Prevalence of *Ixodes dammini* near the homes of Lyme disease patients in Westchester County, New York. *Am J Epidemiol* 1988;127:826–830.

170. Maupin GO, Fish D, Zultowsky J, et al. Landscape ecology of Lyme disease in a residential area of Westchester County, New York. *Am J Epidemiol* 1991;133:1105–1113.

171. Dister SW, Fish D, Bros SM, et al. Landscape characterization of peridomestic risk for Lyme disease using satellite imagery. *Am J Trop Med Hyg* 1997;57:687–692.

172. Kitron U, Kazmierczak JJ. Spatial analysis of the distribution of Lyme disease in Wisconsin. *Am J Epidemiol* 1997;145:558–566.

173. Schulze TL, Taylor GC, Jordan RA, et al. Effectiveness of selected granular acaricide formulations in suppressing populations of *Ixodes dammini* (Acari: Ixodidae): short-term control of nymphs and larvae. *J Med Entomol* 1991;28:624–629.

174. Schulze TL, Jordan RA, Vasvary LM, et al. Suppression of *Ixodes scapularis* (Acari: Ixodidae) nymphs in a large residential community. *J Med Entomol* 1994;31:206–211.

175. Schulze TL, Jordan RA, Hung RW, et al. Efficacy of granular deltamethrin against *Ixodes scapularis* and *Amblyomma americanum* (Acari: Ixodidae) nymphs. *J Med Entomol* 2001;38:344–346.

176. Curran KL, Fish D, Piesman J. Reduction of nymphal *Ixodes dammini* (Acari: Ixodidae) in a residential suburban landscape by area application of insecticides. *J Med Entomol* 1993;30:107–113.

177. Maupin GO, Piesman J. Acaricide susceptibility of immature *Ixodes scapularis* (Acari: Ixodidae) as determined by the disposable pipet method. *J Med Entomol* 1994;31:319–321.

178. Stafford KC 3rd. Effectiveness of carbaryl applications for the control of *Ixodes dammini* (Acari: Ixodidae) nymphs in an endemic residential area. *J Med Entomol* 1991;28:32–36.

179. Daniels TJ, Fish D, Schwartz I. Reduced abundance of *Ixodes scapularis* (Acari: Ixodidae) and Lyme disease risk by deer exclusion. *J Med Entomol* 1993;30:1043–1049.

180. Stafford KC 3rd. Reduced abundance of *Ixodes scapularis* (Acari: Ixodidae) with exclusion of deer by electric fencing. *J Med Entomol* 1993;30:986–996.

181. Mather TN, Ribeiro JM, Spielman A. Lyme disease and babesiosis: acaricide focused on potentially infected ticks. *Am J Trop Med Hyg* 1987;36:609–614.

182. Daniels TJ, Fish D, Falco RC. Evaluation of host-targeted acaricide for reducing risk of Lyme disease in southern New York State. *J Med Entomol* 1991;28:537–543.

183. Stafford KC 3rd. Third-year evaluation of host-targeted permethrin for the control of *Ixodes dammini* (Acari: Ixodidae) in southeastern Connecticut. *J Med Entomol* 1992;29:717–720.

184. Stafford KC 3rd. Effectiveness of host-targeted permethrin in the control of *Ixodes dammini* (Acari: Ixodidae). *J Med Entomol* 1991;28:611–617.

185. Hayes EB, Maupin GO, Mount GA, et al. Assessing the prevention effectiveness of local Lyme disease control. *J Public Health Manag Pract* 1999;5:84–92.

186. Schulze TL, Jordan RA, Hung RW. Suppression of subadult *Ixodes scapularis* (Acari: Ixodidae) following removal of leaf litter. *J Med Entomol* 1995;32:730–733.

187. Stafford KC 3rd. Survival of immature *Ixodes scapularis* (Acari: Ixodidae) at different relative humidities. *J Med Entomol* 1994;31:310–314.

188. Wilson ML. Reduced abundance of adult *Ixodes dammini* (Acari: Ixodidae) following destruction of vegetation. *J Econ Entomol* 1986;79:693–696.

189. Lane RS, Anderson JR. Efficacy of permethrin as a repellent and toxicant for personal protection against the Pacific Coast tick and the Pajaroello tick (Acari: Ixodidae and Argasidae). *J Med Entomol* 1984;21:692–702.

190. Schreck CE, Fish D, McGovern T. Activity of repellents applied to skin for protection against *Amblyomma americanum* and *Ixodes scapularis* ticks (Acari: Ixodidae). *J Am Mosq Control Assoc* 1995;11:136–140.

191. Fradin MS. Mosquitoes and mosquito repellents: a clinician's guide. *Ann Intern Med* 1998;28:931–940.

192. U.S. Environmental Protection Agency, Office of Pesticide Programs. *Using insect repellents safely*. Publication EPA-735/F-93-052R. Washington, DC: U.S. Environmental Protection Agency, 1996.

193. Needham GR. Evaluation of five popular methods for tick removal. *Pediatrics* 1985;75:997–1002.

194. Schwartz I, Fish D, Daniels TJ. Prevalence of the rickettsial agent of human granulocytic ehrlichiosis in ticks from a hyperendemic focus of Lyme disease. *N Engl J Med* 1997;337:49–50.

195. Piesman J, Mather TN, Donahue JG, et al. Comparative prevalence of *Babesia microti* and *Borrelia burgdorferi* in four populations of *Ixodes dammini* in eastern Massachusetts. *Acta Tropica* 1986;43:263–270.

196. Curran KL, Fish D. Increased risk of Lyme disease for cat owners. *N Engl J Med* 1989;320:183.

197. Taylor MA. Recent developments in ectoparasiticides. *Vet J* 2001;161:253–268.

198. Shapiro ED, Gerber MA, Holabird NB, et al. A controlled trial of antimicrobial prophylaxis for Lyme disease after deer-tick bites. *N Engl J Med* 1992;327:1769–1773.

199. Agre F, Schwartz R. The value of early treatment of deer tick bites for the prevention of Lyme disease. *Am J Dis Child* 1993;147:945–947.

200. Costello CM, Steere AC, Pinkerton RE, et al. A prospective study of tick bites in an endemic area for Lyme disease. *J Infect Dis* 1989;159:136–139.

201. Nadelman RB, Nowakowski J, Fish D, et al. Prophylaxis with single-dose doxycycline for the prevention of Lyme disease after an *Ixodes scapularis* tick bite. *N Engl J Med* 2001;345:79–86.

202. Piesman J, Mather TN, Sinsky RJ, et al. Duration of tick attachment and *Borrelia burgdorferi* transmission. *J Clin Microbiol* 1987;25:557–558.

203. Piesman J, Maupin GO, Campos EG, et al. Duration of adult female *Ixodes dammini* attachment and transmission of *Borrelia burgdorferi* with description of a needle aspiration isolation method. *J Infect Dis* 1991;163:895–897.

204. Ribeiro JM, Mather TN, Piesman J, et al. Dissemination and salivary delivery of Lyme disease spirochetes in vector ticks (Acari: Ixodidae). *J Med Entomol* 1987;24:201–205.

205. des Vignes F, Piesman J, Heffernan R, et al. Effect of tick removal on transmission of *Borrelia burgdorferi* and *Ehrlichia phagocytophila* by *Ixodes scapularis* nymphs. *J Infect Dis* 2001;183:773–778.

206. Sood SK, Salzman MB, Johnson BJB, et al. Duration of tick attachment as a predictor of the risk of Lyme disease in an area in which Lyme disease is endemic. *J Infect Dis* 1997;175:996–999.

207. Falco RC, Fish D, Piesman J. Duration of tick bites in a Lyme disease-endemic area. *Am J Epidemiol* 1996;143:187–192.

208. Falco RC, McKenna DF, Daniels TJ, et al. Temporal relation between *Ixodes scapularis* abundance and risk for Lyme disease associated with erythema migrans. *Am J Epidemiol* 1999;149:771–776.

209. Magid D, Schwartz B, Craft J, et al. Prevention of Lyme disease after tick bites: a cost-effectiveness analysis. *N Engl J Med* 1992;327:534–541.

210. Wormser GP, Nadelman RB, Dattwyler RJ, et al. Practice guidelines for the treatment of Lyme disease. *Clin Infect Dis* 2000;31[Suppl 1]:S1–14.

211. Wormser GP, Ramanathan R, Nowakowski J, et al. Duration of antibiotic therapy for early Lyme disease. A randomized, double-blind, placebo-controlled trial. *Ann Intern Med* 2003;138:697–706.

212. Schroeter AL, Turner RH, Lucas JB, et al. Therapy for incubating syphilis: effectiveness of gonorrhea treatment. *JAMA* 1971;218:711–713.

213. Takafuji ET, Kirkpatrick JW, Miller RN, et al. An efficacy trial of doxycycline chemoprophylaxis against leptospirosis. *N Engl J Med* 1984;310:497–500.

214. Clover JR, Lane RS. Evidence implicating nymphal *Ixodes pacificus* (*Acari: Ixodidae*) in the epidemiology of Lyme disease in California. *Am J Trop Med Hyg* 1995;53:237–240.

215. Lane RS, Piesman J, Burgdorfer W. Lyme borreliosis: relation of its causative agent to its vectors and hosts in North America and Europe. *Annu Rev Entomol* 1991;36:587–609.

216. Li X, Peavey CA, Lane RS. Density and spatial distribution of *Ixodes pacificus* (*Acari: Ixodidae*) in two recreational areas in north coastal California. *Am J Trop Med Hyg* 2000;62:415–422.

217. Burkot TR, Clover JR, Happ CM, et al. Isolation of *Borrelia burgdorferi* from *Neotoma fuscipes, Peromyscus maniculatus, Peromyscus boylii* and *Ixodes pacificus* in Oregon. *Am J Trop Med Hyg* 1999;60:453–457.

218. Baradaran-Dilmaghani R, Stanek G. In vitro susceptibility of thirty *Borrelia* strains from various sources against eight antimicrobial chemotherapeutics. *Infection* 1996;24:60–63.

219. Piesman J, Donahue JG, Mather TN, et al. Transovarially acquired Lyme disease spirochetes (*Borrelia burgdorferi*) in field-collected larval *Ixodes dammini* (*Acari: Ixodidae*). *J Med Entomol* 1986;23:219.

220. Nadelman RB, Nowakowski J, Forseter G, et al. The clinical spectrum of early Lyme borreliosis in patients with culture-confirmed erythema migrans. *Am J Med* 1996;100:502–508.

221. Falco RC, Fish D, D'Amico V. Accuracy of tick identification in a Lyme disease endemic area. *JAMA* 1998;280:602–603.

222. Simon MM, Schaible UE, Kramer MD, et al. Recombinant outer surface protein A from *Borrelia burgdorferi* induces antibodies protective against spirochetal infection in mice. *J Infect Dis* 1991;164:123–132.

223. Schaible UE, Wallich R, Kramer MD, et al. Immune sera to individual *Borrelia burgdorferi* isolates or recombinant OspA thereof protect SCID mice against infection with homologous strains but only partially, or not at all against those of different OspA/OspB genotype. *Vaccine* 1993;11:1049–1054.

224. Schaible UE, Kramer MD, Eichmann K, et al. Monoclonal antibodies specific for the outer surface protein A (OspA) of *Borrelia burgdorferi* prevent Lyme borreliosis in severe combined immunodeficiency (scid) mice. *Proc Natl Acad Sci U S A* 1990;87:3768–3772.

225. Hansen MS, Cassatt DR, Guo BP, et al. Active and passive immunity against *Borrelia burgdorferi* decorin binding protein A (DbpA) protects against infection. *Infect Immun* 1998;66:2143–2153.

226. Zhong W, Stehle T, Museteanu C, et al. Therapeutic passive vaccination against chronic Lyme disease in mice. *Proc Natl Acad Sci U S A* 1997;94:12533–12538.

227. Zhong W, Gem L, Stehle T, et al. Resolution of experimental and tick-borne *Borrelia burgdorferi* infection in mice by passive, but not active immunization using recombinant Osp C. *Eur J Immunol* 1999;29:946–957.

228. Barthold SW, de Souza M, Feng S. Serum-mediated resolution of Lyme arthritis in mice. *Lab Invest* 1996;74:57–67.

229. Onrust SV, Goa KL. Adjuvanted Lyme disease vaccine: a review of its use in the management of Lyme disease. *Drugs* 2000;59:281–299.

230. Johnson RC, Kodner C, Russell M. In vitro and in vivo susceptibility of the Lyme disease spirochete, *Borrelia burgdorferi*, to four antimicrobial agents. *Antimicrob Agents Chemother* 1987;31:164–167.

231. Nowakowski J, McKenna D, Nadelman RB, et al. Failure of treatment with cephalexin for Lyme disease. *Arch Fam Med* 2000;9:563–567.

232. Kraiczy P, Weigand J, Wichelhaus TA, et al. In vitro activities of fluoroquinolones against the spirochete *Borrelia burgdorferi*. *Antimicrob Agents Chemother* 2001;45(9):2486–2494.

233. Steere AC, Hutchinson GJ, Rahn DW, et al. Treatment of early manifestations of Lyme disease. *Ann Intern Med* 1983;99:22–26.

234. Dattwyler RJ, Volkman DJ, Conaty SM, et al. Amoxicillin plus probenecid versus doxycycline for treatment of erythema migrans borreliosis. *Lancet* 1990;336:1404–1406.

235. Massarotti EM, Luger SW, Rahn DW, et al. Treatment of early Lyme disease. *Am J Med* 1992;92:396–403.

236. Nadelman RB, Luger SW, Frank E, et al. Comparison of cefuroxime axetil and doxycycline in the treatment of early Lyme disease. *Ann Intern Med* 1992;117:273–280.

237. Luger SW, Paparone P, Wormser GP, et al. Comparison of cefuroxime axetil and doxycycline in treatment of patients with early Lyme disease associated with erythema migrans. *Antimicrob Agents Chemother* 1995;39:661–667.

238. Dever LL, Jorgensen JH, Barbour AG. Comparative in vitro activities of clarithromycin, azithromycin, and erythromycin against *Borrelia burgdorferi*. *Antimicrob Agents Chemother* 1993;37:1704–1706.

239. Hansen K, Hovmark A, Lebech A-M, et al. Roxithromycin in Lyme borreliosis: discrepant results of an in vitro and in vivo animal susceptibility study and a clinical trial in patients with erythema migrans. *Acta Derm Venerol* 1992;72:297–300.

240. Barsic B, Maretic T, Majerus L, et al. Comparison of azithromycin and doxycycline in the treatment of erythema migrans. *Infection* 2000;28:153–156.

241. Strle F, Maraspin V, Lotric-Furlan S, et al. Azithromycin and doxycycline for treatment of *Borrelia* culture positive erythema migrans. *Infection* 1996;24:64–68.

242. Weber K, Wilske B, Preac-Mursic V, et al. Azithromycin versus penicillin V for treatment of early Lyme borreliosis. *Infection* 1993;21:367–372.

243. Strle F, Ruzic E, Cimperman J. Erythema migrans: comparison of treatment with azithromycin, doxycycline and phenoxymethyl penicillin. *J Antimicrob Chemother* 1992;30:543–550.

244. Strle F, Preac-Mursic V, Cimperman J, et al. Azithromycin versus doxycycline for treatment of erythema migrans: clinical and microbiologic findings. *Infection* 1993;21:83–88.

245. Dattwyler RJ, Grunwaldt E, Luft BJ. Clarithromycin in treatment of early Lyme disease: a pilot study. *Antimicrob Agents Chemother* 1996;;40:468–469.

246. Nowakowski J, Nadelman RB, Sell R, et al. Long-term follow-up of patients with culture-confirmed Lyme disease. *Am J Med* 2003;115:91–96.

247. Nadelman RB, Wormser GP. Lyme borreliosis. *Lancet* 1998;352:557–565.

248. Nadelman RB, Horowitz HW, Hsieh T-C, et al. Simultaneous human ehrlichiosis and Lyme borreliosis. *N Engl J Med* 1997;337:27–30.

249. Duffy J, Pittlekow MR, Kolbert P, et al. Coinfection with *Borrelia burgdorferi* and the agent of human granulocytic ehrlichiosis. *Lancet* 1997;349:399.

250. Maraspin V, Cimperman J, Lotric-Furlan S, et al. Treatment of erythema migrans in pregnancy. *Clin Infect Dis* 1996;22:788–793.

251. Williams CL, Strobino B, Weinstein A, et al. Maternal Lyme disease and congenital malformation: a cord blood serosurvey in endemic and control areas. *Paediatr Perinat Epidemiol* 1995;9:320–330.

252. Strobino BA, Williams CL, Abid S, et al. Lyme disease and pregnancy outcome: a prospective study of 2000 prenatal patients. *Am J Obstet Gynecol* 1993;169:367–374.

253. Pfister HW, Einhaupl KM, Garner C, et al. Corticosteroids versus penicillin in the treatment of meningoradiculitis of Bannwarth (Bannwarth's syndrome). *J Neurol(Suppl)* 1985;231:293.

254. Steere AC, Pachner AR, Malawista SE. Neurologic abnormalities of Lyme disease: successful treatment with high-dose intravenous penicillin. *Ann Intern Med* 1983;99:767–772.

255. Clark JR, Carlson RD, Sasaki CT, et al. Facial paralysis in Lyme disease. *Laryngoscope* 1985;95:1341–1345.

256. Kruger H, Kohlhepp W, Konig S. Follow-up of antibiotically treated and untreated neuroborreliosis. *Acta Neurol Scand* 1990;82:59–67.

257. Pfister HW, Einhaupl KM, Franz P, et al. Corticosteroids for radicular pain in BannwarthAs syndrome: a double-blind, randomized, placebo-controlled trial. *Ann N Y Acad Sci* 1988;539:485–487.

258. Kristoferitsch W. *Neuropathien bei Lyme-borreliose*. Berlin: Springer-Verlag, 1989.

259. Wormser GP. Treatment and prevention of Lyme disease, with emphasis on antimicrobial therapy for neuroborreliosis and vaccination. *Semin Neurol* 1997;17:45–52.

260. Reik L, Steere AC, Bartenhagen NH, et al. Neurologic abnormalities of Lyme disease. *Medicine* 1979;58:281–294.

261. Pfister H-W, Preac-Mursic V, Wilske B, et al. Randomized comparison of ceftriaxone and cefotaxime in Lyme neuroborreliosis. *J Infect Dis* 1991;163:311–318.

262. Roberg M, Forsberg P, Fryden A, et al. Long-term findings in patients with facial palsy and antibodies against *Borrelia burgdorferi*. *Scand J Infect Dis* 1994;26(5):559–567.

263. Steere AC, Batsford WP, Weinberg M, et al. Lyme carditis: cardiac abnormalities of Lyme disease. *Ann Intern Med* 1980;93:8–16.

264. Steere AC, Schoen R, Taylor E. The clinical evolution of Lyme arthritis. *Ann Intern Med* 1987;107:725–731.

265. Steere AC, Green J, Schoen RT, et al. Successful parenteral penicillin therapy of established Lyme arthritis. *N Engl J Med* 1985;312:869–874.

266. Dattwyler RJ, Halperin JJ, Pass H, et al. Ceftriaxone as effective therapy for refractory Lyme disease. *J Infect Dis* 1987;155:1322–1325.

267. Dattwyler RJ, Halperin JJ, Volkman DJ, et al. Treatment of late Lyme borreliosis: randomized comparison of ceftriaxone and penicillin. *Lancet* 1988;1:1191–1194.

268. Dattwyler RJ, Luft BJ, Maladorno D, et al. *Treatment of late Lyme disease: a comparison of 2 weeks vs 4 weeks of ceftriaxone* [Abstract 662]. In: Proceedings of the 7th International Congress on Lyme Borreliosis (San Francisco), June 16—21, 1996.

269. Eichenfield AH, Goldsmith DP, Benach JL, et al. Childhood Lyme arthritis: experience in an endemic area. *J Pediatr* 1986;109:753–758.
270. Nocton JJ, Dressler F, Rutledge BJ, et al. Detection of *Borrelia burgdorferi* by polymerase chain reaction in synovial fluid from patients with Lyme arthritis. *N Engl J Med* 1994;330:229–234.
271. Eckman MH, Steere AC, Kalish RA, et al. Cost effectiveness of oral as compared with intravenous antibiotic treatment for patients with early Lyme disease or Lyme arthritis. *N Engl J Med* 1997;337:357–363.
272. Steere AC, Levin RE, Molloy PJ, et al. Treatment of Lyme arthritis. *Arthritis Rheum* 1994;37:878–888.
273. Schoen RT, Aversa JM, Rahn DW, et al. Treatment of refractory chronic Lyme arthritis with arthroscopic synovectomy. *Arthritis Rheum* 1991;34:1056–1060.
274. Logigian EL, Kaplan RF, Steere AC. Successful treatment of Lyme encephalopathy with intravenous ceftriaxone. *J Infect Dis* 1999;180:377–383.
275. Dattwyler RJ, Halperin JJ, Volkman DJ, et al. Treatment of late Lyme borreliosis: a randomized study of ceftriaxone vs penicillin. *Lancet* 1988;1:1191–1194.
276. Hassler D, Zoller L, Haude A, et al. Cefotaxime versus penicillin in the late stage of Lyme disease: prospective, randomized therapeutic approach. *Infection* 1990;18:16–20.
277. Bloom BJ, Wyckoff PM, Meissner HC, et al. Neurocognitive abnormalities in children after classic manifestations of Lyme disease. *Pediatr Infect Dis J* 1998;17:189–196.
278. Seltzer EG, Gerber MA, Canter ML, et al. Long-term outcomes of persons with Lyme disease. *JAMA* 2000;283:609–616.
279. Klempner MS, Hu LT, Evans J, et al. Two controlled trials of antibiotic treatment in patients with persistent symptoms and a history of Lyme disease. *N Engl J Med* 2001;345:85–92.
280. Nadelman RB, Nowakowski J, Forseter G, et al. Failure to isolate *Borrelia burgdorferi* after antimicrobial therapy in culture-documented Lyme borreliosis associated with erythema migrans: report of a prospective study. *Am J Med* 1993;94:583–588.
281. Berger BW, Johnson RC, Kodner C, et al. Failure of *Borrelia burgdorferi* to survive in the skin of patients with antibiotic-treated Lyme disease. *J Am Acad Dermatol* 1992;27:34–37.
282. Preac-Mursic V, Weber K, Pfister HW, et al. Survival of *Borrelia burgdorferi* in antibiotically treated patients with Lyme disease. *Infection* 1989;17:355–359.

CHAPTER 215

Borrelia *Species and* Spirillum minus

Thomas Butler

The genus *Borrelia* comprises spirochetal bacteria that cause the human diseases relapsing fever and Lyme disease. *Borrelia recurrentis* causes louse-borne relapsing fever and *Borrelia hermsii*, *Borrelia turicatae*, *Borrelia parkeri*, and other species cause tick-borne relapsing fever. *Borrelia burgdorferi* is the cause of Lyme disease and is described in Chapter 214. Animal borrelioses include bovine borreliosis (*Borrelia thelleri*), epizootic bovine abortion (*Borrelia coriaceae*), and avian borreliosis (*Borrelia anserina*). Another pathogenic spirochete that is considered in this chapter is *Spirillum minus*, a cause of rat-bite fever.

HISTORY

Borrelia organisms were discovered in 1873 by Obermeier, who observed them with a microscope in the blood of a person with relapsing fever. The transmission of *Borrelia* spirochetes by arthropod vectors was suggested in 1891 by Flugge, who postulated the body louse as a vector. In 1905, Dutton and Todd demonstrated the infection in the *Ornithodoros* ticks of Africa. The genus name *Borrelia* was proposed in 1907, to honor the French bacteriologist Borrel. Successful cultivation of *Borrelia in vitro* was reported by Kelly in 1971. The discovery of *B. burgdorferi* as the cause of Lyme disease was made in 1982. A spiral organism, later named

S. minor, and subsequently *S. minus*, was shown to be a cause of rat-bite fever (*sodoku* in Japanese) in 1908.

CHARACTERISTICS OF THE PATHOGEN

Borrelia organisms are spiral shaped and vary in length from 5 to 40 μm and in width from 0.2 to 0.5 μm. Like other bacteria, these organisms possess an outer cell wall (outer envelope) and an inner cytoplasmic membrane that contains muramic acid. Between the cell wall and cytoplasmic membrane are 7 to 20 flagella, which are anchored to the ends of the spirochete and wrap around its body until they meet near the middle. In three dimensions, the spirochetes have a helical configuration consisting of about 4 to 10 coils with "amplitudes" of about 1 to 4 μm. Under dark-field or phase-contrast microscopy, *Borrelia* spirochetes display an active corkscrew-like motility. Inside the cytoplasmic membrane are ribosomes, DNA, and RNA. These prokaryotic organisms divide by transverse binary fission.

Borrelia organisms are microaerophilic and fermentative in their growth characteristics. Like other pathogenic spirochetes, they require long-chain fatty acids for growth. They are cultivatable in Kelly medium (1), a complex broth containing proteose peptone, tryptone, bovine serum albumin, rabbit serum, N-acetylglucosamine, citric acid, and pyruvate, in addition to glucose and salts. *B. recurrentis* is more fastidious than the tick-borne *Borrelia* species and requires the further addition of asparagine and choline to Kelly medium. *Borrelia* organisms grow slowly in Kelly medium (doubling time, 18 to 26 hours).

Antigenic variation of *Borrelia* occurs in the course of relapsing fever, giving rise to relapse strains that are not recognized by antibody that develops against the initial infecting serotype. In *B. hermsii* infection, 25 different serotypes have been identified with different outer membrane proteins. Barbour (2) showed that switches among serotypes follow from recombination between linear plasmids that carry the genes for these antigens. Genes controlling serotypes that are expressed while spirochetes are in mice are not expressed in ticks (3).

S. minus is fundamentally different from *Borrelia* spirochetes in structure, being a tightly coiled gram-negative rod with external polar flagella. The organisms are 2 to 5 μm long and have two to six spirals. They cannot be propagated in artificial culture media.

EPIDEMIOLOGY

In louse-borne relapsing fever, the vector for *B. recurrentis* is the human body louse, *Pediculus humanus humanus*, and the only known natural reservoir is humans. Thus, the cycle of infection is simply from person to person through the louse. Body lice acquire the infection by feeding on a spirochetemic person, and they remain infected for their entire life span, 10 to 61 days under laboratory conditions (3). The ingested spirochetes pass through the esophagus to the midgut, where they penetrate the gut epithelium to reach the hemolymph, in which they will multiply. Infection is believed to be transmitted to humans after lice are crushed on the skin, which allows liberated spirochetes to penetrate through a bite site or through intact skin. Body lice prefer the normal human body temperature of 37°C over higher temperatures; hence, lice are likely to leave the skin of a febrile person to go to another person. This may in part explain the rapid transmission of infection during epidemics.

The vectors of tick-borne relapsing fever are argasid ticks of the genus *Ornithodoros*. The major reservoirs of the tick-borne relapsing fevers are wild rodents. The infection is passed between the reservoir animals by tick bites, and humans are accidental hosts when they come into contact with infected animal ticks. The exception to the animal reservoirs may be *Borrelia duttonii* in East Africa, which is carried by the domestic tick *Ornithodoros moubata*, for which humans appear to be the reservoir. Neonates have acquired infection from their mother's blood by either transplacental infection or exchange of blood at the time of birth.

Ticks acquire the infection by biting and sucking blood from a spirochetemic animal. After entering the hemocele, the spirochetes invade other tissues of the tick, including the salivary glands, coxal glands on the legs, and ovaries. Transmission of the infection to animals or humans follows injection of either infected saliva or coxal fluid through the bite site or intact skin. Ticks are more durable vectors than are body lice, being able to survive as long as 15 years between blood meals and to harbor viable spirochetes for years. In addition, female ticks can pass *Borrelia* spirochetes transovarially to their offspring; thus, ticks can be infective without having bitten an infected host.

Infections with *S. minus* are rare because of the rarity of rodent bites in the general population. *S. minus* is one cause of rat-bite fever; the other is *Streptobacillus moniliformis*, which can also cause a febrile illness without antecedent rat bites known as Haverhill fever.

PATHOGENESIS AND CLINICAL MANIFESTATIONS

After a bite by a *Borrelia*-infected tick or louse, during an incubation period of 3 to 32 days, the spirochetes migrate outward in the skin and multiply. They are also disseminated through the lymph and blood to other skin sites and to other organs, including the heart and brain.

In relapsing fever, the fever is caused by a nonendotoxic pyrogen in the spirochete that elicits interleukin-1 production by mononuclear phagocytes. Disseminated intravascular coagulation with thrombocytopenia leads to a petechial rash in some patients. The relapsing nature of the disease has been attributed to antigenic variation in the infecting population of spirochetes.

Most patients with relapsing fever recover from their illness with or without antibiotic treatment. (For a more clinical description, see Chapter 167.) Patients develop antibodies against *Borrelia*, which can agglutinate, kill, or opsonize the spirochetes. These antibodies also participate in rendering patients immune to future infection with *Borrelia* of the same serotype.

In rat-bite fever, there is an incubation period of 1 to 4 weeks from the bite to the appearance of inflammation at the bite site. The disease starts with fever. A red-brown macular rash spreads outward on the skin and has been described to recede and sometimes to relapse. A purulent ulcer at the bite site is common, and patients may develop lymphangitis and regional lymphadenitis (4,5). The disease resolves spontaneously in 1 to 2 months. Antibodies against *S. minus* arise during the disease and may cause a false-positive Venereal Disease Research Laboratory test result.

DIAGNOSIS

Culture of the causative spirochetes in these diseases is not feasible in routine laboratories. The diagnosis of relapsing fever is made by demonstrating spirochetemia using Wright-stained blood smears. In *S. minus* infections, the spirochetes may be visualized by dark-field microscopy of skin lesion or lymph node specimens and, sometimes, blood. Intraperitoneal inoculation of clinical specimens into guinea pigs or mice has been used to demonstrate the organism in the animal's blood. Serology is not routinely available, but a recently described antigen, GlpG, present in *Borrelia* species other than *B. burgdorferi* could be used to differentiate between relapsing fever and Lyme disease (6).

TREATMENT

Antibiotic treatment is effective against these infections. For relapsing fever, a single dose of tetracycline or erythromycin is recommended. Procaine penicillin G is also effective but results in relapses more often than does tetracycline (see Chapter 167). *S. minus* infections are treatable with intramuscular procaine penicillin G for 10 days or oral ampicillin or penicillin V for 10 days. (6)

PREVENTION

No vaccine is available against *Borrelia* spirochetes and *S. minus*. Prevention of these infections can be achieved by avoiding exposure to ticks and lice in endemic areas. Useful measures include wearing garments that cover arms and legs completely and applying tick repellants to the skin.

REFERENCES

1. Cutler SJ, Akintunde COK, Moss J, et al. Successful in vitro cultivation of *Borrelia duttoni* and its comparison with *Borrelia recurrentis. Int J Syst Bacteriol* 1999;49:2793.
2. Barbour AG. Antigenic variation of a relapsing fever *Borrelia* species. *Annu Rev Microbiol* 1990;44:155.
3. Schwan TG, Hinnebusch BJ. Bloodstream-versus tick-associated variants of a relapsing fever bacterium. *Science* 1998;280:1938.
4. Centers for Disease Control. Rat bite fever: New Mexico, 1996. *JAMA* 1998; 279:740.
5. Cunningham BB, Paller AS, Katz BZ. Rat bite fever in a pet lover. *J Am Acad Dermatol* 1998;38:330.
6. Schwan TG, Schrumpf ME, Hinnebusch BJ, et al. GIpQ: an antigen for serological discrimination between relapsing fever and Lyme borreliosis. *J Clin Microbiol* 1996;34:2483.

CHAPTER 216
Leptospira

Patrick W. Kelley

Human infections with pathogenic members of the genus *Leptospira* can cause serious clinical manifestations—jaundice, hemorrhage, renal failure, and death—or no symptoms at all. Among domestic animals, *Leptospira* organisms are economically important causes of morbidity and mortality; manifestations of infection can include loss of milk production, abortion, stillbirth, infertility, death, and chronic urinary shedding of viable organisms. Leptospiral infections are among the most widespread zoonoses, being transmitted by both wild and domestic animals through direct or indirect contact with their urine. Humans are accidental hosts.

CHARACTERISTICS OF THE PATHOGEN

Classification and Antigenic Characteristics

Before 1989, classification within the genus *Leptospira* was based on cross-agglutination assays that divided the genus into pathogenic *Leptospira interrogans* and nonpathogenic *Leptospira biflexa* species (1,2). Eventually, another free-living saprophytic strain, *Leptospira parva*, was added. Within these species, about 60 serogroups and 265 serovars were identified. Over time, DNA hybridization techniques have demonstrated extreme heterogeneity within these species. This heterogeneity is independent of the grouping of serovars into serogroups, in that serovars from antigenically defined serogroups may belong to different genetically defined categories (3,4). Ensuing molecular studies have led to the official replacement of the traditional serologically based classification schema with one based more correctly on genetic relatedness (2,3,5). The new schema has resulted in many new species classifications that do not relate to the traditional serogroupings based on the microagglutination test (MAT). Taxonomic divisions now include at least 12 species of *Leptospira*: *L. alexanderi, L. biflexa, L. borgpetersenii, L. fainei, L. inadai, L. interrogans, L. kirschneri, L. noguchii, L. santarosai, L. weilii, L. meyeri,* and *L. wolbachii* (2,5,6).

Restriction endonuclease analysis has also been applied to *Leptospira* (7–9). Monoclonal antibody techniques may eventually find applications not only in classification but also in diagnosis and immunization (1). Polymerase chain reaction (PCR) methods are also being used to classify leptospires; however, these methods cannot specify serovars, which is of public health value (2,10). Despite the new official nomenclature, the traditional taxonomic groupings for serologically distinct strains, serogroup and serovar, remain of practical value and in common use, especially because simple DNA-based identification methods are not readily available. Reflecting the utility and common use of the prior nomenclature, in this chapter, the use of "*L. interrogans*" and "*L. biflexa*" will refer to serogroups and serovars grouped under those former species classifications.

The method for categorizing *Leptospira* in one of the serovar categories is the MAT with cross-agglutinin absorption. Two strains are said to belong to different serovars if, after cross-absorption with adequate amounts of heterologous antigen, more than 10% of the homologous titer regularly remains in at least one of the two antiserum samples in repeated tests (1). This technique is time-consuming and exacting. The more than 200 serovars of *L. interrogans* are grouped into about 24 serogroups on the basis of shared major agglutinogens; *L. biflexa* contains about 65 serovars divided into about 38 serogroups (11). Serogrouping is useful for defining the composition of screening batteries used to test sera or identify isolates.

Structure

Leptospira organisms are motile, flexible, tightly coiled (18 or more coils per cell) helicoid rods about 0.1 µm in diameter and 6 to 20 µm in length (Fig. 216.1). Their narrow diameters allow them to pass through 0.2-µm membrane filters. One or both ends of the cell are usually hooked. Morphologically, *Leptospira* species are indistinguishable. *Leptospira* organisms have two independent, periplasmic, axial filaments that are attached subterminally at each end of the cell; the filaments' free ends extend down the axis of the coil toward the middle, where they may overlap a bit. The helicoid body has a cytoplasmic membrane–cell wall complex similar to that of gram-negative bacteria. A three- to five-layered outer envelope or sheath surrounds the protoplasmic cylinder and axial filaments. Even with staining, because

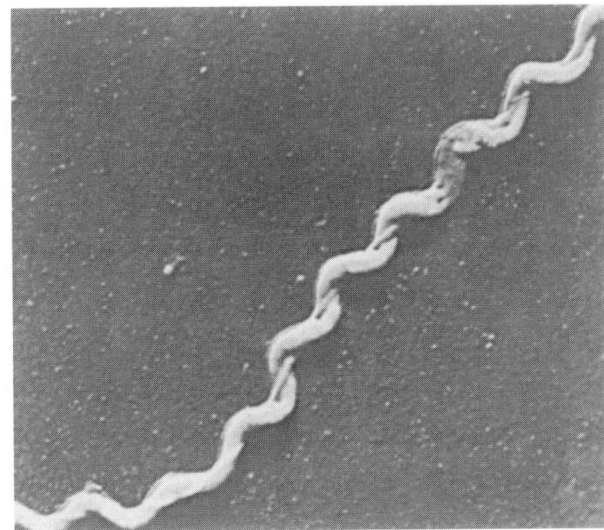

Figure 216.1. Electron micrograph of *Leptospira interrogans* (serovar *canicola*) showing the tightly coiled helicoid rod with the periplasmic axial filament. (From Armed Forces Institute of Pathology, AFIP No. 60-10941, with permission.)

of the thinness of the organism and its motility, dark-field microscopy is necessary for optimal visualization. The motion of *Leptospira* is characteristic and appears in liquid environments as an alternating rotation around the long axis and translation in the direction of the unhooked cell end. In environments of higher viscosity, flexing, boring, and serpentine movements have also been described. There are a few strains without hooked ends, which have little or no translational motility (11).

Biologic and Biochemical Properties

Leptospira organisms are obligate aerobes. Their nutritional requirements are simple but unique. They use long-chain fatty acids or fatty alcohols (15 carbons or more) rather than carbohydrates or amino acids as a source of energy and carbon. Because they cannot synthesize fatty acids, exogenous supplies are also the source of cellular lipids. Because free fatty acids are inherently toxic, in artificial media they are usually supplied bound to albumin or in a detoxified, esterified form. Nitrogen requirements can be met by urea or ammonium salts but not by amino acids. Unlike other spirochetes, *Leptospira* can use exogenous purines but not pyrimidines for DNA synthesis. This fact permits the use in culture media of the pyrimidine analog 5-fluorouracil as a means of selectively preventing the overgrowth of potential contaminants. *Leptospira* organisms also differ from other spirochetes in their ability to synthesize whatever amino acids they require (12). In addition to the fatty acids, vitamin B_1 (thiamine), vitamin B_{12} (cyanocobalamin), iron, and other trace elements are absolute nutritional requirements. Pyruvate enhances the growth of *Leptospira*, particularly the *hardjo* and *ballum* serovars. *Leptospira* organisms have been shown to possess cytochrome enzymes and catalase as well as enzymes of the citric acid cycle and glycolytic and pentose pathways; they also have an acyl coenzyme A dehydrogenase for the β-oxidation of fatty acids (13). They are oxidase positive. Hyaluronidase produced by pathogenic *Leptospira* species may account for their invasive capability (e.g., into the cerebrospinal fluid). Potentially toxic components or products of *Leptospira* have been identified, but their role in the pathogenesis of the disease remains ill defined (2).

Leptospira organisms can live free or in association with human and animal hosts. A key characteristic of pathogenic leptospires is their ability to survive for long periods in the proximal convoluted tubules of the kidney of some animals. On being shed, leptospires can survive under favorable conditions in the environment as long as 6 months. The optimal temperature for survival is 28° to 32°C, although they can also survive subzero temperatures, including freezing in liquid nitrogen (14). Acid environments or concentrated acid urine significantly reduces survival. Tropical, unpolluted, nonsaline waters that are slightly alkaline (pH, 7.2 to 8.0) provide an ideal environment. Survival is less favored in tropical areas where rainfall is low to moderate and seasonal. Under dry conditions, *Leptospira* may die within minutes (14). The nonpathogenic, free-living strains (the former *L. biflexa*) can be found in soil or surface waters; several *L. biflexa* strains have also been isolated from seawater. Survival of *L. interrogans* in seawater is short (15). In addition to its pathogenicity and its more fastidious growth requirements, *L. interrogans* can be differentiated from *L. biflexa* in other ways. Unlike *L. biflexa*, *L. interrogans* does not grow at 13°C or in the presence of 8-azaguanine (225 μg/mL). All *L. interrogans* cells convert to spherical forms in the presence of 1 M sodium chloride; *L. biflexa* serovars do not. There is no genetic homology between *L. interrogans* and *L. biflexa* (11).

Replication

Pathogenic *Leptospira* organisms can be isolated from water, blood, urine, cerebrospinal fluid (CSF), the anterior chamber of the eye, peritoneal fluid, amniotic fluid, and various tissues. Successful isolation from a particular human source depends on the phase of the infection. The optimal time to isolate *Leptospira* from blood and CSF is during the first week of symptoms; isolation from urine is best after the first week. *Leptospira* organisms are effectively cultivated in a variety of media that meet the essential nutritional and other conditions. Modifications of the formulations of Ellinghausen-McCullough-Johnson-Harris (EMJH or Tween 80 albumin) or Fletcher are especially effective (15,16). When properly inoculated with a minimal amount of material, kept in the dark, and aerated at 28° to 30°C, these media can support generation times of about 7 to 12 hours and yield 6 to 8 $\times$ 10^9 cells per mL (15). Cultures should be kept for up to 4 months and examined weekly for growth by dark-field microscopy. When growth is observed, subcultures of fresh media should be made as primary cultures may become nonviable.

Liquid media are used for cultures employed in serodiagnostic techniques and for typing isolates. For the purpose of obtaining isolates from body fluids or tissues, a semisolid medium is made by incorporating 0.2% agar. Growth may be visualized as one or more dense rings several millimeters to centimeters below the surface of the medium (15). Absence of rings does not preclude the presence of *Leptospira*. Solid media (made by adding 1% or 2% agar to the liquid) are useful for making isolations from contaminated sources or for cloning leptospires. Colonies on 1% agar solid media are diffuse to discrete and are usually below the surface. Colonies grown on 2% agar are usually turbid to clear and are located on the surface. Some strains on 1% and 2% agar can be either on or below the surface (11). Some pathogenic strains tend to lose their virulence and immunogenicity after a series of passages in media. Animal passage is better for maintaining these characteristics, and weanling hamsters are best for this purpose (11). Baby guinea pigs, baby rabbits, or gerbils are acceptable although inferior because they are less susceptible to *Leptospira*.

EPIDEMIOLOGY

Transmission

Humans usually become infected when, in the course of occupational, recreational, or even activities around home, pathogens in animal urine or urine-contaminated water, soil, or other surfaces enter through the skin or mucous membranes. Through urination and consequent contamination of soil and surface waters, animals that shed *Leptospira* can also infect others of their species, and other species. Animals may shed *Leptospira* for months or even years, continuously or sporadically. Pigs and other herbivores that have alkaline urine tend to excrete greater numbers of organisms and thus may pose a greater risk than animals with more acid urine, such as dogs. The infection in animals can be transmitted to offspring transplacentally, venereally, or through milk (15,17,18).

Distribution

Leptospira organisms can be found in virtually all tropical and temperate areas of the world. Their density in the environment depends on the presence of suitable domestic and wild animal carriers and on environmental variables, including season and moisture conditions. If carrier animals come into close contact with humans and other animals, even relatively arid regions can develop endemic foci of leptospirosis. The number of serovars tends to be greater in wet tropical regions than in temperate areas. This may reflect the variety and density of animals in the tropics. Classically, specific serovars have been associated with specific animal species (e.g., rats and *Leptospira icterohaemorrhagiae* or dogs and *Leptospira canicola*), although host–serovar associations are dynamic and can vary between geographic areas and over time. Surveillance can show previously "alien" serovars adapting for carriage in a particular species (19). Virulence or transmissibility of a specific serovar for animals and humans is not necessarily constant either and may be influenced by intermediate host factors (14,15). Alterations in the local ecology (e.g., increased contact between farm animals and rodents) probably contribute to some alterations of distribution and risk to humans. Because patterns of morbidity may vary by serovar, knowledge of the prevailing serovars and their hosts is important so that evolving transmission patterns may be documented and appropriate preventive interventions employed. Also, animal vaccines against leptospirosis are serovar specific and must be periodically reevaluated.

Prevalence

Evidence of past or current leptospiral infection in both animals and humans may be quite high in various subpopulations. The chronic carrier state is a common finding in animals, including asymptomatic ones. In 1977, Thiermann (20) found that more than 90% of Norway rats (*Rattus norvegicus*) collected in Detroit were carriers of *Leptospira*. In 1995, PCR evidence of leptospirosis infection was found in 19 of 21 rats trapped in an inner-city Baltimore setting (21). A 1984 survey of six small-mammal species that live in an area of Panamanian jungle that had been associated with many cases of leptospirosis in U.S. troops there showed that 42% of 139 animals caught carried leptospires (Takafuji ET, unpublished data). Alston and Broom (22) reviewed 19 *Leptospira* prevalence studies in dogs and noted that 30% to 40% of the apparently healthy dogs in some areas of the world showed infection.

Traditionally, leptospirosis has been described as an occupationally transmitted infection though recreational, inner-city, and peridomestic transmission has also been noteworthy. Occupational groups with a high incidence of infection include agriculture and aquaculture workers; abattoir workers; persons employed in rat-infested environments such as various fish or poultry processors; those involved in animal husbandry or veterinary medicine; sewer, construction, and mine workers; certain laboratory workers; and military personnel. Recreational activities that bring people into contact with leptospiruric animals or with contaminated soil or bodies of water are increasingly reported as a risk factor for human leptospirosis (23).

PATHOGENESIS

After *Leptospira* organisms enter humans, usually through breaks in the skin or through mucous membranes, they circulate in the bloodstream and spread to various target organs. The primary pathologic lesion is damage to the endothelium of small blood vessels. This is associated with localized ischemic damage to the renal tubules, liver, meninges, muscle, and placenta. The mechanism by which *Leptospira* organisms cause vascular damage is not fully understood, although elaborated toxins may play a role with at least some serovars (2). The immune response to leptospirosis depends on the production of specific antibody, opsonization, and subsequent phagocytosis. The immunoglobulin M (IgM) antibody becomes detectable late in the first week of illness. Titers reach maximum by the third or fourth week. Low agglutinin titers may be measurable for months or years. Secondary infections with an unrelated serovar are possible. Among survivors of leptospirosis, target organ damage usually resolves, and chronic sequelae are relatively uncommon.

CLINICAL MANIFESTATIONS

Human infections by the pathogenic *Leptospira* usually present as influenza-like illness characterized by sudden onset of fever, headache, profound myalgias, chills, back pain, joint pain, neck stiffness, conjunctival suffusion, and prostration. Most cases with this presentation are self-limited and last less than 10 days. Some patients experience relapse after a brief asymptomatic period, with fever and frequently headache. The relapse tends to last only a few days. A minority of patients with leptospirosis develop severe disease associated with a variety of manifestations, which can include renal failure, jaundice, skin and mucosal hemorrhage, hemoptysis, myocarditis, liver failure, and death. The renal failure appears to be most highly correlated with a fatal outcome; dialysis is frequently life saving. Recovery in survivors is usually complete, even in severe cases. The clinical manifestations of human leptospiral infections are described in more detail in Chapter 166.

Leptospiral infections in animals can also vary significantly within and between species (15). Typically, animal leptospirosis is also associated with symptoms of an acute febrile illness, including malaise, depression, anorexia, and conjunctivitis. Signs of bleeding, jaundice, central nervous system involvement, and liver and renal failure may also be noted. Acute leptospirosis in animals may also result in abortion, stillbirth, and mastitis. Some species of animals may develop a chronic kidney infection and shed *Leptospira* intermittently or continuously for months or years. These animals may or may not have had a detectable clinical illness.

DIAGNOSIS

The diagnosis of leptospirosis in humans is typically based on clinical, epidemiologic, and serologic grounds. The initial test customarily employed to evaluate suspected cases of leptospirosis is an IgM enzyme-linked immunosorbent assay (ELISA). Determination of the pathogenic serovar requires specific procedures, such as culture and the MAT (15). The MAT, which is the traditional method used for serologic confirmation, is complicated and time-consuming, requires a dark-field microscope, and is somewhat hazardous; unlike the ELISA or many other assays, it usually employs a battery of live *Leptospira* organisms for antigen (a safer and easier although less sensitive MAT method using formalized antigens has been described) (2). The MAT is best when the organisms in the battery are fresh and represent the serovars that are endemic in the area of possible transmission. In general, three weekly serum specimens should be collected for serologic testing. A serologically confirmed case of leptospirosis is defined by a MAT that shows either seroconversion from a titer of less than 1:50 to at least 1:200 or a fourfold or greater change in the titer between acute- and convalescent-phase serum specimens at least 2 weeks apart and studied at the same laboratory. In the United States, a probable case of leptospirosis can be defined by clinical compatibility and an MAT titer of at least 1:200 on a single specimen obtained after the onset of symptoms (24). Demonstration of *Leptospira* in a clinical specimen by immunofluorescence also meets laboratory criteria for diagnosis (24). A titer of at least 1:800 in the presence of compatible symptoms is strong evidence of recent or current leptospirosis (17,25). In populations where the background risk for exposure is higher than in the United States, such as most tropical countries, a higher cutoff MAT titer than 1:200 should be considered to establish a probable case (2). Rapid, simple dipstick forms of the ELISA are commercially available and possess favorable operating characteristics (26). Indirect hemagglutination and immunofluorescent antibody tests and gold immunoblot and PCR assays have also been evaluated (10,27–31). Where available, PCR may be especially valuable for diagnosis during the first few days of illness. False-negative serologic results may reflect antibiotic treatment, suboptimal timing of specimen collection, or suboptimal composition of the antigen pool used in the various tests.

Vigorous attempts should be made to culture the organism from blood, urine, and (when indicated) CSF fluid or tissue specimens. One reason for this is that the highest MAT titer observed among individual serovars in the test panel does not necessarily indicate the infecting serovar. "Paradoxical" reactions and "anamnestic" responses to prior infections with different serovars are a factor. As early as possible during the first week of symptoms (and before antibiotic administration), patients who have an appropriate clinical and epidemiologic history should have multiple blood specimens taken aseptically for culture on Fletcher, EMJH, or a similar, commercially prepared semisolid medium (15). Cultures should be inoculated at the bedside. If special media are not immediately available, blood should be collected aseptically in a tube containing either sodium oxalate or sodium heparin as the anticoagulant, held at room temperature, and inoculated onto media as soon as possible. Some commercial blood culture systems preserve viability of leptospires for weeks if the bottles are kept at 30°C (32). Because large amounts of blood can inhibit leptospiral growth, serial dilutions are essential. Impressive recovery rates have been achieved by adding 1 mL of fresh, unclotted blood to 10 mL of medium in a tube and then serially diluting the cultures to yield three cultures with concentrations of 1:10, 1:100, and 1:1,000. Several more blood specimens for culture should be taken during the first week of illness.

After the first several days of illness, *Leptospira* may be recoverable from the urine of infected humans and may persist for 30 days or longer. Because leptospiral shedding may be intermittent, several urine specimens for culture should be obtained. Patients whose urine is not alkaline should be given an alkalinizing regimen. Aseptically collected midstream urine should be inoculated promptly, as just described, to produce three tubes with 1:10, 1:100, and 1:1000 dilutions. The addition of 5-fluorouracil (100 to 200 μg/mL of media) to each tube can help control bacterial contamination. Tubes are incubated in the dark at 28° to 30°C for up to four months. Cultures should be examined every few days by inspection and, if necessary, by dark-field examination of a loopful of medium.

Under certain conditions, it is possible to visualize *Leptospira* organisms in tissues by dark-field or phase-contrast (but not bright-field) microscopy. Silver-deposition techniques can enhance visualization of organisms; aniline dyes cannot. Nevertheless, failure to visualize the pathogen is never conclusive evidence. Fluorescent antibody staining techniques are useful if cultural or serologic techniques are not possible (15). In some cases, differential centrifugation of body fluids is useful for removing cellular fibrils, extrusions, or fibrin strains that can resemble *Leptospira*. Close microscopic observation for both the characteristic morphology and mobility is necessary, but confirmation of the diagnosis requires serologic proof, demonstration of *Leptospira* in a clinical specimen by immunofluorescence, or isolation in culture. Direct microscopic examination of blood or tissues is most useful in situations in which the concentration of pathogens is high (e.g., in blood or liver suspensions from animals used for passage or in the examination of urine or kidney suspensions from natural animal hosts).

TREATMENT

Both penicillin and doxycycline are effective for the early treatment of leptospirosis, but the efficacy of these antibiotics after the first 4 or 5 days of illness has been controversial (33–35). Details on relevant treatment studies are provided in Chapter 166.

PREVENTION

A good medical surveillance program for both humans and animals is invaluable in providing information on circulating serovars and other transmission-related issues. This can guide the institution of specific preventive behaviors. Annual immunizations with appropriate serovars can significantly reduce the risk for disease in domestic animals. Secondarily, immunized animals may be less likely to infect their human caretakers. Animal vaccines do not necessarily prevent infection and subsequent shedding of viable *Leptospira* organisms. Laboratory workers should be cognizant of the risk associated with handling leptospiral isolates and infectious tissues. Appropriate measures are indicated to disinfect contaminated surfaces and to prevent mucous membrane or needlestick exposures to the agent. In certain groups of people with short-term exposure to *Leptospira*, 200 mg of doxycycline weekly may be used for prophylaxis (36). In the United States, there are no licensed human vaccines against leptospirosis, but in some other countries, human vaccines against leptospirosis have been used.

REFERENCES

1. Stallman GND. The International Committee on Systematic Bacteriology: Subcommittee on the Taxonomy of *Leptospira*. *Int J Syst Bacteriol* 1987;37:472.
2. Levett PN. Leptospirosis. *Clin Microbiol Rev* 2001;14:296–326.
3. Yasuda PH, Steigerwalt AG, Sulzer KR, et al. Deoxyribonucleic acid relatedness between serogroups and serovars in the family Leptospiraceae with proposals for seven new *Leptospira* species. *Int J Syst Bacteriol* 1987;37:407.
4. Brendel JJ, Rogul M, Alexander AD. Deoxyribonucleic acid hybridization among selected leptospiral serotypes. *Int J Syst Bacteriol* 1974;24:205.
5. Brenner DJ, Kaufmann AF, Sulzer KR, et al. Further determination of DNA relatedness between serogroups and serovars in the family *Leptospiraceae* with a proposal for *Leptospira alexanderi* sp. nov. and four new *Leptospira* genomospecies. *Int J Sys Bacteriol* 1999;49:839–858.
6. Plank R, Dean D. Overview of the epidemiology, microbiology, and pathogenesis of *Leptospira* spp. in humans. *Microbes Infect* 2000;2:1265–1276.
7. Terpstra WJ. Serodiagnosis of bacterial diseases: problems and developments. *Scand J Immunol* 1992;36[Suppl 11]:91.
8. Hookey JV. Characterization of Leptospiraceae by 16S DNA restriction fragment length polymorphisms. *J Gen Microbiol* 1993;139:1681.
9. Hookey JV, Bryden J, Gatehouse L. The use of 16S rDNA sequence analysis to investigate the phylogeny of Leptospiraceae and related spirochaetes. *J Gen Microbiol* 1993;139:2585.
10. Merien F, Amouriaux P, Perolat P, et al. Polymerase chain reaction for detection of *Leptospira* spp. in clinical samples. *J Clin Microbiol* 1992;30:2219.
11. Johnson RC, Faine S. Family II. Leptospiraceae Hovind-Hougen. In: Krieg NR, Holt JG, eds. *Bergey's manual of systematic bacteriology*, Vol 1. Baltimore: Williams & Wilkins, 1984:62–67.
12. Johnson RC. Comparative spirochete physiology and cellular composition. In: Johnson RC, ed. *The biology of parasitic spirochetes*. New York: Academic Press, 1976:39–48.
13. Smibert RM. Spirochaetales: a review. *Crit Rev Microbiol* 1973;2:491.
14. Torten M. Leptospirosis. In: Steele JH, ed. *Handbook series in zoonoses*, Vol 1. Boca Raton, FL: CRC Press, 1979:363–421.
15. Faine S, ed. *Guidelines for the control of leptospirosis*. Geneva: World Health Organization, 1982.
16. Ellinghausen HC, McCullough WG. Nutrition of *Leptospira pomona* and growth of 13 other serotypes: fractionation of oleic albumin complex and a medium of bovine albumin and polysorbate 80. *Am J Vet Res* 1965;26:45.
17. Feigin RD, Anderson DC. Human leptospirosis. *Crit Rev Clin Lab Sci* 1975;5:413.
18. Bolin CA, Koellner P. Human-to-human transmission of *Leptospira interrogans* by milk. *J Infect Dis* 1988;158:246.
19. Shenberg E, Birnbaum S, Rodrig E, et al. Dynamic changes in the epidemiology of canicola fever in Israel: natural adaptation of an established serotype to a new reservoir host. *Am J Epidemiol* 1977;105:42.
20. Thiermann AB. Incidence of leptospirosis in the Detroit rat population. *Am J Trop Med Hyg* 1977;26:970.
21. Vinetz JM, Glass GE, Flexner CE, et al. Sporadic urban leptospirosis. *Ann Intern Med* 1996;125:794–798.
22. Alston JM, Broom JC. *Leptospirosis in man and animals*. Edinburgh: E & S Livingstone, 1958.
23. Kaufmann AF. Epidemiologic trends of leptospirosis in the United States, 1965–1974. In: Johnson RC, ed. *The biology of parasitic spirochetes*. New York: Academic Press, 1976:177–190.
24. Centers for Disease Control. Case definitions for infectious conditions under public health surveillance. *MMWR Morb Mortal Wkly Rep* 1997;46:1–55.
25. Faine S. Leptospirosis. In: Balows A, Hausler WA, Ohashi M, et al., eds. *Laboratory diagnosis of infectious diseases: principles and practice*, Vol 1. New York: Springer-Verlag, 1988:344–352.
26. Levett PN, Branch SL, Whittington CU, et al. Two methods for rapid serological diagnosis of acute leptospirosis. *Clin Diagn Lab Immunol* 2001;8:349–351.
27. Merien F, Baranton G, Perolat P. Comparison of polymerase chain reaction with microagglutination test and culture for diagnosis of leptospirosis. *J Infect Dis* 1995;172:281–285.
28. Brown PD, Gravekamp C, Carrington DG, et al. Evaluation of the polymerase chain reaction for early diagnosis of leptospirosis. *J Med Microbiol* 1995;43:110–114.
29. Petchclai B, Hiranras S, Kunakorn M, et al. Enzyme-linked immunosorbent assay for leptospirosis immunoglobulin M specific antibody using surface antigen from a pathogenic *Leptospira*: a comparison with indirect hemagglutination and microagglutination tests. *J Med Assoc Thai* 1992;75:203.
30. Appassakij H, Silpapojakul K, Wansit R, et al. Evaluation of the immunofluorescent antibody test for the diagnosis of human leptospirosis. *Am J Trop Med Hyg* 1995;52:340.
31. Petchclai B, Hiranras S, Potha U. Gold immunoblot analysis of IgM-specific antibody in the diagnosis of human leptospirosis. *Am J Trop Med Hyg* 1991;45:672.
32. Palmer MF, Zochowski WJ. Survival of leptospires in commercial culture systems revisited. *J Clin Pathol* 2000;53:713–714.
33. McClain JB, Ballou WR, Harrison SM, et al. Doxycycline therapy for leptospirosis. *Ann Intern Med* 1984;100:696.
34. Watt G, Padre LP, Tuazon ML, et al. Placebo-controlled trial of intravenous penicillin for severe and late leptospirosis. *Lancet* 1988;1:433.
35. Edwards CN, Nicholson GD, Hassell TA, et al. Penicillin therapy in icteric leptospirosis. *Am J Trop Med Hyg* 1988;39:388.
36. Takafuji ET, Kirkpatrick JW, Miller RN, et al. An efficacy trial of doxycycline chemoprophylaxis against leptospirosis. *N Engl J Med* 1984;310:497.

CHAPTER 217
Helicobacter*

Julie Parsonnet

Spiral gastric bacteria have been recognized in the human stomach since 1906 (1). It was not until 1982, however, that *Helicobacter pylori* was isolated and speciated for the first time. Today, *Helicobacter* is a rapidly expanding genus of bacterium that encompasses dozens of species, seven of which cause disease in humans. These human *Helicobacter* species can be divided into two types: the gastric, urease producers [*H. pylori* and *Helicobacter heilmannii* (also known as *Gastrospirillum hominis*)] and the enteric nonurease producers [*Helicobacter cinaedi, Helicobacter fennelliae, Helicobacter rappini* (formerly *Flexispira rappini*), *Helicobacter canis,* and *Helicobacter westmeadii*]. Case reports of human infection with other gastric *Helicobacter* species (*Helicobacter felis*), and enterohepatic *Helicobacter* species (*Helicobacter pullorum, Helicobacter canadensis,* and *Helicobacter winghamensis*) have not been fully enough substantiated to classify them definitively as human pathogens (2). With the exception of *H. pylori*, human *Helicobacter* infections are unusual. *H. pylori*, on the other hand, is one of the most common bacterial infections of humans. Moreover, the diseases attributed to *H. pylori* infection, peptic ulcer disease and gastric malignancy, are major causes of morbidity and mortality worldwide. Consequently, the past two decades have witnessed furious research into diagnosis, treatment, and prevention of this infection. Because of its clinical importance relative to other *Helicobacter* species, this chapter focuses predominantly on *H. pylori*.

MICROBIOLOGY

Helicobacter species are microaerophilic, spiral, gram-negative rods that are phylogenetically closest to *Wolinella, Arcobacter,* and *Campylobacter* species (3,4). All species are motile and typically have multiple flagellae. *H. pylori* is 2.5 to 5.0 μm long with four to eight unipolar flagellae providing a corkscrew motility. The enteric *Helicobacter* species, in contrast, typically have one or two bipolar flagellae (with the exception of *H. rappini*, which has numerous flagellae). Chemical characteristics of the most common human *Helicobacter* species can be seen in Table 217.1. *H. heilmannii* organisms, which are longer (3.5 to 7.5 μm) and much more tightly coiled than *H. pylori*, may represent several genetically distinct species. The chemical characteristics of *H. heilmannii* are largely unknown because it has only once been cultured from a human gastric biopsy (5). The cultured strain appeared to be identical to a common dog *Helicobacter* species—*Helicobacter bizzozeronii* (6).

Helicobacter species are relatively fastidious organisms. To culture *H. pylori* from the stomach, biopsies should be immediately placed in transport medium to prevent desiccation. As soon as possible, the ground specimens should be plated on solid agar (7). Recovery of enteric *Helicobacter* species from stool or blood is conducted much the same way as culture of *Campylobacter* species except at 37°C instead of 42°C. Many agar bases will sustain *Helicobacter* species if supplemented with blood or serum; antimicrobial supplements in the medium minimizes overgrowth of competing organisms and increases culture sensitivity (7). Plates should be incubated under microaerophilic conditions at 37°C. *Helicobacter* species grow slowly, and plates and s bottles may require 7 days of incubation to develop recognizable colonies. Because of their indolent growth, positive blood cultures may be missed unless an automated growth detection system is used. Presumptive identification can be made if organisms have typical gram-negative, curved morphology on Gram stain and produce both catalase and oxidase.

HELICOBACTER PYLORI

Pathology, Pathogenesis, and Immunity

H. pylori resides beneath the mucous layer, adjacent to the surface and pit epithelial cells of the gastric antrum and body. Aside from ectopic gastric mucosa (e.g., Meckel's diverticula), no other tissue besides the stomach is known to be infectable with *H. pylori*. Motility appears to be critical for this colonization (8). About one fifth of the organisms are adherent to the mucosal surface, whereas the remainder appear to be free living within the mucus layer (9). Adherence is species specific and is related to features of both the host (e.g., blood group type) and the bacterium (e.g., production of specific outer membrane proteins) (10,11). The process of adherence allows entry of virulence factors into the epithelial cell and precipitates a cascade of cytoplasmic and nuclear events that may mediate infection outcome (12).

H. pylori produces urease at a constitutively high level. This enzyme, a 300- to 625-kd nickel-containing hexamer, is located is largely within the cytoplasm, with only a small proportion excreted (13). Urease is essential for *H. pylori* colonization of the stomach but is not required for survival after colonization (9,14). The precise physiologic role of urease has not been definitively established (15,16). By hydrolyzing urea to carbon dioxide and ammonia, urease may surround the organism with a cloud of ammonia, protecting it from the stomach's acid environment (13). Damage to the gastric mucosa induced by urease and ammonia may also provide the organism with the necessary nutrients and an appropriate environment for attachment and growth. Alternatively, urease-activity may facilitate nitrogen assimilation by the organism.

H. pylori exhibits enormous genetic diversity. Using molecular typing methods (restriction fragment length polymorphisms, arbitrary primer polymerase chain reaction, or gene sequencing), it is unusual to find identical strains in different subjects, even married couples (17); some family members, however, share similar strains (18,19). The genetic variability between strains translates into variability in the presence, expression or activity of virulence factors. The best studied of the variable virulence factors is the *cag* pathogenicity island (PAI)—a cassette of 31 genes, found in 60% of isolates. The *cag* PAI encodes a type IV secretion system that injects the CagA protein into epithelial cells. There, CagA is tyrosine phosphorylated, resulting in cytoskeletal changes. Presence of an intact *cag* PAI is associated with enhanced cytokine expression [particularly of interleukin-8 (IL-8)] and increased inflammation (20,21). Another variable virulence factor is a vacuolating cytotoxin (VacA) that causes host cell vacuolation, altered lysosomal function, and formation of pores that passively transport urea into the cell (22,23). Although the *vacA* gene is present in all *H. pylori* organisms, its gene sequence varies from strain to strain, and expression of functional protein is quite variable. Other putative virulence factors that have variable expression or activity are a blood group antigen-binding adhesin (BabA) (24); an outer membrane protein termed *outer inflammatory protein A*

---

*Editor's note: Microorganisms belonging to the genus *Helicobacter* are helicoid (spiral-shaped) and spirochete-like, but they are not spirochetes. This chapter was placed in the section on spirochetes because of a tendency among scientists to group together all spiral-shaped microorganisms. The mistake was discovered too late in the production process for the chapter to be moved.

TABLE 217.1. Bacteriologic Characteristics of Human *Helicobacter* Species Infections

Characteristic	Enteric *Helicobacter* species				Gastric *Helicobacter* species	
	H. cinaedi	*H. fennelliae*	*H. pullorum*	*H. rappini*	*H. heilmannii*	*H. pylori*
Urease production	−	−	−	+	+	+
Oxidase production	+	+			NA	+
Catalase production	+	+	+	+	NA	+
Nitrate reduction	+	−	+	−	NA	−
Alkaline phosphatase hydrolysis	−	+	−	−	NA	+
Indoxyl acetate hydrolyxis	−	+	−	NA	NA	−
Growth at 42°C	−	−	+	+	NA	−
Susceptibility to:						
Nalidixic acid	S	S	R	R	NA	R
Cephalothin	S	S	S	R	NA	S

S, sensitive; I, intermediate sensitivity; R, resistant; NA, not available.
From Fox JG. The non-*H. pylori* helicobacters: their expanding role in gastrointestinal and systemic diseases. *Gut* 2002;50:273–283.

(OipA) (25); and a protein expressed upon bacterial adhesion to the mucosa, IceA (26).

Infection with *H. pylori* is always accompanied by acute and chronic inflammation in the submucosa (27). Lymphoid follicles (mucosal-associated lymphoid tissue) similar to Peyer's patches are also evident in all patients and are pathognomonic of *H. pylori* infection; these follicles may be particularly prominent in children. Gastric inflammation is accompanied by elevations in bacterium-specific immunoglobulin G (IgG) and IgA (28); these antibodies can be opsonizing but do not appear to be effective in eliminating infection. Moreover, there is some evidence that *H. pylori* antibodies may induce autoimmunity to gastric epithelial cell, augmenting bacterial pathogenicity. Analysis of mucosal CD4 cells indicate a prominent helper T-cell subtype 1 (T$_H$1) response, with pronounced expression of IL-12 and interferon-γ (IFN-γ) (29). The degree of *H. pylori*–related inflammation is thought to be mediated by bacterial factors—including the virulence factors mentioned previously—as well as host genotype. Population-based studies suggest that host polymorphisms in IL-1β (30)—which has acid-suppressive as well as inflammatory effects—and tumor necrosis factor (TNF) may in part determine infection outcome (31).

Little is known about host and bacterial factors required for establishing infection. Given the high, but not universal, prevalence of *H. pylori* throughout the world, it seems likely that many exposures do not result in chronic infection. "Windows of opportunity" (such as periods of hypochlorhydria) may exist when the stomach permits infection. *In vivo* experiments support this finding; in two human inoculation experiments, infection could not be established without altering the gastric pH with histamine antagonists (32,33). Moreover, circumstantial data in children and in people infected during endoscopy suggest that infections can be transient (34,35). However, once established, infection with *H. pylori* persists as long as normal gastric epithelial cells line the stomach (*H. pylori* does not thrive in an atrophic or metaplastic epithelium). For many people, this probably means the organism remains for a lifetime.

People with *H. pylori*–related gastritis can progress to a variety of clinical diseases. The pathogenic mechanisms for the variable outcome of infection (i.e., asymptomatic, ulcer, lymphoma, or cancer) are largely unknown. The pathogeneses of ulcers and of cancer, however, appear to be distinct; the two diseases rarely occur in the same individual (36). People who develop atrophic gastritis in association with *H. pylori* infection are at increased risk for gastric cancer but are largely protected from peptic ulcer disease (37,38). It is assumed that differences in outcome can be explained by a combination of bacterial, environmental, and host

factors (such as host IL-1β genotype) and their effects on gastric acidity (30,39–41). Even in the setting of *H. pylori* infection, the age-old dogma "no acid, no ulcer" remains true. In contrast, "yes acid, no cancer" also appears to be true.

Pathogenesis of cancer may in part depend on the chronicity of inflammation and decreased acid secretion, typically in the setting of atrophic gastritis. Inflammation results in increased cell proliferation, enhancing the likelihood of mutation. Inflammation also induces oxidative bursts of free radicals that can potentially damage DNA (42,43). The loss of acid is thought to enhance gastric carcinogenesis by promoting hypergastrinemia (gastrin is a trophic factor for gastric epithelial cells), increasing gastric superinfection in the stomach with nitrosating microorganisms, and decreasing local concentrations of antioxidants (44). Given these factors, the likelihood of a carcinogenic combination of mutations to occur would almost certainly be higher in infected than in uninfected hosts.

Epidemiology

H. pylori infection is common worldwide. Between and within population groups, however, prevalence can vary widely. In some developing populations, a large majority is infected by 10 years of age, and infection is universal by midlife (45). In industrialized countries, on the other hand, prevalence of infection is considerably lower, although still far from rare. In the United States, at least one third of the population is likely to be infected. Overall, *H. pylori* incidence is decreasing in industrialized countries with time (46,47). In children, incidence of infection is higher than in adults.

Virtually all studies to date have shown an inverse relationship between *H. pylori* infection and socioeconomic status. Socioeconomic status during childhood may serve as a particularly good indicator of *H. pylori* risk (48). In the United States, African Americans and Hispanics exhibit higher rates of infection than do non-Hispanic whites (49). Outside of the United States, racial and ethnic variations in *H. pylori* prevalence have also been observed (50,51). Strains with the *cag* PAI also vary in their distributions within populations (52). The reasons for racial and ethnic differences are not understood. Poor socioeconomic conditions during childhood, as measured by household crowding and parental income, are thought to play an important role. These cannot, however, completely explain observed differences, and a genetic component to infection has been posited (53).

Person-to-person spread is widely considered to be the most prevalent means of *H. pylori* transmission (54). Both fecal–oral and oral–oral transmission are probable. *H. pylori* has been cultured from vomitus and stools—particularly from diarrheal stools (55). *H. pylori* has less frequently been cultured from saliva and dental plaque, suggesting at least a transient presence in the mouth (55,56). Infection is most likely to occur in populations in which person-to-person transmission is common, such as institutions for the disabled or families with young children. Infection with *H. pylori* has also been related to other markers of person-to-person transmission, such as sibship size, birth order, and current number of children in the family. Household crowding particularly engenders greater risk for infection; sharing of beds during childhood is an especially hazardous practice (54).

Iatrogenic transmission of *H. pylori* by endoscopy has been well documented through the isolation of identical strains of *H. pylori* from patients undergoing endoscopy in the same suite. Transmission has been estimated to occur in 0.3% of endoscopies when the endoscope is mechanically cleaned with detergent and ethanol alone (57). More rigorous cleansing methods prevent transmission (58). Not surprisingly, gastroenterologists appear to be at particularly high risk for infection (59).

Although the preponderance of evidence supports direct person-to-person spread of infection, there are some data to suggest other transmission modalities. In particular, two epidemiologic studies from Latin America suggest that water and water-contaminated food might be vehicles for *H. pylori* (60,61). Many investigators have amplified *H. pylori* DNA from environmental water sources, but only one group has successfully cultured the organism; in that instance, untreated municipal waste water from a city in Mexico yielded viable organisms (62). It is plausible, then, that waterborne transmission of *H. pylori* can occur in areas where human water sources are not appropriately treated.

Clinical Disease

The clinical syndrome of acute *H. pylori* infection is not specific and is never diagnosed in clinical practice. Experimental human inoculations, laboratory-acquired infections, and epidemics related to improperly cleansed endoscopy equipment, however, indicate that acute infection causes bloating, epigastric pain, vomiting, and irritability 3 to 7 days after exposure in about half of the infected patients (32–34,63). About 1 to 2 weeks after infection, symptoms remit despite persistence of the organism (33). Chronic infection with *H. pylori* is typically asymptomatic. Although 20% to 30% of *H. pylori*–infected subjects report dyspepsia-like symptoms, these symptoms are equally common in uninfected populations. Thus, any role for *H. pylori* in nonulcer dyspepsia remains hotly debated (64).

Although most *H. pylori*–infected subjects are symptom free, in a subset of infected hosts, *H. pylori* causes life-threatening disease. *H. pylori* infection has been linked to both gastric and extragastric diseases. Among the former are duodenal ulcer disease, gastric ulcer disease, gastric adenocarcinoma, gastric lymphoma, nonulcer dyspepsia, and hypertrophic gastropathy. The extragastric diseases include hepatic encephalopathy, pancreatic cancer, atherosclerosis, autoimmune diseases, parkinsonism, urticaria, rosacia, diabetes mellitus, and migraine headache (65). Many investigators also believe that *H. pylori* infection protects against two diseases of the distal esophagus: gastroesophageal reflux and adenocarcinoma. The data supporting these associations is variable, and only peptic ulcer disease, gastric adenocarcinoma, and gastric lymphoma are widely held to be *H. pylori* related. Consequently, these diseases are presented in more detail later. Accumulating data on atherosclerosis and on protection from esophageal diseases make these associations also worthy of further mention.

H. pylori is the single most important cause of both duodenal and gastric ulcer diseases. Duodenal ulcers should now be assumed to be *H. pylori* related unless other predisposing conditions, such as nonsteroidal antiinflammatory drug (NSAID) use, Zollinger-Ellison syndrome, or Crohn's disease, are present (66). Moreover, persons treated with antimicrobial agents have much lower rates of ulcer relapse than persons treated with acid inhibitory therapy alone (67,68). In support of a causal relationship, if *H. pylori* infection is not successfully eradicated, antibiotics provide no additional benefit over acid inhibition alone. However, only a minority (perhaps 20%) of infected persons develop duodenal ulcer within a 10-year period (69).

The proportion of ulcers that is attributable to *H. pylori* varies from population to population with *H. pylori* prevalence. In areas with high *H. pylori* prevalence, more than 90% of ulcers may be attributable to infection; in the United States and other countries where *H. pylori* prevalence is decreasing, attributable risk estimates range between 40% and 80% (70,71). *H. pylori* is more likely to be a factor in young adult patients with ulcer disease than in elderly patients in whom other factors (e.g., NSAID use) may play a more prominent role (72). Those at highest risk have duodenitis and gastric metaplasia of the duodenal mucosa (73). Environmental cofactors, including cigarette and alcohol use, use of NSAIDs, male gender, blood group O, and other hereditary factors, may also magnify ulcer risk (70,74).

Clinical trials similar to those conducted for duodenal ulcers also support a role for *H. pylori* in gastric ulcer disease (67). The percentage of gastric disease attributable to *H. pylori*, however, is lower than for duodenal ulcers. In the United States, a substantial proportion of gastric ulcers (about 35%) are caused by use of NSAIDs (75). Of the remaining 65%, *H. pylori* must be considered the preeminent cause.

In 1994, the World Health Organization declared *H. pylori* infection to be a Type I Carcinogen, a definite cause of cancer in humans (76). Support for this declaration came from pathologic and epidemiologic studies. Together, these studies show that: (a) chronic gastritis is an important cancer precursor, (b) gastric cancer occurs at an increased rate in regions with high prevalence of *H. pylori* infection, (c) people with *H. pylori* infection are at significantly higher risk for cancer than those without infection, (d) *H. pylori* infection precedes cancer by many years. Although most gastric adenocarcinomas occurring in the gastric body and antrum are due to *H. pylori* infection, less than 1% of infected persons can be expected to develop malignancy. The progression of mucosal changes from superficial gastritis to carcinoma probably requires decades. Therefore, individuals who acquire *H. pylori* infection early in life have the highest risk for malignancy, whereas those infected later in life are unlikely to develop cancer (77). Other factors influencing the development of cancer include dietary exposures (nitrates and salts increase risk, fruits and vegetables decrease risk), genetic predisposition, and infection with cytotoxin-producing strains (78,79). Gastric adenocarcinoma remains a highly lethal disease, with less than 20% of affected individuals surviving 5 years (80).

Gastric lymphoma is a rare disease afflicting only 7 cases per 1 million population per year (81). These tumors almost invariably arise in mucosa-associated lymphoid tissue (MALT) resultant from *H. pylori* infection. Thus, it is not surprising that *H. pylori* infection has been found to increase risk for gastric lymphoma sixfold (82). The remarkable feature of these MALT lymphomas is that 80% will completely regress if *H. pylori* infection is cured. Despite gross and histologic tumor regression, many patients still have molecular evidence of the monoclonal B-cell clone in the mucosal. Although the significance of this finding is unclear, annually 5% of regressed tumors will recur, sometimes in a more aggressive form (83). A translocation mutation [t(11;18)] appears to be an indicator of this poor prognostic form of the tumor. Why a scattered few people with *H. pylori* infection develop these rare lymphomas is presently unknown.

A diversity of evidence links *H. pylori* to atherosclerosis, coronary artery disease, and stroke. Pathophysiologically, several pathways have been entertained for *H. pylori*–induced atherogenesis, including decreasing homocysteine (84), altering lipid profiles (85), increasing production of mediators of vascular inflammation (86), direct bacterial action on blood vessels (*H. pylori* DNA has been amplified from atherosclerotic plaque) (87), and antigenic mimicry of structural peptides of blood vessels (88). Epidemiologic, clinical, and laboratory data to date, however, are conflicting, with no resulting consensus that *H. pylori* does cause atherosclerotic disease (89,90). One strong confounder in all population studies is socioeconomic status, a strong risk factor for both *H. pylori* and for atherosclerosis. Thus, a role of *H. pylori* remains hotly debated and tantalizing, but far from proven.

Another controversial clinical question regarding *H. pylori* infection is whether the organism imparts benefits to the host. In particular, some studies indicate that *H. pylori* infection coincides with a low risk for symptomatic esophageal reflux disease. Moreover, in ulcer patients previously without reflux, eradication of *H. pylori* infection appears to increase reflux symptoms (91). Chronic *H. pylori* infection can cause decreased acid production through destruction of glandular tissue (atrophy); the increased reflux attributed to *H. pylori* treatment is thought to reflect a reversal of this process. Because esophageal reflux disease predisposes to both Barrett's esophagus and esophageal adenocarcinoma—one of the most rapidly increasing tumors in the United States—there is concern that indiscriminate treatment of *H. pylori* infection will bring with it an epidemic of esophageal tumors. Data to support this latter conclusion are limited and conflicting (92,93). Moreover, the clinical significance of any true association is disputed; will putative and potentially treatable esophageal risks outweigh the known risks to the stomach? Additionally, new treatments for gastroesophageal reflux disease and screening methods for Barrett's esophagus may render interest in *H. pylori* moot.

Diagnosis

For patients undergoing endoscopy, a rapid urease test is the diagnostic test of choice. A biopsy of the stomach is obtained and placed in a urea-containing medium with a pH indicator. Production of ammonia turns the indicator red and confirms the presence of the organism. The rapid urease test can often be interpreted in less than 1 hour and is substantially less expensive than histology. It has 90% sensitive, with even greater specificity for *H. pylori* infection (94–97). For patients in whom evaluation of underlying gastric pathology is essential, histologic examination may be preferable to the rapid urease test. Because *H. pylori* is not evenly distributed throughout the gastric mucosa, however, at least two biopsies need to be performed to diagnose infection sensitively (97,98). Routine hematoxylin and eosin or Giemsa staining will usually reveal the organism; the more sensitive but more expensive silver stains should be reserved for inconclusive examinations (99). Culture is the least sensitive but most specific endoscopic method for diagnosis of *H. pylori*. Because other diagnostic tests are less expensive and more widely available, however, culture is best reserved for research laboratories.

For patients in whom endoscopy is not necessary, serology is currently the simplest option for diagnosis. At their best, serologic assays have sensitivity and specificity for active infection exceeding 90% and sometimes exceeding 95% (100). In-office,

qualitative serologic assays are also now available. Like the commercial enzyme-linked immunosorbent assays (ELISAs), these appear to have excellent accuracy in the untreated patient. Unfortunately, although the titers drop, sera obtained following successful therapy will not necessarily be quantitatively negative. Thus, comparison of pretreatment and posttreatment titers is necessary for treatment follow-up. Carbon-labeled urea breath tests and stool antigen tests, obtained at least 4 weeks after completion of therapy, are the best assays for assessing cure of infection (101,102). With the exception of biopsy with histology, no diagnostic test has proven reliability in young children (103).

Treatment

H. pylori infection is curable with antimicrobial therapy. The most widely accepted therapy includes combinations of two antibiotics (usually clarithromycin with either amoxicillin or metronidazole) and either a proton pump inhibitor or a ranitidine-bismuth combination for 10 days to 2 weeks. Cure rates with this regimen range between 80% and 90%. Increasing resistance to clarithromycin and metronidazole diminish the success of therapy (104). Should treatment fail, four-drug therapy containing a proton pump inhibitor, bismuth, tetracycline, and high-dose metronidazole can be used (105). Reinfection following successful treatment is rare (less than 1% per year in industrialized countries) (106). Eradication of the *H. pylori* is associated with slow improvement in submucosal inflammation. One year after successful treatment, neutrophil infiltration will resolve; lymphocyte infiltration and lymphoid follicles improve but persist (107).

The National Institutes of Health recommend treating only persons with active ulcer disease (gastric or duodenal) or persons on maintenance antihistamine therapy for recurrent ulcer disease (66). The European Consensus Conference in 2000, on the other hand, offered much broader recommendations for treatment, including not only patients with ulcer disease but also those with gastric MALT lymphoma, atrophic gastritis, partial gastric resection, family history of gastric cancer, and in many instances, dyspepsia or simply a desire to be treated (108). Other groups have reported that broad-based screening and treatment could be a cost-effective approach to preventing ulcer disease, dyspepsia, and cancer in populations at high risk (109–111). Still others argue that eradicating infection in all infected persons, regardless of symptoms, is the correct approach (112). As new information accumulates, it is likely that diagnosis and therapy will be offered to a wider segment of the U.S. population in order to prevent adverse outcomes of infection. For now, however, there are no recommendations for diagnostic testing or treatment in asymptomatic people or those with dyspepsia of unknown etiology.

HELICOBACTER HEILMANNII

H. heilmannii, like *H. pylori*, is thought to cause acute and chronic gastritis. It has also been anecdotally reported in cases of gastric MALT lymphoma, gastric cancer, and gastric erosion. MALT lymphoma in particular—although still rare—may occur more frequently with *H. heilmannii* than with *H. pylori* infection (83). *H. heilmannii* is considerably less common than *H. pylori*. In one Italian series, *H. heilmannii* was identified endoscopically in only eight (0.1%) of 7,926 symptomatic patients (113). It may be somewhat more common (up to 8% prevalence) in Asia (114). Some data suggest direct transmission of *H. heilmannii* to humans from domestic animals, although this is not firmly established (115,116).

Unlike *H. pylori* infection, colonization and inflammation with *H. heilmannii* appear to be restricted to the acid-secreting portion of the mucosa (114). Pathogenic mechanisms are unknown. Because *H. heilmannii*, like *H. pylori*, does produce urease, some tissue destruction may be similarly related to this enzyme and its toxic metabolites.

HELICOBACTER FENNELLIAE AND HELICOBACTER CINAEDI

H. cinaedi and *H. fennelliae* are unusual pathogens that cause a varied spectrum of clinical disease. Both were identified in the mid-1980s in homosexual men with proctitis and colitis (117,118). Recent data indicate that these organisms more typically cause mild noninflammatory diarrhea. This diarrhea is self-limited in normal hosts but prolonged in immunocompromised patients (119). *H. cinaedi* and *H. fennelliae* have also been reported to cause recurrent bacteremia in immunocompromised patients (120,121). Patients with bacteremia are typically febrile with temperatures higher than 38.5°C and without a leukocytosis. They do not typically appear septic. Accompanying cellulitis—frequent with *H. cinaedi* bacteremia—may be multifocal with a distinctive copper or red-brown color and absence of warmth. Endocarditis and arthritis have also been reported.

The most common predisposing factor for *H. cinaedi* or *H. fennelliae* infection is human immunodeficiency virus (HIV) infection (at least 60% of cases), although *H. cinaedi* and *H. fennelliae* have also been observed in alcoholic patients as well as in immunocompetent hosts. Sexual transmission of both *H. fennelliae* and *H. cinaedi* seems likely because these infections occur predominantly in homosexual men (117,120). Sixteen percent of homosexual men with intestinal symptoms and 8% of those without symptoms have been found to harbor these organisms (118). The reservoir for enteric *Helicobacter* species is unknown. *H. cinaedi* has also been recovered from hamsters, but it is far from clear whether hamsters have any role as a disease vector (122).

Pathogenic mechanisms for *H. fennelliae* and *H. cinaedi* have not yet been identified. In experiments performed in monkeys, infection with *H. fennelliae* or *H. cinaedi* caused noninflammatory diarrhea invariably associated with bacteremia. No mucosal disruption was observed, suggesting that the colitis seen in humans may indicate co-infection with other enteric pathogens (123). Carriage of enteric *Helicobacter* species in monkeys was sustained well after resolution of symptoms despite a brisk serologic response to organism-specific antigens (123). Humans, too, develop specific IgG against the enteric *Helicobacter* species following either bacteremic or enteric infection (124).

H. cinaedi and *H. fennelliae* should be considered in patients with HIV, diarrhea, and unexplained fever. Clinical laboratories should be informed if suspicion is high so that blood and stool cultures are appropriately processed. As yet, there are no clinical series addressing treatment. Case reports and studies of minimal inhibitory concentrations suggest that amoxicillin-clavulanate, tetracycline, or aminoglycosides would be the best choice for bacteremic disease (120,125). Cephalosporins and quinolones appear to be less successful, and bacteremia may recur.

REFERENCES

1. Kreinitz W. Ueber das Auftreten von Spirochaeten verschiedener Form im Mageninhalt bei Carcinoma ventriculi. *Deutsche Med Wochenschr* 1906;32:872–872.
2. Fox JG. The non-H pylori helicobacters: their expanding role in gastrointestinal and systemic diseases. *Gut* 2002;50:273–283.
3. Stanley J, Linton D, Burnens AP, et al. *Helicobacter pullorum* sp. nov.: genotype and phenotype of a new species isolated from poultry and from human patients with gastroenteritis. *Microbiology* 1994;140:3441–3449.
4. Fox JG, Yan LL, Dewhirst FE, et al. *Helicobacter bilis* sp. nov., a novel *Helicobacter* species isolated from bile livers and intestines of aged, inbred mice. *J Clin Microbiol* 1995;33:445–454.
5. Andersen LP, Boye K, Blom J, et al. Characterization of a culturable "Gastrospirillum hominis" (*Helicobacter heilmannii*) strain isolated from human gastric mucosa. *J Clin Microbiol* 1999;37:1069–1076.
6. Jalava K, On SL, Harrington CS, et al. A cultured strain of "*Helicobacter heilmannii*," a human gastric pathogen, identified as *H. bizzozeronii*: evidence for zoonotic potential of *Helicobacter*. *Emerg Infect Dis* 2001;7:1036–1038.
7. Hazell SL. Cultural techniques for the growth and isolation of *Helicobacter pylori*. In: Goodwin CS, Worsley BW, eds. *Helicobacter pylori*: biology and clinical practice. Boca Raton, FL: CRC Press, 1993:273–283.
8. Eaton KA, Morgan DR, Krakowka S. Motility as a factor in the colonisation of gnotobiotic piglets by *Helicobacter pylori*. *J Med Microbiol* 1992;37:123–127.
9. Lee A, Fox J, Hazell S. Pathogenicity of *Helicobacter pylori*: a perspective. *Infect Immun* 1993;61:1601–1610.
10. Ilver D, Arnqvist A, Ogren J, et al. *Helicobacter pylori* adhesin binding fucosylated histo-blood group antigens revealed by retagging. *Science* 1998;279 (5349):373–377.
11. Odenbreit S, Till M, Hofreuter D, et al. Genetic and functional characterization of the alpAB gene locus essential for the adhesion of *Helicobacter pylori* to human gastric tissue. *Mol Microbiol* 1999;31:1537–1548.
12. Jones NL, Sherman PM. *Helicobacter pylori*–epithelial cell interactions: from adhesion to apoptosis. *Can J Gastroenterol* 1999;13:563–566.
13. Weeks DL, Eskandari S, Scott DR, et al. A H⁺-gated urea channel: the link between *Helicobacter pylori* urease and gastric colonization. *Science* 2000;287:482–485.
14. Eaton KA, Brooks CL, Morgan DR, et al. Essential role of urease in pathogenesis of gastritis induced by *Helicobacter pylori* in gnotobiotic piglets. *Infect Immun* 1991;59:2470–2475.
15. Ferrero RL, Labigne A. The organization and expression of the *Helicobacter pylori* urease gene cluster. In: Goodwin CS, Worsley BW, eds. *Helicobacter pylori*: biology and clinical practice. Boca Raton, FL: CRC Press, 1993:171–190.
16. Hazell SL, Mendz GL. The metabolism and enzymes of *Helicobacter pylori*: function and potential virulence effects. In: Goodwin CS, Worsley BW, eds. *Helicobacter pylori*: biology and clinical practice. Boca Raton, FL: CRC Press, 1993:115–142.
17. Kuo CH, Poon SK, Su YC, et al. Heterogeneous *Helicobacter pylori* isolates from *H. pylori*–infected couples in Taiwan. *J Infect Dis* 1999;180:2064–2068.
18. Bamford KB, Bickley J, Collins JS, et al. *Helicobacter pylori*: comparison of DNA fingerprints provides evidence for intrafamilial infection. *Gut* 1993;34:1348–1350.
19. Sugiyama T, Naka H, Yachi A, et al. Direct evidence by DNA fingerprinting that endoscopic cross-infection of *Helicobacter pylori* is a cause of postendoscopic acute gastritis. *J Clin Microbiol* 2000;38:2381–2382.
20. Segal ED, Cha J, Lo J, et al. Altered states: involvement of phosphorylated CagA in the induction of host cellular growth changes by *Helicobacter pylori*. *Proc Natl Acad Sci U S A* 1999;96(25):14559–14564.
21. Stein M, Rappuoli R, Covacci A. Tyrosine phosphorylation of the *Helicobacter pylori* CagA antigen after cag-driven host cell translocation. *Proc Natl Acad Sci U S A* 2000;97(3):1263–1268.
22. Papini E, Zoratti M, Cover TL. In search of the *Helicobacter pylori* VacA mechanism of action. *Toxicon* 2001;39:1757–1767.
23. Tombola F, Morbiato L, Del Giudice G, et al. The *Helicobacter pylori* VacA toxin is a urea permease that promotes urea diffusion across epithelia. *J Clin Invest* 2001;108:929–937.
24. Rad R, Gerhard M, Lang R, et al. The *Helicobacter pylori* blood group antigen-binding adhesin facilitates bacterial colonization and augments a nonspecific immune response. *J Immunol* 2002;168:3033–3041.
25. Yamaoka Y, Kwon DH, Graham DY. A M(r) 34,000 proinflammatory outer membrane protein (oipA) of *Helicobacter pylori*. *Proc Natl Acad Sci USA* 2000; 97:7533–7538.
26. Peek RM Jr, Thompson SA, Donahue JP, et al. Adherence to gastric epithelial cells induces expression of a *Helicobacter pylori* gene, iceA, that is associated with clinical outcome. *Proc Assoc Am Physicians* 1998;110:531–544.
27. Dixon MF, Genta RM, Yardley JH, et al. Classification and grading of gastritis. The updated Sydney System. International Workshop on the Histopathology of Gastritis, Houston 1994. *Am J Surg Pathol* 1996;20:1161–1181.
28. Zevering Y, Jacob L, Meyer TF. Naturally acquired human immune responses against *Helicobacter pylori* and implications for vaccine development. *Gut* 1999;45:465–474.
29. Del Giudice G, Covacci A, Telford JL, et al. The design of vaccines against *Helicobacter pylori* and their development. *Annu Rev Immunol* 2001;19:523–563.
30. El Omar EM, Carrington M, Chow WH, et al. Interleukin-1 polymorphisms associated with increased risk of gastric cancer. *Nature* 2000;404:398–402.
31. Lanas A, Garcia-Gonzalez MA, Santolaria S, et al. TNF and LTA gene polymorphisms reveal different risk in gastric and duodenal ulcer patients. *Genes Immun* 2001;2:415–421.

32. Marshall BJ, Armstrong JA, McGeche DB, et al. Attempt to fulfill Koch's postulates for pyloric Campylobacter. *Med J Aust* 1985;142:436–439.

33. Morris A, Nicholson G. Ingestion of *Campylobacter pylori* causes gastritis and raised fasting gastric pH. *Gastroenterology* 1987;82:192–194.

34. Moriai T, Hirahara N. Clinical course of acute gastric mucosal lesions caused by acute infection with *Helicobacter pylori*. *N Engl J Med* 1999;341:456–457.

35. Klein PD, Gilman RH, Leon-Barua R, et al. The epidemiology of *Helicobacter pylori* in Peruvian children between 6 and 30 months of age. *Am J Gastroenterol* 1994;89:2196–2200.

36. Hansson L-E, Nyren O, Hsing AW, et al. Risk of stomach cancer in patients with gastric or duodenal ulcer disease. *N Engl J Med* 1996;335:242–249.

37. Sipponen P, Kekki M, Haapakoski J, et al. Gastric cancer risk in chronic atrophic gastritis: statistical calculations on cross-sectional data. *Cancer* 1985;35:173–177.

38. Sipponen P, Seppala K. Gastric carcinoma: failed adaptation to *Helicobacter pylori*. *Scand J Gastroenterol* 1992;27[Suppl]:33–38.

39. Israel DA, Salama N, Arnold CN, et al. *Helicobacter pylori* strain-specific differences in genetic content, identified by microarray, influence host inflammatory responses. *J Clin Invest* 2001;107:611–620.

40. Hirai M, Azuma T, Ito S, et al. High prevalence of neutralizing activity to *Helicobacter pylori* cytotoxin in serum of gastric-carcinoma patients. *Int J Cancer* 1994;56:56–60.

41. Fox JG, Correa P, Taylor NS, et al. High prevalence and persistence of cytotoxin-positive *Helicobacter pylori* strains in a population with high prevalence of atrophic gastritis. *Am J Gastroenterol* 1992;87:1554–1560.

42. Davies GR, Simmonds NJ, Stevens TRJ, et al. *Helicobacter pylori* stimulates antral mucosal reactive oxygen metabolite production in vivo. *Gut* 1994;35:179–185.

43. Lynch DA, Mapstone NP, Clarke AM, et al. Cell proliferation in *Helicobacter pylori* associated gastritis and the effect of eradication therapy. *Gut* 1995;36:346–350.

44. Sipponen P, Hyvarinen H, Seppala K, et al. Review article: pathogenesis of the transformation from gastritis to malignancy. *Aliment Pharmacol Ther* 1998; 12[Suppl 1]:61–71.

45. Taylor DN, Parsonnet J. The epidemiology and natural history of *Helicobacter pylori* infection. In: Blaser MJ, Smith PD, Ravdin JI, et al., eds. *Infections of the gastrointestinal tract*, 1st ed. New York: Raven Press, 1995.

46. Parsonnet J, Blaser MJ, Perez-Perez GI, et al. Symptoms and risk factors of *Helicobacter pylori* infection in a cohort of epidemiologists. *Gastroenterology* 1992;102:41–46.

47. Roosendaal R, Kuipers EJ, Buitenwerf J, et al. *Helicobacter pylori* and the birth cohort effect: evidence of a continuous decrease of infection rates in childhood. *Am J Gastroenterol* 1997;92:1480–1482.

48. Malaty HM, Graham DY. Importance of childhood socioeconomic status on the current prevalence of *Helicobacter pylori* infection. *Gut* 1994;35:742–745.

49. Everhart JE, Kruszon-Moran D, Perez-Perez GI, et al. Seroprevalence and ethnic differences in *Helicobacter pylori* infection among adults in the United States. *J Infect Dis* 2000;181:1359–1363.

50. Goh KL, Parasakthi N. The racial cohort phenomenon: seroepidemiology of *Helicobacter pylori* infection in a multiracial South-East Asian country. *Eur J Gastroenterol Hepatol* 2001;13:177–183.

51. Rothenbacher D, Bode G, Berg G, et al. Prevalence and determinants of *Helicobacter pylori* infection in preschool children: a population-based study from Germany. *Int J Epidemiol* 1998;27:135–141.

52. Parsonnet J, Replogle M, Yang S, et al. Seroprevalence of CagA-positive strains among *Helicobacter pylori*–infected, healthy young adults. *J Infect Dis* 1997;175:1240–1242.

53. Malaty HM, Engstrand L, Pedersen NL, et al. *Helicobacter pylori* infection: genetic and environmental influences. *Ann Intern Med* 1994;120:982–986.

54. Brown LM. *Helicobacter pylori*: epidemiology and routes of transmission. *Epidemiol Rev* 2000;22:283–297.

55. Parsonnet J, Shmuely H, Haggerty T. Fecal and oral shedding of *Helicobacter pylori* from healthy, infected adults. *JAMA* 1999;282:2240–2245.

56. Nguyen AM, el Zaatari FA, Graham DY. *Helicobacter pylori* in the oral cavity: a critical review of the literature. *Oral Surg Oral Med Oral Pathol Oral Radiol Endod* 1995;79:705–709.

57. Langenberg W, Rauws EA, Oudbier JH, et al. Patient-to-patient transmission of *Campylobacter pylori* infection by fiberoptic gastroduodenoscopy and biopsy. *J Infect Dis* 1990;161:507–511.

58. Fantry GT, Zheng QX, James SP. Conventional cleaning and disinfection techniques eliminate the risk of endoscopic transmission of *Helicobacter pylori*. *Am J Gastroenterol* 1995;90:227–232.

59. Hildebrand P, Meyer-Wyss BM, Mossi S, et al. Risk among gastroenterologists of acquiring *Helicobacter pylori* infection: case-control study. *BMJ* 2000; 321:149.

60. Klein PD, Graham DY, Gaillour A, et al. Gastrointestinal Physiology Working Group. Water source as risk factor for *Helicobacter pylori* infection in Peruvian children. *Lancet* 1991;337:1503–1506.

61. Hopkins RJ, Vial PA, Ferreccio C, et al. Seroprevalence of *Helicobacter pylori* in Chile: vegetables may serve as one route of transmission. *J Infect Dis* 1993; 168:222–226.

62. Lu Y, Redlinger TE, Avitia R, et al. Isolation and genotyping of *Helicobacter pylori* from untreated municipal wastewater. *Appl Environ Microbiol* 2002; 68:1436–1439.

63. Sobala GM, Crabtree JE, Dixon MF, et al. Acute *Helicobacter pylori* infection: clinical features, local and systemic immune response, gastric mucosal histology and gastric juice ascorbic acid concentrations. *Gut* 1991;32:1415–1418.

64. Talley NJ, Quan C. Review article: *Helicobacter pylori* and nonulcer dyspepsia. *Aliment Pharmacol Ther* 2002;16[Suppl 1]:58–65.

65. De Koster E, De B I, Langlet P, et al. Evidence based medicine and extradigestive manifestations of *Helicobacter pylori*. *Acta Gastroenterol Belg* 2000;63:388–392.

66. NIH Consensus Development Panel on *Helicobacter pylori* in Peptic Ulcer Disease. *Helicobacter pylori* in peptic ulcer disease. *JAMA* 1994;272:65–69.

67. Graham DY, Lew GM, Klein PD, et al. Effect of treatment of *Helicobacter pylori* infection on the long-term recurrence of gastric or duodenal ulcer. A randomized, controlled study. *Ann Intern Med* 1992;116:705–708.

68. Hentschel E, Brandstatter G, Dragosics B, et al. Effect of ranitidine and amoxicillin plus metronidazole on the eradication of *Helicobacter pylori* and the recurrence of duodenal ulcer. *N Engl J Med* 1993;328:308–312.

69. Sipponen P. Natural history of gastritis and its relationship to peptic ulcer disease. *Digestion* 1992;5:70–75.

70. Kurata JH, Nogawa AN. Meta-analysis of risk factors for peptic ulcer. Nonsteroidal antiinflammatory drugs, *Helicobacter pylori*, and smoking. *J Clin Gastroenterol* 1997;24:2–17.

71. Parsonnet J. *Helicobacter pylori*: the size of the problem. *Gut* 1998;43[Suppl 1]:S6–S9.

72. Meucci G, Di Battista R, Abbiati C, et al. Prevalence and risk factors of *Helicobacter pylori*–negative peptic ulcer: a multicenter study. *J Clin Gastroenterol* 2000;31:42–47.

73. Graham DY. Treatment of peptic ulcers caused by *Helicobacter pylori*. *N Engl J Med* 1993;328:349–350.

74. Sipponen P, Aarynen M, Kaariainen I, et al. Chronic antral gastritis, Lewis(a)+ phenotype, and male sex as factors in predicting coexisting duodenal ulcer. *Scand J Gastroenterol* 1989;24:581–588.

75. Marshall BJ. *Helicobacter pylori*. *Am J Gastroenterol* 1994;89:S116–S128.

76. IARC Working Group on the Evaluation of Carcinogenic Risks to Humans. *Helicobacter pylori*. *Schistosomes, liver flukes and Helicobacter pylori: views and expert opinions of an IARC Working Group on the Evaluation of Carcinogenic Risks to Humans*. Lyon: IARC, 1994:177–240.

77. Blaser MJ, Chyou PH, Nomura A. Age at establishment of *Helicobacter pylori* infection and gastric carcinoma, gastric ulcer, and duodenal ulcer risk. *Cancer Res* 1995;55:562–565.

78. Howson C, Hiyama T, Wynder E. The decline in gastric cancer: epidemiology of an unplanned triumph. *Epidemiol Rev* 1986;8:1–27.

79. Blaser MJ, Perez-Perez GI, Kleanthous H, et al. Infection with *Helicobacter pylori* strains possessing cagA is associated with an increased risk of developing adenocarcinoma of the stomach. *Cancer Res* 1995;55:2111–2115.

80. National Cancer Institute, DCCPS Surveillance Research Program Cancer Statistics Branch. *Surveillance, Epidemiology, and End Results (SEER) Program public-use data (1973–1999)*. Available online: http://seer.cancer.gov/.

81. Severson RK, Davis S. Increasing incidence of primary gastric lymphoma. *Cancer* 1990;66:1283–1287.

82. Parsonnet J, Hansen S, Rodriguez L, et al. *Helicobacter pylori* infection and gastric lymphoma. *N Engl J Med* 1994;330:1267–1271.

83. Stolte M, Bayerdorffer E, Morgner A, et al. *Helicobacter* and gastric MALT lymphoma. *Gut* 2002;50[Suppl 3]:III19–III24.

84. Tamura A, Fujioka T, Nasu M. Relation of *Helicobacter pylori* infection to plasma vitamin B12, folic acid, and homocysteine levels in patients who underwent diagnostic coronary arteriography. *Am J Gastroenterol* 2002;97:861–866.

85. Hoffmeister A, Rothenbacher D, Bode G, et al. Current infection with *Helicobacter pylori*, but not seropositivity to *Chlamydia pneumoniae* or cytomegalovirus, is associated with an atherogenic, modified lipid profile. *Arterioscler Thromb Vasc Biol* 2001;21:427–432.

86. Leinonen M, Saikku P. Evidence for infectious agents in cardiovascular disease and atherosclerosis. *Lancet* 2002;2:11–17.

87. Hartge P, Devesa SS. Quantification of the impact of known risk factors on time trends in non-Hodgkin's lymphoma incidence. *Cancer Res* 1992;52:5566s–5569s.

88. Cammarota G, Figura N, Cianci R, et al. Is there an antigenic mimicry between arteriosclerotic lesions and *H. pylori* antigens? *Clin Biochem* 2000;33:419–421.

89. Libby P, Ridker PM, Maseri A. Inflammation and atherosclerosis. *Circulation* 2002;105:1135–1143.

90. Danesh J, Peto R. Risk factors for coronary heart disease and infection with *Helicobacter pylori*: meta-analysis of 18 studies. *BMJ* 1998;316:1130–1132.

91. Vakil NB. Review article: gastro-oesophageal reflux disease and *Helicobacter pylori* infection. *Aliment Pharmacol Ther* 2002;16[Suppl 1]:47–51.

92. Chow WH, Blaser MJ, Blot WJ, et al. An inverse relation between cagA(+) strains of *Helicobacter pylori* infection and risk of esophageal and gastric cardia adenocarcinoma. *Cancer Res* 1998;58(4):588–590.

93. *Helicobacter* and Cancer Collaborative Group. Gastric cancer and *Helicobacter pylori*: a combined analysis of 12 case control studies nested within prospective cohorts. *Gut* 2001;49:347–353.

94. McNulty CA, Dent JC, Uff JS, et al. Detection of *Campylobacter pylori* by the biopsy urease test: an assessment of 1445 patients. *Gut* 1989;30:1058–1062.

95. Marshall BJ, Warren JR, Francis GJ, et al. Rapid urease test in the management of *Campylobacter pylori*–associated gastritis. *Am J Gastroenterol* 1987;82:200–210.

96. Lee N, Lee TT, Fang KM. Assessment of four rapid urease test systems for detection of *Helicobacter pylori* in gastric biopsy specimens. *Diagn Microbiol Infect Dis* 1994;18:69–74.

97. Nedenskov-Sorensen P, Aase S, Bjorneklett A, et al. Sampling efficiency in the diagnosis of *Helicobacter pylori* infection and chronic active gastritis. *J Clin Microbiol* 1991;29:672–675.

98. Morris A, Ali MR, Brown P, et al. *Campylobacter pylori* infection in biopsy specimens of gastric antrum: laboratory diagnosis and estimation of sampling error. *J Clin Pathol* 1989;42:727–732.

99. Brown KE, Peura DA. Diagnosis of *Helicobacter pylori* infection. *Gastroenterol Clin North Am* 1993;22:105–115.

100. Andersen LP. The antibody response to *Helicobacter pylori* infection, and the value of serologic tests to detect *H. pylori* and for post-treatment monitoring. In: Goodwin CS, Worsley BW, eds. *Helicobacter pylori:* biology and clinical practice. Boca Raton, FL: CRC Press, 1993:285–305.

101. Nakamura RM. Laboratory tests for the evaluation of *Helicobacter pylori* infections. *J Clin Lab Anal* 2001;15:301–307.

102. Gisbert JP, Pajares JM. Diagnosis of *Helicobacter pylori* infection by stool antigen determination: a systematic review. *Am J Gastroenterol* 2001;96:2829–2838.

103. Gold BD. *Helicobacter pylori* infection in children. *Curr Probl Pediatr* 2001;31:247–266.

104. van der Wouden EJ, Thijs JC, Kusters JG, et al. Mechanism and clinical significance of metronidazole resistance in *Helicobacter pylori*. *Scand J Gastroenterol Suppl* 2001:10–14.

105. Miehlke S, Bayerdorffer E, Graham DY. Treatment of *Helicobacter pylori* infection. *Semin Gastrointest Dis* 2001;12:167–179.

106. Parsonnet J. The incidence of *Helicobacter pylori* infection. *Aliment Pharmacol Ther* 1995;9[Suppl 2]:45–52.

107. Genta RM, Lew GM, Graham DY. Changes in the gastric mucosa following eradication of *Helicobacter pylori*. *Mod Pathol* 1993;6:281–289.

108. Malfertheiner P, Megraud F, O'Morain C, et al. Current concepts in the management of *Helicobacter pylori* infection—the Maastricht 2-2000 Consensus Report. *Aliment Pharmacol Ther* 2002;16:167–180.

109. Parsonnet J, Harris RA, Hack HM, et al. Modeling cost-effectiveness of *Helicobacter pylori* screening to prevent gastric cancer: a mandate for clinical trials. *Lancet* 1996;348:150–154.

110. Mason J, Axon AT, Forman D, et al. The cost-effectiveness of population *Helicobacter pylori* screening and treatment: a Markov model using economic data from a randomized controlled trial. *Aliment Pharmacol Ther* 2002;16:559–568.

111. Moayyedi P, Soo S, Deeks J, et al. Systematic review and economic evaluation of *Helicobacter pylori* eradication treatment for non-ulcer dyspepsia. Dyspepsia Review Group. *BMJ* 2000;321:659–664.

112. Graham DY. Benefits from elimination of *Helicobacter pylori* infection include major reduction in the incidence of peptic ulcer disease, gastric cancer, and primary gastric lymphoma. *Prev Med* 1994;23:712–716.

113. Ierardi E, Monno RA, Gentile A, et al. *Helicobacter heilmannii* gastritis: a histological and immunohistochemical trait. *J Clin Pathol* 2001;54:774–777.

114. Dubois A. Spiral bacteria in the human stomach: the gastric *Helicobacters*. *Emerging Infect Dis* 1995;1:79–85.

115. Thomson MA, Storey P, Greer R, et al. Canine-human transmission of *Gastrospirillum hominis*. *Lancet* 1994;343:1605–1607.

116. Stolte M, Wellens E, Bethke B, et al. *Helicobacter heilmannii* (formerly *Gastrospirillum hominis*) gastritis: an infection transmitted by animals? *Scand J Gastroenterol* 1995;29:1061–1064.

117. Totten PA, Fennell CL, Tenover FC, et al. *Campylobacter cinaedi* (sp. nov.) and *Campylobacter fennelliae* (sp. nov.): two new *Campylobacter* species associated with enteric disease in homosexual men. *J Infect Dis* 1985;151:131–139.

118. Quinn TC, Goodell SG, Fennell C, et al. Infections with *Campylobacter jejuni* and *Campylobacter*-like infections in homosexual men. *Ann Intern Med* 1985;101:187–92.

119. Mishu Allos B, Lastovica AJ, Blaser MJ. Atypical *Campylobacters* and related organisms. In: Blaser MJ, Smith PD, Ravdin JI, et al., eds. *Infections of the gastrointestinal tract.* New York: Raven Press, 1995:849–866.

120. Kiehlbauch JA, Tauxe RV, Baker CN, et al. *Helicobacter cinaedi*–associated bacteremia and cellulitis in immunocompromised patients. *Ann Intern Med* 1994;121:90–93.

121. Kemper CA, Mickelsen P, Morton A, et al. *Helicobacter (Campylobacter) fennelliae*–like organisms as an important but occult cause of bacteraemia in a patient with AIDS. *J Infect* 1993;26:97–101.

122. Gebhart CJ, Fennell CL, Murtaugh MP, et al. *Campylobacter cinaedi* is normal intestinal flora in hamsters. *J Clin Microbiol* 1989;27:1692–1694.

123. Flores BM, Fennell CL, Kuller L, et al. Experimental infection of pig-tailed macaques (*Macaca nemestrina*) with *Campylobacter cinaedi* and *Campylobacter fennelliae*. *Infect Immun* 1990;58:3947–3953.

124. Flores BM, Fennell CL, Stamm WE. Characterization of *Campylobacter cinaedi* and *C. fennelliae* antigens and analysis of the human immune response. *J Infect Dis* 1989;159:635–640.

125. Kiehlbauch JA, Brenner DJ, Cameron DN, et al. Genotypic and phenotypic characterization of *Helicobacter cinaedi* and *Helicobacter fennelliae* strains isolated from humans and animals. *J Clin Microbiol* 1995;33:2940–2947.

Miscellaneous Microorganisms

CHAPTER 218
Bartonella *Species*

Jennifer S. Daly

HISTORY

The genus *Bartonella* contains not only its original member, *Bartonella bacilliformis*, the etiologic agent of Oroya fever and verruga peruana, but also the organisms previously classified as *Rochalimaea* and *Grahamella* species (Table 218.1). *Bartonella* species produce a variety of clinical manifestations from endocarditis to vascular proliferative lesions, lymphadenopathy and reticuloendothelial system lesions (1). The members of the genus are cultivable on cell free blood- or hemin-containing bacteriologic media and have been determined by 16S ribosomal RNA (rRNA) sequencing studies, DNA-relatedness data, guanine-plus-cytosine content, and phenotypic characteristics to be closely related to *B. bacilliformis*. Not only are these organisms related in the laboratory, but also the clinical characteristics of the diseases produced in humans and animals, as well as the prolonged bacteremia occurring in animals, are similar within the genus. With the description of *Bartonella schoenbuchii* in 2001 (2) and inclusion of the *Rochalimaea* and *Grahamella* species, there are 17 described species in the genus *Bartonella* (3,4) (Table 218.2). One of the species, *Bartonella vinsonii*, has three subspecies, and there are several other isolates that may represent new species but have not been described formally (3). Although the genus *Bartonella* has been classified in the family Bartonellaceae within the order Rickettsiales, some of the closest relatives to the expanded genus *Bartonella* are the *Brucella* species, a fact that has prompted taxonomists to propose that the family Bartonellaceae be removed from the order Rickettsiales (5).

Classic Bartonellosis

The oldest recognized species, *B. bacilliformis*, causes two distinct syndromes (an acute febrile illness and a chronic skin eruption) that are characteristic of the genus. The chronic form of the bartonellosis is verruga peruana or "warts of the Andes." Fever, bacteremia, and hemolysis characterize the acute form, called Oroya fever. The first records of these verrucous lesions are represented on ceramic pottery from the pre-Inca era, and medical description of these lesions can be traced back to the year 1630 (6). In 1871, an epidemic of bartonellosis occurred in workers building a railroad line between Lima and La Oroya, Peru. Nearly 7,000 workers developed fever and massive hemolysis and died, and the disease was given the name Oroya fever, a misnomer because transmission occurs only in the mountainous area near La Oroya and not in the city at its lower elevation. In 1885, a Peruvian medical student, Daniel Carrion, showed that the indolent skin disease, verruga peruana, and highly lethal Oroya fever were caused by the same pathogen when he performed a foolhardy experiment (7). In an attempt to study the skin disease, he tried to inoculate himself with material from the verruga of

TABLE 218.1.   Characteristics of *Bartonella* Species

Species	Reservoir/Host	Known vector	Documented geographic distribution	Human
B. alsatica	Rabbit		France	
B. bacilliformis	Human	Sand fly	Peru, Ecuador, Columbia	Yes
B. birtlesii	Wild rodent		Europe	
B. clarridgeiae	Cat		USA, Europe	Yes
B. doshiae	Vole		UK	
B. elizabethae	Rat	Flea	USA, Peru	Yes
B. grahamii	Vole		UK, Netherlands	Yes
B. henselae	Cat	Cat flea	USA	Yes
B. koehlerae	Cat		USA, Europe	
B. peromysci[a]	Deer mouse			
B. quintana	Human/?	Louse	Worldwide	Yes
B. schoenbuchii	Roe deer		Western Europe	
B. talpae[a]	Mole		Europe	
B. taylorii	Rat		UK	
B. tribocorum	Rat		France	
B. vinsonii subsp. arupensis	Mice		USA	Yes
B. vinsonii subsp. berkhoffii	Coyote/dog	Tick	USA, Europe	Yes
B. vinsonii subsp. vinsonii	Vole	Vole ear mite	Canada	
B. washoenii	Cow		USA	

[a]Historical species (strains not available in any collection).

a patient. He was assisted by a classmate despite the warnings of the older clinicians and developed fever, followed by massive hemolysis. Before he died, he recognized that he was suffering from Oroya fever, and the disease has been known as Carrion's disease since that time (7).

B. bacilliformis is transmitted by phlebotomine sand flies of the genus *Lutzomyia* and related species and geographically limited to the western slopes of the Andes Mountains at elevations between 500 and 3,375 meters in Columbia, Ecuador, Peru, Chile, Bolivia, and probably Guatemala (6,8). Serologic studies suggest that there may be other, related vectors and that there are rodents that serve as reservoirs (9,10). In 1909, Barton demonstrated the organism in red cells, and it was cultured in 1925 by Noguchi (11,12). *B. bacilliformis* was the sole member of this genus until 1993 when the agent of trench fever and related organisms were added.

TABLE 218.2.   Previous Designation of Older *Bartonella* Species

Current name	Previous designations
Human Pathogens	
B. bacilliformis	
B. quintana	Rochalimaea quintana
	Rickettsia quintana
	Rickettsia pediculi
B. henselae	Rochalimaea henselae
B. elizabethae	Rochalimaea elizabethae
Animal Associated	
B. vinsonii	Vole agent
	Rochalimaea vinsonii
B. talpae[a]	Grahamella talpae
B. peromysci[a]	Grahamella peromysci

[a]These strains are not available for comparison to newer species.

As recorded in modern times, in many patients, *B. bacilliformis* produces a biphasic illness, in that over months, the patients experience both the acute and chronic manifestations. Chronic bartonellosis is characterized by vascular proliferation (verruga peruana), which is histologically similar to bacillary angiomatosis, an illness caused by *Bartonella quintana* and *Bartonella henselae*. The organism grows in the vascular epithelium of the skin. Skin lesions consist of nodules exhibiting active proliferation of newly formed capillaries, dilated venules, and precapillary vessels with endothelial hyperplasia (13) and may be found in bone, mucous membranes, lung, liver, spleen, brain, and lymph nodes and may undergo spontaneous regression. The organism is associated with erythrocytes and infiltrates the reticuloendothelial system. The acute-phase illness (Oroya fever) is characterized by high fever and intravascular hemolysis. In the preantibiotic era, mortality was high, with 40% of patients dying of bacterial superinfection, particularly bacteremic salmonellosis. Treatment with chloramphenicol appears to be beneficial (14), but a recent analysis of an epidemic suggests that there are many more mild or asymptomatic cases than previously described (1). Only 4.8% of the patients in this outbreak developed skin lesions (the chronic form of the disease) weeks to months after presenting with the acute febrile phase. In other studies, up to 15% of patients may exhibit prolonged, asymptomatic bacteremia, similar to that seen with the more recently described species in humans and animals. Physicians need to consider the diagnosis in travelers, who may develop skin lesions weeks to months after return from an endemic area.

Trench Fever (*Bartonella quintana*)

Trench fever, caused by *B. quintana*, was first recognized during World War I and affected more than 1 million soldiers involved in trench warfare in Europe. Transmitted by the body louse, the disease reappeared in epidemic form in World War II, particularly in Germany and the eastern front. The organism originally was designated *Rickettsia quintana* by Schmincke (15) in 1917 when he isolated it in cell culture. Sikora, who propagated the organism on human blood agar in 1921 (16), did not realize he had grown the pathogen of trench fever and thought it to be a harmless parasite of lice. He called it *Rickettsia pediculi*. Later, *B. quintana* was cultured from the blood of a patient in Yugoslavia in 1948 (17) and propagated by Vinson and Fuller in 1961 (16); the "Fuller" strain currently is in use in immunologic studies (18). In 1969, Varela and Vinson showed that the organism could be propagated from the blood of patients with trench fever and could be inoculated into volunteers and produce the disease (19,20). Volunteer patients had prolonged bacteremia with the organism, and the lice that fed on these patients would exhibit organisms in their feces. The organism initially was named *Rochalimaea* to honor Henrique da Rocha-Lima and for the fifth day, or quintan fever (*quintana*), which is seen frequently with the disease. Trench fever had been known as wolhynian fever, His-Werner disease, shin fever, and shank fever. After World War II, small epidemics and sporadic cases of trench fever were noted in Europe, but epidemics were not recognized in the United States until 1994. A modern description of this illness involved eight patients with *B. quintana* bacteremia, who had febrile illnesses compatible with trench fever, and two patients with endocarditis (21). Many of these patients were homeless, used alcoholic beverages, and had lice or scabies. The organism has been found in several different geographic areas, including Europe, North America, Ethiopia, and China. In addition to its role as an etiologic agent in cases of trench fever and cases of fever of unknown origin, *B. quintana* has been isolated from skin lesions of patients with bacillary angiomatosis, detected in the liver of patients with peliosis hepatitis, and cultured from the blood of patients with endocarditis.

Bacillary Angiomatosis

Bacillary angiomatosis is a vasculoproliferative disease primarily affecting immunocompromised patients and first diagnosed in 1983 in an HIV-infected man with subcutaneous nodules, fever, and weight loss. Clinical manifestations of the illness are similar to those seen in patients with *B. bacilliformis* infection and those with cat-scratch disease (CSD) (22). Patients most commonly present with multiple, angiomatous, tender papules or subcutaneous nodules. Patients with peliosis often complain of fever, abdominal pain, and weight loss and exhibit hepatomegaly, splenomegaly, or both. Bone lesions, which are lytic in nature, most frequently involve the long bones. Lesions may occur in the mouth, stomach, large or small intestines, and respiratory tract. Patients with bacillary angiomatosis may have prolonged bacteremia that can be documented by processing the blood cultures to detect *Bartonella* species. Systemic signs and symptoms include fever, chills, malaise, headache, anorexia, and weight loss and may be present weeks to months before the diagnosis is made. Occasional patients relapse with fever, bacteremia, or skin lesions when treatment is stopped. Both *B. quintana* and *B. henselae* have been found in patients with bacillary angiomatosis and endocarditis.

Bartonella henselae and *Bartonella clarridgeiae* (Cat-Scratch Disease)

Bartonella species, most commonly *B. henselae* and sometimes *B. clarridgeiae*, cause most cases of cat-scratch disease (CSD). *Bartonella henselae* was first isolated in 1986 from the blood of two patients with fever and symptomatic human immunodeficiency virus type 1 (HIV-1) infection (23). Slater and colleagues determined that the organism resembled *B. quintana* or *Brucella*

species and reported their findings in 1990. In the same issue of the *New England Journal of Medicine*, Relman and others reported identification of the agent of bacillary angiomatosis using polymerase chain reaction (PCR) amplification of the 16S ribosomal RNA gene from tissue specimens (24). The organism remained unnamed until 1992 when Welch and colleagues (25) and Regnery and co-workers (26) formally described the species and proposed the name *Rochalimaea henselae*. Included in the report by Welch and colleagues were patients with prolonged fever and bacteremia or vascular proliferative lesions, including bacillary peliosis hepatitis and bacillary angiomatosis. In 1992, Koehler and co-workers cultured *B. henselae* and *B. quintana* directly from the skin lesions of patients with bacillary angiomatosis (27). The organism was named *R. henselae* for Diane Hensel, a microbiologist from Oklahoma, who contributed to the isolation and identification of the species and in 1993 was transferred to the genus *Bartonella* (5). It was found in patients with bacillary angiomatosis, typical CSD (see Chapter 171), and endocarditis (22). The similarity between bacillary angiomatosis and CSD was first noted in HIV-infected patients, and serologic studies provided confirmation of this association (28). *Bartonella*-specific sequences have been detected in the material used for the CSD skin test.

The role of *Bartonella* species in CSD has unfolded as more techniques become available to detect infection with organisms in this genus. *B. clarridgeiae* was first isolated from the blood of a cat whose owner had an infection with *B. henselae* (29). Both *B. henselae* and *B. clarridgeiae* have been isolated from the blood of cats, and antibody to *B. henselae* has been found in cats owned by patients with CSD (4). *B. clarridgeiae* has been shown to cause classic CSD in some patients (30), but the extent of disease due to *B. clarridgeiae* has not been determined. This species has polar flagella, and hopefully with the use of a specific antibody test using antigen from the polar flagella (not present in *B. henselae*), more information will become available (31). In addition to these two species that are thought to cause most cases of CSD, *B. quintana* has been cultured from the lymph node of a patient with chronic lymphadenopathy who had contact with cats but has not been isolated from patients with the classic findings of CSD (32). Other *Bartonella* species may produce syndromes similar to CSD (33), but further research is needed. Experimental models of *Bartonella* infection in animals have revealed that the organisms in this genus can cause many of the pathologic changes that are suspected or confirmed in humans with *Bartonella* species infections, including lymphadenopathy, prolonged bacteremia, granulomatous lesions, lymphocytic hepatitis, hyperplasia of the spleen, cholangitis or pericholangitis, interstitial lymphocytic nephritis, endocarditis, and myocarditis (34,35). The organisms can be found in the placenta and fetus in pregnant bacteremic animals and may lead to reproductive failure or placental or fetal abnormalities (36–38).

Endocarditis and Heart Disease

Bartonella species have been shown to cause endocarditis in humans and in animals. Cases are difficult to diagnose because the organisms grow slowly, and standard blood cultures are frequently negative (39,40). An example of the difficulty in diagnosis of cases of endocarditis is the history of the discovery of *Bartonella elizabethae*, a species that could not be identified when first isolated in 1986 from a patient with endocarditis treated at Saint Elizabeth's Hospital in Boston (41). The organism was initially subcultured from Bactec blood culture bottles with the subculture plates incubated for 10 days in 5% carbon dioxide. In 1992, after the microbiologic and molecular characteristics of *B. henselae* had been reported, it was found to be a unique organism related to the *Bartonella* species by phenotypic characteristics, cellular fatty acid contents, DNA-relatedness data, and 16S rRNA sequence analysis. Other isolates of this species have been found in rats in the United States and in Peru, and serologic responses to this organism have been detected in patients using intravenous drugs, a patient with retinitis, and a patient with fatal myocarditis (42–47).

In humans, *B. henselae, B. quintana, B. elizabethae,* and several *B. vinsonii* subspecies have been proven to cause endocarditis (40,41,48,49). Patients often have abnormal heart valves and are difficult to cure without surgery (48). Treatment with a variety of antimicrobials has been effective in some cases, and current consensus based on experience and *in vitro* data suggests that aminoglycosides plus ampicillin or ceftriaxone, possibly followed by doxycycline or a macrolide for a prolonged course, may be the best option (49,50). Because organisms of this genus are difficult to culture, diagnosis relies on high clinical suspicion, serology, culture and PCR techniques, and examination of removed tissue. Pathology (including use of the Gimenez stain) and immunohistochemistry studies of heart valves removed at surgery may be the only way to identify the pathogen in some cases (39,51). Diagnosis is further complicated by the fact that serologic studies have shown that some patients with endocarditis due to *B. henselae* fail to demonstrate antibody to the type strain of *B. henselae* (52), strain differences occur within the *B. quintana* serotypes, and cross-reactions between *Bartonella* species and with *Chlamydia* species and *Coxiella burnetti* occur (53). Patients classified as having culture-negative endocarditis and those in some well-described case series of patients reported to have Q fever or *Chlamydia* endocarditis may have had disease caused by *Bartonella* species (53–55).

Experimental models in animals and improvement of methods to culture or detect infection with members of this genus have led to the implications of *Bartonella* species as a cause of previously considered idiopathic myocarditis as well as culture-negative endocarditis. Recently, subspecies of *B. vinsonii* have been shown to cause endocarditis first in a dog and then in humans (56,57). Chronic infections in cats and dogs have been associated with lymphoplasmocytic myocarditis (34,35), and Wesslen and colleagues discovered evidence of subacute *Bartonella* infection in Swedish orienteers with myocarditis, arrhythmias, or sudden death using serology and direct detection of the *Bartonella* sequences in tissue obtained at autopsy (58,59).

Neuroretinitis and Neurologic Disease

Central nervous system and retinal lesions have been documented in classic cases with CSD, in HIV-infected patients with bacillary angiomatosis, and in patients with no other evidence of *Bartonella*-associated disease. Cases have been described of neuroretinitis, or Leber's stellate neuroretinitis, a form of optic neuropathy manifest as optic nerve swelling with a macular star of exudate, similar to that seen in CSD, and in immunocompromised patients and normal hosts (60–63). Many of these patients have serologic evidence of *Bartonella* infection, and the retinitis resolved with or without therapy and often with little visual damage (64,65).

Animal Species

B. vinsonii subspecies *vinsonii,* a species also previously classified in the *Rochalimaea* group, has not been shown to be associated with disease in humans. Baker isolated the organism from voles on Grosse Isle, Quebec, Canada (66). During World War II, Baker, a Captain in the Veterinary Corps of the U.S. Army, was

stationed at the War Disease Control Station on this small island that had served one century earlier as a quarantine station and mass graveyard for thousands of Irish immigrants who had died of typhus. On the island, Baker had the company of U.S. and Canadian scientists, a few species of small animals, two families who were caretakers, and their domestic cats. Baker trapped and performed autopsies on voles living on the island and found that many had enlarged spleens. Baker attempted to isolate a Rickettsiaceae to determine whether the agent of typhus had persisted in the small rodents. He grew an organism in yolk sac cultures from multiple animals and found that almost all of the wild voles were infected. He inoculated hamsters, mice, and guinea pigs intraperitoneally and was able to recover the organism from their blood. The organism, when later examined by researchers, was found to grow on cell-free media and was related to *B. quintana* (67). It was formally described in 1982 and named after J. William Vinson, who had done extensive work with the agent of trench fever (68). Recently, *B. vinsonii* subspecies *berkhoffii* (57,69) was cultured form the blood of dogs and coyotes (70) and is a cause of granulomatous infections (71), myocarditis and endocarditis in dogs (34), and endocarditis in humans. *B. vinsonii* subspecies *arupensis* has been cultured from the blood of a cattle rancher with a febrile syndrome and from mice (72). The animal-associated *Bartonella* species are shown in Table 218.2. The members of this genus have been found in a wide variety of animals all over the world (4). Some species were previously classified as *Grahamella* species, and others have been discovered recently. *Bartonella tribocorum* was isolated from wild rats and characterized in 1988. *Bartonella koehlerae* was isolated form the blood of domestic cats (73) and is often found along with *B. henselae* or *B. clarridgeiae* in the same animal. *Bartonella washoensis* has been found in ticks in California (74).

Like *B. vinsonii* subspecies *vinsonii* (previously *Rochalimaea vinsonii*), the organisms originally classified as *Grahamella* species (*Bartonella talpae, Bartonella peromysci, Bartonella grahamii, Bartonella taylorii,* and *B. doshiae*) have been found only in animals and in the past were named for the animal host (75). *B. talpae* and *B. peromysci* are historical in the sense that there are no culturable strains available for comparison. These organisms are erythrocyte-associated bacteria that were first observed in 1905 by G. S. Graham-Smith in moles. They have been found most commonly in rodents, were first cultured in 1932, and were poorly characterized until 1994 when Birtles and co-workers reported isolation of several species from the blood of two thirds of small mammals trapped in Shropshire, United Kingdom (75). Birtles found the same species, *B. grahamii,* in five different small woodland mammals. He found only one species in each individual animal. The new species, *Bartonella alsatica,* was found in rabbits in the Alsace region of France (76,77), and *Bartonella schoenbuchii* was found in wild roe deer in France (2). These organisms are related genetically but are distinct from the *Bartonella* species that have been isolated from humans up to the present time. Because of the ubiquitous nature of these organisms and the growing list of manifestations associated with infection, the clinician should search for evidence of *Bartonella* infection in patients who have contact with any animals and who have unexplained febrile syndromes.

CHARACTERISTICS OF THE PATHOGENS

Diagnosis and Microbiology

The members of this genus are thin, aerobic, slightly curved rods that stain weakly gram-negative but can be stained with the Warthin-Starry, Giemsa, and Gimenez stains. *B. bacilliformis*

TABLE 218.3. *Bartonella* Species Causing Human Disease and Treatment

Organism	Major human diseases	Possible treatment
B. bacilliformis	Veruga peruana	Chloramphenicol
		Rifampin
	Oroya fever (Carrion's disease)	
B. quintana	Trench fever	Doxycycline
		Chloramphenicol
	Bacillary angiomatosis/visceral peliosis	Macrolides
	Fever/bacteremia	Doxycycline
	Endocarditis	?Ampicillin/gentamicin
		Ceftriaxone/gentamicin
		Plus doxycycline
	Lymphadenopathy	Unknown
B. henselae	Fever/bacteremia	Doxycycline or macrolides
	Bacillary angiomatosis/visceral peliosis	Doxycycline or macrolides
	Cat-scratch disease	None vs. azithromycin or various other agents
	Endocarditis	?Ampicillin/gentamicin
		Ceftriaxone/gentamicin
		Plus doxycycline
B. elizabethae	Endocarditis	Unknown
B. clarridgeiae	Cat-scratch disease	None/unknown
B. vinsonii subsp. *berkhoffi*	Endocarditis	Unknown
B. vinsonii subsp. *arupensis*	Fever	Unknown
B. grahamii	Neuroretinitis	Unknown

grows best at 25°C, and the other species grow at 32° to 37°C. Isolation of these nutritionally fastidious organisms from the blood of patients can be accomplished using commercially available blood culture systems and subculture with prolonged incubation of subculture plates (chocolate agar, anaerobic blood agar, and freshly prepared brain heart infusion agar with 5% rabbit blood) in an atmosphere of 5% carbon dioxide with high humidity (29,78,79). Isolation of the organism from tissue is more difficult than from blood (80). Co-cultivation with an endothelial cell monolayer has been use to aid recovery. Direct plating of tissue has yielded *B. henselae* but in some cases only after up to 60 days of incubation (81). After initial isolation, the organisms will grow in *Haemophilus* test media and specially prepared blood-free media. After several passages, incubation time decreases, and colonies become larger and less adherent. If the Kovacs modification of the standard oxidase test is employed, some of the species may have a weakly positive reaction. *Bartonella* species are catalase, urea, and indole negative (5,41). The previous classified *Grahamella* species are Voges-Proskauer (acetoin from glucose) test positive, and several species may be distinguished from each other using commercial tests to detect specific preformed enzymes (49,82–84). A MicroScan Rapid Anaerobe Identification Panel can be used along with phenotypic characteristics to suggest to the technologist that *Bartonella* species have been isolated, but determination of cellular fatty acids or molecular techniques are needed to confirm the identification. Techniques available in research labs include reactivity with specific antiserum; cellular fatty acid analysis; 16S rRNA gene sequencing; restriction fragment length polymorphism after PCR amplification of the citrate synthase gene, the riboflavin synthetase gene, and the 16S–23S rRNA gene intergenic spacer region (ITS); and pulsed-field gel electrophoresis (85,86). The organisms parasitize the erythrocytes of their hosts (*B. bacilliformis* and animal species), and smears are used for direct detection of *B. bacilliformis* in endemic areas. *B. bacilliformis*, *B. clarridgeiae*, and *B. schoenbuchii* are the only members of the genus that have polar flagella, but others may demonstrate twitching motility (2,30,31).

Epidemiology

A number of epidemiologic associations with insect vectors and animals are known (Table 218.2). Eight species have been found pathogenic for humans (Table 218.3). The other species have been grown only in animals, including rats, voles, moles, mice, cats, cows, rabbits, deer, coyotes, and dogs (49). *B. bacilliformis* infection is associated with transmission by the bite of the sand fly, *B. quintana* has been culture from wild body lice, *B. henselae* can be transmitted from cat to cat by fleas (87), *B. vinsonii* subspecies *berkhoffii* has been found in domestic dogs and wild coyotes (70), and *B. elizabethae* has been cultured from rats (44). There may be more than one vector for each species. Five of the 10 patients bacteremic with *B. quintana* in the report by Spach and co-workers had scabies, and 1 had lice (21). Prevalence of the *Bartonella* bacteremia in animals is most common in summer and early autumn when flea infestations are heaviest, and there seems to be a parallel seasonal increase in the incidence of CSD in humans. Several *Bartonella* species have been found in ticks (74). *B. bacilliformis* is found in a limited geographic region, whereas *B. quintana* and *B. henselae* are found worldwide. Both chronically infected humans and animals serve as a reservoir for these organisms.

In the report by Koehler and others, one patient with *B. quintana*–associated bacillary angiomatosis owned a pet rat (27). Voles were common in the trenches in World War I, and evidence for the transmission of *Grahamella* species in mammals by fleas has been reported (88). CSD is associated with the acquisition of young cats (less commonly, dogs) in the households of patients with this disease (see Chapter 171). Genetic variability in *Bartonella* species, especially *B. henselae* (which may possess bacteriophage-like particles), allows differentiation of isolates for epidemiologic analyses (89).

Diagnosis and Serology

Serologic tests are available to aid in the diagnosis of infection with these organisms and have been used in patients with bacillary angiomatosis, fever or bacteremia, and CSD (53,90–92). Indirect fluorescent-antibody tests are available from the Centers for Disease Control and Prevention, and a commercial enzyme immunoassay for the detection of antibodies to *B. henselae* is available from the Specialty Laboratories, Santa Monica, California. An immunoblot technique that can detect both immunoglobulin M (IgM) and IgG to *B. henselae* has been developed, and new antibody tests for differentiation of the species remain to be validated clinically. Serum from patients with CSD shows both antibodies against *B. quintana* and *B. henselae*, probably owing to cross-reactivity. Patients with *B. bacilliformis* infection may have reactions to serology for brucellosis (40%). Further epidemiologic study, including studies of the rate of antibody response to these organisms, is needed. A genus-specific test has been developed, but the details of the human response in various types of infection or disease have not been quantified (93). Using available tests, the initial serology may be negative, but patients may exhibit a rise in titer over time (94).

Diagnosis and Histology

The diagnosis can be suggested by histologic findings in tissue from skin lesions, lymph nodes, spleen, or liver. In chronic bartonellosis due to *B. bacilliformis*, lesions consist of nodules that exhibit active proliferation of newly formed capillaries, dilated venules, and precapillary vessels with endothelial hyperplasia (13) and may be found in bones, mucous membranes, lungs, liver, spleen, brain, and lymph nodes. In patients with bacillary angiomatosis, nodules show proliferating endothelial and histiocytic cells in a framework of weakly formed capillaries. The lesions contain bacteria that stain with the Warthin-Starry stain and may be few in number or widely disseminated (95). Some patients may have only skin mucosal lesions, and others have histologically similar lesions in bone, lung, liver, spleen, lymph nodes, and the central nervous system. Bacillary angiomatosis–associated lesions in the liver and spleen, bacillary peliosis hepatitis, and bacillary peliosis splenitis show cystic, blood filled spaces, foci of necrosis, or granulation-like tissue. In contrast, immunocompetent patients with CSD are often diagnosed clinically or by serologic tests. If a biopsy is done, the histology of the lesions reflects the host response to the organism. Initially, there is a neutrophilic response, and bacteria can be seen around vessels and in microabscesses. Later in the disease, as the node enlarges, lymphoid hyperplasia occurs, with stellate necrotizing granulomata. Some lymph nodes have caseous necrosis. Few organisms are found with the silver stain in the tissue in the later stages. The pathologic findings are nonspecific, and without the finding of the organism on Warthin-Starry staining or probing of the tissue with a *Bartonella*-specific primer, the diagnosis can only be suggested.

TREATMENT

Antibiotics are known to decrease mortality in Oroya fever. Chloramphenicol, penicillins, and aminoglycosides have been used, but it is not known whether the improved outcome has been due to therapy of the *Bartonella* infection or efficacy against secondary pathogens such as *Salmonella* species. Antibiotics (a macrolide or a tetracycline) appear to be beneficial in patients with bacillary angiomatosis, peliosis hepatis, and bacteremia or fever, but not in most patients with CSD. One study suggests a decrease in volume of affected lymph nodes during therapy with azithromycin compared with controls receiving no treatment. Other agents have appeared to be successful, although

penicillins and first-generation cephalosporins appear to be the least active (96–98). Various agents have been tried in patients with CSD, including trimethoprim-sulfamethoxazole, rifampin, ciprofloxacin, and gentamicin. Only aminoglycosides have bactericidal activity, a similarity the *Bartonella* species share with the closely related *Brucella* species (97).

The optimal duration of therapy is not known, but prolonged treatment from weeks to months, even lifelong, may be needed in HIV-infected patients. Fever and bacteremia in immunocompetent persons initially appeared to be cured after relatively brief courses (7 to 10 days) of antibiotics. However, Lucey and colleagues reported two immunocompetent patients (one with aseptic meningitis) with clinical relapses after treatment who were cured after retreatment (99). This spectrum of clinical disease is similar to that seen in patients with trench fever and infection with *B. bacilliformis*, and the influence of antibiotic treatment on the course and duration of chronic disease is not well understood. *In vitro* testing reveals that the organisms are susceptible to several classes of antimicrobials and does not reflect clearly clinical experience. It is thought that the intracellular growth of bacteria and perhaps inhibitory rather than bactericidal activity of the agents may explain clinical relapses and failure.

PREVENTION

Infection with these organisms can be prevented by avoidance of contact with the vectors. Insecticide spraying of area inhabited by the sand flies, the use of insect netting and repellents, and avoidance of outdoor activities at night have been useful in decreasing the incidence of disease in areas endemic for *B. bacilliformis*. The issuance of new clothing to British soldiers returning from the trenches is credited with preventing spread of *B. quintana* to the civilian population after World War I. Programs to rid individuals of lice and to provide better nourishment to homeless people might decrease transmission in settings such as those described in the recent report from Seattle (21). Avoidance of contact with cats, a recommendation that cannot be made generally because of the large number of cat owners and cat fanciers, should be considered for individuals infected with HIV.

SUMMARY

As laboratories become aware of the growth characteristics of *Bartonella* species and physicians better understand the illnesses caused by these pathogens, it is likely that more cases will be recognized (100). With the increase in detection, more *in vitro* information about antimicrobial susceptibility and *in vivo* data about clinical risk factors for infection will emerge to help clinicians correctly diagnose and treat patients infected by these organisms.

REFERENCES

1. Kosek M, Lavarello R, Gilman RH, et al. Natural history of infection with *Bartonella bacilliformis* in a nonendemic population. *J Infect Dis* 2000;182:865.
2. Dehio C, Lanz C, Pohl R, et al. *Bartonella schoenbuchii* sp. nov., isolated from the blood of wild roe deer. *Intern J Sys Evol Microbiol* 2001;51:1557.
3. Birtles RJ, Hazel S, Bown K, et al. Subtyping of uncultured bartonellae using sequence comparison of 16 S/23 S rRNA intergenic spacer regions amplified directly from infected blood. *Mol Cell Probes* 2000;14:79.
4. Breitschwerdt EB, Kordick DL. *Bartonella* infection in animals: carriership, reservoir potential, pathogenicity, and zoonotic potential for human infection. *Clin Microbiol Rev* 2000;13:428.
5. Brenner DJ, SP OC, Winkler HH, et al. Proposals to unify the genera Bartonella and *Rochalimaea*, with descriptions of *Bartonella quintana* comb. nov., icomb.

nov., *Bartonella henselae* comb. nov., and *Bartonella elizabethae* comb. nov., and to remove the family *Bartonellaceae* from the order *Rickettsiales*. *Int J Syst Bacteriol* 1993;43:777.

6. Alexander B. A review of bartonellosis in Ecuador and Colombia. *Am J Trop Med Hyg* 1995;52:354.

7. Schultz MG. Daniel Carrion's experiment. *N Engl J Med* 1968;278:1323.

8. Amano Y, Rumbea J, Knobloch J, et al. Bartonellosis in Ecuador: serosurvey and current status of cutaneous verrucous disease. *Am J Trop Med Hyg* 1997;57:174.

9. Caceres AG. [Geographic distribution of *Lutzomyia verrucarum* (Townsend, 1913) (Diptera, Psychodidae, Phlebotominae), vector of human bartonellosis in Peru]. *Rev Inst Med Trop Sao Paulo* 1993;35:485.

10. Cooper P, Guderian R, Orellana P, et al. An outbreak of bartonellosis in Zamora Chinchipe Province in Ecuador. *Trans R Soc Trop Med Hyg* 1997;91:544.

11. Noguchi H. Etiology of Oroya fever. I. Cultivation of *Bartonella bacilliformis*. *J Exp Med* 1926;4:851.

12. Weiman D, Kreier J. *Bartonella* and *Grahamella*. In: Kreier JP, ed. *Parasitic protozoa*, Vol 4. New York: Academic Press, 1977:197.

13. Arias-Stella J, Lieberman PH, Erlandson RA, et al. Histology, immunohistochemistry, and ultrastructure of the verruga in Carrion's disease. *Am J Surg Pathol* 1986;10:595.

14. Gray GC, Johnson AA, Thornton SA, et al. An epidemic of Oroya fever in the Peruvian Andes. *Am J Trop Med Hyg* 1990;42:215.

15. Schmincke A. Histopathologischer Befund in Roseolen der haut bei wolhynischem feiber. *Munch Med Wochschr* 1917;64:91.

16. Vinson J. *In vitro* cultivation of the rickettsial agent of trench fever. *Bull W H O* 1966;35:155.

17. Mooser H, Leeman A, Chao SH, et al. Beobach tungen an funftagefieber. *Schweiz Zeitschrift fur Allg Path u Bakt* 1948;11:513.

18. Maurin M, Roux V, Stein A, et al. Isolation and characterization by immunofluorescence, sodium dodecyl sulfate-polyacrylamide gel electrophoresis, Western blot, restriction fragment length polymorphism-PCR, 16S rRNA gene sequencing, and pulsed-field gel electrophoresis of *Rochalimaea quintana* from a patient with bacillary angiomatosis. *J Clin Microbiol* 1994;32:1166.

19. Varela G, Vinson J, Molina-Pasquel C. Trench fever. II. Propagation of *Rickettsia quintana* on cell-free medium from the blood of two patients. *Am J Trop Med Hyg* 1969;18:708.

20. Vinson JW, Varela G, Molina-Pasquel C. Trench fever. III. Induction of clinical disease in volunteers inoculated with *Rickettsia quintana* propagated on blood agar. *Am J Trop Med Hyg* 1969;18:713.

21. Spach DH, Kanter AS, Dougherty MJ, et al. *Bartonella (Rochalimaea) quintana* bacteremia in inner-city patients with chronic alcoholism [see Comments]. *N Engl J Med* 1995;332:424.

22. Adal KA, Cockerell CJ, Petri WA. Cat scratch disease, bacillary angiomatosis, and other infections due to *Rochalimaea*. *N Engl J Med* 1994;330:1509.

23. Slater L, Welch D, Hensel D, et al. A newly recognized fastidious gram-negative pathogen as a cause of fever and bacteremia. *N Engl J Med* 1990; 323:1587.

24. Relman DA, Loutit JS, Schmidt TM, et al. The agent of bacillary angiomatosis: an approach to the identification of uncultured pathogens. *N Engl J Med* 1990;323:1573.

25. Welch DF, Pickett DA, Slater LN, et al. *Rochalimaea henselae* sp. nov., a cause of septicemia, bacillary angiomatosis, and parenchymal bacillary peliosis. *J Clin Microbiol* 1992;30:275.

26. Regnery RL, Anderson BE, Clarridge JE 3rd, et al. Characterization of a novel *Rochalimaea* species, *R. henselae* sp. nov., isolated from blood of a febrile, human immunodeficiency virus-positive patient. *J Clin Microbiol* 1992;30:265.

27. Koehler JE, Quinn FD, Berger TG, et al. Isolation of *Rochalimaea* species from cutaneous and osseous lesions of bacillary angiomatosis. *N Engl J Med* 1992;327:1625.

28. Regnery R, Tappero J. Unraveling mysteries associated with cat-scratch disease, bacillary angiomatosis, and related syndromes. *Emerg Infect Dis* 1995;1:16.

29. Clarridge JE 3rd, Raich TJ, Pirwani D, et al. Strategy to detect and identify *Bartonella* species in routine clinical laboratory yields *Bartonella henselae* from human immunodeficiency virus-positive patient and unique *Bartonella* strain from his cat. *J Clin Microbiol* 1995;33:2107.

30. Kordick DL, Hilyard EJ, Hadfield TL, et al. *Bartonella clarridgeiae*, a newly recognized zoonotic pathogen causing inoculation papules, fever, and lymphadenopathy (cat scratch disease). *J Clin Microbiol* 1997;35:1813.

31. Sander A, Zagrosek A, Bredt W, et al. Characterization of *Bartonella clarridgeiae* flagellin (FlaA) and detection of antiflagellin antibodies in patients with lymphadenopathy. *J Clin Microbiol* 2000;38:2943.

32. Raoult D, Drancourt M, Carta A, et al. *Bartonella (Rochalimaea) quintana* isolation in patient with chronic adenopathy, lymphopenia, and a cat [Letter]. *Lancet* 1994;343:977.

33. Anonymous. Case records of the Massachusetts General Hospital. Weekly clinicopathological exercises. Case 1-1998. An 11-year-old boy with a seizure (clinical conference). *N Engl J Med* 1998;338:112.

34. Breitschwerdt EB, Atkins CE, Brown TT, et al. *Bartonella vinsonii* subsp.berkhoffii and related members of the alpha subdivision of the Proteobacteria in dogs with cardiac arrhythmias, endocarditis, or myocarditis. *J Clin Microbiol* 1999;37:3618.

35. Kordick DL, Brown TT, Shin K, et al. Clinical and pathologic evaluation of chronic *Bartonella henselae* or *Bartonella clarridgeiae* infection in cats. *J Clin Microbiol* 1999;37:1536.

36. Boulouis HJ, Barrat F, Bermond D, et al. Kinetics of *Bartonella birtlesii* infection in experimentally infected mice and pathogenic effect on reproductive functions. *Infect Immun* 2001;69:5313.

37. Guptill L, Slater LN, Wu CC, et al. Evidence of reproductive failure and lack of perinatal transmission of *Bartonella henselae* in experimentally infected cats. *Vet Immunol Immunopathol* 1998;65:177.

38. Kosoy MY, Regnery RL, Kosaya OI, et al. Isolation of *Bartonella* spp. from embryos and neonates of naturally infected rodents. *J Wildl Dis* 1998;34: 305.

39. Bruneval P, Choucair J, Paraf F, et al. Detection of fastidious bacteria in cardiac valves in cases of blood culture negative endocarditis. *J Clin Pathol* 2001;54:238.

40. Spach DH, Kanter AS, Daniels NA, et al. *Bartonella (Rochalimaea)* species as a cause of apparent "culture-negative" endocarditis. *Clin Infect Dis* 1995;20: 1044.

41. Daly JS, Worthington MG, Brenner DJ, et al. *Rochalimaea elizabethae* sp. nov. isolated from a patient with endocarditis. *J Clin Microbiol* 1993;31:872.

42. Birtles RJ, Canales J, Ventosilla P, et al. Survey of *Bartonella* species infecting intradomicillary animals in the Huayllacall Valley, Ancash, Peru, a region endemic for human bartonellosis. *Am J Trop Med Hyg* 1999;60:799.

43. Comer JA, Flynn C, Regnery RL, et al. Antibodies to *Bartonella* species in inner-city intravenous drug users in Baltimore, Md. *Arch Intern Med* 1996;156: 2491.

44. Ellis BA, Regnery RL, Beati L, et al. Rats of the genus *Rattus* are reservoir hosts for pathogenic *Bartonella* species: an Old World origin for a New World disease? *J Infect Dis* 1999;180:220.

45. Holmberg M, McGill S, Ehrenborg C, et al. Evaluation of human seroreactivity to *Bartonella* species in Sweden. *J Clin Microbiol* 1999;37:1381.

46. O'Halloran H, Draud K, Minix M, et al. Leber's neuroretinitis in a patient with serologic evidence of *Bartonella elizabethae*. *Retina* 1998;18:276.

47. Wesslen L, Ehrenborg C, Holmberg M, et al. Subacute *Bartonella* infection in Swedish orienteers succumbing to sudden unexpected cardiac death or having malignant arrhythmias. *Scand J Infect Dis* 2001;33:429.

48. James EA, Hill J, Uppal R, et al. *Bartonella* infection: a significant cause of native valve endocarditis necessitating surgical management. *J Thorac Cardiovasc Surg* 2000;119:171.

49. Maurin M, Birtles R, Raoult D. Current knowledge of *Bartonella* species. *Eur J Clin Microbiol Infect Dis* 1997;16:487.

50. Ohl ME, Spach DH. *Bartonella quintana* and urban trench fever. *Clin Infect Dis* 2000;31:131.

51. Lepidi H, Fournier PE, Raoult D. Quantitative analysis of valvular lesions during *Bartonella* endocarditis. *Am J Clin Pathol* 2000;114:880.

52. Drancourt M, Birtles R, Chaumentin G, et al. New serotype of *Bartonella henselae* in endocarditis and cat-scratch disease. *Lancet* 1996;347:441.

53. Maurin M, Eb F, Etienne J, et al. Serological cross-reactions between *Bartonella* and *Chlamydia* species: implications for diagnosis. *J Clin Microbiol* 1997;35:2283.

54. Breathnach AS, Hoare JM, Eykyn SJ. Culture-negative endocarditis: contribution of *Bartonella* infections. *Heart* 1997;77:474.

55. La Scola B, Raoult D. Serological cross-reactions between *Bartonella quintana*, *Bartonella henselae*, and *Coxiella burnetii*. *J Clin Microbiol* 1996;34:2270.

56. Breitschwerdt EB, Kordick DL, Malarkey DE, et al. Endocarditis in a dog due to infection with a novel *Bartonella* subspecies. *J Clin Microbiol* 1995;33: 154.

57. Roux V, Eykyn SJ, Wyllie S, et al. *Bartonella vinsonii* subsp. *berkhoffii* as an agent of afebrile blood culture-negative endocarditis in a human. *J Clin Microbiol* 2000;38:1698.

58. McGill S, Wesslen L, Hjelm E, et al. Serological and epidemiological analysis of the prevalence of *Bartonella* spp. antibodies in Swedish elite orienteers 1992–93. *Scand J Infect Dis* 2001;33:423.

59. Meininger GR, Nadasdy T, Hruban R et al. Chronic active myocarditis following acute *Bartonella henselae* infection (cat scratch disease). *Am J Surg Pathol* 2001;25:1211.

60. Carithers HA, Margileth AM. Cat-scratch disease: acute encephalopathy and other neurologic manifestations. *Am J Dis Child* 1991;145:98.

61. Kerkhoff FT, Bergmans AM, van Der Zee A, et al. Demonstration of *Bartonella grahamii* DNA in ocular fluids of a patient with neuroretinitis. *J Clin Microbiol* 1999;37:4034.

62. Rosen BS, Barry CJ, Nicoll AM, et al. Conservative management of documented neuroretinitis in cat scratch disease associated with *Bartonella henselae* infection. *Aust N Z J Ophthalmol* 1999;27:153.

63. Wong MT, Dolan MJ, Lattuada CP Jr, et al. Neuroretinitis, aseptic meningitis, and lymphadenitis associated with *Bartonella (Rochalimaea) henselae* infection in immunocompetent patients and patients infected with human immunodeficiency virus type 1. *Clin Infect Dis* 1995;21:352.

64. Chrousos GA, Drack AV, Young M, et al. Neuroretinitis in cat scratch disease. *J Clin Neuroopthalmol* 1990;10:92.

65. Earhart KC, Power MH. *Bartonella* neuroretinitis. *N Engl J Med* 2000;343:1459.

66. Baker J. A rickettsial infection in Canadian voles. *J Exp Med* 1946;84:37.

67. Weiss E, Dasch G. Vole agent identified as a strain of the trench fever rickettsia, *Rochalemaea quintana*. *Infect Immun* 1982;19:1013.

68. Weiss E, Dasch G. Differential characteristics of strains of *Rochalimaea: Rochalimaea vinsonii* sp. nov., the Canadian vole agent. *Int J Syst Bacteriol* 1982;32:305.

69. Kordick DL, Swaminathan B, Greene CE, et al. *Bartonella vinsonii* subsp. *berkhoffii* subsp. nov., isolated from dogs; *Bartonella vinsonii* subsp. *vinsonii*; and emended description of *Bartonella vinsonii*. *Int J Syst Bacteriol* 1996;46:704.

70. Chang CC, Kasten RW, Chomel BB, et al. Coyotes (*Canis latrans*) as the reservoir for a human pathogenic *Bartonella* sp.: molecular epidemiology of *Bartonella vinsonii* subsp. *berkhoffii* infection in coyotes from central coastal California. *J Clin Microbiol* 2000;38:4193.

71. Pappalardo BL, Brown T, Gookin JL, et al. Granulomatous disease associated with *Bartonella* infection in 2 dogs. *J Vet Intern Med* 2000;14:37.

72. Welch DF, Carroll KC, Hofmeister EK, et al. Isolation of a new subspecies, *Bartonella vinsonii* subsp. *arupensis*, from a cattle rancher: identity with isolates found in conjunction with *Borrelia burgdorferi* and *Babesia microti* among naturally infected mice. *J Clin Microbiol* 1999;37:2598.

73. Droz S, Chi B, Horn E, et al. *Bartonella koehlerae* sp. nov., isolated from cats. *J Clin Microbiol* 1999;37:1117.

74. Chang CC, Chomel BB, Kasten RW, et al. Molecular evidence of *Bartonella* spp. in questing adult *Ixodes pacificus* ticks in California. *J Clin Microbiol* 2001;39:1221.

75. Birtles RJ, Harrison TG, Saunders NA, et al. Proposals to unify the genera *Grahamella* and *Bartonella*, with descriptions of *Bartonella talpae* comb. nov., *Bartonella peromysci* comb. nov., and three new species, *Bartonella grahamii* sp. nov., *Bartonella taylorii* sp. nov., and *Bartonella doshiae* sp. nov. *Int J Syst Bacteriol* 1995;45:1.

76. Heller R, Kubina M, Mariet P, et al. *Bartonella alsatica* sp. nov., a new *Bartonella* species isolated from the blood of wild rabbits. *Int J Syst Bacteriol* 1999;49:283.

77. Houpikian PRD. 16S/23S rRNA intergenic spacer regions for phylogenetic analysis, identification, and subtyping of *Bartonella* species. *J Clin Microbiol* 2001;39:2768.

78. La Scola B, Raoult D. Culture of *Bartonella quintana* and *Bartonella henselae* from human samples: a 5-year experience (1993 to 1998). *J Clin Microbiol* 1999;37:1899.

79. Maass M, Schreiber M, Knobloch J. Detection of *Bartonella bacilliformis* in cultures, blood, and formalin preserved skin biopsies by use of the polymerase chain reaction. *Trop Med Parisitol* 1992;43:191.

80. Brenner SA, Rooney JA, Manzewitsch P, et al. Isolation of *Bartonella* (*Rochalimaea*) *henselae*: effects of methods of blood collection and handling. *J Clin Microbiol* 1997;35:544.

81. Wong MT, Thornton DC, Kennedy RC, et al. A chemically defined liquid medium that supports primary isolation of *Rochalimaea* (*Bartonella*) *henselae* from blood and tissue specimens. *J Clin Microbiol* 1995;33:742.

82. Drancourt M. Proposed tests for the routine identification of *Rochalimaea* species. *Eur J Clin Microbiol Infect Dis* 1993;12:710.

83. Welch DF, Hensel DM, Pickett DA, et al. Bacteremia due to *Rochalimaea henselae* in a child: practical identification of isolates in the clinical laboratory. *J Clin Microbiol* 1993;31:2381.

84. Wong MT, Thornton DC, Kennedy RC, et al. A chemically defined liquid medium that supports primary isolation of *Rochalimaea* (*Bartonella*) *henselae* from blood and tissue specimens. *J Clin Microbiol* 1995;33:742.

85. Joblet C, Roux V, Drancourt M, et al. Identification of *Bartonella* (*Rochalimaea*) species among fastidious gram-negative bacteria on the basis of the partial sequence of the citrate-synthase gene. *J Clin Microbiol* 1995;33:1879.

86. Renesto P, Gouvernet J, Drancourt M, et al. Use of rpoB gene analysis for detection and identification of *Bartonella* species. *J Clin Microbiol* 2001;39:430.

87. Higgins JA, Radulovic S, Jaworski DC, et al. Acquisition of the cat scratch disease agent *Bartonella henselae* by cat fleas (*Siphonaptera: Pulicidae*). *J Med Entomol* 1996;33:490.

88. Birtles R, Harrison T. *Grahamella* in small woodland mammals in the U.K.: isolation, prevalence and host specificity. *Ann Trop Med Parasitol* 1994;88:317.

89. Roux V, Raoult D. Inter- and intraspecies identification of *Bartonella* (*Rochalimaea*) species. *J Clin Microbiol* 1995;33:1573.

90. Del Prete R, Fumarola D, Fumarola L, et al. Prevalence of antibodies to *Bartonella henselae* in patients with suspected cat scratch disease (CSD) in Italy. *Eur J Epidemiol* 1999;15:583.

91. Guibal F, de La Salmoniere P, Rybojad M, et al. High seroprevalence to *Bartonella quintana* in homeless patients with cutaneous parasitic infestations in downtown Paris. *J Am Acad Dermatol* 2001;44:219.

92. Nadal D, Zbinden R. Serology to *Bartonella* (*Rochalimaea*) *henselae* may replace traditional diagnostic criteria for cat-scratch disease. *Eur J Pediatr* 1995;154:906.

93. Liang Z, La Scola B, Lepidi H, et al. Production of *Bartonella* genus–specific monoclonal antibodies. *Clin Diagn Lab Immunol* 2001;8:847.

94. Karem KL: Immune aspects of *Bartonella*. *Crit Rev Microbiol* 2000;26:133.

95. Perkocha L, Geaghan S, Benedict Yen T, et al. Clinical and pathological features of bacillary peliosis hepatis in association with human immunodeficiency virus infection. *N Engl J Med* 1990;323:1581.

96. Maurin M, Gasquet S, Ducco C, et al. MICs of 28 antibiotic compounds for 14 *Bartonella* (formerly *Rochalimaea*) isolates. *Antimicrob Agents Chemother* 1995;39:2387.

97. Rolain JM, Maurin M, Raoult D. Bactericidal effect of antibiotics on *Bartonella* and *Brucella* spp.:clinical implications. *J Antimicrob Chemother* 2000;46:811.

98. Sobraques M, Maurin M, Birtles RJ, et al. In vitro susceptibilities of four *Bartonella bacilliformis* strains to 30 antibiotic compounds. *Antimicrob Agents Chemother* 1999;43:2090.

99. Lucey D, Dolan MJ, Moss CW, et al. Relapsing illness due to *Rochalimaea henselae* in immunocompetent hosts: implication for therapy and new epidemiological associations. *Clin Infect Dis* 1992;14:683.

100. Massei F, Messina F, Talini I, et al. Widening of the clinical spectrum of *Bartonella henselae* infection as recognized through serodiagnostics. *Eur J Pediatr* 2000;159:416.

CHAPTER 219
Calymmatobacterium granulomatis

Gary Doern

HISTORY

Donovanosis, or granuloma inguinale, was first described by McLeod (1) in 1882, when he noted "serpiginous ulcerations associated with more or less thickening of tissues" in patients living in Calcutta, India. The causative agent of the disease was initially recognized by Donovan in 1905 (2). Microscopic examination of tissue biopsy specimens revealed intracellular organisms originally thought to be protozoa, which were named *Donovan bodies*. Subsequently, the agent of donovanosis was determined to be a bacterium and was named *Donovania granulomatis* (3). It is now referred to as *Calymmatobacterium granulomatis*.

CHARACTERISTICS OF THE PATHOGEN

C. granulomatis is a gram-negative, nonmotile, non–spore-forming coccobacillus that measures 0.5 to 1.0 $\times$ 1.5 to 20 μm. It is generally categorized as a bacterium of uncertain affiliation; however, it bears many genotypic and phenotypic similarities to members of the family Enterobacteriaceae, in particular *Klebsiella* species and *Enterobacter* species (4–6). The organism possesses a cytoplasmic membrane, a typical gram-negative cell wall, and in many instances, a sharply delineated capsule (7). Surface projections, which appear to be fimbriae or pili, have been observed by electron microscopy (8).

C. granulomatis has been propagated in yolk sacs of chick embryos (3) and in cell culture (9,10). Growing the organisms in cell-free, defined media has been more difficult. Although there have been sporadic reports of propagation, or at least maintenance, using specialized media (11) and on slants composed of coagulated egg yolk (12), for practical purposes, the organism cannot be grown on standard laboratory media. Indeed, currently, there are no cultures of this organism in existence.

EPIDEMIOLOGY

Donovanosis is often referred to as one of the classic ulcerative sexually transmitted diseases, along with syphilis, herpes simplex virus infection, chancroid, and lymphogranuloma venereum. In reality, the role of sexual transmission remains controversial. The high frequency of infection in persons between 20 and 40 years old, the years of greatest sexual activity; the fact that rectal lesions are found in male homosexuals who engage in anal intercourse and whose partners have penile lesions; and the predilection for lesions to occur on the genitalia support the notion of venereal transmission (13). Conversely, in certain parts of the world, donovanosis occurs with great frequency in young children who have no history of sexual contact (14). Furthermore, it is uncommon to find evidence of infection in the heterosexual partners of patients with well-defined genital lesions of *C. granulomatis* infection (15,16). Finally, although infrequently, primary donovanian lesions have been described on skin surfaces such as the trunk and proximal upper extremities, for which sexual contact is an implausible explanation for transmission. It is likely, therefore, that *C. granulomatis* can be transmitted by direct sexual contact as well as by indirect means. An example of the latter mode of transmission is the frequently cited but largely unproven assertion that fecal soilage of the perineal skin and vagina can lead to infection of these sites, presumably by traumatic inoculation of organisms normally present in stool (17). This, of course, presupposes that *C. granulomatis* is a commensal organism in stool, something that also has not been proved.

Donovanosis occurs primarily in tropical and subtropical areas of the world. It used to be more common in the United States, particularly among black persons in the southeastern Atlantic coast region. Today, fewer than 100 cases occur annually. Autochthonous infection by *C. granulomatis* is also nearly unheard of in the developed countries of Western Europe and in Japan. At present, donovanosis is endemic in parts of India; the arid and semiarid regions of central, northern, and western Australia; western New Guinea; southern China; and parts of southwest Asia and Africa. In the Western Hemisphere, endemic donovanosis may be found in Brazil and in some of the Caribbean islands (8,11–13).

In endemic areas, the prevalence of donovanosis may be quite high. For instance, a 1971 surveillance study performed in Papua New Guinea revealed overall infection rates of nearly 5% (14). In male patients attending a venereal disease clinic, the prevalence of donovanosis was 23.5% (18). Men are more often found to be infected than are women (2.5:1) (19). Historically, a preponderance of cases of donovanosis has been observed in black persons. This is probably explained by socioeconomic factors and the geography of endemicity rather than a racial predisposition. There exists a clear association between infection due to *C. granulomatis* and human immunodeficiency virus (HIV) in certain parts of the world (20–22).

PATHOGENESIS AND CLINICAL MANIFESTATIONS

Organisms gain entrance into infected tissue by direct traumatic inoculation through the skin. The incubation period is extremely variable, ranging from 8 to 80 days (mean, 17 days) (13). A dense accumulation of mononuclear cells forms within the affected dermis. Occasional clusters of neutrophils and histiocytes are also found. Acanthosis may be present in the surrounding epithelium. In addition, areas of pseudoepitheliomatous hyperplasia may be found to envelop the granulomatous lesion. The pathognomonic cells of donovanosis are found scattered throughout the lesion but are usually more numerous and conspicuous at the margins. These cells consist of enlarged histocytes with intracytoplasmic vacuoles containing variable numbers of the infectious agent, *C. granulomatis*. More than one cytoplasmic inclusion may be found per histiocyte. As noted later, the appearance of the organism within what are apparently phagocytic vacuoles is quite characteristic. These inclusions have been termed Donovan bodies.

Grossly, the lesions usually begin as solitary, superficial, small, firm papules, which eventually evolve into ulcers as the overlying skin breaks down. Although the actual appearance of the ulcer may be variable, the most common form is a painless, fleshy, beefy-red granulomatous lesion that is neither tender nor indurated and that bleeds profusely when touched. Lesions may take on a verrucous appearance at the periphery when epithelial hyperplasia has occurred. Secondarily infected lesions may become tender and necrotic and show evidence of a purulent exudate. Surrounding cellulitis is rare. Multiple adjacent lesions may coalesce as they enlarge, forming large single lesions. Although there is little tendency to spread locally or disseminate

systemically, secondary donovanian lesions have been noted in the uterus, fallopian tubes, ovaries, and epididymis (contiguous spread) (13,23) and in the liver and skeletal system (systemic spread) (24). Systemic dissemination is most likely the result of hematogenous seeding.

Ninety percent of primary lesions are found on the skin of the genitalia (14): in men, on the prepuce, coronal sulcus, shaft, glans, and frenum (13); in women, usually on the labia minora and majora and the fourchette (23). In 10% of cases, lesions appear on the inguinal skin (14). The perianal skin is involved in 5% to 10% of cases (24). Primary lesions do occur in other sites, such as the rectum and oral cavity, but much less frequently. Inguinal lymphadenopathy, a common finding in patients with syphilis, chancroid, herpes simplex virus infection, or lymphogranuloma venereum, is typically absent in patients with donovanosis unless lesions become superinfected. "Pseudobuboes" may occur, but rather than representing enlarged inguinal lymph nodes, they are subcutaneous granulation tissue that arises as a result of secondary foci of infection formed from local extension.

There are two major consequences of untreated infections: fibrosis and scarring of involved tissue can result in loss of function, and, if the lymphatics are involved, lymph stasis and lymphedema are possible. A second concern pertains to the relationship between donovanosis and squamous cell carcinoma of the penis and vulva (25). This relationship is supported by the following observations. The incidence of genital carcinoma is greater than normal in areas where donovanosis is endemic. Squamous cell carcinomas have been observed within healed *C. granulomatis* lesions. The two conditions have often been found to occur concurrently. Finally, in one investigation, 9 of 62 patients with squamous cell carcinoma of the penis were noted to have circulating antibody reactive with *C. granulomatis* (25). These observations certainly do not prove a role for *C. granulomatis* as a cause of genital carcinoma, but they do justify further investigation of this possibility.

DIAGNOSIS

An accurate clinical diagnosis of donovanosis can be achieved in about 63% of men and 83% of women by experienced clinicians working in an endemic area (26). A definitive diagnosis of *C. granulomatis* infections, however, is best accomplished by microscopic visualization of characteristic Donovan bodies in tissue biopsy material. Biopsies should be obtained from the advancing margins of the base of ulcers. A portion of the specimen should be fixed in formalin and submitted for sectioning and histologic examination. The remainder should be placed between two cleaned glass microscope slides and then crushed and smeared across the slides to produce a thin film of macerated tissue (27). The slides are air dried, and then one is stained with either Wright (28) or Giemsa (27) stain, and the other is processed with either the Dieterle silver impregnation stain or Warthin-Starry stain (29).

A diagnosis of donovanosis is made when clusters of coccobacillus-shaped organisms are observed within phagocytic vacuoles in histiocytes. The organisms possess a distinct bipolar staining characteristic that gives the appearance of two adjacent coccal forms (i.e., a closed safety pin appearance). This results from the accumulation of condensed chromatin material at the poles of the cell. All four of the stains just noted stain the organisms dark blue to black. Organisms examined with the Wright or Giemsa stain may be surrounded by pink capsular material (30).

Crush preparations are usually more rewarding than histologic sections. Culture is of no practical value because of the difficulties of propagating the organism. Similarly, no serologic procedures of proven utility in diagnosing donovanosis are currently available. Molecular diagnosis by polymerase chain reaction performed directly on genital tract specimens has been described recently and shows promise as a diagnostic modality (31,32).

TREATMENT

Numerous antimicrobial agents have been used successfully to treat donovanosis: antimony salts, tetracyclines, streptomycin, trimethoprim-sulfamethoxazole, chloramphenicol, erythromycin, azithromycin, various penicillins, ceftriaxone, and aminoglycosides. Because no controlled comparative clinical trials have been performed, there is little objective basis for defining optimal therapy. In view of this, tetracycline appears to be the drug of first choice; it is certainly the agent with which the greatest clinical experience treating donovanosis has been accumulated (33). Tetracycline should be administered orally in 500-mg doses every 6 hours (34). A clinical response should be evident within about 1 week, as lesions begin to regress. Therapy should be continued until the lesions disappear completely. In some cases, this takes 2 to 3 months. Discontinuing therapy before lesions have healed completely often results in recrudescence of disease. For pregnant women and children with deciduous teeth, trimethoprim-sulfamethoxazole, two single-strength tablets every 12 hours, is adequate alternative therapy (35).

PREVENTION

Preventive measures for reducing the incidence of donovanosis include prompt treatment of recognized cases and improving the personal hygiene and sanitation facilities of persons in areas where the disease is endemic.

REFERENCES

1. McLeod K. Precis of operations by Major McLeod. *Indian Med Gaz* 1882;15:113.
2. Donovan C. Medical cases from Madras General Hospital: ulcerating granuloma of the pudenda. *Indian Med Gaz* 1905;40:414.
3. Anderson K, DeMonbreaun WA, Goodpasture EW. An etiologic consideration of *Donovania granulomatis* cultivated from granuloma inguinale (three cases) in embryonic yolk. *J Exp Med* 1943;81:25.
4. Goldberg J. Studies on granuloma inguinale. IV. Growth requirements of *Donovania granulomatis* and its relationship to the natural habitat of the organism. *Br J Vener Dis* 1959;35:266.
5. Carter JS, Bowden FJ, Bastian I, et al. Phylogenetic evidence for reclassification of *Calymmatobacterium granulomatis* as *Klebsiella granulomatis* comb. nov. *Int J Syst Bacteriol* 1999;49:1695.
6. Kharsany AB, Hoosen AA, Kiepiela P, et al. Phylogenetic analysis of *Calymmatobacterium granulomatis* based on 16S rRNA gene sequences. *J Med Microbiol* 1999;48:841.
7. Davis CM, Collins C. An ultrastructural study of *Calymmatobacterium granulomatis*. *J Invest Dermatol* 1969;53:315.
8. Hart G. Donovanosis. In: Holmes KK, Mardh P-A, Sparling PF, et al., eds. *Sexually transmitted disease.* New York: McGraw-Hill, 1984:393–395.
9. Carter J, Hutton S, Sriprakash KS, et al. Culture of the causative organism of donovanosis (*Calymmatobacterium granulomatis*) in Hep-2 cells. *J Clin Microbiol* 1997;35:2915.
10. Kharsany AB, Hoosen AA, Kiepiela P, et al. Culture of *Calymmatobacterium granulomatis*. *Clin Infect Dis* 1996;22:391.
11. Dunham W, Rake G. Cultural and serologic studies on granuloma inguinale. *Am J Syphilol* 1948;32:145.
12. Goldberg J, Weaver RH, Packer H. Studies on granuloma inguinale. I. Bacteriologic behavior of *Donovania granulomatis*. *Am J Syphilol* 1953;12:57.
13. Sehgal VN, Shyan Prasad AL. Donovanosis: current concepts. *Int J Dermatol* 1986;25:8.
14. Zigas V. Medicine from the past: donovanosis project in Goilala (1951–1954). *Papua New Guinea Med J* 1971;14:148.
15. Hart G. Chancroid, donovanosis, lymphogranuloma venereum. Washington, DC: U.S. Department of Health Education and Welfare publication (CDC), 1975:75-8302.
16. O'Farrell N. Clinico-epidemiological study of donovanosis in Durban, South Africa. *Genitourin Med* 1993;69:108.
17. Goldberg J. Studies on granuloma inguinale. VII. Some epidemiological considerations of the disease. *Br J Vener Dis* 1964;40:140.
18. Hart G. Psychological and social aspects of venereal disease in Papua New Guinea. *Br J Vener Dis* 1974;50:453.
19. Canizares O. Nontreponemal veneral infections. In: Moschella SL, Pillsbury DM, Hurley HJ, eds. *Dermatology,* Vol 1. Philadelphia: WB Saunders, 1975:741–744.
20. Jamkhedkar PP, Hira SK, Shroff HJ, et al. Clinico-epidemiologic features of granuloma inguinale in the era of acquired immune deficiency syndrome. *Sex Transm Dis* 1998;25:196.
21. O'Farrell N. Global eradication of donovanosis: an opportunity for limiting the spread of HIV-1 infection. *Genitourin Med* 1995;71:27.
22. Sanders CJ. Extragenital donovanosis in patients with AIDS. *Sex Transm Infect* 1998;74:142.
23. Wysoki RS, Majmudar B, Willis D. Granuloma inguinale (donovanosis) in women. *J Reprod Med* 1988;33:709.
24. Kirkpatrick DJ. Donovanosis (granuloma inguinale): a rare cause of osteolytic bone lesions. *Clin Radiol* 1970;21:101.
25. Goldberg J, Annamunthodo H. Studies on granuloma inguinale. VIII. Serologic reactivity of sera from patients with carcinoma of the penis when tested with *Donovania* antigens. *Br J Vener Dis* 1966;42:205.
26. O'Farrell N, Hoosen AA, Coetzee KD, et al. Genital ulcer disease: accuracy of clinical diagnosis and strategies to improve control in Durban, South Africa. *Genitourin Med* 1994;70:7.
27. Cannefax GR. The technic of tissue spread method for demonstrating Donovan bodies. *J Vener Dis Infect* 1948;29:201.
28. Greenblatt RB, Dienst RD, West RM. A simple stain for Donovan bodies in diagnosis of granuloma inguinale. *Am J Syphilol* 1951;35:291.
29. Greenblatt RF, Barfield WE. Newer methods in diagnosis and treatment of granuloma inguinale. *Br J Vener Dis* 1952;28:123.
30. Sehgal VN, Prasad ALS, Bechar PC. The histopathology of donovanosis. *Br J Vener Dis* 1984;60:145.
31. Carter JS, Kemp DJ. A colorimetric detection system for *Calymmatobacterium granulomatis*. *Sex Transm Infect* 2000;76:134.
32. Carter J, Bowden FJ, Sriprakash KS, et al. Diagnostic polymerase chain reaction for donovanosis. *Clin Infect Dis* 1999;28:1168.
33. Nongonococcal urethritis and other sexually transmitted diseases of public health importance. Report of a WHO Scientific Group. *W H O Tech Rep Ser* 1981;660:1.
34. Robinson HM. The treatment of granuloma inguinale, lymphogranuloma venereum, chancroid and gonorrhea. *Arch Dermatol Syphilol* 1951;64:284.
35. Lal S, Garg BR. Further evidence of the efficacy of co-trimoxazole in granuloma venereum. *Br J Vener Dis* 1980;56:412.

CHAPTER 220
Nocardia

Dimitrios P. Kontoyiannis

Nocardia was first described by the French veterinarian Edmond Nocard in 1889 when he investigated an outbreak of granulomatous disease in cattle on the island of Guadeloupe. These animals developed multiple draining cutaneous abscesses and eventually pneumonia followed by death. Nocard isolated an aerobic actinomycete, which he named *Streptothrix farcini*, as the cause of this bovine farcy. The first human isolate of *Nocardia* was described by Eppinger in 1891 in a patient who had pneumonia and a brain abscess.

CLASSIFICATION

Nocardia is classified in the order Actinomycetales along with the genera *Actinomyces* and *Streptomyces* (1) (Table 220.1). Furthermore, it is in the family Nocardiaceae with the non—acid-fast genus *Actinomadura*, which is a cause of chronically draining sinuses in the extremities (1,2). Although *Nocardia* exhibits the classic fungal characteristics of true aerial hyphae, it is considered a higher bacterium rather than a fungus because its cell wall consists of peptidoglycans and does not contain either

TABLE 220.1. Characteristics of Actinomycetales

Characteristic	*Actinomyces*	*Nocardia*	*Streptomyces*
Requires oxygen	No	Yes	Yes
Acid-fast (Ziehl-Neelsen)	No	No	No
Weakly acid-fast (Kinyoun)	No	Yes	No

chitin or cellulose. Structurally, *Nocardia* appears as a thin (0.5 to 1.0 μm), branching, often beaded gram-positive rod (Fig. 220.1). Although not acid-fast in the standard acid-alcohol decolorization when using the Ziehl-Neelsen method, *Nocardia* is weakly acid fast when decolorized with 1% sulfuric acid using the Kinyoun carbolfuchsin stain, which helps distinguish it from the anaerobic *Actinomyces* group of organisms. Additionally, *Nocardia* is a hardy aerobe because it can be cultivated on simple media and tolerate temperatures of up to 50°C. Also, 10% carbon dioxide will encourage its growth. It grows slowly, however, because often 4 to 5 days elapse before visible colonies appear on the culture medium.

EPIDEMIOLOGY AND RISK FACTORS

Nocardia species are ubiquitous, found primarily in soil, plants, and organic matter (1–3). The upper aerodigestive tract is the major portal of entry of these species into the body, with the lung being the most common site of infection. The gastrointestinal tract may be an alternative route, with organisms entering the bloodstream or lymphatics through breaks in the gut mucosa. Traumatic inoculation through the skin or eye is also a mechanism of *Nocardia* implantation. Even though nocardiosis is typically recognized as a sporadic, community-acquired infection, nosocomial transmission and temporal clustering have been reported (1). Nosocomial postoperative surgical wound infections caused by *Nocardia* also have been reported, although rarely (1,4). Newer molecular typing techniques, such as pulsed-field electrophoresis, may be helpful in investigating both true outbreaks and pseudo-outbreaks of nocardiosis (4,5).

It is estimated that at least 1,000 new cases of nocardiosis occur every year in the United States (1,3,6). In most reports of nocardiosis, male patients predominate over female patients at ratios of 2:1 to 3:1. Even though nocardiosis may affect normal hosts (1,7), this infection is an increasingly recognized problem in immunosuppressed patients (1–3,6–13). Patients with the highest risk of this serious infection include those undergoing transplantation (8–10) or steroid therapy (1–3,8–11), those with cancer (1,12,13), and those with chronic granulomatous disease, chronic alcoholism, sarcoidosis, or systemic lupus erythematosus (1). In addition, the use of new antineoplastic agents that affect T-cell function, such as the purine analogs, has been described to result in severe nocardiosis (14). Interestingly, nocardiosis has been found as a complication in only 0.2% to 0.3% of acquired immunodeficiency syndrome (AIDS) patients (1–3,11,15–18). The low incidence of nocardiosis in this patient population may reflect the common use of trimethoprim-sulfamethoxazole (TMP-SMX) as *Pneumocystis carinii* pneumonia prophylaxis because TMP-SMX has very good activity against *Nocardia* species (1,3,11). In addition, most AIDS patients with nocardiosis have advanced immunosuppression with a mean CD4 count of 110 cells/mm^3 (1,16–18). Finally, the presence of an endovascular foreign body, such as a prosthetic valve or central venous catheter, and intravenous drug use are predisposing factors for bacteremic nocardiosis (19–22). Specifically, *Nocardia* species have been cultured from the injection paraphernalia of drug users (20). However, the potential of pseudo-outbreaks of bacteremic nocardiosis due to contamination of blood cultures is well recognized (1,5,23).

Finally, outdoor activities, such as farming and gardening, as well as exposure to cats have been linked with cutaneous infections by *Nocardia brasiliensis* (24,25). It is also thought that underlying lung disease, such as bronchiectasis or alveolar proteinosis, may result in increased risk for pulmonary nocardiosis (1–3,11,26). However, transient colonization in the sputum by *Nocardia* species has been reported in patients having underlying lung disease (1–3,11).

PATHOGENESIS

Infection by *Nocardia* species elicits a brisk inflammatory response in the host (1–3,11,27). Specifically, both polymorphonuclear leukocytes and activated lymphocytes are involved in the cellular response to the infection. Histologically, necrosis and abscess formation are common (1–3,11,27,28). Also, it

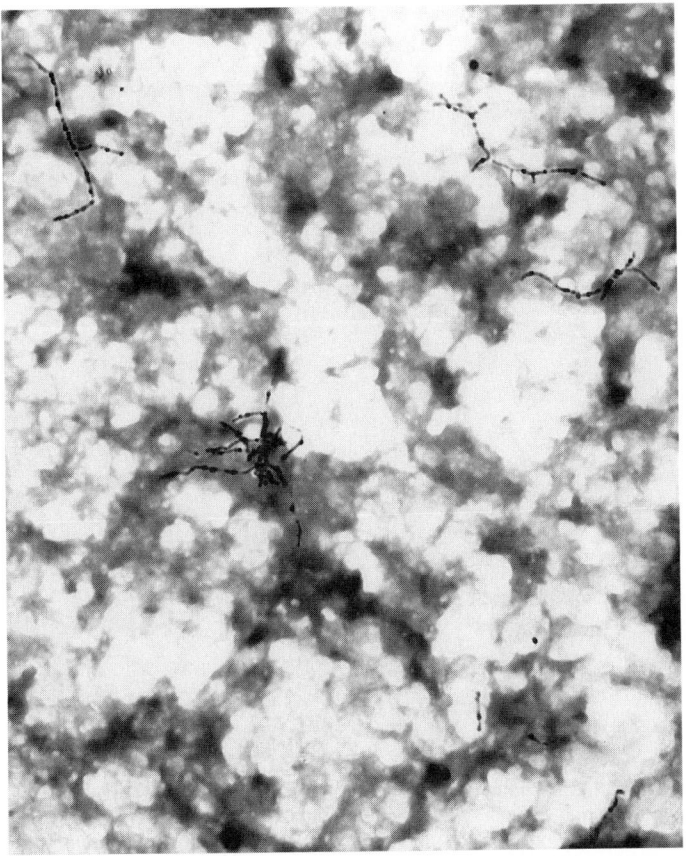

Figure 220.1. Gram stain of a sputum specimen obtained from a patient with *Nocardia asteroides* pneumonia (×1,000).

appears that there are virulence differences among the various *Nocardia* species (1–3,11,27,29,30). Although members of the *Nocardia asteroides* complex are the dominant pathogens in immunosuppressed patients, *N. brasiliensis* and its minocycline-resistant counterpart, *Nocardia pseudobrasiliensis* (11), cause predominantly primary cutaneous disease, mainly in immunocompetent individuals (1,25). The higher virulence of *N. brasiliensis* is also suggested in cases of animal footpad inoculation (25). Other less common species, such as *Nocardia nova*, *Nocardia farcinica*, *Nocardia otitidis-caviarum*, and *Nocardia transvaliensis*, can also cause severe infections (1,3,11,31,32). *N. farcinica* in particular has been recognized recently for its propensity for causing disseminated disease (1–3,11,33).

Efforts to clarify the host response to infection by *Nocardia* species have begun (1–3,11,27). In particular, the male predominance and animal infection by this organism have been seen (2,29). The reasons for this distribution are unclear, but it may be related to hormonal effects on the virulence and growth of *Nocardia* species. In addition, polymorphonuclear leukocytes alone are not sufficient to eradicate these organisms despite the fact that histologic examinations of infected tissues have revealed large numbers of them. Evidence now suggests that neutrophils may delay the growth of *Nocardia* species, allowing time for the recruitment and activation of macrophages. This delay involves both phagocytosis and temporary inhibition of filament formation (11,28). Furthermore, although the oxidative metabolic burst has not been shown to inhibit filament formation *in vitro*, the observation that patients with chronic granulomatous disease appear to be more susceptible to *Nocardia* infection suggests that another mechanism may be operative (34). However, cell-mediated immunity appears to be the most important host-defense mechanism against *Nocardia* infection (1–3,11). This mechanism begins with phagocytosis by macrophages and then lysosomal enzyme release, resulting in destruction of the organism. Virulent organisms appear to be more resistant to phagocytosis and better able both to inhibit the phagosome–lysosome fusion and produce catalase and superoxide dismutase, thus inactivating the myeloperoxidase system of those phagocytic cells (1–3,11,30).

CLINICAL MANIFESTATIONS

Nocardia infection is most commonly seen in the lung, where the organism causes acute, often necrotizing, pneumonia commonly associated with cavitation (1–3,11) (Fig. 220.2). Other presentations may include a slowly enlarging pulmonary nodule or pneumonia with an associated empyema. Infected patients are usually systemically ill, having fever, a cough, and weight loss. Additionally, pleuritic chest pain often precedes or accompanies the development of an empyema. The infection spreads by contiguous extension to involve the pericardium, resulting in suppurative pericarditis; the infection may progress slowly, however, thus mimicking a chronic granulomatous infection such as tuberculosis or a neoplastic disease such as bronchogenic carcinoma. It is unclear whether the presence of *Nocardia* could result in a self-limiting or subclinical pulmonary infection. Hence, isolation of *Nocardia* in the sputum of an asymptomatic patient who has a structural underlying lung disease, such as cavitary tuberculosis, cystic fibrosis, or emphysema, could cause diagnostic uncertainty because there are no reliable clinical criteria to differentiate colonization from early or subclinical infection (1,11).

Because of its propensity for hematogenous dissemination, *Nocardia* infection often produces metastatic spread, most commonly to the brain (Fig. 220.3) because *Nocardia* species have increased tropism for neuroinvasion (1,3,11). However, organs

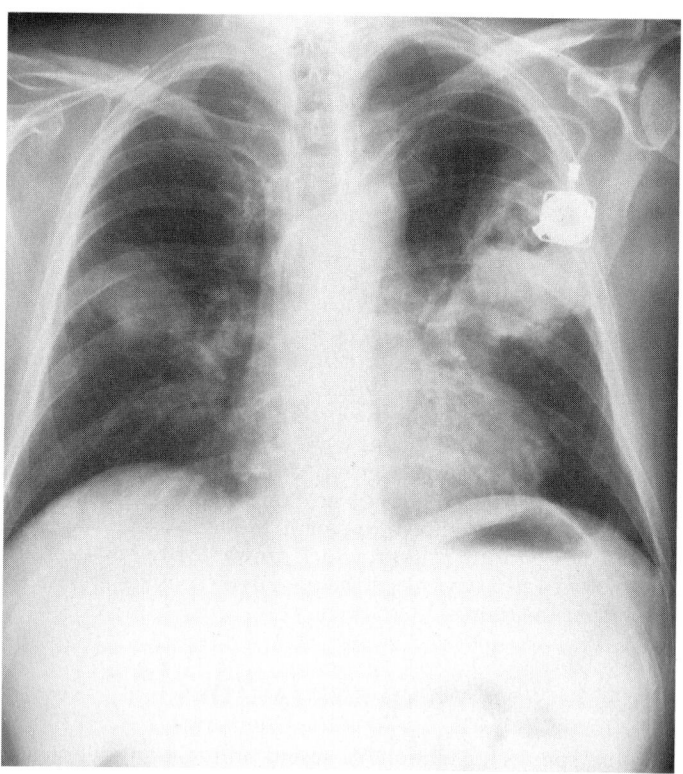

Figure 220.2. Cavitating pneumonia due to *Nocardia asteroides* in a chronic smoker.

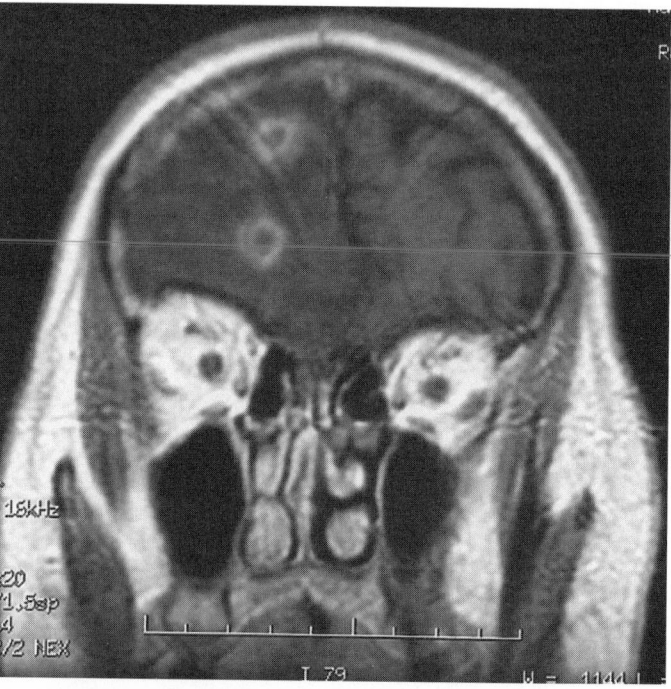

Figure 220.3. Computed tomography scan of the brain showing multiple ring-enhancing frontal-lobe abscesses with surrounding edema in a patient with chronic lymphocytic leukemia who had received fludarabine and steroids. A brain biopsy showed a multilobulated necrotic abscess. Stains confirmed the presence of filamentous branching organisms, and a culture grew *Nocardia asteroides*.

such as the kidneys, spleen, liver, thyroid, adrenal, prostate, testicles, and, rarely, bone may also be involved (1–3,11). The metastatic foci may be clinically silent early on, and patients may develop neurologic signs while receiving therapy for their pulmonary infection. Furthermore, it is believed that up to 55% of the cases of disseminated disease result in secondary central nervous system infection (1,2,6). Brain involvement most commonly consists of a solitary abscess or multiple abscesses. Severely immunocompromised patients who have central nervous system nocardiosis may have prolonged latency (up to 3 years) (1,9). However, nocardial meningitis is rare and typically occurs in the setting of evacuation of an abscess to a subarachnoid space.

Additionally, *Nocardia* infection can occur by direct inoculation through the skin (1–3). In the United States, most cases are due to *N. brasiliensis* and occur in southern states (25). Clinically, this infection appears as a chronically draining ulcerative lesion or slowly expanding nodule, often with minimal systemic symptoms. In addition, a sporotrichoid pattern of lesions has been seen (35). The infection may present as a mycetoma with sinus tracts, and occasionally, sulfur granules can be observed in the exudate. However, one should not always attribute a cutaneous lesion to inoculation because disseminated disease can result in secondary seeding of the skin (Fig. 220.4). Thus, all patients who have cutaneous nocardiosis, especially those who also have

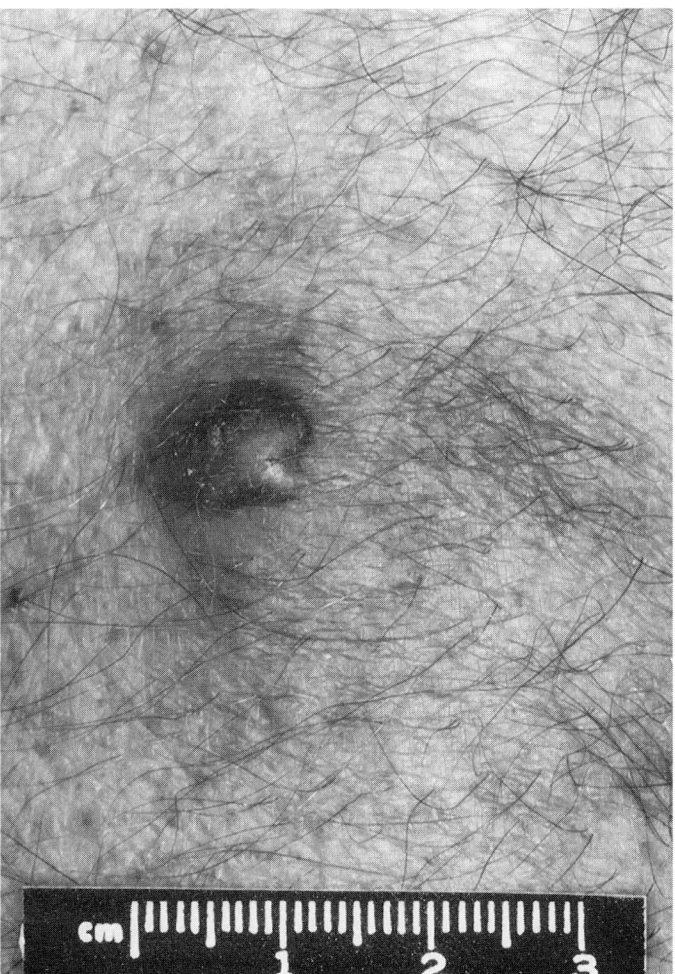

Figure 220.4. Skin lesion in a renal transplant recipient receiving chronic corticosteroids who developed a disseminated infection due to *Nocardia asteroides*.

immunosuppression, initially should be evaluated for disseminated disease. Similarly, *Nocardia* keratitis is the result of direct inoculation following trauma or cataract surgery and mimics fungal keratitis clinically (36).

Even though hematogenous dissemination must occur, isolation of *Nocardia* species from blood cultures is very rare (19). Bacteremic nocardiosis has been seen in patients who have prosthetic valve endocarditis or endovascular catheters or who are intravenous drug users. Conversely, not all cases of nocardial prosthetic valve endocarditis result in documented bacteremia (22). Thus, *Nocardia* infection can be a cause of culture-negative endocarditis. Isolation of *Nocardia* species from one of several blood cultures from a patient who has no endovascular foreign bodies or signs of sepsis or pneumonia probably represents a contaminant.

DIAGNOSIS

Nocardia species are easily missed upon direct examination of clinical samples (1–3,11). A Gram stain of secretions from the infected area provides useful clues, however, because it alerts one early on to the possibility of infection due to *Nocardia* species. Because these organisms grow slowly, the microbiology laboratory should be alerted to their possible presence so that the culture plates will be held for 7 to 10 days. This is important because *Nocardia* species grouped in pure colonies appear after only 48 hours of incubation. Therefore, in mixed infections or contaminated clinical specimens, overgrowth of more rapidly growing bacteria could obscure the small *Nocardia* colonies. In culture, *Nocardia* colonies are chalky and raised, varying in color from white to pink to orange; they are also crumbly and have a characteristic odor. Furthermore, the colonies have a cotton-ball–like appearance owing to the presence of delicate filamentous structures. This macroscopic characteristic is helpful in distinguishing them from mycobacteria and other nocardioform bacteria, such as *Rhodococcus*, *Gordona*, and *Corynebacterium* species (1,2). Finally, the Grocott-Gomori methenamine-silver nitrate and Giemsa stains show these organisms well histologically, but the hematoxylin-eosin and periodic acid–Schiff stains do not.

Nocardia species can grow in a variety of blood culture media; moreover, the average incubation time in positive blood cultures is often relatively short. Therefore, if *Nocardia* endocarditis is suspected, recovery of the *Nocardia* species should be optimized by modifying the routine blood culture procedures, for example, using the Bactec system with an incubation period beyond the usual 5 days and with frequent, terminal subculturing (19).

Finally, serologic diagnosis of nocardiosis has been hampered by a lack of suitable antigens and cross-reactivity with related organisms, such as actinomycetes, rhodococci, and mycobacteria. Even though serology is not currently a clinically useful tool, progress has been made in that area recently (27).

SPECIATION AND SUSCEPTIBILITY TESTING OF *NOCARDIA* SPECIES ORGANISMS

Species identification can be accomplished using a combination of morphologic tests, hydrolysis, and a variety of biochemical tests (1–3,11). Additional species have been characterized by their antimicrobial resistance patterns, thus giving rise to use of the term *N. asteroides* complex (11) (Table 220.2). This heterogeneous group of microorganisms consists of *N. asteroides* sensu stricto, *N. nova*, and *N. farcinica*, the last of which appears

TABLE 220.2.   *In Vitro* Antimicrobial Susceptibility of the *Nocardia asteroides* Complex

Drug	*Nocardia asteroides*	*Nocardia farcinica*	*Nocardia nova*
Cefotaxime	S	R	S
Imipenem	S	R	S
Erythromycin	R	R	S
Ampicillin	V	R	S
Amikacin	S	S	S
Minocycline	S	V	S

S, sensitive; V, variable sensitivity; R, resistant.

to be a highly virulent species because it is often seen with disseminated infection and is characteristically resistant to cefotaxime, tobramycin, and erythromycin (1–3,11). Additionally, the latter two species may make up 10% to 20% of the *N. asteroides* complex. However, the routine *Nocardia* identification procedures used in the clinical laboratory are time-consuming and not always reliable. Therefore, new rapid molecular diagnostic techniques, such as polymerase chain reaction amplification of the 16S ribosomal gene and restriction endonuclease analysis are being introduced to clinical practice (38,39).

Susceptibility testing is important in both guiding therapy and differentiating between members of the *N. asteroides* complex (1,3,11,40–46). Because primary drug resistance is an important reason for treatment failure, significant clinical isolates should be tested for antibiotic susceptibility, thus allowing rational alternative drug selection. Susceptibility testing is also important because of the expected long duration of therapy for nocardiosis and possibility of intolerance of the initial drug used. However, susceptibility testing of *Nocardia* species is not yet standardized due to a lack of bactericidal end points and differences in the media and inocula used. Furthermore, no studies have systematically correlated *in vitro* susceptibility with clinical outcomes in this frequently chronic infection (1,3,11,44). Therefore, the National Committee for Clinical Laboratory Standards recently published a working document to standardize susceptibility testing of *Nocardia* species using a broth microdilution method (47). Also, it has been recommended that clinical isolates be sent to a reference laboratory for optimal susceptibility testing (11,41).

DIFFERENTIAL DIAGNOSIS

Because nocardiosis can progress rapidly in immunocompromised patients, it should be considered in the differential diagnosis of acute pulmonary infections in these patients. Pulmonary nocardiosis can result in a gradually progressive indolent process and may mimic tuberculosis, fungal disease, *Rhodococcus equi* pneumonia, sarcoidosis, and malignancy (1). To complicate the issue further, other copathogens, such as mycobacteria (e.g., tuberculosis and atypical mycobacteria) and invasive molds, have been described in a subset of immunosuppressed patients who have pulmonary nocardiosis (1,10). Additionally, cutaneous nocardiosis should be considered in the differential diagnosis of lymphocutaneous syndrome caused by organisms such as *Sporothrix schenckii*, *Francisella tularensis*, *Mycobacterium chelonei*, *Mycobacterium marinum*, and *Leishmania brasiliensis* (35). Regarding the central nervous system, nocardiosis in the differential diagnosis is similarly broad, including brain abscesses caused by pyogenic bacteria, fungi, and mycobacteria (1–3,11). Finally, because bacteremic nocardiosis

may develop after prolonged hospitalization for other infectious problems (19), one should consider *Nocardia* infection in the differential diagnosis of aerobic gram-positive bacteremia and not dismiss such cases as contaminants due to *Corynebacterium* species.

TREATMENT

The mainstay of therapy for nocardiosis has been the sulfonamides (1–3,11,41,45,46). Despite the suboptimal correlation of the *in vitro* susceptibility testing with outcome, the response of *Nocardia* infection to sulfonamide therapy is generally very good. However, evaluation of optimal therapy using sulfonamides as well as alternative regimens (41) either alone or in combination is hampered by the small number and heterogeneity of cases. The optimal duration of therapy is not well defined for the same reasons.

There is usually good clinical improvement in a patient with nocardiosis within 7 to 10 days after the initiation of therapy. However, the route of administration depends on the patient's overall clinical status. In patients receiving a sulfa-based regimen, it has been customary to measure blood levels of the drug at least once early on to be sure that the patient is absorbing the recommended doses of the drug; if necessary, the dosage should be adjusted to achieve a blood level of 100 to 150 μg/mL about 2 hours after administration of an oral dose. This may be particularly important in patients who have unreliable gastrointestinal absorption and in those who do not have a clinical response to an oral sulfa-based regimen. Although TMP-SMX has been used in many cases, good evidence that it is more effective than sulfonamides alone does not exist.

For *Nocardia* strains that are clinically resistant to sulfonamides and for patients who develop toxic effects of or intolerance to sulfonamides, a number of acceptable alternative therapies are available (Table 220.3). For example, minocycline, a potent tetracycline analog, has excellent *in vitro* efficacy against most *Nocardia* strains and has been shown to be clinically effective. Minocycline is also more active than doxycycline (1,11,48,49). Specifically, in patients who do not develop dizziness or vertigo, it is a good alternative form of therapy.

In addition, in patients who are acutely ill, have acute toxic effects, or are severely immunocompromised and require bactericidal therapy for rapid control of their infection, imipenem and cefotaxime have been shown to be effective (41). Synergism has been shown *in vitro* and in animal models when these two agents are used together, even though the difference is probably not significant compared with using imipenem alone (50). Also, amikacin, an aminoglycoside, has been shown to have very potent activity against *Nocardia* infection *in vitro* (51) and may be used in combination with imipenem or cefotaxime until the

TABLE 220.3. Therapy for *Nocardia* Species Infection

Drug	Dosage	Duration	Side effects
Sulfisoxazole	2 g q6h	6 mo	Rash, fever, leukopenia, crystalluria
Trimethoprim-sulfamethoxazole	1 double-strength tablet b.i.d.	6 mo	Rash fever, leukopenia, *Candida* species infection
Minocycline	100 mg b.i.d.	6 mo	Dizziness, rash
Imipenem-cilastatin[a]	500 mg i.v. q6h	Until change to oral therapy	Rash, seizures with high blood levels
Cefotaxime[a]	1 g i.v. q8h	Until change to oral therapy	Rash
Amikacin[a]	7.5 mg/kg i.v. q12h	Until change to oral therapy	Nephrotoxicity, eighth cranial nerve toxicity

[a]Shows *in vitro* synergism.

patient shows clinical improvement (41). However, it is important to remember the varying susceptibility of the *N. asteroides* complex and to watch carefully the patient's response to therapy. Finally, linezolid, an oxazolidinone, was recently shown to have potent *in vitro* activity against a variety of *Nocardia* species (52). Even though further clinical data are lacking, this drug shows promise as an alternative therapeutic agent, especially against multiresistant *Nocardia* isolates.

When a patient with nocardiosis remains febrile while receiving therapy, the possible causes include a resistant isolate, drug-induced fever, a sequestered abscess that may require drainage, or even a second opportunistic pathogen. Furthermore, because of the tendency for relapses to occur, a therapy duration of at least 12 months is appropriate for disseminated bacteremic disease, especially in patients who have continued immunosuppression. Finally, removal of infected endovascular foreign bodies in the treatment of endovascular *Nocardia* infections and drainage of abscess collections are crucial determinants of a successful outcome.

Finally, the data regarding prophylaxis in patients at high risk for nocardiosis are scant. In one study, intermittent use of TMP-SMX did not appear to protect bone marrow transplant recipients (10).

PROGNOSIS

An average mortality rate as high as 44% has been reported in patients with disseminated nocardiosis (1,53). However, among severely immunocompromised patients, mortality rates as high as 85% have been reported in those with the disseminated form of the disease (1). In addition, because of comorbid underlying illnesses in many patients with *Nocardia* bacteremia, it is difficult to define mortality attributable to the *Nocardia* infection itself without performing matched-control comparisons. Finally, acute disease and involvement of two or more noncontiguous organs carry a poor prognosis (1,53).

REFERENCES

1. McNeil MM, Brown JM. The medically important aerobic actinomycetes: epidemiology and microbiology. *Clin Microbiol Rev* 1994;7:357–417.
2. Beaman BL, Saubolle MA, Wallace RJ. *Nocardia, Rhodococcus, Streptomyces, Oerskovia* and other aerobic actinomycetes of medical importance. In: Murray PR, Baron EJ, Pfaller MA, et al., eds. *Manual of clinical microbiology,* 6th ed. Washington, DC: American Society for Microbiology, 1995.
3. Lerner PI. Nocardiosis. *Clin Infect Dis* 1996;22:891–905.
4. Blumel J, Blumel E, Yasdsin AF, et al. Typing of *Nocardia farcinica* by pulsed-field gel electrophoresis reveals an endemic strain as source of hospital infections. *J Clin Microbiol* 1998;36:118–122.
5. Louie L, Louie M, Simor AE. Investigation of a pseudo-outbreak of *Nocardia asteroides* infection by pulsed-field gel electrophoresis and randomly amplified polymorphic DNA PCR. *J Clin Microbiol* 1997;35:1582–1584.
6. Beaman BL, Burnside J, Edwards B, et al. Nocardial infections in the United States, 1972–1974. *J Infect Dis* 1974;134:286–289.
7. Curry WA. Human nocardiosis: a clinical review with selected case reports. *Arch Intern Med* 1980;140:818–826.
8. Wilson JP, Turner HR, Kirchner KA, et al. Nocardial infections in renal transplant recipients. *Medicine* (Baltimore) 1989;68:38–57.
9. Simpson GL, Stinson EB, Egger MJ, et al. Nocardial infections in the immunocompromised host: a detailed study in a defined population. *Rev Infect Dis* 1981;3:492–507.
10. Choucino C, Goodman SA, Greer JP, et al. Nocardial infections in bone marrow transplant recipients. *Clin Infect Dis* 1996;23:1012–1019.
11. Sorrell TC, Iredell JR, Mitchell DH. *Nocardia* species. In: Mandell GL, Bennett JE, Dolin R, eds. *Mandell, Douglas and Bennett's principles and practice of infectious diseases,* 5th ed. Philadelphia: Churchill Livingstone, 2000:2637–2645.
12. Berkey P, Bodey GP. Nocardial infection in patients with neoplastic diseases. *Rev Infect Dis* 1989;11:407–412.
13. Torres HA, Reddy BT, Raad II, et al. Nocardiosis in cancer patients. *Medicine* (Baltimore) 2002;81:388–397.
14. Samonis G, Kontoyiannis DP. Infectious complications of purine analog therapy: an update. *Curr Opin Infect Dis* 2001;14:409–413.
15. Holtz HA, Lavery DP, Kapila R. Actinomycetales infection in acquired immunodeficiency syndrome. *Ann Intern Med* 1992;102:203–205.
16. Javaly K, Horowitz HW, Wormser GP. Nocardiosis in patients with human immunodeficiency virus infection: report of 2 cases and review of the literature. *Medicine* (Baltimore) 1992;71:128–138.
17. Kim J, Minamoto GY, Grieco MH. Nocardial infection as a complication of AIDS: report of six cases and review. *Rev Infect Dis* 1991;13:624–629.
18. Uttamchandani RB, Daikos GL, Reyes RR, et al. Nocardiosis in 30 patients with advanced human immunodeficiency virus infection: clinical features and outcome. *Clin Infect Dis* 1994;18:348–353.
19. Kontoyiannis DP, Ruoff K, Hooper DC. Nocardia bacteremia: report of four cases and review. *Medicine* (Baltimore) 1998;77:255–267.
20. Vanderstrigel M, Leclercq R, Brun-Buisson C, et al. Blood-borne pulmonary infection with *Nocardia asteroides* in a heroin addict. *J Clin Microbiol* 1986;23:175–176.
21. Kontoyiannis DP, Jacobson K, Whimbey E, et al. Central venous catheter-associated *Nocardia* bacteremia: an unusual manifestation of nocardiosis. *Clin Infect Dis* 2000;31:617–618.
22. Falk RH, Dimock FR, Sharkey J. Prosthetic valve endocarditis resulting from *Nocardia asteroides.* *Br Heart J* 1979;41:125–127.
23. Patterson JE, Chapin-Robertson K, Waycott S, et al. Pseudoepidemic of *Nocardia asteroides* associated with a mycobacterial culture system. *J Clin Microbiol* 1992;320:1357–1360.
24. Bates RR, Rifkind D. *Nocardia brasiliensis* lymphocutaneous syndrome. *Am J Dis Child* 1971;121:246–247.
25. Smego RA, Gallis HA. The clinical spectrum of *Nocardia brasiliensis* infection in the United States. *Rev Infect Dis* 1984;6:164–180.
26. Cremades MJ, Menendez R, Santos M, et al. Repeated pulmonary infection by *Nocardia asteroides* complex in a patient with bronchiectasis. *Respiration* 1998;65:211–213.
27. Beaman BL, Beaman L. *Nocardia* species: host-parasite relationships. *Clin Microbiol Rev* 1994;7:213–264.

28. Filice GA. Inhibition of *Nocardia asteroides* by neutrophils. *J Infect Dis* 1985;151: 47–56.

29. Beaman BL, Sugar AM. *Nocardia* in naturally acquired and experimental animals. *J Hyg* (Lond) 1983;91:393–419.

30. Black CM, Beauman BL, Donovan RM, et al. Effect of virulent and less virulent strains of *Nocardia asteroides* on acid phosphatase activity in alveolar and peritoneal macrophages maintained in vitro. *J Infect Dis* 1983;148:117–124.

31. Causey W. *Nocardia caviae*: a report of 13 new isolations with clinical correlation. *Appl Microbiol* 1974;28:193–198.

32. Wallace RJ Jr, Brown BA, Tsukamura M, et al. Clinical and laboratory features of *Nocardia nova*. *J Clin Microbiol* 1991;29:2407–2417.

33. Peters BR, Saubolle MA, Costantino JM. Disseminated and cerebral infection due to *Nocardia farcinica*: diagnosis by blood culture and cure with antibiotics alone. *Clin Infect Dis* 1996;23:1165–1167.

34. Idriss ZH, Cunningham RJ, Wilfert CM. Nocardiosis in children: report of three cases and review of the literature. *Pediatrics* 1975;55:479–484.

35. Smego RA Jr, Castiglia M, Asperilla MO. Lymphocutaneous syndrome: a review of non-sporothrix causes. *Medicine* (Baltimore) 1999;78:38–63.

36. Rao SK, Madhavan HN, Sitalakshmi G, et al. *Nocardia asteroides* keratitis: report of seven patients and literature review. *Indian J Ophthalmol* 2000;38:217–221.

37. Sugar AM, Schoolnik GK, Stevens DA. Antibody response in human nocardiosis: identification of two immunodominant culture-filtrate antigens derived from *Nocardia asteroides*. *J Infect Dis* 1985;151:895–901.

38. Laurent FJ, Provost F, Boiron P. Rapid identification of clinically relevant *Nocardia* species to genus level by 16S rRNA gene PCR. *J Clin Microbiol* 1999;37:99–102.

39. Conville PS, Fischer SH, Cartwright CP, et al. Identification of *Nocardia* species by restriction endonuclease analysis of an amplified portion of the 16S rRNA gene. *J Clin Microbiol* 2000;38:158–164.

40. Wallace RJ Jr, Tsukamura M, Brown BA, et al. Cefotazime-resistant *Nocardia asteroides* strains are isolates of the controversial species *Nocardia farcinica*. *J Clin Microbiol* 1990;28:2726–2732.

41. Threlkeld SC, Hooper DC. Update on management of patients with Nocardia infection. In: Remington J, Swartz M, eds. *Current topics in infectious diseases,* Vol 17. New York: McGraw-Hill, 1997:1–23.

42. Gombert ME. Susceptibility of *Nocardia asteroides* to various antibiotics, including newer β-lactams, trimethoprim-sulfamethoxazole, amikacin and N-formimidoyl thienamycin. *Antimicrob Agents Chemother* 1982;21:1011.

43. Gutmann L, Goldstein FW, Kitzis MD, et al. Susceptibility of *Nocardia asteroides* to 46 antibiotics including 22 β-lactams. *Antimicrob Agents Chemother* 1983;23:248–252.

44. Wallace RJ, Steele LC. Susceptibility testing of *Nocardia* species for the clinical laboratory. *Diagn Microbiol Infect Dis* 1988;9:155–166.

45. Palmer DL, Harvey RL, Wheeler JK. Diagnostic and therapeutic considerations in *Nocardia asteroides* infection. *Medicine* (Baltimore) 1974;53:391–401.

46. Filice GA, Simpson GL. Management of *Nocardia* infections. In: Remington JS, Swartz MN, eds. *Current clinical topics in infectious diseases,* Vol 5. New York: McGraw-Hill, 1984:49–64.

47. National Committee for Clinical Laboratory Standards. Susceptibility testing of Mycobacteria, Nocardia, and other aerobic Actinomycetes, 2nd ed. Tentative standard M24-T2. Wayne, PA: National Committee for Clinical Laboratory Standards, 2000.

48. Bach MC, Gold O, Finland M. Activity of minocycline against *Nocardia asteroides*: comparison with tetracycline in agar-dilution and standard disc diffusion tests and with sulfadiazine in an experimental infection of mice. *J Lab Clin Med* 1973;81:787–793.

49. Petersen EA, Nash ML, Mammana RB, et al. Minocycline treatment of pulmonary nocardiosis. *JAMA* 1983;250:930–932.

50. Gombert ME, Aulicino TM. Synergism of imipenem and amikacin in combination with other antibiotics against *Nocardia asteroides*. *Antimicrob Agents Chemother* 1983;24:810–811.

51. Wallace RJ, Septimus E, Musher DM, et al. Treatment of experimental nocardiosis in mice: comparison of amikacin and sulfonamide. *J Infect Dis* 1979;140:244–248.

52. Brown-Elliott BA, Ward SC, Crist CJ, et al. In vitro activities of linezolid against multiple *Nocardia* species. *Antimicrob Agents Chemother* 2000;45:1295–1297.

53. Presant CA, Wiernik PH, Serpick AA. Factors affecting survival in nocardiosis. *Am Rev Respir Dis* 1973;108:1444–1448.

CHAPTER 221

Agents of Actinomycosis

John G. Bartlett

Actinomycosis is a relatively unusual infection caused primarily by higher bacteria from the genus *Actinomyces*. The most commonly recognized form is cervicofacial actinomycosis, but multiple other anatomic sites may be involved as well. Clinical features include a chronic, often woody-hard induration that forms external sinuses that drain characteristic "sulfur granules" (grains) and spreads to contiguous sites without regard to anatomic barriers. The term *actinomycosis* is derived from the Greek *aktinos*, in reference to radiating organisms in the sulfur granule, and *mykes*, indicating fungus. Thus, the term indicates "ray fungus" on the basis of the erroneous impression that this was a mycotic infection. Actinomycetes are microaerophilic or anaerobic bacteria found primarily as part of the endogenous flora of the mouth. Infection involving any of the six agents of actinomycosis is characterized by terms based on anatomic location: cervicofacial, thoracic, abdominal, pelvic, musculoskeletal, central nervous system, or disseminated. Nearly all infections involve companion bacteria to the agents of actinomycosis, especially *Actinobacillus actinomycetemcomitans* (so named because of this association), oral *Bacteroides* and *Prevotella* species, fusobacteria, streptococci, and *Eikenella corrodens*. The specific associated organisms depend to a large extent on the anatomic site of the lesion and the normal flora of the adjacent mucosal surface.

HISTORY

The first possible case is traced to circa AD 230 (1,2), but the best descriptions begin with Bollinger (3), who reported *Actinomyces bovis* as the cause of "lumpy jaw" in cattle in 1877. This investigator was responsible for the appellation *actinomyces* (ray fungus) based on the microscopic appearance of granules from tongue lesions (4). Actinomycosis in patients was first described by Israel (5) in 1879. In 1891, Wolff and Israel successfully cultivated the anaerobe that was subsequently named *Actinomyces israelii*. For a long time, *A. bovis* and *A. israelii* were considered identical bacteria isolated from two different host species, but it is now recognized that they are distinctive (6). *A. bovis* has not been found in humans, although *A. israelii* has been found in cattle (7). Wolff and Israel (8) postulated the endogenous infection theory on the basis of the observation that the putative agent was a delicate anaerobe found only in animals or humans and never in nature. The opposing theory postulated by Bostroem in 1890 was that *Actinomyces* was found in nature, primarily on grass and grains (7). This led to the misconception that chewing grass or straw was the cause of cervicofacial actinomycosis, and this represented an occupational hazard to farmers. The evidence in favor of an endogenous source of *Actinomyces* was well supported, especially with the work by Wright (9) in 1905, and is now generally accepted.

EPIDEMIOLOGY

Actinomycosis is a relatively rare infection. The number of annual reported deaths from the disease in the United States from 1930 to 1936 was about 60 (10). The annual incidence during the antibiotic era has been estimated at 1 per 100,000 population in the Netherlands (11) and 1 per 300,000 population in Cleveland (12). The disease is worldwide in distribution with equal frequency in urban and rural dwellers. There is an unexplained 3:1 ratio of infected men to women (12–18); the obvious exception is pelvic actinomycosis. Most cases are seen in adolescents and middle-aged adults. *Actinomyces* becomes a component of the normal oral flora at about 3 years of age, and *Actinomyces* in younger children is rare (19). The most common form of actinomycosis is cervicofacial, followed by thoracic and abdominal (1,7,13–18). The frequency of pelvic actinomycosis is related to usage rates of intrauterine contraceptive devices (IUDs), and its frequency depends to a large extent on criteria used for this diagnosis.

MICROBIAL AGENTS OF ACTINOMYCOSIS

The agents of actinomycosis include *A. israelii*, *Actinomyces naeslundii*, *Actinomyces odontolyticus*, *Actinomyces viscosus*, *Actinomyces meyeri*, and *Propionibacterium propionicum* (previously classified as *Arachnia propionica*) (1,19–24). *Actinomyces pyogenes* (*Corynebacterium pyogenes*) has also been proposed as an agent of actinomycosis (25). The most frequent is *A. israelii*; less frequent in rank order are *P. propionicum*, *A. naeslundii*, *A. viscosus*, *A. odontolyticus*, and *A. meyeri* (26). All grow best in anaerobic conditions at 37°C with the exception of *A. viscosus*, which grows aerobically. These organisms are slow-growing, gram-positive, branching bacilli (Fig. 221.1A). A selective medium containing mupirocin and metronidazole facilitates recovery of *Actinomyces* species from specimens with a mixed flora (27). All are normally present in the oral flora, including the gingival crevice, dental plaque, and tonsillar crypts; they are less frequently found as a component of the colonic flora and are found in the vaginal flora of 5% of women without an IUD (7).

A. israelii grows optimally under anaerobic conditions, but many strains are microaerophilic. Mature colonies, after 5 to 10 days of incubation, show large, white, rough colonies giving a characteristic "molar tooth" appearance (Fig. 221.1B). The organisms appear as gram-positive filaments, sometimes with branching in early lesions. Late lesions usually show the characteristic features of sulfur granules. *P. propionicum* appears identical to *A. israelii* on Gram stain, resembles this organism biochemically, and was originally named *Actinomyces propionicus*. Colonies are smoother and not molar tooth in character. This organism was assigned to a distinct genus, *Arachnia*, in 1969 (26) and has more

recently been reclassified as *P. propionicum* (1). *A. naeslundii* is found in virtually all forms of actinomycosis; it grows both anaerobically and in microaerophilic conditions and is more likely to show free filamentous forms in tissue (26). *A. viscosus* grows well aerobically, is a prominent component of dental plaque, and has primarily been associated with orodental and thoracic infections. *A. odontolyticus* has been involved in all forms of actinomycosis but less frequently than the other species noted. *A. meyeri* is a relatively recent addition to the agents of actinomycosis and is a relatively infrequent cause of disease (23). *A. pyogenes* is a proposed agent (25), but this is not yet clearly accepted (1).

There are other diverse organisms within the genera *Actinomyces* that are periodically encountered in diverse infections, but usually not infections with the characteristic features of actinomycosis. A review of 294 *Actinomyces*-like organisms that proved difficult to identify showed that 128 could be speciated (28). Most were *Actinomyces turicensis*; less common were *Actinomyces radingae* and *Actinomyces europeus*. *A. turicensis* proved relatively easy to identify and was found most frequently in genital infections, followed by urinary tract infections and skin infections. *Actinomyces bernardiae*, *Actinomyces neuii*, and *Actinomyces funkei* are additional species occasionally found in clinical specimens (29–33). Phylogenic analysis of these organisms indicates an urgent need for taxonomic revision and requires subdivision into several genera (34). This includes the proposal to reassign *A. bernardiae* and *A. pyogenes* to the species *Actinomyces reanobacterium*.

PATHOLOGY AND PATHOGENESIS

The characteristic feature of actinomycosis is disruption of the mucosal barrier to permit entry of normal flora. Common associated conditions for cervicofacial lesions are dental disease, jaw trauma, and oral surgery; for abdominal infections, the usual associated conditions are surgery, other inflammatory conditions of the gut, and foreign bodies. In thoracic actinomycosis, the presumed pathogenic mechanism is aspiration. With pelvic infections, the usual associated condition is IUD use. In many cases, the predisposing event is in the remote past because of the indolent nature of actinomycosis. One of the most striking examples illustrating this point is the case of abdominal actinomycosis in Jerry Kramer, the all-pro guard of the Super Bowl champion Green Bay Packers football team. As related in his autobiography *Instant Replay*, he presented to training camp with enigmatic

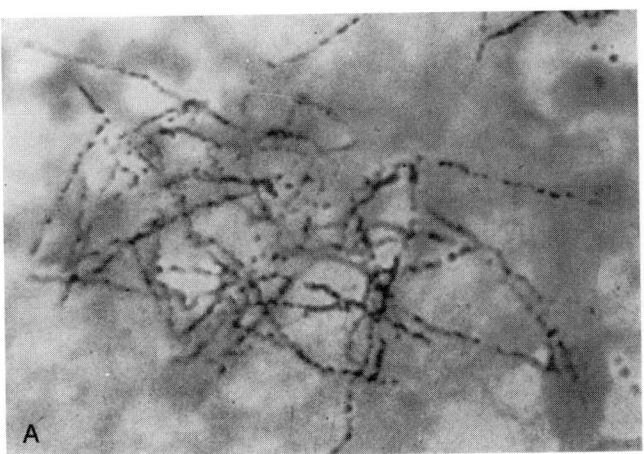
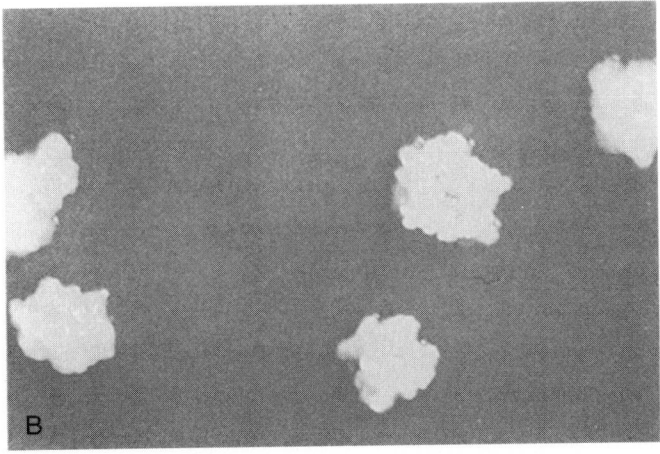

Figure 221.1. A: Gram-stain appearance of agents of actinomycosis: branching "beaded" gram-positive bacilli. **B:** Colonies of *Actinomyces israelii* showing the molar tooth appearance.

fevers, abdominal pain, and an abdominal mass; laparotomy showed an indurated, inflammatory mass with a wood splinter in the center that was traced to penetrating abdominal trauma 20 years previously (35).

Nearly all cases are polymicrobial, and some think that synergy is an essential component of pathogenesis (11,36). This issue is not trivial because of the implications regarding selection of antimicrobial agents. The most frequent companions reflect, to a large extent, the site of infection. Most frequent are *A. actinomycetemcomitans*, various anaerobic bacteria (*Bacteroides, Prevotella, Fusobacterium,* and *Peptostreptococcus*), *E. corrodens, Haemophilus* species, aerobic and microaerophilic streptococci, staphylococci, and (in abdominal actinomycosis) Enterobacteriaceae.

Although the association with a breach in the mucosal integrity is common, there may be an important role for foreign bodies. This is most striking with the IUD-associated form of actinomycosis but has also been seen with fish bones in the abdomen, 12 root fillings (37,38), and wire sutures (39).

Actinomycosis is not clearly associated with the immunocompromised state. Occasional cases are reported in patients with human immunodeficiency virus infection (40–43) or in patients receiving corticosteroids (17), but these are unusual. This is in distinct contrast to *Nocardia*, which resembles the agents of actinomycosis morphologically. The family Actinomycetaceae previously included both aerobic and anaerobic strains. The aerobic nocardioform actinomycetes have subsequently been placed in the genus *Nocardia* and now constitute the family Nocardiaceae (44). Nocardiosis resembles actinomycosis, but the putative agent is aerobic; the infection is clearly associated with the immunocompromised state, is usually exogenously acquired, is usually monomicrobial, and is treated with completely different antimicrobial agents (Table 221.1).

Actinomycosis is characterized by an acute inflammatory phase of infection that may be associated with pain, erythema, edema, and tenderness as with other common infections of soft tissue. More frequently, the disease is indolent with gradual evolution over a period of weeks, months, or even years. The early lesion may be soft and fluctuant with central suppuration (Fig. 221.1). With maturation, the lesion becomes extremely fibrous, which gives it a "wooden" character. With cervicofacial actinomycosis, the acute inflammatory phase of the disease may appear similar to other types of acute soft tissue infections along the mandible. The more characteristic indurated, woody-hard

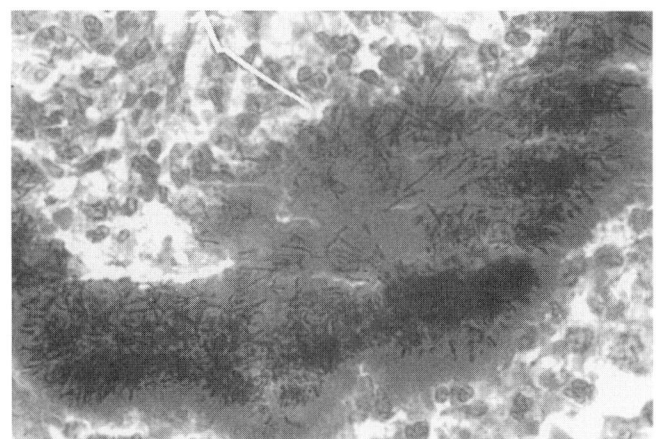

Figure 221.2. Sulfur granule or grain showing amorphous material with a rosette of filamentous radiating gram-positive bacilli.

lesion is often mistaken for a neoplasm. Highly characteristic is the formation of sinus tracts that often drain sulfur granules (in reference to the macroscopic, hard, yellow particles that resemble elemental sulfur particles previously used in pharmaceuticals) (7). Microscopic examination of typical lesions shows an outer zone of fibrous tissue and central foci of acute inflammation with polymorphonuclear cells. The sulfur granules consist of an amorphic central area surrounded with a rosette of filamentous organisms that often show branching (Fig. 221.2). Most lesions show multiple loculations of suppuration with intervening granulation tissue that shows collagen fibers, fibroblasts, lymphocytes, and occasionally multinucleated giant cells (45).

DIAGNOSIS

The diagnosis of actinomycosis is based on the typical clinical features of this disease, preferably combined with recovery of an agent of actinomycosis. Clinical features include an indolent progressive inflammatory mass with sinus tracts, fistulae, fever, leukocytosis, weight loss, and elevated erythrocyte sedimentation rate. The recovery of an agent of actinomycosis may be

TABLE 221.1. Comparison of Actinomycosis and Nocardiosis

Parameter	Actinomycosis	Nocardiosis
Agents	*Actinomyces israelii, Actinomyces naeslundii, Actinomyces odontolyticus, Actinomyces viscosus, Actinomyces meyeri, Propionibacterium propionicum*	*Nocardia asteroides*
Culture	Anaerobic (except *A. viscosus*)	Aerobic
Gram stain	Thin, branching, gram-positive bacilli	Thin, branching, gram-positive bacilli
Modified acid-fast stain	Negative	Positive
Source	Mouth, colon, genital tract	Soil
Host	Usually previously healthy young adult	Immunocompromised, especially reduced cell-mediated immunity
Pathophysiologic process	Endogenous infection starting in oral cavity, lung (aspiration), abdomen, or genital tract	Pneumonia presumably by inhalation; dissemination to extrapulmonary sites
Characteristic of infection	Indurated, draining sinuses, sulfur granules, penetration through tissue	No sulfur granules, penetration through tissue is unusual
Course	Indolent, chronic	Acute, subacute, or asymptomatic

difficult to achieve owing to the fastidious growth requirements of actinomycetes and *P. propionica*. These organisms may be particularly difficult to recover in the presence of antibiotic exposure. An alternative is identification of the specific species by immunofluorescent stains. Species-specific antisera conjugated with fluorescein are available for the four major species of *Actinomyces* and for *P. propionicum* (46,47). Cultivation of an agent of actinomycosis or its detection with fluorescent antibody stain is most meaningful with sulfur granules or in a specimen from a normally sterile site (48). These organisms are components of the normal flora; hence, recovery from specimens subject to contamination, such as expectorated sputum, bronchoscopy aspirates, genital tract specimens, and swabs from the oral cavity, is meaningless (49). Gram stains of lesions show filamentous, gram-positive bacilli that often show branching. Among gram-positive bacilli, *Actinomyces* and *Nocardia* are the only organisms that show branching in tissue.

Sulfur granules are pathognomonic when they are recovered from a typical lesion other than on tonsils (1). These may be microscopic or macroscopic concretions consisting of a mineralized mass with calcium phosphate and radiating filamentous organisms on the surface (50). The granules may drain through sinus tracts and may be seen on covering bandages. Exudate placed on a vertical glass often shows granules adherent to the glass. Sulfur granules may also be seen in microabscesses.

Other infections that may be associated with the production of granules are mycetoma and botryomycosis. Botryomycosis is a chronic bacterial infection of soft tissue caused by *Staphylococcus aureus*, streptococcus, and selected gram-negative bacilli. These organisms and the fungal agents of mycetoma show distinctive morphologic characteristics with Gram stain. A possible exception is *Nocardia* when it is responsible for mycetoma because this organism may be indistinguishable from *Actinomyces* with Gram stain. The distinction may be made with immunofluorescent staining for the agents of actinomycosis or by the Fite-modified acid-fast stain to detect *Nocardia*.

Nocardiosis may resemble actinomycosis with clinical features that include an indolent course with indurated lesions that progresses without respect to anatomic boundaries. Tuberculosis may occasionally show these features as well. Visceral forms of nocardiosis do not have granules, but these may be seen with the mycetoma form of nocardiosis. Other characteristic features of nocardiosis are summarized in Table 221.1.

Granules, when identified, should be washed and crushed between slides for examination using Gram stain and immunofluorescent stains.

Cervicofacial and Oral Actinomycosis

Cervicofacial and oral actinomycosis is the most frequently recognized form of actinomycosis and accounts for about 50% of reported cases (1). Cervicofacial actinomycosis should be considered in any acute, subacute, or chronic infection involving the head and neck. The most frequent presentation is a soft tissue swelling that progresses slowly without regard to tissue planes and without involvement of adjacent lymph nodes (Fig. 221.3). Polar extremes include, at one end, a painless, indurated, slowly expanding lesion, often with a bluish hue, along the mandible or neck that may suggest neoplasm; the other extreme resembles an acute pyogenic infection along the mandible that may seem like parotitis, a perimandibular space infection, or cervical adenitis. The infection at the portal of entry may no longer be obvious, and the initial presentation may be at a relatively distant site, such as the scalp, orbit, tongue, larynx, or sinuses. Many patients are treated for more common types of bacterial infection, and actinomycosis will often respond temporarily but recur when antibiotics are discontinued (51). Fever and leukocytosis are variable (18,51). Most cases are restricted to soft tissue, although there may be osteomyelitis. Dental infections often involve actinomycetes, especially periapical abscesses (52); these are often treated sufficiently early in the course to preclude advancement to the more characteristic, indurated form. Infection at sites of tooth extraction is common, especially at third molars. A dental portal of entry is implicated even with sites that are distant, and most patients show periodontal disease or gingivitis (53). When bone is involved, it is usually the mandible rather than the maxilla (54). Other forms of actinomycosis in the head and neck region include lacrimal caniculitis (55), postoperative endophthalmitis (56), sinusitis (57), parotitis (58), thyroid infections (59), middle-ear infections (60), and osteomyelitis of the mandible (61).

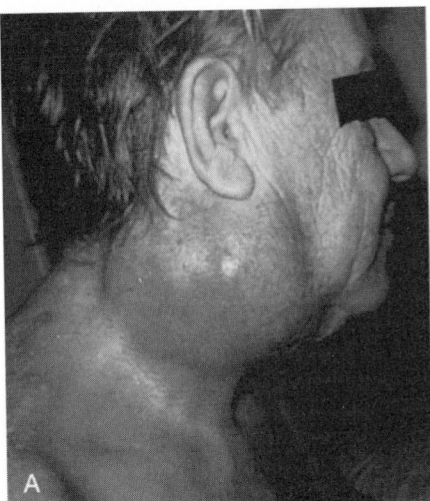 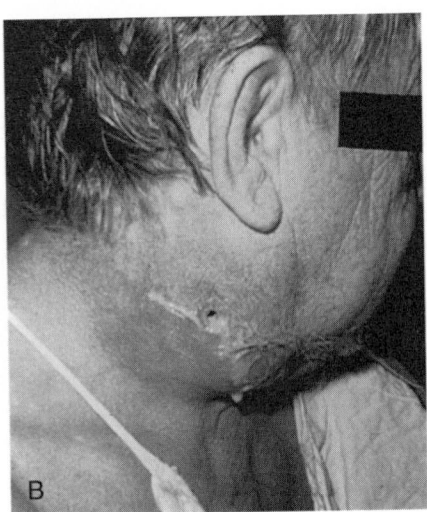 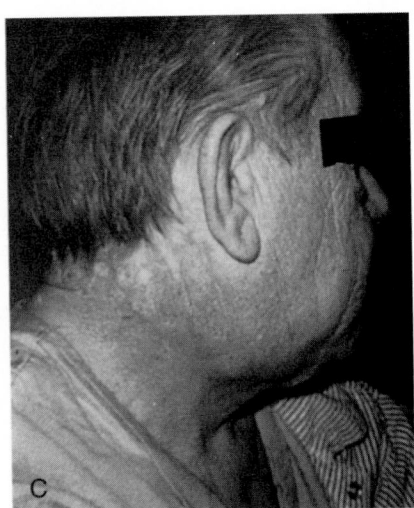

Figure 221.3. Cervicofacial actinomycosis with a large mass at the angle of the jaw. **A:** Initial presentation as a large, fluctuant mass. **B:** Later in the course with induration and a sinus tract. **C:** The lesion after a 6-month course of penicillin.

Thoracic Actinomycosis

Thoracic actinomycosis accounts for about 15% of cases of actinomycosis (62). There may be involvement of the lungs, pleura, mediastinum, and chest wall. The presumed mechanism in most cases is aspiration, and many patients have suggestive dental disease. Less frequent are direct extension from oral infections, hematogenous dissemination, and extension from an abdominal site.

The diagnosis is often not made until relatively late in the course. The usual presentation is a slowly progressive pneumonia with fever, chest pain, weight loss, and cough (62–65). Pleural involvement is common. There may be hemoptysis, hilar adenopathy, bone involvement, pulmonary cavities, cardiac involvement, or mediastinal involvement (63,65–69).

The classic presentation is extension to the chest wall with the development of a soft tissue mass or a draining sinus, although this late form has become uncommon in the antibiotic era (Fig. 221.4). Radiographic changes and computed tomographic findings are often nonspecific, but they may be highly suggestive with pulmonary lesions that extend to and through the chest wall, often with pleural involvement and destruction of adjacent bones (70,71). One or more small cavities are found in about half of cases, but large cavities are unusual (70). Cardiac involvement is common, especially of the pericardium; nevertheless, clinical features of pericarditis are rarely seen (72). Endocarditis is rare.

The diagnosis is infrequently suspected except for patients with the classic presentation of a penetrating chest infection with a chest wall mass or draining sinus, which is found in less than 2% of cases (7). Occasional cases are detected with cytologic examination showing sulfur granules (73). Agents of actinomycosis are not usually recovered from expectorated sputum or bronchoscopy aspirates because these specimens should not be cultured anaerobically and the aerotolerant forms are often too fastidious; even with recovery from these specimens, these results are considered nondiagnostic. Recovery of these agents from pleural fluid or a transthoracic needle aspirate would be considered diagnostic in the presence of an appropriate clinical presentation. In many cases, the diagnosis is made histologically after resection for a suspected neoplasm or with bronchoscopic biopsy (65). This is a chronic, indolent disease with involvement of the pulmonary parenchyma so that the usual diagnostic considerations are tuberculosis, nocardiosis, endemic fungal infection, cryptococcosis, anaerobic pulmonary infection, lymphoma, and bronchogenic cancer.

Abdominal Actinomycosis

Abdominal actinomycosis accounts for about 20% of all cases of actinomycosis (14,15,20,74–80). The usual mechanism is entry through the gut wall, but there may be extension from the thorax or female genital tract or abdominal involvement after hematogenous dissemination. Most patients have had previous abdominal surgery, penetrating abdominal trauma, or a foreign body in the gastrointestinal tract. When there is antecedent surgery or trauma, the latent period may be several years.

The most common presentation, accounting for about two thirds of cases of abdominal actinomycosis, is appendicitis, usually with a periappendiceal mass. Less common sites of involvement include the colon, stomach, liver, gallbladder, pancreas, small bowel, anorectal area, pelvis, and abdominal wall (18). No predisposing factors are noted in up to 50% of cases (17,18,74). Hepatic involvement accounts for 5% to 15% of abdominal actinomycosis cases (20). Some patients present with an intramural gastric lesion that simulates gastric carcinoma (77). In these cases, liver function test results are often normal, neoplasm is often suspected, and there are often multiple small liver abscesses (81–83). Retroperitoneal involvement may result from hematogenous dissemination or direct extension; presentations include pyelonephritis, renal abscess, perinephric abscess, and a mass simulating a bladder tumor (84,85). The diagnosis could conceivably be made with recovery of the agents of actinomycosis in urine culture, but it is not customary to process these specimens anaerobically (86). Obstruction of the ureters with hydronephrosis is sometimes noted with mass lesions of the abdomen or pelvis.

Characteristic features of abdominal actinomycosis are similar to those noted earlier. Most patients have a slowly evolving inflammatory mass with microabscesses, abscesses, draining sinuses, or fistulous tracks. An extremely indurated or woody

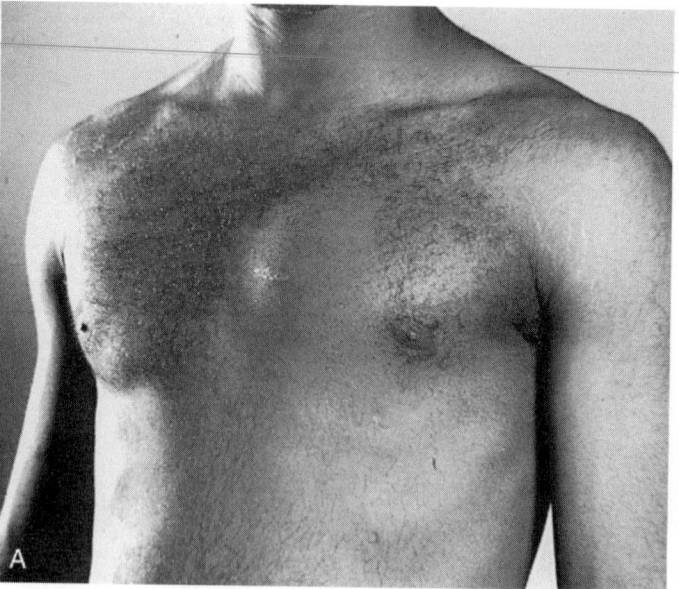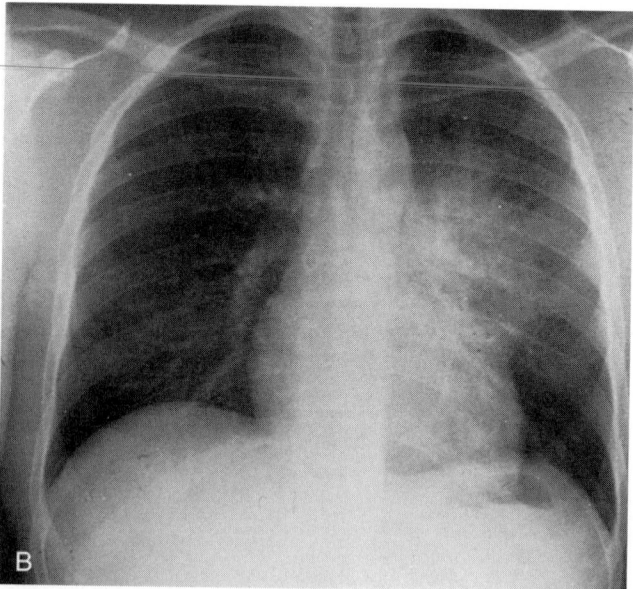

Figure 221.4. Thoracic actinomycosis. **A:** Initial presentation with a bulging mass lesion in the left chest wall with a central sinus tract. **B:** The chest radiograph with the associated pulmonary infiltrate.

mass or actinomycetoma is often suggestive of a neoplasm (87). Characteristic clinical features include fever, weight loss, palpable indurated masses, draining sinuses through the abdominal wall, and computed tomographic evidence of a multicystic contrast-enhancing mass (18,74,75). In many cases, the diagnosis is established with an unnecessary laparotomy and histopathologic examination or recognition of characteristic features intraoperatively (75). Needle aspiration with cytologic examination is an alternative method for establishing this diagnosis (74). For patients who undergo surgery, an intraoperative frozen section will distinguish an inflammatory mass from carcinoma (87).

Pelvic Actinomycosis

Most cases of pelvic actinomycosis are found in association with IUDs. This association was originally noted in 1973 and subsequently popularized by Gupta and colleagues (88–94) with use of Papanicolaou (Pap) smears for detection of the agents of actinomycosis. The Pap smear proved to be a relatively easy, inexpensive, and rapid method for detection of the agents of actinomycosis, but the major controversy concerns the implication of this observation in terms of management decisions. Two methods have been used: (a) the fast smears for detection of Gupta bodies consisting of amorphous material with radiating filaments (90); and (b) the fluorescent antibody conjugate stain for detection of specific agents of actinomycosis (91–93). A survey of Pap smears from 69,925 women screened for *A. israelii* by use of the fluorescent antibody stain showed that this organism was not found in the absence of IUD use; the reported prevalence of *A. israelii* among IUD users is 1.6% to 5.3% (95). In one report, 2 of 112 women with evidence of *A. israelii* had significant clinical infections, and the authors concluded that most patients with this organism had only superficial infections. In a comprehensive review in 1978, Gupta and coworkers (93) reported identification of agents of actinomycosis in 540 vaginal-pancervical (fast) smears from 520 women. Of these, 517 women used IUDs; the other 3 women had infections associated with other foreign bodies. Fluorescent antibody stains in 266 specimens showing cytologic evidence of actinomycosis indicated that *A. israelii* accounted for 250 cases (93). Most patients had IUD use of more than 2 years. These and other investigators have shown that culture is far less sensitive for detection, not an unexpected finding on the basis of the experience with microbial detection by culture at other anatomic sites (96–98).

Pelvic actinomycosis associated with IUDs is highly variable and sometimes controversial. The range of clinical conditions includes vaginal discharge, pelvic inflammatory disease, tuboovarian abscess, and endometritis. In its most advanced and characteristic form, the consequences can be devastating: a frozen pelvis; urinary obstruction; and fistulas that extend to contiguous sites including gut, bladder, skin, or even a distant anatomic site (75). In many cases, the nature of the infection simulates an advanced neoplasm.

The data summarized here have led to a somewhat controversial issue regarding management strategies. The detection of *Actinomyces* on smears appears to be relatively sensitive but not particularly specific for actinomycosis. IUDs are almost always implicated, although other foreign bodies account for a small portion of cases. Among IUD users, the prevalence of *Actinomyces* is relatively high, usually reported at 1% to 10%, but pelvic actinomycosis is rare (89–99). The unknown factor in this association is whether the positive results by smear simply represent early infection or inconsequential colonization. Many authorities believe that this observation represents a contraindication to continued IUD use even in the absence of symptoms.

The alternative option is counseling of the patient and careful follow-up.

Musculoskeletal Actinomycosis

The musculoskeletal system is a relatively unusual primary site of involvement, although direct extension from multiple contiguous sites with involvement of muscle and bone is relatively common. Infection of soft tissue may be associated with trauma, including bite wounds (100). Involvement of soft tissue including muscle may also result from hematogenous dissemination. The usual presentation is an indolent infection with induration and draining sinuses and typical granules. With involvement of feet, this is considered a mycetoma but should be called *actinomycetoma*. Osteomyelitis usually results when a bone is in the direction of contiguous spread. The most common bones are the mandible and vertebrae. With vertebral involvement, there is destruction of the vertebrae and adjacent ribs, but unlike with tuberculosis, there is usually sparing of the disk space and no vertebral collapse (54). Joint involvement is unusual, although agents of actinomycosis have been implicated in prosthetic joint infections (101).

Central Nervous System Actinomycosis

Central nervous system cases account for less than 5% of all cases of actinomycosis. Most represent hematogenous extension (102–105). In a review of 70 reported cases of central nervous system actinomycosis, brain abscess accounted for 67%, meningitis or meningoencephalitis accounted for 13%, actinomycetomas accounted for 7%, subdural empyemas accounted for 6%, and epidural abscesses accounted for 6%. The primary site of infection in these cases was usually the lung, oral cavity, abdomen, or pelvis, and this includes cases associated with IUD use (102). As noted, brain abscess is the most frequent presentation; the usual clinical features are headache and focal neurologic findings with or without fever, and the computed tomographic scan generally shows a ring-enhancing lesion that may easily be mistaken for a neoplasm or pyogenic brain abscess. An actinomycetoma presents as a solid mass (103). Cases classified as chronic meningitis often represent a parameningeal focus. Analysis of the cerebrospinal fluid usually shows an elevated protein level, lymphocytic cells, normal or low glucose level, and negative Gram stain and culture. The agents of actinomycosis are rarely grown from cerebrospinal fluid (104). The diagnosis is usually made by neurosurgery; draining sinuses, sulfur granules, and other characteristic features of actinomycosis at alternative anatomic sites are not seen with central nervous system disease.

Endocarditis

There are multiple case reports of endocarditis caused by *Actinomyces* species (106–108). There is nothing especially unique about these cases, and they generally respond well to penicillin or cephalosporins.

TREATMENT

Antibiotics have revolutionized the outcome of actinomycosis. Antimicrobial agents active *in vitro* include penicillin, ampicillin, antipseudomonad penicillins, most cephalosporins, macrolides, tetracyclines, rifampin, imipenem, and any combination of a β-lactam and β-lactamase inhibitor. Drugs that are less active and should not be used for actinomycosis include metronidazole, aminoglycosides, antistaphylococcal penicillins, cephalexin, ceftazidime, trimethoprim-sulfamethoxazole, and fluoroquinolones (109–112). The lack of activity of metronidazole is curious in view of the nearly universal activity of this agent against obligate anaerobes. On the basis of these observations, it is difficult to go wrong in terms of antibiotic selection. The main problems are dose, duration, the necessity of treating companion organisms, and the role of surgery.

The standard treatment based on decades of experience for most cases of actinomycosis at any anatomic site is high-dose intravenous penicillin (10 to 20 million units per day) for 2 to 6 weeks followed by oral penicillin V or amoxicillin for 6 to 12 months (1,7). The need for high doses is based on the difficulty of achieving therapeutic levels in dense tissue with extensive fibrosis. Consequently, early infections associated with less extensive lesions in terms of size and induration may probably be treated with less aggressive antibiotic treatment. For patients who cannot receive penicillin, the alternative drugs that have had most extensive use are clindamycin and tetracycline or imipenem (65,113). The necessity of treating companion organisms is arbitrary, and most studies indicate that penicillin alone is adequate.

The role of surgery is often controversial. Procedures sometimes advocated include incision and drainage of abscesses; debulking of large, inflammatory masses; and excision of sinus tracts. Some have reported impressive results with antibiotic treatment alone in patients with extensive disease (114,115). Percutaneous drainage of abscesses is another option (112). In many instances, the most appropriate approach is aggressive antibiotic treatment, with surgery reserved for patients who fail to respond and who have the type of lesion or anatomic site of infection that suggests a successful surgical outcome.

REFERENCES

1. Russo TA. Agents of actinomycosis. In: Mandell GL, Bennett JE, Dolin R, eds. *Principles and practice of infectious diseases,* 4th ed. New York: Churchill Livingstone, 1995:2280–2288.
2. Molto JE. Differential diagnosis of rib lesions: a case study from Middle Woodland Southern Ontario circa 230 A.D. *Am J Phys Anthropol* 1990;83:439.
3. Bollinger O. Uber eine neue Pilzkrankheit beim Rinde. *Zentralbl Med Wiss* 1877;15:481.
4. Harz C. *Actinomyces bovis*, ein neuer Schimmel in den Geweben des Rinder. In: *Jahresbuch des Königlich Zentral-Thierarzneischule zu München 1877–1878.* 1879:5:125.
5. Israel J. Neue Beobachtungen auf dem Gebiete der Mykosen des Menschen. *Arch Pathol Anat Physiol* 1879;74:15.
6. Erikson D. Pathogenic anaerobic organisms of the *Actinomyces* group. *Br Med Res Council Spec Rep Ser* 1940;240:1.
7. Lerner PI. *Actinomyces and Arachnia.* In: Gorbach S, Bartlett JG, Blacklow NR, eds. *Infectious diseases.* Philadelphia: WB Saunders, 1992:1626–1632.
8. Wolff M, Israel J. Über Reincultur des *Actinomyces* und seine Obertragbarkeit auf Thiere. *Virchows Arch Pathol Anat* 1891;126:11.
9. Wright JH. The biology of the micro-organism of actinomycosis. *J Med Res* 1905;13:349.
10. Kolouch F, Peltier LF. Actinomycosis. *Surgery* 1946;20:401.
11. Pulverer G. Problems of human actinomycosis. *Postepy Hig Med Dosw* 1974;28:253.
12. Bennhoff D. Actinomycosis: diagnostic and therapeutic considerations and a review of 32 cases. *Laryngoscope* 1984;94:1198.
13. Harvey JC, Cantrell JR, Fisher AM. Actinomycosis: its recognition and treatment. *Ann Intern Med* 1957;46:868.
14. Eastridge C, Prather J, Hughes F, et al. Actinomycosis: a 24-year experience. *South Med J* 1972;65:839.
15. Davis MIJ. Analysis of forty-six cases of actinomycosis with special reference to its etiology. *Am J Surg* 1941;52:447.
16. Putman HC, Dockerty MB, Waugh JM. Abdominal actinomycosis: an analysis of 122 cases. *Surgery* 1950;28:781.
17. Weese WC, Smith IM. A study of 57 cases of actinomycosis over a 36-year period: a diagnostic 'failure' with good prognosis after treatment. *Arch Intern Med* 1975;135:1562.
18. Berardi RS. Abdominal actinomycosis. *Surg Gynecol Obstet* 1979;149:257.
19. Drake DP, Holt RJ. Childhood actinomycosis: report of three recent cases. *Arch Dis Child* 1976;51:979.
20. Coleman RM, Georg LK, Rozzell AR. *Actinomyces naeslundii* as an agent in human actinomycosis. *Appl Microbiol* 1969;18:420.
21. Morris J, Kilbourn P. Systemic actinomycosis caused by *Actinomyces odontolyticus. Ann Intern Med* 1974;81:700.
22. Eng R, Corrado M, Cleri D, et al. Infections caused by *Actinomyces viscosus. Am J Clin Pathol* 1981;75:113.
23. Pordy R. Lumpy jaw due to *Actinomyces meyerii*: report of the first case and review of the literature. *Mt Sinai J Med* 1988;55:190.
24. Brock D, Georg L, Brown JM, et al. Actinomycosis caused by *Arachnia propionica*: report of 11 cases. *Am J Clin Pathol* 1973;59:66.
25. Gahrn-Hansen B, Frederiksen W. Human infections with *Actinomyces pyogenes* (*Corynebacterium pyogenes*). *Diagn Microbiol Infect Dis* 1992;15:349.
26. Georg LK. The agents of human actinomycosis. In: Balows A, eds. *Anaerobic bacteria: role in disease.* Springfield, IL: Charles C Thomas, 1974:237–256.
27. Lewis R, McKenzie D, Bagg J, et al. Experience with a novel selective medium for isolation of *Actinomyces* spp. from medical and dental specimens. *J Clin Microbiol* 1995;33:1613.
28. Sabbe LJ, Van de Merwe D, Schouls L, et al. Clinical spectrum of infections due to the newly described *Actinomyces* species *A. turicensis, A. radingae,* and *A. europaeus. J Clin Microbiol* 1999;37:8.
29. Lawson PA, Nikolaitchouk N, Falsen E, et al. *Actinomyces funkei* sp. nov., isolated from human clinical specimens. *Int J Syst Evol Microbiol* 2001;51:853.
30. Funke G, Alvarez N, Pascual C, et al. *Actinomyces europaeus* sp. nov. isolated from human clinical specimens. *Int J Syst Bacteriol* 1997;47:687.
31. Ieven M, Verhoeven J, Gentens P, et al. Severe infection due to *Actinomyces bernardiae*: case report. *Clin Infect Dis* 1996;22:157.
32. Funke G, von Graevenitz A. Infections due to *Actinomyces neuii* (former "CDC coryneform group 1" bacteria). *Infection* 1995;23:73.
33. Brunner S, Graf S, Riegel P, et al. Catalase-negative *Actinomyces neuii* subsp.*neuii* isolated from an infected mammary prosthesis. *Int J Med Microbiol* 2000;290:285.
34. Ramos CP, Foster G, Collins MD. Phylogenetic analysis of the genus *Actinomyces* based on 16S rRNA gene sequences: description of *Arcanobacterium phocae* sp. nov., *Arcanobacterium bernardiae* comb. nov., *Arcanobacterium pyogenes* comb. nov. *Int J Syst Bacteriol* 1997;47:46.
35. Kramer J. *Instant replay: the Green Bay diary of Jerry Kramer.* New York: World Publishing Company, 1968:48–50.
36. Holm P. Studies on aetiology of human actinomycosis. *Acta Pathol Microbiol Scand* 1950;27:736 and 1951;28:391.
37. Figures K, Douglas C. Actinomycosis associated with a root treated tooth: report of a case. *Int Endodont J* 1991;24:326.
38. Harvey J, Cantrell J, Fisher A. Actinomycosis: its recognition and treatment. *Ann Intern Med* 1957;46:868.
39. Silbermann M, Chiminello F, Doku H, et al. Mandibular actinomycosis: report of a case. *J Am Dent Assoc* 1975;90:162.
40. Klapholz A, Talavera W, Rorat E, et al. Pulmonary actinomycosis in a patient with HIV infection. *Mt Sinai J Med* 1989;56:300.
41. Yeager B, Hoxie J, Weisman R, et al. Actinomycosis in the acquired immunodeficiency syndrome-related complex. *Arch Otolaryngol Head Neck Surg* 1986;112:1293.
42. Chaudhry SI, Greenspan JS. Actinomycosis in HIV infection: a review of a rare complication. *Int J STD AIDS* 2000;11:349.
43. Manfredi R, Mazzoni A, Marinacci G. Progressive intractable actinomycosis in patients with AIDS. *Scand J Infect Dis* 1995;27:405.
44. Waksman SA, Henrici AT. The nomenclature and classification of the actinomycetes. *J Bacteriol* 1943;46:337.
45. Brown J. Human actinomycosis: a study of 181 subjects. *Hum Pathol* 1973;4:319.
46. Hillier S, Moncla B. Anaerobic gram-positive nonsporeforming bacilli and cocci. In: Balows A, ed. *Manual of clinical microbiology.* Washington, DC: American Society for Microbiology, 1991:522–533.
47. Happonen RP, Viander M. Comparison of fluorescent antibody technique and conventional staining methods in diagnosis of cervicofacial actinomycosis. *J Oral Pathol* 1982;11:417.
48. Holmberg K. Diagnostic methods for human actinomycosis. *Microbiol Sci* 1987;4:72.
49. Slack J. The source of infection in actinomycosis. *J Bacteriol* 1942;43:193.
50. Pine L, Overman JR. Determination of the structure and composition of the sulphur granules of *Actinomyces bovis. J Gen Microbiol* 1963;32:209.
51. Spilsbury B, Johnstone F. The clinical course of actinomycotic infections: a report of 14 cases. *Can J Surg* 1962;5:33.
52. Weir J, Buck W. Periapical actinomycosis: report of a case and review of the literature. *Oral Surg* 1982;54:336.
53. Benhoff DF. Actinomycosis: diagnostic and therapeutic considerations and a review of 32 cases. *Laryngoscope* 1984;94:1198.
54. Lewis RP, Sutter VL, Finegold SM. Bone infections involving anaerobic bacteria. *Medicine(Baltimore)* 1978;57:279.
55. Smith R, Henderson P. Actinomycotic canaliculitis. *Aust J Ophthalmol* 1980;8:75.
56. Roussel T, Olson R, Rice T, et al. Chronic postoperative endophthalmitis associated with *Actinomyces* species. *Arch Ophthalmol* 1991;109:60.
57. Har-el G, Prager D, De Soto F, et al. Actinomycotic granuloma masquerading as an infraorbital nerve neoplasm. *Head Neck* 1990;12:261.
58. Chuong R, Goldberg M. CPC, case 60: preauricular mass. *J Oral Maxillofac Surg* 1986;44:214.

59. Arfeen S, Boast M, Large D. Unilateral thyroid swelling due to actinomycosis. *Postgrad Med J* 1986;62:847.
60. Shelton C, Brackmann D. Actinomycosis otitis media. *Arch Otolaryngol Head Neck Surg* 1988;114:88.
61. Bartkowski SB, Zapala J, Heczko P, et al. Actinomycotic osteomyelitis of the mandible: a review of 15 cases. *J Craniomaxillofac Surg* 1998;26:63.
62. Kinnear W, MacFarlane J. A survey of thoracic actinomycosis. *Respir Med* 1990;84:57.
63. Bates M, Cruickshank G. Thoracic actinomycosis. *Thorax* 1957;12:99.
64. Heffner J. Pleuropulmonary manifestations of actinomycosis and nocardiosis. *Semin Respir Infect* 1988;3:352.
65. Yew WW, Wong PC, Lee J, et al. Report of eight cases of pulmonary actinomycosis and their treatment with imipenem-cilastatin. *Monaldi Arch Chest Dis* 1999;54:126.
66. Prather J, Eastridge C, Hughes FA, et al. Actinomycosis of the thorax. *Ann Thorac Surg* 1970;9:307.
67. Morgan D, Nath H, Sanders C, et al. Mediastinal actinomycosis. *AJR Am J Roentgenol* 1990;155:735.
68. Fife T, Finegold S, Grennan T. Pericardial actinomycosis: case report and review. *Rev Infect Dis* 1991;13:120.
69. McQuarrie D, Hall W. Actinomycosis of the lung and chest wall. *Surgery* 1968;64:905.
70. Flynn M, Felson B. The roentgen manifestations of thoracic actinomycosis. *AJR Am J Roentgenol* 1970;110:707.
71. Kwong J, Muller N, Godwin J, et al. Thoracic actinomycosis: CT findings in eight patients. *Radiology* 1992;183:189.
72. Cole FH, Jarrett CL. Primary actinomycosis of the pericardium. *South Med J* 1982;75:1028.
73. Lazzari G, Vineis C, Cugini A. Cytologic diagnosis of primary pulmonary actinomycosis: report of two cases. *Acta Cytol* 1981;25:299.
74. Cintron JR, Del Pino A, Duarte B, et al. Abdominal actinomycosis. *Dis Colon Rectum* 1996;39:105.
75. Kaya E, Yilmazlar T, Emiroglu Z, et al. Colonic actinomycosis: report of a case and review of the literature. *Surg Today* 1995;25:923.
76. Brown JR. Human actinomycosis: a study of 181 subjects. *Hum Pathol* 1973;4:319.
77. Skoutelis A, Panagopoulos C, Kalfarentzos F, et al. Intramural gastric actinomycosis. *South Med J* 1995;88:647.
78. Putman H, Dockerty M, Waugh J. Abdominal actinomycosis: an analysis of 122 cases. *Surgery* 1950;28:781.
79. Stringer M, Cameron A. Abdominal actinomycosis: a forgotten disease? *Br J Hosp Med* 1987;38:125.
80. Deshmukh N, Heaney S. Actinomycosis at multiple colonic sites. *Am J Gastroenterol* 1986;81:1212.
81. Cedermark B, Sundblad R, Willems JS. Suspected neoplasm of the liver with pulmonary metastases cured by surgery and penicillin: disseminated actinomycosis revisited. *Am J Surg* 1981;141:384.
82. Mongiardo M, DeRienzo B, Zanchetta G, et al. Primary hepatic actinomycosis. *J Infect* 1986;12:65.
83. Smithers B, Wall D, Weedon D. Actinomycosis of the gallbladder. *Aust N Z J Surg* 1983;53:587.
84. Ellis L, Kenny G, Nellans R. Urogenital aspects of actinomycosis. *J Urol* 1979;122:132.
85. Ozyurt C, Yurtseven O, Kocak I, et al. Actinomycosis simulating bladder tumour. *Br J Urol* 1995;76:263.
86. Piper J, Stoner B, Mitra SK, et al. Ileo-vesical fistula associated with pelvic actinomycosis. *Br J Clin Pract* 1969;23:341.
87. Veguez JF, Martinez SA, Sands LR, et al. Pelvic actinomycosis presenting as malignant large bowel obstruction: case report and a review of the literature. *Am Surg* 2000;66:85.
88. Muller-Holzner E, Ruth NR, Abfalter E, et al. IUD-associated pelvic actinomycosis: a report of five cases. *Int J Gynecol Pathol* 1995;14:70.
89. Henderson S. Pelvic actinomycosis associated with an intrauterine device. *Obstet Gynecol* 1973;41:726.
90. Gupta PK, Hollander DH, Frost JK. Actinomycetes in cervicovaginal smears: an association with IUD usage. *Acta Cytol* 1976;20:295.
91. Bhagavan BS, Gupta PK. Genital actinomycosis and intrauterine contraceptive devices: cytopathologic diagnosis and clinical significance. *Hum Pathol* 1978;9:567.
92. Spence MR, Gupta PK, Frost JK, et al. Cytologic detection and clinical significance of *Actinomyces israelii* in women using intrauterine contraceptive devices. *Am J Obstet Gynecol* 1978;131:295.
93. Gupta PK, Erozan YS, Frost JK. Actinomycetes and the IUD: an update. *Acta Cytol* 1978;22:281.
94. Fiorino AS. Intrauterine contraceptive device-associated actinomycotic abscess and *Actinomyces* detection on cervical smear. *Obstet Gynecol* 1996;87:142.
95. Valicenti JF, Pappas AA, Graber CD, et al. Detection and prevalence of IUD-associated *Actinomyces* colonization and related morbidity. *JAMA* 1982;247:1149.
96. Mali B, Joshi J, Wagle U, et al. *Actinomyces* in cervical smears of women using intrauterine contraceptive devices. *Acta Cytol* 1986;30:367.
97. Leslie D, Garland S. Comparison of immunofluorescence and culture for the detection of *Actinomyces israelii* in wearers of infra-uterine contraceptive devices. *J Med Microbiol* 1991;35:224.
98. Jarvis D. Isolation and identification of actinomycetes from women using intrauterine contraceptive devices. *J Infect* 1985;10:121.
99. Persson E. Genital actinomycosis and *Actinomyces israelii* in the female genital tract. *Adv Contracept* 1987;3:115.
100. Reiner SL, Harrelson JM, Miller SE, et al. Primary actinomycosis of an extremity: a case report and review. *Rev Infect Dis* 1987;9:581.
101. Cohen O, Keiser J, Pollner J, et al. Prosthetic joint infection with *Actinomyces viscosus*. *Infect Dis Clin Pract* 1993;2:349.
102. Smego RA Jr. Actinomycosis of the central nervous system. *Rev Infect Dis* 1987;9:855.
103. Sharma B, Banerjee A, Sobti M, et al. Actinomycotic brain abscess. *Clin Neurol Neurosurg* 1990;92:373.
104. Bolton C, Ashenhurst E. Actinomycosis of the brain. *Can Med Assoc J* 1964;90:922.
105. Tsai MS, Tam JJ, Liu KS, et al. Multiple brain abscesses: case report. *J Clin Neurosci* 2001;8:183.
106. Huang KL, Beutler SM, Want C. Endocarditis due to *Actinomyces meyeri*. *Clin Infect Dis*. 1998;27:909.
107. Hamed KA. Successful treatment of primary *Actinomyces viscosus* endocarditis with third-generation cephalosporins. *Clin Infect Dis* 1998;26:211.
108. Reddy I, Ferguson DA Jr, Sarubbi FA. Endocarditis due to *Actinomyces pyogenes*. *Clin Infect Dis* 1997;25:1476.
109. Lerner PI. Susceptibility of pathogenic actinomycetes to antimicrobial compounds. *Antimicrob Agents Chemother* 1974;5:302.
110. Holmberg K, Nord C, Dornbusch K. Antimicrobial in vitro susceptibility of *Actinomyces israelii* and *Arachnia propionica*. *Scand J Infect Dis* 1977;9:40.
111. Lerner P. Susceptibility of pathogenic actinomycetes to antimicrobial compounds. *Antimicrob Agents Chemother* 1974;5:302.
112. Martin M. Antibiotic treatment of cervicofacial actinomycosis for patients allergic to penicillin: a clinical and in vitro study. *Br J Oral Maxillofac Surg* 1985;23:428.
113. Schleck W, Gelfand M, Alper B, et al. Medical management of visceral actinomycosis. *South Med J* 1983;76:921.
114. Wohlgemuth S, Gaddy M. Surgical implications of actinomycosis. *South Med J* 1986;79:1574.
115. Goldwag S, Abbitt P, Watts B. Case report: percutaneous drainage of periappendiceal actinomycosis. *Clin Radiol* 1991;44:422.

CHAPTER 222
Chlamydia

Julius Schachter

HISTORY

Chlamydia trachomatis was first visualized in 1907 by Halberstaedter and Prowazek in stained conjunctival scrapings from orangutans that had been inoculated with human trachomatous material (1). Similar inclusions were then seen in conjunctival scrapings from trachoma cases, infants with inclusion blennorrhea, cervical cells of their mothers, and urethral cells of the fathers. By 1910, these inclusions were associated with nongonococcal urethritis (2).

C. trachomatis was first isolated from patients with lymphogranuloma venereum (LGV). In the 1930s, the growth cycle of the LGV organism *in vitro* was noted to be similar to that of *Chlamydia psittaci*, which had been isolated during the psittacosis pandemic of 1929 to 1930. The trachoma agent proved more difficult to recover, not being infective for mice. It was isolated by yolk sac inoculation of embryonated hens' eggs in the 1950s. The first isolate of *Chlamydia* (other than LGV agents) from the genital tract was made in 1959 from the cervix of the mother of an infant with ophthalmia neonatorum. In 1964, *Chlamydia* was isolated from the urethras of men. In 1965, the introduction of a tissue culture isolation method for *C. trachomatis* made it possible to screen large numbers of specimens and to get the result of an isolation attempt in 48 to 72 hours. This made the diagnosis clinically useful and led to identification of a broader clinical spectrum.

C. psittaci disease was first recognized in the late 19th century (1). Sporadic outbreaks were associated with exposure to psittacine birds. Psittacosis attracted considerable attention during a pandemic in 1929 to 1930. The organism was seen in smears from infected birds and human autopsy material and was subsequently isolated. In the preantibiotic era, the case-fatality rate approached 20%. In the 1950s, a major reservoir in poultry was recognized (1). Psittacosis is an occupational hazard to those exposed to infected turkeys in poultry processing plants. *C. psittaci* is also an important pathogen in domestic mammals, causing a number of diseases, such as abortion and arthritis, that have considerable economic impact.

Chlamydia pneumoniae was initially isolated from conjunctival specimens during trachoma studies in Iran and Taiwan (3). Seroepidemiologic studies indicate most adults have been infected (4). Infections begin relatively early in childhood. The organism has been associated with a wide variety of respiratory diseases (5). Severe and fatal cases have been observed in adults with underlying disease and in children in developing countries. This organism has also been implicated as a possible cause of coronary artery disease (6). A fourth species, *Chlamydia pecorum*, is a pathogen of mammals and is not considered an important cause of human disease.

CHARACTERISTICS OF THE PATHOGEN

Taxonomy

The genus *Chlamydia* comprises four species, *C. trachomatis*, *C. psittaci*, *C. pneumoniae*, and *C. pecorum* (Table 222.1). These obligate intracellular bacteria have their own order and family (Chlamydiales, Chlamydiaceae). They are differentiated from other bacteria by a unique developmental cycle involving two morphologic forms—one adapted to extracellular survival and the other to intracellular multiplication. Because *Chlamydia* are small and multiply only within cells, they were long thought to be viruses. However, their cellular organization, mechanisms of macromolecular synthesis and cell division, and antibiotic susceptibility are typically bacterial. *Chlamydia* can be seen with the light microscope.

Different areas of the biology of these organisms have recently been reviewed (7). There is strong DNA homology within each species but surprisingly little among the four. Within species, biovars and serovars may be distinguished on the basis of host range, disease pattern, and antigenic composition. *C. trachomatis* can be divided into four biovars (Table 222.2). Two cause human diseases and can be differentiated serologically and by invasive properties. The LGV biovar infects cultured cells efficiently, whereas the trachoma biovar requires mechanical assistance, such as centrifugation of the inoculum. In naturally occurring disease, the LGV biovar appears to infect endothelial and lymphoid cells, and the trachoma biovar infects squamocolumnar cells. The murine and swine biovars are not known to infect humans.

C. psittaci is virtually ubiquitous among avian species and is a common pathogen of mammals. It infects humans only as zoonoses. There is no systematic schema for differentiating its many biovars and serovars. No animal reservoir has been identified for *C. pneumoniae*, although similar organisms have been isolated from a horse and a koala. It appears to be primarily a respiratory pathogen of humans.

Developmental Cycle

The developmental cycle of *Chlamydia* sets them apart from all other bacteria. There are some differences in inclusion morphology, but the species appear to have essentially identical developmental cycles. The cycle may be divided into several steps: (a) initial attachment of the elementary body (EB) to the host cell, (b) entry into the cell, (c) morphologic change to the reticulate body (RB) with intracellular growth and replication, (d) morphologic change of RBs to EBs, and finally (e) release of infectious particles.

ATTACHMENT

The attachment of *C. psittaci* and the LGV biovar of *C. trachomatis* to cells is highly efficient, as is penetration. In contrast, the trachoma biovar attaches inefficiently. Attachment appears to be mediated by heparin sulfate–like molecules that act as a bridge between a specific receptor on the chlamydial particle and another on the susceptible host cell (8). It is likely that this attachment process initiates a receptor-mediated endocytosis. The attachment of *Chlamydia* to host cells and inhibition of phagolysosomal fusion are inhibited by specific antibody, mild heat treatment (56°C for 30 minutes), or trypsinization.

CELL ENTRY

Once attached, the EB is rapidly internalized by the host cell. If a mixture of EBs and *Escherichia coli* or yeast is presented to susceptible host cells, *Chlamydia* are preferentially ingested. Moulder (9)

TABLE 222.1. Characteristics of *Chlamydia* Species

Species	Elementary body	Sulfa sensitivity	Iodine stain
C. trachomatis	Coccoid	+	+
C. psittaci	Coccoid	−	−
C. pneumoniae	Pear shaped	−	−
C. pecorum	Coccoid	−	−

TABLE 222.2. Natural Host Ranges of *Chlamydia* Species and Human Diseases

Species	Natural hosts	Human diseases
C. psittaci	Birds, lower mammals	Psittacosis
C. pneumoniae	Humans	Respiratory
C. trachomatis		
Trachoma biovar	Humans	Trachoma, conjunctivitis, genital diseases, infant pneumonia
LGV biovar	Humans	LGV
Murine biovar	Mice	None known
Swine biovar	Swine	None known

LGV, lymphogranuloma venereum.

stressed that *Chlamydia* induces phagocytosis by nonprofessional phagocytes. The mechanism of chlamydial uptake is controversial. Ultrastructural studies suggest that *Chlamydia* organisms enter through clathrin-coated pits, through a pathway similar to that for receptor-mediated endocytosis.

MORPHOLOGIC CHANGE AND REPLICATION

The infectious EB is not metabolically active. EBs are 350 nm in diameter and have an electron-dense center (Fig. 222.1). The EB changes to the metabolically active and dividing form, the RB, within 6 to 8 hours. RBs are 1 μm in diameter and are not electron dense. Using the host cell pool of precursors, the RBs synthesize RNA, DNA, and protein. The RBs divide by binary fission from 8 to about 18 to 24 hours. This is the stage of greatest metabolic activity, when the organisms are most sensitive to inhibitors of cell wall synthesis and bacterial metabolic activity. At 18 to 24 hours, some RBs begin to reorganize into EBs (Fig. 222.2). This entire cycle takes place within the phagosome. The development and functions of the inclusion membrane has been perplexing. Obviously, it grows as the number of EBs and RBs within the inclusion increase, and it must be involved in transport of nutrients into the *Chlamydia* and export of degradation products from the inclusion. It also could play a role in evading fusion. The demonstration of specific inclusion proteins that are apparently phosphorylated by the host cell promises to provide important information on the membrane function.

At some time between 48 and 72 hours, the cell ruptures, releasing the infectious EBs. Phagolysosomal fusion does not occur until the death of the cell is imminent. Inhibition is specific to the chlamydial phagosome because other phagosomes in the same cell can fuse.

RBs are not stable outside the host cell. Thus, as part of their unique growth cycle, the *Chlamydia* strains have evolved two morphologic entities: the compact stable EB successfully persists in the extracellular environment and is responsible for cell-to-cell and host-to-host transmission, and the highly labile, noninfective

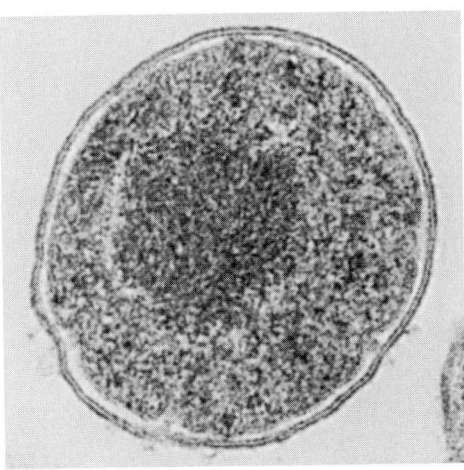

Figure 222.1. Electron micrograph of chlamydial elementary body showing inner and outer membranes and lack of peptidoglycan layer. Electron-dense centers also noted (×118,000). (From Caldwell HD, Kromhout J, Schachter J. Purification and partial characterization of the major outer membrane protein of *Chlamydia trachomatis. Infect Immun* 1981;31: 1161–1176, with permission.)

RB is a metabolically active and vegetative form that does not survive outside the host cell.

Structure

The EB is a spherical particle with projections of the envelope (of unknown function) on one hemisphere (10) (Fig. 222.3). Electron microscopy reveals an outer membrane and an inner membrane. There is no peptidoglycan layer with muramic acid, but the presence of penicillin-binding proteins suggests a related cross-linked structure. The EB envelope is rigid and is relatively impermeable to macromolecules. The outer membrane contains lipopolysaccharide (LPS) and has a major outer membrane

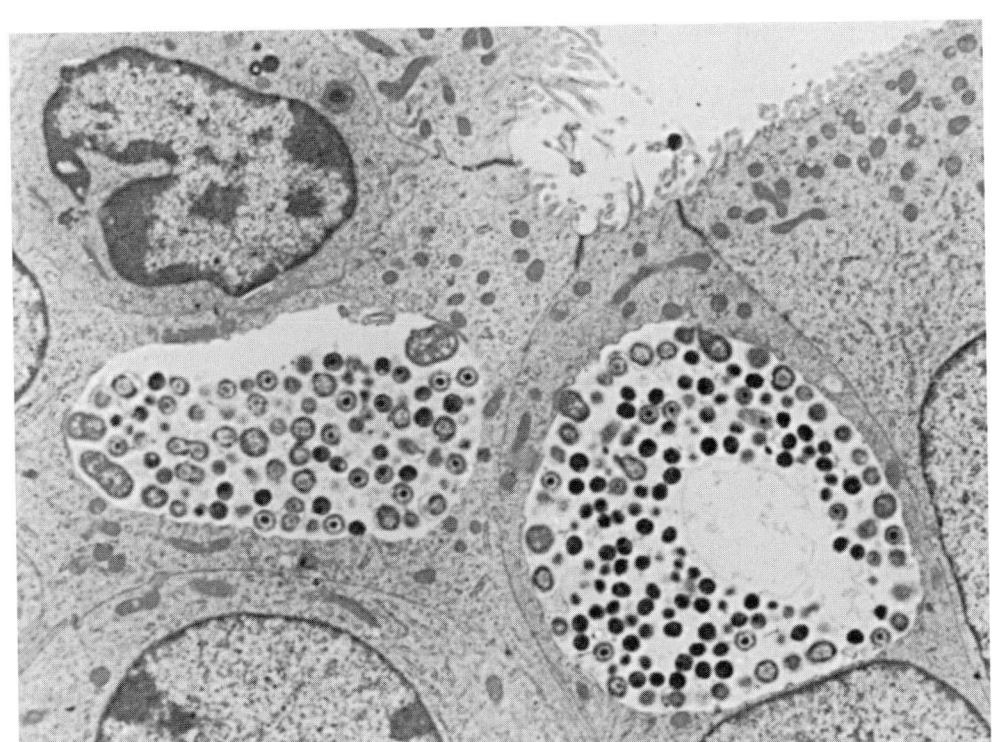

Figure 222.2. Chlamydial inclusions produced by the mouse pneumonitis agent in nonciliated cells in the murine oviduct (×7,000). (From Phillips DM, Swenson CE, Schachter J. Ultrastructure of *Chlamydia trachomatis* infection of the mouse oviduct. *J Ultrastruct Res* 1984;88:244–256, with permission.)

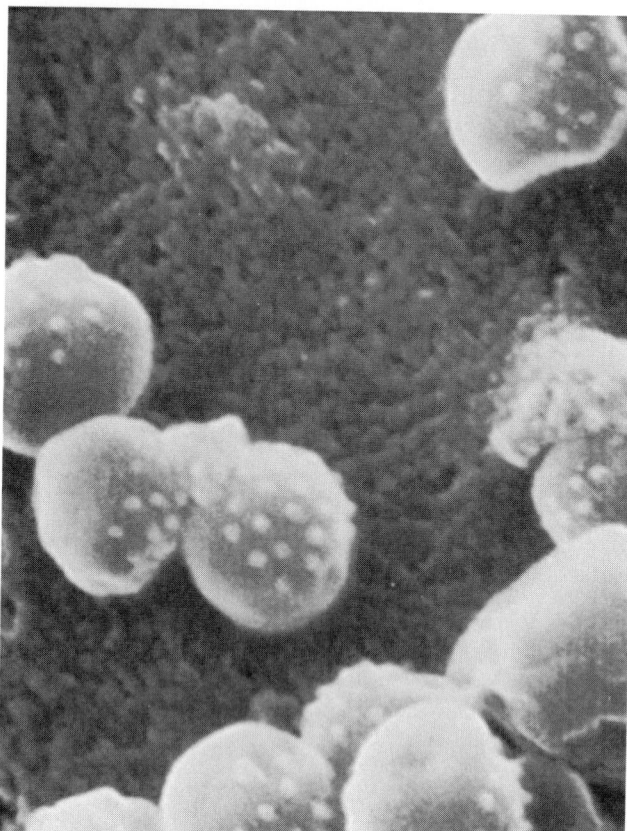

Figure 222.3. Electron micrograph of chlamydial particles showing hemispheric projections. (From Gregory WW, Gardner M, Byrne GI, et al. Arrays of hemispheric surface projections on *Chlamydia psittaci* and *Chlamydia trachomatis* observed by scanning electron microscopy. *J Bacteriol* 1979;138:241–244, with permission.)

protein (MOMP) of 39,000 to 45,000 daltons (11). MOMP is 60% of the weight of the outer membrane. Structural rigidity of the EB appears to depend on disulfide cross-linking of MOMP molecules with each other and with other cysteine-rich proteins. Soon after the EB enters the phagosome, its envelope loses its rigidity, and the subunit layer is disrupted and disappears. This reorganization to the more flexible and fragile structure of the RB probably involves reduction of the cross-linked disulfide bonds, and likely porin formation. The RB cell envelope is highly permeable.

Antigens

Chlamydia organisms contain a heat-stable LPS that is serologically common to the genus. It is quite similar in structure to the LPS of such gram-negative bacteria as *Acinetobacter calcoaceticus* and Re mutants of *Salmonella typhimurium*. There are also heat-labile genus-, species- and serovar-specific antigens. The human *C. trachomatis* pathogens can be divided into at least 15 serovars by a microimmunofluorescence (micro-IF) test (12). The A, B, Ba, and C serotypes are associated with hyperendemic blinding trachoma, and the D to K serovars are commonly associated with sexually transmitted disease. The L1, L2, and L3 serovars represent the LGV biovar (13). Antigens of species, serogroup (closely related serovars), and serovar specificity can be found on the MOMP molecule (14). Only one serovar has been identified among *C. pneumoniae* isolates. There are many different serovars among *C. psittaci*.

Metabolic Properties and Nucleic Acids

Chlamydia have been termed *energy parasites* because they do not generate their own adenosine triphosphate (ATP). In a sense, the endosome containing them functions as a reverse mitochondrion, taking in host cell–produced ATP and releasing adenosine diphosphate (ADP) (15). Typically, *Chlamydia* require well-nourished host cells for their replication. They use the pool of host cell metabolites for their own synthesis.

At 6×10^5 to 8.5×10^5 base pairs, *Chlamydia* have one of the smallest bacterial genomes (one half the size of neisserial or rickettsial DNA). The sequence of the 16S RNA genes of *C. psittaci* and *C. trachomatis* has been determined, and there is only a 5% difference between the two species. The sequence is similar to that of other eubacteria.

The complete genomes of the important human pathogens, the trachoma biovar of *C. trachomatis*, and *C. pneumoniae* have been sequenced (16). This is particularly important because we have no laboratory systems for manipulating chlamydial DNA. Harvesting the riches of this achievement promises to revolutionize our understanding of chlamydial biology.

All *C. trachomatis* serovars contain a 4.4-megadalton plasmid (17). Functions of the plasmid genes are not known, although some of the gene products are expressed during infection. Presence of a plasmid in *C. psittaci* strains appears to be variable; some have bacteriophages.

Chlamydial LPS has been successfully cloned into *Escherichia coli* and is expressed in the outer membrane (18). Because of its important structural and antigenic role, the genes responsible for MOMP have been of particular interest. The amino acid sequence of MOMP is now known for all serovars. There are five conserved and four variable domains within the genes (19). The most variable segments are about 11 amino acids long and occur one each in the N-terminal half and in the C-terminal half of MOMP. These sites are responsible for antigenic reactivity (20).

EPIDEMIOLOGY

Sexually Transmitted Chlamydial Infection

There appear to be two major modes of transmission of *C. trachomatis*. In industrialized Western society, virtually all *C. trachomatis* infections are sexually transmitted. *C. trachomatis* is the most common sexually transmitted bacterial pathogen. In the United States, it is estimated that more than 3 million new infections occur each year (21). These infections are just as important in the developing countries (22). Men who acquire the infection usually develop nongonococcal urethritis 1 to 3 weeks after infection (23). Women have cervical infection, often asymptomatic. Inapparent infections are common. If untreated, infections can persist for years.

The highest rates of chlamydial infections are found in sexually active teenagers. Many studies have found that about 1 in 6 female adolescents and 1 in 10 male adolescents are infected (24,25). Risk factors for chlamydial infection include age, low socioeconomic status, recent change of partner, use of oral contraceptives, and prior chlamydial infection (26,27). Use of barrier methods of contraception is protective.

Ascending genital infections are common. The risk of men developing epididymitis is not known but is probably about 1%. About 10% of young women with lower genital tract chlamydial infection have an episode of pelvic inflammatory disease (28). Even more are likely to develop subclinical salpingitis.

Infants exposed to *Chlamydia* by passage through the infected birth canal may acquire the infection and can develop a number of diseases, including conjunctivitis and pneumonia (29). At least

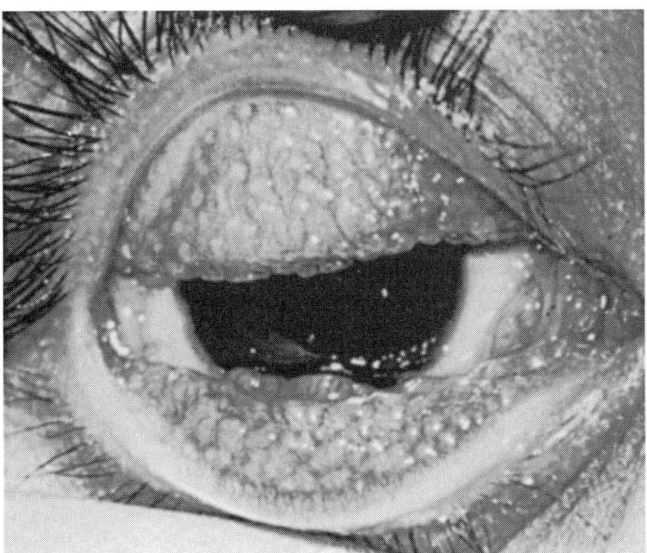

Figure 222.4. Severe active trachoma. This stage is characterized by marked follicular reaction and papillary hypertrophy.

60% to 70% of exposed infants are infected. In adults, if infective genital tract discharges are inoculated into the eye either during sexual activity or by hand-to-eye contact, inclusion conjunctivitis may develop (1).

Endemic Trachoma

In trachoma-endemic areas, *C. trachomatis* is usually spread from child to child (1). In many developing countries, trachoma is endemic, and in some areas, it is hyperendemic or holoendemic. Millions have been blinded (30). In holoendemic areas, children acquire the infection early. In some communities, all are infected by 2 years of age (31). Poor hygiene and unsanitary conditions contribute to the spread of the organism. Flies act as mechanical vectors in spreading infective ocular discharges. The disease begins as an acute mucopurulent conjunctivitis (often complicated by secondary bacterial infections; Fig. 222.4) that becomes a chronic follicular keratoconjunctivitis, sometimes accompanied by pannus (corneal neovascularization) formation. Active disease usually wanes when the children are 6 to 10 years old. Most children have only minor sequelae when the disease becomes inactive, and there is no effect on vision. Some children with moderate to severe trachoma develop badly scarred conjunctivae. This scarring of the upper conjunctiva may, with time, result in distortion of the upper eyelid. The in-turned upper lid margin causes the eyelashes to abrade and ultimately break down the corneal epithelium. It may take 25 or 30 years for this process to evolve fully because the scars contract with age. The blindness seen in adults older than 40 years of age reflects early childhood trachoma. In a hyperendemic area, age-specific blindness rates at age 60 years may be 20% or more. Once common throughout the world, trachoma is now a major problem only in certain developing countries. Still, trachoma is the world's leading preventable cause of blindness (30).

Psittacosis (Ornithosis)

Human psittacosis is a disease contracted from exposure to avian species infected with *C. psittaci* (1). The term ornithosis is also used because the infection is not restricted to psittacines. The organism is ubiquitous among avian species, usually infecting the intestinal tract. It is also common in domestic mammals, but

they are seldom a source of human infection. This zoonosis is relatively uncommon, with only a few hundred cases occurring each year in the United States, and many of these cases have been misattributed due to serologic cross-reactions with the far more common *C. pneumoniae*.

Chlamydia pneumoniae Infection

C. pneumoniae infections appear to occur relatively early in childhood (4,5). Serologic studies indicate an annual incidence of infection of at least 1% to 2%. Seroprevalence may reach 70% to 80% and peaks at 60 years. Infection has been associated with severe pneumonia and epidemics of mild pneumonia. It is likely that most infections cause mild respiratory symptoms or are asymptomatic. Asymptomatic infections have been documented by recovery of the organism from healthy individuals. In Finland, epidemics of mild pneumonias have occurred in military trainees, and 6% to 8% of the soldiers were affected (32).

PATHOGENESIS

The pathogenesis of any of the infections with *C. trachomatis* has not been elucidated. It is clear that LGV is a systemic infection involving lymphoid tissues. The organisms are capable of replicating within macrophages. The trachoma biovar has a limited host range *in vivo*. It appears to be almost exclusively a parasite of squamocolumnar epithelial cells. The disease process and clinical manifestations of chlamydial infections probably represent the combined effects of tissue damage resulting from chlamydial replication and the inflammatory responses caused by the presence of *Chlamydia* and necrotic material from the destroyed host cells. There is an abundant immune response to chlamydial infection (in terms of humoral or cell-mediated responses). There is evidence that chlamydial diseases result in part from hypersensitivity or are diseases of immunopathology (13,33).

LGV is a truly lymphoproliferative disease. The trachoma biovar causes a more localized lymphoproliferative response in the sense that it can induce follicle formation in the mucous membranes. Although such a response is best known for the conjunctiva (trachoma and inclusion conjunctivitis), follicular cervicitis, proctitis, and probably follicular urethritis are recognized. Follicles induced by *C. trachomatis* are true lymphoid follicles with germinal centers.

Trachoma has long been considered a disease in which re-infection is important (13). In nonhuman primates, repeated (weekly) conjunctival instillation of *C. trachomatis* results in a disease with many of the manifestations of trachoma, including conjunctival scarring (34). Similarly severe experimental salpingitis in nonhuman primates was also in part dependent on previous exposure to *Chlamydia* (35). A common pathologic end point of chlamydial infection is scarring of mucous membranes. This is what ultimately leads to the blindness in trachoma and to infertility and ectopic pregnancy after acute salpingitis.

Current theory suggests that it is hypersensitivity to a heat-shock protein (HSP60) that is specifically responsible for much of the chlamydial disease. It is known that this antigen is broadly cross-reactive and is secreted by infected cells, and antibodies to it are found in high levels in women suffering from tubal factor infertility and ectopic pregnancy (36,37).

Immunology

Chlamydia species are highly complex organisms with antigens of genus, species, subspecies, and serovar specificity. The most easily detected antigen is the genus-specific LPS antigen. It is responsible for the complement-fixing reactions commonly used to diagnose psittacosis or LGV (38). Chlamydial LPS has two antigen sites. One is identical to that of other bacteria, and the other is *Chlamydia* specific.

Species-specific antigens are shared by all members of a chlamydial species. Subspecies- or serovar-specific antigens are common only to selected strains within chlamydial species. These antigens have been the basis for a variety of serologic tests used for the classification of *C. trachomatis* (13). The responsible antigens appear to be on the MOMP molecule. The serovars fall into two broad complexes (B and C) by micro-IF (12). Each complex shows extensive cross-reaction within the complex but little reaction with the other complex. Serovar-specific monoclonal antibodies are available for typing purposes. It is likely that immunity to infection, although relatively weak, is serovar specific.

The MOMP molecule is cross-linked to 15- and 60-kd proteins. The 60-kd proteins are important immunogens. Although MOMP appears to be the immunodominant antigen, there may be a more selective response to the 60-kd cystine-rich protein that is surface exposed and has species-specific antigens. The 15-kd proteins are not on the EB surface and have antigens of species and biovar specificity. Monoclonal antibodies directed against MOMP can neutralize infectivity in cell culture and prevent ocular infection in subhuman primates (39).

Control of Chlamydial Infection by the Host

In the majority of chlamydial infections, only a small proportion of cells at affected sites are infected. Because each inclusion releases hundreds of viable EBs and relatively few nearby cells are infected, there must be control mechanisms that limit infectivity. The mechanisms are not clear. Lymphokines have been shown to have an inhibitory effect on *Chlamydia* (40). *C. trachomatis* is sensitive to interferon-α, -β, and -γ. The latter appears to be most active. The lymphokine that inhibits *Chlamydia* in human macrophages and in mice has been identified as interferon-γ (41,42). It appears to delay the developmental cycle at the RB stage. This may result in persistent inapparent infection and may also play a role in immunopathogenesis. The mode of action appears to be, as in other systems, depletion of tryptophan, making it unavailable to the *Chlamydia* organisms (43). Thus, clearance of infection is dependant on a helper T-cell subtype 1 (T$_H$1) response, but the mechanism of resistance to reinfection, which appears to be serovar specific, is not clear.

DESCRIPTION

Chlamydia trachomatis Infection

TRACHOMA

Although onset can be insidious, the disease begins as a mucopurulent conjunctivitis, developing into a follicular keratoconjunctivitis (1). Over time, some of the follicles necrose, resulting in scarring of the conjunctivae. The scars may slowly contract, distorting the eyelid and causing an in-turning of the eyelashes so that they abrade the cornea (Fig. 222.5). This complex represents the blinding lesions of trachoma, called *trichiasis* and *entropion*. Severe lid deformity may not develop until 30 or 40 years after active disease has waned. Trachoma often occurs in areas of the world where seasonal outbreaks of bacterial conjunctivitis make the disease worse.

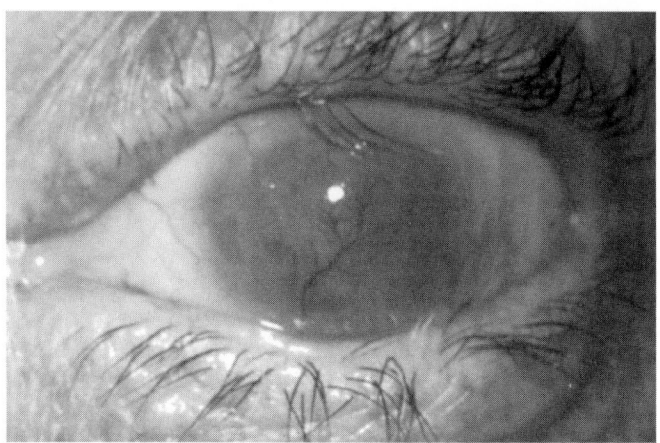

Figure 222.5. Trichiasis and entropion in late trachoma. Eyelashes abrade the cornea, ultimately causing a leukoma and blindness.

GENITAL TRACT INFECTION

In men, *C. trachomatis* causes 35% to 50% of cases of nongonococcal urethritis (2,23). There is usually a mucopurulent discharge and dysuria. Ascending infections can occur. *C. trachomatis* is now recognized as the leading cause of epididymitis in sexually active young men. Chlamydial proctitis is relatively common among homosexual men.

In women, the most commonly affected site is the cervix, where the organism can cause a mucopurulent endocervicitis (23). This condition is characterized by a mucopurulent endocervical discharge. Urethral infections occur and can cause a "sterile" pyuria in young women. Ascending genital infection is common. *C. trachomatis* is found in the endometrium or fallopian tubes of about 25% of acute salpingitis cases in the United States. Chlamydiae cause tubal damage, resulting in infertility and ectopic pregnancy (44). Unfortunately, the preceding chlamydial salpingitis can be clinically mild or even inapparent and thus may not be treated.

NEONATAL INFECTION

About one in three of the exposed infants develops inclusion conjunctivitis of the newborn. It is a mucopurulent conjunctivitis with an incubation period of 5 to 21 days and usually resolves in a few months without treatment. About one in six exposed infants develops a characteristic pneumonia syndrome (45). The age at onset is usually between 2 and 12 weeks. The infants often have a prodrome of rhinitis, and many have conjunctivitis. Affected infants are usually afebrile, are markedly tachypneic and occasionally apneic, and have a staccato cough. Vaginal and gastrointestinal infections also occur but have no known consequences.

Human Infection with *Chlamydia psittaci*

Psittacosis usually occurs in a respiratory or a typhoidal form (1). Respiratory disease can be a mild influenza disease, or it can develop into a severe and fatal (if untreated) pneumonia. The incubation period is typically 1 to 3 weeks. Fever, chills, and severe headache usually occur (Table 222.3). Radiographs may show more extensive lung involvement than is expected from the respiratory difficulty. The typhoidal form of the disease involves a general toxic febrile state without respiratory findings. Person-to-person transmission is uncommon but has occurred.

Most human infections with *C. psittaci* from domestic mammals appear to be subclinical. They have been detected by

TABLE 222.3. Clinical Findings in Confirmed Human Psittacosis

Sign or symptom	Cases (%)
Fever	>95
Headache	>95
Chills	>95
Myalgias	>90
Sweats	50
Conjunctivitis or photophobia	50
Cough	50
Diarrhea or constipation	35
Leukopenia	25

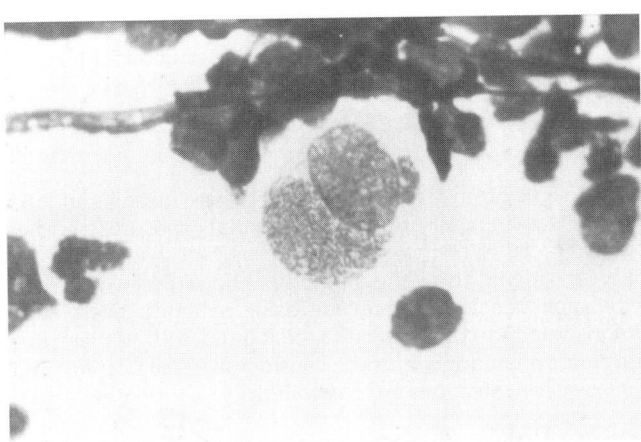

Figure 222.6. *C. trachomatis* inclusion in a conjunctival smear from a patient with trachoma (Giemsa stain; approximately ×1,000).

serologic surveys. *C. psittaci* causing abortions in lower mammals may also cause abortions in humans (46).

Chlamydia pneumoniae Infection

C. pneumoniae has been associated with relatively mild pneumonias in young adults. The clinical picture is similar to that seen with mycoplasmal pneumonia (4,5). More severe disease is recognized but appears to be a function of underlying disease. This is clearly an emerging area in infectious diseases, and the clinical spectrum of *C. pneumoniae* infection is not clear. The spectrum is likely to range from inapparent infection to pharyngitis, bronchiolitis, and pneumonia. Chlamydia infection has also been associated with chronic respiratory disease, including asthma in children and adult-onset asthma.

This organism's possible role in coronary artery disease is currently an active area of research (5,47). There is abundant evidence that *C. pneumoniae* is involved in coronary artery disease. This includes excess antibody levels seen in patients with coronary artery disease as compared with controls, the visualization of the organism within lesions, and isolation of the organism from diseased arteries (6,48). In addition, the organism has been shown capable of growth within vascular endothelial cells and *in vitro* can induce development of foam cells (cholesterol-laden macrophages) by a mechanism likely mediated by LPS (49). None of this evidence constitutes proof of an etiologic association with coronary artery disease. Prospectively designed treatment trials to reduce secondary coronary artery events are currently in progress.

It is unknown whether many of the apparent late-onset conditions that have been associated with *C. pneumoniae* infection reflect responses to a reinfection or to a persistent infection. It is likely that early infection occurs in the lung, and then macrophages distribute the organism to other sites. Some have postulated that infection may be chronic and nonproductive, but still sensitizing, due to immune suppression and concurrent immunopathology.

DIAGNOSIS

Chlamydia trachomatis Infection

TRACHOMA
Trachoma diagnosis is based mainly on clinical findings: identification of follicular reaction, papillary hypertrophy, and scars within the conjunctiva. Laboratory diagnosis was often based on demonstration of chlamydial inclusions in conjunctival smears

(Fig. 222.6). *Chlamydia* organisms may be readily isolated from active cases in cell culture systems (Fig. 222.7). A nucleic acid amplification test (NAAT) is the most sensitive laboratory test for diagnosing chlamydial genes. Serologic tests are not useful.

GENITAL TRACT INFECTION
NAATs (polymerase chain reaction, ligase chain reaction, transcription-mediated amplification, and strand displacement are commercially available) are much more sensitive than previous testing methods. They are the methods of choice (50,51). Serology does not play a role in diagnosing lower genital tract infections. The higher antibody levels seen by micro-IF in complications (e.g., epididymitis, salpingitis) may provide some support for a clinical diagnosis.

NEONATAL INFECTION
Conjunctivitis may be diagnosed readily by any of the cytologic tests. Giemsa stain is adequate in diagnosing severe cases, and the fluorescent antibody techniques are quite sensitive. The agent may be readily isolated, but NAATs will be more sensitive.

A specific diagnosis for pneumonia may be more difficult because of sampling problems, but the organism can usually be isolated from the nasopharynx or tracheobronchial aspirates. Infants with chlamydial pneumonia almost always develop high immunoglobulin M (IgM) antibody levels, and because of their

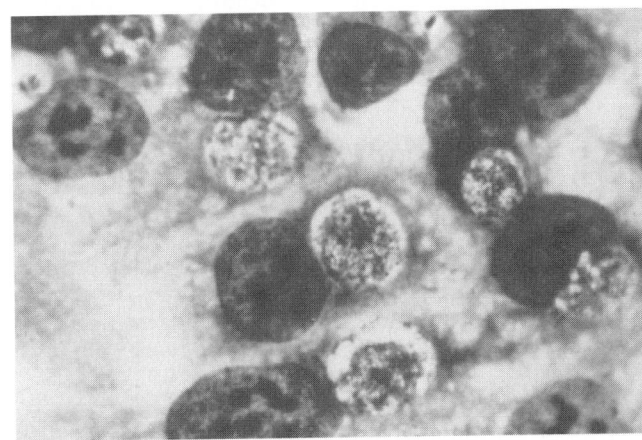

Figure 222.7. *C. trachomatis* inclusions in HeLa cells inoculated with a genital tract specimen (Giemsa stain; approximately ×1,000).

defined exposure (at birth), the diagnosis may be readily established by a single-point determination of specific antichlamydial IgM antibodies of more than 1:32 by micro-IF (52).

Psittacosis

Clinical signs are not pathognomonic. The clinician's index of suspicion (asking questions about potential exposure to birds) is usually crucial to arriving at a diagnosis. Serodiagnosis is generally considered to be the method of choice because isolation of the agent is seldom achieved. Rising antibody levels can be demonstrated by complement fixation or micro-IF. Other causes of atypical pneumonia must be considered when *C. psittaci* and *C. pneumoniae* infections are possibilities.

Chlamydia pneumoniae Infection

Specific serologic tests are available using modification of the micro-IF test with a *C. pneumoniae* antigen (4). Seroconversion can also be demonstrated by the complement fixation test in about half the cases. A presumptive diagnosis for pneumonia may be made if the initial serum specimen has a *C. pneumoniae*–specific IgM titer of more than 1:32 or an IgG titer of more than 1:512. Seroconversion can be delayed, taking more than 4 weeks. The organism can be isolated, with some difficulty, from respiratory tract specimens. Use of HL or HEp-2 cells provides a more sensitive culture system for *C. pneumoniae* than do the McCoy or HeLa cells that are commonly used for culture of *C. trachomatis* (53). Many "home-brewed" NAATs have been described, and a standardized commercial test is sorely needed.

TREATMENT

Azithromycin given in a single 1-g dose is the treatment of choice for uncomplicated lower genital tract infection with *C. trachomatis* (21). This regimen is as effective as a 1-week course of doxycycline (54). Historically, and for financial considerations, tetracyclines are often considered the drugs of choice for chlamydial infections, except when they are contraindicated or not tolerated. In those cases, the alternative is erythromycin. Ofloxacin is also effective. Aminoglycosides and cephalosporins are not active against *Chlamydia*.

Although there are documented treatment failures in which *Chlamydia* organisms have been isolated from patients after treatment, the recovered agents have been found to be susceptible to the antibiotics. There is a suggestion that relative resistance to erythromycin has been developing, but no data suggest that this has reached clinically relevant levels. Rifampin, which is highly active *in vitro*, has not been widely used to treat human chlamydial infections. Rifampin resistance is easily developed in the laboratory, as is quinolone resistance (55,56).

Chlamydia trachomatis Infection

TRACHOMA
To treat trachoma, single-dose azithromycin is the most effective regimen, replacing the 6-week course of 1% tetracycline ointment previously used (57). Community-wide treatment with azithromycin is a part of efforts to control trachoma (58).

GENITAL TRACT INFECTION
Treatment of uncomplicated genital tract infection is relatively easy. Oral azithromycin in a 1-g single dose is the treatment of choice for uncomplicated genital tract infection; this results in

cure rates of more than 95%. It is a coequal treatment of choice with a less expensive 7-day course of oral doxycycline (100 mg 2 × daily). Erythromycin, 500 mg 4 × daily for 7 days, is considered the treatment of choice for pregnant women and for those who are tetracycline intolerant. Ofloxacin is also effective. Upper genital tract infections call for longer courses of therapy.

NEONATAL INFECTION
Chlamydial infection in the infant calls for systemic therapy with erythromycin (50 mg/kg in divided doses each day), 7 to 14 days for conjunctivitis and 14 to 21 days for pneumonia. Topical therapy is not recommended because of relatively high failure rates and the need to eradicate extraocular infection and prevent subsequent development of pneumonia.

Psittacosis and *Chlamydia pneumoniae* Infection

Psittacosis is usually treated with tetracycline, 2 g daily for at least 10 to 14 days. Doxycycline, 100 mg twice daily for the same duration is probably equally effective. Erythromycin is the alternative. Relapses are common if the duration of treatment is inadequate. Regimens for *C. pneumoniae* are likely to be similar, but sufficient experience with controlled trials is not yet available.

PREVENTION

Chlamydia trachomatis Infection

TRACHOMA
Community-wide treatment with oral azithromycin has been shown to reduce dramatically both chlamydial infection and clinical disease (58). As part of an integrated control program, such treatment programs offer the hope of eliminating blinding trachoma as a major public health problem. Current efforts are based on the SAFE strategy: **s**urgery to correct lid deformity; **a**ntibiotics to treat chlamydial infection; **f**acial cleanliness to reduce transmission; and **e**nvironmental improvement to remove conditions conducive to transmission. Experimental vaccines have induced a short-lived immune response, but some vaccinees developed more severe disease, suggesting hypersensitivity to the organism (1,13).

GENITAL TRACT INFECTION
No program for prevention of sexually transmitted chlamydial infection is in effect. Guidelines for such a program have been developed, but economic considerations have prevented their implementation (59). Screening and treatment programs reduce prevalence, prevent complications, and are cost-effective (60). Sensitive and specific NAATs allow diagnosis using noninvasively collected specimens and allow screening of asymptomatic individuals (51). Effective single-dose treatment is available. Lack of a program is a national disgrace.

Psittacosis

Psittacosis is an occupational hazard for those in the poultry or pet bird industries. Chemoprophylaxis for exotic birds is available, and clean premises can be maintained by avoiding introduction of untreated birds.

Immunity

Immunity induced by chlamydial infection is not well understood. It is clear that single infections do not result in solid immunity to reinfection. Repeated infections are common. Some relative immunity probably develops after initial or serial infection. The only human chlamydial infection that has been subjected to extensive vaccine studies is trachoma (1,13). The results from field studies, vaccine trials, and infection of volunteers and subhuman primates indicate that there is a short-lived relative immunity to reinfection with homotypic challenge. No vaccine is available. Many *in vitro* studies indicate that cell-mediated immune response plays an important role in clearing infection.

Neonatal Infection

Pregnant women can be screened for chlamydial infection; treatment of those found to be infected prevents perinatal transmission (61).

REFERENCES

1. Schachter J, Dawson CR. *Human chlamydial infections*. Littleton, MA: Publishing Sciences Group, 1978.
2. Schachter J. Chlamydial infections (in three parts). *N Engl J Med* 1978;298:428–435, 490–495, 540–549.
3. Grayston JT, Kuo C-C, Campbell LA, et al. *Chlamydia pneumoniae* sp. nov. for *Chlamydia* sp. strain TWAR. *Int J Syst Bacteriol* 1989;39:88–90.
4. Grayston JT. *Chlamydia pneumoniae*, strain TWAR pneumonia. *Annu Rev Med* 1992;43:317–323.
5. Saikku P. *Chlamydia pneumoniae*: clinical spectrum. In: Stephens RS, Byrne GI, Christiansen G, et al., eds. *Chlamydial infections: proceedings of the Ninth International Symposium on Human Chlamydial Infection*. San Francisco: International Chlamydia Symposium, 1998:145–154.
6. Saikku P, Leinonen M, Mattila K, et al. Serological evidence of an association of a novel *Chlamydia*, TWAR, with chronic coronary heart disease and acute myocardial infarction. *Lancet* 1988;2:983–986.
7. Stephens RS, ed. *Chlamydia: intracellular biology, pathogenesis, and immunity*. Washington, DC: American Society for Microbiology, 1999.
8. Zhang JP, Stephens RS. Mechanism of *C. trachomatis* attachment to eukaryotic host cells. *Cell* 1992;69:861–869.
9. Moulder JW. Comparative biology of intracellular parasitism. *Microbiol Rev* 1985;49:298–337.
10. Gregory WW, Gardner M, Byrne GI, et al. Arrays of hemispheric surface projections on *Chlamydia psittaci* and *Chlamydia trachomatis* observed by scanning electron microscopy. *J Bacteriol* 1979;138:241–244.
11. Caldwell HD, Kromhout J, Schachter J. Purification and partial characterization of the major outer membrane protein of *Chlamydia trachomatis*. *Infect Immun* 1981;31:1161–1176.
12. Wang SP, Grayston JT. Immunologic relationship between genital TRIC, lymphogranuloma venereum, and related organisms in a new microtiter indirect immunofluorescence test. *Am J Ophthalmol* 1970;70:367–374.
13. Grayston JT, Wang S. New knowledge of chlamydiae and the diseases they cause. *J Infect Dis* 1975;132:87–105.
14. Caldwell HD, Schachter J. Antigenic analysis of the major outer membrane protein of *Chlamydia* spp. *Infect Immun* 1982;35:1024–1031.
15. Hatch TP, Al-Hossainy E, Silverman JA. Adenine nucleotide and lysine transport in Chlamydia psittaci. *J Bacteriol* 1982;150:662–670.
16. Stephens R, Kalman S, Fenner C, et al. *Chlamydia* Genome Project. Available online: http://chlamydia-www.berkeley.edu:4231/.
17. Palmer L, Falkow S. A common plasmid of *Chlamydia trachomatis*. *Plasmid* 1986;16:52–62.
18. Nano FE, Caldwell HD. Expression of the chlamydial genus-specific lipopolysaccharide epitope in *Escherichia coli*. *Science* 1985;228:742–744.
19. Stephens RS, Sanchez-Pescador R, Wagar EA, et al. Diversity of *Chlamydia trachomatis* major outer membrane protein genes. *J Bacteriol* 1987;169:3879–3885.
20. Stephens RS, Wagar EA, Schoolnik GK. High-resolution mapping of serovar-specific and common antigenic determinants of the major outer membrane protein of Chlamydia trachomatis. *J Exp Med* 1988;167:817–831.
21. Centers for Disease Control. 1998 Guidelines for treatment of sexually transmitted diseases. *MMWR Morb Mortal Wkly Rep* 1998;47:1–111.
22. Gerbase AC, Rowley JT, Mertens TE. Global epidemiology of sexually transmitted diseases. *Lancet* 1998;351[Suppl 3]:2–4.
23. Stamm WE. *Chlamydia trachomatis* infections of the adult. In: Holmes KK, Sparling PF, March P-A, et al., eds. *Sexually transmitted diseases*, 3rd ed. New York: McGraw Hill, 1999:407–422.
24. Shafer MA, Prager V, Shalwitz J, et al. Prevalence of urethral *Chlamydia trachomatis* and *Neisseria gonorrhoeae* among asymptomatic, sexually active adolescent boys. *J Infect Dis* 1987;156:223–224.
25. Schachter J, Stoner E, Moncada J. Screening for chlamydial infections in women attending family planning clinics. *West J Med* 1983;138:375–379.
26. Handsfield HH, Jasman LL, Roberts PL, et al. Criteria for selective screening for *Chlamydia trachomatis* infection in women attending family planning clinics. *JAMA* 1986;255:1730–1734.
27. Burstein GR, Gaydos CA, Diener-West M, et al. Incident *Chlamydia trachomatis* infections among inner-city adolescent females. *JAMA* 1998;280:521–526.
28. Westrom L, Eschenbach D. Pelvic inflammatory diseases. In: Holmes KK, Sparling PF, Mardh P-A, et al., eds. *Sexually transmitted diseases*, 3rd ed. New York: McGraw-Hill, 1999:783–810.
29. Alexander ER, Harrison HR. Role of *Chlamydia trachomatis* in perinatal infection. *Rev Infect Dis* 1983;5:713–719.
30. Thylefors B, Negrel AD, Pararajasegaram R, et al. Global data on blindness. *Bull W H O* 1995;73:115–121.
31. Dawson CR, Daghfous T, Messadi M, et al. Severe endemic trachoma in Tunisia. *Br J Ophthalmol* 1976;60:245–252.
32. Kleemola M, Saikku P, Visakorpi R, et al. Epidemics of pneumonia caused by TWAR, a new *Chlamydia* organism, in military trainees in Finland. *J Infect Dis* 1988;157:230–236.
33. Taylor HR, Johnson SL, Schachter J, et al. Pathogenesis of trachoma: the stimulus for inflammation. *J Immunol* 1987;138:3023–3027.
34. Taylor HR, Johnson SL, Prendergast RA, et al. An animal model of trachoma II. The importance of repeated reinfection. *Invest Ophthalmol Vis Sci* 1982;23:507–515.
35. Patton DL, Kuo CC, Wang SP, et al. Distal tubal obstruction induced by repeated *Chlamydia trachomatis* salpingeal infections in pig-tailed macaques. *J Infect Dis* 1987;155:1292–1299.
36. Wagar EA, Schachter J, Bavoil P, et al. Differential human serologic response to two 60,000 molecular weight *Chlamydia trachomatis* antigens. *J Infect Dis* 1990;162:922–927.
37. Toye B, Laferriere C, Claman P, et al. Association between antibody to the chlamydial heat-shock protein and tubal infertility. *J Infect Dis* 1993;168:1236–1240.
38. Schachter J. Chlamydiae. In: Rose NR, Conway de Macario E, Folds JD, et al., eds. *Manual of clinical laboratory immunology*, 5th ed. Washington, DC: ASM Press, 1997:552–557.
39. Zhang YX, Stewart S, Joseph T, et al. Protective monoclonal antibodies recognize epitopes located on the major outer membrane protein of Chlamydia trachomatis. *J Immunol* 1987;138:575–581.
40. Byrne GI, Faubion CL. Lymphokine-mediated microbistatic mechanisms restrict *Chlamydia psittaci* growth in macrophages. *J Immunol* 1982;128:469–474.
41. Rothermel CD, Rubin BY, Murray HW. Gamma-interferon is the factor in lymphokine that activates human macrophages to inhibit intracellular *Chlamydia psittaci* replication. *J Immunol* 1983;131:2542–2544.
42. Byrne GI, Kreuger DA. Lymphokine-mediated inhibition of *Chlamydia* replication in mouse fibroblasts is neutralized by anti-gamma interferon immunoglobulin. *Infect Immun* 1983;42:1152–1158.
43. Byrne GI, Lehmann LK, Landry GJ. Introduction of tryptophan catabolism is the mechanism for gamma-interferon-mediated inhibition of intracellular *Chlamydia psittaci* replication. *Infect Immun* 1986;53:347–351.
44. Westrom L, Joesoef R, Reynolds G, et al. Pelvic inflammatory disease and fertility: a cohort study of 1,844 women with laparoscopically verified disease and 657 control women with normal laparoscopic results. *Sex Transm Dis* 1992;19:185–192.
45. Schachter J, Grossman M, Sweet RL, et al. Prospective study of perinatal transmission of *Chlamydia trachomatis*. *JAMA* 1986;255:3374–3377.
46. Johnson FW, Matheson BA, Williams H, et al. Abortion due to infection with *Chlamydia psittaci* in a sheep farmer's wife. *Br Med J (Clin Res Ed)* 1985;290:592–594.
47. Grayston JT. Antibiotic treatment of *Chlamydia pneumoniae* for secondary prevention of cardiovascular events. In: Stephens RS, Byrne GI, Christiansen G, et al., eds. *Chlamydial infections: proceedings of the Ninth International Symposium on Human Chlamydial Infection*. San Francisco: International Chlamydia Symposium, 1998:187–190.
48. Kuo CC, Shor A, Campbell LA, et al. Demonstration of *Chlamydia pneumoniae* in atherosclerotic lesions of coronary arteries. *J Infect Dis* 1993;167:841–849.
49. Kalayoglu M, Byrne GI. *C. pneumoniae* induces foam cell formation in macrophages. In: Stephens RS, Byrne GI, Christiansen G, et al., eds. *Chlamydial infections: proceedings of the Ninth International Symposium on Human Chlamydial Infection*. San Francisco: International Chlamydia Symposium, 1998:430–433.
50. Schachter J, Stamm WE. Chlamydia. In: Murray PR, Baron EJ, Pfaller MA, et al., eds. *Manual of clinical microbiology*, 7th ed. Washington, DC: American Society for Microbiology, 1999:795–806.
51. Schachter J. NAATs to diagnose *Chlamydia trachomatis* genital infection: a promise still unfulfilled. *Expert Review of Molecular Diagnostics* 2001;1:137–144.
52. Schachter J, Grossman M, Azimi PH. Serology of *Chlamydia trachomatis* in infants. *J Infect Dis* 1982;146:530–535.
53. Cles LD, Stamm WE. Use of HL cells for improved isolation and passage of *Chlamydia pneumoniae*. *J Clin Microbiol* 1990;28:938–940.
54. Martin DH, Mroczkowski TF, Dalu ZA, et al. A controlled trial of a single dose of azithromycin for the treatment of chlamydial urethritis and cervicitis. The Azithromycin for Chlamydial Infections Study Group. *N Engl J Med* 1992;327:921–925.
55. Schachter J. Rifampin in chlamydial infections. *Rev Infect Dis* 1983;5[Suppl 3]:S562–S564.

56. Dessus-Babus S, Bebear CM, Charron A, et al. Alteration in DNA gyrase of fluoroquinolone-resistant mutants of *Chlamydia trachomatis* obtained *in vitro*. In: Stephens RS, Byrne GI, Christiansen G, et al., eds. *Chlamydial infections: proceedings of the Ninth International Symposium on Human Chlamydial Infection.* San Francisco: International Chlamydia Symposium, 1998:309–312.

57. Bailey RL, Arullendran P, Whittle HC, et al. Randomised controlled trial of single-dose azithromycin in treatment of trachoma. *Lancet* 1993;342:453–456.

58. Schachter J, West S, Mabey D, et al. Azithromycin in control of trachoma. *Lancet* 1999;354:630–635.

59. Centers for Disease Control. 1993 Sexually transmitted disease guidelines. *MMWR Morb Mortal Wkly Rep* 1993;42:1–102.

60. Scholes D, Stergachis A, Heidrich FE, et al. Prevention of pelvic inflammatory disease by screening for cervical chlamydial infection. *N Engl J Med* 1996;334:1362–1366.

61. Schachter J, Sweet RL, Grossman M, et al. Experience with the routine use of erythromycin for chlamydial infections in pregnancy. *N Engl J Med* 1986;314:276–279.

CHAPTER 223
Mycoplasmas and Ureaplasmas

William M. McCormack

HISTORY

Mycoplasmal species were first encountered in diseases of animals. By the end of the nineteenth century, the first known member of the group had been identified as the etiologic agent of contagious bovine pleuropneumonia, an important disease of cattle. This agent, now called *Mycoplasma mycoides*, was cultivated by Nocard and Roux in 1898 on serum-enriched, cell-free medium (1). Similar organisms subsequently isolated from various species were called pleuropneumonia-like organisms (PPLO). In 1937, Dienes and Edsall were first to report the isolation from a human of a mycoplasma (most likely *Mycoplasma hominis*), in a Bartholin's gland abscess (2).

Several mycoplasmal species have been isolated from human sources, mainly from the mucous membranes of the urogenital and upper respiratory tracts. Four of the human mycoplasmal species, *M. pneumoniae, M. hominis, Mycoplasma genitalium,* and *Ureaplasma urealyticum,* have been shown to be pathogenic and will be dealt with in detail. The other species are commensals. Mycoplasmal species have been recovered from patients with human immunodeficiency virus (HIV) infection (3–6). Recent studies indicate that these organisms (*Mycoplasma fermentans, Mycoplasma penetrans,* and *Mycoplasma pirum*) do not have an important role in the pathogenesis of HIV or HIV-associated conditions. Table 223.1 lists the human mycoplasmas, indicates their usual habitats, and lists prominent features of each species (1,7).

CHARACTERISTICS OF THE PATHOGEN

Mycoplasmas are small pleomorphic organisms, 0.3 to 0.8 μm in diameter, that lack a cell wall. They are bounded only by a plasma membrane. They belong to the class Mollicutes, order Mycoplasmatales, family Mycoplasmataceae. *Mycoplasma* and *Ureaplasma* species of the family Mycoplasmataceae infect only animals. Mycoplasmataceae require sterols for growth and differ widely in their metabolic activities. Some degrade glucose by the glycolytic pathway; some convert arginine to citrulline or ornithine by the arginine dihydrolase pathway. The ability of the genus *Ureaplasma* to hydrolyze urea sets it apart from the genus *Mycoplasma* (7).

Mycoplasmas differ from viruses in that they contain both RNA and DNA. They resemble chlamydiae, rickettsiae, and viruses in filterability through a 45-μm filter, but they differ in being able to grow on cell-free media. Although cell wall–deficient bacterial variants (L forms, spheroplasts, protoplasts) form colonies that resemble those of mycoplasmas, and although they share some other properties with the mycoplasmas, the two are unrelated. The filterability of mycoplasmas is the result not only of their small size but also of the flexibility of their plasma membrane (1).

On solid medium, most mycoplasmas form small colonies, 50 to 600 μm in diameter, which can be seen only with a hand lens or under low power of a microscope. The classic fried-egg appearance of the usual colony is due to an opaque granular central zone of growth down into the agar and a flat translucent peripheral zone of growth on the surface. Not all mycoplasmas produce fried-egg colonies, and variations in colonial morphology are frequently dependent on the constituents of the medium as well as on atmosphere and inoculum size (7). Ureaplasmas were originally called tiny, or T, strains because they form small (15 to 30 μm) colonies that lack a peripheral area of surface growth (1).

By reason of their limited biosynthetic abilities, these organisms are highly fastidious and require complex enriched culture media for growth. Media ordinarily contain a peptone, a cholesterol, or a related sterol supplied by animal serum; preformed nucleic acid precursors supplied by yeast extract; and a metabolite, such as glucose, arginine, or urea (8). The optimal temperature for growth of all mycoplasmal and ureaplasmal species is 37°C. Most mycoplasmas are facultatively anaerobic, but the growth of some is enhanced by incubation in air with 5% carbon dioxide (2).

Mycoplasmataceae are the simplest and smallest self-replicating prokaryotes. The 500-megadalton (700 kilobase pairs) genome characterizing *Mycoplasma* and *Ureaplasma* and its extremely low guanine-plus-cytosine content impose considerable restrictions on coding capacity, explaining the small number of cell proteins produced, the scarcity of metabolic pathways, and the complex nutritional requirements (9). Like other prokaryotes, these organisms divide by binary fission, but cytoplasmic division and genomic replication are not precisely synchronized and are easily dissociated (7).

Mycoplasmas and ureaplasmas have a circular genome of double-stranded DNA, one fifth to one half as large as that of most bacteria. They generally grow more slowly than bacteria, with a mean generation time of 1 to 3 hours (1).

Classification of mycoplasmas is based primarily on serologic reactions. Tests that detect membrane antigens, such as growth inhibition, metabolism inhibition, and immunofluorescence, are specific enough to detect serologic differences within species. In the growth inhibition test, growth of the organism on agar is inhibited in a zone around a filter paper disk impregnated with specific antiserum. The metabolism inhibition test is unique to mycoplasmas and is based on the premise that inhibition of the growth of the organism by specific antibody is reflected by the failure of the organism to produce normal metabolic end products (1). The advantage of this test is that only a few organisms are required. However, the organisms must be living, and the end points change over time. The direct identification of mycoplasmal colonies on agar by immunofluorescence is rapid and specific and has the further advantage of detecting a mixture of mycoplasmas of different serotypes in the same culture.

Immunoassays have been used to detect antigens of various mycoplasmal species. Diagnosis is relatively inexpensive, and

TABLE 223.1. Properties of Human Mycoplasmas and Ureaplasmas

Species	Substrates metabolized			Usual habitat	Disease association
	Glucose	Arginine	Urea		
Ureaplasma urealyticum	−	−	+	Genital tract	Nongonococcal urethritis Infertility and reproductive failure
Mycoplasma hominis	−	+	−	Genital tract	Pelvic inflammatory disease Postpartum fever
Mycoplasma genitalium	+	−	−	Genital tract	Nongonococcal urethritis
Mycoplasma fermentans	+	+	−	Genital tract	None
Mycoplasma pneumoniae	+	−	−	Respiratory tract	Upper respiratory and lower respiratory infections
Mycoplasma salivarium	−	+	−	Oropharynx	None
Mycoplasma orale	−	+	−	Oropharynx	None
Mycoplasma buccale	−	+	−	Oropharynx	None
Mycoplasma faucium	−	+	−	Oropharynx	None
Mycoplasma lipophilum	−	+	−	Oropharynx	None
Mycoplasma primatum	−	+	−	Genital tract (rare)	None
Acholeplasma laidlawii	+	−	−	Respiratory tract (rare)	None
Mycoplasma pirum	+	+	−	Unknown	Possibly human immunodeficiency virus (HIV) associated
Mycoplasma penetrans	+	+	−	Unknown	Possibly HIV associated

Adapted from Chanock RM, Tully JG. Mycoplasmas. In: Davis BD, et al., eds. *Microbiology,* 3rd ed. New York: Harper & Row, 1980: 785–795; and Velleca WM, Bird BR. *Laboratory diagnosis of mycoplasma infections.* Course 8226-C Washington, DC: U.S. Department of Health and Human Services, Public Health Science Center for Disease Control, October 1980, with permission.

results are obtained quickly. These tests, however, are not sensitive enough to replace culture. Sensitive and specific nucleic acid amplifications tests have been developed for human pathogens and are available in research laboratories.

EPIDEMIOLOGY

An unusual feature of symptomatic infection with *M. pneumoniae* is its peak incidence in children 5 to 15 years of age. The organism accounts for 15% to 50% of all pneumonias in this age group. Infections occur throughout the year, with a predilection for late summer and early fall. Intensive exposure to infected persons appears to be required for transmission of *M. pneumoniae*. The organism is usually introduced into a household by a school-aged child. Spread of the organism from person to person is quite slow and generally not achieved through casual contact. The incubation period is 2 to 3 weeks (1,10,11).

The genital mycoplasmas, *M. hominis* and *U. urealyticum*, are common inhabitants of the genitourinary mucous membranes of humans. Infants presumably become colonized with genital mycoplasmas during passage through the birth canal. Infants delivered by cesarean section are colonized less often than those delivered vaginally (12). Ureaplasmas have been isolated from the genitalia of up to one third of infant girls and *M. hominis* from a smaller proportion (12). Mycoplasmas are recovered less frequently from infant boys (13).

Neonatal colonization tends not to persist. These organisms are seldom recovered from prepubertal boys. From 5% to 22% of prepubertal girls are colonized with *U. urealyticum* and 8% to 17% with *M. hominis* (14). After puberty, colonization is closely associated with sexual experience (15). With increasing sexual experience, colonization increases more rapidly in women than in men, suggesting that it is easier to transmit the organisms from men to women than from women to men. Colonization rates with both *M. hominis* and *U. urealyticum* are higher among clinic populations than among the patients of private obstetricians and gynecologists. In Boston, *M. hominis* was isolated from 53.6% and

ureaplasmas from 76.3% of clinic patients at a municipal hospital, compared with 21.3% and 52.9%, respectively, of patients visiting private obstetricians and gynecologists in the same area (16,17).

Thus, these organisms can be isolated from a significant proportion of heterosexually active men and women. It is against this background that the role of *M. hominis* and *U. urealyticum* in human disease must be viewed. Little is known about the epidemiology of *M. genitalium*.

PATHOGENESIS

Mycoplasmas are surface parasites that adhere to and colonize the mucous membranes of the host (18). They only rarely invade tissue or the bloodstream. Efficient adherence mechanisms are therefore a prerequisite for their survival and pathogenicity. Adherence must be firm enough to prevent detachment by mucous secretions or by the urinary stream. The absence of a cell wall makes possible close contact of the plasma membrane with the host cell membrane. The acquisition of host cell antigens by mycoplasmas, as suggested by Wise and co-workers (19), may help them avoid or alter the host immunologic response. On the other hand, the acquisition of mycoplasmal antigens by the host membrane may trigger autoimmune reactions, which are common in some mycoplasmal infections (20).

M. pneumoniae can attach to the surface of the respiratory epithelium, binding to neuraminic acid receptors. The organism does not enter host cells, nor does it penetrate beneath the epithelial surface. In tracheal organ cultures, its attachment leads to direct damage to the epithelium, with loss of cilia and finally cell death. This cell damage may be produced by hydrogen peroxide released by the organism. Children 2 to 5 years of age often possess mycoplasmacidal antibodies, although the disease appears most often at age 5 to 15 years. Thus, it has been suggested that the pathogenic effects of *M. pneumoniae* may include an immunopathologic reaction in a host sensitized by prior subclinical infection (1).

CLINICAL MANIFESTATIONS

In humans, *M. pneumoniae* causes mild upper respiratory disease more often than it does pneumonia. The onset of pneumonia is generally gradual, and the symptoms may be mild or moderately severe. Involvement is usually interstitial, often limited to one of the lower lobes. The course of the pneumonia is variable, with remittent fever, cough, and headache lasting for several weeks. Convalescence may extend for 4 to 6 weeks even in the absence of complications (1,10,11).

M. hominis and *U. urealyticum* are both commonly isolated from women who have bacterial vaginosis; these organisms appear to be part of the abnormal polymicrobial flora of this condition (21). *M. hominis* and, less often, *U. urealyticum* have been isolated from upper genital tract specimens from some patients with pelvic inflammatory disease. This is probably a reflection of the association of bacterial vaginosis with pelvic inflammatory disease. It is clear that most cases of pelvic inflammatory disease are caused by *Chlamydia trachomatis* and *Neisseria gonorrhoeae* (22).

M. hominis has been shown to cause fever after abortion and postpartum endometritis (23). *M. hominis* may act as an opportunist, causing infections outside the genitourinary tract, including wound, joint, and central nervous system infections (24). *U. urealyticum* has been shown to cause some cases of nongonococcal urethritis (25) and has been associated in some studies with chorioamnionitis (26), low birth weight (27), and neonatal infection (28,29).

M. genitalium plays a role in nongonococcal urethritis. Recent studies using DNA probes and polymerase chain reaction (PCR) have associated this organism with acute and recurrent episodes of urethritis (30–33).

M. genitalium has also been implicated in pelvic inflammatory disease (34).

Both *M. hominis* and *U. urealyticum* have been shown to have multiple serotypes (35). Although the data are scanty, none of the work to date has suggested that any particular serotype is associated with any particular disease process (36).

DIAGNOSIS

Tracheal aspirates, nasopharyngeal swabs, throat swabs, or a sputum specimen should be obtained for *M. pneumoniae* culture (7). *M. hominis* and *U. urealyticum* organisms should be sought in urethral cultures from men (37). In women, vaginal specimens are more likely to contain *M. hominis* and *U. urealyticum* than are specimens from the endocervical canal, posterior fornix, or urethra (38). Urine culture is useful for large epidemiologic studies but is an indirect means of sampling and yields fewer isolates than do cultures obtained directly from the genital mucosa (39).

Swabs are immersed in 2 mL of cold sterile transport medium immediately after collection. Urine specimens are centrifuged, and the sediment is used for culture. Specimens should be kept on wet ice or at 4°C and transported to the laboratory as soon as possible. Specimens that cannot be delivered to the laboratory and inoculated within 24 hours of collection should be frozen at −70°C.

Methylene blue glucose diphasic medium and glucose agar medium are used to cultivate *M. pneumoniae*. The diphasic medium is prepared by using a mycoplasma broth base and a mycoplasma agar base, both of which are supplemented with 20% horse serum, 10% fresh yeast extract, 50% glucose, 0.4% phenol red, 1% methylene blue, 100,000 U/mL penicillin, and 10% thallium acetate. The pH of the medium is adjusted to 7.8 with sterile 1 N NaOH. Once the agar has solidified in 1-mL aliquots

in 13 × 100 mm screw-cap test tubes or 1-dram screw-cap vials, it is overlaid with the broth (7). Glucose agar medium is prepared by combining mycoplasma agar base with 20% horse serum, 10% fresh yeast extract, 50% glucose, 100,000 U/mL penicillin, and 10% thallium acetate. The pH is adjusted to 7.8 with sterile 1 N NaOH (7).

A 0.3-mL aliquot of each specimen is inoculated into the diphasic medium, which is incubated at 36°C and examined daily for color change from blue to yellow. The color change usually begins along the interface of the agar and broth. A color change during the first week of incubation is usually due to a bacterial contaminant, but thereafter, it is almost always caused by growth of *M. pneumoniae*. The diphasic medium must be subcultured to glucose agar as soon as the color begins to change because the organism will lose viability as the medium becomes more acidic. A 0.1-mL aliquot of the diphasic medium is inoculated onto two of more glucose agar plates (7).

Presumptive identification of colonies of *M. pneumoniae* on agar can be accomplished using hemadsorption or β-hemolysis. *M. pneumoniae* colonies adsorb guinea pig erythrocytes, whereas other mycoplasmas do not. The red blood cells can be seen adhering to the colonies under the microscope at × 100. *M. pneumoniae* produces a β-hemolysin (peroxide) that causes complete lysis of guinea pig and sheep erythrocytes. No other mycoplasma will cause complete hemolysis of red blood cells from these species (7).

Available serologic tests include complement fixation and enzyme immunoassay. Serum samples obtained from patients early in their illness and 1 to 3 weeks later usually show a fourfold or greater rise in titer (40).

Cold agglutinins are immunoglobulin M autoantibodies that agglutinate human red blood cells at 4°C. Serum cold agglutinins are positive, in titers greater than 1:32, in 33% to 76% of patients with *M. pneumoniae* pneumonia. Cold agglutinins usually appear at the end of the first week of illness and disappear in 2 to 3 months. The height of the cold agglutinin response is usually directly proportional to the severity of pulmonary involvement. Cold agglutinins may also be present in measles and other infections, but titers are unlikely to be higher than 1:32 (40).

Differences in metabolic activity provide a useful means of identification of genital mycoplasmas. *M. hominis* organisms convert arginine to ornithine, whereas ureaplasmas utilize urea. Both these reactions are associated with a rise in pH. From tubes showing a change in color of the pH indicator, an aliquot is subcultured onto agar for definitive identification (7).

M. hominis and *U. urealyticum* are grown in mycoplasma broth or agar supplemented with 20% horse serum, 10% fresh yeast extract, and phenol red. Penicillin, polymyxin B, and amphotericin B are added to inhibit other organisms (41).

Ureaplasmal medium contains lincomycin, to inhibit *M. hominis*, and 0.1% urea. The pH is adjusted to 6.0. *U. urealyticum* agar is prepared with the same supplements as the broth plus manganous sulfate, cysteine HCl, and putrescine. Medium used to isolate *M. hominis* contains erythromycin, to inhibit ureaplasmas, and arginine. The pH is adjusted to 7.0.

An aliquot of the original specimen is inoculated into 1.0 mL of each specific broth. After inoculation, pH is recorded. Tubes are incubated and read for 8 days; they are discarded as negative if there is no significant pH change. Once a rise in pH is noted, an aliquot is plated onto the appropriate agar.

After the inoculum has dried, a disk containing 15 μg of erythromycin is placed on the ureaplasma agar. Similarly, a disk impregnated with specific antiserum is placed on *M. hominis* agar. Plates are incubated for a minimum of 48 hours in an anaerobic jar in an atmosphere containing 10% carbon dioxide and 90% nitrogen.

Plates are read with a microscope under low power (×10). Colonies of *M. hominis* usually have a classic fried-egg appearance. There is a zone of inhibition around the disk impregnated with specific antiserum. The addition of manganous sulfate to ureaplasma agar causes the colonies to appear quite dark, golden brown to chestnut, with a well-defined periphery (42).

M. hominis will produce nonhemolytic pinpoint colonies on blood agar, but the organisms cannot be visualized in Gram-stained smears of these colonies. *M. hominis* will also grow in some routine blood culture media (43). *Ureaplasma* and *M. genitalium* will not grow in ordinary microbiologic media.

M. genitalium has been isolated in SP4 medium (44). *M. genitalium* is a glucose fermenter. It is more fastidious than either *M. hominis* or *U. urealyticum* and will not grow in conventional mycoplasmal media. These organisms require other supplements, such as CMRL 1066 tissue culture supplement with glutamine, yeastolate, and fetal bovine serum. Modification of SP4 media with polymyxin B and amphotericin prevents contamination. Commercially available culture media for the genital mycoplasmas are available (45,46).

Nucleic acid amplification tests such as PCR have been developed for pathogenic mycoplasmas. These tests have high specificity and are usually more sensitive than culture.

TREATMENT AND PREVENTION

Mycoplasmas are not sensitive to inhibitors of cell wall synthesis. The organisms are not susceptible to sulfonamides and trimethoprim because they do not synthesize folic acid. Protein synthesis in mycoplasmas is prokaryotic; antibiotics that inhibit protein synthesis may be effective (47,48). Mycoplasmas are usually sensitive to tetracyclines, aminoglycosides, and macrolides, but individual strains and species vary. Tetracyclines and erythromycins are effective in the treatment of infections caused by *M. pneumoniae*; clinical improvement occurs even though the organisms persist.

M. hominis organisms are susceptible to clindamycin, moderately susceptible to chloramphenicol, and resistant to erythromycin, rifampin, and azithromycin (49). Tetracycline is the antibiotic that is most frequently used to treat infections caused by *M. hominis*; however, with the emergence of tetracycline-resistant *M. hominis* strains (50,51), other agents, such as clindamycin, should be considered.

U. urealyticum and possibly *M. genitalium* are causes of nongonococcal urethritis; treatment with tetracycline or doxycycline is usually effective in these species, but 10% of *U. urealyticum* strains are resistant to tetracycline (51–53). Patients who have nongonococcal urethritis and show no response to tetracycline should be tested, if possible, for *U. urealyticum* and treated with erythromycin or a quinolone (54).

There are no immunizing preparations available for the genital mycoplasmas. Use of barrier methods of contraception retards colonization with mycoplasmas (17), but because the organisms are so widespread, a significant number of sexually experienced adults eventually become colonized.

REFERENCES

1. Chanock RM, Tully JG. Mycoplasmas. In: Davis BD, et al., eds. *Microbiology*, 3rd ed. New York: Harper & Row, 1980:785–795.
2. Dienes L, Edsall G. Observations on the L-organism of Klieneberger. *Proc Soc Exp Biol Med* 1937;36:740.
3. Montagnier L, Blanchard A. Mycoplasmas as cofactors in infection due to the human immunodeficiency virus [Review]. *Clin Infect Dis* 1993;17[Suppl 1]: S309.
4. Chirgwin KD, Cummings MC, DeMeo LR, et al. Identification of mycoplasmas in urine from persons infected with human immunodeficiency virus. *Clin Infect Dis* 1993;17[Suppl 1]:S264.
5. Bauer FA, Wear DJ, Angritt P, et al. *Mycoplasma fermentans* (incognitus strain) infection in the kidneys of patients with acquired immunodeficiency syndrome and associated nephropathy: a light microscopic, immunohistochemical, and ultrastructural study. *Hum Pathol* 1991;22:63.
6. Wang RY-H, Shih JW-K, Weiss SH, et al. *Mycoplasma penetrans* infection in male homosexuals with AIDS: high seroprevalence and association with Kaposi's sarcoma. *Clin Infect Dis* 1993;17:724.
7. Valleca WM, Bird BR. *Laboratory diagnosis of mycoplasma infections*. Course 8226-C Washington, DC: U.S. Department of Health and Human Services, Public Health Service Center for Disease Control, October 1980.
8. Kenny GE. Mycoplasmas. In: Lennette EH, Balows A, Hausler WJ, et al., eds. *Manual of clinical microbiology*, 4th ed. Washington DC: American Society for Microbiology, 1985:407–411.
9. Razin S. Molecular biology and genetics of mycoplasmas (molecules). *Microbiol Rev* 1985;49:419.
10. Park DR, Sherbin VL, Goodman MS, et al. The etiology of community-acquired pneumonia in an urban public hospital. *J Infect Dis* 2001;184:268.
11. Principi N, Esposito S, Blasi F, et al. Role of *Mycoplasma pneumoniae* and *Chlamydia pneumoniae* in children with community-acquired lower respiratory tract infections. *Clin Infect Dis* 2001;32:1281.
12. Klein JO, Buckland D, Finland M. Colonization of newborn infants by mycoplasmas. *N Engl J Med* 1969;280:1025.
13. Foy HM, Kenny GE, Levinsohn EM, et al. Acquisition of mycoplasmata and T-strains during infancy. *J Infect Dis* 1970;121:579.
14. Hammerschlag MR, Alpert S, Rosner I, et al. Microbiology of the vagina in children: normal and potentially pathogenic organisms. *Pediatrics* 1978; 62:57.
15. McCormack WM, Almeida PC, Bailey PE, et al. Sexual activity and vaginal colonization with genital mycoplasmas. *JAMA* 1972;221:1375.
16. McCormack WM, Rosner B, Lee Y. Colonization with genital mycoplasmas in women. *Am J Epidemiol* 1973;97:240.
17. McCormack WM, Rosner B, Alpert S, et al. Vaginal colonization with *Mycoplasma hominis* and *Ureaplasma urealyticum*. *Sex Transm Dis* 1986;13:67.
18. Razin S. Mycoplasma adherence. In: Razin S, Barile MF, eds. *The Mycoplasmas*, Vol IV. New York: Academic Press, 1985:161–202.
19. Wise KS, Cassell GH, Acton RT. Selective association of murine T lymphoblastoid cell surface alloantigens with *Mycoplasma hyorhinis*. *Proc Natl Acad Sci U S A* 1978;75:4479.
20. Fernald GW. Immunologic interactions between host cells and mycoplasmas: an introduction. *Rev Infect Dis* 1982;4[Suppl]:201.
21. Gravett MG, Eschenbach DA. Possible role of *Ureaplasma urealyticum* in preterm premature rupture of the fetal membrane. *Pediatr Infect Dis* 1986;5[Suppl]: S253.
22. Moller BR. The role of mycoplasmas in the upper genital tract of women. *Sex Transm Dis* 1983;10[Suppl]:281.
23. Plummer DC, Garland SM, Gilbert GL. Bacteremia and pelvic infection in women due to *Ureaplasma urealyticum* and *Mycoplasma hominis*. *Med J Aust* 1987;146:135.
24. Madoff S, Hooper DC. Nongenitourinary infections caused by *Mycoplasma hominis* in adults. *Rev Infect Dis* 1988;10:602.
25. Brunner H, Wolfgang W, Hans-Gerd S. Quantitative studies on the role of *Ureaplasma urealyticum* in non-gonococcal urethritis and chronic prostatitis. *Yale J Med Biol* 1983;56:545.
26. Hillier SL, Krohn MJ, Kiviat N, et al. The association of *Ureaplasma urealyticum* with preterm birth, chorioamnionitis, post partum fever, intrapartum fever and bacterial vaginosis. *Pediatr Infect Dis* 1986;5[Suppl]:S349.
27. Braun P, Lee YH, Klein JO, et al. Birth weight and genital mycoplasmas in pregnancy. *N Engl J Med* 1971;284:167.
28. Waites KB, Crouse DT, Nelson KG, et al. Chronic *Ureaplasma urealyticum* and *Mycoplasma hominis* infections of central nervous system in preterm infants. *Lancet* 1988;1:17.
29. Valencia GB, Banzon F, Cummings M, et al. *Mycoplasma hominis* and *Ureaplasma urealyticum* in neonates with suspected infection. *Pediatr Infect Dis J* 1993;12:571.
30. Totten PA, Schwartz MA, Sjostrom KE, et al. Association of *Mycoplasma genitalium* with nongonococcal urethritis in heterosexual men. *J Infect Dis* 2001;183:269.
31. Horner P, Thomas B, Gilroy CB, et al. Role of *Mycoplasma genitalium* and *Ureaplasma urealyticum* in acute and chronic nongonococcal urethritis. *Clin Infect Dis* 2001;32:995.
32. Maeda S-I, Tamaki M, Kojima K, et al. Association of *Mycoplasma genitalium* persistence in the urethra with recurrence of nongonococcal urethritis. *Sex Transm Dis* 2001;28:472.
33. Hooton TM, Roberts PL, Stamm WE, et al. Prevalence of *Mycoplasma genitalium* determined by DNA probe in men with urethritis. *Lancet* 1988; 1:266.
34. Moller BR, Taylor-Robinson D, Furr PM. Serological evidence implicating *Mycoplasma genitalium* in PID. *Lancet* 1984;1:1102.
35. Lin J-S, Kass EH. Serological reactions of *Mycoplasma hominis*: differences among mycoplasmacidal, metabolic inhibition, and growth agglutination tests. *Infect Immun* 1974;10:535.
36. Lin JS. Human mycoplasmal infections: serologic observations. *Rev Infect Dis* 1985;7:216.

37. Tarr PI, Lee Y-H, Alpert S, et al. Comparison of methods for the isolation of genital mycoplasmas from men. *J Infect Dis* 1976;133:419.
38. McCormack WM, Rankin JS, Lee YH. Localization of genital mycoplasmas in women. *Am J Obstet Gynecol* 1972;112:920.
39. Taylor-Robinson D, McCormack WM. Mycoplasmas in human genitourinary infections. In: Tully JG, Whitcomb RF, eds. *The mycoplasmas,* Vol 2. New York: Academic Press, 1979:307–366.
40. Broughton RA. Infections due to *Mycoplasma pneumoniae* in childhood. *Pediatr Infect Dis* 1986;5:71.
41. Freundt EA. Culture media for classical mycoplasmas. In: Tully JG, Razin S, eds. *Methods in mycoplasmology,* Section C7, Vol 1. New York: Academic Press, 1983.
42. Razin S. Urea hydrolysis. In: Tully JG, Razin S, eds. *Methods in mycoplasmology,* Section E4, Vol 1. New York: Academic Press, 1983.
43. Wallace RJ, Alpert S, Browne K, et al. Isolation of *Mycoplasma hominis* from blood cultures in patients with post partum fever. *Obstet Gynecol* 1978;51:181.
44. Tully JG, Cole RM, Taylor-Robinson D, et al. A newly discovered mycoplasma in the human urogenital tract. *Lancet* 1981;1:1288.
45. Broitman NL, Floyd CM, Johnson CA, et al. Comparison of commercially available media for detection and isolation of *Ureaplasma urealyticum* and *Mycoplasma hominis. J Clin Microbiol* 1992;30:1335.
46. Sillis M. Genital mycoplasmas revisited: an evaluation of a new culture medium. *Br J Biomed Sci* 1993;50:89.
47. Stanbridge EJ, The molecular biology of mycoplasmas. In: Reff ME. Barile MF, Razin S, eds. *The Mycoplasmas,* Vol 1, Cell Biology. New York: Academic Press, 1979:157–185.
48. McCormack WM. Susceptibility of mycoplasmas to antimicrobial agents: clinical implications. *Clin Infect Dis* 1993;17[Suppl 1]:5200.
49. Rumpianesi F, Morandotti G, Sperning R, et al. In vitro activity of azithromycin against *Chlamydia trachomatis, Ureaplasma urealyticum* and *Mycoplasma hominis* in comparison with erythromycin, roxithromycin and minocycline. *J Chemother* 1993;5:155.
50. Koutsky LA, Stamm WE, Brunham RC, et al. Persistence of *Mycoplasma hominis* after therapy: importance of tetracycline resistance and co-existing vaginal flora. *Sex Transm Dis* 1983;10:374.
51. Cummings MC, McCormack WM. Increase in resistance of *Mycoplasma hominis* to tetracyclines. *Antimicrob Agents Chemother* 1990;34:2297.
52. Evans RT, Taylor-Robinson D. The incidence of tetracycline resistant strains of *Ureaplasma urealyticum. J Antimicrob Chemother* 1978;4:57.
53. Taylor-Robinson D, Furr PM. Clinical antibiotic resistance of *Ureaplasma urealyticum. Pediatr Infect Dis* 1986;5[Suppl]:5335.
54. Glatt AE, McCormack WM, Taylor-Robinson D. Genital mycoplasmas. In: Holmes KK, Mardh P-A, Sparling PF, et al., eds. *Sexually transmitted diseases.* New York: McGraw-Hill, 1990:279–293.

Rickettsia

CHAPTER 224

Rickettsia rickettsii (*Rocky Mountain Spotted Fever*)

J. Stephen Dumler

HISTORY

The pioneering work of Howard Taylor Ricketts in his study of the "spotted fever" of the Rocky Mountains in the early 1900s still stands as a model for scientific investigation of infectious diseases (1). He rapidly identified the causative agent and showed transmission by the wood tick, *Dermacentor andersoni*. S. Burt Wolbach described the pathologic findings and provided initial explanations of the pathophysiology of clinical rickettsial illness. Although thought limited to the Rocky Mountains, retrospective studies now clearly show that Rocky Mountain spotted fever (RMSF) caused severe and fatal illness in the eastern United States as early as 1901 (2). Because of Ricketts' contributions and in tribute to his death while studying epidemic typhus,

the genus and species of the bacterium that causes RMSF now bear his name.

CHARACTERISTICS OF THE PATHOGEN

Classification

Rickettsia rickettsii is an obligate intracellular bacterium that has a life cycle partly within mammalian cells and partly within tick cells. Rickettsiae are true bacteria that have evolved within the cytoplasm of host cells and have lost the ability to survive in extracellular niches. Classification of rickettsiae is increasingly based on nucleic acid sequence divergence in the 16S ribosomal RNA genes, and *R. rickettsii* has a phylogenetic position within the alpha subdivision of proteobacteria (3,4). Other genetically close genera include *Orientia, Bartonella, Ehrlichia, Anaplasma,* and *Neorickettsia. Coxiella burnetii,* which causes Q fever, occupies a distant phylogenetic position in the gamma subdivision, closely related to the genus *Legionella.*

Structure and Function of *Rickettsia rickettsii*

R. rickettsii contains DNA, RNA, and ribosomes, enzymes involved in glycolysis and lipid A synthesis, and divides by binary fission (5). The organisms are small, about $0.3 \times 1.5 \ \mu m$, and stain poorly with the Gram stain and well with Giemsa and Gimenez stains. Ultrastructural studies reveal a gram-negative–type cell wall with an inner cell membrane separated from the inner cell wall leaflet by a periplasmic space and surrounded by a microcapsular layer that may contain the spotted fever group lipopolysaccharides and an electron-lucent slime layer (6). Because of the intracellular environment, *R. rickettsii* has evolved mechanisms to obtain host cell nutrients, including an adenosine triphosphate–adenosine diphosphate translocase that shuttles host cell energy-rich phosphate molecules into the bacterium (7).

Members of the *Rickettsia* genus are divided into spotted fever and typhus groups but share at least some antigens and possess lipopolysaccharide antigens that are conserved and define the serologic groups (8–11). All spotted fever group rickettsiae contain these cross-reactive antigens identified by the indirect fluorescent antibody serologic test, so that routine species differentiation within the serologic group can be difficult or impossible (11). *R. rickettsii* contains species-specific epitopes that can be identified by monoclonal antibodies (9,12).

R. rickettsii also contains several immunodominant outer membrane proteins (Omps), including a 190-kd OmpA, a 120-kd OmpB, and a 17-kd lipoprotein that appears to be conserved throughout the genus (12–16). OmpA is unique to the spotted fever group rickettsiae and has a predicted molecular structure that is consistent with a surface-exposed ligand because the gene that encodes the protein has several tandem repeats (15), a motif recognized frequently in cell–cell adherence. Monoclonal antibodies reactive with the OmpA of the related spotted fever group *Rickettsia conorii* inhibit binding of spotted fever group rickettsiae to host cells, further supporting the role of this protein as the major rickettsial ligand for adherence to host cells (17). Recombinant OmpA was tested as an immunogen in mice and in guinea pigs and showed promise as a potential vaccine (18,19). The function of OmpB that is present in both spotted fever group and typhus group *Rickettsia* species is still not certain, but it is the major component of a paracrystalline surface array, or S layer, that may play an important role in maintenance of rickettsial structure (20). OmpB is processed by proteolysis of a larger precursor to yield an accessory 32-kd β fragment that may serve as a membrane anchor domain. However, a *R. rickettsii* OmpB mutant appears to have diminished *in vitro* ability to form plaques, suggesting a role for OmpB in host cell lysis (21). Monoclonal antibodies reactive with OmpB protect mice from lethal rickettsial challenge (22). Data suggest that the rickettsial OmpA and OmpB are differentially expressed when the promoters from the encoding genes are cloned into *Escherichia coli*. This results in 28-fold higher transcription and expression from *ompB* promoters, partly explaining the 9:1 predominance of OmpB to OmpA in *R. rickettsii* (23).

Whether *R. rickettsii* contains a phospholipase has been an important question for several years. Experimental data implicate the rickettsia itself as a source of phospholipase-mediated host cell membrane lysis because phospholipase A and phospholipase C antigens and activity have been localized within *R. rickettsii* (24,25).

Genes for many of these protein antigens and metabolic enzymes have been identified, sequenced, and cloned. Several appear to be useful markers with sufficiently unique sequences to serve as targets for nucleic acid diagnostic methods (26). Genetic manipulation has only recently been successful but will allow an extensive evaluation of molecular pathogenesis (27,28).

PATHOGENESIS OF SPOTTED FEVER GROUP RICKETTSIOSES

Pathogenetic mechanisms in mammalian host cells directly attributable to the rickettsiae are difficult to elucidate given the intimate nature of the relationship between the infectious agent and its obligatory host cell. Like other bacteria that may be intracellular pathogens, *R. rickettsii* attaches to the surface of a eukaryotic cell and is internalized to occupy a niche within the cytoplasmic compartment (17). The predominant host cell *in vivo* is the endothelial cell, although vascular smooth muscle and macrophages may be infected. *In vitro*, infection is easily established in a variety of cell types, including endothelial cells, macrophages, and fibroblasts.

It has been proposed that after attachment of *R. rickettsii* to the surface of the endothelial cell, rickettsial phospholipases focally damage the host cell membrane (24,25,29,30). The focal injury results in endocytic internalization of the damaged host cell membrane, taking with it the attached rickettsiae. Continued phospholipase activity further degrades the endocytic vacuole to allow the rickettsiae free access to the cytoplasmic compartment of the host cell. Rickettsiae are freely mobile in the cytoplasm of the host cell by virtue of directional actin polymerization at one pole of the bacterium (31). This mobility often leads to entry into the nucleus for *R. rickettsii* but not for other *Rickettsia* species, and extrusion of the agent from the infected cell into adjacent uninfected cells furthers the local infection without exposing the rickettsiae to the external milieu. Within the cytoplasm of the infected host cell, *R. rickettsii* divides by binary fission with a generation time of about 9 hours under optimal circumstances.

The rickettsiae greatly affect the host cell by inducing free radical–mediated peroxidation of lipids in host cell membranes (32), continued phospholipase activity (24,30), and protease activity (30), although virulence with regard to these features varies among rickettsial isolates (33). The net result of these pathologic cellular insults is that the infected cell undergoes morphologic changes seen by light microscopy that include cell swelling, necrosis, karyorrhexis, and lysis. Ultrastructural evaluation indicates that these findings correspond to swelling of the endoplasmic reticulum, loss of the Golgi apparatus, and dissolution of cell membranes, probably leading to loss of cellular osmoregulation and cell lysis (34) (Fig. 224.1). The infectious agent may exit the cell propelled by polymerization of actin tails or may be released as the cell finally lyses. *In vitro*, infected endothelial cells have an up-regulated expression of (a) interleukin-1α (35), (b) surface procoagulant activity including tissue factor (36) and release of large von Willebrand factor multimers (37), and (c) E-selectin (38), which may partly contribute to the recruitment of inflammatory cells leading to the pathologic lesion characteristic of the vasculotropic rickettsioses and RMSF vasculitis. These endothelial responses are apparently not related to rickettsial lipopolysaccharide or endotoxin because the lipopolysaccharide of *R. rickettsii* has few or no endotoxic effects *in vivo* (39). In fact, *R. rickettsii* directly activates NFκB independent of the proteasome, allowing increased transcriptional activity of many proinflammatory genes, and inhibits endothelial cell apoptosis, allowing longer survival of cell and pathogen (40,41). The occurrence of fulminant (less than 5 days) RMSF in glucose phosphate

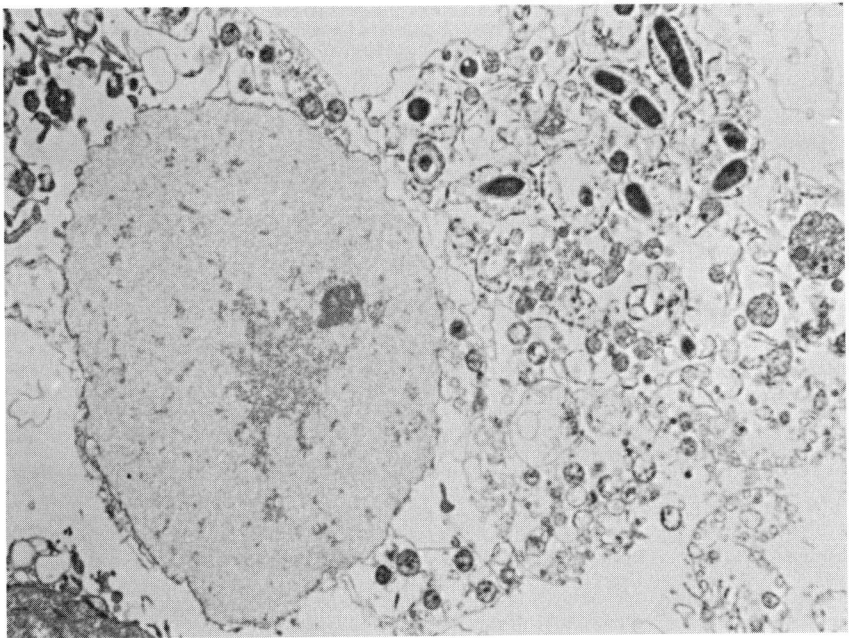

Figure 224.1. *Rickettsia rickettsii*–infected human umbilical vein endothelial cell with advanced cytopathologic changes. The rickettsiae appear in the cytoplasm as dark bacilli surrounded by a clear halo. The infected cell has lost osmoregulatory control and is near lysis. The rickettsiae may be freed from infected cells by lysis when the cell is severely injured or by propulsion with actin filament polymerization when the cell is less completely infected and damaged. Other characteristics here include nuclear condensation, which is a terminal effect of cell death. (From Silverman DJ. *Rickettsia rickettsii*–induced cellular injury of human vascular endothelium in vitro. *Infect Immun* 1984;44:545–553, with permission.)

dehydrogenase–deficient individuals in the absence of host inflammatory or immune responses indicates that *R. rickettsii* alone is sufficient to cause RMSF (42).

Other host responses clearly influence the course of RMSF. Immune suppression, particularly lack of interferon-γ, results in more severe or lethal infection (43). Animal models of spotted fever group rickettsiosis indicate that the proinflammatory cytokines interleukin-1 and tumor necrosis factor and interferon-γ and interleukin-6 appear within 5 days of intravenous inoculation and diminish as the infection becomes lethal (44,45). The antirickettsial protective effects of interferon-γ and tumor necrosis factor-α are synergistic and are mediated by induction of nitric oxide synthase and the resultant increases in nitric oxide in murine endothelial cells and by a process involving tryptophan limitation and hydrogen peroxide production in human endothelial cells (44,45,46). Critical cellular effectors of immunity include NK cells early in infection and CD8 cells throughout the infection, both likely sources of interferon-γ, but also operative by other mechanisms, including perforin production (46,47).

ECOLOGY OF *RICKETTSIA RICKETTSII*

The human is an accidental and dead-end host for *R. rickettsii*. In nature, *R. rickettsii* occupies at least part of its life cycle within a tick vector and part within the tissues and blood of small mammal hosts. Uninfected ticks acquire the infectious agent when a blood meal is taken from a rickettsemic animal, usually an infected small mammal (48). The rickettsiae attach to and infect the gut epithelial cells of the feeding tick and disseminate to infect most tick tissues, including salivary gland, while the tick is molting into its next life stage. Infected ticks may pass *R. rickettsii* from generation to generation (transovarial or vertical transmission) because of ovarian infection in adult female ticks; however, the infectious agent has a markedly deleterious effect by reducing the number of progeny that emerge in the next generation (49). Thus, a critical part of the natural maintenance of *R. rickettsii* depends on tick–mammal–tick transmission. Infected ticks transmit the rickettsiae to an uninfected mammalian host by regurgitation of salivary contents during feeding.

Because the rickettsiae require a short interval of reactivation by exposure to blood or increased temperature associated with the blood meal (48), and a short interval is required before regurgitation of infected tick saliva, there is a "grace period" of about 48 hours or more during which there is a low likelihood of *R. rickettsii* transmission. A variety of new proteins are expressed by the rickettsiae in tick cells with a high multiplicity of infection or when temperature is increased from 28° to 34°C, as would happen with a fresh blood meal. (50). After inoculation of the mammal by the bite of an infected tick, the animal may develop a period of rickettsemia, with or without overt clinical signs, which may last as long as several weeks before immunologic control of the infectious agent supervenes. During this interval, uninfected ticks feeding on the recently infected mammal may acquire the rickettsiae to renew the cycle. Transmission may occur by the bite of a tick at any life stage; however, it is predominantly the adult *Dermacentor* species ticks in the United States that bite large mammals and are responsible for the occasional inadvertent transmission to humans.

REFERENCES

1. Harden VA. Koch's postulates and the etiology of rickettsial diseases. *J Hist Med Allied Sci* 1987;42:277.
2. Dumler JS. Fatal Rocky Mountain spotted fever in Maryland—1901. *JAMA* 1991;265:718.
3. Weisburg WG, Dobson ME, Samuel JE, et al. Phylogenetic diversity of the rickettsiae. *J Bacteriol* 1989;171:4202.
4. Stothard DR, Clark JB, Fuerst PA. Ancestral divergence of *Rickettsia bellii* from the spotted fever and typhus groups of *Rickettsia* and antiquity of the genus *Rickettsia*. *Int J Syst Bacteriol* 1994;44:798.
5. Shaw EL, Wood DO. Characterization of a *Rickettsia rickettsii* DNA fragment analogous to the *firA-ORF17-lpxA* region of *Escherichia coli*. *Gene* 1994;140:109.
6. Silverman DJ, Wisseman CL Jr. Comparative ultrastructural study on the cell envelopes of *Rickettsia prowazekii*, *Rickettsia rickettsii*, and *Rickettsia tsutsugamushi*. *Infect Immun* 1978;21:1020.
7. Winkler HH. Rickettsial permeability: an ADP-ATP transport system. *J Biol Chem* 1976;251:389.
8. Ormsbee R, Peacock M, Philip R, et al. Antigenic relationships between the typhus and spotted fever groups of rickettsiae. *Am J Epidemiol* 1978;108:53.
9. Anacker RL, Mann RE, Gonzales C. Reactivity of monoclonal antibodies to *Rickettsia rickettsii* with spotted fever and typhus group rickettsiae. *J Clin Microbiol* 1987;25:167.
10. Walker DH, Gile JC, Feng H-M, et al. Diagnosis of spotted fever group rickettsioses by immunohistology with a group specific anti-lipopolysaccharide monoclonal antibody. *Mod Pathol* 1994;7:128A.
11. Philip RN, Casper EA, Ormsbee RA, et al. Microimmunofluorescence test for the serological study of Rocky Mountain spotted fever and typhus. *J Clin Microbiol* 1976;3:51.
12. Li H, Lenz B, Walker DH. Protective monoclonal antibodies recognize heatlabile epitopes on surface proteins of spotted fever group rickettsiae. *Infect Immun* 1988;56:2587.
13. Gilmore RD Jr, Joste N, McDonald GA. Cloning, expression and sequence analysis of the gene encoding the 120 kD surface-exposed protein of *Rickettsia rickettsii*. *Mol Microbiol* 1989;3:1579.
14. Gilmore RD Jr. Comparison of the *rompA* gene repeat regions of rickettsiae reveals species-specific arrangements of individual repeating units. *Gene* 1993;125:97.
15. Anderson BE, McDonald GA, Jones DC, et al. A protective protein antigen of *Rickettsia rickettsii* has tandemly repeated, near-identical sequences. *Infect Immun* 1990;58:2760.
16. Anderson BE, Tzianabos T. Comparative sequence analysis of a genus-common rickettsial antigen gene. *J Bacteriol* 1989;171:5199.
17. Li H, Walker DH. Characterization of rickettsial attachment to host cells by flow cytometry. *Infect Immun* 1992;60:2030.
18. McDonald GA, Anacker RL, Garjian K. Cloned gene of *Rickettsia rickettsii* surface antigen: candidate vaccine for Rocky Mountain spotted fever. *Science* 1987;235:83.
19. McDonald GA, Anacker RL, Mann RE, et al. Protection of guinea pigs from experimental Rocky Mountain spotted fever with a cloned antigen of *Rickettsia rickettsii*. *J Infect Dis* 1988;158:228.
20. Ching W-M, Dasch GA, Carl M, et al. Structural analyses of the 120-kDa serotype protein antigens of typhus group rickettsiae. *Ann N Y Acad Sci* 1990;590:334.
21. Hackstadt T, Messer R, Cieplak W, et al. Evidence for proteolytic cleavage of the 120-kilodalton outer membrane protein of rickettsiae: identification of an avirulent mutant deficient in processing. *Infect Immun* 1992;60:159.
22. Anacker RL, McDonald GA, List RH, et al. Neutralizing activity of monoclonal antibodies to heat-sensitive and heat-resistant epitopes of *Rickettsia rickettsii* surface proteins. *Infect Immun* 1987;55:825.
23. Policastro PF, Hackstadt T. Differential activity of *Rickettsia rickettsii ompA* and *ompB* promoter regions in a heterologous reporter gene system. *Microbiology* 1994;140:2941.
24. Silverman DJ, Santucci L, Meyers N, et al. Penetration of host cells by *Rickettsia rickettsii* appears to be mediated by a phospholipase of rickettsial origin. *Infect Immun* 1992;60:2733.
25. Manor E, Carbonetti NH, Silverman DJ. *Rickettsia rickettsii* has proteins with cross-reacting epitopes to eukaryotic phospholipase A2 and phospholipase C. *Microb Pathog* 1994;17:99.
26. Sexton DJ, Kanj SS, Wilson K, et al. The use of a polymerase chain reaction as a diagnostic test for Rocky Mountain spotted fever. *Am J Trop Med Hyg* 1994;50:59.
27. Rachek LI, Hines A, Tucker AM, et al. Transformation of *Rickettsia prowazekii* to erythromycin resistance encoded by the *Escherichia coli ereB* gene. *J Bacteriol* 2000;182:3289.
28. Troyer JM, Radulovic S, Azad AF. Green fluorescent protein as a marker in *Rickettsia typhi* transformation. *Infect Immun* 1999;67:3308.
29. Winkler HH, Miller ET. Phospholipase A and the interaction of *Rickettsia prowazekii* and mouse fibroblasts (L-929 cells). *Infect Immun* 1982;38:109.
30. Walker DH, Firth WT, Ballard JG, et al. Role of phospholipase-associated penetration mechanism in cell injury by *Rickettsia rickettsii*. *Infect Immun* 1983;40:840.
31. Heinzen RA, Hayes SF, Peacock MG, et al. Directional actin polymerization associated with spotted fever group rickettsia infection of Vero cells. *Infect Immun* 1993;61:1926.
32. Eremeeva ME, Silverman DJ. *Rickettsia rickettsii* infection of the EA.hy 926 endothelial cell line: morphological response to infection and evidence for oxidative injury. *Microbiology* 1998;144:2037.
33. Eremeeva ME, Dasch GA, Silverman DJ. Quantitative analyses of variations in the injury of endothelial cells elicited by 11 isolates of *Rickettsia rickettsii*. *Clin Diagn Lab Immunol* 2001;8:788.
34. Silverman DJ. *Rickettsia rickettsii*–induced cellular injury of human vascular endothelium in vitro. *Infect Immun* 1984;44:545.

35. Sporn LA, Marder VJ. Interleukin-1 alpha production during *Rickettsia rickettsii* infection of cultured endothelial cells: potential role in autocrine cell stimulation. *Infect Immun* 1996;64:1609.
36. Sporn LA Haidaris PJ, Rui-Jin S, et al. *Rickettsia rickettsii* infection of cultured human endothelial cells induces tissue factor expression. *Blood* 1994;83:1527.
37. Sporn LA, Rui-Jin S, Lawrence SO, et al. *Rickettsia rickettsii* infection of cultured endothelial cells induces release of large von Willebrand factor multimers from Weibel-Palade bodies. *Blood* 1991;78:2595.
38. Sporn LA, Lawrence SO, Silverman DJ, et al. E-selectin-dependent neutrophil adhesion to *Rickettsia rickettsii*–infected endothelial cells. *Blood* 1993;81:2406.
39. Kaplowitz LG, Lange JV, Fischer JJ, et al. Correlation of rickettsial titers, circulating endotoxin, and clinical features in Rocky Mountain spotted fever. *Arch Intern Med* 1983;143:1149.
40. Sahni SK, Van Antwerp DJ, Eremeeva ME, et al. Proteasome-independent activation of nuclear factor kappaB in cytoplasmic extracts from human endothelial cells by *Rickettsia rickettsii*. *Infect Immun* 1998;66:1827.
41. Clifton DR, Goss RA, Sahni SK, et al. NF-kappa B-dependent inhibition of apoptosis is essential for host cell survival during *Rickettsia rickettsii* infection. *Proc Natl Acad Sci U S A* 1998;95:4646.
42. Walker DH, Hawkins HK, Hudson P. Fulminant Rocky Mountain spotted fever: its pathologic characteristics associated with glucose-6-phosphate dehydrogenase deficiency. *Arch Pathol Lab Med* 1983;107:121.
43. Li H, Jerrells TR, Spitalny GL, et al. Gamma interferon as a crucial host defense against *Rickettsia conorii* in vivo. *Infect Immun* 1987;55:1252.
44. Feng H-M, Wen J, Walker DH. *Rickettsia australis* infection: a murine model of a highly invasive vasculopathic rickettsiosis. *Am J Pathol* 1993;142:1471.
45. Feng H-M, Walker DH. Interferon-γ and tumor necrosis factor-α exert their antirickettsial effect via induction of synthesis of nitric oxide. *Am J Pathol* 1993;143:1016.
46. Feng HM, Walker DH. Mechanisms of intracellular killing of *Rickettsia conorii* in infected human endothelial cells, hepatocytes, and macrophages. *Infect Immun* 2000;68:6729.
47. Walker DH, Olano JP, Feng HM. Critical role of cytotoxic T lymphocytes in immune clearance of rickettsial infection. *Infect Immun* 2001;69:1841.
48. Hayes SF, Burgdorfer W. Reactivation of *Rickettsia rickettsii* in *Dermacentor andersoni* ticks: an ultrastructural analysis. *Infect Immun* 1982;37:779.
49. Niebylski ML, Peacock MG, Schwan TG. Lethal effect of *Rickettsia rickettsii* on its tick vector (*Dermacentor andersoni*). *Appl Environ Microbiol* 1999;65:773.
50. Policastro PF, Munderloh UG, Fischer ER, et al. *Rickettsia rickettsii* growth and temperature-inducible protein expression in embryonic tick cell lines. *J Med Microbiol* 1997;46:839.

CHAPTER 225
Rickettsia typhi *and* Rickettsia prowazekii

Joseph E. McDade and James G. Olson

PROPERTIES OF *RICKETTSIA* ORGANISMS

Rickettsia species are gram-negative, obligate intracellular bacteria. All species are associated with a mammalian host at some stage of their natural life cycles and are transmitted by arthropod vectors. For some species of *Rickettsia*, arthropods are both reservoirs and vectors. With the exception of epidemic typhus rickettsiae (*Rickettsia prowazekii*), humans are not normal hosts in the life cycle of these organisms.

Rickettsiae are rod-shaped or coccobacillary microorganisms, ranging from 0.3 to 0.5 μm in diameter and from 0.8 to 2.0 μm in length. They do not possess flagella or pili (Fig. 225.1). Ultrastructurally, the outer envelope of a *Rickettsia* organism is typical of gram-negative bacteria (1). The outer membrane contains 2-keto-3-deoxyoctonate, a marker of bacterial lipopolysaccharide (2). Rickettsiae also contain a peptidoglycan layer that is presumed to be located between the outer leaflet of the cytoplasmic membrane and the inner leaflet of the cell wall (1). The peptidoglycan is insoluble in sodium dodecyl sulfate, is sensitive to lysozyme, and contains glutamic acid, alanine, and diaminopimelic acid in a molar ratio of 1.0:2.3:1.0, which is characteristic of gram-negative bacteria. The peptidoglycan also contains lysine, which

could provide a linkage site for lipoproteins (3). Rickettsiae are surrounded by a polysaccharide slime layer that can be visualized by special stains (4). The cytosol of rickettsiae contains nuclear structures, ribosomes, and other subcellular organelles typical of most bacteria. Multiplication occurs by binary fission.

Rickettsiae are capable of some independent metabolic activity, both energy producing and synthetic (5). In addition, rickettsiae possess numerous transport systems, which allow them to use metabolites present in host cells (6). Perhaps most notable is the adenosine triphosphate–adenosine diphosphate translocase system that incorporates high-energy phosphate molecules. Rickettsiae are quite unstable outside their hosts, however, and are incapable of independent replication on synthetic or semisynthetic media.

R. prowazekii and *Rickettsia typhi* (formerly *Rickettsia mooseri*) are closely related phylogenetically and have common phenotypic characteristics (7–10). The guanine-plus-cytosine content of their DNA has been estimated at 29% to 30%; interspecies DNA-to-DNA hybridization studies indicate 70% to 77% genetic relatedness (8). The two species are virtually identical when compared by sequence analysis of DNA coding for 16S ribosomal RNA (9). The size of the genomes of *R. typhi* and *R. prowazekii* has been estimated by pulsed-field gel electrophoresis as about 1,100 kb (11). Historically, *R. prowazekii* and *R. typhi* have been distinguished by their association with vectors and pathogenicity for certain experimental animals (10). Human body lice are the vector for *R. prowazekii*, whereas fleas typically transmit *R. typhi*. Laboratory mice are susceptible to infection with *R. typhi* but generally are refractory to *R. prowazekii*. Both species share common antigens, but they can be distinguished by monoclonal antibodies (12). *R. typhi* and *R. prowazekii* also contain specific protein antigens that facilitate identification of the respective microorganisms. Purified specific antigens have also been used in the research laboratory for serodiagnosis of patients with epidemic or murine typhus, but they are not available commercially (13,14). Comparative properties of *R. prowazekii* and *R. typhi* are summarized in Table 225.1.

Rickettsiae can be cultivated in virtually any type of cell culture system; most species also grow extremely well in embryonated hens' eggs (10). These organisms enter cells by induced phagocytosis and multiply within the cytosol unbounded by a phagosome (15). As few as two microorganisms constitute a 50% infectious dose for *R. typhi* or *R. prowazekii* (16). After a short lag phase, growth is exponential: the doubling time is about 9 hours (17). Reasons for the slow growth rate are not known. *R. typhi* apparently moves freely from cell to cell in infected fleas (18), whereas *R. prowazekii* accumulates within a single cell until it bursts (17). Movement of rickettsiae within host cells appears to be directed by actin filaments (19).

NATURAL HISTORY OF *RICKETTSIA TYPHI*

Commensal rats (*Rattus rattus* and *Rattus norvegicus*) are considered the primary reservoir of *R. typhi*, although numerous other rodents, including bandicoot rats (*Bandicota bengalensis* and *Bandicota indica*), the house mouse (*Mus musculus*), the African giant pouched rat (*Cricetomys gambianus*), and the house shrew (*Suncus murinus*), have been reported as reservoirs. Isolation of *R. typhi* has also been reported from domestic and peridomestic animals, such as cats and opossums, and numerous other animals have been infected experimentally. Infection with *R. typhi* apparently does not adversely affect mammalian reservoirs, although rodents remain rickettsemic for days to weeks

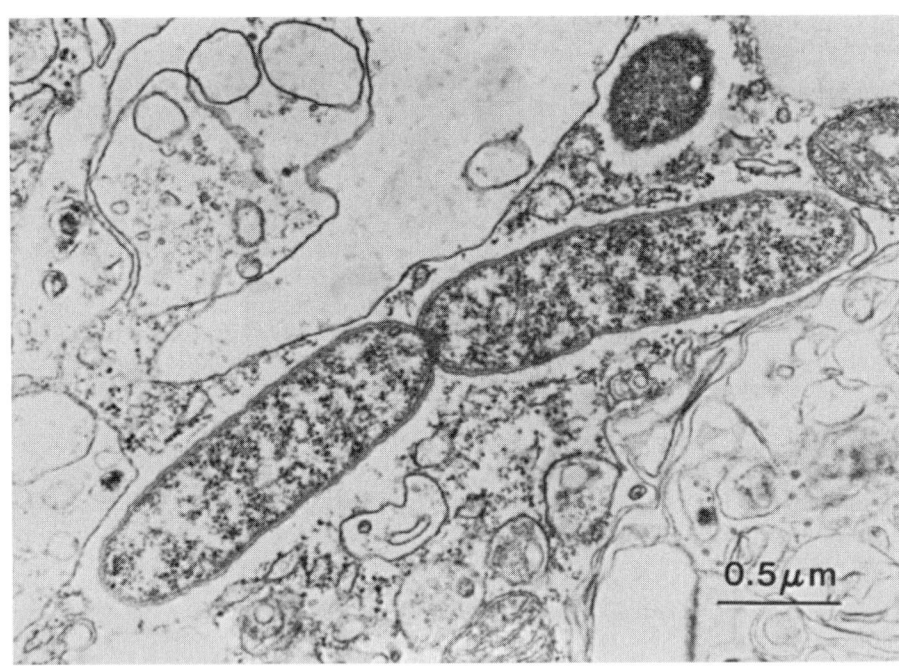

Figure 225.1. Electron photomicrograph of *Rickettsia prowazekii* cultivated on chick embryo cells. (Courtesy of Dr. David Silverman, University of Maryland School of Medicine, Baltimore, MD.)

and provide a source of typhus rickettsiae for ectoparasites during feeding (18,20).

The Asian rat flea (*Xenopsylla cheopis*) is the primary vector among *Rattus* species; humans are accidental hosts in the transmission cycle (Fig. 225.2). Except as noted in the following, *X. cheopis* is considered a vector and not a reservoir of murine typhus rickettsiae. Fleas acquire *R. typhi* when feeding on infected rodent hosts. The rickettsiae multiply primarily within epithelial cells lining the midgut region of the fleas. Results of experimental infection studies indicate that *R. typhi* multiplies exponentially in *X. cheopis* during the first and second weeks after infectious feeding. Murine typhus rickettsiae are then released from infected midgut cells and accumulate in the gut lumen and in flea feces. High titers of *R. typhi* accumulate (10^5 to 10^7 plaque-forming units per flea) and persist indefinitely (21). The growth rate in fleas is temperature dependent (22): titers at 24°C and 30°C are two to three times higher than in fleas held at 18°C. Infection apparently is not harmful to fleas. They presumably remain infective for life (up to 1 year). Infection

of humans and rodent hosts occurs by contamination of the bite site; in addition, irritation of the bite site induces scratching, allowing infection to occur through abraded skin. *X. cheopis* feeds rapidly and intermittently on hosts, facilitating transfer of *R. typhi* (18).

During the third week after infectious feeding, *R. typhi* is also found in foregut tissue of *X. cheopis*, suggesting that *R. typhi* can be transmitted directly by flea bite. Under experimental conditions, transmission of infection occurs by bite at a rate of 20%, probably as a result of regurgitation of rickettsiae in the foregut but not through salivary secretions (23). How frequently infection occurs by bite under natural conditions has not been determined.

Experimental infectivity studies indicate that transovarial transmission of *R. typhi* occurs at a low rate in *X. cheopis* and that fleas in the first filial generation are capable of transmitting *R. typhi* to other rodents (24). Thus, fleas may be a secondary reservoir of *R. typhi* but with limited capability for maintaining this microorganism in nature.

TABLE 225.1. Selected Properties of Typhus *Rickettsia* Species

Species	*Rickettsia prowazekii*	*Rickettsia typhi*
Diseases	Louse-borne typhus, recrudescent typhus (Brill-Zinsser disease), flying squirrel–associated typhus fever	Murine typhus
Geographic distribution	Louse-borne typhus occurs in areas of Africa and of Central and South America where louse infestation is common. Recrudescent typhus occurs worldwide; follows the distribution of former typhus patients. Flying squirrel–associated typhus reported only in the United States, principally east of the Mississippi	Worldwide; usually follows the distribution of *Rattus* species rats
Reservoirs	Humans primary; significance of flying squirrels as reservoirs not entirely clear	*Rattus* species primarily; other rodents secondarily; fleas (*Xenopsylla cheopis*) also a possible reservoir
Vector	For epidemic typhus, body lice; method of transmission of flying squirrel–associated typhus fever uncertain	Asian rat flea (*Xenopsylla cheopis*) principal victor; cat flea (*Ctenocephalides felis*) also a vector
Strain variation	Strains remarkably similar, but flying squirrel isolates distinguishable from classic typhus strains by molecular techniques	No significant differences among strains

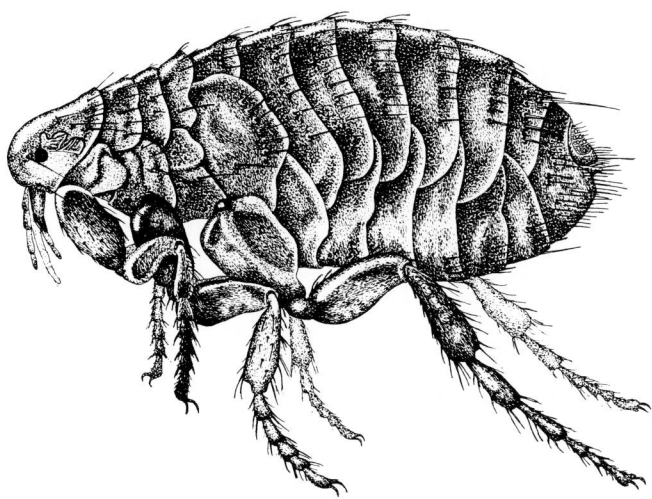

Figure 225.2. Schematic illustration of the Asian rat flea (*Xenopsylla cheopis*), principal vector of murine typhus.

Ten species of flea, three species of lice, and three species of mites have been implicated as actual or potential vectors of murine typhus (18,20). However, most of these ectoparasites have been discounted as vectors of murine typhus on epidemiologic grounds because they are unlikely to feed on humans. For example, comparative infectivity studies indicate that *R. typhi* accumulates to high titers in the mouse flea (*Leptopsylla segnis*) (21) and the cat flea (*Ctenocephalides felis*) (25). However, the mouse flea is presumed to be only a vector between mice because it is sessile and relatively host specific. In contrast, the high infectivity of *R. typhi* for *C. felis*, together with the broad host range of this flea, indicates that it may be a vector to humans. Cases of murine typhus have been reported in Los Angeles in association with seropositive domestic cats and peridomestic opossums, some of which were shown to be infested with cat fleas (26,27).

NATURAL HISTORY OF *RICKETTSIA PROWAZEKII*

R. prowazekii is the etiologic agent of epidemic typhus. It is unique among the rickettsiae in that humans are the principal reservoir. *R. prowazekii* is transmitted from person to person by infected body lice (*Pediculus humanus corporis*). Lice acquire the organism when they imbibe a blood meal from an infected person. Typhus rickettsiae infect cells lining the louse midgut, proliferate there, and progressively destroy the host cells in the process. *R. prowazekii* is then shed in louse feces. Humans become infected when contaminated feces come into contact with abraded skin.

Patients with epidemic typhus develop a nonsterile immunity after infection with *R. prowazekii*. Recrudescence of disease can occur from months to years after the primary infection, and if the ill person and contacts are infested with lice, another cycle of transmission can occur (28). Exactly how *R. prowazekii* remains sequestered in humans is not known, although it has reportedly been isolated from the lymph nodes of former typhus patients during the course of elective surgery that was performed 20 years after their primary infection (29). The digestive processes of lice may facilitate transmission of this organism from former typhus patients. Experimental data indicate that, in the course of digesting a blood meal, enzymes in the louse midgut modify or destroy antibody molecules and presumably render them incapable of neutralizing rickettsiae (30).

Although humans are considered the primary reservoir, *R. prowazekii* has also been isolated from eastern flying squirrels (*Glaucomys volans volans*) captured in Florida and Virginia (31). Numerous types of ectoparasites are known to infest flying squirrels, but lice (*Neohaematopinus sciuropteri*) and fleas (*Orchopeas howardii*) are the most likely vectors of *R. prowazekii* between animals. It has been isolated repeatedly from these ectoparasites but not from others. However, only squirrel lice become persistently infected with *R. prowazekii* under experimental conditions and transmit infection among flying squirrels (32). Presumably, the sylvan cycle of typhus infection is maintained by lice in a manner analogous to epidemic typhus infection in humans. Serologic studies of flying squirrels indicate that most seroconversions to *R. prowazekii* occur in the autumn and early winter, when these animals are infested with the maximal number of ectoparasites. Apparently, infection persists for an indefinite period in a given focus; new infections occur each year among young, nonimmune animals (33).

When the biologic and biochemical properties of flying squirrel isolates of *R. prowazekii* are compared with strains obtained from persons with louse-borne typhus, no significant differences are noted. Strains are 100% identical when compared by DNA-to-DNA hybridization studies (8). In addition, the ability of different strains to form plaques on chicken embryo cell monolayers, to grow in embryonated hens' eggs, or to use glutamate as a substrate is the same. Susceptibility to erythromycin and electrophoretic properties of solubilized proteins of different isolates are also similar (34,35). However, isolates of *R. prowazekii* from humans and from flying squirrels can be distinguished by restriction endonuclease digestion of their respective DNAs (36).

Human infections have been documented in the United States after known or suspected exposure to flying squirrels (37,38). Because patients did not report exposure to fleas, lice, or other vectors, the precise mode of transmission is uncertain. Infection is presumed to have occurred by inhalation of aerosolized feces from infected squirrel lice or fleas. The relative importance of flying squirrels in maintaining *R. prowazekii* in nature is uncertain.

REFERENCES

1. Silverman DJ, Wisseman CL Jr. Comparative ultrastructural study on the cell envelopes of *Rickettsia prowazekii*, *Rickettsia rickettsii*, and *Rickettsia tsutsugamushi*. *Infect Immun* 1978;21:1020.
2. Smith DK, Winkler HH. Separation of inner and outer membranes of *Rickettsia prowazekii* and characterization of their polypeptide composition. *J Bacteriol* 1979;137:963.
3. Pang H, Winkler HH. Analysis of the peptidoglycan of *Rickettsia prowazekii*. *J Bacteriol* 1994;176:923.
4. Silverman DJ, Wisseman CL Jr, Waddell AD, et al. External layers of *Rickettsia prowazekii* and *Rickettsia rickettsii*: occurrence of a slime layer. *Infect Immun* 1978;22:233.
5. Wisseman CL Jr. Some biologic properties of rickettsiae pathogenic for man. *Zentralbl Bakteriol Parasitenkd Infektionskr Hyg* 1968;206:299.
6. Winkler HH. *Rickettsia species* (as organisms). *Annu Rev Microbiol* 1990;44:131.
7. Tyeryar FJ Jr, Weiss E, Miller DB, et al. DNA base composition of rickettsiae. *Science* 1973;180:415.
8. Myers WF, Wisseman CL Jr. Genetic relatedness among the typhus group of rickettsiae. *Int J Syst Bacteriol* 1980;30:143.
9. Weisburg WG, Dobson ME, Samuel JE, et al. Phylogenetic diversity of the rickettsiae. *J Bacteriol* 1989;171:4202.
10. Weiss E, Moulder JW. Order I. Rickettsiales Grieszczkiewicz 1939, 25. In: Krieg NR, Holt JG, eds. *Bergey's manual of systematic bacteriology*, Vol 1. Baltimore, Williams & Wilkins, 1984:687–704.
11. Eremeeva ME, Roux V, Raoult D. Determination of the genome size and restriction pattern polymorphism of *Rickettsia prowazekii* and *Rickettsia typhi* by pulsed field gel electrophoresis. *FEMS Microbiol Lett* 1993;112:105.

12. Black C, Tzianabos T, Roumillat LF, et al. Detection and characterization of mouse monoclonal antibodies to epidemic typhus rickettsiae. *J Clin Microbiol* 1983;18:561.

13. Dasch GA. Isolation of species-specific protein antigens of *Rickettsia typhi* and *Rickettsia prowazekii* for immunodiagnosis and immunoprophylaxis. *J Clin Microbiol* 1981;14:333.

14. Halle S, Dasch GA, Weiss E. Sensitive enzyme-linked immunosorbent assay for detection of antibodies against typhus rickettsiae, *Rickettsia prowazekii* and *Rickettsia typhi*. *J Clin Microbiol* 1977;6:101.

15. Walker TS, Winkler HH. Penetration of cultured mouse fibroblasts (L cells) by *Rickettsia prowazekii*. *Infect Immun* 1978;22:200.

16. Ormsbee R, Peacock M, Gerloff R, et al. Limits of rickettsial infectivity. *Infect Immun* 1978;19:239.

17. Wisseman CL Jr, Waddell AD. In vitro studies on *Rickettsia*–host cell interactions: intracellular growth cycle of virulent and attenuated *Rickettsia prowazekii* in chicken embryo cells in slide chamber cultures. *Infect Immun* 1975;11:1391.

18. Azad AF. Epidemiology of murine typhus. *Annu Rev Entomol* 1990;35:553.

19. Teysseire N, Chiche-Portiche C, Raoult D. Intracellular movements of *Rickettsia conorii* and *R. typhi* based on actin polymerization. *Res Microbiol* 1992;143:821.

20. Traub R, Wisseman CL Jr, Farhang-Azad A. The ecology of murine typhus: a critical review. *Trop Dis Bull* 1978;75:237.

21. Farhang-Azad A, Traub R, Wisseman CL Jr. *Rickettsia mooseri* infection in the fleas *Leptopsylla segnis* and *Xenopsylla cheopis*. *Am J Trop Med Hyg* 1983;32:1392.

22. Farhang-Azad A, Traub R. Transmission of murine typhus rickettsiae by *Xenopsylla cheopis*, with notes on experimental infection and effects of temperature. *Am J Trop Med Hyg* 1985;34:555.

23. Azad AF, Traub R. Experimental transmission of murine typhus by *Xenopsylla cheopis* flea bites. *Med Vet Entomol* 1989;3:429.

24. Farhang-Azad A, Traub R, Baqar S. Transovarial transmission of murine typhus rickettsiae in *Xenopsylla cheopis* fleas. *Science* 1985;227:543.

25. Farhang-Azad A, Traub R, Sofi M, et al. Experimental murine typhus infection in the cat flea *Ctenocephalides felis* (Siphonaptera: Pulicidae). *J Med Entomol* 1984;21:675.

26. Adams WH, Emmons RW, Brooks JE. The changing ecology of murine (endemic) typhus in southern California. *Am J Trop Med Hyg* 1970;19:311.

27. Sorvillo FJ, Gondo B, Emmons R, et al. A suburban focus of endemic typhus in Los Angeles County: association with seropositive domestic cats and opossums. *Am J Trop Med Hyg* 1993;48:269.

28. Murray ES, Snyder JC. Brill's disease: etiology. *Am J Hyg* 1951;53:22.

29. Price WH. Studies on interepidemic survival of louse-borne epidemic typhus fever. *J Bacteriol* 1955;69:106.

30. Wisseman CL Jr, Boese JL, Waddell AD, et al. Modification of antityphus antibodies on passage through the gut of the human body louse with discussion of some epidemiologic and evolutionary implications. *Ann N Y Acad Sci* 1975;266:6.

31. Bozeman FM, Masiello SA, Williams MS, et al. Epidemic typhus rickettsiae isolated from flying squirrels. *Nature* 1975;255:545.

32. Bozeman FM, Sonenshine DE, Williams MS, et al. Experimental infection of ectoparasitic arthropods with *Rickettsia prowazekii* (GVF-16 strain) and transmission to flying squirrels. *Am J Trop Med Hyg* 1981;30:253.

33. Sonenshine DE, Bozeman FM, Williams MS, et al. Epizootiology of epidemic typhus (*Rickettsia prowazekii*) in flying squirrels. *Am J Trop Med Hyg* 1978;27:339.

34. Woodman DR, Weiss E, Dasch GA, et al. Biological properties of *Rickettsia prowazekii* strains isolated from flying squirrels. *Infect Immun* 1977;16:853.

35. Dasch GA, Samms JR, Weiss E. Biochemical characteristics of typhus group rickettsiae with special attention to the *Rickettsia prowazekii* strains isolated from flying squirrels. *Infect Immun* 1978;19:676.

36. Regnery RL, Zhang YF, Spruill CL. Flying squirrel–associated *Rickettsia prowazekii* (epidemic typhus rickettsiae) characterized by a specific DNA fragment produced by restriction endonuclease digestion. *J Clin Microbiol* 1986;23:189.

37. Duma RJ, Sonenshine DE, Bozeman FM, et al. Epidemic typhus in the United States associated with flying squirrels. *JAMA* 1981;245:2318.

38. McDade JE, Shepard CC, Redus MA, et al. Evidence of *Rickettsia prowazekii* infections in the United States. *Am J Trop Med Hyg* 1980;29:277.

CHAPTER 226
Rickettsia tsutsugamushi *and* Rickettsia akari

James G. Olson and Joseph E. McDade

RICKETTSIA TSUTSUGAMUSHI

History of the Microorganism

Scrub typhus (chigger-borne rickettsiosis) can be traced to the third century AD, when the Chinese physician Keh-Hung provided the earliest known description of the disease (1). Westerners became aware of scrub typhus in the mid-nineteenth century, after Commodore Perry's visit to Japan opened the door to scientific and social interchange. Scrub typhus gained prominence in World War II when tens of thousands of soldiers in the Asiatic-Pacific theaters contracted the disease, with case-fatality rates ranging as high as 35%. Thousands of cases still occur each year in the endemic areas (see Chapter 169).

Characteristics of the Pathogen

R. tsutsugamushi is a small (0.5 to 1.2 μm), gram-negative, obligate intracellular bacterium. Like other rickettsiae, it has an arthropod vector (trombiculid mites) as part of its life cycle. Mice are the preferred laboratory hosts, although *R. tsutsugamushi* can also be cultivated in cell culture and in the yolk sac of embryonated eggs. Optimal growth is obtained at 32°C. In contrast to other rickettsiae, which grow optimally *in vitro* when the air is enriched (5%) for carbon dioxide, *R. tsutsugamushi* does not require carbon dioxide enrichment (2). *R. tsutsugamushi* is best visualized when it is stained by a modification of the Gimenez technique (3).

Evidence suggests that *R. tsutsugamushi* may be sufficiently different from other members of the genus *Rickettsia* to be assigned to a new genus (4). Genetic analyses of 16S ribosomal RNA sequences show that *R. tsutsugamushi* is between 90.2% and 90.6% similar to *Rickettsia rickettsii, Rickettsia sibirica, Rickettsia prowazekii*, and *Rickettsia typhi*. The last four species share 98.1% similarity (5). *R. tsutsugamushi* also differs morphologically from other members of the genus. The outer leaflet of its cell wall is much thicker than the inner leaflet; the opposite is true for the rest of the genus (6). *R. tsutsugamushi* lacks peptidoglycan and lipopolysaccharide, substances found in all other members of the genus (7). *R. tsutsugamushi* is soft and fragile, which also reflects its lack of peptidoglycan (8,9). Finally, *R. tsutsugamushi* is more resistant to penicillin than are other members of the genus (10).

R. tsutsugamushi penetrates the plasma membrane of the host cell by active phagocytosis (11), escapes from the phagosome, and then grows freely within the cytoplasm. Organisms then move to the cell periphery and occasionally bud from the surface enclosed in host cell membrane (12,13) (Fig. 226.1). Most observers have concluded that *R. tsutsugamushi*, like other rickettsiae, multiplies by transverse binary fission. Different isolates of *R. tsutsugamushi*, even strains collected in a limited geographic area, exhibit considerable antigenic diversity (14). Group-specific antigens can be extracted from scrub typhus rickettsiae with ether, leaving the strain-specific antigens associated with the

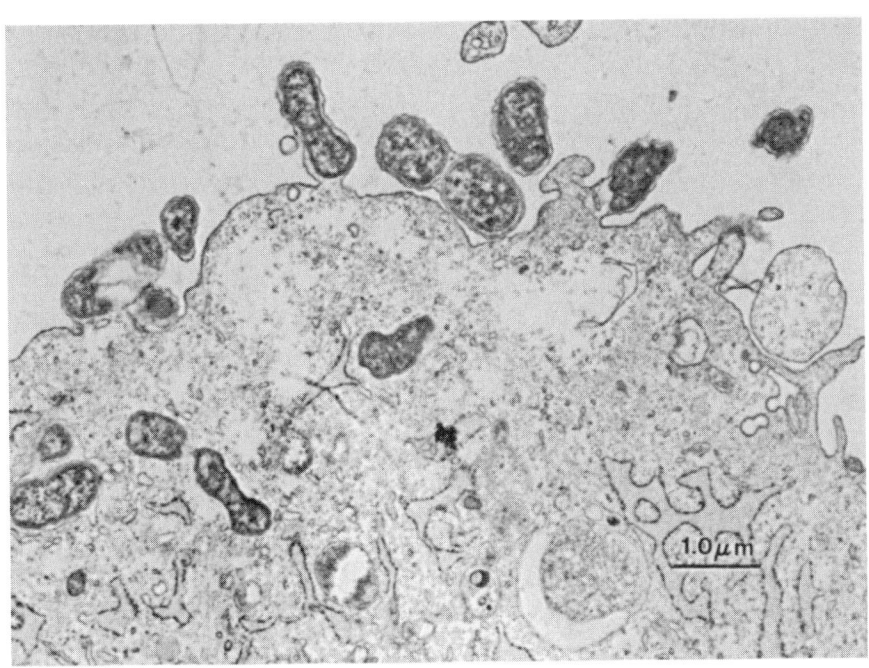

Figure 226.1. Electron micrograph of chick embryo cells infected with *Rickettsia tsutsugamushi*, the etiologic agent of scrub typhus. Note that the rickettsiae appear to bud from the chick cells enclosed in host cell membranes. (Courtesy of Dr. David Silverman, University of Maryland School of Medicine, Baltimore, MD.)

extracted organisms (15,16). Serologic and biochemical analyses of three prototype strains of *R. tsutsugamushi* (Karp, Gilliam, and Kato) have identified several quantitatively dominant antigenic proteins ranging in size from 50 to 63 kd (17). Analysis of one polypeptide with monoclonal antibodies showed that it contained both strain- and species-specific epitopes (17). Both inbred and outbred strains of mice differ in their susceptibility to a given strain of *R. tsutsugamushi* inoculated intraperitoneally; of 15 strains of inbred mice, 9 strains were susceptible and 6 strains were resistant (18). Subsequent genetic analyses of the inbred mice revealed that resistance was correlated with an autosomal dominant gene located on mouse chromosome 5 (19).

Natural History, Reservoirs, and Vectors

Leptotrombidium species mites are both reservoirs and vectors of *R. tsutsugamushi*; infection is transmitted transovarially by females to their progeny. Although several species of rodents become infected with *R. tsutsugamushi* and maintain rickettsemia for several months (20–22), there is no evidence that uninfected chiggers acquire *R. tsutsugamushi* from infected mammals (23). The lack of horizontal transmission of *R. tsutsugamushi* is based on experimental investigations in which three species of *Leptotrombidium* failed to become infected while feeding on infected mammals (23). Only larval mites (chiggers) feed on hosts; humans become infected when they intrude on areas that contain infected chiggers.

Field studies have shown a close correlation between the incidence of scrub typhus cases in humans and the population density of *Leptotrombidium deliense* collected from *Suncus murinus* and *Rattus* species (24). In some geographic areas, there is an association between the species of mite and the serotype of *R. tsutsugamushi* it transmits. *Leptotrombidium scutellare* from Mount Fuji, Japan was responsible for transmitting the Kawasaki serotype; *Leptotrombidium pallidum* transmitted the Karp serotype (25).

RICKETTSIA AKARI

History of the Microorganism, Natural History, Reservoirs, and Vectors

R. akari is the etiologic agent of rickettsialpox. It was first isolated in 1946 in association with an outbreak of rickettsialpox at a housing development in New York City. *R. akari* was isolated from the blood of two patients, from a house mouse (*Mus musculus*) trapped on the premises, and from two pools of rodent mites (*Liponyssoides sanguineus*) that were collected at the same site. The investigation also revealed a strong association between mite exposure and rickettsialpox, further incriminating mites as vectors of the disease (26–29). The relative contribution of mice and mites for maintaining *R. akari* in nature is not clear. *R. akari* has also been isolated from voles and may exist in other ecosystems (30).

Characteristics of the Pathogen

R. akari is a small (0.6 × 1.0 μm), gram-negative, obligate intracellular bacterium. Mice are the preferred laboratory hosts, but guinea pigs are also susceptible. Outbred strains of mice are all susceptible to *R. akari*; inbred strains differ significantly in susceptibility (31). Susceptibility or resistance in inbred mice has been correlated with the ability of their macrophages to phagocytose and kill *R. akari* (32,33). *R. akari* also grows well in tissue culture and the yolk sac of embryonated eggs.

R. akari grows primarily within the cytoplasm of the host cell, although it has also been observed within the nucleus. It can be visualized in infected tissue stained by the Gimenez, Giemsa, or Macchiavello methods (3). *R. akari* is a member of the spotted fever group of rickettsiae. The guanine-plus-cytosine content of *R. akari* DNA, like other spotted fever group rickettsiae, is about 32% to 33% (34). In DNA-to-DNA hybridization studies, 46% relatedness was observed between *R. akari* and *R. rickettsii*, the etiologic agent of Rocky Mountain spotted fever; other spotted fever rickettsiae are more closely related (35). Antigenic analyses of *R. akari*, performed with convalescent human and guinea pig serum samples, have shown that *R. akari* possesses determinants that are common to all spotted fever group rickettsiae (36). However, tests with polyvalent mouse antisera (37) and monoclonal antibodies (38) indicate that *R. akari* also contains species-specific antigens.

REFERENCES

1. Famer DS, Katsampes CP. Tsutsugamushi disease. *U S Naval Med Bull* 1944;43: 800.
2. Kopmans-Gargantiel AI, Wisseman CL Jr. Differential requirements for enriched atmospheric carbon dioxide content for intracellular growth in cell culture among selected members of the genus *Rickettsia*. *Infect Immun* 1981;31: 1277.
3. Elisberg BL, Bozeman FM. The rickettsiae. In: Lennette EH, Schmidt NJ, eds. *Diagnostic procedures for viral, rickettsial and chlamydial infections*. Washington, DC: American Public Health Association, 1979:1061–1108.
4. Tamura A, Ohashi N, Urakami H, et al. Classification of *Rickettsia tsutsugamushi* in a new genus, *Orientia* gen. nov., as *Orientia tsutsugamushi* comb. nov. *Int J Syst Bacteriol* 1995;45:589.
5. Ohashi N, Fukuhara M, Shimada M, et al. Phylogenetic position of *Rickettsia tsutsugamushi* and relationship among its antigenic variants by analyses of 168 rRNA gene sequences. *FEMS Microbiol Lett* 1995;125:299.
6. Silverman DJ, Wisseman CL Jr. Comparative ultrastructural study on the cell envelopes of *Rickettsia prowazekii*, *Rickettsia rickettsii*, and *Rickettsia tsutsugamushi*. *Infect Immun* 1978;21:1020.
7. Amano K, Tamura A, Ohashi N, et al. Deficiency of peptidoglycan and lipopolysaccharide components in *Rickettsia tsutsugamushi*. *Infect Immun* 1987;55:2290.
8. Takahashi M, Urakami H, Tamura A. Purification of cell envelopes of *Rickettsia tsutsugamushi*. *Microbiol Immunol* 1985;29:475.
9. Tamura A, Urakami H, Tsuruhara T. Purification of *Rickettsia tsutsugamushi* by Percoll density gradient centrifugation. *Microbiol Immunol* 1982;26:321.
10. Raoult D, Drancourt M. Antimicrobial therapy of rickettsial diseases. *Antimicrob Agents Chemother* 1991;35:2457.
11. Cohn ZA, Bozeman FM, Campbell JH, et al. Study of growth of rickettsiae. V. Penetration of *Rickettsia tsutsugamushi* into mammalian cells in vitro. *J Exp Med* 1959;109:271.
12. Ewing EP Jr, Takeuchi A, Shirai A, et al. Experimental infection of mouse peritoneal mesothelium with scrub typhus rickettsiae: an ultrastructural study. *Infect Immun* 1978;19:1068.
13. Rikihisa Y, Ito S. Intracellular localization of *Rickettsia tsutsugamushi* in polymorphonuclear leukocytes. *J Exp Med* 1979;150:703.
14. Traub R, Wisseman CL Jr. The ecology of chigger-borne rickettsiosis (scrub typhus). *J Med Entomol* 1974;11:237.
15. Kobayashi Y, Nagai K, Tachibana N. Purification of complement fixing antigens of *Rickettsia orientalis* by ether extraction. *Am J Trop Med Hyg* 1969;18:942.
16. Shishido A, Hikita M, Sat T, et al. Particulate and soluble antigens of *Rickettsia tsutsugamushi* in the complement fixation test. *J Immunol* 1969;113:480.
17. Hanson B. Identification and partial characterization of *Rickettsia tsutsugamushi* major protein immunogens. *Infect Immun* 1985;50:603.
18. Groves MG, Osterman JV. Host defenses in experimental scrub typhus: genetics of natural resistance to infection. *Infect Immun* 1978;19:583.
19. Groves MG, Rosenstreich DL, Taylor BA, et al. Host defenses in experimental scrub typhus: mapping the gene that controls natural resistance in mice. *J Immunol* 1980;125:1395.
20. Traub R, Wisseman CL Jr, Jones MR, et al. The acquisition of *Rickettsia tsutsugamushi* by chiggers (trombiculid mites) during the feeding process. *Ann N Y Acad Sci* 1975;266:91.
21. Strickman D, Smith CD, Corcoran KD, et al. Pathology of *Rickettsia tsutsugamushi* in *Bandicota savilei*, a natural host in Thailand. *Am J Trop Med Hyg* 1994;51:416.
22. Van Peenen PFD, Ho CM, Bourgeois AL. Indirect immunofluorescence antibodies in natural and acquired *Rickettsia tsutsugamushi* infections of Philippine rodents. *Infect Immun* 1977;15:813.
23. Walker JS, Chan CT, Manikumaran C, et al. Attempts to infect and demonstrate transovarial transmission of *R. tsutsugamushi* in three species of *Leptotrombidium* mites. *Ann N Y Acad Sci* 1975;266:80.
24. Olson JG, Bourgeois AL, Fang RCY. Population indices of chiggers (*Leptotrombidium deliense*) and incidence of scrub typhus in Chinese military personnel, Pescadores Islands of Taiwan, 1976–1977. *Trans R Soc Trop Med Hyg* 1982; 76:85.
25. Kawamori F, Akiyama M, Sugeida M, et al. Epidemiology of tsutsugamushi disease in relation to the serotypes of *Rickettsia tsutsugamushi* isolated from patients, field mice, and unfed chiggers on the eastern slope of Mount Fuji, Shizuoka Prefecture, Japan. *J Clin Microbiol* 1992;30:2842.
26. Huebner RJ, Jellison WL, Armstrong C. Rickettsialpox: a newly recognized rickettsial disease. V. Recovery of *Rickettsia akari* from a house mouse (*Mus musculus*). *Public Health Rep* 1947;62:777.
27. Huebner RJ, Jellison WL, Pomerantz C. Rickettsialpox: a newly recognized rickettsial disease. IV. Isolation of a rickettsia apparently identical with the causative agent of rickettsialpox from *Allodermanyssus sanguineus*, a rodent mite. *Public Health Rep* 1946;61:1677.
28. Huebner RJ, Stamps P, Armstrong C. Rickettsialpox: a newly recognized rickettsial disease. I. Isolation of the etiologic agent. *Public Health Rep* 1946;61: 1605.
29. Greenberg M, Pellitteri OJ, Jellison WL. Rickettsialpox: a newly recognized rickettsial disease. III. Epidemiology. *Am J Public Health* 1947;37:860.
30. Jackson EB, Danauskas JX, Coale MC, et al. Recovery of *R. akari* from the Korean vole *Microtus fortis pelliceus*. *Am J Hyg* 1957;66:301.
31. Anderson GW Jr, Osterman JV. Host defenses in experimental rickettsialpox: genetics of natural resistance to infection. *Infect Immun* 1980;28:132.
32. Nacy CA, Meltzer MS. Macrophages in resistance to rickettsial infection: strains of mice susceptible to the lethal effects of *Rickettsia akari* show defective macrophage rickettsiocidal activity in vitro. *Infect Immun* 1982;36: 1096.
33. Kokorin IN, Kabanova EA, Kyet CD, et al. Differences in the susceptibility of mouse cell lines to the rickettsia pox agent. *Acta Virol* 1978;22:497.
34. Tyeryar FJJ, Weiss E, Millar DB, et al. DNA base composition of rickettsiae. *Science* 1973;180:415.
35. Myers WF, Wisseman CL Jr. *Genetic relationships within the spotted fever biotype of the genus Rickettsia* [Abstract]. Third National Meeting, American Society for Rickettsiology and Rickettsial Diseases, Atlanta, GA, March 12–14, 1982.
36. Bell EJ, Stoenner HG. Immunologic relationships among the spotted fever group of rickettsias determined by toxin neutralization tests in mice with convalescent animal serums. *J Immunol* 1960;84:171.
37. Pickens EG, Bell EJ, Lackmen DB, et al. Use of mouse serum in identification and serologic classification of *Rickettsia akari* and *Rickettsia australis*. *J Immunol* 1965;94:883.
38. McDade JE, Black CM, Roumillat LF, et al. Addition of monoclonal antibodies specific for *Rickettsia akari* to the rickettsial diagnostic panel. *J Clin Microbiol* 1988;26:2221.

CHAPTER 227

Coxiella burnetii (*Q Fever*)

Paul D. Holtom and John M. Leedom

HISTORY

Q fever is a protean disease caused by an infection with the obligate intracellular organism *Coxiella burnetii*. Humans are usually infected by inhalation of aerosols from infected domestic animals, mainly cattle, sheep, and goats. Q fever can present as an acute infection with an influenza-like illness with fever and sometimes pulmonary and hepatic involvement, or it can develop into a chronic form characterized by endocarditis or chronic hepatitis. Q fever (for *query*, to indicate the uncertain cause of the disease at the time of its description) was first described in 1936 by Derrick in Australia (1). He reported detailed clinical data on nine abattoir workers who presented with febrile illnesses, and he successfully isolated the causal agent from human blood and urine by passage into guinea pigs. Burnet and Freeman (2) identified the organism as a rickettsia. Davis and Cox (3) independently isolated the same organism from ticks collected near Nine Mile Creek in Montana. In 1940, Cox proved that infection with this agent occurred in humans in the western United States. Subsequently, *C. burnetii* has been shown to have a worldwide distribution.

CHARACTERISTICS OF THE PATHOGEN

Coxiella burnetii has been classified as a member of the tribe Rickettsiaceae since it is a short (0.3 to 0.7 μm long), pleomorphic gram-negative rod that is an obligate intracellular parasite. However, studies have shown that *C. burnetii* is closest to *Legionella* phylogenetically and far removed from the Rickettsiae (4,5). It can be isolated by intraperitoneal injection into guinea pigs, inoculation into the yolk sacs of embryonated chicken eggs, or tissue culture.

C. burnetii differs from the other rickettsiae in staining properties, DNA composition, energy production, antigen solubility and heat stability, antibiotic susceptibility and mode of transmission (6). Unlike the other rickettsiae, *C. burnetii* grows in the acidic environment of the phagolysosome of the cell rather than the cytoplasm or the nucleus (7). It is very resistant to inactivation and can survive for long periods in the environment (8). The reason for this resistance may be the formation of an endospore-like cell variant (9).

In passage through cell cultures or embryonated eggs, the lipopolysaccharide of *C. burnetii* undergoes antigenic shift that is called phase variation (10). Phase I is found in fresh isolates and is highly infectious. Conversion to phase II occurs after repeated passage through embryonated chicken eggs, although there is reversion to phase I with passage through laboratory animals. Although there is no morphologic difference between the two phases, there are differences in antigenic components, sugar composition of their lipopolysaccharides (11), buoyant density, agglutinability, staining properties and resistance to phagocytosis. A major difference is the presence of glucuronic acid on the surface antigen of the phase I organisms but not phase II (12). Plasmids have been identified in both phase I and phase II organisms, and some investigators have suggested a correlation between plasmid profile and clinical manifestations (acute or chronic infection), but this theory has not been confirmed on subsequent investigation (13–15).

EPIDEMIOLOGY

C. burnetii is an extremely infectious organism. In fact, a single inhaled organism is sufficient to initiate infection (16). It is endemic worldwide, with the exception of New Zealand (17). *C. burnetii* infects many species of animals, and in animals the infection usually results in long-lasting parasitism. Mammals (both wild and domestic), birds, fish and arthropods have all been found to be infected with the organism (18). Although many species of ticks have been found to be infected and there may be tick-borne transmission among animals, ticks apparently are not a source of infection in humans.

Q fever in man is usually caused by the inhalation of aerosolized particles, which can be airborne even over long distances, although it is often said to result from the ingestion of contaminated raw milk. A report from France (19) involved Q fever infection associated with goat milk in patients and staff of a psychiatric institution living in rural France. Some of the patients had direct contacts with goats, while others living 5 kilometers away ingested raw milk products from the goats. Serologic evidence of *C. burnetii* infection and/or history of compatible illness was significantly more common in persons who had tended goats, tended goats and ingested raw milk products, or only ingested raw milk products, as compared with persons at the institution who were in none of the three above risk groups. Most reports associating Q fever with ingestion of raw dairy products are similar (19,20). That is, they occur in rural settings where the possibility of inhalation of *C. burnetii*, dust borne from the vicinity, cannot reasonably be excluded. It is of interest that direct studies of individuals ingesting contaminated milk in environments away from rural areas show either seroconversions without disease (21,22) or are totally negative for evidence of *C. burnetii* infection (23).

Large numbers of *C. burnetii* organisms can be present in the parturient fluids of sheep, cattle and cats, and can also be shed in the urine, feces and milk. Q fever is mainly an occupational or geographic disease associated with contact with farm animals such as cattle, sheep and goats, although recently contacts with infected cats have been sources of urban outbreaks (24,25). There have been outbreaks among laboratory workers and workers in buildings where *C. burnetii* has been cultured (26–28). Transmission of infection by blood transfusion (29) and during an autopsy (30) have been documented, but there have been no reports of transmission to health care providers caring for infected persons. Person-to-person transmission of Q fever is unusual but does occur (31,32), including one report of sexual transmission (33). Although isolation and quarantine of patients with Q fever is not recommended, it should be remembered that such transmission has been documented.

CLINICAL MANIFESTATIONS

Infection with *C. burnetii* can cause a wide spectrum of clinical findings, dependent at least in part on different host factors (34). Many people who are infected with *C. burnetii* are asymptomatic; in a series from Switzerland, 54% of serologically diagnosed "cases" with a known exposure were asymptomatic (35). In patients who have clinical illness, the most common presentations are an acute febrile systemic illness, pneumonia, hepatitis or a meningoencephalitis (36). Patients can go on to develop a chronic illness characterized by endocarditis and a granulomatous hepatitis.

The incubation period for Q fever can be as short as 4 to 5 days (37), but it typically ranges from 9 to 39 days. Fever is the most common symptom, occurring in 90% (38) to 100% (39) of patients, and the temperature often spikes to 40.0° to 40.5°C (104° to 105°F). Other signs and symptoms include chills, headache (often severe), retrobulbar pain, myalgias and arthralgias, neck pain and stiffness, pleuritic chest pain, cough, nausea and vomiting, diarrhea, jaundice, hepatomegaly and splenomegaly. Unlike the other rickettsial diseases, Q fever does not usually present with a rash, although a transient erythematous macular rash has been noted in about 4% of patients. The manifestations of Q fever usually resolve within 2 to 4 weeks, although in some patients the fever has lasted as long as 9 weeks (39). Case fatality rates from acute Q fever are very low (0% in most series), but in a recent French series of 323 hospitalized patients the case fatality rate was 2.4% (40).

The incidence of pulmonary involvement in patients with Q fever varies between 0 and 90 per cent (41). The reason for this wide variation is not known; possible explanations include geographic strain variation or the source, route or dose of the infectious agent. In patients with pulmonary involvement the chest radiograph can have patchy infiltrates resembling *Mycoplasma pneumoniae* infection or may show actual lobar consolidation.

Hepatic involvement in acute Q fever may range from minimal elevations of the hepatic transaminase values to a presentation indistinguishable from that of acute viral hepatitis. The incidence of hepatomegaly ranges from 11% to 65% in patients with acute Q fever; the reason for this reported variability is not known. Actual jaundice is uncommon and occurs in 4 to 5 per cent of cases. Liver biopsy examinations in patients with Q fever hepatitis show a wide range of lesions, ranging from focal necrosis to severe, widespread liver cell necrosis with noncaseating granulomas. A characteristic granuloma has been described that consists of a clear central space surrounded by inflammatory cells and a fibrin ring (42,43).

In addition to the common manifestations of fever, pulmonary involvement and hepatic involvement, there are many less common complications of Q fever. These include meningitis, encephalitis (44,45), optic neuritis (46), Guillain-Barre syndrome (47), myelopathy (48), hemolytic anemia (49), bone marrow necrosis (50), glomerulonephritis (51), arthritis, polyserositis, acute pleuropericarditis, myocarditis, thrombophlebitis, inflammatory pseudotumor of the lung, nephritis, orchitis and epididymitis, and hemolytic uremic syndrome (52).

Chronic Q fever is usually manifested by endocarditis, although other manifestations have been described such as chronic hepatitis, infections of vascular prostheses and aneurisms (53), osteomyelitis and interstitial pulmonary fibrosis (54). Q fever endocarditis is usually accompanied by liver involvement and is a rare, severe, and often fatal complication of *C. burnetii* infection. The incidence of Q fever endocarditis appears to be increasing, but this may be due to improved diagnosis rather than a true change in epidemiology. In most of the cases, there is a history of preexisting valvular heart disease, and often patients have a prosthetic valve. The aortic valve is the most common site of infection (55). The illness evolves slowly, presenting any time from 1 to 20 years after the acute infection, and presents clinically as a culture-negative endocarditis, although fever is often absent in Q fever endocarditis. Other findings include hepatomegaly, abnormal liver function tests, splenomegaly, anemia, microscopic hematuria, hyperglobulinemia and thrombocytopenia. Chronic liver involvement in the absence of endocarditis has been reported but is uncommon.

DIAGNOSIS

The clinical presentation of Q fever can resemble that of nearly any infectious disease. The diagnosis can only be made by the isolation of *C. burnetii* from a clinical sample or by serologic demonstration of infection. The other laboratory findings in acute and chronic Q fever are nonspecific. Although isolation of the organism is possible, it is seldom done because of the high risk of infection to laboratory personnel and serologic tests are usually used to confirm the diagnosis.

Several tests are available to detect antibodies specific for *C. burnetii* in patients' sera. Complement fixation (CF) and indirect fluorescent antibody (IFA) are the procedures most commonly used. The enzyme-linked immunosorbent assay (ELISA) has also been proposed as a method of diagnosing Q fever (56). All three methods are highly specific.

In acute *Coxiella burnetii* infection in humans, antibodies to *C. burnetii* phase II antigen are produced, which generally become detectable 8 to 14 days after the onset of illness and peak around week 4 to 8 for IFA titers or week 12 to 13 for CF titers. Although a phase II CF titer of 1:8 is considered significant, confirmation of the diagnosis rests on demonstrating a fourfold or greater rise in CF titer in paired serum specimens. IFA titers for IgG of 1:200 and IgM of 1:50 are predictive of evolving acute or chronic infection (57).

In chronic Q fever, the phase I antibody level becomes elevated. Phase I CF antibody titer greater than 1:200 is considered diagnostic for chronic Q fever (58), although some patients with endocarditis may have lower titers.

TREATMENT

Most acute Q fever infections resolve spontaneously, and symptoms respond to nonspecific therapy such as antipyretics and hydration. However, because of the concern for the development of chronic Q fever, and because some studies suggest that therapy shortens the duration of fever, specific antimicrobial therapy for acute Q fever is advisable. Tetracycline and its analogs are the mainstay of therapy. Tetracycline for 2 weeks at 25 mg/kg per day in four divided doses or doxycycline, 100 mg twice a day for

15 to 21 days, are recommended therapies for adults. The fluoroquinolones are active in vitro against *C. burnetti* (59,60), although resistant strains have been identified (61).

The treatment of chronic Q fever has never been the subject of controlled studies. No antibiotics have been found to be bactericidal for *C. burnetii*, although several (including tetracycline, doxycycline, trimethoprim-sulfamethoxazole, rifampin and ciprofloxacin) have been shown to be bacteriostatic. The combination of rifampin with either doxycycline or trimethoprim-sulfamethoxazole has been recommended in the treatment of Q fever endocarditis. The ideal duration of therapy is also unknown; recommended treatment periods range from 12 months to an indefinite term (62). Valve replacement surgery in Q fever endocarditis is indicated only for significant hemodynamic problems.

PREVENTION

Because *C. burnetii* organisms are widespread in the environment and relatively resistant to inactivation, control of the major reservoirs of the organism is impractical. There is a commercial vaccine available in Australia and in some European countries that is a formalin-inactivated whole cell vaccine. The vaccine is made from phase-I organisms and is highly effective (63). At this time no vaccine is commercially available in the United States.

REFERENCES

1. Derrick EH. "Q" fever, a new fever entity: clinical features, diagnosis and laboratory investigation. *Med J Aust* 1937;2:281.
2. Burnet FM, Freeman M. Experimental studies on the virus of Q fever. *Med J Aust* 1937;2:299.
3. Davis GE, Cox HR. A filter-passing infectious agent isolated form ticks. I. Isolation from *Dermacentor andersoni*, reactions in animals, and filtration experiments. *Public Health Rep* 1938;53:2259.
4. Stein A, Saunders NA, Taylor AG, et al. Phylogenic homogeneity of *Coxiella burnetii* strains as determinated by 16S ribosomal RNA sequencing. *FEMS Microbiol Lett* 1993;113:339.
5. Raoult D, Marrie T. Q fever. *Clin Infect Dis* 20:489, 1995.
6. Ormsbee RA. Rickettsiae (as organisms). *Annu Rev Microbiol* 1969;23:275.
7. Baca OG, Li YP, Kumar H. Survival of the Q fever agent *Coxiella burnetii* in the phagolysosome. *Trends Microbiol* 1994;2:476.
8. Sawyer LA, Fishvein DB, McDade JE. Q fever: current concepts. *Rev Infect Dis* 1987;9:935.
9. McCaul TF, Williams JC. Developmental cycle of *Coxiella burnetii*: structure and morphogenesis of vegatative and sporogenic differentiations. *J Bacteriol* 1981;147:1063.
10. Leedom JM. Q fever: an update. *Curr Clin Top Infect Dis* 1980;1:304.
11. Schramek S, Mayer H. Different sugar compositions of lipopolysaccharides isolated from phase I and pure phase II cells of *Coxiella burnetii*. *Infect Immun* 1982;38:53.
12. Jerrels JR, Hinricks DJ, Mallavia LP. Cell envelope analysis of *Coxiella burnetii* phase I and phase II. *Can J Microbiol* 1974;20:1465.
13. Frazier ME, Mallavia LP, Samuel JE, et al. DNA probes for the identification of *Coxiella burnetii* strains. *Ann N Y Acad Sci* 1990;590:445.
14. Stein A. Lack of pathotype specific gene in human *Coxiella burnetii*. *Microb Pathog* 1993;15:177.
15. Thiele D, Willems H. Is plasmid based differentiation of *Coxiella burnetii* in 'acute' and 'chronic' isolates still valid? *Eur J Epidemiol* 1994;10:427.
16. Tigertt WD, Benenson AS, Bochenour WS. Airborne Q fever. *Bacteriol Rev* 1961;25:285.
17. Kazar J. Q fever is absent from New Zealand. *Int J Epidemiol* 1993;22:945–949.
18. Baca OG, Paretsky D. Q fever and *Coxiella burnetii*: a model for host-parasite interaction. *Microbiol Rev* 1983;47:127.
19. Fishbein DB, Raoult D. A cluster of *Coxiella burnetii* infections associated with exposure to vaccinated goats and their unpasteurized dairy products. *Am J Trop Med Hyg* 1992;47:35.
20. Brown GL, Colwell DC, Hooper WL. An outbreak of Q fever in Staffordshire. *J Hyg* 1968;66:649.
21. Benson WW, Brock DW, Mather J. Serologic analysis of a penitentiary group using raw milk from a Q fever-infected herd. *Public Health Rep* 1963;78:707.
22. Experimental Q fever in man [Editorial]. *Br Med J* 1950;1:1000.
23. Krumbiegel EF, Wisniewski HJ. Q fever in Milwaukee. II. Consumption of raw milk by human volunteers. *Arch Environ Health* 1970;21:63.

24. Langley JM, Marrie TJ, Covert A, et al. Poker players' pneumonia. *N Engl J Med* 1988;319:354.
25. Marrie TJ, Durant H, Williams JC, et al. Exposure to parturient cats is a rick factor for acquisition of Q fever in Maritime Canada. *J Infect Dis* 1988;158:101.
26. Meiklejohn G, Reimer LG, Graves PS, et al. Cryptic epidemic of Q fever in a medical school. *J Infect Dis* 1981;144:107.
27. Bernard KW, Parham GL, Winkler WG, et al. Q fever control measures: recommendations for research facilities using sheep. *Infect Control* 1982;3:461.
28. Ruppanner R, Brooks D, Morrish D, et al. Q fever hazards from sheep and goats used in research. *Arch Enviorn Health* 1982;37:103.
29. Heard SR, Ronalds CJ, Hearth RB. *Coxiella burnetii* infection in immunocompromised hosts. *J Infect* 1985;11:15.
30. Harman JB. Q fever in Great Britain: clinical account of eight cases. *Lancet* 1949;2:1028.
31. Leedom JM. Q fever. In: Spittle JA Jr, ed. *Practice of medicine*, Vol 2. Hagerstown, MD: Harper & Row, 1981.
32. Mann, JS, Douglas JG, Inglis JN, et al. Q fever: person to person transmission within a family. *Thorax* 1985;41:974.
33. Milazzo A, Hall R, Storm PA, et al. Sexually transmitted Q fever. *Clin Infect Dis* 2001;33:399–402.
34. Raoult D. Host factors in the severity of Q fever. *Ann N Y Acad Sci* 1990;590:33.
35. Dupuis G, Petite J, Peter O, et al. An important outbreak of human Q fever in a Swiss alpine valley. *Int J Epidemiol* 1987;16:282.
36. Raoult D, Tissot-Dupont H, Foucault C, et al. Q fever 1985–1998: clinical and epidemiologic features of 1,383 infections. *Medicine* 2000;79:109–123.
37. Young FW. Q fever in Artesia, California. *Calif Med* 1948;69:89.
38. Tselentis Y, Gikas A, Kofteridis D, et al. Q fever in the Greek island of Crete: epidemiologic, clinical and therapeutic data from 98 cases. *Clin Infect Dis* 1995;20:1311.
39. Clark WH, Lennette EH, Railsback OC, et al. Q fever in California. VII. Clinical features in 180 cases. *Arch Intern Med* 1951;88:155.
40. Dupont HT, Raoult D, Brouqui P, et al. Epidemiologic features and clinical presentation of acute Q fever in hospitalized patients: 323 French cases. *Am J Med* 1992;93:427.
41. Murray HW, Tuazon C. Atypical pneumonias. *Med Clin North Am* 1980;64:507.
42. Hoffman CE, Heaton JW. Q fever hepatitis. *Gastroenterology* 1982;83:474.
43. Travis LB, Travis WB, Li C-Y, et al. Q fever: a clinicopathologic study of five cases. *Arch Pathol Lab Med* 1986;110:1017.
44. Ferrante MA, Dolan MJ. Q fever meningoencephalitis in a soldier returning from the Presian Gulf War. *Clin Infect Dis* 1993;16:489.
45. Sempere AP, Elizaga J, Duarte J, et al. Q fever mimicking herpetic encephalitis. *Neurology* 1993;43:2713.
46. Schuil J, Richardus JH, Baarsma GS, et al. Q fever as a possible cause of bilateral optic neuritis. *Br J Ophthalmol* 1985;69:580.
47. Bernard E, Carles M, Laffant C, et al. Guillain-Barré syndrome associated with acute Q fever. *Eur J Clin Microbiol Infect Dis* 13:658, 1994.
48. Hwang YM, Lee MC, Suh DC, et al. Coxiella (Q fever)–associated myelopathy. *Neurology* 1993;43:338.
49. Cardellach F, Font J, Agusti AGN, et al. Q fever and hemolytic anemia. *J Infect Dis* 1983;148:769.
50. Branda M, Bellingham AJ. Bone marrow necrosis and Q fever. *Br Med J* 1980;210:148.
51. Korman TM, Spelman DW, Perry GJ, et al. Acute glomerulonephritis associated with acute Q fever: case report and review of the renal complications of *Coxiella burnetii* infection. *Clin Infect Dis* 1997;26:359–364.
52. Maltezou HC, Kallergi C, Kavazarakis E, et al. Hemolytic-uremic syndrome associated with *Coxiella burnetii* infection. *Pediatr Infect Dis J* 2001;20:811–813.
53. Piquet P, Raoult D, Tranier P, et al. *Coxiella burnetii* infection of pseudoaneurysm of an aortic bypass graft with contiguous vertebral osteomyelitis. *J Vasc Surg* 1994;19:165.
54. Brouqui P, Dupont HT, Drancourt M, et al. Chronic Q fever: ninety-two cases from France; including 27 cases without endocarditis. *Arch Intern Med* 1993;153:642.
55. Sawyer LA, Fishbein DB, McDade JE. Q fever: current concepts. *Rev Infect Dis* 1987;9:935.
56. Peter O, Dupuis G, Peacock MG, et al. Comparison of enzyme-linked immunosorbent assay and complement fixation and indirect fluorescent antibocy tests for detection of *Coxiella burnetii* antibody. *J Clin Microbiol* 1987;25:1063.
57. Tissot-Dupont H, Thirion X, Raoult D. Q fever serology: cutoff determination for microimmunofluorescence. *Clin Diagn Lab Immunol* 1994;1:189.
58. Turck WP, Howitt G, Turnberg LA, et al. Chronic Q fever. *Q J Med* 1976;45:193.
59. Maurin M, Raoult D. Bacteriostatic and bactericidal activity of levofloxacin against *Rickettsia rickettsii, Rickettsia conorii*, "Israeli spotted fever group rickettsia" and *Coxiella burnetii*. *J Antimicrob Chemother* 1997;39:725–730.
60. Gikas A, Spyridaki I, Psaroulaki A, et al. In vitro susceptibility of *Coxiella burnetii* to trovafloxacin in comparison with susceptibilities to pefloxacin, ciprofloxacin, ofloxacin, doxycycline, and clarithromycin. *Antimicrob Agents Chemother* 1998;42(10):2747–2748.
61. Spyridaki I, Psaroulaki A, Aransay A, et al. Diagnosis of quinolone-resistant *Coxiella burnetii* strains by PCR-RFLP. *J Clin Lab Anal* 2000;14:59–63.
62. Tobin MJ, Cahill N, Gearty, G, et al. Q fever endocarditis. *Am J Med* 1982;72:396.
63. Ackland JR, Worswick DA, Marmion BP. Vaccine prophylaxis of Q fever: a follow-up study of the efficacy of Qvac (CSL) 1985–1990. *Med J Aust* 1994;160:704.

PART

VII

Viruses

CHAPTER 228

Virus Classification

Neil R. Blacklow

Viruses are not independently living microorganisms; they require host cells for their replication. This is because unlike all other forms of microorganisms—bacteria, fungi, protozoa, mycoplasmas, rickettsiae, and chlamydiae—viruses do not contain both DNA and RNA. Instead, they possess either DNA or RNA, and this feature represents the starting point for classification. Human virology in this textbook is therefore divided into the two categories of DNA and RNA viruses.

The presentation of human virology in an infectious diseases textbook should not only take into account principles of virus classification but also maintain a clinical orientation of epidemiology and pathogenesis. Thus, our coverage of human viruses follows virus classification where possible but deviates in a few areas in which characteristic diseases occur. In this chapter, I first cover basic information on the classification of human viruses relevant to readers who are working in or interested in the field of infectious diseases; then I explain how and why the book deviates in a few instances from this classification in its virology section.

SPECIFICS OF VIRUS CLASSIFICATION

After being divided into DNA and RNA categories, viruses are divided into families, which are designated by terms with the suffix *-viridae*. There are 21 families of viruses that contain human pathogens. Seven families contain DNA and the remainder RNA (Table 228.1). A few viruses remain unclassified owing to insufficient information about their morphologic characteristics or nucleic acid.

Viruses are classified on the basis of shared biologic characteristics. Classification is based principally on (a) morphologic features and (b) genome (nucleic acid) structure and strategy of its replication. Morphologic features are determined predominantly by electron microscopy: virion size, shape, nucleocapsid symmetry, and presence or absence of an envelope (Fig. 228.1). Genome characteristics include predominantly molecular weight, "strandedness," polarity, and structure. The important properties of virions belonging to families of DNA viruses are outlined in Table 228.2 and those of RNA viruses in Table 228.3.

The highest taxonomic group for virus classification is the family, as just outlined. Further subdivisions into subfamilies,

genera, and species are less clearcut and agreed on, although schema exist. These subdivisions are based predominantly on antigenic differences between viruses. Interested readers are directed to other virology references for more details on viral taxonomy and nomenclature (1–3). It should be noted that it is still customary and accepted virologic practice to use vernacular terms for virus species (e.g., mumps virus).

EPIDEMIOLOGIC CLASSIFICATION

In a less formal way, many viruses can be grouped clinically into four categories based on their modes of transmission.

1. *Enteric viruses.* Enteric viruses are normally acquired by ingestion (fecal-oral route) and localize to the intestinal tract. Examples are in the families Adenoviridae, Picornaviridae, Reoviridae, Astroviridae, and Caliciviridae.
2. *Respiratory viruses.* Respiratory viruses are usually acquired by inhalation (respiratory) or by fomites (hand to nose or mouth or eye) and typically localize to the respiratory tract. Examples are in the families Adenoviridae, Orthomyxoviridae, Paramyxoviridae, Coronaviridae, and Picornaviridae.
3. *Arboviruses* (arthropod-borne viruses). Arboviruses replicate in arthropods that feed on the blood of humans. Examples are in the families Reoviridae, Togaviridae, Flaviviridae, and Bunyaviridae.
4. *Oncogenic viruses.* Oncogenic viruses are acquired by close contact or injection and typically become persistent and may progress to malignancy. Viruses that show these characteristics in experimental animals or humans are in the families Adenoviridae, Herpesviridae, Papovaviridae, Hepadnaviridae, and Retroviridae.

IMPORTANT VIRUS FEATURES DISTINCT FROM FORMAL CLASSIFICATION

Although viruses are classified into families, it is important to recognize that the epidemiologic or pathogenic characteristics of some virus infections are so distinctive that these viruses are best discussed either separately or in relation to viruses from a different family. Furthermore, viruses from one family can produce diverse clinical manifestations. The features of viruses that are distinct from their formal classification are covered in the subsequent three categories.

Viruses in a Family Can Produce Diverse Diseases

Good examples of these viruses can be found in the families Picornaviridae, Reoviridae, and Togaviridae (Table 228.1). Clearly,

TABLE 228.1.   Families of Human Viruses, with Important Examples

Family	Examples
DNA Viruses	
Adenoviridae	Adenovirus
Herpesviridae	Herpes simplex, Epstein-Barr, varicella-zoster viruses, cytomegalovirus, human herpes virus types 6 to 8
Poxviridae	Vaccinia, variola (smallpox), molluscum contagiosum viruses
Parvoviridae	Parvovirus B19
Papillomaviridae	Papillomavirus
Polyomaviridae	BK virus, JC virus
Hepadnaviridae	Hepatitis B virus
RNA Viruses	
Orthomyxoviridae	Influenza virus
Paramyxoviridae	Mumps, measles, parainfluenza, respiratory syncytial viruses
Coronaviridae	Coronavirus, SARS virus
Picornaviridae	Poliovirus, coxsackievirus, echovirus, other enteroviruses, hepatitis A virus, rhinovirus
Reoviridae	Rotavirus, reovirus, Colorado tick fever virus
Retroviridae	Human immunodeficiency virus (HIV) type 1, HIV-2, human T-cell lymphotrophic virus (HTLV) type I, HTLV-II
Togaviridae	Rubella virus; arthropod-borne viruses: eastern equine encephalitis, western equine encephalitis, Venezuelan equine encephalitis, chikungunya viruses
Flaviviridae	Arthropod-borne viruses: yellow fever, dengue, St. Louis encephalitis, Japanese encephalitis, Murray Valley encephalitis, tick-borne encephalitis, hepatitis C viruses, West Nile virus
Bunyaviridae	Hantaan virus; arthropod-borne viruses: California encephalitis, sand fly fever, Rift Valley fever, Crimean-Congo hemorrhagic fever viruses
Arenaviridae	Rodent-borne viruses: lymphocytic choriomeningitis, Lassa fever, Machupo, Junin viruses
Filoviridae	Marburg, Ebola viruses
Rhabdoviridae	Rabies virus
Caliciviridae	Norwalk virus
Astroviridae	Astrovirus
Unclassified Agents	
Agent causing Creutzfeldt-Jakob disease, kuru agents—spongiform encephalopathies, prions	
Hepatitis D (delta) virus (a defective RNA-containing satellite of hepatitis B)	
Hepatitis E virus	

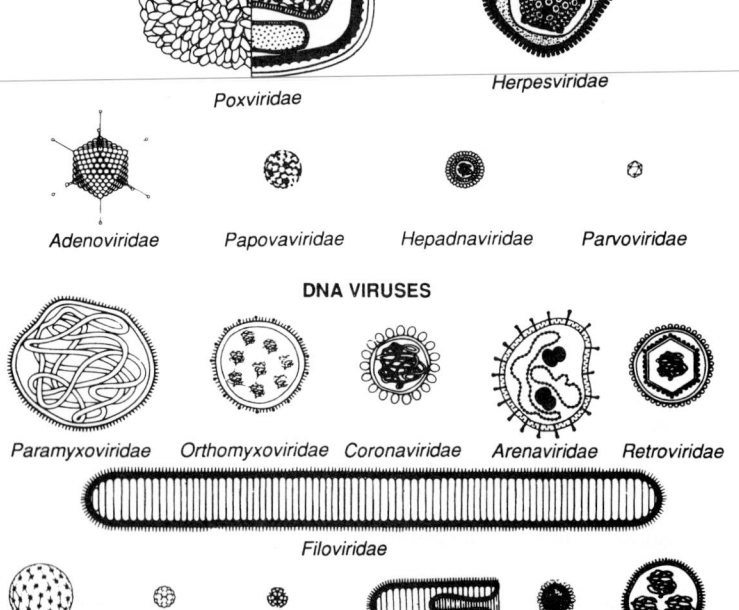

Figure 228.1. Shapes and sizes of viruses of families that include human pathogens. The virions are drawn to scale, but artistic license has been used in representing their structure. In some, the cross-sectional structure of capsid and envelope is shown, with a representation of the genome; with the extremely small virions, only size and symmetry are depicted. Not depicted are the Astroviridae (similar in size and shape to the Picornaviridae and Caliciviridae) and the Papillomaviridae and Polyomaviridae (newly named derivatives of the former Papovaviridae shown in the figure). (From White DO, Fenner FJ. Classification and nomenclature of viruses. In: White DO, Fenner FJ, eds. *Medical virology*, 4th ed. San Diego: Academic Press, 1994:16–29, with permission.)

TABLE 228.2.   Properties of Virions of Families of DNA Viruses Infecting Humans

Family	Virion Diameter (nm)	Envelope	Nucleocapsid Symmetry	Nucleocapsid Capsomers	Nucleocapsid Transcriptase	Genome Nature[a]	Genome Size[b] (kb, kbp)
Parvoviridae	20	−	Icosahedral	32	−	ss, −, linear	5
Papillomaviridae	55	−	Icosahedral	72	−	ds, circular	8
Polyomaviridae	40	−	Icosahedral	72	−	ds, circular	5
Adenoviridae	70	−	Icosahedral	252	−	ds, linear	36–38
Herpesviridae	150	+	Icosahedral	162	−	ds, linear	125–229
Poxviridae	250 × 200 × 200[c]	+[d]	Complex	—	+	ds, linear	130–250
Hepadnaviridae	42		Icosahedral	?	+[e]	ds, circular[f]	3.2

[a]All DNA virus genomes comprise a single molecule. ds, Double stranded; ss, single stranded; + or − indicates sense of single-stranded nucleic acid.
[b]For species that cause human infections
[c]Orthopoxvirus, brick shaped; Parapoxvirus, ovoid, 260 × 160 run.
[d]Not essential for infectivity.
[e]Reverse transcriptase.
[f]Circular molecule is double stranded for most of its length but contains a single-stranded region.
From White DO, Fenner FJ. Classification and nomenclature of viruses. In: White DO, Fenner FJ, eds. *Medical virology;* 4th ed. San Diego: Academic Press, 1994:16–29, with permission.

in the Picornaviridae, rhinovirus produces an epidemiologic and pathogenic form of infection that is different from that of poliovirus or hepatitis A virus. In the Reoviridae, rotavirus infection differs markedly from that produced by the virus of Colorado tick fever. In the Togaviridae, rubella is quite distinct clinically from the other members, which are arthropod-borne viruses.

Epidemiology and Pathogenesis of Disease Syndromes Can Be Indistinguishable Between Viruses Belonging to Different Families

Two examples of these viruses are encephalitis viruses and hemorrhagic fever viruses. As Table 228.1 shows, viruses that produce clinically similar types of encephalitis by an

TABLE 228.3.   Properties of Virions of Families of RNA Viruses Infecting Humans

Family	Virion Diameter (nm)[a]	Envelope	Nucleocapsid Symmetry	Nucleocapsid Capsomers	Nucleocapsid Transcriptase	Genome Nature[b]	Genome Size (kb, kbp)
Picornaviridae	25–30	−	Icosahedral	60	−	ss, +	7.5–8.5
Caliciviridae	35–40	−	Icosahedral	32	−	ss, +	8.0
Astroviridae	28–30	−	Icosahedral	?	−	ss, +	7.5
Togaviridae	60–70	+[c]	Icosahedral	60	−	ss, +	12
Flaviviridae	40–50	+[c]	Icosahedral	?	−	ss, +	10
Coronaviridae	75–160	+[c]	Helical	?	−	ss, +	27–33
Paramyxoviridae	150–300	+	Helical	?	+	ss, −	15–16
Rhabdoviridae	180 × 75	+	Helical	?	+	ss, −	13–16
Filoviridae	790–970 × 80	+	Helical	?	+	ss, −	12.7
Orthomyxoviridae	80–120	+	Helical	?	+	ss, 7–8, −	13.6
Arenaviridae	110–130	+[c]	Helical	?	+	ss, 2, −	10–14
Bunyaviridae	90–120	+[c]	Helical	?	+	ss, 3 −	13.5–21
Reoviridae	60–80	−	Icosahedral	32, 92[d]	+	ds, 10–12[e]	18–27
Retroviridae	80–100	+[c]	Icosahedral	?	+[f]	ss, +	7–10[g]
Deltavirus[h]	32	−	Icosahedral	?	−	ss, −, circular	1.7

[a]Some enveloped viruses are quite pleomorphic and sometimes filamentous.
[b]All genomes except that of deltavirus are linear; ss, single stranded; ds, double stranded; 2–12, number of segments in segmented genomes; + or −, indicates sense of single-stranded nucleic acid.
[c]No matrix protein.
[d]The 32 indicates the inner capsid of *Orbivirus, Rotavirus,* and *Orthoreovirus;* 92, outer capsid of *Orthoreovirus.*
[e]*Orthoreovirus* and *Orbivirus,* 10; *Rotavirus,* 11; *Coltivirus,* 12.
[f]Reverse transcriptase.
[g]Genome is diploid—two identical molecules being held together by hydrogen bonds at their 5′ ends.
[h]Currently unclassified as a family but does contain RNA and is a satellite of hepatitis B.
From White DO, Fenner FJ. Classification and nomenclature of viruses. In: White DO, Fenner FJ, eds. *Medical virology,* 4th ed. San Diego: Academic Press, 1994:16–29, with permission.

arthropod-borne route belong to the Togaviridae, Flaviviridae, and Bunyaviridae families. Viruses that typically produce hemorrhagic fever belong to the Flaviviridae (dengue), Arenaviridae, and Filoviridae families.

Some Individual Viruses Produce Medically Distinctive Disease Syndromes

Some viruses produce a distinct clinical syndrome that is normally quite different from syndromes produced by other members of their taxonomic family. Examples of this are yellow fever virus, rubella virus, poliovirus, and mumps virus (Table 228.1). These are typical examples of viruses that retain the use of vernacular terms for species identification.

CONCLUSION

As a result of these important virus features that are distinct from formal classification, our coverage in the virology section of this book does not follow strictly the formal classification of viruses into families. The virology chapters are arranged in the order of the families as outlined in Table 228.1; however, some viruses from one family have individual chapters because of their medical importance (e.g., herpes simplex, Epstein-Barr, varicella-zoster virus, and cytomegalovirus), other viruses are gathered together from different families because of their common clinical features (e.g., encephalitis viruses, hemorrhagic fever viruses), and still others are handled separately because of their distinctive clinical features (e.g., poliovirus, yellow fever virus). Our overriding goal is to present human virology in an organized but clinically relevant way for readers interested in the field of infectious diseases.

REFERENCES

1. van Regenmortel MHV, Fauquet CM, Bishop DHL, et al. *Virus taxonomy, classification and nomenclature of viruses: seventh report of the International Committee on Taxonomy of Viruses.* San Diego: Academic Press, 2000.
2. Murphy FA. Virus taxonomy and nomenclature. In: Lennette EH, Halonen P, Murphy FA, eds. *Laboratory diagnosis of infectious diseases: principles and practice,* Vol II. New York: Springer-Verlag, 1988:153–176.
3. White DO, Fenner FJ. Classification and nomenclature of viruses. In: White DO, Fenner FJ, eds. *Medical virology,* 4th ed. San Diego: Academic Press, 1994:16–29.

DNA Viruses

CHAPTER 229
Adenoviruses

Tsoline Kojaoghlanian and Marshall S. Horwitz

Adenoviruses are responsible for a variety of infections in the respiratory tract, conjunctiva, urinary tract, intestine, and occasionally other sites. Genetically altered adenoviruses are currently being studied intensively as vectors to deliver foreign genes both for gene therapy and for immunization against other pathogens (1,2). In addition to the importance of adenoviruses as infectious agents, some members of this large family of viruses were the first human viruses shown to be oncogenic in rodents (3,4) in which they have served as excellent models to understand viral transformation, oncogenes, and anti-oncogenes (5); however, there is no evidence that adenoviruses are oncogenic in humans (6). With the increasing numbers of patients with immunodeficiency caused by disease or by iatrogenic manipulations of the immune system, newer manifestations of adenovirus infections, such as a serious form of hepatitis and myocarditis, have been recognized (7–10).

HISTORY

Adenoviruses were discovered serendipitously in 1953 when an endogenous transmissible cytopathic agent emerged during attempts to establish tissue cultures of tonsils and adenoids from children undergoing surgical removal of these tissues (11). The same agents were found in respiratory secretions obtained from febrile military recruits (12,13). With the availability of a culture system for adenoviruses, it was appreciated rapidly that a large number of acute respiratory diseases, including pneumonia (14,15), were caused by this family of viruses, which now includes 51 recognized distinct serotypes (16). The association of some adenoviruses with keratoconjunctivitis helped explain previously reported epidemics of this clinical disease. Among shipyard workers whose occupational exposure frequently traumatized their eyes and required medical evaluation, ocular instruments contaminated with adenoviruses spread this disease iatrogenically (17).

CHARACTERISTICS OF THE PATHOGEN

Structure

All human adenoviruses share similar structural features, an icosahedron with fiber-like projections from each of the 12 vertices (18) (Fig. 229.1). The enteric adenoviruses have two fibers projecting from each vertex (19). The length of the fiber, a trimer of identical subunits, varies between subgroups (see later) and depends on the number of repeating subunits in the shaft (20–22). The fiber has a knoblike structure at its tip, which is the attachment site to the cell receptor, named *coxsackie adenovirus receptor* (CAR) (23,24). As the name implies, CAR is the receptor for two very different classes of viruses. The fiber is attached noncovalently to the icosahedron by a pentomeric polypeptide, named *penton base*, at each of the vertices. The major surface capsomere of the icosahedron is the trimeric polypeptide, the hexon, so named because it has six neighboring capsomeres on the face of the virus. There are other proteins (IIIa, VI, VIII and IX; Fig. 229.1A) necessary to hold the capsid together and to attach it to the linear genomic double-stranded DNA protected by both the capsid and two additional core basic proteins (V and VII; Fig. 229.1A). The viral DNA is about 35 kb in length for most serotypes and has a terminal protein (TP) covalently linked to each 5′ end (25). Figure 229.2 shows the viral DNA, some of the viral messenger RNA (mRNA) spliced transcripts, and the coding positions for both the early (E) viral regulatory proteins and several of the structural proteins. Major type-specific neutralizing epitopes appear both on the fiber and hexon, with minor sites on the penton base (26). However, all of these large surface proteins also have epitopes shared within the entire adenovirus family. For example, hexon has group-specific antigenic sites that are helpful in diagnostic virology. Thus, a single reference serum is capable of recognizing most of the human and

Polypeptide SDS-gel   Structural Unit

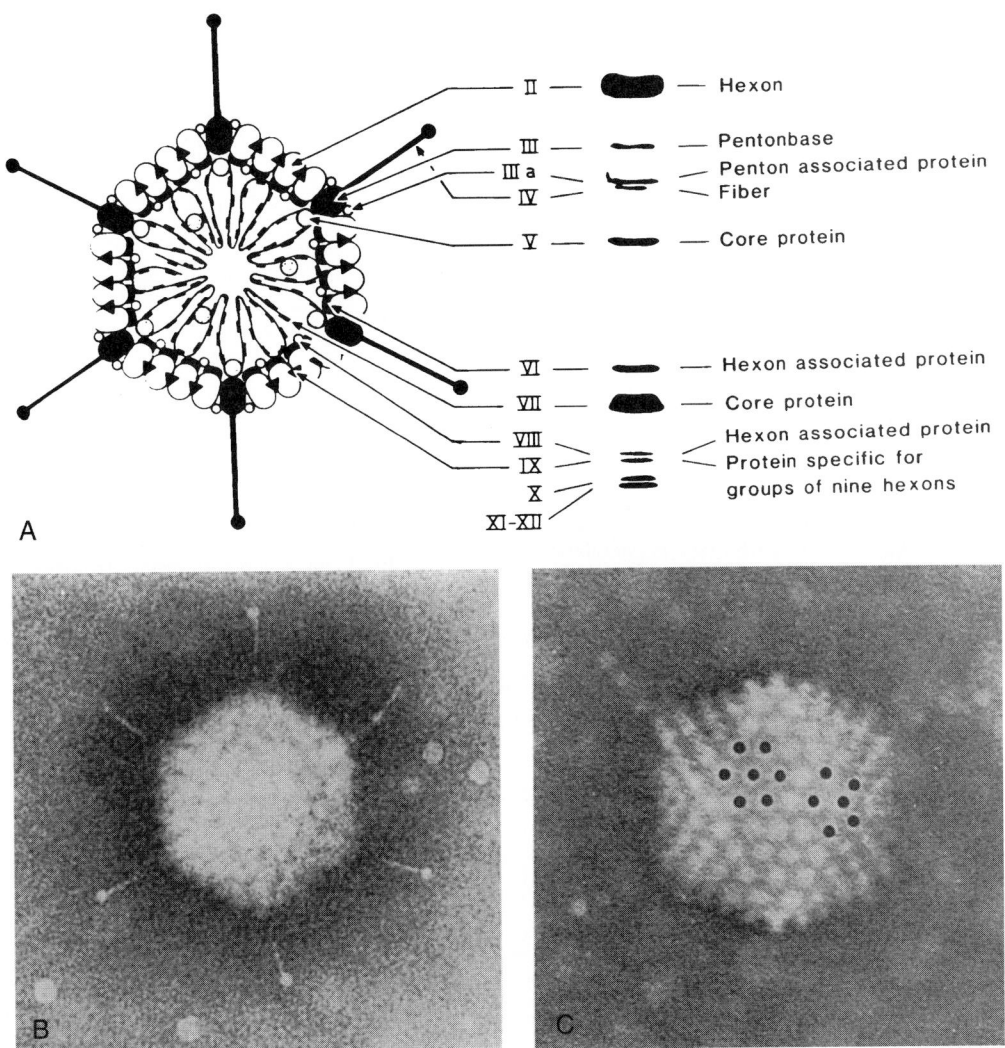

Figure 229.1. Adenovirus morphology and polypeptide composition. **A:** Schematic representation of the virion is shown together with a denaturing polyacrylamide gel stained with Coomassie blue to display the mobility and amount of each of the viral proteins (polypeptide I was an aggregate of some of the others and is not shown) (20,22). Polypeptides II, III, IIIA, IV, VI, VIII, and IX are components of the capsid, and the core proteins are V and VII. The terminal protein covalently linked to each 5′ end of the DNA is not shown. **B:** An electron micrograph of an adenovirus type 5, demonstrating 6 of the 12 vertices (penton base plus fiber). **C:** The six-fold symmetry around each hexon and the five-fold capsomere configuration around each penton base are highlighted. (**A** from Persson H, Philipson L. Regulation of adenovirus. *Curr Top Microbiol Immunol* 1982; **B** and **C** from Valentine RC, Periera HG. Antigens and structure of the adenovirus. *J Mol Biol* 1965;13:13–20 and Horwitz MS. Adenoviridae and their replication. In: Fields B, Knipe DM, Chanock R, et al., eds. *Virology*, 2nd ed. New York: Raven Press, 1990:1679–1721, with permission.)

animal adenoviruses. This group-specific antigen was classically measured by complementation fixation tests, which have been supplemented recently by other serologic tests, such as enzyme-linked immunosorbent assay (ELISA) (27). Many of the adenoviruses hemagglutinate rat or rhesus red blood cells or those of various other species (28). The hemagglutination (HA) test has led to a classification scheme of subgroups from A to F. The HA is a property of the fiber protein, and there is usually a good correlation between the neutralization and hemagglutination inhibition (HI) tests. However, there are an increasing number of field isolates, especially in subgroups B and D (29,30), for which the neutralization and HI tests are divergent, probably because of recombination among different adenovirus isolates within sub-

groups. More distantly related adenoviruses appear to recombine infrequently (31).

Biology

After adenovirus fibers attach to the CAR receptor, the virus–cell interaction is augmented by the binding of penton base to cellular integrins, $\alpha_v\beta_3$ and $\alpha_v\beta_5$ (32). The virus is internalized in endosomes, where it undergoes initial uncoating during acidification of this structure (33). Subsequent uncoating occurs in a stepwise fashion during transit of the particle to the nucleus, where viral DNA is internalized and transcribed into early mRNA (34). The

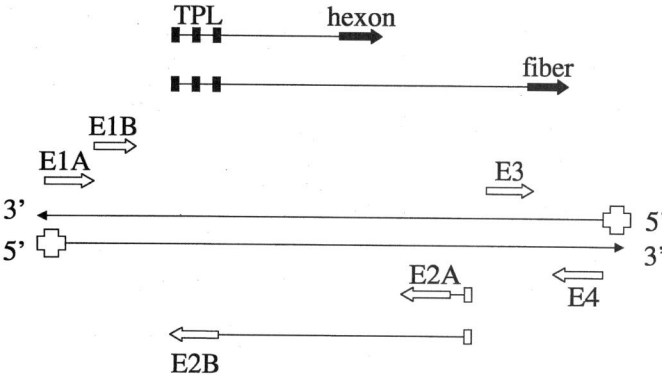

Figure 229.2. Transcription and translation map of early and late messenger RNA (mRNA) and protein products of Ad2. The *open arrows* represent early (E) transcripts, and the *black arrows* are two examples of many late (L) transcripts that direct the synthesis of the structural proteins of the virus. Each of these arrows represents multiple spliced forms of mRNAs encoded in the region designated. L transcripts start at 16.3 map units (numbered from the left of the genome) and use the tripartite leader (TPL), which is a component that increases the translation of all late mRNAs. The L mRNAs are shown for two structural proteins, hexon and fiber, which are components of the viral capsid, as shown in Figure 229.1. The *thin lines* joining the arrows to the *small rectangles* in the mRNA precursor molecules are introns removed by splicing. The *arrows* indicate the direction of transcription, which occurs from each DNA strand, *shown as thin lines with cruciate structure* representing the terminal proteins at each 5′ end. Further details of the transcription and translation maps are provided by Shenk (5).

early proteins synthesized before viral DNA replication begins include the following:

1. A family of transforming and transactivating proteins from the E1A and E1B regions at the left end of the genome (5) (Fig 229.2). The transforming proteins are responsible for some adenovirus serotypes being oncogenic in rodents (35).
2. Three proteins from the E2A and E2B regions, needed for replication of the viral genome: a 140-kd DNA polymerase (pol), an 87-kd precursor to the terminal protein (pTP), and a DNA-binding protein (DBP) (36).
3. A group of proteins synthesized from early region 3 (E3) that controls the host immune and cytokine response to infection (37,38) (see the section "Pathogenesis").
4. A family of early region 4 (E4) proteins, one of which (E4 34-kd) binds to the E1B 55-kd protein. This complex inhibits cellular mRNA accumulation in the cytoplasm but facilitates viral mRNA transcription (39).

One of the adenovirus E1A proteins binds to the anti-oncogene retinoblastoma protein (Rb) (40,41), freeing the transcription factor E2F from its association with Rb and allowing E2F to transactivate other early viral genes such as E2. During the transformation cycle in rodent cells, this process alters transcription of mRNAs for proteins required for control of the cell cycle (42). The function of E1A is augmented by proteins from the E1B region whose major function is to interact with the *p53* anti-oncogene and prevent apoptosis (43,44). Inhibition of apoptosis early in infection could contribute to the survival of the cell until viral progeny are produced during the lytic cycle. During the transformation process in rodents, E1B could promote the immortalization of cells whose cell cycle control had been dysregulated by the E1A functions. The adenovirus structural proteins are synthesized primarily after viral DNA replication has been initiated. Viral DNA enters preformed empty capsids, assembled in the nucleus, to produce new progeny virus. Most of the structural proteins are synthesized from "late" mRNAs that originate at the strong major late promoter at 16.3 map units (Fig. 229.2) and undergo multiple splices before functional mRNA is

TABLE 229.1.   Classification of Human Adenoviruses (Mastadenovirus)

Subgroup	Serotypes	Hemagglutination (HA) species of red cells
A	12, 18, 31	R
B	3, 7, 16, 21, 50 (B1)[a]	My
	11, 14, 34, 35 (B2)	My
C	1, 2, 5, 6	R
D	8, 9, 37	R, Mo, H, Gp, D
	10, 19, 26, 27, 36, 38, 39	R, Mo, H
	13, 43	R, Mo, H, My
	10, 19, 26, 27, 36, 38, 39	R, Mo, H
	15, 22, 23, 30, 44, 45, 46, 47	R, Mo, My
	17, 24, 32, 33, 42	R, My
	48, 49, 51	R
E	4	R
F	40, 41	R

R, rat; My, monkey; Mo, mouse; H, human; GP, guinea pig; D, dog.
[a]B1, B2 subgroups based on differences in DNA restriction sites.
Adapted and modified from Horwitz MS. Adenovirus. In: Knipe DM, Howley PM, eds. *Fields virology.* New York: Lippincott Williams & Wilkins, 2001:2301–2326; and Hierholzer JC. Adenoviruses. In: Lennette EH, Lennette DA, Lennette ET, eds. *Diagnostic procedures for viral rickettsial and chlamydial infections.* Washington, DC: American Public Health Association, 1995:169–188.

formed (5,45). In fact, splicing of eukaryotic mRNAs was discovered in the adenovirus system (46,47).

Classification

Human adenoviruses are classified into subgroups by the hemagglutination pattern of red blood cells, the ability to cause tumors in rodents, or the percentage of guanine-plus-cytosine (G + C) content of their DNA (48) (Table 229.1). These viruses are included in the genus *Mastadenovirus,* which contains other viruses that infect simian, bovine, canine, and other mammals (49). Aviadenoviruses contain additional members that naturally infect birds. Adenoviruses remain species specific in their natural patterns of infection and induction of disease; however, human sera have been shown to have antibodies to some simian, canine, and bovine adenoviruses (50). The G + C content of DNA is also reflected in sequence homology, which should be greater than 50% by hybridization of the entire viral genome for adenoviruses to be classified in the same subgroup (48). Adenoviruses from all subgroups except for Group B bind to the CAR receptor. Very recently, Group B2 Ad35 was shown to bind CD46, a membrane cofactor belonging to the complement regulating family of proteins (50a). There is some clinical significance to the classification scheme in that the manifestations of adenovirus diseases often correlate with the subgroup (Table 229.2). For example, when adenoviruses cause upper respiratory infections in children, they are usually group C agents, types 1, 2, 5, or 6. Adenoviruses related to lower respiratory infection and pneumonia are often group B, types 3, 7, and 21, or group E, type 4. Epidemic keratoconjunctivitis is most often associated with group D adenoviruses, types 8, 19, or 37. Hemorrhagic cystitis in normal children is often a subgroup B adenovirus, type 11 or 21; whereas persistence of adenoviruses in the urinary tract in immunosuppressed patients is also commonly group B, but serotypes 34 and 35. Although adenoviruses of a variety of subgroups can be isolated from fecal samples, only subgroup F, types 40 and 41, appear to cause diarrhea. Subgroup A is also commonly isolated from stool specimens but is not often associated with any disease syndrome other than an occasional case of meningoencephalitis in humans; however, it is highly oncogenic after experimental infection of

TABLE 229.2. Illnesses Associated with Adenovirus Infections

Disease	Individuals most at risk	Principal serotypes
Acute febrile pharyngitis	Infants, young children	1, 2, 5, 6(C); 3, 7(B)
Pharyngoconjunctival fever	School-aged children	3, 7, 14(B)
Acute respiratory disease	Military recruits, adults	3, 7, 14, 21(B); 4(E)
Pneumonia	Infants, young children	1, 2(C); 3, 7(B)
Pneumonia	Military recruits	4(E) 7(B)
Epidemic keratoconjunctivitis	Any age group	8, 19, 37(D)
Pertussis-like syndrome	Infants, young children	5(C)
Acute hemorrhagic cystitis	Young children	11, 21(B)
Gastroenteritis	Infants, young children	40, 41(F)
Meningoencephalitis	Children and immunocompromised hosts	7(B); 12(A); 32(D)
Hepatitis	Infants and children with liver transplants	1, 2, 5(C)
Myocarditis	Children	Unknown
Persistence of virus:	Bone marrow transplant recipients, patients with acquired immunodeficiency or other immunosuppression syndromes	
In urinary tract		34, 35(B)
In colon		42–49(D)

Adapted and modified from Wadell G, Allard A, Hierholzer JC. Adenoviruses. In: Murray P, Baron E, eds. *Manual of clinical microbiology.* Washington, DC: ASM Press, 1999:970–982; and Horwitz MS. Adenoviruses. In: Knipe DM, Howley PM, eds. *Fields virology.* New York: Lippincott Williams & Wilkins, 2001:2301–2326.

hamsters. Group D adenoviruses of higher serotypes are often found in the large intestine of patients with acquired immunodeficiency syndrome (AIDS). These patterns are not absolute, and exceptions to these serotype patterns do occur. About two thirds of all adenovirus serotypes are uncommonly isolated, and their relationship with diseases is poorly defined. Human adenoviruses show a strong preference for growth in human tissue culture, as described in the later section "Diagnosis."

PATHOGENESIS

The most common portal of entry for the adenovirus is through the respiratory and conjunctival mucosa. Contiguous spread then may occur in some patients to the lungs, and viremia is implicated in fatal disease. Enteric disease appears to be acquired by the fecal-oral route. Adenovirus latency in donor organ cells from kidney and heart has been postulated to be the cause of infection in some solid organ transplant recipients (51,52).

Manifestations of adenovirus diseases are probably the results of the cytolytic properties of the virus as well as the immunologic and cytokine responses of the host. In tissue-cultured cells, adenoviruses can lyse cells by inhibiting both host macromolecular synthesis (53) and transport of cellular mRNA to the cytoplasm (54). The initial immune response probably is natural killer (NK) cell and monocyte recognition of infected cells, which evokes an interleukin-1 (IL-1), IL-6, and tumor-necrosis factor-α (TNFα) cytokine response, as demonstrated in animal models (55,56). This phase is followed by the induction of cytotoxic T cells (57) and the appearance of a variety of neutralizing and nonneutralizing antibodies to viral components such as hexon, fiber, and penton base. Elevated levels of IL-6, IL-8, and TNF-α in serum during adenovirus infection correlate with more severe adenovirus infections in humans (58). Adenoviruses also elaborate excess amounts of their penton base protein, which causes cells to round up and detach from tissue culture monolayers (59). Such effects may be cytotoxic *in vivo,* and penton base protein has been demonstrated in the blood obtained from a few patients with fatal adenovirus pneumonia (60); however, the significance of this mechanism in most adenovirus-infected patients has not been further clarified.

Adenoviruses contain genes whose products can affect the immune response (37,61). The viral-associated (VA) RNA can inhibit the action of interferons (62,63), and the E1b proteins inhibit apoptosis (44) that otherwise might abort the production of adenoviruses in infected cells. An adenovirus E3 gene codes for a 19-kd glycoprotein that retains the class I major histocompatibility complex (MHC) in the endoplasmic reticulum and inhibits the tapasin transporter (TAP), which processes peptides for presentation by MHC (64). Inhibition of both of these processes reduces the amount of MHC on the plasma membrane and inhibits the signals for activation of cytotoxic T cell lysis (CTL) (61). Because various herpesviruses also have been demonstrated to have comparable mechanisms for reducing CTL by inhibiting the cellular TAP transporters of peptides to class I MHC (65), this general process to prevent immune cytolysis may be important in viral pathogenesis. Other E3 proteins inhibit TNF-α–mediated cytolysis and reduce chemokine synthesis while inhibiting the proinflammatory transcription factor, NFκB (65a,65b). These processes probably are directed at preventing destruction of infected cells before the full amount of adenoviruses is produced (38,66). Although the structural differences between these E3 genes from various adenovirus serotypes have not yet been correlated with differences in pathogenesis (67), the concept that adenoviruses may control the manifestations of disease by altering the immune response is being actively pursued in animal models (56,68–70). Some of the histologic findings in adenoviral disease may be due to immunopathology (56). The effectiveness of the adenovirus E3 genes as antiinflammatory immunomodulators even when removed from the context of the virus has been shown in a number of animal models, including one in which functional E3 genes, placed into pancreatic islets, permitted the allogeneic transplantation of these immunologically altered donor cells (71). In addition, the Ad E3 transgenes expressed in murine islets prevented autoimmune diabetes in two mouse models of type I diabetes (72,73).

Although adenoviruses do not cause transformation or tumors during infections of humans, they can remain latent or persistent within the human host. In addition to the intermittent shedding of adenoviruses for several years after a primary infection even in the presence of a neutralizing antibody response (74), adenovirus sequences have been found in human lymphocytes

(75) and tonsils (76); however, more recent studies using nested polymerase chain reaction (PCR) failed to show Ad DNA in peripheral blood mononuclear cells (PBMCS) of healthy individuals. In these same studies, viral DNA did appear in PBMCs of infected immunosuppressed patients and correlated with active disease (77). There also has been a report of adenovirus sequences found in lung tissue from patients with chronic obstructive pulmonary disease (78).

CLINICAL FEATURES

Respiratory Diseases

CHILDREN

About 5% of all upper respiratory infections in children younger than 5 years of age (79) and 10% of pneumonias of childhood (80) are caused by adenoviruses. Coryza, cough, and a follicular distribution of exudate on the tonsils may be confused with other respiratory viruses (parainfluenza, influenza, and respiratory syncytial virus) or group A streptococcal infection (81,82). Systemic manifestations, such as fever, malaise, myalgia, and headache, may accompany these infections, which are commonly due to serotypes 1, 2, 5, or 6 (subgroup C) or occasionally serotype 3 (subgroup B). When pneumonia occurs with these agents, it is usually mild to moderate in severity with subsequent recovery in most patients. However, there have been severe cases of adenovirus type 7 or 21 pneumonias with residual pulmonary damage such as bronchiectasis or fatalities (83,84). The relationship between adenovirus infection and the whooping cough syndrome has received considerable attention. Although adenovirus infection can occasionally be accompanied by a severe cough and lymphocytosis (85), whooping cough is caused by *Bordetella pertussis* and does not require an adenovirus co-infection (86). However, it has been noted that during *B. pertussis* infections, adenoviruses are isolated more frequently than from controls (87). Whether the extensive cough or putative cytokine release during *Bordetella* infection facilitates the isolation of adenoviruses has not been resolved.

ADULTS

Adults can develop similar respiratory symptoms with manifestations limited to the upper respiratory tract or extension to the lungs in the form of pneumonia (88). The serotypes involved are usually Ad4, Ad7, and occasionally Ad3. The change in serotypes reflects the immunity that most individuals develop to types 1, 2, 5, and 6 during childhood. Adenovirus disease in military recruits, especially early after induction into the armed services with the accompanying crowding, fatigue, or new exposures to infectious diseases, was called *acute respiratory disease* (ARD) (89). ARD often affected many of the new recruits causing tracheobronchitis and pneumonia requiring hospitalization. Although complete recovery was usual following 3 to 5 days of illness from adenovirus-induced ARD, the disruption of military maneuvers and occasional deaths prompted the development of vaccines against Ad4 and Ad7 (see later).

Pharyngoconjunctival Fever

Although adenoviral pharngoconjunctival (APC) fever can occur sporadically, it usually appears as small outbreaks in children, especially in summer camps (90). A granular palpebral and bulbar conjunctivitis, which may sequentially affect both eyes, is often accompanied by a febrile pharyngitis, cervical adenitis, and rhinitis (91,92). The incubation period is 6 to 9 days but was shorter in experimentally infected volunteers (93,94). Symptoms last 3 to 5 days, and there are usually no sequelae. Adenovirus serotypes most commonly involved, especially when a common source such as a pool or lake were incriminated in "swimming pool conjunctivitis," were Ad3 and Ad7 (95); however, many other serotypes from subgroups B, C, D, and E have been implicated in this disease. Although the epidemiologic association with a common source has been very strong, and adenoviruses are isolated from conjunctival swabs of infected patients, the virus has not been isolated from water samples from the implicated source.

Epidemic Keratoconjunctivitis

Epidemic keratoconjunctivitis (EKC) is a more serious adenovirus infection of the eye that is highly contagious. It is caused by Ad8, Ad19, or Ad37 (predominant cause since 1977) and begins after an 8- to 10-day incubation period (96–98). A follicular conjunctivitis accompanied by lid edema, photophobia, lacrimation, and pain is commonly followed by corneal infiltration of the subepithelial layer. Preauricular adenopathy is a common finding, and the unilateral disease often spreads to the other eye. If the disease progresses to a hemorrhagic conjunctivitis, it may be difficult to distinguish from that caused by enterovirus type 70. Although the inflammatory phase may last several weeks before resolution, corneal opacities may require months or even years to resolve completely. In adults, constitutional symptoms are not common, but children may have generalized adenopathy and fever.

Acute Hemorrhagic Cystitis

Hemorrhagic cystitis in the immunocompetent host is usually a self-limited infection with Ad11 or Ad21 and is more common in males (99,100). The gross hematuria must be distinguished from more serious renal diseases and bacterial infections of the urinary tract. Children between the ages of 6 and 15 years are more commonly affected. They usually are afebrile and do not have any renal functional abnormalities. This disease also occurs in immunosuppressed patients, such as renal transplant recipients in whom the infectious adenoviruses, including types Ad34 and Ad35, may have been latent in the transplanted kidney (101,102). Cytotoxic immunosuppressive drugs in the latter setting may also cause red cells to appear in the urine, and some patients have hematuria from both of these processes (103).

Gastrointestinal Disease

Although many adenovirus serotypes can be isolated from the intestine during respiratory adenovirus infections or even from asymptomatic children, only Ad40 and Ad41 (subgroup F) appear to be associated with diarrhea (104–106). Nosocomial infections have been reported from pediatric wards in patients younger than 4 years of age, and respiratory symptoms often accompany the gastrointestinal disease (106). The incidence of diarrhea caused by adenoviruses varies greatly in the various reports of its contribution to this disease; however, rotaviruses usually are more common as the etiologic agent in most of these studies (107). During outbreaks of adenovirus diarrhea in day care settings, many unaffected children are also found to have the agent in their stool samples (108). By the age of 4 years, 50% of children have antibodies to the enteric adenoviruses (109,110).

Intussusception has also been linked to adenovirus infection but not to the "enteric" types (111,112). Ad1, Ad2, Ad5, and Ad6 (subgroup C) have been isolated from children with intussusception both from intestinal lymph nodes removed during surgery for bowel resection and from stool samples. Whether the enlarged mesenteric lymph nodes that might accompany an adenovirus infection could serve as a lead point for the intussusception, or the hypermotility of irritated bowel is more likely to cause telescoping of the intestine, has not been clarified (113).

Because most patients with intussusception do not have evidence of adenovirus infection, the role of viral infection in this syndrome has not been elucidated further.

Because there is some structural homology between the adenovirus type 12 E1B protein and A-gliadin, which is a component of wheat proteins known to activate celiac disease, a role of viral infection in inducing or aggravating this malabsorption syndrome has been proposed. Molecular mimicry can result in cross-reacting antibodies between A-gliadin and the adenovirus E1b protein (114). Although Ad12 can persist in the intestine for long periods, its relationship with gluten-induced enteropathy has not been resolved (115,116).

Meningoencephalitis

Adenoviruses have been isolated from brain and spinal fluid obtained from cases of meningoencephalitis but are not a common etiology of this disease (117,118). Meningoencephalitis has accompanied outbreaks of Ad7 pneumonia, but in most of these cases, the virus was isolated from extraneural sites (119). There are no pathognomonic findings to distinguish adenovirus infections of the central nervous system from other etiologic agents.

Adenovirus Infections in Immunocompromised Hosts

Adenovirus infections of various organs and by different serotypes are usually more severe in immunocompromised patients (120–122), even those with isolated hypogammaglobulinemia (123). However, several situations deserve further elaboration. Hepatitis due to common group C serotypes (1, 2, and 5) is a problem after pediatric liver transplantation (8,124). It is not clear in individual cases whether the infection is acute or results from reactivation of latent virus in the transplant or the tissues of the host. Of 484 pediatric hepatic transplantation patients, 49 had adenoviruses isolated from at least one sampled site, 20 had invasive disease, and 9 died (8). Discontinuation of immunosuppressive therapy at the time of severe adenovirus infection has not always been successful in reversing the effects of the infection. Adenovirus hepatitis has also ended fatally in patients with severe combined immunodeficiency syndrome, AIDS, and bone marrow transplantation.

In 21% of bone marrow transplant recipients, subgroup B adenoviruses (primarily Ad34 and Ad35) were isolated, and significant disease occurred in 6.5% (51); however, full evaluation of these latter agents revealed that some of them had hemagglutinins of other group B serotypes, indicating that there had been intrasubgroup recombination (125,126). Risk factors for disease after infection include younger age, multiple sites of virus isolation, and the severity of graft-versus-host disease (127). The biggest challenge for the physician is to differentiate infection alone from adenoviral disease. Isolation of adenoviruses from multiple sites or the presence of a positive PCR on peripheral blood mononuclear cells usually correlates with adenoviral disease. Reactivation of latent virus is the most common mechanism, but primary infection may be responsible for higher numbers in the pediatric population (52). The most common manifestation of disease after transplantation is late-onset hemorrhagic cystitis, but fatalities are mostly secondary to pneumonitis, hepatitis, and nephritis. Ad35 is often isolated in this setting but rarely from normal hosts. This results in low levels of Ad35 antibodies in the commercially available immunoglobulin pool.

Recently, Shirali and colleagues (10) found adenovirus by PCR in 6% of 533 endomyocardial biopsies from 149 pediatric cardiac transplantation patients. None of these patients had isolation of adenovirus by culture, but the serotypes were described as primarily Ad2. The presence of adenovirus-positive PCR correlated with an increased incidence of adverse cardiac events, including graft loss and coronary artery vasculopathy. The 5-year graft survival rate in adenovirus-positive PCR patients decreased to 62% from 96% in the adenovirus-negative PCR controls.

In AIDS patients, subgroup B adenoviruses were found in 12% of urine samples (29), and subgroup D adenoviruses of multiple serotypes have been isolated from numerous stool samples. The presence of adenovirus in stool samples and at the site of colonic damage in AIDS patients has suggested that these agents might be responsible for some of the cases of chronic diarrhea (128,129). However, most of the gastrointestinal problems in AIDS patients are probably due to other causes.

EPIDEMIOLOGY

Adenoviruses are ubiquitous agents that cause both sporadic and epidemic diseases. Each mammalian species has distinct adenovirus serotypes that share structural and some antigenic cross-reactivity with human adenoviruses (49); however, there is no significant crossover of infectivity from animals to humans (50). From longitudinal epidemiologic observations (79,130) and "virus watch" studies performed in New York and Seattle (74,131), a number of seminal observations have been made: (a) many adenovirus infections documented by virus isolation or serology are asymptomatic; (b) there is a high degree of intermittent adenovirus shedding, especially in stool specimens; and (c) 7% of febrile illnesses in children are due to adenovirus infection. Group C serotypes 1, 2, and 5 are most common during childhood, and 40% to 60% of older children have antibodies to these types (79,132); infection with types 3, 4, and 7 are uncommon in childhood, and thus these serotypes are more usual as causes of respiratory disease in adults. Group B serotypes 11, 21, 34, and 35 have a predilection for the urinary tract (99,100,126) but can also cause pneumonias (122). Group F serotypes 40 and 41 cause diarrhea in young children (104–106), but group D serotypes are often isolated from stool samples of adult AIDS patients (133). Group D adenoviruses of three serotypes (8, 19, and 37) are responsible for most cases of EKC (96–98). EKC formerly followed infections that could be traced to contaminated ophthalmologic equipment, when tonometers that contacted the corneas were used. However, as a highly transmissible infection, direct person-to-person spread and spread from contaminated objects such as shared towels are currently more common.

The biochemical basis of relative serotype specificity for each of these disease syndromes or sites of adenovirus replication have not been elucidated (see section "Pathogenesis"). The unique occurrence during World War II of ARD in new military recruits and its failure to spread to their civilian contacts was contrasted to influenza outbreaks during which there was no such discrimination of involved individuals (13,134,135). This is even more surprising because controlled studies showed that during Ad4 and Ad7 experimental infections, the infection was airborne (136). Most other adenovirus transmissions are contact infections (from person to person, waterborne for adenoviral pharyngoconjunctival fever, or by contaminated instruments for some cases of epidemic keratoconjunctivitis. Additional information about the epidemiology appears in previous sections describing each of the adenovirus syndromes.

DIAGNOSIS

Except for keratoconjunctivitis, adenovirus syndromes are difficult to diagnose by clinical criteria without the help of the laboratory. Laboratory diagnosis may be required for epidemiologic

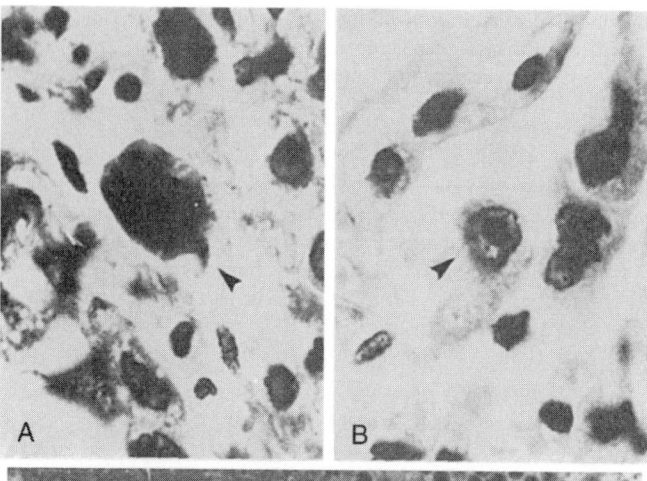

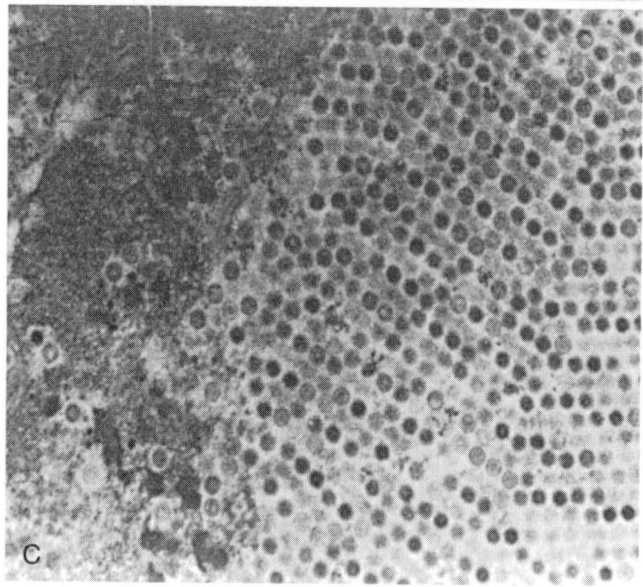

Figure 229.3. Adenovirus cytopathology in human tissue. A "smudge cell" (**A**) designated by an *arrow* is shown in lung tissue from a fatal case of adenovirus pneumonia; a basophilic inclusion fills the nucleus and obliterates the nuclear membrane of a desquamated alveolar cell. A smaller intranuclear inclusion (**B**) contains many virions (**C**), as illustrated by electron microscopy. (Adapted from Myerowitz R, Stalder H, Oxman M, et al. Fatal disseminated adenovirus infection in a renal transplant recipient. *Am J Med* 1975;59:591–598, with permission from the *American Journal of Medicine*.)

characterization of outbreaks, such as hospital-acquired adenovirus gastroenteritis, serious cases of pneumonia that can occur even in immunocompetent hosts, and the hepatitis that complicates therapy of immunosuppressed patients including liver transplant recipients. Tissue biopsy specimens or exfoliated cells may show intranuclear inclusions, characteristically without giant cell formation or cell degeneration, described as "smudge cell" formation, particularly in pulmonary tissue (Fig. 229.3). Viral isolation is more reliable than histology and begins with inoculation of patient samples into tissue culture cells of human origins. Primary human embryonic kidney (HEK) is optimal but expensive and is often replaced by a human continuous lung line, A549 (137). The "293 cell," which was derived by transformation of HEK cells with the adenovirus E1 genes (138), is often used when isolation of enteric adenoviruses is attempted (139,140). The E1B 55-kd gene appears to facilitate the isolation of enteric adenoviruses (141). Although a variety of antigen detection techniques are available for examining exfoliated cells (142,143), and latex agglutination tests have been developed for stool sample diagnosis of enteric adenovirus infections (144), both appear to be

inferior to the sensitivity and specificity of PCR-based techniques (145–147). PCR primers have been made from the hexon, VA1, and E1A regions, for which there is extensive homology among serotypes. E1B-region sequences have been used for the enteric viruses. False-positive results with enteric and false-negative results with group B Ad35 have been shown using hexon primers (77). Quantitative real-time PCR detection of conserved regions of the hexon have been developed and await prospective trials. This method is highly sensitive and levels seem to correlate with disease severity and dissemination (148,149,149a). Once an adenovirus suspected because of typical tissue culture cytopathology has been isolated, it is usually confirmed by group-specific reference sera (150). Subsequently, serotype can be determined by first grouping the isolate by HA pattern with rat and rhesus red blood cells and then by HI. Further characterization by neutralization of growth with type-specific sera prepared in various animals can be done (28). When there is a discrepancy between serum neutralization (SN) and HI typing, the isolate is classified by numbers corresponding to SN and HI (expressed as SN/HI), which usually indicates recombination of adenoviruses within a subgroup (126,151). This can be further clarified by looking at the entire viral genome using restriction endonuclease digestion to indicate the pattern of sequence-specific sites of cleavage. If SmaI digestion is supplemented by the use of several other restriction endonucleases, differences between serotypes and the presence of recombinants usually can be detected (126,152,153). Serologic diagnosis on paired sera looking for rising antibody titers between the acute and convalescence phase of an illness can also be done by a variety of techniques (27), including complement fixation, HI (154), SN (155), and ELISA (156).

TREATMENT

There are no proven effective antiviral agents, either for systemic use or for topical administration to the eyes, that have been shown to benefit patients with any of the adenovirus syndromes; however, there are many antiviral compounds that inhibit adenovirus replication in tissue culture, and some of these have been used in human disease (157–160). Ribavirin has been used to treat hemorrhagic cystitis in several human bone marrow transplant patients, but no controlled trials are available to judge its efficacy (103). Cidofovir, a nucleoside analog, has been reported to be a potent inhibitor of adenovirus replication in human embryonic fibroblast tissue culture and has been used with some success in the rabbit ocular model (161). In clinical settings, there are several reports of successes with cidofovir in a small number of patients who had adenoviruses isolated from the site of their symptoms and histopathologic evidence of infection (162). Treatment of adenovirus infections in most infected patients is thus symptomatic and supportive necessitating cessation of immunosuppressive drugs. Recovery occurring in most cases except for immunosuppressed patients with hepatitis and some cases of pneumonia. There are fatalities reported from adenovirus type 7 pneumonia even in immunocompetent patients, and a particularly virulent form, adenovirus type 7h circulating in South America, was reported in 1993 (163).

PREVENTION

Oral enteric-coated Ad4 and Ad7 live vaccines existed for prevention of ARD in military recruits and were effective (164,165). These adenovirus serotypes have been attenuated only by physically coating the infectious agent to bypass the oropharynx and be displayed first in the intestine. They are not available for civilian populations because the diseases they prevent are not as dramatic as ARD epidemics, and most are self-limited. In addition, there has been some reluctance to use adenovirus vaccines in the general population because these vaccine viruses can cause symptomatic infection in young children and spread to other contacts. In addition, the adenoviruses have transforming genes (3,5); however, after several decades of use in young adults in the military, there is no evidence that these vaccine viruses are harmful to humans (48). Early batches of these adenovirus vaccines were contaminated by recombinant adenovirus–simian virus 40 (Ad-SV40) hybrid strains (166,167), and SV40 is oncogenic in rodents. However, this problem of SV40 contamination introduced by using monkey kidney tissue culture has been completely eliminated by newer tissue culture and detection techniques.

Since 1996, the sole manufacturer of the vaccine has stopped producing it because of problems in the production of new batches (168,169). Subsequently, the reappearance of ARD in the military has once again proved that the vaccine had been highly effective. During the current hiatus in the availability of the adenovirus vaccine, there have even been many cases of ARD at multiple military bases and even two deaths that appeared to be due to adenovirus pneumonia (170).

ADENOVIRUSES AS VECTORS FOR DELIVERY OF THERAPEUTIC GENES

Adenoviruses are currently being explored intensively as tools for the delivery of foreign DNA (1,171). The goals of introducing DNA in such vectors are to (a) overexpress epitopes for immunization against a variety of other infectious agents (172); (b) correct genetic defects in recipient cells, animals (173,174), or humans (175,176); (c) introduce a cytotoxic gene for the treatment of cancer or for the prevention of restenosis after angioplasty (177); and (d) promote angiogenesis (178). Some of the advantages of adenovirus vectors (in contrast to retrovirus vectors) are that they can infect and express genes in nondividing cells as well as be grown to very high titers for the production of large quantities for subsequent use. The disadvantages of adenovirus vectors to correct genetic defects are that they do not efficiently transduce some cell types and are highly immunogenic, eliciting both humoral and cell-mediated responses. The immune response results in transient gene expression and the need for immunosuppression for the prolongation of expression of the foreign gene inserted in an adenovirus gene-therapy vector. Most of the foreign DNA delivered in adenoviruses used to produce immunogenic proteins has been inserted in place of the E3 region, which is not essential for viral growth in tissue culture. This strategy results in replication-competent viral vectors that can expand the epitopes used for immunization. Proteins such as the hepatitis B surface antigen (172) or core protein; the glycoprotein of rabies; Ebola (179); various human immunodeficiency virus type 1 proteins, such as gp120 env, gag, and p24 (180); and numerous others have been expressed as immunogens in the E3 region of adenoviruses.

In contrast, adenoviruses used as vectors for gene therapy usually are deleted of both the E3 and E1 regions to make the vectors replication incompetent in the recipient host and to accommodate large inserts, up to 8.3 kb of foreign DNA within the capsid. These defective adenoviruses can be grown in HEK 293 cells, which constitutively express the adenovirus E1A and E1B genes missing from the virus and complement the defect during the growth of adenoviruses in tissue culture. Numerous genes have been inserted into such defective adenovirus E1 region. Some of the animal studies with adenoviruses expressing ornithine transcarbamylase, blood clotting factors VIII and IX (181), bilirubin uridine diphosphoglucuronate glucuronosyl-

transferase, dystrophin, and erythropoietin (182) have gone quite well in mice and rats. However, the *CFTR* gene, which is defective in cystic fibrosis, has been inserted into adenovirus vectors and has shown some toxicity in limited safety trials in patients with cystic fibrosis (176,183,184). In addition, it has been difficult to infect human tracheobronchial cells *in vivo* with adenoviruses, probably because of the lack of the CAR receptor on the ciliated apical surface. The expression of CAR primarily on the basolateral surfaces has made it more difficult to access with adenovirus vectors (185). Other problems encountered were exemplified by a trial of adenovirus carrying the ornithine transcarbamylase (*OTC*) gene to correct the congenital deficiency in this ammonium ion–detoxifying enzyme. Probably because the human liver has low levels of CAR, it was necessary to use large amounts of Ad-OTC for transfection in a dose escalation trial in humans with this enzymatic defect. As the dose of Ad-OTC vector was escalated in an intrahepatic artery administration protocol, significant toxicity and a fatality resulted probably from excessive cytokine release during such a study (186). Another problem with the use of adenovirus delivery systems is the type-specific immune response to the vector itself. It appears that both humoral and T-cell–based immunity decrease the longevity of foreign gene expression from adenovirus vectors (187). The identification of CD46 as the receptor for Ad35 opens new possibilities for development of Ad35 as a vector (187a). Although recloning an immunogenic foreign protein into two or three distinct adenovirus serotypes might overcome the problem of repeated administration of such a protein to elicit an immune response (188,189), such an approach would appear impractical when considering lifelong administration of a gene product to correct a genetic defect. The design of replication-defective adenoviruses has been extended to produce helper-dependent (HD) vectors devoid of all coding regions for viral proteins but retaining the origins of DNA replication at each end of the DNA and a site for insertion of the foreign gene. These defective adenoviruses require conditionally replication-defective helper viruses such as temperature-sensitive adenovirus mutants to complement in *trans* for the structural proteins and replication enzymes for viral DNA (190,191). However, the immunogenicity of the capsid, into which the HD DNA is packaged, remains. There are several reports that introduction of adenovirus capsids, even without any replication, induces chemokines in the infected cell (192).

Another use of adenoviruses is to make replication-selective vectors that are toxic only to malignant cells. Many strategies in addition to the three that follow have been used for this purpose:

1. Deletion of adenovirus genes that are necessary for replication in normal cells but expendable in tumor cells. The first such virus used in humans was Onyx-015, which has a deletion of the E1B 55-kd region needed to inactivate *p53* to permit the replication of adenoviruses in normal cells. Expression of *p53* is already lost in many human tumors, and the E1B 55-kd region is not needed for replication in some of these cells (193).
2. Engineer tumor-specific promoter and enhancer elements to drive the expression of the early viral genes controlling the replication of adenoviruses containing cytotoxic genes. One good example is CN787, which is specific to prostate-specific antigen–positive prostatic cancer cells, even those that have metastasized (194).
3. Targeted adenovirus therapy involving the inhibition of binding to the CAR and integrin receptors and replacement by a ligand binding to a tumor-target site (195).

The studies with Onyx-015 have entered phase 3 trials, with some promise from the small number of patients with head and neck tumors who have benefited from local tumor injection with this altered adenovirus. Adenovirus therapy was effective in reducing the size of head and neck squamous cell carcinomas in 15% of cases, and repeated intratumoral injections induced antiviral humoral antibody (193). A potentially synergistic interaction with chemotherapy was noted, and most of the patients were treated concurrently with Onyx-015 and chemotherapy. Furthermore, the correlation between Onyx-015 replicating only in *p53*-negative cells clearly is imperfect (196). However, the ability of Onyx-015 to shrink some of the head and neck tumors merits further study of this conditionally dependent, replicating adenovirus (197,198). Other research directed to improving the efficacy of oncolytic viruses includes "arming" the virus to express exogenous therapeutic genes like cytokines and prodrug-activating enzymes.

The reinsertion of the E3 region, which might abrogate some class I cytotoxic T-cell– and TNF-mediated responses (see section "Pathogenesis") is under active investigation to decrease the immunogenicity of adenovectors. Our previous work has shown that the adenovirus E3 region expressed as transgenes can abrogate allogeneic transplantation and autoimmune response to islets (71,72,73). Current experiments are attempting to extend these immunoprotective effects of the E3 region delivered in viral vectors.

REFERENCES

1. Grunhaus A, Horwitz MS. Adenoviruses as cloning vectors. In: Rice C, ed. *Seminars in virology.* London: Saunders Scientific Publications, 1992:237–252.
2. Danthinne X, Imperiale MJ. Production of first generation adenovirus vectors: a review. *Gene Ther* 2000;7(20):1707–1714.
3. Trentin JJ, Yabe Y, Taylor G. The quest for human cancer viruses. *Science* 1962;137:835–849.
4. Huebner RJ, Casey MJ, Chanock RM, et al. Tumors induced in hamsters by a strain of adenovirus type 3. Sharing of tumor antigens and "neoantigens" with those produced by adenovirus type 7 tumors. *Proc Natl Acad Sci U S A* 1965;54:381–388.
5. Shenk T. Adenoviridae. In: Knipe DM, Howley PM, eds. *Fields virology.* New York: Lippincott Williams & Wilkins, 2001:2265–2228.
6. Wold WSM, Mackey JK, Rigden P, et al. Analysis of human cancer DNAs for DNA sequences of human adenovirus serotypes 3, 7, 11, 14, 16, and 21 in group B. *Cancer Res* 1979;39:3479–3484.
7. Krilov LR, Rubin LG, Frogel M, et al. Disseminated adenovirus infection with hepatic necrosis in patients with human immunodeficiency virus infection and other immunodeficiency states. *Rev Infect Dis* 1990;12:303–307.
8. Michaels MG, Green M, Wald ER, et al. Adenovirus infection in pediatric liver transplant recipients. *J Infect Dis* 1992;165:170–174.
9. Bowles NE, Kearney DL, Ni J, et al. The detection of viral genomes by polymerase chain reaction in the myocardium of pediatric patients with advanced HIV disease. *J Am Coll Cardiol* 1999;34(3):857–865.
10. Shirali GS, Ni J, Chinnock RE, et al. Association of viral genome with graft loss in children after cardiac transplantation. *N Engl J Med* 2001;344(20):1498–1503.
11. Rowe WP, Huebner RJ, Gillmore LK, et al. Isolation of a cytopathogenic agent from human adenoids undergoing spontaneous degeneration in tissue culture. *Proc Soc Exp Biol Med* 1953;84:570–573.
12. Hilleman MR, Werner JH. Recovery of new agents from patients with acute respiratory illness. *Proc Soc Exp Biol Med* 1954;85:183–188.
13. Hilleman MR. Epidemiology of adenovirus respiratory infections in military recruit populations. *Ann N Y Acad Sci* 1957;67:262–272.
14. Dingle J, Langmuir AD. Epidemiology of acute respiratory disease in military recruits. *Am Rev Respir Dis* 1968;97:1–65.
15. Commission on Acute Respiratory Disease. Experimental transmission of minor respiratory illness to human volunteers by filter-passing agents. Demonstration of two illness characterized by long and short incubation periods and different clinical features. *J Clin Invest* 1947;26:957–973.
16. De Jong JC, Wermenbol AG, Verweij-Uijterwaal MW, et al. Adenoviruses from human immunodeficiency virus-infected individuals, including two strains that represent new candidate serotypes Ad50 and Ad51 of species B1 and D, respectively. *J Clin Microbiol* 1999;37(12):3940–3945.
17. Jawetz E. The story of shipyard eye. *Br Med J* 1959;1:873–878.
18. Stewart PL, Fuller SD, Burnett RM. Difference imaging of adenovirus: bridging the resolution gap between X-ray crystallography and electron microscopy. *EMBO J* 1993;12:2589–2599.
19. Kidd AH, Chroboczek J, Cusack S, et al. Adenovirus type 40 virions contain two distinct fibers. *Virology* 1993;192:73–84.
20. Green NM, Wrigley NG, Russell WC, et al. Evidence for a repeating cross-b sheet structure in the adenovirus fibre. *EMBO J* 1983;2:1357–1365.
21. Maizel JV Jr, White DO, Scharff MD. The polypeptides of adenovirus. II. Soluble proteins, cores, top components and structure of the virion. *Virology* 1968;36:126–136.
22. Maizel JVJr, White DO, Scharff MD. The polypeptides of adenoviruses. I. Evidence for multiple protein components in the virion and a comparison of types 2,7,12. *Virology* 1968;36:115–125.
23. Devaux C, Caillet-Boudin ML, Jacrot B, et al. Crystallization, enzymatic cleavage, and the polarity of the adenovirus type 2 fiber. *Virology* 1987;161:121–128.
24. Bergelson JM, Cunningham JA, Kurt-Jones E, et al. Isolation of a common receptor for coxsackie B viruses and adenoviruses 2 and 5. *Science* 1997;275:1320–1323.
25. Friefeld BR, Lichy J, Field J, et al. The in vitro replication of adenovirus DNA in the molecular biology of adenoviruses. In: Doerfler W, ed. *Current topics in microbiology and immunology.* New York: Springer Verlag, 1984:221–255.
26. Pirofski L, Horwitz MS. Adenovirus, infection, and immunity. In: Roitt IM, Delves PS, eds. *Encyclopedia of immunology.* San Diego: Academic Press, 1998;2:1514–1516.
27. Wadell G, Allard A, Hierholzer JC. Adenoviruses. In: Murray P, Baron E, eds. *Manual of clinical microbiology.* Washington, DC: ASM Press, 1999:970–982.
28. Hierholzer JC. Further subgrouping of the human adenoviruses by differential hemagglutination. *J Infect Dis* 1973;128:541–550.
29. Horwitz MS, Valderrama G, Hatcher V, et al. Characterization of adenovirus isolates from AIDS patients. *Ann N Y Acad Sci* 1985;437:161–174.
30. Hierholzer JC, Wigand R, Anderson LJ, et al. Adenoviruses from patients with AIDS: a plethora of serotypes and a description of five new serotypes of subgenus D (types 43–47). *J Infect Dis* 1988;158:804–813.
31. Gruber WC, Russell DJ, Tibbetts C. Fiber gene and genomic origin of human adenovirus type 4. *Virology* 1993;196:603–611.
32. Wickham TJ, Mathias P, Cheresch DA, et al. Integrins of a_vb_3 and a_vb_5 promote adenovirus internalization but not virus attachment. *Cell* 1993;73:309–319.
33. Pastan I, Seth P, FitzGerald D, et al. Adenovirus entry into cells; some new observations on an old problem. In: Notkins AL, Oldstone MBA, eds. *Concepts in viral pathogenesis II.* New York: Springer-Verlag, 1986:141–146.
34. Greber UF, Willetts M, Webster P, et al. Stepwise dismantling of adenovirus 2 during entry into cells. *Cell* 1993;75:477–486.
35. Gallimore PH. Tumour production in immunosuppressed rats with cells transformed in vitro by adenovirus type 2. *J Gen Virol* 1972;16:99–102.
36. Chen M, Mermod N, Horwitz MS. Protein-protein interactions between adenovirus DNA polymerase and nuclear factor I mediate formation of the DNA replication preinitiation complexes. *J Biol Chem* 1990;265:18634–18642.
37. Wold WSM, Tollefson AE, Hermiston TW. The E3 transcription unit of adenovirus. In: Doerfler W, ed. *The molecular repertoire of adenoviruses in current topics in microbiology and immunology.* New York: Springer-Verlag, 1995:237–274.
38. Horwitz MS. Adenovirus immunoregulatory genes and their cellular targets. *Virology* 2001;279(1):1–8.
39. Babiss LE, Ginsberg HS, Darnell JE Jr. Adenovirus E1B proteins are required for accumulation of late viral mRNA and for effects on cellular mRNA translation and transport. *Mol Cell Biol* 1985;5:2552–2558.
40. Whyte P, Buchkovich KJ, Horowitz JM, et al. Association between an oncogene and an anti-oncogene: the adenovirus E1A proteins bind to the retinoblastoma gene product. *Nature* 1988;334:124–129.
41. Howe JA, Bayley ST. Effects of Ad5 E1A mutant viruses on the cell cycle in relation to the binding of cellular proteins including the retinoblastoma protein and cyclin A. *Virology* 1992;186:15–24.
42. Faha B, Harlow E, Lees E. The adenovirus E1A-associated kinase consists of cyclin E-p33cdk2 and cyclin A-p33cdk2. *J Virol* 1993;67:2456–2465.
43. White E, Sabbatini P, Debbas M, et al. The 19-kilodalton adenovirus E1B transforming protein inhibits programmed cell death and prevents cytolysis by tumor necrosis factor alpha. *Mol Cell Biol* 1992;12:2570–2580.
44. Rao L, Debbas M, Sabbatini P, et al. The adenovirus E1A proteins induce apoptosis, which is inhibited by the E1B 19-kDa and Bcl-2 proteins [published erratum appears in *Proc Natl Acad Sci U S A* 1992;89(20):9974]. *Proc Natl Acad Sci U S A* 1992;89:7742–7746.
45. Philipson L. Adenovirus assembly. In: Ginsberg H, ed. *The adenoviruses.* New York: Plenum, 1981.
46. Berget SM, Moore C, Sharp PA. Spliced segments at the 5′ terminus of adenovirus 2 late mRNA. *Proc Natl Acad Sci U S A* 1977;74:3171–3175.
47. Chow LT, Roberts JM, Lewis JB, et al. A map of cytoplasmic RNA transcripts from lytic adenovirus type 2, determined by electron microscopy of RNA: DNA hybrids. *Cell* 1977;11:819–836.
48. Horwitz M.S. Adenoviruses. In: Knipe DM, Howley PM, eds. *Fields virology.* New York: Lippincott Williams & Wilkins, 2001:2301–2326.
49. Ishibashi M, Yasue H. Adenoviruses of animals. In: Ginsberg HS, ed. *The adenoviruses.* New York: Plenum, 1984: 497–562.
50. Taylor PE. Adenoviruses: diagnosis of infections. In: Kurstak E, Kurstak C, eds. *Comparative diagnosis of viral disease.* New York: Academic Press, 1977:86–170.
50a. Gaggar A, Shayakhmetov DM, Lieber A. Identification of a cellular receptor for group B2 adenoviruses. *Mol Ther* 2003;7:S164 (abstract).
51. Flomenberg P, Babbitt J, Drobyski WR, et al. Increasing incidence of adenovirus disease in bone marrow transplant recipients. *J Infect Dis* 1994;169:775–781.
52. Foster CB, Choi EH, Chanock SJ. Adenovirus and marrow transplantation in children. *Pediatr Pathol Mol Med* 2000;19:97–114.

53. Horwitz MS. Intermediates in the synthesis of type 2 adenovirus deoxyribonucleic acid. *J Virol* 1971;8:675–683.

54. Pilder S, More M, Logan J, et al. The adenovirus E1B-55K transforming polypeptide modulates transport or cytoplasmic stabilization of viral and host cell mRNAs. *Mol Cell Biol* 1986;6:470–476.

55. Ginsberg HS, Moldawer LL, Sehgal PB, et al. A mouse model for investigating the molecular pathogenesis of adenovirus pneumonia. *Proc Natl Acad Sci U S A* 1991;88:1651–1655.

56. Prince GA, Porter DD, Jenson AB, et al. Pathogenesis of adenovirus type 5 pneumonia in cotton rats (*Sigmodon hispidus*). *J Virol* 1993;67:101–111.

57. Olive M, Eisenlohr L, Flomenberg N, et al. The adenovirus capsid protein hexon contains a highly conserved human CD4+ T-cell epitope. *Hum Gene Ther* 2002;13:1167–1178.

58. Mistchenko AS, Diez RA, Mariani AL, et al. Cytokines in adenoviral disease in children: association of interleukin-6, interleukin-8, and tumor necrosis factor alpha levels with clinical outcome. *J Pediatr* 1994;124:714–719.

59. Bai M, Harfe B, Freimuth P. Mutations that alter an arg-gly-asp (RGD) sequence in the adenovirus type 2 penton base protein abolish its cell-rounding activity and delay virus reproduction in flat cells. *J Virol* 1993;67:5198–5205.

60. Ladisch S, Lovejoy FH, Hierholzer JC, et al. Extrapulmonary manifestations of adenovirus type 7 pneumonia simulating Reye syndrome and the possible role of adenovirus toxin. *J Pediatr* 1979;95:348–355.

61. Wold WSM, Hermiston TW, Tollefson AE. Adenovirus proteins that subvert host defenses.[Review]. *Trends Microbiol* 1994;2:437–443.

62. Kitajewski J, Schneider RJ, Safer B, et al. Adenovirus VAI RNA antagonizes the antiviral action of interferon by preventing activation of the interferon-induced eIF-2 alpha kinase. *Cell* 1986;45:195–200.

63. Mathews MB, Shenk T. Adenovirus virus-associated RNA and translation control. *J Virol* 1991;65:5657–5662.

64. Bennett EM, Bennink JR, Yewdell JW, et al. Cutting edge: adenovirus E19 has two mechanisms for affecting class I MHC expression. *J Immunol* 1999;162(9):5049–5052.

65. Hill A, Jugovic P, York I, et al. Herpes simplex virus turns off the TAP to evade host immunity. *Nature* 1995;375:411–415.

65a. Friedman JM, Horwitz MS. Inhibition of tumor necrosis factor alpha-induced NF-kappa B activation by the adenovirus E3-10.4/14.5K complex. *J Virol* 2002;76:5515–5521.

65b. Lesokhin AM, Delgado-Lopez F, Horwitz MS. Inhibition of chemokine expression by adenovirus early region three (E3) genes. *J Virol* 2002;76:8236–8243.

66. Wold WSM. Adenovirus genes that modulate the sensitivity of virus-infected cells to lysis by TNF. *J Cell Biochem* 1993;53:329–335.

67. Flomenberg PR, Chen M, Horwitz MS. Characterization of a major histocompatibility complex class I antigen-binding glycoprotein from adenovirus type 35, a type associated with immunocompromised hosts. *J Virol* 1987;61:3665–3671.

68. Ginsberg HS, Moldawer LL, Sehgal PB, et al. A mouse model for investigating the molecular pathogenesis of adenovirus pneumonia. *Proc Natl Acad Sci U S A* 1991;88:1651–1655.

69. Tufariello J, Cho S, Horwitz MS. The adenovirus E3 14.7K protein, an antagonist of tumor necrosis factor cytolysis, increases the virulence of vaccinia virus in SCID mice. *Proc Natl Acad Sci U S A* 1994;91:10987–10991.

70. Fejer G, Gyory I, Tufariello J, et al. Characterization of transgenic mice containing the adenovirus early region 3 genomic DNA. *J Virol* 1994;68:5871–5881.

71. Efrat S, Fejer G, Brownlee M, et al. Prolonged survival of pancreatic islet allografts mediated by adenovirus immunoregulatory transgenes. *Proc Natl Acad Sci U S A* 1995;92:6947–6951.

72. von Herrath M, Efrat S, Oldstone MBA, et al. Expression of adenoviral E3 transgenes in B cells prevents autoimmune diabetes. *Proc Natl Acad Sci U S A* 1997;94:9808–9813.

73. Efrat S, Serreze DV, Svetlanov A, et al. Adenovirus early region 3 (E3) immunomodulatory genes decrease the incidence of autoimmune diabetes in nonobese diabetic (NOD) mice. *Diabetes* 2001;50:980–984.

74. Fox JP, Brandt CD, Wassermann FE, et al. The Virus Watch Program: a continuing surveillance of viral infections in metropolitan New York families. VI. Observations of adenovirus infections: virus excretion patterns, antibody response, efficiency of surveillance, patterns of infection and relation to illness. *Am J Epidemiol* 1969;89:25–50.

75. Horvath J, Palkonyay L, Weber J. Group C adenovirus DNA sequences in human lymphoid cell. *J Virol* 1986;59:189–192.

76. Neumann R, Genersch E, Eggers HJ. Detection of adenovirus nucleic acid sequences in human tonsils in the absence of infectious virus. *Virus Res* 1987;7:93–97.

77. Flomenberg P, Gutierrez E, Piaskowski VA, et al. Detection of adenovirus DNA in peripheral blood mononuclear cells by polymerase chain reaction. *J Med Virol* 1997;51(3):182–188.

78. Matsuse T, Hayashi S, Kuwano K, et al. Latent adenoviral infection in the pathogenesis of chronic airways obstruction. *Am Rev Respir Dis* 1992;146:177–184.

79. Brandt CD, Kim HW, Vargosdo AJ. Infections in 18,000 infants and children in a controlled study of respiratory tract disease. I. Adenovirus pathogenicity in relation to serologic type and illness syndrome. *Am J Epidemiol* 1969;90:484–500.

80. Mallet R, Riberre M, Bonnenfant F, et al. Les pneumopathies graves a adenovirus. *Arch Fr Pediatr* 1966;23:1057–1073.

81. Ginsberg HS, Gold E, Jordan WS Jr, et al. Relation of the new respiratory agents to acute respiratory diseases. *Am J Public Health* 1955;45:915–922.

82. Harris DJ, Wulff R, Ray CG, et al. Viruses and disease. III. An outbreak of adenovirus type 7A in a children's home. *Am J Epidemiol* 1971;93:399–402.

83. Lang WR, Howden CW, Laws J, et al. Bronchopneumonia with serious sequelae in children with evidence of adenovirus type 21 infection. *BMJ* 1969;1:73–79.

84. Simila S, Ylikorkala O, Wasz-Hockert O. Type 7 adenovirus pneumonia. *J Pediatr* 1971;79:605–611.

85. Collier AM, Connor JD, Irving WR Jr. Generalized type 5 adenovirus infection associated with pertussis syndrome. *J Pediatr* 1966;69:1073–1078.

86. Sturdy PM, Court SDM, Gardner PS. Viruses and whooping cough. *Lancet* 1971;2:978–979.

87. Nelson KE, Gavitt F, Batt MD, et al. The role of adenoviruses in the pertussis syndrome. *J Pediatr* 1975;86:335–341.

88. Mogabgab WJ. Mycoplasma pneumonia and adenovirus respiratory illnesses in military and university personnel, 1959–1966. *Am Rev Respir Dis* 1968;97:345–358.

89. Miller LF, Rytel M, Pierce WE, et al. Epidemiology of nonbacterial pneumonia among naval recruits. *JAMA* 1963;185:92–99.

90. Bell JA, Rowe WP, Engler JI, et al. Pharyngoconjunctival fever: epidemiological studies of a recently recognized disease entity. *JAMA* 1955;175:1083–1092.

91. Bennett FM, Law BB, Hamilton W, et al. Adenovirus eye infections in Aberdeen. *Lancet* 1957;2:670–673.

92. Murray ES, Chang RS, Bell SD Jr, et al. Agents recovered from acute conjunctivitis cases in Saudi Arabia. *Am J Ophthalmol* 1957;43:32–35.

93. Kaji M, Kimura M, Kamiya S, et al. An epidemic of pharyngoconjunctival fever among school children in an elementary school in Fukuoka Prefecture. *Kyushu J Med Sci* 1961;12:1–8.

94. Bell JA, Ward TG, Huebner RJ, et al. Studies of adenoviruses (APC) in volunteers. *Am J Public Health* 1956;46:1130–1146.

95. Foy HM, Cooney MK, Hatlen JG. Adenovirus type 3 epidemic associated with intermittent chlorination of a swimming pool. *Arch Environ Health* 1968;17:795–802.

96. Dawson CR, O'Day D, Vastine D. Adenovirus 19, a cause of epidemic keratoconjunctivitis, not acute hemorrhagic conjunctivitis. *N Engl J Med* 1975;293:45–46.

97. Dawson CR, Hanna L, Wood TR, et al. Adenovirus type 8 keratoconjunctivitis in the United States. *Am J Ophthalmol* 1970;69:473–480.

98. Kemp MC, Hierholzer JC, Cabradilla CP, et al. The changing etiology of epidemic keratoconjunctivitis: antigenic and restriction enzyme analysis of adenovirus types 19 and 37 isolated over a 10 year period. *J Infect Dis* 1983;148:29–33.

99. Numazaki Y, Kumasaka T, Yano N, et al. Further study of acute hemorrhagic cystitis due to adenovirus type 11. *N Engl J Med* 1973;289:344–347.

100. Mufson MA, Belshe RB, Horrigan TJ, et al. Cause of acute hemorrhagic cystitis in children. *Am J Dis Child* 1973;126:605–609.

101. Harnett GB, Buckens MR, Clay SJ, et al. Acute hemorrhagic cystitis caused by adenovirus type 11 in a recipient of a transplanted kidney. *Med J Aust* 1982;1:565–567.

102. Koga S, Shindo K, Matsuya F, et al. Acute hemorrhagic cystitis caused by adenovirus following renal transplantation: review of the literature. *J Urol* 1993;149:838–839.

103. Murphy GF, Wood DP Jr, McRoberts JW, et al. Adenovirus-associated hemorrhagic cystitis treated with intravenous ribavirin. *J Urol* 1993;149:565–566.

104. Wigand R, Baumeister HG, Maass G, et al. Isolation and identification of enteric adenoviruses. *J Med Virol* 1983;11:233–240.

105. Wood DJ. Adenovirus gastroenteritis. *BMJ* 1988;296:229–230.

106. Yolken RH, Lawrence F, Leister F, et al. Gastroenteritis associated with enteric type adenovirus in hospitalized infants. *J Pediatr* 1982;101:21–26.

107. Reina J, Hervas J, Ros MJ. [Differential clinical characteristics among pediatric patients with gastroenteritis caused by rotavirus and adenovirus] [Spanish]. *Enfermedades Infecciosas y Microbiologia Clinica* 1994;12:378–384.

108. Van R, Wun CC, O'Ryan ML, et al. Outbreaks of human enteric adenovirus types 40 and 41 in Houston day care centers. *J Pediatr* 1992;120:516–521.

109. Shinozaki T, Araki K, Ushijima H, et al. Antibody response to enteric adenovirus types 40 and 41 in sera from people in various age groups. *J Clin Microbiol* 1987;25:1679–1682.

110. Lew JF, Moe CL, Monroe SS, et al. Astrovirus and adenovirus associated with diarrhea in children in day care settings. *J Infect Dis* 1991;164:673–678.

111. Bhisitkul DM, Todd KM, Listernick R. Adenovirus infection and childhood intussusception. *Am J Dis Child* 1992;146:1331–1333.

112. Yunis EJ, Atchison RW, Michaels RH, et al. Adenovirus and iliocecal intussusception. *Lab Invest* 1975;33:347–351.

113. Yunis EJ, Hashida Y. Electron microscopic demonstration of adenovirus in appendix vermiformis in a case of ileocecal intussusception. *Pediatrics* 1973;51:566–570.

114. Kagnoff MF, Paterson VJ, Kumar PJ, et al. Evidence for the role of a human intestinal adenovirus in the pathogenesis of coeliac disease. *Gut* 1987;28:995–1001.

115. Mahon J, Blair GE, Wood GM, et al. Is persistent adenovirus 12 infection involved in coeliac disease? A search for viral DNA using the polymerase chain reaction. *Gut* 1991;32:1114–1116.

116. Vesy CJ, Greenson JK, Papp AC, et al. Evaluation of celiac disease biopsies for adenovirus 12 DNA using a multiplex polymerase chain reaction. *Mod Pathol* 1993;6:61–64.

117. Chou SM, Roos R, Burrell R, et al. Subacute focal adenovirus encephalitis. *J Neuropathol Exp Neurol* 1973;32:34–50.
118. Kelsey DS. Adenovirus meningoencephalitis. *Pediatrics* 1978;61:291–293.
119. Simila S, Jouppila R, Salmi A, et al. Encephalomeningitis in children associated with an adenovirus type 7 epidemic. *Acta Pediatr Scand* 1970;59:310–316.
120. Zahradnik JM, Spencer MJ, Parker DD. Adenovirus infection in the immunocompromised patient. *Am J Med* 1980;68:725–732.
121. Kojaoghlanian T, Flomenberg P, Horwitz MS. The impact of adenovirus infection on the immunocompromised host. *Rev Med Virol* 2003;13:155–171.
122. Myerowitz RL, Stadler H, Oxman MN, et al. Fatal disseminated adenovirus infection in a renal transplant recipient. *Am J Med* 1975;59:591–598.
123. Siegal FP, Dikman SH, Arayata RB, et al. Fatal disseminated adenovirus 11 pneumonia in an agammaglobulinemic patient. *Am J Med* 1981;71:1062–1067.
124. Cames B, Rahier J, Burtomboy G, et al. Acute adenovirus hepatitis in liver transplant recipients. *J Pediatr* 1992;120:33–37.
125. Shields AF, Hackman RC, Fife KH, et al. Adenovirus infections in patients undergoing bone-marrow transplantation. *N Engl J Med* 1985;312:529–533.
126. Flomenberg PR, Chen P, Munk G, et al. The molecular epidemiology of adenovirus type 35 isolates from immunocompromised hosts. *J Infect Dis* 1987;155:1127–1134.
127. Baldwin A, Kingman H, Darville M, et al. Outcome and clinical course of 100 patients with adenovirus infection following bone marrow transplantation. *Bone Marrow Transplant* 2000;26(12):1333–1338.
128. Durepaire N, Ranger-Rogez S, Gandji JA, et al. Enteric prevalence of adenovirus in human immunodeficiency virus seropositive patients. *J Med Virol* 1995;45(1):56–60.
129. Sabin CA, Clewley GS, Deayton JR, et al. Shorter survival in HIV-positive patients with diarrhoea who excrete adenovirus from the GI tract. *J Med Virol* 1999;58(3):280–285.
130. Vihma L. Surveillance of acute viral respiratory disease in children. *Acta Paediatr Scand* 1969;92:8–52.
131. Fox JP, Hall CE, Cooney MK. The Seattle virus watch. VII. Observations of adenovirus infections. *Am J Epidemiol* 1977;105:362–396.
132. Jordan WS Jr, Badger GF, Curtiss C, et al. A study of illness in a group of Cleveland families. X. The occurrence of adenovirus infections. *Am J Hyg* 1956;64:336–348.
133. Janoff EN, Orenstein JM, Manischewitz JF, et al. Adenovirus colitis in the acquired immunodeficiency syndrome. *Gastroenterology* 1991;100:976–979.
134. Hilleman MR, Werner JH, Dascomb HE, et al. Epidemiology of RI (RI-67) group respiratory virus infections in recruit populations. *Am J Hyg* 1955;62:29–43.
135. Rowe WP, Hartley JW, Huebner RJ. Additional serotypes of the APC virus group. *Proc Soc Exp Biol Med* 1956;91:260–262.
136. Couch RB, Cate TR, Douglas RG Jr, et al. Effect of route of inoculation of experimental volunteers and evidence for airborne transmission. *Bacteriol Rev* 1966;30:517–529.
137. Krisher KK, Menegus MA. Evaluation of three types of cell culture for recovery of adenovirus from clinical specimens. *J Clin Microbiol* 1987;25:1323–1324.
138. Graham FL, Smiley J, Russell WC, et al. Characteristics of a human cell line transformed by DNA from human adenovirus type 5. *J Gen Virol* 1977;36:59–72.
139. Takiff HE, Strauss SE, Garon CF. Propagation and in vitro studies of previously non-cultivable enteral adenoviruses in 293 cells. *Lancet* 1981;2:832–834.
140. Shinozaki T, Araki K, Ushijima H, et al. Use of Graham 293 cells in suspension for isolating enteric adenoviruses form the stools of patients with acute gastroenteritis. *J Infect Dis* 1987;156:246.
141. Mautner V, MacKay N, Steinthorsdottir V. Complementation of enteric adenovirus type 40 for lytic growth in tissue culture by E1B 55K function of adenovirus types 5 and 12. *Virology* 1989;171:619–622.
142. Gardner PS, McQuillin J. Adenoviruses. In: Gardner PS, ed. *Rapid virus diagnosis: application of immunofluorescence*. London: Butterworth, 1974:181–193.
143. Grandien M, Pettersson CA, Gardner PS, et al. Rapid viral diagnosis of acute respiratory infections: comparison of enzyme-linked immunosorbent assay and the immunofluorescence technique for detection of viral antigens in nasopharyngeal secretions. *J Clin Microbiol* 1985;22:757–760.
144. Grandien M, Pettersson CA, Svensson L, et al. Latex agglutination test for adenovirus diagnosis in diarrheal disease. *J Med Virol* 1987;23:311–316.
145. Turner PC, Bailey AS, Cooper RJ, et al. The polymerase chain reaction for detecting adenovirus DNA in formalin-fixed, paraffin-embedded tissue obtained post mortem. *J Infect* 1993;27:43–46.
146. Hierholzer JC, Halonen PE, Dahlen PO, et al. Detection of adenovirus in clinical specimens by polymerase chain reaction and liquid-phase hybridization quantitated by time-resolved fluorometry. *J Clin Microbiol* 1993;31:1886–1891.
147. Xu W, McDonough MC, Erdman DD. Species-specific identification of human adenoviruses by a multiplex PCR assay. *J Clin Microbiol* 2000;38(11):4114–4120.
148. Echavarria M, Forman M, van Tol MJ, et al. Prediction of severe disseminated adenovirus infection by serum PCR. *Lancet* 2001;358:384–385.
149. Lankester AC, van Tol MJ, Claas EC, et al. Quantification of adenovirus DNA in plasma for management of infection in stem cell graft recipients. *Clin Infect Dis* 2002;34:864–867.
149a. Heim A, Ebnet C, Harste G, Pring-Akerblom P. Rapid and quantitative detection of human adenovirus DNA by real-time PCR. *J Med Virol* 2003;70:228–239.
150. Hierholzer JC. Adenoviruses. In: Lennette EH, Lennette DA, Lennette ET, eds. *Diagnostic procedures for viral rickettsial and chlamydial infections*. Washington, DC: American Public Health Association, 1995:169–188.
151. Hierholzer JC, Torrence AC, Wright PR. Generalized viral illness caused by an intermediate strain of adenovirus 21/H21+35). *J Infect Dis* 1980;14:281–288.
152. DeJong PJ, Valderrama G, Spigland I, et al. Adenovirus isolates from the urines of patients with the acquired immunodeficiency syndrome. *Lancet* 1983;1:1293–1296.
153. Wadell G, Hammarskjold ML, Winberg G, et al. Genetic variability of adenoviruses. *Ann N Y Acad Sci* 1980;354:16–42.
154. Mei YF, Wadell G. Hemagglutination properties and nucleotide sequence analysis of the fiber gene of adenovirus genome types 11p and 11a. *Virology* 1993;194:453–462.
155. Toogood CI, Crompton J, Hay RT. Antipeptide antisera define neutralizing epitopes on the adenovirus hexon. *J Gen Virol* 1992;73:1429–1435.
156. Herrmann JE, Perron-Henry DM, Blacklow NR. Antigen detection with monoclonal antibodies for the diagnosis of adenovirus gastroenteritis. *J Infect Dis* 1987;155:1167–1171.
157. Dudgeon J, Bhargara SK, Ross CA. Treatment of adenovirus infection of the eye with 5′-iodo-2′-deoxyuridine: a double blind trial. *Br J Ophthalmol* 1969;53:530–533.
158. Waring GO, Laibson PR, Satz JE, et al. Use of vidarabine in epidemic keratoconjunctivitis due to adenovirus types 3, 7, 8 and 19. *Am J Ophthalmol* 1976;82:781–785.
159. Baba M, Mori S, Shigeta S, et al. Selective inhibitory effect of (S)-9-3-(3-hydroxy-2-phosphonylmethozyrpopyl)adenine and 2′-nor-cyclic GMP on adenovirus replication in vitro. *Antimicrob Agents* 1987;31:337–339.
160. Gordon YJ, Romanowski E, Araullo-Cruz T, et al. Inhibitory effect of (S)-HPMPC, (S)-HPMPA, and 2′-nor-cyclic GMP on clinical ocular adenoviral isolates is serotype-dependent in vitro. *Antiviral Res* 1991;16:11–16.
161. Romanowski EG, Gordon YJ. Effects of diclofenac or ketorolac on the inhibitory activity of cidofovir in the Ad5/NZW rabbit model. *Invest Ophthalmol Vis Sci* 2001;42(1):158–162.
162. Legrand F, Berrebi D, Houhou N, et al. Early diagnosis of adenovirus infection and treatment with cidofovir after bone marrow transplantation in children. *Bone Marrow Transplant* 2001;27(6):621–626.
163. Murtagh P, Cerqueiro C, Halac A, et al. Adenovirus type 7h respiratory infections: a report of 29 cases of acute lower respiratory disease. *Acta Paediatr* 1993;82:557–561.
164. Top FH Jr. Control of adenovirus acute respiratory disease in U.S. army trainees. *Yale J Biol Med* 1975;48:185–195.
165. Top FH Jr, Buescher EL, Bancroft WH, et al. Immunization with live types 7 and 4 adenovirus vaccines. II. Antibody response and protective effect against acute respiratory disease due to adenovirus type 7. *J Infect Dis* 1971;124:155–160.
166. Heubner RJ, Chanock RM, Rubin BA, et al. Induction by adenovirus type 7 of tumor in hamster having the antigenic characteristics of SV40 virus. *Proc Natl Acad Sci U S A* 1964;52:1333–1349.
167. Rowe WP, Baum SG. Studies of adenovirus SV40 hybrid viruses. II. Defectiveness of the hybrid particles. *J Exp Med* 1965;122:955–966.
168. Barraza EM, Ludwig SL, Gaydos JC, et al. Reemergence of adenovirus type 4 acute respiratory disease in military trainees: report of an outbreak during a lapse in vaccination. *J Infect Dis* 1999;179(6):1531–1533.
169. Gaydos CA, Gaydos JC. Adenovirus vaccines in the U.S. military. *Milit Med* 1995;160:300–304.
170. Two fatal cases of adenovirus-related illness in previously healthy young adults. *MMWR Morb Mortal Wkly Rep* 2001;6.
171. Hitt MM, Graham FL. Adenovirus vectors for human gene therapy. *Adv Virus Res* 2000;55:479–505.
172. Morin JE, Lubeck MD, Barton JE, et al. Recombinant adenovirus induces antibody response to hepatitis B virus surface antigen in hampsters. *Proc Natl Acad Sci U S A* 1987;84:4626–4630.
173. Jaffe HA, Danel C, Longenecker G, et al. Adenovirus-mediated in vivo gene transfer and expression in normal rat liver. *Nat Genet* 1992;1:372–378.
174. Rosenfeld MA, Siegfried W, Yoshimura K, et al. Adenovirus-mediated transfer of a recombinant alpha 1-antitrypsin gene to the lung epithelium in vivo. *Science* 1991;252:431–434.
175. Crystal RG, McElvaney NG, Rosenfeld MA, et al. Administration of an adenovirus containing the human CFTR cDNA to the respiratory tract of individuals with cystic fibrosis. *Nat Genet* 1994;8:42–51.
176. Knowles MR, Hohneker KW, Zhou Z, et al. A controlled study of adenoviral-vector-mediated gene transfer in the nasal epithelium of patients with cystic fibrosis. *N Engl J Med* 1995;333(13):823–831.
177. Tio RA, Isner JM, Walsh K. Gene therapy to prevent restenosis, the Boston experience. *Semin Interv Cardiol* 1998;3(3–4):205–210.
178. Hammond HK, McKirnan MD. Angiogenic gene therapy for heart disease: a review of animal studies and clinical trials. *Cardiovasc Res* 2001;49(3):561–567.
179. Yang ZY, Wyatt LS, Kong WP, et al. Overcoming immunity to a viral vaccine by DNA priming before vector boosting. *J Virol* 2003;77:799–803.

180. Yoshida T, Okuda K, Xin KQ, et al. Activation of HIV-1-specific immune responses to an HIV-1 vaccine constructed from a replication-defective adenovirus vector using various combinations of immunization protocols. *Clin Exp Immunol* 2001;124(3):445–452.

181. Schneider H, Adebakin S, Themis M, et al. Therapeutic plasma concentrations of human factor IX in mice after gene delivery into the amniotic cavity: a model for the prenatal treatment of haemophilia B. *J Gene Med* 1999;1(6):424–432.

182. Osada S, Ebihara I, Setoguchi Y, et al. Gene therapy for renal anemia in mice with polycystic kidney using an adenovirus vector encoding the human erythropoietin gene. *Kidney Int* 1999;55(4):1234–1240.

183. Crystal RG, McElvaney NG, Rosenfeld MA, et al. Administration of an adenovirus containing the human CFTR cDNA to the respiratory tract of individuals with cystic fibrosis. *Nat Genet* 1994;8:42–50.

184. Zuckerman JB, Robinson CB, McCoy KS, et al. A phase I study of adenovirus-mediated transfer of the human cystic fibrosis transmembrane conductance regulator gene to a lung segment of individuals with cystic fibrosis. *Hum Gene Ther* 1999;10(18):2973–2985.

185. Walters RW, Grunst T, Bergelson JM, et al. Basolateral localization of fiber receptors limits adenovirus infection from the apical surface of airway epithelia. *J Biol Chem* 1999;274(15):10219–10226.

186. Raper SE, Yudkoff M, Chirmule N, et al. A pilot study of in vivo liver-directed gene transfer with an adenoviral vector in partial ornithine transcarbamylase deficiency. *Hum Gene Ther* 2002;13:163–175.

187. Yang Y, Li Q, Ertl HC, et al. Cellular and humoral immune responses to viral antigens create barriers to lung-directed gene therapy with recombinant adenoviruses. *J Virol* 1995;69:2004–2015.

187a. Reddy PS, Ganesh S, Limbach MP, et al. Development of adenovirus serotype 35 as a gene transfer vector. *Virol* 2003;311:384–393.

188. Kass-Eisler A, Leinwand L, Gall J, et al. Circumventing the immune response to adenovirus-mediated gene therapy. *Gene Ther* 1996;3(2):154–162.

189. Mastrangeli A, Harvey BG, Yao J, et al. "Sero-switch" adenovirus-mediated in vivo gene transfer: circumvention of anti-adenovirus humoral immune defenses against repeat adenovirus vector administration by changing the adenovirus serotype. *Hum Gene Ther* 1996;7(1):79–87.

190. Morsy MA, Gu M, Motzel S, et al. An adenoviral vector deleted for all viral coding sequences results in enhanced safety and extended expression of a leptin transgene. *Proc Natl Acad Sci U S A* 1998;95:7866–7871.

191. Parks R, Evelegh C, Graham F. Use of helper-dependent adenoviral vectors of alternative serotypes permits repeat vector administration. *Gene Ther* 1999;6(9):1565–1573.

192. Borgland SL, Bowen GP, Wong NC, et al. Adenovirus vector-induced expression of the C-X-C chemokine IP-10 is mediated through capsid-dependent activation of NF-kappaB. *J Virol* 2000;74(9):3941–3947.

193. Nemunaitis J, Ganly I, Khuri F, et al. Selective replication and oncolysis in p53 mutant tumors with ONYX-015, an E1B-55kD gene-deleted adenovirus, in patients with advanced head and neck cancer: a phase II trial. *Cancer Res* 2000;60(22):6359–6366.

194. Yu DC, Chen Y, Seng M, et al. The addition of adenovirus type 5 region E3 enables calydon virus 787 to eliminate distant prostate tumor xenografts. *Cancer Res* 1999;59(17):4200–4203.

195. Wickham TJ. Targeting adenovirus. *Gene Ther* 2000;7(2):110–114.

196. Rothmann T, Hengstermann A, Whitaker NJ, et al. Replication of ONYX-015, a potential anticancer adenovirus, is independent of p53 status in tumor cells. *J Virol* 1998;72(12):9470–9478.

197. Kirn D. Clinical research results with dl1520 (Onyx-015), a replication-selective adenovirus for the treatment of cancer: what have we learned? *Gene Ther* 2001;8(2):89–98.

198. Nemunaitis J, Cunningham C, Buchanan A, et al. Intravenous infusion of a replication-selective adenovirus (ONYX-015) in cancer patients: safety, feasibility and biological activity. *Gene Ther* 2001;8(10):746–759.

CHAPTER 230
Herpes Simplex Viruses

Lawrence R. Stanberry, Michael N. Oxman, and Anthony Simmons

Primary herpes simplex virus (HSV) infection is usually asymptomatic or causes only mild signs and symptoms. The acute infection is generally self-limited, but virus evades total clearance by entering a latent or dormant state in sensory ganglion neurons. The significance of latency is that it is a reservoir of infection that reactivates periodically, causing either recurrent disease or asymptomatic virus shedding. Transmission to new hosts during periods of reactivation ensures long-term survival of HSV in the human population. There are two different though closely related herpes simplex viruses, type 1 (HSV-1) and type 2 (HSV-2). HSV-1 is transmitted chiefly by contact with contaminated oral secretions, whereas HSV-2 transmission generally requires anogenital contact. In otherwise healthy persons, severe disease is rare, but HSV is frequently life threatening to newborns and immunocompromised persons.

CHARACTERISTICS OF THE PATHOGEN

HSV-1 and HSV-2 are members of the family Herpesviridae and are classified as α herpesviruses. They are neurotropic and have the capacity to cause acute and latent infection in neural tissue (1–4). HSV virions comprise a linear double-stranded DNA molecule packaged into an icosahedral capsid and enclosed in a lipid envelope derived from host cell membranes. The capsid (Fig. 230.1) is composed of 162 identical capsomers. Between the capsid and envelope is an amorphous tegument of viral proteins that are carried into the cell on infection, where they have important regulatory functions. The complete virion is roughly spherical, with a diameter of 150 to 200 nm.

The HSV genome is a linear, double-stranded DNA of approximately 150 kb, comprising covalently linked L (long) and S (short) segments (Fig. 230.2). Each segment contains a stretch of unique sequences bracketed by inverted repeats (5,6). The genomes of HSV-1 and HSV-2 share about half their nucleotide sequences (7). Strains belonging to a single HSV serotype also exhibit genetic variation, but the differences observed are much smaller than those that distinguish HSV-1 from HSV-2 (8). These variations result in restriction endonuclease polymorphisms that can be detected among epidemiologically unrelated strains of HSV-1 and HSV-2 and serve as useful markers for epidemiologic investigations (9).

Biologic Properties

Relevant to the biology of HSV is its ability to replicate in cutaneous tissues (e.g., skin and mucous membranes), to enter and traffic within sensory nerve fibers, and to establish, maintain, and reactivate from latency (10). The HSV genome encodes about 90 transcriptional units, at least 84 of which encode proteins. At least 47 of the viral encoded proteins are not essential for replication in cell culture, suggesting that they play specialized roles in the pathogenesis of infection in the host (2).

Most HSV infections are clinically unrecognized, and virus is shed in secretions, thus facilitating transmission to the unsuspecting (11,12). Only a minority of infections result in the development of clinically overt signs or symptoms. HSV-1 and HSV-2 cause a variety of clinical syndromes that are determined by the anatomic site involved, the immune status of the host, and whether the infection is primary or recurrent (Table 230.1). Infections caused by the two viruses cannot generally be distinguished by clinical signs or symptoms; however, for recurrent mucocutaneous HSV infections, the frequency of recurrences is substantially higher when genital herpes is caused by HSV-2 rather than by HSV-1, whereas the recurrence rate of herpes labialis is substantially higher when it is caused by HSV-1 than by HSV-2 (13,14).

Replication

HSV is characterized by a rapid replication cycle that results in the death of the productively infected cell (2). The viral genes

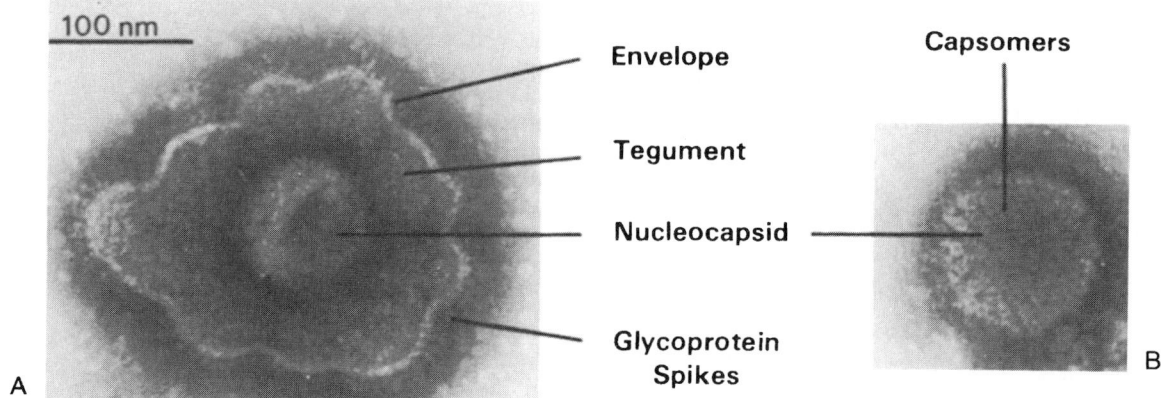

Figure 230.1. A typical herpesvirus negatively stained with phosphotungstic acid. **A:** The complete virion. **B:** The nucleocapsid (original magnification ×40,000). (From Straus SE, Ostrove JM, Inchauspe G, et al. Varicella zoster virus infections: biology, natural history, treatment, and prevention. *Ann Intern Med* 1988;108:221–237, with permission.)

are transcribed in a regulated and sequentially ordered cascade controlled by viral regulatory proteins (2,15). Classically, HSV genes are divided into three major classes on the basis of the temporal sequence of their transcription. First to be expressed are five immediate early (α) genes, which are transcribed in the absence of viral protein synthesis. Four of the α genes encode regulatory proteins, one of which, infected cell polypeptide 4 (ICP4), is required for transcription of early (β) and late (γ) genes (2). Another immediate early gene product, ICP0, transactivates a wide range of viral promoters and enhances the function of ICP4. Although not essential for HSV replication in cell culture, defects in ICP0 delay expression of β and γ genes and impair virus replication (2,16). It has been postulated that ICP0 may be important for reactivation of latent HSV (16).

Another α gene product, ICP47, appears to have an important role in modulating the immune response to infection. It blocks the presentation to CD8$^+$ cells of antigenic peptides, presumably with the exception of virion proteins that are introduced into the cell cytoplasm before ICP47 expression (17). Other gene products also appear to facilitate replication by interfering with immune function (18). Early (β) genes encode enzymes involved in HSV

DNA replication (2). Late, or γ, genes are defined by their transcription only after α and β gene expression, and they encode most of the virion proteins and glycoproteins (2).

After synthesis in the cytoplasm, most of the viral proteins are processed and transported to the nucleus, where they serve as regulatory factors, enzymes involved in DNA replication, or structural components of progeny virions (Fig. 230.3). The HSV glycoproteins are transported to cell membranes. In the nucleus, viral DNA appears to be replicated by a rolling circle mechanism that yields long head-to-tail concatemers. These concatemers are then cleaved into monomers that are packaged into empty capsids previously assembled in the nucleus (19). The nucleocapsid then buds through the inner nuclear membrane, the precise route of virion egress from the space between the inner and outer nuclear membrane is uncertain (2). Assembly of virions in infected neurons may be somewhat different, with the virus nucleocapsids coated with tegument proteins being transported separately from glycoproteins and final assembly of enveloped virus occurring at the axon terminus (20).

Herpes Simplex Virus Latency

Latency is a reversible interruption of the virus replication cycle in sensory neurons. The establishment and maintenance of the latent state appears to be a passive process in so far as no virus gene products are required (21); however, the host response may play a role (22). Latently infected neurons do not express viral antigens and most do not show evidence of transcription of the viral genome. Transcripts from a limited region of the genome are detectable in a subpopulation of latently infected neurons (latency-associated transcripts) (LATs) (Fig. 230.4) (23–26). Latency associated transcription appears to facilitate reactivation from latency (27–29). Latent HSV-1 reactivates most efficiently and frequently from trigeminal ganglia, causing recurrent ocular and orofacial lesions, while latent HSV-2 reactivates primarily from sacral ganglia causing recurrent genital lesions. These characteristic site-specific reactivation phenotypes appear to depend on the latency-associated transcript region (30).

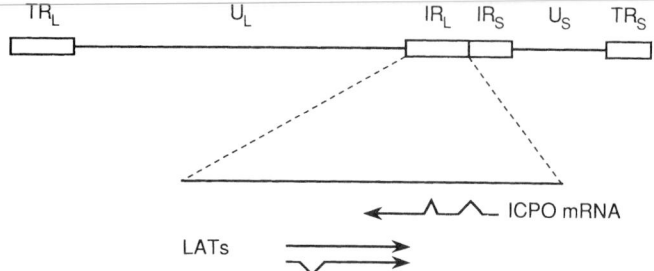

Figure 230.2. Organization of the herpes simplex virus type 1 (HSV-1) and HSV-2 genomes (not to scale). Long (*UL*) and short (*Us*) unique sequences are flanked by internal (*IR$_L$* and *IR$_S$*) and terminal (*TR$_L$* and *TR$_S$*) repeats. IR$_L$ and TR$_L$ are inverted copies of one another, as are IR$_S$ and TR$_S$. The location and orientation of the immediate early gene α0 in IR$_L$ is indicated by the location and orientation of its messenger RNA (*mRNA*), which encodes infected cell protein 0 (*ICP0*). The location and orientation of the latency-associated transcripts (*LATs*) are also indicated. The sequences encoding ICP0 and LATs are repeated in the opposite orientation in TR$_L$. (Modified from Croen KD, Ostrove JM, Dragovic L, et al. Characterization of herpes simplex type 2 latency-associated transcription in human sacral ganglia and in cell culture. *J Infect Dis* 1991;163:23–28, with permission.)

EPIDEMIOLOGY

Humans are the only natural reservoir, and no vectors are involved in transmission. There is no evidence of significant seasonal variation in the incidence of clinically overt disease. For

TABLE 230.1. Clinical Syndromes Caused by Herpes Simplex Virus (HSV) Infection

Category	Syndrome	Predominant virus type	Anatomic site(s)	Primary or recurrent	Immune status or predisposing condition
Mucocutaneous and cutaneous infections	Herpes gingivostomatitis	HSV-1	Oral cavity	Primary	Immunocompetent
	Herpes pharyngitis/tonsillitis	HSV-1	Pharynx and tonsils	Primary	Immunocompetent
	Herpes labialis	HSV-1	Lips predominant site but can occur at other facial or oral sites	Recurrent	Immunocompetent
	Herpes gladiatorum	HSV-1	Any cutaneous site; virus usually enters via abraded skin	Primary or recurrent	Immunocompetent
	Herpes whitlow	HSV-1	Paronychia	Primary or recurrent	Immunocompetent
	Herpes genitalis	HSV-2 (HSV-1 is predominant type in some geographic areas)	Anogenital region, also buttocks and thighs	Primary or recurrent	Immunocompetent
	Eczema herpeticum	HSV-1	Any cutaneous site	Primary or recurrent	Disorders of the skin
	Erythema multiforme	HSV-1 or HSV-2	Skin	Primary or recurrent	Immunocompetent
Ocular infections	Herpes keratitis or keratoconjunctivititis	HSV-1	Cornea	Primary or recurrent	Immunocompetent
	Herpes retinitis	HSV-1	Retina and anterior segment	Primary or recurrent	Immunocompetent
Neural infections	Herpes encephalitis	HSV-1	Central nervous system	Primary or recurrent	Immunocompetent
	Herpes meningitis (including Mollaret's meningitis)	HSV-1 or HSV-2	Meninges	Primary or recurrent	Immunocompetent
	Bell's palsy	HSV-1	Seventh cranial nerve	Primary or recurrent	Immunocompetent
Disseminated infections	Disseminated herpes	HSV-1 and rarely HSV-2	Skin and visceral organs, commonly liver	Primary or recurrent	Immunocompromised
Neonatal infection	Neonatal herpes	HSV-2 but HSV-1 occurs commonly	Skin, eye, or mouth Central nervous system Lungs and visceral organs	Primary	Immuno-immature

nongenital HSV infections there is no evidence of differing gender-related susceptibility; however, for genital HSV infections women appear to be more susceptible (31). The principal mode of transmission is direct contact between mucocutaneous surfaces. As a consequence of its lability, there is no documented transmission from inanimate objects (such as toilet seats) or via swimming pools or hot tubs, and there is no evidence of natural transmission by aerosols (32–36).

Epidemiologic studies (37–39) have been complicated by the prevalence of unrecognized HSV infections. Most new HSV-1 and HSV-2 infections result from contact with persons who are shedding HSV in the absence of recognized symptoms or lesions (11,12). Likewise, most (>80%) new mucocutaneous HSV infections are unrecognized (11,12,40,41); hence, clinical surveys greatly underestimate the incidence and prevalence of infection. Epidemiologic studies have been further complicated by the capacity of HSV-1 and HSV-2 to elicit cross-reactive immune responses (42,43). The development of accurate type-specific serologic testing has facilitated seroepidemiologic studies (38,39).

The different epidemiologic patterns of HSV-1 and HSV-2 infections reflect differences in the mode of transmission. Because HSV-1 is transmitted principally by contact with infected oral secretions or lesions, the incidence and prevalence of infection are influenced by factors that affect the degree of exposure to these sources of infection, such as crowding, poor hygiene, and age. Thus, the rate of acquisition of HSV-1 infection is inversely related to socioeconomic status. Predictably, the age-specific prevalence of antibodies to HSV-1 has been decreasing during the past 40 years in Western industrialized countries, especially in middle-class populations, as the standard of living has improved (33). Primary HSV-1 infections are largely confined to early childhood in developing countries, and even in poor urban populations in the United States, the majority of middle- and upper-income children in Western societies escape HSV-1 infections during childhood and experience a second peak of infections in adolescence and early adult life (33). The clinical manifestations of primary oropharyngeal HSV infection differ in young children (gingivostomatitis) and adults (pharyngotonsillitis). This epidemiologic change has resulted in the appearance of acute herpetic pharyngotonsillitis as a previously unrecognized disease in young adults (44). Moreover, the increasing proportion of the population now reaching puberty without having been infected with HSV-1, which induces partial immunity to subsequent HSV-2 infection, is an important factor in the current epidemic of genital herpes (see Chapter 106).

Clinical surveys have indicated a wide range of prevalence of herpes labialis in Western countries, typically on the order of 20% to 30% (46–49). Seropositive children and adults, including

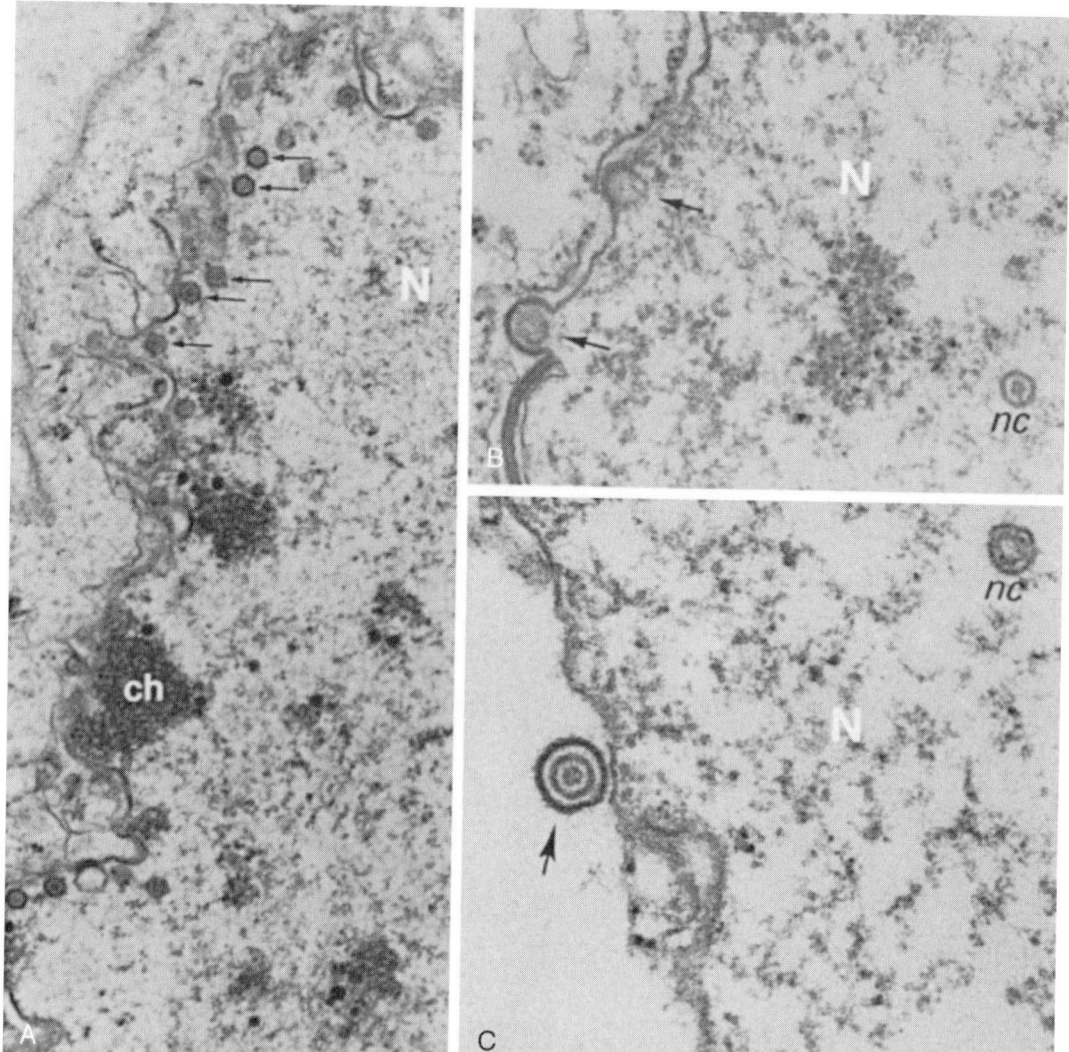

Figure 230.3. Assembly and maturation of herpes simplex virus (HSV). **A:** An infected neuron from the brain of a patient with herpes simplex encephalitis shows the nucleus (*N*) with many HSV nucleocapsids adjacent to the inner surface of the nuclear membrane (*arrows*). Also seen along the inner surface of the nuclear membrane are collections of condensed marginated chromatin (*ch*) (original magnification ×30,000). **B:** Higher magnification (×50,000) showing HSV nucleocapsids in the process of budding through the inner lamella of the nuclear membrane in areas thickened by the incorporation of HSV glycoproteins and the aggregation of tegument proteins on the inner surface (*arrows*); *nc*, nucleocapsids within the nucleus. **C:** The process of budding completed, a mature enveloped HSV virion (*arrow*) is seen in the perinuclear space adjacent to the nuclear membrane (original magnification ×75,000). (From Oxman MN. Herpes simplex encephalitis and meningitis. In: Braude AI, Davis CE, Fierer J, eds. *Infectious diseases and medical microbiology,* 2nd ed. Philadelphia: WB Saunders, 1986:1114–1132, with permission.)

those with no history of symptomatic primary or recurrent infections, periodically shed HSV asymptomatically in their saliva and are the major source of virus that causes new HSV-1 infections (12,50).

Neonatal HSV infections (see Chapter 106), two thirds of which are caused by HSV-2, are usually acquired during passage through the infected birth canal of a mother with asymptomatic genital herpes (51). Infection may also be acquired postnatally from the mother or another adult with nongenital HSV infection or by nosocomial transmission in the nursery. The risk for infection is much greater for infants born to mothers with primary than with recurrent genital HSV infections. The incidence of neonatal HSV infection in the United States is estimated to be between 1 in 3,000 and 1 in 5,000 live births, and it may be increas-

ing in some populations because of the increasing incidence of genital herpes and the decreasing prevalence of prior HSV-1 infection, which may reduce the risk for transmission from mother to infant.

PATHOGENESIS

Successful infection by HSV involves interactions between not only the virus and epithelial cells but also virus and neurons and virus and the host immune system (10,52–55). HSV infection is usually cytolytic, and the resulting pathologic process is a consequence of necrosis of infected epithelial cells plus local inflammatory responses. HSV replicates at the portal of entry in cells

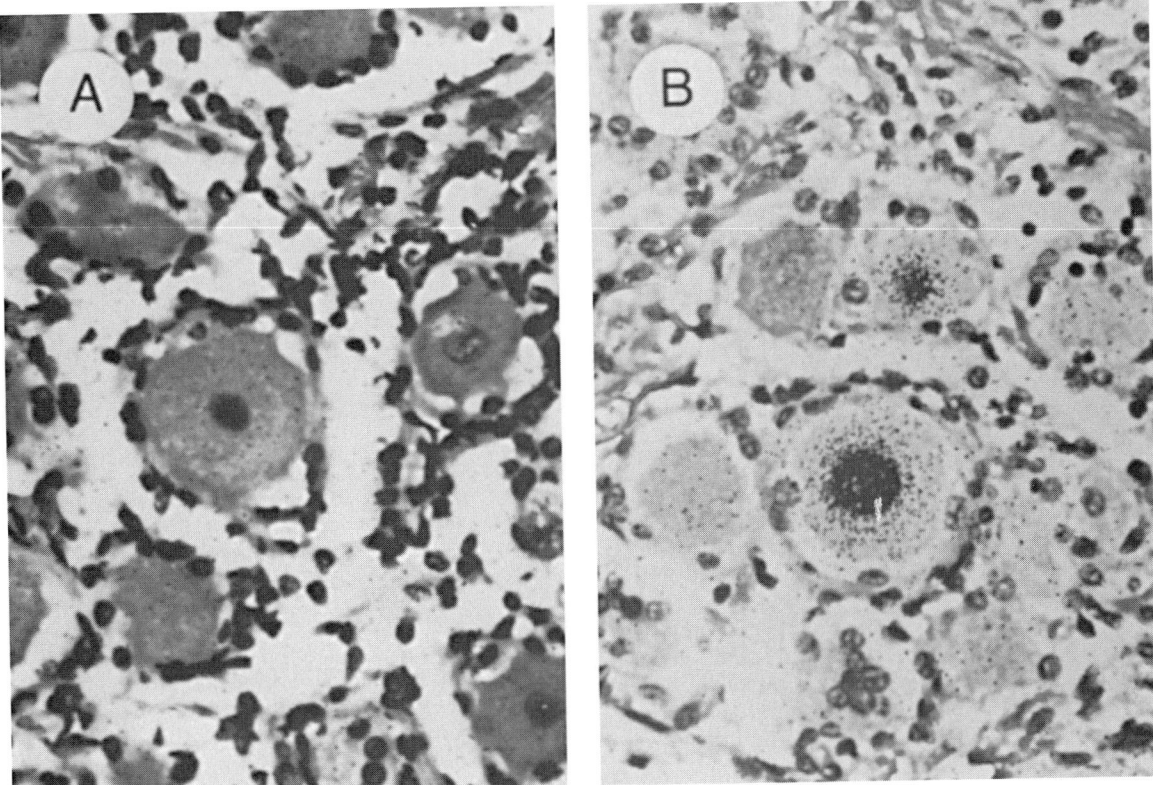

Figure 230.4. Detection of herpes simplex virus (HSV) latency-associated transcripts (LATs) in human sensory ganglia by *in situ* hybridization (original magnification ×200). **A:** Absence of infected cell polypeptide 0 (ICP0) messenger RNA. Hybridization with sulfur 35–labeled RNA complementary to ICP0 messenger RNA reveals no hybridization signal. **B:** Presence of LATs in the nuclei of two sensory neurons. Hybridization with ^{35}S-labeled RNA complementary to LATs reveals a dense accumulation of silver grains over two neuronal nuclei. (From Croen KID, Ostrove JM, Dragovic L, et al. Characterization of herpes simplex type 2 latency-associated transcription in human sacral ganglia and in cell culture. *J Infect Dis* 1991;163:230–28, with permission.)

of the stratum spinosum. Replication at the site of inoculation is generally terminated rapidly by innate immunity and timely development of an adaptive immune response. Hence, the infection usually remains unrecognized. When cell destruction is more extensive, disease may result. Viremia does not play a significant role in the pathogenesis of mucocutaneous HSV infections in the immunocompetent host, but neuronal spread does. Soon after exposure, virus enters nerve endings at the portal of entry and ascends via axonal transport processes to sensory ganglion neurons, where latency is established. The incubation period for symptomatic infections is usually 3 to 7 days (range 1 day to >2 weeks). Recurrent infections involve reactivation from latency and anterograde transport of virus to the original dermatome, where lesions may develop or shedding may occur. In the normal host, reactivations are terminated rapidly by the host's immune response.

Host Defenses

The normal cornified epithelium is an important nonspecific barrier to the initiation and spread of HSV infection. In patients with defects in this host defense (e.g., those who have atopic eczema, Darier's disease, pemphigus, and burns), HSV infections are frequently severe, widespread, and occasionally disseminated (56,57).

Once primary HSV infection is initiated at a mucocutaneous site, a number of nonadaptive defenses enhance local inflammatory responses. Important chemical mediators include complement and interferon-α and cell types include macrophages and monocytes, neutrophils, and natural killer (NK) cells. Together these defenses slow HSV replication and limit its spread.

IgG and IgM antibodies to HSV are first detected several days after the onset of primary infection. IgG antibodies persist for life, while IgM antibodies are transient; however, unlike for some other viruses, detection of IgM antibodies is not a reliable indicator of recent primary infection because reactivation can trigger an anamnestic IgM response (58,59).

During the second week of primary infection, HSV-immune T-lymphocytes can be detected. These include lymphocytes that proliferate and produce interferon-γ and other lymphokines in response to HSV antigens and lymphocytes that are cytolytic for HSV-infected cells (53).

Observations in humans with various deficiencies in host defenses and experiments in animal models identify several critically important host defense mechanisms. The natural resistance of the normal epithelium and the virucidal and cytolytic capacities of macrophages and NK cells play a crucial role in localizing infection at the portal of entry and slowing virus replication during the first few days, before specific immune responses have developed. When these defenses are deficient, as they are in patients with eczema or extensive burns and in newborns, there is risk for early virus dissemination and overwhelming systemic infection (56,57,60). HSV-specific T-lymphocytes are required to eradicate virus from mucocutaneous sites of infection

(53,61–65). Patients with deficient T-lymphocyte function (e.g., patients with acquired immunodeficiency syndrome [AIDS]) develop severe, persistent, locally progressive herpetic lesions but rarely have hematogenous dissemination (66,67). CD4+ T cells are the predominant inflammatory cells infiltrating early recurrent herpetic lesions (68–72). Although patients with deficient cell-mediated immunity are subject to more frequent and more severe HSV recurrences, as well as a much greater frequency of asymptomatic shedding, no specific defect has been consistently identified in otherwise healthy persons who suffer frequent episodes of recurrent genital or labial herpes. However, peripheral blood mononuclear cells from healthy persons infected with HSV-1 who have infrequent episodes of herpes labialis produce higher levels of interferon-γ and interleukin-2 when stimulated with HSV antigen than do peripheral blood mononuclear cells from persons who experience frequent episodes of herpes labialis (73).

A characteristic of HSV is its ability to exploit the immune system to the advantage of the virus and host. Defenses that might otherwise eradicate the virus are modulated by an array of viral gene products (e.g., HSV glycoprotein C, ICP47, glycoprotein E/glycoprotein I) (72–76).

The extensive antigenic cross-reactivity of HSV-1 and HSV-2 results in heterologous humoral and cellular immunity. Consequently, infection with one HSV serotype reduces susceptibility to infection by the other and moderates the severity of those infections that do occur (41,77,78). Site-specific immunity may also afford significant protection against reinfection (79).

CLINICAL MANIFESTATIONS AND TREATMENT

The clinical manifestations of HSV infection are determined by the portal of virus entry, whether the infection is initial or recurrent, immunocompetence, nutritional status, and presence or absence of conditions like eczema or burns that compromise the normal resistance of the skin. The major clinical syndromes caused by HSV are listed in Table 230.1.

Genital and Neonatal Infections

These are discussed in detail in Chapter 106.

Primary Oropharyngeal Infections

Acute herpetic gingivostomatitis (80–86) most often affects children between 6 months and 5 years of age, but it is being reported with increasing frequency in older children and adults. Onset is abrupt, with fever, anorexia, and listlessness. The gums become markedly swollen, and infants become restless, irritable, and unwilling to eat or drink. Mucosal vesicles, which often coalesce to form indurated ulcers, are most common on the tongue, the inner surface of the lips, and the buccal and sublingual mucosa (Fig. 230.5). The submandibular and anterior cervical lymph nodes are enlarged and tender, drooling is marked, and the breath may be fetid owing to overgrowth of anaerobic oral bacteria. In normal children, the disease is self-limited. Without treatment, symptoms subside after an average of 12 to 14 days, but gingivitis may resolve more slowly, and adenopathy often persists for several weeks. For laboratory diagnosis, HSV can be isolated readily from saliva and stool during the acute illness and often from saliva for weeks after recovery.

The proposed treatment of HSV gingivostomatitis in children is acyclovir, 15 mg/kg/dose, 5 times daily for 5 to 7 days (87).

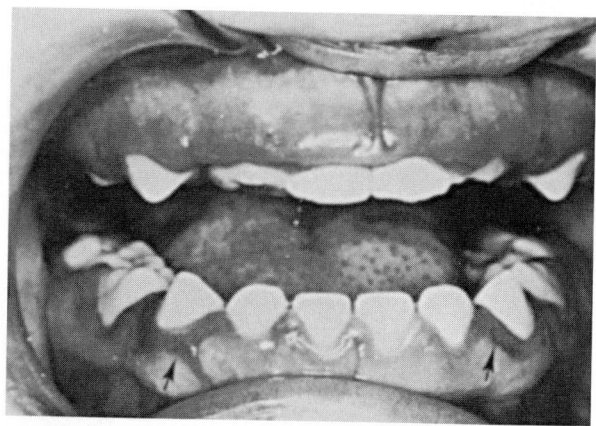

Figure 230.5. Acute herpetic gingivostomatitis/gingivitis. In this child with acute herpetic gingivostomatitis, the gums are tender, swollen, and hyperemic, and there is a bright red line (*arrows*) along the dental margin. (From Oxman MN/Herpes stomatitis. In: Braude AI, Davis CE, Fierer J, eds. *Infectious diseases and medical microbiology*, 2nd ed. Philadelphia: WB Saunders, 1986:752–772, with permission.)

In adults, primary HSV infection causes pharyngitis and tonsillitis (44,88) much more frequently than gingivostomatitis. The illness begins with fever, malaise, headache, and sore throat. It is usually indistinguishable clinically from pharyngotonsillitis caused by the group A β-hemolytic streptococcus. Laboratory diagnosis is required to ensure timely and adequate treatment. In college and university students, HSV is a major cause of pharyngitis and tonsillitis. Persons who have had herpetic pharyngotonsillitis may subsequently develop herpes labialis and asymptomatic shedding of HSV in saliva. However, the incidence of recurrent HSV pharyngotonsillitis remains unknown.

Although there are no data on the treatment of HSV pharyngotonsillitis in adults, it is likely that patients would benefit from treatment with an antiviral regimen similar to that used for primary genital herpes. The proposed treatment for primary genital herpes is acyclovir 400 mg orally three times a day for 7 to 10 days, or acyclovir 200 mg orally five times a day for 7 to 10 days, or famciclovir 250 mg orally three times a day for 7 to 10 days, or valacyclovir 1 g orally twice a day for 7 to 10 days (89).

Herpes Labialis

Herpes labialis (40,45,90) (cold sore, fever blister) is the most common manifestation of recurrent HSV-1 infection. Most patients have a prodrome of pain, burning, tingling, or itching at the site of the subsequent eruption, which usually precedes its onset by 6 hours or less but occasionally lasts 24 to 48 hours. This is followed by the appearance of a small cluster of erythematous papules that rapidly develop into tiny, thin-walled, intraepidermal vesicles (Fig. 230.6). These generally become pustular and then either burst, leaving shallow ulcers, or dry and form a scab. Left undisturbed, the scab is displaced by the regrowth of epithelium. The evolution of the lesions is generally rapid, the papular stage lasting only a few hours and the vesicles crusting within 2 days. Lesion area (usually <100 mm²) and pain are maximal during the vesicular stage and decline rapidly thereafter. Healing is completed, with loss of scabs and without scarring, in 6 to 10 days. Patients sometimes have local lymphadenopathy but no constitutional symptoms. The most common site of herpes labialis is the vermilion border of the lip (95%). Other sites include the nose, the chin, the cheek, and rarely the oral mucosa.

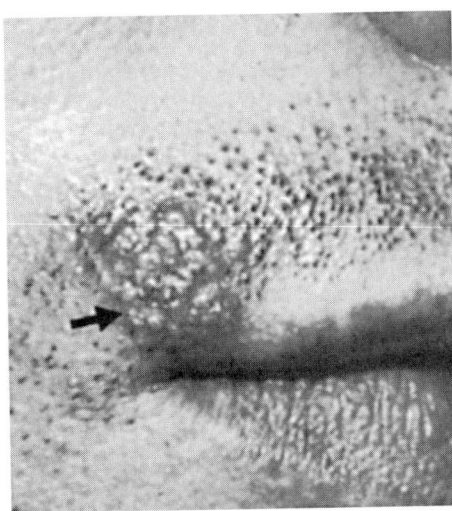

Figure 230.6. Herpes labialis. After a 12-hour prodrome of localized itching and burning, this medical student developed a small group of erythematous papules that quickly evolved into a typical cluster of vesicles (*arrow*) on an erythematous base. (From Oxman MN. Herpes stomatitis. In: Braude AI, Davis CE, Fierer J, eds. *Infectious diseases and medical microbiology*, 2nd ed. Philadelphia: WB Saunders, 1986:752–772, with permission.)

Oral is superior to topical antiviral therapy (91). For acute treatment, oral acyclovir (200–400 mg five times daily for 5 days), famciclovir (500 mg three times daily for 5 days), or valacyclovir (2,000 mg twice daily for 1 day) may be used to shorten the duration of the episode (91). Long-term antiviral prophylaxis with oral acyclovir 400 mg twice daily, or valacyclovir 500 mg once daily, can be considered to prevent recurrences in patients with severe or frequent disease (91).

Ocular Infections

HSV ocular infections may be primary or recurrent and may involve the cornea or anterior segment (92–98). Symptomatic primary ocular HSV infection is usually manifested as unilateral follicular conjunctivitis, often accompanied by blepharitis and preauricular lymphadenopathy. There may be herpetic vesicles on the lid margins and periorbital skin. Many patients have fever and other constitutional symptoms. In the majority of cases, there is no obvious corneal involvement, and the infection resolves spontaneously and completely in 2 to 3 weeks. Some primary infections cause acute herpetic keratoconjunctivitis. Characteristically, ulcers are dendritic in appearance or less often ameboid or "geographic." The stroma underlying the corneal epithelium is generally not involved during primary infection, except in newborns and in patients inadvertently treated with corticosteroids. Primary infection therefore tends to resolve spontaneously without obvious sequelae. When infection does involve the underlying stroma, it may result in corneal edema, infection of other intraocular tissues, extensive scarring, and corneal perforation. Most but not all episodes of ocular reactivation are asymptomatic, with shedding of HSV in tears. However, ocular HSV may recur in the form of keratitis, blepharitis, or keratoconjunctivitis. Recurrent infections tend to involve the underlying stroma; with repeated recurrences, there may be progressive corneal scarring and neovascularization, with eventual loss of vision. HSV is the leading infectious cause of blindness in the United States. Damage appears to be caused by an immunopathologic inflammatory response to viral antigens. Corneal transplantation is frequently performed for end-stage corneal scarring caused by HSV. Unfortunately, some recipients

develop recurrent HSV infection of the graft, which is easily confused with allograft rejection.

HSV ocular infections can result in blindness; hence, management should involve the advice of an ophthalmologist. Treatment options depend on the nature of the ocular infection and have been reviewed in a recent publication (99).

In newborns, HSV infections of the eye are caused by HSV-2 more often than by HSV-1, reflecting the maternal genital source of most infections. Keratoconjunctivitis may progress by direct extension to chorioretinitis, but retinal involvement is usually a consequence of viremia, which occurs, generally in the absence of corneal involvement, in neonates and in immunosuppressed children and adults with disseminated HSV infections. HSV may also reach the retina by direct extension from the brain in patients with HSV encephalitis. Neonatal herpes simplex is considered in greater detail in Chapter 106.

Infections of the Skin

Isolated exogenous HSV infections of the skin are uncommon in normal adults. When they do occur, they are usually associated with cutaneous trauma and exposure to contaminated secretions (e.g., nosocomial; 100) and may occur in some sports such as wrestling (herpes gladiatorum) or rugby (scrumpox) (101–105). Regardless of their location or pathogenesis, cutaneous HSV infections result in the establishment of latency in corresponding sensory ganglia, and the patient is subject to recurrences. Because the virus responsible for recurrent infections originates in sensory ganglia and is transported to the skin by sensory nerves, the lesions of recurrent cutaneous herpes may assume a segmental or dermatomal distribution that resembles that of herpes zoster, and they generally appear as grouped vesicles. A prodrome of pain, burning, itching, or tingling usually heralds the herpetic eruption, preceding it by 2 or 3 hours to 2 or 3 days. Lesions begin as grouped, erythematous papules that progress to vesicles, pustules, and crusts and then heal without scarring in 6 to 10 days. There is often regional lymphadenopathy, but constitutional symptoms are rare. Recurrent cutaneous herpes is sometimes associated with severe local neuralgia, and recurrences on the extremities may be accompanied by local edema and lymphangitis.

There are no clinical trial data upon which to base a recommendation regarding the treatment of isolated cutaneous HSV infections such as herpes gladiatorum or scrumpox. Anecdotal reports suggest that episodic antiviral treatment can be used to shorten an outbreak of herpes gladiatorum (91). Herpes gladiatorum can be treated with oral acyclovir (200 mg five times daily) or valacyclovir (500 mg twice daily) for 7 to 10 days, beginning at the first signs of prodrome (91). For patients with a history of recurrent herpes gladiatorum, valacyclovir 500 mg daily has been reported to suppress recurrent outbreaks (105).

Cutaneous HSV is often severe and potentially life threatening when it occurs in patients with disorders of the skin, such as eczema, Darier's disease, pemphigus, or burns (57,106–114) or following laser resurfacing (115). The lesions are often ulcerative and nonspecific in appearance, although careful examination may reveal vesicles, especially in adjacent normal skin. Diagnosis requires a high index of suspicion, with prompt collection of a sample for HSV detection. Without specific antiviral therapy, the infection may be very severe and patients may die with widespread visceral dissemination. Recurrences are common, and although they may be extensive, they are usually less severe than the primary infection.

Both oral and intravenous acyclovir have been used in the treatment of HSV infections in patients with skin disorders. A study of patients with eczema herpeticum showed that oral acyclovir, 200 mg five times per day for 5 days, altered the course of the illness (91,116,117). For severe or life-threatening HSV infections as occur in burn patients, intravenous acyclovir at doses of 10 to 20 mg/kg per day given every 8 hours has been used (91,118). For patients undergoing laser resurfacing, treatment with either famciclovir (250–500 mg twice daily for 10 days) or valacyclovir (500 mg twice daily for 10–14 days) beginning the day before the procedure has been reported to be effective in preventing cutaneous HSV infections (115,119,120).

HSV infections of the digits are often mistakenly grouped under the umbrella of herpetic whitlow, although this term is appropriate when the condition presents as paronychia (121–125). In adults, it is sometimes an occupational disease of medical and dental personnel exposed to oropharyngeal secretions containing HSV-1. However, adult cases can be caused by HSV-2, acquired by exposure to contaminated genital secretions (126–128). Itching, pain, and erythema begin 2 to 7 days after exposure. As the lesion develops there often appears to be pus under the cuticle, but incision discloses only a little clear fluid or, at a later stage, thick, yellow, necrotic debris (Fig. 230.7). Intense local pain is always present. Regional lymphadenopathy is common, and lymphangitis and neuralgia may occur. Lesions tend to progress for about 10 days, during which time pain persists unabated. There is then abrupt improvement, and resolution is usually complete in 18 to 20 days. Incising the lesion prolongs the period of disability and increases the risk for secondary bacterial infection.

Recurrent herpetic whitlows are often as painful as the primary infection, but they tend to be somewhat shorter in duration and are rarely accompanied by constitutional symptoms. The recurrent whitlow is frequently heralded and accompanied by severe neuralgic pain in the hand and arm, and it is often associated with swelling and edema of the hand, lymphangitis, and regional lymphadenopathy.

It is unknown whether antiviral treatment is beneficial for established herpetic whitlow. High-dose oral acyclovir (1,600–2,000 mg per day for 10 days in two or three doses) at first signs of prodrome has been reported to abort episodes of recurrent herpetic whitlow lesions and significantly reduces symptom duration (91,129,130).

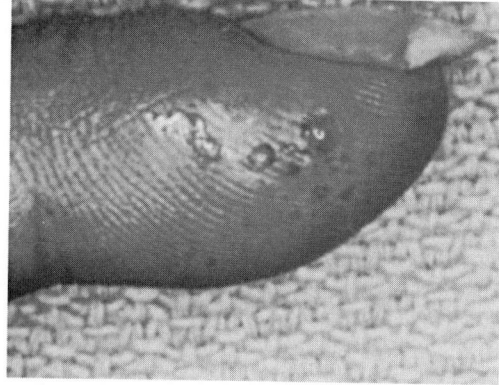

Figure 230.7. Herpetic whitlow. The terminal phalanx of the index finger of a respiratory therapist is exquisitely painful, swollen, and erythematous, with multiple deep and superficial vesicles. Herpes simplex virus type 1 was isolated from vesicle fluid. (From Oxman MN. Herpes stomatitis. In: Braude AI, Davis CE, Fierer J, eds. *Infectious diseases and medical microbiology*, 2nd ed. Philadelphia: WB Saunders, 1986:752–772, with permission.)

Central Nervous System Infections

Herpes simplex encephalitis (131–140) is an acute necrotizing viral encephalitis that, beyond the neonatal period, is nearly always caused by HSV-1. It has a higher mortality rate than most other forms of viral encephalitis (>70% in the absence of specific antiviral therapy). Although rare, it is the most common cause of sporadic acute necrotizing encephalitis in the United States; there are probably more than 1,000 cases each year. Serologic data indicate that herpes simplex encephalitis occurs as a primary infection in about 50% of patients and as a recurrent infection in the remainder, but there is no obvious difference between the two groups in presentation, clinical course, or outcome.

The mode of presentation, clinical manifestations, and sequelae are determined largely by the nature and distribution of the pathologic process—acute asymmetric necrotizing encephalitis that involves primarily the orbitofrontal and temporal cortex and the limbic system. Although the manifestations and rate of progression are variable, most patients present with two recognizable groups of findings: (a) nonspecific changes seen in most forms of encephalitis, which include fever, headache, signs of meningeal irritation, nausea, vomiting, global confusion, generalized seizures, and alteration of consciousness; and (b) changes referable to focal necrosis of the orbitofrontal and temporal cortex and the limbic system, which include anosmia, memory loss, peculiar behavior, defects of speech (especially expressive aphasia), hallucinations (particularly olfactory and gustatory hallucinations), and focal seizures. There is rapid progression in some cases, with the appearance of reflex asymmetry, focal paralysis, hemiparesis, and coma. Cerebral edema contributes to these manifestations and plays an important role in the outcome of the disease. Other patients have a more protracted course, with several days of mild, nonspecific illness punctuated by intermittent periods of bizarre behavior alternating with lethargy or sleep. These patients may present a picture of acute psychosis or delirium tremens and be admitted to hospital for psychiatric care until the appearance of localizing neurologic signs, seizures, and coma alerts their physicians to the severe organic nature of their disease. Cerebrospinal fluid examination usually reveals a moderate pleocytosis with mononuclear cells and polymorphonuclear leukocytes, mildly elevated protein concentration, normal glucose concentration, and often a moderate number of erythrocytes. HSV is rarely isolated from the cerebrospinal fluid. Magnetic resonance imaging appears to be the most sensitive imaging procedure (141,142). Detection of HSV DNA in cerebrospinal fluid after PCR amplification provides a rapid and definitive diagnosis (143–145). Sensitivity and specificity of this technique approach 100%, and it has replaced brain biopsy as the primary means of establishing the diagnosis of herpes simplex encephalitis. Mortality and morbidity can be reduced by early initiation of antiviral therapy, but 5% or more of patients suffer a clinical relapse after antiviral therapy has been discontinued.

Patients over 3 months of age with herpes encephalitis should be promptly treated with intravenous acyclovir (10 mg/kg every 8 hours) for 14 to 21 days (146–148).

Miscellaneous Infections

Herpes simplex may cause an acute, generally benign lymphocytic meningitis (149–160) in otherwise normal adults, often in association with primary genital herpes. Most documented cases have been caused by HSV-2, which can frequently be detected by PCR or culture cerebrospinal fluid. Symptoms, which include headache, fever, photophobia, nausea and vomiting, myalgia, and nuchal rigidity, usually resolve in about a week, but

15% to 25% of patients experience one or more recurrences, sometimes in association with an episode of recurrent genital herpes.

Significant cutaneous or visceral dissemination is a rare but documented consequence of HSV infections in apparently normal hosts (161–184). This may even occur during otherwise asymptomatic primary infections, in the absence of signs or symptoms of disease at the portal of entry. In most cases, clinically significant dissemination is confined to the skin, producing an illness that is virtually indistinguishable from varicella (except when oropharyngeal or genital lesions are present). The illness is self-limited and resolves in 7 to 14 days. Rarely, however, there is severe, often fatal visceral dissemination, which may or may not be accompanied by vesicular lesions in the skin. Multiple organs are involved, but fulminant HSV hepatitis is usually clinically predominant, and it is generally accompanied by leukopenia, thrombocytopenia, and disseminated intravascular coagulation. This syndrome, which is fatal in the majority of cases, occurs with greatest frequency in pregnant women, usually during the third trimester. Disseminated HSV-1 and HSV-2 infections in apparently normal children and adults have also been associated with herpetic esophagitis, adrenal necrosis, interstitial HSV pneumonitis, HSV cystitis, monarticular HSV arthritis, HSV meningitis, and rarely HSV encephalitis.

Herpes simplex infections of the respiratory tract and gastrointestinal tract have also been documented in otherwise apparently normal hosts (185–204). Recurrent HSV infections may be associated with allergic cutaneous and mucocutaneous disorders, especially erythema multiforme (205–211). In many patients, suppressing HSV recurrences with long-term acyclovir prophylaxis has reduced the frequency of attacks (91).

It is becoming increasingly apparent that HSV is responsible for many cases of the condition previously known as idiopathic facial (Bell's) palsy (212).

Herpes Simplex Virus Infections in Immunocompromised Hosts

Patients whose host defenses are compromised by congenital immunodeficiencies, malnutrition, immunosuppressive diseases (including hematologic and lymphoreticular malignant neoplasms and AIDS), iatrogenic immunosuppression, and certain diseases of the skin are at increased risk for severe and even fatal HSV infections (32,34,90,213–242). Hematogenous dissemination generally does not occur in the immunocompetent patient, whereas viremia with dissemination occurs frequently in HSV infections in patients with impaired immunity (162,243–245). The frequency and severity of HSV infections are markedly increased in patients with hematologic and lymphoreticular malignant neoplasms, in patients with AIDS, and in organ and bone marrow allograft recipients, particularly during the first 4 to 6 weeks after transplantation when immunosuppression is greatest. HSV infections in immunocompromised patients are most often reactivation infections rather than primary infections. Asymptomatic HSV shedding from the oropharynx or genital tract commonly occurs. Recurrent symptomatic mucocutaneous infections (e.g., herpes labialis, recurrent genital herpes) often behave normally and resolve without complications. Sometimes, however, the local lesions do not resolve but slowly enlarge, ulcerate, become necrotic, and extend to deeper tissues. Satellite lesions develop, and mucous membrane involvement is often extensive, with ulcerative, sometimes nodular, lesions on the lips, buccal mucosa, tongue, and palate. Pain and chronicity are hallmarks of the disease; lesions may persist for 10 weeks or more, during which time the saliva and involved tissues contain large amounts of virus. These chronic atypical mucocutaneous HSV infections, which involve the perioral or anogenital region, are a major cause of morbidity in profoundly immunosuppressed patients. Latent HSV is also reactivated during postchemotherapy mucositis; the majority of patients who develop stomatitis after cancer chemotherapy shed HSV in saliva, and it is generally difficult to assess the relative contribution of chemotherapy and HSV to the mucosal disease (241). Herpetic esophagitis is a common but often unrecognized complication of oropharyngeal HSV infection in immunocompromised and debilitated patients, especially in the presence of a nasogastric tube (168,195,246). The lungs may also be infected by HSV, either by direct extension of infection from the oropharynx or as a consequence of viremia. Direct extension is facilitated by injury to the respiratory epithelium (e.g., by endotracheal intubation, chemotherapy, radiation, or burn injury). This probably explains the high incidence of herpetic tracheobronchitis in hospitalized burn victims and the frequency of local HSV infection in patients intubated for adult respiratory distress syndrome. In these settings, most patients have focal or multifocal pneumonia, and concurrent HSV esophagitis is common.

Antiviral drugs (acyclovir, valacyclovir, and famciclovir) are frequently used for prophylaxis of HSV infections in transplant patients (247,248). Immunocompromised patients with HSV infections should be treated aggressively with oral or intravenous antiviral drugs (249–253). Drug resistance does occur more frequently in immunocompromised patients (254–265). Individuals not responding to antiviral drug therapy should have their viral isolates tested to determine their sensitivity to antiviral drugs. Strains of virus resistant to acyclovir are often also resistant to famciclovir but may be sensitive to cidofovir or foscarnet (266,267).

DIAGNOSIS

Laboratory diagnosis is frequently necessary, and it is always desirable. For mucocutaneous lesions, the specimen of choice is a swab from the base of a freshly erupted lesion, transported to the laboratory without delay. The availability of specific antiviral therapy now places a high premium on early and reliable diagnosis. Virus isolation remains the gold standard for the diagnosis of most HSV infections because it is widely available and offers good sensitivity and specificity (268–270). Many therapeutic decisions require diagnostic information in minutes to hours rather than days, and several methods for rapid diagnosis are available. Rapid direct detection and identification of HSV antigens or nucleic acids in clinical specimens is the best approach in this regard (269–277). These techniques are specific and sensitive when they are applied to the evaluation of herpetic lesions, and they can even detect viral proteins and nucleic acids late in the course of disease when infectious virus may not be recovered; however, they often lack the sensitivity required to detect the small quantities of virus shed during asymptomatic recurrences, which, for example, are responsible for about 50% of neonatal HSV infections. Other limitations of virus detection include frequent presentation of patients after lesions have healed and receipt of an inadequate specimen by the laboratory. For these reasons the possibility of diagnosing herpes with a blood test is an attractive prospect. There are now several commercially available tests for detection of type-specific antibodies, and currently their sensitivity and selectivity makes them reliable in selected populations with a high prevalence of the infection. This is particularly relevant when attempting to determine whether a patient has been infected with HSV-2. Finally, because of its extraordinary sensitivity, PCR is revolutionizing the diagnosis of HSV infections

(275–277). In particular, for herpes simplex encephalitis it provides a noninvasive diagnostic technique that has replaced brain biopsy.

REFERENCES

1. Roizman B, Pellett PE. The family Herpesviridae: a brief introduction. In: Knipe DM, Howley PM, eds. *Fields virology,* 4th ed. Philadelphia: Lippincott Williams & Wilkins, 2001:2381–2398.
2. Roizman B, Knipe DM. Herpes simplex viruses and their replication. In: Knipe DM, Howley PM, eds. *Fields virology,* 4th ed. Philadelphia: Lippincott Williams & Wilkins, 2001:2399–2459.
3. Taylor TJ, Brockman MA, McNamee EE, et al. Herpes simplex virus. *Front Biosci* 2002;7:752.
4. Cohrs RJ, Gilden DH. Human herpesvirus latency. *Brain Pathol* 2001;11:465.
5. Sheldrick P, Berthelot N. Inverted repetitions in the chromosome of herpes simplex virus. *Cold Spring Harb Symp Quant Biol* 1975;39:667.
6. Wadsworth S, Jacob RJ, Roizman B. Anatomy of herpes simplex virus DNA. II. Size, composition and arrangement of inverted terminal repetitions. *J Virol* 1975;15:1487.
7. Kieff ED, Bachenheimer SL, Roizman B. Size, composition and structure of the DNA of subtypes 1 and 2 herpes simplex virus. *J Virol* 1971;8:125.
8. Hayward GS, Frenkel N, Roizman B. The anatomy of herpes simplex virus DNA: strain differences and heterogeneity in the locations of restriction endonuclease cleavage sites. *Proc Natl Acad Sci U S A* 1975;72:1768.
9. Roizman B, Tognon M. Restriction endonuclease patterns of herpes simplex virus DNA: application to diagnosis and molecular epidemiology. *Curr Top Microbiol Immunol* 1983;104:275.
10. Stanberry LR. The pathogenesis of herpes simplex virus infections. In: Stanberry LR, ed. *Genital and neonatal herpes.* London: John Wiley & Sons, 1996:31–48.
11. Koelle DM, Wald A. Herpes simplex virus: the importance of asymptomatic shedding. *J Antimicrob Chemother* 2000;45(suppl T3):1.
12. Scott DA, Coulter WA, Lamey PJ. Oral shedding of herpes simplex virus type 1: a review. *J Oral Pathol Med* 1997;26:441.
13. Reeves WC, Corey L, Adams HG, et al. Risk of recurrence after first episodes of genital herpes: relation to HSV type and antibody response. *N Engl J Med* 1981;305:315.
14. Lafferty WE, Coombs RW, Benedetti J, et al. Recurrences after oral and genital herpes simplex virus infection. Influence of site of infection and viral type. *N Engl J Med* 1987;316:1444.
15. Honess RW, Roizman B. Regulation of herpesvirus macromolecular synthesis. I. Cascade regulation of the synthesis of three groups of viral proteins. *J Virol* 1974;14:8.
16. Everett RD. ICP0, a regulator of herpes simplex virus during lytic and latent infection. *Bioessays* 2000;22:761.
17. Ahn K, Meyer TH, Uebel S, et al. Molecular mechanism and species specificity of TAP inhibition by herpes simplex virus ICP47. *EMBO J* 1996;15:3247.
18. Favoreel HW, Nauwynck HJ, Pensaert MB. Immunological hiding of herpesvirus-infected cells. *Arch Virol* 2000;145:1269.
19. Knopf CW. Molecular mechanisms of replication of herpes simplex virus 1. *Acta Virol* 2000;44:289.
20. Holland DJ, Miranda-Saksena M, Boadle RA, et al. Anterograde transport of herpes simplex virus proteins in axons of peripheral human fetal neurons: an immunoelectron microscopy study. *J Virol* 1999;73:8503.
21. Wagner EK, Bloom DC. Experimental investigation of herpes simplex virus latency. *Clin Microbiol Rev* 1997;10:419.
22. Pereira RA, Scalzo A, Simmons A. Cutting edge: a NK complex-linked locus governs acute versus latent herpes simplex virus infection of neurons. *J Immunol* 2001;166:5869.
23. Stevens JG, Wagner EK, Devi-Rao GB, et al. RNA complementary to a herpesvirus alpha gene mRNA is prominent in latently infected neurons. *Science* 1987;253:1056.
24. Croen KL, Ostrove JD, Dragovic LJ, et al. Latent herpes simplex virus in human trigeminal ganglia: detection of an immediate early gene "anti-sense" transcript by *in situ* hybridization. *N Engl J Med* 1987;317:1427.
25. Millhouse S, Wigdahl B. Molecular circuitry regulating herpes simplex virus type 1 latency in neurons. *J Neurovirol* 2000;6:6.
26. Preston CM. Repression of viral transcription during herpes simplex virus latency. *J Gen Virol* 2000;81(part 1):1.
27. Leib DA, Bogard CI, Kosz-Vnenchak M, et al. A deletion mutant of the latency-associated transcript of herpes simplex virus type 1 reactivates from the latent state with reduced frequency. *J Virol* 1989;63:2893.
28. Hill JM, Sedarati F, Javier RT, et al. Herpes simplex virus latent phase transcription facilitates *in vivo* reactivation. *Virology* 1990;174:117.
29. Krause PR, Stanberry LR, Bourne N, et al. Expression of the herpes simplex virus type 2 latency-associated transcript enhances spontaneous reactivation of genital herpes in latently infected guinea pigs. *J Exp Med* 1995;181:297.
30. Yoshikawa T, Hill JM, Stanberry LR, et al. The characteristic site-specific reactivation phenotypes of HSV-1 and HSV-2 depend upon the latency-associated transcript region. *J Exp Med* 1996;184:659.
31. Fleming DT, McQuillan GM, Johnson RE, et al. Herpes simplex virus type 2 in the United States, 1976 to 1994. *N Engl J Med* 1997;337:1105.
32. Oxman MN. Genital herpes. In: Braude AI, Davis CE, Fierer J, eds. *Infectious diseases and medical microbiology,* 2nd ed. Philadelphia: WB Saunders, 1986:1041–1054.
33. Stanberry LR, Jorgensen DM, Nahmias AJ. Herpes simplex viruses 1 and 2. In: Evans AS, Kaslow RA, eds. *Viral infections of humans: epidemiology and control,* 4th ed. New York: Plenum, 1997:419–454.
34. Whitley RJ. Herpes simplex viruses. In: Knipe DM, Howley PM, eds. *Fields virology,* 4th ed. Philadelphia: Lippincott Williams & Wilkins, 2001:2461–2509.
35. Nerurkar LS, West F, May M, et al. Survival of herpes simplex virus in water specimens collected from hot tubs in spa facilities and on plastic surfaces. *JAMA* 1983;250:3081.
36. Douglas JM, Corey L. Fomites and herpes simplex viruses: a case for nonvenereal transmission? *JAMA* 1983;250:3093.
37. Plummer G. Serological comparison of the herpesvirus. *Br J Exp Pathol* 1964;45:135.
38. Bergstrom T, Trybala E. Antigenic differences between HSV-1 and HSV-2 glycoproteins and their importance for type-specific serology. *Intervirology* 1996;39:176.
39. Ashley RL, Wald A. Genital herpes: review of the epidemic and potential use of type-specific serology. *Clin Microbiol Rev* 1999;12:1.
40. Spruance SL. The natural history of recurrent oral-facial herpes simplex virus infection. *Semin Dermatol* 1992;11:200.
41. Langenberg AG, Corey L, Ashley RL, et al. A prospective study of new infections with herpes simplex virus type 1 and type 2. Chiron HSV Vaccine Study Group. *N Engl J Med* 1999;341:1432.
42. Schneweis KE. Serologische Untersuchungen zur Typendifferenzierung des Herpesvirus hominis. *Z Immunitätsforsch Exp Ther* 1962;124:24.
43. McClung H, Seth P, Rawls WE. Relative concentrations in human sera of antibodies to cross-reacting and specific antigens of herpes simplex virus types 1 and 2. *Am J Epidemiol* 1976;104:192.
44. McMillan JA, Weiner LB, Higgins AM, et al. Pharyngitis associated with herpes simplex virus in college students. *Pediatr Infect Dis J* 1993;12:280.
45. Spruance SL. Herpes simplex labialis. In: Sacks SL, Straus SE, Whitley RJ, et al., eds. *Clinical management of herpes viruses.* New York: IOS Press, 1995:3–12.
46. Axell T, Liedholm R. Occurrence of recurrent herpes labialis in an adult Swedish population. *Acta Odontol Scand* 1990;48:119.
47. Scully C. Orofacial herpes simplex virus infections: current concepts in the epidemiology, pathogenesis, and treatment, and disorders in which the virus may be implicated. *Oral Surg Oral Med Oral Pathol* 1989;68:701.
48. Reichart PA. Oral mucosal lesions in a representative cross-sectional study of aging Germans. *Commun Dent Oral Epidemiol* 2000;28:390.
49. Kovac-Kovacic M, Skaleric U. The prevalence of oral mucosal lesions in a population in Ljubljana, Slovenia. *J Oral Pathol Med* 2000;29:331.
50. Kameyama T, Sujaku C, Yamamoto S, et al. Shedding of herpes simplex virus type 1 into saliva. *J Oral Pathol* 1988;17:478.
51. Kimberlin DW, Lin CY, Jacobs RF, et al. Natural history of neonatal herpes simplex virus infections in the acyclovir era. *Pediatrics* 2001;108:223.
52. Simmons A. Molecular biology of HSV latency. *Herpes* 1995;2:37.
53. Simmons A, Tscharke D, Speck P. The role of immune mechanisms in control of herpes simplex virus infection of the peripheral nervous system. *Curr Top Microbiol Immunol* 1992;179:31.
54. Cunningham AL, Mikloska Z. The Holy Grail: immune control of human herpes simplex virus infection and disease. *Herpes* 2001;8(suppl 1):6A.
55. Daheshia M, Feldman LT, Rouse BT. Herpes simplex virus latency and the immune response. *Curr Opin Microbiol* 1998;1:430.
56. Goodyear HM, McLeish P, Randall S, et al. Immunological studies of herpes simplex virus infection in children with atopic eczema. *Br J Dermatol* 1996;134:85.
57. Hayden FG, Himel HN, Heggers JP. Herpesvirus infections in burn patients. *Chest* 1994;106(suppl):15.
58. Juto P, Settergren B. Specific serum IgA, IgG and IgM antibody determination by a modified indirect ELISA-technique in primary and recurrent herpes simplex virus infection. *J Virol Methods* 1988;20:45.
59. Hashido M, Kawana T. Herpes simplex virus-specific IgM, IgA and IgG subclass antibody responses in primary and nonprimary genital herpes patients. *Microbiol Immunol* 1997;41:415.
60. Burchett SK, Corey L, Mohan KM, et al. Diminished interferon-gamma and lymphocyte proliferation in neonatal and postpartum primary herpes simplex virus infection. *J Infect Dis* 1992;165:813.
61. Meyers JD, Flournoy N, Thomas ED. Infection with herpes simplex virus and cell-mediated immunity after marrow transplant. *J Infect Dis* 1980;142:338.
62. Merigan TC, Stevens DA. Viral infections in man associated with acquired immunological deficiency states. *Fed Proc* 1971;30:1858.
63. Simmons A, Nash AA. Zosteriform spread of herpes simplex virus as a model of recrudescence and its use to investigate the role of immune cells in prevention of recurrent disease. *J Virol* 1984;52:816.
64. Schmid DS, Rouse BT. The role of T-cell immunity in control of herpes simplex virus. *Curr Top Microbiol Immunol* 1992;179:961.
65. Milligan GN, Bernstein DI, Bourne N. T lymphocytes are required for protection of the vaginal mucosae and sensory ganglia of immune mice against reinfection with herpes simplex virus type 2. *J Immunol* 1998;160:6093.
66. Siegal FP, Lopez C, Hammer GS, et al. Severe acquired immunodeficiency in male homosexuals, manifested by chronic perianal ulcerative herpes simplex lesions. *N Engl J Med* 1981;305:1039.

67. Aoki FY. Management of genital herpes in HIV-infected patients. *Herpes* 2001;8:41.
68. Cunningham AL, Turner RR, Miller AC, et al. Evolution of recurrent herpes simplex lesions: an immunohistologic study. *J Clin Invest* 1985;75:226.
69. Koelle DM, Abbo H, Peck A, et al. Direct recovery of herpes simplex virus (HSV)-specific T lymphocyte clones from recurrent genital HSV-2 lesions. *J Infect Dis* 1994;169:956.
70. Koelle DM, Corey L, Burke RL, et al. Antigenic specificities of human CD4$^+$ T-cell clones recovered from recurrent genital herpes simplex virus type 2 lesions. *J Virol* 1994;68:2803.
71. Koelle DM, Schomogyi M, McClurkan C, et al. CD4 T-cell responses to herpes simplex virus type 2 major capsid protein VP5: comparison with responses to tegument and envelope glycoproteins. *J Virol* 2000;74:11422.
72. Koelle DM, Reymond SN, Chen H, et al. Tegument-specific, virus-reactive CD4 T cells localize to the cornea in herpes simplex virus interstitial keratitis in humans. *J Virol* 2000;74(23):10930.
73. Torseth JW, Merigan TC. Significance of local γ-interferon in recurrent herpes simplex infection. *J Infect Dis* 1986;153:979.
74. Lubinski JM, Wang L, Soulika AM, et al. Herpes simplex virus type 1 glycoprotein gC mediates immune evasion *in vivo*. *J Virol* 1998;72:8257.
75. Hill A, Jugovic P, York I, et al. Herpes simplex virus turns off the TAP to evade host immunity. *Nature* 1995;375(6530):411.
76. Nagashunmugam T, Lubinski J, Wang L, et al. *In vivo* immune evasion mediated by the herpes simplex virus type 1 immunoglobulin G Fc receptor. *J Virol* 1998;72:5351.
77. Mertz GJ, Coombs RW, Ashley R, et al. Transmission of genital herpes in couples with one symptomatic and one asymptomatic partner: a prospective study. *J Infect Dis* 1988;157:1169.
78. Bryson YJ, Dillon M, Bernstein DI, et al. Risk of acquisition of genital herpes simplex virus type 2 in sex partners of persons with genital herpes: a prospective couple study. *J Infect Dis* 1993;167:942.
79. Klein RJ. Reinfections and site-specific immunity in herpes simplex virus infections. *Vaccine* 1989;7:380.
80. Dodd K, Johnston LM, Buddingh GJ. Herpetic stomatitis. *J Pediatr* 1938;12:95.
81. Black WC. Acute infectious gingivostomatitis ("Vincent's stomatitis"). *Am J Dis Child* 1938;56:126.
82. Burnet FM, Williams SW. Herpes simplex: a new point of view. *Med J Aust* 1939;1:637.
83. Scott TF, Steigman AJ, Convey JH. Acute infectious gingivostomatitis: etiology, epidemiology, and clinical pictures of a common disorder caused by the virus of herpes simplex. *JAMA* 1941;117:999.
84. Buddingh GJ, Schrum DI, Lanier JC, et al. Studies of the natural history of herpes simplex infections. *Pediatrics* 1953;11:595.
85. Juretic M. Natural history of herpetic infection. *Helv Paediatr Acta* 1966;21:356.
86. Cesario TC, Poland JD, Wulff H, et al. Six years' experiences with herpes simplex virus in a children's home. *Am J Epidemiol* 1969;90:416.
87. Amir J. Clinical aspects and antiviral therapy in primary herpetic gingivostomatitis. *Paediatr Drugs* 2001;3:593.
88. Evans AS, Dick EC. Acute pharyngitis and tonsillitis in University of Wisconsin students. *JAMA* 1964;190:699.
89. Centers for Diseases Control and Prevention. 2002 Sexually transmitted diseases treatment guidelines. *MMWR* 2002;51(RR-6).
90. Oxman MN. Herpes stomatitis. In: Braude AI, ed. *Infectious diseases and medical microbiology,* 2nd ed. Philadelphia: WB Saunders, 1986:752–772.
91. International Herpesvirus Management Forum. The Management of HSV-1 and Ocular HSV Diseases. 2002. *www.ihmf.org/guidelines/rcmmnd1.asp.*
92. Binder PA. Herpes simplex keratitis. *Surv Ophthalmol* 1977;21:313.
93. Darougar S, Wishart MS, Viswalingam ND. Epidemiological and clinical features of primary herpes simplex virus ocular infection. *Br J Ophthalmol* 1985;69:2.
94. Wilhelmus KR, Coster DJ, Donovan HC, et al. Prognostic indicators of herpetic keratitis. Analysis of a five-year observation period after corneal ulceration. *Arch Ophthalmol* 1981;99:1578.
95. Shuster JJ, Kaufman HE, Nesburn AB. Statistical analysis of the rate of recurrence of herpes virus ocular epithelial disease. *Am J Ophthalmol* 1981;91:328.
96. Dawson C. Management of herpes simplex eye diseases. In: Sacks SL, Straus SE, Whitley RJ, et al., eds. *Clinical management of herpes viruses.* New York: IOS Press, 1995:127–136.
97. Sudesh S, Laibson PR. The impact of the herpetic eye disease studies on the management of herpes simplex virus ocular infections. *Curr Opin Ophthalmol* 1999;10:230.
98. Pavan-Langston D. Herpes simplex of the ocular anterior segment. *Curr Clin Top Infect Dis* 2000;20:298.
99. Kaufman HE. Treatment of viral diseases of the cornea and external eye. *Prog Retin Eye Res* 2000;19:69.
100. Stern H, Elek SD, Miller DM, et al. Herpetic whitlow, a form of cross-infection in hospitals. *Lancet* 1959;2:871.
101. Shute P, Jeffries DJ, Maddocks AC. Scrumpox caused by herpes simplex virus. *BMJ* 1979;2:1629.
102. White WB, Grant-Kels JM. Transmission of herpes simplex virus type 1 infection in rugby players. *JAMA* 1984;252:533.
103. Belongia EA, Goodman JL, Holland EJ, et al. An outbreak of herpes gladiatorum at a high-school wrestling camp. *N Engl J Med* 1991;325:906.
104. Becker TM. Herpes gladiatorum: a growing problem in sports medicine. *Cutis* 1992;50:150.
105. Anderson BJ. The effectiveness of valacyclovir in preventing reactivation of herpes gladiatorum in wrestlers. *Clin J Sport Med* 1999;9:86.
106. Wenner HA. Complications of infantile eczema caused by the virus of herpes simplex: description of the clinical characteristics of an unusual eruption and identification of an associated filterable virus. *Am J Dis Child* 1944;67:247.
107. Ruchman I, Welsh AL, Dodd K. Kaposi's varicelliform eruption: isolation of the virus of herpes simplex from cutaneous lesions of three adults and one infant. *Arch Dermatol Syphilol* 1947;56:846.
108. Foley FD, Greenwald KA, Nash G, et al. Herpesvirus infection in burned patients. *N Engl J Med* 1970;282:652.
109. Orenstein JM, Castadot MJ, Wilens ST. Fatal herpes hepatitis associated with pemphigus vulgaris and steroids in an adult. *Hum Pathol* 1974;5:489.
110. Hazen PG, Eppes RB. Eczema herpeticum caused by herpes virus type 2, a case in a patient with Darier's disease. *Arch Dermatol* 1977;113:1085.
111. Terezhalmy GT, Tyler MT, Ross GR. Eczema herpeticum: atopic dermatitis complicated by primary herpetic gingivostomatitis. *Oral Surg Oral Med Oral Pathol* 1979;48:513.
112. Bork K, Brauninger W. Increasing incidence of eczema herpeticum: analysis of seventy-five cases. *J Am Acad Dermatol* 1988;19:1024.
113. Bartralot R, Garcia-Patos V, Rodriguez-Cano L, et al. Kaposi's varicelliform eruption in a patient with healing second degree burns. *Clin Exp Dermatol* 1996;21:127.
114. Harindra V, Paffett MC. Recurrent eczema herpeticum: an underrecognised condition. *Sex Transm Infect* 2001;77:76.
115. Beeson WH, Rachel JD. Valacyclovir prophylaxis for herpes simplex virus infection or infection recurrence following laser skin resurfacing. *Dermatol Surg* 2002;28:331.
116. Muelleman PJ, Doyle JA, House RF Jr. Eczema herpeticum treated with oral acyclovir. *J Am Acad Dermatol* 1986;15:716.
117. Niimura M, Nishikawa T. Treatment of eczema herpeticum with oral acyclovir. *Am J Med* 1988;(2A):49.
118. Sheridan RL, Schulz JT, Weber JM, et al. Cutaneous herpetic infections complicating burns. *Burns* 2000;26:621.
119. Alster TS, Nanni CA. Famciclovir prophylaxis of herpes simplex virus reactivation after laser skin resurfacing. *Dermatol Surg* 1999;25:242.
120. Gilbert S, McBurney E. Use of valacyclovir for herpes simplex virus-1 (HSV-1) prophylaxis after facial resurfacing: a randomized clinical trial of dosing regimens. *Dermatol Surg* 2000;26:50–54.
121. Rosato FE, Rosato EF, Plotkin SA. Herpetic paronychia: an occupational hazard of medical personnel. *N Engl J Med* 1970;283:804.
122. Greaves WL, Kaiser AB, Alford RH, et al. The problem of herpetic whitlow among hospital personnel. *Infect Control* 1980;1:381.
123. Fedler HM, Long SS. Herpetic whitlow: epidemiology, clinical characteristics, diagnosis and treatment. *Am J Dis Child* 1983;137:861.
124. Gill MJ, Arlette J, Buchan K. Herpes simplex virus infection of the hand. *Am J Med* 1988;84:89.
125. Szinnai G, Schaad UB, Heininger U. Multiple herpetic whitlow lesions in a 4-year-old girl: case report and review of the literature. *Eur J Pediatr* 2001;160:528.
126. Glogau R, Hanna L, Jawetz E. Herpetic whitlow as part of genital virus infection. *J Infect Dis* 1977;136:689.
127. Egan LJ, Bylander JM, Agerter DC, et al. Herpetic whitlow of the toe: an unusual manifestation of infection with herpes simplex virus type 2. *Clin Infect Dis* 1998;26:196.
128. Gill MJ, Denhollander C. DNA restriction enzyme analysis of digital and genital isolates of herpes simplex virus from three patients. *J Infect Dis* 1988;158:242.
129. Gill MJ, Arlette J, Buchan K. Herpes simplex virus infection of the hand. A profile of 79 cases. *Am J Med* 1988;84:89.
130. Gill MJ, Bryant HE. Oral acyclovir therapy of recurrent herpes simplex virus type 2 infection of the hand. *Antimicrob Agents Chemother* 1991;35:382.
131. Oxman MN. Herpes simplex encephalitis and meningitis. In: Braude AI, Davis CE, Fierer J, eds. *Infectious diseases and medical microbiology,* 2nd ed. Philadelphia: WB Saunders, 1986:1114–1132.
132. Whitley RJ, Soong SJ, Dolin R, et al. The NIAID Collaborative Antiviral Study Group. Adenine arabinoside therapy of biopsy-proven herpes simplex encephalitis. *N Engl J Med* 1977;297:289.
133. Whitley RJ, Soong SJ, Hirsch MS, et al. The NIAID Collaborative Antiviral Study Group. Herpes simplex encephalitis: vidarabine therapy and diagnostic problems. *N Engl J Med* 1981;304:313.
134. Whitley RJ, Soong SJ, Linneman C, et al. The NIAID Collaborative Antiviral Study Group. Herpes simplex encephalitis. Clinical assessment. *JAMA* 1982;247:317.
135. Nahmias AJ, Whitley RJ, Visintine AN, et al. Herpes simplex virus encephalitis: laboratory evaluations and their diagnostic significance. *J Infect Dis* 1982;145:829.
136. Sköldenberg B. Herpes simplex encephalitis. *Scand J Infect* 1991;78:40.
137. Rose JW, Stroop WG, Matsuo F, et al. Atypical herpes simplex encephalitis: clinical, virologic, and neuropathologic evaluation. *Neurology* 1992;42:1809.
138. Whitley RJ, Lakeman F. Herpes simplex virus infections of the central nervous system: therapeutic and diagnostic considerations. *Clin Infect Dis* 1995;20:414.
139. Lakeman FD, Whitley RJ. Diagnosis of herpes simplex encephalitis: application of polymerase chain reaction to cerebrospinal fluid from brain-biopsied patients and correlation with disease. *J Infect Dis* 1995;171:857.

140. Marton R, Gotlieb-Steimatsky T, Klein C, et al. Acute herpes simplex encephalitis: clinical assessment and prognostic data. *Acta Neurol Scand* 1996;93:149.

141. Demaerel PH, Wilms G, Robberecht W, et al. MRI of herpes simplex encephalitis. *Neuroradiology* 1992;34:490.

142. Burke JW, Mathews VP, Elster AD, et al. Contrast-enhanced magnetization transfer saturation imaging improves MR detection of herpes simplex encephalitis. *Am J Neuroradiol* 1996;17:773.

143. Aurelius E, Johansson B, Sköldenberg B, et al. Rapid diagnosis of herpes simplex encephalitis by nested polymerase chain reaction assay of cerebrospinal fluid. *Lancet* 1991;337:189.

144. Domingues RB, Lakeman FD, Pannuti CS, et al. Advantage of polymerase chain reaction in the diagnosis of herpes simplex encephalitis: presentation of 5 atypical cases. *Scand J Infect Dis* 1997;29:229.

145. Atkins JT. HSV PCR for CNS infections: pearls and pitfalls. *Pediatr Infect Dis J* 1999;18:823.

146. Skoldenberg B, Forsgren M, Alestig K, et al. Acyclovir versus vidarabine in herpes simplex encephalitis. Randomised multicentre study in consecutive Swedish patients. *Lancet* 1984;2(8405):707.

147. Whitley RJ, Alford CA, Hirsch MS, et al. Vidarabine versus acyclovir therapy in herpes simplex encephalitis. *N Engl J Med* 1986;314:144.

148. Whitley RJ, Kimberlin DW. Viral encephalitis. *Pediatr Rev* 1999;20:192.

149. Terni M, Caccialanza P, Cassai E, et al. Aseptic meningitis in association with herpes progenitalis. *N Engl J Med* 1971;285:503.

150. Corey L, Adams HG, Brown ZA, et al. Genital herpes simplex virus infections: clinical manifestations, course, and complications. *Ann Intern Med* 1983;98:958.

151. Craig CP, Nahmias AJ. Different patterns of neurologic involvement with herpes simplex virus type 1 and 2: isolation of herpes simplex virus type 2 from the buffy coat of two adults with meningitis. *J Infect Dis* 1973;127:365.

152. Stalder H, Oxman MN, Dawson DM, et al. Herpes simplex meningitis: isolation of herpes simplex virus type 2 from cerebrospinal fluid. *N Engl J Med* 1973;289:1296.

153. Skoldenberg B, Jeansson S, Wolontis S. Herpes simplex virus type 2 and acute aseptic meningitis: atypical features of cases with isolation of herpes simplex virus from cerebrospinal fluids. *Scand J Infect Dis* 1975;7:227.

154. Bergström T, Vahlne A, Alestig K, et al. Primary and recurrent herpes simplex virus type 2-induced meningitis. *J Infect Dis* 1990;162:322.

155. Sawanobori S, Onishi S, Matsuyama S, et al. HSV-1 and acute aseptic meningitis. *Lancet* 1974;1:756.

156. Harford CG, Wellinghoff W, Weinstein RA. Isolation of herpes simplex virus from the cerebrospinal fluid in viral meningitis. *Neurology* 1975;25:198.

157. Tedder DG, Ashley R, Tyler KL, et al. Herpes simplex virus infection as a cause of benign recurrent lymphocytic meningitis. *Ann Intern Med* 1994;121:334.

158. Yamato LJ, Tedder DG, Ashley R, et al. Herpes simplex virus type 1 DNA in cerebrospinal fluid of a patient with Mollaret's meningitis. *N Engl J Med* 1991;325:1082.

159. Najioullah F, Bosshard S, Thouvenot D, et al. Diagnosis and surveillance of herpes simplex virus infection of the central nervous system. *J Med Virol* 2000;61:468.

160. Jensenius M, Myrvang B, Storvold G, et al. Herpes simplex virus type 2 DNA detected in cerebrospinal fluid of 9 patients with Mollaret's meningitis. *Acta Neurol Scand* 1998;98:209.

161. Prober CG, Arvin AM. Genital herpes and the pregnant woman. *Curr Clin Top Infect Dis* 1989;10:1.

162. Stanberry LIZ, Floyd-Reising SA, Connelly BL, et al. Herpes simplex viremia: report of eight pediatric cases and review of the literature. *Clin Infect Dis* 1994;18:401.

163. Young EJ, Chafizadeh E, Oliveira VL, et al. Disseminated herpesvirus infection during pregnancy. *Clin Infect Dis* 1996;22:51.

164. Auch Moedy JL, Lerman SJ, White RJ. Fatal disseminated herpes simplex infection in a healthy child. *Am J Dis Child* 1981;135:45.

165. Connor RW, Lorts G, Gilbert DN. Lethal herpes simplex virus type 1 hepatitis in a normal adult. *Gastroenterology* 1979;76:590.

166. Flewett TH, Parker RGF, Philip WM. Acute hepatitis due to herpes simplex virus in an adult. *J Clin Pathol* 1969;22:60.

167. Schneider V, Behm FG, Mumaw VR. Ascending herpetic endometritis. *Obstet Gynecol* 1982;59:259.

168. Buss DH, Scharyj M. Herpesvirus infection of the esophagus and other visceral organs in adults. Incidence and clinical significance. *Am J Med* 1979;66:457.

169. Eron L, Kosinski K, Hirsch MS. Hepatitis in an adult caused by herpes simplex virus type 1. *Gastroenterology* 1976;71:500.

170. Joseph TJ, Vogt PJ. Disseminated herpes with hepatoadrenal necrosis in an adult. *Am J Med* 1974;56:735.

171. Whorton CM, Thomas DM, Denham SW. Fatal systemic herpes simplex virus type 2 infection in a healthy young woman. *South Med J* 1983;76:81.

172. Long JC, Wheeler CE, Briggaman RA. Varicella-like infection due to herpes simplex. *Arch Dermatol* 1978;114:406.

173. Francis TJ, Osuntokun BO, Kemp GE. Fulminant hepatitis due to herpes hominis in an adult human. *J Gastroenterol* 1972;57:329.

174. Goyette RE, Donowho EM, Hieger LIZ, et al. Fulminant herpesvirus hominis hepatitis during pregnancy. *Obstet Gynecol* 1974;43:191.

175. Young EJ, Killam AP, Greene JF. Disseminated herpesvirus infection associated with primary genital herpes in pregnancy. *JAMA* 1976;235:2731.

176. Hensleigh PA, Glover DB, Cannon M. Systemic herpesvirus hominis in pregnancy. *J Reprod Med* 1979;22:171.

177. Kobbermann T, Clark L, Griffin WT. Maternal death secondary to disseminated herpesvirus hominis. *Am J Obstet Gynecol* 1980;6:742.

178. Peacock JE Jr, Sarubbi FA. Disseminated herpes simplex virus infection during pregnancy. *Obstet Gynecol* 1983;61(suppl):13.

179. Chase RA, Pottage JC Jr, Haber MH, et al. Herpes simplex virus hepatitis in adults: two case reports and review of the literature. *Rev Infect Dis* 1987;9:329.

180. Lagrew DC, Furlow TG, Hager D, et al. Disseminated herpes simplex virus infection in pregnancy. Successful treatment with acyclovir. *JAMA* 1984;252:2058.

181. Gelven PL, Gruber KK, Swiger FK, et al. Fatal disseminated herpes simplex in pregnancy with maternal and neonatal death. *South Med J* 1996;89:732.

182. Naraqi W, Jackson GG, Jonasson OM. Viremia with herpes simplex type 1 in adults: four nonfatal cases, one with features of chickenpox. *Ann Intern Med* 1976;85:165.

183. Remafedi G, Muldoon RL. Acute monarticular arthritis caused by herpes simplex virus type 1. *Pediatrics* 1983;72:882.

184. Whittaker JA, Hardson MD. Severe thrombocytopenia after generalized HSV-2 infection. *South Med J* 1978;72:864.

185. Schuller D, Spessert C, Fraser VJ, et al. Herpes simplex virus from respiratory tract secretions: epidemiology, clinical characteristics, and outcome in immunocompromised and nonimmunocompromised hosts. *Am J Med* 1993;94:29.

186. Nash G, Major MC, Foley FD. Herpetic infection of the middle and lower respiratory tract. *Am J Clin Pathol* 1970;54:857.

187. Ramsey PG, Fife KH, Hackman RC, et al. Herpes simplex virus pneumonia: clinical, virologic and pathologic features in 20 patients. *Ann Intern Med* 1982;97:813.

188. Graham BS, Snell JD Jr. Herpes simplex virus infection of the adult lower respiratory tract. *Medicine (Baltimore)* 1983;62:384.

189. Herout F, Vortel V, Vondrackova A. Herpes simplex involvement of the lower respiratory tract. *Am J Clin Pathol* 1966;46:411.

190. Tuxen DV, Cade JF, McDonald MI, et al. Herpes simplex virus from the lower respiratory tract in adult respiratory distress syndrome. *Am Rev Respir Dis* 1982;126:416.

191. Bastian JF, Kaufman IA. Herpes simplex esophagitis in a healthy 10-year-old boy. *J Pediatr* 1982;100:426.

192. Deprew WT, Prentice RSA, Beck IT, et al. Herpes simplex ulcerative esophagitis in a healthy subject. *Am J Gastroenterol* 1977;68:381.

193. Pazin GJ. Herpes simplex esophagitis after trigeminal nerve surgery. *Gastroenterology* 1978;74:741.

194. Owensby LC, Stammer JL. Esophagitis associated with herpes simplex infection in an immunocompetent host. *Gastroenterology* 1978;74:1305.

195. Nash G, Ross JS. Herpetic esophagitis. A common cause of esophageal ulceration. *Hum Pathol* 1974;5:339.

196. Buss DH, Scharyj M. Herpesvirus infection of the esophagus and other visceral organs in adults. Incidence and clinical significance. *Am J Med* 1979;66:457.

197. Camazine B, Antkowiak JG, Nava MER, et al. Herpes simplex viral pneumonia in the postthoracotomy patient. *Chest* 1995;108:876.

198. Greenberg SB. Respiratory herpesvirus infections: an overview. *Chest* 1994;106:15.

199. Klainer AS, Oud L, Randazzo J, et al. Herpes simplex virus involvement of the lower respiratory tract following surgery. *Chest* 1994;106(suppl):8.

200. Prellner T, Flamholc L, Haidl S, et al. Herpes simplex virus—the most frequently isolated pathogen in the lungs of patients with severe respiratory distress. *Scand J Infect Dis* 1992;24:283.

201. Sofer S, Pagtakha RD, Hoogstratten J. Fatal lower respiratory tract infection due to herpes simplex virus in a previously healthy child. *Clin Pediatr* 1984;23:406.

202. Flowers RH, Kernodle DS. Vagal mononeuritis caused by herpes simplex virus: association with unilateral vocal cord paralysis. *Am J Med* 1990;88:686.

203. Miyazato A, Kishimoto H, Tamaki K, et al. Herpes simplex virus bronchopneumonia in a non-immunocompromised individual. *Intern Med* 2001;40:836.

204. Ramanathan J, Rammouni M, Baran J Jr, et al. Herpes simplex virus esophagitis in the immunocompetent host: an overview. *Am J Gastroenterol* 2000;95:2171.

205. Shelly WB. Herpes simplex virus as a cause of erythema multiforme. *JAMA* 1967;201:153.

206. Britz M, Sibulkin D. Recurrent erythema multiforme and herpes genitalis (type 2). *JAMA* 1975;233:812.

207. Kazmierowski JA, Peizner DS, Wuepper KR. Herpes simplex antigen in immune complexes of patients with erythema multiforme: presence following recurrent herpes simplex infection. *JAMA* 1982;247:2547.

208. Fiumara NJ, Solomon J. Recurrent herpes simplex virus infections and erythema multiforme: a report of three patients. *Sex Transm Dis* 1983;10:144.

209. Orton PW, Huff JC, Tonnesen MG, et al. Detection of a herpes simplex viral antigen in skin lesions of erythema multiforme. *Ann Intern Med* 1984;101:48.

210. Weston WL, Brice SL, Jester JD, et al. Herpes simplex virus in childhood erythema multiforme. *Pediatrics* 1992;89:32.

211. Aurelian L, Kokuba H, Burnett JW. Understanding the pathogenesis of HSV-associated erythema multiforme. *Dermatology* 1998;197:219.

212. McCormick DP. Herpes simplex virus as a cause of Bell's palsy. *Rev Med Virol* 2000;10:285.

213. Templeton AC. Generalized herpes simplex in malnourished children. *J Clin Pathol* 1970;23:24.

214. Becker WB, Kipps A, McKenzie D. Disseminated herpes simplex virus infection: its pathogenesis based on virological and pathological studies in 33 cases. *Am J Dis Child* 1968;115:1.

215. Ruchman J, Dodd K. Recovery of herpes simplex virus from the blood of a patient with herpetic rhinitis. *J Lab Clin Med* 1950;35:434.

216. Taylor RJ, Saul SH, Dowling JN, et al. Primary disseminated herpes simplex infection with fulminant hepatitis following renal transplantation. *Arch Intern Med* 1981;141:1519.

217. Keane JR, Malkinson FD, Bryant J, et al. Herpesvirus hominis hepatitis and disseminated intravascular coagulation. *Arch Intern Med* 1976;136:1312.

218. Anuras S, Summers R. Fulminant herpes simplex hepatitis in an adult: report of a case in a renal transplant recipient. *Gastroenterology* 1976;70:425.

219. Muller SA, Hermann EC, Winkilmann RK. Herpes simplex infections in hematologic malignancies. *Am J Med* 1972;52:102.

220. Montgomerie JZ, Becroft DMO, Croxson MC, et al. Herpes simplex virus infection after renal transplantation. *Lancet* 1969;2:867.

221. Korsager B, Spencer ES, Mordhorst C-H, et al. Herpesvirus hominis infections in renal transplant patients. *Scand J Infect Dis* 1975;7:11.

222. Lopyan L, Young AW, Menegus M. Generalized acute mucocutaneous herpes simplex type 2 with fatal outcome. *Arch Dermatol* 1977;113:816.

223. Elliott WC, Houghton DC, Bryant RE, et al. Herpes simplex type 1 hepatitis in renal transplantation. *Arch Intern Med* 1980;140:1656.

224. Walker DP, Longson M, Lawler W, et al. Disseminated herpes simplex virus infection with hepatitis in an adult renal transplant recipient. *J Clin Pathol* 1981;34:1044.

225. Meyers JD, Flournoy N, Thomas ED. Infection with herpes simplex virus and cell-mediated immunity after marrow transplant. *J Infect Dis* 1980;142:338.

226. Rand KH, Rasmussen LE, Pollard RB, et al. Cellular immunity and herpesvirus infections in cardiac-transplant patients. *N Engl J Med* 1977;296:1372.

227. Pollard RB, Arvin AM, Gamberg P, et al. Specific cell-mediated immunity and infections with herpes viruses in cardiac transplant recipients. *Am J Med* 1982;73:679.

228. Stewart JA, Reef SE, Pellett PE, et al. Herpesvirus infections in persons infected with human immunodeficiency virus. *Clin Infect Dis* 1995;21(suppl 1):114.

229. Kusne S, Schwartz M, Breinig MK, et al. Herpes simplex virus hepatitis after solid organ transplantation in adults. *J Infect Dis* 1991;163:1001.

230. Siegal FP, Lopez C, Hammer GS, et al. Severe acquired immunodeficiency in male homosexuals, manifested by chronic perianal ulcerative herpes simplex lesions. *N Engl J Med* 1981;305:1039.

231. Pass RF, Whitley RJ, Whelchel JD, et al. Identification of patients with increased risk of infection with herpes simplex virus after renal transplantation. *J Infect Dis* 1979;140:487.

232. Naraqi W, Jackson GG, Jonasson O, et al. Prospective study of prevalence, incidence and source of herpes-virus infection in patients with renal allografts. *J Infect Dis* 1977;136:531.

233. Arvin AM, Pollard RB, Rasmussen LE, et al. Cellular and humoral immunity in the pathogenesis of recurrent herpes viral infections in patients with lymphoma. *J Clin Invest* 1980;65:869.

234. Wade JC, Day LM, Crowley JJ, et al. Recurrent infection with herpes simplex virus after marrow transplant: role of the specific immune response and acyclovir treatment. *J Infect Dis* 1984;149:750.

235. Logan WS, Tindall JP, Elson MI. Chronic cutaneous herpes simplex. *Arch Dermatol* 1971;103:606.

236. Schneidman DW, Barr RJ, Graham JH. Chronic cutaneous herpes simplex. *JAMA* 1979;241:592.

237. Lam TM, Pazin GJ, Armstrong JA, et al. Herpes simplex infection in acute myelogenous leukemia and other hematologic malignancies: a prospective study. *Cancer* 1981;48:2168.

238. Wade JC, Newton B, McLaren C, et al. Intravenous acyclovir to treat mucocutaneous herpes simplex virus infection after marrow transplantation. *Ann Intern Med* 1982;96:265.

239. Whitley R, Barton N, Collins E, et al. Mucocutaneous herpes simplex virus infections in immunocompromised patients. A model for evaluation of topical antiviral agents. *Am J Med* 1982;73:236.

240. Whitley RJ, Levin M, Barton N, et al. Infections caused by herpes simplex virus in the immunocompromised host. Natural history and topical acyclovir therapy. *J Infect Dis* 1984;150:323.

241. Rand KH, Kramer B, Johnson AC. Cancer chemotherapy associated symptomatic stomatitis. Role of herpes simplex virus (HSV). *Cancer* 1982;50:1262.

242. Neiman PE, Reeves W, Ray G, et al. A prospective analysis of interstitial pneumonia and opportunistic viral infection among recipients of allogeneic bone marrow grafts. *J Infect Dis* 1977;136:754.

243. Halperin SA, Shehab Z, Thacker D, et al. Absence of viremia in primary herpetic gingivostomatitis. *Pediatr Infect Dis* 1983;2:452.

244. Golden SE. Neonatal herpes simplex viremia. *Pediatr Infect Dis J* 1998;7:425.

245. Diamond C, Mohan K, Hobson A, et al. Viremia in neonatal herpes simplex virus infections. *Pediatr Infect Dis J* 1999;18:487.

246. Cirillo NW, Lyon DT, Schuller AM. Tracheoesophageal fistula complicating herpes esophagitis in AIDS. *Am J Gastroenterol* 1992;88:587.

247. Ljungman P. Prophylaxis against herpesvirus infections in transplant recipients. *Drugs* 2001;61:187.

248. Leflore S, Anderson PL, Fletcher CV. A risk-benefit evaluation of aciclovir for the treatment and prophylaxis of herpes simplex virus infections. *Drug Saf* 2000;23:131.

249. Snoeck R. Antiviral therapy of herpes simplex. *Int J Antimicrob Agents* 2000;16:157.

250. Scoular A, Barton S. Therapy for genital herpes in immunocompromised patients: a national survey. The Herpes Simplex Advisory Panel. *Genitourin Med* 1997;73:391.

251. Lazarus HM, Belanger R, Candoni A, et al. Intravenous penciclovir for treatment of herpes simplex infections in immunocompromised patients: results of a multicenter, acyclovir-controlled trial. The Penciclovir Immunocompromised Study Group. *Antimicrob Agents Chemother* 1999;43:1192.

252. Conant MA, Schacker TW, Murphy RL, et al. Valaciclovir versus aciclovir for herpes simplex virus infection in HIV-infected individuals: two randomized trials. *Int J STD AIDS* 2002;13:12.

253. Romanowski B, Aoki FY, Martel AY, et al. Efficacy and safety of famciclovir for treating mucocutaneous herpes simplex infection in HIV-infected individuals. Collaborative Famciclovir HIV Study Group. *AIDS* 2000;14:1211.

254. Chatis PA, Miller CH, Schrager LE, et al. Successful treatment with foscarnet of an acyclovir-resistant mucocutaneous infection with herpes simplex virus in a patient with acquired immunodeficiency syndrome. *N Engl J Med* 1989;320:297.

255. Erlich KS, Mills J, Chatis P, et al. Acyclovir-resistant herpes simplex virus infections in patients with the acquired immunodeficiency syndrome. *N Engl J Med* 1989;320:293.

256. Gately A, Gander RM, Johnson PC, et al. Herpes simplex virus type 2 meningoencephalitis resistant to acyclovir in a patient with AIDS. *J Infect Dis* 1990;161:711.

257. Birch CJ, Tachedjian G, Doherty RR, et al. Altered sensitivity to antiviral drugs of herpes simplex virus isolated from a patient with acquired immunodeficiency syndrome. *J Infect Dis* 1990;162:731.

258. Collins P, Larder BA, Oliver NM, et al. Characterization of a DNA polymerase mutant of herpes simplex virus from a severely immunocompromised patient receiving acyclovir. *J Gen Virol* 1989;70:375.

259. Balfour HH, Benson C, Braun J, et al. Management of acyclovir-resistant herpes simplex and varicella-zoster virus infections. *J AIDS* 1994;7:254.

260. Chatis PA, Crumpacker CS. Resistance of herpesviruses to antiviral drugs. *Antimicrob Agents Chemother* 1992;36:1589.

261. Coen DM. Antiviral drug resistance in herpes simplex virus. *Adv Exp Med Biol* 1996;394:49.

262. Laufer DS, Starr SE. Resistance to antivirals. *Pediatr Clin North Am* 1995;42:583.

263. Pottage JC, Kessler HA. Herpes simplex virus resistance to acyclovir: clinical relevance. *Infect Agents Dis* 1995;4:115.

264. Gaudreau A, Hill E, Balfour HH Jr, et al. Phenotypic and genotypic characterization of acyclovir-resistant herpes simplex viruses from immunocompromised patients. *J Infect Dis* 1998;178:297.

265. Venard V, Dauendorffer JN, Carret AS, et al. Infection due to acyclovir resistant herpes simplex virus in patients undergoing allogeneic hematopoietic stem cell transplantation. *Pathol Biol (Paris)* 2001;49:553.

266. Safrin S. Treatment of acyclovir-resistant herpes simplex and varicella zoster virus infections. *Adv Exp Med Biol* 1996;394:59.

267. Reusser P. Herpesvirus resistance to antiviral drugs: a review of the mechanisms, clinical importance and therapeutic options. *J Hosp Infect* 1996;33:235.

268. Erlich KS. Laboratory diagnosis of herpesvirus infections. *Clin Lab Med* 1987;7:759.

269. Ashley R. Laboratory techniques in the diagnosis of herpes simplex infection. *Genitourin Med* 1993;69:174.

270. Ashley R. Current concepts in laboratory diagnosis of herpes simplex infection. In: Sacks SL, Straus SE, Whitley RJ, et al., eds. *Clinical management of herpes viruses.* New York: IOS Press, 1995:137–174.

271. Richman DD, Cleveland PH, Redfield DC, et al. Rapid viral diagnosis. *J Infect Dis* 1984;149:298.

272. Verano L, Michalski FJ. Herpes simplex virus antigen direct detection in standard transport medium by DuPont Herpchek enzyme-linked immunosorbent assay. *J Clin Microbiol* 1990;28:2555.

273. Kudesia G, Van Hegan A, Wake S, et al. Comparison of cell culture with an amplified enzyme immunoassay for diagnosing genital herpes simplex infection. *J Clin Pathol* 1991;44:778.

274. MacPhail LA, Hilton JF, Heinic GS, et al. Direct immunofluorescence vs. culture for detecting HSV in oral ulcers: a comparison. *J Am Dent Assoc* 1995;126:74.

275. Whitley RJ, Lakeman F. Herpes simplex virus infections of the central nervous system: therapeutic and diagnostic considerations. *Clin Infect Dis* 1995;20:414.

276. Kleinschmidt-DeMasters BK, DeBiasi RL, Tyler KL. Polymerase chain reaction as a diagnostic adjunct in herpesvirus infections of the nervous system. *Brain Pathol* 2001;11:452.

277. Scoular A, Gillespie G, Carman WF. Polymerase chain reaction for diagnosis of genital herpes in a genitourinary medicine clinic. *Sex Transm Infect* 2002;78:21.

CHAPTER 231
Roseoloviruses: Human Herpesviruses 6 and 7

Kathleen M. Neuzil and Donald H. Rubin

Advances in molecular biology have linked specific microbiologic agents to the pathogenesis of clinical syndromes, ranging from childhood exanthems to cancer and peptic ulcer disease. No group of organisms better exemplifies these advances than the human herpesvirus group. In the past decade, three new members, the roseoloviruses: human herpesvirus 6 types A and B (HHV-6), and human herpesvirus 7 (HHV-7), and human herpesvirus 8 (HHV-8) (or Kaposi's sarcoma–associated herpesvirus), have been added to the family previously composed of herpes simplex virus types 1 and 2, cytomegalovirus, Epstein-Barr virus, and varicella-zoster virus. Although the diverse manifestations of these organisms continue to be defined, epidemiologic, clinical, and virologic studies indicate that these viruses have roles in some human disease and are implicated as causal agents in others.

HUMAN HERPESVIRUS 6

History

A virus morphologically and genetically similar to human herpesviruses was originally isolated in 1986 from the peripheral blood leukocytes of patients with human immunodeficiency virus (HIV) infection and lymphoproliferative malignancies and was designated human B-lymphotropic virus (1,2). Subsequently, the virus was shown to have a marked tropism for T-lymphocytes bearing the CD4 antigen, and it was renamed HHV-6 (3). In 1988, Yamanishi and colleagues (4) isolated HHV-6 from the peripheral blood lymphocytes of patients with exanthem subitum (roseola infantum, sixth disease). Since that time, epidemiologic and clinical studies have linked this virus to common febrile illnesses in children, including exanthem subitum, as well as less common maladies in children and adults (Table 231.1), from which the name of this genus of herpesviruses is derived.

Characteristics of the Pathogen

HHV-6 has been classified as a member of the β herpesvirus subfamily, and the genus roseolovirus based on its morphologic, genomic, and lymphotropic characteristics. By serology, there are two variants of HHV-6, designated A and B. It is a large virus with a total diameter of 160 to 200 nm, and a 20- to 40-nm thick envelope that is acquired from the nuclear and cytoplasmic membranes of the host cell (1). The characteristic icosahedral symmetry of the viral nucleocapsid, approximately 90 to 100 nm in diameter, can be seen in the nucleus and cytoplasm of infected cells. Mature virions are released by exocytosis. The double-stranded 160- to 170-kb DNA genome has a guanine plus cytosine content of 43% to 44%, which is lower than that of other human herpesviruses (2). HHV-6 is most closely related to cytomegalovirus, based on its hybridization to a fragment of the cytomegalovirus genome (5). Primary human lymphocytes from peripheral or cord blood readily support the growth of HHV-6,

as does the human diploid lung fibroblast cell line MRC-5 (6). CD4+ T cells are the most readily affected cells in tissue cultures. Growth in primary lymphocytes requires stimulation by phytohemagglutinin and interleukin-2 (7). Tissue culture–adapted HHV-6 grows in diverse cell lines of hematologic, epithelial, and neurologic origin. CD4+ T cells are also the primary target in acute HHV-6 infection *in vivo*, although other hematopoietic cells, liver cells, kidney cells, salivary and bronchial gland cells, and brain cells may be infected (8,9). In primary cell cultures, infection with HHV-6 produces large refractile cells with intranuclear or intracytoplasmic inclusion bodies, resulting in virus production and cell death (1).

Similar to the other human herpesviruses, HHV-6 establishes lifelong latent infection in the host. Peripheral blood mononuclear cells, cerebrospinal fluid, and saliva are all potential reservoirs for latent virus (10,11). HHV-6 possesses the ability to transform human epidermal cells and lymphocytes (12–14) and to affect gene transcription of other human viruses, including papillomaviruses and human immunodeficiency virus (15,16).

Epidemiology

Primary infection with HHV-6 is almost universal. Seroprevalence studies indicate that 95% to 100% of cord blood samples have antibody to HHV-6 (17). This maternally derived antibody declines in the ensuing months, with the lowest antibody levels detected in infants between 4 and 7 months of age. Seroconversion occurs between 6 months and 2 years of age in most children (18–20). Eighty to 100% of healthy adults under 40 years of age have antibodies to HHV-6; thereafter, titers decline (17,21,22). Antibody is acquired at an earlier age and is more prevalent in the Far East compared with Western countries (17,22,23).

The widespread occurrence of HHV-6 in childhood suggests a facile and efficient means of transmission. Oral virus shedding may be the predominant mode of spread, because HHV-6 can be detected in the saliva of more than 85% of adults (9,11,22,24,25). In addition, isolates from the saliva of mothers and the peripheral blood of their infants were genetically related, as determined by restriction enzyme analysis of purified DNA (26). There is a high prevalence of HHV-6 DNA in peripheral blood mononuclear cells of healthy adults (11,27,28). The relevance of this finding to blood product safety is uncertain (29). Perinatal transmission occurs, and viral DNA detected by polymerase chain reaction (PCR) in the vaginal secretions of healthy women suggests the possibility for sexual transmission as well (20). The virus has not been detected in human breast milk (30). HHV-6 can infect renal and hepatic tissues and has caused primary infection in seronegative kidney and liver transplant recipients (31,32).

HHV-6 type B is the predominant type in infants with primary HHV-6 infection, as well as in healthy adult blood donors (33,34). In contrast, either type or both types have been isolated from adult bone marrow transplant recipients (35–37). The reasons for these epidemiologic differences are unclear; type A infection may occur later in life, may be clinically inapparent, or may have a higher propensity for reactivation.

Our understanding of the relationship of HHV-6 to malignancy is evolving. Seroepidemiologic surveys report a greater HHV-6 seropositivity among patients with Hodgkin's lymphoma compared with control subjects (38–41). Furthermore, PCR detects HHV-6 DNA in the peripheral blood and lymph nodes of patients with Hodgkin's disease at rates greater than those found in the healthy population, but less than is seen in populations with reactive lymphadenopathies (34,39,42). Further studies are needed to determine if HHV-6 has a role in

TABLE 231.1.   Clinical Manifestations of Human Herpesvirus 6/7 Infection

Children	Adults	Immunocompromised persons
Fever and rash[a]	Fever, lymphadenopathy	Fever[a]
Fever and otitis[a]	Mononucleosis-like syndrome	Fever and rash[a]
Febrile seizures[a]	Hepatitis	Meningoencephalitis
Hepatitis	Meningoencephalitis	Pneumonitis[b]
Meningoencephalitis	Multiple sclerosis[b]	Bone marrow
Intussusception	Demyelinating encephalomyelitis	suppression[b]
Idiopathic thrombocytopenic	Pityriasis rosea[b]	
purpura		

[a]Common manifestation.
[b]Causation not established.

the pathogenesis of Hodgkin's disease or if the immune status of Hodgkin's disease patients allows for the reactivation of latent virus. There is no evidence for an etiologic role of HHV-6 in the development of other lymphoproliferative malignancies (42). Because HHV-6 can activate transcription of human papillomavirus-transforming genes, it may be a cofactor in the development of cervical cancer (43). In one study, four of six patients with HPV-6–related cervical neoplasias also had HHV-6 in cervical tissue detected by PCR. None of the 30 normal cervical specimens had HHV-6 DNA (15). Patients with oral cancers have a higher seroprevalence to HHV-6 compared with healthy control persons; the significance of these findings remains to be determined (38,44).

Pathogenesis

In acute infection with HHV-6, the virus replicates in peripheral blood mononuclear cells, salivary glands, and neuronal tissue, from which it is readily isolated (20,45). The wide tissue range of infection may relate to the presence of its putative cellular receptor, CD46 antigen, on many cell types (46). *In vitro*, only activated, mature T-lymphocytes support virus replication (7,47). The clinical consequences of acute infection are presumed secondary to direct cytotoxicity, although some manifestations, such as idiopathic thrombocytopenic purpura, may be immune mediated. The roseoloviruses most likely alter their cellular environment during lytic infection by elaboration of several viral proteins that mimic host cytokines or down-regulate important host genes (e.g., interleukin-18) (48,49). After primary infection, the virus establishes latency in several organs, including the lymph nodes, kidneys, liver, salivary glands, and peripheral blood mononuclear cells (25,32,50). Viral DNA can be detected by PCR techniques in the peripheral blood of healthy subjects during clinical latency (20,27). The virus reactivates in recipients of bone marrow and solid organ transplants and in children in the early convalescent stage of measles infection, suggesting a role for T-lymphocytes in the suppression of endogenous replication in healthy persons (51,52). HHV-6 infection induces antibodies to a number of structural and nonstructural viral proteins that persist for many years (53–56). Although neutralizing antibody is present in cord blood in high titer, the duration and degree of protection conferred from passive antibody is uncertain, because primary HHV-6 infection is not rare in the first 6 months of life (17,20). Serum from patients in the convalescent stage of exanthem subitum acquires neutralizing antibody, and the neutralizing antibody titer remains high throughout life (17,57). Second episodes of exanthem subitum are rare, supporting the

correlation of antibody production with immunity and further suggesting that HHV-6 is the predominant virus producing this syndrome.

Clinical Manifestations

CHILDREN

Primary HHV-6 infection in children is almost universal by age 3, being most common between 6 and 12 months of age (18,20,58,59). The illness does not have a seasonal predilection (20,58). Children with primary HHV-6 infection generally have a febrile illness with or without rash; although primary illness without fever and asymptomatic seroconversions have been reported (59–61). Otitis and irritability are common components of the febrile illness. Fever lasts an average of 4 days. Children under 6 months of age have more diarrhea than older children and are more likely to require hospitalization (20,58). Although exanthem subitum is a common manifestation of primary HHV-6 infection in Japan, it accounts for a minority of symptomatic infections in the United States (20,58).

Seizures are the most common complication of primary HHV-6 infection in children, occurring in up to 25% of cases (10,62,63). In patients with exanthem subitum, all seizures occur before the development of the rash (62,64). Status epilepticus has been reported (64). Up to one third of all febrile seizures in children under 2 years of age are associated with primary HHV-6 infection. Meningoencephalitis has also been reported as a manifestation of primary infection (62,65). HHV-6 viral DNA in the cerebrospinal fluid can be detected by PCR in the majority of children with neurologic symptoms. HHV-6 has been implicated in the etiology of recurrent seizures in children, based on the persistence of viral genome in the cerebrospinal fluid (10,66). Other complications of primary HHV-6 infection in childhood include intussusception, thought to be secondary to enlarged mesenteric lymph nodes, and idiopathic thrombocytopenic purpura (67–70).

ADULTS

Information regarding the clinical manifestations of primary HHV-6 infection in immunocompetent adults is limited but parallels that seen with primary cytomegalovirus or Epstein-Barr infection in adulthood. Several clinical syndromes have been reported, and include a nonspecific illness with lymphadenopathy, a mononucleosis-type syndrome, and hepatitis (71–77). A feature of the mononucleosis-like syndrome in a subset of these patients is the presence of a generalized erythematous rash. A skin biopsy from such a patient showed lymphocytes infected with HHV-6 by immunohistochemistry and *in situ* hybridization

(71). There have been case reports of severe neurologic disease associated with HHV-6 infection, including fatal demyelinating encephalomyelitis (78).

IMMUNOCOMPROMISED HOSTS

Recipients of bone marrow and kidney transplants may reactivate HHV-6, typically B, in the early posttransplant period, usually between weeks 2 and 4 (32,52,79–81). The type of immunosuppressive therapy may correlate with reactivation, because therapy with anti-CD3 monoclonal antibody increases the risk (82). Most patients develop fever. In bone marrow transplant recipients, an erythematous papular rash, similar to the rash seen with graft-versus-host disease, may accompany the fever (52,83,84). HHV-6 DNA has been detected in the skin biopsy specimens of these patients by use of the PCR technique (83,84). A bone marrow transplant recipient died of encephalitis with viral replication in neuronal cells (37). HHV-6 DNA has been detected in the lungs of all seropositive bone marrow transplant patients with idiopathic pneumonitis at higher levels than are found in healthy control persons; causality has not been established (11). Likewise, HHV-6 DNA levels in the peripheral blood of bone marrow transplant recipients correlate with the development of graft-versus-host disease and bone marrow suppression (36,85,86). Whether HHV-6 causes the immune system abnormalities or is reactivated secondary to them has not been determined.

The relationship between HIV and HHV-6 infection is equally enigmatic. HHV-6 has been proposed as a cofactor for progression of HIV infection based on the viruses' common tropism for CD4+ T-lymphocytes, their synergistic cytopathic effects, and the ability of HHV-6 to transactivate HIV regulatory genes (16,87). Moreover, infection of peripheral blood mononuclear cells by HHV-6 in vitro results in immunosuppression characterized by reduced interleukin-2 synthesis and diminished CD4+ and CD8+ T-lymphocyte proliferation (88). However, clinical data to support this hypothesis are limited. HHV-6 is widely disseminated at autopsy in patients with end-stage acquired immunodeficiency syndrome, affecting lung, lymph node, spleen, liver, kidney, and brain tissue (89,90). Lymphocytes and lymphatic tissue are disproportionately affected (89,91). It has been postulated that HHV-6 may contribute to disease in these patients based on its presence in tissue and the pathogenicity of other herpesviruses in HIV-infected persons. One study has raised the possibility that roseoloviruses have a synergistic role in the pathogenesis of progressive multifocal leukoencephalopathy, a syndrome due to reactivation of the JC strain of polyomavirus (92). However, the finding that a herpesvirus is present in lesions does not prove causality, because the altered cellular environment may favor herpesvirus replication. Prospective studies of large numbers of HIV-infected patients are needed to determine the relationship of disease to HHV-6 infection.

OTHER CLINICAL SYNDROMES

The prevalence of neuronal infection with involvement of white matter seen in immunocompromised children and adults has raised the possibility that HHV-6 may play a causative role in chronic neurologic diseases. In several studies, the presence of active systemic infection with, evidence of profound immune responses to, or biopsy presence of roseolovirus in the lesions of patients with multiple sclerosis has suggested a causal link to this disease (92,93). However these data are highly controversial, because other studies have not been able to replicate the results (94; see also review in reference 95). Because it is only

one of several infectious diseases that has been similarly linked (see Chapter 56), it is likely that this controversy will require additional studies and more rigorous proof. In addition to multiple sclerosis, adherents to HHV-6 have a role in chronic fatigue syndrome.

Diagnosis

Primary infection with HHV-6 can be diagnosed by isolation of the virus from blood or by serology. Serologic diagnosis of primary HHV-6 infection is based on the presence of immunoglobulin M antibody, which appears about 5 days after onset of disease and persists for approximately 1 month, or a fourfold increase in HHV-6–specific immunoglobulin G antibody. Enzyme-linked immunosorbent assays correlate well with the results of traditional immunofluorescent assays (96,97). The HHV-6 anticomplement immunofluorescent assay and enzyme-linked immunosorbent assay are specific, demonstrating no cross-reactivity to other herpesviruses, including cytomegalovirus (98). Virus isolation from peripheral blood mononuclear cells, although cumbersome, is a useful confirmatory test for primary infection or reactivation. PCR methods are available for the detection of HHV-6 DNA, but these do not distinguish between active and latent infections (11,27). Recently, utilization of reverse PCR has been able to differentiate latent versus active infection (99). This technique holds more promise in helping to establish whether the presence of replicating HHV-6 is clinically important.

HUMAN HERPESVIRUS 7

HHV-7 is a prevalent human herpesvirus that infects during childhood but at a later age than that documented for HHV-6. Like HHV-6, the prevalence of HHV-7 antibody is high at birth and declines in the first 6 months of life. There is an increased prevalence of antibody by the end of the first year, consistent with seroconversion. The seroprevalence to HHV-7 plateaus between the ages of 4 and 10 years (100,101). HHV-7 seroconversion may occur in the presence of high titers of HHV-6 antibody, suggesting lack of protection of HHV-6 against HHV-7 (102). HHV-7 is a T-lymphotropic virus that infects CD4+ and CD8+ lymphocytes (103,104). It is frequently shed in the saliva of healthy adults, providing a potential mode of transmission (105–108). HHV-7 is another causal agent of exanthem subitum; however, infection may occur earlier with HHV-6, thereby resulting in a predominance of cases of exanthem subitum having evidence of HHV-6 infection (109,110). There are some data linking HHV-7 to the cutaneous disease pityriasis rosea (111). However, recovery of HHV-7 is also found in normal skin, and the initial studies have not been reproducible (112–114). Therefore, while features of pityriasis rosea are suggestive of an infectious etiology, the search for a causative agent is not over. Finally, transplant patients with symptomatic disease related to cytomegalovirus also have a statistically significant increase in the recovery of either HHV-6 or HHV-7, suggesting that active infection of the roseolovirus is an independent risk factor (115,116). Alternatively, these results may indicate a more profound level of immunosuppression that provides an environment in which multiple β herpesviruses can replicate.

Therapy

There have been no clinical trials of antiviral therapy for HHV-6 infection. HHV-6 replication is readily inhibited by foscarnet and ganciclovir *in vitro* (53,117,118). Reports on the susceptibility of HHV-6 to acyclovir are discrepant and may reflect differences in virus strains or lack of assay standards. However, HHV-6 appears similar to cytomegalovirus in its susceptibility to acyclovir, requiring high doses in most studies to inhibit replication (117–122). Treatment of patients with foscarnet or ganciclovir decreases the recovery of HHV-6 and HHV-7 and reduces the risk for symptomatic disease (123).

High-dose (>10 units/mL) recombinant interleukin-2 eliminates the cytopathic effect and the presence of extracellular virions in peripheral blood mononuclear cells infected with HHV-6 (47). Likewise, exogenous interferon-α suppresses HHV-6 replication in peripheral blood mononuclear cells *in vitro* (124). Although interleukin-2 has been shown to increase the number of CD4$^+$ cells in HIV-infected hosts, interferon-α therapy has been disappointing (125). Whether either of these immunoregulators used in HIV infection affects concomitant HHV-6 infection has not been determined. Therefore, whether early intervention to decrease HHV-6 replication in the setting of concomitant HIV infection would affect HIV progression remains unknown.

REFERENCES

1. Salahuddin SZ, et al. Isolation of a new virus, HBLV, in patients with lymphoproliferative disorders. *Science* 1986;234(4776):596–601.
2. Josephs SF, et al. Genomic analysis of the human B-lymphotropic virus (HBLV). *Science* 1986;234(4776):601–603.
3. Lusso P, et al. In vitro cellular tropism of human B-lymphotropic virus (human herpesvirus-6). *J Exp Med* 1988;167(5):1659–1670.
4. Yamanishi K, et al. Identification of human herpesvirus-6 as a causal agent for exanthem subitum. *Lancet* 1988;1(8594):1065–1067.
5. Lawrence GL, et al. Human herpesvirus 6 is closely related to human cytomegalovirus. *J Virol* 1990;64(1):287–299.
6. Luka J, Okano M, Thiele G. Isolation of human herpesvirus-6 from clinical specimens using human fibroblast cultures. *J Clin Lab Anal* 1990;4(6):483–486.
7. Frenkel N, et al. T-cell activation is required for efficient replication of human herpesvirus 6. *J Virol* 1990;64(9):4598–4602.
8. Asano Y, et al. Human herpesvirus type 6 infection (exanthem subitum) without fever. *J Pediatr* 1989;115(2):264–265.
9. Jarrett RF, et al. Detection of human herpesvirus-6 DNA in peripheral blood and saliva. *J Med Virol* 1990;32(1):73–76.
10. Caserta MT, et al. Neuroinvasion and persistence of human herpesvirus 6 in children. *J Infect Dis* 1994;170(6):1586–1589.
11. Cone RW, et al. Human herpesvirus 6 DNA in peripheral blood cells and saliva from immunocompetent individuals. *J Clin Microbiol* 1993;31(5):1262–1267.
12. Razzaque A. Oncogenic potential of human herpesvirus-6 DNA. *Oncogene* 1990;5(9):1365–1370.
13. Razzaque A, et al. Neoplastic transformation of immortalized human epidermal keratinocytes by two HHV-6 DNA clones. *Virology* 1993;195(1):113–120.
14. Puri RK, Leland P, Razzaque A. Antigen(s)-specific tumour-infiltrating lymphocytes from tumour induced by human herpes virus-6 (HHV-6) DNA transfected NIH 3T3 transformants. *Clin Exp Immunol* 1991;83(1):96–101.
15. Chen M, et al. Detection of human herpesvirus 6 and human papillomavirus 16 in cervical carcinoma. *Am J Pathol* 1994;145(6):1509–1516.
16. Horvat RT, Wood C, Balachandran N. Transactivation of human immunodeficiency virus promoter by human herpesvirus 6. *J Virol* 1989;63(2):970–973.
17. Yoshikawa T, et al. Neutralizing antibodies to human herpesvirus-6 in healthy individuals. *Pediatr Infect Dis J* 1990;9(8):589–590.
18. Yanagi K, et al. High prevalence of antibody to human herpesvirus-6 and decrease in titer with increase in age in Japan. *J Infect Dis* 1990;161(1):153–154.
19. Asano Y, et al. Fatal fulminant hepatitis in an infant with human herpesvirus-6 infection. *Lancet* 1990;335(8693):862–863.
20. Hall CB, et al. Human herpesvirus-6 infection in children—a prospective study of complications and reactivation. *N Engl J Med* 1994;331(7):432–438.
21. Brown NA, et al. Fall in human herpesvirus 6 seropositivity with age. *Lancet* 1988;2(8607):396.
22. Levy JA, et al. Frequent isolation of HHV-6 from saliva and high seroprevalence of the virus in the population. *Lancet* 1990;335(8697):1047–1050.
23. Kangro HO, et al. Seroprevalence of antibodies to human herpesviruses in England and Hong Kong. *J Med Virol* 1994;43(1):91–96.
24. Harnett GB, et al. Frequent shedding of human herpesvirus 6 in saliva. *J Med Virol* 1990;30(2):128–130.
25. Fox JD, et al. Production of IgM antibody to HHV6 in reactivation and primary infection. *Epidemiol Infect* 1990;104(2):289–296.
26. Mukai T, et al. Molecular epidemiological studies of human herpesvirus 6 in families. *J Med Virol* 1994;42(3):224–227.
27. Cuende JI, et al. High prevalence of HHV-6 DNA in peripheral blood mononuclear cells of healthy individuals detected by nested-PCR. *J Med Virol* 1994;43(2):115–118.
28. Luppi M, et al. Human herpesvirus-6 (HHV-6) in blood donors. *Br J Haematol* 1995;89(4):943–945.
29. Sayers MH. Transfusion-transmitted viral infections other than hepatitis and human immunodeficiency virus infection. Cytomegalovirus, Epstein-Barr virus, human herpesvirus 6, and human parvovirus B19. *Arch Pathol Lab Med* 1994;118(4):346–349.
30. Dunne WM Jr, Jevon M. Examination of human breast milk for evidence of human herpesvirus 6 by polymerase chain reaction. *J Infect Dis* 1993;168(1):250.
31. Ward KN, Gray JJ, Efstathiou S. Brief report: primary human herpesvirus 6 infection in a patient following liver transplantation from a seropositive donor. *J Med Virol* 1989;28(2):69–72.
32. Okuno T, et al. Human herpesvirus 6 infection in renal transplantation. *Transplantation* 1990;49(3):519–522.
33. Dewhurst S, et al. Human herpesvirus 6 (HHV-6) variant B accounts for the majority of symptomatic primary HHV-6 infections in a population of U.S. infants. *J Clin Microbiol* 1993;31(2):416–418.
34. Di Luca D, et al. Human herpesvirus 6: a survey of presence and variant distribution in normal peripheral lymphocytes and lymphoproliferative disorders. *J Infect Dis* 1994;170(1):211–215.
35. Drobyski WR, et al. Prevalence of human herpesvirus 6 variant A and B infections in bone marrow transplant recipients as determined by polymerase chain reaction and sequence-specific oligonucleotide probe hybridization. *J Clin Microbiol* 1993;31(6):1515–1520.
36. Drobyski WR, et al. Human herpesvirus-6 (HHV-6) infection in allogeneic bone marrow transplant recipients: evidence of a marrow-suppressive role for HHV-6 *in vivo*. *J Infect Dis* 1993;167(3):735–739.
37. Drobyski WR, et al. Brief report: fatal encephalitis due to variant B human herpesvirus-6 infection in a bone marrow-transplant recipient. *N Engl J Med* 1994;330(19):1356–1360.
38. Shanavas KR, et al. Anti-HHV-6 antibodies in normal population and in cancer patients in India. *J Exp Pathol* 1992;6(1–2):95–105.
39. Torelli G, et al. Human herpesvirus 6 in non-AIDS related Hodgkin's and non-Hodgkin's lymphomas. *Leukemia* 1992;6(suppl 3):46–48.
40. Clark DA, et al. The seroepidemiology of human herpesvirus-6 (HHV-6) from a case-control study of leukaemia and lymphoma. *Int J Cancer* 1990;45(5):829–833.
41. Levine PH, et al. Antibodies to human herpes virus-6 and clinical course in patients with Hodgkin's disease. *Int J Cancer* 1992;51(1):53–57.
42. Sumiyoshi Y, et al. Analysis of human herpes virus-6 genomes in lymphoid malignancy in Japan. *J Clin Pathol* 1993;46(12):1137–1138.
43. Di Paolo JA, et al. Multistage carcinogenesis utilizing human genital cells and human papillomaviruses. *Toxicol Lett* 1994;72(1–3):7–11.
44. Yadav M, et al. Frequent detection of human herpesvirus 6 in oral carcinoma. *J Natl Cancer Inst* 1994;86(23):1792–1794.
45. Luppi M, et al. Human herpesvirus 6 infection in normal human brain tissue. *J Infect Dis* 1994;169(4):943–944.
46. Santoro F, et al. CD46 is a cellular receptor for human herpesvirus 6. *Cell* 1999;99(7):817–827.
47. Roffman E, Frenkel N. Interleukin-2 inhibits the replication of human herpesvirus-6 in mature thymocytes. *Virology* 1990;175(2):591–594.
48. Arena A, et al. Role of interleukin-18 in peripheral blood mononuclear cells infected with human herpes virus type 6. *Intervirology* 2001;44(4):250–254.
49. Murphy PM. Viral exploitation and subversion of the immune system through chemokine mimicry. *Nat Immunol* 2001;2(2):116–122.
50. Yoshikawa T, et al. A prospective study of human herpesvirus-6 infection in renal transplantation. *Transplantation* 1992;54(5):879–883.
51. Suga S, et al. Activation of human herpesvirus-6 in children with acute measles. *J Med Virol* 1992;38(4):278–282.
52. Yoshikawa T, et al. Human herpesvirus-6 infection in bone marrow transplantation. *Blood* 1991;78(5):1381–1384.
53. Shiraki K, et al. Virion and nonstructural polypeptides of human herpesvirus-6. *Virus Res* 1989;13(2):173–178.
54. Balachandran N, et al. Identification of proteins specific for human herpesvirus 6-infected human T cells. *J Virol* 1989;63(6):2835–2840.
55. Littler E, et al. Identification, cloning, and expression of the major capsid protein gene of human herpesvirus 6. *J Virol* 1990;64(2):714–722.
56. Yamamoto M, et al. Identification of a nucleocapsid protein as a specific serological marker of human herpesvirus 6 infection. *J Clin Microbiol* 1990;28(9):1957–1962.
57. Asada H, et al. Establishment of titration system for human herpesvirus 6 and evaluation of neutralizing antibody response to the virus. *J Clin Microbiol* 1989;27(10):2204–2207.
58. Asano Y, et al. Clinical features of infants with primary human herpesvirus 6 infection (exanthem subitum, roseola infantum). *Pediatrics* 1994;93(1):104–108.
59. Pruksananonda P, et al. Primary human herpesvirus 6 infection in young children. *N Engl J Med* 1992;326(22):1445–1450.
60. Suga S, et al. Human herpesvirus-6 infection (exanthem subitum) without rash. *Pediatrics* 1989;83(6):1003–1006.
61. Yoshiyama H, et al. Role of human herpesvirus 6 infection in infants with exanthema subitum. *Pediatr Infect Dis J* 1990;9(2):71–74.

62. Suga S, et al. Clinical and virological analyses of 21 infants with exanthem subitum (roseola infantum) and central nervous system complications. *Ann Neurol* 1993;33(6):597–603.

63. Ward KN, Gray JJ. Primary human herpesvirus-6 infection is frequently over-looked as a cause of febrile fits in young children. *J Med Virol* 1994;42(2):119–123.

64. Jones CM, et al. Acute encephalopathy and status epilepticus associated with human herpes virus 6 infection. *Dev Med Child Neurol* 1994;36(7):646–650.

65. Ishiguro N, et al. Meningo-encephalitis associated with HHV-6 related exanthem subitum. *Acta Paediatr Scand* 1990;79(10):987–989.

66. Kondo K, et al. Detection by polymerase chain reaction amplification of human herpesvirus 6 DNA in peripheral blood of patients with exanthem subitum. *J Clin Microbiol* 1990;28(5):970–974.

67. Komura E, et al. Human herpesvirus 6 and intussusception. *Pediatr Infect Dis J* 1993;12(9):788–789.

68. Kitamura K, et al. Idiopathic thrombocytopenic purpura after human herpesvirus 6 infection. *Lancet* 1994;344(8925):830.

69. Asano Y, et al. Simultaneous occurrence of human herpesvirus 6 infection and intussusception in three infants. *Pediatr Infect Dis J* 1991;10(4):335–337.

70. Yoshikawa T, et al. Exacerbation of idiopathic thrombocytopenic purpura by primary human herpesvirus 6 infection. *Pediatr Infect Dis J* 1993;12(5):409–410.

71. Sumiyoshi Y, Akashi K, Kikuchi M. Detection of human herpes virus 6 (HHV 6) in the skin of a patient with primary HHV 6 infection and erythroderma. *J Clin Pathol* 1994;47(8):762–763.

72. Akashi K, et al. Brief report: severe infectious mononucleosis-like syndrome and primary human herpesvirus 6 infection in an adult. *N Engl J Med* 1993;329(3):168–171.

73. Sobue R, et al. Fulminant hepatitis in primary human herpesvirus-6 infection. *N Engl J Med* 1991;324(18):1290.

74. Read R, et al. Clinical and laboratory findings in the Paul-Bunnell negative glandular fever-fatigue syndrome. *J Infect* 1990;21(2):157–165.

75. Goedhard JG, Galama JM, Wagenvoort JH. Active human herpesvirus 6 infection in an adolescent male. *Clin Infect Dis* 1995;20(4):1070–1071.

76. Niederman JC, et al. Clinical and serological features of human herpesvirus-6 infection in three adults. *Lancet* 1988;2(8615):817–819.

77. Steeper TA, et al. The spectrum of clinical and laboratory findings resulting from human herpesvirus-6 (HHV-6) in patients with mononucleosis-like illnesses not resulting from Epstein-Barr virus or cytomegalovirus. *Am J Clin Pathol* 1990;93(6):776–783.

78. Novoa LJ, et al. Fulminant demyelinating encephalomyelitis associated with productive HHV-6 infection in an immunocompetent adult. *J Med Virol* 1997;52(3):301–308.

79. Yoshikawa T, Kojima S, Asano Y. Human herpesvirus-6 infection and bone marrow transplantation. *Leuk Lymphoma* 1992;8(1–2):65–73.

80. Asano Y, et al. Reactivation of herpesvirus type 6 in children receiving bone marrow transplants for leukemia. *N Engl J Med* 1991;324(9):634–635.

81. Singh N, Carrigan DR. Human herpesvirus-6 in transplantation: an emerging pathogen. *Ann Intern Med* 1996;124(12):1065–1071.

82. Zerr DM, et al. Human herpesvirus 6 reactivation and encephalitis in allogeneic bone marrow transplant recipients. *Clin Infect Dis* 2001;33(6):763–771.

83. Appleton AL, et al. Human herpesvirus 6 DNA in skin biopsy tissue from marrow graft recipients with severe combined immunodeficiency. *Lancet* 1994;344(8933):1361–1362.

84. Michel D, et al. Human herpesvirus 6 DNA in exanthematous skin in BMT patient. *Lancet* 1994;344(8923):686.

85. Carrigan DR, Knox KK. Human herpesvirus 6 (HHV-6) isolation from bone marrow: HHV-6- associated bone marrow suppression in bone marrow transplant patients. *Blood* 1994;84(10):3307–3310.

86. Wilborn F, et al. Herpesvirus type 6 in patients undergoing bone marrow transplantation: serologic features and detection by polymerase chain reaction. *Blood* 1994;83(10):3052–3058.

87. Levy JA, Landay A, Lennette ET. Human herpesvirus 6 inhibits human immunodeficiency virus type 1 replication in cell culture. *J Clin Microbiol* 1990;28(10):2362–2364.

88. Flamand L, et al. Immunosuppressive effect of human herpesvirus 6 on T-cell functions: suppression of interleukin-2 synthesis and cell proliferation. *Blood* 1995;85(5):1263–1271.

89. Knox KK, Carrigan DR. Disseminated active HHV-6 infections in patients with AIDS. *Lancet* 1994;343(8897):577–578.

90. Corbellino M, et al. Disseminated human herpesvirus 6 infection in AIDS. *Lancet* 1993;342(8881):1242.

91. Dolcetti R, et al. Frequent detection of human herpesvirus 6 DNA in HIV-associated lymphadenopathy. *Lancet* 1994;344(8921):543.

92. Blumberg BM, et al. The HHV6 paradox: ubiquitous commensal or insidious pathogen? A two-step *in situ* PCR approach. *J Clin Virol* 2000;16(3):159–178.

93. Kim JS, et al. Detection of human herpesvirus 6 variant A in peripheral blood mononuclear cells from multiple sclerosis patients. *Eur Neurol* 2000;43(3):170–173.

94. Mirandola P, et al. Absence of human herpesvirus 6 and 7 from spinal fluid and serum of multiple sclerosis patients. *Neurology* 1999;53(6):1367–1368.

95. Enbom M. Human herpesvirus 6 in the pathogenesis of multiple sclerosis. *APMIS* 2001;109(6):401–411.

96. Robert C, et al. Detection of antibodies to human herpesvirus-6 using immunofluorescence assay. *Res Virol* 1990;141(5):545–555.

97. Cermelli C, et al. Comparison between immunofluorescence and enzyme-linked-immunosorbent assay in the determination of serum HHV-6 IgG. *New Microbiol* 1994;17(2):69–73.

98. Asano Y, et al. Enzyme-linked immunosorbent assay for detection of IgG antibody to human herpesvirus 6. *J Med Virol* 1990;32(2):119–123.

99. Van den Bosch G, et al. Development of reverse transcriptase PCR assays for detection of active human herpesvirus 6 infection. *J Clin Microbiol* 2001;39(6):2308–2310.

100. Clark DA, et al. Prevalence of antibody to human herpesvirus 7 by age. *J Infect Dis* 1993;168(1):251–252.

101. Yoshikawa T, et al. Seroepidemiology of human herpesvirus 7 in healthy children and adults in Japan. *J Med Virol* 1993;41(4):319–323.

102. Wyatt LS, et al. Human herpesvirus 7: antigenic properties and prevalence in children and adults. *J Virol* 1991;65(11):6260–6265.

103. Berneman ZN, et al. Human herpesvirus 7 is a T-lymphotropic virus and is related to, but significantly different from, human herpesvirus 6 and human cytomegalovirus. *Proc Natl Acad Sci U S A* 1992;89(21):10552–10556.

104. Frenkel N, et al. Isolation of a new herpesvirus from human CD4⁺ T cells. *Proc Natl Acad Sci U S A* 1990;87(2):748–752.

105. Wyatt LS, Frenkel N. Human herpesvirus 7 is a constitutive inhabitant of adult human saliva. *J Virol* 1992;66(5):3206–3209.

106. Ueda K, et al. Primary human herpesvirus 7 infection and exanthema subitum. *Pediatr Infect Dis J* 1994;13(2):167–168.

107. Hidaka Y, et al. Frequent isolation of human herpesvirus 7 from saliva samples. *J Med Virol* 1993;40(4):343–346.

108. Di Luca D, et al. Human herpesviruses 6 and 7 in salivary glands and shedding in saliva of healthy and human immunodeficiency virus positive individuals. *J Med Virol* 1995;45(4):462–468.

109. Tanaka K, et al. Human herpesvirus 7: another causal agent for roseola (exanthem subitum). *J Pediatr* 1994;125(1):1–5.

110. Asano Y, et al. Clinical features and viral excretion in an infant with primary human herpesvirus 7 infection. *Pediatrics* 1995;95(2):187–190.

111. Drago F, et al. Human herpesvirus 7 in patients with pityriasis rosea. Electron microscopy investigations and polymerase chain reaction in mononuclear cells, plasma and skin. *Dermatology* 1997;195(4):374–378.

112. Kempf W, et al. Pityriasis rosea is not associated with human herpesvirus 7. *Arch Dermatol* 1999;135(9):1070–1072.

113. Bergstrom T. [HHV 6,7 and 8. Recently discovered herpesviruses explain the etiology of well-known diseases]. *Lakartidningen* 1999;96(26–27):3161–3165.

114. Wong WR, et al. Association of pityriasis rosea with human herpesvirus-6 and human herpesvirus-7 in Taipei. *J Formos Med Assoc* 2001;100(7):478–483.

115. DesJardin JA, et al. Association of human herpesvirus 6 reactivation with severe cytomegalovirus-associated disease in orthotopic liver transplant recipients. *Clin Infect Dis* 2001;33(8):1358–1362.

116. Chan PK, et al. Human herpesvirus-6 and human herpesvirus-7 infections in bone marrow transplant recipients. *J Med Virol* 1997;53(3):295–305.

117. Agut H, et al. *In vitro* sensitivity of human herpesvirus-6 to antiviral drugs. *Res Virol* 1989;140(3):219–228.

118. Agut H, et al. Susceptibility of human herpesvirus 6 to acyclovir and ganciclovir. *Lancet* 1989;2(8663):626.

119. Burns WH, Sandford GR. Susceptibility of human herpesvirus 6 to antivirals in vitro. *J Infect Dis* 1990;162(3):634–637.

120. Russler SK, Tapper MA, Carrigan DR. Susceptibility of human herpesvirus 6 to acyclovir and ganciclovir. *Lancet* 1989;2(8659):382.

121. Di Luca D, et al. The replication of viral and cellular DNA in human herpesvirus 6- infected cells. *Virology* 1990;175(1):199–210.

122. Kikuta H, Lu H, Matsumoto S. Susceptibility of human herpesvirus 6 to acyclovir. *Lancet* 1989;2(8667):861.

123. Mendez JC, et al. Human beta-herpesvirus interactions in solid organ transplant recipients. *J Infect Dis* 2001;183(2):179–184.

124. Kikuta H, et al. Interferon induction by human herpesvirus 6 in human mononuclear cells. *J Infect Dis* 1990;162(1):35–38.

125. Kovacs JA, et al. Increases in CD4 T lymphocytes with intermittent courses of interleukin-2 in patients with human immunodeficiency virus infection. A preliminary study. *N Engl J Med* 1995;332(9):567–575.

CHAPTER 232

Kaposi's Sarcoma–Associated Herpesvirus/Human Herpesvirus-8

Joyce Fingeroth

Kaposi's sarcoma-associated herpesvirus (KSHV), also known as human herpesvirus-8 (HHV-8), is the most recently discovered member of the human herpesvirus family (1). As with other herpesviruses, the KSHV life cycle is a complex mixture of both lytic and latent phases that allows the virus to persist indefinitely in the infected host (2). KSHV is a member of the γ herpesvirus subfamily, and although similar to the human lymphocryptovirus (γ1) Epstein-Barr virus (EBV), it was the first rhabdinovirus (γ2) found in humans (1). Like EBV (3), serious disease is associated with unrestricted growth of virus-infected cells and is compounded by defective cellular (T-cell) immunity (4–6). However, the strategies used by KSHV to achieve cell cycle dysregulation appear to be distinct (7). The clinical manifestations of primary infection are not fully known (8–11). However, KSHV is causally associated with three proliferative disorders: Kaposi's sarcoma (KS) (1), primary effusion lymphoma (PEL) (12), and the plasmablastic variant of multicentric Castleman's disease (MCD) (13). Studies of virus evolution suggest that KSHV may be more ancient than EBV (14); however, serologic evidence demonstrates it is not nearly as widespread in the human population (15,16). The reasons are not well understood. The acquired immunodeficiency syndrome (AIDS) epidemic in Africa has provided an impetus to the spread of KSHV (17,18); thus, worldwide dissemination may be only a matter of time.

HISTORY

The existence of a virus as the causative agent of KS was suspected for many years (19–22). This was based on the unusual epidemiology and natural history of this indolent tumor, as well as on intermittent visualization of herpesvirus-like particles in cultured tissue from KS biopsy samples (22,23). In the early the 1980s, an epidemic of aggressive KS in male patients with AIDS (24) greatly stimulated the search for an infectious cause for this disease. Thus, the 1994 demonstration by representational difference analysis (1) that DNA from a novel herpesvirus was present in KS biopsy specimens was long awaited and produced a burst of scientific investigation. Although 30 years had elapsed since the electron microscopical discovery of EBV in Burkitt's lymphoma cells (25), the interim revolution in molecular biology greatly accelerated study of KSHV. Sequencing of the viral genome, cloning and characterization of diverse viral gene products, development of serologic assays, and the identification of two additional KSHV-associated diseases—PEL and plasmablastic MCD—rapidly followed the discovery of KSHV (7). In addition, the recent identification and sequence analysis of several related primate herpesviruses has provided insight into the molecular evolution of KSHV and yielded valuable information about how KSHV causes disease (14,26).

CHARACTERISTICS OF THE PATHOGEN

Classification and Structure

KSHV is a herpesvirus of the γ2 subfamily. The classification of herpesviruses into α, β, and γ subfamilies was introduced by Roizman in the 1970s to distinguish differences in biologic behavior between various family members (27). The classification was validated when the respective genomes were sequenced, their organization revealed, and their relatedness demonstrated by the construction of phylogenetic trees (2,28). The human α viruses [herpes simplex virus type 1 (HSV-1), HSV-2, and varicella-zoster virus (VZV)] and β viruses [cytomegalovirus (CMV), HHV-6A, HHV-6B, HHV-7] replicate productively in cells in culture, persist poorly in tissue culture systems, and cause disease by lytic replication and destruction of infected tissue. In contrast, the γ herpesviruses propagate readily in tissue culture as virus-immortalized lymphoid lines. Their ability to replicate lytically in cultured cells generally ranges from modest (primate rhabdinoviruses) to almost nonexistent (EBV). Importantly, the diseases associated with γ herpesvirus infection result from the ability of virus (a) to persist in cells that can proliferate, (b) to enhance the survival and outgrowth of these cells, and (c) to promote the development of cellular genetic alterations that lead to multistep tumorigenesis. Therefore, as a γ herpesvirus, KSHV is a human tumor virus.

The γ herpesviruses have been further subdivided into the γ1 (lymphocryptovirus) and γ2 (rhabdinovirus) genera. The recent discovery and sequencing of a large number of related viruses from both new and old world primates has provided valuable information about when these lineage's diverged (~80 million years ago, preceding the division of the continents) and also about how they differ in achieving latency and cellular transformation (2,14,26). Comparative studies suggest that although the γ1 and γ2 viruses use different strategies to initiate immortalization, they share a final common pathway that links functional alteration of key cell cycle regulatory proteins (Rb, p53, telomerase) (7) to constitutive activation of the dominant lymphoid transcription factor, nuclear factor-κB (NF-κB) (29–31). EBV and the related γ1 primate viruses alter cell cycle control by expression of a small, unique set of virus-specific genes, namely EBV nuclear antigens (EBNAs): EBNAs 1, 2, 3ABC and leader protein (LP) that tether the virus genome to host cell chromatin (EBNA-1) and activate transcription of both viral proteins (latent membrane protein [LMP]-1, LMP-2) and cell proteins, which in turn are able to modulate cellular signal transduction (reviewed in reference 32). Although the γ2 herpesviruses encode positional and functional homologs of EBNA-1 (latency-associated nuclear antigen [LANA]), LMP-1 (K1), and LMP-2 (latency-associated membrane protein [LAMP]) (33), the additional expression of a subset of "pirated" mammalian genes is believed to be critical for these γ2 viruses to dysregulate the cell cycle (reviewed in references 7 and 34). Thus, viral proteins that are homologs of mammalian genes incorporated into the viral genome and modified during evolution (viral cyclin [vCYC], viral FLICE inhibitory protein [FLIP]) directly interact with cellular proteins to alter cell cycle regulation/cellular proliferation and survival. Whereas the γ1 herpesvirus EBNAs are generated by a complex splicing mechanism that spans almost the entire virus genome (32,35), the pirated γ2 genes are unspliced and therefore may have been incorporated into the genome from cyclic DNAs (7). The mechanism by which this may have occurred cannot be readily explained based on existing knowledge. Although progress in elucidating the functions of KSHV genes has been rapid, additional investigation is needed to clearly identify the key regulators of KSHV latency and immortalization and to uncover how molecular piracy could have come about.

Just as the identification of KSHV brings to a close another chapter in tumor virology, it is remarkable that the investigations stimulated by discovery of this virus have raised new suspicion that a second $\gamma 2$ herpesvirus is present in the human population. Based on recent studies demonstrating that two separate phylogenetic groupings of $\gamma 2$ herpesvirus—RV1 and RV2, or retroperitoneal fibromatosis herpesvirus (RFHV)—co-infect several old world primates (macaques, African green monkeys, chimpanzees) and given the greater similarity of KSHV to RV2mac or RFHV, it has been proposed that a second rhabdinovirus may also infect humans (14,26,36,37).

The morphologic appearance of KSHV is indistinguishable from that of other herpesviruses (38,39). The virion consists of a linear double-stranded DNA-protein core encased by an icosadeltahedral capsid, and surrounded by a robust protein-laden tegument, a typical feature of herpesvirus family members (2). A lipid membrane containing viral transmembrane glycoproteins that project from the virion surface into the extracellular space envelops these elements. Membrane glycoproteins mediate virion attachment, fusion, entry, and possibly egress (40–44). The intact virion is approximately 110 nm long, although considerable size variation has been described (44).

Genome Organization and Variation

The 170-kbp genome is organized in a manner that is typical for members of the γ herpesvirus family and forms a class C herpesvirus sequence arrangement (2), similar to the related primate $\gamma 2$ herpesvirus, herpesvirus saimiri (HVS). KSHV encodes over 85 independent gene products that have been named based on their colinear similarity to HVS. Genes that are unique to KSHV are designated by a separate prefix of K (7). There is a long region of unique sequence in the center of the genome (140–145 kbp) that is flanked by left- and right-side GC-rich terminal repeats. In addition, less prominent repeat elements are also scattered throughout the unique region (45). The unique central region contains seven blocks composed of 26 highly conserved genes that belong to an ancestral core of mammalian herpesvirus genes, which function in virion replication and assembly. Among the most conserved genes are the major DNA binding protein, the DNA packaging function/terminase, virion glycoprotein B, the catalytic subunit of DNA polymerase, the major capsid protein, the DNA-packaging protein, the DNA helicase, and uracil-DNA glycosylase (2). Approximately 42 conserved gene products localize to this central region and comprise about half of the complement of KSHV genes (14). Eight of the genes found in the KSHV genome contain sequences that can be identified in all members of the $\gamma 2$ herpesvirus subfamily (14). At present, little is known about their precise function, with the exception of gene 50, a positional and functional homolog of EBV BRLF1-encoded transcriptional activator or RTA. Similar to RTA, gene 50 is an immediate early transcription factor that appears to play a critical role in initiating lytic replication of KSHV (46–49).

All $\gamma 2$ herpesviruses contain a large number of homologs of mammalian genes; however, these "pirated" genes have undergone significant mutation and are substantially diverged from their mammalian precursors (7,34). Eighteen separate classes of cell homologous genes have been found distributed in the diverse $\gamma 2$ herpesviruses, and others may exist. KSHV is rich in orthologs and contains 12 of the 18 gene classes described, including G-coupled protein receptor, dihydrofolate reductase (DHFR), α-N-formylglycineamide ribonucleotide aminotransferase (FGARAT), complement control protein, interleukin-6 (IL-6), CC chemokines, bcl-2/FLIP, interferon regulatory factors, thymidine kinase and thymidylate synthase, apoptotic protease

inhibitor, cyclin D, and OX-2 cell surface protein (14). Many of the cellular homologs and γ-specific genes localize to regions adjacent to the terminal repeats, where they appear to form functional clusters of genes involved in cell cycle regulation and cell survival (50). Latent gene expression from a gene cluster on the right end of the genome consisting of T0.7, LANA, vCYC, and vFLIP has been detected in all of the virus-associated proliferative diseases (7). Some regulatory genes are dispersed in the unique region of the genome, although they also tend to cluster at just a few genomic loci (50).

Comparison of different isolates of KSHV indicate that overall genomic variation is quite limited (0.4%) (7). However, the K1 gene, localized to the left end of the genome, is hypervariable and contains many nucleotide substitutions in sequences that correspond to the extracellular domain of this transmembrane protein. The K15 (LAMP) gene, localized to the right end of the genome, also displays significant variation, although the more limited nature of these changes is consistent with allelic polymorphism (14). The selective pressures driving high rates of localized mutation are not understood. In fact, K1 is the most variable of any herpesvirus gene studied to date. Importantly, comparison of variant K1 regions among different KSHV isolates has permitted separation of the virus into four major clades with distinct geographic distributions (51,52). Clade B predominates in Africa and may be the most ancient form of the virus. Clade D is found in southern Asia. Clades A and C are most closely related to one another and are seen largely in Europe and North America. Accumulating data suggest that as many as seven major subtypes exist (53). However, this division has yielded no insight into the selective pressures driving K1 evolution. Furthermore, no differences in disease pathogenesis have been associated with infection by the different clades.

Virus Life Cycle

Establishment of a robust tissue culture system in which purified KSHV is able to infect primary cells in culture and efficiently maintain either a latent/immortalizing or lytic infection has been met with limited success in spite of diverse efforts (44,54–62). KSHV can infect primary endothelial cells, particularly microvascular endothelial cells, epithelial cells, monocyte/macrophages, and foreskin fibroblasts in cell culture systems. Virus entry and initiation of both latent and lytic infection appear to be relatively efficient; however, infection rapidly aborts for reasons that are poorly understood (62). Primary B cells do not form lymphoblastoid cells lines upon infection (58), although B-cell infection is well documented *in vivo* and B cells are thought to comprise the reservoir of persistent infection. In addition, viral infection is not maintained in cultured endothelial cells derived from KS biopsy (63), and MCD has not been successfully explanted. One working hypothesis is that a critical inflammatory cytokine provided in trans (i.e., a paracrine growth factor) is needed to support survival of the virus-infected cell. This cytokine is absent in tissue culture systems, but present *in vivo* (64). KSHV infection of certain virus-immortalized endothelial cell lines appears to be more stable than infection of the cognate primary cells (57,62). However, these lines may not be ideal for analyzing the unique effects of KSHV gene expression on cell cycle regulation. Therefore, much remains to be learned about how KSHV initiates natural infection and achieves cellular immortalization.

PATHOGEN ATTACHMENT AND ENTRY: VIRAL PROTEINS AND CELLULAR RECEPTORS

The virion membrane glycoproteins (gp) K8.1 and glycoprotein B(gB) have been implicated in virus attachment and entry

(40–43). Additional viral glycoproteins are also likely to be important. K8.1 shares several properties with EBV gp350/220, the major EBV attachment protein, although the two ligands are structurally unrelated. K8.1 resides in the same relative position in the viral genome as gp350/220 (65) and is similarly expressed as two in-frame splice variants (K8.1A/K8.1B) (66). As with gp350/220, antibodies to K8.1 are neutralizing even in the absence of complement (66). Both K8.1 and gB have been reported to bind heparan sulfate (40–42); however, it is not yet clear whether heparan sulfate is the major cell surface attachment molecule for either of these proteins. KSHV gB is unique among herpesvirus orthologs in containing an N-terminal RGD motif (67). This motif is present in the attachment site of many proteins that bind integrins, and a specific interaction between KSHV gB and the integrin $\alpha 3\beta 1$ (CD49c/CD29) has recently been reported to play a role in virus entry (67). The molecular details of how the virion gains access to the nucleus and begins to replicate—including virus fusion, intracellular transport, and nuclear entry—are currently unknown, although major features are likely to be shared with other herpesvirus family members.

LATENT INFECTION AND LYTIC INFECTION

In contrast to the inability of KSHV to be maintained in primary cell lines or lines derived from explanted KS, B-cell lines that are stably infected with KSHV can be readily derived from PELs (68,69). As a result, most studies of the virus life cycle are based on investigation of PEL lines complemented with biopsy samples from the different KSHV-associated diseases (48,70–74). KSHV-infected tumor cells from PELs grow readily and persist in tissue culture. KSHV is in a latent state in these cells, the circular genome is attached to the host chromosome by LANA (open reading frame [ORF] 73), and few viral gene products are definitively synthesized (LANA, vCYC, vFLIP, T0.7, K10) (48,70,71,73). These latent gene products, which colocalize on the right end of the genome, function to maintain the viral episome, drive the cell cycle, and protect the cell from apoptosis (7,73,75–80) (Table 232.1). The role of additional gene products, such as K1 and K15, that likely also play a role in the initiation or maintenance of latent or immortalizing infection remains to be identified.

Treatment of PEL lines with chemical inducing agents such as phorbol esters and sodium butyrate has been empirically observed to result in induction of the virus lytic cycle and production of virions that can be used to infect new cells (81). How closely chemical induction mimics the physiologic signal to initiate virus replication is unknown, since the physiologic lytic switch signal has not been identified. Northern blot (48,70) and more recently microarray analysis (73) of induced PEL lines has provided insight into the temporal regulation of virus gene expression in the course of virus lytic replication (48,70,73). These studies document the conserved features of immediate early (primary, <10 hours), early (secondary, 10–24 hours), and late (tertiary, 48–72 hours) gene expression resulting in virion replication and assembly, properties shared by all herpesvirus family members. However, they also reveal that the temporal regulation of several genes that are unique to KSHV or to γ herpesviruses appear to be transcribed in a more complex manner that does not strictly fit established definitions (7,70). This has been observed in particular for several of the pirated mammalian genes that are expressed very early after lytic cycle induction, before the conserved viral regulatory genes can be detected. Recently, based on a hierarchical cluster analysis of lytic genes induced in a PEL line, Jenner et al. proposed that KSHV lytic transcripts could be divided into five functional-temporal classes: (a) homologs of cellular regulatory or signal transduction genes, less than 4 hours; (b) virus gene regulators, 4 to 10 hours; (c) DNA replication genes, approximately 10 hours; (d) DNA repair and nucleotide metabolism genes, approximately 14 hours; and (e) virion formation and structural genes, greater than 34 to 72 hours, to more accurately reflect the biology of productive γ herpesvirus infection (7,73,75) (Table 232.2).

Although current knowledge about KSHV latent and lytic cycle gene expression is largely based on study of PEL lines, it is likely that, as in the case of EBV, specific viral gene expression patterns will emerge linked to each of the KSHV-associated diseases (82). For example, although LANA, vCYC, and vFLIP can be detected in all virus-associated disease, the complex regulation of their joint transcription unit suggests that they may nonetheless be differentially expressed in different diseases or in normal latency (71,83). The ORF K10.5 (LANA2) latent transcript prominent in PEL and also detected in MCD appears to be B cell specific and thus far has not been detected in KS (76). Moreover, although vIL-6 is a lytic transcript in PEL lines, expression of vIL-6 can be detected in 10% to 30% of primary PEL tumors as well as in MCD (10%–15% of plasmablasts in most lesions) (84) (variably and less in KS), raising the possibility that it is also expressed during latent infection *in vivo* (82,85–88). With

---

TABLE 232.1.   Latent Gene Expression in Primary Effusion Lymphoma (PEL) Cell Lines

Strictly latent genes expressed in PEL cell lines
  LANA-1 (ORF 73): Tethers Kaposi's sarcoma–associated herpesvirus to the host chromosome, thereby maintaining the virus episome. Conserved among γ herpesvirus family members. Transcriptional regulator (Epstein-Barr virus genes, nuclear factor-κB[NF-κB], telomerase), interacts with multiple cell proteins (p53, RB1, CBP, RING3).
  vCYC (ORF 72): Homolog of cellular cyclin D2. Expressed in cell cycle–dependent manner. Associates with cdk6 to phosphorylate RB and maintain the cell in cycle. Resistant to inhibition by cyclin-dependent kinase inhibitors p16, 21, and 27.
  vFLIP (ORF K13): Homologous to the cellular antiapoptotic protein FLIP. Binds FADD and TRADD.
  LANA-2 (ORF K10.5): Homolog of cellular IRF-4, also known as vIRF-3, abundant nuclear protein, potential inhibitor of p53 mediated apoptosis, appears to be B cell specific.
Latent (inducible) genes expressed in PEL cell lines
  Kaposin complex (T0.7/ORFK12 and vicinity): Abundant complex transcripts expressed in latently infected cells. Translation products include kaposin A, B, and C. Kaposin A induces cellular transformation of Rat-3 cells *in vitro* and *in vivo* (nude mice).
  ORF K15: Transmembrane protein, positional and possibly functional equivalent of LMP-2A. Complex RNA and protein products. Cytoplasmic domain is constitutively tyrosine phosphorylated. Binds TRAFs 1, 2 and 3. Interacts with the HAX-1 protein, an inhibitor of apoptosis. Activates NF-κB.
  Others: vIRFs (ORF K10.1) (ORF K11.1)

TABLE 232.2.   Lytic Gene Expression in a Primary Effusion Lymphoma (PEL) Cell Line (Microassay Analysis)

Primary lytic (0–10 h)	Secondary lytic (10–24 h)	Tertiary lytic (48–72 h)		Unknown	Latent
Homologs of cell regulatory/signal transduction genes	DNA replication	Virion formation and structure		T0.7 RNA	ORF72 (v-cyclin)
K2 (vIL-6)	ORF9 (DNA polymerase)	K8.1 (glycoprotein gp35-37)		T1.1/nut-1/PAN RNA	ORF73 (LANA-1)
K14 (vOx-2/vAdh)	ORF6 (ssDNA binding protein)	ORF67 (tegument protein)		ORF35	ORF K13 (vFLIP)
K4 (vMIP-II/vMIP-1alpha)	ORF59 (processivity factor, PF-8)	ORF17 (protease/assembly protein)		ORF67.5	ORF K10.5 (LANA -2)
K6 (vMIP-I/vMIP-1alpha)	ORF56 (primase)	ORF8 (glycoprotein B)			Latent/lytic
ORF16 (vBCL-2)	ORF40 (helicase/primase subunit)	ORF38 (putative tegument protein)			K10.7 (putative ORF)
ORF74 (vGCR/vIL-8 receptor homolog)	ORF41 (helicase/primase subunit)	ORF39 (glycoprotein M)			K10
K9 (vIRF-1)	ORF44 (helicase/primase subunit)	ORF65 (small viral capsid antigen, sVCA)			K11
K4.1 (vMIP-III/vMIP-1beta)	DNA repair and nucleotide metabolism	ORF64 (tegument protein)			K15 (EXONS 2-3)
IRF homolog (vIRF-2)	ORF61 (ribonucleotide reductase large su)	ORF48 (putative glycoprotein)			K15 (EXONS 4-6)
ORF4 (Complement binding protein)	ORF46 (thymidylate synthase)	ORF47 (glycoprotein L)			K12 (Kaposin)
Virus gene regulation	ORF2 (DHFR)	ORF66 (putative capsid protein)			
K8/K8.1 shared exon	ORF21 (thymidine kinase)	ORF26 (minor capsid protein)			
K8 (k-bZIP)	ORF54 (dUTPase)	ORF19 (tegument protein)			
ORF45	ORF37 (alkaline exonuclease)	ORF62 (assembly/DNA maturation protein)			
ORF57 (KS-SM)	ORF36 (phosphotransferase/protein kinase)	ORF63 (tegument protein)			
ORF 50		ORF25 (major capsid protein)			
Other		ORF29a (packaging protein)			
K5		ORF75 (tegument protein/FGARAT)			
K7		ORF43 (minor capsid protein)			
ORF10		ORF29b (packaging protein)			
ORF11		ORF32 (putative tegument protein)			
ORF7		ORF22 (glycoprotein H)			
ORF58		ORF20 (Putative fusion protein)			
ORF55		Other			
ORF69		ORF27	K1		
		ORF28	K3 (IE-1B)		
		ORF18	K4.2		
		ORF23	K10.1		
		ORF24	K14.1		
		ORF31			
		ORF34	ORF52		
		ORF30	ORF53		
		ORF49	ORF70		
		ORF33	ORF42		

Based on a TPA induction of a PEL cell line, BC-3.

the acquisition of additional knowledge, distinct patterns of gene expression definitively linked to each of the KSHV-associated disease states are likely to be identified.

PIRATED MAMMALIAN GENES

The pirated mammalian genes have been a focus of intense interest. vCYC and vFLIP are conserved among the γ herpesvirus family and are detected in all the known forms of latent disease (KS, PEL, MDC) (7). Although it was suspected that the other pirated proteins would also function in promoting robust latency and immortalization, studies thus far have indicated a greater role for these human homologs in the productive cycle of the virion. Specific lytic life cycle functions include (a) preventing intercurrent apoptosis and death in a cell that is replicating virus, (b) maintaining a nutrient-rich microenvironment for the replicating cell, and (c) protecting the cell from immune system destruction before efficient transmission can occur. Isolation and study of the individual proteins have demonstrated important roles in angiogenesis (G-protein coupled receptor [GCR]), cell migration (macrophage inflammatory proteins [MIPs]), anti-apoptosis (Bcl-2), and immune evasion (interferon regulatory factor [IRFs]) (7,34,75,89,90) (Table 232.3). These functions are often conceptually associated with immortalization. However, in the case of KSHV and similar to several other lytic viruses (i.e., vaccinia, α and β herpesviruses, dengue), many of these viral proteins appear to function by fostering transient cell survival, which promotes efficient virus replication and transmission, rather than by directly contributing to cellular immortalization per se. As research becomes more sophisticated, these views may change. *In vivo*, infection may have a more substantial lytic

component than studies of PEL lines in culture would suggest, particularly in the case of MCD (84,91). It has been proposed that more than one cell type is required for the development of KS (92) and possibly MCD (87), and that some of the pirated genes may function in creating a local milieu that supports migration and survival of additional inflammatory cell types, yet protects the virus-infected cell.

PATHOGENESIS

Epidemiology

The rapid development of serologic tests (15,93–96) that are able to reliably detect antibody to KSHV in different populations has provided critical information about the epidemiology, transmission, and natural history of KSHV (97,98). The recently accumulated seroprevalence data have clarified many of the puzzling features of KSHV pathogenesis that were based solely on observational studies of KS. These studies provide evidence that KSHV is an emerging infection, spurred by the AIDS epidemic, but with an independent pattern of spread (99,100).

Before the onset of global human immunodeficiency virus (HIV) infection, KS was recognized as a rare and usually indolent neoplasm that occurred primarily in elderly men of Mediterranean or Eastern European origin (classic KS) as well as among central African men of younger age groups (endemic KS) (101). In 1979, Penn reported an unusually high incidence of KS among immunosuppressed transplant patients in the United States (transplant KS) (102), noting that disease often

TABLE 232.3.   Pirated Mammalian Genes

ORF	Gene product	Experimental evidence	Putative function in infection or viral persistence	Possible role in KS pathogenesis	Expression pattern
ORF71	vFLIP	See Table 232.1			Latent
ORF72	vcyclin	See Table 232.1			Latent
K10.5	LANA-2 (IRF-4 homolog)	See Table 232.1			Latent
K15	Viral immunoreceptor	See Table 232.1			Latent/productive
K1	Viral immunoreceptor ITAM-like motif	Downregulates surface expression of the BCR, constitutive calcium signaling	Immune evasion, proliferation	Persistent infection	Productive
K2	Viral IL-6	Prevents apoptosis IL-6 dependent plasma cells, only gp130 required	Control para/autocrine amplification in host	Paracine growth stimulation of cells	Productive
K3/K5	Zinc finger membrane protein	Downregulate MHC 1, B7, ICAM-1 Homolog in human ESTs	Immune evasion block CTL and NK	Persistent infection	Productive
K4, K4.1, K6	vMIPs-II,-III,-I	Binding to both CC and CXC receptors attraction of eosinophils, chemotaxis T helper cells, induction of angiogenesis	Amplification in infected host	Angiogenesis	Productive
K9, K11.5	vIRF-1, vIRF-2	K9 transformation, inhibition of p300 and p53 K11.5 inhibits IFN-α promoter	Counteracting IFN-mediated antiviral activity	Interfering with the anti-proliferative action of celluler IRF	Productive
K14	Viral adhesin (vADH or vOX-2)	Attraction of myeloid lineage cells and cytokine induction	Stimulates local production of inflammatory cytokines	Angiogenic proliferation	Productive
ORF4	vCBP		Immune evasion prevents attack by complement	Preventing rapid destruction virus/virus-infected cell by C	Productive
ORF16	vbcl-2	Antiapoptotic activity, Bcl-2 and Bax binding	Counteracting elimination of persistently infected cells	Stabilizing productively infected cells	Productive
ORF74	vGCR, vIL-8R	Constitutively active; induces VEGF secretion, transformation in animals	Amplification in infected host	Angiogenesis, transformation of endothelial cells	Productive
ORFs 2, 9, 21, 60, 61, 70, 75, others	Viral homologs of cell genes that function in nucleic acid synthesis and repair		Provide substrates for viral DNA replication	Synthesis of large quantity of viral DNA for virion assembly	Productive

waned when immunosuppression was withdrawn (103). Soon thereafter the incidence of aggressive KS in the United States soared, concurrent with epidemic HIV infection, and AIDS-associated KS became the most common HIV-associated neoplasm (104,105). Nevertheless, the pattern of disease remained distinctive. Not only was KS far more common in men (15:1 to 2:1 excess risk), consistent with previous observations (101), but the incidence of disease was far greater in HIV-positive men who have sex with men (MSMs) than in HIV-positive hemophiliacs (106,107). These observations suggested that despite its tumor-like behavior, KS was caused by an infectious agent, disease susceptibility was markedly increased by T-cell immuno-compromise, infection was sexually acquired, and transmission was enhanced by a behavior or practice more prevalent among MSMs.

The discovery of a novel herpesvirus and demonstration that the virus was present in all forms of KS confirmed the infectious etiology of this tumor (1). However, because herpesvirus infection is associated with life-long latency, primarily in the absence of frank disease, the relationship between infection, disease, and prevalence in the general population remained obscure. The rapid development of serologic assays (LANA, lytic antigen detection assays) to assess the prevalence of KSHV antibody and polymerase chain reaction (PCR) assays to detect virus in various tissues and body fluids provided rapid and often unexpected answers about KSHV infection in humans (95,97,98,108). The seroprevalence data available to date (16,109) indicate that although KSHV is indeed global in occurrence, the frequency of infection varies greatly in different populations, with pockets of high incidence identifiable even in isolated populations such as the Amerindians of Brazil. Prevalence is high in central and southern Africa (45%–85%), intermediate in regions surrounding

the Mediterranean and in Eastern Europe (15%–45%), and low in the United States, Western Europe, and Asia (0%–5%). Notably, KSHV is not nearly as prevalent as the highly successful γ herpesvirus EBV, which infects more than 90% of the world's population (110), although some data suggest that KSHV is more ancient (111).

The geographic distribution of pre-AIDS KS correlates well with regions of high KSHV prevalence (15), but the high male-to-female ratio characteristic of disease is not concordant with the prevalence of infection (99). In a large study of South African cancer patients, virus infection was equally distributed among men and women, and even more surprisingly, equally distributed between HIV-positive and HIV-negative individuals (99). Although profound T-cell suppression is a definite risk factor for development of KS, the higher incidence of KS in men compared with women cannot be explained on this basis alone. Furthermore, although the AIDS epidemic has stimulated dissemination of KSHV, the epidemiologic relationships leading to spread are complex. Retrospective analyses indicate that the epidemic of KS coordinate with the AIDS epidemic in U.S. MSMs was the result of concomitant introduction of the two viruses, HIV and KSHV, into this population (100). Thus, although transmission of HIV has decreased, transmission of KSHV has remained stable in this cohort. However, the incidence of KS disease has markedly diminished in this population in association with decreased HIV-induced immunosuppression through decreased HIV infection and increased treatment with highly active antiretroviral therapy (HAART) (100).

In Africa and coordinate with the spread of AIDS, the incidence of KS has greatly increased (20-fold in Uganda and Zimbabwe) and is now the most common tumor in adults and the second most common childhood tumor in many parts of

Africa (18,112). Pockets of highly prevalent KSHV infection, however, may have already been present in East and Central Africa (113) before the AIDS epidemic because KS was frequently observed and was estimated to account for 8% of adult cancers (112). Because of limited data collection from sub-Saharan Africa, there are few specimens, and little information is available about the changes in KSHV seroprevalence in the course of the HIV epidemic. Based on recent studies, it is clear that seroprevalence increases rapidly during childhood and adolescence in some areas, reaching 30% to 60% by age 15. Seroprevalence then increases more slowly, reaching levels as high as 50% to 85% in adult populations (114–120). The high rates of transmission within families (mother and siblings) and between other young children demonstrate that sexual transmission is not the major route of infection (115,116,121,122). Nevertheless, a trend toward increasing seroprevalence has been observed with increasing sexual partners and decreasing education (99,114). Notably, the high KSHV prevalence in both HIV-positive and HIV-negative individuals, in the setting of epidemic HIV infection, suggests that while the immunocompromised host can facilitate KSHV spread, transmission occurs independently of HIV infection. KSHV in saliva and blood is frequently detected in an immunocompromised host (123–128). Therefore, it is plausible that increased virus shedding by the immunocompromised host may facilitate spread to all susceptible individuals in their close environment, accounting for the more rapid and ostensibly coordinate emergence of KSHV in regions of Africa with high rates of AIDS.

Transmission

The 1980s epidemic of KS in HIV-positive MSMs strongly suggested that KS was a sexually transmitted disease (106), leading to speculation that semen or possibly feces or blood was the major vehicle for transmission. However, several studies have suggested that oral exposure to infectious saliva, similar to the other human herpesviruses, is likely to be the major route by which infection is spread (123). In KSHV-positive MSMs, shedding of virus is common in saliva, but rare in anal and genital samples (127). Furthermore, the median titer is 2.5 logs higher in saliva than in sources from any other site. Viral DNA and RNA can be readily detected in shed oral epithelial cells in persons that are infected with KSHV. In addition, increases both in virus titer and the frequency of detection occur in persons with frank KS. These findings support a major oral route of transmission, not only among children and between family members, but even among MSMs (129). Thus, a recent study has identified deep kissing as a risk factor associated with sexual transmission (127), although orogenital contact cannot be entirely ruled out (130). Saliva likely constitutes the most significant route of transmission, but other routes of infection can also occur. Virus can be detected by PCR of peripheral blood mononuclear cells (PBMCs) in approximately 50% of latently infected individuals (108), and although transmission by blood transfusion appears to be rare (131,132), organ transplantation (10,133) and to a lesser extent intravenous drug abuse (134) have been clearly associated with acquisition of new KSHV infection.

These recent studies of KSHV epidemiology have provided rapid answers relevant to disease pathogenesis; however, they have also raised additional questions that for now remain unanswered. If KSHV is ancient with origins in Africa, why is it not ubiquitous, like EBV? If KSHV is spread by a mechanism similar to other herpesviruses (saliva), then what accounts for its unusual geographic distribution? Is it much less stable? Is KSHV less able to efficiently replicate? Is this virus less contagious because the cellular target of infection is less accessible? Is

it ancient in primates, but recent in humans (109)? As infection becomes ubiquitous in Africa, what is the risk of rapid global dissemination?

Natural History

The discovery of KSHV coincident with the AIDS pandemic and accompanied by an ostensible KS epidemic led to rapid appreciation of the role of the host immune system in regulating clinical manifestations (135). All known forms of KSHV-associated (KS, MCD, and PEL) proliferative disease appear to be intimately linked to the cellular immune response. This finding is consistent with the observation that much of the human T-cell repertoire is dedicated to control of latent viruses, particularly herpesviruses (5,89,110,136). However, in contrast to several other herpesvirus family members, intercurrent disease associated with KSHV appears to be unusual in the absence of very profound T-cell compromise, perhaps accounting for its comparatively delayed discovery. Similar to EBV-associated lymphoproliferative disease, it has been observed in the case of KS that subtle and transient improvements in cellular immune function can produce regression of lesions, as noted in transplant patients in whom immunosuppression can be tapered (103) and in AIDS patients who receive HAART (137,138).

The long-term risk for developing KS varies with the seroprevalence of KSHV and with the cellular immune status of the population under study (16). In untreated patients co-infected with HIV and KSHV, the likelihood of developing AIDS-associated KS within 10 years was 35% (139,140). Patients who became infected with KSHV before HIV were less likely to develop disease than patients who were infected with HIV first (135,141). Coordinate with the African HIV epidemic, KS has become the most common malignancy of men (accounting for 50% of male malignancies) and second most common malignancy of women and children in parts of Africa (17,18,101,112,142). In HIV-negative patients from areas of intermediate seroprevalence (35%), such as Sardinia and Sicily, the prevalence of classical KS per 100,000 population was 3.2 for men and 0.77 for women. Thus, disease is rare (143,144). The risk of developing KS in the solid organ transplant setting is relatively high (0.5%–5%, depending on geographic location and seroprevalence) (145,146), whether the patient is already seropositive for KSHV or acquires disease at the time of transplantation. The risk for developing KS is greatest 3 to 124 months (median 30 months) after transplantation (147,148).

The plasmablastic variant of MCD and PEL are both inordinately rare malignancies that can occur together with KS (149–152) or with each other (153) and have primarily been observed among patients infected with HIV.

Recent data suggest that primary and additional reactivation syndromes associated with KSHV exist. Aggressive KS of infancy had been observed in young children in Africa predating the AIDS epidemic, and in retrospect it is suspected that this form of KS may identify children with congenital T-cell deficiency (17,154,155). Transient angiolymphoid hyperlasia has been reported in an HIV-positive patient during primary infection (156). More recently, two cases of bone marrow aplasia with plasmacytosis have been reported in association with KSHV infection, one in a renal transplant recipient after primary infection and one in an autologous bone marrow transplant patient known to be seropositive (10). In each case, other viral causes of bone marrow aplasia were ruled out, and KSHV-positive precursor cells were observed in the bone marrow (10).

The natural history of KSHV infection in the immunocompetent host is not yet known. A limited study of HIV-seronegative men suggested that primary infection in adults was associated with fatigue, diarrhea, rash, and lymphadenopathy (8). A study of children (1–4 years old) in Egypt, where seroprevalence is high, showed that 42% of children presenting to an emergency department with fever of unclear etiology were already KSHV antibody positive (9). Contact with greater than two other children in the community was significantly associated with seroconversion. New development of antibody was convincingly documented in 3 of 86 children, and all 3 presented febrile, without adenopathy, but with a craniocaudal maculopapular rash and symptoms of upper respiratory tract infection. Disease manifestations were self-limited, and based on the high seroprevalence in this population, the researchers speculated that most disease acquired in childhood may be asymptomatic (157).

Spectrum of Disease

KAPOSI'S SARCOMA

All forms of KS are associated with KSHV infection. The disease has been classified into four major types, namely classical KS, endemic (African) KS, AIDS-associated KS, and transplant KS (16,101). Whereas classical KS is usually an indolent disease manifest by cutaneous lesions on the lower extremities, the forms of KS associated with profound immunosuppression may be extremely aggressive and involve multiple visceral organs and lymph nodes in addition to skin and mucous membranes (143,158). Indirect markers of profound T-cell compromise such as high plasma virus load and high lytic antibody titers are documented to predict the onset of frank KS in the setting of HIV infection (128). However, the clinical manifestations even of advanced disease may spontaneously wane when T-cell function is restored (103). These observations are underscored by the striking decrease of KS in Western countries after the introduction of HAART (138,139). Increases in CD4 and CD8 T-cell populations and in CD8$^+$ spot-forming cells with specificity for K8.1 and K12 has been associated with control of KS among patients receiving HAART (5,159).

KS lesions are complex, vascular, and consist of multiple cell types. Spindle-shaped cells probably derived from precursors of lymphatic endothelium contain viral genomes and form the major component of the tumor. While most cells express a latent program, a small percentage of these cells (~1%) appear to be lytically infected (160–162). A robust inflammatory cell infiltrate is routinely present, and monocytes/macrophages may also be lytically infected (64,163). Many inflammatory cytokines can be detected in the local milieu, and these are believed to exert direct effects on initiation and maintenance of infection in endothelial cells (64). The absence of specific inflammatory cytokines and the cells that produce them *in vitro* may provide an explanation for the inability of these cells to maintain virus infection in tissue culture systems. The clonality of KS has been much debated (7). That is, does the tumor arise from a single transformed cell or are the proliferating cells oligo- or polyclonal (164)? Despite analysis of both X chromosome inactivation patterns and viral terminal repeat sequences (91,165–167), the issue remains to be resolved. When disease progresses to more advanced stages (i.e., from patch stage to plaque stage to nodular stage), the tumor mass is more clearly monoclonal (91,168). Based on these observations it has been suggested that, as in the case of EBV lymphoproliferative disease, clonal evolution can occur *in vivo* as cells that develop secondary genetic events that enhance proliferation and survival are selected (91).

PRIMARY EFFUSION LYMPHOMA

Primary effusion lymphomas, also known as body cavity–based lymphomas (BCBLs), are unusual neoplasms in which mono-clonal B-lymphocytes proliferate in effusion fluid and occasionally in the peripheral blood (12,169–171). In contrast to other lymphomas, the tumor rarely forms solid masses or causes significant lymphadenopathy. PELS are uniformly KSHV positive, and the majority (70%) are also EBV positive—the first example of a dually infected virus-associated human neoplasm (12,170). The cells are latently infected, and compared with KS spindle cells, derived lines contain a high viral copy number (20–200 genomes per cell) (172,173). When present, EBV is also in a latent state and few viral proteins can be detected. The cells express minimal B-cell activation markers or B-cell adhesion proteins, although they are HLA class II and CD30 positive (169). The phenotype observed is most consistent with a near terminally differentiated B cell, and accordingly tumor cells express the late B-cell differentiation marker CD138/syndecan-1 (174). The B-cell receptor (BCR) is rearranged and somatic mutations are present, which is also consistent with a late stage of B-cell differentiation (175). Common translocations and rearrangements associated with B-cell malignancies have not been identified (169), although frequent mutations in the 5'-untranslated region of the silent Bcl-6 gene have been found (176). Most but not all PELS occur in patients with AIDS, and advanced immunocompromise is associated with disease (170). In these patients, PELS respond poorly to therapy, and death within 5 to 7 month is common (169). Despite the aggressive behavior and monoclonal nature of this tumor, however, spontaneous remissions have sometimes been observed in the setting of rapid immune reconstitution (177).

MULTICENTRIC CASTLEMAN'S DISEASE

Multicentric Castleman's disease was the third major proliferative disorder found to be associated with KSHV infection (13,178). Although considered a reactive lymphadenopathy rather than a bonafide malignancy, MCD is associated with subsequent development of non-Hodgkin's lymphoma and KS (179–181). IL-6 is believed to be a major mediator of disease pathogenesis (182,183). MCD occurs as two major variants (180,184), a hyaline vascular variant that is not KSHV infected and a plasmablastic variant that is (185,186). HIV-associated MCD is almost always KSHV infected, and in normal hosts about 40% to 50% of MCD contains virus (187). Plasmablastic MCD is often accompanied by hyperglobulinemia and autoimmune hemolytic anemia (180,188) and can progress to frank plasmablastic lymphoma (186).

Although both PEL and MCD result from KSHV infection of B-lymphocytes in the setting of HIV infection and profound immunocompromise, the immunobiology of the two diseases is distinct. In contrast to PEL, MCD is characterized by greatly enlarged lymph nodes in which plasmablast-like cells localize to the mantle zone of germinal centers, where they proliferate in small clusters, sometimes forming areas referred to as microlymphomas (186). Both vIL-6 and cellular IL-6 are enriched in the local environment and are believed to contribute to the proliferation of KSHV-infected and -uninfected B cells (183,188). Remarkably, although the B-lymphocytes have the appearance of differentiated plasmablasts, genetic studies reveal that these KSHV-infected cells are rich in cytoplasmic immunoglobulin M and that they that lack evidence of class switching or somatic mutation, indicating the absence of typical B-cell maturation (84). Moreover, the virus-infected cells appear to express only λ light chain, a unique observation among all B-cell malignancies and proliferative disorders (84). This suggests that rapid phenotypic maturation, perhaps driven by IL-6/vIL-6, is not accompanied by genetic differentiation. The clinical behavior of MCD is similarly atypical. On the basis of histopathology MCD is the least tumorigenic of KSHV-associated lesions and is classified as a reactive hyperplasia rather than neoplasia. Disease usually

TABLE 232.4.   Clinical Spectrum of Kaposi's Sarcoma–Associated Herpesvirus Infection

Primary infection syndromes
  Asymptomatic Infection
  Fever and rash (? upper respiratory tract infection, diarrhea, lymphadenopathy)
  Bone marrow aplasia (cytopenia with plasmacytosis)
  Angiolymphoid hyperplasia
  Runaway (rapidly disseminated) Kaposi's sarcoma
Reactivated infection syndromes
  Fever and rash (? hepatitis)
  Bone marrow aplasia (cytopenia with plasmacytosis)
  Kaposi's sarcoma
    Classical
    Endemic
    Transplant-associated
    AIDS-associated
  Multicentric Castleman's disease (plasmablastic variant)
  Plasmablastic lymphoma
  Primary effusion lymphoma
  Other lymphomas (rare)?

AIDS, acquired immunodeficiency syndrome.

progresses to death within 2 years of diagnosis. HAART therapy and immune reconstitution seldom modify the clinical course of MCD (186,189). See Table 232.4 (9,10,16,101,156,190) for a review of the spectrum of disease.

The Role of Other Viruses in KSHV-Associated Disease

One of the most interesting features of KSHV infection is evidence that infection with other viruses and expression of their respective gene products may play a significant role in the development of KSHV-associated disease. EBV, CMV, and HIV have all been implicated as potential copathogens. As noted, EBV is present along with KSHV in the majority of PELs (reviewed in reference 170). EBV alone is not associated with PEL, although KSHV alone may be (68). Both infections are latent, and EBV gene expression is limited to expression of EBNA-1 and EBV-encoded small nuclear RNA (EBERs) (small nonpolyadenylated RNAs), with low detection of LMP1 and LMP2A, consistent with restricted latency (type 2 or a mixture of types 1 and 2) (191,192). EBV-infected B-lymphoblastoid cell lines are not readily infected with KSHV (16). It has been suggested that viral gene products can directly interact (193,194). The advantage conferred by co-infection is not currently understood.

Active CMV infection is also reported to have a significant effect on KSHV replication and the development of KS. Both indirect (immunomodulatory) and direct effects have been proposed. *In vivo* high levels of CMV replication are associated with and may further exacerbate T-cell suppression, increasing the risk for EBV lymphoproliferative disease and other opportunistic infections (195). In a cohort of AIDS patients with CMV retinitis, effective ganciclovir prophylaxis was noted to also decrease the expected incidence of KS, presumably though control of CMV replication, although drug effects on KSHV-infected cells may also have contributed (196). *In vitro*, CMV co-infection of KSHV-infected cells can stimulate lytic replication of KSHV (197); however, whether relevant cells *in vivo* are likely to be co-infected and contribute significantly to disease remains to be established.

Although T-cell suppression predicts all forms of KS, the inordinately aggressive course of AIDS KS has raised suspicion that factors in addition to immunosuppression may affect the natural history of the disease (164). Because the cytokine-rich environment generated within KS lesions may be integral to the pathogenesis of disease and due to the similarity of HIV tat protein to inflammatory cytokines (198–200), a direct role for tat has been proposed in stimulating angiogenesis (reviewed in references 44, 201, and 202), and in the proliferation and survival (203,204) of endothelial cells in KS. In addition, several *in vitro* studies have shown direct effects of purified tat (205,206) or other HIV proteins (207) on KSHV replication, potentially increasing the likelihood of KS development. HIV neither co-infects KS spindle cells nor is HIV significantly present in the microenvironment of KS lesions, although local detection of tat has been reported in some studies (208). The physiologic relevance of these observations still remains to be established.

Diagnosis and Detection

The diagnosis of KS is usually made on the basis of pathologic examination of biopsy specimens from a patient that presents with skin, mucous membrane, lymph node, or visceral (including pulmonary) mass lesions detected by physical examination or imaging techniques. The diagnosis is based on demonstration of classic histopathologic features. MCD is similarly diagnosed on the basis of presentation with a characteristic constellation of symptoms including fever and lymphadenopathy, followed by lymph node biopsy and detection of plasmablastic foci in the mantle zone surrounding germinal centers. PEL is usually diagnosed on the basis of pathologic examination of pleural fluid, ascites, or occasionally solid tumor masses and demonstration of a monoclonal neoplastic B-cell population with a typical cell surface phenotype. Because a patient with one form of KSHV-associated disease may also have another form of disease (149–153) careful investigation to assess whether concurrent disease is present is warranted.

Because KSHV can be detected in all of these lesions, there is increasing utilization of molecular diagnostic techniques, including PCR, DNA and RNA *in situ* hybridization, and various immunohistochemical techniques to demonstrate viral antigens such as LANA in the tumor tissue. Clinical laboratory variation in the use of these techniques, however, is considerable.

Serologic documentation of KSHV infection can help to assure the correct diagnosis has been made, particularly in populations where the seroprevalence is low. Serologic assays have not been entirely standardized. At present, for optimal assessment of the antibody status it is recommended that both latent and lytic antigen binding assays be performed, because the combined tests will detect antibody in more than 90% of infected immunocompetent individuals. Most latent detection assays involve detection of LANA (ORF 73) expressed from PEL cell lines by indirect immunofluorescent assay (IFA). Lytic antibody detection assays are more variable. The highly immunogenic lytic proteins characterized to date include those encoded by K8.1, ORF 26, and ORF 65. Assay techniques detecting antibody to these antigens by IFA, enzyme-linked immunosorbent assay (ELISA), and immunoblot have been developed using either lytically induced PEL cell lines or recombinant synthetic proteins. In general, LANA assays have proved more specific, whereas the lytic antigen assays have higher sensitivity (~80% vs. 95%) (reviewed in references 7 and 98), although cross-reactivity can be a problem (209). An ELISA that detects recombinant ORFs 65 and K8.1A is reported to be highly concordant with LANA detection (101).

In patients who are known to be infected with KSHV and who are at risk for KS, an increasing KSHV load in PBMCs and elevation of antibody titers, particularly titers to lytic antigens, have been shown to predict the onset or recurrence of disease (128,210,211). However, in very advanced AIDS, antibody responses may be blunted (15). High viral DNA loads are also reported to correlate with exacerbation of MCD (212,213). The utilization of viral load and serology to predict and to follow disease, particularly in the seropositive and immunocompromised host, is not routine but may become so in the future (214).

Treatment

As with the other members of the herpesvirus family, persistent (latent) KSHV infection cannot be eliminated. Immune reconstitution (HAART, withdrawal of immunosuppressive drugs) without specific tumor-directed therapy can in some cases lead to regression of KS and PEL (103,138,177,215), whereas MCD appears to be more resistant (186,189). The massive lymphadenopathy characteristic of MCD may transiently respond to steroids and chemotherapeutic regimens used for lymphoma and myeloma (180), but durable responses are rare. Antibodies to IL-6 have been reported to alleviate symptoms of fever and malaise when used on a research basis (16,216,217). Based on the rationale that a lytic component contributes to many lesions, phosphorylated antivirals such as cidofovir have been used as well (218). KSHV thymidine kinase and protein kinase phosphorylate guanine nucleoside analogs (ganciclovir, acyclovir) poorly if at all, although thymidine nucleoside analogs such as azidothymidine (AZT) hold promise (219,220). Recently anti-CD20 antibody (rituximab) therapy was reported to produce a prolonged remission in a patient who had failed to achieve a therapeutic response with combined chemotherapy, antiviral, and anti–IL-6 therapy, as well as HAART (218).

PELs can similarly be treated with B lymphoma chemotherapy (221,222) and transient responses maintained if accompanied by immune reconstitution (177). PELS do not typically express CD20, although some variation has been seen (223). Experimental studies are in progress with interferon-α and high-dose AZT (224) or cidofovir (221), potentially more benign and specific forms of therapy.

Treatment of KS varies with the stage and degree of dissemination of disease and the immunologic competence of the host. Several therapeutic options are available (reviewed in references 101, 225, and 226). Limited lesions of the skin can be treated with excision, radiation, intralesional interferon-α2b, topical aliretinoin gel, intralesional vinblastine, or laser or cryotherapy. Aggressive nodular lesions and visceral disease may respond to liposomal anthracyclines (doxirubicin and daunorubicin) and paclitaxel. Oral etoposide can be effective. Long-term remissions with prolonged administration of interferon-α2b (subcutaneous, intravenous, and intramuscular) in HIV-positive and HIV-negative patients even with advanced disease (227) have been reported. Antiangiogenic drugs such as thalidomide and COL-3 can be used. Many new approaches are under investigation for treatment of the various KSHV-associated proliferative disorders, including agents that target viral genes as well as cellular genes involved in the pathogenesis of disease such as NF-κB (29).

Prevention

Several studies have documented that an increasing KSHV load in plasma and increasing titers to lytic antigens predict an increased risk for developing KS. Responses to therapy and recurrences can also be monitored in this manner. However, definitive studies to determine whether and which form of prophylactic antiviral therapy may be indicated remain to be performed (101,219). Novel cell-based immune therapies (i.e., cytotoxic lymphocyte infusions) may also be used in the future (159).

Progress has been inordinately rapid in the short time since the 1994 discovery of KSHV. The entire genome was sequenced in less than 2 years. Many viral genes have been characterized and an understanding of virus epidemiology developed. However, there is still no cell culture system that adequately recapitulates the early events of virus infection or establishment of latency, or mimics the lesions of KS and MCD. Although T-cell responses are critically important for preventing disease, the specificity of those responses remains unknown. More knowledge regarding how the virus attaches to and enters cells, initiates and maintains latency, and causes immortalization and disease is needed before safe and effective immunization strategies can be developed.

ACKNOWLEDGMENTS

This research was supported by National Institutes of Health awards K24 and ROI DE12186, and by the CFAR. Dr. Fingeroth is an established investigator of the AHA.

REFERENCES

1. Chang Y, Cesarman E, Pessin MS, et al. Identification of herpesvirus-like DNA sequences in AIDS-associated Kaposi's sarcoma [see comments]. *Science* 1994;266:1865–1869.
2. Roizman B, Pellett PE. The family Herpesviridae: a brief introduction. In: Knipe DM, Howley PM, eds. *Field's virology*. Philadelphia: Lippincott Williams & Wilkins, 2001:2381–2397.
3. Cohen JI. Epstein-Barr virus infection. *N Engl J Med* 2000;343:481–492.
4. Strickler HD, Goedert JJ, Bethke FR, et al. Human herpesvirus 8 cellular immune responses in homosexual men. *J Infect Dis* 1999;180:1682–1685.
5. Osman M, Kubo T, Gill J, et al. Identification of human herpesvirus 8-specific cytotoxic T-cell responses. *J Virol* 1999;73:6136–6140.
6. Wang QJ, Jenkins FJ, Jacobson LP, et al. CD8⁺ cytotoxic T lymphocyte responses to lytic proteins of human herpes virus 8 in human immunodeficiency virus type 1–infected and –uninfected individuals. *J Infect Dis* 2000;182:928–932.
7. Moore P, Chang Y. Kaposi's sarcoma–associated herpesvirus. In: Knipe DM, Howley PM, eds. *Fields virology*. Philadelphia: Lippincott-Raven, 2001:2803–2833.
8. Wang QJ, Jenkins FJ, Jacobson LP, et al. Primary human herpesvirus 8 infection generates a broadly specific CD8(+) T-cell response to viral lytic cycle proteins. *Blood* 2001;97:2366–2373.
9. Andreoni M, Sarmati L, Nicastri E, et al. Primary human herpesvirus 8 infection in immunocompetent children. *JAMA* 2002;287:1295–300.
10. Luppi M, Barozzi P, Schulz TF, et al. Bone marrow failure associated with human herpesvirus 8 infection after transplantation. *N Engl J Med* 2000;343:1378–1385.
11. Jenkins FJ, Hoffman LJ, Liegey-Dougall A. Reactivation of and primary infection with human herpesvirus 8 among solid-organ transplant recipients. *J Infect Dis* 2002;185:1238–1243.
12. Cesarman E, Chang Y, Moore PS, et al. Kaposi's sarcoma–associated herpesvirus-like DNA sequences in AIDS-related body-cavity-based lymphomas [see comments]. *N Engl J Med* 1995;332:1186–1191.
13. Soulier J, Grollet L, Oksenhendler E, et al. Kaposi's sarcoma-associated herpesvirus-like DNA sequences in multicentric Castleman's disease. *Blood* 1995;86:1276–1280.
14. McGeoch DJ. Molecular evolution of the gamma-Herpesvirinae. *Philos Trans R Soc Lond B Biol Sci* 2001;356:421–435.
15. Gao SJ, Kingsley L, Li M, et al. KSHV antibodies among Americans, Italians and Ugandans with and without Kaposi's sarcoma. *Nat Med* 1996;2:925–928.
16. Boshoff C, Weiss RA. Epidemiology and pathogenesis of Kaposi's sarcoma-associated herpesvirus. *Philos Trans R Soc Lond B Biol Sci* 2001;356:517–534.
17. Ziegler JL, Katongole-Mbidde E. Kaposi's sarcoma in childhood: an analysis of 100 cases from Uganda and relationship to HIV infection. *Int J Cancer* 1996;65:200–203.

18. Cook-Mozaffari P, Newton R, Beral V, et al. The geographical distribution of Kaposi's sarcoma and of lymphomas in Africa before the AIDS epidemic. *Br J Cancer* 1998;78:1521–1528.

19. Dayan AD, Lewis PD. Origin of Kaposi's sarcoma from the reticulo-endothelial system. *Nature* 1967;213:889–890.

20. Giraldo G, Beth E, Coeur P, et al. Kaposi's sarcoma: a new model in the search for viruses associated with human malignancies. *J Natl Cancer Inst* 1972;49:1495–1507.

21. Beurey J, Weber M, Mazet J, et al. [Association of Kaposi's sarcoma and Hodgkin's disease]. *Ann Dermatol Syphiligr* 1976;103:151–159.

22. Glaser R, Geder L, St Jeor S, et al. Partial characterization of a herpes-type virus (K9V) derived from Kaposi's sarcoma. *J Natl Cancer Inst* 1977;59:55–60.

23. Giraldo G, Beth E, Haguenau F. Herpes-type virus particles in tissue culture of Kaposi's sarcoma from different geographic regions. *J Natl Cancer Inst* 1972;49:1509–1526.

24. Jaffe HW, Choi K, Thomas PA, et al. National case-control study of Kaposi's sarcoma and *Pneumocystis carinii* pneumonia in homosexual men: Part 1. Epidemiologic results. *Ann Intern Med* 1983;99:145–151.

25. Epstein MA, Barr YM, Achong BG. Virus particles in cultured lymphoblasts from Burkitt's lymphoma. *Lancet* 1964;1:702–703.

26. Damania B, Desrosiers RC. Simian homologues of human herpesvirus 8. *Philos Trans R Soc Lond B Biol Sci* 2001;356:535–543.

27. Roizman B, Carmichael LE, Deinhardt F, et al. Herpesviridae. Definition, provisional nomenclature, and taxonomy. The Herpesvirus Study Group, the International Committee on Taxonomy of Viruses. *Intervirology* 1981;16:201–217.

28. Roizman B, Baines J. The diversity and unity of Herpesviridae. *Comp Immunol Microbiol Infect Dis* 1991;14:63–79.

29. Keller SA, Schattner EJ, Cesarman E. Inhibition of NF-kappaB induces apoptosis of KSHV-infected primary effusion lymphoma cells. *Blood* 2000;96:2537–2542.

30. Liu L, Eby MT, Rathore N, et al. The human herpes virus 8-encoded viral FLICE inhibitory protein physically associates with and persistently activates the Ikappa B kinase complex. *J Biol Chem* 2002;277:13745–13751.

31. An J, Lichtenstein AK, Brent G, et al. The Kaposi sarcoma–associated herpesvirus (KSHV) induces cellular interleukin 6 expression: role of the KSHV latency-associated nuclear antigen and the AP1 response element. *Blood* 2002;99:649–654.

32. Kieff E, Rickinson AB. Epstein-Barr virus and its replication. In: Knipe DM, Howley PM, eds. *Fields virology*. Philadelphia: Lippincott Williams & Wilkins, 2001:2511–2573.

33. Nicholas J. Non-conserved proteins of human herpesvirus-8: their possible roles in virus biology and pathogenesis. *Epstein-Barr Virus Report* 2001;8:137–149.

34. Choi J, Means RE, Damania B, et al. Molecular piracy of Kaposi's sarcoma associated herpesvirus. *Cytokine Growth Factor Rev* 2001;12:245–257.

35. Speck SH, Strominger JL. Analysis of the transcript encoding the latent Epstein-Barr virus nuclear antigen I: a potentially polycistronic message generated by long-range splicing of several exons. *Proc Natl Acad Sci U S A* 1985;82:8305–8309.

36. Greensill J, Schulz TF. Rhabdinoviruses (gamma2-herpesviruses) of Old World primates: models for KSHV/HHV8-associated disease? *AIDS* 2000;14(suppl):11–19.

37. Schultz ER, Rankin GW Jr, Blanc MP, et al. Characterization of two divergent lineages of macaque rhabdinoviruses related to Kaposi's sarcoma-associated herpesvirus. *J Virol* 2000;74:4919–4928.

38. Renne R, Zhong W, Herndier B, et al. Lytic growth of Kaposi's sarcoma-associated herpesvirus (human herpesvirus 8) in culture. *Nat Med* 1996;2:342–346.

39. Orenstein JM, Alkan S, Blauvelt A, et al. Visualization of human herpesvirus type 8 in Kaposi's sarcoma by light and transmission electron microscopy. *AIDS* 1997;11:F35–F45.

40. Wang FZ, Akula SM, Pramod NP, et al. Human herpesvirus 8 envelope glycoprotein K8.1A interaction with the target cells involves heparan sulfate. *J Virol* 2001;75:7517–7527.

41. Birkmann A, Mahr K, Ensser A, et al. Cell surface heparan sulfate is a receptor for human herpesvirus 8 and interacts with envelope glycoprotein K8.1. *J Virol* 2001;75:11583–11593.

42. Akula SM, Pramod NP, Wang FZ, et al. Human herpesvirus 8 envelope-associated glycoprotein B interacts with heparan sulfate-like moieties. *Virology* 2001;284:235–249.

43. Pertel PE. Human herpesvirus 8 glycoprotein B (gB), gH, and gL can mediate cell fusion. *J Virol* 2002;76:4390–4400.

44. Dezube BJ, Zambela M, Sage DR, et al. Characterization of Kaposi sarcoma-associated herpesvirus/human herpesvirus-8 infection of human vascular endothelial cells:early events. *Blood* 2002;100:888–896.

45. Lagunoff M, Ganem D. The structure and coding organization of the genomic termini of Kaposi's sarcoma-associated herpesvirus. *Virology* 1997;236:147–154.

46. Lukac DM, Renne R, Kirshner JR, et al. Reactivation of Kaposi's sarcoma-associated herpesvirus infection from latency by expression of the ORF 50 transactivator, a homolog of the EBV R protein. *Virology* 1998;252:304–312.

47. Lukac DM, Kirshner JR, Ganem D. Transcriptional activation by the product of open reading frame 50 of Kaposi's sarcoma-associated herpesvirus is required for lytic viral reactivation in B cells. *J Virol* 1999;73:9348–9361.

48. Sun R, Lin SF, Staskus K, et al. Kinetics of Kaposi's sarcoma-associated herpesvirus gene expression. *J Virol* 1999;73:2232–2242.

49. Gradoville L, Gerlach J, Grogan E, et al. Kaposi's sarcoma–associated herpesvirus open reading frame 50/Rta protein activates the entire viral lytic cycle in the HH-B2 primary effusion lymphoma cell line. *J Virol* 2000;74:6207–6212.

50. Nicholas J, Zong JC, Alcendor DJ, et al. Novel organizational features, captured cellular genes, and strain variability within the genome of KSHV/HHV8. *J Natl Cancer Inst Monogr* 1998;23:79–88.

51. Zong JC, Ciufo DM, Alcendor DJ, et al. High-level variability in the ORF-K1 membrane protein gene at the left end of the Kaposi's sarcoma–associated herpesvirus genome defines four major virus subtypes and multiple variants or clades in different human populations. *J Virol* 1999;73:4156–70.

52. Meng YX, Sata T, Stamey FR, et al. Molecular characterization of strains of Human herpesvirus 8 from Japan, Argentina and Kuwait. *J Gen Virol* 2001;82:499–506.

53. Zong J, Ciufo DM, Viscidi R, et al. Genotypic analysis at multiple loci across Kaposi's sarcoma herpesvirus (KSHV) DNA molecules: clustering patterns, novel variants and chimerism. *J Clin Virol* 2002;23:119–148.

54. Renne R, Blackbourn D, Whitby D, et al. Limited transmission of Kaposi's sarcoma-associated herpesvirus in cultured cells. *J Virol* 1998;72:5182–5188.

55. Flore O, Rafii S, Ely S, et al. Transformation of primary human endothelial cells by Kaposi's sarcoma–associated herpesvirus. *Nature* 1998;394:588–592.

56. Panyutich EA, Said JW, Miles SA. Infection of primary dermal microvascular endothelial cells by Kaposi's sarcoma–associated herpesvirus. *AIDS* 1998;12:467–472.

57. Moses AV, Fish KN, Ruhl R, et al. Long-term infection and transformation of dermal microvascular endothelial cells by human herpesvirus 8. *J Virol* 1999;73:6892–6902.

58. Blackbourn DJ, Lennette E, Klencke B, et al. The restricted cellular host range of human herpesvirus 8. *AIDS* 2000;14:1123–1133.

59. Cerimele F, Curreli F, Ely S, et al. Kaposi's sarcoma-associated herpesvirus can productively infect primary human keratinocytes and alter their growth properties. *J Virol* 2001;75:2435–2443.

60. Sakurada S, Katano H, Sata T, et al. Effective human herpesvirus 8 infection of human umbilical vein endothelial cells by cell-mediated transmission. *J Virol* 2001;75:7717–7722.

61. Ciufo DM, Cannon JS, Poole LJ, et al. Spindle cell conversion by Kaposi's sarcoma-associated herpesvirus: formation of colonies and plaques with mixed lytic and latent gene expression in infected primary dermal microvascular endothelial cell cultures. *J Virol* 2001;75:5614–5626.

62. Lagunoff M, Bechtel J, Venetsanakos E, et al. *De novo* infection and serial transmission of Kaposi's sarcoma–associated herpesvirus in cultured endothelial cells. *J Virol* 2002;76:2440–2448.

63. Flamand L, Zeman RA, Bryant JL, et al. Absence of human herpesvirus 8 DNA sequences in neoplastic Kaposi's sarcoma cell lines. *J Acquir Immune Defic Syndr Hum Retrovirol* 1996;13:194–197.

64. Ensoli B, Sturzl M, Monini P. Reactivation and role of HHV-8 in Kaposi's sarcoma initiation. *Adv Cancer Res* 2001;81:161–200.

65. Li M, MacKey J, Czajak SC, et al. Identification and characterization of Kaposi's sarcoma–associated herpesvirus K8.1 virion glycoprotein. *J Virol* 1999;73:1341–1349.

66. Chandran B, Bloomer C, Chan SR, et al. Human herpesvirus-8 ORF K8.1 gene encodes immunogenic glycoproteins generated by spliced transcripts. *Virology* 1998;249:140–149.

67. Akula SM, Pramod NP, Wang FZ, et al. Integrin alpha3beta1 (CD 49c/29) is a cellular receptor for Kaposi's sarcoma–associated herpesvirus (KSHV/HHV-8) entry into the target cells. *Cell* 2002;108:407–419.

68. Arvanitakis L, Mesri EA, Nador RG, et al. Establishment and characterization of a primary effusion (body cavity–based) lymphoma cell line (BC-3) harboring Kaposi's sarcoma–associated herpesvirus (KSHV/HHV-8) in the absence of Epstein-Barr virus. *Blood* 1996;88:2648–2654.

69. Said W, Chien K, Takeuchi S, et al. Kaposi's sarcoma–associated herpesvirus (KSHV or HHV8) in primary effusion lymphoma: ultrastructural demonstration of herpesvirus in lymphoma cells. *Blood* 1996;87:4937–4943.

70. Sarid R, Flore O, Bohenzky RA, et al. Transcription mapping of the Kaposi's sarcoma-associated herpesvirus (human herpesvirus 8) genome in a body cavity–based lymphoma cell line (BC-1). *J Virol* 1998;72:1005–1012.

71. Sarid R, Wiezorek JS, Moore PS, et al. Characterization and cell cycle regulation of the major Kaposi's sarcoma–associated herpesvirus (human herpesvirus 8) latent genes and their promoter. *J Virol* 1999;73:1438–1446.

72. Parravicini C, Chandran B, Corbellino M, et al. Differential viral protein expression in Kaposi's sarcoma–associated herpesvirus-infected diseases: Kaposi's sarcoma, primary effusion lymphoma, and multicentric Castleman's disease. *Am J Pathol* 2000;156:743–749.

73. Jenner RG, Alba MM, Boshoff C, et al. Kaposi's sarcoma–associated herpesvirus latent and lytic gene expression as revealed by DNA arrays. *J Virol* 2001;75:891–902.

74. Staskus KA, Zhong W, Gebhard K, et al. Kaposi's sarcoma–associated herpesvirus gene expression in endothelial (spindle) tumor cells. *J Virol* 1997;71:715–719.

75. Jenner RG, Boshoff C. The molecular pathology of Kaposi's sarcoma–associated herpesvirus. *Biochim Biophys Acta* 2002;1602:1–22.

76. Rivas C, Thlick AE, Parravicini C, et al. Kaposi's sarcoma–associated herpesvirus LANA2 is a B-cell-specific latent viral protein that inhibits p53. *J Virol* 2001;75:429–438.

77. Fakhari FD, Dittmer DP. Charting latency transcripts in Kaposi's sarcoma–associated herpesvirus by whole-genome real-time quantitative PCR. *J Virol* 2002;76:6213–6223.

78. Sharp TV, Wang HW, Koumi A, et al. K15 protein of Kaposi's sarcoma–associated herpesvirus is latently expressed and binds to HAX-1, a protein with antiapoptotic function. *J Virol* 2002;76:802–816.

79. Muralidhar S, Pumfery AM, Hassani M, et al. Identification of kaposin (open reading frame K12) as a human herpesvirus 8 (Kaposi's sarcoma–associated herpesvirus) transforming gene. *J Virol* 1998;72:4980–4988.

80. Sadler R, Wu L, Forghani B, et al. A complex translational program generates multiple novel proteins from the latently expressed kaposin (K12) locus of Kaposi's sarcoma–associated herpesvirus. *J Virol* 1999;73:5722–5730.

81. Yu Y, Black JB, Goldsmith CS, et al. Induction of human herpesvirus-8 DNA replication and transcription by butyrate and TPA in BCBL-1 cells. *J Gen Virol* 1999;80:83–90.

82. Staskus KA, Sun R, Miller G, et al. Cellular tropism and viral interleukin-6 expression distinguish human herpesvirus 8 involvement in Kaposi's sarcoma, primary effusion lymphoma, and multicentric Castleman's disease. *J Virol* 1999;73:4181–4187.

83. Dittmer D, Lagunoff M, Renne R, et al. A cluster of latently expressed genes in Kaposi's sarcoma–associated herpesvirus. *J Virol* 1998;72:8309–8315.

84. Du MQ, Liu H, Diss TC, et al. Kaposi sarcoma–associated herpesvirus infects monotypic (IgM lambda) but polyclonal naive B cells in Castleman disease and associated lymphoproliferative disorders. *Blood* 2001;97:2130–2136.

85. Cannon JS, Nicholas J, Orenstein JM, et al. Heterogeneity of viral IL-6 expression in HHV-8–associated diseases. *J Infect Dis* 1999;180:824–828.

86. Aoki Y, Yarchoan R, Braun J, et al. Viral and cellular cytokines in AIDS-related malignant lymphomatous effusions. *Blood* 2000;96:1599–1601.

87. Brousset P, Cesarman E, Meggetto F, et al. Colocalization of the viral interleukin-6 with latent nuclear antigen-1 of human herpesvirus-8 in endothelial spindle cells of Kaposi's sarcoma and lymphoid cells of multicentric Castleman's disease. *Hum Pathol* 2001;32:95–100.

88. Menke DM, Chadbum A, Cesarman E, et al. Analysis of the human herpesvirus 8 (HHV-8) genome and HHV-8 vIL-6 expression in archival cases of Castleman disease at low risk for HIV infection. *Am J Clin Pathol* 2002;117:268–275.

89. Cesarman E. The role of Kaposi's sarcoma–associated herpesvirus (KSHV/HHV-8) in lymphoproliferative diseases. *Recent Results Cancer Res* 2002;159:27–37.

90. Chung YH, Means RE, Choi JK, et al. Kaposi's sarcoma–associated herpesvirus OX2 glycoprotein activates myeloid-lineage cells to induce inflammatory cytokine production. *J Virol* 2002;76:4688–4698.

91. Judde JG, Lacoste V, Briere J, et al. Monoclonality or oligoclonality of human herpesvirus 8 terminal repeat sequences in Kaposi's sarcoma and other diseases. *J Natl Cancer Inst* 2000;92:729–736.

92. Sturzl M, Zietz C, Monini P, et al. Human herpesvirus-8 and Kaposi's sarcoma: relationship with the multistep concept of tumorigenesis. *Adv Cancer Res* 2001;81:125–159.

93. Kedes DH, Operskalski E, Busch M, et al. The seroepidemiology of human herpesvirus 8 (Kaposi's sarcoma–associated herpesvirus): distribution of infection in KS risk groups and evidence for sexual transmission. *Nat Med* 1996;2:918–924.

94. Miller G, Rigsby MO, Heston L, et al. Antibodies to butyrate-inducible antigens of Kaposi's sarcoma–associated herpesvirus in patients with HIV-1 infection. *N Engl J Med* 1996;334:1292–1297.

95. Simpson GR, Schulz TF, Whitby D, et al. Prevalence of Kaposi's sarcoma associated herpesvirus infection measured by antibodies to recombinant capsid protein and latent immunofluorescence antigen. *Lancet* 1996;348:1133–1138.

96. Lennette ET, Blackbourn DJ, Levy JA. Antibodies to human herpesvirus type 8 in the general population and in Kaposi's sarcoma patients. *Lancet* 1996;348:858–861.

97. Spira TJ, Lam L, Dollard SC, et al. Comparison of serologic assays and PCR for diagnosis of human herpesvirus 8 infection. *J Clin Microbiol* 2000;38:2174–2180.

98. Schatz O, Monini P, Bugarini R, et al. Kaposi's sarcoma–associated herpesvirus serology in Europe and Uganda: multicentre study with multiple and novel assays. *J Med Virol* 2001;65:123–132.

99. Sitas F, Carrara H, Beral V, et al. Antibodies against human herpesvirus 8 in black South African patients with cancer [see comments]. *N Engl J Med* 1999;340:1863–1871.

100. Osmond DH, Buchbinder S, Cheng A, et al. Prevalence of Kaposi sarcoma–associated herpesvirus infection in homosexual men at beginning of and during the HIV epidemic. *JAMA* 2002;287:221–225.

101. Antman K, Chang Y. Kaposi's sarcoma. *N Engl J Med* 2000;342:1027–1038.

102. Penn I. Kaposi's sarcoma in organ transplant recipients: report of 20 cases. *Transplantation* 1979;27:8–11.

103. Doutrelepont JM, De Pauw L, Gruber SA, et al. Renal transplantation exposes patients with previous Kaposi's sarcoma to a high risk of recurrence. *Transplantation* 1996;62:463–466.

104. O'Brien TR, Kedes D, Ganem D, et al. Evidence for concurrent epidemics of human herpesvirus 8 and human immunodeficiency virus type 1 in US homosexual men: rates, risk factors, and relationship to Kaposi's sarcoma. *J Infect Dis* 1999;180:1010–1017.

105. Goedert JJ. The epidemiology of acquired immunodeficiency syndrome malignancies. *Semin Oncol* 2000;27:390–401.

106. Beral V, Peterman TA, Berkelman RL, et al. Kaposi's sarcoma among persons with AIDS: a sexually transmitted infection? [see comments]. *Lancet* 1990;335:123–128.

107. Rabkin CS, Goedert JJ, Biggar RJ, et al. Kaposi's sarcoma in three HIV-1-infected cohorts. *J Acquir Immune Defic Syndr Hum Retrovirol* 1990;3: S38–43.

108. Whitby D, Howard MR, Tenant-Flowers M, et al. Detection of Kaposi sarcoma associated herpesvirus in peripheral blood of HIV-infected individuals and progression to Kaposi's sarcoma. *Lancet* 1995;346:799–802.

109. Moore PS. The emergence of Kaposi's sarcoma–associated herpesvirus (human herpesvirus 8). *N Engl J Med* 2000;343:1411–1413.

110. Kieff E, Rickinson AB. Epstein-Barr virus. In: Knipe DM, Howley PM, eds. *Field's virology.* Philadelphia: Lippincott Williams & Wilkins, 2001:2575–2627.

111. Hayward GS. KSHV strains: the origins and global spread of the virus. *Semin Cancer Biol* 1999;9:187–199.

112. Thomas JO. Acquired immunodeficiency syndrome-associated cancers in Sub-Saharan Africa. *Semin Oncol* 2001;28:198–206.

113. de-The G, Bestetti G, van Beveren M, et al. Prevalence of human herpesvirus 8 infection before the acquired immunodeficiency disease syndrome–related epidemic of Kaposi's sarcoma in East Africa. *J Natl Cancer Inst* 1999;91:1888–1889.

114. Olsen SJ, Chang Y, Moore PS, et al. Increasing Kaposi's sarcoma–associated herpesvirus seroprevalence with age in a highly Kaposi's sarcoma endemic region, Zambia in 1985. *AIDS* 1998;12:1921–1925.

115. He J, Bhat G, Kankasa C, et al. Seroprevalence of human herpesvirus 8 among Zambian women of childbearing age without Kaposi's sarcoma (KS) and mother-child pairs with KS. *J Infect Dis* 1998;178:1787–1790.

116. Gessain A, Mauclere P, van Beveren M, et al. Human herpesvirus 8 primary infection occurs during childhood in Cameroon, Central Africa. *Int J Cancer* 1999;81:189–192.

117. Andreoni M, El-Sawaf G, Rezza G, et al. High seroprevalence of antibodies to human herpesvirus-8 in Egyptian children: evidence of nonsexual transmission. *J Natl Cancer Inst* 1999;91:465–469.

118. Wilkinson D, Sheldon J, Gilks CF, et al. Prevalence of infection with human herpesvirus 8/Kaposi's sarcoma herpesvirus in rural South Africa. *S Afr Med J* 1999;89:554–557.

119. Rezza G, Tchangmena OB, Andreoni M, et al. Prevalence and risk factors for human herpesvirus 8 infection in northern Cameroon. *Sex Transm Dis* 2000;27:159–164.

120. Wawer MJ, Eng SM, Serwadda D, et al. Prevalence of Kaposi sarcoma–associated herpesvirus compared with selected sexually transmitted diseases in adolescents and young adults in rural Rakai District, Uganda. *Sex Transm Dis* 2001;28:77–81.

121. Bourboulia D, Whitby D, Boshoff C, et al. Serologic evidence for mother-to-child transmission of Kaposi sarcoma–associated herpesvirus infection. *JAMA* 1998;280:31–32.

122. Plancoulaine S, Abel L, van Beveren M, et al. Human herpesvirus 8 transmission from mother to child and between siblings in an endemic population. *Lancet* 2000;356:1062–1065.

123. Koelle DM, Huang ML, Chandran B, et al. Frequent detection of Kaposi's sarcoma-associated herpesvirus (human herpesvirus 8) DNA in saliva of human immunodeficiency virus-infected men: clinical and immunologic correlates. *J Infect Dis* 1997;176:94–102.

124. Blackbourn DJ, Lennette ET, Ambroziak J, et al. Human herpesvirus 8 detection in nasal secretions and saliva. *J Infect Dis* 1998;177:213–216.

125. Lucht E, Brytting M, Bjerregaard L, et al. Shedding of cytomegalovirus and herpesviruses 6, 7, and 8 in saliva of human immunodeficiency virus type 1–infected patients and healthy controls. *Clin Infect Dis* 1998;27:137–141.

126. Sitas F, Newton R, Boshoff C. Increasing probability of mother-to-child transmission of HHV-8 with increasing maternal antibody titer for HHV-8. *N Engl J Med* 1999;340:1923.

127. Pauk J, Huang ML, Brodie SJ, et al. Mucosal shedding of human herpesvirus 8 in men. *N Engl J Med* 2000;343:1369–1377.

128. Tedeschi R, Enbom M, Bidoli E, et al. Viral load of human herpesvirus 8 in peripheral blood of human immunodeficiency virus–infected patients with Kaposi's sarcoma. *J Clin Microbiol* 2001;39:4269–4273.

129. Corey L, Brodie S, Huang ML, et al. HHV-8 infection: a model for reactivation and transmission. *Rev Med Virol* 2002;12:47–63.

130. Dukers NH, Renwick N, Prins M, et al. Risk factors for human herpesvirus 8 seropositivity and seroconversion in a cohort of homosexual men. *Am J Epidemiol* 2000;151:213–224.

131. Challine D, Roudot-Thoraval F, Sarah T, et al. Seroprevalence of human herpes virus 8 antibody in populations at high or low risk of transfusion, graft, or sexual transmission of viruses. *Transfusion* 2001;41:1120–1125.

132. Herve P. [Transfusion safety: emergent or hypothetical risks]. *Transfus Clin Biol* 2000;7:30–38.

133. Regamey N, Tamm M, Wernli M, et al. Transmission of human herpesvirus 8 infection from renal-transplant donors to recipients [see comments]. *N Engl J Med* 1998;339:1358–1363.

134. Cannon MJ, Dollard SC, Smith DK, et al. Blood-borne and sexual transmission of human herpesvirus 8 in women with or at risk for human immunodeficiency virus infection. *N Engl J Med* 2001;344:637–643.

135. Renwick N, Halaby T, Weverling GJ, et al. Seroconversion for human herpesvirus 8 during HIV infection is highly predictive of Kaposi's sarcoma. *AIDS* 1998;12:2481–2488.

136. Khanna R, Burrows SR. Role of cytotoxic T lymphocytes in Epstein-Barr virus-associated diseases. *Annu Rev Microbiol* 2000;54:19–48.

137. Gnann JW Jr, Pellett PE, Jaffe HW. Human herpesvirus 8 and Kaposi's sarcoma in persons infected with human immunodeficiency virus. *Clin Infect Dis* 2000;30(suppl 1):72–76.

138. Cattelan A, Calabro M, Gasperini P, et al. Acquired immunodeficiency syndrome-related Kaposi's sarcoma regression after highly active antiretroviral therapy: biologic correlates of clinical outcome. *J Natl Cancer Inst Monogr* 2001;28:44–49.

139. Biggar RJ, Rabkin CS. The epidemiology of AIDS-related neoplasms. *Hematol Oncol Clin North Am* 1996;10:997–1010.

140. Rezza G, Dorrucci M, Serraino D, et al. Incidence of Kaposi's sarcoma and HHV-8 seroprevalence among homosexual men with known dates of HIV seroconversion. Italian Seroconversion Study. *AIDS* 2000;14:1647–1653.

141. Jacobson LP, Jenkins FJ, Springer G, et al. Interaction of human immunodeficiency virus type 1 and human herpesvirus type 8 infections on the incidence of Kaposi's sarcoma. *J Infect Dis* 2000;181:1940–1949.

142. Wabinga HR, Parkin DM, Wabwire-Mangen F, et al. Cancer in Kampala, Uganda, in 1989–91: changes in incidence in the era of AIDS. *Int J Cancer* 1993;54:26–36.

143. Iscovich J, Boffetta P, Franceschi S, et al. Classic Kaposi sarcoma: epidemiology and risk factors. *Cancer* 2000;88:500–517.

144. Santarelli R, De Marco R, Masala MV, et al. Direct correlation between human herpesvirus-8 seroprevalence and classic Kaposi's sarcoma incidence in Northern Sardinia. *J Med Virol* 2001;65:368–372.

145. Farge D. Kaposi's sarcoma in organ transplant recipients. The Collaborative Transplantation Research Group of Ile de France. *Eur J Med* 1993;2:339–343.

146. Qunibi W, Akhtar M, Sheth K, et al. Kaposi's sarcoma: the most common tumor after renal transplantation in Saudi Arabia. *Am J Med* 1988;84:225–232.

147. Montagnino G, Bencini PL, Tarantino A, et al. Clinical features and course of Kaposi's sarcoma in kidney transplant patients: report of 13 cases. *Am J Nephrol* 1994;14:121–126.

148. Lesnoni La, Parola I, Masini C, Nanni G, et al. Kaposi's sarcoma in renal-transplant recipients: experience at the Catholic University in Rome, 1988–1996. *Dermatology* 1997;194:229–233.

149. Said JW, Tasaka T, Takeuchi S, et al. Primary effusion lymphoma in women: report of two cases of Kaposi's sarcoma herpes virus–associated effusion-based lymphoma in human immunodeficiency virus-negative women. *Blood* 1996;88:3124–3128.

150. Jones D, Ballestas ME, Kaye KM, et al. Primary-effusion lymphoma and Kaposi's sarcoma in a cardiac-transplant recipient. *N Engl J Med* 1998;339:444–449.

151. Saif MW. Castleman disease in an HIV-infected patient with Kaposi sarcoma. *AIDS Read* 2001;11:572–576.

152. Codish S, Abu-Shakra M, Ariad S, et al. Manifestations of three HHV-8-related diseases in an HIV-negative patient: immunoblastic variant multicentric Castleman's disease, primary effusion lymphoma, and Kaposi's sarcoma. *Am J Hematol* 2000;65:310–314.

153. Ascoli V, Signoretti S, Onetti-Muda A, et al. Primary effusion lymphoma in HIV-infected patients with multicentric Castleman's disease. *J Pathol* 2001;193:200–209.

154. Gigase PL. [Epidemiology of Kaposi's sarcoma in Africa]. *Bull Soc Pathol Exot Filiales* 1984;77:546–559.

155. Sanchez-Velasco P, Ocejo-Vinyals JG, Flores R, et al. Simultaneous multiorgan presence of human herpesvirus 8 and restricted lymphotropism of Epstein-Barr virus DNA sequences in a human immunodeficiency virus–negative immunodeficient infant. *J Infect Dis* 2001;183:338–342.

156. Oksenhendler E, Cazals-Hatem D, Schulz TF, et al. Transient angiolymphoid hyperplasia and Kaposi's sarcoma after primary infection with human herpesvirus 8 in a patient with human immunodeficiency virus infection. *N Engl J Med* 1998;338:1585–1590.

157. Andreoni M, Goletti D, Pezzotti P, et al. Prevalence, incidence and correlates of HHV-8/KSHV infection and Kaposi's sarcoma in renal and liver transplant recipients. *J Infect* 2001;43:195–199.

158. Kaposi M. Idiopathisches multiples pigmentsarcom der haut. *Arch Dermatol Syphilis* 1872;4:265–273.

159. Wilkinson J, Cope A, Gill J, et al. Identification of Kaposi's sarcoma–associated herpesvirus (KSHV)-specific cytotoxic T-lymphocyte epitopes and evaluation of reconstitution of KSHV-specific responses in human immunodeficiency virus type 1–infected patients receiving highly active antiretroviral therapy. *J Virol* 2002;76:2634–2640.

160. Zhong W, Wang H, Herndier B, et al. Restricted expression of Kaposi sarcoma–associated herpesvirus (human herpesvirus 8) genes in Kaposi sarcoma. *Proc Natl Acad Sci U S A* 1996;93:6641–6646.

161. Dupin N, Fisher C, Kellam P, et al. Distribution of human herpesvirus-8 latently infected cells in Kaposi's sarcoma, multicentric Castleman's disease, and primary effusion lymphoma. *Proc Natl Acad Sci U S A* 1999;96:4546–4551.

162. Ascherl G, Hohenadl C, Monini P, et al. Expression of human herpesvirus-8 (HHV-8) encoded pathogenic genes in Kaposi's sarcoma (KS) primary lesions. *Adv Enzyme Regul* 1999;39:331–339.

163. Blasig C, Zietz C, Haar B, et al. Monocytes in Kaposi's sarcoma lesions are productively infected by human herpesvirus 8. *J Virol* 1997;71:7963–7968.

164. Gallo RC. The enigmas of Kaposi's sarcoma. *Science* 1998;282:1837–1839.

165. Rabkin CS, Bedi G, Musaba E, et al. AIDS-related Kaposi's sarcoma is a clonal neoplasm. *Clin Cancer Res* 1995;1:257–260.

166. Delabesse E, Oksenhendler E, Lebbe C, et al. Molecular analysis of clonality in Kaposi's sarcoma. *J Clin Pathol* 1997;50:664–668.

167. Gill PS, Tsai YC, Rao AP, et al. Evidence for multiclonality in multicentric Kaposi's sarcoma. *Proc Natl Acad Sci U S A* 1998;95:8257–8261.

168. Rabkin CS, Janz S, Lash A, et al. Monoclonal origin of multicentric Kaposi's sarcoma lesions. *N Engl J Med* 1997;336:988–993.

169. Nador RG, Cesarman E, Chadburn A, et al. Primary effusion lymphoma: a distinct clinicopathologic entity associated with the Kaposi's sarcoma–associated herpes virus. *Blood* 1996;88:645–656.

170. Gaidano G, Carbone A. Primary effusion lymphoma: a liquid phase lymphoma of fluid-filled body cavities. *Adv Cancer Res* 2001;80:115–146.

171. Boshoff C, Gao SJ, Healy LE, et al. Establishing a KSHV$^+$ cell line (BCP-1) from peripheral blood and characterizing its growth in Nod/SCID mice. *Blood* 1998;91:1671–1679.

172. Cesarman E, Moore PS, Rao PH, et al. *In vitro* establishment and characterization of two acquired immunodeficiency syndrome–related lymphoma cell lines (BC-1 and BC-2) containing Kaposi's sarcoma–associated herpesvirus-like (KSHV) DNA sequences. *Blood* 1995;86:2708–2714.

173. Lacoste V, Judde JG, Bestett G, et al. Virological and molecular characterisation of a new B lymphoid cell line, established from an AIDS patient with primary effusion lymphoma, harbouring both KSHV/HHV8 and EBV viruses. *Leuk Lymphoma* 2000;38:401–409.

174. Carbone A, Gaidano G, Gloghini A, et al. Differential expression of BCL-6, CD138/syndecan-1, and Epstein-Barr virus-encoded latent membrane protein-1 identifies distinct histogenetic subsets of acquired immunodeficiency syndrome-related non-Hodgkin's lymphomas. *Blood* 1998;91:747–755.

175. Matolcsy A, Nador RG, Cesarman E, et al. Immunoglobulin VH gene mutational analysis suggests that primary effusion lymphomas derive from different stages of B cell maturation. *Am J Pathol* 1998;153:1609–1614.

176. Gaidano G, Capello D, Cilia AM, et al. Genetic characterization of HHV-8/KSHV-positive primary effusion lymphoma reveals frequent mutations of BCL6: implications for disease pathogenesis and histogenesis. *Genes Chromosomes Cancer* 1999;24:16–23.

177. Winceslaus J. Regression of AIDS-related pleural effusion with HAART. Highly active antiretroviral therapy. *Int J STD AIDS* 1998;9:368–370.

178. Chadburn A, Cesarman E, Nador RG, et al. Kaposi's sarcoma–associated herpesvirus sequences in benign lymphoid proliferations not associated with human immunodeficiency virus. *Cancer* 1997;80:788–797.

179. Frizzera G. Castleman's disease and related disorders. *Semin Diagn Pathol* 1988;5:346–364.

180. Herrada J, Cabanillas F, Rice L, et al. The clinical behavior of localized and multicentric Castleman disease. *Ann Intern Med* 1998;128:657–662.

181. Larroche C, Cacoub P, Soulier J, et al. Castleman's disease and lymphoma: report of eight cases in HIV-negative patients and literature review. *Am J Hematol* 2002;69:119–126.

182. Brandt SJ, Bodine DM, Dunbar CE, et al. Dysregulated interleukin 6 expression produces a syndrome resembling Castleman's disease in mice. *J Clin Invest* 1990;86:592–599.

183. Schwarze MM, Hawley RG. Prevention of myeloma cell apoptosis by ectopic bcl-2 expression or interleukin 6-mediated up-regulation of bcl-xL. *Cancer Res* 1995;55:2262–2265.

184. Keller AR, Hochholzer L, Castleman B. Hyaline-vascular and plasma-cell types of giant lymph node hyperplasia of the mediastinum and other locations. *Cancer* 1972;29:670–683.

185. Corbellino M, Poirel L, Aubin JT, et al. The role of human herpesvirus 8 and Epstein-Barr virus in the pathogenesis of giant lymph node hyperplasia (Castleman's disease). *Clin Infect Dis* 1996;22:1120–1121.

186. Dupin N, Diss TL, Kellam P, et al. HHV-8 is associated with a plasmablastic variant of Castleman disease that is linked to HHV-8–positive plasmablastic lymphoma. *Blood* 2000;95:1406–1412.

187. Soulier J, Grollet L, Oksenhendler E, et al. Kaposi's sarcoma–associated herpesvirus-like DNA sequences in multicentric Castleman's disease [see comments]. *Blood* 1995;86:1276–1280.

188. Parravicini C, Corbellino M, Paulli M, et al. Expression of a virus-derived cytokine, KSHV vIL-6, in HIV-seronegative Castleman's disease. *Am J Pathol* 1997;151:1517–1522.

189. Zietz C, Bogner JR, Goebel FD, et al. An unusual cluster of cases of Castleman's disease during highly active antiretroviral therapy for AIDS. *N Engl J Med* 1999;340:1923–1924.

190. Luppi M, Barozzi P, Schulz TF, et al. Nonmalignant disease associated with human herpesvirus 8 reactivation in patients who have undergone autologous peripheral blood stem cell transplantation. *Blood* 2000;96:2355–2357.

191. Horenstein MG, Nador RG, Chadburn A, et al. Epstein-Barr virus latent gene expression in primary effusion lymphomas containing Kaposi's sarcoma–associated herpesvirus/human herpesvirus-8. *Blood* 1997;90:1186–1191.

192. Fassone L, Bhatia K, Gutierrez M, et al. Molecular profile of Epstein-Barr virus infection in HHV-8-positive primary effusion lymphoma. *Leukemia* 2000;14:271–277.

193. Krithivas A, Young DB, Liao G, et al. Human herpesvirus 8 LANA interacts with proteins of the mSin3 corepressor complex and negatively regulates Epstein-Barr virus gene expression in dually infected PEL cells. *J Virol* 2000;74:9637–9645.

194. Groves AK, Cotter MA, Subramanian C, et al. The latency-associated nuclear antigen encoded by Kaposi's sarcoma–associated herpesvirus activates

two major essential Epstein-Barr virus latent promoters. *J Virol* 2001;75:9446–9457.

195. Walker RC, Marshall WF, Strickler JG, et al. Pretransplantation assessment of the risk of lymphoproliferative disorder. *Clin Infect Dis* 1995;20:1346–1353.
196. Martin DF, Kuppermann BD, Wolitz RA, et al. Oral ganciclovir for patients with cytomegalovirus retinitis treated with a ganciclovir implant. Roche Ganciclovir Study Group [see comments]. *N Engl J Med* 1999;340:1063–1070.
197. Vieira J, O'Hearn P, Kimball L, et al. Activation of Kaposi's sarcoma–associated herpesvirus (human herpesvirus 8) lytic replication by human cytomegalovirus. *J Virol* 2001;75:1378–1386.
198. Barillari G, Gendelman R, Gallo RC, et al. The Tat protein of human immunodeficiency virus type 1, a growth factor for AIDS Kaposi sarcoma and cytokine-activated vascular cells, induces adhesion of the same cell types by using integrin receptors recognizing the RGD amino acid sequence. *Proc Natl Acad Sci U S A* 1993;90:7941–7945.
199. Albini A, Benelli R, Presta M, et al. HIV-tat protein is a heparin-binding angiogenic growth factor. *Oncogene* 1996;12:289–297.
200. Albini A, Soldi R, Giunciuglio D, et al. The angiogenesis induced by HIV-1 tat protein is mediated by the Flk-1/KDR receptor on vascular endothelial cells. *Nat Med* 1996;2:1371–1375.
201. Barillari G, Ensoli B. Angiogenic effects of extracellular human immunodeficiency virus type 1 Tat protein and its role in the pathogenesis of AIDS-associated Kaposi's sarcoma. *Clin Microbiol Rev* 2002;15:310–326.
202. Yen-Moore A, Hudnall SD, Rady PL, et al. Differential expression of the HHV-8 vGCR cellular homolog gene in AIDS-associated and classic Kaposi's sarcoma: potential role of HIV-1 Tat. *Virology* 2000;267:247–251.
203. Cantaluppi V, Biancone L, Boccellino M, et al. HIV type 1 Tat protein is a survival factor for Kaposi's sarcoma and endothelial cells. *AIDS Res Hum Retrovir* 2001;17:965–976.
204. Huang LM, Chao MF, Chen MY, et al. Reciprocal regulatory interaction between human herpesvirus 8 and human immunodeficiency virus type 1. *J Biol Chem* 2001;276:13427–13432.
205. Harrington W Jr, Sieczkowski L, Sosa C, et al. Activation of HHV-8 by HIV-1 tat. *Lancet* 1997;349:774–775.
206. Merat R, Amara A, Lebbe C, et al. HIV-1 infection of primary effusion lymphoma cell line triggers Kaposi's sarcoma–associated herpesvirus (KSHV) reactivation. *Int J Cancer* 2002;97:791–795.
207. Varthakavi V, Smith RM, Deng H, et al. Human immunodeficiency virus type-1 activates lytic cycle replication of Kaposi's sarcoma–associated herpesvirus through induction of KSHV Rta. *Virology* 2002;297:270–280.
208. McGrath MS, Shiramizu BT, Herndier BG. Identification of a clonal form of HIV in early Kaposi's sarcoma: evidence for a novel model of oncogenesis, "sequential neoplasia." *J Acquir Immune Defic Syndr Hum Retrovirol* 1995;8:379–385.
209. Corchero JL, Mar EC, Spira TJ, et al. Comparison of serologic assays for detection of antibodies against human herpesvirus 8. *Clin Diagn Lab Immunol* 2001;8:913–921.
210. Campbell TB, Borok M, Gwanzura L, et al. Relationship of human herpesvirus 8 peripheral blood virus load and Kaposi's sarcoma clinical stage. *AIDS* 2000;14:2109–2116.
211. Rezza G, Andreoni M, Dorrucci M, et al. Human herpesvirus 8 seropositivity and risk of Kaposi's sarcoma and other acquired immunodeficiency syndrome-related diseases. *J Natl Cancer Inst* 1999;91:1468–1474.
212. Grandadam M, Dupin N, Calvez V, et al. Exacerbations of clinical symptoms in human immunodeficiency virus type 1–infected patients with multicentric Castleman's disease are associated with a high increase in Kaposi's sarcoma herpesvirus DNA load in peripheral blood mononuclear cells. *J Infect Dis* 1997;175:1198–1201.
213. Oksenhendler E, Carcelain G, Aoki Y, et al. High levels of human herpesvirus 8 viral load, human interleukin-6, interleukin-10, and C reactive protein correlate with exacerbation of multicentric Castleman disease in HIV-infected patients. *Blood* 2000;96:2069–2073.
214. Lallemand F, Desire N, Rozenbaum W, et al. Quantitative analysis of human herpesvirus 8 viral load using a real-time PCR assay. *J Clin Microbiol* 2000;38:1404–1408.
215. Aboulafia DM. Regression of acquired immunodeficiency syndrome–related pulmonary Kaposi's sarcoma after highly active antiretroviral therapy. *Mayo Clin Proc* 1998;73:439–443.
216. Beck JT, Hsu SM, Wijdenes J, et al. Brief report: alleviation of systemic manifestations of Castleman's disease by monoclonal anti-interleukin-6 antibody. *N Engl J Med* 1994;330:602–605.
217. Nishimoto N, Sasai M, Shima Y, et al. Improvement in Castleman's disease by humanized anti-interleukin-6 receptor antibody therapy. *Blood* 2000;95:56–61.
218. Corbellino M, Bestetti G, Scalamogna C, et al. Long-term remission of Kaposi sarcoma–associated herpesvirus-related multicentric Castleman disease with anti-CD20 monoclonal antibody therapy. *Blood* 2001;98:3473–3475.
219. Gustafson EA, Schinazi RF, Fingeroth JD. Human herpesvirus 8 open reading frame 21 is a thymidine and thymidylate kinase of narrow substrate specificity that efficiently phosphorylates zidovudine but not ganciclovir. *J Virol* 2000;74:684–692.
220. Lock MJ, Thorley N, Teo J, et al. Azidodeoxythymidine and didehydrodeoxythymidine as inhibitors and substrates of the human herpesvirus 8 thymidine kinase. *J Antimicrob Chemother* 2002;49:359–366.
221. Boulanger E, Agbalika F, Maarek O, et al. A clinical, molecular and cytogenetic study of 12 cases of human herpesvirus 8 associated primary effusion lymphoma in HIV-infected patients. *Hematol J* 2001;2:172–179.
222. Okada T, Katano H, Tsutsumi H, et al. Body-cavity-based lymphoma in an elderly AIDS-unrelated male. *Int J Hematol* 1998;67:417–422.
223. Perez CL, Rudoy S. Anti-CD20 monoclonal antibody treatment of human herpesvirus 8–associated, body cavity-based lymphoma with an unusual phenotype in a human immunodeficiency virus-negative patient. *Clin Diagn Lab Immunol* 2001;8:993–996.
224. Toomey NL, Deyev VV, Wood C, et al. Induction of a TRAIL-mediated suicide program by interferon alpha in primary effusion lymphoma. *Oncogene* 2001;20:7029–7040.
225. McGarvey ME, Tulpule A, Cai J, et al. Emerging treatments for epidemic (AIDS-related) Kaposi's sarcoma. *Curr Opin Oncol* 1998;10:413–421.
226. Dezube BJ. New therapies for the treatment of AIDS-related Kaposi sarcoma. *Curr Opin Oncol* 2000;12:445–449.
227. Monini P, Sirianni MC, Franco M, et al. Clearance of human herpesvirus 8 from blood and regression of leukopenia-associated aggressive classic Kaposi's sarcoma during interferon-alpha therapy: a case report. *Clin Infect Dis* 2001;33:1782–1785.

CHAPTER 233
Epstein-Barr Virus

Elliott Kieff

CLASSIFICATION

Epstein Barr virus (EBV) and Kaposi's sarcoma–associated herpesvirus (KSHV) are the two human γ herpesviruses (1). EBV is also known as human herpes virus 4 (HHV-4) and KSHV is also known as HHV-8. Humans are the only natural host for EBV and KSHV. The EBV and KSHV genomes are more closely related to each other than to the genomes of the α herpes viruses, herpes simplex virus type 1 (HSV-1), HSV-2, and varicella-zoster (VZV), or the β herpes viruses, cytomegalovirus (CMV), HHV-6, and HHV-7.

VIRUS STRUCTURE

Herpes viruses have nearly identical virion structures and consist of a core of protein and DNA, which is enclosed in an icosohedral nucleocapsid. The nucleocapsid is covered by "tegument" proteins, and the entire virion is enclosed in an envelope. The virion envelope is composed of host cell lipids and proteins, with most of the cellular proteins having been displaced by viral proteins and glycoproteins. The viral glycoproteins are at least partially oligomeric spike-like structures. Unlike most herpes viruses, EBV has one predominant glycoprotein in the outer envelope (1–9). The most abundant EBV envelope and tegument proteins (350/220 and 152 kd, respectively) differ in size from the major envelope and tegument proteins of HSV-1 (3,10–16). However, the size of the major EBV capsid proteins are 160, 47, and 28 kd, similar to those of HSV-1.

GENOME

The EBV genome is 172 kilobase pairs (kbp) and is composed 60% of guanine and cytosine (17–26). The EBV genome is mostly unique DNA, but also includes terminal repeats (TR) and internal direct repeats (IR) (17–31) (Fig. 233.1). Upon infection, the terminal repeats at the ends of the DNA are ligated together to form a circular episome in infected cell nuclei. Different EBV

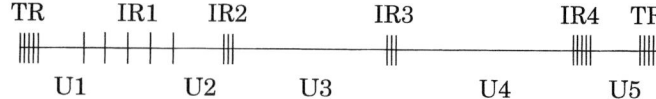

Figure 233.1. Schematic diagram of the Epstein-Barr virus genome in linear form. *TR*, terminal repeat elements; *IR*, internal repeat elements; *U1-5*, unique coding regions.

isolates differ in their number of terminal and internal repeats. The number of repeat elements is evaluated by Southern blot analysis of the size of the DNA fragment that contains the repeat element after restriction endonuclease digestion at unique sequence sites that flank the repeat.

The terminal repeats are often used to study EBV latently infected cell clonality (32–36). The number of terminal repeats varies among the progeny virus from a single virus-infected cell. The variation is due to cleavage within a TR at each end of the genome as a "heedful" genome is packaged into the nucleocapsid (37). When limited virus progeny infect a relatively large number of cells, each cell is infected with one virus. The viral genome circularizes in the infected cell and has a characteristic number of terminal repeats. If the infected cell is latently infected and proliferates, all progeny infected cells tend to have virus genomes with the same number of repeats as the parent infected cell. The limited divergence is partially due to the smaller number of DNA replications that take place in latent versus productive virus infection. Tumors that emerge from a single virus-infected cell tend to have viral genomes with the same number of terminal repeats. EBV-infected Burkitt's lymphoma, nasopharyngeal carcinoma, and Hodgkin's disease tumors are usually proliferations of a single latently infected cell, consistent with the hypothesis that EBV infection is an early event in the evolution of these malignancies.

EBV was the first herpesvirus to be cloned and sequenced (17,18). Since the *Bam*HI restriction enzyme was used to generate the initial library that was sequenced, EBV open reading frames are frequently referred to by their *Bam*H1 fragments (17,38). Thus, the EBV DNA polymerase gene is frequently referred to as BALF3 (*Bam*H1 A fragment, leftward open reading frame number 3). The DNA of the initially cloned strain (termed B95-8) is deleted for a wild-type EBV DNA segment (39–45).

When other herpesviruses were later sequenced, blocks of similarity and homology with EBV proteins were noted despite large differences in base composition (43% guanine plus cytosine for VZV; 71% guanine plus cytosine for HSV) (17,46–55). These blocks encode genes involved in lytic replication. There is little cross-hybridization or antigenic cross-reactivity between different herpesviruses. EBV DNA does not hybridize to HSV, VZV, or CMV DNA. In contrast to most EBV lytic infection genes, EBV latent infection genes have almost no similarity or homology to other herpesvirus genes, with the exception of EBV latent infection membrane protein genes, which are similar to genes of KSHV (51). The EBV nuclear antigen 1 (EBNA1) protein has a glycine alanine repeat domain that is homologous to open reading frames in cell DNA (56). Two cellular proteins can specifically bind to the EBNA1 cognate DNA sequence, consistent with the possibility that EBNA1 may have evolved from one of these cellular proteins (57).

Some EBV lytic infection genes are also related to cellular genes. For instance, the EBV immediate early gene BZLF1 is related to the jun/fos transcriptional activators (58). Also, the early lytic gene BHRF1 is distantly homologous to the Bcl 2 protooncogene that inhibits cellular apoptosis (59,60), whereas the late lytic gene BCRF1 is highly homologous to human interleukin-10 (IL-10) (61,62).

Two EBV types have been identified, and are termed types 1 and 2 or types A and B. The two types differ significantly in genes that encode nuclear antigens, which are expressed in latent infection (33,34,63–76). The type 1 and 2 genes for EBNA2, 3A, 3B and 3C differ in amino acid sequence by 47%, 16%, 20%, and 28%, respectively (63,65,69). EBNALP differs by even less (65,77). In contrast, the integral membrane proteins expressed in latent infection, LMP1 or 2, differ as little between types 1 and 2 as between isolates of type 1 and 2 (36,78–83). EBV type 1 is more common in the Western world, whereas both types 1 and 2 are prevalent in Africa (68,72–74). Almost half of the African Burkitt's lymphomas are latently infected with EBV type 2 (70,72–74,83).

VIRUS INFECTION

Adsorption, Penetration, Uncoating, and Early Intracellular Events in Infection

The EBV receptor on B-lymphocytes is the type 2 complement receptor, which is usually referred to as CD21 (1,14,84–87). The EBV envelope glycoprotein, gp350/220, binds to CD21 with an affinity of 1.2×10^{-8} M (88–91). The core gp350/220 amino acid sequence EDPGFFNVEI that binds to CD21 is similar to the sequence EDPGKQLYNVEA through which the C3d component of complement binds to CD21 (88–92). The gp350/220 designation arises because the gp350 open reading frame has an internal splice donor and acceptor site that results in a second mRNA that encodes an in-frame variant of gp350 (93–95). CD21 is also expressed on basal epithelial cells and may be an EBV receptor on epithelial cells (96). Nasopharyngeal carcinoma (NPC) epithelial cells also express CD21 (97). EBV is likely to have a second receptor on epithelial cells and B-lymphocytes because EBV can infect epithelial cells that lack CD21. Furthermore, a gp350/220 null mutant EBV has residual infectivity (98). Nevertheless, gp350/220 is the most abundant glycoprotein on the EBV envelope, and most human neutralizing antibody responses to EBV are directed to gp350/220 (99).

After adsorbing to the B cell via CD21, EBV causes CD21 and surface immunoglobulin (sIg) to aggregate in the plasma membrane. This results in receptor-associated src family tyrosine kinase signaling and is followed by internalization of virus into cytoplasmic vesicles (14,91,100). The virus envelope then fuses with the vesicle membrane. EBV nucleocapsid and tegument are released into the cytoplasm. B cells can similarly process gp350/220 coated beads into the cytoplasm. Although it is possible that gp350/220 is involved in the fusion of the virus envelope with the vesicle (91), gp85 (gH) is a key mediator of fusion of the EBV envelope with the vesicle membrane (101–105). Monoclonal antibodies to gp85 (gH) inhibit fusion of the EBV envelope and cell membranes (102). Furthermore, a null mutant virus in gH is deficient in entry and the defect can be cured with polyethylene glycol treatment to facilitate membrane fusion (103). The gH null mutant virus was also defective in adsorption to epithelial cells, implicating gH as a component of the ligand for a putative epithelial cell receptor (103). EBV gH is part of heterodimeric gH/gL complexes and heterotrimeric gH, gL, gp42 complexes. The latter are important for EBV interaction with major histocompatibility complex (MHC) class II molecules, which can serve as a coreceptor on B lymphocytes (103–105).

Compared to the better studied herpesviruses, much remains to be discovered regarding EBV capsid dissolution or DNA transport to the nucleus. By 16 hours after infection in B-lymphocytes, the EBV genome circularizes (106–109). Cellular factors determine the frequency with which latent or lytic infection follows.

Lytic EBV Infection

In vitro, EBV infection of B cells is efficient, but usually results in latent infection. In contrast, infection of epithelial cells is inefficient, but usually results in lytic infection. Because of the inefficiency of epithelial cell infection, the ease of growing large quantities of B cells that maintain latent EBV infection, and the ease with which some latently infected B cell lines can be induced to become permissive for lytic EBV infection, lytic infection has been primarily studied under the condition of induction of lytic infection in latently infected B-cell lines (110–115). Phorbol esters (such as tumor-promoting agent) are often used to induce lytic infection and likely induce replication through protein kinase C activation of jun-fos transactivation via AP-1 sites upstream of immediate early EBV genes such as BZLF1 and BRLF1 (38,115–120). A latently infected B-lymphoma cell line termed Akata can be induced for lytic EBV replication in 20% to 50% of cells by cross-linking sIg (121,122). SIg cross-linking induces activation of phospholipase C, which produces IP3 and diacylglycerol, leading to mobilization of free calcium and activation of protein kinase C (123,124). SIg cross-linking may be similar to the physiologic stresses that activate lytic EBV infection in latently infected B cells *in vivo*.

As with other herpesviruses, EBV gene expression proceeds in a cascade of immediate early, followed by early, and then late gene expression (125). Immediate early gene expression is independent of new protein synthesis and in the context of initial viral infection would be turned on by a virion-associated transactivator that is packaged in the tegument. In the instance of induction from latency, the immediate early genes are turned on by the specific inducer of lytic infection. The EBV BZLF1, BRLF1, and BILF4 immediate early genes are transcriptional activators that turn on the early genes (77,117–124,126–149).

Some early genes encode the seven protein components of the DNA replication complex (150). Early gene expression is not dependent on ongoing viral DNA synthesis, is not altered by inhibition of viral DNA synthesis, and is distinct from late gene expression, which ceases in response to inhibitors of viral DNA synthesis. Late genes encode most of the structural components of the virion. Cellular protein synthesis is inhibited early in viral infection (151).

EBV DNA is synthesized in the center of the nucleus. Nucleocapsids assemble at the periphery of the nucleus. Viral DNA extending from one terminal repeat through a genome size length to the next terminal repeat is clipped and packaged from concatenated copies of the viral genome (125). Mature nucleocapsids become enveloped by budding through the inner nuclear membrane (152). The enveloped virus is then nearly mature. A process of definitive envelopment occurs at cytoplasmic or plasma membranes, in which the glycoproteins that are on the initial envelope are replaced by Golgi-processed glycoproteins (152).

IMMEDIATE EARLY GENES

The BZLF1 mRNA consists of three exons, each of which encodes a functional domain (131–139). The first exon (amino acids 1–167) encodes a transactivating domain (131–134). The second exon (amino acids 168–202) encodes a basic domain homologous to the fos/jun transcription factors (135–137,140,141). The basic domain interacts with AP1 DNA sites and targets BZLF1 to the nucleus. The third exon (amino acids 203–245) encodes a coiled coil leucine or isoleucine repeat capable of dimer formation (118,132,135,138,139). BZLF1 phosphorylation on serine 336 appears to regulate DNA binding (141). BZLF1 also associates with the cellular p53 and may inhibit p53-mediated apoptosis in lytic EBV infection (142). BZLF1 also interacts with the p65 nuclear factor κB (NF-κB) subunit (143). BRLF1 binds specifically to

DNA and has distant homology to the cellular c-myb gene (144). Amino acids 520 to 605 contain a potent acidic transactivating domain (133,134).

EARLY GENES

At least 30 EBV early genes and late genes are interspersed throughout the EBV genome (1,17,38,145–149,153). The functions of many of these genes are postulated based on homology to other herpesvirus genes that have previously been described. The BALF2 protein is homologous to the HSV DNA binding protein ICP8 and is important in DNA replication (146). BHRF1, another EBV early gene (60), is homologous to the cellular protooncogene Bcl-2, which inhibits apoptotic cell death. BHRF1 likely prevents apoptotic cell death during lytic infection and thereby allows the production of infectious virions. Other EBV early genes include several linked to DNA replication, including BALF5, the DNA polymerase; BALF2, the major DNA binding protein; BORF2 and BARF1, ribonucleotide reductase; BXLF1, thymidine kinase; and BGLF5, alkaline exonuclease (145–150).

LATE GENES

EBV late genes encode structural proteins or proteins involved in virus envelopment or budding from the cell. Nonglycoprotein late genes include BCLF1, the major nucleocapsid protein, which is homologous to the major HSV capsid protein (50); BNRF1, the major virion external nonglycoprotein and likely a tegument protein (153); and BXRF1, a basic core protein that is homologous to the VZV basic virion core protein (46,47).

Glycoprotein late genes include BLLF1 (gp350/220), BALF4 (gp110), BXLF2 (gp85), ILF2 (gp55/80), and BDLF3 (gp42) (93–105,152–160). BALF4 is homologous to HSV-1 gB, a major HSV virus glycoprotein, but a minor EBV virion glycoprotein. BLLF1 and BXLF2 are found on virus and in the plasma membrane of lytically infected cells.

The EBV late gene BCRF1 is homologous to the cellular IL-10 gene (61,62,161,162). Although IL-10 can stimulate B-cell growth, BCRF1 has no obvious effect on the ability of EBV to transform B-lymphocytes because EBV mutants null for BCRF1 expression can fully transform B-lymphocytes *in vitro* (163). Instead, BCRF1 may function during lytic EBV infection *in vivo* as a negative regulator of cytotoxic T-lymphocytes (62,164). BCRF1 may blunt release of interferon-γ because the initiation of B-cell growth transformation is sensitive to interferon.

Latent Infection Genes

EBV infection of normal human B-lymphocytes usually results in latent infection (1,2). The EBV genome enters the cell nucleus, where it circularizes and usually persists as an episome throughout latent infection (106–108). Rarely, the EBV genome integrates into cell DNA and can still maintain latent infection gene expression (109). At least 11 EBV genes are expressed in latent infection, and the products of these genes work in concert to convert B-lymphocytes into immortalized lymphoblastoid cells capable of continuous growth. These genes include two small, nonpolyadenylated RNAs (EBER 1 and EBER 2), six nuclear proteins (EBNA1, 2, 3A, 3B, 3C, and LP) and three latent infection integral membrane proteins (LMP1, 2A, and 2B). Some researchers use different nomenclatures for EBNA3A, 3B, and 3C, and LMP2A and 2B, referring to EBNA3B and 3C as EBNA 4, 5, or 6, (depending on the researcher), and LMP2A and 2B as TP1 and TP2.

EBNALP and EBNA2 are the first two genes expressed from the EBV genome in B-lymphocytes (106,107). They are products of alternatively spliced mRNAs (Fig. 233.1). EBNALP or leader protein is encoded in multiple exons from the IR1 repeat and in two short unique exons. Because the number of IR1 repeat elements differs among EBV isolates, the size of EBNALP varies among isolates (165,166). EBNALP is expressed throughout the cell nucleus, but is also concentrated in small nuclear granules (166,167). Genetic analysis of EBNALP in recombinant EBV has demonstrated that deletion of the last two unique exons results in reduced transformed cell outgrowth after plating in soft agarose. Fibroblast feeder layers can partially complement the deficient growth of B-lymphocytes infected with the mutant EBV recombinant (168,169).

EBNALP up-regulates EBNA2-mediated transcriptional activation of all viral and cellular promoters that have been tested (170). EBNA2 activates transcription of the cell CD21, CD23, c-fgr, and c-myc promoters and of the EBV EBNA and LMP promoters (170–186), and although only some of these promoters have been formally evaluated in EBNALP coactivation experiments, EBNALP almost certainly participates in these transcriptional activations given its biochemical effects through the EBNA2 acidic domain. Expression of EBNALP and EBNA2 in B cells costimulated with gp350 induced G0 to G1 cell cycle transition, probably because of c-myc up-regulation (171).

The EBNA2 gene is essential for EBV-induced growth transformation of B-lymphocytes (168,172,177). The experimental proof that EBNA2 is essential for LCL outgrowth took advantage of an EBV mutant termed P3HR-1, which is not competent for transformation but is carried in a latently infected B-lymphoma cell line in which it can be induced to replicate (187). P3HR-1 is a type 2 EBV strain that is deleted for EBNA2 and the last two exons of EBNALP. When wild-type EBV DNA that spans the deletion is transfected into P3HR-1 cells and lytic infection is induced, 1 in 105 progeny viruses are restored for the deleted DNA via homologous recombination and are then competent to growth transform primary B-lymphocytes into LCLs, whereas nonrecombinant P3HR-1 EBV does not give rise to LCLs (168,172,177,178). Every LCL clone that is derived from such an experiment is infected with an EBNA2-positive recombinant.

EBNA2 localizes to the cell nucleus within large nuclear granules (167) and transactivates cell and viral gene expression (179–186). EBNA2 induces expression of cellular CD23, CD21, and c-fgr, and of EBV EBNAs, LMP1, and LMP2 (Fig. 233.2). Recombinant molecular genetic analyses of EBNA2 demonstrate that there are three regions required for B-cell transformation

and that at least two of these regions are critical for transactivation activity. Of the 484 EBNA2 amino acids, the essential regions include amino acids 95 to 110, 280 to 337, and 425 to 462 (172,177,178). Amino acids 425 to 462 have acidic transactivating characteristics (188–192) and amino acids 280 to 337 interact with DNA sequence-specific binding proteins that bring EBNA2 in proximity to its response elements (193–195). Amino acids 95 to 110 are probably critical because of the adjacent domains that mediate homodimerization (178). The EBNA2 acidic transactivating domain (amino acids 425–462) is similar to the prototype HSV VP16 acidic domain (188–192). Both the EBNA2 and VP16 acidic domains have affinity for TFIIB, TAF40, TFIIH, RPA70, and p300/CBP and likely recruit TFIIB, TAF40, and TFIIH to responsive promoters. EBNALP up-regulates the activity of the EBNA2 acidic domain (170).

EBNA2 associates with DNA by stably associating with the cellular protein recombination signal sequence binding protein Jk, which binds to the consensus double-stranded DNA sequence GTGGGAA (193–195). Jk association with EBNA2 accounts for only part of EBNA2 transactivation of the LMP1 promoter because mutation of EBNA2 amino acid W319W320, which inactivates Jk interaction, only reduces EBNA2 responsiveness 50%. PU.1, another EBNA2 interacting cellular transcription factor that recognizes a site in the LMP1 promoter, can still mediate EBNA2 activation in transient transfection analyses (195). Thus, EBNA2 is recruited to responsive promoters by Jk and PU.1 and then recruits EBNALP and the transcription factors TFIIB, TAF40, TFIIH, p100, p300/CBP, and RNA Pol II, resulting in transcriptional activation.

The EBNA3A, 3B, and 3C genes encode proteins of 944, 938, and 992 amino acids, respectively, and are located consecutively in the EBV genome (69,196–203). Each gene consists of two exons and a short intron and has repeat elements near the 3' end of the open reading frame. The EBNA3 genes encode hydrophilic proteins containing approximately 20% charged amino acids. EBNA3A, 3B, and 3C accumulate in B-cell nuclei, localize to large clumps, but spare the nucleolus (167).

Analysis of the EBNA3 genes in recombinant EBV has demonstrated that EBNA3A and EBNA3C are essential for EBV-mediated transformation of primary B-lymphocytes, but that EBNA3B is dispensable for transformation (204,205). EBV recombinants that are null for EBNA3A or 3C are not competent to transform primary B-lymphocytes unless the wild-type EBNA3 gene is provided to the infected cell by means of a helper virus. In contrast, EBV recombinants that are null for EBNA3B are fully competent to transform B-lymphocytes in vitro. EBNA3C induces expression of cellular CD21 (Fig. 233.2). EBNA3C competes with EBNA2 for binding to the Jk protein and modulates the ability of the Jk–EBNA2 complex to transactivate the LMP1 promoter (206–208). Furthermore, when EBNA3C binds to Jk, it inhibits the ability of Jk to bind to its consensus DNA binding sequence. EBNA3C can also substitute for EBNALP in coactivating the LMP1 promoter (207,208). Therefore, EBNA3C likely has an important role in modulating EBNA2 transactivation in EBV-transformed LCLs. EBNA3A and EBNA3B also bind to Jk, inhibit its binding to DNA, and are likely involved in regulation of EBNA2 transactivation (206).

The EBNA1 gene encodes 641 amino acids (175,176) and binds specifically to a DNA partial palindrome (209–212). The EBNA1 binding sequences are located at three different sites in EBV (211). The site with highest EBNA1 binding affinity is located at the left end of the EBV genome and contains 20 tandem direct 30-bp repeats. The binding site with the next highest affinity contains two binding sequences in dyad symmetry and two in tandem and is located approximately 1 kbp to the right of the first binding site.

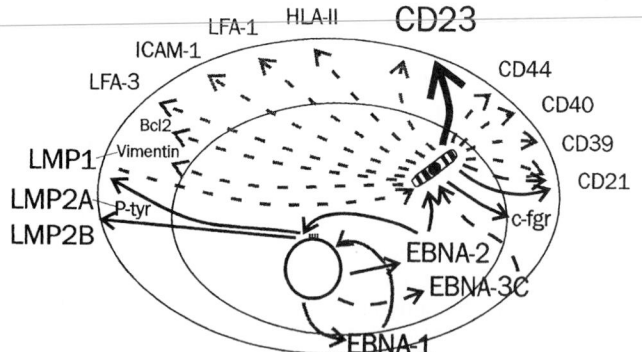

Figure 233.2. Induction of cellular and viral genes by Epstein-Barr virus latent genes. EBNA2 induces expression of CD21, CD23, c-fgr, c-myc, LMP1, and LMP2. EBNA3C can also induce CD21 expression. LMP1 induces expression of vimentin, ICAM-1, ICAM-3, LFA3, bcl 2, HLA II, CD21, CD23, CD39, CD40, and CD44. (Reproduced from Kieff E, Rinkinson A. Epstein-Barr virus and its replication. In: Knipe DM, Howley PM, et al., eds. *Fields virology,* 4th ed. Philadelphia: Lippincott Williams & Wilkins, 2001:2511–2574, with permission.)

The third binding site is located about 10 kbp downstream of the EBNA2 gene. The first two EBNA1 binding sites enable covalently closed circular DNA molecules to replicate as episomes in cells expressing EBNA1 and are important for EBV maintenance in an episomal state in latently infected cells (213–219). For this reason, the DNA encoding these regions is referred to as "ori p" (plasmid DNA replication origin). *In vivo*, EBV episomes use a broader region of the EBV genome to initiate DNA replication (220).

LMP1 is a dominant transforming gene expressed in latent EBV infection. LMP1 is a 386–amino acid protein that consists of an amino-terminal 25–amino acid cytoplasmic domain, six hydrophobic 20–amino acid transmembrane segments separated by five reverse turns, and a 200–amino acid cytoplasmic carboxy-terminus (221). When expressed in cells, LMP1 constitutively forms patches that coalesce into caps in the plasma membrane, similar to activated growth factor receptors (222,223). LMP1 has transforming effects when expressed in many different cell lines, including rodent fibroblast cells (224–226). In rodent fibroblast cell lines, LMP1 causes cells to have altered morphology, allows cells to grow in medium with low serum, causes cells to lose contact inhibition so that they heap up on one another, induces loss of anchorage dependence so cells are able to grow as colonies in soft agar, and causes Rat-1 fibroblast cells to be tumorigenic in nude mice. Expression of LMP1 in EBV-negative B-lymphoma cells induces many of the changes seen when EBV transforms primary B-lymphocytes (180,226–233). These include cell clumping, increased villous projections, and increased cell surface expression of B-cell activation markers and adhesion molecules such as CD23, CD39, CD40, CD44, class II MHC, leukocyte function–associated antigen 1 (LFA-1), intracellular adhesion molecule-1 (ICAM-1), and LFA-3 (Fig. 233.2). LMP1 also protects B cells from apoptosis through induction of expression of the cellular bcl-2 protooncogene. LMP1 induces NF-κB, which up-regulates expression of the antiapoptotic zinc finger

protein A20; A20 protects cells from tumor necrosis factor-α (TNF-α) toxicity (234,235). When expressed in epithelial cells, LMP1 causes cells to have altered morphology and blocks terminal differentiation in a cell line that can be induced to differentiate (236–238). Mice transgenic for LMP1 expression in epithelial cells have epidermal hyperplasia and altered expression of keratin (238), whereas mice transgenic for LMP1 expression in B-lymphocytes have an increased incidence of B-cell hyperplasias and lymphomas (239).

Reverse genetic analyses of LMP1 in recombinant EBV conversion of primary human B-lymphocytes to LCLs indicate that LMP1 is essential for EBV-mediated primary B-lymphocyte growth transformation (240–243). The LMP1 short cytoplasmic amino terminus is not essential for transformation and likely serves to anchor the first LMP1 transmembrane domain (241). In contrast, the carboxy-terminal cytoplasmic domain is essential for LMP1 function, because EBV recombinants lacking this domain are not competent to transform primary B-lymphocytes. Further analyses of the carboxy-terminal domain indicated that deletion of all but the first 44 amino acids of the carboxy terminus results in the ability to transform primary B-lymphocytes, but with diminished capacity and with abnormal LCL growth (242). Furthermore, beyond the first 44 amino acids of the C-terminal cytoplasmic domain, only the last 11 amino acids are critical for LCL outgrowth (243). Thus, there appear to be at least two functional components within the carboxy terminus, one located within the first 44 amino acids of the carboxy terminus and one within the last 11 amino acids. The first 44 amino acids of the LMP1 cytoplasmic carboxy terminus interact with TNF-associated factors 1, 3, 2, and 5 (244,245). The TRAF proteins transmit signals for NF-κB, JNK, and p38 activation from many TNF receptors, including CD40, which, when stimulated causes B cell–activating effects, many of which are similar to the effects of LMP1. LMP1 mimics a constitutively stimulated CD40 receptor (Fig. 233.3). The similarity to TNF receptor signaling

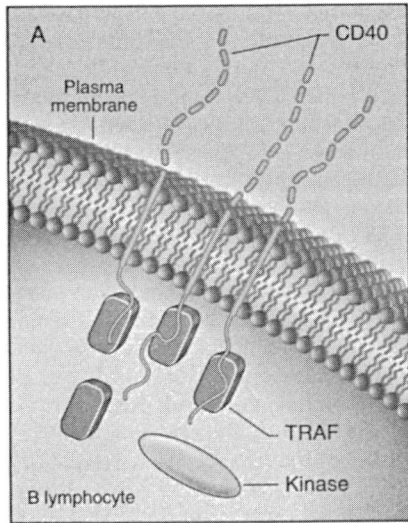
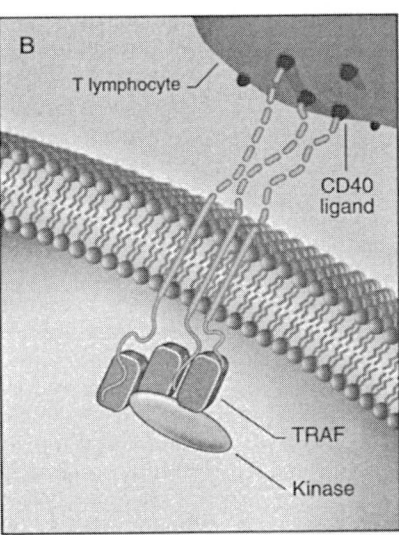
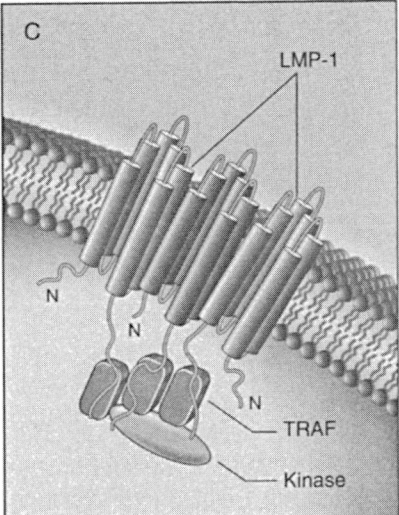

Figure 233.3. Model of LMP1 transforming function. **A:** In unstimulated B cells, CD40 receptor is distributed homogeneously throughout the plasma membrane. **B:** T cells expressing CD40 ligand on their surface cause aggregation of CD40 receptors, bringing TRAF molecules together, which transmit signals through the cell cytoplasm, activating IKK, JNK, and p38 kinases and their downstream transcription factors, NF-κB, Jun/Fos, and AP1. **C:** In Epstein-Barr virus–infected B cells, LMP1 constitutively forms patches in the plasma membrane and brings TRAF molecules together to transmit persistent growth and survival signals to the cell. [Reproduced from Wang F, Marchini A, Kieff E. Epstein-Barr virus (EBV) recombinants: use of positive selection markers to rescue mutants in EBV-negative B-lymphoma cells. *J Virol* 1991;65(4):1701–1709, with permission.]

extends to even the C-terminal 11 amino acids, which engage TNF-associated death domain proteins, including TRADD and RIP, while propagating only nondeath signals (246). In the context of initial EBV infection of primary B-lymphocytes, LMP1 expression has reached substantial levels in response to EBNALP and EBNA2 coactivation before the first round of cell DNA synthesis (106).

In contrast to LMP1, LMP2A and 2B are expressed in latent infection, but do not have a critical role in EBV conversion of primary B-lymphocytes to LCLs. LMP2A and B differ only in their first exon, which for LMP2A encodes a 119 residue amino-terminal cytoplasmic domain, whereas for 2B the first exon is noncoding (247–249). The rest of LMP2A and 2B are 12 hydrophobic integral membrane sequences separated by short reverse turns and a short 27 residue cytoplasmic carboxy-terminal domain. LMP2 colocalizes with LMP1 in LCL plasma membrane patches (249,250). Recombinant EBV null for LMP2A or for LMP2A and 2B are fully competent to transform primary B cells *in vitro* (250–253).

LMP2A has three tyrosine that are in appropriate primary amino acid sequence contexts for binding and phosphorylation by src family tyrosine kinases; two of these are separated by seven amino acids so as to be an ideal syk70 or zap70 binding site (249). Indeed, LMP2A is an excellent substrate for src family tyrosine kinases *in vivo* and associates with src family kinases, including syk, fyn, and lyn (249,254–257). As a consequence of its constitutive phosphorylation and engagement of src and syk family kinases, LMP2 mimics a constitutively activated B-cell receptor (BCR); LMP2A induces a low-level forward signaling and globally desensitizes LCL membranes to BCR or similar signals (254–257). LMP2 blocks the calcium flux normally seen following cross-linking sIgM or class II MHC in B cells. Since BCR cross-linking induces EBV replication and LMP2A blocks BCR signaling in LCLs, LMP2A is a negative regulator of lytic EBV replication (256). The low level of forward signaling from LMP2 may under some circumstances enable cell survival, although such effects are not evident in an LCL background (257,258).

After the first round of cellular DNA synthesis in latent infection, EBV expresses two very abundant small nonpolyadenylated RNAs, EBER1 and 2 (106,259–263). The EBERs are similar in predicted structure to adenovirus VAI and II RNAs, which inhibit the protein kinase PKR and thereby block interferon inhibition of cell and viral protein synthesis. *In vitro*, EBERs can bind to and inactivate PKR (264), and expression of the EBERs in B-lymphoma cells can inhibit apoptosis induced by interferon-α (265). However, the ability of EBERs to inhibit PKR is substantially lower than that of VA RNA, and unlike adenovirus VA RNAs, the EBERs largely localize to the nucleus (261). The EBERs are also transcribed by both RNA Pol II and Pol III (262). The EBERs are complexed with cell proteins, but the significance of these complexes is uncertain (263). Recombinant reverse genetic experiments indicate that EBER-deleted EBV is fully wild type in conversion of primary B-lymphocytes to LCLs; the EBER-positive and -negative LCLs are indistinguishable in their growth (266). Furthermore, although EBV conversion of primary B-lymphocytes to LCLs is sensitive to interferon, EBER-positive virus is as sensitive to interferon as EBER-negative virus in primary B-cell conversion to LCLs (267). Although the putative effects of EBERs on PKR and interferon sensitivity are not evident in primary B-cell conversion to LCL type assays, the EBERs almost certainly have an important role in EBV infection *in vivo*, and the role could be partly related to PKR. Due to their high abundance in the nuclei of most types of latently infected cells, EBERs have served as useful markers for evidence of latent EBV infection in tumors.

EPSTEIN-BARR VIRUS RECOMBINANT GENETICS

EBV recombinant genetics has lagged behind recombinant genetics in other herpesviruses due to the limitation of *in vitro* EBV infection to human B-lymphocytes. B-lymphocytes are nonpermissive or partially permissive for EBV replication. However, some latently infected B-cell lines can be induced to become more permissive by forced expression of the EBV immediate early transactivators of lytic replication or by treatment of cells with activators of PKC, calcium ionophores, histone deacetylase inhibitors, DNA methylation inhibitors, or antibodies to the BCR. P3HR-1 EBV-infected cells have been particularly useful because of their partial permissivity for lytic infection and the defectiveness of the P3HR-1 EBV for transformation due to deletion of DNA encoding part of the critical EBV latent genes EBNALP and EBNA2. P3HR-1–infected cells can be transfected with cloned EBV DNA that contains the full EBNALP and EBNA2 genes, and recombinant EBVs can be marker rescued by the unique ability of recombinants to transform primary B-lymphocytes into LCLs (168,172). The discovery that a second cotransfected EBV DNA fragment will frequently recombine with the DNA that has recombined with the EBNA2 and EBNALP DNA enables the introduction of mutations anywhere in the EBV genome (266,268). Recombinant virus can then be cloned and characterized because of its ability to cause growth of a primary B-lymphocyte into LCLs. In a typical experiment, 10% of the recombinants will have incorporated a marker on the cotransfected EBV DNA. (268–277).

EPSTEIN-BARR VIRUS INFECTION *IN VIVO*

Primary EBV infection initiates in the oropharyngeal epithelium and gains entry to B cells, probably in the tonsils and adenoids (2). EBV-infected B-lymphocytes with typical latency III EBNALP, 2, 3A, 3B, 3C, 1, LMP1, LMP2, and EBER expression appear to multiply in the peripheral blood and tonsils and seed multiple lymphoid organs. The initial B-cell infection is probably inhibited by interferon and other aspects of the nonspecific host immune response. Within 2 weeks, the fraction of EBV-infected B cells in the peripheral blood may reach 10% of all B cells. This results in massive EBV-specific CD4 and CD8 responses, with more than a few percent of the total CD4s and CD8s recognizing each of multiple EBV epitopes from EBNA3A, 3B, 3C, 2, LMP1, LMP2, and EBNA1 (278–281). EBNA1 largely escapes CD8 recognition by escaping primary proteosome degradation. In the normal host, the number of latency III EBV-infected B cells rapidly decreases to less than 0.0001% and remains at that level. A larger fraction of EBV-infected B-lymphocytes persists in the tonsils and other oropharyngeal lymphatics (281,282). The CD4 and CD8 response wanes over time, but persists at the level of several percent EBV commitment for life in normal people (278–280). The persisting latently EBV-infected B-lymphocytes have altered forms of latent infection, wherein they express EBNA1, LMP1, LMP2, and EBERs (latency II) or EBNA1 and EBERs (latency I) (282).

EPSTEIN-BARR VIRUS–ASSOCIATED MALIGNANCIES

EBV infection is etiologically associated with lymphoproliferative disease in immunocompromised hosts, African Burkitt's lymphoma, rare T-cell lymphomas, Hodgkin's disease, anaplastic nasopharyngeal carcinoma, and gastric carcinomas (2,283–314) (Table 233.1). The associations of EBV with these malignancies is based on higher titers of anti-EBV antibodies in patients

TABLE 233.1. Epstein-Barr Virus (EBV)-Associated Malignancies

Malignancy	%EBV associated	EBV latent antigens expressed
African Burkitt's lymphoma	~98	EBNA 1
Hodgkin's disease	~50	EBNA 1, LMP1, LMP2
Lymphoproliferative disease (immunocompromised hosts)	~96	EBNA 1, 2, 3A, 3B, 3C, P, LMP1, LMP2
Nasopharyngeal carcinoma	~98	EBNA 1, LMP1, LMP2

Adapted from Rickinson A, Kieff E. Epstein-Barr virus. In: Knipe DM, Howley PM, et al., eds. *Fields virology,* 4th ed. Philadelphia: Lippincott Williams & Wilkins, 2001, with permission.

with these malignancies; EBV DNA, RNA, or proteins in all tumor cells; uniclonality of the tumor cells with respect to virus infection as judged by the lack of variation in the numbers of terminal repeats; and the expression of LMP1 and LMP2 EBV-encoded proteins that can enhanced cell growth and survival. EBV latent gene expression varies in different tumor types (Table 233.1).

Some of the lymphoproliferative diseases that occur in bone marrow, small bowel, pancreas, liver, heart, or lung—or even in kidney transplant recipients who are on cyclosporine A or FK506 and acquire primary EBV infection with rampant progress into polyclonal EBV-infected cell malignant proliferation—appear to be simply the *in vivo* counterpart of EBV-induced lymphoblastoid cell outgrowth (299–305). Similarly, people infected with the human immunodeficiency virus who have very low CD4 counts, EBV-infected B-lymphocytes that express all of the EBNAs, LMPs, and EBERs are able to escape immune destruction and proliferate as poly- or oligoclonal lymphomas in the lymphatic system, in solid organs, or in the central nervous system (285,301,304,305,311–314). For bone transplant recipients of EBV-infected donors, donor T-lymphocytes are highly therapeutic in causing regression of EBV lymphoproliferative diseases (309). *In vitro,* expansion of the EBV-specific CD4s and CD8s appears to increase specificity, with fewer graft-versus-host–related complications (310). For solid organ transplants, lower doses of immune suppressive drugs can enable a sufficient host immune response (307). Anti–B cell monoclonal antibodies have also been of therapeutic benefit (308).

An EBV-infected cell in lymphoproliferative disease can also undergo a c-myc translocation or amplification, gain malignant potential, and have the characteristics of a Burkitt's lymphoma (283,285,299,303,306). Burkitt's lymphoma cells usually express EBNA1, which is essential for EBV episome persistence, and EBERs *in vivo.* African children with higher EBV antibody titers after initial infection have a high incidence of later onset of Burkitt's lymphoma, suggesting that increased EBV replication is a risk factor for tumor development. While in the holoendemic malaria regions of Africa, New Guinea, and Brazil, EBV is associated with almost all Burkitt's lymphomas, Burkitt's tumors occurring in other parts of the world are uncommon and are less frequently EBV infected. The role of EBV as a major etiologic factor in the high incidence of African Burkitt's lymphoma is probably linked to a cofactor role for holoendemic malaria, which can cause T-cell immune depression and promote B-cell proliferation.

EBV is also associated with approximately 50% of cases of Hodgkin's disease, most commonly in nonlymphocyte predominant forms, in younger and in Hispanic patients (284,286,287). The pattern of EBV latent gene expression in Hodgkin's disease differs from Burkitt's lymphoma in that EBNA1, LMP1, and LMP2 are expressed. EBV DNA and gene expression are found in

Reed-Sternberg cells, which are the malignant cells of Hodgkin's disease. In addition, in EBV-associated Hodgkin's disease, the Reed-Sternberg cells are monoclonally infected with EBV, indicating that EBV infection occurred prior to the onset of tumor formation. Irrespective of EBV infection, Hodgkin's disease Reed-Sternberg cells are B-lymphocytes with rearranged, mutated, and nonproductive Ig genes and very high-level expression of the TNF receptors CD30 and CD40. LMP1 likely provides constitutive activation of many of the CD30 and CD40 signaling pathways and essential survival signals that enable EBV to be an etiologic agent in Hodgkin's disease.

The most common EBV-associated malignancy is anaplastic nasopharyngeal carcinoma (NPC), which is among the most common malignancies in Southern Chinese peoples and Aleut Indians (288,289,291–297). Evidence for particularly carcinogenic strains of EBV or for a toxin cofactor exposure in high-risk populations is not compelling. Host genetic factors remain the most likely cocarcinogenic factor in the high incidence of NPC in Southern Chinese.

With regard to the underlying association of EBV with NPC, patients with NPC have higher titers of EBV antibodies than controls (289,291–293). Antibodies to EBV replication proteins identify people within high-risk populations who are at highest risk for NPC development and recurrences (291–293). EBV DNA is almost always in every NPC tumor cell, and the tumors are clonal with regard to EBV infection (288,294). EBNA1, LMP1, LMP2, and EBERs are usually expressed in the tumor cells (294–298). LMP1 and LMP2 may have a critical role in the development of NPC since they can effect differentiation and survival in epithelial cell cultures and in transgenic models.

REFERENCES

1. Kieff E, Rickinson A. Epstein-Barr virus and its replication. In: Knipe DM, Howley PM, et al., eds. *Fields virology,* 4th ed. Philadelphia: Lippincott Williams & Wilkins, 2001:2511–2574.
2. Rickinson A, Kieff E. Epstein-Barr virus. In: Knipe DM, Howley PM, et al., eds. *Fields virology,* 4th ed. Philadelphia: Lippincott Williams & Wilkins, 2001:2575–2628.
3. Dolyniuk M, Wolff E, Kieff E. Proteins of Epstein-Barr Virus. II. Electrophoretic analysis of the polypeptides of the nucleocapsid and the glucosamine- and polysaccharide-containing components of enveloped virus. *J Virol* 1976;18(1):289–297.
4. Epstein M, Achong B, Barr Y. Morphological and biological studies on a virus in cultured lymphoblasts from Burkitt's lymphoma. *J Exp Med* 1965;121:761–770.
5. Epstein M, Achong B, Barr Y. Virus particles in cultured lymphoblasts from Burkitt's lymphoma. *Lancet* 1964;1:702–703.
6. Pope JH, Achong BG, Epstein MA. Cultivation and fine structure of virus-bearing lymphoblasts from a second New Guinea Burkitt lymphoma: establishment of sublines with unusual cultural properties. *Int J Cancer* 1968;3(2):171–182.
7. Epstein MA, Achong BG. Discovery and general biology of the virus. In: Epstein M, Achong B, eds. *The Epstein-Barr virus.* Heidelberg: Springer-Verlag, 1979:1–22.

8. Epstein M, Achong B. *The Epstein-Barr virus, recent advances.* London: Heinemann, 1986.
9. Epstein M, Achong B. The Epstein Barr virus. *Ann Rev Microbiol* 1973;27:413–436.
10. Mueller-Lantzsch N, Georg B, Yamamoto N, et al. Epstein-Barr virus-induced proteins. II. Analysis of surface polypeptides from EBV-producing and -superinfected cells by immunoprecipitation. *Virology* 1980;102(2):401–411.
11. Qualtiere LF, Pearson GR: Epstein-Barr virus-induced membrane antigens: immunochemical characterization of Triton X-100 solubilized viral membrane antigens from EBV-superinfected Raji cells. *Int J Cancer* 1979;23(6):808–817.
12. Qualtiere LF, Pearson GR. Radioimmune precipitation study comparing the Epstein-Barr virus membrane antigens expressed on P3HR-1 virus–superinfected Raji cells to those expressed on cells in a B-95 virus–transformed producer culture activated with tumor-promoting agent (TPA). *Virology* 1980;102(2):360–369.
13. Taylor N, Countryman J, Rooney C, et al. Expression of the BZLF1 latency-disrupting gene differs in standard and defective Epstein-Barr viruses. *J Virol* 1989;63(4):1721–1728.
14. Tedder TF, Weis JJ, Clement LT, et al. The role of receptors for complement in the induction of polyclonal B-cell proliferation and differentiation. *J Clin Immunol* 1986;6(1):65–73.
15. Thorley-Lawson DA. Characterization of cross-reacting antigens on the Epstein-Barr virus envelope and plasma membranes of producer cells. *Cell* 1979;16(1):33–42.
16. Thorley-Lawson DA, Edson CM. Polypeptides of the Epstein-Barr virus membrane antigen complex. *J Virol* 1979;32(2):458–467.
17. Baer R, Bankier AT, Biggin MD, et al. DNA sequence and expression of the B95-8 Epstein-Barr virus genome. *Nature* 1984;310(5974):207–211.
18. Dambaugh T, Beisel C, Hummel M, et al. Epstein-Barr virus (B95-8) DNA VII: molecular cloning and detailed mapping. *Proc Natl Acad Sci U S A* 1980;77(5):2999–3003.
19. Given D, Kieff E. DNA of Epstein-Barr virus. VI. Mapping of the internal tandem reiteration. *J Virol* 1979;31(2):315–324.
20. Given D, Kieff E. DNA of Epstein-Barr virus. IV. Linkage map of restriction enzyme fragments of the B95-8 and W91 strains of Epstein-Barr Virus. *J Virol* 1978;28(2):524–542.
21. Given D, Yee D, Griem K, et al. DNA of Epstein-Barr virus. V. Direct repeats of the ends of Epstein-Barr virus DNA. *J Virol* 1979;30(3):852–862.
22. Jehn U, Lindahl T, Klein C. Fate of virus DNA in the abortive infection of human lymphoid cell lines by Epstein-Barr virus. *J Gen Virol* 1972;16(3):409–412.
23. Kawai Y, Nonoyama M, Pagano JS. Reassociation kinetics for Epstein-Barr virus DNA: nonhomology to mammalian DNA and homology of viral DNA in various diseases. *J Virol* 1973;12(5):1006–1012.
24. Pritchett R, Pendersen M, Kieff E. Complexity of EBV homologous DNA in continuous lymphoblastoid cell lines. *Virology* 1976;74(1):227–231.
25. Pritchett RF, Hayward SD, Kieff ED. DNA of Epstein-Barr virus. I. Comparative studies of the DNA of Epstein-Barr virus from HR-1 and B95-8 cells: size, structure, and relatedness. *J Virol* 1975;15(3):556–559.
26. Wagner EK, Roizman B, Savage T, et al. Characterization of the DNA of herpesviruses associated with Lucke adenocarcinoma of the frog and Burkitt lymphoma of man. *Virology* 1970;42(1):257–261.
27. Hayward SD, Kieff E. DNA of Epstein-Barr virus. II. Comparison of the molecular weights of restriction endonuclease fragments of the DNA of Epstein-Barr virus strains and identification of end fragments of the B95-8 strain. *J Virol* 1977;23(2):421–429.
28. Kintner CR, Sugden B. The structure of the termini of the DNA of Epstein-Barr virus. *Cell* 1979;17:661–671.
29. Cheung A, Kieff E. Epstein-Barr virus DNA. X. Direct repeat within the internal direct repeat of Epstein-Barr virus DNA. *J Virol* 1981;40(2):501–507.
30. Cheung A, Kieff E. Long internal direct repeat in Epstein-Barr virus DNA. *J Virol* 1982;44(1):286–294.
31. Hayward SD, Nogee L, Hayward GS. Organization of repeated regions within the Epstein-Barr virus DNA molecule. *J Virol* 1980;33(1):507–521.
32. Brown NA, Liu C, Garcia CR, et al. Clonal origins of lymphoproliferative disease induced by Epstein-Barr virus. *J Virol* 1986;58(3):975–978.
33. Dambaugh T, Raab-Traub N, Heller M, et al. Variations among isolates of Epstein-Barr virus. *Ann N Y Acad Sci* 1980;354:309–325.
34. Heller M, Dambaugh T, Kieff E. Epstein-Barr virus DNA. IX. Variation among viral DNAs from producer and nonproducer infected cells. *J Virol* 1981;38(2):632–648.
35. Raab-Traub N, Flynn K. The structure of the termini of the Epstein-Barr virus as a marker of clonal cellular proliferation. *Cell* 1986;47(6):883–889.
36. Miller WE, Edwards RH, Walling DM, et al. Sequence variation in the Epstein-Barr virus latent membrane protein 1. *J Gen Virol* 1994;75:2729–2740.
37. Spaete RR, Mocarski ES. The alpha sequence of the cytomegalovirus genome functions as a cleavage/packaging signal for herpes simplex virus defective genomes. *J Virol* 1985;54(3):817–824.
38. Farrell PJ. Epstein-Barr virus. In: O Brien SJ, ed. *Genetic maps*, 6th ed. New York: Cold Spring Harbor Press, 1993:120–133.
39. Raab-Traub N, Dambaugh T, Kieff E. DNA of Epstein-Barr virus VIII: B95-8, the previous prototype, is an unusual deletion derivative. *Cell* 1980;22(1 part 1):257–267.
40. Arrand JR, Rymo L, Walsh JE, et al. Molecular cloning of the complete Epstein-Barr virus genome as a set of overlapping restriction endonuclease fragments. *Nucleic Acids Res* 1981;9(13):2999–3014.
41. Buell GN, Reisman D, Kintner C, et al. Cloning overlapping DNA fragments from the B95-8 strain of Epstein-Barr virus reveals a site of homology to the internal repetition. *J Virol* 1981;40(3):977–982.
42. Fischer DK, Miller G, Gradoville L, et al. Genome of a mononucleosis Epstein-Barr virus contains DNA fragments previously regarded to be unique to Burkitt's lymphoma isolates. *Cell* 1981;24(2):543–553.
43. Polack A, Hartl G, Zimber U, et al. A complete set of overlapping cosmid clones of M-ABA virus derived from nasopharyngeal carcinoma and its similarity to other Epstein-Barr virus isolates. *Gene* 1984;27(3):279–288.
44. Skare J, Strominger JL. Cloning and mapping of BamHI endonuclease fragments of DNA from the transforming B95-8 strain of Epstein-Barr virus. *Proc Natl Acad Sci U S A* 1980;77(7):3860–3864.
45. Cho MS, Bornkamm GW, zur Hausen H. Structure of defective DNA molecules in Epstein-Barr virus preparations from P3HR-1 cells. *J Virol* 1984;51(1):199–207.
46. Davison AJ, Scott JE. The complete DNA sequence of varicella-zoster virus. *J Gen Virol* 1986;67(part 9):1759–1816.
47. Davison AJ, Taylor P. Genetic relations between varicella-zoster virus and Epstein-Barr virus. *J Gen Virol* 1987;68(part 4):1067–1079.
48. Davison AJ, Wilkie NM. Nucleotide sequences of the joint between the L and S segments of herpes simplex virus types 1 and 2. *J Gen Virol* 1981;55(part 2):315–331.
49. Kouzarides T, Bankier AT, Satchwell SC, et al. Large-scale rearrangement of homologous regions in the genomes of HCMV and EBV. *Virology* 1987;157(2):397–413.
50. Dolan A, Jamieson FE, Cunningham C, et al. The genome sequence of herpes simplex virus type 2. *J Virol* 1998;72:2010–2021.
51. Russo JJ, Bohenzky RA, Chien MC, et al. . Nucleotide sequence of the Kaposi sarcoma-associated herpesvirus (HHV8). *Proc Natl Acad Sci U S A* 1996;93:14862–14867.
52. Nicholas J, Cameron KR, Coleman H, et al. Analysis of nucleotide sequence of the rightmost 43 kbp of herpesvirus saimiri (HVS) L-DNA: general conservation of genetic organization between HVS and Epstein-Barr virus. *Virology* 1992;188(1):296–310.
53. Cameron KR, Stamminger T, Craxton M, et al. The 160,000-Mr virion protein encoded at the right end of the herpesvirus saimiri genome is homologous to the 140,000-Mr membrane antigen encoded at the left end of the Epstein-Barr virus genome. *J Virol* 1987;61(7):2063–2070.
54. Costa RH, Draper KG, Kelly TJ, et al. An unusual spliced herpes simplex virus type 1 transcript with sequence homology to Epstein-Barr virus DNA. *J Virol* 1985;54(2):317–328.
55. Pellett PE, Biggin MD, Barrell B, et al. Epstein-Barr virus genome may encode a protein showing significant amino acid and predicted secondary structure homology with glycoprotein B of herpes simplex virus 1. *J Virol* 1985;56(3):807–813.
56. Luka J, Kreofsky T, Pearson GR, et al. Partial purification and characterization of a cellular protein crossreacting with the 72K EBNA. *J Virol* 1984;52:833–838.
57. Wen LT, Lai PK, Bradley G, et al. Interaction of Epstein-Barr viral (EBV) origin of replication (oriP) with EBNA-1 and cellular anti-EBNA-1 proteins. *Virology* 1990;178(1):293–296.
58. Packham G, Economou A, Rooney CM, et al. Structure and function of the Epstein-Barr virus BZLF1 protein. *J Virol* 1990;64(5):2110–2116.
59. Cleary ML, Smith SD, Sklar J. Cloning and structural analysis of cDNAs for bcl-2 and a hybrid bcl-2/immunoglobulin transcript resulting from the t(14;18) translocation. *Cell* 1986;47(1):19–28.
60. Pearson GR, Luka J, Petti L, et al. Identification of an Epstein-Barr virus early gene encoding a second component of the restricted early antigen complex. *Virology* 1987;160(1):151–161.
61. Moore KW, O'Garra A, de Waal Malefyt R, et al. Interleukin-10. *Annu Rev Immunol* 1993;11:165–190.
62. Moore KW, Vieira P, Fiorentino DF, et al. Homology of cytokine synthesis inhibitory factor (IL-10) to the Epstein-Barr virus gene BCRFI [published erratum appears in *Science* 1990;250(4980):494]. *Science* 1990;248(4960):1230–1234.
63. Adldinger HK, Delius H, Freese UK, et al. A putative transforming gene of Jijoye virus differs from that of Epstein-Barr virus prototypes. *Virology* 1985;141(2):221–234.
64. Apolloni A, Sculley TB. Detection of A-type and B-type Epstein-Barr virus in throat washings and lymphocytes. *Virology* 1994;202(2):978–981.
65. Dambaugh T, Hennessy K, Chamnankit L, et al. U2 region of Epstein-Barr virus DNA may encode Epstein-Barr nuclear antigen 2. *Proc Natl Acad Sci U S A* 1984;81(23):7632–7636.
66. Gerber P, Nkrumah FK, Pritchett R, et al. Comparative studies of Epstein-Barr virus strains from Ghana and the United States. *Int J Cancer* 1976;17(1):71–81.
67. King W, Dambaugh T, Heller M, et al. Epstein-Barr virus DNA XII. A variable region of the Epstein-Barr virus genome is included in the P3HR-1 deletion. *J Virol* 1982;43(3):979–986.
68. Rowe M, Young LS, Cadwallader K, et al. Distinction between Epstein-Barr virus type A (EBNA2A) and type B (EBNA2B) isolates extends to the EBNA 3 family of nuclear proteins. *J Virol* 1989;63(3):1031–1039.
69. Sample J, Young L, Martin B, et al. Epstein-Barr virus types 1 and 2 differ in their EBNA-3A, EBNA-3B, and EBNA-3C genes. *J Virol* 1990;64(9):4084–4092.

70. Sculley TB, Sculley DG, Pope JH, Bornkamm GW, Lenoir GM, Rickinson AB: Epstein-Barr virus nuclear antigens 1 and 2 in Burkitt lymphoma cell lines containing either "A" - or "B" -type virus. *Intervirology* 1988;29(2):77–85.

71. Seibl R, Motz M, Wolf H. Strain-specific transcription and translation of the BamHI Z area of Epstein-Barr virus. *J Virol* 1986;60(3):902–909.

72. Sixbey JW, Shirley P, Chesney PJ, et al. Detection of a second widespread strain of Epstein-Barr virus. *Lancet* 1989;2(8666):761–765.

73. Young LS, Yao QY, Rooney CM, et al. New type B isolates of Epstein-Barr virus from Burkitt's lymphoma and from normal individuals in endemic areas. *J Gen Virol* 1987;68(part 11):2853–2862.

74. Zimber U, Adldinger HK, Lenoir GM, et al. Geographical prevalence of two types of Epstein-Barr virus. *Virology* 1986;154(1):56–66.

75. Levy JA, Levy SB, Hirshaut Y, et al. Presence of EBV antibodies in sera from wild chimpanzees. *Nature* 1971;233(5321):559–560.

76. Nonoyama M, Pagano JS. Homology between Epstein-Barr virus DNA and viral DNA from Burkitt's lymphoma and nasopharyngeal carcinoma determined by DNA-DNA reassociation kinetics. *Nature* 1973;242(5392): 44–47.

77. Jenson HB, Farrell PJ, Miller G. Sequences of the Epstein-Barr virus (EBV) large internal repeat form the center of a 16-kilobase-pair palindrome of EBV (P3HR-1) heterogeneous DNA [published erratum appears in *J Virol* 1987;61(9):2950]. *J Virol* 1987;61(5):1495–1506.

78. Hu LF, Zabarovsky ER, Chen F, et al. Isolation and sequencing of the Epstein-Barr virus BNLF-1 gene (LMP1) from a Chinese nasopharyngeal carcinoma. *J Gen Virol* 1991;72(part 10):2399–2409.

79. Sample J, Kieff EF, Kieff ED. Epstein-Barr virus types 1 and 2 have nearly identical LMP-1 transforming genes. *J Gen Virol* 1994;75(part 10):2741–2746.

80. Dambaugh T, Hennessy K, Chamasukit L, et al. The Epstein-Barr virus genome and its expression in latent infection. In: Epstein M, Achong B, eds. *The Epstein-Barr virus: recent advances.* London: William Heinemann, 1986: 13–45.

81. Rymo L, Lindahl T, Adams A. Sites of sequence variability in Epstein-Barr virus DNA from different sources. *Proc Natl Acad Sci U S A* 1979;76(6):2794–2798.

82. Rymo L, Lindahl T, Povey S, et al. Analysis of restriction endonuclease fragments of intracellular Epstein-Barr virus DNA and isoenzymes indicate a common origin of the Raji, NC-37, and F-265 human lymphoid cell lines. *Virology* 1981;115(1):115–124.

83. Bornkamm GW, von Knebel-Doeberitz M, Lenoir GM. No evidence for differences in the Epstein-Barr virus genome carried in Burkitt lymphoma cells and nonmalignant lymphoblastoid cells from the same patients. *Proc Natl Acad Sci U S A* 1984;81(15):4930–4834.

84. Fingeroth JD, Weis JJ, Tedder TF, et al. Epstein-Barr virus receptor of human B lymphocytes is the C3d receptor CR2. *Proc Natl Acad Sci U S A* 1984;81(14):4510–4514.

85. Frade R, Barel M, Ehlin-Henriksson B, et al. gp140, the C3d receptor of human B lymphocytes, is also the Epstein-Barr virus receptor. *Proc Natl Acad Sci U S A* 1985;82(5):1490–1493.

86. Nemerow GR, Wolfert R, McNaughton ME, et al. Identification and characterization of the Epstein-Barr virus receptor on human B lymphocytes and its relationship to the C3d complement receptor (CR2). *J Virol* 1985;55(2):347–351.

87. Weis JJ, Tedder TF, Fearon DT. Identification of a 145,000 Mr membrane protein as the C3d receptor (CR2) of human B lymphocytes. *Proc Natl Acad Sci U S A* 1984;81(3):881–885.

88. Nemerow GR, Houghten RA, Moore MD, et al. Identification of an epitope in the major envelope protein of Epstein-Barr virus that mediates viral binding to the B lymphocyte EBV receptor (CR2). *Cell* 1989;56(3):369–377.

89. Nemerow GR, Mold C, Schwend VK, et al. Identification of gp350 as the viral glycoprotein mediating attachment of Epstein-Barr virus (EBV) to the EBV/C3d receptor of B cells: sequence homology of gp350 and C3 complement fragment C3d. *J Virol* 1987;61(5):1416–1420.

90. Tanner J, Whang Y, Sample J, et al. Soluble gp350/220 and deletion mutant glycoproteins block Epstein-Barr virus adsorption to lymphocytes. *J Virol* 1988;62:4452–4464.

91. Tanner J, Weis J, Fearon D, et al. Epstein-Barr virus gp350/220 binding to the B lymphocyte C3d receptor mediates adsorption, capping, and endocytosis. *Cell* 1987;50(2):203–213.

92. Lambris JD, Ganu VS, Hirani S, et al. Mapping of the C3d receptor (CR2)-binding site and a neoantigenic site in the C3d domain of the third component of complement. *Proc Natl Acad Sci U S A* 1985;82(12):4235–4239.

93. Beisel C, Tanner J, Matsuo T, et al. Two major outer envelope glycoproteins of Epstein-Barr virus are encoded by the same gene. *J Virol* 1985;54(3):665–674.

94. Biggin M, Farrell PJ, Barrell BG. Transcription and DNA sequence of the BamHI L fragment of B95-8 Epstein-Barr virus. *EMBO J* 1984;3(5):1083–1090.

95. Whang Y, Silberklang M, Morgan A, et al. Expression of the Epstein-Barr virus gp350/220 gene in rodent and primate cells. *J Virol* 1987;61(6):1796–1807.

96. Birkenbach M, Tong X, Bradbury LE, et al. Characterization of an Epstein-Barr virus receptor on human epithelial cells. *J Exp Med* 1992;176(5):1405–1414.

97. Martin DR, Yuryev A, Kalli KR, et al. Determination of the structural basis for selective binding of Epstein-Barr virus to human complement receptor type 2. *J Exp Med* 1991;174(6):1299–1311.

98. Janz A, Oezel M, Kurzeder C, et al. Infectious Epstein-Barr virus lacking major glycoprotein BLLF1 (gp350/220) demonstrates the existence of additional viral ligands. *J Virol* 2000;74(21):10142–10152.

99. Thorley-Lawson DA, Poodry CA. Identification and isolation of the main component (gp350-gp220) of Epstein-Barr virus responsible for generating neutralizing antibodies *in vivo*. *J Virol* 1982;43(2):730–736.

100. Nemerow GR, Cooper NR. Early events in the infection of human B lymphocytes by Epstein-Barr virus: the internalization process. *Virology* 1984;132(1):186–198.

101. Heineman T, Gong M, Sample J, et al. Identification of the Epstein-Barr virus gp85 gene. *J Virol* 1988;62(4):1101–1107.

102. Miller N, Hutt-Fletcher LM. A monoclonal antibody to glycoprotein gp85 inhibits fusion but not attachment of Epstein-Barr virus. *J Virol* 1988;62(7):2366–2372.

103. Wang X, Kenyon WJ, Li Q, et al. Epstein-Barr virus uses different complexes of glycoproteins gH and gL to infect B lymphocytes and epithelial cells. *J Virol* 1998;72(7):5552–5558.

104. Haan KM, Longnecker R. Coreceptor restriction within the HLA-DQ locus for Epstein-Barr virus infection. *Proc Natl Acad Sci U S A* 2000;97(16):9252–9257.

105. Molesworth SJ, Lake CM, Borza CM, et al. Epstein-Barr virus gH is essential for penetration of B cells but also plays a role in attachment of virus to epithelial cells. *J Virol* 2000;74(14):6324–6332.

106. Alfieri C, Birkenbach M, Kieff E. Early events in Epstein-Barr virus infection of human B lymphocytes [published erratum appears in *Virology* 1991;185(2):946]. *Virology* 1991;181(2):595–608.

107. Hurley EA, Thorley-Lawson DA. B cell activation and the establishment of Epstein-Barr virus latency. *J Exp Med* 1988;168(6):2059–2075.

108. Adams A, Lindahl T. Epstein-Barr virus genomes with properties of circular DNA molecules in carrier cells. *Proc Natl Acad Sci U S A* 1975;72(4):1477–1481.

109. Matsuo T, Heller M, Petti L, et al. Persistence of the entire Epstein-Barr virus genome integrated into human lymphocyte DNA. *Science* 1984;226(4680):1322–1325.

110. Hudewentz J, Bornkamm GW, Zur Hausen H. Effect of the diterpene ester TPA on Epstein-Barr virus antigen and DNA synthesis in producer and nonproducer cell lines. *Virology* 1980;100(1):175–178.

111. Luka J, Kallin B, Klein G. Induction of the Epstein-Barr virus (EBV) cycle in latently infected cells by n-butyrate. *Virology* 1979;94(1):228–231.

112. Ragona G, Ernberg I, Klein G. Induction and biological characterization of the Epstein-Barr virus (EBV) carried by the Jijoye lymphoma line. *Virology* 1980;101(2):553–557.

113. Ben-Sasson SA, Klein G. Activation of the Epstein-Barr virus genome by 5-azacytidine in latently infected human lymphoid lines. *Int J Cancer* 1981;28(2):131–135.

114. Saemundsen AK, Kallin B, Klein G. Effect of n-butyrate on cellular and viral DNA synthesis in cells latently infected with Epstein-Barr virus. *Virology* 1980;107(2):557–561.

115. zur Hausen H, O'Neill F, Freese U, et al. Persisting oncogenic herpesvirus induced by tumor promoter TPA. *Nature* 1978;272:373–375.

116. Lee W, Mitchell P, Tjian R. Purified transcription factor AP-1 interacts with TPA-inducible enhancer elements. *Cell* 1987;49(6):741–752.

117. Farrell P, Rowe D, Rooney C, et al. Latent and lytic cycle promoters of the Epstein-Barr virus. *EMBO J* 1983;2:1331–1338.

118. Farrell PJ, Rowe DT, Rooney CM, et al. Epstein-Barr virus BZLF1 transactivator specifically binds to a consensus AP-1 site and is related to c-fos. *EMBO J* 1989;8(1):127–132.

119. Flemington E, Speck SH. Identification of phorbol ester response elements in the promoter of Epstein-Barr virus putative lytic switch gene BZLF1. *J Virol* 1990;64(3):1217–1226.

120. Laux G, Freese UK, Fischer R, et al. TPA-inducible Epstein-Barr virus genes in Raji cells and their regulation. *Virology* 1988;162(2):503–507.

121. Takada K. Cross-linking of cell surface immunoglobulins induces Epstein-Barr virus in Burkitt lymphoma lines. *Int J Cancer* 1984;33(1):27–32.

122. Takada K, Ono Y. Synchronous and sequential activation of latently infected Epstein-Barr virus genomes. *J Virol* 1989;63(1):445–449.

123. Daibata M, Humphreys RE, Sairenji T. Phosphorylation of the Epstein-Barr virus BZLF1 immediate-early gene product ZEBRA. *Virology* 1992;188(2):916–920.

124. Daibata M, Humphreys RE, Takada K, et al. Activation of latent EBV via anti-IgG-triggered, second messenger pathways in the Burkitt's lymphoma cell line Akata. *J Immunol* 1990;144(12):4788–4793.

125. Roizman B, Pellett PE. The family Herpesviridae: a brief introduction. In: Knipe DM, Howley PM, et al., eds. *Field's virology,* 4th ed. Philadelphia: Lippincott Williams & Wilkins, 2001:2381–2397.

126. Marschall M, Schwarzmann F, Leser U, et al. The BI'LF4 trans-activator of Epstein-Barr virus is modulated by type and differentiation of the host cell. *Virology* 1991;181(1):172–179.

127. Grogan E, Jenson H, Countryman J, et al. Transfection of a rearranged viral DNA fragment, WZhet, stably converts latent Epstein-Barr viral infection to productive infection in lymphoid cells. *Proc Natl Acad Sci U S A* 1987;84(5):1332–1336.

128. Jenson HB, Miller G. Polymorphisms of the region of the Epstein-Barr virus genome which disrupts latency. *Virology* 1988;165(2):549–564.

129. Jenson HB, Rabson MS, Miller G. Palindromic structure and polypeptide expression of 36 kilobase pairs of heterogeneous Epstein-Barr virus (P3HR-1) DNA. *J Virol* 1986;58(2):475–486.

130. Miller G, Rabson M, Heston L. Epstein-Barr virus with heterogeneous DNA disrupts latency. *J Virol* 1984;50(1):174–182.

131. Lieberman PM, Berk AJ. *In vitro* transcriptional activation, dimerization,

and DNA-binding specificity of the Epstein-Barr virus Zta protein *J Virol* 1990;64(6):2560–2568.

132. Chi T, Carey M. The ZEBRA activation domain: modular organization and mechanism of action. *Mol Cell Biol* 1993;13(11):7045–7055.

133. Flemington EK, Borras AM, Lytle JP, et al. Characterization of the Epstein-Barr virus BZLF1 protein transactivation domain. *J Virol* 1992;66(2):922–929.

134. Lieberman PM, Berk AJ. The Zta trans-activator protein stabilizes TFIID association with promoter DNA by direct protein-protein interaction. *Genes Dev* 1991;5(12B):2441–2454.

135. Chang YN, Dong DL, Hayward GS, et al. The Epstein-Barr virus Zta trans-activator: a member of the bZIP family with unique DNA-binding specificity and a dimerization domain that lacks the characteristic heptad leucine zipper motif. *J Virol* 1990;64(7):3358–3369.

136. Flemington EK, Lytle JP, Cayrol C, et al. DNA-binding-defective mutants of the Epstein-Barr virus lytic switch activator Zta transactivate with altered specificities. *Mol Cell Biol* 1994;14(5):3041–3052.

137. Mikaelian I, Drouet E, Marechal V, et al. The DNA-binding domain of two bZIP transcription factors, the Epstein-Barr virus switch gene product EB1 and Jun, is a bipartite nuclear targeting sequence. *J Virol* 1993;67(2):734–742.

138. Kouzarides T, Packham G, Cook A, et al. The BZLF1 protein of EBV has a coiled coil dimerisation domain without a heptad leucine repeat but with homology to the C/EBP leucine zipper. *Oncogene* 1991;6(2):195–204.

139. Flemington E, Speck SH. Evidence for coiled-coil dimer formation by an Epstein-Barr virus transactivator that lacks a heptad repeat of leucine residues. *Proc Natl Acad Sci U S A* 1990;87(23):9459–9463.

140. Lieberman PM, Hardwick JM, Sample J, et al. The zta transactivator involved in induction of lytic cycle gene expression in Epstein-Barr virus–infected lymphocytes binds to both AP-1 and ZRE sites in target promoter and enhancer regions. *J Virol* 1990;64(3):1143–1155.

141. Kolman JL, Taylor N, Marshak DR, et al. Serine-173 of the Epstein-Barr virus ZEBRA protein is required for DNA binding and is a target for casein kinase II phosphorylation. *Proc Natl Acad Sci U S A* 1993;90(21):10115–10119.

142. Zhang Q, Gutsch D, Kenney S. Functional and physical interaction between p53 and BZLF1: implications for Epstein-Barr virus latency. *Mol Cell Biol* 1994;14(3):1929–1938.

143. Gutsch DE, Holley-Guthrie EA, Zhang Q, et al. The bZIP transactivator of Epstein-Barr virus, BZLF1, functionally and physically interacts with the p65 subunit of NF-kappa B. *Mol Cell Biol* 1994;14(3):1939–1948.

144. Gruffat H, Sergeant A. Characterization of the DNA-binding site repertoire for the Epstein-Barr virus transcription factor R. *Nucleic Acids Res* 1994;22(7):1172–1178.

145. Bankier AT, Deininger PL, Satchwell SC, et al. DNA sequence analysis of the EcoRI Dhet fragment of B95-8 Epstein-Barr virus containing the terminal repeat sequences. *Mol Biol Med* 1983;1(4):425–445.

146. Biggin M, Bodescot M, Perricaudet M, et al. Epstein-Barr virus gene expression in P3HR1-superinfected Raji cells. *J Virol* 1987;61(10):3120–3132.

147. Gibson T, Stockwell P, Ginsburg M, et al. Homology between two EBV early genes and HSV ribonucleotide reductase and 38K genes. *Nucleic Acids Res* 1984;12(12):5087–5099.

148. Gibson TJ, Barrell BG, Farrell PJ. Coding content and expression of the EBV B95-8 genome in the region from base 62,248 to base 82,920. *Virology* 1986;152(1):136–148.

149. Hatfull G, Bankier AT, Barrell BG, et al. Sequence analysis of Raji Epstein-Barr virus DNA. *Virology* 1988;164(2):334–340.

150. Fixman ED, Hayward GS, Hayward SD. trans-acting requirements for replication of Epstein-Barr virus ori- Lyt. *J Virol* 1992;66(8):5030–5039.

151. Gergely L, Klein G, Ernberg I. Host cell macromolecular synthesis in cells containing EBV-induced early antigens, studied by combined immunofluorescence and radioautography. *Virology* 1971;45(1):22–29.

152. Gong M, Kieff E. Intracellular trafficking of two major Epstein-Barr virus glycoproteins, gp350/220 and gp110. *J Virol* 1990;64(4):1507–1516.

153. Hummel M, Kieff E. Mapping of polypeptides encoded by the Epstein-Barr virus genome in productive infection. *Proc Natl Acad Sci U S A* 1982;79(18):5698–5702.

154. Gong M, Ooka T, Matsuo T, et al. Epstein-Barr virus glycoprotein homologous to herpes simplex virus gB. *J Virol* 1987;61(2):499–508.

155. Hummel M, Thorley-Lawson D, Kieff E. An Epstein-Barr virus DNA fragment encodes messages for the two major envelope glycoproteins (gp350/300 and gp220/200). *J Virol* 1984;49(2):413–417.

156. Mackett M, Conway MJ, Arrand JR, et al. Characterization and expression of a glycoprotein encoded by the Epstein-Barr virus BamHI I fragment. *J Virol* 1990;64(6):2545–2552.

157. Emini EA, Luka J, Armstrong ME, et al. Identification of an Epstein-Barr virus glycoprotein which is antigenically homologous to the varicella-zoster virus glycoprotein II and the herpes simplex virus glycoprotein B. *Virology* 1987;157(2):552–555.

158. Hoffman GJ, Lazarowitz SG, Hayward SD. Monoclonal antibody against a 250,000-dalton glycoprotein of Epstein-Barr virus identifies a membrane antigen and a neutralizing antigen. *Proc Natl Acad Sci U S A* 1980;77(5):2979–2983.

159. Strnad BC, Neubauer RH, Rabin H, et al. Correlation between Epstein-Barr virus membrane antigen and three large cell surface glycoproteins. *J Virol* 1979;32(3):885–894.

160. Thorley-Lawson DA, Geilinger K. Monoclonal antibodies against the major glycoprotein (gp350/220) of Epstein-Barr virus neutralize infectivity. *Proc Natl Acad Sci U S A* 1980;77(9):5307–5311.

161. Hsu DH, de Waal Malefyt R, Fiorentino DF, et al. Expression of interleukin-10 activity by Epstein-Barr virus protein BCRF1. *Science* 1990;250(4982):830–832.

162. Vieira P, de Waal-Malefyt R, Dang MN, et al. Isolation and expression of human cytokine synthesis inhibitory factor cDNA clones: homology to Epstein-Barr virus open reading frame BCRFI. *Proc Natl Acad Sci U S A* 1991;88(4):1172–1176.

163. Swaminathan S, Hesselton R, Sullivan J, et al. Epstein-Barr virus recombinants with specifically mutated BCRF1 genes. *J Virol* 1993;67(12):7406–7413.

164. Kurilla MG, Swaminathan S, Welsh RM, et al. Effects of virally expressed interleukin-10 on vaccinia virus infection in mice. *J Virol* 1993;67(12):7623–7628.

165. Finke J, Rowe M, Kallin B, et al. Monoclonal and polyclonal antibodies against Epstein-Barr virus nuclear antigen 5 (EBNA-5) detect multiple protein species in Burkitt's lymphoma and lymphoblastoid cell lines. *J Virol* 1987;61(12):3870–3878.

166. Wang F, Petti L, Braun D, Seung S, et al. A bicistronic Epstein-Barr virus mRNA encodes two nuclear proteins in latently infected, growth-transformed lymphocytes. *J Virol* 1987;61(4):945–954.

167. Petti L, Sample C, Kieff E. Subnuclear localization and phosphorylation of Epstein-Barr virus latent infection nuclear proteins. *Virology* 1990;176(2):563–574.

168. Hammerschmidt W, Sugden B. Genetic analysis of immortalizing functions of Epstein-Barr virus in human B lymphocytes. *Nature* 1989;340(6232):393–397.

169. Mannick JB, Cohen JI, Birkenbach M, et al. The Epstein-Barr virus nuclear protein encoded by the leader of the EBNA RNAs is important in B-lymphocyte transformation. *J Virol* 1991;65(12):6826–6837.

170. Harada S, Kieff E. Epstein-Barr virus nuclear protein LP stimulates EBNA-2 acidic domain-mediated transcriptional activation. *J Virol* 1997;71(9):6611–6618.

171. Sinclair AJ, Palmero I, Peters G, et al. EBNA-2 and EBNA-LP cooperate to cause G0 to G1 transition during immortalization of resting human B lymphocytes by Epstein-Barr virus. *EMBO J* 1994;13(14):3321–3328.

172. Cohen JI, Wang F, Mannick J, et al. Epstein-Barr virus nuclear protein 2 is a key determinant of lymphocyte transformation. *Proc Natl Acad Sci U S A* 1989; 86(23):9558–9562.

173. Miller G, Robinson J, Heston L, et al. Differences between laboratory strains of Epstein-Barr virus based on immortalization, abortive infection, and interference. *Proc Natl Acad Sci U S A* 1974;71(10):4006–4010.

174. Hennessy K, Kieff E. A second nuclear protein is encoded by Epstein-Barr virus in latent infection. *Science* 1985;8;227(4691):1238–1240.

175. Hennessy K, Kieff E. One of two Epstein-Barr virus nuclear antigens contains a glycine-alanine copolymer domain. *Proc Natl Acad Sci U S A* 1983;80(18):5665–5669.

176. Hennessy K, Heller M, van Santen V, et al. Simple repeat array in Epstein-Barr virus DNA encodes part of the Epstein-Barr nuclear antigen. *Science* 1983;220(4604):1396–1398.

177. Cohen JI, Wang F, Kieff E. Epstein-Barr virus nuclear protein 2 mutations define essential domains for transformation and transactivation. *J Virol* 1991; 65(5):2545–2554.

178. Harada S, Yalamanchili R, Kieff E. Epstein-Barr virus nuclear protein 2 has at least two N-terminal domains that mediate self-association. *J Virol* 2001;75(5):2482–2487.

179. Wang F, Gregory CD, Rowe M, et al. Epstein-Barr virus nuclear antigen 2 specifically induces expression of the B-cell activation antigen CD23. *Proc Natl Acad Sci U S A* 1987;84(10):3452–3456.

180. Wang F, Gregory C, Sample C, et al. Epstein-Barr virus latent membrane protein (LMP1) and nuclear proteins 2 and 3C are effectors of phenotypic changes in B lymphocytes: EBNA-2 and LMP1 cooperatively induce CD23. *J Virol* 1990;64(5):2309–2318.

181. Knutson JC. The level of c-fgr RNA is increased by EBNA-2, an Epstein-Barr virus gene required for B-cell immortalization. *J Virol* 1990;64(6):2530–2536.

182. Abbot SD, Rowe M, Cadwallader K, et al. Epstein-Barr virus nuclear antigen 2 induces expression of the virus-encoded latent membrane protein. *J Virol* 1990;64(5):2126–2134.

183. Wang F, Tsang SF, Kurilla MG, et al. Epstein-Barr virus nuclear antigen 2 transactivates latent membrane protein LMP1. *J Virol* 1990;64(7):3407–3416.

184. Fahraeus R, Jansson A, Ricksten A, et al. Epstein-Barr virus–encoded nuclear antigen 2 activates the viral latent membrane protein promoter by modulating the activity of a negative regulatory element. *Proc Natl Acad Sci U S A* 1990;87(19):7390–7394.

185. Tsang SF, Wang F, Izumi KM, et al. Delineation of the cis-acting element mediating EBNA-2 transactivation of latent infection membrane protein expression. *J Virol* 1991;65(12):6765–6771.

186. Zimber-Strobl U, Kremmer E, Grasser F, et al. The Epstein-Barr virus nuclear antigen 2 interacts with an EBNA2 responsive cis-element of the terminal protein 1 gene promoter. *EMBO J* 1993;12(1):167–175.

187. Hinuma Y, Konn M, Yamaguchi J, et al. Immunofluorescence and herpes-type virus particles in the P3HR-1 Burkitt lymphoma cell line. *J Virol* 1967;1(5):1045–1051.

188. Cohen JI, Kieff E. An Epstein-Barr virus nuclear protein 2 domain essential for transformation is a direct transcriptional activator. *J Virol* 1991;65(11):5880–5885.

189. Cohen JI. A region of herpes simplex virus VP16 can substitute for a

transforming domain of Epstein-Barr virus nuclear protein 2. *Proc Natl Acad Sci U S A* 1992;89(17):8030–8034.

190. Tong X, Wang F, Thut CJ, et al. The Epstein-Barr virus nuclear protein 2 acidic domain can interact with TFIIB, TAF40, and RPA70 but not with TATA-binding protein. *J Virol* 1995;69(1):585–588.

191. Tong X, Drapkin R, Yalamanchili R, et al. The Epstein-Barr virus nuclear protein 2 acidic domain forms a complex with a novel cellular coactivator that can interact with TFIIE. *Mol Cell Biol* 1995;15(9):4735–4744.

192. Wang L, Grossman SR, Kieff E. Epstein-Barr virus nuclear protein 2 interacts with p300, CBP, and PCAF histone acetyltransferases in activation of the LMP1 promoter. *Proc Natl Acad Sci U S A* 2000;97(1):430–435.

193. Grossman SR, Johannsen E, Tong X, et al. The Epstein-Barr virus nuclear antigen 2 transactivator is directed to response elements by the J kappa recombination signal binding protein. *Proc Natl Acad Sci U S A* 1994;91(16):7568–7572.

194. Henkel T, Ling PD, Hayward SD, et al. Mediation of Epstein-Barr virus EBNA2 transactivation by recombination signal-binding protein J kappa. *Science* 1994;265(5168):92–95.

195. Johannsen E, Koh E, Mosialos G, et al. Epstein-Barr virus nuclear protein 2 transactivation of the latent membrane protein 1 promoter is mediated by J kappa and PU.1. *J Virol* 1995;69(1):253–262.

196. Joab I, Rowe DT, Bodescot M, et al. Mapping of the gene coding for Epstein-Barr virus–determined nuclear antigen EBNA3 and its transient overexpression in a human cell line by using an adenovirus expression vector. *J Virol* 1987;61(10):3340–3344.

197. Kallin B, Dillner J, Ernberg I, et al. Four virally determined nuclear antigens are expressed in Epstein- Barr virus-transformed cells. *Proc Natl Acad Sci U S A* 1986;83(5):1499–1503.

198. Kerdiles B, Walls D, Triki H, et al. cDNA cloning and transient expression of the Epstein-Barr virus–determined nuclear antigen Ebna3b in human cells and identification of novel transcripts from its coding region. *J Virol* 1990;64(4):1812–1816.

199. Petti L, Kieff E. A sixth Epstein-Barr virus nuclear protein (EBNA3B) is expressed in latently infected growth-transformed lymphocytes. *J Virol* 1988; 62(6):2173–2178.

200. Petti L, Sample J, Wang F, et al. A fifth Epstein-Barr virus nuclear protein (EBNA3C) is expressed in latently infected growth-transformed lymphocytes. *J Virol* 1988;62(4):1330–1338.

201. Ricksten A, Kallin B, Alexander H, et al. BamHI E region of the Epstein-Barr virus genome encodes three transformation-associated nuclear proteins. *Proc Natl Acad Sci U S A* 1988;85(4):995–999.

202. Bodescot M, Brison O, Perricaudet M. An Epstein-Barr virus transcription unit is at least 84 kilobases long. *Nucleic Acids Res* 1986;14(6):2611–2620.

203. Bodescot M, Perricaudet M. Epstein-Barr virus mRNAs produced by alternative splicing. *Nucleic Acids Res* 1986;14(17):7103–7114.

204. Tomkinson B, Kieff E. Use of second-site homologous recombination to demonstrate that Epstein-Barr virus nuclear protein 3B is not important for lymphocyte infection or growth transformation *in vitro*. *J Virol* 1992;66(5):2893–2903.

205. Tomkinson B, Robertson E, Kieff E. Epstein-Barr virus nuclear proteins EBNA-3A and EBNA-3C are essential for B-lymphocyte growth transformation. *J Virol* 1993;67(4):2014–2025.

206. Robertson ES, Lin J, Kieff E. The amino-terminal domains of Epstein-Barr virus nuclear proteins 3A, 3B, and 3C interact with RBPJ(kappa). *J Virol* 1996;70(5):3068–3074.

207. Allday MJ, Farrell PJ. Epstein-Barr virus nuclear antigen EBNA3C/6 expression maintains the level of latent membrane protein 1 in G1-arrested cells. *J Virol* 1994;68(9):3491–3498.

208. Lin J, Johannsen E, Robertson E, et al. Epstein-Barr virus nuclear antigen 3C putative repression domain mediates coactivation of the LMP1 promoter with EBNA-2. *J Virol* 2002;76(1):232–242.

209. Jones CH, Hayward SD, Rawlins DR. Interaction of the lymphocyte-derived Epstein-Barr virus nuclear antigen EBNA-1 with its DNA-binding sites. *J Virol* 1989;63(1):101–110.

210. Ambinder RF, Shah WA, Rawlins DR, et al. Definition of the sequence requirements for binding of the EBNA-1 protein to its palindromic target sites in Epstein-Barr virus DNA. *J Virol* 1990;64(5):2369–2379.

211. Rawlins DR, Milman G, Hayward SD, et al. Sequence-specific DNA binding of the Epstein-Barr virus nuclear antigen (EBNA-1) to clustered sites in the plasmid maintenance region. *Cell* 1985;42(3):859–868.

212. Kimball AS, Milman G, Tullius TD. High-resolution footprints of the DNA-binding domain of Epstein-Barr virus nuclear antigen 1. *Mol Cell Biol* 1989;9(6):2738–2742.

213. Yates J, Warren N, Reisman D, et al. A cis-acting element from the Epstein-Barr viral genome that permits stable replication of recombinant plasmids in latently infected cells. *Proc Natl Acad Sci U S A* 1984;81(12):3806–3810.

214. Yates JL, Warren N, Sugden B. Stable replication of plasmids derived from Epstein-Barr virus in various mammalian cells. *Nature* 1985;313(6005):812–815.

215. Reisman D, Yates J, Sugden B. A putative origin of replication of plasmids derived from Epstein-Barr virus is composed of two cis-acting components. *Mol Cell Biol* 1985;5(8):1822–1832.

216. Sugden B, Marsh K, Yates J. A vector that replicates as a plasmid and can be efficiently selected in B-lymphoblasts transformed by Epstein-Barr virus. *Mol Cell Biol* 1985;5(2):410–413.

217. Chittenden T, Lupton S, Levine AJ. Functional limits of oriP, the Epstein-Barr virus plasmid origin of replication. *J Virol* 1989;63(7):3016–3025.

218. Yates JL, Guan N. Epstein-Barr virus-derived plasmids replicate only once per cell cycle and are not amplified after entry into cells. *J Virol* 1991;65(1):483–438.

219. Su W, Middleton T, Sugden B, et al. DNA looping between the origin of replication of Epstein-Barr virus and its enhancer site: stabilization of an origin complex with Epstein-Barr nuclear antigen 1. *Proc Natl Acad Sci U S A* 1991;88(23):10870–10874.

220. Norio P, Schildkraut CL. Visualization of DNA replication on individual Epstein-Barr virus episomes. *Science* 2001;294(5550):2361–2364.

221. Fennewald S, van Santen V, Kieff E. Nucleotide sequence of an mRNA transcribed in latent growth-transforming virus infection indicates that it may encode a membrane protein. *J Virol* 1984;51(2):411–419.

222. Hennessy K, Fennewald S, Hummel M, et al. A membrane protein encoded by Epstein-Barr virus in latent growth-transforming infection. *Proc Natl Acad Sci U S A* 1984;81(22):7207–7211.

223. Liebowitz D, Wang D, Kieff E. Orientation and patching of the latent infection membrane protein encoded by Epstein-Barr virus. *J Virol* 1986;58(1):233–237.

224. Wang D, Liebowitz D, Kieff E. An EBV membrane protein expressed in immortalized lymphocytes transforms established rodent cells. *Cell* 1985;43(3 part 2):831–840.

225. Wang D, Liebowitz D, Kieff E. The truncated form of the Epstein-Barr virus latent-infection membrane protein expressed in virus replication does not transform rodent fibroblasts. *J Virol* 1988;62(7):2337–2346.

226. Wang D, Liebowitz D, Wang F, et al. Epstein-Barr virus latent infection membrane protein alters the human B-lymphocyte phenotype: deletion of the amino terminus abolishes activity. *J Virol* 1988;62(11):4173–4184.

227. Liebowitz D, Mannick J, Takada K, et al. Phenotypes of Epstein-Barr virus LMP1 deletion mutants indicate transmembrane and amino-terminal cytoplasmic domains necessary for effects in B-lymphoma cells. *J Virol* 1992;66(7):4612–4616.

228. Peng M, Lundgren E. Transient expression of the Epstein-Barr virus LMP1 gene in human primary B cells induces cellular activation and DNA synthesis. *Oncogene* 1992;7(9):1775–1782.

229. Rowe M, Peng-Pilon M, Huen DS, et al. Upregulation of bcl-2 by the Epstein-Barr virus latent membrane protein LMP1: a B-cell-specific response that is delayed relative to NF-kappa B activation and to induction of cell surface markers. *J Virol* 1994;68(9):5602–5612.

230. Zhang Q, Brooks L, Busson P, et al. Epstein-Barr virus (EBV) latent membrane protein 1 increases HLA class II expression in an EBV-negative B cell line. *Eur J Immunol* 1994;24(6):1467–1470.

231. Gregory CD, Dive C, Henderson S, et al. Activation of Epstein-Barr virus latent genes protects human B cells from death by apoptosis. *Nature* 1991;349(6310):612–614.

232. Henderson S, Rowe M, Gregory C, et al. Induction of bcl-2 expression by Epstein-Barr virus latent membrane protein 1 protects infected B cells from programmed cell death. *Cell* 1991;65(7):1107–1115.

233. Martin JM, Veis D, Korsmeyer SJ, et al. Latent membrane protein of Epstein-Barr virus induces cellular phenotypes independently of expression of Bcl-2. *J Virol* 1993;67(9):5269–5278.

234. Laherty CD, Hu HM, Opipari AW, et al. The Epstein-Barr virus LMP1 gene product induces A20 zinc finger protein expression by activating nuclear factor kappa B. *J Biol Chem* 1992;267(34):24157–24160.

235. Hammarskjold ML, Simurda MC. Epstein-Barr virus latent membrane protein transactivates the human immunodeficiency virus type 1 long terminal repeat through induction of NF-kappa B activity. *J Virol* 1992;66(11):6496–6501.

236. Dawson CW, Rickinson AB, Young LS. Epstein-Barr virus latent membrane protein inhibits human epithelial cell differentiation. *Nature* 1990;344(6268):777–780.

237. Fahraeus R, Rymo L, Rhim JS, et al. Morphological transformation of human keratinocytes expressing the LMP gene of Epstein-Barr virus. *Nature* 1990;345(6274):447–449.

238. Wilson JB, Weinberg W, Johnson R, et al. Expression of the BNLF-1 oncogene of Epstein-Barr virus in the skin of transgenic mice induces hyperplasia and aberrant expression of keratin 6. *Cell* 1990;61(7):1315–1327.

239. Kulwichit W, Edwards RH, Davenport EM, et al. Expression of the Epstein-Barr virus latent membrane protein 1 induces B cell lymphoma in transgenic mice. *Proc Natl Acad Sci U S A* 1998;95(20):11963–11968.

240. Kaye KM, Izumi KM, Kieff E. Epstein-Barr virus latent membrane protein 1 is essential for B-lymphocyte growth transformation. *Proc Natl Acad Sci U S A* 1993;90(19):9150–9154.

241. Izumi KM, Kaye KM, Kieff ED. Epstein-Barr virus recombinant molecular genetic analysis of the LMP1 amino-terminal cytoplasmic domain reveals a probable structural role, with no component essential for primary B-lymphocyte growth transformation. *J Virol* 1994;68(7):4369–4376.

242. Kaye KM, Izumi KM, Li H, et al. An Epstein-Barr virus that expresses only the first 231 LMP1 amino acids efficiently initiates primary B-lymphocyte growth transformation. *J Virol* 1999;73(12):10525–10530.

243. Izumi KM, Cahir McFarland ED, Riley EA, et al. The residues between the two transformation effector sites of Epstein-Barr virus latent membrane protein 1 are not critical for B-lymphocyte growth transformation. *J Virol* 1999;73(12):9908–9916.

244. Mosialos G, Birkenbach M, Yalamanchili R, et al. The Epstein-Barr virus transforming protein LMP1 engages signaling proteins for the tumor necrosis factor receptor family. *Cell* 1995;80:389–399.

245. Devergne O, Cahir McFarland ED, Mosialos G, et al. Role of the TRAF binding

site and NF-kappaB activation in Epstein-Barr virus latent membrane protein 1-induced cell gene expression. *J Virol* 1998;72(10):7900–7908.

246. Izumi KM, Cahir McFarland ED, Ting AT, et al. The Epstein-Barr virus oncoprotein latent membrane protein 1 engages the tumor necrosis factor receptor-associated proteins TRADD and receptor-interacting protein (RIP) but does not induce apoptosis or require RIP for NF-kappaB activation. *Mol Cell Biol* 1999;19(8):5759–5767.

247. Laux G, Perricaudet M, Farrell PJ. A spliced Epstein-Barr virus gene expressed in immortalized lymphocytes is created by circularization of the linear viral genome. *EMBO J* 1988;7(3):769–774.

248. Sample J, Liebowitz D, Kieff E. Two related Epstein-Barr virus membrane proteins are encoded by separate genes. *J Virol* 1989;63(2):933–937.

249. Longnecker R, Druker B, Roberts TM, et al. An Epstein-Barr virus protein associated with cell growth transformation interacts with a tyrosine kinase. *J Virol* 1991;65(7):3681–3692.

250. Longnecker R, Miller CL, Miao XQ, et al. The only domain which distinguishes Epstein-Barr virus latent membrane protein 2A (LMP2A) from LMP2B is dispensable for lymphocyte infection and growth transformation *in vitro*; LMP2A is therefore nonessential. *J Virol* 1992;66(11):6461–6469.

251. Kim OJ, Yates JL. Mutants of Epstein-Barr virus with a selective marker disrupting the TP gene transform B cells and replicate normally in culture. *J Virol* 1993;67(12):7634–7640.

252. Longnecker R, Miller CL, Miao XQ, et al. The last seven transmembrane and carboxy-terminal cytoplasmic domains of Epstein-Barr virus latent membrane protein 2 (LMP2) are dispensable for lymphocyte infection and growth transformation *in vitro*. *J Virol* 1993;67(4):2006–2013.

253. Longnecker R, Miller CL, Tomkinson B, et al. Deletion of DNA encoding the first five transmembrane domains of Epstein-Barr virus latent membrane proteins 2A and 2B. *J Virol* 1993;67(8):5068–5074.

254. Burkhardt AL, Bolen JB, Kieff E, et al. An Epstein-Barr virus transformation-associated membrane protein interacts with src family tyrosine kinases. *J Virol* 1992;66(8):5161–5167.

255. Miller CL, Longnecker R, Kieff E. Epstein-Barr virus latent membrane protein 2A blocks calcium mobilization in B lymphocytes. *J Virol* 1993;67(6):3087–3094.

256. Miller CL, Lee JH, Kieff E, et al. An integral membrane protein (LMP2) blocks reactivation of Epstein-Barr virus from latency following surface immunoglobulin crosslinking. *Proc Natl Acad Sci U S A* 1994;91(2):772–776.

257. Miller CL, Burkhardt AL, Lee JH, et al. Integral membrane protein 2 of Epstein-Barr virus regulates reactivation from latency through dominant negative effects on protein-tyrosine kinases. *Immunity* 1995;2(2):155–166.

258. Merchant M, Caldwell RG, Longnecker R. The LMP2A ITAM is essential for providing B cells with development and survival signals *in vivo*. *J Virol* 2000;74(19):9115–9124.

259. Lerner MR, Andrews NC, Miller G, et al. Two small RNAs encoded by Epstein-Barr virus and complexed with protein are precipitated by antibodies from patients with systemic lupus erythematosus. *Proc Natl Acad Sci U S A* 1981;78(2):805–809.

260. Rosa MD, Gottlieb E, Lerner MR, et al. Striking similarities are exhibited by two small Epstein-Barr virus-encoded ribonucleic acids and the adenovirus-associated ribonucleic acids VAI and VAII. *Mol Cell Biol* 1981;1(9):785–796.

261. Howe JG, Steitz JA. Localization of Epstein-Barr virus–encoded small RNAs by *in situ* hybridization. *Proc Natl Acad Sci U S A* 1986;83(23):9006–9010.

262. Howe JG, Shu MD. Epstein-Barr virus small RNA (EBER) genes: unique transcription units that combine RNA polymerase II and III promoter elements. *Cell* 1989;57(5):825–834.

263. Glickman JN, Howe JG, Steitz JA. Structural analyses of EBER1 and EBER2 ribonucleoprotein particles present in Epstein-Barr virus–infected cells. *J Virol* 1988;62(3):902–911.

264. Laing KG, Elia A, Jeffrey IW, et al. Analysis of RNA-protein interactions of the EBV-encoded small RNAs, the EBERs. *In vitro* assays. *Methods Mol Biol* 2001;174:297–310.

265. Nanbo A, Inoue K, Adachi-Takasawa K, et al. Epstein-Barr virus RNA confers resistance to interferon-alpha-induced apoptosis in Burkitt's lymphoma. *EMBO J* 2002;21(5):954–965.

266. Swaminathan S, Tomkinson B, Kieff E. Recombinant Epstein-Barr virus with small RNA (EBER) genes deleted transforms lymphocytes and replicates in vitro. *Proc Natl Acad Sci U S A* 1991;88(4):1546–1572.

267. Swaminathan S, Huneycutt BS, Reiss CS, et al. Epstein-Barr virus–encoded small RNAs (EBERs) do not modulate interferon effects in infected lymphocytes. *J Virol* 1992;66(8):5133–5136.

268. Tomkinson B, Kieff E. Second-site homologous recombination in Epstein-Barr virus: insertion of type 1 EBNA 3 genes in place of type 2 has no effect on *in vitro* infection. *J Virol* 1992;66(2):780–789.

269. Lee MA, Kim OJ, Yates JL. Targeted gene disruption in Epstein-Barr virus. *Virology* 1992;189(1):253–265.

270. Lee MA, Yates JL. BHRF1 of Epstein-Barr virus, which is homologous to human proto-oncogene bcl2, is not essential for transformation of B cells or for virus replication *in vitro*. *J Virol* 1992;66(4):1899–1906.

271. Marchini A, Cohen JI, Wang F, et al. A selectable marker allows investigation of a nontransforming Epstein-Barr virus mutant. *J Virol* 1992;66(5):3214–3219.

272. Marchini A, Kieff E, Longnecker R. Marker rescue of a transformation-negative Epstein-Barr virus recombinant from an infected Burkitt lymphoma cell line: a method useful for analysis of genes essential for transformation. *J Virol* 1993;67(1):606–609.

273. Marchini A, Longnecker R, Kieff E. Epstein-Barr virus (EBV)-negative B-lymphoma cell lines for clonal isolation and replication of EBV recombinants. *J Virol* 1992;66(8):4972–4981.

274. Marchini A, Tomkinson B, Cohen JI, et al. BHRF1, the Epstein-Barr virus gene with homology to Bcl2, is dispensable for B-lymphocyte transformation and virus replication. *J Virol* 1991;65(11):5991–6000.

275. Robertson ES, Tomkinson B, Kieff E. An Epstein-Barr virus with a 58-kilobase-pair deletion that includes BARF0 transforms B lymphocytes *in vitro*. *J Virol* 1994;68(3):1449–1458.

276. Tomkinson B, Robertson E, Yalamanchili R, et al. Epstein-Barr virus recombinants from overlapping cosmid fragments. *J Virol* 1993;67(12):7298–7306.

277. Wang F, Marchini A, Kieff E. Epstein-Barr virus (EBV) recombinants: use of positive selection markers to rescue mutants in EBV-negative B-lymphoma cells. *J Virol* 1991;65(4):1701–1709.

278. Appay V, Dunbar PR, Callan M, et al. Memory CD8+ T cells vary in differentiation phenotype in different persistent virus infections. *Nat Med* 2002;8(4):379–385.

279. Bickham K, Munz C, Tsang ML, et al. EBNA1-specific CD4+ T cells in healthy carriers of Epstein-Barr virus are primarily Th1 in function. *J Clin Invest* 2001;107(1):121–130.

280. Hislop AD, Annels NE, Gudgeon NH, et al. Epitope-specific evolution of human CD8(+) T cell responses from primary to persistent phases of Epstein-Barr virus infection. *J Exp Med* 2002;195(7):893–905.

281. Kurth J, Spieker T, Wustrow J, et al. EBV-infected B cells in infectious mononucleosis: viral strategies for spreading in the B cell compartment and establishing latency. *Immunity* 2000;13(4):485–495.

282. Babcock GJ, Thorley-Lawson DA. Tonsillar memory B cells, latently infected with Epstein-Barr virus, express the restricted pattern of latent genes previously found only in Epstein-Barr virus-associated tumors. *Proc Natl Acad Sci U S A* 2000;97(22):12250–12255.

283. Rowe M, Rowe DT, Gregory CD, et al. Differences in B cell growth phenotype reflect novel patterns of Epstein-Barr virus latent gene expression in Burkitt's lymphoma cells. *EMBO J* 1987;6(9):2743–2751.

284. Herbst H, Dallenbach F, Hummel M, et al. Epstein-Barr virus latent membrane protein expression in Hodgkin and Reed-Sternberg cells. *Proc Natl Acad Sci U S A* 1991;88(11):4766–4770.

285. Pallesen G, Hamilton-Dutoit SJ, Rowe M, et al. Expression of Epstein-Barr virus replicative proteins in AIDS-related non-Hodgkin's lymphoma cells. *J Pathol* 1991;165(4):289–299.

286. Jarrett RF, Gallagher A, Jones DB, et al. Detection of Epstein-Barr virus genomes in Hodgkin's disease: relation to age [see comments]. *J Clin Pathol* 1991;44(10):844–848.

287. Pallesen G, Hamilton-Dutoit SJ, Rowe M, et al. Expression of Epstein-Barr virus latent gene products in tumour cells of Hodgkin's disease [see comments]. *Lancet* 1991;337(8737):320–322.

288. Zur Hausen H, Schulte-Holthauzen H, Klein G, et al. EBV DNA in biopsies of Burkitt tumours and anaplastic carcinomas of the nasopharynx. *Nature* 1970;228:1956–1958.

289. Henle W, Henle G, Ho HC, et al. Antibodies to Epstein-Barr virus in nasopharyngeal carcinoma, other head and neck neoplasms, and control groups. *J Natl Cancer Inst* 1970;44(1):225–231.

290. Old L, Clifford P, Boyse E, et al. Precipitating antibody in human serum to an antigen present in cultured Burkitt's lymphoma cells. *Proc Natl Acad Sci U S A* 1966;56:1699–1704.

291. Chien YC, Chen JY, Liu MY, et al. Serologic markers of Epstein-Barr virus infection and nasopharyngeal carcinoma in Taiwanese men. *N Engl J Med* 2001;345(26):1877–1882

292. Henle G, Henle W. Epstein-Barr virus-specific IgA serum antibodies as an outstanding feature of nasopharyngeal carcinoma. *Int J Cancer* 1976;17(1):1–7.

293. Zeng Y. Seroepidemiological studies on nasopharyngeal carcinoma in China. *Adv Cancer Res* 1985;44:121–138.

294. Pathmanathan R, Prasad U, Sadler R, et al. Clonal proliferations of cells infected with Epstein-Barr virus in preinvasive lesions related to nasopharyngeal carcinoma. *N Engl J Med* 1995;333(11):693–698.

295. Brooks L, Yao QY, Rickinson AB, et al. Epstein-Barr virus latent gene transcription in nasopharyngeal carcinoma cells: coexpression of EBNA1, LMP1, and LMP2 transcripts. *J Virol* 1992;66(5):2689–2697.

296. Busson P, McCoy R, Sadler R, et al. Consistent transcription of the Epstein-Barr virus LMP2 gene in nasopharyngeal carcinoma. *J Virol* 1992;66(5):3257–3262.

297. Fahraeus R, Fu HL, Ernberg I, et al. Expression of Epstein-Barr virus–encoded proteins in nasopharyngeal carcinoma. *Int J Cancer* 1988;42(3):329–338.

298. Young LS, Dawson CW, Clark D, et al. Epstein-Barr virus gene expression in nasopharyngeal carcinoma. *J Gen Virol* 1988;69(part 5):1051–1065.

299. Locker J, Nalesnik M. Molecular genetic analysis of lymphoid tumours arising after organ transplantation. *Am J Pathol* 1989;135:977–987.

300. Shapiro RS, McClain K, Frizzera G, et al. Epstein-Barr virus associated B cell lymphoproliferative disorders following bone marrow transplantation. *Blood* 1988;71(5):1234–1243.

301. Weiss LM, Movahed LA. *In situ* demonstration of Epstein-Barr viral genomes in viral-associated B cell lymphoproliferations. *Am J Pathol* 1989;134(3):651–659.

302. Zutter MM, Martin PJ, Sale GE, et al. Epstein-Barr virus lymphoproliferation after bone marrow transplantation. *Blood* 1988;72(2):520–529.

303. Gratama JW, Zutter MM, Minarovits J, et al. Expression of Epstein-Barr virus–encoded growth-transformation–associated proteins in lymphoproliferations of bone-marrow transplant recipients. *Int J Cancer* 1991;47(2):188–192.

304. Thomas JA, Hotchin NA, Allday MJ, et al. Immunohistology of Epstein-Barr virus–associated antigens in B cell disorders from immunocompromised individuals. *Transplantation* 1990;49(5):944–953.

305. Young L, Alfieri C, Hennessy K, et al. Expression of Epstein-Barr virus transformation–associated genes in tissues of patients with EBV lymphoproliferative disease. *N Engl J Med* 1989;321(16):1080–1085.

306. Purtilo D, DeFlorio DJ, Huff L, et al. Variable phenotypic expression of an X-linked lymphoproliferative syndrome. *N Engl J Med* 1977;297:1077–1081.

307. Starzl T, Nalesnik M, Porter K, et al. Reversibility of lymphomas and lymphoproliferative lesions developing under cyclosporin A-steroid therapy. *Lancet* 1984;1:583–587.

308. Fischer A, Blanche S, Le Bidois J, et al. Anti–B-cell monoclonal antibodies in the treatment of severe B-cell lymphoproliferative syndrome following bone marrow and organ transplantation. *N Engl J Med* 1991;324:1451–1456.

309. Papadopoulos EB, Ladanyi M, Emanuel D, et al. Infusions of donor leukocytes to treat Epstein-Barr virus–associated lymphoproliferative disorders after allogeneic bone marrow transplantation [see comments]. *N Engl J Med* 1994;330(17):1185–1191.

310. Savoldo B, Cubbage ML, Durett AG, et al. Generation of EBV-specific CD4+ cytotoxic T cells from virus naive individuals. *J Immunol* 2002;168(2):909–918.

311. Pedersen C, Gerstoft J, Lundgren JD, et al. HIV-associated lymphoma: histopathology and association with Epstein-Barr virus genome related to clinical, immunological and prognostic features. *Eur J Cancer* 1991;27(11):1416–1423.

312. Hamilton-Dutoit SJ, Rea D, Raphael M, et al. Epstein-Barr virus–latent gene expression and tumor cell phenotype in acquired immunodeficiency syndrome–related non-Hodgkin's lymphoma. Correlation of lymphoma phenotype with three distinct patterns of viral latency. *Am J Pathol* 1993;143(4):1072–1085.

313. Hamilton-Dutoit SJ, Raphael M, Audouin J, et al. *In situ* demonstration of Epstein-Barr virus small RNAs (EBER 1) in acquired immunodeficiency syndrome–related lymphomas: correlation with tumor morphology and primary site. *Blood* 1993;82(2):619–624.

314. MacMahon EM, Glass JD, Hayward SD, et al. Epstein-Barr virus in AIDS-related primary central nervous system lymphoma. *Lancet* 1991;338(8773):969–973.

CHAPTER 234
Varicella-Zoster Virus

Charles Grose and John A. Zaia

STRUCTURE OF THE VIRUS AND ITS GENOME

Varicella-zoster virus (VZV) is one of the eight human herpesviruses; the other seven are herpes simplex virus (HSV) types 1 and 2, human cytomegalovirus, Epstein-Barr virus, and human herpesvirus types 6, 7, and 8 (also called Kaposi's human herpesvirus). Like the other members of the herpesvirus family, VZV is an enveloped virus that contains double-stranded DNA within its protein core. The viral particle is an icosahedron. The complete enveloped virion is 150 to 200 nm in diameter; the naked particle is about 95 nm in diameter (Fig. 234.1).

The linear duplex VZV DNA has a buoyant density of 1.705 g/cm³ in cesium chloride (1). When measured by electron microscopy and compared with a known standard, the relative mass was found to be 80×10^6 daltons, and this result has been confirmed by electrophoretic analyses. The viral DNA exists predominantly as two isomers (2,3). In the conventional arrangement established for the DNA of the prototype HSV, VZV DNA can be divided into two segments, long (L) and short (S), separated by a joint region. The long segment is composed almost entirely of a unique sequence (UL). In contrast, the short segment contains a central unique sequence (US) flanked by internal and terminal inverted repeated sequences (IRs and TRs). Because of the presence of these repeated sequences, the short segment can be found in either of two equimolar orientations relative to the long segment of the VZV genome. These two arrangements are the basis for the two isomers of VZV DNA, in contrast to HSV, which, because both UL and US can invert relative to each other, exists as four isomers (4).

The entire sequence of the VZV genome has been determined by M13-dideoxynucleotide technology (5). The sequence includes 124,884 base pairs. The sequence data imply that the VZV genome contains 71 open reading frames, including several VZV glycoprotein genes. These glycoprotein genes have been designated gB, gC, gE, gH, gI, and gL (6). In contrast to other herpesviruses, VZV gE is the predominant glycoprotein. Comprehensive reviews of the VZV glycoproteins have been published elsewhere (7,8).

REPLICATION OF THE VIRUS IN TISSUE CULTURE

Before the development of adequate virologic methods for isolation of VZV in tissue culture, clinical observation suggested that the causative agents of chickenpox and herpes zoster were similar (9). Varicella was observed to occur not only after exposure to zoster but also after inoculation of susceptible children with vesicle fluid from persons with acute herpes zoster. The major significant advance in understanding the nature of these agents, however, was contributed by the Nobel laureate Weller, who demonstrated the method for isolation and propagation of VZV (10). To study virus replication, growth kinetic experiments have been conducted in cell culture. One of the peculiar properties of VZV is its propensity to remain cell associated (i.e., the viral particle remains attached to the outer cell membrane and is not released into the cell culture medium). Therefore, cell-free virus is difficult to prepare, and viral infectivity titers are invariably low (10,11).

The spread of virus from cell to cell has also been documented by fluorescent antibody staining. Viral antigens are first detected in the nucleus of the newly infected cell within 4 hours of infection. Subsequently, the pattern of virus-specific fluorescence spreads to the cytoplasm by 14 hours and to neighboring cells by 18 hours after infection. Thus, a single VZV replication cycle is estimated to last approximately 18 hours. To obtain maximal titers of infectivity in an infected monolayer, the virus appears to pass through two or three replication cycles.

The regulatory mechanisms affecting VZV replication have not been well delineated, but they probably resemble those already described for HSV replication (12). Based on an operational definition, this regulatory cycle is divided into a minimum of three phases, which have been designated immediate early, early, and late. The synthesis of proteins in each phase is said to be coordinately regulated and sequentially ordered in a cascade pattern; otherwise stated, groups of viral peptides appear in an infected cell in a predictable pattern, and the synthesis of the later-appearing proteins is dependent on the prior synthesis of earlier proteins. The last viral proteins to be synthesized during the late phase are the structural components of the virion.

The cytopathic effect of VZV infection is shown in Fig. 234.2. In tissue culture, the virus spreads through the cell monolayer at a slower rate than HSV, presumably because of the relatively small amount of extracellular virus. Infected cells contain an intranuclear inclusion body indistinguishable from the Cowdry type A inclusions first described in HSV infection.

Electron micrographic analysis of vesicle fluid from children with chickenpox demonstrates cell-free enveloped virions (Fig. 234.1). The mechanism by which the VZV particle becomes enveloped and exits from an infected cell is not known. Based on

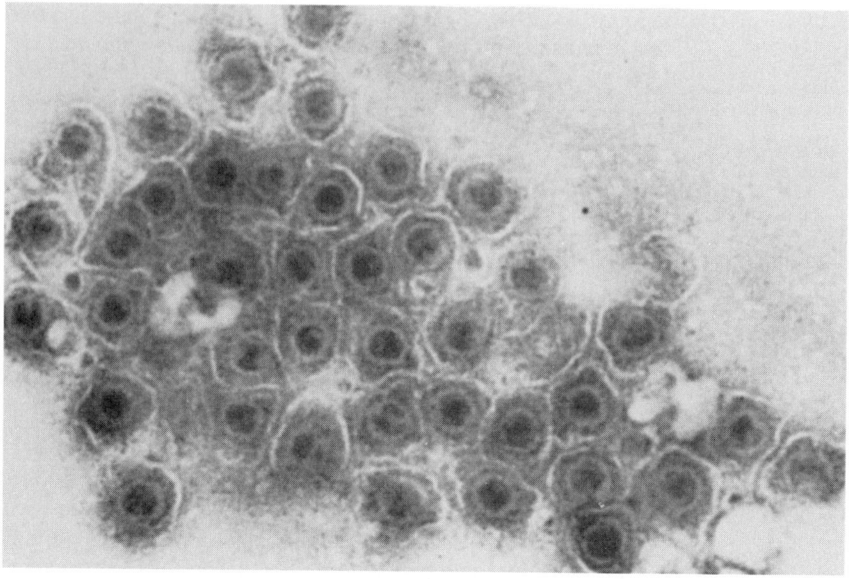

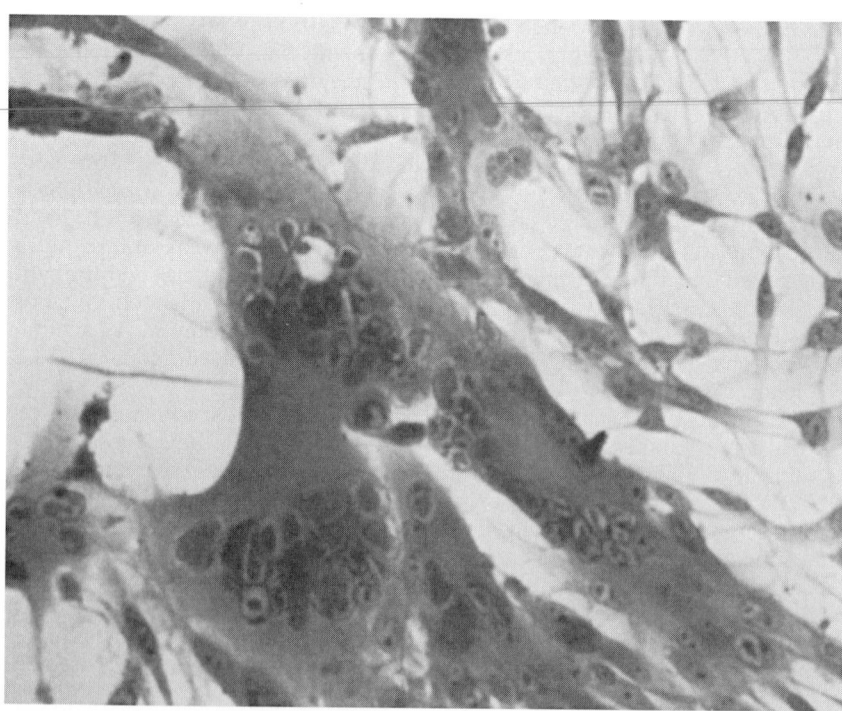

Figure 234.1. Varicella-zoster virus in vesicle fluid. Fluid was removed from a vesicle of a child with chickenpox. Examination of the vesicular fluid by electron microscopy (original magnification ×75,000) demonstrated numerous enveloped virus particles.

the presence of enveloped virions within cytoplasmic vesicles, it is presumed that VZV does not acquire its envelope by budding through the outer cell membrane as do RNA viruses (13). Instead, the nucleocapsid is formed in the nucleus and surrounds the newly synthesized viral DNA; it acquires an envelope after it exits the nucleus and buds into a cytoplasmic vacuole. These cytoplasmic vacuoles, which are thought to be derived from the trans Golgi network, carry the enveloped virions to the outer cell membrane, where exocytosis occurs (13).

HOST IMMUNE RESPONSE TO INFECTION

Acute VZV infection in the human causes the disease chickenpox. The virus spreads through the body during two viremic phases (14). During the second viremic phase, the immune response is detectable. The antibody response to VZV has been measured by several methods with various degrees of sensitivity. In the 1950s and 1960s, the usual procedure was the complement fixation (CF) test. When serum samples from persons with chickenpox were assayed for CF antibody, it was observed that almost all children developed VZV antibody by the second week of illness. Within 1 year after chickenpox, VZV antibody was no longer detectable in 75% of the subjects. Thus, the VZV CF test is a poor assay for determining humoral immune status in the general population.

This deficiency was overcome in the 1970s by the development of an indirect fluorescent method (15,16). In this assay, human serum is incubated with an infected cell monolayer, after which a fluorescein-tagged antihuman globulin is added to the

Figure 234.2. Cytopathic effect induced by varicella-zoster virus infection in a human cell culture monolayer. A large syncytium (polykaryon) is visible in the center. Within each syncytium are numerous clustered nuclei, each containing a large inclusion body.

mixture. This test has been called by the acronym FAMA (fluorescent antibody to membrane antigen). Because the FAMA test is more sensitive than the CF test, it can detect low levels of VZV-specific antibody in the serum of persons who had chickenpox long ago. With this test, it is possible to determine the humoral immune status in populations at high risk, such as children with leukemia or adult health care providers exposed to chickenpox (17).

A major portion of the immune response is directed against the VZV glycoproteins, especially gE, gB and gH (18). The humoral immune response to the individual VZV glycoprotein antigens can be assessed by immunoprecipitation reactions between radiolabeled VZV antigens and human serum samples (Fig. 234.3). By this method, antibody to at least one of the major VZV glycoproteins is easily demonstrable within 1 week after onset of chickenpox. By 2 weeks, antibodies to two more viral glycoproteins are present.

Cellular immunity is measured by lymphocyte proliferation assays and cytotoxicity assays. Susceptible persons have no proliferative response *in vitro* to VZV antigens, while those with acute chickenpox develop a cell-mediated immune response to the individual VZV glycoproteins. Similarly, both major histocompatibility complex (MHC) class I restricted CD8+ T-lymphocytes and MHC class II restricted CD4+ T-lymphocytes are sensitized to VZV antigens during primary infection (19). As with the antibody responses, most T-cell responses are directed against the viral glycoproteins. These immunologic analyses affirm that viral glycoproteins are important for induction of a protective immune response to VZV.

MUTANT VARICELLA-ZOSTER VIRUS IN NORTH AMERICA

In 1998, a report about the unexpected discovery of a mutant VZV was published in the United States (20). The virus was isolated from a 6-year-old boy living in the Minneapolis-St. Paul area of Minnesota. The child had been hospitalized for treatment of chickenpox because he had leukemia; a virus culture was taken as part of a routine admission assessment. The virus isolate was difficult to type as VZV because the virus did not stain well with a commercial diagnostic kit (see later section on Laboratory Diagnosis). Therefore, the virus was further analyzed in a research laboratory. Extensive DNA sequence analysis firmly established that the community virus, designated VZV-MSP, had a missense mutation in the structural gene encoding glycoprotein gE. The mutation led to a codon change from aspartic acid to asparagine in the ectodomain of the gE glycoprotein. In turn, this amino acid mutation resulted in the loss of a B-cell epitope on the gE protein.

Subsequent characterization of the mutant virus in three research laboratories has documented that VZV-MSP exhibited an accelerated cell-to-cell phenotype in both cell culture and an animal model of VZV infection (21). Thus, VZV-MSP represents a second VZV genotype/phenotype. The prevalence of this variant virus in North America is not known. However, a detailed genetic analysis of the viral genomes of several VZV strains collected from North America, Europe, and Japan has uncovered more single nucleotide polymorphisms than expected (22). In other words, it is now possible to differentiate one VZV strain from a second VZV strain because of their genetic differences. For example, the Oka vaccine strain has genetic differences that distinguish it from community strains. The above results suggest that other mutant VZV strains will be found in the future.

LABORATORY DIAGNOSIS

Several methods are available for diagnosing VZV infection (23). Diagnosis can reliably be made on clinical grounds alone when there is a history of close exposure to chickenpox or herpes zoster in the past 10 to 21 days and a vesicular eruption consistent with chickenpox. In many situations, particularly those involving immunocompromised persons, often there are no clear historical data to support the diagnosis. In this situation, because treatment is of paramount importance, laboratory diagnosis is necessary. The earliest method for diagnosis was light microscopic examination of the vesicle contents stained with Wright-Giemsa stain to demonstrate multinucleated giant cells (Tzanck test). The presence of these giant cells strongly suggests a herpesvirus infection but not specifically VZV; for example, HSV infection causes similar cytopathology. Electron microscopic visualization of vesicular fluid also demonstrates VZV particles (Fig. 234.1). Again, VZV particles cannot be differentiated from other herpesviruses by this diagnostic procedure.

In many virology laboratories, VZV infection is diagnosed by virus isolation in cell culture. Vesicular fluid is usually collected in sterile capillary tubes or tuberculin syringes, which are subsequently evacuated into culture medium. The medium is then layered over cultured cells, and in 3 to 5 days the cytopathic effect is visible in the monolayer (11). In human melanoma cells, an excellent substrate for VZV isolation, the virus induces characteristic large syncytial foci whose nuclei are filled with inclusions (Fig. 234.2).

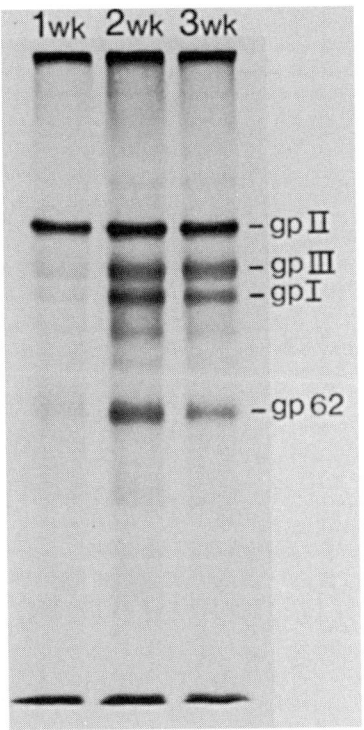

Figure 234.3. The human antibody response to the varicella-zoster virus (VZV) glycoproteins during chickenpox. Serum from a healthy child with chickenpox was collected weekly, and all three samples were analyzed for immunoglobulin G antibodies to VZV glycoproteins by radioimmunoprecipitation methods. The autoradiographic profiles indicated the presence of antibody to VZV gpII during the first week (*wk*) of chickenpox (lane 1), whereas antibodies to gpI and gpIII appeared during the second week of illness (lanes 2 and 3). The current nomenclature for the VZV glycoproteins is as follows: gpI is now gE; gpII, gB; gpIII, gH; and gp62, gI. (From Grose C, Litwin V. Immunology of the varicella-zoster viral glycoproteins. *J Infect Dis* 1988;157:877–881, with permission.)

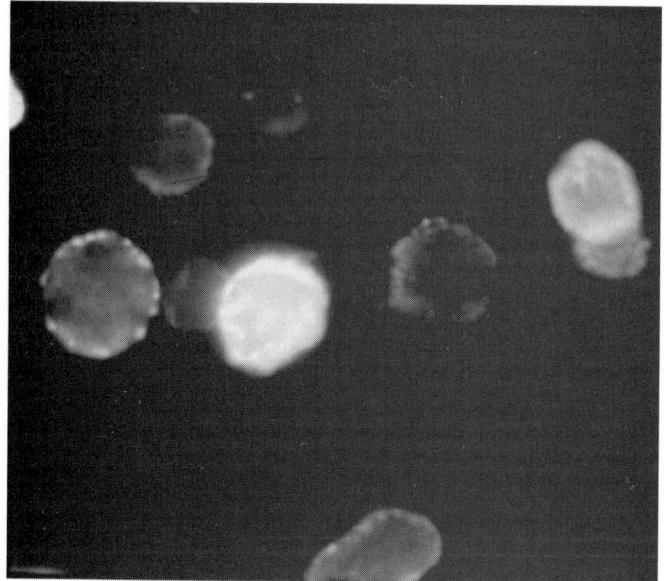

Figure 234.4. A positive rapid varicella-zoster virus (VZV) antigen test. Human cells infected with VZV were dried on a glass slide. The cells were covered with a VZV-specific monoclonal antibody to the gE protein tagged with fluorescein. Bright surface staining is easily seen on several cells. Because the VZV rapid antigen test is more sensitive and specific, it should replace the Tzanck test.

Commercial kits for rapid diagnosis of VZV infection use one or more fluorescein-conjugated VZV monoclonal antibodies (23). Samples of cells are obtained from the base of the vesicle lesion and dried onto a glass slide. The cells are then probed with the conjugated VZV-specific monoclonal antibody. Infected cells that contain VZV antigens fluoresce brightly and are easily detectable. Rapid diagnosis by antigen detection can also quickly differentiate between vesicular rashes caused by VZV and HSV infection. Most kits use antibody to VZV gE, because gE is the major cell surface antigen produced in infected cells (Fig. 234.4). Finally, some commercial laboratories now offer polymerase chain reaction amplification for detection of VZV DNA in clinical samples.

Serologic methods can be used to confirm the diagnosis, but because this requires acute- and convalescent-phase serum specimens, it is clearly not a method for rapid diagnosis (22). Serum samples are obtained during the acute illness and then 14 to 28 days later. Titration of the level of VZV antibodies shows a fourfold or greater increase in titer. Advances in serologic techniques to measure VZV antibody include the development of enzyme-linked immunosorbent assays by commercial laboratories.

Because they are so sensitive, the FAMA or enzyme-linked immunosorbent assays are reliable methods for demonstrating prior chickenpox infection. For this reason, these tests are widely used as presumptive evidence of immunity in health care personnel. It should be noted, however, that these commercial testing kits often do not detect VZV antibody titers following varicella vaccination, because the titers in vaccinees may be lower than titers following natural chickenpox infection (false negative).

ACKNOWLEDGMENT

Research by the authors was supported by grants from the National Institutes of Health and the VZV Research Foundation.

REFERENCES

1. Dumas AM, Geelen JLMC, Maris W, et al. Infectivity and molecular weight of varicella-zoster virus DNA. *J Gen Virol* 1980;47:233.
2. Straus SE, Aulakh HS, Ruyechan WT, et al. Structure of varicella-zoster virus DNA. *J Virol* 1981;40:516.
3. Ecker JR, Hyman RW. Varicella zoster virus DNA exists as two isomers. *Proc Natl Acad Sci U S A* 1982;79:156.
4. Roizman B. The structure and isomerization of herpes simplex virus genomes. *Cell* 1979;16:481.
5. Davison AJ, Scott JE. The complete DNA sequence of varicella-zoster virus. *J Gen Virol* 1986;67:1759.
6. Davison AJ, Edson CM, Ellis RW, et al. New common nomenclature for glycoprotein genes of varicella-zoster virus and their glycosylated products. *J Virol* 1986;57:1195.
7. Grose C. Glycoproteins encoded by varicella-zoster virus: biosynthesis, phosphorylation, and intracellular trafficking. *Annu Rev Microbiol* 1990;44:59.
8. Grose C. The predominant varicella-zoster virus gE and gI glycoprotein complex. In: Bogner E, Holzenburg A, eds. *Structure function relationships of human pathogenic viruses.* London: Kluwer Academic, 2002;195–224.
9. Zaia JA. Clinical spectrum of varicella-zoster virus infection. In: Nahmias AJ, et al., eds. *The human herpesviruses.* Amsterdam: Elsevier North Holland, 1981.
10. Weller TH. Serial propagation *in vitro* of agents producing inclusion bodies derived from varicella and herpes zoster. *Proc Soc Exp Biol Med* 1953;83:340.
11. Grose C, Perrotta DM, Brunell PA, et al. Cell-free varicella-zoster virus in cultured human melanoma cells. *J Gen Virol* 1979;43:15.
12. Honess RW, Roizman B. Regulation of herpesvirus macromolecular synthesis. I. Cascade regulation of the synthesis of three groups of viral proteins. *J Virol* 1974;14:8.
13. Harson R, Grose C. Egress of varicella-zoster virus from the melanoma cell: A tropism for the melanocyte. *J Virol* 1995;69:4994.
14. Grose C, Ye M, Padilla J. Pathogenesis of primary infection. In: Arvin AM, Gershon AA, eds. *Varicella-zoster virus.* Cambridge, UK: Cambridge University Press, 2000:105–122.
15. Williams V, Gershon A, Brunell PA. Serologic response to varicella-zoster membrane antigens measured by indirect immunofluorescence. *J Infect Dis* 1971;130:669.
16. Zaia JA, Oxman MN. Antibody to varicella-zoster virus–induced membrane antigen: immunofluorescence assay using monodisperse glutaraldehyde-fixed target cells. *J Infect Dis* 1977;136:519.
17. Gershon AA, Steinberg SP. Antibody response to varicella-zoster virus and the role of antibody in host defense. *Am J Med Sci* 1981;282:12.
18. Grose C, Litwin V. Immunology of the varicella-zoster viral glycoproteins. *J Infect Dis* 1988;157:877.
19. Abendroth A, Arvin AM. Host response to primary infection. In: Arvin AM, Gershon AA, eds. *Varicella-zoster virus.* Cambridge, UK: Cambridge University Press, 2000:142–156.
20. Santos RA, Padilla JA, Hatfield C, et al. Antigenic variation of varicella-zoster virus Fc receptor gE: loss of a major B cell epitope in the ectodomain. *Virology* 1998;249:21.
21. Santos RA, Hatfield C, Cole NL, et al. Varicella-zoster virus gE escape mutant VZV-MSP exhibits an accelerated cell spread phenotype in both infected cell culture and SCID-hu mice. *Virology* 2000;275:306.
22. Wagenaar TR, Chow VT, Buranathai C, et al. The out of Africa model of varicella-zoster virus evolution: polymorphisms distinguish Asian clades from European/North American clades. *Vaccine* 2003;21:1072.
23. Forghani B. Laboratory diagnosis of infection. In: Arvin AM, Gershon AA, eds. *Varicella-zoster virus.* Cambridge, UK: Cambridge University Press, 2000:351–382.

CHAPTER 235
Cytomegalovirus

Laura L. Gibson and Sarah H. Cheeseman

HISTORY

Human cytomegalovirus (CMV), originally called human salivary gland virus, was described in 1956 by three independent investigators. The organism was isolated by Rowe and colleagues (1) from resected adenoid glands of normal children, by Smith (2) from salivary glands of a child with disseminated disease and another child dying of an unrelated tumor, and by Weller and colleagues (3) from a liver biopsy specimen from a child with a congenital infection syndrome.

CLASSIFICATION AND STRUCTURE

CMV belongs to the family Herpesviridae, whose members share a similar genome and virion structure as well as the ability to establish persistent infection with intermittent reactivation. CMV is classified in the subfamily Betaherpesviridae, along with human herpesviruses 6 and 7, based on a restricted host range and long replication cycle. The virus particle is approximately 200 nm in diameter and consists of a DNA core within an icosahedral nucleocapsid embedded in a phosphoprotein tegument and surrounded by a lipid envelope studded with a variety of glycoproteins. Highly immunogenic tegument phosphoproteins make up an estimated 40% of the virion protein mass (4). In addition to typical mature virions, noninfectious variants are also produced within CMV-infected cells. They include dense bodies that lack a DNA core and capsid, and enveloped particles that lack only a DNA core.

The mature CMV particle contains a linear double-stranded DNA genome consisting of approximately 230 kilobase pairs (kbp), including long (U_L, 190 kbp) and short (U_S, 40 kbp) unique regions. Each unique region is framed by inverted terminal repeating sequences with mirror symmetry (called TRL and IRL for the long, and TRS and IRS for the short unique regions). Consequently, four isomers of the CMV genome may occur. The genome sequences of laboratory strains AD169 and Towne, as well as many clinical isolates, show at least 208 open reading frames (5). However, the products and function of many of these genes have not been defined for CMV or have been deduced based on homology with other herpesvirus gene products of known function.

Viral components previously identified by their location, structure, or molecular weight have been renamed based on the unique region of the genome and the map unit at which the open reading frame begins (6). A prefix identifying the gene product as a protein (p), glycoprotein (gp), or phosphoprotein (pp) is included if applicable. For example, lower matrix pp65 is now designated ppUL83, while envelope glycoprotein gB is designated gpUL55.

The CMV genome encodes at least 30 capsid, tegument, and envelope proteins with molecular weights from 20 to more than 200 kd (6). The capsid consists of two predominant proteins, the major (pUL86, 90% of the capsid protein mass) and minor (pUL85) capsid proteins. These and other capsid proteins are thought to be involved in DNA anchoring and capsid assembly (4). The tegument layer contains at least 20 proteins, including the lower matrix protein (pp65 or ppUL83, 95% of the tegument protein mass) and the basic phosphoprotein (pp150 or ppUL32). These and other tegument proteins are phosphate acceptors for the viral protein kinase, but little else is know about their function (4,7). They are highly immunogenic as major targets of the CD8$^+$ T-lymphocyte immune response (ppUL83) and the humoral immune response (ppUL32). In addition, ppUL83 is the predominant CMV antigen detected in leukocytes of actively infected patients (8). The viral envelope contains up to eight glycoproteins, including gpUL55 (gB) and gpUL75 (gH). These molecules mediate virus entry into host cells and virus transmission from infected to uninfected cells via attachment, fusion, and penetration. The host cell receptors for these glycoproteins are unknown, but likely involve heparin sulfate or other host cell surface proteoglycans (William Britt, personal communication). Envelope glycoproteins are major targets of the humoral immune response to CMV (Table 235.1).

LIFE CYCLE

Human CMV is highly species specific. The laboratory-attenuated Towne strain replicates in skin fibroblasts of chim-

TABLE 235.1. Nomenclature of Cytomegalovirus Genes and Proteins

Gene	Protein	Alternate protein designation
UL 32	ppUL32	pp150
UL 54	pUL54	DNA polymerase
UL 55	gpUL55	glycoprotein B (gB)
UL 75	gpUL75	glycoprotein H (gH)
UL 83	ppUL83	pp65
UL 122	ppUL122	immediate early 1 (IE1)
UL 123	ppUL123	immediate early 2 (IE2)

panzees but not other nonhuman primates (201). Several cell types are permissive for CMV replication during natural infection, including endothelial and epithelial cells, fibroblasts, monocytes, and dendritic cells (9). Laboratory strains of CMV are propagated in human skin or lung fibroblasts, but primary clinical isolates can replicate in endothelial cells that do not support the laboratory strains (10,11). However, clinical strains of CMV may differ in tropism for endothelial cells, a variation that may depend on transport of viral DNA to the cell nucleus after viral penetration (12). The virus displays a preference for differentiated cells (13,14).

Attachment and Entry

During acute infection, CMV attaches to target cells by the interaction of viral envelope glycoproteins (primarily gpUL55 or glycoprotein B) with a ubiquitous nonspecific receptor found on host cells both permissive and nonpermissive to infection. Inhibition studies suggest that the cell surface proteoglycan heparan sulfate mediates this interaction (15). However, CMV-specific binding and fusion occur by unknown host cell receptors unrelated to heparin sulfate. The presence of certain host cell receptors appears to affect the efficiency of this process (202). A variety of these receptors have been studied, but none have proven to be indispensable for viral replication. A 30- to 36-kd protein binds to CMV gpUL55 (203,204) but may not be essential for viral entry (16). Similarly, a larger 92-kd protein that binds to CMV gpUL75 (glycoprotein H) (17) and may mediate fusion (18) has recently been cloned (19). Other possible factors have been suggested (20) but were later shown by viral mutant models to be nonessential (21).

Viral Gene Expression

After viral entry, nucleocapsids and tegument proteins migrate to the nucleus where tegument protein ppUL83 (pp65) can be detected shortly after infection (6,22). Viral gene expression subsequently occurs throughout the 48- to 72-hour life cycle of CMV. Genes are categorized based primarily on timing of expression after initial viral infection of host cells: immediate early (α) genes begin within 30 to 60 minutes, early (β) genes within 4 to 12 hours, and late (γ) genes more than 24 hours. Information about CMV genes and their products has been gathered primarily by studying viral mutants that do not express the gene under investigation as well as by comparison with other herpesviruses.

Immediate early α genes are transcribed directly from the inoculating viral genome, and do not require the expression of other viral genes (23). They transcribe gene products critical to successful production of viral progeny as well as modulation of host cell functions that facilitate this production. Four α genes have been identified, including UL36-38, TRS1-IRS1, US3, and UL122-123 (ie1/ie2 or MIE gene), but most activity occurs at the latter gene. The major immediate early (MIE) gene encodes a product that is subsequently spliced into immediate early protein 1 (ppUL123 or pp72 or IE1) and immediate early protein 2 (ppUL122 or pp80 or IE2) as well as other proteins. Expression of IE1 in the nucleus may be the only evidence of infection in cells in which the virus does not complete its replicative cycle (205). IE1 promotes further MIE gene expression (24) and efficient β and γ gene expression (25), while IE2 controls the transition from α to later gene expression and the down-regulation of α genes late in viral replication (26). Other α genes similarly encode products that perform functions important early in the viral life cycle. Products include those of the US3 gene, which inhibit host cell major histocompatibility complex (MHC) class I expression and therefore antigen presentation (27,28); the TRS1-IRS1 gene, which regulates viral gene expression (29); and the UL36-38 gene, which inhibits apoptosis (30).

Expression of β and γ genes depends primarily on the successful generation of α gene products, including IE1 and IE2. While several early or β genes have been used extensively in studies on gene regulation, their products are poorly understood (31). For example, while the $\beta_{1.2}$ and $\beta_{2.7}$ genes generate 20% to 40% of all viral transcripts, their gene products are known only for their 1.2- and 2.7-kbp size, respectively (31). Other β genes include several involved in viral DNA replication, namely UL54 and UL44 (DNA polymerase and its processivity factor, respectively) and UL112-113 (a group of phosphoproteins that regulate DNA replication), as well as US11, the gene product of which inhibits host cell MHC class I expression (32,33). Relatively little is known about late or γ genes. Tegument proteins ppUL83 (or pp65) and ppUL99 (or pp28) are products of these genes.

Production of Progeny Virus

DNA replication occurs within compartments in the host cell nucleus, beginning early and peaking late in the viral life cycle (34–36). Thousands of genome copies are generated from circularized, unintegrated viral DNA (37). Although its purpose is unclear, progeny genome inversion produces four possible isomers depending on L and S region orientation (35). DNA is packaged into capsids that form "owl's eye" inclusions in the nucleus. In addition, viral RNA transcripts can be detected in both infectious virions and host cells immediately after infection, suggesting that some viral gene products can be synthesized upon host cell entry without transcription of the viral genome (38). These viral RNA transcripts may be incorporated into the virion nonspecifically (39). The maturing virion acquires tegument proteins as well as the envelope with glycoproteins (derived from the nuclear or cytoplasmic membranes) during migration to the cell surface via the Golgi apparatus. Aggregates of capsids and dense bodies in the Golgi may deform the nucleus into the typical "kidney bean" shape.

Cytomegalovirus and Host Cell Functions

CMV influences the normal function of its host cell throughout productive infection. First, CMV stimulates host cell gene expression and therefore RNA and protein synthesis (40). Several classes of host genes seem to be targeted by the virus, including interferon-responsive genes and those regulating cell cycle, apoptosis, and immune response (41–45). However, some genes with antiviral roles may be down-regulated, especially during the first few hours of infection. Second, CMV inhibits DNA synthesis and other processes associated with cell division. For example, CMV-infected fibroblasts in the resting G_0 phase of the cell cycle do not progress to the S phase, and in fact seem to re-

main in G_1/S arrest (46–48). Similarly, fibroblasts in the S or G_2 phase may remain in G2/M arrest (48). The mechanism underlying the interaction between CMV and its host cell has not been precisely defined. Several viral factors appear to influence host cell RNA and protein synthesis and cell cycle arrest, including virion components present at attachment and entry (41,43–45,49) as well as regulatory proteins synthesized after entry (42).

VIRUS AND HOST INTERACTION

Portals of entry include mucosal surfaces of the upper respiratory, gastrointestinal, and genital tracts after exposure to infectious secretions. The virus disseminates widely via polymorphonuclear leukocytes (PMNLs) (50), although circulating endothelial cells have been shown to carry CMV in immunocompromised individuals (51). Noninfectious viral DNA can also be detected in the plasma of immunocompromised patients (52,53). CMV preferentially infects a variety of cell types within both solid and hematopoietic tissues, including endothelial and epithelial cells as well as myeloid-lineage cells of the bone marrow and peripheral blood (54). Ductal epithelial cells support productive infection resulting in release of infectious virus into secretions such as saliva, breast milk, urine, and genital fluids. The host immune response clears viremia within months of primary infection in normal adults (55,56). However, CMV remains latent for the lifetime of the host, reactivating intermittently. The natural history of CMV infection depends primarily on the degree of homeostasis between the virus and host.

Evasion of the Host Immune Response

CMV uses several means by which to evade the host immune response after primary infection in order to establish latency, replicate, and spread to the next susceptible host. Genes controlling these functions are not required for propagation in cell culture where the host immune response does not affect CMV survival. These genes encode products that alter normal immune recognition of CMV-infected cells by disguising them with markers homologous to the host, hindering their expression of molecules essential for elimination by T cells, and decreasing their ability to secrete cytokines, mature successfully, and self-destruct in response to infection. In fact, genes dedicated to host immune evasion may comprise 10% to 20% of the total CMV genome (57).

The products of at least nine CMV genes show genetic homology with immunomodulatory host proteins (57). For example, the UL18 gene product resembles the human MHC class I molecule essential for communication between a variety of cells of the immune system (58). Like MHC class I heavy chain, gpUL18 binds $\beta 2$ microglobulin (59) and peptide (60). As an MHC class I homologue, gpUL18 may disguise CMV-infected cells from elimination by natural killer (NK) cells that recognize the lack of self class I expression as a stimulus for cytotoxicity (61). Lymphocyte inhibitory receptor-1 (LIR-1) is a major NK cell ligand that binds gpUL18 with a higher affinity than human MHC class I molecules, allowing recognition of gpUL18 despite a lower concentration on the cell surface (62,63). However, the complex interaction between CMV-infected cells and NK cells has not been fully elucidated (64–66). Similarly, products of the UL27, UL28, UL33, and UL78 genes show homology with human chemokine receptors (67). Although the function of these viral molecules has not been determined, they may play a role in attracting uninfected leukocytes to CMV-infected cells, clearing chemokines from the local environment of CMV-infected cells, or affecting intracellular signaling within CMV-infected cells

(68–70). A homolog of interleukin-10 (IL-10), possibly a product of the UL111A gene, decreases both surface expression of MHC class II molecules and synthesis of proinflammatory cytokines (71).

Many CMV genes, each expressed at a particular time in the viral life cycle, also contribute to host immune evasion by limiting the appearance of MHC molecules on the surface of CMV infected cells (72), including antigen-presenting cells and endothelial cells (73). CMV encodes proteins that affect expression of both class I and class II molecules on the cell surface (27,74). The US2 gene encodes an early β product that elicits degradation of both class I and class II molecules in the endoplasmic reticulum (ER) shortly after synthesis (75,76), most likely by reducing their half-life from hours to minutes (77). The US3 gene encodes an immediate early α product that prevents egress of class I molecules from the ER (28,78). The US6 gene encodes a γ product that hinders the association of peptide with the MHC class I molecule and the transporter of antigen processing (TAP) (79–82). Like US2, the US11 gene encodes an early β product that contributes to class I molecule degradation, but using a different mechanism (83–85). CMV can also inhibit constitutive (by antigen-presenting cells) and inducible (by endothelial and epithelial cells) MHC class II expression via mechanisms involving signal transduction pathways and gene regulation (86).

CMV uses a variety of other immune evasion strategies. The virus can decrease secretion of proinflammatory chemokines and cytokines by infected cells, including RANTES secretion by endothelial cells (87) and interferon secretion by fibroblasts and epithelial cells (88). In addition, CMV can hinder maturation of antigen-presenting cells such as dendritic cells, thereby reducing the efficiency with which these cells stimulate CD8$^+$ T-lymphocytes (89). Finally, CMV genes UL36 and UL37 encode products that inhibit apoptosis, or cell death, induced by stimuli such as viral infection. These gene products act by separate mechanisms within the apoptosis pathway (30,90).

Viral Latency

CMV evasion of the host immune response contributes to the establishment of viral latency. The risk of CMV transmission to recipients of solid organ transplants donated by seropositive individuals has long been observed. However, one report of infectious virus isolation from normal blood donors has not been repeated despite testing of more than 1,500 specimens (91). The difficulty in supporting the full cycle of CMV replication *in vitro*, despite production of immediate early gene products as evidence of infection (92–97), focused attention on the likelihood that CMV survives in a latent state in hematopoietic cells in healthy seropositive donors. The CMV genome exists as a circular plasmid within peripheral CD14$^+$ mononuclear cells of healthy donors (37). Viral DNA can be detected in both cultured precursors of granulocyte-monocyte (GM) lineage cells (98–100) and mononuclear cells of seropositive subjects (101–104). Viral RNA in latently infected cells derives primarily from the UL122/123 immediate early genes (105). Using polymerase chain reaction (PCR) with *in situ* hybridization and quantitative competitive PCR, Slobedman and Mocarski determined that 0.004% to 0.01% of mononuclear cells mobilized from peripheral blood or bone marrow from seropositive individuals carry the CMV genome at 2 to 13 copies per infected cell (54). Primitive CD34$^+$ bone marrow cells also support latent CMV infection (106) and adhere to CMV-infected bone marrow stromal cells (107).

CMV has also been isolated from a variety of other cell types. In studies of immunocompromised patients with active infection, the virus has been found primarily in PMNLs (50,108,109),

unlike the mononuclear cell localization of the virus in latent infection (102). Vascular endothelial cells also support CMV replication and appear to be an important source of CMV transmission to PMNLs (51,110).

Reactivation from latency occurs routinely in CMV-infected individuals. In latently infected, cultured GM precursors, productive viral replication can be induced in the presence of permissive cells (99) or cytokines (98). Latent virus can also be reactivated from mononuclear cells obtained from CMV-seropositive donors by allogeneic stimulation (111) and addition of cytokines, especially interferon-γ (112). Thus, reactivation from latency seems to require host cell differentiation in the context of an inflammatory response (14,106,113).

Host Immune Response

Despite attempts to avoid clearance, CMV remains the object of a vigorous immune response that serves to control the virus during both acute and latent infection. Antibodies to a variety of CMV antigens can be detected in sera of infected individuals, including envelope glycoproteins gpUL55 (gB) and gpUL75 (gH) found in more than 95% of subjects (114–116), tegument proteins ppUL99 (pp28) and ppUL32 (pp150) (117,118), and ppUL54 (DNA polymerase) (119). While CMV-specific antibodies do not protect against CMV infection, they are associated with partial but significant protection from disease. For example, maternal seropositivity is associated with protection from congenital CMV infection, but does not completely prevent reinfection during pregnancy or neonatal CMV disease (120–122).

Cell-mediated immunity remains the primary means by which the host controls CMV infection. Clinical experience reveals that patients with impairments of cellular immunity exhibit the most severe CMV disease, including those with solid or hematopoietic tissue transplants or immunodeficiency syndromes. Moreover, transfer of donor CMV-specific CD8$^+$ T-cell clones to bone marrow transplant recipients can prevent CMV disease (123,124). NK cells recognize and eliminate CMV-infected cells during nonspecific immunosurveillance (64). However, a coordinated response by CMV-specific T cells serves as the major defense against CMV disease. CMV-specific CD4$^+$ and CD8$^+$ T cells have been detected at high frequencies during both acute (125,126) and convalescent phases of infection (127–129). The frequency of CMV-specific CD8$^+$ T cells in seropositive individuals determined by staining with MHC class I–peptide tetrameric complexes varies from 0.03% to 5% (129). T-cell responses are directed primarily at the UL83 (pp65) and UL122 (immediate early 1) gene products (130–133), which show infrequent mutations within the genes coding for immunodominant peptide epitopes (134). CMV-specific CD8$^+$ T cells undergo clonal expansion following CMV infection as defined by T-cell receptor (TCR) repertoire. Further evaluation of these memory T cell clones in healthy CMV-infected donors reveals limited TCR usage within individuals but a high diversity of usage between donors (131,135,136). Moreover, a variety of phenotypes defined by surface markers can be identified within the CMV-specific CD8$^+$ T-cell memory pool. These cells express CD57 but not CD28, as well as varying levels of CD45RO and CD45RA isoforms (137–139).

CMV-specific T-cell responses have also been studied in immunocompromised patient populations. These cells can be quantified by MHC class I–peptide tetrameric complexes in order to monitor recovery of CMV-specific immunity following allogeneic stem cell transplantation (140,141). For example, the percentage of CMV-specific CD8$^+$ T cells in donor cells given to seropositive patients is inversely related to the frequency of recurrent CMV infection requiring preemptive ganciclovir. Moreover, those CMV-seropositive patients who fail to recover CMV-specific immunity are more likely to develop clinical CMV disease following viremia (141). Although HIV-infected patients with CD4 counts above 200 cells/μL on antiretroviral therapy can maintain strong CMV-specific CD4$^+$ and CD8$^+$ T-cell responses over time (142), these responses may remain lower than in HIV-uninfected controls (143). However, a decline in CMV-specific CD4$^+$ T-cell responses is associated with a failure to sustain CMV-specific CD8$^+$ T cell frequencies and function. CMV-specific CD8$^+$ T cells may persist even in patients with few circulating CD4$^+$ T cells, but these cells do not exhibit cytolytic function (144). CD4$^+$ T-cell count may not correlate with functional activity of CMV-specific CD4$^+$ T cells (145). CMV-specific T-cell responses have also been shown to be important in solid organ transplant recipients (146,147).

DIAGNOSIS

Virus Isolation

Virus isolation in cell culture demonstrates productive infection. CMV has traditionally been cultured in human diploid fibroblasts, such as human embryonic lung and human foreskin fibroblasts. This method produces the best virus yield when subconfluent monolayers are used, and may be augmented by blind passage (trypsinization, division, and reseeding of the cells). Live virus is detected by its cytopathic effect on the cell line, namely foci of enlarged, refractile, oval to round cells, often with a dirty pigmentary deposit, that appear as a hole in the monolayer. While most CMV isolates are recognized in the second week of incubation, cytopathic effect may appear in 5 to 6 weeks with some specimens or in 24 hours with others, such as urine from congenitally infected infants or lung samples from patients with severe interstitial pneumonitis. Due to the need for prolonged incubation, conventional viral culture has been replaced by the shell vial assay (148). This method uses centrifugation to enhance infectivity through a mechanism not yet understood (149) followed by immunofluorescent staining for the major immediate early antigen. Cultures processed by this technique yield results within 24 hours, and show nearly complete concordance with conventional cultures performed in parallel.

Serology

CMV-specific immunoglobulin G (IgG) antibodies are measured to determine past infection or, using acute and convalescent samples, recent infection with CMV. The vast majority of serologic assays use the AD169 strain of CMV to identify antibodies in a clinical specimen, although this method may fail to detect antibodies that do not cross-react with this laboratory strain (150). The level of complement-fixing antibody has long been known to rise and fall in sequential blood samples from normal healthy persons (151). Alternative methods are now widely available, including enzyme-linked immunosorbent assays, indirect hemagglutination, and a latex agglutination test (152–157).

The presence of immunoglobulin M (IgM) antibodies does not reliably identify recent or acute infection. This test may be positive as a result of nonspecific binding of immunoglobulin heavy chains or rheumatoid factor to Fc receptors on CMV-infected cells used as antigen. Even assays that control stringently for rheumatoid factor detect IgM in some subjects who had CMV infection in the past (158–160). The accuracy of antibody testing for primary CMV infection in pregnant women may be improved by determining IgG avidity and antigen specificity (118,161). Because the avidity of IgG antibodies for CMV antigens increases over time, the detection of low-avidity antibodies suggests recent infection. Antibody to ppUL83 (pp65) peaks early and declines, while antibody to ppUL32 (pp150) may remain in circulation (118,162). The development of antibodies to gpUL55 (gB) and gpUL75 (gH) may be delayed relative to other proteins (116).

Antigenemia

The antigenemia assay quantitates CMV in blood by detection of the UL83 gene product in PMNLs (8,163,164). Cells are separated from whole blood, fixed on a slide, stained with monoclonal antibodies to ppUL83, and counted by examination of the slide. For each specimen, two to three slides are made using 1.5 to 2.0 $\times$ 10^6 cells per slide. Results of this assay are expressed as the number of cells positive for ppUL83 per number of input cells on the slide. The ppUL83 protein is deposited into PMNLs from input virions rather than viral DNA replication (163). As a predictor of CMV disease, the antigenemia assay is more sensitive than viral culture, but less sensitive that PCR in most studies (165–167). While levels of CMV in blood measured by antigenemia and PCR tend to correlate in both hematopoietic and solid organ transplant patients, CMV is usually detected by PCR earlier than by antigenemia (168,169). The threshold value of antigenemia predicting CMV disease varies widely by patient population, and ranges from more than 2 positive cells per 50,000 PMNLs for allogeneic bone marrow transplant recipients to 100 to 200 positive cells per 50,000 PMNLs for heart or liver transplant recipients (170). Since the antigenemia assay requires a significant number of PMNLs for CMV detection, this method is not sufficiently sensitive in neutropenic patients (166,171).

Polymerase Chain Reaction

PCR uses sequential amplification of a target DNA sequence, allowing detection and quantitation of small amounts of DNA. Protocols differ in many respects, including DNA extraction, target DNA sequences, PCR cycle temperatures, and PCR product detection methods (172). Commercial PCR kits using plasma samples have been evaluated in HIV-positive patients (173), allogeneic stem cell transplant recipients (167), and renal transplant recipients (52). Compared with kits using plasma samples, those using leukocyte samples have shown higher sensitivity as well as earlier first positive result before development of CMV disease symptoms (174–176). Real-time PCR, which amplifies DNA and detects the products of amplification simultaneously, eliminates the need to detect products in a separate step, thereby reducing the risk for contamination and the amount of time required to perform the assay. Real-time and standard PCR using leukocyte specimens show a high degree of correlation and equivalent sensitivities and specificities in both hematopoietic and solid organ transplant patients (177–179). Schafer et al. (180) recently proposed a novel approach to interpreting results of leukocyte PCR and antigenemia assays. The area under the curve (AUC) representing the level and duration of viremia may predict CMV disease more accurately compared with the standard viral load when used in immunocompromised patients.

Studies comparing multiple methods of detecting CMV in both hematopoietic (166) and solid organ (176) transplant recipients conclude that molecular detection of CMV DNA in leukocytes is the preferred approach to evaluation and management of CMV disease in these populations. However, no standard protocol has been adopted for this purpose or for screening donated blood for latent CMV infection.

VACCINE DEVELOPMENT

The Institute of Medicine has rated the development and utilization of a CMV vaccine as a top priority for the twenty-first century (181). Mathematical modeling of a CMV vaccine with 80% to 90% efficacy in preventing primary infection suggests that only 66% to 75% of the population would need to be immunized in order to eradicate the virus (182). In contrast, vaccination rates greater than 90% are required to eradicate measles, mumps, and rubella. A CMV vaccine may be most beneficial for seronegative women of child-bearing age, seronegative organ transplant recipients, and young children who are reservoirs for infection of susceptible adults.

The first vaccine candidates employed the live Towne strain of CMV. About 50% of recipients experienced a local reaction, with soreness and induration in the arm. Humoral and cellular immune responses were detected in cytotoxic and lymphoproliferative assays (183,184). Challenge of healthy vaccinees with CMV 1 year after immunization failed to produce serologic or clinical evidence of infection using 10 plaque-forming units of wild-type virus, but vaccine seemed less protective than natural immunity against challenge with 100 plaque-forming units (185). In seronegative patients who received vaccine or placebo while awaiting renal transplantation, there was no difference in the rate of CMV infection or disease (186). In the group at highest risk for serious CMV disease, seronegative (prevaccine) recipients of kidneys from seropositive donors, severe disease appeared to be more frequent among placebo recipients. A study in CMV-seronegative mothers of CMV-shedding children in day care showed no protection against primary infection in those who received Towne strain vaccine compared with placebo recipients (187). A new lot of the Towne strain vaccine showed that the vaccine was well tolerated and elicited detectable humoral and cellular immune responses in adults, including women of child-bearing age, and children (188).

Because of concerns about the use of live virus preparations in potentially pregnant or immunocompromised hosts, viral subunit vaccines have also been proposed. These vaccines have primarily used the envelope glycoprotein gpUL55 (gB) to induce significant neutralizing antibody titers (189,190). Recombinant baclovirus-infected cells expressing a modified gpUL55 protein elicit a high-titer antibody response to neutralizing epitopes in vaccinees comparable with naturally seropositive individuals (190). Phase I clinical trials of a gpUL55 subunit vaccine incorporating a novel adjuvant given to adults (191,192) and children (193) show safety and immunogenicity.

However, control of CMV infection requires a strong cellular immune response from both CD4$^+$ and CD8$^+$ T cells in addition to antibodies. Several vaccine prototypes have incorporated the UL83 gene product, an immunodominant target of T-cell responses (194). Point mutations in the UL83 gene may decrease the toxicity of a vaccine without altering its immunogenicity (195). Target proteins of the cellular or humoral immune response can be introduced into the vaccinee using a variety of vehicles. A canarypox vector expressing the UL83 gene has been evaluated in a randomized, placebo-controlled phase I clinical trial with seronegative adults (196). This vaccine, given in a four-dose series, elicited ppUL83-specific CD8$^+$ T-cell responses after only two doses, and these responses remained detectable up to 26 months after the initial dose. A canarypox vector vaccine expressing the UL55 gene also elicits a significant humoral immune response, especially when given as a primer for the Towne strain live attenuated vaccine (197). DNA can also be injected directly in the form of plasmids expressing CMV genes (198,199). Peptide-based vaccines use immunodominant epitopes to elicit protective cellular immune responses in recipients with the appropriate HLA type (200).

REFERENCES

1. Rowe WP, Hartley JW, Waterman S, et al. Cytopathogenic agent resembling human salivary gland virus recovered from tissue cultures of human adenoids. *Proc Soc Exp Biol Med* 1956;92:418.
2. Smith MG. Propagation in tissue cultures of a cytopathogenic virus from human salivary gland virus (SGV) disease. *Proc Soc Exp Biol Med* 1956;92:424.
3. Weller TH, Macauley IC, Craig JM, et al. Isolation of intranuclear inclusion producing agents from infants with illnesses resembling cytomegalic inclusion disease. *Proc Soc Exp Biol Med* 1957;94:4.
4. Gibson W. Structure and assembly of the virion. *Intervirology* 1996;39:389.
5. Bankier AT, Beck S, Bohni R, et al. The DNA sequence of the human cytomegalovirus genome. *J DNA Sequencing Mapp* 1991;2:1.
6. Spaete RR, Gehrz RC, Landini MP. Human cytomegalovirus structural proteins. *J Gen Virol* 1994;75:3287.
7. Roby C, Gibson W. Characterization of phosphoproteins and protein kinase activity of virons, noninfectious enveloped particles, and dense bodies of human cytomegalovirus. *J Virol* 1986;59:714.
8. Gerna G, Revello MG, Percivalle E, et al. Quantification of human cytomegalovirus viremia by using monoclonal antibodies to different viral proteins. *J Clin Microbiol* 1990;28:2681.
9. Riegler S, Hebart H, Einsele H, et al. Monocyte-derived dendritic cells are permissive to the complete replicative cycle of human cytomegalovirus. *J Gen Virol* 2000;81:393.
10. Waldman WJ, Roberts WH, Davis DH, et al. Preservation of natural endothelial cytopathogenicity of cytomegalovirus by propagation in endothelial cells. *Arch Virol* 1991;117:143.
11. Sinzger C, Schmidt K, Knapp J, et al. Modification of human cytomegalovirus tropism through propagation *in vitro* is associated with changes in the viral genome. *J Gen Virol* 1999;80:2867.
12. Sinzger C, Kahl M, Laib K, et al. Tropism of human cytomegalovirus for endothelial cells is determined by a post-entry step dependent on efficient translocation to the nucleus. *J Gen Virol* 2000;81:3021.
13. Poland sd, Bambrick LL, Dekaban GA, et al. The extent of human cytomegalovirus replication in primary neurons is dependent on host cell differentiation. *J Infect Dis* 1994;170:1267.
14. Taylor-Wiedeman J, Sissons P, Sinclair J. Induction of endogenous human cytomegalovirus gene expression after differentiation of monocytes from healthy carriers. *J Virol* 1994;68:1597.
15. Compton T, Nowlin DM, Cooper NR. Initiation of human cytomegalovirus infection requires initial interaction with cell surface heparan sulfate. *Virology* 1993;193:834.
16. Pietropaolo R, Compton T. Interference with annexin II has no effect on entry of cytomegalovirus into fibroblast cells. *J Gen Virol* 1999;80:1807.
17. Keay S, Merigan TC, Rasmussen L. Identification of cell surface receptors for the 86-kilodalton glycoprotein of human cytomegalovirus. *Proc Natl Acad Sci U S A* 1989;86:10100.
18. Keay S, Baldwin B. Anti-idiotype antibodies that mimic gp86 of human cytomegalovirus inhibit viral fusion but not attachment. *J Virol* 1991;65:5124.
19. Baldwin BR, Zhang CO, Keay S. Cloning and epitope mapping of a functional partial fusion receptor for human cytomegalovirus gH. *J Gen Virol* 2000;81:27.
20. Grundy JE, McKeating JA, Ward PJ, et al. Beta 2 microglobulin enhances the infectivity of cytomegalovirus and when bound to the virus enables class I HLA molecules to be used as a virus receptor. *J Gen Virol* 1987;68:793.
21. Browne H, Churcher M, Minson T. Construction and characterization of a human cytomegalovirus mutant with the UL18 (class I homologue) gene deleted. *J Virol* 1992;66:6784.
22. Dal Monte P, Bessia C, Landini MP, et al. Expression of human cytomegalovirus ppUL83 (pp65) in a stable cell line and its association with metaphase chromosomes. *J Gen Virol* 1996;77:2591.
23. Iwayama S, Yamamoto T, Furuya T. et al. Intracellular localization and DNA-binding activity of a class of viral early phosphoproteins in human fibroblasts infected with human cytomegalovirus (Towne strain). *J Gen Virol* 1994;75:3309.
24. Mocarski ES, Kemble GW, Lyle JM, et al. A deletion mutant in the human cytomegalovirus gene encoding IE1 (491aa) is replication defective due to a failure in autoregulation. *Proc Natl Acad Sci U S A* 1996;93:11321.
25. Greaves RF, Mocarski ES. Defective growth correlates with reduced accumulation of a viral DNA replication protein after low multiplicity infection by a human cytomegalovirus *ie* 1 mutant. *J Virol* 1998;72:366.
26. Stenberg RM. The human cytomegalovirus major immediate early gene. *Intervirology* 1996;39:343.
27. Ahn K, Angulo A, Ghazal P. Human cytomegalovirus inhibits antigen presentation by a sequential multistep process. *Proc Natl Acad Sci U S A* 1996;93:10990.
28. Jones TR, Wiertz EJHJ, Sun L, et al. Human cytomegalovirus US3 impairs transport and maturation of major histocompatibility complex class I heavy chains. *Proc Natl Acad Sci U S A* 1996;93:11327.
29. Romanowski MJ, Shenk T. Characterization of the human cytomegalovirus

irs1 and trs1 genes: a second immediate-early transcription unit within irs1 whose product antagonizes transcriptional activation. *J Virol* 1997;71:1485.

30. Skaletskaya A, Bartle LM, Chittenden T, et al. A cytomegalovirus-encoded inhibitor of apoptosis that suppresses caspase-8 activation. *Proc Natl Acad Sci U S A* 2001;98:7829.

31. Spector DH. Activation and regulation of human cytomegalovirus early genes. *Intervirology* 1996;39:361.

32. Shamu CE, Story CM, Rapoport TA, et al. The pathway of US11-dependent degradation of MHC class I heavy chains involves a ubiquitin-conjugated intermediate. *J Cell Biol* 1999;147:45.

33. Wiertz EJ, Jones TR, Sun L, et al. The human cytomegalovirus US11 gene product dislocates MHC class I heavy chains from the endoplasmic reticulum to the cytosol. *Cell* 1996;84:769.

34. Penfold ME, Mocarski ES. Formation of cytomegalovirus DNA replication compartments defined by localization of viral proteins and DNA synthesis. *Virology* 1997;239:46.

35. McVoy MA, Adler SP. Human cytomegalovirus DNA replicates after early circularization by concatemer formation, and inversion occurs within the concatemer. *J Virol* 1994;68:1040.

36. Anders DG. The human cytomegalovirus genes and proteins required for DNA synthesis. *Intervirology* 1996;39:378.

37. Bolovan-Fritts CA, Mocarski ES, Wiedeman JA. Peripheral blood CD14+ cells from healthy subjects carry a circular conformation of latent cytomegalovirus genome. *Blood* 1999;93:394.

38. Bresnahan WA, Shenk T. A subset of viral transcripts packaged within human cytomegalovirus particles. *Science* 2000;288:2373.

39. Greijer AE, Dekkers CAJ, Middeldorp JM. Human cytomegalovirus virions differentially incorporate viral and host cell RNA during the assembly process. *J Virol* 2000;74:9078.

40. Yurochko AD, Huang ES. Human cytomegalovirus binding to human monocytes induces immunoregulatory gene expression. *J Immunol* 1999;162:4806.

41. Zhu H, Cong JP, Mamtora G, et al. Cellular gene expression altered by human cytomegalovirus: global monitoring with oligonucleotide arrays. *Proc Natl Acad Sci U S A* 1998;95:14470.

42. Browne EP, Wing B, Coleman D, et al. Altered cellular mRNA levels in human cytomegalovirus-infected fibroblasts: viral block to the accumulation of antiviral mRNAs. *J Virol* 2001;75:12319.

43. Nicholl MJ, Robinson LH, Preston CM. Activation of cellular interferon-responsive genes after infection of human cells with herpes simplex virus type 1. *J Gen Virol* 2000;81:2215.

44. Preston CM, Harman AN, Nicholl MJ. Activation of interferon response factor-3 in human cells infected with herpes simplex virus type 1 or human cytomegalovirus. *J Virol* 2001;75:8909.

45. Simmen KA, Singh J, Mattias Luukkonen BG, et al. Global modulation of cellular transcription by human cytomegalovirus is initiated by viral glycoprotein B. *Proc Natl Acad Sci U S A* 2001;98:7140.

46. Bresnahan WA, Boldogh I, Thompson EA, et al. Human cytomegalovirus inhibits cellular DNA synthesis and arrests productively infected cells in late G1. *Virology* 1996;224:150.

47. Dittmer D, Mocarski ES. Human cytomegalovirus infection inhibits G1/S transition. *J Virol* 1997;71:1629.

48. Lu M, Shenk T, Human cytomegalovirus infection inhibits cell cycle progression at multiple points, including the transition from G1 to S. *J Virol* 1996;70:8850.

49. Boyle KA, Pietropaolo RL, Compton T. Engagement of the cellular receptor for glycoprotein B of human cytomegalovirus activates the interferon-responsive pathway. *Mol Cell Biol* 1999;19:3607.

50. Gerna G, Percivalle E, Baldanti F, et al. Human cytomegalovirus replicates abortively in polymorphonuclear leukocytes after transfer from infected endothelial cells via transient microfusion events. *J Virol* 2000;74:5629.

51. Gerna G, Zavattoni M, Baldanti F, et al. Circulating cytomegalic endothelial cells are associated with high human cytomegalovirus (HCMV) load in AIDS patients with late-stage disseminated HCMV disease. *J Med Virol* 1998;55:64.

52. Aitken C, Barrett-Muir W, Millar C, et al. Use of molecular assays in diagnosis and monitoring of cytomegalovirus disease following renal transplantation. *J Clin Microbiol* 1999;37:2804.

53. Boivin G, Handfield J, Toma E, et al. Evaluation of the AMPLICOR cytomegalovirus test with specimens from human immunodeficiency virus-infected subjects. *J Clin Microbiol* 1998;36:2509.

54. Slobedman B, Mocarski ES. Quantitative analysis of latent human cytomegalovirus. *J Virol* 1999;73:4806.

55. Revello MG, Zavattoni M, Sarasini A. et al. Human cytomegalovirus in blood of immunocompetent persons during primary infection: prognostic implications for pregnancy. *J Infect Dis* 1998;177:1170.

56. Zaghellini F, Boppana SB, Emery VC, et al. Asymptomatic primary cytomegalovirus infection: virologic and immunologic features. *J Infect Dis* 1999;180:702.

57. Leonon WAM, Bruggeman CA, Wiertz EJHJ. Immune evasion by human cytomegalovirus: lessons in immunology and cell biology. *Semin Immunol* 2001;13:41.

58. Beck S, Barrell BG. Human cytomegalovirus encodes glycoprotein homologous to MHC class-I antigens. *Nature* 1988;331:269.

59. Browne H, Smith G, Beck S, et al. A complex between the MHC class I homologue encoded by human cytomegalovirus and β2 microblobulin. *Nature* 1990;347:770.

60. Fahnestock ML, Johnson JL, Feldman RM. et al. The MHC class homolog encoded by human cytomegalovirus binds endogenous peptides. *Immunity* 1995;3:583.

61. Reyburn HT, Mandelboim O, Vales-Gomez M, et al. The class I MHC homologue of human cytomegalovirus inhibits attack by natural killer cells. *Nature* 1997;386:514.

62. Cosman D, Fanger N, Borges L. Human cytomegalovirus, MHC class I and inhibitory signaling receptors: more questions than answers. *Immunol Rev* 1999;168:177.

63. Chapman TL, Heikema AP, Bjorkman PJ. The inhibitory receptor LIR-1 uses a common binding interaction to recognize class I MHC molecules and the viral homolog UL18. *Immunity* 1999;11:603.

64. Lopez-Botet M, Llano M, Ortega M, et al. Human cytomegalovirus and natural killer-mediated surveillance of HLA class I expression: a paradigm of host-pathogen adaptation. *Immunol Rev* 2001;181:193.

65. Sutherland CL, Chalupny NJ, Cosman D. The UL16-binding proteins, a novel family of MHC class I-related ligands for NKG2D, activate natural killer cell functions. *Immunol Rev* 2001;181:185.

66. Farrell HE, Degli-Esposti MA, Davis-Poynter NJ. Cytomegalovirus evasion of natural killer cell responses. *Immunol Rev* 1999;168:187.

67. Lalani AS, Barrett JW, McFadden G. Modulating chemokines: more lessons from viruses. *Immunol Today* 2000;21:100.

68. Chee MS, Satchwell SC, Preddie E, et al. Human cytomegalovirus encodes three G protein-coupled receptor homologues. *Nature* 1990;344:774.

69. Billstrom MA, Johnson GL, Avdi NJ, et al. Intracellular signaling by the chemokine receptor US28 during human cytomegalovirus infection. *J Virol* 1998;72:5535.

70. Bodaghi B, Jones TR, Zipeto D, et al. Chemokine sequestration by viral chemoreceptors as a novel viral escape strategy: withdrawal of chemokines from the environment of cytomegalovirus-infected cells. *J Exp Med* 1998; 188:855.

71. Spencer JV, Lockridge KM, Barry PA, et al. Potent immunosuppressive activities of cytomegalovirus-encoded interleukin-10. *J Virol* 2002;76: 1285.

72. Yamashita Y, Shimokata K, Mizuno S, et al. Down-regulation of the surface expression of class I MHC antigens by human cytomegalovirus. *Virology* 1993;193:727.

73. Benz C, Reusch U, Muranyi W, et al. Efficient downregulation of major histocompatibility complex class I molecules in human epithelial cells infected with cytomegalovirus. *J Gen Virol* 2001;82:2061.

74. Jones TR, Hanson HI, Sun L, et al. Multiple independent loci within the human cytomegalovirus unique short region down-regulate expression of major histocompatibility complex class I heavy chains. *J Virol* 1995;69:4830.

75. Jones TR, Sun L. Human cytomegalovirus US2 destabilizes major histocompatibility complex class I heavy chains. *J Virol* 1997;71:2970.

76. Tomazin R, Boname J, Hegde NR, et al. Cytomegalovirus US2 destroys two components of the MHC class II pathway, preventing recognition by CD4+ T cells. *Nat Med* 1999;5:1039.

77. Wiertz EJ, Tortorella D, Bogyo M, et al. Sec61-mediated transfer of a membrane protein from the endoplasmic reticulum to the proteosome for destruction. *Nature* 1996;384:432.

78. Gruhler A, Peterson PR, Fruh K. Human cytomegalovirus immediate early glycoprotein US3 retains MHC class I molecules by transient association. *Traffic* 2000;1:318.

79. Ahn K, Gruhler A, Galocha B, et al. The ER-luminal domain of the HCMV glycoprotein US6 inhibits peptide translocation by TAP. *Immunity* 1997;6:613.

80. Hengel H, Koopmann JO, Flohr T, et al. A viral ER-resident glycoprotein inactivates the MHC-encoded peptide transporter. *Immunity* 1997;6:623.

81. Lehner PJ, Karttunen JT, Wilkinson GWG, et al. The human cytomegalovirus US6 glycoprotein inhibits transporter associated with antigen processing-dependent peptide translocation. *Proc Natl Acad Sci U S A* 1997;94:6904.

82. Hengel H, Flohr T, Hammerling GJ, et al. Human cytomegalovirus inhibits peptide translocation into the endoplasmic reticulum for MHC class I assembly. *J Gen Virol* 1996;77:2287.

83. Shamu CE, Story CM, Rapoport TA, et al. The pathway of US11-dependent degradation of MHC class I heavy chains involves a ubiquitin-conjugated intermediate. *J Cell Biol* 1999;147:45.

84. Story CM, Furman MH, Ploegh HL. The cytosolic tail of class I MHC heavy chain is required for its dislocation by the human cytomegalovirus US2 and US11 gene products. *Proc Natl Acad Sci U S A* 1999;96:8516.

85. Wiertz EJHJ, Jones TR, Sun L, et al. The human cytomegalovirus US11 gene product dislocates MHC class I heavy chains from the endoplasmic reticulum to the cytosol. *Cell* 1996;84:769.

86. Miller DM, Cebulla CM, Rahill BM, et al. Cytomegalovirus and transcriptional down-regulation of major histocompatibility complex class II expression. *Semin Immunol* 2001;13:11.

87. Billstrom Schroeder M, Worthen GS. Viral regulation of RANTES expression during human cytomegalovirus infection of endothelial cells. *J Virol* 2001;75:3383.

88. Miller DM, Zhang Y, Rahill BM, et al. Human cytomegalovirus inhibits IFN-stimulated antiviral and immunoregulatory responses by blocking multiple levels of IFN-signal transduction. *J Immunol* 1999;162:6107.

89. Arrode G, Boccaccio C, Abastado JP, et al. Cross-presentation of human cytomegalovirus pp65 (UL83) to CD8+ T cells is regulated by virus-induced, soluble-mediator-dependent maturation of dendritic cells. *J Virol* 2002;76:142.

90. Goldmacher VS, Bartle LM, Skaletskaya A, et al. A cytomegalovirus-encoded

mitochondria-localized inhibitor of apoptosis structurally unrelated to Bcl-2. *Proc Natl Acad Sci U S A* 1999;96:12536.

91. Adler SP. Transfusion-associated cytomegalovirus infections. *Rev Infect Dis* 1983;5:977.

92. Rice GPA, Schrier RD, Oldstone MBA. Cytomegalovirus infects human lymphocytes and monocytes: virus expression is restricted to immediate-early gene products. *Proc Natl Acad Sci U S A* 1984;81:6134.

93. Einhorn L, Ost A. Cytomegalovirus infection of human blood cells. *J Infect Dis* 1984;149:207.

94. Reiser H, Kuhn J, Doerr HW, et al. Human cytomegalovirus replicates in primary human bone marrow cells. *J Gen Virol* 1986;67:2595.

95. Schrier RD, Nelson JA, Oldstone MBA. Detection of human cytomegalovirus in peripheral blood lymphocytes in a natural infection. *Science* 1985;230:1048.

96. Maciejewski JP, Bruening EE, Donahue RE, et al. Infection of hematopoietic progenitor cells by human cytomegalovirus. *Blood* 1992;80:170.

97. Soderberg C, Larsson S, Bergstedt-Lindqvist S, et al. Definition of a subset of human peripheral blood mononuclear cells that are permissive to human cytomegalovirus infection. *J Virol* 1993;67:3166.

98. Hahn G, Jores R, Mocarski ES. Cytomegalovirus remains latent in a common precursor of dendritic and myeloid cells. *Proc Natl Acac Sci U S A* 1998;95:3937.

99. Kondo K, Kaneshima H, Mocarski ES. Human cytomegalovirus latent infection of granulocyte-macrophage progenitors. *Proc Natl Acad Sci U S A* 1994;91:11879.

100. Kondo K, Xu J, Mocarski ES. Human cytomegalovirus latent gene expression in granulocyte-macrophage progenitors in culture and in seropositive individuals. *Proc Natl Acad Sci U S A* 1996;93:11137.

101. Mendelson M, Monard S, Sissons P, et al. Detection of endogenous human cytomegalovirus in CD34+ bone marrow progenitors. *J Gen Virol* 1996;77:3099.

102. Taylor-Wiedeman J, Hayhurst GP, Sissons JG, et al. Polymorphonuclear cells are not sites of persistence of human cytomegalovirus in healthy individuals. *J Gen Virol* 1993;74:265.

103. Taylor-Wiedeman J, Sissons JG, Borysiewicz LK, et al. Monocytes are a major site of persistence of human cytomegalovirus in peripheral blood mononuclear cells. *J Gen Virol* 1991;72:2059.

104. Sindre H, Tjoonnfjord GE, Rollag H, et al. Human cytomegalovirus suppression of and latency in early hematopoietic progenitor cells. *Blood* 1996;88:4526.

105. Lunetta JM, Wiedeman JA. Latency-associated sense transcripts are expressed during *in vitro* human cytomegalovirus productive infection. *Virology* 2000;278:467.

106. Zhuravskaya T, Maciejewski JP, Netski DM, et al. Spread of human cytomegalovirus (HCMV) after infection of human hematopoietic progenitor cells: model of HCMV latency. *Blood* 1997;90:2482.

107. Michelson S, Rohrlich P, Beisser P, et al. Human cytomegalovirus infection of bone marrow myofibroblasts enhances myeloid progenitor adhesion and elicits viral transmission. *Microbes Infect* 2001;3:1005.

108. Hassan-Walker AF, Mattes FM, Griffiths PD, et al. Quantity of cytomegalovirus DNA in different leukocyte populations during active infection in vivo and the presence of gB and UL18 transcripts. *J Med Virol* 2001;64:283.

109. Revello MG, Percivalle E, Arbustini E, et al. *In vitro* generation of human cytomegalovirus pp65 antigenemia, viremia, and leukoDNAemia. *J Clin Invest* 1998;101:2686.

110. Grundy JE, Lawson KM, MacCormac LP, et al. Cytomegalovirus-infected endothelial cells recruit neutrophils by the secretion of C-X-C chemokines and transmit virus by direct neutrophil-endothelial cell contact and during neutrophil transendothelial migration. *J Infect Dis* 1998;177:1465.

111. Söderberg-Nauclér C, Fish KN, Nelson JA. Reactivation of latent human cytomegalovirus by allogeneic stimulation of blood cells from healthy donors. *Cell* 1997;91:119.

112. Söderberg-Nauclér C, Streblow DN, Fish KN, et al. Reactivation of latent human cytomegalovirus in CD14+ monocytes is differentiation dependent. *J Virol* 2001;75:7543.

113. Hummel M, Zhang Z, Yan S, et al. Allogeneic transplantation induces expression of cytomegalovirus immediate-early genes *in vivo*: a model for reactivation from latency. *J Virol* 2001;75:4814.

114. Urban M, Klein M, Britt WJ, et al. Glycoprotein H of human cytomegalovirus is a major antigen for the neutralizing humoral immune response. *J Gen Virol* 1996;77:1537.

115. Ohlin M, Sundqvist VA, Mach M, et al. Fine specificity of the human immune response to the major neutralization epitopes expressed on cytomegalovirus gp58/116 (gB), as determined with human monoclonal antibodies. *J Virol* 1993;67:703.

116. Schoppel K, Kropff B, Schmidt C, et al. The humoral immune response against human cytomegalovirus is characterized by a delayed synthesis of glycoprotein-specific antibodies. *J Infect Dis* 1997;175:533.

117. Giugni TD, Churchill MA, Pande H, et al. Expression in insect cells and immune reactivity of a 28K tegument protein of human cytomegalovirus. *J Gen Virol* 1992;73:2367.

118. Greijer AE, van de Crommert JMG, Stevens SJC, et al. Molecular finespecificity analysis of antibody responses to human cytomegalovirus and design of novel synthetic-peptide-based serodiagnostic assays. *J Clin Microbiol* 1999;37:179.

119. Landini MP, Lazzarotto T, Ertl PF. Humoral immune response to human cytomegalovirus DNA polymerase. *J Clin Microbiol* 1993;31:724.

120. Boppana SB, Rivera LB, Fowler KB, et al. Intrauterine transmission of cytomegalovirus to infants of women with preconceptional immunity. *N Engl J Med* 2001;344:1366.

121. Fowler KB, Stagno S, Pass RF, et al. The outcome of congenital cytomegalovirus infection in relation to maternal antibody status. *N Engl J Med* 1992;326:663

122. Adler SP, Starr SE, Plotkin SA, et al. Immunity induced by primary human cytomegalovirus infection protects against secondary infection among women of childbearing age. *J Infect Dis* 1995;171:26.

123. Steffens HP, Kurz S, Holtappels R, et al. Preemptive CD8 T-cell immunotherapy of acute cytomegalovirus infection prevents lethal disease, limits the burden of latent viral genomes, and reduces the risk of virus recurrence. *J Virol* 1998;72:1797.

124. Walter EA, Greenberg PD, Gilbert MJ, et al. Reconstitution of cellular immunity against cytomegalovirus in recipients of allogeneic bone marrow by transfer of T-cell clones from the donor. *N Engl J Med* 1995;333:1038.

125. Jin X, Demoitie MA, Donahoe SM, et al. High frequency of cytomegalovirus-specific cytotoxic T-effector cells in HLA-A*0201 positive subjects during multiple viral coinfections. *J Infect Dis* 2000;181:165.

126. Zanghellini F, Boppana SB, Emery VC, et al. Asymptomatic primary cytomegalovirus infection: virologic and immunologic features. *J Infect Dis* 1999;180:702.

127. Bitmansour AD, Waldrop SL, Pitcher CJ, et al. Clonotypic structure of the human CD4+ memory T cell response to cytomegalovirus. *J Immunol* 2001;167:1151.

128. Asanuma H, Sharp M, Maecker HT, et al. Frequencies of memory T cells specific for varicella-zoster virus, herpes simplex virus, and cytomegalovirus by intracellular detection of cytokine expression. *J Infect Dis* 2000;181:859.

129. Gillespie GMA, Wills MR, Appay V, et al. Functional heterogeneity and high frequencies of cytomegalovirus-specific CD8+ T lymphocytes in healthy seropositive donors. *J Virol* 2000;74:8140.

130. Wills MR, Carmichael AJ, Mynard K, et al. The human cytotoxic T-lymphocyte (CTL) response to cytomegalovirus is dominated by structural protein pp65: frequency, specificity, and T-cell receptor usage of pp65-specific CTL. *J Virol* 1996;70:7569.

131. Peggs K, Verfuerth S, Pizzey A, et al. Characterization of human cytomegalovirus peptide-specific CD8+ T-cell repertoire diversity following *in vitro* restimulation by antigen-pulsed dendritic cells. *Blood* 2002;99:213.

132. Vaz-Santiago J, Lulé J, Rohrlich P, et al. *Ex vivo* stimulation and expansion of both CD4+ and CD8+ T cells from peripheral blood mononuclear cells of human cytomegalovirus-seropositive blood donors by using a soluble recombinant chimeric protein, IE1-pp65. *J Virol* 2001;75:7840.

133. Kern F, Surel IP, Faulhaber N, et al. Target structures of the CD8+ T-cell response to human cytomegalovirus: the 72-kilodalton major immediate-early protein revisited. *J Virol* 1999;73:8179.

134. Zaia JA, Gallez-Hawkins G, Li X, et al. Infrequent occurrence of natural mutations in the pp65$_{495-503}$ epitope sequence presented by the HLA A*0201 allele among human cytomegalovirus isolates. *J Virol* 2001;75:2472.

135. Weekes MP, Wills MR, Mynard K, et al. The memory cytotoxic T-lymphocyte (CTL) response to human cytomegalovirus infection contains individual peptide-specific CTL clones that have undergone extensive expansion *in vivo*. *J Virol* 1999;73:2099.

136. Weekes MP, Carmichael AJ, Wills MR, et al. Human CD28-CD8+ T cells contain greatly expanded functional virus-specific memory CTL clones. *J Immunol* 1999;162:7569.

137. Vargas AL, Lechner F, Kantzanou M, et al. *Ex vivo* analysis of phenotype and TCR usage in relation to CD45 isoform expression on cytomegalovirus-specific CD8+ T lymphocytes. *Clin Exp Immunol* 2001;125:432.

138. Wills MR, Carmichael AJ, Weekes MP, et al. Human virus-specific CD8+ CTL clones revert from CD45ROhigh to CD45RAhigh *in vivo*: CD45RAhighCD8+ T cells comprise both naive and memory cells. *J Immunol* 1999;162:7080.

139. Weekes MP, Wills MR, Mynard K, et al. Large clonal expansions of human virus specific memory cytotoxic T lymphocytes within the CD57+CD28−CD8+ T cell population. *Immunology* 1999;98:443.

140. Aubert G, Hassan-Walker AF, Madrigal JA, et al. Cytomegalovirus-specific cellular immune responses and viremia in recipients of allogeneic stem cell transplants. *J Infect Dis* 2001;184:955.

141. Gratama JW, van Esser JWJ, Lamers CHJ, et al. Tetramer-based quantification of cytomegalovirus (CMV)-specific CD8+ T lymphocytes in T-cell-depleted stem cell grafts and after transplantation may identify patients at risk for progressive CMV infection. *Blood* 2001;98:1358.

142. Komanduri KV, Donahoe SM, Moretto WJ, et al. Direct measurement of CD4+ and CD8+ T-cell responses to CMV in HIV-1-infected subjects. *Virology* 2001;279:459.

143. Villacres MC, Lacey SF, La Rosa C, et al. Human immunodeficiency virus infected patients receiving highly active antiretroviral therapy maintain activated CD8+ T cell subsets as a strong adaptive immune response to cytomegalovirus. *J Infect Dis* 2001;184:256.

144. Spiegel HML, Ogg GS, DeFalcon E, et al. Human immunodeficiency virus type 1- and cytomegalovirus-specific cytotoxic T lymphocytes can persist at high frequency for prolonged periods in the absence of circulating peripheral CD4+ T cells. *J Virol* 2000;74:1018.

145. Piccinini G, Comolli G, Genini E, et al. Comparative analysis of human cytomegalovirus-specific CD4+ T-cell frequency and lymphoproliferative response in human immunodeficiency virus–positive patients. *Clin Diagn Lab Immunol* 2001;8:1225.

146. Gamadia LE, Rentenaar RJ, Baars PA, et al. Differentiation of cytomegalovirus-specific CD8+ T cells in healthy and immunosuppressed virus carriers. *Blood* 2001;98:754.

147. Hassan-Walker AF, Vargas Cuero AL, Mattes FM, et al. CD8+ cytotoxic lymphocyte responses against cytomegalovirus after liver transplantation: correlation with time from transplant to receipt of tacrolimus. *J Infect Dis* 2001;183:835.

148. Gleaves CA, Smith TF, Shuster EA, et al. Rapid detection of cytomegalovirus in MRC-5 cells inoculated with urine specimens by using low-speed centrifugation and monoclonal antibody to an early antigen. *J Clin Microbiol* 1984;19:917.

149. Hudson JB. Further studies on the mechanism of centrifugal enhancement of cytomegalovirus infectivity. *J Virol Methods* 1988;19:97.

150. Faix RG. Cytomegalovirus antigenic heterogeneity can cause false negative results in indirect hemagglutination and complement-fixation antibody assay. *J Clin Microbiol* 1985;22:768.

151. Warier J, Weller TH, Kevy SV. Patterns of cytomegaloviral complement-fixing antibody activity: a longitudinal study of blood donors. *J Infect Dis* 1973;127:538.

152. Yeager AS. Improved indirect hemagglutination test for cytomegalovirus using human O erythrocytes in lysine. *J Clin Microbiol* 1979;10:64.

153. Kettering JD, Schmidt NJ, Galls D, et al. Anti-complement immunofluorescence test for antibodies to human cytomegalovirus. *J Clin Microbiol* 1977;6:627.

154. Beckwith DG, Halstead DC, Alpaugh K, et al. Comparison of a latex agglutination test with five other methods for determining the presence of antibody against cytomegalovirus. *J Clin Microbiol* 1985;21:328.

155. McHugh TM, Casavant CH, Wilber JC, et al. Comparison of six methods for the detection of antibody to cytomegalovirus. *J Clin Microbiol* 1985;22:1014.

156. Sererat MN, Schifano JV, Lau P, et al. Evaluation of cytomegalovirus (CMV) antibody screening tests for blood donors. *Am J Clin Pathol* 1986;86:523.

157. Leland DS, Barth KA, Cunningham EB, et al. Evaluation of four methods for cytomegalovirus antibody detection for use by a bone marrow transplantation service. *J Clin Microbiol* 1989;27:176.

158. Rasmussen L, Kelsall D, Nelson R, et al. Virus-specific IgG and IgM antibodies in normal and immunocompromised subjects infected with cytomegalovirus. *J Infect Dis* 1982;145:191.

159. Stagno S, Tinker MK, Elrod C, et al. Immunoglobulin M antibodies detected by enzyme-linked immunosorbent assay and radioimmunoassay in the diagnosis of cytomegalovirus infections in pregnant women and newborn infants. *J Clin Microbiol* 1985;21:930.

160. Chou S, Kim DY, Scott KM, et al. Immunoglobulin M to cytomegalovirus in primary and reactivation infections in renal transplant recipients. *J Clin Microbiol* 1987;25:52.

161. Lazzarotto T, Spezzacatena P, Varani S, et al. Anticytomegalovirus (anti-CMV) immunoglobulin G avidity in identification of pregnant women at risk of transmitting congenital CMV infection. *Clin Diagn Lab Immunol* 1999;6:127.

162. Ohlin M, Plachter B, Sundqvist VA, et al. Human antibody reactivity against the lower matrix protein (pp65) produced by cytomegalovirus. *Clin Diagn Lab Immunol* 1995;2:325.

163. Revello MG, Percivalle E, Di Matteo A, et al. Nuclear expression of the lower matrix protein of human cytomegalovirus in peripheral blood leukocytes of immunocompromised viraemic patients. *J Gen Virol* 1992;73:437.

164. Grefte JM, van der Gun BT, Schmolke S, et al. The lower matrix protein pp65 is the principal viral antigen present in peripheral blood leukocytes during an active cytomegalovirus infection. *J Gen Virol* 1992;73:2923.

165. Landry ML, Ferguson D. Comparison of quantitative cytomegalovirus antigenemia assay with culture methods and correlation with clinical disease. *J Clin Microbiol* 1993;31:2851.

166. Preiser W, Brauninger S, Schwerdtfeger R, et al. Evaluation of diagnostic methods for the detection of cytomegalovirus in recipients of allogeneic stem cell transplants. *J Clin Virol* 2001;20:59.

167. Solano C, Muñoz I, Gutiérrez A, et al. Qualitative plasma PCR assay (AMPLICOR CMV Test) versus pp65 antigenemia assay for monitoring cytomegalovirus viremia and guiding preemptive ganciclovir therapy in allogeneic stem cell transplantation *J Clin Microbiol* 2001;39:3938.

168. Guiver M, Fox AJ, Mutton K, et al. Evaluation of CMV viral load using TaqMan(tm) CMV quantitative PCR and comparison with CMV antigenemia in heart and lung transplant recipients. *Transplantation* 2001;71:1609.

169. Griscelli F, Barrois M, Chauvin S, et al. Quantification of human cytomegalovirus DNA in bone marrow transplant recipients by real-time PCR. *J Clin Microbiol* 2001;39:4362.

170. Boeckh M, Boivin G. Quantitation of cytomegalovirus: methodologic aspects and clinical applications. *Clin Microbiol Rev* 1998;11:533.

171. Flexman J, Kay I, Fonte R, et al. Differences between the quantitative antigenemia assay and the COBAS AMPLICOR MONITOR quantitative PCR assay for detecting CMV viraemia in bone marrow and solid organ transplant patients. *J Med Virol* 2001;64:275.

172. Roback JD, Hillyer CD, Drew WL, et al. Multicenter evaluation of PCR methods for detecting CMV DNA in blood donors. *Transfusion* 2001;41:1249.

173. Caliendo AM, Schuurman R, Yen-Lieberman B, et al. Comparison of quantitative and qualitative PCR assays for cytomegalovirus DNA in plasma. *J Clin Microbiol* 2001;39:1334.

174. Sia IG, Wilson JA, Espy MJ, et al. Evaluation of the COBAS AMPLICOR CMV MONITOR test for detection of viral DNA in specimens taken from patients after liver transplantation. *J Clin Microbiol* 2000;38:600.

175. Boivin G, Bélanger R, Delage, R, et al. Quantitative analysis of cytomegalovirus (CMV) viremia using the pp65 antigenemia assay and the COBAS AMPLICOR CMV MONITOR PCR test after blood and marrow allogeneic transplantation. *J Clin Microbiol* 2000;38:4356.

176. Pellegrin I, Garrigue I, Ekouevi D, et al. New molecular assays to predict occurrence of cytomegalovirus disease in renal transplant recipients. *J Infect Dis* 2000;182:36.

177. Schaade L, Kockelkorn P, Ritter K, et al. Detection of cytomegalovirus DNA in human specimens by LightCycler PCR. *J Clin Microbiol* 2000;38:4006.

178. Yun Z, Lewensohn-Fuchs I, Ljungman P, et al. Real-time monitoring of cytomegalovirus infections after stem cell transplantation using the TaqMan polymerase chain reaction assays. *Transplantation* 2000;69:1733.

179. Razonable RR, Brown RA, Espy MJ, et al. Comparative quantitation of cytomegalovirus (CMV) DNA in solid organ transplant recipients with CMV infection by using two high-throughput automated systems. *J Clin Microbiol* 2001;39:4472.

180. Shafer P, Tenschert W, Cremaschi L, et al. Area under the viraemia curve versus absolute viral load: utility for predicting symptomatic cytomegalovirus infections in kidney transplant patients. *J Med Virol* 2001;65:85.

181. Stratton KR, Durch JS, Lawrence RS, eds. *Vaccines for the 21st century: a tool for decision making.* Washington, DC: National Academy Press, 2001.

182. Griffiths PD, McLean A, Emery VC. Encouraging prospects for immunisation against primary cytomegalovirus infection. *Vaccine* 2001;19:1356.

183. Quinnan GV, Delery M, Rook AH, et al. Comparative virulence and immunogenicity of the Towne strain and a nonattenuated strain of cytomegalovirus. *Ann Intern Med* 1984;101:478.

184. Gehrz RC, Christianson WR, Linner KM, et al. Cytomegalovirus vaccine. Specific humoral and cellular immune responses in human volunteers. *Arch Intern Med* 1980;140:936.

185. Plotkin SA, Starr SE, Friedman HM, et al. Protective effects of Towne cytomegalovirus vaccine against low-passage cytomegalovirus administered as a challenge. *J Infect Dis* 1989;159:860.

186. Brayman KL, Dafoe DC, Smythe WR, et al. Prophylaxis of serious cytomegalovirus infection in renal transplant candidates using live human cytomegalovirus vaccine: interim results of a randomized controlled trial. *Arch Surg* 1988;123:1502.

187. Adler SP, Starr SE, Plotkin SA, et al. Immunity induced by primary human cytomegalovirus infection protects against secondary infection among women of childbearing age. *J Infect Dis* 1995;171:26.

188. Adler SP, Hempfling SH, Starr SE, et al. Safety and immunogenicity of the Towne strain cytomegalovirus vaccine. *Pediatr Infect Dis J* 1998;17:200.

189. Britt W, Fay J, Seals J, et al. Formulation of an immunogenic human cytomegalovirus vaccine: responses in mice. *J Infect Dis* 1995;171:18.

190. Marshall GS, Li M, Stout GG, et al. Antibodies to the major linear neutralizing domains of cytomegalovirus glycoprotein B among natural seropositives and CMV subunit vaccine recipients. *Viral Immunol* 2000;13:329.

191. Frey SE, Harrison C, Pass RF, et al. Effects of antigen dose and immunization regimens on antibody responses to a cytomegalovirus glycoprotein B subunit vaccine. *J Infect Dis* 1999;180:1700.

192. Pass RF, Duliegè AM, Boppana S, et al. A subunit cytomegalovirus vaccine based on recombinant envelope glycoprotein B and a new adjuvant. *J Infect Dis* 1999;180:970.

193. Mitchell DK, Holmes SJ, Burke RL, et al. Immunogenicity of a recombinant human cytomegalovirus gB vaccine in seronegative toddlers. *Pediatr Infect Dis J* 2002;21:133.

194. Gonczol E, Plotkin S. Development of a cytomegalovirus vaccine: lessons from recent clinical trials. *Expert Opin Biol Ther* 2001;1:401.

195. Yao ZQ, Gallez-Hawkins G, Lomeli NA, et al. Site-directed mutation in a conserved kinase domain of human cytomegalovirus-pp65 with preservation of cytotoxic T lymphocyte targeting. *Vaccine* 2001;19:1628.

196. Berencsi K, Gyulai Z, Gönczöl E, et al Canarypox vector expressing cytomegalovirus (CMV) phosphoprotein 65 induces long-lasting cytotoxic T cell responses in human CMV-seronegative subjects. *J Infect Dis* 2001;183:1171.

197. Adler SP, Plotkin SA, Gönczöl E, et al. A canarypox vector expressing cytomegalovirus (CMV) glycoprotein B primes for antibody responses to a live attenuated CMV vaccine (Towne). *J infect Dis* 1999;180:843.

198. Endrész V, Burián K, Berencsi K, et al. Optimization of DNA immunization against human cytomegalovirus. *Vaccine* 2001;19:3972.

199. Endrész V, Kari L, Berencsi K, et al. Induction of human cytomegalovirus (HCMV)-glycoprotein B (gB)-specific neutralizing antibody and phosphoprotein 65 (pp65)-specific cytotoxic T lymphocyte responses by naked DNA immunization. *Vaccine* 1999;17:50.

200. Diamond DJ, York J, Sun JY, et al. Development of a candidate HLA A*0201 Restricted peptide-based vaccine against human cytomegalovirus infection. *Blood* 1997;90:1751.

201. Perot K, Walker CM. Primary chimpanzee skin fibroblast cells are fully permissive for human cytomegalovirus replication. *J Gen Virol* 1992;72:3281.

202. Nowlin DM, Cooper NR, Compton T. Expression of a human cytomegalovirus receptor correlates with infectibility of cells. *J Virol* 1991;65:3114.

203. Adlish JD, Lahijani RS, St. Jeor SC. Identification of a putative cell receptor for human cytomegalovirus. *Virology* 1990;176:337.

204. Taylor HP, Cooper NR. The human cytomegalovirus receptor on fibroblasts is a 30-kilodalton membrane protein. *J Virol* 1990;64:2484.

205. Mocarski ES, Stinski MF. Persistence of the cytomegalovirus genome in human cells. *J Virol* 1979;31:761.

CHAPTER 236
Human Parvovirus

Neal S. Young

HISTORY

Although parvoviruses commonly cause disease in animals, it was only in 1975 that the first human pathogen of this family was discovered by Cossart and colleagues (5) in screening normal blood bank donors' sera for hepatitis antigen (one of the donor's serum samples was coded B19). Epidemiologic surveys established that serum from approximately half of the adult population contained immunoglobulin G (IgG) antibodies to this virus (6–8), suggesting acquisition of immunity during childhood. Evidence of recent infection (viral antigen, IgM antibody to virus) was first found in the blood of Jamaican children residing in London, all of whom had presented with transient aplastic crisis of sickle cell disease (9), and the close association of parvovirus and aplastic crisis was confirmed in a large retrospective study of serum from sickle cell disease patients with this complication (10). Later, B19 parvovirus was shown to be the etiologic agent of fifth disease in hematologically normal persons (11) and, when infection of the mother occurred during pregnancy, of some cases of nonimmune hydrops fetalis (12). B19 parvovirus infection can persist and cause chronic bone marrow failure (13). B19 parvovirus also has been implicated in rheumatic syndromes and in vasculitis. The virus' biology and the clinical consequences of infection have been well reviewed (1–4).

CHARACTERISTICS OF THE PATHOGEN

Classification and Structure

A typical member of the Parvoviridae family has about 5,000 nucleotides of single-stranded DNA encapsidated in a small (~20 nm in diameter) icosahedrally symmetric and unenveloped structure (14–18) (Fig. 236.1). The subfamily Parvovirinae contains the autonomous animal parvoviruses (genus *Parvovirus*), viruses that require a helper virus for replication (genus *Dependovirus*), and B19 and its simian relatives (genus *Erythrovirus*) (19). B19 shares basic morphologic and DNA structural features (20,21) with other members of the Parvoviridae. Minor variants of B19 have been cloned and sequenced (22,23); however, parallel epidemic curves (24) and the illness produced in normal volunteers (25) strongly suggest that a single parvovirus species is responsible for all clinical manifestations of B19 parvovirus infection.

Although B19 is the only known human pathogenic parvovirus, there are other human parvoviruses. The adeno-associated viruses were discovered in tissue culture, but the prevalence of antibodies to them in humans indicates the occurrence of natural infection (16–18). They have also been isolated from throat and anal swab specimens from healthy children. More closely related to B19 is simian parvovirus, which can cause fatal anemia in cynomolgus monkeys (26).

Genomic Organization

B19 parvovirus has been cloned (27) and sequenced (28) and its pattern of transcription mapped (21) (Fig. 236.2). The two structural proteins of the capsid are encoded in overlapping transcriptional frames on the right side of the genome, and a single non-

structural protein is encoded on the left side (29,30). The smaller structural protein (58 kd, vP2) is the major constituent of the capsid, and the larger protein (83 kd, VP1), which differs by only 227 amino acids from VP2, is the minor (31). The structural proteins can self-assemble into capsids, into which the DNA is inserted (32). In contrast, expression of the nonstructural protein is lethal in cells in which the gene has been transfected (33). The functions of the B19 nonstructural protein are unknown, although the nonstructural proteins of other parvoviruses have been shown to act as replication competence factors and enhancer elements and to bind DNA. Selective expression of the B19 nonstructural protein can lead to apoptosis (34) in the absence of viral replication. In addition to nonstructural protein, small proteins of unknown function, encoded on the left side of the genome, are expressed during infection (35).

Although the genomic organization of B19 is similar to that of other Parvoviridae organisms, it is much more complex and differs in significant features, including the presence of a single strong promoter at the left side, failure of all transcripts to coterminate at the right side, and extensive splicing of all but the nonstructural protein RNA (29). RNA expression occurs in early and late stages: nonstructural protein transcription, followed by capsid protein RNA expression (36). B19 parvovirus' genomic organization and the identical sequence of the left- and right-hand terminal repeats place it close to human adeno-associated virus, and the extreme tissue specificity of B19 parvovirus may be analogous to the defective nature of the dependoviruses.

Replication

The limited size of their genome makes parvoviruses dependent on actively cycling populations of cells for their own replication. Adeno-associated viruses need helper functions provided by other viruses, particularly adenovirus and herpesvirus (16–18,37). Nuclear helper functions are also important in tissue tropism: minute virus of mice variants enter nonpermissive cells

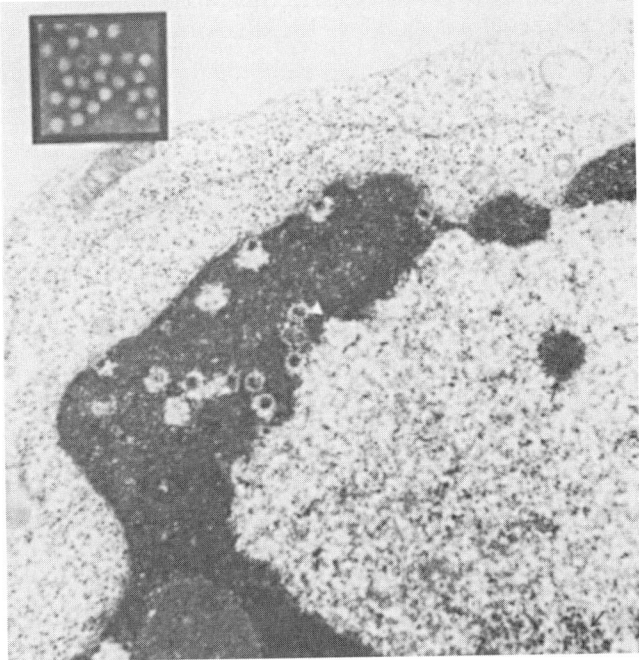

Figure 236.1. Electron micrographs of B19 parvovirus in a human erythroid progenitor cell infected *in vitro* and in serum (**inset**).

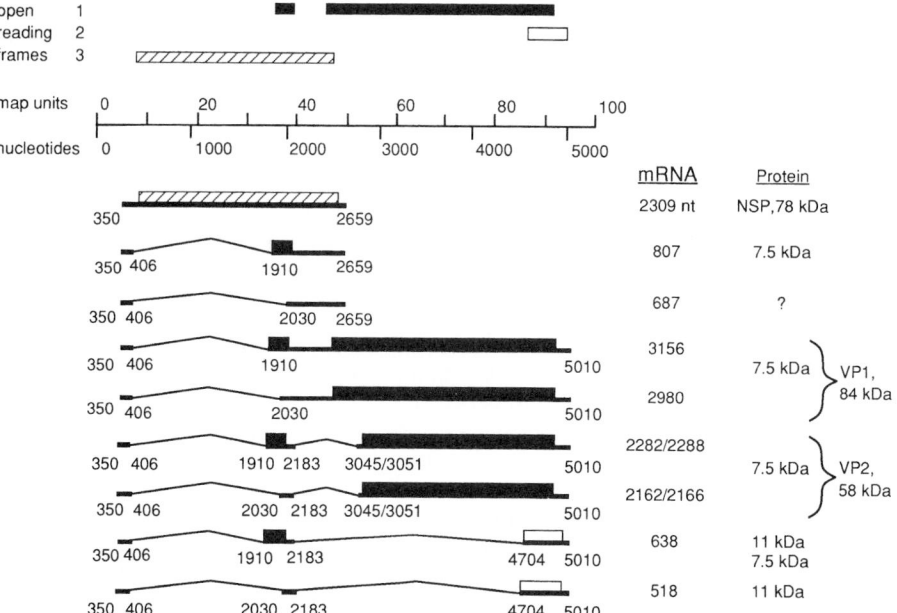

Figure 236.2. B19 parvovirus genomic organization. The 5,400 nucleotides are divided into 100 map units for convenience. The molecular mass of the RNA transcripts is indicated on the left. The major capsid protein (*VP2*), minor capsid protein (*VP1*), and nonstructural protein (*NSP*) and their molecular masses are indicated on the right. The coding sequences are shown by the open boxes, with reading frames indicated by the numeral. All transcription begins at a single promoter on the far left-hand side of the genome. (Adapted from Luo W, Astell CR. A novel protein encoded by small RNAs of parvovirus B19. *Virology* 1993;195:448–455, with permission.)

but are unable to complete their replicative cycle (38) (a difference encoded, surprisingly, within the capsid genes) (39). Natural infections of parvoviruses usually occur in mitotically active tissues: this predilection results in infection of fetuses and young growing animals and in "embryonic" tissues of the lymphoid and hematopoietic systems (40,41). Three examples are worth citing: outbreaks of spontaneous abortions of pig litters caused by porcine parvovirus (42), fatal myocarditis in puppies caused by canine parvovirus (43), and infection of lymphocytes and bone marrow cells caused by feline parvovirus (44).

Like that of other parvoviruses (45–47), the replication strategy of B19 is based on the inverted terminal repeat structures (27,28). Replication of the single-stranded DNA of the Parvoviridae is initiated from these brief regions of double-strandedness, with formation of higher molecular weight intermediates visible on Southern blot analysis (47). Thus, in clinical samples, not only the presence of virus but also active viral replication can be detected (48–50).

PATHOGENESIS

Host Cell

The bone marrow is a mitotically active tissue, and the only known natural host cell of B19 is the human erythroid progenitor cell (Figs. 236.3 and 236.4). The virus also replicates in tissue culture of fetal liver (51) and peripheral blood cells (52). B19 parvovirus can be propagated in some human megakaryocytoblastoid cell lines grown in the presence of erythropoietin (53,54). B19 inhibits erythroid, but not myeloid, colony formations (55–57), and virus inoculation depletes suspension cultures of bone marrow of erythroid precursor cells (58). B19 is cytotoxic to both early and late erythroid progenitors (55,57), inducing *in vitro* characteristic morphologic changes observed by light and electron microscopy (58,59) similar to the appearance of bone marrow from patients with parvovirus infection.

Cellular Receptor and Tissue Specificity

Tissue specificity is largely determined by the nature of the cellular receptor, erythrocyte P antigen or globoside, a glycolipid tetrohexoseceramide (60). Virus binds with high affinity to P antigen, and infectivity *in vitro* can be blocked by either an excess of soluble globoside or monoclonal antibody to P antigen. Remarkably, rare individuals who lack globoside on the red blood cell surface (p phenotype) cannot be infected with B19 (61). Globoside is abundant on the red blood cell surface but is also found on megakaryocytes, endothelial cells, some placental cells, and fetal liver and heart (62).

In addition to the P receptor, permissivity requires intracellular factors. The pattern of transcription of B19 parvovirus RNA differs between marrow cells and nonpermissive cell lines, suggestive of a transcription factor that enables capsid gene RNA expression (63).

Cytotoxicity

Productive parvovirus infection is cytotoxic. The renewable nature of the erythroid progenitor target cell population is an

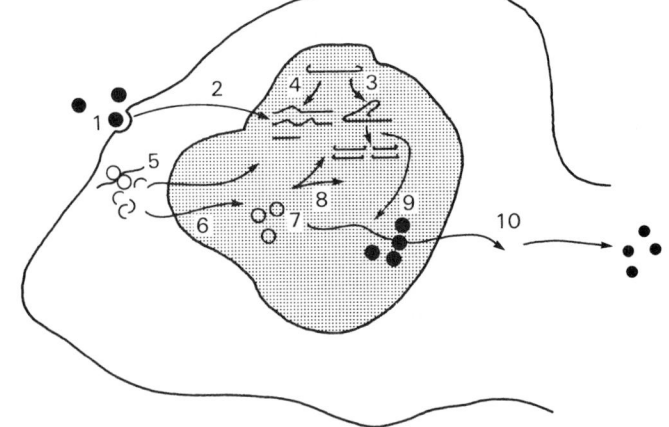

Figure 236.3. Life cycle of the B19 parvovirus: *1*, binding to P antigen, the cellular receptor; *2*, translocation to nucleus and encoding; *3*, DNA replication; *4*, RNA transcription; *5*, protein translation; *6*, protein trafficking to nucleus; *7*, empty capsid assembly; *8*, nonstructural protein effects; *9*, DNA insertion; and *10*, cell lysis and virus release.

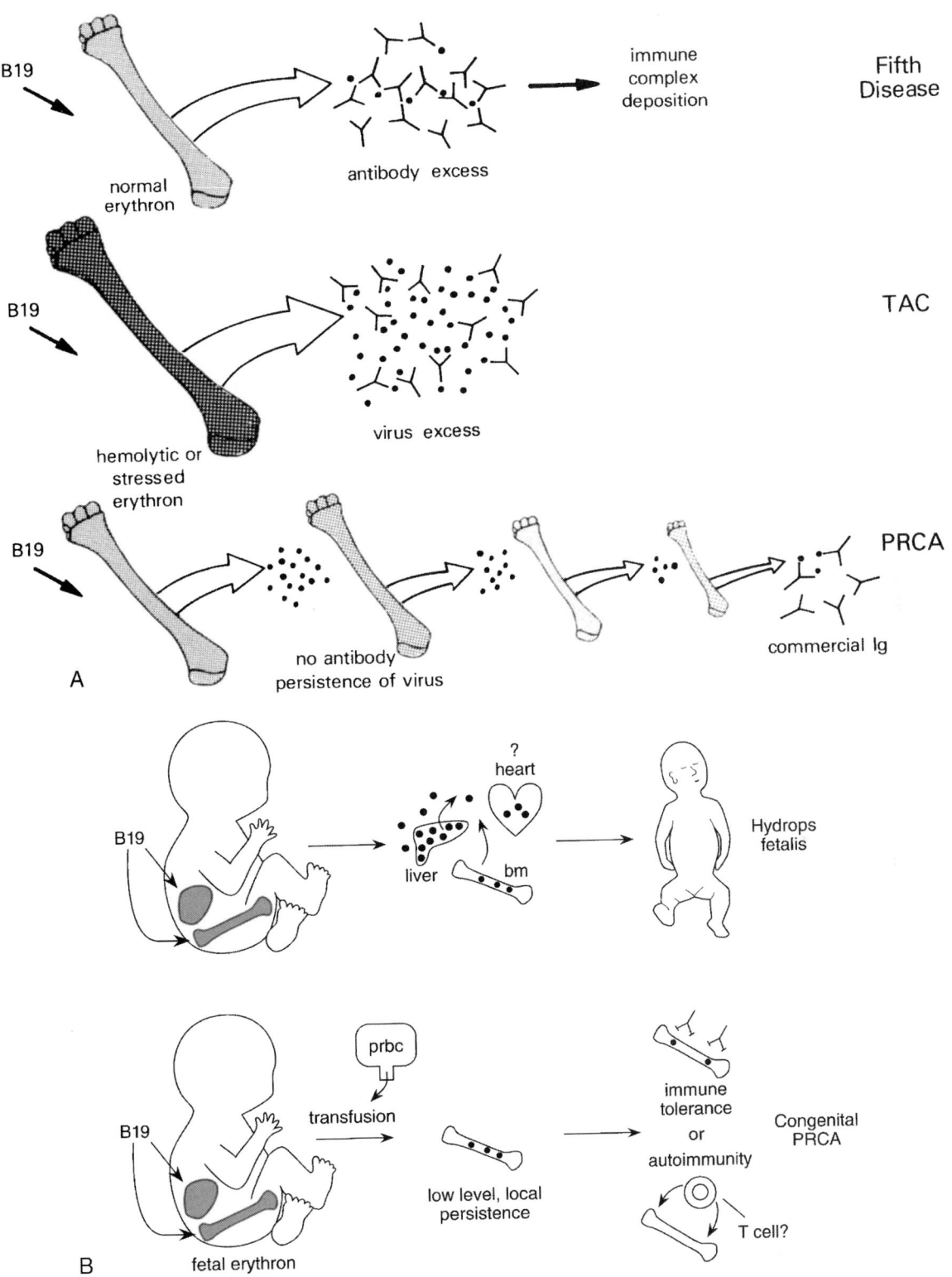

Figure 236.4. A: Patterns of B19 parvovirus disease, emphasizing the balance among target cell number, virus production, and immune response. *TAC,* transient aplastic crisis; *PRCA,* pure red (blood) cell aplasia. **B:** Patterns of B19 parvovirus infection of the fetus, resulting in either death *in utero* or at birth or, when treated by transfusion of packed red blood cells (*prbc*), in PRCA. *bm,* bone marrow.

important variable in clinical infection. Study of persistently infected patients over time has suggested that virus propagation and cell regeneration may alternate in cycles to achieve equilibrium between target cells and virus production (49,50). Lower titers of virus in persistently infected patients are com-

patible with depletion of erythroid cells (64). As with other viruses, irreversible organ damage may be the only "footprint" of parvovirus infection. For example, feline parvovirus infection of cerebellar cells results in atrophy of this organ, and the persistence of ataxia in developing kittens is evidence of intrauterine infection (65). Similar mechanisms might exist for congenital bone marrow failure syndromes in humans (13).

Persistence

Parvoviruses can persist in tissue culture (66) and in animals (41). Adeno-associated virus has been shown to integrate as concatemers at a specific chromosomal site in cell lines (67). Aleutian disease virus persists in minks, and the sustained and exaggerated humoral immune response leads to hypergammaglobulinemia and immune complex disease (68). Latent virus infection is also apparent in the pattern of virus excretion in young pigs (42) and kittens (69). While B19 parvovirus persists in patients, neither persistence nor integration of this virus has been demonstrated in cells.

Immune Response

Antibodies specific for B19 are made after natural exposure (70) and experimental inoculation (25), with IgM rising at the end of the second week and IgG rising a few days later. Serum containing antibodies neutralizes viral cytotoxicity for human bone marrow cells (55,71). A cellular proliferative response to the virus has not been reproducibly demonstrated *in vitro* (71). Immediately after infection, the immune response is directed primarily to the common sequences of the major and minor capsid species, but late in convalescence and in random serum samples, the dominant antibody specificity is directed to the minor capsid protein (71).

Failure to produce IgG that binds capsid proteins on immunoblot and that can neutralize virus activity is a feature of the aberrant immune response of persistently infected patients (49,50,64,71).

B19 Pathogenesis

Marrow failure is an early event after virus infection, often coincident with viremia and preceding the appearance of antiparvovirus IgG (4,24,70); in normal volunteers, viremia and the disappearance of reticulocytes from the circulation occur 5 days after inoculation, when the only symptoms are nonspecific rash and malaise (24). These data are consistent with hematopoietic cells' serving as the major site of virus replication. On the other hand, fifth disease, the manifestation of parvovirus infection in hematologically normal persons, occurs late in respect to inoculation or exposure (24,71) and is almost certainly an immune complex disorder. The serum of children with a clinical diagnosis of fifth disease contains IgM antibody to B19 parvovirus but rarely virus (11,72,73). In normal volunteers, both the cutaneous and the rheumatic symptoms and signs of fifth disease occur 17 to 18 days after inoculation, when there are increasing titers of specific antiviral immunoglobulins in the blood. Fifth disease can also be produced by infusion of immunoglobulins into chronically viremic patients (50). Although patients with fifth disease are rarely viremic and probably not contagious, low concentrations of virus may be detectable for months after infection by polymerase chain reaction amplification (64). A rash illness, even when anticipated, is rare enough after aplastic crisis to be reportable (74), perhaps owing to larger quantities of virus and smaller amounts of antibody produced during infection of an expanded erythroid marrow.

EPIDEMIOLOGY

Stability, Contagion, and Transmission

Parvoviruses are notoriously contagious. They are relatively resistant to heat and stable to 60°C for at least 16 hours, probably because they lack a labile envelope. In addition, extremely high titers of virus may be present in the blood during acute infection (as many as 10^{16} genomic copies per milliliter). Parvovirus has been detected in throat swabbings (70) and respiratory secretions (25), but the usual route of transmission under natural conditions is unknown. Parvovirus may be acquired as a nosocomial (75–77) or laboratory (78) infection. Parvovirus may be transmitted by clotting factor concentrate and other plasma derivatives (79,80). Nucleic acid testing has been proposed to screen for and remove potentially infectious lots (81). Because it is present in circulating cells (37), parvovirus has been acquired from cellular blood products, including during bone marrow transplantation (82).

Distribution and Prevalence

IgG to B19 is present in about half of the adult population worldwide, and seroepidemiologic surveys have suggested that most people acquire immunity between the ages of 5 and 19 years (2,6–8). Seropositivity rates increase with age, consistent with continuing exposure to virus throughout adult life.

CLINICAL MANIFESTATIONS

Fifth Disease

Fifth disease, or erythema infectiosum, is the common manifestation of acute B19 parvovirus infection. Fifth disease was first categorized and separated from other related rash illnesses of childhood like rubella, rubeola, and scarlet fever at the end of the nineteenth century. The high rate of contagion and its clinical features strongly suggested a virus. Because virtually all affected children with fifth disease have serologic evidence of recent infection with parvovirus (11,72,73), the illness is more accurately termed acute parvovirus infection. In children, fifth disease manifests as an exanthem, typically involving the face ("slapped cheek"), trunk, and proximal extremities with a lacy, reticular, erythematous eruption (83–88). The macular or maculopapular appearance may mimic measles, although a vesiculopustular eruption in fifth disease has been described (89). The rash may be evanescent and recurrent for weeks. Children with fifth disease are usually not extremely ill and may not be febrile. Although typical cases are easily diagnosed, fifth disease is often recognized by its epidemic character.

Fifth disease in adults is often a rheumatic syndrome (83,90). In experimentally inoculated adult volunteers, joint pain and swelling were the major symptoms, and the pattern of cutaneous eruption was not specific (24). About 15% of adults with newly diagnosed arthritis had evidence of recent parvovirus infection (91,92). Polyarthralgia and frank arthritis may be acute, or the syndrome may persist for months and resemble rheumatoid arthritis in the pattern of joint involvement. Some patients have rheumatoid factor in the blood (93), and B19 antigen has been detected in the synovial fluid (94). However, B19 parvovirus does not have a general role in the etiology of rheumatoid arthritis (95,96).

Other rheumatic illnesses associated with B19 parvovirus infection include fibromyalgia (97) and a systemic lupus erythematosus–like syndrome (98,99). Infection has also been associated with some cases of vasculitis, including Wegener's granulomatosis (100) and Kawasaki disease (101).

Parvovirus infection has been associated with mild serum transaminase elevations and much more occasionally with frank severe hepatitis (102); its role in true fulminant hepatitis is dubious, and the virus does not appear to be a major etiology of seronegative hepatitis (103).

Transient Aplastic Crisis

Transient aplastic crisis is a unique event in the life of persons with hemolytic disease, characterized by abrupt cessation of bone marrow erythropoiesis, reticulocytopenia, and severe but temporary anemia (4,10,70,101). Aplastic crisis occurs in virtually every hemolytic state, including sickle cell disease, hereditary spherocytosis, erythrocyte enzyme deficiencies, autoimmune hemolysis, paroxysmal nocturnal hemoglobinuria, and the thalassemias (4). Although readily treated by red blood cell transfusions, anemia may precipitate fatal heart failure (104). Virtually all cases of typical transient aplastic crisis are caused by B19 parvovirus infection (4,10), but erythroid marrow failure in these patients can also accompany serious systemic bacterial or mycobacterial infections (104). Occasionally, parvovirus infection in a patient with underlying hemolysis is not followed by transient aplasia (105).

The bone marrow of transient aplastic crisis shows an absence of erythroid precursor cells and the presence of striking giant pronormoblasts; rarely, necrosis of marrow may occur (106). Reticulocytopenia and a decrease in hemoglobin level are the sequelae of inoculation of parvovirus into hematologically normal volunteers (24) associated with temporary cessation of marrow erythropoiesis (107). Because of the 120-day average life span of a red blood cell in the circulation, this regular effect of B19 infection has hematologic consequences only for persons who have a heightened demand for red blood cells, usually owing to hemolysis. In cases of compensated hemolysis, in which a normal hemoglobin level is maintained by increased marrow activity, transient aplastic crisis can unmask the underlying hematologic disease (108–110). Aplastic crisis caused by B19 infection can occur in persons with erythropoietic stress due to blood loss or iron deficiency. Neutrophil and platelet numbers commonly decrease during transient aplastic crisis (104,111–113), and parvovirus infection has been cited in cases of isolated thrombocytopenia (114) as well as transient (111–113) and permanent (115) pancytopenia. B19 parvovirus is a cause of hemophagocytic syndrome, in which variable pancytopenia occurs with characteristic bone marrow morphologic features (116). However, transient erythroblastopenia of childhood has not been associated by serologic studies with recent parvovirus infection (117).

Chronic Bone Marrow Failure

B19 parvovirus can persist in immunosuppressed patients and cause chronic transfusion-dependent anemia, sometimes with severe neutropenia (49,50,64,118,119). Anemia is commonly the only evidence of persistent B19 infection. About 15% of cases of "idiopathic" pure red blood cell aplasia represent persistent parvovirus infection (120). Persistent infection has been documented in congenital (49,64) and acquired immunodeficiency syndrome, including with human immunodeficiency virus type 1 infection (121), and in children with acute lymphocytic leukemia in remission who are receiving chemotherapy (50,118,119). The congenital immunodeficiency state that predis-poses to persistent infection has not been well characterized, although there are usually defects in both T- and B-cell function (Nezelof's syndrome); anemia due to B19 may be the major clinical manifestation of the immunodeficiency state. Anemia may remit during periods in which virus is not present in the circulation (49,50,64).

Hydrops Fetalis and Congenital Infection

B19 infection is a cause of nonimmune hydrops fetalis, in which death of the term fetus is due to severe anemia and congestive heart failure (2,12,122–131). Parvovirus has been demonstrated in fetal tissue by *in situ* hybridization, electron microscopy, and immunoblotting for proteins (127–131). Similar to children and adults, the erythron appears to be the major target of virus infection, with characteristic morphologic changes and virus most consistently present in the liver, the major blood-producing organ of the fetus. Most women have been infected in the second trimester, so infection in the fetus is also presumably chronic. The role of B19 infection in early pregnancy in producing spontaneous abortions is unknown (2,132). Maternal fifth disease is not usually followed by a poor fetal outcome, and the risk of hydrops is probably around 9% with documented exposure (2,127,133).

Occasionally, parvovirus infection acquired during pregnancy can persist in the infant (134). Hydropic infants treated *in utero* or at birth by red blood cell transfusions may remain anemic. The marrow may show red blood cell aplasia or dysplastic changes. Virus does not circulate and can be detected only by gene amplification of marrow. In contrast to persistent infection in later life, congenital infection does not respond to immunoglobulin therapy. There is little evidence to suggest that parvovirus is otherwise teratogenic in humans (135). The virus has been detected in myocardial cells (136) that bear P antigen (and the puppy heart is a site of attack of canine parvovirus).

DIAGNOSIS

Both capture radioimmunoassays (6,137) and enzyme-linked immunoassays (7) have been used to measure anti-B19 IgG and IgM in serum. The presence of IgM to B19 in serum is evidence of recent infection; the quantity of IgG in exposed persons varies widely, and increasing titers cannot be used to infer recent exposure. As described earlier, patients with persistent B19 parvovirus infection may not have serum antibodies to virus (50), or antibodies that react by immunoassay but not on immunoblot to capsid proteins (49,71), or a pattern of antibody typical of early convalescence (IgM, and IgG directed mainly to the 58-kd capsid protein) (64,71).

The diagnosis of persistent B19 parvovirus infection depends on detecting virus itself rather than virus-specific antibody (49,50). Virus alone will also be present in serum from patients with transient aplastic crisis obtained at the onset of illness. DNA hybridization methods allow quantitation of virus as genome copy number (137–141). In acute infection, the period of viremia is brief but often intense; there may be as many as 10^{16} genome copies per milliliter of serum. In persistent infection, 10^5 to 10^8 genome copies are more usual. Amplification of viral DNA by polymerase chain reaction is far more sensitive than direct hybridization methods, and viremia is more prolonged, even in acute infection, than was previously suspected (142). The results of polymerase chain reaction studies should be interpreted cautiously—the sensitivity of the technique makes it susceptible to contamination and false-positive results. Replicating virus can be detected by Southern blot hybridization after restriction enzyme digestion. Parvovirus has been detected by blot and *in situ* hybridization and by immunofluorescence studies of bone marrow, spleen, and a variety of fetal organs.

TREATMENT

In normal children, fifth disease is a mild illness and no treatment is required. The polyarthralgia-arthritis syndrome in adults is usually a brief episode; more chronic rheumatic symptoms are treated with antiinflammatory drugs. The severity of anemia in transient aplastic crisis usually requires erythrocyte transfusion, but hospitalization is not mandatory. Hydrops fetalis can be diagnosed noninvasively *in utero*, and it may be possible to salvage the fetus by intrauterine transfusions (141).

As described earlier, the defect in persistent parvovirus infection is humoral. Commercial immunoglobulin preparations contain anti-B19 parvovirus IgG (70). Anemia due to persistent infection responds to infusions of commercial immunoglobulin (64), and this treatment is recommended for immunodeficient anemic patients with evidence of B19 DNA in the blood. Fifth disease symptoms may result from formation of immune complexes between circulating virus and the administered immunoglobulin.

PREVENTION

Viremia accompanies transient aplastic crisis, and patients in crisis as well as persistently infected patients should be considered infectious, and, if hospitalized, separated from susceptible persons likely to suffer complications of parvovirus infection: patients who are immunosuppressed or who have underlying hemolysis, and pregnant staff. Susceptibility can be predicted by the presence or absence of IgG antibody to virus in serum. The risk of contagion in typical fifth disease in the community likely is highest during the early phases of infection, when symptoms are least specific and the disease is most difficult to diagnose; the viremic patient can also be entirely asymptomatic, making control of spread of infection problematic. There is little rationale for excluding children with fifth disease exanthem from school (2).

Animal parvovirus infections can be prevented by active immunization (40,41). Capsid proteins expressed in animal cells (31) or in a baculovirus system (143) self-assemble into empty capsids. These capsids are immunogenic in animals (144), especially if enriched for VP1, the minor capsid protein that contains most of the linear neutralizing epitopes (145). Such recombinant capsids have been administered safely to normal volunteers, in whom they elicited production of high titers of neutralizing antibodies (146,147).

REFERENCES

1. Young NS. Parvoviruses. In: Fields BM, Knipe DM, Howley PM, eds. *Fields virology*, 3rd ed. Philadelphia: Lippincott-Raven, 1996:2199–2220.
2. Centers for Disease Control and Prevention. Risks associated with human parvovirus B19 infection. *MMWR* 1989;38:81.
3. Anderson LJ. Role of parvovirus B19 in human disease. *Pediatr Infect Dis J* 1987;6:711.
4. Young NS. Hematologic and hematopoietic consequences of B19 parvovirus infection. *Semin Hematol* 1988;25:159.
5. Cossart YE, Field AM, Cant B, et al. Parvovirus-like particles in human sera. *Lancet* 1975;1:72.
6. Cohen BJ, Mortimer PP, Pereira MS. Diagnostic assays with monoclonal antibodies for the human serum parvovirus-like virus (SPLV). *J Hyg* 1983;91:113.
7. Anderson LJ, Tsou C, Parker RA, et al. Detection of antibodies and antigens of human parvovirus B19 by enzyme-linked immunoabsorbent assays. *J Clin Microbiol* 1986;24:533.
8. Cohen BJ, Buckley MM. The prevalence of antibody to human parvovirus B19 in England and Wales. *J Med Microbiol* 1988;25:151.
9. Pattison JR, Jones SE, Hodgson J, et al. Parvovirus infections and hypoplastic crisis in sick-cell anaemia [Letter]. *Lancet* 1981;1:664.
10. Serjeant GR, Topley JM, Mason K, et al. Outbreak of aplastic crises in sickle cell anaemia associated with parvovirus-like agent. *Lancet* 1981;2:595.
11. Anderson MJ, Lewis E Kidd IM, et al. An outbreak of erythema infectiosum associated with human parvovirus infection. *J Hyg* 1984;93:85.
12. Anderson LJ, Hurwitz ES. Human parvovirus B19 and pregnancy. *Clin Perinatol* 1988;15:273.
13. Frickhofen N, Young NS. Persistent human parvovirus infection. *Microb Pathogen* 1989;7:319.
14. Tattersall P, Cotmore SF. The nature of parvoviruses. In: Pattison JR, ed. *Parvoviruses and human diseases*. Boca Raton, FL: CRC Press, 1988:5–41.
15. Cotmore S, Tattersall P. The autonomously replicating parvoviruses of vertebrates. *Adv Virus Res* 1987;33:91.
16. Blacklow NR. Adeno-associated viruses of humans. In: Pattison JR, ed. *Parvoviruses and human diseases*. Boca Raton, FL: CRC Press, 1988:165–174.
17. Berns KI, Bohenzky RA. Adeno-associated viruses: an update. *Adv Virus Res* 1987;32:243.
18. Cukor G, Blacklow NR, Hoggan MD, et al. Biology of adenoassociated virus. In: Berns KI, ed. *The parvoviruses*. New York: Plenum, 1984:33–66.
19. Pringle CR. Virus taxonomy update. Taxonomic decisions ratified at the plenary meeting of the ICTV at the 9th International Congress of Virology held in Glasgow on the 10th of August 1993. *Arch Virol* 1993;133:491.
20. Summers J, Jones SE, Anderson MJ. Characterization of the genome of the agent of erythrocyte aplasia permits its classification as a human parvovirus. *J Gen Virol* 1983;64:2527.
21. Clewley JP. Biochemical characterization of a human parvovirus. *J Gen Virol* 1984;65:241.
22. Nguyen QT, Sifer C, Schneider V, et al. Novel human erythrovirus associated with transient aplastic anemia. *J Clin Microbiol* 1999;37:2483–2487.
23. Nguyen QT, Wong S, Heegaard ED, Brown KE. Identification and characterization of a second novel human erythrovirus variant, A6. *Virology* 2002;301:374–380.
24. Chorba TL, Coccia P, Holman RC, et al. The role of parvovirus B19 in aplastic crisis and erythema infectiosum (fifth disease). *J Infect Dis* 1986;154:383.
25. Anderson MJ, Higgins PG, Davis LIZ, et al. Experimental parvoviral infection in humans. *J Infect Dis* 1985;152:257.
26. O'Sullivan MG, Anderson DC, Fikes JD, et al. Identification of a novel simian parvovirus in cynomolgus monkeys with severe anemia: a paradigm of human B19 parvovirus infection. *J Clin Invest* 1993;93:1571.
27. Cotmore SF, Tattersall P. Characterization and molecular cloning of a human parvovirus genome. *Science* 1984;226:1161.
28. Shade RO, Blundell MC, Cotmore SF, et al. Nucleotide sequence and genome organization of human parvovirus B19 isolated from the serum of a child during aplastic crisis. *J Virol* 1986;58:921.
29. Ozawa K, Ayub J, Hao Y-S, et al. Novel transcription map for the B19 (human) pathogenic parvovirus. *J Virol* 1987;61:2395.
30. Cotmore SF, McKie VC, Anderson LJ, et al. Identification of the major structural and nonstructural proteins encoded by human parvovirus B19 and mapping of their genes by procaryotic expression of isolated genomic fragments. *J Virol* 1986;60:548.
31. Ozawa K, Young NS. Characterization of capsid and noncapsid proteins of B19 parvovirus propagated in human erythroid bone marrow cell cultures. *J Virol* 1987;61:2627.
32. Kajigaya S, Shimada T, Fujita S, et al. A genetically engineered cell line that produces empty capsids of B19 (human) parvovirus. *Proc Natl Acad Sci U S A* 1989;86:7601.
33. Ozawa K, Ayub J, Kajigaya S, et al. The gene encoding the nonstructural protein of B19 (human) parvovirus may be lethal in transfected cells. *J Virol* 1988;62:2884.
34. Sol N, LeJunger J, Vassias I, et al. Possible interactions between the NS-1 protein and tumor necrosis factor alpha pathways in erythroid cell apoptosis induced by human parvorius B19. *J Virol* 1999;73:8762–8770.
35. Luo W, Astell CR. A novel protein encoded by small RNAs of parvovirus B19. *Virology* 1993;195:448.
36. Shimomura S, Wong S, Komatsu N, et al. Early and late gene expression in UT-7 cells infected with B19 parvovirus. *Virology* 1993;194:149.
37. Carter BJ, Laughlin CA. Adeno-associated virus defectiveness and the nature of the adenovirus helper function. In: Berns KI, ed. *The parvoviruses*. New York: Plenum, 1984:67–128.
38. Spalholz BA, Tattersall P. Interaction of minute virus of mice with differentiated cells: strain-dependent target cell specificity is mediated by intracellular factors. *J Virol* 1983;46:937.
39. Antonietti JP, Sahli R, Beard P, et al. Characterization of the cell type-specific determinant in the genome of minute virus of mice. *J Virol* 1988;62:552.
40. Siegl G. Biology of pathogenicity of autonomous parvoviruses. In: Berns KI, ed. *The parvoviruses*. New York: Plenum, 1984:297–362.

41. Siegl G. Patterns of parvovirus disease in animals. In: Pattison JR, ed. *Parvoviruses and human diseases*. Boca Raton, FL: CRC Press, 1988:43–67.

42. Johnson RH, Collings DF. Transplacental infection of piglets with a porcine parvovirus. *Res Vet Sci* 1971;12:570.

43. Siegl G. Canine parvovirus: origin and significance of a "new" pathogen. In: Berns KI, ed. *The parvoviruses*. New York: Plenum, 1984:363–388.

44. Kurtzman GJ, Platanias L, Lustig L, et al. Feline parvovirus propagates in cat bone marrow cultures and inhibits hematopoietic colony formation. *Blood* 1989;74:71.

45. Ozawa K, Kurtzman G, Young N. Replication of the B19 parvovirus in human bone marrow cell cultures. *Science* 1986;233:883.

46. Hauswirth WW. Autonomous parvovirus DNA structure and replication. In: Berns KI, ed. *The parvoviruses*. New York: Plenum, 1984:129–152.

47. Berns KI, Hauswirth WW. Adeno-associated virus DNA structure and replication. In: Berns KI, ed. *The parvoviruses*. New York: Plenum, 1984:1–31.

48. Kurtzman GJ, Gascon P, Caras M, et al. B19 Parvovirus replicates in circulating cells of acutely infected patients. *Blood* 1988;71:1448.

49. Kurtzman GJ, Ozawa K, Hanson GR, et al. Chronic bone marrow failure due to persistent B19 parvovirus infection. *N Engl J Med* 1987;317:287.

50. Kurtzman GJ, Cohen B, Meyers P, et al. Persistent B19 parvovirus infection as a cause of severe chronic anaemia in children with acute lymphocytic leukaemia. *Lancet* 1988;2:1159.

51. Yaegashi N, Shiraishi H, Takeshita T, et al. Propagation of human parvovirus B19 in primary culture of erythroid lineage cells derived from fetal liver. *J Virol* 1989;63:2422.

52. Schwarz TF, Serke S, Hottentrager B, et al. Replication of parvovirus B19 in hematopoietic progenitor cells generated *in vitro* from normal human peripheral blood. *J Gen Virol* 1992;66:1273.

53. Shimomura S, Komatsu N, Frickhofen N, et al. First continuous propagation of B19 parvovirus in a cell line. *Blood* 1992;79:18.

54. Munshi NC, Zhou S, Woody MJ, et al. Successful replication of parvovirus B19 in the human megakaryocytic cell line MB-02. *J Virol* 1993;67:562.

55. Mortimer PP, Humphries RK, Moore JG, et al. A human parvovirus-like virus inhibits hematopoietic colony formation *in vitro*. *Nature* 1983;302:426.

56. Takahashi T, Ozawa K, Takahashi K, et al. Susceptibility of human erythropoietic cells to B19 parvovirus *in vitro* increases with differentiation. *Blood* 1990;75:603.

57. Srivastava A, Lu L. Replication of B19 parvovirus in highly enriched hematopoietic progenitor cells from normal human bone marrow. *J Virol* 1988;62:3059.

58. Ozawa K, Kurtzman G, Young NS. Productive infection by B19 parvovirus of human erythroid bone marrow cells *in vitro*. *Blood* 1987;70:384.

59. Young NS, Harrison M, Moore JG, et al. Direct demonstration of the human parvovirus in erythroid progenitor cells infected *in vitro*. *J Clin Invest* 1984;74:2024.

60. Brown KE, Anderson SM, Young NS. Erythrocyte P antigen: cellular receptor for B19 parvovirus. *Science* 1993;262:114.

61. Brown KE, Hibbs JR, Gallinella G, et al. Resistance to parvovirus B19 due to lack of virus receptor (erythrocyte P antigen). *N Engl J Med* 1994;330:1192.

62. Marcus DM, Kundu SK, Suzuki A. The P blood group system: recent progress in immunochemistry and genetics. *Semin Hematol* 1981;18:63.

63. Liu J, Green S, Shimada T, et al. A block in full-length transcript maturation in cells nonpermissive for B19 parvovirus. *J Virol* 1992;66:4686.

64. Kurtzman GJ, Frickhofen N, Kimball J, et al. Pure red cell aplasia of ten years' duration due to B19 parvovirus infection and its cure with immunoglobulin therapy. *N Engl J Med* 1989;321:519.

65. Kilham L, Margolis G. Viral etiology of spontaneous ataxia of cats. *Am J Pathol* 1966;48:991.

66. Cheung AKM, Hoggan MD, Hauswirth WW, et al. Integration of the adeno-associated virus genome into cellular DNA in latently infected human Detroit 6 cells. *J Virol* 1980;33:739.

67. Kotin RM, Siniscalco M, Samulski RJ, et al. Site-specific interaction by adeno-associated virus. *Proc Natl Acad Sci U S A* 1990;87:2211.

68. Porter DD. Aleutian disease: a persistent parvovirus infection of mink with maximal but ineffective host humoral immune response. *Prog Med Virol* 1986;33:42.

69. Csiza CK, Scott FW, de Lahunta A, et al. Immune carrier state of feline panleukopenia virus-infected cats. *Am J Vet Sci* 1971;32:419.

70. Saarinen UM, Chorba TL, Tattersall P, et al. Human parvovirus B19–induced epidemic red cell aplasia in patients with hereditary hemolytic anemia. *Blood* 1986;67:1411.

71. Kurtzman GJ, Blaese M, Oseas R, et al. Immune response to B19 parvovirus infection. *J Clin Invest* 1989;84:1114.

72. Plummer FA, Hammond GW, Forward K, et al. An erythema infectiosum–like illness caused by human parvovirus infection. *N Engl J Med* 1985;313:74.

73. Okabe N, Kobayashi S, Tatsuzawa O, et al. Detection of antibodies to human parvovirus in erythema infectiosum (fifth disease). *Arch Dis Child* 1984;59:1016.

74. Nunoue T, Koike T, Koike R, et al. Infection with human parvovirus (B19), aplasia of the bone marrow and a rash in hereditary spherocytosis. *J Infect* 1987;14:67.

75. Evans JPM, Rossiter MA, Kumaran TO, et al. Human parvovirus aplasia: case due to cross infection in a ward. *BMJ* 1984;288:681.

76. Pell LM, Naides SJ, Stollmon P, et al. Human parvovirus B19 infection among hospital staff members after contact with infected patients. *N Engl J Med* 1989;321:485.

77. Seng C, Watkins P, Morse D, et al. Parvovirus B19 outbreak on an adult ward. *Epidemiol Infect* 1994;113:345.

78. Cohen BJ, Courouce AM, Schwartz TF, et al. Laboratory infection with parvovirus B19 [Letter]. *J Clin Pathol* 1988;41:1027.

79. Mortimer PP, Luban NLC, Kelleher JF, et al. Transmission of serum parvovirus-like by clotting factor concentrates. *Lancet* 1983;2:482.

80. Bartolomei Corsi O, Assi A, et al. Human parvovirus infection in haemophiliacs first infused with treated clotting factor concentrates. *J Med Virol* 1988;25:165.

81. Willkommen H, Schmid I, Lower J. Safety issues for plasma derivatives and benefit from NAT testing. *Biologicals* 1999;27(4):325–331.

82. Heegaard EK, Petersen BL. Parvovirus B19 transmitted by bone marrow. *Br J Haematol* 2000;111:659–661.

83. Ager EA, Chin TKY, Poland JP. Epidemic erythema infectiosum. *N Engl J Med* 1966;275:1326.

84. Anderson MJ. Rash illness due to B19 virus. In: Pattison JR, ed. *Parvoviruses and human diseases*. Boca Raton, FL: CRC Press, 1988.

85. Balfour HH Jr. Erythema infectiosum (fifth disease): clinical review and description of 91 cases seen in an epidemic. *Clin Pediatr* 1969;8:721.

86. Brass C, Elliott L, Stevens DA. Academy rash. A probable epidemic of erythema infectiosum ("fifth disease"). *JAMA* 1982;248:568.

87. Cramp HE, Armstrong BDJ. Erythema infectiosum: an outbreak of "slapped cheek" disease in north Devon. *BMJ* 1976;1:885.

88. Lauer BA, MacCormack JN, Wilfert C. Erythema infectiosum. An elementary school outbreak. *Am J Dis Child* 1976;130:252.

89. Naides SJ, Piette W, Veach LA, et al. Human parvovirus B19-induced vesiculopustular skin eruption. *Am J Med* 1988;84:968.

90. Moore TL. Parvovirus-associated arthritis [Review]. *Curr Opin Rheumatol* 2000;12(4):289–294.

91. Reid DM, Reid TMS, Brown T, et al. Human parvovirus-associated arthropathy. *Lancet* 1985;1:419.

92. White DG, Woolf AD, Mortimer PP, et al. Human parvovirus arthropathy. *Lancet* 1984;1:422.

93. Cohen BJ, Buckley MM, Clewley JP, et al. Human parvovirus infection in early rheumatoid and inflammatory arthritis. *Ann Rheum Dis* 1986;45:832.

94. Stierle G, Brown KA, Rainsford SG, et al. Parvovirus associated antigen in the synovial membrane of patients with rheumatoid arthritis. *Ann Rheum Dis* 1987;46:21.

95. Mimori A, Misaki Y, Hachiya T, et al. Prevalence of antihuman parvovirus B19 IgG antibodies in patients with refractory rheumatoid arthritis and polyarticular juvenile rheumatoid arthritis. *Rheumatol Int* 1994;14:87.

96. Nikkari S, Luukkainen R, Mottonen T, et al. Does parvovirus B19 have a role in rheumatoid arthritis? *Ann Rheum Dis* 1994;53:106.

97. Leventhal LJ, Naides SJ, Freundlich B. Fibromyalgia and parvovirus infection. *Arthritis Rheum* 1991;34:1319.

98. Cope AP, Jones A, Brozovic M, et al. Possible induction of systemic lupus erythematosus by human parvovirus. *Ann Rheum Dis* 1992;51:803.

99. Kalish RA, Knopf AN, Gary GW, et al. Lupus-like presentation of human parvovirus B19 infection. *J Rheumatol* 1992;19:169.

100. Finkel TH, Török TJ, Ferguson PJ, et al. Chronic parvovirus B19 infection and systemic necrotising vasculitis: opportunistic infection or aetiological agent? *Lancet* 1994;343:1255.

101. Nigro G, Zerbini M, Krzysztofiak A, et al. Active or recent parvovirus B19 infection in children with Kawasaki disease. *Lancet* 1994;343:1260.

102. Sokal EM, Melchior M, Cornu C, et al. Acute parvovirus B19 infection associated with fulminant hepatitis of favourable prognosis in young children. *Lancet* 1998;352(9142):1739–1741.

103. Wong S, Young NS, Brown KE. Prevalence of parvovirus B19 in liver tissue: no association with fulminant hepatitis or hepatitis-associated aplastic anemia. *J Infect Dis* 2003;187:1581–1586.

104. Notari EP 4th, Orton SL, Cable RG, et al. Seroprevalence of known and putative hepatitis markers in United States blood donors with ALT levels at least 120 IU per L. *Transfusion* 2001;41(6):751–755.

105. Anderson MJ, Davis LIZ, Hodgson J, et al. Occurrence of infection with a parvovirus-like agent in children with sickle cell anaemia during a two-year period. *J Clin Pathol* 1982;35:744.

106. Conrad ME, Studdard H, Anderson LJ. Case report: aplastic crisis in sickle cell disorders: bone marrow necrosis and human parvovirus infection. *Am J Med Sci* 1988;295:212.

107. Potter CG, Potter AC, Hatton CSR, et al. Variation of erythroid and myeloid precursors in the marrow and peripheral blood of volunteer subjects infected with human parvovirus (B19). *J Clin Invest* 1987;79:1486.

108. Lefrere JJ, Courouce A-M, Girot R, et al. Six cases of hereditary spherocytosis revealed by human parvovirus infection. *Br J Haematol* 1986;62:653.

109. McLellan NJ, Rutter N. Hereditary spherocytosis in sisters unmasked by parvovirus infection. *Postgrad Med J* 1987;63:49.

110. Bertrand Y, Lefrere JJ, Leverger G, et al. Autoimmune hemolytic anaemia revealed by human parvovirus linked erythroblastopenia. *Lancet* 1985;2:382.

111. Frickhofen N, Raghavachar A, Heit W, et al. Human parvovirus infection [Letter]. *N Engl J Med* 1986;314:646.

112. Saunders PWG, Reid MM, Cohen BJ. Human parvovirus induced cytopenias: a report of five cases [Letter]. *Br J Haematol* 1986;63:407.

113. Hanada T, Koike K, Takaya T, et al. Human parvovirus B19–induced transient pancytopenia in a child with hereditary spherocytosis. *Br J Haematol* 1988;70:113.

114. Lefrere JJ, Got D. Peripheral thrombocytopenia in human parvovirus infection [Letter]. *J Clin Pathol* 1987;40:469.
115. Hamon MD, Newland AC, Anderson MJ. Severe aplastic anemia after parvovirus infection in the absence of underlying hemolytic anemia [Letter]. *J Clin Pathol* 1988;41:1242.
116. Shirono K, Tsuda H. Parvovirus B19–associated haemophagocytic syndrome in healthy adults. *Br J Haematol* 1995;89:923.
117. Young NS, Mortimer PP, Moore JG, et al. Characterization of a virus that causes transient aplastic crisis. *J Clin Invest* 1984;73:224.
118. Van Horn DK, Mortimer PP, Young N, et al. Human parvovirus associated red cell aplasia in the absence of underlying hemolytic anemia. *Am J Pediatr Hematol Oncol* 1986;8:235.
119. Smith MA, Shah NR, Lobel JS, et al. Severe anemia caused by human parvovirus in a leukemia patient on maintenance chemotherapy. *Clin Pediatr* 1988;27:383.
120. Frickhofen N, Chen ZJ, Young NS, et al. Parvovirus B19 as a cause of acquired chronic pure red cell aplasia. *Br J Haematol* 1994;87:818.
121. Frickhofen N, Abkowitz JL, Safford M, et al. Persistent B19 parvovirus infection in patients infected with human immunodeficiency virus-1: a treatable cause of anemia in AIDS. *Ann Intern Med* 1990;113:926.
122. Rodis JF, Hovick TJ Jr, Quinn DL, et al. Human parvovirus infection in pregnancy. *Obstet Gynecol* 1988;72:733.
123. Brown T, Anand A, Ritchie LD, et al. Intrauterine parvovirus infection associated with hydrops fetalis. *Lancet* 1984;2:1033.
124. Knott PD, Welply GAC, Anderson MJ. Serologically proved intrauterine infection with parvovirus. *BMJ* 1984;289:1660.
125. Anand A, Gray ES, Brown T, et al. Human parvovirus infection in pregnancy and hydrops fetalis. *N Engl J Med* 1987;316:183.
126. Franciosi RA, Tattersall P. Fetal infection with human parvovirus B19. *Hum Pathol* 1988;19:489.
127. Maeda H, Shimokawa H, Satoh S, et al. Nonimmunologic hydrops fetalis resulting from intrauterine human parvovirus B19 infection: report of two cases. *Obstet Gynecol* 1988;72:482.
128. Clewley JP, Cohen BJ, Field AM. Detection of parvovirus B19 DNA, antigen, and particles in the human fetus. *J Med Virol* 1987;23:367.
129. Porter HJ, Khong TY, Evans MF, et al. Parvovirus as a cause of hydrops fetalis: detection by *in situ* DNA hybridization. *J Clin Pathol* 1988;41:381.
130. Knisely AS, O'Shea PA, McMillan P, et al. Electron microscopic identification of parvovirus virions in erythroid-line cells in fatal hydrops fetalis. *Pediatr Pathol* 1988;8:163.
131. Caul EO, Usher MJ, Burton PA. Intrauterine infection with human parvovirus B19: a light and electron microscopy study. *J Med Virol* 1988;24:55.
132. Kinney JS, Anderson LJ, Farrar J, et al. Risk of adverse outcomes of pregnancy after human parvovirus B19 infection. *J Infect Dis* 1988;157:663.
133. Miller E, Fairley CK, Cohen BJ, et al. Immediate and long term outcome of human parvovirus B19 infection in pregnancy. *Br J Obstet Gynaecol* 1998;105:174–178.
134. Brown KE, Green SW, Antunez de Mayolo J, et al. Congenital anaemia following transplacental B19 parvovirus infection. *Lancet* 1994;343:895.
135. Weiland HT, Vermey-Keers C, Salimans MM, et al. Parvovirus B19 associated with fetal abnormality [Letter]. *Lancet* 1987;1:682.
136. Porter HJ, Quantrill AM, Fleming KA: B19 Parvovirus infection of myocardial cells [Letter]. *Lancet* 1988;1:535.
137. Cohen BJ. Laboratory tests for the diagnosis of infection with B19 virus. In: Pattison JR, ed. *Parvoviruses and human diseases.* Boca Raton, FL: CRC Press, 1988:69–83.
138. Anderson MJ, Jones SE, Minson AC. Diagnosis of human parvovirus infection by dot-blot analysis using cloned viral DNA. *J Med Virol* 1985;15:163.
139. Clewley JP. Detection of human parvovirus using a molecularly cloned probe. *J Med Virol* 1985;15:173.
140. Cunningham DA, Pattison JR, Craig RK. Detection of parvovirus DNA in human serum using biotinylated RNA hybridisation probes. *J Virol Methods* 1988;19:279.
141. Schwarz TF, Roggendorf M, Hottentrager B, et al. Human parvovirus B19 infection in pregnancy [Letter]. *Lancet* 1988;2:566.
142. Clewley JP. Polymerase chain reaction assay of parvovirus B19 DNA in clinical specimens. *J Clin Microbiol* 1989;27:2647.
143. Kajigaya S, Fujii H, Field A, et al. Self-assembled parvovirus capsids, produced in a baculovirus system, are antigenically and immunogenically similar to virions. *Proc Natl Acad Sci U S A* 1991;88:4646.
144. Bansal GP, Hatfield JA, Dunn FE, et al. Candidate recombinant vaccine for human B19 parvovirus. *J Infect Dis* 1993;167:1034.
145. Saikawa T, Momoeda M, Anderson S, et al. Neutralizing linear epitopes of B19 parvovirus cluster in the VP1 unique and VP1-VP2 junction region. *J Virol* 1993;67:3004.
146. Bostic JR, Brown KE, Young NS, et al. Quantitative analysis of neutralizing immune responses to human parvovirus B19 using a novel reverse transcriptase-polymerase chain reaction–based assay. *J Infect Dis* 1999;179:19–26.
147. Ballon WR, Reed JL, Noble W, et al. Safety and immunogenicity of a recombinant parvovirus B19 vaccine formulated with MF59C.1. *J Infect Dis* 2003;187:675–678.

CHAPTER 237
Human Papillomaviruses

Keerti V. Shah

HISTORY

The viral cause of human skin warts was established early in the twentieth century by experimental transmission of disease to susceptible persons with cell-free filtrate of wart extract. In the 1930s, the studies of the cottontail rabbit papillomavirus provided the first example of a mammalian tumor virus, but further progress in the characterization of papillomaviruses was hampered because they could not be propagated in tissue culture or transmitted to laboratory animals. This difficulty was bypassed to some extent by the advent of molecular cloning in the 1970s, when viral genomes in affected tissues were cloned directly in plasmid vectors. More than 100 individually distinct human papillomaviruses (HPVs) have been described to date.

HPVs infect the squamous epithelia of the skin and the mucous membranes. Genital tract infections with HPVs are highly prevalent; infections with high-risk HPVs (e.g., HPV-16 and HPV-18) contribute to the occurrence of lower genital tract cancers and are linked etiologically to cancer of the cervix. Low-risk HPV types 6 and 11 are responsible for genital warts, and intrapartum transmission of these HPVs from an infected mother to the offspring sometimes results in the production of respiratory papilloma in the exposed children. Cutaneous HPVs largely produce benign, self-limited warts; however, progression of warty lesions to squamous cell carcinomas may occur in the rare dermatologic disorder epidermodysplasia verruciformis. Cutaneous HPV sequences are frequently detected in normal skin.

CHARACTERISTICS OF THE PATHOGEN

Papillomaviruses are small, nonenveloped viruses with icosahedral symmetry, 72 capsomers, double-stranded circular DNA genome, and nucleus as the site of viral multiplication. The viral genome is divided into an early region (~4.5 kb), which is necessary for transformation; a late region (~2.5 kb), which codes for the capsid proteins; and a regulatory region (~1 kb), which contains the origin of replication and many of the control elements for transformation and replication (Fig. 237.1). There are eight ORFs (E1 to E8) in the early region and two in the late region (ORFs L1 and L2), all of which are located on the same strand (1,2). Their functions are indicated in Table 237.1.

Papillomaviruses are classified on the basis of species of origin (e.g., human, bovine, rabbit) and the extent of genetic relatedness with other papillomaviruses from the same species. New types are defined on the basis of sequence variation from the known types in specific regions of the genome. The papillomavirus virion contains a major capsid protein of 57 kd and a minor capsid protein of 70 kd. Species-specific and genus-specific determinants are located on the major capsid protein.

Papillomaviruses have not yet been propagated in conventional tissue culture to yield virus particles, probably because full cellular differentiation required for virus production is not achieved in cultured cells. Infectious virus is produced when

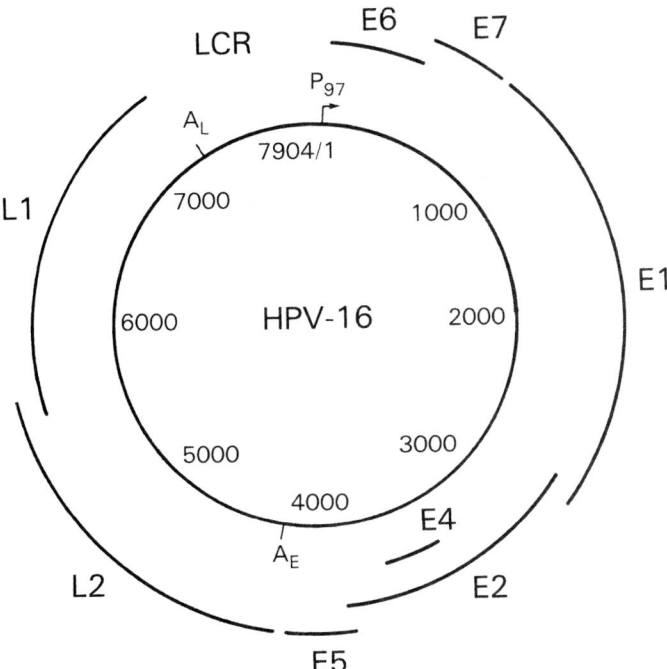

Figure 237.1. Genomic map of human papillomavirus (HPV)-16 determined from the DNA sequence. The genome is a double-stranded circular DNA molecule of 7,904 base pairs. Transcription occurs in a clockwise manner; the only transcriptional promoter mapped yet for HPV-16 is designated P97. The ORFs deduced from the DNA sequence are designated E1 to E7, L1, and L2 and are indicated outside the circular genome. AE and AL represent the early and late polyadenylation sites. The viral long control region (*LCR*) contains transcriptional and replication regulatory elements. (From Shah KV, Howley PM. Papillomaviruses. In: Fields BN, Knipe DM, Howley PM, et al., eds. *Virology*. Philadelphia: Lippincott-Raven, 1996:2077–2109, with permission.)

fragments of susceptible tissue are exposed to a condyloma extract that contains HPV-11 and transplanted beneath the renal capsule of athymic nude mice or when HPV-infected keratinocytes are allowed to differentiate fully in the organotypic "raft" system.

Papillomaviruses are highly species specific and display a marked degree of cellular tropism. Mucosal HPVs are rarely detected on the skin (except in the genital area), and cutaneous HPVs are rarely detected at mucosal sites. All HPVs are strictly epitheliotropic, but a subset of animal papillomaviruses induces both dermal and epithelial proliferation to produce fibropapillo-

TABLE 237.1. Functions of Papillomavirus Open Reading Frames

Open reading frame	Function
E1	Plasmid replication
E2	Regulation of transcription; plasmid replication
E3, E8	Not known
E4	Coding for late cytoplasmic protein
E5, E6	Transformation (bovine papillomavirus)
E6, E7	Transformation (human papillomavirus)
L1	Coding for major capsid protein
L2	Coding for minor capsid protein

mas. Warts are thought to be of monoclonal origin, arising from the proliferation of a single infected basal cell. Basal cells are presumably exposed to infectious virus after minor trauma to the epithelium, as would occur during sexual intercourse or after minor skin abrasions. All cells of a wart contain the viral genome, but the expression of viral genes is tightly linked to the state of cellular differentiation. Only the upper layers of the epithelium (which contain the differentiating and keratinizing cells) permit late gene expression and synthesis of viral particles. Virus multiplication is confined to the nucleus. Koilocytosis (cytoplasmic vacuolization) with an abnormal nucleus is a characteristic feature of productive papillomavirus infection.

Papillomaviruses are associated with naturally occurring cancers in humans and other animals (Table 237.2). These cancers share several characteristics. First, only some of the papillomavirus types that infect a species are associated with cancers in that species. In humans this is exemplified by the association of HPV-16 and HPV-18 with genital tract cancers and of HPV-5 and HPV-8 with cancers arising in the warty lesions of patients with epidermodysplasia verruciformis. Second, the time interval between the initial infection and development of invasive cancer may be long. In human genital tract cancers, this period spans several decades. Third, cofactors are required for progression to malignancy—sunlight, x-irradiation, diet, or a genetic defect (Table 237.2). Cofactors have not been identified for all papillomavirus-related cancers. The viral genome in these cancers may be present in an integrated state (as in most human genital tract cancers), or in an extrachromosomal state (as in rabbit carcinomas), or it may be lost altogether with progression (as in bovine papillomavirus type 4–associated alimentary carcinomas of cattle).

Animal papillomaviruses that induce fibropapillomas in nature (e.g., bovine papillomavirus types 1 and 2) readily transform rodent cells in culture. The transformed cells are tumorigenic in syngeneic animals. In contrast, HPVs can transform rodent cells only in cooperation with an activated *ras* oncogene. The transforming activity of HPV types *in vitro* is correlated with their role in naturally occurring cancers. HPV-16 and HPV-18, which are associated with genital tract cancers, display greater transforming activity than HPV-6 and HPV-11, which are seldom found in genital tract cancers. Human keratinocytes transfected with HPV-16 and HPV-18 become immortal and carry the viral genome in an integrated state (3). These cells are not tumorigenic in nude mice. In the collagen raft system, which permits epithelial cell differentiation, HPV-16– and HPV-18–transfected human keratinocytes stratify and show the morphologic features of intraepithelial neoplasia (4). In quantitative assays of keratinocyte transformation by HPV DNAs, both oncogenic and nononcogenic HPVs induce transient cellular proliferation, but only the oncogenic HPVs give rise to immortalized cell lines. The transforming activity of bovine papillomavirus type 1 is localized to the E5 and E6 ORFs, whereas that of HPVs is localized to the E6 and E7 ORFs.

IMMUNE RESPONSE

Clinical observations have shown that conditions in which T-cell response is depressed (e.g., immunosuppressive therapy, organ transplantation, acquired immunodeficiency syndrome) are associated with a high prevalence and exacerbation of warts. Also, regressing flat skin warts show histologic evidence of a cell-mediated immune response. Infection appears to produce a low-titered antibody response to capsid proteins as measured by enzyme-linked immunosorbent assay with

TABLE 237.2. Papillomaviruses and Naturally Occurring Cancers

Species	Cancer	Predominant viral types	State of viral genome in cancers	Cofactors
Humans	Skin carcinomas in EV patients	HPV-5, -8	Extrachromosomal	Sunlight; genetic defect
	Cervical, vulvar, penile carcinomas	HPV-16, -18	Integrated or extrachromosomal	Not known
	Malignant progression of respiratory papillomas	HPV-6, -11	Extrachromosomal	X-irradiation or not known
Cattle	Alimentary tract carcinoma	BPV-4	Absent	Bracken fern
	Eye and skin carcinoma	Not characterized	Not known	Sunlight
Sheep	Skin carcinoma	Not characterized	Not known	Sunlight
Cottontail rabbit	Skin carcinoma	CRPV	Extrachromosomal	Not known

EV, epidermodysplasia verruciformis; HPV, human papillomavirus; BPV, bovine papillomavirus; CRPV, cottontail rabbit papillomavirus.

virus-like particles synthesized in recombinant baculovirus or vaccinia virus systems (5). Antibodies to the transforming proteins E6 and E7 are markers of HPV-associated invasive cervical cancer (6).

EPIDEMIOLOGY AND CLINICAL FEATURES

The HPVs fall naturally into two groups, cutaneous HPVs and mucosal HPVs. The major clinical associations of HPV infections are shown in Table 237.3. About 20 cutaneous HPVs have been recovered, almost exclusively from patients with epidermodysplasia verruciformis. Most of the mucosal HPVs reside in the genital tract, but two HPVs, HPV-13 and HPV-32, appear to infect the oral cavity exclusively. Genital tract

HPVs also infect other mucosal sites, such as the respiratory tract, the oral cavity, and the conjunctiva. Infection is acquired through minor skin abrasions (cutaneous warts), by sexual intercourse (genital warts), or by transmission at birth from the genital tract of an infected mother to the offspring (respiratory papillomas).

Cutaneous Human Papillomavirus Infections

Skin warts are acquired by direct contact with an infected person or by contact with contaminated objects. Recreational activities (e.g., swimming), in which wet, bare skin is exposed in communally used facilities, increases the risk for acquiring plantar warts. Meat handlers, butchers, and abattoir personnel have a high prevalence of warts on their hands. These warts are caused

TABLE 237.3. Clinical Associations of Human Papillomavirus Types

Clinical condition	Human papillomavirus type
Skin	
Plantar warts	1
Common warts	2, 4
Mosaic warts (superficial spreading wart)	2
Flat warts	3, 10, 28, 41
Macular plaques of epidermodysplasia verruciformis	5, 8, 9, 12, 14, 15, 17, 19, 20, 21, 22, 23, 24, 25, 36, 47, 50
Butchers' warts	7
Mucosa	
Exophytic condyloma (any site)	6, 11
Flat condyloma (especially cervix)	6, 11, 16, 18, 31, others
Bowenoid papulosis	16
Giant condyloma (Buschke-Löwenstein tumor)	6, 11
Cervical cancer	
Strong association	16, 18
Moderate association	31, 33, 35, 45, 51, 52, 56
Weak association or none	6, 11, 42, 43, 44
Vulvar cancer	16
Oropharyngeal cancer	16
Respiratory papillomas	6, 11
Conjunctival papillomas	6, 11
Oral cavity	
Focal epithelial hyperplasia	13, 32
Mucosal warty lesions	6, 11, 16
Warts on lips	2

Human papillomavirus types for which information is limited are not listed.

by HPV infections and not by transmission of animal papillomaviruses. Skin warts are most common in older children and young adults and are rare before age 5 years. A majority of warts regress spontaneously within 2 years. There is a strong correlation between site and morphology of the wart and infecting HPV type (Table 237.3).

Epidermodysplasia verruciformis is a rare dermatologic disorder of worldwide distribution in which a wart virus infection does not resolve (7). The disease has a genetic basis; it is often familial, and patients frequently give a history of parental consanguinity. The lesions are either flat warts or reddish-brown macular plaques. In about a third of the cases, multiple foci of malignant transformation arise in the reddish brown plaques, most often in lesions that are exposed to sunlight and are caused by HPV-5 and HPV-8. The viral genome is present as multiple copies of unintegrated DNA.

The role of HPV infections in nonmelanoma skin cancers is an area of intense investigation (8,9). Genomic sequences of a heterogeneous group of HPVs have been found in normal skin, and in nonmelanoma skin cancers in immunocompetent and immunodeficient patients. The prevalence of HPV sequences is higher in cancer tissues than in normal skin, and highest in cancers in immunodeficient individuals.

Mucosal Human Papillomavirus Infections

Genital tract infections with HPVs are highly prevalent. Between 10% and 20% of men and women in the age group 15 to 49 years (12–24 million persons) in the United States may have prevalent HPV infection. A large majority of these infections are clinically inapparent and show no cytologic or colposcopic abnormalities. The genital tract is frequently infected at multiple sites. Apparently normal epithelium adjacent to clinical lesions contains the viral genome.

The most clearly recognized clinical manifestations of HPV infection are genital warts (condylomata). The incidence of genital warts has increased more than fivefold between 1966 and 1986 (10). Exophytic condylomata are largely the result of infections with HPV-6 and HPV-11.

Relationship to Cancers in the Genital Tract

SQUAMOUS CELL CARCINOMA OF THE CERVIX
Worldwide, about one-half million cases of cancer of the cervix are diagnosed annually. Cervical cancer accounts for about one fourth of all cancers in women in the developing world and for about 7% of cancers in women in the industrialized nations. The lifetime risk for developing cancer of the cervix varies as much as 10-fold in different geographic areas of the world. Squamous cell carcinoma of the cervix (~85% of all cervical cancers) is associated with multiple sexual partners and has the characteristics of a sexually transmitted disease. Invasive cancer is preceded by a progressive series of abnormalities of the cervical epithelium that are classified as cervical intraepithelial neoplasia grades 1, 2, or 3. The interval between mild cervical abnormalities and invasive cancer may be several decades.

The evidence linking HPV infections and cervical cancer has been reviewed extensively (11) and is summarized in Table 237.4. The epidemiologic evidence is strongly reinforced by laboratory studies, and together they make a compelling case for HPV as the cause of invasive cervical cancer.

HPV infections by themselves are not sufficient to lead to cancer of the cervix. It is thought that HPVs increase the life span of the affected cells and produce genetic instability that other cellular events (e.g., oncogene activation, inactivation of tumor suppressors, mutations) eventually lead to malignancy (1,2). Epidemiologic studies have suggested that smoking and oral contraceptive use may be independent risk factors for cervical cancer.

OTHER CANCERS
Adenocarcinoma of the cervix, which constitutes about 10% to 15% of cervical cancers, is also associated with HPVs, especially

---

TABLE 237.4. Evidence Linking Human Papillomavirus (HPV) Infections with Cervical Cancer

HPV infections have the same risk factors as cervical cancer

HPV infections precede the precursor lesions of cervical cancer

HPVs are recovered from a large proportion of invasive cervical cancers as well as from CIN-1, -2, and -3, the precursor lesions of cancer (11, 22).

HPV-16 and HPV-18 (and some other HPV types) are preferentially associated with cancers. Between 50% and 60% of invasive cancers yield HPV-16 or HPV-18. Many other types (e.g., HPV-6 and HPV-11) are frequently found in mild cervical lesions and in inapparent infections but are virtually absent from invasive cancer. The viral genome in HPV-associated cancers is present in the cancer cells themselves in the primary tumor (as shown by hybridization studies *in situ*) as well as in metastatic tumors. The viruses found in cancer tissues are the ones that have transforming activity in studies *in vitro*.

The viral genome not only is present but also is transcriptionally active. ORFs E6 and E7 are consistently expressed in cancer tissues. Studies *in vitro* show that these ORFs code for the transforming proteins of HPVs.

In many invasive cancers, the viral genome is integrated into the cellular chromosomes. The integration appears to facilitate expression of E6 and E7. The circular viral genome breaks most often in the E1/E2 region for integration. This leaves intact the E6 and E7 ORFs and also removes the repressive effect, which E2 probably exercises on the promoter for E6 and E7.

Most of the cell lines derived from invasive cervical cancers contain HPV-16 or HPV-18. The viral genome is integrated in most HPV-associated cell lines and expresses E6 and E7 ORFs.

The viral transforming proteins E6 and E7 dysregulate the cell cycle by complexing, respectively, with cellular tumor suppressor proteins p53 and Rb. This leads to genetic instability and additional chromosmal changes, which underlie the development of invasive cancer.

CIN, Cervical intraepithelial neoplasia; ORFs, open reading frames.

HPV-18. Many cancers of the penis, the vulva, the vagina, the anus, and the perineum are also HPV associated, but these cancers are much less common than cancer of the cervix. The lower incidence of malignancy at extracervical sites is ascribed to the absence at these sites of an area as susceptible to oncogenic transformation as the transformation zone at the squamocolumnar junction of the cervix.

Cancers of the oropharynx, especially tonsillar cancer, appear to be linked etiologically to HPV infections (12).

Human Papillomaviruses in the Respiratory Tract, Oral Cavity, and Conjunctiva

Adult-onset as well as juvenile-onset respiratory papillomas are caused by genital tract HPV-6 and HPV-11. It is likely that intrapartum transmission of HPV from infected mother to offspring is responsible for most of the cases of juvenile-onset respiratory papillomas. It has been estimated that only one of many children born to infected mothers develops respiratory papillomas (13). The manner in which adult-onset respiratory HPV infection is acquired is not known. Most of the conjunctival papillomas are also caused by HPV-6 or HPV-11.

The oral cavity mucosa may be infected with HPVs that have a reservoir in the oral cavity (HPV-13 and HPV-32) and by genital tract HPVs (HPV-6, -11, and -16). HPV-13 and HPV-32 are associated with a clinical condition called focal epithelial hyperplasia, which is common in indigenous populations of Central and South America and of Alaska and Greenland but is rare in whites.

HPV-6 and HPV-11 are associated with the rare cases of severe dysplasia and malignant progression that occur in respiratory papillomas.

DIAGNOSIS

Diagnosis of HPVs requires nucleic acid hybridization studies. HPV sequences are detected by methods based on gene amplification by polymerase chain reaction or by direct hybridization of the genomes in the specimens, without prior amplification. The most commonly used polymerase chain reaction tests utilize consensus primers, which are capable of amplifying a large number of HPVs, and type-specific probes to identify the sequences in the polymerase chain reaction products (14,15). These tests have a high degree of analytic specificity and sensitivity. A U.S. Food and Drug Administration–approved, commercially available assay that screens for 14 genital HPV types by direct hybridization is also available (16). HPV diagnosis may be useful, as an adjunct to the Papanicolaou smear, in identifying women with low-grade cervical cytologic abnormalities who harbor high-risk HPVs and may therefore be at risk for disease progression (17).

TREATMENT

Interferons administered into the lesions or given parenterally have been used successfully in treating refractory genital warts but have been only marginally useful in the treatment of respiratory papillomas. Traditional therapies include application of caustic agents (e.g., podophyllin, trichloroacetic acid), application of a DNA inhibitor (5-fluorouracil), cryotherapy, and surgical therapy. Cure rates of more than 90% are achieved in the treatment of cervical intraepithelial neoplasia lesions by any one of several treatment modalities, but the viruses may persist in a latent state.

PREVENTION

It is anticipated that HPV-based strategies will bring about the reduction of cervical cancer burden in the world. Tests for high-risk HPV DNAs in genital tract specimens have the potential to improve primary cervical cancer screening (18). These tests can be performed on specimens self-collected by the women (19). Prophylactic vaccines based on L1 protein expressed by recombinant DNA technology produced high titers of antibodies in human volunteers (20). The effectiveness of several such vaccine formulations for preventing cervical cancer precursor lesions is being examined in phase 3 trials. In addition, immunotherapy of preinvasive and invasive HPV-associated diseases, targeting the viral E6 and E7 oncoproteins, is being investigated in animal models and in humans (21).

REFERENCES

1. Lowy DR, Howley PM. Papillomaviruses. In: Knipe DM, Howley PM, eds. *Fields virology.* Philadelphia: Lippincott Williams & Wilkins, 2001:2231–2264.
2. Howley PM, Lowy DR. Papillomaviruses and their replication. In: Knipe DM, Howley PM, eds. *Fields virology.* Philadelphia: Lippincott Williams & Wilkins, 2001:2197–2229.
3. Durst M, Dzarlieva-Petrusevzka P, Boukamp P, et al. Molecular and cytogenetic analysis of immortalized human primary keratinocytes obtained after transfection with human papillomavirus type 16 DNA. *Oncogene* 1987;1:251.
4. McCance DJ, Kopan R, Fuchs E, et al. Human papillomavirus type 16 alters human epithelial cell differentiation *in vitro. Proc Natl Acad Sci U S A* 1988;85:7169.
5. Kirnbauer R, Hubbert N, Wheeler CM. A virus-like particle enzyme-linked immunosorbent assay detects serum antibodies in a majority of women infected with human papillomavirus type 16. *J Natl Cancer Inst* 1994;86:494.
6. Sun Y, Eluf-Neto J, Muñoz N, et al. Human papillomavirus-related serological marker of invasive cervical carcinoma in Brazil. *Cancer Epidemiol Biomarkers Prev* 1994;3:341–347.
7. Orth G. Epidermodysplasia verruciformis. In: Salzman NP, Howley PM, eds. *The Papovaviridae.* Vol. 2. The papillomaviruses. New York: Plenum, 1987:199–243.
8. Pfister H, ter Schegget J. Role of HPV in cutaneous premalignant and malignant tumors. *Clin Dermatol* 1997;15:335–347.
9. de Villiers EM. Papillomavirus and HPV typing. *Clin Dermatol* 1997;15:199–206.
10. Becker TM, Stone KM, Alexander ER. Genital human papillomavirus infection: a growing concern. *Obstet Gynecol Clin North Am* 1987;14:389.
11. International Agency for Research on Cancer. *IARC monograph on the evaluation of carcinogenic risks to humans.* Vol. 64. Human papillomaviruses. Lyon: International Agency for Research on Cancer, 1995.
12. Gillison ML, Koch WM, Capone RB, et al. Evidence for a causal association between human papillomavirus and a subset of head and neck cancers. *J Natl Cancer Inst* 2000;92:709–720.
13. Shah KV, Howley PM. Papillomaviruses. In: Fields BN, Knipe DM, Howley PM, et al., eds. *Virology.* Philadelphia: Lippincott-Raven, 1996:2077–2109.
14. Hildesheim A, Schiffman MH, Gravitt PE, et al. Persistence of type-specific human papillomavirus infection among cytologically normal women in Portland, Oregon. *J Infect Dis* 1994;169:235–240.
15. Jacobs MV, de Roda Husman AM, van den Brule AJC, et al. Group specific differentiation between high- and low-risk human papillomavirus genotypes by general primers-mediated polymerase chain reaction and two cocktails of oligonucleotide-probes. *J Clin Microbiol* 1995;33:901–905.
16. Cox JT, Lorincz AT, Schiffman MH, et al. Human papillomavirus testing by hybrid capture appears to be useful in triaging women with a cytologic diagnosis of atypical squamous cells of undetermined significance. *Am J Obstet Gynecol* 1995;172:946–954.
17. Solomon D, Schiffman M, Tarone R, for the ALTS Group. Comparison of three management strategies for patients with atypical squamous cells of undetermined significance: baseline results from a randomized trial. *J Natl Cancer Inst* 2001;93:293–299.
18. Wright TC Jr, Denny L, Kuhn L, et al. HPV DNA testing of self-collected vaginal samples compared with cytologic screening to detect cervical cancer. *JAMA* 2000;283:81–86.
19. Moscicki AB. Comparison between methods for human papillomavirus DNA testing: a model for self-testing in young women. *J Infect Dis* 1993;167:723–725.
20. Harro CD, Pang Y-YS, Roden RBS, et al. Safety and immunogenicity trial in adult volunteers of an HPV 16 L1 virus-like particle vaccine. *J Natl Cancer Inst* 2001;93:284–292.
21. Chen CH, Wang TL, Hung CF, et al. Enhancement of DNA vaccine potency by linkage of antigen gene to an HSP70 gene. *Cancer Res* 2000;60:1035–1042.
22. Bosch FX, Manos MM, Muñoz N, et al. Prevalence of human papillomavirus in cervical cancer: a worldwide perspective. *J Natl Cancer Inst* 1995;87:796–802.

CHAPTER 238
Human Polyomavirus

Keerti V. Shah

Polyomavirus infections of humans were not recognized until 1971, when two polyomaviruses, BK virus (BKV) and JC virus (JCV), were isolated from immunosuppressed patients (1,2). JCV is the etiologic agent of progressive multifocal leukoencephalopathy (PML), a degenerative disease of the central nervous system (3). BKV infection is associated with some urinary tract illnesses, including a recently recognized syndrome of nephropathy in renal transplant recipients (4,5). Millions of U.S. residents were inadvertently exposed to simian virus 40 (SV40), an oncogenic polyomavirus of Asian macaques, because this virus was a frequent and unrecognized contaminant of inactivated poliovirus vaccines that were administered between 1955 and 1961. There is no firm evidence that SV40 produced any ill effects in the exposed population (6). Polyomaviruses are widely distributed in nature and cause a variety of illnesses in their natural hosts, affecting kidney, brain, lung, and other organs (Table 238.1). The viruses are species specific and infect only one or a few closely related species.

CHARACTERISTICS OF THE PATHOGEN

The viral particle is small (diameter 45 nm), is nonenveloped, and has an icosahedral capsid with 72 capsomers. The structure and functions of polyomavirus genomes are known in great detail (7). The viral genome is a small, double-stranded, circular DNA molecule of about 5,000 base pairs. It is functionally divided into an early region (2.3 kb) that codes for large and small T proteins, a late region (2.3 kb) that codes for viral capsid proteins, and a noncoding regulatory region (0.4 kb) that contains the origin of DNA replication and transcription control sequences. Viral DNA replication occurs bidirectionally starting from the origin of replication. The early and late regions are transcribed from different strands of the DNA molecule. The proteins coded by the viral genome are listed in Table 238.2. The large T antigen is a multifunctional, regulatory early protein. It binds to specific sites in the regulatory region of the viral genome and initiates viral DNA replication, activates cellular genes that mediate cellular DNA synthesis, and modulates early and late viral transcription. The major viral polypeptide VP1, a late protein, is the main component of the viral capsid, is involved in viral attachment to cellular receptors, and contains type-specific and type-common epitopes.

BKV and JCV are closely related and their DNAs have an overall nucleotide sequence homology of 75%. The amino acid sequence homology between BKV and JCV proteins ranges from a high of 83% for large T protein to a low of 59% for the agnoprotein. Both viruses are propagated in cell cultures of human origin. Primary human embryonic kidney cells and human diploid fibroblasts are suitable for primary isolation of BKV, whereas primary glial cells derived from fetal brains are suitable for primary isolation of JCV. Even in susceptible cells, the growth of BKV and JCV is inefficient and inconsistent. Both viruses transform cells from a variety of rodent species. Ultraviolet-irradiated noninfectious BKV can transform human embryonic kidney cells. The BKV genome remains episomal in BKV-transformed human cells but is integrated in BKV-transformed rodent cells. Both viruses are oncogenic for newborn hamsters and produce brain tumors of many histologic types in intracerebrally inoculated animals. After intracerebral inoculation, BKV produces largely tumors of ventricular surfaces (e.g., ependymoma, choroid plexus papilloma) and JCV produces tumors of neural origin. Intravenous inoculation of BKV into hamsters produces insulinomas, osteosarcomas, and ependymomas. Intracerebral inoculation of JCV into owl and squirrel monkeys results in brain tumors, the only known example of a virus-induced central nervous system tumor in primates (8).

PATHOGENESIS

The respiratory tract may be the site of entry of BKV and JCV. Mild respiratory illness may accompany primary BKV infection (9). It is likely that the viruses multiply at the site of entry and are transported to the kidney in the bloodstream. After primary infection, the virus may remain latent in the kidney of the immunocompetent host for an indefinite period of time and produce no ill effects. Viral genomic sequences have been detected in cadaver kidneys, B-lymphocytes (10,11), and normal human brain (12). Immunologic impairment, especially conditions that affect T-cell functions, bring about virus reactivation and result in virus-associated pathology.

The viruses multiply exclusively in the nucleus of the infected cell. Productive infection in permissive cells is associated with a variety of nuclear changes (increase in size, occurrence of basophilic inclusions, and others) and results in cell death. The pathologic consequences of polyomavirus infections can be attributed to virus-induced destruction of infected cells. For example, infection and destruction of oligodendrocytes by JCV, and the resulting demyelination, account for the pathologic and clinical features of PML. Immunopathologic factors have not been implicated in diseases caused by polyomaviruses.

BKV and JCV differ in their biologic behavior and disease potential. BKV-related pathology is confined largely to the urinary tract and JCV-related pathology exclusively to the central nervous system. JCV shedding in urine is frequent in immunocompetent individuals and increases in older individuals (13). Human immunodeficiency virus (HIV)-induced immunosuppression leads to a marked increase in BKV shedding, but does not affect JCV shedding (14).

EPIDEMIOLOGY AND CLINICAL FEATURES

Infections with BKV and JCV occur in childhood (7). Serologic studies have shown that 50% of children in the United States are infected with BKV by age 3 or 4 years and with JCV by age 10 to 14 years. Although BKV and JCV have been recovered most often from urine, the rapid acquisition of antibodies in childhood is more consistent with an infection disseminated from the respiratory tract than from the urinary tract. With rare exceptions, illnesses caused by BKV and JCV are confined to immunocompromised persons.

PROGRESSIVE MULTIFOCAL LEUKOENCEPHALOPATHY

PML is a rare, subacute, fatal demyelinating disease of the central nervous system of worldwide distribution. It occurs on a

TABLE 238.1. Natural Hosts and Principal Characteristics of Polyomaviruses

Natural host	Viruses	Tropism	Associated illness
Humans	BK virus	Kidney epithelium	Hemorrhagic cystitis, ureteral stenosis, allograft failure
	JC virus	Kidney epithelium and brain oligodenodrocytes	Progressive multifocal leukoencephalopathy (PML)
Monkeys	Simian virus 40 of Asian macaques	Kidney epithelium	PML-like illness in some colonies
	Simian agent 12 of baboons	Kidney epithelium	None recognized
	Lymphotropic polyomavirus of African green monkeys	B-lymphocytes	None recognized
	Cynomolgus polyomavirus	Kidney epithelium	Interstitial nephritis; ureteritis
Cattle	Bovine polyomavirus	Not known	None recognized
Rabbit	Rabbit kidney vacuolating virus	Kidney epithelium	None recognized
Mouse	Mouse polyoma virus	Kidney epithelium	Tumors in athymic mice
Hamster	K virus	Lung endothelium	Respiratory illness
	Hamster papovavirus	Not known	Cutaneous tumors
Athymic rat	Rat polyomavirus	Not known	Parotid gland abnormalities
Parakeet	Budgerigar fledgling disease virus	Many organs	Fatal illness in fledgling birds

background of illnesses known to depress T-cell functions, for example, in patients with acquired immunodeficiency syndrome (AIDS) or with lymphoproliferative and chronic diseases, organ transplant recipients taking immunosuppressive therapy, and persons who have primary immunodeficiency diseases. PML in patients with AIDS is reported to occur in nearly 4% of those with neurologic abnormalities, and it accounts for the large majority of PML cases in the United States (15). The age distribution of PML cases has changed from that in the past. A few years ago it was predominantly a disease of the fifth and sixth decades of life, but it is now found increasingly in younger persons, including children.

The onset of the disease is insidious. Early signs and symptoms suggest multifocal and asymmetric lesions in the brain. Impaired speech and vision and mental deterioration are common. As the disease progresses, paralysis of limbs, cortical blindness, and sensory abnormalities occur. Death usually occurs 3 to 6 months after onset. Throughout the illness, the patient remains afebrile, with normal cerebrospinal fluid and without signs of increased intracranial pressure. Electroencephalograms show non-specific changes. Until a few years ago, the diagnosis of PML could be established only by pathologic examination of a brain biopsy sample; however, more recently, noninvasive techniques such as computed tomography and magnetic resonance imaging have been effective in the diagnosis of PML.

The pathognomonic lesions of PML are the foci of demyelination surrounded by affected oligodendrocytes, which have inclusion-bearing, enlarged nuclei. In addition, many foci of demyelination contain within them abnormal astrocytes of greatly increased size and with bizarre nuclear changes. The demyelinating lesions are most frequent in the subcortical white matter, and the cerebrum is almost always affected. An inflammatory response is absent or mild.

Both viral particles and viral DNA are found in large quantities in PML brains. JCV is often detected in the cerebrospinal fluid of patients with acquired immunodeficiency syndrome (16). The nuclei of affected oligodendrocytes contain abundant amounts of viral particles, often seen as dense crystalline arrays. Affected astrocytes only rarely contain viral particles but display JCV T antigen when they are cultured from PML patients' brains.

TABLE 238.2. Functions of Virus-Coded Polyomavirus Proteins

Protein	No. of amino acids[a]	Functions
Early region		
Large T	708	Initiation of viral DNA replication, stimulation of host DNA synthesis, regulation of early and late transcription, establishment and maintenance of transformation
Middle T[b]	421[c]	Cell transformation
Small T	174	Efficient viral DNA replication
Late region		
VP1	362	Major capsid protein, attaches to cellular receptors, mediates hemagglutination, has type-specific and type-common epitopes
VP2	352	Minor capsid protein
VP3	234	Minor capsid protein, subset of VP2
Agnoprotein	62	Not known

[a]For simian virus 40, except for middle T, as deduced from nucleotide sequence data.
[b]Middle T is found in mouse and hamster polyomaviruses but not in BKV, JCV, and simian virus 40.
[c]For mouse polyomavirus.

It has been suggested that the oligodendrocytes and the astrocytes represent, respectively, productive infection and transformation by JCV. Patients who die with PML are found to have small amounts of virus at extraneural sites (kidney, liver, lung). The multifocal distribution of the discrete demyelinating foci in the brain suggests that the virus is seeded into the brain through the blood (8).

DNA of JCV isolates from PML cases shows characteristic rearrangements in the regulatory region (17). It is probable that these rearrangements are adaptive for the multiplication of JCV in the central nervous system.

BK VIRUS–ASSOCIATED ILLNESSES

BKV reactivation and viruria occur frequently in pregnant women, in recipients of kidney and bone marrow allografts, in HIV-infected individuals, and in others whose immunity is depressed. Reactivation in pregnancy has not been associated with any ill effect or with transmission of the infection to the newborn. BKV infection has been associated with ureteral stenosis, an infrequent and late complication of renal transplantation, with hemorrhagic cystitis in bone marrow transplant recipients (18), as well as with occasional cases of cystitis in otherwise healthy, immunocompetent children. Atypical primary BKV infection in an immunologically defenseless child can lead to tubulointerstitial nephritis and irreversible renal damage (19).

A new syndrome, BKV nephropathy, has been recently identified in renal transplant recipients. In these patients, extensive BKV multiplication in the tubular epithelium results in a loss of allograft function (5,20). The patient sheds large numbers of BKV-infected epithelial cells in the urine and has BKV DNA in the serum. The disease occurs in about 2% to 3% of renal transplant recipients and may be related to the introduction of new immunosuppressive drugs (21). BKV-related vasculopathy, a new tropism for BKV, has been described recently, in which a fatal case of disseminated BKV infection in a renal transplant recipient was associated with BKV multiplication in endothelial cells (22).

BK VIRUS, JC VIRUS, AND SIMIAN VIRUS 40 IN HUMAN TUMORS

Genomic sequences of polyomaviruses have been reported from a wide variety of human tumors, including pediatric brain tumors, osteosarcomas, and mesotheliomas (23). JCV sequences have been reported from a majority of pediatric medulloblastomas (24). The significance of these observations is not clear (25).

DIAGNOSIS

Serologic tests for BKV and JCV antibodies are not helpful for clinical diagnosis. Cytomorphology of urinary epithelial cells may be useful as an indicator of polyomavirus excretion in urine. The presence of virus in the urine or the brain can be demonstrated by a variety of techniques, including electron microscopy, isolation in tissue culture, enzyme-linked immunosorbent assay for viral antigens, nucleic acid hybridization assays for viral genomes, and gene amplification by polymerase chain reaction.

TREATMENT

Treatment of PML by administration of nucleic acid analogs in an attempt to inhibit virus multiplication has been generally unsuccessful, although occasional remissions have been reported (3). It is thought that reduction or elimination of iatrogenic immunosuppression in PML patients who have relatively intact immune functions (e.g., renal transplant recipients) may be beneficial.

PREVENTION

No efforts have been made to develop preventive measures against BKV and JCV infections.

ACKNOWLEDGMENT

This work was partially supported by Public Health Service Grant P01 A115969.

REFERENCES

1. Gardner SD, Field AM, Coleman DV, et al. New human papovirus (B.K.) isolated from urine after renal transplantation. *Lancet* 1971;1:1253–1257.
2. Padgett BL, Walker DL, Zu Rhein GM, et al. Cultivation of papova-like virus from human brain with progressive multifocal leucoencephalopathy. *Lancet* 1971;1:1257–1260.
3. Walker D, Padgett B. Progressive multifocal leukoencephalopathy. In: Fraenkel-Conrat H, Wagner RR, eds. *Comprehensive virology*. Vol. 18. New York: Plenum, 1983:161–193.
4. Arthur RR, Shah KV. The occurrence and significance of papovaviruses Bk and JC in the urine. *Prog Med Virol* 1989;36:42–61.
5. Nickeleit V, Hirsch HH, Zeiler M, et al. BK-virus nephropathy in renal transplants: tubular necrosis, MHC-class II expression and rejection in a puzzling game. *Nephrol Dial Transplant* 2000;15:323–331.
6. Shah KV. Does SV40 infection contribute to the development of human cancers? *Rev Med Virol* 2000;10:31–43.
7. Major E. Human polyomavirus. In: Knipe DM, Howley PM, eds. *Fields virology*. Philadelphia: Lippincott Williams & Wilkins, 2001:2175–2195.
8. Houff SA, London W, ZuRhein GM, et al. New world primates as a model of virus-induced astrocytomas. In: Sever JL, Madden DL, eds. *Polyomaviruses and human neurological diseases*. New York: Alan R Liss, 1983:223–226.
9. Sundsfjord A, Spein AR, Lucht E, et al. Detection of human polyomavirus BK DNA in nasopharyngeal aspirates from children with respiratory infections but not in saliva from immunodeficient and immunocompetent patients. *J Clin Microbiol* 1994;32:1390–1394.
10. Dorries K, Vogel E, Gunther S, et al. Infection of human polyomaviruses JC and BK in peripheral blood leuckotyes from immmunocompetent individuals. *Virology* 1994;198:59–70.
11. Tornatore C, Berger JR, Houff SA, et al. Detection of JC virus DNA in peripheral lymphocytes from patients with and without progressive multifocal leukoencephalopathy. *Ann Neurol* 1992;31:454–462.
12. White FA III, Ishaq M, Stoner GL, et al. JC virus DNA is present in many human brain samples from patients without progressive multifocal leukoencephalopathy. *J Virol* 1992;66:5726–5734.
13. Kitamura T, Kunitake T, Guo J, et al. Transmission of the human polyomavirus JC virus occurs both within the family and outside the family. *J Clin Microbiol* 1994;32:2359–2363.
14. Markowitz RB, Thompson HC, Mueller JF, et al. Incidence of BK virus and JC virus viruria in human immunodeficiency virus-infected and -uninfected subjects. *J Infect Dis* 1993;167:13–20.
15. Berger JR, Levy RM. The neurologic complications of human immunodeficiency virus infections. *Med Clin North Am* 1993;77:1–23.
16. Holman RC, Torok RJ, Belay ED, et al. Progressive multifocal leukoencephalopathy in the United States, 1979–1994: increased mortality associated with HIV infection. *Neuroepidemiology* 1998;17:303–309.
17. Iida T, Kitamura T, Guo J, et al. Origin of JC polyomavirus variants associated with progressive multifocal leukoencephalopathy. *Proc Natl Acad Sci U S A* 1993;90:5062–5065.
18. Arthur RR, Shah KV, Baust SJ, et al. Association of BK viruria with hemorrhagic cystitis in recipients of bone marrow transplants. *N Engl J Med* 1986;315:230–234.
19. Rosen S, Harmon W, Krensky A, et al. Tubulo-interstitial nephritis associated with polyomavirus (BK type) infection. *N Engl J Med* 1983;308:1192–1196.

20. Randhawa PS, Finkelstein S, Scantlebury V, et al. Human polyoma virus–associated interstitial nephritis in the allograft kidney. *Transplantation* 1999;67:103–109.
21. Binet I, Nickeleit V, Hirsch HH, et al. Polyomavirus disease under new immunosuppressive drugs. *Transplantation* 1999;67:918–922.
22. Petrogiannis-Haliotis T, Sakoulas G, Kirby J, et al. BK-type polyomavirus vasculopathy in a renal-transplant patient. *N Engl J Med* 2001;345:1250–1255.
23. Carbone M, Fisher S, Powers A, et al. New molecular and epidemiological issues in mesothelioma: role of SV40. *J Cell Physiol* 1999;180:167–172.
24. Khalili K, Krynska B, Del Valle L, et al. Medulloblastomas and the human neurotropic polyomavirus JC virus [Letter]. *Lancet* 1999;353:1152–1153.
25. Shah KV. Polyoma viruses (JC virus, BK virus and simian virus 40) and human cancer, In: Goedert JJ, ed. *Infectious causes of cancer: targets for intervention.* Totowa, NJ: Humana Press, 2000:461–474.

CHAPTER 239
Hepatitis B Virus and Hepatitis D Virus

Raymond S. Koff

HEPATITIS B VIRUS

On a global basis, human hepatitis B virus (HBV) is the most common cause of persistent viremia and the most important cause of chronic liver disease and hepatocellular carcinoma. Clinically apparent HBV infections may have been extant for several millennia, but virologic characterization of the responsible agent was achieved only 35 years ago (1). HBV belongs to a family of genetically related but distinct hepatotropic DNA-containing animal viruses, the hepadnaviruses; the family name is Hepadnaviridae. The host range of these agents appears to be restricted to mammalian and avian species. The terms *orthohepadnavirus* and *avihepadnavirus* are applied to the mammalian and avian genera, respectively.

Phylogenetic Relationships and Host Range

Human HBV and the other members of the family Hepadnaviridae are morphologically and antigenically similar, but the sequelae of infection are variable. The viruses are double shelled, with a diameter of about 42 nm (Fig. 239.1). Each virus contains a small, partially double-stranded, circular DNA genome with long, minus strands of nearly equal nucleotide length (Table 239.1). HBV is one of the smallest human viruses identified; it has a compact genome with a size of about 3.2 kb.

Because HBV and the other hepadnaviruses use reverse transcription during genome replication and may share some nucleotide sequences with the retroviruses, an evolutionary relationship had been suggested but remains speculative (2). An evolutionary relationship among the avian and mammalian hepadnaviruses also has been postulated on the basis of examination of specific genomic sequences, a limited number of which are shared. Human HBV, currently classified as hepadnavirus type 1, was the first recognized member of the orthohepadnavirus family. In addition to HBV, orthohepadnaviruses have been described in the Eastern woodchuck, the Beechey ground squirrel, the tree squirrel, the tree shrew, the wooley monkey, gibbons, orangutans, and gorillas. Only some of these are well characterized. An indigenous chimpanzee HBV also has been reported (3). Avihepadnaviruses have been identified in the gray heron and in the domestic Pekin duck. Chronic infections with human HBV, with woodchuck hepatitis virus, with ground squir-rel hepatitis virus, and with duck hepatitis B virus have been linked to the development of hepatocellular carcinoma (4).

The host range of the known hepadnaviruses has been extended to other species (e.g., geese and chipmunks), but humans probably cannot be infected by the nonhuman hepadnaviruses, and the human HBV host range appears to be limited to humans and some nonhuman primate species. Experimental transmission of HBV to chimpanzees has served as a model for the study of infection; other nonhuman primates may also be susceptible, but infection in these animals has been inconsistent, and they have not proved useful for laboratory investigation.

Hepatitis B Virus Variants

Human HBV strains have been classified into seven genotypes, designated A through G, based on nucleotide divergences greater than 8% in the complete genome or 4% in the S gene, which encodes the hepatitis B surface antigen (HBsAg). The genotypes have a characteristic geographic distribution despite the observation that homologous recombination has been described (5). Genotypes A and D are common in the United States (6).

As indicated earlier, HBV uses a reverse transcription step in genomic replication. As a consequence of the poor proofreading ability of the HBV DNA polymerase protein, mutations are common (2×10^{-5} nucleotides per year) in chronic HBV infection, are distributed over the entire genome, and lead to a number of HBV genetic variants (HBV mutants) (7). Most of these arise during the period in chronic infection when the immune response is strongest, whereas in the early stages of infection, the genome appears to be very stable (8). Statistical analysis indicates an increasing frequency of mutations from the S gene (the lowest) to the C (core) gene, to the P (pol or polymerase) gene, to region X, to the precore (pre-C) region, and finally to the pre-S2/pre-S1 regions (9). These variants may differ in their biologic behavior compared with wild-type HBV; however, their role in the biology of HBV infection remains incompletely understood (7). Some of the variants have been associated with increased pathogenicity (e.g., the precore mutant), whereas others may have lower pathogenicity (e.g., the X deletion mutants).

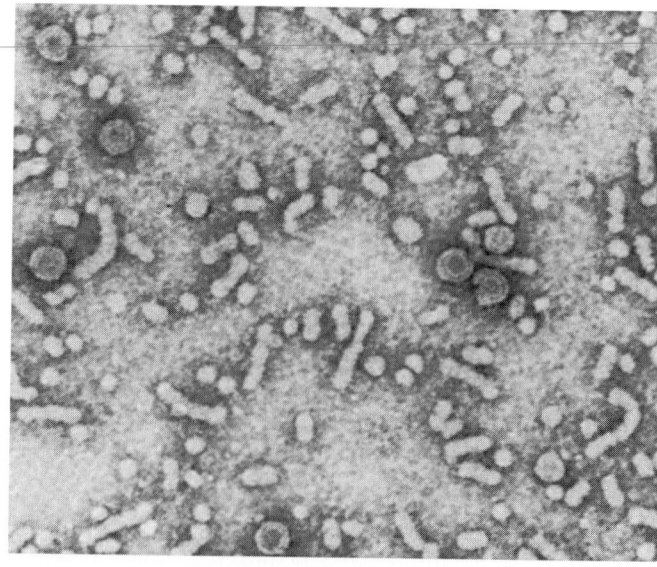

Figure 239.1. Electron micrograph of serum sample showing the 42-nm hepatitis B virus particle and the smaller 22-nm spheres and tubules containing hepatitis B surface antigen envelope proteins and lipid.

TABLE 239.1. Genome Length of Representative Members of the Hepadnaviridae Family

Agent	Minus strand nucleotide length
Human hepatitis B virus	3,188
Woodchuck hepatitis virus	3,320
Ground squirrel hepatitis virus	3,311
Duck hepatitis B virus	3,021

Some may be associated with reduced viral replication and suppression of HBV gene product expression. Some of the more commonly detected variants are listed in Table 239.2.

Structure

HBV is a double-shelled, spherical particle, 42 nm in diameter, composed of a 27-nm diameter, spherical, icosahedral nucleocapsid core and a surrounding envelope 7 nm in width (10). HBV is associated with three circulating particles that are readily visualized by electron microscopy (Fig. 239.1). These include the complete 42-nm HBV particle, smaller spherical particles about 22 nm (range of 15 to 25 nm) in diameter, and tubular particles with an average width of about 22 nm and a variable length of up to 200 nm. The small spherical and tubular particles are present in quantities far in excess of the 42-nm HBV particles. The 22-nm spherical and tubular particles are composed of the proteins, carbohydrate, and lipid of the envelope (surface or coat) of HBV but lack DNA or RNA transcripts and DNA polymerase activity.

HBV's structural integrity and infectivity can be destroyed by heating up to 98°C and by exposure to chemical agents such as glutaraldehyde. Even low-level quaternary ammonium germicides may be effective (11).

ENVELOPE

The principal protein and antigenic material of the HBV envelope is the small (major) protein of HBsAg, comprising 226 amino acids, encoded by the S open reading frame of HBV DNA. A group-specific determinant, labeled *a*, and a set of subtype determinants, labeled *d*, *y*, *w*, and *r*, are also encoded by the S open reading frame and are present on the small HBsAg protein. The *a* determinant has been found in all HBV isolates and elicits protective immunity against infection by all HBV serotypes except in the case of the uncommon vaccine-induced escape mutant (12). In addition to the small HBsAg protein, two other proteins, namely, the middle protein, encoded by the pre-S2 region and

TABLE 239.2. Hepatitis B Virus Variants

Precore mutation at codon 28
Core deletion
Core point mutation at codons 48–60, 84–101, 147–155
Core promoter mutation
Encapsidation mutant
S point mutation at codons 145, 126, 131, 132
S deletion
Pre-S1/2 junction deletion
Pre-S1 deletion
Pre-S2/S promoter deletion
X deletion
Truncated X
Polymerase region mutation

S open reading frame, and the large protein, encoded by pre-S1, pre-S2, and S, are expressed on the envelope of the HBV particle (Table 239.3). The large protein is present on the 22-nm spherical and tubular particles in a much smaller proportion than on the HBV particle. The small, middle, and large HBsAg proteins are present in both glycosylated and nonglycosylated forms. Interactions among the three HBsAg proteins appear to affect the biosynthesis, processing, and transport of the proteins. In addition to the glycosylated proteins, other carbohydrate components of the envelope may be present. Approximately one third of the content of the 22-nm particles appears to be host-derived lipid. An additional structural protein, a novel polymerase-surface fusion glycoprotein (encoded by a spliced RNA) similar to the large HBsAg protein has been reported in the 22-nm spherical particle and the HBV particle (13). Confirmation of its existence is not yet available.

NUCLEOCAPSID (CORE)

The nucleocapsid consists of about 180 repeating subunits of its core protein, which contains C-terminal packaging signals and nuclear localization signals. Nucleocapsid particles can be released from intact HBV particles by treatment with nonionic detergents, which strip away the envelope, exposing free core particles and their associated antigens. The HBV nucleocapsid contains the circular DNA, a covalently attached primer protein, HBV DNA polymerase, reverse transcriptase, RNase, and protein kinase activity. The last serves to phosphorylate the core-associated proteins. The core protein expresses a major antigenic reactivity, the hepatitis B core antigen (HBcAg) and self-assembles into a capsid-like structure. HBcAg has been localized either to the surface or to internal locations of the

TABLE 239.3. Hepatitis B Virus Open Reading Frames, Gene Products, and Amino Acid Residues of Identified Proteins

Open reading frame	Gene product	Amino acid residues of identified protein
Pre-S1, pre-S2, S	Large HBsAg protein	400
Pre-S2, S	Middle HBsAg protein	281
S	Small (major) HBsAg protein	226
Pre-C, C	HBeAg	189
C	HBcAg	212
P	DNA polymerase	844
X	HBxAg	154

HBsAg, hepatitis B surface antigen; HBeAg, hepatitis B e antigen; HBcAg, hepatitis B core antigen; HBxAg, hepatitis B x antigen.

nucleocapsid particle. A related antigenic reactivity known as the hepatitis B e antigen (HBeAg) is a nonparticulate, soluble antigen derived from HBcAg by proteolytic self-cleavage at the endoplasmic reticulum and is released into the circulation from infected hepatocytes. It differs from HBcAg in the antigen processing pathway (14). Whereas the presence of HBeAg in blood is generally correlated with active HBV replication, mutations in the precore and core region may result in a replicating HBV variant in which HBeAg is not expressed. The function of HBeAg in the life cycle of HBV remains incompletely understood, but it appears to be immunoregulatory, playing a role in immune clearance of the virus and in the *in utero* induction of T-lymphocyte tolerance (15).

Genomic Structure of Hepatitis B Virus

OPEN READING FRAMES

The long, minus DNA strand of HBV is organized into four overlapping open reading frames: S, C (Core), X, and P (Pol) (Fig. 239.2). S and C have associated upstream regions termed pre-S and pre-C, respectively. The open reading frames, their gene products, and the amino acid residues of the products are listed in Table 239.3. The S open reading frame codes for the small (major) HBsAg protein. The upstream pre-S2 region and the S open reading frame encode the middle-sized HBsAg protein; the pre-S1, pre-S2, and S encode the large HBsAg protein.

The pre-C region (containing a signal sequence) and the C open reading frame serve to specify the HBeAg; the C open reading frame encodes the HBcAg protein. Derived from the precore protein that harbors sequences essential for its secretion (16), HBeAg contains an additional 10 amino acid residues at its N-terminal end but is truncated by about 35 amino acids at its C-terminal end. Mutations in the pre-C region abort translation of the HBeAg precursor, and mutations in the core promoter affect transcription of the HBeAg coding region. In both cases, HBV infections occur without detectable HBeAg.

The longest open reading frame of the HBV genome is the P (pol or polymerase) open reading frame, which overlaps the others. P specifies a multifunctional polypeptide with RNA- and DNA-dependent DNA polymerase, reverse transcriptase, ribonuclease H (RNase H), pyrophophorolysis, and protein-priming activities, and at its N-terminal end it contains the protein required for replication and packaging (17).

The X open reading frame encodes the X proteins (a full-length and shorter forms), which serve as transcriptional trans-activators, enhancing the transcription and replication of HBV, other viruses, and host cell genes, possibly acting as a tumor promoter (18), as well as promoting the resistance of infected hepatocytes to immune-mediated apoptosis (19). The mechanism by which the X proteins activate transcription is not fully understood, but interactions with nuclear proteins are involved (20).

PROMOTERS AND ENHANCERS

At least four promoters and two transcriptional enhancer elements have been recognized on the HBV genome (21). Two separate promoters, the pre-S1 promoter and the S promoter, are used to code for the three HBsAg proteins. The pre-S1 produces a single transcript that codes for the large HBsAg 2.4-kb transcript, whereas the S promoter produces a 2.1-kb transcript that codes for the middle and small HBsAg proteins. The third promoter, the core promoter, is associated with the open reading frame of HBcAg and codes for the 3.5-kb transcript that yields the core protein, serves as the template for translation of the polymerase protein, and serves as the pregenomic RNA from which HBV DNA is reverse transcribed. The fourth promoter is associated with the X open reading frame and gives rise to a 0.8-kb transcript that codes for the full-length and shorter X proteins. Binding sites for a number of transcription factors have been identified within the HBV promoters. Two enhancer elements, enhancer I and enhancer II, which stimulate the transcriptional activity of the promoters, have also been identified. The enhancer I element is governed by cooperative interactions between enhancer binding proteins (e.g., nuclear receptors and liver-specific factors) and can up-regulate each of the promoters. The enhancer II element is also capable of binding with multiple hepatocyte-specific transcription factors (22). Mutations in the enhancer II element result in a dramatic reduction in HBV replication (23). In addition, a glucocorticosteroid response element has been identified in the S open reading frame; it may increase expression of HBsAg in the presence of glucocorticoids. Other presently unidentified elements may also regulate the activity of HBV enhancers and promoters.

Replication *In Vitro*

Cloned, tandemly repeated multimers of HBV DNA have been used to transfect human hepatocellular carcinoma or hepatoblastoma cell lines, which then secrete HBsAg, HBeAg, HBV DNA polymerase activity, and HBV DNA associated with virus-like particles with the physical characteristics of HBV. The tandem nature of the DNA inserts permits the production of the 2.2- and 3.5-kb RNA replicative intermediates of HBV. The HBV produced by transfected cell lines has been shown to be capable of causing acute HBV infection in chimpanzees. Primary adult and fetal human hepatocytes also have been shown to support HBV infection and replication, but only a proportion of these cells are susceptible, and they gradually lose their susceptibility over time. Replication of HBV also has been reported in primary hepatocytes of the tree shrew (24). Efficient replication of HBV and secretion of infectious HBV particles has been reported to have been achieved by insertion of HBV genome into an adenovirus vector transferred to the livers of mice *in vivo* (25).

The tropism of HBV for the hepatocyte is likely to be related to the existence of a specific hepatocyte receptor for HBV as well as the presence of nuclear hormone receptors, which serve as essential transcription factors for synthesis of pregenomic RNA and for viral replication (26). Strict restriction to the hepatocyte seems unlikely, however, because infection *in vivo* has been

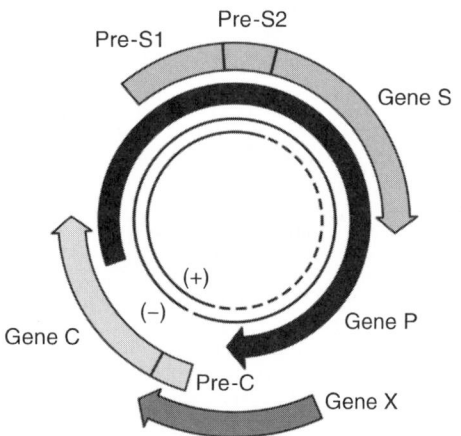

Figure 239.2. The circular configuration of the four open reading frames on the long, minus strand of the hepatitis B virus genome and the upstream regions of the S and C genes are depicted. (From the American Gastroenterological Association, Bethesda, MD, with permission.)

demonstrated in extrahepatic sites. Suspension cultures of human bone marrow cells have been infected by HBV; both progenitor and stromal cells support HBV replication. Unfortunately, none of the hepatocyte, hepatocyte-derived, or bone marrow cell tissue culture systems studied to date has permitted consistently high levels of HBV replication. In addition to mammalian cells, the HBV genome has been cloned in a variety of vectors, including bacterial and yeast cells.

Replication *In Vivo*

TARGETING TO HEPATOCYTES

The initiating events of HBV infection are poorly understood. HBV attachment to a specific cell-surface hepatocyte-specific viral receptor has been postulated to involve binding affinity sites on the pre-S1 and pre-S2 proteins of the HBV envelope, but the nature of the receptor remains speculative. Regardless of the exact mechanism of initial attachment, HBV entry into the hepatocyte probably results from fusion of viral and hepatocyte membranes. Subsequently the nucleocapsid is transferred to the cell nucleus and HBV DNA is released in an open, relaxed, circular form. In some instances, further processing of HBV DNA may be inhibited, and the infection remains latent without evidence of viral replication or the production of viral gene products. However, most infections lead to HBV replication. Integration of subgenomic fragments of HBV DNA or the intact HBV genome into the host genome of some hepatocytes may occur during HBV infection, but is not a required step in the replicative cycle of HBV (see the later section on Integration of Hepatitis B Virus DNA). An episomal form of HBV DNA has been infrequently detected in liver as long as 30 years after apparent recovery from infection (27,28).

SITE OF REPLICATION

The liver appears to be the major target organ of HBV infection and the principal site of HBV replication. Other hepadnaviruses (e.g., duck hepatitis B virus and woodchuck hepatitis virus) have been shown to be capable of replication in extrahepatic tissues. These sites may serve as a reservoir of latent hepadnavirus infection, which may lead under specific circumstances to viral reactivation and amplification. The presence of HBV DNA, HBV RNA, HBV replicative intermediates, and HBV proteins has now been described in a large number of extrahepatic organs and in a variety of cell types of individuals with chronic HBV infection (29) (Table 239.4). It is noteworthy that active replication of HBV and gene expression in these cells are not associated with injury or inflammation at these sites. The precise importance of extrahepatic replication of HBV remains uncertain. Although it seems likely that replication at these sites contributes minimally to the large viral burden of infected individuals, it may play a role in HBV reactivation and in HBV recurrence after liver transplantation for chronic hepatitis B.

MECHANISM

In the hepatocyte nucleus, the relaxed, circular HBV DNA is converted to a covalently closed circular DNA by repair of the positive DNA strand. This fully double-stranded DNA serves as a template for the synthesis of a series of RNA transcripts that include a longer than genome RNA (pregenomic RNA) with about 3,500 nucleotides and smaller RNA transcripts (30). After translation the HBV reverse transcriptase is bound to the pregenomic RNA, which will serve as a template for reverse transcription, leading to production of full-length (about 3,200 nucleotides) minus DNA strands of HBV as well as the messenger RNA (mRNA) for the core and polymerase proteins. The pregenomic RNA tran-

TABLE 239.4. Hepatitis B Virus Replication-Competent Tissues and Cell Types

Tissues	Cell types
Liver	Hepatocytes, Kupffer cells, endothelial cells
Blood	Mononuclear cells/monocytes/lymphocytes
Spleen	Macrophage/monocyte, endothelial cells
Lymph node	Macrophage/monocyte, endothelial cells
Periadrenal ganglion	Neuronal cells, sustentacular cells
Skin	Basal keratinocytes, dermal stromal fibroblasts
Intestine	Mucosal endothelial cells, stromal fibroblasts, endothelial cells
Pancreas	Acinar cells, endothelial cells
Kidney	Endothelial cells
Bone marrow	Progenitor cells, stromal cells
Testes	Intertubular stromal fibroblasts

Adapted from Mason A, Wick M, White H, et al. Hepatitis B virus replication in diverse cell types during chronic hepatitis B virus infection. *Hepatology* 1993;18: 781–789, with permission.

script and the HBV reverse transcriptase are encapsidated in core particles; it is within these particles within the cytoplasm of the cell that the minus DNA strand is catalyzed by reverse transcription and the polymerization of deoxynucleotides triphosphates onto the growing DNA chain occurs. Phosphorylation of the core protein occurs within the core particles during a later stage of viral genome maturation, possibly after transport back to the nucleus. Simultaneously, the RNA template is degraded. The structural and nonstructural viral proteins are translated from the smaller RNA transcripts, which vary in size from 700 to 2,400 nucleotides. In contrast to reverse transcription of the long strand, the short positive-sense strands, which vary between 1,700 and 2,800 nucleotides in length, are believed to be generated from templates of negative-stranded DNA.

In addition to HBV DNA and HBV-specific RNA, superhelical, closed circular duplex DNA and intermediates in HBV biosynthesis, namely incomplete HBV DNA forms comprising protein-linked minus strands with or without plus strands and HBV RNA-DNA hybrids, may be detected in infected hepatocytes. Current evidence suggests that the HBsAg envelope, with its posttranslationally modified HBsAg envelope proteins, is formed, at least in part, as a transmembrane polypeptide of the endoplasmic reticulum and is added to the core particle in the endoplasmic reticulum. Oligosaccharide trimming, namely, the removal of terminal glucose residues from HBsAg glycoproteins, is believed to play a role in the transport of particles from the endoplasmic reticulum to the Golgi apparatus. The intact nascent HBV particle is then exported from the hepatocyte by a poorly understood process.

Integration of Hepatitis B Virus DNA

Integration of HBV DNA into the DNA of the host hepatocyte is not a requisite step in the replicative cycle. Nonetheless, it may occur randomly throughout the early phases of HBV infection, and most HBV DNA integrations are subgenomic. Hepatocytes with integrated HBV genomic fragments may express gene products but do not support genomic replication. The mechanisms subserving and controlling HBV DNA integration and the proportion of affected hepatocytes have yet to be established. Presumably, nearly all hepatocytes in which integration occurs are destroyed during the immune attack on infected cells. Those hepatocytes that survive may undergo clonal expansion, and some may be transformed into the malignant cells of hepatocellular carcinoma. The mechanisms by which HBV DNA integration leads to tumor development remain incompletely understood. Transformation may due to the presence of chromosome abnormalities (deletions, duplications, and translocations) at the sites of HBV DNA integration, insertional mutagenesis, activation of cellular oncogenes, or an effect of the hepatitis B X protein (31,32).

HEPATITIS D VIRUS

History

The existence of the hepatitis D (delta) virus (HDV) as a distinct agent of viral hepatitis was recognized just over 25 years ago (33). The HDV antigen was discovered in the livers of patients with severe chronic hepatitis B. HDV is a defective, transmissible, RNA-containing satellite virus of HBV. It requires the helper or rescue function of the HBsAg of HBV or other hepadnaviruses for its expression, assembly, and pathogenicity. Nonetheless, HDV replication may occur in the absence of hepadnavirus infection (34). HDV appears to interfere with the synthesis of the helper HBV in most if not all dual HDV-HBV infections. HDV is not thought to be directly cytopathic.

Interaction of Hepatitis D and B Viruses

HDV infection is limited to persons who are infected by HBV: either HBV-infected individuals superinfected with HDV or those who simultaneously contract primary infections with HBV and HDV, a circumstance termed co-infection. In the former case, the HBV of the persistently infected host serves the helper functions required by HDV. In co-infections, the helper functions are assumed by the infecting HBV accompanying HDV. Superimposition of HDV on chronic HBV infection often leads to chronic HDV infection. In contrast, because HDV infection cannot outlive infection with HBV, and because more than 95% of acute HBV infections in adults resolve spontaneously with clearance of HBV, HDV infection and expression tend to be self-limited during co-infection with HBV.

Replicative Interactions

By transcapsidation, newly synthesized HDV acquires the HBsAg subtype of its host in superinfections or the HBsAg subtype of its accompanying HBV in co-infections. Coincident with this process, the synthesis of preexisting HBV gene products (HBsAg and HBeAg) may diminish, and HBV replication may be transiently inhibited in most patients with HDV superinfections (35). In a few instances, HBsAg may be permanently lost; however, in some patients, presumably a minority, replication of HBV and HDV occurs concurrently without mutual inhibition (35).

Morphology and Characteristics

HDV particles are 35 to 37 nm in diameter (Fig. 239.3) and are coated with HBsAg and small amounts of the pre-S proteins, similar in composition to the small 22-nm HBsAg particles found in the circulation of HBV-infected persons. However, the large HBsAg protein is present in lower concentrations in HDV coat material. It has been suggested that HDV carries the pre-S HBV receptor in its coat material to attach to or exit from the plasma membrane of the hepatocyte. Within the virus particle, ribonucleoprotein cores, consisting of HDV RNA complexed to about 70 copies of the HDV antigens, appear to have a diameter of about 19 nm (36).

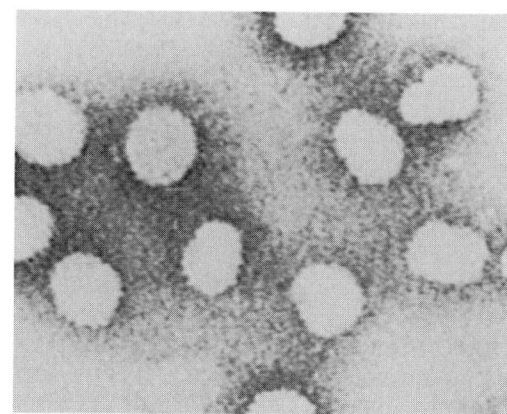

Figure 239.3. Electron micrograph of 35- to 37-nm hepatitis D virus particles in serum.

The HDV antigens that complex with HDV RNA are nuclear phosphoproteins that exist in two phosphorylated isoforms, a 195–amino acid and a 214–amino acid protein (37), which also interact with nucleolar phosphoproteins to regulate HDV RNA replication (38). The HDV antigens are produced from an 800-nucleotide polyadenylated mRNA of antigenomic sense (39) (Fig. 239.4), and in addition to the ability to bind RNA, they possess a nuclear localization signal and the ability to self-associate into multimers that are probably necessary for HDV assembly. The smaller HDV antigen participates in the transport of RNA into the nucleus and is essential for HDV replication. The larger antigen is isoprenylated, a posttranslational change that enhances targeting to the nucleus and aids in its inhibition of HDV RNA replication (40). Small amounts of the larger antigen inhibit genomic RNA synthesis from the antigenomic RNA template but not the synthesis of the antigenomic RNA from the genomic-sense RNA (41). The larger antigen also is required for the envelopment of HDV RNA by HBsAg and the secretion of the assembled HDV particles out of the host cell. It also enhances intracellular signal transduction pathways (42).

RNA Genome

The HDV RNA genome is single stranded, covalently closed, and circular, with slightly less than 1,680 nucleotides (43). It is the smallest RNA genome known to infect humans, the only circular RNA found in the animal viruses, and it has structural

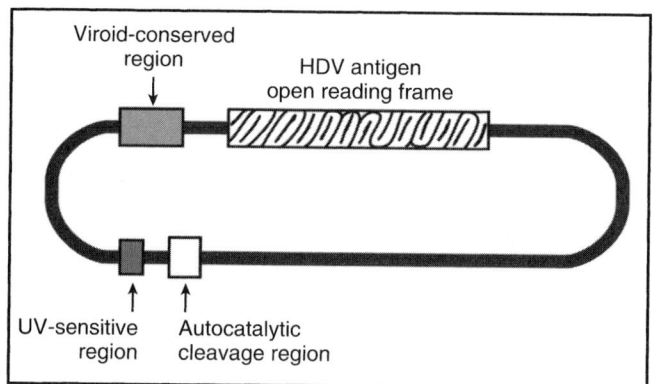

Figure 239.4. Schematic illustration of the hepatitis D virus antigenome and identified regions. *UV,* ultraviolet light. (From the American Gastroenterological Association, Bethesda, MD, with permission.)

and replicative similarities to certain infectious RNAs found in plants. Despite its association with HBV infection, the RNA of HDV is not homologous to the DNA of HBV. Genetic heterogeneity among HDV isolates is well known; at least three genotypes with different geographic distributions and possibly distinct associations with disease severity have been identified, but the mechanisms responsible for these differences remain ill defined. Despite its circular conformation, the RNA of HDV can form an unbranched rodlike structure by folding on itself through intramolecular base pairing, affecting 70% of the bases. A catalytic domain present on the genome is thought to represent a ribozyme that has a nested double pseudoknot secondary structure (44), which may also serve to stabilize downstream transcripts after polyadenylation (45). The HDV antigenome (Fig. 239.4) is a genome-complementary, circular RNA present in the infected hepatocyte and, to a lesser extent, in purified HDV particles. It contains, in addition to the open reading frame for HDV antigen, an autocatalytic cleavage region, a viroid-conserved region, and an ultraviolet light–sensitive region.

Classification

The HDV RNA genome resembles those of viroid RNAs, virusoids, and the RNAs of the circular plant satellite viruses, but they are smaller and contain no open reading frames. Hence, although similarities to the plant satellite viruses exist, HDV remains unclassified.

Mechanisms of Replication

HDV replication is limited to mammalian cells (46) and is presumed to occur solely in the hepatocyte. HDV is thought to replicate efficiently *in vivo*, producing as many as 300,000 genomic copies in the average hepatocyte and as many as 2×10^{12} HDV particles per milliliter of serum. The precise mechanism of replication remains to be established; however, it is clear that HDV RNA does not encode an RNA-dependent RNA polymerase. Therefore, genomic replication is thought to involve the redirection of host RNA polymerase II. HDV antigen binds to this polymerase, promotes its elongation, and thereby regulates mRNA synthesis and HDV genomic RNA replication (47). The synthesis of the antigenomic RNA appears to be independent of host RNA polymerase II (48), suggesting that other host polymerases may be responsible. Although HBsAg is not required for the replication of HDV RNA, it is necessary for the packaging, release, and pathogenicity of HDV. HDV is thought to replicate by a "double rolling circle" mechanism (43), in which RNA-directed RNA transcription from the circular RNA genome leads to the formation of a multimeric length RNA intermediate, which is then self-cleaved into monomers (49). Self-ligation of these monomers forms the circular antigenome, which through another cycle of the rolling circle mechanism produces nascent, progeny-genomic RNA.

Propagation

A variety of cell lines (primary chimpanzee or woodchuck hepatocytes and human hepatocellular carcinoma cells) have been transfected with HDV complementary DNA constructs and transiently express HDV RNA and HDV antigens. Replication of HDV appears to be noncytopathic in cultured cells (50) or transgenic mice (51). HDV has been experimentally transmitted to chimpanzees infected with HBV (52) but few studies of infection in this model are available.

REFERENCES

1. Purcell RH. The discovery of the hepatitis viruses. *Gastroenterology* 1993;104:955–963.
2. Miller RH, Robinson WS. Common evolutionary origin of hepatitis B virus and retroviruses. *Proc Natl Acad Sci U S A* 1986;83:2531–2535.
3. Takahashi K, Brotman B, Usuda S, et al. Full-genome sequence analyses of hepatitis B virus (HBV) strains recovered from chimpanzees infected in the wild: implications for an origin of HBV. *Virology* 2000;267:58–64.
4. Duflot A, Mehrotra R, Yu S-Z, et al. Spectrum of liver disease and duck hepatitis B virus infection in a large series of Chinese ducks with hepatocellular carcinoma. *Hepatology* 1995;21:1483–1491.
5. Morozov V, Pisareva M, Groudin M. Homologous recombination between different genotypes of hepatitis B virus. *Gene* 2000;260:55–65.
6. Swenson PD, Van Geyt C, Alexander ER, et al. Hepatitis B virus genotypes and HBsAg subtypes in refugees and injection drug users in the United States determined by LiPA and monoclonal EIA. *J Med Virol* 2001;64:305–311.
7. Gunther S, Fischer L, Pult I, et al. Naturally occurring variants of hepatitis B virus. *Adv Viral Res* 1999;52:25–137.
8. Hannoun C, Horal P, Lindh M. Long-term mutation rates in the hepatitis B virus genome. *J Gen Virol* 2000;81:75–83.
9. Lauder IJ, Lin H-J, Lau JYN, et al. The variability of the hepatitis B virus genome: statistical analysis and biological implications. *Mol Biol Evol* 1993;10:457–470.
10. Tiollais P, Pourcel C, Dejean A. The hepatitis B virus. *Nature* 1985;317:489–495.
11. Prince DL, Prince HN, Thraenhart O, et al. Methodological approaches to disinfection of human hepatitis B virus. *J Clin Microbiol* 1993;31:3296–3304.
12. Carman WF, Zanetti AR, Karayiannis P, et al. Vaccine induced escape mutant of hepatitis B virus. *Lancet* 1990;326:325–329.
13. Huang H-L, Jeng K-S, Hu C-P, et al. Identification and characterization of a structural protein of hepatitis B virus: a polymerase and surface fusion protein encoded by a spliced RNA. *Virology* 2000;275:398–410.
14. Diepolder HM, Ries G, Jung MC, et al. Differential antigen-processing pathways of the hepatitis B e and core proteins. *Gastroenterology* 1999;116:650–657.
15. Milich DR, Jones JE, Hughes JL, et al. Is a function of the secreted hepatitis B e antigen to induce immunological tolerance in utero? *Proc Natl Acad Sci U S A* 1990;87:6599–6603.
16. Carlier D, Jean-Jean O, Fouillot N, et al. Importance of the C terminus of the hepatitis B virus precore protein in secretion of HBe antigen. *J Gen Virol* 1995;76:1041–1045.
17. Urban S, Urban S, Fischer KP, et al. Efficient pyrophosphorolysis by a hepatitis B virus polymerase may be a primer-unblocking mechanism. *Proc Natl Acad Sci U S A* 2001;98:4984–4989.
18. Madden CR, Finegold MJ, Slagle BL. Hepatitis B virus X protein acts as a tumor promoter in development of diethylnitrosamine-induced preneoplastic lesions. *J Virol* 2001;75:3851–3858.
19. Pan J, Duan L-X, Sun BS, et al. Hepatitis B virus X protein protects against anti–FAS-mediated apoptosis in human liver cells by inducing NF-κB. *J Gen Virol* 2001;82:171–182.
20. Hoare J, Henkler F, Dowling JJ, et al. Subcellular localisation of the X protein in HBV infected hepatocytes. *J Med Virol* 2001;64:419–426.
21. Yen TSB. Regulation of hepatitis B virus gene expression. *Semin Virol* 1993;4:33–42.
22. Ishida H, Ueda K, Ohkawa K, et al. Identification of multiple transcription factors, HLF, FTF, and E4BP4, controlling hepatitis B virus enhancer II. *J Virol* 2000;74:1241–1251.
23. Xie Y, Li M, Wang Y, et al. Site-specific mutation of the hepatitis B virus enhancer II B1 element: effect of virus transcription and replication. *J Gen Virol* 2001;82:531–535.
24. Kock J, Nassal M, MacNelly S, et al. Efficient infection of primary tupaia hepatocytes with purified human and woolly monkey hepatitis B virus. *J Virol* 2001;75:5084–5089.
25. Sprinzl MF, Oberwinkler H, Schaller H, et al. Transfer of hepatitis B virus genome by adenovirus vectors in cultured cells and mice: crossing the species barrier. *J Virol* 2001;75:5108–5118.
26. Tang H, McLachlan A. Transcriptional regulation of hepatitis B virus by nuclear hormone receptors is a critical determinant of viral tropism. *Proc Natl Acad Sci U S A* 2001;98:1841–1846.
27. Blackberg J, Kidd-Ljunggren K. Occult hepatitis B virus after acute self-limited infection persisting for 30 years without sequence variation. *J Hepatol* 2000;33:992–997.
28. Marasuwa H, Uemoto S, Hijikata M, et al. Latent hepatitis B virus infection in healthy individuals with antibodies to hepatitis B core antigen. *Hepatology* 2000;31:488–495.
29. Mason A, Wick M, White H, et al. Hepatitis B virus replication in diverse cell types during chronic hepatitis B virus infection. *Hepatology* 1993;18:781–789.
30. Ganem D, Varmus HE. The molecular biology of the hepatitis B virus. *Annu Rev Biochem* 1987;56:651–693.
31. Paterlini P, Poussin K, Kew M, et al. Selective accumulation of the X transcript of hepatitis B virus in patients negative for hepatitis B surface antigen with hepatocellular carcinoma. *Hepatology* 1995;21:313–321.
32. Kim CM, Koike K, Saito I, et al. HBx gene of hepatitis B virus induces liver cancer in transgenic mice. *Nature* 1991;351:317–320.

33. Rizzetto M, Canese MG, Arico S, et al. Immunofluorescence detection of new antigen-antibody system (delta/anti-delta) associated to hepatitis B virus in liver and serum of HBsAg carriers. *Gut* 1977;18:997–1003.

34. Taylor J, Mason W, Summers J, et al. Replication of human hepatitis delta virus in primary cultures of woodchuck hepatocytes. *J Virol* 1987;61:2891–2895.

35. Bas C, Bartolome J, La Banda F, et al. Assessment of hepatitis B virus DNA levels in chronic HBsAg carriers with or without hepatitis delta virus superinfection. *J Hepatol* 1988;6:208–213.

36. Ryu W-S, Netter HJ, Bayer M, et al. Ribonucleoprotein complexes of hepatitis delta virus. *J Virol* 1993;67:3281–3287.

37. Mu J-J, Wu H-L, Chiang B-L, et al. Characterization of the phosphorylated forms and the phosphorylated residues of hepatitis delta virus delta antigens. *J Virol* 1999;73:10540–10545.

38. Huang WH, Yung BY, Syu WJ, et al. The nucleolar phosphoprotein B23 interacts with hepatitis delta antigens and modulates the hepatitis delta virus RNA replication. *J Biol Chem* 2001;276:25166–25175.

39. Gudima S, Wu SY, Chiang CM, et al. Origin of hepatitis delta virus mRNA. *J Virol* 2000;74:7204–7210.

40. Shih KN, Lo SJ. The HDV large-delta antigen fused with gfp remains functional and provides for studying its dynamic distribution. *Virology* 2001;285:138–152.

41. Modahl LE, Lai MMC. The large delta antigen of hepatitis delta virus potently inhibits genomic but not antigenomic RNA synthesis: a mechanism enabling initiation of viral replication. *J Virol* 2000;74:7375–7380.

42. Goto T, Kato N, Ono-Nita SK, et al. Large isoform of hepatitis delta antigen activates serum response factor-associated transcription. *J Biol Chem* 2000;275:37311–37316.

43. Taylor JM. Hepatitis delta virus. *Intervirology* 1999;42:173–178.

44. Nishikawa F, Nishikawa S. Requirement for canonical base pairing in the short pseudoknot structure of genomic hepatitis delta virus ribozyme. *Nucleic Acids Res* 2000;28:925–931.

45. Tanner NK, Schaff S, Thill G, et al. A three-dimensional model of hepatitis delta virus ribozyme based on biochemical and mutational analyses. *Curr Biol* 1994;4:488–498.

46. Liu YT, Brazas R, Ganem D. Efficient hepatitis delta virus RNA replication in avian cells requires a permissive factor(s) from mammalian cells. *J Virol* 2001;75:7489–7493.

47. Yamaguchi Y, Filipovska J, Yano K, et al. Stimulation of RNA polymerase II elongation by hepatitis delta antigen. *Science* 2001;293:124–127.

48. Modahl LE, Macnaughton TB, Zhu N, et al. RNA-dependent replication and transcription of hepatitis delta virus RNA involve distinct cellular RNA polymerases. *Mol Cell Biol* 2000;20:6030–6039.

49. Diegelman AM, Kool ET. Mimicry of the hepatitis delta virus replication cycle mediated by synthetic circular oligodeoxynucleotides. *Chem Biol* 1999;6:569–576.

50. Wang D, Pearlberg J, Liu YT, et al. Deleterious effects of hepatitis delta virus replication on host cell proliferation. *J Virol* 2001;75:3600–3604.

51. Guilhot S, Huang S-N, Xia YP, et al. Expression of the hepatitis delta virus large and small antigens in transgenic mice. *J Virol* 1994;68:1052–1058.

52. Rizzetto M, Canese MG, Gerin JL, et al. Transmission of the hepatitis B virus–associated delta antigen to chimpanzees. *J Infect Dis* 1980;141:590–602.

CHAPTER 240
Poxviruses

Bernard Moss

The poxviruses constitute a large family of complex DNA viruses that are distinguished by their replication within the cytoplasm of infected cells (1,2). Of the nine poxviruses that have been associated with human disease, only variola virus and molluscum contagiosum virus (MCV) are specific for humans; the other infections are zoonoses (Table 240.1). The devastating effects of smallpox, caused by variola virus, and its successful eradication by immunization with vaccinia virus have been recorded in detail (3). Nevertheless, variola virus still exists in two registered laboratories and perhaps elsewhere. Because routine smallpox vaccination ceased more than 20 years ago, large populations are now susceptible to variola virus, and its reintroduction could have grave consequences. Cessation of vaccination also increased susceptibility to other orthopoxviruses. Of the latter, monkeypox virus is of greatest concern because it continues to cause a sporadic smallpox-like disease in humans of Central and West Africa (4). As a precautionary measure, the United States government has commissioned production of a new tissue culture–derived smallpox vaccine. Considerable efforts are also going into the development of recombinant vaccinia virus and avian poxviruses as live vaccines against other pathogenic microorganisms and cancer (5).

CHARACTERISTICS OF POXVIRUSES

Classification

Poxviruses are large double-stranded DNA viruses that replicate in the cytoplasm of infected cells (1). The vertebrate poxviruses have been placed into eight genera: *Avipoxvirus*, *Capripoxvirus*, *Leporipoxvirus*, *Molluscipoxvirus*, *Orthopoxvirus*, *Parapoxvirus*, *Suipoxvirus*, and *Yatapoxvirus* (6). Members of the same genus are antigenically and genetically related and have similar morphologies. Complete genome sequences have been obtained for the following chordopoxviruses: vaccinia virus (7,8), variola virus (9,10), molluscum contagiosum virus (11), myxoma virus (12), rabbit fibroma virus (13), lumpy skin disease virus (14), Yaba-like disease virus (15), and fowlpox virus (16). Many of the remaining species are likely to be sequenced in the near future.

Structure of the Virion

The infectious virus particles appear in electron microscopic images as oval or brick-shaped bodies between 200 and 400 nm long with a complex internal structure (17,18). Thin sections of vertebrate poxviruses reveal a characteristic biconcave core flanked by lateral bodies. Intracellular mature virions (IMVs) have two closely opposed membranes that may be derived from the endoplasmic reticulum or intermediate cellular compartment (18), although this has been debated (19). Some of the IMVs become wrapped by additional membranes derived from the Golgi network (Fig. 240.1) and are called intracellular enveloped virions (IEVs) (20,21). The extracellular enveloped virions (EEVs) lose the outer of the two IEV membranes during their exit from the cell. All three forms—IMVs, IEVs and EEVs—are infectious.

Biochemical Components of the Virion

DNA, packaged within the virus core, consists of a linear duplex molecule with a hairpin loop at each end connecting the strands

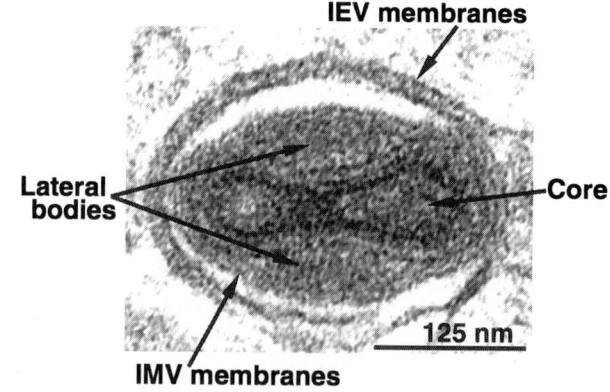

Figure 240.1. Electron micrograph of a thin-sectioned infected cell showing an intracellular enveloped vaccinia virus particle. (Kindly provided by A. Weisberg.)

TABLE 240.1. Poxviruses That Cause Human Disease

Genus	Disease	Common names and characteristics of diseases
Orthopoxvirus	Variola	Smallpox; systemic; general rash; extinct
	Monkeypox	Systemic; general rash; rare zoonosis
	Vaccinia	Smallpox vaccine; local skin lesion
	Cowpox	Local skin lesion; rare zoonosis
Parapoxvirus	Orf	Local skin lesion; rare zoonosis
	Paravaccinia	Milker's nodules; rare zoonosis
Yatapoxvirus	Tanapox	Local skin lesion; rare zoonosis
	Yabapox	Local skin lesion; rare accidental infection
Molluscipoxvirus	Molluscum contagiosum	Multiple skin lesions; human transmission

(22,23). Identical sequences with inverted orientations, usually containing blocks of short repeats and a few or no genes, are present at the two ends of the genome (24,25). Most of the DNA consists of closely spaced protein coding regions separated by transcriptional regulatory sequences. The essential genes map within the conserved central region of the genome, whereas many of those dispensable for replication in tissue culture are nearer the ends (1).

Proteins constitute 90% of the dry weight of vaccinia virions, and more than 100 polypeptides have been resolved by two-dimensional polyacrylamide gel electrophoresis (26). In addition to structural proteins, more than a dozen enzymes are packaged in the virion (1). Many of these, including a DNA-dependent RNA polymerase, capping and methylating enzymes, and poly(A) polymerase, are involved in messenger RNA (mRNA) synthesis. The IMV and EEV surface membranes contain at least 12 and 5 unique polypeptides, respectively.

Lipids, mostly cholesterol and phospholipids, account for about 3% of the dry weight of vaccinia virus (27–29). Fowlpox virus, however, has a much higher amount of lipid, including squalene and cholesterol esters (30).

VIRUS REPLICATION

Most of the detailed information regarding replication has been obtained with orthopoxviruses, especially vaccinia virus. Nevertheless, the main features are likely to be conserved among all members of the family.

Virus Entry

Little is know about how poxviruses enter cells, and both conventional membrane fusion (31) and unspecified nonfusion (32) mechanisms have been proposed. Heparin- and chondroitin-binding proteins of IMVs may contribute to cell attachment (33–35). Because IMVs and EEVs have unique surface proteins, they presumably use different cellular receptors (36). Antibodies to the L1R (37), A27L (38), and H3L (34) IMV proteins are neutralizing, suggesting that the latter are involved in cell attachment or penetration. Antibodies to the B5R and A33R EEV proteins were protective in animal models, though only the former were neutralizing (39).

Uncoating

The release of the core into the cytoplasm, constituting the first stage of uncoating, requires neither RNA nor protein synthesis (40). The second stage of uncoating, resulting in the susceptibility

of the genome to DNase, begins within 2 hours after infection and is dependent on viral RNA and protein synthesis. Neither of these steps are well defined.

Prereplicative Gene Expression

Expression of the poxvirus genome is regulated by a cascade mechanism that is divided into prereplicative (early) and postreplicative (intermediate and late) phases (41) (Fig. 240.2). Regulation occurs primarily at the transcriptional level, and early-, intermediate-, and late-stage genes have distinctive promoter sequences (42–44).

Transcription of the early genes occurs soon after virus entry, coincident with the first stage of uncoating, by enzymes packaged in the virus core (45,46). The viral DNA-dependent RNA polymerase resembles its eukaryotic counterpart with regard to the number of subunits, of which the two largest are homologous (47). An additional RNA polymerase-associated polypeptide, RAP94 (48), and a heterodimeric protein known as vaccinia virus early transcription factor (49,50) provide specificity for transcription of early genes. This transcription factor binds to vaccinia virus early promoters, which are approximately 30 base pairs in length (42,51). The sequence UUUUUNU, in which N can be any nucleotide, in the nascent RNA signals termination about 50 nucleotides downstream (52,53) in conjunction with at least two virus-coded proteins (54,55). The enzymes that cap (56), methylate (56,57), and polyadenylylate (58) viral mRNAs are also virus encoded (59–62). Some enzymes have multiple functions. For example, the capping enzyme also methylates the guanosine cap (56), and is an early transcription termination factor (54) and an intermediate transcription factor (63). A second RNA methyltransferase is also a subunit of the poly(A) polymerase (62). The steps in initiation, elongation, and termination have been partially elucidated (64–66).

Postreplicative Gene Expression

Intermediate and late gene expression occur after initiation of viral DNA replication. The intermediate and late mRNAs can be distinguished from the majority of early mRNAs by their heterogeneous length and presence of a 5' capped poly(A) leader of unknown function (41,67–69). The enzymes and factors needed for intermediate transcription are synthesized early after infection (70,71). At least three virus-encoded proteins, namely RNA polymerase, capping enzyme, and an intermediate transcription factor (63,72), and one cellular protein (73) are required for transcription of intermediate genes. The promoters recognized by the intermediate factors are similar in length but differ in sequence from early promoters (44).

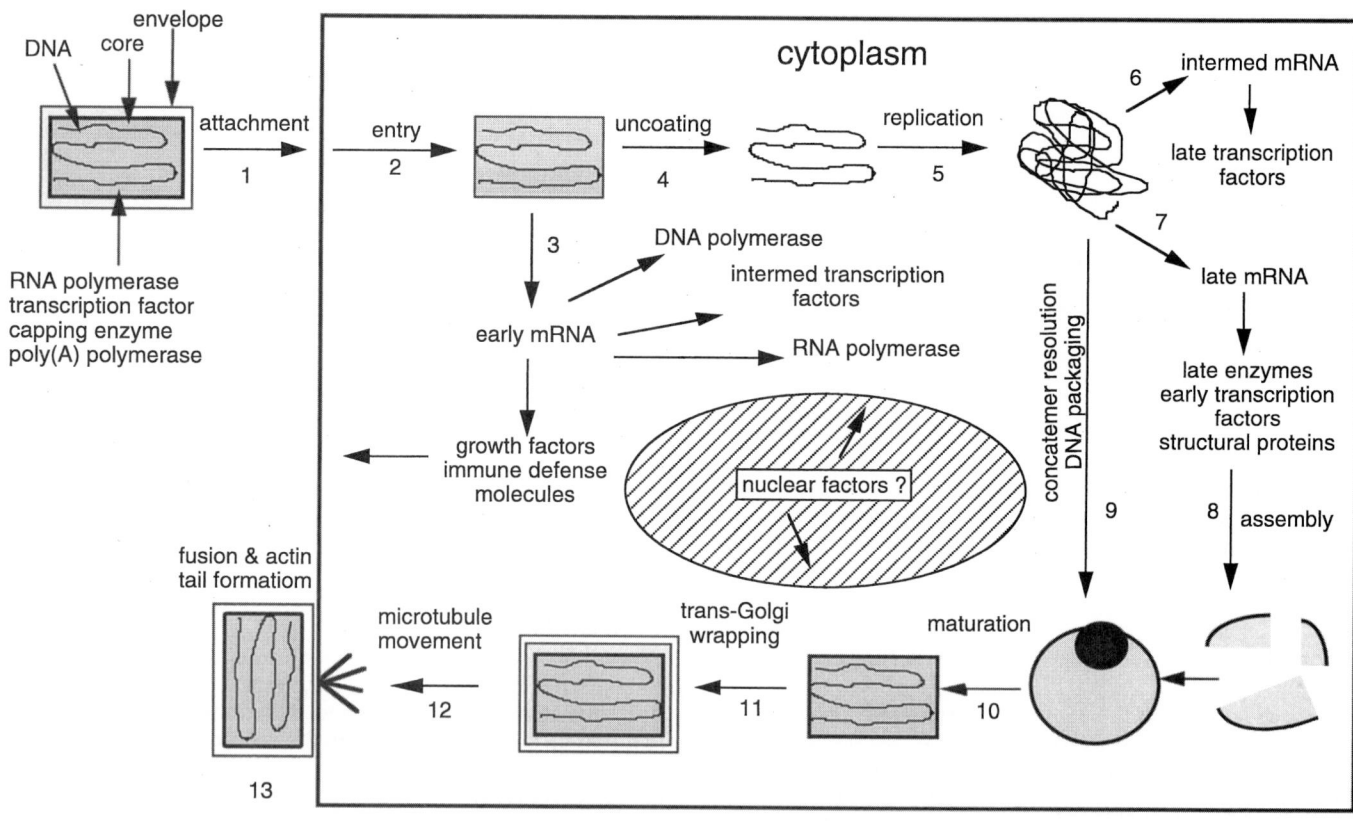

Figure 240.2. Outline of the replication cycle of an orthopoxvirus. Virions, containing a double-stranded DNA genome, enzymes, and transcription factors, attach to cells (*1*) and fuse with the cell membrane, releasing cores into the cytoplasm (*2*). The cores synthesize early messenger RNAs that are translated into a variety of proteins, including growth factors, immune defense molecules, enzymes, and factors for DNA replication and intermediate transcription (*3*). Uncoating occurs (*4*), and the DNA is replicated to form concatemeric molecules (*5*). Intermediate genes in the progeny DNA are transcribed and the messenger RNAs are translated to form late transcription factors (*6*). The late genes are transcribed and the messenger RNAs are translated to form virion structural proteins, enzymes, and early transcription factors (*7*). Assembly begins with the formation of discrete membrane structures (*8*). The concatemeric DNA intermediates are resolved into unit genomes and packaged in immature virions (*9*). Maturation proceeds to the formation of infectious intracellular mature virions (*10*). The virions are wrapped by modified Golgi membranes (*11*) and transported via microtubules to the periphery of the cell (*12*). Fusion of the wrapped virions with the plasma membrane results in release of extracellular enveloped virus (*13*). Although replication occurs entirely in the cytoplasm, nuclear factors may be involved in transcription and assembly. (From Moss B. Poxviridae: the viruses and their replication. In: Knipe DM, Howley PM, eds. *Fields virology*, 4th ed. Vol. 2. Philadelphia: Lippincott Williams & Wilkins, 2001:2849–2883, with permission.)

Three viral intermediate genes encode transcription factors for late genes (71). These and an additional cellular protein can reconstitute transcription *in vitro* (74). Additional viral proteins appear to stimulate RNA initiation, elongation, or transcript release (75–78). Late promoters differ in sequence from both early and intermediate promoters (43). However, both intermediate and late promoters have an AAA triplet at the transcriptional start site, which accounts for the generation of a novel 5' poly(A) leader by slippage of the RNA polymerase (44,79). The AAA sequence is occasionally found at the initiation site of early genes and then also leads to formation of a poly(A) leader (80,81). The early transcription termination signal is not recognized during transcription of either intermediate or late genes, resulting in RNAs of heterogeneous length. However, the ends of some late transcripts are formed by cleavage (82).

DNA Replication

Poxvirus DNA is replicated in the cytoplasm by a virus-encoded polymerase (83,84) and at least three additional proteins: a nu-

cleic acid-independent nucleoside triphosphatase (85), a serine/threonine protein kinase (86), a uracil DNA glycosylase (87,88), and a protein encoded by the A20R open reading frame (89,90). During replication, concatemeric DNA structures are formed (91,92) and resolved into unit-size genomes by a site-specific mechanism (93,94) that requires one or more late viral proteins (95,96). A topoisomerase (97) and a Holliday junction resolvase (98,99) have been proposed as concatemer resolving enzymes.

Virus Assembly

Electron microscopic images suggest a sequence of developmental events (Fig. 240.2) that begins in circumscribed granular regions of the cytoplasm with the formation of spicule-covered crescent membranes within which a dense nucleoprotein mass forms and undergoes internal differentiation (18,29,100–102). Morphogenesis involves proteolytic cleavages (103,104) and the formation of disulfide bonds (105) by a novel cytoplasmic pathway (106). The resulting infectious IMVs can be efficiently released only by cell lysis. As the IMVs move out of the assembly areas, some are enveloped by trans-Golgi or endosomal cisternae (20,21) and transported via microtubules to the cell periphery where budding through the plasma membrane occurs (107–109). Two viral proteins are known to be required for the wrapping step: one is palmitylated and contains an essential phospholipase motif (110,111); the other is a glycosylated type 1 integral membrane protein (112,113). Many of the extracellular virions remain associated with the cell membrane and have been called cell-associated enveloped virions (CEVs) (114). Some of the CEVs acquire actin tails and are propelled at the tips of long microvilli to enhance infection of neighboring cells. Three proteins, encoded by the A33R, A34R, and A36R genes, are required for actin tail formation (115–118). The nucleation of actin tails is dependent on tyrosine phosphorylation of the A36R protein and is mediated by cellular proteins (119). Although CEVs mediate cell-to-cell spread, released extracellular-associated virions (EEVs) may be important for long-range virus spread within the host (120). The virions of certain poxviruses, such as cowpox virus, become embedded in dense occlusions, which may protect them from the environment (121,122).

IMMUNE DEFENSE MECHANISMS

Poxviruses are not known to have a latent phase, although some, such as MCV, persist for many months. Instead, poxviruses encode a variety of proteins that suppress or subvert the immune response. These immune defense proteins, some of which are cellular homologs, protect against the actions of complement, interferons, tumor necrosis factor, numerous cytokines, and inducers of apoptosis (123,124).

EPIDEMIOLOGY

Although at least nine poxviruses can cause disease, human-to-human transmission is uncommon except with variola virus and MCV. Variola virus spreads primarily by direct transfer of infective droplets to the oropharyngeal or respiratory mucosa (3). Less commonly, spread was from scabs or fomites. The absence of natural new cases of smallpox during the past two decades confirms the lack of environmental or animal reservoirs of variola virus.

Vaccinia virus is normally transmitted by vaccination, but spread by direct contact to secondary sites on the vaccinee or to others occurs occasionally. Buffalopox in India appears to be an endemic infection of buffalo, caused by subspecies of vaccinia virus that can be transmitted to milkers (125). Transmission of vaccinia virus from cattle to humans has been reported in Brazil (126).

MCV causes benign skin tumors in humans but has not been reliably isolated from other species or propagated in tissue culture or laboratory animals (127,128), although there are reports of minimal replication in human skin grafts in immunodeficient mice (129,130). The disease occurs worldwide, including the United States, and the genital form appears to be increasing in incidence. A survey in Australia revealed that 23% of the general population is seropositive, probably a low estimate of past infection since not even all with active infections were seropositive. The lowest antibody prevalence was in children 6 months to 2 years of age (3%), and seropositivity increased with age to reach 39% in persons greater than or equal to 50 years of age. These findings indicate that subclinical MCV infections are more common in the general community than pre-

viously suspected (131). MCV appears to spread by direct contact (132). Analysis of the genome by restriction endonuclease analysis indicated two major and at least one minor clinically indistinguishable variant (133–138). MVC infections are common in patients with acquired immunodeficiency syndrome, and type II MCV infection may be proportionally higher than in the general population (139).

Human monkeypox, a disease clinically resembling smallpox, was discovered in tropical rainforest areas of central and western Africa during the smallpox eradication campaign (140). Monkeypox virus has been isolated from chimpanzees and several species of monkeys and squirrels, although the latter are considered the most important reservoir. Human infections occur sporadically and affect mainly children in remote villages whose population has frequent wild animal contacts. Usually, single cases occur but the virus can be transmitted with low frequency from human to human. From 1970 to 1995, 388 of the 418 cases of human monkeypox recorded occurred in Zaire (now the Democratic Republic of the Congo) (141). The number of suspected cases exceeded 500 in 1996 and 1997, and the Congo health authorities reported several hundred new cases in January 1999 (4). Because smallpox vaccination provided protection against monkeypox, there is concern of increasing human susceptibility.

Although human cowpox infection can occur by milking of cows, bovine cowpox is uncommon. Cowpox virus has been isolated from cats and zoo animals, but rodents are thought to be the principal reservoir in Europe and Asia (142,143). Domestic cats are frequently implicated in human transmission (144,145).

Parapoxviruses infect domesticated animals, including sheep, goats, cattle, and camels; humans are infected through skin abrasions. The skin disease acquired from sheep or goats is called orf, and that from cows is called milker's nodules, paravaccinia, or pseudocowpox (146–148).

Tanapox virus, Yaba monkey tumor poxvirus, and Yaba disease–like virus belong to the genus *Yatapoxvirus*. Epidemics of human tanapox occurred in 1957 and 1962 among people living in the flood plain of the Tana River in Kenya (149). Many cases were seen in Zaire (now the Democratic Republic of the Congo) (150) and the disease probably occurs throughout tropical Africa. Monkeys are infected, and there have been tanapox epizootics in primate centers in the United States (151). The reservoir species for tanapox virus is not known, but arthropods may act as mechanical vectors for transmission. Yabapox virus was isolated from captive rhesus monkeys in Nigeria; humans have been infected only accidentally (152).

CLINICAL SYMPTOMS AND PATHOGENESIS

Variola and monkeypox viruses are the only poxviruses that regularly cause an acute systemic infection with a generalized rash in humans (3). Other poxviruses generally produce local ulcerative or proliferative skin lesions. Tanapox may present as an acute febrile illness associated with localized skin nodules (150). Yabapox virus produces subcutaneous tumors in primates (153). Cowpox occurs most frequently on the hands; the lesions resemble those produced by a primary smallpox vaccination and may be accompanied by lymphangitis, lymphadenitis, and fever (154). Milker's nodules, caused by parapoxvirus, are usually small indolent papules on the hands. The proliferative umbilicated skin lesions produced by orf frequently ulcerate before healing (155). In molluscum contagiosum, firm, raised, flesh-colored nodules about 2 to 5 mm in diameter may occur singly or in clusters (156). The lesions may occur anywhere on the body, but infrequently on the hands or soles, and may persist for months and years with little inflammatory reaction. The virus grows only in the epidermis, and no systemic spread occurs even when there is an immunodeficiency.

The importance of cell-mediated immunity in the control of orthopoxvirus infection in humans was demonstrated by the progressive spread of vaccinia virus in infants and children who suffered from such deficiencies (157,158). By contrast, children with specific defects in antibody production usually reacted normally to vaccination.

DIAGNOSIS

Poxvirus infection is usually suggested by the characteristic proliferative or ulcerative skin lesions and the clinical history. Confirmation can be obtained by biopsy, electron microscopy of negatively stained material from scabs or vesicular fluid, detection of viral antigen, or virus isolation except in the case of MCV. Differentiation between poxviruses has been made on the basis of biologic properties, specific serologic tests, or DNA analysis (159–165). Additional rapid diagnostic tests are under development.

PREVENTION AND TREATMENT

Variola virus was eradicated by inoculation with infectious vaccinia virus (3) which can elicit both humoral and cellular immunity. Laboratory studies indicated that inactivated virus failed to elicit antibodies that neutralized extracellular enveloped virions and gave lower levels of protection (166,167). Inactivated vaccines were not used for prevention of smallpox. Vaccinia immune globulin, however, provided some protection when given during the incubation period and was beneficial for the treatment of vaccine complications. Recent studies have demonstrated that DNA vaccines can protect mice against vaccinia virus (168). Methisazone (N-methylisatin β-thiosemicarbazone) was not effective in treating smallpox but probably had a beneficial effect when given prophylactically (3,169). A variety of other compounds, cidofovir in particular, show promise as chemotherapeutic agents against poxviruses (170,171).

REFERENCES

1. Moss B. Poxviridae: the viruses and their replication. In: Knipe DM, Howley PM, eds. *Fields virology.* Philadelphia: Lippincott Williams & Wilkins, 2001:2849–2883.
2. Esposito LJ, Fenner F. Poxviruses. In: Knipe DM, Howley PM, eds. *Fields virology.* Philadelphia: Lippincott Williams & Wilkins, 2001:2885–2921.
3. Fenner F, Henderson DA, Arita I, et al. *Smallpox and its eradication.* Geneva: World Health Organization, 1988.
4. Breman JG. Monkeypox: an emerging infection of humans? In: Scheid WM, Craig WA, Hughes JM, eds. *Emerging infections.* Washington, DC: ASM Press, 2000:45–67.
5. Moss B. Genetically engineered poxviruses for recombinant gene expression, vaccination, and safety. *Proc Natl Acad Sci U S A* 1996;93:11341–11348.
6. Murphy FA, Fauquet CM, Bishop DHL, et al. Virus taxonomy. Classification and nomenclature of viruses. *Arch Virol* 1995;(suppl 10):1–586.
7. Goebel SJ, Johnson GP, Perkus ME, et al. The complete DNA sequence of vaccinia virus. *Virology* 1990;179:247–266, 517–563.
8. Antoine G, Scheiflinger F, Dorner F, et al. The complete genomic sequence of the modified vaccinia virus Ankara strain: comparison with other orthopoxviruses. *Virology* 1998;244:365–396.
9. Massung RF, Liu L-I, Qi J, et al. Analysis of the complete genome of smallpox Variola major virus strain Bangladesh-1975. *Virology* 1994;201:215–240.
10. Shchelkunov SN, Massung RF, Esposito JJ. Comparison of the genome DNA sequences of Bangladesh-1975 and India-1967 variola viruses. *Virus Res* 1995;36:107–118.
11. Senkevich TG, Koonin EV, Bugert JJ, et al. The genome of molluscum contagiosum virus: analysis and comparison with other poxviruses. *Virology* 1997;233:19–42.
12. Cameron C, Hota-Mitchell S, Chen L, et al. The complete DNA sequence of myxoma virus. *Virology* 1999;264:298–318.
13. Willer DO, McFadden G, Evans DH. The complete genome sequence of Shope (rabbit) fibroma virus. *Virology* 1999;264:319–343.
14. Tulman ER, Afonso CL, Lu Z, et al. Genome of lumpy skin disease virus. *J Virol* 2001;75:7122–7130.
15. Lee HJ, Essani K, Smith GL. The genome sequence of Yaba-like disease virus, a yatapoxvirus. *Virology* 2001;281:170–192.
16. Afonso CL, Tulman ER, Lu Z, et al. The genome of fowlpox virus. *J Virol* 2000;74:3815–3831.
17. Griffiths G, Wepf R, Wendt T, et al. Structure and assembly of intracellular mature vaccinia virus: isolated-particle analysis. *J Virol* 2001;75:11034–11055.
18. Griffiths G, Roos N, Schleich S, et al. Structure and assembly of intracellular mature vaccinia virus: thin-section analyses. *J Virol* 2001;75:11056–11070.
19. Hollinshead M, Vanderplasschen A, Smith GL, et al. Vaccinia virus intracellular mature virions contain only one lipid membrane. *J Virol* 1999;73:1503–1517.
20. Hiller G, Weber K. Golgi-derived membranes that contain an acylated viral polypeptide are used for vaccinia virus envelopment. *J Virol* 1985;55:651–659.
21. Schmelz M, Sodeik B, Ericsson M, et al. Assembly of vaccinia virus: the second wrapping cisterna is derived from the trans Golgi network. *J Virol* 1994;68:130–147.
22. Geshelin P, Berns KI. Characterization and localization of the naturally occurring cross-links in vaccinia virus DNA. *J Mol Biol* 1974;88:785–796.
23. Baroudy BM, Venkatesan S, Moss B. Incompletely base-paired flip-flop terminal loops link the two DNA strands of the vaccinia virus genome into one uninterrupted polynucleotide chain. *Cell* 1982;28:315–324.
24. Garon CF, Barbosa E, Moss B. Visualization of an inverted terminal repetition in vaccinia virus DNA. *Proc Natl Acad Sci U S A* 1978;75:4863–4867.
25. Wittek R, Moss B. Tandem repeats within the inverted terminal repetition of vaccinia virus DNA. *Cell* 1980;21:277–284.
26. Essani K, Dales S. Biogenesis of vaccinia: evidence for more than 100 polypeptides in the virion. *Virology* 1979;95:385–394.
27. Stern W, Dales S. Biogenesis of vaccinia: concerning the origin of the envelope phospholipids. *Virology* 1974;62:293–306.
28. Hiller G, Eibl H, Weber K. Acyl bis(monoacylglycero)phosphate, assumed to be a marker for lysosomes is a major phospholipid of vaccinia virus. *Virology* 1981;113:761–764.
29. Sodeik B, Doms RW, Ericsson M, et al. Assembly of vaccinia virus: role of the intermediate compartment between the endoplasmic reticulum and the Golgi stacks. *J Cell Biol* 1993;121:521–541.
30. Lyles DS, Randall CC, Gafford LG, et al. Cellular fatty acids during fowlpox virus infection of three different host systems. *Virology* 1976;70:227–229.
31. Doms RW, Blumenthal R, Moss B. Fusion of intra- and extracellular forms of vaccinia virus with the cell membrane. *J Virol* 1990;64:4884–4892.
32. Locker JK, Kuehn A, Schleich S, et al. Entry of the two infectious forms of vaccinia virus at the plasma membrane is signaling-dependent for the IMV but not the EEV. *Mol Biol Cell* 2000;11:2497–2511.
33. Chung C-S, Hsiao J-C, Chang Y-S, et al. A27L protein mediates vaccinia virus interaction with cell surface heparin sulfate. *J Virol* 1998;72:1577–1585.
34. Lin CL, Chung CS, Heine HG, et al. Vaccinia virus envelope H3L protein binds to cell surface heparan sulfate and is important for intracellular mature virion morphogenesis and virus infection *in vitro* and *in vivo. J Virol* 2000;74:3353–3365.
35. Hsiao JC, Chung CS, Chang W. Vaccinia virus envelope D8L protein binds to cell surface chondroitin sulfate and mediates the adsorption of intracellular mature virions to cells. *J Virol* 1999;73:8750–8761.
36. Vanderplasschen A, Smith GL. A novel virus binding assay using confocal microscopy: demonstration that intracellular and extracellular vaccinia virions bind to different cellular receptors. *J Virol* 1997;71:4032–4041.
37. Wolffe EJ, Vijaya S, Moss B. A myristylated membrane protein encoded by the vaccinia virus L1R open reading frame is the target of potent neutralizing monoclonal antibodies. *Virology* 1995;211:53–63.
38. Rodriguez JF, Esteban M. Mapping and nucleotide sequence of the vaccinia virus gene that encodes a 14-kilodalton fusion protein. *J Virol* 1987;61:3550–3554.
39. Galmiche MC, Goenaga J, Wittek R, et al. Neutralizing and protective antibodies directed against vaccinia virus envelope antigens. *Virology* 1999;254:71–80.
40. Joklik WK. The intracellular uncoating of poxvirus DNA. I. The fate of radioactively-labeled rabbitpox virus. *J Mol Biol* 1964;8:263–276.
41. Baldick CJ Jr, Moss B. Characterization and temporal regulation of mRNAs encoded by vaccinia virus intermediate stage genes. *J Virol* 1993;67:3515–3527.
42. Davison AJ, Moss B. The structure of vaccinia virus early promoters. *J Mol Biol* 1989;210:749–769.
43. Davison AJ, Moss B. The structure of vaccinia virus late promoters. *J Mol Biol* 1989;210:771–784.
44. Baldick CJ, Keck JG, Moss B. Mutational analysis of the core, spacer and

initiator regions of vaccinia virus intermediate class promoters. *J Virol* 1992;66:4710–4719.

45. Kates JR, McAuslan BR. Poxvirus DNA-dependent RNA polymerase. *Proc Natl Acad Sci U S A* 1967;58:134–141.

46. Munyon WE, Paoletti E, Grace JT Jr. RNA polymerase activity in purified infectious vaccinia virus. *Proc Natl Acad Sci U S A* 1967;58:2280–2288.

47. Moss B, Ahn BY, Amegadzie B, et al. Cytoplasmic transcription system encoded by vaccinia virus. *J Biol Chem* 1991;266:1355–1358.

48. Ahn B-Y, Moss B. RNA polymerase-associated transcription specificity factor encoded by vaccinia virus. *Proc Natl Acad Sci U S A* 1992;89:3536–3540.

49. Broyles SS, Yuen L, Shuman S, et al. Purification of a factor required for transcription of vaccinia virus early genes. *J Biol Chem* 1988;263:10754–10760.

50. Gershon PD, Moss B. Early transcription factor subunits are encoded by vaccinia virus late genes. *Proc Natl Acad Sci U S A* 1990;87:4401–4405.

51. Cassetti MC, Moss B. Interaction of the 82-kDa subunit of the vaccinia virus early transcription factor heterodimer with the promoter core sequence directs downstream DNA binding of the 70-kDa subunit. *Proc Natl Acad Sci U S A* 1996;93:7540–7545.

52. Yuen L, Moss B. Oligonucleotide sequence signaling transcriptional termination of vaccinia virus early genes. *Proc Natl Acad Sci U S A* 1987;84:6417–6421.

53. Shuman S, Moss B. Bromouridine triphosphate inhibits transcription termination and mRNA release by vaccinia virions. *J Biol Chem* 1989;264:21356–21360.

54. Shuman S, Broyles SS, and Moss B. Purification and characterization of a transcription termination factor from vaccinia virions. *J Biol Chem* 1987;262:12372–12380.

55. Deng L, Shuman S. Vaccinia NPH-I, a DExH-box ATPase, is the energy coupling factor for mRNA transcription termination. *Genes Dev* 1998;12:538–546.

56. Martin SA, Paoletti E, Moss B. Purification of mRNA guanylyltransferase and mRNA (guanine 7-)methyltransferase from vaccinia virus. *J Biol Chem* 1975;250:9322–9329.

57. Barbosa E, Moss B. mRNA (nucleoside-2′-)-methyltransferase from vaccinia virus. Purification and physical properties. *J Biol Chem* 1978;253:7692–7697.

58. Moss B, Rosenblum EN, Paoletti E. Polyadenylate polymerase from vaccinia virions. *Nature (New Biol)* 1973;245:59–63.

59. Morgan JR, Cohen LK, Roberts BE. Identification of the DNA sequences encoding the large subunit of the mRNA capping enzyme of vaccinia virus. *J Virol* 1984;52:206–214.

60. Niles EG, Lee-Chen G-J, Shuman S, et al. Vaccinia virus gene D12L encodes the small subunit of the viral mRNA capping enzyme. *Virology* 1989;172:513–522.

61. Gershon PD, Ahn BY, Garfield M, et al. Poly(A) polymerase and a dissociable polyadenylation stimulatory factor encoded by vaccinia virus. *Cell* 1991;66:1269–1278.

62. Schnierle BS, Gershon PD, Moss B. Cap-specific mRNA (nucleoside-O$^{2'}$-)-methyltransferase and poly(A) polymerase stimulatory activities of vaccinia virus are mediated by a single protein. *Proc Natl Acad Sci U S A* 1992;89:2897–2901.

63. Vos JC, Sasker M, Stunnenberg HG. Vaccinia virus capping enzyme is a transcription initiation factor. *EMBO J* 1991;10:2553–2558.

64. Baldick CJ, Cassetti MC, Harris N, et al. Ordered assembly of a functional preinitiation transcription complex, containing vaccinia virus early transcription factor and RNA polymerase, on an immobilized template. *J Virol* 1994;68:6052–6056.

65. Hagler J, Shuman S. A freeze-frame view of eukaryotic transcription during elongation and capping of nascent mRNA. *Science* 1992;255:983–986.

66. Li J, Broyles SS. The DNA-dependent ATPase activity of vaccinia virus early gene transcription factor is essential for its transcription activation function. *J Biol Chem* 1993;268:20016–20021.

67. Schwer B, Visca P, Vos JC, et al. Discontinuous transcription or RNA processing of vaccinia virus late messengers results in a 5′ poly(A) leader. *Cell* 1987;50:163–169.

68. Bertholet C, Van Meir E, ten Heggeler-Bordier B, et al. Vaccinia virus produces late mRNAs by discontinuous synthesis. *Cell* 1987;50:153–162.

69. Ahn B-Y, Moss B. Capped poly(A) leader of variable lengths at the 5′ ends of vaccinia virus late mRNAs. *J Virol* 1989;63:226–232.

70. Vos JC, Stunnenberg HG. Derepression of a novel class of vaccinia virus genes upon DNA replication. *EMBO J* 1988;7:3487–3492.

71. Keck JG, Baldick CJ, Moss B. Role of DNA replication in vaccinia virus gene expression: a naked template is required for transcription of three late transactivator genes. *Cell* 1990;61:801–809.

72. Sanz P, Moss B. Identification of a transcription factor, encoded by two vaccinia virus early genes, that regulates the intermediate stage of viral gene expression. *Proc Natl Acad Sci U S A* 1999;96:2692–2697.

73. Rosales R, Sutter G, Moss B. A cellular factor is required for transcription of vaccinia viral intermediate stage genes. *Proc Natl Acad Sci U S A* 1994;91:3794–3798.

74. Wright CF, Oswald BW, Dellis S. Vaccinia virus late transcription is activated *in vitro* by cellular heterogeneous nuclear ribonucleoproteins. *J Biol Chem* 2001;276:40680–40686.

75. Kovacs GR, Rosales R, Keck JG, et al. Modulation of the cascade model for regulation of vaccinia virus gene expression: purification of a prereplicative, late-stage-specific transcription factor. *J Virol* 1994;68:3443–3447.

76. Black EP, Condit RC. Phenotypic characterization of mutants in vaccinia virus gene G2R, a putative transcription elongation factor. *J Virol* 1996;70:47–54.

77. Lackner CA, Condit RC. Vaccinia virus gene A18R DNA helicase is a transcript release factor. *J Biol Chem* 2000;275:1485–1494.

78. Xiang Y, Latner DR, Niles EG, et al. Transcription elongation activity of the vaccinia virus J3 protein *in vivo* is independent of poly(A) polymerase stimulation. *Virology* 2000;269:356–369.

79. Stunnenberg HG, de Magistris L, Schwer B. The generation of poly(A) heads on vaccinia late mRNA: a proposal of a slippage mechanism. In: Cech TR, ed. *Molecular biology of RNA.* New York: Alan R Liss, 1989:199–208.

80. Ink BS, Pickup DJ. Vaccinia virus directs the synthesis of early mRNAs containing 5′ poly(A) sequences. *Proc Natl Acad Sci U S A* 1990;87:1536–1540.

81. Ahn B-Y, Jones EV, Moss B. Identification of the vaccinia virus gene encoding an 18-kilodalton subunit of RNA polymerase and demonstration of a 5′ poly(A) leader on its early transcript. *J Virol* 1990;64:3019–3024.

82. Antczak JB, Patel DD, Ray CA, et al. Site-specific RNA cleavage generates the 3′ end of a poxvirus late mRNA. *Proc Natl Acad Sci U S A* 1992;89:12033–12037.

83. Earl PL, Jones EV, Moss B. Homology between DNA polymerases of poxviruses, herpesviruses, and adenoviruses: nucleotide sequence of the vaccinia virus DNA polymerase gene. *Proc Natl Acad Sci U S A* 1986;83:3659–3663.

84. Traktman P. Molecular genetic and biochemical analysis of poxvirus DNA replication. *Semin Virol* 1991;2:291–304.

85. Evans E, Klemperer N, Ghosh R, et al. The vaccinia virus D5 protein, which is required for DNA replication, is a nucleic acid-independent nucleotide triphosphatase. *J Virol* 1995;69:5353–5361.

86. Rempel RE, Traktman P. Vaccinia virus–B1 kinase–phenotypic analysis of temperature-sensitive mutants and enzymatic characterization of recombinant proteins. *J Virol* 1992;66:4413–4426.

87. Millns AK, Carpenter MS, DeLange AM. The vaccinia virus–encoded uracil DNA glycosylase has an essential role in viral DNA replication. *Virology* 1994;198:504–513.

88. Stuart DT, Upton C, Higman MA, et al. A poxvirus-encoded uracil DNA glycosylase is essential for virus viability. *J Virol* 1993;67:2503–2512.

89. Ishii K, Moss B. Role of vaccinia virus A20R protein in DNA replication: construction and characterization of temperature-sensitive mutants. *J Virol* 2001;75:1656–1663.

90. Klemperer N, McDonald W, Boyle K, et al. The A20R protein is a stoichiometric component of the processive form of vaccinia virus DNA polymerase. *J Virol* 2001;75:12298–12307.

91. Moyer RW, Graves RL. The mechanism of cytoplasmic orthopoxvirus DNA replication. *Cell* 1981;27:391–401.

92. Merchlinsky M, Garon C, Moss B. Molecular cloning and sequence of the concatemer junction from vaccinia virus replicative DNA: viral nuclease cleavage sites in cruciform structures. *J Mol Biol* 1988;199:399–413.

93. Merchlinsky M, Moss B. Resolution of linear minichromosomes with hairpin ends from circular plasmids containing vaccinia virus concatemer junctions. *Cell* 1986;45:879–884.

94. DeLange AM, McFadden G. Efficient resolution of replicated poxvirus telomeres to native hairpin structures requires two inverted symmetrical copies of a core target DNA sequence. *J Virol* 1987;61:1957–1963.

95. Merchlinsky M, Moss B. Resolution of vaccinia virus DNA concatemer junctions requires late gene expression. *J Virol* 1989;63:1595–1603.

96. DeLange AM. Identification of temperature-sensitive mutants of vaccinia virus that are defective in conversion of concatemeric replicative intermediates to the mature linear DNA genome. *J Virol* 1989;63:2437–2444.

97. Sekiguchi J, Cheng C, Shuman S. Resolution of a Holliday junction by vaccinia topoisomerase requires a spacer DNA segment 3′ of the CCCTT downward arrow cleavage sites. *Nucleic Acids Res* 2000;28:2658–2663.

98. Garcia AD, Aravind L, Koonin EV, et al. Bacterial-type DNA Holliday junction resolvases in eukaryotic viruses. *Proc Natl Acad Sci U S A* 2000;97:8926–8931.

99. Garcia AD, Moss B. Repression of vaccinia virus Holliday junction resolvase inhibits processing of viral DNA into unit-length genomes. *J Virol* 2001;75:6460–6471.

100. Dales S, Pogo BGT. *Biology of poxviruses.* New York: Springer-Verlag, 1981.

101. Grimley PM, Rosenblum EN, Mims SJ, et al. Interruption by rifampin of an early stage in vaccinia virus morphogenesis: accumulation of membranes which are precursors of virus envelopes. *J Virol* 1970;6:519–533.

102. Morgan C. Vaccinia virus reexamined: development and release. *Virology* 1976;73:43–58.

103. Moss B, Rosenblum EN. Protein cleavage and poxvirus morphogenesis: tryptic peptide analysis of core precursors accumulated by blocking assembly with rifampicin. *J Mol Biol* 1973;81:267–269.

104. Lee P, Hruby DE. Proteolytic cleavage of vaccinia virus virion proteins. Mutational analysis of the specificity determinants. *J Biol Chem* 1994;269:8616–8622.

105. Locker JK, Griffiths G. An unconventional role for cytoplasmic disulfide bonds in vaccinia virus proteins. *J Cell Biol* 1999;144:267–279.

106. Senkevich TG, White CL, Koonin EV, et al. A viral member of the ERV1/ALR protein family participates in a cytoplasmic pathway of disulfide bond formation. *Proc Natl Acad Sci U S A* 2000;97:12068–12073.

107. Ward BM, Moss B. Visualization of intracellular movement of vaccinia virus virions containing a green fluorescent protein-B5R membrane protein chimera. *J Virol* 2001;75:4802–4813.

108. Ward BM, Moss B. Vaccinia virus intracellular movement is associated with microtubules and independent of actin tails. *J Virol* 2001;75:11651–11663.

109. Hollinshead M, Rodger G, Van Eijl H, et al. Vaccinia virus utilizes microtubules for movement to the cell surface. *J Cell Biol* 2001;154:389–402.

110. Blasco R, Moss B. Extracellular vaccinia virus formation and cell-to-cell virus transmission are prevented by deletion of the gene encoding the 37,000 Dalton outer envelope protein. *J Virol* 1991;65:5910–5920.

111. Roper RL, Moss B. Envelope formation is blocked by mutation of a sequence related to the HKD phospholipid metabolism motif in the vaccinia virus F13L protein. *J Virol* 1999;73:1108–1117.

112. Wolffe EJ, Isaacs SN, Moss B. Deletion of the vaccinia virus B5R gene encoding a 42-kilodalton membrane glycoprotein inhibits extracellular virus envelope formation and dissemination. *J Virol* 1993;67:4732–4741.

113. Engelstad M, Smith GL. The vaccinia virus 42-kDa envelope protein is required for the envelopment and egress of extracellular virus and for virus virulence. *Virology* 1993;194:627–637.

114. Blasco R, Moss B. Role of cell-associated enveloped vaccinia virus in cell-to-cell spread. *J Virol* 1992;66:4170–4179.

115. Roper R, Wolffe EJ, Weisberg A, et al. The envelope protein encoded by the A33R gene is required for formation of actin-containing microvilli and efficient cell-to-cell spread of vaccinia virus. *J Virol* 1998;72:4192–4204.

116. Wolffe EJ, Katz E, Weisberg A, et al. The A34R glycoprotein gene is required for induction of specialized actin-containing microvilli and efficient cell-to-cell transmission of vaccinia virus. *J Virol* 1997;71:3904–3915.

117. Wolffe EJ, Weisberg AS, Moss B. Role for the vaccinia virus A36R outer envelope protein in the formation of virus-tipped actin-containing microvilli and cell-to-cell virus spread. *Virology* 1998;244:20–26.

118. Sanderson CM, Frischknecht F, Way M, et al. Roles of vaccinia virus EEV-specific proteins in intracellular actin tail formation and low pH-induced cell-cell fusion. *J Gen Virol* 1998;79:1415–1425.

119. Moreau V, Frischknecht F, Reckmann I, et al. A complex of N-WASP and WIP integrates signalling cascades that lead to actin polymerization. *Nat Cell Biol* 2000;2:441–448.

120. Boulter EA, Appleyard G. Differences between extracellular and intracellular forms of poxvirus and their implications. *Prog Med Virol* 1973;16:86–108.

121. Ichihashi Y, Matsumoto S, Dales S. Biogenesis of poxviruses: role of A-type inclusions and host cell membranes in virus dissemination. *Virology* 1971;46:507–532.

122. Funahashi S, Sato T, Shida H. Cloning and characterization of the gene encoding the major protein of the A-type inclusion body of cowpox virus. *J Gen Virol* 1988;69:35–47.

123. Moss B, Shisler JL. Immunology 101 at poxvirus U: immune evasion genes. *Semin Immunol* 2001;13:59–66.

124. Shisler JL, Moss B. Immunology 102 at poxvirus U: avoiding apoptosis. *Semin Immunol* 2001;13:67–72.

125. Dumbell K, Richardson M. Virological investigations of specimens from buffaloes affected by buffalopox in Maharashtra State, India between 1985 and 1987. *Arch Virol* 1993;128:257–267.

126. Damaso CRA, Esposito JJ, Condit RC, et al. An emergent poxvirus from humans and cattle in Rio de Janeiro State: Cantagalo virus may derive from Brazilian smallpox vaccine. *Virology* 2000;277:439–449.

127. Epstein WL. Molluscum contagiosum. *Semin Dermatol* 1992;11:184–189.

128. Porter CD, Blake NW, Cream JJ, et al. Molluscum contagiosum virus. *Mol Cell Biol Hum Dis* 1992;1:233–257.

129. Buller RML, Chen JBW, Kreider J. Replication of molluscum contagiosum virus. *Virology* 1995;213:655–659.

130. Fife KH, Whitfeld M, Faust H, et al. Growth of molluscum contagiosum virus in a human foreskin xenograft model. *Virology* 1996;226:95–112.

131. Konya J, Thompson CH. Molluscum contagiosum virus: antibody responses in persons with clinical lesions and seroepidemiology in a representative Australian population. *J Infect Dis* 1999;179:701–704.

132. Brown ST, Nalley JF, Kraus SJ. Molluscum contagiosum. *Sex Transm Dis* 1981;8:227–234.

133. Darai G, Reisner H, Scholz J, et al. Analysis of the genome of molluscum contagiosum virus by restriction endonuclease analysis and molecular cloning. *J Med Virol* 1986;18:29–39.

134. Scholz J, Rosen-Wolff A, Bugert J, et al. Epidemiology of molluscum contagiosum using genetic analysis of the viral DNA. *J Med Virol* 1989;27:87–90.

135. Porter CD, Muhlemann MF, Cream JJ, et al. Molluscum contagiosum: characterization of viral DNA and clinical features. *Epidemiol Infect* 1987;99:563–567.

136. Porter CD, Archard LC. Characterisation by restriction mapping of three subtypes of molluscum-contagiosum virus. *J Med Virol* 1992;38:1–6.

137. Thompson CH, De Zwart-Steffe RT, Biggs IM. Molecular epidemiology of Australian isolates of molluscum contagiosum. *J Med Virol* 1990;32:1–9.

138. Nakamura J, Arao Y, Yoshida M, et al. Molecular epidemiological study of molluscum contagiosum virus in 2 urban areas of western Japan by the in-gel endonuclease digestion method. *Arch Virol* 1992;125:339–345.

139. Thompson CH, de Zwart-Steffe RT, Donovan B. Clinical and molecular aspects of molluscum contagiosum infection in HIV-1 positive patients. *Int J STD AIDS* 1992;3:101–106.

140. Jezek Z, Fenner F. Human monkeypox. *Monogr Virol* 1988;17:1–140.

141. Mukinda VB, Mwema G, Kilundu M, et al. Re-emergence of human monkeypox in Zaire in 1996. Monkeypox Epidemiologic Working Group. *Lancet* 1997;349:1449–1450.

142. Marennikova SS, Ladnyj ID, Ogorodnikova SI, et al. Identification and study of a poxvirus isolated from wild rodents in Turkmenia. *Arch Virol* 1978;56:7–14.

143. Bennett M, Gaskell CJ, Baxby D, et al. Feline cowpox virus infection. A review. *J Small Anim Pract* 1990;14:167–173.

144. Baxby D, Bennett M, Getty B. Human cowpox 1969–93: a review based on 54 cases. *Br J Dermatol* 1994;131:598–607.

145. Zhukova OA, Tsanava SA, Marennikova SS. Experimental infection of domestic cats by cowpox virus. *Acta Virol* 1992;36:329–331.

146. Mayr A, Büttner M. Ecthyma (orf) virus. In: Dinter Z, Morein B, eds. *Virus infections of ruminants.* Amsterdam: Elsevier, 1990:33–42.

147. Mayr A, Büttner M. Milker's node virus. In: Dinter Z, Morein B, eds. *Virus infections of ruminants.* Amsterdam: Elsevier, 1990:29–32.

148. Mayr A, Büttner M. Bovine papular stomatitis virus. In: Dinter Z, Morein B, eds. *Virus infections of ruminants.* Amsterdam: Elsevier, 1990:23–28.

149. Downie AW, Taylor-Robinson CH, Caunt AE, et al. Tanapox: a new disease caused by a poxvirus. *BMJ* 1971;1:363–368.

150. Jezek Z, Arita I, Szczeniowski M, et al. Human tanapox in Zaire: clinical and epidemiological observations on cases confirmed by laboratory studies. *Bull WHO* 1985;63:1027–1035.

151. Downie AW, España C. Comparison of Tanapox virus and Yaba-like viruses causing epidemic disease in monkeys. *J Hyg (London)* 1972;70:23–32.

152. Grace JT, Mirand EA. Human susceptibility to a simian tumor virus. *Ann NY Acad Sci* 1963;108:1123–1128.

153. Niven JSF, Armstrong JA, Andrewes CH, et al. Subcutaneous "growths" in monkeys produced by a poxvirus. *J Pathol Bacteriol* 1961;81:1–10.

154. Downie AW. A study of the lesions produced experimentally by cowpox virus. *J Pathol Bact* 1939;48:361–379.

155. Johannessen JV, Krogh H-K, Solberg I, et al. Human orf. *J Cutan Pathol* 1975;2:265–283.

156. Gottlieb SL, Myskowski PL. Molluscum contagiosum. *Int J Dermatol* 1994;33:453–461.

157. Freed ER, Duma RJ, Escobar MR. Vaccinia necrosum and its relationship to impaired immunologic responsiveness. *Am J Med* 1972;52:411–420.

158. Fulginiti VA, Kempe CH, Hathaway EE, et al. Progressive vaccinia in immunologically deficient individuals. *Birth Defects* 1968;4:129–145.

159. Fenner F, Nakanao JH. Poxviridae: the poxviruses. In: Lennette EH, Halonen P, Murphy FA, eds. *The laboratory diagnosis of infectious diseases: principles and practice.* New York: Springer-Verlag, 1988:177–210.

160. Ropp SL, Jin Q, Knight JC, et al. PCR strategy for identification and differentiation of small pox and other orthopoxviruses. *J Clin Microbiol* 1995;33:2069–2076.

161. Esposito JJ, Obijeski JF, Nakano JH. Orthopoxvirus DNA: strain differentiation by electrophoresis of restriction endonuclease fragmented virion DNA. *Virology* 1978;89:53–66.

162. Pfeffer M, Meyer H, Wiedmann M. A ligase chain reaction targeting two adjacent nucleotides allows the differentiation of cowpox virus from other Orthopoxvirus species. *J Virol Methods* 1994;49:353–360.

163. Meyer H, Pfeffer M, Rziha H-J. Sequence alterations within and downstream of the A-type inclusion protein gene allows differentiation of *Orthopoxvirus* species by polymerase chain reaction. *J Gen Virol* 1994;75:1975–1981.

164. Meyer H, Osterrieder N, Pfeffer M. Differentiation of species of the genus Orthopoxvirus in a dot blot assay using digoxigenin-labeled DNA-probes. *Vet Microbiol* 1993;34:333–344.

165. Loparev VN, Massung RF, Esposito JJ, et al. Detection and differentiation of Old World orthopoxviruses: restriction fragment length polymorphism of the crmB gene region. *J Clin Microbiol* 2001;39:94–100.

166. Appleyard G, Hapel AJ, Boulter EA. An antigenic difference between intracellular and extracellular rabbitpox virus. *J Gen Virol* 1971;13:9–17.

167. Boulter EA, Zwartouw HT, Titmuss DHJ, Maber HB. The nature of the immune state produced by inactivated vaccinia virus in rabbits. *Am J Epidemiol* 1971;94:612–620.

168. Hooper JW, Custer DM, Schmaljohn CS, et al. DNA vaccination with vaccinia virus L1R and A33R genes protects mice against a lethal poxvirus challenge. *Virology* 2000;266:329–339.

169. Brainerd HD, Hanna L, Jawetz E. Methisazone in progressive vaccinia. *N Engl J Med* 1967;276:620–622.

170. De Clercq E. Vaccinia virus inhibitors as a paradigm for the chemotherapy of poxvirus infections. *Clin Microbiol Rev* 2001;14:382–397.

171. Bray M, Martinez M, Smee DF, et al. Cidofovir protects mice against lethal aerosol or intranasal cowpox virus challenge. *J Infect Dis* 2000;181:10–19.

RNA Viruses

CHAPTER 241
Influenza Viruses

Peter F. Wright and Kathleen M. Neuzil

HISTORY

The highly contagious, acute respiratory illness known as influenza has afflicted humans since ancient times. The sudden appearance of febrile, respiratory disease that persists within a community for a 3- to 4-week period is sufficiently characteristic to permit identification of a number of major epidemics stretching into the distant past. Historical data have permitted us to establish that epidemics of varying severity have occurred almost yearly, causing the greatest mortality in the very young, those with cardiopulmonary disease, and the elderly. Historical and current emergence of epidemics has often been traced to the Far East.

While influenza has killed untold millions throughout the centuries, the pandemic of 1918 to 1919 was particularly severe. The Spanish influenza, as it was called, killed between 20 and 40 million people worldwide. The severity of the pandemic of 1918 to 1919 greatly accelerated the search for the causative agent of influenza. In 1933, a virus was isolated from humans by Smith, Andrewes, and Laidlaw of the National Institute for Medical Research in London (1). Subsequently, influenza has been an intense area of molecular, epidemiologic, vaccine, and therapeutic studies that have vastly enhanced our understanding of this pathogen and our capacity to respond to the influenza infection. Nevertheless, influenza remains a major annual winter scourge with the capacity for pandemic spread and great resultant illness.

CHARACTERISTICS OF THE PATHOGEN

Influenza viruses, the causative agents of influenza, belong to the Orthomyxoviridae family of RNA viruses and has three genera of importance in human disease; influenza A, B, and C viruses. Of these, influenza A is the dominant pathogen. Influenza A viruses are divided into subtypes, and the current nomenclature system (2) includes the host of origin, geographic location of first isolation, strain number, and year of isolation. The antigenic description of the two surface proteins that dictate humoral immunity, the hemagglutinin (HA) and neuraminidase (NA), is given parenthetically, for example, A/Puerto Rico/8/34 (H1N1). There are 15 HA and 9 NA subtypes. No new subtypes have been isolated since 1983, suggesting that there is a finite number of distinct influenza A viruses circulating, with the largest reservoir being in aquatic birds.

When influenza virus is examined by electron microscopy, irregularly shaped spherical particles approximately 120 nm in diameter are seen. The most striking feature of the influenza virion is a layer of spikes projecting radially outward over the surface (3). These surface spikes on influenza A viruses are of two distinct types, corresponding to the HA and NA. The HA spike appears rod shaped, and the NA spike is mushroom shaped. The HA and NA glycoproteins are attached by short sequences of hydrophobic amino acids to a lipid envelope derived from the plasma membrane of the host cell. Within the lipid envelope lays the matrix protein (M1), which is structural in function. Inside the matrix shell are eight single-stranded RNA molecules of negative sense (i.e., the virion RNA is complementary to the messenger RNA) associated with the nucleocapsid protein (NP) and three large proteins (PB1, PB2, and PA) responsible for RNA replication and transcription. Two virus-coded nonstructural proteins (NS1 and N52) are found in infected cells. The packaging of the eight single-stranded RNA segments within the virion is poorly understood. What is clear is that the segmented genome allows gene reassortment between influenza viruses infecting the same cell and hence tremendous capacity for exchange of gene segments between viruses.

EPIDEMIOLOGY

The influenza viruses are unique among the respiratory tract viruses in that they undergo significant antigenic variation. Both of the surface antigens of the influenza A viruses undergo two types of antigenic variation: antigenic drift and antigenic shift. Antigenic drift involves minor antigenic changes in the HA and NA, while shift involves major antigenic changes in these molecules resulting from replacement of a gene segment.

Antigenic drift occurs by accumulation of a series of point mutations resulting in amino acid substitutions in sites recognized by antibodies in the HA, thus preventing binding of antibodies induced by the previous infection and permitting the virus to infect the host. The NA is the second most abundant spike protein on influenza virus and with the HA determines serotype specificity.

Since the first human influenza virus was isolated in 1933, antigenic shifts in type A influenza viruses have occurred in 1957 when the H2N2 subtype (Asian influenza) replaced the H1N1 subtype, in 1968 when the Hong Kong (H3N2) virus appeared replacing H2N2, and in 1977 when the H1N1 virus reappeared. Each of these major antigenic shifts have several characteristics in common: (a) their appearance was sudden, (b) they first were recognized in China, (c) they were antigenically distinct from the influenza viruses then circulating in humans, and (d) they were confined to the H1, H2, and H3 subtypes.

Each of these new pandemic strains in humans was derived from avian influenza viruses by reassortment of avian genes with the currently circulating human strain. However, transmission of H5N1 influenza viruses to humans in 1997 in Hong Kong confirmed the direct transmission of avian influenza to humans apparently without an intermediate host. The avian H5N1 influenza virus caused high mortality in both poultry, killing 70% to 100% of chickens, and in humans, with 6 of 18 infected patients dying (4–6). The slaughter of approximately 1.6 million poultry in Hong Kong in December 1997 stopped the spread of H5N1 influenza viruses to humans. The failure of H5N1 to transmit from human to human, and the slaughter of poultry before the human A/Sydney/05/95 (H3N2) strain began circulating in humans in Hong Kong probably prevented the generation of reassortants. Subsequently, in 1998 and 1999, H9N2 avian influenza viruses were reported from five human cases in southern China (7) and a further two children in March 1999 in Hong Kong. The children had typical influenza and recovered.

From the above discussion it is apparent that there are several ways in which pandemic influenza viruses can arise, and each has probably played a role in the evolution of the influenza viruses currently found in humans.

In the United States influenza virus epidemics generally occur between January and April, with occasional epidemics in

December or May (8). The temporal curves of individual influenza epidemics are similar. The seeding of a community with virus is followed by a relatively sharp, single peak of virus activity as indicated by school and industrial absenteeism and, slightly later, excess mortality (8). The appearance of an epidemic in any given year represents a subtle interplay between intrinsic properties of the virus, the extent of antigenic drift of the virus, and the level of immunity in the population (9).

Influenza viruses have a major impact on morbidity, with increases in hospitalizations and visits to health care providers accompanying almost every epidemic. Using large databases, the morbidity has recently been defined in children (10), in women of all ages with high-risk conditions (11), and in pregnant women (12). In the elderly, the group at highest risk, the impact of influenza has been shown to extend beyond influenza and pneumonia illnesses to other acute and chronic respiratory conditions and to congestive heart failure (13). High rates of hospitalization are also observed in children under 5 years of age, with the highest rates in children being in those under 1 year of age (14). The observations that influenza virus infects 14% to 16% of children seeking medical care for febrile respiratory illness reinforces influenza's contribution to outpatient morbidity (15–18). Preschool- and school-aged children are also major vectors in transmission of influenza A viruses in the community (19).

The major factor that diminishes morbidity following exposure to influenza A virus is the level of preexisting immunity from past exposure, through vaccination or natural infection, to viruses bearing related surface glycoproteins. The more severe illness seen in naive individuals explains the high morbidity seen in infants and young children undergoing first infection (14) and the high morbidity seen in all age groups following the introduction of new pandemic viruses such as in 1918 (H1N1), 1957 (H2N2), and 1968 (H3N2) (20).

Influenza virus is uniquely important among respiratory viruses as a cause of excess mortality. A recent paper has created a severity index for judging the impact of influenza epidemics (21). The researchers found that epidemics associated with the circulation of influenza A H3N2 viruses have higher mortality than those seen with H1N1 or B strains. Their estimate of the total mortality attributable to influenza in the United States for the 20-year period from 1972 to 1992 was 426,000 deaths.

In fewer years, influenza B infections can be a serious problem (e.g. 1990).

PATHOGENESIS

Influenza A virus is most effectively spread from person to person by the aerosol route (22). It is probable that most influenza A virus infections are transmitted via droplets formed during coughing or sneezing. The incubation period for influenza illness is about 3 days for influenza A virus and 4 days for influenza B viruses (23).

Influenza virus replicates throughout the respiratory tract, with virus being recoverable from the upper and lower tracts of people naturally or experimentally infected with virus. Human influenza viruses replicate exclusively in superficial epithelial cells of the respiratory tract. The pattern of virus replication in 13 adult volunteers administered an influenza A/HK/68-like H3N2 virus, in relationship to the onset of clinical symptoms, interferon response, and serum and nasal wash antibody responses, is presented in Fig. 241.1. Virus replication peaks at about 48 hours after inoculation and declines somewhat slowly thereafter, with little shedding after days 6 to 8 (24). In children naturally infected with influenza viruses, virus is most frequently recovered 1 to 2 days after the onset of symptoms and can be found for up to 13 days thereafter (25). The peak titer is achieved on the first day of illness and averages $10^{4.0}$, 50% tissue culture infections dose $(TCID_{50})/mL$ of nasal wash (26).

Influenza A virus induces pathologic changes throughout the respiratory tract, but the most significant pathology is present in the lower respiratory tract (27). During bronchoscopy of persons with uncomplicated influenza infections, acute diffuse inflammation of the larynx, trachea, and bronchi were observed with mucosal inflammation and edema. Light microscopic studies of infected cells reveal that the columnar ciliated cells become vacuolated, edematous, and lose cilia before being desquamating. Within 1 day after the onset of symptoms, desquamation of the ciliated and mucus-producing epithelial cells down to a one-cell-thick basal layer is observed; in other areas the thickened and hyalinized basement membrane is exposed. From the third to fifth day after onset of illness, mitoses appear in the basal cell layer, and regeneration of the epithelium begins. During this

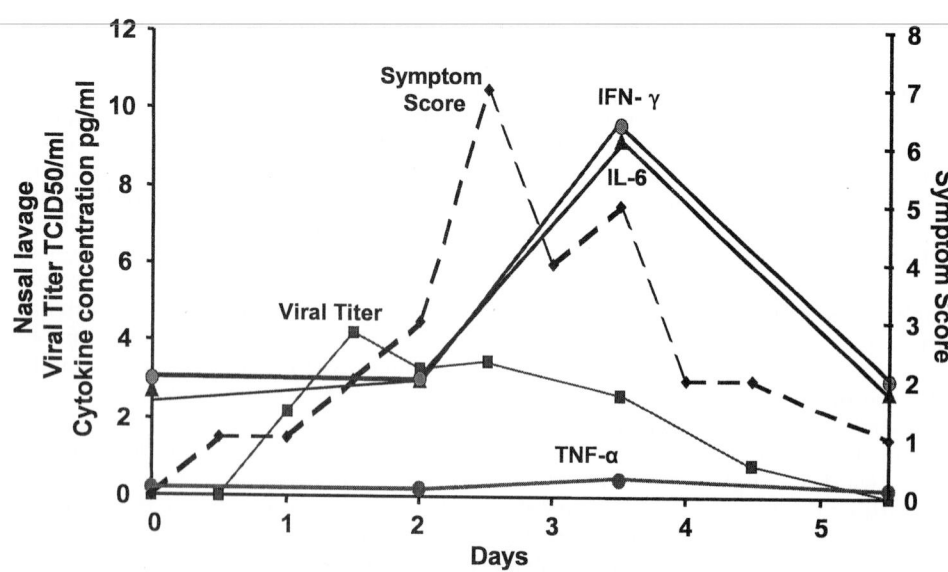

Figure 241.1. The clinical, virologic, and cytokine response to experimental influenza virus A infection. The symptom score was cumulative and based on the graded severity of 14 respiratory and systemic symptoms as described by Hayden et al. (104). (Composite figure derived from data presented in Hayden FG, et al. Inhaled zanamivir for the prevention of influenza in families. Zanamivir Family Study Group. *N Engl J Med* 2001;343:1282–1289.)

time, reparative and destructive processes may be present simultaneously. Complete resolution of the epithelial necrosis probably takes up to a month because pulmonary function abnormalities persist beyond the period of symptomatic recovery from the acute phase (28).

The extremely short incubation period between infection and clinical illness implies that innate immunity or preformed cognate recognition components are important. The respiratory tract has a series of such innate protective mechanisms against influenza infection, including the mucin layer, ciliary action, and protease inhibitors that may prevent effective cell entry and virus uncoating. Once the epithelial cell is infected, proinflammatory cytokines, notably interleukin-6 and interferon-α, are induced and released from these cells. These cytokines reach their peak by day 3 after experimental infection (29). These two cytokines correspond in their release with the highest clinical symptom score, mucus production, fever, and viral load. The importance of interferon in regulation of influenza replication is suggested by the observation that the NS-1 protein is an interferon antagonist. Deletion of NS-1 leads to increased induction of interferon and a virus that is highly attenuated except in a mouse with an interruption in the interferon induction pathway (30).

During infection of humans with influenza A virus, antibodies to the HA, NA, NP, and M proteins are produced (31). Antibodies to the HA and NA glycoproteins are associated with resistance to infection or illness in humans and in laboratory animals, whereas antibodies to the internal M1 and NP proteins are not (32). Studies of vaccinia-recombinant viruses expressing each of 10 gene products of the influenza A virus clearly identified the HA and NA glycoproteins as primary protective antigens, and the primary mediators of the resistance to virus challenge induced by these glycoproteins were antibodies (33). HA antibodies can prevent infection by neutralizing the infectivity of the virus (34), whereas NA antibodies mediate their antiviral effect primarily after infection has been initiated by restricting spread of virus within the respiratory tract of the host (35).

The role of cellular immunity in clearance of influenza virus has been well defined in the murine model but less well in humans (36). There are two subsets of effector lymphocytes in humans. The first subset consists of cells that mediate cytoxicity that is restricted by class I histocompatibility antigens and has the CD8$^+$ phenotype. These cytotoxic lymphocytes (CTLs) appear in the blood of infected or vaccinated individuals on days 6 to 14 and disappear by day 21 (37). Subsequently they can be recalled after *in vitro* stimulation as memory CTLs. The prechallenge level of memory CTLs does not correlate with susceptibility to infection or illness following experimental administration of wild-type virus, but is correlated with accelerated clearance of virus from the respiratory tract of humans (38).

CD4$^+$ T-cells can also contribute to immunity to influenza A virus infection. The important role of CD4$^+$ T cells in immunity to influenza virus infection has been defined from studies in CD8$^+$ T-cell deficient animals that can clear influenza A virus by a CD4$^+$ T cell–dependent mechanism (39). The primary antiviral activity of the CD4$^+$ T cell is to provide help to B cells to produce antiviral antibodies. Animals deficient in both CD4$^+$ and CD8$^+$ T cells succumb to infection, indicating that nonspecific mediators of immunity are not sufficient in the absence of T cells to significantly restrict influenza A virus infection (40).

Francis was the first to detect neutralizing activity to influenza virus in nasal secretions and, subsequently, that resistance to experimental influenza A virus infection in the mouse is mediated primarily by antibody present in bronchial secretions (41). The neutralizing antibody in nasal secretions of humans is primarily of the immunoglobulin A (IgA) isotype (42) and is locally produced (43).

Local IgA antibody stimulated by natural infection is detectable for 3 to 5 months after infection, and there is local IgA memory for influenza antigen (44,45). When detectable, nasal wash IgG appears to be predominantly a transudate from serum with a serum-to-nasal-wash concentration gradient of 350:1 (46). The presence of local IgA antibody induced by infection with an attenuated virus correlated with resistance of volunteers to infection and illness after challenge with a virulent wild-type virus (47). Challenge of children with an attenuated live vaccine showed similar findings (48). Also, resistance to experimental wild-type infection correlated with the level of local HA antibody present at the time of virus administration, with IgG as well as IgA each contributing to resistance (49).

CLINICAL MANIFESTATIONS

Infection with influenza A viruses results in a spectrum of clinical responses ranging from an asymptomatic infection to a primary viral pneumonia that rapidly progresses to a fatal outcome. The typical uncomplicated influenza syndrome is a tracheobronchitis, with the additional involvement of small airways (50). The incubation period can be as short as 24 hours or up to 4 or 5 days, depending in part on the dose of virus and the immune status of the host. The onset of illness is usually abrupt, with the occurrence of headache, chills, and dry cough, which is rapidly followed by high fever, significant myalgias, malaise, and anorexia (Fig. 241.1). Substernal tightness and soreness can accompany the cough. The most prominent sign of infection is fever that often peaks within 24 hours, commonly in the 38 to 40°C range. The fever usually begins to decline on the second or third day of illness and is usually gone by the sixth day; the median duration is 3 days (51). The elderly can present without high fever, lassitude, and confusion without respiratory signs (52). Other than fever, the physical findings in influenza are usually confined to the respiratory tract, although patients can appear quite toxic. Nasal obstruction, rhinorrhea, and sneezing often occur, and pharyngeal inflammation without exudate is common. Conjunctival inflammation and excessive tearing may occur. Chest x-ray and auscultatory findings are usually normal, although occasionally patchy rales and rhonchi are heard.

As the fever is declining, the respiratory signs and symptoms such as rhinorrhea and coughing may become more intense. The cough frequently changes from a dry, hacking nature to one that is productive of small amounts of sputum that are usually mucoid but can be purulent. After the fever and upper respiratory tract symptoms resolve, cough and weakness can persist for 1 to 2 additional weeks. The loss of the mucociliary blanket is a factor in a predisposition to secondary bacterial pneumonia seen following influenza infection. Although significant abnormalities in large and small airways can be demonstrated during acute infection and early convalescence, uncomplicated influenza appears to cause little permanent damage in the lung, even in patients with chronic obstructive lung disease (53).

The clinical manifestations of influenza in children are similar to those seen in adults, but there are some distinct differences between these two age groups. Children have higher fever, and febrile convulsions can occur (16). Influenza viruses cause at least 14% febrile respiratory illnesses that result in a visit to a pediatrician (15). Otitis media, croup, pneumonia, and myositis are more frequent in children (54). Influenza A and B virus infections increase the risk for developing otitis media (54). Approximately

12% of naturally infected seronegative children develop otitis media (55).

It is important to emphasize that influenza A and B viruses are important causes of serious lower respiratory tract disease in children (18,56). In a prospective study of 121 susceptible (seronegative) young children seen in a clinic during an H3N2 virus outbreak in 1974, 5 of 60 infected infants had clinical and x-ray evidence of pneumonia (57). In the H2N2 era, influenza A virus infection was associated with 8% of all croup requiring hospitalization and in the H3N2 era with 24% of all such croup. Croup occurred predominantly in children less than 1 year of age. Influenza-associated croup can be especially severe and occasionally requires intubation (58). In addition, influenza A virus infection has been shown to exacerbate asthma (59).

RESPIRATORY COMPLICATIONS OF INFLUENZA

Three distinct syndromes of severe pneumonia can follow influenza infection in children or adults. Such complications are most common in the elderly.

Primary Viral Pneumonia

Primary influenza virus pneumonia was first described in 1959 (60) in fatal cases caused by the 1957 Asian influenza A virus (H2N2), though retrospectively it had been observed during previous influenza A epidemics (61,62). Primary viral pneumonia occurs predominantly in individuals at high risk for the complications of influenza virus infection (i.e., the elderly or patients with cardiopulmonary disease), but 25% of the cases are in normal individuals and an additional 13% in pregnant women. The typical case of primary viral pneumonia develops abruptly following the onset of influenza illness. It progresses within 6 to 24 hours to a severe pneumonia with a rapid respiratory rate (30–60 respirations per minute), tachycardia (>120 beats/min), cyanosis (in 80% of patients), high fever (average of 39°C), and hypotension. Auscultatory findings include bilateral crepitant inspiratory rales. Radiographic examinations reveal mottled densities in two or more lobes and diffuse symmetric interstitial infiltrates or areas of consolidation; cavitation or pleural effusion suggests bacterial superinfection. Electrocardiographic abnormalities occur but are not those consistent with myocarditis. Pathologic findings in the trachea and bronchi are similar to those previously described during acute uncomplicated disease, but bronchiolitis is also present.

In nonfatal cases initial improvement occurs from 5 to 16 days after onset of pneumonia with resolution of x-ray changes taking up to 4 months (63). Survivors can develop diffuse interstitial fibrosis with a decrease in diffusion capacity of carbon monoxide and a decrease in arterial oxygen tension (64). Influenza B virus can cause severe disease but has not been reported to be associated with fatal primary viral pneumonia in normal individuals (65).

Combined Viral-Bacterial Pneumonia

A combined viral-bacterial pneumonia is approximately three times more common than primary viral pneumonia. The bacteria most commonly involved are *Streptococcus pneumoniae, Staphylococcus aureus, and Hemophilus influenzae,* although other microorganisms can play a role (60,66–70). Clinically, this syndrome may be indistinguishable from primary viral pneumonia, except that the symptoms of pneumonia appear somewhat later after onset of influenza symptoms and chest radiographs taken early in

the course of pneumonia are more apt to reveal the presence of pleural effusion. The erythrocyte sedimentation rate is elevated more frequently than in primary viral pneumonia. Because there is no effective distinction between the two syndromes, the diagnosis depends solely on the demonstration of bacteria in the sputum, in fluid obtained at bronchoscopy, or in the pleural fluid. The case-fatality rate for combined viral-bacterial pneumonia is about 10% to 12% (60,66,69). However, co-infection with influenza and *Staphylococcus aureus* has a higher fatality rate of up to 42% (71).

There are strains of *Staphylococcus aureus* that secrete proteases capable of activating the infectivity of influenza virus by proteolytic cleavage of the HA. These strains play a synergistic role in experimental pneumonia in mice (72). Such protease-secreting bacterial strains could well be an added pathogenic factor in combined viral-bacterial pneumonias in humans.

Influenza Infection Followed by a Secondary Bacterial Pneumonia

In this syndrome, an individual has a typical influenzal illness and is beginning to improve but then develops shaking chills, pleuritic chest pain, and an increase in cough productive of bloody or purulent sputum (60). Cyanosis and a marked increase in respiratory rate are less common than with a primary viral pneumonia. Examination by x-ray reveals local areas of lung consolidation but not diffuse pneumonia. Often influenza A virus is not recovered from the upper or lower respiratory tract, leukocytosis is common, and the erythrocyte sedimentation rate is elevated. This is generally a milder form of pneumonia, although a case-fatality rate of about 7% has been described (61).

NONRESPIRATORY COMPLICATIONS OF INFLUENZA

Systemic

In children and adults, a diffuse form of the disease occurs with generalized pain, tenderness, and weakness of muscles, increased serum levels of muscle enzymes, myoglobinemia, and myoglobinuria (73). Fatal acute renal failure can follow this form of the disease. The pathogenesis of the myositis remains uncertain. Muscle cell necrosis with or without inflammation can occur, and although influenza virus has been recovered from muscle, the relationship between the virus and the myositis remains unclear (73).

Reye's syndrome, which is a neurologic and metabolic disease of children and adolescents, is characterized by a rapidly progressive noninflammatory encephalopathy and fatty infiltration of the viscera, especially the liver, resulting in severe hepatic dysfunction as indicated by elevated serum transaminase and ammonia levels. This syndrome has followed respiratory viruses, varicella virus, and gastrointestinal infections (74). Histologically there is electron microscopic evidence of mitochondrial swelling (75). Influenza B, in particular, but also influenza A H1N1 and H3N2 viruses, have been identified as antecedent infections (74). The administration of therapeutic doses of salicylates is a risk factor in the development of Reye's syndrome (76). The onset of the central nervous system (CNS) and hepatic symptoms usually begins as respiratory tract symptoms wane. The case-fatality rate varies and has been estimated to be between 22% and 42% (74). The disease associated with influenza B virus occurs in children 0 to 18 years of age (median age 11 years) and is more frequently seen in a rural than in an urban environment (74). The etiology and pathogenesis of this syndrome are unknown. There has been a dramatic decrease in Reye's syndrome cases in the United States in both varicella-associated and nonvaricella-associated cases related to reduced use of salicylates that are contraindicated for use in influenza infection (76).

Central Nervous System Manifestations

Two specific CNS syndromes have been suggested to accompany influenza infection: influenzal encephalopathy and postinfluenzal encephalitis. Encephalopathy occurs at the height of influenza illness and may progress to death (77–79). There are recent reports of encephalitis from Japan (80). The cerebrospinal fluid (CSF) is usually normal, the brain at autopsy shows severe congestion, and histologic changes are minimal. Lungs of such patients show changes typical of influenza and can yield virus in high titer. The postencephalitic syndrome is extremely rare and occurs from 2 to 3 weeks after recovery from influenza. The CSF findings indicate inflammatory changes, and recovery occurs in the majority of cases.

It has been suggested that the syndrome of encephalitis lethargica followed by postencephalitic Parkinson's disease was associated with the influenza epidemics of 1918 and the epidemics following shortly thereafter (81). The epidemics of encephalitis lethargica followed 1 year after the epidemics of influenza, and these were followed in turn by postencephalitic Parkinson's disease about one decade later.

Febrile convulsions leading to hospitalization occur in children with and without underlying CNS abnormalities. An increase in the incidence of the Guillain-Barré syndrome has not been seen following influenza A or B virus epidemics.

INFLUENZA IN PREGNANCY

Pregnant women in the second or third trimester have an increased risk for developing fatal influenza disease (12). The increased mortality is generally seen during the years after introduction of a new pandemic strain, as in 1918 and 1957 (82–84), although using a large data set, the impact can be appreciated in the interpandemic period (12). The virus itself has not been implicated as a cause of congenital defects (85).

INFLUENZA IN IMMUNOCOMPROMISED PATIENTS

Influenza viruses can infect and cause severe disease in immunocompromised individuals (86), but more often the illness resembles that seen in fully immunocompetent persons. Prolonged shedding of virus occurs in immunosuppressed persons (86).

INFLUENZA B AND C

Influenza B virus can cause the same spectrum of disease as that seen following influenza A virus infection, and severe illness can occur (87). The frequency of serious influenza B virus infections requiring hospitalization is about fourfold less than that of influenza A virus (54a). Influenza B virus illness occurs in epidemic form and predominantly involves adolescents and school-aged children, but adults and the elderly can also be affected (15). Myositis and gastrointestinal symptoms are more common manifestations of influenza B than A virus infection (88,89).

Influenza C virus causes sporadic upper respiratory tract illness and is rarely associated with severe lower respiratory tract disease (41). By early adulthood most individuals (96%) have antibody to influenza C virus (90). Administration of influenza C virus to volunteers induced mild coryza with some systemic symptoms (91).

DIAGNOSIS

The respiratory tract manifestations of influenza virus infections are not specific and can be seen during infection with other respiratory tract pathogens, including mycoplasma, respiratory syncytial virus, parainfluenza viruses, coronaviruses, adenoviruses, rhinoviruses, *Mycoplasma pneumoniae* and *Bacillus anthracis* (92). Since the severe forms of viral pneumonia are extremely rare with other respiratory viruses in adults, it is reasonable to assume that during an epidemic of influenza A virus in the community, diffuse interstitial viral pneumonia in an adult is likely to be due to influenza virus. The recent documentation that another wintertime virus, respiratory syncytial virus, can cause equally severe illness in the elderly makes even this assumption tenuous (93). The protean manifestations of influenza A virus demand that influenza virus be considered in the differential diagnosis of fever in neonates and of myositis, febrile convulsions, and encephalopathies occurring in the general population during influenza epidemics. The diagnosis can be established only by recovery of virus, by demonstration of the presence of viral antigen or viral genetic material in clinical specimens, or by detection of an increase in specific antibody titer in serum or nasal secretions (94–96).

TREATMENT AND PREVENTION USING ANTIVIRALS

Amantadine hydrochloride and rimantadine, an analog of amantadine, are currently licensed for prophylactic and therapeutic use against influenza A virus in humans in the United States. Both have a tricyclic structure with an amine side group and have antiviral properties against all subtypes of influenza A virus, but not against influenza B or C viruses (97). The primary antiviral action of these compounds results from blocking the flow of hydrogen ions from the acidified endosome into the interior of the virion, a process necessary for release of the transcriptionally active ribonucleoprotein complex for transport to the nucleus.

At the recommended adult dose of amantadine or rimantadine (i.e., 200 mg orally), side effects are unusual in young and middle-aged adults (Table 241.1). At dosages of 300 to 400 mg per day, significant symptoms referable to the CNS such as depression, difficulty concentrating, nervousness, sleep disturbances, and gastrointestinal complaints occur. These effects are more frequently observed in recipients of amantadine than rimantadine and are more evident in the elderly, in whom a reduced dose of 100 mg orally is recommended. The kidneys clear amantadine and the dose must be adjusted with renal impairment, whereas the liver metabolizes rimantadine. Compared with amantadine, rimantadine has the desirable properties of (a) fewer side effects; (b) one dose can be administered daily rather than two; and (c) renal function does not affect clearance of drug.

Amantadine and rimantadine are useful for prophylaxis against H1N1, H2N2, and H3N2 influenza A virus infections in adults and children. During an epidemic involving both influenza A H1N1 and H3N2 viruses, amantadine and rimantadine protected against influenza-like illness (78% and 65%, respectively), documented influenza illness (91% and 85%), and

TABLE 241.1. Antiviral Agents for the Prevention and Treatment of Influenza

	Amantadine	Rimantadine	Oseltamivir	Zanamivir
Spectrum of activity	Influenza A	Influenza A	Influenza A and B	Influenza A and B
Route of administration	Oral (tablet, capsule, syrup)	Oral (tablet, syrup)	Oral (capsule, oral suspension)	Oral inhalation
Ages approved for prophylaxis	≥1 yr	≥1 yr	≥13 yr	Not approved
Ages approved for treatment	≥1 yr	≥18 yr[a]	≥1 yr	≥7 yr
Major adverse effects	Anxiety, poor concentration, confusion, seizures	Same as amantadine, but less frequent	Nausea, vomiting	Possible bronchospasm in those with hyperactive airways disease
Dose in healthy adults[b]	100 mg twice daily age <65 yr ≤100 mg daily age ≥65	100 mg twice daily age <65 yr 100 or 200 mg daily age ≥65	75 mg twice daily	2 inhalations twice daily, 12 h apart

[a]Many experts believe it is appropriate for treatment of children >1 year of age.
[b]See package inserts for dose adjustments for creatinine clearance, liver disease, and pediatric or elderly patients.
Source: From Neuzil KM. Treatment for influenzavirus infection. *Curr Treat Options Infect Dis* 2002;4:37–42, with permission.

influenza infection (74% and 66%) (98). Lower efficacy rates against documented illness (70%) and infection (39%) were observed for amantadine prophylaxis during an H1N1 virus epidemic.

Amantadine or rimantadine is also useful in the therapy of illness caused by influenza H1N1, H2N2, and H3N2 viruses. Symptomatic improvement, including accelerated clearance of local symptoms and fever, occurs about 1 day earlier in treated patients, and peripheral airway dysfunction also resolves more quickly. Accelerated clearance of symptoms is seen in children infected with an H3N2 virus treated with rimantadine compared with control children receiving an antipyretic (99). Virus was cleared more rapidly in such treated individuals than in controls. Development of serum and nasal wash influenza antibodies was not inhibited by amantadine treatment.

Recommendations for prophylactic and therapeutic uses of amantadine include prophylactic use in individuals at high risk who have not been vaccinated, as well as hospital personnel who could spread infection in the hospital. Therapeutic use includes individuals with uncomplicated influenza who have a high temperature of less than 48 hours' duration. It would be helpful to know that amantadine is useful in treating primary viral pneumonia, but efficacy in this clinical setting remains to be established. Resistant strains of influenza A virus can be isolated *in vitro* and *in vivo*. Updated recommendations for use of these compounds by the Advisory Committee on Immunization Practices are published yearly (100).

The creation of compounds that block the active site of neuraminidase are a more recent development. The first licensed was zanamivir, which is a specific inhibitor of the NA of all influenza A and B viruses. Zanamivir has to be administered intranasally or inhaled for optimal effect. An additional NA inhibitor, oseltamivir, has been developed that can be taken orally. This was achieved through the discovery and utilization of a hydrophobic pocket in the enzyme-active center that could accommodate lipophilic groups necessary to improve the inhibitor's oral bioavailability (101).

Both zanamivir and oseltamivir are well tolerated in humans and are efficacious for prophylaxis and treatment of influenza in humans. Both zanamivir and oseltamivir of these NA inhibitors have been approved for use in humans. For all zanamivir recipients, prophylaxis was 96% effective against viral shedding, 82% effective against infection, and 95% effective in preventing febrile illness ($p < 0.001$); it reduced peak viral titers by 2.0 log $TCID_{50}/mL$ ($p < 0.001$) and reduced the median duration of vi-

ral shedding by 3 days ($p < 0.001$); and the frequency of febrile illness by 85% ($p < 0.01$) (102).

The efficacy of zanamivir against acute influenza has been shown in double-blind placebo-controlled field trials. For all infected patients, the median time to alleviation of all major influenza symptoms (i.e., headache, myalgia, cough, and sore throat) was 4 days compared with 5 days for the placebo group (103). When treatment was started within 30 hours after infection, the treated group recovered 3 days earlier, and if treatment was started less than 30 hours after infection, the alleviation of symptoms was up to 4 days. Thus, early diagnosis and treatment are necessary. Similar efficacy has recently been shown for oseltamivir (104). While both drugs significantly reduce secondary complications and antibiotic use compared with placebo, the studies were not powered to show a reduction in severe complications such as pneumonia. Recommendations for the use of each compound have recently been published by the Centers for Disease Control and Prevention (100). Oseltamavir can be used in children over 1 year of age and zanamivir in children over 7 years of age.

The neuraminidase inhibitors are generally well tolerated, although oseltamivir may cause nausea and vomiting, and zanamivir should be used with caution in those with hyperactive airways disease, because it has been associated with bronchospasm.

Resistant variants to the NA inhibitors have been selected under drug pressure *in vitro* but only with difficulty and at a much lower frequency than amantadine. Future large-scale studies are needed to determine if resistant mutants can be detected after *in vivo* use in humans. Now that zanamivir and oseltamivir have been approved for use in humans it is important to monitor for the emergence of resistance to these inhibitors under field conditions.

PREVENTION THROUGH IMMUNIZATION

Inactivated influenza A and B virus vaccines are licensed for parenteral administration in humans. The strains to be included each year for the annual vaccination program and recommendations for usage are made by the Public Health Service (Table 241.2). The quantity of immunoreactive HA in each dose is standardized to contain the amount recommended by the Advisory Committee on Immunization Practices (98), which is

TABLE 241.2. Recommendations for the Use of Influenza Vaccine: Target Groups for Vaccination

Persons at increased risk for complications
  Persons age ≥65 yr
  Residents of nursing homes and other chronic care facilities that house persons of any age who
    have chronic medical conditions
  Adults and children who have chronic disorders of the pulmonary or cardiovascular systems
    including asthma
  Adults and children who have required medical follow-up or hospitalization during the preceding
    year because of chronic metabolic diseases (including diabetes mellitus), renal dysfunction,
    hemoglobinopathies, or immunosuppression (including immunosuppression caused by
    medications or by human immunodeficiency [HIV] virus)
  Children and teenagers (aged 6 mo–18 yr) who are receiving long-term aspirin therapy and there
    might be at risk for developing Reye's syndrome after influenza infection
  Women who will be in the second or third trimester of pregnancy during the influenza season
Persons aged 50–64 yr
  Vaccination is recommended for persons ages 50–64 years because this group has an increased
    prevalence of persons with high-risk conditions.
Persons who can transmit influenza to those at high risk
  Physicians, nurses, and other personnel in both hospital and outpatient care settings, including
    emergency response workers
  Employees of nursing homes and chronic care facilities who have contact with patients or residents
  Employees of assisted living and other residences for persons in groups at high risk
  Persons who provide home care to persons in groups at high risk and household members
    (including children) of persons in groups at high risk

From the Centers for Disease Control and Prevention. Prevention and control of influenza: recommendations of the advisory committee on immunization practices (ACIP). *MMWR* 2001;50(RR04):1–46, with permission.

usually 15 mg per component for older children (3 years of age) or 7.5 mg for children not over 3 years of age (Table 241.3). The quantity of NA is not standardized because this glycoprotein is quite labile during the process of purification and storage (105). Each 0.5-mL dose of vaccine contains approximately 10 billion virus particles, and one egg yields one to three doses of vaccine. Vaccine also contains variable but small quantities of endotoxin, egg-derived protein, free formaldehyde, and preservative that do not appear to contribute to the reactogenicity of the vaccines for humans. The route of immunization is intramuscular.

The vaccines potentially available are designated whole-virus (WV) vaccine or subvirion (SV) (split or purified surface antigen are alternative terms) virus vaccine. The WV vaccine (not currently available in the United States) contains intact, inactivated virus, whereas the SV vaccine contains purified virus disrupted with detergents that solubilize the lipid-containing viral envelope, followed by chemical inactivation of residual virus.

Immunogenicity and reactogenicity of vaccines has been evaluated in four large-scale, placebo-controlled trials in adults and children (100). Satisfactory serologic responses were achieved in children and adults with doses of vaccine that caused minimal clinical reactions. Reactions generally occurred within the first 24 hours and lasted for 1 to 2 days; these included systemic manifestations such as fever, malaise, myalgia, and headache, as well as local manifestations such as pain, erythema, induration, and tenderness at the site of vaccination. In adults, the frequency of systemic reactions to monovalent or trivalent WV or SV vaccines was not different from recipients of placebo. Local reactions occurred in 3% to 5% of adults and rarely caused significant morbidity. The reactogenicity of influenza B virus vaccine is similar to that of influenza A virus.

In children, a difference in reactogenicity of WV or SV vaccine was apparent. WV vaccinees exhibited significantly more systemic reactions than SV vaccinees. These observations form

TABLE 241.3. Influenza Vaccine Dosage, by Age Group—United States

Age group	Product[a]	Dose	No. of doses	Route[b]
6–35 mo	Split virus only	0.25 mL	1 or 2[c]	Intramuscular
3–8 yr	Split virus only	0.50 mL	1 or 2[c]	Intramuscular
9–12 yr	Split virus only	0.50 mL	1	Intramuscular
>12 yr	Whole or split virus[d]	0.50 ml	1	Intramuscular

[a]Because of their decreased potential for causing febrile reactions, only split-virus vaccines should be used for children. The vaccines might be labeled as "split," "subvirion," or "purified-surface-antigen" vaccine. Immunogenicity and side effects of split- and whole-virus vaccines are similar among adults when vaccines are administered at the recommended dosage.
[b]For adults and older children, the recommended site of vaccination is the deltoid muscle. The preferred site for infants and young child is the anterolateral aspect of the thigh.
[c]Two doses administered ≥1 months apart are recommended for children aged <9 years who are receiving influenza vaccine for the first time.
[d]No whole-virus vaccine was distributed in the United States during the 2001–2002 influenza season.
From the Centers for Disease Control and Prevention. Prevention and control of influenza: recommendations of the advisory committee on immunization practices (ACIP). *MMWR* 2001;50(RR04):1–46, with permission.

the basis for recommending that only SV vaccine be used in children under 12 years of age.

Local or systemic allergic reactions to vaccine components occur rarely. It is believed that the majority of these reactions are due to residual egg protein (100). High-risk patients who have egg allergies may be immunized using a specific protocol (106).

An increase in the number of reported cases of the Guillain-Barré syndrome (GBS) occurred following the National Influenza Immunization Program in 1976 to 1977 (107). About 1 in 100,000 individuals who received the swine influenza virus vaccine developed GBS, with a relative risk in vaccinees about four- to eightfold greater than unvaccinated subjects. Influenza virus vaccine produced after 1977 had not been associated with an increased risk for GBS, until a recent report implicated a low but definable excess risk (1 to 2 cases per million vaccinees) with the 1992 to 1993 and 1993 to 1994 vaccines (108).

The serum antibody response of elderly subjects to inactivated virus vaccines is variable but is generally lower than that of younger subjects (109). The antibody response of children over 6 months of age was similar to that of unprimed adults, but with two doses of SV vaccine needed to achieve a satisfactory level of antibody on primary immunization of children up to 8 years of age. In infants under 6 months of age, inactivated vaccines are less immunogenic than in older infants and children (110). The serum antibody responses of the young seronegative vaccinee can be quite strain specific, which is an important property to bear in mind when antigenically distinct viruses of the same type or subtype are cocirculating (111).

The level of antibody induced in unprimed or primed individuals given two doses of SV vaccine decreased 75% over an 8-month period. The rate of decline of antibody following SV vaccine administration is faster than that observed following infection in young children.

Antibody responses in patients with renal failure or with cancer are less than those in control individuals. Vaccine responses in high-risk patients with pulmonary or heart disease not receiving immunosuppressive drugs do not differ from controls. Immunization of immunocompromised individuals can induce antibody responses dependent on the level of immunocompetence (100).

Parenteral vaccination with influenza A and B viruses consistently induces resistance to illness and, to a lesser extent, infection with influenza A and B viruses. The resistance induced is manifested by a reduction in the frequency and severity of the illness, including otitis media in children (112). Efficacy ranges from 60% to 80%, with the higher value seen following challenge with homologous virus and the lower value following challenge with virus that has undergone antigenic drift.

Resistance to experimental or natural challenge correlates with the level of serum HAI antibody induced to the infecting strain. In those situations in which vaccine efficacy was low or not detectable, surface antigens of the epidemic virus differed significantly from those of the vaccine virus, or vaccines were of low potency and thus did not stimulate sufficient antibody to the epidemic virus. Vaccine is effective in the elderly who are at high risk for morbidity and mortality, but the level of efficacy is often less than that seen in young adults (113). Vaccination not only protects the vaccinee, but unvaccinated individuals can also benefit if the extent of vaccination is sufficient to dampen the epidemic spread of virus in the community (114). The duration of immunity following vaccination has not been evaluated systematically, but the relatively rapid decline in antibody levels suggests that protective immunity is of short duration. At any rate, antigenic changes in the influenza virus predicate annual immunization with current vaccines.

Annual vaccination is recommended for persons over 6 months of age who have chronic conditions, such as (a) heart disease, (b) bronchopulmonary disease, (c) renal disease, (d) diabetes or other metabolic disorders, (e) children on long-term aspirin therapy, and (f) women in the second or third trimester of pregnancy (98). In addition, individuals over the age of 50 should be vaccinated annually. Health care providers should be vaccinated as well as others in contact with high-risk groups. Influenza vaccine may be administered to any person who wishes to reduce the chance of becoming infected with influenza.

A live influenza virus vaccine has just been licensed for ages 5–50 years (Flu Mist, MedImmune, Gaithersburg, Md.). Similar experimental live vaccines have been developed and evaluated for their usefulness in the immunoprophylaxis of influenza illness in adults (115) and in children (116). There are two major reasons for continued interest in the use of live vaccines in humans. First, the current inactivated vaccines are recommended primarily for those at high risk for influenza virus infection and even in those groups offer only partial protection. In contrast, live vaccines appear to have the potential to broaden the indications for influenza vaccine and hence to have an impact on the overall morbidity and perhaps spread of the disease. Second, local immunity is increasingly recognized to play a major role in resistance to most respiratory pathogens (117). Respiratory tract infection with a live attenuated vaccine has been found to be the most efficient method of stimulating such immunity. Since infection of the respiratory tract stimulates systemic as well as local immunity, and theoretically is the optimal way of stimulating cell mediated immunity, all components of the host's immune response are brought into play.

As previously indicated, influenza A viruses (and to a lesser extent, influenza B viruses) are unique among viruses that infect the respiratory tract in that they undergo significant antigenic variation on virtually a yearly basis. The strategy for developing a live virus vaccine must take this property into account. It is not feasible to attenuate each new variant of influenza virus that appears in nature by multiple passages in a heterologous host, a method that has been successfully used to attenuate viruses that do not show antigenic variation. Therefore, a strategy is needed in which attenuation can be achieved in a single step by transfer of attenuating genes from an attenuated donor virus to each new epidemic or pandemic virulent virus (118).

Because resistance to influenza A virus is mediated by the development of an immune response to the HA and NA glycoproteins, the genes coding for these surface antigens must come from the epidemic virus, while the attenuating genes are derived from the attenuated parent. This scheme is possible because of the segmented nature of the influenza genome in which the HA and NA genes are derived from the virulent wild-type virus and the other genes are derived from the attenuated donor virus. In this approach, it is necessary that the genes that confer attenuation not code for the HA and NA glycoproteins, because these genes must be derived from the new epidemic or pandemic virus. Several donor viruses have been evaluated for their ability to reproducibly attenuate new epidemic influenza A viruses, including significant work in Russia with the A/Leningrad strains (119). The A/Ann Arbor/6/60 (H2N2) cold-adapted (ca) donor virus developed by John Maassab shows the most immediate promise as a vaccine candidate (120).

The influenza A/AA/6/60 (H2N2) ca donor virus was developed by passage of the wild-type virus at progressively lower temperatures in primary chick kidney cell cultures until a mutant was identified that replicated efficiently at 25°C, a temperature restrictive for the replication of wild-type virus (120). New live, attenuated reassortant virus vaccines are generated by mating the ca donor virus with a virulent wild-type virus and then selecting reassortant progeny at 25°C (restrictive for replication of wild-type virus) in the presence of an H2N2 antiserum, which inhibits replication of the viruses bearing the surface antigens of the attenuated A/AA/6/60 (H2N2) ca donor virus. A large series of H1N1 and H3N2 reassortants has been evaluated in humans and found to be satisfactorily (a) infectious, (b) attenuated for seronegative children and immunologically primed adults, (c) immunogenic, and (d) genetically stable. The viruses are poorly transmissible. The attenuation manifested by ca reassortants was accompanied by markedly reduced replication of virus in the upper respiratory tract of susceptible adults compared with that of volunteers infected with wild-type virus. Similar studies in other age groups revealed that the replication of ca reassortant viruses is (a) greatest in seronegative infants or children because viral growth is not limited by immunity induced by prior infection with influenza viruses; (b) intermediate in children and young adults who have had prior experience with related influenza A viruses; and (c) lowest in the elderly who have been infected many times with related influenza A viruses. Despite the efficient replication of ca reassortant viruses in young, fully susceptible, seronegative pediatric subjects, the vaccinees experience few symptoms, and those that occur are confined to the upper respiratory tract.

The ca reassortant vaccines induce resistance to experimental or natural challenge with wild-type influenza A viruses in adult and pediatric subjects who have had some prior experience with influenza A viruses (115,121). In addition, they are highly immunogenic in seronegative subjects, and this suggests that the vaccine would be efficacious in this population (46). Recently, very impressive efficacy, 93% overall, against culture confirmed influenza A/H3N2 and B was shown in a pediatric population 15 to 71 months of age following either one or two doses of trivalent ca reassortant vaccine given as a nasal spray (116). In the elderly, coadministration of live ca virus vaccine and inactivated virus vaccine may be more efficacious than inactivated virus vaccine alone against natural infection with influenza A virus (122).

Because the populations to be immunized have such disparate past experience with influenza A viruses, it is not surprising that different vaccines (i.e., live vs. inactivated virus vaccine) or different vaccine schedules would be needed for each population. The suggested usage and schedule of annual immunization with ca reassortant and inactivated virus vaccines and the reasons for the choice of vaccine in the pediatric, young adult, and elderly adult population are as follows: (a) the seronegative pediatric population over 6 months of age may preferentially get live vaccine because this type of vaccine has been shown to be more immunogenic in this population; (b) previously primed children and adults under 65 years of age may get either vaccine because efficacy of live and inactivated vaccines are comparable for this population, although a live virus vaccine may be better accepted because of an easier route of delivery; and (c) elderly individuals (>65 years of age) may get live plus inactivated virus vaccine if this combination proves more efficacious in this population. Additional studies are being done to support this suggested usage, and licensure of the live vaccine is hoped for in the next few years.

REFERENCES

1. Smith W, Andrewes CH, Laidlaw PP, et al. A virus obtained from influenza patients. *Lancet* 1933;2:66–68.
2. Memorandum W, et al. A revised system of nomenclature for influenza viruses. *Bull WHO* 1980;58:585–591.
3. Murti KG, Webster RG, et al. Distribution of hemagglutinin and neuraminidase on influenza virions as revealed by immunoelectron microscopy. *Virology* 1986;149:36–43.
4. Subbarao K, et al. Characterization of an avian influenza A (HSNJ) virus isolated from a child with a fatal respiratory illness. *Science* 1998;279:393–396.
5. Suarez DL, et al. Comparisons of highly virulent HSNI influenza A viruses isolated from humans and chickens from Hong Kong. *J Virol* 1998;72:6678–6688.
6. Yuen KY, et al. Clinical features and rapid viral diagnosis of human disease associated with avian influenza A HSNJ virus. *Lancet* 1998;351:467–471.
7. Guo YJ, Li JW, Cheng I, et al. Discovery of humans infected by avian influenza A (H9N2) virus. *Chin J Exp Clin Virol* 1999;15:105–108.
8. Noble GR, et al. Epidemiological and clinical aspects of influenza. In: Beare AS, ed. *Basic and applied influenza research*. Boca Raton, FL: CRC Press, 1982: 1–50.
9. Daly JM, Wood JM, Robertson JS, et al. Cocirculation and divergence of human influenza viruses. Oxford, UK: Blackwell Science, 1998:168–177.
10. Neuzil KM, et al. The effect of influenza on hospitalizations, outpatient visits, and courses of antibiotics in children. *N Engl J Med* 2000;342:225–231.
11. Neuzil KM, et al. Influenza-associated morbidity and mortality in young and middle-aged women. *JAMA* 1999;281:901–907.
12. Neuzil KM, et al. Impact of influenza on acute cardiopulmonary hospitalizations in pregnant women. *Am J Epidemiol* 1998;148:1094–1102.
13. Nichol KL, et al. The efficacy and cost effectiveness of vaccination against influenza among elderly persons living in the community. *N Engl J Med* 1994;331:778–784.
14. Perrotta DM, Decker M, Glezen WP, et al. Acute respiratory disease hospitalizations as a measure of impact of epidemic influenza. *Am J Epidemiol* 1985;122:468–476.
15. Glezen WP, Paredes A, Taber LH, et al. Influenza in children. Relationship to other respiratory agents. *JAMA* 1980;243:1345–1349.
16. Wright PF, et al. Patterns of illness in the highly febrile young child: epidemiologic, clinical, and laboratory correlates. *Pediatrics* 1981;67:694–700.
17. Fox JP, et al. Influenzavirus infections in Seattle families, 1975–1979. II. Pattern of infection in invaded households and relation of age and prior antibody to occurrence of infection and related illness. *Am J Epidemiol* 1982;116:228–242.
18. Neuzil KM, et al. Burden of interpandemic influenza in children younger than 5 years. A 25-year prospective study. *J Infect Dis* 2002;147–152.
19. Monto AS, Kioumehr F, et al. The Tecumseh Study of Respiratory Illness. IX. Occurrence of influenza in the community, 1966–1971. *Am J Epidemiol* 1975;102:553–563.
20. Jordan WS Jr, et al. The mechanism of spread of Asian influenza. *Am Rev Respir Dis* 1961;83:29–40.
21. Siinonsen L, et al. The impact of influenza epidemics on mortality: introducing a severity index. *Am J Public Health* 1997;87:1944–1950.
22. Moser MR, et al. An outbreak of influenza aboard a commercial airliner. *Am J Epidemiol* 1979;110:1–6.
23. Foy HM, et al. Influenza B in households. virus shedding without symptoms or antibody response. *Am J Epidemiol* 1987;126:506–515.
24. Richmond DD, et al. Three strains of influenza virus (H3N2): interferon sensitivity *in vitro* and interferon production in volunteers. *J Chin Microbiol* 1976;3:223–226.
25. Frank AL, et al. Patterns of shedding of myxoviruses and paramyxoviruses in children. *J Infect Dis* 1981;144:433–441.
26. Hall GB, et al. Viral shedding patterns of children with influenza B infection. *J Infect Dis* 1979;140:610–613.
27. Hers JF, et al. Disturbances of the ciliated epithelium due to influenza virus. *Am Rev Respir Dis* 1966;93:162–171.
28. Hall WJ, et al. Pulmonary mechanics after uncomplicated influenza A infection. *Am Rev Respir Dis* 1976;113:141–17.
29. Hayden FG, et al. Local and systemic cytokine responses during experimental human influenza A virus infection: relation to symptom formation and host defense. *J Chin Invest* 1998;101:643–649.
30. Garcia-Sastre A, et al. Influenza A virus lacking the NSJ gene replicates in interferon-deficient systems. *Virology* 1998;252:324–330.
31. Potter CW, Oxford JS, et al. Determinants of immunity to influenza infection in man. *Br Med Bull* 1979;35:69–75.
32. Askonas BA, McMichael AJ, Webster RG, et al. The immune response to influenza viruses and the problem of protection against infection. In: Beare AS, ed. *Basic and applied influenza research*. Boca Raton, FL: CRC Press, 1982:77–83.
33. Epstein SL, et al. Beta 2-microglobulin–deficient mice can be protected against influenza A infection by vaccination with vaccinia-influenza recombinants expressing hemagglutinin and neuraminidase. *J Immunol* 1993;150:5484–5493.
34. Virelizier JL, et al. Host defenses against influenza virus: the role of anti-hemagglutinin antibody. *J Immunol* 1975;115:434–439.
35. Schulman JL, Khakpour M, Kilbourne ED, et al. Protective effects of specific immunity to viral neuraminidase on influenza virus infection of mice. *J Virol* 1968;2:778–786.
36. Karzon DT, et al. Cytotoxic T cells in influenza immunity. *Semin Virol* 1996;7:265–271.
37. Ennis FA, et al. HLA restricted virus-specific cytotoxic T-lymphocyte responses to live and inactivated influenza vaccines. *Lancet* 1981;2:887–891.
38. McMichael AJ, et al. Cytotoxic T-cell immunity to influenza. *N Engl J Med* 1983;309:13–17.

39. Bender BS, et al. Transgenic mice lacking class I major histocompatibility complex-restricted T cells have delayed viral clearance and increased mortality after influenza virus challenge. *J Exp Med* 1992;175:1143–1145.

40. Lightman S, et al. Do L3T4⁺ T cells act as effector cells in protection against influenza virus infection? *Immunology* 1987;62:139–144.

41. Francis TJ, Quilligan JJJ, Minuse E, et al. Identification of another epidemic respiratory disease. *Science* 1950;112:495–497.

42. Artenstein MS, Bellanti JA, Buescher EL, et al. Identification of the antiviral substances in nasal secretions. *Proc Soc Exp Biol Med* 1964;117:558–564.

43. Rossen RD, et al. The proteins in nasal secretion. II. A longitudinal study of IgA and neutralizing antibody levels in nasal washings from men infected with influenza virus. *JAMA* 1970;211:1157–1161.

44. Murphy BR, Clements ML, et al. The systemic and mucosal immune response of humans to influenza A virus. *Curr Top Microbiol Immunol* 1989;146:107–116.

45. Wright PF, et al. Secretory immunological response after intranasal inactivated influenza A virus vaccinations: evidence for immunoglobulin A memory. *Infect Immun* 1983;40:1092–1095.

46. Murphy BR, et al. Secretory and systemic immunological response in children infected with live attenuated influenza A virus vaccines. *Infect Immun* 1982;36:1102–1108.

47. Johnson PR, et al. Immunity to influenza A virus infection in young children: a comparison of natural infection, live cold-adapted vaccine, and inactivated vaccine. *J Infect Dis* 1986;154:121–127.

48. Boyce TG, et al. Mucosal immune response to trivalent live attenuated intranasal influenza vaccine in children. *Vaccine* 1999;18:82–88.

49. Clements ML, et al. Serum and nasal wash antibodies associated with resistance to experimental challenge with influenza A wild-type virus. *J Clin Microbiol* 1986;24:157–160.

50. Walsh JJ, et al. Bronchotracheal response in human influenza. Type A, Asian strain, as studied by light and electron microscopic examination of bronchoscopic biopsies. *Arch Intern Med* 1961;108:376–388.

51. Douglas RG, et al. In: Kilbourne ED, ed. Influenza in man. Orlando, FL: Academic Press, 1975:395–447.

52. Govaert TME, et al. The predictive value of influenza symptomatology in elderly people. *Family Pract* 1997;15:16–22.

53. Smith GE, et al. Effect of viral infections on pulmonary function in patients with chronic obstructive pulmonary diseases. *J Infect Dis* 1980;141:271–280.

54. Henderson FW, et al. A longitudinal study of respiratory viruses and bacteria in the etiology of acute otitis media with effusion. *N Engl J Med* 1980;306:1377–1383.

55. Glezen WP, Decker M, Perrotta DM, et al. Survey of underlying conditions of persons hospitalized with acute respiratory disease during influenza epidemics in Houston, 1978–1981. *Am Rev Respir Dis* 1987;136:550–555.

56. Kim HW. Influenza A and B infections in infants and young children during the years 1957–1976. *Am J Epidemiol* 1979;109:464–479.

57. Wright PF, et al. Influenza A infections in young children. Primary natural infection and protective efficacy of live vaccine-induced or naturally acquired immunity. *N Engl J Med* 1977;296:829–834.

58. Buchan KA, Marten KW, et al. An etiology and epidemiology of viral croup in Glasgow, 1966–1972. *J Hyg (Lond)* 1974;73:143–150.

59. Kondo S, Abe K, et al. The effects of influenza virus infection on FEVJ in asthmatic children. The time-course study. *Chest* 1991;100:1235–1238.

60. Louria DB, et al. Studies on influenza in the pandemic of 1957–1958. II. Pulmonary complications of influenza. *J Chin Invest* 1959;38:213–265.

61. Mulder J, Hers JF, et al. Influenza. Groningen, The Netherlands: Wolters-Noordhoff, 1979.

62. Goodpasture EW, et al. The significance of certain pulmonary lesions in relation to the etiology of influenza. *Am J Med Sci* 1919;158:863–870.

63. Winterbauer RH, Ludwig WR, Hammar SP, et al. Clinical course, management, and long-term sequelae of respiratory failure due to influenza viral pneumonia. *Johns Hopkins Med* 1977;141:148–155.

64. Pinsker KL. Unusual interstitial pneumonia following Texas A2 influenza infection. *Chest* 1981;80:123–126.

65. Finland M, et al. Excursions into epidemiology: selected studies during the past four decades at Boston City Hospital. *J Infect Dis* 1973;128:76–124.

66. Bisno AL, et al. Pneumonia and Hong Kong influenza: a prospective study of the 1968–1969 epidemic. *Am J Med Sci* 1971;261:251–263.

67. Gerber GJ, Farmer WG, Fulkerson LL, et al. Hemolytic streptococcal pneumonia following influenza. *JAMA* 1987;240:242–243.

68. Martin GM, et al. Asian influenza A in Boston, 1957–1958. I. Observations in thirty-two influenza-associated fatal cases. *Arch Intern Med* 1959;103:515–531.

69. Petersdorf RG, et al. Pulmonary infections complicating Asian influenza. *AMA Arch Intern Med (Chicago)* 1959;103:262–272.

70. Schwarzmann SW, et al. Bacterial pneumonia during the Hong Kong influenza epidemic of 1968–1969. Experience in a city-county hospital. *Arch Intern Med* 1971;127:1037–1041.

71. Robertson L, Galey JP, Moore J, et al. Importance of *Staphylococcus aureus* in pneumonia in the 1957 epidemic of influenza A. *Lancet* 1958;2:2333–2336.

72. Tashiro M, Klenk HD, Rott R, et al. Inhibitory effect of a protease inhibitor, leupeptin, on the development of influenza pneumonia, mediated by concomitant bacteria. *J Gen Virol* 1987;68:2039–2041.

73. Minow RA, et al. Myoglobinuria associated with influenza A infection. *Am Intern Med* 1974;80:359–361.

74. Hurwitz ES, et al. National surveillance for Reye syndrome: a five-year review. *Pediatrics* 1982;70:895–900.

75. Partin JG, et al. Isolation of influenza virus from liver and muscle biopsy specimens from a surviving case of Reye's syndrome. *Lancet* 1976;2:599–602.

76. Barrett MJ, et al. Changing epidemiology of Reyes syndrome in the United States. *Pediatrics* 1986;77:598–602.

77. Delorme L, Middleton PJ, et al. Influenza A virus associated with acute encephalopathy. *Am J Dis Child* 1979;133:822–824.

78. Flewett TH, Hoult JG, et al. Influenzal encephalopathy and post-influenzal encephalitis. *Lancet* 1958;2:11–15.

79. Hoult JG, Flewett TH, et al. Influenzal encephalopathy and post-influenzal encephalitis. *BMJ* 1958;1:1847–1850.

80. Ito Y, et al. Detection of influenza virus RNA by reverse transcription-PCR and proinflammatory cytokines in influenza-virus–associated encephalopathy. *J Med Virol* 1999;58:420–425.

81. Ravenholt RT, Foege WH, et al. 1918 influenza, encephalitis lethargica, parkinsonism. *Lancet* 1982;2:860–864.

82. Greenberg M, et al. Maternal mortality in the epidemic of Asian influenza, New York City, 1957. *Am J Obstet Gynecol* 1958;76:897–902.

83. Schoenbaum SC, Weinstein L, et al. Respiratory infection in pregnancy. *Clin Obstet Gynecol* 1979;22:293–300.

84. Woolston WJ, Gonley DO, et al. Epidemic pneumonia (Spanish influenza) in pregnancy. Effect in one hundred and one cases. *JAMA* 1918;71:1898–1899.

85. MacKenzie JS, Houghton M, et al. Influenza infections during pregnancy: association with congenital malformations and with subsequent neoplasms in children, and potential hazards of live virus vaccines. *Bacteriol Rev* 1974;38:356–370.

86. Whimbey E, Bodey GP, et al. Viral pneumonia in the immunocompromised adult with neoplastic disease: the role of common community respiratory viruses. *Semin Respir Infect* 1992;7:122–131.

87. Wright PF, Bryant JD, Karzon DT, et al. Comparison of influenza B/Hong Kong virus infections among infants, children, and young adults. *J Infect Dis* 1980;141:430–435.

88. Farrell MK, Partin JG, Bove KE, et al. Epidemic influenza myopathy in Cincinnati in 1977. *J Pediatr* 1980;96:545–551.

89. Kerr AA, et al. Gastric flu influenza B causing abdominal symptoms in children. *Lancet* 1975;1:291–295.

90. O'Callaghan RJ, Gohd RS, Labat DD, et al. Human antibody to influenza C virus: its age-related distribution and distinction from receptor analogs. *Infect Immun* 1980;30:500–505.

91. Joosting AG, et al. Production of common colds in human volunteers by influenza C virus. *BMJ* 1968;4:153–154.

92. Centers for Disease Control and Prevention, et al. Clinical issues in the prophylaxis, diagnosis, and treatment of anthrax. *Emerg Infect Dis* 2002;8:222–225.

93. Falsey AR, et al. Respiratory syncytial virus and influenza A infection in the hospitalized elderly: clinical and epidemiologic findings. *J Infect Dis* 1995;172:389–394.

94. Claas EG, et al. Prospective application of reverse transcriptase polymerase chain reaction for diagnosing influenza infections in respiratory samples from a children's hospital. *J Clin Microbial* 1993;31:2218–2221.

95. Schepetiuk SK, Kok T, et al. The use of MDCK, MEK and LLC-MK2 cell lines with enzyme immunoassay for the isolation of influenza and parainfluenza viruses from clinical specimens. *J Virol Methods* 1993;42:241–250.

96. Waner JL, et al. Comparison of Directigen FLU-A with viral isolation and direct immunofluorescence for the rapid detection and identification of influenza A virus. *J Clin Microbiol* 1991;29:479–482.

97. Van Voris LP, Newell PM, et al. Antivirals for the chemoprophylaxis and treatment of influenza. *Semin Respir Infect* 1992;7:61–70.

98. Dolin R, et al. A controlled trial of amantadine and rimantadine in the prophylaxis of influenza A infection. *N Engl J Med* 1982;307:580–584.

99. Hall GB, et al. Children with influenza A infection: treatment with rimantadine. *Pediatrics* 1987;80:275–282.

100. Centers for Disease Control and Prevention, et al. Prevention and control of influenza: recommendations of the advisory committee on immunization practices (ACIP). *MMWR* 2001;50(RRO4):1–46.

101. Kim CU. Influenza neuraminidase inhibitors possessing a novel hydrophobic interaction in the enzyme active site: design, synthesis, and structural analysis of carbo cyclic sialic acid analogous with potent anti-influenza activity. *J Am Chem Soc* 1997;119:681–690.

102. Hayden FG, et al. Safety and efficacy of the neuraminidase inhibitor GG167 in experimental human influenza. *JAMA* 1996;275:295–299.

103. Hayden FG, et al. Efficacy and safety of the neuraminidase inhibitor zanamivir in the treatment of influenzavirus infections. *N Engl J Med* 1997;337:874–880.

104. Hayden FG, et al. Use of the selective oral neuraminidase inhibitor oseltamivir to prevent influenza. *N Engl J Med* 1999;341:1336–1343.

105. Kendal AP, Bozeman FM, Ennis FA, et al. Further studies of the neuraminidase content of inactivated influenza vaccines and the neuraminidase antibody responses after vaccination of immunologically primed and unprimed populations. *Infect Immun* 1980;29:966–971.

106. Murphy KR, Stunk RG, et al. Safe administration of influenza vaccine in asthmatic children hypersensitive to egg proteins. *J Pediatr* 1985;106:931–933.

107. Safranek TJ, et al. Reassessment of the association between Guillain-Barré

syndrome and receipt of swine influenza vaccine in 1976–1977. Results of a two-state study. Expert Neurology Group. *Am J Epidemiol* 1991;133:940–951.

108. Lasky T, et al. The Guillain-Barré syndrome and the 1992–1993 and 1993–1994 influenza vaccines. *N Engl J Med* 1998;339:1797–1802.

109. Palache AM, et al. Antibody response after influenza immunization with various vaccine doses: a double-blind, placebo-controlled, multi-centre, dose-response study in elderly nursing-home residents and young volunteers. *Vaccine* 1993;11:3–9.

110. Groothuis JR, et al. Immunization of high-risk infants younger than 18 months of age with split-product influenza vaccine. *Pediatrics* 1991;87:823–828.

111. Levandowski RA, et al. Antibody responses to influenza B viruses in immunologically unprimed children. *Pediatrics* 1991;88:1031–1036.

112. Heikkinen T, et al. Influenza vaccination in the prevention of acute otitis media in children. *Am J Dis Child* 1991;145:445–448.

113. Nichol KL, Wuorenma I, von Steinberg T, et al. Benefits of influenza vaccination for low-, intermediate-, and high-risk senior citizens. *Arch Intern Med* 1998;158:1769–1776.

114. Monto AS, et al. Effect of vaccination of a school-age population upon the course of an A2-Hong Kong influenza epidemic. *Bull WHO* 1969;41:537–542.

115. Nichol KL, et al. Effectiveness of live, attenuated intranasal influenza virus vaccine in healthy, working adults: a randomized controlled trial. *JAMA* 1999;282:137–144.

116. Belshe RB, et al. The efficacy of live attenuated, cold-adapted, trivalent, intranasal influenzavirus vaccine in children. *N Engl J Med* 1998;338:1405–1412.

117. Boyce TG, et al. Safety and immunogenicity of adjuvanted and unadjuvanted subunit influenza vaccines administered intranasally to healthy adults. *Vaccine* 1999;18:82–88.

118. Murphy BR, et al. Use of live attenuated cold-adapted influenza A reassortant virus vaccines in infants, children, young adults, and elderly adults. *Infect Dis Clin Pract* 1993;2:174–181.

119. Kendal AP, et al. Cold-adapted live attenuated influenza vaccines developed in Russia: can they contribute to meeting the needs for influenza control in other countries? *Eur J Epidemiol* 1997;13:591–609.

120. Maassab HF, Bryant ML, et al. The development of live attenuated cold-adapted influenza virus vaccine for humans. *Rev Med Virol* 1999;9:237–244.

121. Edwards KM, et al. A randomized controlled trial of cold-adapted and inactivated vaccines for the prevention of influenza A disease. *J Infect Dis* 1994;169:68–76.

122. Treanor JJ, et al. Protective efficacy of combined live intranasal and inactivated influenza A virus vaccines in the elderly. *Am Intern Med* 1992;117:625–633.

123. Neuzil KM. Treatment for influenzavirus infection. *Curr Treat Options Infect Dis* 2002;4:37–42.

CHAPTER 242
Human Parainfluenza Viruses

Kelly J. Henrickson

INTRODUCTION

The Paramyxoviridae family is a large rapidly growing group of viruses that cause significant human and veterinary disease (Table 242.1). In fact, this virus family is one of the most costly in terms of disease burden and economic impact to our planet. Recently discovered Paramyxoviridae (Megamyxoviruses: Hendra, Nipah; and Metapneumovirus [hMPV]) emphasize this point (1–4).

Between 1955 and 1957, three viruses with some myxovirus-like properties were isolated from children with lower respiratory tract infections. However, these three viruses proved to be easily separated from other myxoviruses by their poor growth in embryonated eggs and lack of antigenic relationship to the influenza viruses. In 1959 a fourth virus was found that met these same criteria, and a new taxonomic group was created called "parainfluenza viruses" (see Table 242.1).

Human parainfluenza viruses (HPIV) now belong to two genera (*Respirovirus* and *Rubulavirus*). There are four major virus groups within HPIV (types 1–4). Until recently, these belonged

to one genus (*Paramyxovirus*). Further major subtypes of HPIV-4 (5) and subgroups/genotypes of HPIV-1 (6–9) and HPIV-3 (10) have been described. HPIV types 1-3 are major causes of lower respiratory infections in infants and young children (11–15). Together, HPIV is one of the most common respiratory viral groups infecting mankind. A typical virus has a single negative strand of ribonucleic acid (RNA) in its genome and is surrounded by a lipid envelope of host cell origin. These medium-size viruses (150–200 nm) are all very similar in their structural, physiochemical, and biologic characteristics. However, they each have different host ranges and epidemiology that help make them unique.

CLINICAL ASPECTS AND EPIDEMIOLOGY

HPIV are ubiquitous respiratory pathogens that have been found throughout the world. Malnutrition, overcrowding, vitamin A deficiency, lack of breast-feeding, and environmental smoke or toxins may predispose to these infections (11,12,16–18). There are greater then 5 million lower respiratory infections (LRI) each year in the United States in children younger than 5 years of age (13,14). Approximately one third of these are caused by HPIV-1, 2, and 3 (13–15). Also, these viruses cause upper respiratory infections (URI) in infants, children, and adults, and to a lesser extent, LRI in the immunocompromised and elderly. HPIV-4 can cause disease in young infants and children but is rarely isolated. Antibody to HPIV-4 is detectable in most children between 6 to 10 years of age, suggesting mild or asymptomatic infections (19). Three percent to 18% of admissions to pediatric hospitals can be for acute respiratory infections and HPIV can be detected in 9% to 30%, depending on the time of year (15,18,20,21). There are between 500,000 and 800,000 LRI hospitalizations (patients younger than 18 years of age) in the United States each year with approximately 12% being for HPIV-1, 2, and 3 (21,22). This is second only to respiratory syncytial virus (RSV) as a cause of hospitalization for viral LRI. The majority of the clinical discussion will focus out of necessity on children.

HPIV-1 occurs in biennial epidemics during the fall in both hemispheres (15,18,21,23). At least 50% of croup cases in the United States can be linked to this virus (14,23,24). It has been estimated that in the United States between 18,000 and 35,000 children younger than 5 years of age are hospitalized during each HPIV-1 epidemic (13,14,23–28). Also, HPIV-1 causes bronchiolitis, tracheobronchitis, pneumonia, and febrile and afebrile wheezing, predominantly in children seven to 36 months of age with a peak incidence in the second and third year of life (21). HPIV-1 can cause LRI in young infants but is rare below the age of 1 month. The full burden of HPIV-1 in adults and the elderly has not been determined, but several studies have shown this virus to cause yearly hospitalizations in healthy adults and perhaps play a role in bacterial pneumonias and deaths in nursing home residents (29–31). HPIV-1, 2, and 3 have all been found to occur at low levels in most months of the year similar to RSV and influenza (21,32).

Infection with HPIV-2 has been reported to occur biennially with HPIV-1 or alternate years with HPIV-1. However, more recently in some locations HPIV-2 has occurred in yearly outbreaks (15,20,27). The majority of respiratory tract infections caused by this virus appear in the fall to early winter. Croup is the most frequent LRI caused by HPIV-2 but all of the respiratory syndromes have been described. LRI caused by this virus has been reported much less frequently than with HPIV-I and HPIV-3. This may be due to difficulties in isolation and detection. As many as 6,000 children younger than 18 years of age may be hospitalized each year in the United States because of HPIV-2 (21). The peak incidence of HPIV-2 occurs in the second year of

TABLE 242.1.   Taxonomic Relationships of Human Parainfluenza Viruses: Paramyxoviridae Family

	Human	Animal
Paramyxovirinae (subfamily)		
Respirovirus (genus)	PIV-1 and 3	Sendai (MOUSE PIV-1)
		Bovine PIV-3
		Simian PIV-10
Rubulavirus (genus)	PIV-2 and 4A, 4B Mumps	NDV (1)
		Yucaipa (2)
		Kunitachi (5)
		Avian PIV 3, 4, 6-9
		La-Piedad-Michoacan-Mexico (Porcine)
		Simian PIV 5 and 41
Morbillivirus (genus)	Measles	Canine distemper
		Rinderpest (bovine)
		Pest-Des-Petits-ruminants
		Dolphin distemper
		Porpoise distemper
		Phocine distemper
Megamyxovirus (genus)	Hendra	HeV (equine) bats
	Nipah	NIPAH (porcine) bats
Pneumovirinae (subfamily)		
Pneumovirus (genus)	RSV	Bovine RSV
		Pneumonia virus of mice
Metapneumovirus (genus)	hMPV (HUMAN)	Avian pneumovirus

hMPV, Human metapneumovirus; PIV, parainfluenza virus; RSV, respiratory syncytial virus.

life, but significant numbers of infections take place in infants younger than 1 year of age. Approximately 60% of HPIV-2 infections take place in a child's first 5 years. Although frequently overshadowed by HPIV-1 and HPIV-3, HPIV-2 can in any one year be the predominate cause of LRI in young children.

HPIV-3 is unique among the parainfluenza viruses in its propensity to infect infants younger than 6 months of age. This virus causes the majority of its infections in the first 12 months of life (approximately 40%) with bronchiolitis and pneumonia being the most common clinical syndromes. It is second only to RSV as a cause of LRI in neonates and young infants and has caused outbreaks within neonatal intensive care units (32). Approximately 18,000 infants and children are hospitalized each year in the United States because of LRI caused by HPIV-3 (21). Although endemic throughout the world, this virus also occurs in spring/summer epidemics in North America. These epidemics may be dependent on ambient climate conditions (33,34).

HPIV-4 has been isolated from a very small number of children and adults, and there have been few epidemiologic reports (5,19,35–37). Approximately one third of cases have been in infants younger than 1 year of age, one third in preschool children, and one third in school age children and adults. Seroprevalence studies have demonstrated 60% to 84% of infants have significant antibody levels after birth (presumably maternal in origin). These levels drop to 7% to 9% by 7 to 12 months of age and stay low for several years before increasing to about 50% by 3 to 5 years of age. Antibody levels to HPIV-4 continue to rise throughout childhood until approximately 95% of adults have antibody to HPIV-4 A, and 75% have antibody to HPIV-4 B (19). Interestingly, the majority of HPIV-4 clinical isolates appear to be subtype B. All of the different respiratory tract syndromes can be caused by HPIV-4. Severe LRI and pneumonia has been associated with hospitalization of infants and young children (38). However, based on the seroprevalence data, because infection with HPIV-4 is almost universal, serious disease is either rare or difficult to diagnose.

Several investigators have suggested that some animal parainfluenza viruses can on occasion infect humans. The majority of evidence to support this hypothesis is serologic and because of the antigenic relatedness of the *Respirovirus* and *Rubulavirus* genera, it is difficult to substantiate. However, closely related Megamyxoviruses (*Hendra, Nipah*), whose natural host appear to be bats, have recently caused serious epidemics of encephalitis in humans (2–4). Also, Newcastle disease virus (NDV) clearly causes human disease and is discussed under animal pathogenesis. In addition, Bovine PIV-3 can infect humans, HPIV-1 can infect mice, and mouse PIV-1 (Sendai) can infect African green monkeys (39–41). Usually these infections are asymptomatic.

Clinical Syndromes

Every upper and lower respiratory tract illness has been described for HPIV. However, there is a strong relationship between HPIV-1, HPIV-2, and HPIV-3 and specific clinical syndromes, age of child, and time of year. HPIV-4 has not demonstrated such a relationship, but this may simply reflect our lack of epidemiologic data on this virus.

CROUP

Symptoms of acute laryngotracheobronchitis include hoarseness, cough, inspiratory stridor with laryngeal obstruction, and fever. It is more common in boys and has a peak incidence between the first and second year of life. In Milwaukee, white children have had a much higher incidence than African-American children for over a decade (21,42). This clinical entity accounts for between 10% and 25% of LRI in preschool children (depending on age). Etiologic agents have been isolated from 36% to 74% of symptomatic children averaging around 50% (14,15,21,24,38). HPIV have made up between 56% and 74% of these cases of croup (24). HPIV-1 is the most frequently isolated virus in croup, accounting for 26% to 74% (average approximately 50%) of identified causes. HPIV-2 and HPIV-3 average around 10% each as etiologic agents. Sampling of national databases (0.5% of total) and community based estimates has suggested between 27,000 and 66,000 hospitalizations each year in the United States for croup (21,23,42). In years where HPIV-1 is not epidemic, HPIV-2 has been shown to sometimes cause outbreaks. In 1991, during a peak HPIV-1 year, Milwaukee, Wisconsin experienced an HPIV-2 outbreak in which this virus made up two thirds of the identified agents (23). HPIV-3 has been demonstrated to cause severe croup in an adult (43). RSV, influenza A and B, adenoviruses, rhinoviruses, hMPV, and, in school age children, mycoplasma have all been shown to cause croup. A recent retrospective review suggested that influenza croup was more severe than parainfluenza croup (44).

TRACHEOBRONCHITIS

This is a clinical "wastebasket" for patients who have lower respiratory signs and symptoms but do not fit into any of the three well-described syndromes. Typically, these patients have cough and large airway noise on auscultation (rhonchi), but also may have fever and URI. Approximately 20% to 30% of children with LRI receive this diagnosis. The incidence decreases somewhat in the first 5 years of life but is fairly evenly diagnosed throughout childhood and adolescence. Viral agents make up the majority of etiologies in children (14). HPIV make up greater than 25% of the etiologic agents that have been reported to cause tracheobronchitis. Also, this diagnosis is found more commonly in patients with chronic diseases (21). HPIV-3 is most frequently isolated followed by HPIV-1 and HPIV-2. Several studies have recorded this as the most common diagnosis in patients with HPIV-4 infections.

BRONCHIOLITIS

This is usually defined as expiratory wheezing with tachypnea, air trapping, and the use of accessory respiratory muscles (retractions). Infants and children often have fever, and rales may be present. Bronchiolitis peaks in the first year of life (81% younger than 1 year old) and then dramatically declines until it is unusual in school age children (21). Overall, approximately 25% to 30% of LRI in childhood are diagnosed as bronchiolitis. At least 90% of bronchiolitis is thought to be viral in origin and a viral identification rate as high as 83% has been reported (14,15).

Hospitalizations for bronchiolitis have been dramatically increasing over the past 20 years in the United States (21,22). All four types of HPIV can cause bronchiolitis, but HPIV-1 and HPIV-3 have been reported most commonly. Each of these two groups appears to cause 10% to 15% of bronchiolitis in non-hospitalized children. However, in hospitalized children, HPIV-3 causes many more cases than HPIV-1 (three or four to one) and is second only to RSV as a cause of bronchiolitis and pneumonia in young infants.

PNEUMONIA

Fever, rales, and evidence of pulmonary consolidation on physical examination or radiography is the classic method of diagnosing pneumonia. It represents on average 29% to 38% of pediatric inpatient admissions for LRI and 23% of children treated as outpatients (14,15,21,27,45,46). Pneumonia causes 83% of hospitalizations for children with LRI who were older than 5 years of age in Milwaukee (21). The peak incidence for pneumonia is in the second and third year of life. Recently, approximately one third of pneumonia hospitalizations have been in children with chronic diseases (21). Viruses have been shown to cause up to 90% of these LRI, especially in the first year (14,47–51), and this percentage decreases to approximately 50% by school age (14,45,51). After 9 to 10 years of age, viruses cause a decreasing

but still significant amount of pneumonia in immunocompetent individuals. The percentage of pneumonias with a viral etiology eventually declines to about 12% by adulthood (31,53,54). HPIV-1 and HPIV-3 each cause about 10% of outpatient pneumonias. However, HPIV-3 causes a greater percentage of hospitalized cases. HPIV-2 and HPIV-4 have both been reported to cause pneumonia but the exact proportion of disease caused by these viruses is unclear. HPIV-1 infection has been associated with secondary bacterial pneumonias in the elderly (30).

Several of these LRI syndromes can occur simultaneously or progressively in the same child, but if this occurs, they are usually caused by a single virus. Two or more respiratory viruses are isolated in 5% to 20% of acute LRIs, and may be associated with more severe disease (54). HPIV routinely cause otitis media, pharyngitis, conjunctivitis, and coryza (common cold). These URI can occur singularly or in any combination with the previously mentioned LRI. Otitis media has been shown to be associated with viral respiratory tract infections in 30% to 60% of cases. Although only a small number of otitis media is caused solely by viruses, they may act synergistically with bacteria to initiate infection or prolong symptoms during antimicrobial therapy (55). In children with acute otitis media, HPIV have been found in 1% of middle ear effusions and in 2% of nasopharyngeal secretions (56). HPIV-3 has been reported more frequently than other types (28).

IMMUNOCOMPROMISED HOSTS

HPIV have been reported to cause serious and fatal LRI in immunocompromised children and adults. Giant-cell pneumonia with HPIV-2 has been reported in severe combined immunodeficiency syndrome (SCIDS) (57) and with HPIV-3 in SCIDS (58–62), acute myelomonocytic leukemia (63), and after bone marrow transplantation (64). Many of these patients had dual infections with other pathogens. Persistent respiratory tract infection and viral excretion of HPIV-1, HPIV-2, and HPIV-3 have been described in SCIDS (57,60,61), with HPIV-3 in a child with DiGeorge syndrome after thymic transplant (65), and in HIV infected children (66–68). HIV infected children do not appear to have more severe disease with these viruses until they are significantly T-cell deficient, but the epidemiology of HPIV in this population still needs to be studied (69). HPIV-3 has been associated with acute rejection episodes in renal and liver transplant recipients (70,71). HPIV upper and lower respiratory tract infections, including consolidated and interstitial pneumonia, have been reported in organ and bone marrow transplant patients (64,72–77). HPIV-3 has been the most frequent parainfluenza virus isolated from immunocompromised patients with LRI and is a common cause of fever and neutropenia in children with cancer (78–80). This virus has been found to be persistently shed from bone marrow transplant patients for up to 4 months without accumulating any mutations (81). HPIV-1, 2, and 3 infect between 5% and 7% of adult bone marrow transplant recipients and leukemia patients (76–80); pneumonia will develop in approximately 24% to 50%, and 22% to 75% of these patients will die. In the pediatric bone marrow transplant population, a retrospective study found that pneumonia developed in 41% of those with HPIV infection (47% of viral respiratory infections) and 6% died (79). HPIV has been shown to cause serious LRI and death (8%) in lung transplant recipients up to 5 years after transplantation (82). Children with SCIDS and common variable hypogammaglobulinemia have been reported with parotitis caused by HPIV-3 (83). Other non-respiratory sites of infection in immunocompromised patients have included cerebrospinal fluid (CSF), pericardial fluid, white blood cells, liver (60), and in postmortem cultures, myocardium and liver (84).

NEUROLOGIC DISEASE

There has been an association between parainfluenza viruses and acute and chronic neurologic disease for several decades. Febrile seizures have been reported in up to 62% of children hospitalized with HPIV-4B compared to only 17% for HPIV-3 and 7% for HPIV-1 (20). HPIV-1 viruses were isolated from two patients with multiple sclerosis (MS) (85,86), but evidence of antibody to HPIV-1 in the serum or CSF of MS patients has been lacking (87,88). One report demonstrated that two of 25 CSF samples from MS patients had low positive hemagglutinin inhibition titers to HPIV-1 but three of 25 had positive titers to measles virus (89). Similarly, virus cultures and electron microscopy of other MS patients failed to find evidence of HPIV-1. However, recent evidence using the polymerase chain reaction (PCR) has demonstrated that both HPIV-1 and Sendai virus can infect olfactory bulbs of mice for prolonged periods (90,91). Animal parainfluenza viruses related to HPIV-2 have been found in patients with MS and subacute sclerosing panencephalitis (92,93). Two closely related paramyxoviruses (*Hendra, Nipaha*) have been shown to cause severe encephalitis and death in children and adults (2–4). HPIV-3 has been isolated from the CSF of a patient with Guillain-Barré syndrome (94) and adults with demyelinization syndromes (95), and has rarely been shown to cause meningitis in children (95–97) and adults (95). HPIV-1, 2, and 3 have been isolated from the respiratory tract of children with acute encephalitis (98). In addition; A) encephalitis, ventriculitis, and pneumonia leading to fetal hydrops and death; and B) cluster headaches in an adult; have been serologically linked to HPIV-3 (99,100). These anecdotal reports and many animal studies suggest the possibility that some strains of HPIV may have neurotropism in certain hosts. Much more work needs to be done to clarify the role HPIV plays in human neurologic disease, but at the present time this appears to be very minor compared to the significant role these viruses play in respiratory disease.

OTHER SYNDROMES

Preterm and full-term neonates with HPIV-3 respiratory tract infection have developed apnea and bradycardia (99,101–103). HPIV-1 has been cultured from two children with adult respiratory distress syndrome (104). HPIV-3 has been implicated in supraglottitis and bronchiolitis obliterans (105,106). HPIV-1 and HPIV-3 have been isolated in cases of parotitis in otherwise healthy children (107,108), in immunocompromised children (76), and in a patient with cystic fibrosis (109). Also, bacterial tracheitis has been associated with viral croup, and HPIV infections (110). Exacerbations of nephrotic syndrome in children have been linked to viral respiratory infections in general (111). It is extremely unusual to have non-respiratory tissues infected with HPIV. However, viremia and disseminated infection have been documented in immunocompromised patients and children with croup (112). Paramyxovirus-like nucleocapsids have been seen in acute non-A,B,C syncytial giant-cell hepatitis in children and adults (113). It is possible that one of the HPIV groups may play a role in this disease. HPIV-3 has been cultured from a 37-year-old man with myopericarditis and other HPIV diagnosed serologically in patients with myocarditis or pericarditis (114). Elevated levels of antibodies to HPIV-1 have been reported in systemic lupus erythematosus and Reiter's syndrome (115). However, the differences between the mean antibody titers of the controls and the subjects were only one to two dilutions. Recent work using RT-PCR has demonstrated no evidence of mumps P or HN genes in patients with inflammatory bowel disease (116). There does not yet appear to be a clear link established between HPIV and inflammatory or connective tissue disease. There is a relationship between infection with common respiratory pathogens and myalgias and rhabdomyolysis. HPIV-3

has been cultured from a child who died with rhabdomyolysis (117). Also, HPIV-2 has been serologically linked to myalgias and myoglobinuria in an adult (118). An adult patient with bloody diarrhea had HPIV-3 cultured from throat and rectal cultures (119). Subsequent to this report, the role of rotavirus, adenovirus, and other previously uncultured agents has become recognized in acute gastroenteritis. Approximately 11% of young children with rotavirus gastroenteritis may have a concurrent viral respiratory tract infection (120). Therefore, HPIV does not have a firmly established etiologic role in gastroenteritis.

Nosocomial Infections

Respiratory viruses are frequently transmitted inside of medical institutions, including doctor's offices, hospitals, and chronic care facilities. Nosocomial transmission of HPIV is most significant in young preschool age children, the immunocompromised, and the elderly (81). Approximately 20% of uninfected control children residing on the same ward with HPIV-3 infected children will excrete virus during their hospital stay (121). Mild respiratory symptoms will develop in about one third of these, but some will experience serious LRI and even death (20,121). Serious sequelae are most common in patients with underlying medical problems. Even in those with only mild symptoms, the mean length of hospitalization was increased by many days because of unnecessary tests and therapies due to their new signs and symptoms. Isolation of all children admitted to hospitals with respiratory signs and symptoms clearly is not practical. However, enforcing strict handwashing between patients, placing high-risk patients away from those with respiratory infections, and limiting potentially infected visitors (children and adults) or staff may help to decrease nosocomial HPIV infections.

Economic Burden

The ultimate cost of HPIV infection is dependent on the socioeconomic conditions within a country. In a developed country like the United States, cost is mostly in hospitalization, lost productivity for parents, and perhaps, in long-term respiratory tract sequela in children. Rate of hospitalization has already been discussed and time lost from work for parents with HPIV infected infants and children is difficult to estimate but is considerable. Extrapolation of hospitalization rates at the Children's Hospital of Wisconsin (CHW) indicate that the cost of HPIV-1 and HPIV-2 infection during the fall of 1991 could exceed 186 million dollars nationally (25). Another estimate based on a computer generated sampling of a national database (0.5%) for croup caused by HPIV-1 resulted in an estimate of 30 million dollars per epidemic for this specific disease and virus (23). Separate and independent extrapolations using more recent data from CHW suggest that the yearly cost of hospitalizations for HPIV infections in the United States exceeds $200 million (21). In addition, this estimate does not take into account URI caused by these viruses, the fact that HPIV-3 causes longer and more costly stays than HPIV-1 or 2, nor the economic burden of infections in adults and immunocompromised patients.

Morbidity and Mortality

Increased bronchial reactivity has been reported in children who were tested years after having croup (122). Also, long-term pulmonary abnormalities have been found in children after RSV LRI including decreased gas exchange (123,124), restrictive lung disease (125,126), obstructive lung disease, and hyperreactivity (123–125,127). Even adults have been reported with chronic lung disease following HPIV LRI (128). These viruses clearly cause acute inflammatory changes directly to airways, and also are capable of inducing responses in the immune system (e.g., humeral, cellular, cytokine production, interaction with allergens) that lead to acute pulmonary changes (127). The exact role of HPIV or other common respiratory viruses in chronic respiratory illness (e.g., asthma, COPD, etc.) is still being determined. This includes looking at the question of biased selection of susceptible or "at risk" individuals (phenotype expression) in long-term follow-up studies. However, parainfluenza LRI in animal models have shown persistent changes in lung mechanics and hyperresponsiveness (129,130), suggesting that HPIV LRI may lead to chronic pulmonary damage in some people.

HPIV induced mortality is unusual in developed countries and is seen almost entirely in young infants, the immunocompromised, and the elderly. However, in developing countries, significant mortality takes place in preschool children. It has been estimated that between 25% and 30% of all deaths in this age group are caused by LRI with HPIV causing about 10% of these deaths (11). Also, HPIV may contribute to mortality in the developing world by facilitating secondary bacterial infections in children.

Mode of Transmission

There have been very few studies specifically investigating HPIV transmission. It has been shown that in only two out of 40 HPIV-1 infected children could virus be recovered from air sampled 60 cm away from the patient (131). This makes small particle aerosol spread an unlikely mode of transmission. Studies in RSV have shown that aerosolization of large droplets may be important for close contact transmission and for contaminating surfaces. Furthermore, these surfaces may then lead to direct self-inoculation (132). It is thought that HPIV is transmitted by similar modalities. HPIV-1, HPIV-2 and HPIV-3 have all been shown to survive up to 10 hours on nonporous surfaces and four hours on porous surfaces (133). However HPIV-3 experimentally placed on fingers has been shown to lose greater than 90% of its infectivity in the first 10 minutes and could not be transferred to other fingers (134). Person-to-person spread by direct hand contact appears to be an unlikely means of transmission. However, the amount of virus excreted from an acutely infected child may be more than 10 times higher then that tested (135). Most common disinfectants or antiseptic agents effectively remove HPIV from surfaces. Alcohol and water are least effective (133).

Pathogenesis

The mechanisms of pathogenesis for HPIV are still being investigated. As stated previously, HPIV infect respiratory epithelium almost exclusively. However, recent studies in mice have demonstrated that Sendai virus may gain access to the CNS via the olfactory neurons during intranasal infection (91). Tissue tropism for HPIVs is known to be directed by the hemagglutinin-neuraminidase (HN) protein (see section on structure). There may be differences between these viruses in where and how they are absorbed and released from respiratory epithelium (polarity)(136). HPIV-3 appears to be absorbed and released greater from the apical then the basolateral domains of A549 cells. Viral antigen has been localized to the apical portion of epithelial cells in infected cotton rats (137). Actin and the cytoskeleton have been reported to play roles in transcription, maturation, and the movement of viral glycoproteins to the surface of infected cells. HPIV-3 needs functioning microtubules for efficient release (136). Similarly, HPIV-2 forms filamentous shapes 5 to

15 um long in polarized epithelial cells and this formation is dependent on actin (138). HPIV-3 and mouse PIV-1 do not form these shapes. More work needs to be done to better understand these important relationships.

After HPIV have infected a cell, the cell may exhibit focal rounding and increase in size of the cytoplasm and nucleus. HPIV decreases host cell mitotic activity as soon as 24 hours after inoculation (139). Other changes that can be observed include single or multilocular cytoplasmic vacuoles, basophilic or eosinophilic inclusions, and the formation of multinucleated giant cells (139,140). These giant cells (fusion cells) usually occur late in infection and contain between two and seven nuclei. Paramyxoviruses are known to induce apoptosis in tissue culture cells (141). The focal tissue destruction caused by HPIV is usually mild, rapidly repaired, and in many infections may not even be detectable. Infection in immunocompromised hosts is an exception where giant-cell pneumonia can lead to death. Disease severity has been correlated with HPIV shedding in children (135), but not in adults (142). Species specific down regulation of mouse smooth muscle receptors have been reported following Sendai virus infection (143). However, viral-induced pathologic features and hyperresponsiveness still occurred in rats even without down regulation. Airway hyperresponsiveness in guinea pigs has been associated with sensory neuropeptide depletion (144).

Persistent infection with active viral replication has been demonstrated in tissue culture and during human infection (145–154). The majority of persistent infections with HPIV do not seem to cause morphologic changes or symptoms (e.g., HPIV-2) (154). However, genetic alterations in HPIV and host cells have been reported (146,147,152) as well as decreased amounts of host cell surface sialic acid HN receptors (145). The immune response, or lack thereof, in an infected patient clearly affects the clearance of HPIV and the development of persistent infection (59,63,70,150). It is not known what percentage of HPIV infections lead to persistent infection or how persistence is maintained in human hosts.

Both the HN and the fusion (F) proteins have been demonstrated to be involved with cell membrane fusion, but this appears to be virus (type)–specific with some paramyxoviruses needing only the F protein (145,155). Furthermore, fusion may demonstrate different kinetics depending on whether it takes place virus-to-cell or cell-to-cell (145). Certainly, HPIV host range and virulence are determined in part by the ability of host epithelial cell to enzymatically activate the F protein. Also, the neuraminidase activity of the HN protein may play a role in altering muscarinic receptors leading to vagal induced bronchospasm, and can cause HPIV infected cells to resist infection when challenged with HPIV (viral interference) (156–158).

The role that immune mechanisms play in local cell injury and tissue damage is largely unknown. HPIV-specific IgE and histamine may contribute to disease severity in infants (159). Increased numbers of inflammatory cells, airway hyperreactivity, and decreased bronchoalveolar cellular superoxide production are found during acute infection in guinea pigs (160–162). In other animal studies, antibody to formalin-inactivated HPIV-3 has been shown to enhance pulmonary inflammation upon challenge (163). In this same animal model, HPIV-3 induced greater peribronchiolar lymphocyte aggregation and histologic change in one species of rat than in another (141). This implies that HPIV pathogenesis may be mediated by an organism's genetically programmed immunologic responses.

HPIV can activate the initial components of complement directly independent of antibody (164). This may decrease viral attachment to host cell receptors. Also, complement has been shown to participate directly in virus membrane destruction via the terminal attack complex, but the extent of this form of viral neutralization in vivo is unclear. HPIV-1 and other respiratory viruses have been shown to have procoagulant activity that may play a role in cardiovascular disease (165). Also, parainfluenza viruses have been shown to enhance the appearance of pulmonary edema in hypoxic rats suggesting they may be a cause of high altitude pulmonary edema (166).

Immunologic Aspects

Previous studies have shown that humoral immunity to the two surface glycoproteins ([HN] and [F]) is important in host protection (167,168). The majority of children are born with neutralizing antibody to all four types of HPIV, but this quickly falls during the first 6 months of life. Serologic and culture surveys have shown that approximately two thirds of children will have been infected with HPIV-3 during the first year of life (at least one third will have been symptomatic). Almost all children have antibody by 3 years of age. Animal studies have shown that antibody to either the HN or the F protein can protect against HPIV-3 challenge but anti-HN antibodies may play a larger role (168). However, high levels of anti-HN antibody alone do not fully protect infants from LRI (167). Repeated infections are often needed before protection develops. It is not known whether it is the concomitant increase in anti-F antibody, improved cellular immunity, or both that helps protect children. Antibody mediated virus neutralization of progeny virus may be more important than antibody reacting with infected host cells (169). The majority of antibody response appears to be IgG1, but 30% of adults will have significant increases in IgG3, IgG4, serum IgA, and IgM (170). The majority of children under the age of six demonstrate IgM antibody during or shortly following acute HPIV infection (171). Immunity to HPIV-1 and HPIV-2 develops later than HPIV-3, increasing more rapidly during the second and third years of life. HPIV-4 antibody levels in the general population do not go up dramatically until approximately school age.

The protective role of secretory IgA in natural infections with parainfluenza viruses is not well defined. Most children and adults develop measurable levels of secretory IgA following natural infection with HPIV (172–175). In adults this has been shown to be correlated with disease prevention and amelioration (173,176). However, no correlation was found between secretory IgA levels in infants and the ability of nasal secretions to neutralize virus or decrease disease severity (174). Cytotoxic T-lymphocyte (CTL) responses appear to be important in the clearance of virus from the lower respiratory tract during infections with HPIV-3 (177–179) and mouse PIV-1 (180–183). T-cells with alpha-beta receptors appear to play a major role in this viral clearance, but gamma-delta T cells and natural killer cells may also be involved (181,184,185). Human CTL response has been shown to be directed to determinants on the HN, P, and NP proteins of HPIV-1 and 3 (186,187). However, the viral epitopes important in stimulating this line of defense are still largely unknown. More recently, the cytokines produced by CD4 and CD8 T-cells have been described during acute LRI caused by Sendai virus in a mouse model. IL-2, IFN (gamma), tumor necrosis factor (TNF), IL-6, and IL-10 were all detected in the lungs (188). Similarly, human peripheral blood leukocytes stimulated by Sendai virus have been shown to produce macrophage inflammatory protein-1 alpha, monocyte chemotactic protein 1, TNF-α, IL-6 and IL-8 (189). Interferon may inhibit HPIV-3 primary transcription (190) and likewise HPIV-3 may inhibit interferon mediated pathways in T-cells including MHC class II antigen expression (191). Another inflammatory mediator induced by Sendai virus is inter-

cellular adhesion molecule-1 (ICAM-1) this has been shown to be responsible for neutrophil and lymphocyte migration into the lung (192).

HPIV-3 has been shown to induce IL-10 production in T-cells. IL-10 then contributes to decreased T-cell proliferation and protected the t-cells from viral-mediated apoptosis (193). In addition, HPIV-3 stimulates IL-II from stromal cells, which can be detected *in vivo* during urinary tract infections (URIs) in children, and correlates with clinical bronchospasm (194). No long-lasting immunity to URI caused by HPIV develops, and infections continue throughout life.

Prevention and Treatment

Approximately 35 years ago, field trials of formalin-killed whole HPIV-1, HPIV-2, and HPIV-3 vaccines failed to protect children against natural infection (195,196). Although there were significant seroconversion rates for all three virus types, antibody levels following vaccination were considerably lower than those following natural infection (195). Furthermore, HPIV vaccination did not appear to stimulate good mucosal immunity, and some of the antibody produced may not have neutralized native virus (197). Current approaches to HPIV vaccines include intranasal administration of live attenuated strains, subunit strategies using the HN and F proteins, recombinant bovine/human viruses, and strains engineered using "reverse genetics."

Bovine PIV-3 (BPIV-3) has antigenic similarities to the human virus and induces resistance in rats and primates to challenge with HPIV-3 (198). Although, this Jennerian approach did not produce significant immune responses in seropositive adult volunteers (199), it was quite effective in infecting and inducing antibody responses in seronegative volunteers (200). Vaccine studies in young infants and children have demonstrated these same promising results (39). Further studies evaluating the safety and efficacy of BPIV-3 when given as multiple doses and simultaneously with routine childhood immunizations are underway (201). A new approach using recombinant Bovine PIV-3 with human F and HN genes and human RSV G and F genes has induced good antibody titers and protection in hamsters and rhesus monkeys (202–204). Another Jennerian approach being studied is the use of Sendai virus (mouse PIV-1) to protect against HPIV-1. So far initial results demonstrated that two doses of Sendai virus vaccine protected primates from infection by HPIV-1 (41).

Cold-adapted (CA) strains of HPIV-3 have been shown to be stable and demonstrate multiple markers of attenuation in tissue culture (205). These CA strains have shown protection in weanling hamsters and chimpanzees but poor infectivity in older children and adults (199,206). Also, evidence of reversion toward wild type has been reported in low passage strains (199). Higher passage CA HPIV-3 strains have demonstrated immunogenicty and attenuation in younger infants, but symptoms still developed (207). Additional clinical studies on CA strains of HPIV-3 with greater attenuation demonstrated good infectivity, immunogenicity, attenuation (no diseases), and stability (208–210). In addition, CA HPIV-3 appears to be more immunogenic then BPIV-3. Cold-adapted strains of HPIV-1 and HPIV-2 have also been developed, and initial investigation demonstrates attenuation in tissue culture and animal models.

Another approach toward developing attenuated strains of HPIV is the use of protease activation mutants.

The F protein must be cleaved by a trypsin-like protease for strains to be infected. HPIV strains that are resistant to trypsin cleavage but sensitive to cleavage by another protease may be attenuated in humans (211). Studies using Sendai virus (mouse PIV-1) have demonstrated that protease activation mutants can protect mice from lethal infections (212,213).

Subunit vaccines containing envelope glycoproteins of HPIV-3 have demonstrated efficacy in rats, lambs, mice, and hamsters (214–217). Immunizations have been subcutaneous, intramuscular, and intranasal. No human trials have yet been reported. Vaccinia and baculovirus have been used as vector systems to produce cloned HN or F proteins for immunization in rats and primates (168,218,219). Viral shedding and peak titer have both been reduced upon subsequent challenge. Reverse genetics are now being used to develop systems able to evaluate current live HPIV-3 vaccines in terms of specific mutations and hopefully introduce specific mutations into wild type strains in the future (220,221). An example of this is the production of a recombinant HPIV-3 that contains the HN and F for HPIV-1 and the specific mutations for cold adaption found in the L gene of HPIV-3 (222). This vaccine has been found to be protective in hamsters. There are no HPIV vaccines currently licensed for use but several may become available during the next decade.

Many different agents have been found to have antiviral activity against paramyxoviruses including neuraminidase inhibitors (e.g., Zanamivir), protein synthesis inhibitors (puromycin), nucleic acid synthesis inhibitors, benzthiazole derivatives, 1, 3, 4-thiadiazol-2-ylcyanamide, carbocyclic 3-deezaadenosine (Cc3Ado), ascorbic acid, calcium elenolate, extracts of sanicula europaea leaves, etc. (223–235). None of these agents have yet found clinical applications. Recently, synthetic peptides to a specific domain on the F protein of HPIV-3 or mouse PIV-1 (Sendai virus) were found to be highly sensitive and specific inhibitors of syncytium formation in tissue culture (236–238). These peptides may provide a novel approach to the development of antiviral therapies for HPIV. Amantadine has anti-HPIV activity only at very high concentrations and has been found not to be effective in protecting adult volunteers from HPIV-1 induced URI (173). However, ribavirin has both in vitro and in vivo activity against HPIV (239, 240). Furthermore, there have been anecdotal reports of decreased HPIV shedding and clinical improvement when infected immunocompromised patients have been treated with aerosolized and oral ribavirin (241–244). However, a recent review at Fred Hutchinson Cancer center demonstrated that established HPIV-3 pneumonias responded poorly to aerosolized ribavirin (245). There are no current antiviral drugs with proven clinical efficacy against HPIV.

Nonspecific immunostimulators such as dihydroheptaprenol (DHP), N-acetylglucosaminylmuramyl tri- or tetrapeptides (GM), imiquimod, and polyriboinosinic/polyribocytidylic acids have been shown to help protect against challenge infections with paramyxoviruses (246–249). Some of this protective effect is due to stimulation of endogenous cytokines. The administration of cytokines themselves has been found to be protective in animal models (246,250). Cytokines tested have included interferon (alpha and gama), human granulocyte colony-stimulating factor, and human IL-1 β (251). Numerous studies as summarized in a recent meta-analysis have demonstrated that oral or systemic steroids are effective at improving symptoms of croup as early as 6 hours after treatment (252).

Passive transfer of viral specific antibodies has been shown to protect against RSV and other respiratory pathogens (253,254). There is some evidence that this might be useful in other paramyxovirus induced LRI (255–257), but little has been reported concerning the use of immunotherapy in HPIV disease. Combined immunotherapy and steroids have been demonstrated to decrease pulmonary virus titer and inflammation in a cotton rat model (258). Until safe and effective vaccines and antiviral drugs are available, immunotherapy may be an effective alternative in patients with severe disease.

DESCRIPTION AND NATURE OF THE AGENT

HPIV have recently been split into two genera, respirovirus (HPIV 1,3) and rubulavirus (HPIV-2,4). Both genera belong to the paramyxoviridae family (see Table 242.1) and are separated morphologically from other myxoviruses (e.g., influenza) by their non-segmented thick nucleocapsids (17 nm vs. 9 nm) (259,260). Parainfluenza viruses are further separated from other paramyxoviridae by the presence of a neuraminidase which morbilliviruses (e.g., measles, distemper) do not have and a thicker nucleocapsid than the pneumoviruses (e.g., RSV).

Physical Properties and Structure

The HPIV are pleomorphic enveloped viruses which have an average diameter of 150 to 250 nm (Fig. 242.1). Much larger parainfluenza virions or aggregates have often been reported (260–262). The majority of virus particles contain single stranded RNA with negative polarity (complementary to messenger RNA). Some virions may contain positive sense RNA, but these are presumed to be non-infectious (260). There are approximately 15,000 nucleotides in the HPIV genome (263,264). All HPIV vRNA encode at least six structural proteins [3'-NP-P-C -M-F-HN-L-5'] (265). Recent work using reverse genetic systems have demonstrated a "rule of six" for HPIV. The most efficient replication and transcription takes place when the genome is divisible by six although it is not absolute (220,221,266).

There is great similarity in protein size by electrophoresis between the four major HPIV types except for the phosphoprotein (P). HPIV-2 and HPIV-4 have a P protein with a molecular weight (MW) of 49 to 53 Kdal vs 83 to 90 Kdal for HPIV-1 and HPIV-3 (263–265, 267-271). The nucleocapsid protein (N) (MW, 66 to 70 Kdal), " large" nucleocapsid protein-[polymerase] (L) (MW, 175 to 251 Kdal), and the P protein are all closely associated with the vRNA. The hemagglutinin-neuraminidase (HN) (MW, 69 to 82 Kdal) and fusion protein (Fo) (MW, 60 to 66 Kdal) are glycoproteins that project as spikes from the viral lipid envelope. Finally, the membrane protein (M) (MW, 28 to 40 Kdal) is strongly associated with and found just beneath the viral membrane. The MW as calculated from cloning and sequencing data can differ considerably from that seen on gel electrophoresis for viral proteins that undergo extensive post-translational modification (e.g., glycosylation or phosphorylation). Many small nonstructural proteins are produced from multiple overlapping reading frames within the P gene of some paramyxoviruses. Many of these require editing of the mRNA. HPIV-1, HPIV-2, and HPIV-3 encode for a nonstructural protein labeled (C) (265,272,273). HPIV-2 (and maybe HPIV-3) has an additional nonstructural protein (V), which HPIV-1 does not contain (272,274,275). This protein appears to have several actions. It binds N and may play a role in regulating viral replication (276). However, the V protein distribution (nuclei and cytoplasm) does not appear to be similar to the N or P protein (cytoplasmic granules) within virus infected cells (277). Recent work suggests that slowing the cell cycle might be one way the V protein favors viral replication (278). In addition it may be involved in *Rubulavirus* inhibition of the interferon response by inducing degradation of STAT1, STAT2, or both (140,279–281). The C protein PIV-1 (Sendai virus) may perform the same function (279). HPIV-3 appears to have a unique nonstructural protein D,

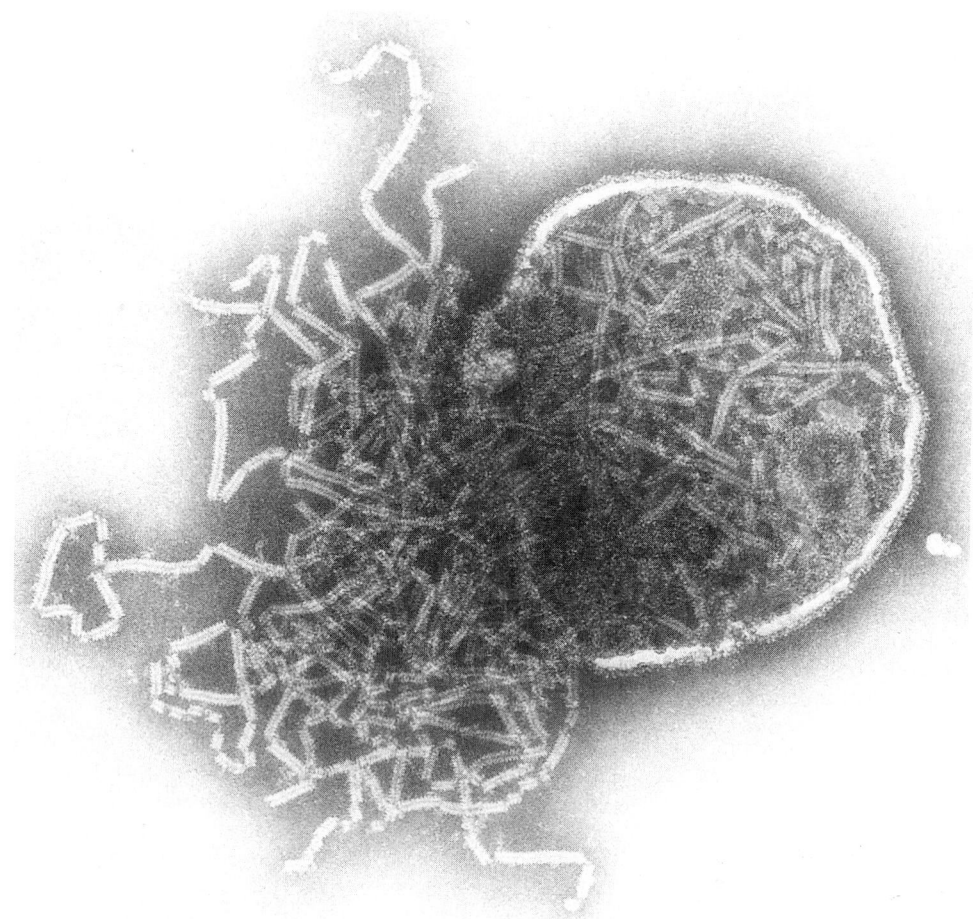

Figure 242.1. Electron micrograph of human parainfluenza virus type 1. Surface glycoproteins and nucleocapsid core being extruded are both visualized.

which is a chimera between the upstream half of P and a second internal ORF (282).

The N, L, and P proteins together with vRNA form the nucleocapsid core of HPIV. The N binds to the vRNA (1 N protein to 6 nucleotides) making a template that allows the L (RNA dependent RNA polymerase) and P proteins to transcribe and eventually replicate the HPIV genome (259). The P protein of HPIV is probably a homotrimer (283). The M protein interacts with the surface glycoproteins (HN and F) and may be involved in their insertion and aggregation at specific cell membrane locations. This protein also appears to play a role in attracting completed nucleocapsids to those areas of infected cell membrane that will soon become viral envelope and may be involved in viral budding (282,284–286).

The HN protein most likely exists as a tetramer on the lipid envelope of HPIV (6,287,288). There it functions in virus-host cell attachment via sialic acid receptors and has neuraminidase activity (important for virus release from cells). The terminal sialic acid sequences important for HN binding of HPIVs are just beginning to be worked out (289). It appears that HPIV-1 HN is more limited in its binding than HPIV-3 HN which may be important for host/tissue range. The HN protein similarly attaches to receptors on red blood cells allowing the well recognized "hemagglutination" or hemadsorption of paramyxoviruses. Elegant work by Moscona has demonstrated that the HN- cell receptor interaction is specific and complex. The affinity of the HPIV-3 HN to its receptor(s) affects subsequent F protein–mediated cell fusion (290). Also, cell to cell fusion requires a minimum density of receptors which

is greater than the density needed for virus membrane-cell membrane fusion (infection). Persistently infected tissue cultures may be created by the enzymatic removal of a certain number of Sailic acid receptors. This is one explanation for HPIV-3 persistence in vitro but in vivo persistence may have additional mechanisms. Persistent infection with HPIV-2 appears to use a different mechanism (154). There are significant differences in the number of HN glycosylation sites between HPIV types and among strains within one type (7–9). This may be part of the strategy HPIV use to escape immune detection.

The F protein is involved in virus-host cell membrane fusion, which is required for nucleocapsid entry and host cell infection. Also, it is integral in membrane fusion between host cells (syncytial formation) and causes hemolysis. This protein is originally made as an inactive precursor (Fo) which must be cleaved by an endopeptidase to yield the active fusion protein composed of two disulfide-linked molecules (F1 and F2). The new N-terminus on F1 is highly hydrophobic and is thought to make the first contact with the lipid membrane during virus-cell fusion. Furin and Kex2 have recently been proposed as the enzymes responsible for this proteolytic cleavage in humans (291) but trypsin is most frequently used *in vitro*. Cleavage of each HPIV Fo is a major determinant of host range and virulence. The ability of the F protein to independently induce both fusion and hemolysis varies among the different parainfluenza viruses. HPIV-1, 2, and 3 in vitro require both HN and F for fusion and hemolysis (292–294). The actual location and structure of the domains on the HN protein responsible for F protein interaction, fusion promotion, oligomer formation, and cell surface expression are still being determined (9,295–297).

REPLICATION

The nucleocapsid gains entry into the cytoplasm of a host cell via fusion of virus-host lipid membranes. Once in the cytoplasm, transcription takes place utilizing virus specific RNA-dependent RNA polymerase (L protein). This produces messenger RNA, which is translated by cellular ribosomal machinery into viral proteins. These then direct the full-length replication of the virus genome, first into a positive strand and then into the appropriate negative strand. Thus produced, the negative strands are encapsidated with NP and may proceed to further rounds of transcription/replication or be packaged for export as a new virion (260,261).

Resistance and Sensitivity to Physiochemical Agents

HPIV are relatively sensitive to temperature, humidity, pH, and the composition of the storage fluid. Temperatures above 37°C markedly decrease HPIV survival until at 50°C almost all virus is inactivated within 15 minutes (298). At room temperature, myxovirus titers have been reported to decrease by greater then 50% within 2 hours to 1 week, but this rate averages closer to hours then days (135,298–301). HPIV is most stable at 4°C or frozen (e.g., −70°C). Freezing clearly causes loss of infectivity and virus destruction. This loss can be considerable (greater than 90%) (298,302). However, the small amount of infectivity that is left must be sufficient for virus recovery. HPIV-1 can be recovered even after 26 years of being frozen (−70°C) with a recovery rate greater then 90% (Henrickson KJ, unpublished observation,1992). The addition of 0.5% bovine serum albumin, skim milk, 5% DMSO, or 2% chicken serum prolongs HPIV survival (298,303,304). HPIV survive best in a pH range of 7.4 to 8.0. Infectivity is rapidly lost at pH 3.0 to 3.4 (301,305), low humidity (306), and with virus desiccation (133,134). Like all myxoviruses, HPIV is sensitive to inactivation by ether (307).

Serotypes

There are four predominant HPIV serotypes. These serotypes and the other species within the paramyxovirinae subfamily (Table 242.1) can be serologically and antigenically divided into three genera: a) HPIV-1, HPIV-3, sendai virus, BPIV-3; b) HPIV-2, HPIV-4, mumps, simian virus 5 and 41; and c) measles (6,308–310). The human parainfluenza viruses all share common antigens and variable levels of heterotypic antibody that are often detected during infection. It is usually impossible to determine whether the heterotypic responses are amnestic in nature or simply crossreactions to similar antigens during serologic testing. However, specific hyperimmune animal serum (e.g., hamster or guinea pig) can usually differentiate between these viruses in standard hemagglutinin-inhibition (HI), hemadsorption-inhibition (HAdI), complement fixation, neutralization, or enzyme linked immunosorbent assay (37,311).

Shortly after being identified, HPIV-4 was found to have two major subtypes (A and B). These subtypes could be distinguished by HAdI and neutralization assays but not by complement fixation (1). During that same decade, several HPIV-2 strains were isolated that could be differentiated serologically from the type stain (312). More recent studies have demonstrated significant antigenic variation between different clinical isolates (313). Also, strains of HPIV-1 have been reported that could be separated from the type strain by HI, neutralization assays, and ELISA

(61). Recent molecular analysis of all four types have demonstrated more antigenic and genetic heterogeneity than had been previously appreciated (6–9,308,314–317). It appears that at different periods, all four major HPIV types have virus subgroups that have unique antigenic and genetic characteristics. This includes variability even within HPIV-4 subtypes (316). The evolution of these viruses appears to be most similar in pattern to influenza B. Most of these HPIV strains still have enough common "type" antigens that they will react in polyclonal serologic testing as previously described. However, subgroups of HPIV-1 (A, C, and D) and HPIV-3 have been reported with progressive antigenic change taking place (9). Furthermore, HPIV-1 strains isolated over the past 10 years demonstrate persistent antigenic and genetic differences compared to the 1957 type strain including differences between genotypes within the same epidemic and same geographic location (6–9,317). Because of this, standard reference sera raised to HPIV isolates from the 1950s, or antigen prepared from these same "type" strains may not react with all stains in routine serologic assays in the future. This has already occurred with an HPIV-3 variant, which failed to react with two commercial monoclonal antibodies (318).

Pathogenicity in Animals

There are a number of non-human parainfluenza viruses antigenically related to HPIV. Sendai virus infects mice, hamsters, and pigs and is related to HPIV-1 (304,318,319). Simian virus 5 and 41 are related to HPIV-2 and infect primates (309,320,321). Dogs develop croup and LRI when infected with canine parainfluenza virus (CP2), which is closely related to SV5 (322,323). Bovine PIV-3 has been associated with shipping fever in cattle, and is antigenically related to HPIV-3 (324). It or similar viruses may also infect horses, sheep, goats, water buffaloes, deer, dogs, cats, monkeys, guinea pigs, rats, and pigs (141,325–327). Newcastle disease virus (NDV) infects poultry, penguins and other birds (328,329). NDV has been responsible for conjunctivitis in bird handlers and laboratory workers (330). Human infections by some of the other non-human parainfluenza viruses have been reported but have not been well established (309,320,324,331).

Many different animals can be infected with HPIV. This can occur both naturally or under experimental conditions. HPIV-I, HPIV-2, HPIV-3, and HPIV-4 can cause asymptomatic infection in hamsters, guinea pigs, and adult ferrets (37,304,332–334). HPIV-I, HPIV-2, and HPIV-3 cause fatal disease in newborn ferrets (333). HPIV-3 causes asymptomatic infection in cotton rats, but demonstrates significant respiratory pathology and virus replication (141). Similarly, HPIV-3 induces hyperreactivity in the trachea of guinea pigs (335). Neonatal hydrocephalus has been reported in hamsters whose mothers were intervenously inoculated with HPIV-3 (336). Most primates can be infected with HPIV but are asymptomatic. Chimpanzees, macaques, squirrel, owl, patas, and rhesus monkeys have been asymptomatically infected with HPIV-3 or HPIV-4 (337–339) and marmosets have developed symptomatic URI with HPIV-3 and Sendai virus (340).

Growth in Cell Culture

HPIV grow in a number of primary and secondary cell lines. These include LLC-MK2, Vero, CV-I, primary cynomologus and rhesus monkey kidney, Wish, HMV-II, HEp-2, MDCK, BHK, HeLa, primary human embryo, KB, Am, HEB' L929, HEF, and others (147, 205, 293, 341–346). Also, parainfluenza viruses can multiply in organ cultures from mouse, guinea pig, ferret, and human fetal respiratory epithelium (139). Primary monkey kidney tissue culture is more sensitive to initial isolation of HPIV-I and HPIV-2 than LLC-MK2 but must be watched for foamy virus contamination. This contamination does not appear to interfere with HPIV detection.

In general, epithelial cell lines are superior to fibroblast cell lines in the isolation of HPIV. Some serotypes and strains of HPIV require the addition of an exogenous protease (trypsin) to the cell culture maintenance medium to facilitate efficient virus recovery. This need varies depending on the cells being used and their ability to produce appropriate proteases. HPIV-3 grows efficiently in PMK cells and to high titer in LLC-MK2 cells with serum-free medium, but the addition of trypsin allows increased infectivity in HEp-2 cells (341). HPIV-1, HPIV-2, and HPIV-4 demonstrate greater replication in Vero cells using trypsin (347,348). HPIV-1 has a strict and specific requirement for trypsin or a trypsin-like protease in LLC-MK2 cells. HPIV-1, HPIV-2, and HPIV-3 all can be recovered in PMK cells (e.g., cynomologus, rhesus) without trypsin, and there is evidence that the F protein of HPIV-2 is efficiently cleaved in PMK cells (349). However, the species of monkey was not stated in this latter study and there is great variability between species of PMK cells and the ability to efficiently grow HPIV (25). The addition of trypsin increases recovery rates of HPIV in some PMK cell lines (e.g. Africangreen).

CYTOPATHIC EFFECTS

The majority of HPIV isolates recovered in PMK cells show no cytopathic effects. HPIV-2 and HPIV-3 are the serotypes most likely to demonstrate focal rounding and destruction, elongated cells, and rare syncytia on initial isolation. After adaption to a particular cell line, all HPIV demonstrate greater CPE with HPIV-3 still being the most aggressive. Well adapted strains of HPIV-3 can destroy greater than 50% of a tissue culture monolayer by the third day.

IMMUNE REAGENTS

Virus and Viral Antigens

HPIV can be used whole or it can be disrupted chemically or physically to yield many useful antigens. Treatment with various detergents (or ether) and ultracentrifugation will allow separation of the membrane associated proteins HN, F, and M from the nucleocapsid (N, L, P, and RNA). Further purification and separation can then be accomplished using dialysis and column chromatography. Also, many of the structural proteins of HPIV have been genetically cloned and produced in appropriate expression vectors but are not available commercially. Antigen prepared in any of the above ways can be used in most assays. However, HPIV with its membrane disrupted by buffer with 0.5% triton-X100 yields an antigenic preparation that works well in ELISA. Whole virus treated with SDS works well in PAGE and western blot analysis. Radioimmune precipitation can be easily performed on HPIV using the detergent NP40 to disrupt the viral membrane. The HN and F proteins are on the surface of the viral membrane such that whole virus preparations without detergent work well when trying to detect antigenic sites on these molecules (e.g., HA, Hl, HAdl, neuraminidase assay).

Preparation and Use of Antibodies

Any portion of HPIV can be used to make polyclonal or monoclonal antibodies. Whole virus intranasally inoculated into guinea pigs or hamsters makes virus specific hyperimmune sera that reacts well in standard serologic tests (37). Immunized animals always need to be screened for naturally occurring parainfluenza antibody before immunization and kept isolated. Intramuscular booster immunization should be accomplished 2 to 3 weeks following the initial immunization. Some heterotypic antibody will be produced but usually is of a low level. Goat antisera to HPIV-1 and HPIV-3 is available commercially, but the latter cross reacts with HPIV-2. If viral subunits are being used to make more specific antisera, then adjuvants may need to be used and immunizations are usually intermuscular, intradermal, or intravenous. Monoclonal antibodies (MAbs) have been produced to all four major serotypes of HPIV and are commercially available. In general, MAbs to one HPIV serotype do not cross react with another. However, there have been some limited cross-reactions between MAbs to HPIV and similar non-human parainfluenza viruses (6). Polyclonal and monoclonal antibodies can be used for virus detection in ELISA, immunofluorescent assays, Hl, HAdl, complement fixation, western blot, radioimmune precipitation, and neutralization assays. A modification of the ELISA technique using time-resolved fluorometry may be more sensitive than ELISA in HPIV antigen detection (350). However, antigenic variation and evolution is taking place within HPIV so that many MAbs no longer bind and/or function in ELISA, Hl, or neutralization assays. Future detection assays using MAbs may need to routinely contain multiple different antibodies for maximum sensitivity.

COLLECTION AND PREPARATION OF SPECIMENS

HPIV are usually shed from the naso and oropharynx. The highest titer of virus is shed early in an infection and decreases quickly thereafter. In adult volunteers illness usually starts about 3 to 4 days after inoculation and lasts from 3 to 17 days with an average of 4 days for HPIV-1 and 6 to 13 days for HPIV-2 and HPIV-4 (173,351). Virus recovery in adults is often difficult compared to children. In children, virus is shed usually from 3 to 4 days before the onset of clinical symptoms until approximately 10 days afterward (352). However, HPIV-3 has been isolated in children from as early as 6 days, before 6 weeks past the first symptom. Persistent viral shedding of HPIV-I, HPIV-2, and HPIV-3 lasting many months has been documented in immunocompromised patients and in adults with normal and abnormal respiratory tracts (353,354). Throat swabs, nasopharyngeal swabs, nasal wash, and nasal aspiration have all been used successfully to recover HPIV (13,135,346,355,356). There has been very little work published on the optimal methods for parainfluenza virus specimen collection. Only nasal wash and nasal aspirates have been shown to yield high numbers and percentages of HPIV 1 and HPIV-3, respectively (135,357) and are recommended even in young infants for viral isolation.

As previously mentioned, HPIV lose infectivity rapidly at room temperature or higher. Specimens (swabs or 2- to 4-mL nasal wash aspirates) should be collected and placed in viral transport medium (2 to 3 mL), either veal infusion broth (VIB) or minimum essential medium (MEM) supplemented with some protein source (not serum) such as 0.5% bovine serum albumin. This transport medium should be buffered so that after the specimen is added the pH is between 7.5 and 8.0. Also, the addition of antibiotics and antifungal agents is recommended to decrease contamination of tissue culture. The specimen in transport medium should then be kept at 4°C until tissue culture inoculation. Centrifugation at 1,000X before inoculation is also helpful in removing debris.

HPIV have only rarely been isolated from nonrespiratory secretions. Cerebrospinal fluid can be directly plated onto tissue culture cells. Rectal swabs can be agitated in transport medium that contains additional antibiotics. Tissues can be homogenized in a dounce and then added to the standard transport medium prior to inoculation.

Serum for Serologic Tests

Acute serum should be collected as soon into the person's HPIV illness as possible. Peak neutralizing antibody titers occur between the third and fifth weeks after infection. Convalescent serum should be drawn during this period. Both samples should have the serum removed as quickly as possible and then be stored at either −70°C or at −20°C in a non–frost-free freezer. Serologic testing should be performed simultaneously in both the acute and convalescent samples.

LABORATORY DIAGNOSIS

Direct Examination for Viruses

HPIV can be easily visualized by electron microscopy (see Fig 242.1). However, it is impossible to differentiate these viruses from other paramyxoviruses (e.g., mumps). No large study looking at the diagnostic utility of electron microscopy for HPIV infection has been published (358,359), and less expensive methods of diagnosis have been developed.

Enzyme linked, radio, and fluoro immunoassays (i.e., enzyme immunoassay [EIA], radioimmunoassay [RIA], fluorescent immunoassay [FIA]) have all been developed to detect HPIV antigens (303,350,360–362), but none of these are available commercially in the United States. Using polyclonal sera, EIA, RIA, and FIA have reported sensitivities between 75% and 95% with the MAb-FIA demonstrating slightly higher detection of HPIV-1 and HPIV-2 (94% to 100%) (350). Until widely and easily available, this method of HPIV detection will be difficult for most clinical virology laboratories to perform.

Immunofluorescence (IF) has been used to detect HPIV in nasopharyngeal specimens for more than two decades (355,357,363–372). The majority of these techniques involved the production of serotype specific antisera in various animal species by each individual laboratory and subsequent conjugation to fluorescein isothiocyanate (FITC). Direct detection of HPIV has been highly variable. Some studies have shown virtually 100% sensitivity when compared to tissue culture while others have had very poor detection. HPIV-3 has been detected best using IF with sensitivities ranging between 31% and 100% while most studies report between 50% and 75%. Comparison of direct IF antigen detection for HPIV-1 has demonstrated sensitivities between 0% and 92% with a range of 50% to 100% for HPIV-2. The most common reported sensitivities for these latter two viruses range between 50% and 83%. The variability is caused by differences in the specimen collection, specimen processing, antibody production, and testing procedure. Specificity appears to be uniformly excellent, and treatment of nasopharyngeal specimens with a mucolytic (N-acetylcysteine) may improve sensitivity using polyclonal sera. HPIV-3 has demonstrated a rate of 16% for IF positive/culture negative specimens. It is not known whether these are all false-positive results or specimens without viable virus. Commercially available MAbs in direct detection of HPIV-3 have been able to detect between 31% and 93% of culture positive specimens. Results recently presented by Leland using MAbs for direct detection of HPIV demonstrated a sensitivity of 80% (HPIV-1), 83% (HPIV-2), and 72% (HPIV-3) when compared to tissue culture. This same antigen detection using IF was also shown to have 20% false-positive and 15% false-negative results (373).

Another method for the rapid identification of HPIV is a shell vial assay. This involves the centrifugation of inoculated tissue culture to speed viral absorption and cell infection followed by IF detection typically at 48 hours and 5 days. Although variable results have been reported, the majority of data appear to demonstrate improved detection using this method (374). Most data concern RSV and influenza. Published sensitivities for HPIV compared to standard tissue culture average 84% but the majority of viruses tested have been HPIV-3 (375–377).

A new shell vial technique using a mixture of two cell lines, mink lung cells, and A549 cells (R-mix; Diagnostic Hybrids, Athens, OH) has been compared to standard tissue culture and rapid antigen tests for detecting community acquired respiratory viruses but including very few HPIV positive samples (378–386). Little has been published but abstract data have demonstrated mixed results when the R-Mix cells were stained at 2 or 5 days. Some investigators have shown decreased sensitivity compared to direct IF or tissue culture. The largest study demonstrated a sensitivity for HPIV of 77% (23 of 30) compared to standard tissue culture (386).

Standard IF detection is done visually using a fluorescent microscope with appropriate mirrors and filters for FITC. Another method of detecting fluorescence is by using flow cytometry (FACS) analysis. This method allows for quantitative interpretation of fluorescent antibody binding to cell surfaces. It is limited by the minimum number of cells needed (2,000), extra time, and cost. These limitations make this technique most useful in the research setting. Careful microscopic examination by an experienced observer gives comparable qualitative results to FACS analysis.

The RNA genome of HPIV can be detected by several means. One method is to perform a Northern hybridization or a dot blot using virus specific DNA probes. This takes many hours to complete, yields less uniform results, and even with sensitive detection methods appears to be most useful as a research tool. However, the polymerase chain reaction (PCR) can be used easily and efficiently to detect low numbers of virus in different fluids. Several studies demonstrating PCR to be sensitive and specific in detecting HPIV have been published (387–390). Currently, there is one commercial multiplex PCR assay available for detecting HPIV-1, 2,3 along with RSV A, RSV B, influenza A, and influenza B (Fig. 242.2). This RT-PCR-EHA has a reported sensitivity of 95% to 100% and a specificity of 97% to 100% compared to tissue culture (392–402).

Virus Isolation

TISSUE CULTURE

Primary monkey kidney is the preferred cell line for the growth of HPIV. Rhesus is the most popular cell line but may not be the most sensitive, especially for HPIV-2 (343). Cynomolgus and African green are also used. A secondary monkey kidney cell line (LLC-MK2) is almost as good for primary isolation and excellent for continued passage. Trypsin (2 to 3 ug/mL) must be added to maintenance medium for LLC-MK2 cells to recover all HPIV serotypes and may be helpful even for PMK cell lines. Optimal isolation of HPIV may need to include both PMK and LLC-MK2. Some strains of HPIV-2 and HPIV-3 and most strains of HPIV-4 are detected ten days or longer after inoculation. PMK cells may start to degenerate between 10 and 14 days, especially if trypsin is in the medium. This means that if HPIV has not been detected in PMK tissue culture by 10 days, further testing might not be possible. Therefore, for maximum yield, both PMK and LLC-MK2 cell lines should be infected and initial detection methods (IF, HAd) performed on the PMK cells while holding the MK2 cells in reverse for testing at 14 and 21 days if needed.

IN ANIMALS

HPIV grow very poorly in eggs. It is only after many repeated passages and much presumed antigenic change that HPIV can

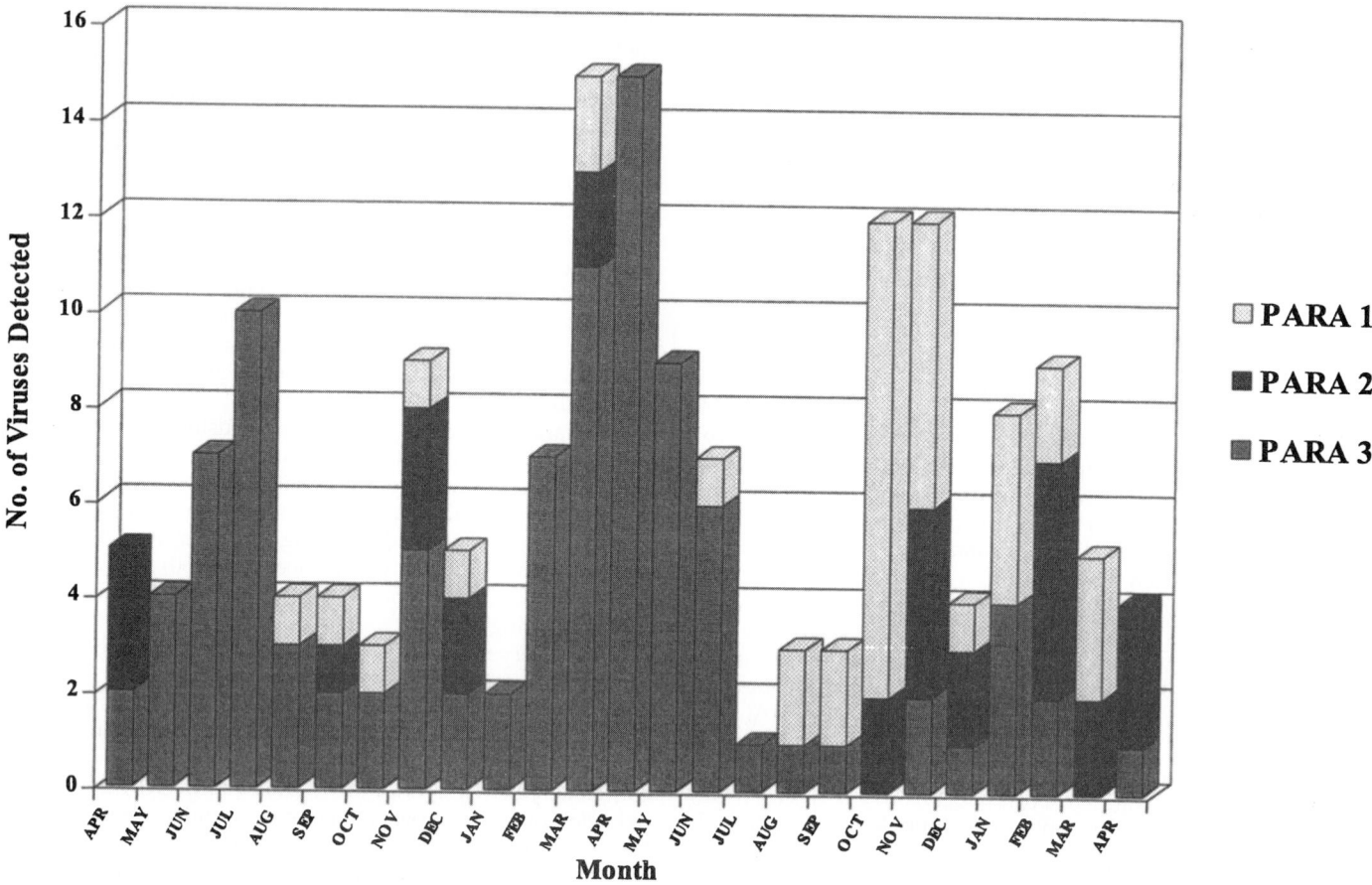

Figure 242.2. HPIV-1, 2, and 3 detected by multiplex RT-PCR-EHA (Hexaplex, Prodesse, Waukesha, Wisconsin) at Children's Hospital of Wisconsin during 2002.

be detected in embryonated eggs. Primary isolation in eggs has only been reported for three isolates of HPIV-2 (403).

DETECTION AND TYPING

HPIV rarely demonstrates CPE during primary isolation in tissue culture such that this is not a reliable or useful method to detect positive cultures. The most common method to detect the presence of HPIV is by hemadsorption (HAd) of guinea pig red blood cells directly onto the tissue culture monolayer. Most isolates of HPIV-1 can be detected using HAd by the fourth day (25), but HPIV-3 may take slightly longer (5,37,404). Only 35% of HPIV-2 isolates are HAd positive by the seventh day (25), and HPIV-4 may take 3 weeks or longer (5). Also, HPIV-4 hemadsorbs better at room temperature or 37°C, while all of the other serotypes react well at 4°C (37, 405).

The most rapid and accurate method currently available to detect and type HPIV in tissue culture is IF (364,365,372). This technique allows for earlier diagnosis of HPIV-1, HPIV-2, and HPIV-3 then traditional HAd and detects many positive cultures that are HAd negative. This is especially true for HPIV-2 (25). Furthermore, use of IF eliminates the need for further typing and thus saves considerable time and money. During peak seasons, in high risk populations (e.g., preschool children), IF detection could be performed on all inoculated PMK tissue culture cells on days 2 or 3, 4 or 5, and 10; and on MK2 cells, on days 14 and 21. It could be accomplished with a MAb pool necessitating only a single test per culture (372). HAd could be coupled with this or during off-season months HAd could be performed first and then IF only if these test results were pos-

itive. If HAd is the primary screening method for detection of HPIV, then some HPIV-positive cultures will be missed because of poor or no HAd. Also, the addition of centrifugation (e.g., shell vial) to the above IF schedule may speed HPIV detection one or more days (406). Other useful methods of detecting and typing HPIV in tissue culture include hemadsorption inhibition (HAdI), hemagglutinin-inhibition (HI), complement fixation, and neutralization (5,6,407). All of these methods (except HI) are time consuming and costly compared to IF and are currently more useful for research purposes. HAdI was the method of choice for HPIV serotype identification until commercial MAb IF reagents became widely available. The great disadvantage to HAdI is that it took an additional 3 to 5 days after the culture was HAd positive before a specific HPIV type was identified (37). HI assay is fast and easy to perform, but on primary isolation most HPIV strains do not release enough free virus into the supernatant to react. Although tissue culture is the current gold standard, the new molecular assays like PCR are rapidly replacing this time-honored method in clinical virology.

Serologic Diagnosis

Antibodies to HPIV can be detected by ELISA, RIAs, HI, complement-fixation, western-blot, and neutralization assays. Serologic diagnosis for acute HPIV infection is difficult because of the corresponding elevations in heterologous antibodies (407,408). HPIV-1 and HPIV-3 have the greatest copositivity rate, but mumps antibody also cross reacts with these viruses (409–412). A large number of children's sera that test positive by ELISA and HI to HPIV-3 will have similar titers to HPIV-1. Complement fixation titers are the least sensitive to acute infection but appear to be the most specific (410). ELISA, on the other hand, are the least specific with many dual rises in antibody titer, but ELISA detects the greatest number of titer rises in patients with respiratory illness. The least amount of serologic cross-reactivity occurs with HPIV-2 (410,411).

Serologic testing should always be done on paired, acute, and convalescent serum. It should be done at the same time for both serum samples and a four-fold or greater rise in titer is generally thought to be significant. A positive serologic increase in titer to any of the HPIV (even if without heterologous antibody demonstrated) only indicates infection with HPIV (304). It does not accurately predict the serotype and should not be used to determine type of infection. Virus isolation and typing with MAbs is the best and most accurate method for establishing the serotype of HPIV. Antigen detection and molecular techniques, including PCR, will hopefully soon add to our ability to diagnose this group of viruses.

REFERENCES

1. Van den Hoogen B, De Jong JC, et al. A newly discovered human pneumovirus isolated from young children with respiratory tract disease. *Nat Med* 2001;7(6):719–724.
2. Mounts AW, Kaur H, Parashar UD, et al. A cohort study of health care workers to assess nosocomial transmissibility of Nipah virus, Malaysia, 1999. *J Infect Dis* 2001;183:810–813.
3. Nichol ST, Arikawa J, Kawaoka Y. Emerging viral diseases. *Proc Natl Acad Sci USA* 2000;97:12411–12412.
4. Chua KB, Lam SK, Tan CT, et al. High mortality in nipah encephalitis is associated with presence of virus in cerebrospinal fluid. *Ann Neurol* 2000;48:802–805.
5. Canchola J, Vargosko AJ, Kim HW, et al. Antigenic variation among newly isolated strains of parainfluenza type 4 virus. *Am J Hyg* 1964;79:357–364.
6. Henrickson KJ. Monoclonal antibodies to human parainfluenza virus type 1 detect major antigenic changes in clinical isolates. *J Infect Dis* 1991;164:1128–1134.
7. Henrickson KJ, Savatski L. Genetic variation and evolution of human parain-tiuenza virus type 1 hemagglutinin neuraminidase: analysis of 12 clinical isolates. *J Infect Dis* 1992;166:995–1005.
8. Henrickson KJ, Savatski LL. Two distinct human parainfluenza virus type one genotypes detected during the 1991 epidemic. *J Clin Microbiol* 1996;34:695–700.
9. Henrickson KJ, Savatski LL. Antigenic structure, function, and evolution of the hemagglutinin-neuraminidase protein of human parainfluenza virus type 1. *J Infect Dis* 1997;176:867–875.
10. Prinoski K, Cote MJ, Kang CY, Dimock K. Evolution of the fusion protein gene of human parainfluenza virus 3. *Virus Res* 1992;22:55–69.
11. Berman S. Epidemiology of acute respiratory infections in children of developing countries. *Rev Infect Dis* 1991;13:S454–S462.
12. Mcintosh K. Pathogenesis of severe acute respiratory infections in the developing world: respiratory syncytial virus and parainfluenza viruses. *Rev Infect Dis* 1991;13:S492–S500.
13. Glezen HP, Loda FA, Clyde HA Jr, et al. Epidemiologic patterns of acute lower respiratory disease of children in a pediatric group practice. *J Pediatr* 1971;78:397–406.
14. Denny FW, Clyde WA Jr. Acute lower respiratory infections in nonhospitalized children. *J Pediatr* 1986;108:635–646.
15. Murphy B, Phelan PD, Jack I, Uren E. Seasonal pattern in childhood viral lower respiratory tract infections in Melbourne. *Med J Aust* 1980;1:22–24.
16. Kim MR, Lee HR, Lee GM. Epidemiology of acute viral respiratory tract infections in Korean children. *J Infect* 2000;41:152–158.
17. Tsai HP, Kuo PPH, Liu CC, Wang JR. Respiratory viral infections among pediatric inpatients and outpatients in Taiwan from 1997 to1999. *J Clin Microbiol* 2001;39:111–118.
18. Carballal G, Videla CM, Espinosa A, et al. Multicentered study of viral acute lower respiratory infections in children from four cities of Argentina, 1993–1994. *J Med Virol* 2001;64:167–174.
19. Gardner SD. The isolation of parainfluenza 4 subtypes A and B in England and serological studies of their prevalence. *J Hyg (Camb)* 1969;67:545–550.
20. Downham MA, McDuillin J, Gardner PS. Diagnosis and clinical significance of parainfluenza virus infections in children. *Arch Dis Child* 1974;49:8–15.
21. Henrickson KJ, Hoover SH, Kehl KS, Hua W. Epidemiology of respiratory viruses detected in hospitalized children using PCR. *Southern Med J* (submitted).
22. Shay DK, Holman RC, Newman RD, et al. Bronchiolitis-associated hospitalization among US children, 1980-1996. *JAMA* 1999;282:1440–1446.
23. Marx A, Torok TJ, Holman RC, et al. Pediatric hospitalizations for croup (laryngotracheobronchitis): biennial increases associated with human parainfluenza virus 1 epidemics. *J Infect Dis* 1997;1423–1427.
24. Denny FH, Murphy TF, Clyde WA Jr, et al. Croup: an 11-year study in a pediatric practice. *Pediatrics* 1983;71:871–876.
25. Henrickson KJ, Kuhn SM, Savatski LL, Sedmak J. Recovery of human parainfluenza virus types one and two. *J Virol Meth* 1994;46:189–206.
26. Skolnik NS. Treatment of croup. A critical review. *Am J Dis Child* 1989;143:1045–1049.
27. Belshe RB, Van Voris LP, Mufson MA. Impact of viral respiratory diseases on infants and young children in a rural and urban area of southern West Virginia. *Am J Epidemiol* 1983;117:467–474.
28. Wright P. Parainfluenza viruses. In: Belshe RB, ed. *Textbook of human virology.* Littleton. MA: PSG Publishing, 1984:299–310.
29. Falsey AR. Noninfluenza respiratory infection in long-term care facilities. *Infect Control Hosp Epidemiol* 1991;12:602–608.
30. Fiore AE, Iverson C, Messmer T, et al. Outbreak of pneumonia in a long-term care facility: antecedent human parainfluenza virus 1 infection may predispose to bacterial pneumonia. *J Am Geriatr Soc* 1998;46:1112–1117.
31. Marx A, Gary HE, Marston BJ, et al. Parainfluenza virus infection among adults hospitalized for lower respiratory tract infection. *Clin Infect Dis* 1999;29:134–140.
32. Washburne JF, Bocchini JA, Jamison RM. Summertime respiratory syncytial virus infection: Epidemiology and clinical manifestations. *South Med J* 1992;85:579–583.
33. de Silva LH, Cloonan MJ. Brief report: parainfluenza virus type 3 infections: findings in Sydney and some observations on variations in seasonality worldwide. *J Med Virol* 1991;35:19–21.
34. Glezen HP, Frank AL, Taber LH, Kasel JA. Parainfluenza virus type 3: seasonality and risk of infection and reinfection in young children. *J Infect Dis* 1984;150:851–857.
35. Kiligore GE, Dowdle WR. Antigenic characterization of parainfluenza 4A and 4B by the hemagglutination-inhibition test and distribution of HI amibody in human sera. *Am J Epidemiol* 1970;91:308–316.
36. Chanock RM, Parrott RH. Acute respiratory disease in infancy and childhood: present understanding and prospects for prevention. E. Mead Johnson Address, October, 1964. *Pediatrics* 1965;6:21–39.
37. Canchola JG, Chanock RM, Jeffries BC, et al. Recovery and identification of human myxoviruses. *Bacteriol Rev* 1965;29:496–503.
38. Lindquist SW, Darnule A, Istas A, Demmler GJ. Parainfluenza virus type 4 infections in pediatric patients. *Pediatr Infect Dis J* 1997;16:34–38.
39. Karron RA, Makhene M, Gay K. Evaluation of a live attenuated bovine parainfluenza type 3 vaccine in two-to six-month old infants. *Pediatr Infect Dis J* 1996;15:650–654.
40. Sangster M, Smith FS, Coleclough C, Hurwitz JL. Human parainfluenza virus type 1 immunization of infant mice protects from subsequent sendai virus infection. *Virology* 1995;212:13–19.
41. Horowitz JL, Soike KF, Sangster MY, et al. Intranasal sendai virus vaccine protects African green monkeys from infection with human parainfluenza virus-type one. *Vaccine* 1997;15:533–540.
42. Henrickson KJ, Kuhm SM, Savatski LL. Epidemiology and cost of human parainfluenza virus type one and two infections in young children. *Clin Infect Dis* 1994;18:770–779.
43. Woo PCY, Young K, Tsang KWT, et al. Adult croup: a rare but more severe condition. *Respiration* 2000;67:684–688.
44. Peltola V, Heikkinen T, Ruuskanen O. Clinical courses of croup caused by influenza and parainfluenza viruses. *Pediatr Infect Dis J* 2002;21:76–78.
45. Jennings LC, Oawson KP, Abbott GO, Allan J. Acute respiratory tract infections of children inhospital: a viral and mycoplasma pneumoniae profile. *NZ Med J* 1985;98:582–585.
46. Kellner G, Popow-Kraupp T, Kundi M, et al. Contribution of rhinoviruses to respiratory viral infections in childhood. A prospective study in a mainly hospitalized infant population. *J Med Virol* 1988;25:455–469.
47. Murphy TF, Henderson FW, Clyde WA, et al. Pneumonia: an eleven year study in a pediatric practice. *Am J Epidemiol* 1981;113:12–21.
48. Nohynek H, Eskola J, Laine E, et al. The causes of hospital-treated acute lower respiratory tract infection in children. *Am J Dis Child* 1991;145:618–622.
49. Hortal M, Suarez A, Deleon C, et al. Etiology and severity of community acquired pneumonia in children from Uruguay: a 4 year study. *Rev Inst Med Trop Sao Paulo* 1994;36:255–264.
50. Davies HD, Wang EEL, Manson D, et al. Reliability of the chest radiograph in the diagnosis of lower respiratory infections in young children. *Pediatr Infect Dis J* 1996;15:600–604.
51. Korppi M, Halonen P, Kleemola M, Launiala K. Viral findings in children under the age of two years with expiratory difficulties. *Acta Paediatr Scand* 1986;75:457–464.
52. Dowell SF, Anderson LJ, Gary HE, et al. Respiratory syncytial virus is an important cause of community-acquired lower respiratory infection among hospitalized adults. *J Infect Dis* 1996;174:456–462.
53. Greenberg SB. Viral pneumonia. *Infect Dis Clin North Am* 1991;5:603–621.
54. Drews AL, Atmar BL, Glezen WP, et al. Dual respiratory virus infections. *Clin Infect Dis* 1997;25:1421–1429.

55. Chonmaitree T, Owen MJ, Howie VM. Respiratory viruses interfere with bacteriologic response to antibiotic in children with acute otitis media. *J Infect Dis* 1990;162:546–549.

56. Ruuskanen O, Arola M, Heikkinen T, Ziegler T. Viruses in acute otitis media: increasing evidencefor clinical significance. *Pediatr Infect Dis J* 1991;10:425–427.

57. Karp O, Willis J, Wilfert CM. Parainfluenza virus II and the immunocompromised host. *Am J Dis Child* 1974;127:592–593.

58. Delage G, Brochu P, Pelletier M, et al. Giant-cell pneumonia caused by parainfluenza virus. *J Pediatr* 1979;94:426–429.

59. Mcintosh K, Kurachek SC, Cairns LM, et al. Treatment of respirator viral infection in an immunodeficient infant with ribavirin aerosol. *Am J Dis Child* 1934;138:305a.

60. Frank JA Jr, Warren RW, Tucker JA, et al. Disseminated parainfluenza infection in a child with severe combined immunodeficiency. *Am J Dis Child* 1983;137:1172–1174.

61. Jarvis WR, Middleton PJ, Gelfand CW. Parainfluenza pneumonia in severe combined immunodeficiency. *J Pediatr* 1979;94:423–425.

62. Little BW, Tihen WS, Dickerman JO, Craighead JE. Giant cell pneumonia associated with parainfluenza virus type 3 infection. *Hum Pathol* 1981;12:478–481.

63. Weintrub PS, Sullender WM, Lombard C, et al. Giant cell pneumonia caused by parainfluenza type 3 in a patient with acute myelomonocytic leukemia. *Arch Pathol Lab Med* 1987;111:569–570.

64. Wendt CH, Weisdorf DJ, Jordan MC, et al. Parainfluenza virus respiratory infection after bone marrow transplantation. *N Engl J Med* 1992;326:921–926.

65. Beard LJ, Robertson EF, Thong YH. Parainfluenza pneumonia in DiGeorge syndrome two years after thymic epithelial transplantation. *Acta Paediatr Scand* 1980;69:403–406.

66. Josephs S, Kim HW, Brandt CD, Parrott RH. Parainfluenza 3 virus and other common respiratory pathogens in children with human immunodeficiency virus infection. *Pediatr Infect Dis J* 1988;7:207–209.

67. King JC, Burke AR, Clemens JD, et al. Respiratory syncytial virus illnesses in human immunodeficiency virus and noninfected children. *Pediatr Infect Dis J* 1993;12:733–739.

68. King JC. Community respiratory viruses in individuals with human immunodeficiency virus infection. *Am J Med* 1997;102(3A):19–24.

69. McSherry GD. Human immunodeficiency-virus-related pulmonary infections in children. *Sem Respir Infect* 1996;11:173–183.

70. DeFabritus AM, Riggio RR, Oavid OS, et al. Parainfluenza type 3 in a transplant unit. *JAMA* 1979;241:384–386.

71. Herzog KD, Ounn SP, Langham MR Jr., Marmon LM. Association of parainfluenza virus type 3 infection with allograft rejection in a liver transplant recipient. *Pediatr Infect Dis J* 1989;8:534–536.

72. Wasserman R, August CS, Plotkin SA. Viral infections in pediatric bone marrow transplant patients. *Pediatr Infect Dis J* 1988;7:109–115.

73. Ljungman CA, Gleaves CA, Meyers JD. Respiratory virus infection in immunocompromised patients. *Bone Marrow Transplantation* 1989;4:35–40.

74. Apalsch AM, Green M, Wald ER. Influenza and parainfluenza virus infections in pediatric organ transplant recipients. *Clin Infect Dis* 1995;20:394–399.

75. Whimberg E, Vartivarian S, Chamolin R, et al. Parainfluenza virus infection among adult bone marrow transplant (BMT) patients, 1992 (ICAAC Abstract).

76. Whimbey E, Englund JA, Ljungman P. Community respiratory viral infections in the immunocompromised host. Proceedings of a symposium. *Am J Med* 1997;102:1–80.

77. Lewis VA, Champlin R, Englund J. Respiratory disease due to parainfluenza virus in adult bone marrow transplant recipients. *Clin Infect Dis* 1996;23:1033–1037.

78. Arola M, Ruuskanen O, Ziegler T, et al. Respiratory virus infections during anticancer treatment in children. *Pediatr Infect Dis J* 1995;14:690–694.

79. Lujan-Zilbermann J, Benaim E, Tong X, et al. Respiratory virus infections in pediatric hematopoietic stem cell transplantation. *Clin Infect Dis* 2001;33:962–968.

80. Nicholas WG, Corey L, Gooley T, et al. Parainfluenza virus infections after hematopoietic stem cell transplantation: risk factors, response to antiviral therapy, and effect on transplant outcome. *Blood* 2001;98:573–578.

81. Zambon M, Bull T, Sadler CJ, et al. Molecular epidemiology of two consecutive outbreaks of parainfluenza 3 in a bone marrow transplant unit. *J Clin Microbiol* 1998;36:2289–2293.

82. Vilchez RA, McCurry K, Dauber J, et al. The epidemiology of parainfluenza virus infection in lung transplant recipients. *Clin Infect Dis* 2001;33:2004–2008.

83. Cullen SJ, Baublis JV. Parainfluenza type 3 parotitis in two immunodeficient children. *J Pediatr* 1980;96:437–438.

84. Fishaut M, Tubergen O, Mcintosh K. Cellular response to respiratory viruses with particular reference to children with disorders of cell-mediated immunity. *J Pediatr* 1980;96:179–186.

85. Meolen V, Koprowski H, Iwasaki Y, et al. Etrusion of cultured multiple-sclerosis brain cells with indicator cells: presence of nucleocapsids and virions and isolation of parainfluenza-type virus. *Lancet* 1972;2:1–5.

86. Lewandowski LJ, Lief FS, Verini A, et al. Analysis of a viral agent isolated from multiple sclerosis brain tissue: characterization as a parainfluenza virus type1. *J Virol* 1974;13:1037–1045.

87. Lehrich JR, Arnason DG, Fuller TC, Wray SH. Parainfluenza, histocompatibility, and multiple sclerosis. Association of parainfluenza antibodies and histocompatibility types in 115 and optic neuritis. *Arch Neurol* 1974;30:327–329.

88. Brown P, Cathala F, Gajdusek DC. Further studies of viral antibodies in the cerebrospinal fluid of patients with multiple sclerosis: vaccinia and parainfluenza type 1 (37422). *Proc Soc Exp Biol Med* 1973;143:828–829.

89. Barbosa LH, Hamilton R. Virological studies with multiple-sclerosis brain tissues. *Lancet* 1973;1:1415–1417.

90. Mori I, Komatsu T, Takeuchi K, et al. Parainfluenza virus type 1 infects olfactory neurons and establishes long-term persistence in the nerve tissue. *J Gen Virol* 1995;76:1251–1254.

91. Mori I, Nakakuki K, Kimura Y. Temperature-sensitive parainfluenza type 1 vaccine virus directly accesses the central nervous system by infecting olfactory neurons. *J Gen Virol* 1996;77:2121–2124.

92. Goswami KK, Cameron KR, Russell WC, et al. Evidence for the persistence of paramyxoviruses in human bone marrows. *J Gen Virol* 1984;65:1:81–88.

93. Robbins SJ, Wrzos H, Kline AL, et al. Rescue of a cytopathic paramyxovirus from peripheral blood leukocytes in subacute sclerosing panencephalitis. *J Infect Dis* 1981;143:396–403.

94. Roman G, Phillips CA, Poser CM. Parainfluenza virus type 3: isolation from CSF of a patient with Gullain-Barre syndrome. *JAMA* 1978;240:1613–1615.

95. Vreede RW, Schellekens H, Jluiderwijk M. Isolation of parainfluenza virus type 3 from cerebrospinal fluid. *J Infect Dis* 1992;165:1166.

96. Wong VK, Steinberg E, Warford A. Parainfluenza virus type 3 meningitis in an 11-montn-old infant. *Pediatr Infect Dis J* 1988;7:300–301.

97. Arguedas A, Stutman HR, Blanding JG. Parainfluenza type 3 meningitis. Report of two cases and review of the literature. *Clin Pediatr* 1990;29:175–178.

98. Bitnun A, Ford-Jones EL, Petric M, et al. Acute childhood encephalitis and Mycoplasma pneumoniae. *Clin Infect Dis* 2001;32:1674–1684.

99. Seidman DS, Nass D, Mendelson E, et al. Prenatal ultrasonographic diagnosis sof fetal hydrocephalus due to infection with parainfluenza virus type 3. *Ultrasound Obstet Gynecol* 1996;7:52–54.

100. Blanchard BM. Cluster headache associated with parainfluenza virus, preceded and succeeded by migraine. *Headache* 1998;38:132–134.

101. Singh-Naz N, Willy M, Riggs N. Outbreak of parainfluenza virus type 3 in a neonatal nursery. *Pediatr Infect Dis J* 1990;9:31–33.

102. McCarthy VP, Carlile JR, Reichelderfer PS, Clark JS. Parainfluenza type 3 in newborns. *Pediatr Infect Dis J* 1987;6:217–218.

103. Meissner HC, Murray SA, Kiernan MA, et al. A simultaneous outhreak of respiratory syncytial virus and parainfluenza virus type 3 in a newborn nursery. *J Pediatr* 1984;104:680–684.

104. Hotez PJ, Goldstein B, Ziegler J, et al. Adult respiratory distress syndrome associated with parainfluenza virus type I in children. *Pediatr Infect Dis J* 1990;9:750–752.

105. Grattan-Smith T, Forer M, Kilham H, Gillis J. Viral supraglottitis. *J Pediatr* 1987;110:434–435.

106. Peramaki E, Salmi I, Kava T, et al. Unilateral bronchiolitis obliterans organizing pneumonia and bronchoalveolar lavage neutrophilia in a patient with parainfluenza 3 virus infection. *Respir Med* 1991;85:159–161.

107. Zollar LM, Mufson MA. Acute parotitis associated with parainfluenza 3 virus infection. *Am J Dis Child* 1970;199:147–148.

108. Bloom HH, Johnson KM, Jacobsen R, Chanock RM. Recovery of parainfluenza viruses from adults with upper respiratory illness. *Am J Hyg* 1961;74:50–59.

109. Buckley JM, Poche P, Mcintosh K. Parotitis and parainfluenza 3 virus. *Am J Dis Child* 1972:124:789.

110. Liston SL, Gehrz RC, Siegel LC, Tilelli J. Bacterial tracheitis. *Am J Dis Child* 1983;137:764–767.

111. MacDonald NE, Wolfish N, McLaine P, et al. Role of respiratory viruses in exacerbations of primary nephrotic syndrome. *J Pediatr* 1986;108:378–382.

112. Rocchi G, Arangio-Ruiz G, Giannini V, et al. Detection of viraemia inacute respiratory disease of man. *Acta Virol* 1970;14:405–407.

113. Phillips MJ, Blendis LM, Poucell S, et al. Syncytial giant-cell hepatitis. Sporadic hepatitis with distinctive pathological features, a severe clinical course, and paramyxoviral features. *N Engl J Med* 1991;324:455–460.

114. Wilks D, Burns SM. Myopericarditis associated with parainfluenza virus type 3 infection. *Eur J Clin Microbiol Infect Dis* 1998;17:363–365.

115. Phillips PE, Christian CL. Myxovirus antibody increases in human connective tissue disease. *Science* 1970;168:982–984.

116. Iizuka M, Saito H, Yukawa M, et al. No evidence of persistent mumps virus infection in inflammatory bowel disease. *Gut* 2001;48:637–641.

117. Ueda K, Robbins DA, Iitaka K, Linnemann CC Jr. Fatal rhabdomyolysis associated with parainfluenza type 3 infection. *Hiroshima J Med Sci* 1978;27:99–103.

118. O'Connor JV, Iyer SK. Myoglobinuria associated with parainfluenza type 2 infection. *NY State J Med* 1982;82:1469–1470.

119. Aronson MD, Kaminsky D, Phillips CA. Parainfluenza virus type 3 isolates in a case of bloody diarrhea [Letter]. *Ann Intern Med* 1974;81:856–857.

120. Brandt CD, Kim HW, Rodriguez WJ, et al. Simultaneous infections with different enteric and respiratory tract viruses. *J Clin Microbiol* 1986;23:177–179.

121. Mufson MA, Mocega HE, Krause HE. Acquisition of parainfluenza 3 virus infection by hospitalized children. I. Frequencies, rates and temporal data. *J Infect Dis* 1973;128:141–147.

122. Louqhlin GM, Taussig LM. Pulmonary function in children with a history of laryngotracheobronchitis. *J Pediatr* 1979;94:365–369.

123. Hall CB, Hall WJ, Gala CL, et al. Long-term prospective study in children after respiratory syncytial virus infection. *J Pediatr* 1984;105:358–364.

124. Kattan M, Keens TG, Lapierre JG, et al. Pulmonary function abnormalities in symptom-free children after bronchiolitis. *Pediatrics* 1977;59:683–688.

125. Henry RL, Hodqes IG, Milner AO, Stokes GM. Respiratory problems 2 years after acute bronchiolitis in infancy. *Arch Dis Child* 1983;58:713–716.

126. Stokes GM, Milner AD, Hodges IGC, Groggins RC. Lung function abnormalities after acute bronchiolitis. *J Pediatr* 1981;98:871–874.

127. Tuffaha A, Gern JE, Lemanske RF. The pathobiology of asthma: implications for treatment. *Clin Chest Med* 2000;21.

128. O'Reilly JF. Adult bronchiolitis and parainfluenza type 2. *Postgrad Med J* 1930;56:787a.

129. Sorkness R, Lemanske RFJ, Castleman WL. Persistent airway hyperresponsiveness after neonatal viral bronchiolitis in rats. *J Appl Physiol* 1991;70:375–383.

130. Quan SF, Lemen RJ, Witten ML, et al. Changes in lung mechanics and reactivity with age after viral bronchiolitis in beagle puppies. *J Appl Physiol* 1990;69:2034–2042.

131. McLean OM, Bannatyne RM, Givan KF. Myxovirus dissemination by air. *Can Med Assoc J* 1967;96:1449–1453.

132. Hall CB, Douglas RG Jr. Modes of transmission of respiratory syncytial virus. *J Pediatr* 1981;99:100–103.

133. Brady MT, Evans J, Cuartas J. Survival and disinfection of parainfluenza viruses on environmental surfaces. *Am J Infect Control* 1990;18:18–23.

134. Ansari SA, Springthorpe VS, Sattar SA, et al. Potential role of hands in the spread of respiratory viral infections: studies with human parainfluenza virus 3 and rhinovirus 14. *J Clin Microbiol* 1991;29:2115–2119.

135. Hall CB, Geiman JM, Breese BB, Douglas RG Jr. Parainfluenza viral infections in children: correlation of shedding with clinical manifestations. *J Pediatr* 1977;91:194–198.

136. Bose S, Malur A, Banerjee AK. Polarity of human parainfluenza virus type 3 infection in polarized human lung epithelial A549 cells: role of microfilament and microtubule. *J Virol* 2001;75:1984–1989.

137. Porter DD, Prince GA, Hemming VG, Porter HG. Pathogenesis of human parainfluenza virus 3 infection in two species of cotton rats: *Sigmodon hispidus* develops bronchiolitis, while *Sigmodon fulviventer* develops interstitial pneumonia. *J Virol* 1991;65:103–111.

138. Yao Q, Compans RW. Filamentous particle formation by human parainfluenza virus type 2. *J Gen Virol* 2000;81:1305–1312.

139. Konovalova NG, Blyumkin VN, Zakstelskaya LY. Action of parainfluenza viruses on the mitotic activity of primary trypsinized human embryo kidney cell cultures. *Acta Virol* 1967;11:564.

140. Craighead JE, Brennan BJ. Cytopathic effects of parainfluenza virus type 3 in organ cultures of human respiratory tract tissue. *Am J Pathol* 1968;52:287–300.

141. He B, Lin GY, Durbin JE, et al. The SH integral membrane protein of the paramyxovirus simian virus 5 is required to block apoptosis in MDBK cells. *J Virol* 2001;75:4068–4079.

142. Tremonti LP, Lin JS, Jackson GG. Neutralizing activity in nasal secretions and serum in resistance of volunteers to parainfluenza virus type 2. *J Immunol* 1968;101:572–577.

143. Knott PG, Henry PJ, McWilliam AS, et al. Influence of parainfluenza-1 respiratory tract viral infection on endothelin receptor-effector systems in mouse and rat tracheal smooth muscle. *Br J Pharmacol* 1996;119:291–298.

144. Riedel F, Benden C, Philippou S, et al. Role of sensory neuropeptides in PIV-3-infection-induced airway hyperresponsiveness in guinea pigs. *Respiration* 1997;64:211–219.

145. Moscona A, Peluso RW. Fusion properties of cells infected with human parainfluenza virus type 3: receptor requirements for viral spread and virus-mediated membrane fusion. *J Virol* 1992;66:6280–6287.

146. Murphy DG, Dimock K, Kang CY. Numerous transitions in human parainfluenza virus 3 RNA recovered from persistently infected cells. *Virology* 1991;181:760–763.

147. Genest P. Daniel P. Genomic modifications in cell line cultures chronically infected with a myxovirus. *Proc Soc Exp Biol Med* 1966;123:722–725.

148. Muchmore HG, Parkinson AJ, Humphries JE, et al. Persistent parainfluenza virus shedding during isolation at the South Pole. *Nature* 1981;289:187–189.

149. Gross PA, Green RH, Curnen MG. Persistent infection with parainfluenza type 3 virus in man. *Am Rev Respir Dis* 1973;108:894–898.

150. Gross PS, Green RH, Lerner E, Curnen MG. Immune response in persistent infection. Further studies on persistent respiratory infection in man with parainfluenza type 3 virus. *Am Rev Respir Dis* 1974;110:676–681.

151. Fraser KB, Anderson J. Persistent non-cytocidal infection of BHK 21 cells by human parainfluenza type 2 virus. *J Gen Microbiol* 1966;44:47–58.

152. Ebina T, Kamo I, Homma M, Ishida N. Autoradiographic studies of HeLa-S3 cells persistently infected with hemadsorption type 2 virus. *Exp Cell Res* 1969;57:359–364.

153. Iwata H, Tagaya M, Matsumoto K, et al. Aerosol vaccination with a sendai virus temperature-sensitive mutant (HVJ-pB) derived from persistently infected cells. *J Infect Dis* 1990;162:402–407.

154. Ah-Tye C, Schwartz S, Huberman K, et al. Virus-receptor interactions of human parainfluenza viruses types 1, 2, and 3. *Microb Pathogen* 1999;27:329–336.

155. Hu XL, Ray R, Compans RW. Functional interactions between the fusion Protein andhemagglutinin-neuraminidase of human parainfluenza viruses. *J Virol* 1992;66:1528–1534.

156. Horga MA, Gusella GL, Greengard O, et al. Mechanism of interference mediated by human parainfluenza virus type 3 infection. *J Virol* 2000;74:11792–11799.

157. Fryer AD, el-Fakahany EE, Jacoby OB. Parainfluenza virus type 1 reduces the affinity of agonists for muscarinic receptors in guinea pig lung and heart. *Eur J Pharmacol* 1990;181:51–58.

158. Fryer AD, Jacoby OB. Parainfluenza virus infection damages inhibitory Mz muscarinic receptors on pulmonary parasympathetic nerves in the guinea-pig. *Br J Pharmacol* 1991;102:267–271.

159. Welliver RC, Wong DT, Middleton EJ, et al. Role or parainfluenza virus-specific IgE in pathogenesis of croup and wheezing subsequent to infection. *J Pediatr* 1982;101:889–896.

160. Folkerts G, van Esch B, Janssen M, Nijkamp FP. Superoxide production by broncho-alveolar cells is diminished in parainfluenza-3 virus treated guinea pigs. *Agents Actions [Suppl]* 1990;31:139–142.

161. Folkerts G, Janssen M, Nijkamp FP. Parainfluenza-3 induced hyperreactivity or the guinea Di9 trachea coincides with an increased number of bronchoalveolar cells. *Br J Clin Pharmacol* 1990;30:159S–161S.

162. Riedel F, Krause A, Slenczyka W, Rieger CHL. Parainfluenza-3-virus infection enhances allergic sensitization in the guinea-pig. *Clin Exp Allergy* 1996;26:603–609.

163. Ottolini M, et al. Enhanced pulmonary inflammation in cotton rats exposed to parainfluenza type 3 (PIV3) after immunization with a formalin-inactivated vaccine, 1992 (ICAAC Abstract).

164. Vasantha S, Coelingh KL, Murphy BR, et al. Interactions of a nonneutralizing IgM antibody and complement in parainfluenza virus neutralization. *Virology* 1988;167:433–441.

165. Visseren FLJ, Bouwman JJM, Bouter KP, et al. Procoagulant activity of endothelial cells after infection with respiratory viruses. *Thromb Haemost* 2000;84:319–324.

166. Carpenter TC, Reeves JT, Durmowicz AG. Viral respiratory infection increases susceptibility of young rats to hypoxia-induced pulmonary edema. *J Appl Physiol* 1998;84:1048–1054.

167. Kasel JA, Frank AL, Keitel WA, et al. Aquisition of serum antibodies to specific viral glycoproteins of parainfluenza virus 3 in children. *J Virol* 1984;52:828–832.

168. Spriggs MK, Murphy BR, Prince GA, et al. Expression of the F and HN glycoproteins of human parainfluenza virus type 3 by recombinant vaccinia viruses: contributions or the individual proteins to host immunity. *J Virol* 1987;61:3416–3423.

169. Mozdzanowska K, Furchner M, Washko G, et al. A pulmonary influenza virus infection in SCID mice can be cured by treatment with hemagglutinin-specific antibodies that display very low virus-neutralizing activity in vivo. *J Virol* 1997;71:4347–4355

170. Julkunen I, Hovi T, Seppala I, Makela O. Immunoglobulin G subclass antibody responses in influenza A and parainfluenza type 1 virus infection. *Clin Exp Immunol* 1985;60:130–138.

171. van der Logt JT, van Loon AM, van der Veen J. Detection of parainfluenza IgM antibody by hemadsorption immunosorbent technique. *J Med Virol* 1982;10:213–221.

172. Welliver R, Wong DT, Choi TS, Ogra PL. Natural history of parainfluenza virus infection in childhood. *J Pediatr* 1982;101:180–187.

173. Smith CB, Purcell RH, Bellanti JA, Chanock RM. Protective effect of antibody to parainfluenza type 1 virus. *N Engl J Med* 1966;275:1145–1152.

174. Yanagihara R, Mcintosh K. Secretory immunological response in infants and children to parainfluenza virus types 1 and 2. *Infect Immun* 1980;30:23–28.

175. Hruskova J, Fedova D, Syrucek L, et al. Haemagglutination inhibition antibodies in nasal secretions of persons after natural parainfluenza virus infection. *Acta Virol* 1978;22:203–208.

176. Tremonti LP, Lin JS, Jackson GG. Neutralizing activity in nasal secretions and serum in resistance of volunteers to parainfluenza virus type 2. *J Immunol* 1968;101:572–577.

177. Henderson FW. Pulmonary cell-mediated cytotoxicity in hamsters with parainfluenza virus type 3 pneumonia. *Am Rev Respir Dis* 1979;120:41–47.

178. Kimmel KA, Wyde PR, Glezen WP. Evidence of a T-cell-mediated cytotoxic response to parainfluenza virus type 3 pneumonia in hamsters. *J Reticuloendothel Soc* 1982;31:71–83.

179. Hou S, Doherty PC, Zijlstra M, Katz JM. Delayed clearance of Sendai virus in mice lacking class I MHC-restricted CD8+ T cells. *J Immunol* 1992;149:1319–1325.

180. Kast WM, Bronihorst AH, DeWaal P, Melief CJ. Cooperation between cytotoxic and helper T lymphocytes in protection against lethal Sendai virus infection. Protection by T cells is MHC restricted and MHC regulated: a model for MHC-disease associations. *J Exp Med* 1986;164:723.

181. Kast WM, Bluestone JA, Heemskerk MH, et al. Treatment with monoclonal anti-CD3 antibody protects against lethal Sendai virus infection by induction of natural killer cells. *J Immunol* 1990;145:2254–2259.

182. Hogan RJ, Usherwood EJ, Zhong W, et al. Activated antigen-specific CD8+ T cells persist in the lungs following recovery from respiratory virus infections. *J Immunol* 2001;166:1813–1822.

183. Hogan RJ, Zhong W, Usherwood EJ, et al. Protection from respiratory virus infections can be mediated by antigen-specific CD4+ T cells that persist in the lungs. *J Exp Med* 2001;193:981–986.

184. Doherty PC, Allan W, Eichelberger M, et al. Involvement of gamma delta T cells in respiratory virus infections. *Curr Top Microbiol Immunol* 1991;173:291–296.

185. Mandelbolm O, Lieberman N, Lev M, et al. Recognition of haemagglutinins on virus-infected cells by NKp46 activates lysis by human NK cells. *Nature* 2001;409:1055–1060.

186. Dave V, Allan JE, Slobod KS, et al. Viral cross-reactivity and antigenic determinants recognized by human parainfluenza virus type 1-specific cytotoxic T-cells. *Virology* 1994;199:376–383.

187. Cole GA, Katz JM, Hogg TL, et al. Analysis of the primary T-cell response to Sendai virus infection in C57BL/6 mice CD4+ T-cell recognition is directed predominantly to the hemagglutinin-neuraminidase glycoprotein. *J Virol* 1994;68:6863–6870.

188. Mo XY, Sarawar SR, Doherty PC. Induction of cytokines in mice with parainfluenza pneumonia. *J Virol* 1995;69:1288–1291.

189. Hua J, Liao MJ, Rashidbaigi A. Cytokines induced by Sendai virus in human peripheral blood leukocytes. *J Leukocyte Biol* 1996;60:125–128.

190. Choudhary S, Gao J, Leaman DW, De BP. Interferon action against human parainfluenza virus type 3: involvement of a novel antiviral pathway in the inhibition of transcription. *J Virol* 2001;75:4823–4831.

191. Gao J, De BP, Han Y, et al. Human parainfluenza virus type 3 inhibits gamma interferon induced major histocompatibility complex class II expression directly and by inducing alpha/beta interferon. *J Virol* 2001;75:1124–1131.

192. Sorkness RL, Mehta H, Kaplan MR, et al. Effect of ICAM-1 blockade on lung inflammation and physiology during acute viral bronchiolitis in rats. *Pediatr Res* 2000;47:819–824.

193. Sieg S, King C, Huang Y, Kaplan D. The role of interleukin-10 in the inhibition of T-cell proliferation and apoptosis mediated by parainfluenza virus type 3. *J Virol* 1996;70:4845–4848.

194. Einarson C, Geba GP, Zhu Z, et al. Interleukin-11: stimulation in vivo and in vitro by respiratory viruses and induction of airways hyperresponsiveness. *J Clin Invest* 1996;97:915–924.

195. Fulginiti VA, Eller JJ, Sieber OF, et al. Respiratory virus immunization. 1. A field trial of two inactivated respiratory virus vaccines; an aqueous trivalent parainfluenza virus vaccine and an alum-precipitated respiratory syncytial virus vaccine. *Am J Epidemiol* 1969;89:435–448.

196. Chin J, Magoffin RL, Shearer LA, et al. Field evaluation of a respiratory syncytial virus vaccine and a trivalent parainfluenza virus vaccine in a pediatric population. *Am J Epidemiol* 1969;89:449–463.

197. Murphy BR, Graham BS, Prince GA, et al. Serum and nasal-wash immunoglobulin G and A antibody response of infants and children to respiratory syncytial virus F and G glycoproteins following primary infection. *J Clin Microbiol* 1986;23:1009–1014.

198. van Vyke Coelingh KL, Hinter CC, Tierney EL, et al. Attenuation of bovine parainfluenza virus type 3 in nonhuman primates and its ability to confer immunity to human parainfluenza virus type 3 challenge. *J Infect Dis* 1988;157:655–662.

199. Clements ML. Belshe RB, King J, et al. Evaluation of bovine, cold-adapted human and wild-type human parinfluenza type 3 viruses in adult volunteers and in chimpanzees. *J Clin Microbiol* 1991;29:1175–1182.

200. Crowe JE. Current approaches to the development of vaccines against disease caused by respiratory syncytial virus (RSV) and parainfluenza virus (PIV). *Vaccine* 1995;13:415–421.

201. Lee MS, Greenberg DP, Yey SH, et al. Antibody responses to bovine parainfluenza virus type 3 (PIV3) vaccination and human PIV3 infection in young infants. *J Infect Dis* 2001;184:909–913.

202. Schmidt AC, McAuliffe JM, Huang A, et al. Bovine parainfluenza virus type 3 (BPIV3) fusion and hemagglutinin-neuraminidase glycoproteins make an important contribution to the restricted replication of BPIV3 in primates. *J Virol* 2000;74:8922–8929.

203. Schmidt AC, McAuliffe JM, Murphy BR, Collins PL. Recombinant bovine/human parainfluenza virus type 3 (B/HPIV3) expressing the respiratory syncytial virus (RSV) G and F proteins can be used to achieve simultaneous mucosal immunization against RSV and HPIV3. *J Virol* 2001;75:4594–4603.

204. Haller AA, Miller T, Mitiku M, Coelingh K. Expression of the surface glycoproteins of human parainfluenza virus type 3 by bovine parainfluenza virus type 3, a novel attenuated virus vaccine vector. *J Virol* 2000;74:11626–11635.

205. Belshe RB, Hissom FK. Cold adaptation of parainfluenza virus type 3: induction of three phenotypic markers. *J Med Virol* 1982;10:235–242.

206. Crookshanks-Newman FK, Belshe RB. Protection of weanling hamsters from experimental infection with wild-type parainfluenza virus type 3 (para 3) by cold adapted mutants of para 3. *J Med Virol* 1986;18:131–137.

207. Belshe RB, Karron RA, Newman FK, et al. Evaluation of a live attenuated, cold-adapted parainfluenza virus type 3 in children. *J Clin Microbiol* 1992;30:2064–2070.

208. Karron RA, Wright PF, Newman FK. A live human parainfluenza type 3 virus vaccine is attenuated and immunogenic in healthy infants and children. *J Infect Dis* 1995;172:1445–1450.

209. Yao Q, Compans RW. Peptides corresponding to the heptad repeat sequence of human parainfluenza virus fusion protein are potent inhibitors of virus infection. *Virology* 1996;223:103–112.

210. Durbin AP, Cho J, Elkins WR, et al. Comparison of the immunogenicity and efficacy of a replication-defective vaccinia virus expressing antigens of human parainfluenza virus type 3 (HPIV3) with those of a live attenuated HPIV3 vaccine candidate in rhesus monkeys passively immunized with PIV3 antibodies. *J Infect Dis* 1999;179:1345–1351.

211. Scheid A, Choppin PN. Protease activation mutants of Sendai virus: Activation of biological properties by specific proteases. *Virology* 1976;69:265–277.

212. Tashiro M, Tobita K, Seto JT, Rott R. Comparison of protective effects of serum antibody on respiratory and systemic infection of Sendai virus in mice. *Arch Virol* 1989;107:85–96.

213. Maru M, Haraguchi M, Sato K, et al. Evaluation of a protease activation mutant of Sendai virus as a potent live vaccine. *Vet Microbiol* 1992;30:1–12.

214. Morein B, Sharp M, Sundquist B, Simons K. Protein subunit vaccines of parainfluenza type 2 virus: immunogenic effect in lambs and mice. *J Gen Virol* 1983;64:1557–1569.

215. Ray R, Brown VE, Compans RW. Glycoproteins of human parainfluenza virus type 3: characterization and evaluation as a subunit vaccine. *J Infect Dis* 1985;152:1219–1230.

216. Ray R, Glaze BJ, Moldoveanu Z, Compans RW. Intranasal immunization of hamsters with envelope glycoproteins of human parainfluenza virus type 3. *J Infect Dis* 1988;157:648–654.

217. Ambrose MW, Wyde PR, Ewasyshyn M, et al. Evaluation of the immunogenicity and protective efficacy of a candidate parainfluenza virus type 3 subunit vaccine in cotton rats. *Vaccine* 1991;9:505–511.

218. Spriggs MK, Collins PL, Tierney E, et al. Immunization with vaccinia virus recombinants that express the surface glycoproteins of human parainfluenza virus type 3 (PIV3) protects pates monkeys against PIV3 infection. *J Virol* 1988;62:1293–1296.

219. van Wyke Coelingh KL, Winter CC, Jorgensen ED, Murphy BR. Antigenic and structural properties of the hemagglutinin-neuraminidase glycoprotein of human parainfluenza virus type 3: sequence analysis of variants selected with monoclonal antibodies which inhibit infectivity, hemagglutination, and neuraminidase activities. *J Virol* 1987;61:1473–1477.

220. Durbin A, Slew JW, Murphy BR, Collins PL. Minimum protein requirements for transcription and RNA replication of a minigenome of human parainfluenza virus type 3 and evaluation of the rule of six. *Virology* 1997;234:74–83.

221. Hoffman MA, Banerjee AK. An infectious clone of human parainfluenza virus type 3. *J Virol* 1997;71:4272–4277.

222. Tao T, Skiadopoulos MH, Durbin AP, et al. A live attenuated chimeric recombinant parainfluenza virus (PIV) encoding the internal proteins of PIV type 3 and the surface glycoproteins of PIV type 1 induces complete resistance to PIV1 challenge and partial resistance to PIV3 challenge. *Vaccine* 1999;17:1100–1108.

223. White LA, Freeman CY, Forrester BD, Chappell WA. In vitro effect of ascorbic acid on infectivity of herpesviruses and paramyxoviruses. *J Clin Microbiol* 1986;24:527–531.

224. Wyde PR, Ambrose MN, Meyer HL, Gilbert AE. Toxicity and antiviral activity of LY253963 against respiratory syncytial and parainfluenza type 3 viruses in tissue culture and in cotton rats. *Antiviral Res* 1990;14:237–247.

225. Wyde PR, Ambrose NN, Meyer HL, et al. Evaluation of the toxicity and antiviral activity of carbocyclic 3-deazaadenosine against respiratory syncytial and parainfluenza type 3 viruses in tissue culture and in cotton rats. *Antiviral Res* 1990;14:215–225.

226. Gergely L, Toth FD, Hadhazy GY. Examination in vitro of the virus inhibitory action of a new benzthiazide derivative. *Acta Microbiol Acad Sci Hung* 1968;15:145–150.

227. Luczak M, Korbecki M, Kobus M, Hankiewicz W. Puromycin as an inhibitor of parainfluenza 3 virus multiplication. *Acta Virol* 1971;15:374–380.

228. Meindl P, Bodo G, Palese P, et al. Inhibition of neuraminidase activity by derivatives of 2-deoxy-2, 3-debydro-N-acetyineurmaminic acid. *Virology* 1974;58:457–463.

229. Soret MG. Antiviral activity of calcium elenlate on parainfluenza infection of hamsters. *Antimicrob Agents Chemother* 1969;9:160–166.

230. Wyde PR, Moore DK, Pimentel M, et al. Evaluation of the antiviral activity of N-(phosphonoacetyl)-L-aspartate against paramyxoviruses in tissue culture and against respiratory syncytial virus in cotton rats. *Antiviral Res* 1995;27:59–69.

231. Murrell MT, Porotto M, Greengard O, et al. A single amino acid alteration in the human parainfluenza virus type 3 hemagglutinin-neuraminidase glycoprotein confers resistance to the inhibitory effects of zanamivir on receptor binding and neuraminidase activity. *J Virol* 2001;75:6310–6320.

232. Karagoz A, Arda N, Goren N, et al. Antiviral activity of Sanicula europaea L. extracts on multiplication of human parainfluenza virus type 2. *Phytother Res* 1999;13:436–438.

233. Saladino R, Crestini C, Palamara AT, et al. Synthesis, biological evaluation, and pharmacophore generation of uracil, 4(3H)-pyrimidinone, and uridine derivatives as potent and selective inhibitors of parainfluenza 1 (Sendae) virus. *J Med Chem* 2001;44:4554–4562.

234. Greengard O, Poltoratskaia P, Leikina E, et al. The anti-influenza virus agent 4-GU-DANA (Zanamivir) inhibits cell fusion mediated by human parainfluenza virus and influenza virus HA. *J Virol* 2000;74:11108–11114.

235. Porotto M, Greengard O, Poltoratskaia N, et al. Human parainfluenza virus type 3 HN-receptor interaction: effect of 4-guanidino-neu5Ac2en on a neuraminidase-deficient variant. *J Virol* 2001;75:7481–7488.

236. Lambert DM, Barney S, Lambert AL, et al. Peptides from conserved regions of paramyxovirus fusion (F) proteins are potent inhibitors of viral fusion. *Proc Natl Acad Sci USA* 1996;93:2186–2191.

237. Pastey M, Gower TL, Spearman PW, et al. A rhoA-derived peptide inhibits syncytium formation induced by respiratory syncytial virus and parainfluenza virus type 3. *Nat Med* 2000;6:35–40.

238. Ghosh JK, Shae Y. A peptide derived from a conserved domain of sendai virus fusion protein inhibits virus-cell fusion. *J Biol Chem* 1998;273:7252–7259.

239. Sidwell RN, Khare GP, Allen LB, et al. In vitro and in vivo effect of 1-beta-D-ribofuranosyl-1,-2,4-triazole-3-carboxamide (ribavirin) on types 1 and 3 parainfluenza virus infections. *Chemotherapy* 1975;21:205–220.

240. Browne MJ. Comparative inhibition of influenza and parainfluenza virus replication by ribavirin cells. *Antimicrob Agents Chemother* 1981;19:712–715.

241. Sparrelid E, Ljungman P, Ekelof-Andstrom E, et al. Ribavirin therapy in bone marrow transplant recipients with viral respiratory tract infections. *Bone Marrow Transplant* 1987;19:905–908.

242. Chakrabarti S, Collingham KE, Holder K, et al. Parainfluenza virus type 3 infections in hematopoetic stem cell transplant recipients: response to ribavirin therapy. *Clin Infect Dis* 2000;31:1516–1518.

243. Malinowski MD, Hostoffer RW. Home care based treatment with short course inhaled ribavirin of parainfluenza in a patient with severe combined immunodeficiency. *J Allergy Clin Immunol* 2001;107:663.

244. Chakrabarti S, Collingham KE, Holder K, et al. Pre-emptive oral ribavirin therapy of paramyxovirus infections after haematopoietic stem cell transplantation: a pilot study. *Bone Marrow Transplant* 2001;28:759–763.

245. Nichols WG, Gooley T, Boeckh M. Community acquired respiratory syncytial virus and parainfluenza virus infections after hematopoietic stem cell transplantation: The Fred Hutchinson Cancer Research Center Experience. *Biol Blood Marrow Transplant* 2001;7:11S–15S.

246. Iida J, Saiki I, Ishihara C, Azuma I. Prophylactic activity against Sendai virus infection and macrophage activation with lipophilic derivatives of H-acetylglucosaminylmuramyl tri- or tetrapeptides. *Vaccine* 1989;7:225–228.

247. Iida J, Ishihara C, MizuLoshi M, et al. Prophylactic activity of dihydroheptatrenoi, a synthetic polyprenol derivative, against Sendai virus infection in mice. *Vaccine* 1990;8:376–380.

248. Hill DA, Baron S, Chanock RM. Sensitivity of common respiratory viruses to in interferon inducer in human cells. *Lancet* 1969;2:187–188.

249. Stokes JR, Sorkness RL, Kaplan MR, et al. Attenuation of virus-induced airway dysfunction in rats treated with imiquimod. *Eur Respir J* 1998;11:324–329.

250. Fulton RN, Burge LJ, McCraken JS. Effect of recombinant DNA-derived bovine and human interferons on replication of bovine herpesvirus-1, parainfluenza-3, and respiratory syncytial virus. *Am J Vet Res* 1986;47:751–753.

251. Zhao H, De BP, Das T, Banerjee AK. Inhibition of human parainfluenza virus-3 replication by interferon and human MxA. *Virology* 1996;220:330–338.

252. Somani R, Evans MJ. Role of glucocorticoids in treating croup. *Can Fam Physician* 2001;47:733–735.

253. Connor E, PREVENT Study Group. Reduction of RSV hospitalization among premature infants and infants with bronchopulmonary dysplasia using respiratory syncytial virus immune globulin prophylaxis. *Pediatrics* 1997;99:93–99.

254. Siber GR, Leszcynski J, Pena-Cruz V, et al. Protective activity of a human respiratory syncytial virus immune globulin prepared from donors screened by microneutralization assay. *J Infect Dis* 1992:165:456–463.

255. Tashiro M, Homma H. Protection of mice from wild-type Sendai virus infection by a trypsin-resistant mutant, TR-2. *J Virol* 1985;53:228–234.

256. Carthew P, Riley J, Dinsdale O. Amelioration of established Sendai viral pneumonia in the nude mouse using a monoclonal antibody to the virus fusion protein. *Br J Exp Pathol* 1989;70:727–735.

257. Piga N, Kessler N, Layani MP, Aymard M. Correlation between the reactivity patterns of monoclonal antibodies to distinct antigenic sites on HN glycoprotein and their protective abilities in Sendai (6/94) virus infection. *Arch Virol* 1990;110:179–193.

258. Prince GA, Porter DD. Treatment of parainfluenza virus type 3 bronchiolitis and pneumonia in a cotton rat model using topical antibody and glucocorticosteroid. *J Infect Dis* 1996;173:598–608.

259. Chanock RM, McKintosh K. Parainfluenza viruses. In: Fields BN, ed. *Virology.* New York: Raven Press, 1985:1241.

260. Kingsbury DW. Paramyxoviruses. In: Nayak DP, eds. *The molecular biology of animal viruses.* New York: Marcel Decker, 1977:349–382.

261. Kingsbury DW. Orthomyxo- and Paramyxoviruses and their replication. In: Fields BN, ed. *Virology.* New York, Raven Press, 1985:1157.

262. Howe C, Morgan C, de Vaux St. et al. Morphogenesis of type 2 parainfluenza virus examined by light and electron microscopy. *J Virol* 1967;1:215–237.

263. Storey DG, Dimock K, Kang CY. Structural characterization of virion proteins and genomic RHA pf human parainfluenza virus 3. *J Virol* 1984;52:761–766.

264. Wechsler SL, Lambert DM, Galinski MS, et al. Human parainfluenza virus 3: purification and characterization of subviral components, viral proteins and viral RNA. *Virus Res* 1985;3:339–351.

265. Spriggs MK, Collins PL. Human parainfluenza virus type 3: messenger RNAs, polypeptide coding assignments, intergenic sequences, and genetic map. *J Virol* 1986;59:646–654.

266. Kolakofsky D, Pelet T, Garcin D, et al. Paramyxovirus RNA synthesis and the requirement for hexamer genome length: the rule of six revisited. *J Virol* 1998;72:891–899.

267. Sanchez A, Banerjee AK. Studies on human parainfluenza virus 3: characterization of the structural proteins and in vitro synthesized proteins coded by mRNAs isolated from infected cells. *Virology* 1985;143:45–54.

268. Jambou RC, Elango N, Venkatesan S. Proteins associated with human parainfluenza virus type 3. *J Virol* 1985,56:298–302.

269. Cowley JA, Barry RD. Characterization of human parainfluenza viruses. I. The structural proteins of influenza and parainfluenza viruses involving adsorption to erythrocytes. *J Gen Virol* 1983;64:2117–2125.

270. Yoshida T, Nakayama Y, Toyoda T, et al. The polypeptides of human parainfluenza 1 (HA-2) virus and their antigenic relationships to those of Sendai virus (HVJ). *Microbiol Immunol* 1985;29:577–582.

271. Komada H, Tsurudome M, Bando H, et al. Immunological response of monkeys infected intranasally with human parainfluenza virus type 4. *J Gen Virol* 1989;70:3487–3492.

272. Matsuoka Y, Curran J, Pelet T, et al. The P gene of human parainfluenza virus type 1 encodes P and C proteins but not a cysteine-rich V protein. *J Virol* 1991;65:3406–3410.

273. Ohgimoto S, Sando H, Kawano M, et al. Sequence analysis of P gene of human parainfluenza type 2 virus: P and cysteine-rich proteins are translated by two mRNAs that differ by two nontemplited G residues. *Virology* 1990;177:116–123.

274. Southern JA, Precious O, Randall RE. Two nonplated nucleotide additions are required to generate the P mRNA of parainfluenza virus type 2 since the RNA genome encodes protein V. *Virology* 1990;177:38:3–90.

275. Durbin AP, McAuliffe JM, Collins PL, Murphy BR. Mutations in the C, D, and V open reading frames of human parainfluenza virus type 3 attenuate replication in rodents and primates. *Virology* 1999;261:319–330.

276. Watanabe N, Kawano M, Tsurudome M, et al. Binding of the V proteins to the nucleocapsid proteins of human parainfluenza type 2 virus. *Scand Microbiol Immunol* 1996;185:89–94.

277. Nishio M, Tsurudome M, Ito M, et al. Isolation of monoclonal antibodies directed against the V protein of human parainfluenza virus type 2 and localization of the V protein in virus-infected cells. *Med Microbiol Immunol* 1999;188:79–82.

278. Lin GY, Lamb RA. The paramyxovirus simian virus 5 V protein slows progression of the cell cycle. *J Virol* 2000;74:9152–9166.

279. Nishio M, Tsurudome M, Ito M, et al. High resistance of human parainfluenza type 2 virus protein expressing cells to the antiviral and anti-cell proliferative activities of alpha/beta interferons: cystein-rich V-specific domain is required for high resistance to the interferons. *J Virol* 2001;75:9165–9176.

280. Kawano M, Kaito M, Kozuka Y, et al. Recovery of infectious human parainfluenza type 2 virus from cDNA clones and properties of the defective virus without V-specific cysteine-rich domain. *Virology* 2001;284:99–112.

281. Gotoh B, Komatsu T, Takeuchi K, Yokoo J. Paramyxovirus accessory proteins as interferon antagonists. *Microbiol Immunol* 2001;45:787–800.

282. Langedijk JP, Daus FJ, van Oirschot JT. Sequence and structure alignment of Paramyxoviridae attachment proteins and discovery of enzymatic activity for a morbillivirus hemagglutinin. *J Virol* 1997;71:6155–6167.

283. Curran J. A role for the Sendai virus P protein trimer in RNA synthesis. *J Virol* 1998;72:4274–4280.

284. Choppin PW, Richardson CD, Merz CD, et al. The functions and inhibition of the membrane glycoproteins of paramyxoviruses and myxoviruses and the role of the measles virus 11 protein in subacute sclerosing panencphalitis. *J Infect Dis* 1981;143:352–362.

285. Patterson S, Gross J, Oxford JS. The intracellular distribution of influenza virus matrix protein and nucleoprotein in infected cells and their relationship to haemagglutinin in the plasma membrane. *J Gen Virol* 1988;69:1859–1872.

286. Coronel EC, Takimoto T, Murti G, et al. Nucleocapsid incorporation into parainfluenza virus is regulated by specific interaction with matrix protein. *J Virol* 2001;75:1117–1123.

287. Parks GD, Lamb RA. Effective assembly and intracellular transport of mutant paramyxovirus hemagglutinin-neuraminidase proteins containing altered cytoplasmic domans. *J Virol* 1990;64:3605–3616.

288. Thompson SD, Laver WG, Murti KG, Portner A. Isolation of a biologically active soluble form of the hemagglutinin-neuraminidase protein of Sendai virus. *J Virol* 1983;62:4653–4660.

289. Suzuki T, Portner A, Scroggs RA, et al. Receptor specificities of human-respiroviruses. *J Virol* 2001;75:4604–4613.

290. Moscona A. Interaction of human parainfluenza virus type 3 with the host cell surface. *Pediatr Infect Dis J* 1997;16:917–924.

291. Ortmann D, Ohuchi M, Angliker H, et al. Proteolytic cleavage of wild type and mutants of the F protein of human parainfluenza virus type 3 by two subtilisin-like endoproteases, furin and Kex2. *J Virol* 1994;68:2772–2776.

292. Yao Q, Hu X, Compans RW. Association of the parainfluenza virus fusion and hemagglutinin-neuraminidase glycoproteins on cell surfaces. *J Virol* 1997;71:650–656.

293. Moscona A, Peluso RW. Fusion properties of cells persistently infected with human parainfluenza virus type 3: participation of hemagglutinin-neuraminidase in membrane fusion. *J Virol* 1991;65:2773–2777.

294. Ebata SN, Cote MJ, Kang CY, Dimock K. The fusion and hemagglutinin-neuraminidase glycoproteins or human parainfluenza virus 3 are both required for fusion. *Virology* 1991;183:437–441.

295. Tanabayashi K, Compans RW. Functional interaction of paramyxovirus glycoproteins: identification of a domain in Sendai virus HN which promotes cell fusion. *J Virol* 1996;70:6112–6118.

296. Okamoto K, Tsurudome M, Ohgimoto S, et al. An anti-fusion regulatory protein-1 monoclonal antibody suppresses human parainfluenza virus type 2-induced cell fusion. *J Gen Virol* 1997;78:83–89.

297. Yuasa T, Kawano M, Tabata N, et al. A cell fusion-inhibiting monoclonal antibody binds to the presumed stalk domain of the human parainfluenza type 2 virus hemagglutinin-neuraminidase protein. *Virology* 1995;206:1117–1125.

298. Zielinska-Jenczylik J. The influence of environment on parainfluenza 3 virus anc its replication in tissue cultures. *Arch Immunol Ther Exp* 1972;20:525–542.

299. Baxter BO, Couch RB, Greenberg SB, Kasel JA. Maintenance of viability and comparison of identification methods for influenza and other respiratory viruses of humans. *J Clin Microbiol* 1977;6:19–22.

300. Treuhaft MW, Soulup JM, Sullivan BJ. Practical recommendations for the detection of pediatric respiratory syncytial virus infections. *J Cl in Microbiol* 1985;22:270–273.

301. Hambling MH. Survival of the respiratory syncytial virus during storage under various conditions. *Br J Exp Pathol* 1964;45:647–655.

302. Parkinson AJ, Muchmore HG, Scott LV, Miles JA. Parainfluenza virus isolation enhancement utilizing a portable cell culture system in the field. *J Clin Microbiol* 1980;11:535–536.

303. Hurrell JM. Methods of storing viruses at low temperatures with particular reference to the Myxovirus group. *J Med Lab Tech* 1967;24:30–41.

304. Chanock RM. Parainfluenza viruses. In: Lennette EH, ed. *Diagnostic procedures for viral, rickettsial and chlamydial infections.* Washington, D.C.: American Public Health Association, 1979:611–633.

305. Hamparian VV, Hilleman MR, Ketler A. Contributions to characterization and classification of animal viruses. *Proc Soc Exp Biol Med* 1963;112:1040–1050.

306. Miller WS, Artenstein MS. Aerosol stability of three acute respiratory disease viruses. *Proc Soc Exp Med* 1967;125:222–227.

307. Andrewes CH, Bang FB, Burnet FM. A short description of the myxovirus group (Influenza and related items). *Virology* 1955;1:176–184.

308. Tsurudome M, Nishio M, Komada H, et al. Extensive antigenic diversity among human parainfluenza type 2 virus isolates and immunological relationships among pararnyxoviruses revealed by monoclonalantibodies. *Virology* 1989;171:38–48.

309. Randall RE, Young DF. Comparison between parainfluenza virus type 2 and simian virus S: monoclonal antibodies reveal major antigenic differences. *J Gen Virol* 1988;69:2051–2060.

310. Ray R, Compans RW. Monoclonal antibodies reveal extensive antigenic differences between the hemagglutinin-neuraminidase glycoproteins of human and bovine parainfluenza 3 viruses. *Virology* 1986;148:232–236.

311. Sarkkinen HK, Haionen PE, Salmi M. Type-specific detection of parainfluenza viruses by enzyme immuncassay and radioimmunoassay in nasopharyngeal specimens of parents wtih acute respiratory disease. *J Gen Virol* 1981;56:49–57.

312. Numazaki Y, Shigeta S, Yano N, et al. A variant of parainfluenza type 2 virus. *Proc Soc Exp Biol Med* 1968;127:992–996.

313. Ray R, Duncan J, Quinn R, Matsuoka Y. Distinct hemaggutinin and neuraminidase epitopes involved in antigenic variation of recent human parainfluenza virus type 2 isolates. *Virus Res* 1992;24:107–113.

314. Yurlova Tl, Sverkunova MV, Furaeva VA, et al. Studies of natural population variability of parainfluenza viruses during their epidemic circulation. *Acta Virol* 1991;25:64–70.

315. van Hyke Coelingh KL, Winter CC, Murphy BR. Antigenic variation in the hemagglutinin-neuraminidase protein of human parainfluenza type 3 virus. *Virology* 1985;143:569–582.

316. Komada H, Orstavik I, Ito Y, Nornby E. Strain variation in parainfluenza virus type 4. *J Gen Virol* 1990;71:1581–1583.

317. Komada H, Kusagawa S, Orvell C, et al. Antigenic diversity of human parainfluenza virus type 1 isolates and their immunological relationship with Sendai virus revealed by monoclonal antibodies. *J Gen Virol* 1992;73:875–884.

318. Iwata H, Tagaya M, Matsunoto K, et al. Aerosol vaccination with a sendai virus temperature sensitive mutant (HVJ-pB) derived from persistently infected cells. *J Infect Dis* 1990;162:402–407.

319. Profeta ML, Lief FS, Plotkin SA. Enzootic sendai infection in laboratory hamsters. *Am J Epidemiol* 1969;89:316–324.

320. Hsiung GD. Parainfluenza-5 virus. Infection of man and animal. *Prog Med Virol* 1972;14:241–274.

321. Miller RH, Pursell AR, Mitchell FE, Johnson KM. A newly discovered myxovirus (S.V.$_{41}$) isolated from cell cultures of cynomolqus monkey kidney. *Am J Hyg* 1964;80:365–376.

322. Paterson RG, Lamb RA, Moss B, Murphy BR. Comparison of the relative roles of the F anG Hh surface glycoproteins of the paramyxovirus simian virus 5 in inducing protective immunity. *J Virol* 1987;61:1972–1977.

323. Baumqartner W, Krakowka S, Gorham JR. Canine parainfluenza virus-induced encephalitis in ferrets. *J Comp Pathol* 1989;100:67–76.

324. Woods GT, Mansfield ME, Cmarik G, Sibinovic K. Effect of vaccination against bovine myxovirus parainfluenza-3 before weaning and at the time of weaning on the natural history of respiratory disease in beef calves. *Am Rev Respir Dis* 1967;95:278–284.

325. Lyon M, Leroux C, Greenland T, et al. Presence of a unique parainfluenza virus 3 strain identified by RT-PCR in visna-maedi virus infected sheep. *Vet Microbiol* 1997;51:95–104.

326. Afshar A. The occurence of antibodies to parainfluenza 3 virus in sera of farm animals and man in Iran. *Br Vet J* 1969;125:529–533.

327. Fenner F, Bacbmann PA, Gibbs EPJ, et al. In: Fenner F, ed. *Veterinary virology.* Orlando, Fla: Academic Press, 1987:492.

328. Alexander DJ, Manvell QJ, Collins MS, et al. Characterization of paramyxoviruses isolated from penguins in Antarctica and sub-Antarctica during 1976–1979. *Arch Virol* 1989;109:135–143.

329. Box PG, Furminger IG, Robertson WW. Immunising turkeys against Newcastle disease with oil emulsion killed vaccine. *Vet Rec* 1974;95:371–372.

330. Nelson CB, Pomeroy BS, Schrall K, et al. An outbreak of conjunctivitis due to newcastle disease virus (NDV) occurring in poultry workers. *Am J Pub Health* 1962;42:672.

331. Ben-Ishai Z, Naftali V, Avram A, Yatziv S. Human infection by a bovine strain of parainfluenza virus type 3. *J Med Virol* 1980;6:165–168.

332. Johnson DP, Green RH. Viremia during parainfluenza type 3 virus infection of hamsters. *Proc Soc Exp Med* 1973;144:745–748.

333. Mascoli CC, Gower TA, Capilupo FA, Metzger DP. Further studies in the neonatal ferret model of infection and immunity to and attenuation of human parainfluenza viruses. *Dev Biol Scand* 1976;33:384–390.

334. Ray R, Matsuoka R, Burnett TL, et al. Human parainfluenza virus induces a type-specific protective immune response. *J Infect Dis* 1990;162:746–749.

335. Buckner CK, Songsiridej V, Dick EC, Busse WW. In vivo and in vitro studies on the use of the guinea pig as a model for virus-provoked airway hyperreactivity. *Am Rev Respir Dis* 1985;132:305–310.

336. Takano T, Ohno M, Yamano T, Shimada M. Congenital hydrocephalus in suckling hamsters caused by transplacental infection with parainfluenza virus type 3. *Brain Dev* 1991;13:371–373.

337. Spriggs MK, Collins PL, Tierney E, et al. Immunization with vaccinia virus recombinants that express the surface glycoproteins of human parainrluenza virus type 3; (PIV3) protects pates monkeys against PIU3 infection. *J Virol* 1988;62:1233–1236.

338. Komada H, Tsurudome M, Ueda M, et al. Isolation and characterization of monoclonal antibodies to human parainfluenza virus type 4 and their use in revealing antigenic relation between subtypes 1A and 4B. *Virology* 1989;171:28–37.

339. Van Hyke Coelingh KL, Winter CC, et al. Antibody responses of humans and nonhuman primates to individual antigenic sites of the hemagglutinin-neuraminidase and fusion glycoproteins after primary infection or reinfection with parainfluenza type 3 virus. *J Virol* 1990;64:3833–3843.

340. Hawthorne JD, Lorenz D, Albrecht P. Infection of marmosets with parainfluenza virus types 1 and 3. *Infect Immun* 1982;37:1037–1041.

341. Sabina LR, Munro TW. Effects of trypsin on replication of parainfluenza-3 virus in HEp-2 cell cultures. *Can J Microbiol* 1969;15:577–582.

342. Luczak M, Korbecki M. Comparitive studies on susceptibility of established cell lines to parainfluenza 3 virus. *Acta Virol (Praha)* 1970;14:279–284.

343. Frank AL, Couch RB, Griffin CA, Baxter BD. Comparison of different tissue cultures for isolation and quantitation of influenza ana parainfluenza viruses. *J Clin Microbiol* 1973;10:2–6.

344. Shimokata K, Ito Y, Nishiyama Y, Kimura Y. Plaque formation by human-origin parainfluenza type 2 virus in established cell lines. *Arch Virol* 1981;67:355–360.

345. Numazaki Y, Oshima T, Ohmi A, et al. A microplate method for isolation of viruses from infants and children with acute respiratory infections. *Microbiol Immunol* 1987;31:1085–1095.

346. Moriucki H, Oshima T, Nishimura H, et al. Human malignant melanoma cell line (HMV-II) for isolation of influenza C and parainfluenza viruses. *J Clin Microbiol* 1990;28:1147–1150.

347. Morimoto Y, Doi Y, Itoh H. Effect of trypsin on reproduction of type 4 parainfluenza virus in vero cell cultures under fluid overlay. *Jpn J Med Sci Biol* 1970;23:1–11.

348. Shimokata K, Ito Y, Nishiyama Y, Kimura Y. Influence of trypsin on the infectivity and bolological properties of parainfluenza type 2 (croup-associated) virus in Vero cells. *J Gen Virol* 1980;48:407–410.

349. Bando H, Kawano M, Kondo K, et al. Growth properties and F protein cleavage site sequences of naturally occurring human parainfluenza type 2 viruses. *Virology* 1991;184:87–92.

350. Hierholzer JC, Binglam PG, Coombs RA, et al. Comparison of monoclonal antibody time-resolved fluoroimmunoassay with monoclonal antibody capture-biotinylated detector enzyme immunoassay for respiratory syncytial virus and parainfluenza virus antigen detection. *J Clin Microbiol* 1989;27:1243–1249.

351. Tyrrell DA, Bynoe ML. Studies on parainfluenza type 2 and 4 viruses obtained from patients with common colds. *BMJ* 1969;1:471–474.

352. Frank AL, Taber LH, Wells CR, et al. Patterns of shedding myxoviruses and paramyxoviruses in children. *J Infect Dis* 1981;144:433–441.

353. Gross PA, Green RH, Curnen MG. Persistent infection with parainfluenza type 3 virus in man. *Am Rev Resp Dis* 1973;108:894–898.

354. Muchoore HG, Parkinson AJ, Humphries JE, et al. Persistent parainfluenza virus shedding during isolation at the South Pole. *Nature* 1981;289:187–189.

355. Marks MI, Nagahama H, Eller JJ. Parainfluenza virus immunofluorescence. In vitro and clinical application of the direct method. *Pediatrics* 1971;48:73–78.

356. Frayha J, Castriciano S, Mahony J, Chenesky M. Nasopharyngeal swabs and nasopharyngeal aspirates equally effective for the diagnosis of viral respiratory disease in hospitalized children. *J Clin Microbiol* 1939;27:1387–1389.

357. Wong DT, Welliver RC, Riddlesberger KR, et al. Rapid diagnosis of parainfluenza virus infection in children. *J Clin Microbiol* 1982;16:164–167.

358. Doane FW, Anderson N, Chatiyanonda K, et al. Rapid laboratory diagnosis of paramyxovirus infections by electron microscopy. *Lancet* 1967;2:751–753.

359. Joncas J, Berthiaume L, Pavilanis V. The structure of the respiratory syncytial virus. *Virology* 1969;38:493–496.

360. Hietala J, Uhari M, Tuokko H. Antigen detection in the diagnosis of viral infections. *Scand J Infect Dis* 1988;20:595–599.

361. Sarikinen HK, Halonen PE, Salmi AA. Type-specific detection of parainfluenza viruses by enzynne-immunoassay and radioimmnunoassay in nasopharyngeai specimens of patients with acute respiratory disease. *J Gen Virol* 1981;56:49–57.

362. Sarkkinen HK, Halonen PE, Arstiia PP, Salmi AA. Detection of respiratory syncytial. parainfluenza type 2, and adenovirus antigens by radioimmunoassay and enzyme immunoassay on nasopharyngeal specimens from children with acute respiratory disease. *J Clin Microbiol* 1981;13:258–265.

363. Ray CG, Minnich LL. Efficiency of immunofluorescence for rapid detection of common respiratory viruses. *J Clin Microbiol* 1987;25:355–357.

364. Gardner PS, McQuillin J, MccGuckin R, Ditchburn RK. Observations on clinical and immunofluorescent diagnosis of parainfluenza virus infections. *BMJ* 1971;2:7–12.

365. Waner JL. Whitehurst NJ, Downs T, Graves OG. Production of monoclonal antibodies against parainfluenza 3 virus and their use in diagnosis by immunofluorescence. *J Clin Microbiol* 1985;22:535–538.

366. Grauballe PC, Johnsen llJ, Hornsleth A. Rapid diagnosis by immunofluorescence of viral infections associated with the croup syndrome in children. *Acta Pathol Microbiol Scand* 1974;82:41–47.

367. Puthavathana P, Wasi C, Kositanont U, et al. A hospital-based study of acute viral infections of the respiratory tract in Thai children, w.ith emphasis on laboratory diagnosis. *Rev Infect Dis* 1990;12:S988–S994.

368. Hallsworth PG, McDonald PJ. Rapid diagnosis of viral infections with fluorescent antisera. *Pathology* 1985;17:629–632.

369. Fedova DO, Pecenkova-Plachtova I, et al. Application of the fluorescent antibody method in the diagnosis of M. parainfluenzae. 3. Isolation and identification of *M. parainfluenzae* on monkey kidney tissue cultures and in nasal and nasopharyngeal swabs. *J Hyg Epidmiol Microbiol Immunol* 1971;15:82–92.

370. Fulton RE, Middleton PJ. Comparison of immunofluorescence and isolation techniques in the diagnosis of respiratory viral infections in children. *Infect Immun* 1974;l0:92–101.

371. Blanding JG, Hoshiko MG, Stutrnan HR. Routine viral culture for pediatric respiratory specimens submitted for direct immunofluorescence testing. *J Clin Microbiol* 1989;27:1438.

372. Stout C, Murphy MD, Lawrence S, Julian S. Evaluation of a monoclonal antibody pool for rapid diagnosis of respiratory viral infections. *J Clin Microbiol* 1989;27:448–452.

373. Leland DS. Direct detection for viral diagnosis. 13th Annual Clinical Virology Symposium, Clearwater Beach, Florida, April 27–30, 1997.

374. Hughes JH. Physical and chemical methods for enhancing rapid detection of viruses and other agents. *Clin Mirobiol Rev* 1993;6:150–175.

375. Maurer CC, Klepspies SL, Igel HJ. The rapid detection of five respiratory viruses in Hep-2 and primary rhesus monkey kidney shell vial cultures using pooled and individual monoclonal antibodies. Abstract M11, 9th Annual Clinical Virology Symposium.

376. Olsen MA, Shuck KM, Sambol SM, et al. Isolation of seven respiratory viruses in shell vials: a practical and highly sensitive method. *J Clin Microbiol* 1993;31:422–425.

377. Rabalais GP, Stout GG, Ladd KL, Cost KM. Rapid diagnosis of respiratory viral infections by using a shell vial assay and monoclonal antibody pool. *J Clin Microbiol* 1992;30:1505–1508.

378. Barenfanger J, Drake C, Mueller T, et al. R-mix cells are faster, at least as sensitive, and marginally more costly than conventional cell lines for the detection of respiratory viruses. *J Clin Virol* 2001;22(1):101–110.

379. Castriciano S, Smieja M, Chernesky M. Comparison of direct chemicon DFA, with or without diagnostic hybrids R-mix cell culture, to bartels' IFA, for the rapid detection of respiratory viruses. Eighteenth Annual Clinical Virology Symposium and Annual Meeting Pan American Society of Clinical Virology, Clearwater, Florida, April 28–May 1, 2002.

380. Chua R, Cruz R, Mazzulli T. The utilization of R-mix Freshcells® in tube culture for the detection of respiratory viruses. Eighteenth Annual Clinical Virology Symposium and Annual Meeting Pan American Society of Clinical Virology, Clearwater, Florida, April 28–May 1, 2002.

381. Chua R, Cruz R, Mazzulli T. Comparison of 24 hours versus 48 hours R-mixed Freshcell® shell vial methods for the detection of respiratory syncytial virus (RSV), influenza A (Influenza A), and influenza B (Influenza B) viruses. Eighteenth Annual Clinical Virology Symposium and Annual Meeting Pan American Society of Clinical Virology, Clearwater, Florida, April 28–May 1, 2002.

382. Kampert M, Carey RB. Comparison of R-Mix® shell vials to MRC-5 shell vials for isolation of respiratory viruses. Eighteenth Annual Clinical Virology Symposium and Annual Meeting Pan American Society of Clinical Virology, Clearwater, Florida, April 28–May 1, 2002

383. Langer J, Kelley C, Dunn J, Carroll K. Comparison of individual mink lung and A549 shell vials to the R-mix (Diagnostic Hybrids Inc) fresh cells™ shell vial for the rapid detection of respiratory viruses. Eighteenth Annual Clinical Virology Symposium and Annual Meeting Pan American Society of Clinical Virology, Clearwater, Florida, April 28–May 1, 2002.

384. Mitchell RJ. Rapid detection and identification of respiratory viruses from clinical specimens using R-mix shell vials. Eighteenth Annual Clinical Virology Symposium and Annual Meeting Pan American Society of Clinical Virology, Clearwater, Florida, April 28–May 1, 2002.

385. Ostermann D, Jestila CM, Saubolle MA. R-mix culture for detection of respiratory viral pathogens. Eighteenth Annual Clinical Virology Symposium and Annual Meeting Pan American Society of Clinical Virology, Clearwater, Florida, April 28–May 1, 2002.

386. Dunn J, Woolstenhulme D, Kelley C, Carroll KC. Evaluation of the impact of routine incorporation of R-mix (Diagnostic Hybrids Inc.) fresh cells™ into respiratory virus cultures over a two year period. Eighteenth Annual Clinical Virology Symposium and Annual Meeting Pan American Society of Clinical Virology, Clearwater, Florida, April 28–May 1, 2002.

387. Fan J, Henrickson KJ. Rapid diagnosis of human parainfluenza virus type I infection by quantitative reverse transcription-PCR-enzyme hybridization assay. *J Clin Microbiol* 1996;34:1914–1917.

388. Karron RA, Froehlich JL, Bobo L, et al. Rapid detection of parainfluenza virus type 3 RNA in respiratory specimens: use of reverse transcription-PCR-enzyme immunoassay. *J Clin Microbiol* 1994;32:484–488.

389. Eugene-Ruellan G, Freymuth F, Bahloul C, et al. Detection of respiratory syncytial virus A and B and parainfluenza 3 sequences in respiratory tracts of infants by a single PCR with primers targeted to the L-polymerase gene and differntial hybridization. *J Clin Microbiol* 1998;36:796–801.

390. Echevarria JE, Erdman DD, Meissner HC, Anderson L. Rapid molecular epidemiologic studies of human parainfluenza viruses based on detect sequencing of amplified DNA from a multiplex RT-PCR assay. *J Virol Meth* 2000;88:105–109.

391. Freymuth F, Vabret A, Galateau-Salle F, et al. Detection of respiratory syncytial virus, parainfluenzavirus 3, adenovirus and rhinovirus sequences in respiratory tract of infants by polymerase chain reaction and hybridization. *Clin Diag Virol* 1997;8:31–40.

392. Fan J, Henrickson KJ, Savatski LL. Rapid simultaneous diagnosis of infections with respiratory syncytial viruses A and B, influenza viruses A and B, and human parainfluenza virus types 1, 2, and 3 by multiplex quantitative reverse transcription-polymerase chain reaction-enzyme hybridization assay (Hexaplex). *Clin Infect Dis* 1998;26:397–402.

393. Henrickson KJ. Viral pneumonia in children. *Semin Pediatr Infect Dis* 1998;9:227–233.

394. Covalciuc KA, et al. Comparison of four clinical specimen types for detection of influenza A and B viruses by optical immunoassay (FLU OIA Test) and cell culture methods. *J Clin Microbiol* 1999;27:2971–2974.

395. Buckingham SC, Henrickson KJ, Fan J, et al. Comparison of respiratory syncytial virus (RSV) quantification by plaque assay and Hexaplex PCR. Presented at the 2nd International Symposium for influenza and other respiratory viruses, December 20, 1999.

396. Chonmaitree T, Henrickson KJ. Detection of respiratory viruses in the middle ear fluids of children with acute otitis media by multiple reverse transcription: polymerase chain reaction assay. *Pediatr Infect Dis J* 2000;19:258–260.

397. Barenfranger J, et al. Clinical and financial benefits of rapid detection of respiratory viruses: an outcomes study. *J Clin Microbiol* 2000;38:2824–2828.

398. Kehl SC, Henrickson KJ. Evaluation of the Hexaplex assay for detection of respiratory viruses in children. *J Clin Microbiol* 2001;39:1696–1701.

399. Hindiyeh M, Hillyard D, Carroll K. Evaluation of the Prodesse Hexaplex multiplex PCR assay for direct detection of seven respiratory viruses in clinical specimens. *Am J Clin Pathol* 2001;116:218–224.

400. Liolios L, Jenney A, Spelman D, et al. Comparison of a multiplex reverse transcription-PCR-enzyme hybridization assay with conventional viral culture and immunofluorescence techniques for the detection of seven viral respiratory pathogens. *J Clin Microbiol* 2001;39:2779–2783.

401. Henrickson KJ, Werch H, Rohwedder A. Comparison of Hexaplex (Multiplex-RT-PCR) and tissue culture (TC) to detect common respiratory viruses in children in Germany during 1999-2000 (PRIDE). Diagnostic Approaches for Infectious Diseases, IDSA, FDA, CDC, April 29–May 1, 2001, Orlando, Florida.

402. Kehl S, Henrickson KJ. Cost effective utilization of a multiplex RT-PCR assay (Hexaplex-R) for respiratory virus detection at a Children's Hospital. Diagnostic Approaches for Infectious Diseases, IDSA, FDA, CDC, April 29–May 1, 2001, Orlando, Florida.

403. Von Euler L, Kantor FS, Hsiung GD. Studies of parainfluenza viruses. 1. Clinical, pathological and virological observations. *Yale J Biol Med* 1963;35:523–533.

404. Herrmann EC, Hable KA. Experiences in laboratory diagnosis of parainfluenza viruses in routine medical practice. *Mayo Clin Proc* 1970;45:177–188.

405. Gardner SO. The isolation of parainfluenza 4 subtypes A and B in England and serological studies of their prevalence. *J Hyg (Camb)* 1969;67:545–550.

406. Rabalais GP, Stout GG, Ladd KL, Cost KM. Rapid diagnosis of respiratory viral infections by using a shell vial assay and monoclonal antibody pool. *J Clin Microbiol* 1992;30:1505–1508.

407. Chanock RM, Parrott RH, Cook KM, et al. Newly recognized myxoviruses from children with respiratory disease. *N Engl J Med* 1958;258:207–213.

408. Chanock RM, Parrott RH, Bell JA, et al. New viruses observed in children with respiratory diseases. *Public Health Rep* 1958;73:193–195.

409. Lennette EH, Jensen FW, Guenther RW, Magoffin RL. Serologic responses to parainfluenza viruses in patients with mumps virus infection. *J Lab Clin Med* 1963;61:780–788.

410. Julkunen I. Serological diagnosis of parainfluenza virus infections by enzyme immunoassay with special emphasis on purity of viral antigens. *J Med Virol* 1984;14:177–187.

411. Vuorinen T, Meurman O. Enzyme immunoassays for detection of IgG and IgM antibodies to parainfluenza types 1, 2, and 3. *J Virol Methods* 1989;23:63–70.

CHAPTER 243
Mumps Virus

Hillel Janai, Adriano Arguedas,
and Melvin I. Marks

HISTORY AND EPIDEMIOLOGY

Mumps, derived from the English verb "to mump," meaning "to grimace," obtained its name from the most frequently associated physical finding—painful parotid swelling. Until the current era of virologic and serologic diagnostic capabilities, mumps was called epidemic parotitis. Although the mumps virus is the most common pathogen causing parotitis, other viruses have been identified as a cause of parotid swelling (1).

A virus was first described as a cause of epidemic parotitis in 1934 (2). The authors of this elegant study showed that when saliva from patients with epidemic parotitis was inoculated into the parotid glands of monkeys, the monkeys developed parotitis. The parotid tissues were then excised, filtered, and inoculated into parotid glands of other monkeys. Identical parotid inflammation occurred.

As techniques of viral culture improved, the mumps virus was cultivated in embryonated chicken eggs. By using this technique to isolate the antigen, serologic and skin tests for delayed hypersensitivity to mumps virus were developed (3). Virus inactivation with formalin and vaccine production proved to be effective in disease prevention; however, the protective period was short and this preparation was never widely used as a vaccine (4). A live, attenuated mumps vaccine was developed by virus attenuation through passage in tissue culture and was licensed in 1967 (5).

Mumps is a contagious disease, and 90% of infections occur in the pediatric age group. Infectivity rates are difficult to evaluate because 30% to 40% of infections are subclinical. It is endemic throughout the year, with epidemics occurring among unvaccinated children and young adults, usually congregated in a kindergarten, school, or military camp.

CLINICAL MANIFESTATIONS AND COMPLICATIONS

Clinical manifestations of mumps in early childhood are mild, the most common being fever and painful parotid swelling. In older children and young adults, complications of mumps occur more often (6). (For details, see Chapter 141.)

VIRUS STRUCTURE

Mumps virus belongs to the Paramyxoviridae family. Other viruses in this family include human pathogens, parainfluenza and measles viruses, as well as animal pathogens, such as Newcastle disease virus and simian viruses. Viruses from this family are usually spherical and measure 150 to 200 nm in diameter. Pleomorphism may exist with variant viral dimensions ranging between 100 and 700 nm (7).

The genetic material of mumps virus is encoded in a single-stranded ribonucleic acid (RNA). After infecting a cell, messenger RNA (mRNA) is transcribed from the viral RNA by polymerase enzymes of viral origin. The core of the viral particle is helical and contains RNA incorporated with capsid proteins. This core is surrounded by an envelope composed of lipid and glycoprotein projections. The glycoproteins have two distinct properties. One has both hemagglutinin and neuraminidase activity, and the other, fusion and hemolysin properties (8).

Mumps virus produces inclusion bodies in the cytoplasm of infected human cells in vivo but, unlike other paramyxoviruses, the mumps virus also produces intranuclear inclusions in infected tissue culture cells. These inclusions are called nucleocapsid antigen or soluble antigen. Antibodies directed against this soluble antigen persist for only a short period, and their detection may represent a recent infection. Cross-reactions may occur due to the presence of similar binding sites to other paramyxoviruses (simian virus 5, parainfluenza virus, Newcastle disease virus).

Infected cells can be identified by the appearance of two surface glycoproteins on their cell membrane, the hemagglutinin and the hemolysin-fusion antigens. The hemagglutinin is responsible for the hemadsorption phenomenon (adherence of erythrocytes to mumps-infected cells) and is used in the hemagglutination inhibition test, which quantitates specific mumps antibodies. The hemolysin-fusion glycoprotein causes fusion of cell membranes and the creation of multinucleated giant cells both in vivo and in vitro. The hemolysin-fusion glycoprotein also has an important pathogenic role in central nervous system manifestations of mumps. Monoclonal antibodies against this particular antigen prevent mumps-induced encephalitis and brain necrosis in animal models injected with the mumps virus intracerebrally (9).

IMMUNE RESPONSE

Mumps virus induces host immune responses primarily by humoral antibody formation and secondary cellular T lymphocyte activation. The immune response does not differ between natural mumps infection and vaccine-induced immunity. Immunoglobulin G (IgG) is the major quantitative isotope followed by IgM, IgA, and IgE. IgG2 and IgG4 play almost no role in human immune response to mumps virus (10).

The dynamics of immunoglobulin production in the cerebrospinal fluid of children with mumps meningitis are of interest. In children with meningoencephalitis, specific mumps immunoglobulin levels are detected earlier and remain higher than in children with meningitis alone. There is no shift from IgM to IgG as observed in the humoral response (11). After infection, neutralizing antibodies maintain low but protective concentrations. Most persons have clinically apparent mumps only once in a lifetime. It is possible that subclinical mumps infections may occur after protective levels of neutralizing antibodies decline, thereby boosting immune response and protecting patients from clinical illness (12).

Although a striking feature of mumps is parotid gland swelling, clinical infection with mumps can occur in its absence. Moreover, even with the lack of meningeal findings, cerebrospinal pleocytosis may frequently be found (13).

Like other viruses, mumps virus activates lymphocytes. Studies in mice have shown that mumps virus induces production of helper T cells and killer cells, some of which have tumoricidal activity. Human studies in Japan have used mumps virus as immunotherapy in some types of advanced gynecologic cancers (14). Patients were sensitized subcutaneously with mumps virus and later injected locally or systemically with the virus. Clinical improvement and tumor regression were observed in the majority of patients. The T-cell response to mumps virus is regulated by human leukocyte antigen restriction elements (15).

TABLE 243.1.   Diagnostic Tests for Mumps Virus

Virus isolation
    Viral culture (urine, saliva, cerebrospinal fluid)
    Direct fluorescent antibody test (urine, saliva)
Serologic methods
    Complement fixation for soluble antigen
    Indirect fluorescent antibody test
    Enzyme-linked immunosorbent assay
Antibody capture enzyme immunoassay

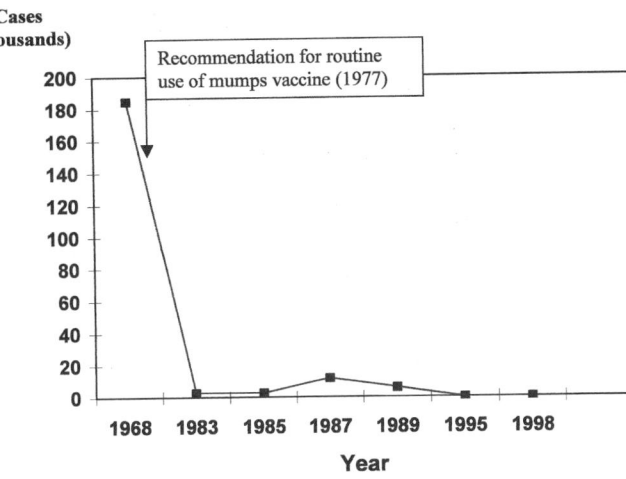

Figure 243.1. Mumps: reported cases, by year, in the United States, 1968 to 1998.

The fact that mumps infection may induce islet cell antibodies has led to hypotheses linking mumps virus to the cause of type I diabetes mellitus (16). Despite this, however, Schulz and colleagues (17) did not find any relationship between mumps infection and type I diabetes mellitus in a well-designed prospective study.

DIAGNOSIS

The diagnosis of mumps is usually made on clinical grounds. A child with the typical appearance of swollen parotid glands and fever and a negative history of mumps immunization does not usually require serodiagnosis. If required, however, additional diagnostic methods are available (Table 243.1).

Mumps virus can be isolated from clinical specimens of patients with mumps, with or without parotitis. Saliva, urine, and cerebrospinal fluid specimens can be cultivated on a variety of cell line cultures. Syncytium formation can be pathognomonic, but hemadsorption and indirect immunofluorescence are both more sensitive (18). Serologic tests for mumps virus have used different methods with variable sensitivity and specificity, mainly because of cross-reactivity with other paramyxovirus antigens. For example, complement fixation of V and S antigens may cross-react with parainfluenza and other viral antigens. The hemagglutination inhibition test has the same cross-reactivity problems. The viral neutralization test, although specific, is complex and time-consuming.

Current laboratory methods for determining infection with mumps virus include measurement of the serum IgG component using an enzyme-linked immunoabsorbent assay in both acute and convalescent serum samples. Techniques have become available that allow measurement of IgM by a variation of the enzyme-linked immunosorbent assay known as antibody capture. By using this method, the assay can be performed in 6 hours, yielding results that are both highly sensitive and highly specific (19,20) Also, polymerase chain reaction is available as a rapid method for detecting mumps virus within 48 hours (21).

PREVENTION

No effective anti-mumps virus therapy exists, and passive immunization attempts have failed. Primary prevention with live, attenuated mumps virus has proved to be effective. Although antibody levels are eight- to tenfold lower in postvaccination serum than in convalescent serum, neutralization of the clinical infection rate is high (22).

Mumps became a nationally reportable disease in the United States in 1968. As current immunization provides high, long-term protection, complications of mumps are now rarely encountered. In the United States between 1968 and 1998, a major

decrease in the annual number of cases has been observed; however, in 1986 and 1987, the reported cases of mumps more than doubled with the highest number of patients being among older school-age and college age youth who were born before the recommendations for routine vaccination were established (23,24). Since 1989, there has been a steady decline in reported cases of mumps from 5,712 cases at that time to 606 cases in 1998. This decrease in mumps observed in recent years is most likely the result of the implementation of the second dose scheme for measles as measles-mumps-rubella vaccination (25) (Fig. 243.1).

Questions about long-term efficacy of the vaccine have been raised. Cochi and colleagues (26) reviewed the data available on mumps vaccine since its introduction. Their survey pointed out that, after licensure, a decade elapsed before mumps vaccine was accepted as a routine immunization. Therefore, children born between 1967 and 1977 were not fully immunized, resulting in outbreaks within this high-risk group, especially in states that did not enforce vaccine administration before children entered school. Without enforcement of vaccine requirements, such epidemics may occur and may also affect part of the previously immunized population (in which vaccine efficacy ranges from 40% to 100%) (27–29).

Measles-mumps-rubella vaccine is commercially available, is safe and highly immunogenic, and provides protection. There are some fears of side effects because these vaccines contain animal and avian proteins with potential for allergic reactions, however, a new vaccine, prepared with only human tissue provides similar antibody response and safety and is now commercially available (28–30). (For more information, see Chapter 141.)

REFERENCES

1. Tolpin MD, Schauf V. Mumps virus. In: Belshe R, ed. *Textbook of human virology.* Littleton, MA: PSG Publishing, 1985:311–331.
2. Johnson CD, Goodpasture EW. An investigation of the etiology of mumps. *J Exp Med* 1934;59:1.
3. Enders JF. Mumps: techniques of laboratory diagnosis, tests for susceptibility, and experiments on specific prophylaxis. *J Pediatr* 1946;29:129.
4. Habel K. Vaccination of human beings against mumps: vaccine administration at start of epidemic. I. Incidence and severity of mumps in vaccinated and control groups. *Am J Hyg* 1951;54:295.
5. Hilleman MR, Buynak EB, Weibel RE, et al. Live, attenuated mumps-virus vaccine. *N Engl J Med* 1968;278:227.
6. Young NA. Chickenpox, measles and mumps. In: Remington JS, Klein JO, eds.

Infectious diseases of the fetus and newborn infant. Philadelphia: WB Saunders, 1976:521–586.

7. Choppin PW, Scheid A. The role of viral glycoproteins in adsorption, penetration, and pathogenicity of virus. *Rev Infect Dis* 1980;2:40.
8. Lerner AM. Guide to immunization against mumps. *J Infect Dis* 1970;122:116.
9. Love A, Rydbeck R, Utter G, et al. Monoclonal antibodies against the fusion protein are protective in necrotizing mumps meningoencephalitis. *J Virol* 1986;58:220.
10. Sarnesto A, Julkunen I, Makela O. Proportions of Ig classes and subclasses in mumps antibodies. *Scand J Immunol* 1985;22:345.
11. Statz A, Felgenhauer K. Differentiation of cerebrospinal immunoglobulins in mumps meningoencephalitis. *Monatsschr Kinderheilkd* 1987;135:265.
12. Chang TW. Recurrent viral infection (reinfection). *N Engl J Med* 1971;284:765.
13. Bank HO, Bang J. Involvement of the central nervous system in mumps. *Acta Med Scand* 1943;113:487.
14. Shimizu Y, Hasumi K, Okudaira Y, et al. Immunotherapy of advanced gynecologic cancer patients utilizing mumps virus. *Cancer Detect Prev* 1988;12:487.
15. Bruserud O, Paulsen G, Thorsby E. The mumps-specific T-cell response in healthy individuals and insulin-dependent diabetics: preferential restriction by DR4-associated elements. *Acta Pathol Microbiol Immunol Scand* 1087;95:173.
16. Hyoty H, Hiltunen M, Reunanen A, et al. Decline of mumps antibodies in type 1 (insulin-dependent) children and a plateau in the rising incidence of type 1 diabetes after introduction of the mumps-measles-rubella vaccine in Finland. *Diabetologia* 1993;12:1303.
17. Schulz B, Michaelis D, Hildmann W, et al. Islet cell surface antibodies (ICSA) in subjects with a previous mumps injection-A prospective study over a 4 year period. *Exp Clin Endocrinol* 1987;90:62.
18. Due-Nguyer H. Hemadsorption of mumps virus examined by light and electron microscopy. *J Virol* 1968;2:494, 1968.
19. Sakata H, Tsurudome M, Hishiyama M, et al. Enzyme-linked immunosorbent assay for mumps IgM antibody: comparison of IgM capture and indirect IgM assay. *J Virol Methods* 1985;12:303.
20. Glikmann G, Pedersen M, Mordhorst CH. Detection of specific immunoglobulin M to mumps virus in serum and cerebrospinal fluid samples from patients with acute mumps infection, using an antibody-capture enzyme immunoassay. *Acta Pathol Microbiol Immunol Scand* 1986;94:145.
21. Boriskin Y, Booth JC, Yamada A. Rapid detection of mumps virus by the polymerase chain reaction. *J Virol Methods* 1993;42:23.
22. Fedova D, Bruckova M, Plesnik V, et al. Detection of post vaccination mumps virus antibody by neutralization test, enzyme linked immunosorbent assay and sensitive hemagglutination inhibition test. *J Hyg Epidemiol Microbiol Immunol* 1987;31:409.
23. Wharton M, Cochi SL, Hutcheson RH, et al. A large outbreak of mumps in the postvaccine era. *J Infect Dis* 1988;158:1253.
24. Kaplan KM, Marder DC, Cochi SL, et al. Mumps in the workplace. Further evidence of the changing epidemiology of a childhood vaccine-preventable disease. *JAMA* 1988;260:1434.
25. CDC. Measles, Mumps and rubella—vaccine use and strategies for elimination of measles, rubella and congenital rubella syndrome and control of mumps: recommendations of the Advisory Committee on Immunization Practices (ACIP). *MMWR* 1998;47(RR-8):1–57.
26. Cochi SL, Preblud SR, Orenstein WA. Perspectives on the relative resurgence of mumps in the United States. *Am J Dis Child* 1988;142:499.
27. Fahlgren K. Two doses of MMR vaccine-Sufficient to eradicate measles, mumps and rubella? *Scand J Soc Med* 1988;16:129.
28. Forsey T. Mumps vaccines—current status [Editorial]. *J Med Microbiol* 1994;4:1.
29. Hersh BS, Fine PEM, Kent WK, et al. Mumps outbreak in a highly vaccinated population. *J Pediatr* 1991;119:187.
30. Just M, Berger R, Gluck R, et al. Evaluation of combined vaccine against measles-mumps-rubella produced on human diploid cells. *Dev Biol Scand* 1986;65:25.

CHAPTER 244
Rubeola (Measles) and Subacute Sclerosing Panencephalitis Virus

Gilbert M. Schiff

RUBEOLA

Measles virus causes a highly contagious, relatively distinct exanthematous disease featuring a prodrome of fever, cough, coryza, and conjunctivitis followed by an erythematous, maculopapular, confluent rash and a pathognomonic enanthema (Koplik spots). Because of its highly contagious nature and high morbidity, measles (rubeola) was recognized in early civilizations, although it was frequently confused with smallpox and other exanthematous diseases (1). Since the introduction of effective vaccines, serious complications involving the respiratory tract and central nervous system (CNS) now occur only rarely in developed countries, but they were common earlier and remain a major cause of mortality and morbidity in underdeveloped countries.

History

Rhazes, a tenth century Persian physician, first described measles as an entity distinct from smallpox (2) but it was not until the early 17th century that the distinction between the two diseases was relatively clear (3). John Hall was the first to describe measles in America, during a 1657 epidemic in Boston (4). The pathognomonic enanthema of measles was first reported by Koplik (5) in 1896, although Koplik spots were recognized about a century earlier. The extraordinary work and report of Panum (6) on an epidemic in the Faroe Islands defined the 14-day incubation period and lifetime immunity.

Measles was first transmitted to monkeys by Josias in 1898; Anderson and Goldberger (in 1911) and Blake and Trask (in 1921) demonstrated that monkeys could be infected with blood and nasopharyngeal secretions obtained from measles patients (7). Plotz in 1938, and Rake and Shaffer in 1942 reported the adaptation of measles virus to chick embryos, although reliable tissue culture methods did not become available until a decade later (3). In 1954, Enders and Peebles (8) reported isolating measles virus in human and rhesus monkey kidney tissue culture and the neutralization of the cytopathic effect by measles convalescent-phase serum. During the 1960s, the relationship between acute measles and the rare development of late progressive encephalitis (subacute sclerosing panencephalitis [SSPE]) was uncovered (9).

The further adaptation of measles virus to grow in chicken embryo tissue culture (10) led the way for the development of measles vaccines. Extensive trials of killed and attenuated (live) measles vaccines were conducted from 1958 to 1962. In 1963, both became available for general use, followed by the development and widespread use after 1965 of live, further attenuated measles vaccines. Since the Childhood Immunization Initiative and the Measles Elimination Program, which began in 1978, the incidence of measles in the United States has fallen dramatically. However, continued outbreaks of measles in the United States (11,12) demonstrate that elimination of measles remains a difficult goal, and various global strategies are being formulated (13).

Characteristics of the Pathogen

CLASSIFICATION

Measles virus is a member of the genus *Morbillivirus* in the family Paramyxoviridae. Included in this genus are canine distemper and rinderpest viruses, which share close immunologic relationships to measles (14). Morbilliviruses differ from other paramyxoviruses in that they lack detectable neuraminidase activity and interact with cellular receptors that are insensitive to neuraminidase treatment (15). Measles virus is a relatively large enveloped ribonucleic acid (RNA) virus with a spherical but pleomorphic shape. The diameter of the particle varies between 100 and 250 nm (mean, approximately 150 nm).

STRUCTURE

The measles virus is composed of an outer lipoprotein envelope surrounding a helical nucleocapsid (14). Six viral structural proteins and one nonstructural protein have been identified (16) (Fig. 244.1). The nucleocapsid is a coiled rod that contains the viral genome RNA. Approximately 5% of the nucleocapsid is RNA (molecular mass approximately 4.8 MDa). The outer envelope is 10- to 22-nm thick and contains the H (hemagglutinin) and F (fusion) factors, which are inserted into the lipid envelope as short surface projections or spikes, as well as the M (matrix) protein. The H and F proteins are glycosylated. The H protein is responsible for hemagglutination and mediates the adsorption of virus to the host cell. The H peplomers are formed by more than one and possibly three H molecules. The H and F proteins appear to function together for cell fusion of virus and host cell (17). The F protein is synthesized as a 55- to 60-kDa glycoprotein; the fusion activity is generated by cleavage into a nonglycosylated F_1 part and a glycosylated F_2 part. The M protein is nonglycosylated

and is associated with the inner lipid bilayer of the envelope. It appears to play a role in assembly of the virus.

The virus genome is linear, negative-sense RNA that is complexed with three viral proteins. Thus, the genome RNA must first be transcribed into message sense before production of virus-coded proteins. Sequence data are available for much of the genome. The linear order of genes is 3'-N-P/C-M-F-H-L-5', the same as for Sendai virus (15). The NP (nucleoprotein) is the major internal protein. It is phosphorylated and protects the viral RNA. The other internal virion components are the L, large protein, and the P, polymerase (phospho) protein. Both are believed to be part of the transcription complex. In addition to these six structural proteins, there is a nonstructural protein, C protein. Measles virions also contain an internal RNA-dependent RNA polymerase like other negative-sense RNA viruses (18).

BIOLOGIC AND BIOCHEMICAL PROPERTIES

Only a small fraction of virions produced in culture are infectious (14). Infectious virions are rapidly inactivated by heat, ultraviolet light, lipid solvents, and extremes of acidity and alkalinity (pH below 5 or above 10) (19). Their lability at room temperature is of major importance in the handling of vaccines. Measles virus suspensions that have been stabilized with protein can be stored at −70°C for years without significant loss of infectivity.

REPLICATION

Measles virus can infect a broad range of nucleated cells, although it is not easily isolated from infected patients (20). The human (membrane cofactor protein) CD46 and CD150 are major measles virus receptors that mediate binding and entry and determine viral tropism (21). Recovery of virus from infected persons occurs best with primary human and monkey kidney culture (20). Isolation of virus from patients with SSPE requires cocultivation of explant cultures of brain tissue with cells susceptible to measles virus, although the viruses recovered by this method are often defective replicating viruses.

Two distinct types of cytopathic effects occur in tissue culture (14). Syncytium formation, or giant cells, form when boundaries of adjoining cells are lost and nuclei aggregate to the center. Ten to 50 nuclei containing intranuclear inclusion bodies may be present. The second form of cytopathic effect is characterized by a change of individual polygonal-looking cells into a spindle or stellate form that is often refractile. The proportion of the various changes depends on the virus strain, passage conditions, and host cells. Replication in tissue culture proceeds through an attachment phase followed by the adsorption of virus and an eclipse phase of 6 to 12 hours. Measles antigen can first be detected at about 12 hours. Most virus remains cell associated. Persistent infection can also develop readily in cells that are usually lysed by infection (14). Giant cell formation can also occur during measles infection. Giant cells in lymphoid tissue are called Warthin-Finkeldey cells. Giant cells can also be formed by fusion of epithelial cells in the upper and lower respiratory tract, causing syncytium formation. These may be found in the nasal secretions.

Humans are the only natural host for measles virus, although primates can be infected by contact with measles patients. Infection of primates is usually subclinical, with the exception of the marmoset, which may develop severe symptoms. Laboratory strains of measles virus have been adapted for experimental studies in calves, lambs, dogs, ferrets, and rats but have been studied most extensively in hamsters and mice.

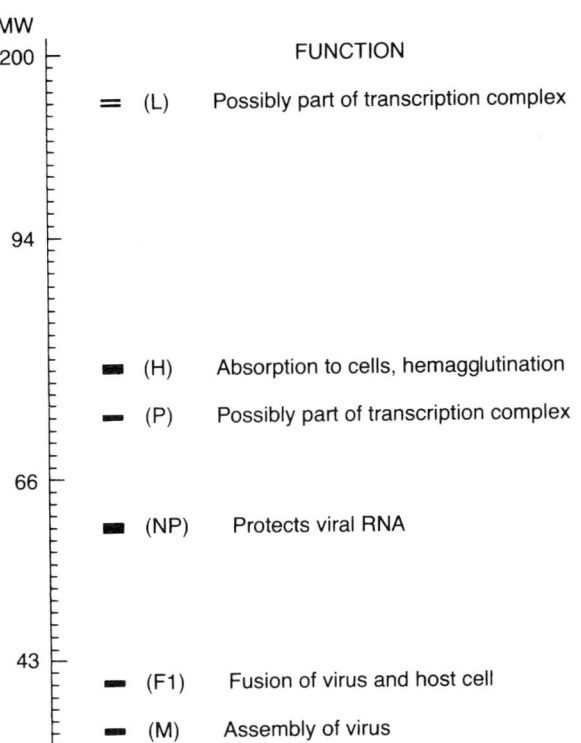

Figure 244.1. Schematic representation of sodium dodecyl sulfate-polyacrylamide gel electrophoresis pattern of measles virus proteins and their corresponding function. On the left are molecular weight standards (X10^{-3}).

ANTIGENIC CHARACTERISTICS

Although the measles virus is considered a monotypic, antigenically stable virus, nucleotide sequence analysis of the genes of the measles virus has identified distinct differences in the N, H, P, and M genes of the wild-type measles virus, and the establishment of distinct genetic groups (22). In contrast, the sequence of vaccine virus differed by less than 0.6%. Antigenic variations in the H and F proteins have also been demonstrated by use of monoclonal antibodies (14). Cross reactivity has been demonstrated with the three members of the *Morbillivirus* genus but not with other members of the Paramyxoviridae family (23). The F component of measles and canine distemper virus are highly conserved, whereas the M and NP, and possibly the P, components show moderate antigenic relationships. The H protein of measles appears to be more closely related to rinderpest than to canine distemper virus.

Epidemiology

Measles is highly communicable and is found worldwide (3). It appears that infection is spread predominately by the respiratory route through aerosolized droplets of respiratory secretions from ill patients (24). Spread from mild, atypical, or asymptomatic infections may exist.

During epidemics in densely vaccinated populations, mild cases of measles may be missed because they do not meet typical clinical criteria. Infected persons are most contagious during the catarrhal stage of illness, which is marked by extensive virus excretion in respiratory secretions. Patients should be considered contagious from 1 to 2 days before the onset of symptoms (3 to 5 days before the rash) to at least 7 days after the onset of symptoms or 4 days after the appearance of the rash. Patients with SSPE are not infectious.

The prevalence of measles is affected by population density and, in more recent years, by the availability of measles vaccine. In the temperate zones among unimmunized populations, measles usually occurs in winter-spring epidemics in 2- or 5-year cycles that last 3 or 4 months. In rural settings or among isolated communities, populations can reach adult life without having been exposed. When measles virus is introduced into these communities, the results can be devastating. A classic description of such an outbreak in 1846 in the Faroe Islands was reported by Panum (6).

In the prevaccine era, measles was a disease of children, the highest rate being among those 5 to 10 years of age (24). Between 1960 and 1964, about half of all measles patients were in this age group. In developing countries, measles generally occurs before age 5 years. Because of protection from maternal antibody, infection before the age of 6 months is, however, rare. In many developing countries, measles is the most important cause of death from age 1 through 5 years and accounts for between 1 and 2 million deaths per year worldwide (25). The frequency of measles is the same in males and females, although the complication rate may be higher among males (including the frequency of SSPE) (3,24). Measles susceptibility does not differ by race.

The introduction of measles vaccine has markedly altered the age incidence of measles. The prevaccine incidence of measles in those older than 10 years of age was less than 10%. In 1985, however, more than 60% of measles cases occurred in persons older than 10 years, and approximately half occurred in adolescents and young adults (3). More recently, outbreaks on college campuses account for a significant proportion of all reported cases (11,13). Two main patterns of outbreaks in the United States have been seen. Outbreaks have been detected in highly immunized populations who had received one dose of vaccine; other outbreaks occurred in unvaccinated children of ethnic or racial minorities (13,26). Nucleotide sequencing of the measles virus has led to the development of new tools to determine the epidemiology of measles, the surveillance of measles locally and globally, and the design and evaluation of measles control programs (27).

Pathogenesis

Infection occurs as a result of contact by nasopharyngeal or possibly conjunctival epithelial surfaces with measles-contaminated respiratory droplets (3,13). The virus initially spreads to regional lymphatics, followed by a primary viremia, replication in the regional and distant reticuloendothelial system and in the respiratory epithelium at the site of initial infection. A secondary viremia occurs on the fifth to seventh day after inoculation, which produces a more extensive and prolonged infection, that seeds virus to lymphatic cells throughout the body.

The characteristic feature of virus multiplication in lymphoid tissues is the formation of multinucleated giant cells similar to those seen in tissue culture (3,13). Warthin-Finkeldey giant cells are found in reticuloendothelial cells, including the adenoids, tonsils, Peyer patches, appendix, lymph nodes, spleen, and thymus. Giant cells are readily detected on respiratory and other epithelial surfaces (including Koplik spots).

The viral content of the blood and respiratory tract is greatest between the 11th and 14th days after inoculation. By the time prodromal symptoms appear, virus is widely disseminated in epithelial membranes, small blood vessels, lymphocytes, and in many cases the CNS as manifested by pleocytosis in the cerebrospinal fluid and/or electroencephalogram changes (28,29). Clinical encephalitis occurs in 0.5 to 1 in 1,000 measles cases. Studies indicate a direct role for the virus in the pathogenic process, although immune mechanisms are probably involved (30). Specific interactions between the measles virus and cellular receptors have been shown to determine the type of CNS involvement (21).

A distinct clinical syndrome of measles (atypical measles) has been observed in some persons who were previously immunized with inactivated measles vaccine (see Measles, Chapter 137). Although the pathogenic mechanisms responsible for this syndrome are still unclear, patients with atypical measles lack antibody to the F protein (probably because the antigenic properties of this protein were destroyed by formalin inactivity) and have exaggerated or altered cellular responses to measles antigens with a predominance of Th1-type response (3). Thus, the infecting virus replicated and spread, initiating pathologic immune reactions of the Arthus type.

Immune Response

Measles virus infection induces both humoral and cell-mediated immunity and provides lifelong immunity. Primary infection initially induces a humoral immunoglobulin M response that is short-lived and then an immunoglobulin G response that persists for life. A local immunoglobulin A response also occurs in nasal secretions. Neutralizing antibody and hemagglutination inhibitory antibody appear in serum about the 14th day and peak 4 to 6 weeks after either natural infection or immunization. Complement-fixing antibody appears slightly later than hemagglutination inhibitory antibody.

Cell-mediated immune responses appear to be especially important in limiting the initial infection. Thus, persons with defects in cell-mediated immunity seem susceptible to fatal disseminated infections, whereas agammaglobulinemic patients can recover from their infections (30). The specificities of cellular immune responses are poorly understood. After infection, a lymphoproliferative response to measles can be demonstrated (31). T-cell clones of both CD4$^+$ class II-restricted helper cytotoxic T cells and CD8$^+$ class I-restricted cytotoxic T cells have been established from healthy seropositive adults (32), although cytotoxic T cells appear to be primarily restricted to class II (33). Clones specific for the H, F, M, and NP proteins have been demonstrated (32,33). Increased levels of interferon-γ are seen during the rash of measles, but as the rash subsides, interleukin-4 levels increase and remain elevated for weeks, indicating a predominant Th2-type response (25,30). It has been suggested that measles infection initially produces a CD8$^+$ T-cell response that decreases virus replication, followed by a Th2-type CD4$^+$ T-cell response that is required for optimal antibody production (34).

Measles infection also induces a number of immune dysfunctions. Leukopenia is readily observed after infection and can also be seen after vaccination. Numbers of both neutrophils and lymphocytes are reduced, including T, B, and null cells, although the ratio between helper and suppressor cytotoxic T cells appears to be unchanged. Delayed hypersensitivity responses are also suppressed after both natural infection and measles vaccination. This includes skin test reactivity to common antigens and measured blastogenic responses to mitogens and specific antigens *in vitro*. Further natural killer cell activity and immunoglobulin synthesis of B cells are also impaired. It is still unclear, however, what the basic mechanisms of inhibition are. Monocytes are also affected during measles, and levels of tumor necrosis factor-α are decreased (34). Deficiencies of tumor necrosis factor-α could contribute to a decrease in lymphoproliferative or other cell-related responses. Similarly, increased levels of interleukin-4 found in measles-infected patients could down-regulate macrophage-activated lymphoproliferative and delayed-type hypersensitivity responses (34). During an outbreak of measles in Gambia, interleukin-12 production by peripheral blood monocytes was significantly suppressed in patients, and may be the mechanism responsible for the prolonged cell-mediated immune suppression found in measles infection (35).

Clinical Manifestations

After an incubation period of 10 to 14 days and a prodromal stage characterized by cough, coryza, conjunctivitis, and fever, the typical rash appears (3). The pathognomonic Koplik spots can be seen before the rash as 1- to 3-mm pale bluish white spots on an erythematous background on the lateral buccal mucosa. The characteristic macular or maculopapular rash first appears on the forehead and behind the ears and then spreads over the face, neck, trunk, and limbs within 24 to 48 hours.

Respiratory tract involvement is common after measles infection. Manifestations include laryngitis, tracheobronchitis, bronchiolitis, and pneumonia. Secondary bacterial pneumonia and otitis media, caused by typical respiratory pathogens, are not uncommon. Other complications, including cardiac, acute neurologic involvement, and acute renal failure may be seen (36).

The diagnosis of measles in an epidemic setting can usually be made by history and physical findings, although as the number of physicians trained who have not regularly seen measles increases and the number of epidemics decreases, laboratory confirmation becomes more important. Although virus isolation and identification of measles antigens in nasopharyngeal secretions are possible, laboratory confirmation is usually accomplished by serologic determination of an elevation of measles antibody titer (see Chapter 137).

SUBACUTE SCLEROSING PANENCEPHALITIS

SSPE is a rare chronic degenerative neurologic disease of children and adolescents produced by persistent measles virus infection of the CNS. Viral inclusions, measles virus antigens, and a measles-like virus have been found and cultivated from patient's brain tissue (3).

Pathogenesis and Pathology

The seeding of the CNS with measles virus probably occurs during natural infection. Half to one third of children who acquire measles infections naturally have CSF pleocytosis and transient electroencephalographic changes (37), and disease is more severe in younger children. Neither infectious virus nor viral particles are detectable within the CNS, but viral nucleoprotein structures are seen as inclusion bodies by electron microscopy. This is accompanied by a strong inflammatory response. When SSPE first appears, measles virus ribonucleocapsids have begun to spread to the entire CNS without formation of viral particles, despite humoral and cellular immune responses.

The inability of SSPE virus (measles virus that is recovered from SSPE patients) to produce infectious virus was initially attributed to the absence of the M protein. Subsequent studies have shown transcriptional and translational changes that affect the expression, stability, and formation of the H, F, and especially M genes. Other studies have shown that several measles genes are affected by mutation (38–40). The M gene is most affected, but deletion in the cytoplasmic domain of the F protein may also be important in the altered growth properties of the virus. It is still unclear how SSPE virus can spread throughout the CNS without formation of infectious viral particles in the presence of a strong immune response. It is also unclear whether the pathologic changes are due to virus-mediated cell destruction or to immune or autoimmune responses.

In the assessment of the SSPE pathophysiologic process, it is important to recognize the dynamic nature of this disease; inflammation leads to necrosis and destruction, then to reparative or gliotic changes, and these dynamic processes move in a rostro-caudad direction (41).

Epidemiology

The incidence of SSPE is estimated to be between 0.6 and 2.2 cases for every 100,000 cases of measles (3,24). The risk of SSPE is greater for children who acquire the disease at an early age; half of SSPE patients have a history for measles infection before age 2 years and three fourths before age 4 years. Males outnumber females by 2 to 1. The lack of any consistent association with human leukocyte antigens suggests that variability in disease occurrence by ethnic group probably does not reflect genetic predisposition to the disease. Use of measles vaccine has resulted in a marked decline in SSPE cases.

Clinical Symptoms

The initial clinical manifestations of SSPE typically appear 6 to 8 years after measles infection. The onset of disease (stage 1) is insidious, the first symptoms being progressive behavioral and intellectual deterioration. Stage 2 disease appears with the onset of myoclonic spasms that are characteristically repetitive with rapid onset and a delayed relaxation phase. Ocular abnormalities, ataxia, dyskinesia, focal neurologic deficits, and visual and speech impairment are noted during this stage. Progression leads to stage 3 disease, with stupor, dementia, mutism, coma, and decerebrate rigidity. Patients with stage 4 disease show diminished muscle tone, central blindness, and decorticate rigidity and have difficulty chewing, and swallowing. At this advanced stage, unexplained episodes of hyperthermia and profuse diaphoresis are seen and myoclonus may disappear. Deterioration continues, and the majority of patients die in 1 to 3 years (37).

Laboratory Diagnosis

The diagnosis of SSPE is based on a combination of clinical and laboratory factors, including the electroencephalogram and measles antibody titers. An electroencephalogram with typical burst-suppression pattern-paroxysmal complexes of two to three per second synchronous spike wave discharges with interim suppression of electrical activity occurring at 5- to 8-second intervals is diagnostic of SSPE. This pattern is characteristic of stage 2 disease before the onset of dementia, and it deteriorates in later stages. Patients have unusually high serum and CSF measles antibody titers. The CSF commonly shows no abnormalities of pressure cell count, total protein, or glucose level but does contain abnormal oligoclonal immunoglobulin G bands (42). This oligoclonal immunoglobulin G is antibody directed against measles antigens and is present in CSF/serum ratios that indicate intrathecal measles antibody synthesis usually not found in acute infection. Computed tomography and magnetic resonance imaging can be used to confirm the clinical picture. As the disease progresses, the computed tomographic scan is more predictive, showing enlarging ventricles and widened sulci with multi-focal low-density lesions probably indicating cerebral atrophy with areas of demyelination and encephalitis (43).

Treatment

No specific treatment is of proven benefit. The rarity of the disease makes it difficult to perform randomized prospective controlled studies although many agents have been evaluated (3,44). Palliative treatments of importance include anticonvulsants, nutritional supplements antibiotics when needed, physical therapy, and mental and behavioral control therapies.

REFERENCES

1. Babbott FL Jr, Gordon JE. Modern measles. *Am J Med Sci* 1954;228:334.
2. Black FL. Measles. In: Evans AS, ed. *Viral infections of humans: epidemiology and control.* New York: Plenum Publishing, 1976:297–316.
3. Cherry JD. Measles. In: Feigin RD, Cherry JR, eds. *Textbook of pediatric infectious diseases,* 4th ed. Philadelphia: WB Saunders, 1998:2054–2074.
4. Caulfield E. Early measles epidemics in America. *Yale J Biol Med* 1943;15:531.
5. Koplik H. The diagnosis of the invasion of measles from a study of the exanthema as it appears in the buccal mucous membrane. *Arch Pediatr* 1896;13:918.
6. Panum PL. Observations made during the epidemic of measles on the Faroe Islands in the year 1846. *Med Classics* 1039;3:829.
7. Measles (rubeola). In: Krugman S, Katz SL, Gershon AA, et al., eds. *Infectious diseases of children,* 9th ed. St. Louis: CV Mosby, 1992:223–245.
8. Enders JF, Peebles TC. Propagation in tissue cultures of cytopathogenic agents from patients with measles. *Proc Soc Exp Biol Med* 1954;86:277.
9. Sever JL, Zenman W, eds. Proceedings of symposium on measles virus and subacute sclerosing panencephalitis. *Neurology* 1968;18:1.
10. Katz SL, Milovanovic MV, Enders JF. Propagation of measles virus in cultures of chick embryo cells. *Proc Soc Exp Biol Med* 1958;97:23.
11. Markowitz LE, Preblud SR, Orenstein WA, et al. Patterns of transmission in measles outbreaks in the United States 1985–1986. *N Engl J Med* 1989;320:75.
12. Centers for Disease Control. Measles-Los Angeles County, California, 1989. *MMWR* 1989;38:49.
13. Redd SC, Markowitz LE, Katz SL. Measles vaccine. In: Plotkin SA, Orenstein WA, eds. *Vaccines,* 3rd ed. Philadelphia: WB Saunders, 1999:222–266.
14. Norrby E. Measles virus. In: Fields BN, Knipe DM, eds. *Fields virology,* 2nd ed. New York: Raven Press, 1990:1013–1044.
15. Barrett T. The molecular biology of the morbillivirus (measles) group. *Biochem Soc Symp* 1987;53:25.
16. Tyrrell DLJ, Norrby E. Structural polypeptides of measles virus. *J Gen Virol* 1978;39:219.
17. Wild TF, Malvoisin E, Buckland R. Measles virus: Both the haemagglutinin and fusion glycoproteins are required for fusion. *J Gen Virol* 1991;72:439.
18. Seifried AS, Albrecht P, Milstien JB. Characterization of an RNA dependent RNA polymerase activity associated with measles virus. *J Virol* 1978;25:781.
19. Musser SJ, Underwood GE. Studies on measles virus. II. Physical properties and inactivation studies of measles virus. *J Immunol* 1960;85:292.
20. Fuccillo DA, Sever JL. Measles virus. In: Schmidt NJ, Emmons RW, eds. *Diagnostic procedures for viral rickettsial and chlamydial infections,* 6th ed. Washington, DC: American Public Health Association, 1989:713–730.
21. Schneider-Schaulies J, ter Meulen V, Schneider-Schaulies S. Measles virus interactions with cellular receptors: Consequences for viral pathogenesis. *J NeuroVirol* 2001;7:391–399.
22. Bellini WJ, Rota JS, Rota PA. Virology of measles virus. *J Infect Dis* 1994;170(Suppl):S15.
23. Sheshberadaran H, Norrby E, McCullough KC, et al. The antigenic relationship between measles, canine distemper and rinderpest viruses studied with monoclonal antibodies. *J Gen Virol* 1986;67:1381.
24. Oxman MN. Measles. In: Richman DD, Whitley RJ, Hayden FG, eds. *Clinical virology.* New York: Churchill Livingston, 1997:821–861.
25. Li H, Hickman CJ, Helfand RF, et al. Induction of cytokine mRNA in peripheral blood mononuclear cells of infants after the first dose of measles vaccine. *Vaccine* 2001;19:4896–4900.
26. Gustafson TL, Brunell PA, Lievens AW, et al. Measles outbreak in a "fully immunized" secondary school population. *N Engl J Med* 1987;316:771.
27. Bellini WJ, Rota PA. Genetic diversity of wild-type measles viruses: Implications for global measles elimination programs. *Emerging Infect Dis* 1998;4:29–35.
28. Ojala A. On changes in the cerebrospinal fluid during measles. *Ann Med Fenn* 1947;36:321.
29. Gibbs FA, Gibbs EL, Carpenter PR, et al. Electroencephalographic abnormality in "uncomplicated" childhood diseases. *JAMA* 1959;171:1050.
30. Griffin DE. Immune responses during measles virus infection. *Curr Top Microbiol Immunol* 1995;191:117.
31. Greenstein JI, McFarland HF. Response of human lymphocytes to measles virus after natural infection. *Infect Immun* 1983;40:198.
32. van Binnendijk RS, Poelen MCM, deVries P. Measles virus specific human T cell clones. *J Immunol* 1989;142:2847.
33. Jacobson S, Sekaly RP, Jacobson CL, et al. HLA class II restricted presentation of cytoplasmic measles virus antigen to cytotoxic T cells. *J Virol* 1989;63:1756.
34. Griffin DE, Ward BJ, Esolen LM. Pathogenesis of measles virus infection: an hypothesis for altered immune responses. *J Infect Dis* 1994;170:524.
35. Atabani SF, Byrnes AA, Jaye A, et al. Natural measles causes prolonged suppression of interleukin-12 production. *J Infect Dis* 2001;184:1–9.
36. Wairagkar NS, Gandhi BV, Katrak SM, et al. Acute renal failure with neurological involvement in adults associated with measles virus isolation. *Lancet* 1999;354:992–995.
37. Groves MC. Subacute sclerosing panencephalitis. *Neurol Clin* 1984;2:267.
38. Hirano A, Ayata M, Wang AH, Wong TO. Functional analysis of matrix proteins expressed from cloned genes of measles virus variants that cause subacute sclerosing panencephalitis reveals a common defect in nucleocapsid binding. *J Virol* 1993;67:1848.
39. Schmid A, Spielhofer P, Cattaneo R, et al. Subacute sclerosing panencephalitis is typically characterized by alterations in the fusion protein cytoplasmic domain of the persisting measles virus. *Virology* 1992;188:910.
40. Billeter MA, Cattaneo R, Spielhofer P, et al. Generation and properties of measles virus mutations typically associated with subacute sclerosing panencephalitis. *Ann NY Acad Sci* 1994;724:367.
41. Dyken PR. Subacute sclerosing panencephalitis. *Neurol Clin* 1985;3:179.
42. Mehta PD, Patrick BA, Thormar H. Identification of virus-specific oligoclonal bands in subacute sclerosing panencephalitis by immunofixation after isoelectric focusing and peroxidase staining. *J Clin Microbiol* 1982;16:985.
43. Bohlega S, al-Kawi MZ. Subacute sclerosing panencephalitis. Imaging and clinical correlation. *J Neuroimaging* 1994;4:71.
44. Taylor WJ, DuPont RH, Dyken PR. Treatment of subacute sclerosing panencephalitis. *Drug Intell Clin Pharmacol* 1984;18:375.

CHAPTER 245
Hantaviruses

Frederick Koster and Brian Hjelle

Human Hantavirus infections cause two distinct syndromes. Acute infection with the Eurasian Hantaviruses causes the hemorrhagic fever renal syndrome (HFRS) (1–3), and acute infection with the North and South American hantaviruses causes the hantavirus pulmonary syndrome (HPS; also called hantavirus cardiopulmonary syndrome, or HCPS) (4–7). In North America one hantavirus, Sin Nombre virus, causes the vast majority of HCPS (Table 245.1), whereas in South America a greater diversity of hantaviruses cause HCPS with a wider diversity of manifestations (8–12). HCPS was recognized first in a cluster of cases that occurred in the Four Corners region of the southwestern United States in the spring and summer of 1993 (13). Prominent disease characteristics included rapidly progressive respiratory insufficiency due to noncardiogenic pulmonary edema, and cardiogenic shock (4,14), representing a new syndrome with a mortality rate initially exceeding 50%.

CHARACTERISTICS OF THE PATHOGEN

Hantavirus is a genus of enveloped ribonucleic acid (RNA) viruses in the family Bunyaviridae (15). The genus includes the pathogenic Hantaan (HTN), Seoul (SEO), Puumala (PUU), Dobrava/Belgrade (DOB), Andes (AND), Laguna Negra (LN), Choclo (CHO), and Sin Nombre (SN) viruses. There is a larger number of species that are either less well characterized agents of human infection or known only from their rodent reservoirs. Hantavirus virions consist of an RNA nucleocapsid surrounded by an outer lipid envelope (16–19). The RNA genome includes three segments called L (large), M (middle), and S (short). The nucleocapsid is comprised of a complex of nucleocapsid (N) protein and the viral RNA segments. The lipid envelope contains two glycoproteins (G1 and G2) encoded by the medium segment. The long segment encodes the viral RNA-dependent RNA polymerase.

Hantaviruses normally infect rodents, and human infections result from incidental rodent-to-human transmission. Each *hantavirus* species normally infects a single rodent species, although "spillover" infections of numerous other rodent species are recognized. The prototypic hantavirus, HTN, is associated with the Asian striped field mouse (*Apodemus agrarius*) and is the etiologic agent of Korean hemorrhagic fever in humans (20). SEO infects the urban rat (*Rattus norvegicus*) and causes a human disease that is similar to Korean hemorrhagic fever (21). SEO, like its rodent host, is cosmopolitan and infects rats in some coastal cities of the United States (22). DOB causes severe HFRS in Europe, primarily in the Balkans, and is enzootic among the yellow-necked field mouse *Apodemus flavicolis* (23). PUU, which is enzootic among bank voles (*Clethrionomys glareolus*) in northern Europe, causes a relatively mild form of hemorrhagic fever called nephropathia epidemica (24–28). The diseases caused by HTN, SEO, and PUU share many features and are now known collectively as HFRS.

SNV, the first identified agent of HCPS, infects the deer mouse (*Peromyscus maniculatus*) (5,29–31). *P. maniculatus*, a member subfamily Sigmodontinae, family Muridae, is distributed throughout most of North America. SNV has been implicated in the large majority of cases of HCPS in North America for which the viral

etiology has been ascertained. Small numbers of cases of HCPS acquired in the eastern United States were caused by unique hantaviruses of other sigmodontine rodent species, including the white-footed mouse *Peromyscus leucopus* (New York virus) (32,33) and the cotton rat *Sigmodon hispidus* (Black Creek Canal virus) (34). Three cases of HCPS that occurred in Louisiana and eastern Texas were caused by a unique hantavirus (Bayou virus), which is carried by the rice rat *Oryzomys palustris* (35–37). SNV, New York virus, Black Creek Canal virus, Bayou virus, Choclo virus, Andes virus and Laguna Negra constitute a monophyletic genetic lineage that includes all of the known North and South American agents of HCPS (8). These viruses, which are all associated with sigmodontine rodents, are most closely related to one another, followed by Prospect Hill virus (PHV) and PUU, and are more distantly related to SEO and HTN.

Nucleotide sequence analysis of SNV complementary deoxyribonucleic acids (DNAs) showed that SNV was a unique hantavirus (30,31). Each of the three SNV genomic segments was diverged by a similar extent from the homologous genomic segments of other hantaviruses. Genetic analysis of SNV complementary DNA clones from throughout the western United States and Canada indicated that although nucleotide sequence variations existed regionally, SNV amino acid sequences were highly conserved (5,38). The phylogenetic relatedness of different hantaviruses parallels the phylogenetic relatedness of their rodent hosts, suggesting that the hantaviruses are coevolving with their hosts (39); this holds true for SNV and its rodent host *P. maniculatus*. Therefore, there is no evidence that the 1993 outbreak in Four Corners resulted from the sudden emergence of a new human pathogen through mutation or gene segment reassortment. Indeed, SNV infections among *P. maniculatus* and HCPS cases in humans that occurred decades before the 1993 HCPS outbreak have been documented (40,41).

EPIDEMIOLOGY OF HEMORRHAGIC FEVER RENAL SYNDROME AND HANTAVIRUS CARDIOPULMONARY SYNDROME

Most human hantavirus infections appear to result from exposure to wild rodents or their habitats (20,22,29,38). Rodents develop chronic hantavirus infections that do not appear to result in tissue damage or disease (42–46). Experimental infection models have verified the suggestion of field experiments that infection of rodents is persistent despite the presence of a strong immune response (42–46). Rodent urine and feces contain infectious virus, and humans may acquire infection through inhaling airborne particles of rodent excreta that contain viable virus. Studies with Hantaan virus suggest that virus may remain infectious in urine for at least several days (47). Indoor exposures are nearly always identifiable when sought, and outdoor exposures appear to be very uncommon (48). The most compelling evidence for airborne transmission is found in experimental rodent colonies; in research laboratories a 10-minute exposure without direct contact to caged infected rodents resulted in human infection (49–51). Transmission may also occur by rodent bite, although it is difficult to decisively distinguish exposure by bite from more conventional exposures through the air (52). Unlike other *Bunyaviridae* members, no arthropod vector has been implicated in the transmission of hantaviruses. However this possibility deserves further investigation, as hantaviruses have been identified with polymerase chain reaction (PCR) in trombiculid mites (chiggers) in eastern Texas (53).

HTN virus infects more than 100,000 people in China each year, with a case-fatality ratio of approximately 1% to 5%. The frequency of HTN infection is highest among workers in certain

TABLE 245.1. The Hantaviruses

Hantavirus strain	Host rodent (species)	Geographic range	Syndrome in humans	Mortality rate
Hantaan	Striped field mouse (*Apodemus agrarius*)	Eastern, central Asia	HFRS	1%–5%
Seoul	Common rat (*Rattus norvegicus*)	Urban worldwide	HFRS	1%–2%
Puumala	Bank vole (*Clethrionomys glareolus*)	Northern, central Europe	Nephropathia epidemica	0.1%–1.0%
Dobrava	Yellow-necked field mouse (*Apodemus falvicollis*)	Balkans	HFRS	15%
Sin Nombre	Deer mouse (*Peromyscus maniculatus*)	Western North America	HCPS	35%–45%
New York	White-footed mouse (*Peromyscus leucopus*)	Eastern North America	HCPS	3 cases, 1 fatal
Black Creek Canal	Cotton rat (*Sigmodon hispidus*)	Florida	HCPS with hemorrhage	1 case
Bayou	Rice rat (*Oryzomys palustris*)	Louisiana	HCPS with hemorrhage	5 cases, 1 fatal
Andes	Long-tailed rice rat (*Oligoryzomys longicaudatus*)	Argentina, Chile	HCPS with hemorrhage	44%
Laguna Negra	(*Calomys laucha*)	Western Paraguay	HCPS	9%
Choclo	Costa Rican rice rat (*Oligoryzomys fulvesens*)	Panama	HCPS	20%

HFRS, Hemorrhagic fever renal syndrome; HCPS, hantavirus pulmonary syndrome.

agricultural occupations (54,55), who are more likely to come into close contact with the striped field mouse in houses or food storage buildings. HCPS is much less common, with approximately 300 North American cases and 400 South American cases documented since 1993. Similar to HTNV infections, human SNV and AND infections occur almost exclusively in rural settings (56,57). Patients in whom HCPS develops often reported having entered or disturbed a dwelling, agricultural building, or automobile that was infested with mice (48,57). Person-to-person transmission has not been documented for either Hantaan (58) or SN infection (59), but compelling evidence for Andes virus has been described by cluster and molecular epidemiology in Argentina (60,61) and Chile. HCPS patients have ranged in age from 10 to 75 years of age, with a mean of 35 years (4,62). There is a slight excess of males and a relative overrepresentation of Native Americans among Sin Nombre HCPS case patients.

Prediction of outbreaks of Hantavirus infection would have public health implications. In the American Southwest there is a five-fold variation in annual case incidence between 1993 and 2001. The 1993 to 1994 outbreak followed an El Niño Southern Oscillation (ENSO) event that resulted in increased precipitation in the Four Corners states, resulting in increased abundance of deer mice (63). A strong ENSO of 1997 to 1998 with increased local precipitation was followed by a fivefold increase in case incidence in 1998 to 1999 (48). Similar increases in cases of AND infection in Chile have occurred during the La Niña phase of the ENSO cycle during 1995 to 1996 and 2001. Accurate predictions will depend on improved understanding of the ecologic characteristics that favor proliferation of reservoir rodents and events that favor human exposure to rodents (64).

CLINICAL FEATURES

Hemorrhagic Fever with Renal Syndrome

Whereas the clinical features of infection by HTN, Dobrava, SEO, and PUU viruses clearly define HFRS, morbidity and mor-

tality vary considerably among the different viral strains (65–72) (see Table 245.1). The incubation period ranges from 12 to 21 days, with incubation as long as 6 weeks noted (65). The ratio of infection to illness is 5:1 (54). The syndrome is divided into five phases: febrile, shock, oliguria, diuresis, and convalescence (Fig. 245.1). In the febrile phase, common nonspecific symptoms include high temperature, chills, dizziness, headache, myalgias, abdominal pain, back pain, nausea, vomiting and blurred vision (Table 245.2). A dry cough and shortness of breath precede the onset of mild pulmonary edema in 10% to 20% of the cases (73). The physical examination is notable for conjunctival effusion without marked erythema and an erythematous flush over the face, neck, chest, and nail beds. Petechiae may appear before the shock phase on the palate, face, chest, hips, thighs, and skin folds. Flank tenderness may be prominent in severe cases.

After the petechiae appear, the hematocrit increases, and plasma volume falls as plasma fluid is leaking through the injured capillaries into tissue spaces. Death from primary shock accounts for one third of the fatalities. Proteinuria becomes massive, and oliguria progresses from irregularly present to well established to mark the oliguric phase (1). Renal failure persists for 1 to 6 days, and dialysis may be required until diuresis begins. Recovery is impaired primarily by subcortical hemorrhage (74). The hematocrit decreases as extravascular edema fluid is reabsorbed into the circulation. Spontaneous diuresis of 4 to 8 L/day leads to a rapid decrease in azotemia but may be complicated by electrolyte disorders requiring careful monitoring (1).

The clinical course extends for 2 to 4 weeks, with slow recovery in the majority. There is evidence of only slight residual tubule injury after recovery from acute renal failure in Korean hemorrhagic fever and nephropathia epidemica (75,76). Fatal hemorrhage, particularly in the central nervous system, remains rare, usually occurring in the shock and oliguric phases. Hematologic changes include elevated leukocyte count with marked left shift to the myeloid precursors, severe thrombocytopenia, and circulating atypical lymphocytes. Evidence for a

Severe Hantavirus Pulmonary Syndrome
(Sin Nombre Virus)

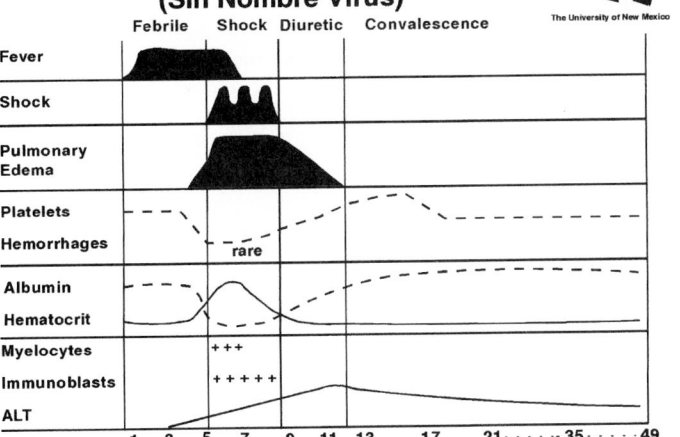

Severe Hemorrhagic Fever Renal Syndrome
(Hantaan Virus)

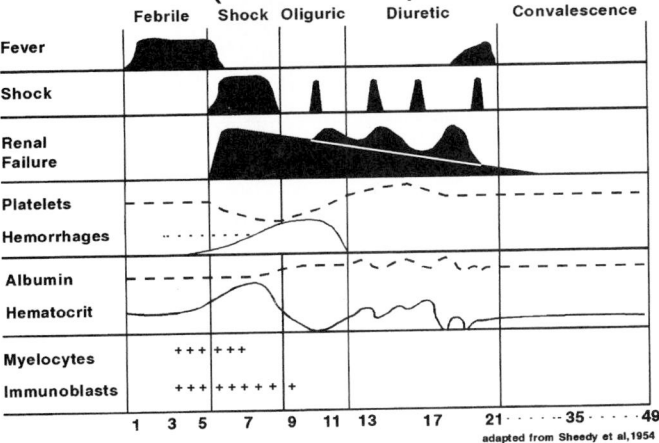

Figure 245.1. Evolution of hantavirus pulmonary syndrome (HCPS) and hemorrhagic fever renal syndrome (HFRS), comparing organ-specific and laboratory abnormalities for each phase of illness. ALT, Alanine aminotransferase. (Adapted and reprinted by permission of the publisher from Sheedy JA, Froeb HF, Batson HA, et al. The clinical course of epidemic hemorrhagic fever. *Am J Med* 1954;16:619. Copyright 1954 by Excerpta Medica, Inc.)

consumptive coagulopathy includes prolonged bleeding time, prolonged prothrombin and activated partial thromboplastin times, circulating D-dimer, and decreased fibrinogen levels (77,78).

Hantavirus Cardiopulmonary Syndrome

The clinical course of HCPS bears both similarities and striking differences compared with HFRS. The incubation period of HCPS has been calculated to be 9 to 33 days, median 14 to 17 days, in 11 cases for which exposure was clearly defined (79). Subclinical infections and uncomplicated febrile illnesses appear to be very uncommon in SN infection (80) and Andes infection, as indicated by low seroprevalence rates. Two Hantaviruses, Laguna Negra in Paraguay (81) and Choclo virus in Panama (38), are associated with high seroprevalence rates without history of associated pulmonary syndrome in seropositive individuals. In North America no children younger than 10 years have been diagnosed with HCPS and younger children have a febrile illness only rarely (82). In South America, severe HCPS has been doc-

umented among children (83) and antibody reactivity against hantaviruses is not uncommon among children in Panama (B. Armien, unpublished data).

HCPS is divided into four phases: febrile prodrome, pulmonary edema and shock, diuresis, and convalescence (see Fig. 245.1) (4). HCPS begins with a febrile prodrome phase, lasting 1 to 12 days, characterized by the abrupt onset of fever, chills, intense myalgias, malaise, nausea and vomiting, headache, and dizziness (see Table 245.2). Because the early symptoms of HCPS mimic a host of other viral and bacterial infections, the clinician is faced with a difficult task to recognize HCPS before the onset of pulmonary edema. Abdominal pain, diarrhea, nausea, and vomiting may mimic acute appendicitis. The physical examination reveals an acutely ill person with tachypnea and tachycardia, but additional features such as pulmonary rales, abdominal tenderness, and conjunctival effusion are seen during the prodrome phase only in the minority of patients. HCPS due to Andes virus is more commonly associated with conjunctival effusion, facial flushing, and pharyngeal congestion (11). After 1 to 5 days of high temperature, the appearance of dry cough and tachypnea heralds the onset of pulmonary edema.

The second phase, or pulmonary edema/shock phase, is characterized by the abrupt onset of shortness of breath and hypoxemia due to pulmonary edema, progressing during a 6- to 12-hour period to severe hypoxemia requiring mechanical ventilation in 50% to 75% of cases. Bronchiolar cuffing and Kerley B lines characterize early pulmonary edema, with rapid progression to bilateral interstitial edema and alveolar flooding 6 to 12 hours later (84). In spite of its severity, pulmonary edema persists only 4 to 6 days and is followed by a spontaneous diuresis lasting 3 to 4 days in patients who survive the shock phase. Initial hypotension is often secondary to hypovolemia associated with vomiting and with fluid shifts of the pulmonary capillary leak, and is readily corrected with several liters of intravenous fluids. Cardiogenic shock, however, is diagnosed by a cardiac index of less than 2.2 L/min per m² and a plasma lactate value of greater than 6.0 mmol/L, and is a grave prognostic sign (85). Cardiogenic shock in HCPS is characterized by a low cardiac index and normal to elevated systemic vascular resistance (85), in contrast to typical septic shock in which the cardiac index is elevated and systemic vascular resistance is diminished. Even in infections with lower mortality rates such as Laguna Negra virus, cardiogenic hypotension requiring inotropic medication may occur in up to 40% of hospitalized patients (9).

In contrast to HFRS, HCPS due to SN infection rarely has significant proteinuria, and elevations of creatinine values reflect volume depletion and prerenal azotemia only. In South America, proteinuria and elevated serum creatinine occurs in most patients, but rarely requires dialysis or results in a nephrotic syndrome. Consistently abnormal laboratory findings include elevated serum lactate dehydrogenase primarily from the lung, elevated serum aspartate aminotransferase levels secondary to mild hepatic triaditis, and decreased serum albumin levels related to the severity of the pulmonary capillary leak (4,11).

The platelet count begins to decrease during the prodrome phase and is the earliest laboratory abnormality that would distinguish HCPS from the host of other influenza-like syndromes. Hematologic changes are distinguished by a leukocytosis with marked left shift and by the appearance of circulating immunoblasts (atypical lymphocytes) coincident with the development of pulmonary edema (4,86). The triad of thrombocytopenia, circulating myelocytes, and circulating immunoblasts is highly specific and sensitive for the presumptive diagnosis of HCPS (87). This triad of hematologic findings is not always

TABLE 245.2. Comparison of the Clinical Features of Four Major Pathogenic Hantaviruses Worldwide

Clinical feature	Sin nombre	Andes	Hantaan	Puumala
Fever	100	100	100	100
Myalgias	95	76	69–78	20
Chills	80	48	92	60
Nausea and vomiting	71	44	72–82	78
Backache	29	24	95	82
Abdominal pain	24	20	23–25	67
Diarrhea	59	8	11–37	12
Dizziness, vertigo	41	16	41–100	12
Headache	71	72	83–86	90
Conjunctival suffusion	18	42	23–64	18
Cough	71	64	40	10
Dyspnea	95	64	<10	<10
Lymphadenopathy	0	12	3–38	15
Petechiae	0	12	32–56	12
Hemorrhage	2	8	31–72	10
Platelets <100,000/mm^3	100	55	54–78	80
White cell count >10,000/mm^3	88	75	92	57
Hypotension (MAP <70 mm Hg)	40–65	72	42–80	40
Pulmonary edema	97	98	20	10
Ventilator dependent	71	60	5	2
Creatinine >2.0 mg/dL	17	69	94–100	70
Proteinuria >1+	17	100	96	100

present during the febrile prodrome phase, and serologic diagnosis is always required at any stage of the disease. A mild coagulopathy is demonstrable in all cases of HCPS (4,86), yet petechiae, ecchymoses, and frank hemorrhage in the pulmonary tree are rare. Disseminated intravascular coagulation and arterial thromboses have occurred, but in most cases the coagulopathy is manifest only as minor gastrointestinal hemorrhage and bleeding from venipuncture sites. Manifestations of hemorrhage are common in HCPS due to Andes virus, with pulmonary hemorrhage and hemothorax as significant causes of death (10,11).

During the convalescent phase postexertional fatigue and dyspnea is very common for several months. Some patients, however, have significant persistent exertional dyspnea which appears to be related to pulmonary function findings of diminished small airways flow and reduced diffusion capacity. These observations have been documented after infection with SN, Andes, and Choclo virus infection, and are not clearly related to the severity of the acute Hantavirus pneumonitis. Observations during convalescence also note complaints of weakness, insomnia, myalgias, arthralgias, proteinuria, scarring after retinal hemorrhage (Andes), and sexual dysfunction (D Goade, unpublished data). The pathogenesis of these problems is not known.

PATHOGENESIS

The clinical features of both HCPS and HFRS are largely the result of a capillary leak syndrome, myocardial dysfunction, and coagulopathy. Whether each of these entities share common pathophysiologic pathways, or whether each entity has a unique pathogenesis, is unknown. With respect to the pulmonary pathology, evidence for T cell–mediated immunopathology has been accumulated. In both HCPS and HFRS, inhalation of virus into the lungs appears to initiate the infection. A viremia is detected by RT-PCR assay of serum collected at the onset of pulmonary edema in HCPS, and the level of viremia

is high in some patients (88,89). Viremia detected by tissue culture has been accomplished only for Andes virus among the HCPS-causing pathogens in the Americas. Viral nucleocapsid antigen is identified in capillary endothelial cells in many organs by immunohistochemistry, but staining is most intense in the lung (90,91). The kidneys from patients dying in the acute phase of Korean hemorrhagic fever contain dense precipitates, typical inclusion bodies, and Hantaan virion-like structures (92). The lungs from patients dying of acute HCPS contain typical inclusion bodies, but hantavirus-like virions are uncommon (86,90).

The evidence for altered vascular permeability in HFRS is widespread capillary engorgement, focal hemorrhage, and interstitial edema in many organs (93). Retroperitoneal edema is massive in some cases, with histologic evidence for renal medullary congestion, pituitary necrosis, and adrenal hemorrhage and necrosis in many fatal cases. In HCPS, the most striking finding at autopsy is edematous lungs with pleural effusions as large as 8 L (86,90). The pulmonary alveoli are filled with acellular proteinaceous fluid with hyaline-like membranes. The modestly thickened septa contain primarily large mononuclear cells, including immunoblasts, monocytes, and plasma cells but few polymorphonuclear leukocytes. The alveolar epithelial cells are intact. This is in marked contrast to acute respiratory distress syndrome, characterized by thickened septa, hyaline membranes, and neutrophilic inflammatory infiltrate in the septa and alveoli.

The heart, kidneys, brain, and adrenals are grossly and histologically normal in SN infection, but in Andes and Choclo virus infection perivascular lymphocytic infiltrate is found in the heart and brain in some patients. The liver may be slightly enlarged and has microscopic evidence of triaditis. The spleen is slightly enlarged, displays immunoblast infiltration of the periarteriolar white pulp, and is the site of intense virus infection by immunohistochemistry (90).

Cellular immune responses appear to play a role in the pathogenesis of both HFRS and HCPS. In HFRS, the presence of activated T cells, soluble interleukin-2 receptors, and interferon-γ–producing cells in peripheral blood is evidence of highly activated T cells (94). The immunoblasts populating the lung, pleural effusion, liver, spleen, lymph nodes, and bloodstream are a striking feature of HCPS. However, immunoblastic cells are not found infiltrating the kidney, heart, and most other tissues, suggesting that the myocardial dysfunction is not related to the immunopathology in the lung (86,90). Immunoperoxidase studies document activated T cells in lung parenchyma (86,90). Flow cytometry studies identified the large blastlike cells in blood and pleural fluid as predominantly activated CD8+ and CD4+ T cells. Cell lines generated from acutely ill HCPS patients are predominantly CD8+ and CD4+ phenotype, secrete interferon-γ (IFN-γ) but not interleukin-4 (IL-4), and derived clones display marked epitope specificity (95). Elevated plasma levels of IL-2, IL-2 receptors, IL-6, tumor necrosis factor-α (TNF-α), and soluble receptors for tumor necrosis factor suggest marked cytokine activation (96–98). Severe HCPS was distinguished from mild HCPS by higher and more persistent plasma levels of TNF-α and TNF receptors and high levels of the chemokine IL-8 (F. Koster, unpublished data).

In HFRS, circulating immune complexes are detected (99) and the classical complement pathway is activated (100). Moreover, the kidney in the acute phase of nephropathia epidemica contains deposits of immunoglobulin and complement beneath the basement membrane (101), suggesting that immune complexes may have a role in the immunopathogenesis of the renal lesion in HFRS. In HCPS circulating immune complexes are detected, but serum levels of activated complement components are normal or only modestly decreased.

Genetic susceptibility to severe Hantavirus infection has been suggested, both for Puumala and SN infection. A common HLA haplotype associated with autoimmune diseases in Northern Europe has been associated with severe nephropathia epidemica (102), and another common B locus allele B27 has been associated with a benign clinical course (103). A severe course of SN infection has been associated with a different HLA haplotype in the Southwestern United States (104), while B27 is associated with a benign clinical course. Whether the pathogenesis associations are due to the class I and II gene products themselves, or to other gene products in linkage disequilibrium with the HLA haplotypes, is not known.

The aggregate observations suggest that immunopathologic mechanisms may mediate the capillary leak syndrome in both HFRS and HCPS. In this hypothesis, hantavirus-infected endothelial cells may be the target of attack by virus-specific cytolytic T cells, which appear in the circulation several days after virus-specific IgM and immunoglobulin G antibody, both of which are present at onset of symptoms. Local secretion of cytokines, particularly TNF, may control viral replication but induces collateral injury in the endothelial cell, creating temporary paracellular gaps that permit the escape of plasma fluid, but not cells, out of the capillary into the interstitium and alveolus, a scenario suggested by *in vitro* models (105). Disturbances in the immune response accounting for unbridled collateral damage in fatal cases are unclear, but the higher levels of TNF-α may play a role. More importantly, significantly lower neutralizing antibody titer at admission in severe cases of HCPS, compared to mild cases, suggests an impaired humoral response failing to control viral proliferation (106). The role of the virus and viral products is unclear. To enter host cells, Hantaviruses use the $\beta3$ integrins, which are present on the surface of endothelial cells, platelets and macrophages (107). Although Hantaviruses are not cytolytic (108), infection of vascular endothelial cells and other cells may mediate the altered vascular permeability and platelet consumption seen in HFRS and HCPS.

DIAGNOSIS OF HANTAVIRUS INFECTIONS

Acute Hantavirus infections are diagnosed by detecting immunoglobulin G and IgM antibodies in serum that react with Hantavirus antigens (109–114). In acute SNV infections, SNV RNA can be detected in peripheral blood mononuclear cells, and frequently in plasma, by reverse transcriptase–polymerase chain reaction (RT-PCR) (88). The propagation of Hantaviruses in cell culture or in laboratory animals is not currently a practical diagnostic modality (20,111).

Hantavirus nucleocapsid proteins are highly antigenic, and high titers of IgM and immunoglobulin G N antibodies are detected in serum at the onset of symptoms in HFRS and in HCPS (106,109,110,112,113). N IgG antibodies reach high titers and persist for decades (39,109,113,115). N polyclonal responses include antibodies that cross-react with the N proteins of related hantaviruses, and the strength of the cross-reactivity varies with the closeness of the evolutionary relatedness of the viruses (116). In both human and *P. maniculatus* SNV infections, an immunodominant region has been localized within the N-terminal 59 amino acids of SNV N (110,112,117). Antibodies that react within this region cross-react strongly with PUU N and PHV N and cross-react weakly with SEO N and HTN N. Therefore, the detection of hantavirus N antibody responses is a sensitive indicator of current or past hantavirus infection but generally cannot differentiate between infections caused by different hantavirus species.

In contrast, envelope glycoprotein (G1 and G2) responses tend to be more virus type specific and include neutralizing antibodies that block virus infectivity in vitro and in laboratory animals (106,110,115–120). The observation that G1 and G2 antibodies neutralize virus infectivity in vitro forms the basis for the plaque reduction neutralization test, a time-consuming assay for detecting hantavirus species-specific antibody reactivities (17,115,116,121). In SNV infections, species-specific linear antibodies directed against SNV G1 antigens occur, but attempts to identify similar reactivities in a limited set of other etiologic agents of HCPS have been unsuccessful (112). The detection of these SNV G1 reactivities permits the virus type-specific diagnosis of SNV infections (110). IgG antibodies against SNV G1 are detected at onset of disease symptoms, but IgM antibodies are sometimes present at low or undetectable levels. Most of the serum reactivity against the linear form of G1 is directed against an N-proximal portion of the protein (between amino acids 58 and 88) (110,122). N and G1 reactivities arise at similar times after infection, and reach approximately similar endpoint titers, but both IgG and IgM antibodies against G1 fade more rapidly than do antibodies against N, often disappearing within 6 mo after infection (106,112). Despite the diagnostic advantage to using both antigens, many commonly used tests for antibodies to SNV utilize only the N antigen.

In nephropathia epidemica, PUU G1 antibodies are detected in acute and early convalescent serum samples, lagging somewhat behind PUU responses (109,113,114). PUU G2 antibody reactivities are not detected within the first 5 weeks after infection but rise gradually to high titers in subsequent weeks. IgG and/or IgM antibodies against SNV G1 are detected at onset of disease symptoms (109,113).

Hantavirus recombinant proteins have commonly been used as antigen targets in serodiagnostic assays because of the difficulty in obtaining adequate amounts of native viral proteins (110,114). In the SNV strip immunoblot assay (SIA), serum

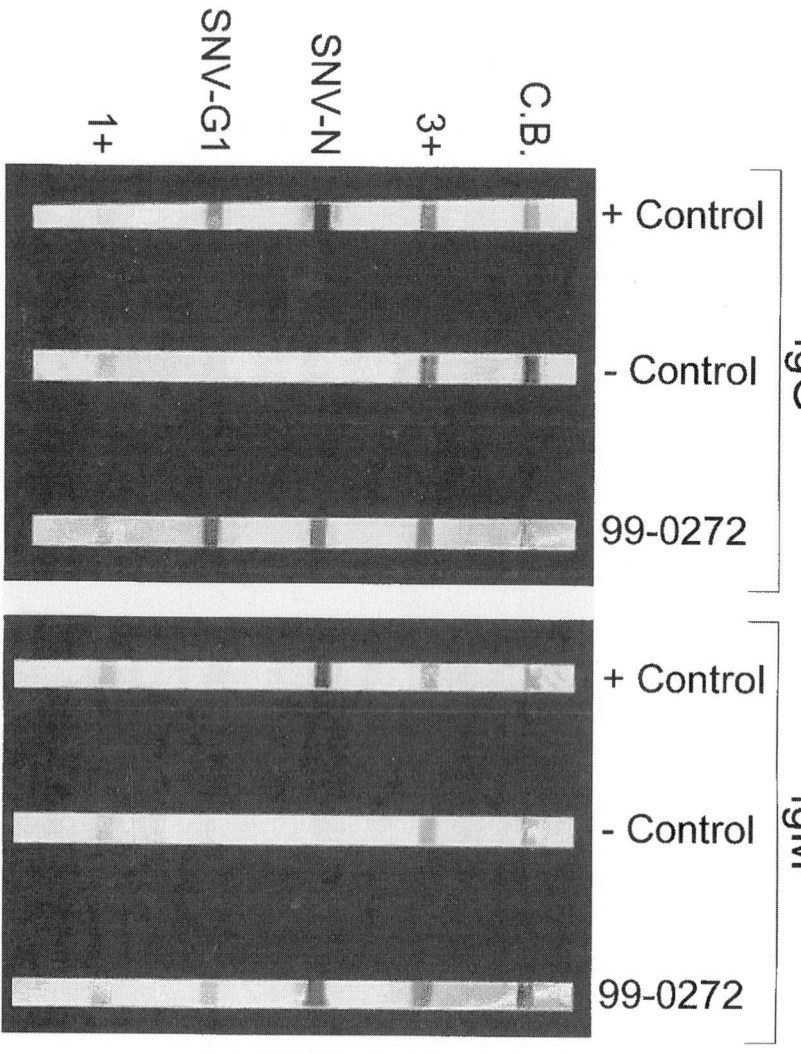

Figure 245.2. Representative strip immunoblot assay (SIA) for antibodies to Sin Nombre virus (SNV) conducted by TriCore Reference Laboratory (Albuquerque, NM). The patient sample, serum sample 99-0272, was used to probe SIA strips that were coated with recombinant N and G1 antigens. Bound immunoglobulin G (IgG) and M (IgM) were then detected with enzyme-linked conjugates directed against those antibodies. That the clinical sample had IgG and IgM reactivities against SNV N and G1 antigens is evident by the dark bands at the appropriate locations on the strips. Control bands used to verify the correct function of the strips are designated *C.B.* (Coomassie Blue), *3+* and *1+*. Control studies were conducted with serum samples known to come from infected (+*Control*) and uninfected (−*Control*) patients, respectively.

samples are tested for the presence of IgG and IgM antibodies that react with recombinant SNV N and G1 proteins (Fig. 245.2) (110).

SNV RNA can be detected in the peripheral blood or in virtually any solid organ of patients with acute HCPS by RT-PCR (88). Hantavirus genomic RNAs can be amplified by RT-PCR by use of oligonucleotide primers. SNV RNA becomes undetectable in blood during convalescence, and it is presumed that the virus has been cleared from the body. In cases in which the identity of the infecting Hantavirus is in doubt, due to ambiguous serologic results, RT-PCR and nucleotide sequencing can provide a definitive identification (88).

In fatal cases of Hantavirus infections in which serum and fresh tissue samples are not available for study, Hantavirus antigens can be detected by immunohistochemical staining of paraffin-embedded tissue sections (90,91). High densities of Hantavirus antigens are observed in renal endothelial and in pulmonary endothelial cells in fatal cases of either HFRS or HCPS. Renal sections are preferred, followed by lung sections (90,123).

MANAGEMENT

The management of HFRS focuses on restoring fluid balance, correcting electrolyte disorders, treating hypovolemic hypotension with judicious fluid replacement, and treating cardiogenic shock with inotropic agents (1,124,125). Peritoneal dialysis or hemodialysis is essential for acute renal failure. Corticosteroids may predispose the patient to nosocomial pneumonia and are not recommended. Intravenous ribavirin has been shown in a placebo-controlled, randomized trial to reduce morbidity and mortality of HFRS in China for patients receiving at least 5 days of therapy (126).

The management of HCPS also focuses on supportive care (127). Since the transition from nondescript febrile prodrome to profound shock is frequently rapid, the prompt recognition of the syndrome and transfer of the patient to an intensive care unit is recommended (14,85). Inspection of the peripheral blood smear to obtain a rapid presumptive diagnosis may aid in decision making prior to the availability of diagnostic serology results (87). In the hypotensive patient, placement of a pulmonary artery catheter to measure pulmonary wedge pressures will help avoid excessive fluid replacement and exacerbation of alveolar flooding. The use of diuretics may exacerbate the volume depletion and shock, without alleviating the pulmonary edema. Pressors for inotropic support should be used to restore blood pressure, urine output, and peripheral circulation, and dobutamine should be initiated prior to the onset of shock. For patients with severe gas exchange abnormalities with a partial pressure of arterial oxygen/fraction of inspired oxygen (PaO_2/FIO_2) of less than 100, mechanical ventilation with high levels of positive end-expiratory pressure, and conventional volume-controlled ventilation are necessary. Complete paralysis with vecuronium bromide, and the experimental reversed ratio ventilation, may be necessary in selected patients. Indicators of a high risk for mortality include admission serum lactate level above 4.0 $\mu g/dL$ and a cardiac index less than 2.1 L/minute per m^2 (85). Experience with critically ill HCPS patients treated with extracorporeal membrane oxygenation suggests that this experimental modality should be considered when it is available for patients with a high risk for mortality (128). Until HCPS is diagnosed by serology, presumptive antibiotic therapy for common causes of sepsis should be instituted in every patient. Available uncontrolled data on ribavirin (129) and corticosteroids in HCPS do not permit conclusions on efficacy until trials in North America, and Chile, respectively, are completed.

PREVENTION

The Centers for Disease Control and Prevention has issued interim guidelines for reducing the risk for transmission of Hantavirus infections (130). These guidelines emphasize practical recommendations for preventing rodent infestations, for cleaning up rodent-infested sites, and for trapping and disposing of rodents. The information is available from state and local health departments as well as on the worldwide web at: *www.cdc.gov/ncidod/diseases/hanta/hantvrus.htm*.

Recombinant protein vaccines have been developed for HTN, and rodent brain vaccines have been used in Korea and China (131–134). Studies indicate that immunization with Hantavirus glycoproteins (G1 and G2) induces neutralizing antibody responses (120,131). It is conceivable that recombinant SNV glycoprotein vaccines could be useful when the risk for SNV transmission is high. Gene fragments of the SNV glycoproteins that elicit strong immune responses in rodent models have recently been shown to be capable of preventing infection in the deer mouse model (Hjelle et al., unpublished data) (135).

REFERENCES

1. Earle DP. Symposium on epidemic hemorrhagic fever. *Am J Med* 1954;16:617.
2. Lee HW, Lee PW, Lahdevirta J, Brummer-Korventkotio M. Aetiological relation between Korean haemorrhagic fever and nephropathia epidemica. *Lancet* 1979;1:186.
3. Mertz GJ, Hjelle BL, Bryan RT. Hantavirus infection. *Adv Intern Med* 1997;42:369–421.
4. Duchin JS, Koster FT, Peters CJ, et al. Hantavirus pulmonary syndrome: a clinical description of 17 patients with a newly recognized disease. *N Engl J Med* 1994;330:949.
5. Nichol ST, Spiropoulou CF, Morzunov S, et al. Genetic identification of a novel hantavirus associated with an outbreak of acute respiratory illness in the southwestern United States. *Science* 1993;262:914.
6. Schmaljohn C, Hjelle B. Hantaviruses: a global disease problem. *Emerg Infect Dis* 1997;3:85–87.
7. Young JC, Mills JN, Enria DA, et al. New World Hantaviruses. *Br Med Bull* 1998;54:659–673.
8. Levis S, Morzunov S, Rowe JE, et al. Genetic diversity and epidemiology of hantaviruses in Argentina. *J Infect Dis* 1998;177:529–538.
9. Williams RJ, Bryan RT, Mills JN, et al. An outbreak of hantavirus pulmonary syndrome in western Paraguay. *Am J Trop Med Hyg* 1997;57:274–282.
10. Toro J, Vega JD, Khan AS, et al. An outbreak of hantavirus pulmonary syndrome, Chile, 1997. *Emerg Infect Dis* 1998;4:687–694.
11. Lazaro ME, Resa AJ, Barclay CM, et al. Hantavirus pulmonary syndrome in Southern Argentina. *Medicina (Buenos Aires)* 2000;60:289–301.
12. Vincent MJ, Quiroz E, Gracia F, et al. Hantavirus pulmonary syndrome in Panama: identification of novel hantaviruses and their likely reservoirs. *Virology* 2000;277:14–19.
13. Centers for Disease Control and Prevention. Outbreak of acute illness—Southwestern United States, 1993. *MMWR* 1993;42:421.
14. Levy H, Simpson SQ. Hantavirus pulmonary syndrome. *Am J Respir Crit Care Med* 1994;149:1710.
15. Schmaljohn CS, Dalrymple JM. Analysis of Hantaan virus RNA: evidence for a new genus of Bunyaviridae. *Virology* 1983;131:482.
16. Elliott LH, Kiley MP, McCormick JB. Hantaan virus: identification of virion proteins. *J Gen Virol* 1984;65:1285.
17. Schmaljohn CS, Hasty SE, Dalrymple JM, et al. Antigenic and genetic properties of viruses linked to hemorrhagic fever with renal syndrome. *Science* 1985;227:1041.
18. Schmaljohn CS, Jennings JB, Hay J, et al. Coding strategy of the S genome segment of Hantaan virus. *Virology* 1986;155:633.
19. Schmaljohn CS, Schmaljohn AL, Dalrymple JM. Hantaan virus M RNA: coding strategy, nucleotide sequence, and gene order. *Virology* 1987;157:31.
20. Lee HW, Lee PW, Johnson KM. Isolation of the etiologic agent of Korean hemorrhagic fever. *J Infect Dis* 1978;137:298.
21. LeDuc JW, Smith GA, Johnson KM. Hantaan-like viruses from domestic rats captured in the United States. *Am J Trop Med Hyg* 1984;33:992.
22. Childs JE, Korch GW, Glass GE, et al. Epizootiology of hantavirus infections in Baltimore: isolation of a virus from Norway rats, and characteristics of infected rat populations. *Am J Epidemiol* 1987;126:55.
23. Avsic-Zupanc T, Toney A, Anderson K, et al. Genetic and antigenic properties of Dobrava virus: unique member of the *Hantavirus* genus, family *Bunyaviridae*. *J Gen Virol* 1995;76:2801–2808.
24. Brummer-Korvenkontio M, Vaheri A, von Bonsdorff C-H, et al. Nephropathia epidemica: detection of antigen in bank voles and serologic diagnosis of human infection. *J Infect Dis* 1980;141:131.
25. Mustonen J, Brummer-Korvenkontio M, Hedman K, et al. Nephropathia epidemica in Finland: A retrospective study of 126 cases. *Scand J Infect Dis* 1994;26:7.
26. Niklasson B, LeDuc JW. Epidemiology of nephropathia epidemica in Sweden. *J Infect Dis* 1987;155:269.
27. Settergren B. Nephropathia epidemica (hemorrhagic fever with renal syndrome) in Scandinavia. *Rev Infect Dis* 1991;13:736.
28. Vapalahti O, Kallio-Kokko H, Salonen EM, et al. Cloning and sequencing of Puumala virus Sotkamo strain S and M segments: evidence for strain variation in hantaviruses and expression of the nucleocapsid protein. *J Gen Virol* 1992;73:829.
29. Childs JE, Ksiazek TG, Spiropoulou CF, et al. Serologic and genetic identification of Peromyscus maniculatus as the primary rodent reservoir for a new hantavirus in the southwestern United States. *J Infect Dis* 1994;169:1271.
30. Hjelle B, Jenison S, Torrez-Martinez N, et al. A novel hantavirus associated with an outbreak of fatal respiratory disease in the southwestern United States: evolutionary relationships to known hantaviruses. *J Virol* 1994;68:592.
31. Spiropoulou CF, Morzunov S, Feldmann H, et al. Genome structure and variability of a virus causing hantavirus pulmonary syndrome. *Virology* 1994;200:715.
32. Brackett LE, Rotenberg J, Sherman CB. Hantavirus pulmonary syndrome in New England and Europe. *N Engl J Med* 1994;331:545.
33. Hjelle B, Krolikowski J, Torrez-Martinez N, et al. Phylogenetically distinct hantavirus implicated in a case of hantavirus pulmonary syndrome in the northeastern United States. *J Med Virol* 1995;46:21.
34. Centers for Disease Control and Prevention. Newly identified hantavirus-Florida. *MMWR* 1994;43:99.
35. Morzunov SP, Feldmann H, Spiropoulou CF, et al. A newly recognized virus associated with a fatal case of hantavirus pulmonary syndrome in Louisiana. *J Virol* 1995;69:1980.
36. Torrez-Martinez N, Bharadwaj M, Goade D, et al. Bayou virus-associated hantavirus pulmonary syndrome in Eastern Texas: identification of the rice rat, *Oryzomys palustris*, as reservoir host. *Emerg Infect Dis* 1998;4:105–111.
37. Hjelle B, Goade D, Torrez-Martinez N, et al. Hantavirus pulmonary syndrome, renal insufficiency, and myositis associated with infection by Bayou hantavirus. *Clin Infect Dis* 1996;23:495–500.
38. Hjelle B, Chavez-Giles F, Torrez-Martinez N, et al. Dominant glycoprotein epitope of Four Corners hantavirus is conserved across a wide geographical area. *J Gen Virol* 1994;75:2881.
39. Xiao S-Y, LeDuc JW, Chu Y-K, et al. Phylogenetic analysis of virus isolates of the genus *Hantavirus*, family Bunyaviridae. *Virology* 1994;198:205.
40. Nerurkar VR, Song K-J, Song J-W, et al. Genetic evidence for a hantavirus enzootic in deer mice (*Peromyscus maniculatus*) a decade before the recognition of hantavirus pulmonary syndrome. *Virology* 1994;204:563.
41. Wilson C, Hjelle B, Jenison S. A probable case of hantavirus pulmonary syndrome that occurred in New Mexico in 1975. *Ann Intern Med* 1994;120:813.
42. Botten J, Mirowsky K, Kusewitt D, et al. Experimental infection model for Sin Nombre hantavirus in the deer mouse (*Peromyscus maniculatus*). *Proc Natl Acad Sci USA* 2000;97:10578–10583.
43. Hutchinson KL, Rollin PE, Peters CJ. Pathogenesis of a North American hantavirus, Black Creek Canal virus, in experimentally infected *Sigmodon hispidus*. *Am J Trop Med Hyg* 1998;59:58–65.
44. Lee HW, Lee PW, Baek LJ, et al. Intraspecific transmission of Hantaan virus, etiologic agent of Korean hemorrhagic fever, in the rodent *Apodemus agrarius*. *Am J Trop Med Hyg* 1981;30:1106–1112.
45. Bernshtein AD, Apekina NS, Mikhailova TV, et al. Dynamics of Puumala hantavirus infection in naturally infected bank voles (*Clethrinomys glareolus*). *Arch Virol* 1999;144:2415–2428.

46. Gavrilovskaya IN, Apekina NS, Myasnikov Y, et al. Features of circulation of hemorrhagic fever with renal syndrome (HFRS) virus among small mammals in the European U.S.S.R. *Arch Virol* 1983;75:313–316.

47. Schmaljohn CS. Molecular biology of hantaviruses. In: Elliott RM, ed. *The bunyaviridae.* New York: Plenum Press, 1996:63–86.

48. Hjelle B, Glass GE. Outbreak of hantavirus infection in the four corners region of the United States in the wake of the 1997–1998 El Niño-southern oscillation. *J Infect Dis* 2000;181:1569–1573.

49. Umenai T, Lee HW, Lee PW, et al. Korean haemorrhagic fever in staff in an animal laboratory. *Lancet* 1979;1:1314.

50. Lee HW, Johnson KM. Laboratory-acquired infections with Hantaan virus, the etiologic agent of Korean hemorrhagic fever. *J Infect Dis* 1982;146:645.

51. Kawamata J, Yamanouchi T, Dohmae K, et al. Control of laboratory acquired hemorrhagic fever with renal syndrome. *Lab Anim Sci* 1987;37:431.

52. Dournon E, Moriniere B, Matheron S, et al. HFRS after a wild rodent bite in the Haute-Savoie and risk of exposure to Hantaan-like virus in a Paris laboratory. *Lancet* 1984;1:676.

53. Houck MA, Qin H, Roberts HR. Hantavirus transmission: potential role of ectoparasites. *Vector Borne Zoonotic Dis* 2001;1:75–79.

54. Ruo SL, Li YL, Tong Z, et al. Retrospective and prospective studies of hemorrhagic fever with renal syndrome in rural China. *J Infect Dis* 1994;70:527.

55. Xu Z-Y, Guo C-S, Wu Y-L, et al. Epidemiological studies of hemorrhagic fever with renal syndrome: analysis of risk factors and mode of transmission. *J Infect Dis* 1985;152:137.

56. Flood J, Mintz L, Jay M, et al. Hantavirus infection following wilderness camping in Washington State and northeastern California. *West J Med* 1995;163:162.

57. Zeitz PS, Butler JC, Cheek JE, et al. A case-control study of hantavirus pulmonary syndrome during an outbreak in the southwestern United States. *J Infect Dis* 1995;171:864.

58. Gauld RL, Craig JP. Epidemiological pattern of localized outbreaks of epidemic hemorrhagic fever. *Am J Hyg* 1954;59(1):32–38.

59. Vitek CR, Breiman RF, Ksiazek TG, et al. Evidence against person-to-person transmission of hantavirus to health care workers. *Clin Infect Dis* 1996;22:824–826.

60. Enria D, Padula P, Segura EL, et al. Hantavirus pulmonary syndrome in Argentina. Possibility of person to person transmission. *Medicina (B Aires)* 1996;56:709–711.

61. Padula PJ, Edelstein A, Miguel SD, et al. Hantavirus pulmonary syndrome outbreak in Argentina: molecular evidence for person-to-person transmission of Andes virus. *Virology* 1998;241:323–330.

62. Khan AS, Khabbaz RF, Armstrong LR, et al. Hantavirus pulmonary syndrome: the first 100 U.S. cases. *J Infect Dis* 1996;173:1297–1303.

63. Hjelle B, Jenison S, Mertz G, et al. Emergence of hantaviral disease in the southwestern United States. *West J Med* 1994;161:467–473.

64. Engelthaler DM, Mosley DG, Cheek JE, et al. Climatic and environmental patterns associated with hantavirus pulmonary syndrome, four corners region, United States. *Emerg Infect Dis* 1999;5:87–94.

65. Counts EF, Seltzer R. The early diagnosis of endemic hemorrhagic fever. *Ann Intern Med* 1953;38:67.

66. Powell GM. Hemorrhagic fever: a study of 300 cases. *Medicine (Baltimore)* 1954;33:97.

67. Lee HW, van der Groen G. Hemorrhagic fever with renal syndrome. *Prog Med Virol* 1989;36:62.

68. Lee JS, Lee MC, Choi SJ, et al. Clinical features of serologically proven Korean hemorrhagic fever patients. *Seoul J Med* 1980;21:163.

69. Kim YS, Ahn C, Han JS, et al. Hemorrhagic fever with renal syndrome caused by the Seoul virus. *Nephron* 1995;71:419–427.

70. Lahdevirta J. Nephropathia epidemica in Finland: a clinical, serological and epidemiological study. *Ann Clin Res* 1971;3[Suppl 8]:1.

71. Antoniadis A, LeDuc JW, Acritidis N, et al. Hemorrhagic fever with renal syndrome in Greece: clinical and laboratory characteristics. *Rev Infect Dis* 1989;11[Suppl 4]:S891.

72. Avsic-Zupanc T, Petrovec M, Furlan P, et al. Hemorrhagic fever with renal syndrome in the Dolenjska region of Slovenia—a 10-year survey. *Clin Infect Dis* 1999;28:860–865.

73. Linderholm M, Sandstrom T, Rinnstrom O, et al. Impaired pulmonary function in patients with hemorrhagic fever with renal syndrome. *Clin Infect Dis* 1997;25:1084–1089.

74. Oliver J, MacDowell M. The renal lesion in epidemic hemorrhagic fever. *J Clin Invest* 1957;36:99.

75. Rubini ME, Jablon S, McDowell ME. Renal residuals of acute epidemic hemorrhagic fever. *Arch Intern Med* 1960;128:378.

76. Lahdevirta J, Collan Y, Jokinen EJ, Hiltunen R. Renal sequelae to nephropathia epidemica. *Acta Pathol Microbiol Scand A* 1978;86:265.

77. Settergren B, Juto P, Trollifors B. Hemorrhagic complications and other clinical findings in nephropathia epidemica in Sweden. A study of 355 serologically verified cases. *J Infect Dis* 1988;157:380.

78. Guang MY, Liu GZ, Cosgriff TM. Hemorrhage in hemorrhagic fever with renal syndrome in China. *Rev Infect Dis* 1989;11[Suppl 4]:S884.

79. Young JC, Hansen GR, Graves TK, et al. The incubation period of hantavirus pulmonary syndrome. *Am J Trop Med Hyg* 2000;62:714–717.

80. Zavasky DM, Hjelle B, Peterson MC, et al. Acute infection with Sin Nombre hantavirus without pulmonary edema. *Clin Infect Dis* 1999;29:664–666.

81. Ferrer JF, Jonsson C, Esteban E, et al. High prevalence of hantavirus antibodies in Indian communities of the Paraguayan and Argentinean Gran Chaco. *Am J Trop Med Hyg* 1998;59:438–444.

82. Armstrong L, Bryan RT, Sarisky J, et al. Mild hantaviral disease due to Sin Nombre virus in a four-year-old child. *Pediatr Infect Dis J* 1995;14:1108–1110.

83. Pini N, Resa A, Laime G, et al. Hantavirus infection in children in Argentina. *Emerg Infect Dis* 1998;4:85–87.

84. Ketai LH, Williamson MR, Telepak RJ, et al. Hantavirus pulmonary syndrome (HCPS): radiographic findings in 16 patients. *Radiology* 1994;191:665.

85. Hallin GW, Simpson SQ, Crowell RE, et al. Hantavirus pulmonary syndrome: experience at the University of New Mexico Hospital. *Crit Care Med* 1996;24:252.

86. Nolte KB, Feddersen RM, Foucar K, et al. Hantavirus pulmonary syndrome in the United States: pathologic description of a disease caused by a new agent. *Hum Pathol* 1995;26:110.

87. Koster F, Foucar K, Hjelle B, et al. Rapid presumptive diagnosis of hantavirus cardiopulmonary syndrome by peripheral blood smear review. *Am J Clin Pathol* 2001;116:665–672.

88. Hjelle B, Spiropoulou CF, Torrez-Martinez N, et al. Detection of Muerto Canyon virus RNA in peripheral blood mononuclear cells from patients with hantavirus pulmonary syndrome. *J Infect Dis* 1994;170:1013.

89. Terajima M, Hendershot JD, Kariwa H, et al. High levels of viremia in patients with the hantavirus pulmonary syndrome. *J Infect Dis* 1999;180:2030–2034.

90. Zaki SR, Greer PW, Coffield LM, et al. Hantavirus pulmonary syndrome-Pathogenesis of an emerging infectious disease. *Am J Pathol* 1995;146:552.

91. Green W, Feddersen R, Yousef O, et al. Tissue distribution of hantavirus antigen in naturally infected humans and deer mice. *J Infect Dis* 1998;177:1696–1700.

92. Tao H, Jing-Yi Z, Yun-Ming T, et al. Identification of Hantaan virus-related structures in kidneys of cadavers with haemorrhagic fever with renal syndrome. *Arch Virol* 1992;122:187.

93. Lukes RJ. The pathology of thirty-nine fatal cases of epidemic hemorrhagic fever. *Am J Med* 1954;16:639.

94. Huang C, Jin B, Wang M, et al. Hemorrhagic fever with renal syndrome: relationship between pathogenesis and cellular immunity. *J Infect Dis* 1994;169:868.

95. Ennis FA, Cruz J, Spiropoulou CF, et al. Hantavirus pulmonary syndrome: CD8+ and CD4+ cytotoxic T lymphocytes to epitopes on sin nombre virus nucleocapsid protein isolated during acute illness. *Virology* 1997;238:380–390.

96. Simpson SQ, Mapel V, Koster FT, et al. Evidence for tumor necrosis factor activation in the hantavirus pulmonary syndrome. *Crit Care Med* 1996;24:A26.

97. Krakauer T, LeDuc JW, Krakauer H. Serum levels of tumor necrosis-α, interleukin-1, and interleukin-6 in hemorrhagic fever with renal syndrome. *Viral Immunol* 1995;8:12.

98. Linderholm M, Ahlm C, Settergren B, et al. Elevated plasma levels of tumor necrosis factor (TNF)-α, soluble TNF receptor, interleukin (IL)-6, and IL-10 in patients with hemorrhagic fever with renal syndrome. *J Infect Dis* 1996;173:38–43.

99. Luo DD, Wang XH, Jin WE, Fan JZ. Detection and analysis of specific circulating immune complexes in epidemic hemorrhagic fever. *Chin J Infect Dis* 1985;3:86.

100. Yan D, Gu X, Wang D, Yang S. Studies on immunopathogenesis in epidemic hemorrhagic fever: Sequential observations on activation of the first complement component in sera from patients with epidemic hemorrhagic fever. *J Immunol* 1981;127:1064.

101. Jokinen EJ, Lahdevirta J, Collan Y. Nephropathia epidemica: immunohistochemical study of pathogenesis. *Clin Nephrol* 1978;9:1.

102. Mustonen J, Partanen J, Kanerva M, et al. Genetic susceptibility to severe course of nephropathia epidemica caused by Puumala hantavirus. *Kidney Int* 1996;49:217–221.

103. Mustonen J, Partanen J, Kanerva M, et al. Association of HLA B27 with benign clinical course of nephropathia epidemica caused by Puumala hantavirus. *Scand J Immunol* 1998;47:277–279.

104. Mertz GJ, Hjelle BL, Williams TM, Koster FT. Host responses in the hantavirus cardiopulmonary syndrome. In: Saluzzo JF, Dodet B, eds. *Factors in the emergence and control of rodent-borne viral diseases (hantaviral and arenal diseases).* Amsterdam: Elsevier, 1999:133–137.

105. Goldblum SE, Hennig B, Jay M, et al. Tumor necrosis factor-induced pulmonary vascular endothelial injury. *Infect Immun* 1989;57:1218.

106. Bharadwaj M, Nofchissey R, Goade D, et al. Humoral immune responses in the hantavirus cardiopulmonary syndrome. *J Infect Dis* 2000;182:43–48.

107. Gavrilovskaya IN, Shepley M, Shaw R, et al. β_3 integrins mediate the cellular entry of hantaviruses that cause respiratory failure. *Proc Natl Acad Sci USA* 1998;95:7074–7079.

108. Pensiero MN, Sharefkin JB, Dieffenbach CW, Hay J. Hantaan virus infection of human endothelial cells. *J Virol* 1992;66:5929–5936.

109. Groen J, Dalrymple J, Fisher-Hoch S, et al. Serum antibodies to structural proteins of hantavirus arise at different times after infection. *J Med Virol* 1992;37:283.

110. Jenison S, Yamada T, Morris C, et al. Characterization of human antibody responses to four corners hantavirus infections among patients with hantavirus pulmonary syndrome. *J Virol* 1994;68:3000.

111. Elliott LH, Ksiazek TG, Rollin PE, et al. Isolation of the causative agent of hantavirus pulmonary syndrome. *Am J Trop Med Hyg* 1994;51:102.

112. Hjelle B, Jenison S, Torrez-Martinez N, et al. Rapid and specific detection of Sin Nombre virus antibodies in patients with hantavirus pulmonary syndrome by a strip immunoblot assay suitable for field diagnosis. *J Clin Microbiol* 1997;35:600–608.
113. Lundkvist AA, Horling J, Niklasson B. The humoral response to Puumala virus infection (nephropathia epidemica) investigated by viral protein specific immunoassays. *Arch Virol* 1993;130:121.
114. Zöller LG, Yang S, Gott P, et al. A novel mu-capture enzyme linked immunosorbent assay based on recombinant proteins for sensitive and specific diagnosis of hemorrhagic fever with renal syndrome. *J Clin Microbiol* 1993;31:1194.
115. Settergren B, Ahlm C, Juto P, et al. Specific Puumala IgG virus half a century after haemorrhagic fever with renal syndrome. *Lancet* 1991;338:66.
116. Chu YK, Lee HW, LeDuc JW, et al. Serological relationships among viruses in the Hantavirus genus, family Bunyaviridae. *Virology* 1994;198:196.
117. Yamada T, Hjelle B, Lanzi R, et al. Antibody responses to Four Corners hantavirus infections in the deer mouse (*Peromyscus maniculatus*): identification of an immunodominant region of the viral nucleocapsid protein. *J Virol* 1995;69:1939.
118. Arikawa J, Schmaljohn AL, Dalrymple JM, et al. Characterization of Hantaan virus envelope glycoprotein antigenic determinants defined by monoclonal antibodies. *J Gen Virol* 1989;70:615.
119. Lundkvist AA, Niklasson B. Bank vole monoclonal antibodies against Puumala virus envelope glycoproteins: identification of epitopes involved in neutralization. *Arch Virol* 1992;126:93.
120. Wang M, Pennock DG, Spik KW, et al. Epitope mapping studies with neutralizing and non-neutralizing monoclonal antibodies to the G1 and G2 envelope glycoproteins of Hantaan virus. *Virology* 1993;197:757.
121. Chu YK, Jennings G, Schmaljohn A, et al. Cross-neutralization of hantaviruses with immune sera from experimentally infected animals and from HFRS or HCPS patients. *J Infect Dis* 1995;172:1581.
122. Hjelle B, Chavez-Giles F, Torrez-Martinez N, et al. Dominant glycoprotein epitope of Four Corners hantavirus is conserved across a wide geographical area. *J Gen Virol* 1994;75(Pt 11):2881–2888.
123. Ruo SL, Sanchez A, Elliott LH, et al. Monoclonal antibodies to three strains of hantaviruses: Hantaan, R22, and Puumala. *Arch Virol* 1991;119:1.
124. Lee JS. Clinical manifestations and treatment of HFRS (Hantaan and Seoul viruses). In: Lee HW, Calisher C, Schmaljohn C, eds. *Manual of hemorrhagic fever with renal syndrome and hantavirus pulmonary syndrome.* Seoul: WHO Collaborating Center for Virus Reference and Research (Hantaviruses), Asian Institute for Life Sciences, 1999:18–27.
125. Lahdevirta J. Clinical Manifestations and treatment of HFRS (Puumala virus). In: Lee HW, Calisher C, Schmaljohn C, eds. *Manual of hemorrhagic fever with renal syndrome and hantavirus pulmonary syndrome.* Seoul: WHO Collaborating Center for Virus Reference and Research (Hantaviruses), Asian Institute for Life Sciences, 1999:28–32.
126. Huggins JW, Hsiang CM, Cosgriff TM, et al. Prospective, double-blind, concurrent, placebo-controlled clinical trial of intravenous ribavirin therapy for hemorrhagic fever with renal syndrome. *J Infect Dis* 1991;164:119.
127. Koster F, Levy H. Clinical manifestations and treatment of HCPS. In: Lee HW, Calisher C, Schmaljohn C, eds. *Manual of hemorrhagic fever with renal syndrome and hantavirus pulmonary syndrome.* Seoul: WHO Collaborating Center for Virus Reference and Research (Hantaviruses), Asian Institute for Life Sciences, 1999:33–38.
128. Crowley MR, Katz RW, Kessler R, et al. Successful treatment of adults with severe hantavirus pulmonary syndrome with extracorporeal membrane oxygenation. *Crit Care Med* 1998;26:409–414.
129. Chapman LE, Mertz GJ, Peters CJ, et al. Intravenous ribavirin for Hantavirus Pulmonary syndrome: Safety and tolerance during one year of open label experience. *Antiviral Ther* 1999;4:211–219.
130. Centers for Disease Control and Prevention. Hantavirus infection in the southwestern United States: interim recommendations for risk reduction. *MMWR* 1993;42(RR-11):1.
131. Schmaljohn CS, Chu YK, Schmaljohn AL, et al. Antigenic subunits of Hantaan virus expressed by baculovirus and vaccinia virus recombinants. *J Virol* 1990;64:3162.
132. McClain DJ, Summers PL, Harrison SA, et al. Clinical evaluation of a vaccinia-vectored Hantaan virus vaccine. *J Med Virol* 2000;60:77–85.
133. Kamrud KI, Hooper JW, Elgh F, Schmaljohn CS. Comparison of the protective efficacy of naked DNA, DNA-based Sindbis replicon, and packaged Sindbis replicon vectors expressing Hantavirus structural genes in hamsters. *Virology* 1999;263:209–219.
134. Cho HW, Howard CR. Antibody responses in humans to an inactivated hantavirus vaccine (Hantavax). *Vaccine* 1999;17:2569–2575.
135. Bharadwaj M, Lyons CR, Wortman IA, Hjelle B. Intramuscular inoculation of Sin Nombre hantavirus cDNAs induces cellular and humoral immune responses in BALB/c mice. *Vaccine* 1999;17:2836–2843.

CHAPTER 246
Respiratory Syncytial Virus

Robert C. Welliver and Pearay L. Ogra

Respiratory syncytial virus (RSV) is the single most common cause of severe lower respiratory tract infections in infancy. Its worldwide distribution and unique seasonal occurrence in temperate climates, its potential for causing life-threatening or fatal respiratory illness, the possible role of the immune system in the pathogenesis of pulmonary disease, and its ability to cause reinfection in the presence of preexisting immunity have stimulated considerable investigative interest. Available modes of specific and nonspecific treatment do not yield impressive therapeutic outcomes, making the development of effective means of prevention a high priority.

CHARACTERISTICS OF THE PATHOGEN

Classification

RSV is a member of the paramyxovirus family and has been assigned to the genus *Pneumovirus* because of certain differences from other paramyxoviruses, principally the lack of a hemagglutinin (1). The virus contains a single, unsegmented strand of ribonucleic acid (RNA) of negative polarity.

Structure

RSV is an enveloped virus with a diameter of 300 to 350 nm, exhibiting spherical and filamentous forms (2). It is currently believed that the genome of RSV codes for the synthesis of at least ten viral proteins (3), depicted in Table 246.1. Two nonglycosylated proteins are associated with the inner virion membrane, but, much more important, two glycoproteins are also found extending from the surface of the virion (4,5). One of these glycoproteins has a molecular mass of 68 kDa and functions as the fusion protein after proteolytic cleavage into subunits with molecular masses of 48 kDa (F_1) and 20 kDa (F_2) (6). The larger G glycoprotein has a molecular mass of approximately 90 kDa and has been identified as the attachment protein of RSV (7). Within the envelope is a helical nucleocapsid.

Replication

Replication of viral nucleic acid appears to proceed in a manner similar to that of other paramyxoviruses and is inhibited by 6-azauridine, an inhibitor of RNA replication (8), but not by actinomycin D (9).

Antigenic Characteristics

In the past it was believed that only one serotype of RSV existed; with animal serum, neutralizing titers vary somewhat against various strains of RSV However, human convalescent serum seems to manifest essentially equivalent neutralizing antibody titers against all strains tested (10). Panels of monoclonal antibodies have been developed against multiple epitopes on various viral proteins. Analysis of RSV strains using these antibodies in enzyme-linked immunosorbent assay (ELISA) and immunofluorescence assays has demonstrated that there is considerable homology among RSV proteins produced by most strains of the

TABLE 246.1. Major Proteins Associated with Respiratory Syncytial Virus

Envelope (host cell membrane derived)
  Matrix (M), 28 kDa
  Large glycoprotein (G), 90 kDa
  Fusion protein (F), 70 kDa
    F_1 subunit, 50 kDa
    F_2 subunit, 20 kDa
  Other, 22 kDa
Internal viral nucleocapsid (RNA)
  Nucleoprotein (NP), 42 kDa
  Phosphoprotein (P), 34 kDa
  Large protein (L), 200 kDa
Other proteins
  Virion-associated (1A), 9.5 kDa
  Nonstructural
    1B, 11 kDa
    1C, 14 kDa

TABLE 246.2. Survival of Respiratory Syncytial Virus in Patients' Secretions on Fomites

Object inoculated	Time until no virus recoverable (h)
Skin	0.5
Cloth	1
Paper tissue	1
Gloves	2
Countertop	7

Data from Hall CB, Douglas RG Jr, Geiman JM. Possible transmission by fomites of respiratory syncytial virus. *J Infect Dis* 1980;141:98–102.

virus but that some variability in the antigenic structure of the G protein is evident among different strains (11). On the basis of this type of analysis, two distinct subtypes of human RSV have been identified—subtype A and subtype B (12). It has also been demonstrated that the degree of antigenic relatedness between the G proteins of the two subgroups is only about 5% whereas the relatedness between the fusion (F) proteins of the two subgroups is nearly 50% (13). A further analysis of strains within each subgroup was carried out by determining the antigenic characteristics and size of structural proteins of 20 subgroup A and 43 subgroup B strains. Subgroup A strains are relatively uniform, whereas subgroup B strains vary to a much greater extent and have tentatively been divided into 131 and B2 variants on the basis of differences residing principally in the G and P proteins (14). The clinical significance of this degree of antigenic variability is unknown. That is, it has not yet been demonstrated that individuals infected with one subtype are either more or less resistant to reinfections with the other subtype.

EPIDEMIOLOGY

Distribution

Serologic surveys from essentially all areas of the world indicate that infection with RSV occurs commonly in all geographic and climatic areas (15). In the United States and other countries in the temperate zones, sharp annual outbreaks of RSV occur during the colder months, in both the Northern and the Southern hemispheres (16–18). It is apparent that both subtype A and subtype B strains may be present simultaneously or follow each other by several weeks in one epidemic season (19–21). In the tropics and subtropical areas, outbreaks of RSV may be spread over several months and have less obvious peaks of activity. Interestingly, outbreaks in these areas occur during the hotter rainy seasons (22). This peculiar epidemiologic pattern may be related to an increased amount of time spent indoors and to greater crowding during cold or rainy seasons. Other attempts to explain the onset and termination of RSV outbreaks on the basis of climatic conditions, such as temperature and hours of sunlight, have been generally unsuccessful (23).

Prevalence

Most estimates of the prevalence of RSV infection have used hospitalization rates for bronchiolitis caused by RSV as the principal indicator of disease activity. This is because RSV infections

in older persons are generally, but certainly not always, mild enough that they do not require medical attention. The risk of hospitalization for RSV bronchiolitis in infancy has been estimated to be between one and seven per thousand (15,24,25). Increased rates of hospitalization are observed in younger infants and those from lower socioeconomic circumstances. In one study, the rate of hospitalization for RSV infection of infants 1 to 3 months old in industrialized areas was 24.5 per thousand (26). Estimates of the frequency with which RSV infects older persons are not easily obtained.

Among children in daycare centers, 75% were reinfected during their second exposure to virus in the classroom, and 65% were infected during the third exposure (27). Adults are readily infected when RSV is introduced into a household (28) or during occupational exposure to infants with RSV (29). Serologic evidence of previous RSV infection is almost uniform among older children and adults (30,31), suggesting that reinfection occurs with sufficient frequency to maintain serum antibody titers at high levels.

Transmission

RSV is spread by self-inoculation after contact with virus, in secretions or on fomites, and possibly by large-droplet inoculation. In one study, five of seven persons who had direct physical contact with infected infants for 2 to 4 hours became infected, whereas none of 14 persons who sat at a distance of 6 feet or more from an infant's bed for 3 hours became infected. Ten other volunteers entered a patient's room only after the infant had been removed and then touched the bed and other objects that had been contaminated with secretions. Four of them became infected after touching the mucous membranes of their nose or eyes upon leaving the room (29). Despite its reputation as an extraordinarily labile virus, RSV is capable of surviving on hands and inanimate objects as long as several hours after inoculation (12) (Table 246.2).

PATHOGENESIS

Antibody-Mediated Immunity

Antibody responses in the immunoglobulin (1g) G, IgM, and IgA isotypes develop in serum and secretions after primary RSV infection (33,34). In some studies (35), the appearance of secretory IgA antibody to RSV in the nasopharynx was associated with termination of virus shedding, while in another study (34) antibody was present in the respiratory tract at a time when virus shedding would be expected to be ongoing. Therefore, the role of secretory antibody in termination of RSV infection remains controversial.

Repeated infections with RSV result in progressively milder forms of clinical illness (27), suggesting that some component of the immune system may provide partial protection against reinfection. Secretory antibody responses have been shown to be enhanced after secondary RSV infection (34). Because virus shedding decreases with repeated infection, it may be true that enhanced secretory antibody responses with repeated infection account for partial immunity seen in older individuals. In addition, there is a correlation between the quantity of serum antibody acquired transplacentally and protection against illness caused by RSV infection in the first few months of life (25). Nevertheless, infection occurs readily in the presence of reasonably large quantities of antibody acquired transplacentally or from a previous infection (25,30,31). The method by which RSV escapes neutralization by preexisting antibody is unclear. Subtype differences in RSV do not completely account for this phenomenon, because consecutive infections with virus strains of the same subtype have also been observed (36).

The development of RSV specific IgE antibody has been demonstrated in both the nasopharyngeal secretions and the serum of infants with acute RSV infection. Titers of this antibody were significantly higher in patients with wheezing than in patients who had RSV infection without wheezing (37,38), and the titer seemed to correlate with the severity of illness (37). Airway obstruction may be related to the IgE-directed release of chemical mediators that cause bronchoconstriction or excessive mucus secretion, such as histamine (37) or leukotriene C4 (39). Alternatively, the detection of RSV-specific IgE antibody may be an indication of a quantitatively greater overall immune response in certain individuals.

Cell-Mediated Immunity

Cell-mediated immune mechanisms presumably play a role in limiting RSV infection, because it has been shown that RSV infections are particularly prolonged or severe in persons who have defects of cell-mediated immunity (40,41). In contrast, cell-mediated immune hypersensitivity, whether a result of previous immunization with inactivated vaccines (42) or natural infection (43) has been associated with more severe forms of illness. RSV-specific cytotoxic T lymphocytes have been demonstrated, and their role in termination or enhancement of infection remains to be determined (44,45). These RSV specific cells seem to recognize several different viral proteins, including nucleoprotein, which are thought to be constant between different strains. Specific T cells may therefore be able to respond equally to infection with different viral subtypes (46).

Asthma is characterized by the production of interleukins 4 and 5, which promote many of the characteristic immune changes seen in asthma (47). RSV infection is also associated with IgE responses, eosinophil degranulation and the release of mediators such as histamine and leukotrienes in secretions at the time of infection. However the immune pathway leading to these changes appears to be different in RSV infection than in asthma (48).

Other Defense Mechanisms

Cells infected with RSV have been shown to activate the complement cascade as well as neutrophil-mediated cytotoxicity mechanisms (49,50). The role of these mechanisms in limiting infection or in disease pathogenesis is unknown at present.

CLINICAL MANIFESTATIONS

The major clinical manifestations associated with RSV infection are shown in Table 246.3.

TABLE 246.3. Major Clinical Syndromes Associated with Respiratory Syncytial Virus Infection

Bronchiolitis in infancy
Asthma in children and adults
Pneumonia
Croup
Otitis media
Apnea in early infancy
Sudden infant death syndrome

Bronchiolitis

The most common form of severe illness caused by RSV infection is bronchiolitis. This illness most frequently affects infants from 2 to 6 months old, infrequently younger ones, and is progressively less frequent after 6 months of age. Illness generally begins with symptoms of mild upper respiratory tract infection, with progression of cough and the development of wheezing. Fever is usually of low grade, but dyspnea and respiratory distress may be quite prominent. Auscultation of the chest reveals coarse inspiratory rales with rhonchi and wheezing on expiration. Significant hypoxemia may be present. Clinical improvement usually occurs in 3 to 4 days despite continued virus shedding. Fatalities are extremely uncommon (probably fewer than 500 fatal cases annually in the United States) (51,52) with good supportive care and in the absence of underlying cardiac or pulmonary disease (53), in which fatality rates may approach 3% to 5%. Recurrent episodes of wheezing (resulting from repeated RSV infection and other causes) occur commonly throughout infancy and early childhood, and evidence of pulmonary dysfunction has frequently been demonstrated on long-term follow-up of patients who had bronchiolitis in infancy (54,55). Whether these long-term abnormalities are the result of damage to the airway at a critical time in development or a manifestation, an immunologic alteration resulting in greater allergic responses to environmental antigens, or an inborn tendency toward small-airway dysfunction that is first signaled by the development of RSV bronchiolitis remains uncertain.

Pneumonia

RSV has been implicated as a frequent cause of pneumonia in infants and young children, particularly in those admitted to the hospital. Curves reflecting the incidence of pneumonia in infants and young children parallel the seasonal incidence of bronchiolitis as well as the frequency of isolation of RSV from inpatients. In fact, pneumonia and bronchiolitis are often diagnosed concurrently and are difficult to separate clinically in RSV infected infants (56).

Although RSV pneumonia is a rare event in immunocompetent older children and adults, it is becoming recognized as an important problem in recipients of organ transplantation (57). Prolonged shedding of the virus is the rule, and some deaths appear to have been caused by RSV pneumonia in this population.

Croup

RSV can be recovered from approximately 10% of children with croup, especially during the first few years of life (58). Croup caused by RSV may be milder in nature but otherwise indistinguishable from croup caused by the parainfluenza viruses, which are the most common causes of this illness.

Otitis Media

Viral agents are rarely recovered from the middle-ear cavities of children with acute otitis media, although this may be because viruses are responsible only for obstruction of the eustachian tube without direct invasion of the middle-ear cavity. In children who have acute otitis media during the RSV season, evidence of concurrent RSV infection has been found in up to 40% of cases (59).

Apnea

Infants younger than 6 months old who have RSV infection may present with apnea early in the course of illness. It has been demonstrated that apnea caused by RSV may be followed by mild upper respiratory tract infection alone, or lower respiratory tract disease may develop later (60). In our experience, RSV may be recovered from the respiratory tract of infants who present with idiopathic apnea in the total absence of any symptoms of respiratory infection.

Sudden Infant Death Syndrome

RSV and other viral agents may be identified in the lungs of as many as 30% of infants with sudden infant death syndrome. It is unclear how fairly minor infections with these agents may contribute to the development of sudden infant death (61).

Clinical Course

As noted previously, most RSV infections resolve spontaneously or with supportive therapy during several days. Infections that are more severe or more persistent may occur in immunocompromised children (41) and adults (62) or in infants with bronchopulmonary dysplasia (63) or cyanotic congenital heart disease (64). Even in otherwise healthy adults, RSV infection may result in pneumonia (65), primary episodes of obstructive airway disease, and abnormalities on pulmonary function tests that may last for up to 8 weeks after infection (66). Studies performed on institutionalized adults or those in adult day care situations indicate that as much as 5% of community-acquired pneumonia (including that resulting in hospitalization) is due to RSV infection (67).

LABORATORY FINDINGS

The results of routine laboratory investigations are so nonspecific in RSV infection as to be useless in identifying a specific agent. The usual findings at chest radiography include diffusely increased interstitial markings, areas of consolidation, which may vary considerably in size, and, most consistently, hyperinflation (68,69). The presence of wheezing clinically, and diffuse interstitial infiltrates with hyperinflation radiographically, often makes it possible to distinguish RSV pneumonia from bacterial pneumonia.

DIAGNOSIS

The specific diagnosis of RSV infection is best made by isolation of the virus in tissue culture, by detection of viral antigen in exfoliated airway cells or secretions, or by specific serologic procedures.

Cell Culture

RSV can be recognized in cell culture by the formation of characteristic syncytia. These may be evident as early as a few days after inoculation of cell culture if conditions are optimal (70). Maximal sensitivity is achieved by using low-passage human epithelial (HEp-2) cell lines. RSV is recovered much more frequently if clinical specimens are obtained by nasal washing or aspiration than if throat swabs or nasopharyngeal swabs are used (71).

Shell vial procedures have replaced standard cell culture techniques in many diagnostic laboratories. Samples of respiratory secretions are centrifuged (700X) onto monolayers of culture cells in tubes, fresh medium is added, and the cell sheet is examined at various intervals for a cytopathic effect. The cell sheet can also be stained using immunofluorescence techniques for RSV antigen (72,73). In general, shell vial assays have proved to be as accurate as cell culture, with results available in 1 to 2 days, compared with an average of 4 to 5 days for cell culture. Cell culture using a variety of cell lines may identify the presence of other viral agents more frequently (Table 246.4).

Rapid Diagnostic Tests

ANTIGEN DETECTION TECHNIQUES

The diagnosis of RSV infection has been greatly facilitated by the development of rapid diagnostic tests for identification of viral antigen in nasopharyngeal secretions, in bronchoalveolar lavage specimens, or in tissues obtained by biopsy or at autopsy. The accuracy of several commercially available kits that use indirect immunofluorescence, ELISA, or enzyme immunoassay procedures, is shown in Table 246.5. When compared with cell culture, there are probably no major differences in the sensitivity and specificity of each of these kits for diagnosis of RSV infection. There is considerable evidence that the rapid diagnostic assays are, in fact, far more sensitive for the detection of RSV infection than cell culture or shell vial assays (70,74–76). This is because as much as 40% of infectivity of a specimen may be lost even during storage in transport media at 4°C (72) and because antigen detection assays can still identify viral antigen in secretions or on the surface of exfoliated epithelial cells obtained several days into the course of illness, at a time when virus is no longer being shed. In the vast majority of instances when antigen detection assays yield positive results and the virus isolation assay is negative, appropriate blocking experiments have confirmed that positive results in antigen detection techniques represent true positive findings (74–76). It should be noted that specimens obtained by nasopharyngeal aspiration also yield positive results by antigen detection techniques more commonly than specimens obtained by swabbing (77).

Commercially available kits often employ monoclonal antibodies as the detector antibody, because the background reactivity is quite low using monoclonal, versus polyclonal, antibodies. Some concern has arisen that highly specific monoclonal antibodies might not have broad enough reactivity to identify antigenically variant strains of RSV; however, antigen detection kits that utilize pools of monoclonal antibodies to RSV containing antibodies to the fusion (F) protein and nucleoprotein react quite well with strains from either nucleoprotein subtype A or B (77).

POLYMERASE CHAIN REACTION TECHNOLOGY

The polymerase chain reaction technique has also been adapted for the diagnosis of RSV infection (78). A reverse transcription method proved to be approximately as sensitive and specific

TABLE 246.4. Features of Various Diagnostic Tests for Respiratory Syncytial Virus Infection

Technique	Time until definitive result	Comment
Antigen detection using enzyme immunoassay or immunofluorescence	Several hours	Fastest and most sensitive assays False-positive results must be excluded Live virus not required
Polymerase chain reaction	4–12 h	Approximately as sensitive as cell culture
Shell vial assays	16–10 h	As accurate as cell culture, with earlier availability of results False-negative results later in illness Specimens must be handled carefully and promptly to avoid loss of infectivity
Cell culture	4–5 d on average	Highest specificity Identifies the presence of viruses other than respiratory syncytial virus Specimens must be handled carefully and promptly to avoid loss of infectivity

as conventional cell culture. Results were available with polymerase chain reaction in 8 to 24 hours, versus several days for cell culture. The polymerase chain reaction assay amplified a 243-base pair segment of the genome that codes for the F, subunit of the fusion protein, which is identical in subtype A and B strains. The lower limit of detection was ten median tissue culture infectious doses. In general, PCR has not proved superior to other methods of detecting the presence of RSV in infants, although PCR may be considerably more sensitive in older children and adults.

Serologic Diagnosis

A variety of serologic techniques have been used in attempts to diagnose RSV infection. Of these, complement fixation techniques have been shown to be insensitive to RSV infection in infants, the age group in which the most severe form of illness occurs (79). Immunofluorescence can be adapted to demonstrate RSV specific responses in the IgG, IgM, and IgA isotypes, and increased sensitivity of the immunofluorescent technique in comparison with complement fixation techniques has been demonstrated in the diagnosis of RSV infection in infancy (79). ELISAs have also been used to determine isotype-specific antibody responses to RSV. Although extensive evaluations have not been carried out, the sensitivity of ELISAs in infancy appears to be greater than that of complement fixation assays and

approximately equal to that of immunofluorescent assays. Neutralization assays using standard techniques have approximately the same sensitivity as ELISA or immunofluorescent assays (80). Complement-enhanced neutralization assays (80) are probably the most sensitive method for detection of RSV antibody in general use, but all neutralization assays have the disadvantage of being tedious and they also do not provide information on isotype-specific responses.

None of the foregoing assay systems yields evidence of seroconversion to RSV reliably in patients in the age group at which serious RSV infections occur most commonly, that is, 1 to 3 months. Each is probably equally useful in diagnosis of RSV infection in older children and adults.

Differential Diagnosis

Illness caused by RSV does not seem to be clinically distinguishable from that related to infections caused by other viruses (81,82), with the exception that the most severe forms of bronchiolitis are almost always associated with RSV infection. Parainfluenza and influenza virus bronchiolitis most closely mimics the severity of RSV-related disease, although respiratory failure in bronchiolitis is almost never caused by infection with these agents. It is nearly impossible to distinguish RSV bronchiolitis from the first episode of true infantile asthma. In fact, RSV infection may provoke the first asthmatic episode in many children.

TABLE 246.5. Accuracy of Commercial Rapid Diagnostic Kits for Identification of Respiratory Syncytial Virus Infection

Technique	Manufacturer	Sensitivity (%)[a]	Specificity (%)[a]	Reference
IFA	Burroughs-Wellcome	92[b]	94	65
IFA	Burroughs-Wellcome	61	89	72
ELISA	Ortho	88[c]	94	71
ELISA	Ortho	69	100	72
EIA	Abbott	96[c]	96	70
EIA	Abbott	88	95	69

IFA, Indirect immunofluorescence assay; ELISA, enzyme-linked immunosorbent assay; EIA, enzyme immunoassay.
[a]Versus tissue culture.
[b]Immunofluorescence performed on tissue culture to confirm IFA-positive, culture-negative tests as true-positive results.
[c]Blocking assays used to confirm ELISA or EIA-positive, culture-negative result.

TREATMENT

Specific Antiviral Therapy

Ribavirin is a synthetic nucleoside that possesses *in vitro* antiviral properties against a variety of RNA and DNA viruses. When given by aerosol to infants with RSV infection, ribavirin has been associated with more rapid improvement in clinical illness scores and in oxygenation when compared with those of patients inhaling water as a control (83,84). Although there was initially some concern that ribavirin, because of its tendency to precipitate in the circuits of mechanical ventilators, could not be used to treat infants who needed mechanically assisted ventilation, the drug can nevertheless be administered safely to such patients provided that filters are placed and changed appropriately in the ventilatory circuits (85).

The adequacy of the experimental design and methods of data evaluation in studies of the efficacy of ribavirin have been challenged (86). The greatest benefit of ribavirin therapy was reported in a study of infants and young children who required mechanically assisted ventilation because of RSV infection (87). In this study, in which water was used as the placebo, the time of ventilation and the duration of oxygen therapy were reduced by approximately one half in ribavirin recipients. Nevertheless, inhalation of water may cause bronchospasm or changes in diffusion capacity. A second study, using saline as a placebo, showed only slight differences favoring ribavirin use, which were not statistically significant (88). Most studies have demonstrated a mild degree of improvement when ribavirin is administered early in the course of infection. Given the limited benefits and high costs of ribavirin, it should be used for only the most seriously ill infants with respiratory failure, if it is to be used at all. The effectiveness of ribavirin in transplant recipients who have RSV pneumonia has not been studied adequately.

Nonspecific Therapy

Most patients hospitalized for mild-to-moderate forms of RSV infection recover within a few days with supportive therapy alone. This includes administration of supplemental oxygen and replacement of fluid deficits. Unfortunately, there is not much to offer those with more severe forms of RSV infection. Despite continuing controversy, there is little convincing evidence that aerosolized bronchodilators (89–910), theophylline (92), or corticosteroids (93) are beneficial to the majority of patients with bronchiolitis. A small percentage of infants with bronchiolitis may respond favorably to the first dose of aerosol therapy with β-adrenergic agents, but it appears impossible to identify them in advance. Repeated doses do not produce the same beneficial response.

PREVENTION

Nosocomial Infection

Hospital-acquired RSV infections are common on pediatric wards. Although these infections are usually not severe, they often prolong hospital stays unnecessarily. Occasionally, however, severe or fatal illness does occur (94,95). Hospital staff play a significant role in the spread of these infections. The use of protective coverings such as gowns, masks, and goggles has not been effective in reducing the rate of infection of health care workers (96,97). Adequate protection of patients and medical staff from nosocomial infection can be attained by compliance with simple hand-washing procedures that remove RSV from the hands of health care providers (98,99).

Immunization

ACTIVE

There is a clear need for effective immunoprophylaxis of RSV infection both in the United States and throughout the world. Because the major impact of the virus is expressed during the first half-year of life, programs for immunization against RSV face the considerable challenges of developing a vaccine that can be given in a single dose and is safe for this quite young, relatively unstable population. Prevention of spread of infection to infants might seem achievable by vaccination of adults and older children, but reinfection is common in these age groups, even in the presence of preexisting immunity. In all likelihood, secondary spread to infants could not be prevented.

A formalin-inactivated RSV vaccine evaluated in the 1960s did not provide protection against infection, and actually enhanced disease in many vaccine recipients (100). The focus of RSV vaccine development therefore switched to the development of live, attenuated vaccines. Temperature-sensitive mutant strains of RSV were produced, with the expectation that virus could grow at the relatively lower temperature of the nasopharynx but not in the lungs. Infection of seronegative children with these candidate vaccines resulted in shedding of virus strains that had reverted back to the virulent (wild-type) strains, and otitis media occurred in some recipients (101). Investigation of live vaccines with further mutations inducing temperature-sensitivity is in progress, although the use of these live vaccines is made more difficult by the variable amounts of maternal antibody present in the serum of infants (102).

An inactivated vaccine consisting of purified preparations of the RSV F protein or attachment protein has been under investigation in humans. Adequate responses developed in seropositive children 18 to 36 months of age but not in younger infants (103). Another strategy being evaluated is that of immunizing women in the third trimester of pregnancy with inactivated RSV vaccines, to enhance the titer of antibody crossing the placenta to the infant. A variety of nucleic acid vaccines, animal strains of RSV, human strains with gene deletions and subunit vaccines also are under investigation, but the development of a safe and effective vaccine is not imminent.

Neutralizing antibody induced by natural infection (and antibody against either the F or attachment glycoprotein) does not provide complete protection against infection (104). The contribution of cell-mediated immunity to protection against infection is unknown. Further information about the exact mechanism of resistance to RSV infection may be required before an effective vaccine can be developed.

PASSIVE

An interesting development is the use of a hyperimmune human globulin (105) and a monoclonal antibody against the fusion protein (106) in the prevention of RSV infection in infants and children with a history of premature birth, lung disease of prematurity and, perhaps, congenital heart disease. These children are at high risk for severe illness at the time of RSV infection. Extensive studies indicate that the rate of hospitalization of infants with these high-risk conditions is reduced by approximately 50% when either of these compounds is administered throughout the RSV epidemic season (105,106). The use of standard intravenous immune globulin preparations is not effective.

REFERENCES

1. Kingsbury DW, Bratt MA, Choppin PW, et al. Paramyxoviridae. *Intervirology* 1978;10:137.
2. Berthiaume L, Joncas J, Pavilanis V. Comparative structure, morphogenesis and biological characteristics of the respiratory syncytial virus and the pneumonia virus of mice (PVM). *Arch Gesamte Virusforsch* 1974;45:39.
3. Huang YT, Collins PL, Wertz GW. Characterization of the 10 proteins of human respiratory syncytial virus: identification of a fourth envelope-associated protein. *Virus Res* 1985;2:157.
4. Routledge EG, Willcocks MM, Morgan L, et al. Expression of the respiratory syncytial virus 22K protein on the surface of infected HeLa cells. *J Gen Virol* 1987;68:1217.
5. Ueba O. Respiratory syncytial virus. II. Isolation and morphology of the glycoproteins. *Acta Med Okayama* 1980;34:245.
6. Gruber C, Levine S. Respiratory syncytial virus polypeptides. III. The envelope-associated proteins. *J Gen Virol* 1983;64:825.
7. Levine S, Klaiber-Franco R, Paradiso PR. Demonstration that glycoprotein G is the attachment protein of respiratory syncytial virus. *J Gen Virol* 1987;68:2521.
8. Levine S, Peeples M, Hamilton R. Effective respiratory syncytial virus infection of HeLa cells macro-molecular synthesis. *J Gen Virol* 1977;37:53.
9. Lambert DM, Pons MW, Mbuy GN, et al. Nucleic acids of respiratory syncytial virus. *J Virol* 1980;36:837.
10. Coates HV, Aping DW, Channock RM. An antigenic analysis of respiratory syncytial virus isolates by a plaque reduction neutralization test. *Am J Epidemiol* 1966;83:299.
11. Anderson LJ, Hierholzer JC, Tsou C, et al. Antigenic characterization of respiratory syncytial virus strains with monoclonal antibodies. *J Infect Dis* 1985;151:626.
12. Mufson MA, Orvell C, Rafnar B, et al. Two distinct subtypes of human respiratory syncytial virus. *J Gen Virol* 1985;66:2111.
13. Johnson PR Jr, Olmsted RA, Prince GA, et al. Antigenic relatedness between the glycoproteins of human respiratory syncytial virus subgroups A and B: evaluation of the contributions of F and G glycoproteins to immunity. *J Virol* 1987;61:3163.
14. Akerlind B, Norrby E, Orvell C, et al. Respiratory syncytial virus: heterogeneity of subgroup B strains. *J Gen Virol* 1988;69:2145.
15. Channock RM, Kim HW, Brandt CD, et al. Respiratory syncytial virus. In: Evans AS, ed. *Viral infections of humans, epidemiology and control*, 2nd ed. New York: Plenum, 1983:471–490.
16. Kim HW, Arrobio JA, Brandt CD, et al. Epidemiology of respiratory syncytial virus infection in Washington, DC. *Am J Epidemiol* 1973;98:216.
17. Florman AL, McLaren LC. The effect of altitude and weather on the occurrence of outbreaks of respiratory syncytial virus infections. *J Infect Dis* 1988;158:1401.
18. DeSilva LM, Hanlon MG. Respiratory syncytial virus: a report of a 5 year study at a children's hospital. *J Med Virol* 1986;19:299.
19. Mufson MA, Belshe RB, Orvell C, et al. Respiratory syncytial virus epidemics: Variable dominance of subgroups A and B strains among children, 1981–1986. *J Infect Dis* 1988;157:143.
20. Akerlind B, Norrby E. Occurrence of respiratory syncytial virus subtypes A and B strains in Sweden. *J Med Virol* 1986;19:241.
21. Hendry RM, Talis AL, Godfrey E, et al. Concurrent circulation of antigenically distinct strains of respiratory syncytial virus during community outbreaks. *J Infect Dis* 1986;153:291.
22. Spence L, Barratt N. Respiratory syncytial virus associated with acute respiratory infections in Trinidadian patients. *Am J Epidemiol* 1968;88:256.
23. Sung RYT, Murray HGS, Chan RCK, et al. Seasonal patterns of respiratory syncytial virus infection in Hong Kong: a preliminary report. *J Infect Dis* 1987;156:527.
24. Glezen WP. Pathogenesis of bronchiolitis—epidemiologic considerations. *Pediatr Res* 1977;11:239.
25. Glezen WP, Paredes A, Allison JE, et al. Risk of respiratory syncytial virus infection for infants from low-income families in relationship to age, sex, ethnic group, and maternal antibody level. *J Pediatr* 1981;98:708.
26. Respiratory syncytial virus infection: Admissions to hospital in industrial, urban, and rural areas. Report to the Medical Research Council Subcommittee on Respiratory Syncytial Virus Vaccines. *BMJ* 1978;2:796.
27. Henderson FW, Collier AM, Clyde WA Jr, et al. Respiratory syncytial virus infections, reinfections and immunity. *N Engl J Med* 1979;300:530.
28. Hall CB, Geiman JM, Biggar R, et al. Respiratory syncytial virus infections within families. *N Engl J Med* 1976;294:414.
29. Hall CB, Douglas RG Jr. Modes of transmission of respiratory syncytial virus. *J Pediatr* 1981;99:100.
30. Beem M, Egerer R, Anderson J. Respiratory syncytial virus neutralizing antibodies in persons residing in Chicago, Illinois. *Pediatrics* 1964;34:761.
31. Johnson KM, Bloom HH, Mufson MA, et al. Natural reinfection of adults by respiratory syncytial virus. *N Engl J Med* 1962;267:68.
32. Hall CB, Douglas RG Jr, Geiman JM. Possible transmission by fomites of respiratory syncytial virus. *J Infect Dis* 1980;141:98.
33. Welliver RC, Kaul TN, Putnam TI, et al. The antibody response to primary and secondary infection with respiratory syncytial virus: kinetics of class-specific responses. *J Pediatr* 1980;96:808.
34. Kaul TN, Welliver RC, Wong DT, et al. Secretory antibody response to respiratory syncytial virus infection. *Am J Dis Child* 1981;135:1013.
35. McIntosh K. Interferon in nasal secretions from infants with viral respiratory tract infections. *J Pediatr* 1978;93:33.
36. Mufson MA, Belshe RB, Orvell C, et al. Subgroup characteristics of respiratory syncytial virus strains recovered from children with two consecutive infections. *J Clin Microbiol* 1987;25:1535.
37. Welliver RC, Wong DT, Sun M, et al. The development of respiratory syncytial virus-specific IgE and the release of histamine in nasopharyngeal secretions after infection. *N Engl J Med* 1981;305:841.
38. Bui RHD, Monilaro GA, Kettering JD, et al. Virus-specific IgE and IgG4 antibodies in serum of children infected with respiratory syncytial virus. *J Pediatr* 1987;110:87.
39. Volovitz B, Welliver RC, DeCastro G, et al. The release of leukotrienes in the respiratory tract during infection with respiratory syncytial virus: role in obstructive airway disease. *Pediatr Res* 1988;24:504.
40. Fishaut M, Tubergen D, McIntosh K. Cellular response to respiratory viruses with particular reference to children with disorders of cell-mediated immunity. *J Pediatr* 1980;96:179.
41. Hall CB, Powell KR, MacDonald NE, et al. Respiratory syncytial viral infection in children with compromised immune function. *N Engl J Med* 1986;315:77.
42. Kim HW, Leikin SL, Arrobio J, et al. Cell-mediated immunity to respiratory syncytial virus induced by inactivated vaccine or by infection. *Pediatr Res* 1976;10:75.
43. Welliver RC, Kaul A, Ogra PL. Cell-mediated immune response to respiratory syncytial virus infection: relationship to the development of reactive airway disease. *J Pediatr* 1979;94:370.
44. Bangham CRM, McMichael AJ. Specific human cytotoxic T cells recognize B-cell lines persistently infected with respiratory syncytial virus. *Proc Natl Acad Sci USA* 1986;83:9183.
45. Isaacs D, Bangham CRM, McMichael AJ. Cell-mediated cytotoxic response to respiratory syncytial virus in infants with bronchiolitis. *Lancet* 1987;2:769.
46. Bangham CRM, Openshaw PJM, Ball LA, et al. Human and murine cytotoxic T cells specific to respiratory syncytial virus recognize the viral nucleoprotein (N), but not the major glycoprotein (G), expressed by vaccinia virus recombinants. *J Immunol* 1986;137:3973.
47. Robinson DS, Hamid Q, Ying S, et al. Predominant TH2-like bronchoalveolar T-lymphocyte population in atopic asthma. *N Engl J Med* 1992;326:298–304.
48. Garofalo RP, Patti J, Hintz KA, et al. Macrophage inflammatory protein-1α (not T helper type 2 cytokines) is associated with severe forms of respiratory syncytial virus bronchiolitis. *J Infect Dis* 2001;184:393–399.
49. Kaul TN, Faden H, Baker R, et al. Virus-induced complement activation and neutrophil-mediated cytotoxicity against respiratory syncytial virus (RSV). *Clin Exp Immunol* 1984;56:501.
50. Smith TH, McIntosh K, Fishaut M, et al. Activation of complement by cells infected with respiratory syncytial virus. *Infect Immun* 1981;33:43.
51. Shay DK, Holman RC, Newman RD, et al. Bronchiolitis-associated hospitalizations among US children, 1980–1996. *JAMA* 1999;282:1440–1446.
52. Shay DK, Holman RC, Roosevelt GE, et al. Bronchiolitis-associated mortality and estimates of respiratory syncytial virus-associated deaths among US children, 1979–1997. *J Infect Dis* 2001;183:16–22.
53. Wohl MEB, Chernick V. Bronchiolitis. *Am Rev Respir Dis* 1978;118:759.
54. Gurwitz D, Mindorff C, Levison H. Increased incidence of bronchio-reactivity in children with a history of bronchiolitis. *J Pediatr* 1981;98:551.
55. Kattan M, Keenes TG, Lapierre JG, et al. Pulmonary function abnormalities in symptom-free children after bronchiolitis. *Pediatrics* 1977;59:683.
56. Murphy TF, Henderson FW, Clyde WA Jr, et al. Pneumonia: an 11 year study in a pediatric practice. *Am J Epidemiol* 1981;113:12.
57. Whimbey E, Champlin RE, Couch RB, et al. Community respiratory virus infections among hospitalized adult bone marrow transplant recipients. *Clin Infect Dis* 1996;22:778.
58. Denny FW, Murphy TF, Clyde WA Jr, et al. Croup: an 11 year study in a pediatric practice. *Pediatrics* 1983;71:871.
59. Berglund B, Salmivalli A, Toivanen P, et al. Isolation of respiratory syncytial virus from middle ear exudates of infants. *Arch Dis Child* 1966;41:554.
60. Bruhn FW, Mokrohisky ST, McIntosh K. Apnea associated with respiratory syncytial virus infection in young infants. *J Pediatr* 1977;90:382.
61. Uren EC, Williams AL, Jack I, et al. Association of respiratory virus infection with sudden infant death syndrome. *Med J Aust* 1980;1:417.
62. Englund JA, Sullivan CJ, Jordan MC, et al. Respiratory syncytial virus infection in immunocompromised adults. *Ann Intern Med* 1988;109:203.
63. Groothuis JR, Gutierrez KM, Lauer BA. Respiratory syncytial virus infection in children with bronchopulmonary dysplasia. *Pediatrics* 1988;82:199.
64. MacDonald NE, Hall CB, Suffin SC, et al. Respiratory syncytial viral infection in infants with congenital heart disease. *N Engl J Med* 1982;307:397.
65. Vikerfors T, Grandien M, Olcen P. Respiratory syncytial virus infections in adults. *Am Rev Respir Dis* 1987;136:561.
66. Hall WJ, Hall CB, Speers DM. Respiratory syncytial virus infection in adults: clinical, virologic and serial pulmonary function studies. *Ann Intern Med* 1978;88:203.
67. Falsey AR, Cunningham CK, Barker WH, et al. Respiratory syncytial virus and influenza A infections in the hospitalized elderly. *J Infect Dis* 1995;172:389–394.

68. Simpson W, Hacking PM, Court SDM, et al. The radiologic findings in respiratory syncytial virus infection in children. II. The correlation of radiological categories with clinical and virological findings. *Pediatr Radiol* 1974;2: 155.

69. Rice RP, Loda F. A roentgenographic analysis of respiratory syncytial virus pneumonia in infants. *Radiology* 1966;87:1021.

70. Kaul A, Scott R, Gallagher M, et al. Respiratory syncytial virus infection: rapid diagnosis in children by use of indirect immunofluorescence. *Am J Dis Child* 1978;132:1088.

71. Treuhaft MW, Soukup JM, Sullivan BJ. Practical recommendations for the detection of pediatric respiratory virus infections. *J Clin Microbiol* 1985;22: 270.

72. Smith MC, Creutz C, Huang YT. Detection of respiratory syncytial virus in nasopharyngeal secretions by shell vial technique. *J Clin Microbiol* 1991;29: 463.

73. Pedneault L, Robillard L, Turgeon JP. Validation of respiratory syncytial virus enzyme immunoassay and shell vial assay results. *J Clin Microbiol* 1994;32:2861.

74. Swenson PD, Kaplan MH. Rapid detection of respiratory syncytial virus in nasopharyngeal aspirates by a commercial enzyme immunoassay. *J Clin Microbiol* 1986;23:485.

75. Bromberg K, Tannis G, Daidone B, et al. Comparison of HEp-2 cell culture and Abbot respiratory syncytial virus enzyme immunoassay. *J Clin Microbiol* 1987;24:434.

76. Lauer BA, Masters HA, Wren CG, et al. Rapid detection of respiratory syncytial virus in nasopharyngeal secretions by enzyme-linked immunosorbent assay. *J Clin Microbiol* 1985;22:782.

77. Ahluwalia G, Embree J, McNicol P, et al. Comparison of nasopharyngeal aspirate and nasopharyngeal swab specimens for respiratory syncytial virus diagnosis by cell culture, indirect immunofluorescence assay, and enzyme-linked immunosorbent assay. *J Clin Microbiol* 1987;25: 763.

78. Gottschalk J, Zbinden R, Kaempf L, Heinzer I. Discrimination of respiratory syncytial virus subgroups A and B by reverse transcription-PCR. *J Clin Microbiol* 1996;34:41.

79. Richardson LS, Yolken RH, Belshe RB, et al. Enzyme-linked immunosorbent assay for measurement of serologic response to respiratory syncytial virus infection. *Infect Immun* 1978;20:660.

80. Kaul TN, Welliver RC, Ogra PL. Comparison of fluorescent antibody, neutralizing antibody, and complement-enhanced neutralizing antibody assays for detection of serum antibody to respiratory syncytial virus. *J Clin Microbiol* 1981;13:957.

81. Valenti WM, Clarke TA, Hall CB, et al. Concurrent outbreaks of rhinovirus and respiratory syncytial virus in an intensive care nursery: epidemiology and associated risk factors. *J Pediatr* 1982;100:722.

82. Caul EO, Waller DK, Clarke SKR. A comparison of influenza and respiratory syncytial virus infections among infants admitted to hospital with acute respiratory infections. *J Hyg (Lond)* 1976;77:383.

83. Hall CB, McBride JT, Walsh EE, et al. Aerosolized ribavirin treatment of infants with respiratory syncytial viral infection. *N Engl J Med* 1983;308: 1443.

84. Rodriguez WJ, Kim HW, Brandt CD, et al. Aerosolized ribavirin in the treatment of patients with respiratory syncytial virus disease. *Pediatr Infect Dis J* 1987;6:159.

85. Outwater KM, Meissner C, Peterson MB. Ribavirin administration to infants receiving mechanical ventilation. *Am J Dis Child* 1988;142:512.

86. Wald ER, Dashefsky B, Green M. In re ribavirin: a case of premature adjudication? *J Pediatr* 1988;112:154.

87. Smith DW, Frankel LIZ, Mathers LH, et al. A controlled trial of aerosolized ribavirin in infants receiving mechanical ventilation for severe respiratory syncytial virus infection. *N Engl J Med* 1991;325:24.

88. Meert KL, Sarnaik AP, Gelmini MJ, et al. Aerosolized ribavirin in mechanically ventilated children with respiratory syncytial virus lower respiratory tract disease: a prospective, double blind, randomized trial. *Crit Care Med* 1994;22:566.

89. Rutter N, Milner AD, Hiller EJ. Effect of bronchodilators on respiratory resistance in infants and young children with bronchiolitis and wheezy bronchitis. *Arch Dis Child* 1975;50:719.

90. Lenney W, Milner AD. Alpha and beta adrenergic stimulants in bronchiolitis and wheezy bronchitis in children under 18 months of age. *Arch Dis Child* 1978;53:707.

91. Hughes DM, Lesouef PN, Landau LL. Effect of salbutamol on respiratory mechanics in bronchiolitis. *Pediatr Res* 1987;22:83.

92. Brooks LJ, Cropp GJA. Theophylline therapy in bronchiolitis: a retrospective study. *Am J Dis Child* 1981;135:934.

93. American Academy of Pediatrics Committee on Drugs. Should steroids be used in treating bronchiolitis? *Pediatrics* 1970;46:640.

94. Simms DG, Downham MA, Webb JK, et al. Hospital cross infection on children's wards with respiratory syncytial virus and the role of adult carriage. *Acta Paediatr Scand* 1975;64:541.

95. Hall CB, Douglas RG Jr, Geiman JM, et al. Nosocomial respiratory syncytial virus infections. *N Engl J Med* 1975;293:1343.

96. Murphy D, Todd JK, Chao RK, et al. The use of gowns and masks to control respiratory illness in pediatric hospital personnel. *J Pediatr* 1981;99: 746.

97. Agah R, Cherry JD, Garakian AJ, et al. Respiratory syncytial virus (RSV) infec-

98. Leclair JM, Freeman J, Sullivan BF, et al. Prevention of nosocomial respiratory syncytial virus infections through compliance with glove and gown isolation precautions. *N Engl J Med* 1987;317:329.

99. Albert RK, Condie F. Hand washing patterns in medical intensive care units. *N Engl J Med* 1981;304:1465.

100. Kapikian AZ, Mitchell RH, Chanock RM, et al. An epidemiologic study of altered clinical reactivity to respiratory syncytial (RS) virus infection in children previously vaccinated with an inactivated RS virus vaccine. *Am J Epidemiol* 1969;89:405.

101. Hodes DS, Kim HW, Parrott RH, et al. Genetic alteration in a temperature sensitive mutant of respiratory syncytial virus after replication in vivo. *Proc Soc Exp Biol Med* 1974;145:1158.

102. Wright PF, Karron RA, Belshe RB, et al. Evaluation of a live, cold-passaged, temperature-sensitive, respiratory syncytial virus vaccine candidate in infancy. *J Infect Dis* 2000;182:1331–1342.

103. Tristram DA, Welliver RC, Mohar CK, et al. Immunogenicity and safety of respiratory syncytial virus subunit vaccine in seropositive children 18–36 months old. *J Infect Dis* 1993;167:191.

104. Hendry RM, Burns JC, Walsh EE, et al. Strain-specific serum antibody responses in infants undergoing primary infection with respiratory syncytial virus. *J Infect Dis* 1988;157:640.

105. Groothuis JR, Simoes EAF, Levin MJ, et al. Prophylactic administration of respiratory syncytial virus immune globulin to high risk infants and young children. *N Engl J Med* 1993;329:1524.

106. The IM-pact RSV Study Group. Palivizumab, a humanized respiratory syncytial virus monoclonal antibody, reduces hospitalization from respiratory syncytial virus infection in high-risk infants. *Pediatrics* 1998;102:531–537.

tion rate in personnel caring for children with RSV infections. *Am J Dis Child* 1987;141:695.

CHAPTER 247
Coronaviruses

C. George Ray

HISTORY

Diseases caused by animal coronaviruses have been recognized since the 1930s. The first human coronaviruses (HCVs) were reported in 1965, when respiratory specimens from patients with common colds that had been inoculated into organ cultures (OCs) of human fetal tracheal or nasal epithelium yielded cytopathic agents that were designated OC43 and OC38 (1). The 229E virus was subsequently isolated during studies of medical students with acute upper respiratory tract illnesses (2). The designation of these agents as coronaviruses was proposed in 1968, because their fringe of petal-shaped spikes resembled a "crown like the corona spinarum in religious art" (3). In November, 2002, a new, novel coronavirus appeared in southern China, causing a severe, acute respiratory syndrome (SARS) that has now spread globally (3a). Coronavirus-like particles in human feces have also been described (4) and subsequently associated with diarrheal diseases.

CHARACTERISTICS OF THE PATHOGEN

The family Coronaviridae has been divided into two genera: coronaviruses and toroviruses (5,6). The genus *Coronavirus* consists of enveloped, generally spherical virions with helical nucleocapsids, ranging from 100 to 120 nm in diameter. They are distinguished by prominent petal-shaped spikes (peplomers) up to 20 nm in length that cover the entire envelope surface and give them the coronal appearance (Fig. 247.1). The single, large positive-polarity ribonucleic acid (RNA) genome functions as a messenger for the translation of protein. The major structural proteins include the S or spike glycoprotein, composed

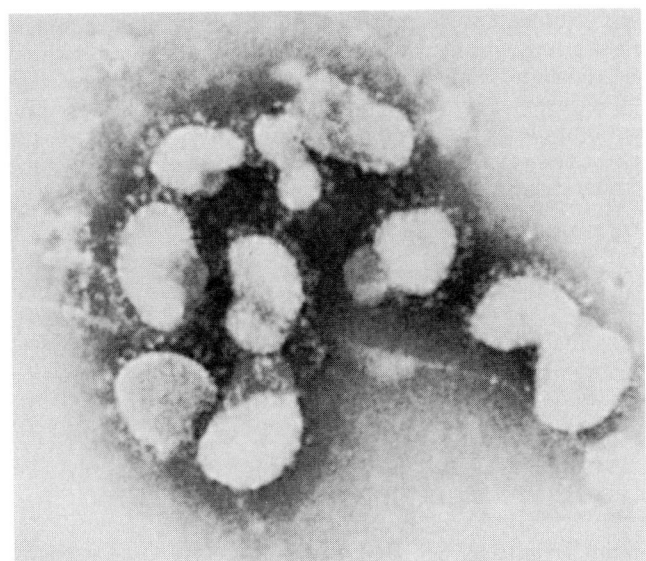

Figure 247.1. Electron micrograph of HCV 229E demonstrates the petal-shaped peplomers projecting from the envelope surfaces. (Courtesy of Dr. Claire M. Payne, University of Arizona College of Medicine, Tucson, AZ.)

TABLE 247.1. Antigenic Groups of Coronaviridae

Group	Representative strains	Host
1	HCV 229E	Human
	Canine coronavirus	Dog
	Feline infectious peritonitis virus	Cat
	Porcine transmissible gastroenteritis virus	Pig
2	HCV OC43	Human
	Mouse hepatitis virus	Mouse
	Bovine coronavirus	Cattle
3	Avian infectious bronchitis virus	Chicken
4	SARS-CoV	Human

of peplomers on the virion envelope; the matrix glycoprotein, designated M; the E (envelope) protein; the hemagglutinin-esterase (HE) glycoprotein, which is found in the envelope of some antigenic group 2 viruses, including HCV OC43; and the nucleocapsid phosphoprotein, N, which binds to virion RNA, providing the structural basis for the helical nucleocapsid (6).

The S glycoprotein mediates attachment to sialic acid–containing residues in the plasma membrane of host cells leading to infection and induces cell fusion (6,7); cell-mediated cytotoxicity against mouse hepatitis virus-infected cells is directed against S glycoprotein. Antibody to S glycoprotein neutralizes viral infectivity and inhibits the fusion-inducing ability of the virus. The M glycoprotein and E protein form the viral envelope and determine virion budding from the rough endoplasmic reticulum and Golgi membranes. Antibodies to the M glycoprotein can neutralize the virus only in the presence of complement (6). The HE glycoprotein, found only on some coronaviruses, shares some sequence homology with hemagglutinin of influenza C virus. It exhibits hemagglutinating and esterase activities, which permits elution of virus adsorbed to erythrocytes. Antibody to HE glycoprotein neutralizes viral infectivity (8).

Coronaviruses bind to cells via S glycoprotein and possibly HE glycoprotein, if present. A cellular receptor for coronavirus 229E, human aminopeptidase N, has been described (9). After entry of the virus into the cell, replication and assembly occur entirely in the cytoplasm. Virions assemble by budding at the Golgi apparatus or rough endoplasmic reticulum and are released by cell lysis or via cellular secretory mechanisms (6).

Coronaviruses have been divided into antigenic groups based on serologic comparisons. There is a diversity of agents that affect birds and mammals, many of which are important in veterinary medicine and agriculture (Table 247.1). The prototypic human strains, 229E and OC43, are in groups 1 and 2, respectively, along with other mammalian strains. Extensive genetic variation within strains is well recognized for the mammalian agents; this also occurs with those among humans, but the extent and significance are not yet well defined. The SARS agent

(SARS-CoV) has been placed in a new group, based on phylogenetic analysis (6a).

EPIDEMIOLOGY

Respiratory transmission from person to person is apparently common. Serologic surveys from different areas of the world have shown antibody prevalences among adults of 87% to 100% for HCV OC43, and 86% to 94% for HCV 229E.

Infections with HCV have been reported to account for a significant proportion of respiratory infections in adults and children (10,11). With the exception of SARS-CoV, their overall importance and possible sequelae are not well understood, principally owing to the lack of reliable cell culture and other systems that can be conveniently used for their detection.

Coronaviruses have been determined to be responsible for approximately 15% of upper respiratory tract infections in adults (12). On the other hand, SARS-CoV can cause severe pneumonia with mortality approaching 10% (13).

One study used an enzyme immunoassay with polyclonal antibodies to detect HCV antigens in nasal secretions of infants and children 6 months to 6 years of age (14). Antigens were detected in 30% of 108 acute respiratory episodes experienced by 30 children with a history of recurrent respiratory infections, and in 29% of 51 acute respiratory illnesses among their siblings. Most infections were due to HCV 229E; incidences peaked in the late fall or early winter and early summer. In contrast, other studies have shown that the highest frequency of antibody rises to both agents occurred during the winter months. Serologic evidence suggesting reinfection was frequently observed during a 3-year period (15). In a group of frail, elderly persons, HCV 229E was determined to be a cause of at least 8% of moderately debilitating acute respiratory illnesses (16).

Nosocomial spread can also occur. HCV 229E has been shown to retain infectivity for at least 3 hours on surfaces such as surgical gloves; HCV OC43 survived for only 1 hour or less. Both were susceptible to chemical disinfectants, such as povidone-iodine (17).

PATHOGENESIS

Studies in HCV infected human embryonic tracheal organ cultures (1,12) and exfoliated cells from the nasopharynx of experimentally inoculated volunteers indicate that a cytolytic effect on ciliated epithelial cells occurs and that this likely results in an inflammatory host response. Immunologic injury mediates feline infectious peritonitis (18), an animal coronavirus infection, and mouse hepatitis virus induces autoimmune-mediated demyelination in rodents (19), but the importance of immune factors or viral persistence in the pathogenesis of HCV remains unknown.

Neurotropism of murine strains of coronaviruses is well recognized, and there is a close analogy between rodent demyelinating disease and multiple sclerosis (20). Numerous studies have reported an association of HCV with multiple sclerosis (21–23) and coronavirus antigen and RNA sequences have been detected in brain tissue of patients with multiple sclerosis (24). However, these data do not establish coronavirus as the cause of multiple sclerosis.

A high frequency of mutation and recombination has been observed among animal coronaviruses and may contribute to the large number of serotypes (6). The number of serotypes of HCV has not been determined primarily because of the difficulty in culture adapting these viruses, but strain differences have been observed among HCVs (25). Immunity is serotype-specific.

CLINICAL MANIFESTATIONS

The incubation period of HCV infection ranges from 2 to 7 days, and the usual illness lasts 3 to 18 days (mean, 7 days). In adults, HCV usually produces an illness resembling that associated with rhinovirus infections. Symptoms of nasal discharge and malaise seem to be more prominent in coronavirus infections and cough more common in rhinovirus infections (12). SARS-CoV illnesses are far more severe, with fever >38.0°C at onset, followed by chills, myalgia, dry cough, and respiratory distress (6a).

The exact role of HCV in lower respiratory tract infections is less clear. It appears that HCV OC43 infections can produce cough as well as nasal symptoms in adults (26,27) and HCV infection has been associated with pneumonia and pleural reaction in military recruits (28). In children, sore throat, cough, coryza, and fever are common, and pulmonary crackles have been noted in 5% of patients (26). Acute attacks of wheezing can also occur, particularly among those known to be asthmatic or disposed to recurrent lower respiratory tract infections (14,29). Exacerbations of symptoms among persons with chronic obstructive pulmonary disease have also been reported (30).

DIAGNOSIS

Primary isolation of HCV is difficult. HCV 229E can be cultivated in several human diploid fibroblast cell strains or lines, but organ cultures remain the system of choice for HCV OC43. Both viruses can be adapted to replicate in a variety of diploid and heteroploid cell lines, and OC43 strains have been adapted *in vivo* in suckling mouse brains. SARS-CoV can be readily isolated in several cell lines derived from primate kidneys (3a). Diagnoses have usually been made serologically, using enzyme immunoassay or indirect immunofluorescence (10,11,15,26–30). An indirect enzyme immunoassay for the detection of antibody has been found to be highly specific (3a,31).

Antigen detection methods that use monoclonal antibody immunofluorescence of infected cells or enzyme immunoassay of respiratory secretions have been reported (17,36). Nucleic acid hybridization and reverse transcription-polymerase chain reaction (RT-PCR) have also been applied to the detection of HCV 229E RNA sequences (32,33). Of these, RT-PCR currently shows the greatest promise for rapid diagnosis.

The differential diagnosis of HCV infections encompasses the spectrum of agents that can affect the respiratory tract. These include rhinoviruses, myxoviruses, paramyxoviruses, adenoviruses, respiratory syncytial virus, Epstein-Barr virus; herpes simplex virus, some enteroviruses, and *Streptococcus pyogenes*. The severe coryza and occasional wheezing sometimes encountered can also mimic acute allergic rhinitis or asthma.

TREATMENT AND PREVENTION

Symptomatic supportive care is all that is available. No specific preventive measures other than good hygiene and respiratory precautions are known.

ENTERIC CORONAVIRUS-LIKE PARTICLES

Coronavirus-like particles have been observed by direct electron microscopy of stool samples from patients with epidemic sprue, neonatal necrotizing enterocolitis, and gastroenteritis, particularly among premature infants and young children (4,34–36). A particularly high frequency of occurrence of these particles in diarrheal stool specimens submitted for electron microscopic examination has been noted in southern Arizona (37); however, high rates of asymptomatic virus shedding have also been noted in some areas of the world (38).

It is not yet clear whether this agent (or agents) belongs to the family Coronaviridae. Isolation in cell cultures has been reported but not confirmed, but some strains have been propagated with difficulty in human fetal intestinal organ cultures (35).

REFERENCES

1. Tyrrell DAJ, Bynoe ML. Cultivation of a novel type of common-cold virus in organ cultures. *BMJ* 1965;1:1467.
2. Hamre D, Procknow JJ. A new virus isolated from the human respiratory tract. *Proc Soc Exp Biol Med* 1966;121:190.
3. Tyrrell DAJ, Almeida JD, Berry DM, et al. Coronaviruses. *Nature* 1968;220:650.
3a. Kziazek TG, Erdman D, Goldsmith CS, et al. A novel coronavirus associated with severe acute respiratory syndrome. *N Engl J Med* 2003;348:1953–1966.
4. Mathan M, Mathan VI, Swaminathan SP, et al. Pleomorphic virus-like particles in human faeces. *Lancet* 1975;1:1068.
5. Snijder EJ, Horzinek MC, Spaan WJM. The Coronavirus-like superfamily. *Adv Exp Med Biol* 1993;342:235.
6. Lai MC, Holmes KV. Coronaviridae: the viruses and their replication. In: Knipe DM, Howley PM, eds. *Fields virology*, 4th ed. Philadelphia: Lippincott, Williams & Wilkins, 2001:1163–1185.
6a. Rota PA, Oberste MS, Monroe SS, et al. Characterization of a novel coronavirus associated with severe acute respiratory syndrome. *Science* 2003;300:1394–1399.
7. Holmes KV. Coronaviruses. In: Knipe DM, Howley PM, eds. *Fields virology*, 4th ed. Philadelphia: Lippincott, Williams & Wilkins, 2001:1187–1203.
8. Deregt D, Babiuk LA. Monoclonal antibodies to bovine coronavirus: characteristics and topographical mapping of neutralizing epitopes on the E2 and E3 glycoproteins. *Virology* 1987;161:410.
9. Yeager CL, Ashmun RA, Williams RK, et al. Human aminopeptidase N is a receptor for human coronavirus 229E. *Nature* 1992;357:420.
10. Hamre D, Beem M. Virologic studies of acute respiratory disease in young adults. V. Coronavirus 229E infections during six years of surveillance. *Am J Epidemiol* 1972;96:94.
11. Monto AS, Lim SK. The Tecumseh study of respiratory illness. VIII. Acute infection in chronic respiratory disease and comparison groups. *Am Rev Respir Dis* 1985;111:27.
12. Bradburne AF, Bynoe ML, Tyrrell DAJ. Effects of the "new" human respiratory virus in volunteers. *BMJ* 1967;3:767.
13. Centers for Disease Control. Update: Severe acute respiratory syndrome—United States. *MMWR* 2003;52:550–551.
14. Isaacs D, Flowers D, Clarke JR, et al. Epidemiology of coronavirus respiratory infections. *Arch Dis Child* 1983;59:500.

15. Schmidt OW, Allan ID, Cooney MK, et al. Rises in titers of antibody to human coronaviruses OC43 and 229E in Seattle families during 1975–1979. *Am J Epidemiol* 1986;123:862.

16. Falsey AR, McCann RM, Hall WJ, et al. The "common cold" in frail, older persons: impact of rhinovirus and coronavirus in a senior daycare center. *J Am Geriatr Soc* 1997;45:706.

17. Sizun J, Yu MW, Talbot PJ. Survival of human coronaviruses 229E and OC43 in suspension and after drying on surfaces: a possible source of hospital-acquired infections. *J Hosp Infect* 2000;46:55.

18. Jacobse-Geels H, Daha MR, Horinek M. Isolation and characterization of feline C3 and evidence for the immune complex pathogenesis of feline infectious peritonitis. *J Immunol* 1980;125:1606.

19. Watanabe R, Wege H, ter Meulen V. Adoptive transfer of EAE-like lesions from rats with coronavirus-induced demyelinating encephalomyelitis. *Nature* 1983;305:150.

20. ter Meulen V, Masa PT, Dörries R. Coronaviruses. In: McKendall RR, ed. *Handbook of clinical neurology*, vol 12, *Viral disease*. New York: Elsevier, 1989:439–451.

21. Tanaka R, Iwaskai Y, Koprowski H: Intracisternal virus-like particles in brain of multiple sclerosis patient. *J Neurol Sci* 1976;28:121.

22. Burks JS, DeVald BL, Jankovsky LD, et al. Two coronaviruses isolated from central nervous system tissue of two multiple sclerosis patients. *Science* 1980;209:933.

23. Fleming JO, El Zaatari FAK, Gilmore W, et al. Antigenic assessment of coronaviruses isolated from patients with multiple sclerosis. *Arch Neurol* 1988;45:629.

24. Murray RS, Brown B, Brian D, et al. Detection of coronavirus RNA and antigen in multiple sclerosis brain. *Ann Neurol* 1992;31:525.

25. Reed SE. The behavior of recent isolates of human respiratory coronaviruses in vitro and in volunteers: evidence of heterogeneity among 229E-related strains. *J Med Virol* 1984;13:179.

26. Kaye HS, Marsh HB, Dowdle WR. Seroepidemiologic survey of coronavirus (strain OC43)-related infection in a children's population. *Am J Epidemiol* 1971;94:43.

27. Hendley JO, Fishburne HB, Gwaltney JM Jr. Coronavirus infections in working adults: Eight year study with 229E and OC43. *Am Rev Respir Dis* 1972;105:805.

28. Wenzel RP, Hendley JO, Davies JA, et al. Coronavirus infections in military recruits. *Am Rev Respir Dis* 1974;109:621.

29. McIntosh K, Ellis EF, Hoffman LS, et al. The association of viral and bacterial respiratory infections with exacerbations of wheezing in young asthmatic children. *J Pediatr* 1973;82:578.

30. Smith CB, Golden CA, Kanner RE, et al. Association of viral and *Mycoplasma pneumoniae* infections with acute respiratory illness in patients with chronic obstructive pulmonary diseases. *Am Rev Respir Dis* 1980;121:225.

31. Gill EP, Dominguez EA, Greenberg SB, et al. Development and application of an enzyme immunoassay for coronavirus OC43 antibody in acute respiratory illness. *J Clin Microbiol* 1994;32:2372.

32. Pilkaranka A, Jero J, Arruda D, et al. Polymerase chain reaction-based detection of rhinovirus, respiratory syncytial virus and coronavirus in otitis media with effusion. *J Pediatr* 1998;133:390.

33. Sizun J, Arbour N, Talbot PJ. Comparison of immunofluorescence with monoclonal antibodies and RT-PCR for the detection of human coronaviruses 229E and OC43 in cell culture. *J Virol Methods* 1998;72:145.

34. Vaucher YE, Ray CG, Minnich LL, et al. Pleomorphic, enveloped, virus-like particles associated with gastrointestinal illness in neonates. *J Infect Dis* 1982;145:27.

35. Resta S, Luby JP, Rosenfield CR, et al. Isolation and propagation of a human enteric coronavirus. *Science* 1985;229:978.

36. Mortensen ML, Ray CG, Payne CM, et al. Coronavirus-like particles in human gastrointestinal disease. *Am J Dis Child* 1985;139:928.

37. Payne CM, Ray CG, Borduin V, et al. An eight year study of the viral agents of acute gastroenteritis in humans: ultrastructural observations and seasonal distribution with a major emphasis on coronavirus-like particles. *Diagn Microbiol Infect Dis* 1986;5:39.

38. Sitbom M. Human enteric coronavirus-like particles (CVLP) with different epidemiological characteristics. *J Med Virol* 1985;16:67.

CHAPTER 248
Poliovirus

Cara C. Burns, Mark A. Pallansch, and Olen M. Kew

HISTORY

Poliomyelitis is a disease of great antiquity. Perhaps the earliest evidence is on an Egyptian stele from around 1350 BC depicting a young man with typical asymmetric flaccid paralysis and atrophy of the leg. Several scattered reports of the disease also appear in the literature from the 17th and 18th centuries. By the mid-19th century, the Industrial Revolution had brought increased urbanization to Europe and North America and with it significant changes and improvements in living conditions. Coincident with these massive changes was the advent of larger and more frequent outbreaks of poliomyelitis in these regions. From the late 1800s, outbreaks were occurring in several European countries and in the United States, and they remained a dominant public health problem in the developed world for the first half of the 20th century (1).

Major landmarks in the study of poliomyelitis include the successful passage of the virus to nonhuman primates in 1909 (2) and the development of cell culture systems for *in vitro* propagation of the virus in 1949 (3). These advances and the recognition of three distinct serotypes (4) opened the way for all subsequent work on vaccines and study of the biochemical and biophysical properties of polioviruses.

By the 1950s, two different approaches to the prevention of poliomyelitis by vaccination were developed. The first successful poliovaccine, the inactivated poliovaccine (IPV), was produced by Salk and Youngner in 1954 by formaldehyde inactivation of cell culture-propagated virus (5). This vaccine was completely noninfectious, yet following injection elicited an immune response that was protective against paralytic disease. During the same period, many laboratories sought to produce live, attenuated poliovaccines. The oral poliovaccine (OPV) strains of Sabin were licensed in 1961 and widespread mass immunization campaigns in the United States began in 1962 (6). Both IPV and OPV contain three components, one for each immunologically distinct serotype of poliovirus.

Widespread immunization with IPV, and since 1962 with OPV, has virtually eliminated poliomyelitis throughout most of the world, most recently through the efforts of the Poliovirus Eradication Initiative (7). To achieve high vaccine coverage in all regions of the world, the Poliovirus Eradication Initiative relies upon supplemental immunization campaigns and aggressive investigation of all suspect cases of acute flaccid paralysis to identify wild poliovirus circulation (8). The eradication goal is attainable because humans are the only known reservoir for poliovirus. The annual number of paralytic poliomyelitis cases has been reduced more than 99% since the start of the World Health Assembly Eradication Initiative in 1988 (7). Figure 248.1 shows the extent of recent progress, where the number of reported polio cases has decreased from approximately 35,000 (estimated cases worldwide: 310,000) in 1988 to approximately 500 in 2001 (9) (*www.polio-eradication.org*).

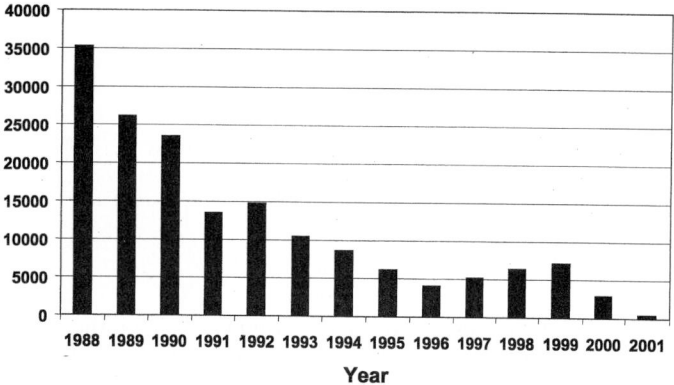

Figure 248.1. Global annual reported polio cases from 1988 to 2001. Apparent increase in 1999 mostly reflects improved surveillance. (Figure derived from World Health Organization. Global poliovirus update. Geneva: World Health Organization, 2002. Available at: *www.polio-eradication.org.*)

CHARACTERIZATION OF THE PATHOGEN

Polioviruses belong to the genus *Enterovirus* in the family Picornaviridae (10). All are small, round 30 nm particles with icosahedral symmetry. Polioviruses share most of their biochemical and biophysical characteristics with the other enteroviruses (11) and differ from some of the other picornaviruses (Table 248.1). The infectious particles are relatively heat-resistant (when stabilized by magnesium cations), resistant to acid pH (pH 3 to 5 for 1 to 3 hours), and also resistant to many common detergents and disinfectants, including most soaps, nonionic detergents, ethanol, ether, chloroform, and other lipid solvents (12,13). The virus is stable for weeks or more at 4°C and for days at room temperature. Desiccation, ultraviolet light, heat (in the absence of magnesium cation), formaldehyde, and free chlorine, however, readily inactivate the virus.

The poliovirion consists of 60 copies each of four polypeptide chains that form a very highly structured capsid shell. Located inside the capsid shell, the viral genome consists of a single molecule of ribonucleic acid (RNA), which is about 7,500 nucleotides long. The four capsid polypeptides are produced by the proteolytic cleavage of a single polyprotein precursor. In addition, one small protein, VPg, is covalently linked to the 5′ end of the virion RNA. A major advance in studies on the structure of polioviruses was the solution of the crystal structure to high resolution (14). Three-dimensional visualization of the molecular details of the virion surface has been particularly useful in understanding the neutralization of poliovirus by antibodies and binding of the virus to its cellular receptor. The observed structure of the three distinct antigenic sites explains why antigenicity of the virus is destroyed by disruption of the virion structure (15). In addition, there are other antigenic sites that elicit an immune response that is not neutralizing. The poliovirus receptor binds to a canyon-like channel on the virion surface (14).

The poliovirus-neutralizing antibody response is serotype-specific, with the exception of some minor cross-reaction between poliovirus types 1 and 2. Heat-disrupted virions, particularly those heated in the presence of detergent, induce antibodies that react with many enteroviruses (16,17). These broadly reacting antibodies are generally not neutralizing. Antisera raised in animals to each of the viruses are largely type-specific and are used for the determination of serotype in neutralization assays. The virus also contains more than one T-cell epitope (18), although the role of cell-mediated immunity in controlling infection is not well defined.

Polioviruses are among the simplest viruses in terms of genetic complexity and size. The RNA genomes from all three serotypes of poliovirus have been sequenced (19). The genomic RNA is infectious and serves as messenger RNA for viral protein synthesis. The RNA is translated in a single open reading frame into one large polyprotein, which is then processed through proteolytic cleavage by two distinct virus-encoded proteases into the functional viral proteins (20).

Despite much research and the simple genetic organization of the virus, the details of RNA replication have been elucidated slowly. The process begins with a protein-mediated priming reaction when the viral polymerase covalently links uridylic acid residues to a precursor of the VPg protein (21). RNA chain elongation of the uridylylated VPg generates a complementary RNA (cRNA). In the next step, the progeny viral RNA is synthesized from the cRNA. The newly synthesized viral RNA is covalently linked to the VPg protein at the 5′ end of the RNA. Only the positive sense strand of RNA is encapsidated in the viral structural proteins to form infectious viral particles (22). The extensive studies into virus replication and assembly have resulted in the remarkable accomplishment of complete cell-free replication of poliovirus starting only with the viral RNA template (23).

EPIDEMIOLOGY

There are several routes of poliovirus transmission (24). The fecal-oral route is probably the most important in most developing countries. The virus replicates efficiently in the intestinal tract and is shed in the stool for 2 to 4 weeks, and sometimes for several weeks longer (25). Shedding may be intermittent and is

TABLE 248.1.	**Comparative Physical and Biochemical Properties of Picornaviruses**			
Property	Poliovirus	Nonpolio enterovirus	Rhinovirus	Hepatitis A virus
Acid stability[a]	+	+	−	+
Buoyant density[b]	1.34	1.34	1.40	1.34
Stable at 50°C[c]	−	−	+	+
Stable at 65°C	−	−	−	+
Serotypes	3	61	100	1

[a]Incubation at pH 3.0 for 1 hour.
[b]Cesium chloride equilibrium density expressed as g/mL.
[c]Infectivity stable for 1 hour in the absence of magnesium cations.
Data from Melnick JL. Portraits of viruses: the picornaviruses. *Intervirology* 1983;20:61–100, and Melnick JL, Wenner HA, Phillips CA. Enteroviruses. In: Lennette EH, Schmidt NJ, eds. *Viral Rickettsial and Chlamydial Infections.* Washington, DC: American Public Health Association, 1979:471–534.

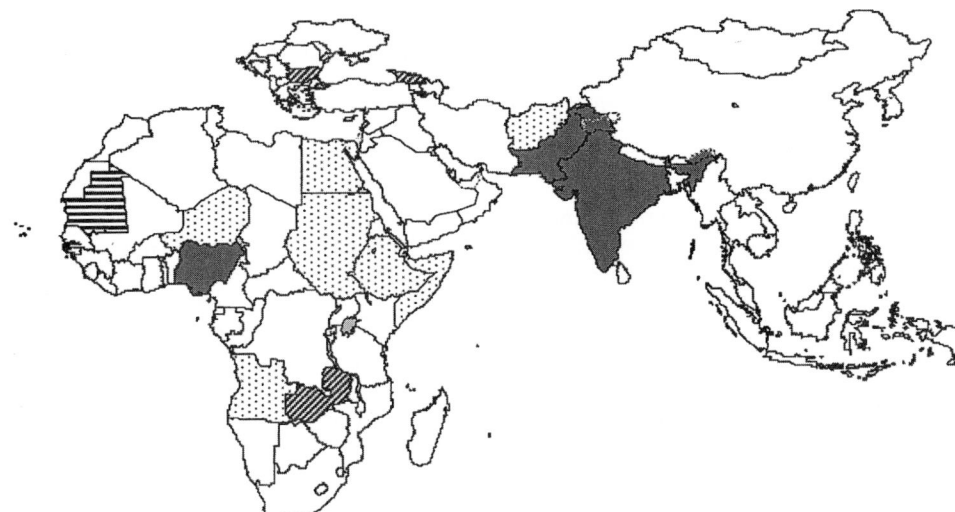

Figure 248.2. Worldwide distribution of wild poliovirus, 2001–2002. Countries that have high incidence of wild poliovirus (*n* = 20) are shown in grey shading. Countries that have low incidence of wild poliovirus (less than 20) are stippled, and those countries that did not have wild poliovirus are unshaded. Poliovirus importations are denoted by diagonal bars, and a country that had a wild virus of uncertain origin is shaded with horizontal bars. Data are presented from the 12-month period prior to March 12, 2002. (Figure derived from World Health Organization. Global poliovirus update. Geneva: World Health Organization, 2002. Available at: *www.polio-eradication.org.*)

affected by the immune status of the individual. Past natural infection with wild poliovirus and vaccination with OPV serve to significantly reduce the extent and duration of poliovirus shedding. IPV and competing enteric infections may also reduce the extent and duration of stool shedding to a lesser degree (26,27).

Since virus also replicates in the upper respiratory tract, polioviruses are also spread through upper respiratory tract secretions. Virus can be recovered from throat swabs and washings during the early acute phases of infection. Factors that affect transmission of the virus include extent of crowding, levels of hygiene, water quality, and sewage handling facilities. In areas with poor sanitary conditions and contaminated surface water or water supplies, the most important route of transmission is probably fecal-oral. In areas with good sanitary conditions and uncontaminated drinking water, other routes of transmission are probably more important. Studies with nonpolio enteroviruses suggest that respiratory tract secretions are infectious and may provide a source of virus for close contact spread through direct person-to-person contact, large-particle aerosols, or fomites.

The epidemiology of poliovirus infection has been radically altered by the widespread use of both IPV and OPV. The recent activities of the Polio Eradication Initiative have eliminated endemic poliovirus from most of the world. Since 1988, poliomyelitis from wild poliovirus has declined dramatically, and in the year 2001 only occurs in approximately ten countries in Africa, the Middle East, and Southern Asia (Fig. 248.2). Three regions of the world, the Americas, the Western Pacific, and Europe, have been certified to be free of endemic poliovirus transmission (7).

All cases of poliomyelitis reported since 1979 in the United States have been associated with exposure to OPV, either among vaccine recipients (usually with the first dose) or their contacts (28). The incidence of disease associated with use of OPV is estimated to be one case for every 1.4 million doses among first-dose recipients and 1 case for every 6.4 million doses (all doses) among contacts (29). Beginning in January 2000, only IPV has been used in the United States, and as a result, vaccine-associated paralytic poliomyelitis has disappeared. Occasionally, paralytic illness clinically indistinguishable from poliomyelitis has occurred after infection with other enteroviruses, particularly enterovirus 71. Such cases are infrequent and are discussed further in Chapter 249.

Any area with endemic wild polioviruses can serve as a reservoir for reintroduction of poliovirus to areas that have no endemic poliovirus circulation (30). In addition to several docu-

mented long-range importations over the past 25 years (30), wild poliovirus has recently been imported from India to China in 1999 (31), from Angola to the Cape Verde Islands in 2000 (32), and from the Asian subcontinent to Bulgaria (33) and Georgia in 2001. The frequency and ease of international travel probably results in frequent introduction of wild poliovirus into all regions of the world. High rates of poliovaccine coverage are necessary to prevent poliomyelitis epidemics.

Molecular Epidemiology

A powerful tool for tracking the circulation of wild poliovirus strains is the genomic sequence characterization of poliovirus isolates. By comparing the genetic changes among poliovirus isolates, their geographic and temporal origins can be determined (30). For example, sequence analysis has traced the circulation of a particular poliovirus type 1 strain throughout China from 1991 to 1993 (34), elucidated pathways of transmission during outbreaks (35), and documented importations from endemic regions into polio-free countries (31,33). The World Health Organization (WHO) Poliovirus Laboratory Network of 147 formally accredited poliovirus labs provides critical information about wild poliovirus circulation, allowing immunization efforts to be targeted to the virus reservoir areas (36). In addition, improved sequencing technology has facilitated the analysis of complete genomes of circulating polioviruses. This has expanded our understanding of the types of mutations that occur in human populations, including the frequent exchange of genetic material between poliovirus and its closest relatives (34,37).

PATHOGENESIS

Disease associated with poliovirus infection results from tissue-specific cell destruction. Polioviruses are cytolytic both *in vivo* and in cell culture. Upon entering a cell via specific receptors, the virus rapidly takes over cellular protein synthesis and inhibits cellular RNA transcription and deoxyribonucleic acid replication. Consequently, the cells degenerate and lyse, releasing the progeny virus. In culture, several thousand infectious progeny viruses are released from each infected cell. Because an infection cycle takes about 6 hours, a small inoculum can be amplified rapidly and spread quickly through the host.

The site of virus replication is dependent on the presence of virus-specific receptors. The poliovirus receptor is a member of the immunoglobulin (Ig) superfamily (38) encoded by a gene on chromosome 19 (39). Studies with transgenic mice that express the human poliovirus receptor have provided insights into the pathogenesis of poliomyelitis (40–42).

In humans, the initial sites of infection are epithelial cells in the intestinal and respiratory tracts. Following primary infection, more extensive virus replication occurs in lymphoid tissue of the tonsils and Peyer's patches, and from there enters the blood, and infects other tissues, occasionally including motor neurons. Paralytic illness follows directly from the lytic infection of motor neurons: in the anterior horn for spinal poliomyelitis, or in the medulla for bulbar poliomyelitis (43). Sensory neurons are spared. Several factors are associated with an increased risk of paralytic disease (including strenuous exercise, intramuscular injection, tonsillectomy, and pregnancy), presumably by increasing the chance of the virus infecting and lysing motor neurons (44–46).

A fundamental question about the pathogenesis of poliomyelitis is identification of the viral determinants of neurovirulence, a property that distinguishes wild polioviruses from other enteroviruses and the attenuated poliovaccine strains. The specific determinants of poliovirus neurovirulence map to the capsid, as neurovirulent recombinants having 5′-noncoding region and noncapsid sequences derived from other enteroviruses are frequently isolated from poliomyelitis patients (37). An important distinguishing function of the poliovirus capsid is to bind the specific poliovirus receptor on the surfaces of neural and lymphoid cells. Other enteroviruses do not use the poliovirus receptor. The molecular basis of attenuation of the Sabin OPV strains has been intensively studied. The primary determinants of attenuation map to a small number of nucleotide substitutions in the 5′-noncoding and capsid regions (reviewed in [47,48]). The substitutions in the 5′-noncoding region that are characteristic of the OPV strains reduce the efficiency of translation of poliovirus proteins (48). The role of the capsid mutations is less well defined. In studies conducted with transgenic mice, increased neurologic disease has been associated with axonal transport from peripheral nerves and possibly with an increased expression of the poliovirus receptor (49). Further studies may improve our understanding of the pathogenesis of poliomyelitis and the virus functions modified in the attenuated vaccine strains.

Primary infection induces a strong humoral immune response. Typically this includes the production of an IgM response within 7 to 10 days of infection, followed by an IgG response beginning about 14 days after infection. Because the first symptoms occur 3 to 14 days after infection, serum specimens taken early in the clinical illness often already contain poliovirus antibody. Within a few months of initial infection the titer of IgM antibody begins to fall; however, the neutralizing IgG antibodies persist, providing long-term protection from viremia and disease. Infection with one serotype of poliovirus does not protect against infection or disease with other poliovirus serotypes, and patients have had successive episodes of paralytic disease from different serotypes. Therefore, immunization of patients with acute poliomyelitis is appropriate, because disease indicates susceptibility to poliovirus because of the absence of or ineffective previous immunization. For these patients, however, immunization should be given only after specimens have been obtained for laboratory confirmation of poliovirus infection.

CLINICAL MANIFESTATIONS

The sequence of clinical symptoms follows the sequence of sites of viral replication (24,43). The primary site of infection in ep-

ithelial and lymphoid tissue of the pharynx and gut may be associated with no specific symptoms or with mild systemic symptoms such as fever, headache, malaise, and occasionally mild gastrointestinal symptoms. If the virus secondarily infects the central nervous system, a second phase of illness (aseptic meningitis, paralysis, or both) occurs 3 to 10 days after the first phase of mild systemic symptoms. The clinical course of poliovirus aseptic meningitis is identical to that associated with the other enteroviruses and is described in Chapter 249. The much greater tendency of poliovirus to infect motor neurons distinguishes its clinical picture from that of other enteroviruses.

Paralysis is usually associated with fever, stiff neck, muscle aches, and headaches; it develops rapidly and is typically asymmetric. It is a flaccid paralysis that most often affects the lower extremities and is associated with reduced or absent deep tendon reflexes and no sensory defects. During the period immediately following the primary illness, some recovery of function can be noted and complete functional recovery can occur. The permanent loss of motor neurons results in denervation atrophy of the affected muscles.

Poliomyelitis should be considered in all cases of pure motor paralysis and is usually associated with a normal or slightly elevated value for protein, normal sugar value, and moderate mononuclear pleocytosis in cerebrospinal fluid (CSF). Early in the illness polymorphonuclear cells may predominate in the CSF, followed by a shift to mononuclear cells. Defects in the ventral horns of the spinal cord can be observed by magnetic resonance imaging (MRI). The MRI lesion corresponds to the innervation pattern of the affected extremity. Electromyography and nerve conduction velocities (NCV) generally fail to show evidence of a conduction block.

The differential diagnosis includes spinal cord compression, stroke, neuropathy, and Guillain-Barré syndrome (GBS). Spinal cord compression is unlikely in the absence of central involvement in neural imaging. Lack of sensory involvement would exclude neuropathies. For stroke in the setting of meningoencephalitis, flaccid paralysis sometimes occurs, but the classic spasticity of upper motor lesions should follow. In GBS, protein concentration is markedly elevated in the CSF and pleocytosis is mild or absent. Fever is usually absent, and paralysis is usually symmetric and ascending with evidence of conduction block by NCV (Table 248.2).

Delayed progression of neuromuscular symptoms (postpolio syndrome) may occur 20 years or longer after the initial paralysis due to poliovirus (50). Postpolio syndrome is characterized by new muscle weakness associated with dysfunction of surviving motor neurons. The illness is usually associated with deterioration of those nerves involved in reinnervation during recovery from the original poliovirus infection. Inflammation is sometimes present in association with degenerating neurons (51). It is believed that the life span of these nerves has been shortened

TABLE 248.2. Differential Diagnosis of Poliomyelitis and Guillain-Barré Syndrome

Sign	Poliomyelitis	Guillain-Barré syndrome
Paralysis	Asymmetric	Symmetric, ascending
Fever	Present	Absent
Protein in CSF	Normal	Elevated
Pleocytosis	Yes	Mild or absent
NCV[a]	No block	Block

[a]Electromyography: nerve conduction velocities.

by the process of reinnervation. This syndrome is not a form of amyotrophic lateral sclerosis. It does not appear that reactivation or replication of poliovirus is involved, but current data are inconclusive (52,53).

DIAGNOSIS

The key to laboratory confirmation of poliovirus infection is the collection of appropriate clinical specimens (11,54). Isolation of the virus also makes it possible to determine whether the virus is wild or vaccine-related. In areas considered to be free of wild poliovirus this information may be important to public health officials, who must decide whether intervention is needed to prevent further cases of poliomyelitis. Laboratory studies can also be used to support the diagnosis of poliovirus infection when the patient has no knowledge of exposure or has an atypical disease presentation.

Poliovirus infection is most definitively demonstrated by isolation of poliovirus from clinical specimens (11). Virus is most frequently detected from stool specimens (preferred) or rectal swabs, less frequently in throat swabs or throat washings, and rarely from CSF. Stool specimens for viral isolation should always be obtained from suspect cases, since the virus is shed the longest and in highest titer from the intestinal tract. Early in the acute phase of the illness, virus is frequently isolated from the throat. Isolation of virus from CSF could provide the most direct link to disease, but isolation rates are low. Methods have been developed using the polymerase chain reaction (PCR) assay for rapid detection and characterization of polioviruses (55), including determination of the virus serotype (56). Nucleic acid probes, polymerase chain reaction, enzyme-linked immunosorbent assay, and monoclonal antibodies can be used to determine whether the isolate is vaccine-derived or wild poliovirus (57). The different methods have different sensitivities and specificities for the different strains of viruses. Poliovirus infection may occasionally be confirmed by demonstrating a rise in titers of neutralizing antibody to one of the poliovirus serotypes. The most common infectious agents that can mimic poliovirus disease are other enteroviruses, which are discussed further in Chapter 249.

TREATMENT

Treatment of acute poliomyelitis consists principally of supportive therapy and reduced physical activity. Mechanical ventilation is sometimes required in severe cases. Although specific antiviral treatment for poliovirus has been pursued for many years, there is no currently available drug treatment for polioviral (enteroviral) infections in clinical use. Several classes of compounds have been identified that exhibit antiviral activity against poliovirus in cell culture and experimental animals (58–60).

PREVENTION

Immunization is the primary means of poliomyelitis prevention. Two highly effective vaccines are available, and immunization with one or the other is part of routine childhood immunization schedules in most of the world. Recommended vaccination schedules vary among countries, and debate continues on the relative merits of the two vaccines (61–63). In the United States, OPV was used successfully for many years. After a 2-year pe-

riod of sequential IPV-OPV vaccination, an all-IPV schedule was adopted in the United States in early 2000 (64). Current recommendations are for four doses of IPV at ages 2, 4, and 6 to 18 months, and 4 to 6 years. Several European countries have used IPV as the sole vaccine for routine childhood immunization for many years (5,65).

The WHO recommends for developing countries three routine doses of OPV be given at 6, 10, and 14 weeks of age and an additional dose at birth in endemic regions where exposure of very young infants to wild virus can be expected (66). Supplementary pulse immunization through national immunization days have proven to be the most effective means to break the chains of wild virus transmission in endemic areas (8).

There have been at least three poliomyelitis outbreaks associated with circulating vaccine-derived polioviruses (cVDPV): on the island of Hispaniola in the Americas in 2000 to 2001 (37), in the Philippines in 2001 (67), and in Egypt from at least 1988 to 1993 (68). The outbreak strains were unusual because their capsid sequences (encoding antigenic properties) were derived from OPV, whereas most of the other genomic sequences were of non-vaccine origin. These viruses had recovered the capacity to cause paralytic poliomyelitis in humans and to be transmitted efficiently among human populations (37). Intense investigations suggest that circulation of vaccine-derived virus is a rare event, occurring only in populations with low immunization rates and high population densities. The recent discovery of cVDPVs has created an urgency in planning a comprehensive post-eradication immunization strategy.

The presence of a patient hospitalized with poliomyelitis has elicited concerns from hospital personnel who are unfamiliar with the risks associated with poliovirus infection. High rates of vaccine coverage and the rarity of wild poliovirus infections have essentially eliminated the risk of nosocomial poliomyelitis in the developed world. Since paralytic disease can also be caused by other infectious agents, such as enterovirus 71 and rabies virus, infection control practices should be appropriate to all potential agents until clinical, epidemiologic, or laboratory data have identified the likely agent. All immunocompetent patients with suspected or confirmed poliomyelitis should be placed in contact isolation, and in a private room if hygiene is poor, during the first 7 days of their illness. Staff should wear gowns and gloves if contact with infectious material (primarily feces) is likely (69). Staff should also be aware of the risk of transmitting virus to other patients who may not be immunized or are at increased risk of paralytic disease because of immune deficiency. The immunization status of staff should also be reviewed and staff with a history of inadequate vaccination should be excluded from caring for patients with poliomyelitis until completion of the appropriate immunization regimen. Public health officials should be notified immediately, so they can determine whether wild poliovirus may be involved and community prevention programs are warranted.

REFERENCES

1. Paul JR. *A history of poliomyelitis.* New Haven: Yale University Press, 1971.
2. Landsteiner K, Popper E. Uebertragung der poliomyelitis acuta auf Affen. *Xtschr Immunitatsfors Exp Ther* 1909;2:377.
3. Enders JF, Weller TH, Robbins FC. Cultivation of the Lansing strain of poliomyelitis virus in cultures of various human embryonic tissues. *Science* 1949;109:85.
4. Bodian D, Morgan IM, Howe HA. Differentiation of three types of poliomyelitis viruses. III. The grouping of fourteen strains into three immunological types. *Am J Hyg* 1949;49:234.
5. Salk J, Salk D. Control of influenza and poliomyelitis with killed virus vaccines. *Science* 1977;195(4281):834–847.
6. Sabin AB. Oral poliovirus vaccine: history of its development and use and

current challenge to eliminate poliomyelitis from the world. *J Infect Dis* 1985;151(3):420–436.

7. Centers for Disease Control and Prevention. Progress toward global eradication of poliomyelitis, 2001. *MMWR* 2002;51:253–256.

8. Hull HF, Ward NA, Hull BP, et al. Paralytic poliomyelitis: seasoned strategies, disappearing disease. *Lancet* 1994;343(8909):1331–1337.

9. World Health Organization. Global poliovirus update. Geneva: World Health Organization, 2002. Available at: *www.polio-eradication.org*

10. Melnick JL. Portraits of viruses: the picornaviruses. *Intervirology* 1983;20(2–3): 61–100.

11. Melnick JL, Wenner HA, Phillips CA. Enteroviruses. In: Lennette EH, Schmidt NJ, eds. *Viral, rickettsial and chlamydial infections.* Washington, DC: American Public Health Association, 1979:471–534.

12. Mbithi JN, Springthorpe VS, Sattar SA. Comparative in vivo efficiencies of hand-washing agents against hepatitis A virus (HM-175) and poliovirus type 1 (Sabin). *Appl Environ Microbiol* 1993;59(10):3463–3469.

13. Schurmann W, Eggers HJ. An experimental study on the epidemiology of enteroviruses: water and soap washing of poliovirus 1–contaminated hands, its effectiveness and kinetics. *Med Microbiol Immunol* 1985;174(5):221–236.

14. Hogle JM, Chow M, Filman DJ. Three-dimensional structure of poliovirus at 2.9 A resolution. *Science* 1985;229(4720):1358–1365.

15. Page GS, Mosser AG, Hogle JM, et al. Three-dimensional structure of poliovirus serotype 1 neutralizing determinants. *J Virol* 1988;62(5):1781–1794.

16. Mertens T, Pika U, Eggers HJ. Cross antigenicity among enteroviruses as revealed by immunoblot technique. *Virology* 1983;129(2):431–442.

17. Emini EA, Schleif WA, Colonno RJ, et al. Antigenic conservation and divergence between the viral-specific proteins of poliovirus type 1 and various picornaviruses. *Virology* 1985;140(1):13–20.

18. Graham S, Wang EC, Jenkins O, et al. Analysis of the human T-cell response to picornaviruses: identification of T-cell epitopes close to B-cell epitopes in poliovirus. *J Virol* 1993;67(3):1627–1637.

19. Toyoda H, Kohara M, Kataoka Y, et al. Complete nucleotide sequences of all three poliovirus serotype genomes. Implication for genetic relationship, gene function and antigenic determinants. *J Mol Biol* 1984;174(4):561–585.

20. Pallansch MA, Kew OM, Semler BL, et al. Protein processing map of poliovirus. *J Virol* 1984;49(3):873–880.

21. Paul AV, van Boom JH, Filippov D, et al. Protein-primed RNA synthesis by purified poliovirus RNA polymerase. *Nature* 1998;393(6682):280–284.

22. Novak JE, Kirkegaard K. Improved method for detecting poliovirus negative strands used to demonstrate specificity of positive-strand encapsidation and the ratio of positive to negative strands in infected cells. *J Virol* 1991;65(6):3384–3387.

23. Molla A, Paul AV, Wimmer E. Cell-free, de novo synthesis of poliovirus. *Science* 1991;254(5038):1647–1651.

24. Melnick JL. Enteroviruses. In: Evans AS, ed. *Viral infections of humans: epidemiology and control.* New York: Plenum Publishing: 1982:187–251.

25. Alexander JP Jr, Gary HE Jr, Pallansch MA. Duration of poliovirus excretion and its implications for acute flaccid paralysis surveillance: a review of the literature. *J Infect Dis* 1997;175[Suppl 1]:S176–S182.

26. Chin TD. Immunity induced by inactivated poliovirus vaccine and excretion of virus. *Rev Infect Dis* 1984;6[Suppl 2]:S369–S370.

27. Domok I, Balayan MS, Fayinka OA, et al. Factors affecting the efficacy of live poliovirus vaccine in warm climates. Efficacy of type 1 Sabin vaccine administered together with antihuman gamma-globulin horse serum to breast-fed and artificially fed infants in Uganda. *Bull World Health Organ* 1974;51(4):333–347.

28. Sutter RW, Brink EW, Cochi SL, et al. A new epidemiologic and laboratory classification system for paralytic poliomyelitis cases. *Am J Public Health* 1989;79(4):495–498.

29. Strebel PM, Sutter RW, Cochi SL, et al. Epidemiology of poliomyelitis in the United States one decade after the last reported case of indigenous wild virus-associated disease. *Clin Infect Dis* 1992;14(2):568–579.

30. Kew OM, Mulders MN, Lipskaya GY, et al. Molecular epidemiology of polioviruses. *Semin Virol* 1995;6:401–414.

31. Chiba Y, Murakami H, Kobayashi M, et al. A case of poliomyelitis associated with infection of wild poliovirus in Qinghai province, China, in October 1999. *Jpn J Infect Dis* 2000;53(3):135–136.

32. Centers for Disease Control and Prevention. Public health dispatch: outbreak of poliomyelitis—Cape Verde, 2000. *MMWR* 2000;49:1070.

33. Centers for Disease Control and Prevention. Imported wild poliovirus causing poliomyelitis—Bulgaria, 2001. *MMWR* 2001;50:1033–1035.

34. Liu HM, Zheng DP, Zhang LB, et al. Molecular evolution of a type 1 wild-vaccine poliovirus recombinant during widespread circulation in China. *J Virol* 2000;74(23):11153–11161.

35. Shulman LM, Handsher R, Yang CF, et al. Resolution of the pathways of poliovirus type 1 transmission during an outbreak. *J Clin Microbiol* 2000;38(3):945–952.

36. Centers for Disease Control and Prevention. Laboratory surveillance for wild poliovirus and vaccine-derived poliovirus, 2000–2001. *MMWR* 2002;51:369–371.

37. Kew O, Morris-Glasgow V, Landaverde M, et al. Outbreak of poliomyelitis in Hispaniola associated with circulating type 1 vaccine-derived poliovirus. *Science* 2002;296(5566):356–359.

38. Mendelsohn CL, Wimmer E, Racaniello VR. Cellular receptor for poliovirus:

39. Bernhardt G, Bibb JA, Bradley J, et al. Molecular characterization of the cellular receptor for poliovirus. *Virology* 1994;199(1):105–113.

40. Horie H, Koike S, Kurata T, et al. Transgenic mice carrying the human poliovirus receptor: new animal models for study of poliovirus neurovirulence. *J Virol* 1994;68(2):681–688.

41. Racaniello VR, Ren R, Bouchard M. Poliovirus attenuation and pathogenesis in a transgenic mouse model for poliomyelitis. *Dev Biol Stand* 1993;78:109–116.

42. Gromeier M, Solecki D, Patel DD, et al. Expression of the human poliovirus receptor/CD155 gene during development of the central nervous system: implications for the pathogenesis of poliomyelitis. *Virology* 2000;273(2):248–257.

43. Sabin AB. Paralytic poliomyelitis: old dogmas and new perspectives. *Rev Infect Dis* 1981;3(3):543–564.

44. Russell WR. The pre-paralytic stage and the effect of physical activity on the severity of paralysis. *BMJ* 1947;2:1023.

45. Wyatt HV. Provocation of poliomyelitis by multiple injections. *Trans R Soc Trop Med Hyg* 1985;79(3):355–358.

46. Strebel PM, Ion-Nedelcu N, Baughman AL, et al. Intramuscular injections within 30 days of immunization with oral poliovirus vaccine—a risk factor for vaccine-associated paralytic poliomyelitis. *N Engl J Med* 1995;332(8):500–506.

47. Racaniello VR, Ren R. Poliovirus biology and pathogenesis. *Curr Top Microbiol Immunol* 1996;206:305–325.

48. Gromeier M, Bossert B, Arita M, et al. Dual stem loops within the poliovirus internal ribosomal entry site control neurovirulence. *J Virol* 1999;73(2):958–964.

49. Gromeier M, Wimmer E. Mechanism of injury-provoked poliomyelitis. *J Virol* 1998;72(6):5056–5060.

50. Wiechers DO. Late effects of polio: historical perspectives. *Birth Defects Orig Artic Ser* 1987;23(4):1–11.

51. Dalakas MC. New neuromuscular symptoms after old polio ("the post-polio syndrome"): clinical studies and pathogenetic mechanisms. *Birth Defects Orig Artic Ser* 1987;23(4):241–264.

52. Melchers W, de Visser M, Jongen P, et al. The postpolio syndrome: no evidence for poliovirus persistence. *Ann Neurol* 1992;32(6):728–732.

53. Sharief MK. Poliovirus persistence in the postpolio syndrome. *Ann Neurol* 1993;34(3):415–417.

54. Kapsenberg JG. Picornaviridae: the enteroviruses (polioviruses, coxsackieviruses, echoviruses). In: Lennette EH, Halonen P, Murphy FA, eds. *Laboratory diagnosis of infectious diseases: principles and practices.* New York: Springer-Verlag, 1988:692–722.

55. Kilpatrick DR, Nottay B, Yang CF, et al. Group-specific identification of polioviruses by PCR using primers containing mixed-base or deoxyinosine residue at positions of codon degeneracy. *J Clin Microbiol* 1996;34(12):2990–2996.

56. Kilpatrick DR, Nottay B, Yang CF, et al. Serotype-specific identification of polioviruses by PCR using primers containing mixed-base or deoxyinosine residues at positions of codon degeneracy. *J Clin Microbiol* 1998;36(2):352–357.

57. van der Avoort HG, Hull BP, Hovi T, et al. Comparative study of five methods for intratypic differentiation of polioviruses. *J Clin Microbiol* 1995;33(10):2562–2566.

58. De Meyer N, Haemers A, Mishra L, et al. 4′-Hydroxy-3-methoxyflavones with potent antipicornavirus activity. *J Med Chem* 1991;34(2):736–746.

59. Garozzo A, Pinizzotto F, Guerrera J, et al. Antipoliovirus activity of isothiazole derivatives: mode of action of 5,5′-diphenyl-3,3′-diisothiazole disulfide (DID). *Arch Virol* 1994;135(1–2):1–11.

60. Rombaut B, Andries K, Boeye A. A comparison of WIN 51711 and R 78206 as stabilizers of poliovirus virions and procapsids. *J Gen Virol* 1991;72(Pt 9):2153–2157.

61. Salk J. Poliomyelitis vaccination—choosing a wise policy. *Pediatr Infect Dis J* 1987;6(10):889–893.

62. Amren DP, Mayer TR. National immunization policymaking: a controversial endeavor. *Postgrad Med* 1985;77:93.

63. Sabin AB. Is there a need for a change in poliomyelitis immunization policy? *Pediatr Infect Dis J* 1987;6(10):887–889.

64. Immunization Practices Advisory Committee. Poliomyelitis prevention in the United States. *MMWR* 2000;49(RR05):1–22.

65. Immunization Practices Advisory Committee. Poliomyelitis prevention: enhanced-potency inactivated poliomyelitis vaccine—supplementary statement. *MMWR* 1987;36:795.

66. Sutter RW, Cochi SL, Melnick JL. Live attenuated poliovirus vaccines. In: Plotkin SA, Orenstein WA, eds. *Vaccines.* Philadelphia: WB Saunders, 1999:364–408.

67. Centers for Disease Control and Prevention. Public health dispatch: acute flaccid paralysis associated with circulating vaccine-derived poliovirus—Philippines 2001. *MMWR* 2001;50:874–875.

68. Centers for Disease Control and Prevention. Circulation of a type 2 vaccine-derived poliovirus—Egypt, 1982–1993. *MMWR* 2001;50:41–42,51.

69. Garner JS, Simmons BP. Guideline for isolation precautions in hospitals. *Infect Control* 1983;4[4 Suppl]:245–325.

CHAPTER 249
Coxsackievirus, Echovirus, and Other Enteroviruses

Mark A. Pallansch and M. Steven Oberste

HISTORY

The development of better systems for growing poliovirus resulted in the detection of numerous agents that are pathogenic for laboratory animals or cytopathic for cultured cells (1). Many of these agents are presently classified as non-polio enteroviruses and are associated with a variety of clinical diseases.

In searching for suitable animals to replace monkeys for poliomyelitis studies, Dalldorf and Sickles (2) inoculated suckling mice with fecal suspensions from two suspected cases of poliomyelitis. The mice became paralyzed, not with poliovirus, but with the first isolate of a new virus group that subsequently was named for the patient's home town, Coxsackie, New York. Further isolation studies with mice identified several additional members of this group. With some isolates, however, the mice developed a spastic rather than the typical flaccid paralysis. These differences in pathogenicity in mice led to isolates being classified as either group A viruses (flaccid paralysis) or group B (spastic paralysis). The discovery of these agents led to the realization that some cases of "nonparalytic poliomyelitis" or aseptic meningitis were due to these agents and not necessarily to poliovirus. Many other illnesses, including herpangina, rash, pleurodynia, and myocarditis, were soon recognized as being related to infection with the coxsackieviruses.

Cell culture studies led to the isolation of other enteroviruses from the stools of persons with aseptic meningitis and from asymptomatic persons. The viruses caused cytopathic effects in cell culture but did not kill suckling mice. Since they were isolated from stool specimens, cytopathic for cell culture, and not initially linked to disease, they were called *e*nteric *c*ytopathic *h*uman *o*rphan viruses, which eventually evolved to the designation echoviruses. The fundamental similarities among the coxsackieviruses, echoviruses, and polioviruses caused them to be grouped in the genus *Enterovirus*, in the family *Picornaviridae*. Enteroviruses have also been isolated from cattle, swine, and non-human primates.

During the next 20 years, more than 60 antigenically distinct virus isolates were described. The isolates were numbered sequentially as they were described within the three groups, Coxsackie A, Coxsackie B, or echovirus (e.g., echovirus 11). Eventually it was discovered that virus isolates of the same serotype could have different degrees of pathogenicity in mice. Using this classification scheme, some isolates of the same serotype would be classified as coxsackievirus and other isolates as echovirus. Consequently, all new enterovirus serotypes isolated since 1967 have been assigned to the enterovirus group and numbered sequentially, beginning with enterovirus 68.

Just as the discovery of this large group of viruses followed from isolation studies of polioviruses, much of our understanding of the structure, mode of transmission, and biology of these viruses is based on studies of poliovirus. The reader is referred to Chapter 248 for a review of this information.

CHARACTERIZATION OF THE PATHOGEN

The genus *Enterovirus* in the family *Picornaviridae* consists of 64 recognized viruses (3,4), including the three serotypes of poliovirus described in Chapter 248. One additional non-polio enterovirus serotype has been identified by molecular means, and more new serotypes may exist (5). The ribonucleic acid (RNA) genomes from several enteroviruses have been cloned, sequenced, and found to have similar genetic organization to poliovirus (6–9). Molecular characterization of echoviruses 22 and 23 has demonstrated that these two viruses are genetically distinct from the enteroviruses. This finding has resulted in their reclassification as members of the new picornavirus genus, *Parechovirus* and the viruses have been renamed human *Parechovirus* 1 and 2, respectively (10). Molecular genetic analysis has resulted in a reclassification of the human enteroviruses into five species, A–D and poliovirus (10) (Table 249.1). It should be emphasized that the great diversity of serotypes of non-polio enteroviruses presents considerable problems for laboratory diagnosis and epidemiologic investigations, but the serotype usually has minimal relevance to the diagnosis and clinical management of an individual patient.

The structure and physical properties of enteroviruses are very similar to those of poliovirus. Many parallels between structural components of poliovirus and the other enteroviruses are evident from biochemical and structural studies. Antisera to each of the viruses raised in animals are usually type specific and provide reference reagents for the serotype determination of the enterovirus isolates (11). These antigenic differences are the primary means of distinguishing different enterovirus isolates. Infection with one serotype provides long-term protection from infection by that serotype but little protection, if any, from infection by other serotypes. Antigenic differences among isolates in the same serotype can be very complex, but variation at one or several epitopes does not change the serotype as determined by polyclonal antibodies or host response.

EPIDEMIOLOGY

The patterns of virus shedding and routes of transmission for enteroviruses are mostly the same as those for poliovirus. The virus is isolated in the highest titer and for the longest time in stool specimens but can also be isolated from respiratory secretions. Therefore, both fecal-oral transmission and spread by contact with respiratory secretions (person-to-person, fomites, and possibly large particle aerosol) are considered the most important modes of transmission for these viruses. The relative importance of the different modes probably varies with the virus and the environmental setting. In addition, enteroviruses that cause a vesicular exanthem can, presumably, be spread by direct or indirect contact with vesicular fluid that contains infectious virus (12). Exceptions to the usual modes of enterovirus transmission are the agents of acute hemorrhagic conjunctivitis, enterovirus 70 (EV70) and coxsackievirus A24 variant (CA24v). These two viruses are seldom isolated from respiratory tract or stool specimens and are probably spread primarily by direct or indirect contact with eye secretions (12).

An important concept in understanding the epidemiology of the enteroviruses is variation by serotype, by time, by geographic location, and by disease. This concept is illustrated in surveillance studies of non-polio enterovirus infections (13). For example, Fig. 249.1 summarizes the data for the 32 years from 1970 to 2001 for echovirus 9 (E9), echovirus 30 (E30), and coxsackievirus

TABLE 249.1.   Classification of Enteroviruses

Species	Serotypes	Mice	Culture
A	CAV2-8, 10, 12, 14, 16, EV71	+[a]	+/−[b]
B	CBV1-6, E1-7, 9, 11-21, 24-27, 29-33, EV69, EV73	+[c]	+
C	CAV1, 11, 13, 15, 17-22, 24	+	+/−[b]
D	EV68, EV70	−	+
Poliovirus[d]	PV1-3	−	+

[a]EV71 is not usually pathogenic for suckling mice.
[b]All coxsackie A viruses except serotypes 1, 19, and 22 have been isolated or propagated in some cell culture.
[c]The coxsackie B viruses are pathogenic for suckling mice, but the majority of echovirus isolates are not.
[d]Polioviruses are closely related to members of species C.

B3 (CB3) isolates in the United States collected and analyzed by the Centers for Disease Control and Prevention (14–18). These data illustrate two patterns of enterovirus prevalence: endemic and epidemic. The epidemic pattern, as typified by E9, is characterized by sharp peaks in numbers of isolations followed by periods with few isolations. During the study period, major epidemics of E9 occurred in the United States every 3 to 4 years, in 1971, 1975, 1978, 1981, 1984, 1988 to 1989, 1992, 1995, and 1998.

E30 also exhibited an epidemic pattern, but with much broader peaks, spanning 1978 to 1985, 1990 to 1993, and 1997 to 1998. By contrast, CB3 was isolated in about the same numbers every year, with only one major peak (in 1980). Similar endemic and epidemic patterns are seen for other enteroviruses.

Many studies have examined the prevalence of antibodies to the enteroviruses in specific populations (19–26). Several important conclusions can be drawn from these serosurveys. First, the

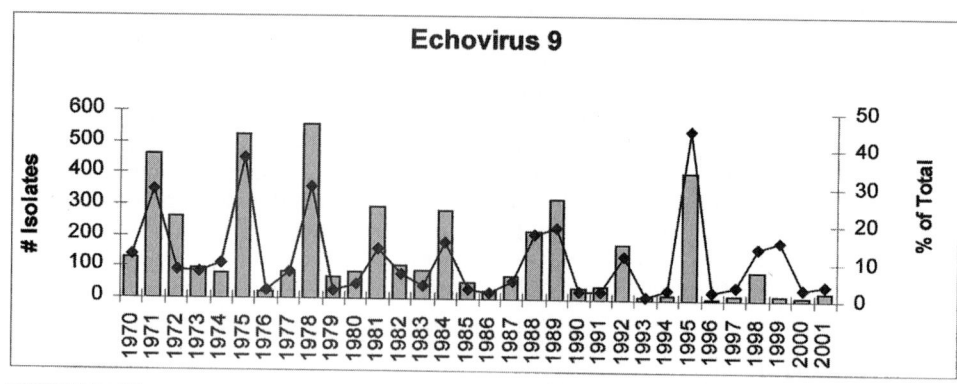

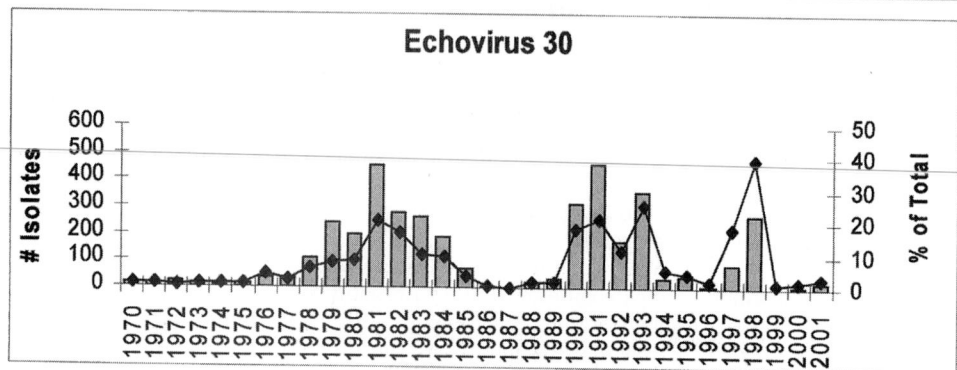

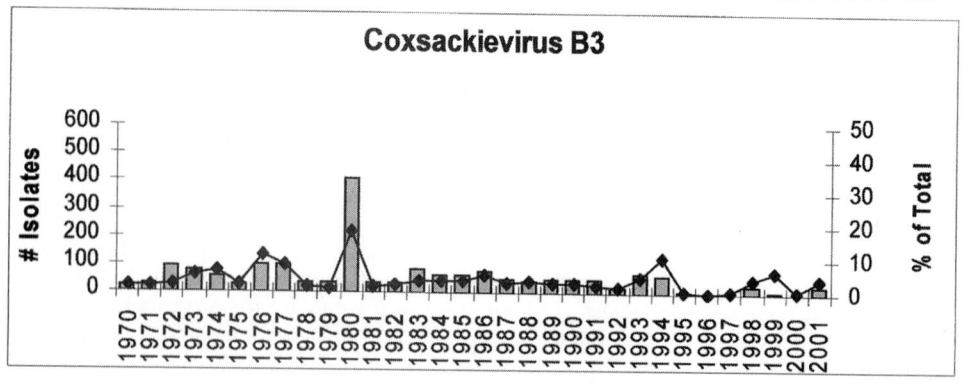

Figure 249.1. Temporal prevalence of echovirus 9, echovirus 30, and coxsackievirus B3 in the United States from 1970 to 2001. The graph shows the number of isolates (*bar graph*) and the fraction of all non-polio enteroviruses (*line graph*) that each of the serotypes represents in each year.

number of persons who have neutralizing antibody to any given enterovirus is large, indicating a high incidence of past infection. A high incidence of recent infection is also suggested by immunoglobulin M (IgM) surveys, which typically show 4% to 6% positivity. Second, infections with one serotype of enterovirus can boost the antibody titers to other enterovirus serotypes as measured by either IgM or neutralization. The pattern of the heterotypic response varies by serotype and among individuals. Third, the pattern of antibody prevalence by serotype varies by geographic location, by time, and by age. Thus prevalence data from different years and locations are not directly comparable. These three points must be considered when interpreting the findings of serologic studies of associations between enterovirus infection and disease.

PATHOGENESIS

Enteroviruses are cytopathic, and much of the associated disease presumably results from tissue-specific cell destruction. Some disease manifestations, enteroviral exanthems and myocarditis, for example (3,4,27), are thought to result from the host immune response to the infection. The actual mechanisms of virus-induced disease, however, have not been well characterized. Some insight into human myocarditis has been gained from recent studies using animal model systems (28–32). Typically, the primary site of infection is the epithelial cells of the respiratory or gastrointestinal tract, followed by a viremia that may lead to a secondary site of tissue infection. Secondary infection of the central nervous system results in aseptic meningitis or, rarely, encephalitis or paralysis. Other tissue-specific infection can result in pleurodynia or myocarditis. Disseminated infection can lead to exanthems, nonspecific myalgias, or severe multiple-organ disease in neonates.

Virus infection is dependent on the presence of specific receptors. Four distinct receptors for different non-polio enteroviruses have been identified from human cells, an integrin, decay-accelerating factor (DAF), the "coxsackievirus-adenovirus receptor" (CAR), and intracellular adhesion molecule 1 (ICAM-1) (33). Some enteroviruses are able to use more than one receptor and other unidentified receptors for this group of viruses may also exist. Studies of the virus-receptor interactions should improve our understanding of the pathogenesis of enteroviral disease and, possibly, help develop prevention or treatment strategies.

Infection with enteroviruses elicits a strong humoral immune response. Often this response is heterotypic; that is, infection with one serotype induces an immune response to several other serotypes (34,35). Young children develop a more homotypic response, whereas older children and adults develop a more heterotypic response. This age difference in the specificity of the antibody response to an enterovirus infection probably reflects exposure to a greater number of serotypes with advancing age. The basis of this heterotypic response is not known, but it may reflect shared epitopes present in multiple serotypes.

CLINICAL MANIFESTATIONS

Enterovirus infections can result in a wide variety of disease syndromes. A summary of these syndromes is given in Table 249.2 and details of viral meningitis, encephalitis, pericarditis, myocarditis, and conjunctivitis can be found in other chapters. The most common result of enterovirus infection is either no symp-

TABLE 249.2. Clinical Syndromes Associated with Enterovirus Infection

Central nervous system
  Aseptic meningitis
  Encephalitis
  Flaccid paralysis
Respiratory
  Mild upper respiratory tract
  Lymphonodular pharyngitis
Exanthems
  Hand, foot, and mouth disease
  Herpangina
Cardiac
  Myocarditis
  Pericarditis
Other
  Pleurodynia
  Acute hemorrhagic conjunctivitis
  Neonatal disseminated disease
  Chronic infection of agammaglobulinemic patients

Data from references 2, 3, 13, 15.

toms or mild upper respiratory tract symptoms (3,13,36). Other mild enteroviral illness, consisting of fever, headache, malaise, and occasionally mild gastrointestinal symptoms, may also occur. Much less frequently, serious illness brings the patient to the attention of a physician.

It is important to remember that the link between an enterovirus infection and a disease syndrome should be made with caution. Inapparent infections and prolonged excretion of virus, especially in stools, are common. A link cannot be made between infection and disease based solely on isolating virus from the stool of an individual patient. A link can be inferred if the virus is isolated from a site that corresponds to the clinical symptoms and if that site is normally sterile. The association between infection and disease has most often been made from studies of outbreaks in which a large number of persons with the same clinical signs and symptoms have evidence of infection with the same serotype. Such studies have clearly demonstrated that enterovirus infection can cause aseptic meningitis, pericarditis, pleurodynia, myocarditis, and encephalitis. When an individual patient has a disease syndrome shown clearly to be associated with enterovirus infection and there is no evidence for involvement by another agent, infection implies probable causation.

The most commonly recognized serious manifestation of enterovirus infection is central nervous system disease, usually aseptic meningitis, but sometimes, encephalitis or paralysis (3,13,36); the clinical descriptions are found in Chapter 149. Acute myocarditis and pericarditis are also discussed, in Chapter 64, and enterovirus involvement is reviewed elsewhere (37,38). Although the association between myocarditis and pericarditis and enterovirus infection is clearly established, it is not yet clear how often enterovirus infections are responsible for the disease syndromes. One study has shown CB virus IgM in a group of patients with acute myocarditis is significantly higher than in controls (39). Enterovirus RNA has also been detected in myocardial biopsy specimens from patients with myocarditis (40,41). These and other studies suggest, but do not clearly show, that CB virus infection may be associated with a large fraction of cases of acute myocarditis. By contrast, different studies have failed to show conclusive evidence for the involvement of enterovirus infection in idiopathic dilated cardiomyopathies (42–44).

A number of enterovirus serotypes have been associated with severe illness in neonates, including sepsis and generalized disseminated infection. The most systematic study of such illness, reported by Kaplan and coworkers, covered records for a 10-year period in Nassau County, New York (45). Among hospitalized neonates were 77 patients with CB virus infection documented by isolation and six died. The investigators estimated that one of every 2,000 infants in that area was hospitalized during the first 3 months of life. This probably underestimates the true rate, because virus isolation studies miss some infections and other enteroviruses can also cause this syndrome (46).

Two enterovirus serotypes, enterovirus 70 and coxsackievirus A24 variant, are associated with acute hemorrhagic conjunctivitis. This disease is different from other enteroviral illnesses, having occurred in global pandemics since its introduction around 1969. The incubation period for these agents is shorter than for other enteroviruses (24 to 72 hours), systemic illness much less common, and conjunctival replication the rule. The disease is characterized by acute onset of lacrimation, severe pain, chemosis and periorbital edema, photophobia, conjunctival hyperemia, and mild to severe subconjunctival hemorrhages. The disease is usually bilateral. It is generally self-limiting, but may lead to secondary bacterial infection.

Association between enterovirus infection and other disease syndromes is less clearly defined. Of considerable interest is the possible association with several chronic diseases: diabetes mellitus, cardiomyopathies, and arthritis. The most significant potential association is with juvenile-onset insulin-dependent diabetes mellitus (IDDM) (47,48). Several case-control studies and individual case reports suggest that enteroviruses can cause IDDM, but it is not yet known if they are a common or uncommon cause of IDDM (49–53).

Although there are few studies that examine the relationship between enterovirus infection and adverse effects on the fetus, one study found serologic evidence of CNS infection with CB virus in ventricular fluid from 4 of 28 newborns with congenital neural tube defects (54). The infants had neutralizing antibody to only one CB serotype in the ventricular fluid, but to several in serum. The unique distribution of antibodies in the ventricular fluid compared to that in serum supports the purported association. The mothers had antibodies to the same serotype as well as some other CB serotypes. No virus was isolated from infants or mothers. Two other studies have documented an association between enterovirus infection and miscarriages and stillbirths (55,56). Further studies are needed to assess the possibility of enterovirus infection of the fetus.

DIAGNOSIS

The key to laboratory confirmation of enterovirus infection is the collection of appropriate clinical specimens for direct detection, virus isolation or serologic studies (11). Enterovirus infection cannot be inferred from the clinical syndrome alone, since many other infectious agents can cause similar illness.

Virus isolation is accomplished by inoculation of appropriate specimens onto susceptible cultured cells. The best specimens for isolation of virus are, in order of preference, stool specimens or rectal swabs, throat swabs or washings, and cerebrospinal fluid. Fecal specimens should always be obtained, since virus is excreted longest and in the highest titer from the intestinal tract. Throat swabs or washings and cerebrospinal fluid are most likely to yield virus isolates if they are obtained early in the acute phase of the illness. For cases of acute hemorrhagic conjunctivitis the best specimens, in order of sensitivity, are conjunctival swabs and tears. The virus is detected in cell culture by its cytopathic effect and identified as a specific enterovirus by neutralization

with type-specific antisera (57), but serotyping remains a time-consuming and expensive procedure (11).

The use of the polymerase chain reaction to detect enterovirus genomes in cell culture, clinical specimens, and tissues promises to significantly improve the detection of enteroviruses (58–61). This technique is more rapid than isolation and has the potential for providing diagnostic answers in a timely way for clinical patient management. Molecular serotyping systems offer many advantages (62–66) and may eventually supplant antigenic typing as global stocks of serotype-specific antisera are depleted.

Serologic studies can be used in certain circumstances for detecting infection. Classically, infection has been demonstrated by a rise in titers of neutralizing antibody between acute and convalescent serum pairs. Enzyme immunoassays have been developed, such as those to detect CB virus-specific IgM antibodies (34,67–69). In most cases, the IgM antibody tests are not serotype specific (35). Depending on the configuration and sensitivity of the test, from 10% to nearly 70% of serum samples show a heterotypic response due to other enterovirus infections. A positive result with this method indicates recent enteroviral infection, although with IgM assays the infecting serotype may not be the same one determined by the assay.

TREATMENT

Because no antiviral therapy is presently available for enterovirus infections, treatment is directed toward alleviating symptoms. Drugs have been identified that exhibit antiviral activity against several enteroviruses including poliovirus in tissue culture and experimental animals (70–73). These drugs, however, have not completed clinical trials. Interferon has been proposed for treatment of acute hemorrhagic conjunctivitis, but this awaits further evaluation.

In patients with agammaglobulinemia, chronic enterovirus infections have been treated with γ-globulin, and in some cases this has controlled the infection (74). Use of γ-globulin in other clinical illness has not been systematically evaluated.

PREVENTION

There are no vaccines available for non-polio enteroviruses. General preventive measures include enteric precautions and good personal hygiene. Enteroviruses can be a cause of nosocomial infection. Serious infection is most common in newborns, although persons with compromised immune systems are also at high risk. Hospital staff can inadvertently carry the virus between patients or become infected themselves and spread the virus. Patients with suspected enterovirus infection should be managed with enteric precautions (75). Patients and staff can be cohorted during outbreaks, and during several newborn outbreaks, neonatal nurseries were closed to new admissions.

REFERENCES

1. Melnick JL. Portraits of viruses: the picornaviruses. *Intervirology* 1983;20:61–100.
2. Dalldorf G, Sickles GM. An unidentified, filtrible agent isolated from the feces of children with paralysis. *Science* 1948;108:61–62.
3. Pallansch MA, Roos RP. Enteroviruses: polioviruses, coxsackieviruses, echoviruses, and newer enteroviruses. In: Knipe DM, et al, eds. *Fields virology*. Philadelphia: Lippincott Williams & Wilkins, 2000:723–775.
4. Modlin JF. Coxsackieviruses, echoviruses, and newer enteroviruses. In: Mandell GL, Douglas RGJ, Bennett JE, eds. *Principles and practices of infectious diseases*. New York: John Wiley and Sons, 1999:1367–1383.
5. Oberste MS, et al. Molecular identification of new picornaviruses and characterization of a proposed enterovirus 73 serotype. *J Gen Virol* 2001;82:409–416.

6. Jenkins O, et al. The complete nucleotide sequence of coxsackievirus B4 and its comparison to other members of the Picornaviridae. *J Gen Virol* 1987;68(Pt 7):1835–1848.

7. Iizuka N, Kuge S, Nomoto A. Complete nucleotide sequence of the genome of coxsackievirus B1. *Virology* 1987;156(1):64–73.

8. Lindberg AM, Stalhandske PO, Pettersson U. Genome of coxsackievirus B3. *Virology* 1987;156(1):50–63.

9. Zhang G, et al. Complete nucleotide sequence of a coxsackie B5 virus and its relationship to swine vesicular disease virus. *J Gen Virol* 1993;74:845–853.

10. King AMQ, et al. Picornaviridae. In: Van Regenmortel MHV, et al., eds. *Virus taxonomy. Seventh report of the international committee on taxonomy of viruses.* San Diego: Academic Press, 2000:657–678.

11. Grandien M, Forsgren M, Erhrnst A. Enteroviruses. In: Lennette EH, Lennette DA, Lennette ET, eds. *Diagnostic procedures for viral, rickettsial, and chlamydial infections.* Washington, DC: American Public Health Association, 1995:279–297.

12. Pallansch MA. Acute hemorrhagic conjunctivitis. In: Strickland GT, ed. *Hunter's tropical medicine.* Philadelphia: WB Saunders, 2000:226–227.

13. Morens DM, Pallansch MA. Epidemiology. In: Rotbart HA, ed. *Human enterovirus infections.* Washington, DC: ASM Press, 1995:3–23.

14. Morens DM, Zweighaft RM, Bryan JM. Non-polio enterovirus disease in the United States, 1971–1975. *Int J Epidemiol* 1979;8(1):49–54.

15. Centers for Disease Control and Prevention. Nonpolio enterovirus surveillance—United States, 1993–1996. *MMWR* 1997;46:748–750.

16. Centers for Disease Control and Prevention. Enterovirus surveillance—United States, 1997–1999. *MMWR* 2000;49:913–916.

17. Moore M. Centers for Disease Control. Enteroviral disease in the United States, 1970–1979. *J Infect Dis* 1982;146(1):103–108.

18. Strikas RA, Anderson LJ, Parker RA. Temporal and geographic patterns of isolates of nonpolio enterovirus in the United States, 1970–1983. *J Infect Dis* 1986;153:346–351.

19. Bell EJ, McCartney RA. A study of Coxsackie B virus infections, 1972–1983. *J Hyg* 1984;93(2):197–203.

20. Danes L, Jaresova I. Neutralization microtest with human coxsackievirus and echovirus serotypes. *J Hyg Epidemiol Microbiol Immunol* 1985;29(4):399–408.

21. Manjunath N, Balaya S, Seth P. Serologic survey for neutralizing antibodies against group B coxsackieviruses in normal population in Delhi area. *Ind J Med Res* 1982;76:656–661.

22. Mukundan P, John TJ. Prevalence and titres of neutralising antibodies to group B coxsackieviruses. *Ind J Med Res* 1983;77:577–589.

23. Santhanam S, Choudhury DS. Antibodies against coxsackie B2 virus in infants and children in Delhi. *J Commun Dis* 1984;16(4):304–306.

24. Morag A, et al. Acquisition of antibodies to various Coxsackie and Echo viruses and hepatitis A virus in agricultural communal settlements in Israel. *J Med Virol* 1984;14(1):39–47.

25. Margalith M, et al. Prevalence of antibodies to enteroviruses and varicella-zoster virus among residents and overseas volunteers at agricultural settlements in Israel. *J Med Virol* 1986;20(2):189–197.

26. Lau RC. Coxsackie B virus infections in New Zealand patients with cardiac and non-cardiac diseases. *J Med Virol* 1983;11(2):131–137.

27. Woodruff JF. Viral myocarditis. A review. *Am J Pathol* 1980;101(2):425–484.

28. Klingel K, et al. Pathogenesis of murine enterovirus myocarditis: virus dissemination and immune cell targets. *J Virol* 1996;70(12):8888–8895.

29. Gauntt CJ. Roles of the humoral response in coxsackievirus B-induced disease. *Curr Topics Microbiol Immunol* 1997;223:259–282.

30. Kandolf R. (Myocarditis and cardiomyopathy). *Verhandlungen Deutsch Gesellschaft Pathol* 1996;80:127–138.

31. Kim K-S, et al. The group B coxsackieviruses and myocarditis. *Rev Med Virol* 2001;11:355–368.

32. Tracy S, et al. Group B coxsackievirus myocarditis and pancreatitis: connection between viral virulence phenotypes in mice. *J Med Virol* 2000;62(1):70–81.

33. Schneider-Schaulies J. Cellular receptors for viruses: links to tropism and pathogenesis. *J Gen Virol* 2000;81(Pt 6):1413–1429.

34. Dorries R, ter Meulen V. Specificity of IgM antibodies in acute human coxsackievirus B infections, analysed by indirect solid phase enzyme immunoassay and immunoblot technique. *J Gen Virol* 1983;64(Pt 1):159–167.

35. Pattison JR. Tests for coxsackie B virus-specific IgM. *J Hyg* 1983;90(3):327–332.

36. Melnick JL. Enteroviruses. In: Evans AS, ed. *Viral infections of humans: epidemiology and control.* New York: Plenum, 1982:187–251.

37. Reyes MP, Lerner AM. Coxsackievirus myocarditis—with special reference to acute and chronic effects. *Progr Cardiovasc Dis* 1985;27(6):373–394.

38. Martino TA, et al. Enteroviral myocarditis and cardiomyopathy: a review of clinical and experimental studies. In: Rotbart HA, ed. *Human enterovirus infections.* Washington, DC: ASM Press, 1995:291–351.

39. Frisk G, Torfason EG, Diderholm H. Reverse radioimmunoassays of IgM and IgG antibodies to Coxsackie B viruses in patients with acute myopericarditis. *J Med Virol* 1984;14(3):191–200.

40. Bowles NE, et al. The detection of cardiotropic viruses in the myocardium of patients with arrhythmogenic right ventricular dysplasia/cardiomyopathy. *J Am Coll Cardiol* 2002;39(5):892–895.

41. Grumbach IM, et al. Adenoviruses and enteroviruses as pathogens in myocarditis and dilated cardiomyopathy. *Acta Cardiol* 1999;54(2):83–88.

42. Arola A, et al. Identification of enteroviruses in clinical specimens by competitive PCR followed by genetic typing using sequence analysis. *J Clin Microbiol* 1996;34(2):313–318.

43. Giacca M, et al. Low frequency of detection by nested polymerase chain reaction of enterovirus ribonucleic acid in endomyocardial tissue of patients with idiopathic dilated cardiomyopathy. *J Am Coll Cardiol* 1994;24(4):1033–1040.

44. Keeling PJ, et al. Similar prevalence of enteroviral genome within the myocardium from patients with idiopathic dilated cardiomyopathy and controls by the polymerase chain reaction. *Br Heart J* 1992;68(6):554–559.

45. Kaplan MH, et al. Group B coxsackievirus infections in infants younger than three months of age: a serious childhood illness. *Rev Infect Dis* 1983;5(6):1019–1032.

46. Modlin JF. Perinatal echovirus infection: insights from a literature review of 61 cases of serious infection and 16 outbreaks in nurseries. *Rev Infect Dis* 1986;8(6):918–926.

47. von Herrath MG, et al. Is activation of autoreactive lymphocytes always detrimental. Viral infections and regulatory circuits in autoimmunity. In: von Herrath MG, ed. *Molecular pathology of type 1 diabetes mellitus.* Basel: Karger, 2001:91–122.

48. Rewers M, Atkinson M. The possible role of enteroviruses in diabetes mellitus. In: Rotbart HA, ed. *Human enterovirus infections.* Washington, DC: ASM Press, 1995:353–385.

49. Roivainen M, et al. Several different enterovirus serotypes can be associated with prediabetic autoimmune episodes and onset of overt IDDM. Childhood Diabetes in Finland (DiMe) Study Group. *J Med Virol* 1998;56(1):74–78.

50. Lonnrot M, et al. Enterovirus infection as a risk factor for beta-cell autoimmunity in a prospectively observed birth cohort: the Finnish Diabetes Prediction and Prevention Study. *Diabetes* 2000;49(8):1314–1318.

51. Lonnrot M, et al. Enterovirus RNA in serum is a risk factor for beta-cell autoimmunity and clinical type 1 diabetes: a prospective study. Childhood Diabetes in Finland (DiMe) Study Group. *J Med Virol* 2000;61(2):214–220.

52. Helfand RF, et al. Serologic evidence of an association between enteroviruses and the onset of type 1 diabetes mellitus. Pittsburgh Diabetes Research Group. *J Infect Dis* 1995;172(5):1206–1211.

53. Sadeharju K, et al. Enterovirus antibody levels during the first two years of life in prediabetic autoantibody-positive children. *Diabetologia* 2001;44(7):818–823.

54. Gauntt CJ, et al. Coxsackievirus group B antibodies in the ventricular fluid of infants with severe anatomic defects in the central nervous system. *Pediatrics* 1985;76(1):64–68.

55. Frisk G, Diderholm H. Increased frequency of coxsackie B virus IgM in women with spontaneous abortion. *J Infect* 1992;24(2):141–145.

56. Axelsson C, et al. Coxsackie B virus infections in women with miscarriage. *J Med Virol* 1993;39(4):282–285.

57. Lim KA, Benyesh-Melnick M. Typing of viruses by combinations of antiserum pools. Application to typing of enteroviruses (coxsackie and ECHO). *J Immunol* 1960;84:309–317.

58. Rotbart HA, et al. Diagnosis of enterovirus infection by polymerase chain reaction of multiple specimen types. *Pediatr Infect Dis J* 1997;16(4):409–411.

59. Rotbart HA, et al. Diagnosis of enteroviral meningitis by using PCR with a colorimetric microwell detection assay. *J Clin Virol* 1994;32(10):2590–2592.

60. Rotbart HA. Enzymatic RNA amplification of the enteroviruses. *J Clin Microbiol* 1990;28(3):438–442.

61. Nicholson F, et al. Detection of enterovirus RNA in clinical samples by nested polymerase chain reaction for rapid diagnosis of enterovirus infection. *J Virol Meth* 1994;48(2–3):155–166.

62. Oberste MS, et al. Typing of human enteroviruses by partial sequencing of VP1. *J Clin Microbiol* 1999;37(5):1288–1293.

63. Oberste MS, et al. Comparison of classic and molecular approaches for the identification of "untypable" enteroviruses. *J Clin Microbiol* 2000;38:1170–1174.

64. Caro V, et al. Molecular strategy for 'serotyping' of human enteroviruses. *J Gen Virol* 2001;82:79–91.

65. Casas I, et al. Molecular characterization of human enteroviruses in clinical samples: comparison between VP2, VP1, and RNA polymerase regions using RT nested PCR assays and direct sequencing of products. *J Med Virol* 2001;65:138–148.

66. Norder H, Bjerregaard L, Magnius LO. Homotypic echoviruses share aminoterminal VP1 sequence homology applicable for typing. *J Med Virol* 2001;63:35–44.

67. Chan D, Hammond GW. Comparison of serodiagnosis of group B coxsackievirus infections by an immunoglobulin M capture enzyme immunoassay versus microneutralization. *J Clin Microbiol* 1985;21(5):830–834.

68. Boman J, Nilsson B, Juto P. Serum IgA, IgG, and IgM responses to different enteroviruses as measured by a coxsackie B5-based indirect ELISA. *J Med Virol* 1992;38(1):32–35.

69. McCartney RA, Banatvala JE, Bell EJ. Routine use of mu-antibody-capture ELISA for the serological diagnosis of Coxsackie B virus infections. *J Med Virol* 1986;19(3):205–212.

70. See DM, Tilles JG. Treatment of Coxsackievirus A9 myocarditis in mice with WIN 54954. *Antimicrob Agents Chemother* 1992;36(2):425–428.

71. Andries K, et al. In vitro activity of pirodavir (R 77975), a substituted phenoxy-pyridazinamine with broad-spectrum antipicornaviral activity. *Antimicrob Agents Chemother* 1992;36(1):100–107.

72. Pevear DC, et al. Activity of pleconaril against enteroviruses. *Antimicrob Agents Chemother* 1999;43(9):2109–2115.

73. Rotbart HA. Antiviral therapy for enteroviruses and rhinoviruses. *Antiviral Chem Chemother* 2000;11(4):261–271.

74. O'Neill HJ, et al. Isolation of viruses from clinical specimens in microtitre plates with cells inoculated in suspension. *J Virol Methods* 1996;62(2):169–178.

75. Garner JS, Simmons BP. Guideline for isolation precautions in hospitals. *Infection Control* 1983;4[4 Suppl]:245–325.

CHAPTER 250
Rhinoviruses

Roland A. Levandowski

The rhinoviruses are picornaviruses that infect the respiratory tract of humans to produce the syndrome known as the common cold. Since the first strains were isolated in tissue cultures in the 1950s, more than 100 individual serotypes have been identified and numbered on the basis of a panel of specific neutralizing antibodies (1–5). The numbering system for rhinovirus serotypes roughly reflects the chronology of isolation of the prototypic strains of each serotype: the lowest numbered strains were isolated and submitted for typing earliest. However, shared properties of rhinoviruses are becoming better understood as more serotypes are examined with biochemical and molecular techniques. Morphologic and structural information has been correlated with the effects of antiviral agents to place rhinoviruses into two genetically related groups of rhinoviruses, Genus A and Genus B. (Table 250.1) (6–8). In addition, cellular receptors have been identified for all but one of the numbered serotypes (9,10). Although the diversity of serotypes has been an obstacle to the production and implementation of a simple vaccine for rhinoviruses, common properties such as receptor binding domains and the effect of rhinoviruses on the host's inflammatory responses continue to be targets for potentially broad applications to prevent and treat rhinovirus infections.

CHARACTERISTICS OF THE PATHOGEN

The rhinovirus, like other picornaviruses, consists of a single-stranded ribonucleic acid (RNA) genome (in positive, or message, sense in the intact virion) surrounded by a non-lipid–enveloped protein capsid. The virion has a total molecular mass of approximately 8 MDa and a diameter of 30 nm. The capsid is composed of 60 identical subunits arranged as 12 pentamers in an icosahedron (10–15) (Fig. 250.1). Each subunit includes one strand of each of the four structural proteins (VP1 to VP4). VP1, VP2, and VP3 have exterior projections, or loops, that interact with neutralizing antibodies and correspond to the portions of the viral genome that demonstrate the greatest variability (16–18). A depression, or "canyon," approximately 15 Å deep in the surface of the capsid exists around the fivefold axis. The floor of the "canyon" is composed of well-conserved amino acids (10–15,19,20). Associated with the "canyon" is a more internally located hydrophobic pocket that functions as a control on conformational changes during replication of the rhinovirus (20,21). Rhinoviruses in Genus B have been shown to have a small (eight or 12 carbon) fatty acid, termed "pocket factor," inserted in the hydrophobic pocket, and the occupancy of the hydrophobic pocket by "pocket factor" is associated with greater resistance to conformational change induced by temperature and acidification (10,15,20). Rhinoviruses in Genus A lack "pocket factor." Stabilization of rhinoviruses (both Genus A and Genus B) by antiviral agents appears to result from occupancy of the hydrophobic pocket by portions of the antiviral agents (22–24). The relative affinity of the antiviral activity is affected by changes in the amino acid residues of the hydrophobic pocket, and these changes possibly influence the replicative vigor and pathogenicity of rhinovirus serotypes (6).

Thirty percent of the molecular weight of the virion is contributed by the viral RNA, which is shown schematically in Fig 250.2. The viral RNA is composed of approximately 7,200 nucleotides with highly conserved nontranslated nucleotides at the 5′ and 3′ ends of the genome (25–29). The nontranslated region of 550 to 600 nucleotides at the 5′ end of the genome contains secondary structure that directs ribosomal entry and binding to an internal location to initiate translation of the message (30–35). The 3′-nontranslated end of the RNA contains a conserved stem loop structure of 72 nucleotides between the translated open reading frame and the polyadenylated terminus. The 3′ stem loop functions in RNA replication, but substantial modifications can be introduced without eliminating viral replication, even though replication efficiency is reduced (36–38). Although much of the rest of the genome also shows evolutionary conservation, differences between serotypes can be demonstrated and hypervariable regions located in the domain of the structural proteins (VP0-VP1) correspond to the antigenic sites where neutralizing antibodies attach to the rhinovirus capsid proteins (16,21).

For initiation of infection, rhinoviruses attach to specific cellular receptors. Two glycoproteins that bind rhinoviruses have been identified on the surface of human cells (39,40) (see Table 250.1). At least one serotype does not appear to bind to either of the identified glycoproteins, and data from other studies suggest that other cellular receptors may yet be identified (9,41,42). More than 80% of serotypes tested bind to a receptor that has been identified as a leukocyte attachment protein known as intercellular adhesion molecule 1 (ICAM-1) (43–46). ICAM-1 has been detected on most cells of human origin including HeLa cells, fibroblasts, and cells in the respiratory epithelium. A minority of serotypes bind to a second receptor on human cells identified as the low-density lipoprotein receptor (41,47–50). Unlike the serotypes binding to ICAM-1 (often referred to as the "major group"), rhinoviruses binding to the low-density lipoprotein (LDL) receptor (referred to as the "minor receptor group") also bind to a receptor on cells of murine origin (47). In the case of rhinoviruses binding to ICAM-1, antiviral agents occupying the hydrophobic pocket also prevent attachment of the receptor to the rhinovirus, consistent with the observation that the ICAM-1 binding site is located within the "canyon" (21). In the case of rhinoviruses binding to the LDL receptor, the receptor binding site is located external to the "canyon" and near the apex of the fivefold axis (51).

Neutralization by antibodies results from interference with receptor binding. The antigenic sites for the attachment of strong neutralizing antibodies (corresponding to surface loop projections from VP1, VP2, and VP3) border the receptor binding sites (16,52). Antibodies with strong binding affinity, whether by monovalent or bivalent interaction with the rhinovirus capsid, neutralize viruses more efficiently and may interact directly with amino acid residues within the receptor sites, even some of those in the "canyon" (53–54a). The epitopes recognized by neutralizing antibodies include both linear and conformational amino acid sequences (52–57). Permissible variation in the surface loop projections is potentially great, since antigens foreign to the rhinovirus capsid can be incorporated in the loop structures by site-directed mutagenesis, and deletions in loop structures can result in infectious escape mutants (55,58).

Penetration and uncoating of the virion remain incompletely understood but different pathways have been suggested for viruses in the two defined receptor groups (59–62). Paradoxically, it has been shown that a rhinovirus using the LDL receptor for attachment can enter the cell without need for a clathrin coated pit, even though the LDL receptor has a signal to target clathrin mediated endocytosis and it seems likely that this mechanism is operative under physiologic conditions (62). Likewise

TABLE 250.1.   Numbered Human Rhinovirus Serotypes Categorized by Antiviral Susceptibility (Genus A and B) and by Cellular Receptor

	Serotypes	
Receptor	**Genus A**	**Genus B**
ICAM-1	3–6, 8, 13, 14, 17, 26, 27, 32, 35, 37, 42, 43, 45, 48, 52, 54, 69, 70, 72, 79, 83, 84, 86, 91–93, 95, 97, 99	7, 9, 10–12, 15, 16, 18–25, 28, 33, 34, 36, 38, 39–41, 46, 50, 51, 53, 55–61, 63–68, 71, 73–78, 80–82, 85, 88–90, 94, 96, 100
LDL-receptor[a]		1A, 1B, 2, 29–31, 44, 47, 49, 62
Uncertain	87	

[a]Viruses in this receptor group bind to cells of mouse and human origin.
Data from Andries K, Dewindt B, Snoeks J, et al. Two groups of rhinoviruses revealed by a panel of antiviral compounds present sequence divergence and differential pathogenicity. *J Virol* 1990;64:1117, and Uncapher DR, DeWitt CM, Colonno RJ: The major and minor group receptor families contain all but one human rhinovirus serotype. *Virology* 1991;180:814, and Verdaguer N, Blaas D, and Fita I. Structure of human rhinovirus serotype 2 (HRV2). *J Mol Biol* 2000;300:1179.

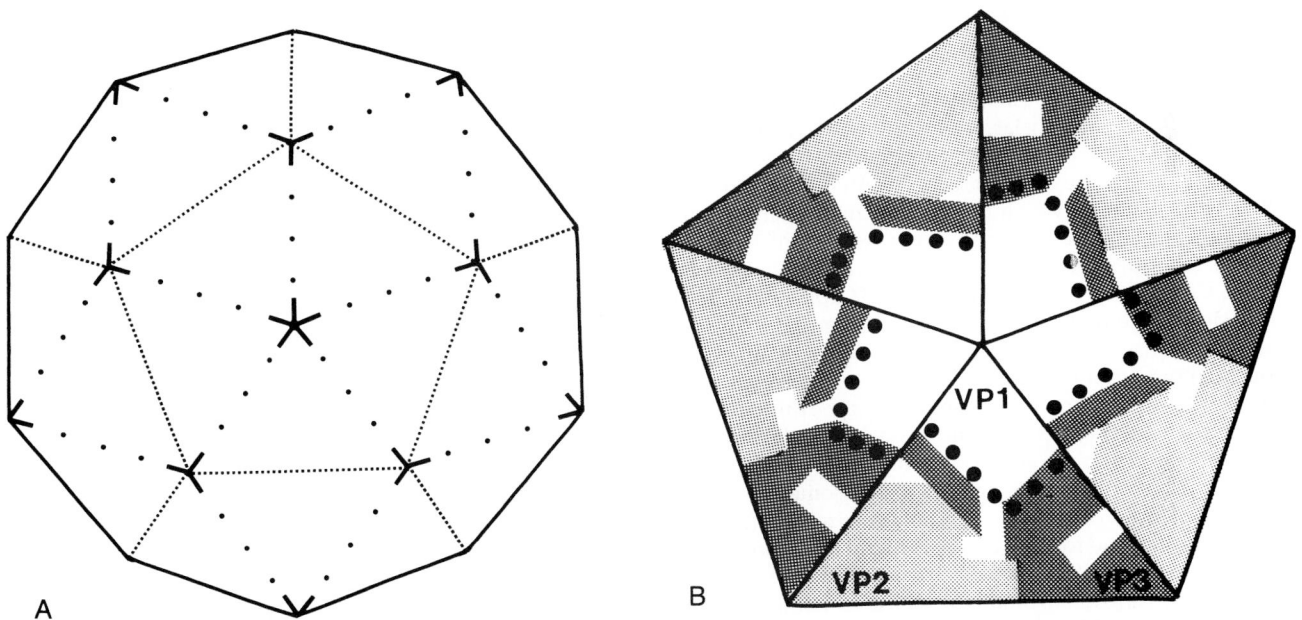

Figure 250.1. A, Schematic diagram of a rhinovirus capsid. The capsid consists of 60 capsomers arranged as 12 pentamers in an icosahedron. The fivefold axes extend through the apices of pentamers (*); threefold axes extend through meeting of three pentamers (Y); twofold axes pass through meeting of two pentamers (....). **B,** Arrangement of rhinovirus capsid proteins (VP1, white; VP2, light gray; and VP3, dark gray) in one pentamer. The dotted line around the fivefold axis of the pentamer indicates the relative location of a depression in the capsid surface, or "canyon." Interior to the "canyon" is a hydrophobic pocket. Receptor binding occurs in either the "canyon" (ICAM 1) or around the fivefold axis (LDL receptor family).

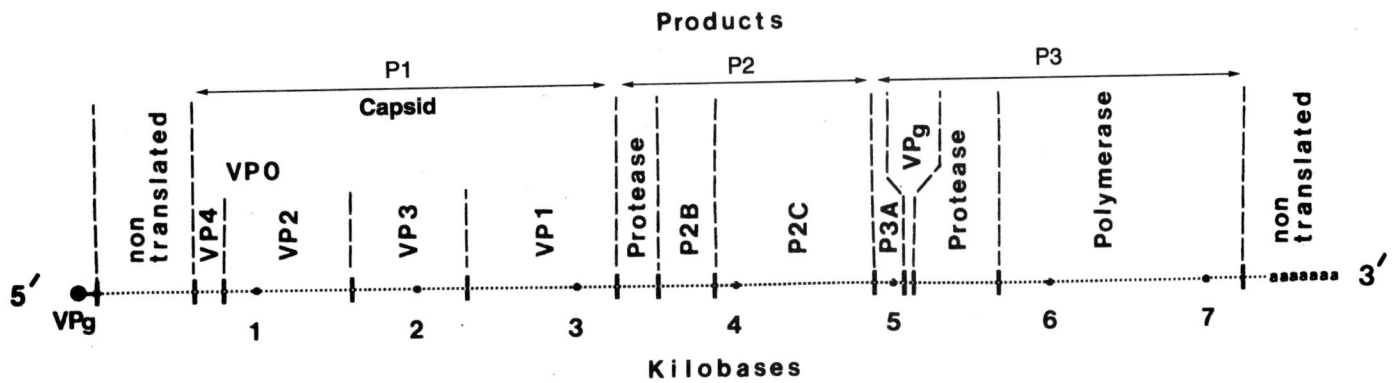

Figure 250.2. Sequence and sizes of genes from a representative rhinovirus. Products are labeled according to convention, as given by Rueckert and Wimmer (25).

paradoxically, it has been shown that a rhinovirus using ICAM-1 for attachment may be dependent on clathrin-mediated endocytosis, even though ICAM-1 does not target clathrin-mediated endocytosis (60). This has led to the suggestion that other, as yet undefined, factors may participate in the process of internalization of rhinoviruses. Although the uncoating process appears to require an endosomal compartment, attachment of ICAM-1 alone at neutral pH is sufficient to complete the conformational change and release viral RNA for rhinoviruses using ICAM-1 as receptor while viruses binding LDL-receptor must undergo acidification in the endosomal environment for the conformational change to be effected (59,63). The differences in uncoating may relate partly to the location on the rhinovirus of the receptor interaction. For ICAM-1, receptor binding on the rhinovirus capsid occurs in and around the "canyon" near the hydrophobic pocket and may produce conformational alterations by interaction with the amino acid residues of the receptor binding site (15). However, binding of the LDL receptor occurs externally near the fivefold axis of the rhinovirus capsid, which may induce less molecular distortion of the capsids of the "minor receptor group" viruses, so that acidification becomes crucial to the uncoating process (51).

Translation of the genome is monocistronic and requires no cap, consistent with the internal initiation of ribosomal binding at a site within the 5′ nontranslated region (30–33). As the translation product extends from the ribosome, viral proteases cleave the message to release the capsid precursors VP0, VP1 and VP3 (27). VP4, which is exclusively internal in the mature, infectious viral particle, and VP2 result from a precursor (VP0) cleaved autocatalytically during encapsidation of the RNA (25,64) (see Fig. 250.2). Cleavage of VP0 to VP4 and VP2 appears to be a necessary step in the replication cycle, because mutation at the cleavage site results in a defective virus incapable of establishing infection even though it binds to receptors and undergoes conformational alterations similar to those of wild-type rhinoviruses (65). The nonstructural proteins of the message include two proteases with specific cleavage sites (one protease in the P2 region and the other protease in the P3 region of the genome), an RNA-dependent RNA polymerase, and a small protein, VPg (66–69). VPg is covalently bound to the 5′ end of the viral RNA, and it has been found on both positive- and negative-stranded intermediates where it may function to bind viral RNAs to membranes for transcription (69). In addition to a function in viral protein processing, the P2 protease also cleaves eukaryotic initiation factor 4G (eIF4G) (35,70,71). Cleavage of eIF4G inactivates the complex required for binding of the host cell messenger RNAs to ribosomes, and reduces competition of the viral message for translation. Genomic products of the P2BC region are partly responsible for host restriction; mutations have been identified in this region during adaptation of a rhinovirus to replicate in cells of murine origin (72,73). However, under most conditions, human rhinoviruses are restricted mainly by availability of an appropriate cellular receptor which may be found on cells of primate or human origin.

The rhinovirus particle is variably susceptible to physical agents. The virion is not inactivated by organic solvents such as ether and chloroform because the capsid is not enveloped by a lipid membrane. Rhinoviruses are also resistant to trichlorofluoromethane, ethanol, and weak phenol (74). Although acid-resistant rhinoviruses have been selected from wild-type virus populations by repeated passage after exposure to low pH, the capsids of extracellular rhinoviruses normally undergo an irreversible conformational change and are inactivated when the pH is less than 5 (75,76). Human enteroviruses (poliovirus, coxsackievirus, and echovirus) are not inactivated by exposure to acidic conditions, which is used to differentiate the rhinoviruses from the other human picornaviruses (77). Rhinoviruses also undergo

conformational changes at increased temperature. The infectivity of most rhinoviruses is indefinitely stable at −70°C. At 37°C the half-life of inactivation is on the order of hours to a day, and at 56°C it is minutes to a few hours. In some circumstances the virion may be temperature stabilized by divalent cations, although the effect is variable for different serotypes (78). The antiviral agents that bind to the hydrophobic pocket near the receptor binding site also stabilize the viral capsid and prevent the conformational changes that normally occur during exposure of rhinoviruses to heat or acid (20,21). Rhinoviruses are inactivated by exposure to ultraviolet light, particularly when replication of the virus takes place in the presence of photoactive materials such as neutral red.

CLINICAL EXPERIENCE

There is no human population in which rhinovirus infection cannot occur. Of all common colds, rhinoviruses account for 30% to 50%, but they may account for close to 100% of viral respiratory infections during certain periods and in outbreak situations (79–84). Under natural conditions, multiple serotypes circulate in a given geographic location (85–89) (Table 250.2). Some serotypes persist to cause infection during subsequent seasons, whereas others disappear or are replaced by new serotypes. The cyclic replacement of serotypes reflects the interaction of the host and virus with the immune status of the host population resulting in the temporary elimination of some circulating serotypes and permitting the introduction of new serotypes.

The family unit is basic to rhinovirus transmission (80). Rhinovirus infection is often introduced by a school-age child or one in daycare to other siblings and parents at home. Mothers are more often infected than fathers, presumably because of the increased intensity of personal contact with greater exposure and opportunity for transmission. Although susceptibility to rhinovirus infections decreases in adults because of multiple exposures over the years, the protection afforded by neutralizing antibody is incomplete, and infection on more than one occasion with the same serotype is possible if the infecting inoculum is adequately large (90).

Fall and spring peaks have been documented for the occurrence of rhinovirus infection in temperate climates (80,91,92) (Fig. 250.3). The fall peak may be related partly to social events, because return to school means many more opportunities for transmission of rhinoviruses among larger groups of children. During the winter months of most years, the occurrence of rhinovirus infections in industrial countries is reduced (although not absent). It is possible that the reduced occurrence of rhinovirus infection in winter months reflects direct interference by influenza virus and other more efficiently spread viruses; alternatively, the induction of interferon by influenza and other respiratory viruses may also prevent or mask some rhinovirus infections (93). However, the lower relative humidity during winter months may contribute to the inactivation of rhinoviruses, and reduce their transmission (94).

The nasopharynx is the major source of rhinovirus during the acute infection (95,96). The quantity of virus present in nasopharyngeal secretions varies from person to person and from day to day in the same infected person. Generally, the peak of shedding of a rhinovirus is on the second to fourth day after inoculation and parallels the severity of clinical symptoms (Fig. 250.4). Virus is usually shed for 7 to 10 days, but instances of shedding for several weeks are documented (80,95). Although the secretions of the nasopharynx may traverse the posterior oropharynx, little infectious rhinovirus is found in oral secretions. The paucity of virus in oral secretions at least partly explains the inefficiency of oral secretions in transmitting infection (96,97). In families, the

TABLE 250.2. Rhinovirus Serotypes Isolated in More Than 1 Year from Adult Medical Center Students and Personnel with Naturally Acquired Common Colds in Chicago[a]

Serotype[b]	Year									
	1968	1969	1970	1971	1972	1973	1974	1975	1976	1977
7	+			+						
8				+	+					
9	+	+								
19			+		+	+				
21		+	+	+	+	+				+
25	+		+	+	+					
40			+			+				
41				+				+		
51			+							+
62									+	+
Total serotypes	11	9	9	11	6	4	ND[c]	3	5	5

[a]Some serotypes appear in consecutive years. Other serotypes appear only sporadically. Serotypes isolated in only 1 year are included in the total number of serotypes for each year.
[b]All nontypeable strains counted as one serotype for each year. Typing done with specific antisera for serotypes 1A and 1B through 89.
[c]ND, No data available.
Courtesy of Jackson GG, Rubenis M, Levandowski RA. University of Illinois, Chicago, IL.

interval between the initial infection and subsequent ones is related to the quantity and duration of the shedding of virus and ranges up to 10 days with an average of 3 days (96–99).

The transmission of rhinoviruses has been studied in experimental conditions examining person-to-person contact, exposure to fomites, and exposure to aerosols. Which of these is the predominant natural mode of transmission has not been definitively demonstrated. Although rhinoviruses may persist on inanimate surfaces for several hours after application, infection after contact with rhinovirus-contaminated objects often does not occur (94,97,100,101). Transfer of rhinovirus from an infected person to a susceptible one can occur through hand touching of only a few seconds' duration (102). In this setting, infection of the respiratory tract is achieved by direct self-inoculation of se-

cretions containing rhinovirus onto the nasopharyngeal mucosa by rubbing the nares or by way of the lacrimal canals by rubbing the eyes with secretion-laden fingers. Under conditions in which person-to-person contact is precluded and susceptible persons are long exposed to infected persons shedding large quantities of rhinovirus, aerosol transmission may occur (100). The ease of demonstration, the high percentage of infections achieved in experimental conditions, and an observed natural tendency of humans to touch the eyes and nose combine to suggest that person-to-person contact is the more powerful route of transmission; however, in some circumstances, aerosol transmission may be favored (97,98,100).

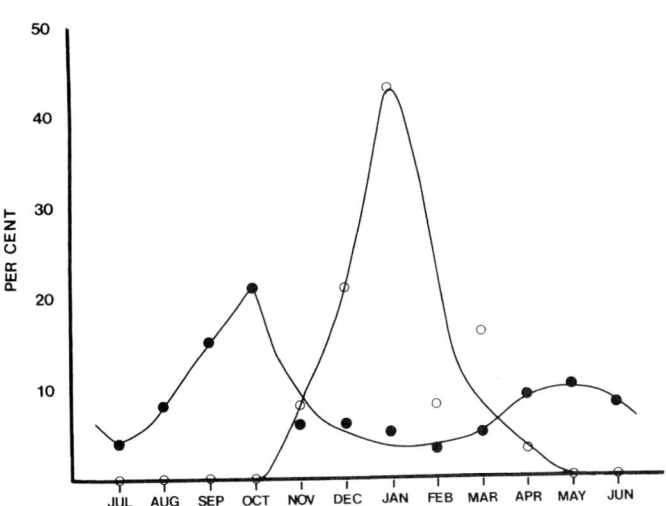

Figure 250.3. Monthly isolation of rhinoviruses as a percentage of all rhinovirus infections (•) and influenza virus isolates as a percentage of all influenza virus infections (○) during 20 years among adult medical center students and personnel in Chicago. The nadir of rhinovirus isolation in winter months between the fall and spring peaks coincides with the peak of influenza activity. Although influenza virus infection is absent between May and October, rhinovirus infections are observed throughout the year. (Courtesy of G. G. Jackson, M. Rubenis, and R. A. Levandowski, University of Illinois, Chicago, IL.)

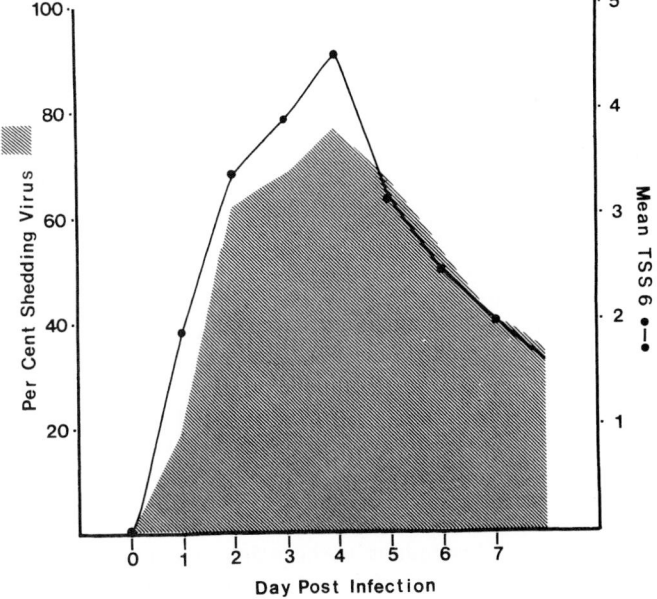

Figure 250.4. Percentage of volunteers shedding virus in nasal secretions and daily mean total symptom scores for six symptoms (TSS6) during the 7 days after experimental infection with rhinovirus serotype 25. The six symptoms are nasal obstruction, nasal discharge, sneezing, sore throat, cough, and headache graded to reflect the severity above the baseline day (day 0).

A number of factors influence susceptibility to rhinovirus infection. Probably the most important factor is the immunologic experience of the host. Over a lifetime, people are exposed to and infected by many rhinovirus serotypes. The secretory immunoglobulin A of the respiratory tract and the systemic immunoglobulin G responses that provide serotype-specific neutralizing antibodies are correlated with one another to an extent, and the detection of either suggests that an individual is likely to be protected from infection (80). The protection afforded is relative, because the neutralizing capacity of antibodies can be overwhelmed by a large inoculum of rhinovirus (90). Although rhinovirus and rhinovirus serotype-specific lymphocyte proliferative responses have been detected (even in the absence of neutralizing antibodies), the implications for susceptibility to infection and the direct contribution of cellular immune functions to prevention or clearance of rhinovirus infections are unknown (103–107). Women have been shown in some studies to exhibit increased susceptibility to respiratory virus infection at the midpoint of the menstrual cycle (108). Contrary to popular myth, susceptibility to rhinovirus infection is not increased by exposure to cold, as demonstrated in volunteers and in polar settlements (84,109,110). Temporary resistance to infection after respiratory virus infections occurs and is the result of local production of interferon and possibly other mediators such as nitric oxide (111–114). Although there is little direct evidence to associate psychological stress with neuro-hormonal-immunological alterations, some clinical studies suggest that psychological stress predisposes to increased symptoms, if not increased susceptibility to infection (115).

The replication of rhinoviruses occurs predominantly in the upper airways, partly because the replication of rhinoviruses is maximal at nasal temperature, 33°C to 34°C (116). However, rhinoviruses have been recovered from warmer body sites including the middle ear during acute otitis media and from paranasal sinuses during acute sinusitis under circumstances that suggest the virus is the primary etiology in the pathogenesis of illness (117,118). Rhinovirus replication has been shown in the lower airways of infected volunteers by a number of methods including methods that eliminate the possibility of contamination of the lower respiratory tract by infected secretions from the upper airways (119–122). Although it is often difficult to demonstrate morphologic or functional abnormalities of the tissues involved, infected nasopharyngeal and bronchial epithelial cells can be identified by a number of methods including immunologic staining methods, in situ hybridization, and in situ polymerase chain reaction (PCR) (120–128). Rhinovirus has been recovered from heart blood at necropsy, but rhinoviremia has never been demonstrated ante mortem (129). Although large volumes of the nasal secretions enter the gastrointestinal tract, rhinoviruses have rarely been recovered from the gastrointestinal contents. However, the apparent lack of replication of rhinoviruses in the gut is not related simply to gastric acidity, because gastric aspirates inconsistently inactivate rhinoviruses (130).

A multitude of interacting factors are implicated in the production of the respiratory tract symptoms during rhinovirus infection in the typical human host. Reflex mechanisms may account for some of the nasal discharge, as anticholinergic compounds reduce the quantity of nasal secretions (131,132). Increased levels of histamine have been detected in the upper and lower airways during rhinovirus infection (133,134). Kinins have been identified in the nasal secretions during acute rhinovirus infection and correlate with measures of vascular permeability and symptoms (135). Exogenous kinins applied to the nasopharynx produce sore throat and stimulate nasal obstruction and discharge. Nitric oxide produced in response to rhinovirus infection in vitro and in vivo has protective effects by directly inhibiting rhinovirus replication and by reducing cytokine production (113,114,136).

The spectrum of inflammatory and immune mediators produced by mononuclear leukocytes and epithelial cells in response to rhinovirus infection is not fully determined, but many including RANTES, GM-CSF, interleukin-1, interleukin-6, interleukin-8, interleukin-11, interleukin-16, tumor necrosis factor-α, interferon-α, interferon-γ, and eotaxin have been found, and their contributions to the evolution of symptoms and airway reactivity are being investigated (121,137–144). The origin of the interferon found in nasal secretions during rhinovirus infection is presumably the cells of the nasopharyngeal tissues and may include the lymphocytes of the submucosa, because rhinoviruses potently induce interferon when cultured with mononuclear leukocytes in vitro (145–147). Although interferon may limit the extent of viral replication, it may also modify the local inflammatory response and recruit lymphocytes from the blood pool for interactions in the respiratory mucosal environment (148). Eotaxin, which is increased during acute rhinovirus infection, is a cytokine that selectively increases the chemotaxis of eosinophils (143). Interleukin-8, which is produced by peripheral blood mononuclear leukocytes on exposure to rhinoviruses, is found in nasal secretions during rhinovirus infection and is a potent chemoattractant for polymorphonuclear leukocytes (142,149). The presence of interleukin-8 correlates with the appearance of polymorphonuclear leukocytes in nasal secretions and with the severity of symptoms during rhinovirus infections (149). Interleukin-11 is released by rhinovirus-infected epithelial cells, produces increased airways responsiveness when administered to mice, and it is found in increased quantities in the nasal secretions of children with clinical wheezing during acute respiratory virus infections (138).

During the first few days of rhinovirus infection, changes in leukocyte populations can be identified in the peripheral blood and in the tissues of the airways. The majority of studies examining leukocyte populations have identified a transient increase in the number of circulating polymorphonuclear leukocytes, while lymphocyte populations, particularly the T lymphocytes, decline in the blood compartment during first 2 to 3 days after initiation of infection (106,145,150–154). As the acute phase of the infection progresses, polymorphonuclear leukocytes migrate into the nasal secretions in increasing numbers (155,156). The destination of the lymphocytes leaving the peripheral blood is less certain, but lymphocytes and other mononuclear leukocytes can be found in nasal secretions and increased numbers of lymphocytes, particularly T lymphocytes, and eosinophils migrate to submucosal and epithelial sites in the lower airways (153–155). Although rhinoviruses attach to specific receptors on mononuclear leukocytes and certainly interact with them by inducing a number of cytokine cell products, replication, if it occurs at all, is quite limited (140,142,147). Chemoattractants produced by infected and/or immunologically activated cells of the airways seem likely to account for the migration of leukocytes in response to rhinovirus infection (143,149,156,157). Although the severity of symptoms in rhinovirus infections can be correlated with the magnitude of change in numbers of leukocytes and with the presence of cytokines, much remains to be learned of the role of specific leukocytes either directly or by way of cytokine products in the pathophysiology of rhinovirus infection (137–144,147,149,156).

The typical illness associated with rhinovirus infection begins by 24 to 72 hours following the deposition of virus in the nasopharynx (158). Sore throat and sneezing often herald the onset of a rhinovirus cold. Nasal discharge and nasal obstruction, the symptoms most typical of a cold, reach their peak within a day or two of onset of symptoms and gradually recede over the next several days. The nasal discharge in a rhinovirus cold is initially clear and watery but becomes variably mucopurulent and viscous in later days. The consistency of the secretions relates to the origins: in early infection local histamine production increases vascular permeability while during later infection secretions from the glandular cells of the mucosa predominate (133). The color of the secretions does not result from changes in the bacterial flora of the nose but from the increased number of leukocytes, overwhelmingly polymorphonuclear neutrophils, in nasopharyngeal secretions (123,155,156). Thickening of mucosal linings of the paranasal sinuses and fluid levels may be detected in paranasal sinuses by noninvasive imaging techniques (159,160). Headache as a result of sinusitis or inflammation involving the ostia of paranasal sinuses may appear early or late. Cough, when it occurs, is a rather persistent symptom and is often productive of sputum. Whether cough is reflexive or compensates for alterations in airway clearance mechanisms is unclear. Clearance of material from the nasopharynx and lung may be disordered by rhinovirus infection (124,161). However, ciliary function in the trachea does not appear to be appreciably affected in otherwise healthy adults, which is perhaps consistent with the relatively low numbers of infected epithelial cells shed from the airways (162). When cough occurs, the total duration of symptoms may be prolonged by several days. With the symptoms considered together, the typical rhinovirus cold lasts 5 to 7 days: 1 or 2 days of mild malaise, headache, sneezing, and sore throat; 3 to 6 days of moderate nasal discharge and obstruction; and 2 to 4 days of mild coughing.

However, symptom severity is highly variable. Some persons have symptoms that suggest and may be confused with allergic rhinitis. Some rhinovirus colds are so mild that infection with a rhinovirus may not be suspected on clinical grounds. There are reports associating rhinoviruses with clinical pneumonia during profound immunosuppression; however, even in this setting the predominant illness associated with rhinovirus is the typical common cold (163,164). The illness associated with rhinovirus infection can be more severe in persons who have underlying bronchopulmonary disorders. Exacerbation of airway obstruction after rhinovirus infections has been documented in a number of studies in patients with asthma and chronic obstructive lung disease, and changes in airways function may be detected in otherwise healthy people with special pulmonary function maneuvers (165–171).

A complex host interaction with rhinoviruses is being defined in asthmatic responses associated with rhinovirus infections (122,134,153,154). During rhinovirus infections in both non-asthmatic and asthmatic persons, production of histamine, inflammatory mediators, and many cytokines occurs, and migration of leukocytes to the airways has been documented. The increased airways responsiveness to histamine (or methacholine) observed in asthmatics as the result of rhinovirus infection is accompanied by an increase in the numbers of lymphocytes (predominantly T lymphocytes) and eosinophils in the lower respiratory tract (134,154). Eosinophilia, airway sensitivity to histamine challenge, and histamine release triggered by antigen exposure persist in asthmatics beyond the acute illness associated with rhinovirus infection (134,154). One cytokine suggested as a possible factor contributing to acute exacerbations of asthma following rhinovirus infections is interleukin-11, which is increased during rhinovirus infection, produces increased methacholine (and probably histamine) responsiveness in the airways of mice, and is associated with clinical wheezing in children with respiratory virus infections (138). Possibly counteracting any contribution of other mediators, nitric oxide, which is produced in response to rhinovirus infection *in vitro* and *in vivo*, not only inhibits rhinovirus replication, but may also exert a protective effect by reducing the production

of cytokines and by reducing sensitivity to histamine in the asthmatic (136). While steroids may be useful in the treatment of asthma, steroids do not appear to reduce the typical symptoms specific for rhinovirus infection, and may prolong viral shedding (172).

LABORATORY ASPECTS

Newer methods such as polymerase chain reaction following reverse transcription (RT-PCR) are gaining acceptance and wider use. However, tissue cultures inoculated with secretions still provide a direct and practical way for most clinical laboratories to identify rhinoviruses as agents of common colds. The yield is improved when nasal secretions are collected directly or are washed from the mucosal surface with a physiologic salt solution (95). Oral secretions contain fewer infectious virions, and nasal swabs sample a smaller portion of the secretions than nasal washing. Collecting several samples daily and early from an infected person improves recovery, because the maximal titer of shed virus and the greatest proportion of shedders are found during the first days of infection (96) (see Fig. 250.4).

Rhinoviruses replicate in many tissue types, including human diploid fibroblasts (WI-38, MRC-5, foreskin), HeLa, KB, HEp-2, WISH, monkey kidney, human fetal tonsil, and nasal polyp explants (4,75,80,147,173–179). Permissive HeLa strains provide high titers of rhinovirus, and diploid fibroblasts provide a system that facilitates identification of virus replication (4,75,177,178). Agitation and incubation at 33°C (the optimal temperature that mimics nasal conditions) encourage replication (116). The cytopathologic appearance of the infected monolayer of tissue culture by itself is strongly suggestive of rhinovirus infection and is confirmed by acid lability and ether resistance of the isolate. Intersecting pools of sera may facilitate serotyping efforts, although cross-reactivity among serotypes is noted (180,181). The most widely used method for detecting antibodies to a specific rhinovirus is neutralization of virus using a standardized input of the median tissue culture infectious dose ($TCID_{50}$). The assay is maximally sensitive with a low viral inoculum of 10 to 100 $TCID_{50}$ (182). Acute- and convalescent-phase serum samples collected 2 to 6 weeks apart are used to determine whether antibody titer has risen significantly. Neither of the foregoing methods for identifying rhinovirus infection is optimal for implementation of therapeutic intervention with antiviral agents, because isolation of a rhinovirus from clinical samples may require up to 2 weeks and serodiagnosis of rhinovirus infection by specific neutralizing antibody is cumbersome, not only because of the multitude of serotypes, but also because the antibody response requires several weeks to develop fully.

Potential means of rapid rhinovirus detection include methods employed for other agents, such as immunoassays or probing with labeled DNA complementary to the viral genome (183,184). The detection of specific rhinovirus enzymes is also conceivable if appropriate substrates can be devised (185). However, amplification of viral nucleic acid by RT-PCR is now within the reach of most clinical laboratories, and it appears to be a promising means of detecting rhinoviruses. Several well-conserved portions of the rhinovirus genome have been successfully targeted to produce generally useful primers for reverse transcription and for amplification (Table 250.3) (128,186–196). The sensitivity (theoretically a single genome copy) makes RT-PCR a potentially powerful tool for clinical detection of rhinoviruses (186,187,189–191,194,195). Because the primers shown in Table 250.3 may also amplify enteroviruses, other steps may be needed to ensure specificity in identifying rhinoviruses. Specific identification is achieved by performing DNA sequencing or hybridization with specific oligonucleotide

TABLE 250.3.   Some Primers Used for Detection and Amplification of Rhinovirus RNA Sequences by Polymerase Chain Reaction

Product size (bp)	Anti-message sense primer[a]	Message sense primer
524	OL68-1 5'GGTAAQTTCCACCACCANCC 3' (1065-1046[b])	OL24 5'CTACTTTGGGTGTCC G 3' (542-557[b])
388	OL27 5'CGGACACCCAAAGTAG 3' (557-542[b])	OL26 5'GCACTTCTGTTTCCC C 3' (170-185[b])
120	4− 5'GAAACACGGACACCCAAAGTA 3' (553-533[c])	3+ 5'TCCTCCGGCCCCTGAATG 3' (434-451[c])

(Q=T or C; N=A,G,T or C)

[a]Primer used for reverse transcription of message sense rhinovirus RNA.
[b]Nucleotide numbering from HRV 1B.
[c]Nucleotide numbering from HRV 2.
Data from Gama RE, Horsnell PR, Hughes PJ, et al. Amplification of rhinovirus specific nucleic acids from clinical samples using the polymerase chain reaction. *J Med Virol* 1989;28:73, Olive DM, Al-Mufti S, Al-Mulla, et al. Detection and differentiation of picornaviruses in clinical samples following genomic amplification. *J Gen Virol* 1990;71:2141, Halonen P, Rocha E, Hierholzer J, et al. Detection of enteroviruses and rhinoviruses in clinical specimens by PCR and liquid-phase hybridization. *J Clin Microbiol* 1995;33:648, and Santti J, Hyypia T, Halonen P. Comparison of PCR primer pairs in the detection of human rhinoviruses in nasopharyngeal aspirates. *J Virol Meth* 1997;66:139.

probes (192,193). In addition, restriction fragment length polymorphisms related to even single base differences in genomes of picornaviruses can be exploited to differentiate rhinoviruses from enteroviruses and can even be used to identify specific rhinovirus serotypes (187,188,196). Although RT-PCR is a very sensitive method of detecting viral nucleic acids, an amplification step of replication in tissue cultures can be considered to increase the probability of detection.

TREATMENT AND PREVENTION

Inactivated rhinoviruses produce immunity in volunteers after parenteral or intranasal inoculation (197–199); however, the rhinovirus vaccines tested have conferred homotypic, but not heterotypic, protection. Animal studies with synthetic rhinovirus peptides suggest that a heterotypic antibody response may be induced, but it is not known whether the response is protective (200,201). Use of a multivalent rhinovirus vaccine in humans suggests that a variable response to the contained antigens occurs and that heterotypic immunity is not sufficiently increased (202). Although serum antibody titers decline after natural infection, the durability of antibody after immunization is not defined, but is probably shorter lived if consistent with responses to other vaccines. At present there is no useful vaccine to prevent infections caused by rhinoviruses, and there has been no recent significant development in recent years (203).

Interruption of transmission of rhinoviruses from person to person can be achieved in some measure by awareness that rhinovirus-containing secretions are the main source of transmission, and that hand washing and proper disposal of contaminated articles such as paper handkerchiefs can help to reduce exposures. In the laboratory and in field trials, the use of paper handkerchiefs permeated with chemical inactivating agents such as citric acid and iodine has reduced transmission and might be considered for circumstances of high transmission or severe consequences of infection (204–206).

The evaluation of rhinovirus specific antiviral treatments is progressing in a number of areas. Although a monoclonal antibody directed against ICAM-1 on the cells of the nasal epithelium did little to prevent infection and reduce symptoms (207), a sol-

uble form of ICAM-1 has been produced as a purified protein and has been shown to be capable of preventing infection of tissue cultures by most rhinovirus serotypes that bind to ICAM-1 (208,209). In clinical trials, soluble ICAM-1 did not eliminate infectivity, but it did reduce virus shedding by approximately 15% (210). However, when it was given up to 12 hours after exposure of susceptible volunteers to rhinovirus, soluble ICAM-1 reduced overall common cold symptoms, nasal discharge and interluekin-8 production. Although the results are highly favorable to this approach, not all serotypes previously identified as being in the "major receptor group" (e.g., serotypes 23 and 25) by studies with monoclonal antibodies are well inhibited by soluble ICAM-1. In addition, some serotypes may develop reduced affinity for ICAM-1, presumably by clonal selection or genetic mutation on exposure to ICAM-1 (42). Furthermore, not all rhinovirus receptors have been identified (see Table 250.1) However, discovery of the LDL receptor family suggests that receptor blockade for the "minor receptor group" rhinoviruses should also be expected (41,48–51). Further clinical trials will help to determine the general applicability of receptor blockade for the prevention and treatment of rhinovirus infections.

Many antiviral agents that are active against rhinoviruses have been identified and some have undergone clinical trials (6,23,211–225). Some are unacceptable because of toxicity. Others studied in clinical trials have had limited antiviral effects. Although some drugs have shown prophylactic effects in preventing rhinovirus infections, none has been shown to be beneficial after infection is established. In general, the best strategy for delivery of many of the drugs has been direct delivery via intranasal administration of powdered or dissolved drug. A limiting feature in some instances appears to be maintenance of adequate concentrations of drug at the target nasopharyngeal tissues, which are protected by complex clearance mechanisms. As an example, pirodavir when given as a nasal spray six times per day reduced infection rates by approximately half as compared with placebo but had no effect when given three times per day (223). As another example, enviroxime, which is one of the most potent chemical inhibitors of rhinoviruses in tissue culture, had inconsistent effects in volunteer challenge studies, possibly because of the poor water solubility of the compound (212–214). However, alternative formulations designed to bypass solubility barriers and to improve retention of the drug at the intranasal site may help to improve effectiveness of antiviral chemicals (215).

Many studies have shown the efficacy of interferon alpha or interferon inducers applied locally in the nasopharynx in preventing rhinovirus infection (146,226–233). Strategies for use are based on the observed seasonality and family clustering of infections with rhinoviruses. Administration of interferon alpha on a long-term basis results in infiltration of the nasal mucosa with increased numbers of lymphocytes and causes nasal bleeding (usually not sufficient to result in epistaxis) in 5% to 10% of recipients (232,233). Limiting the duration of use of interferon to a week or two after introduction of a respiratory virus into a family reduces some of the undesirable aspects of administration; however, when this approach is used rhinovirus infections are fewer but other common cold viruses such as parainfluenza virus are relatively unaffected (228). The paucity of symptoms in many infected persons suggests that subclinical infections could also reduce the efficacy of interferon alpha used in this manner (99). Preparations of interferon beta and interferon gamma have been less well studied. Although some reduction in symptoms caused by rhinovirus infection has been demonstrated, interferon beta does not appear to prevent acquisition of the infection either experimentally or naturally (234,235). Human interferon gamma not only fails to prevent rhinovirus infection but also may augment the symptomatic response (236). No study with interferon has shown a therapeutic effect once infection has been established and symptoms have begun.

Some of the nonspecific remedies that have received much popular attention as potential remedies for the common cold include ascorbic acid and zinc (237–245). However, neither ascorbic acid nor zinc has been shown to prevent rhinovirus infection in volunteer challenge studies (237,241,242). Although symptomatic benefits of administration of ascorbic acid or zinc have been described in studies of naturally occurring respiratory infections, the results have shown no consistent, reproducible pattern for the type of symptoms affected, the degree of relief, or the duration of symptoms. These inconsistencies may be attributed in some instances to the failure of "blinding" (because both ascorbic acid and zinc can be readily discerned by taste). In other instances, positive outcomes may reflect a statistical artifact. The current data, however, indicate a modest effect at best and are insufficient to prompt a strong recommendation in favor of ascorbic acid or zinc. Nevertheless, interest in ascorbic acid and zinc has continued because it seems to offer a simple, benign treatment for an infectious disease lacking a well-defined, specific remedy. Another recently popularized remedy for respiratory viral infections is Echinacea. However, a controlled clinical trial in volunteers infected experimentally with a rhinovirus demonstrated no effect of Echinacea on either infection or illness (246).

In the absence of specific antiviral therapy, several simple measures may be readily undertaken in alleviating symptoms. Maintenance of hydration to keep secretions loose and the judicious use of nasal decongestant medications offer the most convenient combination for treatment. The nasal wash maneuver with room temperature physiologic salt solution is surprisingly pleasant and provides temporary opening of nasal passages by removing tenacious secretions and causing detumescence of the mucosa. Aspirin and other nonsteroidal anti-inflammatory agents may improve systemic symptoms such as malaise but are of no clear benefit to local inflammatory symptoms (247). Aspirin should be used cautiously and should not be given to children. Acetaminophen is preferred as the anti-inflammatory agent for children, because many respiratory viruses can cause the common cold, the etiology of respiratory infection may not

be determined easily, and aspirin administration has been implicated in the development of Reye's syndrome related to respiratory virus infection (248). Although the symptoms may result from immuno-inflammatory responses, steroids do not prevent symptoms and may prolong viral shedding during rhinovirus infection (172). Antihistamines such as brompheniramine maleate and clemastine fumarate have been demonstrated to reduce sneezing and nasal discharge (249–252). Some side effects of antihistamine use (e.g., dry nose and mouth) may offset perceived benefits, and injudicious use may lead to rebound symptoms at discontinuation. Pseudoephedrine has shown a benefit in relieving nasal congestion and anticholinergic agents have also demonstrated some effect in reducing nasal discharge (131,132,253,254). A combination of several of these modalities has been suggested as a potential therapeutic approach. In a study of volunteers infected with a rhinovirus 1 day before beginning treatment, the combination of interferon alpha to reduce virus replication, naproxen as an antiinflammatory agent to reduce systemic symptoms, and ipratropium as an anticholinergic medication to reduce nasal secretions was effective in reducing symptoms without impairing immune responses to the infecting strain (254).

The promising effectiveness of specific antiviral treatments (e.g., receptor blockade) and combined nonspecific medical interventions suggest that continued investigation of similar regimens may be useful. In addition, the mediators of the inflammatory and cytokine responses to rhinovirus infections are emerging as potential targets for the development of other remedies for preventing or treating the rhinovirus common cold.

REFERENCES

1. Rhinoviruses: a numbering system. *Nature* 1967;213:761.
2. A collaborative report. Rhinoviruses—extension of the numbering system. *Virology* 1971;43:524–526.
3. Hamparian VV, Colonno RJ, Cooney MK, et al. A collaborative report. Rhinoviruses—extension of the numbering system from 89 to 100. *Virology* 1987;159:191–192.
4. Conant RM, Hamparian VV. Rhinoviruses: basis for a numbering system. I. HeLa cells for propagation and serologic procedures. *J Immunol* 1968;100:107.
5. Conant RM, Hamparian VV. Rhinoviruses: basis for a numbering system. II. Serologic characterization of prototype strains. *J Immunol* 1968;100:114.
6. Andries K, Dewindt B, Snoeks J, et al. Two groups of rhinoviruses revealed by a panel of antiviral compounds present sequence divergence and differential pathogenicity. *J Virol* 1990;64:1117.
7. Horsnell C, Gama RE, Hughes PJ, et al. Molecular relationships between 21 human rhinovirus serotypes. *J Gen Virol* 1995;76:2549.
8. King AMQ, Brown F, Christian P, et al. Picornaviridae. In: Van Regenmortel MHV, Fauquet CM, Bishop DHL, et al., eds. *Virus taxonomy: Seventh report of the international committee for the taxonomy of viruses.* New York: Academic Press, 2000:996.
9. Uncapher CR, DeWitt CM, Colonno RJ. The major and minor group receptor families contain all but one human rhinovirus serotype. *Virology* 1991;180:814.
10. Verdaguer N, Blaas D, Fita I. Structure of human rhinovirus serotype 2 (HRV2). *J Mol Biol* 2000;300:1179.
11. Rossmann MG, Arnold E, Erickson JW, et al. Structure of a human common cold virus and functional relationship to other picornaviruses. *Nature* 1985;317:146.
12. Kim S, Smith TJ, Chapman MS, et al. The crystal structure of human rhinovirus serotype 1A (HRV1A). *J Mol Biol* 1989;210:91.
13. Arnold E, Rossmann MG. Analysis of the structure of a common cold virus, human rhinovirus-14, refined at a resolution of 3.0 Å. *J Mol Biol* 1990;211:763.
14. Oliviera MA, Thao R, Lee WM, et al. The structure of human rhinovirus 16. *Structure* 1993;1:51.
15. Zhao R, Pevear DC, Kremer MJ, et al. Human rhinovirus 3 at 3.0 A resolution. *Structure* 1996;4:1205.
16. Sherry B, Mosser AG, Colonno RJ, et al. Use of monoclonal antibodies to identify four neutralization immunogens on a common cold picornavirus, human rhinovirus 14. *J Virol* 1986;57:246.
17. Smith TJ, Olson NH, Cheng RH, et al. Structure of a human rhinovirus-bivalently bound antibody complex: implications for viral neutralization and antibody flexibility. *Proc Natl Acad Sci USA* 1993;90:7015.

18. Barnett PV, Rowlands DJ, Parry NR. Characterization of monoclonal antibodies raised against a synthetic peptide capable of inducing a neutralizing response to human rhinovirus type 2. *J Gen Virol* 1993;74:1295.

19. Rossmann MG, Palmenberg AC. Conservation of the putative receptor attachment site in picornaviruses. *Virology* 1988;164:373.

20. Rossmann MG, Bella J, Kolatkar PR, et al. Cell recognition and entry by rhino- and enteroviruses. *Virology* 2000;269:239.

21. Bibler-Muckelbauer JK, Kremer MJ, Rossmann MG, et al. Human rhinovirus 14 complexed with fragments of active antiviral compounds. *Virology* 1994;202:360.

22. Smith TJ, Kremer MJ, Luo M, et al. The site of attachment in human rhinovirus 14 for antiviral agents that inhibit uncoating. *Science* 1986;233:1286.

23. Badger J, Minor I, Kremer MJ, et al. Structural analysis of a series of antiviral agents complexed with human rhinovirus 14. *Proc Natl Acad Sci USA* 1988;85:3304.

24. Ismail-Cassim N, Chezzi C, Newman JFE. Inhibition of the uncoating of bovine enterovirus by short chain fatty acids. *J Gen Virol* 1990;71:2283.

25. Rueckert RR, Wimmer E. Systematic nomenclature of picornavirus proteins. *J Virol* 1984;50:957.

26. Stanway G, Hughes PJ, Mountford RC, et al. The complete nucleotide sequence of a common cold virus: human rhinovirus 14. *Nucleic Acids Res* 1984;12:7859.

27. Skern T, Sommergruber W, Blaas D, et al. Human rhinovirus 2: complete nucleotide sequence and proteolytic processing signals in the capsid protein region. *Nucleic Acids Res* 1985;13:2111.

28. Duechler M, Skern T, Sommergruber W, et al. Evolutionary relationships within the human rhinovirus genus: comparison of serotypes 89, 2, and 14. *Proc Natl Acad Sci USA* 1987;84:2605.

29. Hughes PJ, North C, Jellis CH, et al. The nucleotide sequence of human rhinovirus 113: molecular relationships within the rhinovirus genus. *J Gen Virol* 1988;69:49.

30. Trono D, Andino R, Baltimore D. An RNA sequence of hundreds of nucleotides at the 5' end of poliovirus RNA is involved in allowing viral protein synthesis. *J Virol* 1988;62:2291.

31. Jackson RJ. RNA translation: picornaviruses break the rules. *Nature* 1988;334:292.

32. Rivera VM, Welsh JD, Maizel JV Jr. Comparative sequence analysis of the 5' noncoding region of the enteroviruses and rhinoviruses. *Virology* 1988;165:42.

33. Pilipenko EV, Blinov VM, Romanova LI, et al. Conserved structural domains in the 5' untranslated region of picornaviral genomes: an analysis of the segment controlling translation and neurovirulence. *Virology* 1989;168:201.

34. Rohll JB, Percy N, Ley R, et al. The 5'-untranslated regions of picornavirus RNAs contain independent functional domains essential for RNA replication and translation. *J Virol* 1994;68:4384.

35. Belsham GJ, Sonenberg N. RNA-protein interactions in regulation of picornavirus RNA translation. *Microbiol Rev* 1996;60:499.

36. Rohll J, Moon DH, Evans DJ, et al. The 3' untranslated region of picornavirus RNA: features required for efficient genome replication. *J Virol* 1995;69:7835.

37. Todd S, Semler BL. Structure-infectivity analysis of the human rhinovirus genomic RNA 3' non-coding region. *Nucleic Acids Res* 1996;24:2133.

38. Mellits KH, Meredith JM, Rohll JB, et al. Binding of a cellular factor to the 3' untranslated region of the RNA of entero- and rhinoviruses plays a role in virus replication. *J Gen Virol* 1998;79:1715.

39. Tomassini JE, Colonno RJ. Isolation of a receptor protein involved in attachment of human rhinoviruses. *J Virol* 1986;58:290.

40. Mischak H, Neubauer C, Kuechler E, et al. Characteristics of the minor group receptor of human rhinoviruses. *Virology* 1988;163:19.

41. Hofer F, Gruenberger M, Kowalski H, et al. Members of the low density lipoprotein receptor family mediate cell entry of a minor-group common cold virus. *Proc Natl Acad Sci USA* 1994;91:1839.

42. Crump CE, Arruda E, Hayden FG. In vitro inhibitory activity of soluble ICAM-1 for the numbered serotypes of human rhinovirus. *Antiviral Chem Chemother* 1993;4:323.

43. Colonno RJ, Callahan PL, Long WJ. Isolation of a monoclonal antibody that blocks attachment of the major group of human rhinoviruses. *J Virol* 1986;57:7.

44. Greve JM, Davis G, Meyer AM, et al. The major human rhinovirus receptor is ICAM-1. *Cell* 1989;56:839.

45. Staunton DE, Merluzzi VJ, Rothlein R, et al. A cell adhesion molecule, ICAM-1, is the major surface receptor for rhinoviruses. *Cell* 1989;56:849.

46. Lineberger DW, Uncapher CR, Graham DJ, et al. Domains 1 and 2 of ICAM-1 are sufficient to bind human rhinoviruses. *Virus Res* 1992;24:173.

47. Yin FH, Lomax NB. Host range mutants of human rhinovirus in which non-structural proteins are altered. *J Virol* 1983;48:410.

48. Marlovits TC, Abrahamsberg C, Blaas D. Soluble LDL minireceptors: minimal structure requirements for recognition of minor group human rhinovirus. *J Biol Chem* 1998;273:33835.

49. Ronacher B, Marlovits TC, Moser R, et al. Expression and folding of human very-low-density lipoprotein receptor fragments: neutralization capacity toward human rhinovirus HRV 2. *Virology* 2000;278:541.

50. Marlovits TC, Abrahamsberg C, Blaas D. Very-low-density lipoprotein receptor fragment shed from HeLa cells inhibits human rhinovirus infection. *J Virol* 1998;72:10246.

51. Hewat EA, Neumann E, Conway JF, et al. The cellular receptor to human rhinovirus 2 binds around the 5-fold axis and not in the canyon: a structural view. *EMBO J* 2000;19:6317.

52. Appleyard G, Russell SM, Clarke BE, et al. Neutralization epitopes of human rhinovirus type 2. *J Gen Virol* 1990;71:1275.

53. Hewat EA, Blaas D. Structure of a neutralizing antibody bound bivalently to human rhinovirus 2. *EMBO J* 1996;15:1515.

54. Smith TJ, Chase ES, Schmidt TJ, et al. Neutralizing antibody to human rhinovirus 14 penetrates the receptor-binding canyon. *Nature* 383:350, 1996.

54a. Colonno RJ, Callahan PL, Long WJ. Isolation of a monoclonal antibody that blocks attachment of the major group of human rhinoviruses. *J Virol* 1986;57:7.

55. Hewat EA, Marlovits TC, Blaas D. Structure of a neutralizing antibody bound monovalently to human rhinovirus 2. *J Virol* 1998;72:4396.

56. Tormo J, Blaas D, Parry NR, et al. Crystal structure of a human rhinovirus neutralizing antibody complexed with a peptide derived from viral capsid protein VP2. *EMBO J* 1994;13:2247.

57. Speller SA, Sangar DV, Clarke BE, et al. The nature and spatial distribution of amino acid substitutions conferring resistance to neutralizing monoclonal antibodies in human rhinovirus type 2. *J Gen Virol* 1993;74:193.

58. Resnick DA, Smith AD, Geisler SC, et al. Chimera from a human rhinovirus 14-human immunodeficiency virus type 1 (HIV-1) V3 loop seroprevalence library induce neutralizing responses against HIV-1. *J Virol* 1995;69:2406.

59. Schober D, Kroneneberger P, Prchla E, et al. Major and minor receptor group human rhinoviruses penetrate from endosomes by different mechanisms. *J Virol* 1998;72:1354.

60. DeTulleo L, Kirchhausen T. The clathrin endocytic pathway in viral infection. *EMBO J* 1998;17:4585.

61. Bayer N, Prchla E, Schwab M, et al. Human rhinovirus HRV14 uncoats from early endosomes in the presence of bafilomycin. *FEBS Lett* 1999;463:175.

62. Bayer N, Schober D, Huttinger M, et al. Inhibition of clathrin-dependent endocytosis has multiple effects on human rhinovirus serotype 2 cell entry. *J Biol Chem* 2001;276:3952.

63. Prchla E, Kuechler E, Blaas D, et al. Uncoating of human rhinovirus serotype 2 from late endosomes. *J Virol* 1994;68:3713.

64. Arnold E, Luo M, Vriend G, et al. Implications of the picornavirus capsid structure for polyprotein processing. *Proc Natl Acad Sci USA* 1987;84:21.

65. Lee WM, Monroe SS, Rueckert RR. Role of maturation cleavage in infectivity of picornaviruses: activation of an infectosome. *J Virol* 1993;67:2110.

66. Ivanoff L, Towatari T, Ray J, et al. Expression and site-specific mutagenesis of the poliovirus 3C protease in E. coli. *Proc Natl Acad Sci USA* 1986;83:5392.

67. Sommergruber W, Zorn M, Blaas D, et al. Polypeptide 2A of human rhinovirus type 2: identification as a protease and characterization by mutational analysis. *Virology* 1989;169:68.

68. Korant BD, Lonberg-Holm K, LaColla P. Picornaviruses and togaviruses: targets for design of antivirals. In: De Clerq E, Walker RT, eds. *Targets for the design of antiviral agents.* New York: Plenum Publishing, 1984:61–98.

69. Semler BL, Anderson CL, Hanecak R, et al. A membrane-associated precursor to poliovirus VPg identified by immunoprecipitation with antibodies directed against a synthetic heptapeptide. *Cell* 1982;28:405.

70. Krausslich HG, Nicklin MJ, Toyoda H, et al. Poliovirus proteinase 2A induces cleavage of eukaryotic initiation factor 4F polypeptide p220. *J Virol* 1987;61:2711.

71. Glaser W, Skern T. Extremely efficient cleavage of eIF4G by picornaviral proteinases L and 2A in vitro. *FEBS Lett* 2000;480:151.

72. Yin FH, Lomax NB. Establishment of a mouse model for human rhinovirus infection. *J Gen Virol* 1986;67:2335.

73. Lomax NB, Yin FH. Evidence for the role of the P2 protein of human rhinovirus in its host range change. *J Virol* 1989;63:2396.

74. Hamparian VV, Ketler A, Hilleman MR. Recovery of new viruses (coryzavirus) from cases of common cold in human adults. *Proc Soc Exp Biol Med* 1961;108:444.

75. Korant BD, Lonberg-Holm K, Noble J, et al. Naturally occurring and artificially produced components of three rhinoviruses. *Virology* 1972;48:71.

76. Skern T, Torgersen H, Auer H, et al. Human rhinovirus mutants resistant to low pH. *Virology* 1991;183:757.

77. Tyrrell DAJ, Chanock RM. Rhinoviruses: a description. *Science* 1963;141:152.

78. Dimmock NJ, Tyrrell DAJ. Some physicochemical properties of rhinoviruses. *Br J Exp Pathol* 1964;45:271.

79. Cooney MK, Hall CE, Fox JP. The Seattle virus watch. III. Evaluation of isolation methods and summary of infections detected by virus isolations. *Am J Epidemiol* 1972;96:286.

80. Fox JP, Cooney MK, Hall CE. The Seattle virus watch. V. Epidemiologic observations of rhinovirus infections, 1965–1969, in families with young children. *Am J Epidemiol* 1975;101:122.

81. Wulff H, Noble GR, Maynard JE, et al. An outbreak of respiratory infection in children with rhinovirus serotypes 16 and 29. *Am J Epidemiol* 1969;90:304.

82. Phillips CA, Melnick JL, Grim CA. Rhinovirus infections in a student population: isolation of five new serotypes. *Am J Epidemiol* 1968;87:447.

83. Hamre D, Connelly AP Jr, Procknow JJ. Virologic studies of acute respiratory disease in young adults. III. Some biologic and serologic characteristics of

seventeen rhinovirus serotypes isolated October, 1960 to June, 1961. *J Lab Clin Med* 1964;64:450.

84. Warshauer DM, Dick EC, Mandel AD, et al. Rhinovirus infections in an isolated Antarctic station. Transmission of the viruses and susceptibility of the population. *Am J Epidemiol* 1989;129:319.

85. Gwaltney JM Jr, Hendley JO, Simon G, et al. Rhinovirus infections in an industrial population. III. Number and prevalence of serotypes. *Am J Epidemiol* 1968;87:158.

86. Calhoun AM, Jordan WS Jr, Gwaltney JM Jr. Rhinovirus infections in an industrial population. V. Change in distribution of serotypes. *Am J Epidemiol* 1974;99:58.

87. Monto AS, Cavallaro JJ. The Tecumseh study of respiratory illness. IV. Prevalence of rhinovirus serotypes, 1966–1969. *Am J Epidemiol* 1972;96:352.

88. Monto AS, Bryan ER, Ohmit S. Rhinovirus infections in Tecumseh, Michigan: frequency of illness and number of serotypes. *J Infect Dis* 1987;156:43.

89. Thwing CJ, Arruda E, Vieira Filho JPB, et al. Rhinovirus antibodies in an isolated Amazon Indian tribe. *Am J Trop Med Hyg* 1993;48:771.

90. Hendley JO, Edmondson WP Jr, Gwaltney JM Jr. Relation between naturally acquired immunity and infectivity of two rhinoviruses in volunteers. *J Infect Dis* 1972;125:243.

91. Monto AS, Sullivan KM. Acute respiratory illness in the community. Frequency of illness and the agents involved. *Epidemiol Infect* 1993;110:145.

92. Aymard M, Chomel JJ, Allard JP, et al. Epidemiology of viral infections and evaluation of the potential benefit of OM-85 BV on the virologic status of children attending day-care centers. *Respiration* 1994;61[Suppl 1]:24.

93. Holmes MJ, Reed SE, Stott EJ, et al. Studies of experimental rhinovirus type 2 infections in polar isolation and in England. *J Hyg (Lond)* 1976;76:379.

94. Reed SE. An investigation of the possible transmission of rhinovirus colds through indirect contact. *J Hyg (Lond)* 1975;75:249.

95. Douglas RG Jr, Cate TR, Gerone PJ, et al. Quantitative rhinovirus shedding patterns in volunteers. *Am Rev Respir Dis* 1966;94:159.

96. D'Alessio DJ, Peterson JA, Dick CR, et al. Transmission of experimental rhinovirus colds in volunteer married couples. *J Infect Dis* 1976;233:28.

97. Hendley JO, Wenzel RP, Gwaltney JM Jr. Transmission of rhinovirus colds by self-inoculation. *N Engl J Med* 1973;288:1361.

98. Gwaltney JM Jr, Hendley JO. Rhinovirus transmission: one if by air, and two if by hand. *Am J Epidemiol* 1978;107:357.

99. Foy HM, Cooney MK, Hall C, et al. Case-to-case intervals of rhinovirus and influenza virus infections in households. *J Infect Dis* 1988;157:180.

100. Dick EC, Jennings LC, Mink KA, et al. Aerosol transmission of rhinovirus colds. *J Infect Dis* 1987;156:442.

101. Jennings LC, Dick EC, Mink KA, et al. Near disappearance of rhinovirus along a fomite transmission chain. *J Infect Dis* 1988;158:888.

102. Gwaltney JM Jr, Moskalski PB, Hendley JO. Hand-to-hand transmission of rhinovirus colds. *Ann Intern Med* 1978;88:463.

103. Levandowski RA, Pachucki CT, Rubenis M. Specific mononuclear cell response to rhinovirus. *J Infect Dis* 1983;148:1125.

104. Hsia J, Goldstein AL, Smith GL, et al. Peripheral blood mononuclear cells, interleukin-2 and interferon-gamma production, cytotoxicity and antigen-stimulated blastogenesis during experimental rhinovirus infection. *J Infect Dis* 1990;162:591–597.

105. Hastings GZ, Francis MJ, Rowlands DJ, et al. Antigen processing and presentation of human rhinovirus to CD4 T cells is facilitated by binding to cellular receptors for virus. *Eur J Immunol* 1993;23:1340.

106. Skoner DP, Whiteside TL, Wilson JW, et al. Effect of rhinovirus 39 infection on cellular and immune parameters in allergic and nonallergic subjects. *J Allergy Clin Immunol* 1993;92:732.

107. Gern JE, Dick EC, Kelly EAB, et al. Rhinovirus-specific T cells recognize both shared and serotype-specific epitopes. *J Infect Dis* 1997;175:1108.

108. Dowling HF, Jackson GG, Inouye T. Transmission of the experimental common cold in volunteers. II. The effect of certain host factors upon susceptibility. *J Lab Clin Med* 1957;50:516.

109. Dowling HF, Jackson GG, Spiesman IG, et al. Transmission of the common cold to volunteers under controlled conditions. III. The effect of chilling of the subjects upon susceptibility. *Am J Hyg* 1958;68:59.

110. Douglas RG Jr, Lindgren KM, Couch RB. Exposure to cold environment and rhinovirus common cold. Failure to demonstrate effect. *N Engl J Med* 1968;279:742.

111. Fleet WF, Couch RB, Cate TR, et al. Homologous and heterologous resistance to rhinovirus common cold. *Am J Epidemiol* 1965;82:185.

112. Cate TR, Rossen RD, Douglas RG Jr, et al. The role of nasal secretion and serum antibody in the rhinovirus common cold. *Am J Epidemiol* 1966;84:352.

113. Sanders SP, Siekierski ES, Porter JD, et al. Nitric oxide inhibits rhinovirus-induced cytokine production and viral replication in a human respiratory epithelial cell line. *J Virol* 1998;72:934.

114. Sanders SP, Siekierski ES, Richards SM, et al. Rhinovirus infection induces expression of type 2 nitric oxide synthase in human respiratory epithelial cells in vitro and in vivo. *J Allergy Clin Immunol* 2001;107:235.

115. Cohen S. Psychological stress and susceptibility to upper respiratory infections. *Am J Respir Crit Care Med* 1995;152:S53.

116. Tyrrell DAJ. Common cold viruses. *Int Rev Exp Pathol* 1962;1:209.

117. Arola M, Ziegler T, Ruuskanen O, et al. Rhinovirus in acute otitis media. *J Pediatr* 1988;113:693.

118. Hamory BH, Sande MA, Sydnor A Jr, et al. Etiology and antimicrobial therapy of acute maxillary sinusitis. *J Infect Dis* 1979;139:197.

119. Halperin SA, Eggleston PA, Hendley JO, et al. Pathogenesis of lower respiratory tract symptoms in experimental rhinovirus infection. *Am Rev Respir Dis* 1983;128:806.

120. Gern JE, Galagan DW, Jarjour NN, et al. Detection of rhinovirus RNA in lower airway cells during experimentally induced infection. *Am J Respir Crit Care Med* 1997;155:1159.

121. Papadopoulos NG, Bates PJ, Bardin PG, et al. Rhinoviruses infect the lower airways. *J Infect Dis* 2000;181:1875.

122. Johnston SL. Natural and experimental rhinovirus infections of the lower respiratory tract. *Am J Respir Crit Care Med* 1995;152:S46.

123. Turner RB, Hendley JO, Gwaltney JM Jr. Shedding of infected ciliated epithelial cells in rhinovirus colds. *J Infect Dis* 1982;145:849.

124. Wilson R, Alton E, Rutman A, et al. Upper respiratory tract viral infection and mucociliary clearance. *Eur J Respir Dis* 1987;70:272.

125. Hamory BH, Hendley JO, Gwaltney JM Jr. Rhinovirus growth in nasal polyp organ culture. *Proc Soc Exp Biol Med* 1977;155:577.

126. Bruce C, Chadwick P, Al-Nakib W. Detection of rhinovirus RNA in nasal epithelial cells by in situ hybridization. *J Virol Methods* 1990;30:115.

127. Arruda E, Mifflin TE, Gwaltney JM Jr, et al. Localization of rhinovirus replication in vitro with in situ hybridization. *J Med Virol* 1991;34:38.

128. Bates PJ, Sanderson G, Holgate ST, et al. A comparison of RT-PCR, in-situ hybridization and in-situ RT-PCR for the detection of rhinovirus infection in paraffin sections. *J Virol Methods* 1997;67:153.

129. Urquhart GED, Stott EJ. Rhinoviraemia. *BMJ* 1970;2:28.

130. Cate TR, Douglas RG Jr, Johnson KM, et al. Studies on the inability of rhinovirus to survive and replicate in the intestinal tract of volunteers. *Proc Soc Exp Biol Med* 1967;124:1290.

131. Borum P, Olsen L, Winther B, et al. Ipratropium nasal spray: a new treatment for rhinorrhea in the common cold. *Am Rev Respir Dis* 1981;123:418.

132. Gaffey MJ, Gwaltney JM Jr, Dressler WE, et al. Intranasally administered atropine methonitrate treatment of experimental rhinovirus colds. *Am Rev Respir Dis* 1987;135:241.

133. Igrashi YI, Skoner DP, Doyle WJ, et al. Analysis of nasal secretions during experimental rhinovirus upper respiratory infections. *J Allergy Clin Immunol* 1993;92:722.

134. Calhoun WJ, Dick EC, Schwartz LB, et al. A common cold virus, rhinovirus 16, potentiates airway inflammation after segmental antigen bronchoprovocation in allergic subjects. *J Clin Invest* 1994;94:2200.

135. Naclerio RM, Proud D, Lichentenstein LM, et al. Kinins are generated during experimental rhinovirus colds. *J Infect Dis* 1988;157:133.

136. deGouw HWFM, Grunberg K, Schot R, et al. Relationship between exhaled nitric oxide and airway hyperresponsiveness following experimental rhinovirus infection in asthmatic subjects. *Eur Respir J* 1998;11:126.

137. Proud D, Gwaltney J Jr, Hendley JO, et al. Increased levels of interleukin-1 are detected in nasal secretions of volunteers during experimental rhinovirus colds. *J Infect Dis* 1994;169:1007.

138. Einarsson O, Geba GP, Zhu Z, et al. Interleukin-11: stimulation in vivo and in vitro by respiratory viruses and induction of airways hyperresponsiveness. *J Clin Invest* 1996;97:915.

139. Gern JE, Vrtis R, Kelly EAB, et al. Rhinovirus produces nonspecific activation of lymphocytes through a monocyte dependent mechanism. *J Immunol* 1996;157:1605.

140. Gem JE, Dick EC, Lee WM, et al. Rhinovirus enters but does not replicate inside monocytes and airway macrophages. *J Immunol* 1996;156:621.

141. Zhu Z, Tang W, Ray A, et al. Rhinovirus stimulation of interleukin-6 in vivo and in vitro: evidence for nuclear factor kB-dependent transcriptional activation. *J Clin Invest* 1996;97:421.

142. Johnston SL, Papi A, Monick MM, et al. Rhinoviruses induce interleukin-8 mRNA and protein production in human monocytes. *J Infect Dis* 1997;175:323.

143. Greiff L , Andersson M, Andersson E, et al. Experimental common cold increases mucosal output of eotaxin in atopic individuals. *Allergy* 1999;54:1204.

144. Schroth MK, Grimm E, Frindt P, et al. Rhinovirus replication causes RANTES production in primary bronchial epithelial cells. *Am J Respir Cell Mol Biol* 1999;20:1220.

145. Cate TR, Couch RB, Johnson KM. Studies with rhinoviruses in volunteers, production of illness, effect of naturally acquired antibody, and demonstration of a protective effect not associated with serum antibody. *J Clin Invest* 1964;43:56.

146. Panusarn C, Stanley ED, Dirda V, et al. Prevention of illness from rhinovirus infection by a topical interferon inducer. *N Engl J Med* 1974;291:57.

147. Levandowski RA, Horohov DW. Rhinovirus induces natural killer-like cytotoxic cells and interferon alpha in mononuclear leukocytes. *J Med Virol* 1991;35:116.

148. Hayden FG, Winther B, Donowitz GR, et al. Human nasal mucosal responses to topically applied recombinant leukocyte A interferon. *J Infect Dis* 1987;156:64.

149. Turner RB, Weingand KW, Yeh C-H, et al. Association between interleukin-8 concentration in nasal secretins and severity of symptoms of experimental rhinovirus colds. *Clin Infect Dis* 1998;26:840.

150. Douglas RG Jr, Alford RH, Cate TR, et al. The leukocyte response during viral respiratory illness in man. *Ann Intern Med* 1966;64:521.

151. Levandowski RA, Ou DW, Jackson GG. Acute-phase decrease of T-lymphocyte subsets in rhinovirus infection. *J Infect Dis* 1986;153:743.

152. Thomas LH, Fraenkel DJ, Bardin PG, et al. Leukocyte responses to experimental infection with human rhinovirus. *J Allergy Clin Immunol* 1994;94:1255.

153. Cheung D, Dick EC, Timmers MC, et al. Rhinovirus inhalation causes long-lasting excessive airway narrowing in response to methacholine in asthmatic subjects in vivo. *Am J Resp Crit Care Med* 1995;152:1490.

154. Fraenkel DJ, Bardin PG, Sanderson G, et al. Lower airways inflammation during rhinovirus colds in normal and in asthmatic subjects. *Am J Respir Crit Care Med* 1995;151:879.

155. Levandowski RA, Weaver CW, Jackson GG. Nasal secretion leukocyte populations determined by flow cytometry during acute rhinovirus infection. *J Med Virol* 1988;25:423.

156. Turner RB. The role of neutrophils in the pathogenesis of rhinovirus infections. *Pediatr Infect Dis J* 1990;9:832.

157. Turner RB. Rhinovirus infection of human embryonic lung fibroblasts induces the production of a chemoattractant for polymorphonuclear leukocytes. *J Infect Dis* 1988;157:346.

158. Jackson GG, Dowling HF, Spiesman IG, et al. Transmission of the common cold to volunteers under controlled conditions. I. The common cold as a clinical entity. *Arch Intern Med* 1958;101:267.

159. Turner BW, Cail WS, Hendley JO, et al. Physiologic abnormalities in the paranasal sinuses during experimental rhinovirus colds. *J Allergy Clin Immunol* 1992;90:474.

160. Gwaltney JM Jr, Phillips CD, Miller RD, et al. Computed tomographic study of the common cold. *N Engl J Med* 1994;330:25.

161. Lourenço RV, Stanley ED, Gatmaitan B, et al. Abnormal deposition and clearance of inhaled particles during upper respiratory viral infections. *J Clin Invest* 1971;50:62a.

162. Garrard CS, Levandowski RA, Gerrity TR, et al. The effects of acute respiratory virus infection upon tracheal mucus transport. *Arch Environ Health* 1985;40:322.

163. Ghosh S, Champlin R, Couch R, et al. Rhinovirus infections in myelosuppressed adult blood and bone marrow transplant. *Clin Infect Dis* 1999;29:528.

164. Crooks BNA, Taylor CE, Turner AJL, et al. Respiratory viral infections in primary immune deficiencies: significance and relevance to clinical outcome in a single BMT unit. *Bone Marrow Transplant* 2000;26:1097.

165. Minor TE, Dick EC, Baker JW, et al. Rhinovirus and influenza A infections as precipitants of asthma. *Am Rev Respir Dis* 1976;113:149.

166. Lemanske RF Jr, Dick EC, Swenson CA, et al. Rhinovirus upper respiratory infection increases airway hyperreactivity and late asthmatic reactions. *J Clin Invest* 1989;83:1.

167. Stenhouse AC. Rhinovirus infection in acute exacerbations of chronic bronchitis: a controlled prospective study. *BMJ* 1967;3:461.

168. Nicholson KG, Kent J, Ireland DC. Respiratory viruses and exacerbations of asthma in adults. *BMJ* 1993;307:982.

169. Johnston SL, Pattemore PK, Sanderson G, et al. Community study of role of viral infections in exacerbations of asthma in 9–11 year old children. *BMJ* 1995;310:1225.

170. Fridy WW Jr, Ingram RH Jr, Hierholzer JC, et al. Airways function during mild viral respiratory illnesses: the effect of rhinoviruses on cigarette smokers. *Ann Intern Med* 1974;80:150.

171. Blair HT, Greenberg SB, Stevens PM, et al. Effects of rhinovirus infection on pulmonary function of healthy human volunteers. *Am Rev Respir Dis* 1976;114:95.

172. Gustafson LM, Proud D, Hendley JO, et al. Oral prednisone therapy in experimental rhinovirus infections. *J Allergy Clin Immunol* 1996;97:1009.

173. Price WH. The isolation of a new virus associated with respiratory clinical disease in humans. *Proc Natl Acad Sci USA* 1956;42:546.

174. Pelon W, Mogabgab WJ, Phillips IA, et al. A cytopathogenic agent isolated from naval recruits with mild respiratory illness. *Proc Soc Exp Biol Med* 1957;94:262.

175. Mogabgab WJ, Felon W. Problems in characterizing and identifying an apparently new virus found in association with mild respiratory disease in recruits. *Ann NY Acad Sci* 1957;67:403.

176. Half RF, Wohlsen B, Force EE, et al. Growth characteristics of two rhinovirus strains in WI-26 and monkey kidney cells. *J Bacteriol* 1966;91:2339.

177. Stott EJ, Tyrrell DAJ. Some improved techniques for the study of rhinoviruses using HeLa cells. *Arch Gesamte Virusforsch* 1968;23:236.

178. Lewis FA, Kennet ML. Comparison of rhinovirus-sensitive HeLa cells and human embryo fibroblasts for isolation of rhinoviruses from patients with respiratory disease. *J Clin Microbiol* 1976;3:528.

179. Hamory BH, Hendley JO, Gwaltney JM Jr. Rhinovirus growth in nasal polyp organ culture. *Proc Soc Exp Biol Med* 1977;155:577.

180. Kenney GE, Cooney MK, Thompson DJ. Analysis of serum pooling schemes for identification of large numbers of viruses. *Am J Epidemiol* 1970;91:439.

181. Cooney MK, Wise JA, Kenney GE, et al. Broad antigenic relationships among rhinovirus serotypes revealed by cross-immunization of rabbits with different serotypes. *J Immunol* 1975;114:635.

182. Douglas RG Jr, Fleet WF, Cater TR, et al. Antibody to rhinovirus in human sera. I. Standardization of a neutralization test. *Proc Soc Exp Biol Med* 1968;127:497.

183. Dearden CJ, Al-Nakib W. Direct detection of rhinoviruses by an enzyme-linked immunosorbent assay. *J Med Virol* 1987;23:179.

184. Bruce CB, Al-Nakib W, Tyrrell DAJ, et al. Synthetic oligonucleotides as diagnostic probes for rhinoviruses. *Lancet* 1988;2:53.

185. Korant BD. Viral proteases—an emerging therapeutic target. *Crit Rev Biotechnol* 1988;8:149.

186. Gama RE, Hughes PJ, Bruce CB, et al. Polymerase chain reaction amplification of rhinovirus nucleic acids from clinical material. *Nucleic Acids Res* 1988;16:9346.

187. Gama RE, Horsnell PR, Hughes PJ, et al. Amplification of rhinovirus specific nucleic acids from clinical samples using the polymerase chain reaction. *J Med Virol* 1989;28:73.

188. Torgersen H, Skern T, Blaas D. Typing of human rhinoviruses based on sequence variations in the 5' non-coding region. *J Gen Virol* 1989;70:3111.

189. Olive DM, Al-Mufti S, Al-Mulla, et al. Detection and differentiation of picornaviruses in clinical samples following genomic amplification. *J Gen Virol* 1990;71:2141.

190. Atmar RL, Georghiou PR. Classification of respiratory tract picornavirus isolates as enteroviruses or rhinoviruses by using reverse transcription-polymerase chain reaction. *J Clin Microbiol* 1993;31:2544.

191. Johnston SL, Sanderson G, Pattemore PK, et al. Use of polymerase chain reaction for diagnosis of picornavirus infection in subjects with and without respiratory symptoms. *J Clin Microbiol* 1993;31:111.

192. Mori J, Clewley JP. Polymerase chain reaction and sequencing for typing rhinovirus RNA. *J Med Virol* 1994;44:323.

193. Halonen P, Rocha E, Hierholzer J, et al. Detection of enteroviruses and rhinoviruses in clinical specimens by PCR and liquid-phase hybridization. *J Clin Microbiol* 1995;33:648.

194. Santti J, Hyypia T, Halonen P. Comparison of PCR primer pairs in the detection of human rhinoviruses in nasopharyngeal aspirates. *J Virol Methods* 1997;66:139.

195. Blomqvist S, Skytta A, Roivainen M, et al. Rapid detection of human rhinoviruses in nasopharyngeal aspirates by a microwell reverse transcription-PCR-hybridization assay. *J Clin Microbiol* 1999;37:2813.

196. Papadopoulos NG, Hunter J, Sanderson G, et al. Rhinovirus identification by BglI digestion of picornavirus RT-PCR amplicons. *J Virol Methods* 1999;80:179.

197. Price WH. Vaccine for the prevention in humans of coldlike symptoms associated with the JH virus. *Proc Natl Acad Sci USA* 1957;43:790.

198. Andrewes CH, Tyrrell DAJ, Stones PB, et al. Prevention of colds by vaccination against a rhinovirus. *BMJ* 1965;1:1344.

199. Perkins JC, Tucker DN, Knopf HLS, et al. Evidence of protective effect of an inactivated rhinovirus vaccine administered by the nasal route. *Am J Epidemiol* 1969;90:319.

200. McCray J, Werner G. Different rhinovirus serotypes neutralized by antipeptide antibodies. *Nature* 1987;329:736.

201. Francis MJ, Hastings GZ, Sangar DV, et al. A synthetic peptide which elicits neutralizing antibody against rhinovirus type 2. *J Gen Virol* 1987;68:2687.

202. Hamory BH, Hamparian VV, Conant RM, et al. Human responses to two decavalent rhinovirus vaccines. *J Infect Dis* 1975;132:623.

203. Fox JP. Is a rhinovirus vaccine possible? *Am J Epidemiol* 1976;103:345.

204. Gwaltney JM Jr, Moskalski PB, Hendley JO. Interruption of experimental rhinovirus transmission. *J Infect Dis* 1980;142:811.

205. Dick EC, Hossain SU, Mink KA, et al. Interruption of transmission of rhinovirus colds among human volunteers using virucidal paper handkerchiefs. *J Infect Dis* 1986;153:352.

206. Longhini IM Jr, Monto AS. Efficacy of virucidal nasal tissues in interrupting familial transmission of respiratory agents. A field trial in Tecumseh, Michigan. *Am J Epidemiol* 1988;128:639.

207. Hayden FG, Gwaltney JM Jr, Colonno RJ. Modification of experimental rhinovirus colds by receptor blockade. *Antiviral Res* 1988;9:233.

208. Ohlin A, Hoover-Litty H, Sanderson G, et al. Spectrum of activity of soluble intercellular adhesion molecule-1 against rhinovirus reference strains and field isolates. *Antimicrob Agents Chemother* 1994;38:1413.

209. Crump CE, Arruda E, Hayden FG. Comparative antirhinoviral activities of soluble intercellular adhesion molecule-1 (sICAM-1) and chimeric ICAM-1/immunoglobulin A molecule. *Antimicrob Agents Chemother* 1994;38:1425.

210. Turner RB, Wecker MT, Pohl G, et al. Efficacy of tremacamra, a soluble intercellular adhesion molecule 1, for experimental rhinovirus infection. *JAMA* 1999;281:1797.

211. DeLong DC, Reed SE. Inhibition of rhinovirus replication in organ cultures by a potential antiviral drug. *J Infect Dis* 1980;141:87.

212. Phillpotts RJ, DeLong DC, Wallace J, et al. The activity of enviroxime against rhinovirus infection in man. *Lancet* 1981;1:1342.

213. Hayden FG, Gwaltney JM Jr. Prophylactic activity of intranasal enviroxime against experimentally induced rhinovirus type 39 infection. *Antimicrob Agents Chemother* 1982;21:892.

214. Levandowski RA, Pachucki CT, Rubenis M, et al. Topical enviroxime against rhinovirus infection. *Antimicrob Agents Chemother* 1982;22:1004.

215. Wyde PR, Six HR, Wilson SZ, et al. Activity against rhinoviruses, toxicity, and delivery in aerosol of enviroxime in liposomes. *Antimicrob Agents Chemother* 1988;32:890.

216. Zerial A, Werner GH, Phillpotts RJ, et al. Studies on 44 081 R.P., a new antirhinovirus compound, in cell cultures and in volunteers. *Antimicrob Agents Chemother* 1985;27:846.

217. Diana GD, Oglesby RC, Akullian V, et al. Structure-activity studies of 5-[[4-(4,5-dihydro-2-oxazolyl)phenoxy]alkyl]-3-methylisoxazoles: inhibitors of picornavirus uncoating. *J Med Chem* 1987;30:383.

218. Al-Nakib W, Willman J, Higgins PG, et al. Failure of intranasally administered 4',6-dichloroflavan to protect against rhinovirus infection in man. *Arch Virol* 1987;92:255.

219. Kenny MT, Torney HL, Dulworth JK. Mechanism of action of the antiviral compound MDL 20,610. *Antiviral Res* 1988;9:249.

220. Al-Nakib W, Higgins PG, Barrow I, et al. Intranasal chalcone, Ro 09-0410, as prophylaxis against rhinovirus infection in human volunteers. *J Antimicrob Chemother* 1987;20:887.

221. Fox MP, Otto MJ, McKinlay MA. The prevention of rhinovirus and poliovirus uncoating by WIN 51711: a new antiviral drug. *Antimicrob Agents Chemother* 1986;30:110.

222. Al-Nakib W, Higgins PG, Barrow GI, et al. Suppression of colds in human volunteers challenged with rhinovirus by a new synthetic drug (R61837). *Antimicrob Agents Chemother* 1989;33:522.

223. Hayden FG, Andries K, Janssen PAJ. Safety and efficacy of intranasal pirodavir (R77975) in experimental rhinovirus infection. *Antimicrob Agents Chemother* 1992;36:727.

224. Denyer C, Jackson P, Loakes DM, et al. Isolation of antirhinoviral sesquiterpenes from ginger (*Zingiber officinale*). *J Nat Prod* 1994;57:658.

225. Oren DA, Zhang A, Nesvadba H, et al. Synthesis and activity of piperazine-containing antirhinoviral agents and crystal structure of SDZ 880-061 bound to human rhinovirus 14. *J Mol Biol* 1996;259:120.

226. Stanley ED, Jackson GG, Dirda V, et al. Effect of a topical interferon inducer on rhinovirus infections in volunteers. *J Infect Dis* 1976;133[Suppl]:A121.

227. Scott GM, Wallace J, Greiner J, et al. Prevention of rhinovirus colds by human interferon-α_2 from *Escherichia coli*. *Lancet* 1982;2:186.

228. Monto AS, Shope TC, Schwartz SA, et al. Intranasal interferonaze for seasonal prophylaxis of respiratory infection. *J Infect Dis* 1986;154:128.

229. Douglas RM, Moore BW, Miles HB, et al. Prophylactic efficacy of intranasal α_2-interferon against rhinovirus infections in the family setting. *N Engl J Med* 1986;314:65.

230. Hayden FG, Albrecht JK, Kaiser DL, et al. Prevention of natural colds by contact prophylaxis with intranasal α_2-interferon. *N Engl J Med* 1986;314:71.

231. Foy HM, Fox JP, Cooney MK. Efficacy of α_2-interferon against the common cold. *N Engl J Med* 1986;315:513.

232. Douglas RM, Albrecht JK, Miles HB, et al. Intranasal interferon-α_2 prophylaxis of natural respiratory virus infection. *J Infect Dis* 1985;151:731.

233. Hayden FG, Mills SE, Johns ME. Human tolerance and histopathologic effects of long-term administration of intranasal interferon-α_2. *J Infect Dis* 1983;148:914.

234. Sperber SJ, Levine PA, Innes DJ, et al. Tolerance and efficacy of intranasal administration of recombinant β-serine interferon in healthy adults. *J Infect Dis* 1988;158:166.

235. Sperber SJ, Levine PA, Sorrentino JV, et al. Ineffectiveness of recombinant interferon-beta serine nasal drops for prophylaxis of natural colds. *J Infect Dis* 1989;160:700.

236. Higgins PG, Al-Nakib W, Barrow GI, et al. Recombinant human interferon-γ as prophylaxis against rhinovirus colds in volunteers. *J Interferon Res* 1988;8:591.

237. Schwartz AR, Togo Y, Hornick RB, et al. Evaluation of the efficacy of ascorbic acid in prophylaxis of induced rhinovirus 44 infection in man. *J Infect Dis* 1973;128:500.

238. Coulehan JL. Ascorbic acid and the common cold: reviewing the evidence. *Postgrad Med* 1979;66:153.

239. Eby GA, Davis DR, Halcomb WW. Reduction in duration of common colds by zinc gluconate lozenges in a double-blind study. *Antimicrob Agents Chemother* 1984;25:20.

240. Douglas RM, Miles HB, Moore BW, et al. Failure of effervescent zinc acetate lozenges to alter the course of upper respiratory tract infections in Australian adults. *Antimicrob Agents Chemother* 1987;31:1263.

241. Al-Nakib W, Higgins PG, Barrow I, et al. Prophylaxis and treatment of rhinovirus colds with zinc gluconate lozenges. *J Antimicrob Chemother* 1987;20:893.

242. Farr BM, Conner EM, Betts RF, et al. Two randomized controlled trials of zinc gluconate lozenge therapy of experimentally induced rhinovirus colds. *Antimicrob Agents Chemother* 1987;31:1183.

243. Mink KA, Dick EC, Jennings LC, et al. Amelioration of rhinovirus colds by vitamin C (ascorbic acid) supplementation. *Med Virol* 1988;7:356.

244. Hemila H. Does vitamin C alleviate the symptoms of the common cold? A review of current evidence. *Scand J Infect Dis* 1994;26:1.

245. Jackson JL, Peterson C, Lesho E. A meta-analysis of zinc salts lozenges and the common cold. *Arch Intern Med* 1997;3373.

246. Turner RB, Riker DK, Gangemi JD. Ineffectiveness of Echinacea for prevention of experimental rhinovirus colds. *Antimicrob Agents Chemother* 2000;44:1708.

247. Stanley ED, Jackson GG, Panusarn C, et al. Increased virus shedding with aspirin treatment of rhinovirus infection. *JAMA* 1975;231:1248.

248. Fulginiti VA, Committee on Infectious Diseases. Special report: aspirin and Reye's syndrome. *Pediatrics* 1982;69:810.

249. Gaffey MJ, Gwaltney JM Jr, Sastre A, et al. Intranasally and orally administered antihistamine treatment of experimental rhinovirus colds. *Am Rev Respir Dis* 1987;136:556.

250. Gwaltney JM Jr, Park J, Paul RA, et al. Randomized controlled trial of clemastine fumarate for treatment of experimental rhinovirus colds. *Clin Infect Dis* 1996;22:656.

251. Turner RB, Sperber SJ, Sorrentino JV, et al. Effectiveness of clemastine fumarate for treatment of rhinorrhea and sneezing associated with the common cold. *Clin Infect Dis* 1997;25:824.

252. Gwaltney JM Jr, Druce HM. Efficacy of brompheniramine maleate for the treatment of rhinovirus colds. *Clin Infect Dis* 1997;25:1188.

253. Sperber SJ, Gwaltney JM Jr, Sorrentino JV, et al. Pseudoephedrine alone or combined with ibuprofen as treatment for experimental rhinovirus colds. In: *Program and abstracts of the 27th interscience conference on antimicrobial agents and chemotherapy*. Washington, DC: American Society for Microbiology, 1987:184.

254. Gwaltney JM Jr. Combined antiviral and antimediator treatment of rhinovirus colds. *J Infect Dis* 1992;166:776.

CHAPTER 251
Hepatitis A Virus

Stanley M. Lemon and Annette Martin

HISTORY

Although records dating as far back as Hippocrates describe epidemic jaundice, it wasn't until the early twentieth century that "catarrhal jaundice" was suggested by Cockayne to result from an infection of the liver (1). He proposed the term *infective hepatitis* for what we now know as type A viral hepatitis. The infectious, non-bacterial nature of the responsible agent was firmly established by the transmission of disease to human volunteers during World War II (2). At that time, two forms of viral hepatitis, designated *infectious hepatitis* and *homologous serum hepatitis*, were differentiated based on their epidemiology, incubation periods, and lack of protection in cross-challenge studies. The terms *hepatitis A* and *hepatitis B* were proposed shortly thereafter and are still used today. Hepatitis A virus (HAV) was first identified in 1973 by Feinstone et al., who applied immune electron microscopy to the examination of fecal suspensions collected from human volunteers (3) (Fig. 251.1). Definitive propagation of hepatitis A virus (HAV) in cell culture followed approximately 6 years later (4). In the interim, however, much had been learned about the biology of this virus and the pathogenesis of type A hepatitis by experimental inoculation of chimpanzees and several other species of higher primates (5–8). These animals remain the only available animal models for the disease. These studies have been complemented by the molecular cloning of cDNA that was reverse-transcribed from the ribonucleic acid (RNA) genome of the virus (9,10). The molecular cloning of the viral genome led to the proper classification of HAV among the picornaviruses, and has also provided much indirect information about the biology of the virus.

The general structure and genomic organization of HAV is similar in many respects to other picornaviruses. However, HAV has several unique features that distinguish it from other human and animal viruses. Although the virus was originally classified as enterovirus type 72, these distinctive features of HAV, coupled with the fact that it shares only very limited nucleotide homology with other picornaviruses (10), has resulted in its classification within a unique genus, the genus *Hepatovirus*, within the family Picornaviridae (11). Only a single other species of virus, an avian virus (avian encephalomyelitis virus), which appears to have a remarkably close phylogenetic relationship to HAV, is classified within this genus.

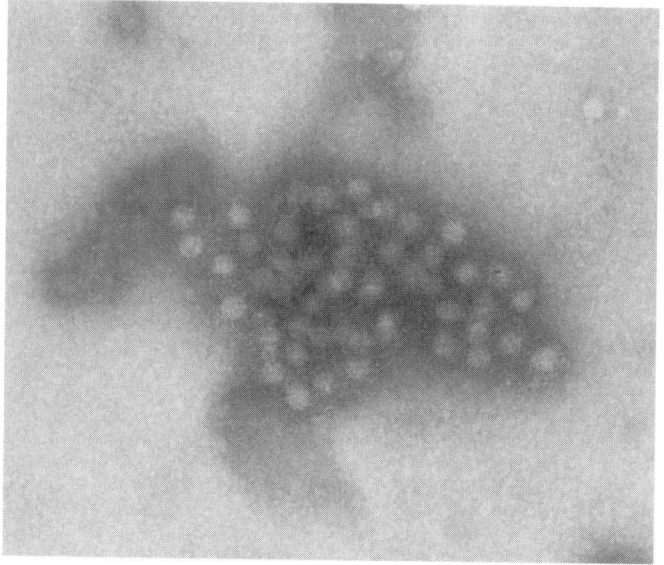

Figure 251.1. Hepatitis A virus. Negatively stained virions as seen by immune electron microscopy. Purified cell culture-derived virus has been aggregated by specific antibody. 100,000X magnification. (Courtesy of S.M. Feinstone.)

CHARACTERISTICS OF THE PATHOGEN

The infectious HAV particle is small, non-enveloped, icosahedral, and approximately 27 nm in diameter. It possesses a highly stable protein capsid with an RNA genome consisting of a single, messenger-sense molecule approximately 7.5 kb in length. There is a small viral protein (VPg) linked to the 5′ terminus of the RNA and a lengthy, templated poly-A track at its 3′ end. The genome organization resembles that of other picornaviruses, as detailed below. The virus particle contains no enzymatic activities, and the virion RNA acts directly as the messenger RNA for viral protein synthesis. This leads to the production of a single, large viral polyprotein that is subsequently cleaved by viral and cellular proteases into at least 10 unique proteins that function in genome replication and the assembly of new virus particles. Viral replication takes place in the cytoplasm of the infected hepatocyte, and most likely occurs by a protein-primed mechanism of RNA replication similar to that which has been proposed for poliovirus (12). The assembly of new virus particles occurs within membranous vesicles, which appear to be transported to the plasma membrane where it interfaces with the hepatic canaliculi, resulting ultimately in the secretion of virus into the biliary system. A detailed review of the biology and molecular virology of HAV is available elsewhere (13).

Physical Characteristics

The majority of infectious HAV particles sediment at 156S and band at a density of 1.325 g/cm³ in cesium chloride (14). However, infectious dense particles banding at 1.40 to 1.44 g/cm³ in cesium comprise a small percentage of all virions, and presumably represent virions with capsids that are permeable to cesium cations. Virus particles which band at much lower densities and which are resistant to antibody-mediated neutralization probably represent virions which are complexed with lipid-containing cellular materials (15,16).

Like the enteroviruses, hepatitis A is stable at low pH (less than pH 3.0) (17). However, the thermal stability of HAV is considerably greater than that of other picornaviruses, placing the virus among the most stable of all human viral pathogens (18–20). Incubation of the virus for 4 weeks at room temperature results in only a 100-fold decrease in infectivity. Held at high temperatures for short periods (10 minutes), significant loss of infectivity does not occur until 60°C (19). The virus capsid is significantly stabilized in the presence of 1 M Mg²⁺, resulting in only a 100-fold decrease in infectivity upon heating to 80°C for 10 minutes (18). However, infectivity is destroyed almost instantaneously by heating above 90°C. HAV is highly resistant to drying, and infectious virus has been recovered from acetone-fixed cell sheets. It is also highly resistant to detergents, surviving a 1% concentration of sodium dodecyl sulfate. Significantly, the infectivity of HAV is not reduced by solvent-detergent inactivation procedures applied to blood products, explaining in part the recent occurrence of hepatitis A transmission following administration of HAV-contaminated clotting factor concentrates (21).

Capsid Composition

At present, our understanding of the physical structure of the HAV particle is based largely on analogy with other picornaviruses, and limited biochemical studies. The highly stable capsid of HAV is thought to be composed of 60 copies each of three major structural proteins, VP1, VP2, and VP3, which are approximately 273, 222, and 246 amino acids in length, respectively (10,22). Although detailed, atomic-level resolution models of the structure of poliovirus and other important picornaviruses have been deduced from X-ray crystallographic studies (23,24), no such model exists at present for HAV. However, recent cryoelectron microscopy studies suggest that HAV has a structure that is similar to that of other members of this viral family, and shows promise of providing more detailed information concerning unique features of the virus structure in the future (25).

The largest of the HAV capsid proteins, VP1, is sometimes found to be present in particles as an immature precursor protein, VP1-2A, otherwise known as the "pX" protein (26). Although details are lacking, it appears that the carboxy-terminal 2A extension on the VP1 protein may play a critical role in defining the conformation and/or assembly of the capsid proteins (27,28). A fourth, and much smaller structural protein, VP4, with a predicted length of 23 amino acids is suggested by the genomic RNA sequence (see below) but has not been demonstrated in polyacrylamide gels (29). If a consensus myristylation signal that is present within the putative VP4 coding region is used like in other picornaviruses, this protein would be only 17 amino acids in length. However, data exist that suggest that this site is not utilized in HAV (30,31). In this respect, HAV differs significantly from other picornaviruses, which have considerably larger and universally myristylated VP4 structural proteins (32).

Antigenic Structure

Complementary deoxyribonucleic acid (cDNA) prepared from several strains of HAV recovered from humans has been molecularly cloned; the complete nucleotide sequences of these different viruses are known (9,10,33–35). Analysis of the amino acid sequences of the HAV capsid proteins deduced from the nucleotide sequences revealed approximately 97% amino acid conservation in the sequences of VP1, VP2, and VP3. In contrast, these protein sequences demonstrate very little relatedness to the capsid protein sequences of group C enteroviruses or other human picornaviruses. Few strains of hepatitis A have been well studied for antigenic variation. However, available evidence suggests that there is only one known serotype of HAV (as defined by classical virus neutralization studies), and that this is antigenically distinct from all other picornaviruses (36,37). Classical polyclonal antibody cross-neutralization studies of human HAV (HM175 strain) and an owl monkey-derived viral isolate (PA21) have suggested no significant differences in the neutralization antigen(s) of these two disparate strains (36). While some monoclonal antibodies are capable of distinguishing between human strains of HAV and several strains which have been isolated from naturally infected nonhuman primates (cynomolgus and African green monkeys) (38,39), all simian and human strains of HAV demonstrate significant antigenic cross-reactivity and probably stimulate cross-protective antibodies. Thus, there is good evidence for high level antigenic conservation among HAV strains.

The analysis of mutant HAVs, selected in cell culture for resistance to neutralization by murine monoclonal antibodies to the virus, suggests that there is an array of closely spaced epitopes comprising an immunodominant neutralization site on the capsid surface (40,41). Several pieces of evidence indicate that these epitopes are assembled (that is, conformationally derived) structures rather than linear epitopes that would be accurately modeled by an oligopeptide. First, neutralizing murine monoclonal antibodies do not recognize denatured capsid proteins separated by SDS-PAGE. Second, antibody elicited to purified HAV capsid polypeptides only weakly recognizes native capsids and has limited neutralization activity (42). Third, HAV proteins expressed from recombinant DNA as fusion proteins in *Escherichia coli* are capable of eliciting antibodies reactive with denatured capsid polypeptides, but these antibodies do not react with or neutralize native virus. These facts have made difficult the development of a vaccine based on recombinant DNA technology, which is unfortunate because growth of HAV in cell culture is relatively inefficient, making the production of conventional, inactivated whole virus vaccines relatively expensive (see below and Chapter 85).

Virion Ribonucleic Acid: The Hepatitis A Virus Genome

The HAV genome is a single-stranded 35S RNA of positive polarity, approximately 7,478 bases in length and terminating in a 3′ poly-(A) tract (Fig. 251.2) (10,29). As with other positive-strand viruses, purified genomic RNA is itself infectious and will regenerate virus following transfection of permissive cells. Synthetic *in vitro* RNA transcripts synthesized from genome-length cloned cDNAs are also infectious following transfection of permissive cells, or direct inoculation into the liver of susceptible primates (43,44).

The genome contains a relatively lengthy 5′ nontranslated region (5′NTR), approximately 734 bases long, and a short 3′NTR. Both NTRs have substantial secondary RNA structure composed of several complex stem-loop structures (45). Like other picornaviruses, the 5′NTR contains a highly structured, approximately 0.6-kb RNA segment that functions as an "internal ribosomal binding site" (IRES), directing the binding of 40S ribosomal subunits to the viral RNA and causing the initiation of viral translation in a 5′ cap-independent fashion (46,47). Most studies suggest that the IRES of HAV is less active than the IRES of other picornaviruses, resulting in inefficient translation of the viral message and possibly contributing to the slow growth of the virus (48,49). IRES-directed translation uses one or more cell-specific translation initiation factors (50–52), and the affinity of the 5′NTR for these and other cellular proteins probably plays

a role in defining cellular tropisms of the virus (49,53–56). Remarkably, the HAV IRES differs from the IRES elements of other picornaviruses in having a specific requirement for intact cellular translation initiation factor eIF-4G (48,57). This cellular protein is proteolytically digested by proteinases expressed by several other picornaviruses (including poliovirus), resulting in shutdown of host cell translation, a feature that is not observed in HAV-infected cells.

The noncoding regions flank a single large open reading frame which encodes a polyprotein that is processed into both structural (P1-2A region) and nonstructural viral proteins (2BC and P3 genomic regions) (see Fig. 251.2). The primary cleavage of the polyprotein occurs between these two segments of the polyprotein, under the direction of the only proteinase encoded by the virus, the 3C^{pro} protein (58–60). Thus, HAV differs from poliovirus and many other human and animal picornaviruses in that the 2A protein lacks proteinase activity and, as discussed above, remains attached to some fully formed virions (26). Proteins 2B and 2C (possibly also the precursor 2BC) are believed to have a role in RNA replication and most probably contribute to host range specificity (61,62). Protein 2B is very hydrophobic, and may play a role in anchoring replicase complexes to intracellular membranes (63). On the other hand, 2C has NTPase activity and contains a helicase sequence motif. The overexpression of these proteins leads to rearrangements in intracellular membranes, presumably mimicking an early step in assembly of the replicase complex (63,64). The P3 nonstructural proteins include a putative RNA-dependent RNA polymerase (3Dpol) and a cysteine proteinase (3Cpro) (65), which is responsible for most cleavages in the processing of the viral polyprotein (66) (see Fig. 251.2).

THE VIRAL REPLICATION CYCLE

The first step in replication of HAV is likely to be its binding to a specific cellular receptor. One candidate receptor (HAVcr-1), a mucin-like glycoprotein has been identified in cultured cells (69). This receptor is widely distributed in different tissues, and may or may not be involved in virus attachment and penetration of hepatocytes *in vivo*. Although mature virus particles undergo uncoating with release of viral RNA into the cytoplasm approximately 4 hours after infection in cultured cells (70), further details of the cellular penetration and uncoating of HAV are unknown. Subsequent steps in the viral life cycle, however, include (i) the translation of the large open reading frame within the virion RNA, leading to the synthesis of a giant polyprotein, (ii) the transcription of a negative-strand copy of the viral genome, (iii) the synthesis of new, positive-strand RNA molecules from this negative-strand intermediate, (iv) the packaging of these new viral RNAs into assembled virus particles, and (v) the release of virus from the hepatocyte into the biliary canaliculi (Fig. 251.3). Many aspects of this highly coordinated process of viral protein expression and RNA replication remain poorly understood.

The positive-sense virion RNA acts directly as messenger for the synthesis of the large polyprotein following its release into the cytoplasmic compartment and elimination of the small virally-encoded peptide (VPg), which is covalently linked to its 5′ end (71). As indicated above, protein translation is initiated in a 5′ cap-independent fashion under the control of the IRES located within the 5′ nontranslated RNA segment of the genome. The resulting polyprotein is co- and post-translationally processed by the virus-specified 3C^{pro} proteinase (65) into both structural and nonstructural proteins (see Fig. 251.2) (58,66,72). The initial cleavage of the polyprotein by 3C^{pro} releases the amino

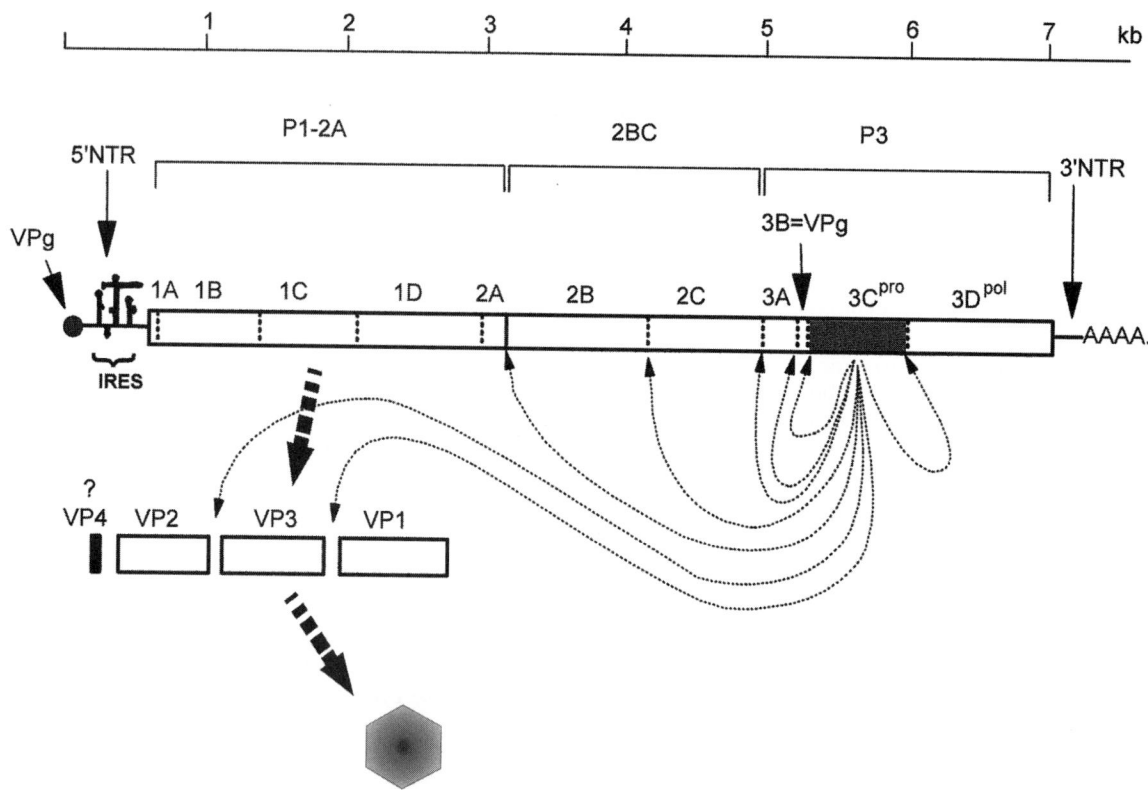

Figure 251.2. Organization of the HAV genome. The virion RNA is 7.5 kb in length, positive-sense and thus able to function directly as messenger. It contains three major regions: the 5′ and 3′ nontranslated regions (5′NTR and 3′NTR), and a single large open reading frame encoding the viral polyprotein (shown as the *large rectangular box*). The 5′ terminal nucleotide of the 5′NTR is covalently attached to a small viral protein (3B, otherwise known as VPg). The 3′NTR has a 3′ terminal poly(A) tract. The 5′NTR contains substantial RNA secondary structure which forms the viral internal ribosomal entry site (IRES) that directs the cap-independent translation of the viral polyprotein. This polyprotein can be divided into three (P1-2A, 2BC and P3) domains: each of these domains is proteolytically processed to yield smaller viral proteins (1A, 1B, 1C, etc.). The capsid proteins, VP1, VP2, VP3 (and possibly VP4), are encoded by the P1 region, while nonstructural proteins involved in replication are encoded by the 2BC and P3 regions. These include an NTPase (2C) with possible helicase activity, VPg (3B) which may play a role in priming for new RNA synthesis, a viral specific protease (3C^pro, *shaded region*), and an RNA-dependent RNA polymerase (3D^pol). Proteolytic processing of the polyprotein is directed entirely by 3C^pro (*dotted lines* indicate cleavage activities of this protease), which also has RNA-binding activity and plays a role in RNA replication. Primary cleavage occurs between the 2A and 2B proteins. Replication of viral RNA proceeds asymmetrically, as with poliovirus, resulting in production of a large excess of positive-sense over negative-sense RNAs. Only positive-sense RNA molecules are packaged in progeny virions.

terminal approximately 40% of the polyprotein (P1-2A segment), containing the structural proteins that comprise the viral capsid. This segment undergoes subsequent processing by 3C^pro, producing VP0 (VP4-VP2, otherwise known as 1A1B, which is itself a precursor protein), VP3 (1C), and VP1-2A (1D2A, or pX) (see Fig. 251.2). VP4-VP2 is cleaved into its two constituent polypeptides after the assembly of the virus particle and packaging of the viral RNA, and occurs by an as yet undetermined mechanism. This is called the "maturation cleavage," and probably results in an increased stability of the virus particle. The 2A polypeptide segment is cleaved from the VP1-2A precursor protein in late virus assembly intermediates, presumably via the action of a cellular proteinase (22,73). The 1A-2A structural segment of the genome appears to play no role in viral RNA replication, since various RNA genomes bearing large deletions within this region are capable of replication in cultured cells (27,74,75).

All of the polypeptides located downstream of 2A in the polyprotein play essential, although poorly defined, roles in RNA replication, and many if not all are likely to have mul-

tiple functions in viral replication. The further processing of the 2BC-P3 segment of the polyprotein appears to be completely directed by 3C^pro. Based on studies with other picornaviruses, some polypeptides which seem abundant in HAV infected cells may have unique functions as partially uncleaved processing intermediates (such as 3ABC) that differ significantly from their functions as fully cleaved, mature proteins (13). The 3D^pol RNA-dependent, RNA polymerase of HAV serves as the catalytic core of a large, membrane-bound macromolecular complex that acts as an RNA replicase (63). The 3A protein is likely to play a role in anchoring this replicase complex to cellular membranes via a hydrophobic sequence located near its amino terminus (76).

Within this replicase complex, the virion RNA serves as template for negative-strand RNA synthesis (see Fig. 251.3). This negative-strand intermediate then acts in turn as template for synthesis of more positive-strand RNA, that can either be translated into protein (reinitiating the replication cycle) or packaged into new virions. 3B (VPg), the small genome linked protein, is likely to function in the priming of viral RNA synthesis in

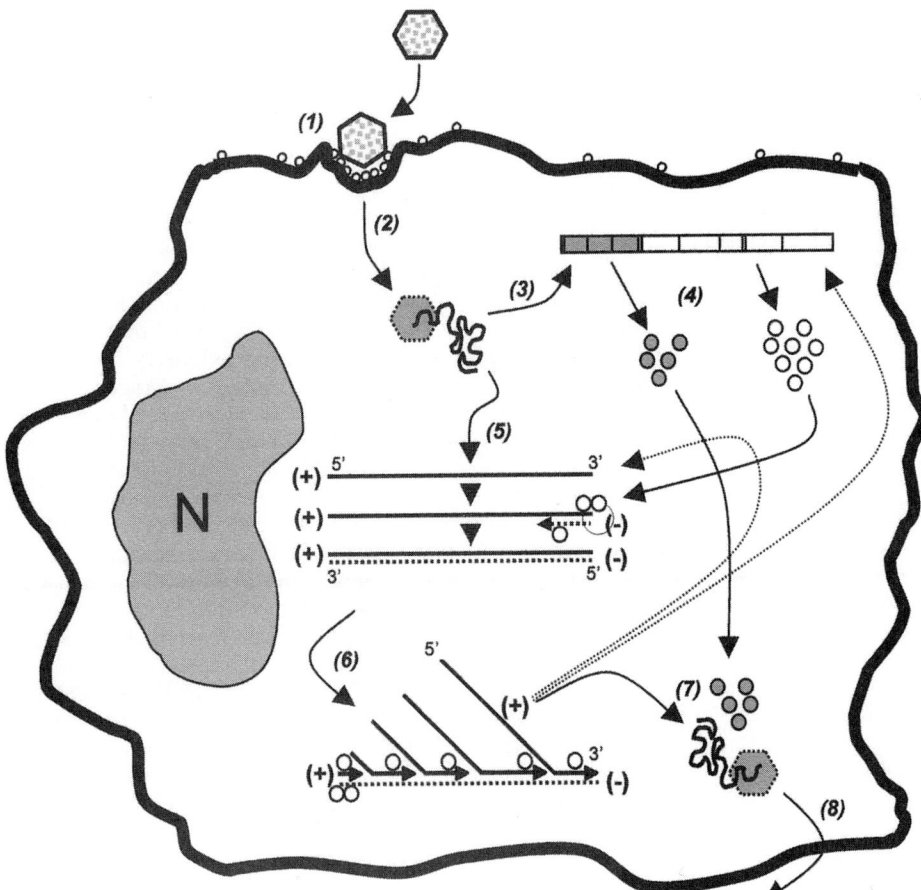

Figure 251.3. Schematic showing major features of the replication cycle of HAV. *(1)* Virus attachment occurs at a specific cellular receptor on the basolateral surface of the hepatocyte, within the space of Disse, and is followed by *(2)* penetration and uncoating of the virus particle. Subsequent events take place exclusively within the cytoplasm of the cell, and do not disrupt cellular homeostasis. These events include *(3)* translation of the polyprotein by a 5′ cap independent mechanism, *(4)* cotranslational processing of the polyprotein by the 3C^pro proteinase, as shown in Fig. 251.2, *(5)* synthesis of a negative-strand intermediate RNA molecule by a membrane-bound viral replicase complex, *(6)* synthesis of new positive-strand progeny RNA genomes, which can either reinitiate the cycle by undergoing translation *(dotted lines)* or *(7)* be packaged into new virus particles. *(8)* Newly formed virus particles are transported to the apical surface of the cell and exported into the biliary canaliculus.

these reactions (12), and remains covalently coupled to the 5′ ends of both strands of RNA. Not much is known about the molecular determinants of RNA replication that are probably present within the extremities of the 5′ and 3′NTRs (77,78). The poly(A) tail following the 3′NTR appears to be elongated during RNA replication in cells transfected with RNA transcripts, indicating that its length may be important for genome replication (79). RNA amplification is asymmetric, with much more of the positive-sense, genomic RNA present in infected cells than the negative-strand intermediate (13). Newly synthesized positive-strand RNA is either used for further rounds of replication, or packaged within the capsid proteins for export from the hepatocyte across the apical canalicular membrane into the bile. Only the positive-strand RNA is packaged into new virions. A number of mutations that have been shown to confer important adaptive properties related to the replication of the virus in cultured cells have been mapped to 2B (62). Their importance in determining the efficiency of RNA replication also has been demonstrated in the context of subgenomic replicons, indicating that their effect is on RNA replication and not on other steps in the virus life cycle (75).

PROPAGATION OF HEPATITIS A VIRUS IN CULTURED CELLS

Investigators have known since the 1940s that both serum and fecal specimens could transmit hepatitis A to humans, but attempts to grow the virus in a variety of primary cell cultures and continuous cell lines were unsuccessful for many years. These

efforts probably failed because the virus grows slowly *in vitro* and usually does not induce a cytopathic effect (CPE) in infected cells. With the advent of serologic tests for viral antigen and the availability of various assays to detect viral antigen or nucleic acid, it has been possible to monitor the replication of virus in cell cultures.

HAV was first isolated in marmoset liver explant cultures and was subsequently propagated in continuous fetal rhesus monkey kidney cells (4,80). Subsequent studies have demonstrated that the virus may be directly isolated from clinical materials in primary African green monkey kidney (AGMK) cells, or, with somewhat greater difficulty, in several continuous cell lines including BS-C-1 cells, PLC/PRF-5 (human hepatoma cells), and others (81–83). More recent evidence indicates that the virus replicates in a broader diversity of mammalian-derived cell types including cells of guinea-pig or dolphin origin (84). Wild-type virus usually replicates very slowly and to relatively low titers in cultured cells. With *in vitro* passage, however, virus becomes progressively adapted to growth in cell culture, replicating more rapidly and to higher titers (85). Virus infection does not shut down host-cell macromolecular synthesis, nor usually result in death of the infected cell. Rather, *in vitro* infection uniformly leads to persistent infections. The virus requires several days to weeks to reach maximal titers in cell cultures, and usually requires immunological or hybridization techniques to be detected because of a lack of virus-induced cytopathic effect (CPE). Well-adapted variants of the virus that replicate rapidly (replication cycle less than 18 to 24 hours) and to higher than usual titers in cultured cells do cause a CPE, however, and have been shown to induce apoptosis in infected cells (19,63,86). This virus allow the use of conventional plaque assays for viral quantitation. *In vitro* replication is blocked by guanidine and brefeldin A (75,87,88), which are both known to inhibit the replication of other picornaviruses.

The molecular basis underlying the adaptation of HAV to cell culture has been studied in detail and has been shown to be due to changes in the 2BC proteins and viral IRES element which facilitate interactions with host cell–specific factors involved in viral translation and RNA replication (49,53,61,62,89–91). Highly cell culture–adapted viruses are often attenuated (or no longer even infectious) when used to challenge susceptible primates and have been studied as candidate attenuated vaccines (92,93) (see below).

MOLECULAR EPIDEMIOLOGY

Classical features of the epidemiology of type A viral hepatitis are described in Chapter 85 and are not repeated here in detail. HAV has a world-wide distribution characterized by fecal-oral transmission, usually through close personal contact or contaminated food or water, with rare episodes of apparent transmission from blood or blood products (94). The molecular epidemiology of HAV has been investigated by determining the partial genomic nucleotide sequences of a large number of human HAV strains recovered from diverse sources (95–97). These studies have shown that circulating human strains of HAV are relatively closely related genetically, especially when compared to the genetic diversity evident among other picornaviruses such as poliovirus. Two major human HAV "genotypes" (genotypes I and III) have been documented, the sequences of which differ from each other at greater than 15% of the bases studied. At least two other human HAV isolates belong to other, much less common genotypes (II and VII). This genetic classification is of epidemiologic interest, but it is not of clinical significance with respect to severity of symptoms or other manifestations of hepatitis A.

Viruses from geographic regions in which hepatitis A is endemic (e.g., China) or intermediate in prevalence (e.g., the United States) are often closely related to each other genetically, while viruses isolated from cases recognized in Northern Europe (where hepatitis A is a relatively rare event) demonstrate greater genomic heterogeneity. These observations are consistent with the idea that most infections in Northern Europe are imported by travelers returning from lesser developed regions (95). An important exception was observed among parenteral drug users in Sweden, among which a genetically distinct virus strain was observed to circulate over a number of years. This suggests that there may be small "pockets" of virus circulation among certain high risk groups. In these Swedish individuals, it is likely that virus was transmitted by contaminated needles as with other agents of viral hepatitis. Partial genomic sequencing of virus strains has also been useful in identifying the source of virus in other epidemiologic studies, including demonstration of the transmission of HAV to hemophilic patients via high purity, solvent-detergent inactivated factor VIII preparations (98).

Strains of virus recovered from naturally infected nonhuman primates represent three additional genotypes (IV, V, VI) and, unlike the human genotypes, demonstrate subtle antigenic differences as described above. The simian viruses are likely to have low pathogenicity for humans (38,39). Evidence suggests that they constitute a biologically distinct group of viruses which are capable of causing liver disease in infected cynomolgus and African green monkeys, but not chimpanzees which, like New World owl monkeys and certain tamarin species, develop acute hepatitis following challenge with human strains of HAV (67). In contrast, human strains of HAV generally do not cause disease in the former primate species. These differences in virus host range could be due, at least in part, to differences in the cellular receptors utilized by these viruses (37,68).

PATHOGENESIS

Experimental infections involving humans and susceptible nonhuman primates have provided an understanding of the events occurring during HAV infection (for a more detailed description, see Chapter 85) (5–8,68,99,100). The incubation period of hepatitis A is approximately 28 days (considerably shorter than hepatitis B or non-A non-B hepatitis) but may range from 2 to 6 weeks. The early virologic events remain shrouded in mystery, but data support the existence of viral replication within intestinal epithelial cells (101). Presumably, the virus spreads from this source to reach the liver via a hematogenous route. In cultured polarized, colonic carcinoma (CaCo-2) cells, however, the release of progeny virus occurs exclusively through the apical (lumenal) surface, suggesting the possibility that initial steps in viral invasion are more complex (88). The dominant site of replication is the hepatocyte, from which virus reaches the intestinal contents and is shed in feces via the bile (5). Viremia and fecal shedding of virus precede abnormalities in liver function, and are maximal late in the incubation period, just before the onset of liver disease. Viremia persists for several weeks during the prodromal and symptomatic periods of the infection (68,100), during which bloodborne transmission of the virus is a possibility.

Liver biopsy specimens obtained from experimentally infected primates reveal mononuclear cell infiltration of the portal and periportal regions and swollen hepatocytes with 10% or more containing HAV antigen by immunofluorescence (99,102–106). Hepatocellular necrosis is usually focal but can span entire lobules of the liver. Abnormalities of liver function often persist for several months after the onset of acute illness, rarely longer. Chronic fecal shedding of HAV has not been observed, suggesting that persistent hepatitis A infection does not occur. It is not known whether the virus replicates in tissues other than the liver and intestinal epithelia, although HAV antigen has been demonstrated in the germinal centers of the spleen, lymph nodes, and kidneys of animals inoculated intravenously with the virus (99). This may reflect the deposition of immune complexes.

During acute disease there is a nonspecific increase in total serum immunoglobulins coincident with acute liver necrosis. However, specific antiviral antibodies are almost always present at the time of onset of liver disease (107–109). The humoral response includes IgM, IgG and IgA antibodies. IgM anti-HAV is short lived, generally becoming undetectable after 6 months, and is used as a diagnostic marker for infection (108,110). IgG anti-HAV is present early in the acute illness, generally remains at detectable levels for years, and is thought to confer lifelong immunity. The protective role of secretory antibodies is uncertain: such antibodies have been demonstrated by immunoassays, but fecal suspensions and saliva samples from naturally infected humans or experimentally infected primates are usually devoid of virus neutralizing activity (111,112). One interpretation of this result is that viral replication in intestinal tissues may be quite limited, but the consensus is that secretory IgA antibodies are not important for prevention of hepatitis A. While neutralizing serum antibody appears to play a critical role in protection against reinfection (109,113), other immune mechanisms such as natural killer cells, HLA-restricted T-cell-mediated cytotoxicity, and induction of interferons are very likely to be important in clearing acute HAV infection (114–116).

CLINICAL MANIFESTATIONS OF HEPATITIS A VIRUS INFECTION

The clinical manifestations of HAV infection are reviewed in detail in Chapter 85. In the individual patient, clinical features of hepatitis A are indistinguishable from those of other types of viral hepatitis. In young children (younger than age 2) most infections are anicteric and not recognized as due to a hepatitis virus; in contrast, overt hepatitis develops in the majority of infected adults (94,117). The severity of disease increases with age, but mortality is low (less than 0.2% of hospitalized cases) (118–120). HAV does not cause chronic viral hepatitis.

DIAGNOSIS OF HEPATITIS A VIRUS INFECTION

Marked elevations of serum aspartate and alanine aminotransferase (AST and ALT) activities coupled with malaise, nausea, vomiting, abdominal pain, and fever suggest the possibility of viral hepatitis, but do not point to a specific virus etiology. The specific diagnosis of HAV infection rests on demonstration of serum IgM anti-HAV (108,110). This antibody is readily detected using any of a variety of commercially available assays that are based on an IgM capture technology. Such tests are very sensitive. However, because the serum is diluted prior to testing, IgM usually is no longer detectable after 6 months. In occasional cases it may persist for up to 1 year. The other commonly used antibody test is a competitive inhibition immunoassay that is not specific for any single immunoglobulin isotype (107,121). This test is not specific for acute infection, but is useful in determining prior infection (and hence immunity). In general, these tests are not very sensitive and usually fail to detect protective levels of antibody conferred by passive immunization with pooled immune globulins (113,122). They also may not detect protective levels of antibody conferred by active immunization with inactivated HAV vaccines (see Chapter 85). Although solid-phase immunoassays for HAV antigen have been developed, they are of little diagnostic value since most HAV shedding occurs prior to acute liver injury. Similarly, tissue culture isolation of the virus as described above is not achieved easily and its use is restricted to research laboratories. Reverse transcription of viral RNA to yield cDNA, followed by polymerase chain reaction amplification of the cDNA (RT-PCR assay) permits detection of HAV in feces and serum, and may also provide information concerning the virus genotype (95,96). While potentially useful in epidemiologic studies, this will likely remain a research procedure.

PREVENTION OF HEPATITIS A VIRUS INFECTION

Inasmuch as HAV is generally transmitted via the fecal-oral route, one of the most effective methods of control is the maintenance of high standards of hygiene. This includes public sanitation measures to protect drinking water supplies and proper collection, treatment, and disposal of sewage. However, two forms of specific immunoprophylaxis are available for prevention of hepatitis A: immunization with inactivated hepatitis A vaccines, or passive prophylaxis with pooled human immune globulins (123). Passive immunoprophylaxis has existed as a method of controlling the infection for many decades, whereas successful

inactivated vaccines have only become available relatively recently due to the development of methods for the propagation of virus in cultured cells. These vaccines are prepared by formalin-inactivation of virus that has been purified from infected cell cultures, with alum added as adjuvant. They are very immunogenic in both adults and children, and have been shown to induce a high level of protection against hepatitis A (122,124,125). The use of inactivated vaccines and immune globulins to prevent hepatitis A is described in detail in Chapter 85.

While the inactivated vaccine is both safe and effective (123,126,127), it remains relatively expensive. The cost of the vaccine continues to limit its use, especially among children in HAV-endemic regions. An attenuated virus vaccine might be much less expensive to produce, but early attempts to produce an attenuated Sabin poliovirus-like vaccine for HAV were unsuccessful. Some cell culture-adapted strains of HAV (see above) have been found to be attenuated. These viruses demonstrated a reduced capacity to cause liver injury in inoculated primates and in human volunteers (92,93,128,129). Attenuation is likely to be due to mutations in the 2BC proteins and possibly also the 5′ nontranslated region of the viral genome that accumulated during the adaptation and passage of the virus in cell culture (61,130). However, these virus variants had significantly reduced immunogenicity for humans and generally induced only low levels of protective antibodies. They were not infectious by the oral route. Thus, although an attenuated vaccine has been used quite widely in China (131), no vaccine candidate has been clearly demonstrated to be acceptable in terms of both attenuation and immunogenicity. Chimeric viruses containing sequences derived from both a simian and a human strain of HAV have been suggested as possible candidates for a live attenuated vaccine, and have been studied in animal models (132). Some chimeras retain a good balance between replication efficiency in cell culture and attenuation, but their immunogenicity remains to be demonstrated.

REFERENCES

1. Cockayne EA. Catarrhal jaundice, sporadic and epidemic, and its relation to acute yellow atrophy of the liver. *Q J Med* 1912;6:1–29.
2. MacCallum FO, Bradley WH. Transmission of infective hepatitis to human volunteers: effect on rheumatoid arthritis. *Lancet* 1944;ii:228.
3. Feinstone SM, Kapikian AZ, Purcell RH. Hepatitis A: detection by immune electron microscopy of a viruslike antigen associated with acute illness. *Science* 1973;182:1026–1028.
4. Provost PJ, Hilleman MR. Propagation of human hepatitis A virus in cell culture *in vitro*. *Proc Soc Exp Biol Med* 1979;160:213–221.
5. Schulman AN, Dienstag JL, Jackson DR, et al. Hepatitis A antigen particles in liver, bile, and stool of chimpanzees. *J Infect Dis* 1976;134:80–84.
6. Dienstag JL, Feinstone SM, Purcell RH, et al. Experimental infection of chimpanzees with hepatitis A virus. *J Infect Dis* 1975;132:532–545.
7. Holmes AW, Deinhardt F, Wolfe L, et al. Specific neutralization of human hepatitis type A in marmoset monkeys. *Nature* 1973;243:419–420.
8. Provost PJ, Villarejos VM, Hilleman MR. Suitability of the rufiventer marmoset as a host animal for human hepatitis A virus. *Proc Soc Exp Biol Med* 1977;155:283–286.
9. Najarian R, Caput D, Gee W, et al. Primary structure and gene organization of human hepatitis A virus. *Proc Natl Acad Sci USA* 1985;82:2627–2631.
10. Cohen JI, Ticehurst JR, Purcell RH, et al. Complete nucleotide sequence of wild-type hepatitis A virus: comparison with different strains of hepatitis A virus and other picornaviruses. *J Virol* 1987;61:50–59.
11. Regenmortel MHV, Fauquet CM, Bishop DL, et al. *Virus taxonomy: the classification and nomenclature of viruses. The seventh report of the international committee on taxonomy of viruses*. San Diego: Academic Press, 2000.
12. Paul AV, Van Boom JH, Filippov D, Wimmer E. Protein-primed RNA synthesis by purified poliovirus RNA polymerase. *Nature* 1998;393:280–284.
13. Martin A, Lemon SM. The molecular biology of hepatitis A virus. In: Ou J-H, ed. *Hepatitis viruses*. Norwell, MA: Kluwer Academic Publishers, 2002:23–50.
14. Lemon SM, Jansen RW, Newbold JE. Infectious hepatitis A virus particles produced in cell culture consist of three distinct types with different buoyant densities in CsCl. *J Virol* 1985;54:78–85.

15. Lemon SM, Binn LN. Incomplete neutralization of hepatitis A virus *in vitro* due to lipid-associated virions. *J Gen Virol* 1985;66:2501–2505.

16. Provost PJ, Wolanski BS, Miller WJ, et al. Biophysical and biochemical properties of CR326 human hepatitis A virus. *Am J Med Sci* 1975;270:87–92.

17. Scholz E, Heinricy U, Flehmig B. Acid stability of hepatitis A virus. *J Gen Virol* 1989;70:2481–2485.

18. Siegl G, Weitz M, Kronauer G. Stability of hepatitis A virus. *Intervirology* 1984;22:218–226.

19. Lemon SM, Murphy PC, Shields PA, et al. Antigenic and genetic variation in cytopathic hepatitis A virus variants arising during persistent infection: evidence for genetic recombination. *J Virol* 1991;65:2056–2065.

20. Murphy P, Nowak T, Lemon SM, Hilfenhaus J. Inactivation of hepatitis A virus by heat treatment in aqueous solution. *J Med Virol* 1993;41:61–64.

21. Lemon SM, Murphy PC, Smith A, et al. Removal/neutralization of hepatitis A virus during manufacture of high purity, solvent/detergent factor VIII concentrate. *J Med Virol* 1994;43:44–49.

22. Martin A, Benichou D, Chao SF, et al. Maturation of the hepatitis A virus capsid protein VP1 is not dependent on processing by the 3Cpro proteinase. *J Virol* 1999;73:6220–6227.

23. Hogle JM, Chow M, Filman DJ. Three-dimensional structure of poliovirus at 2.9 - resolution. *Science* 1985;229:1358–1365.

24. Rossmann MG, Arnold E, Erickson JW, et al. Structure of a human common cold virus and functional relationship to other picornaviruses. *Nature* 1985;317:145–153.

25. Cheng H. Pleomorphic and symmetrical organizations of viral capsids in virus assembly and entry. Symposium on positive-strand RNA viruses. Paris, France: 2001.

26. Anderson DA, Ross BC. Morphogenesis of hepatitis A virus: Isolation and characterization of subviral particles. *J Virol* 1990;64:5284–5289.

27. Cohen L, Benichou D, Martin A. Analysis of deletion mutants indicate that the 2A polypeptide of hepatitis A virus is involved in virion morphogenesis. *J Virol* 2002;76:7495–7505.

28. Probst C, Jecht M, Gauss-Muller V. Intrinsic signals for the assembly of hepatitis A virus particles. Role of structural proteins VP4 and 2A. *J Biol Chem* 1999;274:4527–4531.

29. Lemon SM, Robertson BH. Current perspectives in the virology and molecular biology of hepatitis A virus. *Semin Virol* 1993;4:285–295.

30. Tesar M, Harmon SA, Summers DF, Ehrenfeld E. Hepatitis A virus polyprotein synthesis initiates from two alternative AUG codons. *Virology* 1992;186:609–618.

31. Tesar M, Jia X-Y, Summers DF, Ehrenfeld E. Analysis of a potential myristoylation site in hepatitis A virus capsid protein VP4. *Virology* 1993;194:616–626.

32. Chow M, Newman JFE, Filman DJ, et al. Myristylation of picornavirus capsid protein VP4 and its structural significance. *Nature* 1987;327:482–486.

33. Baroudy BM, Ticehurst JR, Miele TA, et al. Sequence analysis of hepatitis A virus cDNA coding for capsid proteins and RNA polymerase. *Proc Natl Acad Sci USA* 1985;82:2143–2147.

34. Linemeyer DL, Menke JG, Martin-Gallardo A, et al. Molecular cloning and partial sequencing of hepatitis A viral cDNA. *J Virol* 1985;54:247–255.

35. Paul AV, Tada H, von der Helm K, et al. The entire nucleotide sequence of the genome of human hepatitis A virus isolate MBB. *Virus Res* 1987;8:153–171.

36. Lemon SM, Binn LN. Antigenic relatedness of two strains of hepatitis A virus determined by cross-neutralization. *Infect Immun* 1983;42:418–420.

37. Lemon SM, Jansen RW, Brown EA. Genetic, antigenic, and biologic differences between strains of hepatitis A virus. *Vaccine* 1992;10:S40–S44.

38. Tsarev SA, Emerson SU, Balayan MS, et al. Simian hepatitis A virus HAV. strain AGM-27: comparison of genome structure and growth in cell culture with other HAV strains. *J Gen Virol* 1991;72:1677–1683.

39. Nainan OV, Margolis HS, Robertson BH, et al. Sequence analysis of a new hepatitis A virus naturally infecting cynomolgus macaques *Macaca fascicularis*. *J Gen Virol* 1991;72:1685–1689.

40. Ping L-H, Jansen RW, Stapleton JT, et al. Identification of an immunodominant antigenic site involving the capsid protein VP3 of hepatitis A virus. *Proc Natl Acad Sci USA* 1988;85:8281–8285.

41. Ping L-H, Lemon SM. Antigenic structure of human hepatitis A virus defined by analysis of escape mutants selected against murine monoclonal antibodies. *J Virol* 1992;66:2208–2216.

42. Hughes JV, Bennett C, Stanton LW, et al. Hepatitis-A virus structural proteins: sequencing and ability to induce virus-neutralizing antibody responses. In: Lerner RA, Chanock RM, Brown F, eds. *Vaccines 85: molecular and chemical basis of resistance to parasitic, bacterial and viral diseases.* Cold Spring Harbor, NY: Cold Spring Harbor Laboratory, 1985:255–259.

43. Cohen JI, Ticehurst JR, Feinstone SM, et al. Hepatitis A virus cDNA and its RNA transcripts are infectious in cell culture. *J Virol* 1987;61:3035–3039.

44. Emerson SU, Lewis M, Govindarajan S, et al. cDNA clone of hepatitis A virus encoding a virulent virus: induction of viral hepatitis by direct nucleic acid transfection of marmosets. *J Virol* 1992;66:6649–6654.

45. Brown EA, Day SP, Jansen RW, Lemon SM. The 5′ nontranslated region of hepatitis A virus: secondary structure and elements required for translation in vitro. *J Virol* 1991;65:5828–5838.

46. Brown EA, Zajac AJ, Lemon SM. In vitro characterization of an internal ribosomal entry site IRES present within the 5′ nontranslated region of hepatitis A virus RNA: comparison with the IRES of encephalomyocarditis virus. *J Virol* 1994;68:1066–1074.

47. Glass MJ, Summers DF. A *cis*-acting element within the hepatitis A virus 5′-non- coding region required for in vitro translation. *Virus Res* 1992;26:15–31.

48. Whetter LE, Day SP, Elroy-Stein O, et al. Low efficiency of the 5′ nontranslated region of hepatitis A virus RNA in directing cap-independent translation in permissive monkey kidney cells. *J Virol* 1994;68:5253–5263.

49. Funkhouser AW, Schultz DE, Lemon SM, et al. Hepatitis A virus translation is rate-limiting for virus replication in MRC-5 cells. *Virology* 1999;254:268–278.

50. Chang KH, Brown EA, Lemon SM. Cell type-specific proteins which interact with the 5′ nontranslated region of hepatitis A virus RNA. *J Virol* 1993;67:6716–6725.

51. Gosert R, Chang KH, Rijnbrand R, et al. Transient expression of cellular polypyrimidine-tract binding protein stimulates cap-independent translation directed by both picornaviral and flaviviral internal ribosome entry sites in vivo. *Mol Cell Biol* 2000;20:1583–1595.

52. Graff J, Cha J, Blyn LB, Ehrenfeld E. Interaction of polyrC. binding protein 2 with the 5′ noncoding region of hepatitis A virus RNA and its effects on translation. *J Virol* 1998;72:9668–9675.

53. Day SP, Murphy P, Brown EA, Lemon SM. Mutations within the 5′ nontranslated region of hepatitis A virus RNA which enhance replication in BS-C-1 cells. *J Virol* 1992;66:6533–6540.

54. Schultz DE, Honda M, Whetter LE, et al. Mutations within the 5′ nontranslated RNA of cell culture-adapted hepatitis A virus which enhance cap-independent translation in cultured African green monkey kidney cells. *J Virol* 1996;70:1041–1049.

55. Yi M, Schultz DE, Lemon SM. Functional significance of the interaction of hepatitis A virus RNA with glyceraldehyde 3-phosphate dehydrogenase GAPDH.:opposing effects of GAPDH and polypyrimidine tract binding protein on internal ribosome entry site function. *J Virol* 2000;74:6459–6468.

56. Graff J, Normann A, Flehmig B. Influence of the 5′ noncoding region of hepatitis A virus strain GBM on its growth in different cell lines. *J Gen Virol* 1997;78:1841–1849.

57. Borman AM, Kean KM. Intact eukaryotic initiation factor 4G is required for hepatitis A virus internal initiation of translation. *Virology* 1997;237:129–136.

58. Martin A, Escriou N, Chao S-F, et al. Identification and site-direct mutagenesis of the primary 2A/2B. cleavage site of the hepatitis A virus polyprotein: functional impact on the infectivity of HAV transcripts. *Virology* 1995;213:213–222.

59. Jia XY, Summers DF, Ehrenfeld E. Primary cleavage of the HAV capsid protein precursor in the middle of the proposed 2A coding region. *Virology* 1993;193:515–519.

60. Gosert R, Cassinotti P, Siegl G, Weitz M. Identification of hepatitis A virus non-structural protein 2B and its release by the major virus protease 3C. *J Gen Virol* 1996;77:247–255.

61. Emerson SU, Huang YK, McRill C, et al. Mutations in both the 2B and 2C genes of hepatitis A virus are involved in adaptation to growth in cell culture. *J Virol* 1992;66:650–654.

62. Emerson SU, Huang YK, Purcell RH. 2B and 2C mutations are essential but mutations throughout the genome of HAV contribute to adaptation to cell culture. *Virology* 1993;194:475–480.

63. Gosert R, Egger D, Bienz K. A cytopathic and a cell culture adapted hepatitis A virus strain differ in cell killing but not in intracellular membrane rearrangements. *Virology* 2000;266:157–169.

64. Teterina NL, Bienz K, Egger D, et al. Induction of intracellular membrane rearrangements by HAV proteins 2C and 2BC. *Virology* 1997;237:66–77.

65. Allaire M, Chernaia MM, Malcolm BA, James MNG. Picornaviral 3C cysteine proteinases have a fold similar to chymotrypsin-like serine proteinases. *Nature* 1994;369:72–76.

66. Schultheiss T, Sommergruber W, Kusov Y, Gauss-Müller V. Cleavage specificity of purified recombinant hepatitis A virus 3C proteinase on natural substrates. *J Virol* 1995;69:1727–1733.

67. Purcell RH. Approaches to immunization against hepatitis A virus. In: Hollinger FB, Lemon SM, Margolis HS, eds. *Viral hepatitis and liver disease.* Baltimore: Williams & Wilkins, 1991:41–46.

68. Lemon SM, Binn LN, Marchwicki R, et al. In vivo replication and reversion to wild-type of a neutralization-resistant variant of hepatitis A virus. *J Infect Dis* 1990;161:7–13.

69. Kaplan G, Totsuka A, Thompson P, et al. Identification of a surface glycoprotein on African green monkey kidney cells as a receptor for hepatitis A virus. *EMBO J* 1996;15:4282–4296.

70. Bishop NE, Anderson DA. Uncoating kinetics of hepatitis A virus virions and provirions. *J Virol* 2000;74:3423–3426.

71. Weitz M, Baroudy BM, Maloy WL, et al. Detection of a genome-linked protein VPg. of hepatitis A virus and its comparison with other picornaviral VPgs. *J Virol* 1986;60:124–130.

72. Jia X-Y, Ehrenfeld E, Summers DF. Proteolytic activity of hepatitis A virus 3C protein. *J Virol* 1991;65:2595–2600.

73. Graff J, Richards OC, Swiderek KM, et al. Hepatitis A virus capsid protein VP1 has a heterogeneous C terminus. *J Virol* 1999;73:6015–6023.

74. Harmon SA, Emerson SU, Huang YK, et al. Hepatitis A viruses with deletions

in the 2A gene are infectious in cultured cells and marmosets. *J Virol* 1995;69:5576–5581.

75. Yi M, Lemon SM. Replication of subgenomic hepatitis A virus RNAs expressing firefly luciferase is enhanced by mutations associated with adaptation of virus to growth in cultured cells. *J Virol* 2002;76:1171–1180.

76. Beneduce F, Ciervo A, Morace G. Site-directed mutagenesis of hepatitis A virus protein 3A: Effects on membrane interaction. *Biochim Biophys Acta Biomembr* 1997;1326:157–165.

77. Kusov YY, Gauss-Muller V. In vitro RNA binding of the hepatitis A virus proteinase 3C HAV 3Cpro. to secondary structure elements within the 5′ terminus of the HAV genome. *RNA* 1997;3:291–302.

78. Kusov Y, Weitz M, Dollenmeier G, et al. RNA-protein interactions at the 3′ end of the hepatitis A virus RNA. *J Virol* 1996;70:1890–1897.

79. Kusov YY, Shatirishvili G, Dzagurov G, Gauss-Muller V. A new G-tailing method for the determination of the polyA. tail length applied to hepatitis A virus RNA. *Nucleic Acids Res* 2001;29:E57.

80. Deinhardt F, Scheid R, Gauss-Muller V, et al. Propagation of human hepatitis A virus in cell lines of primary human hepatocellular carcinomas. *Prog Med Virol* 1981;27:109–113.

81. Daemer RJ, Feinstone SM, Gust ID, Purcell RH. Propagation of human hepatitis A virus in African Green Monkey kidney cell culture: primary isolation and serial passage. *Infect Immun* 1981;32:388–393.

82. Binn LN, Lemon SM, Marchwicki RH, et al. Primary isolation and serial passage of hepatitis A virus strains in primate cell cultures. *J Clin Microbiol* 1984;20:28–33.

83. Flehmig B, Vallbracht A, Wurster G. Hepatitis A virus in cell culture: III. Propagation of hepatitis A virus in human embryo kidney cells and human embryo fibroblast strains. *Med Microbiol Immunol* 1981;170:83–89.

84. Dotzauer A, Feinstone SM, Kaplan G. Susceptibility of nonprimate cell lines to hepatitis A virus infection. *J Virol* 1994;68:6064–6068.

85. Jansen RW, Newbold JE, Lemon SM. Complete nucleotide sequence of a cell culture-adapted variant of hepatitis A virus: comparison with wild-type virus with restricted capacity for *in vitro* replication. *Virology* 1988;163:299–307.

86. Brack K, Frings W, Dotzauer A, Vallbracht A. A cytopathogenic, apoptosis-inducing variant of hepatitis A virus. *J Virol* 1998;72:3370–3376.

87. Cho MW, Ehrenfeld E. Rapid completion of the replication cycle of hepatitis A virus subsequent to reversal of guanidine inhibition. *Virology* 1991;180:770–780.

88. Blank CA, Anderson DA, Beard M, Lemon SM. Infection of polarized cultures of human intestinal epithelial cells with hepatitis A virus: vectorial release of progeny virions through apical cellular membranes. *J Virol* 2000;74:6476–6484.

89. Funkhouser AW, Purcell RH, D'Hondt E, Emerson SU. Attenuated hepatitis A virus: genetic determinants of adaptation to growth in MRC-5 cells. *J Virol* 1994;68:148–157.

90. Graff J, Normann A, Feinstone SM, Flehmig B. Nucleotide sequence of wild-type hepatitis A virus GBM in comparison with two cell culture-adapted variants. *J Virol* 1994;68:548–554.

91. Zhang HC, Chao SF, Ping LH, et al. An infectious cDNA clone of a cytopathic hepatitis A virus: genomic regions associated with rapid replication and cytopathic effect. *Virology* 1995;212:686–697.

92. Midthun K, Ellerbeck E, Gershman K, et al. Safety and immunogenicity of a live attenuated hepatitis A virus vaccine in seronegative volunteers. *J Infect Dis* 1991;163:735–739.

93. Sjogren MH, Purcell RH, McKee K, et al. Clinical and laboratory observations following oral or intramuscular administration of a live, attenuated hepatitis A vaccine candidate. *Vaccine* 1992;10[Suppl 1]:S135–S137.

94. Lemon SM. Type A viral hepatitis: new developments in an old disease. *N Engl J Med* 1985;313:1059–1067.

95. Jansen RW, Siegl G, Lemon SM. Molecular epidemiology of human hepatitis A virus defined by an antigen-capture polymerase chain reaction method. *Proc Natl Acad Sci USA* 1990;87:2867–2871.

96. Robertson BH, Khanna B, Nainan OV, Margolis HS. Epidemiologic patterns of wild-type hepatitis A virus determined by genetic variation. *J Infect Dis* 1991;163:286–292.

97. Robertson BH, Jansen RW, Khanna B, et al. Genetic relatedness of hepatitis A virus strains recovered from different geographic regions. *J Gen Virol* 1992;73:1365–1377.

98. Mannucci PM, Gdovin S, Gringeri A, et al. Transmission of hepatitis A to patients with hemophilia by factor VIII concentrates treated with organic solvent and detergent to inactivate viruses. *Ann Intern Med* 1994;120:1–7.

99. Mathiesen LR, Drucker J, Lorenz D, et al. Localization of hepatitis A antigen in marmoset organs during acute infection with hepatitis A virus. *J Infect Dis* 1978;138:369–377.

100. Cohen JI, Feinstone S, Purcell RH. Hepatitis A virus infection in a chimpanzee: duration of viremia and detection of virus in saliva and throat swabs. *J Infect Dis* 1989;160:887–890.

101. Asher LVS, Binn LN, Mensing TL, et al. Pathogenesis of hepatitis A in orally inoculated owl monkeys *Aotus trivergatus*. *J Med Virol* 1995;47:260–268.

102. Dienstag JL, Popper H, Purcell RH. The pathology of viral hepatitis types A and B in chimpanzees. *Am J Pathol* 1976;85:131–144.

103. Shimizu YK, Shikata T, Beninger PR, et al. Detection of hepatitis A antigen in human liver. *Infect Immun* 1982;36:320–324.

104. Murphy BL, Maynard JE, Bradley DW, et al. Immunofluorescence of hepatitis A virus antigen in chimpanzees. *Infect Immun* 1978;21:663–665.

105. Teixera MR Jr, Weller IVD, Murray A, et al. The pathology of hepatitis A in man. *Liver* 1982;2:53–60.

106. Keenan CM, Lemon SM, LeDuc JW, et al. Pathology of hepatitis A infection in the owl monkey *Aotus trivirgatus*. *Am J Pathol* 1984;115:1–8.

107. Mathiesen LR, Feinstone SM, Wong DC, et al. Enzyme-linked immunosorbent assay for detection of hepatitis A antigen in stool and antibody to hepatitis A antigen in sera: comparison with solid-phase radioimmunoassay, immune electron microscopy, and immune adherence hemagglutination assay. *J Clin Microbiol* 1978;7:184–193.

108. Lemon SM, Brown CD, Brooks DS, et al. Specific immunoglobulin M response to hepatitis A virus determined by solid-phase radioimmunoassay. *Infect Immun* 1980;28:927–936.

109. Lemon SM, Binn LN. Serum neutralizing antibody response to hepatitis A virus. *J Infect Dis* 1983;148:1033–1039.

110. Decker RH, Kosakowski SM, Vanderbilt AS, et al. Diagnosis of acute hepatitis A by HAVAB^R-M, a direct radioimmunoassay for IgM anti-HAV. *Am J Clin Pathol* 1981;76:140–147.

111. Coulepis AG, Locarnini SA, Lehmann NI, Gust ID. Detection of hepatitis A virus in the feces of patients with naturally acquired infections. *J Infect Dis* 1980;141:151–156.

112. Stapleton JT, Lange DK, LeDuc JW, et al. The role of secretory immunity in hepatitis A virus infection. *J Infect Dis* 1991;163:7–11.

113. Stapleton JT, Jansen RW, Lemon SM. Neutralizing antibody to hepatitis A virus in immune serum globulin and in the sera of human recipients of immune serum globulin. *Gastroenterology* 1985;89:637–642.

114. Vallbracht A, Gabriel P, Maier K, et al. Cell-mediated cytotoxicity in hepatitis A virus infection. *Hepatology* 1986;6:1308–1314.

115. Maier K, Gabriel P, Koscielniak E, et al. Human gamma interferon production by cytotoxic T lymphocytes sensitized during hepatitis A virus infection. *J Virol* 1988;62:3756–3763.

116. Vallbracht A, Maier K, Stierhof Y-D, et al. Liver-derived cytotoxic T cells in hepatitis A virus infection. *J Infect Dis* 1989;160:209–217.

117. Hadler SC, Webster HM, Erben JJ, et al. Hepatitis A in day-care centers: a community-wide assessment. *N Engl J Med* 1980;302:1222–1227.

118. Rakela J, Redeker AG, Edwards VM, et al. Hepatitis A virus infection in fulminant hepatitis and chronic active hepatitis. *Gastroenterology* 1978;74:879–882.

119. Forbes A, Williams R. Changing epidemiology and clinical aspects of hepatitis A. *Br Med Bull* 1990;46:303–318.

120. Hadler SC. Global impact of hepatitis A virus infection: changing patterns. In: Hollinger FB, Lemon SM, Margolis HS, eds. *Viral hepatitis and liver disease.* Baltimore: Williams and Wilkins, 1991:14–20.

121. Purcell RH, Wong DC, Moritsugu Y, et al. A microtiter solid-phase radioimmunoassay for hepatitis A antigen and antibody. *J Immunol* 1976;116:349–356.

122. Lemon SM, Murphy PC, Provost PJ, et al. Immunoprecipitation and virus neutralization assays demonstrate qualitative differences between protective antibody responses to inactivated hepatitis A vaccine and passive immunization with immune globulin. *J Infect Dis* 1997;176:9–19.

123. Prevention of hepatitis A through active or passive immunization: recommendations of the Advisory Committee on Immunization Practices ACIP. *MMWR* 1999;48.

124. Innis BL, Snitbhan R, Kunasol P, et al. Protection against hepatitis A by an inactivated vaccine. *JAMA* 1994;271:1328–1334.

125. Werzberger A, Mensch B, Kuter B, et al. A controlled trial of a formalin-inactivated hepatitis A vaccine in healthy children. *N Engl J Med* 1992;327:453–457.

126. Lemon SM, Shapiro CN. The value of immunization against hepatitis A. *Infect Agents Dis* 1994;3:38–49.

127. Lemon SM, Thomas DL. Vaccines to prevent viral hepatitis. *N Engl J Med* 1997;336:196–204.

128. Provost PJ, Bishop RP, Gerety RJ, et al. New findings in live, attenuated hepatitis A vaccine development. *J Med Virol* 1986;20:165–175.

129. Karron RA, Daemer RJ, Ticehurst JR, et al. Studies of prototype live hepatitis A virus vaccine in primate models. *J Infect Dis* 1988;157:338–345.

130. Cohen JI, Rosenblum B, Feinstone SM, et al. Attenuation and cell culture adaptation of hepatitis A virus HAV: a genetic analysis with HAV cDNA. *J Virol* 1989;63:5364–5370.

131. Mao JS, Dong DX, Zhang HY, et al. Primary study of attenuated live hepatitis A vaccine H2 strain. in humans. *J Infect Dis* 1989;159:621–624.

132. Raychaudhuri G, Govindarajan S, Shapiro M, et al. Utilization of chimeras between human HM-175. and simian AGM-27. strains of hepatitis A virus to study the molecular basis of virulence. *J Virol* 1998;72:7467–7475.

CHAPTER 252
Hepatitis C Virus

Raymond S. Koff

HISTORY

By the mid-1970s, the development of serologic tests for hepatitis A and hepatitis B virus infections made it clear that another etiologic form of viral hepatitis existed: non-A, non-B hepatitis. Molecular cloning of the hepatitis C virus (HCV), the major responsible bloodborne pathogen of non-A, non-B hepatitis, was reported in 1989 along with the development of serologic tests to identify HCV infection (1). In succeeding years, the association of HCV with acute and chronic hepatitis, with the development of cirrhosis and hepatocellular carcinoma, and with a variety of extrahepatic disorders, has established the importance of HCV as a pathogenic agent. With a global prevalence of 3%, in excess of 175 million people are actively infected worldwide, and close to 3 million patients in the United States.

MORPHOLOGY

HCV is a lipoprotein-enveloped, ribonucleic acid (RNA)–containing virus with a buoyant density in sucrose estimated to be 1.08 g/dL and a nucleocapsid buoyant density estimated to be 1.25 g/cm^3. Classic filtration studies suggested a diameter of between 38 and 60 nm for the HCV particle and electron microscopy of an enriched plasma sample revealed the presence of spherical, enveloped 55-nm to 65 nm virus-like particles (2,3), which are probably the actual virions. Treatment with detergent liberated 30-nm to 35-nm icosahedral particles presumed to be associated with the HCV nucleocapsid. Envelope projections observed on the virus-like particles have included spikes, knobs, or neither.

CHARACTERISTICS

HCV contains a positive-sense, single-stranded RNA molecule that is infectious (4). The genome has a length of approximately 9,600 nucleotides and contains a 5′-nontranslated region of about 332 to 342 nucleotides, which is well conserved in the different strains that have been studied, and a single, large open reading frame that encodes a large polyprotein of approximately 3,000 amino acids. The putative structure of the HCV genome is shown in Fig. 252.1, and the probable function and gene products of the genomic regions are shown in Table 252.1. The highly conserved 5′ nontranslated region contains an internal ribosomal entry site at which translation of the HCV polyprotein is initiated (5). Small hairpin structures, multiple stem-loops, a pseudoknot, three to six AUG codons, and a six-nucleotide motif that may be involved in modulating viral transcription have been described in the 5′ nontranslated region. After the large open reading frame, a short but variable in length 3′-nontranslated region containing poly(U) or poly(A) sequences is thought to be involved in RNA replication, HCV packaging, and infectivity (6).

The large polyprotein encoded by the HCV open reading frame is subjected to co-translational and posttranslational cleavage through the action of cellular signal peptidases and virus-specific proteinases (7). Approximately one third of the polyprotein, after the 5′-nontranslated region, comprises a number of structural proteins. These are recognized to include an internal viral structural protein called the nucleocapsid or core (C) protein and two glycosylated proteins, termed El and E2, which are present in the lipid-containing envelope of the virus and may generate neutralizing antibodies. The envelope glycoproteins and the core protein are cleaved from the polyprotein by the action of the cellular signalase. The HCV core protein is processed in vivo by cleavage of its C-terminal hydrophobic segment to generate the mature core protein (a phosphoprotein) that can bind RNA, is membrane associated, and may function as a transcriptional transactivator. Sequencing of the core gene has revealed the presence of two nuclear localization signals, a DNA-binding motif, a phosphorylation site, and hydrophilic domains containing immunogenic epitopes (8). An HCV encoded cleavage product, termed p7, located between the E2 and NS2 proteins may have an immunoregulatory function (9). It is preceded by a hydrophobic sequence in E2 that may direct translocation into the endoplasmic reticulum.

The remaining two thirds of the polyprotein is also cleaved into distinct nonstructural proteins (termed NS2, NS3, NS4A, NS4B, NS5A, and NS5B) that are involved in the replication of HCV and have metalloproteinase, protease, helicase, and RNA polymerase activities (see Table 252.1). Processing of the nonstructural polyprotein involves at least two virus-encoded proteinases: one at NS2/3 and one at NS3. The NS2/3 enzyme is a zinc-dependent metalloproteinase; the NS3 enzyme carries two enzymatic activities: a chymotrypsin-like serine proteinase that appears to function in both cis and trans cleavage modes and a nucleoside triphosphatase/helicase (8). NS4A sequences appear to be important in the polyprotein processing, particularly for the NS4B/5A cleavage site (8). The function of NS4B is unknown but it appears to be a cytoplasmically-oriented integral endoplasmic reticulum membrane protein (10). NS5A is thought to suppress interferon-induced cellular double-stranded RNA-activated protein kinase (PKR) activity and it may function as a transcriptional modulator. The RNA-dependent RNA polymerase and RNA-binding protein required for HCV RNA synthesis is encoded by the NS5B region (11). The nonstructural proteins may form complex interactions with one another, may form dimers, and may recruit cellular proteins for some components of viral replication and production of virions.

CLASSIFICATION

HCV is currently classified as a separate third genus, termed *Hepacivirus*, in the Flaviviridae family, which includes both the flaviviruses and the animal pestiviruses.

GENETIC VARIATION

A high degrees of HCV variability, which may favor viral persistence, has been attributed to a high rate of viral replication coupled with poor or absent proofreading ability of the RNA polymerase leading to failure to detect transcription errors. More than 10^{12} virions with a virion half-life of 2.7 hours are produced daily (12) and the rate of HCV mutation has been calculated to be 10^{-3} to 10^{-4} base substitutions per genome site per year. The most variable region of the HCV genome, located at the N-terminus of the E2 gene, is a domain of 31 amino acids, defined as the hypervariable region-1 (HVR1); it may play a role in attachment to the hepatocyte. Increasing diversity in HVR1 quasispecies (see

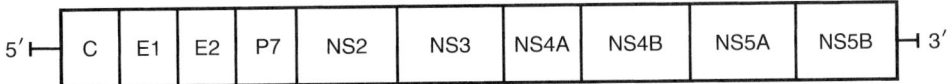

Figure 252.1. Genomic map of HCV RNA depicting the regions encoding the structural and nonstructural proteins. The 5'-nontranslated region and the shorter 3'-nontranslated region containing poly (U) or poly (A) sequences are indicated by the horizontal lines preceding the C (core) region (on the left side) and following the NS5B region (on the right side).

below) has been linked with the development of chronic infection (13) but diversity in other regions may also contribute. The role of host immune pressure on genetic drift of HCV remains controversial.

Comparison of HCV isolates has revealed marked differences among the sequenced nucleotides. Currently, all known HCV isolates are phylogenetically divided into six distinct classes comprising 11 genotypes and as many as 80 subtypes. By general agreement, HCV genotypes have nucleotide divergence of more than 30%; within genotypes, nucleotide divergence does not exceed 20% and in subtypes, up to 10%. In any single infected individual, HCV circulates as a family of closely related viruses, termed quasispecies.

The worldwide distribution of genotypes is variable: HCV genotypes 1, 2, and subtype 3a appear to be the most prevalent in North America, Europe, and Japan. Among patients in the United States with chronic hepatitis C, nearly 75% have HCV genotype 1; three fourths are 1a and one fourth are 1b (14). Genotypes 1 and 4 have been linked to relative resistance to interferon treatment.

PROPAGATION

HCV has been transmitted to and serially passaged in chimpanzees but other susceptible mammalian or non-mammalian species, with the possible exception of the tree shrew (15), have yet to be identified. Hence, the host range of HCV appears to be restricted.

Many cell culture systems expressing HCV gene products or supporting low levels of HCV replication have been reported using human lymphocytic cell lines, hepatocellular carcinoma cell lines, primary adult and fetal chimpanzee and human hepatocyte cultures, Chinese hamster ovary cells, and other non-hepatic cells (16). The establishment of a transfection system producing subgenomic RNA replicons that efficiently replicate autonomously in human hepatocellular carcinoma cells appears to be a major advance in the field that may prove useful in the study of HCV biology and infectivity and in the screening of antiviral drugs (17). However, infectious HCV particles have not been produced in these systems.

REPLICATION

The life cycle and precise replicative mechanisms of HCV remain poorly understood and the receptor(s) for HCV attachment and entry remains uncertain. Candidates have included a cell surface molecule (CD81), the low-density lipoprotein receptor, and glycosaminoglycans (8). After attachment, membrane fusion and endocytosis presumably result in HCV entry and uncoating of the HCV envelope. The nucleocapsid is thought to disaggregate freeing the HCV RNA which is then translated into the large polyprotein that is lead by internally located signal peptides to the endoplasmic reticulum for further processing into the envelope, nucleocapsid, and non-structural proteins. Through the catalytic actions of the RNA-dependent RNA polymerase, the positive-stranded RNA genome is transcribed into a negative strand, which then serves as a template for the transcription of a nascent positive RNA strand. The progeny positive strands are subsequently encapsidated within the nucleocapsid and acquire the envelope glycoproteins that have accumulated in the endoplasmic reticulum, the presumed site of HCV particle assembly and budding from the hepatocyte.

TABLE 252.1. Hepatitis C Virus Genomic Regions: Functional Role and Gene Products

Genomic regions	Functional role and gene products
5' Nontranslated	Internal ribosomal entry site ? Modulation of virus transcription
C (core)	Nuclear localization signals DNA-binding motif Phosphorylation site Hydrophilic domains containing immunogenic epitopes Nucleocapsid phosphoprotein binds RNA, membrane associated, transcriptional transactivator
E1	Envelope glycoprotein (epitope)
E2	Envelope glycoprotein (epitope), role in cell attachment, translocation signal to endoplasmic reticulum, interaction with RNA-activated protein kinase (PKR) induced by interferon
P7	? Immunoregulatory function
NS2/3	Zinc-dependent metalloproteinase
NS3	Chymotrypsin-like serine proteinase Nucleoside triphosphatase/helicase
NS4A	Involved in polyprotein processing, at NS4B/5A cleavage site
NS4B	Unknown
NS5A	Inhibition of PKR induced by interferon Transcriptional modulation
NS5B	RNA-dependent RNA polymerase RNA-binding
3' Nontranslated	Required for infectivity, RNA replication, packaging Interacts with ribosomal proteins

DNA, deoxyribonucleic acid; RNA, ribonucleic acid.

Site of Replication

The totality of tissue sites at which HCV RNA replication occurs has yet to be fully determined. HCV replication occurs in hepatocytes and probably in hematopoietic cells, such as peripheral blood mononuclear cells (18). Replicative forms may be present in B-lymphocytes but the contribution of hematopoietic cells to total HCV production is likely to be minimal. HCV proteins have been detected in bile duct epithelial cells but proof of replication is lacking (19). Whether other cell types support replication remains uncertain.

REFERENCES

1. Choo Q-L, Kuo G, Weiner AJ, et al. Isolation of a cDNA clone derived from a blood-borne non-A, non-B viral hepatitis genome. *Science* 1989;244:359–362.
2. Takahashi K, Kishimoti S, Yoshizawa H, et al. p26 protein and 33-nm particle associated with nucleocapsid of hepatitis C virus recovered from the circulation of infected hosts. *Virology* 1992;191:431–434.
3. Kaito M, Watanabe S, Tsukiyama-Kohara K, et al. Hepatitis C virus particle detected by immunoelectron microscopic study. *J Gen Virol* 1994;75:1755–1760.
4. Kolyhakov AA, Agapov EV, Blight KJ, et al. Transmission of hepatitis C by intrahepatic inoculation with transcribed RNA. *Science* 1997;277:570–574.
5. Tsukiyama-Kohara K, Iizuka N, Kohara M, et al. Internal ribosome entry site within hepatitis C virus RNA. *J Virol* 1992;66:1476–1483.
6. Yanagi M, St. Claire M, Emerson SU, et al. In vivo analysis of the 3′ untranslated region of the hepatitis C virus after in vitro mutagenesis of an infectious cDNA clone. *Proc Natl Acad Sci U S A* 1999;96:2291–2295.
7. Bartenschlager R, Lohmann V. Replication of hepatitis C virus. *J Gen Virol* 2000;81:1631–1648.
8. Lin C, Lindenbach BD, Pragai BM, et al. Processing in the hepatitis C virus E2-NS2 region: Identification of p7 and two distinct E2-specific products with different C termini. *J Virol* 1994;68:5063–5073.
9. Lechmann M, Murata K, Satoi J, et al. Hepatitis C virus-like particles induce virus-specific humoral and cellular immune responses in mice. *Hepatology* 2001;34:417–423.
10. Hugle T, Fehrmann F, BieckE, et al. The hepatitis C virus nonstructural protein 4B is an integral endoplasmic reticulum membrane protein. *Virology* 2001;284:70–81.
11. Qin W, Yamashita T, Shirota Y, et al. Mutational analysis of the structure and functions of hepatitis C virus RNA-dependent RNA polymerase. *Hepatology* 2001;33:728–737.
12. Neumann AU, Lam NP, Dahari H, et al. Hepatitis C viral dynamics in vivo and the antiviral efficacy of interferon-alpha therapy. *Science* 1998;282:103–107.
13. Farci P, Shimoda A, Coiana A, et al. The outcome of acute hepatitis C predicted by the evolution of the viral quasispecies. *Science* 2000;288:339–344.
14. Alter MJ, Kruszon-Moran D, Nainan OV, et al. The prevalence of hepatitis C virus infection in the United States, 1988 through 1994. *N Engl J Med* 1999;341:556–562.
15. Xie ZC, Riezu JL, Lasarte JJ, et al. Transmission of hepatitis C virus infection to tree shews. *Virology* 1998;244:513–520.
16. Kato N, Shimotohno K. Systems to culture hepatitis C virus. *Curr Top Microbiol Immunol* 2000;242:261–278.
17. Blight KJ, Kolyhakov AA, Rice CM. Efficient initiation of HCV RNA replication in cell culture. *Science* 2000;290:1972–1974.
18. Muller HM, Pfaff E, Goeser T, et al. Peripheral blood leukocytes serve as a possible extrahepatic site for hepatitis C virus replication. *J Gen Virol* 1993;74:669–676.
19. Haruna Y, Kanda T, Honda M, et al. Detection of hepatitis C virus in the bile and bile duct epithelial cells of hepatitis C virus-infected patients. *Hepatology* 2001;33:977–980.

CHAPTER 253

Hepatitis E Virus

Raymond S. Koff

HISTORY

An enterically transmitted agent of viral hepatitis, resembling hepatitis A virus in its epidemiologic behavior and serologically distinct from all other known hepatitis viruses, has been responsible for outbreaks of predominantly waterborne hepatitis in the Indian subcontinent; central and Southeast Asia, including the central Asian republics of the former Soviet Union; the Middle East; northern Africa; and, in the Americas, Mexico (1). The etiologic agent, designated hepatitis E virus (HEV), has defied taxonomic classification although a common evolutionary origin to specific plant and animal viruses has been suggested (2). HEV has been placed in a separate family called hepatitis E–like viruses. It is a non-enveloped agent with a polyadenylated,

positive-sense, single-stranded ribonucleic acid (RNA) genome (3). Serologically documented epidemics of hepatitis E have been extant at least since the mid-1950s (4,5), but it is likely that this infection has a considerably longer history. HEV is now thought to be the major agent of sporadic hepatitis among young individuals in developing countries. The host range includes human and nonhuman primates, and possibly swine. Although definitive data are not yet available, the host range also may include a wide range of other domestic animals and rodents.

MORPHOLOGY AND CHARACTERISTICS OF THE AGENT

Spherical virus-like particles with icosahedral symmetry, 27 to 34 nm in diameter, (Fig.253.1), have been visualized by electron microscopy or immunoelectron microscopy of stool samples of naturally infected patients and experimentally infected human volunteers and nonhuman primates (1). Isolates of these HEV particles, recovered from stool samples, have induced hepatitis in inoculated marmosets, cynomolgus, rhesus and owl monkeys, and chimpanzees. HEV appears to be labile and can be inactivated by cycles of freeze-thawing or heating to 100°C but is relatively stable to acid and mild alkaline states. A sedimentation coefficient of 183S and a buoyant density of 1.29 g/cm in a potassium tartrate-glycerol gradient have been reported. A poorly defined and characterized HEV antigen may be present on the surface of HEV particles; it has been identified in the cytoplasm of hepatocytes of experimentally infected nonhuman primates (6).

HEPATITIS E VIRUS GENOME

The complete RNA genome is approximately 7.2 long (3). Transfection studies have indicated that the full-length RNA genome is infectious (7). A capped 27 to 35 nucleotide untranslated

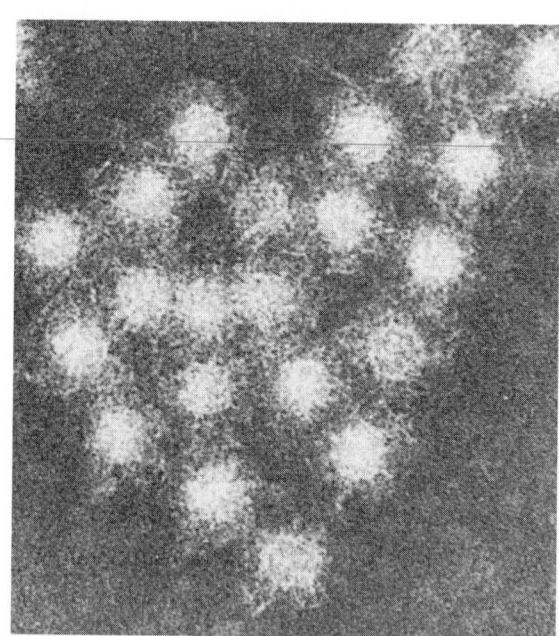

Figure 253.1. HEV particles, approximately 32 nm in diameter, isolated from stool and aggregated by anti-HEV in acute-phase serum (222X, 566X). (Courtesy of Daniel Bradley.)

TABLE 253.1. Hepatitis E Virus Open Reading Frames

Open reading frame number	Encoded amino acids	Function
1	1690	RNA-dependent RNA polymerase (RNA replicase)
		Helicase
		Cysteine protease
		Methyltransferase
		"Y" and "X" domains
		Proline-rich "hinge" region
2	660	Capsid protein with immunodominant epitope
3	123	Immunodominant epitope
		Membrane anchor region
		Signal transduction

RNA, ribonucleic acid.

region has been identified at the 5′ end and a 65 to 74 nucleotide poly (A) tail at the 3′ end. The 3′ end of the genome appears to interact with the RNA-dependent RNA polymerase and may serve as a site for the initiation of replication (8). Three discontinuous, partially overlapping open reading frames (ORF-1, ORF-2, and ORF-3) (Table 253.1) encoding nonstructural proteins at the 5′ end, and structural proteins at the 3′ end have been identified (9).

The first open reading frame (ORF-1), the longest, encodes a 1,690-amino acid protein that is cleaved into a number of nonstructural replicative proteins, including a RNA-dependent RNA polymerase (RNA replicase) and others shown in Table 253.1. The second open reading frame (ORF-2) encodes a protein of 660 amino acids that is the major structural, capsid protein of HEV. It is expressed intracellularly and on the cell surface and contains immunodominant epitopes (10). The ORF-2 protein has been shown to self-assemble into virus-like particles in the absence of either ORF-1 or ORF-3 (11). The smallest open reading frame (ORF-3) encodes a structural phosphoprotein of 123 amino acids which also contains epitopes and may serve a membrane anchor function and play a role in the signal transduction pathway (12).

Genetic Variation

Only one human serotype of HEV has been identified and homologous immunity seems likely despite the fact that at least four, and possibly as many as 9 main genotypes and multiple subtypes have been identified (13). Novel human HEV variants have been reported from non-endemic areas as well as endemic ones. A swine HEV sharing nearly identical amino acid homology with some human isolates has been identified and one of the human HEV strains closely related to the swine HEV has been experimentally transmitted to pigs (14). In general, isolates from patients infected during outbreaks show a high degree of identity as do isolates recovered from a given geographic area. Isolates recovered from geographically more distant areas tend to show greater diversity.

PROPAGATION

HEV has been propagated in continuous cell lines derived from human lung or liver and in primary macaque hepatocytes. Cell line-dependent, antibody-neutralizable cytopathic effects have been reported (15,16). The utility of these cell lines in studies of HEV replication and in the development of antiviral therapy or a HEV vaccine remains uncertain.

REPLICATION

Replication of HEV is probably limited to the hepatocyte and possibly bile duct epithelium. Direct studies of the replication strategies utilized by HEV in infected human beings are not available. It has been postulated that after HEV enters the hepatocyte, the positive-sense HEV RNA is translated to produce the nonstructural proteins, including the RNA-dependent RNA polymerase. By itself or in association with cell proteins, the RNA polymerase directs the generation of negative-stranded pregenomic RNA from the 3′ end of the genome (17). In experimentally infected nonhuman primates, HEV RNA–negative strands were found in hepatocytes during the incubation period (18). Subsequently, positive-strand RNA synthesis takes place with the negative-strand RNA serving as the template. The positive-sense RNA and subgenomic RNAs produce the structural proteins that encapsidate the positive-sense RNA to form nascent viral particles. Extensive investigations of the morphogenesis, packaging, and transfer of HEV from the hepatocyte to the bile duct epithelium and secretion into the bile remain to be undertaken.

REFERENCES

1. Krawczynski K. Hepatitis E. *Hepatology* 1993;17:932–941.
2. Magden J, Takeda N, Li T, et al. Virus-specific mRNA capping enzyme encoded by hepatitis E virus. *J Virol* 2001;75:6249–6255.
3. Reyes GR, Purdy MA, Kim JP, et al. Isolation of a cDNA from the virus responsible for enterically transmitted non-A, non-B hepatitis. *Science* 1990;247:1335–1339.
4. Wong DC, Purcell RH Sreenivasan MA, et al. Epidemic and endemic hepatitis in India: Evidence for a non-A, non-B hepatitis virus aetiology. *Lancet* 1980;2:876–878.
5. Khuroo MS. Study of an epidemic of non-A, non-B hepatitis: possibility of another human hepatitis virus distinct from posttransfusion non-A, non-B type. *Am J Med* 1980;68:818–824.
6. Krawczynski K, Bradley DW. Enterically transmitted non-A, non-B hepatitis: identification of virus-associated antigen in experimentally infected cynomolgus macaques. *J Infect Dis* 1989;159:1042–1049.
7. Panda SK, Ansari IH, Durgapal H, et al. The in vitro-synthesized RNA from a cDNA clone of hepatitis E virus is infectious. *J Virol* 2000;74:2430–2437.
8. Agrawal S, Gupta D, Panda SK. The 3′ end of hepatitis E virus (HEV) genome binds specifically to the viral RNA-dependent RNA polymerase (RdRp). *Virology* 2001;282:87–101.
9. Tam AW, Smith MM, Guerra ME, et al: Hepatitis E virus (HEV): molecular cloning and sequencing of the full-length viral genome. *Virology* 1991;185:120–131.
10. Khudyakov YE, Favorov MO, Jue DL, et al. Immunodominant antigenic regions in a structural protein of the hepatitis E virus. *Virology* 1994;198:390–393.
11. Xing L, Kato K Tiancheng L, et al. Recombinant hepatitis E capsid protein self-assembles into a dual-domain *TA* particle presenting native virus epitopes. *Virology* 1999;265:35–45.
12. Tyagi S, Jameel S, Lal SK. Self-association and mapping of the interaction domain of hepatitis E virus ORF3 protein. *J Virol* 2001;75:2493–2498.
13. Schlauder GG, Desai SM, Zanetti AR, et al. Novel hepatitis E virus (HEV) isolates from Europe: evidence for additional genotypes of HEV. *J Med Virol* 1999;57:243–251.
14. Halbur PG, Kasorndorkbua C, Gilber C, et al. Comparative pathogenesis of infection of pigs with hepatitis E virus recovered from a pig and human. *J Clin Microbiol* 2001;39:918–923.
15. Huang R, Li D, Wei T, et al. Cell culture of sporadic hepatitis E virus in China. *Clin Diag Lab Immunol* 1999;6:729–733.
16. Divizia M, Gabrielli R, Degener AM, et al. Evidence of hepatitis E virus replication on cell cultures. *Microbiologica* 1999;22:77–83.
17. Reyes GR, Huang C-C, Tam AW, Purdy MA. Molecular organization and replication of hepatitis E virus (HEV). *Arch Virol Suppl* 1993;7:15–25.
18. Kawai HF, Koji T, Iida F, et al. Shift of hepatitis E RNA from hepatocytes to biliary epithelial cells during acute infection of rhesus monkey. *J Viral Hepatitis* 1999;6:287–297.

CHAPTER 254

Rotaviruses and Other Reoviridae

John E. Herrmann

The family Reoviridae consists of four genera that infect humans: *Orthoreovirus*, *Coltivirus*, *Orbivirus*, and *Rotavirus*. Additional genera of viruses infect insects, plants, fish, and other animals but these genera will not be discussed. The reoviruses (respiratory enteric orphan viruses) were the first to be described. They are the type genus of the family and are the prototype viruses of the genus *Orthoreovirus*. All four of the Reoviridae genera share similar physiochemical characteristics in that they have nonenveloped virions approximately 60 to 80 nm in diameter with inner and outer capsids, and they are unique among viruses in containing double-stranded ribonucleic acid (RNA). The diseases caused by each genus, however, are markedly different. The most important agents of human disease are the group A rotaviruses, which are the major cause of gastroenteritis in infants and young children. The reoviruses, although they were the first to be recognized and are widespread among animal species and humans, have not been clearly implicated as etiologic agents for any specific disease. The orbiviruses are more important as veterinary pathogens but cause febrile illnesses and possibly other illnesses in humans. Colorado tick fever virus is the important pathogen in the *Coltivirus* genus.

ROTAVIRUS

Group A rotaviruses are the most important cause of severe, acute diarrhea in children younger than 2 years of age. The number of deaths due to rotavirus infections is not known, but some estimates are in the hundreds of thousands per year in developing countries (1). Deaths resulting from rotavirus infections are uncommon in developed countries but the morbidity is similar to that of developing countries. In the United States, rotaviruses cause approximately 50,000 hospitalizations per year, with an estimated cost of $274 million in medical care (1).

Non-group A rotaviruses have been associated with diarrheal disease but have been implicated in disease far less frequently. Group B rotaviruses have been associated with epidemics of gastroenteritis in China, primarily in older children and adults (2). Group C rotaviruses have been implicated in occasional cases of diarrhea in many countries, including the United States (3).

Characteristics of the Pathogen

Rotaviruses contain double-stranded RNA enclosed in a triple-layered icosahedral protein capsid, an outer shell, an intermediate layer, and an inner core that can be seen by viral degradation. Complete triple-layered (previously called double-shelled) particles are approximately 70 mm in diameter. Incomplete double-layered (previously called single-shelled) particles of approximately 55 run in diameter are also found. The intact complete particles as seen by negative-stain electron microscopy (Fig. 254.1) have a characteristic wheel (Latin *rota*) shape. Triple layered and double layered single-shelled particles have a density in cesium chloride of 1.36 g/cm^3 and 1.38 g/cm^3, respectively (4,5). The viral genome is composed of 11 segments of double-stranded RNA as shown by electrophoretic analysis. The segments have an estimated total mass of 1.1×10^7 daltons in cesium chloride (4,5).

Group A rotaviruses contain a group-specific common antigen designated VP6, a protein on the surface of the first inner capsid protein. The more recently recognized non-group A rotaviruses, which currently include groups B to G and possibly others, are morphologically the same as group A rotaviruses but lack the group A common antigen. Group B through G rotaviruses have also been referred to in past studies as non-group A rotaviruses, atypical rotaviruses, or pararotaviruses. These rotaviruses have been detected in pigs (6,7), calves, lambs (8), and chickens (9) as well as in humans (10).

Serotypes of group A rotaviruses are based on differences in two outer capsid proteins that elicit neutralizing antibodies, VP4 and VP7. Serotypes based on VP7 are designated G types (for glycoprotein), and serotypes based on VP4 are designated P types (for protease-sensitive protein) (5, 11, 12). Because of cross-reactivities seen with antibodies to VP4, P types have also been distinguished on the basis of gene sequences (genotypes). There are currently 14 G serotypes, 17 P serotypes, and 20 P genotypes. Human rotavirus isolates are most commonly in G serotypes 1 to 4 but are also found in G serotypes 5, 6, 8, 9, 10, and 12. Eight human P serotypes have been described: 1A, 113, 2, 3A, 3B, 4, 5, and 8. There have also been two subgroups described, based on antigenic differences in VP6, and numerous electropherotypes based on migration patterns of rotaviral RNA segments in gels.

Rotavirus strains have been shown to retain infectivity at pH 3.5 or pH 10.0 and after treatment with ether, chloroform, fluorocarbons, or proteases (13). The most effective disinfectants for rotaviruses are 95% ethanol, formalin, and Lysol (14,15). Sodium hypochlorite may (16) or may not (15) be effective, and rotaviruses have been shown to survive chlorine treatment in community water supplies (17).

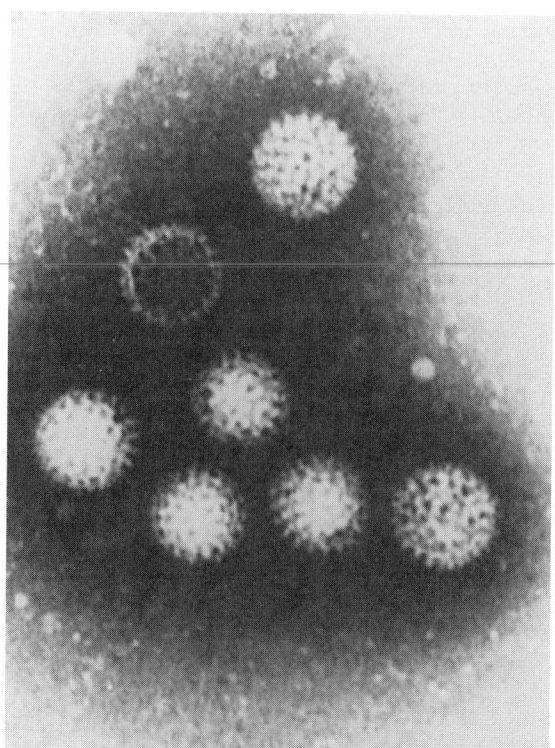

Figure 254.1. Rotavirus particles observed by negative-stain electron microscopy in a stool suspension of a child with diarrhea. (Courtesy of Dr. W. D. Cubitt, Institute of Child Health, London.)

Epidemiology

Although group A rotavirus gastroenteritis occurs primarily in infants and young children, outbreaks in adults have been reported (18,19) but do not appear to be common. In temperate climates, rotavirus infections increase sharply during the winter months, whereas in tropical climates, infections usually occur year-round. Transmission of the virus is thought to be by the fecal-oral route, although transmission through food and water has been suggested. The incubation period is estimated to be 2 days. Maximal virus shedding occurs in stools 2 to 5 days after the onset of diarrhea, but there may be no correlation between the amount of virus excreted in the stools and the severity of the diarrhea (20). Detection of virus-specific immunoglobulin A in pharyngeal secretions of patients with rotavirus gastroenteritis (20) and detection of rotavirus antigen in respiratory secretions of children with pneumonia (21) suggest that transmission by virus aerosols may occur. The frequency of disease is highest in the 6- to 24-month-old age group, and rotavirus is not thought to be a major factor in infant mortality in developing countries but has been reported (22).

Diarrheal diseases due to rotavirus infections are also important in young farm animals, and rotaviruses have been identified in a number of species including monkeys, apes (23–25), dogs (26,27), cats (28), rabbits (29), mice (30), chickens, turkeys (31,32), and deer (31). There is no evidence that natural virus transmission from humans to animals or animals to humans occurs, but experimental infection of newborn animals with human rotavirus strains may result in symptomatic infection (34).

Nosocomial infections are not uncommon, and it has been reported that approximately 20% of rotavirus infections in hospitals were considered nosocomial (35,36). Thus, appropriate infection control measures should be undertaken when patients with suspected viral gastroenteritis are admitted.

Pathogenesis

Rotavirus-induced diarrhea appears to be due to decreased absorption of salt and water related to selective infection of the absorptive intestinal villus cells, which results in net fluid secretion. Depressed levels of disaccharidases (37) and impaired D-xylose absorption have been observed (38). Pale, fatty stools have been associated with rotaviral diarrhea, suggesting that rotavirus infection may interfere with digestion of fats and pigmentation of feces (39). Villus shortening, reticular cell enlargement, mitochondrial swelling, lymphocyte infiltration of the villous lamina propria, and irregular microvilli have been observed in histopathologic studies. Intestinal fluid loss may also be due to activation of the enteric nervous system. Drugs that inhibit the enteric nervous system have been shown to inhibit rotavirus-induced diarrhea in 4 to 6 day old mice, which supports this concept (40). It further suggests that this system may be a target for therapy of rotavirus infection. The enteric nervous system could also be activated by toxins (40). The demonstration that purified preparations of the rotavirus non-structural protein NSP4 caused diarrhea in mice suggested that this protein acts as an enterotoxin, and it was further shown that specific peptide regions of NSP4 were responsible for the toxic effect (41). In addition, it was found that immunization with NSP4 gave protection against rotavirus diarrhea in neonatal mice (41). However, the role of NSP4 in pathogenesis of rotavirus infection remains to be determined. In comparisons of attenuated and virulent strains, some have shown that rotavirus virulence was related to mutations in the NSP4 protein gene (42), whereas others have not (43–45). It has also been questioned whether the cytotoxic function of NSP4 are operant during natural rotavirus infection (46). The pathogenesis of non-group A rotavirus diarrhea appears to be similar, although the occurrence of syncytia on the surface of villi has been detected in a number of animal species and may be a pathognomonic lesion for non-group A rotavirus infections (47).

Clinical Manifestations

Common clinical findings usually include vomiting, abdominal distress, diarrhea, and mild dehydration. Fever and vomiting frequently precede diarrhea. In one study of children with confirmed rotavirus gastroenteritis, temperature of 37.9°C to 39°C was found in 46% and greater than 39°C in 31% of these patients (48). Other findings may include irritability and pharyngeal or tympanic membrane erythema. Stools are typically watery and usually do not contain blood or leukocytes. Dehydration and associated electrolyte imbalance may occur in severe cases, requiring hospitalization. Fatalities are rare in developed nations but are common in developing nations, where rotavirus produces more severe dehydration than bacterial diarrheas do. The course of rotavirus disease is generally 3 to 9 days, and the mean time of hospitalization when required is 4 days (49).

Rotavirus infections have been associated with a variety of conditions such as intussusception, Reye's syndrome, hemolytic-uremic syndrome, and Kawasaki syndrome, but prior to the vaccine-associated intussusception discussed below under prevention, disease association with rotavirus is strongest for some cases of neonatal necrotizing enterocolitis (50). Chronic symptomatic infections occur in patients with primary immunodeficiency diseases, and severe disease may occur in those who are immunosuppressed for bone marrow transplantation.

Asymptomatic rotavirus infections are common, especially in newborn children, and the association of illness with rotavirus infection increases with the age of the child up to the age of 2 years. Virus shedding was associated with diarrhea in 29% of neonates, in 50% of children age 1 to 6 months, and in 74% of children 7 to 24 months old (51). Infection in adults is usually asymptomatic, but severe illness has been reported both in elderly patients (18) and in apparently normal young adults (19). Severe gastroenteritis in adults due to non-group A rotaviruses has been reported in China (2). In a comparison of rotavirus illness in children and adults in families, the infection rate was 32% in children compared with 17% for adults, and 70% of infected children were symptomatic, whereas only 40% of the infected adults were symptomatic (52). The strains that infect newborns asymptomatically may not be different from the strains causing illness in older infants (53).

Diagnosis

Before virus cultivation techniques and immunoassays were developed for rotavirus detection, electron microscopy was the major technique used. For isolation of rotavirus from clinical materials, the use of primary African green monkey kidney or cynomolgus monkey kidney cells appears to be more effective than MA104 cells (54–56) but isolation of human strains is still considered to be inefficient, and the methods are time-consuming.

Several tests have been developed for diagnosis of rotavirus infection, but antigen detection by enzyme-linked immunosorbent assay (ELISA) is now the preferred method, and tests are available from a number of manufacturers. Commercially produced tests that use polyclonal serum may give false-positive results, especially in stool samples from neonates (57–59). The use of monoclonal antibody to the rotaviral group antigen in ELISA has been found to give higher sensitivity than polyclonal antibodies, and it eliminates the problems of nonspecificity (60,61). An ELISA that uses sensitized latex particles on membrane filters is more rapid than standard ELISAs are, but the test has been found unreliable for use with frozen stool samples (62). An ELISA for non-group A rotaviruses has been described (63), but is not widely available. Whether routine testing for the non-group A rotaviruses will become necessary depends on the results of future epidemiologic studies. Latex agglutination tests for detection of rotavirus antigen in stool samples are also available from several commercial sources. Most use polystyrene particles sensitized with polyclonal antibody, although monoclonal antibody-based tests have been reported (64). The tests are convenient to use and can usually be done more rapidly than ELISA but are generally less sensitive than ELISA (65–67).

The preferred specimen for viral antigen detection is a freshly collected undiluted stool sample, although other specimens such as anal swabs can be used. Samples to be assayed for rotavirus may be shipped on wet ice, and stored for a few days at 4°C, but the preferred method for handling virus samples is to send them on dry ice, with subsequent storage at −70°C.

Additional tests may be necessary for confirmation if a definitive diagnosis cannot be obtained with commercially produced or other rotavirus assays. The best method is gel electrophoresis; electron microscopy or immunoelectron microscopy can also be used, if available.

The availability of monoclonal antibodies to subgroup antigens (68,69) and to specific G and P serotypes (70,71) permits diagnosis of rotaviruses as to specific subgroup and serotype, but this is not routinely done or required because the disease produced by different subgroups or serogroups is indistinguishable. Use of these antibodies does, however, facilitate classification of rotavirus isolates in epidemiologic studies. The use of polymerase chain reaction may not result in increased sensitivity over other methods, but permits serotype identification (72).

Treatment

There is presently no specific antiviral therapy for rotavirus infections. Ribavirin has been shown to inhibit animal rotaviruses *in vitro*, but it was not effective against murine rotavirus infection *in vivo* (73). Treatment with rotavirus-specific neutralizing antibodies given orally to infants with acute gastroenteritis was not effective (74), but it was effective in resolving chronic rotavirus diarrhea in immunodeficient children (75). Treatment, therefore, is usually directed at prevention of severe dehydration and electrolyte imbalance. Use of oral rehydration salt solutions containing glucose or sucrose has been shown to be as effective as intravenous fluid therapy for mild to moderately severe dehydrating rotavirus gastroenteritis (76). The standard World Health Organization formula consists, per liter of water, of glucose 20 g, sodium chloride 3.5 g, sodium bicarbonate 2.5 g, and potassium chloride 1.5 g. Oral rehydration solutions are also commercially available. Intravenous therapy must be administered if oral rehydration is not successful in replacing fluids and electrolytes or if the patient is in shock or is severely dehydrated.

Prevention

Because the morbidity in developed countries is similar to that in developing countries, it is thought that diarrhea in developing countries is not likely to be reduced by improved sanitation and water supplies; thus, control measures will require effective vaccines (77). The principal approach taken in the past as well as in more recent years has been active immunization with live, attenuated rotavirus. The first series of studies were done with orally administered animal strains of rotavirus, and three vaccines were used the most in field trials. One used the Nebraska calf diarrhea virus strain of bovine rotavirus, another the WC3 bovine rotavirus strain, and the third was a rhesus rotavirus strain.

Field trials in Finland with the Nebraska calf diarrhea virus vaccine, designated RIT 4237, indicated that a high level of protection was obtained in infants vaccinated at age 6 to 12 months. Infants vaccinated at age 7 days were also found to be protected in two of three studies (78). Seroconversion occurred in approximately 50% of the vaccine recipients. The RIT 4237 vaccine was also found efficacious in protecting children in Lima, Peru (79). Studies in Butare, Rwanda, with the same vaccine, however, did not show any protective effect or in rates of seroconversion (80). Lack of protection was also found in a study of Gambian children (81). After these vaccine failures, the manufacturer withdrew RIT 4237 from further studies. There were no clear reasons for the failure of the vaccine in either study. It has been suggested that breast-feeding could interfere with vaccines owing to antirotavirus antibody and nonspecific rotavirus inhibitors (82–85). Also, interference by other enteric viruses might be a factor (82,83). In this regard it was found in a later study that co-administration of oral poliovirus vaccine with an oral rotavirus vaccine (using a parenteral poliovirus vaccine as a control) to children at ages 2, 4, and 6 months of age caused a decrease in the rate of development of serum antibodies to rotavirus. However, by age 7 months there were no significant differences in antibody levels obtained (86).

The rhesus rotavirus vaccine has been found to be more immunogenic than vaccines based on bovine rotavirus strain (87). In clinical trials with the rhesus rotavirus vaccine, a study involving children in the United States found no significant differences in the frequency of rotavirus diarrhea among vaccine or placebo recipients (88). Other studies have shown protection to vary from year to year (89,90). The WC3 bovine rotavirus vaccine has also shown variable rates of protection (91,92) and was particularly ineffective in developing countries (93).

The most recent approach has been use of human-animal reassortant vaccines that express human G proteins but retain the attenuated characteristics of the animal strains (94,95). Both rhesus rotavirus and bovine rotavirus reassortant vaccines containing gene segments coding for neutralization proteins for human G serotypes have been prepared. The most attention has been given to the tetravalent rhesus-human reassortant tetravalent vaccine (RRV-TV). This vaccine contains rhesus rotavirus G3 and human rotavirus G1, 2, and 4. In studies in the United States and Finland the efficacy of the vaccine in preventing all rotavirus diarrhea was 49–68% and was 61 to 100% in preventing severe disease (96–99). In rural areas of Venezuela the efficacy in preventing all rotavirus diarrhea was 48% and 88% effective in preventing severe disease (100). In studies in Peru and Brazil (101,102), the overall efficacy was 18% to 35% and 0% to 56% in preventing severe disease. Based on these findings, the RRV-TV vaccine was licensed by the U.S. Food and Drug administration in August of 1998. However, as the vaccine became more widely distributed, adverse effects were reported (103) and the recommendation for its use was withdrawn (104). Subsequently, the manufacturer withdrew the vaccine. The most serious adverse effect was intussusception (103). Analyses of the rates of intussusception show that those receiving the vaccine were several times as likely to develop intussusception as those not receiving the vaccine, most frequently after the first dose (105–107).

Rotavirus strains of human origin have also been evaluated for use as live, orally administered vaccines. A naturally attenuated nursery strain vaccine that cross-reacts with G serotypes 1 through 4 has been tested but did not provide protection against rotavirus disease (108). A more recent nursery strain (RV3) has been tested in a phase I clinical trial in Australia (109). In initial studies in the US, an attenuated human rotavirus strain designated 89-12 gave a protective efficacy of 89% and adverse reactions, when noted, were mild (110).

Methods for passive immunization have been investigated as well. Human breast milk contains rotavirus-specific immunoglobulin, and this immunoglobulin A can be transferred to neonates and detected in the neonates' feces (111). This may account, in part, for the protective, anti-infective properties of breast milk (112). Passive immunization by artificial means has been successfully demonstrated to prevent rotavirus illness in animals, as has oral administration of rotavirus-specific antibodies to neonates (113) or children (114). Current interest in prevention, however, has concentrated on vaccine development. Because the vaccines produced to date do not provide complete protection and may have adverse effects associated with them, new approaches to immunization will continue to be needed. New approaches that have shown promise in animal models of rotavirus infection include the use of virus-like particles prepared from recombinant rotavirus proteins (115–117), chimeric rotavirus proteins (118,119), and plasmid DNA vaccines encoding specific rotavirus proteins (120–122).

REOVIRUS

Serologic surveys indicate that reovirus infections in humans are common and widespread, but most of these infections appear either to be inapparent or to result in mild symptoms. At one time, these viruses were included among the echoviruses (enteric cytopathic human orphan viruses) before more complete characterization. When they were reclassified as reoviruses (123) the orphan label was retained to indicate the lack of association with specific diseases.

Characteristics of the Pathogen

Reoviruses (which are also called orthoreoviruses to avoid confusion with the family Reoviridae) are nonenveloped viruses of approximately 75 nm in diameter. Complete particles have a double capsid, and the virions contain double-stranded RNA that has ten segments. Reoviruses can be inactivated by treatment with 70% ethanol for 1 hour at room temperature, but they may not be inactivated by other commonly used disinfectants (124,125). There are three distinct serotypes of human reoviruses, but all three share a common group antigen as detected by complement fixation or immunodiffusion (123,126). A more extensive review of reovirus biology is available (127).

Epidemiology

Reoviruses have frequently been isolated from the stool samples of infants and children, and seroepidemiologic studies indicate that more than 70% of children acquire antibodies to reovirus before the age of 5 years (128). Thus, it appears that reovirus infections occur primarily in younger children, although no definitive association with disease has been established. The mode of transmission has also not been established, but the ability to isolate these viruses from stools and respiratory secretions along with their relatively stable nature suggests that reoviruses are transmitted by a fecal-oral route, and possibly by a respiratory route, in a manner similar to that proposed for enteroviruses and rotaviruses.

Reovirus infections have also been reported in a variety of animal species, including farm animals, cats, dogs, and nonhuman primates (127). There are avian strains that do not share mammalian reovirus group antigens. There is no evidence of transmission of reoviruses between humans and animals.

Clinical Manifestations

Reovirus infections in avian and mammalian animal species are clearly associated with respiratory illnesses (129,130) but no specific clinical manifestations are well documented for human infections. However, there has been some correlation of minor respiratory symptoms both in children and in adult volunteers (131,132). An association of reovirus type 3 with biliary atresia in infants has been reported (133,134) and reoviruses have also been associated with exanthemal and neurologic illnesses (129,134), including aseptic meningitis (135) but the significance of these findings remains to be clearly established.

Diagnosis

Detection of either reovirus antigen or antibody can be used to diagnose reovirus infections. Isolation of virus in primary Macaca kidney cell cultures or in mouse L cells is usually from fecal samples or from throat and nasal swabs. Direct detection of antigen in fixed tissues by immunofluorescent or immunoperoxidase staining can also be done. Paired acute- and convalescent-phase serum samples can be used to detect seroconversion by hemagglutination inhibition, complement fixation, ELISA, or virus neutralization. Details of methods for detection of reovirus and antibodies are available elsewhere (127,136).

Treatment and Prevention

No specific treatment or prevention measures have been recommended for reovirus infections in humans because of the lack of definitive association with disease. Vaccine preparations are available for veterinary use (129).

ORBIVIRUS

Orbiviruses are arthropod-borne viruses classified as a genus of the family Reoviridae; the genus contains viruses that cause infections in animals and in humans. The most important diseases in animals are bluetongue in sheep and other ruminants and African horse sickness. The importance and epidemiology of orbiviruses in humans are not well defined, but several have been associated with disease. Tickborne viruses of the Kemerovo serogroup have caused severe febrile illness in Eastern Europe and in the western United States (137). Other orbiviruses that have been implicated in febrile illnesses include Changuinola virus (Panama), Lebombo virus (Africa), and Orungo virus (Africa).

Characteristics of the Pathogen

All of the orbiviruses have nonenveloped virions of approximately 80 run in diameter with a double capsid. The inner capsid contains circular capsomers, hence the genus name (Latin *orbis*, meaning "orbit" or "circle"). The double-stranded RNA contains ten segments. There are more than 100 subtypes as distinguished by virus neutralization tests, but orbiviruses do not share a group antigen.

Coltivirus

There are two recognized serotypes (Eyach and Colorado tick fever viruses) and nine probable serotypes in this genus (137). Colorado tick fever virus was originally classified as an orbivirus, but because it has 12 rather than ten genome segments, it is now classified in the *Coltivirus* genus (137). Colorado tick fever is the only well-defined disease caused by coltiviruses and is the only one discussed here.

Epidemiology

The geographic distribution of Colorado tick fever virus is similar to that of its tick vector, *Dermacentor andersoni*, and includes the western United States and parts of Alberta and British Columbia in Canada. The virus is transmitted to humans by infected ticks; the major occurrence is in spring and early summer. Other tick species may be infected but have not been shown to be a vector for human disease. Rodents, especially ground squirrels and chipmunks, are important reservoirs for the virus. Infections of humans are associated with occupational or recreational exposure to infected ticks in epidemic areas. There are approximately 100 to 200 cases reported per year, although the true incidence is thought to be several times higher (138). Infection of *D. andersoni* ticks may be as high as 20% in some areas (139).

Pathogenesis and Clinical Manifestations

Colorado tick fever virus infects erythrocyte precursors in bone marrow and may persist in erythrocytes for up to 20 weeks (140) without apparent lysis or damage of the cells. Pathogenesis in humans is not well characterized, but infection may cause pathologic changes, especially in the myocardium and liver (141,142).

After an incubation period of 3 to 6 days, illness may include high fever, chills, lethargy, nausea, myalgia, and ocular pain. Fever is biphasic in approximately 50% of cases. A macular rash may or may not be present. Neurological symptoms may also occur. The disease is rarely fatal, and recovery is usually complete after 7 to 10 days, although convalescence may be prolonged (143). A rapid drop in the peripheral leukocyte count to 2,000 to 3,000/mm^3 is the major laboratory finding.

Diagnosis

Viral antigen can be detected directly by immunofluorescent staining of blood smears (144) or by immunofluorescent staining of blood smears after inoculation of suckling mice with patients' blood. Colorado tick fever virus can be cultivated in cell culture, but the technique is not considered sensitive enough for primary virus isolation. Detection in blood with polymerase chain reaction has also been reported (145). If paired acute- and convalescent-phase serum samples are available, an indirect immunofluorescent test with cell culture infected with high-titer virus stocks can be used to demonstrate seroconversion to Colorado tick fever virus (146). ELISA procedures for detection of immunoglobulin G and immunoglobulin M antibodies to Colorado tick fever virus have also been described (147).

Treatment and Prevention

Specific antiviral therapy is not available, and treatment for the disease is symptomatic (antipyretic, analgesic). There are no vaccines available for general use, although experimental vaccines have been reported (148), so prevention is accomplished by avoidance of tick-infested areas, use of tick repellents, and rapid removal of ticks before they become attached. To prevent possible Colorado tick fever virus transmission by transfusion, patients should not donate blood for 6 months after recovery.

REFERENCES

1. Parashar UD, Bresee JS, Gentsch JR, Glass RI. Rotavirus. *Emerging Infect Dis* 1998;4:561.
2. Hung T, Chen G, Wang C, et al. Waterborne outbreak of rotavirus diarrhoea in adults in China caused by a novel rotavirus. *Lancet* 1984;1:1139.
3. Jiang B, Dennehy PH, Spangenberger S, et al. First detection of group C rotavirus in fecal specimens of children with diarrhea in the United States. *J Infect Dis* 1995;172:45.
4. Kapikian AZ, Kalica AR, Shih JW, et al. Buoyant density in cesium chloride of the human reovirus-like agent of infantile gastroenteritis by ultracentrifugation, electron microscopy, and complement fixation. *Virology* 1976;70:564.
5. Estes MK, Cohen J. Rotavirus gene structure and function. *Microbiol Rev* 1989;53:410.
6. Bohl EH, Saif LJ, Theil KW, et al. Porcine pararotavirus: detection, differentiation from rotavirus and pathogenesis in gnotobiotic piglets. *J Clin Microbiol* 1982;15:312.
7. Bridger JC, Clarke IN, McCrae MA. Characterization of an antigenically distinct porcine rotavirus. *Infect Immun* 1982;35:1058.
8. Snodgrass DR, Herring AJ, Campbell JM, et al. Comparison of atypical rotaviruses from calves, piglets, lambs and man. *J Gen Virol* 1984;65:909.
9. McNulty MS, Allan GM, Todd D, et al. Isolation from chickens of a rotavirus lacking the group antigen. *J Gen Virol* 1981;55:405.
10. Espejo RT, Puerto F, Soler C, et al. Characterization of human pararotavirus. *Infect Immun* 1984;44:112.
11. Gorziglia M, Larralde G, Kapikian AZ, Chanock RM. Antigenic relationships among human rotaviruses as determined by outer capsid protein VP4. *Proc Natl Acad Sci USA* 1990;87:7155.
12. Larralde G, Gorziglia M. Distribution of conserved and specific epitopes on the VP8 subunit of rotavirus VP4. *J Virol* 1992;66:7438.
13. Estes MK, Palmer EL, Obijeski JF. Rotaviruses: a review. *Curr Top Microbiol Immunol* 1985;105:123.
14. Tan JA, Schnagl RD. Inactivation of a rotavirus by disinfectants. *Med J Aust* 1981;1:19.
15. Snodgrass DR, Herring JA. The activity of disinfectant on lamb rotavirus. *Vet Rec* 1977;101:81.
16. Tan JA, Schnagl RD. Rotavirus inactivated by a hypochlorite-based disinfectant: A reappraisal. *Med J Aust* 1983;1:550.
17. Smith EM, Gerba CP. Development of a method for detection of human rotavirus in water and sewage. *Appl Environ Microbiol* 1982;43:1440.
18. Marrie TJ, Lee SHS, Faulkner RS, et al. Rotavirus infection in a geriatric population. *Arch Intern Med* 1982;142:313.
19. Echeverria P, Blacklow NR, Cukor G, et al. Rotavirus as a cause of severe gastroenteritis in adults. *J Clin Microbiol* 1983;18:663.
20. Stals F, Walther FJ, Bruggeman CA. Faecal and pharyngeal shedding of rotavirus and rotavirus IgA in children with diarrhoea. *J Med Virol* 1984;14:333.
21. Santocham M, Yolken RH, Quiroz E, et al. Detection of rotavirus in respiratory secretions of children with pneumonia. *J Pediatr* 1983;103:583.
22. Carlson JAK, Middleton PJ, Szymanski M, et al. Fatal rotavirus gastroenteritis: an analysis of 21 cases. *Am J Dis Child* 1978;132:477.
23. Malherbe HH, Strickland-Cholmley M. Simian virus SA-11 and the related "O" agent. *Arch Ges Virusforsch* 1967;22:235.
24. Stuker G, Oshiro LS, Schmidt NJ, et al. Virus detection in monkeys with diarrhea: the association of adenoviruses with diarrhea and the possible role of rotaviruses. *Lab Animal Sci* 1979;29:610.
25. Ashley CR, Caul EO, Clark SKR, et al. Rotavirus infections of apes. *Lancet* 1978;2:477.
26. Roseto A, Lema F, Sitbon M, et al. Detection of rotavirus in dogs. *Soc Occup Med* 1979;7:478.
27. England JJ, Poston RP. Electron microscopic identification and subsequent isolation of a rotavirus from a dog with fatal neonatal diarrhea. *Am J Vet Res* 1980;41:782.
28. Snodgrass DR, Angus KW, Gray EW. A rotavirus from kittens. *Vet Rec* 1979;104:222.
29. Bryden AS, Thouless ME, Flewett TH. A rabbit rotavirus. *Vet Rec* 1976;99:323.
30. Much D, Zajac I. Purification and characterization of epizootic diarrhea of infant mice virus. *Infect Immun* 1972;6:1019.

31. Jones RC, Hughes CS, Henry RR. Rotavirus infection in commercial laying hens. *Vet Rec* 1979;104:22.

32. McNulty MS, Allan GM, Todd D, et al. Isolation and cell culture propagation of rotaviruses from turkeys and chickens. *Arch Virol* 1979;61:13.

33. Tzipori S, Caple TW, Butler R. Isolation of a rotavirus from deer. *Vet Rec* 1976;99:398.

34. Wyatt RG, Mebus CA, Yolken RH, et al. Rotaviral immunity in gnotobiotic calves: heterologous resistance to human virus induced by bovine virus. *Science* 1979;203:548.

35. Ryder RW, McGowan JE, Hatch MH, et al. Reovirus-like agent as a cause of nosocomial diarrhea in infants. *J Pediatr* 1977;90:698.

36. Black RE, Merson MH, Rahman ASMM, et al. A two-year study of bacterial, viral and parasitic agents associated with diarrhea in rural Bangladesh. *J Infect Dis* 1980;142:660.

37. Bishop RF, Davidson GP, Holmes IH, et al. Virus particles in epithelial cells of duodenal mucosa from children with viral gastroenteritis. *Lancet* 1973;2:1281.

38. Mavromichalis J, Evans N, McNeish AS, et al. Intestinal damage in rotavirus and adenovirus gastroenteritis assessed by D-xylose malabsorption. *Arch Dis Child* 1977;52:589.

39. Thomas MEM, Luton P, Matimer JY. Virus diarrhoea associated with pale fatty faeces. *J Hyg (Lond)* 1981;87:313.

40. Lundgren O, Peregrin AT, Persson K, et al. Role of the enteric nervous system in the fluid and electrolyte secretion of rotavirus diarrhea. *Science* 2000;287:491.

41. Ball JM, Tian P, Zeng CQ-Y, et al. Age-dependent diarrhea induced by a rotaviral nonstructural glycoprotein. *Science* 1996;272:101.

42. Zhang M, Zeng CQ, Dong Y, et al. Mutations in rotavirus nonstructural glycoprotein NSP4 are associated with altered virus virulence. *J Virol* 1998;72:333–366.

43. Ward RL, Mason BB, Bernstein DI, et al. Attenuation of a human rotavirus vaccine candidate did not correlate with mutations in the NSP4 protein gene. *J Virol* 1997;71:62–67.

44. Lee CN, Wang YL, Kao CL, et al. NSP4 gene analysis of rotaviruses recovered from infected children with and without diarrhea. *J Clin Microbiol* 2000;38:4471.

45. Oka T, Nakagomi T, Nakagomi O. A lack of consistent amino acid substitution in NSP4 between rotaviruses derived from diarrheal and asymptomatically-infected kittens. *Microbiol Immunol* 2001;45:173.

46. Mohan KV, Dermody TS, Atreya CD. Mutations selected in rotavirus enterotoxin NSP4 depend on the context of its expression. *Virology* 2000;275:125.

47. Hall GA. Comparative pathology of infection by novel diarrhoea viruses. *Ciba Found Symp* 1987;128:218.

48. Rodriguez WJ, Kim HW, Arrobio JO, et al. Clinical features of acute gastroenteritis associated with human reovirus-like agent in infants and young children. *J Pediatr* 1977;91:188.

49. Middleton PJ, Szymanski MT, Petric M. Viruses associated with acute gastroenteritis in young children. *Am J Dis Child* 1977;131:733.

50. Rotbart HA, Nelson WL, Glode MP, et al. Neonatal rotavirus associated necrotizing enterocolitis: case control study and prospective surveillance during an outbreak. *J Pediatr* 1988;112:87.

51. Champsaur H, Questiaux E, Prevot J, et al. Rotavirus carriage, asymptomatic infection and disease in the first years of life. I. Virus shedding. *J Infect Dis* 1984;149:667.

52. Wenman WM, Hinde D, Feltham S, et al. Rotavirus infection in adults: Result of a prospective family study. *N Engl J Med* 1979;301:303.

53. Vial PA, Kotloff KL, Losonsky GA. Molecular epidemiology of rotavirus infection in a room for convalescing newborns. *J Infect Dis* 1988;157:668.

54. Hasegaws A, Matsuno S, Inouye S, et al. Isolation of human rotavirus in primary cultures of monkey kidney cells. *J Clin Microbiol* 1982;16:387.

55. Ward RL, Knowlton DR, Pierce MJ. Efficiency of human rotavirus propagation in cell culture. *J Clin Microbiol* 1984;19:748.

56. Naguib T, Wyatt RG, Mohieldin MS, et al. Cultivation and subgroup determination of human rotaviruses from Egyptian infants and young children. *J Clin Microbiol* 1984;19:210.

57. Krause PJ, Hyams JS, Middleton PJ, et al. Unreliability of Rotazyme ELISA test in neonates. *J Pediatr* 1983;103:259.

58. Chrystie IL, Totterdell BM, Banatvala JE. False positive Rotazyme tests on faecal samples from babies. *Lancet* 1983;2:1028.

59. Rotbart HA, Yolken RH, Nelson WL, et al. Confirmatory testing of Rotazyme results in neonates. *J Pediatr* 1985;107:289.

60. Herrmann JE, Blacklow NR, Perron DM, et al. Monoclonal antibody enzyme immunoassays for the detection of rotavirus in stool specimens. *J Infect Dis* 1985;152:830.

61. Dennehy PH, Gauntlet DR, Tente WE. Comparison of nine commercial immunoassays for the detection of rotavirus in fecal specimens. *J Clin Microbiol* 1988;26:1630.

62. Brooks RG, Brown L, Franklin RB. Comparison of a new rapid test (test pack rotavirus) with standard enzyme immunoassay and electron microscopy for the detection of rotavirus in symptomatic hospitalized children. *J Clin Microbiol* 1989;27:775.

63. Brown DWG, Beards GM, Guang-Mu C, et al. Prevalence of antibody to group B (atypical) rotavirus in humans and animals. *J Clin Microbiol* 1987;25:316.

64. Pothier P, Limone F, Kohli E, et al. Development and preliminary evaluation of a latex agglutination test using a monoclonal antibody for rotavirus detection in stool specimens. *Ann Inst Pasteur* 1987;138:523.

65. Morinet F, Ferchal F, Colimon R, et al. Comparison of six methods for detecting human rotavirus in stools. *Eur J Clin Microbiol* 1984;3:136.

66. Knisley CV, Bednarz-Prashad AJ, Pickering LK. Detection of rotavirus in stool specimens and monoclonal and polyclonal antibody-based assay system. *J Clin Microbiol* 1986;23:897.

67. Doern GV, Herrmann JE, Henderson P, et al. Detection of rotavirus with a new polyclonal antibody enzyme immunoassay (Rotazyme II) and a commercial latex agglutination test (Rotalex): comparison with a monoclonal antibody enzyme immunoassay. *J Clin Microbiol* 1986;23:226.

68. Lambert KP, Marbehant P, Marissens D, et al. Monoclonal antibodies directed against different antigenic determinants of rotavirus. *J Virol* 1984;51:47.

69. Taniguchi K, Urasawa T, Urasawa S, et al. Production of subgroup-specific monoclonal antibodies against human rotavirus and their application to an enzyme-linked immunosorbent assay for subgroup determination. *J Med Virol* 1984;14:115.

70. Coulson BS, Unicomb LE, Pitson GA, et al. Simple and specific enzyme immunoassay using monoclonal antibodies for serotyping human rotaviruses. *J Clin Microbiol* 1987;25:509.

71. Taniguchi K, Urasawa T, Morita Y, et al. Direct serotyping of human rotaviruses in stools by an enzyme-linked immunosorbent assay using serotype 1-, 2-, 3- and 4-specific monoclonal antibodies to VP7. *J Infect Dis* 1987;155:1159.

72. Gouveau V, Glass P, Woods K, et al. Polymerase chain reaction amplification and typing of rotavirus nucleic acids from stool specimens. *J Clin Microbiol* 1990;28:276.

73. Schoub BD, Prozesky DW. Antiviral activity of ribavirin in rotavirus gastroenteritis in mice. *Antimicrob Agents Chemother* 1977;12:543.

74. Hilpert H, Brussow H, Mieten C, et al. Use of bovine milk concentrate containing antibody to rotavirus to treat rotavirus gastroenteritis in infants. *J Infect Dis* 1987;156:158.

75. Guarino A, Guandalini S, Albano F, et al. Enteral immunoglobulins for treatment of protracted rotaviral diarrhea. *Pediatr Infect Dis* 1991;10:612.

76. Santosham M, Daun RS, Dillman L, et al. Oral rehydration therapy of infantile diarrhea. A controlled study of well-nourished children hospitalized in the United States and Panama. *N Engl J Med* 1985;306:159.

77. Bishop RF. Development of candidate rotavirus vaccines. *Vaccine* 1993;11:247.

78. Vesikari T. Clinical trials of live oral rotavirus vaccines: the Finnish experience. *Vaccine* 1993;2:255.

79. Lanata CF, Black RE, del Aguila R, et al. Protection of peruvian children against rotavirus diarrhea of specific serotypes by one, two, or three doses of the RIT 4237 attenuated bovine rotavirus vaccine. *J Infect Dis* 1989;159:453.

80. DeMol P, Zissis G, Butzler JP, et al. Failure of live, attenuated oral rotavirus vaccine. *Lancet* 1986;2:108.

81. Hanlon P, Marsh V, Shenton F, et al. Trial of an attenuated bovine rotavirus vaccine (RIT 4237) in Gambian infants. *Lancet* 1986;1:1342.

82. Edelman R. Perspective on the development and deployment of rotavirus vaccine. *Pediatr Infect Dis J* 1987;6:704.

83. Albert MG. Failure of live, oral vaccine in developing countries. *J Infect Dis* 1987;155:1350.

84. McLean BS, Holmes IH. Effects of antibodies, trypsin and trypsin inhibitors on susceptibility of neonates to rotavirus infection. *J Clin Microbiol* 1981;13:33.

85. Berger R, Hadziselimovic F, Just M, Reigel F. Influence of breast milk on nosocomial rotavirus infection in infants. *Infection* 1984;12:171.

86. Migasena S, Simasathien S, Samakoses R, et al. Simultaneous administration of oral rhesus-human reassortant tetravalent (RRV-TV) rotavirus vaccine and oral poliovirus vaccine (OPV) in Thai infants. *Vaccine* 1995;13:168.

87. Vesikari T, Kapikian AZ, Delem A, et al. A comparative trial of rhesus monkey (RRV-1) and bovine (RIT 4237) oral rotavirus vaccines in young child. *J Infect Dis* 1986;153:832.

88. Wright PF, Tajima T, Thompson J, et al. Candidate rotavirus vaccine (rhesus rotavirus strain) in children: an evaluation. *Pediatrics* 1987;80:473.

89. Christy C, Madore HP, Pichichero ME, et al. Field trial of rhesus rotavirus vaccines in infants. *Pediatr Infect Dis J* 1988;7:647.

90. Madore HP, Christy C, Pichichero M, et al. Field trial of rhesus rotavirus or human-rhesus rotavirus reassortant vaccine of VP7 serotype 3 or 1 specificity in infants. *J Infect Dis* 1992;166:235.

91. Clark HF, Borian FE, Bell LM, et al. Protective effect of WC3 vaccine against rotavirus diarrhea in infants during a predominantly serotype 1 rotavirus season. *J Infect Dis* 1988;158:570.

92. Bernstein DI, Smith VE, Sander DS, et al. Evaluation of WC3 rotavirus vaccine and correlates of protection in healthy infants. *J Infect Dis* 1990;162:1055.

93. Georges-Courbot MC, Monges J, Siopathis MR, et al. Evaluation of the efficacy of a low passage bovine rotavirus vaccine (strain WC3) in children in Central Africa. *Res Virol* 1991;142:405.

94. Midthun K, Greenberg B, Hoshino Y, et al. Reassortant rotaviruses as potential live rotavirus vaccine candidates. *J Virol* 1985;53:949.

95. Clark HF, Offit PA, Ellis RW, et al. The development of multivalent bovine rotavirus (strain WC3) reassortant vaccine for infants. *J Infect Dis* 1996;174[Suppl 1]:S73.

96. Bernstein DI, Glass RI, Rodgers G, et al. Evaluation of rhesus rotavirus

monovalent and tetravalent reassortant vaccines in US children. US Rotavirus Vaccine Efficacy Group. *JAMA* 1995;273:1191.

97. Rennels MB, Glass RI, Dennehy PH, et al. Safety and efficacy of high-dose rhesus-human reassortant rotavirus vaccines-report of the National Multicenter Trial. United States rotavirus vaccine efficacy group. *Pediatrics* 1996;97:7.

98. Santosham M, Moulton LH, Reid R, et al. Efficacy and safety of high-dose rhesus-human reassortant rotavirus vaccine in Native American populations. *J Pediatr* 1997;131:632.

99. Joensuu J, Koskenniemi E, Pang XL, Vesikari T. Randomised placebo-controlled trial of rhesus-human reassortant rotavirus vaccine for prevention of severe rotavirus gastroenteritis. *Lancet* 1997;350:1205–1209.

100. Pérez-Schael I, Guntinas MJ, Perez M, et al. Efficacy of the rhesus rotavirus-based quadrivalent vaccine in infants and young children in Venezuela. *N Engl J Med* 1997;337:181.

101. Lanata CF, Midthun K, Black RE, et al. Safety, immunogenicity, and protective efficacy of one and three doses of the tetravalent rhesus-human, reassortant rotavirus vaccine in infants in Lima, Peru. *J Infect Dis* 1996;174:268.

102. Linhares AC, Gabbay YB, Mascarenhas JD, et al. Immunogenicity, safety and efficacy of tetravalent rhesus-human, reassortant rotavirus vaccine in Belem, Brazil. *Bull WHO* 1996;74:491.

103. Centers for Disease Control and Prevention. Intussusception among recipients of rotavirus vaccine, United States, 1998–1999. *MMWR* 1999;48:577.

104. Centers for Disease Control and Prevention. Withdrawal of rotavirus vaccine recommendation. *MMWR* 1999;48:1007.

105. Kramarz P, France EK, Destefano F, et al. Population-based study of rotavirus vaccination and intussusception. *Pediatr Infect Dis J* 2001;20:410.

106. Murphy TV, Gargiullo PM, Massoudi MS, et al. Intussusception among infants given an oral rotavirus vaccine. *N Engl J Med* 2001;344:564.

107. Zanardi LR, Haber, P, Moottrey GT, et al. Intussusception among recipients of rotavirus vaccine: reports to the vaccine adverse event reporting system. *Pediatrics* 2001;107(6).

108. Vesikari T, Ruuska T, Koivu H-P, et al. Evaluation of the M37 human rotavirus vaccine in 2- to 6-month-old infants. *Pediatr Infect Dis J* 1991;10:912.

109. Barnes GL, Lund JS, Adams L, et al. Phase I trial of a candidate rotavirus vaccine (RV3) derived from a human neonate. *J Paediatr Child Health* 1997;33:300.

110. Bernstein DI, Sack DA, Rothstein E, et al. Efficacy of live, attenuated human rotavirus vaccine 89-12: a randomised placebo-controlled trial. *Lancet* 1999;354:287.

111. Rahmen MM, Yamauchi M, Hanada N, et al. Local production of rotavirus-specific IgA in breast tissue and transfer to neonates. *Arch Dis Child* 1987;62:401.

112. Welsh JK, May TT. Anti-infective properties of breast milk. *J Pediatr* 1979;94:1.

113. Barnes GL, Doyle IW, Hewson PH, et al. A randomised trial of oral gammaglobulin in low-birth-weight infants infected with rotavirus. *Lancet* 1983;1:1371.

114. Ebina T, Sato A, Umezu K, et al. Prevention of rotavirus infection by cow colostrum containing antibody against human rotavirus. *Lancet* 1983;2:1029.

115. Conner ME, Crawford SE, Barone C, et al. Rotavirus subunit vaccines. *Arch Virol Suppl* 1996;12:199.

116. Fernandez FM, Conner ME, Hodgins DC, et al. Passive immunity to bovine rotavirus in newborn calves fed colostrum supplements from cows immunized with recombinant SA11 rotavirus core-like particle (CLP) or virus-like particle (VLP) vaccines. *Vaccine* 1998;16:507.

117. Crawford SE, Estes MK, Ciarlet M, et al. Heterotypic protection and induction of a broad heterotypic neutralization response by rotavirus-like particles. *J Virol* 1999;73:4813.

118. Choi AH, Basu M, McNeal MM, Clements JD, Ward RL. Antibody-independent protection against rotavirus infection of mice stimulated by intranasal immunization with chimeric VP4 or VP6 protein. *J Virol* 1999;73:7574.

119. Choi AH, Basu M, McNeal MM, et al. Functional mapping of protective domains and epitopes in the rotavirus VP6 protein. *J Virol* 2001;74:11574.

120. Herrmann JE, Chen SC, Fynan EF, et al. DNA vaccines against rotavirus infections. *Arch Virol Suppl* 1996;12:207.

121. Chen SC, Jones DH, Fynan EF, et al. Protective immunity induced by oral immunization with a rotavirus DNA vaccine encapsulated in microparticles. *J Virol* 1998;72:5757.

122. Herrmann JE, Chen SC, Jones DH, et al. Immune responses and protection obtained by oral immunization with rotavirus VP4 and VP7 DNA vaccines encapsulated in microparticles. *Virology* 1999;259:148.

123. Sabin AB. Reoviruses, a new group of respiratory and enteric viruses formerly classified as ECHO type 10 is described. *Science* 1959;103:1387.

124. Stanley NF, Dorman DC, Ponsford J. Studies on the pathogenesis of a hitherto undescribed virus (hepatoencephalomyelitis) producing unusual symptoms in suckling mice. *Aust J Exp Biol* 1953;31:147.

125. Stanley NF, Dorman DC, Ponsford J. Studies on the hepatoencephalomyelitis virus. *Aust J Exp Biol* 1954;32:543.

126. Leers WD, Rozee KR, Wardlow HC. Immunodiffusion and immunoelectrophoretic studies of reovirus antigens. *Can J Microbiol* 1968;14:161.

127. Tyler KL: Mammalian reoviruses. In: Knipe DM, Howley PM, eds. *Fields virology*, 4th ed. Philadelphia: Lippincott Williams & Wilkins, 2001:1729–1745.

128. Lerner AM, Cherry JD, Klein JO, et al. Infections with reoviruses. *N Engl J Med* 1962;267:947.

129. Thein P, Scheid R. Reoviral infections. In: Steele, ed. *CRC handbook series in zoonoses, section B, viral zoonoses,* vol II. Boca Raton, FL: CRC Press, 1981:191–216.

130. Stanley NF. Diagnosis of reovirus infections: comparative aspects. In: Kurstak E, Kurstak K, eds. *Comparative diagnosis of viral diseases.* New York: Academic Press, 1977:385–421.

131. Rosen L, Hovis JF, Mastrota FM, et al. An outbreak of infection with a type 1 reovirus among children in an institution. *Am J Hyg* 1960;71:266.

132. Rosen L, Evans HE, Spickard A. Reovirus infections in human volunteers. *Am J Hyg* 1963;77:29.

133. Morecki R, Glaser JH, Cho S, et al. Biliary atresia and reovirus type 3 infection. *N Engl J Med* 1982;307:481.

134. Glaser JH, Balistreri WF, Morecki R. Role of reovirus type 3 in persistent infantile cholestasis. *J Pediatr* 1984;105:912.

135. Johansson PJ, Sveger T, Ahlfors K, et al. Reovirus type 1 associated with meningitis. *Scand J Infect Dis* 1996;28:117.

136. Rosen L. Reoviruses. In: Lennette EH, Schmidt NJ, eds. *Diagnostic procedures for viral, rickettsial, and chlamydial infections,* 5th ed. Washington, DC: American Public Health Association, 1979:577–584.

137. Calisher CH. Medically important arboviruses of the United States and Canada. *Clin Microbiol Rev* 1994;7:89.

138. Emmons RW. Reoviridae: the orbiviruses (Colorado tick fever). In: Lennette EH, Halonen P, Murphy FA, eds. *Laboratory diagnosis of infectious diseases, principles and practice,* vol II. New York: Springer-Verlag, 1988:375–383.

139. Monath TP. Orbivirus (Colorado tick fever). In: Mandell GL, Douglas RG, Bennett JE, eds. *Principles and practice of infectious diseases,* 2nd ed. New York: John Wiley & Sons, 1985:931–932.

140. Philip RN, Casper EA, Cory J, et al. The potential for transmission of arboviruses by blood transfusion with particular references to Colorado tick fever. In: Greenwalt TJ, Jamieson GA, eds. *Transmissible disease and blood transfusion.* New York: Grime & Stratton, 1975:175–195.

141. Emmons RW, Schade HI. Colorado tick fever simulating acute myocardial infarction. *JAMA* 1972;222:87.

142. Loge RV. Acute hepatitis associated with Colorado tick fever. *West J Med* 1985;142:91.

143. Goodpasture HC, Poland JD, Francy DB, et al. Colorado tick fever: clinical, epidemiologic, and laboratory aspects of 228 cases in Colorado in 1973–1974. *Ann Intern Med* 1978;88:303.

144. Emmons RW, Lennette EH. Immunofluorescent staining in the laboratory diagnosis of Colorado tick fever. *J Lab Clin Med* 1966;68:923.

145. Johnson AJ, Karabatsos N, Lanciotti RS. Detection of Colorado tick fever virus by using reverse transcriptase PCR and application of the technique in laboratory diagnosis. *J Clin Microbiol* 1997;35:1203.

146. Emmons RW, Dondero DV, Devlin V, et al. Serologic diagnosis of Colorado tick fever. A comparison of complement-fixation, immunofluorescence, and plaque-reduction methods. *Am J Trop Med Hyg* 1969;18:796.

147. Calisher CH, Poland JD, Calisher SB, et al. Diagnosis of Colorado tick fever virus infection by enzyme immunoassays for immunoglobulin M and G antibodies. *J Clin Microbiol* 1985;22:84.

148. Thomas LA, Philip RN, Patzer E, et al. Long duration of neutralizing-antibody response after immunization of man with a formalinized Colorado tick fever vaccine. *Am J Trop Med Hyg* 1967;16:60.

CHAPTER 255

Human Retroviruses

Vladimir Novitsky, Roger Shapiro, and Max Essex

HISTORICAL BACKGROUND

Mammalian retroviruses were first identified by Gross in the early 1950s, through careful selection of inbred strains of mice prone to leukemia (1). By the mid-1960s, a retrovirus was also identified in association with leukemia in outbred domestic cats (2). A decade later, it was recognized that such feline retroviruses often caused lethal immune suppression (3).

The first human retrovirus—human T-cell lymphotropic virus type I (HTLV-1)—was described in 1980 by Gallo and colleagues (4). This agent was associated with a characteristic type of hematopoietic malignancy called adult T-cell leukemia (ATL); a syndrome described a few years earlier by Takatsuki and colleagues (5). In 1981, the same virus was independently described by Hinuma and colleagues (6) as the ATL virus. It soon became apparent that HTLV-I was regularly associated with ATL, a disease that was more common in areas such as southwestern Japan.

The second human retrovirus, HTLV-II, was identified in a patient who had hairy cell leukemia (7). It was immediately recognized as related to but distinct from HTLV-I. Attempts to find the cause of acquired immunodeficiency syndrome (AIDS) revealed a third human retrovirus, human immunodeficiency virus type 1 (HIV-1). Although AIDS was recognized as a new disease (8), most early hypotheses suggested that it was caused by drugs or alloantigenic stimulation (9). When cases of AIDS were observed in blood transfusion recipients and hemophiliacs, hypotheses of an infectious agent emerged. The first identification by Barre-Sinoussi and colleagues (10) of a retrovirus in a homosexual patient with lymphadenopathy—initially designated lymphadenopathy-associated virus (LAV)—combined with other reports (11,12), focused attention on retroviruses. Extensive analysis by Gallo and colleagues (13,14) later provided conclusive evidence that this virus was the cause of AIDS. Initially referred to as LAV (10), HTLV-III (14), AIDS-related virus (15), and HTLV-III/LAV, this virus is now designated HIV-1.

Human immunodeficiency virus type 2 (HIV-2) was identified in West Africa as a virus related to, but distinct from, HIV-1 (16). Initially designated HTLV-IV, it is much more closely related to a simian immunodeficiency virus (SIV) of monkeys (17) than to HIV-1. Largely restricted to West Africa (18), HIV-2, although biologically similar to HIV-1, has reduced pathogenicity compared with HIV-1 (19).

RETROVIRUSES

In 2000, the International Committee on the Taxonomy of Viruses updated the classification of Retroviruses by subdividing the family Retroviridae into seven genera (20): Alpharetroviruses, Betaretroviruses, Gammaretroviruses, Deltaretroviruses, Epsilonretroviruses, Lentiviruses and Spumaviruses (foamy viruses). Genus Deltaretroviruses includes human T-cell lymphotropic virus 1 and 2 (HTLV-1 and HTLV-2), while human immunodeficiency virus belongs to the Lentiviruses.

Retroviruses have a similar genetic organization (Fig. 255.1A). The retroviral genome is approximately 10 kb in length and utilizes two identical RNA molecules (with a cap structure at the 5'-end and a poly-A tail at the 3'-end). Retroviruses replicate via a

A. Genomic organization of retroviruses:

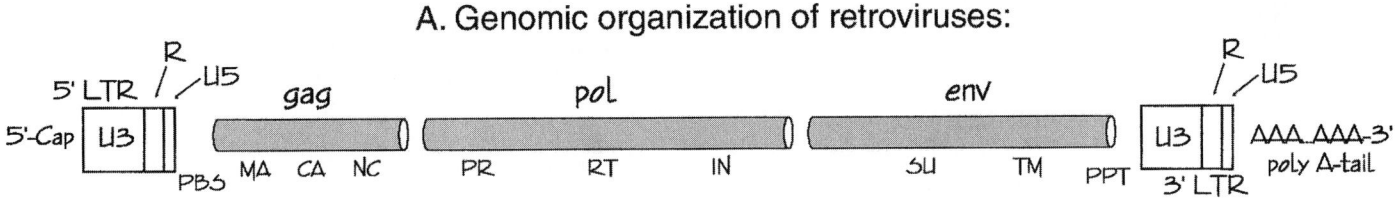

B. Genomic organization of human retroviruses:

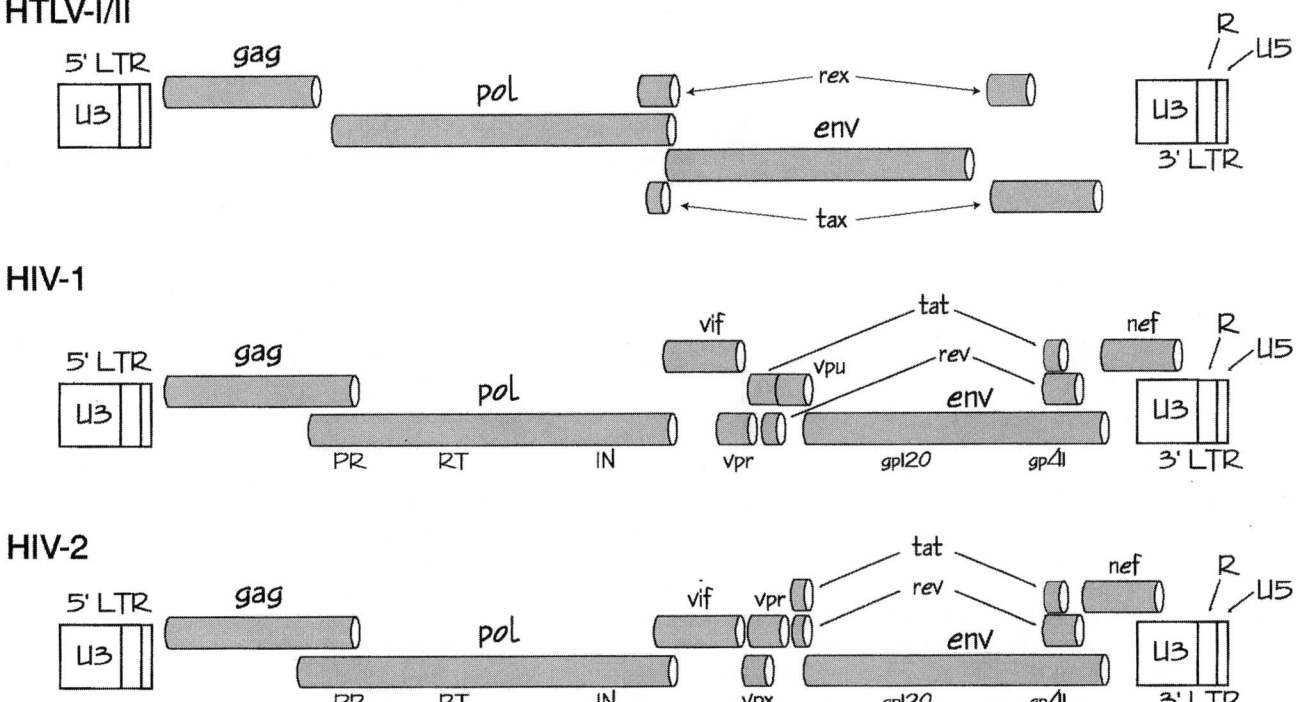

Figure 255.1. **A:** Genomic organization of retroviruses. **B:** Genomic organization of human retroviruses.

transitional deoxyribonucleic acid (DNA; provirus) and have the promoter sequence that initiates the expression of RNA. Some simple retroviruses (i.e., murine or avian leukemia virus) contain only three main gene-encoding regions: gag ("group-specific antigen"), pol ("polymerase") and env ("envelope") flanked by two LTR ("long terminal repeats"). More complex retroviruses (i.e., HIV or HTLV) in addition to the main regions have a number of accessory and regulatory genes (Fig. 255.1B). The structural proteins are first synthesized as precursor polyproteins and are processed into mature products by proteolytic cleavage. Proteolytic processing of Gag and Pol is catalyzed by a protease encoded by the virus, and processing of Env is catalyzed by cellular proteases.

The *gag* gene encodes the Gag polyprotein, the precursor for the internal viral core, which is proteolytically processed into the mature protein's MA (matrix), CA (capsid), NC (nucleocapsid) and some other domains (i.e., p6 in primate retroviruses). The *pol* gene encodes multiple enzymes required for the virus life cycle such as reverse transcriptase, ribonuclease (RNase) H, integrase and protease. The Gag-Pol polyprotein is translated from full-length messenger RNA (mRNA), which also serves as the genomic RNA. The *pol* products are translated as a Gag-Pol fusion protein by frameshifting because *pol* of human retroviruses does not have an initiation codon and it is encoded in a different frame than *gag*. The frameshift regulates the ratio of *gag* and *pol* products. The *env* gene encodes an external surface protein (SU, gp120) and a transmembrane protein (TM, gp41).

The retrovirus life cycle starts with the infection of a susceptible cell by interaction of viral envelope with receptors and co-receptors on the cell surface, followed by entering of the viral core into the cell and conversion of the viral genomic RNA into a linear double-stranded proviral DNA.

The provirus is transported into the nucleus of the cell, where it is spliced at the end of its LTR, which results in viral integration into the host genome. Reverse transcription and integration are two unique characteristics of retroviruses, catalyzed by reverse transcriptase (RT) and integrase, respectively (reviewed in [21] and [22]). The enzymatic activity of RT includes a DNA polymerization of either an RNA or a DNA template, and an RNase H activity, which cleaves RNA if it is a part of an RNA/DNA complex. Reverse transcription is initiated from a host transfer RNA (tRNA) annealed to the primer binding site (PBS) near the 5' end of the viral RNA (Fig. 255.2). First-strand DNA synthesis creates an RNA/DNA duplex, which serves as a substrate for RNase H. After the DNA synthesis reaches the end of the viral RNA (a minus DNA strand), RNase H degrades the 5' end of RNA, and DNA synthesis transfers to the 3' end of the viral genome, which is mediated by identical repeated (R) sequences. Subsequent to minus-strand DNA synthesis, RNase H degradation occurs for all the RNA template except the purine-rich polypurine tract (PPT), which is resistant to the RNase H cleavage and serves as a primer for second-strand DNA synthesis. Following the RNase H degradation of tRNA and PPT, the second strand transfer results in the annealing of the newly generated PBS DNA to the PBS from the first DNA strand. Completion of second-strand synthesis produces a linear DNA duplex with complete LTRs (U3, R and U5) at both ends and serves as a substrate for the viral integrase enzyme that inserts the linear viral DNA in the host genome. Viral mRNAs are transcribed from the integrated provirus by host transcription machinery. Retroviruses carry a specific transcription activator on their own LTR. After posttranscriptional processing, transcribed mRNAs are transported to the cytoplasm and translated to produce viral proteins.

Human Immunodeficiency Virus Type 1 and Human Immunodeficiency Virus Type 2

VIRAL STRUCTURE AND LIFE CYCLE

The HIVs are spherical viruses of approximately 100 nm in diameter. The core or nucleocapsid is condensed into a cylindrical, trapezoidal, or triangular shape instead of the spherical shape as for the HTLVs. HIV-1 and HIV-2 may be distinguishable from each other by the degree of condensation of the nucleocapsid, particularly as it separates from the envelope. Gag proteins compile the conical core of the mature HIV virion. MA protein lies underneath the lipid membrane and makes contact with it via the amino-terminal myristylated and positively charged segment (21). CA protein forms the capsid, the outer layer of the core. The complex of NC protein and viral RNA is in the center of the core. RT and IN molecules are associated with this complex by binding to the nucleic acid. Some host-cell proteins, such as MHC class I proteins, may be incorporated in the viral membrane (21).

The HIV has a sophisticated replication cycle, involving at least nine functional genes with identified products. The rate of replication may vary in different cell types. The HIV envelope glycoprotein, Env, binds to CD4 and a coreceptor, which is a member of the chemokine receptor family (attachment of viral particle). Fusion of the viral and cell membrane results in the entry of a viral core carrying the HIV genome into the cytoplasm (entry or penetration). Reverse transcription follows the entry, and the resulting proviral DNA is transported to the nucleus, where it integrates into the host genome. Transcription and splicing of the various messages occur in the nucleus, using the integrated chromosomal provirus as template. Both genomic and nongenomic forms of RNA are transported to the cytoplasm, where translation occurs. Viral genomes and newly produced structural proteins are transported to assembly sites at the cytoplasmic membrane, where morphogenesis and budding of progeny virus occur. Both HIV-1 and HIV-2 bud from cytoplasmic membranes and perhaps from vacuolar membranes. Whereas the budding of most retroviruses has no deleterious effects on infected cells, the production of large amounts of HIV can cause the lysis of lymphocytes. In vitro, HIV may cause cell lysis or multinuclear cell (syncytium) formation.

GENES OF HUMAN IMMUNODEFICIENCY VIRUS

During the initial phase of HIV-1 and HIV-2 research, most of the viral gene products were classified into three categories (Table 255.1). The first category included viral structural genes, *gag*, *pol*, and *env*. The second group contained regulatory genes *tat* (transactivator of transcription) and *rev* (regulator of viral gene expression). The third category embraced accessory genes *vif* (virus infectivity factor), nef (negative regulatory factor), *vpr* (virus protein R), *vpu* (virus protein U, unique for HIV-1), and *vpx* (viral protein X, unique for HIV-2). Mutations within accessory genes did not abolish virus replication in established cell lines. Given the similarity of HIV-1 and HIV-2 genomic organization and their homology in primary structures, it is generally assumed that the functions of their corresponding accessory genes are similar to each other.

Structural Genes

The HIV-1 *gag* gene encodes the Gag polyprotein, the precursor for the internal structural machinery of the virion, namely the matrix (MA), capsid (CA), nucleocapsid (NC), and p6 domain. The Gag polyprotein is responsible for the late stages of viral replication, such as assembly and release of viral particles

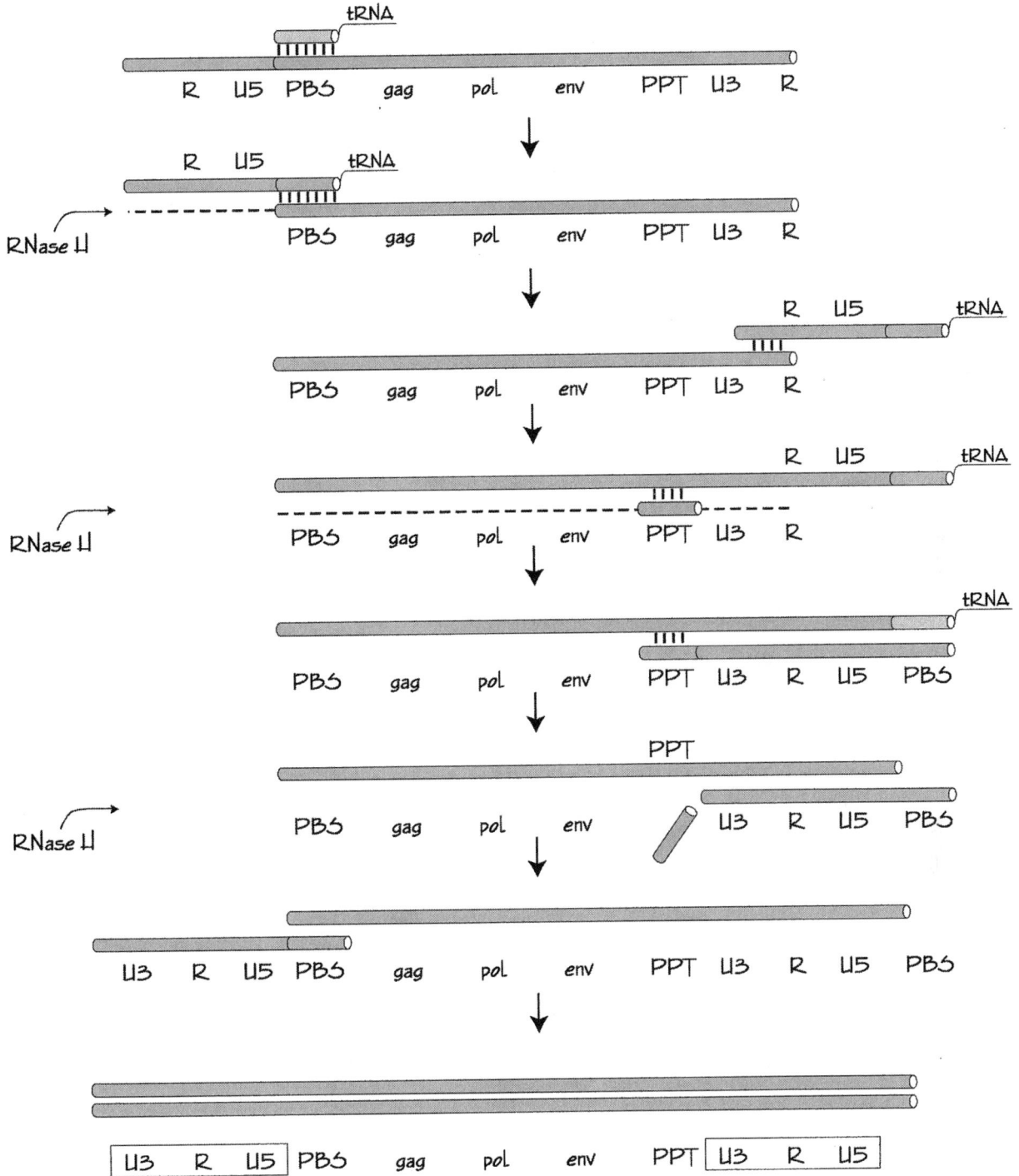

Figure 255.2. The process of reverse transcription.

(budding). For the virion to be mature and become infectious, the Gag polyprotein needs to be cleaved by the viral protease (23,24). Two essential functions of the MA domain include membrane targeting and incorporation of the envelope glycoprotein spikes into assembling particles. The N-terminal domain of MA is myristylated, which is essential for virus particle formation and viral replication (25–27). The consensus sequence for myristylation is Met-Gly-X-X-Ser/Thr. After the initiating methionyl residue is removed, the fatty acid is linked via an amide bond to the free amino group of the glycyl residue (21). The three-dimensional structure of

HIV-1 MA disclosed a globular "head" formed by four α-helices and a C-terminal α-helix aside from the core domain (28–30). The HIV-1 MA interaction with membranes is regulated by a myristyl switch mechanism (31–33). Gag membrane targeting and incorporation of the HIV-1 envelope (Env) glycoprotein spikes are essential functions of MA. The MA-Env interaction can significantly influence the cell tropism of HIV-1.

The capsid (CA) forms the core of the mature HIV-1 virion. The CA has two distinct α-helical domains connected through a flexible linker region (34–36). The CA domains have different roles in virus morphogenesis (23). The N-terminal domain is

TABLE 255.1. HIV-1/HIV-2 Genes and Their Products

Gene		Protein	Function
Structural	gag	Gag MA, p17	Membrane anchoring; env interaction; nuclear transport of viral core
		Gag CA, p24	Core capsid
		Gag NC, p7	Nucleocapsid, binds RNA
		Gag p6 domain	Binds Vpr
	pol	Protease, p15	Cleavage and maturation
		Reverse transcriptase/RNase H, p66/p51	Reverse transcription, ribonuclease H activity
		Integrase	Provirus integration
	env	gp120	External glycoproteins
		gp41	
Regulatory	Tat	Tat, p16/p14	Transcriptional transactivator
	Rev	Rev, p19	RNA transport, stability, and utilization factor
Accessory	Nef	Nef p27-p25	CD4 and MHC class I downregulation
	Vif	Vif p23	Promotes viral maturation and infectivity
	Vpr	Vpr, p10-p15	Facilitates nuclear localization of the preintegration complex, arrests infected cells at G2/M phase
	Vpu (HIV-1 only)	Vpu, p16	Promotes production of extracellular viral particles; degrades CD4 in the ER
	Vpx (HIV-2 only)	Vpx, p12-16	Analog HIV-1 Vpu

responsible for the formation of the cone-shaped core of the mature virion but is not essential for the assembly of immature viral particles, while the C-terminal domain is critical for Gag polyprotein multimerization and virion particle assembly (23,36–39).

The nucleocapsid, NC has two specific motifs created by spaced cysteine and histidine residues called "zinc fingers," that coordinate a Zn^{2+} ion and that have a role in the binding of certain proteins to nucleic acids. The HIV Cys-His motif has the structure $CX_2CX_4 HX_4C$, where Xs are not conserved residues. One of the motifs has the paramount role in RNA encapsidation. Stretches of basic residues within NC are required for assembly or budding of the virion (21).

The HIV p6 domain is a polypeptide that is cleaved from the Gag protein downstream from NC. It is responsible for release of virus in the final steps of budding and for incorporation of Vpr and Vpx proteins into the virion (21).

The *pol* products provide various essential enzyme functions. In addition to protease, which is at the N-terminus, the *pol* gene encodes reverse transcriptase, ribonuclease H, and integrase. The HIV-1 protease is responsible for the post-translational processing of the viral Gag and Gag-Pol polyproteins. Protease is an aspartic protease composed of two non-covalently associated structurally identical monomers of 99 amino acids in length. Its active site contains the conserved triad, Asp-Thr-Gly, at positions 25 to 27. The hydrophobic substrate cleft recognizes and cleaves nine different sequences to produce the matrix, capsid, nucleocapsid, and p6 proteins from the Gag polyprotein and the protease, RT, and integrase proteins from the Gag-Pol polyprotein (40–42). Reverse transcriptase and associated ribonuclease H activity make the first proviral DNA strand. After the DNA provirus is made, the integrase or endonuclease integrates the provirus into the chromosomal DNA of the cell. RT is a heterodimer comprised of p66 and p51 subunits.

The *env* gene encodes a polyprotein, gp160, which is cleaved to the external glycoprotein, gp120, and the transmembrane protein, gp41. The gp120 molecule is highly glycosylated, with a mean of 24 different sites harboring residues of either mannose or other complex sugars. As a result, more than half of the mass of the molecule is carbohydrate. Env glycoproteins exist as a trimolecular complex of gp120-gp41 heterodimers (43–46).

Regulatory and Accessory Genes

Along with the replication and assembly of the virus and its components, a major activity of HIV is the regulation of viral replication. There are two essential regulatory genes in primate lentiviruses, *tat* and *rev*, that are clearly required for viral replication.

The Tat is the trans-activator protein, which efficiently controls HIV transcription. Tat regulates viral gene expression through the control of elongation. The subunit CDK9 of Tat-associated kinase, cyclin T1 and Spt5 are critical components of the Tat-dependent elongation mechanism (47). Tat interacts with the bulge of TAR. The presence of cellular cofactor cyclin T1 is important for conformational changes and for recognition of TAR RNA by Tat. Tat is subdivided into several distinct regions that are essential for protein function: a N-terminal activation region, a cysteine-rich domain, a core region, a basic region, and a glutamine-rich region. The last three regions are involved in RNA binding. Additionally, the basic region performs as a nuclear localization signal.

The *rev* gene, the viral RNA nuclear export factor, is another essential regulator of posttranscriptional events. The *rev* gene is required for the expression of virus structural proteins. Rev gene alleviates the negative effects of a *cis*-acting repression sequence via binding to *rev*-responsive elements, which are located within the *env* gene.

HIV-1 and HIV-2 have three common accessory genes, *vif*, *vpr*, and *nef* that are nonessential for viral growth in cell culture suggesting that their functions are specialized for viral persistence *in vivo* (48). In addition, HIV-1 contains *vpu*, while HIV-2 contains *vpx*.

The *vif* gene of HIV-1 encodes a 23-kDa protein. The *vif* gene is responsible for efficient replication of HIV in CD4$^+$ cells and in some cell lines. Vif affects the infectivity of released viral particles by modifying virions (49). The mechanism of action of the *vif* gene remains unknown.

The *vpr* gene encodes a protein of approximately 12 kDa that is present in viral particles and in infected cells. Most of Vpr is in the nucleus, although when viral particles are produced at the plasma membrane, Vpr is efficiently recruited into them (49). The carboxy-terminal segment of HIV-1 Gag (p6) is responsible for interacting with Vpr. Vpr facilitates the transport of a preintegration complex to the nucleus together with MA. HIV-1 Vpr manifests pleiotropic effects such as transactivation of several promoters and arrest of the cell cycle at the G_2/M phase. The *vpx* gene in HIV-2 is an analog of the HIV-1 *vpr* gene.

The *nef* gene encodes a myristylated p27 protein and plays multiple roles in HIV pathogenesis, although initially it was described as a negative effector of viral transcription. Nef downregulates cell surface CD4 through direct bridging of the cytoplasmic tail of CD4 to an adapter protein (50,51) as well as the expression of major histocompatability complex class I molecules. Enhancement of virion infectivity and modulation of cellular activation were also attributed to the Nef function.

The *vpu* gene in HIV-1 encodes a 16-kDa product, an integral membrane phosphoprotein that forms multimers. Vpu downregulates the levels of the CD4 receptor by accelerating its destruction (49). This activity is carried out in association with the endoplasmic reticulum and/or other membranes. Vpu also facilitates the release of virus particles from the surface of infected cells (52).

IMMUNE RESPONSES

Both humoral and cell-mediated immune responses occur in the course of natural HIV infection (Fig. 255.3). Although the immune system plays a key role in determining the viral set point and delaying disease progression, the overall HIV-specific immune responses fail to eradicate integrated virus, and without efficient therapy cannot prevent the progression of HIV infection and development of AIDS.

CD8$^+$ T-cells are an important component of an HIV-1-specific immune response and play an essential role in the immune-mediated containment of HIV-1 infection. Viral-specific CD8$^+$ T-cells are able to kill HIV-1-infected cells directly or indirectly through the secretion of a variety of cytokines and chemokines (53–56). The HIV-1-specific cytotoxic T-lymphocyte (CTL) responses are involved in the control of viral infection (54,57) including acute (58–61) and chronic (62,63) infection, as described for rapid progressors (64,65), long-term non-progressors (66,67), and perhaps exposed uninfected individuals (68–73). An expansion of virus-specific CD8$^+$ T-cell responses chronologically follows the first peak of viremia and

massive dissemination of HIV during acute infection. The CD8$^+$ CTLs are detectable by 2 to 3 weeks after the initial infection, reach a peak by 9 to 12 weeks, and are largely responsible for the declining viral load in plasma and thus for partial control of the virus. To be recognized by virus-specific CTLs, viral peptides are presented in a complex of the major histocompatibility complex (MHC) class I HLA molecules on the cell surface.

The killing function of CD8$^+$ T-cells is usually more efficient before the infected cell produces new virions (74). However the immune selection pressure and the frequently impaired function of CD8$^+$ T-cells might result in generation of viral mutants and subsequent viral escape from the immune response (see Replication and Heterogeneity section). Even a single amino acid change within a CTL epitope may abrogate presentation by the MHC class I molecules on the cell surface, which might result in more rapid viral replication.

Differentiation of CD8$^+$ T cells requires cytokines produced by CD4$^+$ T-helper cells and/or costimulators expressed on infected cells (75). Therefore, CD4$^+$ T-cell help is a necessary component of the efficient CTL response (reviewed in [74]), including priming (76), memory (77), and function maturing (78). CD4$^+$ T-cells can trigger dendritic cells to produce IL-12, which is crucial in initiating the CTL response (76). Lack of another cytokine provided by CD4$^+$ T-helper cells, IL-2, might have a negative effect on survival of CTL memory cells.

Although CD4$^+$ T-cell function might be impaired early in HIV infection, CD4$^+$ T-helper cells are involved in both innate and adaptive immune responses to HIV through abundant cell-to-cell interactions and release of cytokines. CD4$^+$ T-helper cells are MHC class II–restricted, stimulated by exogenous antigen, and require the presence of antigen-presenting cells (APC). CD4$^+$ T cells can be activated by properly processed HIV peptides that are expressed on the surface of APC in the context of MHC class II presentation.

Antibody responses to HIV develop within 6 to 9 weeks after infection and usually peak at week 12 following the identification of CD8$^+$ CTLs, although the increased titers of antibodies found later on in the natural course of HIV infection cannot efficiently control and/or contain the virus. Neutralizing antibodies can directly neutralize free virus and target envelope glycoproteins or epitopes within gp120 and gp41, namely the V3 loop and the CD4 binding domain (79,80). Neutralizing antibodies can block gp120 from binding to the cellular receptor CD4$^+$ or coreceptors (CCR5 and/or CXCR4) and prevent gp41 fusion with the target cell membrane (81–86). Antibodies are also directed against linear or 3-dimensional conformation segments of the envelope protein, as well as against virion debris. Gp120 exhibits a high degree of sequence variation, and can escape relatively easily from recognition by neutralizing antibodies through the evolution of viral mutants. Usually neutralizing antibodies are able to neutralize earlier clones of isolated virus but fail to neutralize the current or later isolates (87–89). Antibodies in the sera of HIV-infected patients effectively neutralize the autologous (completely matched) viral variant but not heterologous viruses (90–95). Antibody can directly neutralize HIV or eliminate infected cells through the alternative mechanism of antibody-dependent cellular cytotoxicity.

The apparent detection of HIV-specific immune responses in individuals exposed to HIV infection but persistently uninfected suggests the possibility of transient abortive infection and highlights an important role for immune-mediated protection in the course of HIV infection. Detectable CTL responses in seronegative persons might suggest an efficient clearance of HIV or control of the virus below the detectable level. However, there are a number of factors limiting the efficient immune control of HIV infection that include immune exhaustion, lack of adequate

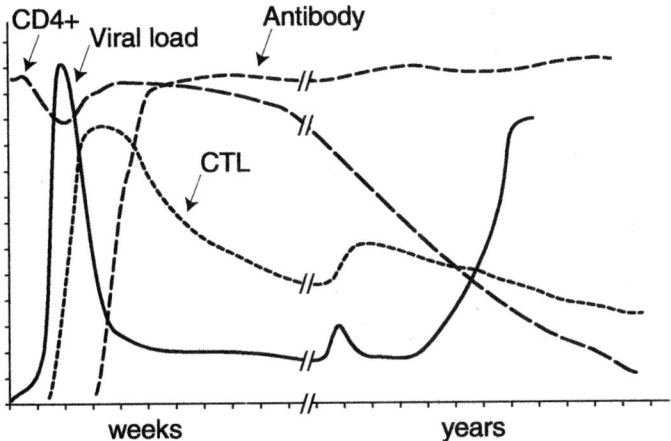

Figure 255.3. Immune responses in the natural course of HIV-1 infection.

T-helper function, escape from immune recognition, host genetics, protected viral reservoirs, potential infection of CD8$^+$ cells, and defects in antigen-presenting cells (reviewed in [96] and [97]).

HUMAN IMMUNODEFICIENCY VIRUS TROPISM AND CORECEPTORS

Viral entry into target cells, which is a critical first step of viral replication, starts when HIV-1 interacts with both the CD4 and the coreceptor. The principal coreceptors of HIV-1 entry are CCR5 and CXCR4 (98, 99). Binding of the HIV-1 Env gp120 to CD4 induces conformational changes in gp120 that create or expose a binding site for a co-receptor (85,86,100). Use of the CCR5 or CXCR4 coreceptors helps in understanding the cellular tropism of different HIV-1 isolates. Based on phenotypic categorization of HIV-1 isolates and selective use of the CCR5 or CXCR4 coreceptors, isolates were classified into R5 and/or X4 viruses (101,102). CCR5 coreceptor is the principal coreceptor for HIV-1 that is transmitted sexually and has the monocyte-macrophage phenotype (100,103). CXCR4 coreceptor is used by T-tropic viruses, or by dual tropic R5X4 virus variants (103). The phenotypic switch from R5 to X4 occurs after several years of infection in about a half of all HIV-1 infections. Noteworthy, in contrast to other HIV-1 subtypes, subtype C uses almost exclusively CCR5 coreceptors without switching to the X4 phenotype.

HIV-1 coreceptors belong to the seven transmembrane G-protein–coupled chemokine receptor family. The CCR5 amino-terminal domain plays an important role in virus fusion and entry. The determinants of CCR5 coreceptor function were precisely mapped in recent studies (reviewed in [103]) and include (i) Asp-2, Tyr-3, Tyr-10, Asp-11, Tyr-14, Tyr-15, and Glu-18 that are critical for CD4-induced gp120-CCR5 binding; (ii) Ser-6, Ser-7, Ile-9, Asn-13, Gln-21 and Lys-22 that are involved in coreceptor function; and (iii) Gln-93, Gly-163, Tyr-184, Ser-185, Arg-197, Asp-276, and Gln-280 that are located in the CCR5 extracellular loops and were found to influence coreceptor function. The CCR5 amino-terminal domain interacts only with gp120 proteins from isolates that use this coreceptor (103). The CCR5 amino-terminal sulphopeptides bind to conserved residues in the C4/V3 stem region of gp120, while residues in the V3 crown are important for gp120 binding to cell surface CCR5 but not to the amino-terminal sulfopeptides (104). To enter into target cells all R5 isolates use the same negatively charged and sulfotyrosine residues in the amino-terminal domain of CCR5, while X4 isolates use different subsets of amino acids from the negatively charged and tyrosine residues in the extracellular domain of CXCR4 (103). Coreceptors in general and CCR5 in particular

represent viable drug targets aimed at slowing HIV-1 replication and progression to AIDS (100).

REPLICATION AND HETEROGENEITY

HIV is able to replicate in the presence of host immune responses, and has a highly error-prone reverse transcriptase. Reverse transcriptase can rapidly produce an enormous number of viral mutants. The accumulation of proviral variants during HIV-1 infection together with genetic recombination results in accumulation of genetically distinct viral variants that are known as viral quasispecies that are a hallmark of HIV-1 infection. The HIV-1 quasispecies undergo continuous genetic variation and selection. Variety within the quasispecies allows virus to evade immune selection pressure from the host or develop drug resistance through generations of viral escape mutants.

Mutations in HIV occur at a rate more than 100 times the rate of mutations seen in eukaryotic DNA resulting in a 10^6-fold faster rate of evolution (105). The evolution rate of viruses within the HIV-1 M group was estimated as 0.0024 (0.0018 to 0.0028) substitutions per base pair per year in the *env* gp160 gene region and 0.0019 (0.0009 to 0.0027) substitutions per base pair per year in the *gag* gene region (106). Despite the high evolution rate of the HIV there are conserved regions across the viral genome that include the Lys-tRNA primer binding site (PBS), the polypurine tract, Rev-responsive element (RRE), and other elements involved in replication and packaging of the viral genome. The protein-coding regions of the HIV genome are moderately conserved, while the catalytic and functional domains within the viral protein are highly conserved. Overall, the *gag* and *pol* are more conserved than *tat, env* or *nef*. The highly variable *env* gene may include many insertions and deletions. However, the coiled structure of the Env is more conserved, as are structures and key residues in the catalytic sites of polymerase and protease. The HIV protein structures are reviewed in (107). Table 255.2 shows the nucleotide and amino acid diversity within HIV-1 subtype C, which is one of the most diversified subtypes of HIV.

MOLECULAR PHYLOGENY OF HUMAN IMMUNODEFICIENCY VIRUS

HIV-1 and HIV-2 presumably entered the human population through multiple zoonotic infections from nonhuman primates infected with simian immunodeficiency viruses (SIV) (108). HIV-1 is closely related to SIVcpz isolated from the chimpanzee *Pan troglodytes*, while HIV-2 is most closely related to SIVsm isolated from sooty mangabeys (108–111). HIV-1 has been categorized in three groups: the HIV-1 main (M), outlier (O), and N

TABLE 255.2.   HIV-1 Subtype C Nucleotide and Amino Acid Diversity, Percent of Nucleotide and Amino Acid Distances in *Gag, Pol, Vif, Vpr, Tat, Rev, Vpu, Env,* and *Nef*

Gene	Nucleotide diversity	Amino acid diversity
Gag	7.78 ± 1.22 (2.07–10.98)	9.50 ± 1.84 (2.61–15.40)
Pol	6.01 ± 0.89 (1.45–9.63)	6.42 ± 1.01 (0.15–10.17)
Vif	6.98 ± 1.56 (1.22–13.89)	11.62 ± 2.61 (0.54–22.06)
Vpr	9.39 ± 2.27 (1.74–17.71)	11.94 ± 3.45 (1.04–24.53)
Tat	9.87 ± 2.44 (2.68–20.23)	18.27 ± 5.36 (4.15–39.11)
Rev	10.10 ± 2.30 (2.75–18.99)	17.35 ± 5.98 (2.73–46.84)
Vpu	14.78 ± 3.48 (2.73–27.09)	25.20 ± 6.89 (2.45–49.97)
Env	12.82 ± 1.39 (4.43–16.71)	20.02 ± 2.28 (7.43–26.35)
Nef	11.88 ± 2.15 (3.28–22.51)	18.56 ± 3.28 (5.11–30.57)
LTR	9.0 ± 1.79 (2.97–17.06)	N/A

Mean value ± standard deviation, range in brackets.

(non-M, non-O). The spread and contribution of HIV-1 groups to the global AIDS epidemic is uneven. The HIV-1 M group dominates worldwide, while N and O groups are endemic to Cameroon and neighboring countries in West Central Africa, but there only occur at low rates. Based on the phylogenetic relationships between viral isolates, the HIV-1 M group was further subdivided into genetic subtypes, named A through K, namely A1, A2, B, C, D, F1, F2, G, H, J and K (112) (Fig. 255.4). Several of the HIV-1 M group subtypes are thought to have diverged from a single ape to human transmission event.

Historically, some isolates within the HIV-1 M group were assigned to particular subtypes based on a relatively short region of their sequence. Subsequent analyses revealed that viral isolates designated initially as HIV-1 subtypes E and I shared a portion of their sequence with other HIV-1 subtypes and actually have a recombinant origin. Thus, former subtype E is now referred to as CRF01_AE (see next section) to reflect that it is an A/E recombinant. Former subtype I was found to be a mosaic with regions associated with subtypes A, G, H, K as well as unclassified regions (112). Pure viruses with subtype E or I across the entire viral genome have not been found.

The dynamic character of the AIDS epidemic and the non-uniform historical distribution of HIV-1 subtypes worldwide have been exemplified by an unprecedented increase in prevalence of HIV-1 subtype C (HIV-1C). In recent years HIV-1C has become the predominant virus in different regions of the world including southern Africa, the horn of Africa, and South/Southeast Asia. HIV-1C now represents at least 56% of all circulating group M infections (113) and was predicted to dominate in the coming years (113,114). Distinguishing features of the HIV-1C epidemics include but are not limited to: (i) a high prevalence rate—up to 20% to 40%—in the general population (115,116); (ii) higher rates of vertical transmission (117); (iii) high viral load (118); (iv) high levels of viral diversity (119–121); (v) preferential CCR5-coreceptor usage (122–125); and (vi) a number of unique subtype signatures across the viral genome (119,126–128).

Subtype A is the second most prevalent genetic variant of HIV-1, which is largely represented by CRF02_AG (see next section) and is predominant in countries along the central belt of Africa (114), where prevalence among the general population varies from 1.5% to 14.5% (115). Similar to subtype C, the transmission mode of subtype A is mainly heterosexual, although it has spread rapidly among injection drug users in eastern Europe (i.e., Russia and Ukraine). Subtype A infections were also reported in East Asia, the Pacific, in western Europe, and North America.

Subtype B is considered to be the third most common HIV-1 subtype accounting for a significant number of infections in the world AIDS epidemic (12.3% of global cases in 2000) (114). The

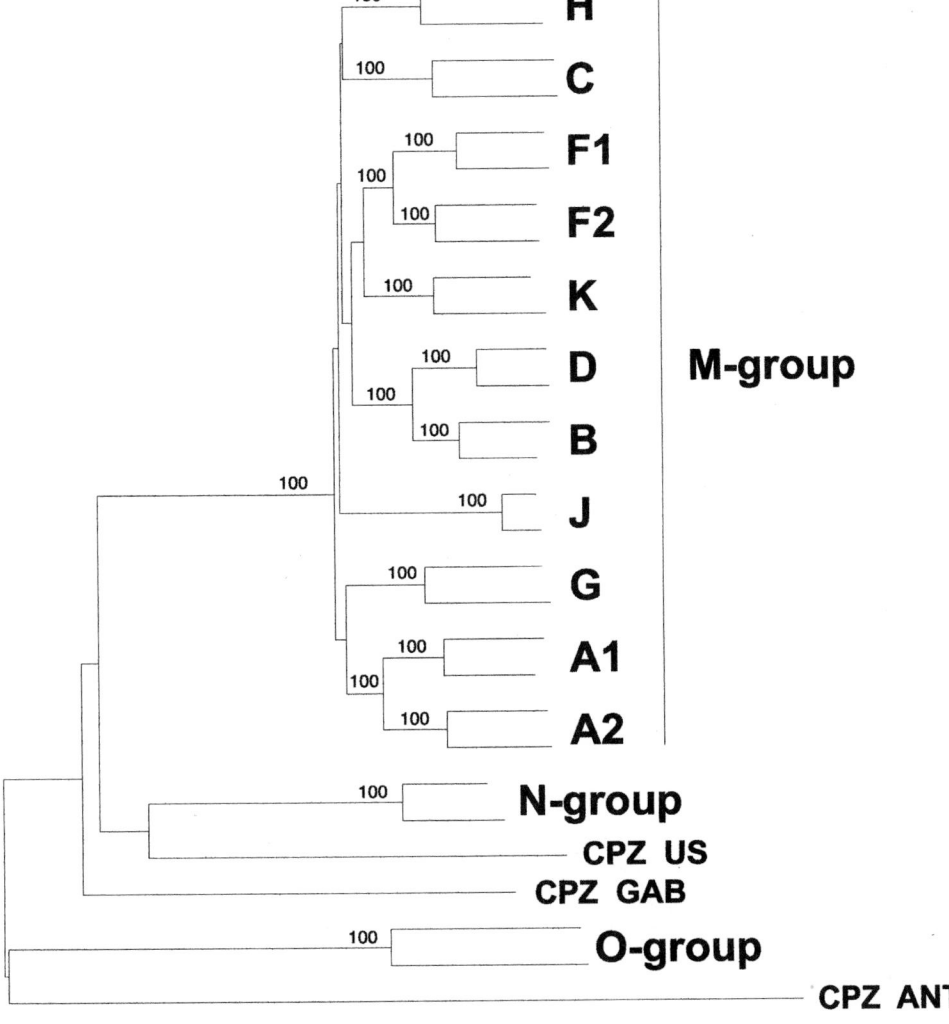

Figure 255.4. Phylogenetic relationships between representative strains of HIV-1 group M subtypes A1, A2, B, C, D, F1, F2, G, H, J and K, groups N and O, and SIVcpz derived from the near full-length genome nucleotide sequences. The alignment was gap-stripped. The neighbor-joining phylogenetic tree is shown. The numbers indicate percentage bootstrap replicates. The scale bar indicates 5% nucleotide sequence divergence.

HIV-1 subtype B is predominant in North America, Western Europe, and Australia.

None of the other subtypes is responsible for more than 6% of global HIV-1 infections (114). The relationship between viral genotype and biologic phenotype of HIV-1 isolates is complex. Both cross-clade immunity (129–133) and subtype-specific immune responses have been reported (70,134,135), which indicates that the relative importance of cross-reactive versus clade-specific immunity remains unknown and requires further studies. The genetic classification of HIV-1 strains continues to be useful for epidemiologic tracking of the pandemic, vaccine design, and for providing a foundation for detecting potential biological differences (112).

RECOMBINATION

If two different HIV strains simultaneously infect the same cell, the resulting virions might be heterozygous, i.e., include different RNA transcripts. In the later infection the RT can jump between the two RNA templates generating a recombinant or "mosaic" proviral DNA. The recombination is a common event among diverse strains of HIV. Although recombination is most obvious among viral isolates of different subtypes, it is also likely to occur among members of the same subtype, although current methods fail to reliably detect such intra-subtype recombination (136).

Mosaic HIV-1 genomes with similar (or even identical) structure could be identified in unlinked individuals and may play a significant role in the global AIDS epidemic. These HIV-1 recombinants that have similar breakpoints reflecting common ancestry from the same recombination event(s) are designated as circulating recombinant forms, or CRF (137). There are 11 CRF as currently defined (Table 255.3). The predominant recombinant forms in the global epidemic are CRF01-AE and CRF02-AG. The HIV-1 CRF01-AE (referred to as former env/subtype E) is circulating in Southeast Asia. The proportion of CRF01-AE has been estimated as 63% of all new infections in the region (114). The HIV-1 CRF02-AG represents a large proportion of subtype A cases, which caused 27% of all global HIV-1 infections in 2000 (114). In countries with cocirculating multiple HIV-1 subtypes the proportion of CRF might exceed 35%.

HOST GENETIC FACTORS

Factors that influence susceptibility or resistance to HIV-1 infection and rate of disease progression are a combination of viral, host, and environmental determinants (138). A mutation in the chemokine receptor gene, CCR5, provides strong protection from HIV-1 infection (139–141), although the frequency of the genotype CCR5Δ32/CCR5Δ32 is relatively low (overall 1%) and differs between different ethnic groups ranging from near 0% in Africans to approximately 15% in Northern Europeans. The deletion begins in the region encoding the third extracellular domain of CCR5, and results in a frame shift and premature stop codon in the fifth transmembrane domain. The truncated protein is not expressed on the cell surface, which blocks viral interaction with CCR5 and does not allow virus to enter the cell. Heterozygous individuals (CCR5Δ32/CCR5) are not protected from the HIV infection but progress to AIDS more slowly. The CCR5 promoter polymorphisms might change the level of CCR5 expression on the cell surface and alter infectability by R5 variants of HIV-1.

CCR5 is in strong linkage disequilibrium with another chemokine receptor, CCR2. A variant of the CCR2 gene with a conservative change from valine to isoleucine at position 64 (CCR2-64I) was associated with slow progress to AIDS and potentially lower viral load. The CCR2-64I variant is relatively frequent: 10% in whites, 15% in African Americans, 17% in Hispanics, and 25% in Asians (138).

A delayed progression to AIDS was also associated with polymorphism at position 801 in the SDF1, a chemokine ligand for CXCR4 (142).

IL10, a TH-2 cell cytokine, may control HIV proliferation through the inhibition of macrophage growth and secretion of T-cell cytokines (143, 144). A C → A transversion within the promoter of IL10 at position −592 upstream of the translation start (designed as IL10-5'A) was associated with reduced production of IL10 and accelerated progression to AIDS (138,142,145). The frequency of IL10-5'A is relatively high among most ethnic groups: 23.6% in whites, 40% in African Americans, 33% in Hispanics, and 60% in Asians (138).

Individuals who are heterozygous at HLA loci are capable of presenting a larger variety of antigenic peptides than homozygous individuals, which results in more efficient immune responses to numerous viral pathogens (overdominant selection or heterozygote advantage). In contrast, individuals who are homozygous at HLA loci present a limited repertoire of antigenic epitopes and progress more rapidly to develop AIDS (138).

A number of MHC class I and class II HLA alleles and haplotypes were associated with protection or faster progression to AIDS. The B*35-Cw*04 haplotype was linked with rapid progression of HIV infection (146). In contrast, B*27 and B*57 were shown to have a protective effect on progression to AIDS (147–149). HLA-A29 and -B22 were associated with rapid progression, while B14 and C8 were associated with slow progression (150).

TABLE 255.3. Circulating Recombinant Forms of HIV-1 Group M

CRF name	Subtypes	Predominance (geographic distribution)
CRF01-AE	A, E	Southeast Asia, sporadic in Central Africa
CRF02-AG	A, G	West and West Central Africa
CRF03-AB	A, B	Russia (Kaliningrad)
CRF04-cpx	A, G, H, K, U	Greece, Cyprus
CRF05-DF	D, F	Democratic Republic of Congo
CRF06-cpx	A, G, J, K	West Africa (Mali, Senegal, Nigeria, Burkina Faso, Niger)
CRF07-BC	B, C	Northwest China
CRF08-BC	B, C	Southeast China
CRF09-cpx		Senegal, United States
CRF10-CD	C, D	Tanzania
CRF11-cpx	A, E, G, J	Central Africa (Cameroon, Central African Republic, Gabon)

CRF, circulating recombinant forms.

Many other suggested associations still need to be confirmed in multiple cohort studies.

An inverse correlation between the levels of RANTES and MIP-1β secretion and disease progression was documented (151,152). Polymorphisms in the promoter region of RANTES ($-403A/-28G$) were associated with slower rates of CD4$^+$ cell depletion (153). Tumor necrosis factor-α (TNF-α) and lymphotoxin (TNF-β) are strong inducers of HIV replication through activation of the transcription factor NF-κB (154,155). Increased levels of TNF-α have been reported in patients with AIDS, while polymorphisms in the promoter region of the TNF-α were associated with disease progression (156). The MHC class II HLA-DR3 and DR4 were linked with higher levels of TNF-α, while HLA-DR2 was associated with low TNF-α production (157–159).

Overall, host genetics together with viral variation and environmental factors contribute significantly to HIV pathogenesis, disease susceptibility, and the rate of progression to AIDS.

DIAGNOSTICS AND DRUG-RESISTANCE TESTING

Techniques for HIV diagnostics range from direct isolation of virus to detection of viral antigens, viral transcripts (mRNA), proviral DNA, and host antibody responses to viral antigens. HIV-1 antigen or nucleic acid may be detected in early HIV infection during the period from exposure to seroconversion. Later, in the period after seroconversion, the antibody responses become detectable in serum or plasma. Standard screening protocols for the HIV diagnostics include enzyme-linked immunoassay (ELISA) or immunofluorescent assay (IFA) for the detection of anti-HIV antibodies in sera or plasma. These most commonly used screening tests use extracellular virus, recombinant viral proteins or synthetic peptides as an antigen source to detect circulating antibodies to HIV. The viral antigens most often used in the tests are portions of envelope gp120. Western blot (WB) is used as confirmatory test. A detuned assay (160) or an ELISA that detects increasing levels of anti-HIV IgG after seroconversion (161) can be used for detecting recent HIV-1 infections and identification of incident cases within the population.

Current ELISA format tests have greater than 98% sensitivity and specificity for HIV infection. Positive predictive value is greater than 99% for strongly reactive samples from persons at high risk. False-positive results occur at higher frequency with samples from people with alcoholic hepatitis, neoplasms, immune abnormalities, multiple transfusions, multiparity, leprosy, and malaria. A combined HIV-1/HIV-2 screening assay may be useful in geographic areas where both viruses are circulating. A confirmatory WB identifies bands of HIV-specific antibodies to discrete viral antigens that are electrophoretically separated and transferred to nitrocellulose paper. Criteria for a positive WB result differ between manufacturers but usually include the presence of bands for at least two viral gene products. Negative WB samples should have no bands. Indeterminate patterns with fewer bands may indicate an early stage of seroconversion, loss of p24 antibodies in progression to AIDS, or HIV-2 infection. Isolated faint reactivity to p24 is often nonspecific.

PCR, a method of DNA or RNA amplification, uses blood cells or plasma to detect as few as one or several copies of the viral genome. The method is highly sensitive and useful for confirming HIV in indeterminate or antibody-negative samples or perinatal infection and detecting HIV in tissue samples. Quantitative PCR was developed to detect viral load in infected individuals. Viral load (VL) has become a common clinical tool for determining when to initiate therapy, and whether treatment is effective or drug resistance has developed. There are at least three commercially available assays for measuring HIV RNA in plasma: (i) a quantitative PCR-based assay (Amplicor HIV-1 Monitor, Roche

Diagnostics), which uses a standard or ultrasensitive protocol; (ii) a branched-chain DNA (bDNA) assay (Quantiplex, Chiron Corp.), and (iii) a nucleic acid sequence-based amplification assay (NASBA, Organon Technika).

Virus isolation may be performed using peripheral blood, bone marrow, genital secretions, brain or CSF by cocultivation of the specimen with uninfected, mitogen-stimulated peripheral blood mononuclear cells. Isolation takes several weeks and is based on elevation of p24 antigen or reverse transcriptase in the supernatant of infected cells. Isolated virus can be further studied including phenotypic and genotypic analysis.

Detection and quantification of CD4$^+$ and CD8$^+$ cells has become a routine lab technique in the course of natural HIV infection. A relative and absolute reduction of CD4 cells or T cells is routinely done to monitor clinical progression of AIDS and to decide when to initiate therapy. Methods for evaluation of virus-specific T-cell responses in the course of HIV infection, including the ^{51}Cr-release assay, limiting dilution assay and proliferation assay are often used in research protocols. More sophisticated methods include enzyme-linked immunospot (ELISPOT), intracellular cytokine staining (ICS), and tetramer staining (reviewed in [162]).

Drug resistance testing is an important part of patient clinical management. The International AIDS Society regularly updates HIV drug resistance testing guidelines (163,164) to assist clinicians in better use of the resistance tests (see *www.IASUSA.org*). The phenotypic and genotypic resistance assays are two basic methods to measure the susceptibility of HIV to drug therapy and can be applied in aiding both short-term and long-term antiretroviral treatment planning.

Phenotypic tests assess the actual response of a patient's viral isolate to individual antiretroviral drugs in culture. Phenotypic assays measure the susceptibility of a patient's viral isolate to the antiretroviral drug by measuring the ability of HIV-1 to grow in the presence of a different antiretroviral agent over a fixed period. Various drug-resistant HIV phenotypes are identified by measuring an increase in the 50% inhibitory concentration (IC$_{50}$) of a drug relative to a reference strain of HIV-1. Phenotypic testing can be done (i) by traditional culturing of the virus from the patient's PBMC and measuring the effects of different concentrations of a drug on viral replication, or (ii) by a recombinant assay, where a region of the viral genome containing the determinants of drug resistance (i.e., protease and reverse transcriptase) is amplified and inserted into an HIV vector that is deleted for the protease or reverse transcriptase. There are two phenotypic assays based on the recombinant virus approach that are currently available to clinicians: PhenoSense (ViroLogic, San Francisco) and Antivirogram (Virco, Mechelen, Belgium).

Genotypic assays test viral sequence, providing an indirect measure of resistance based on knowledge of established HIV-1 genetic mutations for resistance to a particular antiretroviral drug. Two sequencing kits detect resistance mutations in HIV-1 protease and reverse transcriptase: ViroSeq HIV-1 Genotyping System (Celera Diagnostics, Alameda, California) and TRUGENE Genotyping Kit (Visible Genetics, Toronto, Ontario, Canada). A number of in-house genotypic assays have also been used for the genotyping of drug-resistant mutations. An array-based hybridization assay is also being developed for use in detecting HIV protease and RT resistance mutations. Most of genotyping methods are based on (i) initial amplification (PCR or RT-PCR) of PR and/or RT; (ii) sequencing; and (iii) analysis of the sequences.

The limitations of drug-resistant testing include but are not limited to: (i) samples with low viral copy number might be difficult or impossible to amplify (threshold varies from 10^2 to 10^4 copies/mL); (ii) amplification or sequencing primers might mismatch with the patient's virus; (iii) specimens for analysis must be prepared in a precise manner; and (iv) the methods do not allow the quantification of viruses that vary at ambiguous positions.

Nevertheless, drug-resistance testing is a powerful scientific tool for physicians that improves short-term patient outcomes by allowing better selection of the most effective antiretroviral agents, and allows earlier switching to a more sensitive medication.

VACCINE DEVELOPMENT

The "first generation" of experimental HIV vaccines were focused on the induction of humoral responses to HIV envelope proteins. The first vaccine candidate was a monomeric HIV-1 envelope gp120 that originated from lab-adapted HIV-1 strains and was used to generate neutralizing antibody (165,166). Although the gp120 antibodies induced could successfully neutralize lab-adapted strains, antibodies induced by the recombinant gp120 were unable to neutralize primary viral isolates (95). The results of the first phase III vaccine trials of the recombinant gp120 vaccine AIDSVAX showed no protection overall in the trials, but showed a startling efficacy among a few ethnic subsets. Attempts to make trimeric molecules by inserting disulfide bonds into the gp120/gp41 complex (167) or by preventing gp120/gp41 cleavage (168) resulted in slightly improved immunogenicity but the vaccine constructs were not able to induce broadly neutralizing antibodies. The "second-generation" HIV vaccines shifted toward cell-mediated immunity by targeting CD8$^+$ and CD4$^+$ immune responses induced by a variety of structural, regulatory and accessory HIV proteins.

Entire viral genes or their parts, as well as individual protective epitopes are often utilized as antigenic components of experimental HIV vaccines designed to elicit cytolytic T-cell responses. A consensus approach to the design of the immunogenic component has been suggested recently to potentially overcome the high genetic diversity of HIV (169,170). The immunogenic element of the vaccine might be augmented by cytokines, adjuvants, or costimulatory molecules that can enhance immune responses (171–174).

To increase immunogenicity of the native HIV envelope numerous modifications have been proposed including: (i) deglycosylation of the envelope protein by removing glycosyl moieties (175); (ii) removing variable loops from gp120 (176); (iii) fusing gp120 to CD4 to change morphology (177); and (iv) generating a CD4-independent virus.

The *gag* gene has become the most attractive component of the vaccine constructs aimed at inducing CD8+ CTL responses. The *pol* or *nef* genes have also been used in HIV vaccine designs. The Tat protein was also shown to be a promising immunogen in the primate model (178,179).

Advances in biotechnology opened a new era for DNA vaccines. A "codon-optimization" or "humanized" sequence modification of the DNA vaccine designs results in increased expression of HIV genes and more immunogenicity.

Recombinant vaccinia was the first major vector used in the field of HIV vaccine development. Vaccinia can readily express different HIV genes (i.e., *gag–pol*, or *env*). It grows well and recombinant constructs can be produced in sufficient quantity. A protein boost immunization usually strengthens the antibody response induced by the vaccinia construct. However, there are safety concerns for replication competent vaccinia. Modified vaccinia Ankara (MVA) and canarypox are representative poxviruses that cannot produce progeny in human cells but can initiate infection and efficiently express recombinant HIV genes. Both MVA and canarypox-based vaccines are currently in human vaccine trials.

Alphaviruses and adenoviruses are used as vaccine vectors that have been modified to be avirulent because their genes encoding structural proteins were deleted and substituted by the heterologous HIV gene of interest, i.e., *gag*, *pol*, or *env*, etc. The resulting recombinant constructs can produce viral replicons, or virus-like particles, and package vaccine genes inside the replicon if their deleted genes are supplied in trans by a helper packaging system. The alphaviruses Venezuelan equine encephalitis virus (VEE), Sindbis virus, and Semliki forest virus have been used. A comparatively large adenovirus with a deleted E1 gene provides a very attractive packaging system that was successfully developed by Merck (West Point, PA) in a series of primate experiments (180).

Bacterial vectors expressing HIV antigens that are administered orally may also provide specific CTL and T-helper responses including efficient mucosal immunity. Salmonella, Listeria, *Streptococcus gordonii* and *Mycobacterium*-based vectors were demonstrated to be efficient vaccine vehicles that are able to induce HIV-specific immune responses.

Comprehensive vaccine efficacy trials are urgently needed to test a growing number of promising vaccine candidates. Preliminary results of vaccine trials strongly suggest that to achieve protection an efficient vaccine will require both cell-mediated and humoral immunity.

Human T-Cell Leukemia Virus 1 and 2

The HTLV contains two identical RNA strands that are linked at their 5' end and form a dimeric structure, which is important for viral infectivity. Generally, HTLV infection by free virions is inefficient, and requires presence of HTLV-1 or HTLV-2 infected cells. The HTLV-1 genome contains a unique region at the 3' end, designated the pX region, which encodes regulatory proteins, such as Tax and Rex (181). The virions are approximate 100 nm spheres with a condensed core that is round but not cone-shaped as is the core of HIV. The genome is approximately 9 kb long. HTLV-1 and HTLV-2 are approximately 60% to 70% related at the primary nucleotide sequence level and the proteins show substantial antigenic cross-reactivity. Virus production appears to be much less efficient for the HTLVs, and transmission between cells is primarily with cell-associated virus.

GENES AND STRUCTURE

HTLV-1 has a myristylated Gag precursor, responsible for the binding to the plasma membrane (182,183). The globular MA structure consists of five helices, packed together to form a hydrophobic core (184,185). The 19-kd MA has 11 basic amino acids spread across the protein and involved in cell-to-cell transmission (183). The structure of the 24-kd CA has been determined to be the major capsid protein (186). A 15-kd nucleocapsid has also been defined.

HTLV reverse transcriptase is synthesized from a Gag-Pro-Pol precursor, and requires two successful frameshifts (187), which might be associated with the relatively low infectivity of the virus. The protease catalyzes cleavage of the Gag and Pol polyproteins. A single protein of approximately 860 amino acids appears to encode the reverse transcriptase, integrase, and RNase H functions. The reverse transcriptase works most efficiently with Mg^{2+} as the required cation.

HTLV envelope glycoproteins are synthesized and incorporated into the virion in a fusion-incompetent form. In order to achieve fusion they require a major conformation change (185). The major Env product is glycosylated but not as heavily as the analogous HIV protein. It undergoes cleavage to form the outer and transmembrane proteins. The SU gp46 of HTLV-1 is the principal target for neutralizing antibodies and it is associated with receptor attachment, pore formation and necrosis (188). The p21 TM protein is linked to syncytia formation and fusion (189).

The HTLV encodes two regulatory proteins, Rex and Tax. The Rex protein is similar to the HIV Rev protein (reviewed in [21]). Rex is required for the cytoplasmic expression of large unspliced or singly spliced RNAs and contains an arginine-rich nucleolar localization signal that mediates binding to the Rex response element (RexRE). Rex may also promote the stability and/or expression of cellular RNAs (21). Rex may occur as a 27-kd protein and a 21-kd protein. The p27 is associated with the expression of RNA for the structural genes. Tax protein is an efficient trans-activator (reviewed in [190]). Tax is a phosphoprotein, which is encoded by a multiply spliced RNA and located in the nucleus of infected cells. At the N-terminal, Tax contains zinc-finger-like cysteine-rich and histidine-rich motifs that are important for trans-activation. Tax activates HTLV transcription through the LTR promoter and modulates the transcription of a number of cellular genes that contribute to the role of HTLV in oncogenesis (21). The Tax protein is approximately 40 kd.

The pX region also encodes several small proteins; p12, p13, and p30 (181). These proteins are not required for virus replication or transformation.

IMMUNE RESPONSES

As with HIV, the major core and envelope proteins of the HTLVs induce readily detectable antibodies in most infections. For the Gag protein p24, the antibodies induced are highly cross-reactive between HTLV-1 and HTLV-2. Antibodies to Tax are also detectable in a significant fraction of HTLV-1–infected persons (191). Some reports also claim that antibodies to Tax may be present in the case of tumors such as cutaneous T-cell lymphoma when antibodies to Gag or Env are not detectable (192).

Antibodies to the major envelope glycoprotein, gp46, can be readily detected and are directed to both linear and conformational epitopes (193). Such antibodies may be important to restrict transmission of free virus. Cytolytic T-cell responses have also been described, but much less is known about the range of epitopes for HTLV as compared to HIV.

VIRUS REPLICATION AND CELL TROPISM

HTLVs have a replication cycle that seems similar to other retroviruses. While B cells and some non-lymphoid cells appear to be able to produce virus at low levels, only T cells can be transformed. The cellular receptor for HTLV 1 has been localized to section q21 to q23 of the long arm of chromosome 17 (194). Based on syncytia induction experiments, it has been speculated that HTLV-1 and HTLV-2 use the same receptor (195).

Virtually all proviral DNA in peripheral blood cells from infected persons is found in T cells. However, it is primarily in T4 cells in the case of HTLV-1 (196) and T8 cells in the case of HTLV-2 (197).

MOLECULAR PHYLOGENY AND VARIATION

A wide spectrum of apes and monkeys has been shown to harbor simian T cell leukemia viruses (STLV) that are closely related to the HTLVs. These STLV viruses are widespread in both Asia and Africa. The most common progenitor may be an STLV found in the pygmy chimpanzee (198).

HTLVs show much less variation than HIVs. This is probably due to a combination of lower rates of replication combined with lower rates of transmission and selection pressure. HTLV 1 and 2 appear to share approximate 60% to 70% homology at the primary nucleotide level and the different subtypes of HTLV-1 appear to share 95% to 99% homology, whether found in Asia or Africa. HTLV-1A, for example, also called the cosmopolitan type, is distributed in Asia, Africa, and the new world with all isolates appearing to be at least 98% related to each other. A second subtype, B, appears distributed primarily in central Africa. Subtype C, distributed in Papua New Guinea and Melanesia, apparently has a different STLV origin. HTLV-1D has been associated primarily with pygmies in central Africa. HTLV-2 viruses appear to have a historical distribution in both Amazon Indians and African Pygmies (199).

TRANSFORMATION AND ONCOGENESIS

HTLV-1 immortalizes T4 lymphoblasts through some combination of mitogenic stimulation by viral surface proteins and the immortalizing effects of the Tax protein. This is the same cell population that becomes highly malignant in the case of adult T-cell leukemia or lymphoma (ATL).

While most retroviruses transform cells by either the transduction and representation of an oncogene, or by insertion next to the promoter of a proto-oncogene, HTLV does not appear to act by either of these mechanisms. Although transformed and malignant cells contain HTLV proviral sequences, the integration sites are randomly distributed. Cells immortalized by HTLV-1 have an activation of the Jak/STAT pathway. Tax, which inhibits the expression of p53 (200), is essential for transformation (201).

DIAGNOSIS AND VACCINE DEVELOPMENT

Several different screening tests are available for detecting HTLV-1 and HTLV-2. Most blood banks in the west and in Japan use an enzyme linked immunosorbent assay to detect antibodies to the virus envelope glycoprotein, or to whole disrupted virus. For confirmation, a western blot analysis or PCR is usually done. Antibody titers are generally lower than those for HIV (202), and mucosal fluids such as saliva are usually negative (203).

No vaccine for HTLV is currently available. It is generally expected that developing a vaccine for HTLV-1 would be easier than making a vaccine for HIV. This is partly because HTLV shows much less genomic variation, and also because antibodies to HTLV appear to be highly protective in animal models (204).

PATHOGENESIS OF HUMAN IMMUNODEFICIENCY VIRUS INFECTION

Human Immunodeficiency Virus–Induced Immunopathogenesis

HIV-1 infection of two critical components of the immune system, lymphocytes and macrophages, results in a cascade of predictable quantitative and qualitative defects in cellular and humoral immunity. Through $CD4^+$ T lymphocyte depletion and dysfunction, HIV infection disrupts the immune system's ability to activate macrophages, secrete IL-2 and other cytokines for lymphoid and hematopoietic growth and differentiation, and induce cytotoxic and suppressor T cells and B cells. In addition, HIV probably disrupts many of the essential activities of the macrophage, including phagocytosis and destruction of foreign antigens, presentation of antigens to lymphocytes, and secretion of cytokines (205–207). Data suggest that monocyte chemotaxis is frequently impaired and that many of the functional defects seen in HIV-infected monocytes are the result of failure of $CD4^+$ cells to signal cytokine induction. For example, in vitro, addition of one of these deficient cytokines, interferon-γ, partially reconstitutes the defective monocyte respiratory burst that is important in eliminating foreign organisms (206–208).

Characteristic immunologic abnormalities of HIV infection include lymphopenia with depletion of $CD4^+$ helper T cells; impaired delayed-type hypersensitivity reactions; polyclonal

B-cell activation and increased immunoglobulin production; decreased humoral responses to immunization; decreased T- and B-cell (209) proliferative responses; decreased production of interferon-γ, IL-2, and tumor necrosis factor-α (TNF-α); increased levels of acid-labile interferon; and diminished cell-mediated cytotoxicity (210–213). The consequences of a defective humoral response are particularly severe in persons who were not previously exposed to a bacterial pathogen and who therefore depend on the primary immunoglobulin M response for immune protection (214,215). Selective immune defects make HIV-infected persons susceptible to a wide range of opportunistic infections and tumors that may differ depending on the individual's route of HIV infection and endemic geographic exposures to other infections (216–218). Although HIV-2–associated AIDS is uncommon, similar forms of immune compromise may occur (219,220).

The mechanism of HIV immune system pathogenesis involves high viral production and rapid T-cell turnover (221,222). More than 10^9 viral particles and T cells are produced each day, resulting in an immunologic standoff between virus and host. Eventually, immunologic escape occurs through the development of viral variation and quasi-species, and declining immunologic function results. The decline in CD4$^+$ cells that occurs with disease progression may be the combined result of direct T-cell destruction through altered cellular processes among infected cells (223,224), syncytium formation between infected and uninfected cells (225), immune-mediated destruction of infected cells (226), loss of T-cell regeneration capacity (227,228), superantigen production and cellular destruction (229), and activation-induced apoptosis (230).

In vitro, both HIV-1 and HIV-2 infect cells of monocyte/macrophage lineage without significant cytopathic effects. The lack of cytopathicity may be related to the propensity of HIV in these cells to bud into and accumulate in intracytoplasmic vacuoles where HIV remains immunologically sequestered (231). In humans, noncytopathic, latent infection of monocyte/macrophage lineage cells (including bone marrow precursors) and microglial cells in the nervous system may thus provide a reservoir where HIV can persist and be reactivated (232,233). It is believed that this reservoir is established soon after infection, during the acute phase of illness (234). In vitro, silently infected cells can be activated to produce virus by a variety of agents, including specific antigens and mitogens, ultraviolet light, coinfecting viruses (herpesviruses, hepatitis B virus, HTLV-1), and cytokines (granulocyte-macrophage colony-stimulating factor [GM-CSF] and TNF-α) (210). Enhanced HIV expression (by cytokines and other agents) may involve the effect of a DNA binding protein on the HIV promoter region (235).

Langerhans and other dendritic cells are also infected by HIV, and are believed to be the point of entry when HIV is transmitted sexually (236). Dendritic cells are able to form syncytia with CD4$^+$ T cells either at the mucosal surface or in lymph nodes (237,238), resulting in amplified viral production and eventual spread throughout the body (239).

Human Immunodeficiency Virus–Induced Neuropathogenesis

Neurologic involvement of HIV-1 infection is common. Nearly 30% of untreated patients develop neurologic complications directly related to HIV, primarily in the form of dementia, neuropathy, and myelopathy (240,241). Autopsy studies indicate that HIV infection of the nervous system is evident in approximately 90% of symptomatic HIV-infected persons and may involve the brain, spinal cord, or peripheral nerves (242). These studies often uncover evidence of disease that was not clinically evident, and high viral loads have been demonstrated in the CNS independent of the serum viral load (243). Neuropathologic evaluation reveals multinucleated giant cells (syncytia), white matter gliosis and demyelination, microglial nodules, focal necrosis of neurons, and perivascular inflammation (244,245). Data obtained by immunochemical staining and hybridization methods for HIV-1 antigen and nucleic acids in brain tissue indicate that most HIV in the nervous system of infected patients is present in monocyte/macrophages and in related cells such as microglial cells and multinucleated giant cells of monocyte origin (246,247). Neurons and vascular endothelial cells, which have relatively few CD4 receptors, rarely contain HIV (248).

Several mechanisms of pathogenesis have been proposed for the development of HIV-related neurologic disease. HIV-infected macrophages may play an indirect role in pathogenesis, as in vitro data indicate that macrophages express a low density of CD4 on their cell surface and are susceptible to infection but are refractory to syncytium formation and cell killing (249). HIV-infected monocyte/macrophages may initiate central nervous system damage by releasing cytokines or proteolytic enzymes toxic to adjacent neuronal cells (the "innocent bystanders"), including endothelial cells, astrocytes, and neurons. Disruption of the blood-brain barrier by injury to endothelial cells (or by direct infection of these cells) may allow toxic agents to enter from the blood stream, which cause further damage. Another potential mechanism for CNS pathogenesis is direct HIV infection of neurons and glial cells, resulting in cell killing by the virus itself and by CTL recognition and killing of infected cells (250). It has also been proposed that neurotoxic effects of viral products such as gp120 may play a role in neuropathogenesis by causing destruction of adjacent cells, which induces release of mediators of inflammation and neurotoxic cytokines such as TNF and IL-1 (251). The relative contributions of these mechanisms of neuropathogenesis of HIV await further study. Combination antiretroviral therapy, particularly with agents that cross the blood-brain barrier such as zidovudine (252) may be effective in reversing some of the clinical features of AIDS-related dementia.

Natural History of Infection

ACUTE INFECTION

Within days of infection, HIV can be detected in local lymph nodes, from which it soon spreads throughout the lymphatic system and to the CNS (234). High viral loads are typically seen in primary infection, and may rise to more than 10^6 copies (253). Approximately 50% to 90% of persons infected with HIV-1 recall a mild to severe mononucleosis-like syndrome after a time of possible HIV exposure, consisting of fever, myalgia, headache, sore throat, and rash (253,254). This illness typically occurs two to four weeks after HIV-1 exposure, although incubation periods of ten months have been reported (255). The median time from infection to laboratory evidence of seroconversion is estimated to be 2.1 months, with 95% of persons seroconverting by 5.8 months. Following seroconversion, immunologic control of the virus is established and a viral "set point" is reached; in one study, the mean CD4 count 6 months after seroconversion was 780/mm^3, and fell to 670/mm^3 after 1 year (256). Viral load set points typically nadir between 12,000 and 60,000 copies, and those with higher set points progress more rapidly to AIDS (257–259).

Once an adult is infected with HIV, the virus is virtually always detectable; in a few rare cases of reversion from seropositive status to seronegative status, PCR techniques have demonstrated continued evidence of HIV genome (260). Silent HIV infection—a prolonged seronegative state in which virus can be cultured and viral nucleotide can be detected by PCR methods—is unusual (261,262). Studies of uninfected commercial sex workers in Nairobi, Kenya with regular frequent exposure to HIV-1 suggest that a few people may become infected locally and develop a Th1-mediated cellular immune response without developing antibodies or systemic infection (69). A strong HIV-specific $CD8^+$ T cell response in the genital mucosa of these women may play a role in providing protective immunity (263).

DISEASE PROGRESSION

Clinical progression of HIV infection to AIDS, regardless of route of transmission, involves a prolonged but variable incubation period with a median time of approximately 10 years in seroincident adult cohorts in industrialized countries (264,265). CD4 counts decline by approximately $50/mm^3$ per year, with a range of 30 to $90/mm^3$ per year (256,258,266,267). Progression to AIDS is more variable among African cohorts, where some studies demonstrate similar rates of progression to industrialized countries (216,268,269), and others report a more rapid clinical course (270,271). The incubation period is substantially shorter in mother-to-infant cases (272). Current theories on causes of individual differences in rates of progression to AIDS include host genetics (205,273), virulence of viral strains (274), nutritional factors (275), and immune activation related to coinfections (217,276). A small fraction of infected individuals, perhaps 1% to 4%, become long-term nonprogressors, showing no reduction in CD4 cell count or immune function until at least 10 years after infection (65,277). Although HIV-2 infection may progress to AIDS in some persons, viral load set points are substantially lower than those in HIV-1 (278) and a benign clinical course occurs in a significant fraction of infected persons (19).

Epidemiology of Human Immunodeficiency Virus Infection

SEXUAL TRANSMISSION

Heterosexual transmission is the dominant mode of HIV spread throughout the world, accounting for more than 80% of all transmission (279). Heterosexual HIV transmission is also becoming increasingly common in the United States, where about 33% of new HIV infections are acquired by heterosexual contact, compared with 42% by homosexual contact and 25% from intravenous drug use. Women, most of whom have acquired HIV through sexual transmission, now account for approximately 30% of HIV infections in the United States and 47% of all infections worldwide.

Data on heterosexual HIV transmission efficiency from spouses of hemophiliacs and transfusion recipients have revealed a rate of male-to-female HIV transmission estimated to be less than 0.2% per contact (280). Several reports in the developed world indicate lower sexual transmission efficiency from a female infected index case than from a male, a characteristic seen with other sexually transmitted diseases (281,282). However, in the Rakai District of Uganda, transmission among serodiscordant couples was found to be equivalent for male and female index cases (283). Differences in male circumcision rates, or in other biologic factors, may account for these findings. The overall transmission among serodiscordant monogamous couples in the Rakai District was 0.11% per sexual act, a rate similar to developed countries (284).

Sexual behaviors that lead to contact with more virus increase the chance of transmission, which is likely responsible for the increased risk from anal sex and the decreased risk from oral sex, as compared with vaginal sex (285,286). Although sexual contact with fluid exchange is a necessary component of sexual HIV transmission, biologic factors of both host and virus may significantly alter transmission efficiency and play a substantial role in the dynamics of the HIV epidemic. In a multisite study of risk factors for HIV in high and low prevalence areas of sub-Saharan Africa, sexual behavior alone did not account for differences in regional HIV prevalence (287). Multiple risk factors for transmission have been identified, and these include:

1. Viral load: High viral load, seen among individuals either near the time of seroconversion or late in the disease when symptoms are present, increases the risk of HIV transmission. The amount of virus present in body tissues and fluids during sexual contact, which is usually proportional to viral load (288), probably contributes to this finding. In Uganda, Quinn et al. have demonstrated that viral load was the most important determinant of transmission among serodiscordant couples (283). These findings suggest a potential role for viral suppression through the use of antiretroviral agents to reduce sexual transmission, and there is some evidence of decreased transmission among those on therapy (289); however, this strategy is unlikely to be reliably effective (290) and evidence of HIV is still found in semen and cervical secretions of those on effective therapy (291,292).

2. Sexually transmitted diseases (STDs): STDs may act to enhance host infectiousness or to increase susceptibility to HIV by genital tract inflammation, which disrupts epithelial integrity and brings more susceptible cells in contact with infective secretions. Breaks in the integrity of the mucosal barrier (vaginal, oral, rectal) or of penile squamous epithelium facilitate HIV transmission to exposed persons. Increased risk of HIV transmission results from contact with more virus, either free virus or cell-associated virus in infective secretions (286,293). Local inflammation increases the numbers of all types of white blood cells in semen and may activate lymphocytes and macrophages to produce HIV (294). Thus, both STDs and other chronic infections may also increase HIV transmission indirectly through the recruitment of infected $CD4^+$ cells and the production of cytokines, which may elevate HIV levels in blood and bodily fluids (295,296). Data from both the developed and the developing world clearly document a greater risk of HIV seroconversion associated with prior or coexisting genital ulceration from chancroid, syphilis, or herpes simplex (297–300).

3. Viral subtype: HIV-1 group M virus has at least 10 known subtypes that circulate in different areas of the planet. Subtype B predominates in North America and Europe, subtypes A, D, C, and others predominate in Africa. There are potential differences in transmissibility and use of coreceptors among subtypes *in vitro* (122,123) and differences may exist in the response of subtypes to cytokine stimulation from co-infections (301). However, several subtypes have shown themselves capable of extremely high prevalence given the right conditions, and more epidemiologic work is needed to understand any true differences in transmissibility between subtypes.

4. Male circumcision: There is abundant evidence that male circumcision reduces risk of HIV infection. Multiple studies have demonstrated increased HIV risk (ranging from two- to eightfold) among uncircumcised men (302,303). The proposed mechanism for this protective effect is that the foreskin is lined by Langerhans cells, which contain $CD4^+$ and CCR5 receptors (304), and that it may be more prone to trauma during sex than the rest of the penis.

5. Immunologic or genetic factors: Failure to transmit HIV to longstanding sexual partners suggests that some hosts may be

minimally infectious or that their partners may be resistant to infection. Persons with certain HLA types may be less likely to acquire HIV and to progress to AIDS (273), and those homozygous for a deletion in the CCR5 coreceptor are relatively resistant to infection (140,305). Persons with poor immunologic control of HIV in early and late infection are probably more likely to transmit HIV because of the resulting elevation in viral load (283).

PARENTERAL TRANSMISSION

HIV is transmitted by both cell-free and cell-associated blood products. Before the institution of routine blood screening for HIV in the spring of 1985, substantial numbers of transfusion recipients and hemophiliacs were infected by HIV-contaminated blood products. Nearly 100% of transfusion recipients of HIV-contaminated blood exhibit seroconversion (306,307). Needle sharing among HIV-infected injection drug users is a particularly risky and efficient route of spread (308). It is estimated that one fourth of new HIV infections in the United States occur through injection drug use.

PERINATAL TRANSMISSION

Perinatal transmission causes almost all of the pediatric HIV infections in the world, and is common in areas with significant seroprevalence of HIV-1 among women of childbearing age. Untreated, HIV-1-infected women transmit infection to their infants at rates ranging from 13% to over 50% (309–311) but diagnosis is usually delayed because antibodies found in newborns do not distinguish between active infection and passively acquired maternal antibodies until after 12 to 15 months (312). Enzyme-linked immunosorbent assay (ELISA) p24 antigen testing, viral culture, and especially DNA PCR analysis are useful for earlier detection in infants. A positive PCR result in an infant should be confirmed with repeat testing, especially in the first month of life when small numbers of positive cells in a PCR assay might represent infected maternal cells carried over to the infant. Studies from the developing world suggest that HIV-infected infants are more likely to suffer from prematurity and low birth weight (313,314), and many die of AIDS within their first 2 years if untreated (315). Although few data are available, perinatal transmission of HIV-2 appears to be rare (316).

Among infants who were breast-fed for 18 to 24 months, approximately 20% to 25% of overall HIV perinatal transmission occurs in utero, 35% to 50% intrapartum, and 40% to 50% postpartum from breast feeding (317,318). Improved specificity of PCR testing at birth and in the first month of life have helped to establish the important role of intrapartum and postpartum transmission. Reported risk factors for in utero and intrapartum transmission include high maternal viral load (319,320); advanced maternal immunodeficiency, prolonged rupture of membranes, chorioamnionitis, and other obstetrical factors (321,322); and vitamin A deficiency (323). Duration of breast feeding (324), viral load (325), mastitis (326), and, potentially, mixed feeding rather than exclusive breast feeding (327) are reported risk factors for transmission through breast milk.

In 1994, ACTG 076 demonstrated that the administration of zidovudine to HIV-infected mothers for an extended period during pregnancy, delivery, and postpartum can reduce the rate of infection in infants by 67% (328). Since that time, shorter and less expensive zidovudine regimens have reduced in utero and intrapartum transmission by up to 50% in the developing world (329), and the HIVNET 012 trial in Uganda demonstrated 47% transmission reduction relative to very short-course zidovudine using a single pill of nevirapine to mothers during labor and to infants at birth (330). Since the advent of effective combination antiretroviral therapy used in pregnancy, perinatal trans-

mission rates have declined drastically in the developed world. Strong correlation exists between maternal viral load reduction and decreased perinatal transmission, although transmission has been documented even with undetectable viral loads (331,332).

Postpartum HIV transmission through breast milk remains a significant challenge for the developing world, where breast milk substitutes may not be appropriate, acceptable, or available for infant feeding. Breast feeding transmission may eliminate hard-won gains in transmission reduction from short-course antiretroviral programs. For example, in the PETRA study conducted in South Africa, Uganda, and Tanzania, transmission was reduced by up to 51% at 6 weeks postpartum through the use of peripartum antiretroviral agents, but this fell to only 21% at the end of 18 months because of breast feeding (333). Nduati et al. demonstrated that formula feeding significantly improved HIV-free infant survival compared to breast feeding in a randomized trial among women in Nairobi, Kenya with access to clean water (318). Exclusive breast feeding (rather than mixed feeding) with early weaning has also been promoted as a means to limit postpartum HIV transmission while allowing infants to derive the benefits of breast milk (327). The availability of safe water sources and breast milk substitutes, and regional data regarding infant mortality rates from diarrheal and respiratory diseases, must be factored into breast feeding decisions. Determining optimal strategies for feeding infants born to HIV-infected women in the developing world is an important scientific objective for the next decade.

Diagnosis and Prognosis of Infection with Human Immunodeficiency Virus Types 1 and 2

MARKERS OF ACQUIRED IMMUNODEFICIENCY SYNDROME PROGRESSION

The most useful clinical predictors of progression to AIDS are a decrease in the $CD4^+$ lymphocyte count and a decrease in the ratio of $CD4^+$ to $CD8^+$ cells (which is not dependent on leukocyte count and therefore varies less than the total $CD4^+$ cell count). Using a nonspecific indicator of immune stimulation—elevation in either β_2-microglobulin or neopterin—in conjunction with either of these markers further improves prediction of prognosis. Serum levels of immunoglobulin A, IL-2 receptor, and p24 antigen provide only scant additional information (334).

Plasma HIV RNA is a useful clinical marker that indicates both long-term prognosis and response to effective antiretroviral therapies. HIV RNA levels provide an important clinical indication of the speed of disease progression, with higher viral loads predictive of more rapid progression (257,335). A 10-year prospective study among injection drug users found that each increase of 1 log in the initial viral load after seroconversion increased the hazard ratio for progression to AIDS by 1.55 (95% confidence interval, 0.97 to 2.47) among men and 1.43 (95% confidence interval, 0.76 to 2.69) among women (336).

Although doing so is technically difficult, HIV-1 can be isolated from both cell-free plasma and peripheral blood mononuclear cells from most infected persons. Patients with Centers for Disease Control and Prevention stage 4 disease or with AIDS have 10 to 100 times greater levels of both plasma viremia (free virus) and cell-associated virus than do healthy HIV-seropositive persons (337). Viral titers *in vivo* are not closely linked to either p24 antibody or p24 antigen, both of which may be difficult to measure in circulating immune complexes (338). The titer of antibodies to p24 appears to follow a pattern reciprocal to that of p24 antigen. Levels of p24 antigen correlate with virus replication in vitro and in primary infection. Antibodies to p24 increase and remain high during latency, often in association with a drop in measurable free p24 antigen, and may fall as HIV symptoms develop and p24 antigenemia increases. Viral heterogeneity, circulating immune complexes, or other factors may underlie problems with use of currently available ELISAs as potential prognostic markers.

HIV-2–associated AIDS appears to have an immune profile comparable to that of HIV-1 AIDS—skin test anergy, diminishing CD4+ cell count, and elevated β_2-microglobulin and neopterin levels. In persons followed prospectively, HIV-2 infection appears to induce progressive decreases in CD4$^+$ lymphocytes, although less rapidly than does HIV-1 (19).

BIOMEDICAL PREVENTION AND CONTROL STRATEGIES AND PROSPECTS FOR HUMAN IMMUNODEFICIENCY VIRUS DISEASE

Approaches to Antiretroviral Therapy

Current HIV therapies aim to prevent HIV-related disease by attacking actively replicating virus and enhancing the host immune system. These strategies identify or target HIV-infected cells that express viral gene products within the cell or on its surface. Besides these approaches against already infected cells, strategies to protect uninfected cells from being infected by HIVs are also important. Characteristics of the ideal antiretroviral agent include high viral inhibitory activity with low toxicity during prolonged use and excellent penetration into lymphocytes, macrophages, the nervous system, and other immunologically privileged cells or tissues that may harbor virus. Future therapies will most likely use both antiviral agents and immunomodulators for long-term control of HIV infection.

Advances in combination chemotherapy have been responsible for dramatic declines in HIV-associated morbidity and mortality in the developed world (339). Optimal combinations of drugs and strategies with different mechanisms of action and synergistic anti-HIV effects are required not only to minimize toxicity but also to prevent the emergence of drug resistance. At present, no single antiviral agent has been demonstrated to prevent progression to AIDS except for brief periods. The major cause of the failure is the presence of viral mutant quasi species, which results in the growth of the clone that is resistant to that particular drug. Drug resistance mutations are specific to each of the major drug classes, and cross-resistance between the classes does not occur. Viral resistance testing through either genotyping or phenotyping, which are optimally used while a patient is receiving a failing regimen, can facilitate the selection of salvage therapy and lead to improved outcomes (340,341).

Antiretroviral Therapies

Antiretroviral agents can be classified into two major categories on the basis of their molecular weight. Agents with a low molecular weight include several enzyme inhibitors, peptides, or other compounds. These agents are usually administered as drugs and do not need a special delivery system. Another group of agents are molecules with higher molecular weight. These include recombinant proteins and nucleic acid derivatives. These agents may be administered as they are or delivered via special transfer techniques.

ENZYME INHIBITORS

Inhibitors of enzymes that are required for HIV replication control HIV infection by interfering at critical steps in the viral life cycle. Currently these represent the major group of antiviral drugs. Potential target enzymes are reverse transcriptase, protease, and integrase. The development of inhibitors of integrase is still in an early stage. The enzyme inhibitors that have successfully been developed into antiretroviral agents are reviewed in detail in Chapter 127, and include:

1. Nucleoside/nucleotide reverse transcriptase inhibitors: Nucleoside analogs, which are phosphorylated by cellular kinases, were the first class of antiretroviral agents developed and act to competitively inhibit viral reverse transcriptase and terminate DNA chain synthesis. Nucleotide reverse transcriptase inhibitors act in a similar manner as nucleoside analogs to inhibit reverse transcriptase, but have an abbreviated intracellular activation pathway allowing more rapid and complete conversion to the active agent. Nucleotide analogs may also generate a non-overlapping spectrum of resistance mutations with nucleoside analogs, and can therefore retain activity among patients heavily treated with nucleoside analogs.
2. Non-nucleoside reverse transcriptase inhibitors: The reverse transcriptase gene may also be inhibited by non-nucleoside inhibitors, which interact with a specific 'pocket' site of HIV-1 reverse transcriptase that is closely associated with, but distinct from, the nucleoside reverse transcriptase inhibitor binding site. When used in combination therapy, newer non-nucleoside agents have demonstrated similar potency to protease inhibitors but with fewer side effects (342). Resistance mutations to non-nucleoside agents often affect the entire class.
3. Protease inhibitors: HIV protease is another major target of enzyme inhibitors. The structure of protease was used to guide the development of these drugs, which prevent the cleavage of viral protease into a functional enzyme. Protease inhibitors do not require intracellular processing to become activated, and have activity against both HIV-1 and HIV-2. Drug-drug interactions are significant with this class of agents because of their extensive metabolism by the hepatic cytochrome P-450 complex (a property which has been used to advantage to boost drug levels through selective combination treatment), and metabolic and other side effects are associated with long-term usage.

THERAPEUTIC MACROMOLECULES

This group contains a broad range of molecules aimed at various steps of virus replication. Advances in knowledge of the HIV-1 life cycle and the introduction of the concept of intracellular immunization guided this approach (343). Candidate therapeutic molecules range from proteins to nucleic acids. Entry and fusion inhibitors are a promising group of agents, and drugs are in development to prevent the binding of gp120 to the CD4 molecule, to prevent binding of the protein envelope with the chemokine coreceptors (CCR5 or CXCR4), and to block the fusion of viral and cellular membranes. Fusion inhibitors are currently in clinical trials; an agent called T-20, which binds near the fusion domain of the viral envelope protein gp41 and prevents interactions with the cellular membrane, has demonstrated efficacy as part of a salvage antiretroviral regimen (344).

An approach of gene therapy can be utilized to transduce therapeutic trans-dominant negative mutants of viral genes, ribozymes, and antisense oligonucleotides into infected as well as uninfected target cells (345). Depending on the kind of molecules and the genes targeted, a variety of steps of virus replication can be attacked. Although some of the agents are quite effective in vitro, a major problem is the low efficiency of delivery and the difficulty of specific targeting to appropriate cell populations.

BIOLOGY OF HUMAN T-CELL LEUKEMIA VIRUS INFECTION

Pathogenesis of Adult T-Cell Leukemia/Lymphoma

Only a small fraction of HTLV-1 infections, perhaps 1% to 5%, lead to the development of adult T cell leukemia/lymphoma (ATL). Most of the estimates of HTLV disease outcome are based on southern Japan or the Caribbean, as these are the only geographical sites in the developed world with high prevalence rates of infection. ATL only develops decades after infection, with a mean onset at 50 years of age.

While HTLV-1 infection causes immortalization of T cells in most infected people, progression is infrequent. A stage-wise transformation occurs in a minority with "flower cells" and/or oligoclonal integration (346), but even this stage does not always progress to ATL.

When ATL develops, it is associated with monoclonal integration of HTLV-1 and rapid death. A minority of patients has smoldering, less aggressive disease. Hypercalcemia and skin lesions are often associated with ATL. Malignant T cells in ATL patients express high levels of the IL2 receptor due to autocrine stimulation, and granulocytosis and eosinophilia may occur from increased production of GM-CSF. ATL is sometimes difficult to distinguish from other T cell malignancies such as non-Hodgkin's lymphoma and T cell lymphocytic leukemia. Some HLA alleles have been associated with development of ATL, perhaps because of an inability to respond immunologically to Tax (347).

When ATL develops, the deregulation of T-helper cells can also result in immune compromise with opportunistic infections and other tumors similar to those seen in AIDS patients (348).

Pathogenesis of Tropical Spastic Paraparesis or Human T-Cell Leukemia Virus–Associated Myelopathy

As with ATL, only approximately 1% of HTLV-1 infected people develop TSP/HAM. Unlike ATL, TSP/HAM sometimes occurs within a few years after exposure to the virus. Individuals with TSP/HAM usually have higher copy numbers of HTLV DNA as compared to asymptomatic seropositive carriers (349,350). Patients may also have higher antibody titers (351), antibodies in cerebrospinal fluid (352), and immune complexes (353). TSP/HAM clearly has different mechanisms of pathogenesis than ATL. The clinical response of many TSP/HAM patients to steroid therapy is compatible with a mechanism of immune activation. The disease has also been associated with an interaction between the *tax* gene product and neurofilaments (354) as well as dysregulation of cytokine production (355). The *tax* gene of one subgroup of HTLV-1 (A), has been more frequently associated with TSP/HAM (356). The disease is manifested as a slowly progressive weakness, spasticity of the limbs, and incontinence.

Other Manifestations of Human T-Cell Leukemia Virus-1 Infection

One group has persistently claimed an association between HTLV-1 and certain other T-cell tumors, such as mycosis fungoides and cutaneous T-cell lymphoma, even though patients are usually seronegative for antibodies to HTLV structural protein antigens (192). Occasionally chronic lymphocytic leukemias of B-cell origin have been linked to HTLV-1, proposed to be related to activation of a B-cell clone responding to HTLV antigens (357). In addition to immunosuppression; rare cases of arthritis (358) and uveitis (359) have also been weakly associated with HTLV-1.

Various interactions between HTLV-1 and HIV-1 have been reported. These include upregulation of HTLV-1 by HIV-1 *tax* transactivation (360) and HTLV-1 Tax activation of CXCR4, the coreceptor of syncytia-inducing HIVs (361). However, one report observed no correlation between proviral loads of HTLV and HIV in individuals who were coinfected (362).

Human T-Cell Leukemia Virus-2

Although HTLV-2 was originally detected in a case of hairy cell leukemia, no convincing link has yet been made between infection and this or any other disease.

Epidemiology of Human T-Cell Leukemia Virus

The highest rates of HTLV-1 are found on the islands of southwestern Japan and on the Caribbean islands, such as Trinidad and Jamaica. Elevated rates also occur in the northwestern regions of South and Central America and in some regions of Africa. Because the infection causes disease and death in only a small fraction of those infected, prevalence increases with increasing age. In the United States, rates of HTLV-1 are highest in the southeastern part of the country, but even there, rates are much lower than in southwestern Japan. Indigenous Indian populations of both North and South America may have elevated rates of HTLV-1 or HTLV-2 (363). Within the United States and Europe, injection drug users (IDU) have the highest rates of HTLV infections, but it is usually with HTLV-1. Except for IDUs, rates of HTLV infection are low in Europe, especially in northern Europe where they are extremely low (209).

HTLVs are highly cell associated, and transmission occurs most effectively with HTLV-1 contaminated cell products. Noncellular blood products do not appear to cause transmission (364). Epithelial cells in milk of HTLV-1 positive women are often genome positive and such cells can presumably mediate transmission to breast-feeding infants (365).

Overall, transmission of HTLV-1 and HTLV-2 appears to occur by the same routes as for the HIVs: sexual contact, blood, and perinatal exposure. The major differences would appear to be that the HTLVs are not as efficiently transmitted in cell free blood products as is HIV, and mother to infant infections occur primarily by breast feeding in the case of the HTLVs. The significant risks for HIV-1 infection in utero and by passage through the birth canal do not appear to be present for the HTLVs. As with the HIVs, sexual transmission appears to be more efficient from the male partner for HTLV-1, and genome positive cells can be found in semen. There is some evidence that antibodies to the Tax protein may serve as indicators for risk of sexual transmission (366).

Diagnosis and Prognosis of Human T-Cell Leukemia Virus Infections

The screening of blood for the HTLVs has been in place for about 15 years in most developed countries. However, in some places where rates are very low only new donors are screened (367). Blood screening is usually done by assaying for antibodies to envelope antigens using recombinant proteins or peptides or in some instances whole disrupted virus. Since most tests are made with HTLV-1 only and cross-reactivity in the envelope proteins is not complete, a small fraction of HTLV-2 infected people will score as false negatives. Enzyme linked immunosorbent assays (ELISA) or agglutination tests are usually used for screening. Western blotting or PCR tests are usually used for confirmation.

A small percentage of HTLV 1 carriers who have antibodies to Tax may score negative for antibodies to structural proteins (368).

Because only a small number of HTLV-1 infected individuals develop disease, the prognosis of infection is usually good. Diagnosis of ATL or TSP/HAM usually indicates a very grave prognosis. Because HTLV-2 has not been associated with disease, infection with this virus should not be cause for great concern.

Prevention and Control of Human T-Cell Leukemia Virus Infection

Routine blood screening for HTLV has already resulted in substantial reductions in new infections for transfusion recipients. Pregnant women should also be screened in high incidence areas, and breastfeeding should be avoided when the woman is known to be HTLV-1 positive.

THERAPY

Once an individual is infected with HTLV-1 or HTLV-2, there is no known therapy that can rid the body of the virus. Although some antiretroviral drugs may control replication of the virus, their use seems unnecessary and inappropriate as virus replication rates are low (unlike HIV) and most infected individuals will not develop disease.

Most patients with ATL cannot be successfully treated. Occasionally patients have shown temporary remission when treated with interferons (369,370), selected chemotherapeutics (371, 372), or antibody to the IL 2 receptor (373). Patients with TSP/HAM have been treated with corticosteroids (374,375) and alpha-interferons (376) with variable results.

REFERENCES

1. Gross L. "Spontaneous" leukemia developing in C3H mice following inoculation in infancy with AK-leukemic extracts or A-K embryos. *Proc Soc Exp Biol Med* 1953;78:27.
2. Jarrett B, Crawford E, Martin WB, et al. Leukemias in the cat: a virus-like particle associated with leukemia (lymphosarcoma). *Nature* 1964;202:567.
3. Essex M. Horizontally and vertically transmitted oncornavirus of cats. *Adv Cancer Res* 1975;21:175–248.
4. Poiesz BJ, Ruscetti FW, Gazdar AF, et al. Detection and isolation of type C retrovirus particles from fresh and cultured lymphocytes of a patient with cutaneous T-cell lymphoma. *Proc Natl Acad Sci USA* 1980;77:7415–7419.
5. Takatsuki K, Uchiyama T, Sagawa K, et al. Adult T-cell leukemia in Japan. *Excerpta Med Int Congr Ser* 1977;415:73.
6. Hinuma Y, Nagata K, Hanaoka M, et al. Adult T-cell leukemia: antigen in an ATL cell line and detection of antibodies to the antigen in human sera. *Proc Natl Acad Sci USA* 1981;78:6476–6480.
7. Kalyanaraman VS, Sarngadharan MG, Robert-Guroff M, et al. A new subtype of human T-cell leukemia virus (HTLV-II) associated with a T-cell variant of hairy cell leukemia. *Science* 1982;218:571–573.
8. Gottlieb, M., Schroff R, Schanker HM, et al. Pneumocystis carinii pneumonia and mucosal candidiasis in previously healthy homosexual men: evidence of a new acquired cellular immunodeficiency. *N Engl J Med* 1981;305:1425–1431.
9. Francis, D.P., Curran JW, Essex M. Epidemic acquired immune deficiency syndrome: Epidemiologic evidence for a transmissible agent. *J Natl Cancer Inst* 1983;71:1–4.
10. Barre-Sinoussi F, Chermann JC, Rey F, et al. Isolation of a T-lymphotropic retrovirus from a patient at risk for acquired immune deficiency syndrome (AIDS). *Science* 1983;220:868–871.
11. Essex M, McLane MF, Lee TH, et al. Antibodies to cell membrane antigens associated with human T-cell leukemia virus in patients with AIDS. *Science* 1983;220:859–862.
12. Gelmann E, Popovic M, Blayney D, et al. Proviral DNA of a retrovirus, human T–cell leukemia virus, in two patients with AIDS. *Science* 1983;220:862–865.
13. Popovic M, Sarngadharan MG, Read E, et al. Detection, isolation, and continuous production of cytopathic retroviruses (HTLV-III) from patients with AIDS and pre-AIDS. *Science* 1984;224:497–500.
14. Gallo R, Salahuddin SZ, Popovic M, et al. Frequent detection and isolation of cytopathic retroviruses (HTLV-III) from patients with AIDS and at risk for AIDS. *Science* 1984;224:500–503.
15. Levy J, Hoffman AD, Kramer SM, et al. Isolation of lymphocytopathic retroviruses from San Francisco patients with AIDS. *Science* 1984;225:840–842.
16. Barin F, M'Boup S, Denis F, et al. Serological evidence for virus related to simian T-lymphotropic retrovirus III in residents of West Africa. *Lancet* 1985;2:1387–1389.
17. Kanki P, McLan MF, King NW Jr, et al. Serologic identification and characterization of a macaque T-lymphotropic retrovirus closely related to HTLV-III. *Science* 1985;228:1199–1201.
18. Romieu I, Marlink R, Kanki P, et al,. HIV-2 link to AIDS in West Africa. *J Acquir Immune Defic Syndr* 1990;3:220–230.
19. Marlink R, et al. Reduced rate of disease development after HIV-2 infection as compared to HIV-1. *Science* 1994;265:1587–1590.
20. Hunter E, et al. Family Retroviridae In: van Regenmortel MHV, et al, eds. *Virus taxonomy, VII report of the ICTV.* San Diego: Academic Press, 2000:369–387.
21. Coffin JM, Hughes SA, Varmus HE. Retroviruses. Cold Spring Harbor, NY: Cold Spring Laboratory Press, 1997.
22. Whitcomb JM, Hughes SH. Retroviral reverse transcription and integration: progress and problems. *Annu Rev Cell Biol* 1992;7:275–306.
23. Gottlinger HG. The HIV-1 assembly machine. *AIDS* 2001;15[Suppl 5]:S13–S20.
24. Garnier L, Bowzard JB, Wills JW. Recent advances and remaining problems in HIV assembly. *AIDS* 1998;12[Suppl A]:S5–S16.
25. Gottlinger HG, Sodroski JG, Haseltine WA. Role of capsid precursor processing and myristoylation in morphogenesis and infectivity of human immunodeficiency virus type 1. *Proc Natl Acad Sci USA* 1989;86(15):5781–5785.
26. Bryant M, Ratner L. Myristoylation-dependent replication and assembly of human immunodeficiency virus 1. *Proc Natl Acad Sci USA* 1990;87(2):523–527.
27. Pal R, et al. Myristoylation of gag proteins of HIV-1 plays an important role in virus assembly. *AIDS Res Hum Retroviruses* 1990;6(6):721–730.
28. Massiah MA, et al. Three-dimensional structure of the human immunodeficiency virus type 1 matrix protein. *J Mol Biol* 1994;244(2):198–223.
29. Matthews S, et al. Refined solution structure of p17, the HIV matrix protein. *Biochem Soc Trans* 1995;23(4):725–729.
30. Hill CP, et al. Crystal structures of the trimeric human immunodeficiency virus type 1 matrix protein: implications for membrane association and assembly. *Proc Natl Acad Sci USA* 1996;93(7):3099–3104.
31. Spearman P, et al. Membrane binding of human immunodeficiency virus type 1 matrix protein in vivo supports a conformational myristyl switch mechanism. *J Virol* 1997;71(9):6582–6592.
32. Hermida-Matsumoto L, Resh MD. Human immunodeficiency virus type 1 protease triggers a myristoyl switch that modulates membrane binding of Pr55(gag) and p17MA. *J Virol* 1999;73(3):1902–1908.
33. Paillart JC, Gottlinger HG. Opposing effects of human immunodeficiency virus type 1 matrix mutations support a myristyl switch model of gag membrane targeting. *J Virol* 1999;73(4):2604–2612.
34. Gitti RK, et al. Structure of the amino-terminal core domain of the HIV-1 capsid protein. *Science* 1996;273(5272):231–235.
35. Momany C, et al. Crystal structure of dimeric HIV-1 capsid protein. *Nat Struct Biol* 1996;3(9):763–770.
36. Gamble TR, et al. Structure of the carboxyl-terminal dimerization domain of the HIV-1 capsid protein. *Science* 1997;278(5339):849–853.
37. Dorfman T, et al. Functional domains of the capsid protein of human immunodeficiency virus type 1. *J Virol* 1994;68(12):8180–8187.
38. Borsetti A, Ohagen A, Gottlinger HG. The C-terminal half of the human immunodeficiency virus type 1 Gag precursor is sufficient for efficient particle assembly. *J Virol* 1998;72(11):9313–9317.
39. Mammano F, et al. Role of the major homology region of human immunodeficiency virus type 1 in virion morphogenesis. *J Virol* 1994;68(8):4927–4936.
40. Erickson JW, Gulnik SV, Markowitz M. Protease inhibitors: resistance, cross-resistance, fitness and the choice of initial and salvage therapies. *AIDS* 1999;13[Suppl A]:S189–S204.
41. Miller V. Resistance to protease inhibitors. *J Acquir Immune Defic Syndr* 2001;26[Suppl 1]:S34–S50.
42. Shafer RW, et al. A Guide to HIV-1 reverse transcriptase and protease sequencing for drug resistance studies. In: Kuiken C, et al, eds. *HIV Sequence Compendium 2001.* Los Alamos, NM: Theoretical Biology and Biophysics, Los Alamos National Laboratory; 2001:1–51.
43. Chan DC, et al. Core structure of gp41 from the HIV envelope glycoprotein. *Vaccine* 1997;89(2):263–73.
44. Earl PL, Doms RW, Moss B. Oligomeric structure of the human immunodeficiency virus type 1 envelope glycoprotein. *Proc Natl Acad Sci USA* 1990;87(2):648–652.
45. Lu M, Blacklow SC, Kim PS. A trimeric structural domain of the HIV-1 transmembrane glycoprotein. *Nat Struct Biol* 1995;2(12):1075–1082.
46. Weissenhorn W, et al. Atomic structure of the ectodomain from HIV-1 gp41. *Nature* 1997;387(6631):426–430.

47. Karn J. Tat, a novel regulator of HIV transcription and latency. In: Kuiken C, et al, eds. *HIV Sequence Compendium 2001*. Los Alamos, NM: Theoretical Biology and Biophysics, Los Alamos National Laboratory; 2000: 2–18.

48. Cullen BR. HIV-1 auxiliary proteins: making connections in a dying cell. *Cell* 1998;93:685–692.

49. Coffin J. Retroviridae and their replication. In: Fields B, ed. *Virology*. New York: Raven, 1990:1437–1500.

50. Aiken C, et al. Nef induces CD4 endocytosis: requirement for a critical dileucine motif in the membrane-proximal CD4 cytoplasmic domain. *Cell* 1994;76:853–864.

51. Bandres JC, Shaw AS, Ratner L. HIV-1 Nef protein downregulation of CD4 surface expression: relevance of the lck binding domain of CD4. *Virology* 1995;207:338–341.

52. Gottlinger HG, et al. Vpu protein of human immunodeficiency virus type 1 enhances the release of capsids produced by gag gene constructs of widely divergent retroviruses. *Proc Natl Acad Sci USA* 1993;90(15):7381–7385.

53. Walker CM, et al. CD8+ lymphocytes can control HIV infection in vitro by suppressing virus replication. *Science* 1986;234(4783):1563–1566.

54. Walker BD, et al. HIV-specific cytotoxic T lymphocytes in seropositive individuals. *Nature* 1987;328(6128):345–348.

55. Cocchi F, et al. Identification of RANTES, MIP-1 alpha, and MIP-1 beta as the major HIV-suppressive factors produced by CD8+ T cells. *Science* 1995;270(5243):1811–1815.

56. Baier M, et al. HIV suppression by interleukin-16. *Nature* 1995;378(6557):563.

57. Plata F, et al. AIDS virus-specific cytotoxic T lymphocytes in lung disorders. *Nature* 1987;328(6128):348–351.

58. Borrow P, et al. Virus-specific CD8+ cytotoxic T-lymphocyte activity associated with control of viremia in primary human immunodeficiency virus type 1 infection. *J Virol* 1994;68:6103–6110.

59. Koup RA, et al. Temporal association of cellular immune responses with the initial control of viremia in primary human immunodeficiency virus type 1 syndrome. *J Virol* 1994;68:4650–4655.

60. Altfeld M, et al. Cellular immune responses and viral diversity in individuals treated during acute and early HIV-1 infection. *J Exp Med* 2001;193(2):169–180.

61. Pantaleo G, et al. Major expansion of CD8+ T cells with a predominant V beta usage during the primary immune response to HIV. *Nature* 1994;370:463–467.

62. Ogg GS, et al. Quantitation of HIV-1–specific cytotoxic T lymphocytes and plasma load of viral RNA. *Science* 1998;279:2103–2106.

63. Goulder PJ, et al. Substantial differences in specificity of HIV-specific cytotoxic T cells in acute and chronic HIV infection. *J Exp Med* 2001;193(2):181–194.

64. Klein MR, et al. Kinetics of Gag-specific cytotoxic T lymphocyte responses during the clinical course of HIV-1 infection: a longitudinal analysis of rapid progressors and long-term asymptomatics. *J Exp Med* 1995;181(4):1365–1372.

65. Pantaleo G, et al. Studies in subjects with long-term nonprogressive human immunodeficiency virus infection. *N Engl J Med* 1995;332(4):209–216.

66. Rinaldo C, et al. High levels of anti-human immunodeficiency virus type 1 (HIV-1) memory cytotoxic T-lymphocyte activity and low viral load are associated with lack of disease in HIV-1 infected long-term nonprogressors. *J Virol* 1995;69:5838–5842.

67. Harrer T, et al. Strong cytotoxic T cell and weak neutralizing antibody responses in a subset of persons with stable nonprogressing HIV type 1 infection. *AIDS Res Hum Retroviruses* 1996;12(7):585–592.

68. Langlade-Demoyen P, et al. Human immunodeficiency virus (HIV) nef-specific cytotoxic T lymphocytes in noninfected heterosexual contact of HIV-infected patients. *J Clin Invest* 1994;93(3):1293–1297.

69. Rowland-Jones S, et al. HIV-specific cytotoxic T-cells in HIV-exposed but uninfected Gambian women. *Nat Med* 1995;1:59–64.

70. Rowland-Jones SL, et al. Cytotoxic T cell responses to multiple conserved HIV epitopes in HIV-resistant prostitutes in Nairobi. *J Clin Invest* 1998;102(9):1758–1765.

71. Lucchiari-Hartz M, et al. Human immune response to HIV-1 Nef. II. Induction of HIV-1/HIV-2 Nef cross-reactive cytotoxic T lymphocytes in peripheral blood lymphocytes of non-infected healthy individuals. *Int Immunol* 1996;8(4):577–584.

72. Bernard NF, et al. Human immunodeficiency virus (HIV)-specific cytotoxic T lymphocyte activity in HIV-exposed seronegative persons. *J Infect Dis* 1999;179(3):538–547.

73. Trask SA, et al. Molecular epidemiology of human immunodeficiency virus type 1 transmission in a heterosexual cohort of discordant couples in Zambia. *J Virol* 2002;76(1):397–405.

74. McMichael AJ, Rowland-Jones SL. Cellular immune responses to HIV. *Nature* 2001;410(6831):980–987.

75. Abbas AK, Lichtman AH, Pober JS. *Cellular and molecular immunology*, 4th ed. Philadelphia: WB Saunders, 2000:–.

76. Ridge JP, Di Rosa F, Matzinger P. A conditioned dendritic cell can be a temporal bridge between a CD4+ T-helper and a T-killer cell. *Nature* 1998;393(6684):474–478.

77. Walter EA, et al. Reconstitution of cellular immunity against cytomegalovirus in recipients of allogeneic bone marrow by transfer of T-cell clones from the donor. *N Engl J Med* 1995;333(16):1038–1044.

78. Zajac AJ, et al. Viral immune evasion due to persistence of activated T cells without effector function. *J Exp Med* 1998;188(12):2205–2213.

79. Parren PW, et al. The neutralizing antibody response to HIV-1: viral evasion and escape from humoral immunity. *AIDS* 1999;13[Suppl A]:S137–S162.

80. Poignard P, Klasse PJ, Sattentau QJ. Antibody neutralization of HIV-1. *Immunol Today* 1996;17(5):239–246.

81. Alkhatib G, et al. CC CKR5: a RANTES, MIP-1alpha, MIP-1beta receptor as a fusion cofactor for macrophage-tropic HIV-1. *Science* 1996;272(5270):1955–1958.

82. Dragic T, et al. HIV-1 entry into CD4+ cells is mediated by the chemokine receptor CC-CKR-5. *Nature* 1996;381(6584):667–673.

83. Feng Y, et al. HIV-1 entry cofactor: functional cDNA cloning of a seven transmembrane, G protein-coupled receptor. *Science* 1996;272:872–877.

84. Kowalski M, et al. Functional regions of the envelope glycoprotein of human immunodeficiency virus type 1. *Science* 1987;237(4820):1351–1355.

85. Trkola A, et al. CD4-dependent, antibody-sensitive interactions between HIV-1 and its co-receptor CCR-5. *Nature* 1996;384(6605):184–187.

86. Wu L, et al. CD4-induced interaction of primary HIV-1 gp120 glycoproteins with the chemokine receptor CCR-5. *Nature* 1996;384(6605):179–183.

87. Albert J, et al. Rapid development of isolate-specific neutralizing antibodies after primary HIV-1 infection and consequent emergence of virus variants which resist neutralization by autologous sera. *AIDS* 1990.;4(2):107–112.

88. Arendrup M, et al. Autologous HIV-1 neutralizing antibodies: emergence of neutralization-resistant escape virus and subsequent development of escape virus neutralizing antibodies. *J Acquir Immune Defic Syndr* 1992;5(3):303–307.

89. Bradney AP, et al. Neutralization escape in human immunodeficiency virus type 1-infected long-term nonprogressors. *J Infect Dis* 1999;179(5):1264–1267.

90. Graham BS. Serological responses to candidate AIDS vaccines. *AIDS Res Hum Retroviruses* 1994;10[Suppl 2]:S145–S148.

91. Moog C, et al. Autologous and heterologous neutralizing antibody responses following initial seroconversion in human immunodeficiency virus type 1-infected individuals. *J Virol* 1997;71(5):3734–3741.

92. Mulligan MJ, Weber J. Human trials of HIV-1 vaccines. *AIDS* 1999; 13[Suppl A]:S105–S112.

93. Pilgrim AK, et al. Neutralizing antibody responses to human immunodeficiency virus type 1 in primary infection and long-term-nonprogressive infection. *J Infect Dis* 1997;176(4):924–932.

94. Bures R, et al. Immunization with recombinant canarypox vectors expressing membrane-anchored glycoprotein 120 followed by glycoprotein 160 boosting fails to generate antibodies that neutralize R5 primary isolates of human immunodeficiency virus type 1. *AIDS Res Hum Retroviruses* 2000;16(18):2019–2035.

95. Mascola JR, et al. Immunization with envelope subunit vaccine products elicits neutralizing antibodies against laboratory-adapted but not primary isolates of human immunodeficiency virus type 1. The National Institute of Allergy and Infectious Diseases AIDS Vaccine Evaluation Group. *J Infect Dis* 1996;173(2):340–348.

96. Walker BD. Immune reconstitution and immunotherapy in HIV infection. Available at: *www.medscape.com/Medscape/HIV/ClinicalMgmt/CM.v15/CM.v15/public/CM.v15-toc.html* Accessed 2001.

97. Lieberman J, et al. Dressed to kill? A review of why antiviral CD8 T lymphocytes fail to prevent progressive immunodeficiency in HIV-1 infection. *Blood* 2001;98(6):1667–1677.

98. Zhang YJ, Moore JP. Will multiple coreceptors need to be targeted by inhibitors of human immunodeficiency virus type 1 entry? *J Virol* 1999;73(4):3443–3448.

99. Zhang Y, et al. Use of inhibitors to evaluate coreceptor usage by simian and simian/human immunodeficiency viruses and human immunodeficiency virus type 2 in primary cells. *J Virol* 2000;74(15):6893–6910.

100. Cormier EG, Dragic T. An overview of HIV-1 co-receptor function and its inhibitors. In: Kuiken C, et al, eds. *HIV sequence compendium 2000*. Los Alamos, NM: Theoretical Biology and Biophysics, Los Alamos National Laboratory; 2000:19–34.

101. Berger EA, et al. A new classification for HIV-1 [letter]. *Nature* 1998; 391(6664):240.

102. Doms RW, Moore JP. HIV-1 coreceptor use: a molecular window into viral tropism. In: Korber B, et al, eds. *HIV molecular immunology database*. Los Alamos, NM: Los Alamos National Laboratory: Theoretical Biology and Biophysics; 1997:III-1–III-12.

103. Dragic T. An overview of the determinants of CCR5 and CXCR4 co–receptor function. *J Gen Virol* 2001;82(Pt 8):1807–1814.

104. Cormier EG, et al. Mapping the determinants of the CCR5 amino-terminal sulfopeptide interaction with soluble human immunodeficiency virus type 1 gp120-CD4 complexes. *J Virol* 2001;75(12):5541–5549.

105. Foley BT. An overview of the molecular phylogeny of lentiviruses. In: Kuiken C, et al, eds. *HIV sequence compendium 2000*. Los Alamos, NM: Theoretical Biology and Biophysics, Los Alamos National Laboratory; 2000:35–43.

106. Korber B, et al. Timing the ancestor of the HIV-1 pandemic strains. *Science* 2000;288(5472):1789–1796.

107. Turner BG, Summers M. Structural biology of HIV. *J Mol Biol* 1999;285(1):1–32.

108. Hahn BH, et al. AIDS as a zoonosis: scientific and public health implications. *Science* 2000;287(5453):607–614.

109. Peeters M, et al. Isolation and partial characterization of an HIV-related virus occurring naturally in chimpanzees in Gabon. *AIDS* 1989;3(10):625–630.

110. Gao F, et al. Human infection by genetically diverse SIVSM-related HIV-2 in west Africa. *Nature* 1992;358(6386):495–499.

111. Hirsch VM, et al. An African primate lentivirus (SIVsm) closely related to HIV-2. *Nature* 1989;339(6223):389–392.

112. Robertson DL, et al. HIV-1 nomenclature proposal. *Science* 2000;288(5463):55–56.

113. Esparza J, Bhamarapravati N. Accelerating the development and future availability of HIV-1 vaccines: why, when, where, and how? *Lancet* 2000;355(9220):2061–2066.

114. Osmanov S, et al. Estimated global distribution and regional spread of HIV-1 genetic subtypes in the year 2000. *J Acquir Immune Defic Syndr Hum Retrovirol* 2002;29(2):184–190.

115. UNAIDS and WHO. Global HIV/AIDS and STD surveillance. Epidemiological fact sheets by country. Available at: *www.who.int/emc-hiv/fact_sheets/*. Accessed 2000.

116. UNAIDS. AIDS epidemic update. December 2001. Available at: *www.unaids.org/worldaidsday/2001/Epiupdate2001/Epiupdate2001_en.pdf* Accessed 2001.

117. Renjifo B, et al. Differences in perinatal transmission among human immunodeficiency virus type 1 genotypes. *J Hum Virol* 2001;4(1):16–25.

118. Neilson JR, et al. Subtypes of human immunodeficiency virus type 1 and disease stage among women in Nairobi, Kenya. *J Virol* 1999;73(5):4393–4403.

119. Novitsky VA, et al. Molecular cloning and phylogenetic analysis of HIV-1 subtype C: a set of 23 full-length clones from Botswana. *J Virol* 1999;73(5):4427–4432.

120. van Harmelen J, et al. Characterization of full length HIV-1 subtype C sequences from South Africa. *AIDS Res Hum Retroviruses* 2001;17(16):1527–1531.

121. Choudhury S, et al. Increased promoter diversity reveals a complex phylogeny of human immunodeficiency virus type 1 subtype C in India. *J Hum Virol* 2000;3(1):35–43.

122. Peeters M, et al. Evidence for differences in MT2 cell tropism according to genetic subtypes of HIV-1: syncytium-inducing variants seem rare among subtype C HIV-1 viruses. *J Acquir Immune Defic Syndr Hum Retrovirol* 1999;20(2):115–121.

123. Tscherning C, et al. Differences in chemokine coreceptor usage between genetic subtypes of HIV-1. *Virology* 1998;241(2):181–188.

124. Björnal Å et al. Phenotypic characteristics of human immunodeficiency virus type 1 subtype c isolates of Ethiopian AIDS patients. *Aids Research Hum Retroviruses* 1999;15(7):647–653.

125. Abebe A, et al. HIV-1 subtype C syncytium- and non-syncytium–inducing phenotypes and coreceptor usage among Ethiopian patients with AIDS. *AIDS* 1999;13(11):1305–1311.

126. Salminen MO, et al. Full-length sequence of an Ethiopian human immunodeficiency virus type 1 (HIV-1) isolate of genetic subtype C. *AIDS Res Hum Retroviruses* 1996;12(14):1329–1339.

127. Gao F, et al. A comprehensive panel of near-full-length clones and reference sequences for non-subtype B isolates of human immunodeficiency virus type 1. *J Virol* 1998;72(7):5680–5698.

128. Rodenburg CM, et al. Near full-length clones and reference sequences for subtype C isolates of HIV type 1 from three different continents. *AIDS Res Hum Retroviruses* 2001;17(2):161–168.

129. Betts MR, et al. Cross-class human immunodeficiency virus (HIV)–specific cytotoxic T-lymphocyte responses in HIV-infected Zambians. *J Virol* 1997;71(11):8908–8911.

130. Cao H, et al. Cytotoxic T—lymphocyte cross-reactivity among different human immunodeficiency virus type 1 clades: implications for vaccine development. *J Virol* 1997;71(11):8615–8623.

131. Durali D, et al. Cross-reactions between the cytotoxic T-lymphocyte responses of human immunodeficiency virus-infected African and European patients. *J Virol* 1998;72(5):3547–3553.

132. McAdam S, et al. Cross-clade recognition of p55 by cytotoxic T lymphocytes in HIV-1 infection. *AIDS* 1998;12:571–579.

133. Wilson SE, et al. Cross-clade envelope glycoprotein 160–specific CD8+ cytotoxic T lymphocyte responses in early HIV type 1 clade B infection. *AIDS Res Hum Retroviruses* 1998;14(11):925–937.

134. Cao H, et al. Cellular immunity to human immunodeficiency virus type 1 (HIV-1) clades: relevance to HIV-1 vaccine trials in Uganda. *J Infect Dis* 2000;182(5):1350–1356.

135. Dorrell L, et al. Distinct recognition of non-clade B human immunodeficiency virus type 1 epitopes by cytotoxic T lymphocytes generated from donors infected in Africa. *J Virol* 1999;73(2):1708–1714.

136. Peeters M. Recombinant HIV sequences: their role in the global epidemic. In: Kuiken C, et al, eds. *HIV sequence compendium 2000*. Los Alamos, NM: Theoretical Biology and Biophysics, Los Alamos National Laboratory; 2000:54–72.

137. Carr JK, et al. Reference sequences representing the principal genetic diversity of HIV-1 in the pandemic. In: Korber B, et al, eds. *Human Retroviruses and AIDS 1998*. Los Alamos, NM: Theoretical Biology and Biophysics, Group T-10, Los Alamos National Laboratory: 1998:III-10–III-19.

138. Carrington M, Nelson G, O'Brien SJ. Considering genetic profiles in functional studies of immune responsiveness to HIV-1. *Immunol Lett* 2001;79(1-2):131–140.

139. Dean M, et al. Genetic restriction of HIV-1 infection and progression to AIDS by a deletion allele of the CKR5 structural gene. Hemophilia Growth and Development Study, Multicenter AIDS Cohort Study, Multicenter Hemophilia Cohort Study, San Francisco City Cohort, ALIVE Study. *Science* 1996;273(5283):1856–1862.

140. Liu R, et al. Homozygous defect in HIV-1 coreceptor accounts for resistance of some multiply-exposed individuals to HIV-1 infection. *Cell* 1996;86(3):367–377.

141. Samson M, et al. Resistance to HIV-1 infection in caucasian individuals bearing mutant alleles of the CCR-5 chemokine receptor gene. *Nature* 1996;382(6593):722–725.

142. Winkler C, et al. Genetic restriction of AIDS pathogenesis by an SDF-1 chemokine gene variant. ALIVE Study, Hemophilia Growth and Development Study (HGDS), Multicenter AIDS Cohort Study (MACS), Multicenter Hemophilia Cohort Study (MHCS), San Francisco City Cohort (SFCC). *Science* 1998;279(5349):389–393.

143. Fiorentino DF, Bond MW, Mosmann TR. Two types of mouse T helper cell. IV. Th2 clones secrete a factor that inhibits cytokine production by Th1 clones. *J Exp Med* 1989;170(6):2081–2095.

144. Fiorentino DF, et al. IL-10 inhibits cytokine production by activated macrophages. *J Immunol* 1991;147(11):3815–3822.

145. Crawley E, et al. Polymorphic haplotypes of the interleukin-10 5′ flanking region determine variable interleukin-10 transcription and are associated with particular phenotypes of juvenile rheumatoid arthritis. *Arthritis Rheum* 1999;42(6):1101–1108.

146. Carrington M, et al. HLA and HIV-1: heterozygote advantage and B*35-Cw*04 disadvantage. *Science* 1999;283(5408):1748–1752.

147. Goulder PJ, et al. Late escape from an immunodominant cytotoxic T-lymphocyte response associated with progression to AIDS. *Nat Med* 1997;3:212–217.

148. Migueles SA, et al. HLA B*5701 is highly associated with restriction of virus replication in a subgroup of HIV-infected long term nonprogressors. *Proc Natl Acad Sci USA* 2000;97(6):2709–2714.

149. Phillips RE, et al. Human immunodeficiency virus genetic variation that can escape cytotoxic T cell recognition. *Nature* 1991;354(6353):453–459.

150. Hendel H, et al. New class I and II HLA alleles strongly associated with opposite patterns of progression to AIDS. *J Immunol* 1999;162(11):6942–6946.

151. Paxton WA, et al. Reduced HIV-1 infectability of CD4+ lymphocytes from exposed-uninfected individuals: association with low expression of CCR5 and high production of beta-chemokines. *Virology* 1998;244(1):66–73.

152. Xiao L, et al. Adaptation to promiscuous usage of CC and CXC-chemokine coreceptors in vivo correlates with HIV-1 disease progression. *AIDS* 1998;12(13):F137–F143.

153. Liu H, et al. Polymorphism in RANTES chemokine promoter affects HIV–1 disease progression. *Proc Natl Acad Sci USA* 1999;96(8):4581–4585.

154. Matsuyama T, Nobuyuki K, Yamamoto N. Cytokines and HIV infection: is AIDS a tumor necrosis factor disease? *AIDS* 1991;5:1405–1417.

155. Duh EJ, et al. Tumor necrosis factor alpha activates human immunodeficiency virus type 1 through induction of nuclear factor binding to the NF-kappa B sites in the long terminal repeat. *Proc Natl Acad Sci USA* 1989;86(15):5974–5978.

156. Brinkman BM, et al. Polymorphisms within the human tumor necrosis factor-alpha promoter region in human immunodeficiency virus type 1-seropositive persons. *J Infect Dis* 1997;175(1):188–190.

157. Jacob CO, et al. Heritable major histocompatibility complex class II-associated differences in production of tumor necrosis factor alpha: relevance to genetic predisposition to systemic lupus erythematosus. *Proc Natl Acad Sci USA* 1990;87(3):1233–1237.

158. Abraham LJ, French MA, Dawkins RL. Polymorphic MHC ancestral haplotypes affect the activity of tumour necrosis factor-alpha. *Clin Exp Immunol* 1993;92(1):14–18.

159. Bendtzen K, et al. Association between HLA-DR2 and production of tumour necrosis factor alpha and interleukin 1 by mononuclear cells activated by lipopolysaccharide. *Scand J Immunol* 1988;28(5):599–606.

160. Janssen RS, et al. New testing strategy to detect early HIV-1 infection for use in incidence estimates and for clinical and prevention purposes. *JAMA* 1998;280(1):42–48.

161. Parekh BS, et al. Quantitative detection of increasing HIV type 1 antibodies after seroconversion: a simple assay for detecting recent HIV infection and estimating incidence. *AIDS Res Hum Retroviruses* 2002;18(4):295–307.

162. Allen TM, Watkins DI. New insights into evaluating effective T-cell responses to HIV. *AIDS* 2001;15[Suppl 5]:S117–S126.

163. Hirsch MS, et al. Antiretroviral drug resistance testing in adults with HIV infection: implications for clinical management. International AIDS Society—USA Panel. *JAMA* 1998;279(24):1984–1991.

164. Hirsch MS, et al. Antiretroviral drug resistance testing in adult HIV-1 infection: recommendations of an International AIDS Society—USA Panel. *JAMA* 2000;283(18):2417–2426.

165. Schwartz DH, et al. Induction of HIV-1–neutralising and syncytium-inhibiting antibodies in uninfected recipients of HIV-1IIIB rgp120 subunit vaccine. *Lancet* 1993;342(8863):69–73.

166. Berman PW, et al. Human immunodeficiency virus type 1 challenge of chimpanzees immunized with recombinant envelope glycoprotein gp120. *Proc Natl Acad Sci USA* 1988;85(14):5200–5204.

167. Binley JM, et al. A recombinant human immunodeficiency virus type 1 envelope glycoprotein complex stabilized by an intermolecular disulfide bond between the gp120 and gp41 subunits is an antigenic mimic of the trimeric virion-associated structure. *J Virol* 2000;74(2):627–643.

168. Yang X, et al. Modifications that stabilize human immunodeficiency virus envelope glycoprotein trimers in solution. *J Virol* 2000;74(10):4746–4754.

169. Novitsky V, et al. HIV-1 subtype C molecular phylogeny: consensus sequence for an AIDS vaccine design? *J Virol* 2002;76(11):5435–5451.

170. Gaschen B, et al. Diversity considerations in HIV-1 vaccine selection. *Science* 2002;296(5577):2354–2360.

171. Iwasaki A, et al. Enhanced CTL responses mediated by plasmid DNA immunogens encoding costimulatory molecules and cytokines. *J Immunol* 1997;158(10):4591–4601.

172. Barouch DH, et al. Control of viremia and prevention of clinical AIDS in rhesus monkeys by cytokine-augmented DNA vaccination. *Science* 2000;290(5491):486–492.

173. Barouch DH, et al. Augmentation of immune responses to HIV-1 and simian immunodeficiency virus DNA vaccines by IL-2/Ig plasmid administration in rhesus monkeys. *Proc Natl Acad Sci USA* 2000;97(8):4192–4197.

174. O'Hagan DT, MacKichan ML, Singh M. Recent developments in adjuvants for vaccines against infectious diseases. *Biomol Eng* 2001;18(3):69–85.

175. Reitter JN, Desrosiers RC. Identification of replication-competent strains of simian immunodeficiency virus lacking multiple attachment sites for N-linked carbohydrates in variable regions 1 and 2 of the surface envelope protein. *J Virol* 1998;72(7):5399–5407.

176. Cherpelis S, et al. DNA vaccination with the human immunodeficiency virus type 1 SF162DeltaV2 envelope elicits immune responses that offer partial protection from simian/human immunodeficiency virus infection to CD8(+) T-cell-depleted rhesus macaques. *J Virol* 2001;75(3):1547–1550.

177. Devico A, et al. Covalently crosslinked complexes of human immunodeficiency virus type 1 (HIV-1) gp120 and CD4 receptor elicit a neutralizing immune response that includes antibodies selective for primary virus isolates. *Virology* 1996;18(1):258–263.

178. Cafaro A, et al. Control of SHIV-89.6P-infection of cynomolgus monkeys by HIV-1 Tat protein vaccine. *Nat Med* 1999;5(6):643–650.

179. Pauza CD, et al. Vaccination with tat toxoid attenuates disease in simian/HIV-challenged macaques. *Proc Natl Acad Sci USA* 2000;97(7):3515–3519.

180. Shiver JW, et al. Replication-incompetent adenoviral vaccine vector elicits effective anti-immunodeficiency-virus immunity. *Nature* 2002;415(6869):331–335.

181. Johnson JM, Harrod R, Franchini G. Molecular biology and pathogenesis of the human T-cell leukaemia/lymphotropic virus type-1 (HTLV-1). *Int J Exp Pathol* 2001;82(3):135–147.

182. Ootsuyama Y, et al. Myristylation of gag protein in human T-cell leukemia virus type-I and type-II. *Jpn J Cancer Res* 1985;76(12):1132–1135.

183. Le Blanc I, Rosenberg AR, Dokhelar MC. Multiple functions for the basic amino acids of the human T-cell leukemia virus type 1 matrix protein in viral transmission. *J Virol* 1999;73(3):1860–1867.

184. Christensen AM, et al. Three-dimensional structure of the HTLV-II matrix protein and comparative analysis of matrix proteins from the different classes of pathogenic human retroviruses. *J Mol Biol* 1996;264(5):1117–1131.

185. Le Blanc I, et al. HTLV-1 structural proteins. *Virus Res* 2001;78(1-2):5–16.

186. Khorasanizadeh S, Campos-Olivas R, Summers MF. Solution structure of the capsid protein from the human T-cell leukemia virus type-I. *J Mol Biol* 1999;291(2):491–505.

187. Nam SH, et al. Characterization of ribosomal frameshifting for expression of pol gene products of human T-cell leukemia virus type I. *J Virol* 1993;67(1):196–203.

188. Sagara Y, et al. HTLV type 1 envelope glycoprotein gp46 evokes necrosis by binding to receptor complex. *AIDS Res Hum Retroviruses* 2000;16(16):1701–1704.

189. Poon B, Chen IS. Identification of a domain within the human T-cell leukemia virus type 2 envelope required for syncytium induction and replication. *J Virol* 1998;72(3):1959–1966.

190. Cullen BR. Mechanism of action of regulatory proteins encoded by complex retroviruses. *Microbiol Rev* 1992;56:375–394.

191. Yokota T, Chou MJ, Tachibana N, et al. The prevalence of antibody to p42 of HTLV-I among ATLL patients in comparison with healthy carriers in Japan. *Int J Cancer* 1989;43:970–974.

192. Pancake B, Wassef EH, Zucker-Franklin D. Demonstration of antibodies to human T-cell lymphotropic virus-I tax in patients with the cutaneous T-cell lymphoma, mycosis fungoides, who are seronegative for antibodies to the structural proteins of the virus. *Blood* 1996;88(8):3004–3009.

193. Hadlock K, Rowe J, Foung SK. The humoral immune response to human T-cell lymphotropic virus type 1 envelope glycoprotein gp46 is directed primarily against conformational epitopes. *J Virol* 1999;73(3):1205–1212.

194. Tajima Y, Tashiro K, Camerini D. Assignment of the possible HTLV receptor gene to chromosome 17q21-q23. *Somat Cell Mol Genet* 1997;23(3):225–227.

195. Sommerfelt M, Williams BP, Clapham PR, et al. Human T cell leukemia viruses use a receptor determined by human chromosome 17. *Science* 1988;242:1557–1559.

196. Richardson J, Edwards AJ, Cruickshank JK, et al. In vivo cellular tropism of human T-cell leukemia virus type 1. *J Virol* 1990;64:5682–5687.

197. Ijichi S, Ramundo MB, Takahashi H, Hall WW. In vivo cellular tropism of human T-cell leukemia virus type II (HTLV-II). *J Exp Med* 1992;176:293–296.

198. Vandamme A, Liu HF, Van Brussel M, De Meurichy W, Desmyter J, Goubau P. The presence of a divergent T-lymphotropic virus in a wild-caught pygmy chimpanzee (*Pan paniscus*) supports an African origin for the human T-lymphotropic/simian T-lymphotropic group of viruses. *J Gen Virol* 1996;77:1089–1099.

199. Slattery J, Franchini G, Gessain A. Genomic evolution, patterns of global dissemination, and interspecies transmission of human and simian T-cell leukemia/lymphotropic viruses. *Genome Res* 1999;9(6):525–540.

200. Pise-Masison C, Mahieux R, Radonovich M, et al. Insights into the molecular mechanism of p53 inhibition by HTLV type 1 Tax. *AIDS Res Hum Retroviruses* 2000;16(16):1669–1675.

201. Ross T, Pettiford SM, Green PL. The tax gene of human T-cell leukemia virus type 2 is essential for transformation of human T lymphocytes. *J Virol* 1996;70(8):5194–5202.

202. Zehender G, Girotto M, De Maddalena C, Francisco G, Moroni M, Galli M. HTLV infection in ELISA-negative blood donors. *AIDS Res Hum Retroviruses* 1996;12(8):737–740.

203. Belec L, Jean Georges A, Hallouin MC, Si Mohamed A, Morand-Joubert L, Georges-Courbot MC. Human T-lymphotropic virus type I excretion and specific antibody response in paired saliva and cervicovaginal secretions. *AIDS Res Hum Retroviruses* 1996;12(2):157–167.

204. Kataoka R, Takehara N, Iwahara Y, et al. Transmission of HTLV-1 blood transfusion and its prevention by passive immunization. *Blood* 1990;76:1657–1661.

205. Spear GT, et al. Decreased oxidative burst activity of monocytes from asymptomatic HIV-infected individuals. *Clin Immunol Immunopathol* 1990.;54(2):184–191.

206. Smith PD, et al. Monocyte function in the acquired immune deficiency syndrome. Defective chemotaxis. *J Clin Invest* 1984;74(6):2121–2128.

207. Pennington JE, et al. Effect of intravenous recombinant gamma-interferon on the respiratory burst of blood monocytes from patients with AIDS. *J Infect Dis* 1986;153(3):609–612.

208. Poli G, et al. Monocyte function in intravenous drug abusers with lymphadenopathy syndrome and in patients with acquired immunodeficiency syndrome: selective impairment of chemotaxis. *Clin Exp Immunol* 1985;62(1):136–142.

209. Seroepidemiology of the human T-cell leukaemia/lymphoma viruses in Europe. The HTLV European Research Network. *J Acquir Immune Defic Syndr Hum Retrovirol* 1996;13(1):68–77.

210. Hirsch MS, Curran J. Human immunodeficiency viruses. In: Fields KD, ed. *Fields virology*, 2nd ed. New York: Raven, 1990:1545–1570.

211. Lane HC, et al. Abnormalities of B-cell activation and immunoregulation in patients with the acquired immunodeficiency syndrome. *N Engl J Med* 1983;309(8):453–458.

212. Pahwa SG, et al. Defective B-lymphocyte function in homosexual men in relation to the acquired immunodeficiency syndrome. *Ann Intern Med* 1984;101(6):757–763.

213. Redfield RR, Wright DC, Tramont EC. The Walter Reed staging classification for HTLV-III/LAV infection. *N Engl J Med* 1986;314(2):131–132.

214. Ammann AJ, et al. B-cell immunodeficiency in acquired immune deficiency syndrome. *JAMA* 1984;251(11):1447–1449.

215. Polsky B, et al. Bacterial pneumonia in patients with the acquired immunodeficiency syndrome. *Ann Intern Med* 1986;104(1):38–41.

216. Piot P, et al. AIDS: an international perspective. *Science* 1988;239(4840):573–579.

217. Quinn TC, et al. Serologic and immunologic studies in patients with AIDS in North America and Africa. The potential role of infectious agents as cofactors in human immunodeficiency virus infection. *JAMA* 1987;257(19):2617–2621.

218. Marlink RG, Essex M. Africa and the biology of human immunodeficiency virus. *JAMA* 1987;257(19):2632–2633.

219. Clavel F, et al. Human immunodeficiency virus type 2 infection associated with AIDS in West Africa. *N Engl J Med* 1987;316(19):1180–1185.

220. Naucler A, et al. HIV-2–associated AIDS and HIV-2 seroprevalence in Bissau, Guinea-Bissau. *J Acquir Immune Defic Syndr* 1989;2(1):88–93.

221. Wei X, et al. Viral dynamics in human immunodeficiency virus type 1 infection. *Nature* 1995;373(6510):117–122.

222. Ho DD, et al. Rapid turnover of plasma virions and CD4 lymphocytes in HIV-1 infection. *Nature* 1995;373(6510):123–126.

223. Fisher AG, et al. Infectious mutants of HTLV-III with changes in the 3′ region and markedly reduced cytopathic effects. *Science* 1986;233(4764):655–659.

224. Hoxie JA, et al. Alterations in T4 (CD4) protein and mRNA synthesis in cells infected with HIV. *Science* 1986;234(4780):1123–1127.

225. Narayan O, Kennedy-Stoskopf S, Zink MC. Lentivirus-host interactions: lessons from visna and caprine arthritis-encephalitis viruses. *Ann Neurol* 1988;23[Suppl]:S95–S100.

226. Lyerly HK, et al. Human T-cell lymphotropic virus IIIB glycoprotein (gp120) bound to CD4 determinants on normal lymphocytes and expressed by infected cells serves as target for immune attack. *Proc Natl Acad Sci USA* 1987;84(13):4601–4605.

227. Fauci AS. The human immunodeficiency virus: infectivity and mechanisms of pathogenesis. *Science* 1988;239(4840):617–622.

228. Schnittman SM, et al. Evidence for susceptibility of intrathymic T-cell precursors and their progeny carrying T-cell antigen receptor phenotypes TCR alpha beta + and TCR gamma delta + to human immunodeficiency virus infection:

a mechanism for CD4+ (T4) lymphocyte depletion. *Proc Natl Acad Sci USA* 1990;87(19):7727–7731.

229. Pantaleo G, Graziosi C, Fauci AS. New concepts in the immunopathogenesis of human immunodeficiency virus infection. *N Engl J Med* 1993;328(5):327–335.

230. Amadori A, et al. CD4 epitope masking by gp120/anti-gp120 antibody complexes. A potential mechanism for CD4+ cell function down-regulation in AIDS patients. *J Immunol* 1992;148(9):2709–2716.

231. Gendelman HE, et al. Efficient isolation and propagation of human immunodeficiency virus on recombinant colony-stimulating factor 1–treated monocytes. *J Exp Med* 1988;167(4):1428–1441.

232. Klatzmann D, et al. Selective tropism of lymphadenopathy associated virus (LAV) for helper-inducer T lymphocytes. *Science* 1984;225(4657):59–63.

233. Folks TM, et al. Infection and replication of HIV-1 in purified progenitor cells of normal human bone marrow. *Science* 1988;242(4880):919–922.

234. Kahn JO, Walker BD. Acute human immunodeficiency virus type 1 infection. *N Engl J Med* 1998;339(1):33–39.

235. Nelbock P, et al. A cDNA for a protein that interacts with the human immunodeficiency virus Tat transactivator. *Science* 1990;248(4963):1650–1653.

236. Blauvelt A. The role of skin dendritic cells in the initiation of human immunodeficiency virus infection. *Am J Med* 1997;102(5B):16–20.

237. Rowland-Jones SL. HIV: the deadly passenger in dendritic cells. *Curr Biol* 1999;9(7):R248–R250.

238. Grouard G, Clark EA. Role of dendritic and follicular dendritic cells in HIV infection and pathogenesis. *Curr Opin Immunol* 1997;9(4):563–567.

239. Pope M. Mucosal dendritic cells and immunodeficiency viruses. *J Infect Dis* 1999;179[Suppl 3]:S427–S430.

240. Nakagawa M, et al. Nationwide survey of neurologic manifestations of acquired immunodeficiency syndrome in Japan. *Intern Med* 1997;36(3):175–178.

241. Simpson DM, Tagliati M. Neurologic manifestations of HIV infection. *Ann Intern Med* 1994;121(10):769–785.

242. Budka H. Neuropathology of human immunodeficiency virus infection. *Brain Pathol* 1991;1(3):163–175.

243. Wiley CA, et al. Distribution of brain HIV load in AIDS. *Brain Pathol* 1998;8(2):277–284.

244. Petito CK, et al. Neuropathology of acquired immunodeficiency syndrome (AIDS): an autopsy review. *J Neuropathol Exp Neurol* 1986;45(6):635–646.

245. Lantos PL, et al. Neuropathology of the brain in HIV infection. *Lancet* 1989;1(8633):309–311.

246. Koenig S, et al. Detection of AIDS virus in macrophages in brain tissue from AIDS patients with encephalopathy. *Science* 1986;233(4768):1089–1093.

247. Nuovo GJ, et al. In situ detection of polymerase chain reaction-amplified HIV-1 nucleic acids and tumor necrosis factor-alpha RNA in the central nervous system. *Am J Pathol* 1994;144(4):659–666.

248. Wiley CA, et al. Cellular localization of human immunodeficiency virus infection within the brains of acquired immune deficiency syndrome patients. *Proc Natl Acad Sci USA* 1986;83(18):7089–7093.

249. Ho DD, Rota TR, Hirsch MS. Infection of monocyte/macrophages by human T lymphotropic virus type III. *J Clin Invest* 1986;77(5):1712–1715.

250. Sethi KK, Naher H, Stroehmann I. Phenotypic heterogeneity of cerebrospinal fluid–derived HIV-specific and HLA-restricted cytotoxic T-cell clones. *Nature* 1988;335(6186):178–181.

251. Brenneman DE, et al. Neuronal cell killing by the envelope protein of HIV and its prevention by vasoactive intestinal peptide. *Nature* 1988;335(6191):639–642.

252. Sidtis JJ, et al. Zidovudine treatment of the AIDS dementia complex: results of a placebo-controlled trial. AIDS Clinical Trials Group. *Ann Neurol* 1993;33(4):343–349.

253. Schacker T, et al. Clinical and epidemiologic features of primary HIV infection. *Ann Intern Med* 1996;125(4):257–264.

254. Tindall B, Cooper DA. Primary HIV infection: host responses and intervention strategies. *AIDS* 1991;5(1):1–14.

255. Ridzon R, et al. Simultaneous transmission of human immunodeficiency virus and hepatitis C virus from a needle-stick injury. *N Engl J Med* 1997;336(13):919–922.

256. Stein DS, Korvick JA, Vermund SA. CD4+ lymphocyte cell enumeration for prediction of clinical course of human immunodeficiency virus disease: a review. *J Infect Dis* 1992;165(2):352–363.

257. Lyles RH, et al. Natural history of human immunodeficiency virus type 1 viremia after seroconversion and proximal to AIDS in a large cohort of homosexual men. Multicenter AIDS Cohort Study. *J Infect Dis* 2000;181(3):872–880.

258. Schacker TW, et al. Biological and virologic characteristics of primary HIV infection. *Ann Intern Med* 1998;128(8):613–620.

259. Mellors JW, et al. Prognosis in HIV-1 infection predicted by the quantity of virus in plasma. *Science* 1996;272(5265):1167–1170.

260. Farzadegan H, et al. Loss of human immunodeficiency virus type 1 (HIV-1) antibodies with evidence of viral infection in asymptomatic homosexual men. A report from the Multicenter AIDS Cohort Study. *Ann Intern Med* 1988;108(6):785–790.

261. Loche M, Mach B. Identification of HIV-infected seronegative individuals by

a direct diagnostic test based on hybridisation to amplified viral DNA. *Lancet* 1988;2(8608):418–421.

262. Imagawa DT, et al. Human immunodeficiency virus type 1 infection in homosexual men who remain seronegative for prolonged periods. *N Engl J Med* 1989;320(22):1458–1462.

263. Kaul R, et al. HIV-1–specific mucosal CD8+ lymphocyte responses in the cervix of HIV-1– resistant prostitutes in Nairobi. *J Immunol* 2000;164(3):1602–1611.

264. Rutherford GW, et al. Course of HIV-I infection in a cohort of homosexual and bisexual men: an 11 year follow up study. *BMJ* 1990;301(6762):1183–1188.

265. Hessol NA, et al. Progression of human immunodeficiency virus type 1 (HIV-1) infection among homosexual men in hepatitis B vaccine trial cohorts in Amsterdam, New York City, and San Francisco, 1978–1991. *Am J Epidemiol* 1994;139(11):1077–1087.

266. Lang W, et al. Patterns of T lymphocyte changes with human immunodeficiency virus infection: from seroconversion to the development of AIDS. *J Acquir Immune Defic Syndr* 1989;2(1):63–69.

267. Hughes MD, et al. Within-subject variation in CD4 lymphocyte count in asymptomatic human immunodeficiency virus infection: implications for patient monitoring. *J Infect Dis* 1994;169(1):28–36.

268. Leroy V, et al. Four years of natural history of HIV-1 infection in african women: a prospective cohort study in Kigali (Rwanda), 1988–1993. *J Acquir Immune Defic Syndr Hum Retrovirol* 1995;9(4):415–421.

269. Mann JM, et al. Natural history of human immunodeficiency virus infection in Zaire. *Lancet* 1986;2(8509):707–709.

270. Morgan D, et al. Progression to symptomatic disease in people infected with HIV-1 in rural Uganda: prospective cohort study. *BMJ* 2002;324(7331):193–197.

271. Grant AD, Djomand G, De Cock KM. Natural history and spectrum of disease in adults with HIV/AIDS in Africa. *AIDS* 1997;11[Suppl B]:S43–S54.

272. Rogers MF, et al. Acquired immunodeficiency syndrome in children: report of the Centers for Disease Control National Surveillance, 1982 to 1985. *Pediatrics* 1987;79(6):1008–1014.

273. Kaslow RA, McNicholl JM. Genetic determinants of HIV-1 infection and its manifestations. *Proc Assoc Am Physicians* 1999;111(4):299–307.

274. Kanki PJ, et al. Human immunodeficiency virus type 1 subtypes differ in disease progression. *J Infect Dis* 1999;179(1):68–73.

275. Moseson M, et al. The potential role of nutritional factors in the induction of immunologic abnormalities in HIV-positive homosexual men. *J Acquir Immune Defic Syndr* 1989;2(3):235–247.

276. Gendelman HE, et al. Trans-activation of the human immunodeficiency virus long terminal repeat sequence by DNA viruses. *Proc Natl Acad Sci USA* 1986;83(24):9759–9763.

277. Cao Y, et al. Virologic and immunologic characterization of long-term survivors of human immunodeficiency virus type 1 infection. *N Engl J Med* 1995;332(4):201–208.

278. Andersson S, et al. Plasma viral load in HIV-1 and HIV-2 singly and dually infected individuals in Guinea-Bissau, West Africa: significantly lower plasma virus set point in HIV-2 infection than in HIV-1 infection. *Arch Intern Med* 2000;160(21):3286–3293.

279. UNAIDS. Report on the global HIV/AIDS epidemic. June 2000. 2000, Joint United Nations Programme on HIV/AIDS.

280. Peterman TA, et al. Risk of human immunodeficiency virus transmission from heterosexual adults with transfusion-associated infections. *JAMA* 1988;259(1):55–58.

281. Holmberg SD, et al. Biologic factors in the sexual transmission of human immunodeficiency virus. *J Infect Dis* 1989;160(1):116–125.

282. Johnson AM. Heterosexual transmission of human immunodeficiency virus. *BMJ* 1988;296(6628):1017–1020.

283. Quinn TC, et al. Viral load and heterosexual transmission of human immunodeficiency virus type 1. Rakai Project Study Group. *N Engl J Med* 2000;342(13):921–929.

284. Gray RH, et al. Probability of HIV-1 transmission per coital act in monogamous, heterosexual, HIV-1–discordant couples in Rakai, Uganda. *Lancet* 2001;357(9263):1149–1153.

285. Samuel MC, et al. Factors associated with human immunodeficiency virus seroconversion in homosexual men in three San Francisco cohort studies, 1984–1989. *J Acquir Immune Defic Syndr* 1993;6(3):303–312.

286. Padian NS, Shiboski SC, Jewell NP. The effect of number of exposures on the risk of heterosexual HIV transmission. *J Infect Dis* 1990;161(5):883–887.

287. Ferry B, et al. Comparison of key parameters of sexual behaviour in four African urban populations with different levels of HIV infection. *AIDS* 2001;15[Suppl 4]:S41–S50.

288. Merigan TC. Use of PCR to measure HIV viral changes in drug-resistant genes in genital fluids. *J Reprod Immunol* 1998;41(1-2):177–185.

289. Musicco M, et al. Antiretroviral treatment of men infected with human immunodeficiency virus type 1 reduces the incidence of heterosexual transmission. Italian Study Group on HIV Heterosexual Transmission. *Arch Intern Med* 1994;154(17):1971–1976.

290. Haase AT, Schacker TW. Potential for the transmission of HIV-1 despite highly active antiretroviral therapy. *N Engl J Med* 1998;339(25):1846–1848.

291. Zhang H, et al. Human immunodeficiency virus type 1 in the semen of men receiving highly active antiretroviral therapy. *N Engl J Med* 1998;339(25):1803–1809.

292. Rasheed S, et al. Presence of cell-free human immunodeficiency virus in cervicovaginal secretions is independent of viral load in the blood of human immunodeficiency virus-infected women. *Am J Obstet Gynecol* 1996;175(1):122–129.

293. Kreiss JK, et al. AIDS virus infection in Nairobi prostitutes. Spread of the epidemic to East Africa. *N Engl J Med* 1986;314(7):414–418.

294. Wolff H, Anderson DJ. Male genital tract inflammation associated with increased numbers of potential human immunodeficiency virus host cells in semen. *Andrologia* 1988;20(5):404–410.

295. Nkengasong JN, et al. Human immunodeficiency virus type 1 (HIV-1) plasma virus load and markers of immune activation among HIV-infected female sex workers with sexually transmitted diseases in Abidjan, Cote d'Ivoire. *J Infect Dis* 2001;183(9):1405–1408.

296. Rotchford K, Strum AW, Wilkinson D. Effect of coinfection with STDs and of STD treatment on HIV shedding in genital-tract secretions: systematic review and data synthesis. *Sex Transm Dis* 2000;27(5):243–248.

297. Cameron DW, et al. Female to male transmission of human immunodeficiency virus type 1: risk factors for seroconversion in men. *Lancet* 1989;2(8660):403–407.

298. Simonsen JN, et al. Human immunodeficiency virus infection among men with sexually transmitted diseases. Experience from a center in Africa. *N Engl J Med* 1988;319(5):274–278.

299. Holmberg SD, et al. Prior herpes simplex virus type 2 infection as a risk factor for HIV infection. *JAMA* 1988;259(7):1048–1050.

300. Wald A, Link K. Risk of human immunodeficiency virus infection in herpes simplex virus type 2–seropositive persons: a meta-analysis. *J Infect Dis* 2002;185(1):45–52.

301. Montano MA, et al. Elevated tumor necrosis factor-alpha activation of human immunodeficiency virus type 1 subtype C in Southern Africa is associated with an NF-kappaB enhancer gain-of-function. *J Infect Dis* 2000;181(1):76–81.

302. Halperin DT, Bailey RC. Male circumcision and HIV infection: 10 years and counting. *Lancet* 1999;354(9192):1813–1815.

303. Moses S, Nagelkerke NJ, Blanchard J. Analysis of the scientific literature on male circumcision and risk for HIV infection. *Int J STD AIDS* 1999;10(9):626–628.

304. Szabo R, Short RV. How does male circumcision protect against HIV infection? *BMJ* 2000;320(7249):1592–1594.

305. Paxton WA, et al. Relative resistance to HIV-1 infection of CD4 lymphocytes from persons who remain uninfected despite multiple high-risk sexual exposure. *Nat Med* 1996;2(4):412–417.

306. Anderson KC, et al. Transfusion-acquired human immunodeficiency virus infection among immunocompromised persons. *Ann Intern Med* 1986;105(4):519–527.

307. Ward JW, et al. Risk of human immunodeficiency virus infection from blood donors who later developed the acquired immunodeficiency syndrome. *Ann Intern Med* 1987;106(1):61–62.

308. Chaisson RE, et al. Human immunodeficiency virus infection in heterosexual intravenous drug users in San Francisco. *Am J Public Health* 1987;77(2):169–72.

309. Blanche S, et al. A prospective study of infants born to women seropositive for human immunodeficiency virus type 1. HIV Infection in Newborns French Collaborative Study Group. *N Engl J Med* 1989;320(25):1643–1648.

310. Ryder RW, et al. Perinatal transmission of the human immunodeficiency virus type 1 to infants of seropositive women in Zaire. *N Engl J Med* 1989;320(25):1637–1642.

311. Hira SK, et al. Perinatal transmission of HIV-1 in Zambia. *BMJ* 1989;299(6710):1250–1252.

312. Pyun KH, et al. Perinatal infection with human immunodeficiency virus. Specific antibody responses by the neonate. *N Engl J Med* 1987;317(10):611–614.

313. Coley JL, et al. The association between maternal HIV-1 infection and pregnancy outcomes in Dar es Salaam, Tanzania. *BJOG* 2001;108(11):1125–1133.

314. Temmerman M, et al. Maternal human immunodeficiency virus-1 infection and pregnancy outcome. *Obstet Gynecol* 1994;83(4):495–501.

315. Lallemant M, et al. Mother-child transmission of HIV-1 and infant survival in Brazzaville, Congo. *AIDS* 1989;3(10):643–646.

316. Adjorlolo-Johnson G, et al. Prospective comparison of mother-to-child transmission of HIV-1 and HIV-2 in Abidjan, Ivory Coast. *JAMA* 1994;272(6):462–466.

317. De Cock KM, et al. Prevention of mother-to-child HIV transmission in resource-poor countries: translating research into policy and practice. *JAMA* 2000;283(9):1175–1182.

318. Nduati R, et al. Effect of breastfeeding and formula feeding on transmission of HIV-1: a randomized clinical trial. *JAMA* 2000;283(9):1167–1174.

319. Mofenson LM, et al. Risk factors for perinatal transmission of human immunodeficiency virus type 1 in women treated with zidovudine. Pediatric AIDS Clinical Trials Group Study 185 Team. *N Engl J Med* 1999;341(6):385–393.

320. Garcia PM, et al. Maternal levels of plasma human immunodeficiency virus type 1 RNA and the risk of perinatal transmission. Women and Infants Transmission Study Group. *N Engl J Med* 1999;341(6):394–402.

321. Landesman SH, et al. Obstetrical factors and the transmission of human immunodeficiency virus type 1 from mother to child. The Women and Infants Transmission Study. *N Engl J Med* 1996;334(25):1617–1623.

322. Zorrilla CD. Obstetric factors and mother-to-infant transmission of HIV-1. *Infect Dis Clin North Am* 1997;11(1):109–118.

323. Semba RD, et al. Maternal vitamin A deficiency and mother-to-child transmission of HIV-1. *Lancet* 1994;343(8913):1593–1597.

324. Nduati RW, et al. Human immunodeficiency virus type 1–infected cells in breast milk: association with immunosuppression and vitamin A deficiency. *J Infect Dis* 1995;172:1461–1468.

325. John GC, et al. Correlates of mother-to-child human immunodeficiency virus type 1 (HIV-1) transmission: association with maternal plasma HIV-1 RNA load, genital HIV-1 DNA shedding, and breast infections. *J Infect Dis* 2001;183(2):206–212.

326. Semba RD, et al. Human immunodeficiency virus load in breast milk, mastitis, and mother-to-child transmission of human immunodeficiency virus type 1. *J Infect Dis* 1999;180(1):93–98.

327. Coutsoudis A, et al. Influence of infant-feeding patterns on early mother-to-child transmission of HIV-1 in Durban, South Africa: a prospective cohort study. South African Vitamin A Study Group. *Lancet* 1999;354(9177):471–476.

328. Connor EM, et al. Reduction of maternal-infant transmission of human immunodeficiency virus type 1 with zidovudine treatment. Pediatric AIDS Clinical Trials Group Protocol 076 Study Group. *N Engl J Med* 1994;331(18):1173–1180.

329. Shaffer N, et al. Short-course zidovudine for perinatal HIV-1 transmission in Bangkok, Thailand: a randomised controlled trial. Bangkok Collaborative Perinatal HIV Transmission Study Group. *Lancet* 1999;353(9155):773–780.

330. Guay LA, et al. Intrapartum and neonatal single-dose nevirapine compared with zidovudine for prevention of mother-to-child transmission of HIV-1 in Kampala, Uganda: HIVNET 012 randomised trial. *Lancet* 1999;354(9181):795–802.

331. Contopoulos-Ioannidis DG, Ioannidis JP. Maternal cell-free viremia in the natural history of perinatal HIV-1 transmission: a meta-analysis. *J Acquir Immune Defic Syndr Hum Retrovirol* 1998;18(2):126–135.

332. Cao Y, et al. Maternal HIV-1 viral load and vertical transmission of infection: the Ariel project for the prevention of HIV transmission from mother to infant. *Nat Med* 1997;3(5):549–552.

333. Gray G. The PETRA study: early and late efficacy of three short ZDV/3TC combination regimens to prevent mother-to-child transmission of HIV-1 (LbOr5). In: 13th International AIDS Conference, 2000. Durban, South Africa.

334. Fahey JL, et al. The prognostic value of cellular and serologic markers in infection with human immunodeficiency virus type 1. *N Engl J Med* 1990;322(3):166–172.

335. Mellors JW, et al. Plasma viral load and CD4+ lymphocytes as prognostic markers of HIV-1 infection. *Ann Intern Med* 1997;126(12):946–954.

336. Sterling TR, et al. Initial plasma HIV-1 RNA levels and progression to AIDS in women and men. *N Engl J Med* 2001;344(10):720–725.

337. Ho DD, Moudgil T, Alam M. Quantitation of human immunodeficiency virus type 1 in the blood of infected persons. *N Engl J Med* 1989;321(24):1621–1625.

338. Allain JP, et al. Long-term evaluation of HIV antigen and antibodies to p24 and gp41 in patients with hemophilia. Potential clinical importance. *N Engl J Med* 1987;317(18):1114–1121.

339. Marschner IC, et al. Use of changes in plasma levels of human immunodeficiency virus type 1 RNA to assess the clinical benefit of antiretroviral therapy. *J Infect Dis* 1998;177(1):40–47.

340. Tural C, et al. Clinical utility of HIV-1 genotyping and expert advice: the Havana trial. *AIDS* 2002;16(2):209–218.

341. Clevenbergh P, et al. Persisting long-term benefit of genotype-guided treatment for HIV-infected patients failing HAART. The Viradapt study: week 48 follow-up. *Antivir Ther* 2000;5(1):65–70.

342. Staszewski S, et al. Efavirenz plus zidovudine and lamivudine, efavirenz plus indinavir, and indinavir plus zidovudine and lamivudine in the treatment of HIV-1 infection in adults. Study 006 team. *N Engl J Med* 1999;341(25):1865–1873.

343. Baltimore D. Gene therapy. Intracellular immunization. *Nature* 1988;335(6189):395–396.

344. Lalezari J, et al. Forty eight week analysis of patients receiving T-20 as a component of multidrug salvage therapy. Abstract LbPp116. In: XIII International AIDS Conference; July 9–14, 2000. 2000. Durban, South Africa.

345. Morgan RA, Anderson WF. Human gene therapy. *Annu Rev Biochem* 1993;62:191–217.

346. Cavrois M, Wain-Hobson S, Gessain A, Plumelle Y, Wattel E. Adult T-cell leukemia/lymphoma on a background of clonally expanding human T-cell leukemia virus type-1-positive cells. *Blood* 1996;88(12):4646–4650.

347. Yashiki S, Fujiyoshi T, Arima N, et al. HLA-A*26, HLA-B*4002, HLA-B*4006, and HLA-B*4801 alleles predispose to adult T cell leukemia: the limited recognition of HTLV type 1 tax peptide anchor motifs and epitopes to generate anti-HTLV type 1 tax CD8(+) cytotoxic T lymphocytes. *AIDS Res Hum Retroviruses* 2001;17(11):1047–1061.

348. Kozuru M, Uike N, Muta K, Goto T, Suehiro Y, Nagano M. High occurrence of primary malignant neoplasms in patients with adult T-cell leukemia/lymphoma, their siblings, and their mothers. *Cancer* 1996;78(5):1119–1124.

349. Bhagavati S, Ehrlich G, Kula RW, et al. Detection of human T-cell lymphoma/leukemia virus type I DNA and antigen in spinal fluid and blood

of patients with chronic progressive myelopathy. *N Engl J Med* 1988;318:1141–1147.

350. Nagai M, Usuku K, Matsumoto W, et al. Analysis of HTLV-I proviral load in 202 HAM/TSP patients and 243 asymptomatic HTLV-I carriers: high proviral load strongly predisposes to HAM/TSP. *J Neurovirol* 1998;4:586–593.

351. Osame M, Usuku K, Izumo S, et al. HTLV-I associated myelopathy, a new clinical entity. *Lancet* 1986;1:1031–1032.

352. Osame M, Igata A, Matsumoto M, et al. HTLV-1 associated myelopathy: a report of 85 cases. *Ann Neurol* 1987;22:116.

353. Shimada K, Koh CS, Yanagisawa N, et al. Anti-lymphocyte antibodies and circulating immune complexes in the sera of patients with myelopathy associated with human T lymphotropic virus type-I. *Neuroimmunology* 1993;42:161–166.

354. Reddy T, Li X, Jones Y, Ellisman MH, Ching GY, Liem RK, Wong-Staal F. Specific interaction of HTLV tax protein and a human type IV neuronal intermediate filament protein. *Proc Natl Acad Sci USA* 1998;95(2):702–707.

355. Wrzesinski S, Seguin R, Liu Y, et al. HTLV type 1 tax transduction in microglial cells and astrocytes by lentiviral vectors. *AIDS Res Hum Retroviruses* 2000;16(16):1771–1776.

356. Furukawa Y, Yamashita M, Usuku K, Izumo S, Nakagawa M, Osame M. Phylogenetic subgroups of human T cell lymphotropic virus (HTLV) type I in the tax gene and their association with different risks for HTLV-I–associated myelopathy/tropical spastic paraparesis. *J Infect Dis* 2000;182(5):1343–1349.

357. Mann K, DeSantis P, Mark G, et al. HTLV-I–associated B-cell CLL: indirect role for retrovirus in leukemogenesis. *Science* 1987;236:1103–1106.

358. Sato K, Maruyama I, Maruyama Y, et al. Arthritis in patients infected with human T lymphotropic virus type I. Clinical and immunopathologic features. *Arthritis Rheum* 1991;34:714–721.

359. Mochizuki M, Ono A, Ikeda E, et al. HTLV-I uveitis. *J AIDS Hum Retroviruses* 1996;13[suppl]:50–56.

360. Szabo J, Beck Z, Csoman E, et al. Differential patterns of interaction between HIV type 1 and HTLV type I in moncyte-derived macrophages cultured in vitro: implications for in vivo coinfection with HIV type I and HTLV type I. *AIDS Res Hum Retroviruses* 1999;15(18):1653–1666.

361. Moriuchi M, Moriuchi H, Fauci AS. HTLV type I tax activation of the CXCR4 promoter by association with nuclear respiratory factor 1. *AIDS Res Hum Retroviruses* 1999;15(9):821–827.

362. Cesaire R, Dehee A, Lezin A, et al. Quantification of HTLV type I and HIV type I DNA load in coinfected patients: HIV type 1 infection does not alter HTLV type I proviral amount in the peripheral blood compartment. *AIDS Res Hum Retroviruses* 2001;17(9):799–805.

363. Fujiyoshi T, Li HC, Lou H, et al. Characteristic distribution of HTLV type I and HTLV type II carriers among native ethnic groups in South America. *AIDS Res Hum Retroviruses* 1999;15(14):1235–1239.

364. Lairmore M, Jason JM, Hartley TM, et al. Absence of human T-cell lymphotropic virus type I coinfection in human immunodeficiency virus–infected hemophilic men. *Blood* 1989;74:2596–2599.

365. Southern S, Southern PJ. Persistent HTLV-I infection of breast luminal epithelial cells: a role in HTLV transmission? *Virology* 1998;241(2):200–214.

366. Chen Y, Okayama A, Lee TH, Tachibana N, Mueller N, Essex M: Sexual transmission of human T-cell leukemia virus type I associated with the presence of anti-tax antibody. *Proc Natl Acad Sci USA* 1991;88:1182–1186.

367. Tynell E, Andersson S, Lithander E, et al. Screening for human T cell leukaemia/lymphoma virus among blood donors in Sweden. Cost effectiveness analysis. *BMJ* 1998;316:1417–1422.

368. Zucker-Franklin D, Pancake BA, Marmor M, Legler PM. Reexamination of human T cell lymphotropic virus (HTLV-I/II) prevalence. *Proc Natl Acad Sci USA* 1997;94(12):6403–6407.

369. Matsushima M, Yoneyama A, Nakamura T, et al. A first case of complete remission of beta interferon sensitive adult T cell leukemia. *Eur J Haematol* 1987;39:282–287.

370. Tamura K, Makino S, Araki Y, et al. A case of CD4+/CD8-adult T cell leukemia with good response to interferon beta terminating as a CD4+/CD8+ adult T cell lymphoma. *Leuk Res* 1987;11:665–668.

371. Uike N, Choi I, Tokoro A, et al. Adult T-cell leukemia-lymphoma successfully treated with 2-chlorodeoxyadenosin. *Intern Med* 1998;37:411–413.

372. Okamura T, Shibuya T, Harada M, Niho Y. Successful treatment of chronic adult T-cell leukemia with Ubenimex. *Acta Haematol* 1992;87:94–97.

373. Waldmann T, Goldman CK. Therapy of patients with human T-cell lymphotropic virus type I induced adult T-cell leukemia with anti Tac, a monoclonal antibody to the receptor for interleukin 2. *Blood* 1988;72:1805–1816.

374. Osame M, Igata A, Matsumoto M, et al. HTLV-I–associated myelopathy (HAM) treatment trials, retrospective survey and clinical and laboratory findings. *Hematol Rev Commun* 1989;3:271–284.

375. Waclawik A, Fadic R, Lotz BP, et al. CD8 and CD4 T cell–mediated polymyositis complicating the HTLV-1 associated myelopathy. Quantitative evaluation of corticosteroid treatment. *Acta Neurol Scand* 1996;94:115–119.

376. Yamasaki K, Kira J, Koyanagi Y, et al. The long-term, high dose interferon-alpha treatment in HTLV-I–associated myelopathy/tropical spastic paraparesis: a combined clinical, virological and immunological study. *J Neurol Sci* 1997;147:135–144.

CHAPTER 256
Rubella Virus

Hans M. L. Spiegel and John L. Sever

HISTORY

It appears that rubella was known to the early Arabian physicians under the name *al-hamikah*. First described clinically as a variant of measles or scarlet fever by de Bergen in 1752 and Orlow in 1758, it was named roetheln (1). Manton (2) in 1815 first described the illness as a separate clinical entity. The English term rubella was first used in 1861 by Veale (3). In 1881 at the International Congress of Medicine in London, rubella was officially recognized as a distinct illness, and a complete description of acquired rubella infection was known by the early twentieth century (1). However, it was thought to be a mild, self-limited illness that rarely produced complications. This view was changed in 1941 when Gregg (4), an Australian ophthalmologist, published a paper in which he noted an association between maternal rubella infection and congenital defects. Although this association was initially doubted, by 1944, Gregg's observations were confirmed by fellow Australians Swan and colleagues and by investigators in the United States (1). Verification of the viral agent did not occur until 1962, when two separate teams, Weller and Neva (5) at Harvard University and Parkman and co-workers (6) at Walter Reed Hospital, independently isolated the virus in cell culture.

CHARACTERISTICS OF THE PATHOGEN

Classification

Rubella virus belongs to the Togaviridae family and is the only member of the genus *Rubivirus*. Only one immunologically distinct serotype has been described, and no common serologic relationship exists between the rubella virus and other viruses. Humans are the only known host (1).

Structure

The rubella virus is round to ovoid, measuring 60 to 70 nm in diameter, with a central nucleoid measuring 30 nm, and contained within a host-derived lipid bilayer, acquired during the process of viral budding into cytoplasmic vesicles or through the plasma membrane. The envelope is lipoprotein in nature and, being nonrigid, gives rise to pleomorphic viral particles. E1 and E2 glycoprotein spikes protrude from the virion surface and are 5 to 6 nm in size (7).

RUBELLA VIRUS GENOME

The rubella virus genome consists of a single-stranded, plus-sense RNA genome of 9,762 nucleotides that is capped on its 5′ end and polyadenylated on its 3′ end. The RNA-dependent RNA polymerase, together with other nonstructural proteins, is encoded in the 5′ proximal open reading frame, whereas the viral structural proteins, the capsid protein, and the E1 and E2 envelope glycoproteins, are encoded in the 3′ proximal open reading frame (7). DNA has not been detected in wild virus preparation; however, after growth in baby hamster kidney cells, viral variants that are recombinants between rubella and a latent retrovirus have been detected (8).

Biologic and Biochemical Properties

The virus is heat labile and has a half-life of 1 hour at 37°C. Infectivity is lost within 2 minutes at 100°C (6), but Kistler and Sapatino (9) have noted that even after heating at 70°C for 60 minutes, some infectivity persists. In regard to colder temperatures, infectivity is rapidly lost during storage at −10° to −20°C. However, in the presence of 2% albumin, infectivity is maintained for a week or more at 4°C and indefinitely at −60°C. Heat inactivation can be prevented through stabilization by the addition of magnesium sulfate to the viral suspension; protein stabilization allows survival of rapid freeze–thaw cycles (1).

Infectivity is also lost at pH levels below 6.8 or above 8.1, in the presence of ultraviolet light, lipid-active solvents, or other chemicals such as formalin, ethylene oxide, deoxycholate, proteolytic enzymes (trypsin), and β-propiolactone. Thimerosal does not inactivate the virus (1).

In cell culture, rubella virus infectivity is inhibited by amantadine, but clinical efficacy of this drug has not been proved (10). Attenuated virus strains show decreased infectivity in some laboratory animals owing to the failure of attenuated virus to multiply at 39°C, the body temperature of rabbits.

ANTIGENIC CHARACTERISTICS

E1 and E2 Glycoproteins

The virion envelope proteins, E1 and E2, are type 1 membrane glycoproteins. Both proteins contain a presumptive transmembrane domain (7).

The E1 protein contains three N-linked glycosylation sites, whereas the number of glycosylation sites for the E2 protein was found to vary between three and four, depending on the type of rubella virus strain (11). Glycosylation of E1 glycoprotein appears to be required for the correct folding and expression of antigenic and immunogenic epitopes (12,13), and the N-linked glycosylation sites in E2 are as well required for the stability of this protein (14).

E1 protein contains at least six non-overlapping epitopes, some of which are associated with hemagglutination and neutralization (15). E1 appears to be the main surface protein, with domains involved in the attachment of the virus to the cell. More recent studies have revealed that a 28-residue internal hydrophobic domain of E1 is responsible for the fusogenic activity of rubella virus. In addition, this region is involved in the binding to E2 for heterodimer formation (16).

The exact function of E2 is not yet completely known, but it appears to play a role in the cell surface expression of E1 (17–20). E2 is disulfide-linked to E1 in the mature virion and is topologically hidden behind E1, which makes it less accessible to the host's immune response (21). Viral strain-specific as well as partial hemagglutination and neutralizing epitopes of E2 have been identified, however (22), and both E1 and E2 have demonstrated viral neutralizing activity (17–20).

Capsid Protein

The capsid protein is a disulfide-linked homodimer with a molecular mass of 33 to 38 kd. It is phosphorylated, but nonglycosylated (17,23,24). Clusters of proline and arginine residues within the capsid protein interact with nucleotide 347 to 375 of the rubella virus genome and are thought to be important for the packaging of the genome (7,25).

Two precipitating antigens have been identified, designated theta and iota, and these are associated with the viral envelope and core, respectively. Natural infection with rubella virus leads to the formation of antibody against both of these precipitating antigens. Earlier vaccines led to antibody formation against the theta component only; the presently used vaccine (the RA 27/3 vaccine) produces a strong response to the theta component and a weak response to the iota component (18–20). The antigenic sites responsible for complement fixation and platelet aggregation have not yet been identified, although there now appear to be two distinct rubella complement-fixing antigens.

Culture Techniques

Rubella virus grows in a wide variety of primary cell cultures (such as human, simian, bovine, rabbit, canine, and duck) but does not produce a cytopathic effect (26). Instead, the rubella virus is detected by its ability to produce interference to superinfection by a wide variety of viruses, with this effect being due to interferon production. The African green monkey kidney cell culture is the best suited and is the one most frequently used in clinical laboratories for isolation of the rubella virus by the interference technique.

When grown in continuous cell lines (hamster, rabbit, simian, human), rubella virus can lead to a wide variety of cytopathic effects. The continuous cell lines RK-13 (rabbit kidney line) and Vero (vervet kidney line) produce a good cytopathic effect uncomplicated by adventitious simian agents, provided that conditions are well controlled (27). Because of the inability of the continuous cell lines BHK-21 and Vero to produce interferon, high titers of rubella virus are produced, and this allows the use of these cell lines for antigen production (to be used in serologic testing). Viral plaquing, which is the basis for the neutralization assays, can be performed with RK-13, BHK-21, SIRC (rabbit cornea), or Vero cells (28).

IMMUNE RESPONSES TO RUBELLA VIRUS

Immune Response to Acquired Infection

HUMORAL IMMUNE RESPONSES

Multiple antibody measurement techniques have been developed for use in rubella virus infections. The earliest two described were the neutralizing antibody in 1964 (29) and the hemagglutination inhibition (HAI) test in 1967 (30). Both techniques can detect immunoglobulin G (IgG) 2 to 3 days after onset of rash (about 2 weeks after becoming infected). IgG peaks within a month, and persists, although with decreasing titers, for years and possibly lifelong (29,30). The distinguishing feature of the two antibody measurement techniques is that they measure the inhibition of the infectivity of the rubella virus. The neutralizing antibody test has the best correlation with protective immunity of all the available antibody measurement techniques, but the HAI test also correlates well (31).

Because the neutralizing antibody and HAI tests are time-consuming, expensive, and difficult to perform, other techniques were developed. These include latex agglutination, immunofluorescence, radioimmunoassay, dot immunoassay, and enzyme immunoassay (EIA) (32). By these techniques, IgG typically becomes detectable within 5 to 15 days after rash onset, peaks at 15 to 30 days, and then gradually declines to a persistent titer. In most cases, there is persistence for life. In addition, passive hemagglutination can be used to measure IgG antibody (33). However, the passive hemagglutination antibody is first detectable 15 to 20 days after rash onset and peaks by 200 days (33). This is followed by persistence of antibody. Overall, IgG1 appears to be the predominant IgG subclass involved (1).

Of all these techniques, the most commonly used in clinical laboratories are the EIAs because of their ease and low cost. However, IgG titers detected by these methods, compared with the neutralizing antibody and HAI tests, do not necessarily equate with protective immunity. High titers of IgG (by EIA and similar techniques) appear to indicate true protection, but it is well recognized that reinfection can occur in subjects with even moderate IgG levels but no antibody titer by either the neutralizing antibody or HAI test (31,34).

Rubella-specific IgM antibody response can also be measured by HAI, radioimmunoassay, immunofluorescence, or EIA (35). IgM antibodies are detectable 5 to 10 days after the onset of rash, peak at 20 days, and then disappear within 50 to 70 days. In some subjects, low levels of IgM can persist longer, with up to 4 years being documented.

Complement fixation antibodies and precipitins are also detectable (36,37). Of the precipitins, the theta titer rises promptly, persists, and is seen after both natural infection and administration of any of the approved rubella vaccines. The iota titer rises slowly and is induced only by the RA 27/3 vaccine. The complement fixation and iota titers become detectable 10 days after onset of rash and slowly rise to a peak between 30 and 90 days out. The iota precipitins are present for only a few months.

IgA mediates the local nasopharyngeal immune response and appears within 10 days after infection. With natural infection, the IgA antibody persists for up to 1 year and at times longer (38). On the contrary, after rubella vaccination, a lack of local nasopharyngeal IgA is usually seen (39), except in cases in which the vaccine is administered intranasally. This method of administration is not done, however, because of a weaker systemic response. IgD and IgE antibodies become detectable within 6 to 9 days after infection; IgE peaks earlier than IgD, remains elevated for about 2 months, and then declines by 6 months. Synthetic peptides might be used to develop vaccines with lower complication rates than those of the vaccines presently used, and could be used to create antigens for EIAs (18–20).

CELLULAR IMMUNE RESPONSES

Acute natural rubella infection is associated with a CD8$^+$ T-cell expansion (40). Cell-mediated immunity usually precedes humoral immunity by a week. Peak activity of cell-mediated immunity is concurrent with peak antibody responses and may persist for life. Cellular immune response to rubella virus can be measured by lymphocyte transformation response, levels of interferon and macrophage inhibitory factor, response of delayed hypersensitivity to skin testing, and release of lymphokines by lymphocytes (41).

T-cell–mediated immune responses are needed to clear rubella virus infection. The E1 polypeptide and the virus capsid have been identified as targets of rubella virus–specific T-cell responses (18–20,41). A sequence within the amino terminus of the capsid protein C1 to C29 has been identified, which contains both class I and II major histocompatibility complex (MHC)–restricted epitopes (41).

Rubella virus capsid protein residues 263 to 275 have been shown to elicit a CD4$^+$ cytotoxic T-lymphocyte response, whereas the nonamer capsid protein sequence residues 264 to 272 constitute an optimal peptide epitope for HLA-A11 and HLA-A3–restricted rubella virus–specific CD8$^+$ cytotoxic T lymphocytes (CTLs) (42). Rubella virus surface glycoprotein E1 residues 273 to 284 have been shown to be recognized by a class II MHC

(HLA-DR4)–restricted CTL response. This T-cell epitope overlaps with a virus neutralizing antibody-binding site previously identified with human antibodies (43).

Two further non-overlapping T-cell peptide epitopes were identified in E1, which are restricted by HLA-DRB1 (44).

Three minimal helper T-cell epitopes are located at amino acid positions 280 to 287 (VIGSQARK), 385 to 393 (KFVTAALLN), and 412 to 419 (RVIDPAAQ) within rubella virus envelope glycoprotein E1 (45). Further lymphoproliferative responses can be elicited against the following peptide epitopes in rubella virus envelope glycoprotein: E1, amino acid residues 254 to 285, 301 to 314, 389 to 408, and 462 to 481 rubella virus envelope glycoprotein; and E2: amino acid residues 134 to 150, 140 to 156, 168 to 179, and rubella virus capsid protein amino acid residues 1 to 29 and 88 to 111. Six of these residues also contain rubella virus–neutralizing antibody domains (46).

Several studies appear to indicate that the development of chronic arthritis after natural infection is secondary to altered T-cell recognition of the appropriate rubella virus antigens (47–49). If there is a poor recognition, the virus can possibly persist and lead to joint complications in this manner. If the recognition triggers a hyperimmune response, the joint complications are caused by an immune mechanism. Several studies have examined the efficacy of using either saliva or oral fluid to measure an immune response to rubella. Both IgA and IgG can be measured in these fluids, and results indicate good correlation with the standard serum EIA to determine the immune status of a subject (50,51).

Immune Response to Congenital Infection

HUMORAL IMMUNE RESPONSES

Transplacental maternal antibody transfer is poor during the first half of gestation, and the fetal humoral immune response is also minimal during this time. Thus, measurements of either IgG or IgM levels in fetal blood samples before 16 weeks of gestation are difficult to determine (52). As the pregnancy progresses, IgG is transferred to the child, and IgM is produced by the fetal immune system. At birth, presence of an IgM level in an infant indicates (with high probability, assuming minimal blood exchange at birth) an intrauterine rubella infection (34).

There are several complications of the humoral immune system related to congenital rubella infection. Hypogammaglobulinemia can occur, with only IgA being affected typically. Also, there is a persistence of rubella-specific IgM, with the mechanism for this not being clear. The IgM levels remain elevated in 60% of infants during the first 4 months of life and in 40% of infected infants aged 8 to 12 months. When measured by sensitive serologic tests, such as radioimmunoassay and immunofluorescence, IgM levels may persist beyond 1 year of life (53,54). Finally, there is a slow maturation of IgG1 avidity. After an acquired rubella infection, the IgG1 antibody initially has a low avidity or functional affinity (54). However, this quickly changes to high-avidity rubella-specific IgG1 antibody production. After congenital infection, the avidity of the IgG1 antibodies remains low for a prolonged time; up to 40% of congenitally infected infants in one study still produced low-avidity IgG1 antibodies 3 years after birth (54,55).

Children with congenital rubella syndrome and their mothers, however, have further low or undetectable levels of E2-specific antibodies and deficient antibody responses against the major neutralizing domain SP15 on E1, whereas these responses were shown to be normal in asymptomatic infants born to mothers with primary rubella virus infection during pregnancy.

Hence, detection of high-avidity IgG, neutralizing antibodies directed against SP15, and specific responses directed against conformational epitopes in E2 can possibly predict a benign outcome of intrauterine rubella virus infection (56).

CELLULAR IMMUNE RESPONSES

The cellular immune response in congenitally infected children may also be impaired. Studies have shown selective tolerance to the E1 protein of the rubella virus, leading to inadequate T-cell response and persistence of live virus. This persistence of a low level of active infection leads to the development of the delayed manifestations seen in congenitally infected infants. The etiology of this selective tolerance is not clear (18).

CONCLUSIONS

Patients with congenital rubella infection pose an immunologic paradox. They have high levels of rubella-specific IgG and persistence of high levels of rubella-specific IgM and yet present with complications indicative of persistent active infection. Fetal hepatitis B surface antigen vaccination studies in nonhuman primates have recently established evidence for the capacity of the fetal immune system to respond to *in utero* vaccination, with no immunologic tolerance induction by prior fetal immunization (57).

The differences in the overall immune response of children with congenital rubella syndrome and their mothers, compared with asymptomatic controls, could be due to the early time of exposure during gestation, the specific effects of the pathogen on the developing immune system of the fetus, and possible interferences with the maternal immune response. This subsequently leads to the observed slow maturation of the avidity of the IgG1 subclass, low or undetectable levels of E2-specific antibodies and deficient antibody responses against the major neutralizing domain SP15 on E1 in the infant and mother, and the selective tolerance of T cells to the E1 antigen.

REFERENCES

1. Cherry JD. Rubella. In: Feigin RD, Cherry JD, eds. *Textbook of pediatric infectious diseases*, 4th ed. Philadelphia: WB Saunders, 1998:1922–1941.
2. Manton WG. Some accounts of rash liable to be mistaken for scarlatina. *Med Trans R Coll Physicians (Lond)* 1815;5:149.
3. Veale H. History of epidemic Rotheln, with observations on its pathology. *Edinb Med J* 1866;12:404.
4. Gregg NM. Congenital cataracts following German measles in the mother. *Trans Ophthalmol Soc Aust* 1941;3:35.
5. Weller TH, Neva FA. Propagation in tissue culture of cytopathic agents from patients with rubella-like illness. *Proc Soc Exp Biol Med* 1962;111:225.
6. Parkman PD, Buescher EL, Artenstein MS, et al. Studies of rubella. I. Properties of the virus. *J Immunol* 1964;93:595.
7. Frey TK. Molecular biology of rubella virus. *Adv Virus Res* 1994;44:69–160.
8. Bardeletti G, Kessler N, Aymard-Henry M. Morphology, biochemical analysis and neuraminidase activity of rubella virus. *Arch Virol* 1975;49:175.
9. Kistler GS, Sapatino V. Temperature- and UV-light resistance of rubella virus infectivity. *Arch Ges Virusforsch* 1972;38:11.
10. Gershon A. Rubella virus (German measles). In: Mandell G, Bennett J, Dolin R, eds. *Principles and practice of infectious diseases*, 5th ed. New York: Churchill Livingstone, 2000:1708–1714.
11. Qiu Z, Tufaro F, Gillam S. The influence of N-linked glycosylation on the antigenicity and immunogenicity of rubella virus E1 glycoprotein. *Virology* 1992;190:876–881.
12. Terry GM, Ho-Terry L, Londesborough P, Rees KR. A bio-engineered rubella E1 antigen. *Virology* 1989;190:63–75.
13. Lee JY, Bowden DS. Rubella virus replication and links to teratogenicity. *Clin Microbiol Rev* 2000;13:571–587.
14. Qiu Z, Tufaro F, Gillam S. The influence of N-linked glyco-sylation on the antigenicity and immunogenicity of rubella virus E1 glyco-protein. *Virology* 1992;190:876–888.
15. Wolinsky JS, Sukholutsky E, Moore WT, et al. An antibody and synthetic peptide-defined rubella virus E1 glycoprotein and neutralization domain. *J Virol* 1993;67:961–968.
16. Yang D, Hwang D, Qiu Z, et al. Effects in the mutation in the rubella virus E1 glycoproteins on E1-E2 interaction and membrane fusion activity. *J Virol* 1998;72:8747–8755.
17. Bowden DS, Westway EG. Rubella virus: structural and non-structural proteins. *J Gen Virol* 1984;65:933.
18. Mauracher CA, Mitchell LA, Tingle AJ. Selective tolerance to the E1 protein of rubella virus in congenital rubella syndrome. *J Immunol* 1993;151:2041.
19. Chaye H, Ou D, Chong P, et al. Human T- and B-cell epitopes of E1 glycoprotein of rubella virus. *J Clin Immunol* 1993;13:93.
20. Ou D, Chong P, Tingle AJ. Mapping T-cell epitopes of rubella virus structural proteins E1, E2, and C recognized by T-cell lines and clones derived from infected and immunized populations. *J Med Virol* 1993;40:175.
21. Waxham MN, Wolinsky J. Detailed immunologic analysis of the structural polypeptides of rubella virus using monoclonal antibodies. *Virology* 1985;143:153–165.
22. Green KY, Dorsett PH. Rubella virus antigens: localization epitopes involved in hemagglutination and neutralization by using monoclonal antibodies. *J Virol* 1986;57:893–898.
23. Marr LD, Sanchez A, Frey TK. Efficient in vitro translation and processing of the rubella virus structural proteins in the presence of microsomes. *Virology* 1991;180:400–405.
24. Oker-Blom C, Kalkkinen N, Kaeaeriaeinen L, et al. Rubella virus contains one capsid protein and three envelope glycoproteins, E1, E2a, and E2b. *J Virol* 1983;46:964–973.
25. Liu Z, Yang D, Qiu Z, et al. Identification of domains in rubella virus genomic RNA and capsid protein necessary for specific interaction. *J Virol* 1996;70:2184–2190.
26. Parkman PD, Buescher EL, Artenstein MS. Recovery of rubella virus from army recruits. *Proc Soc Exp Biol Med* 1962;111:225.
27. McCarthy K, Taylor-Robinson CH. Rubella. *Br Med Bull* 1967;23:185.
28. Hermann KL. Rubella virus. In: Lennette EH, Schmidt NJ, eds. *Diagnostic procedures for viral, rickettsial and chlamydial infections*. Washington, DC: American Public Health Association, 1979:725.
29. Parkman PD, Mundon FK, McCown JM, et al. Studies of rubella. II. Neutralization of the virus. *J Immunol* 1964;93:608.
30. Stewart GL, Parkman PD, Hopps HE, et al. Rubella virus hemagglutination inhibition test. *N Engl J Med* 1967;276:554.
31. Zrein M, Joncas JH, Pedneault L, et al. Comparison of a whole-virus enzyme immunoassay (EIA) with a peptide-based EIA for detecting rubella virus immunoglobulin G antibodies following rubella vaccination. *J Clin Microbiol* 1993;31:1521.
32. Hermann KL. Available rubella serologic tests. *Rev Infect Dis* 1985;7[Suppl 1]:S108.
33. Hauknes G. Experience with an indirect (passive) hemagglutination test for the demonstration of rubella virus antibody. *Acta Pathol Microbiol Scand* 1980;88:85.
34. The American College of Obstetricians and Gynecologists (ACOG). Rubella and pregnancy: ACOG technical bulletin number 171-August 1992. *Int J Gynecol Obstet* 1993;42:60.
35. Cubie H, Edmond E. Comparison of five different methods of rubella IgM antibody testing. *J Clin Pathol* 1985;38:203.
36. Sever JL, Huebner RJ, Castellano GA, et al. Rubella complement fixation test. *Science* 1965;148:385.
37. Cappel R, Schluederberg A, Horstmann DM. Large-scale production of rubella precipitinogens and their use in the diagnostic laboratory. *J Clin Microbiol* 1975;1:201.
38. Salonen EM Hove T, Meurman O, et al. Kinetics of specific IgA, IgD, IgE IgG, and IgM antibody responses in rubella. *J Med Virol* 1985;16:1.
39. Saule H, Enders G, Zeller J, et al. Congenital rubella infection after previous immunity of the mother. *Eur J Pediatr* 1988;147:195.
40. Ueno Y, Katow S, Tanaka T, et al. Natural rubella infection with CD8+ T cell expansion and failure to detect viral genome in synovial fluid. *J Rheumatol* 1999;26(1):229–231.
41. Lovett AE, Hahn CS, Rice CM, et al. Rubella virus-specific cytotoxic T-lymphocyte responses: identification of the capsid as a target of major histocompatibility complex class I- restricted lysis and definition of two epitopes. *J Virol* 1993;67:5849–5858.
42. Ou D, Mitchell LA, Decarie D, et al. Characterization of an overlapping CD8+ and CD4+ T-cell epitope on rubella capsid protein. *Virology* 1997;235(2):286–292.
43. Ou D, Mitchell LA, Ho M, et al. Analysis of overlapping T- and B-cell antigenic sites on rubella virus E1 envelope protein: influence of HLA-DR4 polymorphism on T-cell clonal recognition. *Hum Immunol* 1994;39:177–187.
44. Nepom GT, Domeier ME, Ou D, et al. Recognition of contiguous allele-specific peptide elements in the rubella virus E1 envelope protein. *Vaccine* 1997;15:648–652.
45. Marttila J, Ilonen J, Lehtinen M, et al. Definition of three minimal T helper cell epitopes of rubella virus E1 glycoprotein. *Clin Exp Immunol* 1996;104:394–397.
46. Mitchell LA, Tingle AJ, Decarie D, et al. Identification of rubella virus T-cell epitopes recognized in anamnestic response to RA27/3 vaccine: associations with boost in neutralizing antibody titer. *Vaccine* 1999;17:2356–2365.
47. Ueno Y. Rubella arthritis: an outbreak in Kyoto. *J Rheumatol* 1994;21:874.
48. Mitchell LA, Decarie D, Shukin R, et al. Cellular hyperimmunoreactivity to

rubella virus synthetic peptides in chronic rubella associated arthritis. *Ann Rheum Dis* 1993;52:590.

49. Mitchell LA, Tingle AJ, Shukin R, et al. Chronic rubella vaccine-associated arthropathy. *Arch Intern Med* 1993;153:2268.
50. Thieme T, Piacentini S, Davidson S, et al. Determination of measles, mumps, and rubella immunization status using oral fluid samples. *JAMA* 1994;272:219.
51. Perry KR, Brown DWG Parry JV, et al. Detection of measles, mumps, and rubella antibodies in saliva using antibody capture radioimmunoassay. *J Med Virol* 1993;40:235.
52. Valente P, Sever JL. In utero diagnosis of congenital infections by direct fetal sampling. *Israel J Med Sci* 1994;30:416.
53. Cooper LZ, Alford A. Rubella. In: Remington JS, Klein JO, eds. *Infections of the fetus and newborn infant*, 5th ed. Philadelphia: WB Saunders, 2001:347–388.
54. Thomas HIJ, Morgan-Capner P, Cradock-Watson JE, et al. Slow maturation of IgG1 avidity and persistence of specific IgM in congenital rubella: implications for diagnosis and immunopathology. *J Med Virol* 1993;41:196.
55. Williams LL, Shannon BT, Leguire LE, et al. Persistently altered T cell immunity in high school students with the congenital rubella syndrome and profound hearing loss. *Pediatr Infect Dis J* 1993;12:831.
56. Pustowoit B, Liebert UG. Predictive value of serological tests in rubella virus infection during pregnancy. *Intervirology* 1998;41:170–177.
57. Watts AM, Stanley JR, Shearer MH, et al. Fetal immunization of baboons induces a fetal-specific antibody response. *Nat Med* 1999;5:427–430.

CHAPTER 257
Yellow Fever Virus

Theodore F. Tsai

HISTORY

Yellow fever virus arose in Africa and was spread, with its mosquito vector, *Aedes aegypti*, to the new world on trading ships. In the eighteenth and nineteenth centuries, epidemics plagued Europe and America, reaching coastal and river port cities as far north as Swansea, Wales, Boston, and St. Louis in epidemics that were associated with attack rates as high as 30% and mortality rates of 10%. The last yellow fever outbreaks in the United States occurred in 1905 in the Mississippi delta. The mosquito-borne transmission of yellow fever, championed by Carlos Finlay, was proved in 1900 by a U.S. Army commission led by Walter Reed. This understanding made it possible to prevent the disease through the control of vector mosquitoes prior to the isolation of the viral etiologic agent in 1928 (1,2).

CHARACTERISTICS OF THE PATHOGEN

Yellow fever virus is the type species of RNA viruses in the family Flaviviridae (3). Virions are enveloped and spherical, with a diameter of about 40 nm. The lipid bilayer envelope contains a matrix (M) protein and the envelope (E) protein, which is variably glycosylated. The genome, a single segment of positive-sense RNA, is bound into a nucleocapsid with a basic capsid (C) protein. Virions enter host cells by receptor-mediated endocytosis. Viral RNA synthesis occurs in the cytoplasm, and protein synthesis proceeds in the endoplasmic reticulum, from which mature virions are released through the plasma membrane by exocytotic fusion.

The 11-kb viral genome has a single open reading frame of 10,233 nucleotides, which is translated into a polyprotein that is cleaved into the three structural proteins (C, M, and E) and several nonstructural proteins with replicative functions. NS1, a glycosylated protein found within the cell and in soluble form extracellularly also induces protective complement-fixing antibodies. NS1 and other nonstructural proteins (NS2b and NS3) contain epitopes recognized by cytotoxic lymphocytes (4).

The E protein (53 to 54 kd) has a major role in virion attachment to host cells, hemagglutination, and virus neutralization. Differences between the consensus-complete nucleotide sequence of yellow fever 17D vaccine and its wild-type Asibi virus parent are scattered throughout the genome and have been associated with virulence properties and other phenotypic attributes.

Yellow fever virus is classified antigenically in a distinct serocomplex with cross-reactivity to several African flaviviruses, including Uganda S, Bouboui, Wesselsbron, Banzi, and Zika viruses. Molecular taxonomic studies have differentiated yellow fever strains into several African and two South American genotypes, with a close relationship between New World and West African lineages (4).

EPIDEMIOLOGY

Yellow fever occurs in tropical America and in Africa in endemic zones bounded by about 15 degrees north latitude and 15 degrees south latitude (Fig. 257.1). Epidemic (urban) yellow fever is transmitted in an interhuman cycle by *A. aegypti* mosquitoes, which after feeding on viremic humans can transmit infections to other hosts for 1 to 2 weeks. Although Asia is a receptive area for the virus because of the widespread abundance of *A. aegypti* vector mosquitoes, the disease has never been reported from the region.

Sylvatic yellow fever, in which the virus is transmitted between forest mosquitoes and monkeys, and incidentally infects persons who work in or who visit forested areas, predominates in South America. Three fatal cases have been reported among unvaccinated American travelers to forested locations in South America since 1996 (5–7). Sporadic cases and outbreaks occur principally during the late rainy season (January to May), when vector *Haemagogus* species mosquitoes are most abundant. However, improved transportation between previously isolated forest areas and human settlements and the encroachment of towns upon sylvatic habitats that support enzootic viral transmission have increased the likelihood of the virus insertion into an epidemic urban *A. aegypti*–borne transmission cycle. Several suspected urban cases have been reported recently in Bolivia and Brazil, leading to mass vaccination in the cities at risk; in Brazil, 45 million doses of vaccine were administered between 1997 and 2000 after a series of outbreaks occurred in a nearly nationwide distribution (8–11). Other countries reporting cases between 1991 and 2000 were Peru (1,094 cases), Bolivia (382 cases), Brazil (335 cases), Ecuador (81 cases), Colombia (32 cases), Venezuela (16 cases), and French Guiana (1 case).

In Africa, recurrent viral activity during the rainy season leads to a high level of enzootic and endemic transmission among monkeys and humans and periodically to outbreaks in forest and moist savanna regions. Cases originating in these emergence zones may spread to villages in the dry savanna and to urban areas where there is a risk for interhuman *A. aegypti*–borne epidemic transmission (Fig. 257.1). In the past decade, epidemics were recognized in Benin (192 cases), Cote d'Ivoire (12 cases), Ghana (306 cases), Guinea-Bissau (4 cases), Liberia (522 cases), Burkina Faso (6 cases), Cameroon (10 cases), Gabon (44 cases), Guinea (445 cases), Nigeria (3,096 cases), Senegal (no official reports), and in Kenya (72 cases) in East Africa (11).

Official notifications significantly underreport cases in both Africa and South America. In many instances, only fatal cases are recognized, and the several hundred officially reported cases from South America and several thousand from Africa may represent only 1% of true morbidity.

Resistance to acquiring yellow fever may be associated with cross-immunity to dengue fever virus and other flaviviruses.

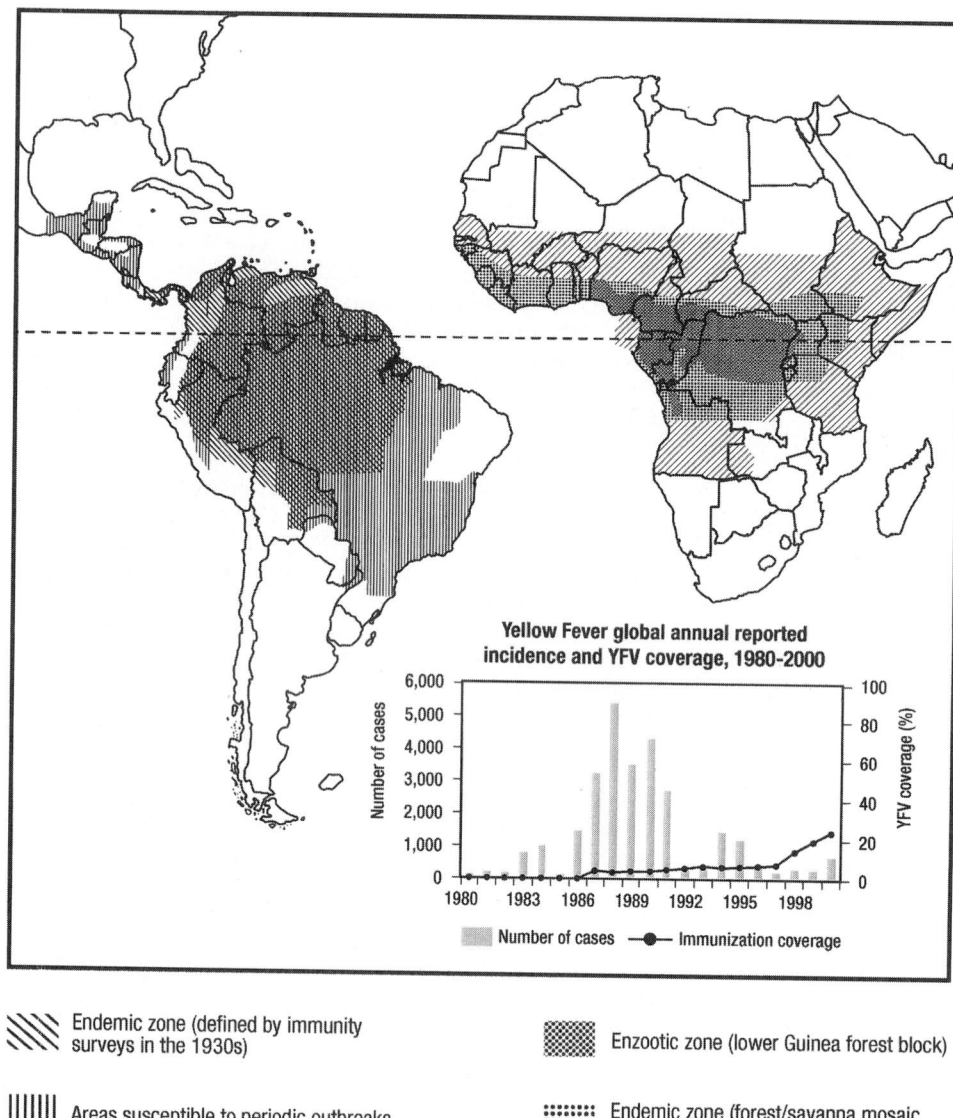

Endemic zone (defined by immunity surveys in the 1930s)

Areas susceptible to periodic outbreaks

Enzootic zone (lower Guinea forest block)

Endemic zone (forest/savanna mosaic, humid and semi-humid savannas)

Epidemic zone (dry savanna)

Figure 257.1. Geoecologic distribution of yellow fever, and reported cases, 1980 to 2000.

This cross-reactive immunity may provide a barrier to the introduction of yellow fever to Asia.

CLINICAL FEATURES

Classic yellow fever is a biphasic illness progressing through three stages: infection, remission, and intoxication. Infection may result in subclinical infection, a self-limited influenza-like syndrome, or in 15% to 25% of cases, fulminating illness that leads to death within days (12–14). After an incubation period of 3 to 6 days, an abrupt onset of fever and chills is followed rapidly by headache, backache, generalized myalgias, nausea, and vomiting. Few physical signs are present other than flushing of the face and conjunctivae and Faget's sign, a relative bradycardia. After 3 to 4 days, symptoms and fever remit for a period of hours to 1 or 2 days, only to recur and intensify in patients who progress to the fulminant stage of intoxication. The illness evolves into a secure multisystem hemorrhagic fever characterized notably by jaundice, the clinical sign for which the disease is named, renal dysfunction, and clinical manifestations of a hem-

orrhagic diathesis and ultimately hypotension and potentially fatal shock. Mucosal bleeding petechiae and ecchymoses, bleeding from venipuncture sites and gastrointestinal hemorrhage, the black vomit mentioned in early descriptions of the disease, may be severe and reflect reduced hepatic synthesis of clotting factors, platelet dysfunction, and disseminated intravascular coagulation. Transaminases are elevated, reflecting principally hepatocellular damage, which can lead to hepatorenal syndrome in severe cases. Oliguria and azotemia may represent prerenal volume depletion, due to vomiting, and extravascular extravasation, but albuminuria is a key feature of the disease, and in severe cases, oligoanuria and elevated creatinine develop, possibly due to primary glomerular and interstitial nephritis. Acute tubular necrosis may follow as a late event associated with hypotension. Myocarditis may be detected in electrographic abnormalities and less frequently may be manifested clinically by cardiac dysfunction and arrhythmias after occurring late in the illness. Signs and symptoms of encephalopathy associated with hepatic and renal failure reflect cerebral edema. Secondary bacterial infections, including pneumonia and bacteremia, frequently complicate the course of illness and can contribute to death. The overall case-fatality rate is 5% to 10%, but 20% to 50% of patients entering the stage of intoxication may die.

Clinical laboratory abnormalities include leukopenia, albuminuria, prolonged prothrombin time, and elevations in serum transaminase and indirect and direct bilirubin values and in serum urea nitrogen and creatinine. Early and marked transaminase and bilirubin elevations signal a poor outcome. Mild chemical disturbances in liver function may be present in anicteric cases. Thrombocytopenia and other signs of consumptive coagulopathy are present in some cases. Hepatic damage may lead to hypoglycemia. The cerebrospinal fluid may be under pressure and exhibits a pattern of elevated protein without pleocytosis, most consistent with encephalopathy and cerebral edema.

The differential diagnosis of mild cases includes malaria, dengue, and other self-limited but prostrating grippes. Severe cases must be differentiated from leptospirosis, louse-borne relapsing fever, typhoid fever, acute viral hepatitis, and other viral hemorrhagic fevers produced by Lassa, Ebola, Marburg, Congo-Crimean hemorrhagic fever, dengue, and Rift Valley fever viruses. Intoxications, sometimes associated with traditional medicines, also should be considered (15).

LABORATORY DIAGNOSIS

In locations where yellow fever is potentially epidemic, rapid and definitive diagnosis of suspected cases is essential to the implementation of control measures. Direct detection of viral antigen and polymerase chain reaction (PCR) analysis of acute serum samples have been used successfully in anecdotal cases or small series and should be applied more systematically (12,16).

The diagnosis of yellow fever frequently is confirmed serologically by demonstrating fourfold or greater increases in complement-fixing or neutralizing antibodies or by detecting specific immunoglobulin M in a single serum sample by immunoglobulin M capture enzyme immunoassay. Patients with previous flavivirus infections or immunization develop heterologous antibodies that limit the interpretation of serologic reactions to yellow fever virus, especially in broadly reactive assays such as hemagglutination inhibition. In patients who have had numerous flavivirus infections, serologic assays may be uninterpretable.

Isolation of virus from the blood of viremic cases (during the initial acute phase of illness and before virus is cleared in the period of transmission) typically is deferred to high-security laboratories because the differential diagnosis includes other viral hemorrhagic fever viruses with a potential for laboratory-acquired infection. MOS61 (Aedes pseudoscutellaris) mosquito cell cultures are the most sensitive substrate, but the virus also can be isolated in Toxorhynchites species mosquitoes, suckling mice, and Vero, C6/36, or LLCMK$_2$ cell cultures. In fatal cases, viral antigen and genome should be sought in liver tissue by immunohistochemical staining or in situ hybridization, respectively (16,17). Ordinary histopathologic examination of viscerotomy samples is a widely used approach to surveillance, but it is contraindicated for critically ill patients; moreover, histopathologic diagnosis is nonspecific because other toxic and infectious agents, especially other hemorrhagic fever viruses, can produce similar pathologic patterns.

PATHOLOGY AND PATHOPHYSIOLOGY

The initial replicative sites are reticuloendothelial cells of local lymph nodes, bone marrow, spleen, and Kupffer's cells (12), from which virions disseminate hematogenously to multiple sites during the early period of infection. The principal pathologic finding is a patchy, primarily midzonal eosinophilic degeneration of hepatocytes with minimal inflammatory or proliferative responses, reflecting apoptotic cell death (12,17–19). Hepatocytes surrounding the central vein and portal areas are spared to a greater degree, and the reticular architecture is largely preserved. Hepatocytes undergo an acidophilic degeneration progressing from a cloudy appearance to progressive shrinkage of the cytoplasm and formation of Councilman's bodies. Accumulation of ceroid pigment and microvesicular fat is prominent. Torres' bodies, intranuclear inclusions, are found occasionally. Viral antigen can be identified in hepatocytes and within Councilman's bodies. Transient nonspecific changes of hepatitis are found after the acute stages of illness, and healing proceeds without fibrosis; anecdotal cases of chronic active hepatitis have been reported. The kidneys are enlarged and edematous. Glomeruli may show mesangial proliferation and capillary endothelial swelling, whereas the interstitium is edematous with swollen tubular epithelial cells that may contain viral antigen. Degeneration and necrosis of the myocardium and lesions in the conduction system may be present. Viral antigen can be detected in occasional myocardial fibers. The absence of an inflammatory response and the cellular morphology of degenerating kidney and cardiac cells suggest an apoptotic mechanism of all deaths in the organs as well. Depletion of lymphocytes in B-cell areas of lymph nodes and spleen may compromise the immune response.

Viral clearance results from a combination of humoral and cellular responses. Viremia disappears within about 5 days after the acute onset of illness with the elaboration of neutralizing antibodies and nonneutralizing antibodies to NS1. Cytokines released in the course of cellular responses to infected parenchymal and monocytic cells may account for the vascular instability shock and other elements of a systemic inflammatory response-like syndrome (12).

The immunoglobulin M antibody titer remains elevated for years in some patients and in vaccinees, suggesting the possibility of viral persistence.

TREATMENT

No specific therapy is available (12). Ribavirin therapy has been shown to be ineffective in animal models of infection. Therapy with neutralizing monoclonal antibody was given late in the illness of an imported case that ultimately was fatal. It is unclear whether such therapy administered earlier in the course of illness could modify the disease. Supportive therapy should be directed at correcting fluid losses and maintaining hemodynamic stability with pressors if needed. Prevention and treatment of hypoglycemia with intravenous drips and of gastrointestinal bleeding with H$_2$ antagonists or proton pump inhibitors have been recommended as well as surveillance and treatment of secondary bacterial infection. The pathogenesis of the bleeding diathesis in yellow fever is not clear, but in one small study, administration of heparin led to improvement of patients shown to have disseminated intravascular coagulation. Vitamin K and fresh-frozen plasma are recommended to replenish liver-dependent clotting factors. Dialysis may be needed to treat renal failure. Liver transplantation was considered as an option in a case imported to Europe. Nosocomial infection from direct contact with patient blood or fluids is not considered a risk; however, mosquito-borne transmission is possible for about the first 5 days of acute illness, when patients should be isolated by bed nets and other means.

PREVENTION

A live attenuated virus (17D) has been used safely and effectively as a vaccine for 50 years (20). The strain was derived from a human isolate (Asibi) and was attenuated by serial passages in mouse and chick embryo cells (16,17). Vaccine-related adverse events are generally mild and occur in less than 5% of vaccinees.

Anaphylactic reactions (to gelatin or egg proteins in the vaccine) have been estimated to occur in 1 in 130,000 vaccinees (21). Skin testing with diluted vaccine has led to an antibody response in some persons. A residual neurotropic potential is seen in an age-related encephalitis that occurs exclusively in children, especially infants younger than 4 months. Eighteen cases, one fatal, have been reported, and for this reason, the vaccine is contraindicated in infants younger than 4 months, and immunization of children aged 4 to 6 months is recommended only if they cannot avoid epidemic areas. After age 6 months, infants may be immunized if they reside in rural areas of endemic zones. Immunization should be deferred until age 9 to 12 months for residents of urban areas. Yellow fever and measles vaccine have been given together at 6 to 9 months of age in many World Health Organization Expanded Program on Immunization (EPI) programs in Africa without signals of central nervous system adverse events (Fig. 257.1). Congenital infection without malformation was demonstrated in one case after inadvertent immunization during the first trimester of pregnancy, but other studies have shown no risk for congenital infections.

A series of severe and some fatal cases of illness mimicking natural yellow fever following vaccination of persons in the United States and Australia where no possibility of natural infection exists, as well as in Brazil, constitute the first reports that the attenuated vaccine strain can, in some adults, produce a virulent infection. Although cases in Australia and Brazil occurred in young persons, all reported cases from the United States were in elderly individuals, and a travel clinic survey suggested an association of risk with advanced age. Although severe, the extremely low incidence of these events has not suggested a rationale to modify existing recommendations for use of the vaccine in travelers, other than to reinforce that the vaccine be given only to travelers to a yellow fever endemic zone (one of the travelers was vaccinated unnecessarily for a trip to Asia). The recent occurrence of three fatal yellow fever cases in unvaccinated U.S. travelers to South America underscores the need to question carefully the itinerary and vaccination history of all travelers to Africa and South America (22–24). The protection afforded by immunization to mildly immunosuppressed persons, to asymptomatic human immunodeficiency virus (HIV)-seropositive persons, and to pregnant women may outweigh the risks of the vaccine if the potential for exposure to yellow fever is judged to be high.

Immunogenicity and safety of yellow fever vaccine were shown in several studies of HIV-infected adults with CD4$^+$ cell counts greater than 200 cells/mm^3. However, infants with HIV infection without acquired immunodeficiency syndrome (AIDS) have responded poorly to the vaccine when it was given at 1 year of age (25). When important, antibody responses to vaccination should be determined in persons with HIV infection or other immunosuppressive conditions. No significant adverse events after vaccination were reported in the study participants or from the vaccines administration to large numbers of infants in EPI programs in Africa or South America.

A single 0.5-mL subcutaneous dose confers long-lasting immunity after 7 to 10 days. Measurable neutralizing antibody may persist for more than 40 years, but reimmunization at 10-year intervals is required for international travelers. Yellow fever vaccine can be given concurrently with immune serum globulin, chloroquine, and other vaccines, such as group A/C meningopolysaccharide vaccine, DTP, measles vaccinia, hepatitis A and B vaccine, and oral or intramuscular typhoid vaccine. Coadministration of the last may have an adjuvant effect.

Protective measures against mosquito bites, such as application of repellents to skin and clothing and the use of bed netting, are well advised.

REFERENCES

1. Duffy J: Yellow fever in the continental United States during the nineteenth century. *Bull N Y Acad Med* 1968;44:687.
2. Smith HH, Downs WG. Historical perspectives on yellow fever vector research. *Curr Top Vector Res* 1983;1:1.
3. Co MD, Terajima M, Cruz J, et al. Human cytotoxic T lymphocyte responses to live attenuated 17D yellow fever vaccine: identification of HLA-B35-restricted CTL epitopes on nonstructural proteins NS1, NS2b, NS3, and the structural protein E. *Virology* 2002;293:151–163.
4. Mutebi JP, Wang H, Li L, et al. Phylogenetic and evolutionary relationships among yellow fever virus isolates in Africa. *J Virol* 2001;75:6999–7008.
5. McFarland JM, Baddour LM, Nelson JE, et al. Imported yellow fever in a United States citizen. *Clin Infect Dis* 1997;25:1143–1147.
6. Centers for Disease Control and Prevention. Fatal yellow fever in a traveler returning from Venezuela, 1999. *MMWR Morb Mortal Wkly Rep* 2000;49:303–305.
7. Centers for Disease Control and Prevention. Fatal yellow fever in a traveler returning from Amazonas, Brazil, 2002. *MMWR Morb Mortal Wkly Rep* 2002;51:324–325.
8. Mondet B. Yellow fever epidemiology in Brazil. *Bull Soc Pathol Exot* 2001;943:260–267.
9. Vasconcelos PF, Costa ZG, Travassos Da Rosa ES, et al. Epidemic of jungle yellow fever in Brazil 2000: implications of climatic alterations in disease spread. *J Med Virol* 2001;65:598–604.
10. Van der Stuyft P, Gianella A, Priard M, et al. Urbanisation of yellow fever in Santa Cruz, Bolivia. *Lancet* 1999;353:1558–1562.
11. Yellow fever, 1998–1999. *Wkly Epidemiol Rec* 2000;75:321–328.
12. Monath TP. Yellow fever: an update [Review]. *Lancet Infect Dis* 2001;1:11–20.
13. Kerr JA. The clinical aspects and diagnosis of yellow fever. In: Strode GK, ed. *Yellow fever.* New York: McGraw-Hill, 1951:385.
14. Monath TP. Yellow fever: a medically neglected disease. Report on a seminar. *Rev Infect Dis* 1987;9:165.
15. Issaacson M. Viral hemorrhagic fever hazards for travelers in Africa [Review]. *Clin Infect Dis* 2001;15;33:1707–1712.
16. Deubel V, Huerre M, Cathomas G, et al. Molecular detection and characterization of yellow fever virus in blood and liver specimens of a non-vaccinated fatal human case. *J Med Virol* 1997;53:212–217.
17. deBrito T, Sigueira SAC, Santos RTM, et al. Human fatal yellow fever: immunohistochemical detection of viral antigens in the liver, kidney and heart. *Pathol Res Pract* 1992;188:177.
18. Francis TI, Moore DL, Edington GM, et al. A clinicopathological study of human yellow fever. *Bull W H O* 1972;46:659.
19. Huerre MR, Lan NT, Marianneau P, et al. Liver histopathology and biological correlates in five cases of fatal dengue fever in Vietnamese children. *Virchows Arch* 2001;438:107–115.
20. Monath TP. Yellow fever. In: Plotkin SA, Orenstein WA, eds. *Vaccines,* 3rd ed. Philadelphia: WB Saunders, 1999:815–879.
21. Kelso JM, Mootrey GT, Tsai TF. Anaphylaxis from yellow fever vaccine. *J Allergy Clin Immunol* 1999;103:698–701.
22. Marianneau P, Georges-Courbot M, Deubel V. Rarity of adverse effects after 17D yellow-fever vaccination [Review]. *Lancet* 2001;358:84–85.
23. Martin M, Weld LH, Tsai TF, et al. Advanced age a risk factor for illness temporally associated with yellow fever vaccination. *Emerg Infect Dis* 2001;7:945–951.
24. Centers for Disease Control and Prevention. Yellow fever vaccine recommendations of the Advisory Committee on Immunization Practices (ACIP), 2002. *MMWR* 2002;51(RR-17):1–11.
25. Sibailly TS, Wiktor SZ, Tsai TF, et al. Poor antibody response to yellow fever vaccination in children infected with human immunodeficiency virus type 1. *Pediatr Infect Dis J* 1997;16:1177–1179.

CHAPTER 258
Dengue Viruses

Scott B. Halstead

HISTORY

The dengue syndrome is an acute febrile viral exanthem accompanied by headache, myalgia, anorexia, gastrointestinal disturbances, and prostration caused by viruses transmitted by mosquitoes. Before the etiologic agent was identified and during the period of European colonization, outbreaks of febrile exanthems thought to be dengue were reported widely. Classic dengue fever was described first by Benjamin Rush, who treated cases during the 1780 outbreak in Philadelphia. An earlier account of a dengue-like disease in Batavia (Jakarta, Indonesia) by David Bylon appears to have been caused by chikungunya, a togavirus also transmitted to humans by the bite of *Aedes aegypti* (1). Four types are known: dengue types 1 and 2 were isolated during World War II by Japanese and U.S. workers (2); types 3 and 4 were recovered in the Philippines in 1956 (3). Dengue syndromes caused by dengue viruses and those caused by chikungunya, O'nyong-nyong, and West Nile viruses, although often temporarily incapacitating, were generally known to have a good prognosis. This view changed in Manila in 1956, with the recognition of the dengue hemorrhagic fever and dengue shock syndrome (DHF-DSS). Since that time, more than 5 million children have been hospitalized, and 68,000 have died with this syndrome, principally in tropical Asia, but more recently in Caribbean and South American countries (4).

CHARACTERISTICS OF THE PATHOGEN

The four dengue viruses are single-stranded, enveloped, positive-sense RNA viruses of the family of Flaviviridae (type species, yellow fever virus). The family is composed of 54 serologically related viruses (5,6). Dengue viruses are spherical, 50-nm virions consisting of a nucleocapsid core about 30 nm in diameter surrounded by a lipoprotein envelope. Virions contain three structural proteins. The capsid protein surrounds the genome. The envelope (E) contains replicates of the E and matrix (M) proteins embedded in a lipid bilayer. The lipid is derived from host cell membranes. When assembled into a virion, the E protein bears epitopes that are specific for the virus serotype. Presumably, these serve as sites for viral attachment to plasma membranes and entry into host cells (7,8). Other epitopes are shared between dengue viruses (dengue subgroup antigens) or nondengue flaviviruses (flavivirus group antigens). Neutralization can be achieved only when antibody attaches conformationally to the virion surface at several discontinuous segments of the E protein (8).

Complete gene sequences are known for many strains of all types of dengue viruses. Flavivirus genomes are 11 kb long and contain a single, long open reading frame with short, nontranslated portions at the 3' and 5' ends (9). The gene is translated as a single polyprotein with structural proteins at the 5' end. Once in the cytosol, like other RNA viruses, dengue viruses use cellular cytoplasmic ribosomes to produce proteins that, together with positive RNA copies, are assembled into complete virions in cytoplasmic vacuoles. Virions are thought to be exfoliated by reverse pinocytosis.

Dengue viruses have a narrow biologic range *in vivo*. Viremia follows subcutaneous inoculation only in primate species. Virus replication in primates appears to involve cells of mononuclear phagocyte lineage (10). *In vitro*, dengue viruses replicate in a wide range of cell cultures of vertebrate and nonvertebrate origin. In addition, dengue viruses of all four types can be selected for their ability to replicate in central nervous system tissues of laboratory animals, such as mice, rats, and hamsters. Passage in mice and in some tissue cultures (e.g., primary dog kidney) places selective pressure on dengue viruses that reduces their ability to produce viremia in monkeys and clinical disease in humans. Flavivirus antibodies, when present at subneutralizing concentrations and incubated with dengue viruses in the presence of primate monocytes, result in enhanced infection, a phenomenon called *antibody-dependent enhancement* (ADE) (10–12).

Nucleotide sequence data reveal geographic homologies (genotypes) among dengue viruses (13). Currently, two genotypes have been described for dengue virus strain 1, five for dengue 2, four for dengue 3, and two for dengue 4. In dengue 1–immune individuals, infections with the American genotype of dengue 2 did not produce DHF-DSS (14), although for Asian genotype dengue 2 viruses, this same epidemiologic setting reliably produced DHF-DSS (15,16). Apparently, the American dengue 2 virus has not been under selective pressure from other dengue serotypes and is highly neutralized by anti–dengue 1 sera (17). The requirement to replicate in mosquitoes as well as humans may slow mutational change. Dengue 2 viruses recovered from the same region at an interval of 20 years showed less genetic variation than is generally predicted for RNA viruses (18).

EPIDEMIOLOGY

Dengue viruses are transmitted by mosquitoes of the daytime-biting Stegomyia family, principally *A. aegypti*. In most tropical areas, *A. aegypti* is highly urbanized, breeding in water stored for drinking or bathing or in rainwater collected in manufactured or natural containers. In Africa and tropical Asia, a jungle cycle exists with high rates of dengue virus transmission among several species of monkeys. In Malaysia, dengue viruses may be maintained in a cycle involving *Aedes niveus*, which feed on both monkeys and humans (19). Viruses from the urban and jungle cycles are genetically distinct, suggesting that discrete transmission cycles (20). Human dengue viruses evolved separately from monkey dengue 1 to 4 viruses beginning about 1,000 years ago (20). In suburban and rural areas, limited transmission from person to person may be sustained by *Aedes albopictus*. Outbreaks attributed solely to *A. albopictus* occurred in Japan during World War II and more recently in the Seychelles and in Hawaii (21). Dengue 1 transmission was reported in the state of Hawaii in 2001 for the first time since 1943. An indolent outbreak occurred in a rural population on the island of Maui that followed visits by tourists from Tahiti where an epidemic was in progress (Gubler DJ, personal communication) In most circumstances, *A. albopictus* is insufficiently anthropophilic to serve as an efficient epidemic vector. This is evidenced by the absence of dengue outbreaks in areas of Japan, Korea, the northern portion of Taiwan, China, and 25 other United States where *A. albopictus* is present but *A. aegypti* is absent (22). Because dengue is common among tourists from these countries, it is likely that viruses have been introduced frequently but without local transmission.

Currently, *A. aegypti* is almost universally distributed in the tropics between 30 degrees north and 20 degrees south latitude, an area in which nearly half of the world's populations live (23). Dengue viruses have spread throughout this range. Most transmission occurs at altitudes below 2,000 feet and during the rainy season. Frosts or sustained cold weather destroys adult mosquitoes and interrupts transmission. *A. aegypti* has a short flight range, and the dispersal of dengue viruses is almost entirely due to the movement of viremic humans (24). Under epidemic conditions, dengue usually spreads along major transportation arteries. Typically, it exhibits the epidemiologic features of a respiratory tract disease. An infected index case introduces virus into a household infested with *A. aegypti*, and after the combined extrinsic (mosquito) and intrinsic (host) incubation periods, secondary cases occur. As a result, dengue transmission is intense in crowded, urban areas. In some countries, middle- and upper-income housing provides more mosquito-breeding sites than does that of the urban poor.

Nonimmune populations support outbreaks of classic dengue fever. In certain areas where multiple dengue types are endemic, outbreaks of DHF-DSS are common. Between 250,000 and 500,000 DHF-DSS cases occur throughout the world annually; the case-fatality rate is 1% to 5%. Countries principally involved are China (Hainan), the Philippines, Vietnam, Laos, Cambodia, Thailand, Malaysia, Indonesia, Myanmar, Bangladesh, India, and Sri Lanka. Small outbreaks have been reported from Pakistan (4,22). In the American hemisphere, DHF-DSS first occurred in 1981, when Cuba experienced a sharp outbreak (25). After an absence of dengue transmission for 40 years, dengue 1 virus was introduced in 1977, producing high infection rates. In 1981, a Southeast Asian genotype dengue 2 resulted in an estimated 10,000 cases of DHF-DSS (15). Subsequent spread of Southeast Asian dengue 2 viruses has resulted in endemic DHF-DSS in Central America, Venezuela, Colombia, Guyana, and Brazil. In 1997, a Southeast Asian genotype dengue 2 was introduced into Santiago de Cuba, producing a sharp outbreak of DHF-DSS in adults infected with dengue 1 as children in 1977 (26). An important observation in the Cuban outbreaks was that blacks, although infected by dengue 1 and 2 viruses at the same frequency as whites, experienced DHF-DSS only one fifth as often (25). This observation was confirmed in Haiti where multiple dengue viruses are endemic, resulting in high rates of secondary dengue infections but little or no detectable DHF-DSS (27). These observations imply that the severity of secondary dengue virus infections is under host genetic control. Human dengue virus infections in Africa have been unusually mild (28). In the past, dengue viruses of multiple serotypes have circulated in Bangladesh, India, and Sri Lanka, with DHF-DSS cases reported only sporadically (29). From 1988, major outbreaks have been reported in each of these countries, suggesting that new dengue strains have been introduced into the region (4). Unfortunately, viral populations were not well characterized during the prolonged period of silent transmission that preceded DHF-DSS outbreaks.

PATHOGENESIS

Retrospective and prospective epidemiologic data show that DHF-DSS occurs in two immunologic settings: infections in infants born to dengue-immune mothers and second infections in children older than 1 year of age (30–33). In the latter category, all four dengue viruses result in DHF-DSS. In Thailand, where all four dengue viruses are endemic, second infections with dengue 2 and 3 account for three fourths of all studied hospitalized disease (34). Dengue viruses differ in their inherent ability to cause disease. In Cuban studies, primary dengue 2 infections (Southeast Asian genotype) were almost always inapparent, in

adults as well as children (26). The global absence of reports of virgin-soil dengue 4 epidemics suggests that primary infections with this virus are also usually inapparent. In island epidemics as well as human volunteer studies, dengue 1 viruses uniformly produce overt dengue fever in susceptible adults (2,35). Primary dengue 3 infections may also usually be clinically overt (36).

Host factors, such as age, ethnicity, and sex, influence the severity of dengue illness. For example, primary dengue infections are milder in children than in adults. The severity of secondary dengue infections, however, is inversely related to age; the youngest children are at highest risk for developing acute vascular permeability and the DHF-DSS syndrome (37). Females are at higher risk for severe disease and death than males. Blacks are intrinsically less susceptible to severe and fatal disease accompanying second dengue infections (38).

The circulation of infection-enhancing antibodies, passively or actively acquired, is the pathogenic mechanism common to the two immunologic settings. Children who are at risk for DHF appear to circulate infection-enhancing but not neutralizing antibodies (39). Functionally, ADE antibodies are raised by the large number of dengue-group and flavivirus-group E protein determinants common to the four dengue viruses. ADE antibodies form infectious complexes that promote attachment to Fc receptors (FcR). Once a virus–antibody complex attaches to the FcR, virus quickly gains entry to the cell by normal cell receptor and virus entry mechanisms (40,41). Studies on autopsy materials suggest that FcR-bearing cells of mononuclear phagocyte lineage, including dendritic cells, are major replicative hosts for dengue viruses (10,42). The 1997 epidemic in Santiago proved that ADE antibodies circulate for many years after infection. In fact, dengue 2 infections were 40 times more likely to result in severe disease and death at a 20-year interval compared with a 4-year interval after dengue 1 infection (43). Only a small percentage, 2% to 4%, of dengue-infected children are at risk for DHF-DSS during a second dengue infection (44). Prospective studies have shown that if a child circulates cross-reactive neutralizing antibodies raised as the result of a first dengue infection, these do not prevent infection, but they do protect against DHF-DSS (39). This phenomenon also explains the failure of American genotype dengue 2 viruses to cause DHF. This virus is highly neutralized by human anti–dengue 1 antibodies (17). People who have experienced two different dengue virus infections are at reduced risk for DHF-DSS, and higher-parity infections do not result in severe disease.

In monkeys, and from limited experimental and autopsy studies of human cases, it appears that dengue viruses replicated in Langerhans' (dendritic) cells in the skin at sites of injection. Virus spreads to macrophages in draining lymph nodes, then to macrophages in the spleen, lung, thymus, Kupffer's cells in the liver, bone marrow mononuclear cells, blood monocytes, and finally in mononuclear phagocytes—possibly dendritic cells in the skin (42,45). In monkeys, virus infects these cells at the time of the late maculopapular rash. It is hypothesized that ADE increases the number of infected cells but also might drive virus into cells not involved during first infections. *In vivo* evidence of ADE in an animal model was obtained when rhesus monkeys circulated higher-peak viremias during second compared with first dengue 2 infections (46). This phenomenon has been confirmed in human beings. Peak viremia titers of dengue 1, 2, and 3 viruses were significantly higher in children with DHF than in children who experienced dengue fever during a second dengue infection (47,48).

The late and sudden appearance of increased vascular permeability suggests that early interactions between elements of the immune response and dengue virus–infected cells result

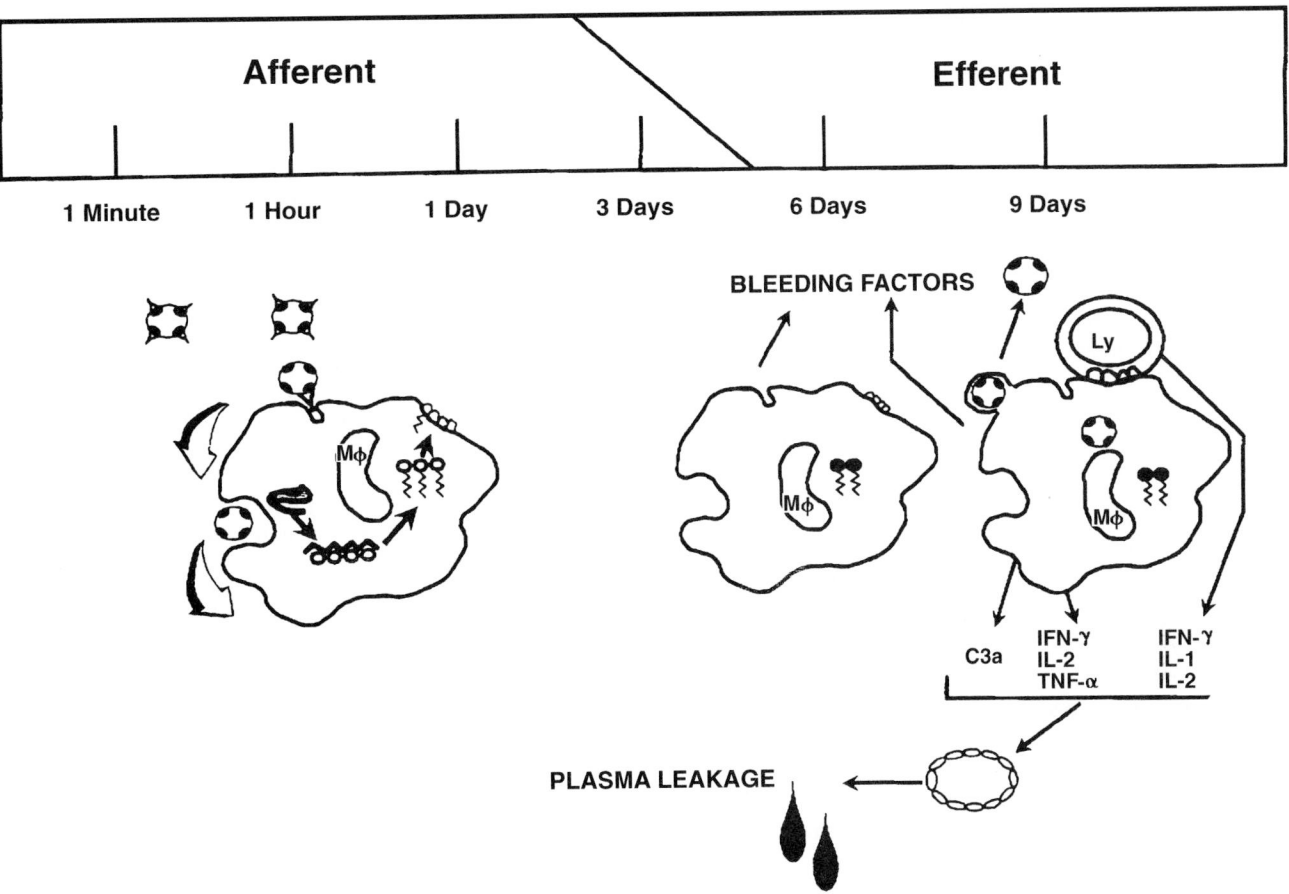

Figure 258.1. Hypothesized model of early (afferent) and late (efferent) events in the pathogenesis of dengue virus infection. Antibody-dependent enhancement of infection of mononuclear phagocytes is an afferent event that regulates the production of cytokines, which results in the signs and symptoms of dengue hemorrhagic fever-dengue shock syndrome.

in the activation of complement and release of cytokines that, in turn, activate the coagulation system and mediate vascular permeability (Fig. 258.1). No single-shock mediator has been found. Blood concentrations of tumor necrosis factor-α, interferon-γ, and interleukin-2 are elevated during the shock stage and may act synergistically (49).

CLINICAL MANIFESTATIONS

Dengue Fever

Manifestations vary with age and from patient to patient. In infants and young children, the disease may be undifferentiated or characterized by a 1- to 5-day fever, pharyngeal inflammation, rhinitis, and mild cough (50). In outbreaks, the majority of infected older children and adults exhibit most of the findings described here (51).

After an incubation period of 1 to 7 days, there is sudden onset of fever; the temperature rapidly rises to 39.4° to 41.1°C (100° to 106°F), usually accompanied by frontal or retroorbital headache. Occasionally, back pain antedates the fever. A transient, macular, generalized rash that blanches under pressure may appear. The pulse may be slow relative to the degree of fever. Myalgia or arthralgia occurs soon after the onset and increases in severity. Involvement of the joints may be particularly severe in patients with chikungunya or O'nyong-nyong infection. From the second

to the sixth days of fever, nausea and vomiting are apt to occur, and generalized lymphadenopathy, cutaneous hyperesthesia or hyperalgesia, taste aberrations, and pronounced anorexia may develop.

One to 2 days after defervescence, a generalized, morbilliform, maculopapular rash appears that spares the palms and soles. It disappears in 1 to 5 days; desquamation may occur. Rarely, there is edema of the palms and soles. About the time this second rash appears, the body temperature, which had dropped to normal, may become slightly elevated, establishing the biphasic temperature curve.

Epistaxis, petechiae, and purpuric lesions are uncommon but may occur at any stage. Swallowed blood from epistaxis, vomited or passed per rectum, may be erroneously interpreted as evidence of gastrointestinal bleeding. In adults and possibly in children, underlying lesions, such as peptic ulcer, may lead to clinically significant bleeding (52). Convulsions may occur during high temperature, especially with chikungunya fever.

Dengue Hemorrhagic Fever

The incubation period of DHF is presumed to be that of dengue fever. The course is characteristic in severely ill children (53). A relatively mild first phase of abrupt onset of fever, malaise, vomiting, headache, anorexia, and cough is followed after 2 to 5 days by rapid clinical deterioration and collapse. In this second phase, the patient usually has cold and clammy extremities, warm trunk, flushed face, diaphoresis, restlessness, irritability, and mid-epigastric pain. Shock is evidenced by a pulse pressure of 20 mm Hg or less. Prognosis and treatment should be based on pulse pressure (54). Frequently, there are scattered petechiae on the forehead and extremities; spontaneous ecchymosis may appear, and easy bruisability and bleeding at sites of venipuncture are common. A macular or maculopapular rash may appear, and there may be circumoral and peripheral cyanosis. Respirations are rapid and often labored. The pulse is weak, rapid, and thready, and the heart sounds are faint. There is delayed venous filling time. The patient is anuric. Around the time of defervescence, the liver may enlarge to extend to 4 to 6 cm below the costal margin, and it is usually firm and somewhat tender. Less than 10% of patients have gross ecchymosis or gastrointestinal bleeding, usually after a period of uncorrected shock.

After a 24- to 36-hour period of crisis, convalescence is fairly rapid for the children who recover. The temperature may return to normal before or during the stage of shock. Bradycardia and ventricular extrasystoles are common during convalescence. Infrequently, there is residual brain damage due to prolonged shock, or occasionally to intracranial hemorrhage.

LABORATORY FINDINGS

The most common hematologic abnormalities during clinical shock are a 20% or greater increase in hematocrit value over the recovery value (53), thrombocytopenia, mild leukocytosis (the cell count values seldom exceeding 10,000/mm^3), prolonged bleeding time, and moderately decreased prothrombin level (seldom less than 40% of control values) (55). Fibrinogen levels may be subnormal, and fibrin split products elevated (56).

Other abnormalities include hypocomplementemia; moderate elevations of serum transaminase values; mild metabolic acidosis with hyponatremia, and, at times, hypochloremia; slight elevation of serum urea nitrogen; and hypoalbuminemia (53,57). Radiographs of the chest reveal pleural effusions in nearly all patients (36). Sonograms may reveal pleural and pericardial effusions, ascites, and peri-gallbladder edema.

DIAGNOSIS

Clinical

The World Health Organization defines DHF as a disease with acute onset of high fever accompanied by evidence of hemostatic abnormality, most frequently a positive tourniquet test, by thrombocytopenia (100,000 mm^3 or less) and a hematocrit elevated to at least 20% above recovery value. DSS includes the above plus evidence of hypotension or a pulse pressure of 20 mm Hg or less. DHF without shock is divided into two grades without and with spontaneous hemorrhagic phenomena (58).

Virus Isolation

Blood should be obtained during the febrile period, preferably before the fifth day after onset of illness. The acute-phase serum or plasma sample may be frozen, optimally at −65°C or colder. Because of large quantities of antibody, virus is isolated from blood only rarely during hospitalization for a secondary dengue virus infection (59). Results may be improved by collecting blood samples early in the disease and by using mosquito inoculation, fluid overlay cell cultures, or mosquito cell lines as virus recovery systems (47,60,61).

Serologic Diagnosis

Etiologic diagnosis can be made on properly collected acute- and convalescent-phase serum samples or, using the immunoglobulin M capture technique, on a single sample collected within 6 weeks of the onset of illness (62). When a secondary dengue infection is suspected, paired serum samples should be collected during the period of hospitalization at an interval of at least 1 day. If a primary infection is suspected, paired sera should be obtained during the febrile period before the fifth day of illness, and a second sample at least 2 weeks after onset (58). In paired sera, diagnosis depends on demonstrating a fourfold or greater increase in antibody titer by the hemagglutination inhibition, complement fixation, enzyme-linked immunosorbent assay (ELISA), fluorescent antibody, or neutralization test (58). The most widely used test is the immunoglobulin M (IgM) capture ELISA. Dengue IgM antibodies, if present more than 5 days and less than 90 days after onset of fever, are found with both primary and secondary dengue infections (62). Differentiation of a primary antibody response from a secondary one can be accomplished using the hemagglutination inhibition, neutralization, or immunoglobulin capture techniques. In the hemagglutination inhibition test, the evolution of a primary antibody response is relatively slow, and the titer achieved is relatively low (58,62). Thus, the titer is generally less than 1:20 if measured before the fifth day and not more than 1:1280 if measured 2 weeks or more after onset. In a secondary response, the hemagglutination inhibition titer is generally greater than 1:20 before the fifth day after onset and rises to 1:2,560 or higher, often so rapidly that high fixed titers are observed. In neutralization tests, primary infections result in relatively dengue type–specific responses in convalescent-phase serum, whereas a broadly reactive response, usually involving all four types, characterizes a secondary-type antibody responses. In the ELISA, the ratio of IgM to IgG is greater than 1:1 in the acute phase of primary infections and less than 1:1 in secondary infections (58,62).

Differential Diagnosis

DENGUE FEVER

Clinical diagnosis derives from a high index of suspicion and knowledge of the geographic distribution and environmental cycles of causal viruses. Tourists may be exposed to dengue in hotels and during daytime shopping trips in epidemic or endemic areas. The differential diagnosis includes a number of viral respiratory tract and influenza-like diseases plus the early stages of malaria, scrub typhus, hepatitis, and leptospirosis. Abortive forms of each of these diseases modified by therapy or vaccine may never evolve beyond a dengue-like stage.

Clinical dengue fever may be caused by chikungunya, O'nyong-nyong, or West Nile virus. Chikungunya, a togavirus, is distributed in Africa and throughout Southeast Asia. The period of fever lasts a mean of 3 days, and infection is usually accompanied by arthralgia (63). O'nyong-nyong, also a togavirus, transmitted by *Anopheles* species, produced a sizable epidemic in Tanzania in 1952 (64). West Nile virus, a flavivirus distributed in western India, East Africa, and the United States, in addition to encephalitis in elderly people, has produced a milder syndrome indistinguishable from that caused by dengue viruses (65).

Four arboviral diseases have dengue-like courses but without rash: Colorado tick fever, sand fly fever, Rift Valley fever, and Ross River fever. Colorado tick fever occurs sporadically among campers and hunters in the western United States; sand fly fever, in the Mediterranean region, the Middle East, southern Russia, and parts of the Indian subcontinent; Rift Valley fever, in North, East, Central, and South Africa; and Ross River fever is endemic in much of eastern Australia with epidemic extension to Fiji. In adults, Ross River fever often produces protracted and crippling arthralgia involving weight-bearing joints. Because clinical findings vary and there are many possible agents, the term *dengue-like disease* should be used until a specific diagnosis is established.

DENGUE HEMORRHAGIC FEVER

In endemic areas, hemorrhagic fever should be suspected in children who have a febrile illness and exhibit hemoconcentration and thrombocytopenia with or without hemorrhagic manifestations, and with or without shock in confirmed dengue infections (66). A hypodynamic, hypovolemic acute infectious shock syndrome is pathognomonic. In DHF, there is reduced microvascular flow, increased postcapillary pressure, raised local capillary pressure, and reduced capillary flow (67). Because many rickettsial diseases, meningococcemia, and other severe illnesses caused by a variety of agents may produce hemorrhagic phenomena, the term DHF-DSS should be used only when epidemiologic, virologic, or serologic evidence suggests the possibility of dengue infection. Hemorrhagic manifestations have been described in other diseases known or presumed to be viral, including the clinically distinguishable hemorrhagic fevers described in Chapter 261.

TREATMENT

Dengue Fever

Treatment is supportive. Bed rest is recommended during the febrile period. Antipyretic drugs or cold-water sponging should be used to keep body temperature below 40°C (104°F). Analgesics or mild sedation may be required to control pain. Because of its effects on hemostasis, aspirin should not be given. Fluid and electrolyte replacement is required when there are deficits due to sweating, fasting, thirst, vomiting, or diarrhea.

Dengue Hemorrhagic Fever and Dengue Shock Syndrome

Management requires immediate evaluation of vital signs and of the degree of hemoconcentration, dehydration, and electrolyte imbalance (53,58,68). Close monitoring is essential for at least 48 hours because shock may occur or recur precipitously early in the disease. Patients who are cyanotic or have labored breathing should be given oxygen. Rapid intravenous replacement of fluids and electrolytes can frequently sustain patients until spontaneous recovery occurs. When elevation of the hematocrit persists after replacement of fluids, plasma or plasma colloid preparations are indicated (68,69). Care must be taken to avoid overhydration, which may contribute to cardiac failure. Transfusions of fresh blood or of platelets suspended in plasma may be necessary to control bleeding; they should not be given during hemoconcentration but only after evaluation of hemoglobin or hematocrit values. Salicylates are contraindicated because of their effect on blood clotting.

Paraldehyde or chloral hydrate may be required for children who are markedly agitated. Use of pressor amines, β-adrenergic-blocking agents, and aldosterone has not significantly reduced the mortality rate compared with simple supportive therapy.

Steroids do not shorten the duration of disease or improve prognosis for children receiving conscientious supportive therapy (70).

Hypervolemia during the fluid reabsorptive phase may be life threatening and is heralded by a drop in hematocrit with wide pulse pressure. Diuretics may be necessary.

PREVENTION

Chimeric and live-attenuated vaccines for dengue virus types 1, 2, 3, and 4 are under development (71–73). A killed vaccine for chikungunya is efficacious but not generally available (74). Prophylaxis consists of avoiding mosquito bites by use of insecticides, repellents, protective clothing, screening in houses, and destruction of *A. aegypti* breeding sites (58,74). If water storage is mandatory, a tight-fitting lid or a thin layer of oil on all containers may prevent egg laying or hatching. A larvicide, such as temephos [Abate: *O,O'*-(thiodi-4,1-phenylene)phosphorothioic acid *O,O,O,O'*-tetramethyl ester], available as a 1% sand-granule formulation and effective at a concentration of one part per million, may be added safely to drinking water. Ultra-low-volume spray equipment effectively dispenses malathion from truck or airplane for rapid killing of adult mosquitoes during an epidemic. Only personal antimosquito measures are effective against mosquitoes in the field, forest, or jungle.

REFERENCES

1. Carey DE. Chikungunya and dengue: a case of mistaken identity? *J Hist Med Allied Sci* 1971;26:243–262.
2. Sabin AB. Research on dengue during World War II. *Am J Trop Med Hyg* 1952;1:30–50.
3. Hammon WM, Rudnick A, Sather GE. Viruses associated with epidemic hemorrhagic fevers of the Philippines and Thailand. *Science* 1960;131:1102–1103.
4. Halstead SB. Epidemiology of dengue and dengue hemorrhagic fever. In: Gubler DJ, Kuno G, ed. *Dengue and dengue hemorrhagic fever*. Wallingford, UK: CAB, 1997;23–44.
5. Westaway EG, Brinton MA, Gaidamovich SY, et al. Flaviviridae. *Intervirology* 1985;24:183–192.
6. Karabatsos N. *International catalog of arboviruses*. Ft. Collins, CO: American Society of Tropical Medicine and Hygiene, 1985.
7. Mason PW, Dalrymple JM, Gentry MK, et al. Molecular characterization of a neutralizing domain of the Japanese encephalitis virus structural glycoprotein. *J Gen Virol* 1989;70:2037–2049.
8. Anderson R, King AD, Innis BL. Correlation of E protein binding with cell susceptibility to dengue 4 virus infection. *J Gen Virol* 1992;73:2155–2159.
9. Hahn YS, Galler R, Hunkapiller T, et al. Nucleotide sequence of dengue 2 RNA and comparison of the encoded proteins with those of other flaviviruses. *Virology* 1988;162:167–180.
10. Halstead SB. Pathogenesis of dengue: challenges to molecular biology. *Science* 1988;239:476–481.
11. Halstead SB, O'Rourke EJ. Dengue viruses and mononuclear phagocytes. I. Infection enhancement by non-neutralizing antibody. *J Exp Med* 1977;146:201–217.
12. Halstead SB, O'Rourke EJ, Allison AC. Dengue viruses and mononuclear phagocytes. II. identity of blood and tissue leukocytes supporting in vitro infection. *J Exp Med* 1977;146:218–228.
13. Rico-Hesse R. Molecular evolution and distribution of dengue viruses type 1 and 2 in nature. *Virology* 1990;174:479–493.
14. Watts DM, Porter KR, Putvatana P, et al. Failure of secondary infection with American genotype dengue 2 to cause dengue haemorrhagic fever [see Comments]. *Lancet* 1999;354:1431–1434.
15. Guzman MG, Deubel V, Pelegrino JL, et al. Partial nucleotide and amino acid sequences of the envelope and the envelope/nonstructural protein-1 gene junction of four dengue-2 virus strains isolated during the 1981 Cuban epidemic. *Am J Trop Med Hyg* 1995;52:241–246.
16. Rico-Hesse R, Harrison LM, Salas RA, et al. Origins of dengue type 2 viruses associated with increased pathogenicity in the Americas. *Virology* 1997;230:244–251.
17. Kochel TJ, Watts DM, Halstead SB, et al. Neutralization of American genotype dengue 2 viral infection by dengue 1 antibodies may have prevented dengue hemorrhagic fever in Iquitos, Peru. *Lancet* 2002;360:310–312.

18. Trent DW, Grant JA, Monath TP, et al. Genetic variation and microevolution of dengue 2 virus in Southeast Asia. *Virology* 1989;172:523–535.

19. Rudnick A. Ecology of dengue virus. *Asian J Infect Dis* 1978;2:156–160.

20. Wang E, Ni H, Xu R, et al. Evolutionary relationships of endemic/epidemic and sylvatic dengue viruses. *J Virol* 2000;74:3227–3234.

21. Metsalaar D, Grainger CR, Oei KG, et al. An outbreak of type 2 dengue fever in the Seychelles, probably transmitted by Aedes albopictus (Skuse). *Bull W H O* 1980;58:937–943.

22. Gubler DJ. Dengue and dengue hemorrhagic fever: its history and resurgence as a global public health problem. In: Gubler DJ, Kuno G, eds. *Dengue and dengue hemorrhagic fever*. New York: CAB International, 1997:1–22.

23. Division Vector-Borne Disease Control. *Geographical distribution of arthropod-borne diseases and their principal vectors*. Geneva: World Health Organization, 1989.

24. Sheppard PM, MacDonald WW, Tonn RJ, et al. The dynamics of an adult population of *Aedes aegypti* in relation to dengue hemorrhagic fever in Bangkok. *J Animal Ecol* 1969;38:661–702.

25. Kouri GP, Guzman MG, Bravo JR, Triana C. Dengue haemorrhagic fever/dengue shock syndrome: lessons from the Cuban epidemic, 1981. *Bull W H O* 1989;67:375–380.

26. Guzman MG, Kouri G, Valdes L, et al. Epidemiologic studies on dengue in Santiago de Cuba, 1997. *Am J Epidemiol* 2000;152:793–799.

27. Halstead SB, Streit TG, Lafontant JG, et al. Haiti: absence of dengue hemorrhagic fever despite hyperendemic dengue virus transmission. *Am J Trop Med Hyg* 2001;65:180–183.

28. Saluzzo JF, Cornet M, Castagnet P, et al. Isolation of dengue 2 and dengue 4 viruses from patients in Senegal. *Trans R Soc Trop Med Hyg* 1986;80:5.

29. Carey DE, Myers RM, Reuben R, et al. Studies on dengue in Vellore, South India. *Am J Trop Med Hyg* 1966;15:580–587.

30. Halstead SB, Nimmannitya S, Cohen SN. Observations related to pathogenesis of dengue hemorrhagic fever. IV. Relation of disease severity to antibody response and virus recovered. *Yale J Biol Med* 1970;42:311–328.

31. Kliks SC, Nimmannitya S, Nisalak A, et al. Evidence that maternal dengue antibodies are important in the development of dengue hemorrhagic fever in infants. *Am J Trop Med Hyg* 1988;38:411–419.

32. Sangkawibha N, Rojanasuphot S, Ahandrik S, et al. Risk factors in dengue shock syndrome: a prospective epidemiologic study in Rayong, Thailand. I. The 1980 outbreak. *Am J Epidemiol* 1984;120:653–669.

33. Thein S, Aung MM, Shwe TN, et al. Risk factors in dengue shock syndrome. *Am J Trop Med Hyg* 1997;56:566–572.

34. Vaughn DW, Green S, Kalayanarooj S, et al. Dengue in the early febrile phase: viremia and antibody responses. *J Infect Dis* 1997;176:322–330.

35. Simmons JS, St. John JH, Reynolds FHK. Experimental studies of dengue. *Philippine J Sci* 1931;44:1–252.

36. Kalayanarooj S, Vaughn DW, Nimmannitya S, et al. Early clinical and laboratory indicators of acute dengue illness. *J Infect Dis* 1997;176:313–321.

37. Guzman MG, Kouri G, Bravo J, et al. Effect of age on outcome of secondary dengue 2 infections. *Int J Infect Dis* 2002;6:118–124.

38. Guzman MG, Kouri GP, Bravo J, et al. Dengue hemorrhagic fever in Cuba, 1981: a retrospective seroepidemiologic study. *Am J Trop Med Hyg* 1990;42:179–184.

39. Kliks SC, Nisalak A, Brandt WE, et al. Antibody-dependent enhancement of dengue virus growth in human monocytes as a risk factor for dengue hemorrhagic fever. *Am J Trop Med Hyg* 1989;40:444–451.

40. Gollins SW, Porterfield JS. Flavivirus infection enhancement in macrophages: an electron microscopic study of viral cellular entry. *J Gen Virol* 1985;66:1969–1982.

41. Hase T, Summers PL, Eckels KH. Flavivirus entry into cultured mosquito cells and human peripheral blood monocytes. *Arch Virol* 1989;104:129–143.

42. Wu SJ, Grouard-Vogel G, Sun W, et al. Human skin Langerhans cells are targets of dengue virus infection [see Comments]. *Nat Med* 2000;6:816–820.

43. Guzman MG, Kouri G, Valdes L, et al. Enhanced severity of secondary dengue 2 infections occurring at an interval of 20 compared with 4 years after dengue 1 infection. *Panamerican J Epidemiol* (in press).

44. Halstead SB. Immunological parameters of Togavirus disease syndromes. In: Schlesinger RW, ed. *The togaviruses: biology, structure, replication*. New York: Academic Press, 1980:107–173.

45. Marchette NJ, Halstead SB, Falkler WA Jr, et al. Studies on the pathogenesis of dengue infection in monkeys. 3. Sequential distribution of virus in primary and heterologous infections. *J Infect Dis* 1973;128:23–30.

46. Halstead SB, Shotwell H, Casals J. Studies on the pathogenesis of dengue infection in monkeys. II. clinical laboratory responses to heterologous infection. *J Infect Dis* 1973;128:15–22.

47. Vaughn DW, Green S, Kalayanarooj S, et al. Dengue viremia titer, antibody response pattern, and virus serotype correlate with disease severity. *J Infect Dis* 2000;181:2–9.

48. Sudiro TM, Zivny J, Ishiko H, et al. Analysis of plasma viral RNA levels during acute dengue virus infection using quantitative competitor reverse transcription-polymerase chain reaction. *J Med Virol* 2001;63:29–34.

49. Rothman AL, Ennis FA. Immunopathogenesis of dengue hemorrhagic fever. *Virology* 1999;257:1–6.

50. Halstead SB, Nimmannitya S, Margiotta MR. Dengue and Chikungunya virus infection in man in Thailand, 1962–1964. II. Observations on disease in outpatients. *Am J Trop Med Hyg* 1969;18:972–983.

51. Simmon JS, St John JH, Reynolds FHK. Experimental studies of dengue. *Philippine J Sci* 1931;44:1–252.

52. Tsai CJ, Kuo CH, Chen PC, et al. Upper gastrointestinal bleeding in dengue fever. *Am J Gastroenterol* 1991;86:33–35.

53. Cohen SN, Halstead SB. Shock associated with dengue infection. I. Clinical and physiologic observations of dengue hemorrhagic fever in Thailand, 1964. *J Pediatr* 1966;68:448–456.

54. Bethell DB, Flobbe K, Cao XT, et al. Pathophysiologic and prognostic role of cytokines in dengue hemorrhagic fever. *J Infect Dis* 1998;177:778–782.

55. Weiss HJ, Halstead SB. Studies of hemostasis in Thai hemorrhagic fever. *J Pediatr* 1965;66:918–926.

56. Bokisch VA, Top FH Jr, Russell PK, et al. The potential pathogenic role of complement in dengue hemorrhagic shock syndrome. *N Engl J Med* 1973;289:996–1000.

57. Memoranda. Pathogenic mechanisms in dengue hemorrhagic fever. Report of an international collaborative study. *Bull W H O* 1973;48:117–132.

58. Anonymous. *Dengue haemorrhagic fever: diagnosis, treatment, prevention and control*, 2nd ed. Geneva: World Health Organization, 1997.

59. Nisalak A, Halstead SB, Singharaj P, et al. Observations related to pathogenesis of dengue hemorrhagic fever. III. Virologic studies of fatal disease. *Yale J Biol Med* 1970;42:293–310.

60. Rosen L, Gubler DJ. The use of mosquitoes to detect and propagate dengue viruses. *Am J Trop Med Hyg* 1974;23:1153–1160.

61. Igarashi A. Isolation of a Singh's *Aedes albopictus* cell clone sensitive to dengue and Chikungunya viruses. *J Gen Virol* 1978;40:531–544.

62. Innis BL, Nisalak A, Nimmannitya S, et al. An enzyme-linked immunosorbent assay to characterize dengue infections where dengue and Japanese encephalitis co-circulate. *Am J Trop Med Hyg* 1989;40:418–427.

63. Carey DE, Myers RM, DeRanitz CM, et al. The 1964 Chikungunya Epidemic at Vellore, South India, including observations on Concurrent Dengue. *Trans R Soc Trop Med Hyg* 1969;63:434–445.

64. Robinson MC. An epidemic of virus disease in Southern Province, Tanganyika Territory in 1952–1953. I. Clinical features. *Trans R Soc Trop Med Hyg* 1955;49:28–32.

65. Carey DE, Rodrigues FM, Myers RM, et al. Arthropod-borne viral infections in children in Vellore, South India, with particular reference to dengue and West Nile viruses. *Indian Pediatr* 1968;5:285–296.

66. Nimmannitya S, Halstead SB, Cohen S, et al. Dengue and chikungunya virus infection in man in Thailand, 1962–1964. I. Observations on hospitalized patients with hemorrhagic fever. *Am J Trop Med Hyg* 1969;18:954–971.

67. Bethell DB, Gamble J, Pham PL, et al. Noninvasive measurement of microvascular leakage in patients with dengue hemorrhagic fever. *Clin Infect Dis* 2001;32:243–53.

68. Ngo NT, Cao XT, Kneen R, et al. Acute management of dengue shock syndrome: a randomized double-blind comparison of 4 intravenous fluid regimens in the first hour. *Clin Infect Dis* 2001;32:204–213.

69. Dung NM, Day NPJ, Tam DTH, et al. Fluid replacement in dengue shock syndrome: a randomized, double-blind comparison of four intravenous-fluid regimens. *Clin Infect Dis* 1999;29:787–794.

70. Tassniyom S, Vasanawathana S, Chirawatkul A, et al. Failure of high-dose methylprednisolone in established dengue shock syndrome: a placebo-controlled, double-blind study. *Pediatrics* 1993;92:111–115.

71. Bhamarapravati N, Yoksan S, Chayaniyayothin T, et al. Immunization with a live attenuated dengue-2-virus candidate vaccine (16681-PDK 53): clinical, immunological and biological responses in adult volunteers. *Bull W H O* 1987;65:189–195.

72. Kinney RM, Huang CY. Development of new vaccines against dengue fever and Japanese encephalitis. *Intervirology* 2001;44:176–197.

73. Guirakhoo F, Arroyo J, Pugachev KV, et al. Construction, safety, and immunogenicity in nonhuman primates of a chimeric yellow fever-dengue virus tetravalent vaccine. *J Virol* 2001;75:7290–304.

74. Harrison VR, Binn LN, Randall, R. Comparative immunogenicities of chikungunya vaccines prepared in avian a mammalian tissues. *Am J Trop Med Hyg* 1967;16:786–791.

75. Halstead SB. Selective primary health care: strategies for control of disease in the developing world. XI. Dengue. *Rev Infect Dis* 1984;6:251–264.

CHAPTER 259

Encephalitis Viruses Belonging to the Families Flaviviridae, Togaviridae, and Bunyaviridae

Charles H. Hoke, Jr.

HISTORY

Seven families of viruses contain pathogens that cause encephalitis in humans. Four of those families contain the bulk of these pathogens: the Flaviviridae, Togaviridae, Bunyaviridae, and Herpesviridae (Table 259.1). The first three of these families are discussed in this chapter. A new paramyxovirus, Nipah virus, is covered briefly. Viruses of the family Flaviridae that cause encephalitis include West Nile, St. Louis encephalitis, Japanese encephalitis (JE), Murray Valley encephalitis (MVE), tick-borne encephalitis (including Central European and Russian spring-summer encephalitis), and Powassan (1). Viruses of the genus *Alphavirus* of the family Togaviridae that cause encephalitis include eastern equine encephalitis (EEE), western equine encephalitis (WEE), and Venezuelan equine encephalitis (VEE). Encephalitogenic members of the Bunyaviridae family include California, La Crosse, Jamestown Canyon, and Rift Valley fever viruses. St. Louis encephalitis virus, the first viral agent of encephalitis to be isolated, was isolated in 1933 from a patient who died in an outbreak that occurred in St. Louis and Kansas City, Missouri (2). In relatively quick succession, most of the known agents of other types of viral encephalitis were discovered (3–14). In 1986, infection by human immunodeficiency virus (HIV) was demonstrated to be a cause of viral encephalitis (15). Additional causes of acute viral encephalitis may exist, and viruses may spread suddenly far beyond the areas in which they are known to circulate. For clinical and public health reasons, it is imperative to pursue the diagnosis of every case of viral encephalitis, especially fatal cases. Pursuing isolations of virus from animals affected by fatal epizootics may yield clues to the etiology of human epidemics. Blood and cerebrospinal fluid rarely yield virus isolates. Brain tissue may be required. In fatal cases of viral encephalitis, postmortem tissue should be sought. The laboratory evaluation of viral encephalitis must be carefully planned in coordination with public health authorities and available microbiologic services. Because the capability to isolate etiologic agents is highly specialized, evaluations may require participation of state and national laboratories. A wide range of cells and animals may be required for virus isolation. Serologic confirmation of many etiologies can be made by virus-specific immunoglobulin M (IgM) capture assays and other types of serologic tests. Broadly reactive serologic tests and polymerase chain reaction (PCR)-based assays with carefully chosen sets of primers may provide clues to the taxonomic classification of etiologic agents in puzzling cases.

Recent dramatic increases in the areas of the world affected by JE (now in Australia), West Nile virus (now in the United States) and Rift Valley fever (now in Saudi Arabia and Yemen), as well as an outbreak of a new type of encephalitis (due to Nipah virus) in Malaysia and Singapore, suggest that clinicians should think broadly of the possible etiologies of all cases of viral encephalitis, even when travel histories do not suggest exposure in the traditional areas affected by the various viral agents. Encephalitis viruses may infect humans far from the areas normally associated with viral transmission. Surveillance and control measures are specific for vectors and viruses. Therefore, an etiology should be sought for every case of suspected viral encephalitis (16).

CHARACTERISTICS OF THE PATHOGENS

Flaviviridae

JAPANESE ENCEPHALITIS VIRUS

History and Geographic Location. JE virus was isolated from a human in 1935 (3) and from the vector mosquito, *Culex tritaeniorhynchus*, in 1938. Numerous summertime epidemics of encephalitis had occurred in Japan and Korea in the preceding decades. Once a virus was isolated, subsequent encephalitis epidemics were clearly associated with the JE virus. After World War II, intensive study of the ecology of the virus in Japan and Korea was undertaken. A great deal was learned about the role of birds, pigs, and other animals as amplifying hosts and about the many mosquito species that served as vectors. Vaccines were developed for U.S. soldiers during and after the war by combined efforts of the Army and the National Institutes of Health. Vaccine technology was transferred to Japan after World War II for use in Japanese children, and a purified version was introduced in 1966. Widespread use of the vaccine, along with improved living standards, was associated with a reduction in the annual incidence from several thousand cases to about 10. In 1988, the vaccine was proved efficacious under field conditions in Thailand (17). JE is important in many Asian countries. China probably has between 10,000 and 50,000 cases per year. Morbidity and mortality are considerable in Nepal, Thailand, Sri Lanka, India, the Philippines, Malaysia, and Vietnam. In addition to Japan, the nations China, Taiwan, Korea, Thailand, Sri Lanka, and India also have JE immunization programs, programs that have been associated with distinct reductions in attack rates in humans, despite continued enzootic transmission (18). The World Health Organization provides standardization of JE vaccines manufactured in different countries. In 1995, JE spread into the Torres Strait, Northern Queensland Australia, probably from New Guinea (19). Continued cases suggest establishment of transmission in this new region (20).

Classification. JE virus is a member of the family Flaviviridae, along with the agents of yellow fever, dengue fever, and MVE, St. Louis encephalitis, and West Nile encephalitis. Groupings based on genotypic analysis are useful in tracking evolutionary and geographic movement of the virus. The relative similarity of the genetic information in large collections of isolates suggests that JE viruses may belong to a single serotype (21).

Structure. The Flaviviridae have a spherical nucleocapsid surrounded by a lipid-containing envelope with surface projections. The particles are 40 to 70 nm in diameter and contain a single molecule of single-stranded RNA, which is positive sense (the genome and the messenger RNA are the same). The entire genome has been sequenced many times. The genome contains about 10,000 base pairs. There are three structural polypeptides: the envelope (E), the matrix (M), and the capsid (C), which are glycosylated, and several nonstructural proteins. The three-dimensional structure of the envelope glycoprotein has been

TABLE 259.1.   Initial Isolations of Flaviviridae, Togaviridae, and Bunyaviridae Associated with Viral Encephalitis

Virus and encephalitis type	Animal host		Humans		Vector		
	Animal	Year	Location	Year	Location	Species	Year
Family Flaviviridae							
St. Louis	Birds	1955	St. Louis Kansas City, MO	1933	Yakima, WA	*Culex pipiens* *Culex tarsalis*	1941
Japanese	Horses	1937	Nagasaki, Japan Tokyo	1934 1938	Japan	*Culex tritaeniorhynchnus*	1930
Tick-borne	Insectivores, rodents, birds	1939(?)	Far Eastern Russia Former Czechoslovakia	1937 1948	Far Eastern Russia	*Ixodes persulcatus*	1937
Murray Valley	Horses	1984	Australia	1951	Australia	*Culex annulirostris*	1960
West Nile	Horses	1968	West Nile Province, Uganda	1937	Egypt	*Culex* species	1952
Powassan	Squirrels	1968	Ontario, Canada	1958	Colorado	*Dermacentor andersoni*	1952
Rocio	Sparrows	1975	Rural Sao Paolo, Brazil	1975	Brazil	*Psorophora ferox*	1978
Family Togaviridae, genus *Alphavirus*							
Eastern equine	Horses	1933	Massachusetts	1938	Georgia	*Coquillettidia perturbans*	1949
Western equine	Horses	1930	California	1938	Washington State	*Aedes aegypti* *Culex tarsalis*	1941
Venezuelan equine	Horses	1936	Trinidad	1944	Trinidad	*Mansonia titillans*	1944
Members of the family Bunyaviridae, California serogroup							
California	Unknown		San Joaquin, CA	1945	California	*Aedes malanimon*	1943
La Crosse	Squirrels	1970	La Crosse, WI	1964	Wisconsin	*Aedes triseriatus*	1972
Jamestown Canyon	White-tailed deer	1973	Wisconsin	1965	Colorado	*Culiseta inornata*	1962

predicted, allowing analysis of the location of important epitopes (22). The structure of these epitopes depends on appropriate disulfide linkages (23). The mutations responsible for attenuation may be in genes that code for viral proteases or those coding for the envelope protein. Convincing evidence localizing an attenuating mutation to residue 138 of the envelope glycoprotein has been demonstrated (24,25).

Biologic and Biochemical Properties. JE virus replicates to high titer in a number of vertebrate and insect cell lines, causing a cytopathic effect (CPE) (26). The virus readily infects the brain of many animals, when inoculated directly into the brain, into the blood followed by mechanical disruption of the blood–brain barrier, or across the cribriform plate after intranasal instillation. Exposure of monkeys by the latter route has led to development of a model for evaluation of protection afforded by new vaccines (27,28). The proteins of the virus, especially the envelope protein and the NS1 nonstructural protein, can be readily observed in antigenically reactive form on polyacrylamide gel electrophoresis. The complete genome has been cloned, sequenced, and expressed in a number of prokaryotic and eukaryotic expression systems (29,30). Infectious complementary DNA has been made, and mutants with reduced neurovirulence have been recovered (31).

Replication. The virus replicates in inoculated mosquitoes, in cell lines derived from them, and in vertebrates and their cells (32). The virus membrane fuses with the cell membrane and penetrates the cytoplasm, where replication of the positive-sense genome and synthesis of both structural and nonstructural proteins takes place. The structural proteins are assembled into virion particles, which then bud from the surface of infected cells (33).

Antigenic Characteristics

JE virus was originally classified with yellow fever and dengue viruses as a group B arbovirus. This assignment was based on cross-reactions observed using the hemagglutination inhibition test (34). This classification was, unfortunately, a confusing coincidence because this B is unrelated to the B originally used in the now obsolete term *Japanese B encephalitis*. The B in this term was used to distinguish encephalitis caused by JE virus from von Economo encephalitis lethargica, which was called type A. Neutralization of the virus using specific monkey or mouse serum confirms its identity. Specific monoclonal antibodies have been developed that are now in wide use for unequivocal identification of JE virus. Nucleotide sequence amplification techniques have been used to determine the genetic relatedness of isolates. Manipulation of the genes of JE has led to construction of a number of candidate vaccines. Recombinants of JE envelope protein genes and the NYVAC vector stimulate neutralizing antibody, but only in volunteers who have not previously received small pox vaccine (vaccinia). Similarly engineered recombinant viruses based on the ALVAC platform were not immunogenic (35). Engineered chimeras between yellow fever and JE virus have been more promising (36). DNA plasmids containing JE genes stimulate neutralizing antibodies in mice, but protection is inferior to that afforded by commercially available vaccines (37). JE virus replicates to high enough titers that inactivated cell culture–derived vaccine may be possible (38).

Laboratory Demonstration of Infection

The diagnosis can be made by demonstrating virus-specific antiviral IgM antibody in the cerebrospinal fluid or serum, which was present in the specimens of 80% of patients collected at the time of admission to a hospital in rural Thailand. One hundred percent of specimens collected 3 days later contained virus-specific IgM antibody (39,40). For use in regions where diagnostic support is limited, an IgM antibody capture dot enzyme-linked immunosorbent assay (ELISA) with adequate sensitivity and specificity may be used (41,42). Commercially manufactured tests for diagnosis of JE have been developed and tested (43), although none is currently licensed in the United States. Application by the manufacturers and licensure by the U.S. Food and Drug Administration are needed before such tests can be made available for use in diagnosing U.S. travelers suspected of having JE. Occasionally, the virus can be isolated from cerebrospinal fluid, particularly in fulminant disease when there is abundant virus replication. In fatal cases, the virus can be isolated from virtually any site in the brain, although specimens from several sites should be cultivated. Cultures derived from hamster, porcine, chicken, monkey, and mosquito cells (AP61 or C6/36) are useful for isolating the virus. Once a CPE is observed, the virus' identity may be confirmed by use of an ELISA. Alternatively, the virus may be identified by demonstration of a reduction in the number of virus plaques after treatment with virus-specific antiserum. PCR may be used to diagnose JE infections (44); however, diagnoses made using PCR do not yield virus for further study, and thus cultivation is encouraged.

In 1998 to 1999, an alarming outbreak of encephalitis occurred in pig handlers in Malaysia and in pig slaughterhouse workers in Singapore. Because of the association between pig farming and encephalitis in Southeast Asia, the etiologic agent of the outbreak was initially suspected to be JE virus. However, because many of the handlers had been immunized against JE, other etiologies were suspected. The outbreak turned out to be due to Nipah virus, a newly discovered paramyxovirus related to Hendra virus. Because encephalitis due to Nipah virus appears to be transmitted by nasal secretions from pig to human, the possibility of human-to-human transmission is within the realm of imagination. Should transmission from human to human occur and become sustained, truly alarming outbreaks might result. ELISA tests are available that may be useful in diagnosing Nipah virus infection. Magnetic resonance imaging may help distinguish Nipah infections from JE (45,46). Electron microscopical examination of cerebrospinal fluid may reveal paramyxovirus-like particles (47).

ST. LOUIS ENCEPHALITIS VIRUS

History and Geographic Location. St. Louis encephalitis virus is an important cause of epidemic viral encephalitis in the United States. St. Louis encephalitis virus was isolated from a human brain in 1933 (2), and proof of natural infection of *Culex tarsalis* mosquito vectors came during study of an outbreak in 1941 (48). Since 1933, both urban and rural outbreaks have occurred, some focal and some widespread. Urban outbreaks have occurred in many cities. Notable outbreaks have occurred in Missouri, Illinois, Kentucky, Texas, Arizona, Colorado, New Jersey, California, and Florida; significant outbreaks occurred in 1932, 1937, 1954, 1962, 1972, 1980, 1984, and 1990. The virus has been detected across much of North America and in much of South America. In Florida in 1990 and 1991, 222 cases were documented, with the most serious in older age groups and in those with prolonged evening exposure (49). Outbreaks in Florida between 1990 and 1999 varied greatly in magnitude, with increased transmission occurring after periods with conditions that favored the presence of abundant vector (*Culex nigripalpus*) and avian host species (50). Analysis of St. Louis encephalitis virus isolates collected between 1986 and 1999 in Harris County, Texas, demonstrated that multiple genotypes coexist in the same location, with particular genotypes associated with focal areas (51).

Classification. St. Louis encephalitis virus is a member of the family Flaviviridae. It is grouped in the JE complex.

Structure. St. Louis encephalitis virus is structurally identical to other flaviviruses: they have a single strand of RNA of positive polarity about 11,000 base pairs long. The nucleotide sequence of the RNA is known, and the genes are arranged in the following order: capsid, pre-M, E, NS1, NS1a, NS2b, NS3, NS4a, NS4b, NS5. The virus particle is constructed only from the first three proteins. The NS, or nonstructural, proteins are involved in the replication of RNA or the transport and assembly of the virus but are not included in the final structure. A single long open reading frame (contains no natural stopping codons) allows the protein to be transcribed as a single amino acid chain, which is later cleaved into individual proteins (52). The RNA is complexed with a highly basic capsid protein. The nucleocapsid is surrounded by a lipid bilayer. Two proteins, the M and the E protein, surround the lipid bilayer.

Biologic and Biochemical Properties. The virus can be grown in a number of cell lines [BHK-21 (baby hamster kidney), Vero, LLC-MK$_2$, MA-104, and porcine kidney] in which a CPE occurs, and under proper conditions, plaques are formed (53). Baby mice and hamsters are highly susceptible to intracerebral infection. The virus can be identified by its susceptibility to neutralization by specific monkey or human serum or in ELISAs using appropriate reagents. The life cycle of the virus includes birds and several species of mosquito (*Culex pipiens, C. nigripalpus, C. tarsalis,* and *Culex quinquefasciatus*) that are capable of transmitting the virus to humans.

Replication. After the virus enters the cell, the nucleocapsid is uncoated. The nucleus is an important site of early RNA replication steps (54). Translation of the RNA into a long protein begins at a single site. Individual proteins are cut from the long polyprotein. The RNA is also transcribed into complementary (negative-sense) RNA strands, which in turn are transcribed into more full-length genomes, which can be either translated or assembled as genome into new viral particles. The RNA and the proteins are assembled into viral packages in a poorly understood process that aligns the membrane proteins together around the nucleocapsid and ultimately allows budding from the cell membrane.

Antigenic Characteristics. St. Louis encephalitis virus is most closely related to the JE, MVE, and West Nile viruses, and these viruses have been grouped using mouse hyperimmune ascites fluid in the JE antigenic complex, along with several other viruses (55). With monoclonal antibodies, some variation in St. Louis encephalitis virus isolates has been detected. Eight antigenic epitopes on the envelope glycoprotein have been characterized. Monoclonal antibody that mediates *in vitro* biologic functions of hemagglutination and neutralization also is most protective against lethal *in vivo* challenge with intraperitoneally administered St. Louis encephalitis virus (56).

Laboratory Demonstration of Infection. As with JE virus, isolation is most often successful with postmortem tissue. Virus antigen can be demonstrated by specific staining methods. IgM antibody capture ELISA can be used to establish the diagnosis. IgM antibodies are detectable in the serum of encephalitis patients drawn between days 4 and 21 of illness in 99% of cases. The titer of IgM antibody wanes over several weeks, so that diagnosis may be based on falling virus-specific IgM levels (57). Other forms of antibody tests (complement fixation, hemagglutination inhibition, neutralization) have been used. An antigen capture enzyme immunoassay capable of detecting St. Louis encephalitis in pools of infectious mosquitoes facilitates surveillance for the presence of St. Louis encephalitis in vector populations (58).

CENTRAL EUROPEAN ENCEPHALITIS (TICK-BORNE AND RUSSIAN SPRING-SUMMER ENCEPHALITIS) VIRUS

History and Geographic Location. Central European encephalitis was first recognized in 1932 in Far Eastern Russia. The virus was isolated from human brain in 1937 and that same year was shown to be transmissible by ticks (59,60). In 1948, the disease was described in the Strakonice District of Czechoslovakia. A virus isolated from a patient with the disease was shown to be similar to the one that had been isolated from the cases in Far Eastern Russia (61). Most affected persons are exposed to ticks in woodland areas between May and October, although the disease may occasionally be acquired by consuming raw milk. Central European encephalitis occurs across Europe and Russia, with occasional cases being reported in Japan (62). The ecology of Central European encephalitis virus in many areas of Europe and Asia has been studied in detail and interrelationships between vectors and virus analyzed. The prevalence of tick-borne encephalitis in Europe led to development and manufacture of inactivated vaccines that are licensed in Europe. Because the virus is the principal cause of arbovirus encephalitis in Europe, a vigorous research effort to describe the virus molecular biology has flourished at several European universities (63). Studies of the crystallographic structure of the Central European encephalitis virus envelope glycoprotein yielded models that have served as the standards against which the structure of other flaviviruses have been compared. In recent years, the virus has assumed importance for military travelers to Europe. Many missile silos in the former Soviet Union were located in wooded areas. Inspectors of these silos were felt to be at risk, as were U.S. forces deployed to Bosnia and French forces in Kosovo. European vaccines have been used intermittently to immunize these forces (64).

Classification. Formerly, the names *Russian spring-summer encephalitis* and *tick-borne encephalitis virus* were widely used. Because no virus named tick-borne encephalitis virus has been entered in the *International Catalog of Arboviruses*, Calisher (65) proposed that the complex be referred to as *Central European encephalitis virus*.

Structure. The structure of viruses of this complex is the same as that of other flaviviruses. Crystallographic analysis of the major envelope glycoprotein demonstrated that the surface protein forms a dimer that lies in a rather flat orientation to the viral surface. Numerous antigenically important sites have been identified (66).

Biologic and Biochemical Properties. Flaviviruses are generally stable between pH 7.0 and 9.0, but Central European encephalitis virus is stable at lower pH (67). This property may account for its infectiousness when ingested orally.

The virus replicates in a large range of cells, including human, chicken (egg and cell culture), cow, pig, monkey, reptile, and amphibian (68). It also replicates in ticks: *Ixodes persulcatus* and *Ixodes ricinus* have been shown experimentally to be competent vectors (59,69). Virus disseminates in the ticks after a meal of infected blood and is subsequently transmissible when the tick feeds. Many small mammals, including shrews, moles, voles, hamsters, and mice, are highly susceptible to infection and are heavily infested by vector ticks in the wild. These mammals serve as maintenance hosts for the virus. Cows and mice become viremic after being bitten by infected ticks and subsequently shed virus in milk (70). Animals may be infected for long periods. Intracerebral in-

oculation of sheep and monkeys causes encephalitis (71). The genetic sequence of Central European encephalitis virus is highly homologous with the sequences of other flaviviruses (72). The binding sites of monoclonal antibodies to component proteins and the location of disulfide cross-links in the envelope glycoprotein have been determined. The genetic changes responsible for developing resistance to neutralizing monoclonal antibodies and of attenuation have been identified (73). Analysis of the binding of monoclonal antibodies suggests that the virus antigens in strains isolated over a wide range in Austria have been stable during a 14-year period (74). Using site-directed mutagenesis, site 310, normally containing a threonine residue, has been identified as having an important role in attenuation of the virus (75).

Replication. Replication of Central European encephalitis virus is similar to that of other flaviviruses.

Antigenic Characteristics. The hemagglutination inhibition test shows Central European encephalitis virus to be antigenically related to the other members of the family Flaviviridae. Neutralization tests afford serologic identification of infecting flaviviruses. Through studies of the antigen sites on the envelope glycoprotein, the binding of a number of monoclonal antibodies to a series of important epitopes has been mapped. Other studies using various molecular fragments or disrupted molecular structures have contributed to the development of a widely accepted two-dimensional diagram of this protein. Glycosylation appears to have no effect on the immunoreactive structures (76). Isolates from across Europe and Asia are similar enough that the vaccine made in Europe protects immunized mice against lethal challenge with a wide range of isolates. In addition, serum from human recipients of the European vaccine neutralizes strains from Siberia and other far-eastern areas (77).

Laboratory Demonstration of Infection. Early in the illness, virus may be isolated from the blood. In fatal cases, it can be isolated from brain tissue in infant mice and a number of types of cell culture (61). As for other flaviviruses, IgM capture ELISA has replaced older serologic tests (78).

MURRAY VALLEY ENCEPHALITIS VIRUS

History and Geographic Location. Although outbreaks of MVE had been noted as early as 1917, the virus was not characterized until 1951 (10). Epidemics occurred between 1917 and 1925 and again in 1950 to 1951. Most cases occurred in the Murray Valley of Australia, giving the virus its name. Outbreaks occurred in 1956, 1971, 1974, 1978, 1981, and 1984 (61). Cases have been confirmed in New Guinea (79). MVE virus is closely related to Kunjin virus, another flavivirus that occasionally causes encephalitis (80).

Classification. MVE virus is antigenically and genetically similar to JE virus. It is classified as a member of the JE virus complex (55).

Structure. MVE virus is similar in structure to that of the other flaviviruses.

Biologic and Biochemical Properties. MVE virus grows in a variety of cells (81) and in infant mice, hamsters, and chickens.

Replication. MVE virus replicates in a manner similar to that of other flaviviruses.

Antigenic Characteristics. The virus is antigenically similar to other flaviviruses. Consequently, antibody detected by hemagglutination inhibition may cross-react with those viruses.

Laboratory Demonstration of Infection. The virus can be isolated from the brain postmortem in cultures of chick embryo and infant mice cells. Hemagglutination inhibition, complement fixation, and neutralizing antibody tests can be used to confirm infection by demonstrating at least a fourfold increase in antibody titer from acute- to convalescent-phase specimens. Detection of virus-specific IgM is useful in diagnosis (82).

WEST NILE VIRUS

History and Geographic Location. West Nile virus was first isolated in 1937 from a febrile patient who became ill in the town of West Nile in Uganda. The virus was recognized as a cause of encephalitis in 1957. Before 1999, the West Nile virus was widespread in an area that included eastern Africa, southern Europe, the Middle East, and the western half of India. Outbreaks of infection due to this virus have occurred in many countries in East Africa and the Middle East, especially Egypt and Israel. A dramatic urban outbreak occurred in 1996 and 1997 in Romania. In 1999, an outbreak of West Nile encephalitis occurred in Israel. Four hundred seventeen cases were confirmed, of which nearly 60% were encephalitis. Significant mortality occurred among elderly patients (83). In 2000, West Nile virus was introduced into the United States, where an initial outbreak in the Staten Island area of New York was recognized by astute clinicians and public health personnel. Early in the outbreak, the etiologic virus was thought to be St. Louis encephalitis virus. However, careful study demonstrated that the virus was, in fact, West Nile virus, nearly identical in sequence to a virus that had been isolated from a patient in Israel. The virus also caused many avian deaths, both in zoo-housed birds and in wild living birds. The virus was found to be transmissible by a number of vector mosquitoes present in the United States. Intensive surveillance efforts were established to deal with this new threat (84). These surveillance efforts demonstrated the rapid spread of the virus up and down the eastern coastal region of the United States. Spread of the virus was followed by surveillance for dead crows and other birds and subsequent isolation of West Nile virus from the dead birds. On Staten Island, during 2000, 10 human neurologic cases and 2 equine cases were identified (85). In 2001, 48 human cases from many states on the east coast of the United States were identified between July and October; 4,607 infected crows and 189 infected horses were detected during this period. West Nile virus was detected in animals as far west as Iowa, Arkansas, and Missouri (86). The sudden introduction of West Nile virus into the United States, the suggestion of dramatically increased neurovirulence, and its rapid spread among humans, mosquitoes, birds, and animals all point out the degree to which populations may be vulnerable to threats formerly thought to be limited in distribution to remote lands (87,88). Elderly patients with febrile illnesses, neurologic symptoms, and gastrointestinal complaints or muscle weakness might be suspected of having West Nile infection (89). Identification of new or newly moved agents of encephalitis may lead to implementation of the specific control measures needed to control transmission of each new agent identified.

Classification. West Nile virus is classified in the family Flaviviridae. Serologically it is a member of the Japanese encephalitis virus complex. Viruses recently isolated from patients in New York appear nearly identical to isolates from Israel from an outbreak in 2000 (90,91).

Biologic and Biochemical Properties. West Nile virus is morphologically indistinguishable from other flaviviruses. Viral particles are 40 to 60 nm in diameter, and enveloped. They contain positive-sense, single-stranded RNA about 10,000 to 11,000 base pairs in length. Virus has been isolated from numerous mosquito species in the New York area (*Aedes vexans, C. pipiens, Culex salinarius, Ochlerotatus triseriatus,* and *Psorophora ferox*). The persistence of the virus in over-wintering mosquitoes suggests that, once introduced into a region, the virus may persist (92). By comparing viruses with varying degrees of neuroinvasiveness, molecular determinants of attenuation include sites on the envelope protein, although other genetic determinants may exist as well (93).

Replication. The virus grows readily in Vero cells. Infectious clones of West Nile virus have been established, and these appear more stable than the clones of other flaviviruses (94). Although no antiviral medication is approved for treatment of West Nile infection, high levels of ribavirin do inhibit replication in cultured neural cells (95).

Antigenic Characteristics. The gene coding for the envelope protein has been expressed in an *Escherichia coli* system and found to be authentic enough both to be recognized by antibodies from virus-infected humans and to stimulate antibody and protection in mice. Expressed, purified E protein may provide the basis for a candidate vaccine for West Nile (96). Humanized mouse monoclonal antibodies directed against the envelope glycoprotein of West Nile virus have been proposed as possible therapeutic or passive prophylactic reagents (97). Genes coding for West Nile envelope protein have been inserted in a DNA plasmid and administered to horses and mice with subsequent protection against West Nile challenge. In addition, COS-1 cells, transformed by insertion of this plasmid, secrete West Nile envelope protein into the culture medium, from which it can be purified to serve as a highly standardizable reagent for serologic tests or for vaccine (98). Capitalizing on progress in using a yellow fever virus backbone for making chimeric live attenuated flavivirus vaccines, a West Nile vaccine–yellow fever chimeric virus has been developed as a potential candidate for attenuated vaccine against West Nile virus (99).

Laboratory Demonstration of Infection. Numerous serologic and virologic assays have been developed for diagnosis of West Nile infection. Older hemagglutination inhibition tests, immunofluorescence antibody tests, and various IgG- and IgM-specific ELISA tests have been developed. Virus may be detected in mosquito pools, tissues, or cerebrospinal fluid using virus isolation, TaqMan reverse transcription PCR, or antigen capture ELISA tests. Diagnosis is best coordinated through local and state public health laboratories. Virus genome may be detected in equine and avian tissues using a reverse transcriptase nested PCR procedure (100).

POWASSAN VIRUS
First isolated in 1959, Powassan is a tick-borne encephalitis flavivirus that infects people in North America. Only about 30 cases have been diagnosed (101).

Togaviridae

The Togaviridae that cause encephalitis—EEE, WEE, and VEE viruses—are all members of the genus *Alphavirus*. EEE virus readily causes serious brain infection. All three viruses are associated with outbreaks of encephalitis in equine populations, with VEE causing massive epizootics on occasion. WEE virus tends to cause encephalitis in very young children. In humans, VEE virus generally causes only a debilitating febrile disease with severe headache. Actual encephalitis occurs only in a small fraction of cases. Alphaviruses are 60 to 65 nm in diameter and spherical. The single-stranded RNA genome is contained in a nucleocapsid core. A glycoprotein shell surrounds a lipid bilayer (102) from which glycoprotein spikes protrude. The genome is about 11,700 bases long. The genome codes for four nonstructural proteins of unknown function. All members of the genus have a similarly organized genome. There are strong antigenic cross-reactions among the alphaviruses, and many serologic assays cross-react. Hemagglutination inhibition is somewhat more specific. The alphaviruses replicate and produce CPE in a wide variety of vertebrate cells. Plaque assays sensitive to a single infectious particle can be performed readily on a variety of cells. CPE is much less notable in invertebrate cell lines. Animals may be readily infected. Horses develop encephalitis after inoculation with WEE, EEE, or VEE virus. Inoculated infant mice develop fatal encephalitis (5).

EASTERN EQUINE ENCEPHALITIS VIRUS

History and Geographic Location. EEE virus was first isolated in 1933 (6). It is transmitted between birds and humans by the mosquito vector. It causes fatal encephalitis in humans along the east coast of the United States and in some inland locations in New York, Michigan, and South Dakota (5).

Classification. EEE is a member of the genus *Alphavirus* of the Togaviridae family.

Structure. The structure of EEE is that described earlier for members of the *Alphavirus* genus of Togaviridae.

Biologic and Biochemical Properties. EEE virus replicates well in BHK cells, Vero cells, and avian embryo cells. It causes a CPE and can be plaqued on these cells. The molecular basis of its invasiveness and virulence for children is not known.

Replication. The virus attaches to specific receptors on the surface of target cells and undergoes endocytosis (103). RNA serves as the template for both new protein synthesis and RNA synthesis. Replication takes place in the cytoplasm.

Antigenic Characteristics. EEE shares antigenic determinants with other alphaviruses as determined by immunofluorescence, ELISA, and radioimmunoassays or complement fixation tests. It can be distinguished from other strains by neutralization or modified hemagglutination inhibition tests (104).

Laboratory Demonstration of Infection. Virus may be isolated from serum collected early in infection (105) and from the brain of fatal cases. Serologic tests are used to demonstrate development of specific antibody during acute illness. An IgM capture ELISA can be used to confirm infection with a single specimen (106).

WESTERN EQUINE ENCEPHALITIS VIRUS

History and Geographic Location. WEE virus was first isolated from the brain of a horse that became ill in a major epizootic outbreak in the San Joaquin Valley of California (4). It was isolated in 1938 from the brain of a child who had died of encephalitis and in 1941 from mosquitoes (107). It is found in western North and South America.

Classification. WEE is a member of the genus *Alphavirus* in the family Togaviridae.

Structure. The structure of WEE is similar to that of EEE and other alphaviruses.

Biologic and Biochemical Properties. WEE is less neuroinvasive than EEE (107) but infects similar cells. It grows especially well in suckling mice and embryonated eggs. Analysis of the genomes of WEE, EEE, and Sindbis virus, an alphavirus from the Old World, has led to the suggestion that WEE was derived from a recombination of genetic material from EEE and Sindbis virus (108).

Replication. Replication is similar to that of EEE.

Antigenic Characteristics. WEE may be distinguished from other alphaviruses on the basis of the hemagglutination inhibition test or neutralization tests with specific antisera or monoclonal antibodies.

Laboratory Demonstration of Infection. Virus may be isolated postmortem from brain tissue. The antibody tests described for EEE may be used to demonstrate increased antibody titer or the presence of virus-specific IgM (106). Occasionally, it can be isolated from throat swab samples or cerebrospinal fluid (109).

VENEZUELAN EQUINE ENCEPHALITIS VIRUS

History and Geographic Location. VEE virus was isolated from the brain of a horse in an outbreak of fatal encephalomyelitis in Venezuela in 1936 (110). Having been distinguished from the already isolated EEE and WEE viruses, it was named for that country (111). The first recognized human cases were reported in 1944 in Trinidad. Epizootic infections occurred between 1955 and 1972 with associated epidemics. In 1979, disease in humans and horses spread through northern Central America and into Texas (112,113). VEE has the capability to cause massive epizootics in horses. Vaccines for horses exist. On occasion, large numbers of horses have been immunized to control outbreaks. No human vaccine is licensed in the United States. However, a vaccine designed to protect laboratory workers against VEE has been administered under an investigational new drug (IND) exemption for some years. Once aerosolized, VEE is highly contagious. As interest in VEE virus increases, particularly as a potential agent of biologic warfare or as a replicon vector for other antigens, laboratory-associated infections are likely.

Classification. VEE virus is a member of the genus *Alphavirus* of the family Togaviridae.

Structure. VEE virus is, like other alphaviruses, a spherical particle about 60 nm in diameter. A nucleocapsid core containing genomic RNA and nucleocapsid protein is contained within a lipid bilayer and an outer glycoprotein shell. Glycoprotein spikes on the surface are made up of trimers of the proteins E1 and E2. The genome of the virus is contained on a single strand of RNA (102). The genome contains about 11,700 bases, which contain the genes for eight proteins: four nonstructural proteins, a capsid, a p62 (or E2) protein, 6K, and E1. The last four proteins, along with new RNA, are assembled into the final particle (114).

Biologic and Biochemical Properties. VEE viruses grow well in newborn mice and in cultures of mammalian and insect cells.

Replication. Replication of VEE probably begins in lymph nodes draining the site of inoculation and, when the central nervous system is invaded, in neural cells. The virus enters cells by a process called *adsorptive endocytosis.* Nucleocapsids are released, and viral RNA is uncoated for replication. Viral RNA serves as messenger RNA, and the resulting nonstructural proteins serve as catalysts for subsequent RNA transcription. The genomic RNA is also transcribed into a full-length negative-sense RNA, which in turn is transcribed into a genomic positive-sense RNA. Viral structural proteins are produced by translation of a subgenomic piece of the RNA (called *subgenomic RNA* because it contains only the portion of the genome that codes for the structural proteins). The structural proteins are assembled into viral particles by a physical process that is driven by the nature of the proteins, their proximity to one another, and their insertion into internal cell membranes (114).

Antigenic Characteristics. Isolates of VEE virus have been grouped into a complex containing several subtypes (I through VI) based on distinctions detectable in the hemagglutination inhibition test. Subtype I has been subdivided into variants A through F, and variants IA, IB, and IC are associated with epizootics and human cases (5). Cross-protection by vaccine containing a single variant may be limited, suggesting significant antigenic diversity.

Laboratory Demonstration of Infection. Virus may be isolated by inoculating specimens from serum and throat swabs into suckling mice or Vero cells. Virus may be identified by plaque reduction using specific sera. Serologic diagnosis can be made using hemagglutination inhibition and neutralization tests or an IgM capture ELISA (106,115–117).

Bunyaviridae

The family Bunyaviridae (the name of which was derived from the name of the town in Uganda where the prototype virus, Bunyamwera virus, was isolated from mosquitoes) contains more than 250 individual species in five genera. The encephalitis viruses, members of the California serogroup, cause California, Jamestown Canyon, and La Crosse encephalitis. Rift Valley fever virus has been associated with encephalitis and hemorrhagic fever in an increasing area.

History and Geographic Location. The California encephalitis virus was isolated during studies of arbovirus encephalitis in Kern County, California, in 1943. Serologic studies confirmed that it had caused three cases of viral encephalitis (13,118). Further cases of encephalitis caused by this virus have not been observed, but a serologically related virus, La Crosse virus, was first isolated from a fatal human case in Wisconsin in 1960 (14), and this virus has been associated with human disease across the midwestern United States (119). Jamestown Canyon virus, discovered subsequently, has caused occasional cases of encephalitis (120,121). In 1997 and 1998, an outbreak of Rift Valley fever occurred in Kenya. Infections were associated with both hemorrhagic fever and encephalitis (122). In 2000 and 2001, outbreaks occurred in Saudi Arabia and Yemen, suggesting that this disease, like West Nile, may be increasing its geographic scope. Because of the large number of potential vector mosquitoes and susceptible livestock, further spread may occur.

Classification. Viruses of the Bunyaviridae family have been classified on the basis of complement fixation analysis. Cross-neutralization and hemagglutination inhibition tests have been used to develop the serogroups. Comparing different members,

genomes are organized similarly, and protein-coding mechanisms are similar. Molecular characteristics are used to define the genera (123). Rift Valley fever virus is a member of the genus phlebovirus.

Structure. Bunyavirus lipid-enveloped particles contain two glycoproteins. Glycoprotein spikes, which bear type-specific antigenic determinants, protrude from a lipid membrane. Contained within the particles are three negative-sense (proteins are translated from complementary messenger RNA), single-stranded RNA molecules, each one contained in a viral nucleoprotein, and an enzyme with transcriptase activity. The virions are between 80 and 120 nm in diameter. The RNA genome has a small, a medium-sized, and a large segment. The M segment codes for the two structural glycoproteins, G1 and G2. The large, small, and medium-sized segments also code for nonstructural proteins (123).

Biologic and Biochemical Properties. Most of these viruses are transmitted to animal hosts by arthropods (124). They may be isolated in cell culture, in which a CPE is observed, or by suckling mouse brain inoculation. California encephalitis virus is found in the western United States and Canada and may be isolated from the principal mosquito vector, *Aedes melanimon.* The principal vertebrate hosts are rodents and rabbits. Isolation from humans is uncommon. Cultures may be propagated in mice or BHK-21 cells. La Crosse virus, which occurs in the central and eastern United States, is transmitted by *Aedes triseriatus.* The principal vertebrate hosts are chipmunks and squirrels. The virus may be isolated by inoculation of suckling mouse brains or cultivation in BHK-21 cells. Jamestown Canyon virus occurs in North America. The animal host is the white-tailed deer. Although many human infections have occurred, only a few cases of human encephalitis have been identified (125).

Replication. Bunyaviruses attach to the surface of host cells by means of interactions between surface glycoproteins and host cells. After fusion of cell and virion membranes, the virus is uncoated. The genome RNA is transcribed into complementary messenger RNA using virion-associated polymerase. The large and small segments are translated by free ribosomes, and the medium-sized segment is translated by membrane-bound ribosomes. The genome is replicated using the previously synthesized complementary RNA. G1 and G2 proteins are glycosylated. As they accumulate in the Golgi apparatus, modified host membrane is acquired as particles bud into the Golgi cisternae. Finally, cytoplasmic vesicles fuse with the plasma membrane and virus particles are released from the cell. Virus replication slows cell protein synthesis and may or may not destroy the host cell (123).

Antigenic Characteristics. Immune response is directed principally against the G1 and G2 glycoproteins on the surface of the particles and the nucleoprotein capsid protein. Bunyaviruses share complement fixation antigens (126). Blocking of viral hemagglutination by antibody forms the basis of the hemagglutination inhibition assay. Antibody that neutralizes the ability to form plaques is stimulated by infection. Monoclonal antibodies have proved useful for distinguishing isolates (127).

Laboratory Demonstration of Infection. Rising antibody titers during the course of acute infection indicate infection by a suspected virus. Virus may be isolated postmortem from brain tissue by inoculating suckling mouse brain or by cultivating specimens in cell lines such as the BHK-21 cell line. Isolates are identified serologically (128). IgG- and IgM-specific antibody ELISA tests, virus isolation, reverse transcription PCR with sequencing of DNA product, and immunohistochemical procedures may be used to diagnose Rift Valley fever virus infections.

REFERENCES

1. Westaway EG, Brinton MA, Gaidamovich SY, et al. Flaviviridae. *Intervirology* 1985;24:183.
2. Webster LT, Fite GL. A virus encountered in the study from cases of encephalitis in the St. Louis and Kansas City epidemic of 1933. *Science* 1933;78:463.
3. Mitamura T, Kitaoka M, Watanabe M, et al. Study on Japanese encephalitis virus: animal experiments and mosquito transmission experiments. *Kansai Iji* 1936;1:260.
4. Meyer KF, Harting CM, Howitt B. The etiology of epizootic encephalomyelitis of horses in the San Joaquin Valley, 1930. *Science* 1931;74:227.
5. Peters CJ, Dalrymple JM. Alphaviruses. In: Fields BN, Knipe DM, eds. *Fields virology,* 2nd ed. New York: Raven Press, 1990:713–761.
6. TenBroeck C, Merrell MH. A serological difference between eastern and western equine encephalomyelitis virus. *Proc Soc Exp Biol Med* 1933;31:217.
7. Farber S, Hill A, Connerley ML, et al. Encephalitis in infants and children caused by the virus of eastern variety of equine encephalitis. *JAMA* 1940;114:1725.
8. Randall R, Mills JW. Fatal encephalitis in man due to the Venezuelan virus of equine encephalomyelitis in Trinidad. *Science* 1944;99:225.
9. Smorodintsev AA. Tick-borne spring-summer encephalitis. *Prog Med Virol* 1958;1:210.
10. French EL. Murray Valley encephalitis: isolation and characterization of the etiological agent. *Med J Aust* 1952;1:100.
11. McLean CM, Donohue WL. Powassan virus: isolation of virus from a fatal case of encephalitis. *Can Med Assoc J* 1959;80:708.
12. Lopes O, Coimbra TLM, Sacchetta L de A, et al. Emergence of a new arbovirus disease in Brazil. I. Isolation and characterization of the etiologic agent, Rocio virus. *Am J Epidemiol* 1978;107:444.
13. Reeves WC, Hammon WMcD. Epidemiology of the arthropod-borne viral encephalitides in Kern County, California, 1943–1952. *Univ Calif Public Health* 1962;4:1.
14. Thompson WH, Kahlfayan B, Anslow RO. Isolation of California encephalitis group virus from a fatal human illness. *Am J Epidemiol* 1965;81:245.
15. Bigger RJ, Johnson BK, Mrisoke SS, et al. Severe illness associated with appearance of antibody to human immunodeficiency virus in an African. *Br Med J* 1986;293:1210.
16. Thomson RB Jr, Bertram H. Laboratory diagnosis of central nervous system infections. *Infect Dis Clin North Am* 2001;15:1047.
17. Hoke CH, Nisalak A, Sangawhipa N, et al. Protection against Japanese encephalitis by formalin-inactivated vaccines. *N Engl J Med* 1988;319:608.
18. Wu YC, Huang YS, Chien LJ, et al. The epidemiology of Japanese encephalitis on Taiwan during 1966–1997. *Am J Trop Med Hyg* 1999;61:78.
19. Johansen CA, van den Hurk AF, Pyke AT, et al. Entomological investigations of an outbreak of Japanese encephalitis virus in the Torres Strait, Australia, in 1998. *J Med Entomol* 2001;38:581.
20. Hanna JN, Ritchie SA, Phillips DA, et al. Japanese encephalitis in north Queensland, Australia, 1998. *Med J Aust* 1999;170:533.
21. Tsarev SA, Sanders ML, Vaughn DW, et al. Phylogenetic analysis suggests only one serotype of Japanese encephalitis virus. *Vaccine* 2000;18[Suppl 2]:36.
22. Kolaskar AS, Kulkarni-Kale U. Prediction of three-dimensional structure and mapping of conformational epitopes of envelope glycoprotein of Japanese encephalitis virus. *Virology* 1999;261:31.
23. Srivastava AK, Aira Y, Mori C, et al. Antigenicity of Japanese encephalitis virus envelope glycoprotein V3 (E) and its cyanogen bromide cleaved fragments examined by monoclonal antibodies and Western blotting. *Arch Virol* 1987;96:97.
24. Ni H, Chang GJ, Xie H. Molecular basis of attenuation of neurovirulence of wild-type Japanese encephalitis virus strain SA14. *J Gen Virol* 1995;76:409.
25. Sumiyoshi H, Tignor GH, Shope RE. Characterization of a highly attenuated Japanese encephalitis virus generated from molecularly cloned cDNA. *J Infect Dis* 1995;171:1144.
26. Leake CJ, Burke DS, Nisalak A, et al. Isolation of Japanese encephalitis virus from clinical specimens using a continuous mosquito cell line. *Am J Trop Med Hyg* 1986;35:1045.
27. Raengsakulrach B, Nisalak A, Gettayacamin M, et al. An intranasal challenge model for testing Japanese encephalitis vaccines in rhesus monkeys. *Am J Trop Med Hyg* 1999;60:329.
28. Myint KS, Raengsakulrach B, Young GD, et al. Production of lethal infection that resembles fatal human disease by intranasal inoculation of macaques with Japanese encephalitis virus. *Am J Trop Med Hyg* 1999;60:338.
29. McAda PC, Mason PW, Schmaljohn CS, et al. Partial nucleotide sequence of the Japanese encephalitis virus genome. *Virology* 1987;158:348.
30. Sumiyoshi H, Mori C, Fuke I, et al. Complete nucleotide sequence of the Japanese encephalitis virus genome RNA. *Virology* 1987;161:497.
31. Sumiyoshi H, Tignor GH, Shope RE. Characterization of a highly attenuated Japanese encephalitis virus generated from molecularly cloned cDNA. *J Infect Dis* 1995;171:1144.
32. Beatty BJ, Calisher CH, Shope RE. Arboviruses. In: Schmidt NJ, Emmons RW, eds. *Diagnostic procedures for viral, rickettsial and chlamydial infections.* Washington, DC: American Public Health Association, 1989:797–856.
33. Hase T, Summers PL, Dubois DR. Ultrastructural changes of mouse brain neurons infected by Japanese encephalitis virus. *Int J Exp Pathol* 1990;71:493.
34. Casals J, Brown LV. Hemagglutination with arthropod-borne viruses. *J Exp Med* 195499:429.
35. Kanesa-thasan N, Smucny JJ, Hoke CH, et al. Safety and immunogenicity of NYVAC-JEV and ALVAC-JEV attenuated recombinant Japanese encephalitis virus—poxvirus vaccines in vaccinia-nonimmune and vaccinia-immune humans. *Vaccine* 2000;19:483.
36. Guirakhoo F, Zhang ZX, Chambers TJ, et al. Immunogenicity, genetic stability, and protective efficacy of a recombinant, chimeric yellow fever-Japanese encephalitis virus (ChimeriVax-JE) as a live, attenuated vaccine candidate against Japanese encephalitis. *Virology* 1999;257:363.
37. Kaur R, Sachdeva G, Vrati S. Plasmid DNA immunization against Japanese encephalitis virus: immunogenicity of membrane-anchored and secretory envelope protein. *J Infect Dis* 2002;185:1.
38. Srivastava AK, Putnak JR, Lee SH. A purified inactivated Japanese encephalitis virus vaccine made in Vero cells. *Vaccine* 2001;19:4557.
39. Burke DS, Nisalak A, Ussery MA, et al. Kinetics of IgM and IgG responses to Japanese encephalitis virus in human serum and cerebrospinal fluid. *J Infect Dis* 1985;151:1093.
40. Burke DS, Nisalak A, Hoke CH Jr. Field trial of a Japanese encephalitis diagnostic kit. *J Med Virol* 1986;18:41.
41. Solomon T, Thao LT, Dung NM, et al. Rapid diagnosis of Japanese encephalitis by using an immunoglobulin M dot enzyme immunoassay. *J Clin Microbiol* 1998;36:2030.
42. Gajanana A, Samuel PP, Thenmozhi V. An appraisal of some recent diagnostic assays for Japanese encephalitis. *Southeast Asian J Trop Med Public Health* 1996;27:673.
43. Cuzzubbo AJ, Endy TP, Vaughn DW, et al. Evaluation of a new commercially available immunoglobulin M capture enzyme-linked immunosorbent assay for diagnosis of Japanese encephalitis infections. *J Clin Microbiol* 1999;37:3738.
44. Meiyu F, Huosheng C, Cuihua C, et al. Detection of flaviviruses by reverse transcriptase-polymerase chain reaction with the universal primer set. *Microbiol Immunol* 1997;41:209.
45. Wong SC, Ooi MH, Wong MN, et al. Late presentation of Nipah virus encephalitis and kinetics of the humoral immune response. *J Neurol Neurosurg Psychiatry* 2001;71:552.
46. Lim CC, Sitoh YY, Hui F, et al. Nipah viral encephalitis or Japanese encephalitis? MR findings in a new zoonotic disease. *Am J Neuroradiol* 2000;21:455.
47. Chow VT, Tambyah PA, Yeo WM, et al. Diagnosis of Nipah virus encephalitis by electron microscopy of cerebrospinal fluid. *J Clin Virol* 2000;19:143.
48. Hammon W McD, Reeves, WC, Brookman B, et al. Mosquitoes and encephalitis in the Yakima Valley Washington. V. Summary of case against *Culex tarsalis* Coquillet as a vector of the St. Louis and western equine viruses. *J Infect Dis* 1942;70:278.
49. Meehan PJ, Wells DL, Paul W, et al. Epidemiological features of and public health response to a St. Louis encephalitis epidemic in Florida, 1990–1. *Epidemiol Infect* 2000;125:181.
50. Day JF, Stark LM. Frequency of Saint Louis encephalitis virus in humans from Florida, USA: 1990–1999. *J Med Entomol* 2000;37:626.
51. Chandler LJ, Parsons R, Randle Y. Multiple genotypes of St. Louis encephalitis virus (Flaviviridae: *Flavivirus*) circulate in Harris County, Texas. *Am J Trop Med Hyg* 2001;64:12.
52. Trent DW, Kinney RM, Johnson BJ, et al. Partial nucleotide sequence of St. Louis encephalitis virus RNA: structural proteins, NS1, ns2a, and ns2b. *Virology* 1987;156:293.
53. Karabatsos N. General characteristics and antigenic relationships. In: Monath TP, eds. *St. Louis encephalitis.* Washington, DC: American Public Health Association, 1980:105–158.
54. Brawner IA, Trousdale MD, Trent DW. Cellular localization of Saint Louis encephalitis virus replication. *J Virol* 1979;23:284.
55. Calisher CH, Karabatsos N, Dalrymple JM, et al. Antigenic relationships between flaviviruses as determined by cross-neutralization tests with polyclonal antisera. *J Gen Virol* 1989;70:37.
56. Mathews JH, Roehrig JT. Elucidation of the topography and determination of the protective epitopes on the E glycoprotein of Saint Louis encephalitis virus by passive transfer with monoclonal antibodies. *J Immunol* 1984;132:1533.
57. Monath TP, Nystrom RR, Bailey RE, et al. Immunoglobulin M antibody capture enzyme-linked immunosorbent assay for diagnosis of St. Louis encephalitis. *J Clin Microbiol* 1984;20:784.
58. Tsai TF, Bolin RA, Montoya M, et al. Detection of St. Louis encephalitis virus antigen in mosquitoes by capture enzyme immunoassay. *J Clin Microbiol* 1987;25:370.
59. Zilber LA, Soloviev VD. Far Eastern tick-borne spring-summer (spring) encephalitis. *Annu Rev Sov Med Spec* 1946;5[Suppl]:1.
60. Smorodintsev AA. Tick-borne spring-summer encephalitis. *Prog Med Virol* 1958;1:210.

61. Monath TP, Heinz FX. Flaviviruses. In: Fields BN, Knipe DM, Howley PM, et al., eds. *Fields virology,* 3rd ed. Philadelphia: Lippincott-Raven, 1996:961–1034.
62. Takashima I. Epidemiology of tick-borne encephalitis in Japan. *Comp Immunol Microbiol Infect Dis* 1998;21:81.
63. Heinz FX, Mandl CW. The molecular biology of tick-borne encephalitis virus. *APMIS* 1993;101:735.
64. Desjeux G, Lemardeley P, Colin C, et al. Cost-benefit ratio of tick-borne encephalitis vaccination of French troops based in Kosovo. *Rev Epidemiol Sante Publique* 2001;49:249.
65. Calisher CH. Antigenic classification and taxonomy of flaviviruses (family Flaviviridae) emphasizing a universal system for the taxonomy. *Acta Virol* 1988;32:469.
66. Rey FA, Heinz FX, Mandl C, et al. The envelope glycoprotein from tick-borne encephalitis virus at 2 A resolution. *Nature* 1995;375:275.
67. Pogodina VV. The resistance of tick-borne encephalitis virus to the effects of gastric juice. *Vopr Virusol* 1958;3:295.
68. Pudney M, Varma MGR. The growth of some tick-borne arboviruses in cell cultures derived from tadpoles of the common frog, *Rana temporaria. J Gen Virol* 1971;10:131.
69. Rampas J, Gallia F. The isolation of encephalitis virus from *Ixodes ricinus* ticks. *Cas Lek Cesk* 1949;88:1179.
70. Pogodina VV. Experimental study of the pathogenesis of tick-borne encephalitis on alimentary infection. 11. Study of pathways of excretion of virus from white mice. *Probl Virol* 1960;5:304.
71. Zilber LA. Pathogenicity of Far Eastern and Western (European) tick-borne encephalitis viruses in sheep and monkeys. In: Libikova H, ed. *Biology of viruses of the tick-borne encephalitis complex.* New York: Academic Press, 1960:260–265.
72. Mandl CW, Heinz FX, Kunz C. Sequence of the structural proteins of tick-borne encephalitis virus (western subtype) and comparative analysis with other flaviviruses. *Virology* 1988;166:197.
73. Heinz FX, Kunz C. Molecular epidemiology of tick-borne encephalitis virus: peptide mapping of large nonstructural proteins of European isolates and comparison with other flaviviruses. *J Gen Virol* 1982;62:271.
74. Guirakhoo F, Radda AC, Heinz FX, et al. Evidence for antigenic stability of tick-borne encephalitis virus by the analysis of natural isolates. *J Gen Virol* 1987;68:859.
75. Mandl CW, Allison SL, Holzmann H, et al. Attenuation of tick-borne encephalitis virus by structure-based site-specific mutagenesis of a putative flavivirus receptor binding site. *J Virol* 2000;74:9601.
76. Winkler G, Heinz FX, Kunz C. Studies on the glycosylation of flavivirus E proteins and the role of carbohydrate in antigenic structure. *Virology* 1987;159:237.
77. Hayasaka D, Goto A, Yoshii K, et al. Evaluation of European tick-borne encephalitis virus vaccine against recent Siberian and far-eastern subtype strains. *Vaccine* 2001;19:4774.
78. Heinz FX, Roggendorf M, Hofmann H, et al. Comparison of two different enzyme immunoassays for detection of immunoglobulin M antibodies against tick-borne encephalitis virus in serum and cerebrospinal fluid. *J Clin Microbiol* 1981;14:141.
79. French EL, Anderson SG, Price AVG, et al. Murray Valley encephalitis in New Guinea. I. Isolation of Murray Valley encephalitis virus from the brain of a fatal case of encephalitis occurring in a Papuan native. *Am J Trop Med Hyg* 1957;6:827.
80. Mackenzie JS, Broom AK. Australian X disease, Murray Valley encephalitis and the French connection. *Vet Microbiol* 1995;46:79.
81. Westaway EG. Assessment and application of a cell line from pig kidney for plaque assay and neutralization tests with twelve group B arboviruses. *Am J Epidemiol* 1966;84:439.
82. Marshall ID. Murray Valley and Kunjin encephalitis. In: Monath TP, ed. *The arboviruses: epidemiology and ecology.* Boca Raton, FL: CRC Press, 1988:151–190.
83. Chowers MY, Lang R, Nassar F, et al. Clinical characteristics of the West Nile fever outbreak, Israel, 2000. *Emerg Infect Dis* 2001;7:675.
84. Anonymous. West Nile virus activity—eastern United States, 2001. *MMWR Morb Mortal Wkly Rep* 2001;50:617.
85. Kulasekera VL, Kramer L, Nasci RS, et al. West Nile virus infection in mosquitoes, birds, horses, and humans, Staten Island, New York, 2000. *Emerg Infect Dis* 2001;7:722.
86. Anonymous, Weekly update: West Nile virus activity—United States, November 14–20, 2001. *MMWR Morb Mortal Wkly Rep* 2001;50:1061.
87. Marfin AA, Gubler DJ. West Nile encephalitis: an emerging disease in the United States. *Clin Infect Dis* 2001;33:1713.
88. Hayes CG. West Nile virus: Uganda, 1937, to New York City, 1999. *Ann N Y Acad Sci* 2001;951:25.
89. Weiss D, Carr D, Kellachan J, et al. West Nile Virus Outbreak Response Working Group: clinical findings of West Nile virus infection in hospitalized patients, New York and New Jersey, 2000. *Emerg Infect Dis* 2001;7:654.
90. Hindiyeh M, Shulman LM, Mendelson E, et al. Isolation and characterization of West Nile virus from the blood of viremic patients during the 2000 outbreak in Israel. *Emerg Infect Dis* 2001;7:748.
91. Giladi M, Metzkor-Cotter E, Martin DA, et al. West Nile encephalitis in Israel, 1999: the New York connection. *Emerg Infect Dis* 2001;7:659.
92. Nasci RS, Savage HM, White DJ, et al. West Nile virus in overwintering *Culex* mosquitoes, New York City, 2000. *Emerg Infect Dis* 2001;7:742.
93. Chambers TJ, Halevy M, Nestorowicz A, et al. West Nile virus envelope proteins: nucleotide sequence analysis of strains differing in mouse neuroinvasiveness. *J Gen Virol* 1998;79:2375.
94. Yamshchikov VF, Wengler G, Perelygin AA, et al. An infectious clone of the West Nile flavivirus. *Virology* 2001;281:294.
95. Jordan I, Briese T, Fischer N, et al. Ribavirin inhibits West Nile virus replication and cytopathic effect in neural cells. *J Infect Dis* 2000;182:1214.
96. Wang T, Anderson JF, Magnarelli LA, et al. Immunization of mice against West Nile virus with recombinant envelope protein. *J Immunol* 2001;167:5273.
97. Roehrig JT, Staudinger LA, Hunt AR, et al. Antibody prophylaxis and therapy for flavivirus encephalitis infections. *Ann N Y Acad Sci* 2001;951:286.
98. Davis BS, Chang GJ, Cropp B, et al. West Nile virus recombinant DNA vaccine protects mouse and horse from virus challenge and expresses in vitro a noninfectious recombinant antigen that can be used in enzyme-linked immunosorbent assays. *J Virol* 2001;75:4040.
99. Arroyo J, Miller CA, Catalan J, et al. Yellow fever vector live-virus vaccines: West Nile virus vaccine development. *Trends Mol Med* 2001;7:350.
100. Johnson DJ, Ostlund EN, Pedersen DD, et al. Detection of North American West Nile virus in animal tissue by a reverse transcription-nested polymerase chain reaction assay. *Emerg Infect Dis* 2001;7:739.
101. Anonymous. Outbreak of Powassan encephalitis—Maine and Vermont, 1999–2001. *MMWR Morb Mortal Wkly Rep* 2001;50:761.
102. Harrison SC. Alphavirus structure. In: Schlesinger S, Schlesinger MJ, eds. *The Togaviridae and Flaviviridae.* New York: 1986:21–34.
103. Kielian M, Helenius A. Entry of alphavirus. In: Schlesinger S, Schlesinger MJ, eds. *The Togaviridae and Flaviviridae.* New York: Plenum Publishing, 1986:91–119.
104. Karabatsos N. Antigenic relationships of group A arboviruses by plaque reduction neutralization testing. *Am J Trop Med Hyg* 1975;24:527.
105. Clarke DH. Two nonfatal human infections with the virus of eastern encephalitis. *Am J Trop Med Hyg* 1961;10:67.
106. Calisher CH, El-Kafrawi AO, Al-Deen Mahmud MI, et al. Complex-specific immunoglobulin M antibody patterns in humans infected with alphaviruses. *J Clin Microbiol* 1986;23:155.
107. Hayes RO. Eastern and western encephalitis. In: Beran GW, ed. *Handbook series in zoonoses, section B, viral zoonoses,* Vol 1. Boca Raton FL: CRC Press, 1981:29–57.
108. Hahn CS, Lustig S, Strauss EG, et al. Western equine encephalitis virus is a recombinant virus. *Proc Natl Acad Sci USA* 1988;85:5997.
109. Rozdilsky B, Robertson HE, Chorney J. Western encephalitis. Report of eight fatal cases: Saskatchewan epidemic, 1965. *Can Med Assoc J* 1968;98:79.
110. Kubes V, Rios FA. The causative agent of infectious equine encephalomyelitis in Venezuela. *Science* 1939;90:20.
111. Beck CE, Wyckoff RWG: Venezuelan equine encephalitis. *Science* 1938;88:530.
112. Venezuelan encephalitis. In: *Proceedings of the Workshop-Symposium on Venezuelan Encephalitis Virus.* Washington, DC: Pan American Health Organization, 1972. Scientific publication 243.
113. Walton TE, Grayson MA. Venezuelan equine encephalomyelitis. In: Monath TP, eds. *The arboviruses: epidemiology and ecology.* Boca Raton, FL: CRC Press, 1988.
114. Schlesinger S, Schlesinger MJ. Replication of Togaviridae and Flaviviridae. In: Fields BN, Knipe DM, eds. *Fields virology,* 2nd ed. New York: Raven Press, 1990:697–711.
115. Briceno Rossi AL. Rural epidemic encephalitis in Venezuela caused by a group A arbovirus (VEE). In: Melnick JL, eds. *Progress in medical virology,* Vol 9. Basel: S Karger, 1967:176–203.
116. Dietz WH Jr, Peralta PH, Johnson KM. Ten clinical cases of human infection with Venezuelan equine encephalomyelitis virus, subtype ID. *Am J Trop Med Hyg* 1979;28:329.
117. Sanchez JL, Lednar WM, Macasaet FF, et al. Venezuelan equine encephalomyelitis: report of an outbreak associated with jungle exposure. *Milit Med* 1984;149:618.
118. Hammon W McD, Reeves WC. California encephalitis virus: a newly described agent. I. Evidence of natural infection in man and other animals. *Calif Med* 1952;77:303.
119. Kappus KD, Monath TP, Kaminski RM, et al. Reported encephalitis associated with California serogroup virus infections in the United States, 1963–1981. In: Calisher CH, Thompson WH, eds. *California serogroup viruses.* New York: Alan R Liss, 1983:31–41.
120. Deibel R, Srihongse S, Grayson MA, et al. Jamestown Canyon virus: the etiologic agent of an emerging human disease? In: Calisher CH, Thompson WH, eds. *California serogroup viruses.* New York: Alan R Liss, 1983:313–328.
121. Srihongse S, Grayson MA, Deibel R. California serogroup viruses in New York State: the role of subtypes in human infections. *Am J Trop Med Hyg* 1984;33:1218.
122. Woods CW, Karpati AM, Grein T, et al. An outbreak of Rift Valley Fever in Northeastern Kenya, 1997–1998. *Emerg Infect Dis* 2002;8:138.
123. Schmaljohn C. Bunyaviridae: the viruses and their replication. In: Fields BN, Knipe DM, Howley PM, eds. *Fields virology,* 3rd ed. Philadelphia: Lippincott-Raven, 1996:1447–1471.
124. Bishop DHL, Calisher C, Casals J, et al. Bunyaviridae. *Intervirology* 1980;14:125.
125. Grimstad PR, Calisher CH, Haroff RN, et al. Jamestown Canyon virus (California serogroup) is the etiologic agent of widespread infection in Michigan humans. *Am J Trop Med Hyg* 1984;35:376.

126. Shope RE, Causey OR. Further studies on the serological relationships of group C arthropod-borne viruses and the application of these relationships to rapid identification of types. *Am J Trop Med Hyg* 1962;11:886.

127. Gonzalez-Scarano F, Shope RE, et al. Characterization of monoclonal antibodies against the G1 and N proteins of La Crosse and Tahyna, two California serogroup bunyaviruses. *Virology* 1982;120:42.

128. Calisher CH, Monath TP, Karabatsos N, et al. Arbovirus subtyping: applications to epidemiologic studies, availability of reagents, and testing services. *Am J Epidemiol* 1981;114:619.

CHAPTER 260
West Nile Virus

Sharone Green and Alan L. Rothman

HISTORY

West Nile virus was first isolated from a woman in Uganda in 1937. The virus was identified as the etiology of West Nile fever in Israeli military troops in the 1950s and later was determined to be the cause of meningoencephalitis in that region (1,2). Subsequent outbreaks followed in the Middle East and Eastern Europe (Table 260.1). A hallmark of recent outbreaks in Israel and the United States has been the finding of significant bird morbidity and mortality (geese and crows, respectively), which had not been previously described (3). In 1999, exotic birds at the Bronx and Queens Zoos in New York became ill and died (4). A concomitant cluster of meningoencephalitis associated with muscle weakness in Flushing Hospital, Queens, New York was reported (5). The human cases were initially diagnosed as the related flavivirus, St. Louis encephalitis virus. A diagnosis of West Nile virus infection in birds confirmed the etiology of the disease in humans and the emergence of this virus into North America.

CHARACTERISTICS OF THE PATHOGEN

West Nile virus is a positive-strand RNA virus and belongs to the family Flaviviridae. It is a member of the Japanese encephalitis (JE) serogroup, which includes JE virus, St. Louis encephalitis virus, Murray Valley encephalitis virus, and Kunjin virus. The virus contains a lipid bilayer that contains the envelope (E) protein. The genome is about 11 kb and encodes a single open reading frame of 11,029 nucleotides that is translated as a single polyprotein with subsequent posttranslational cleavages to produce three structural (core, premembrane, and envelope) and seven nonstructural proteins (NS1-2a, -2b, -3, -4a, -4b, and -5) (6). NS1 is involved in viral replication, although its precise role is unknown (7). NS5 is believed to be the viral RNA polymerase (8). NS3 contains both the protease and helicase (9).

The E protein binds to the host cell and permits virus entry through an unknown viral receptor. It also has a major role in the induction of neutralizing and hemagglutination-inhibiting antibodies. Amino acid changes in the E protein have been associated with virulence and attenuation in related flaviviruses such as yellow fever virus and JE virus (10,11). Genomic sequencing studies have revealed that there are two lineages of West Nile virus. The strain introduced into North America is from lineage 1. Although most closely related to a virus isolated from a goose in Israel in 1998, this strain is also closely related to recently isolated West Nile viruses from North Africa, Romania, Kenya, Italy, and the Middle East (12).

EPIDEMIOLOGY

The primary enzootic cycle for West Nile virus is mosquito–bird–mosquito. Ornithophilic mosquitoes of the *Culex pipiens* complex are believed to be the primary vectors for West Nile virus in North America, Europe, and Africa. West Nile virus has been isolated from other mosquito species as well as several tick species, but there is no evidence that they play a role in viral transmission (13). Birds are the predominant reservoir worldwide (14). Migrating birds infected with West Nile virus have been hypothesized to enable the spread of the virus (15,16). West Nile disease (myocarditis and encephalitis) and mortality in birds is a particular finding of recent outbreaks in Israel and the United States (4,17). Since the introduction of West Nile virus into New York in 1999, the range of the virus has rapidly expanded south and west (Fig. 260.1). In 2002, human cases were diagnosed in 39 states (Fig. 260.1 and Table 260.2). Humans and horses both exhibit neurologic disease due to West Nile virus infection and are considered to be incidental and dead-end hosts for the virus. Other mammals that can be infected with West Nile virus include domestic animals (dogs, camels, cows, donkeys, water buffalo, and sheep) and small wild mammals (bats, chipmunks, squirrels, rabbits, rats, and skunks) (18–20). Recent experimental infection studies of horses with West Nile virus have demonstrated that the level of viremia is insufficient to transmit the virus back to mosquitoes (21). A study in dogs using an African strain of West Nile virus yielded similar results (22). Recent experimental evidence demonstrates that avian species may be capable of transmitting virus without a requirement for vector (23).

After the 1996 West Nile outbreak in Bucharest, Romania, serosurveys demonstrated that 4.1% of 959 people had antibodies to West Nile virus and an estimated 70,000 had probably been infected during the epidemic. It was estimated that 1 in 140 to 320 infections resulted in central nervous system illness. The attack rate increased with increasing age (24). Similar results were found after the 1999 New York City outbreak with a seroprevalence of 2.6% in the affected area of Queens and a subclinical-to-clinical infection ratio of 1 in 140. Over the age of 65 years, the risk for encephalitis increased to 1 in 50. Twenty-one percent of seropositive individuals had a febrile illness, with muscle ache, fatigue, headache, or joint pain (25). Sera from healthy Israeli soldiers collected between 1982 and 1987 demonstrated seroprevalence rates of 7% in soldiers aged 18 to 20 years to 41.9% in soldiers aged 40 to 55 years, underscoring the fact that milder illness due to West Nile virus infection is largely underreported (26).

Risk factors for infection with West Nile virus relate to activities that predispose to mosquito exposure (e.g., gardening, sitting on porch at dawn or dusk) (27). Older age is associated with a higher risk for developing neurologic disease in West Nile virus–infected individuals and is a risk factor for death due to West Nile virus infection (24,28,29). In the New York City outbreak, the presence of diabetes was also found to be a significant risk factor, whereas during the 2000 Israel epidemic, change in level of consciousness and anemia on admission were associated with a higher mortality rate (28,29).

CLINICAL FEATURES

The incubation period of West Nile virus is typically 3 to 6 days (14). Most infections are asymptomatic. West Nile virus can cause a systemic febrile illness associated with rash, myalgia, and lymphadenopathy (West Nile fever), or central nervous system illness (meningitis, meningoencephalitis, encephalitis). West Nile fever was initially recognized in Israel in 1951 to 1953 with initial reports of fever, headache, rash, and lymphadenopathy as the predominant features (30). Virus was

TABLE 260.1.   Selected Reports of West Nile Virus Epidemics

Year(s)	Country	Species	References
1951–1954, 1957	Israel	Human	2, 30
1962–1964	France	Human, equine	63
1974	South Africa	Human	40
1980	Israel	Human	64
1984	South Africa	Human	65
1994	Algeria	Human	66
1996	Morocco	Equine	63
1996	Romania	Human	24
1997	Tunisia	Human	63
1998	Italy	Equine	63
1998	Israel	Avian	67
1999	Volgograd, Russia	Human	68
1999	United States	Human, avian, equine	5
2000	United States	Human, avian, equine	48
2000	France	Equine	63
2000	Israel	Human	29, 67
2001	United States	Human, avian, equine	69

also isolated from febrile children in Egypt during the same period (18). In 1957, an outbreak in a nursing home in Hadera, Israel led to the recognition of West Nile virus as an etiologic agent for encephalitis (2).

Symptoms of West Nile fever consist of fever, headache, myalgias, weakness, and backache and may include conjunctival injection and pharyngitis. When present, the rash is typically nonpruritic, roseolar, or maculopapular; is distributed over the chest, back, and arms; and may last up to a week. The sentinel cluster of West Nile encephalitis cases in Queens, New York in 1999 consisted of eight patients (six with encephalitis, two with meningitis) in whom a higher frequency of gastrointestinal symptoms (nausea, vomiting, diarrhea) was noted when compared with other published series (31). In addition, four of six patients with encephalitis exhibited neuromuscular weakness or flaccid paralysis associated with electromyographic findings of axonal polyneuropathy without sensory involvement, initially attributed to Guillaine-Barré syndrome. Subsequent clinical and electrodiagnostic findings from West Nile virus–infected patients presenting with acute flaccid paralysis (asymmetric weakness and areflexia, no sensory abnormalities, in the presence

or absence of fever) are more suggestive of anterior horn cell involvement resulting in a poliomyelitis-like syndrome (31a). Others have reported optic neuritis, polyradiculitis, and acute anterior myelitis (32,33). Extraneurologic complications include pancreatitis, myocarditis, and hepatitis (34–36). Encephalitis is a more common manifestation in the very young and the very old (28,37). The frequencies of clinical syndromes, signs, and symptoms of West Nile virus infection are shown in Table 260.3.

Laboratory findings may include leukocytosis or leukopenia; lymphocytopenia has been reported to persist up to 52 days (31,38). In patients with central nervous system signs, lymphocyte-predominant pleocytosis and mildly elevated protein levels may be seen in the cerebrospinal fluid (CSF). Radiologic imaging of brain is reported to be abnormal in a high percentage of patients, but these changes are believed to be age related rather than specific for West Nile virus infection (29).

LABORATORY DIAGNOSIS

Virus Isolation and Detection

West Nile virus has been reported to be isolated from the blood of immunocompetent individuals for up to 10 days after onset of

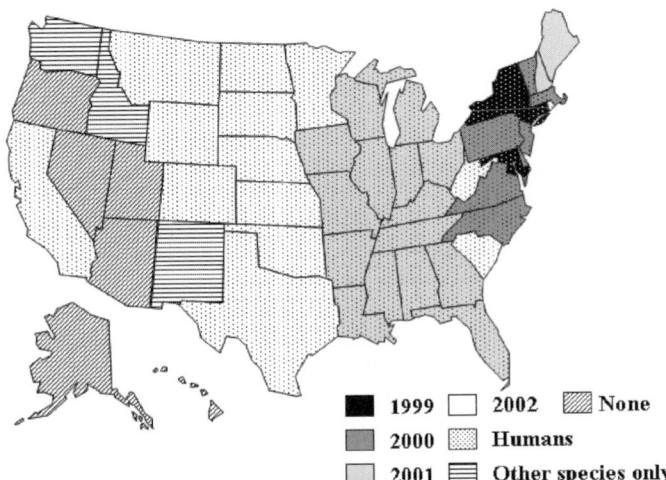

Figure 260.1. Yearly distribution of West Nile virus in the United States, 1999–2002. (Adapted from Centers for Disease Control and Prevention. Provisional surveillance of the West Nile virus epidemic—United States, January–November 2002. *MMWR Morb Mortal Wkly Rep* 2002;51:1129–1130.)

TABLE 260.2.   Expansion of Geographic Location of Human Cases (n) in the United States, 1999–2002[a]

1999	2000	2001
New York (62)	New York (14)	New York (14)
	New Jersey (6)	Florida (12)
	Connecticut (1)	New Jersey (9)
		Connecticut (6)
		Maryland (6)
		Georgia (6)
		Massachusetts (3)
		Pennsylvania (3)
		Alabama (2)
		Louisiana (1)
TOTAL = 6	TOTAL = 21	TOTAL = 62

[a] In 2002, 4156 human cases of West Nile virus infection were reported. (Data may be accessed at http://www.cdd.gov/ncidod/dvbid/westnile/surv&controlcasecount 02.htm)

TABLE 260.3. Reported Frequencies (%) of Clinical Syndromes, Signs, and Symptoms in Selected West Nile Virus Outbreaks

	Israel—1953[a] (n = 50)	New York—1999 (n = 59)[b]	Israel—2000[c] Hospitalized (n = 233)	Israel—2000[c] Ambulatory (n = 37)
Syndrome				
Febrile illness	98	8	27	92
Aseptic Meningitis	2	29	16	0
Encephalitis	0	63	57	8
Case-fatality rate	0	12	14	0
Symptoms				
Fever	100	90	98	—
Headache	80	47	58	—
Weakness	—[d]	56	—	—
Nuchal rigidity	2	19	29	—
Confusion	—	—	40	—
Change in level of consciousness	—	46	47	—
Coma	—	—	17	—
Tremor	—	12	—	—
Slurred speech	—	8	—	—
Focal sensory change	—	7	—	—
Seizures	—	3	—	—
Backache	40	—	—	—
Chills	35	—	—	—
Muscle pains	25	17	15	—
Ocular pain or photophobia	45	14	—	—
Lack of appetite	55	—	—	—
Nausea	25	53	—	—
Vomiting	10	51	31	—
Abdominal pain	20	7	19	—
Diarrhea	30	27	—	—
Sore Throat	30	5	—	—
Cough	8	19	—	—
Signs				
Flushed face	55	—	—	—
Conjunctival injection	60	3	—	—
Coating of tongue	50	—	—	—
Injection of throat	40	—	—	—
Gladular swelling of:		2	4	—
Occipital region	75			
Axillary region	90			
Inguinal region	85			
Rash	50	19	22	—
Splenomegaly	20	—	—	—
Hepatomegaly	10	—	—	—
Focal neurologic signs	—	7	9	—

[a]Study of 50 soldiers with serologically or virologically confirmed West Nile illness (70).
[b]Clinical data reported for 59 hospitalized patients (28).
[c]Clinical data reported for 233 and 37 serologically confirmed West Nile virus illnesses in hospitalized and ambulatory patients, respectively (29,67).
[d]Data not reported.

illness, although in most studies, viremia is of shorter duration (1 to 6 days) (14,39,40). West Nile virus was isolated from 13 of 34 (38%) patients with West Nile fever in Israel; virus isolation rates were highest on the first day of illness (77%), and virus was not recovered from blood by the fifth day of illness (39). Two healthy individuals from whom virus was isolated subsequently developed West Nile fever. Viremia may last as long as 28 days in the immunocompromised host (41). Peak viremia in cancer patients experimentally inoculated with West Nile virus (Egypt 101) occurred between days 4 and 9 after inoculation, with peak titers ranging from 10^2 to 10^5 LD$_{50}$ in mice (41). West Nile virus

could not be isolated from feces, urine, or throat swabs (42). Virus can be isolated from CSF in patients with encephalitis (42). However, because West Nile virus is classified as a biosafety level 3 agent, it is not feasible for most diagnostic laboratories to perform such testing.

Reverse transcription polymerase chain reaction (PCR), TaqMan PCR, and nucleic acid sequence-based amplification (NASBA) assays have been developed for detection of West Nile viral RNA and permit rapid, high-throughput diagnostic capability (43–45). These assays can be performed within 24 hours if a laboratory with capability for performing the assay is nearby.

CSF specimens are likely to contain viral RNA early in the course of illness; persistently positive CSF specimens may be associated with poor outcome (44,46). The experience to date demonstrates that serum samples in encephalitis cases are infrequently positive in serologically confirmed cases of West Nile virus infection (16 of 28 CSF specimens versus 4 of 28 serum specimens positive using TaqMan PCR), most likely due to the relatively short-lived viremia (42,44). The NASBA assay appears to be the most sensitive assay and can be performed in less than 1 hour (45).

Serologic Diagnosis

West Nile virus can be diagnosed serologically by immunoglobulin M (IgM) or IgG enzyme-linked immunosorbent assay (ELISA), but serologic cross-reactivity among the flaviviruses may complicate the diagnosis (13). Because the ELISA may cross-react between flaviviruses (e.g., St. Louis encephalitis, dengue), it should be used as a screening test only. To confirm West Nile virus as the etiologic agent, plaque reduction neutralization testing on acute and convalescent sera should be performed (13). Serum IgM to West Nile virus may be detected as early as the second day of illness, with about 70% of sera found to be positive by the seventh day of illness (47). However, persistence of West Nile virus–specific serum IgM for up to 500 days has been documented, necessitating paired specimens to document a fourfold rise in titer to rule out previous infection (47–49). In patients with symptoms of encephalitis, CSF IgM may be detectable early in the illness, with 50% of specimens found to be positive by the third day of illness (47).

PATHOLOGY AND PATHOPHYSIOLOGY

The incubation period for West Nile virus is believed to be 3 to 6 days (14). Virus can be recovered from blood only during the first few days of illness (39). A hamster model of the related flavivirus, St. Louis encephalitis virus, suggests that central nervous system extension occurs through viral replication in the olfactory bulb with dissemination through neuronal processes, rather than direct hematogenous seeding (50). Viremia precedes the onset of neurologic symptoms in that model. Alternatively, West Nile virus may infect vascular endothelial cells and "grow" across the blood–brain barrier (51). As mentioned earlier, most West Nile virus infections appear to be subclinical. The observation of more severe central nervous system disease due to West Nile virus in elderly people may be related to immunosenescence, with a diminished ability of the host to clear virus peripherally.

Histopathologic examination of brain tissues in fatal encephalitis cases has demonstrated microglial nodules composed mainly of lymphocytes and histiocytes in the gray and white matter, with a predilection for the brainstem. Cerebellum, thalamus, and cortex are less frequently involved. A mononuclear perivascular infiltrate may also be present. Inflammation of the leptomeninges was demonstrated in two of four autopsy cases in New York City. Viral antigen is present in the neurons, neuronal processes, and areas of brain necrosis. No antigen staining has been detected in other major organs. Immunohistochemical staining shows numerous CD8+ T cells within microglial nodules, in the perivascular infiltrates, in the meninges, and in the cranial roots. CD4+ T cells are present but in far fewer numbers. CD20+ B cells are prominent around the blood vessels (52). West Nile virus was inoculated into 84 terminal cancer patients in an attempt to induce tumor lysis (42). Eleven percent of patients developed encephalitis. Individuals with hematologic malignancies had a longer duration of viremia and a 5.5-fold

higher incidence of encephalitis. At autopsy, virus was isolated most frequently from lymph nodes, spleen, lung, and liver, and less often from brain or spinal cord, lung, heart, muscle, and pancreas.

The role of preexisting immunity to other flaviviruses in the setting of West Nile virus infection is unknown. Hamsters immune to dengue, JE virus, or St. Louis encephalitis virus were protected from clinical illness from West Nile virus challenge (53,54).

Chronic neurologic infections due to West Nile virus have been demonstrated in monkeys (55). The persistence of IgM antibodies in certain individuals after West Nile virus encephalitis is suggestive of persistent infection in humans (47–49).

TREATMENT

Supportive care, including airway support for decreased mental status and control of seizures, as clinically indicated, is the mainstay of therapy. There is no specific antiviral therapy available for the treatment of West Nile virus infection. *In vitro* data demonstrate suppression of West Nile virus replication by ribavirin, but only at doses that would have significant toxicity in humans (56). In an anecdotal report, pooled intravenous immune globulin (IVIG) was given to one individual who recovered in Israel (57). Subsequent testing of the IVIG demonstrated high levels of neutralizing antibodies to West Nile virus.

PREVENTION

There is currently no vaccine approved for use in humans. An equine vaccine was recently approved for use in the United States. Several candidate West Nile virus vaccines are currently under development, including DNA vaccines and chimeric vaccines (yellow fever or dengue virus backbone with structural gene components of West Nile virus), but these are many years away from use in humans (58–60). A live-attenuated JE virus vaccine, available only in China, has been shown to protect hamsters from clinical illness after West Nile virus challenge, although low-level viremia was detected (54).

Sentinel birds have long been used in the United States to alert local public health departments that various arboviruses are circulating (e.g., St. Louis encephalitis, equine encephalitis virus) (61). Although significant bird mortality, in particular crows, has been associated with recent West Nile virus outbreaks, the density of dead birds has not always correlated with human disease. Sentinel chickens have been successfully used for early warning of West Nile virus activity in Africa, but they did not predict human disease in the northeastern United States in 2000 (13). Studies are ongoing to determine whether other sentinel birds, such as recaptured tagged wild-range birds, will be more predictive of the spread of the virus into the human population (62).

Preventive measures against infection with West Nile virus include personal protection from mosquito vectors and vector control. Individuals should avoid being outdoors at dawn and dusk, wear long sleeves and trousers, and use mosquito repellent containing DEET when mosquito exposure is unavoidable. In the United States, state and local health departments have implemented mosquito and dead bird or sentinel bird surveillance systems. At present, it is unclear the precise role of avian surveillance in predicting human disease outbreaks in North America. When birds or mosquito pools test positive for West Nile virus, it is the decision of local health officials to determine whether targeted vector control measures (spraying, larvicides) should be implemented.

REFERENCES

1. Goldblum N, Sterk VV, Paderski B. West Nile fever. The clinical features of the disease and isolation of West Nile virus from the blood of human cases. *Am J Hyg* 1954;59:89–103.

2. Spigland I, Jasinska-Klingberg W, Hofshi E, et al. Clinical and laboratory observations in an outbreak of West Nile fever in Israel. *Harefuah* 1958;54.

3. Centers for Disease Control and Prevention. Update: West Nile-like viral encephalitis—New York, 1999. *MMWR Morb Mortal Wkly Rep* 1999;48:890–892.

4. Steele KE, Linn MJ, Schoepp RJ, et al. Pathology of fatal West Nile virus infections in native and exotic birds during the 1999 outbreak in New York City, New York. *Vet Pathol* 2000;37:208–224.

5. Centers for Disease Control and Prevention. Outbreak of West Nile-like viral encephalitis—New York, 1999. *MMWR Morb Mortal Wkly Rep* 1999;48:845–849.

6. Chambers TJ, Hahn CS, Galler R, et al. Flavivirus genome organization, expression, and replication. *Annu Rev Microbiol* 1990;44:649–688.

7. Hall RA, Khromykh AA, Mackenzie JM, et al. Loss of dimerisation of the nonstructural protein NS1 of Kunjin virus delays viral replication and reduces virulence in mice, but still allows secretion of NS1. *Virology* 1999;264:66–75.

8. Khromykh AA, Sedlak PL, Westaway EG. Cis- and trans-acting elements in flavivirus RNA replication. *J Virol* 2000;74:3253–3263.

9. Ryan MD, Monaghan S, Flint M. Virus-encoded proteinases of the Flaviviridae. *J Gen Virol* 1998;79:947–959.

10. Ryman KD, Ledger TN, Campbell GA, et al. Mutation in a 17D-204 vaccine substrain-specific envelope protein epitope alters the pathogenesis of yellow fever virus in mice. *Virology* 1998;244:59–65.

11. Monath TP, Arroyo J, Levenbook I, et al. Single mutation in the flavivirus envelope protein hinge region increases neurovirulence for mice and monkeys but decreases viscerotropism for monkeys: relevance to development and safety testing of live, attenuated vaccines. *J Virol* 2002;76:1932–1943.

12. Lanciotti RS, Roehrig JT, Deubel V, et al. Origin of the West Nile virus responsible for an outbreak of encephalitis in the northeastern United States. *Science* 1999;286:2333–2337.

13. Kramer LD, Bernard KA. West Nile virus in the western hemisphere. *Curr Opin Infect Dis* 2001;14:519–525.

14. Hubalek Z, Halouzka J. West Nile fever—a reemerging mosquito-borne viral disease in Europe. *Emerg Infect Dis* 1999;5:643–650.

15. Rappole JH, Derrickson SR, Hubalek Z. Migratory birds and spread of West Nile virus in the Western Hemisphere. *Emerg Infect Dis* 2000;6:319–328.

16. Malkinson M, Banet C, Weisman Y, et al. Introduction of West Nile virus in the Middle East by migrating white storks. *Emerg Infect Dis* 2002;8:392–397.

17. Bin H, Grossman Z, Pokamunski S, et al. West Nile fever in Israel 1999–2000: from geese to humans. *Ann N Y Acad Sci* 2001;951:127–142.

18. Taylor RM, Work TH, Hurlbut HS, et al. A study of the ecology of West Nile virus in Egypt. *Am J Trop Med Hyg* 1956;5:579–620.

19. Komar N, Panella NA, Boyce E. Exposure of domestic mammals to West Nile virus during an outbreak of human encephalitis, New York City, 1999. *Emerg Infect Dis* 2001;7:736–738.

20. Marfin AA, Petersen LR, Eidson M, et al. Widespread West Nile virus activity, eastern United States, 2000. *Emerg Infect Dis* 2001;7:730–735.

21. Bunning ML, Bowen RA, Cropp B, et al. Experimental infection of horses with West Nile virus and their potential to infect mosquitoes and serve as amplifying hosts. *Ann N Y Acad Sci* 2001;951:338–339.

22. Blackburn NK, Reyers F, Berry WL, et al. Susceptibility of dogs to West Nile virus: a survey and pathogenicity trial. *J Comp Pathol* 1989;100:59–66.

23. McLean RG, Ubico SR, Docherty DE, et al. West Nile virus transmission and ecology in birds. *Ann N Y Acad Sci* 2001;951:54–57.

24. Tsai TF, Popovici F, Cernescu C, et al. West Nile encephalitis epidemic in southeastern Romania. *Lancet* 1998;352:767–771.

25. Mostashari F, Bunning ML, Kitsutani PT, et al. Epidemic West Nile encephalitis, New York, 1999: results of a household-based seroepidemiological survey. *Lancet* 2001;358:261–264.

26. Cohen D, Zaide Y, Karasenty E, et al. Prevalence of antibodies to West Nile fever, sandfly fever Sicilian, and sandfly fever Naples viruses in healthy adults in Israel. *Public Health Rev* 1999;27:217–230.

27. Han LL, Popovici F, Alexander JP Jr, et al. Risk factors for West Nile virus infection and meningoencephalitis, Romania, 1996. *J Infect Dis* 1999;179:230–233.

28. Nash D, Mostashari F, Fine A, et al. The outbreak of West Nile virus infection in the New York City area in 1999. *N Engl J Med* 2001;344:1807–1814.

29. Chowers MY, Lang R, Nassar F, et al. Clinical characteristics of the West Nile fever outbreak, Israel, 2000. *Emerg Infect Dis* 2001;7:675–678.

30. Radt P. Clinical observations on patients with West Nile fever during outbreaks of the disease in 1950–1953. *Harefuah* 1955;49:41–44.

31. Asnis DS, Conetta R, Teixeira AA, et al. The West Nile virus outbreak of 1999 in New York: the Flushing Hospital experience. *Clin Infect Dis* 2000;30:413–418.

31a. Sejvar JJ, Leis AA, Stokic DS, et al. Acute flaccid paralysis and West Nile virus infection. *Emerg Infect Dis* 2003;9:788–793.

32. Vaispapir V, Blum A, Soboh S, et al. West Nile virus meningoencephalitis with optic neuritis. *Arch Intern Med* 2002;162:606–607.

33. Gadoth N, Weitzman S, Lehmann EE. Acute anterior myelitis complicating West Nile fever. *Arch Neurol* 1979;36:172–173.

34. Perelman A, Stern J. Acute pancreatitis in West Nile Fever. *Am J Trop Med Hyg* 1974;23:1150–1152.

35. Albagalic CR. A case of West Nile myocarditis. *J Med Assoc Isr* 1959;57:274–275.

36. Georges AJ, Lesbordes JL, Georges-Courbet MC, et al. Fatal hepatitis from West Nile virus. *Ann Inst Pasteur* 1987;138:237–244.

37. George S, Gourie-Devi M, Rao JA, et al. Isolation of West Nile virus from the brains of children who had died of encephalitis. *Bull WHO* 1984;62:879–882.

38. Cunha BA, Minnaganti V, Johnson DH, et al. Profound and prolonged lymphocytopenia with West Nile encephalitis. *Clin Infect Dis* 2000;31:1116–1117.

39. Goldblum N, Sterk VV, Jasinska-Klingberg W. The natural history of West Nile fever. II. Virological findings and the development of homologous and heterologous antibodies in West Nile infection in man. *Am J Hyg* 1957;66:363–380.

40. McIntosh BM, Jupp PG, Dos Santos I, et al. Epidemics of West Nile and Sindbis viruses in South Africa with *Culex (Culex) univittatus* Theobald as vector. *S Afr J Sci* 1976;72:295–300.

41. Southam CM, Moore AE. Clinical studies of viruses as antineoplastic agents, with particular reference to Egypt 101 virus. *Cancer* 1952;5:1025–1034.

42. Southam CM, Moore AE. Induced virus infections in man by the Egypt isolates of West Nile virus. *Am J Trop Med Hyg* 1954;3:19–50.

43. Shi PY, Kauffman EB, Ren P, et al. High-throughput detection of West Nile virus RNA. *J Clin Microbiol* 2001;39:1264–1271.

44. Lanciotti RS, Kerst AJ, Nasci RS, et al. Rapid detection of West Nile virus from human clinical specimens, field-collected mosquitoes, and avian samples by a TaqMan reverse transcriptase-PCR assay. *J Clin Microbiol* 2000;38:4066–4071.

45. Lanciotti RS, Kerst AJ. Nucleic acid sequence-based amplification assays for rapid detection of West Nile and St. Louis encephalitis viruses. *J Clin Microbiol* 2001;39:4506–4513.

46. Briese T, Glass WG, Lipkin WI. Detection of West Nile virus sequences in cerebrospinal fluid. *Lancet* 2000;355:1614–1615.

47. Tardei G, Ruta S, Chitu V, et al. Evaluation of immunoglobulin M (IgM) and IgG enzyme immunoassays in serologic diagnosis of West Nile Virus infection. *J Clin Microbiol* 2000;38:2232–2239.

48. Centers for Disease Control and Prevention. Update: West Nile virus activity—Northeastern United States, January–August 7, 2000. *MMWR Morb Mortal Wkly Rep* 2000;49:714–718.

49. Roehrig JT, Nash D, Maldin B, et al. Persistence of virus-reactive immunoglobulin M antibody in confirmed West Nile virus encephalitis cases. *Emerg Infect Dis* 2003;9:376–379.

50. Monath TP, Cropp B, Harrison AK. Mode of entry of a neurotropic arbovirus into the central nervous system. Reinvestigation of an old controversy. *Lab Invest* 1983;48:399–410.

51. Albrecht P. Pathogenesis of neurotropic arbovirus infections. *Curr Top Microbiol Immunol* 1968;43:44–91.

52. Sampson BA, Ambrosi C, Charlot A, et al. The pathology of human West Nile virus infection. *Hum Pathol* 2000;31:527–531.

53. Price WH, Thind IS. Protection against West Nile virus induced by a previous injection with dengue virus. *Am J Epidemiol* 1971;94:596–607.

54. Tesh RB, Travassos da Rosa AP, Guzman H, et al. Immunization with heterologous flaviviruses protective against fatal West Nile encephalitis. *Emerg Infect Dis* 2002;8:245–251.

55. Pogodina VV, Frolova MP, Malenko GV, et al. Study on West Nile virus persistence in monkeys. *Arch Virol* 1983;75:71–86.

56. Jordan I, Briese T, Fischer N, et al. Ribavirin inhibits West Nile virus replication and cytopathic effect in neural cells. *J Infect Dis* 2000;182:1214–1217.

57. Shimoni Z, Niven MJ, Pitlick S, et al. Treatment of West Nile virus encephalitis with intravenous immunoglobulin. *Emerg Infect Dis* 2001;7:759.

58. Davis BS, Chang GJ, Cropp B, et al. West Nile virus recombinant DNA vaccine protects mouse and horse from virus challenge and expresses in vitro a noninfectious recombinant antigen that can be used in enzyme-linked immunosorbent assays. *J Virol* 2001;75:4040–4047.

59. Monath TP. Prospects for development of a vaccine against the West Nile virus. *Ann NY Acad Sci* 2001;951:1–12.

60. Pletnev AG, Putnak R, Speicher J, et al. West Nile virus/dengue type 4 virus chimeras that are reduced in neurovirulence and peripheral virulence without loss of immunogenicity or protective efficacy. *Proc Natl Acad Sci USA* 2002;99:3036–3041.

61. Bernard KA, Kramer LD. West Nile virus activity in the United States, 2001. *Viral Immunol* 2001;14:319–338.

62. Komar N. West Nile virus surveillance using sentinel birds. *Ann NY Acad Sci* 2001;951:58–73.

63. Murgue B, Murri S, Zientara S, et al. West Nile outbreak in horses in southern France, 2000: the return after 35 years. *Emerg Infect Dis* 2001;7:692–696.

64. Katz G, Rannon L, Nili E, et al. West Nile fever—occurrence in a new endemic site in the Negev. *Isr J Med Sci* 1989;25:39–41.

65. Jupp PG, Blackburn NK, Thompson DL, et al. Sindbis and West Nile virus infections in the Witwatersrand-Pretoria region. *S Afr Med J* 1986;70:218–220.

66. Le Guenno B, Bougermouth A, Azzam T, et al. West Nile: a deadly virus? *Lancet* 1996;348:1315.

67. Weinberger M, Pitlik SD, Gandacu D, et al. West Nile fever outbreak, Israel, 2000: epidemiologic aspects. *Emerg Infect Dis* 2001;7:686–691.

68. Lvov DK, Butenko AM, Gromashevsky VL, et al. Isolation of two strains of West Nile virus during an outbreak in southern Russia, 1999. *Emerg Infect Dis* 2000;6:373–376.

69. Centers for Disease Control and Prevention. West Nile virus activity—United States, November 14–20, 2001. *MMWR Morb Mortal Wkly Rep* 2001;50:1061–1062.

70. Marberg K, Goldblum N, Sterk VV, et al. The natural history of West Nile fever. I. Clinical observations during an epidemic in Israel. *Am J Hyg* 1956;64:259–269.

CHAPTER 261

Hemorrhagic Fever Viruses Belonging to the Families Arenaviridae, Filoviridae, and Bunyaviridae[1]

Kelly T. McKee, Jr. and Ali S. Khan

The viral hemorrhagic fevers are a group of geographically diverse diseases with generally similar clinical, pathologic, and epidemiologic features. All are caused by RNA viruses, and those covered in this chapter derive from three taxonomic families (Table 261.1). Hemorrhagic fevers caused by flaviviruses (e.g., yellow fever, dengue hemorrhagic fever, Omsk hemorrhagic fever, Kyasanur Forest disease) are considered in Chapters 257, 258, and 259.

As a group, hemorrhagic fever viruses cause severe, often fatal, infections in humans. They are zoonoses whose distribution is closely tied to the ecology and population biology of specific rodents or arthropod vectors. The fundamental lesion in the viral hemorrhagic fever syndrome is disruption of the vascular bed; clinical manifestations relate to consequences of microvascular damage and increased vascular permeability. Person-to-person spread has been described for many of these diseases, and clustering of cases or community outbreaks may occur.

ARENAVIRIDAE

Six arenaviruses are known to cause disease in humans after natural exposure: lymphocytic choriomeningitis virus (LCMV), Lassa fever virus (Lassa fever), Junin virus [Argentine hemorrhagic fever (AHF)], Machupo virus [Bolivian hemorrhagic fever (BHF)], Guanarito virus (Venezuelan hemorrhagic fever), and Sabia virus (Brazilian or Sao Paulo hemorrhagic fever) (Table 261.2). Numerous others have been recognized, several of which reportedly have caused illness in laboratory workers. When viewed under the electron microscope, arenaviruses are pleomorphic particles averaging 110 to 130 nm in diameter, with a unit membrane and 10-nm club-shaped projections. Individual virions contain electron-dense particles thought to represent cellular ribosomes captured during the viral maturation process (1). Two virus-specific and two ribosomal (host-derived) RNA species can be isolated from intact virions. The small (S) segment codes for the three major structural proteins of the virus: N (nucleoprotein) and [through a precursor protein (GPC)] the two membrane glycoproteins (G1 and G2). The large (L) segment codes for a protein believed to represent an RNA-dependent RNA polymerase (2). A novel coding strategy has been recognized for arenaviruses. Termed *ambisense*, the 3' half of the S RNA codes for the N protein in the viral complementary sense, whereas the 5' half codes for GPC in the viral sense (3).

[1]The views presented are those of the authors and do not necessarily represent the views of Camber Corporation, the Department of the Army, the Department of Defense, or the United States government.

Epidemiology

All arenaviruses naturally pathogenic for humans are carried by rodents. Each virus is associated with a predominant host species, in which it establishes a chronic, persistent infection (4). Chronically infected rodents shed large quantities of infectious virus in secreta and excreta (particularly saliva and urine). Arenaviruses are spread horizontally and vertically within susceptible reservoir populations. Infection of mature rodents is usually without evident effect, whereas decreased survivorship, growth, and reproduction may result from neonatal infections acquired *in utero* (5,6).

With the exception of *Mus musculus* (the common house mouse, which hosts LCMV), reservoir hosts for arenaviruses occupy rural or semirural habitats. Thus, most naturally acquired arenavirus diseases occur in rural settings. Although mechanisms of transmission have not been precisely defined, evidence strongly suggests that humans become infected through percutaneous or mucous membrane inoculation with infectious virus, or inhalation of contaminated particles.

LYMPHOCYTIC CHORIOMENINGITIS

LCMV is more or less globally distributed. The true extent of human illness worldwide is unknown, however. Early studies established the epidemiologic association of LCMV with feral rodents and subsequently house mice, particularly during the winter months (7,8). There has been a decline in reported human infections, thought to be due to some combination of changing virus–rodent dynamics, improvements in socioeconomic conditions, and underreporting of cases. Most cases of LCMV infection are currently identified through laboratory surveillance of neurotropic virus diseases and through recognition of occasional outbreaks traceable to a specific source.

M. musculus is the natural reservoir for LCMV. Mice infected as newborns develop lifelong infections associated with virus shedding in secretions and excreta. Human infections are believed to occur subsequent to direct contact with infected excreta in aerosols or by inoculation of mucous membranes or abraded skin surfaces. In addition to sporadic commensal rodent-associated cases, mice and hamsters used as laboratory animals and as pets have been repeatedly documented as sources of LCMV epidemics (9–11). Even LCMV-infected tumors, passed in laboratory animals and subsequently infecting them, have provided a source for outbreaks (10,11). Person-to-person transmission of LCMV has not been described.

LASSA FEVER

Lassa fever occurs exclusively in West Africa. Although clinical disease has been documented in Sierra Leone, Liberia, Guinea, and Nigeria, serologic evidence of infection has been reported from virtually all other countries in the region. Lassa fever is an extremely common infection in endemic areas; estimates range from thousands to tens of thousands of cases annually, with no predilection for age or sex. In one study from Sierra Leone, antibody prevalence ranged from 8% to 52% and increased with age (12). Illness-to-infection ratios of 9% to 26% have been suggested, but reinfection and seroreversion occur, complicating these estimates (12). Multimammate rats of the genus *Mastomys* are reservoirs for Lassa virus; at least two species (*Mastomys huberti* and *Mastomys erythroleucus*) are infected (13). *M. huberti* is highly commensal with humans and regularly contaminates houses and peridomestic areas with infectious urine and respiratory secretions. Humans apparently become infected through contact with these infectious excreta as aerosols or fomites. Strongest associations occur for households with high rodent

TABLE 261.1. Viral Hemorrhagic Fevers of Humans

Family	Disease	Geography	Natural transmission	Case fatality	Person-to-person spread
Arenaviridae	South American hemorrhagic fevers	Rural Argentina Rural Bolivia Rural Venezuela Rural (?) Brazil	Rodent to human by inhalation or contact with contaminated secreta or excreta	10%–30% (untreated)	Yes
	Lassa fever	Rural West Africa		1%–3% overall (?); 20% in hospitalized patients (untreated)	Yes
Bunyaviridae	Hemorrhagic fever with renal syndrome	Rural Asia, Far East Rural Balkans Rural Scandinavia and Western Europe Urban centers worldwide	Same as Arenaviridae	<1%–15% (strain and geography dependent)	No
	Hantavirus pulmonary syndrome	Rural Americas	Same as Arenaviridae	About 30%	No[a]
	Crimean-Congo hemorrhagic fever	Rural Africa, west Asia, central Europe	Tick bite; inhalation or contact with blood of infected mammals	Highly variable; 15%–40% in recognized cases	Yes
Filoviridae	Ebola hemorrhagic fever, Marburg virus disease	Rural sub-Saharan Africa	Unknown	30%–90%	Yes

[a]Person-to-person spread documented with Andes strain hantavirus (South America) only.

populations, indiscriminate food storage, and direct rodent contact (14).

Lassa virus is transmitted from rodents to humans and from human to humans, although the relative importance of each mode of spread remains poorly defined (15,16). Clustering of cases and seropositive subjects has been seen, but the presumed common source for exposure is usually unrecognized (15). Person-to-person transmission of Lassa virus is well described. Infections have followed direct contact with febrile patients and have occurred by sexual transmission during incubation and convalescence. The virus has been recovered from breast milk, and transmission from nursing mothers to infants probably occurs. Nosocomial infections are well recognized, and explosive outbreaks, possibly due to airborne spread, although uncommon, have occurred in Nigeria and Liberia (17,18). Ex-perience in endemic areas indicates that application of barrier nursing and isolation practices can significantly reduce the risk for nosocomial spread. Laboratory-acquired infection has been described as well.

Lassa fever is an important cause of morbidity and mortality among adults in parts of West Africa. In Sierra Leone, 10% to 16% of all adult medical hospitalizations, 39% to 47% of adult febrile admissions, and 30% of adult medical deaths were due to Lassa fever (19). The case fatality among hospitalized patients is 16% to 17%. The case fatality among pregnant women is higher, reaching 30% or more during the third trimester (20). In children, Lassa fever is similarly important. Studies suggest that more than 20% of febrile pediatric admissions in endemic areas are due to this disease; the case fatality in children younger than 15 years is estimated at 12% to 14% (21).

TABLE 261.2. Arenaviruses Pathogenic for Humans

Virus	Disease	Geography	Principal reservoir	Current annual incidence	Case fatality (untreated)	Specific treatment
Lymphocytic choriomeningitis (LCM)	LCM	Worldwide	*Mus musculus*	(?)10^3–10^4	<1%	None usually needed
Lassa fever	Lassa fever	West Africa	*Mastomys* species	10^3–10^4	1%–3%; 20% in hospital	Ribavirin
Junin	Argentine hemorrhagic fever (HF)	Argentine pampas	*Calomys musculinus*	10^1–10^2	15%–20%	Immune plasma, (?) ribavirin
Machupo	Bolivian HF	Beni Department, Bolivia	*Calomys callosus*	10^1	20%+	(?) Ribavirin
Guanarito	Venezuelan HF	Central plains of Venezuela	*Zygodontomys brevicauda*	10^1–(?) 10^2	20%–30%	(?) Ribavirin
Sabia	Brazilian HF	Sao Paulo State, Brazil	Unknown	Unknown	Unknown	(?) Ribavirin

SOUTH AMERICAN HEMORRHAGIC FEVERS

AHF is a seasonal disease endemic to the pampas of north-central Argentina. First described in 1955, the disease initially was limited to a 16,000 km² region of Buenos Aires Province. Since that time, however, the endemic area has expanded to the north and west, nearly eight times the area originally described; portions of three additional provinces are now involved (22). During the 1980s, the annual incidence of AHF ranged from 200 to 500 cases, but numbers were higher in earlier decades (23). The etiologic agent, Junin virus, is carried in nature by several field-dwelling rodent species, of which *Calomys musculinus* is the most important. Although cases of AHF are diagnosed year-round, most occur during a well-defined epidemic season lasting from February through July that coincides with autumn grain harvests and maximal rodent population densities. The male-to-female case ratio is 4:1, with a preponderance of cases among 15- to 60-year-old males living or working in rural areas. Rodent-to-human transmission is the principal route of infection; cases are associated with inhalation of aerosols generated by mechanical grain harvesters and with exposure to linear habitats such as roadsides and fence-rows inhabited by *C. musculinus* (24,25). Person-to-person transmission of Junin virus seldom occurs but is documented in sexual partners. Nosocomial transmission is rare. Infections occur in children, but relatively infrequently.

Machupo virus, the cause of BHF, exists in nature only in the Beni Department of northern Amazonian Bolivia. From 1959 to 1962, nearly 500 cases of BHF were reported, with a 30% mortality rate (26); then, between 1962 and 1964, a series of devastating epidemics in and around the community of San Joachin occurred after an influx of the principal virus reservoir, *Calomys callosus*, into the town (27). Effective rodent surveillance and control programs subsequently eliminated epidemic BHF, and only sporadic cases have been recognized since. Although most BHF is thought to follow exposure to aerosolized urine from Machupo virus–infected rodents, case clusters in Cochabamba in 1971 and near the town of Magdalena in 1994, as well as anecdotal reports, provide strong evidence for person-to-person transmission of Machupo virus (28,29).

Venezuelan hemorrhagic fever was first recognized in 1989 and is known to occur only in the rural plains region of central Venezuela. From the time of its discovery until 1992, nearly 100 infections were reported; since then, relatively few cases have been seen (30,31). The epidemiologic aspects of the illness appear to be similar to those of sporadic AHF and BHF. The cane rat (*Zygodontomys brevicauda*) is the reservoir host for Guanarito virus (32). Neither person-to-person nor laboratory-acquired infections with Guanarito virus have yet been reported, although there is no reason to suspect that they could not occur.

Naturally acquired Sabia virus infection has been documented only once, the virus having been recovered from a fatal human case of hemorrhagic fever in São Paulo State, Brazil (33). The epidemiologic aspects remain undefined. Serious illness in laboratory workers exposed to aerosolized virus has validated its pathogenic potential, however (34).

Pathogenesis

The principal targets for arenaviruses appear to be macrophages and, to a lesser extent, vascular endothelium. Clinicopathologic manifestations stem from endogenous mediator release, extravasation of fluid into extravascular spaces, and activation of hematologic and immunologic cascades. Histopathologic findings are typically unimpressive, and, with the exception of LCMV, investigations into possible immunologic mechanisms of damage have yielded unconvincing results.

LYMPHOCYTIC CHORIOMENINGITIS

Neurologic disease in LCMV infection is believed to be immunologically mediated. Patients with aseptic meningitis or other central nervous system lesions develop these manifestations during the second phase of a biphasic illness. Immunosuppressed patients inoculated with LCMV as experimental therapy for malignancy failed to develop neurologic disease despite high viremias and, in one case, high brain tissue titers (35). Autopsy findings in otherwise normal patients have been remarkable for perivascular mononuclear cell infiltrates throughout the leptomeninges and brain substance (36). Viral antigen is observed in the meninges and cortical cells by immunofluorescence (IF), consistent with virus replication in the central nervous system.

LASSA FEVER

Infection with Lassa virus results in widespread dissemination of virus, but damage is limited to focal hepatic necrosis without significant inflammatory response, some evidence of interstitial pneumonitis, and occasional focal adrenal cortical necrosis (37). Liver damage is variable, with concomitant cellular injury, necrosis, and regeneration. Histopathologic changes are insufficient in themselves to account for death, however.

Outcome in Lassa fever correlates with the degree of virus replication (38) (Fig. 261.1). Increases of serum aspartate aminotransferase levels to greater than 150 IU/L, but not of other hepatic enzymes, are also associated with a poor prognosis (19,38) (Fig. 261.1). Levels of interleuken-8 and interferon-inducible protein-10, typically high in patients with acute nonfatal Lassa fever, are low or undetectable in those with fatal disease (39). Cardiac involvement has been limited to hemorrhage and lymphocytic infiltrates in the pericardium and with occasional interstitial myocarditis. The severe retrosternal or epigastric pain present in many patients may be due to pleural or pericardial involvement.

Increased vascular permeability is significant. Important clinical events in fatal disease are a consequence of endothelial and platelet dysfunction (despite adequate numbers of circulating platelets) (40,41). An inhibitor of platelet function has been identified in the serum of nonhuman primates and of patients with severe Lassa fever, specifically inhibiting platelet-dense granule and adenosine triphosphate release (42) and also suppressing

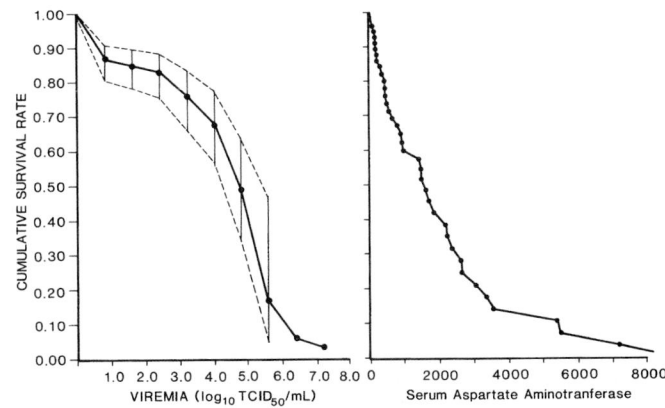

Figure 261.1. Relationship between viremia and aspartate aminotransferase (AST) levels in serum and outcome of Lassa fever by survival analysis. (Data from McCormick JB, King IJ, Webb PA, et al. A case-control study of the clinical diagnosis and course of Lassa fever. *J Infect Dis* 1987;155:445–455; and Johnson KM, McCormick JB, Webb PA, et al. Clinical virology of Lassa fever in hospitalized patients. *J Infect Dis* 1987;155:456–464, with permission.)

superoxide generation in neutrophils (43). Platelet and fibrinogen turnover is normal, and there is no increase in fibrinogen breakdown products (44); therefore, disseminated intravascular coagulation is not significant.

SOUTH AMERICAN HEMORRHAGIC FEVERS

Infection with Junin, Machupo, and Guanarito viruses produces similar lesions in humans. Multiple organs are involved, with changes most evident in the vascular, lymphoreticular, hematologic, and central nervous systems. Bleeding, rash, and extravasation of fluid into the soft tissues of the face implicate vascular damage complicated by thrombocytopenia as an important element in pathogenesis. Proteinuria is common, and renal tubular involvement is seen pathologically (45). Macrophages and lymphocytes contain viral particles and antigen, although the mechanism of their destruction remains undefined (46). Interferon-α levels in AHF are extremely high, ranging from 1,000 to 16,000 IU/mL (47); higher levels correlate with poor prognosis (48). It is likely that the high and prolonged levels of circulating interferon are responsible for many of the clinical and pathologic changes observed, although a variety of other mediators (e.g., tumor necrosis factor-α) are likely candidates as well (49). Involvement of the central nervous system is frequent; both neuroinvasion and neurovirulence have been demonstrated in animal models of these infections, and the occurrence of a late neurologic syndrome in AHF patients after treatment with immune plasma (see later) points to viral invasion of the brain in humans (50).

Clinical Features

LYMPHOCYTIC CHORIOMENINGITIS

LCMV in humans follows an incubation period of 1 to 3 weeks (8). In the largest existing study of human LCMV infections, 33 of 94 (35%) were asymptomatic, 47 (50%) were mild to moderate febrile illnesses without significant central nervous system manifestations, and 14 (15%) were typical LCMV (51). The typical disease begins with fever, malaise, weakness, anorexia, nausea, myalgia, and severe, often retroorbital, headache with photophobia. Fifty percent of patients may have sore throat, vomiting, or arthralgias; chest pain and pneumonitis occur less frequently. Alopecia, parotitis, orchitis, and transient arthritis of the hands have been reported. Physical examination shows pharyngeal inflammation, usually without exudate.

This phase lasts about 1 week, with a remission for a few days, which is then followed by a second and occasionally a third wave of fever. During these later febrile periods, neurologic involvement occurs. Most neurologic disease presents as aseptic meningitis, and about one third of these patients develop encephalopathy. Cerebrospinal fluid from patients with meningeal signs contains several hundred white cells per cubic millimeter, predominantly lymphocytes (more than 80%), with mildly increased protein and occasionally low glucose levels. Virus is often found in cerebrospinal fluid taken during the acute phase of disease (52). Although rarely fatal, the disease can be severe, necessitating hospitalization, and has a prolonged convalescence with persistent fatigue, somnolence, and dizziness. Neurologic sequelae are unusual but have been reported (53), including a single reported case of permanent unilateral deafness similar to that associated with Lassa fever (54). Infection with LCMV in pregnancy can result in fetal or early neonatal death as well as microcephaly, hydrocephalus, chorioretinitis, and psychomotor retardation (55,56). A Lassa fever–like syndrome has been reported once (57).

LASSA FEVER

The onset of Lassa fever is subtle. After an incubation period of 8 to 14 days (3 weeks at most), patients note the gradual onset of fever, malaise, and headache. During a period of several days, sore throat, myalgia, arthralgia, epigastric or retrosternal pain, severe frontal headache, and dry cough develop. By the end of the first week, patients are highly febrile and in a toxic condition. Conjunctivitis, lymphadenopathy, abdominal and muscle tenderness, hypotension, and relative bradycardia may be found at physical examination. A painful purulent pharyngitis is found in about 40% of cases and is sometimes associated with vesicles or ulcers. There is no characteristic rash, and neither cutaneous hemorrhages nor jaundice is seen early in the disease. With disease progression, edema of the face and neck and evidence of fluid buildup in the lungs occur. Hemorrhage is associated with fatal outcome but occurs in only 15% to 20% of patients; most often bleeding is from the gums and nose, less frequently from the gastrointestinal tract or vagina. About one fifth of patients have pleural or pericardial rubs.

Neurologic signs are infrequent; stupor, coma, and convulsions, as well as hemorrhage and severe hypotension, portend a poor prognosis. The duration of illness is typically about 1 month in survivors. Recovery is slow, and convalescence may be complicated by pericarditis, orchitis, uveitis, pleural effusion, or ascites. Acute-onset eighth cranial nerve deafness develops in up to 25% of patients and may be permanent (58).

Lassa fever is particularly hazardous for pregnant women. The risk for death during the third trimester is nearly six times that during the first two (20). Spontaneous or therapeutic abortion improves outcome, but fetal and perinatal wastage is high. Lassa fever in infants and extremely young children may present as swollen baby syndrome due to diffuse edema and abdominal distention (59). In older children, cough and gastrointestinal symptoms may dominate the clinical picture.

Most clinical laboratory studies in Lassa fever are not diagnostically useful. Leukopenia may be present early, but normal or elevated white cell counts are more typical as the disease progresses. Platelet counts are normal or elevated, although platelets themselves are dysfunctional. Proteinuria is inconsistent. High serum viremia [more than $10^{3.6}$ TCID$_{50}$ (median tissue culture infective doses) per milliliter] and aspartate aminotransferase values higher than 150 IU/L are associated with poor outcomes (50% and 73% mortality rates, respectively; 80% if both factors coexist) (38,60).

Differentiating Lassa fever from arbovirus diseases, malaria, typhoid fever, and other febrile illnesses common to West Africa is difficult on clinical grounds. Triads of pharyngitis, retrosternal pain, and proteinuria, or pharyngitis, retrosternal pain, and vomiting, yielded the best combinations of sensitivity, specificity, and positive predictive value in a single published case-control study from Sierra Leone (19).

SOUTH AMERICAN HEMORRHAGIC FEVERS

The clinical features of AHF, BHF, and Venezuelan hemorrhagic fever are remarkably similar (23,25,31,61). Between 1 and 2 weeks after exposure to the virus, patients experience the gradual onset of fever, malaise, anorexia, and myalgia. Shortly afterward, headache, back pain, epigastric pain, dizziness, and gastrointestinal disturbances appear. Vascular phenomena such as flushing of the face and chest, conjunctival injection, and orthostatic hypotension become apparent. Cutaneous petechiae are seen in most patients, most frequently involving the axillae and palate. Congestion and bleeding of the gums are common. The appearance of a hemorrhagic gingival margin at the point of dental insertion is a characteristic finding. Neurologic changes are almost universally present, with diminished deep tendon reflexes, tremors (particularly of the tongue), lethargy, and hyperesthesia seen most often. Most patients improve after 7 to 10 days and go on to an uneventful recovery. However, in the more severely ill patients (about 30% of the total), the disease evolves along one of three fairly distinctive lines: (a) a pronounced hemorrhagic diathesis manifested by diffuse ecchymoses and bleeding from mucous membranes and puncture sites; (b) a neurologic syndrome characterized by delirium, obtundation, coma, and convulsions; or (c) a mixed hemorrhagic-neurologic syndrome with shock. If the disease is untreated, the overall mortality rate may be as high as 20% to 30%.

Leukopenia (less than 4,000 cells/mm³ with lymphocytes and neutrophils proportionally affected) and thrombocytopenia (less than 100,000 cells/mm³) are virtually invariable. Proteinuria is extremely common and may be accompanied by microscopic hematuria. Serum enzyme and renal function studies are not seriously abnormal, and routine clotting studies are within normal ranges except in severe cases. Convalescence is prolonged (3 to 6 weeks) and is characterized by weakness, weight loss, autonomic instability, and occasional alopecia (62).

Diagnosis

Arenavirus infections are traditionally diagnosed by demonstration of a fourfold rise in virus-specific antibody titer, isolation of virus, or demonstration of high-titer immunoglobulin G (IgG) antibody and virus-specific IgM antibody in association with a compatible clinical illness (63). Antigens may be prepared and inactivated so that serologic diagnosis can be performed without high-level safety precautions. Antibodies detectable by IF appear earlier in illness in Lassa fever and lymphocytic choriomeningitis (within 1 to 2 weeks) than in South American hemorrhagic fevers (usually during the third week). In Lassa fever, viral antigen and IgM antibodies detected by enzyme immunoassay (EIA) are useful indicators of acute disease, whereas detection by EIA of IgG is suggestive of past infection (63a). Neutralizing antibodies are reliably detected in AHF and BHF after day 21 but are inconsistent and difficult to detect in Lassa fever and lymphocytic choriomeningitis.

Virus isolation is best performed by inoculation of body fluids or tissue samples onto Vero or other susceptible cell cultures, followed by staining of infected cells at periodic intervals using specific antisera for identification. Virus is readily recovered early in disease from serum in Lassa fever patients (and often from throat washing and urine) but is lower in titer and more difficult to detect in South American arenavirus infections. In patients with AHF, co-cultivation of peripheral blood mononuclear cells with susceptible cell lines improves yields considerably (64). Antigen detection by EIA has proved useful for Lassa fever and Machupo virus infections in humans (28,65). Immunohistochemistry techniques have been applied for postmortem tissue diagnoses. Application of newer technologies such as reverse transcription polymerase chain reaction holds great promise for diagnosis of arenavirus infections in the future (66).

Treatment

Fundamental to management of all arenavirus hemorrhagic fevers is careful attention to and correction of fluid, electrolyte, and osmotic disturbances that accompany these infections. Even vigorous support of these imbalances, however, may be insufficient in itself to prevent progression to death. Administration

TABLE 261.3. Immune Plasma Therapy for Argentine Hemorrhagic Fever

Effect of day of therapy on outcome (fatality rate)	
<8 Day's illness	>8 Day's illness
1%	16%

Effect of dose[a] (fatality rate)		
1,000–2,000 TU	2,000–3,000 TU	>3,000 TU
8.3%	2.5%	0.8%

[a]Therapeutic units (TU): E (neutralizing antibody titer X plasma volume)/body weight (kg).
Data from Maiztegui JI, Fernandez NJ, de Damilano AJ. Efficacy of immune plasma in treatment of Argentine haemorrhagic fever and association between treatment and a late neurological syndrome. *Lancet* 1979;2:1216–1217; and Enria D, France SG, Ambrosio A, et al. Current status of the treatment of Argentine hemorrhagic fever. *Med Microbiol Immunol* 1986;175:173–176, with permission.

of convalescent immune plasma has proved to be effective in treatment of AHF when given within the first 8 days of illness (67). Therapeutic efficacy correlates with the amount of neutralizing antibody delivered (68,69) (Table 261.3). Use of immune plasma has reduced the mortality rate of AHF from 15% to 20% to less than 1% among patients treated within 8 days of disease onset. A curious side effect of immune plasma therapy has been the occurrence of a late neurologic syndrome of uncertain cause in about 10% of treated survivors (67). This condition, characterized by fever, headache, ataxia, and intention tremors, begins 4 to 6 weeks after plasma treatment but is generally benign.

Ribavirin is effective in treating Lassa fever (60). Although dosing by both oral and intravenous routes reduces mortality, parenterally administered drug is more effective. Optimal benefit is derived within the first 6 days of illness (Table 261.4). Preliminary studies of ribavirin in AHF have suggested benefit (70), and the drug has been successfully used under compassionate

TABLE 261.4. Ribavirin Therapy for Lassa Fever

Therapy	Risk factor[a]	
	Admission viremia 10³·⁶ TCID₅₀/mL	Admission AST >150 IU/L
Treatment within 6 Days of Onset of Illness		
None	15/20 (75%)	11/18 (61%)
Ribavirin PO	1/5 (20%)	1/5 (20%)
Ribavirin IV	1/11 (9%)	1/20 (5%)
Plasma	5/9 (56%)	6/16 (38%)
Treatment after 6 Days of Onset of Illness		
None	21/27 (78%)	22/44 (52%)
Ribavirin PO	2/5 (40%)	1/9 (11%)
Ribavirin IV	9/19 (47%)	11/43 (26%)
Plasma	7/12 (58%)	8/66 (66%)

AST, aspartate aminotransferase; TCID₅₀, median tissue culture infective dose; PO, by mouth; IV, intravenously.
[a]Number of deaths/total number of patients (% fatal).
Data from McCormick JB, King IJ, Webb PA, et al. Lassa fever: effective therapy with ribavirin. *N Engl J Med* 1986;314:20–26, with permission.

protocol to treat patients with BHF (28) and Sabia virus infection (34).

Prevention

On the basis of principles developed and implemented during BHF outbreaks of the 1960s (71), surveillance and control of rodents in communities of the Bolivian Beni Department have effectively eliminated epidemic disease. The sylvatic nature of the reservoirs for Junin and Guanarito viruses make rodent population control to prevent AHF and VHF (and sporadic BHF) impractical, however. Similarly, control of rodents outside of living spaces to prevent Lassa fever is not feasible.

A live attenuated vaccine against AHF has been developed and extensively tested in the United States and Argentina (72). This vaccine, Candid-1, proved effective in preventing AHF under conditions of natural exposure in a double-blind, placebo-controlled field trial conducted in the AHF endemic area (73). The vaccine has subsequently been administered to more than 200,000 persons in the endemic area without significant adverse effect (74). Fewer than 10 cases of AHF have occurred to date among Candid-1 vaccinees, and there has been a sharp drop in reported incidence of disease since implementation of widespread immunization (74). Candid-1 also proved effective in prophylaxis against BHF in a rhesus macaque model of this infection (Jahrling PB, unpublished data), but its utility has not yet been assessed for disease prevention in Bolivia. Interestingly, the vaccine was of no benefit in animal model infection with Guanarito virus (Jahrling PB, unpublished data). A vaccinia-vectored Lassa fever virus vaccine has been developed and tested in animal models but has not yet been evaluated in humans (75).

In the event of significant exposure (e.g., needlestick or intimate personal contact) to Lassa virus (or any other pathogenic arenavirus), it has been recommended that oral ribavirin, 500 mg four times daily for 7 days, be administered (76). The efficacy of this prophylactic regimen is unproved, however, and close monitoring of disease contacts for at least one normal incubation period, with initiation of therapy at the first sign of illness, represents an acceptable alternative.

FILOVIRIDAE

The Filoviridae are a family of RNA viruses capable of inducing severe and highly lethal hemorrhagic fevers in primates, including humans. Five viruses have been described: Marburg virus and four Ebola viruses subtypes (Ebola Sudan, Ebola Zaire, Ebola Cote d' Voir, and Ebola Reston) (77–79). These mysterious agents are maintained in nature through unknown mechanisms and have been responsible for sporadic disease and explosive outbreaks that have captured the attention of both the scientific and lay communities (80). A single, negative-sense RNA strand codes for seven polypeptides: a nucleoprotein, a glycoprotein, a polymerase, and four other proteins (81–83). Morphology is unique, with particles assuming long (up to 14,000 nm), filamentous, often bizarre shapes (U, 6, or circular configurations) of constant 80-nm diameter (84). Although biochemically similar in makeup, there is little serologic cross-reactivity between Marburg virus and the various Ebola virus subtypes, whereas all Ebola viruses recognized to date cross-react to varying degrees among themselves (85–87).

Epidemiology

Filoviruses were unknown to science until 1967, when simultaneous outbreaks of hemorrhagic fever occurred in Marburg and Frankfurt, Germany, and Belgrade, Yugoslavia (88). Thirty-two cases (25 primary and 7 secondary) of what came to be known as Marburg virus disease were recognized, 7 of which were fatal. Primary infections were linked to contact with African green monkeys shipped from a primate export facility in Uganda. The virus then disappeared from view until 1975 when a young Australian tourist who had traveled in Zimbabwe contracted Marburg virus infection and died in a Johannesburg, South Africa, hospital (89). His female traveling companion became ill a week after onset in her partner, and a nurse in Johannesburg subsequently became infected, but both survived. In 1980, an expatriate engineer contracted the disease in northwestern Kenya and died; his physician became ill but survived (90). In 1987, a Danish teenager contracted the disease in Kenya and died (91). An extensive outbreak of Marburg fever occurred at Durba in the Democratic Republic of Congo from 1998 to 2000 (with retrospective identification of disease in 1997) (92). A total of 103 cases were diagnosed with 69 deaths in 1998 and 1999, and at least 16 additional cases were diagnosed in 2000 until flooding denied access to a local mine that was the presumptive source of the infection. Despite extensive investigation, no reservoir, vector, or naturally occurring source for any Marburg virus infection has ever been identified.

Two simultaneous explosive, but unrelated, outbreaks of hemorrhagic fever in 1976 in northern Zaire and southern Sudan proved to be the sentinel cases of Ebola virus disease in humans (93). These epidemics lasted for months and affected more than 500 persons. Mortality was quite high (nearly 90% in Zaire and 50% in Sudan), and secondary cases associated with exposure to blood or other body fluids (e.g., reuse of needles and syringes, sexual contacts) were common. Isolated Ebola virus cases in 1972 (one putative nonfatal case retrospectively identified by serology, along with one probable fatal case) (94), 1976 (one nonfatal laboratory infection) (95) and 1977 (a single fatal case in Tandala, Zaire) (96), together with a second outbreak in southern Sudan involving 34 persons (22 fatalities) in 1979 (97), round out the confirmed experience with these viruses in Africa before the 1990s.

In November 1989, an outbreak of hemorrhagic fever occurred among cynomolgus monkeys (*Macaca fascicularis*) housed in a quarantine facility in Reston, Virginia (98). Ebola virus was identified in culture fluids from several pathologic specimens, prompting investigations nationwide to assess the scope and significance of the problem (98,99). Subsequently, Ebola virus was identified at facilities in Texas and Pennsylvania among colonies of sick and dying cynomolgus monkeys, most of which had been procured from a single source in the Philippines. Epidemiologic investigations in the Philippines confirmed the presence of widespread Ebola infections among captured and caged animals in the exporter's facilities but failed to clarify the source or extent of the infection in nature (100). The virus either persisted or was later reintroduced into the Philippine export facility: infected macaques traced to this same source were detected in Italy in 1992 and Alice, Texas, in 1997 (101,102). Despite the high (more than 75%) case fatality documented among these Asian macaques, however, no human illness has occurred among the several individuals shown virologically and serologically to have been infected with this virus strain (103).

In 1994, a Swiss ethnologist developed a hemorrhagic fever syndrome after dissecting one of several chimpanzees that had died of unknown causes in the Ivory Coast (79). The strain of Ebola virus recovered from her blood (Ebola Ivory Coast) proved distinct from previously recognized filoviruses. A 1994 outbreak due to Ebola Zaire was retrospectively diagnosed in Makokou, Gabon; two thirds of the 44 infected individuals died (104).

In 1995, a community-wide epidemic of Ebola hemorrhagic fever due to Ebola Zaire virus was recognized in Kikwit, Zaire, following a deadly nosocomial outbreak in hospitals (105). Over a 7-month period, 315 people were identified with Ebola hemorrhagic fever; the overall case fatality was 80%. About one third of cases occurred among health care workers, in whom infections were associated with inadequate barrier nursing practices (106). Two additional outbreaks due to Ebola Zaire occurred in Gabon during 1996. The first involved the butchery and preparation for consumption of a chimpanzee carcass near Mayibout in which several secondary cases occurred. The second outbreak occurred in the rural Boue area with transport of a patient to the capital city, Libreville. Three fourths of the 60 subsequently infected patients died (104). A fatal nosocomial infection occurred in Johannesburg, South Africa, in conjunction with this outbreak: a nurse caring for a patient who had been unknowingly transported from Gabon was exposed to large volumes of blood in the course of her routine duties, became ill 4 days later, and subsequently died (107). Another epidemic of Ebola hemorrhagic fever occurred in northern Uganda during 2000 and 2001. This community-wide outbreak due to Ebola Sudan virus proved difficult to trace epidemiologically but was clearly associated with cross-infection of health care workers and patients in local hospitals. The case fatality in this epidemic was 50%, similar to that seen in the 1976 Sudan outbreak due to this strain (108). Additional outbreaks with high human and nonhuman primate mortality have continued to occur in central Africa (108a).

The natural history of filoviruses remains enigmatic. That these are zoonotic viruses is strongly suggested by the patterns of human infection, the biologic properties of the agents, and some intriguing epidemiologic associations with exposure to bats (supported by laboratory evidence of virus replication and circulation) (109); despite extensive ecologic study, however, no natural source for any filovirus has been identified. Person-to-person transmission of filoviruses has been documented in association with parenteral or mucous membrane exposure to contaminated body fluids by direct contact, large-particle droplets, or fomites. The role of small-particle aerosol transmission is less clear, however. Experimental aerosol transmission of Marburg and Ebola viruses has been demonstrated (86,87), and aerosol spread of Ebola Reston virus may have occurred among quarantined cynomolgus monkeys (99).

Pathogenesis

Hematogenous spread of Ebola and Marburg viruses to multiple organs follows mucous membrane exposure or direct inoculation of virus. Extensive virus replication is associated with focal necrotic changes in liver, spleen, lymph nodes, kidney, lung, and gonads (88,93,110). The most prominent pathologic changes are observed in the liver, where foci of parenchymal necrosis containing Councilman-like bodies are seen. The presence of virus is strongly correlated with visible necrosis. Few inflammatory cells accompany the hepatic lesions, however, and blood biochemical changes suggest that liver damage is not central to disease outcome. There is also nearly complete obliteration of lymphoid cells in the spleen.

The major manifestation of this usually severe disease is vascular failure. Pathologic features of fatal Marburg and Ebola virus infection typically include hemorrhages in skin, mucous membranes, alimentary luminal surfaces, and viscera (88,93,110,111). These abnormalities are temporally associated with increased vascular permeability. Extravasation of fluid into abdominal viscera, lungs, and kidneys precipitates organ dysfunction. Endothelial cell dysfunction and subsequent loss of vascular integrity appear to be due both to direct (cytopathology) and indirect (mediator induced) virus effects. Ebola virus particles are capable of adhering to a variety of cell types, including vascular endothelium, through a specialized glycoprotein (112). Folate receptor-α has been implicated as a cofactor for cellular entry of both Marburg and Ebola (113), but other cell surface molecules are almost certainly involved as well. Disseminated intravascular coagulation has been observed in primate models of Marburg virus infection, but its role in human pathogenesis is uncertain.

Humans and other primates fatally infected with filoviruses die with high viremias and little or no evidence of an effective humoral immune response. In animal models, both cellular and humoral components of the immune system appear important in protection from lethal infection (86,114–116).

Clinical Features

Clinical disease after infection with Marburg and African Ebola viruses is severe, relentlessly progressive, and frequently fatal (117,118). As of this writing, there have been no reports of human illness after infection with filoviruses of Asian origin. However, experience with these latter agents is extremely limited, and they are closely related antigenically to African filoviruses (87); thus, avirulence of these viruses for humans should not be generally assumed.

The incubation period for African filoviruses in humans typically ranges from 3 to 8 days but can be somewhat longer in secondary exposures. Onset of illness is sudden, with severe frontal headache, fever, chills, myalgias, extreme malaise, and anorexia. Nausea, vomiting, diarrhea, and abdominal pain are common early in disease. Conjunctivitis, hiccups, retrosternal pain, pharyngitis, and oral ulcerations are frequently described as well. Patients appear prostrate and apathetic and may be disoriented. A maculopapular rash that ultimately desquamates in survivors appears on the trunk and back around the 5th day of illness. Gross bleeding is frequent and is most often seen from mucous membranes (including the gastrointestinal tract), nasopharynx, and vagina; petechiae and oozing from venipuncture sites are also commonly observed.

Thrombocytopenia and leukopenia with a left shift are present early in disease. After a few days, significant neutrophilia appears. Serum biochemical studies show elevated enzyme values (aspartate aminotransferase higher than alanine aminotransferase), with normal or only slightly elevated bilirubin values. Viremia is present during acute disease and can persist for weeks in visceral organs and other sites (e.g., semen, anterior chamber of the eye) after apparently normal recovery (88,89,95).

Death due to intractable shock occurs on days 6 to 16 of illness. Infections in pregnancy produce many maternal deaths, and abortion or fetal demise is virtually universal. Convalescence is prolonged for survivors, requiring many weeks for recovery from the severe wasting that typically occurs.

Diagnosis

Historically, serologic diagnosis of recent filovirus infection was based on the indirect IF assay (63,119). Because of concerns over specificity of IF, particularly in epidemiologic studies (86), this assay has been supplanted by enzyme EIAs for IgG and IgM antibodies (63,87,120). Other, more technically demanding, diagnostic tools such as Western blot, immunohistochemistry, and immunoprecipitation assays have been applied to the diagnosis of filoviruses as well (98,119,121–123).

Infectious virus and viral antigen are present in blood and tissues of patients during acute disease and postmortem. However, isolation and other experimental manipulation of filoviruses in animals or cell culture systems are highly hazardous and should be undertaken only under maximal biologic safety (level 4) conditions.

Viral antigen can be detected using antigen capture EIA (124). The ability of this test to detect antigen in samples that have been inactivated using gamma-irradiation or betapropiolactone provides an avenue for acute diagnosis in the absence of elaborate biologic containment facilities.

The unique morphology of the Filoviridae makes electron microscopy potentially useful in examination of patients' specimens (84,87,125). This tool has particular utility for assessment of infection retrospectively in tissues preserved by formalin fixation, where isolation is no longer possible.

A wide range of infectious diseases with similar presentations occur in those parts of sub-Saharan Africa where filovirus infections have occurred. Among these afflictions, malaria, typhoid, rickettsial diseases, and other viral hemorrhagic fevers represent particularly important and potentially treatable entities that must be excluded.

Treatment

No specific treatment exists for hemorrhagic fevers caused by filoviruses. Supportive management of shock, organ failure, clotting disturbances, and volume shifts is most important. There is no effective antiviral therapy for these diseases. Human interferon, in conjunction with convalescent plasma, was used in a patient who survived (95), although experimental studies have shown no *in vitro* sensitivity of filoviruses for interferon. The use of immune serum in animal studies and blood from survivors in two anecdotal reports of Ebola hemorrhagic fever in humans have shown promise (126), but the efficacy of these treatments has not been clearly shown. In the absence of more definitive therapy, infusion of human convalescent plasma containing strain-specific antibodies or whole blood (containing inflammatory mediators) would seem justified (assuming the infusate is free of other infectious agents).

Prevention

Although candidate immunogens have yielded varying degrees of protection in animal models, no Marburg or Ebola virus vaccines have been tested in humans. Poor understanding of mechanisms of protection and recovery from illness has complicated development of effective prophylactic measures. Experience in epidemic settings supports the central role of interruption of person-to-person transmission through early identification of cases and intervention in limiting spread of disease among close personal contacts (76). Prevention of nosocomial spread can be accomplished through use of sterile equipment, adequate decontamination procedures, and application of barrier nursing practices. Absence of identified reservoirs or vectors precludes use of ecologic controls to limit acquisition of disease from natural sources. Recognition of risks to individuals involved in work with wild-caught monkeys or their tissues has resulted in institution of controls pertaining to importation and quarantine of animals (127).

BUNYAVIRIDAE

Bunyaviruses regularly associated with hemorrhagic fever syndromes derive from two of the family's five currently recognized genuses: hantaviruses and nairoviruses. Rift valley fever virus, a member of the phlebovirus genus, is associated with hemorrhagic fever in 1% to 2% of cases. Bunyaviridae are negative-stranded RNA viruses with tripartite genomes (128,129). The medium-sized (M) RNA segment contains the gene encoding two envelope glycoproteins (G1 and G2); the L segment encodes the viral polymerase, and the S segment encodes the nucleoprotein (130,131). Virus particles are typically spherical to oval, with glycoprotein spikes embedded in the lipid envelope; diameters range from 80 to 115 nm (132,133).

Hantavirus Diseases

All hantaviruses described to date are associated with a predominant (murid) rodent host in which they establish a chronic inapparent infection (134). These agents are presently divided into New World and Old World complexes, a scheme that also neatly segregates their rodent reservoirs and clinical presentations. Old World hantaviruses are etiologic agents linked to hemorrhagic fever with renal syndrome (HFRS), whereas New World hantaviruses cause a severe acute febrile illness characterized by noncardiogenic pulmonary edema and shock; this syndrome is referred to as *hantavirus pulmonary syndrome* (HPS) (135–138). At least 23 hantaviruses are currently recognized, 20 of which have been linked to human disease (139) (Table 261.5).

HFRS gained widespread attention as a serious and frequently fatal affliction of United Nations forces during the Korean War (140). However, syndromes of fever, hematologic abnormality, and renal dysfunction had actually been recognized as distinct clinical entities throughout the Far East, Scandinavia, and central Europe for many decades previously. In 1953, Gadjusek noted clinical and epidemiologic similarities among these geographically diverse disorders and proposed a common cause (141). The causative agent of HFRS in Korea, Hantaan virus, was identified by Lee and Lee in 1976 through demonstration of antigen in the lungs of infected reservoir rodents, the striped field mouse (*Apodemus agrarius*) (142,143). In November 1993, a new hantavirus, associated with what is now known as HPS, was identified in deer mice (*Peromyscus maniculatus*) captured in the Four Corners area of the Southwest (136–138,144). This agent, Sin Nombre virus, was the first in a series of New World hantaviruses now known to be well established in various rat and mouse species throughout the Americas (136).

EPIDEMIOLOGY

The epidemiology of hantavirus infections is tightly linked to the ecology, population dynamics, and distribution of the various rodent reservoirs. Within endemic areas, circumscribed foci or microfoci of rodent infection and human disease are seen (145). Chronically infected animals shed large amounts of virus in saliva, urine, and feces. It is thought that humans become infected through contact with these contaminated secreta and excreta by inhalation of small-particle aerosols or contact of mucous membrane or nonintact skin with infectious materials.

Human HFRS cases number in the tens to thousands annually, depending on the infecting virus and the geographic setting. The burden of HPS has yet to be defined, although cases will likely number in the dozens to hundreds annually during most years throughout the Americas.

With the exception of Seoul virus infections, HFRS is a rural disease. Hantaan virus circulates across eastern Russia, China, and the Korean peninsula, carried by the striped field mouse (146). The bank vole (*Clethrionomys glariolus*) serves as principal

TABLE 261.5.   Some Hantaviruses of Medical Importance

Virus	Reservoir	Distribution	Clinical form
Hantaan	*Apodemus agrarius*	East Asia	Severe HFRS
Dobrava	*Apodemus flavicollis*	Balkans, Slovenia, Baltics, other parts of Europe	Severe HFRS
Seoul	*Rattus norvegicus*	East Asia, perhaps worldwide	Mild or moderate HFRS
Puumala	*Clethrionomys glariolus*	Europe, Balkans	Nephropathia epidemica (usually mild HFRS)
Sin Nombre	*Peromyscus maniculatus*	Canada, USA	HPS major cause of HPS in USA and Canada
New York	*Peromyscus leucopus*	Eastern USA	HPS
Monongahela	*Peromyscus maniculatus nubiterrae*	Eastern USA	HPS
Bayou	*Oryzomys palustris*	Southeastern USA	HPS; may have more renal involvement
Black Creek Canal	*Sigmodon hispidus*	Florida	HPS; may have more renal involvement
Laguna Negra	*Calomys laucha*	Paraguay, Bolivia	HPS
Andes	*Oligoryzomys longicaudatus*	Argentina, Chile, Uruguay	HPS; only hantavirus in which person-to-person transmission suggested
Orán	*Oligoryzomys longicaudatus*	Northern Argentina	HPS
Choclo	*Oligoryzomys fulvescens*	Panamá	HPS
Lechiguanas	*Oligoryzomys flavescens*	Argentina	HPS
Castelo dos Sonhos	Unknown	Brazil	HPS
Araraquara	Unknown	Brazil	HPS
Juquitiba	Unknown	Brazil	HPS
Hu39694	Unknown	Argentina	HPS

HFRS, hemorrhagic fever with renal syndrome; HPS, hantavirus pulmonary syndrome.

reservoir for Puumala virus, the etiologic agent of HFRS in Scandinavia, northern Europe, and Russia west of the Ural Mountains (146,147). In the Balkans, HFRS has been associated with two viruses: Puumala and Dobrava (also known as Belgrade), the latter carried primarily by the yellow-necked field mouse *Apodemus flavicollis* (148–150). *Rattus* species are hosts for Seoul-like viruses distributed worldwide; human infections are most frequently seen in eastern Asia. Inapparent infections of laboratory rats with Seoul-like viruses have resulted in outbreaks of severe and sometimes fatal HFRS among animal handlers, scientists, and others exposed to caged housing infected animals (151).

In the United States, numerous hantaviruses are known to circulate. Seoul-like agents have reportedly been associated with human infections in several urban centers, but significant disease has not been recognized despite evocative links to chronic renal disease and hypertension (152–154). Antibodies to Prospect Hill virus, associated with the meadow vole *Microtus pennsylvanicus*, have been found in selected groups (e.g., mammologists), but no association with human illness has been made (155,156). Sin Nombre and related viruses have been linked to more than 350 cases of HPS from at least 30 states and the three western provinces of Canada. However, HPS is a much larger problem in Latin America, with reports of disease from Panama, Argentina, Bolivia, Brazil, Chile, Paraguay, and Uruguay (157,158) (Fig. 261.2).

HFRS is a seasonal disease, although individual cases are seen year-round (147,151). Far Eastern HFRS and Balkan HFRS occur primarily during the late fall and early winter, with smaller peaks in the spring and summer. Most European HFRS occurs between the late summer and early winter. Men 20 to 50 years of age occupationally or recreationally active in rural settings are most often affected, with agricultural workers, foresters, and soldiers in the field being at greatest risk for exposure. Infections due to Seoul (rat-borne) virus tend to occur more frequently during the warmer months and are more evenly distributed among the age and sex classes than are rural hantavirus infections, presumably because the reservoir predominates in peridomestic settings. In the United States, HPS has been seen primarily in rural settings, reflecting the ecology of rodent reservoirs. Most cases occur during the spring and early summer months, with temporal cycles broadly linked to climatic changes (159,160). Infections have been about equally distributed between the sexes, and the ages of those affected has ranged from 12 to 69 years (most being 20 to 40 years old) (159,161). In South America, HPS also occurs in mainly rural or semirural environments that support contact with infected rodents. Although a number of studies suggest a preponderance of disease among young persons, serologic evidence of infection in large segments of select communities has been seen (162,163).

PATHOGENESIS

The portal of viral entry is the respiratory tract (by inhalation) or mucous membranes and nonintact skin (by direct contact or inoculation). Serum antibodies are generally present at clinical presentation, and virus can be detected for up to 7 to 10 days after onset of illness from peripheral blood mononuclear cells (and possibly plasma) (164,165). The renal, hematologic, and cardiovascular systems are most severely affected in HFRS. Pathologic changes in fatal cases of classic HFRS involve multiple organ systems, but a triad of lesions consisting of hemorrhagic necrosis of the renal medulla, anterior pituitary, and cardiac right atrium is characteristic (166). In HPS, few changes in the kidneys, brain, and heart have been observed; rather, the predominant findings at autopsy have involved the lungs. Pulmonary edema with large serous pleural effusions dominate the gross

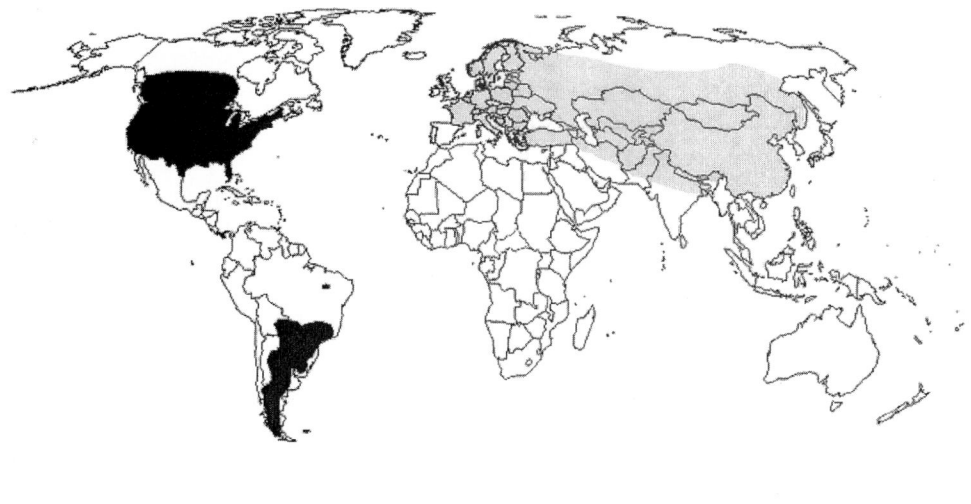

HFRS

HPS

Figure 261.2. Geographic distribution of hemorrhagic fever with renal syndrome (HFRS) and hantavirus pulmonary syndrome (HPS).

findings, with intraalveolar edema, interstitial mononuclear infiltrates, and focal hyaline membrane formation observed microscopically (135,161,167). Interestingly, retroperitoneal effusions seen almost universally in classic HFRS tend to be absent in HPS.

Hantaviruses display an *in vivo* predilection for endothelial cells and macrophages, and it is presumed that inflammatory mediators play a significant role in the vascular damage that underlies the pathologic changes observed clinically in HFRS and HPS. Hantavirus antigens, particles, or both appear to be preferentially distributed in critical target organs (kidney for HFRS and lung for HPS), whereas high numbers of cytokine-producing cells have been seen in lungs and spleen of HPS patients (167). Moreover, cellular entry of some hantaviruses has been shown to be mediated by β_3-integrins, critical receptors on endothelial cells and platelets that regulate vascular permeability and platelet activation and adhesion (168). With endothelial compromise, capillaries and small blood vessels become grossly dilated; this leads to extravasation of fluid and, to a lesser extent, cellular elements, into surrounding tissues. Vascular dysregulation and release of soluble factors acting on hematologic and immunologic systems occur as well. The clinical features of classic HFRS, including flushing, facial edema, conjunctival effusion and injection, pulmonary edema, and petechiae, are manifestations of this generalized capillary and small vessel damage. The peculiar distribution of the triad lesions is poorly understood but

probably reflects susceptibility of these organ sites to the volume shifts, pressure necrosis, and anoxia resulting from multisystem vascular insults. In HPS, cardiac function is depressed without obvious viral invasion of the myocardium, suggesting action by some soluble mediators. The perfusion deficit leading to hypotension appears to be localized because a multiorgan dysfunction syndrome is conspicuously absent. Such localized perfusion deficits may be based on viral target organ specificity and serve to explain, at least in part, the different hantaviral tropisms for HFRS (renal endothelium) and HPS (pulmonary endothelium).

CLINICAL FEATURES

HFRS is a complex, multiphasic disorder (169–171). A spectrum of clinical severity, ranging from asymptomatic or mild disease to fulminant hemorrhagic fever or pulmonary failure and death, may be seen (Table 261.6). The incubation period ranges from 4 to 42 days, but most cases of HFRS (and presumably HPS) occur within 2 to 3 weeks after exposure. In classic HFRS caused by Hantaan virus, five phases of disease have been described: febrile, hypotensive, oliguric, diuretic, and convalescent. The phases often overlap or blend together, however. Prodromal symptoms are infrequent, and illness onset is typically abrupt. Presenting signs and symptoms include high temperature, chills, malaise, myalgias, headache, dizziness, and anorexia. Shortly

TABLE 261.6.   Clinical Features of Human Pathogenic Hantavirus Infections[a]

Virus	Overall severity	Complexity	System affected		Hemorrhagic phenomena	Case fatality (%)
			Renal	Pulmonary		
Hantaan	2+–4+	Multiphasic	4+	1+–2+	1+–4+	1–15
Seoul	1+–3+	Multiphasic (blurred)	2+	0–1+	1+–2+	~1
Puumala	1+–2+[b]	Biphasic	1+–2+	0–1+	0–1+	<1
Dobrava	1+–4+	Multiphasic	4+	1+–2+	>10%	Unknown
Sin Nombre	3+–4+	Biphasic	0–3+	4+	0–1+	~30

[a]Scale 0–4+: assignments based on reported findings relative to other clinical types.
[b]Reports indicate that severe clinical forms of Puumala infection exist.

afterward, severe back and abdominal pain appears, leading often to misdiagnosis as an acute abdomen. Erythematous facial flushing extending often to the neck, shoulders, and upper thorax is characteristic and is accompanied by periorbital swelling and conjunctival, palatal, and pharyngeal injection. Petechiae are frequently present on the soft palate and axillae. As the disease progresses, white cell counts gradually rise, platelet counts begin to drop, and protein becomes increasingly evident in the urine.

Within a week, a period of hypotension ensues, beginning abruptly and coinciding with defervescence. The fall in blood pressure may be accompanied in severe cases by typical signs of hypotensive shock: tachycardia, cold and clammy skin, and mental changes. By this stage, laboratory abnormalities are striking: leukocytosis with a marked shift to the left, profound thrombocytopenia, and massive proteinuria with hematuria. Although potentially serious, the hypotensive phase generally is brief: hours to a few days. Most patients then develop oliguria. The degree of oliguria varies from patient to patient, and output may decrease to the point of anuria in severely affected individuals. Pulmonary edema may suddenly appear. Serum urea nitrogen and creatinine levels may rise to extraordinary levels, accompanied by metabolic changes typical of renal insufficiency. Dialysis at this point may be life saving. A more profound bleeding diathesis may supervene, resulting in potentially lethal pulmonary, gastrointestinal, or intracranial hemorrhages.

After 3 to 7 days, renal function is restored spontaneously, and patients enter a period of diuresis. Urine outputs typically exceed 5 to 6 L per day, and electrolyte disturbances consequent to massive diuresis may hazard recovery. Convalescence is prolonged, with complete clinical recovery often requiring several months. Anemia and hyposthenuria often persist for many months or years. Permanent sequelae of clinical significance are uncommon, but abnormalities in renal function have been described in a number of survivors years after infection, and evidence suggests an association with hypertensive renal disease (154).

Severe HFRS occurring in the Balkan states is similar clinically to Hantaan virus disease. Seoul virus infections generally are somewhat milder than that just described and may be more likely to cause hepatic dysfunction, but fatalities have been reported. The syndrome associated with Puumala virus, nephropathia epidemica, is usually milder still and only rarely fatal; however, severe HFRS associated with Puumala-like strains has been reported from Germany and elsewhere (172).

HPS is a much more serious, life-threatening disorder with considerable morbidity and high mortality. The signs and symptoms of Sin Nombre and related virus infections are primarily referable to the cardiopulmonary system. During the 3- to 6-day prodromal phase of HPS, fever and myalgia are almost universally present. Gastrointestinal distress, headache, and dizziness may be observed, but respiratory symptoms are generally absent early in the disease process. The prodrome is followed by a cardiopulmonary phase, heralded by progressive dyspnea and cough. Tachypnea and tachycardia accompany the preexisting fever, and hypotension occurs. Signs of generalized vascular dysregulation (flushing, injection, petechiae), so typical of classic HFRS, are conspicuously absent (except in some South American HPS cases). Thrombocytopenia typically occurs, but is not always present early. Atypical lymphocytes are visible in peripheral blood smears and are virtually always present at the onset of the cardiopulmonary phase. A left shift in the differential count (with or without leukocytosis) is common. Mild proteinuria is frequent, and mild renal insufficiency is seen in about 15% of patients. With Bayou and Black Creek Canal virus infections in the southern United States, significant renal dysfunction with elevated creatine kinase levels may occur, but frank renal

failure with other New World hantavirus infections is uncommon (173). Other laboratory abnormalities may include mildly elevated transaminases, decreased serum protein, and hyponatremia.

Progressive hypoxemia and pulmonary edema requiring intubation and assisted ventilation have characterized most HPS cases confirmed to date. The case fatality is variable but has stabilized at 30% in the United States (174). Deaths are generally subsequent to cardiac dysrhythmias due to intractable hypotension 2 to 16 days after disease onset (135). Lactic acidosis is a poor prognostic finding. Convalescence among survivors is characterized by an often rapid improvement in oxygenation and return to normal hemodynamic function. Long-term sequelae of HPS include mild fatigue and the presence of clinically insignificant small airway disease (175).

DIAGNOSIS

A high index of suspicion is vital to early recognition of human hantavirus infection. The differential diagnosis of HFRS includes rickettsial, leptospiral, meningococcal, other viral, and poststreptococcal syndromes. Initial signs and symptoms mimic an acute intraabdominal process in some cases. The presentation of HPS may suggest bacterial pneumonia and sepsis, pneumonic plague, tularemia, legionellosis, histoplasmosis (or other fungal pulmonary infection), psittacosis, leptospirosis, or severe rickettsial disease. Laboratory diagnosis is made by demonstration of specific hantavirus IgM antibodies in acute serum by EIA, or by a fourfold or greater rise in virus-specific IgG antibodies by EIA or IF (138,176). Purified recombinant hantavirus antigens have been produced for use in both EIA and Western blot assays, enhancing diagnostic specificity (177–179). Neutralizing antibody tests are highly specific but are impractical for clinical use. Hantaviral antigens can be detected in tissues by immunohistochemical techniques (167), and the availability of nucleic acid primers from several hantavirus strains has enabled amplification of nucleotide sequences from fresh or frozen tissues by reverse transcription polymerase chain reaction (136).

Isolation of hantaviruses from human specimens is difficult, technically demanding, and not useful for diagnosis. Because of their aerosol infectivity, any attempts at isolation of hantaviruses should be made only under appropriately high levels of biocontainment (BSL 3 or 4).

TREATMENT

Close monitoring with emphasis on volume balance and electrolyte status is fundamental to successful treatment of HFRS. Early hospitalization, bed rest, and avoidance of trauma are necessary to minimize disruption of fragile vascular beds. Patients with severe HFRS and all cases of HPS should be managed in an intensive care environment. With HFRS, wide fluctuations in volume requirements often occur. Careful fluid restriction is necessary early in the disease; massive inputs to cover losses may be required later during diuretic periods. Severe renal failure with attendant fluid and metabolic complications should be anticipated in seriously ill patients; peritoneal dialysis or hemodialysis can be life saving (171).

In HPS, the goal of supportive therapy is maintenance of oxygenation and tissue perfusion. Hypoxemia should be managed through oxygen supplementation, with use of mechanical ventilation as necessary. Fluid input should be judicious, and early use of inotropic agents is indicated in lieu of increasing fluids to maintain tissue perfusion (161).

Hantaviruses are susceptible *in vitro* to ribavirin. When given early in disease, intravenous ribavirin has been shown to reduce mortality and to reduce severity of renal dysfunction and hemorrhage in Chinese HFRS patients (180). Although ribavirin has been used to treat patients with HPS through an open-label trial, effectiveness has not been demonstrated (181).

A single hantavirus recovered in Argentina and Chile, Andes virus, has been associated with person-to-person spread (182,183). Otherwise, isolation of patients with HFRS and HPS (except in South America) is unnecessary, even under conditions of severe hemorrhage. Use of standard precautions in handling blood and body fluids from hantavirus-infected patients is prudent, however. Physical barriers and respiratory protection should be employed when clinical procedures or specimen processing is likely to generate aerosols. In South America, droplet and contact precautions are also indicated.

PREVENTION

The prevalence and ubiquity of reservoirs make rodent population control impractical in the field. However, measures to minimize infestations in domestic and peridomestic settings, coupled with general guidelines for avoidance of rodents and their excreta, should reduce exposure risk. Insecticides should be used simultaneously with rodent extermination techniques to control fleas, which may serve as vectors for other human pathogens (e.g., *Yersinia pestis*).

Candidate Hantaan virus vaccines have been developed using both classic and molecular techniques. Cell culture– and mouse brain–derived products have been tested widely in China and Korea, and a vaccinia-vectored recombinant immunogen (expressing M and S gene products from the prototype Hantaan strain) is under study in human volunteers (184). However, no vaccine has yet proved effective in preventing hantavirus infections in controlled clinical trials.

Crimean-Congo Hemorrhagic Fever

Crimean-Congo hemorrhagic fever (CCHF) is a tick-borne viral disease with a wide geographic distribution. Human infections have been recognized in Eastern Europe, the Middle East, across Asia as far east as China, and throughout Africa. The etiologic agent of what had been known since the 1930s as Crimean hemorrhagic fever was identified as a virus in 1947 (185). In 1969, however, a virus that had been recovered from a febrile patient in the Belgian Congo (now the Democratic Republic of the Congo) in 1956 was found to be identical to the Crimean hemorrhagic fever agent, and the nomenclature was revised to reflect the linkage—hence the current name, CCHF (186).

CCHF virus is a member of the genus *Nairovirus* in the family Bunyaviridae. All viruses of this genus are thought to be transmitted by ticks. As with other Bunyaviridae, virions are 90 to 120 nm in diameter, with 10-nm surface projections. The tripartite negative-stranded RNA genome codes for two surface glycoproteins (by the M segment), a nucleoprotein (by the S segment), and a viral polymerase (by the L segment).

EPIDEMIOLOGY

The epidemiology of CCHF is tied to complex relationships that exist between the virus's arthropod vectors and their nonhuman vertebrate hosts (187). The virus is a parasite of at least 24 species of ixodid (hard) ticks, particularly *Hyalomma* species. Transovarial and transstadial transmission of CCHF virus has been documented in several of these tick species, which pre-

sumably serve as both reservoir and vector of the agent. In addition, the ticks feed on (and infect) a wide variety of wild and domestic animals, including birds; specific vertebrate hosts are parasitized (and possibly infected) in both a tick species and a life cycle stage-specific pattern. Although quantitative studies are few, it is clear that vertebrate amplification of CCHF infection is a major contributor to sustainment and spread of the virus in nature. In general, wild hares and large herbivores represent the major vertebrate amplifier reservoirs. Human infections occur secondary to bites from infected ticks; exposure to viremic animal blood, tissues, and excreta; and nosocomially. The last route is particularly significant inasmuch as several serious outbreaks of CCHF have occurred among hospital personnel after exposure to infectious materials from unsuspected cases (188–191).

Seasonality of CCHF depends on local climatic conditions, and peaks correspond to periods of maximal tick infestation. CCHF is a rural disease, and many of the endemic areas are remote; information on incidence and prevalence is consequently variable in quality. Important exceptions are infections among butchers, tanners, and animal handlers in urban centers in the Middle East from either imported animals or acute infection of naive animals or their shed ticks (192). A relatively high range of illness-to-infection ratios have been reported from some countries (from 20% to 50%), but human infections have not been recognized in some areas where infected ticks or seropositive animals and humans have been found [reviewed in Watts and colleagues (190) and Peters and LeDuc (193)]. This variability is unexplained but may relate to geographic differences in virulence among CCHF virus strains, predominant mode of disease acquisition, or density of infection in reservoir or vector populations. Case fatality among hospitalized patients in Eurasia has ranged from 13% to 50%; in southern Africa, the mortality rate is about 30%, despite availability of relatively advanced medical care (187,194).

PATHOGENESIS

CCHF is a multisystem disease (195,196). Generalized vascular damage, endothelial lesions, and scattered focal hemorrhages with edema are typically seen in multiple organs. Immunohistochemical studies have demonstrated the presence of viral antigen concentrated in mononuclear phagocytes, endothelial cells, and hepatocytes. Histologically, focal to massive necrosis of the liver is seen, but the degree of hepatic involvement is generally disproportionate to the amount of antigen present. Although association of parenchymal necrosis in liver with the presence of viral antigen suggests that cell damage may be mediated by direct viral cytopathic effect, it is unclear whether circulating inflammatory mediators play a role in cell damage (197). Disseminated intravascular coagulation is well documented as an early and prominent feature of CCHF, and the resultant microthrombus formation with subsequent infarction is undoubtedly critical in pathogenesis. In contrast to other viral hemorrhagic fevers, gross bleeding in CCHF is quite common, and the volume of blood loss may be significant. Anemia or circulatory collapse may contribute to death in fatal cases.

CLINICAL FEATURES

The incubation period for CCHF is generally 2 to 7 days (194,195). Onset is abrupt, with high temperature, chills, severe headache, myalgia, weakness, epigastric pain, and nausea and vomiting. Conjunctival injection, flushing of the face and chest, pharyngeal hyperemia, and palatal petechiae are frequent. After 3 to 5 days, a brief remission of several hours' duration may be seen in one

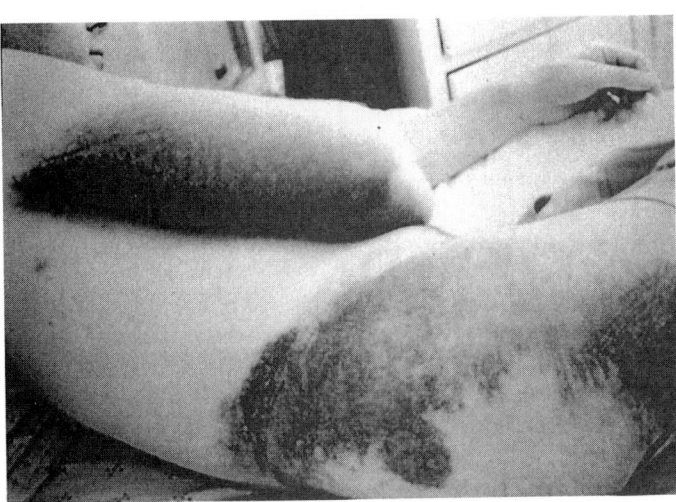

Figure 261.3. Patient with Crimean-Congo hemorrhagic fever virus infection illustrating extensive ecchymoses.

third to two thirds of patients, followed by a second, overtly hemorrhagic, phase of illness. During this latter period, bradycardia, pulmonary edema, and hypovolemic shock occur. Petechiae appear on most patients, distributed over the chest and abdomen. Epistaxis is common, and in more severe cases, uncontrolled bleeding at other mucosal surfaces, as well as venipuncture sites, may occur. In such cases, large pressure-associated ecchymoses frequently are seen (Fig. 261.3). This stage may last 3 to 10 days and is associated with changes in mood and affect.

Leukopenia, thrombocytopenia, and elevated serum transaminase values are generally present at the time of initial clinical consultation. Studies of South African patients showed that leukocytosis (white cell count of 10,000 cells/mm³ or higher), severe thrombocytopenia (platelet count of 20,000 cells/mm³ or lower), or marked abnormalities of serum transaminase levels (aspartate aminotransferase level of at least 200 IU/L, alanine aminotransferase level of at least 150 IU/L) or coagulation (activated partial thromboplastin time of 60 seconds or more, or fibrinogen levels of at least 110 mg/dL) were 90% predictive of a fatal outcome if seen during the first 5 days of illness (195). Recovery in survivors is slow and prolonged.

DIAGNOSIS

CCHF virus is readily recovered from blood after its inoculation into newborn mice or cell cultures. Viral antigen can be demonstrated in many organs of fatal cases by immunohistochemistry and nucleic acid detection (197,198). In most patients, virus-specific IgM and IgG antibodies can be detected by indirect IF or EIA on days 7 to 9 of illness, with IgM falling to low or undetectable levels by 3 to 5 months (199). However, virus-specific IgM and IgG may be absent in early or fatal cases; antigen should be sought by EIA for acute diagnosis (192). Neutralizing antibody appears toward the end of the first week of illness but reaches only modest titer (1:16 to 1:256) and persists only 4 to 5 months in survivors (196).

TREATMENT

As with other viral hemorrhagic fevers, close attention to fluid, electrolyte, and volume status is critical to management. Treatment of CCHF with immune plasma has been generally unsuccessful (199). The virus is sensitive *in vitro* to ribavirin (199), and this drug has been reported to be useful in management of South African and Pakistani CCHF cases (200).

PREVENTION

Avoidance of tick bite is the most effective strategy for preventing infection. This is best done through use of personal protective measures such as repellents and sprays for impregnating clothing. Avoidance of mucous membrane or nonintact skin contact with human or animal blood in endemic areas, as well as avoidance of high-risk behaviors such as crushing ticks by hand, is prudent.

A formalin-inactivated mouse brain CCHF vaccine has been used in the former Soviet Union and Bulgaria, but no data on efficacy are available.

ISOLATION OF PATIENTS

With the exception of most hantaviruses, the viral hemorrhagic fevers addressed in this chapter are renowned for their propensity for person-to-person spread in nosocomial and familial settings. Many of these transmissions can be traced to inoculation of infectious materials (e.g., shared needles) or exchange of body fluids (e.g., sexual transmission); however, not all case clusters or outbreaks are so readily explained. In general, application of standard precautions in handling of body fluids and sharp objects such as needles, scalpel blades, and broken glass implements by clinical and laboratory personnel will minimize the potential for spread of infectious materials in hospital settings. All hemorrhagic fever viruses are relatively stable as droplets and aerosols, however, and the potential for interpersonal spread under conditions other than direct inoculation or close contact exists. Therefore, it would appear prudent to maximize isolation precautions to the greatest extent possible when dealing with a viral hemorrhagic fever patient (other than HFRS and North American HPS), to include use of face shields, personal respirators, disposable gowns impermeable to blood and other fluids, and disposable shoe covers. All samples for laboratory testing should be clearly labeled as biohazards, and equipment and supplies leaving the patient care area should be sterilized using high temperature or gas.

REFERENCES

1. Murphy FA, Whitfield SG. Morphology and morphogenesis of arenaviruses. *Bull W H O* 1975;52:409.
2. Buchmeier MJ, Parekh BS. Protein structure and expression among arenaviruses. *Curr Top Microbiol Immunol* 1987;133:41.
3. Auperin DD, Romanowski V, Galinski M, et al. Sequencing studies of Pichinde arenavirus S RNA indicate a novel coding strategy, an ambisense viral S RNA. *J Virol* 1986;52:897.
4. Murphy FA, Walker DH. Arenaviruses: persistent infection and viral survival in reservoir hosts. In: Kurstak E, Maramorosch K, eds. *Viruses and environment.* New York: Academic Press, 1978:155–180.
5. Webb PA, Justines G, Johnson KM. Infection of wild and laboratory animals with Machupo and Latino viruses. *Bull W H O* 1975;52:493.
6. Vitullo AD, Hodara VL, Merani MS. Effect of persistent infection with Junin virus on growth and reproduction of its natural reservoir, *Calomys musculinus. Am J Trop Med Hyg* 1987;37:663.
7. Armstrong C, Sweet LK. Lymphocytic choriomeningitis. *Public Health Rep* 1939;54:673.
8. Armstrong C. Studies on choriomeningitis and poliomyelitis. *Bull N Y Acad Med* 1941;17:295.
9. Biggar RJ, Woodall JP, Walter PD, et al. Lymphocytic choriomeningitis outbreak associated with pet hamsters: fifty-seven cases from New York State. *JAMA* 1975;232:494.
10. Gregg MB. Recent outbreaks of lymphocytic choriomeningitis in the United States of America. *Bull W H O* 1975;52:549.

11. Dykewicz CA, Data VM, Fisher-Hoch SP, et al. Lymphocytic choriomeningitis outbreak associated with nude mice in a research laboratory. *JAMA* 1992;267:1349.

12. McCormick JB, Webb PA, Krebs JW, et al. A prospective study of the epidemiology and ecology of Lassa fever. *J Infect Dis* 1987;155:437.

13. Salazar-Bravo J, Ruedas LA, Yates TL. Mammalian reservoirs of arenaviruses. *Curr Top Microbiol Immunol* 2002;262:25–63.

14. Monath TP, Newhouse VF, Kemp GE, et al. Lassa virus isolation from *Mastomys natalensis* rodents during an epidemic in Sierra Leone. *Science* 1974;185:263.

15. Fraser DW, Campbell CC, Monath TP, et al. Lassa fever in the eastern province of Sierra Leone, 1970–1972. 1. Epidemiologic studies. *Am J Trop Med Hyg* 1974;23:1131.

16. Keenlyside RA, McCormick JB, Webb PA, et al. Case-control study of *Mastomys natalensis* and humans in Lassa virus-infected households in Sierra Leone. *Am J Trop Med Hyg* 1983;32:829.

17. Carey DE, Kemp GE, White HA, et al. Lassa fever: epidemiological aspects of the 1970 epidemic, Jos, Nigeria. *Trans R Soc Trop Med Hyg* 1972;66:402.

18. Monath TP, Mertens PE, Patton R, et al. A hospital epidemic of Lassa fever in Zorzor, Liberia, March–April 1972. *Am J Trop Med Hyg* 1973;22:773.

19. McCormick JB, King IJ, Webb PA, et al. A case-control study of the clinical diagnosis and course of Lassa fever. *J Infect Dis* 1987;155:445.

20. Price ME, Fisher-Hoch SP, Craven RB, et al. A prospective study of maternal and fetal outcome in acute Lassa fever during pregnancy. *BMJ* 1988;297:584.

21. Webb PA, McCormick JB, King IJ, et al. Lassa fever in children in Sierra Leone, West Africa. *Trans R Soc Trop Med Hyg* 1986;80:577.

22. Maiztegui JI, Feuillade M, Briggiler A. Progressive extension of the endemic area and changing incidence of Argentine hemorrhagic fever. *Med Microbiol Immunol* 1986;175:149.

23. Carballal G, Videla CM, Merani MS. Epidemiology of Argentine hemorrhagic fever. *Eur J Epidemiol* 1988;4:259.

24. Maiztegui JI. Clinical and epidemiological patterns of Argentine haemorrhagic fever. *Bull W H O* 1975;52:567.

25. Mills JN, Ellis BA, McKee KT Jr, et al. A longitudinal study of Junin virus activity in the rodent reservoir of Argentine hemorrhagic fever. *Am J Trop Med Hyg* 1992;47:749.

26. Hemorrhagic Fever Commission of Bolivia. Hemorrhagic fever in Bolivia [in Spanish]. *Bull Pan Am Health Org* 1965;58:93.

27. MacKenzie RB. Epidemiology of Machupo virus infection. I. Pattern of human infection, San Joachin, Bolivia, 1962–1964. *Am J Trop Med Hyg* 1965;14:808.

28. Centers for Disease Control. Bolivian hemorrhagic fever: El Beni Department, Bolivia, 1994. *MMWR Morbid Mortal Wkly Rep* 1994;43:943.

29. Peters CJ, Kuehne RW, Mercado RR, et al. Hemorrhagic fever in Cochabamba, Bolivia, 1971. *Am J Epidemiol* 1974;99:425.

30. Salas R, de Manzione N, Tesh RB, et al. Venezuelan haemorrhagic fever. *Lancet* 1991;338:1033.

31. deManzione N, Salas RA, Paredes H, et al. Venezuelan hemorrhagic fever: clinical and epidemiological studies of 165 cases. *Clin Infect Dis* 1998;26:308.

32. Fulhorst CF, Bowen MD, Salas R, et al. Natural rodent host associations of Guanarito and Pirital viruses (family Arenaviridae) in central Venezuela. *Am J Trop Med Hyg* 1999;61:325.

33. Coimbra TLM, Nassar ES, Burattini MN, et al. New arenavirus isolated in Brazil. *Lancet* 1994;343:391.

34. Barry M, Russi M, Armstrong L, et al. Brief report: Treatment of a laboratory-acquired Sabia virus infection. *N Engl J Med* 1995;333:294.

35. Horton J, Hotchin JE, Olson KB, et al. The effects of MP virus infection in lymphoma. *Cancer Res* 1971;31:1066.

36. Warkel RL, Rinaldi CF, Bancroft WH, et al. Fatal acute meningoencephalitis due to lymphocytic choriomeningitis virus. *Neurology* 1973;23:198.

37. Walker DH, McCormick JB, Johnson KM, et al. Pathologic and virologic study of Lassa fever in man. *Am J Pathol* 1982;107:349.

38. Johnson KM, McCormick JB, Webb PA, et al. Clinical virology of Lassa fever in hospitalized patients. *J Infect Dis* 1987;155:546.

39. Mahanty S, Bausch DG, Thomas RL, et al. Low levels of interleukin-8 and interferon-inducible protein-10 in serum are associated with fatal infections in acute Lassa fever. *J Infect Dis* 2001;183:1713.

40. Fisher-Hoch SP, Mitchell SW, Sasso DR, et al. Physiologic and immunologic disturbances associated with shock in Lassa fever in a primate model. *J Infect Dis* 1987;155:465.

41. Fisher-Hoch SP, McCormick JB, Sasso D, et al. Hematologic dysfunction in Lassa fever. *J Med Virol* 1988;26:127.

42. Cummins D, Fisher-Hoch SP, Walshe KJ, et al. A plasma inhibitor of platelet aggregation in patients with Lassa fever. *Br J Haematol* 1989;72:543.

43. Roberts PJ, Cummins D, Bainton AD, et al. Plasma from patients with severe Lassa fever profoundly modulates f-met-leu-phe induced superoxide generation in neutrophil. *Br J Haematol* 1989;73:152.

44. Lange JV, Mitchell SW, McCormick JB, et al. Kinetic study of platelets and fibrinogen in Lassa virus-infected monkeys and early pathologic events in Mopeia virus-infected monkeys. *Am J Trop Med Hyg* 1985;34:999.

45. Cossio P, Laguens R, Arana R, et al. Ultrastructural and immunochemical study of the human kidney in Argentine haemorrhagic fever. *Virchows Arch* 1975;368:1.

46. Gonzales PH, Cossio PM, Arana R, et al. Lymphatic tissue in Argentine hemorrhagic fever. *Arch Pathol Lab Med* 1980;104:250.

47. Levis SC, Saavedra MC, Ceccoli C, et al. Endogenous interferon in Argentine hemorrhagic fever. *J Infect Dis* 1984;149:428.

48. Levis SC, Saavedra MC, Ceccoli C, et al. Correlation between endogenous interferon and the clinical evolution of patients with Argentine haemorrhagic fever. *J Interferon Res* 1985;5:383.

49. Heller MV, Saavedra MC, Falcoff R, et al. Increased tumor necrosis factor-α levels in Argentine hemorrhagic fever. *J Infect Dis* 1992;166:1203.

50. Peters CJ, Jahrling PB, Liu CT, et al. Experimental studies of arenaviral hemorrhagic fevers. *Curr Top Microbiol Immunol* 1987;132:5.

51. Hinman AR, Fraser DW, Douglas RG, et al. Outbreak of lymphocytic choriomeningitis virus infections in medical center personnel. *Am J Epidemiol* 1975;101:103.

52. Vanzee BE, Douglas RG Jr, Betts RF, et al. Lymphocytic choriomeningitis in university hospital personnel: clinical features. *Am J Med* 1975;58:803.

53. Meyer HM Jr, Johnson RT, Crawford IP, et al. Central nervous syndromes of "viral" etiology. *Am J Med* 1960;29:334.

54. Ormay I, Kovacs P. Lymphocytic choriomeningitis causing unilateral deafness [in Hungarian]. *Orv Hetil* 1989;130:789.

55. Sheinbergas MM. Antibody to lymphocytic choriomeningitis virus in children with congenital hydrocephalus. *Acta Virol* 1975;19:165.

56. Barton LL, Budd SC, Morfitt WS, et al. Congenital lymphocytic choriomeningitis virus infection in twins. *Pediatr Infect Dis J* 1993;12:942.

57. Smadel JE, Green RH, Pahtraul RM, et al. Lymphocytic choriomeningitis: two human fatalities following an unusual febrile illness. *Proc Soc Exp Biol Med* 1942;49:683.

58. Cummins D, McCormick JB, Bennet D, et al. Acute sensorineural deafness in Lassa fever. *JAMA* 1990;264:2093.

59. Monson MH, Cole AK, Frame JD, et al. Pediatric Lassa fever: a review of 33 Liberian cases. *Am J Trop Med Hyg* 1987;36:408.

60. McCormick JB, King IJ, Webb PA, et al. Lassa fever: effective therapy with ribavirin. *N Engl J Med* 1986;314:20.

61. Mackenzie RB, Beye HK, Valverde L, et al. Epidemic hemorrhagic fever in Bolivia. I. A preliminary report of the epidemiologic and clinical findings in a new epidemic area in South America. *Am J Trop Med Hyg* 1964;13:620.

62. Weissenbacher MC, Laguens RP, Coto CE. Argentine hemorrhagic fever. *Curr Top Microbiol Immunol* 1987;134:79.

63. Jahrling PB. Filoviruses and arenaviruses. In: Murray PR, Baron EJ, Pfaller MA, et al., eds. *Manual of clinical microbiology*, 6th ed. Washington, DC: ASM Press, 1995:1068–1081.

63a. Bausch DG, Rollin PE, Demby AH, et al. Diagnosis and clinical virology of Lassa fever as evaluated by enzyme-linked immunosorbent assay, indirect fluorescent-antibody test, and virus isolation. *J Clin Microbiol* 2000;38:2670.

64. Ambrosio AM, Enria DA, Maiztegui JI. Junin virus isolation from lymphomononuclear cells of patients with Argentine hemorrhagic fever. *Intervirology* 1986;25:97.

65. Niklasson BS, Jahrling PB, Peters CJ. Detection of Lassa fever antigens and Lassa-specific immunoglobulin G and M by enzyme-linked immunosorbent assay. *J Clin Microbiol* 1984;20:239.

66. Demby AH, Chamberlain J, Brown DWG, et al. Early diagnosis of Lassa fever by reverse transcription-PCR. *J Clin Microbiol* 1994;32:2898.

67. Maiztegui JI, Fernandez NJ, de Damilano AL. Efficacy of immune plasma in treatment of Argentine haemorrhagic fever and association between treatment and a late neurological syndrome. *Lancet* 1979;2:1216.

68. Enria D, Briggiler AM, Fernandez NJ, et al. Importance of dose of neutralizing antibodies in treatment of Argentine haemorrhagic fever with immune plasma. *Lancet* 1984;2:255.

69. Enria D, Franco SG, Ambrosio A, et al. Current status of the treatment of Argentine hemorrhagic fever. *Med Microbiol Immunol* 1986;175:173.

70. Enria DA, Briggiler AM, Levis S, et al. Preliminary report: tolerance and antiviral effect of ribavirin in patients with Argentine hemorrhagic fever. *Antiviral Res* 1987;7:353.

71. Johnson KM, Webb PA, Justines G. Biology of Tacaribe-complex viruses. In: Lehman-Grube F, ed. *Lymphocytic choriomeningitis virus and other arenaviruses*. Berlin: Springer-Verlag, 1973:241–258.

72. Barrera Oro JG, McKee KT Jr. Toward a vaccine against Argentine hemorrhagic fever. *Bull Pan Am Health Org* 1991;25:118.

73. Maiztegui JI, McKee KT Jr, Barrera Oro JG, et al. Protective efficacy of a live attenuated vaccine against Argentine hemorrhagic fever. *J Infect Dis* 1998;177:277.

74. Enria DA, Feuillade MR, Briggiler AM, et al. *Informe para la Reunion annual del Programa Nacional de Lucha contra la Fiebre Hemorragica Argentina*. Ministerio de Salud, Republica Argentina, 30 June 2000.

75. Fisher-Hoch SP, McCormick JB, Auperin D, et al. Protection of rhesus monkeys from fatal Lassa fever by vaccination with a recombinant vaccinia virus containing the Lassa virus glycoprotein gene. *Proc Natl Acad Sci U S A* 1988;85:1.

76. Centers for Disease Control. Update: management of patients with suspected viral hemorrhagic fever. *MMWR Morb Mortal Wkly Rep* 1995;44:475–479.

77. Kiley MP, Bowen ETW, Eddy GA, et al. Filoviridae: a taxonomic home for Marburg and Ebola viruses? *Intervirology* 1982;18:24.

78. Feldmann H, Klenk H-D, Sanchez A. Molecular biology and evolution of filoviruses. *Arch Virol* 1993;7[Suppl 1]:81.

79. Le Guenno B, Formentry P, Wyers M, et al. Isolation and partial characterization of a new strain of Ebola virus. *Lancet* 1995;345:1271.

80. Preston R. *The hot zone.* New York: Random House, 1994.

81. Kiley MP, Cox NJ, Elliott LH, et al. Physiochemical properties of Marburg virus: evidence for three distinct virus strains and their relationship to Ebola virus. *J Gen Virol* 1988;69:1957.

82. Elliott LH, Kiley MP, McCormick JB. Descriptive analysis of Ebola virus proteins. *Virology* 1985;147:169.

83. Sanchez A, Kiley MP, Holloway BP, et al. Sequence analysis of the Ebola virus genome: organization, genetic elements, and comparison with the genome of Marburg virus. *Virus Res* 1993;29:215.

84. Murphy FA, van der Groen G, Whitfield SG, et al. Ebola and Marburg virus morphology and taxonomy. In: Pattyn SR. *Ebola virus haemorrhagic fever.* Amsterdam: Elsevier North Holland, 1978:61–84.

85. Bowen ETW, Platt GS, Lloyd G, et al. A comparative study of strains of Ebola virus isolated from southern Sudan and northern Zaire in 1976. *J Med Virol* 1980;6:129.

86. Peters CJ, Sanchez A, Rollin PE, et al. Filoviridae: Marburg and Ebola viruses. In: Fields BN, Knipe DM, Howley PM, eds. *Fields virology*, 3rd ed. Philadelphia: Lippincott-Raven, 1996:1161–1176.

87. Peters CJ, Sanchez A, Feldmann H, et al. Filoviruses as emerging pathogens. *Semin Virol* 1994;5:147.

88. Martini GA, Siegert R, eds. *Marburg virus disease.* New York: Springer-Verlag, 1971.

89. Gear JSS, Cassel GA, Gear AJ, et al. Outbreak of Marburg virus disease in Johannesburg. *Br Med J* 1975;4:489.

90. Smith DH, Johnson BK, Isaacson M, et al. Marburg-virus disease in Kenya. *Lancet* 1982;1:816.

91. Johnson ED, Koimet E, Gitau LG, et al. Marburg virus disease: an environmental health threat in Kenya. In: Kinoti SH, Waiyoki PG, Were BO, eds. *The role of man in disease control.* Proceedings of the llth Annual Medical Scientific Conference. African Medical and Research Foundation, 1990.

92. World Health Organization: Viral haemorrhagic fever/Marburg-Democratic Republic of the Congo. *Wkly Epidemiol Rec* 1999;74:157.

93. Pattyn SR, ed. *Ebola virus haemorrhagic fever.* Amsterdam: Elsevier North Holland, 1978.

94. Johnson KM, Scribner CL, McCormick JB. Ecology of Ebola virus: a first clue? *J Infect Dis* 1981;143:749.

95. Emond RTD, Evans B, Bowen ETW, et al. A case of Ebola virus infection. *Br Med J* 1977;2:541.

96. Heymann DL, Weisfeld JS, Webb PA, et al. Ebola hemorrhagic fever: Tandala, Zaire, 1977–1978. *J Infect Dis* 1980;142:372.

97. Baron RC, McCormick JB, Zubeir OA. Ebola hemorrhagic fever in southern Sudan: hospital dissemination and intrafamiliar spread. *Bull W H O* 1983;6:997.

98. Jahrling PB, Geisbert TW, Dalgard DW, et al. Preliminary report: isolation of Ebola virus from monkeys imported to USA. *Lancet* 1990;335:502.

99. Peters CJ, Johnson ED, Jahrling PB, et al. Filoviruses. In: Morse S, eds. *Emerging viruses.* New York: Oxford University Press, 1991:159–175.

100. Hayes CG, Burans JP, Ksiazek TG, et al. Outbreak of fatal illness among captive macaques in the Philippines caused by an Ebola-related filovirus. *Am J Trop Med Hyg* 1992;46:664.

101. World Health Organization. Viral haemorrhagic fever in imported monkeys. *Wkly Epidemiol Rec* 1992;67:142.

102. Rollin PE, Williams RJ, Bressler DS, et al. Ebola (subtype Reston) virus among quarantined nonhuman primates recently imported from the Philippines to the United States. *J Infect Dis* 1999;179[Suppl 1]:S108.

103. Centers for Disease Control. Update: filovirus infection among persons with occupational exposure to nonhuman primates. *MMWR Morb Mortal Wkly Rep* 1990;39:266.

104. Georges AJ, Leroy AM, Renaut AA, et al. Ebola hemorrhagic fever outbreaks in Gabon, 1994–1997: epidemiologic and health control issues. *J Infect Dis* 1999;179[Suppl 1]:S65.

105. World Health Organization. Ebola haemorrhagic fever. *Wkly Epidemiol Rec* 1995;70:149.

106. American Health Consultants. Lack of barrier precautions linked to Ebola spread. *Hosp Infect Control* 1995;22:101.

107. Richards GA, Murphy S, Jobson R, et al. Unexplained Ebola virus in a tertiary setting: clinical and epidemiologic aspects. *Crit Care Med* 2000;28:240.

108. Centers for Disease Control and Prevention. Outbreak of Ebola hemorrhagic fever-Uganda. *MMWR Morb Mortal Wkly Rep* 2001;50:73.

108a. Ebola hemorrhagic fever—Congo Rep. PROMED-mail 2003; 7 May. *www.promedmail.org* Accessed 7 May 2003.

109. Swanepoel R, Leman PA, Burt FJ, et al. Experimental inoculation of plants and animals with Ebola virus. *Emerg Infect Dis* 1996;2:321.

110. Murphy FA. Pathology of Ebola virus infection. In: Pattyn SR, ed. *Ebola virus haemorrhagic fever.* Amsterdam: Elsevier North Holland, 1978:37–42.

111. Fisher-Hoch SP, Platt GS, Neild GH, et al. Pathophysiology of shock and hemorrhage in a fulminating viral infection (Ebola). *J Infect Dis* 1985;152:887.

112. Yang Z, Delgado R, Xu L, et al. Distinct cellular interactions of secreted and transmembrane Ebola virus glycoproteins. *Science* 1998;279:1034.

113. Chan SY, Empig CJ, Welte FJ, et al. Folate receptor-α is a cofactor for cellular entry by Marburg and Ebola viruses. *Cell* 2001;106:117.

114. Wilson JA, Hart MK. Protection from Ebola virus mediated by cytotoxic T lymphocytes specific for the viral nucleoprotein. *J Virol* 2001;75:2660.

115. Leroy EM, Baize S, Volchkov VE, et al. Human asymptomatic Ebola infection and strong inflammatory response. *Lancet* 2000;355:2210.

116. Gupta M, Mahanty S, Bray M, et al. Passive transfer of antibodies protects immunocompetent and immunodeficient mice against lethal Ebola virus infection without complete inhibition of viral replication. *J Virol* 2001;75:4649.

117. Gear JHS. Clinical aspects of African viral hemorrhagic fevers. *Rev Infect Dis* 1989;11[Suppl 4]:S777.

118. Surreau PH. Firsthand clinical observations of hemorrhagic manifestations in Ebola hemorrhagic fever in Zaire. *Rev Infect Dis* 1989;11[Suppl 4]:S790.

119. Elliott LH, Bauer SP, Perez-Oronoz G, et al. Improved specificity of testing methods for filovirus antibodies. *J Virol Methods* 1993;43:85.

120. Ksiazek T. Laboratory diagnosis of filovirus infections in nonhuman primates. *Lab Anim* 1991;20:34.

121. Richman DD, Cleveland PH, McCormick JB, et al. Antigenic analysis of strains of Ebola virus: identification of two Ebola virus serotypes. *J Infect Dis* 1983;147:268.

122. Leroy EM, Baize S, Lu CY, et al. Diagnosis of Ebola haemorrhagic fever by RT-PCR in an epidemic setting. *J Med Virol* 2000;60:463.

123. Zaki SR, Shieh WJ, Greer PW, et al. A novel immunohistochemical assay for the detection of Ebola virus in skin: implications for diagnosis, spread, and surveillance of Ebola hemorrhagic fever. *J Infect Dis* 1999;179[Suppl 1]:S36.

124. Ksiazek TG, Rollin PE, Williams AJ, et al. Clinical virology of Ebola hemorrhagic fever (EHF): virus, virus antigen, and IgG and IgM antibody findings among EHF patients in Kikwit, Democratic Republic of the Congo, 1995. *J Infect Dis* 1999;179[Suppl 1]:S177.

125. Geisbert TW, Jahrling PB. Use of immunoelectron microscopy to show Ebola virus during the 1989 United States epizootic. *J Clin Pathol* 1990;43:813.

126. Mupapa K, Massamba M, Kibadi K, et al. Treatment of Ebola hemorrhagic fever with blood transfusions from convalescent patients. *J Infect Dis* 1999;179[Suppl 1]:S18.

127. Centers for Disease Control. Update: Ebola-related filovirus infection in nonhuman primates and interim guidelines for handling nonhuman primates during transit and quarantine. *MMWR Morb Mortal Wkly Rep* 1990;39:22.

128. Schmaljohn CS, Hasty SE, Dalrymple JM, et al. Antigenic and genetic properties of viruses linked to hemorrhagic fever with renal syndrome. *Science* 1985;227:1041.

129. Schmaljohn CS, Hasty SE, Harrison SA, et al. Characterization of Hantaan virions, the prototype virus of hemorrhagic fever with renal syndrome. *J Infect Dis* 1983;148:1005.

130. Schmaljohn CS, Dalrymple JM. Analysis of Hantaan virus RNA: evidence for a new genus of Bunyaviridae. *Virology* 1983;131:482.

131. Elliott RM, Schmaljohn CS, Collett MS. Bunyaviridae genome structure and gene expression. *Curr Top Microbiol Immunol* 1991;169:91.

132. White JD, Shirey FG, French GR, et al. Hantaan virus, aetiological agent of Korean haemorrhagic fever, has Bunyaviridae-like morphology. *Lancet* 1982;1:768.

133. Hung T, Choi Z, Zhao T, et al. Morphology and morphogenesis of viruses of hemorrhagic fever with renal syndrome (HFRS). I. Some peculiar aspects of the morphogenesis of various strains of HFRS virus. *Intervirology* 1985;23:97.

134. LeDuc JW. Epidemiology of Hantaan and related viruses. *Lab Anim Sci* 1987;37:413.

135. Duchin JS, Koster FT, Peters CJ, et al. Hantavirus pulmonary syndrome: a clinical description of 17 patients with a newly recognized disease. *N Engl J Med* 1994;330:949.

136. Nichol ST, Spiropoulou CF, Morzunov S, et al. Genetic identification of a hantavirus associated with an outbreak of acute respiratory illness. *Science* 1993;262:914.

137. Elliott LH, Ksiazek TG, Rollin PE, et al. Isolation of the causative agent of hantavirus pulmonary syndrome. *Am J Trop Med Hyg* 1994;51:102.

138. Ksiazek TG, Peters CJ, Rollin PE, et al. Identification of a new North American hantavirus that causes acute pulmonary insufficiency. *Am J Trop Med Hyg* 1995;52:117.

139. Xiao S-Y, LeDuc JW, Chu YK, et al. Phylogenetic analysis of virus isolates in the genus *Hantavirus*, family Bunyaviridae. *Virology* 1994;198:205.

140. Earle DP. Symposium on epidemic hemorrhagic fever. *Am J Med* 1954;16:617.

141. Gajdusek DC. *Acute infectious hemorrhagic fevers and mycotoxicoses in the Union of Soviet Socialist Republics.* Washington, DC: Army Medical Service Graduate School, Walter Reed Army Medical Center, 1953. Medical Science publication 2.

142. Lee HW, Lee PW. Korean hemorrhagic fever. I. Demonstration of causative antigen and antibodies. *Korean J Intern Med* 1976;19:371.

143. Lee HW, Lee PW, Johnson KM. Isolation of the etiologic agent of Korean hemorrhagic fever. *J Infect Dis* 1978;137:298.

144. Khan AS, Ksiazek TG, Peters CJ. Hantavirus pulmonary syndrome. *Lancet* 1996;347:739.
145. Yanagihara R. Hantavirus infection in the United States: epizootology and epidemiology. *Rev Infect Dis* 1990;12:449.
146. Lee HW, Lee PW, Baek LJ, et al. Geographical distribution of hemorrhagic fever with renal syndrome and hantaviruses. *Arch Virol* 1990; 115[Suppl 1]:5.
147. Settergren B. Nephropathia epidemica (hemorrhagic fever with renal syndrome) in Scandinavia. *Rev Infect Dis* 1991;13:736.
148. Avsic-Zupanc T, Likar M, Novakovic S, et al. Evidence of the presence of two hantaviruses in Slovenia. *Arch Virol* 1990;115[Suppl 1]:87.
149. Avsic-Zupanc T, Xiao S-Y, Stojanovic R, et al. Characterization of Dobrava virus: a hantavirus from Slovenia. *J Med Virol* 1992;38:132.
150. Gligic A, Dimkovic N, Xiao S-Y, et al. Belgrade virus: a new *Hantavirus* causing severe hemorrhagic fever with renal syndrome in Yugoslavia. *J Infect Dis* 1992;166:113.
151. Lee HW. Epidemiology. In: Lee HW, Dalrymple JM, eds. *Manual of hemorrhagic fever with renal syndrome.* Seoul: World Health Organization Collaborating Center for Virus Reference and Research Institute for Viral Diseases, Korea University, 1989:39–48.
152. Childs JE, Glass GE, Korch GW, et al. Evidence of human infection with a rat-associated *Hantavirus* in Baltimore, Maryland. *Am J Epidemiol* 1988;127:875.
153. Childs JE, Glass GE, Ksiazek TG, et al. Human-rodent contact and infection with lymphocytic choriomeningitis and Seoul viruses in an inner-city population. *Am J Trop Med Hyg* 1991;44:117.
154. Glass GE, Watson AJ, LeDuc JW, et al. Infection with a ratborne Hantavirus in US residents is consistently associated with hypertensive renal disease. *J Infect Dis* 1993;167:614.
155. Yanagihara R, Chin CT, Weiss MB, et al. Serological evidence of *Hantavirus* infection in the United States. *Am J Trop Med Hyg* 1985;34:396.
156. Yanagihara R, Gajdusek DC, Gibbs CJ Jr, et al. Prospect Hill virus: serological evidence for infection in mammologists. *N Engl J Med* 1984;310: 1325.
157. Stephen C, Johnson M, Bell A. First reported cases of hantavirus pulmonary syndrome in Canada. *Can Commun Dis Rep* 1994;20:121.
158. Padula PJ, Colavecchia SB, Martinez VP, et al. Genetic diversity, distribution, and serologic features of hantavirus infection in five countries in South America. *J Clin Microbiol* 2000;38:3029.
159. Chapman LE, Khabbaz RF. Epidemiology and etiology of the Four Corners *hantavirus* outbreak. *Infect Agents Dis* 1994;3:234.
160. Hjelle B, Glass GE. Outbreak of hantavirus infection in the Four Corners region of the United States in the wake of the 1997–1998 El Nino-southern oscillation. *J Infect Dis* 2000;181:1569.
161. Butler JC, Peters CJ. Hantaviruses and hantavirus pulmonary syndrome. *Clin Infect Dis* 1994;19:387.
162. Pini NC, Resa A, del Jesus Laime G, et al. Hantavirus infection in children in Argentina. *Emerg Infect Dis* 1998;4:85.
163. Ferrer JF, Jonsson CB, Esteban E, et al. High prevalence of hantavirus infection in Indian communities of the Paraguayan and Argentinean Gran Chaco. *Am J Trop Med Hyg* 1998;59:438.
164. Hjelle B, Spiropoulou CF, Torrez-Martinez N, et al. Detection of Muerto Canyon virus RNA in peripheral blood mononuclear cells from patients with hantavirus pulmonary syndrome. *J Infect Dis* 1994;170:1013.
165. Horling J, Lundkvist A, Persson K, et al. Detection and subsequent sequencing of Puumala virus from human specimens by PCR. *J Clin Microbiol* 1995;33: 277.
166. Hullinghorst RL, Steer A. Pathology of epidemic hemorrhagic fever. *Ann Intern Med* 1953;38:77.
167. Zaki SR, Greer PW, Coffield LM, et al. Hantavirus pulmonary syndrome: pathogenesis of an emerging infectious disease. *Am J Pathol* 1995;146:552.
168. Mackow ER, Gavrilovskaya IN. Cellular receptors and hantavirus pathogenesis. *Curr Top Microbiol Immunol* 2001;256:91.
169. Chun CH, Laehdevirta J, Lee HW. Clinical manifestations of HFRS. In: Lee HW, Dalrymple JM, eds. *Manual of hemorrhagic fever with renal syndrome.* Seoul: World Health Organization Collaborating Center for Virus Reference and Research Institute for Viral Diseases, Korea University, 1989: 19–38.
170. McKee KT Jr, MacDonald C, LeDuc JW, et al. Hemorrhagic fever with renal syndrome: a clinical perspective. *Milit Med* 1985;150:640.
171. Bruno P, Hassell LH, Brown J, et al. The protean manifestations of hemorrhagic fever with renal syndrome: a retrospective review of 26 cases from Korea. *Ann Intern Med* 1990;113:385.
172. Pilaski J, Feldmann H, Morzunov S, et al. Genetic identification of a new Puumala virus strain causing severe hemorrhagic fever with renal syndrome in Germany. *J Infect Dis* 1994;170:1456.
173. Passaro DJ, Shieh W-J, Hacker JK, et al. Predominant kidney involvement in a fatal case of hantavirus pulmonary syndrome caused by Sin Nombre virus. *Clin Infect Dis* 2001;33:263.
174. Centers for Disease Control. Hantavirus pulmonary syndrome—Vermont, 2000. *MMWR Morb Mortal Wkly Rep* 2001;50:603.
175. Goade DE, Koster FT, Mertz GJ, et al. *Preliminary evidence for pulmonary dysfunction in survivors of hantavirus pulmonary syndrome.* Presented at the Fourth International Conference on HFRS and Hantaviruses. March 5–7, Atlanta, Georgia.
176. Lee PW, Meegan JM, LeDuc JW, et al. Serologic techniques for detection of Hantaan virus infection, related antigens and antibodies. In: Lee HW, Dalrymple JM, eds. *Manual of hemorrhagic fever with renal syndrome.* Seoul: World Health Organization Collaborating Center for Virus Reference and Research Institute for Viral Diseases, Korea University, 1989:36–38.
177. Zoller L, Yang S, Gott P, et al. Use of recombinant nucleocapsid proteins of the Hantaan and nephropathia epidemica serotypes of hantaviruses as immunodiagnostic antigens. *J Med Virol* 1993;39:200.
178. Feldmann H, Sanchez A, Morzunov S, et al. Utilization of autopsy RNA for the synthesis of the nucleocapsid antigen of a newly recognized virus associated with hantavirus pulmonary syndrome. *Virus Res* 1993;30:351.
179. Jenison S, Yamada T, Morris C, et al. Characterization of human antibody responses to four corners hantavirus infections among patients with hantavirus pulmonary syndrome. *J Virol* 1994;68:3000.
180. Huggins JW, Hsiang CM, Cosgriff TM, et al. Prospective, double-blind, concurrent, placebo-controlled clinical trial of intravenous ribavirin therapy of hemorrhagic fever with renal syndrome. *J Infect Dis* 1991;164: 1119.
181. Chapman LE, Mertz GJ, Peters CJ, et al. Intravenous ribavirin for hantavirus pulmonary syndrome: safety and tolerance during 1 year of open-label experience. *Antiviral Ther* 1999;4:211.
182. Padula PJ, Edelstein A, Miguel SD, et al. Hantavirus pulmonary syndrome outbreak in Argentina: molecular evidence for person-to-person transmission of Andes virus. *Virology* 1998;241:323.
183. Toro J, Vega JD, Khan AS, et al. An outbreak of hantavirus pulmonary syndrome, Chile, 1997. *Emerg Infect Dis* 1998;4:687.
184. Hooper JW, Li D. Vaccines against hantaviruses. *Curr Top Microbiol Immunol* 2001;256:171.
185. Chumakov MP. A new virus disease: Crimean hemorrhagic fever [in Russian]. *Nov Med* 1947;4:9.
186. Casals J. Antigenic similarity between the virus causing Crimean hemorrhagic fever and Congo virus. *Proc Soc Exp Biol Med* 1969;131:233.
187. Hoogstral H. The epidemiology of tick-borne Crimean-Congo hemorrhagic fever in Asia, Europe, and Africa. *J Med Entomol* 1979;51:307.
188. Burney MI, Ghafoor A, Sateen M, et al. Nosocomial outbreak of viral hemorrhagic fever caused by Crimean hemorrhagic fever-Congo virus in Pakistan, January 1976. *Am J Trop Med Hyg* 1980;29:941.
189. Simpson DIH, Knight EM, Courtois GH, et al. Congo virus: a hitherto undescribed virus occurring in Africa. I. Human isolations: clinical notes. *East Afr Med J* 1967;44:86.
190. Watts DM, Ksiazek TG, Linthicum KJ, et al. Crimean-Congo hemorrhagic fever. In: Monath TP, ed. *The arboviruses: epidemiology and ecology,* Vol 2. Boca Raton, FL: CRC Press, 1989:177–222.
191. Altaf A, Luby S, Ahmed AJ, et al. Outbreak of Crimean-Congo haemorrhagic fever in Quetta, Pakistan: contact tracing and risk assessment. *Trop Med Int Health* 1998;3:878.
192. Williams RJ, Al-Busaidy S, Mehta FR, et al. Crimean-Congo haemorrhagic fever: a seroepidemiological and tick survey in the Sultanate of Oman. *Trop Med Int Health* 2000;5:99.
193. Peters CJ, LeDuc JW. Bunyaviridae: bunyaviruses, phleboviruses, and related viruses. In: Belshe RB, ed. *Textbook of human virology,* 2nd ed. St. Louis: Mosby-Year Book, 1991:571–614.
194. Swanepoel R, Shepherd At, Leman PA, et al. Epidemiologic and clinical features of Crimean-Congo hemorrhagic fever in Southern Africa. *Am J Trop Med Hyg* 1987;36:120.
195. Swanepoel R, Gill DE, Shepherd AJ, et al. The clinical pathology of Crimean-Congo hemorrhagic fever. *Rev Infect Dis* 1989;11[Suppl 4]:S794.
196. Shepherd AJ, Swanepoel R, Leman PA. Antibody response in Crimean-Congo hemorrhagic fever. *Rev Infect Dis* 1989;11[Suppl 4]:S801.
197. Burt FJ, Swanepoel R, Shieh WJ, et al. Immunohistochemical and in situ localization of Crimean-Congo hemorrhagic fever (CCHF) virus in human tissues and implications for CCHF pathogenesis. *Arch Pathol Lab Med* 1997;121: 839.
198. Burt FJ, Leman PA, Smith JF, et al. The use of a reverse transcription-polymerase chain reaction for the detection of viral nucleic acid in the diagnosis of Crimean-Congo haemorrhagic fever. *J Virol Methods* 1998;70:129–137.
199. Watts DM, Ussery MA, Nash D, et al. Inhibition of Crimean-Congo hemorrhagic fever viral infectivity in vitro by ribavirin. *Am J Trop Med Hyg* 1989;41:581.
200. Fisher-Hoch SP, Khan JA, Rehman S, et al. Crimean-Congo haemorrhagic fever treated with oral ribavirin. *Lancet* 1995;346:472.

CHAPTER 262
Rabies Virus

Charles E. Rupprecht, Lillian Orciari, and James E. Childs

Rabies is an acute, fatal encephalomyelitis. The disease is etiologically attributable to rabies virus and its neurotropic *Lyssavirus* species relatives and occurs on all inhabited continents. Warm-blooded vertebrates are susceptible to experimental infection, but in greatly varying degrees. In nature, mammals form the principal hosts, with distinct reservoirs among the Carnivora and Chiroptera. Owing to its insidious nature and reemergence, the basic ultrastructural, biochemical, molecular, pathobiologic, and immunologic attributes of *Lyssavirus* are receiving increasing attention, despite being one of the oldest recognized maladies (1–5).

CLASSIFICATION

Rabies and rabies-related viruses occur within the family Rhabdoviridae. Together with the Filoviridae, Paramyxoviridae, and Bornaviridae, these families form the order Mononegavirales. The Rhabdoviridae family (associated with vertebrates) consists of the genus *Vesiculovirus* [type species: vesicular stomatitis virus (VSV)], the genus *Ephemerovirus* (type species: bovine ephemeral fever virus), the genus *Novirhabdovirus* (type species: infectious hematopoietic necrosis virus), and the genus *Lyssavirus* (type species: rabies virus). Other members include viruses isolated from a variety of plants and animals, primarily assigned on the basis of their distinctive rod- or bullet-shaped morphology (6). The genus *Lyssavirus* includes rabies virus and a group of antigenically and genetically related Old World lyssaviruses (7). Rabies and the rabies-related viruses had been defined on the basis of morphology, serology, and the ability to cause encephalitis in laboratory animals (8,9). Two rhabdovirus species isolated from insects in Africa, Obodhiang and kotonkan, were seemingly aligned with this group on the basis of serology, but await further characterization. Tentatively, at least six other distinct lyssaviruses are related to rabies virus (9–14) (Fig. 262.1 and Table 262.1). These viruses are easily distinguished by their characteristic antigenic and genetic properties: (a) Lagos bat virus, isolated from straw-colored fruit bats, *Eidolon helvum*, on Lagos Island, Nigeria, in 1956; (b) Mokola virus, isolated from *Crocidura* species shrews in Ibadan, Nigeria, during 1968; (c) Duvenhage virus, isolated from a man bitten on the lip by a bat during 1970, in Warmbaths, South Africa; (d) two different European bat viruses, type 1 and type 2, originally isolated from insectivorous bats throughout Europe during the 1950 to 1970s; (e) and Australia bat virus, recently isolated from flying foxes and insectivorous bats throughout the continent, from 1995 to date.

Originally, the nonrabies lyssaviruses were thought to be little more than biologic curiosities, restricted in their geographic distribution to wildlife in regions of sub-Saharan Africa (8). Although experimental vaccination of laboratory animals with traditional rabies virus vaccine did not provide good cross-reactive immunity to the nonrabies lyssaviruses, such as Mokola or Lagos bat virus, little concern was engendered initially because these viral species appeared limited in host range. Several observations have increased the level of concern of public health workers over the potential significance of the nonrabies lyssaviruses. Mokola and Lagos bat viruses have been isolated from vacci-

nated domestic animals, raising the possibility of more frequent bite transmission to humans in Africa (11,15–17). Moreover, the finding of European bat viruses during the 1970s to 1980s from bats in western Germany, and later from *Eptesicus serotinus* and *Myotis* species bats throughout western Europe, demonstrated that the distribution and incidence of infection were greater than previously believed (18). In 1985, a Finnish bat biologist died with type 2 European bat virus infection, presumably resulting from bat bite, although a definitive source of exposure was not identified. That same year, a child also died of a rabies-like illness in Russia, and the causative agent was later demonstrated to be type 1 European bat virus. Important questions remain to be answered about these rabies-related lyssaviruses: How widely distributed are these nonrabies lyssaviruses? What are their native reservoirs? How are these viruses transmitted among their reservoirs, and how are they transmitted to humans and domestic animals? What is the role of nonbite transmission, if any, in the natural cycles of the African lyssaviruses, such as Mokola? Will it become necessary to develop new vaccines against these rabies-related viruses? What is the likelihood of translocation of lyssaviruses between the Old and New Worlds?

Besides their differentiation from the other lyssaviruses, isolates of rabies virus may be informally categorized as either fixed laboratory or vaccine strains, adapted by passage in animals or cell culture, or street (wild-type) viruses. The use of monoclonal antibodies (MABs) and genetic sequencing to differentiate lyssaviruses has been useful in identifying virus variants originating in major host reservoirs throughout the world (16–34). Such techniques are useful in implicating the likely sources of human exposure when a definitive history of animal bite is unavailable. Great progress has been made since the late 1980s in understanding *Lyssavirus* epidemiology and phylogeny through the application of molecular techniques, particularly rabies virus nucleic acid detection by amplification of complementary DNA by the reverse transcription polymerase chain reaction (RT-PCR), with subsequent generation of viral nucleotide sequences (35). For example, such analyses have provided historical insights into the global dissemination of rabies virus variants by human colonization (27). Moreover, molecular analysis has demonstrated the significance of wildlife translocation in current disease distribution patterns (36,37). However, the extreme sensitivity of the RT-PCR technique also greatly increases the probability of a false-positive diagnosis resulting from laboratory contamination (38). Because of *Lyssavirus* heterogeneity, false-negative results can occur if primer selection is inadequate to compensate for sequence disparity. Universal primers for all known global *Lyssavirus* variants, and samples collected under a variety of circumstances, have not been clearly identified or adequately standardized. In view of these factors, the related costs, and the considerable expertise required for proper analysis and interpretation, such molecular techniques are not recommended for routine rabies diagnosis at present (39).

CHARACTERISTICS OF THE PATHOGEN

Lyssaviruses are single-stranded, negative-sense, unsegmented RNA viruses, with a molecular mass of about 4.6×10^6 daltons (2). Mature virions measure about 75 to 80 nm by 180 to 200 nm, although defective interfering particles may be smaller. The virion is composed of a helically wound internal ribonucleoprotein (RNP) core or nucleocapsid, containing the nucleic acid. An outer envelope contains a lipid bilayer membrane covered with spikes of protein trimers, some projecting 6 to 10 nm in length (40) (Fig. 262.2).

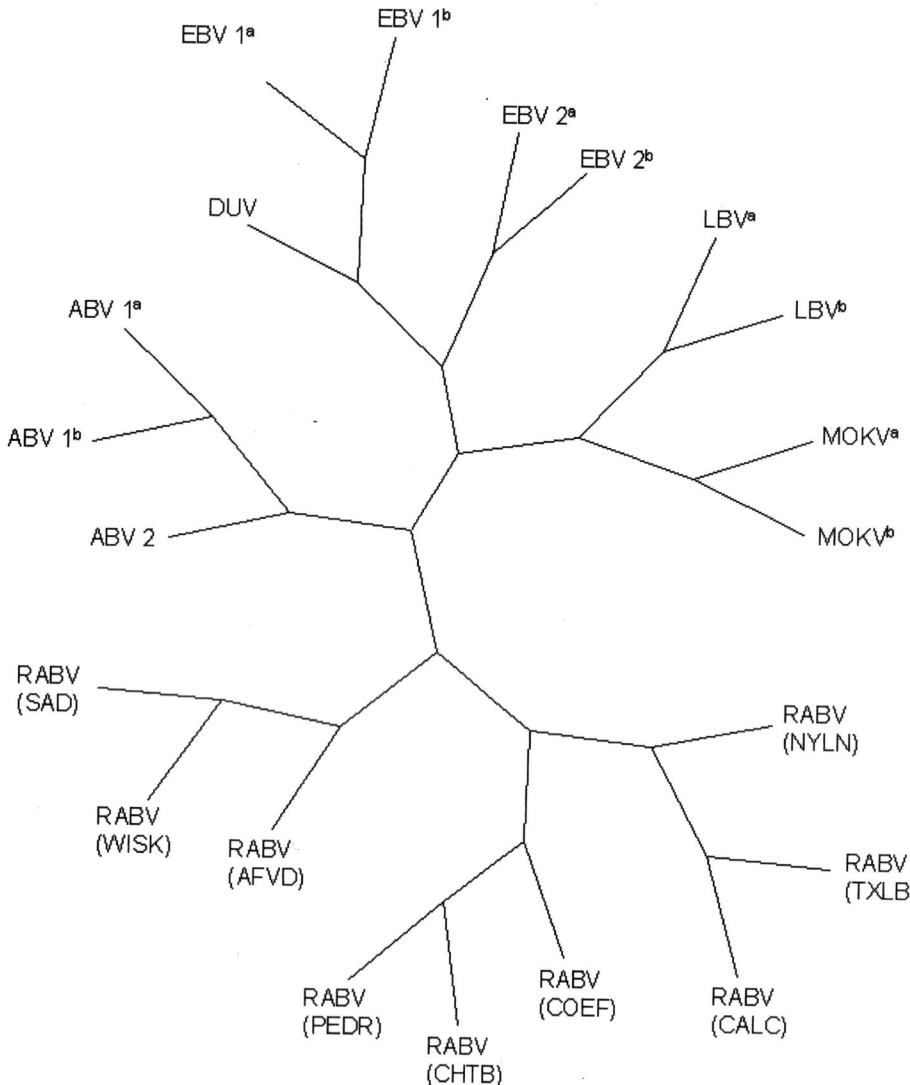

Figure 262.1. Classification and analysis of extant lyssavirus genera. Members of the genus *Lyssavirus* (RABV, rabies virus; ABV 1, Australian bat virus type 1; ABV 2, Australian bat virus type 2; DUV, Duvenhage virus; EBV 1, European bat virus type 1; EBV 2, European bat virus type 2; LBV, Lagos bat virus; MOKV, Mokola virus) are separated by distinct antigenic and genetic properties. The phylogenetic relationships of these viruses are demonstrated by the consensus radial tree generated from the nucleotide sequence analysis (1,350 bp) of the N gene amino acid coding region using maximum parsimony and neighbor joining in Phylip 96. Among these viruses, the Australian bat viruses are most closely related to the rabies viruses; the Mokola viruses and Lagos bat viruses are most distantly related to the rabies viruses. Distances are based percentages of homologies between the lyssaviruses given in Table 262.1.

Isolates included in alignments are: ABV 1[a] (Genbank Af081020), ABV 1[b] (Genbank NC003243), ABV 2 (Genbank Af006497), EBV 1[a] (Genbank U22845), EBV 1[b] (Genbank U22845), EBV 2[a] (Genbank U22846), EBV 2[b] (Genbank U22847), DUV (Genbank U22848), LBV[a] (ref. 16), LBV[b] (Genbank U22842), MOKV[a] (Genbank S59448), MOKV[b] (ref. 16), RAB (SAD) (Genbank M31046), RAB (WISK) (Genbank Af461045), RAB (AFVD) (Genbank Af467949), RAB (PEDR) (Genbank Af070449), RAB (CHTB) (Genbank Af070450), RAB (COEF) (Genbank Af394888), RAB (NYLN) (Genbank Af394880), RAB (TXLB) (Genbank Af394886) RAB (CALC) (Genbank Af394883).

Several nontranslated, intergenic regions divide the 11.9-kb rabies virus genome (Fig. 262.3), which encodes five polypeptides. One region of the genome located between the end of the G (glycoprotein) protein coding sequence and the beginning of the L (large) protein coding sequence was previously suggested as representative of a remnant sixth *Lyssavirus* gene (41). Other data, however, indicate that this region of the genome encodes a G messenger RNA with a long 3'-noncoding region and does not possess evidence of a pseudogene (42). The five expressed virus proteins are associated with either the symmetrically helical nucleocapsid complex or the viral envelope. The L (originally large polymerase protein), the N (nucleoprotein), and the P (nominal phosphoprotein, originally nonstructural transcriptase-associated or M1) proteins constitute, together with the linear viral RNA, the RNP complex. The M (matrix protein, or M2) and G proteins are associated with the envelope of neutral lipids, glycolipids, and phospholipids.

An understanding of the functions of the five *Lyssavirus* proteins continues to evolve (43). The relatively high-molecular-mass (but small-copy-number) L protein (about 185 to 244 kd, about 2,142 amino acids) functions during transcription and replication, with associated RNA-dependent RNA polymerase, methylation, messenger RNA 5'-capping, 3'-poly(A), and protein kinase activities. The G protein (about 58 to 80 kd, about 505 amino acids) forms protrusions that cover the outer surface of the virion envelope and may be *N*-glycosylated at several sites, as a prerequisite for efficient cell surface expression. The G protein is associated with reception at the host cell membrane, induction of pH-mediated endocytosis, and serotype definition within the *Lyssavirus* genus (44). The G protein has received an enhanced degree of biomedical focus because it is the only rabies protein known to induce virus-neutralizing antibody (VNA), in addition to its elicitation of cell-mediated immunity. As supposed "quasi-species," selection of rabies virus G protein point mutants has allowed definition of specific sites in the genome that may serve as prerequisites for virulence (45–47). In contrast to the external G protein, the N protein (about 51 to 62 kd, about 450 amino acids) is the major component of the nucleocapsid and determines the group specificity among lyssaviruses, owing to its considerable antigenic cross-reactivity (48). It is associated with full-length negative- and positive-sense RNA. Although the precise role of the N protein is unclear, it is tightly bound to the viral RNA and may protect against cellular ribonucleases (49). In addition, the N protein can modulate transcription and appears to promote replication. Phosphorylation of the N protein may involve a host cell protein kinase. The P protein (about 33 to 40 kd, about 297 amino acids) is necessary for transcription and may prevent protein aggregation while assisting in the deposition of

TABLE 262.1. Divergence of Lyssaviruses Species

	MOKV[a]	MOKV[b]	LBV[a]	LBV[b]	RABV CALC	RABV TXLB	RABV NYLN	RABV COEF	RABV CHTB	RABV PEDR	RABV SAD	RABV WISK	RABV AFVD	ABV1[a]	ABV1[b]	ABLV2	EBV1[a]	EBV1[b]	EBV2[a]	EBV2[b]	DUV
MOKV[a]	0.00																				
MOKV[b]	12.30	0.00																			
LBV[a]	23.04	22.22	0.00																		
LBV[b]	23.56	23.85	17.11	0.00																	
RABV CALC	27.41	28.00	27.78	26.59	0.00																
RABV TXLB	27.56	28.67	27.19	26.15	2.37	0.00															
RABV NYLN	28.15	28.74	27.41	26.44	5.19	5.48	0.00														
RABV COEF	27.56	28.59	26.67	26.52	9.93	10.07	8.59	0.00													
RABV CHTB	28.52	28.89	26.59	26.59	11.33	12.07	9.56	7.04	0.00												
RABV PEDR	27.93	28.74	26.37	26.15	12.44	12.52	11.19	8.59	7.63	0.00											
RABV SAD	26.74	27.85	26.74	26.81	15.11	14.81	15.56	13.78	14.89	14.96	0.00										
RABV WISK	26.96	28.67	26.37	25.85	15.93	15.33	15.63	13.70	14.81	14.74	5.63	0.00									
RABV AFVD	26.15	28.22	27.11	26.67	17.19	17.04	17.04	15.85	16.67	16.30	11.78	11.48	0.00								
ABV1[a]	27.93	29.11	26.74	27.04	22.89	22.89	23.33	23.63	23.41	22.74	22.89	23.11	24.22	0.00							
ABV1[b]	27.93	29.11	26.74	27.04	22.89	22.89	23.33	23.63	23.41	22.74	22.89	23.11	24.22	0.00	0.00						
ABLV2	27.56	27.63	24.89	27.41	22.37	22.59	22.74	22.81	22.81	22.44	21.63	21.93	22.15	16.07	16.07	0.00					
EBV1[a]	27.93	29.78	27.48	27.48	25.78	26.00	25.33	25.85	25.26	25.85	25.33	24.37	25.26	24.52	24.52	22.81	0.00				
EBV1[b]	27.70	30.00	28.07	26.44	24.81	25.19	24.52	25.48	24.67	25.11	24.96	24.22	24.44	25.04	25.04	23.70	4.00	0.00			
EBV2[a]	26.96	28.52	25.48	25.41	24.44	24.30	24.59	25.33	25.26	24.59	24.15	23.70	24.81	22.81	22.81	22.52	22.89	24.00	0.00		
EBV2[b]	26.96	28.89	26.00	25.56	24.44	24.37	24.44	25.19	25.04	24.22	24.00	24.74	23.26	23.26	23.11	22.00	23.11	23.11	4.30	0.00	
DUV	27.93	27.19	24.74	26.59	25.33	25.19	25.70	25.78	25.63	25.63	25.26	24.44	26.00	23.70	23.70	22.96	24.07	24.22	20.74	20.22	0.00

Differences in nucleotide sequences are described for all the lyssaviruses in Fig. 262.1 after analysis of 1,350 bp.

The numeric values are equal to changes per 100 nucleotides.

The distances demonstrated are unweighed; however, calculation of distances of the data for phylogenetic analysis (Fig. 262.1) was performed using the Kimura two-parameter aligorithim.

Information was highlighted by species for comparision purposes. Mokola viruses in this set differ from the rabies virus isolates by about 26%–29% and from all nonrabies lyssaviruses by 23%–30%.

Divergence within the rabies viruses ranged from 2% to 17%.

Australian bat viruses differ from the rabies viruses by about 14%–29%.

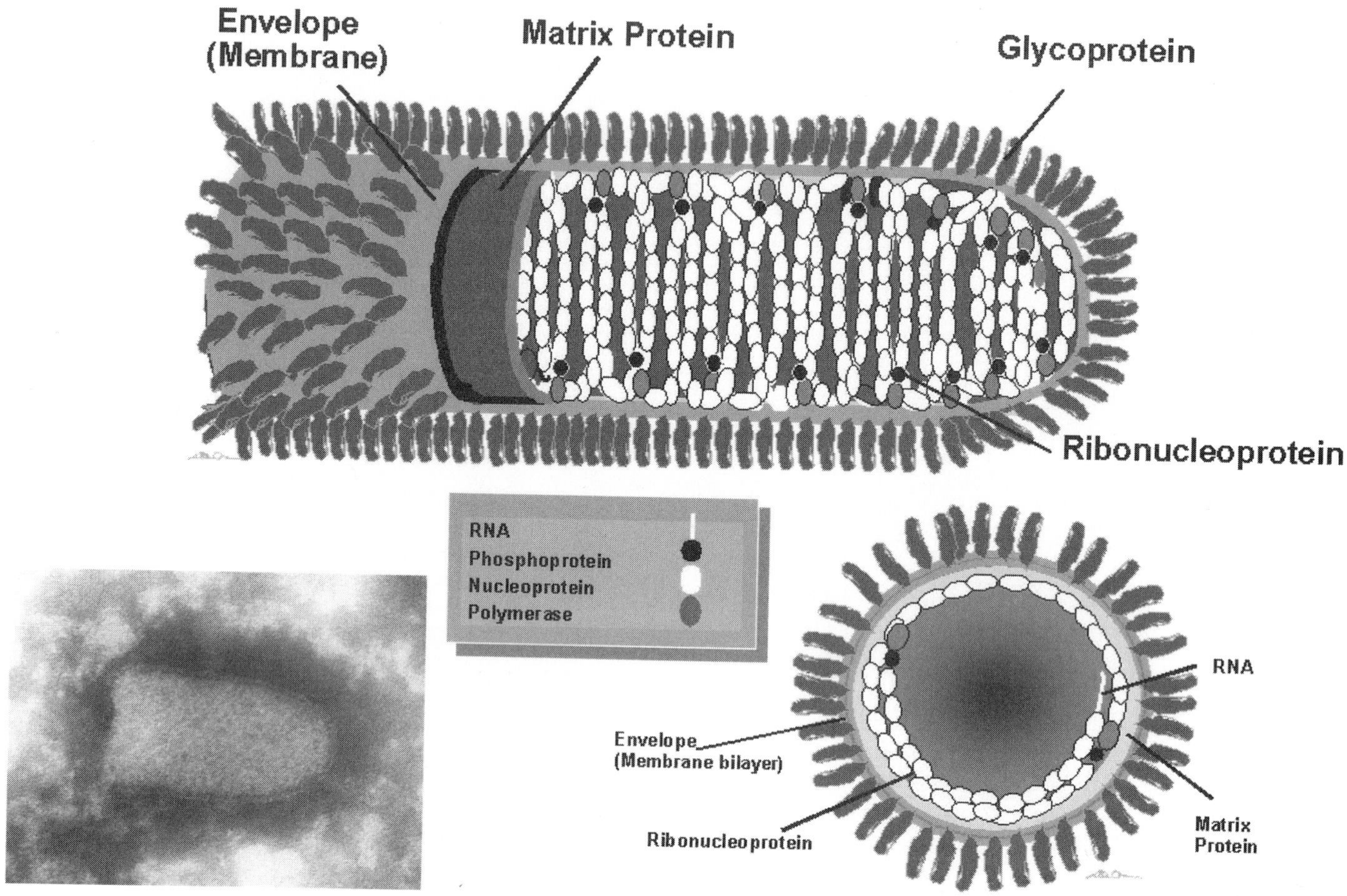

Envelope (Membrane)   **Matrix Protein**   **Glycoprotein**

Ribonucleoprotein

RNA
Phosphoprotein
Nucleoprotein
Polymerase

RNA

Envelope
(Membrane bilayer)

Ribonucleoprotein

Matrix
Protein

Figure 262.2. Lyssavirus morphology. Rabies virions are bullet shaped and measure about 180 nm in length and 75 nm in diameter. The outer surface is covered by 10-nm spike-shaped glycoprotein peplomers inserted into the host cell membrane. The genome RNA encodes for five structural proteins: glycoprotein (G), nucleoprotein (N), phosphoprotein (P), large polymerase (L), and matrix (M) proteins. The N, NS, and L proteins and the genomic RNA form the ribonucleoprotein (RNP) core.

N protein onto RNA (50,51). Its phosphorylation probably involves the L viral protein kinase. The M protein (about 21 to 26 kd, about 202 amino acids) is an integral structural component that appears to bind to the nucleocapsid and the cytoplasmic domain of the G protein. The M protein, positioned beneath the lipid membrane bilayer, probably facilitates the viral assembly and budding process and may also assist in the regulation of RNA genome transcription (52).

Lyssaviruses do not persist in the environment. Susceptibility to chemical and physical agents partly depends on the source and nature of the infectious material, such as brain tissue, a film of saliva, or purified virus. As an enveloped agent, the virus is sensitive to many lipid solvents (53). It is rapidly destroyed by exposure to formalin, strong acids and bases, most detergents,

and ultraviolet irradiation, including sunlight. Repeated freezing and thawing may lead to a loss of infectivity. Viability may last only for minutes at 56°C, hours to days at 4°C, weeks to months at −20°C, and years in the proper diluent and sterile conditions at −70°C or colder.

Laboratory isolation of *Lyssavirus* can readily occur by either animal inoculation or cell culture (54). Newborn, weanling, or young adult rodents (usually mice), are the typical hosts of choice for primary virus isolation. Animals are inoculated intracranially with brain, saliva, or other material. Animals are usually observed for a minimum of 4 weeks, although they may show clinical illness as early as 5 to 7 days after inoculation. A number of susceptible host cells, notably continuous lines of BHK-21 or murine neuroblastoma cells,

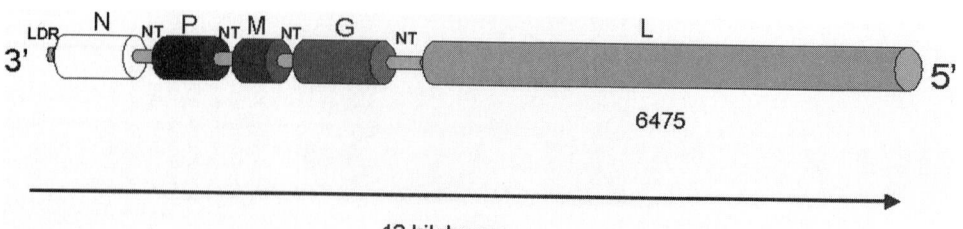

Figure 262.3. A stylized lyssavirus genome. The RNA is single stranded, antisense, and nonsegmented, of about 12 kb. There is a leader of 50 nucleotides followed by N, P, M, G, and L genes, which code for the five structural proteins. The intergenic noncoding regions are considered the most variable, especially the M-G and G-L genes.

have gradually replaced routine animal inoculation for virus isolation.

VIRUS REPRODUCTION

In general, *Lyssavirus* replication (Fig. 262.4) is believed to be similar to that of other negative-stranded RNA viruses that have been studied more intensively, such as VSV. The precise mechanism of viral entry into the neuron is not clear. Some evidence supports the belief that rabies virus binds selectively at or near nicotinic acetylcholine receptors through neuromuscular junctions (55–64). Such sites are close to unsheathed nerves at synaptic clefts, where virus can gain ready access to the axoplasm. This hypothesis does not preclude alternative mechanisms or routes supportive of viral neurotropism because other protein-based

receptors can also bind rabies virus, and acetylcholine receptors are not exclusively found in some sites permissively supportive of rabies virus infection (65–69).

After viral invasion at a host portal of entry (usually a bite wound), viral attachment to host cell membranes may occur through a conformational alteration in the G protein during receptor-mediated endocytosis or by planar fusion. After adsorption, virus particles may penetrate the cell cytoplasm within an endosome. Coated vesicles may fuse with lysosomes and are uncoated to RNP in a low-pH microenvironment, perhaps mediated by a putative fusion domain of the G protein (70,71). In cellular locales rich in ribosomes, such as in the perikaryon or proximal dendrite, the RNP core initiates primary transcription of the five complementary monocistronic messenger RNAs by using the virion-associated RNA-dependent RNA polymerase. Each RNA is translated into an individual viral protein. After

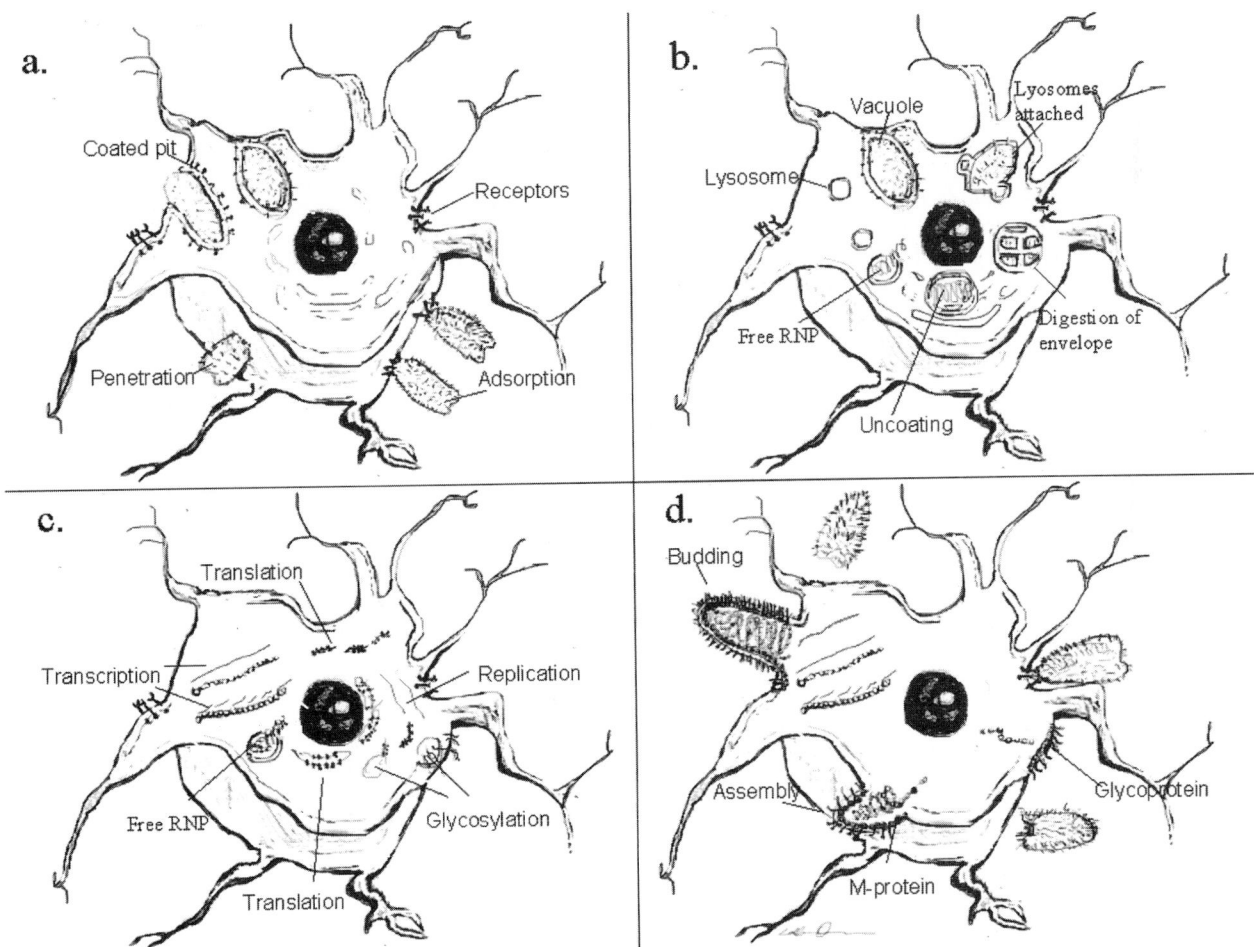

Figure 262.4. Generalized lyssavirus cycle of infection and replication. Typically, it involves adsorption (virus peplomers–host cell receptor interaction); penetration (endocytosis or pinocytosis of the virus through clathrin-coated pits); uncoating [release of the ribonucleoprotein (RNP) into the host cell cytoplasm]; transcription [L + P polymerase transcribe negative-sense RNA to form five capped, methylated, polyadenylated messenger RNAs (mRNAs) and 50-nt leader]; translation (synthesis of N, P, and M proteins on polyribosomes in the rough endoplasmic reticulum); processing (stepwise glycoprotein glycosylation, migration, and insertion into the cytoplasmic membrane); replication (production of positive-strand genome template and complementary negative strand); assembly (binding of the N, P, and L proteins and RNA to form RNP, the formation of M-RNP complex, which binds to the cytoplasmic membrane containing glycoprotein inserts to form complete virus); and budding (release of completed virions). (These figures were designed to depict the stages of the infections cycle components and were not drawn to scale for visualization purposes. The panels were modified from Wagner RR, Thomas JR, McGowan JJ. Rhabdovirus cytopathology: effects on cellular macromolecular synthesis. In: Fraenkel-Courat H, Wagner RR, eds. *Comprehensive virology*, Vol 19. New York: Plenum Publishing, 1984:223–295; and Dubois-Dalco M, Holmes KV, Rentier B. *Assembly of enveloped RNA viruses*. New York: Springer-Verlag, 1984, with permission.)

viral protein synthesis, replication of the genomic RNA continues with full-length, positive-stranded RNA, which acts as a template for the production of progeny negative-stranded RNA. Within the central nervous system (CNS), *Lyssavirus* replication has been associated almost exclusively with neurons. Scant evidence suggests replication in astrocytes, glial cells, oligodendrocytes, or Schwann's cells (1).

Whereas nucleocapsid production commences in the cytosol, the viral G protein appears to be synthesized and glycosylated on the rough endoplasmic reticulum as a 524–amino acid precursor, in which the N-terminal 19–amino acid leader or signal is cleaved, leaving a portion of about 505 amino acids (2). Primary structure of the G protein consists of a C-terminal cytoplasmic endodomain anchor, a transmembrane portion, and an antigenic ectodomain of about 439 amino acids. Removal of the about 44 amino acids of the endodomain and a portion of the transmembrane portion results in a truncated soluble form of the G protein, which is ordinarily unable to induce effective immunity without alteration (72,73). Further G-protein processing may occur by transport through the Golgi apparatus. A specific chemical configuration appears to act in avoidance of nonspecific membrane fusion, until acquisition of a native state at the cell surface (74). Viral assembly of nucleocapsid with membrane components and budding of the virion from the infected cell may occur by the inverse process of initial viral attachment and adsorption. In contrast, the process of envelope formation on cytoplasmic membranes is quite variable and may be exceedingly complex in regard to three-dimensional array (1). A high proportion of amino acid substitutions in the G protein may be tolerated while retaining molecular functions (provided that comparative charge and hydrophobicity or hydrophilicity are conserved). However, even a single amino acid alteration at certain locations may be critical in the determination of relative virulence, in part because of influences on secondary structure, recognition at neural termini, restrictions in conformational epitopes, and subsequent viral clearance (75–78). The generation of viral escape mutants under neutralizing antibody pressure *in vitro* has proved useful in the delineation of operational antigenic sites as well as in the development of attenuated rabies virus vaccines (79). A variety of other viral hydrophobic membrane proteins have been crystallized, and future definition of the three-dimensional structure of the rabies G protein by x-ray crystallography may enable a better topographic localization of operationally defined epitopes. Mapping of the amino acid substitutions of escape virus variants belonging to particular antigenic groups could augment the design novel antiviral agents.

PATHOGENESIS, PATHOPHYSIOLOGY, PATHOLOGY, AND CLINICAL FEATURES

For more than a century, investigators appreciated that rabies was primarily caused by entry of an infectious agent into a wound, usually inflicted by a bite (80). In 1804, the rudimentary pathogenesis of rabies was described by Zinke, who experimentally transmitted infection by swabbing the saliva of rabid dogs onto fresh wounds of rabbits and dogs and showed that saliva contained the agent. He also indirectly confirmed the observations of Morgagni, who in 1769 described the "paresthesia" of early sensory and motor symptoms at the site of bite exposure, as supportive evidence that the agent traveled through the nervous system.

Centripetal spread of virus from the site of entry to the CNS occurs within motor and sensory axons of peripheral nerves. Sectioning of the sciatic nerve after ipsilateral footpad inoculation can prevent the development of rabies, suggesting that

rabies virus spreads to the spinal cord through primary innervation pathways (81). Local application of microtubule-disrupting agents (active on tubulin-containing cytoskeletal structures) to the ischiatic nerve, thereby inhibiting axonal transport, can alter virus propagation, providing additional evidence for axonal transport of rabies virus (82). The neurotropic property of rabies virus provides utility as a microanatomic tracer of neuronal networks *in vivo* (83,84). After primary infection of hypoglossal motor neurons, retrograde transneuronal viral transfer can occur within 2 days after inoculation (unaccompanied by neuronal degeneration), with sequential involvement of second-order neurons and spread to higher-order cortical and subcortical cell groups, but not to adjoining glial cells or uninfected fibers of passage.

The incubation period of rabies in humans and animals may vary from days to years (26,85,86). An unusually slow course of productive infection in the proximate host may ensure rabies virus survival until new susceptible reservoirs achieve a population density necessary for optimal virus transmission (87). Long incubation periods may assist in the selection of a virus population that can reach and multiply in the salivary glands and be excreted in the saliva of an infected individual. A primary difference in rabies infection between reservoir hosts (i.e., species involved in virus transmission and perpetuation in nature, such as mammalian carnivores and bats) and a "dead end" or victim species (i.e., livestock and humans) may have more to do with differential biting behavior of the species in question when rabid, rather than with the nature of the infection itself in any individual animal.

By extension from experimental animal models, rabies virus may replicate in muscle cells during early stages of infection, before entry into nerve endings, and virus may remain at the site of entry for a prolonged time (4,88). Other experiments, however, demonstrate that virus replication in muscle cells before entry of the nerve endings is not necessarily a requirement for the development of CNS infection (89). Obviously, somewhat conflicting observations do not adequately explain the precise location, the form of residual virus, or the mechanism by which virus can exist during this eclipse phase. A number of factors, alone or in combination, may be operative as potential explanations. Virus may be sequestered at the original site of entry, undergoing no, or minimal, replication in muscle or associated tissue, until a future event stimulates a cascade within a distal nerve ending. In contrast, sequestration may not necessarily be nonneural in origin but may be at the level of the dorsal root ganglia and involve RNP with minimal replication owing to some defect in the available biochemical milieu (90). If frank disease has an immunologic basis, incubation periods may equate with a dynamic stasis, perhaps related to delayed immunologic surveillance by antigen-presenting cells (91). In theory, inocula may also contain defective interfering particles that limit neuronal access until after a variable delay. Regardless, unusually long incubation periods, exceeding 6 months, tend to be the exception rather than the rule.

During the centripetal transport of rabies virus locally to the brain, insufficient viral antigen may be detected by the immune system to induce an immune response (5). No reliable diagnostic method is currently available to determine qualitatively a case of rabies in humans or animals during the incubation period, before the prodromal stage. Once CNS neurons are infected, rapid dissemination of the virus occurs along neuronal pathways. Infection spreads to the brainstem and deep cerebellar nuclei, cerebellar Purkinje's cells, and neurons in the cerebral cortex.

Rabies virus spreads to the hippocampus relatively late, mainly infecting the pyramidal neurons with little or no involvement of the dentate gyrus (92). Centrifugal spread of virus from the CNS to peripheral organs is also along neuronal routes. Salivary gland infection is the main source for transmission of rabies virus by the oral fluids of the biting rabid animal.

Late in infection, rabies virus may occasionally be found in tissues other than the CNS and salivary glands, such as the adrenal medulla, tonsils, and nasal glands (4,93). Corneal epithelial cells and cutaneous neuronal elements are also common sites of extra-CNS infection. Detection of rabies virus in the saliva or of viral antigen in corneal epithelial cells and in nuchal skin biopsy specimens is commonly used for the antemortem diagnosis of rabies in humans (94).

Early clinical signs and symptoms of rabies are nonspecific and may begin with fever, malaise, and headache (95). Irritation or pain may be experienced at the wound site, but girdle pain may also be present. One of the most striking symptoms of rabies as it progresses to an acute neurologic phase in humans is hydrophobia, a contraction of the throat muscles after attempts to swallow water. True hydrophobia is rare in viral encephalitis, except rabies. Paresis beginning in the bitten limb may often be accompanied by fibrillary contractions that rapidly increase to complete flaccid paralysis, spreading to other limbs, the trunk, the rectum, and the bladder. Sensory loss, if noted at all, and involvement of the respiratory system occur rather late in the course of the illness. Death usually results from cardiac or respiratory failure. In rabies enzootic areas, any patient who develops an acute neurologic disease of viral cause should be suspected of having rabies. Definitive rabies diagnosis requires a careful evaluation of the epidemiology of animal rabies in the area where the patient may have been exposed, in addition to the clinical examination of the patient.

Rabies is usually considered to be invariably fatal. However, recovery from rabies, usually with severe neurologic sequelae, has been documented in a few naturally infected humans (96,97). Similar observations have also been made in experimentally infected animals (98–103).

Despite its acute onset, striking clinical manifestations, and overt lethality, along with the extensive neuronal involvement of the CNS, the pathologic findings associated with rabies are relatively mild, with little to no cell destruction or cytopathic changes. Typically, no gross pathologic changes are visible other than a variable degree of cerebral edema and meningeal congestion. Nonspecific inflammation of variable severity can be observed in the brain, spinal cord, and ganglia. Inflammatory infiltration, consisting primarily of mononuclear cells, may be detected in the leptomeninges. The severity of infection and to some extent the location of pathologic changes may be directly proportional to the duration of the morbidity period. Long morbidity periods can result in greater pathologic changes and a wider distribution of virus in the CNS and peripheral organs (104). Apoptosis, or programmed cell death in response to viral infection, has an uncertain role in rabies pathogenesis (105,106). Microscopic changes, including perivascular cuffing, neuronophagia, and modest neuronal necrosis, tend to be sparse in relation to the overall extent of viral antigen detection by immunofluorescence tests (107–109).

Light microscopic histopathologic study, focused on identification of the eosinophilic intracytoplasmic pathognomic inclusion body (Negri body) of rabies virus in infected neurons, can underestimate the wider distribution of viral antigen in the brain. Negri bodies are haloed, ovoid cytoplasmic bodies, and their development is usually related to the morbidity period (110,111). Such inclusions are typically detected by light microscopy in only 50% to 75% of specimens otherwise found positive by virus isolation, immunofluorescence, or ultrastructural microscopy (109). Negri bodies are seen most frequently in Purkinje's cells in the cerebellum and pyramidal cells in the hippocampus, and less of-

ten in the medulla spinal cord, cerebral cortex, basal ganglia, and peripheral ganglia. Negri bodies consist of viral nucleocapsid protein, akin to the mass of matrices seen by electron microscopy (112). Matrices correspond to the site of virus replication. Neurons containing viral matrices, accompanied by prolific numbers of viral particles budding from membranes of the rough endoplasmic reticulum and the plasma membrane, are usually seen by ultrastructural microscopy (1). Less commonly appreciated as a pathologic manifestation of rabies, induced spongiform change of the gray matter, affecting the neuropil and neuronal cell bodies of the thalamus and cerebral cortex, has been documented in experimental and naturally occurring cases (113,114).

Rather than physical destruction of microscopic elements, select organic dysfunction, due to pathophysiologic disruption in critical neuronal activities and neurotransmitter imbalance, may ultimately explain the underlying mechanisms of apparent viral virulence (115). Recognition of the functional interaction that exists between the immune system and the CNS during health and disease is also clearly indicated. For example, during rabies virus encephalitis, brain receptors for interleukin-1 may decrease while local interleukin-1 concentrations are increasing (116,117). Moreover, copious amounts of nitric oxide may be produced locally in the brain in response to rabies infection (118,119). A combined, targeted immunopharmacologic rationale, following rapid, accurate diagnosis, may hold the future approach toward any resolution of an otherwise lethal viral encephalomyelitis (120).

HOST IMMUNE MECHANISMS

Immunity to rabies potentially involves the induction of both nonspecific and specific immune responses in the host. Exposure to virus may or may not lead to productive infection, and either outcome may or may not result in detectable immune responses, depending on an interplay of viral and host factors (5,121,122). In the nontreated patient, rabies-specific VNA may be only rarely detected in serum at the onset of illness and usually does not occur, if at all, until later stages of disease. Antibody in high titer in the cerebrospinal fluid of infected individuals, in contrast to the vaccinee, is considered a reliable indication of CNS infection. The immune reaction may be appropriate and protective or may in some instances be detrimental and actually contribute to the pathogenesis of clinical disease (123–125). Administration of humoral antibody alone immediately after exposure may actually prolong the incubation period of rabies infection, as demonstrated by passive immunization in experimental animals. Immunosuppression, either induced or genetic, may also prolong the incubation period. Conversely, administration of rabies VNA may induce what has been termed the *early death phenomenon*, associated with inflammatory neuronal lesions. Primates inoculated with low-potency vaccines after rabies virus exposure died earlier than did nonimmunized rabies-infected control animals, suggesting that clinical rabies may involve immunopathologic mechanisms.

Cytokines such as interferon can also be involved in the immunity or pathogenesis of rabies (126–129). Although rabid patients have relatively low levels of endogenous interferon in the terminal CNS, virus replication can be inhibited by interferon administration early after infection. Nevertheless, experimental administration of interferon was not therapeutic when administered either peripherally or intrathecally 1 to 2 weeks after the onset of disease.

Although rabies virus particles represent complex antigens consisting of five different structural proteins, the induction of protective antiviral immunity has focused primarily on the response to the surface G protein. Historically, rabies VNAs were believed to play the major role in immune protection against rabies (124,125). However, comparison of VNA titers and mortality in laboratory animals immunized with whole-virus vaccine or viral G protein does not always delineate a clear relationship between absolute titer level of VNA and vaccine-induced resistance to rabies (130,131). Rather, some immunization experiments indicate that protective activity may correlate more with a vaccine's ability to induce immunologic memory. This lack of a firm correlation between absolute VNA titers and survivorship in immunized animals suggested that, in addition to the G protein and VNA alone, other antigens and immune effector mechanisms were likely to be involved in the protection against lethal rabies virus infection, in either preexposure or postexposure situations (132,134).

Identification of the relative contribution of the individual *Lyssavirus* antigens in humoral versus cellular immunity has been slowly forthcoming. To this end, the relative role of different *Lyssavirus* antigens in helper T-cell activation has been approached experimentally by measuring antigen-mediated lymphokine release to various rabies structural proteins (134). Intact virus usually induces the highest lymphokine secretion, with the greatest response to purified viral antigens being to the N, G, NS, and M proteins, respectively. In addition, several human T-lymphocyte clones from rabies vaccine recipients have been isolated and characterized (135–139). Most of these rabies-reactive clones were of the helper/inducer class of T lymphocytes. These T-cell clones were tested in proliferation assays for their ability to recognize antigenic determinants in rabies virus and related lyssaviruses. Some cells cross-reacted with fixed rabies viruses, and also with Duvenhage and Mokola viruses. Most of these cross-reactive helper T cells recognized determinants present in the viral RNP. In addition, rabies cytotoxic T-cell responses were evident against antigenic determinants of both the RNP and the G proteins. Those T-cell clones that exhibited different cross-reactivity patterns among several viruses recognized closely situated epitopes, presented in the context of the same major histocompatibility complex molecule. Thus, lack of recognition of a particular *Lyssavirus* by a given clone may be attributable in some cases to amino acid variation in the antigen of question. Moreover, immune responses to rabies virus are apparently restricted by more than a single product of the leukocyte antigen–gene complex. Such data also suggest that besides the external G protein, other antigens are a major target for rabies-specific helper T cells.

Certain internal *Lyssavirus* antigens may possess an inherent capacity to enhance immune responsiveness. In lieu of other antigens, rabies RNP is capable of inducing protection against a peripheral rabies virus challenge, in the absence of VNA (140–143). A single inoculation of RNP prepared from either rabies or Mokola virus resulted in 80% to 90% protection against a peripheral lethal rabies challenge. In addition, administration of Mokola or rabies virus RNP resulted in substantial protection of mice challenged with Duvenhage virus, indicating that immunization with RNP can confer cross-protective immunity against infection to heterologous lyssaviruses. One of the significant functions of these RNP-specific immune responses may be the promotion of viral RNP attachment through Fc receptors to phagocytic cells, which are then stimulated by virus to produce cytokines such as interferon, inhibiting virus replication.

The last century has exploited the small advances made in applied immunology in the development of a plethora of rabies vaccines (144). Ideally, these biologicals should maximize potency, purity, safety, efficacy, and cost. Although a few live virus vaccines were effective in rabies prophylaxis, did not re-

quire adjuvant, and induced a long-lasting immune response that involved the full spectrum of immune effectors, these traditionally carried the risk for vaccine-induced disease, especially in the immunocompromised host (145). Inactivated animal neural vaccines eliminated the potential for vaccine-associated rabies but were hampered by low potency and adverse reactions due to myelin basic proteins (146). The research focus in rabies vaccinology during the past 30 years has been toward inactivated tissue culture rabies vaccines for domestic animal and human use, which vary in the nature of the cell substrate, seed strain, method of concentration and inactivation, adjuvant type, and phase for storage (147). Modern methods of vaccine production are finally able to begin to reach those populations in the developing world most at risk for rabies (148–156).

Human rabies postexposure treatment typically includes the simultaneous administration of vaccine and polyclonal antirabies immunoglobulin. This extremely effective treatment regimen (with relatively few exceptions) (157,158) still presents certain practical obstacles arising from availability, quality assurance, and cost. In addition, passively administered antibodies may interfere with the induction of immune effectors, such as helper T-cell and cytotoxic T-cell responses. Thus, novel biologicals, such as murine antirabies MABs, may fill a niche in the postexposure treatment of humans against rabies (159,160). However, murine MABs may induce an immune response in humans to mouse allotypes, which may later interfere with the use of other mouse MABs (e.g., MABs used for cancer treatment). Recombinant DNA techniques can minimize this problem by "humanizing" mouse MAB genes. Alternatively, hybridomas that secrete rabies virus antigen-specific human MABs have been generated (161–165). Protection experiments in rabies virus–infected animals revealed that MABs may be effective in preventing lethal rabies virus infection even after the virus may have entered the CNS (166). Such an MAB cocktail might offer several distinctive advantages over hyperimmune serum: the specific virus-neutralizing activity and protective activity would be higher than those of rabies immunoglobulin; only relatively small quantities of MABs have to be utilized based on protein content; and use of MABs may be superior for local wound treatment, when only small volumes can be inoculated at the actual bite site (provided they do not interfere with active immunization from vaccine) (167). If selective, cost-effective, panreactive antibodies can be developed, these might form the basis for the development of a more rational treatment protocol, perhaps involving MABs and a next generation of recombinant-derived *Lyssavirus* biologicals (168,169).

Both G- and N-protein genes have now been effectively expressed in a number of prokaryotic and eukaryotic systems for parenteral and oral applications (170–183). The productive analysis of these and other *Lyssavirus* genes may eventually contribute to a better understanding of the precise role of individual proteins in the effective induction of protective immune mechanisms. Clearly, host defense against rabies infection is an extremely complex and still poorly understood phenomenon a century after Pasteur's death. Despite numerous and intensive studies of rabies pathogenesis and immunity, the appreciation of the virus–host interaction in this almost invariably fatal viral infection is far from complete.

REFERENCES

1. Gosztonyi G. Reproduction of lyssaviruses: ultrastructural composition of *Lyssavirus* and functional aspects of pathogenesis. *Curr Top Microbiol Immunol* 1994;187:43.
2. Wunner WH. Rabiesviruses. In: Jackson AC, Wunner WH, eds. *Rabies*. New York: Academic Press, 2002:23.

3. Tordo N, Kouknetzoff A. The rabies virus genome: an overview. *Onderstepoort J Vet Res* 1993;60:263.
4. Charlton KM. The pathogenesis of rabies and other lyssaviral infections: recent studies. *Curr Top Microbiol Immunol* 1994;187:95.
5. Lafon M. Immunobiology. In: Jackson AC, Wunner WH, eds. *Rabies*. New York: Academic Press, 2002:351.
6. Van-Regenmortel MH, Faquet CM, Bishop CM, et al. *Viral taxonomy*. The Seventh Report of the International Committee on Taxonomy of Viruses. San Diego: Academic Press, 2000.
7. Bourhy H, Kissi B, Tordo N. Molecular diversity of the *Lyssavirus* genus. *Virology* 1993;194:70.
8. Shope RE. Rabies-related viruses. *Yale J Biol Med* 1982;55:271.
9. Badrane H, Bahloul C, Perrin P, et al. Evidence of two *Lyssavirus* phylogroups with distinct pathogenicity and immunogenicity. *J Virol* 2001;75:3268–3276.
10. Rupprecht CE, Dietzschold B, Wunner WH, et al. Antigenic relationships of lyssaviruses. In: Baer GM, ed. *The natural history of rabies*, 2nd ed. Boca Raton, FL: CRC Press, 1991:69–100.
11. Swanepoel R, Barnard BJH, Meredith CD, et al. Rabies in southern Africa. *Onderstepoort J Vet Res* 1993;60:325.
12. Schneider LG, Cox JH. Bat lyssaviruses in Europe. *Curr Top Microbiol Immunol* 1994;187:207.
13. King AA, Meredith CD, Thomson GR. The biology of southern African lyssavirus variants. *Curr Top Microbiol Immunol* 1994;187:267.
14. Gould AR, Hyatt AD, Lunt R, et al. Characterisation of a novel lyssavirus isolated from pteropid bats in Australia. *Virus Res* 1998;54:165–187.
15. Foggin CM. Mokola virus infection in cats and a dog in Zimbabwe. *Vet Rec* 1983;113:115.
16. Mebatsion T, Cox JH, Frost JW, et al. Isolation and characterization of 115 street rabies virus isolates from Ethiopia by using monoclonal antibodies: identification of 2 isolates as Mokola and Lagos bat viruses. *J Infect Dis* 1992;166:972–977.
17. Wiktor TJ, Macfarlan RI, Foggin CM, et al. Antigenic analysis of rabies and Mokola virus from Zimbabwe using monoclonal antibodies. *Dev Biol Stand* 1984;57:199.
18. Muller WW. Review of reported rabies case data in Europe to the WHO Collaborating Centre Tübingen from 1977 to 1994. *Rabies Bull Eur* 1994;18:17.
19. Dietzschold B, Tollis M, Rupprecht CE, et al. Antigenic variation in rabies and rabies-related viruses: cross-protection independent of glycoprotein-mediated virus-neutralizing antibody. *J Infect Dis* 1987;156:815.
20. Dietzschold B, Rupprecht CE, Tollis M, et al. Antigenic diversity of the glycoprotein and nucleocapsid proteins of rabies and rabies-related viruses: implications for epidemiology and control of rabies. *Rev Infect Dis* 1988;10[Suppl 4]:S785.
21. Bourhy H, Kissi B, Lafon M, et al. Antigenic and molecular characterization of bat rabies virus in Europe. *J Clin Microbiol* 1992;30:2419.
22. Kissi B, Tordo N, Bourhy H. Genetic polymorphism in the rabies virus nucleoprotein gene. *Virology* 1995;209:526.
23. Bourhy H, Kissi B, Tordo N. Taxonomy and evolutionary studies on lyssaviruses with special reference to Africa. *Onderstepoort J Vet Res* 1993;60:277.
24. Smith JS. Rabies virus epitopic variation: use in ecologic studies. *Adv Virus Res* 1989;36:215.
25. Smith JS, Yager PA, Bigler WJ, et al. Surveillance and epidemiologic mapping of monoclonal antibody-defined rabies variants in Florida. *J Wildl Dis* 1990;26:473.
26. Smith JS, Fishbein DB, Rupprecht CE, et al. Unexplained rabies in three immigrants in the United States: a virologic investigation. *N Engl J Med* 1991;324:205.
27. Smith JS, Orciari LA, Yager PA, et al. Epidemiologic and historical relationships among 87 rabies virus isolates as determined by limited sequence analysis. *J Infect Dis* 1992;166:296.
28. Smith JS, Seidel HD. Rabies: a new look at an old disease. *Prog Med Virol* 1993;40:82.
29. McColl KA, Gould AR, Selleck PW, et al. Polymerase chain reaction and other laboratory techniques in the diagnosis of long incubation rabies in Australia. *Aust Vet J* 1993;70:84.
30. Smith JS, Orciari LA, Yager PA. Molecular epidemiology of rabies in the United States. *Semin Virol* 1995;6:387.
31. Sacramento D, Bourhy H, Tordo N. PCR technique as an alternative method for diagnosis and molecular epidemiology of rabies virus. *Mol Cell Probes* 1991;5:229.
32. Orciari LA. *Genetic analysis of rabies virus isolates from skunks in the United States* [Master's dissertation]. Athens, GA: University of Georgia, 1995.
33. Nadin-Davis SA, Casey GA, Wandeler AI. A molecular epidemiological study of rabies virus in central Ontario and western Quebec. *J Gen Virol* 1994;75:2575.
34. Mebatsion T, Cox JH, Conzelmann KK. Molecular analysis of rabies-related viruses from Ethiopia. *Onderstepoort J Vet Res* 1993;60:289.
35. Ermine A, Larzul D, Ceccaldi PE, et al. Polymerase chain reaction amplification of rabies virus nucleic acids from total mouse brain RNA. *Mol Cell Probes* 1990;4:189.
36. Centers for Disease Control and Prevention. Translocation of coyote rabies-Florida, 1994. *MMWR Morb Mortal Wkly Rep* 1995;44:580.
37. Rupprecht CE, Smith JS, Fekadu M, et al. The ascension of wildlife rabies: a cause for public health concern or intervention? *Emerg Infect Dis* 1995;1:107.
38. Kitchin PA, Bootman JS. Quality of the polymerase chain reaction. *Rev Med Virol* 1993;3:107.
39. World Health Organization. *WHO workshop on genetic and antigenic molecular epidemiology of lyssaviruses*. Geneva: World Health Organization, 1994.
40. Gaudin Y, Ruigrok RW, Tuffereau C, et al. Rabies virus glycoprotein is a trimer. *Virology* 1992;187:627.
41. Tordo N, Poch O, Ermine A, et al. Walking along the rabies genome: is the large G-L intergenic region a remnant gene? *Proc Natl Acad Sci U S A* 1986;83:3914.
42. Ravkov EV, Smith JS, Nichol ST. Rabies virus glycoprotein gene contains a long 3′ noncoding region which lacks pseudogene properties. *Virology* 1995;206:718.
43. Kawai A, Morimoto K. Functional aspects of lyssavirus proteins. *Curr Top Microbiol Immunol* 1994;187:27.
44. Gaudin Y, Ruigrok RW, Knossow M, et al. Low-pH conformational changes of rabies virus glycoprotein and their role in membrane fusion. *J Virol* 1993;67:1365.
45. de la Torre JC, Holland JJ. RNA virus quasispecies populations can suppress vastly superior mutant progeny. *J Virol* 1990;64:6278.
46. Coulon P, Lafay F, Tuffereau C, et al. The molecular basis for altered pathogenicity of lyssavirus variants. *Curr Top Microbiol Immunol* 1994;187:69.
47. Coulon P, Ternaux JP, Flamand A, et al. An avirulent mutant of rabies virus is unable to infect motoneurons in vivo and in vitro. *Virology* 1998;72:273–278.
48. Kissi B, Tordo N, Bourhy H. Genetic polymorphism in the rabies virus nucleoprotein gene. *Virology* 1995;209:526.
49. Kouznetzoff A, Buckle M, Tordo N. Identification of a region of the rabies virus N protein involved in direct binding to the viral RNA. *J Gen Virol* 1998;79:1005–1013.
50. Chenik M, Chebli K, Gaudin Y, et al. In vivo interaction of rabies virus phosphoprotein (P) and nucleoprotein (N): existence of two N-binding sites on P protein. *J Gen Virol* 1994;75:2889.
51. Yang J, Koprowski H, Dietzschold B. Phosphorylation of rabies virus nucleoprotein regulates viral RNA transcription and replication by modulating leader RNA encapsulation. *J Virol* 1999;73:1661–1664.
52. Nakahara K, Ohnuma H, Sugita S, et al. Intracellular behavior of rabies virus matrix protein (M) is determined by the viral glycoprotein (G). *Microbiol Immunol* 1999;43:259–270.
53. Kaplan MM. Safety precautions in handling rabies virus. In: Meslin F-X, Kaplan MM, Koprowski H, eds. *Laboratory techniques in rabies*, 4th ed. Geneva: World Health Organization, 1996:3–8.
54. Sureau P, Ravisse P, Rollin PE. Rabies diagnosis by animal inoculation, identification of Negri bodies, or ELISA. In: Baer GM, ed. *The natural history of rabies*, 2nd ed. Boca Raton, FL: CRC Press, 1991:203–217.
55. Lentz TL, Burrage TG, Smith AL, et al. Is the acetylcholine receptor a rabies virus receptor? *Science* 1982;215:182.
56. Lentz TL, Burrage TG, Smith AL, et al. The acetylcholine receptor as a cellular receptor for rabies virus. *Yale J Biol Med* 1983;56:315.
57. Lentz TL, Wilson PT, Hawrot E, et al. Amino acid sequence similarity between rabies virus glycoprotein and snake venom curaremimetic neurotoxins. *Science* 1984;226:847.
58. Lentz TL, Benson RJ, Klimowicz D, et al. Binding of rabies virus to purified *Torpedo* acetylcholine receptor. *Brain Res* 1986;387:211.
59. Lentz TL, Hawrot E, Wilson PT. Synthetic peptides corresponding to sequences of snake venom neurotoxins and rabies virus glycoprotein bind to the nicotinic acetylcholine receptor. *Proteins* 1987;2:298.
60. Lentz TL, Hawrot E, Donnelly-Roberts D, et al. Synthetic peptides in the study of the interaction of rabies virus and the acetylcholine receptor. *Adv Biochem Psychopharmacol* 1988;44:57.
61. Lentz TL. Rabies virus binding to an acetylcholine receptor alpha-subunit peptide. *J Mol Recognit* 1990;3:82.
62. Baer GM, Shaddock JH, Quirion R, et al. Rabies susceptibility and acetylcholine receptor [Letter]. *Lancet* 1990;335:664.
63. Lentz TL. Structure-function relationships of curaremimetic neurotoxin loop 2 and of a structurally similar segment of rabies virus glycoprotein in their interaction with the nicotinic acetylcholine receptor. *Biochemistry* 1991;30:10949.
64. Gastka M, Horvath J, Lentz TL. Rabies virus binding to the nicotinic acetylcholine receptor al subunit demonstrated by virus overlay protein binding assay. *J Gen Virol* 1996;77:2437–2440.
65. Thoulouze MI, Lafage M, Schachner M, et al. The neural cell adhesion molecule is a receptor for rabies virus. *J Virol* 1998;72:7181–7190.
66. Tuffereau C, Desmezieres E, Benejean J, et al. Interaction of lyssaviruses with the low-affinity nerve-growth factor receptor p75NTR. *J Gen Virol* 2001;82:2861–2867.
67. Reagan KJ, Wunner WH. Rabies virus interaction with various cell lines is independent of the acetylcholine receptor. *Arch Virol* 1985;84:277.
68. Broughan JH, Wunner WH. Characterization of protein involvement in rabies virus binding to BHK-21 cells. *Arch Virol* 1995;140:75.
69. Durrer P, Gaudin Y, Ruigrok RWH, et al. Photolabeling identifies a putative fusion domain in the envelope glycoprotein of rabies and vesicular stomatitis viruses. *J Biol Chem* 1995;270:17575.

70. Gaudin Y. Rabies virus-induced membrane fusion pathway. *J Cell Biol* 2000;150:601–612.
71. Gaudin Y, Tuffereau C, Durrer P, et al. Rabies virus-induced membrane fusion. *Mol Membr Biol* 1999;16:21–31.
72. Dietzschold B, Wiktor TJ, Wunner WH, et al. Chemical and immunological analysis of the rabies soluble glycoprotein. *Virology* 1983;124:330.
73. Wojczyk B, Shakin-Eshleman SH, Doms RW, et al. Stable secretion of a soluble, oligomeric form of rabies virus glycoprotein: influence of *N*-glycan processing on secretion. *Biochemistry* 1995;34:2599.
74. Gaudin Y, Tuffereau C, Durrer P, et al. Biological function of the low-pH, fusion-inactive conformation of rabies virus glycoprotein (G): G is transported in a fusion-inactive state-like conformation. *J Virol* 1995;69:5528.
75. Dietzschold B, Wunner WH, Wiktor TJ, et al. Characterization of an antigenic determinant of the glycoprotein that correlates with pathogenicity of rabies virus. *Proc Natl Acad Sci U S A* 1983;80:70.
76. Dietzschold B, Wiktor TJ, Trojanowski JQ, et al. Differences in cell-to-cell spread of pathogenic and apathogenic rabies virus in vivo and in vitro. *J Virol* 1985;56:12.
77. Dietzschold B, Tollis M, Lafon M, et al. Mechanisms of rabies virus neutralization by glycoprotein-specific monoclonal antibodies. *Virology* 1987;161:29.
78. Flamand A, Coulon P, Gaudin Y, et al. Reversible conformational changes of the rabies glycoprotein that mask or expose epitopes involved in virulence. *J Cell Biochem Suppl* 1995;19A:277.
79. Lafay F, Benejean J, Tuffereau C, et al. Vaccination against rabies: construction and characterization of SAG2, a double avirulent derivative of SADBern. *Vaccine* 1994;12:317.
80. Steele JH, Fernandez PJ. History of rabies and global aspects. In: Baer GM, ed. *The natural history of rabies,* 2nd ed. Boca Raton, FL: CRC Press, 1991:1.
81. Baer GM, Cleary WF, Diaz AM, et al. Characteristics of 11 rabies virus isolates in mice: titers and relative invasiveness of virus, incubation period of infection, and survival of mice with sequelae. *J Infect Dis* 1977;136:336.
82. Tsiang H. Evidence for an intraaxonal transport of fixed and street rabies virus. *J Neuropathol Exp Neurol* 1979;38:286.
83. Ugolini G. Specificity of rabies virus as a transneuronal tracer of motor networks: transfer from hypoglossal motoneurons to connected second-order and higher order central nervous system cell groups. *J Comp Neurol* 1995;356:457.
84. Kelly RM, Strick PL. Rabies as a transneuronal tracer of circuits in the central nervous system. *J Neurosci Methods* 2000;103:63–71.
85. Gratten-Smith PJ, O'Reagan WJ, et al. Rabies: a second Australian case with a long incubation period. *Med J Aust* 1992;156:651–654.
86. Para M. An outbreak of post-vaccinal rabies (rage de laboratoire) in Fortaleza, Brazil, in 1960: residual fixed virus as the etiological agent. *Bull WHO* 1965;33:177.
87. Wandeler AI, Nadin-Davis SA, Tinline RR, et al. Rabies epidemiology: some ecological and evolutionary perspectives. *Curr Top Microbiol Immunol* 1994;187:297.
88. Murphy FA, Bauer SP. Early street rabies virus infection in striated muscle and later progression to the central nervous system. *Intervirology* 1974; 3:256.
89. Shankar V, Dietzschold B, Koprowski H. Direct entry of rabies virus into the central nervous system without prior local replication. *J Virol* 1991;65:2736.
90. Gosztonyi G, Dietzschold B, Kao M, et al. Rabies and borna disease: a comparative pathogenetic study of two neurovirulent agents. *Lab Invest* 1993;68:285.
91. Ray NB, Ewalt LC, Lodmell DL. Rabies virus replication in human and murine macrophage-like cell lines: implications for viral persistence. *J Virol* 1995;69:764.
92. Jackson AC, Reimer DL. Pathogenesis of experimental rabies in mice: an immunohistochemical study. *Acta Neuropathol* (Berl) 1989;78:159.
93. Balachandran A, Charlton KM. Experimental rabies infection of non-nervous tissues in skunks (*Mephitis mephitis*) and foxes (*Vulpes vulpes*). *Vet Pathol* 1994;31:93.
94. Smith JS. Rabies virus. In: Murray PR, Baron EJ, Pfaller MA, et al., eds. *Manual of clinical microbiology,* 6th ed. Washington, DC: ASM Press, 1995:997–1003.
95. Hemachuda T. Rabies. In: Vinken PJ, Bruyn GW, Klawans HL, eds. *Handbook of clinical neurology.* Amsterdam: Elsevier Science Publishers, 1989:383–404.
96. Hattwick MA, Weis TT, Stechschulte CJ, et al. Recovery from rabies: a case report. *Ann Intern Med* 1972;76:931.
97. Alvarez AL, Fajardo R, Lopez ME, et al. Partial recovery from rabies in a nine-year-old boy. *Pediatr Infect Dis J* 1994;13:1154.
98. Miller A, Morse HC III, Winkelstein J, et al. The role of antibody in recovery from experimental rabies. I. Effect of depletion of B and T cells. *J Immunol* 1978;121:321.
99. Fekadu M, Baer GM. Recovery from clinical rabies of 2 dogs inoculated with a rabies virus strain from Ethiopia. *Am J Vet Res* 1980;41:1632.
100. Fekadu M, Shaddock JH, Baer GM. Intermittent excretion of rabies virus in the saliva of a dog two and six months after it had recovered from experimental rabies. *Am J Trop Med Hyg* 1981;30:1113.
101. Prabhakar BS, Fischman HR, Nathanson N. Recovery from experimental rabies by adoptive transfer of immune cells. *J Gen Virol* 1981;56:25.
102. Jackson AC, Reimer DL, Ludwin SK. Spontaneous recovery from the encephalomyelitis in mice caused by street rabies virus. *Neuropathol Appl Neurobiol* 1989;15:459.
103. Fekadu M, Summer JW Shaddock JH, et al. Sickness and recovery of dogs
challenged with a street rabies virus after vaccination with a vaccinia virus recombinant expressing rabies virus N protein. *J Virol* 1992;66:2601.
104. Dupont JR, Earle KM. Human rabies encephalitis: a study of forty-nine fatal cases with a review of the literature. *Neurology* 1965;15:1023.
105. Thoulouze MI, Lafage M, Montano-Hirose JA, et al. Rabies virus infects mouse and human lymphocytes and induces apoptosis. *J Virol* 1997;71:7372–7380.
106. Morimoto K, Hooper DC, Spitsin S, et al. Pathogenicity of different rabies viruses variants inversely correlates with apoptosis and rabies virus glycoprotein expression in infected primary neuron cultures. *J Virol* 1999;73:510–518.
107. Trimarchi CV, Debbie J. The fluorescent antibody in rabies. In: Baer GM, ed. *The natural history of rabies,* 2nd ed. Boca Raton, FL: CRC Press, 1991:219–233.
108. Dean DJ, Abelseth MK. The fluorescent antibody test. In: Kaplan MM, Koprowski H, eds. *Laboratory techniques in rabies.* Geneva: World Health Organization, 1973:73–84.
109. Velleca WM, Forrester FT. *Laboratory methods for detecting rabies.* Washington, DC: U.S. Government Printing Office, 1981.
110. Kristensson K, Dastur DK, Manghani DK, et al. Rabies interactions between neurons and viruses: a review of history of Negri inclusion bodies. *Neuropathol Appl Neurobiol* 1996;22:179–187.
111. Murphy FA, Harrison AK, Winn WC, et al. Comparative pathogenesis of rabies and rabies-like viruses: infection of the central nervous system and centrifugal spread of virus to peripheral tissues. *Lab Invest* 1973;29:1.
112. Matsumoto S. Electron microscopy of nerve cells infected with street rabies virus. *Virology* 1962;17:198.
113. Charlton KM. Rabies: spongiform lesions in the brain. *Acta Neuropathol* (Berl) 1984;63:198.
114. Charlton KM, Casey GA, Webster WA, et al. Experimental rabies in skunks and foxes: pathogenesis of the spongiform lesions. *Lab Invest* 1987;57:634.
115. Tsiang H. Pathophysiology of rabies virus infection of the nervous system. *Adv Virus Res* 1993;42:375.
116. Marquette C, Ceccaldi P-E, Ban E, et al. Alteration of interleukin-1 alpha production and interleukin-1 binding sites during rabies virus infection. *Arch Virol* 1996;141:573–585.
117. Haour F, Marquette C, Ban E, et al. Receptors for interleukin-1 in the central nervous and neuroendocrine systems: role in infection and stress. *Ann Endocrinol* (Paris) 1995;56:173.
118. Koprowski H, Zheng YM, Heber-Katz E, et al. In vivo expression of inducible nitric oxide synthase in experimentally induced neurologic disease. *Proc Natl Acad Sci USA* 1993;90:3024.
119. Koprowski H, Zheng YM, Fu ZF, et al. NOS expression in experimentally induced neurologic diseases. *J Neurochem* 1995;64:S32.
120. Hemachudha T. Human rabies: clinical aspects, pathogenesis, and potential therapy. *Curr Top Microbiol Immunol* 1994;187:121.
121. Peterhans E, Zanoni R, Bertoni G. How to succeed as a virus: strategies for dealing with the immune system. *Vet Immunol Immunopathol* 1999;72:111–117.
122. Follmann EH, Ritter DG, Beller M. Survey of trappers in northern Alaska for rabies antibody. *Epidemiol Infect* 1994;113:137.
123. Prabhakar BS, Nathanson N. Acute rabies death mediated by antibody. *Nature* 1981;290:590.
124. Smith JS, McCelland CL, Reid FL, et al. Dual role of the immune response in street rabiesvirus infection of mice. *Infect Immun* 1982;35:213.
125. Nathanson N, Gonzalez-Scarano F. Immune response to rabies virus. In: Baer GM, ed. The natural history of rabies, 2nd ed. Boca Raton, FL: CRC Press, 1991:145–161.
126. Baer GM, Shaddock JH, Moore SA, et al. Successful prophylaxis against rabies in mice and Rhesus monkeys: the interferon system and vaccine. *J Infect Dis* 1977;136:286.
127. Baer GM, Moore SA, Shaddock JH, et al. An effective rabies treatment in exposed monkeys: a single dose of interferon inducer and vaccine. *Bull W H O* 1979;57:807.
128. Merigan TC, Baer GM, Winkler WG, et al. Human leukocyte interferon administration to patients with symptomatic and suspected rabies. *Ann Neurol* 1984;16:82.
129. Baer GM, Shaddock JH, Levy H, et al. Interferon in rabies postexposure prophylaxis. In: Thraenhart O, Koprowski H, Bogel K, et al., eds. *Progress in rabies control.* Kent, UK: Wells Medical, 1989:245–250.
130. Bunn TO. Canine and feline vaccines, past and present. In: Baer GM, ed. *The natural history of rabies,* 2nd ed. Boca Raton, FL: CRC Press, 1991:415–425.
131. Wunderli PS, Shaddock JH, Schmid DS, et al. The protective role of humoral neutralizing antibody in the NIH potency test for rabies vaccines. *Vaccine* 1991;9:638.
132. Xiang ZQ, Knowles BB, McCarrick JW, et al. Immune mechanisms required for protection to rabies. *Virology* 1995;214:398–404.
133. Rupprecht CE, Dietzschold B. Perspectives on rabies virus pathogenesis. *Lab Invest* 1987;57:603.
134. Ertl HC, Dietzschold B, Gore M, et al. Induction of rabies virus-specific T-helper cells by synthetic peptides that carry dominant T-helper cell epitopes of the viral ribonucleoprotein. *J Virol* 1989;63:2885.
135. Celis E, Ou DW, Dietzschold B, et al. Recognition of rabies and rabies-related viruses by T cells derived from human vaccine recipients. *J Virol* 1988;62:3128.
136. Celis E, Karr RW, Dietzschold B, et al. Genetic restriction and fine specificity of human T cell clones reactive with rabies virus. *J Immunol* 1988;141:2721.
137. Celis E, Ou D, Dietzschold B, et al. Rabies virus-specific T cell hybridomas:

identification of class II MHC-restricted T-cell epitopes using synthetic peptides. *Hybridoma* 1989;8:263.

138. Celis E, Miller RW, Wiktor TJ, et al. Isolation and characterization of human T cell lines and clones reactive to rabies virus: antigen specificity and production of interferon-gamma. *J Immunol* 1986;136:692.

139. Celis E, Larson J, Otvos L Jr, et al. Identification of a rabies virus T cell epitope on the basis of its similarity with a hepatitis B surface antigen peptide presented to T cells by the same MHC molecule (HLA-DPw4). *J Immunol* 1990;145:305–310.

140. Hooper DC, Pierard I, Modelska A, et al. Rabies ribonucleocapsid as an oral immunogen and immunological enhancer. *Proc Natl Acad Sci USA* 1994;91:10908.

141. Lafon M, Scott-Algara D, Marche PN, et al. Neonatal deletion and selective expansion of mouse T cells by exposure to rabies virus nucleocapsid superantigen. *J Exp Med* 1994;180:1207.

142. Dietzschold B, Wang HH, Rupprecht CE, et al. Induction of protective immunity against rabies by immunization with rabies virus ribonucleoprotein. *Proc Natl Acad Sci USA* 1987;84:9165.

143. Tollis M, Dietzschold B, Volia CB, et al. Immunization of monkeys with rabies ribonucleoprotein (RNP) confers protective immunity against rabies. *Vaccine* 1991;9:134.

144. Vodopija I, Clark HF. Human vaccination against rabies. In: Baer GM, ed. The natural history of rabies, 2nd ed. Boca Raton, FL: CRC Press, 1991:571–595.

145. Bingham J, Foggin CM, Gerber H, et al. Pathogenicity of SAD rabies vaccine given orally in chacma baboons (*Papio ursinus*). *Vet Rec* 1992;131:55.

146. Thraenhart O, Marcus I, Kreuzfelder E. Current and future immunoprophylaxis against human rabies: reduction of treatment of failures and errors. *Curr Top Microbiol Immunol* 1994;187:173.

147. Jenkins SR, Austander M, Conti L, et al. Compendium of animal rabies prevention and control, 1995. National Association of State Public Health Veterinarians, Inc. *MMWR Morb Mortal Wkly Rep* 2000;49(RR-8):21.

148. Lin FT. The protective effect of the large-scale use of PHKC rabies vaccine in humans in China. *Bull WHO* 1990;68:449.

149. Chutivongse S, Wilde H, Supich C, et al. Postexposure prophylaxis for rabies with antiserum and intradermal vaccination. *Lancet* 1990;335:896.

150. Chutivongse S, Wilde H, Fishbein DB, et al. One-year study of the 2-1-1 intramuscular postexposure rabies vaccine regimen in 100 severely exposed Thai patients using rabies immune globulin and Vero cell rabies vaccine. *Vaccine* 1991;9:573.

151. Fishbein DB, Miranda NJ, Merrill P, et al. Rabies control in the Republic of the Philippines: benefits and costs of elimination. *Vaccine* 1991;9:581.

152. Sehgal S, Bhattacharya D, Bhardwaj M. Clinical evaluation of purified Vero-cell rabies vaccine in patients bitten by rabid animals in India. *J Commun Dis* 1994;26:139.

153. Dutta JK, Warrell JJ, Dutta TK. Intradermal rabies immunization for pre- and post-exposure prophylaxis. *Nat Med J India* 1994;7:119.

154. Meslin FX, Fishbein DB, Matter HC. Rationale and prospects for rabies elimination in developing countries. *Curr Top Microbiol Immunol* 1994;187:1.

155. Khawplod P, Glueck R, Wilde H, et al. Immunogenicity of purified duck embryo rabies vaccine (Lyssavac-N) with use of the WHO-approved intradermal postexposure regimen. *Clin Infect Dis* 1995;20:646.

156. Wilde H, Glueck R, Khawplod P, et al. Efficacy study of a new albumin-free human diploid cell rabies vaccine (Lyssavac-HDC, Bema) in 100 severely rabies-exposed Thai patients. *Vaccine* 1995;13:593.

157. Wilde H, Choomkasien P, Hemachudha T, et al. Failure of rabies postexposure treatment in Thailand. *Vaccine* 1989;7:49.

158. Tabbara KF, Al-Omar O. Eyelid laceration sustained in an attack by a rabid desert fox. *Am J Ophthalmol* 1995;119:651.

159. Schumacher CL, Dietzschold B, Ertl HC, et al. Use of mouse anti-rabies monoclonal antibodies in postexposure treatment of rabies. *J Clin Invest* 1989;84:971.

160. Montano-Hirose JA, Lafage M, Weber P, et al. Protective activity of a murine monoclonal antibody against European bat lyssavirus 1 (EBL1) infection in mice. *Vaccine* 1993;11:1259.

161. Lafon M, Edelman L, Bouvet JP, et al. Human monoclonal antibodies specific for the rabies virus glycoprotein and N protein. *J Gen Virol* 1990;71:1689.

162. Dietzschold B, Gore M, Casali P, et al. Biological characterization of human monoclonal antibodies to rabies virus. *J Virol* 1990;64:3087.

163. Cheung SC, Dietzschold B, Koprowski H, et al. A recombinant human Fab expressed in *Escherichia coli* neutralizes rabies virus. *J Virol* 1992;66:6714.

164. Dorfman N, Dietzschold B, Kajiyama W, et al. Development of human monoclonal antibodies to rabies. *Hybridoma* 1994;13:397.

165. Rando RF, Notkins AL. Production of human monoclonal antibodies against rabies virus. *Curr Top Microbiol Immunol* 1994;187:195.

166. Dietzschold B, Kao M, Zheng YM, et al. Delineation of putative mechanisms involved in antibody-mediated clearance of rabies virus from the central nervous system. *Proc Natl Acad Sci USA* 1992;89:7252.

167. Schumacher CL, Ertl HC, Koprowski H, et al. Inhibition of immune responses against rabies virus by monoclonal antibodies directed against rabies virus antigens. *Vaccine* 1992;10:754.

168. Schnell MJ, Mebatsion T, Conzelmann K-K. Infectious rabies viruses from cloned cDNA. *EMBO J* 1994;13:4195.

169. Xiang ZQ, Spitalnik S, Tran M, et al. Vaccination with a plasmid vector carrying the rabies virus glycoprotein gene induces protective immunity against rabies virus. *Virology* 1994;199:132.

170. Wiktor TJ, Macfarlan RI, Reagan KJ, et al. Protection from rabies by a vaccinia virus recombinant containing the rabies virus glycoprotein gene. *Proc Natl Acad Sci USA* 1984;81:7194.

171. Prehaud C, Takehara K, Flammand A, et al. Immunogenic and protective properties of rabies virus glycoprotein expressed by baculovirus vectors. *Virology* 1989;173:390.

172. Fekadu M, Shaddock JH, Summer JW, et al. Oral vaccination of skunks with raccoon poxvirus recombinants expressing the rabies glycoprotein or the nucleoprotein. *J Wildl Dis* 1991;27:681.

173. Fu ZF, Dietzschold B, Schumacher CL, et al. Rabies virus nucleoprotein expressed in and purified from insect cells is efficacious as a vaccine. *Proc Natl Acad Sci USA* 1991;88:2001.

174. Sumner JW, Fekadu M, Shaddock JH, et al. Protection of mice with vaccinia virus recombinants that express the rabies nucleoprotein. *Virology* 1991;183:703.

175. Fu ZF, Rupprecht CE, Dietzschold B, et al. Oral vaccination of raccoons (*Procyon lotor*) with baculovirus-expressed rabies virus glycoprotein. *Vaccine* 1993;11:925.

176. Klepfer SR, Debouck C, Uffelman J, et al. Characterization of rabies glycoprotein expressed in yeast. *Arch Virol* 1993;128:269.

177. Goto H, Minamoto N, Ito H, et al. Expression of the nucleoprotein of rabies virus in *Escherichia coli* and mapping of antigenic sites. *Arch Virol* 1995;140:1061.

178. Brochier B, Costy F, Pastoret P-P. Elimination of fox rabies from Belgium using a recombinant vaccinia-rabies vaccine: an update. *Vet Microbiol* 1995;46:269.

179. Aubert MFA, Masson E, Artois M, et al. Oral wildlife rabies vaccination field trials in Europe, with recent emphasis on France. *Curr Top Microbiol Immunol* 1994;187:219.

180. Campbell JB. Oral rabies immunization of wildlife and dogs: challenges to the Americas. *Curr Top Microbiol Immunol* 1994;187:245.

181. Lutze-Wallace C, Sapp T, Sidhu M, et al. In vitro assessments of the genetic stability of alive recombinant human adenovirus vaccine against rabies. *Can J Vet Res* 1995;59:157.

182. Taylor J, Meignier B, Tartaglia J, et al. Biological and immunogenic properties of a canarypox-rabies recombinant, ALVAC-RG (vCP65) in non-avian species. *Vaccine* 1995;13:539.

183. Rupprecht CE, Shankar V, Hanlon CA, et al. Beyond Pasteur to 2001: future trends in lyssavirus research? *Curr Top Microbiol Immunol* 1994;187:325.

CHAPTER 263
Caliciviruses and Astroviruses

Neil R. Blacklow

Viral gastroenteritis is a common, medically important illness that occurs worldwide. Despite its frequency and importance, no pathogens were identified until the early 1970s with the discovery of Norwalk virus (1,2). In the past, electron microscopic (EM) and antigen detection techniques were the prerequisite for the detection in stools and study of Norwalk virus and most other small round gastroenteritis viruses. This is because, despite intensive efforts, the viruses (with the exception of the astroviruses) have remained refractory to cultivation *in vitro* in cell culture. The cloning of the Norwalk virus genome has now established conclusively that the virus is a calicivirus (3,4). The understanding of Norwalk virus molecular virology has clarified the nature of other related small round gastroenteritis viruses that are also caliciviruses. Most of our knowledge of the caliciviruses is derived from the study of Norwalk virus, the prototype and most extensively studied calicivirus. This discussion of caliciviruses therefore concentrates for the most part on Norwalk virus. More recently, other small, round gastroenteritis viruses that are unrelated to caliciviruses have been extensively characterized and form a second major family of diarrheal agents, the astroviruses (5). Less medically relevant information is known about astroviruses than caliciviruses. The syndrome of viral gastroenteritis is also produced by two other virus families that are larger in size than the small, round caliciviruses and astroviruses, namely, the enteric adenoviruses and the rotaviruses (covered in Chapters 229 and 254, respectively).

CLASSIFICATION AND COMPARATIVE VIROLOGY OF SMALL, ROUND GASTROENTERITIS VIRUSES

The small, round viruses that are associated with gastroenteritis are 27 to 40 nm in diameter and can be categorized morphologically into two families–caliciviruses and astroviruses–on the basis of careful EM studies of the agents in stool specimens (5,6). The caliciviruses, such as Norwalk virus and related agents, form a first category. These agents usually possess an amorphous surface structure with a feathery, ragged outline that lacks clearcut geometric symmetry (Fig. 263.1A). On the basis of biochemical and molecular virologic studies (see the section "Caliciviruses"), these agents (previously called *small round structured viruses*) are now known to belong to the family Caliciviridae (4). These viruses share characteristics of density in cesium chloride (1.34 to 1.42 g/cm³), size (27 to 40 nm in diameter), and derivation from epidemics or family outbreaks of gastroenteritis. The individual calicivirus strains are named after the location of the outbreak from which they are derived (e.g., Norwalk, Ohio; Hawaii; Snow Mountain, Colorado; Toronto, Canada; Mexico; Lordsdale, England). These viruses are now classified in the genus *Norovirus* in the family Caliciviridae. At least three of these virus strains

(Norwalk, Hawaii, Snow Mountain) are immunologically distinct on the basis of immunoelectron microscopy (IEM) studies that employ human serum from infected and uninfected persons in the assays. These three viruses have also induced disease in volunteers (they do not produce disease in animals, including primates), and this has provided the necessary human clinical material for development of immunoassays to detect each of them in stools and their antibodies in serum (7–10). In contrast to the Noroviruses, some other calicivirus strains, detected in young children, demonstrate a distinct virion surface structure with cup-shaped indentations or hollows (Latin *calix*, meaning cup) that may form a six-pointed star (star of David, Fig. 263.1B), which is the classic appearance of the virus family Caliciviridae (11,12). These viruses are now classified in the genus *Sapovirus* in the family Caliciviridae, named after Sapporo, Japan where they were initially discovered.

The second category of small, round gastroenteritis viruses consists of the agents belonging to the family Astroviridae. The astroviruses have a definitive, classic surface structure on EM (12). They are 27 to 32 nm in diameter and have a five- or six-pointed star on their surface that consists of a continuous, rounded structure (Fig. 263.1C). This morphologic feature contrasts with that of classic Sapovirus caliciviruses, whose surface is broken by hollows, and with that of Norovirus caliciviruses, whose surface is feathery and ragged. Biochemical and molecular virologic studies (see the section "Astroviruses") also

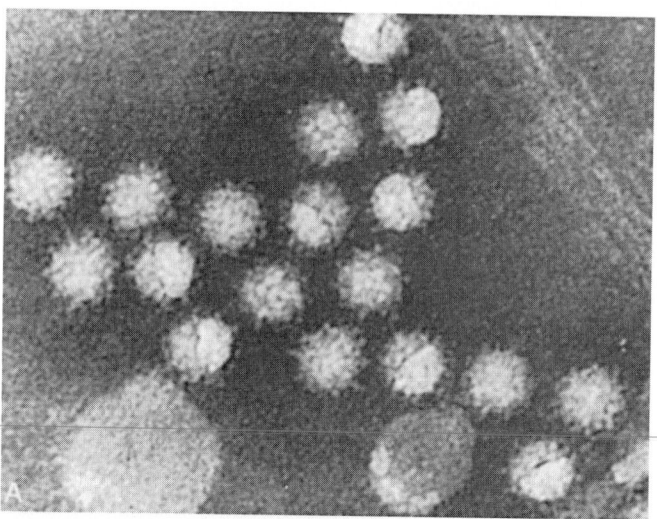
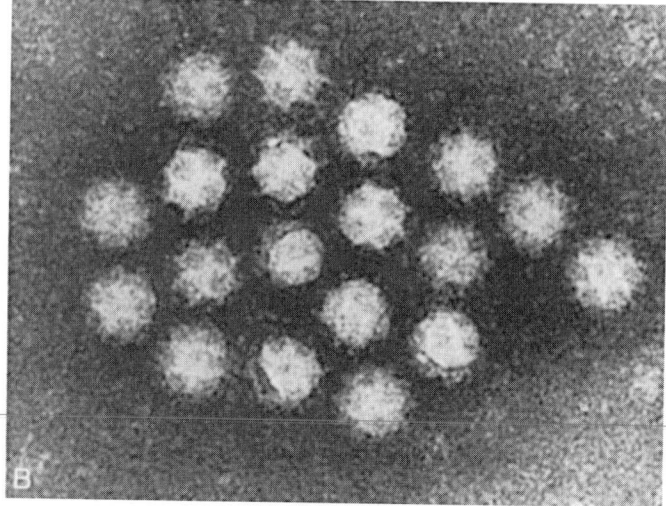
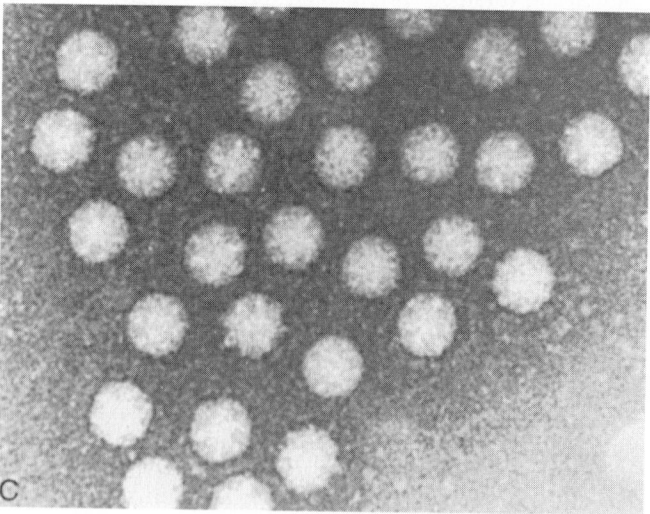

Figure 263.1. Small round gastroenteritis viruses visualized by electron microscopic examination of stool specimens. **A:** Calicivirus belonging to the Norovirus genus from a patient infected during a foodborne outbreak of gastroenteritis. **B:** Calicivirus belonging to the Sapovirus genus from a young child with vomiting and diarrhea. Characteristic hollows are present on the surface of some virions. **C:** Astrovirus from an elderly patient with diarrhea in a nursing home. Particles have a continuous rounded surface structure, and some particles also show a star on their surface. (**A** to **C** courtesy of W. David Cubitt, Department of Virology, Institute of Child Health, London.)

indicate the distinctiveness of astroviruses from caliciviruses. Immunoassays that now detect and quantify astroviruses have revealed their medical importance in the same way that immunoassay earlier permitted recognition of Norwalk virus as an important pathogen (13,14).

CALICIVIRUSES

Characteristics of the Pathogen

Norwalk virus, the prototype calicivirus, is difficult to recognize in stools by direct EM owing to its small size and the fact that it is shed in relatively low titer in feces. It can be visualized by IEM reaction of feces with human convalescent-phase serum that contains Norwalk antibodies, which aggregate viral particles (1). By IEM, the virions are round, nonenveloped, and 27 nm in average diameter; they have a ragged outline in which there is a suggestion of small indentations on the surface (15) (Fig. 263.1A and B). New structural studies, based on recombinant Norwalk virus particles produced in insect cells by a baculovirus recombinant expressing the complementary DNA that encodes the single major Norwalk capsid protein, now clearly demonstrate icosahedral particles with 32 cup-shaped depressions at each icosahedral axis, characteristic of caliciviruses (16).

Norwalk virus and other caliciviruses have not been cultivated *in vitro*, nor do they produce disease in animal model systems. Biochemical studies of Norwalk virus, purified from human stool samples, indicate a single major structural protein of about 60 kd, which is characteristic of caliciviruses (17). The viral genome has been molecularly cloned and completely sequenced; it contains single-stranded RNA of positive polarity, about 7.6 kb in size, permitting definitive classification in the family Caliciviridae (4). The viral genome encodes three open reading frames: the first codes for the 60-kd major structural protein of the viral capsid, the second codes for a minor structural protein, and the third codes for a precursor of nonstructural proteins (18,19).

Norovirus caliciviruses can be categorized into two genogroups on the basis of their nucleotide–amino acid sequence homologies in the polymerase region and in the capsid region of their genomes (20–35). The genogroups include agents such as Norwalk, Southampton, and Desert Shield viruses in group I; and Hawaii, Snow Mountain, Mexico, Toronto, and Lordsdale viruses in group II. Sapovirus caliciviruses consist of a single genogroup including agents such as Sapporo; Manchester, England; and Parkville, United States. Norovirus and Sapovirus genogroups are defined on the basis of arbitrary genetic criteria and do not necessarily relate to immunobiologic characteristics; for example, Hawaii and Snow Mountain viruses, both members of the same genogroup, are distinct on the basis of IEM reactions with defined human serum (36,37). Medically relevant serotypic differences between the various calicivirus strains clearly await further delineation.

Epidemiology

Immunoassay techniques, using defined human clinical reagents, were initially employed to determine the epidemiology of Norwalk virus as a medically important pathogen. Disease usually occurs in epidemic fashion, characterized by acute vomiting and diarrhea with a short incubation period (24 to 48 hours), and sweeps through communities. Forty-two percent of 74 acute nonbacterial gastroenteritis outbreaks studied in the United States were associated with Norwalk virus, and an additional 23% were provisionally associated (a minority of patients

TABLE 263.1. Epidemiologic Settings for Gastroenteritis Outbreaks Caused by Norwalk Virus

Ingestion of fecally contaminated foods (most common)
Community or family locations
Schools (elementary through college)
Military troops
Recreational camps
Athletic teams
Cruise ships
Contaminated drinking or swimming water
Ingestion of incompletely cooked shellfish
Nursing homes

showed seroconversion) with the virus or a related calicivirus. (38) More recently, using more sensitive molecular assays (see the section "Diagnosis"), Noroviruses have been identified as causing 96% of 90 outbreaks of nonbacterial gastroenteritis reported to the Centers for Disease Control and Prevention from January 1996 to June 1997 (39). Outbreaks typically occur in certain settings (Table 263.1), such contaminated drinking or swimming water, ingestion of raw or incompletely cooked shellfish or fecally contaminated foods (most common), recreational camps, cruise ships, nursing homes, schools (elementary through college), and community or family locations (40). Outbreaks occur during all seasons, affecting older (school-aged) children and adults, and seemingly sparing infants and young children; however, there is the suggestion that more sensitive diagnostic assays are revealing outbreaks and endemic disease in very young populations (41).

Sapoviruses typically cause gastroenteritis in infants and young children. Although less is known about their epidemiology than that of Norwalk virus, the illness resembles that produced by rotavirus and may cause 2% to 5% of pediatric diarrhea, including that found in day care centers (11,42–44).

In the United States, antibody prevalence levels to Norwalk virus are low in childhood, as determined by immunoassay using defined human clinical reagents. Antibody prevalence levels rapidly rise during adolescence and early adulthood, paralleling Norwalk disease expression, reaching about 60% of the population by middle age (45). In developing tropical nations, antibody prevalence increases at an earlier age, 2 to 6 years (45). Antibody prevalence levels to Noroviruses in China by immunoassay using recombinant virus capsid proteins as antigens are 90% by 5 years of age, with prevalence levels rising rapidly after the first year (46). Interestingly, a study of Finnish infants and young children provided evidence (seroconversions) for Norwalk virus infection when serum samples were tested in a more sensitive immunoassay containing baculovirus-expressed recombinant Norwalk virus capsid protein as antigen (47). Whether the occurrence of Norwalk virus infection and disease in the very young is actually widespread and common remains to be determined.

Norwalk virus infection has been shown conclusively in volunteer studies to be spread by the fecal-oral route (2). Some epidemiologic data suggest airborne transmission (48–50), which is consistent with its reported presence in vomitus and also with the extremely rapid secondary spread of Norwalk virus infection that is often observed.

Pathogenesis

Volunteer studies performed with Norwalk and Hawaii viruses reveal that gastroenteritis occurs in about half of those administered the virus orally (37). Illness is accompanied by a mucosal lesion of the proximal small intestine that is characterized by damage to villus absorptive cells, infiltration of the lamina propria by polymorphonuclear leukocytes and mononuclear cells, and villus shortening with crypt hypertrophy (51,52). These changes, associated with malabsorption of D-xylose, lactose, and fat, revert to normal within 2 weeks of the onset of illness. In contrast, the rectal mucosa and gastric mucosa are not altered during illness, although there is a marked delay in gastric motor function and emptying that is likely to be responsible for the nausea and vomiting (53).

Norwalk virus illness commonly occurs in the presence of preexisting serum or intestinal antibodies to the virus (8,54–57). Uninfected volunteers are more likely to have absent or lower preexisting antibody titers than infected individuals. Volunteers who have been rechallenged with the virus about 2 to 4 years later develop illness again. Volunteers remain well if they did not become ill on the first challenge, and they usually lack or have low levels of serum or intestinal antibody. Thus, the rise in serum antibody titer seen after Norwalk virus illness appears to be a marker for infection in susceptible persons and can lack a protective role. The explanation for the confusing aspects of clinical immunity seen with Norwalk virus is not clear. It is possible that the unusual pattern of clinical immunity is related to a genetic control of host susceptibility or the need for repeated exposures to the virus to generate illness and immune response. Recent studies have linked Norwalk virus infection to types of ABH histo–blood group antigens, because some antigens such as blood group O are cell receptors for the virus and others are not, such as blood group B (57a). It does seem that immunity to Norwalk virus is not long lasting and that repeated bouts of illness throughout life are possible. After a sufficient number of repeated illnesses due to the virus, it is conceivable that clinical immunity could develop.

Clinical Manifestations

Norwalk virus illness is typically acute and explosive, characterized by rapid onset of vomiting, diarrhea, or both; it is accompanied by a varying spectrum of signs and symptoms, such as abdominal cramps, low-grade fever, nausea, headache, malaise, and myalgia (2). Vomiting is more common in children, and diarrhea is more common in adults. Disease usually resolves spontaneously within 24 to 48 hours. Death is extremely rare; those who succumb are elderly or debilitated. A minority of patients may develop transient leukocytosis, and fecal leukocytes are nearly always absent.

Diagnosis

In an individual patient, a diagnosis of Norwalk virus gastroenteritis cannot be made on clinical grounds alone because the entity can be consistent with other causes of acute noninflammatory infectious diarrhea. A presumptive diagnosis during a disease outbreak can be made if there is an absence of bacterial or parasitic pathogens, the presence of vomiting in most cases, a duration of illness from 0.5 to 5 days, and an incubation period estimated at 1 to 2 days (58).

A specific diagnosis of Norwalk virus gastroenteritis requires demonstration of the virus or its antigen in feces or a rise in specific serum antibody titer to the virus. (Norwalk virus and other caliciviruses are not normally found in the stool of asymptomatic persons.) Immunoassay techniques are developed for the specific diagnosis of several Noroviruses but are not commercially available because they require limited supplies of human clinical diagnostic reagents to perform the tests (7–10,59). Immunoglob-

ulin M antibody responses to Norwalk virus can be detected and indicate recent infection, but the immunoglobulin M assays also require reagents derived from human volunteers (60,61). Use of IEM is impractical because it is too cumbersome for routine or rapid diagnosis. New diagnostic tests include immunoassays that use genetically assembled Norovirus capsid proteins that self-assemble into virus-like particles; these assays have, to date, been virus type–specific and not broadly reactive (19,40). Modification of these assays for serologic testing is also limited by type specificity, although not to the extent of the antigen assays (19,40). Nucleic acid hybridization assays and reverse transcription polymerase chain reaction assays detect Norovirus genomes in clinical specimens (62,63) and are the most sensitive of all diagnostic assays; they are still not sufficiently broadly reactive for widespread diagnostic use and can be subject to difficulties of laboratory contamination. They do, however, offer the most promise for eventual clinically useful diagnostic tests (19,40).

Treatment and Prevention

Because no specific antiviral therapy is available for Norwalk virus gastroenteritis, therapy must be supportive, including replacement of fluid and electrolytes, as for other infectious diarrheas. In one study, it was shown that oral administration of bismuth subsalicylate reduced the severity and duration of abdominal cramps in volunteers ill with Norwalk virus gastroenteritis and reduced the duration of gastrointestinal symptoms from 20 to 14 hours (64). Secondary spread of infection, as in nosocomial settings, can be prevented by standard enteric precautions. The duration of virus shedding can be up to 7 days, which is considerably longer than the length of symptomatic illness; viral antigen can be shed for prolonged periods, but it is not known whether infectious virus is also present (40). Volunteers exposed to the virus who remain asymptomatic may also shed it for up to a week (57). These findings carry implications for infection control practices. It will be difficult to develop a useful vaccine for long-term prevention of Norwalk virus illness because the natural disease does not confer long-term immunity. It is possible that a vaccine could be developed for short-term prevention of illness for travelers, for example, because volunteers who were previously ill remained well when challenged again 4 to 14 weeks later (54). Norwalk virus capsid protein, assembled into virus-like particles, represents a candidate vaccine; it generated modest immune responses in volunteers who were administered this vaccine in transgenic potatoes (65). Current efforts are directed at the study of mucosal adjuvants that could enhance immune responses (66).

ASTROVIRUSES

Characteristics of the Pathogen

Astrovirus can be visualized by direct EM examination of diarrheal stool samples from infants (12). The virus is a 27- to 32-nm diameter round particle that possesses a distinctive ultrastructure, exhibiting a five- or occasionally six-pointed star appearance on its surface and a continuous outer margin that forms a distinct rim (Fig. 263.1C). The virus is named after the star shape that appears on the surface of some particles. The morphologic characteristics of the astroviruses clearly distinguish them from those of the caliciviruses (12).

The virus can be cultivated in cell cultures treated with trypsin (13,67). This has facilitated viral characterization. The virus contains a positive-sense, single-stranded RNA genome of about

7.2 kb (67) that has three open reading frames coding for a viral protease, a polymerase, and a capsid precursor. Several astrovirus structural proteins are described, including an 87-kd protein produced in infected cells that reacts with monoclonal antibody specific for viral capsids (67). This protein may serve as a precursor to three to five smaller icosahedral capsid proteins of about 30 kd (68). Sequence analysis of the viral genome, together with the size and number of structural proteins, as well as the replication strategy characteristics of the virus, led to the official classification of astrovirus as a new family of RNA viruses, the Astroviridae (69).

There are eight viral serotypes, defined by IEM (13,70–72). A monoclonal antibody has been prepared that reacts with a group-specific antigen shared by all viral serotypes (13). When incorporated into an enzyme immunoassay format, the monoclonal antibody detects all astroviral serotypes in stool, thereby providing the framework for understanding the epidemiology and medical importance of the astroviruses (73).

Epidemiology

Astrovirus gastroenteritis is most prominent in young children but also occurs in immunocompromised individuals and elderly institutionalized patients (14,74,75). Peak occurrence is in the winter months in temperate regions and in the rainy season in tropical areas (76,77). Infection is spread person to person by the fecal-oral route and by contaminated food and water (78).

The disease occurs in several clinical settings (Table 263.2). Most noteworthy is endemic childhood diarrhea, typically among children younger than 2 years, for which astrovirus appears to be responsible for about 3% to 9% of cases in studies performed in Asia, Europe, Central America, and the United States (14,77,79–85). Astrovirus is also an important pathogen in day care settings, where it has caused 4% to 7% of cases of diarrhea (86–88). The virus seems to be a common cause of nosocomial outbreaks of infant diarrhea as well as of non-outbreak nosocomial gastroenteritis (89,90). A recent U.S. study revealed it as the cause of 6.8% of community-acquired pediatric diarrhea requiring hospitalization as well as the cause of 16.2% of nosocomial diarrhea (91). An Australian study indicated astrovirus as causing 3% of pediatric diarrhea requiring hospitalization (92). It appears to be an uncommon cause of epidemic diarrhea, unlike calicivirus, with only a few outbreaks reported (93–95). However, astrovirus infection does appear to produce significant clinical illness in elderly and immunocompromised patients in whom immunity may have waned (74,75,96,97). Several disease outbreaks have been diagnosed in residential facilities for the elderly and on geriatric wards (75,96,97). In the most complete study reported to date of the role of enteric viruses in acute diarrhea of patients with acquired immunodeficiency syndrome (that employed a broad repertoire of assays to detect all known human diarrhea viruses), astrovirus was most commonly

identified (12% of cases) (74). Indeed, it produced diarrhea more frequently than any pathogen, whether bacterial, parasitic, or viral. Finally, in one study, astrovirus caused 4% of episodes of diarrhea occurring after bone marrow transplantation, equaling *Clostridium difficile* as the most common identifiable infectious agent (98).

In the United Kingdom, antibody prevalence levels to astroviruses rise rapidly during early childhood, reaching more than 70% of the population by 3 to 4 years of age. (99). Most adults have serum antibodies. Antibodies to all viral serotypes are present in commercial preparations of human γ-globulin in the United States and Japan (94,100). Because most astrovirus disease occurs in the young, but disease outbreaks are found in elderly people, it may be that most young adults are protected by antibody levels that decline with age. Cellular immunity may also be important because helper T cells in the duodenal mucosa of adults have been shown to react with specificity against astrovirus (101).

Pathogenesis

In the only reported histopathologic study to date, astrovirus has been visualized by EM in human intestinal epithelial cells obtained by small intestinal biopsy from two children who also shed the virus in diarrheal stool (102). The only other pathogenesis data in humans are derived from limited volunteer studies. In two studies, a total of 36 adult volunteers were administered astrovirus orally, only 2 of whom developed unequivocal gastroenteritis (75,103). Virus-specific antibody rises (seroconversion) developed in most volunteers, and fecal virus shedding in some. It therefore seems that astrovirus is of relatively low pathogenicity in immunocompetent, healthy young adults, in contrast to the effect of Norwalk virus in volunteers.

Clinical Manifestations

Astrovirus illness typically consists of watery diarrhea lasting 2 to 5 days in immunocompetent patients, with vomiting sometimes less common than that seen with calicivirus illness (14,75,94). Accompanying findings include fever, anorexia, nausea, and abdominal pain. Dehydration in ill infants and young children occurs less commonly than with rotavirus disease (14). Diarrhea may occasionally last 7 to 14 days with prolonged fecal virus shedding, and some patients can develop prolonged lactose intolerance (104). Illness in immunocompromised patients can also be prolonged (98,104).

Diagnosis

The traditional gold standard for diagnosis has been examination of stool specimens by EM (12). However, this technique is cumbersome, expensive, and restricted to highly experienced electron microscopists. A monoclonal antibody–based enzyme immunoassay test detects all astrovirus serotypes in stools with a high degree of sensitivity and specificity and has been the basis for many reported clinicoepidemiologic studies (71,73). This enzyme immunoassay test makes the diagnosis of astrovirus infection much more practical and inexpensive than EM. Detection of astrovirus or its antigen in stool typically indicates symptomatic infection because the virus is not usually found in asymptomatic persons. A reverse transcription polymerase chain reaction test to diagnose astrovirus infection in stools has also been developed, and its findings have closely correlated with and confirmed the enzyme immunoassay diagnostic test results (74,87,92,98,105,106).

TABLE 263.2. Clinical Settings for Astrovirus Infections

Endemic diarrhea of infants and young children
Day care center diarrhea
Nosocomial diarrhea
Epidemic diarrhea of school-aged children and adults
Nursing home diarrhea
Diarrhea in bone marrow transplant recipients
Acute diarrhea in patients with acquired immunodeficiency syndrome

Treatment and Prevention

Therapy is supportive with replacement of fluid and electrolytes. Virus transmission is prevented by standard enteric precautions. Virus shedding in stool can continue for several days after resolution of diarrhea (104). Further understanding of the economic importance of astrovirus diarrhea and of the mechanisms of immunity to the virus is necessary before vaccine development can be considered.

REFERENCES

1. Kapikian AZ, Wyatt RG, Dolin R, et al. Visualization by immune electron microscopy of a 27-nm particle associated with acute infectious nonbacterial gastroenteritis. *J Virol* 1972;10:1075–1081.
2. Blacklow NR, Dolin R, Fedson DS, et al. Acute infectious nonbacterial gastroenteritis: etiology and pathogenesis. *Ann Intern Med* 1972;76:993.
3. Jiang X, Graham DY, Wang K, et al. Norwalk virus genome cloning and characterization. *Science* 1990;250:1580.
4. Jiang X, Wang M, Wang K, et al. Sequence and genomic organization of Norwalk virus. *Virology* 1993;195:51.
5. Caul EO, Appleton H. The electron microscopical and physical characteristics of small round human fecal viruses: an interim scheme for classification. *J Med Virol* 1982;9:257.
6. Caul EO. Small round human fecal viruses. In: Pattison JR, ed. *Parvoviruses and human disease.* Boca Raton, FL: CRC Press, 1988:139–163.
7. Greenberg HB, Wyatt RG, Valdesuso J, et al. Solid-phase microtiter radioimmunoassay for detection of the Norwalk strain of acute nonbacterial epidemic gastroenteritis virus and its antibodies. *J Med Virol* 1978;2:97.
8. Blacklow NR, Cukor G, Bedigian MK, et al. Immune response and prevalence of antibody to Norwalk enteritis virus as determined by radioimmunoassay. *J Clin Microbiol* 1979;10:903.
9. Dolin R, Roessner KD, Treanor JJ, et al. Radioimmunoassay for detection of the Snow Mountain agent of viral gastroenteritis. *J Med Virol* 1986;19:11.
10. Treanor JJ, Madore HP, Dolin R. Development of an enzyme immunoassay for the Hawaii agent of viral gastroenteritis. *J Virol Methods* 1988;22:207.
11. Cubitt WD. The candidate caliciviruses. *Ciba Found Symp* 1987;128:157.
12. Madeley CR. Comparison of the features of astroviruses and caliciviruses seen in samples of feces by electron microscopy. *J Infect Dis* 1979;139:519.
13. Herrmann JE, Hudson RW, Perron-Henry DM, et al. Antigenic characterization of cell-cultivated astrovirus serotypes and development of astrovirus-specific monoclonal antibodies. *J Infect Dis* 1988;158:182.
14. Herrmann JE, Taylor DN, Echeverria P, et al. Astroviruses as a cause of gastroenteritis in children. *N Engl J Med* 1991;324:1757.
15. Kapikian AZ, Chanock RM. Norwalk group of viruses. In: Fields BN, Knipe DM, eds. *Virology.* New York: Raven Press, 1985:1495–1517.
16. Prasad BV, Hardy ME, Dokland T, et al. X-ray crystallographic structure of the Norwalk virus capsid. *Science* 1999;286:287.
17. Greenberg HB, Valdesuso JR, Kalica AR, et al. Proteins of Norwalk virus. *J Virol* 1981;37:994.
18. Glass PJ, White LJ, Ball JM, et al. The Norwalk virus ORF3 encodes a minor structural protein. *J Virol* 2000;74:6581.
19. Atmar RL, Estes MK. Diagnosis of noncultivatable gastroenteritis viruses, the human caliciviruses. *Clin Microbiol Rev* 2001;14:15.
20. Green J, Norcott JP, Lewis D, et al. Norwalk-like viruses: demonstration of genomic diversity by polymerase chain reaction. *J Clin Microbiol* 1991;31:3007.
21. Lambden PR, Carl EO, Ashley CR, et al. Sequence and genome organization of a human small round-structured (Norwalk-like) virus. *Science* 1993;259:516.
22. Moe CL, Gentsch J, Grohmann G, et al. Application of PCR to detect Norwalk virus in fecal specimens from outbreaks of gastroenteritis. *J Clin Microbiol* 1994;32:642.
23. Lew JF, Petric M, Kapikian AZ, et al. Identification of "minireovirus" as a Norwalk-like virus in pediatric patients with gastroenteritis. *J Virol* 1994;68:3391.
24. Lew JF, Kapikian AZ, Jiang X, et al. Molecular characterization and expression of the capsid protein of a Norwalk-like virus recovered from a Desert Shield troop with gastroenteritis. *Virology* 1994;200:319.
25. Lew JF, Kapikian AZ, Valdesuso J, et al. Molecular characterization of Hawaii virus and other Norwalk-like viruses: evidence for genetic polymorphism among human caliciviruses. *J Infect Dis* 1994;170:535.
26. Wang J, Jiang X, Madore HP, et al. Sequence diversity of small round structured viruses. *J Virol* 1994;68:5982.
27. Cubitt WD, Jiang XJ, Wang J, et al. Sequence similarity of human caliciviruses and small round structured viruses. *J Med Virol* 1994;43:252.
28. Green SM, Dingle KE, Lambden PR, et al. Human enteric caliciviridae: a new prevalent SRSV group defined by RNA-dependent RNA polymerase and capsid diversity. *J Gen Virol* 1994;75:1883.
29. Matson DO, Zhong WM, Nakata S, et al. Molecular characterization of a human calicivirus with sequence relationships closer to animal caliciviruses than other known human caliciviruses. *J Med Virol* 1995;45:215.
30. Ando T, Monroe SS, Gentsch JR, et al. Detection and differentiation of antigeni-

31. cally distinct small round-structured viruses (Norwalk-like viruses) by reverse transcription-PCR and Southern hybridization. *J Clin Microbiol* 1995;33:64.
31. Liu BL, Clarke IN, Caul EO, et al. Human enteric caliciviruses have a unique genome structure and are distinct from the Norwalk-like viruses. *Arch Virol* 1995;140:1345.
32. Jiang X, Wang J, Estes MK. Characterization of SRSVs using RT-PCR and a new antigen ELISA. *Arch Virol* 1995;140:363.
33. Yuen LKW, Catton MG, Cox BJ, et al. Heminested multiplex reverse transcription-PCR for detection and differentiation of Norwalk-like virus genogroups 1 and 2 in fecal samples. *J Clin Microbiol* 2001;39:2690.
34. Green KY, Ando T, Balayan MS, et al. Taxonomy of the caliciviruses. *J Infect Dis* 2000;181[Suppl 2]:S322.
35. Ando T, Noel JS, Fankhauser RL. Genetic classification of "Norwalk-like viruses." *J Infect Dis* 2000;181[Suppl 2]:S336.
36. Cubitt WD, Blacklow NR, Herrmann JE, et al. Antigenic relationships between human caliciviruses and Norwalk virus. *J Infect Dis* 1987;156:806.
37. Blacklow NR, Greenberg HB. Viral gastroenteritis. *N Engl J Med* 1991;325:252.
38. Kaplan JE, Gary GW, Baron RC, et al. Epidemiology of Norwalk gastroenteritis and the role of Norwalk virus in outbreaks of acute nonbacterial gastroenteritis. *Ann Intern Med* 1982;96:756.
39. Fankhauser RL, Noel JS, Monroe SS, et al. Molecular epidemiology of "Norwalk-like viruses" in outbreaks of gastroenteritis in the United States. *J Infect Dis* 1998;178:1571.
40. Centers for Disease Control. Norwalk-like viruses: public health consequences and outbreak management. *Morb Mortal Wkly Rep* 2001;50[Suppl].
41. Pang XL, Joensuu J, Vesikari T. Human calicivirus-associated sporadic gastroenteritis in Finnish children less than two years of age followed prospectively during a rotavirus vaccine trial. *Pediatr Infect Dis* 1999;18:420.
42. Nakata S, Honma S, Numata KK, et al. Members of the family Caliciviridae are the most prevalent cause of gastroenteritis outbreaks among infants in Japan. *J Infect Dis* 2000;181:2029.
43. Matson DO, Estes MK, Glass RI, et al. Human calicivirus-associated diarrhea in children attending day care centers. *J Infect Dis* 1989;159:71.
44. Riepenhoff-Talty M, Saif LJ, Barrett HJ, et al. Potential spectrum of etiological agents of viral enteritis in hospitalized infants. *J Clin Microbiol* 1983;17:352.
45. Cukor G, Blacklow NR, Echeverria P, et al. Comparative study of the acquisition of antibody to Norwalk virus in pediatric populations. *Infect Immun* 1980;29:822.
46. Jing Y, Qian Y, Huo Y, et al. Seroprevalence against Norwalk-like human caliciviruses in Beijing, China. *J Med Virol* 2000;60:97.
47. Lew JF, Valdesuso J, Vesikari T, et al. Detection of Norwalk virus or Norwalk-like virus infections in Finnish infants and young children. *J Infect Dis* 1994;169:1364.
48. Sawyer LA, Murphy JJ, Kaplan JE, et al. 25- to 30 nm virus particle associated with a hospital outbreak of acute gastroenteritis with evidence for airborne transmission. *Am J Epidemiol* 1988;127:1261.
49. Marks PJ, Vipond IB, Carlisle D, et al. Evidence for airborne transmission of Norwalk-like virus (NLV) in a hotel restaurant. *Epidemiol Infect* 2000;124:481.
50. Cheesbrough JS, Green J, Gallimore CI, et al. Widespread environmental contamination with Norwalk-like viruses (NLV) detected in a prolonged hotel outbreak of gastroenteritis. *Epidemiol Infect* 2000;125:93.
51. Schreiber DS, Blacklow NR, Trier JS. The mucosal lesion of the proximal small intestine in acute infectious nonbacterial gastroenteritis. *N Engl J Med* 1973;288:1318.
52. Schreiber DS, Blacklow NR, Trier JS. The small intestinal lesion induced by Hawaii agent acute infectious nonbacterial gastroenteritis. *J Infect Dis* 1974;129:705.
53. Meeroff JC, Schreiber DS, Trier JS, et al. Abnormal gastric motor function in viral gastroenteritis. *Ann Intern Med* 1980;92:370.
54. Parrino TA, Schreiber DS, Trier JS, et al. Clinical immunity in acute gastroenteritis caused by Norwalk agent. *N Engl J Med* 1977;297:86.
55. Greenberg HB, Wyatt RG, Kalica AR, et al. New insights in viral gastroenteritis. *Perspect Virol* 1981;11:163.
56. Johnson PC, Mathewson JJ, DuPont HL, et al. Multiple challenge study of host susceptibility to Norwalk gastroenteritis in U.S. adults. *J Infect Dis* 1990;161:18.
57. Graham DY, Jiang X, Tanaka T, et al. Norwalk virus infection of volunteers: new insights based on improved assays. *J Infect Dis* 1994;170:34.
57a. Lindesmith L. Human susceptibility and resistance to Norwalk virus infection. *Nat Med* 2003;9:548.
58. Kaplan JE, Feldman R, Campbell DS, et al. The frequency of a Norwalk-like pattern of illness in outbreaks of acute gastroenteritis. *Am J Public Health* 1982;72:1329.
59. Herrmann JE, Blacklow NR, Matsui SM, et al. Monoclonal antibodies for detection of Norwalk virus antigen in stools. *J Clin Microbiol* 1995;33:2511.
60. Cukor G, Nowak NA, Blacklow NR. Immunoglobulin M responses to the Norwalk virus of gastroenteritis. *Infect Immun* 1982;37:463.
61. Erdman DD, Gary GW, Anderson LJ. Development and evaluation of an IgM capture enzyme immunoassay for diagnosis of recent Norwalk virus infection. *J Virol Methods* 1989;24:57.
62. DeLeon R, Matsui SM, Baric RS, et al. Detection of Norwalk virus in stool specimens by reverse transcriptase-polymerase chain reaction and nonradioactive oligoprobes. *J Clin Microbiol* 1992;30:3151.
63. Jiang X, Wang J, Graham DY, et al. Detection of Norwalk virus in stool by polymerase chain reaction. *J Clin Microbiol* 1992;30:2529.

64. Steinhoff MC, Douglas RG Jr, Greenberg HB, et al. Bismuth subsalicylate therapy of viral gastroenteritis. *Gastroenterology* 1980;78:1495.
65. Tacket CO, Mason MS, Losonsky G, et al. Human immune responses to a novel Norwalk virus vaccine in transgenic potatoes. *J Infect Dis* 2000;182:302.
66. Guerrero RO, Ball JM, Krater SS, et al. Recombinant Norwalk virus-like particles administered intranasally to mice induce systemic and mucosal (fecal and vaginal) immune responses. *J Virol* 2001;75:9713.
67. Lewis TL, Greenberg HB, Herrmann JE, et al. Analysis of astrovirus serotype 1 RNA, identification of the viral RNA-dependent RNA polymerase motif, and expression of a viral structural protein. *J Virol* 1994;68:77.
68. Monroe SS, Stine SE, Goulkin L, et al. Temporal synthesis of proteins and RNAs during human astrovirus infection of cultured cells. *J Virol* 1991;65:641.
69. Monroe SS, Jiang B, Stine SE, et al. Subgenomic RNA sequence of human astrovirus supports classification of Astroviridae as a new family of RNA viruses. *J Virol* 1993;67:3611.
70. Lee TW, Kurtz JB. Prevalence of human astrovirus serotypes in the Oxford region 1976–92, with evidence for two new serotypes. *Epidemiol Infect* 1994;112:187.
71. Glass RI, Noel J, Mitchell DK, et al. The changing epidemiology of astrovirus-associated gastroenteritis: a review. *Arch Virol* 1996;12[Suppl]:287.
72. Taylor MB, Walter J, Berke T, et al. Characterization of a South African human astrovirus as type 8 by antigenic and genetic analyses. *J Med Virol* 2001;64:256.
73. Herrmann JE, Nowak NA, Perron-Henry DM, et al. Diagnosis of astrovirus gastroenteritis by antigen detection with monoclonal antibodies. *J Infect Dis* 1990;161:226.
74. Grohmann GS, Glass RI, Pereira HG, et al. Enteric viruses and diarrhea in HIV-infected patients. *N Engl J Med* 1993;329:14.
75. Midthun K, Greenberg HB, Kurtz JB, et al. Characterization and seroepidemiology of a type 5 astrovirus associated with an outbreak of gastroenteritis in Marin County, California. *J Clin Microbiol* 1993;31:955.
76. Bates PR, Bailey AS, Wood DJ, et al. Comparative epidemiology of rotavirus, subgenus F (types 40 and 41) adenovirus, and astrovirus gastroenteritis in children. *J Med Virol* 1993;39:224.
77. Cruz JR, Bartlett AV, Herrmann JE, et al. Astrovirus-associated diarrhea among Guatemalan ambulatory rural children. *J Clin Microbiol* 1992;30:1140.
78. Appleton H. Small round viruses: classification and role in food-borne infections. *Ciba Found Symp* 1987;128:108.
79. Kurtz JB, Lee TW, Pickering D. Astrovirus-associated gastroenteritis in a children's ward. *J Clin Pathol* 1977;30:948.
80. Madeley CR, Cosgrove BP, Bell EJ, et al. Stool viruses in babies in Glasgow. I. Hospital admission with diarrhea. *J Hyg (Lond)* 1977;78:261.
81. Ashley CR, Caul EO, Paver WK. Astrovirus-associated gastroenteritis in children. *J Clin Pathol* 1978;31:939.
82. Kotloff KL, Herrmann JE, Blacklow NR, et al. The frequency of astrovirus as a cause of diarrhea in Baltimore children. *Pediatr Infect Dis* 1992;11:587.
83. Utagawa ET, Nishizawa S, Sekine S, et al. Astrovirus as a cause of gastroenteritis in Japan. *J Clin Microbiol* 1994;32:1841.
84. Pang XL, Vesikari T. Human astrovirus-associated gastroenteritis in children under 2 years of age followed prospectively during a rotavirus vaccine trial. *Acta Paediatr* 1999;88:532.
85. Naficy AB, Rao MR, Holmes JL, et al. Astrovirus diarrhea in Egyptian children. *J Infect Dis* 2000;182:685.
86. Lew JF, Moe CL, Monroe SS, et al. Astrovirus and adenovirus associated with diarrhea in children in day care settings. *J Infect Dis* 1991;164:673.
87. Mitchell DK, Van R, Morrow AL, et al. Outbreaks of astrovirus gastroenteritis in day care centers. *J Pediatr* 1993;123:725.
88. Mitchell DK, Matson DO, Jiang X, et al. Molecular epidemiology of childhood astrovirus infection in child care centers. *J Infect Dis* 1999;180:514.
89. Esahli H, Breback K, Bennet R, et al. Astroviruses as a cause of nosocomial outbreaks of infant diarrhea. *Pediatr Infect Dis* 1991;10:511.
90. Ford-Jones EL, Mendorff CM, Langley JM, et al. Epidemiologic study of 4684 hospital-acquired infections in pediatric patients. *Pediatr Infect Dis J* 1989;8:668.
91. Dennehy PH, Nelson SM, Spangenberger S, et al. A prospective case-control study of the role of astrovirus in acute diarrhea among hospitalized young children. *J Infect Dis* 2001;184:10.
92. Mustafa H, Palombo EA, Bishop RF. Epidemiology of astrovirus infection in young children hospitalized with acute gastroenteritis in Melbourne, Australia, over a period of four consecutive years, 1995–1998. *J Clin Microbiol* 2000;38:1058.
93. Oishi I, Yamazaki K, Kimoto T, et al. A large outbreak of acute gastroenteritis associated with astrovirus among students and teachers in Osaka, Japan. *J Infect Dis* 1994;170:439.
94. Konno T, Suzuki H, Ishida N, et al. Astrovirus-associated epidemic gastroenteritis in Japan. *J Med Virol* 1982;9:11.
95. Belliot G, Laveran H, Monroe SS. Outbreak of gastroenteritis in military recruits associated with serotype 3 astrovirus infection. *J Med Virol* 1997;51:101.
96. Gray JJ, Wreghitt TG, Cubitt WD, et al. An outbreak of gastroenteritis in a home for the elderly associated with astrovirus type 1 and human calicivirus. *J Med Virol* 1987;23:377.
97. Lewis DC, Lightfoot NF, Cubitt WD, et al. Outbreaks of astrovirus type 1 and rotavirus gastroenteritis in a geriatric inpatient population. *J Hosp Infect* 1989;14:9.
98. Cox GJ, Matsui SM, Lo RS, et al. Etiology and outcome of diarrhea after marrow transplantation: a prospective study. *Gastroenterology* 1994;107:1398.
99. Kurtz J, Lee T. Astrovirus gastroenteritis age distribution of antibody. *Microbiol Immunol* 1978;166:227.
100. LeBaron CW, Furutan NP, Lew JF, et al. Viral agents of gastroenteritis: public health importance and outbreak management. *MMWR Morb Mortal Wkly Rep* 1990;39:1.
101. Molberg O, Nilsen EM, Sollid LM, et al. CD4+ T cells with specific reactivity against astrovirus isolated from normal human small intestine. *Gastroenterology* 1998;114:115.
102. Phillips AD, Rice SJ, Walker-Smith JA. Astrovirus within human small intestinal mucosa. *Gut* 1982;23:A923.
103. Kurtz JB, Lee TW, Craig JW, et al. Astrovirus infection in volunteers. *J Med Virol* 1979;3:221.
104. Kurtz JB, Lee TW. Astroviruses: human and animal. *Ciba Found Symp* 1987;128:92.
105. Sakomoto T, Negishi H, Wang QH, et al. Molecular epidemiology of astroviruses in Japan from 1995 to 1998 by reverse transcription-polymerase chain reaction with serotype-specific primers (1 to 8). *J Med Virol* 2000;61:326.
106. Sakon N, Yamazaki K, Utagawa E, et al. Genomic characterization of human astrovirus type 6 Katano virus and the establishment of a rapid and effective reverse transcription-polymerase chain reaction to detect all serotypes of human astrovirus. *J Med Virol* 2000;61:125.

VIII

Unconventional Agents Causing Slow Infections

CHAPTER 264
Transmissible Spongiform Encephalopathies

David M. Asher

The transmissible spongiform encephalopathies (TSEs) constitute a group of slow infections of the nervous system (see Chapter 153) with unique agents whose nature remains controversial (1). At least five clinically distinct TSEs have been recognized in humans (Table 264.l): kuru (2); Creutzfeldt-Jakob disease (CJD) (3,4), often subdivided into sporadic, iatrogenic, and familial syndromes (5); Gerstmann-Sträussler-Scheinker syndrome (GSS) (6), considered by some to be a familial CJD; and a unique new "variant" of CJD (vCJD) (7,8) in people exposed to the agent of bovine spongiform encephalopathy (BSE). The syndromes of fatal familial insomnia (FFI) (9) and a similar sporadic disease (10) have also been attributed to infection with a TSE agent (10–12).

TSEs also affect a variety of animals: scrapie in sheep and goats (13), transmissible mink encephalopathy (TME) in ranch mink (14–16), and chronic wasting disease (CWD) in American elk and deer (17–19). In 1986, BSE was first recognized among British cattle and zoo ungulates (20); feline spongiform encephalopathy of domestic cats and zoo felines probably originated from BSE (21).

All TSEs share a generally similar clinical and histopathologic picture of progressive neurologic degeneration, differing in some features, including the areas of central nervous system most affected, and all are associated with infectious agents similar in properties. The TSEs take their name (5,22) from a striking neuropathologic change that occurs in each disease to a greater or lesser extent: neuronal vacuolation leading to spongy degeneration of the cerebral cortical gray matter (Fig. 264.l).

ETIOLOGIC AGENTS OF TRANSMISSIBLE SPONGIFORM ENCEPHALOPATHIES

Brain tissues (and other tissues less consistently) of humans and animals with TSEs harbor infectious agents demonstrable by experimental transmission of disease to susceptible animals (23) (Fig. 264.2). The infectious agents replicate in some cell cultures (24–36), but they do not achieve the high titers of infectivity found in brain tissues, nor do they cause recognizable cytopathic effects (37). Although not replacing animals as an assay for infectivity, cell cultures have been useful for studying the synthesis and secretion of abnormal prion protein (PrP)—the protease-resistant protein associated with the agents—and the potential effects of drug treatments on TSEs (28,30–36,38–41). Most studies characterizing the infectious agents and the pathogenesis of infection have employed the agent of sheep scrapie adapted to rodents (42).

Pathogens transmitting TSEs were originally called viruses (23). Titrations of infectivity by serial dilution of suspensions taken from tissues of animals in successive passages clearly demonstrate that the TSE agents replicate. The infectivity of scrapie agent was retained by filters with average pore diameter of 50 nm or less (43,44), suggesting that it has the physical size of a small virus (45,46). However, the TSE agents are much more resistant to inactivation by a variety of chemical and physical treatments, including heat, ultraviolet light, and ionizing radiation than are conventional viruses, stimulating hypotheses that they might be unique pathogens not containing nucleic acid (47–49). The demonstration that infectivity of scrapie was substantially reduced by treatments that denature proteins (50) indicated that the infectious moiety must either contain or be protected by a protein. Prusiner concluded that the pathogens causing TSEs are probably subviral in size, devoid of nucleic acid, and contain protein, and he proposed that they be called *prions* for proteinaceous infectious agent (49,51). Proponents of a rival theory, that the agents are composed of a tiny unique nucleic acid protected by host components, suggested the term *virino* (52,53).

The prion or "all-protein" hypothesis is now widely but not universally accepted (54,55). The unusual resistance of TSE agents to heat and chemical exposures may repose in a tiny resistant fraction, the great bulk of infectivity being destroyed with kinetics of inactivation resembling those of known viruses (45,46). This resistant fraction may be protected from inactivation by host proteins and by aggregation into hydrophobic masses. These anomalies make it difficult to interpret inactivation studies as ruling out a nucleic acid component within the scrapie agent. Irradiation inactivation kinetic studies were reinterpreted as consistent with the hypothesis that the scrapie agent might have a nucleic acid genome of small viral size (56). Even proponents of the prion theory originally allowed for a possibility that the infectious particle might contain a small nucleic acid (57–59).

Studies showed that transgenic mice overexpressing certain transfected recombinant genes for the prion protein (PrP,

TABLE 264.1.   Transmissible Spongiform Encephalopathies (TSEs) Slow Infections of the Nervous System Caused by Unconventional Agents (TSE Agents or Prions)

Disease	Naturally infected hosts	Familial occurrence
Creutzfeldt-Jakob disease (CJD)	Humans	Sometimes
Familial CJD (fCJD)		Yes
Sporadic CJD (sCJD)		No
Iatrogenic CJD (iCJD)		No
Variant CJD (vCJD)		No
Gerstmann-Sträussler-Scheinker syndrome (GSS)	Humans	Yes
Fatal insomnia syndromes[a]	Humans	Usually
Fatal familial		Yes
Sporadic fatal		No
Kuru	Humans	No
Bovine spongiform encephalopathy (BSE)	Cattle, other ungulates, felines as feline spongiform encephalopathy (FSE), humans as vCJD	No
Chronic wasting disease	American and Canadian deer, elk	No
Scrapie	Sheep, goats	No (resistant genotypes)
Transmissible mink encephalopathy	Mink	No

[a]Histologically not spongiform.

discussed later) became ill with a spongiform encephalopathy (60), and extracts of their brain (containing surprisingly little abnormal PrP) were claimed to have transmitted encephalopathy to hamsters and some transgenic mice, although not to ordinary mice (61), in serial passage. Those results would strongly support the prion hypothesis but have never been independently confirmed.

Possible virus-like structures have been described in brain tissues from animals and humans with TSEs. Unique tubulovesicular particles have been regularly seen in thin sections of plastic-embedded infected tissue (62,63) (Fig. 264.3); they have not been demonstrated to contain either prion protein or nucleic acid or to be associated with infectivity (64). No nucleic acids unique to the TSEs have been identified (65,66), although those attempts should be repeated using more powerful molecular methodology now available (67). Until their actual structure is determined

unambiguously and the component encoding the self-replicating pathogenic information identified, it seems less contentious to continue calling them simply TSE agents.

Merz and colleagues (68–70) observed scrapie-associated fibrils (Fig. 263.4), resembling but distinguishable from the amyloid fibrils that accumulate in brains of patients with Alzheimer's disease, in extracts of tissues from patients and animals with TSEs. Prusiner and co-workers described a group of antigenically related low-molecular-weight proteins, relatively resistant to digestion with the enzyme proteinase K (PK) and ranging in mass from about 27 to 30 kd (Fig. 264.5), in brain of animals with scrapie (71) and in patients with CJD (72,73). They postulated that the abnormal proteins might be the prions or a component of them, and they designated the proteins as prion protein 27–30, or PrP27–30 (74). Scrapie-associated fibrils were found to contain PrP27–30 (75–77). PrP27–30—or, more

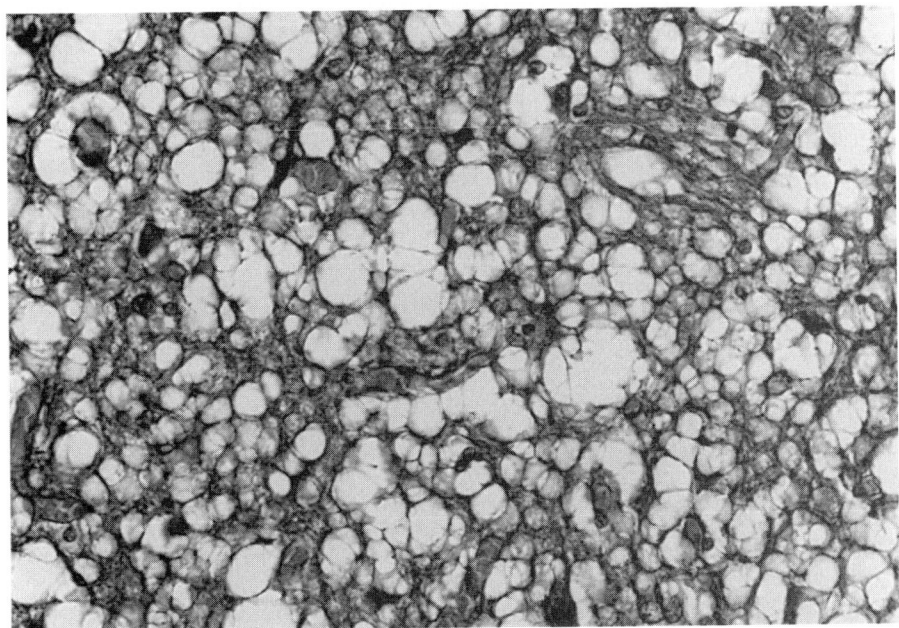

Figure 264.1. Status spongiosus: severe vacuolation in the cerebral cortex of a young man who died with familial CJD. (Hematoxylin and eosin stain.) (From Asher DM. Slow viral infections. In: Scheld WM, Whitley RJ, Durack DT, eds. *Infections of the central nervous system,* 2nd ed. Philadelphia: Lippincott-Raven, 1997:199–221, with permission.)

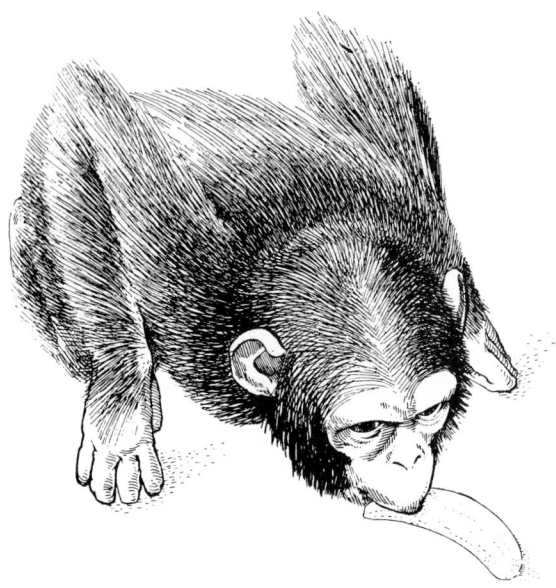

Figure 264.2. A chimpanzee in the intermediate stage of experimental kuru has lost normal prehension and eats directly from the floor. (From Asher DM, Gibbs CJ Jr, David E, et al. Experimental kuru in the chimpanzee. In: Montagna W, McNulty WP, eds. *Symposia of the Fourth International Congress of Primatology, Beaverton, Oregon,* Vol 4. Basel: S Karger, 1973:44, with permission.)

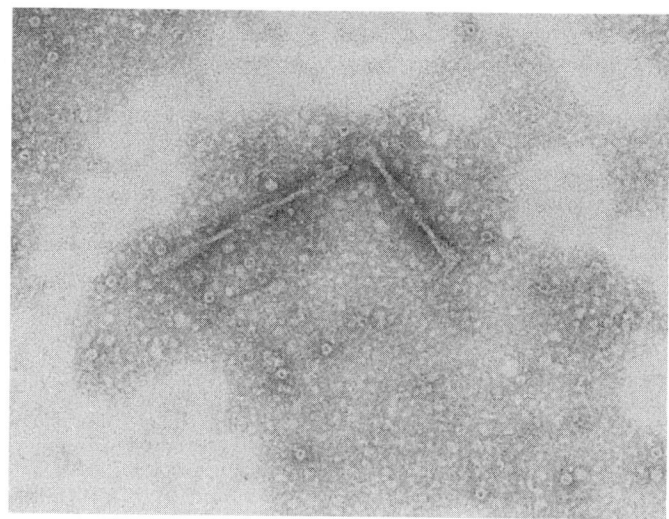

Figure 264.4. Scrapie-associated fibrils extracted from the brain of a hamster with scrapie. (Phosphotungstic acid stain.) (From Asher DM, Gibbs CJ Jr. Chronic neurological diseases caused by slow infections. In: Evans AS, Kaslow R, eds. *Viral infections of humans,* 2nd ed. New York: Plenum, 1997:1027–1051, with permission.)

precisely, a larger protein, also relatively resistant to PK, from which PrP27–30 is cleaved during extraction from tissues—is found consistently in brain of patients and animals with TSEs (78) and in TSE amyloid plaques (76). Abnormal PrP generally co-purifies with infectivity of scrapie (51,79), although several groups claimed to have separated infectivity from PrP (80–82) or found differences between the physical behavior of the infectious entity and that of PrP (83–85). Therefore, it remains controversial whether abnormal PrP constitutes the complete infectious TSE agent or is a component of the agent or simply an important pathologic host protein not usually separated from the agent. The demonstration that PrP is encoded by a normal host gene (86,87) with an amino acid sequence identical to that of the normal gene product (88) seemed to favor the last possibility, as did the recognition that there are distinct strains of scrapie agent.

There are substantial differences in several properties of disease transmitted by isolates of the same TSE to animals—differences in incubation periods (89,90) and in histologic picture, including presence and distribution of amyloid plaques in brain (89,91) and of vacuolation (92). Those properties are determined by the agent and are usually not altered after serial passages in animals or even after passages through animals of another species expressing a different PrP (93). Agent-specific properties have occasionally changed suddenly and then remained stable on subsequent passages in animals, a phenomenon resembling mutation (90). It is not understood how agent-specific information can be transmitted and replicated in the absence of some genetic material independent of the host. Ingenious hypotheses have been proposed to explain how a host-coded protein, the gene for which is present and expressed in all normal subjects, might replicate and transmit pathogenic information (94–97). It was proposed that differences in protein conformation alone might serve to transmit self-replicating pathogenic information (23,97–103). One study found

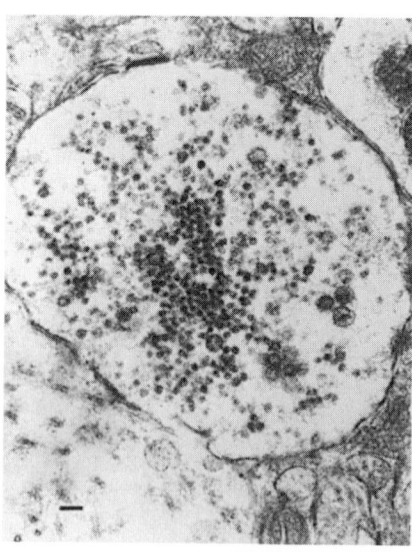

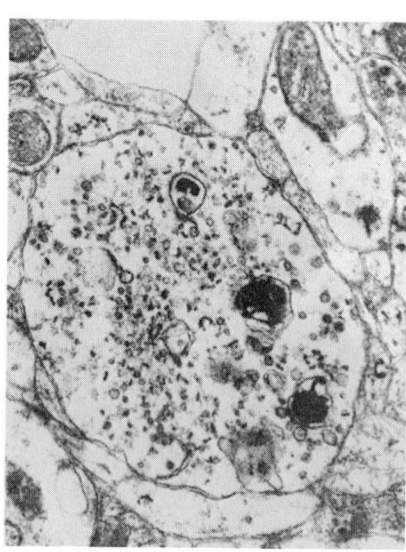

Figure 264.3. Tubulovesicular particles measuring about 23 nm across in the postsynaptic process of a mouse with scrapie (*left*) and a patient with CJD (*right*). (Bar = 100 nm.) (Courtesy of Dr. Harash K. Narang, Public Health Laboratory, Newcastle upon Tyne, England.)

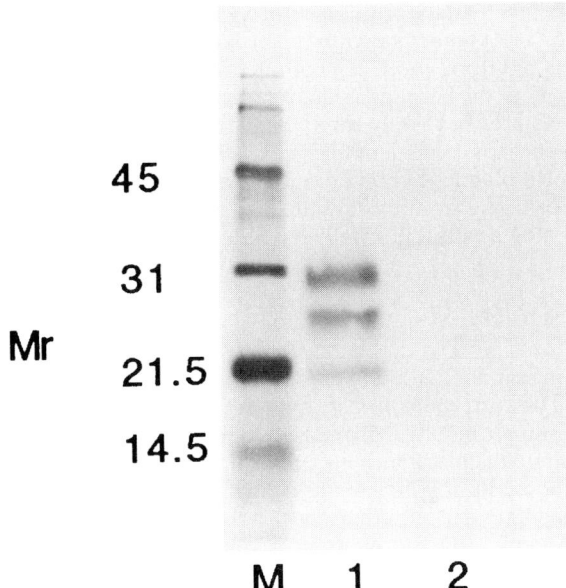

Figure 264.5. Immunoblot of brain extracts with antibodies to PrP27-30. Detergent-protease K extracts of brain tissues from a patient with Gerstmann-Sträussler-Scheinker syndrome (1) and a patient without neurologic disease (2) were fractionated by polyacrylamide gel electrophoresis, transferred to a nitrocellulose membrane, incubated with rabbit antiserum to hamster PrP, and then stained by an indirect immunoperoxidase method. M, molecular weight markers. (From Asher DM, Gibbs CJ Jr. Chronic neurological diseases caused by slow infections. In: Evans AS, Kaslow R, eds. *Viral infections of humans*, 2nd ed. New York: Plenum, 1997:1027–1051, with permission.)

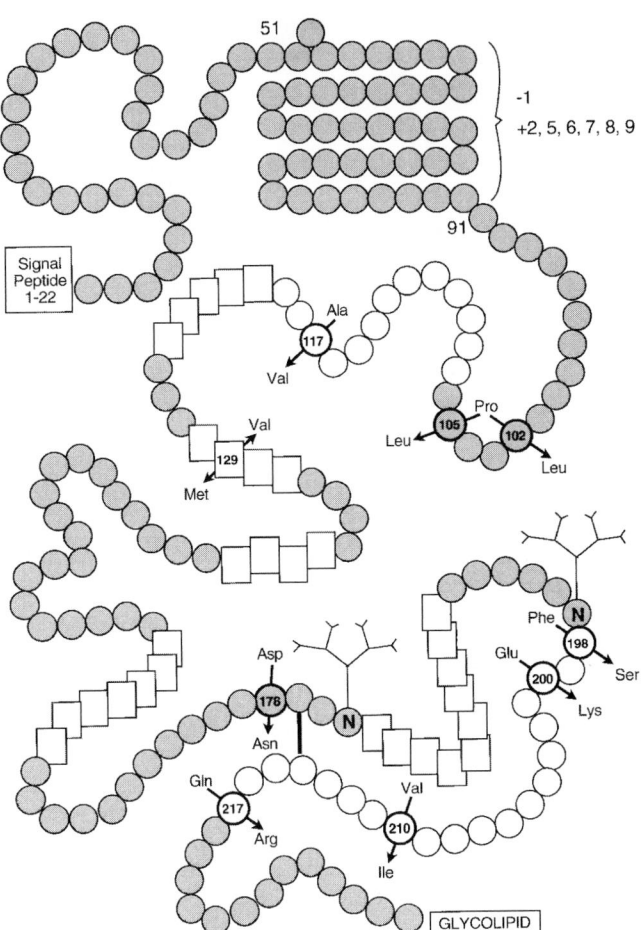

Figure 264.6. Schematic diagram of the amino acid structure of PrP showing mutations associated with familial TSEs. (Courtesy of Dr. Paul Brown, National Institutes of Health, Bethesda, MD.)

agent-associated differences in proteinase cleavage sites of PrP, suggesting that an altered folding might explain strain differences (16,104). Skeptics have continued to suspect that the complete infectious agents more probably contain small unique nucleic acids as the actual self-replicating and pathogenic information-bearing moieties (54,55).

Whatever its relationship to the actual infectious particles, PrP clearly plays a central role in the pathogenesis of TSEs, and its expression in the cell is obligatory for replication of the infectious agent (105). PrP27–30 is a glycoprotein (106) consisting of 55 amino acids (85) with attached carbohydrates, a sialic acid residue (106), and a glycophosphoinositol anchor (28) (Fig. 264.6). It has the physical properties of an amyloid protein (72)—staining with Congo red dye and bi-refringent in polarized light—presumably resulting from its high content of β-pleated sheet structures. The PrPs of several species of animals are similar in amino acid sequence and antigenicity, although not identical (107,108). The host encodes the primary structure of PrP, and the amino acid sequence is not influenced by the source of infectious agent provoking its formation (109), although in chimeric animals expressing PrP genes from two rodent species, the abnormal PrP that accumulated was that of the species to which the infecting strain of agent had been adapted (110). PrP27–30 is cleaved from a larger precursor protein [originally designated PrP33–35 (111)] consisting of about 250 amino acids (112), now abbreviated as PrP. It occurs in tissues of normal humans and animals as well as in those with TSEs. The amino acid sequences of PrPs extracted from normal tissue and the amyloid-staining protein from infected tissues are identical (87), but the two proteins differ in physical properties: the abnormal PrP from infected tissues [now termed PrP(Sc) for scrapie-type PrP, regardless of the TSE or species in which it is found] has a highly β-pleated conformation and is, like PrP27–30, relatively resistant to prote-

olysis with PK, whereas PrP from normal tissue [termed cellular PrP or PrP(C)] has a high content of α-helix and is sensitive to PK digestion (113). [Some authorities prefer the operational designations of PrP-res for the abnormal PK-resistant PrP and PrP-sen for the normal PK-sensitive form (31).] This difference must result from some posttranslational change in conformation, the nature of which remains unknown (100). Intermediate forms of PrP that are PK sensitive but abnormally insoluble in solutions of chaotropes (guanidine salts) have recently been described in extracts of tissues from animals with TSEs (102,103,114,115).

PrP has been detected on cell surfaces (28) as well as within endoplasmic reticulum (116). It was first recognized only in neurons (112), but it was later detected in spleen and lymphoid tissues as well (117). PrP must serve a nonessential function in normal cells because knockout mice not expressing the PrP gene are normal (118). [Some studies found that PrP binds copper ions (119) and may play a role in synaptic transmission (120,121).]

PATHOLOGY

Recognizable histopathologic changes in TSEs occur only in neural tissues (122). Typical changes are vacuolation and loss of neurons (Fig. 264.7) with hypertrophy and proliferation of astrocytes demonstrable by gold stain (Fig. 264.8) or by immunostaining with glial fibrillary acidic protein. Changes are more pronounced

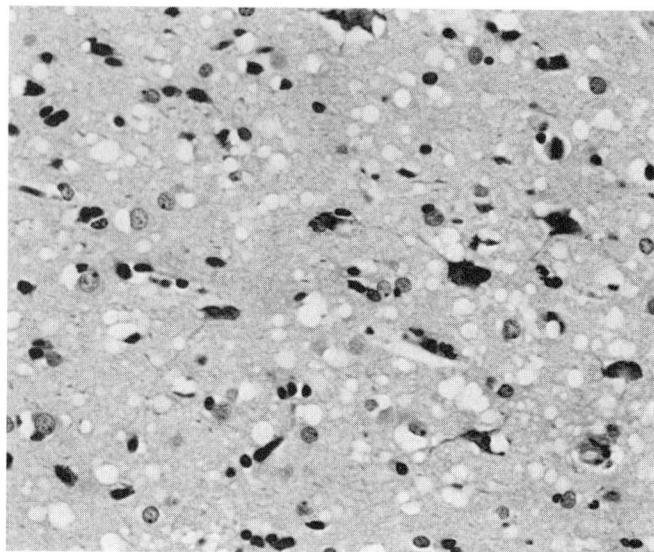

Figure 264.7. Vacuolation and loss of neurons in the cerebral cortex of a patient with Gerstmann-Sträussler-Scheinker syndrome. (Hematoxylin and eosin stain.)

in the cerebral cortex in CJD and GSS and in the cerebellum in kuru and are typically most severe in gray matter. CJD patients with prominent white matter involvement have been described (123,124); some loss of myelin is seen in other cases, probably secondary to degeneration of neurons. There is no inflammation. Vacuoles vary in severity and distribution; they appear to arise by budding from cell membranes into the cytoplasm and later from the walls of existing vacuoles to form multiple vacuolations (125). Amyloid plaques (Fig. 264.9) are found in brain of all patients with GSS and vCJD, in at least 70% of patients with kuru, and less commonly in those with typical sporadic CJD. Amyloid plaques are most common in the cerebellum but occur elsewhere in the brain as well. The plaques react with anti-PrP antibodies (91,116,126,127) but not with antisera to the amyloid A protein found in plaques of Alzheimer's disease (116,128). In TSE brain specimens without typical plaques, PrP(Sc) can usually be detected in the parenchyma by immunostaining (129), which is enhanced by treatment of tissue sections with formic acid (91,130) and by autoclaving (131,132).

In all patients who died with vCJD, unusually prominent "florid" PrP plaques surrounded by halos of spongiform change were noted throughout cerebellum and cerebrum, with smaller numbers in the basal ganglia, hypothalamus, and thalamus (7). Such plaques have only rarely been seen in sporadic CJD (133) and—perhaps coincidentally—in CWD (17). The finding of similar florid plaques in brain of monkeys inoculated with suspensions of tissue from cows with BSE gives additional evidence suggesting a causal link between BSE and vCJD (134).

PATHOGENESIS

Little information is available about the pathogenesis of human TSEs. The kuru agent probably entered the body through lesions in the skin or mouth (23) exposed to infected tissues during ritual cannibalism; mean incubation of kuru has been estimated to be about 10 to 13 years, and maximum incubation periods after a single exposure may be longer than 40 years (135,136). In iatrogenic CJD, the agent is accidentally introduced into the body either directly into nervous system—the brain or eye—by surgery (with incubation periods of 15 months or more) or indirectly by subcutaneous injection of contaminated hormones [with incubation periods from several years (137) to more than 38 years (138)]. In GSS, familial CJD, and sporadic cases of CJD, the portal of entry (if any) of the infectious agent is not known. It is assumed that exposure to BSE agent–contaminated beef transmitted vCJD to humans; ground meat products containing bovine neural tissues are suspected as being the most likely vehicle (139). Concern about the remote theoretical possibility that some vaccines might have been contaminated with the BSE agent (140) prompted precautionary changes in formulation of those products (*www.fda.gov/cber/BSE/BSE.htm*); however, epidemiologic studies found no link between vaccine exposures and vCJD (141).

In sheep naturally exposed to scrapie, the infectious agent was first detected in intestines and mesenteric lymph nodes (142), suggesting that the alimentary tract is a portal of infection in that disease. Contaminated placental tissues have been incriminated as the major vehicle for transmission both to the involved lamb and other animals in contact with infectious material (143,144). Epidemiologic evidence suggests an oral portal for BSE in cattle (145), feline spongiform encephalopathy (146), and TME in mink (15); there is limited evidence suggesting possible

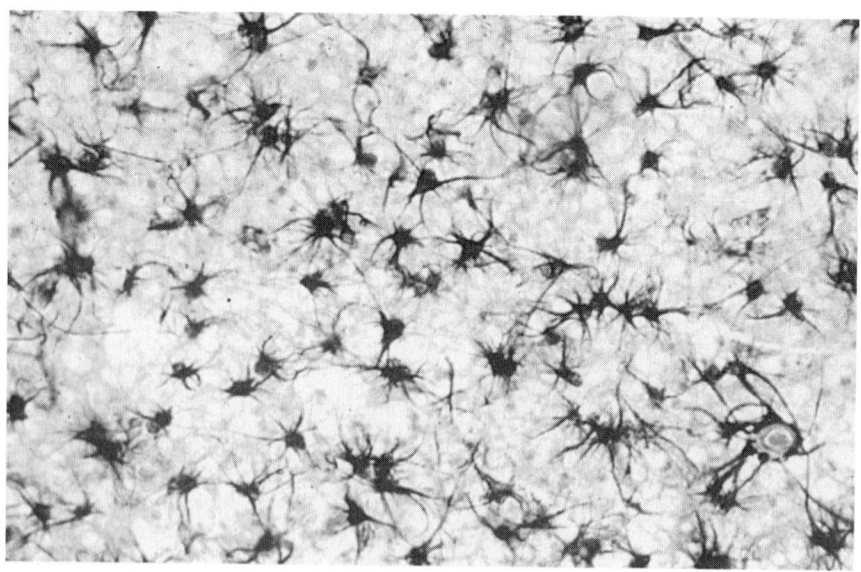

Figure 264.8. Proliferation and hypertrophy of astrocytes in the cerebral cortex of a chimpanzee with experimental kuru. (Cajal gold stain.) (Courtesy of Ms. Elisabeth Beck, Institute of Psychiatry, London, UK.)

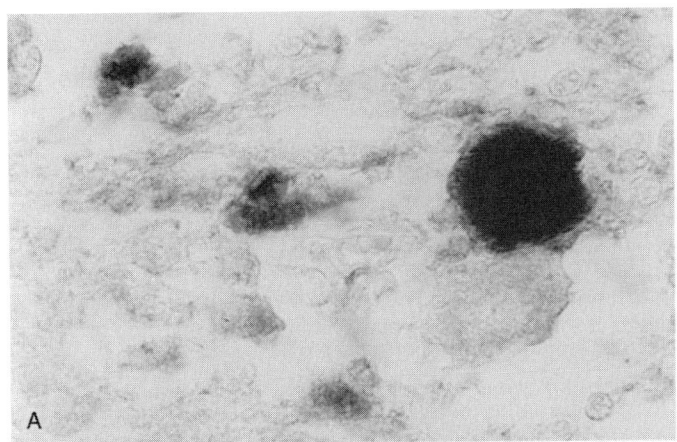

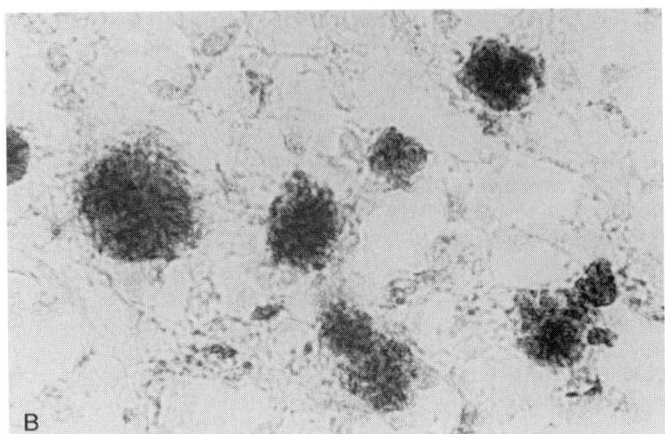

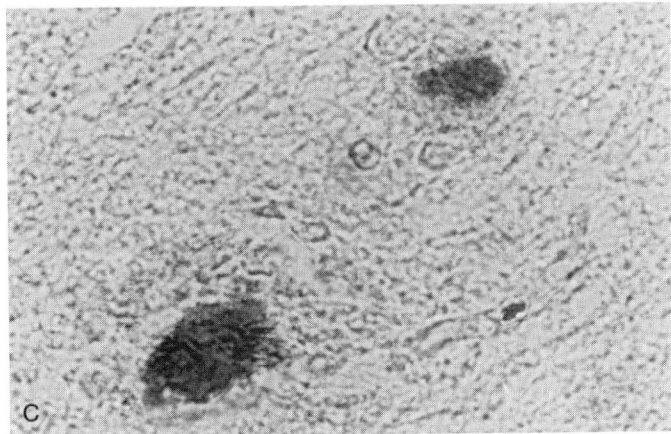

Figure 264.9. Amyloid plaques in the brains of patients with kuru (**A**), Creutzfeldt-Jakob disease (**B**), and Gerstmann-Sträussler-Scheinker syndrome (**C**) incubated with rabbit antiserum to hamster PrP and then stained by an indirect immunoperoxidase method. (**A** to **C** courtesy of Dr. Don Guiroy, National Institutes of Health, Bethesda, MD.)

occasional perinatal transmission of BSE (147) but not TME. (15). Little is known of sources of infection in CWD; its rapid spread suggests transmission by contact with contaminated secretions or excretions. Monkeys were experimentally infected with the agents of scrapie, kuru, and CJD by feeding them contaminated tissue (148).

Spread of the TSE agents within the human body is also poorly understood. In animals inoculated intraperitoneally, subcutaneously, or orally, the first site of replication of the agents appears to be in tissues of the reticuloendothelial system (142,149). The agent has been detected in lymph nodes and spleens of occa-

sional CJD patients at autopsy (150–152) (Table 264.2), suggesting that the same thing may be true in human disease. Recent studies with vCJD suggest that lymphoid tissues, which contain prominent accumulations of PrP(Sc), are even more consistently involved in infection than those in sporadic CJD (153,154); this finding has practical implications for the safety of transfused blood components or transplanted tissues from donors who may have been exposed to the BSE agent.

It has not been determined with certainty whether the agent occurs in human blood during the incubation period or symptomatic illness with CJD. Transmissions of disease to animals

TABLE 264.2. Infectivity of Tissue and Body Fluids from Patients with Creutzfeldt-Jakob Disease and Kuru

Consistently transmit infectious agent (≥50% of attempts)[a]	Sometimes transmit infectious agent (10%–20% of attempts)[a]	Possibly transmit infectious agent (occasional unconfirmed reports)
Brain (234/259)	Lymph node (3/15)	Blood
Eye (4/5)	Kidney (5/28)	Urine
Spinal cord (4/6)	CSF (3/26)	Placenta
Lung (2/4)	Liver (4/35)	
	Spleen (3/31)	

[a]Number of transmissions/number of tissues tested.
Adapted from Brown P, Gibbs C Jr, Rodgers-Johnson P, et al. Human spongiform encephalopathy: the NIH series of 300 cases of experimentally transmitted disease. *Ann Neurol* 1994;35:513; and Asher DM. Slow viral infections of the nervous system. In: Scheld WM, Whitley RJ, Durack DT, eds. *Infections of the central nervous system.* New York: Raven Press, 1991:145–166, with permission.

injected with human blood have been claimed (155–158), although not confirmed, in a limited number of attempts (150,152). Epidemiologic and clinical studies did not support the hypothesis that donors had transmitted CJD to recipients of blood or derivatives (159,160), although an anecdotal report raised that possibility (161,162). However, the agent of CJD has been repeatedly and convincingly demonstrated in blood of experimentally infected rodents (163–166), mainly associated with nucleated cells but also in plasma. Recently, infectivity was also reported in blood of monkeys (167) and sheep experimentally infected with the BSE agent (168,169) and scrapie (169). (A review of concerns and recommendations of the U.S. Food and Drug Administration (FDA) regarding CJD—with special emphasis on vCJD—and the safety of the blood supply can be found through the Internet at *www.fda.gov/cber/gdlns/cjdvcjd.htm*).

In natural scrapie of sheep, the agent first appears in the central nervous system rather late in disease, multiplying there to much higher levels than in lymphoid and other tissues that are infected earlier (142). In experimental infections of mice, the scrapie agent may spread to the central nervous system by ascending peripheral nerves (149,170) rather than through the bloodstream.

In human kuru, it is probable that the only portal of exit of the agent from the body, in quantities sufficient to infect others, was through infected tissues exposed during cannibalism (23); in iatrogenically transmitted CJD, the infected tissues of source patients provided a similar portal of exit (171,172). Brain, spinal cord, and eyes of patients with CJD are consistently infectious (152). Several other human tissues and cerebrospinal fluid (CSF) sometimes contained the agent as well (152) (Table 264.2). A small number of studies failed to find infectious agent in secretions or excretions from patients with CJD (152), although one report, never confirmed, claimed that human urine transmitted disease to mice (156). A recent report that both PrP(Sc) and infectivity were found in some muscle tissues of mice with experimental scrapie (173) suggests that more intensive investigation of tissues previously thought to be uninvolved in TSEs is needed.

No antibodies and no cell-mediated immunity to the infectious agents of the spongiform encephalopathies have been demonstrated in patients or animals at any time during illness (150). [Antibodies to PrP have been reported to free cell cultures of TSE infectivity (40).] This apparent lack of immune response to infection remains unexplained.

EPIDEMIOLOGY AND MECHANISMS OF TRANSMISSION

Kuru once affected many children 4 years of age and older, adolescents, and adults, especially women, among the Fore people (Fig. 264.10) in a restricted area of Papua New Guinea. It became increasingly uncommon (Fig. 264.11) and most recently has affected only older adults (136). Children born to and nursed by affected mothers never developed kuru unless they also participated in cannibalism (135). No evidence indicates spread of kuru by any mechanism except by ritual cannibalism, which ended in the late 1950s (136). In 1999, for the first time since surveillance began, no case of kuru was registered in Papua New Guinea (Alpers MP, personal communication).

The epidemiology of CJD and its variants is more complicated than that of kuru. CJD has been recognized worldwide, at rates of 0.25 to 2 cases per million population per year (174–176), with foci of much higher incidence among Libyan Jews in Israel, in isolated villages of Slovakia, and in other limited areas (23). Hypothetic mechanisms for the origin of sporadic CJD have been proposed, including exposure to a ubiquitous agent with a low transmission rate and rare spontaneous somatic misfolding of normal PrP yielding an infectious protein agent *de novo* (177,178). Except for indirect evidence provided by the iatrogenic spread of CJD (179), which accounts for a relatively small proportion of cases, and the cluster of vCJD cases linked to BSE (7), supporting the hypothesis of exogenous infection, neither hypothesis has convinced opponents. Like kuru, CJD has not occurred in children born to affected mothers (152,172). One unconfirmed study claimed to have transmitted disease to mice inoculated with placenta and cord blood of a mother with CJD (157).

Iatrogenic transmission of CJD from patients to uninfected subjects has been amply documented (179). More than 40 years

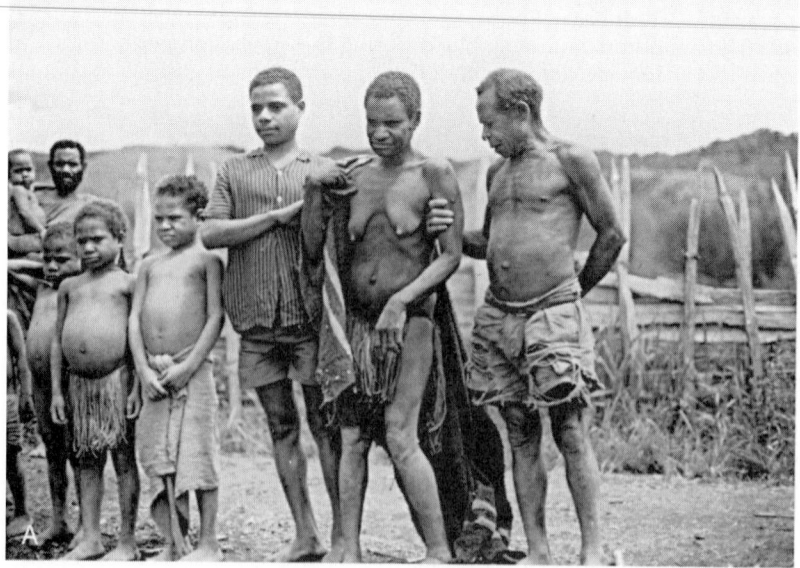
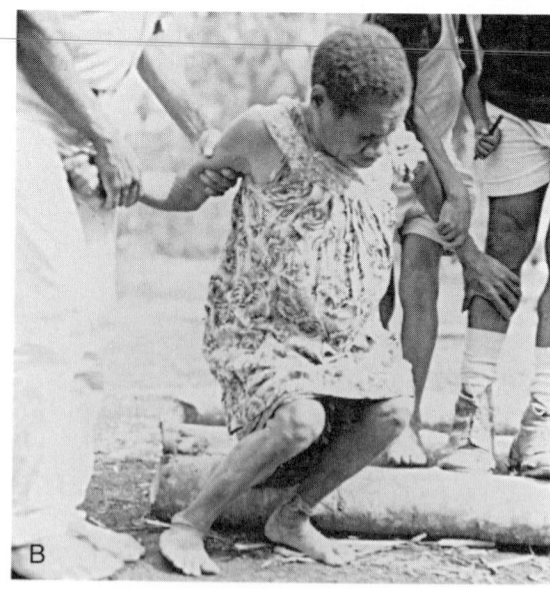

Figure 264.10. Women with kuru unable to stand without support. (**A** and **B** courtesy of Dr. D. Carleton Gajdusek, National Institutes of Health, Bethesda, MD.)

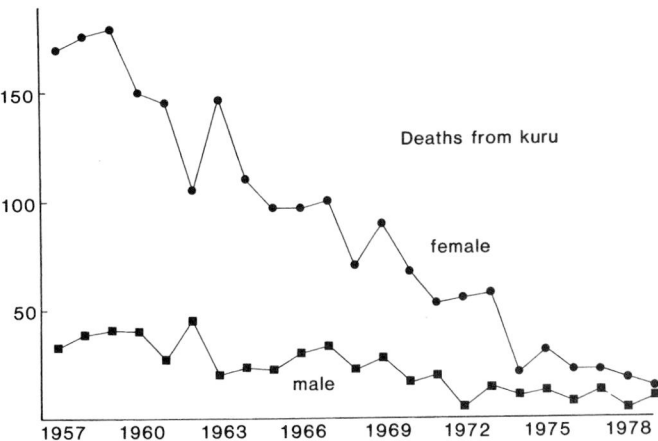

Figure 264.11. Deaths from kuru registered in Okapa, Papua New Guinea during the first 20 years of study. (Courtesy of Dr. D. Carleton Gajdusek, National Institutes of Health, Bethesda, MD.)

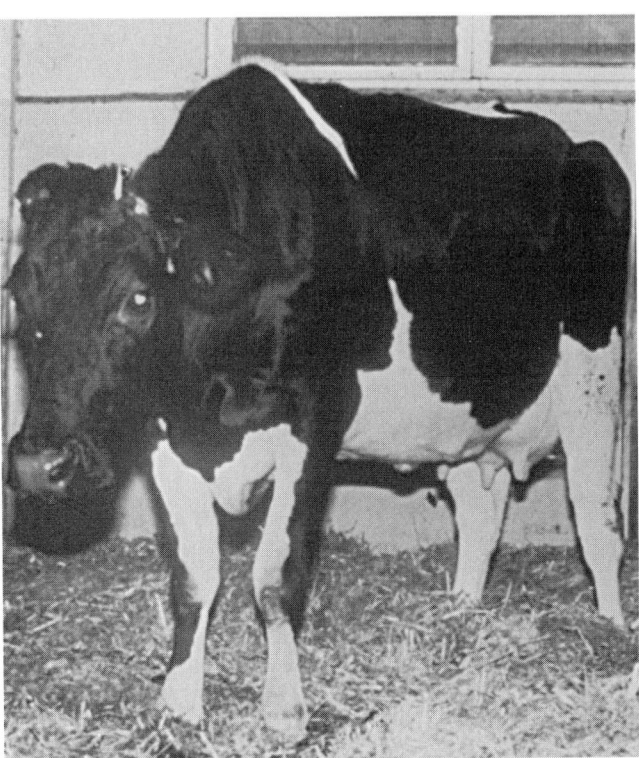

Figure 264.12. A British cow with bovine spongiform encephalopathy. (Courtesy of Dr. C. J. Gibbs, Jr., National Institutes of Health, Bethesda, MD.)

ago, CJD was diagnosed in three patients who had previous neurosurgery performed in the same operating suite (22,180). A similar situation—in which the probable source case of CJD was recognized—occurred in Paris (181). CJD was accidentally transmitted by transplantation of contaminated corneas (182–184) and by contaminated cortical electrodes used during epilepsy surgery (172,185). CJD has affected more than 100 young people who received injections of human cadaver pituitary growth hormone involving at least five contaminated lots in three countries (137,179,186) and four recipients of human pituitary gonadotropin (187) with minimal incubation periods as long as 38 years (138). One sample of cadaver growth hormone among several retained lots transmitted disease to a monkey (171). Cases of CJD also occurred in many patients who received grafts of processed cadaver dura mater allograft (137,188,189,190,191–195). Almost all dura allografts implicated in the transmission of CJD were from one commercial product never cleared for use in the United States; however, a cleared product was involved in a single case (196,197). The FDA has reviewed the risk and recommended precautions for preparation of dura mater allograft to reduce the risk for transmitting CJD (available through the Internet at *www.fda.gov/cdrh/ode/054.html*). Use of human dura mater grafts has been discontinued in a number of other countries.

Most cases of CJD must be considered sporadic, and no probable source of iatrogenic infection—probable exposure to a TSE agent—can be identified.

Spouses and household contacts of patients are at low risk for acquiring CJD, although two conjugal cases have been reported (198,199), each more suggestive of common-source exposure than of case-to-case transmission. It was thought that medical personnel had no increased risk for CJD (176,200); reports of CJD in histopathology technicians (201,202), a neurosurgeon (133), an orthopedist (who had collected dura) (203), a pathologist (204), and at least 15 other health care workers (205) forced reconsideration of that issue, although the risk must be very low.

The recognition in the United Kingdom of BSE among cattle (Fig. 264.12) and of similar TSEs affecting captive ungulates, domestic cats, and felines in zoos—all apparently infected by eating contaminated feed (20,145,206,207)—raised concern that the scrapie agent, never linked to human disease, had crossed a species barrier from sheep to cattle and acquired a broadened range of susceptible hosts, posing a potential danger for humans.

However, recognition of vCJD, a new clinical-histopathologic variant of CJD already affecting more than 125 relatively young people [only one older than 55 years of age (139,208)], forced authorities in the United Kingdom to conclude that a "link with BSE . . . may be the most plausible explanation" (7). Since its original description in 1996, more than 125 definite and probable cases of vCJD have been recognized in the United Kingdom and single cases in long-time U.K. residents living in Canada, Hong Kong, Ireland, and the United States. Cases of vCJD have also occurred in France and Italy, affecting persons who had not been in the United Kingdom. Current information about the status of vCJD in the United Kingdom can be obtained from the Department of Health (at the time of this writing, available through the Internet at *www.doh.gov.uk/cjd/stats/sep02.htm*), and advice for U.S. travelers to BSE countries from the Centers for Disease Control and Prevention (which provide links to other useful information about TSEs at *www.cdc.gov/ncidod/diseases/cjd/cjd.htm*).

After changes in feeding of cattle (prohibition of most nonmilk mammalian proteins in ruminant feeds) and in meat-cutting and rendering procedures were introduced in the United Kingdom, precautions intended to reduce opportunities for exposure of livestock to infection, cases of BSE dropped markedly (Fig. 264.13), especially among younger cattle (145). Those steps, plus prohibition of consumption of bovine brain and spinal cord and any meat product from cattle older than 30 months of age, should also have reduced the likelihood of human exposure. BSE has been found in native cattle of 22 countries besides the United Kingdom and probably occurs in others that fed contaminated meat-and-bone meal to cattle. Current information on the status of BSE in various countries may be obtained through the Internet from the Office International des Epizooties (at the time of this writing at *www.oie.int/eng/info/en_esb.htm*). BSE has never been recognized in the United States despite

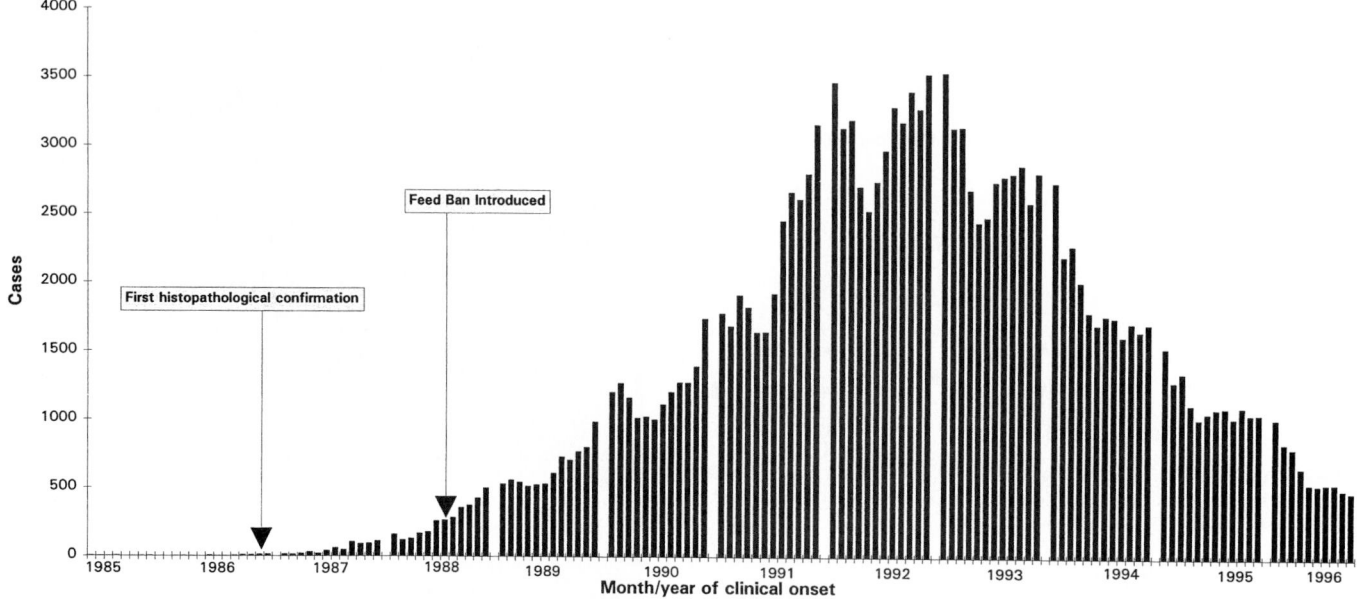

Figure 264.13. Confirmed cases of bovine spongiform encephalopathy registered by month and year of clinical onset. Data are valid to the end of October 1996; produced April 8, 1997. (Courtesy of the Ministry of Agriculture, Food and Fisheries, Hook Rise South, Tolworth, Surbiton, Surrey, UK.)

increasingly intense surveillance (such as examination of brain from thousands of cattle, including many with evidence of central nervous system disease) by the U.S. Department of Agriculture (USDA; recent information currently available through the Internet at *www.fsis.usda.gov/oa/topics/bse.htm* and its links).

Scrapie has been recognized in Great Britain and on the European continent for more than 200 years; it was accidentally imported to the United States in 1947 and gradually spread, especially among sheep of the Suffolk breed (13). Scrapie is transmitted laterally from infected sheep to uninfected sheep and goats exposed to them. Transmission from infected ewe to lamb appears to be especially important in maintaining scrapie in flocks (143). Postnatal infection clearly takes place, and recent data suggest that infected placental tissues may serve as an important vector for transmission (143,209). Although other potential mechanisms for contact transmission of scrapie are not completely understood, it has been proposed that parasites [hay mites (210), and intestinal worms (209)] may also play a role. Neither epidemiologic studies nor anecdotal reports have suggested that human exposure to the scrapie agent is a source of CJD. [It is of some concern, however, that monkeys—although not chimpanzees—have been experimentally infected with scrapie (148).]

TME has occurred only in self-limited outbreaks of ranch mink in the United States (14,15,211,212), none since 1985. Both TME and BSE resemble kuru rather than scrapie in epidemiology; they appear to be mainly if not entirely food borne, and there is little convincing evidence of contagion by animal-to-animal contact or maternal transmission of infection in either disease (15,145). The epidemiology of CWD—its origin, spread through captive and wild herds, and its possible relationship to other TSEs—is not yet understood. CWD has recently spread from its original focus among farmed and wild elk and deer in northeastern Colorado and adjacent parts of Wyoming, west of the Rocky Mountains, east to Nebraska and Wisconsin, and southwest into New Mexico. CWD also affects farmed elk and deer in Canada. The implications of human exposure to the CWD agent are not

known but are of concern; no link between those exposures and CJD has been established (213).

CLINICAL MANIFESTATIONS AND DIAGNOSIS

Kuru, the first human spongiform encephalopathy recognized to be a slow infection (5,214), is a progressive degenerative disease of the cerebellum and brainstem with less marked involvement of the cerebral cortex. The first sign of kuru is usually a cerebellar ataxia, followed by progressive incoordination (Fig. 264.10) and coarse shivering tremors. Variable abnormalities in cranial nerve function appear with frequent impairment in conjugate gaze and swallowing. Patients die of inanition and pneumonia, decubitus ulcers with septicemia, or accidental burns, usually less than a year after onset. Although changes in mentation are common in kuru, there is no frank dementia or progression to coma as in CJD. There are no signs of acute encephalitis—no fever (except during secondary infections), headaches, or convulsions.

CJD occurs throughout the world, affecting mainly middle-aged and older subjects (mean ages in most series from 60 to 69 years) (152) and occurring rarely in older adolescents and young adults (215–222). Patients initially have either sensory disturbances or confusion and inappropriate behavior, progressing in weeks or months to frank dementia and then coma. GSS is a familial disease resembling CJD (6), but with more prominent cerebellar ataxia and later appearance of dementia and amyloid plaques at autopsy.

Mean survival of patients with CJD is less than a year from earliest signs of illness, although about 10% live for more than 2 years (223). Reports of remission have never been confirmed. Recipients of human pituitary hormones who acquired iatrogenic CJD have typically presented with cerebellar ataxia and became demented only late in disease (224). Variant CJD, convincingly attributed to exposure to the BSE agent (7,8), differs in several respects from typical sporadic CJD, most strikingly in younger age at onset (225), frequent early complaints of dysesthesia or pain in the extremities, and absence of periodic electroencephalogram

TABLE 264.3.   U.K. Department of Health Criteria for Diagnosis of Variant Creutzfeldt-Jakob Disease (vCJD) Description of Diagnostic Criteria

Criterion number	Criterion factors
I	A. Progressive neuropsychiatric disorder
	B. Duration of illness > 6 months
	C. Routine investigations suggest no alternative diagnosis
	D. No history of potential iatrogenic exposure
II	A. Early psychiatric symptoms (1)
	B. Persistent painful sensory symptoms (2)
	C. Ataxia
	D. Myoclonus or chorea or dystonia
	E. Dementia
III	A. EEG does not show typical appearance of sporadic CJD (3) (or no EEG performed)
	B. Bilateral high signal in pulvinar on MRI scan
IV	A. Positive tonsil biopsy (accumulation of abnormal prion protein)
Definite vCJD	Criterion I and neuropathologic confirmation of vCJD (4)
Probable vCJD	Criterion I and 4 of 5 factors of criterion II and IIIA and IIIB, or I and IVA

1. Depression, anxiety, apathy, withdrawal, delusions
2. Complaints of frank pain and/or unpleasant dysesthesia
3. Generalized triphasic periodic complexes about once per second
4. Spongiform change and extensive deposition of prion protein with florid plaques throughout cerebrum and cerebellum

EEG, electroencephalogram; MRI, magnetic resonance imaging.
Modified slightly from original, available from the Internet at *www.doh.gov.uk/cjd/stats/sep02.htm*. A slightly different case definition used in the United States by Centers for Disease Control and Prevention is available at *www.fda.gov/cber/gdlns/cjdvcjd.htm*

(EEG) changes (Table 264.3). Most patients with all forms of CJD develop myoclonic jerking movements, frequently with generalized "startle" myoclonus.

Fatal familial insomnia (FFI), an inherited syndrome with an autosomal dominant pattern of occurrence, characterized by progressively severe insomnia and dysautonomia with selective atrophy of two thalamic nuclei, was described in several Italian kindreds (9,226–228). Patients with FFI have ataxia, myoclonus, and other signs resembling those of CJD and GSS. Only a few affected patients had spongiform changes in the cerebral cortex. Those findings suggested that FFI might be a new prion disease; indeed, protease-resistant PrP was detected in brains of patients with FFI, although it apparently differed in location of its protease cleavage site from the PrP found in most patients with CJD or GSS (9). In a small number of attempts, FFI has not been transmitted to primates (152); transmission of encephalopathy from thalamic tissues of FFI patients to mice was claimed by two groups (11,12). Transmission of disease to mice by inoculation of tissues from a patient with a similar sporadic syndrome was also reported (10).

The TSEs of animals (13,15,18,206) are all characterized by progressive incoordination and frequently by inappropriate behavior and inanition; tremors, abnormal movements, and convulsions are less common. Pruritus, not seen in the other TSEs, is often observed in sheep with scrapie, and polydipsia or polyuria appear in deer and elk with CWD (18).

LABORATORY FINDINGS

Most patients with sporadic, iatrogenic, and familial forms of CJD have abnormal EEG findings at some time (152); as disease progresses, the background becomes slow and irregular with diminished amplitude. A variety of paroxysmal changes (slow waves, sharp waves, spike-and-wave complexes) may also appear; these may sometimes be unilateral or focal as well as bilaterally synchronous. Paroxysmal discharges may be precipitated by loud noise. Many patients with CJD have typical periodic suppression–burst complexes of high-voltage slow activity on the EEG (Fig. 264.14) at some time during the illness (229). Patients with vCJD have thus far lacked typical EEG findings.

Computed tomography may show cortical atrophy with large ventricles late in the course of CJD. Cerebral magnetic resonance imaging has been reported to be useful in distinguishing vCJD (increased density in the pulvinar) from sporadic CJD (230,231). There may be some elevation of total CSF protein value. Abnormal liver function studies sometimes suggest hepatic parenchymal disease (232). Results of other clinical laboratory tests are generally normal.

One additional laboratory test has been useful in establishing the diagnosis of CJD. Two abnormal protein spots were detected in the CSF of most patients with CJD using two-dimensional gel electrophoresis-isoelectric focusing (233) (Fig. 264.15). They also occurred in the CSF of some patients with acute viral encephalitides and after cerebral infarctions but generally not in the CSF of patients with Alzheimer's disease. The spots were identified by Western immunoblotting as derived from 14-3-3 protein (234), a ubiquitous protein thought to be involved in signal transduction and the cell cycle (235). The 14-3-3 protein is found in normal brain and other tissues but is usually detected only in trace amounts in CSF (236). Elevated levels of 14-3-3 in the CSF of a patient with appropriate clinical findings and course suggest but cannot conclusively establish the diagnosis of CJD (234,237,238). The 14-3-3 protein is not related to PrP. Recent reports of the finding of noninfectious PrP(Sc) in urine of humans and animals with TSEs (239) and of marked reductions in an unrelated messenger RNA in blood of animals with TSEs (240), although intriguing and potentially useful for ante mortem diagnosis, remain to be confirmed.

None of the tests described earlier has replaced examination of brain tissue from autopsy for establishing the final diagnosis of a TSE. Rapid tests to detect PrP(Sc) in brain (or lymphoid

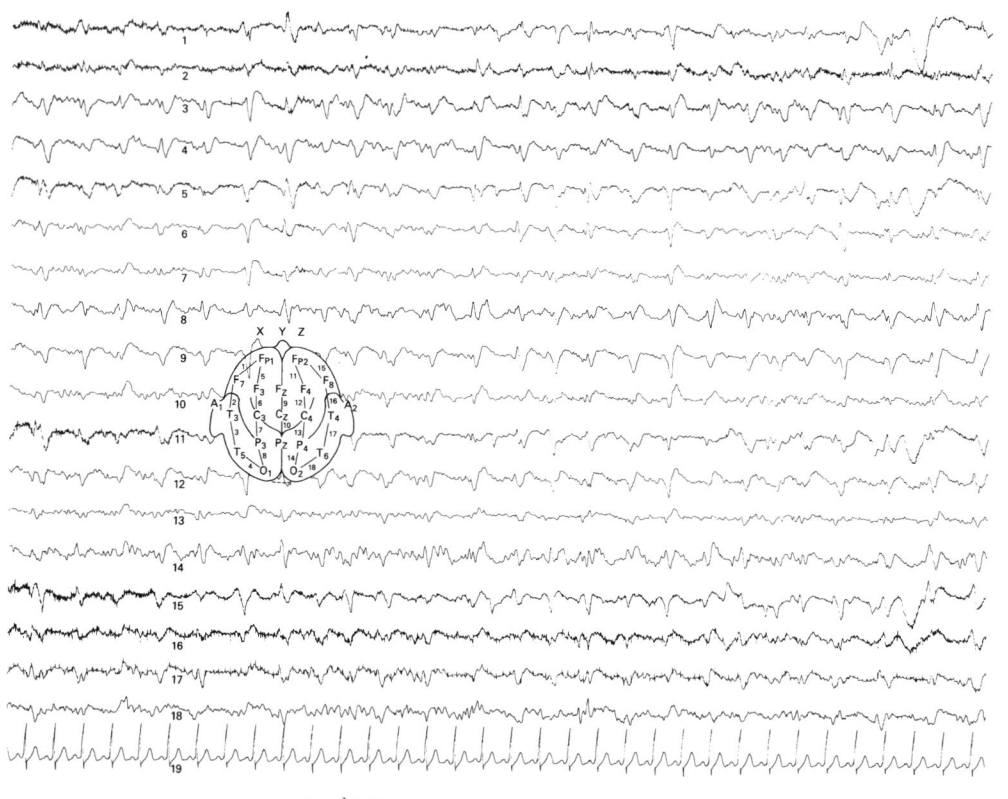

1 sec | 50 μV

Figure 264.14. Electroencephalogram from a patient with Creutzfeldt-Jakob disease. Periodic high-voltage slow-wave complexes are present on a slow, poorly organized background. (Courtesy of Dr. Charles Henry, Department of Neurology, Medical College of Virginia, Richmond, VA.)

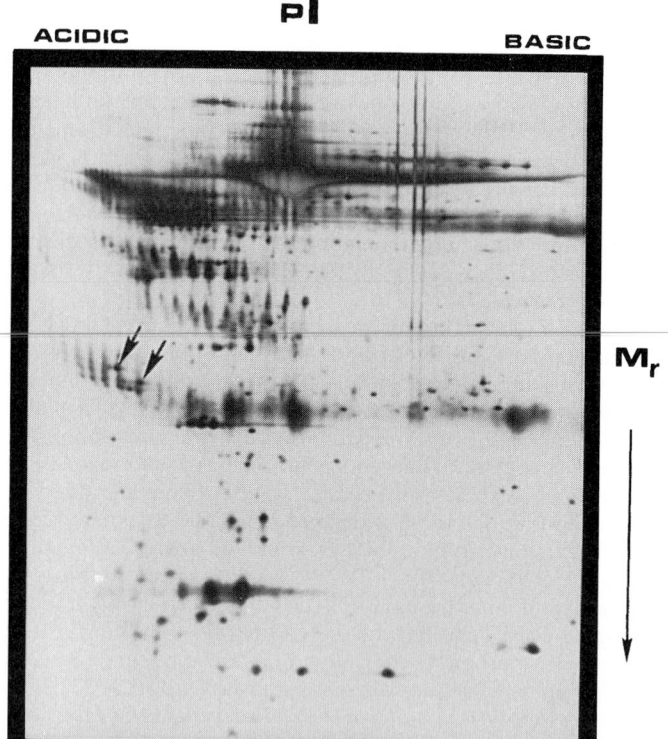

pI

ACIDIC   BASIC

M_r

Figure 264.15. Polypeptides in cerebrospinal fluid (CSF) of a patient with Creutzfeldt-Jakob disease (CJD) demonstrated by two-dimensional separation: electrophoresis-isoelectric focusing and silver staining. Although not unique to CJD, the spots have not been seen in CSF of patients with Alzheimer's disease or healthy older subjects. The image was digitized and computer enhanced. (Courtesy of Dr. Michael Harrington, California Institute of Technology, Pasadena, CA.)

tissues, where appropriate) have been very useful for diagnosis of BSE in cattle (241); there is no obvious reason why similar tests would not serve the same purpose for diagnosis of human TSEs. Several modified tests detecting abnormal PrP with increased sensitivity have recently been described (102,103,115,242); these may eventually aid in the early diagnosis of TSEs.

DIAGNOSIS AND DIFFERENTIAL DIAGNOSIS

The demonstration of scrapie-associated fibrils (70) or PrP (243) in extracts of brain treated with detergent and PK confirms the histopathologic diagnosis, although their absence does not absolutely rule it out. Transmission of disease to susceptible animals by inoculation of brain suspension—although the most sensitive method for detecting TSE agents—is unavailable except in a few research laboratories. Chimpanzees and squirrel monkeys are consistently susceptible to the human TSEs with relatively shorter incubation periods than those of other primates (152,244); animals should be observed for at least 3 years before transmission attempts can be considered tentatively negative. Transgenic mice expressing human PrP sequences are expected to replace monkeys as assay animals eventually but are not yet commercially available.

Unusual cases of CJD may be difficult to distinguish from Alzheimer's disease; the finding of the 14-3-3 proteins in CSF (Fig. 264.15) strongly suggests the former. The two diseases can sometimes be distinguished only at autopsy. The plaques of TSEs, where present, can be differentiated from those of Alzheimer's disease by immunostaining with specific antisera (116,128) (Fig. 264.9).

Although brain biopsy is often diagnostic of TSE (though not always due to patchy distribution of histopathology), this procedure can be recommended only if some other potentially treatable disease remains to be excluded or if rapid diagnosis is justified for reasons of public health.

HOST GENETICS AND TRANSMISSIBLE SPONGIFORM ENCEPHALOPATHIES

In most series of CJD, about 10% of cases have a family history of presenile dementia consistent with the disease (176,245), the pattern of occurrence suggesting an autosomal dominant mode of inheritance. The clinical and histopathologic findings in patients with a family history of CJD (fCJD) resemble those in sporadic cases. GSS is defined as a familial encephalopathy (6). The basis for the familial occurrence of TSEs lies in a series of mutations in the gene coding for PrP (designated *PRNP* gene in humans).

The gene coding for PrP is closely linked or identical to that controlling the incubation periods of scrapie in sheep (246) and both scrapie and CJD in mice (246–248), and amino acid substitutions associated with long incubation periods have been identified (249). The human *PRNP* gene is located on the short arm of chromosome 20 (250). The *PRNP* gene has a single open reading frame of 759 nucleotides (109) in which at least 18 different point mutations (perhaps more than 20) and 11 insertions of varying length (all found in a region of several normal octapeptide repeats) have been linked to the occurrence of familial TSEs. Several of the point mutations are summarized in Table 264.4. A fuller list of PRNP mutations is currently available through the Internet at *www.archive.uwcm.ac.uk/uwcm/mg/ns/1/120720.html* and other sites. Some mutations and insertions were found in only a single patient and may have been incidental, and some cases of neurologic disease associated with mutations were not documented TSEs.

Hsaio and colleagues (250) found a point mutation (single nucleotide change) in codon 102 of the *PRNP* gene [designated 102(Leu) or P102L, changing the encoded amino acid from proline to leucine] linked to GSS, and Goldgaber and co-workers

(251) found another point mutation in PRNP at codon 200 [200(Lys) or E200K] that co-segregated with fCJD. Those appear to be the two most common point mutations associated with familial TSEs.

Patients with kuru had neither mutations nor insertions in their *PRNP* genes (252). In patients with FFI, a mutation was found in the *PRNP* gene at codon 178 [178(Asn)], identical to that found in some kindreds with fCJD. However, the two groups of patients differed in *PRNP* sequences at codon 129 of the abnormal allele. (Codon 129 encodes methionine in about 60% of *PRNP* alleles of normal subjects and valine in the rest.) FFI patients had 129(Val) on the 178(Asn) allele, whereas fCJD patients had 129(Met) (253,254).

Homozygosity at the same 129 locus is much more common in subjects with iatrogenic CJD (iCJD) (255) and sporadic CJD (sCJD) (256) than in general populations, suggesting that it increases susceptibility to infection. Thus far, every vCJD patient tested has been homozygous for 129(Met) (7), although that genotype is expected in less than half of the general population. Homozygosity for 129(Met) is also overrepresented in patients with kuru (257). [A similar association of scrapie with homozygosity of codon 171(Gln) of the PrP gene in Suffolk sheep has been noted (258)].

In addition to the methionine-valine polymorphism at codon 129, there are other normal polymorphisms in the *PRNP* gene at codons 117 and 124 (silent polymorphisms with both variants encoding the same amino acid) and in the octapeptide repeat region between codons 51 and 91, where both deletions and short insertions of less than five extra repeats have been detected in healthy subjects (23). It is not known whether these polymorphisms play any role in neurologic diseases.

Other genes may also influence susceptibility to spongiform encephalopathies; one study purported to show increased frequency of one allele of the apolipoprotein E gene in subjects with CJD compared with normal subjects from the same population (259,260), although that finding is disputed (261,262). Some genetic factors other than the PrP-encoding gene also affect susceptibility of transgenic mice to infection with the CJD agents

---

TABLE 264.4. Point Mutations in *PRNP* Gene Associated with Familial Transmissible Spongiform Encephalopathies (TSEs)[a]

Codon	Normal amino acid	Mutant amino acid	Type of TSE
178	Asp	Asn	fCJD
180	Val	Ile	fCJD
200[b]	Glu	Lys	fCJD
208	His	Arg	fCJD
210	Val	Ile	fCJD
232	Met	Arg	fCJD
102[b]	Pro	Leu	GSS
105	Pro	Leu	GSS
117	Ala	Val	GSS
145[c]	Tyr	Stop	GSS
198	Phe	Ser	GSS
217	Gln	Arg	GSS
129	Met or Val	Met or Val	fCJD/178Asn + 129Val FFI/178Asn + 129Met
117	Ala	Ala	?None
124	Gly	Gly	?None
232	Met	Arg	?None

? None, possible normal polymorphism.
[a]Partial listing. Some information was kindly provided by Dr. L. Cervenakova, American Red Cross. A more complete list with references is available through the Internet at *www.archive.uwcm.ac.uk/uwcm/mg/ns/1/120720.html*
[b]The greatest number of cases of familial spongiform encephalopathies have been associated with these two mutations.
[c]Stop codon (amber mutant)

(263) and incubation period with scrapie (264,265). There is no reason to think that human TSEs are different.

Not all subjects with mutations in the *PRNP* gene have expressed disease, even in affected families. Penetrance appears to be quite high for GSS patients with the 102(Leu) mutation and for fCJD patients with the 178(Asn) mutation; less than 60% of subjects with the 200(Lys) mutation had developed CJD, at least by the usual expected age (266) [although a life table analysis of 13 Libyan Jewish families with the 200(Lys) mutation predicted that penetrance would be close to 100% in carriers surviving past the age of 80 years (267)]. Several members of families with FFI have survived past the age of 60 years without showing signs of illness, although they bore the 178(Asn) mutation. It is not known whether unaffected family members with such mutations in the *PRNP* gene have unapparent infections, perhaps because of exceptionally long incubation periods, or escaped infection with the transmissible agent.

The mechanism by which the mutations act is also in dispute. Those favoring the prion hypothesis (178) postulate that mutations facilitate the folding of protein into an abnormal self-replicating β-sheet of amyloid, perhaps by nucleation (23), whereas those who support the idea that the pathogen may contain a small nucleic acid attribute familial disease to a genetically controlled susceptibility, possibly involving increased affinity of PrP for the agent as a receptor protein on the host cell membrane, or protecting the pathogen from inactivation, or both.

TREATMENT

Several substances—the polyanions HPA-23, carrageenan, and dextran sulfate (268), as well as amphotericin B (269,270) and a derivative compound (271)—interfered with experimental scrapie (prolonging the asymptomatic incubation period and reducing expression of PrP, although not infectivity) in rodents treated before or shortly after inoculation, but no treatment reversed an established infection of the central nervous system. The polyanion Congo red inhibited synthesis of PrP in scrapie-infected cells (29,38,272). More recently, antibodies to PrP(C) (40), branched polyamines (41), and derivatives of acridine (quinacrine) and phenothiazine (chlorpromazine)(39)—the last selected because of their long history of use in treating common human diseases and ability to penetrate the blood-brain barrier—were all found to inhibit formation of PrP(Sc) in persistently infected cell cultures. Clinical trials using these drugs to treat patients with TSEs have begun. More recently, tetracycline treatment of tissue homogenates containing rodent-adapted scrapie agent was found to reduce the content of infectivity (273), and postexposure treatment of mice with immunostimulating CpG oligodeoxynucleotides was reported to prolong the survival of infected rodents (274). It remains to be seen whether any of these experimental therapies is helpful in treating humans. Remission of human CJD after treatment has occasionally been claimed but never confirmed.

PREVENTION OF INFECTION AND DISINFECTION OF CONTAMINATED MATERIALS

Brain tissues of patients with all forms of TSEs—sporadic, iatrogenic and familial—contain the infectious agents (6,176) and pose a potential risk for accidental transmission to other patients and to medical personnel. Other tissues and CSF (Table 264.2) are less often infectious and probably contain smaller amounts of agent (275); those materials must also be treated with caution.

As noted earlier, although human blood has not been convincingly incriminated in transmission of TSEs (276), there has been concern about potential risk, resulting in precautionary deferrals of some blood donors who may be at increased risk for iCJD, fCJD, and vCJD.

Materials and surfaces contaminated with tissues or CSF from patients suspected of having CJD must be treated with care. Adherence to universal precautions for handling blood and body fluids (277) should reduce the chances of accidental exposure. Exposure to the BSE agent must also be considered a potential danger for humans.

Whenever possible, contaminated instruments should be discarded by careful packaging and transported to sites of incineration. Although no method of sterilization can be relied on to remove all infectivity from contaminated surfaces (278), several methods reduce titers of infectivity markedly (279). Contaminated tissues and most biologic products probably cannot be completely freed of infectivity without destroying their structural integrity and biologic activity. (Organic-solvent extraction was reported to free one class of biologic drugs prepared from raw materials experimentally spiked with scrapie infectivity (280). Medical and family histories of individual tissue donors should be carefully reviewed for dementia. Dura allografts should be obtained only from selected donors, pooled grafts avoided, and graft materials of allogeneic human origin replaced with autologous or synthetic materials whenever possible. The preparation of hormones from pools of pituitary glands for use in humans has been discontinued in the United States.

Three treatments are currently recommended for disinfection of objects and surfaces contaminated by TSE agents: heat, sodium hydroxide, and chlorine bleach (281–283). Incineration of disposable items is safest. Steam autoclaving for at least 90 minutes (at 132°C or higher rather than 121°C) should be employed when possible; one study found that some infectivity survived even harsher conditions of heating and actually appeared to be stabilized by treatment with formaldehyde before heating (284). Sodium hydroxide solutions (1N or stronger) are effective in inactivating large amounts of both scrapie and CJD agents (151), especially when combined with autoclaving; contaminated materials should be exposed for at least 1 hour. Aluminum vessels are not suitable for autoclaving NaOH. NaOH solutions are more caustic when hot than at room temperature, and special efforts should be taken to avoid their boiling over in the autoclave. Sodium hypochlorite, at least 5.25% solution (chlorine bleach), had considerable activity in several experimental studies and was more effective than 2N sodium hydroxide in one comparison (278). Sequential, but not simultaneous, treatment of potentially contaminated material with bleach and autoclaving has also been recommended as more effective than either treatment alone. One study suggested that the same formic acid treatment used to enhance the immunostaining of amyloid in tissue sections reduced the infectivity of scrapie agent in the tissue markedly (284); such treatment should be considered by pathology laboratories. One phenolic disinfectant was reported to be effective in eliminating infectivity (281); it is not commercially available in the United States at this time. Attempts to sterilize TSE agents with ethylene oxide gas and with a variety of other commercial liquid disinfectants were ineffective (285). Reliance on traditional methods to sterilize surgical instruments resulted in rare accidental iatrogenic transmissions of CJD. Useful guidelines for TSE infection control in various clinical and laboratory settings have been proposed by consultations of authorities in the United Kingdom (CJD Incidents Panel, Consultation Paper 2001, available through the Internet at www.doh.gov.uk/cjd/consultation) and the World Health

Organization Infection Control Guidelines for TSEs, available at *www.who.int/emc-documents/tse/docs/whocdscsraph2003.pdf*), by the College of American Pathologists (at *www.cap.org/captoday/ cjd.html*), and by the University of California San Francisco (at *www.ehs.ucsf.edu/manuals/BSM/appendix%20L.html#appendixL2*). [Some others (286) do not consider the rigorous treatments recommended by those authorities to be necessary in clinical settings.]

OTHER DEGENERATIVE DISEASES OF THE CENTRAL NERVOUS SYSTEM CAUSED BY UNCONVENTIONAL AGENTS

It was claimed that other human diseases might be caused by infections with agents similar to those causing the TSEs: familial Alzheimer's disease of adults (287) and Alpers' disease (a convulsive disorder with hemiatrophy and status spongiosus of the cerebral gray matter) of young children (288). These claims, as well as an assertion that the blood of many normal subjects contains a TSE agent (289), were not confirmed (290). A later claim that suspensions of brain tissue from subjects with Alzheimer's disease transmitted a similar condition to marmosets (291) remains unsubstantiated (292).

REFERENCES

1. Chesebro B. BSE and prions: uncertainties about the agent. *Science* 1998; 279:42.
2. Gajdusek DC, Gibbs CJ Jr, Alpers M. Experimental transmission of a kuru-like syndrome in chimpanzees. *Nature* 1966;209:794.
3. Jakob A. Ueber eigenartige Erkrankungen des Zentralnervensystems mit bewerkenswertem anatomische Befunde (Spastische Pseudosklerose-Encephalomyelopathie mit disseminierten Degenerationsherden). *Deutsche Zeitschrift fuer Nervenheilkunde* 1921;70:132.
4. Kirschbaum WR. *Jakob-Creutzfeldt disease.* New York: American Elsevier, 1968.
5. Gibbs CJ Jr, Gajdusek DC, Asher DM, et al. Creutzfeldt-Jakob disease (spongiform encephalopathy): transmission to the chimpanzee. *Science* 1968; 161:388.
6. Masters CL, Gajdusek DC, Gibbs CJ Jr. Creutzfeldt-Jakob disease virus isolation from the Gerstmann-Sträussler syndrome, with an analysis of the various forms of amyloid deposition in the virus-induced spongiform encephalopathies. *Brain* 1981;104:559.
7. Will RG, Ironside JW, Zeidler M, et al. A new variant of Creutzfeldt-Jakob disease in the UK. *Lancet* 1996;347:921.
8. Spencer MD, Knight RS, Will RG. First hundred cases of variant Creutzfeldt-Jakob disease: retrospective case note review of early psychiatric and neurological features. *BMJ* 2002;324:1479.
9. Medori R, Tritschler HJ, Leblanc A, et al. Fatal familial insomnia, a prion disease with a mutation at codon-178 of the prion protein gene. *N Engl J Med* 1992;326:444.
10. Mastrianni JA, Nixon R, Layzer R, et al. Prion protein conformation in a patient with sporadic fatal insomnia. *N Engl J Med* 1999;340:1630.
11. Collinge J, Palmer MS, Sidle KC, et al. Transmission of fatal familial insomnia to laboratory animals. *Lancet* 1995;346:569.
12. Tateishi J, Brown P, Kitamoto T, et al. First experimental transmission of fatal familial insomnia. *Nature* 1995;376:434.
13. Detwiler LA. Scrapie. *Rev Sci Tech* (Paris) 1992;11:491.
14. Marsh RF, Burger D, Hanson RP. Transmissible mink encephalopathy: behavior of the disease agent in mink. *Am J Vet Res* 1969;30:1637.
15. Marsh RF, Hanson RP. On the origin of transmissible mink encephalopathy. In: Prusiner SB, Hadlow WJ, eds. *Slow transmissible diseases of the nervous system,* Vol 1. New York: Academic Press, 1979:451–460.
16. Marsh RF, Bessen RA. Physicochemical and biological characterizations of distinct strains of the transmissible mink encephalopathy agent. *Philos Trans R Soc Lond B Biol Sci* 1994;343:413.
17. Williams ES, Young S. Neuropathology of chronic wasting disease of mule deer (*Odocoileus hemionus*) and elk (*Cervus elaphus nelsoni*). *Vet Pathol* 1993; 30:36.
18. Williams ES, Young S. Chronic wasting disease of mule deer: a spongiform encephalopathy. *J Wildl Dis* 1980;16:89.
19. Williams ES, Miller MW. Chronic wasting disease in deer and elk in North America. *Rev Sci Tech* (Paris) 2002;21:305.
20. Wilesmith JW. Epidemiology of bovine spongiform encephalopathy and re-

lated diseases. *Arch Virol* 1993;S7(Unconventional Agents and Unclassified Viruses):245.
21. Pearson GR, Wyatt JM, Gruffydd-Jones TJ, et al. Feline spongiform encephalopathy: fibril and PrP studies. *Vet Rec* 1992;131:307.
22. Nevin S, McMenemy WH, Behrman D, et al. Subacute spongiform encephalopathy: a subacute form of encephalopathy attributed to vascular dysfunction (spongiform cerebral atrophy). *Brain* 1960;83:519.
23. Gajdusek DC. Infectious amyloids: subacute spongiform encephalopathies as transmissible cerebral amyloidoses. In: Fields BN, Knipe DM, eds. *Virology,* Vol 2, 3rd ed. New York: Raven, 1996:2851–2900.
24. Beranger F, Mange A, Solassol J, et al. Cell culture models of transmissible spongiform encephalopathies. *Biochem Biophys Res Commun* 2001;289: 311.
25. Butler DA, Scott MR, Bockman JM, et al. Scrapie-infected murine neuroblastoma cells produce protease-resistant prion proteins. *J Virol* 1988;62: 1558.
26. Caughey B, Race R, Vogel M, et al. In vitro expression of cloned PrP cDNA derived from scrapie-infected mouse brain: lack of transmission of scrapie infectivity. In: Bock G, Marsh J, eds. *Novel infectious agents and the central nervous system.* Ciba Foundation Symposium. 1998;135:197.
27. Caughey B, Race RE, Chesebro B. Detection of prion protein mRNA in normal and scrapie-infected tissues and cell lines. *J Gen Virol* 1988;69:711.
28. Caughey B, Race RE, Ernst D, et al. Prion protein biosynthesis in scrapie-infected and uninfected neuroblastoma cells. *J Virol* 1989;63:175.
29. Caughey B, Raymond GJ. Sulfated polyanion inhibition of scrapie-associated PrP accumulation in cultured cells. *J Virol* 1993;67:643.
30. Oleszak EL, Murdoch G, Manuelidis L, et al. Growth factor production by Creutzfeldt-Jakob disease cell lines. *J Virol* 1992;62:3103.
31. Priola SA, Caughey B, Race RE, et al. Heterologous PrP molecules interfere with accumulation of protease-resistant PrP in scrapie-infected murine neuroblastoma cells. *J Virol* 1994;68:4873.
32. Race RE, Fadness LH, Chesebro B. Characterization of scrapie infection in mouse neuroblastoma cells. *J Gen Virol* 1987;68:1391.
33. Priola SA, Caughey B, Raymond GJ, et al. Prion protein and the scrapie agent: in vitro studies in infected neuroblastoma cells. *Infect Agent Dis* 1994; 3:54.
34. Race RE, Caughey B, Graham K, et al. Analyses of frequency of infection, specific infectivity, and prion protein biosynthesis in scrapie-infected neuroblastoma cell clones. *J Virol* 1988;62:2845.
35. Rubenstein R, Deng H, Race R, et al. Scrapie strain infection in vitro induces changes in neuronal cells. *Mol Neurobiol* 1994;8:129.
36. Scott MR, Butler DA, Bredesen DE, et al. Prion protein gene expression in cultured cells. *Prot Eng* 1988;2:69.
37. Asher DM, Yanagihara RT, Gajdusek DC, et al. Studies of spongiform encephalopathies in cell culture. In: Prusiner S, Hadlow W, eds. *Slow transmissible agents of the nervous system,* Vol 2. New York: Academic Press, 1979:235–242.
38. Caughey B. Scrapie associated PrP accumulation and its prevention: insights from cell culture. *BMJ* 1993;49:860.
39. Korth C, May BC, Cohen FE, et al. Acridine and phenothiazine derivatives as pharmacotherapeutics for prion disease. *Proc Natl Acad Sci U S A* 2001;98:9836.
40. Peretz D, Williamson RA, Kaneko K, et al. Antibodies inhibit prion propagation and clear cell cultures of prion infectivity. *Nature* 2001;412:739.
41. Supattapone S, Wille H, Uyechi L, et al. Branched polyamines cure prion-infected neuroblastoma cells. *J Virol* 2001;75:3453.
42. Kimberlin RH, Walker CA. Pathogenesis of scrapie (strain 263K) in hamsters infected intracerebrally, intraperitoneally or intraocularly. *J Gen Virol* 1986;67:255.
43. Gibbs CJ Jr. Search for infectious etiology in chronic and subacute degenerative diseases of the central nervous system. *Curr Top Microbiol Immunol* 1967;40:44.
44. Gibbs C Jr, Gajdusek D, Latarget R. Unusual resistance to ionizing radiation of the viruses of kuru, Creutzfeldt-Jakob disease and scrapie. *Proc Natl Acad Sci U S A* 1978;75:6268.
45. Rohwer RG. Virus-like sensitivity of scrapie agent to heat inactivation. *Science* 1984;223:600.
46. Rohwer RG. Scrapie infectious agent is virus-like in size and susceptibility to inactivation. *Nature* 1984;308:658.
47. Gibbons RA, Hunter GD. Nature of the scrapie agent. *Nature* 1967;215: 1041.
48. Lewin P. Scrapie: an infective peptide? *Lancet* 1972;1:748.
49. Prusiner SB. Novel proteinaceous infectious particles cause scrapie. *Science* 1982;216:136.
50. Cho H. Requirement of a protein component for scrapie infectivity. *Intervirology* 1980;14:213.
51. Prusiner S. Scrapie prions. *Annu Rev Microbiol* 1989;43:345.
52. Kimberlin R. Scrapie agent: prions or virinos? *Nature* 1982;297:107.
53. Carp RI, Kascsak RJ, Rubenstein R, et al. The puzzle of PrP(Sc) and infectivity: do the pieces fit? *Trends Neurosci* 1994;17:148.
54. Chesebro B, Caughey B. Scrapie replication without the prion protein? *Curr Biol* 1993;3:696.
55. Chesebro B. Prion protein and the transmissible spongiform encephalopathy diseases. *Neuron* 1999;24:503.
56. Rohwer RG. Estimation of scrapie nucleic acid MW from standard curves for virus sensitivity to ionizing radiation. *Nature* 1986;320:381.

57. Riesner D, Kellings K, Wiese U, et al. Prions and nucleic acids: search for residual nucleic acids and screening for mutations in the PrP gene. *Dev Biol Stand* 1993;80:173.

58. Kellings K, Prusiner SB, Riesner D. Nucleic acids in prion preparations: unspecific background or essential component? *Philos Trans R Soc Lond B Biol Sci* 1994;343:425.

59. Bellinger-Kawahara C, Cleaver JE, Diener TO, et al. Purified scrapie prions resist inactivation by UV irradiation. *J Virol* 1987;61:159.

60. Hsiao KK, Scott M, Foster D, et al. Spontaneous neurodegeneration in transgenic mice with mutant prion protein. *Science* 1990;250:1587.

61. Hsiao KK, Groth D, Scott M, et al. Serial transmission in rodents of neurodegeneration from transgenic mice expressing mutant prion protein. *Proc Natl Acad Sci U S A* 1994;9:9126.

62. David-Ferreira JF, David-Ferreira KL, Gibbs CJ Jr, et al. Scrapie in mice: ultrastructural observations in the cerebral cortex. *Proc Soc Exp Biol Med* 1968;28:313.

63. Narang HK, Asher DM, Pomeroy KL, et al. Abnormal tubulovesicular particles in brains of hamsters with scrapie. *Proc Soc Exp Biol Med* 1987;184:504.

64. Liberski PP, Jeffrey M. Tubulovesicular structures: what are they really? *Microsc Res Tech* 2000;50:46.

65. Borras T, Gibbs CJ Jr. Molecular hybridization studies with scrapie brain nucleic acids. I. Search for specific DNA sequences. *Arch Virol* 1986;88:67.

66. Duguid JR, Rohwer RG, Seed B. Isolation of cDNAs of scrapie-modulated RNAs by subtractive hybridization of a cDNA library. *Proc Natl Acad Sci U S A* 1988;85:5738.

67. Lisitsyn N, Wigler M. Cloning the differences between two complex genomes. *Science* 1993;259:946.

68. Merz PA, Somerville RA, Wisniewski HM, et al. Abnormal fibrils from scrapie-infected brain. *Acta Neuropathol* 1981;54:63.

69. Merz PA, Somerville RA, Wisniewski HM, et al. Scrapie-associated fibrils in Creutzfeldt-Jakob disease. *Nature* 1983;306:474.

70. Merz PA, Rohwer RG, Kascsak R, et al. Infection-specific particle from the unconventional slow virus diseases. *Science* 1984;225:437.

71. Bolton DC, McKinley MP, Prusiner SB. Identification of a protein that purifies with the scrapie prion. *Science* 1982;218:1309.

72. Bockman JM, Kingsbury DT, McKinley MP, et al. Creutzfeldt-Jakob disease prion proteins in human brains. *N Engl J Med* 1985;312:73.

73. Bendheim PE, Bockman JM, McKinley MP, et al. Scrapie and Creutzfeldt-Jakob disease prion proteins share physical properties and antigenic determinants. *Proc Natl Acad Sci U S A* 1985;82:997.

74. McKinley MP, Bolton DC, Prusiner SB. A protease-resistant protein is a structural component of the scrapie prion. *Cell* 1983;35:57.

75. Barry RA, McKinley MP, Bendheim PE, et al. Antibodies to the scrapie protein decorate prion rods. *J Immunol* 1985;135:603.

76. DeArmond SJ, McKinley MP, Barry RA, et al. Identification of prion amyloid filaments in scrapie-infected brain. *Cell* 1985;41:221.

77. Diringer H, Gelderblom H, Hilmert H, et al. Scrapie infectivity, fibrils and low molecular weight protein. *Nature* 1983;306:476.

78. Brown P, Coker-Vann M, Pomeroy K, et al. Diagnosis of Creutzfeldt-Jakob disease by Western blot identification of marker protein in human brain tissue. *N Engl J Med* 1986;314:547.

79. Ceroni M, Piccardo P, Safar J, et al. Scrapie infectivity and prion protein are distributed in the same pH range in agarose isoelectric focusing. *Neurology* 1990;40:508–513.

80. Miyamoto T, Sakaguchi S, Katamine S, et al. The infectivity is dissociated from PrP accumulation in salivary gland of Creutzfeldt-Jakob disease agent-inoculated mice. *Ann N Y Acad Sci* 1994;724:310.

81. Xi YG, Ingrosso L, Ladogana A, et al. Amphotericin-B treatment dissociates in vivo replication of the scrapie agent from PrP accumulation. *Nature* 1992;356:598.

82. Lasmézas CI, Deslys JP, Robain O, et al. Transmission of the BSE agent to mice in the absence of detectable abnormal prion protein. *Science* 1997;275:402.

83. Manuelidis L, Manuelidis EE. Creutzfeldt-Jakob disease and dementias. *Microb Pathog* 1989;7:157.

84. Manuelidis L, Sklaviadis T, Akowitz A, et al. Viral particles are required for infection in neurodegenerative Creutzfeldt-Jakob disease. *Proc Natl Acad Sci U S A* 1995;92:5124.

85. Multhaup G, Diringer H, Hilmert H, et al. The protein component of scrapie-associated fibrils is a glycosylated low molecular weight protein. *EMBO J* 1985;4:1495.

86. Chesebro B, Race R, Wehrly K, et al. Identification of scrapie prion protein-specific mRNA in scrapie-infected and uninfected brain. *Nature* 1985;315:331.

87. Basler K, Oesch B, Scott M, et al. Scrapie and cellular PrP isoforms are encoded by the same chromosomal gene. *Cell* 1986;46:417.

88. Hope J, Morton LJ, Farquhar CF, et al. The major polypeptide of scrapie-associated fibrils (SAF) has the same size, charge distribution and N-terminal protein sequence as predicted for the normal brain protein (PrP). *EMBO J* 1986;5:2591.

89. Bruce ME, Dickinson AG. Genetic control of amyloid plaque production and incubation period in scrapie-infected mice. *J Neuropathol Exp Pathol* 1985;44:285.

90. Bruce ME, Dickinson AG. Biological evidence that scrapie agent has an independent genome. *J Gen Virol* 1987;68(Pt 1):79.

91. McBride PA, Bruce ME, Fraser H. Immunostaining of scrapie cerebral amyloid plaques with antisera raised to scrapie-associated fibrils (SAF). *Neuropathol Appl Neurobiol* 1988;14:325.

92. Bruce M, Chree A, McConnell I, et al. Transmission of bovine spongiform encephalopathy and scrapie to mice: strain variation and the species barrier. *Philos Trans R Soc Lond B Biol Sci* 1994;343:405.

93. Kimberlin RH, Walker CA, Fraser H. The genomic identity of different strains of mouse scrapie is expressed in hamsters and preserved on reisolation in mice. *J Gen Virol* 1989;70(Pt 8):2017.

94. Weissmann C. A 'unified theory' of prion propagation. *Nature* 1991;352:679.

95. Wills PR. Potential pseudoknots in the PrP-encoding mRNA. *J Theor Biol* 1992;159:523.

96. Wills PR. Self-organization of genetic coding. *J Theor Biol* 1993;162:267.

97. Prusiner SB, Dearmond SJ. Prion diseases and neurodegeneration. *Annu Rev Neurosci* 1994;17:311.

98. Prusiner SB. Biology and genetics of prion diseases. *Annu Rev Microbiol* 1994;48:655.

99. Safar J, Roller PP, Gajdusek DC, et al. Thermal stability and conformational transitions of scrapie amyloid (prion) protein correlate with infectivity. *Prot Sci* 1993;2:2206.

100. Safar J, Roller PP, Gajdusek DC, et al. Scrapie amyloid (prion) protein has the conformational characteristics of an aggregated molten globule folding intermediate. *Biochemistry* 1994;33:8375.

101. Baldwin MA, Pan KM, Nguyen J, et al. Spectroscopic characterization of conformational differences between PrPc and PrPsc: an alpha-helix to beta-sheet transition. *Philos Trans R Soc Lond B Biol Sci* 1994;343:435.

102. Safar J, Wille H, Itri V, et al. Eight prion strains have PrP(Sc) molecules with different conformations. *Nat Med* 1998;4:1157.

103. Safar J, Cohen FE, Prusiner SB. Quantitative traits of prion strains are enciphered in the conformation of the prion protein. *Arch Virol Suppl* 2000;16:227.

104. Bessen RA, Marsh RF. Distinct PrP properties suggest the molecular basis of strain variation in transmissible mink encephalopathy. *J Virol* 1994;68:7859.

105. Sailer A, Bueler H, Fischer M, et al. No propagation of prions in mice devoid of PrP. *Cell* 1994;77:967.

106. Bolton DC, Meyer RK, Prusiner SB. Scrapie PrP 27-30 is a sialoglycoprotein. *J Virol* 1985;53:596.

107. Bode L, Pocchiari M, Gelderblom H, et al. Characterization of antisera against scrapie-associated fibrils (SAF) from affected hamster and cross-reactivity with SAF from scrapie-affected mice and from patients with Creutzfeldt-Jakob disease. *J Gen Virol* 1985;66:2471.

108. Kretzschmar HA, Stowring LE, Westaway D, et al. Molecular cloning of a human prion protein cDNA. *DNA* 1986;5:315.

109. Bockman JM, Prusiner SB, Tateishi J, et al. Immunoblotting of Creutzfeldt-Jakob disease prion proteins: host species-specific epitopes. *Arch Neurol* 1987;21:589.

110. Prusiner SB, Scott M, Foster D, et al. Transgenetic studies implicate interactions between homologous PrP isoforms in scrapie prion replication. *Cell* 1990;63:673.

111. Braig HR, Diringer H. Scrapie: concept of a virus-induced amyloidosis of the brain. *EMBO J* 1985;4:2309.

112. Kretzschmar HA, Prusiner SB, Stowring LE, et al. Scrapie prion proteins are synthesized in neurons. *Am J Pathol* 1986;122:1.

113. Meyer RK, McKinley MP, Bowman KA, et al. Separation and properties of cellular and scrapie prion proteins. *Proc Natl Acad Sci U S A* 1986;83:2310.

114. MacGregor I, Hope J, Barnard G, et al. Application of a time-resolved fluoroimmunoassay for the analysis of normal prion protein in human blood and its components. *Vox Sang* 1999;77:88.

115. Barnard G, Helmick B, Madden S, et al. The measurement of prion protein in bovine brain tissue using differential extraction and DELFIA as a diagnostic test for BSE. *Luminescence* 2000;15:357.

116. Piccardo P, Safar J, Ceroni M, et al. Immunohistochemical localization of prion protein in spongiform encephalopathies and normal tissue. *Neurology* 1990;40:518.

117. Doi S, Ito M, Shinagawa M, et al. Western blot detection of scrapie-associated fibril protein in tissues outside the central nervous system from preclinical scrapie-infected mice. *J Gen Virol* 1988;69:955.

118. Büeler H, Aguzzi A, Sailer A, et al. Mice devoid of PrP are resistant to scrapie. *Cell* 1993;73:1339.

119. Brown DR. Copper and prion disease. *Brain Res Bull* 2001;55:165.

120. Collinge J, Whittington MA, Sidle KCL, et al. Prion protein is necessary for normal synaptic function. *Nature* 1994;370:295.

121. Whittington MA, Sidle KCL, Gowland I, et al. Rescue of neurophysiological phenotype seen in PrP null mice by transgene encoding human prion protein. *Nat Genet* 1995;9:197.

122. Beck E, Daniel PM, Matthews WB, et al. Creutzfeldt-Jakob disease: the neuropathology of a transmission experiment. *Brain* 1969;92:699.

123. Tateishi J, Ohta M, Koga M, et al. Transmission of chronic spongiform encephalopathy with kuru plaques from humans to small rodents. *Ann Neurol* 1979;5:581.

124. Tateishi J, Sato Y, Koga H, et al. Experimental transmission of human spongiform encephalopathy to small rodents. 1. Clinical and histological observations. *Acta Neuropathol* 1980;51:127.

125. Beck E, Daniel PM, Davey AJ, et al. A note on membrane lamellation. *Brain* 1985;108:153.
126. Baron H, Baron-van Evercooren A, Brucher JM. Antiserum to scrapie-associated fibril protein reacts with amyloid plaques in familial transmissible dementia. *J Neuropathol Exp Neurol* 1988;47:158.
127. Kitamoto T, Tateishi J, Tashima T, et al. Amyloid plaques in Creutzfeldt-Jakob disease stain with prion protein antibodies. *Ann Neurol* 1986;20:204.
128. Bobin SA, Currie JR, Merz PA, et al. The comparative immunoreactivities of brain amyloids in Alzheimer's disease and scrapie. *Acta Neuropathol* 1987;74:313.
129. Kitamoto T, Tateishi J. Immunohistochemical confirmation of Creutzfeldt-Jakob disease with a long clinical course with amyloid plaque core antibodies. *Am J Pathol* 1988;131:435.
130. Kitamoto T, Ogomori K, Tateishi J, et al. Formic acid pretreatment enhances immunostaining of cerebral and systemic amyloids. *Lab Invest* 1987;57:230.
131. Hayward PAR, Bell JE, Ironside JW. Prion protein immunocytochemistry: reliable protocols for the investigation of Creutzfeldt-Jakob disease. *Neuropathol Appl Neurobiol* 1994;20:375.
132. Haritani M, Spencer YI, Wells GAH. Hydrated autoclave pretreatment enhancement of prion protein immunoreactivity in formalin-fixed bovine spongiform encephalopathy-affected brain. *Acta Neuropathol* 1994;87:86.
133. Gajdusek DC, Gibbs CJ Jr, Earle K, et al. Transmission of subacute spongiform encephalopathy to the chimpanzee and squirrel monkey from a patient with papulosis maligna of Köhlmeyer-Degos. *Excerpta Medica International Congress Series* 1974;319:390.
134. Lasmézas CI, Deslys JP, Demaimay R, et al. BSE transmission to macaques. *Nature* 1996;381:743.
135. Klitzman RL, Alpers MP, Gajdusek DC. The natural incubation period of kuru and the episodes of transmission in three clusters of patients. *Neuroepidemiology* 1984;3:3.
136. Huillard d'Aignaux JN, Cousens SN, Maccario J, et al. The incubation period of kuru. *Epidemiology* 2002;13:402.
137. Brown P, Preece M, Brandel JP, et al. Iatrogenic Creutzfeldt-Jakob disease at the millennium. *Neurology* 2000;55:1075.
138. Croes EA, Roks G, Jansen GH, et al. Creutzfeldt-Jakob disease 38 years after diagnostic use of human growth hormone. *J Neurol Neurosurg Psychiatr* 2002;72:792.
139. Brown P, Will RG, Bradley R, et al. Bovine spongiform encephalopathy and variant Creutzfeldt-Jakob disease: background, evolution, and current concerns. *Emerg Infect Dis* 2001;7:6.
140. United States Public Health Service C. Public Health Service recommendations for the use of vaccines manufactured with bovine-derived materials. *MMWR Morb Mortal Wkly Rep* 2000;49:1137.
141. Minor PD, Will RG, Salisbury D. Vaccines and variant CJD. *Vaccine* 2000;19:409.
142. Hadlow WJ, Kennedy RC, Race RE. Natural infection of Suffolk sheep with scrapie virus. *J Infect Dis* 1982;146:657.
143. Race R, Jenny A, Sutton D. Scrapie infectivity and proteinase K-resistant prion protein in sheep placenta, brain, spleen, and lymph node: implications for transmission and antemortem diagnosis. *J Infect Dis* 1998;178:949.
144. Tuo W, O'Rourke KI, Zhuang D, et al. Pregnancy status and fetal prion genetics determine PrPSc accumulation in placentomes of scrapie-infected sheep. *Proc Natl Acad Sci U S A* 2002;99:6310.
145. Wilesmith JW. An epidemiologist's view of bovine spongiform encephalopathy. *Philos Trans R Soc Lond B Biol Sci* 1994;343:357.
146. Ryder SJ, Wells GA, Bradshaw JM, et al. Inconsistent detection of PrP in extraneural tissues of cats with feline spongiform encephalopathy. *Vet Rec* 2001;148:437.
147. Donnelly CA, Ferguson NM, Ghani AC, et al. Analysis of dam-calf pairs of BSE cases: confirmation of a maternal risk enhancement. *Proc R Soc Lond B Biol Sci* 1997;264:1647.
148. Gibbs C Jr, Amyx H, Bacote A, et al. Oral transmission of kuru, Creutzfeldt-Jakob disease, and scrapie to nonhuman primates. *J Infect Dis* 1980;142:205.
149. Kimberlin RH. Scrapie: how much do we really understand? *Neuropathol Appl Neurobiol* 1986;12:131.
150. Asher DM, Gibbs CJ Jr, Gajdusek DC. Pathogenesis of spongiform encephalopathies. *Ann Clin Lab Sci* 1976;6:84.
151. Asher DM. Slow viral infections of the human nervous system. In: Scheld WM, Whitley RJ, Durack DT, eds. *Infections of the nervous system*, 2nd ed. New York: Raven, 1997:199–221.
152. Brown P, Gibbs C Jr, Rodgers-Johnson P, et al. Human spongiform encephalopathy: the NIH series of 300 cases of experimentally transmitted disease. *Ann Neurol* 1994;35:513.
153. Zeidler M, Knight R, Stewart G, et al. Diagnosis of Creutzfeldt-Jakob disease: routine tonsil biopsy for diagnosis of new variant Creutzfeldt-Jakob disease is not justified. *BMJ* 1999;318:538.
154. Hilton DA, Fathers E, Edwards P, et al. Prion immunoreactivity in appendix before clinical onset of variant Creutzfeldt-Jakob disease. *Lancet* 1998;352:703.
155. Manuelidis EE, Kim JH, Mericangas JR, et al. Transmission to animals of Creutzfeldt-Jakob disease from human blood. *Lancet* 1985;2:896.
156. Tateishi J. Transmission of Creutzfeldt-Jakob disease from human blood and urine into mice. *Lancet* 1985;2:1074.
157. Tamai Y, Kojima H, Kitajima R, et al. Demonstration of the transmissible agent in tissue from a pregnant woman with Creutzfeldt-Jakob disease. *N Engl J Med* 1992;327:649.
158. Deslys JP, Lasmézas C, Dormont D. Selection of specific strains in iatrogenic Creutzfeldt-Jakob disease. *Lancet* 1994;343:848.
159. Esmonde TFG, Will RG, Slattery JM, et al. Creutzfeldt-Jakob disease and blood transfusion. *Lancet* 1993;341:205.
160. Heye N, Hensen S, Muller N. Creutzfeldt-Jakob disease and blood transfusion. *Lancet* 1994;343:298.
161. Klein R, Dumble LJ. Transmission of Creutzfeldt-Jakob disease by blood transfusion. *Lancet* 1993;341:768.
162. Créange A, Gray F, Cesaro P, et al. Creutzfeldt-Jakob disease after liver transplantation. *Ann Neurol* 1995;38:269.
163. Kuroda Y, Gibbs CJ Jr, Amyx HL, et al. Creutzfeldt-Jakob disease in mice: persistent viremia and preferential replication of virus in low-density lymphocytes. *Infect Immun* 1983;41:154.
164. Manuelidis EE, Gorgacz EJ, Manuelidis L. Viremia in experimental Creutzfeldt-Jakob disease. *Science* 1978;200:1069.
165. Holada K, Vostal JG, Theisen PW, et al. Scrapie infectivity in hamster blood is not associated with platelets. *J Virol* 2002;76:4649.
166. Brown P, Rohwer RG, Dunstan BC, et al. The distribution of infectivity in blood components and plasma derivatives in experimental models of transmissible spongiform encephalopathy. *Transfusion* 1998;38:810.
167. Bons N, Lehmann S, Mestre-Frances N, et al. Brain and buffy coat transmission of bovine spongiform encephalopathy to the primate *Microcebus murinus*. *Transfusion* 2002;42:513.
168. Houston F, Foster JD, Chong A, et al. Transmission of BSE by blood transfusion in sheep. *Lancet* 2000;356:999.
169. Hunter N, Foster J, Chong A, et al. Transmission of prion diseases by transfusion. *J Gen Virol* 2002;83:2897–2905.
170. Kimberlin RH, Walker CA. Pathogenesis of experimental scrapie. In: Bock G, Marsh J, eds. *Novel infectious agents and the central nervous system.* Ciba Foundation Symposium 1988;135:37.
171. Gibbs CJ Jr, Asher DM, Brown PW, et al. Creutzfeldt-Jakob disease infectivity of growth hormone derived from human pituitary glands. *N Engl J Med* 1993;328:358.
172. Gibbs CJ Jr, Asher DM, Kobrine A, et al. Transmission of Creutzfeldt-Jakob disease to a chimpanzee by electrodes contaminated during neurosurgery. *J Neurol Neurosurg Psychiatr* 1994;57:757.
173. Bosque PJ, Ryou C, Telling G, et al. Prions in skeletal muscle. *Proc Natl Acad Sci U S A* 2002;99:3812.
174. Holman RC, Khan AS, Kent J, et al. Epidemiology of Creutzfeldt-Jakob disease in the United States, 1979–1990: analysis of national mortality data. *Neuroepidemiology* 1995;14:174.
175. Holman RC, Khan AS, Belay ED, et al. Creutzfeldt-Jakob disease in the United States, 1979–1994: using national mortality data to assess the possible occurrence of variant cases. *Emerg Infect Dis* 1996;2:333.
176. Masters CL, Harris JO, Gajdusek DC, et al. Creutzfeldt-Jakob disease: patterns of world wide occurrence and the significance of familial and sporadic clustering. *Ann Neurol* 1979;5:177.
177. Prusiner SB. Genetic and infectious prion diseases. *Arch Neurol* 1993;50:1129.
178. Prusiner SB. Shattuck lecture—neurodegenerative diseases and prions. *N Engl J Med* 2001;344:1516.
179. Brown P, Preece MA, Will RG. Friendly fire in medicine: hormones, homografts, and Creutzfeldt-Jakob disease. *Lancet* 1992;340:24.
180. Will RG, Matthews WB. Evidence for case-to-case transmission of Creutzfeldt-Jakob disease. *J Neurol Neurosurg Psychiatr* 1982;45:235.
181. Foncin JF, Gaches J, Cathala F, et al. Transmission iatrogene interhumaine possible de maladie de Creutzfeldt-Jakob avec atteinte des grains de cervelet. *Rev Neurol (Paris)* 1980;136:280.
182. Duffy P, Collins G, Devoe AG, et al. Possible person-to-person transmission of Creutzfeldt-Jakob disease. *N Engl J Med* 1974;290:693.
183. Hogan RN, Brown P, Heck E, et al. Risk of prion disease transmission from ocular donor tissue transplantation. *Cornea* 1999;18:2.
184. Kennedy RH, Hogan RN, Brown P, et al. Eye banking and screening for Creutzfeldt-Jakob disease. *Arch Ophthalmol* 2001;119:721.
185. Bernoulli C, Siegfried J, Baumgartner G, et al. Danger of accidental person-to-person transmission of Creutzfeldt-Jakob disease by surgery. *Lancet* 1977;1:478.
186. Huillard d'Aignaux J, Costagliola D, Maccario J, et al. Incubation period of Creutzfeldt-Jakob disease in human growth hormone recipients in France. *Neurology* 1999;53:1197.
187. Cochius JI, Hyman N, Esiri MM. Creutzfeldt-Jakob disease in a recipient of human pituitary-derived gonadotrophin: a second case. *J Neurol Neurosurg Psychiatr* 1992;55:1094.
188. Martinez-Lage JF, Poza M, Sola J, et al. Accidental transmission of Creutzfeldt-Jakob disease by dural cadaveric grafts. *J Neurol Neurosurg Psychiatr* 1994;57:1091.
189. Martinez-Lage JF, Poza M, Tortosa JG. Creutzfeldt-Jakob disease in patients who received a cadaveric dura mater graft: Spain, 1985–1992. *MMWR Morb Mortal Wkly Rep* 1993;42:560.
190. Centers for Disease Control. Rapidly progressive dementia in a patient who received a cadaveric dura mater graft. *MMWR Morb Mortal Wkly Rep* 1987;36:49.

191. Nakamura Y, Yanagawa H, Kitamoto T, et al. Epidemiologic features of 65 Creutzfeldt-Jakob disease patients with a history of cadaveric dura mater transplantation in Japan. *Epidemiol Infect* 2000;125:201.

192. Nakamura Y, Oki I, Tanihara S, et al. A case-control study of Creutzfeldt-Jakob disease in Japan: transplantation of cadaveric dura mater was a risk factor. *J Epidemiol* 2000;10:399.

193. Hoshi K, Yoshino H, Urata J, et al. Creutzfeldt-Jakob disease associated with cadaveric dura mater grafts in Japan. *Neurology* 2000;55:718.

194. Masullo C, Pocchiari M, Macche G, et al. Transmission of Creutzfeldt-Jakob disease by dural cadaveric graft. *J Neurosurg* 1989;71:954.

195. Nisbet TJ, MacDonaldson I, Bishara SN. Creutzfeldt-Jakob disease in a second patient who received a cadaveric dura mater graft. *JAMA* 1989;261:1118.

196. Dobbins JG, Belay ED, Malecki J, et al. Creutzfeldt-Jakob disease in a recipient of a dura mater graft processed in the US: cause or coincidence? *Neuroepidemiology* 2000;19:62.

197. Hannah EL, Belay ED, Gambetti P, et al. Creutzfeldt-Jakob disease after receipt of a previously unimplicated brand of dura mater graft. *Neurology* 2001;56:1080.

198. Jellinger K, Seitelberger F, Heiss W-D, et al. Konjugale Form der subakuten spongiöse Enzephalopathie (Jakob-Creutzfeldt Erkrankung). *Wien Klin Wochenschr* 1972;84:245.

199. Matthews WB. Epidemiology of Creutzfeldt-Jakob disease in England and Wales. *J Neurol Neurosurg Psychiatr* 1975;38:210.

200. Gajdusek DC, Gibbs CJ Jr, Asher DM, et al. Precautions in medical care of and in handling materials from patients with transmissible virus dementia (Creutzfeldt-Jakob disease). *N Engl J Med* 1977;297:1253.

201. Miller D. Creutzfeldt-Jakob disease in histopathology technicians. *N Engl J Med* 1988;318:853.

202. Sitwell L, Lach B, Atack E, et al. Creutzfeldt-Jakob disease in histopathology technicians. *N Engl J Med* 1988;318:854.

203. Weber T, Tumani H, Holdorff B, et al. Transmission of Creutzfeldt-Jakob disease by handling of dura mater. *Lancet* 1993;341:123.

204. Gorman DG, Benson DF, Vogel DG, et al. Creutzfeldt-Jakob disease in a pathologist. *Neurology* 1992;42:463.

205. Berger JR, David NJ. Creutzfeldt-Jakob disease in a physician: a review of the disorder in health care workers. *Neurology* 1993;43:205.

206. Bradley R, Wilesmith JW. Epidemiology and control of bovine spongiform encephalopathy (BSE). *BMJ* 1993;49:932.

207. Kimberlin RH. Bovine spongiform encephalopathy: an appraisal of the current epidemic in the United-Kingdom. *Intervirology* 1993;35:208.

208. Lorains JW, Henry C, Agbamu DA, et al. Variant Creutzfeldt-Jakob disease in an elderly patient. *Lancet* 2001;357:1339.

209. Hourrigan J, Klingsporn A, Clark W, et al. *Epidemiology of scrapie in the United States*, Vol 1. New York: Academic Press, 1979.

210. Wisniewski HM, Sigurdarson S, Rubenstein R, et al. Mites as vectors for scrapie. *Lancet* 1996;347:1114.

211. Marsh RF. Bovine spongiform encephalopathy in the United States. *J Am Vet Med Assoc* 1990;196:1677.

212. Marsh RF, Hadlow WJ. Transmissible mink encephalopathy. *Rev Sci Tech (Paris)* 1992;11:539.

213. Belay ED, Gambetti P, Schonberger LB, et al. Creutzfeldt-Jakob disease in unusually young patients who consumed venison. *Arch Neurol* 2001;58:1673.

214. Gajdusek DC, Zigas V. Degenerative disease of the central nervous system in New Guinea: epidemic occurrence of "kuru" in the native population. *N Engl J Med* 1957;257:974.

215. Lacey RW, Dealler SF. Vertical transfer of prion disease. *Hum Reprod* 1994;9:1792.

216. Berman PH, Davidson GS, Becker LE. Progressive neurological deterioration in a 14-year-old girl. *Pediatr Neurosci* 1988;14:42.

217. Brown P, Cathala F, Labauge R, et al. Epidemiologic implications of Creutzfeldt-Jakob disease in a 19 year-old girl. *Eur J Epidemiol* 1985;1:42.

218. Brown P, Cervenakova L, Goldfarb LG, et al. Molecular genetic testing of a fetus at risk of Gerstmann-Sträussler-Scheinker syndrome. *Lancet* 1994;343:181.

219. Brown P. Vertical transmission of prion disease. *Hum Reprod* 1994;9:1796.

220. Monreal J, Collins GH, Masters CL, et al. Creutzfeldt-Jakob disease in an adolescent. *J Neurol Sci* 1981;52:341.

221. Packer RJ, Cornblath DR, Gonatas NK, et al. Creutzfeldt-Jakob disease in a 20-year-old woman. *Neurology* 1980;30:492.

222. Will RG. Response to the article: 'Vertical transfer of prion disease' by Lacey and Dealler. *Hum Reprod* 1994;9:1797.

223. Brown P, Rodgers-Johnson P, Cathala F, et al. Creutzfeldt-Jakob disease of long duration: clinicopathological characteristics, transmissibility, and differential diagnosis. *Ann Neurol* 1984;16:295.

224. Brown P, Cervenakova L, Goldfarb LG, et al. Iatrogenic Creutzfeldt-Jakob disease: an example of the interplay between ancient genes and modern medicine. *Neurology* 1994;44:291.

225. Will RG, Zeidler M, Stewart GE, et al. Diagnosis of new variant Creutzfeldt-Jakob disease. *Ann Neurol* 2000;47:575.

226. Medori R, Montagna P, Tritschler HJ, et al. Fatal familial insomnia: a second kindred with mutation of prion protein gene at codon-178. *Neurology* 1992;42:669.

227. Manetto V, Medori R, Cortelli P, et al. Fatal familial insomnia: clinical and pathologic study of five new cases. *Neurology* 1992;42:312.

228. Gambetti P, Petersen R, Monari L, et al. Fatal familial insomnia and the widening spectrum of prion diseases. *BMJ* 1993;49:980.

229. Gloor P, Kalabay O, Giard N. The electroencephalogram in diffuse encephalopathies: electroencephalographic correlates of grey and white matter lesions. *Brain* 1968;91:779.

230. Zeidler M, Sellar RJ, Collie DA, et al. The pulvinar sign on magnetic resonance imaging in variant Creutzfeldt-Jakob disease. *Lancet* 2000;355:1412.

231. Collie DA, Sellar RJ, Zeidler M, et al. MRI of Creutzfeldt-Jakob disease: imaging features and recommended MRI protocol. *Clin Radiol* 2001;56:726.

232. Roos R, Gajdusek DC, Gibbs CJ Jr. The clinical characteristics of transmissible Creutzfeldt-Jakob disease. *Brain* 1973;96:1.

233. Harrington MG, Merril CR, Asher DM, et al. Abnormal proteins in the cerebrospinal fluid of patients with Creutzfeldt-Jakob disease. *N Engl J Med* 1986;315:279.

234. Hsich G, Kenney K, Gibbs CJ, et al. The 14-3-3 brain protein in cerebrospinal fluid as a marker for transmissible spongiform encephalopathies. *N Engl J Med* 1996;335:924.

235. Burbelo PF, Hall A. Hot numbers in signal transduction. *Curr Biol* 1995;5:95.

236. Boston PF, Jackson P, Thompson RJ. Human 14-3-3 protein: radioimmunoassay, tissue distribution, and cerebrospinal fluid levels in patients with neurological disorders. *J Neurochem* 1982;38:1475.

237. Blisard K, Davis L, Harrington M, et al. Pre-mortem diagnosis of Creutzfeldt-Jakob disease by detection of abnormal cerebrospinal fluid proteins. *J Neurol Sci* 1990;99:75.

238. Yun M, Wu W, Hood L, et al. Human cerebrospinal fluid protein database: edition 1992. *Electrophoresis* 1992;13:1002.

239. Shaked GM, Shaked Y, Kariv-Inbal Z, et al. A protease-resistant prion protein isoform is present in urine of animals and humans affected with prion diseases. *J Biol Chem* 2001;276:31479.

240. Miele G, Manson J, Clinton M. A novel erythroid-specific marker of transmissible spongiform encephalopathies. *Nat Med* 2001;7:361.

241. Moynagh J, Schimmel H. Tests for BSE evaluated: bovine spongiform encephalopathy. *Nature* 1999;400:105.

242. Saborio GP, Permanne B, Soto C. Sensitive detection of pathological prion protein by cyclic amplification of protein misfolding. *Nature* 2001;411:810.

243. Serban D, Taraboulos A, DeArmond SJ, et al. Rapid detection of Creutzfeldt-Jakob disease and scrapie prion proteins. *Neurology* 1990;40:110.

244. Asher DM. Transmission of human spongiform encephalopathies to experimental animals: comparison of the chimpanzee and squirrel monkey. *Dev Biol Stand* 1993;80:9.

245. Asher DM, Masters CL, Gajdusek DC, et al. Familial spongiform encephalopathies. In: Kety S, Rowland L, Sidman R, et al., eds. *Genetics of neurological and psychiatric disorders*. New York: Raven Press, 1983:273–291.

246. Hunter N, Foster JD, Dickinson AG, et al. Linkage of the gene for the scrapie-associated fibril protein (PrP) to the Sip gene in Cheviot sheep. *Vet Rec* 1989;124:364.

247. Carlson GA, Kingsbury DT, Goodman PA, et al. Linkage of prion protein and scrapie incubation time genes. *Cell* 1986;46:503.

248. Westaway D, Goodman PA, Mirenda CA, et al. Distinct prion proteins in short and long scrapie incubation period mice. *Cell* 1987;51:651.

249. Westaway D, Carlson GA, Prusiner SB. Unraveling prion diseases through molecular genetics. *Trends Neurosci* 1989;12:221.

250. Hsiao K, Baker HF, Crow TJ, et al. Linkage of a prion protein missense variant to Gerstmann-Sträussler syndrome. *Nature* 1989;338:342.

251. Goldgaber D, Goldfarb LG, Brown P, et al. Mutations in familial Creutzfeldt-Jakob disease and Gerstmann-Sträussler-Scheinker's syndrome. *Exper Neurol* 1989;106:204.

252. Goldfarb LG, Brown P, Goldgaber DG, et al. Creutzfeldt-Jakob disease and kuru patients lack a mutation consistently found in the Gerstmann-Sträussler-Scheinker syndrome. *Exp Neurol* 1990;108:247.

253. Goldfarb LG, Petersen RB, Tabaton M, et al. Fatal familial insomnia and familial Creutzfeldt-Jakob disease: disease phenotype determined by a DNA polymorphism. *Science* 1992;258:806.

254. Medori R, Tritschler HJ. Prion protein gene analysis in 3 kindreds with fatal familial insomnia (FFI): codon-178 mutation and codon-129 polymorphism. *Am J Hum Genet* 1993;53:822.

255. Collinge J, Palmer MS, Dryden AJ. Genetic predisposition to iatrogenic Creutzfeldt-Jakob disease. *Lancet* 1991;337:1441.

256. Palmer MS, Dryden AJ, Hughes JT, et al. Homozygous prion protein genotype predisposes to sporadic Creutzfeldt-Jakob disease. *Nature* 1991;352:340.

257. Lee HS, Brown P, Cervenakova L, et al. Increased susceptibility to kuru of carriers of the PRNP 129 methionine/methionine genotype. *J Infect Dis* 2001;183:192.

258. Westaway D, Zuliani V, Cooper CM, et al. Homozygosity for prion protein alleles encoding glutamine-171 renders sheep susceptible to natural scrapie. *Genes Dev* (Cold Spring Harbor, NY) 1994;8:959.

259. Amouyel P, Vidal O, Launay JM, et al. The apolipoprotein E alleles as major susceptibility factors for Creutzfeldt-Jakob disease. *Lancet* 1994;344:1315.

260. Amouyel P, Alperovitch A, Delasnerie-Laupretre N, et al. Apolipoprotein E in Creutzfeldt-Jakob disease. *Lancet* 1995;345:595.
261. Roses AD, Saunders AM, Strittmatter WJ, et al. Apolipoprotein E in Creutzfeldt-Jacob disease. *Lancet* 1995;345:69.
262. Zerr I, Helmhold M, Armstrong VW, et al. Apolipoprotein E in Creutzfeldt-Jakob disease. *Lancet* 1995;345:266.
263. Telling GC, Scott M, Mastrianni J, et al. Prion propagation in mice expressing human and chimeric PrP transgenes implicates the interaction of cellular PrP with another protein. *Cell* 1995;83:79.
264. Dickinson AG, Fraser H. An assessment of the genetics of scrapie in sheep and mice. In: Pruisner SB, Hadlow WJ, eds. *Slow transmissible diseases of the nervous system*, Vol 1. New York: Academic Press, 1979:367–385.
265. Lloyd SE, Onwuazor ON, Beck JA, et al. Identification of multiple quantitative trait loci linked to prion disease incubation period in mice. *Proc Natl Acad Sci U S A* 2001;98:6279.
266. Goldfarb LG, Brown P. The transmissible spongiform encephalopathies. *Annu Rev Med* 1995;46:57.
267. Spudich S, Mastrianni JA, Wrensch M, et al. Complete penetrance of Creutzfeldt-Jakob disease in Libyan Jews carrying the E200K mutation in the prion protein gene. *Mol Med* 1995;1:607.
268. Kimberlin RH, Walker CA. Suppression of scrapie infection in mice by heteropolyanion 23, dextran sulfate, and some other polyanions. *Antimicrob Agents Chemother* 1986;30:409.
269. Pocchiari M, Schmittinger S, Masullo C. Amphotericin B delays the incubation period of scrapie in intracerebrally inoculated hamsters. *J Gen Virol* 1987;168:219.
270. Pocchiari M, Casaccia P, Ladogana A. Amphotericin B: a novel class of antiscrapie drugs. *J Infect Dis* 1989;160:795.
271. Demaimay R, Adjou K, Lasmezas C, et al. Pharmacological studies of a new derivative of amphotericin B, MS-8209, in mouse and hamster scrapie. *J Gen Virol* 1994;75:2499.
272. Caughey B, Brown K, Raymond GJ, et al. Binding of the protease-sensitive form of prion protein PrP to sulfated glycosaminoglycan and Congo red. *J Virol* 1994;68:2135.
273. Forloni G, Iussich S, Awan T, et al. Tetracyclines affect prion infectivity. *Proc Natl Acad Sci U S A* 2002;99:10849.
274. Sethi S, Lipford G, Wagner H, et al. Postexposure prophylaxis against prion disease with a stimulator of innate immunity. *Lancet* 2002;360:229.
275. Brown P, Gibbs CJ Jr, Amyx HL, et al. Chemical disinfection of Creutzfeldt-Jakob disease virus. *N Engl J Med* 1982;306:1279.
276. Brown P. Transfusion medicine and spongiform encephalopathy. *Transfusion* 2001;41:433.
277. Occupational Safety and Health Administration US Department of Labor. Occupational exposure to bloodborne pathogens; final rule (29 CFR Part 1910.1030). *Fed Reg* 1991;56:64175.
278. Taylor DM, Fraser H, McConnell I, et al. Decontamination studies with the agents of bovine spongiform encephalopathy and scrapie. *Arch Virol* 1994;139:313.
279. Taylor DM. Inactivation of transmissible degenerative encephalopathy agents: a review. *Vet J* 2000;159:10.
280. DiMartino A, Safar J, Ceroni M, et al. Purification of non-infectious ganglioside preparations from scrapie-infected brain tissue. *Arch Virol* 1992;124:111.
281. Ernst DR, Race RE. Comparative analysis of scrapie agent inactivation methods. *J Virol Methods* 1993;41:193.
282. Brown P, Rohwer R, Gajdusek D. Sodium hydroxide disinfection of Creutzfeldt-Jakob disease virus. *N Engl J Med* 1984;310:727.
283. Taylor DM. Inactivation of SE agents. *BMJ* 1993;49:810.
284. Brown P, Liberski PP, Wolff A, et al. Resistance of scrapie infectivity to steam autoclaving after formaldehyde fixation and limited survival after washing at 360°C: practical and theoretical implications. *J Infect Dis* 1990;161:467.
285. Asher DM, Gibbs CJJ, Gajdusek DC. Slow viral infections: safe handling of the agents of the subacute spongiform encephalopathies. In: Miller B, Gröschel D, Richardson J, et al., eds. *Laboratory safety: principles and practice.* Washington, DC: American Society for Microbiology, 1986:59–71.
286. Rutala WA, Weber DJ. Creutzfeldt-Jakob disease: recommendations for disinfection and sterilization. *Clin Infect Dis* 2001;32:1348.
287. Manuelidis EE, de Figueiredo FJ, Kim JH, et al. Transmission studies from blood of Alzheimer disease patients and healthy relatives. *Proc Natl Acad Sci U S A* 1988;85:4898.
288. Manuelidis EE, Rorke LB. Transmission of Alpers' disease (chronic progressive encephalopathy) produces experimental Creutzfeldt-Jakob disease in hamsters. *Neurology* 1989;39:615.
289. Manuelidis EE, Manuelidis L. A transmissible Creutzfeldt-Jakob disease-like agent is prevalent in the human population. *Proc Natl Acad Sci U S A* 1993;90:7724.
290. Godec MS, Asher DM, Kozachuk WE, et al. Blood buffy coat from Alzheimer's disease patients and their relatives does not transmit spongiform encephalopathy to hamsters. *Neurology* 1994;44:1111.
291. Baker HF, Ridley RM, Duchen LW, et al. Induction of beta(A4)-amyloid in primates by injection of Alzheimer's disease brain homogenate: comparison with transmission of spongiform encephalopathy. *Mol Neurobiol* 1994;8:25.
292. Goudsmit J, Morrow CH, Asher DM, et al. Evidence for and against the transmissibility of Alzheimer's disease. *Neurology* 1980;30:945.

CHAPTER 265

Mycobacterium tuberculosis *and Other Mycobacteria*

Kevin P. Fennelly and Jerrold J. Ellner

The genus *Mycobacterium* is the only member of the family My-cobacteriaceae and consists of slow-growing, rod-shaped, non–spore-forming, nonmotile organisms that are acid fast; that is, once stained, they resist destaining by acid alcohol treatment. This characteristic is attributed to their cell walls that have un-usually high content of lipids (25%), in contrast to 0.5% for gram-positive bacteria and 3% for gram-negative bacteria. Mycolic acids are the principal components of the complex cell walls (1), some of which contribute to virulence. Wax D, a complex of pep-tides, polysaccharides, and mycolic acid, enhances cell-mediated immune responses against mycobacterial proteins. Cord factor is lethal to mice and inhibits polymorphonuclear leukocyte mi-gration. Sulfolipids inhibit activation of macrophages and, thus, production of microbicidal molecules (2).

Mycobacteria are straight or slightly curved bacilli, 0.2 to 0.6 μm wide by 1.0 to 10 μm long, sometimes with branching (3). They are more strongly acid fast than organisms that are weakly acid fast, such as *Nocardia, Rhodococcus, Corynebacterium, Tsukamurella,* and *Gordona* species. Acid fastness is partly or com-pleted lost at some stages of growth in some species and un-der conditions of starvation in *Mycobacterium tuberculosis* (4). On cultivation, colony morphology is variable. Some species grow on simple substrates, others are fastidious, and some are not cultivable (e.g., *Mycobacterium leprae*). Species requiring light to form pigment are called *photochromogens,* and those forming pig-ment with or without light are *scotochromogens.* Growth rates are slow, with generation times ranging from 2 hours to more than 20 hours and with grossly visible colonies appearing at 2 days to 8 weeks. Optimal growth temperatures vary from 30° to 45°C. Previously considered an obligate aerobe, *M. tuberculosis* has been found to survive anaerobic conditions (5).

There are now more than 100 species of mycobacteria identi-fied, and the number continues to grow, largely because of the contribution of molecular genetics to taxonomic studies (6,7). Be-fore these developments, only about 30 culturable species had been previously identified as "mycobacteria other than tuber-culosis," owing to the limitations imposed by biochemical and culture-based tests (8). Mycobacteria are ubiquitous and range from organisms that have no pathogenicity for humans to the highly virulent species of *M. tuberculosis* and *M. leprae.* Between these extremes are species increasingly recognized as oppor-tunistic pathogens in patients with preexisting lung disease or immunosuppressed patients. Although cumbersome, *mycobac-teria other than tuberculosis* (MOTT) is probably the most ap-propriate nomenclature because "nontuberculous mycobacte-ria" (NTM) still form tubercles (9), although *M. leprae* remains a special case. These organisms are also sometimes referred to as "atypical mycobacteria" causing the diseases of "atypical tuber-culosis" to differentiate them from "typical" tuberculosis (TB) or as "environmental mycobacteria" to reflect their ecological niches in soil or water.

MYCOBACTERIUM TUBERCULOSIS

Characteristics of the Pathogen

Robert Koch described *M. tuberculosis* as "The Etiology of Tu-berculosis" in 1882 (10). "They are rod-shaped bacilli...often inside cells" (10). Some taxonomists now consider the five mem-bers of the *M. tuberculosis* complex to be so closely related that they should be regarded as subspecies of *M. tuberculosis* rather than distinct species (6). *M. tuberculosis* and *Mycobacterium bo-vis* cause the most disease in humans. *Mycobacterium africanum* may cause 18% to 49% of TB in Africa (11,12). *Mycobacterium microti* is a pathogen of rodents. *Mycobacterium canetti* is the most recently described member of the complex. Humans are the only natural reservoir for *M. tuberculosis,* despite its abil-ity to infect other primates, elephants, and experimental animal models (6).

M. tuberculosis grows slowly with a doubling time of 12 to 18 hours. On complex solid media, colonies are visible in 3 to 6 weeks. Growth is enhanced by 10% carbon dioxide. Virulent strains form strands or cords in liquid media. *M. tuberculosis* is differentiated from other mycobacteria by its production of niacin, reduction of nitrates, usual production of a heat-labile catalase, and characteristic susceptibility to isoniazid (INH). A radiometric method using Middlebrook 7H12 culture medium with radiolabeled fatty acid (palmitate labeled with carbon 14) as substrate (Bactec) has reduced the time required for isolation and identification of *M. tuberculosis* by half, from 4 weeks to 2 weeks on average. Tubercle bacilli can be distinguished from NTM by their sensitivity to *p*-nitro-*o*-acetylamino-3-hydroxypropiophenone or by nucleic acid amplification tests. A major advance opening the field of molecular epidemiology is DNA fingerprinting by restriction fragment length polymor-phism (RFLP), which has been successfully applied in outbreaks of TB (13). The most widely used system is based on RFLP with detection of the insertion element IS6110, which is present only in isolates of *M. tuberculosis* complex and in high copy numbers (14). The sequencing of the entire genome of *M. tuberculosis* is a landmark achievement that opens the door for major scientific advances in genomics and proteomics in the near future (15).

Epidemiology

There were an estimated 8 million (range, 6.3 to 11.1 million) incident cases of TB in the world in 1997, with 1.9 million (range, 1.4 to 2.8 million) deaths attributed to TB annually (16). Eighty percent of the global burden of TB lies in 22 countries in Southeast Asia, sub-Saharan Africa, and Eastern Europe. Ninety-five percent of all TB cases and 98% of TB deaths occur in developing countries, largely because of the global human immunodeficiency virus (HIV) epidemic as well as to poverty, war, migration, and poor political commitment to TB control. Nearly one third of new TB cases in sub-Saharan Africa now occur in HIV-infected individuals, and 9 of the 10 countries with the highest incidence rates are in Africa. Although only 5% to 10% of individuals with latent infection with tuberculosis (LTBI) develop active disease, one third of the world's population, or 1.86 billion people, is estimated to be infected, an enormous reservoir of potential disease.

Multidrug-resistant tuberculosis (MDR-TB), defined as *in vitro* drug resistance to at least isoniazid and rifampin, continues to be a global public health problem, despite recent significant decreases in prevalence in France and the United States (17). Although the median prevalence among all new cases was only 1.0%, "hot spots" of MDR-TB in Eastern Europe and Asia continue to have rates among new cases of 5 to 14.1%. In Estonia, the prevalence of MDR-TB among all cases increased from 11.7% in 1994 to 18.1% in 1998. Although directly observed short-course chemotherapy has decreased morbidity and mortality in TB (18), it alone does not cure drug-resistant TB (19).

Case rates in the United States had been declining at a rate of 6% per year, but there was a resurgence of TB from 1986 to 1992 attributed to increased immigration, waning of the public health infrastructure, but probably most importantly the HIV epidemic. The principal increase in the number of TB patients occurred in the 25- to 44-year-old age group, and most cases were reported from locations with high HIV prevalence, such as New York City, New Jersey, and Florida. Nosocomial outbreaks involving multidrug-resistant strains of *M. tuberculosis* with transmission to patients and health care professionals (20) were alarming and led to new action and investment in controlling TB (21).

Case rates in the United States have declined steadily since 1992; in 2000, there were 16,377 reported cases for a rate of 5.9 per 100,000, the lowest on record in the United States (22). Racial and ethnic minorities remain disproportionately affected, accounting for 75% of all reported cases. Nearly one third of cases occur in non-Hispanic blacks, 23% in Hispanics, 21% in Asians and Pacific Islanders, and 1% in Native Americans and Alaskan Natives. In 2000, the proportion of TB cases in foreign-born persons increased from 24% to 46% of all cases, owing to increased immigration and improved control of TB in U.S.-born persons. Similar changes have been noted in other high-income countries, suggesting the need for developing a more global approach to TB control. The impact of highly active antiretroviral therapy (HAART) for HIV infection on the epidemiology of TB has been generally favorable in the United States (23), Europe (24), and Brazil (25).

Transmission

After decades of debate about the mode of transmission, Wells and Riley confirmed that most TB is transmitted by the airborne route (26,27). Close contacts of a smear-positive patient are at maximal risk for being infected. Roughly 25% to 50% of those exposed become infected, and the attack rate may be as high as 80% if a sustained, heavy exposure occurs (28–30). The rate of infection for contacts of smear-negative, culture-positive patients (5%) had previously been thought to be similar to the background rate in the community (31). A more recent study in San Francisco using molecular epidemiology (i.e., DNA fingerprinting of isolates using RFLP to assess clustering) found that smear-negative cases accounted for about 17% of recent transmission (32). Transmission by other means is rare. Infection can occur by dermal inoculation of bacilli, occasionally seen in hospital personnel handling infected tissues and cultures. In the developed countries, infection with *M. bovis* through milk from infected cows has been eliminated by pasteurization of milk. Gastrointestinal transmission may still affect those in developing countries, including cross-border travelers (33).

Spread of TB can be rapid in settings of overcrowding. Case rates among prison inmates are among the highest reported prevalence rates (34). In the ex-USSR state of Georgia, there were 448 confirmed TB cases among 7,473 inmates, for a prevalence of 5,995 per 100,000 (35). Nursing home residents also have higher case rates than those of age-matched control subjects who live at home, probably owing to cohabitation with infectious patients with TB and to waning of immunocompetence secondary to aging (36). The prevalence of TB in homeless persons is substantially higher than in the general population, and shelters have been identified as sources of TB outbreaks (37,38).

Pathogenesis

Infectious particles of experimentally nebulized *M. tuberculosis* were estimated to be 1 to 5 μm by Wells (26,39), a size range well suited to deposition of particles in the alveoli (40). Riley and co-workers used infections of guinea pigs exposed to the air from an experimental TB ward to estimate the concentrations of aerosols of *M. tuberculosis* from infectious patients (41), and other exposures have been estimated by modeling data based on those studies (42,43). These data suggest that the production of infectious aerosols in pulmonary TB varies over 3 orders of magnitude from 1.25 to more than 1,500 infectious units per hour (44).

Bacilli that are deposited in the alveoli and that escape clearance mechanisms then encounter a number of innate immune mechanisms, including surfactant proteins (45), toll-like receptors (46), granulysin (47), defensins (48), and other antimicrobial peptides. Tubercle bacilli escaping these defense mechanisms undergo phagocytosis by macrophages. After phagocytosis, mycobacteria are contained within phagosomes. Although killed mycobacteria are found in lysosomes, some mycobacteria appear to block the maturation of the phagosome and to resist delivery to the lysosome (49).

The immune response to *M. tuberculosis* contributes considerably to the pathology and is characterized by a paradoxical mix of immune activation and suppression (50). Acquired cellular immunity develops within 4 to 6 weeks. Subsets of T lymphocytes producing macrophage-activating cytokines, in particular interferon-γ (IFN-γ), enable the phagocytes to destroy intracellular bacilli. Macrophage production of cytokines, such as tumor necrosis factor (TNF), proteases, and lipases, enhances liquefaction of caseous foci, favoring extracellular bacillary growth and cavity formation. Other cytokines, such as transforming growth factor, may favor local bacillary growth, suppress T-cell responses, and promote fibrosis. Although pulmonary infection remains restricted anatomically, organisms spread to the draining hilar lymph nodes and then through the thoracic duct to the bloodstream. On pathologic examination, inflammation, caseation necrosis, cavity formation, and fibrosis occur sequentially (51). However, there may be a mixed response, with various stages occurring in different areas of the lungs at the same time. Spread within the lungs is by bronchial channels (bronchogenic spread) or directly to neighboring alveoli. Progression from minimal disease to advanced disease may occur within months but is accelerated to weeks with HIV co-infection. Extrapulmonary disease occurs when bacillemia results in the seeding of other tissues of the body. Such dissemination occurs more commonly among the immunosuppressed, notably in HIV infection. Bacilli are usually not totally eradicated because a lifelong potential for reactivation remains.

The mechanisms underlying reactivation of latent TB are not well understood. However, a critical role for TNF-α regulation is now recognized. In an experimental murine model of chronic persistent TB, neutralization of TNF-α resulted in fatal reactivation of TB with an increased bacillary burden in the lungs and in severe lung pathology (52). These data are consonant with clinical observations of 70 reported cases of reactivation TB after treatment with infliximab, an antibody against TNF-α used in the treatment of Crohn's disease and rheumatoid arthritis (53). Similarly, the importance of IFN-γ in host defense is supported by increased susceptibility to mycobacterial infections in those with inherited deficiencies of IFN receptors, as discussed later regarding NTM infections.

The pathogenesis of latent infection is even less well understood, but it appears that the bacillus is capable of survival through at least two stages of "nonreplicating persistence," one of which is an anaerobic stage (5). Persistence of *M. tuberculosis* is facilitated by isocitrate lyase, an enzyme essential for fatty acid metabolism, which is expressed more with activation of host macrophages (54). Exposure to chemotherapy induces the *sigF* gene, which is similar to genes involved in bacterial stress responses (55), reflecting the ability of the tubercle bacillus to respond not only to the host response to infection but also to therapy.

Prevention

The most effective methods to prevent TB are (a) rapid, appropriate drug treatment of active pulmonary disease to prevent further transmission; and (b) treatment of latent infection to prevent reactivation. These interventions are discussed in Chapter 156.

VACCINATION

Although bacille Calmette Guérin (BCG) vaccine has been used worldwide for decades except in a few developed countries, the value of BCG vaccination as protection against TB remains unclear, with protection rates varying from 0% to 80%. Genomic analyses of BCG strains reveals numerous differences among strains, but their effects on the variability of effectiveness are unknown (56). BCG vaccination may be beneficial in reducing miliary and meningeal disease in children. BCG should not be administered to children or adults who have symptomatic HIV infection because it may lead to disseminated BCG infection. However, the World Health Organization recommends BCG vaccination for asymptomatic HIV-infected children who are at increased risk for tuberculous infection. The tuberculin skin test (TST) is the mainstay of assessing exposure in contact investigations in developed countries; therefore, BCG vaccination is usually not recommended because it may confuse the interpretation of the TST. Intense efforts are underway to develop better TB vaccines.

TUBERCULOSIS INFECTION CONTROL

In response to outbreaks of nosocomial MDR-TB involving fatalities in both patients and health care workers, the Centers for Disease Control and Prevention issued new "Guidelines for Preventing the Transmission of *Mycobacterium tuberculosis* in Health-Care Facilities, 1994" (57). These guidelines are being revised, but the hierarchy of administrative, engineering, and personal respiratory protection control measures remain the basis for TB infection control. The most important strategy to prevent transmission of *M. tuberculosis* in congregate settings is the rapid identification, isolation, and appropriate treatment of infectious patients, which is the goal of administrative controls.

The foundation of engineering controls is the negative-pressure "airborne infection room." Negative pressure within the room prevents infectious aerosol from being carried outside, whereas dilution ventilation of 6 to 12 air changes per hour (ACH) removes the infectious particles. Adjunctive measures include ultraviolet germicidal irradiation (UVGI) of either upper room air or the inside of ducts and high-efficiency particulate air (HEPA) filtration. Both require expertise in installation and periodic maintenance to be efficacious. The adjunctive measures are probably most effective in high-risk areas where there may be infectious TB patients but where there is inadequate dilution ventilation.

Personal respiratory protection refers to the use of masks designed to protect the wearer from inhalation hazards, such as infectious aerosols. This continues to be the most controversial aspect of the Centers for Disease Control and Prevention guidelines. The most commonly used masks are disposable particulate respirators now certified as N95, meaning that the filter material is 95% efficient at removing test particles. Better markers of infectiousness are needed to prioritize more confidently and to implement such resources, especially in crowded facilities in high-incidence areas.

M. tuberculosis has been transmitted not only by the infectious aerosols generated during bronchoscopies also but directly by contaminated bronchoscopes (58). Pseudoinfections due to poor disinfection have also been reported (58) and can be costly. Improved disinfectants have become available, and rigorous policies and procedures are required to clean and disinfect such equipment (59).

MYCOBACTERIA OTHER THAN *MYCOBACTERIUM TUBERCULOSIS*

Mycobacteria other than *M. tuberculosis* and *M. leprae* are ubiquitous in the environment, usually in water or soil, and have a varied spectrum of pathogenicity for humans. With the greater frequency of disease due to some NTM and the increasing numbers of immunocompromised patients, recognition of these infections is important. As mycobacterial infections other than TB are not reportable to public health departments, the best available data are from national surveys. The most recent data in the U.S. are from 1981 to 1983, before the HIV epidemic, when clinical and laboratory data were collected on 5,469 patients; almost 90% of the isolates were from respiratory tract specimens (60). Prevalence rates were calculated using a diagnostic algorithm, with most disease associated with *Mycobacterium avium* complex (MAC; 1.3 per 100,000), *Mycobacterium kansasii*

(0.3 per 100,000), and *Mycobacterium fortuitum-chelonae* (0.2 per 100,000). The prevalence rate of all NTM infections was estimated to be 1.78 per 100,000, corresponding to 4,201 prevalent cases in the United States. After the onset of the HIV epidemic, the number of infections due to disseminated infections with MAC and other MOTT increased tremendously in the United States and other developed countries (61).

The amount of disease due to MOTT in the developing world is even less well understood, and detection is limited by laboratory capacity and by the high prevalence of TB. In contrast to the United States, there is little to no disease due to *M. avium* in Ugandan patients with acquired immunodeficiency syndrome (AIDS) (62). This is not explained by lack of environmental exposure because *M. avium* has been isolated frequently in soil and water samples in Uganda and other African sites (61). A decreased risk for disseminated MAC infection has been observed among HIV-infected persons with a history of active TB (relative risk, 0.52; $p < 0.001$) (63), suggesting a protective role of TB in preventing disseminated MAC infection. In northern Malawi, IFN-γ responses were highest for *M. avium*, *M. intracellulare*, and *M. scrofulaceum* (the MAIS complex), suggesting prior exposure to these MOTT (64). The investigators found concordance between these results and skin test results, with an additional observation that delayed hypersensitivity to rapidly growing mycobacteria was associated with a decreased risk for TB and leprosy (65).

Although it appears that most NTM are acquired from the environment, there are at least 10 reports in the literature of familial clustering of cases, most often with *M. kansasii* (66–68). In only one of these was there microbiologic testing of the home tap water, which yielded negative results (68). Thus, it is not clear whether these clusters were due to a shared environmental exposure, such as to tap water, or to person-to-person transmission. If the latter occurs, it probably does so rarely given the small number of clusters reported over the past 40 years. The most recently reported family cluster was clearly due to a common environmental source: an indoor hot tub contaminated with multiple mycobacterial species (69). NTM appear to have become part of the ecology of indoor living; 90% of biofilm samples from water-treatment plants, home plumbing, and aquaria were found to contain *M. chelonae*, *Mycobacterium flavescens*, *M. fortuitum*, *Mycobacterium gordonae*, *M. kansasii*, and *Mycobacterium terrae-nonchromogenicum* (70).

Mycobacteria have been implicated with uncertainty for years as causative agents in both sarcoidosis and Crohn's disease. It appears that *Propionibacterium* species are more likely associated with sarcoidosis than the mycobacteria (71). An association between cell wall–deficient forms of *M. avium* subspecies *paratuberculosis* and Crohn's disease has been suggested (72), but the role of mycobacteria in Crohn's disease remains controversial (61,73).

The most clinically important NTM and the clinical infections associated with them are listed in Table 265.1 and discussed

TABLE 265.1. Infections Associated with Mycobacteria

Mycobacterium species	Lungs	Skin, soft tissue	Skeletal, tendon	Lymphadenitis	Disseminated
M. tuberculosis complex					
M. africanum	+	+			+
M. bovis[a]	++		+	+	+
M. tuberculosis[a]	+++	+	+	++	++
M. leprae[a]		+++			
Slowly growing mycobacteria					
M. avium complex[a] (M. avium and M. intracellulare)	++		++	++	++
M. branderi	+				+
M. celatum	+	+			+
M. genavense					+
M. gordonae[b]	+	+			+
M. haemophilum[a]		+	+		+
M. interjectum	+			+	
M. intermedium	+				
M. kanasii[a]	++	+	++		++
M. lentiflavum[a,b]	+		+	+	+
M. malmoense	+			+	+
M. marinum		++	++		+
M. scrofulaceum	+		+	+	+
M. simiae	+				+
M. smegmatis	+	+	+		+
M. szulgai[a]	+	+	+	+	+
M. terrae/chromogenicum complex	+		+		
M. ulcerans		+			
M. xenopi[a]	+				+
Rapidly growing mycobacteria					
M. abscessus[a]	++	++	++	+	++
M. chelonae[a]		++	++		++
M. fortuitum complex (M. fortuitum, M. peregrinum)[a]	+	++	++	+	+
M. mucogenicum					+
M. neoarum					+

+++, more common; ++, less common; +, infrequent/rare.
[a]Nosocomial or iatrogenic infections reported.
[b]Contamination/pseudoinfection most common.

later. Nosocomial transmission and pseudoinfections have been reported most often due to contaminated water supplies, and iatrogenic infections have been associated with contaminated surgical materials. Because of the environmental sources of many MOTT, it is likely that additional species will be associated with nosocomial disease in the future. More detailed coverage of treatment can be found in Chapter 34, and additional clinical information is in Chapter 157.

Pathogenesis

The pathogenesis of mycobacterial infections other than TB is less well understood, although there are some common features. Because these organisms are ubiquitous in the environment but rarely cause disease, host susceptibility factors may be more important determinants of infection than the degree of exposure or the virulence of the organism. The most striking genetic susceptibilities are conferred by deficiencies of IFN-γ receptor, involving both the complete IFN-γ receptor ligand-binding chain (IFN-γR1) and the signaling chain (IFN-γR2). These children are unable to form mature granulomas and are susceptible to severe mycobacterial and salmonella infections. Milder clinical presentations are associated with partial deficiencies of these factors. These deficiencies highlight the essential role of IFN-γ in defense against mycobacterial infections, also supported by the symptomatic and radiographic improvement of seven patients with refractory, disseminated infection with NTM in a small trial of therapeutic IFN-γ given subcutaneously (74).

Acquired deficiency of cell-mediated immunity, most commonly due to HIV infection, is also associated with disseminated MAC infection. Other host factors that predispose to pulmonary mycobacterial infections are preexisting lung disease, including underlying chronic lung diseases such as chronic obstructive pulmonary disease (COPD) and pneumoconioses (75,76); bronchiectasis (77); and cystic fibrosis (78). Pulmonary infections other than MOTT occur in women without recognized risk factors (79) or with pectus excavatum, thoracic scoliosis, and mitral valve prolapse (80). However, the mechanisms underlying the susceptibility in these women are not known.

Mycobacterium avium Complex

Mycobacterium avium and *Mycobacterium intracellulare*, previously differentiated by their virulence for chickens and rabbits, respectively, are similar biochemically and genetically and are referred to as MAC. Growth is slow and optimal at 37°C. Colonies are usually not pigmented and are either opaque and domed or transparent and flat. MAC, like many other MOTT, has been isolated from both water and soil (81,82). In addition, MAC has been isolated from bronchoscopes, raw milk, and cigarettes (61). The source of MAC infection is usually unknown, although cases have been linked to isolates from hospital and municipal tap water (83). Hot tubs are another source of MAC aerosols causing both infection and hypersensitivity pneumonitis in immunocompetent patients (84,85). About 90% of MAC isolates from AIDS patients have been identified as *M. avium* by DNA probe, whereas about 40% of isolates from non–AIDS patients were *M. intracellulare* (61). Infection with more than one strain or species in AIDS patients appears common (61). This is an important consideration because different strains from the same patient may have different drug susceptibility patterns (86).

MAC is the most common MOTT associated with human disease, and its ability to cause human disease has only been recognized since 1943 (87). In a U.S. national survey from 1981 to 1983, the prevalence of MAC disease was estimated to be 1.3 per 100,000. In a study of 670,000 U.S. Navy recruits, delayed hypersensitivity responses to purified protein derivative from MAC (PPD-B or the "Battey" antigen) were 70% or greater in those from the Southeast compared with 10% to 20% in those from the North and West (88). This suggests at least greater exposure to MAC in the southeastern United States, probably from environmental sources.

Risk factors for MAC infection are as suggested earlier: (a) patients with preexisting lung disease, especially COPD, (b) thin middle-aged and elderly women, and (c) patients with HIV infection. The epidemiology may be changing because there are anecdotal reports among clinicians that there appear to be fewer male patients with COPD and more thin women among their non–HIV-infected patients with pulmonary MAC infections. These patients present with symptoms similar to those of persons with underlying lung disease, often with an insidious onset and indolent progression. Disseminated MAC disease affects immunocompromised hosts, specifically AIDS patients (89). Cervical lymphadenitis (especially in children), bone and joint infection, urinary tract involvement, and cutaneous infections, including panniculitis, have been reported.

The diagnosis of pulmonary MAC requires the presence of pulmonary symptoms with chest radiograph abnormalities of infiltrates, nodules, or cavities. MAC may occasionally present as a chest mass. The microbiologic diagnosis requires three positive acid-fast bacilli (AFB) cultures (or two positive cultures and one positive smear) if sputum alone is obtained. If a bronchoscopy is done, one positive culture (2 to 4+) is sufficient on washing or biopsy, or if histopathology demonstrates AFB or granulomatous inflammation, any growth on another specimen is adequate (90).

Chemotherapy for MAC is similar to that for TB in that it requires multiple drugs to avoid the emergence of resistance, except that MAC is usually resistant to isoniazid. Currently recommended therapy for pulmonary MAC without HIV co-infection includes daily treatment with clarithromycin or azithromycin; rifampin or rifabutin; and ethambutol (90). Sputa should be examined monthly for AFB smears and cultures, and treatment should continue for 1 year after conversion to culture negativity. Streptomycin given 2 to 3 times per week may be added for the first 2 months. Treatment of either pulmonary or disseminated MAC infection in the HIV-infected patient is similar, but rifabutin is the preferred rifamycin. AIDS patients with disseminated MAC should receive lifelong therapy with (1) clarithromycin or azithromycin, and (2) ethambutol, with or without rifabutin, unless immune reconstitution occurs due to HAART (91). For HIV-infected patients with CD4 cell counts below 50 cells/μL, the preferred primary prophylaxis regimen is clarithromycin or azithromycin (91). Because of increasing evidence that anti-MAC prophylaxis can usually be stopped safely in AIDS patients responding to HAART (92,93), current recommendations suggest discontinuation if the CD4 count remains above 100 cells/μL for 3 months or more (91). See Chapter 34 for drug dosages and additional recommendations. The utility of drug susceptibility testing for MAC and other NTM has been debated in the literature. Although current recommendations do not suggest routine drug susceptibility testing for all NTM, they do suggest its utility as baseline testing in case the patient does not respond to therapy or in the event of relapse (90). Emergence of drug-resistant mutants in patients with AIDS is likely due to the large numbers of bacilli present, and drug-resistant isolates have been recovered in patients receiving both single- and multiple-drug therapy. Relapse of symptoms has been associated with the emergence of drug resistance (61).

Mycobacterium kansasii

Initially isolated in 1953, *M. kansasii* is most commonly isolated from tap water but not from natural water (90). *M. kansasii* antigens cross-react with PPD-S (from *M. tuberculosis*); hence, delayed hypersensitivity skin testing has little utility. Reports suggest that *M. kansasii* disease is more common in the central United States, England, and Wales. In the United States, the prevalence of *M. kansasii* disease is greatest in the metropolitan areas of the Southeast and Midwest; the male-to-female ratio is 4:1. Eighty percent of patients are white; their median age is 50 years. Chronic obstructive lung disease and pneumoconiosis predispose to infection. Miners, welders, sandblasters, and painters are at highest risk for development of disease. Guinea pigs exposed to *M. kansasii* developed progressive lung disease only if the inoculum contained dust aerosols (94).

The most common form of disease due to *M. kansasii* is a chronic pneumonia, generally milder than TB but associated with more hemoptysis. Extensive unilateral upper lobe disease is more common than with MAC infection, but none of the radiographic features is specific for any of the mycobacterioses, including TB. Cervical lymphadenitis (especially in children), cutaneous abscesses or cellulitis mimicking pyogenic infection, and musculoskeletal involvement including arthritis, fasciitis, tenosynovitis, or osteomyelitis have been reported. Dissemination occurs rarely with far-advanced disease or in immunocompromised hosts such as AIDS patients (95). *M. kansasii* does not cause as much disease in AIDS patients as does MAC, for unknown reasons.

Trained microscopists can sometimes identify *M. kansasii* by virtue of the long, beaded bacilli with Ziehl-Neelsen staining, but culture is always needed for confirmation (96). It is the only mycobacterium that produces a bright-yellow pigment on exposure to light. Although *in vitro* drug resistance may be reported to isoniazid at 0.2 or 1.0 μg/mL and to streptomycin at 1 μg/mL, this may not have clinical relevance as long as rifampin is being used (90). All isolates are resistant to pyrazinamide; thus, it is not recommended for treatment. Although there have been no clinical treatment trials, the current American Thoracic Society (ATS) recommendation is to treat disease due to *M. kansasii* with isoniazid, rifampin, and ethambutol for 18 months, including at least 12 months during which sputum cultures are negative (90). Clarithromycin has excellent *in vitro* activity; hence, it is a reasonable alternative drug.

Rapidly Growing Mycobacteria

Early studies classified the rapidly growing mycobacteria (RGM) by phenotypic characteristics into subspecies of *M. fortuitum* (*M. fortuitum* biovar *fortuitum*, *M. fortuitum* biovar *peregrinum*, and an unnamed biovariant complex) and of *M. chelonae* (*M. chelonae* subspecies *abscessus* and *M. chelonae* subspecies *chelonae*). However, more recent taxonomy studies using molecular biologic tools have classified these as separate species (97). Colonies grow at 25° to 40°C in 7 days on both mycobacterial medium and routine bacteriologic medium. Acid fastness is often negative (98). A number of nosocomial outbreaks have been associated with exposure to tap water (99). This may be due to biofilms, 90% of which may contain mycobacteria (70).

Skin and soft tissue infection, the most common clinical form of disease, is usually secondary to a puncture wound and occurs within 6 weeks to 6 months. Systemic symptoms are absent, and dissemination is extremely unusual. Spontaneous resolution occurs within 1 to 2 years in as many as 20% of cases. Nosocomial infections include skin infections of vaccination sites, surgical wounds (including plastic surgery), and indwelling peri-

toneal or intravenous catheters. Disseminated disease is uncommon in severely immunocompromised persons and is associated with a high rate of mortality. Chronic pneumonia due to RGM presents in a manner indistinct from disease caused by other mycobacteria (100). Most patients are women who have no preexisting lung disease. Risk factors include achalasia, cystic fibrosis, lipoid pneumonia, and healed TB. On radiographic examination, a reticulonodular pattern is seen, usually bilateral, sparing the upper lobes, and rarely associated with cavities. Clinical exacerbations occur during a period of years, but there is no spontaneous resolution. In general, these mycobacteria are resistant to antituberculous drugs, except amikacin, and are sensitive to cefoxitin, clarithromycin, and imipenem. The rapidly growing mycobacteria have varying susceptibility patterns to drugs. A combination of parenteral antibiotics (e.g., amikacin and cefoxitin), followed by treatment with oral drugs for up to 6 months, has been effective. Surgical resection for infection by drug-resistant species (*M. abscessus*) and with unilateral localized disease may be considered.

Other Mycobacteria

M. marinum causes "swimming pool granuloma" with sources from water and aquatic organisms. A photochromogen, *M. marinum* grows optimally at 32°C; colonies appear in 8 to 14 days. Cutaneous disease usually occurs as a result of trauma to skin in contaminated, nonchlorinated fresh, or salty water. Two to 3 weeks after inoculation, a single papulonodular lesion develops, which may later ulcerate. A sporotrichoid pattern, with abscess formation and secondary nodules along the lymphatics, can also occur. Dissemination in immunocompromised hosts, synovitis, and osteomyelitis have been reported.

Mycobacterium simiae is a slow-growing species that may cause pulmonary disease mimicking TB or pulmonary MAC. In some laboratories relying on biochemical testing, it may be confused with *M. tuberculosis* because *M. simiae* is the only NTM that is niacin positive. It is unique in having 16S ribosomal RNA sequences similar to those found in both rapidly growing and slowly growing mycobacteria. Drug resistance is common; thus, *in vitro* susceptibility testing should guide therapy (90).

Mycobacterium scrofulaceum is a cause of cervical lymphadenitis in children 1 to 5 years of age; it must be differentiated from *M. tuberculosis* and MAC. Because of antigenic and drug susceptibility similarities with MAC, some authors have classified it in a group with *M. avium* and *M. intracellulare* as the MAIS complex.

Mycobacterium ulcerans is endemic to Australia, Africa, and Mexico. It causes a chronic necrotizing skin infection known as Bairnsdale ulcer in Australia and Buruli ulcer in Uganda, usually on the distal aspect of an extremity following trauma. Satellite lesions and extensive ulceration requiring wide surgical débridement may develop. Treatment options include dapsone and streptomycin with or without ethambutol (87).

Unique among mycobacteria in its absolute requirement for iron, *Mycobacterium haemophilum* is a fastidious bacillus that grows at temperatures below 32°C. It most often causes nodular, popular, or cystic skin lesions that may progress to painful ulcers in individuals immunocompromised by HIV infection (101), organ or bone marrow transplantation, or lymphoma (102). Osteomyelitis, arthritis, sinusitis, pneumonitis, lymphadenitis, and bacteremia may also occur. Successful treatment regimens have included ciprofloxacin, clarithromycin, and rifampin (103).

Mycobacterium genavense is a slowly growing fastidious organism that fails to grow on conventional solid media but grows slowly in liquid culture. *M. genavense* infection causes a syndrome indistinguishable from MAC and is estimated to be responsible for 10% of disseminated NTM infections (104,105). Fever, weight loss, diarrhea, hepatomegaly, splenomegaly, and anemia are common. Response to antimycobacterial therapy directed against MAC and survival in patients with *M. genavense* infection are similar to those with MAC infection and are dependent on absolute CD4$^+$ cell levels in AIDS patients.

Mycobacterium xenopi grows optimally at 43°C; hence, its isolation from clinical specimens may require prolonged incubation at 37°C or at higher temperatures. It is commonly isolated from tap water and has been implicated in nosocomial pulmonary infections (106) and bronchoscopy-associated pseudoinfections (107). It has been increasingly recognized in Western Europe as a cause of pulmonary disease (108). Extrapulmonary and disseminated disease has been reported. Initial therapy should include a macrolide, a rifamycin, and ethambutol (90).

Mycobacterium szulgai causes lung and extrapulmonary disease indistinguishable from TB (109). It occurs worldwide, but its source is unknown. Most patients respond to treatment with antituberculous therapy (90). *Mycobacterium, malmoense* is slow growing, often requiring at least 6 weeks of incubation (103). It is rare in the United States but increasingly reported from northern Europe, England, and Wales. It may cause pulmonary disease in patients with underlying lung disease as well as extrapulmonary disease in children or immunosuppressed patients. Most isolates are susceptible to ethambutol, rifampin, and streptomycin.

Members of the slowly growing *M. terrae* complex may cause infections of the lungs, skin, bones, and joints. Drug susceptibility testing should be done because patterns vary widely. Surgical excision often is needed. Although the rapidly growing *Mycobacterium smegmatis* is often used in laboratories as an avirulent environmental species, it may cause human disease (110). *M. gordonae* has been called the "tap-water bacillus." Although it may rarely cause infection in patients with and without immunosuppression (111), it is more commonly a source of pseudoinfections (103). *Mycobacterium celatum* may infect patients with AIDS and rarely immunocompetent individuals (112), and it may cause false-positive results on nucleic acid amplification tests for *M. tuberculosis* (113,114).

Largely due to the HIV epidemic and the increasing use of immunosuppressive therapies, infections have been found to be caused by a growing number of mycobacteria that are uncommon, unidentified, or previously unrecognized as pathogens, including the following *Mycobacterium* species: *M. alvei, M. asiaticum, M. bohemicum, M. branderi, M. brumae, M. confluentis, M. conspicuum, M. gastrii, M. flavescens, M. goodi, M. hassiacum, M. heckeshornense, M. heidelbergense, M. intermedium, M. interjectum, M. kubicae, M. lentiflavum, M. mageritense, M. mucogenicum, M. nvocastrense, M. peregrinum, M. phlei, M. septicum, M. shimodei, M. thermoresistibile, M. triplex, M. tusciae,* and *M. wolinskyi* (115).

ACKNOWLEDGMENTS

Dr. Fennelly was supported in this work by an NIH Career Development Award (1K23 AI01676-03).

REFERENCES

1. Chaterjee D. The surface glycopeptidolipds of mycobacteria: structures and biological properties. *Cell Mol Life Sci* 2001;58(14):2018–2042.
2. Pabst MJ, Gross IMS, Brozna JP, et al. Inhibition of macrophage priming by sulfatids from *Mycobacterium tuberculosis*. *J Immunol* 1988;140:634–640.
3. Metchock BG, Nolte FS, Wallace RJJ. Mycobacterium. In: Murray PR, ed. *Manual of clinical microbiology*, 7th ed. Washington, DC: ASM Press, 1999:399–437.
4. Nyka W. Studies of the effect of starvation on mycobacteria. *Infect Immun* 1974;9:843–850.
5. Wayne LG, Hayes LG. An in vitro model for sequential study of shiftdown of Mycobacterium tuberculosis through two stages of nonreplicating persistence. *Infect Immun* 1996;64:2062–2069.
6. Van Soolingen D. Molecular epidemiology of tuberculosis and other mycobacterial infections: main methodologies and achievements. *J Intern Med* 2001;249:1–26.
7. Euzeby JP. List of bacterial names with standing in nomenclature: a folder available on the Internet (URL: http://www.bacterio.cict.fr/). *Int J Syst Bacteriol* 1997;47:590–592.
8. Tortoli E, Nanetti A, Peirsimoni C, et al. Performance assessment of new multiplex probe assay for identification of mycobacteria. *J Clin Microbiol* 2001;39:1079–1084.
9. Iseman MD. The search for consensus on myobacterial nomenclature: a study in chaos (and power). *Am Rev Respir Dis* 1990;142:258.
10. Koch R. The etiology of tuberculosis [Die Aetiologie der Tuberculose]. In: *Berliner klinische Wochenschrift* 1882;19:221–30). Essays of Robert Koch. Westport, CT: Greenwood Press, 1987.
11. Schwander S, Rusch-Gerdes S, Mateega A. A pilot study of antituberculous combinations comparing rifabutin with rifampicin in the treatment of HIV-1 associated tuberculosis. *Tubercle* 1995;76:210–218.
12. Ledru S, Cauchoix B, Yameogo M. Impact of short-course therapy on tuberculosis drug resistance in South-West Burkina Faso. *Tuberc Lung Dis* 1996;77:429–436.
13. Shoemaker SA, Fisher JH, Jones WDJ, et al. Restriction fragment analysis of chromosomal DNA defines different strains of *Mycobacterium tuberculosis*. *Am Rev Respir Dis* 1986;134:210–213.
14. Small PM, Shafer RW, Hopewell PC, et al. Exogenous reinfection with multidrug-resistant *Mycobacterium tuberculosis* in patients with advanced HIV infection. *N Engl J Med* 1993;328:1137–1144.
15. Cole ST, Brosch R, Parkhill J, et al. Deciphering the biology of *Mycobacterium tuberculosis* from the complete genome sequence. *Nature* 1998;393:537–544.
16. Dye C, Scheele S, Dolin P, et al. Consensus statement. Global burden of tuberculosis: estimated incidence, prevalence, and mortality by country. WHO Global Surveillance and Monitoring Project. *JAMA* 1999;282:677–686.
17. Espinal MA, Laszlo A, Simonsen L, et al. Global trends in resistance to antituberculous drugs. World Health Organization-International Union against Tuberculosis and Lung Disease Working Group on Anti-Tuberculosis Drug Resistance Surveillance. *N Engl J Med* 2001;344:1294–1303.
18. Suarez PG, Watt CJ, Alarcon E, et al. The dynamics of tuberculosis in response to 10 years of intensive control effort in Peru. *J Infect Dis* 2001;184:473–478.
19. Espinal MA, Kim SJ, Suarez PG, et al. Standard short-course chemotherapy for drug-resistant tuberculosis: treatment outcomes in 6 countries. *JAMA* 2000;283:2575–2576.
20. Centers for Disease Control and Prevention. Nosocomial transmission of multidrug-resistant tuberculosis among HIV-infected persons-Florida and New York, 1988–91. *MMWR Morb Mortal Wkly Rep* 1991;40:585–591.
21. Frieden TR, Fujiwara PL, Washko RM, et al. Tuberculosis in New York City: turning the tide. *N Engl J Med* 1995;333:229–233.
22. Centers for Disease Control and Prevention, Division of TB Elimination. *Reported tuberculosis in the United States, 2000*. Atlanta, GA: U.S. Department of Health and Human Services, 2001.
23. Jones JL, Hanson DL, Dworkin MS, et al. HIV-associated tuberculosis in the era of highly active antiretroviral therapy. The Adult/Adolescent Spectrum of HIV Disease Group. *Int J Tuberc Lung Dis* 2000;4:1026–1031.
24. Kirk O, Gatell JM, Mocroft A, et al. Infections with *Mycobacterium tuberculosis* and *Mycobacterium avium* among HIV-infected patients after the introduction of highly active antiretroviral therapy. EuroSIDA Study Group. *Am J Respir Crit Care Med* 2000;162:865–872.
25. Santoro-Lopes G, de Pinho A, Harrison LH, et al. Reduced risk of tuberculosis among Brazilian patients with advanced human immunodeficiency virus infection treated with highly active antiretroviral therapy. *Clin Infect Dis* 2002;34:543–546.
26. Wells WF. In: *Airborne contagion and hygiene*. Cambridge, MA: Harvard University Press, 1955.
27. Riley RL, Mills CC, Nyka W, et al. Aerial dissemination of pulmonary tuberculosis: a two year study of contagion in a tuberculosis ward. *Am J Hyg* 1959;70:185–196.
28. Houk VH, Kent DC, Baker JH, et al. The Byrd study: in-depth analysis of a micro-outbreak of tuberculosis in a closed environment. *Arch Environ Health* 1968;16:4–6.
29. Sepkowitz KA. Tuberculin skin testing and the health care worker: lessons of the Prophit Survey. *Tuberc Lung Dis* 1996;77:81–85.
30. Stead WW. Tuberculosis among elderly persons: an outbreak in a nursing home. *Ann Intern Med* 1981;94:606–610.
31. Styblo K. Recent advances in epidemiological research in tuberculosis. *Adv Tuberc Res* 1980;20:1–63.
32. Behr MA, Warren SA, Salamon H, et al. Transmission of *Mycobacterium tuberculosis* from patients smear-negative for acid-fast bacilli. *Lancet* 1999;353:444–449.
33. Besser RE, Pakiz B, Schulte JM, et al. Risk factors for positive Mantoux tuberculin skin tests in children in San Diego, California: evidence for boosting and possible foodborne transmission. *Pediatrics* 2001;108:305–310.

34. Stead WW. Undetected tuberculosis in prison: source of infection for community at large. *JAMA* 1978;240:2544–2547.

35. Aerts A, Habouzit M, Mschiladze L, et al. Pulmonary tuberculosis in prisons of the ex-USSR state Georgia: results of a nation-wide prevalence survey among sentenced inmates. *J Tuberc Lung Dis* 2000;4:1104–1110.

36. Stead WW, Lofgren JP, Warren E, et al. Tuberculosis as an endemic and nosocomial infection among the elderly in nursing homes. *N Engl J Med* 1985;312:1483–1487.

37. Nardell E, McInnis B, Thomas B, et al. Exogenous reinfection with tuberculosis in a shelter for the homeless. *N Engl J Med* 1986;315:1570–1575.

38. Barnes PF, el-Hajj H, Preston-Martin S, et al. Transmission of tuberculosis among the urban homeless. *JAMA* 1996;275:305–307.

39. Calder RA, Duclos P, Wilder MH, et al. *Mycobacterium tuberculosis* transmission in a health clinic. *Bull Int Union Tuberc Lung Dis* 1991;66:103–106.

40. Yeates DB, Mortensen J. Deposition and clearance. In: Murray JF, Nadel JA, eds. *Textbook of respiratory medicine*, Vol 1. Philadelphia: WB Saunders, 2000:349–384.

41. Riley RL, Mills CC, O'Grady F, et al. Infectiousness of air from a tuberculosis ward–ultraviolet irradiation of infected air: comparative infectiousness of different patients. *Am Rev Respir Dis* 1962;85:511–525.

42. Catanzaro A. Nosocomial tuberculosis. *Am Rev Respir Dis* 1982;125:559–562.

43. Nardell EA, Keegan J, Cheney SA, et al. Airborne infection: theoretical limits of protection achievable by building ventilation. *Am Rev Respir Dis* 1991;144:302–306.

44. Fennelly KP, Nardell EA. The relative efficacy of respirators and room ventilation in preventing occupational tuberculosis. *Infect Control Hosp Epidemiol* 1998;19:754–759.

45. Ferguson JS, Schlesinger LS. Pulmonary surfactant in innate immunity and the pathogenesis of tuberculosis. *Tuberc Lung Dis* 2000;80:173–184.

46. Flynn JL, Chan J. Immunology of tuberculosis. *Annu Rev Immunol* 2001;19:93–129.

47. Stenger S, Hanson DA, Teitelbaum R, et al. An antimicrobial activity of cytolytic T cells mediated by granulysin. *Science* 1998;282:121–125.

48. Miyakawa YPR, Rao AG, et al. In vitro activity of the antimicrobial peptides human and rabbit defensins and porcine leukocyte protegrin against *Mycobacterium tuberculosis*. *Infect Immun* 1996;64:926–932.

49. Ferrari G, Langen H, Naito M, et al. A coat protein on phagosomes involved in the intracellular survival of mycobacteria. *Cell* 1999;97:435–447.

50. Vanham G, Toossi Z, Hirsch CS, et al. Examining a paradox in the pathogenesis of human pulmonary tuberculosis: immune activation and suppression/anergy. *Tuberc Lung Dis* 1997;78:145–158.

51. Rich AR. *The pathogenesis of tuberculosis*, 2nd ed. Springfield, IL: Charles C. Thomas, 1951.

52. Mohan VP, Scanga CA, Yu K, et al. Effects of tumor necrosis factor alpha on host immune response in chronic persistent tuberculosis: possible role for limiting pathology. *Infect Immun* 2001;69:1847–1855.

53. Keane J, Gershon S, Wise RP, et al. Tuberculosis associated with infliximab, a tumor necrosis factor alpha-neutralizing agent. *N Engl J Med* 2001;345:1098–1104.

54. McKinney JD, Honer zu Bentrup K, Munoz-Elias EJ, et al. Persistence of *Mycobacterium tuberculosis* in macrophages and mice requires the glyoxalate shunt enzyme isocitrate lyase. *Nature* 2000;406:735–738.

55. Michele TM, Ko C, Bishai WR. Exposure to antibiotics induces expression of the *Mycobacterium tuberculosis sig F* gene: implications for chemotherapy against mycobacterial persistors. *Antimicrob Agents Chemother* 1999;43:218–225.

56. Behr MA. Correlation between BCG genomics and protective efficacy. *Scand J Infect Dis* 2001;33:249–252.

57. Centers for Disease Control and Prevention. Guidelines for preventing the transmission of *Mycobacterium tuberculosis* in health-care facilities, 1994. *MMWR Morb Mortal Wkly Rep* 1994;43(RR-13).

58. Centers for Disease Control and Prevention. Bronchoscopy-related infections and pseudoinfections—New York, 1996 and 1998. *MMWR Morb Mortal Wkly Rep* 1999;48:557–560.

59. Rutala WA, Weber DJ. New disinfection and sterilization methods. *Emerg Infect Dis* 2001;7:348–353.

60. O'Brien RJ, Geiter LJ, Snider DEJ. The epidemiology of nontuberculous mycobacterial disease in the United States. *Am Rev Respir Dis* 1987;135:1007–1014.

61. Falkinham JO. Epidemiology of infection by nontuberculous mycobacteria. *Clin Microbiol Rev* 1996;9:177–215.

62. Morrissey AB, Aisu TO, Falkinham JO, et al. Absence of *Mycobacterium avium* complex disease in patients with AIDS in Uganda. *J Acquir Immune Defic Syndr* 1992;5:477–478.

63. Horsburgh CRJ, Hanson DL, Jones JL, et al. Protection from *Mycobacterium avium* disease in human-immunodeficiency virus-infected persons with a history of tuberculosis. *J Infect Dis* 1996;174:1212–1217.

64. Black GF, Dockrell HM, Crampin AC, et al. Patterns and implications of naturally acquired immune responses to environmental and tuberculous mycobacterial antigens in northern Malawi. *J Infect Dis* 2001;184:322–329.

65. Fine PE, Floyd S, Stanford JL, et al. Environmental mycobacteria in northern Malawi: implications for the epidemiology of tuberculosis and leprosy. *Epidemiol Infect* 2001;126:379–387.

66. Johanson WGJ, Nicholson DP. Pulmonary disease due to *Mycobacterium kansasii*: an analysis of some factors affecting prognosis. *Am Rev Respir Dis* 1969;99:73–85.

67. Onstad GD. Familial aggregations of group I atypical mycobacterial disease. *Am Rev Respir Dis* 1969;99:426–429.

68. Penny ME, Cole RB, Gray J. Two cases of *Mycobacterium kansasii* infection occurring in the same household. *Tubercle* 1982;63:129–131.

69. Mangione EJ, Huitt G, Lenaway D, et al. Nontuberculous mycobacterial disease following hot tub exposure. *Emerg Infect Dis* 2001;7:1039–1042.

70. Schulze-Robbecke R, Janning B, Fischeder R. Occurrence of mycobacteria in biofilm samples. *Tuberc Lung Dis* 1992;73:141.

71. Eishi Y, Suga M, Ishige I, et al. Quantitative analysis of mycobacterial and propionibacterial DNA in lymph nodes of Japanese and European patients with sarcoidosis. *J Clin Microbiol* 2002;40:198–204.

72. Sechi LA, Mura M, Tanda F, et al. Identification of *Mycobacterium avium* subsp. *paratuberculosis* in biopsy specimens from patients with Crohn's disease identified by in situ hybridization. *J Clin Microbiol* 2001;39:4514–4517.

73. Quirke P. Antagonist. *Mycobacterium avium* subspecies *paratuberculosis* is a cause of Crohn's disease. *Gut* 2001;49:755–756.

74. Holland SM, Eisenstein EM, Kuhns DB, et al. Treatment of refractory disseminated nontuberculous mycobacterial infection with interferon gamma: a preliminary report. *N Engl J Med* 1994;330:1348–1355.

75. Rosenzweig DY. Pulmonary mycobacterial infections due to Mycobacterium avium-intracellulare complex: clinical features and course in 100 consecutive cases. *Chest* 1979;75:115–119.

76. Wolinsky E. Nontuberculous mycobacteria and associated diseases. *Am Rev Respir Dis* 1979;119:107–159.

77. Chan CHS, Ho AKC, Chan RCY, et al. Mycobacteria as a cause of infective exacerbation in bronchiectasis. *Postgrad Med J* 1992;68:896–899.

78. Oliver A, Maiz L, Canton R, et al. Nontuberculous mycobacteria in patients with cystic fibrosis. *Clin Infect Dis* 2001;32:1298–1303.

79. Prince DS, Peterson DD, Steiner RM, et al. Infection with *Mycobacterium avium* complex in patients without predisposing conditions. *N Engl J Med* 1989;321:863–868.

80. Iseman MD, Buschman DL, Ackerson LM. Pectus excavatum and scoliosis: thoracic anomalies associated with pulmonary disease caused by *Mycobacterium avium* complex. *Am Rev Respir Dis* 1991;144:914–916.

81. Wolinsky E, Rynearson TK. Mycobacteria in soil and their relation to disease-associated strains. *Am Rev Respir Dis* 1968;97:1032–1037.

82. Collins CH, Grange JM, Yates MD. Mycobacteria in water. *J Appl Bacteriol* 1984;57:193–211.

83. von Reyn CF, Maslow JN, Barber TW, et al. Persistent colonization of potable water as a source of *Mycobacterium avium* infection in AIDS. *Lancet* 1994;343:1137–1141.

84. Khoor A, Leslie KO, Tazelaar HD, et al. Diffuse pulmonary disease caused by nontuberculous mycobacteria in immunocompetent people (hot tub lung). *Am J Clin Pathol* 2001;115:755–762.

85. Embil J, Warren P, Yakrus M, et al. Pulmonary illness associated with exposure to *Mycobacterium-avium* complex in hot tub water. *Chest* 1997;111:813–816.

86. von Reyn CF, Jacobs NJ, Arbeit RD, et al. Polyclonal *Mycobacterium avium* complex in patients with AIDS: variations in antimicrobial susceptibilities of different strains of *M. avium* isolated from the same patient. *J Clin Microbiol* 1995;33:1008–1010.

87. Woods GL, Washington JAI. Mycobacteria other than *Mycobacterium tuberculosis*: review of microbiologic and clinical aspects. *Rev Infect Dis* 1987;9:275–294.

88. Edwards LB, Acquaviva FA, Livesay VT, et al. An atlas of sensitivity to tuberculin, PPD-B, and histoplasmin in the United States. *Am Rev Respir Dis* 1969; 99[Suppl]:1–15.

89. Greene JB, Sidhu GS, Lewin S, et al. *Mycobacterium avium-intracellulare: A* cause of disseminated life-threatening infection in homosexuals and drug abusers. *Ann Intern Med* 1982;97:539–546.

90. ATS. Diagnosis and treatment of disease caused by nontuberculous mycobacteria. *Am J Respir Crit Care Med* 1997;156:S1–S25.

91. Centers for Disease Control and Prevention. Guidelines for preventing opportunistic infections among HIV-infected persons—2002. *MMWR Morb Mortal Wkly Rep* 2002;51(RR-8):1–46.

92. Soriano V, Dona C, Rodriguez-Rosado R, et al. Discontinuation of secondary prophylaxis for opportunistic infections in HIV-infected patients receiving highly active antiretroviral therapy. *AIDS* 2000;14:383–386.

93. Zeller V, Truffot C, Agher R, et al. Discontinuation of secondary prophylaxis against disseminated *Mycobacterium avium* complex infection and toxoplasmic encephalitis. *Clin Infect Dis* 2002;34:662–667.

94. Geruez-Rienx C, Tacquet A, Devulder B, et al. Experimental study of interactions of pneumoconiosis and mycobacterial infections. *Ann N Y Acad Sci* 1972;200:106–126.

95. Sherer R, Sable R, Sonnenberg M, et al. Disseminated infection with *Mycobacterium kansasii* in AIDS. *Ann Intern Med* 1986;105:710–712.

96. Campbell IA, Jenkins PA. *Mycobacterium kansasii*. In: Schlossberg D, ed. *Tuberculosis and nontuberculous mycobacterial infections*, 4th ed. Philadelphia: WB Saunders, 1999:380–385.

97. Wallace RJJ. Recent changes in taxonomy and disease manifestations of the rapidly growing mycobacteria. *Eur J Clin Microbiol Dis* 1994;13: 953.

98. Runyon EH, Karlson AG, Kubica GP, et al. Mycobacterium. In: Lennette

EH, Spaulding EH, Truant JP, eds. *Manual of clinical microbiology*, 2nd ed. Washington, DC: American Society for Microbiology, 1974:148–174.

99. Wallace RJJ, Brown BA. *Mycobacterium fortuitum, chelonae, abscessus*. In: Schlossberg D, ed. *Tuberculosis and nontuberculous mycobacterial infections*, 4th ed. Philadelphia: WB Saunders, 1999:372–379.

100. Griffith DE, Wallace RJ. Pulmonary disease due to rapidly growing mycobacteria. *Semin Respir Med* 1988;9:505.

101. Rogers PL, Walker RE, Lane MC, et al. Disseminated *Mycobacterium haemophilum* infection in two patients with AIDS. *Am J Med* 1988;84:640–642.

102. Straus WL, Ostroff SM, Jernigan DB, et al. Clinical and epidemiologic characteristics of *Mycobacterium haemophilum*, an emerging pathogen in immunocompromised patients. *Ann Intern Med* 1994;120:118–125.

103. Preheim L. Other nontuberculous mycobacteria and *Mycobacterium bovis*. In: Schlossberg D, ed. *Tuberculosis and nontuberculous mycobacterial infections*, 4th ed. Philadelphia: WB Saunders, 1999:398–405.

104. Bessessen MT, Shlay J, Stone-Venohr B, et al. Disseminated *Mycobacterium genavense* infection: clinical and microbiological features and response to therapy. *AIDS* 1993;7:1357–1361.

105. Bottger EC, Teske A, Kirschner P, et al. Disseminated "*Mycobacterium genavense*" infection in patients with AIDS. *Lancet* 1992;340:76–80.

106. Costrini AM, Mahler DA, Gross WM, et al. Clinical and roentgenographic features of nosocomial infection due to *Mycobacterium xenopi*. *Am Rev Respir Dis* 1981;123:104–109.

107. Bennet SN, Peterson DE, Johnson DR, et al. Bronchoscopy-associated *Mycobacterium xenopi* pseudoinfections. *Am J Respir Crit Care Med* 1994;150:245–250.

108. Yates MD, Grange JM, Collins CH. The nature of mycobacterial disease in southeast England, 1977–84. *J Epidemiol Commun Health* 1986;40:295–300.

109. Maloney JM, Gregg CR, Stephens DS, et al. Infections caused by *Mycobacterium szulgai* in humans. *Rev Infect Dis* 1987;9:1120–1126.

110. Wallace RJ, Nash DR, Tsukamura M, et al. Human disease due to *Mycobacterium smegmatis*. *J Infect Dis* 1988;158:52–59.

111. Weinberger M, Berg SL, Feuerstein IM, et al. Disseminated infection with *Mycobacterium gordonae*: report of a case and critical review of the literature. *Clin Infect Dis* 1992;14:1229–1239.

112. Bux-Gewehr I, Hagen HP, Rusch-Gerdes S, et al. Fatal pulmonary infection with *Mycobacterium celatum* in an apparently immunocompetent patient. *J Clin Microbiol* 1998;36:587–588.

113. Butler WR, O'Connor SP, Yakrus MA, et al. Cross-reactivity of genetic probe for detection of *Mycobacterium tuberculosis* with newly described species *Mycobacterium celatum*. *J Clin Microbiol* 1994;32:536–538.

114. Somoskovi A, Hotaling JE, Fitzgerald M, et al. False-positive results for *Mycobacterium celatum* with the AccuProbe *Mycobacterium tuberculosis* assay. *J Clin Microbiol* 2000;38:2743–2745.

115. Hale YM, Pfyffer GE, Salfinger M. Laboratory diagnosis of mycobacterial infections: new tools and lessons learned. *Clin Infect Dis* 2001;33:834–846.

CHAPTER 266

Mycobacterium leprae

Diana N. J. Lockwood and
Keith P. W. J. McAdam

MICROBIAL AGENT

Leprosy is caused by *Mycobacterium leprae*, an acid-fast intracellular organism that has the longest doubling time of all known bacteria and is not cultivatable on artificial media. The *M. leprae* genome was sequenced in 2001, and this is leading to an exciting reevaluation of the organism and its unique biology.

The presence of acid-fast rods in the nodules of lepromatous leprosy patients was first recorded in 1873 by Armauer Hansen, who postulated that these bacilli cause leprosy (1). To his chagrin, he was unable to fulfill Koch's postulates, thereby demonstrating that these organisms caused leprosy, and the postulates remain unproven today because of a continuing inability to grow *M. leprae in vitro*.

M. leprae is a gram positive, acid-fast rod-shaped organism with rounded ends, 1 to 8 μm long and 0.3 μm wide (2). It is an obligate intracellular parasite with a special affinity for skin macrophages and peripheral nerve Schwann cells. In lepromatous patients, uncontrolled growth occurs, and organisms cluster into globi (Fig. 266.1). Uniform acid-fast staining is seen in only a small proportion of *M. leprae* from biopsies. Irregularly stained bacteria are nonviable.

In Vivo Cultivation of *Mycobacterium leprae*

In 1960, the first useful laboratory growth of *M. leprae* was achieved when Shepherd demonstrated bacillary multiplication in the mouse footpad of *M. leprae* derived from nasal washings of lepromatous patients (3). The growth of a typical inoculum of 10^3 acid-fast bacilli (AFB) is slow and limited, with an initial lag phase followed by multiplication to 10^6 organisms over 6 months. *M. leprae* may also be grown in immunodeficient mice (thymectomized-irradiated and congenitally athymic), with yields of up to 10^9 organisms after a year, accompanied by hematogenous spread (4).

The nine-banded armadillo is naturally susceptible to *M. leprae* infection (5), maybe because of the animal's low core temperature. Infection is progressive and systemic, with dissemination of AFBs particularly to the skin, lymph nodes, liver, and spleen. Wild armadillos have been found in Louisiana with naturally occurring *M. leprae* infections (6).

Experimental transmission to rhesus, mangabey, and African green monkeys has been achieved (7). However, unlike the armadillo, these primates do not provide large amounts of antigen. The mouse and armadillo models of *M. leprae* infection have enabled the biologic characteristics of *M. leprae* to be elucidated and banks of purified antigen to be established.

BIOLOGIC CHARACTERISTICS

M. leprae is a stable and remarkably hardy organism (Table 266.1); in a South Indian laboratory, it remained viable after 5 months drying in the shade (8). *M. leprae* has a doubling time of 12 days (compared with 20 minutes for *Escherichia coli*). The optimum growth temperature is 27 to 30°C, which is consistent with the clinical observation of maximal *M. leprae* growth at cool superficial sites (skin, nasal mucosa, and peripheral nerves). The minimal infecting dose in the mouse footpad model is 3 to 40 solid staining bacteria (9,10). There is no change in pathogenicity with serial passaging through mice and armadillos. Previously *M. leprae* appeared to be a single species with isolates having similar biologic characteristics and identical genotypes (using restriction fragment polymorphism analysis) irrespective of the type of leprosy or the race or geographic origin of the patient (11). Now *M. leprae* can be typed on the basis of copy numbers of short tandem repeats. This may be a useful research tool (12).

Mycobacterial Genome

M. leprae has a 3.27-megabase (Mb) genome that displays extreme reductive evolution (13). Less than half the genome contains functional genes, and many pseudogenes are present. One hundred sixty-five genes are unique to *M. leprae*, and functions can be attributed to 29 of them. Comparison of biosynthetic pathways with *M. tuberculosis* shows that for lipolysis, *M. leprae* has only 2 genes (*M. tuberculosis* has 22). *M. leprae* has lost many genes for carbon catabolism, and many carbon sources (e.g., acetate and galactose) are unavailable to it. *M. leprae* growth may be restricted to a few carbon sources on which it can maintain a balanced carbon metabolism. It has also lost anaerobic and micro-aerophilic

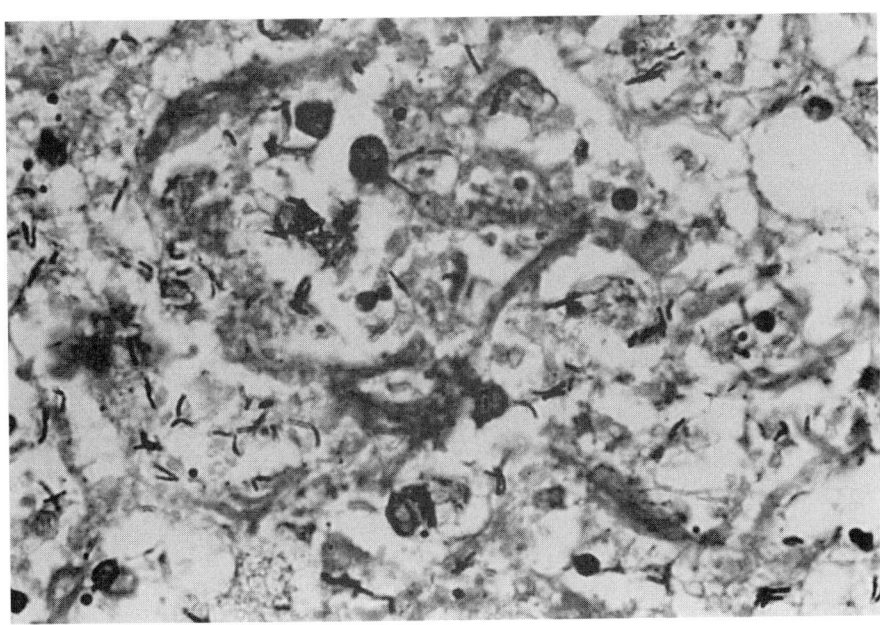

Figure 266.1. A skin biopsy showing numerous intracellular acid fast bacilli clumping into globi. (Wade-Fite stain, ×1,000.)

electron transfer systems. *M. leprae* has many genes for heme- and iron-based proteins, but it is severely limited in its iron uptake capacity because it has lost the ability to produce iron-scavenging sideropores.

MYCOBACTERIAL STRUCTURE

M. leprae is characterized by a thick and lipophilic mycobacterial cell wall giving the organism acid fastness, aggregation of cells, and resistance to many bactericidal agents and possibly retarding nutrient transport into the cell. The cell wall is a complex lipid structure with a phospholipid envelope abutting onto a peptidoglycan backbone, which supports an arabinogalactan matrix (14) (Fig. 266.2). Within this matrix are numerous complex molecules, notably phenolic glycolipid, which is unique to *M. leprae*.

The survival of *M. leprae* within macrophages is partly due to a lipoidal layer, which forms outside the cell wall, containing phenolic glycolipid and other polar mycosides that bind and exclude macrophage produced toxic oxygen metabolites and hydrolytic enzymes (15). Within the macrophage, the leprosy bacillus also inhibits phagosome–lysosome fusion, enabling the bacillus to escape into the cytoplasm and to avoid contact with harmful lysosome enzymes (16). Two enzymes, superoxide dismutase and peroxidase, partially protect *M. leprae* from the toxic oxygen metabolites generated by the macrophage respiratory burst (17). However, *M. leprae* lacks catalase and thus is probably killed by hydrogen peroxide, which it is unable to reduce to a less toxic form (18).

MYCOBACTERIAL PATHOGENESIS

The neurotropism of *M. leprae* may be attributed to its affinity for the G domain of the α-chain of laminin-2, an extracellular

TABLE 266.1.   Biologic Characteristics of *Mycobacterium leprae*

Minimal countable numbers as AFB	5×10^4
Routine infecting dose (total AFB)	5×10^3–10^4
Minimal infecting dose (solid staining AFB)	3–40
Temperature for optimum growth	27°–30°C
Doubling time (logarithmic phase)	12.5 d
Plateau yield	1×10^6
Resistance to 0.5N sodium hydroxide	Exposure < 20 min
Retention of viability in tissues or homogenates at 4°C	7–10 d
Survival in dried nasal discharge at 26.7°C, 77.6% humidity	<14 d
Growth rate and pathogenicity after 26–42 serial mouse passages (over 16–24 years)	Unchanged

AFB, acid-fast bacilli.
Adapted from Rees RJW. The contribution of Charles C. Shepard to leprosy research: from mouse footpad model to new DNA technology. *Lepr Rev* 1986; [Suppl]:10, with permission.

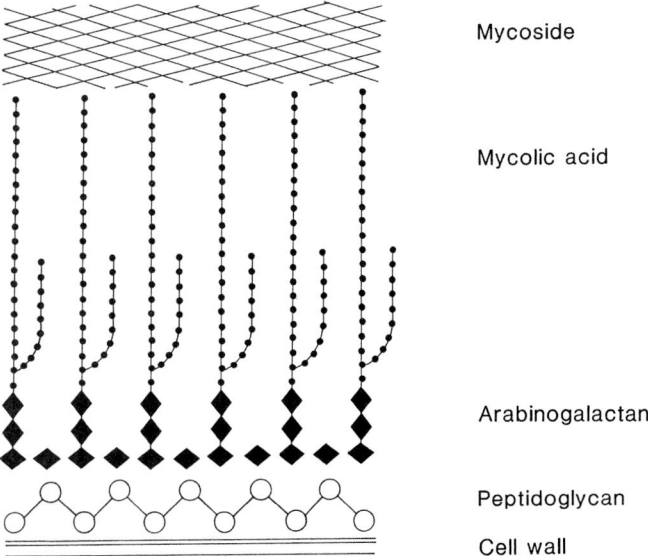

Mycoside

Mycolic acid

Arabinogalactan

Peptidoglycan

Cell wall

Figure 266.2. Diagrammatic section of the mycobacterial cell wall.

matrix protein present in the basal lamina of Schwann cells. In turn, *M. leprae*–laminin-2 complexes bind to α/β-dystroglycan complexes expressed on the surface of Schwann cells. Recently, a 21-kd laminin-biding receptor, a histone-like protein (HLP), has been identified on *M. leprae*. This mycobacterial receptor may function as a critical surface adhesin for the G domain of the laminin-α2 chain (19,20).

MYCOBACTERIAL ANTIGENS

Identifying immunologically important *M. leprae* antigens is crucial for understanding the immune response and for developing vaccine and diagnostic reagents. The two major types of antigens in *M. leprae* are the carbohydrate/lipid group and the protein antigens. The dominant carbohydrate epitopes are in three classes, the phenolic glycolipids, lipoarabinomannan (LAM), and the arabinogalactan–peptidoglycan complex (21). *M. leprae* synthesizes a species-specific lipid, phenolic glycolipid (PGL), which has a unique disaccharide terminal residue (22,23). PGL is an important antigen in the generation of the antibody response to *M. leprae*: high titers of antibodies directed against PGL are found only in leprosy patients, more than 90% of lepromatous leprosy patients have PGL antibodies, and after starting antileprosy treatment, both the PGL antibody titer and PGL antigen levels fall (24,25). In contrast, less than 50% of tuberculoid patients have PGL antibodies, thus limiting the usefulness of PGL antibody in the detection of early leprosy in population surveys. A five-fold rise in immunoglobulin M antibodies to synthetic PGL in patients with bacterial indexes of between 0 and 1 has been demonstrated, suggesting that PGL antibodies may be a good indicator of early bacillary multiplication in close contacts of leprosy patients (26). A dipstick test has been developed for detecting PGL antibodies, and this may be useful for screening household contacts.

The two other major carbohydrate antigens are LAM and the arabinogalactan–peptidoglyglycan complex. LAM has now been recognized to be highly immunogenic, both as a B-cell antigen (27) and in its effects on the cellular immune system. LAM isolated from *M. tuberculosis* has been shown to suppress T-cell activation (28), inhibit interferon-γ (IFN-γ) activation of macrophages (29), induce the release of tumor necrosis factor (30), and mediate a generalized inhibition of antigen presentation (31). LAM also plays a pivotal role in the intracellular survival of mycobacteria within the macrophage because it down-regulates macrophage effector function by scavenging potentially cytotoxic oxygen free radicals, inhibits protein kinase C activity, and may block transcription of inducible IFN-γ genes (32,33).

Polyacrylamide gel electrophoresis of disrupted *M. leprae* separates at least 50 proteins ranging from 10 to 100 kd (34). The relative importance of these proteins has been assessed using several different techniques. First, analysis of murine monoclonals produced from mice immunized with *M. leprae* lysates shows at least six *M. leprae* proteins important in the generation of an immune response (35); second, a genomic library of *M. leprae* has been constructed, and recombinant clones produced from this library have been screened with antibody and oligonucleotide probes (36,37); and third, T-cell responses of leprosy patients to recombinant protein antigens have been measured (38).

Using the murine monoclonal antibodies, six immunodominant *M. leprae* proteins (70, 65, 36, 30, 28, and 18 kd) were identified (39). The 70- and 65-kd proteins stimulate strong cellular immune responses in patients and their contacts (40,41). The 28-kd protein is a superoxide dismutase enzyme with close homology to a human mitochondrial enzyme (42). The 18-kd

protein is clearly a major immunogen, stimulating *M. leprae*–specific T-cell clones and eliciting peripheral blood T-cell and antibody responses in leprosy patients (43). The responses of the contacts of leprosy patients are particularly interesting because these patients are most likely to have encountered *M. leprae* and thus to have developed protective immunity if they are not incubating disease. Potentially protective antigens should stimulate T cells to proliferate and secrete cytokines such as IFN-γ, which would activate macrophages to kill mycobacteria. So far, no single antigen has been shown to be associated with protective immunity. Probably, protective immunity is not determined by a single antigen but results from several antigens that initiate a complex balance of responses.

Cloning mycobacterial genes and expressing the gene product has been a vital step in permitting the analysis of the protein antigens of *M. leprae*. The most successful approach to cloning the *M. leprae* genes has been the cloning of small fragments of *M. leprae* DNA into an *E. coli* λgt11 phage expression vector with resultant expression of *M. leprae* proteins (44).

M. leprae proteins may be classified according to their location: cell wall associated, membrane associated, cytoplasmic, or secreted. Cell wall fractions containing antigenic proteins have been used with some success to protect mice against footpad infection (45). Hunter (46) has isolated two major membrane proteins of 35 and 22 kd. The 35-kd contains *M. leprae*–specific epitopes (47) and T-cell epitopes (48). Rivoire has isolated the major *M. leprae* cytosolic protein of 10 kd and has sequenced and amplified the gene for this protein and produced a promising 10-kd skin test reagent (49). The 36- and 30/31-kd and antigen 85 complex are secreted antigens released by viable mycobacteria. A recombinant 30-kd protein stimulated *M. leprae*–reactive T-cell clones and reacted with sera from lepromatous leprosy patients (50). These antigens have not been extensively studied but may prove to be important in the development of an early protective response because they will be encountered by the immune system at an early stage.

The *M. leprae* 10-, 70-, and 65-kd protein antigens have recently been shown to be structural homologues of heat-shock proteins, which are synthesized by cells in response to hostile environmental conditions (51). Heat-shock proteins may provide some structural function that is necessary for cellular integrity, especially in response to environmental stresses and so constitute an important adaptive survival mechanism. Both antibodies and T cells directed against the 65-kd protein have been demonstrated in people with mycobacterial infections and people immunized with bacille Calmette Guérin (BCG) or heat-killed *M. leprae* (52). The 65-kd gene is highly conserved with the amino acid sequences of this protein in *M. leprae*, *M. tuberculosis*, and *M. bovis* BCG displaying greater than 95% homology, even though the total genomes of these organisms only show a 20% homology (53). Monoclonal antibodies directed against the mycobacterial 65-kd protein detect similar antigens in gram-negative and gram-positive bacteria, spirochetes, and rickettsiae. The widespread cross-species conservation of sequence and structure of this protein suggests that it is biologically important, perhaps a major immune target and contributing to the immune protection conferred by BCG.

MOLECULAR-BASED DIAGNOSTIC TESTS

Several polymerase chain reaction (PCR) primers (18-, 36-, and 65-kd and ribosomal RNA sequences) have been developed for the detection of *M. leprae* DNA. However, these primers have poor sensitivity in paucibacillary cases. In a study from the

United States, PCR was positive in 93% of lepromatous patients, but only 39% of tuberculoid patients. These latter patients are negative for acid fast bacilli and more difficult to diagnose (53a).

Detection of rifampicin resistance takes between 6 and 12 months for *M. leprae*, using the available mouse footpad culture techniques. The molecular basis for rifampicin resistance has now been elucidated in *M. leprae*, and the mutations responsible for resistance have been shown to lie within a region of 23 amino acids. Using a polymerase chain reaction single-strand polymorphism technique, rifampicin-resistant isolates can be identified within hours (54).

Two new approaches are being taken to develop improved skin test antigens. In one, *M. leprae* fractions have been prepared and tested as skin test reagent. The subcellular fraction containing membrane proteins, many unique to *M. leprae*, appears promising and will shortly go into clinical trials in Nepal (55). In the other approach, T-cell response to peptide antigens representing *M. leprae*–specific epitopes have been measured. The evaluation of these antigens should enable the preparation of a cocktail that would be recognizable by people with leprosy, provided that they are capable of making a T-cell response to antigen (56).

VACCINES AGAINST LEPROSY

The substantial cross-reactivity between BCG and *M. leprae* has been exploited in leprosy vaccine development. Trials of BCG as a vaccine against leprosy in Uganda, New Guinea, Burma, and South India showed it to confer statistically significant but variable protection, ranging from 80% in Uganda to 20% in Burma (57). In Northern Malawi, BCG gives 50% protection against leprosy but no significant protection against tuberculosis (58). A case-control study in Venezuela showed BCG vaccination to give 56% protection to the household contacts of leprosy patients (59). The variability and unpredictability of BCG has led to various attempts to improve its protective efficacy. Adding killed *M. leprae* to BCG did not enhance protection in studies in Malawi (60) and Venezuela (61). In a large South Indian trial, the best protection came from an Indian cultivable bacillus ICRC (vaccine efficacy, 65.5%), BCG plus heat-killed *M. leprae* gave 64% protection and BCG alone 34.1% (62). The variable protection induced by BCG may be due to early contact with environmental mycobacteria priming the immune system, and perhaps the immunity toward mycobacterial antigens shared between environmental species and *M. leprae* confers protective immunity against *M. leprae*. Vaccination with BCG after contact with environmental mycobacteria will then contribute little toward inducing improved immunity against *M. leprae* (63).

Assessing a leprosy vaccine is a complex problem because one is vaccinating against a disease of long incubation and low prevalence with differing manifestations. It has been estimated that evaluating a vaccine requires 10 or more years with populations of 80,000 to 100,000 being vaccinated. There is also the fear that the vaccination of people with subclinical infection or undiagnosed disease may potentiate T-cell–mediated responses against infected host cells producing immunopathology and particularly nerve damage. Furthermore, the success of multidrug therapy has reduced the need for a vaccine against leprosy.

The understanding of the structure and metabolism of *M. leprae* is still far from complete, and the steps involved in the development of both immune and pathologic responses to the organism remain unclear. The development of new drugs, new diagnostic tests, and ultimately a rational vaccine remain contingent on a better understanding of the organism and the human immune response to it.

REFERENCES

1. Hansen GA. Undersolgelser angraaende spedalskhedens aasger. *Norsk Mag Laeger* 1874;4:1.
2. Rees RJW, Young DB. The microbiology of leprosy. In: Hasting RC, ed. *Leprosy.* Edinburgh: Churchill Livingstone, 1994:49–86.
3. Shepard CC. Acid-fast bacilli in nasal excretions in leprosy and results of inoculation of mice. *Am J Hyg* 1960;71:147.
4. Colston MJ, Hilson GRF. Growth of *Mycobacterium leprae* and *M. marinum* in congenitally athymic (nude) mice. *Nature* 1976;262:399.
5. Kircheimer WF, Storrs EE. Attempts to establish the armadillo (*Dasypus novemcinctus* Linn) as a model for the study of leprosy. 1. Report of lepromatoid leprosy in an experimentally infected armadillo. *Int J Lepr* 1971;39:693.
6. Walsh GP, Meyers WM, Binford CH. Leprosy: a zoonosis. *Lepr Rev* 1981; 52(Suppl):77.
7. Wolf RN, Gormus BJ, Martin LN. Experimental transmission of *Mycobacterium leprae* to primates. *Science* 1986;227:529.
8. Desikan KV, Sreevatsa. Extended studies on the viability of *M. leprae* outside the human body. *Lepr Rev* 1995;66:287–295.
9. Davey TF, Rees RJW. The nasal discharge in lepros: clinical and bacteriological aspects. *Lepr Rev* 1974;45:121.
10. Rees RJW. The contribution of Charles C. Shepard to leprosy research: from mouse footpad model to new DNA technology. *Lepr Rev* 1986;57[Suppl]:10.
11. Williams DL, Gillis TP. A study of the relatedness of *Mycobacterium leprae* isolates using restriction fragment polymorphism analysis. *Acta Leprol* (Geneve)1989;7[Suppl 1]:226.
12. Young D. Prospects for molecular epidemiology of leprosy. *Lepr Rev* 2003;74: 11–17.
13. Cole ST, Eiglmeier K, Parkhill J, et al. Massive gene decay in the leprosy bacillus. *Nature* 2001;409:1007–1011.
14. Wheeler PR, Ratledge C. Metabolism in *Mycobacterium leprae, Mycobacterium tuberculosis,* and other pathogenic mycobacteria. *Br Med Bull* 1988;44:547–561.
15. Ryter A, Fretel C, Rastogi N, et al. Macrophage interaction with mycobacteria, including *M. leprae. Acta Leprol* (Geneve) 1984;21:2116.
16. Sibley LD, Franzblau SG, Krahenbuhl JL. Intracellular fate of *Mycobacterium leprae* in normal and activated mouse macrophages. *Infect Immun* 1987;55:680–685.
17. Wheeler PR, Gregory D. Superoxide dismutase, peroxidatic activity and catalase in *Mycobacterium leprae* purified from armadillo liver. *J Gen Microbiol* 1980;121:457.
18. Sharp AK, Colston MJ, Banerjee DK. Susceptibility of *Mycobacterium leprae* to the bactericidal activity of mouse macrophages and to hydrogen peroxide. *J Med Microbiol* 1985;19:77.
19. Rambukkana A, Salzer JL, Yurchenco PD, et al. Neural targetting of *Mycobacterium leprae* mediated by the G domain of the laminin alpha 2 chain. *Cell* 1997;88:811–821.
20. Rambukkana A. How does Mycobacterium leprae target the peripheral nervous system? *Trends Microbiol* 2000;8:23–28.
21. Gaylord H, Brennan PJ. Leprosy and the leprosy bacillus: Recent developments in characterization of antigens and immunology of the disease. *Annu Rev Microbiol* 1987;41:645–685.
22. Hunter SW, Fujiwara T, Brennan PJ. Structure and antigenicity of the major specific glycolipid antigen of *Mycobacterium leprae. J Biol Chem* 1982;257: 15072.
23. Young DB, Khanolkar SR, Barg LL. Generation and characterization of monoclonal antibodies to the phenolic glycolipid of *Mycobacterium leprae. Infect Immun* 1984;43:183.
24. Cho S, Yanagihara DI, Hunter SW, et al. Serological specificity of phenolic glycolipid 1 from *Mycobacterium leprae* and use in serodiagnosis of leprosy. *Infect Immun* 1983;41:1077–1083.
25. Cho S, Hunter SW, Gelber RH, et al. Quantitation of the phenolic glycolipid of *Mycobacterium leprae* and relevance to glycolipid antigenemia in leprosy. *J Infect Dis* 1986;153:560–569.
26. Hussain R, Jamil S, Kifayet A. Quantitation of IgM antibodies to the *M. leprae* synthetic disaccharide can predict early bacterial multiplication in leprosy. *Int J Lepr* 1990;58:491.
27. Brennan PJ. The carbohydrate-containing antigens of *M leprae. Lepr Rev* 1986; 57:39.
28. Kaplan G, Ghandhi RR, Weinstein DE, et al. *Mycobacterium leprae* antigen induced suppression of T cell proliferation *in vitro. J Immunol* 1987;138:3028–3034.
29. Sibley LD, Hunter SW, Brennan PJ, et al. Mycobacterial lipoarabinomannan inhibits gamma interferon-mediated activation of macrophages. *Infect Immun* 1988;56:1232–1236.
30. Barnes PF, Fong S, Brennan PJ, et al. Local production of tumour necrosis factor and IFN-g in tuberculous pleuritis. *J Immunol* 1990;145:149–154.
31. Moreno C, Mehlert A, Lamb J. The inhibitory effects of mycobacterial lipoarabinomannan and polysaccharide upon polyclonal and monoclonal human T cell proliferation. *Clin Exp Immunol* 1988;74:206–210.
32. Chan J, Fujiwara T, Brennan PJ, et al. Microbial glycolipids: possible virulence factors that scavenge oxygen radicals. *Proc Natl Acad Sci U S A* 1989;86:2453–2457.
33. Chan J, Fan X, Hunter SW, et al. Lipoarabinomannan, a possible virulence factor involved in persistence of *Mycobacterium tuberculosis* within macrophages. *Infect Immun* 1991;59:1755–1761.

34. Chakrabarty AK, Maire MA, Lambert PH. SDS PAGE analysis of *M. leprae* protein antigens reacting with antibodies from sera from lepromatous patients and infected armadillos. *Clin Exp Immunol* 1982;49:523.

35. Kaufmann SHE, Young DB. Vaccination against tuberculosis and leprosy. *Immunobiology* 1992;184:208–229.

36. Young RA, Mehra V, Sweetser D, et al. Genes for the major protein antigens of the leprosy parasite *Mycobacterium leprae*. *Nature* 1985;316:450–452.

37. Clark-Curtiss JE, Jacobs WR, Docherty MA. Molecular analysis of DNA and construction of genomic libraries of *Mycobacterium leprae*. *J Bacteriol* 1985;161:1093.

38. Dockrell HM, Stoker NG, Lee SP, et al. T-cell recognition of the 18-kilodalton antigen of *Mycobacterium leprae*. *Infect Immun* 1989;57:1979–1983.

39. Engers HD, Abe M, Bloom BR, et al. Results of a World Health Organisation–sponsored workshop on monoclonal antibodies to *Mycobacterium leprae*. *Infect Immun* 1985;48:603–605.

40. Ottenhoff THM, Haanen JBAG, Geluk A, et al. Regulation of mycobacterial heat shock reactive T-cells by HLA class II molecules: lessons from leprosy. *Immunol Rev* 1991;121:171–191.

41. Adams E, Garsia RJ, Hellqvist L, et al. T cell reactivity to the purified mycobacterial antigens P65 and P70 in leprosy patients and their contacts. *Clin Exp Immunol* 1990;80:206–212.

42. Thangaraj HS, Lamb FI, Davis EO, et al. Identification, sequencing and expression of *Mycobacterium leprae* superoxide dismutase, a major antigen. *Infect Immun* 1990;58:1937–1942.

43. Roche PW, Prestige RL, Watson JD, et al. Antibody responses to the 18kD protein of *Mycobacterium leprae* in leprosy and tuberculosis patients. *Int J Lepr* 1992;60:201–207.

44. Eiglmeier K, Honore N, Woods SA, et al. Use of an ordered cosmid library to deduce the genomic organisation of *Mycobacterium leprae*. *Mol Microbiol* 1993;7:197–206.

45. Roche PW, Neupane KD, Britton WJ. Cellular immune response to the cell walls of *Mycobacterium leprae* in leprosy patients and healthy subjects exposed to leprosy. *Clin Exp Immunol* 1992;89:110–114.

46. Hunter SW, Rivoire S, Mehra V, et al. The major native proteins of the leprosy bacillus. *J Biol Chem* 1990;265:14065–14068.

47. Roche PW, Britton WJ, Failbus SS, et al. Operational value of serological measurements in multibacillary leprosy patients: clinical and bacteriological correlates of antibody responses. *Int J Lepr* 1990;58:480–490.

48. Mohagheghpour N, Munn MW, Gelber RH, et al. Identification of an immunostimulatory protein from *Mycobacterium leprae*. *Infect Immun* 1990;58:703–710.

49. Rivoire B, Pessolani MCV, Bozic CM, et al. Chemical definition, cloning and expression of the major protein of the leprosy bacillus. *Infect Immun* 1994;62:2417–2425.

50. Thole JER, Schoringh R, Janson AA, et al. Molecular and immunological analysis of a fibronectin-binding protein secreted by *Mycobacterium leprae*. *Mol Microbiol* 1992;6:153–163.

51. Young DB, Lathigra R, Hendrix R, et al. Stress proteins are immune targets in leprosy and tuberculosis. *Proc Natl Acad Sci U S A* 1988;85:4267–4270.

52. Shinnick TM, Vodkin MH, Williams JC. The *Mycobacterium tuberculosis* 65-kilodalton antigen is a heat shock protein which corresponds to common antigen and to the *Escherichia coli* GroEL protein. *Infect Immun* 1988;56:446–451.

53. Shinnick TM, Sweetser D, Thole J, et al. The etiologic agents of leprosy and tuberculosis share an immunoreactive protein antigen with the vaccine strain *Mycobacterium bovis* BCG. *Infect Immun* 1987;55:1932–1935.

53a. Williams DL, Scollard DM, Gillis TP. PCR-based diagnosis of leprosy in the United States. *Clin Microbiol Newsletter* 2003;25:57–61.

54. Honore N, Perrani E, Telenti A, et al. A simple and rapid technique for the detection of rifampin resistance in *Mycobacterium leprae*. *Int J Lepr* 1993;61:600–604.

55. Brenan PJ. Skin test development: progress with first generation skin test antigens; approach to a second generation. *Lepr Rev* 2000;71[Suppl]:S50–54.

56. Dockrell HM. Diagnostic essays for leprosy based on T cell epitopes. *Lepr Rev* 2000;71[Suppl]:S55–59.

57. Fine PEM, Rodrigues LC. Modern vaccines: mycobacterial diseases. *Lancet* 1990;335:1016–1019.

58. Ponnighaus JM, Fine PEM, Sterne JAC, et al. Efficacy of BCG vaccine against leprosy and tuberculosis in northern Malawi. *Lancet* 1992;339:636–639.

59. Convit J, Smith PG, Zuniga M, et al. BCG vaccination protects against leprosy in Venezuela: a case control study. *Int J Lepr* 1993;61:185–191.

60. Karonga Prevention trial Group. Randomised controlled trial of single BCG, repeated BCG or combined BCG and killed *Mycobacterium leprae* vaccine for prevention of leprosy and tuberculosis in Malawi. *Lancet* 1996;348:17–24.

61. Convit J, Sampson C, Zuniga M, et al. Immunoprophylactic trial with combined *Mycobacterium leprae*/BCG vaccine against leprosy: preliminary results. *Lancet* 1992;339:446–450.

62. Gupte MD, Vallishayee RS, Anantharaman DS, et al. Comparative leprosy vaccine trial in South India. *Ind J Lepr* 1998;70:369–388.

63. Anonymous. Bettering BCG. *Lancet* 1992;339:462–463.

CHAPTER 267
Candida albicans *and Related Species*

Janine R. Maenza and William G. Merz

Candida species are the most common fungal pathogens affecting humans. These organisms cause a wide spectrum of opportunistic diseases, from noninvasive superficial skin infections to deep-seated infections of solid organs. The past few decades have seen increasing numbers of *Candida* infections, both community acquired and nosocomial, reflecting, among other factors, the use of broad-spectrum antibacterials, the use of intravascular devices, and a growing population of high-risk patients.

CHARACTERISTICS OF THE PATHOGEN

There are nearly 200 *Candida* species, of which fewer than 20 are capable of causing disease in humans. Most species may be seen morphologically as budding yeast, hyphal, or pseudohyphal forms, but some, such as *Candida* (*Torulopsis*) *glabrata*, are found only as yeast or hyphae. The genus *Candida* is not a tight taxonomic group based on true phylogenetic relationships but rather a somewhat diverse group of asexual organisms with similar phenotypic characteristics. When the sexual form of a *Candida* species is identified, the organism is classified into the proper sexual species that does reflect phylogenetic relationship. Thus, for example, the sexual form of *Candida krusei* is *Issatchenkia orientalis*, that of *Candida lusitaniae* is *Clavispora lusitaniae*, that of *Candida guilliermondii* is *Yamadazyma guilliermondii*, and that of *Candida kefyr* is *Kluyveromyces marxianus*. This variety of sexual genera attests to the diversity of this group of microorganisms. Therefore, it would seem probable that this diversity contributes to significant differences in virulence and response to antifungal therapy.

Candida albicans is the species most commonly found as both a colonizer and a pathogen. Other frequently encountered species include *C. guilliermondii*, *C. kefyr* (previously known as *Candida pseudotropicalis*), *C. krusei*, *C. lusitaniae*, *Candida parapsilosis*, and *Candida tropicalis*. Most authorities also now recognize the commonly encountered organism *Torulopsis glabrata* as a *Candida* species, thus leading to its renaming as *C. glabrata*. *Candida* species less frequently found as human colonizers or pathogens include *C. lipolytica*, *C. rugosa*, *C. viswanathii*, *C. haemulonii*, *C. norvegensis*, *C. catenulata*, *C. intermedia*, *C. lambica*, and *C. zeylanoides*. *Saccharomyces cerevisiae* and *Hansenula anomala*, although not *Candida* species, are mentioned here because they are yeasts that have similar phenotypic characteristics and can cause some infections that are indistinguishable from those caused by *Candida* species.

Anatomic areas colonized by *Candida* species include skin, mouth, rectum, and vagina, from which *C. albicans* is frequently isolated; other species are not as common and tend to colonize fewer anatomic sites. *C. glabrata* is known to colonize the mouth, rectum, and vagina; *C. parapsilosis* may be found in rectal and skin cultures; and *C. tropicalis* may be isolated from the mouth and skin (1).

PATHOGENESIS

There are significant differences in virulence among different *Candida* species, as evidenced by clinical data and animal models. There is no single fungal factor, however, but multiple factors that contribute to their ability to cause infection (2,3) (Table 267.1). One notable factor associated with the virulence of *C. albicans* is the presence of surface molecules that permit the organism to adhere to epithelial cells, endothelial cells, extracellular matrix, and hardware. Production of surface molecules that mimic host substances and thereby allow avoidance of immune surveillance has been described. An additional factor that may be involved in host invasion is the production of hydrolytic enzymes (including acid proteases and phospholipases). The ability of *C. albicans* to convert rapidly to a hyphal form (with either true hyphae or pseudohyphae) may also contribute to pathogenicity (4). Loss of a single factor does not appear to be sufficient to render an isolate avirulent, although it may restrict its ability to cause all types of infections. Evidence for this comes from mutants of *C. albicans* that produce no or lower levels of acid protease and grow more slowly than wild-type strains but are not completely avirulent (5). In fact, the ability of this genus to cause disease depends as much, if not more, on host defects as on any particular virulence factor inherent to the organism. Structural host defects associated with *Candida* infection include breaks in the integrity of the skin or mucous membranes due to burns, trauma, or occlusion and maceration. Exogenous causes of host defects include the use of antimicrobials that change the normal colonizing flora and procedures, resulting in the presence of prosthetic materials. Endogenous host factors include the extremes of age, diabetes, and immunologic abnormalities, including specific lymphocyte deficiencies and granulocyte and complement abnormalities.

TABLE 267.1.   Virulence Factors of *Candida Albicans*

Adhesion
Ability to transform rapidly from yeast to hyphae
Production of hydrolytic enzymes
   Acid proteinase secretion
   Phospholipase secretion
Phenotypic switching and chromosomal instability
Antigenic variation
Host mimicry
Toxin production

Adapted from Bodey GP. *Candidiasis: pathogenesis, diagnosis, and treatment.* New York: Raven Press, 1993; and Cutler JE. Putative virulence factors of *Candida albicans. Annu Rev Microbiol* 1991;45:187–218; with permission.

EPIDEMIOLOGY

Although *Candida* organisms can be isolated from environmental sources (soil, foods, water, plants), most infections are acquired from endogenous flora (6,7). The evidence for endogenous sources of infection comes from molecular typing systems with use of DNA-based methods, including restriction endonuclease fragment polymorphisms analyzed by electrophoresis (normal or pulsed field), electrophoretic karyotyping, and rapid arbitrarily primed polymerase chain reaction amplification (8). Data support that most patients are colonized with a distinct strain of *Candida*; if a bloodstream or other infection occurs, the infecting strain is frequently the same strain as the colonizers (6,7). An exception to this scenario may be *C. parapsilosis*, which is reported to cause infection from exogenous sources without prior colonization (9) and has been responsible for outbreaks related to intravenous infusions (10). In addition, neonatal *Candida* infections and sexually transmitted cases usually occur by person-to-person transmission, and there are isolated reports of nosocomial transmission of a single *C. albicans* strain between patients in other settings (9,11).

Different types of *Candida* infections are associated with different host populations. Cutaneous *Candida* infections and *Candida* vaginitis may occur in immunologically intact hosts. The many forms of mucocutaneous candidiasis of the oropharynx are usually found in patients with defects of cell-mediated immunity, although it may also be seen in patients with diabetes mellitus and patients receiving broad-spectrum antibacterials. Bloodstream and associated solid organ *Candida* infections are most commonly seen in burn patients, postsurgical patients, and immunocompromised patients. Specific risk factors associated with candidemia and deep tissue infections in these populations include the use of indwelling intravascular catheters, parenteral hyperalimentation, broad-spectrum antibacterials, and intensive chemotherapy regimens leading to prolonged neutropenia (12,13). In addition, among surgical patients, gastrointestinal procedures are associated with an increased rate of candidemia, probably related to disruption of bowel mucosa colonized with *Candida*. Neonatal candidemia is associated with prematurity and low birth weight.

Mortality due to invasive candidiasis in the United States has been tracked by the National Center for Health Statistics (14): From 1980 through 1989, the mortality rate associated with invasive disease climbed steadily to a peak of 0.6 deaths per 100,000 population. In comparison, from 1989 to 1997, the mortality rate declined 50%. The reasons for this decline are unclear but have been postulated to include a larger proportion of less virulent non-*albicans* infections associated with the increasing use of antifungal prophylaxis (14).

CLINICAL DISEASES

The many clinical syndromes associated with *Candida* species are most frequently caused by *C. albicans*. As these clinical entities are described, other species known to be responsible are noted as appropriate.

Cutaneous Candidiasis

Cutaneous candidiasis may be seen in normal as well as in immunocompromised hosts. In normal hosts, risk factors for the development of infection include moist or occluded areas, obesity, friction, burn sites, or skin areas that have been irradiated. Cutaneous candidiasis is more frequent in diabetic than in nondiabetic individuals (15). In adults, cutaneous candidiasis may herald the onset of diabetes mellitus. The infection manifests as intense erythema of intertriginous areas. The erythematous areas may be papular, plaquelike, or confluent. Satellite lesions consisting of pustules or erythematous papules may surround these areas. Commonly involved sites include the axillae, inguinal regions, perineum, skin beneath the breasts, and digital web spaces. *Candida* folliculitis may also be seen, especially in moist or occluded areas.

Sterile lesions, which may be hyperkeratotic, papular, or eczematous, can occur in locations separate from the sites of *Candida* infection. These lesions represent allergic reactions, known as *id reactions*, and have been seen in patients with mucous membrane as well as cutaneous candidiasis (1,16). Resolution of the id reaction is seen with antifungal treatment of the initiating infection. In addition, there may be urticarial reactions to the organism.

Candidiasis may also involve the nails and nail folds. Onychomycosis, with nail discoloration or destruction, may occur in previously damaged nails or with a concomitant paronychial infection. Unlike dermatophyte infections of the nails, *Candida* onychomycosis is often painful (1). *Candida* paronychial infections present as erythematous lesions, often lacking the purulence seen in bacterial infections. Both onychomycosis and paronychial infections are usually found as occupational infections in people whose hands remain wet for long periods (e.g., dish washers and people who come into contact with organic solvents).

Diagnosis of these cutaneous disorders is often made on clinical grounds, although confirmation may be added by detection of the budding yeast and hyphal forms on direct microscopic examination (potassium hydroxide) of skin or nail scrapings. Cultures are not routinely done because they are unlikely to add to the results of the microscopic examination and may reflect only fungal colonization. Skin lesions may also be a manifestation of disseminated candidiasis. These secondary lesions arise from hematogenous spread and may include erythematous macronodular papules, subcutaneous nodules, lesions resembling ecthyma gangrenosum, and rarely purpuric lesions (17–19). These lesions are more common with *C. tropicalis* and *C. krusei* than with *C. albicans*.

Chronic Mucocutaneous Candidiasis

Chronic mucocutaneous candidiasis includes a group of somewhat heterogeneous syndromes in patients with T-cell abnormalities. Anergy may be specifically related to *Candida* only or to other antigens also. Not all patients have the same deficits, but the immunologic abnormalities may include additional abnormalities of T-lymphocyte function as well as occasional dysfunction of B cells, granulocytes, or complement (20).

The clinical manifestations grouped together as chronic mucocutaneous candidiasis are thus varied. Most patients present in infancy or early childhood. The first signs may be oral thrush or perineal candidiasis. Some patients may develop more widespread cutaneous candidiasis and onychomycosis, others may have only localized skin involvement, and others may have disease involving only the nails. Invasive infections are rare in all forms of this disease (21).

In some instances, syndromes of chronic mucocutaneous candidiasis are associated with other disorders, such as multiple endocrine abnormalities (22) and recurrent viral and bacterial pulmonary or sinus infections (23). In patients in whom the diagnosis of chronic mucocutaneous candidiasis is suspected, an initial evaluation should include phenotypic characterization of lymphocyte subsets and investigation of T-cell function (e.g., response to mitogens).

Oral and Esophageal Candidiasis

Systemic factors associated with the development of upper gastrointestinal candidiasis include the use of antibiotics, diabetes, hematologic malignant neoplasms, medication-induced immunosuppression, and human immunodeficiency virus (HIV) infection. Local structural or functional factors may also be associated with disease development; disorders of esophageal motility in particular are associated with *Candida* overgrowth. In the newborn, oral candidiasis may occur as a consequence of colonization or infection from the mother's vaginal flora or other exogenous sources. In immunosuppressed patients with mucositis, oral and esophageal candidiasis must be considered potential sources of disseminated candidiasis. Most cases of oral and esophageal candidiasis are caused by *C. albicans*, but *C. glabrata*, *C. krusei*, *C. tropicalis*, *C. parapsilosis*, *S. cerevisiae*, and *H. anomala* are also reported to cause this disease (24–27).

Oral candidiasis may present with different clinical manifestations. The most common is typical oral thrush, or the pseudomembranous form of oral candidiasis. In this form, white pseudomembranous plaques are seen on the surfaces of the oropharynx. Less commonly seen are erythematous candidiasis (red mucosal patches in the absence of pseudomembranes), hyperplastic candidiasis or *Candida* leukoplakia (rough plaques that cannot be removed by scraping), and angular cheilitis (in which the corners of the lips are involved with erythema and cracking). The diagnosis of oral candidiasis is usually made clinically by noting one of these typical appearances on physical examination. Confirmation can be obtained by direct microscopic examination. Culture is not generally helpful given the high colonization rate of the oropharynx with *Candida* species.

Esophageal candidiasis also has a range of clinical manifestations from superficial infection to deep invasive disease. This diversity is most commonly due to varying host defects, with superficial disease seen in patients with HIV infection and deep infection in neutropenic patients. It may present with or without concomitant oral infection. Symptoms are indistinguishable from those of other infectious and noninfectious causes of esophagitis and include dysphagia, odynophagia, and retrosternal chest pain. Patients may also be asymptomatic even with extensive disease. Complications of esophageal candidiasis include perforation; bleeding; a risk for dissemination; and, in chronic *Candida* esophagitis, esophageal stenosis. The diagnosis of esophageal candidiasis is frequently made on clinical grounds in high-risk populations. For example, a patient with HIV infection, oral thrush, and esophageal symptoms may be treated empirically for *Candida* esophagitis. In neutropenic patients with concomitant thrombocytopenia, the potential bleeding complications of endoscopy may preclude the use of this diagnostic procedure, and empirical treatment may again be used. In instances of esophageal symptoms when the diagnosis is less certain or in patients who do not respond to empirical treatment, a definitive diagnosis can be made by endoscopy and biopsy (Fig. 267.1). Endoscopy may also be useful for obtaining cultures for species identification and susceptibility testing in HIV-infected patients who are refractory to azole treatment.

Oral and esophageal candidiasis that is clinically refractory to ketoconazole, fluconazole, and itraconazole has been documented, most frequently in HIV-infected patients. Fluconazole resistance, in particular, has been well described (28–35) and is more likely to occur in HIV-infected patients with advanced immunosuppression (low CD4$^+$ lymphocyte counts), multiple prior episodes of thrush or esophagitis, and extensive previous exposure to systemic azoles (27,36). Fluconazole-resistant candidiasis represents a significant clinical problem because many patients with this disease require treatment with parenteral

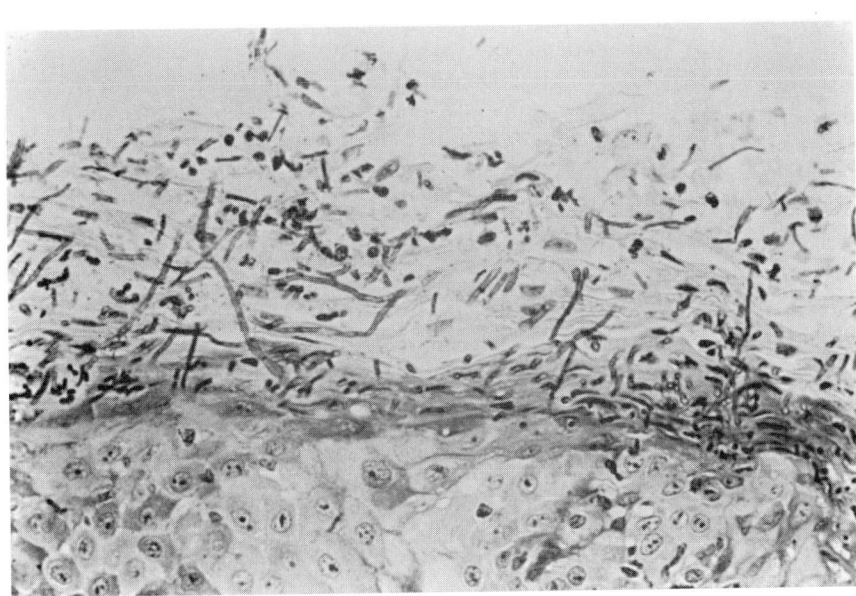

Figure 267.1. Histologic specimen demonstrating candidal esophagitis.

amphotericin B (27,33). Strategies to prevent the development of fluconazole resistance have not been clearly delineated but may include using topical agents as first-line therapy for oral thrush and reserving systemic azoles for patients who are refractory to topical treatment or have esophageal involvement. Treatment of the underlying immunosuppression (use of effective antiretroviral therapy for HIV) may also minimize the occurrence of resistant infection.

Vulvovaginal Candidiasis

Vulvovaginal candidiasis is a common fungal infection both in normal women and in women with deficits of cell-mediated immunity. The infection causes vulvar itching and a thick vaginal discharge. Physical examination usually reveals vulvar erythema and an adherent white discharge. The use of antibacterial agents, which change the normal vaginal flora, is frequently associated with the development of this disease (37,38). Pregnancy (39) and diabetes (40) are also associated with *Candida vaginitis*, and some studies have suggested the use of oral contraceptives as a risk factor (41,42).

C. albicans is the cause of more than 80% of cases of vulvovaginal candidiasis (43), but non-*albicans* species are also reported as pathogens (44). *C. tropicalis* and *C. glabrata* are the most commonly identified non-*albicans* species, although *C. parapsilosis* and *S. cerevisiae* have also been described (45).

Recurrent vulvovaginal candidiasis, usually defined as three or four episodes in a year (1), may be more common in women with immune defects (43,46). A recurrent infection within 3 months is usually due to reinfection with the same *Candida* strain; after 3 months, reinfection with a different strain is more common (47,48). Some data suggest that persistence of vaginal organisms after treatment (49–51), rather than a gastrointestinal reservoir (43,47) or sexual transmission (51–53), is responsible for recurrent episodes. Theories to explain the mechanism of recurrent disease include (a) deficiencies in normal bacterial flora, (b) a *Candida*-specific deficiency in T-lymphocyte activity, and (c) an acquired hypersensitivity reaction to *Candida* (43). Management of recurrent disease may require long courses of antifungal therapy or chronic antifungal prophylaxis (48).

Because *Candida* species may be found as normal vaginal flora in 40% of women (54), the diagnosis of *Candida* vaginitis should not be made in the absence of symptoms. In addition, because the signs and symptoms may overlap those of bacterial vaginitis, history and physical examination alone cannot be relied on with diagnostic certainty. The diagnosis is usually made by consistent clinical findings combined with a microscopic examination of a saline wet preparation to ensure the absence of clue cells and *Trichomonas* organisms and a potassium hydroxide preparation to look for the presence of yeast or hyphal forms. Cultures may be necessary in unusual presentations, in recurrent episodes, or for choosing therapy in selected patients (e.g., HIV-infected or heavily pretreated women, who may have azole-resistant infections) (55–57).

Candidemia

Candidemia is uncommon as a community-acquired infection, except in intravenous drug users, but is a frequent nosocomial complication. Inpatient populations most at risk for the development of candidemia include burn patients, postsurgical patients, oncology patients, and patients who are immunosuppressed after solid organ transplantation. The frequency of nosocomial *Candida* bloodstream infections increased up to fourfold during the 1980s (58,59) and remained at these levels in the 1990s (60,61).

Factors related to the development of candidemia include the use of central venous catheters, parenteral alimentation, broad-spectrum antibacterials, and intensive chemotherapy and immunosuppressive regimens (12,13).

The greatest concern with the patient with candidemia is that the bloodstream infection is a marker for disseminated disease with invasive solid organ infection as well. The attributable mortality of nosocomial candidemia has been shown to be as high as 38% (62). The organs most frequently involved in disseminated infection are eye, kidney, and heart. It is also possible to see gastrointestinal, cutaneous, and joint involvement. Candidemia in the setting of immunosuppression is frequently a sign of disseminated infection with an associated risk for increased mortality. In the immunocompetent patient, candidemia may be less commonly associated with disseminated disease and may frequently be related to an infection of an intravascular catheter. In a study of nonneutropenic patients with candidemia, 72% of all episodes were thought to arise from vascular catheters (63).

Disseminated candidiasis often occurs in the absence of documented candidemia. An autopsy study revealed that only 43% of cases of invasive candidiasis were diagnosed by antemortem blood cultures (64). This presents a difficult situation in a disease with few specific findings in which a diagnosis of disseminated candidiasis must frequently be made on clinical grounds. Diagnostic clues may include skin lesions associated with disseminated candidiasis (see cutaneous candidiasis), endophthalmitis (in nonneutropenic patients), esophagitis, myalgias, and myositis. In any neutropenic or high-risk intensive care unit patient with fever unresponsive to broad-spectrum antibacterial therapy, the diagnosis must be considered likely.

The difficulty of diagnosis of disseminated candidiasis in the absence of positive blood cultures has been a major impetus in the development of nonculture methods. These techniques (discussed later) lack the sensitivity to be uniformly recommended. Specificity of the tests is also variable, but a positive result should be regarded as an additional piece of evidence suggesting disseminated infection.

Fungal surveillance cultures of urine, stool, and respiratory secretions have also been studied as possible predictors of systemic fungal infections in oncology patients. Positive cultures for *C. tropicalis* have been shown to correlate with systemic disease, whereas cultures of *C. albicans* do not (65). A benefit of surveillance cultures is that species identification may be predicted when deep tissue or blood cultures first become positive for yeast. Negative surveillance cultures are predictive of the absence of systemic disease (65).

Although, in general, *C. albicans* remains the most common cause of candidemia, non-*albicans* species cause a substantial number of infections. At Johns Hopkins Hospital, we have observed a clear difference in the frequency of non-*albicans* infections in oncology patients compared with nononcology patients; during the years 1992 to 1995, 47% of candidemia episodes in nononcology patients were caused by non-*albicans* species, compared with 81% of the episodes in oncology patients (66). This frequency of non-*albicans* infections is higher than has been described historically; a review found that 46% of the reported infections in oncology patients during the previous 40 years were due to non-*albicans* species (predominantly *C. tropicalis*, *C. glabrata*, *C. parapsilosis*, and *C. krusei*) (67). Specific associations have been found between patients with leukemia and *C. tropicalis* infections and between bone marrow transplant recipients and *C. krusei* or *C. lusitaniae* infections (67,68). In addition, the prophylactic use of fluconazole in these patients has been associated with the emergence of *C. krusei* and *C. glabrata* infections (69,70).

Urinary Tract Infections

Candida species may colonize the lower urinary tract and cause either lower or upper urinary tract infections. In patients with lower tract infections, symptoms include the classic findings of cystitis: urgency, frequency, and dysuria, indistinguishable from bacterial infections. Upper tract infections may result either from a primary ascending (lower) urinary tract infection or from seeding of the kidney from a hematogenous infection. Multiple microabscesses, perinephric abscess, papillary necrosis, and fungus balls have been seen as manifestations of upper tract *Candida* infections.

Candida urinary infections are most commonly seen in patients with indwelling urinary catheters. Diabetes and the use of broad-spectrum antibacterials or immunosuppressive agents may also be risk factors for infection. *C. albicans* is the most common cause of *Candida* urinary infections, but *C. glabrata, C. guilliermondii, C. kefyr, C. lusitaniae, C. tropicalis,* and *S. cerevisiae* have all been reported to cause cystitis (1).

The finding of candiduria may reflect anything from contamination, to asymptomatic colonization, to a localized lower or upper urinary tract infection, to disseminated candidiasis with the kidney as a target organ. Thus, a urine culture showing *Candida* must be interpreted in light of the clinical picture including the patient's underlying risk factors, symptoms, physical examination findings, and history of urinary catheterization or instrumentation. Unlike the situation with bacteriuria, there is no specific breakpoint at which colony counts are considered significant; there is not necessarily a correlation between severity of disease and colony count in urine (1). To assess for true infection, an indwelling catheter should be changed if one is present, and urinalysis and culture should be repeated. If there is no history of recent genitourinary instrumentation, patients should be evaluated both for the presence of a urinary obstruction or other structural abnormality and for evidence of disseminated candidiasis (71). Candiduria should always be treated in neonates and in patients who are symptomatic, neutropenic, have undergone renal transplantation, or will have a genitourinary procedure (72).

Ocular Infections

Although *Candida* species can cause infection of almost any area of the eye, the most common and serious ocular infection is *Candida* endophthalmitis. Most cases are due to *C. albicans,* but rare cases of *C. parapsilosis* and *C. krusei* infection are reported (73–76). Endophthalmitis can occur either as a primary event, with direct infection of the eye in the setting of trauma or surgery, or as a secondary process in patients with candidemia. The latter is becoming increasingly frequent, and because the disease may be asymptomatic, all patients with candidemia should have an ophthalmoscopic examination to assess for its presence. Ophthalmoscopic examination to assess for the presence of *Candida* endophthalmitis is also useful as a method to detect deep tissue infection in the absence of positive blood cultures. Diagnosis of *Candida* endophthalmitis is usually made clinically by the typical appearance of the retina on ophthalmoscopic examination: a white lesion with indistinct margins. There may be extension into the vitreous or associated hemorrhage. In patients who do have symptoms, both ocular pain and visual disturbances have been reported. Ocular symptoms and the classic findings of *Candida* endophthalmitis are unusual in neutropenic patients (2).

When the clinical picture is uncertain, a definitive diagnosis can be made by either a vitreous tap or a partial vitrectomy. Partial vitrectomy is also used as a therapeutic technique in some patients (77). Early diagnosis is important to avoid disease progression that could require enucleation. Even with early institution of antifungal therapy, however, *Candida* endophthalmitis may lead to vitreal scarring with permanent visual impairment.

Candida keratitis, or keratoconjunctivitis, is an uncommon, exogenous, superficial *Candida* eye infection. The disease most often occurs after trauma or in patients receiving long-term steroid eye drops. The diagnosis of fungal infection may be suggested by physical examination revealing ulcerative lesions with spidery borders or inflammation, but corneal scrapings for histopathologic examination and culture are necessary to establish the specific cause. A specific culture method is employed in which plates are streaked by the ophthalmologist immediately on obtaining cultures. The streaking is done in patterns, and fungal growth that is not in the area of streaking is not interpreted as a positive result.

Candida Endocarditis

Members of the genus *Candida* are the most common cause of fungal endocarditis (78). This infection is increasing in frequency in conjunction with the increased rates of the underlying risk factors for the disease. These risk factors include cardiac surgery, prosthetic heart valves, central venous catheters, and intravenous drug use. *Candida* endocarditis may also occur in the setting of a structurally abnormal native valve or as a secondary infection in patients with bacterial endocarditis. It is an extremely rare occurrence in patients with normal cardiac valves or as a complication of neutropenia.

Although *C. albicans* remains the most common cause of *Candida* endocarditis, non-*albicans* species, especially species that commonly colonize the skin, such as *C. parapsilosis,* are important pathogens, especially in intravenous drug users (79).

Patients with *Candida* endocarditis usually have a symptom complex indistinguishable from that of bacterial endocarditis. Fever, nonspecific systemic symptoms, and congestive heart failure are common. Multiple large arterial emboli occur more frequently than in bacterial endocarditis.

The specific diagnosis of *Candida* endocarditis is usually made when blood cultures are positive for *Candida,* although this may occur late in disease, in conjunction with echocardiographic findings, or by histopathologic examination and cultures taken at the time of surgery. Specific diagnosis may require surgery, which is acceptable since surgical resection, as well as antifungal therapy, is necessary for optimal therapy. As with bacterial endocarditis, transthoracic echocardiograms may be falsely normal; transesophageal echocardiography has better diagnostic sensitivity.

Candida Meningitis

Central nervous system infections with *Candida* are rare, but when they occur, meningitis is the most common manifestation. Other clinical syndromes include mycotic aneurysms and cerebral abscesses. Risk factors for *Candida* central nervous system infections include the presence of a ventriculoperitoneal shunt, recent neurosurgery, and hematologic malignant neoplasms (80). *Candida* meningitis may also be seen in the neonatal period in low-birth-weight or premature infants.

Although patients with *Candida* meningitis may have headache, fever, photophobia, and meningismus, the signs and symptoms of *Candida* meningitis are often more subtle and chronic than these classic findings of bacterial meningitis. Fever may, in fact, be absent and the course indolent. Diagnosis is made by cerebrospinal fluid (CSF) evaluation; nonspecific findings include a CSF pleocytosis (of either neutrophils or lymphocytes), increased protein concentration, and low glucose level. A CSF Gram stain may be positive, but the diagnosis is most often made by culture. It may, however, be necessary to perform repeated CSF analyses before documentation of a positive culture in patients with chronic *Candida* meningitis. In a review of 18 cases of chronic *Candida* meningitis, only 8 patients had a positive culture from the first CSF sample (81). In contrast, cultures may be readily positive with postneurosurgical *Candida* meningitis or shunt infections. In addition to *C. albicans*, *C. tropicalis*, *C. parapsilosis*, *C. lusitaniae*, and *C. glabrata* have been identified as rare causes of postneurosurgical *Candida meningitis* or shunt infections (82,83).

Hepatosplenic Candidiasis

Hepatosplenic candidiasis is a syndrome of disseminated candidiasis found in patients being treated for acute leukemia or bone marrow transplant recipients who have had long periods of severe neutropenia. The disease is most often diagnosed when the neutrophil count is recovering. The patients have multifocal hepatic and splenic abscesses. At this point, patients may be noted to have fever once empirical antifungal therapy is stopped. Signs and symptoms, in addition to fever, usually include right upper quadrant abdominal pain, elevated liver function test results, and hepatosplenomegaly. Blood cultures are rarely positive, and the diagnosis is usually made by the characteristic appearance of multiple focal lesions in the liver and spleen as seen by computed tomography or ultrasonography. Computed tomography has been reported to have a higher sensitivity (93%) than ultrasonography (less than 50%) (84).

Gastrointestinal Candidiasis

Mucosal gastric and duodenal candidiasis may complicate peptic ulcer disease and malignant neoplasms. Peritoneal and other gastrointestinal (mucosal, invasive, and biliary) infections are potential complications of disseminated candidiasis. In addition, deep infections may occur in the setting of peritoneal dialysis or after gastrointestinal tract surgery. The diagnosis may be suggested by imaging studies but often needs to be confirmed with an invasive procedure. In patients undergoing peritoneal dialysis, intraperitoneal amphotericin B has occasionally been used for therapy; this is not generally recommended because it may well cause adhesions leading to a subsequent inability to perform peritoneal dialysis.

Bone and Soft Tissue Infections

Although less common than the previously discussed infections, *Candida* infections of the bone and contiguous soft tissue may also be complications of disseminated infections. Diagnosis usually requires needle aspiration, and treatment may require surgical débridement in addition to antifungal therapy.

LABORATORY DIAGNOSIS

Laboratory diagnosis of superficial *Candida* infections (e.g., cutaneous or vaginal) usually involves demonstrating the organism's presence by direct microscopic examination. Budding yeast cells, hyphae, or pseudohyphae may be seen by use of a wet mount potassium hydroxide preparation, calcofluor white stain for fluorescent examination, Gram stain, or methylene blue stain. However, the sensitivity and specificity of all these techniques are less than 100%.

Cultures play an important part in the diagnosis of invasive forms of candidiasis. However, a positive culture from the gastrointestinal or respiratory tract may represent colonization, and contamination of other specimens may occur; therefore, biopsy for histologic examination is necessary to prove invasion. Cultures from sterile sites, however, need to be interpreted as evidence of disease.

The techniques for culturing blood for *Candida* have improved in more recent years. There has been increased frequency and speed of recovery of yeast from blood by the use of lysis centrifugation techniques and automated continuously monitoring systems. Automated continuously monitoring systems detect the growth of organisms by means of a metabolic signal. Currently available automated systems include Bactec 9240, BacT/Alert, ESP, and Vital. Although the total recovery of yeast and time to recovery are improved with use of these systems, there is some concern for false-negative results with candidemia because there may be instances in which organisms grow in the media but do not produce a metabolic signal (85).

Once a culture is positive, species identification is extremely important and can be made by a number of different methods. *C. albicans* may be identified morphologically by means of the germ tube test (in which hyphae are produced from the yeast cells when the organism is incubated in serum at 37°C for 2 to 3 hours) (1) or by rapid commercially available enzymatic assays. Additional identification involves biochemical reactions done manually or with commercial automated systems. Reactions include urease activity, carbohydrate fermentation reactions, carbon assimilation patterns, and chromogenic enzymatic reactions. CHROMagar Candida is a medium that allows presumptive identification of *Candida* species on the basis of reactions of species-specific enzymes with substrates in the medium that develop into different colors (86). This medium is useful for detection of multiple yeast species in a specimen and for more rapid identification of these species. Finally, DNA-based assays have been shown to be feasible for the detection of *Candida* and are likely to play a larger role in the future for species identification (87).

As noted previously, the lack of sensitivity of blood cultures for the diagnosis of disseminated candidiasis has been a major factor leading to the development of nonculture detection systems. Among studied techniques, enzyme-linked immunosorbent assay and latex agglutination tests have been shown to have low sensitivity in immunocompromised patients and low specificity in immunocompetent patients. Most antigen detection tests (including those for mannan and enolase) also lack the sensitivity and specificity to be clinically relied on (88–90). Detection of fungus-specific metabolites has the potential to be useful for diagnosis. One study has shown that elevated levels of D-arabinitol have a 74% sensitivity for the detection of fungemia and are present earlier than positive blood cultures; thus, D-arabinitol determination may be useful in addition to performing blood cultures (91). DNA-based techniques, using polymerase chain reaction amplification methods, are also being developed as nonculture methods for detection of candidemia. A variety of DNA sequences, including those for 14-α-lanosterol demethylase, actin, and aspartic proteinase, have been studied as potential targets. Compared with cultures, these assays have a sensitivity ranging from 79% to 100% (87); however, their sensitivity and specificity for the diagnosis of disseminated candidiasis, especially in patients with the absence of positive blood cultures, remain to be determined in large clinical trials.

In some situations, antifungal susceptibility testing should be performed to help guide therapeutic decisions. Susceptibility testing may be useful in the clinical setting of oral or esophageal candidiasis that is clinically refractory to systemic azole therapy

TABLE 267.2. Interpretive Breakpoints for *Candida* Species[a] Isolates

	Minimum inhibitory concentration (µg/mL)		
	S	S-DD	R
Fluconazole	≤8	16–32	≥32
Itraconazole	≤0.125	0.25–0.5	≥0.5

S, susceptible; S-DD, susceptible–dose dependent; R, resistant.
[a]*Candida kruseii* is intrinsically resistant to fluconazole: these breakpoints do not apply to this species.
Adapted from Rex JH, Walsh TJ, Sobel JD, et al. Practice guidelines for the treatment of candidiasis. *Clin Infect Dis* 2000;30:662–678, with permission.

(92), with breakthroughs of prophylaxis, for specific species (e.g., *C. lusitaniae*, which may develop resistance to amphotericin B, and *C. glabrata*, which may be resistant, or develop resistance, to fluconazole) (93), and especially for all positive blood cultures in patients for whom fluconazole therapy is contemplated. *In vitro* susceptibility testing has become more standardized in the past few years. Guidelines from the National Committee for Clinical Laboratory Standards (NCCLS) recommend a system of broth macrodilution involving a series of tube dilutions. The minimal inhibitory concentration of an antifungal agent is the lowest concentration of that agent that inhibits the growth of the organism. These end points are clear with amphotericin B but tend to be less sharp with azoles. Nevertheless, amphotericin B resistance is not reliably determined with NCCLS methods, and because the amount of slight turbidity is usually the same for all concentrations above the minimal inhibitory concentration, an 80% inhibition standard is used to define the minimal inhibitory concentration for azoles. This system of susceptibility testing is also notable for use of the description "susceptibility–dose dependent," indicating that optimization of dose may be an important aspect of treatment. Table 267.2 shows the breakpoints for use with the reference broth susceptibility testing.

TREATMENT

Treatment of *Candida* infections varies substantially on the basis of the anatomic location of disease, the patient's underlying risk factors for infection, the specific species responsible for infection, and in some cases the strain's susceptibility to drug (72). In general, the classes of agents used to treat candidiasis include allylamines (terbinafine), azoles (e.g., clotrimazole, ketoconazole, fluconazole, voriconazole, itraconazole), polyenes (e.g., nystatin, amphotericin B), and nucleoside analogs (flucytosine). Newer agents include lipid formulations of amphotericin B (amphotericin B lipid complex, amphotericin B colloidal dispersion, and liposomal amphotericin B). These medications were designed on the basis of the theory that toxicity could be decreased by providing site-specific delivery of amphotericin B by the use of phospholipid membranes or vesicles, thereby directly transferring the drug to the fungal membranes and permitting use of higher concentrations of drug while minimizing toxicity. Available data indicate that the lipid formulations of amphotericin B are less toxic than conventional amphotericin B, but there is also a substantial cost difference. There is a paucity of efficacy data from randomized clinical trials, and it is therefore not entirely clear what the role of these alternative formulations should be. They have, however, been used successfully in some instances

of invasive candidiasis that were refractory to standard therapy and should be considered in patients with nephrotoxicity, in those receiving other concomitant nephrotoxins, and in those with significant infusion-related side effects. Another new class of antifungal agents is the echinocandins, which act by disrupting cell wall synthesis. In this class, micafungin has been shown to have *in vitro* activity against *Candida* (94), and caspofungin has been shown to have *in vitro* activity as well as clinical efficacy for *Candida* esophagitis (95), but neither has not yet been thoroughly studied or approved for the treatment of candidiasis. In addition, a new member of the azole class, voriconazole, appears to provide effective therapy for serious *Candida* infections (96), including non-albicans species (e.g., *C. krusei* and *C. glabrata*) that are resistant to fluconazole.

Superficial cutaneous infections may be treated with any of a number of topical agents, if the infection is localized and lacking nail involvement. Available topical agents include clotrimazole, ketoconazole, miconazole, nystatin, and terbinafine. With extensive cutaneous infection in immunocompromised patients, with folliculitis, or with nail involvement, treatment should usually include a systemic agent (most frequently an oral azole), with or without concomitant topical therapy.

Oral candidiasis may be treated with a topical agent (nystatin, clotrimazole, or amphotericin B oral suspension) or systemically with an oral azole or parenteral amphotericin B (in patients with azole resistance). *Candida* esophagitis requires systemic therapy, usually an oral azole, but parenteral amphotericin B may be similarly needed in patients who do not respond to azole therapy or in whom there is a concern for disseminated candidiasis.

Candida vaginitis is usually treated with a topical agent, but oral azoles have been shown to have clinical and microbiologic efficacy. The oral agents may also be useful in that they decrease gastrointestinal carriage of *Candida*, thought by some to be a reservoir that may lead to recurrent infections. Recurrent vulvovaginal infections do, in fact, often require chronic or prophylactic oral azole therapy for control (48). There is no evidence from controlled trials to indicate that treatment of male sexual partners reduces recurrences in women (43); however, such treatment is recommended by some clinicians.

Candidemia requires treatment in all populations of patients. Candidemia and disseminated candidiasis in neutropenic patients should be treated with parenteral amphotericin B (to a total dose of 0.5 to 1.0 g). *C. albicans* and *C. glabrata* infections may be treated with low to moderate doses of amphotericin B (0.5 to 0.6 mg/kg per day). Treatment with higher doses is often recommended for *C. krusei* and *C. tropicalis* infections (greater than 0.7 mg/kg per day, and often 1.0 mg/kg per day), whereas *C. parapsilosis* may show amphotericin B tolerance requiring moderate to high doses of amphotericin B, often in combination with flucytosine. *C. lusitaniae* may be resistant to amphotericin B; susceptibility testing should be performed on this organism, and optimal therapy is likely to be a combination. Flucytosine should almost never be used alone because of the potential for the rapid development of resistance. When it is used in combination with amphotericin B or fluconazole, serum levels should be monitored (peak, 70 to 80 µg/mL; trough, 30 to 40 µg/mL) to prevent dose-related toxic effects. White blood cell growth factors, both granulocyte colony-stimulating factor and granulocyte-macrophage colony-stimulating factor, are often used to reduce the duration of neutropenia in these patients as an adjunctive measure in the treatment of infectious complications. There are no data on the specific role that these substances play in helping to prevent or treat *Candida* infections (88); however, one study showed that bone marrow transplant patients with invasive candidiasis who received macrophage colony-stimulating factor had improved survival compared with historical control subjects (97). In nonneutropenic patients, fluconazole (400 mg per day for 14 days beyond the time of the last positive blood culture) can be used for the treatment of candidemia in relatively noncritically ill patients (63,98). However, fluconazole should not be used in patients with infections due to *C. glabrata* or *C. krusei* given the lower susceptibility of these organisms to this agent. Studies are also underway to assess the efficacy of itraconazole for bloodstream infections. In addition to antifungal therapy, a crucial component of managing candidemia is the removal of intravenous catheters (99). When intravenous lines cannot be changed (e.g., because of severity of illness, thrombocytopenia, or a coagulopathy), aggressive therapy should be instituted with the realization that cultures remaining positive in this setting herald a poor prognosis.

Treatment of *Candida* urinary tract infections should involve changing the urinary catheter if one is present. Antifungal therapy should be with parenteral amphotericin B or fluconazole (400 mg per day) if there is a concern that candiduria is a manifestation of systemic infection; otherwise, oral azoles (e.g., fluconazole 100 mg per day) or amphotericin B bladder washings (50 mg of amphotericin B in 1 L of sterile water per day) may be used (71,100).

Standard treatment of *Candida* endophthalmitis involves the use of parenteral amphotericin B with or without concomitant flucytosine. Intravitreal injection of antifungals is advocated by some. In some centers, partial vitrectomy is used as a therapeutic modality (77). Although there are reports of successful use of systemic azole therapy (101), none of these agents has been evaluated prospectively for use in endophthalmitis.

There are also case reports of successful medical therapy for *Candida* endocarditis (102,103), but in general, treatment of this disease requires a combined medical-surgical approach. Treatment with amphotericin B (0.6 to 0.8 mg/kg per day) with or without flucytosine should be initiated once the diagnosis is made. Valve replacement should then be performed and amphotericin B continued postoperatively. Recommendations are usually for a total duration of 6 to 10 weeks or a total dose of 1 to 2 g. Some authors recommend following amphotericin B therapy with fluconazole suppression.

Candida meningitis should be treated with amphotericin B (0.6 to 0.8 mg/kg per day), with or without flucytosine. Some patients are treated with intrathecal amphotericin B in addition to systemic therapy. Durations of therapy are not well defined but often extend to 6 weeks. Treatment of meningitis that occurs in the setting of a CSF shunt usually requires removal or replacement of the shunt.

PROPHYLAXIS

Prophylaxis to prevent *Candida* infections has been used mainly in four groups of patients: those with HIV infection, patients who are neutropenic during cancer chemotherapy or after bone marrow transplantation, solid organ transplant recipients, and surgical intensive care unit patients.

In HIV-infected patients, a study comparing systemic fluconazole (200 mg per day) with topical clotrimazole in patients with CD4+ cell counts less than 200 cells/mm^3 showed that fluconazole prevented the development of esophageal candidiasis and other deep fungal infections but had no effect on mortality (104). Nevertheless, because of concerns about cost, drug–drug interactions, and the potential development of azole resistance, fluconazole prophylaxis is still a matter of debate for this group of patients. Prophylaxis may be useful for patients with severe or frequent recurrences.

In neutropenic patients, prophylactic strategies have been considered in light of information that fungal colonization often precedes infection. Oral fluconazole (400 mg per day) has been shown to decrease fungal colonization, superficial and hematogenous infections, and mortality in bone marrow transplant patients and has been used in oncology centers for the purpose of preventing invasive candidiasis (105–107). In patients with leukemia, however, a study comparing fluconazole with placebo during the period of neutropenia failed to show a difference in the rate of invasive fungal infections or mortality (108). In addition, fluconazole has been shown in some studies to change the species responsible for colonization of these patients, with increases in *C. glabrata* and *C. krusei* (69,70).

Antifungal prophylaxis after solid organ transplantation, especially after liver transplantation, has often been recommended because of the high risk for fungal infections immediately after transplantation (109–112). A randomized trial supports the use of fluconazole for this purpose. Compared with nystatin, fluconazole (100 mg per day) has been shown to reduce both *Candida* colonization and infection after liver transplantation (113). The use of antifungal prophylaxis has also been evaluated in other surgical patients. A placebo-controlled trial of prophylactic fluconazole (400 mg per day for 3 days) in critically ill surgical patients showed a significant decrease in candidal infections in the treated group (114). The benefit of antifungal prophylaxis in surgical intensive care units patients was also shown in a large observational study (115) but has not been demonstrated for less severely ill surgical patients (116).

Azole resistance is not commonly reported in *C. albicans* isolated from oncology or organ transplant patients (117). It is likely that the short courses of azole prophylaxis used in these populations lead to a lower risk for the development of resistance than is seen in HIV-infected patients who may receive extended azole therapy.

REFERENCES

1. Odds FC. Candida *and candidiasis: a review and bibliography.* Philadelphia: WB Saunders, 1988.
2. Bodey GP. *Candidiasis: pathogenesis, diagnosis, and treatment.* New York: Raven Press, 1993.
3. Calderone RA, Fonzi WA. Virulence factors of *Candida albicans. Trends Microbiol* 2001;9(7):327–335.
4. Cutler JE. Putative virulence factors of *Candida albicans. Annu Rev Microbiol* 1991;45:187.
5. Edison AM, Manning-Zweerink M. Comparison of the extracellular proteinase activity produced by a low-virulence mutant of *Candida albicans* and its wild-type parent. *Infect Immun* 1988;56:1388.
6. Reagan DR, Pfaller MA, Hollis RJ, et al. Characterization of the sequence of colonization and nosocomial candidemia using DNA fingerprinting and a DNA probe. *J Clin Microbiol* 1990;28:2733.
7. Voss A, Hollis RJ, Pfaller MA, et al. Investigation of the sequence of colonization and candidemia in nonneutropenic patients. *J Clin Microbiol* 1994;32:975.
8. Pfaller MA. Epidemiology of fungal infections: the promise of molecular typing. *Clin Infect Dis* 1995;20:1535.
9. Pfaller MA. Nosocomial candidiasis: emerging species, reservoirs and modes of transmission. *Clin Infect Dis* 1996;22[Suppl 2]:S89.
10. Plouffe JF, Brown DG, Silva J Jr, et al. Nosocomial outbreak of *Candida parapsilosis* fungemia related to intravenous infusions. *Arch Intern Med* 1977;137:1686.
11. Bart-Delabesse E, Van Deventer H, Goessens W, et al. Contribution of molecular typing methods and antifungal susceptibility testing to the study of a candidemia cluster in a burn care unit. *J Clin Microbiol* 1995;33:3278.
12. Fraser VJ, Jones M, Dunkel J, et al. Candidemia in a tertiary care hospital: epidemiology, risk factors, and predictors of mortality. *Clin Infect Dis* 1992;15:414.
13. Wey SB, Mori M, Pfaller MA, et al. Risk factors for hospital-acquired candidemia: a matched case-control study. *Arch Intern Med* 1989;149:2349.
14. McNeil MM, Nash SL, Hajjeh RA, et al. Trends in mortality due to invasive mycotic diseases in the United States, 1980–1997. *Clin Infect Dis* 2001;33:641–647.
15. Vazquez JA, Sobel JD. Fungal infections in diabetes. *Infect Dis Clin North Am* 1995;9:97.

16. Hosen H. Id reactions from focal fungus infections treated by immunological methods. *Tex Med* 1973;69:83.
17. Bodey GP, Luna M. Skin lesions associated with disseminated candidiasis. *JAMA* 1974;229:1466.
18. Jarowski CL, Fialk MA, Murray HW, et al. Fever, rash, and muscle tenderness: a distinctive clinical presentation of disseminated candidiasis. *Arch Intern Med* 1978;138:544.
19. Marcus J, Grossman ME, Yunakov MJ, et al. Disseminated candidiasis, *Candida* arthritis, and unilateral skin lesions. *J Am Acad Dermatol* 1992;26:295.
20. Herrod HG. Chronic mucocutaneous candidiasis in childhood and complications of non-*Candida* infection: a report of the Pediatric Immunodeficiency Collaborative Study Group. *J Pediatr* 1990;116:377.
21. Kauffman CA, Shea MJ, Frame PT. Invasive fungal infections in patients with chronic mucocutaneous candidiasis. *Arch Intern Med* 1981;141:1076.
22. Edwards JE, Lehner RI, Stiehm ER, et al. Severe candidal infections: clinical perspective, immune defense mechanisms, and current concepts of therapy. *Ann Intern Med* 1978;89:91.
23. Chipps BE, Saulsbury FT, Hsu SH, et al. Noncandidal infections in children with chronic mucocutaneous candidiasis. *Johns Hopkins Med J* 1979;122:175.
24. Powderly WG. Mucosal candidiasis caused by non-albicans species of *Candida* in HIV-positive patients. *AIDS* 1992;6:604.
25. Cameron ML, Schell WA, Bruch S, et al. Correlation of in vitro fluconazole resistance of *Candida* isolates in relation to therapy and symptoms of individuals seropositive for human immunodeficiency virus type 1. *Antimicrob Agents Chemother* 1993;37:2449.
26. Chavanet P, Lopez J, Grappin M, et al. Cross-sectional study of the susceptibility of *Candida* isolates to antifungal drugs and in vitro-in vivo correlation in HIV-infected patients. *AIDS* 1994;8:945.
27. Maenza JR, Keruly JC, Moore RD, et al. Risk factors for fluconazole-resistant candidiasis in human immunodeficiency virus-infected patients. *J Infect Dis* 1996;173:219.
28. Vuffray A, Durussel C, Boerlin P, et al. Oropharyngeal candidiasis resistant to single-dose therapy with fluconazole in HIV-infected patients [Letter]. *AIDS* 1994;8:708.
29. Boken DJ, Swindells S, Rinaldi MG. Fluconazole-resistant *Candida albicans*. *Clin Infect Dis* 1993;17:1018.
30. Redding S, Smith J, Farinacci G, et al. Resistance of *Candida albicans* to fluconazole during treatment of oropharyngeal candidiasis in a patient with AIDS: documentation by in vitro susceptibility testing and DNA subtype analysis. *Clin Infect Dis* 1994;18:240.
31. Newman SL, Flanigan TP, Fisher A, et al. Clinically significant mucosal candidiasis resistant to fluconazole treatment in patients with AIDS. *Clin Infect Dis* 1994;19:684.
32. White A, Goetz MB. Azole-resistant *Candida albicans:* report of two cases of resistance to fluconazole and review. *Clin Infect Dis* 1994;19:687.
33. Bailey GG, Perry FM, Denning DW, et al. Fluconazole-resistant candidosis in an HIV cohort. *AIDS* 1994;8:787.
34. Sangeorzan JA, Bradley SF, Xiaogang H, et al. Epidemiology of oral candidiasis in HIV-infected patients: colonization, infection, treatment, and emergence of fluconazole resistance. *Am J Med* 1994;97:339.
35. Sanguineti A, Carmichael K, Campbell K. Fluconazole-resistant *Candida albicans* after long-term suppressive therapy. *Arch Intern Med* 1993;153:1122.
36. Fichtenbaum CJ, Koletar S, Yiannoutsos C, et al. Refractory mucosal candidiasis in advanced human immunodeficiency virus infection. *Clin Infect Dis* 2000;30:749–756.
37. Caruso LJ. Vaginal moniliasis after tetracycline therapy: the effects of amphotericin B. *Am J Obstet Gynecol* 1967;90:374.
38. Oriel JD, Waterworth PM. Effects of minocycline and tetracycline on the vaginal yeast flora. *J Clin Pathol* 1975;28:403.
39. Morton RS, Rashid S. Candidal vaginitis: natural history, predisposing factors, and prevention. *Proc R Soc Med* 1977;70[Suppl 4]:3.
40. Fleury FJ. Adult vaginitis. *Clin Obstet Gynecol* 1981;24:407.
41. Catterall RD. Influence of estrogenic contraceptive pills on candidiasis. *Br J Vener Dis* 1971;47:45.
42. Oriel JD, Partridge BM, Denny MJ, et al. Genital yeast infections. *BMJ* 1972;4:761.
43. Sobel JD. Pathophysiology of vulvovaginal candidiasis. *J Reprod Med* 1989;34[Suppl 8]:572.
44. Horowitz BJ, Giaquinta D, Ito S. Evolving pathogens in vulvovaginal candidiasis: implications for patient care. *J Clin Pharmacol* 1992;32:248.
45. Spinillo A, Michelone G, Cavanna C, et al. Clinical and microbiological characteristics of symptomatic vulvovaginal candidiasis in HIV-seropositive women. *Genitourin Med* 1994;70:268.
46. Monif GRG. Classification and pathogenesis of vulvovaginal candidiasis. *Am J Obstet Gynecol* 1985;152:935.
47. O'Connor MI, Sobel JD. Epidemiology of recurrent vulvovaginal candidiasis: identification and strain differentiation of *Candida albicans*. *J Infect Dis* 1986;154:358.
48. Sobel JD. Recurrent vulvovaginal candidiasis: a prospective study of the efficacy of maintenance ketoconazole therapy. *N Engl J Med* 1986;315:1455.
49. Sobel JD. Epidemiology and pathogenesis of recurrent vulvovaginal candidiasis. *Am J Obstet Gynecol* 1985;152:924.
50. El-Din SS, Reynolds MT, Ashbee HR, et al. An investigation into the pathogenesis of vulvo-vaginal candidosis. *Sex Transm Infect* 2001;77(33):179–183.
51. Calderson-Marquez JJ. Itraconazole in the treatment of vaginal candidiasis and the effect of treatment of the sexual partner. *Rev Infect Dis* 1987;9[Suppl 1]:S143.
52. Buch A, Christensen ES. Treatment of vaginal candidiasis with natamycin and effect of treating the partner at the same time. *Acta Obstet Gynecol Scand* 1982;61:393.
53. Bisschop MP, Merkus JM, Scheygrond H, et al. Cotreatment of the male partner in vaginal candidiasis: a double-blind randomized control study. *Br J Obstet Gynaecol* 1986;93:79.
54. Soll DR, Galask R, Schmid J, et al. Genetic dissimilarity of commensal strains of *Candida* spp. carried in different anatomical locations of the same healthy women. *J Clin Microbiol* 1991;29:1702.
55. Vazquez JA, Peng G, Sobel JD, et al. Evolution of antifungal susceptibility among *Candida* species isolates recovered from human immunodeficiency virus-infected women receiving fluconazole prophylaxis. *Clin Infect Dis* 2001;33:1069–1075.
56. Sobel JD, Ohmit SE, Schuman P, et al. The evolution of *Candida* species and fluconazole susceptibility among oral and vaginal isolates recovered from human immunodeficiency virus (HIV)-seropositive and at-risk HIV-seronegative women. *J Infect Dis* 2001;183:286–293.
57. Mathema B, Cross E, Dun E, et al. Prevalence of vaginal colonization by drug-resistant *Candida* species in college-age women with previous exposure to over-the-counter azole antifungals. *Clin Infect Dis* 2001;33:e23–e27.
58. Banerjee SN, Emori TG, Culver DH, et al. Secular trends in nosocomial primary bloodstream infections in the United States, 1980–1989. *Am J Med* 1991;91[Suppl 3B]:86S.
59. Jarvis WR. Epidemiology of nosocomial fungal infections, with emphasis on *Candida* species. *Clin Infect Dis* 1995;20:1526.
60. Richards MJ, Edwards JR, Culver DH, et al. Nosocomial infections in combined medical-surgical units in the United States. *Infect Control Hosp Epidemiol* 2000;21(8):510–515.
61. Pfaller MA, Diekema DJ, Jones RN, et al. International surveillance of bloodstream infections due to *Candida* species: frequency of occurrence and in vitro susceptibilities to fluconazole, ravuconazole, and voriconazole of isolates collected from 1997 through 1999 in the SENTRY antimicrobial surveillance program. *J Clin Microbiol* 2001;39(9):3254–3259.
62. Wey SB, Mori M, Pfaller MA, et al. Hospital-acquired candidemia: the attributable mortality and excess length of stay. *Arch Intern Med* 1988;148:2642.
63. Rex JH, Bennett JE, Sugar AM, et al. A randomized trial comparing fluconazole with amphotericin B for the treatment of candidemia in patients without neutropenia. *N Engl J Med* 1994;331:1325.
64. Berenguer J, Buck M, Witebsky F, et al. Lysis-centrifugation blood cultures in the detection of tissue-proven invasive candidiasis. *Diagn Microbiol Infect Dis* 1993;17:103.
65. Sanford GR, Merz WG, Wingard JR, et al. The value of fungal surveillance cultures as predictors of systemic fungal infections. *J Infect Dis* 1980;142:503.
66. Maenza JR, Merz WG. Candidemia: epidemiology and laboratory detection. *Infect Dis Clin Pract* 1997;2:83.
67. Wingard JR. Importance of *Candida* species other than *C. albicans* as pathogens in oncology patients. *Clin Infect Dis* 1995;20:115.
68. Kontoyiannis DP, Vaziri I, Hanna HA, et al. Risk factors for *Candida tropicalis* fungemia in patients with cancer. *Clin Infect Dis* 2001;33:1676–1678.
69. Wingard JR, Merz WG, Rinaldi MG, et al. Increase in *Candida krusei* infection among patients with bone marrow transplantation and neutropenia treated prophylactically with fluconazole. *N Engl J Med* 1991;325:1274.
70. Wingard JR, Merz WG, Rinaldi MG, et al. Association of *Torulopsis glabrata* infections with fluconazole prophylaxis in neutropenic bone marrow transplant patients. *Antimicrob Agents Chemother* 1993;37:1847.
71. Fisher JF, Newman CL, Sobel JD. Yeast in the urine: solutions for a budding problem. *Clin Infect Dis* 1995;20:183.
72. Rex JH, Walsh TJ, Sobel JD, et al. Practice guidelines for the treatment of candidiasis. *Clin Infect Dis* 2000;30:662–678.
73. Weens JJ Jr. *Candida parapsilosis:* Epidemiology, pathogenicity, clinical manifestations, and antimicrobial susceptibility. *Clin Infect Dis* 1992;14:756.
74. McQuillen DP, Zingman BS, Meunier F, et al. Invasive infections due to *Candida krusei:* report of ten cases of fungemia that include three cases of endophthalmitis. *Clin Infect Dis* 1992;14:472.
75. Joshi N, Hamory BH. Endophthalmitis caused by non-*albicans* species of *Candida*. *Rev Infect Dis* 1991;13:281.
76. O'Day DM, Head WS, Robinson RD. An outbreak of *Candida parapsilosis* endophthalmitis: analysis of strains by enzyme profile and antifungal susceptibility. *Br J Ophthalmol* 1987;71:126.
77. Snip RC, Michels RG. Pars plana vitrectomy in the management of endogenous *Candida* endophthalmitis. *Am J Ophthalmol* 1976;82:699.
78. Ellis ME, Al-Abdely H, Sandridge A, et al. Fungal endocarditis: evidence in the world literature, 1965–1995. *Clin Infect Dis* 2001;32:50–62.
79. Andriole VT. Endocarditis in the drug user. *Conn Med* 1970;34:327.
80. Bayer AS, Edwards JE Jr, Seidel JS, et al. *Candida* meningitis: report of seven cases and review of the English literature. *Medicine* (Baltimore) 1976;55:477.

81. Voice RA, Bradley SF, Sangeorzan JA, et al. Chronic candidal meningitis: an uncommon manifestation of candidiasis. *Clin Infect Dis* 1994;19:60.
82. Nguyen MH, Yu VL. Meningitis caused by *Candida* species: an emerging problem in neurosurgical patients. *Clin Infect Dis* 1995;21:323.
83. Sánchez-Portocarrero J, Martín-Rabadán, Saldaña CJ. *Candida* cerebrospinal fluid shunt infection. *Diagn Microbiol Infect Dis* 1994;20:33.
84. Anttila Veli-Jukka, Ruutu P, Bondestam S, et al. Hepatosplenic yeast infection in patients with acute leukemia: a diagnostic problem. *Clin Infect Dis* 1994;18:979.
85. Wakefield T, Wagner D, Antik N, et al. Importance of >5 day incubation or terminal subculture of BacT/Alert and BACTEC 460 blood culture systems (Abstr C-72). In: *Abstracts of the General Meeting of the American Society for Microbiology*, Atlanta, May 16–20, 1993:458.
86. Odds FC, Bernaerts R. CHROMagar Candida, a new differential isolation medium for presumptive identification of clinically important *Candida* species. *J Clin Microbiol* 1994;32:1923.
87. Mitchell TG, Sandin RL, Bowman BH, et al. Molecular mycology: DNA probes and applications of PCR technology. *J Med Vet Mycol* 1994;32[Suppl 1]:351.
88. Swerdloff JN, Filler SG, Edwards JE Jr. Severe candidal infections in neutropenic patients. *Clin Infect Dis* 1993;17[Suppl 2]:S457.
89. Harley WB, Dummer JS. Diagnosis of disseminated candidiasis by detection of antigenemia: a critical review. *Infect Dis Clin Pract* 1994;3:168.
90. Ibanez-Nolla J, Torres-Rodriguez JM, Nolla M, et al. The utility of serology in diagnosing candidosis in non-neutropenic critically ill patients. *Mycoses* 2001;44(1–2):47–53.
91. Walsh TJ, Merz WG, Lee JW, et al. Diagnosis and therapeutic monitoring of invasive candidiasis by rapid enzymatic detection of serum D-arabinitol. *Am J Med* 1995;99:164.
92. Walmsley S, King S, McGeer A, et al. Oropharyngeal candidiasis in patients with human immunodeficiency virus: correlation of clinical outcome with in vitro resistance, serum azole levels, and immunosuppression. *Clin Infect Dis* 2001;32:1554–1561.
93. Edwards JE Jr, Filler SG. Current strategies for treating invasive candidiasis: emphasis on infections in nonneutropenic patients. *Clin Infect Dis* 1992;14[Suppl 1]:S106.
94. Mikamo H, Sato Y, Tamaya T. In vitro antifungal activity of FK463, a new water-soluble echinocandin-like lipopeptide. *J Antimicrob Chemother* 2000;46:485–487.
95. Villanueva A, Arathoon EG, Gotuzzo E, et al. A randomized double-blind study of caspofungin versus amphotericin for the treatment of candidal esophagitis. *Clin Infect Dis* 2001;33:1529–1535.
96. Ally R, Schurmann D, Kreisel W, et al. A randomized, double-blind, double-dummy, multicenter trial of voriconazole and fluconazole in the treatment of esophageal candidiasis in immunocompromised patients. *Clin Infect Dis* 2001;33:1447–1454.
97. Nemunaitis J, Shannon-Dorcy K, Appelbaum FR, et al. Long-term follow-up of patients with invasive fungal disease who received adjunctive therapy with recombinant human macrophage colony-stimulating factor. *Blood* 1993;82:1422.
98. Kontoyiannis DP, Bodey GP, Mantzoros CS. Fluconazole vs. amphotericin B for the management of candidemia in adults: a meta-analysis. *Mycoses* 2001;44(5):125–135.
99. Mermel LA, Farr BM, Sheretz RJ, et al. Guidelines for the management of intravascular catheter-related infections. *Clin Infect Dis* 2001;32:1249–1272.
100. Lundstrom T, Sobel J. Nosocomial candiduria: a review. *Clin Infect Dis* 2001;32:1602–1607.
101. Akler ME, Vellend H, McNeely DM, et al. Use of fluconazole in the treatment of candidal endophthalmitis. *Clin Infect Dis* 1995;20:657.
102. Wells CJ, Leech GJ, Lever AML, et al. Treatment of native valve *Candida* endocarditis with fluconazole. *J Infect* 1995;31:233.
103. Zahid MA, Klotz SA, Hinthorn DR. Medical treatment of recurrent candidemia in a patient with probable *Candida parapsilosis* prosthetic valve endocarditis. *Chest* 1994;105:1597.
104. Powderly WG, Finkelstein DM, Feinberg J, et al. A randomized trial comparing fluconazole with clotrimazole troches for the prevention of fungal infections in patients with advanced human immunodeficiency virus infection. *N Engl J Med* 1995;332:700.
105. Uzan O, Anaissie EJ. Antifungal prophylaxis in patients with hematologic malignancies: a reappraisal. *Blood* 1995;86:2063.
106. Goodman JL, Winston DJ, Greenfield RA, et al. A controlled trial of fluconazole to prevent fungal infections in patients undergoing bone marrow transplantation. *N Engl J Med* 1992;326:845.
107. Slavin MA, Osborne B, Adams R, et al. Efficacy and safety of fluconazole prophylaxis for fungal infections after marrow transplantation: a prospective, randomized, double-blind study. *J Infect Dis* 1995;171:1545.
108. Winston DJ, Chandrasekar PH, Lazarus HM. Fluconazole prophylaxis of fungal infections in patients with acute leukemia. *Ann Intern Med* 1993;188:495.
109. Paya CV. Fungal infections in solid-organ transplantation. *Clin Infect Dis* 1993;16:677.
110. Warnock DW. Fungal complications of transplantation: diagnosis, treatment and prevention. *J Antimicrob Chemother* 1995;36[Suppl B]:73.
111. Kung N, Fisher N, Gunson B, et al. Fluconazole prophylaxis for high-risk liver transplant recipients. *Lancet* 1995;345:1234.
112. Rex JH, Sobel JD. Prophylactic antifungal therapy in the intensive care unit. *Clin Infect Dis* 2001;32:1191–1200.
113. Lumbreras C, Cuervas-Mons V, Jara P, et al. Randomized trial of fluconazole versus nystatin for the prophylaxis of *Candida* infection following liver transplantation. *J Infect Dis* 1996;174:583.
114. Pelz RK, Hendrix CW, Swoboda SM, et al. Double-blind placebo-controlled trial of fluconazole to prevent candidal infections in critically ill surgical patients. *Ann Surg* 2001;233(4):542–548.
115. Blumberg HM, Jarvis WR, Soucie JM, et al. Risk factors for candidal bloodstream infections in surgical intensive care unit patients: the NEMIS prospective multicenter study. *Clin Infect Dis* 1995;33:177–186.
116. Sobel JD, Rex JH. Invasive candidiasis: turning risk into a practical prevention policy? *Clin Infect Dis* 2001;33:187–190.
117. Lopez J, Pernot C, Aho S, et al. Decrease in *Candida albicans* strains with reduced susceptibility to fluconazole following changes in prescribing policies. *J Hosp Infect* 2001;48(2):122–128.

CHAPTER 268

Cryptococcus neoformans

John R. Graybill

HISTORY

Cryptococcus neoformans has been recognized as a pathogen in humans since 1894, but it was considered an uncommon cause of disease until recent years.

CHARACTERISTICS OF THE PATHOGEN

C. neoformans is familiar to us as the only encapsulated fungus, a characteristic that is relevant not only to classification but also to pathogenicity. *C. neoformans* was formerly considered an asexually reproducing yeast, but Kwon-Chung (1) was able to identify mating types and convert the organism to its perfect mycelial form, *Filobasidiella neoformans*. When the basidiospores are plated onto routine culture media or inoculated into mice, they convert to typical encapsulated cryptococci within a few days.

When cultured either from the environment or from patients, the fungus appears as small, yeastlike cells with narrow-based budding daughter cells (2). The capsule is composed of α-1,3-mannan with monosaccharide branches of xylose and glucuronic acid (3,4). The presence of a capsule is readily detected by the India ink or nigrosin test, in which a specimen is mixed with either India ink or nigrosin and examined under a microscope. A halo effect about the organism distinguishes the capsule. Capsular material can also be stained in tissues with mucicarmine. Indirectly, the capsular polysaccharide can be identified immunologically with specific antibodies raised against it. This is the basis of the diagnostic latex cryptococcal agglutination test (LCAT) (5). The LCAT has been modified as an enzyme-linked immunosorbent assay (cryptococcal antigen test, CRAG, now more commonly used to reduce the false-positive results commonly associated with latex agglutination tests). Finally, *C. neoformans* colonies can be identified in culture media containing caffeic acid (6). *C. neoformans* can uniquely metabolize caffeic acid to a melanin-like pigment, making the brown cryptococcal colonies readily distinguishable from other fungal colonies.

EPIDEMIOLOGY

C. neoformans has been divided into *C. neoformans* variety *neoformans* (serotypes A and D) and *C. neoformans* variety *gattii* (serotypes B and C). *C. neoformans* variety *gattii* has caused cryptococcosis mainly in patients without acquired immunodeficiency syndrome (AIDS), largely in Australia, with a few cases along the southern California coast and in the tropical Americas. The ecologic niche of the mycelial form of *C. neoformans* variety *gattii* is *Eucalyptus camaldulensis,* the Australian red river gum tree. It is likely that the organism reached the Americas with importation of this tree. All four serotypes are pathogenic to humans, but *C. neoformans* variety *neoformans* causes most human disease, and the most common serotype is A (4).

Among the groups most commonly exposed to *C. neoformans* are pigeon fanciers. These people rarely become ill with cryptococcosis, but they develop delayed-type hypersensitivity to cryptococcal antigens, indicating prior infection. Most of those who become ill with cryptococcosis are immunosuppressed. In the past, this population included mostly patients who had depressed cell-mediated immunity (7–10) as a result of lymphocytic leukemia, lymphomas, steroid therapy, or another underlying disorder. These groups accounted for 300 to 500 cases per year in the United States. At present, by far the most commonly affected group is patients with AIDS. Before the availability of highly active antiretroviral therapy (HAART), 5% to 7% of patients with AIDS in the United States and up to 30% in Africa developed cryptococcosis (11). In 1995, HAART therapy sharply improved immune responses and slowed progression of human immunodeficiency virus (HIV) infection to AIDS, and as a result, the incidence of cryptococcosis in Europe, the United States, and Australia dropped dramatically (12). The organism is thought to be transmitted only by the respiratory route and not directly from one human to another.

PATHOGENESIS

Much of our understanding of the pathogenesis and host defense mechanisms comes from studies of animal models, especially mice. Presumably, after being inhaled, *C. neoformans* is ingested by alveolar macrophages. The efficiency of phagocytosis *in vivo* is not clear and may depend in part on the antiphagocytic properties of the capsule (13). Unencapsulated yeast cells are readily phagocytosed and killed, whereas encapsulated cells are more resistant. Melanin also inhibits phagocytosis, and passive immunization with antimelanin antibodies prolongs survival of infected mice (14). Both macrophages and polymorphonuclear leukocytes can ingest and kill cryptococci, and the process may depend in part on opsonization by complement and antibody directed at the capsule and other cell components (15). Monoclonal antibodies to capsular polysaccharide have been used successfully to passively immunize mice against *C. neoformans.* Antibodies derived from humans immunized with cryptococcal capsular polysaccharide antigens are protective in mice, in part by enhancing clearance of the organism from serum and the brain, and in part by enhancing immune granuloma formation. Thus, humoral immune mechanisms are important in resistance to *C. neoformans.*

Various cell-mediated mechanisms have also been demonstrated in the murine model. Among these, there is evidence that natural killer cells may participate in early killing of cryptococci and that antibody-dependent cell-mediated killing may be operative (16). Within the first week after immunization of mice with cryptococcal antigens, T-lymphocyte activity can be demonstrated. CD4, CD8, and CD56 cells have been demonstrated to be active in the first weeks after infection. Interferon-γ (IFN-γ) and interleukin-2 (IL-2) are also associated with these cells (15). In a successful host response, there is an increase

in helper T-cell activity, skin-test conversion, and reduction of *C. neoformans* organisms in tissue counts. Indeed, augmentation of chemotherapy with IFN-γ has been demonstrated in murine cryptococcosis (17). Therefore, it is clear in mice that T lymphocytes are critical to successful host defenses, and the clinical settings of cryptococcosis strongly support a similar role in humans.

C. neoformans may pass through the lungs clinically unsuspected, with the later development of meningitis being the first indication of disease. Alternatively, if the infection is contained in the lungs, it may cause pneumonia, poorly defined mass lesions, pulmonary nodules, occasional hilar adenopathy, acute respiratory distress syndrome, or pleural effusion (7,8,18). Patients with disease limited to the lungs often have no major defects of cell-mediated immunity, although immune defects are common to patients with disseminated disease. In Australia, *C. neoformans* variety *gattii* continues to cause predominantly pulmonary disease in immune-competent patients. Conversely, *C. neoformans* variety *neoformans,* seen as meningitis in immune-suppressed patients, is decreasing with the increasing use of HAART in Australia (19).

When *C. neoformans* escapes from the lungs, the major secondary site of infection is the meninges. In patients with AIDS, the infection is usually widely distributed and commonly infects the prostate. The prostate and central nervous system are major sources of relapse for patients with AIDS if therapy is interrupted (20).

In patients who do not have AIDS, a chronic lymphocytic inflammatory response is elicited in the cerebrospinal fluid (CSF). There are usually 10 to 100 lymphocytes/mm^3, reduced CSF glucose value, and elevated protein level. As many as two thirds of patients have positive serum CRAG results for antigen. The CRAG test is positive in CSF in more than 95% of patients with AIDS and cryptococcal meningitis. Patients with AIDS and cryptococcal meningitis commonly have a minimal to absent cellular response, protein elevation, and depressed glucose in CSF. Patients with meningeal cryptococcosis produce cytokines in the CSF, including IL-8, IL-6, tumor necrosis factor-α, and IL-10, although these responses are much less than non–HIV-infected patients (21).

Chronic inflammation may involve the aqueduct of Sylvius, producing obstructive hydrocephalus. There may also be vasculitis, with subsequent focal ischemic damage to the brain or cranial nerves. Focal lesions are more commonly seen with variety *gattii* than *neoformans* and are more common in immuno-competent hosts. More often, there may be diffuse inflammation of the meninges, which impairs reabsorption of CSF and causes communicating hydrocephalus. In patients with AIDS, the massive fungal burden rather than inflammation appears to block CSF resorption and cause hydrocephalus. Extracerebral foci of infection may also include the skin, prostate, other soft tissues, and bones.

CLINICAL COURSE OF INFECTION

Although the first encounter of humans with *C. neoformans* occurs in the lungs, it is surprising that cryptococcal pneumonia occurs in less than 15% of patients (Fig. 268.1). Pulmonary infection may be manifested by cough that produces mucoid sputum, by chest pain, and sometimes by fever. Cavitations and calcification are rare. One study of patients with cryptococcal infection confirmed that many of them were either only modestly symptomatic or asymptomatic during their pulmonary infection, but the patients with immune suppression tended to develop

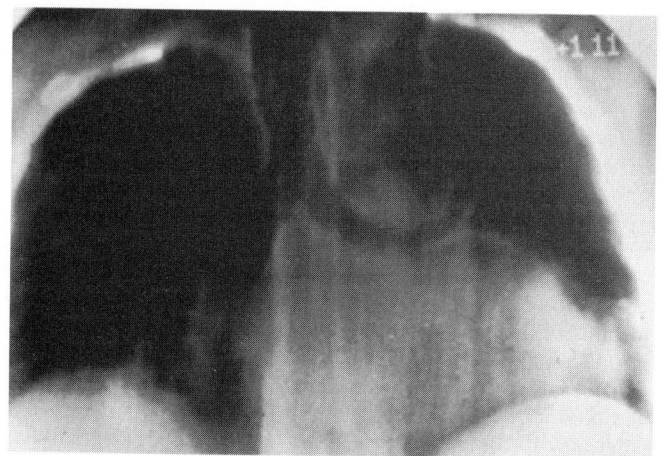

Figure 268.1. Chest radiograph of a patient with cryptococcal pneumonia showing dense homogeneous left lung infiltration.

meningitis, whereas immunocompetent patients have disease confined to the lungs (8). Pulmonary disease may be severe, and in one recent report, 11 of 33 patients with pulmonary cryptococcosis presented with acute respiratory failure (22). Patients with or without AIDS may have acute respiratory distress syndrome caused by cryptococcosis.

The most dangerous form of disease and that most frequently encountered is meningitis. This takes the form of chronic meningitis, with progressive headache, personality changes, dementia, and focal neurologic findings related to vascular or cranial nerve involvement (Table 268.1). Loss of vision may be associated with papilledema and high CSF pressure or may be due to direct involvement of the optic nerve by *C. neoformans*. More than half of the patients have no meningismus or fever. Cryptococcal meningitis may be completely asymptomatic early in the course (23). Less commonly, there may be nodular or ulcerative skin lesions (24). Focal osteomyelitis may also occur.

Intracerebral hypertension causes a potentially lethal syndrome of increased headache, papilledema, obtundation, and coma. In a large series of patients followed by the Mycoses Study Group, the median CSF pressure was about 250 mm H_2O, and the top quartile had pressures more than 350 mm H_2O. Higher pressure was associated with higher CSF antigen titers, papilledema, and increased mortality in the first weeks of treatment (25). The

mechanism for intracerebral hypertension is unclear but may relate to the load of fungal organisms or capsular polysaccharide impeding CSF drainage. Computed tomography rarely showed obstructive hydrocephalus. Pressure may be relieved by serial lumbar punctures with drainage of large volumes of fluid, sufficient to reduce the CSF pressure to 200 mm H_2O or less. Rapid attention to this acute problem may be a major reason for the sharp reduction of early mortality to less than 10% in cryptococcal meningitis. Removal of CSF polysaccharide by formation of antigen–antibody complexes may also be beneficial and is the subject of ongoing investigations by the Mycoses Study Group.

DIAGNOSIS

The diagnosis of cryptococcosis depends on demonstrating the organism or its capsular polysaccharide in tissues or body fluids (5,9). Because *C. neoformans* may be a commensal organism, its recovery from sputum cultures does not establish a diagnosis of invasive cryptococcosis; however, multiple cultures, when associated with pulmonary infiltrates or mass lesions, do support a diagnosis of pulmonary cryptococcal disease (7,18). Recovery of *C. neoformans* from tissue biopsy specimens, urine, blood, bone marrow, or CSF establishes the diagnosis of invasive cryptococcosis. In the case of tissue obtained without cultures, Gomori methenamine silver stain identifies yeast cells, but mucicarmine stain is necessary to confirm that the organism is *C. neoformans*. Unfortunately, some clinical isolates of *C. neoformans* have produced minimal polysaccharide, and the CRAG test may be equivocal (26).

Demonstration of the pathogen on an India ink preparation is specific for *C. neoformans* infection, but the observer must distinguish yeast cells from talc granules (which come from the gloves used during lumbar puncture), erythrocytes, and leukocytes (Table 268.2). The India ink preparation finding is positive in more than half of patients with meningitis who do not have AIDS and in even more of those who do have AIDS.

A positive LCAT or CRAG test result is significant for diagnosis in any titer. Because false-positive LCAT results in serum may be associated with antigen–antibody complexes and rarely with infection caused by *Trichosporon beigelii* (an organism with cell wall antigens similar to those of *C. neoformans*), we have used the CRAG in recent years. The CRAG result is positive in the

TABLE 268.1. Signs and Symptoms of Cryptococcal Meningoencephalitis at the Time of Hospitalization

Sign or symptom	Number	
	Not immunosuppressed	Acquired immunodeficiency syndrome
Headache	91	82
Fever	64	75
Stiff neck	75	33
Nausea and vomiting	55	46
Altered consciousness	50	24
Impaired mentation	41	16
Cranial nerve lesion	50	15
Visual deficits	27	10
Papilledema	27	8
Seizures	7	18
Focal neurologic deficits	11	5

TABLE 268.2. Typical Cerebrospinal Fluid Findings in Cryptococcal Meningitis

Measure	Non-AIDS	AIDS
Leukocytes per mm^3	10–300	<5
Differential	>80% lymphocytes	>80% lymphocytes
Glucose value	<40 mg/dL	>40 mg/dL
Protein level	100–300 mg/dL	20–100 mg/dL
Positive finding on India ink preparation	60%–70%	>90%
Cerebrospinal fluid CRAG titer	1:1–1:512 Usually <1:1000	1:1–1:1,000,000 Frequently >1:1000
Serum CRAG test result positive	70%	>90%

AIDS, acquired immunodeficiency syndrome; CRAG, cryptococcal antigen.
Source: Data from references 5, 9, 12, 29, 30.

serum of about 70% of non-AIDS patients with cryptococcosis and in more than 90% of patients with AIDS and cryptococcosis. The significance of a positive serum antigen test result in non-AIDS patients is not clear. However, there is general agreement that a positive serum antigen test result in patients with AIDS, even with no recovery of organisms from any tissue, is an indication for treatment to prevent meningitis. The CSF CRAG is useful for both diagnosis and prognosis. Whereas there is no correlation of serum titer with outcome, a high initial CSF titer greater than 1:1,024 in patients with AIDS is a predictor of a fatal outcome (Table 268.3). Obtundation, high CSF pressure, and CSF cell counts less than 20 cells/mm^3 are also predictors of a poor outcome. During therapy for acute infection, an unchanged or rising CSF (but not serum) CRAG titer is predictive of treatment failure, and a rise of the titer during long-term suppressive therapy is predictive of relapse (27).

The differential diagnosis of cryptococcosis, particularly meningitis, is broad. It includes chronic infectious meningitis, as from syphilis, brucellosis, tuberculosis, histoplasmosis, coccidioidomycosis, cysticercosis, or even epidural abscess; neoplastic processes, such as lymphoma or carcinomatous meningitis; au-

toimmune diseases, such as systemic lupus erythematosus; and a variety of miscellaneous diseases, including sarcoidosis.

TREATMENT

Treatment of cryptococcal meningitis has undergone dramatic changes, with marked improvement of outcome. Most investigations have been concentrated in patients infected with HIV, who represent the majority of those with cryptococcosis. The traditional therapy for patients without AIDS has been 0.5 to 1.0 mg/kg of amphotericin B per day, given intravenously, and up to 150 mg/kg per day of flucytosine, given orally, for as long as 6 weeks (28). This regimen is curative in up to 75% of non-AIDS patients but because of toxicity of amphotericin B and flucytosine at these doses is now rarely used. Much more is known about treatment response in patients with AIDS and cryptococcosis, and results with cryptococcosis in the setting of HIV have been extended to non-HIV patients with cryptococcal disease. Initial reports in patients with AIDS noted high treatment failure and relapse rates after traditional amphotericin B and flucytosine

TABLE 268.3. Value of Cryptococcal Antigen Measurement in Management of Acquired Immunodeficiency Syndrome-Associated Cryptococcal Meningitis

	Indicated titer change					
	Decrease		No change		Increase	
Group	N	%	N	%	N	%
Initial treatment: Baseline cerebrospinal fluid titer ≥1:8						
Responders (N = 21)	18	86	2	9	1	5
Failures (N = 25)	11	44	12	48	2	8
p < 0.01 for responders versus failures						
Long-term suppression after initial treatment						
Cerebrospinal fluid titer						
Success (N = 126)	74	59	46	36	6	5
Relapse (N = 14)	4	29	4	29	6	43
p = 0.001 for successful suppression versus relapse						
Serum titer						
Success (N = 157)	67	43	68	43	22	14
Relapse (N = 13)	6	46	5	39	2	15
No correlation of serum titer with relapse						

Data from Powderly WG, Cloud GA, Dismukes WA, et al. Measurement of cryptococcal antigen in serum and cerebrospinal fluid: value in the management of AIDS-associated cryptococcal meningitis. *Clin Infect Dis* 1992;18:789–792, with permission.

TABLE 268.4.   Percent Relapses with Long-term Suppressive Therapy

Study	Placebo		Amphotericin B		Fluconazole		Itraconazole	
	N	%	N	%	N	%	N	%
Bozette et al. (20)[a]	27	37			34	3		
Powderly et al. (31)[b]			78	18	111	2		
Mycoses Study Group (35)[c] (unpublished data)					51	4	57	23

[a]Fluconazole at 200 mg/d superior to placebo.
[b]Fluconazole at 200 mg/d superior to amphotericin B at 1 mg/kg/wk.
[c]Fluconazole at 200 mg/d superior to itraconazole at 200 mg/d.

administration was terminated (29,30). Two large randomized studies indicated that long-term fluconazole suppression therapy (2% to 3% relapse) was more effective in preventing relapse than placebo (37%) or weekly amphotericin B (18%) and better tolerated than amphotericin B (20,31). Thus, after initial treatment, there is widespread agreement that fluconazole should be continued indefinitely at 200 mg per day to prevent relapse. Whether late relapses are caused by noncompliance with suppressive treatment or by emergence of fluconazole-resistant isolates is not clear (32) (Table 268.4).

Initial reports of fluconazole and itraconazole were encouraging for clinical responses, in patients with AIDS, but fewer than 50% of patients showed CSF culture result conversion to negative, and there were late microbiologic relapses noted for itraconazole recipients (33–35). One retrospective comparison of HIV-negative patients treated with fluconazole or amphotericin B showed overall responses of about 70% to either drug, but noted that the more seriously ill patients tended to receive amphotericin B (36). In this study, failures from fluconazole were attributed to persistent positive cultures, and those to amphotericin B were attributed to nephrotoxicity. Nevertheless, because of persistent CSF positive cultures, triazoles are now not generally used alone for primary treatment of cryptococcal meningitis.

Based on a large randomized trial, which suggested superiority of the combined regimen of amphotericin B and flucytosine (over amphotericin B alone), the Mycoses Study Group has recommended amphotericin B, 0.7 mg/kg, with flucytosine at 100 mg/kg per day for 2 weeks, followed by fluconazole, 400 mg per day for 8 weeks, then 200 mg per day indefinitely for patients with AIDS and cryptococcosis (37,38). Of 381 patients entered into the study, approximately 80% of either treatment group had clinically improved by 2 weeks of therapy. Those who received amphotericin B alone had 51% negative culture results versus 60% for those receiving combined amphotericin B and flucytosine ($p = 0.06$). Few people left the study because of flucytosine toxic effects, suggesting that flucytosine was well tolerated. In addition, flucytosine was administered without blood level measurement, and dose adjustment was based on renal function and peripheral blood cell counts. At a 1-year follow-up of patients who achieved negative CSF culture results during primary therapy, only 2 flucytosine recipients relapsed, versus 13 of those who had not received flucytosine. On the basis of these findings, 2 weeks of combined amphotericin B and flucytosine therapy is recommended. The Mycoses Study Group recommended a similar amphotericin B–flucytosine induction regimen for patients without AIDS, but suggested consolidation therapy with fluconazole, 400 mg per day for 10 to 12 weeks. In a recent large case study of patients without HIV infection, the response to amphotericin B initiation and fluconazole consolidation regimens was successful for 74% of patients, with attributable mortality to cryptococcosis only 12% (39) (Table 268.5).

An alternative approach was taken by the California Cooperative Treatment Group, which evaluated an oral regimen of fluconazole (400 mg per day) plus flucytosine (150 mg/kg per day) (40). In the initial series by the California Cooperative Treatment Group, 67% of patients had culture result conversion of their CSF during the 8-week course of therapy evaluated. However, the toxic effect of flucytosine was still a problem in some patients at the high dose of 150 mg/kg per day, and for this reason, the oral regimen is seen as a distant second-line treatment.

In addition to chemotherapy, the Mycoses Study Group has recommended that great attention be paid to the opening CSF pressure at the baseline lumbar puncture. In the absence of focal mass lesions, and if the pressure is more than 250 mm H_2O, serial lumbar drainage should be undertaken until the pressure

TABLE 268.5.   Results of Initial Treatment of Cryptococcal Meningitis in Patients with Acquired Immunodeficiency Syndrome[a]

Study	Amphotericin B ± flucytosine		Fluconazole		Fluconazole + flucytosine	
	N	% Success	N	% Success	N	% Success
Larsen Leal, and Chan (34)	6	100	14	43		
Van der Horst et al. (37)	63	40	131	34		
Larsen et al. (40)					32	75

[a]Successful treatment is defined as conversion of cerebrospinal fluid culture results to negative within 10 wk.

is maintained 200 mm H$_2$O or less. With careful observation of CSF pressure and repeated mechanical drainage of CSF for high pressures (few patients had obstructive hydrocephalus at computed tomography), the mortality during the first 2 weeks of treatment was less than 6% (37,38). Rarely, hydrocephalus may require shunting for management (41).

For nonmeningeal cryptococcosis, fluconazole (or itraconazole) at 200 to 400 mg per day is recommended for up to 1 year if no HIV infection is present or indefinitely in the presence of AIDS (38).

There are several unanswered questions remaining. One is whether successful HAART will prompt termination of chronic suppressive therapy in patients with AIDS. CD4 cell counts, titers of cryptococcal antigen, and dose of amphotericin B have all been associated with early treatment failures in patients with AIDS (42). It seems reasonable that recovery of CD4 cell counts would be associated with effective immune response and ability to discontinue therapy. However, there has been some hesitation to this because fluconazole is a relatively benign agent and suppression is so effective. One is a reduction of amphotericin B toxicity by using lipid-associated forms of amphotericin B, such as liposomes (AmBisome, Gilead). AmBisome has been found similarly effective as amphotericin B in a recent large comparative study, and whether reduction of nephrotoxicity will be a sufficient impetus to use this as primary therapy is unclear (43). New triazoles such as voriconazole and posaconazole have also shown some efficacy in open salvage studies of cryptococcosis, but the experience is small and there are no clear advantages over fluconazole or amphotericin B. Cytokine therapy has still to make the jump from animals to clinical studies; given the excellent responses to amphotericin B and flucytosine in severely immune depressed patients, it is unclear what immune modulators would offer.

REFERENCES

1. Kwon-Chung KJ. A new genus, *Filobasidiella*, the perfect state of *Cryptococcus neoformans. Mycologia* 1975;67:1197.
2. Neilson JB, Fromtling RA, Bulmer GS. *Cryptococcus neoformans*: size range of infectious particles from aerosolized soil. *Infect Immun* 1977;17:634.
3. Bhattacharjee AK, Kwon-Chung KJ, Glaudemans CP. On the structure of the capsular polysaccharide from *Cryptococcus neoformans* serotype C. *Immunochemistry* 1978;15:673.
4. Bhattacharjee AK, Bennett JE, Glaudemans CPJ. Capsular polysaccharide from *Cryptococcus neoformans. Rev Infect Dis* 1984;6:619.
5. Kaufman CA, Bergman AG, Severance PJ, et al. Detection of cryptococcal antigen: comparison of two latex agglutination tests. *Am J Clin Pathol* 1980;81:106.
6. Wang HS, Zeimis RT, Roberts GD. Evaluation of a caffeic acid ferric citrate test for rapid identification of *Cryptococcus neoformans. J Clin Microbiol* 1977;6:445.
7. Hammerman KG, Powell KE, Christianson CS, et al. *Cryptococcosis*: clinical forms and treatment. *Am Rev Respir Dis* 1973;108:1116.
8. Kerkering TM, Duma RJ, Shadomy S. The evolution of pulmonary cryptococcosis. *Ann Intern Med* 1981;94:611.
9. Diamond RD, Bennett JE. Prognostic factors in cryptococcal meningitis: a study of 111 cases. *Ann Intern Med* 1974;80:175.
10. Kaplan MH, Rosen PP, Armstrong D. *Cryptococcosis* in a cancer hospital. Clinical and pathological correlates in forty-six patients. *Cancer* 1977;39:2265.
11. Dismukes WE. Cryptococcal meningitis in patients with AIDS. *J Infect Dis* 1988;157:624.
12. van Elden LJR, Walenkamp AME, Lipovsky MM, et al. Declining incidence of patients with cryptococcosis in the Netherlands in the era of highly active antiretroviral therapy. *AIDS* 2000;14:2787.
13. Casadevall A, Perfect J. Virulence factors. In: *Cryptococcus neoformans*. Washington, DC: ASM Press, 1998:145.
14. Rosas A, Nosanchuk JD, Casadevall A. Passive immunization with melanin-binding monoclonal antibodies prolong survival of mice with lethal *Cryptococcus neoformans* infection. *Infect Immun* 2001;69:3410.
15. Casadevall A, Perfect J. Specific immunity and cytokines. In: *Cryptococcus neoformans*. Washington, DC: ASM Press, 1998.
16. Casadevall A, Perfect J. Physical defenses and nonspecific immunity. In: *Cryptococcus neoformans*. ASM Press Washington, DC 1998:177.
17. Lutz JE, Clemons KV, Stevens DA. Enhancement of antifungal chemotherapy by interferon gamma in experimental murine cryptococcosis. *J Antimicrob Chemother* 2000;46:437.
18. Balmes JR, Hawkins JG. Pulmonary cryptococcosis. *Semin Respir Med* 1987;9:180.
19. Chen S, Sorrell T, Nimmo G, et al. Epidemiology and host- and variety-dependent characteristics of infection due to *Cryptococcus neoformans* in Australia and New Zealand. *Clin Infect Dis* 2001;31:499.
20. Bozette SA, Larsen RA, Chiu J, et al. A placebo-controlled trial of maintenance therapy with fluconazole after treatment of cryptococcal meningitis in the acquired immunodeficiency syndrome. *N Engl J Med* 1991;324:580.
21. Lortholary O, Dromer F, Mathoulin-Pelissier S, et al. Immune mediators in cerebrospinal fluid during cryptococcosis are influenced by meningeal involvement and human immunodeficiency virus status. *J Infect Dis* 2001;183:294.
22. Vilchez RA, Linden P, Lacomis J, et al. Acute respiratory failure associated with pulmonary cryptococcosis in non-AIDS patients. *Chest* 2001;119:1865.
23. Liss HP, Rimland D. Asymptomatic cryptococcal meningitis. *Am Rev Respir Dis* 1981;124:88.
24. Schupbach CW, Wheeler CF, Briggaman RA. Cutaneous manifestations of disseminated cryptococcosis. *Arch Dermatol* 1976;112:1734.
25. Graybill JR, Sobel J, Saag M, et al. Diagnosis and management of increased intracranial pressure in patients with AIDS and cryptococcal meningitis. *Clin Infect Dis* 2000;30:47.
26. Tintelnot K, Adler S, Bergmann F, et al. Case reports: disseminated cryptococcoses without cryptococcal antigen detection. *Mycoses* 2000;43:203.
27. Powderly WG, Cloud GA, Dismukes WA, et al. Measurement of cryptococcal antigen in serum and cerebrospinal fluid: value in the management of AIDS-associated cryptococcal meningitis. *Clin Infect Dis* 1992;18:789.
28. Bennett JE, Dismukes WE, Duma RJ, et al. A comparison of amphotericin B alone and combined with flucytosine. *N Engl J Med* 1979;301:126.
29. Kovacs JA, Kovacs AA, Polis M, et al. Cryptococcosis in the acquired immunodeficiency syndrome. *Ann Intern Med* 1985;103:533.
30. Eng RHK, Bishburg E, Smith SM, et al. Cryptococcal infections in patients with the acquired immunodeficiency syndrome. *Am J Med* 1986;81:19.
31. Powderly WG, Saag MS, Cloud GA, et al. A controlled trial of fluconazole or amphotericin B to prevent relapse of cryptococcal meningitis in patients with the acquired immunodeficiency syndrome. *N Engl J Med* 1992;326:83.
32. Aller AI, Martin-Manzuelos E, Lozano F, et al. Correlation of fluconazole MICs with clinical outcome in cryptococcal infection. *Antimicrob Agents Chemother* 2000;44:1544.
33. Saag MS, Powderly WG, Cloud GA, et al. Comparison of amphotericin B with fluconazole in the treatment of acute AIDS-associated cryptococcal meningitis. *N Engl J Med* 1992;326:83.
34. Larsen RA, Leal MA, Chan LS. Fluconazole compared with amphotericin B plus flucytosine for cryptococcal meningitis in AIDS. *Ann Intern Med* 1990;113:183.
35. Saag MS, Cloud GA, Graybill JR, et al. A comparison of itraconazole versus fluconazole as maintenance therapy for AIDS-associated cryptococcal meningitis. *Clin Infect Dis* 1999;28:291.
36. Dromer F, Mathoulin S, Dupont B, et al. Comparison of the efficacy of amphotericin B and fluconazole in the treatment of cryptococcosis in human immunodeficiency virus-negative patients: retrospective analysis of 83 cases. *Clin Infect Dis* 1996;22[Suppl 2]:S154.
37. Van der Horst C, Saag M, Cloud G, et al. Treatment of cryptococcal meningitis associated with the acquired immunodeficiency syndrome. *N Engl J Med* 1997;337:15.
38. Saag MS, Graybill JR, Larsen RA, et al. Practice guidelines for the management of cryptococcal disease. *Clin Infect Dis* 2000;30:710.
39. Pappas PG, Perfect JR, Cloud GA. Cryptococcosis in human immunodeficiency virus-negative patients in the era of effective azole therapy. *Clin Infect Dis* 2001;33:690.
40. Larsen RA, Bozette SA, Jones BE, et al. Fluconazole combined with flucytosine for treatment of cryptococcal meningitis in patients with AIDS. *Clin Infect Dis* 1991;19:745.
41. Park MK, Hospenthal DR, Bennett JE. Treatment of hydrocephalus secondary to cryptococcal meningitis by use of shunting. *Clin Infect Dis* 1999;28:629.
42. Robinson PA, Bauer M, Leal MAE, et al. Early mycological failure in AIDS-associated cryptococcal meningitis. *Clin Infect Dis* 1999;28:82.
43. Hamill RJ, Sobel J, El-Sadr W. Randomized double-blind trial of AmBisome (liposomal amphotericin B) and amphotericin B in acute cryptococcal meningitis in AIDS patients. Paper presented at: Thirty Ninth Interscience Conference on Antimicrobial Agents and Chemotherapy; 1999. Abstract no. 1161.

CHAPTER 269
Aspergillus *Species*

Richard D. Meyer

HISTORY

The term *aspergillosis* refers to a diverse set of conditions that range from intoxication through colonization or provocation of an allergic reaction to either localized or widespread invasive disease. *Aspergillus* species, of which more than 180 have been described, show mycelial morphology whether in a saprophytic state or in invasive disease (1,2). Disease in humans has been related to numerous species, most commonly *Aspergillus fumigatus*, *Aspergillus flavus*, and to lesser extents, *Aspergillus niger*, *Aspergillus terreus*, and *Aspergillus nidulans* (2). Molecular methods have led to taxonomic revisions (1,2).

Aspergillus species were described in the eighteenth century, and then in avian and later in human disease in the mid-nineteenth century. Subsequently, Virchow described aspergillosis in pulmonary disease. By the turn of the late nineteenth century, pulmonary disease in wig cleaners and pigeon breeders had been described and associated with moldy grain. Animal intoxications putatively caused by aflatoxins were described. Various workers then described the saprophytic pulmonary and more recently the allergic forms of human disease; more recently much emphasis has been placed on the well-known importance of the increased incidence of *Aspergillus* species as opportunistic pathogens in invasive infections (1–4).

CHARACTERISTICS OF THE PATHOGEN

Aspergillus species are members of the eumycetes. They grow in nature in the same way that they do on appropriate culture media. Most species reproduce only asexually, but some also have a perfect or sexual phase (teleomorphs) (1). Conidia are produced in both forms; the conidiogenous cell is phialidic (1). *A. fumigatus,* for example, grows into gray-green colonies with a conidial mass and on microscopic examination displays septate hyphae branched at 45-degree angles with conidial heads, composed of a vesicle, phialides, and conidial chains (1). Aflatoxins and other toxins play a role in intoxication. *Aspergillus* species have antigenic moieties that elicit antibody responses in patients with allergic forms of the disease or with mycetoma.

EPIDEMIOLOGY

Aspergillus species are ubiquitous; they are saprobic in soil and water, on various foodstuffs, and in decaying vegetation. The conidia, which under auspicious circumstances will form hyphae, are unevenly distributed, as has been noted in the occupational risks of disease.

Human disease may be community acquired (more common in noninvasive forms of aspergillosis) or nosocomial (more common in invasive disease because of the complex interaction of the amount of inoculum with host defenses). The principal route of transmission is airborne. The pathogen enters the respiratory tract or sometimes an operative site. A secondary transmission route is contact, usually with skin or a wound (5). Invasive aspergillosis is second in frequency to candidiasis among invasive mycoses in patients with leukemia and lymphoma.

Nosocomial point-source acquisition of invasive aspergillosis has been increasingly recognized as an important source of invasive disease. Walsh and Pizzo (5) classified most of those cases as directly hospital acquired by airborne transmission. Subclasses of sources include nonfiltered, nonventilated air as indirectly documented; contaminated intake ducts, exhaust ducts, or filters in ventilation systems (documented in several outbreaks); construction, either installation of contaminated fireproofing materials or inadequate barriers between construction, demolition, or renovation sites and areas for care of patients; and contaminated surfaces and potted plants (1,5). Contact transmission from contaminated dressings to skin or bone or from inadvertent intraperitoneal administration of *Aspergillus* organisms also occurs (5). Use of marijuana contaminated with *A. fumigatus* has also led to infection (6) (Fig. 269.1).

Several typing systems based on phenotypic or genomic features have been described to distinguish *A. fumigatus* strains. The latter include restriction endonuclease analysis of deoxyribonucleic acid (DNA), randomly amplified polymorphic DNA markers, and others; some recent studies have linked invasive isolates to clonal relatives in the environment (7,8).

PATHOGENESIS

Aspergillus organisms may colonize preexisting pulmonary cavities and grow saprobically but subsequently only rarely invade tissue. The greatest risk factor for invasive aspergillosis is granulocytopenia, particularly if it is protracted; patients with T-cell dysfunction are also at increased risk, but in the absence of granulocytopenia, they account for a minority of cases (3–5,9–13). Thus, patients with hematologic and other malignancies, organ allograft (lung, liver, and others) recipients, and those receiving immunosuppressive therapy, for example, for rheumatologic disorders, are all at increased risk. In orthotopic

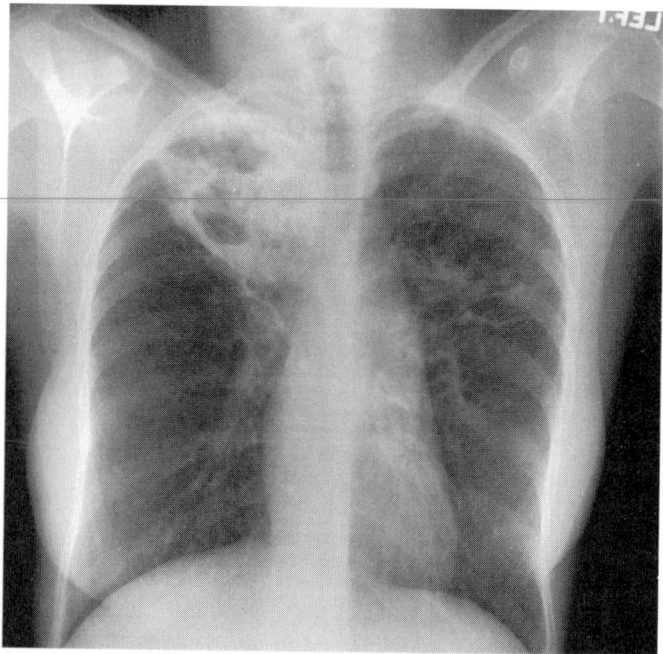

Figure 269.1. Posteroanterior chest radiograph from a 20-year-old female marijuana smoker with *Aspergillus fumigatus* infection in sputum and recurrent wheezing and fever. Bilateral upper lobe infiltrates with prominence on right and cavitation are seen. Antibacterial and prednisone therapy given for allergic bronchopulmonary aspergillosis led to resolution.

liver transplant recipients, risk factors for invasive pulmonary aspergillosis are increased serum creatinine concentration and prior cytomegalovirus infection (11). Autologous bone marrow transplant recipients are at particular risk early after transplantation and allogeneic recipients later during corticosteroid therapy to treat graft-versus-host disease (12,13).

Patients with chronic granulomatous disease of childhood are also at increased risk, particularly for *A. nidulans* infections (14). Invasive aspergillosis is associated with acquired immunodeficiency syndrome (AIDS); it usually occurs late in the course of disease, sometimes as a nosocomial complication. Almost all cases occur in patients with CD4+ lymphocyte counts of less than 50 cells/mm^3 and some with neutropenia. A wide spectrum of pulmonary infections, as well as less common infection at other sites, including the paranasal sinuses and central nervous system (CNS), is noted (16–18). Invasive disease has been associated with the anti–tumor necrosis factor-α (TNF-α) monoclonal antibody infliximab (19).

Many of these associations correlate with the primary importance of the granulocytes and alveolar macrophages in containment of *Aspergillus*. Nonetheless, invasive paranasal sinus, pulmonary, and disseminated aspergillosis in previously normal hosts or those with miscellaneous medical conditions has been described. Some of these "normal" hosts have underlying alcoholic liver disease. Failure to contain *Aspergillus* organisms in the lung is followed by hematogenous dissemination. Invasive pulmonary aspergillosis rarely complicates viral influenza (2,20).

Alveolar, but not peritoneal, macrophages inhibit germination of and then kill spores by a mechanism independent of oxidative killing mechanisms or T-cell activation (21). Normal monocytes can also damage them (22). Granulocytes ingest but may not kill spores, and although they are unable to engulf hyphae of aspergilli because of the size discrepancy, they nonetheless cause damage to the hyphae (23). Granulocytes, like monocytes, damage the hyphal form via an oxidative mechanism (24).

CLINICAL MANIFESTATIONS

Classification of clinical syndromes of aspergillosis sometimes lacks precision because of the frequent overlap in findings. The following schema modified from Pennington (25) applies to pulmonary aspergillosis and demonstrates the wide spectrum of underlying host conditions.

Aspergillus Hypersensitivity Lung Diseases

In extrinsic asthma inhalation of spores from the environment provokes immunoglobulin E (IgE)–mediated sensitized mast cell mechanisms in airways of allergic persons (25).

Aspergillus species spores—on moldy barley, oats, corn, or hay—are among the many precipitants of extrinsic allergic alveolitis, commonly also referred to as *farmer's lung*. Cough, dyspnea, and sometimes fever and chills follow inhalation of spores by a sensitized person. Diffuse pulmonary infiltrates and a restrictive pattern on pulmonary function testing result; eventually pulmonary fibrosis may ensue. Skin testing with *Aspergillus* antigen usually shows an Arthus reaction, *Aspergillus* serum precipitin levels are elevated, and corticosteroid therapy is usually salutary, perhaps because of a role of lymphocyte transformation in pathogenesis (25,26).

Allergic bronchopulmonary aspergillosis (ABPA) principally occurs in previously allergic asthmatic patients, usually adults,

and has been found in patients with cystic fibrosis. Exposure may be environmental or from colonization in the respiratory tract. Clinical features include worsening bronchospasm, and less commonly nonspecific complaints and low-grade fever; up to two thirds of patients have cough with brownish sputum, and sputum shows *Aspergillus* organisms (25–27). Radiographic infiltrates may or may not be present, but they commonly involve upper lobes (Fig. 269.1). Mucoid impaction, nodules, and multilobar bronchiectasis are computer tomographic (CT) scan findings (28). The last is a common result if ABPA is not treated promptly; pulmonary fibrosis is another sequela. IgE and immunoglobulin G (IgG) antibodies, as well as cellular immune mechanisms, are likely to be important in pathogenesis. Criteria for diagnosis include asthma, peripheral eosinophilia, immediate reaction to *Aspergillus* skin testing, serum precipitins against *Aspergillus*, an elevated serum IgE level, elevated levels of serum IgG and IgE against *Aspergillus*, pulmonary infiltrates, and central bronchiectasis (26–28). Systemic therapy with corticosteroids is indicated. Itraconazole has been shown to be beneficial, including allowing reduction of corticosteroid requirements (29). Although ABPA is typically not associated with invasion, *A. fumigatus* has been found in lung parenchyma after corticosteroid therapy, and rarely it has even disseminated (29,30). The ABPA syndrome is rarely associated with other fungal precipitants. More detailed therapeutic recommendations are found in recent guidelines (30a).

Bronchocentric granulomatosis associated with chronic asthma is associated with aspergilli in some cases and may resemble ABPA in an overlap syndrome (31,32). Allergic *Aspergillus* sinusitis affects allergic persons with nasal polyps and shares certain features of ABPA: aspergilli, mucoid impaction and inflammatory debris in paranasal sinuses, and serum antibodies to *A. fumigatus* (26,32).

Mucoid impaction of the bronchi is associated with asthma, ABPA, and eosinophilic pneumonia; the last condition has been ascribed to hypersensitivity to fungi, including aspergilli, and may overlap with ABPA (31,32). Mucoid impaction of bronchi includes obstruction of proximal bronchi by plugs larger than those seen in ABPA, some of which contain aspergilli. Patients usually suffer from asthma or chronic bronchitis. Common presenting features are cough, fever, chest pain, hemoptysis, and expectoration of mucous plugs. By definition, hypersensitivity to *Aspergillus* is not found. Mucolytic agents are used for therapy (31).

Noninvasive Pulmonary Aspergillosis

Aspergillus species are the pathogens of the vast majority of mycetomata or fungus balls, which grow in preexisting cavities, usually from antecedent tuberculosis; fungus balls less commonly develop in other underlying pulmonary disorders, such as cystic cavities (25,26). Mats of hyphae grow saprobically with host material in the cavities, but limited local invasion into the cavity wall may also occur. Hemoptysis is the most common presenting complaint, although cough and weight loss have also been described (25).

A chest radiograph or CT scan of such a patient with hemoptysis (or frequently an asymptomatic patient) shows the fungus ball with a surrounding air-crescent shadow. A similar or even eidetic radiographic appearance may be seen with an entirely different pathogenesis in the evolution of necrotic lung parenchyma into an abscess or sequestrum-like mass (Fig. 269.2). A patient with an aspergilloma generally shows serum IgG precipitins to *Aspergillus* organisms, and sputum cultures usually propagate the organism (25).

The natural history of an aspergilloma is quite variable. Overlap syndrome with ABPA has been reported (33). Opinions on

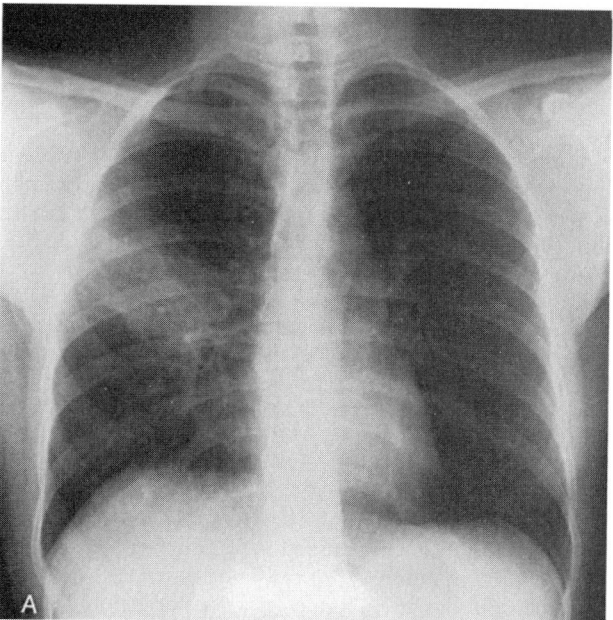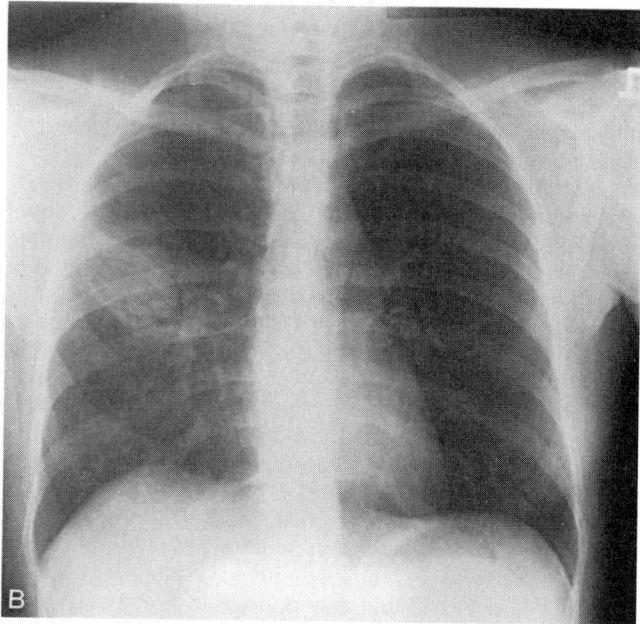

Figure 269.2. Posteroanterior chest radiographs from a 28-year-old woman with acute myelogenous leukemia and granulocytopenia showing wedge-shaped right upper lobe infiltrate **(A)** and air-crescent sign around sequestrum **(B)**. Surgical resection was curative with remission of leukemia. (From Meyer RD, Young LS, Armstrong D, et al. Aspergillosis complicating neoplastic disease. *Am J Med* 1973;54:6–15, with permission.)

management are controversial. Bronchoscopy may be indicated to localize a bleeding source. Systemic antifungal therapy is of benefit if there is overlap into invasion with the chronic necrotizing form of pulmonary aspergillosis (34). Supportive therapy suffices for the vast majority of patients, although those with life-threatening hemoptysis and selected others require surgical intervention (30a). Surgery may be difficult because of underlying disease and may be complicated by inadvertent spillage of fungi into the pleural cavity and subsequent *empyema thoracis*, dissemination, or both (35). Use of either inhalation or direct intracavitary instillation of various antimycotic medicaments (amphotericin B, nystatin, miconazole, iodides) has had limited success (29). Preliminary results with oral itraconazole therapy suggest possible efficacy (30a,36).

Invasive Pulmonary Aspergillosis

The confounded nosology and possibility of overlap syndromes are exemplified by descriptions of a semiinvasive or slowly progressing chronic necrotizing form of aspergillosis. The presence of underlying systemic or lung disease or mild immunosuppressive therapy with radiation, chemotherapy, or corticosteroids precedes development of a smoldering (usually for 1 to 6 months) infection followed by cavity formation, which is often associated with an air-crescent sign (34,37). Necrotizing bronchitis with pseudomembrane formation has been described in patients with AIDS and in others, including lung transplant recipients (2,11).

The lung is the site most commonly involved in invasive disease and is a way station for disseminated disease in at least one fourth of patients with classic invasive pulmonary aspergillosis (3,4,9). In patients at risk (see section "Pathogenesis"), this frequently occurs in the setting of relapse of the underlying condition or immunosuppressive therapy (especially with granulocytopenia) and prior antibacterial therapy without sustained

response. Unremitting fever and new pulmonary infiltrates are common features, as are dyspnea and nonproductive cough. Pleural pain and the findings of a pleural rub occur in a minority of patients and with other findings (hemoptysis, tachycardia) mimic the syndrome of pulmonary embolus with infarction; this results from hemorrhagic infarction secondary to blood vessel invasion by aspergilli (4). Massive hemoptysis is uncommon. Physical examination may also disclose findings of dullness, rales, or pulmonary consolidation.

Radiographic changes are quite varied. They most often show patchy or bronchopneumonic infiltrates, wedge-shaped pleural-based infiltrates, or nodular densities (Figs. 269.2A and 269.3A). Interstitial infiltrates or sequestrum formation (Fig. 269.2B) are less common (4). CT findings include a halo sign around a pulmonary mass early in the course and an air-crescent sign with cavitation later (38). Other patients show a much more fulminant course, with rapidly progressive pulmonary infiltrates, fever, and death. Pneumothorax may develop from a cavity.

Other Forms of Invasive Aspergillosis

Disseminated disease almost always results from a primary pulmonary infection, but it can also occur from skin inoculation or when no likely entry source is identifiable. Virtually any site can be involved as a result of hematogenous dissemination, including the CNS, heart (abscesses or pericarditis), gastrointestinal tract, kidney, liver (resembling hepatosplenic candidiasis), thyroid, or spleen. Clinical findings related to abscesses and infarcts vary according to the involved site and range from dramatic to silent (2–4,16,18).

CNS aspergillosis as part of disseminated disease is usually manifested by infarcts, which are often multiple and associated with vascular invasion and hemorrhage, and occasionally abscess formation (5,18,39). Onset of seizure activity, focal neurologic deficits, and depressed levels of consciousness are

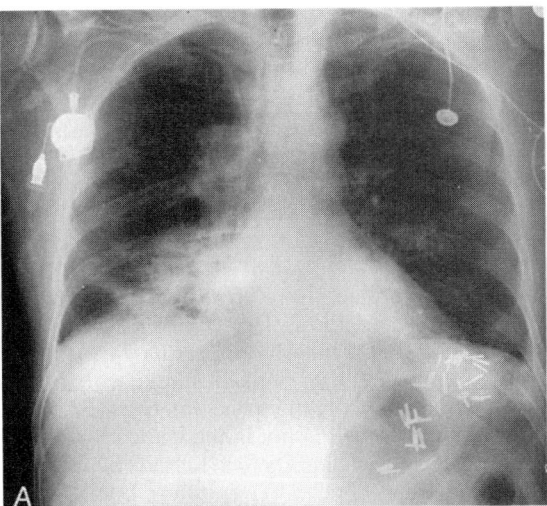

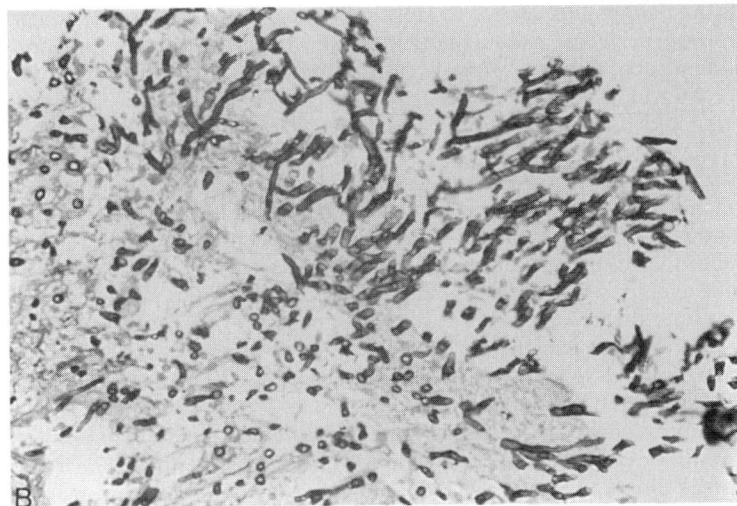

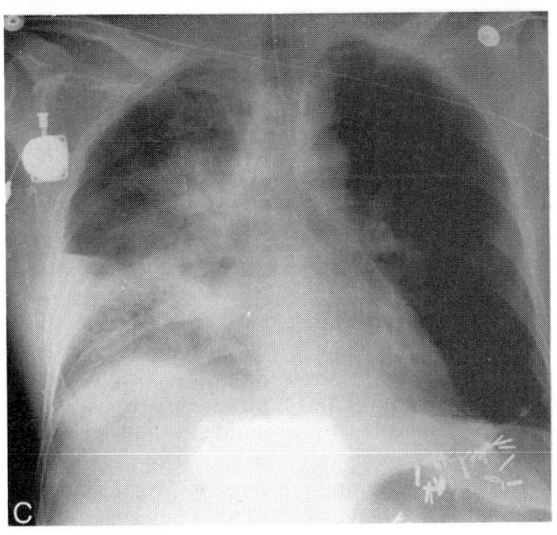

Figure 269.3. A: Posteroanterior chest radiograph from a 57-year-old man with lymphoma (undergoing methylprednisolone therapy) and granulocytopenia shows a hazy nodular right lower lobe and right upper lobe infiltrates that arose over 2 weeks. **B:** Histopathologic examination of a transbronchial biopsy specimen shows hyphae of aspergilli (cytologic preparation of bronchoalveolar lavage specimen also showed hyphae). **C:** Fatal progression of infiltrates followed, despite amphotericin B therapy.

common clinical findings (2,4,18). Chronic meningitis and ventriculitis are unusual findings in immunocompromised patients. Manifestations in intravenous drug abusers include necrotizing vasculitis, granulomata, meningitis, and ventriculitis (40). Endophthalmitis may be secondary to trauma, endogenous (e.g., from intravenous narcotic abuse, endocarditis, or as part of disseminated disease), or from direct extension (2,41,42). *Aspergillus* species, particularly *A. niger,* cause otomycosis, an almost always benign condition of the external ear canal and pinna. On the other hand, severe external otitis with invasion and necrosis from aspergillosis resembles that caused by *Pseudomonas aeruginosa* infection and requires an aggressive surgical approach and systemic therapy (43,44). Mastoiditis may result.

Aspergillosis of the paranasal sinuses has been caused by *A. flavus* in the Sudan and elsewhere by it and other species. One form is a chronic noninvasive form characterized by a luminal mass that may cause inflammation and is primarily treated by surgical removal of the mass. Invasive paranasal sinus disease occurs in immunosuppressed patients including those with granulocytopenia and/or AIDS (2,9,15–17,45). This form, which is either acute (as in granulocytopenic or immunosuppressed patients) or chronic (in healthy or only mildly immunocompromised patients) also requires systemic antifungal chemotherapy (2,16,17,45). Chronic noninvasive disease and chronic invasive

disease are distinguished with CT or magnetic resonance imaging (MRI) or at surgery (46). Nasal and orbitonasal disease with black, necrotic eschars also occurs; epiglottitis has been described in the face of leukemia (2).

Endocarditis on a native or prosthetic valve or in a mural location is characterized by peripheral embolization and almost always negative results of blood cultures (42). Diagnosis is usually made by examination of an embolus. Primary therapy is surgical, with amphotericin B as an adjunct. Mycotic aneurysm with embolization and vascular graft infections have also been reported (47,48).

Pleural aspergillosis, or *empyema thoracis,* usually follows surgery complicated by a bronchopleural or pleurocutaneous fistula, much less commonly follows another episode of aspergillosis, and has rarely been related to silk suture material acting as a nidus (2,35,49,50). Therapy consists of surgical management, removal of foreign bodies, and on an individualized basis, systemic therapy. Local instillation of amphotericin B has been recommended, but its role is not clear (49).

Osteomyelitis in children usually results from contiguous spread from pulmonary infection into rib or vertebra, usually in the setting of chronic granulomatous disease of childhood; a similar process rarely occurs in immunocompromised adults (14,51,52). Sternal infection with *Aspergillus* may follow median sternotomy incisions (53). In immunocompromised adults, hematogenous spread to most commonly the vertebrae occurs; both vertebral osteomyelitis and discitis in drug abusers have been separately reported (51,54,55). Articular aspergillosis is rare and when it does occur is part of hematogenously disseminated disease, usually in immunosuppressed patients (56).

Cutaneous aspergillosis occurs as a result of hematogenous spread in a small number of cases of dissemination; multiple erythematous papules that form pustules and large necrotic lesions resembling ecthyma gangrenosum have been noted (2,9). Similar erythematous to violaceous, edematous, indurated plaques that become eschars probably result from primary cutaneous inoculation (at permanent indwelling intravenous catheters), and some spread distantly (57–59). Biopsy is required for diagnosis. Operative débridement, control of the underlying disorder, and intravenous amphotericin B are recommended therapy, even without documented dissemination. Cutaneous seeding and formation of a nodule have also followed transthoracic needle biopsy in a leukemic patient with pulmonary aspergillosis (60). *Aspergillus* burn wound infections progress rapidly and are treated with wide débridement or amputation. Sources for listings of other miscellaneous anatomic sites involved are available (2–5,11,30a).

DIAGNOSIS

General guidelines for therapy with reference sources for therapy of noninvasive aspergillosis have been listed (30a). The clinical syndrome of neutropenic fever (usually with other immunosuppression) unresponsive to optimal antibacterial therapy, especially with new pulmonary infiltrates, should lead to immediate consideration of performance of diagnostic procedures and empirical use of antifungal therapy, usually amphotericin B (60a). The disappointingly low yield (only 10% or slightly more) of cultures of respiratory tract material taken noninvasively that yield aspergilli in the face of invasive pulmonary or disseminated disease is well known (3,4). Moreover, aspergilli seen on direct examination or cultured from sputum specimens in this setting may represent only colonization (2,4). Isolation of *A. fumigatus* or *A. flavus* alone from sputum cultures of patients at high risk often is not due to contamination and cannot be ignored in them (2,61). Follow-up assessment is required. Ideally, examination of specimens obtained by bronchoalveolar lavage (BAL) or transbronchial biopsy (or percutaneous transthoracic biopsy or open lung biopsy) should be used to confirm tissue invasion (Fig. 269.3B). Microscopy of BAL fluid and other respiratory tract secretions combined with culture has a diagnostic yield of 15% to 20% (2). In patients with acute leukemia, a transbronchial biopsy specimen is likely to add little to findings of examination of BAL and brushing specimens; open lung biopsy is likewise likely to have limited value, unless the underlying disease is controlled (62,63). Other species, such as *A. terreus*, are much less likely to cause invasion but also do so, because even they cannot be summarily dismissed (2,9,11,64).

Definitive diagnosis can be made only by finding tissue invasion by characteristic structures at histopathologic examination with appropriate stains (calcofluor white and others) and confirming the findings by culture. Morphological criteria alone are not totally reliable for diagnosis because of confusion with other fungi. Eumycetes confused with aspergilli on histopathologic examination include *Pseudoallescheria boydii* (*Scedosporium apiospermum* treated with itraconazole or voriconazole rather than amphotericin B), *Fusarium* species, and others (2). Biopsy of skin and other involved sites should be performed whenever possible, together with histopathologic examination and culture of skin scrapings and biopsy specimens.

Blood cultures almost never yield aspergilli in the face of invasive disease. Examination of cerebrospinal fluid in CNS aspergillosis typically shows red blood cells and small numbers of mononuclear cells, but culture of cerebrospinal fluid only rarely yields the organism (4). Persistent neutrophilia in cerebrospinal fluid is unusual (40). CT shows infarcts or abscesses; MRI scans are more sensitive and may show contrast-enhancing lesions (2,16,18).

Serologic tests for antibody have no established value in the diagnosis of invasive aspergillosis. Detection of circulating antigen in serum of patients with invasive disease has been most convincingly shown with an enzyme-linked immunosorbent assay method for detection of circulating galactomannan (38,65,66). It is licensed for use in Europe but not in the United States. Serial chest CT scanning is complementary (66). Reports of polymerase chain reaction techniques applied to respiratory tract specimens or blood indicate that they are promising but are fraught with false-positive results (67,68).

TREATMENT

Surgical drainage, débridement, or resection should generally be carried out whenever feasible for invasive disease such as sinusitis, cutaneous aspergillosis, or *empyema thoracis*. Removal of the catheter is a cornerstone of therapy of aspergillosis complicating chronic peritoneal dialysis. Successful resection for sequestrum formation in invasive pulmonary aspergillosis has been successfully carried out (4,38,69,70).

Amphotericin B usually is the initial choice for systemic therapy for invasive aspergillosis and in pulmonary or disseminated forms is given in daily doses of up to 1.0 mg/kg if tolerated, to a total dose of at least 30 mg/kg. The course of the underlying disorder greatly affects duration of therapy. Less immunocompromised patients have been selected for itraconazole therapy. Long-term survival rates for patients with leukemia or lymphoma, as well as bone marrow transplant recipients, are about 10% but are higher (about 25%) for treated renal allograft recipients (11,70,71). Disseminated and CNS infections have the highest mortality rates (9,72,73). Either flucytosine or rifampin used empirically with amphotericin B is unlikely to be very useful.

Liposomal, lipid complex, and colloidal dispersion preparations of amphotericin B are associated with less nephrotoxicity than amphotericin B deoxycholate and usually are used after it but have not had much if any impact on mortality (73). Higher dose therapy with liposomal amphotericin B is no more effective than use of 1 mg/kg per day (74). Direct injection or instillation of amphotericin B by subconjunctival, intravitreal, intrapleural, or intraperitoneal routes or lavage of paranasal sinuses may be useful in specific patients.

Itraconazole is approved for use in second-line therapy of pulmonary and extrapulmonary aspergillosis, including disseminated disease, in patients who have failed to respond to or are intolerant of amphotericin B therapy (2,75). It may also be tried in patients with relatively less serious infections or greater immunocompetence. Long-term therapy is necessary, and therapy with "off-label" doses greater than 400 mg per day may be required. Suspension preparation is preferred because it leads to higher blood levels than capsule preparations. Caspofungin, an echinocandin, has been approved for intravenous use as salvage therapy (76). Voriconazole, a triazole, has been approved for initial therapy of invasive disease but not for empirical use (77,77a). Other experimental triazoles, including posaconazole, are being developed (2,30a,38,78). Terbinafine has not been investigated for this indication. Granulocyte growth factors are adjunctive agents with little impact (2). Recombinant human interferon-γ given subcutaneously as an adjunct to antifungal chemotherapy has been used in selected patients, for example, chronic granulomatous disease; its role is uncertain (2,79). The importance of *in vitro* susceptibility test results of aspergilli is uncertain, and usually testing versus amphotericin B is not recommended. Resistance to itraconazole has, however, been noted (80). Antifungal agents are described in Chapter 33.

PREVENTION

Environmental control measures to prevent conidia from reaching patients at risk are indicated, including during construction activities (6,81). Additional measures such as laminar airflow units with high-efficiency particulate air filters temporarily reduce the risk but are generally not used because of their expense, lack of tolerance by some patients, and contraction of disease while outside of the units (5,82). Fluconazole is not effective in prophylaxis; data from a control trial using itraconazole are pending (12). An aerosolized spray of topical amphotericin B has been somewhat effective in retrospective but not prospective study (11).

REFERENCES

1. Kwon-Chung KJ Bennett JE. *Medical mycology.* Philadelphia: Lea & Febiger, 1992.
2. Denning DW. Invasive aspergillosis. *Clin Infect Dis* 1998;26:781–805.
3. Young RC, Bennett JE, Vogel CL, et al. Aspergillosis: the spectrum of disease in 98 patients. *Medicine (Baltimore)* 1970;49:147–173.
4. Meyer RD, Young LS, Armstrong D, et al. Aspergillosis complicating neoplastic disease. *Am J Med* 1973;54:6–15.
5. Walsh TJ, Pizzo PA. Nosocomial fungal infections: a classification for hospital-acquired fungal infections and mycoses arising from endogenous flora or reactivation. *Annu Rev Microbiol* 1988;42:517–545.
6. Hamadeh R, Ardehali A, Locksley RM, et al. Fatal aspergillosis associated with smoking contaminated marijuana, in a marrow transplant recipient. *Chest* 1988;94:432–433.
7. Radford SA, Johnson EM, Leeming JP, et al. Molecular epidemiological study of *Aspergillus fumigatus* in a bone marrow transplantation unit by PCR amplification of ribosomal intergenic spacer sequences. *J Clin Microbiol* 1998;36:1294–1299.
8. Leenders ACA, Belkum A, Behrendt M, et al. Density and molecular epidemiology of *Aspergillus* in air and relationship to outbreaks of *Aspergillus* infection. *J Clin Microbiol* 1999;37:1752–1757.
9. Patterson TF, Kirkpatrick WR, White ML, et al. Invasive aspergillosis. Disease spectrum, treatment practices, and outcomes. *Medicine (Baltimore)* 2000;79:250–260.
10. Conesa D, Rello J, Valles J, et al. Invasive aspergillosis: a life-threatening complication of short-term steroid therapy. *Ann Pharmacother* 1995;29:1235–1237.
11. Paterson DL, Singh N. Invasive aspergillosis in transplant recipients. *Medicine (Baltimore)* 1999;78:123–138.
12. Baddley JW, Stroud TP, Salzman D, et al. Invasive mold infections in allogeneic bone marrow transplant recipients. *Clin Infect Dis* 2001;32:1319–1324.
13. Ninin E, Milpied N, Moreau P, et al. Longitudinal study of bacterial, viral, and fungal infections in adult recipients of bone marrow transplants. *Clin Infect Dis* 2001;33:41–47.
14. Segal BH, DeCarlo ES, Kwon-Chung KJ, et al. *Aspergillus nidulans* infection in chronic granulomatous disease. *Medicine (Baltimore)* 1998;77:345–354.
15. Lortholary O, Meyohas M-C, Dupont B, et al. Invasive aspergillosis in patients with acquired immunodeficiency syndrome: report of 33 cases. *Am J Med* 1993;95:177–187.
16. Meyer RD, Gaultier CG, Yamashita JT, et al. Fungal sinusitis in patients with AIDS: Report of four cases and review of the literature. *Medicine (Baltimore)* 1994;73:69–78.
17. Mylonakis E, Barlam TF, Flanigan T, et al. Pulmonary aspergillosis and invasive disease in AIDS. Review of 342 cases. *Chest* 1998;114:251–262.
18. Mylonakis E, Paliou M, Sax PE, et al. Central nervous system aspergillosis in patients with human immunodeficiency virus infection. Report of 6 cases and review. *Medicine (Baltimore)* 2000;79:269–280.
19. Warris A, Bjorneklett A, Gaustad P. Invasive pulmonary aspergillosis associated with infliximab therapy [Letter]. *N Engl J Med* 2001;344:1099–1100.
20. Clancy CJ, Nguyen MH. Acute community-acquired pneumonia due to aspergillus in presumably immunocompetent hosts. Clues for recognition of a rare but fatal disease. *Chest* 1998;114:629–634.
21. Schaffner A, Douglas H, Braude AI. Killing of *Aspergillus* spores depends on the anatomical source of the macrophage. *Infect Immun* 1983;42:1109–1115.
22. Diamond RD, Huber E, Haudenschild CC. Mechanisms of destruction of *Aspergillus fumigatus* hyphae mediated by human monocytes. *J Infect Dis* 1983; 147:474–483.
23. Diamond RD, Krzesicki R, Epstein B, et al. Damage to hyphal forms of fungi by human leukocytes *in vitro. Am J Pathol* 1978;91:313–328.
24. Rex JH, Bennett JE, Gallin JI, et al. Normal and deficient neutrophils can cooperate to damage *Aspergillus fumigatus* hyphae. *J Infect Dis* 1990;162:523–528.
25. Pennington JE. *Aspergillus* lung disease. *Med Clin North Am* 1980;64:475–490.
26. Levitz SM. Aspergillosis. *Infect Dis Clin North Am* 1989;3:1–18.
27. Greenberger PA, Patterson R. Allergic bronchopulmonary aspergillosis: model of bronchopulmonary disease with defined serologic, radiologic, pathologic and clinical findings from asthma to fatal destructive lung disease. *Chest* 1987;91[Suppl]:165S–171S.
28. Ward S, Heyneman L, Lee MJ, et al. Accuracy of CT in the diagnosis of allergic bronchopulmonary aspergillosis in asthmatic patients. *Am J Roentgenol* 1999;173:937–942.
29. Stevens DA, Schwartz HJ, Yee JY, et al. A randomized trial of itraconazole in allergic bronchopulmonary aspergillosis. *N Engl J Med* 2000;342:756–762.
30. Riley DJ, MacKenzie JW, Uhlman WE, et al. Allergic bronchopulmonary aspergillosis: evidence of limited tissue invasion. *Am Rev Respir Dis* 1975;111: 232–236.
30a. Stevens DA, Kan VL, Judson MA, et al. Practice guidelines for diseases caused by *Aspergillus. Clin Infect Dis* 2000;30:696–709.
31. Katzenstein AL, Liebow AA, Friedman PJ. Bronchocentric granulomatosis, mucoid impaction, and hypersensitivity reactions to fungi. *Am Rev Respir Dis* 1975;111:497–537.
32. Case records of the Massachusetts General Hospital (Case 24-2001). *N Engl J Med* 2001;345:443–449.
33. Ein ME, Wallace RJ, Williams TW. Allergic bronchopulmonary aspergillosis-like syndrome consequent to aspergilloma. *Am Rev Respir Dis* 1979;119:811–820.
34. Binder RE, Faling LJ, Pugatch RD, et al. Chronic necrotizing pulmonary aspergillosis: a discrete clinical entity. *Medicine (Baltimore)* 1982;61:109–124.
35. Rosenberg RS, Creviston SA, Schonfeld AJ. Invasive aspergillosis complicating resection of a pulmonary aspergilloma in a nonimmunocompromised host. *Am Rev Respir Dis* 1982;126:1113–1115.
36. Dupont B. Itraconazole therapy in aspergillosis: study in 49 patients. *J Am Acad Dermatol* 1990;23:607–614.
37. Gefter WB, Weingrad TR, Epstein DM, et al. "Semi-invasive" pulmonary aspergillosis. *Radiology* 1980;140:313–321.
38. Caillot D, Casasnovas O, Bernard A, et al. Improved management of invasive pulmonary aspergillosis in neutropenic patients using early thoracic computed tomographic scan and surgery. *J Clin Oncol* 1997;15:139–147.
39. Peacock JE Jr, McGinnis MR, Cohen MS. Persistent neutrophilic meningitis: report of four cases and review of the literature. *Medicine (Baltimore)* 1984;63:379–393.
40. Morrow R, Wong B, Finkelstein WE, et al. Aspergillosis of the cerebral ventricles in a heroin abuser. *Arch Intern Med* 1983;143:161–164.
41. Barr CC, Walsh A, Wainscott B, et al. *Aspergillus* endophthalmitis in intravenous-drug users—Kentucky. *MMWR Morb Mortal Wkly Rep* 1990;39: 48–49.
42. Gumbo T, Taege AJ, Mawhorter S, et al. Aspergillus valve endocarditis in patients without prior cardiac surgery. *Medicine (Baltimore)* 2000;79:261–268.
43. Cunningham M, Yu VL, Turner J, et al. Necrotizing otitis externa due to *Aspergillus* in an immunocompetent patient. *Arch Otolaryngol Head Neck Surg* 1988;114:554–556.
44. Gordon G, Giddings NA. Invasive otitis externa due to *Aspergillus* species: case report and review. *Clin Infect Dis* 1994;19:866–870.
45. Iwen PC, Rupp ME, Hinrichs SH. Invasive mold sinusitis: 17 cases in immunocompromised patients and review of the literature. *Clin Infect Dis* 1997;24:1178–1184.
46. Washburn RG, Kennedy DW, Begley MG, et al. Chronic fungal sinusitis in apparently normal hosts. *Medicine (Baltimore)* 1988;67:231–247.
47. Rose HD, Stuart JL. Mycotic aneurysm of the thoracic aorta caused by *Aspergillus fumigatus. Chest* 1976;70:81–84.
48. Aguado JM, Valle R, Anjons R, et al. Aortic bypass graft infection due to *Aspergillus:* report of a case and review. *Clin Infect Dis* 1992;14:916–921.
49. Stamatis G, Greschuchna D. Surgery for pulmonary aspergilloma and pleural aspergillosis. *Thorac Cardiovasc Surg* 1988;36:356–360.
50. Hendrix WC, Arudo LK, Platts-Mills TAE, et al. *Aspergillus* epidural abscess and hand compression in a patient with aspergillosis and empyema. Survival and response to high dose amphotericin B therapy. *Am Rev Respir Dis* 1992;145:1483–1486.
51. Tack KJ, Rhame FS, Brown B, et al. *Aspergillus* osteomyelitis. *Am J Med* 1982;73:295–300.
52. Caligiuri P, MacMahon H, Courtney J, et al. Opportunistic pulmonary aspergillosis with chest wall invasion. *Arch Intern Med* 1983;143:2323–2324.

53. Barzaghi N, Emmi V, Mencherini S, et al. Sternal osteomyelitis due to *Aspergillus fumigatus* after cardiac surgery. *Chest* 1994;105:1275–1277.
54. Holmes PF, Osterman DW, Tullos HS. *Aspergillus* discitis. *Clin Orthop* 1988;226:240–246.
55. Brown DL, Musher DM, Taffet GE. Hematogenously acquired *Aspergillus* vertebral osteomyelitis in seemingly immunocompetent drug addicts. *West J Med* 1987;147:84–85.
56. Alvarez L, Calvo E, Abril C. Articular aspergillosis. Case report. *Clin Infect Dis* 1995;20:457–460.
57. Prystowsky SD, Vogelstein B, Ettinger DS, et al. Invasive aspergillosis. *N Engl J Med* 1976;295:655–658.
58. McCarty JM, Flam MS, Pullen G, et al. Outbreak of primary cutaneous aspergillosis related to intravenous arm boards. *J Pediatr* 1986;108:721–724.
59. Allo MD, Miller J, Townsend T, et al. Primary cutaneous aspergillosis associated with Hickman intravenous catheters. *N Engl J Med* 1987;317:1105–1108.
60. Jobin EH, Westenfeld F, Dietrich P. Cutaneous infection due to *Aspergillus* species after transthoracic lung biopsy [Letter]. *Clin Infect Dis* 1993;17:955–956.
60a. Hughes WT, Armstrong D, Bodey GP, et al. 2002 guidelines for the use of antimicrobial agents in neutropenic patients with cancer. *Clin Infect Dis* 2002;34:730–751.
61. Horvath JD, Dummer S. The use of respiratory-tract cultures in the diagnosis of invasive pulmonary aspergillosis. *Am J Med* 1996;100:171–178.
62. Albelda SM, Talbot GH, Gierson SL, et al. Role of fiberoptic bronchoscopy in the diagnosis of invasive pulmonary aspergillosis in patients with acute leukemia. *Am J Med* 1984;76:1027–1034.
63. McCabe RE, Brooks RG, Mark JBD, et al. Open lung biopsy in patients with acute leukemia. *Am J Med* 1985;78:609–616.
64. Trite DM, Woods GL. Fatal disseminated infection with *Aspergillus terreus* in immunocompromised hosts. *Clin Infect Dis* 1993;16:118–122.
65. Maertens J, Verhaegen J, Demuynck H, et al. Autopsy-controlled prospective evaluation of serial screening for circulating galactomannan by a sandwich enzyme-linked immunosorbent assay for hematological patients at risk for invasive aspergillosis. *J Clin Microbiol* 1999;37:3223–3228.
66. Denning DW. Early diagnosis of invasive aspergillosis [Editorial]. *Lancet* 2000;355:423–424.
67. Bretagne S, Costa J-M, Marmorat-Khuong A, et al. Detection of *Aspergillus* species DNA in bronchoalveolar lavage samples by competitive PCR. *J Clin Microbiol* 1995;33:1164–1168.
68. Buchheit D, Baust C, Skladny H, et al. Detection of *Aspergillus* species in blood and bronchoalveolar lavage samples from immunocompromised patients by means of 2-step polymerase chain reaction: clinical results. *Clin Infect Dis* 2001;33:428–435.
69. Young VK, Maghur HA, Luke DA, et al. Operation for cavitating invasive pulmonary aspergillosis in immunocompromised patients. *Ann Thorac Surg* 1992;53:621–624.
70. Weiland D, Ferguson RM, Peterson PK, et al. Aspergillosis in 25 renal transplant patients: epidemiology, clinical presentation, diagnosis, and management. *Ann Surg* 1983;198:622–629.
71. Denning DW, Stevens DA. The treatment of invasive aspergillosis: surgery and antifungal therapy of 2121 published cases. *Rev Infect Dis* 1990;12:1147–1201.
72. Denning DW. Therapeutic outcome in invasive aspergillosis. *Clin Infect Dis* 1996;23:608–615.
73. Lin S-J, Schranz J, Teutsch SM. Aspergillosis case-fatality rate: systematic review of the literature. *Clin Infect Dis* 2001;32:358–366.
74. Ellis M, Spence D, de Pauw B, et al. An EORTC international multicenter randomized trial (EORTC number 19923) comparing two dosages of liposomal amphotericin B for treatment of invasive aspergillosis. *Clin Infect Dis* 1998;27:1406–1412.
75. Stevens D, Lee JY. Analysis of compassionate use itraconazole therapy for invasive aspergillosis by the NIAID mycoses study group criteria. *Arch Intern Med* 1997;157:1857–1862.
76. Caspofungin (CANCIDAS) for aspergillosis. *Med Lett Drugs Ther* 2001;43:58–59.
77. Voriconazole. *Med Letter Drugs Ther* 2002;44:63–65.
77a. Powers JH, Diton CA, Goldberger MJ. Voriconazole versus liposomal amphotericin B in patients with neutropenia and persistent fever. [Letter] *New Engl J Med* 2002;346:289–290.
78. Petraitiene R, Petraitis V, Groll AH, et al. Antifungal activity and pharmacokinetics of posaconazole (SCH 56592) in treatment and prevention of experimental invasive pulmonary aspergillosis: correlation with galactomannan antigenemia. *Antimicrob Agents Chemother* 2001;45:857–869.
79. Bernhisel-Broadbent J, Camargo EE, Jaffe HS, et al. Recombinant human interferon-gamma as adjunct therapy for *Aspergillus* infection in a patient with chronic granulomatous disease. *J Infect Dis* 1991;163:908–911.
80. Denning DW, Venkateswarlu K, Oakley KL, et al. Itraconazole resistance in *Aspergillus fumigatus*. *Antimicrob Agents Chemother* 1997;41:1364–1368.
81. Loo VG, Bertrand C, Dixon C, et al. Control of construction-associated nosocomial aspergillosis in an antiquated hematology unit. *Infect Control Hosp Epidemiol* 1996;17:360–364.
82. Sherertz RJ, Belani A, Kramer BS, et al. Impact of air filtration of nosocomial *Aspergillus* infections: unique risk of bone marrow transplant recipients. *Am J Med* 1987;83:709–718.

CHAPTER 270
Histoplasma

Joe Wheat

HISTORY

Darling first described histoplasmosis in 1905 in autopsy material from a case seen in the Panama Canal Zone, identifying the organism to be *Leishmania*. He named these structures *Histoplasma capsulatum* because they resembled "plasmodium"-like organisms within "histocytes" (1). The apparent capsule proved a staining artifact caused by cytoplasmic shrinkage. In 1945, Christie and Peterson (2), recognizing the frequency of pulmonary calcifications in children with negative tuberculin skin-test results, suspected histoplasmosis to be a common but benign pulmonary infection. In 1945, Edwards and colleagues (3) reported the geographic distribution of histoplasmosis in the United States. Emmons (4) isolated the organism from soil in 1949. Furcolow detected the organism in air samples in 1954, supporting earlier suspicions that the disease was acquired when conidia were inhaled. In 1951, Zeidberg and associates (5) reported the importance of bird droppings for growth of *H. capsulatum* in soil.

CHARACTERISTICS OF THE PATHOGEN

H. capsulatum variety *capsulatum* is an Ascomycete of the family Arthrodermataceae (6). Its telemorphic state is *Ajellomyces capsulatus*. *H. capsulatum* grows as a mold in the soil and is found primarily in microfoci containing large amounts of rotted guano where starlings have roosted or bats have inhabited. The mold is composed of hyphae bearing large tuberculate macroconidia (8 to 14 μm in diameter) characteristic of *H. capsulatum* and smaller (2- to 5-μm) microconidia, which are the infectious form of the organism (Fig. 270.1).

At temperatures higher than 35°C, *H. capsulatum* grows as a yeast measuring 2 to 3 by 3 to 4 μm in diameter (Fig. 270.2). The yeast form is typically found in infected tissues; however, hyphal

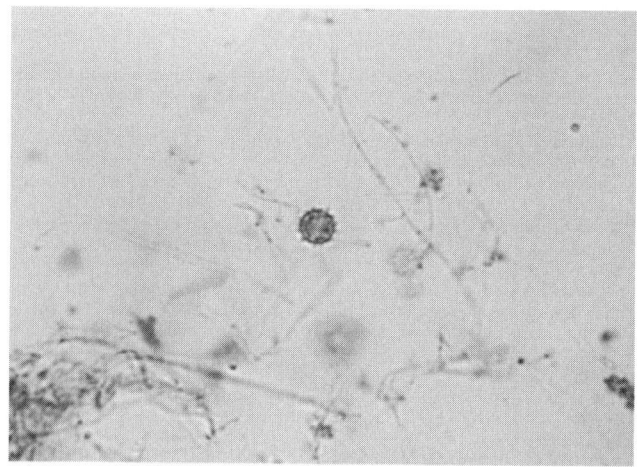

Figure 270.1. Mold phase of *Histoplasma capsulatum* showing tuberculate macroconidia and hyphae bearing microconidia.

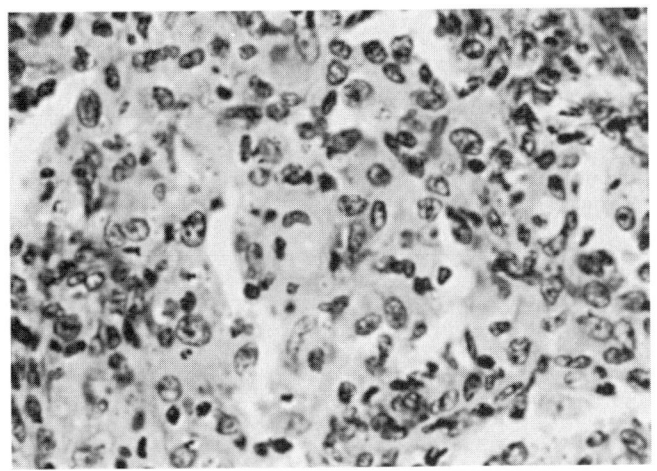

Figure 270.2. Hematoxylin and eosin stain of tissue showing typical yeast–phase organisms demonstrating capsule-like staining artifact surrounding the yeast.

elements have been seen in cardiac vegetations and other sites of intravascular infection (7,8).

Growth on fungal media at room temperature is slow, requiring incubation of 1 to 4 weeks. Definitive identification as *H. capsulatum* variety *capsulatum* requires conversion of the mold to the yeast, demonstration of specific reactivity with anti–*H. capsulatum* antisera (exoantigen tests), or reactivity with deoxyribonucleic acid (DNA) probes specific for *Histoplasma* messenger ribonucleic acid (mRNA) (9).

EPIDEMIOLOGY

Although *H. capsulatum* is recognized as endemic in certain areas of North and Latin America (3), its distribution is much wider. Cases have been reported from Europe and Asia. In the United States, most cases have occurred within the Ohio and Mississippi River valleys (10) (Fig. 270.3). Factors accounting for this distribution are not fully understood, but humid environmental conditions and acidic permeable soil characteristics appear to be important. Bird and bat excrement enhance growth of the organism in soil by accelerating sporulation. Sites harboring *H. capsulatum* and activities causing exposure are shown in Table 270.1. Spores can be blown by the wind for miles, exposing individuals without contact with the contaminated site. Also, sites not visibly contaminated with droppings may harbor the organism.

Attack rates and severity of clinical disease after exposure vary greatly. Exposure in enclosed areas usually causes more severe illnesses than exposure occurring outdoors (11). Attack rates are higher when exposure occurs in schools or other areas involving children, because children are less likely than adults to have developed immunity as a result of previous infection (12).

PATHOGENESIS

The outcome of *H. capsulatum* infection depends on an interplay of host and parasite interactions (13,14). Infection develops when microconidia are inhaled into the lungs. These spores germinate into yeasts, which promote the influx of neutrophils,

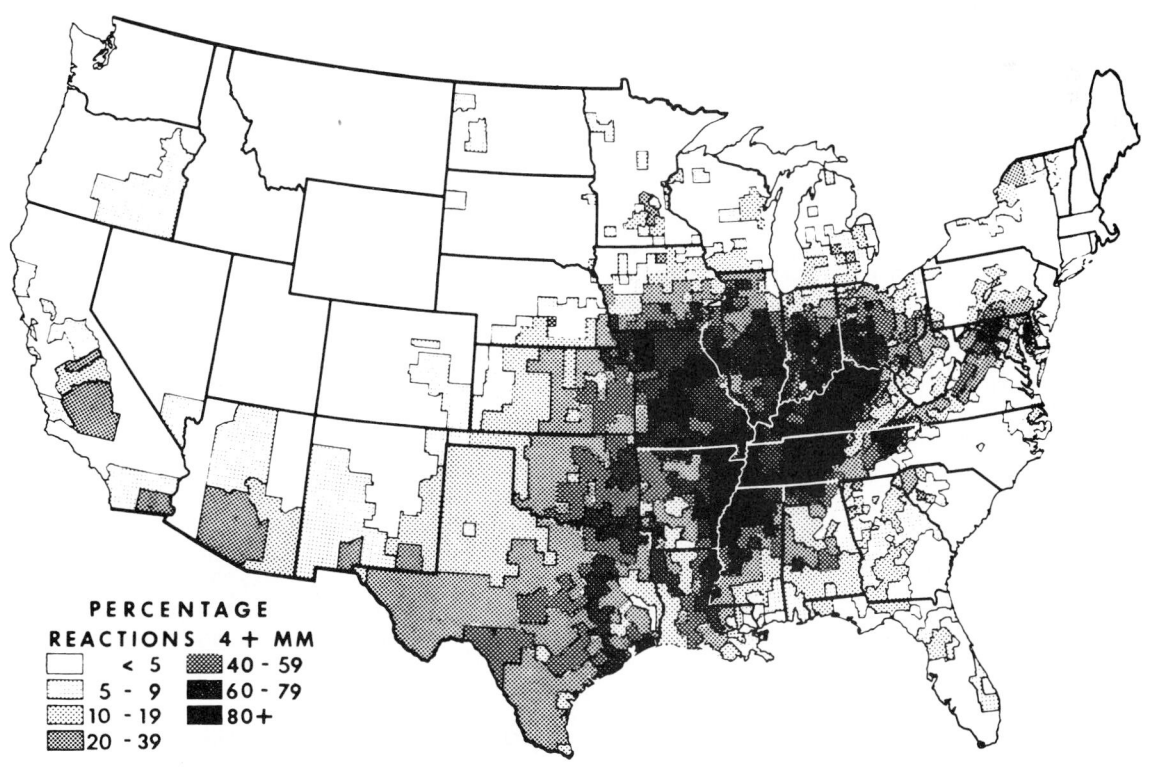

PERCENTAGE
REACTIONS 4 + MM
< 5   40 - 59
5 - 9   60 - 79
10 - 19   80+
20 - 39

Tuberculosis Program U S Public Health Service

Figure 270.3. Endemic distribution of histoplasmosis in the United States based on skin-test results in military recruits. (From Edwards LB, Acquaviva FA, Livesay VT, et al. An atlas of sensitivity to tuberculin, PPD-B and histoplasmin in the United States. *Am Rev Respir Dis* 1969;99:1–18, with permission.)

TABLE 270.1.   Sources of Exposure to *Histoplasma capsulatum*

Microfocus	Activities
Caves	Spelunking
Chicken coops	Cleaning, demolition, use of bird droppings in garden
Bird roosts	Excavation, camping
Bamboo canebrakes	Cutting cane, recreation
School yards	Routine activities, cleaning
Prison grounds	Routine activities, cleaning
Decayed wood piles	Transporting or burning wood
Dead trees	Recreational, cutting wood
Contaminated chimneys	Cleaning, demolition
Old building	Demolition, remodeling, cleaning
Any of above	Epidemiological studies at contaminated microfoci
Laboratories	Research

TABLE 270.2.   Clinical Manifestations of Histoplasmosis

Manifestations	Heavy inoculum (%)	Light inoculum (%)
Asymptomatic	10–50	99
Self-limited	50–90	1
Pulmonary (80% of symptomatic)		
Arthritis erythema nodosum (5%–10%)		
Pericarditis (5%–10%)		
Mediastinal granuloma (unknown)		
Disseminated	Unknown	0.05
Chronic pulmonary	Unknown	0.05
Inflammatory or fibrotic	Unknown	0.02
Fibrosing mediastinitis		
Sarcoid like		
Constrictive pericarditis		
Broncholithiasis		

macrophages, and natural killer (NK) cells, serving to inhibit progression of the infection. *H. capsulatum* parasitizes macrophages, facilitating dissemination throughout the reticuloendothelial system. With development of specific cellular immunity, cytokines arm macrophages to kill the fungus and halt progression of the disease. These defense mechanisms are generally sufficient to control the infection in immunocompetent individuals, explaining the subclinical or self-limited course characteristic of acute histoplasmosis. Individuals with underlying conditions that impair these defenses, such as acquired immunodeficiency syndrome (AIDS), develop progressive disseminated infection.

Reinfection and reactivation of "clinically quiescent" infection also occur in histoplasmosis. T-cell immunity may wane in the absence of occasional reexposure, or exposure to heavy inocula may overcome immune mechanisms, permitting reinfection to occur. Illnesses are thought to be milder after reinfection. Reactivation of latent histoplasmosis may occur in immunocompromised patients (15).

CLINICAL MANIFESTATIONS

After low-inoculum exposure, about 1 in 100 exposed individuals develops symptomatic histoplasmosis, and the remainder experience clinically unrecognized infection (Table 270.2). Underlying host factors, including cellular immunity, prior infection with *H. capsulatum*, emphysema, and extent of exposure, interact to influence the outcome of infection. The attack rate approaches 100% after heavy exposure, particularly in persons not previously exposed to *H. capsulatum*, and the illnesses are more severe.

Acute Pulmonary Histoplasmosis

Acute self-limited illnesses comprise the majority of symptomatic cases (Table 270.2). About 80% present with flu-like, acute pulmonary symptoms of fever, chills, headache, myalgia, anorexia, nonproductive cough, and retrosternal or pleuritic chest pain (16). Chest roentgenograms show enlarged hilar or mediastinal lymph nodes with patchy infiltrates. Rarely cavitation may occur (17,18). Pulmonary complaints improve within a few weeks (12), but fatigue may linger. After heavy exposure, most patients develop symptomatic infection and many present with diffuse pulmonary involvement causing respiratory insufficiency (19) (Table 270.2).

Mediastinal Granuloma

Enlarged lymph nodes can partially obstruct the airways, pulmonary vessels, or vena cava, or the esophagus, occurring in less than 10% of patients. Such findings, the result of smoldering, may be delayed for years after the initial infection. Fistulas can form between necrotic nodes and adjacent mediastinal structures. Computed tomography (CT) scans of the chest define the impingement on adjacent structures. Although enlarged mediastinal nodes usually shrink and symptoms resolve without treatment (20), obstructive syndromes may be severe, and the masses may persist for years (21). Granulomatous mediastinitis is not thought to progress to fibrosing mediastinitis (22).

Rheumatologic Syndromes

Arthritis or prominent arthralgia occurs in 5% to 10% of patients (23). The involvement is usually polyarticular and symmetric, and half of patients exhibit erythema nodosum. Imaging studies of the joints show no abnormalities. The joint symptoms usually resolve over several weeks in response to antiinflammatory therapy. Arthritis rarely may be a manifestation of disseminated infection.

Pericarditis

Pericarditis is another inflammatory complication of histoplasmosis, occurring in 5% to 10% of symptomatic patients (24). Clinical findings resemble those of viral pericarditis, except that chest roentgenograms usually show mediastinal lymphadenopathy. Pericardial fluid often is bloody. These patients typically respond to antiinflammatory treatment but up to one fourth exhibit pericardial tamponade. Late constriction is rare (25). Pericarditis also may be a complication of disseminated histoplasmosis.

Chronic Pulmonary Histoplasmosis

Chronic pulmonary histoplasmosis occurs in patients with underlying emphysema and is characterized by fibrotic apical lung infiltrates with cavitation (26,27). Symptoms include cough, dyspnea, chest pain, hemoptysis, weakness, fatigue, fever, sweats, and weight loss. Upper lobe infiltrates are present in nearly all

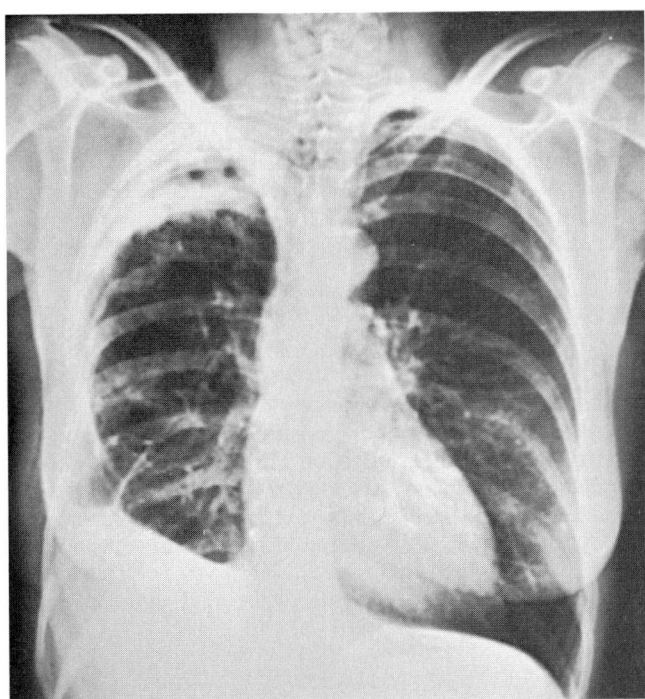

Figure 270.4. Chest roentgenogram showing fibrotic right upper lobe infiltrate with cavitation and diffuse scarring in the right lung with elevation of the right diaphragm in a patient with concurrent sarcoidosis.

patients, and cavities in 65% to 87% (Fig. 270.4). Other radiographic findings include bullae, mediastinal or pulmonary calcifications, pleural thickening, and hilar retraction. Progression in chronic pulmonary histoplasmosis is manifested by formation of new cavities, spread to new areas of the lungs, cavity enlargement, and bronchopleural fistula in rare cases (28).

Progressive Disseminated Histoplasmosis

Progressive disseminated histoplasmosis occurs in about 1 in 2,000 acute infections (29). Underlying immunosuppressive conditions and extremes of age predispose to progressive dissemination (30). Other chronic debilitating diseases also may predispose to dissemination, but cases may occur in persons without recognizable risk factors. Patients may present shortly after the exposure or years later and may experience asymptomatic periods interrupted by symptomatic relapses. Fever and weight loss are the most common symptoms, often accompanied by hepatomegaly or splenomegaly (about 50% of cases) and lymphadenopathy. Shock, respiratory distress, hepatic and renal failure, and coagulopathy may complicate severe cases (31). Other common sites of dissemination include the oropharyngeal or gastrointestinal (GI) tract mucosa and skin. GI tract lesions include ulcerations or polypoid masses, leading to misdiagnoses of colitis or malignancy (32–36). Lesions most often involve the ileal cecal area but may occur from the mouth to the anus. Skin lesions may be erythematous maculopapular, pustulonecrotic, hyperpigmented, or crateriform in character (37–39).

Central nervous system (CNS) involvement occurs in 10% to 20% of cases (40). CNS infection presents either as a manifestation of widely disseminated disease or as an isolated focal infection. The most common manifestation is subacute or chronic meningitis, but focal brain or spinal cord lesions (41,42), stroke syndromes caused by vascular involvement or emboli, and encephalitis also occur. Basilar meningeal involvement is typical

and can lead to nonobstructive (communicating) hydrocephalus in 20% of cases. Cerebrospinal fluid (CSF) abnormalities include lymphocytic pleocytosis, protein elevation, and hypoglycorrhachia. CT scan or magnetic resonance imaging (MRI) shows single or multiple enhancing brain lesions in one third of patients (40).

Adrenal involvement is found in 80% to 90% of autopsied cases, but Addison's disease is uncommon (less than 10% of cases) (43). Physicians should exclude histoplasmosis in patients with adrenal masses or Addison's disease and should rule out adrenal insufficiency in patients with disseminated histoplasmosis who have hyperkalemia, hyponatremia, or hypotension. Other sites of dissemination include the kidneys, bone and joints, sinuses, optic nerve, eye, ears, esophagus, peritoneum, omentum, gallbladder, cystic duct, common bile duct, panniculus, prostate, breast, epididymis, urinary bladder, penis, vagina, testis, ovary, pleura, aorta, and thymus. Hypercalcemia rarely has been described and may cause renal failure (44,45).

Laboratory findings of anemia, leukopenia, and thrombocytopenia suggest bone marrow involvement, and alkaline phosphatase elevation may be a clue to the presence of hepatic involvement. The lactic acid dehydrogenase and ferritin may be markedly elevated. Chest roentgenograms usually show diffuse interstitial or reticulonodular infiltrates (Fig. 270.5) but may be normal; mediastinal adenopathy occurs in 20%, whereas cavitation is rare (29,31,46).

Broncholithiasis

Lymph nodes and pulmonary granulomas calcify within a few years of initial infection (47). Calcified nodes may erode into adjacent bronchi causing hemoptysis or obstruction (48,49). Symptoms include cough, purulent sputum production, and hemoptysis, which may be fatal (49). Patients may expectorate rocklike particles of tissue and experience bronchial obstruction or tracheoesophageal fistula.

Mediastinal Fibrosis

Fibrosing mediastinitis represents a fibrotic response to a prior episode of histoplasmosis. The hypothesis that certain

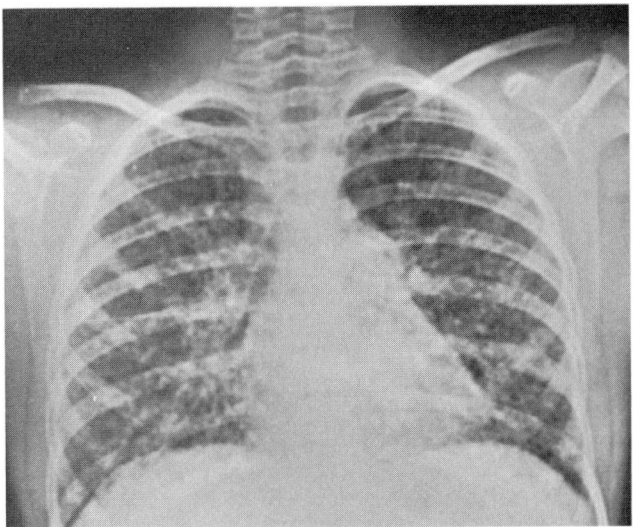

Figure 270.5. Chest roentgenogram of a patient with disseminated histoplasmosis showing diffuse interstitial alveolar infiltrates.

individuals are predisposed to this excessive fibrotic response to *Histoplasma* antigens is plausible, but unproven. Ongoing infection is not felt to play a role in the pathogenesis of fibrosing mediastinitis, based on the rarity of isolation of *H. capsulatum* from the tissues and the lack of response to antifungal therapy. Obstruction may involve the superior vena cava, airways, pulmonary arteries or veins, or esophagus (22,50). Progressive right heart failure and respiratory insufficiency occur in one third of cases (22,50). Recurrent and even massive hemoptysis can result from parenchymal damage caused by airway obstruction and vascular compromise. Subcarinal or superior mediastinal widening is seen on chest radiograph; CT scans reveal restriction and invasion of mediastinal structures (22,50). Pulmonary artery or venous contrast studies may be required to define the extent of obstruction in patients who have severe manifestations of disease.

Presumed Ocular Histoplasmosis

Choroiditis involving the macula and causing visual loss has been attributed to histoplasmosis without convincing scientific evidence. The association has been based on residence in an endemic area for histoplasmosis or histoplasmin skin-test reactivity rather than demonstration of fungus in the eye. In a few cases, yeasts were described in the eyes, but results of cultures were not reported (51). Occurrence of identical clinical findings in nonendemic areas discounts histoplasmosis as a cause for this syndrome (52). Although the eye rarely may be involved in disseminated histoplasmosis (53), "presumed ocular histoplasmosis" represents a different syndrome of unknown etiology.

DIAGNOSIS

Diagnosis of histoplasmosis requires a high index of clinical suspicion and understanding of the uses and limitations of a battery of serologic and mycologic tests (Table 270.3).

Antigen Detection

A rapid diagnosis is important in patients with severe manifestations of histoplasmosis. Detection of *Histoplasma* antigen in the body fluids offers a valuable approach to diagnosis in such cases (54,55), providing results within 24 to 48 hours. Antigen is found in the blood and/or urine of most individuals with disseminated histoplasmosis and in up to 75% of those with diffuse lung involvement during acute pulmonary histoplasmosis.

Antigen may be found in CSF of 25% to 50% of patients with chronic meningitis caused by histoplasmosis (56) and in the alveolar lavage fluid of those with diffuse pulmonary involvement (57). Cross-reacting antigens occur in patients with blastomycosis, paracoccidioidomycosis, coccidioidomycosis, *Penicillium marneffei* infection and African histoplasmosis caused by *H. capsulatum* variety *duboisii*. Antigen levels decline after treatment (58) and increase with relapse (59), providing a tool for monitoring therapy (59). Antigen testing is available at MiraVista Diagnostics (1-866-miravista).

Fungal Stain

Fungal staining of tissue sections or Wright stain of peripheral blood smears permits rapid diagnosis but with a lower sensitivity than culture or antigen detection. Fungal stains are positive in about half of disseminated cases (29). *H. capsulatum* may be seen in peripheral blood smears in severe cases (60,61). Organisms that may be misidentified as *H. capsulatum* include *Pneumocystis carinii*, *Blastomyces dermatitidis*, *Candida glabrata*, *Leishmania donovani*, and *Toxoplasma gondii*. Artifacts also may be mistaken for *H. capsulatum*.

Fungal Cultures

Cultures provide the strongest proof for histoplasmosis but are limited by low sensitivity (10% to 15%) in self-limited infections and slow growth (2 to 4 weeks). In disseminated histoplasmosis, the highest yield is from bone marrow or blood, positive in more than 75% of patients (29). In cavitary histoplasmosis, organisms can be found in sputum of 60% to 85% of patients if multiple specimens are cultured (55,62). Cultures usually are negative in patients with mild acute pulmonary, pericardial, or rheumatologic manifestations and need not be performed (5563) but may be positive in those with extensive pulmonary histoplasmosis.

Serologic Tests

The standard serologic tests for antibodies to *H. capsulatum* are the complement fixation (CF) test using both yeast and mycelial antigens and the immunodiffusion (ID) assay. Enzyme immunoassay methods are poorly standardized, difficult to interpret, and complicated by high background positivity, and thus are not recommended. Serologic tests are positive in more than 90% of patients with pulmonary histoplasmosis (29,63) and about 80% with disseminated disease (64). However, certain

TABLE 270.3. Summary of Diagnostic Test Results in Histoplasmosis

	Self-limited	Cavitary	Disseminated
		(%) Positive	
Antibody			
Immunodiffusion	75	100	63
Complement Fixation	89	93	63
Either immunodiffusion or complement fixation	99	100	71
Antigen detection	40–75	21	92
Culture	15	85	85

limitations of serologic testing should be recognized. First, 4 to 12 weeks are required for antibody production. Second, serologic tests are less sensitive in immunosuppressed patients and titers are lower (31,55). Third, positive serologic test results may result from prior infection and thus incorrectly suggest active histoplasmosis in patients with other diseases. Background rates of seropositivity range from 0.5% by ID to 4% by CF. Antibodies to *H. capsulatum* may be elevated in patients with other fungal infections, most commonly blastomycosis, coccidioidomycosis, and paracoccidioidomycosis (65). The CF test is more sensitive than the ID test (63). In acute pulmonary histoplasmosis, the CF test is positive (titers more than or equal to 1:8) in 90% of patients, whereas ID reveals M bands in 76% and H bands in only 23% (55,63). However, CF assays appear to be less specific than ID assays. Cross-reactions with other fungal infections occur in 5% of cases by ID, 18% by CF, and 49% by radioimmunoassay (66). Antibody titers decline after self-limited infection, reaching low or undetectable levels in 2 to 5 years (63). Antibody levels often remain high in those with chronic pulmonary infection (27), progressive disseminated disease (29), or fibrosing mediastinitis (22,50).

Histoplasmin Skin Test

Skin tests are not useful diagnostically because of high background rates of skin-test positivity (50% to 80%) in endemic areas, false-positive results in patients with other fungal diseases, and false-negative results in patients with disseminated disease (3,67). Furthermore, skin tests boost antibody levels, compromising interpretation of serologic tests (68).

TREATMENT

Treatment guidelines have been recently published (69). In many patients, the disease is self-limited and no treatment is indicated. Chronic pulmonary and disseminated histoplasmosis are progressive, justifying treatment in all cases. Other complications, including fibrosing mediastinitis and broncholithiasis, are caused by the host response to the infection, rather than the infection per se, and do not respond to therapy. The outcome of therapy for other complications, such as granulomatous mediastinitis, is poorly characterized, but treatment appears warranted.

Acute Pulmonary Histoplasmosis

Antifungal therapy is unnecessary in most patients with localized disease because they recover without treatment within 1 month (12). Some patients, however, may remain symptomatic longer (70) and benefit from therapy. Treatment is recommended for patients whose symptoms have not improved after 3 to 4 weeks of observation (Table 270.4). Oral itraconazole for 6 to 12 weeks is recommended in such cases.

Patients with diffuse pulmonary histoplasmosis and who are symptomatic should receive antifungal therapy (19,71). If the patient is left untreated, recovery is slow (70) and the outcome can be fatal (72,73). For severe cases in nonimmunosuppressed individuals, amphotericin B (0.7 to 1.0 mg/kg per day) is recommended, with prednisone (60 mg daily) tapered over 2 weeks (19,71). Patients with less severe manifestations can be treated with itraconazole for 3 months.

TABLE 270.4. Treatment Recommendations for Histoplasmosis

Type histoplasmosis	Severe manifestation	Mild/moderate severe manifestation
Acute, diffuse pulmonary following heavy exposure	Amphotericin B with corticosteroids followed by itraconazole for 12 wk[a]	Itraconazole for 12 wk[a,b]
Subacute, focal pulmonary	Not applicable	None in the usual case, because resolves spontaneously; itraconazole for 6–12 wk in those with persistent symptoms >4 wk
Chronic pulmonary	Amphotericin B followed by itraconazole for 12–24 mo	Itraconazole for 12–24 mo
Disseminated in non–acquired immunodeficiency syndrome (AIDS)	Amphotericin B followed by itraconazole for 6–18 mo[a]	Itraconazole for 6–18 mo[a]
Disseminated in AIDS	Amphotericin B[c] followed by itraconazole for life	Itraconazole for life (study in progress to determine whether can stop after 1 yr if CD4 count >150 cells/mm³)
Meningitis	Amphotericin B for 3 mo followed by fluconazole or itraconazole for 12 mo	Same as severe because of poor outcome
Granulomatous mediastinitis	Amphotericin B followed by itraconazole for 6–12 mo	Itraconazole for 6–12 mo
Fibrosing mediastinitis	Itraconazole for 3 mo[d]	Same as severe
Pericarditis	Corticosteroids 1 mg/kg/d[e] or pericardial drainage procedure	Nonsteroidal antiinflammatory agents for 2–12 wk
Rheumatologic	Nonsteroidal antiinflammatory agents for 2–12 wk	Same as severe

[a]Amphotericin B should be given at a dose of 0.7 mg/kg/d (50 mg/d) and itraconazole 5.0 mg/kg/d (400 mg/d given as 200 mg b.i.d.).
[b]Itraconazole blood concentrations should be measured during the second week of therapy to ensure that detectable concentrations have been achieved. If the concentration is <1 μg/mL, the dose may be insufficient or drug interactions may be impairing absorption or accelerating metabolism, requiring a change in dosage. If the concentrations are >10 μg/mL, the dosage may be reduced.
[c]Liposomal amphotericin B (AmBisome) may be more appropriate for disseminated disease, because it was more effective than the deoxycholate formulation is a study of patients with AIDS. Therapy should continue until *Histoplasma* antigen concentrations are ≤4 units in urine and serum.
[d]Therapy is controversial and probably ineffective except in cases of granulomatous mediastinitis, which are misdiagnosed as fibrosing mediastinitis.
[e]If corticosteroids are administered, concurrent antifungal therapy is recommended.

Chronic Pulmonary Histoplasmosis

Treatment is indicated in all patients with chronic pulmonary histoplasmosis to halt further lung destruction and reduce mortality. Amphotericin B is reasonably effective, with response rates from 59% to 100% (74–77) (Table 270.4). Itraconazole (200 mg daily for at least 3 months) was effective in 80% of cases (78), but relapse occurred in 10% to 15% within 1 year. Similar results have been reported with ketoconazole (79,80). Fluconazole (200 to 400 mg daily) appears to be less effective (64% response rate) (81). Itraconazole (200 mg once or twice daily based on blood concentration) is the preferred therapy and should be given for 12 to 24 months and until the chest CT shows no evidence for ongoing infection.

Granulomatous Mediastinitis

The role of therapy for granulomatous mediastinitis is unclear. Prospective trials, or even retrospective case studies, have not been conducted. Patients may recover without treatment (82), complicating assessment of anecdotal reports of response to medical or surgical therapy. Despite the uncertainty about the role of therapy, a trial of itraconazole for 6 to 12 months is recommended in patients with symptomatic infection and those with significant impingement on mediastinal structures. Amphotericin B may be appropriate initially if the patient is severely ill. Surgical resection of obstructive masses may be indicated if antifungal therapy is not helpful, but not to prevent progression to fibrosing mediastinitis.

Fibrosing Mediastinitis

Fibrosing mediastinitis, a complication of histoplasmosis, has no known effective therapy. Although most authorities believe that neither antifungal nor antiinflammatory treatment ameliorates this disease (22,50), one report suggested benefit from ketoconazole therapy (83). A 3-month trial of itraconazole seems reasonable, particularly if CF titers and the sedimentation rate are elevated. If follow-up CT scans and clinical evaluation show objective evidence for response, treatment should be continued for at least 1 year. Use of corticosteroids or other antiinflammatory agents is not recommended. CT scans should be repeated yearly to identify progression of the fibrosis and assess the indications for surgery.

Surgery is controversial in the management of fibrosing mediastinitis (84). Fewer than 40% of patients benefited and 20% died as a complication of surgery in the largest review of the surgical treatment of this disease (22). Others have recommended earlier referral for surgery but also have reported high operative mortality (about 25%) (85). Surgeons who are experienced in operating on patients with fibrosing mediastinitis should be consulted in view of the difficulty of the procedures and the high mortality rates (22,85). Placement of intravascular stents may be helpful in selected patients with superior vena cava or pulmonary vascular obstruction, and angiographic embolization may relieve pulmonary hemorrhage.

Pericarditis and Rheumatologic Syndromes

Pericarditis and rheumatologic manifestations are caused by an inflammatory response to the infection, not by the infection per se. Antifungal therapy would not be expected to alter the course of this inflammatory manifestation. Symptomatic patients respond to antiinflammatory therapy. If corticosteroids are used for more aggressive antiinflammatory therapy, however, itracona-zole should be given to reduce the possibility of dissemination of *H. capsulatum.*

Disseminated Histoplasmosis

Mortality without treatment is 80% (70), compared with less than 25% with amphotericin B (29,75,86,87). A recent study of patients with AIDS showed that liposomal amphotericin B (AmBisome) was more effective than standard amphotericin B, significantly improving survival (88). Thus, liposomal amphotericin B is preferred for patients with severe or moderately severe disseminated histoplasmosis. Itraconazole is the drug of choice for treatment of disseminated histoplasmosis in patients with less severe illness and for consolidation therapy after an initial response to amphotericin B (69). The intravenous formulation can be used to accelerate achievement of therapeutic concentrations and potentially improve the response to therapy. The recommended dosage of the intravenous formulation is 200 mg twice daily for 3 days as a loading dose, and then 200 mg daily for the first 2 weeks, followed by oral therapy with 200 mg twice daily. Fluconazole is less active than itraconazole against *H. capsulatum,* and less effective as therapy for histoplasmosis. In one study of patients with AIDS, 74% of patients responded to 800 mg daily of fluconazole, but 30% relapsed over the next 6 months while receiving 400 mg daily (89). Resistance to fluconazole developed in more than half of the patients failing therapy (89).

Relapse occurs in 10% to 20% of patients with disseminated histoplasmosis and in as many as 80% of those with AIDS. Until recently, lifelong maintenance therapy with itraconazole was recommended for all patients with AIDS (90). Studies in progress, however, suggest that maintenance therapy may be stopped after 1 year in patients who have responded well to antiretroviral therapy (CD4 counts of more than 150 cells/mm^3 and *Histoplasma* antigen levels of less than 4 units).

Endocarditis

Antifungal therapy combined with resection of the infected valve is recommended (91,92). In one report, five (71%) of seven patients treated with antifungal therapy combined with surgery were cured compared with four (44%) of 9 who received antifungal therapy alone (92). These observations support a recommendation to administer amphotericin B, preferably the liposomal formulation (AmBisome), at maximum doses for 2 to 3 months, followed by itraconazole for another year, and to replace the valve as soon as is feasible. Long-term maintenance therapy with itraconazole is appropriate in those who relapse or who cannot undergo valve replacement.

Central Nervous System Histoplasmosis

Although most patients respond initially to treatment with amphotericin B, half relapse during the next 2 years (40). Whether the liposomal form of amphotericin B, which achieves higher concentrations in brain tissue in animal models (93), would be more effective than the standard formulation is unknown. The poor outcome of *Histoplasma* meningitis supports its use for this indication. Fluconazole achieves high concentrations in the CSF (94) and has been used successfully in four patients with *Histoplasma* meningitis (95–97). Each had previously failed amphotericin B therapy, and one had also failed itraconazole therapy (95). Itraconazole does not penetrate the CSF but has been used successfully in cryptococcal and coccidioidal meningitis. When used in a murine model of *Histoplasma* meningitis, itraconazole was more effective than fluconazole, and addition of either triazole to amphotericin B did not improve the outcome (97a). Other studies show that fluconazole antagonizes the effect of amphotericin B in histoplasmosis (98). Although the best therapy is still not known, it seems reasonable to begin therapy with liposomal amphotericin B, 3 to 5 mg/kg per day for 2 to 3 months and until CSF cultures are negative, followed by itraconazole, 200 mg twice daily, or fluconazole, 800 mg daily, for at least another year. Lifelong maintenance therapy may be needed in patients who relapse or in those whose CSF findings do not return to normal. Patients who fail long-term azole therapy have few options. One approach is direct injection of amphotericin B into the lumbar CSF or the ventricles. However, such treatment is poorly tolerated and marginally effective in *Histoplasma* meningitis (40).

Cerebritis or histoplasmomas in the brain or spinal cord, without meningitis, are perhaps more responsive to antifungal therapy. Parenchymal lesions usually do not require surgical excision (40) and should resolve with antifungal therapy in most cases. Liposomal amphotericin B for 2 to 3 months, followed by itraconazole or fluconazole for at least a year, is recommended (93). MRI scans should be followed to affirm resolution before stopping therapy.

PREVENTION

Prophylaxis with itraconazole, 200 mg daily, in persons with AIDS with CD4 counts less than 150 cells/mm^3 is highly effective and should be considered if the case rate of histoplasmosis exceeds 10 cases per 100 patient-years (99). Persons whose vocation or avocation could potentially expose them to *H. capsulatum* conidia should take appropriate precautions as outlined by the Centers for Disease Control and Prevention (100). Workers involved with soil disruption, building demolition, or refurbishing of old structures that have been known to provide roosts for bats and birds should wear approved respirators. In areas known to contain *H. capsulatum*, the soil or debris can be treated with formalin to inactivate the conidia before construction work. Immunocompromised patients should not undertake activities such as spelunking or renovation projects that might put them at risk for exposure to the conidia of *H. capsulatum*.

REFERENCES

1. Darling ST. A protozoan general infection producing pseudotubercles in the lungs and focal necroses in the liver, spleen, and lymph nodes. *JAMA* 1906;46:1283–1285.
2. Christie A, Peterson JC. Pulmonary calcification in negative reactors to tuberculin. *Am J Public Health* 1945;35:1131–1147.
3. Edwards LB, Acquaviva FA, Livesay VT, et al. An atlas of sensitivity to tuberculin, PPD-B and histoplasmin in the United States. *Am Rev Respir Dis* 1969;99:1–18.
4. Emmons CW. Isolation of *Histoplasma capsulatum* from soil. *Am J Public Health* 1949;64:892–896.
5. Zeidberg LD, Ajello L, Dillon A, et al. Isolation of *Histoplasma capsulatum* from soil. *Am J Public Health* 1952;42:930–935.
6. Bowman BH, Taylor JW, White TJ. Molecular evolution of the fungi: human pathogens. *Mol Biol Evol* 1992;9:893–904.
7. Hutton JP, Durham JB, Miller DP, et al. Hyphal forms of *Histoplasma capsulatum*: a common manifestation of intravascular infections. *Arch Pathol Lab Med* 1985;109:330–332.
8. Svirbely JR, Ayers LW, Buesching WJ. Filamentous *Histoplasma capsulatum* endocarditis involving mitral and aortic valve porcine bioprostheses. *Arch Pathol Lab Med* 1985;109:273–276.
9. Stockman L, Clark KA, Hunt JM, et al. Evaluation of commercially available acridinium ester-labeled chemiluminescent DNA probes for culture identification of *Blastomyces dermatitidis*, *Coccidioides immitis*, *Cryptococcus neoformans*, and *Histoplasma capsulatum*. *J Clin Microbiol* 1993;31:845–850.
10. Cano M, Hajjeh RA. The epidemiology of histoplasmosis; a review. *Semin Respir Infect* 2001;16(2):109–118.
11. Waldman RJ, England AC, Tauxe R, et al. A winter outbreak of acute histoplasmosis in northern Michigan. *Am J Epidemiol* 1983;117:68–75.
12. Brodsky AL, Gregg MB, Kaufman L, et al. Outbreak of histoplasmosis associated with the 1970 Earth Day activities. *Am J Med* 1973;54:333–342.
13. Woods JP, Heinecke EL, Luecke JW, et al. Pathogenesis of *Histoplasma capsulatum*. *Semin Respir Infect* 2001;16(2):91–101.
14. Newman SL. Cell-mediated immunity to *Histoplasma capsulatum*. *Semin Respir Infect* 2001;16(2):102–108.
15. Keath EJ, Kobayashi GS, Medoff G. Typing of *Histoplasma capsulatum* by restriction fragment length polymorphisms in a nuclear gene. *J Clin Microbiol* 1992;30:2104–2107.
16. Wheat LJ, Slama TG, Eitzen HE, et al. A large urban outbreak of histoplasmosis: clinical features. *Ann Intern Med* 1981;94:331–337.
17. Chick EW, Dillon ML, Tahanasab A. Acute cavitary histoplasmosis. *Chest* 1977;71:674–675.
18. Bennish M, Radkowski MA, Rippon JW. Cavitation in acute histoplasmosis. *Chest* 1983;84:496–497.
19. Kataria YP, Campbell PB, Burlingham BT. Acute pulmonary histoplasmosis presenting as adult respiratory distress syndrome: effect of therapy on clinical and laboratory features. *South Med J* 1981;74:534–537.
20. Sakulsky SB, Harrison EG, Dines DE, et al. Mediastinal granuloma. *J Thorac Cardiovasc Surg* 1967;54:280–290.
21. Dovenbarger WV, Tsubura E, Schwarz J, et al. Mediastinal cystic granuloma due to *Histoplasma capsulatum*: a report of three patients treated surgically. *J Thorac Cardiovasc Surg* 1961;42:193–199.
22. Loyd JE, Tillman BF, Atkinson JB, et al. Mediastinal fibrosis complicating histoplasmosis. *Medicine (Baltimore)* 1988;67:295–310.
23. Rosenthal J, Brandt KD, Wheat LJ, et al. Rheumatologic manifestations of histoplasmosis in the recent Indianapolis epidemic. *Arthr Rheum* 1983;26:1065–1070.
24. Wheat LJ, Stein L, Corya BC, et al. Pericarditis as a manifestation of histoplasmosis during two large urban outbreaks. *Medicine (Baltimore)* 1983;62:110–119.
25. Wooley CF, Hosier DM. Constrictive pericarditis due to *Histoplasma capsulatum*. *N Engl J Med* 1961;264:1230–1232.
26. Goodwin RA Jr, Owens FT, Snell JD, et al. Chronic pulmonary histoplasmosis. *Medicine (Baltimore)* 1976;55:413–452.
27. Wheat LJ, Wass J, Norton J, et al. Cavitary histoplasmosis occurring during two large urban outbreaks: analysis of clinical, epidemiologic, roentgenograghic, and laboratory features. *Medicine (Baltimore)* 1984;63:201–209.
28. Furcolow ML. Course and prognosis of untreated histoplasmosis. *JAMA* 1961;177:292–296.
29. Sathapatayavongs B, Batteiger BE, Wheat LJ, et al. Clinical and laboratory features of disseminated histoplasmosis during two large urban outbreaks. *Medicine (Baltimore)* 1983;62:263–270.
30. Wheat LJ, Slama TG, Norton JA, et al. Risk factors for disseminated or fatal histoplasmosis. *Ann Intern Med* 1982;96:159–163.
31. Wheat LJ, Connolly-Stringfield PA, Baker RL, et al. Disseminated histoplasmosis in the acquired immune deficiency syndrome: clinical findings, diagnosis and treatment, and review of the literature. *Medicine (Baltimore)* 1990;69:361–374.
32. Schneider RP, Edwards W. Histoplasmosis presenting as an esophageal tumor. *Gastrointest Endosc* 1977;23:158–159.
33. Cimponeriu D, LoPresti P, Lavelanet M, et al. Gastrointestinal histoplasmosis in HIV infection: two cases of colonic pseudocancer and review of the literature. *Am J Gastroenterol* 1994;89:129–131.
34. Lee KR, Lin F. The radiology corner: gastrointestinal histoplasmosis, roentgenographic, clinical and pathological correlation. *Am J Gastroenterol* 1975;63:255–265.
35. Lee SH, Barnes WG, Hodges GR, et al. Perforated granulomatous colitis caused by *Histoplasma capsulatum*. *Dis Colon Rect* 1985;28:171–176.
36. Morrison YY, Rathbun RC, Huycke MM. Disseminated histoplasmosis mimicking Crohn's disease in a patient with the acquired immunodeficiency syndrome. *Am J Gastroenterol* 1994;89:1255–1257.
37. Hazelhurst JA, Vismer HF. Histoplasmosis presenting with unusual skin lesions in acquired immunodeficiency syndrome (AIDS). *Br Med J* 1985;II3:345–348.
38. Barton EN, Roberts L, Ince WE, et al. Cutaneous histoplasmosis in the acquired immune deficiency syndrome: a report of three cases from Trinidad. *Trop Geogr Med* 1988;40:153–157.
39. Cott GR, Smith TW, Hinthorn DR, et al. Primary cutaneous histoplasmosis in immunosuppressed patients. *JAMA* 1979;242:456–457.
40. Wheat LJ, Batteiger BE, Sathapatayavongs B. *Histoplasma capsulatum* infections of the central nervous system: a clinical review. *Medicine (Baltimore)* 1990;69:244–260.
41. Bazan C 3rd, New PZ. Intramedullary spinal histoplasmosis efficacy of gadolinium enhancement. *Neuroradiology* 1991;33:190.
42. Livas IC, Nechay PS, Nauseef WM. Clinical evidence of spinal and cerebral histoplasmosis twenty years after renal transplantation. *Clin Infect Dis* 1995;20:692–695.

43. Goodwin RA Jr, Shapiro JL, Thurman GH, et al. Disseminated histoplasmosis: clinical and pathologic correlations. *Medicine (Baltimore)* 1980;59:1–33.
44. Walker JV, Baran D, Yakub N, et al. Histoplasmosis with hypercalcemia, renal failure, and papillary necrosis: confusion with sarcoidosis. *JAMA* 1977;237:1350–1352.
45. Murray JJ, Heim CR. Hypercalcemia in disseminated histoplasmosis: aggravated by vitamin D. *Am J Med* 1985;78:881–884.
46. Conces DJ Jr, Stockberger SM, Tarver RD, et al. Disseminated histoplasmosis in AIDS: findings on chest radiographs. *AJR Am J Roentgenol* 1993;160:15–19.
47. Goodwin RA, Loyd JE, des Prez RM. Histoplasmosis in normal hosts. *Medicine (Baltimore)* 1981;60:231–266.
48. Garrett HE Jr, Roper CL. Surgical intervention in histoplasmosis. *Ann Thorac Surg* 1986;42:711–722.
49. Arrigoni MG, Bernatz PE, Donoghue FE. Broncholithiasis. *J Thorac Cardiovasc Surg* 1971;62:231–237.
50. Goodwin RA, Nickell JA, des Prez RM. Mediastinal fibrosis complicating healed primary histoplasmosis and tuberculosis. *Medicine (Baltimore)* 1972;51:227–246.
51. Roth A. *Histoplasma capsulatum* in the presumed ocular histoplasmosis syndrome. *Am J Ophthalmol* 1977;84(3):293–298.
52. Suttorp-Schulten MSA, Bollemeijer JG, Bos PJM, et al. Presumed ocular histoplasmosis in the Netherlands—an area without histoplasmosis. *Br J Ophthalmol* 1997;81(1):7–11.
53. Specht CS, Mitchell KT, Bauman AE, et al. Ocular histoplasmosis with retinitis in a patient with acquired immune deficiency syndrome. *Ophthalmology* 1991;98:1356–1359.
54. Wheat LJ, Kohler RB, Tewari RP. Diagnosis of disseminated histoplasmosis by detection of *Histoplasma capsulatum* antigen in serum and urine specimens. *N Engl J Med* 1986;314:83–88.
55. Williams B, Fojtasek M, Connolly-Stringfield P, et al. Diagnosis of histoplasmosis by antigen detection during an outbreak in Indianapolis, Ind. *Arch Pathol Lab Med* 1994;118:1205–1208.
56. Wheat LJ, Kohler RB, Tewari RP, et al. Significance of *Histoplasma* antigen in the cerebrospinal fluid of patients with meningitis. *Arch Intern Med* 1989;149:302–304.
57. Wheat LJ, Connolly-Stringfield PA, Williams B, et al. Diagnosis of histoplasmosis in patients with the acquired immunodeficiency syndrome by detection of *Histoplasma capsulatum* polysaccharide antigen in bronchoalveolar lavage fluid. *Am Rev Respir Dis* 1992;145:1421–1424.
58. Wheat LJ, Connolly-Stringfield P, Blair R, et al. Effect of successful treatment with amphotericin B on *Histoplasma capsulatum* variety *capsulatum* polysaccharide antigen levels in patients with AIDS and histoplasmosis. *Am J Med* 1992;92:153–160.
59. Wheat LJ, Connolly-Stringfield P, Blair R, et al. Histoplasmosis relapse in patients with AIDS: detection using *Histoplasma capsulatum* variety *capsulatum* antigen levels. *Ann Intern Med* 1991;115:936–941.
60. Kurtin PJ, McKinsey DS, Gupta MR, et al. Histoplasmosis in patients with acquired immunodeficiency syndrome: hematologic and bone marrow manifestations. *Am J Clin Pathol* 1990;93:367–372.
61. Zarabi CM, Thomas R, Adesokan A. Diagnosis of systemic histoplasmosis in patients with AIDS. *South Med J* 1992;85:1171–1175.
62. Sutcliffe MC, Savage AM, Alford RH. Transferrin-dependent growth inhibition of yeast-phase *Histoplasma capsulatum* by human serum and lymph. *J Infect Dis* 1980;142:209–219.
63. Wheat LJ, French MLV, Kohler RB, et al. The diagnostic laboratory tests for histoplasmosis: analysis of experience in a large urban outbreak. *Ann Intern Med* 1982;97:680–685.
64. Wheat LJ. Laboratory diagnosis of histoplasmosis: a review. *Semin Respir Infect* 2001;16(2):131–140.
65. Zimmerman SE, French MLV, Kleiman MB, et al. Evaluation of an enzyme-linked immunosorbent assay that uses ferrous metal beads for determination of antihistoplasmal immunoglobulins G and M. *J Clin Microbiol* 1990;28:59–64.
66. Wheat LJ, French MLV, Kamel S, et al. Evaluation of cross-reactions in *Histoplasma capsulatum* serologic tests. *J Clin Microbiol* 1986;23:493–499.
67. Zeidberg LD, Dillon A, Gass RS. Some factors in the epidemiology of histoplasmin sensitivity in Williamson County, Tennessee. *Am J Public Health* 1951;41:80–89.
68. Kaufman L, Terry RT, Schubert JH, et al. Effects of a single histoplasmin skin test on the serological diagnosis of histoplasmosis. *J Bacteriol* 1967;94:798–803.
69. Wheat J, Sarosi G, McKinsey D, et al. Practice guidelines for the management of patients with histoplasmosis. *Clin Infect Dis* 2000;30(4):688–695.
70. Rubin H, Furcolow ML, Yates JL, et al. The course and prognosis of histoplasmosis. *Am J Med* 1959;27:278–288.
71. Wynne JW, Olsen GN. Acute histoplasmosis presenting as the adult respiratory distress syndrome. *Chest* 1974;66:158–161.
72. Sollod N. Acute fulminating disseminated histoplasmosis. *J South Carol Med Assoc* 1971;67:231–234.
73. Prior JA, Saslaw S, Cole CR. Experiences with histoplasmosis. *Ann Intern Med* 1954;40:221–244.
74. Parker JD, Sarosi GA, Doto IL, et al. Treatment of chronic pulmonary histoplasmosis. *N Engl J Med* 1970;283:225–229.
75. Furcolow ML. Comparison of treated and untreated severe histoplasmosis. *JAMA* 1963;183:121–127.
76. Sutliff WD, Andrews CE, Jones E, et al. Histoplasmosis cooperative study: Veterans Administration-Armed Forces Cooperative Study on histoplasmosis. *Am Rev Respir Dis* 1964;89:641–650.
77. Putnam LR, Sutliff WD, Larkin JC, et al. Histoplasmosis cooperative study: chronic pulmonary histoplasmosis treated with amphotericin B alone and with amphotericin B and triple sulfonamide. *Am Rev Respir Dis* 1968;97:96–102.
78. Dismukes WE, Bradsher RW Jr, Cloud GC, et al. Itraconazole therapy for blastomycosis and histoplasmosis. *Am J Med* 1992;93:489–497.
79. Dismukes WE, Cloud G, Bowles C, et al. Treatment of blastomycosis and histoplasmosis with ketoconazole: results of a prospective randomized clinical trial. *Ann Intern Med* 1985;103:861–872.
80. Slama TG. Treatment of disseminated and progressive cavitary histoplasmosis with ketoconazole. *Am J Med* 1983;70:73.
81. McKinsey DS, Kauffman CA, Pappas PG, et al. Fluconazole therapy for histoplasmosis. *Clin Infect Dis* 1996;23(5):996–1001.
82. Alcorn GL. Clinical problems in cardiopulmonary disease: histoplasmosis with symptomatic lymphadenopathy, clinical evaluation by R.A. Goodwin, M.D. *Chest* 1980;77:213–215.
83. Urschel HC Jr, Razzuk MA, Netto GJ, et al. Sclerosing mediastinitis: improved management with histoplasmosis titer and ketoconazole. *Ann Thorac Surg* 1990;50:215–221.
84. Davis A, Pierson D, Loyd JE. Mediastinal fibrosis. *Semin Respir Infect* 2001;16(2):119–130.
85. Mathisen DJ, Grillo HC. Clinical manifestations of mediastinal fibrosis and histoplasmosis. *Ann Thorac Surg* 1992;54:1053–1058.
86. Wilson DA, Muchmore HG, Tisda RG, et al. Histoplasmosis of the adrenal glands studied by CT. *Radiology* 1984;150:779–783.
87. Sarosi GA, Voth DW, Dahl BA, et al. Disseminated histoplasmosis: results of long-term follow-up. *Ann Intern Med* 1971;75:511–516.
88. Johnson P, Wheat LJ, Cloud G, et al. Safety and efficacy of liposomal amphotericin B compared with conventional amphotericin B for induction therapy of histoplasmosis in patients with AIDS. *Ann Intern Med* 2002;137:105–109.
89. Wheat J, MaWhinney S, Hafner R, et al. Treatment of histoplasmosis with fluconazole in patients with acquired immunodeficiency syndrome. *Am J Med* 1997;103(3):223–232.
90. Wheat J, Hafner R, Wulfson M, et al. Prevention of relapse of histoplasmosis with itraconazole in patients with the acquired immunodeficiency syndrome. *Ann Intern Med* 1993;118:610–616.
91. Gaynes RP, Gardner P, Causey W. Prosthetic value endocarditis caused by *Histoplasma capsulatum*. *Arch Intern Med* 1981;141:1533–1537.
92. Kanawaty DS, Stalker MJB, Munt PW. Nonsurgical treatment of *Histoplasma* endocarditis involving a bioprosthetic valve. *Chest* 1991;99:253–256.
93. Groll AH, Giri N, Petraitis V, et al. Comparative efficacy and distribution of lipid formulations of amphotericin B in experimental *Candida albicans* infection of the central nervous system. *J Infect Dis* 2000;182(1):274–282.
94. Tucker RM, Williams PL, Arathoon EG, et al. Pharmacokinetics of fluconazole in cerebrospinal fluid and serum in human coccidioidal meningitis. *Antimicrob Agents Chemother* 1988;32(3):369–373.
95. Diaz M, Negroni R, Montero-Gei F, et al. A pan-American 5-year study of fluconazole therapy for deep mycoses in the immunocompetent host. *Clin Infect Dis* 1992;14:s68–s76.
96. Rivera I, Curless R, Indacochea F, et al. Chronic progressive CNS histoplasmosis presenting in childhood: response to fluconazole therapy. *Pediatr Neurol* 1992;8:151–153.
97. Tiraboschi I, Casas Parera I, Pikielny R, et al. Chronic *Histoplasma capsulatum* infection of the central nervous system successfully treated with fluconazole. *Eur Neurol* 1992;32:70–73.
97a. Haynes RR, Connolly PA, Durkin MM, et al. Antifungal therapy for central nervous system histoplasmosis, using a newly developed intracranial model of infection. *J Infect Dis* 2002;185:1830–1832.
98. LeMonte A, Washum K, Smedema M, et al. Amphotericin B combined with itraconazole or fluconazole for treatment of histoplasmosis. *J Infect Dis* 2000;(182):545–550.
99. McKinsey DS, Wheat LJ, Cloud GA, et al. Itraconazole prophylaxis for fungal infections in patients with advanced human immunodeficiency virus infection: randomized, placebo-controlled, double-blind study. *Clin Infect Dis* 1999;28(5):1049–1056.
100. Lenhart S. Recommendations for protecting workers from *Histoplasma capsulatum* exposure during bat guano removal from a church's attic. *Appl Occup Environ Hyg* 1994;9:230–236.

CHAPTER 271
Coccidioides immitis

Stanley C. Deresinski, Laurence F. Mirels,
and Carol A. Kemper

HISTORY

In 1892, when Alejandro Posadas reported the case history of an Argentinean soldier named Domingo Escurra afflicted with what he believed to be mycosis fungoides (1–3), Posadas believed that the microorganisms he detected in the lesions were the cause of this malignant disease. Shortly thereafter, Emmet Rixford and T. C. Gilchrist (4,5) reported finding apparently identical organisms in cutaneous lesions of both Joas Furtado Silverra and Jose Teixara Periera, both immigrants to California from the Azores.

All three investigators believed that the organism they had observed was a protozoan, and because of its resemblance to the coccidia, Rixford and Gilchrist named it *Coccidioides*. The isolate from Silverra was given the further appellation, *immitis*, to indicate its apparent virulence. In 1900, Ophüls and Moffitt examined the "white moldy growth" (also observed by Rixford and Gilchrist but discarded by them as a "contaminant") recovered from another Azorean immigrant and rapidly determined that *Coccidioides immitis* (CI) was a fungus, described its life cycle, and satisfied Koch's postulates (6–8). In 1932, the fungus was isolated from soil under the California bunkhouse of four Filipino farm workers who had developed serious coccidioidal infections (9).

Although infections caused by CI seemed to early observers to be almost invariably fatal (8), laboratory, clinical, and epidemiological observations by Dickson and Gifford (10,11) later determined that "valley fever," a usually self-limited disease seen with great frequency in the San Joaquin Valley of California, was also caused by CI and that the respiratory tract was its portal of entry. Charles Smith subsequently developed an effective reagent (coccidioidin) for skin and serologic testing and, by means of clinical observation and enormous skin-test and serologic surveys, further defined much of the nature and geographic distribution of the disease. Smith et al. (12–14) described the predisposition of certain demographic groups to severe disease, demonstrated that self-limited infection appeared to protect individuals from subsequent illness on reexposure, and reported the prognostic values of both skin-test reactivity and the magnitude of the complement-fixing antibody response.

CHARACTERISTICS OF THE PATHOGEN

Classification, Replication, and Structure

CI is a monophyletic dimorphic fungus that has been proposed as a member of the family Onygenaceae, order Onygenales, division Ascomycotina (15,16). Its guanine plus cytosine content is 49.41% to 49.61% (17), and it is variously reported to have three or four pairs of chromosomes (18,19). Sequencing of the CI genome is currently in progress. CI exhibits the mycelial form in its saprophytic state, whereas it exists as an endosporulating spherule in the parasitic (tissue) phase. In contrast to most other pathogenic dimorphs, its morphological state is not simply thermally determined; a key factor in the formation of endosporulating spherules *in vitro* is the maintenance of carbon dioxide tension in the range of 20 to 60 mm Hg (20), values that encompass a range found in human and animal hosts and thus may also be critical for morphological conversion *in vivo*. It has been proposed that polymorphonuclear leukocytes may play an additional role in maintenance of the organism in the spherule-endospore phase *in vivo* (21,22).

CI has a unique mode of reproduction (23–25). Although mating and meiosis have not been directly observed, population genetic and molecular phylogenetic analyses have provided evidence most consistent with genetic recombination, indicating that cryptic sexual reproduction may occur (25). The saprobic phase is seen in soil and under standard methods of cultivation in the laboratory (Fig. 271.1). Within several days of inoculation of culture media with the tissue phase of the organism, conversion to vegetative hyphal growth occurs. Hyphae extend by apical growth and branching to form mycelia. Multiple septa form simultaneously in fertile hyphae, creating cells that divide with subsequent internal (enteroarthric) development of thick-walled multinucleated arthroconidia alternating with thin-walled cells apparently lacking internal structure. The latter cells, called disjunctors, undergo autolysis, and as a result, arthroconidia, the infectious units of CI, readily disarticulate from the colony (in a process called rhexolytic secession) and may become airborne (Fig. 271.2). Subsequent arthroconidial deposition onto soil restart the hyphal growth cycle, whereas inhalation of the airborne arthroconidia by an animal or human may then lead to infection.

In the host, the arthroconidia swell and become uninucleate and, within 48 hours, convert to spherules, which continue to isotropically enlarge, reaching a size of 20 to 150 μm in diameter. The wall simultaneously thickens and the nucleus undergoes repeated synchronous divisions to form a syncytium. After approximately 72 hours, and after cessation of mitosis, the nascent spherule undergoes septation by inward growth of cell wall matrix, initially dividing the internal contents into separate multinucleated protoplasmic compartments. A β-glucosidase that appears identical to a known immunoglobulin M (IgM)–reactive 120-kd antigen detected in the tube precipitin test may be important in spherule morphogenesis, as may ornithine decarboxylase, which is expressed only during isotropic growth and segmentation (26,27). Secondary cleavage further divides the coenocytic (multinucleated) protoplasm into uninucleated endospores (Fig. 271.3). The network of internal cleavage planes, called the *segmentation apparatus,* undergoes autolysis; because this degradative process does not affect spherule or endospore walls, it is presumed to be under both temporal and spatial regulatory control. A 36-kd serine proteinase with broad substrate specificity may be at least partly responsible for this autolysis. This enzyme is present in the cell wall of the mycelial phase and of the spherule phase but reaches its highest concentration in the wall of the segmentation apparatus just before segmentation and may be regulated, at least in part, by a low-molecular-weight proteinase inhibitor (28,29). The mature spherule may contain several hundred endospores, each 2 to 5 μm in diameter. Rupture of the spherule wall leads to release of the endospores in "packets," with individual cells held together by fibrillar material derived from the inner spherule cell wall (30) (Fig. 271.4). Endospores then enlarge, becoming nascent spherules and repeating the parasitic phase reproductive cycle.

Biologic and Biochemical Properties

Approximately half the mycelial cell wall is made up of protein and chitin, a polymer of *N*-acetylglucosamine; the remainder is composed of other large polysaccharides (31–35). The inner

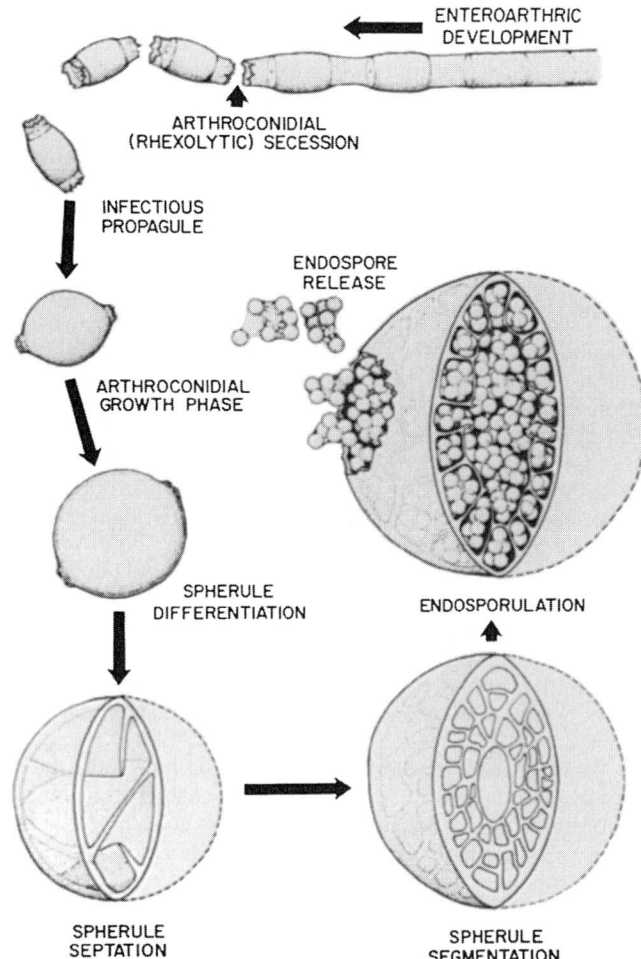

Figure 271.1. Life cycle of *Coccidioides immitis*. (From Cole GT, Sun SH. Arthroconidium-spherule-endospore transformation in *Coccidioides immitis*. In: Szaniszlo PJ, ed. *Fungal dimorphism: with emphasis on fungi pathogenic for humans*. New York: Plenum Publishing, 1985:281–336, with permission.)

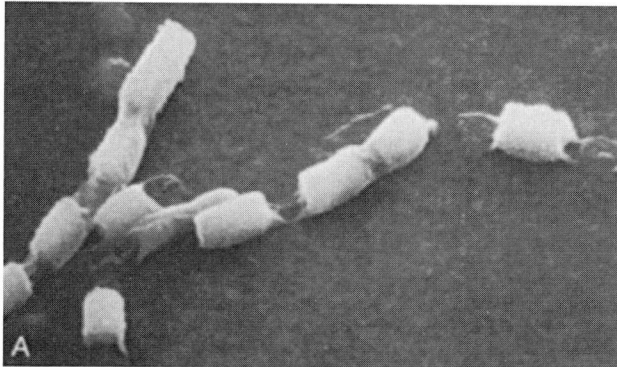

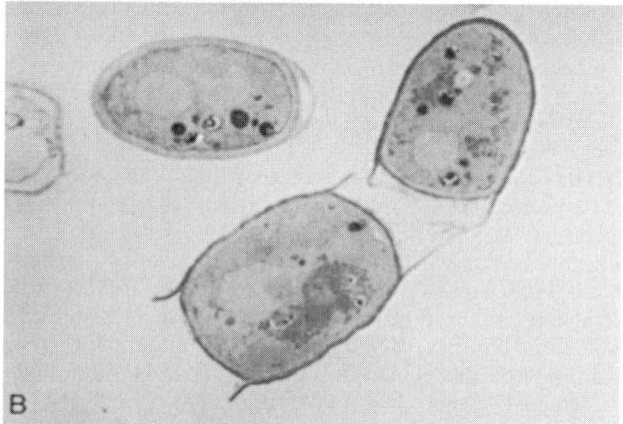

Figure 271.2. A: Scanning electron microscopy of mycelial fragment demonstrating arthroconidia alternating with "clear spaces." B: Transmission electron microscopy of arthroconidia undergoing rhexolytic secession with demonstration of retained hyphal outer wall. (Courtesy Dr. S. H. Sun, Veterans Administration Medical Center, San Antonio, Texas.)

spherule wall consists of a matrix of chitin and β-(1-3)-glucan, whereas the outer part of the wall is primarily made up of the latter (36). The chitin content of spherules is almost twice that of mycelia. Approximately 4% of the spherule wall is made up of lipid; 17% is peptide.

CI is a strict aerobe and produces catalase (35,37). Both morphological forms of the fungus contain most or all of the enzymes of the Krebs, the pentose phosphate, and the Embden-Meyerhof pathways (38). A wide variety of substrates can be used as a carbon source (39,40).

The rate of growth and release of endospores *in vitro* is stimulated via specific binding to cytosolic proteins, by testosterone, 17β-estradiol, and progesterone. In the case of the last two hormones, binding to cytosolic fungal receptors occurs at concentrations that are physiologic during pregnancy (41,42), and it has been proposed that this phenomenon contributes to the increased risk of dissemination during late gestation.

Antigenic Characteristics

"Antigen 2," also known as proline-rich antigen (PRA), is a major immunogen derived from alkaline extracts of mycelial and spherule cell walls and is detected in the IgM tube precip-

itin antibody reaction (43–45). A spherule-derived β-glucosidase also reacts with IgM antibody in the tube precipitin test and a 48-kd chitinase is detected in the complement-fixing antibody and immunodiffusion tests (26,46,47).

Antigenic differences exist between arthrospores and spherules (48). Coccidioidin, prepared from mycelia, contains at least 26 antigenic components, 16 of which are not found in the spherule-derived preparation, Spherulin. Conversely, Spherulin contains at least 16 antigens not present in coccidioidin (49). SOWgp is a major antigen that elicits both humoral and cellular immune responses, that is expressed on the surface of spherules, and that appears to function as an adhesin (50,51).

EPIDEMIOLOGY

Transmission

Infection is almost exclusively initiated by inhalation of airborne arthroconidia. Individuals who are routinely exposed to dust from infected soil, such as farm and construction workers and archeologists are at greatest risk (52,53). Natural phenomena that disturb topsoil and allow it to become airborne may lead to outbreaks of coccidioidomycosis (54). The minimum infective dose in humans is not known, but in animal models, including primates, infection may be established by inhalation of as few as 10 arthroconidia (55). Inhalation of arthroconidia from contaminated fomites may also lead to infection, and in one instance, airborne transmission, presumably of spherule-endospore phase

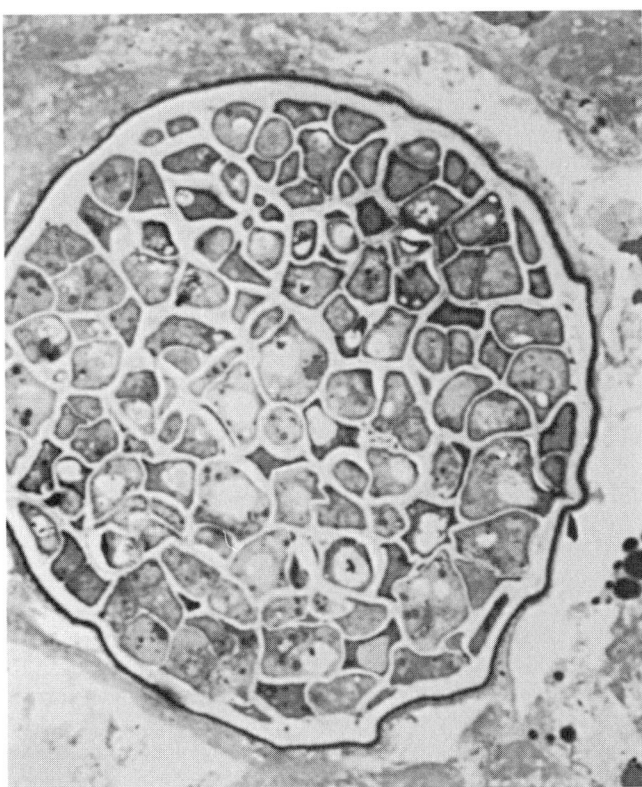

Figure 271.3. Transmission electron microscopy of segmenting spherule *in vivo*. (Courtesy Dr. S. H. Sun, Veterans Administration Medical Center, San Antonio, Texas.)

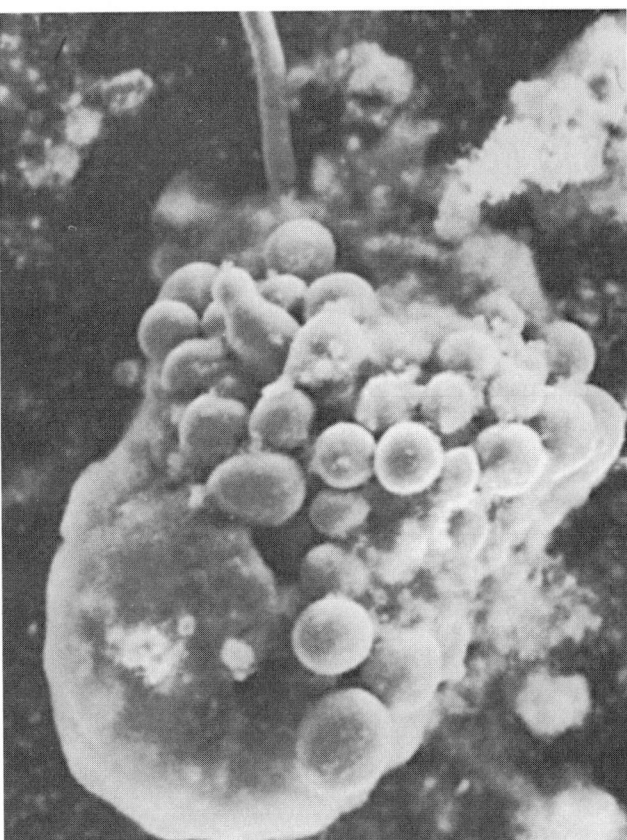

Figure 271.4. Scanning electron microscopy of spherule undergoing cell wall rupture with release of endospores. (Courtesy Dr. S. H. Sun, Veterans Administration Medical Center, San Antonio, Texas.)

organisms, may have resulted from aerosol generated by use of a band saw to cut through a patellar abscess during a postmortem examination (56). Infection may rarely result from direct cutaneous inoculation, which occurs most commonly in agricultural and laboratory workers but has also been reported in an individual who had embalmed the body of an individual who had died with disseminated coccidioidomycosis (57,58). Infection in the neonate is reported, albeit rarely, suggesting vertical transmission either via placental infection or at the time of birth (59,60). Apparent sexual transmission has also been reported (61), as has transmission by transplantation of an infected lung (62).

Transmission via fomite has been invoked to explain some cases of primary coccidioidomycosis occurring outside the endemic area (63–67). However, most presentations of primary coccidioidomycosis in nonendemic areas are the consequence of infection acquired within an endemic area that first becomes symptomatic after a traveler has returned home (67–69). Analyses of transmission have been advanced by the use of multilocus genotyping as an epidemiological tool (68–73), and determination of the geographic source of individual isolates has been facilitated by the recognition that there appear to be two reproductively isolated taxa of CI, one centered in California and one primarily including isolates from outside California (71–73).

Distribution

The ecologic niche of CI is the soil of the lower Sonoran life zone, a semiarid area with hot summers, infrequent winter freezes, and alkaline boron-rich soil (74). The areas of highest endemicity are in the southwestern United States (and northeastern Utah) and northern Mexico, although scattered areas of Central America (the Montagua Valley in Guatemala and the Comayagua Valley

of Honduras) and South America (parts of Venezuela, Colombia, Paraguay, Bolivia, Argentina, and Brazil) also harbor the fungus (75–82) (Fig. 271.5). The distribution of the fungus within these areas is, for incompletely defined reasons, spotty.

Infection may also be acquired outside the usual endemic areas under unusual circumstances such as the occurrence of coccidioidomycosis in epidemic form in nonendemic areas when a dust storm blew out of the Central Valley of California in 1977 and blanketed parts of the coastal region (83). This event did not appear to result in the establishment of new areas of endemicity.

Prevalence and Incidence

Prevalence studies largely rely on skin-test surveys. Some surveys indicate that with an annual rate of new infections of 3% to 5%, as many as 75% to 90% of long-term residents of highly endemic areas such as Tucson, Arizona, have been infected at some time in their lives (12,82). Other studies, however, report a lower prevalence (84). Skin-test surveys may actually underestimate prevalence because some patients with proven coccidioidomycosis never develop dermal sensitivity to antigens of the etiologic agent and because of apparent waning of skin-test reactivity (82,84).

Data from skin-test surveys have led to estimates that 25,000 to 100,000 new infections are acquired annually in the United States (79). The average annual percentage of cases of symptomatic coccidioidomycosis among individuals presenting to the student health service of the University of Arizona in

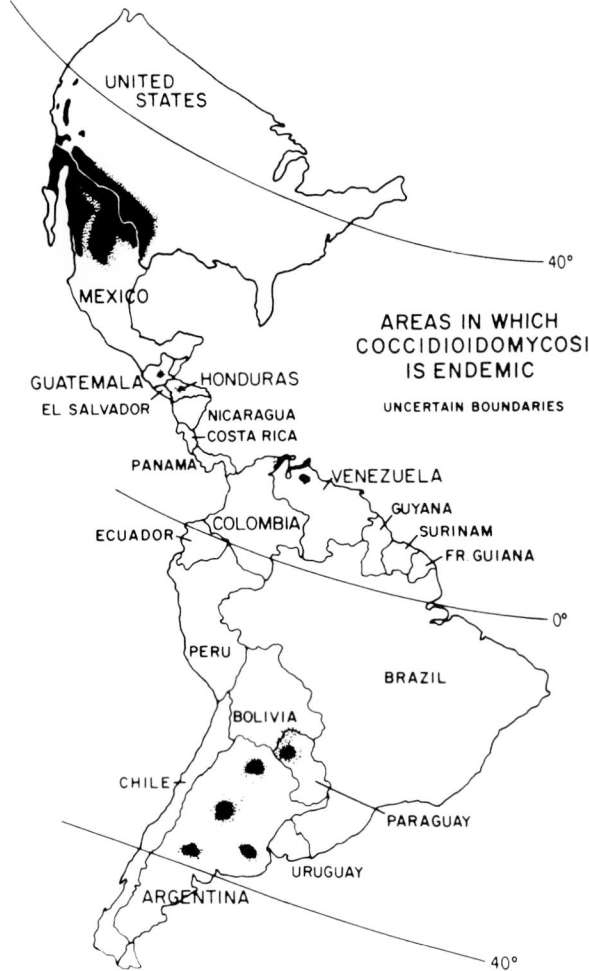

Figure 271.5. This map displays the regions in which coccidioidomycosis is most highly endemic. The stippled areas represent the uncertain boundaries. Not represented are recently identified endemic areas in northeastern Utah in the United States and in northeastern Brazil. (From Pappagianis D. In: Stevens DA, ed. *Coccidioidomycosis*. New York: Plenum Publishing, 1980:64, with permission.)

Tucson between 1979 and 1983 was 0.43% (85). Attack rates of 60% to 93% have been reported in point-source exposures such as have occurred in archeology students and military personnel (86–89). The incidence of reported cases in Arizona doubled from 7.0 per 100,000 population in 1990 to 14.9 per 100,000 in 1995 (90).

The incidence of acute primary infection usually reaches a peak in the dry period from summer to late fall in California, and two seasonal peaks are seen in Arizona (91,92). The annual number of cases reported in California, a statistic that had remained relatively constant for more than a decade, increased almost 10-fold, to approximately 5,000, during the early 1990s, most likely as the result of an unusual sequence of prolonged drought followed by heavy rains (93,94).

Symptoms are reported by approximately 40% of those infected and approximately 5% develop pulmonary residua such as nodules or cavities. Potentially life-threatening acute or chronic disseminated forms of the disease occur in approximately 1%, but this frequency varies widely depending on a number of genetic, demographic, and clinical factors. Severe disease has been associated with both ABO blood group and class II human leukocyte antigen (HLA) loci (95). Filipinos have a risk of dissemination estimated as 10 to 175 times that of non-Hispanic whites. African Americans also have an increased risk

for dissemination, although of lesser magnitude (12,95). More recent studies have found that independent risk factors for severe pulmonary infection include diabetes mellitus, recent cigarette smoking, low income, and older age (96,97), whereas those for dissemination include being African American, being pregnant, and having low income (96).

Pregnancy abrogates the apparent relative protection of non-Hispanic white women from dissemination (98,99), possibly as a result of the trophic effects of estrogen and progesterone on CI and the relative immunocompromise of pregnancy (41,42). Immunosuppressive disease and therapies that blunt the cellular immune response also increase the risk of severe disease (100,101).

PATHOGENESIS AND IMMUNE RESPONSE

Arthroconidia convert to the spherule-endospore phase within 48 to 72 hours of inhalation infection. The initial inflammatory response to arthroconidia, which temporarily retain an antiphagocytic outer wall layer (102) (Fig. 271.2B), consists of an influx of polymorphonuclear leukocytes (103), possibly in response to a complement-dependent chemotaxinogen (104). Coincident with conversion to the spherule phase, the infiltrate develops mononuclear cell predominance and well-formed granulomata may be produced. Spherule rupture with release of endospores is associated with a transient reversion of the infiltrate to one predominantly consisting of polymorphonuclear leukocytes (103), consistent with the observation that spherule lysates are chemotaxigenic for neutrophils (104,105). Normal human polymorphonuclear leukocytes, but not those of patients with chronic granulomatous disease, inhibit the incorporation of N-acetylglucosamine into cell wall chitin of arthroconidia (106). Polymorphonuclear leukocytes also release lysozyme, which may affect the surface of the spherule wall (107). The effect of polymorphonuclear leukocytes on spherules is limited, however, possibly because of the presence of an extracellular glycoprotein fibrillar matrix, as well as the large size of this form of the organism relative to that of the neutrophil (108).

Both murine and primate macrophages readily phagocytose arthroconidia and endospores but fail to kill them, probably as the result of failure of phagosome-lysosome fusion (109,110). *In vitro* activation of murine peritoneal macrophages before infection by incubation with spherule-stimulated lymphocyte culture supernatant is associated with enhanced phagosome-lysosome fusion and killing of CI (111). This effect can be duplicated by incubation with recombinant interferon-γ (IFN-γ) (112). Studies with susceptible and resistant strains of mice also indicate that IFN-γ plays a key role in protection, whereas interleukin-4 (IL-4) diminishes protective immunity against CI (113–118). IL-1α, IL-6, IL-12, and tumor necrosis factor-α (TNF-α) may also play roles in protection in the mouse; IL-10 may be detrimental. Experimental infection in mice is associated with production of not only TNF-α and IL-6, but also IL-4 (118). Pretreatment of human peripheral blood mononuclear cells with either IFN-γ or TNF-α leads to enhanced growth inhibition of ingested endospores but not of arthroconidia (119,120). Mature spherules induce murine peritoneal macrophages to produce TNF-α (121). These observations are consistent with evidence that the primary murine effector cells in resistance to this fungus are polymorphonuclear leukocytes and macrophages (122).

Human dendritic cells pulsed with coccidioidal antigens prime lymphocytes for coccidioidal antigen-specific responses (123,124) and lymphocytes from patients with coccidioidomycosis respond *in vitro* to soluble antigens of CI as well as to intact killed spherules, arthrospores, and endospores (125,126). The *in vitro* response of peripheral blood mononuclear cells from normal individuals with positive skin-test responses to spherule-derived antigens includes enhanced production of IL-2 and IFN-γ, but the correlation of the magnitude of these responses with the intensity of the dermal hypersensitivity reaction to the same antigens is poor (126). Human glass adherent peripheral blood mononuclear cells incubated with killed arthroconidia or spherules produce TNF-α, and these cells ingest killed endospores and can phagocytose arthroconidia and inhibit their growth (127,128). Patients with disseminated disease often have impaired lymphocyte response to coccidioidal antigens, in parallel with defective cutaneous delayed hypersensitivity reactions (13,129–134).

Adoptive transfer of immunity in mice is T-lymphocyte dependent (109) and susceptibility of inbred strains of mice to infection with CI appears to be influenced by a gene whose product is expressed in spleen cells and is associated with an acquired suppression of coccidioidal-specific cell-mediated immunity (110–112). Loss of immunologic responsiveness in mice appears to be due to the activation of a splenic suppressor cell population induced by circulating coccidioidal antigen (132). In humans, suppression of lymphocyte responses may be mediated by immunoglobulin G (IgG), either alone or in immune complexes (133). This is consistent with the observation that serum antibody to CI is not protective. There is, in fact, generally a direct relationship between the magnitude of the complement-fixing antibody response and the extent of extrapulmonary dissemination of the fungus (13,14).

The importance of a robust cellular immune response to CI infection, together with the lack of protection afforded by antibody, suggests that a favorable outcome depends on the development of a dominant helper T cell type 1 (T_H1) response (134,135). The T_H1 cytokine IFN-γ appears to play a key role in protective immunity, whereas the helper T cell type 2 (T_H2) cytokine IL-4 impairs an effective immune response in murine models (117). IL-12 administration to mice significantly ameliorates systemic infection with CI, and this is associated with a shift from a T_H2 to a T_H1 cytokine pattern in pulmonary lymphocytes (135) and coadministration of an IL-12 expression vector enhances protective immunity elicited by vaccination (136). Examination of cytokine production patterns of peripheral blood mononuclear cells obtained from patients with disseminated infection and from coccidioidal-immune control subjects also suggests that inadequate immunologic control of CI is associated with a relatively deficient T_H1 response (137). Furthermore, this hypothesis is also consistent with evidence of a correlation between elevated serum concentrations of immunoglobulin E (IgE) and disease severity, because IL-4, a cytokine that is key to the T_H2-dominant response, facilitates B-cell switching to IgE production (138–140). IL-5, another cytokine associated with the T_H2 response, is a potent regulator of eosinophil production and eosinophilia, sometimes associated with disseminated infection (141). To the extent that T_H1 dominance is important for recovery from infection with CI, cytokine therapy (e.g., IL-12, IL-2, IFN-γ) or anticytokine therapy (e.g., anti–IL-4) may possibly prove therapeutically effective.

The characteristics of CI that account for its virulence are little understood. A surface glycoprotein, SOWgp, produced only by the spherule-endospore form of the organism acts as an adhesin and appears to contribute to the virulence of the organism (50,51). Endospores produce urease and respond to an acid environment by increased production of ammonium. Thus, endospores that have been ingested by phagocytic cells may increase the pH level within the phagosome and thereby avoid degradation by its acid proteases (142). An enzyme with elastase (and lesser collagenase) activity, possibly identical to or a subunit of the serine proteinase

thought to be important in the dissolution of the segmentation apparatus during spherule-endospore reproduction, has been recovered from culture filtrates of the parasitic phase of CI. The activity of this enzyme peaks at the time of endospore release. This ability to enzymatically degrade connective tissue matrix macromolecules may have an important role in the pathogenesis of coccidioidomycosis. Breakdown of pulmonary connective tissue matrix at the time of endospore release may allow intrapulmonary and extrapulmonary spread of the organism and may contribute to progressive loss of pulmonary parenchyma and cavity formation (143). In addition, the enzymatic breakdown products of elastin are chemotactic and may thus further contribute to the inflammatory response (144).

CLINICAL MANIFESTATIONS

Primary Infection

Infection results in symptomatic illness in only approximately 40% of cases. In most of these, it consists of a prolonged and sometimes severe but self-limited influenza-like illness, commonly with pneumonitis (Figs. 271.6 and 271.7). Approximately 5% are left with pulmonary residua such as nodules and cavities (12). Fewer than 1% of patients develop clinically apparent extrapulmonary dissemination.

Symptoms reported by most patients with clinical illness include fatigue, cough, and chest pain. Approximately one half report fever, and one fifth complain of dyspnea, although arthralgia, myalgia, and headache are each also reported by one fifth (145,146). Patients with acute primary infection may develop various presumably immune-mediated complications. Most prominent among these are exanthems, including nonspecific, often evanescent erythematous macular or confluent skin eruptions and erythrodermas, erythema multiforme, and erythema nodosum. Elements of more than one type of eruption may be present simultaneously. Erythema nodosum occurs most commonly in young nongravid female patients and is an indicator of good prognosis (12); this correlation may be strongest when infection occurs during pregnancy (147).

Patients may also develop arthritis ("desert rheumatism"), a manifestation that must be differentiated from joint infection resulting from hematogenous dissemination of CI (145).

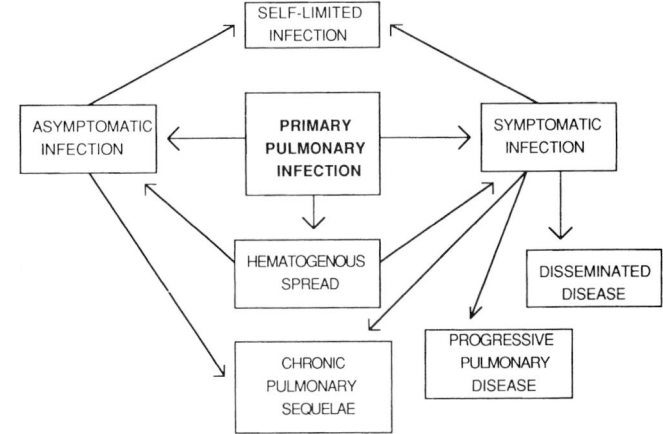

Figure 271.6. Suggested overall schema of infection with *Coccidioides immitis*. The probable occurrence of asymptomatic dissemination is suggested by the frequent finding of chorioretinitis and by recovery of *C. immitis* from the urine in patients without other clinical evidence of dissemination.

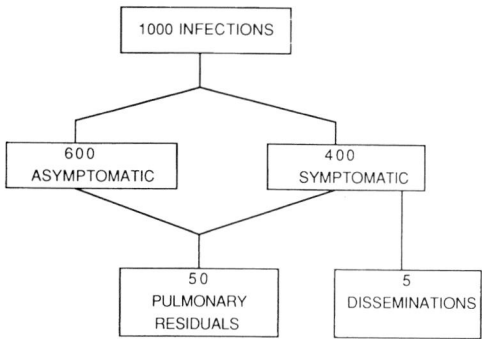

Figure 271.7. Outcome of infection. (Based on data from Smith CE, Beard RR, Whiting EG, et al. Varieties of coccidioidal infection in relation to the epidemiology and control of disease. *Am J Public Health* 1946;36:1394, with permission.)

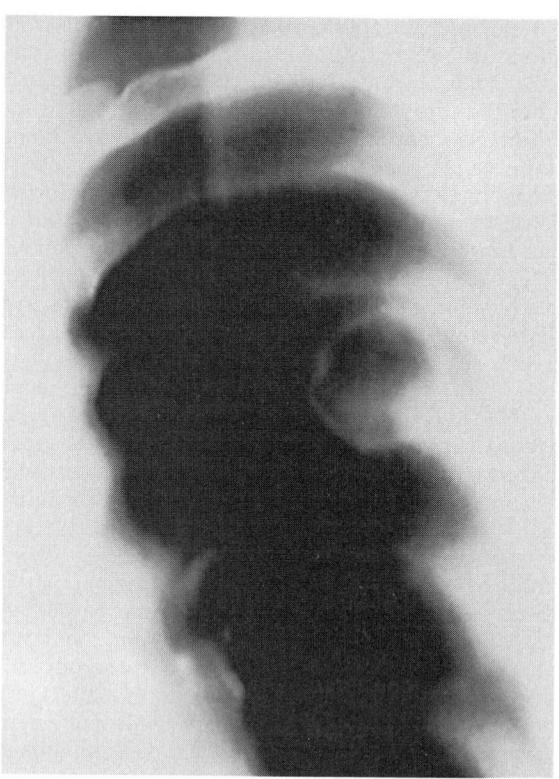

Figure 271.8. Thin-walled pulmonary cavity caused by *Coccidioides immitis.* (Courtesy Dr. David Stevens, Santa Clara Valley Medical Center, San Jose, California.)

Unusual examples of immune-mediated disease in CI infection include glomerulonephritis associated with mixed cryoglobulinemia, and occult pulmonary coccidioidomycosis in which a cold-reacting protein contained anticoccidioidin IgG (148). Although transient eosinophilia is common, especially in patients with these immunologic manifestations, persistent eosinophilia may be indicative of dissemination (149). The total white blood cell count is usually normal (148).

Pulmonary Disease

Pneumonia, though usually self-limited, may become acutely progressive, sometimes leading to respiratory failure; a more indolent chronic progressive form of pneumonitis is also recognized (150–155). Abnormalities on the chest radiograph are evident in approximately half of patients with acute symptomatic infection and consist most often of segmental or lobar consolidation or of nodular or patchy infiltrates. Small pleural effusions and hilar adenopathy are each seen in approximately 20% (156,157). The latter finding is thought to be associated with an increased risk of dissemination.

Acutely progressive pulmonary disease may be associated with a diffuse miliary or reticulonodular radiographic pattern, often together with mediastinal adenopathy (158). Miliary disease with dissemination may be associated with a picture of septic shock (158). Exudative pleural and pericardial effusions may result from serosal involvement (159–161). In one series, 48% of patients with pleural effusion had erythema nodosum or erythema multiforme (161). Airway infection may present with hoarseness in patients with laryngeal involvement and may result, particularly in children, in upper airway obstruction (162–164). Endobronchial lesions occur and may be associated with atelectasis (164). Cavitation, characteristically thin walled, of lung parenchyma (Fig. 271.8) may regress, stabilize, or proceed progressively and inexorably, and the subsequent clinical course may be benign or complicated by hemoptysis, mycetoma, rupture into the pleural space, and bacterial superinfection (165–168). Residual asymptomatic pulmonary nodules, if first discovered at a time remote from the primary infection, may require distinction from malignant neoplasm (169). Other pulmonary residua include fibrosis, bronchiectasis, and calcifications (156,157,169).

Disseminated Infection

At least two observations suggest that subclinical dissemination commonly occurs during the acute phase of infection. Chorio-

retinal lesions have been found in as many as 40% of patients with acute infection in the absence of other clinical or laboratory evidence of dissemination (170,171) and CI can frequently be recovered from urine of patients thought to have only pulmonary disease (172,173). Clinically evident dissemination, which generally declares itself within the first 6 months after primary infection, may be widespread, involving multiple sites, and rarely may be associated with septic shock (174). Most often, however, the clinical disease resulting from dissemination is apparently limited to just a few sites or even just one site. Frequently identified sites of disseminated disease include skin and subcutaneous tissues, bones and joints, lymph nodes, liver, spleen, genitourinary tract (175,176), peritoneal cavity (177), eyes (178,179), thyroid (180,181), and, most devastatingly, the central nervous system. Infection of vascular graft material may occur as the result of dissemination (182). Hypercalcemia has been reported in association with disseminated infection (183).

SKIN

Skin is the most commonly recognized site of dissemination. Manifestations of hematogenous skin infection include plaques, papules (which are often verrucous), pustules, granulomatous lesions, and subcutaneous abscesses (184) (Fig. 271.9). The prognosis for survival in patients with skin lesions depends on the extent of involvement of other organ systems; those with little or no disease at other sites generally experience a relatively benign outcome with treatment. The presence of an ulcerating subcutaneous lesion must lead to consideration of it, representing the egress site of a sinus tract. Such tracts may be remarkably extensive and a reflection of distant disease, most commonly of bone. Direct inoculation into skin results in primary

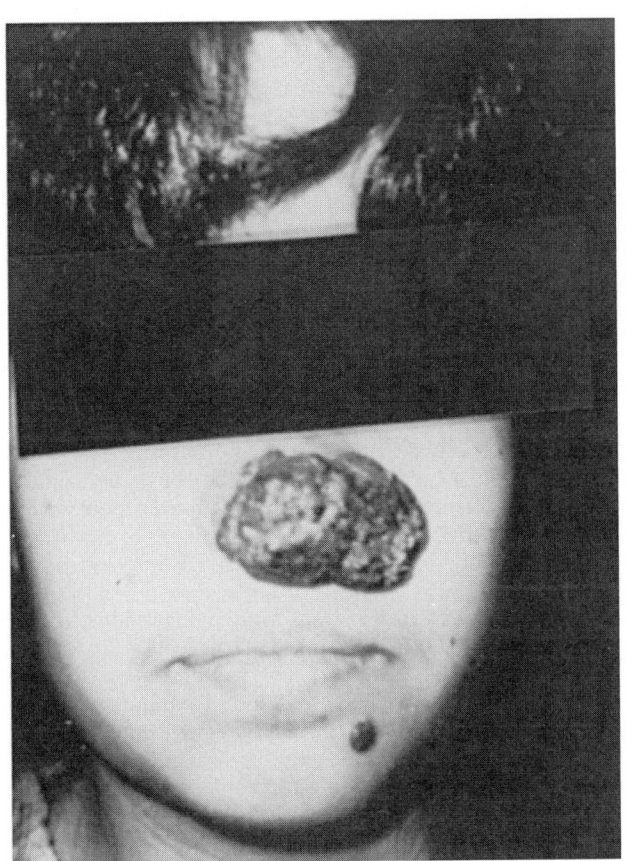

Figure 271.9. Two skin lesions on the face of a child with disseminated coccidioidomycosis: an exuberant verrucous tumor-like lesion of the nose and one of the chin that appears nodular and granulomatous. (Courtesy Dr. Richard Tucker, Wenatchee Valley Clinic, Wenatchee, Washington.)

cutaneous coccidioidomycosis, which may manifest as a chancriform lesion.

CENTRAL NERVOUS SYSTEM

Dissemination to the central nervous system results in clinical and laboratory findings typical of chronic granulomatous meningitis, although unusual presentations, such as anterior spinal artery syndrome or parenchymal abscess, may occur (185–189). Thus, onset is usually gradual with complaints and findings that include headache, vomiting, stiff neck, diplopia, confusion, ataxia, and cranial neuropathies (190). The presence of systemic symptoms is variable and may be absent.

Several neurohistopathologic patterns are described: leptomeningitis, leptomeningitis with cerebritis, leptomeningitis with cerebritis and infarcts (with associated endarteritis obliterans involving small penetrating arteries), and rarely disseminated miliary granulomata (191). Cerebral abscess formation occurs rarely but may do so in the absence of frank meningitis (189,192). Computed tomography, useful in detecting hydrocephalus (193), commonly reveals contrast enhancement of the basilar meninges. Magnetic resonance imaging is more sensitive and may detect intense contrast enhancement of the cervical subarachnoid space, as well as of the basilar, sylvian, and interhemispheric cisterns. In addition, focal parenchymal signal abnormalities consistent with ischemia or infarction may be seen, as may, on occasion, mass lesions that are usually hypodense and enhancing (189,192,194).

Examination of cerebrospinal fluid (CSF) reveals a predominantly mononuclear pleocytosis (with the total white blood cell count generally in the range of 100 to 1,500 cells/mm³), elevated protein concentration, and often low glucose level. CSF eosinophilia is common; approximately one third of patients in one series had more than 10 eosinophils/mm³ of CSF (195), and this finding may be helpful in suggesting the diagnosis. CSF protein concentration is in most cases less than 300 mg/dL; a concentration approaching or exceeding 1,000 mg/dL suggests the presence of obstruction to CSF flow (193). Tests performed on ventricular CSF may be misleading, because in the absence of ventriculitis (an uncommon complication), the abnormalities detected may be minimal or absent. Because the organism is very rarely visualized directly and is recovered in culture from CSF in only a few cases, the etiologic diagnosis usually depends on the detection of IgG antibody to the fungus in CSF. The development of hydrocephalus (most often communicating) is a common complication (196) and may be the result of an ongoing inflammatory response with persisting pleocytosis and elevated CSF concentrations of proinflammatory cytokines (197). Individual ventricles may become trapped (198). Large-vessel vasculitis, which may cause infarction, is associated with high mortality (199–201) and may also be associated with aneurysm formation and subsequent rupture with production of subarachnoid hemorrhage (202). Thrombosis of dural and cerebral veins may occur (203). Meningitis, which is ultimately uniformly fatal in the absence of treatment, remains a highly morbid and potentially lethal disease despite aggressive therapeutic management.

MUSCULOSKELETAL SYSTEM

The most common site of coccidioidal osteomyelitis is the vertebral column, followed by tibia, skull, metacarpals, metatarsals, femur, and ribs (204–211). Infection is polyostotic in 40% of patients. Paraspinal abscesses, often with extensive sinus tract formation, commonly accompany vertebral infection. Lesions of larger bones appear primarily lytic on radiographs, but those of the small bones of the hands and feet often have an irregular moth-eaten appearance (210,212). Magnetic resonance imaging of coccidioidal spondylitis may reveal unifocal or multifocal lesions with usual involvement of intervertebral discs, and vertebral body marrow, as well as of adjacent epidural and soft tissue (213). Technetium pyrophosphate (⁹⁹ᵐTc) methylene diphosphonate bone scans and gallium-67 (⁶⁷Ga) scans are complementary and are more sensitive than radiographic examination (214,215). It has been suggested that all patients with suspected disseminated coccidioidomycosis undergo bone scanning to identify cryptic bone disease (214). Hypercalcemia has been reported in coccidioidomycosis, but not all affected patients have evident infection of bone, suggesting that a humoral or diffusible osteolytic substance is responsible (216–218).

Patients with coccidioidal infection of joints (204–207) represent approximately 20% of those with disseminated disease. Infection also affects extraarticular sites in 25% of patients of coccidioidal arthritis at the time of presentation. Arthritis is monoarticular in 90%, with the large weight-bearing joints most commonly involved in adult patients. Thus, the knee is affected in approximately three fourths of patients and the ankle in 10%; the elbow, wrist, hip, and interphalangeal joints being less commonly involved. The small joints of the hands and feet appear to be involved with greater frequency in children than adults. Synovial effusions are exudative, with protein concentrations in excess of 3.0 g/dL and with total white blood cell counts as high as 50,000/mm³ with a predominantly mononuclear cell pleocytosis. Culture of synovial fluid yields the organism in approximately half the cases; culture and histologic examination of synovial tissue may have a greater yield. Tenosynovitis may occur in the absence of bone or joint infection (219).

OTHER SITES

Disseminated infection may present with coccidioidal lymphadenitis. Any site within the genitourinary tract may be affected, including kidneys, prostate (220,221), testicles, and epididymis (175,222), as well as ovaries, oviducts, and uterus (176,223,224). CI may be recovered from urine in the absence of overt urinary tract disease (172,173). Peritonitis with an exudative peritoneal effusion may occur (177), may present as an omental mass (225), and has been described in patients undergoing continuous ambulatory peritoneal dialysis (226) in whom an eosinophilic effusion may be present. Both liver abscess and biliary tract infection are reported (227,228). Ocular involvement may consist of asymptomatic chorioretinitis, as well as necrotizing conjunctivitis and potentially sight-threatening iridocyclitis (170,171,178,179). Endocrine organs affected have included, in addition to adrenal glands, thyroid and pituitary gland (180,181,229). Infection of the mastoids may occur.

Infection in the Immunocompromised Host

Dissemination in the patient with impaired cellular immunity may occur in the context of recent infection or reactivation of latent infection (230–232). In either case, the clinical presentation may be explosive, rapidly progressive, and often fatal (232–235). Furthermore, serologic test results may be falsely negative (236). One third of patients with hematologic malignancy with coccidioidomycosis had disseminated infection (236). Approximately 5% of cardiac allograft recipients in Arizona developed coccidioidomycosis, with reactivation of past infection being responsible in a number of these (237). The risk of developing coccidioidomycosis in the first year after renal transplantation during maximum immune suppression among patients in Arizona is, however, only 2% to 3% greater than that for subsequent years, suggesting that reactivation of latent infection accounts for only a small proportion of cases in this setting (238). Infection has occurred as the result of transmission via a transplanted lung (62). Whereas the risk of development of coccidioidal disease diminishes after the first posttransplant year, the potential for late reactivation remains significant and accounts for the fact that allograft recipients and other similarly immunocompromised patients may first present in a geographic location outside the endemic area (237,238).

Because persisting antibody (but not skin-test reactivity) appears to be a marker of increased risk of reactivation after immunosuppression, serum coccidioidal antibodies should be measured in any transplant candidate who has been in a coccidioidomycosis-endemic area, even if only briefly or remotely in time (238). Those with serum antibody to CI before transplantation or with a known history of coccidioidomycosis should be considered candidates to receive antifungal therapy during times of peak posttransplantation immunosuppression, although patients with cystic fibrosis may have falsely positive serologic test results for IgM antibody to CI antigens (238a). Posttransplantation serologic surveillance should be performed in these patients (237,238). Coccidioidomycosis was reported with increasing frequency in patients infected with human immunodeficiency virus (HIV) in the era before the availability of highly active antiretroviral therapy (HAART) (101). The estimated cumulative rate of active coccidioidomycosis among HIV-infected patients residing in an endemic area was as high as 25% after 41 months of observation, with those with a diagnosis of acquired immunodeficiency syndrome (AIDS) or a CD4+ lymphocyte count of less than 250 cells/mm³ being at greatest risk (239). Neither a positive skin-test result nor a prior history of coccidioidomycosis contributed significantly to this risk (239,240),

although a history of oropharyngeal or esophageal candidiasis has been identified as increasing the risk of coccidioidal disease, as has being African American (241). As with organ transplant recipients, however, coccidioidal seropositivity may identify a group with increased risk for subsequent active coccidioidomycosis. In one study performed in an endemic area, seropositivity in the absence of contemporaneous active coccidioidomycosis was associated with an approximately 70% risk for active fungal infection at 36 months compared with a previously reported risk of approximately 25% during a similar period among HIV-infected patients who initially had no detectable antibody to coccidioidal antigens (238,240).

This problem is not limited to areas of CI endemicity; almost half of the HIV-infected patients reported to the Centers for Disease Control and Prevention with disseminated coccidioidomycosis resided in nonendemic counties in 35 states (242). This observation, which is most likely the consequence of late reactivation of dormant infection resulting from progressive immunodeficiency, demonstrates the importance of an accurate lifelong travel and residence history in HIV-infected patients (243).

A history of receipt of an azole antifungal for *Candida* infection has been reported to be associated with protection from the development of coccidioidomycosis (241). Whereas consideration has been given to prophylaxis in selected patients (e.g., those with low CD4+ lymphocyte counts resident in or traveling to endemic areas and those with a positive serologic test result), no clinical trial data exist to validate such an approach (244,245).

The presentation and course of CI infection in HIV-infected patients depend to a large extent on the level of immunocompromise as generally reflected by the CD4+ lymphocyte count (246). In patients with relatively intact cellular immunity, coccidioidomycosis most often resembles that observed in the general population. However, in patients with low CD4+ lymphocyte counts, diffuse reticulonodular pulmonary disease and extrapulmonary dissemination appear to occur with increased frequency (244,246). In one series, two thirds had diffuse reticulonodular lung infection, while approximately 15% had focal pulmonary disease or a normal chest radiograph; 15% had meningitis (246). The mortality rate of coccidioidomycosis in HIV-infected patients in the pre-HAART era was reported to be as high as 60% (246). Those presenting with bilateral interstitial pulmonary infection have been reported to have a median survival of only 1 to 2 months, but those with only unilateral focal lung disease often follow a relatively benign clinical course given appropriate therapy (244,246).

The diagnosis of coccidioidomycosis in HIV-infected patients often requires a high index of suspicion. Not only may patients often first present outside endemic areas, but approximately 20% will have negative serologic test results and some have normal chest radiographs (244,246,247). On the other hand, persisting seropositivity may be seen in HIV-infected patients without evidence of active coccidioidomycosis (240). Furthermore, active coccidioidomycosis may coexist with other opportunistic infections. Of particular concern is its occasional simultaneous presentation with *Pneumocystis jiroveci (carinii)* pneumonia. In that circumstance, coccidioidomycosis may first become evident as the result of clinical worsening in the face of adjunctive corticosteroid therapy given for *Pneumocystis* pneumonia (248).

Pregnancy

Pregnancy is an independent risk factor for the development of dissemination consequent to infection with CI (96,249), although the risk may be less than previously believed (147). It has been estimated that the rate of dissemination after infection in the first trimester is 23%; the risks in the second and third trimesters are 59% and 68%, respectively (249), although in one series, dissemination throughout pregnancy occurred in only 9% and no fatalities were observed among 32 patients (147). Analysis of more recent data indicates an increased risk for coccidioidal meningitis in pregnant women relative to those not pregnant but fails to confirm an increased risk of dissemination after infection acquired in the third trimester relative to earlier trimesters (250). The development of erythema nodosum is associated with a favorable outcome in pregnancy; in one series, dissemination occurred in no patients with erythema nodosum, whereas 35% without this manifestation suffered from disseminated infection (251).

Neonatal coccidioidomycosis is rare (252), possibly because the placenta appears to be resistant to infection (253). The normal placenta, however, produces cytokines, such as IL-4 and IL-10, which are associated with a T_H2-like lymphocyte response and which may inhibit local T_H1-like responses that could otherwise be injurious to the fetus (254). Systemic spillover of this effect would be expected to lead to increased susceptibility to intracellular pathogens. The increasing risk for dissemination as pregnancy progresses is consistent with both the trophic effects of estradiol and progesterone on CI, as well as evidence of reduced cellular immunity to antigens of CI near term and in the postpartum period (41,42,255).

LABORATORY DIAGNOSIS

Direct Examination

Histologic or microbiologic identification of CI remains the most reliable means of diagnosis of coccidioidal infection. Direct examination of body tissues, exudates, or respiratory tract secretions may permit visualization of the characteristic parasitic form of CI, the spherule. In cases of widespread dissemination, bone marrow or liver biopsy specimens may, on occasion, provide diagnostic information (256,257). Pus and sputum may be examined by potassium hydroxide preparation with Parker's superchrome ink or lactophenol cotton blue stain added to enhance visualization. Papanicolaou stain of a cytologic preparation of sputum is superior to potassium hydroxide preparation, however (258,259). Fungal stains, such as periodic acid–Schiff, may enhance detection and identification, as may calcofluor white (260). Cytologic examination of bronchoalveolar lavage fluid obtained from patients with pulmonary coccidioidomycosis reveals the organism in approximately half of cases; culture and histologic examination of tissue obtained by transbronchial biopsy may improve diagnostic sensitivity (261). Detection of the characteristic endosporulating spherule is diagnostic. However, some pollens, especially that of the mulberry, cottonwood, and elm trees (262) that may be found in respiratory tract secretions, can resemble the spherules of CI.

Examination of cytologic preparations of specimens obtained by fine-needle aspiration of pulmonary lesions commonly reveals the presence of endosporulating spherules, and granulomata may not be detected, presumably because of the small sample size (263). The organism may be readily identified on histologic examination of biopsy specimens on routine staining with hematoxylin-eosin or Gomori–methenamine silver. The only organisms that produce a tissue phase that may morphologically resemble a mature spherule are *Prototheca westermani* (264) and *Rhinosporidium seeberi* (265), but the internal septations of the former can be distinguished from endospores and the sporangia of

the latter, reaching as much as 350 μm in diameter, are much larger than spherules of CI. Small, immature, nonendosporulating spherules of CI may be confused with yeasts such as *Blastomyces dermatitidis* and *Cryptococcus neoformans*. The mycelial forms of CI are occasionally also visualized in tissue, especially in pulmonary cavities, in which with careful examination they have been reported to be present in up to 75% of specimens and in approximately 30% of pulmonary granulomata (266). Hyphal forms have also been observed in coccidioidal pulmonary mycetomas (167,267) and in CSF obtained from patients with coccidioidal meningitis and central nervous system plastic devices such as shunts on which CI may grow as a biofilm (268–270).

Culture

If coccidioidomycosis is suspected, the microbiology laboratory must be notified when it is sent samples for cultivation because of the significant biohazard represented by the mycelial phase of this organism. Specimens should be inoculated onto slants, rather than plates, to reduce the hazard.

CI may be isolated from a wide variety of clinical sources, including sputum, exudates, prostatic secretions, urine, tissue, bone marrow (271), CSF, and very rarely blood (272). Potentially contaminated specimens, such as sputum, should be processed within 2 hours to minimize overgrowth of bacteria. CI will grow on most routine media, including those containing 0.4 mg/mL of cycloheximide, which inhibits most morphologically similar nonpathogenic fungi. Growth is usually visible within 3 to 6 days of inoculation of Sabouraud's dextrose agar and with incubation at 25°C to 30°C; the agar surface rapidly becomes covered. Colonies may initially appear smooth and moist but soon develop an abundant aerial mycelium. Colonies are initially white but with continued incubation darken to become tan or brown. As many as 20% of isolates may exhibit variations in pigmentation and other atypical morphological features (23).

CI can be recovered from the urine of 9% to 24% of patients with pulmonary coccidioidomycosis when a large volume of the first morning urine is processed by centrifugation with inoculation of the sediment onto appropriate media (172,173). With prostatic involvement, expressed secretions may yield a positive culture. CI may rarely be recovered from blood after inoculation into trypticase soy broth (vented) and incubation for a median of 5 days; positive blood cultures are obtained almost exclusively from severely immunocompromised patients (272). Inoculation of spherules into BACTEC 6B media yields visible growth within several days of inoculation (273).

Microscopic examination of a culture tease preparation will demonstrate branched septate hyphae, approximately 2 μm wide, with alternating barrel-shaped arthroconidia and clear zones termed *disjunctors*. The arthroconidia are 3.0 to 4.5 μm wide and 3 to 12 μm long (274). Although this morphological appearance is strongly suggestive of CI, it is not pathognomonic. More than a dozen keratinophilic soil fungi produce similarly appearing arthroconidia and cannot be readily distinguished from CI morphologically when grown at 25°C (274). These nonpathogenic mimes include *Malbranchea*, *Geotrichum*, *Arthroderma*, *Uncinocarpus*, *Oidiodendron*, and *Auxarthron* (275,276).

Definitive morphological identification of an isolate as CI classically relied on demonstration that the mold recovered on culture media converted to an endosporulating spherule after inoculation into animals. Phase conversion can also be achieved *in vitro* at 37°C to 40°C under increased carbon dioxide tension (277). The identification of exoantigens of CI in culture supernatants by immunodiffusion can obviate the need to demonstrate phase conversion (278,279). A commercially available

Diagnosis of Coccidioidomycosis

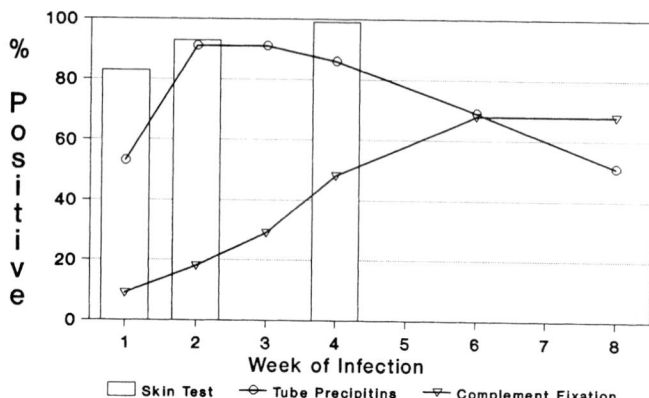

Figure 271.10. Skin-test response to coccidioidin and tube precipitin and complement-fixing antibody responses in the first 8 weeks of symptomatic illness. (Provided by Dr. Richard Tucker and based on data from references 13, 14.)

Diagnosis of Coccidioidomycosis

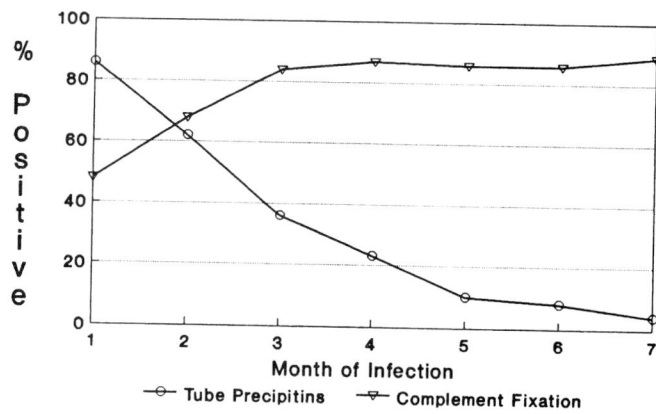

Figure 271.11. Tube precipitin and complement-fixing antibody test results from months 1 through 7 after the onset of symptomatic illness. (Provided by Dr. Richard Tucker and based on data from references 13, 14.)

deoxyribonucleic acid (DNA) probe (Gen-Probe) that specifically identifies CI genomic material is becoming the method of choice for this purpose (276,280).

Skin Test

The demonstration of a delayed dermal reaction to the administration of coccidioidal antigens was previously widely used to detect infection. Skin-test reactivity may be detected as early as 3 days after onset of symptoms. Of those who develop a positive reaction, 83% do so in the first week, 93% by the end of the second week, and 99% by the end of the fourth week (281) (Fig. 271.10). Although reactivity may wane with time, it often persists for life, thus rendering the skin test useless as a tool for the diagnosis of active infection. Repeated skin testing may cause apparent conversion to a positive reaction because of a boosting phenomenon or by sensitization to noncoccidioidal antigens in the preparation (282); as a result, even apparent skin-test conversion may be suspect. The utility of skin testing, therefore, is largely as an epidemiological tool, but it also has prognostic utility. Patients who are anergic to coccidioidal skin-test antigens (such anergy is often specific to antigens of this fungus) are more likely to suffer from disseminated infection (13), to respond poorly to therapy, and to suffer relapses of their disease after discontinuation of therapy (283). Restoration of skin-test reactivity may occur in the course of successful therapy (130).

Two skin-test reagents have been used for detection of delayed dermal sensitivity to CI: coccidioidin, a culture filtrate of the mycelial phase, and Spherulin, a filtrate of the spherule-endospore phase of the organism (284–287). Both represent mixtures of numerous predominantly polysaccharide antigens and require standardization by bioequivalence testing. In each case, induration of at least 5 mm in diameter 24 to 72 hours after intradermal injection is considered a positive reaction. Neither coccidioidin nor Spherulin skin testing elicits antibody responses to coccidioidal antigens (288,289), but coccidioidin may elicit a serologic response to histoplasmin (289). At this time, neither reagent is commercially available.

Serology

Serologic tests are very useful in the diagnosis and management of coccidioidomycosis (290,291) (Figs. 271.10 and Fig. 271.11). The

initial IgM antibody response to infection with CI can be demonstrated in 90% of patients within 1 to 3 weeks after the onset of symptoms of acute primary infection using a tube precipitin test (14). IgM antibody that detects the same antigen (46) can also be detected with somewhat greater sensitivity by an immunodiffusion test. A third test used to detect IgM antibody to CI, the latex particle agglutination test, may become positive before either the tube precipitin or the immunodiffusion assay but has lesser specificity; consequently confirmation of positive latex agglutination test results must be confirmed by one of these alternative methods. IgM antibodies are seldom detectable for more than 6 months after infection, and they have no prognostic value. Their usefulness lies in the ability to detect serologic evidence of coccidioidomycosis soon after infection and in providing an ability to determine the time frame in which an infection had occurred. Tests for the detection of IgM antibody to CI are not, however, useful in the examination of CSF of patients suspected of having coccidioidal meningitis.

IgG antibody to coccidioidin may be detected by sheep red blood cell complement fixation, immunodiffusion, or enzyme immunoassay. The immunodiffusion test detects an antibody that corresponds to the complement-fixing antibody detected by the sheep red blood cell method but has somewhat greater specificity (290–292). Results obtained using a commercially available enzyme immunoassay correlate well with those obtained by complement fixation (293,294). IgG antibody is first detectable by either method several weeks after the onset of infection and after tests that detect IgM antibody to CI antigens have become positive. The complement-fixation test for CI is, in addition to its diagnostic value, extremely useful in estimating the extent of infection (14), prognosis (14,283), and in following the response to therapy (291).

When performed in a reliable reference laboratory, the height of the complement-fixing antibody titer determined by the sheep red blood cell method has a direct correlation with the activity and extent of infection, with titers greater than 1:16 often heralding the presence of extrapulmonary dissemination (14) (Table 271.1). Patients with single-site dissemination (e.g., a solitary bone site) may have a lower titer. The immunodiffusion test with detection of IgG antibody corresponding to complement-fixing antibody gives comparable qualitative results and may also be of value when it is used quantitatively (292). An enzyme-linked immunosorbent assay

TABLE 271.1.	Complement-fixing Antibody Titer and Dissemination of Coccidioidomycosis		
Clinical status		Patients (N)	Complement-fixing antibody titer >1:16 (%)
Not disseminated			
Primary infection (no dissemination)		3,154	5.3
Pulmonary residua (including cavities)		848	1.0
Disseminated			
All disseminated		709	61.0
Single site (not meningeal)		141	15.0
Meningitis		136	49.0
Extensive dissemination (not meningeal)		291	83.0

Source: Adapted from Smith CE, Saito MT, Simmons SA. Pattern of 39,500 serologic tests in coccidioidomycosis. *JAMA* 1956;160:546–552, with permission.

capable of detecting IgM and IgG antibody to CI is also available; results obtained with this test appear to correlate with those obtained with alternative methods (293,294). A practical strategy is to use the immunodiffusion test for initial detection of both IgM and IgG antibodies to CI, including a concentrate of the patient's serum to enhance sensitivity, followed by the complement-fixation test for confirmation and quantification (291).

Despite their clinical value, caution must be exerted in interpretation of these serologic tests. Seropositivity (IgG antibody) may persist after recovery from infection; this may be especially true among HIV-infected patients and allograft recipients (237,240). Fifteen percent of patients with cystic fibrosis are reported to have falsely positive IgM antibody results (238a). Serologic cross-reactions with antigens of other fungi, including *H. capsulatum* and *B. dermatitidis,* have been reported. Sixteen percent of patients with acute histoplasmosis have complement-fixing antibody to CI (295).

Some patients with chronic cavitary coccidioidomycosis may have negative complement-fixing antibody test results. Although most patients who are immunocompromised by virtue of renal failure, underlying malignant neoplasms, or immunosuppressive therapy seem to maintain their ability to mount an antibody response to infection (233), some patients with hematologic malignancies or AIDS who are infected with CI may not (236,246,296). Significant interlaboratory variation in the results of the complement-fixation test, as well as variation in results obtained with different commercially available immunodiffusion kits, presents important additional problems (297).

Both the complement-fixing antibody and the immunodiffusion tests are invaluable in the diagnosis of coccidioidal meningitis, because culture of CSF fails to yield CI in the overwhelming majority of cases. The detection of complement-fixing antibody in nontraumatically obtained CSF is pathognomonic of meningeal coccidioidomycosis in the absence of a parameningeal focus of infection; however, the CSF of as many as 5% of patients will not have detectable antibody, particularly if the sample is obtained very early in the course of disease. Effective therapy is reflected in a reduction of CSF complement-fixing antibody titer, whereas a rising titer is indicative of failing therapy (185–187).

One potential method of circumventing the vagaries of the host antibody response for diagnosis is to detect circulating fungal products. Antigens of CI have been detected in the serum of one half to three fourths of patients with active coccidioidomy-

cosis, but such tests have not been systematically evaluated or made commercially available (298–300).

DIFFERENTIAL DIAGNOSIS

The protean manifestations of coccidioidomycosis compel the consideration of a wide range of alternative diagnoses. When patients present with immunologic manifestations of acute primary infection, consideration must be given to diseases such as acute allergic reactions, serum sickness, rheumatoid arthritis, vasculitis, and many more. The differential diagnosis of acute pneumonia is broad. Patients with chronic cavitary disease or solitary pulmonary nodules must be evaluated for, among other things, the possibility of malignant neoplasm, other granulomatous infections such as tuberculosis, and histoplasmosis, or immunologic diseases, such as Wegener's granulomatosis. Coccidioidomycosis is often misdiagnosed as neoplastic disease, especially in patients with solitary pulmonary nodules (301,302).

The differential diagnosis of chronic meningitis caused by CI encompasses many etiologic considerations (303). These include tuberculosis, cryptococcosis, malignant neoplasm, and immunologic disease, such as Behçet's syndrome. Coccidioidal osteomyelitis or arthritis often resembles that due to *Mycobacterium tuberculosis,* as do cold abscesses due to CI infection (204–206). The extensive sinus tract formation sometimes seen in CI infection may also be seen with some other infections, such as blastomycosis and actinomycosis.

TREATMENT

For an overview of treatments of infection, see references 304 and 305, as well as Table 271.2.

Nonmeningeal Infection

PULMONARY

Most primary coccidioidal infections are self-limited. For that reason, and because of the known toxicities of amphotericin B, treatment has historically been reserved for instances in which the illness is unusually severe, progressive or disseminated, or in which the patient is in a high-risk category for the development of extrapulmonary disease as a result of demographic, clinical, or serologic factors (306,307). With the availability of effective, well-tolerated orally administered azoles, the threshold for initiation of treatment has been lowered, and some clinicians consider the treatment of many patients with uncomplicated primary pulmonary coccidioidomycosis appropriate even in the absence of increased risk of dissemination (308). Pharmacoeconomic analysis suggests that such treatment is cost-effective in all except those with the lowest risk for complications of their infection (309). A case-control study found that receipt of oral antifungal therapy was associated with a reduced risk of development of severe pulmonary disease (96). However, no treatment modality for this form of coccidioidomycosis has been subjected to prospective randomized placebo-controlled trials.

The appropriate duration of treatment of uncomplicated primary pulmonary coccidioidomycosis in the immunologically intact host is unknown, but antifungal administration should probably be continued for 3 to 6 months, including 3 months after all signs and symptoms of the active infection have resolved. The presence of a persistently high or rising complement-fixing antibody titers dictate an even more prolonged duration of therapy. Longer courses may also be considered in patients in risk

TABLE 271.2. Summary Recommendations for Treatment of Coccidioidomycosis

Indication		Treatment
Primary pulmonary infection	Discomfort, superinfection, absent	Observe OR Treat with either fluconazole[a] 400 mg daily or itraconazole 200 mg twice daily for approximately 3–6 mo, including 3 mo after resolution of clinical infection
	Dissemination risk present	Treat with either fluconazole 400 mg/d or itraconazole 200 mg b.i.d. for at least 3–6 mo, including at least 3 mo after resolution of clinical infection
	Diffuse (bilateral reticulonodular or miliary) pulmonary disease	Initiate treatment with amphotericin B; consider substitution of an azole after clinical improvement is achieved; treat for at least 1 yr (longer if patient is immunocompromised)
Pulmonary nodule		Antifungal therapy is unnecessary in the absence of significant immunodeficiency
Pulmonary cavity	Asymptomatic	Observe for 2 or more years; consider chemotherapy and/or resection if it persists, demonstrate progressive enlargement, is immediately adjacent to the pleura, or becomes symptomatic
	Symptomatic (local discomfort, superinfection, hemoptysis)	Chronic or intermittent azole therapy OR Resection
	Ruptured into pleural space	Lobectomy with decortication together with antifungal chemotherapy OR Chest tube drainage with antifungal chemotherapy
Chronic fibrocavitary disease		Azole therapy for at least 1 yr OR Surgical resection (if refractory and localized or if significant hemoptysis is present) plus azole therapy
Nonmeningeal disseminated disease	Immediately life threatening	Amphotericin B 0.6–1.0 mg/kg/d; consider switch to fluconazole or itraconazole when control is achieved, and continue for a minimum of 1–2 yr; lifelong therapy may be required OR fluconazole ≥400 mg/d or itraconazole ≥200 mg b.i.d., usually for a minimum of 1–2 yr; lifelong therapy may be required
	Slowly progressive or stable	Fluconazole ≥400 mg/d or itraconazole ≥200 mg b.i.d., usually for a minimum of 1–2 yr; lifelong therapy may be required in some cases
Meningitis		Fluconazole ≥400 mg/d or itraconazole ≥200 mg b.i.d., lifelong therapy may be required OR (in some cases) Azole orally plus amphotericin B directly into cerebrospinal fluid space

[a]Azoles are teratogenic and must be avoided in pregnancy.
Source: Adapted from Galgiani JN, Ampel NM, Catanzaro A, et al. Practice guideline for treatment of coccidioidomycosis. Infectious Diseases Society of America. *Clin Infect Dis* 2000;30:650–661, with permission.

groups for dissemination. Patients with progressive pulmonary or disseminated infection not involving the central nervous system should continue to receive chemotherapy for at least 1 to 2 years, including at least 6 to 12 months after the disease appears to have been rendered inactive by clinical, microbiologic, and serologic assessments. Treatment of those with ongoing severe immunocompromise may require treatment for the duration of their immune deficiency, which may be lifelong. Asymptomatic solitary pulmonary nodules in the absence of immunocompromise do not require therapeutic intervention. The approach to cavitary and fibrocavitary lung disease is variable (Table 271.2).

Many clinicians continue to consider amphotericin B to be the initial treatment of choice for rapidly progressive or otherwise life-threatening infection. Lipid formulations of amphotericin B have not been subjected to comparative clinical trials in patients with coccidioidomycosis, but they are at least as effective as the conventional deoxycholate formulation in a murine model of infection (310). With stabilization of the infection, consideration of changing therapy from amphotericin B to an orally administered azole may be considered.

Noncomparative trials using ketoconazole indicate that it may be efficacious, although the relapse rate is high; in the absence of randomized trial data, its efficacy relative to other agents is unknown (311–314). Fluconazole is effective in the treatment of chronic pulmonary and nonmeningeal disseminated coccidioidomycosis, although the relapse rate, even after prolonged therapy, remains high (315,317). Noncomparative experience suggested that itraconazole was also efficacious and a subsequent comparative trial confirmed this (316). In that trial, itraconazole (200 mg twice daily) proved at least as effective as fluconazole (400 mg once daily) in the treatment of patients with nonmeningeal progressive coccidioidomycosis involving lung, soft tissue, or skeletal structures after 8 months of therapy, and results at 12 months suggested superiority of itraconazole, especially in patients with skeletal disease (317).

Among agents under investigation, posaconazole appears, based on noncomparative clinical data, to be the most promising (318). Voriconazole is active against CI *in vitro*. Caspofungin has activity in a murine model of CI infection (319).

The response to therapy can be gauged by a falling complement-fixing antibody titer, as well as by clinical and microbiologic assessments. All apparently successful therapies for coccidioidomycosis carry a risk of relapse after discontinuation of drug administration, and thus, careful prolonged follow-up, both clinical and serologic, is necessary. Risk factors for relapse include the presence of immunodeficiency, a negative coccidioidin skin-test result, and a peak complement-fixing antibody titer more than or equal to 1:256 (283).

Immunomodulatory therapy has been attempted in the past with "transfer factor," an ill-defined heterogeneous product of antigen-stimulated peripheral blood mononuclear cells, but its efficacy remains unproven (320). The potential role of cytokines is under investigation. One of these, IL-2, had no effect in a murine model of coccidioidomycosis (321). Other potential candidates for investigation include IL-12, IFN-γ, and granulocyte-macrophage colony-stimulating factor.

Bone and Joint Infection

Coccidioidal infection of joints is difficult to eradicate. Intraarticular amphotericin B produces cartilage damage in experimental animals and thus probably carries some risk in humans. Radical synovectomy, though difficult to accomplish totally, may produce the best chance of cure, when used in combination with systemically administered antifungal chemotherapy. Patients with coccidioidal osteomyelitis may benefit from surgical débridement in combination with systemic chemotherapy (211). Although topical irrigation of osteomyelitic lesions or of associated sinus tracts is commonly used, its role is uncertain (204–206). Randomized trial data suggest that itraconazole may be superior to fluconazole in the treatment of skeletal CI infection (317).

Pulmonary Cavity Infection

Cavitary lung lesions often respond poorly to chemotherapy (322). Stable asymptomatic cavities may best be ignored, but rapidly expanding cavities, life-threatening hemoptysis, recurrent bacterial superinfection, and threatened rupture into the pleural space are indications for surgical resection (323).

Ocular Infection

Ocular infection, such as chorioretinitis, granulomatous conjunctivitis, and iridocyclitis, should be treated with a systemically administered antifungal agent. Amphotericin B has been administered by intraocular injection (178), but the value and safety of this mode of administration is unproven.

Meningitis

The largest experience in the treatment of coccidioidal meningitis has been with amphotericin B deoxycholate, a drug that does not penetrate into CSF after intravenous administration and that is ineffective when given by that route alone for this indication. Treatment of meningitis with this polyene antibiotic therefore requires its delivery directly into the intrathecal or intraventricular space (324,325). The drug may be administered into the lumbar space, into the cisterna magna, by lateral cervical puncture, or into a lateral ventricle after placement of an indwelling catheter with a subcutaneous reservoir (325). Because abnormalities of CSF flow patterns are common in these patients and in fact loculation of fluid may occur, it is important to define flow initially and at intervals thereafter, using radionuclide or other dynamic techniques. An oral azole agent is usually concomitantly administered with intrathecal amphotericin B.

When amphotericin B is administered into the lumbar space, it is probably best to use the so-called hyperbaric method in which the drug is in 10% dextrose in water, together with 20 mg

of hydrocortisone, after which the patient is placed in the Trendelenburg position for approximately 45 minutes. This method has two potential benefits: delivery of the drug to the site of maximal infection, the basal meninges; and rapid removal from the lumbar space, where the drug may cause arachnoiditis, radiculitis, myelitis, and spinal artery thrombosis. Whichever route is used, treatment is initiated with small doses of 0.01 to 0.05 mg. Each dose is administered in dextrose in water together in an attempt to reduce local adverse effects. The dose is gradually increased, on a daily basis, until a maximally tolerated dose of 0.5 to 2.0 mg is reached. CSF protein level, glucose level, and cell counts are monitored after each dose, and CSF CI complement-fixing antibody titers are measured at intervals. The dose of amphotericin and the interval between administrations may need to be altered at times because of toxic effects. As clinical and laboratory improvement occurs, the dosing interval is progressively prolonged. Whereas the desired total duration of this therapeutic modality has not been well defined, one recommended approach is to discontinue treatment when CSF measurements, including the complement-fixing antibody titer, have stably returned to normal or nearly normal and have remained so for at least 12 to 24 months, during which time CSF should be examined and amphotericin B administered every 4 to 6 weeks. Periodic examination of CSF for at least 1 year after discontinuation of intrathecal therapy is probably wise. Relapse may, however, occur many years later (185,324). As a result of the high frequency of relapse, many patients continue to receive an orally administered azole after therapy with intrathecally administered amphotericin B has been discontinued.

Coadministration of an azole may decrease the total amount of intrathecal amphotericin B required for treatment (326). Patients who present with mild meningitis may be treated with azoles alone, although some clinicians favor initiation of intrathecally administered amphotericin B in most patients to rapidly gain control of the infection. Treatment with orally administered fluconazole, a drug with excellent penetration into CSF, is reported, when given alone, to yield response rates comparable to those previously reported with intrathecally administered amphotericin B (324,327–329). The use of higher doses (e.g., 800 mg daily) may hasten the response to therapy but is associated with an increased risk of adverse reactions. Itraconazole therapy, sometimes also in high dose, has also produced clinical and laboratory responses in patients with coccidioidal meningitis, despite the relative lack of penetration of this drug into CSF (330). Treatment of coccidioidal meningitis with azoles may have to be administered for the life of the patient in many cases because of the high risk for relapse when these basically fungistatic therapies are discontinued after apparent resolution of infection (331).

Impairment of CSF flow resulting in hydrocephalus is a common complication of coccidioidal meningitis and is amenable to the placement of a CSF shunt (332,193). Another potential cause for deterioration of the patient is bacterial superinfection of a CSF shunt or intra-CSF catheter, which usually requires removal of the foreign body for cure. Deterioration may also be the result of associated vasculitis (200). Anecdotal experience and experimental animal model evidence indicate promise for systemically administered liposomal amphotericin B in the treatment of coccidioidal meningitis (333).

Special Underlying Conditions

PREGNANCY

The apparent high risk for dissemination of coccidioidomycosis during the second and third trimesters of pregnancy necessitates strong consideration of therapy in all patients whose infection presents during that period. Azoles are not considered safe for use in pregnancy because of their teratogenicity (334,335). There is a reasonable record of safe use of amphotericin B in pregnancy, so this drug remains the systemic antifungal agent of choice for use in pregnancy.

HUMAN IMMUNODEFICIENCY VIRUS INFECTION

Primary nonprogressive pulmonary coccidioidomycosis has resolved without treatment in some HIV-infected patients with relatively high CD4+ lymphocyte counts. Nonetheless, all HIV-infected patients with active coccidioidomycosis should probably receive antifungal chemotherapy. Those with disseminated infection and/or advanced immunodeficiency should receive such therapy indefinitely, although it may prove acceptable, as has been the case with several other opportunistic infections, to discontinue maintenance antifungal therapy in patients who experience immune reconstitution in response to antiretroviral therapy (336).

The absorption of many drugs from the gastrointestinal tract may be reduced in patients with AIDS. Because hypochlorhydria is common in HIV infection (337), drugs such as ketoconazole and itraconazole, which require low gastric pH levels for absorption when administered in capsule form, may have poor bioavailability. An additional concern with regard to the use of the azoles is the potential for pharmacokinetic interactions with other drugs taken by patients with AIDS, such as rifampin, rifabutin, clarithromycin (338,339), efavirenz, buffered preparations of didanosine, and at least some HIV protease inhibitors.

Clinical studies are required to determine whether patients with AIDS with positive serologic test results for coccidioidomycosis in the absence of active fungal infection would benefit from preemptive therapy. Also to be determined is the potential benefit of prophylactic therapy in patients with AIDS resident in or traveling to endemic areas.

PREVENTION

Immunization

While a protective coccidioidal vaccine is feasible and desirable (340), none is currently available. A trial of a relatively crude spherule-derived vaccine in humans yielded disappointing results (341,342). Vaccination with urease, urease DNA (343), or with Ag2/PRA or its N-terminal fragment has demonstrated efficacy in murine models of infection (344–347).

General Preventive Measures

Because no vaccine is available, prevention of infection entails avoidance of exposure to the fungus either in its natural setting or in the laboratory setting. In addition, CI may be temporarily eliminated from small soil foci by the use of fungicides. Patients with pulmonary and other forms of coccidioidomycosis do not require isolation. However, in the health care setting, dressings should be changed daily, and material contaminated with infected body substances should be disposed of promptly. Masks should be worn during procedures that may create aerosols from sites with high-density infection. Disinfection of surfaces can be accomplished with iodophors, phenols, formaldehyde, and hypochlorite (348,349). Although CI is the only human fungal pathogen on the "Select Agent" list, its potential usefulness as a bioweapon is questionable (350).

ACKNOWLEDGMENTS

The authors would like to acknowledge the assistance of Ms. Rebbeca Simmons and Ms. Melanie Della Santina, as well as the bibliographic assistance of Lynn Marsh, librarian at Sequoia Hospital, Redwood City, California.

REFERENCES

1. Fiese MJ. *Coccidioidomycosis.* Springfield, IL: Charles C. Thomas, 1958.
2. Deresinski SC. History of coccidioidomycosis: "dust to dust." In: Stevens DA, ed. *Coccidioidomycosis: a text.* New York, Plenum Publishing, 1980: 1–20.
3. Posada A. Un nuevo caso de micosis fungoidea con psorospermias. *An Circ Med Argent* 1892;15:585–597.
4. Rixford E. A case of protozoic dermatitis. *Occident Med Times* 1894;8:704–707.
5. Rixford E, Gilchrist TC. Two cases of protozoan (coccidioidal) infection of the skin and other organs. *Johns Hopkins Hosp Rep* 1896;1:209–268.
6. Ophüls W, Moffitt HC. A new pathogenic mould (formerly described as a protozoan (*Coccidioides immitis pyogenes*): preliminary report. *Phila Med J* 1900;5:1471–1472.
7. Ophüls W. Further observations on a pathogenic mould formerly described as a protozoan (*Coccidioides immitis, Coccidioides pyogenes*). *J Exp Med* 1905;6:443–486.
8. Ophüls W. Coccidioidal granuloma. *JAMA* 1905;45:1201–1296.
9. Stewart RA, Meyer KF. Isolation of *Coccidioides immitis* from soil. *Proc Soc Exp Biol Med* 1932;29:937–938.
10. Dickson EC. "Valley fever" of the San Joaquin Valley and fungus *Coccidioides. Calif West Med* 1937;47:151–155.
11. Dickson EC, Gifford MA. *Coccidioides* infection (coccidioidomycosis). *Arch Intern Med* 1938;62:853–871.
12. Smith CE, Beard RR, Whiting EG, et al. Varieties of coccidioidal infection in relation to the epidemiology and control of the disease. *Am J Public Health* 1946;36:1394–1402.
13. Smith CE, Whiting EG, Baker EE, et al. The use of coccidioidin. *Am Rev Tuberc* 1948;57:330–360.
14. Smith CE, Saito MT, Simmons SA. Pattern of 39,500 serologic tests in coccidioidomycosis. *JAMA* 1956;160:546–552.
15. Currah RS. Taxonomy of the Onygenales: Arthrodermataceae, Gymnoascaceae, Myxotrichaceae and Onygenaceae. *Mycotaxin* 1985;24:1–216.
16. Bowman BH, Taylor JW, White TJ. Molecular evolution of the fungi: human pathogens. *Mol Biol Evol* 1922;9:893–904.
17. Pappagianis D, Omelas A, Hector R. Guanine plus cytosine content of the DNA of *Coccidioides immitis. Sabouraudia* 1985;23:451–454.
18. Kwon-Chung KJ. *Coccidioides immitis:* Cytological study on the formation of the arthrospores. *Can J Genet Cytol* 1969;11:43–53.
19. Sun SH, Huppert M. A cytological study of morphogenesis in *Coccidioides immitis. Sabouraudia* 1976;14:185–198.
20. Klotz SA, Drutz DJ, Huppert M, et al. The critical role of CO_2 in the morphogenesis of *Coccidioides immitis* in cell-free subcutaneous chambers. *J Infect Dis* 1984;150:127–134.
21. Baker O, Braude AI. A study of stimuli leading to the production of spherules in coccidioidomycosis. *J Lab Clin Med* 1956;47:169–181.
22. Galgiani JN, Hayden R, Payne CM. Leukocyte effects on the dimorphism of *Coccidioides immitis. J Infect Dis* 1982;146:56–63.
23. Huppert M, Sun SH. Overview of mycology and the mycology of *Coccidioides immitis.* In: Stevens DA, ed. *Coccidioidomycosis: a text.* New York: Plenum Publishing, 1980:21–46.
24. Cole GT, Sun SH. Arthroconidium-spherule-endospore transformation in *Coccidioides immitis.* In: Szaniszlo PJ, ed. *Fungal dimorphism: with emphasis on fungi pathogenic for humans.* New York: Plenum Publishing, 1985:281–333.
25. Burt A, Carter DA, Koenig GL, et al. Molecular markers reveal cryptic sex in the human pathogen *Coccidioides immitis. Proc Natl Acad Sci U S A* 1996; 93:770–773.
26. Hung CY, Yu JJ, Lehmann PF, et al. Cloning and expression of the gene which encodes a tube precipitin antigen and wall-associated beta-glucosidase of *Coccidioides immitis. Infect Immun* 2001;69:2211–2222.
27. Guevara-Olvera L, Hung CY, Yu JJ, et al. Sequence, expression and functional analysis of the *Coccidioides immitis* ODC (ornithine decarboxylase) gene. *Gene* 2000;242:437–448.
28. Yuan L, Cole GT, Sun SH. Possible role of a proteinase in endosporulation of *Coccidioides immitis. Infect Immun* 1988;56:1551–1559.
29. Yuan L, Cole GT. Characterization of a proteinase inhibitor isolated from the fungal pathogen *Coccidioides immitis. Biochem J* 1989;257:729–736.
30. Huppert M, Sun SH, Harrison JL. Morphogenesis throughout saprobic and parasitic cycles of *Coccidiodes immitis. Mycopathologia* 1982;78:107–122.
31. Wheat RW, Tritschler C, Conant NF, et al. Comparison of *Coccidioides immitis* arthrospore, mycelium and spherule cell walls, and influence of

growth medium on mycelial cell wall composition. *Infect Immun* 1977;17: 91–97.

32. Wheat RW, Su Chung KS, Ornellas EP, et al. Extraction of skin test activity from *Coccidioides immitis* mycelia by water, perchloric acid and aqueous phenol extraction. *Infect Immun* 1978;19:152–159.

33. Wheat RW, Su Chung KS. Antigenic fractions of *Coccidioides immitis*. In: Ajello L, ed. *Coccidioidomycosis: current clinical and diagnostic status*. Miami, FL: Symposia Specialists, 1977:453–460.

34. Wheat RW, Scheer E. Cell walls of *Coccidioides immitis*: neutral sugars of aqueous alkaline extract polymers. *Infect Immun* 1977;17:91–97.

35. Cole GT, Hung CY. The parasitic cell wall of *Coccidioides immitis*. *Med Mycol* 2001;39[Suppl 1]:31–40.

36. Hector R, Pappagianis D. Enzymatic degradation of the walls of spherules of *Coccidioides immitis*. *Exp Mycol* 1982;6:136–152.

37. Zimmer BL, Pappagianis D. Taxonomic and physiologic characteristics of *Coccidioides immitis*. In: Leive L, ed. *Microbiology*. Washington, DC: American Society for Microbiology, 1986:165–168.

38. Lones G. Studies of intermediary metabolism in *Coccidioides immitis*. In: Ajello L, ed. *Coccidioidomycosis: proceedings of the 2nd symposium on Coccidioidomycosis*. Tucson, AZ: University of Arizona Press, 1965:349–353.

39. Baker EE, Smith CE. Utilization of carbon and nitrogen compounds by *Coccidioides immitis* (Rixford and Gilchrist, 1896). *J Infect Dis* 1942;70: 51–53.

40. Sippel JE, Levine HB. Sugars and amino acids as carbon, nitrogen, or energy sources for *Coccidioides immitis* spherules and endospores. *Appl Microbiol* 1969;18:522–524.

41. Powell BL, Drutz DJ, Huppert M, et al. Relationship of progesterone- and estradiol-binding proteins in *Coccidioides immitis* to coccidioidal dissemination in pregnancy. *Infect Immun* 1983;40:478–485.

42. Powell BL, Drutz DA. Identification of a high-affinity binder for estradiol and a low-affinity binder for testosterone in *Coccidioides immitis*. *Infect Immun* 1984;45:784–786.

43. Cox RA, Huppert M, Starr P, et al. Reactivity of alkali soluble, water-soluble cell wall antigen of *Coccidioides immitis* with anti-*Coccidioides* immunoglobulin M precipitin antibody. *Infect Immun* 1984;43:502–507.

44. Ward ER, Cox RA, Schmitt JA, et al. Delayed-type hypersensitivity responses to cell wall fraction of the mycelial phase of *Coccidioides immitis*. *Infect Immun* 1975;12:1093–1097.

45. Lecara G, Cox RA, Simpson RB. *Coccidioides immitis* vaccine: potential of an alkali-soluble, water-soluble cell wall antigen. *Infect Immun* 1983;39:437–475.

46. Hung CY, Yu JJ, Lehmann PF, et al. Cloning and expression of the gene which encodes a tube precipitin antigen and wall-associated beta-glucosidase of *Coccidioides immitis*. *Infect Immun* 2001;69:2211–2222.

47. Johnson SM, Pappagianis D. The coccidioidal complement fixation and immunodiffusion-complement fixation antigen is a chitinase. *Infect Immun* 1992;60:2588–2592.

48. Landay ME, Wheat RW, Conant NF, et al. Serological comparison of spherules and arthrospores of *Coccidioides immitis*. *J Bacteriol* 1967;94:1400–1405.

49. Huppert M, Spratt NS, Vukovich KR, et al. Antigenic analysis of coccidioidin and Spherulin determined by two dimensional immunoelectrophoresis. *Infect Immun* 1978;20:541–551.

50. Hung CY, Ampel NM, Christian L, et al. A major cell surface antigen of *Coccidioides immitis*, which elicits both humoral and cellular immune responses. *Infect Immun* 2000;68:584–593.

51. Hung CY, Yu JJ, Seshan KR, et al. A parasitic phase-specific adhesin of *Coccidioides immitis* contributes to the virulence of this respiratory fungal pathogen. *Infect Immun* 2002;70:3443–3456.

52. Cairns L, Blythe D, Kao A, et al. Outbreak of coccidioidomycosis in Washington state residents returning from Mexico. *Clin Infect Dis* 2000;30: 61–64.

53. Coccidioidomycosis in workers at an archeologic site—Dinosaur National Monument, Utah, June–July 2001. *MMWR Morb Mortal Wkly Rep* 2001;50:1005–1008.

54. Schneider E, Hajjeh RA, Spiegel RA, et al. A coccidioidomycosis outbreak following the Northridge, Calif, earthquake. *JAMA* 1997;277:904–908.

55. Converse JL, Reed RE. Experimental epidemiology of coccidioidomycosis. *Bacteriol Rev* 1966;30:678–695.

56. Kohn GJ, Linne SR, Smith CM, et al. Acquisition of coccidioidomycosis at necropsy by inhalation of coccidioidal endospores. *Diagn Microbiol Infect Dis* 1992;15:527–530.

57. Pappagianis D. Coccidioidomycosis. In: Demis DJ, ed. *Clinical dermatology*. Hagerstown, MD: Harper & Row, 1973:1–11.

58. Wilson JW, Smith CE, Plunkett OA. Primary cutaneous coccidioidomycosis. *Calif Med* 1953;79:233–239.

59. Bernstein DI, Tipton JR, Schoot SF, et al. Coccidioidomycosis in a neonate: maternal-infant transmission. *J Pediatr* 1981;99:752–754.

60. Spark RP. Does transplacental spread of coccidioidomycosis occur? Report of a neonatal fatality and review of the literature. *Arch Pathol Lab Med* 1981;105:347–350.

61. Perez JA, Abraham J. Coccidioidomycosis: a new sexually transmitted disease? Centennial Conference on Coccidioidomycosis (abstract 28). In: Programs and abstracts of the 5th International Conference on Coccidioidomycosis; August 24–27, 1994; Stanford University; Stanford, Calif.

62. Tripathy U, Yung GL, Kriett JM, et al. Donor transfer of pulmonary coccidioidomycosis in lung transplantation. *Ann Thorac Surg* 2002;73:306–308.

63. Eckmann BH, Schaefer GL, Huppert MH. Bedside transmission of coccidioidomycosis via growth on fomites. *Am Rev Respir Dis* 1964;89:1175–1185.

64. Gehlbach SH, Hamilton JD, Conant NF. Coccidioidomycosis. An occupational disease in cotton mill workers. *Arch Intern Med* 1973;131:254–255.

65. Schwarz J, Kantman CA. Occupational hazards from deep mycoses. *Arch Dermatol* 1977;113:1270–1275.

66. Velasco-Castrejón O, González-Ochoa A. Coccidioidomicosis adquirida en la ciudad de Mexico. Un caso atipico desde el punto de vista epidemiologico. *Rev Invest Salus Publica* 1975;35:97–102.

67. Desai SA, Minai OA, Gordon SM, et al. Coccidioidomycosis in non-endemic areas: a case series. *Respir Med* 2001;95:305–309.

68. Chaturvedi V, Ramani R, Gromadzki S, et al. Coccidioidomycosis in New York State. *Emerg Infect Dis* 2000;6:25–29.

69. Standaert SM, Schaffner W, Galgiani JN, et al. Coccidioidomycosis among visitors to a *Coccidioides immitis*–endemic area: an outbreak in a military reserve unit. *J Infect Dis* 1995;171:1672–1675.

70. Zimmerman CR, Snedker CJ, Pappagianis D. Characterization of *Coccidioides immitis* isolates by restriction fragment length polymorphisms. *J Clin Microbiol* 1994;32:3040–3042.

71. Burt A, Dechairo BM, Koenig GL, et al. Molecular markers reveal differentiation among isolates of *Coccidioides immitis* from California, Arizona and Texas. *Mol Ecol* 1997;6:781–786.

72. Koufopanou V, Burt A, Taylor JW. Concordance of gene genealogies reveals reproductive isolation in the pathogenic fungus *Coccidioides immitis*. *Proc Natl Acad Sci U S A* 1997;94:5478–5482.

73. Fisher MC, Rannala B, Chaturvedi V, et al. Disease surveillance in recombining pathogens: multilocus genotypes identify sources of human *Coccidioides* infections. *Proc Natl Acad Sci* 2002;99:9067–9071.

74. Maddy KT. The geographic distribution of *Coccidioides immitis* and possible ecologic implications. *Ariz Med* 1958;15:178–188.

75. Padua y Gabriel A, Martinez-Ordaz VA, Velasco-Rodriguez VM, et al. Prevalence of skin reactivity to coccidioidin and associated risks factors in subjects living in a northern city of Mexico. *Arch Med Res* 1999;30:388–392.

76. Eulalio KD, de Macedo RL, Cavalcanti MA, et al. *Coccidioides immitis* isolated from armadillos (*Dasypus novemcinctus*) in the state of Piaui, northeast Brazil. *Mycopathologia* 2001;149:57–61.

77. Martins Mdos A, de Araujo Eda M, Kuwakino MH, et al. Coccidioidomycosis in Brazil. A case report. *Rev Inst Med Trop Sao Paulo* 1997;39:299–304.

78. Wanke B, Lazera M, Monteiro PC, et al. Investigation of an outbreak of endemic coccidioidomycosis in Brazil's northeastern state of Piaui with a review of the occurrence and distribution of *Coccidioides immitis* in three other Brazilian states. *Mycopathologia* 1999;148:57–67.

79. Pappagianis D. Epidemiology of coccidioidomycosis. In: Stevens DA, ed. *Coccidioidomycosis: a text*. New York: Plenum Publishing, 1980: 63–85.

80. Rippon JW. *Medical mycology*. Philadelphia: WB Saunders, 1988:435–439.

81. Pappagianis D. Epidemiology of coccidioidomycosis. *Curr Top Med Mycol* 1988;2:199–238.

82. Hicks MJ, Hagaman RM, Barbee RA. The prevalence of cellular immunity to coccidioidomycosis in a highly endemic area. *West J Med* 1986;144:425–428.

83. Pappagianis D, Einstein H. Tempest from Tehachapi takes toll. *West J Med* 1978;129:527–530.

84. Dodge RR, Lebowitz MD, Barbee R, et al. Estimates of *C. immitis* infection by skin test reactivity in an endemic area. *Am J Public Health* 1985;75:863–865.

85. Kerrick SS, Lundergan LL, Galgiani JN. Coccidioidomycosis at a University Health Service. *Am Rev Respir Dis* 1985;131:100–102.

86. Gilman DW, Wehrle PF, Cowper H. Coccidioidomycosis—Canoga Park, California. *MMWR Morb Mortal Wkly Rep* 1965;14:302–303.

87. Lacy GH, Swatek FE. *Coccidioides* in California. In: Ajello L, ed. *Coccidioidomycosis: current clinical and diagnostic status*. Miami, FL: Symposia Specialists, 1977:79–90.

88. Werner SB, Pappagianis D, Heindl I, et al. An epidemic of coccidioidomycosis among archaeology students in northern California. *N Engl J Med* 1972;286:507–512.

89. Crum N, Lamb C, Utz G, et al. Coccidioidomycosis outbreak among United States Navy SEALs training in a *Coccidioides immitis*–endemic area—Coalinga, California. *J Infect Dis* 2002;186:865–868.

90. Ampel NM, Mosley DG, England B, et al. Coccidioidomycosis in Arizona: increase in incidence from 1990 to 1995. *Clin Infect Dis* 1998;27:1528–1530.

91. Smith CE, Beard RR, Rosenberger HG, et al. Effect of season and dust control on coccidioidomycosis. *JAMA* 1946;132:833–838.

92. Hugenholtz P. Climate and coccidioidomycosis. In: Ferguson MS, ed. *Proceedings of the symposium on Coccidioidomycosis*. Atlanta: Communicable Disease Center, 1957:136–143. US Public Health Service publication no. 575.

93. Pappagianis D. Marked increase in cases of coccidioidomycosis in California: 1991, 1992, and 1993. *J Infect Dis* 1994;19[Suppl 1]:S14–S18, 1994.

94. Fisher MC, Koenig GL, White TJ, et al. Pathogenic clones versus environmentally driven population increase: analysis of an epidemic of the human fungal pathogen *Coccidioides immitis*. *J Clin Microbiol* 2000;38:807–813.

95. Louie L, Ng S, Hajjeh R, et al. Influence of host genetics on the severity of coccidioidomycosis. *Emerg Infect Dis* 1999;5:672–680.

96. Rosenstein NE, Emery KW, Werner SB, et al. Risk factors for severe pulmonary and disseminated coccidioidomycosis: Kern County, California, 1995–1996. *Clin Infect Dis* 2001;32:708–715.

97. Leake JA, Mosley DG, England B, et al. Risk factors for acute symptomatic coccidioidomycosis among elderly persons in Arizona, 1996–1997. *J Infect Dis* 2000;181:1435–1440.

98. Smale LE, Birsner JW. Maternal deaths from coccidioidomycosis. *JAMA* 1949;140:1152–1154.

99. Wack EE, Ampel NM, Galgiani JN, et al. Coccidioidomycosis during pregnancy. An analysis of ten cases among 47,120 pregnancies. *Chest* 1988;94:376–379.

100. Cohen IM, Galgiani JN, Potter D, et al. Coccidioidomycosis in renal replacement therapy. *Arch Intern Med* 1982;142:489–494.

101. Bronnimann DA, Adam RD, Galgiani JN, et al. Coccidioidomycosis in the acquired immunodeficiency syndrome. *Ann Intern Med* 1987;106:372–379.

102. Drutz DJ, Huppert M. Coccidioidomycosis: factors affecting the host-parasite interaction. *J Infect Dis* 1983;147:372–390.

103. Savage DC, Madin SH. Cellular responses in lungs of immunized mice to intranasal infection with *Coccidioides immitis*. *Sabouraudia* 1968;6:94–102.

104. Galgiani JN, Isenberg RA, Stevens DA. Chemotaxigenic activity of extracts from the mycelial and spherule phases of *Coccidioides immitis* for human polymorphonuclear leukocytes. *Infect Immun* 1978;21:862–865.

105. Galgiani JN, Yam P, Petz LD, et al. Complement activation by *Coccidioides immitis*: in vitro and clinical studies. *Infect Immun* 1980;28:944–949.

106. Galgiani JN, Payne CM, Jones JF. Human polymorphonuclear leukocyte inhibition of chitin precursors into mycelia of *Coccidioides immitis*. *J Infect Dis* 1984;149:404–411.

107. Collins MS, Pappagianis D. Effects of lysozyme and chitinase on the spherules of *Coccidioides immitis* and *Histoplasma capsulatum*. *Contrib Microbiol Immunol* 1973;3:106–125.

108. Frey CL, Drutz DJ. Influence of fungal surface components on the interaction of *Coccidioides immitis* with polymorphonuclear neutrophils. *J Infect Dis* 1986;153:933–943.

109. Beaman L, Pappagianis D, Benjamini E. Significance of T cells in resistance to experimental murine coccidioidomycosis. *Infect Immun* 1977;17:580–585.

110. Kirkland TN, Fierer J. Inbred mouse strains differ in resistance to lethal *Coccidioides immitis* infection. *Infect Immun* 1983;40:912–916.

111. Kirkland TN, Fierer J. Genetic control of resistance to *Coccidioides immitis*: A single gene that is expressed in spleen cells determines resistance. *J Immunol* 1985;135:548–552.

112. Cox RA, Kennell W, Boncyk L, et al. Induction and expression of cell-mediated immune responses in inbred mice infected with *Coccidioides immitis*. *Infect Immun* 1988;56:13–17.

113. Beaman L, Benjamini E, Pappagianis D. Role of lymphocytes in macrophage-induced killing of *Coccidioides immitis* in vitro. *Infect Immun* 1981;34:347–353.

114. Beaman L, Holmberg CA. In vitro response of alveolar macrophages to infection with *Coccidioides immitis*. *Infect Immun* 1980;28:594–600.

115. Beaman L, Benjamini E, Pappagianis D. Activation of macrophages by lymphokines: enhancement of phagosome-lysosome fusion and killing of *Coccidioides immitis*. *Infect Immun* 1983;39:1201–1207.

116. Beaman L. Fungicidal activation of murine macrophages by recombinant gamma interferon. *Infect Immun* 1987;55:2951–2955.

117. Magee DM, Cox RA. Roles of gamma interferon and interleukin-4 in genetically determined resistance to *Coccidioides immitis*. *Infect Immun* 1995;63:3514–3519.

118. Cox RA, Magee DM. Production of tumor necrosis factor alpha, interleukin-1 alpha, and interleukin-6 during murine coccidioidomycosis. *Infect Immun* 1995;63:4178–4180.

119. Beaman L. Effects of recombinant gamma interferon and tumor necrosis factor on in vitro interactions of human mononuclear phagocytes with *Coccidioides immitis*. *Infect Immun* 1991;59:4427–4429.

120. Ampel NM, Bejarano GC, Galgiani JN. Killing of *Coccidioides immitis* by human peripheral blood mononuclear cells. *Infect Immun* 1992;60:4200–4204.

121. Slagle DC, Cox RA, Kuruganti U. Induction of tumor necrosis factor alpha by spherules of *Coccidioides immitis*. *Infect Immun* 1989;57:1916–1921.

122. Clemons KV, Leathers CR, Lee KW. Systemic *Coccidioides immitis* infection in nude and beige mice. *Infect Immun* 1985;47:814–821.

123. Richards JO, Ampel NM, Galgiani JN, et al. Dendritic cells pulsed with *Coccidioides immitis* lysate induce antigen-specific naive T cell activation. *J Infect Dis* 2001;184:1220–1224.

124. Richards JO, Ampel NM, Lake DF. Reversal of coccidioidal anergy in vitro by dendritic cells from patients with disseminated coccidioidomycosis. *J Immunol* 2002;169:2020–2025.

125. Deresinski SC, Stevens DA, Applegate RJ, et al. Cellular immunity to *Coccidioides immitis*: in vitro lymphocyte response to spherules, arthrospores, and endospores. *Cell Immunol* 1977;32:110–119.

126. Ampel NM, Dols CL, et al. Coccidioidomycosis during human immunodeficiency virus infection: results of a prospective study in a coccidioidal endemic area. *Am J Med* 1993;94:235–240.

127. Deresinski SC, Levine HB, Stevens DA. *Coccidioides immitis* endospores: phagocytosis by human cells. *Mycopathologia* 1978;3:179–181.

128. Ampel NM, Galgiani JN. Interaction of human peripheral blood mononuclear cells with *Coccidioides immitis* arthroconidia. *Cell Immunol* 1991;133:253–262.

129. Ampel NM, Bejarano GC, Salas SD, et al. In vitro assessment of cellular immunity in human coccidioidomycosis: relationship between dermal hypersensitivity, lymphocyte transformation, and lymphokine production by peripheral blood mononuclear cells from healthy adults. *J Infect Dis* 1992;165:710–715.

130. Cox RA, Vivas JR. Spectrum of in vivo and in vitro cell-mediated immune responses in coccidioidomycosis. *Cell Immunol* 1977;31:130–141.

131. Cox RA, Vivas JR, Gross A, et al. In vivo and in vitro cell-mediated immune responses in coccidioidomycosis. I. Immunologic responses of persons with primary, asymptomatic infection. *Am Rev Respir Dis* 1976;114:937–942.

132. Cox RA, Kennell W. Suppression of T-lymphocyte response by *Coccidioides immitis* antigen. *Infect Immun* 1988;56:1424–1429.

133. Cox RA, Pope RM. Serum-mediated suppression of lymphocyte transformation responses in coccidioidomycosis. *Infect Immun* 1987;55:1058–1062.

134. Deresinski SC. The immunology of coccidioidomycosis. In: Friedman H, Chmel H, Bendinelli M, eds. *Pulmonary infections and immunity*. New York: Plenum Publishing, 1994:29–49.

135. Magee DM, Cox RA. Interleukin-12 regulation of host defenses against *Coccidioides immitis*. *Infect Immun* 1996;64:3609–3613.

136. Jiang C, Magee DM, Cox RA. Coadministration of interleukin 12 expression vector with antigen 2 cDNA enhances induction of protective immunity against *Coccidioides immitis*. *Infect Immun* 1999;67:5848–5853.

137. Corry DB, Ampel NM, Christian L, et al. Cytokine production by peripheral blood mononuclear cells in human coccidioidomycosis. *J Infect Dis* 1996;174:440–443.

138. Cox RA, Baker BS, Stevens DA. Specificity of immunoglobulin E in coccidioidomycosis and correlation with disease involvement. *Infect Immun* 1982;37:609–616.

139. Shapira SK, Jabara HH, Thienes CP, et al. Deletional switch recombination occurs in interleukin-4–induced isotype switching to IgE expression by human B cells. *Proc Natl Acad Sci U S A* 1991;88:7528–7532.

140. Scott P. IL-12: initiation cytokine for cell-mediated immunity. *Science* 1993;260:496–497.

141. Sanderson CJ. Interleukin-5, eosinophils, and disease. *Blood* 1992;79:3101–3109.

142. Cole GT. Ammonia production by *Coccidioides immitis* and its significance to the host-fungus interplay (Abstr L29). In: Programs and abstracts of the 5th Symposium on Topics in Mycology: Host-Fungus Interplay; June 27–30, 1995; Stanford University, Stanford, Calif.

143. Resnick S, Pappagianis D, McKerrow JH. Proteinase production by the parasitic cycle of the pathogenic fungus *Coccidioides immitis*. *Infect Immun* 1987;55:2807–2815.

144. Hunninghake GW, Davidson JM, Rennard S, et al. Elastin fragments attract macrophage precursors to diseased sites in pulmonary emphysema. *Science* 1981;212:925–927.

145. Smith CE. Coccidioidomycosis. *Med Clin North Am* 1943;27:790–807.

146. Yozwiak ML, Lundergan LL, Kerrick SS, et al. Symptoms and routine laboratory abnormalities associated with coccidioidomycosis. *West J Med* 1988;149:419–421.

147. Caldwell JW, Arsura EL, Kilgore WB, et al. Coccidioidomycosis in pregnancy during an epidemic in California. *Obstet Gynecol* 2000;95:236–239.

148. Gamble CN, Ruggles SW. The immunopathogenesis of glomerulonephritis associated with mixed cryoglobulinemia. *N Engl J Med* 1978;299:81–84.

149. Schermoly MJ, Hinthorn DR. Eosinophilia in coccidioidomycosis. *Arch Intern Med* 1988;148:895–896.

150. Bayer AS. Fungal pneumonias: pulmonary coccidioidal syndromes (part I). Primary and progressive primary coccidioidal pneumonias—diagnostic, therapeutic, and prognostic considerations. *Chest* 1981;79:575–583.

151. Bayer AS. Fungal pneumonias: pulmonary coccidioidal syndromes (part 2). Miliary, nodular, and cavitary pulmonary coccidioidomycosis: chemotherapeutic and surgical considerations. *Chest* 1981;79:686–691.

152. Larsen RA, Jacobson JA, Morris AH, et al. Acute respiratory failure caused by primary pulmonary coccidioidomycosis. Two case reports and a review of the literature. *Am Rev Respir Dis* 1985;131:797–799.

153. Bayer AS, Yoshikawa TT, Guze LB. Chronic progressive coccidioidal pneumonitis. report of six cases with clinical, roentgenographic, serologic and therapeutic features. *Arch Intern Med* 1979;139:536–540.

154. Feldman BS, Snyder LS. Primary pulmonary coccidioidomycosis. *Semin Respir Infect* 2001;16:231–237.

155. Batra P. Pulmonary coccidioidomycosis. *J Thorac Imaging* 1992;7:29–38, 1992.

156. Cha JM, Jung S, Bahng HS, et al. Multi-organ failure caused by reactivated coccidioidomycosis without dissemination in a patient with renal transplantation. *Respirology* 2000;5:87–90.

157. Birsner JW. The roentgen aspects of five hundred cases of pulmonary coccidioidomycosis. *Am J Roentgenol Radium Ther Nucl Med* 1954;72:4.
158. Arsura EL, Kilgore WB. Miliary coccidioidomycosis in the immunocompetent. *Chest* 2000;117:404–409.
159. Schwartz EL, Waldmann EB, Payne RM, et al. Coccidioidal pericarditis. *Chest* 1976;70:670–672.
160. Amundson DE. Perplexing pericarditis caused by coccidioidomycosis. *South Med J* 1993;86:694–696.
161. Lonky SA, Catanzaro A, Moser KM, et al. Acute coccidioidal pleural effusion. *Am Rev Respir Dis* 1976;114:681–688.
162. Boyle JO, Coulthard SW, Mandel RM. Laryngeal involvement in disseminated coccidioidomycosis. *Arch Otolaryngol Head Neck Surg* 1991;117:433–438.
163. Moskowitz PS, Sue JY, Gooding CA. Tracheal coccidioidomycosis causing upper airway obstruction in children. *AJR Am J Roentgenol* 1982;139:596–600.
164. Polesky A, Kirsch CM, Snyder LS, et al. Airway coccidioidomycosis—report of cases and review. *Clin Infect Dis* 1999;28:1273–1280.
165. Winn WA. A long term study of 300 patients with cavitary-abscess lesions of the lung of coccidioidal origin. An analytical study with special reference to treatment. *Dis Chest* 1968;54[Suppl 1]:12–16.
166. Putnam JS, Harper WK, Greene JF Jr, et al. *Coccidioides immitis:* a rare cause of pulmonary mycetoma. *Am Rev Respir Dis* 1975;112:733–738.
167. Winn RE, Johnson R, Galgiani JN, et al. Cavitary coccidioidomycosis with fungus ball formation. Diagnosis by fiberoptic bronchoscopy with coexistence of hyphae and spherules. *Chest* 1994;105:412–416.
168. Cunningham RT, Einstein H. Coccidioidal pulmonary cavities with rupture. *J Thorac Cardiovasc Surg* 1982;84:172–177.
169. Kim KI, Leung AN, Flint JD, et al. Chronic pulmonary coccidioidomycosis: computed tomographic and pathologic findings in 18 patients. *Can Assoc Radiol J* 1998;49:401–407.
170. Blumenkranz MS, Stevens DA. Endogenous coccidioidal endophthalmitis. *J Ophthalmol* 1980;87:974–984.
171. Rodenbiker HT, Ganley JP, Galgiani JN, et al. Prevalence of chorioretinal scars associated with coccidioidomycosis. *Arch Ophthalmol* 1981;99: 71–75.
172. Petersen EA, Friedman BA, Crowder ED. Coccidioiduria: clinical significance. *Ann Intern Med* 1976;85:34–38.
173. DeFelice R, Wieden MA, Galgiani JN. The incidence and implications of coccidioiduria. *Am Rev Respir Dis* 1982;125:49–52.
174. Arsura EL, Bellinghausen PL, Kilgore WB, et al. Septic shock in coccidioidomycosis. *Crit Care Med* 1998;26:62–65.
175. Liao JC, Reiter RE. Coccidioidomycosis presenting as testicular mass. *J Urol* 2001;166:1396.
176. Chowfin A, Tight R. Female genital coccidioidomycosis (FGC), Addison's disease and sigmoid loop abscess due to *Coccidioides immitis;* case report and review of literature on FGC. *Mycopathologia* 1999;145:121–126.
177. Chen KTK. Coccidioidal peritonitis. *Am J Clin Pathol* 1983;80:514–516.
178. Maguire LJ, Campbell RJ, Edson RS. Coccidioidomycosis with necrotizing granulomatous conjunctivitis. *Cornea* 1994;13:539–542.
179. Moorthys RS, Rao NA, Sidikaro Y, et al. Coccidioidomycosis iridocyclitis. *Ophthalmology* 1994;101:1923–1928.
180. Loeb JM, Livermore BM, Wofsy D. Coccidioidomycosis of the thyroid. *Ann Intern Med* 1979;91:409–412.
181. Smilack JD, Argueta R. Coccidioidal infection of the thyroid. *Arch Intern Med* 1998;158:89–92.
182. Schwartz DN, Film SD, Miller RA. Infection of an arterial prosthesis as the presenting manifestation of disseminated coccidioidomycosis: control of disease with fluconazole. *Clin Infect Dis* 1993;16:486–488.
183. Westphal SA. Disseminated coccidioidomycosis associated with hypercalcemia. *Mayo Clin Proc* 1998;73:893–894.
184. Jacobs PH. Cutaneous coccidioidomycosis. In: Stevens DA, ed. *Coccidioidomycosis: a text.* New York: Plenum Publishing, 1980:213–224.
185. Kelly PC. Coccidioidal meningitis. In: Stevens DA, ed. *Coccidioidomycosis: a text.* New York: Plenum Publishing, 1980:163–194.
186. Galgiani JN, Peng T, Lewis ML, et al. Cerebrospinal fluid antibodies detected by ELISA against a 33-kDa antigen from spherules of *Coccidioides immitis* in patients with coccidioidal meningitis. The National Institute of Allergy and Infectious Diseases Mycoses Study Group. *J Infect Dis* 1996;173:499–502.
187. Bouza E, Dreyer JS, Hewitt WL, et al. Coccidioidal meningitis. An analysis of thirty-one cases and review of the literature. *Medicine (Baltimore)* 1981;60:139–172.
188. Wrobel CJ, Rothrock J. Coccidioidomycosis meningitis presenting as anterior spinal artery syndrome. *Neurology* 1992;42:1840.
189. Bañuelos AF, Williams PF, Johnson RH, et al. Central nervous system abscesses due to *Coccidioides* species. *Clin Infect Dis* 1996;22:240–250.
190. Vincent T, Galgiani JN. The natural history of coccidioidomycosis: VA-Armed Forces Cooperative Studies, 1955–1958. *Clin Infect Dis* 1993;16:247–254.
191. Sobel RA, Ellis WG, Nielsen SL, et al. Central nervous system coccidioidomycosis: a clinicopathologic study of treatment with and without amphotericin B. *Hum Pathol* 1984;15:980–995.
192. Mendel E, Milefchik EN, Ahmadi J, et al. Coccidioidomycosis brain abscess. Case report. *J Neurosurg* 1994;80:140–142.
193. Romeo JH, Rice LB, McQuarrie IG. Hydrocephalus in coccidioidal meningitis: case report and review of the literature. *Neurosurgery* 2000;47:773–777.
194. Wrobel CJ, Meyer S, Johnson RH, et al. MR findings in acute and chronic coccidioidomycosis meningitis. *AJNR Am J Neuroradiol* 1992;13:1241–1245.
195. Ragland AS, Argura EL, Ismail Y, et al. Eosinophilic pleocytosis in coccidioidal meningitis: frequency and significance. *Am J Med* 1993;95:254–257.
196. Shetter AG, Fischer DW, Flom RA. Computed tomography in cases of coccidioidal meningitis, with clinical correlation. *West J Med* 1985;142:782–786.
197. Ampel NM, Ahmann DR, Delgado KL, et al, and the National Institute of Allergy and Infectious Diseases Mycoses Study Group: tumor necrosis factor-alpha and interleukin-1 beta in cerebrospinal fluid of patients with coccidioidal meningitis during therapy with ketoconazole. *J Infect Dis* 1995;171:1675–1678.
198. Harrison HR, Reynolds AF. Trapped fourth ventricle in coccidioidal meningitis. *Surg Neurol* 1982;17:197–199.
199. Hadley MN, Martin NA, Spetzler RF, et al. Multiple intracranial aneurysms due to *Coccidioides immitis* infection. Case report. *J Neurosurg* 1987;66:453–456.
200. Williams PL, Johnson R, Pappagianis D, et al. Vasculitic and encephalitic complications associated with *Coccidioides immitis* infection of the central nervous system in humans: report of 10 cases and review. *Clin Infect Dis* 1992;14:673–682.
201. Williams PL. Vasculitic complications associated with coccidioidal meningitis. *Semin Respir Infect* 2001;16:270–279.
202. Erly WK, Labadie E, Williams PL. Disseminated coccidioidomycosis complicated by vasculitis: a cause of fatal subarachnoid hemorrhage in two cases. *AJNR Am J Neuroradiol* 1999;20:1605–1608.
203. Kleinschmidt-DeMasters BK, Mazowiecki M, Bonds LA, et al. Coccidioidomycosis meningitis with massive dural and cerebral venous thrombosis and tissue arthroconidia. *Arch Pathol Lab Med* 2000;124:310–314.
204. Kemper CA, Deresinski SC. Fungal diseases of bones and joints. In: Kibbler CC, Odds FC, MacKenzie DWR, eds. *Principles and practice of mycology.* Sussex, England: John Wiley & Sons, 1996:49–68.
205. Deresinski SC. Coccidioidomycosis of bone and joints. In: Stevens DA, ed. *Coccidioidomycosis: a text.* New York: Plenum Publishing, 1980:195–212.
206. Bried JM, Galgiani JN. *Coccidioides immitis* infections in bones and joints. *Clin Orthop* 1986;211:235–243.
207. Kemper CA, Deresinski SC. Fungal arthritis. In: Maddison PJ, Isenberg DA, Woo P, et al, eds. *The Oxford textbook of rheumatology.* Oxford: Oxford University Press, 1993:599–607.
208. Wrobel CJ, Chappell ET, Taylor W. Clinical presentation, radiological findings, and treatment results of coccidioidomycosis involving the spine: report on 23 cases. *J Neurosurg* 2001;95:33–39.
209. Kushwaha VP, Shaw BA, Gerardi JA, et al. Musculoskeletal coccidioidomycosis. A review of 25 cases. *Clin Orthop* 1996;(332):190–199.
210. Zeppa MA, Laorr A, Greenspan A, et al. Skeletal coccidioidomycosis: imaging findings in 19 patients. *Skeletal Radiol* 1996;25:337–343.
211. Holley K, Muldoon M, Tasker S. *Coccidioides immitis* osteomyelitis: a case series review. *Orthopedics* 2002;25:831–832.
212. Dalinka MK, Dinnenberg S, Greendyke WH, et al. Roentgenographic features of osseous coccidioidomycosis. *J Bone Joint Surg Am* 1971;53:1157–1164.
213. Olson EM, Duberg AC, Herron LD, et al. Coccidioidal spondylitis: MR findings in 15 patients. *AJR Am J Roentgenol* 1998;171:785–789.
214. Boddicker JH, Fong D, Walsh TE, et al. Bone and gallium scanning in the evaluation of disseminated coccidioidomycosis. *Am Rev Respir Dis* 1980;122:279–287.
215. Moreno AJ, Weisman I, Rodriguez AA, et al. Nuclear imaging in coccidioidal osteomyelitis. *Clin Nucl Med* 1987;12:604–609.
216. Lee JC, Catanzaro A, Parthemore JG, et al. Hypercalcemia in disseminated coccidioidomycosis. *N Engl J Med* 1977;297:431–433.
217. Walter RM Jr, Lawrence RM. Hypercalcemia in disseminated coccidioidomycosis. *Am J Med Sci* 1981;281:97–99.
218. Parker MS, Dokoh S, Woolfenden JM, et al. Hypercalcemia in coccidioidomycosis. *Am J Med* 1984;76:341–344.
219. Reid GD, Klinkhoff A, Bozek C, et al. Coccidioidomycosis tenosynovitis: case report and review of the literature. *J Rheumatol* 1984;11:392–394.
220. Price MJ, Lewis EL, Carmalt JE. Coccidioidomycosis of prostate gland. *Urology* 1982;19:653–655.
221. Lawrence MA, Ginsberg D, Stein JP, et al. Coccidioidomycosis prostatitis associated with prostate cancer. *BJU Int* 1999;84:372–373.
222. Chen KT. Coccidioidomycosis of the epididymis. *J Urol* 1983;130:978–979.
223. Salgia K, Bhatia L, Rajashekaraiah KR, et al. Coccidioidomycosis of the uterus. *South Med J* 1982;75:614–616.
224. Parker P, Adcock LL. Pelvic coccidioidomycosis. *Obstet Gynecol Surv* 1981;36:225–229.
225. Dooley DP, Reddy RK, Smith CE. Coccidioidomycosis presenting as an omental mass. *Clin Infect Dis* 1994;19:802–803.
226. Ampel NM, White JD, Varanasi UR, et al. Coccidioidal peritonitis associated with continuous ambulatory peritoneal dialysis. *Am J Kidney Dis* 1988;11:512–514.

227. Thomas S, Basu S, Dutta R. et al. Coccidioidomycosis presenting as liver abscess. *Indian J Gastroenterol* 2001;20:113–114.

228. Sydorak RM, Albanese CT, Chen Y, et al. Coccidioides immitis in the gallbladder and biliary tree. *J Pediatr Surg* 2001;36:1054–1056.

229. Scanarini M, Rotilio A, Rigobello L, et al. Primary intrasellar coccidioidomycosis simulating a pituitary adenoma. *Neurosurgery* 1991;28:748–751.

230. Logan JL, Blair JE, Galgiani JN. Coccidioidomycosis complicating solid organ transplantation. *Semin Respir Infect* 2001;16:251–256.

231. Blair JE, Logan JL. Coccidioidomycosis in solid organ transplantation. *Clin Infect Dis* 2001;33:1536–1544.

232. Seltzer J, Broaddus VC, Jacobs R, et al. Reactivation of *Coccidioides* infection. *West J Med* 1986;145:96–98.

233. Deresinski SC, Stevens DA. Coccidioidomycosis in compromised hosts. Experience at Stanford University Hospital. *Medicine (Baltimore)* 1974;54:377–395.

234. Rutala PJ, Smith JW. Coccidioidomycosis in potentially compromised hosts: the effect of immunosuppressive therapy in dissemination. *Am J Med Sci* 1982;275:283–295.

235. Holt CD, Winston DJ, Kubak B, et al. Coccidioidomycosis in liver transplant patients. *Clin Infect Dis* 1997;24:216–221.

236. Smilack J, Blair S, Caples S. *Coccidioidomycosis in patients with hematological malignancies. Proceedings of the 42nd Interscience Conference on Antimicrobial Agents and Chemotherapy, September 27–30, 2002, San Diego, California.* M-886, p. 392.

237. Hall KA, Sethi GK, Rosado LJ, et al. Coccidioidomycosis and heart transplantation. *J Heart Lung Transplant* 1993;12:525–526.

238. Hall KA, Copeland JG, Zukoski CF, et al. Markers of coccidioidomycosis before cardiac or renal transplantation and the risk of recurrent infection. *Transplantation* 1993;55:1422–1424.

238a. Dosanjh A, Theodore J, Pappagianis D. Probable false positive coccidioidal serologic results in patients with cystic fibrosis. *Pediatr Transplant* 1998;2:313–317.

239. Ampel NM. Delayed-type hypersensitivity, *in vitro* T-cell responsiveness and risk of active coccidioidomycosis among HIV-infected patients living in the coccidioidal endemic area. *Med Mycol* 1999;37:245–250.

240. Arguinchona HL, Ampel NM, Dols CL, et al. Persistent coccidioidal seropositivity without clinical evidence of active coccidioidomycosis in patients infected with human immunodeficiency virus. *J Infect Dis* 1995;20:1281–1285.

241. Woods CW, McRill C, Plikaytis BD, et al. Coccidioidomycosis in human immunodeficiency virus–infected persons in Arizona, 1994–1997: incidence, risk factors, and prevention. *J Infect Dis* 2000;181:1428–1434.

242. Jones JL, Fleming PL, Cieselski CA, et al. Coccidioidomycosis among persons with AIDS in the United States. *J Infect Dis* 1995;171:961–966.

243. Kemper CA, Linette A, Kane C, et al. Travels with HIV: the effects of travel on the compliance and health of HIV infected adults. *Int J STD AIDS* 1996;7:1–6.

244. Fish DG, Ampel NM, Galgiani JN, et al. Coccidioidomycosis during human immunodeficiency virus infection. A review of 77 patients. *Medicine (Baltimore)* 1990;69:384–391.

245. McNeil MM, Ampel NM. Opportunistic coccidioidomycosis in patients infected with human immunodeficiency virus: prevention issues and priorities. *Clin Infect Dis* 1995;21[Suppl 1]:S111–S113.

246. Singh VR, Smith DK, Lawerence J, et al. Coccidioidomycosis in patients infected with human immunodeficiency virus: review of 91 cases at a single institution. *Clin Infect Dis* 1996;3:563–568.

247. Antoniskis D, Larsen RA, Akil B, et al. Seronegative disseminated coccidioidomycosis in patients with HIV infection. *AIDS* 1990;4:691–693.

248. Mahaffey KW, Hippenmeyer CL, Mandel R, et al. Unrecognized coccidioidomycosis complicating *Pneumocystis carinii* pneumonia in patients infected with the human immunodeficiency virus and treated with corticosteroids. A report of two cases. *Arch Intern Med* 1993;153:1496–1498.

249. Peterson CM, Schuppert K, Kelly PC, et al. Coccidioidomycosis and pregnancy. *Obstet Gynecol Surv* 1993;48:149–156.

250. Einstein H, Johnson R, Caldwell J, et al. Coccidioidomycosis and pregnancy: the Kern County experience. In: Programs and abstracts of the 35th Interscience Conference on Antimicrobial Agents and Chemotherapy; September 17–20, 1995; San Francisco, Calif; p. 324. Abstract no. K202.

251. Arsura EL, Kilgore WB, Ratnayake SN. Erythema nodosum in pregnant patients with coccidioidomycosis. *Clin Infect Dis* 1998;27:1201–1203.

252. Charlton V, Ramsdell K, Sehring S. Intrauterine transmission of coccidioidomycosis. *Pediatr Infect Dis J* 1999;18:561–563.

253. Park RO. Does transplacental spread of coccidioidomycosis occur? Report of a neonatal fatality and review of the literature. *Arch Pathol Lab Med* 1981;105:347–350.

254. Wegmann TG, Lin H, Guilbert LJ, et al. Bidirectional cytokine interactions in the maternal-fetal relationship. Is successful pregnancy a $T_H 2$ phenomenon? *Immunol Today* 1993;14:353–356.

255. Barbee RA, Hicks MJ, Grosso D, et al. The maternal immune response in coccidioidomycosis—is pregnancy a risk factor for serious infection? *Chest* 1991;100:709–715.

256. Howard PF, Smith JW. Diagnosis of disseminated coccidioidomycosis by liver biopsy. *Arch Intern Med* 1983;143:1335–1338.

257. Wolfson D, Lee S. Coccidioidomycosis diagnosed from bone marrow smear. *JAMA* 1991;266:707.

258. Warlick MA, Quan SF, Sobonya RE. Rapid diagnosis of pulmonary coccidioidomycosis. Cytologic v. potassium hydroxide preparations. *Arch Intern Med* 1983;143:723–725.

259. Sarosi GA, Lawrence JP, Smith DK, et al. Rapid diagnostic evaluation of bronchial washings in patients with suspected coccidioidomycosis. *Semin Respir Infect* 2001;16:238–241.

260. Hageage GJ, Harrington BJ. Use of calcofluor white in clinical mycology. *Lab Med* 1984;15:109–112.

261. DiTomasso JP, Ampel NM, Sobonya RE, et al. Bronchoscopic diagnosis of pulmonary coccidioidomycosis. Comparison of cytology, culture, and transbronchial biopsy. *Diagn Microbiol Infect Dis* 1994;18:83–87.

262. Nunez D, Stanley C, Robertstad, et al. Pseudoepidemic of coccidioidomycosis. *Am J Infect Control* 1982;10:68–71.

263. Raab SS, Silverman JF, Zimmerman KG. Fine-needle aspiration biopsy of pulmonary coccidioidomycosis. Spectrum of cytologic findings in 73 patients. *Am J Clin Pathol* 1993;99:582–587.

264. Kaufman L, Valero G, Padhye AA. Misleading manifestations of *Coccidioides immitis in vivo. J Clin Microbiol* 1998;36:3721–3723.

265. Fredricks DN, Jolley JA, Lepp PW, et al. Rhinosporidium seeberi: a human pathogen from a novel group of aquatic protistan parasites. *Emerg Infect Dis* 2000;6:273–282.

266. Puckett TF. Hyphae of *Coccidioides immitis* in tissues of the human host. *Am Rev Tuberc* 1954;70:320–327.

267. Nosanchuk JD, Snedeker J, Nosanchuk JS. Arthroconidia in coccidioidoma: case report and literature review. *Int J Infect Dis* 1998;3:32–35.

268. Hagman HM, Madnick EG, D'Agostino AN, et al. Hyphal forms in the central nervous system of patients with coccidioidomycosis. *Clin Infect Dis* 2000;30:349–353.

269. Wages DS, Helfend L, Finkle H. *Coccidioides immitis* presenting as a hyphal form in a ventriculoperitoneal shunt. *Arch Pathol Lab Med* 1995;119:91–93.

270. Davis LE, Cook G, Costerton JW. Biofilm on ventriculo-peritoneal shunt tubing as a cause of treatment failure in coccidioidal meningitis. *Emerg Infect Dis* 2002;8:376–379.

271. Fainstein V, Hopfer RL, Trier P, et al. Bone marrow cultures: their value in diagnosing fungal and mycobacterial infection in patients with cancer. *J Infect Dis* 1981;144:79.

272. Ampel NM, Ryan KJ, Carry PJ, et al. Fungemia due to *Coccidioides immitis*. An analysis of 16 episodes in 15 patients and a review of the literature. *Medicine (Baltimore)* 1986;65:312–321.

273. Ampel NM, Wieden MA. Discrepancy between growth of *Coccidioides immitis* in bacterial blood culture media and a radiometric growth index. *Diagn Microbiol Infect Dis* 1988;9:7–10.

274. Huppert M, Sun SH, Bailey JW. Natural variability in *Coccidioides immitis*. In: Ajello L, ed. *Coccidioidomycosis: proceedings the 2nd symposium on coccidioidomycosis.* Tucson, AZ: University of Arizona Press, 1965:323–328.

275. Sigler L, Carmichaell JW. Taxonomy of *Malbranchea* and some other hyphomycetes with arthroconidia. *Mycotaxon* 1976;4:349–488.

276. Larone DH, Mitchell TG, Walsh TJ. *Histoplasma, Blastomyces, Coccidioides,* and the dimorphic fungi causing systemic mycoses. In: Murray PR, Baron EJ, Pfaller MA, et al, eds. *Manual of clinical microbiology,* 7th ed. Washington, DC: ASM Press, 1999:1259–1274.

277. Brosbe EA. Use of refined agar for the in vitro propagation of spherule phase of *Coccidioides immitis. J Bacteriol* 1967;93:497–498.

278. Standard PG, Kaufman L. Immunological procedure for the rapid and specific identification of *Coccidioides immitis* in cultures. *J Clin Microbiol* 1977;5:149–153.

279. Kaufman L, Standard PG. Improved version of the exoantigen test for identification of *Coccidioides immitis* and *Histoplasma capsulatum. J Clin Microbiol* 1978;8:42–45.

280. Beard JS, Benson PM, Skillman L. Rapid diagnosis of coccidioidomycosis with a DNA probe to ribosomal RNA. *Arch Dermatol* 1993;129:1589–1593.

281. Smith CE. Diagnosis of pulmonary coccidioidomycosis. *Calif Med* 1951;75:385.

282. Galgiani JN, and the Valley Fever Vaccine Study Group. Development of dermal hypersensitivity to coccidioidal antigens associated with repeated skin testing. *Am Rev Respir Dis* 1986;191:1045–1047.

283. Oldfield EC 3rd, Bone WD, Martin CR, et al. Prediction of relapse after treatment of coccidioidomycosis. *Clin Infect Dis* 1997;25:1205–1210.

284. Levine HB, Gonzalez-Ochoa A, Ten Eyck DR. Dermal sensitivity to *Coccidioides immitis*. A comparison of responses elicited in man by Spherulin and coccidioidin. *Am Rev Respir Dis* 1973;107:379–385.

285. Stevens DA, Levine HB, Deresinski SC, et al. Spherulin in clinical coccidioidomycosis. *Chest* 1975;68:697–702.

286. Gifford J, Catanzaro A. A comparison of coccidioidin and Spherulin skin testing in the diagnosis of coccidioidomycosis. *Am Rev Respir Dis* 1981;124:440–444.

287. Woodruff WW III, Buckley CE III, Gallis HA, et al. Reactivity to spherule-derived coccidioidin in the southeastern United States. *Infect Immun* 1984;43:860–869.

288. Pappagianis D, Smith CE, Campbell CC. Serologic status after positive coccidioidin skin reactions. *Am Rev Respir Dis* 1967;96:520–523.

289. Deresinski SC, Levine HB, Kelly PC, et al. Spherulin skin testing and histoplasmal and coccidioidal serology: lack of effect. *Am Rev Respir Dis* 1977;116:1116–1118.

290. Pappagianis D, Zimmer BL. Serology of coccidioidomycosis. *Clin Microbiol Rev* 1990;3:247–268.

291. Pappagianis D. Serologic studies in coccidioidomycosis. *Semin Respir Infect* 2001;16:242–250.

292. Wieden MA, Galgiani JN, Pappagianis D. Comparison of immunodiffusion techniques with standard complement fixation assay for quantitation of coccidioidal antibodies. *J Clin Microbiol* 1983;18:529–534.

293. Zartarian M, Peterson EM, de la Maza LM. Detection of antibodies to *Coccidioides immitis* by enzyme immunoassay. *Am J Clin Pathol* 1997;107:148–153.

294. Martins TB, Jaskowski TD, Mouritsen CL, et al. Comparison of commercially available enzyme immunoassay with traditional serologic tests for detection of antibodies to *Coccidioides immitis*. *J Clin Microbiol* 1995;33:940–943.

295. Wheat J, French MLV, Kamel S, et al. Evaluation of cross-reactions in *Histoplasma capsulatum* serologic tests. *J Clin Microbiol* 1986;23:493–499.

296. Roberts CJ. Coccidioidomycosis in acquired immune deficiency syndrome. Depressed humoral as well as cellular immunity. *Am J Med* 1984;76:734–736.

297. Johnson JE, Jeffery B, Huppert M. Evaluation of five commercially available immunodiffusion kits for detection of *Coccidioides immitis* and *Histoplasma capsulatum* antibodies. *J Clin Microbiol* 1984;20:530–532.

298. Yoshinoya S, Cox RA, Pope RM. Circulating immune complexes in coccidioidomycosis. Detection and characterization. *J Clin Invest* 1980;66:655–663.

299. Weiner MH. Antigenemia detected in human coccidioidomycosis. *J Clin Microbiol* 1983;18:136–142.

300. Galgiani JN, Dugger KO, Ito JI, et al. Antigenemia in primary coccidioidomycosis. *Am J Trop Med Hyg* 1984;33:645–649.

301. Oldfield EC III, Olson PE, Bone WD, et al. Coccidioidomycosis presenting as neoplasia: another great imitator disease. *Infect Dis Clin Pract* 1995;4:87–92.

302. Deresinski SC. Commentary: the masquerades of coccidioidomycosis. *Infect Dis Clin Pract* 1995;4:93–94.

303. Wilhelm C, Ellner JJ. Chronic meningitis. *Neurol Clin* 1986;4:115–141.

304. Galgiani JN, Ampel NM, Catanzaro A, et al. Practice guideline for the treatment of coccidioidomycosis. Infectious Diseases Society of America. *Clin Infect Dis* 2000;30:658–661.

305. Deresinski SC. Coccidioidomycosis: efficacy of new agents and future prospects. *Curr Opin Infect Dis* 2001;14:693–696.

306. Winn WA. Coccidioidomycosis and amphotericin B. *Med Clin North Am* 1963;47:1131–1148.

307. Stevens DA. Coccidioidomycosis and the indications for chemotherapy. *Drugs* 1983;26:334–336.

308. Caldwell J, Welch G, Johnson R, et al. Evaluation of response to early azole treatment in primary coccidioidomycosis. In: Programs and abstracts of the Centennial Conference on Coccidioidomycosis; 5th International Conference on Coccidioidomycosis; August 24–27, 1994; Stanford University, Stanford, Calif. Abstract no. 43.

309. Bauer R, Caldwell J, Johnson R. The pharmacoeconomics of early azoles in primary coccidioidomycosis. Paper presented at the 35th Interscience Conference on Antimicrobial Agents and Chemotherapy; September 17–20, 1995; San Francisco, Calif; p. 346. Abstract no. N5.

310. Gonzalez GM, Tuerina R, Najvar LK, et al. Therapeutic efficacy of amphotericin B complex (AMBLC), amphotericin B colloidal dispersion (ABCD), liposomal amphotericin B (LAMB), and conventional amphotericin B (AMB) in murine coccidioidomycosis. Paper presented at the 42nd Interscience Conference on Antimicrobial Agents and Chemotherapy; September 27–30, 2002; San Diego, Calif; p. 372. Abstract no. M-194.

311. Galgiani JN, Stevens DA, Graybill JR, et al. Ketoconazole therapy of progressive coccidioidomycosis. Comparison of 400- and 800-mg doses and observations at higher doses. *Am J Med* 1988;84:603–610.

312. Catanzaro A, Friedman PJ, Shillaci R, et al. Treatment of coccidioidomycosis with ketoconazole: an evaluation utilizing a new scoring system. *Am J Med* 1983;74:58–63.

313. Stevens DA, Stiller RL, Williams PL, et al. Experience with ketoconazole in three major manifestations of progressive coccidioidomycosis. *Am J Med* 1983;74:64–69.

314. Dismukes WE, Stamm AM, Graybill JR, et al. Treatment of systemic mycoses with ketoconazole: emphasis on toxicity and clinical response in 52 patients. National Institute of Allergy and Infectious Diseases collaborative antifungal study. *Ann Intern Med* 1983;98:13–20.

315. Catanzaro A, Galgiani JN, Levine BE, et al. Fluconazole in the treatment of chronic pulmonary and nonmeningeal disseminated coccidioidomycosis. *Am J Med* 1995;98:249–256.

316. Graybill JR, Stevens DA, Galgiani JN, et al. Itraconazole treatment of coccidioidomycosis. NIAID Mycoses Study Group. *Am J Med* 1990;89:282–290.

317. Galgiani JN, Catanzaro A, Cloud GA, et al. Comparison of oral fluconazole and itraconazole for progressive, nonmeningeal coccidioidomycosis. A randomized, double-blind trial. NIAID Mycoses Study Group. *Ann Intern Med* 2000;133:676–686.

318. Catanzaro A, Cloud G, Stevens D, et al. Safety and tolerance of posaconazole (SCH 56592) in patients with nonmeningeal disseminated coccidioidomycosis. Paper presented at the 40th Interscience Conference on Antimicrobial Agents and Chemotherapy; September 17–20, 2000; Toronto, Ontario, Canada. Abstract no. 2120.

319. Gonzalez GM, Tijerina R, Najvar LK, et al. Correlation between antifungal susceptibilities of *Coccidioides immitis in vitro* and antifungal treatment with caspofungin in a mouse model. *Antimicrob Agents Chemother* 2001;45:1854–1859.

320. Catanzaro A, Spitler L, Moser KM. Immunotherapy of coccidioidomycosis. *J Clin Invest* 1974;54:690–701.

321. Hoeprich PD, Merry JM. Effect of recombinant human interleukin-2 in experimental murine coccidioidomycosis. *Diagn Microbiol Infect Dis* 1988;9:115–118.

322. Catanzaro A, Drutz DJ. Pulmonary coccidioidomycosis. In Stevens DA, ed. *Coccidioidomycosis: a text.* New York: Plenum Publishing, 1980:147–161.

323. Salomon NW, Osborne R, Copeland JG. Surgical manifestations and results of treatment of pulmonary coccidioidomycosis. *Ann Thorac Surg* 1980;30:433–438.

324. Labadie EL, Hamilton RH. Survival improvement in coccidioidal meningitis by high-dose intrathecal amphotericin B. *Arch Intern Med* 1986;146:2013–2018.

325. Stevens DA, Shatsky SA. Intrathecal amphotericin in the management of coccidioidal meningitis. *Semin Respir Infect* 2001;16:263–269.

326. Craven PC, Graybill JR, Jorgensen JH, et al. High-dose ketoconazole for treatment of fungal infections of the central nervous system. *Ann Intern Med* 1983;98:160–167.

327. Galgiani JN, Catanzaro A, Cloud GA, et al. Fluconazole therapy for coccidioidal meningitis. The NIAID Mycoses Study Group. *Ann Intern Med* 1993;119:28–35.

328. Tucker RM, Galgiani JN, Denning DW, et al. Treatment of coccidioidal meningitis with fluconazole. *Rev Infect Dis* 1990;12[Suppl 3]:S380–S389.

329. Tucker RM, Williams PL, Arathoon EG, et al. Pharmacokinetics of fluconazole in cerebrospinal fluid and serum in human coccidioidal meningitis. *Antimicrob Agents Chemother* 1988;32:369–373.

330. Tucker RM, Denning DW, Dupont B, et al. Itraconazole therapy for chronic coccidioidal meningitis. *Ann Intern Med* 1990;112:108–112.

331. Dewsnup DH, Galgiani JN, Graybill JR, et al. Is it ever safe to stop azole therapy for *Coccidioides immitis* meningitis? *Ann Intern Med* 1996;124:305–310.

332. Young RF, Gade G, Grinnell V. Surgical treatment for fungal infections in the central nervous system. *J Neurosurg* 1985;63:371–381.

333. Clemons KV, Sobel RA, Williams PL, et al. Efficacy of intravenous liposomal amphotericin B (AmBisome) against coccidioidal meningitis in rabbits. *Antimicrob Agents Chemother* 2002;46:2420–2426.

334. Washton H. Review of fluconazole: a new triazole antifungal agent. *Diagn Microbiol Infect Dis* 1989;12:2295–2335.

335. Pursley TJ, Blomquist IK, Abraham J, et al. Fluconazole-induced congenital anomalies in three infants. *Clin Infect Dis* 1996;22:336–340.

336. Ampel NM. Coccidioidomycosis among persons with human immunodeficiency virus infection in the era of highly active antiretroviral therapy (HAART). *Semin Respir Infect* 2001;16:257–262.

337. Lake-Bakaar G, Tom W, Lake-Bakaar D, et al. Gastropathy and ketoconazole malabsorption in the acquired immunodeficiency syndrome (AIDS). *Ann Intern Med* 1988;109:471–473.

338. Marty F, Mylonakis E. Antifungal use in HIV infection. *Expert Opin Pharmacother* 2002;3:91–102.

339. Schafer-Korting M. Pharmacokinetic optimization of oral antifungal therapy. *Clin Pharmacokinet* 1993;25:329–341.

340. Pappagianis D. Seeking a vaccine against *Coccidioides immitis* and serologic studies: expectations and realities. *Fungal Genet Biol* 2001;32:1–9.

341. Williams PL, Sable DL, Sorgen SP, et al. Immunologic responsiveness and safety associated with the *Coccidioides immitis* spherule vaccine in volunteers of white, black, and Filipino ancestry. *Am J Epidemiol* 1984;119:591–602.

342. Pappagianis D, and the Valley Fever Vaccine Study Group. Evaluation of the protective efficacy of the killed *Coccidioides immitis* vaccine in humans. *Am Rev Respir Dis* 1993;148:656–670.

343. Li K, Yu JJ, Hung CY, et al. Recombinant urease and urease DNA of *Coccidioides immitis* elicit an immunoprotective response against coccidioidomycosis in mice. *Infect Immun* 2001;69:2878–2887.

344. Shubitz L, Peng T, Perrill R, et al. Protection of mice against *Coccidioides immitis* intranasal infection by vaccination with recombinant antigen 2/PRA. *Infect Immun* 2002;70:3287–3289.

345. Shubitz L, Peng T, Perrill R, et al. Protection of mice against *Coccidioides immitis* intranasal infection by vaccination with recombinant antigen 2/PRA. *Infect Immun* 2002;70:3287–3289.

346. Jiang C, Magee DM, Cox RA. Coadministration of interleukin 12 expression vector with antigen 2 cDNA enhances induction of protective immunity against *Coccidioides immitis*. *Infect Immun* 1999;67:5848–5853.

347. Jiang C, Magee DM, Ivey FD, et al. Role of signal sequence in vaccine-induced protection against experimental coccidioidomycosis. *Infect Immun* 2002;70:3539–3545.

348. Kruse RH, Green TH, Chambers RC, et al. Disinfection of aerosolized pathogenic fungi on laboratory surfaces. I. Tissue phase. *Appl Microbiol* 1963;11:436–445.

349. Kruse RH, Green TH, Chambers RC, et al. Disinfection of aerosolized pathogenic fungi on laboratory surfaces. II. Culture phase. *Appl Microbiol* 1964;12:155–160.

350. Deresinski SC. *Coccidioides immitis* as a bioweapon. *Semin Respir Infect* (in press).

CHAPTER 272
Sporothrix schenckii

Ronald A. Greenfield

CHARACTERISTICS OF THE PATHOGEN

Sporothrix schenckii is a dimorphic fungus that grows as yeast form at 37°C in culture and infected hosts or as a mold at 25°C. At room temperature, rapidly growing, off-white mold colonies develop that turn yellow, brown, or black with age. Oval hyaline conidia (2 to 3 by 3 to 6 μm) are born on conidiophores, which often form a characteristic flower-like cluster resembling a daisy or palm tree (Fig. 272.1). Although in infected tissues they are usually present in small numbers, when found, *S. schenckii* cells appear as round, oval, or cigar-shaped yeasts that vary in size from 1 to 3 by 3 to 10 μm. A possible pathogenic role for *Sporothrix cyanescens* in a lung lesion in a heart transplant recipient has been reported (1).

EPIDEMIOLOGY

S. schenckii organisms are widely but nonuniformly distributed in nature, growing on plant debris in soils, on tree bark, on shrubs, and on garden plants. They have also been recovered from air, water, and other substrates. The fungus and the disease occur throughout much of the world, principally in temperate and tropical zones, but with great geographic variation (2).

S. schenckii is usually acquired by traumatic inoculation of conidia, often from minor trauma, into and beneath the skin, by splinters, thorns (especially rose thorns), or woody fragments of plants, but any activity involving contact with plants or plant products (e.g., sphagnum moss) and minor skin trauma may be adequate to initiate the infectious process (3–7). In addition, various zoonotic transmissions are reported (8). The most common of these results from human handling of cats or horses that have extensive skin lesions.

Most exposures to *S. schenckii* do not result in clinically apparent disease. Delayed hypersensitivity skin testing and antibody assays for *S. schenckii* have been reported positive in 11% to 26% of individuals tested (9–11).

Osteoarticular and disseminated sporotrichosis develop most commonly in patients with chronic alcoholism or immunosuppression. In particular, persons with human immunodeficiency virus (HIV) infection and the acquired immunodeficiency syndrome (AIDS) have been reported with disseminated cutaneous sporotrichosis and with disseminated sporotrichosis, including sporotrichal meningitis (12–17). The incidence of sporotrichosis in persons with AIDS is not precisely known; however, disseminated sporotrichosis is less common than other endemic mycoses in such persons. Experimental evidence (18) and these observations indicate a role of CD4$^+$ lymphocytes and cell-mediated immunity in protection from disseminated sporotrichosis.

PATHOGENESIS

The primary lesion, a suppurating granuloma occasionally containing an asteroid body, appears 1 to 10 weeks or longer after the penetrating skin injury (19). From the initial lesion, the fungus spreads along local lymphatic channels, forming the chain of indolent nodular and ulcerating lesions that typify lympho-

cutaneous sporotrichosis. The thermal sensitivity of this fungus is a factor in the restriction of lesions to skin and subcutaneous lymphatics. Many *S. schenckii* isolates from the fixed and lymphocutaneous lesions are unable to grow well at temperatures higher than 35°C (20,21).

Bones, joints, tendon sheaths, and bursae are the structures most often involved by the nonlymphocutaneous form of sporotrichosis (osteoarticular sporotrichosis). Pulmonary sporotrichosis is uncommon, and whether it results from inhalation or from hematogenous spread of the fungus is not clear. However, reports of sporotrichal sinusitis lend credence to the role of the inhalation route (22). Central nervous system (CNS) sporotrichosis is rare (14,17,23).

CLINICAL MANIFESTATIONS

Lymphocutaneous Sporotrichosis

The primary lesion develops in the skin at the site of inoculation, typically the hand or fingers, but it can be located on any (exposed) part of the body, including the face. The initial small nodule slowly enlarges, turns red, becomes pustular, and ulcerates, releasing small amounts of purulent material from which the organism is readily cultured. Some patients exhibit no lymphangitic spread, and the disease presents as an indolent, ulcerating plaque that persists for years if it is not treated. This is called *fixed cutaneous* or *plaque sporotrichosis*. The frequency of this form of the disease varies from 10% in some series from the United States (24) to more than 50% in patients reported from other countries (25). The lesions usually are not painful.

In the lymphocutaneous form of the disease, extension along lymphatic channels of the skin is soon apparent, and a chain of nodules develops. The older more distal lesions ulcerate and drain, and the newer more proximal lesions form subcutaneous nodules that attach to the skin as they age and begin to ulcerate (Fig. 272.2). Epitrochlear lymph nodes may be involved, but the axillary and inguinal nodes are usually spared. Spontaneous healing of cutaneous and lymphocutaneous sporotrichosis is reported (26), but without treatment, the lesions usually persist for years.

Extracutaneous Sporotrichosis

The fungus likely spreads to deeper tissues via hematogenous dissemination. Lesions may occur in almost any organ, but

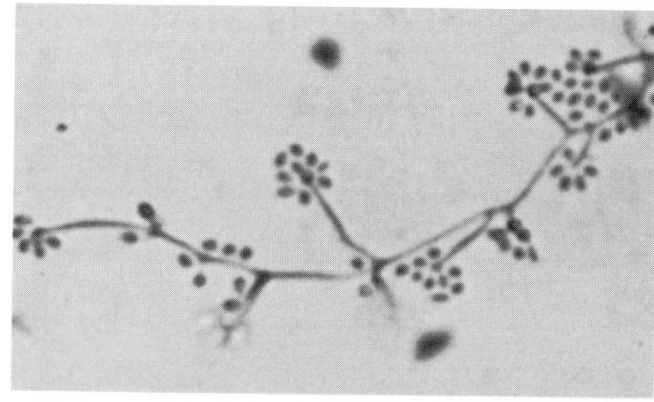

Figure 272.1. Daisy-like clusters of ovoid conidia are born at the tips of slender conidiophores that arise at angles from a single hyphal filament. The photograph was made from a slide culture.

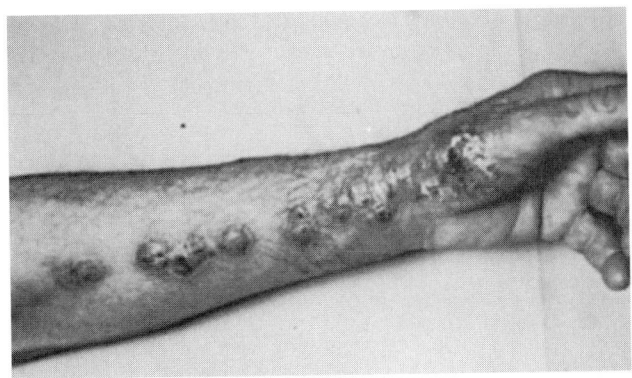

Figure 272.2. The chain of ulcerating nodular skin lesions is typical of the lymphocutaneous form of sporotrichosis. Characteristically, the older distal lesions show more ulceration and the younger proximal lesions have not yet broken down. The "bridges" of normal skin between lesions occur frequently, but a firm swollen lymphatic "cord" connecting the nodules can be felt under the skin.

disease tends to localize in the joints, especially of the extremities, and in the adjacent long bones. The process generally begins as a monoarticular arthritis, but other joints may become involved successively (27). The resulting arthritis is often confused with inflammatory arthritis, often for many months or years, until bone destruction and draining fistulas suggest the need for cultures to establish the cause of the osteomyelitis. Non-AIDS patients with osteoarticular sporotrichosis typically do not have concurrent evident cutaneous or lymphocutaneous disease.

The inflammatory response in sporotrichosis of bones, joints, and tendons is most often low grade and chronic, but the patient usually has pain and the involved areas may be warm and red. Patients with sporotrichal arthritis initially do not have the severe limitation on motion characteristic of bacterial arthritis. Functional impairment from long-standing joint sporotrichosis may become severe.

Pulmonary sporotrichosis typically presents as a chronic pneumonitis with cavitation, usually in the upper lobes, which is clinically indistinguishable from mycobacterial or other fungal infections (28,29). Patients usually have underlying chronic obstructive pulmonary disease. Symptoms are productive cough with often-minimal constitutional symptoms.

Sporotrichosis lesions occasionally develop in a variety of other organs—eye, prostate, oral mucosa, and larynx—and the clinical manifestations then depend on the organ involved. Involvement of the CNS and meninges is more common in patients with AIDS but is still rare (14,15,17,23).

The presentation of sporotrichosis can be atypical and more invasive in patients with HIV infection and particularly with AIDS. Whereas patients with early HIV infection may have typical cutaneous or lymphocutaneous sporotrichosis, widespread often ulcerative cutaneous lesions and multifocal extracutaneous dissemination occurs in patients with CD4$^+$ lymphocyte counts of less than 200 cells/mL (15).

DIAGNOSIS

The characteristic chain of ulcerating skin nodules should stimulate a high degree of clinical suspicion. Individual skin lesions have no diagnostic features, and laboratory diagnosis is required. The extracutaneous forms of the disease are even less distinctive. Recovery of the fungus may be difficult, and repeated attempts

may be necessary. Synovial biopsy is more often positive than synovial fluid culture.

Specific Laboratory Diagnosis

A positive serologic test result provides support for the diagnosis and should stimulate culture and biopsy confirmation. A variety of tests, based on detection of antibody to the peptidorhamnomannan of the outer cell wall of the organism (19), are available commercially and from reference laboratories; considerable interlaboratory variability in sensitivity and specificity seems to exist. Other techniques have been evaluated (23,30), but further data are needed.

Demonstration of *S. schenckii* is necessary for definitive diagnosis, and this is accomplished by recovery on culture from normally sterile body sites and/or identification of the fungus in biopsy specimens with periodic acid–Schiff, Gomori methenamine silver, or immunohistochemical stains.

DIFFERENTIAL DIAGNOSIS

Sporotrichosis is the most common cause of lymphocutaneous syndrome, also called *nodular lymphangitis*, in the United States (31–32). The most common alternative causes of this syndrome are *Nocardia brasiliensis* (and less commonly other *Nocardia* species), *Mycobacterium marinum* (and less commonly *Mycobacterium chelonae* and other *Mycobacterium* species), and *Leishmania brasiliensis* (and less commonly *Leishmania tropica* and *Leishmania major*) (31,32). Less common causes than this group include *Coccidioides immitis* and *Francisella tularensis*.

The differential diagnosis of pulmonary sporotrichosis includes tuberculosis, atypical mycobacteriosis, histoplasmosis, coccidioidomycosis, nocardiosis, and other subacute or chronic cavitary pulmonary infections. The primary differential diagnosis of sporotrichal arthritis includes rheumatoid arthritis and other inflammatory arthritides. Sporotrichal osteomyelitis must be distinguished from bacterial and other fungal etiologies of osteomyelitis.

TREATMENT

Cutaneous and lymphocutaneous sporotrichosis usually respond to treatment with saturated solution of potassium iodide (SSKI), although response rates have not been precisely determined. An initial dose of 10 drops diluted in liquid, preferably fruit juice, to mask its bitter taste, is given three times daily after meals, and increased drop-wise to 120 drops per day or the maximum tolerated by the individual patient (usually less than 60 drops). This last dose is continued for 3 to 6 months to include 1 to 2 months after the lesions appear to be fully healed. Although relatively inexpensive, this form of therapy is poorly accepted by many patients and often complicated by increased lacrimation, increased salivation, salivary gland swelling, gastrointestinal tract upset, hypothyroidism, and an acneiform rash. These side effects can sometimes be managed by temporary cessation of therapy, followed by resumption at a reduced dose. Although still useful in many parts of the world, therapy with SSKI has been supplanted by more tolerable, albeit more expensive, therapies in much of the developed world. The mechanism of action of potassium iodide is unknown; it is ineffective *in vitro* against *S. schenckii* and could not be shown to enhance killing of the organism by neutrophils or monocytes (33).

The azole antifungals have efficacy in cutaneous and lymphocutaneous sporotrichosis. Itraconazole has become the drug of choice, dosed as 100 to 200 mg per day for 3 to 6 months (34). The expected success rate is 90% to 100% (35–37). Fluconazole is second-line treatment for sporotrichosis (34). It is less effective than itraconazole (38,39), and for cutaneous or lymphocutaneous infection, it should be dosed as 400 mg per day in patients who cannot tolerate itraconazole. Ketoconazole is even less effective than fluconazole (40) and should not be used (34). Voriconazole has poor *in vitro* activity against *S. schenckii* (41).

Terbinafine appears to be effective (42) but cannot be recommended for use based on the limited available data. Additional trials are in progress. Amphotericin B preparations are active, but not recommended for cutaneous or lymphocutaneous sporotrichosis because of toxicity in treatment of this localized non–life-threatening infection (34). Amphotericin B is the only agent for treatment when sporotrichosis must be treated during pregnancy (34).

Local application of heat may be useful adjunctively (20,43). Itraconazole at a dose of 200 mg twice daily should be used as initial therapy for most patients with osteoarticular sporotrichosis and continued for 12 months (34). The expected rate of success of this therapy is 60% to 80% (37,44). Fluconazole is less effective (39) but might be used, only in patients intolerant of itraconazole, at a dose of 800 mg daily (34). Amphotericin B preparations may be indicated for treating patients with extensive involvement or for those patients in whom itraconazole therapy fails (34). A total dose of 1 to 2 g is usually used. Success rates appear to be similar to those achieved with itraconazole, but the drug is less well tolerated. As in other bone and joint infections, drainage and débridement are often required in osteoarticular sporotrichosis (27).

Treatment options for pulmonary sporotrichosis are amphotericin B preparations (total dose 1 to 2 g of conventional amphotericin B) and itraconazole (200 mg twice daily). Amphotericin B is indicated for patients with life-threatening or extensive pulmonary sporotrichosis (34). A combination of initial amphotericin B and subsequent surgical resection appears most effective but is unavailable to many patients because of the severity of the underlying pulmonary disease (29). Itraconazole can be used as initial therapy for patients with non–life-threatening pulmonary sporotrichosis or for continued therapy after initial induction with amphotericin B. Protracted therapy is required, although the optimal duration of therapy is undefined.

The preferred treatment for meningeal sporotrichosis is amphotericin B (34). Both flucytosine and rifampin usually show *in vitro* synergism with amphotericin B (34). The role of combination antifungal therapy for sporotrichosis is largely undefined, but these agents may be useful adjuncts in treatment of recalcitrant disease and in treatment of meningitis.

On the basis of case reports, amphotericin B is the drug of choice for treatment of disseminated sporotrichosis in patients with AIDS (17). Itraconazole appears beneficial for long-term (lifelong or until immune reconstitution) maintenance therapy after a course of amphotericin B and can be used as initial therapy for non–immediately life-threatening disease with documented absence of meningitis (34).

PREVENTION

Sporotrichosis can be prevented when specific environmental sources of *S. schenckii* are identified and avoided or eliminated. For the most part, however, the simple precautions needed to prevent infection in agricultural workers are difficult to achieve, because of the inconvenience and cost of the necessary protective clothing for hands, feet, arms, and legs. Protection against avocational exposures is even less likely to be universally achieved.

ACKNOWLEDGMENTS

The author acknowledges the roles of Harold G. Muchmore, M.D., and E. Nan Scott, Ph.D., in authorship of this chapter in previous editions.

REFERENCES

1. Tambini R, Farina C, Fiocchi R, et al. Possible pathogenic role for *Sporothrix cyanescens* isolated from a lung lesion in a heart transplant patient. *J Med Vet Mycol* 1996;34:195–198.
2. Pappas PG, Tellez I, Deep AE. Sporotrichosis in Peru: description of an area of hyperendemicity. *Clin Infect Dis* 2000;30:65–70.
3. Powell KE, Taylor A, Phillips BJ, et al. Cutaneous sporotrichosis in forestry workers. *JAMA* 1978;240:232.
4. Control CFD. Multistate outbreak of sporotrichosis in seedling handlers. *MMWR Morb Mortal Wkly Rep* 1988;37:652.
5. Coles FB, Schuchat A, Hibbs JR. A multistate outbreak of sporotrichosis associated with sphagnum peat moss. *Am J Epidemiol* 1992;136:475–487.
6. Hajjeh R, McDonnell S, Reef S, et al. Outbreak of sporotrichosis among tree nursery workers. *J Infect Dis* 1997;176:499–504.
7. Dooley DP, Bostic PS, Beckius ML. Spook house sporotrichosis: a point-source outbreak of sporotrichosis associated with hay bale props in a Halloween haunted house. *Arch Intern Med* 1997;157:1885–1887.
8. Reed KD, Moore FM, Geiger GE, et al. Zoonotic transmission of sporotrichosis. Case report and review. *Clin Infect Dis* 1993;16:384.
9. Schneidau JD, Lamar LM, Hairston MA. Cutaneous hypersensitivity to sporotrichin in Louisiana. *JAMA* 1964;188:371.
10. Gonzales-Ochoa A, et al. Valoracion comparativa de los antigenos polisacarido y cellular de *Sporothrix schenckii. Rev Invest Salud Publica* 1970;30:303.
11. Scott EN, Muchmore HG, Parkinson AJ. Enzyme and radioimmunoassays in human sporotrichosis. In: Proceedings of the VIIIth Congress of the International Society of Human and Animal Mycology; 1982; Palmerston North, New Zealand: International Society of Human and Animal Mycology.
12. Heller HM, Fuhrer J. Disseminated sporotrichosis in patients with AIDS: case report and review of the literature. *AIDS* 1991;5:1243.
13. Keiser P, Whittle D. Sporotrichosis in human immunodeficiency virus–infected patients: report of a case. *Rev Infect Dis* 1991;13:1027.
14. Penn CC, Goldstein E, Bartholomew WR. *Sporothrix schenckii* meningitis in a patient with AIDS. *Clin Infect Dis* 1992;15:741.
15. Donabedian H, O'Donnell E, Olszewski C, et al. Disseminated cutaneous and meningeal sporotrichosis in an AIDS patient. *Diagn Microbiol Infect Dis* 1994;18:111–115.
16. Bolao F, Podzamezer D, Ventin M, et al. Efficacy of acute phase and maintenance therapy with itraconazole in an AIDS patient with sporotrichosis. *Eur J Clin Microbiol Infect Dis* 1994;13:609.
17. Rotz LD, Slater LN, Wack MF. Disseminated sporotrichosis with meningitis in a patient with AIDS. *Infect Dis Clin Pract* 1996;5:566–568.
18. Tachibana T, Matsuyama T, Mitsuyama M. Involvement of CD4+ T cells and macrophages in acquired protection against infection with *Sporothrix schenckii* in mice. *Med Mycol* 1999;37:397–404.
19. Rippon JW. Sporotrichosis. In: Rippon JW, ed. *Medical mycology: the pathogenic fungi and the pathogenic actinomycetes.* Philadelphia: WB Saunders, 1988:325–352.
20. MacKinnon JE, Conti-Diaz IA. The effect of temperature on sporotrichosis. *Sabouraudia* 1962;2:56.
21. Kwon-Chung J. Comparison of isolates of *Sporothrix schenckii* obtained from fixed cutaneous lesions with isolates from other types of lesions. *J Infect Dis* 1979;139:424.
22. Morgan M, Reves R. Invasive sinusitis due to *Sporothrix schenckii* in a patient with AIDS. *Clin Infect Dis* 1996;23:1319–1320.
23. Scott EN, Kaufman L, Brown AC, et al. Serologic studies in the diagnosis and management of meningitis due to *Sporothrix schenckii. N Engl J Med* 1987;317:935–940.
24. Dellatorre DL, Lattanand A, Buckley HR, et al. Fixed cutaneous sporotrichosis of the face. *Am Acad Dermatol* 1982;6:97.
25. Honbo S, Yamano T, Masaki J, et al. Analytical studies on peculiar cases of sporotrichosis, the lesions of which contained numerous fungal elements. In: Proceedings of the IXth Congress of the International Society of Human and Animal Mycology; 1985. Atlanta: International Society of Human and Animal Mycology.
26. Iwatsu T, Nishimura K, Niyaji M. Spontaneous disappearance of cutaneous sporotrichosis. *Int J Dermatol* 1985;24:524.
27. Bayer AS, Scott VJ, Guze LB. Fungal arthritis. III. Sporotrichoid arthritis. *Semin Arthritis Rhem* 1979;9:66.

28. Zvetina JR, Rippon JW, Daum V. Chronic pulmonary sporotrichosis. *Mycopathologia* 1978;64:53.
29. Pluss JL, Opal SM. Pulmonary sporotrichosis: review of treatment and outcome. *Medicine (Baltimore)* 1986;65:143–153.
30. Scott EN, Muchmore HG. Immunoblot analysis of antibody responses to *Sporothrix schenckii. J Clin Microbiol* 1989;27:300.
31. Smego RA Jr, Castiglia M, Asperilla MO. Lymphocutaneous syndrome: a review of non-sporothrix causes. *Medicine (Baltimore)* 1999;78:38–63.
32. Tobin EH, Jih WW. Sporotrichoid lymphocutaneous infections: etiology, diagnosis, and therapy. *Am Fam Physician* 2001;63:326–332.
33. Rex JH, Bennett JE. Administration of potassium iodide to normal volunteers doe not increase killing of *Sporothrix schenckii* by their neutrophils or monocytes. *J Med Vet Mycol* 1990;28:185–189.
34. Kauffman CA, Hajjeh R, Chapman SW, for the Mycoses Study Group. Practice guidelines for the management of patients with sporotrichosis. *Clin Infect Dis* 2000;30:684–687.
35. Restrepo A, Robledo J, Gomez I, et al. Itraconazole therapy in lymphangitic and cutaneous sporotrichosis. *Arch Dermatol* 1986;122:413.
36. Conti-Diaz IA, Civila E, Gezuele E, et al. Treatment of human cutaneous sporotrichosis with itraconazole. *Mycoses* 1992;35:153–156.
37. Sharkey-Mathis PK, Kauffman CA, Graybill JR, et al. Treatment of sporotrichosis with itraconazole. NIAID Mycoses Study Group. *Am J Med* 1993;95:279–285.
38. Diaz M, Negroni R, Montero-Gei F, et al. A Pan-American 5-year study of fluconazole therapy for deep mycoses in the immunocompetent host. *Clin Infect Dis* 1992;14:S68–S76.
39. Kauffman CA, Pappas PG, McKinsey DS, et al. Treatment of lymphocutaneous and visceral sporotrichosis with fluconazole. *Clin Infect Dis* 1996;22:46–50.
40. Calhoun DL, Waskin H, White MP, et al. Treatment of systemic sporotrichosis with ketoconazole. *Rev Infect Dis* 1991;30:315.
41. Espinel-Ingroff A. *In vitro* activity of the new triazole voriconazole (UK-109,496) against opportunistic filamentous and dimorphic fungi and common and emerging yeast pathogens. *J Clin Microbiol* 1998;36:198.
42. Hull PR, Vismer HF. Treatment of cutaneous sporotrichosis with terbinafine. *Br J Dermatol* 1992;126:51–55.
43. Hiruma M, Katoh T, Yamamoto I, et al. Local hyperthermia in the treatment of sporotrichosis. *Mykosen* 1987;30:315.
44. Winn RE, Anderson J, Piper J, et al. Systemic sporotrichosis treated with itraconazole. *Clin Infect Dis* 1993;17:210–217.

CHAPTER 273

Blastomyces *and* Paracoccidioides

George S. Deepe, Jr.

BLASTOMYCES

George S. Deepe, Jr., and Bruce S. Klein

In 1894, T. C. Gilchrist examined a skin biopsy specimen from the hand of a patient who had been diagnosed with scrofuloderma. He failed to detect tubercle bacilli but noted the presence of protozoan-like organisms that appeared budding and yeast-like (1). Shortly thereafter, Gilchrist and Stokes (2,3) identified a similar organism in the skin of a patient who was thought to have lupus vulgaris. They successfully cultured it on artificial medium and transferred the infection to a dog. Because the microbe resembled blastomycetes morphologically, the new pathogen was called *Blastomyces dermatitidis.*

CHARACTERISTICS OF THE PATHOGEN

B. dermatitidis is a dimorphic fungus that exists as a mycelial form in nature and a yeast form in tissues from infected humans and animals. In culture, the organism grows as a mycelium at room temperature and as a yeast at 37°C. *In vitro* the transition from mycelium to yeast can be divided into three stages. Stage 1 is characterized by uncoupling of oxidative phosphorylation and a decrement in cellular adenosine triphosphate levels. In stage 2, spontaneous respiration terminates. Subsequently, the cells enter stage 3, in which respiration recovers and the fungus transforms to the yeast phase. Cysteine is required during stage 2 for conversion to yeast cells (4). Existence of this pathway in the dimorphic fungi, *Histoplasma capsulatum* and *Paracoccidioides brasiliensis,* suggests a common mechanism for survival *in vivo* (4,5).

On artificial media, such as Sabouraud's, mycelia grow as fluffy white colonies. Conidia range from 2 to 10 μm in diameter. Yeast colonies are wrinkled and folded. Yeast cells are multinucleate and form broad-based buds, and individual ones may vary from 8 to 30 μm in diameter (6). *B. dermatitidis* possesses a sexual stage termed *Ajellomyces dermatitidis.* The organism is heterothallic, and both "positive" (pigmented colonies) and "negative" (white colonies) mating types have been identified (7). Both mating types cause clinical disease, apparently in equal proportions, and both have been isolated from a single patient (7,9).

Two serotypes that differ in the expression of cell wall A antigen, and multiple genotypes, defined by restriction fragment length polymorphisms, have been described (10,11).

EPIDEMIOLOGY

Infection with *B. dermatitidis* has been reported from North and South America, Europe, Africa, and Asia (6). Delineation of the endemic regions, particularly in North America, has relied on case reports of human or animal infection because no widely available test exists to identify asymptomatic infection. In the United States, blastomycosis occurs in the Midwest and southeast (except Florida), western Pennsylvania, and northern New York. Endemic zones are found in the Canadian provinces of Ontario, Quebec, and Alberta.

In the past, *B. dermatitidis* was rarely recovered from soil. Epidemiological studies of outbreaks of blastomycosis in Wisconsin have uncovered a natural habitat in soil along riverbanks where human cases have been exposed. Cultures of soil and organic debris from these sites propagated *B. dermatitidis.* Hence, the environment along waterways may represent an important reservoir for infection (12,13).

Clinical illness caused by *B. dermatitidis* develops nine times more often in men than in women (14), a finding that has been attributed to sex differences in occupation and recreational activities. The vast majority of reported cases have occurred in manual laborers, hunters, and agricultural workers, and in the past, these endeavors have been performed principally by men. In blastomycosis epidemics, documented infection is not more prevalent in men.

Exact information regarding incidence and prevalence of infection does not exist, because the illness is not reportable and a reliable diagnostic test is not widely available. Surveys of hospital discharges performed by the Centers for Disease Control and Prevention during 1970 and 1980 to 1982 indicate that the incidence of blastomycosis is 0.6 per million per year (15). However, this figure underestimates the true occurrence of infection. Most cases are sporadic, but several epidemics have been recognized (12,13,16–18).

With the exception of rare cases of sexual transmission (19,20), blastomycosis is not transmitted from human to human. One report indicated that human blastomycosis resulted from the bite of an actively infected dog (21). Reports of inoculation blastomycosis in pathologists indicate the infection may be an occupational hazard (22).

PATHOGENESIS

Presumably, infection with *B. dermatitidis* develops from accidental inhalation of hyphae and conidia from soil, although definitive proof is lacking (23). Most likely, the inhaled fungal elements settle into respiratory bronchioles or alveoli, where they transform within days into the yeast phase. Upon the transition, BAD1 (previously termed *WI-1*) a 120-kd protein and essential virulence factor gets displayed on the surface of yeast cells (23a,23b). BAD1 binds the fungus to host tissue and inhibits innate immune responses by impeding production of tumor necrosis factor-α (TNF-α) by phagocytes (23b,23c). Surviving organisms disseminate lymphohematogenously to regional lymph nodes and other organ systems. *Blastomyces* organisms induce two distinct inflammatory responses. In visceral organs such as lung, liver, and genitourinary tract, the typical reaction, which is termed *pyogranulomatous*, is an admixture of suppuration and granulomatous inflammation with giant cells (Fig. 273.1). Although granulomata often surround areas of suppurative necrosis, tissue sections may contain fields composed either strictly of neutrophils and necrotic debris or of granulomata. Pyogranulomatous inflammation is also found in tissues of those infected with *Coccidioides immitis* and *P. brasiliensis*. The characteristic histopathologic picture of the skin and squamous mucosa (e.g., trachea, larynx) is that of pseudoepitheliomatous proliferation with intraepithelial microabscesses (23). In visceral organs, the evolution of the inflammatory response to *B. dermatitidis* yeasts has been ascertained from limited autopsy material and experimental models (24–26). The earliest cellular infiltrate (within 24 hours) contains polymorphonuclear leukocytes. By 7 days, granulomata and suppurative necrosis can be detected (25). The incubation period for primary pulmonary blastomycosis is approximately 6 weeks and ranges from 21 to 106 days. It is shorter for occupational blastomycosis (median 14 days, range of 7 to 35 days) (22).

Blastomyces yeasts release a chemotactic factor that induces influx of neutrophils and monocytes (27). The pyogranulomatous

reaction can be elicited by cell walls from virulent yeasts. Phospholipid from this material may be responsible for producing the granulomatous response (28,29).

IMMUNE RESPONSE AND HOST DEFENSES

Detection of antibody in response to infection by *B. dermatitidis* has been hampered by lack of a suitable antigen. Humoral responses to A antigen can be measured in many cases (30). Unfortunately, A antigen contains carbohydrate epitopes that are shared with other dimorphic fungi, which causes the nonspecificity in commercial serologic assays for blastomycosis (31). More recently, the BAD1 antigen has been shown to be a specific target of the humoral response of humans (32). The antibodies are directed against a 25–amino acid repeat arrayed in tandem on this protein and on A antigen (31,33). Specific antibody appears to have no role in host defenses (34).

In vitro, human neutrophils and mononuclear phagocytes kill conidia, but these phagocytes, which are prominent in the inflammatory response, kill yeasts inefficiently (35,36). In cell-free systems, conidia and yeasts are susceptible to products of oxygen metabolism. Conidia are partially eliminated by hydrogen peroxide and are killed completely by hypochlorous acid or a combination of hydrogen peroxide, myeloperoxidase, and halide (36,37). Yeasts are much less susceptible to hydrogen peroxide. Killing by this substance can be augmented by addition of Fe^{2+} and halide (38,39).

Infection activates cell-mediated immunity. The percentage of humans with blastomycosis who mount a skin-test response to blastomycin has ranged from 0% to 50% (40,41). The high incidence of anergy is probably related to the poor antigenicity of blastomycin. *In vitro*, human monocyte-derived macrophages recognize the yeast through binding the BAD1 surface protein with CR3 (CD11b/CD18) and CD14 receptors. Subsequent uptake of the yeast and processing of this and other antigens leads to outgrowth of $CD4^+$ T cells and is associated with development of acquired resistance (42,43). An alkali-soluble, water-soluble antigen (B-ASWS) from the cell wall and the BAD1 antigen share a determinant that induces T-cell proliferative responses by peripheral blood mononuclear cells of persons who

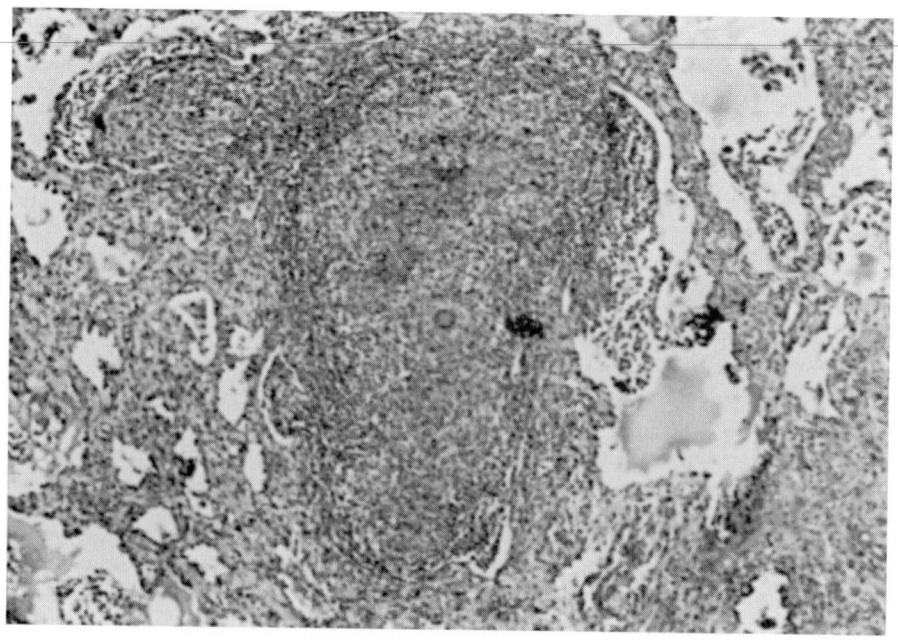

Figure 273.1. Pyogranulomatous response to *Blastomyces dermatitidis* in a lung specimen from a patient with pulmonary blastomycosis. A mantle of mononuclear cells surrounds the area of acute inflammation. A giant cell is seen in the middle of the field (×165). (Courtesy Judith Rhodes, PhD, University of Cincinnati College of Medicine, Cincinnati, Ohio.)

have recovered from blastomycosis (43,44). Both antigens are useful for skin testing *B. dermatitidis*–infected animals but have not been studied in humans. Protective immunity is conferred by antigen-reactive T lymphocytes (34). Interferon-γ (IFN-γ) enhances the anti-*Blastomyces* activity of neutrophils, monocytes, and macrophages (45,46,46a).

CLINICAL MANIFESTATIONS

Like other systemic mycoses, blastomycosis is a spectral disease. Most likely most of these infections are asymptomatic. Clinical features of blastomycosis range from acute, self-limited pneumonia to a disseminated form (Table 273.1).

Pulmonary Disease

Acute pulmonary blastomycosis produces two distinct patterns of illness. One is a systemic, influenza-like illness characterized by fever, chills, myalgias, arthralgias, photophobia, and headache. A nonproductive cough can progress to a cough productive of mucopurulent sputum. The second type of illness consists of pleuritic chest pain of abrupt onset without constitutional symptoms. The pain usually lasts no longer than 48 hours. Occasionally, acute pulmonary infection fails to resolve and advances by bronchogenic spread from a localized pneumonia to widespread involvement of all lung fields (47–49). Frequently, ulcerative bronchitis is present in pulmonary tissues of patients with this form of disease (23). Chest radiographs of acute disease typically reveal segmental airspace disease, which varies from patchy nodular opacities to extensive confluent densities (Fig. 273.2). Less common abnormalities include mass lesions, interstitial infiltrates, cavitation, and miliary pattern (48,50,51).

Chronic pulmonary blastomycosis, defined by the presence of symptoms lasting longer than 3 weeks (48), is clinically indistinguishable from pulmonary tuberculosis, histoplasmosis, or coccidioidomycosis. This illness may be the result of nonhealing acute pneumonia or reactivation of dormant disease foci. Fatigue, low-grade fever, malaise, and weight loss are often observed. Radiographic abnormalities, if present, are similar to those in acute pulmonary infection.

Extrapulmonary Blastomycosis

Evidence of dissemination is common among patients with blastomycosis. Spread of the fungus beyond the lungs (Table 273.2) may result from progression of pulmonary infection or reacti-

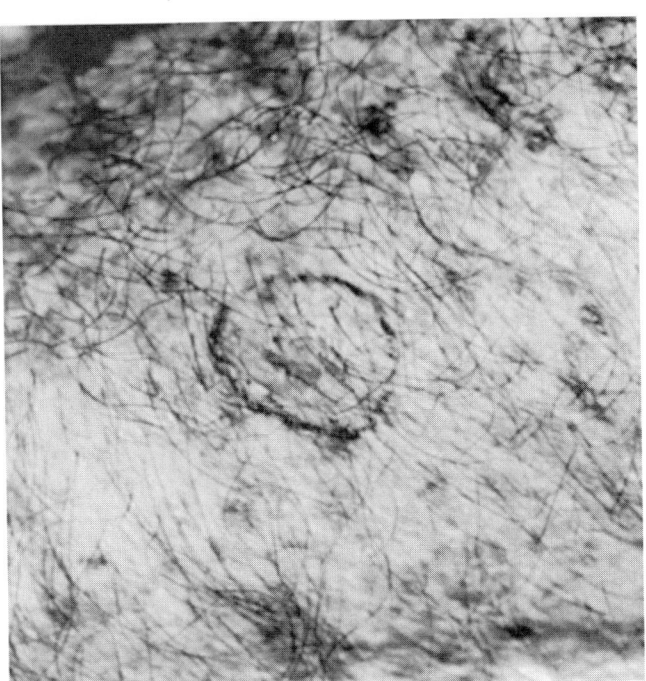

Figure 273.2. Early skin lesion of disseminated blastomycosis. A small papule is present on the forearm of a patient with systemic blastomycosis. (Courtesy Corwin Dunn, MD, Christ Hospital, Cincinnati, Ohio.)

vated disease (48,52). The most common sites of involvement are skin, bone, genitourinary tract, and central nervous system (CNS).

Cutaneous lesions begin as subcutaneous nodules or pustular papules (Fig. 273.3). Untreated, they become ulcerated with verrucous borders. The center is crusted, and "black dots" (degenerated capillaries) (53) are present in the ulcer (Fig. 273.4). These lesions are usually distributed on exposed areas of skin but can also develop on mucocutaneous surfaces and may be misdiagnosed as carcinoma. A second type of skin manifestation is the papule that becomes ulcerated with a granulomatous base.

Bone is a common site of involvement in disseminated blastomycosis. Although any bone may be infected, ribs, vertebrae, long bones, skull, and facial bones are the most common. The lesions are painless and may be manifested only by a draining sinus or subcutaneous abscess. The characteristic radiographic

---

TABLE 273.1. Clinical Manifestations of Blastomycosis

Pulmonary blastomycosis
  Acute (duration of symptoms ≤3 wk)
    Asymptomatic
    Influenza-like illness (fever, chills, cough, myalgias)
    Pleuritic symptoms
  Chronic (duration of symptoms >3 wk)
    Progression by bronchogenic spread from acute pulmonary
      disease
    Endogenous reactivation
Extrapulmonary blastomycosis
  Lymphohematogenous spread from advancing pneumonia
  Endogenous reactivation

TABLE 273.2. Prevalence of Extrapulmonary Blastomycosis by Site

Site	Prevalence[a] (%)
Skin	68.8
Bone and joints	18.7
Genitourinary tract	14.5
Reticuloendothelial system (liver, spleen, lymph nodes, bone marrow)	9.4
Subcutaneous tissue	5.0
Mucosa[b]	4.3
Thyroid	2.2

[a]Percentages based on reviews of references 41, 48, 62, 66–70. Calculations include autopsy studies.
[b]Laryngeal, oropharyngeal, and nasal.

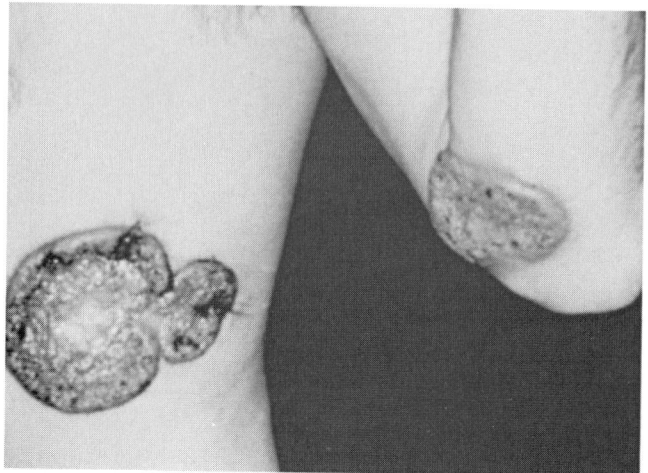

Figure 273.3. Advanced skin lesions of disseminated blastomycosis on the thorax and arm. The patient had an 18-month history of progressive skin disease. Note the verrucous borders and ulcerated center, as well as the numerous black dots on the arm lesion.

feature of osseous disease is a lytic lesion (54). The fungus can spread from bone to joints (55).

Within the genitourinary tract, kidneys, prostate, epididymides, testes, seminal vesicles, and bladder can be infected by *B. dermatitidis*. In kidneys, *Blastomyces* yeasts and pyogranulomatous inflammation are more common in the cortex than in the medulla (56). Involvement of the prostate may cause nonspecific prostatitis and symptoms of obstruction. Epididymitis can be recurrent. The last two diseases can be the presenting symptom of disseminated blastomycosis (23,41,57).

CNS infection has been reported in as many as 33% of autopsies, but clinically apparent disease is less common (see Table 273.2). The fungus elicits a granulomatous or a suppura-

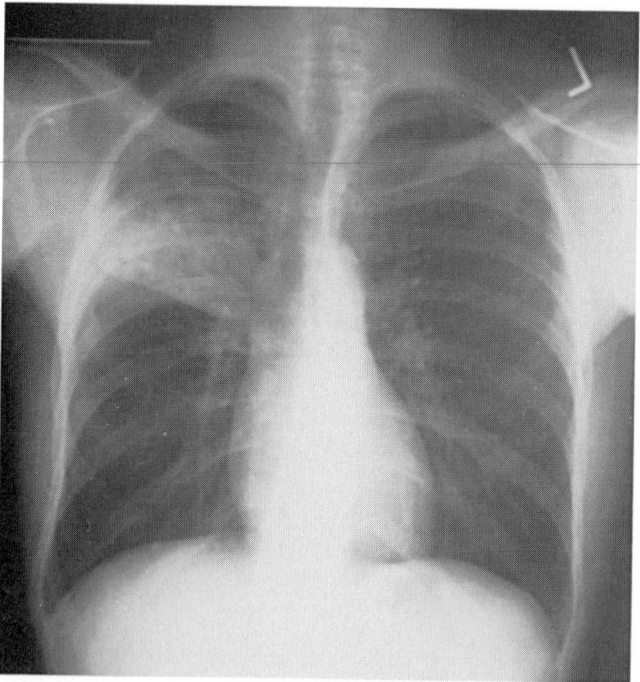

Figure 273.4. Pulmonary blastomycosis. Right upper lobe airspace disease is apparent.

tive mass lesion that may be mistaken for tumor. Chronic basilar meningitis is a late manifestation and is indistinguishable from other causes of this illness. Lymphocytic pleocytosis, hypoglycorrhachia, and elevated protein level are common laboratory findings in cerebrospinal fluid (CSF) of persons with blastomycotic meningitis (58).

Blastomyces organisms may spread to adrenals, larynx, thyroid, gastrointestinal tract, liver, and spleen. Hypoadrenalism is rare. Far fewer children than adults contract blastomycosis, but the spectrum of disease is similar in both (59).

Blastomycosis is predominantly a disease of immunocompetent hosts, although infection does occur in patients who are immunosuppressed. Clinical manifestations of disseminated infection in immunocompromised persons are virtually the same as those in persons whose immune system is putatively intact, except that the disease progresses more rapidly (60–60b).

Laboratory abnormalities can exist in all forms of blastomycosis, but they are nonspecific. Elevated erythrocyte sedimentation rates, leukocytosis with an increase in band forms of neutrophils, and anemia are often present.

DIAGNOSIS

The yeasts can be visualized in specimens from body fluids or aspirated skin lesions. A wet-mount preparation, with or without 10% potassium hydroxide, can be examined by light microscopy (Fig. 273.5). CSF, bronchoalveolar lavage fluid, urine, and pleural fluid specimens should be centrifuged to optimize the chance of detecting the organism. In such specimens, yeasts are characteristic. They are large and possess a broad-based bud and a refractile cell wall. These features help distinguish *B. dermatitidis* from *P. brasiliensis*, which has a narrow bud, and from *Cryptococcus neoformans*, which has a capsule. In skin aspirates, yeasts should not be confused with lipid droplets.

When blastomycosis is suspected, histopathologic examination of tissue specimens should include staining with Gomori methenamine silver because yeasts may not be seen with hematoxylin-eosin stain. The presence of pyogranulomatous inflammation should alert the physician to the possibility of blastomycosis. Periodic acid–Schiff stain colors the cell wall red and can be a useful adjunctive stain, because it allows evaluation of the inflammatory response and morphologic characteristics of the organism. If *Cryptococcus* infection is considered, mucicarmine, which stains the cell wall of *Cryptococcus* but not *Blastomyces*, may be used.

Specimens should be submitted for culture. Material is plated on Sabouraud's glucose agar and cultured at 30°C. Specimens contaminated with bacteria may be plated on agar containing penicillin and streptomycin or chloramphenicol. If the fungus is to be confirmed, the yeast form must be grown, and this is accomplished by culturing on nutrient agar at 37°C.

Serologic tests are performed by immunodiffusion using A antigen. Precipitin antibodies are reported in up to 80% of cases (30). An enzyme immunoassay using A antigen is more sensitive but has a higher frequency of false-positive results (20% to 25%). No reliable skin test is available. Lymphocyte transformation studies *in vitro* with B-ASWS or BAD1 antigens can identify a large proportion of infected patients, but the test is not feasible for most clinical laboratories (12).

The differential diagnosis of acute pulmonary blastomycosis includes other fungal pneumonias acquired from nature and bacterial pneumonias. Disseminated blastomycosis should be distinguished from disseminated coccidioidomycosis and paracoccidioidomycosis.

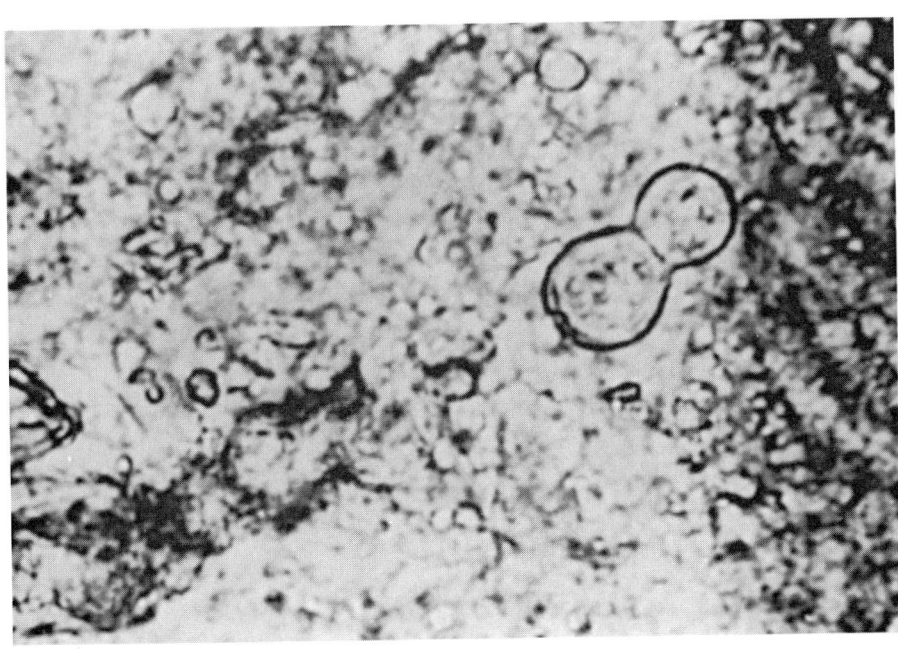

Figure 273.5. *Blastomyces* yeast in potassium hydroxide preparation from skin aspiration. Note the broad-based budding of this fungal form.

TREATMENT

Rarely, patients with acute blastomycosis may not require specific antifungal therapy if they have no significant underlying disease and if symptoms have been present less than 3 weeks, although this approach is controversial (49). No specific indices are available to aid the physician in determining who is at risk for progressive disease. Therefore, the patient should be observed for several months after the initial illness, to ensure that infection has not progressed.

Before the advent of effective antifungal therapy, the mortality rate of blastomycosis exceeded 60%. Amphotericin B has been the mainstay of therapy for the past three decades. The exact amount of amphotericin B required to cure blastomycosis has not been determined, but studies have suggested that a total dose of less than 1.0 g is associated with a higher mortality and a total dose of less than 1.5 g with a higher rate of relapse. Therefore, recommendations for total dose usually range from 2.0 to 2.5 g of amphotericin B or 30 to 35 mg/kg. Even with this dose, 10% to 20% of patients suffer a relapse 5 years after treatment is completed (62). Many relapses respond to a second course of amphotericin B. Numerous schedules for amphotericin B administration have been published, but it is our practice to give 10 mg on the first day and increase the daily dose by 10 to 15 mg to a maximum of 50 mg. If the patient is seriously ill, amphotericin B is given daily until symptoms resolve, then three times a week. Patients who are less ill receive 50 mg three times a week.

Itraconazole and ketoconazole have emerged as important therapeutic options in the treatment of nonmeningeal blastomycosis in immunocompetent hosts. A clinical trial showed that itraconazole therapy produced cure rates of 90% in nonmeningeal and in non–life-threatening forms of blastomycosis and was less toxic than ketoconazole therapy. Many experts now prefer itraconazole to ketoconazole because of its similar efficacy and lower toxicity. The recommended initial dose of itraconazole in adults is 200 mg per day. If disease persists or progresses, the dose should be increased in increments of 100 mg up to a maximum of 400 mg per day. Treatment should be continued for at least 6 months. After that, it can be discontinued when symptoms have dissipated or radiographic abnormalities have improved or stabilized. There is little published clinical experience with the use of itraconazole in children (65).

PARACOCCIDIOIDES

George S. Deepe, Jr.

HISTORY

The first cases of paracoccidioidomycosis were described in Brazil by Adolfo Lutz in 1908 (71). He reported two patients with granulomatous disease of the nasopharynx and cervical lymphadenopathy. He identified in tissues the presence of a budding organism that resembled *C. immitis*. Material removed from the lymph nodes grew a filamentous organism that was indicative of a fungus. Lutz called the infectious process "hyphoblastomycosis." For many years, the illness was believed to be caused by *C. immitis* until Almeida provided evidence that hyphoblastomycosis was caused by a distinct pathogenic fungus (72). Subsequently, the organism was named *P. brasiliensis*.

CHARACTERISTICS OF THE PATHOGEN

The agent of paracoccidioidomycosis is the dimorphic fungus *P. brasiliensis*. In secretions from mucocutaneous lesions, in tissues, and in culture at 37°C, the fungus is found as a double-walled, oval to round yeast cell of 4 to 40 µm in diameter. The yeast may exhibit single or multiple budding (73); a yeast cell surrounded by numerous budding yeasts gives the appearance of a pilot wheel, which is characteristic of this pathogenic fungus (Fig. 273.6).

The fungus is usually grown on Sabouraud's dextrose agar, although other media support its growth. At 37°C, the colonies are soft and cream colored and have a cerebriform, or wrinkled, appearance. At 19°C to 28°C, the fungus grows as a mold; at room temperature, well-formed colonies do not appear

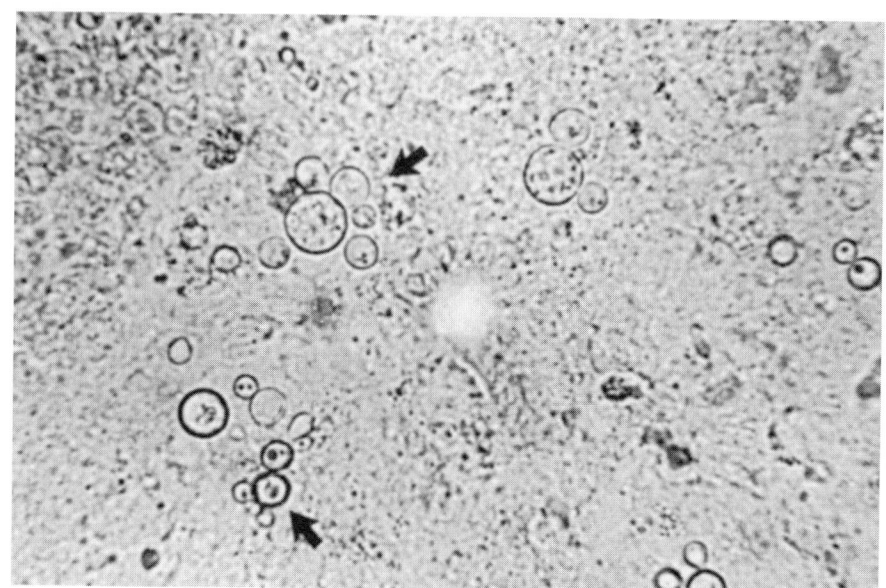

Figure 273.6. *Paracoccidioides brasiliensis* yeasts in potassium hydroxide-treated sputum sample. Note the (*arrows*) pilot-wheel appearance of the fungus. (Courtesy Angela Restrepo, PhD, Mycology Unit, Corporacìon des Investigaciones Biológicas, Medellín, Colombia.)

until 20 to 30 days of incubation (74). The mycelial phase does not sporulate well, especially if the organism is grown on media containing simple or complex carbohydrates, but when grown on yeast extract agar, there is abundant production of conidia, arthroconidia, and arthroaleurioconidium approximately 2 to 5 μm in diameter (74). Unequivocal identification of *P. brasiliensis* depends on the ability to cultivate the yeast phase.

The virulence of isolates of *P. brasiliensis* varies widely, which may account for marked differences in clinical manifestations of disease among individuals. Expression of virulence by *Paracoccidioides* has been correlated directly with glucan content in cell walls of yeasts (75,76).

EPIDEMIOLOGY

Paracoccidioidomycosis is limited geographically to Central and South America, from Mexico to Argentina. No endemic cases have been reported from Belize, Nicaragua, Surinam, Guyana, Chile, or the Caribbean islands (77). Cases have been described in North America, Europe, and Asia, but in each instance, the victim had resided in endemic areas (78,79). Eighty percent of reported cases are from Brazil (80).

Because the fungus has been isolated only rarely from nature, its ecologic niche has been difficult to determine. Case reports and skin-test results have been used to define endemic areas. Based on epidemiological studies, the areas of highest prevalence are the rural and suburban regions of Brazil, Colombia, Venezuela, Ecuador, and Argentina (77). It is thought that regions in these countries possess the climatic and ecologic conditions suitable for fungal growth in soil. This includes the combination of moderate temperatures, relatively high humidity, and rich vegetation (81).

Clinically apparent disease is observed most commonly in men who are in close contact with nature. It is rare in women (male-to-female ratio is 15:1), adolescents, and children, but the prevalence of skin-test reactivity in men and women is equal. In Colombia, Ecuador, and Argentina, the male-to-female ratio is approximately 150:1 (82). In the endemic regions, the estimated annual incidence is 1 to 3 clinical cases per 100,000 inhabitants, or 3,000 to 10,000 new cases per year (77). Most cases are observed in those who work in agriculture.

PATHOGENESIS

Human infection with *P. brasiliensis* is acquired via accidental inhalation of airborne fungal propagables (83). The small fungal elements settle into the small airways of the lungs. Once the mycelial forms have transformed into yeasts, an early neutrophilic response is followed by an influx of mononuclear cells. The yeasts spread from lung parenchyma lymphohematogenously to regional lymph nodes, forming a primary complex (84). The organism can migrate to involve many visceral organs, especially those of the mononuclear phagocyte system. Healed lesions may calcify, but it seems to happen much less frequently than in tuberculosis or histoplasmosis. After spread to distant organs, the organism may become dormant or be completely eliminated from tissues (85).

In visceral organs, the typical inflammatory response is characterized by an admixture of a necrotizing suppurative process and granulomatous inflammation (85). The evolution of the inflammatory response is derived from animal studies (86) that suggest that the earliest infiltrates (within 2 weeks) are composed of neutrophils that produce suppuration; granulomata are present from 2 weeks to 1 month after inoculation.

The increased frequency of disease in adult men suggests that hormonal factors may play a role in the pathogenesis of infection. Indeed, physiologic concentrations of estrogens, but not androgens, inhibit the transformation of mycelia to yeast (87). Estrogens do not alter yeast growth or budding (88). The increased resistance of women to *P. brasiliensis* may be caused by circulating estrogens.

IMMUNE RESPONSE AND HOST DEFENSES

Circulating specific antibody is detected in a large proportion of infected persons, and titers may escalate in progressive disseminated forms of paracoccidioidomycosis (89). Anti–*P. brasiliensis* antibody is an opsonin and enhances phagocytosis by macrophages (90). Yeast cells trigger activation of the alternative pathway of complement, and constituents of the complement cascade can act as opsonins (91).

Human neutrophils ingest yeast cells of *P. brasiliensis*, but it is not clear whether these phagocytes exert fungicidal activity (92). In cell-free systems, large amounts of hydrogen peroxide kill yeasts, and adding a halide to this system reduces the concentration of hydrogen peroxide required to exert fungicidal activity (93). Pulmonary macrophages from mice weakly kill isolates of *P. brasiliensis* yeasts. Exposure to IFN-γ can enhance the antifungal effects of these phagocytes (94). Murine natural killer cells also can limit growth of yeast cells (95).

Most patients with subclinical infection demonstrate cutaneous reactivity to paracoccidioidin, and their peripheral blood mononuclear cells mount a blastogenic response to this antigen *in vitro* (96). In widely disseminated disease, generalized anergy is observed in a large proportion of patients, but cutaneous reactivity may be restored after therapy (97). Mononuclear cells from these persons do not respond to mitogens or antigens *in vitro* and release less IFN-γ (98,99). The underlying causes of the anergic have been attributed to suppressor cells, cytokine dysregulation, and a plasma inhibitory factor (97,99–101).

CLINICAL MANIFESTATIONS

The clinicopathologic and immunologic manifestations of paracoccidioidomycosis, like those of histoplasmosis and tuberculosis, should be considered as occurring along a spectrum (Table 273.3). The clinical features of infection range from an acute pulmonary infection that is self-limited to chronic pulmonary disease to a progressive disseminated form with frequent involvement of mucocutaneous tissues, the reticuloendothelial system, and the adrenals.

Pulmonary Disease

In approximately 80% of adults infected with this fungus, pulmonary disease is evident by radiography, but most infections are asymptomatic (102,103). A smaller proportion of patients exhibit persistent cough, purulent sputum, chest pain, weight loss, weakness, malaise, dyspnea, and fever (104). Auscultatory findings are uncommon. The most common radiographic picture of the lungs in actively infected patients is diffuse interstitial and alveolar infiltrates (Fig. 273.7). The chest radiograph may also demonstrate nodules, cavitation, and hilar adenopathy. Rarely, a large cavitary mass, sometimes referred to as a *paracoccidioidoma*, is detected (104).

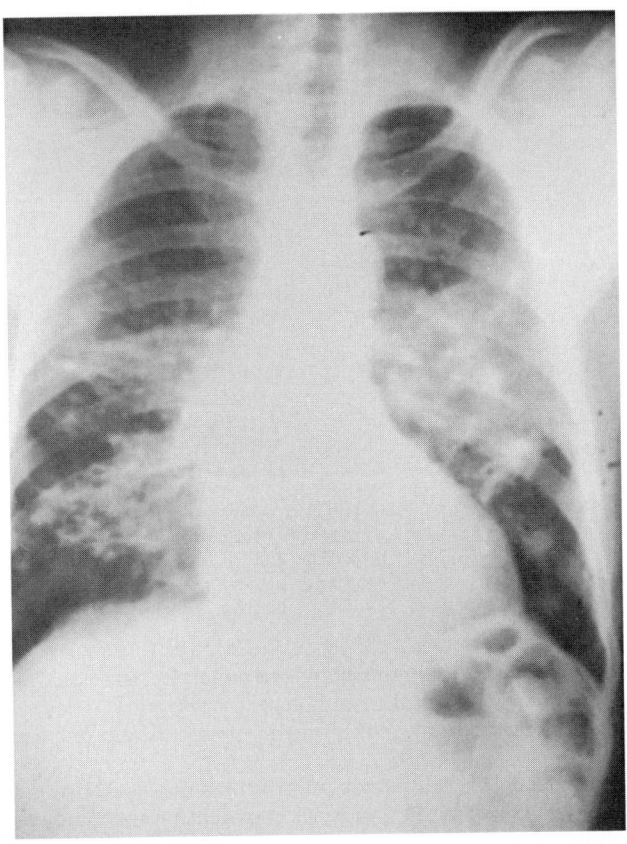

Figure 273.7. Pulmonary paracoccidioidomycosis. The chest radiograph reveals bilateral interstitial and alveolar infiltrates in the middle and lower lobes. The upper lobes are spared. (Courtesy Angela Restrepo, PhD, Mycology Unit, Corporaciòn des Investigaciones Biológicas, Medellín, Colombia.)

TABLE 273.3. Clinicopathologic and Immunologic Manifestations of Paracoccidioidomycosis[a]

Classification	Hyperergic	Intermediate	Anergic
Clinical manifestations	Asymptomatic, paracoccidioidoma	Progressive pulmonary infection, with or without mucocutaneous involvement	Widespread involvement of reticuloendothelial system, lymphadenopathy, miliary lung disease
Immune reactions			
Positive skin test (%)	90–100	42–76	<30
Anti–*Paracoccidioides brasiliensis* antibodies (%)	<5	80–95	70–100
Blastogenic response to antigens and mitogens	+++	++/+++	+/−
Histopathology	Granuloma; rare yeast cells, if any	Granuloma and necrotizing suppuration; few yeast cells	Diffuse infiltration with polymorphonuclear leukocytes and macrophages; abundant yeasts

[a]+++, Stimulation index >10; ++, stimulation index 5–10; +, stimulation index 3–5.
Source: Data from references 85,95,96,102.

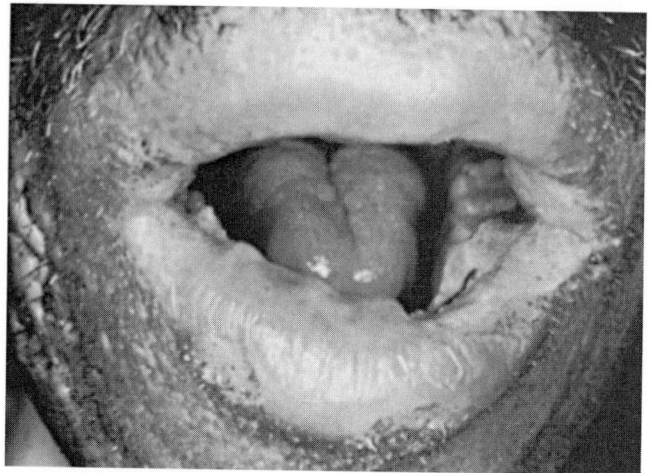

Figure 273.8. Angular cheilitis and lip lesions caused by *Paracoccidioides brasiliensis.* Hemorrhagic spots are evident at both angles of the lips. (Courtesy Angela Restrepo, PhD, Mycology Unit, Corporacìon des Investigaciones Biológicas, Medellín, Colombia.)

Chronic pulmonary infections are generally associated with progressive fibrosis of the pulmonary parenchyma. As a consequence, deterioration of lung function and cor pulmonale may ensue.

The usual sites of dissemination are the mucosal tissues and skin: Approximately 58% and 34% of patients, respectively, have such involvement (104–106). These two sites are often infected concurrently. Oropharyngeal lesions begin as papules, which then progress to form ulcers (Fig. 273.8). The borders are heaped up, the base is infiltrated, and the lesions are typically dark purple. Small hemorrhagic spots can be seen in the base of the ulcer (Fig. 273.9). Skin lesions are often extensions of mucosal lesions, and their morphological appearance is varied. Papules, ulcers, abscesses, and verrucous lesions have been observed.

Other sites of dissemination include lymph nodes, adrenals, liver, spleen, CNS, and bones. Enlarged cervical lymph nodes are associated with mucosal lesions. Involved nodes are firm

and adherent to skin, and draining sinuses may arise from them. In autopsy series, *P. brasiliensis* is present in adrenal glands in as many as 95% of cases (103). Decreased adrenal reserve is detected in as many as 48% of nonfatal cases (107). The proportion of patients with overt Addison's disease is smaller but may be as high as 14% (108).

Children and young adults exhibit an acute or subacute form of the disease, with large numbers of yeasts in the mononuclear phagocyte system and fungemia. Cutaneous lesions are acneiform. The lung radiograph typically shows a miliary pattern (104).

DIAGNOSIS

Specimens such as sputum or pus should be examined directly on a slide with a drop of 10% potassium hydroxide. *P. brasiliensis* yeasts will appear as double-walled yeasts 4 to 40 μm in diameter. Identification of multiple budding yeasts with the pilotwheel appearance is indicative of *Paracoccidioides* infection. Repeated examinations are helpful.

Tissue biopsy examination (excluding mucocutaneous tissue) reveals the typical admixture of necrotizing suppuration and granulomatous inflammation. Yeasts may be detected by hematoxylin-eosin staining (Fig. 273.10), but they are much more readily observed in specimens using silver stains (Fig. 273.11). In contrast, histopathologic examination of the mucocutaneous lesions demonstrates pseudoepitheliomatous hyperplasia and intraepithelial microabscesses with yeast cells. In visceral organs of children with disseminated paracoccidioidomycosis, yeast cells are abundant and tissues contain massive aggregates of macrophages.

Unequivocal confirmation that the illness is caused by *P. brasiliensis* requires that cultures be performed. Material for culture is placed on Sabouraud's dextrose agar or yeast extract agar containing antibiotics and cycloheximide and is incubated at room temperature. Mycelia are usually evident by 20 to 30 days. Because the organism does not produce characteristic conidia, the identity of the fungus must be established by conversion to the yeast phase at 37°C.

The common serologic assays used for diagnosis include immunodiffusion in agar gel and complement fixation. The former is a specific and sensitive assay, and detection of precipitation bands 1 and 2 is suggestive of either recent or remote infection (109). As many as 95% of patients with active disease have antibodies detected by immunodiffusion (74). The complement-fixation test result is positive in 80% to 95% of patients with active disease (110), although there may be crossreactivity with *Histoplasma* antigens. The quantitative nature of this test may provide a means to follow the response to therapy. Other serologic tests include immunoelectrophoresis, counterimmunoelectrophoresis, and enzyme-linked immunosorbent assay, but they are not widely used. A specific exoantigen has been detected in culture filtrates of *P. brasiliensis*. This 43-kd antigen is specific and has properties of a proteinase (111–114). This antigen may provide a specific test for diagnosis of paracoccidioidomycosis.

Skin testing with paracoccidioidin is useful for epidemiological studies but not for clinical diagnosis, because a large proportion of patients with active disease may have negative results on skin tests. Cross-reactivity with histoplasmin may be observed.

The principal differential diagnosis for paracoccidioidomycosis is tuberculosis. Concomitant infections with *P. brasiliensis* and *M. tuberculosis* may be present in as many as 25% of patients

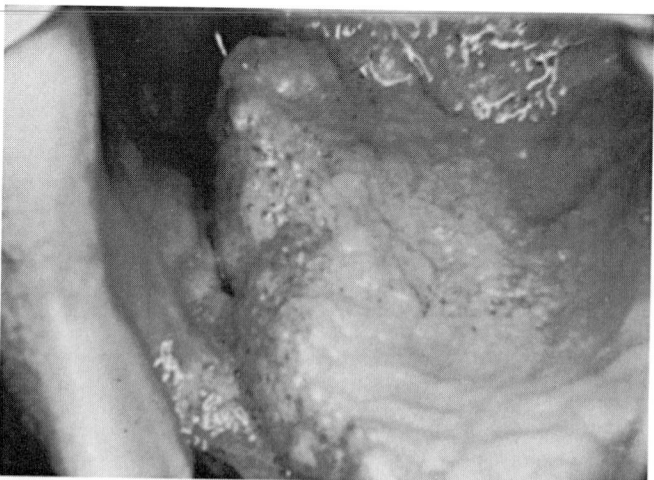

Figure 273.9. Large ulceration of the tongue caused by *Paracoccidioides.* Hemorrhagic spots are widely dispersed. (Courtesy Angela Restrepo, PhD, Mycology Unit, Corporacìon des Investigaciones Biológicas, Medellín, Colombia.)

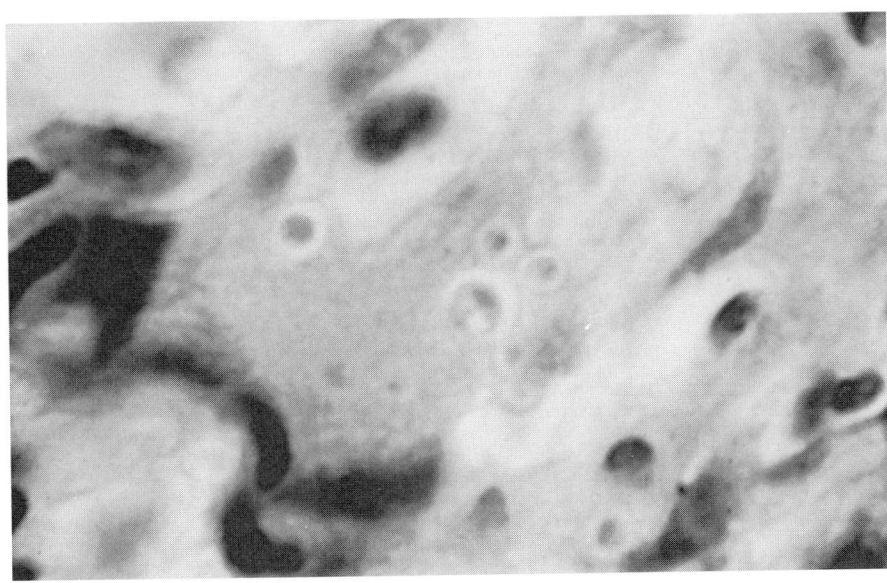

Figure 273.10. Photomicrograph of *Paracoccidioides* yeasts in tissue stained with hematoxylin-eosin. Multiple budding is present in addition to the "Mickey Mouse" configuration of budding yeasts. (Courtesy Angela Restrepo, PhD, Mycology Unit, Corporacion des Investigaciones Biológicas, Medellín, Colombia.)

(115). Other diseases that may mimic paracoccidioidomycosis include histoplasmosis, blastomycosis, leishmaniasis, and chromoblastomycosis. The extensive lymphadenopathy of patients with paracoccidioidomycosis may be misconstrued as lymphoma.

TREATMENT

Before the introduction of ketoconazole, sulfonamides were the primary treatment for paracoccidioidomycosis (115). Sulfadiazine or sulfamerazine, 2 to 6 g per day, is administered daily for 4 weeks or until there is clinical or microbiologic evidence of improvement. Once this is attained, the dose is reduced to 2 to 3 g per day; treatment is continued for 3 to 5 years. Alternatively, long-acting sulfonamides such as sulfamethoxypyridazine may be given, 1 g per day for 1 week initially, followed by 500 mg per day for several years (116). Treatment with sulfonamides is associated with a 15% relapse rate.

The oral azoles have become the mainstay of therapy for all forms of paracoccidioidomycosis because of their efficacy and ease of administration. Although ketoconazole is effective in more than 85% of cases, itraconazole is superior because it is more active and the length of therapy can be reduced to 6 months. Relapse rates are less with itraconazole (3% to 5%) versus ketoconazole (0% to 11%). If ketoconazole is initiated, the dosage should be at least 200 mg per day and continued for at least 6 months. Some physicians routinely use 400 mg per day. This dosage is recommended for disseminated disease (105,106,117,118). If itraconazole is used, a dosage of 100 to 200 mg per day is recommended (119,120).

Amphotericin B is used for life-threatening infections. The dose of amphotericin B ranges from 0.25 to 1.2 mg/kg, either every day if the patient is acutely ill, or every other day. Usually, a total dose of 1 to 3 g is sufficient. All patients who take a course of amphotericin B should be given itraconazole for several months thereafter. Few data exist concerning the lipid-based amphotericin B preparations. One report using amphotericin B colloidal dispersion at 3 mg/kg per day reported that four of four patients relapsed after taking this drug (121). Thus, the efficacy of these forms of amphotericin B requires additional study.

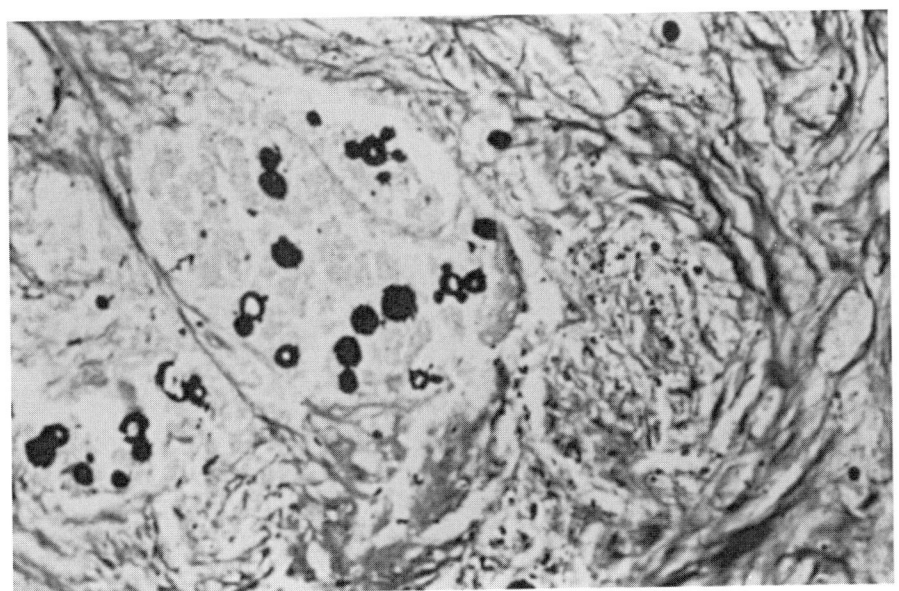

Figure 273.11. *Paracoccidioides* yeasts in tissue stained with Gomori methenamine silver. Multiple budding yeasts are evident. (Courtesy Judith Rhodes, PhD, University of Cincinnati College of Medicine, Cincinnati, Ohio.)

There is little place for surgery in the treatment of paracoccidioidomycosis. Surgical intervention may be necessary to diagnose visceral forms of the disease or to remove paracoccidioidomas or mass lesions caused by *P. brasiliensis*.

REFERENCES

Blastomyces

1. Gilchrist TC. Protozoan dermatitis. *J Cutan Gen Dis* 1894;12:496.
2. Gilchrist TC, Stokes WR. The presence of an oidium in tissues of a case of pseudo-lupus vulgaris. *Johns Hopkins Hosp Rep* 1896;7:129.
3. Gilchrist TC, Stokes WR. Case of pseudo-lupus vulgaris caused by blastomycosis. *J Exp Med* 1896;3:53.
4. Medoff G, Painter A, Kobayashi GS. Mycelial-to-yeast phase transitions of the dimorphic fungi *Blastomyces dermatitidis* and *Paracoccidioides brasiliensis*. *J Bacteriol* 1987;169:4055.
5. Maresca B, Lambowitz AM, Kumar VB, et al. Role of cysteine in regulating morphogenesis and mitochondrial activity in the dimorphic fungus *Histoplasma capsulatum*. *Proc Natl Acad Sci U S A* 1981;78:4596.
6. Rippon JW. Blastomycosis. In: *Medical mycology: the pathogenic fungi and the pathogenic actinomycetes*, 2nd ed. Philadelphia: WB Saunders, 1982:428–458.
7. McDonough ES, Lewis AL. *Blastomyces dermatitidis*: production of a sexual stage. *Science* 1967;156:528.
8. McDonough ES, McNamara WJ, Chan DM, et al. Geographic distribution of "+" and "−" isolates of *Blastomyces (Ajellomyces) dermatitidis* in North America. *Am J Epidemiol* 1973;98:63.
9. McDonough ES, Chan DM, McNamara WJ. Dual infection by + and − mating types of *Ajellomyces (Blastomyces) dermatitidis*. *Am J Epidemiol* 1977;106:67.
10. Kaufman L, Standard PG, Weeks RJ, et al. Detection of two *Blastomyces dermatitidis* serotypes by exoantigen analysis. *J Clin Microbiol* 1983;18:110.
11. Fraser VJ, Keath EJ, Powderly WG. Two cases of blastomycosis from a common source: use of DNA restriction analysis to identify strains. *J Infect Dis* 1991;163:1378.
12. Klein BS, Vergeront JM, Weeks RJ, et al. Isolation of *Blastomyces dermatitidis* in soil associated with a large outbreak of blastomycosis in Wisconsin. *N Engl J Med* 1986;314:529.
13. Klein BS, Vergeront JM, Disalvo AF, et al. Two outbreaks of blastomycosis along rivers in Wisconsin. *Am Rev Respir Dis* 1987;136:1333.
14. Furculow ML, Chick EW, Busey JD, et al. Prevalence and incidence studies of human and canine blastomycosis. I. Cases in the United States, 1885–1968. *Am Rev Respir Dis* 1970;102:60.
15. Reingold AL, Lu XD, Plikaytis BD, et al. Systemic mycoses in the United States, 1980–1982. *J Med Vet Mycol* 1986;24:433.
16. Smith JR Jr, Harris JS, Conant NF, et al. An epidemic of North American blastomycosis. *JAMA* 1970;158:641.
17. Tosh FE, Hammerman KJ, Weeks RJ, et al. A common source epidemic of North American blastomycosis. *Am Rev Respir Dis* 1974;109:525.
18. Kitchen MS, Reiber CG, Eastin GB. An urban epidemic of North American blastomycosis. *Am Rev Respir Dis* 1977;115:1063.
19. Farber ER, Leahy MS, Meadows TR. Endometrial blastomycosis acquired by sexual contact. *Obstet Gynecol* 1968;32:306.
20. Craig MW, Davey WN, Green RA. Conjugal blastomycosis. *Am Rev Respir Dis* 1970;102:86.
21. Gnann JW Jr, Bressler GS, Bodet A III, et al. Human blastomycosis after a dog bite. *Ann Intern Med* 1983;98:48.
22. Klein BS, Vergeront JM, Davis JP. Epidemiologic aspects of blastomycosis, the enigmatic systemic mycosis. *Semin Respir Infect* 1986;1:29.
23. Schwarz J, Baum GL. Blastomycosis. *Am J Clin Pathol* 1951;11:999.
23a. Rooney P, Sullivan T, Klein BS. Selective expression of the virulence factor BAD1 upon morphogenesis to the pathogenic yeast form of *Blastomyces dermatitidis*: evidence for transcriptional regulation by a conserved mechanism. *Mol Microbiol* 2001;39:875.
23b. Brandhorst T, Wuethrich M, Warner T, et al. Targeted gene disruption reveals an adhesin indispensable for pathogenicity of *Blastomyces dermatitidis*. *J Exp Med* 1999;189:1207.
23c. Finkel-Jimenez BE, Wüthrich M, Brandhorst T, et al. Down-regulation of phagocyte TNF-α production by the WI-1 adhesin imparts pathogenicity on *Blastomyces dermatitidis*. *J Immunol* 2001;166:2665.
24. Harvey RP, Schmid ES, Carrington CC, et al. Mouse model of pulmonary blastomycosis: utility, simplicity, and quantitative parameters. *Am Rev Respir Dis* 1978;117:695.
25. Deepe GS Jr, Taylor CL, Bullock WE. Evolution of the inflammatory response and cellular immune responses in a murine model of disseminated blastomycosis. *Infect Immun* 1985;50:183.
26. Williams JE, Moser SA. Chronic murine pulmonary blastomycosis induced by intratracheally inoculated *Blastomyces dermatitidis* conidia. *Am Rev Respir Dis* 1987;135:17.

27. Thurmond LM, Mitchell TG. *Blastomyces dermatitidis* chemotactic factor: kinetics of production and biological characterization evaluated by a modified neutrophil chemotaxis assay. *Infect Immun* 1984;46:87.
28. Cox RA, Mills LR, Best GK, et al. Histologic reaction to cell walls of an avirulent and virulent strain of *Blastomyces dermatitidis*. *J Infect Dis* 1979;129:179.
29. Cox RA, Best GK. Cell wall composition of two strains of *Blastomyces dermatitidis* exhibiting differences in virulence for mice. *Infect Immun* 1972;5:449.
30. Kaufman L, McLaughlin DW, Clark MJ, et al. Specific immunodiffusion test for blastomycosis. *Appl Microbiol* 1973;26:244.
31. Klein BS, Jones JM. Purification and characterization of the major antigen WI-1 from *Blastomyces dermatitidis* yeasts and immunological comparison with A antigen. *Infect Immun* 1994;62:3890.
32. Klein BS, Jones JM. Isolation, purification, and radiolabeling of a novel 120-kD surface protein on *Blastomyces dermatitidis* yeasts to detect antibody in infected patients. *J Clin Invest* 1990;85:152.
33. Klein BS, Hogan LH, Jones JM. Immunological recognition of a 25 amino acid repeat arrayed in tandem on a major antigen of *Blastomyces dermatitidis*. *J Clin Invest* 1993;92:330.
34. Brummer E, Morozumi PA, Vo PT, et al. Protection against pulmonary blastomycosis: adoptive transfer with T lymphocytes, but not serum, from resistant mice. *Cell Immunol* 1982;73:349.
35. Drutz DJ, Frey CL. Intracellular and extracellular defenses of human phagocytes against *Blastomyces dermatitidis* conidia and yeasts. *J Lab Clin Invest* 1985;105:737.
36. Schaffner A, Davis CE, Schaffner T, et al. *In vitro* susceptibility of fungi to killing by neutrophil granulocytes discriminates between primary pathogenicity and opportunism. *J Clin Invest* 1986;78:511.
37. Sugar AM, Picard M. Macrophage- and oxidant-mediated inhibition of the ability of live *Blastomyces dermatitidis* conidia to transform to the pathogenic yeast phase: implications for the pathogenesis of dimorphic fungal infections. *J Infect Dis* 1991;163:371.
38. Sugar AM, Chahal RS, Brummer E. Susceptibility of *Blastomyces dermatitidis* strains to products of oxidative metabolism. *Infect Immun* 1983;41:908.
39. Sugar AM, Chahal RS, Brummer E. The iron-hydrogen peroxide system in fungicidal activity against the yeast phase of *Blastomyces dermatitidis*. *J Leukoc Biol* 1984;36:545.
40. Smith DT. Immunologic types of blastomycosis: a report on 40 cases. *Ann Intern Med* 1949;31:463.
41. Witorsch P, Utz JP. North American blastomycosis: a study of 40 patients. *Medicine (Baltimore)* 1968;47:169.
42. Newman SL, Chatuverdi S, Klein BS. The WI-1 antigen of *Blastomyces dermatitidis* yeasts mediate binding to human macrophage CD11b/CD18 (CR3) and CD14. *J Immunol* 1995;154:753.
43. Klein BS, Sondel PS, Jones JM. WI-1, a 120 kD surface protein on *Blastomyces dermatitidis* yeasts, is a target antigen of cell-mediated immunity in human blastomycosis. *Infect Immun* 1992;60:4291.
44. Bradsher RW, Alford RH. *Blastomyces dermatitidis* antigen-induced lymphocyte reactivity in human blastomycosis. *Infect Immun* 1981;33:485.
45. Brummer E, Morrison CJ, Stevens DA. Recombinant and natural γ-interferon activation of macrophages *in vitro*: different dose requirements for induction of killing activity against phagocytizable and nonphagocytizable fungi. *Infect Immun* 1984;49:787.
46. Morrison CJ, Brummer E, Isenberg RA, et al. Activation of murine polymorphonuclear neutrophils for fungicidal activity by recombinant γ interferon. *J Leukoc Biol* 1987;41:434.
46a. Wuethrich M, Fillutowicz H, Klein B. Mutation at a single genetic locus in *Blastomyces dermatitidis* produces an attenuated vaccine strain that induces type 1 cytokines and resistance to infection. *J Clin Invest* 2000;106:1381.
47. Sarosi GA, Hammerman KJ, Tosh FE, et al. Clinical features of acute pulmonary blastomycosis. *N Engl J Med* 1974;290:540.
48. Sarosi GA, Davies SF. Blastomycosis. *Am Rev Respir Dis* 1979;120:911.
49. Recht, LD, Philips JR, Eckman MR, et al. Self-limited blastomycosis: a report of thirteen cases. *Am Rev Respir Dis* 1979;120:1109.
50. Cush R, Light RW, George RB. Clinical and roentgenographic manifestations of acute and chronic blastomycosis. *Chest* 1976;69:345.
51. Halvorsen RA, Duncan JD, Merten DF. Pulmonary blastomycosis: radiologic manifestations. *Radiology* 1984;150:1.
52. Laskey W, Sarosi GA. Endogenous activation in blastomycosis. *Ann Intern Med* 1978;88:50.
53. Leavell UW. Cutaneous North American blastomycosis and black dots. *Arch Dermatol* 1965;92:155.
54. Gehweiler JA, Capp MP, Chick EW. Observations on the roentgen patterns in blastomycosis of bone. *Am J Roentgenol Radium Ther Nucl Med* 1970;108:497.
55. Bayer AS, Scott VJ, Guze LB. Fungal arthritis. IV. Blastomycotic arthritis. *Semin Arthritis Rheum* 1979;9:145.
56. Schwarz J, Salfelder K. Blastomycosis: a review of 152 cases. *Curr Top Pathol* 1977;65:165.
57. Inoshita T, Youngberg GA, Boelen LJ, et al. Blastomycosis presenting with prostatic involvement: report of two cases and review of the literature. *J Urol* 1982;130:160.
58. Gonyea EF. The spectrum of primary pulmonary blastomycotic meningitis: a review of central nervous system blastomycosis. *Ann Neurol* 1978;3:26.

59. Laskey WL, Sarosi GA. Blastomycosis in children. *Pediatrics* 1980;l65:111.
60. Recht LD, Davies SF, Eckman MR, et al. Blastomycosis in immunosuppressed patients. *Am Rev Respir Dis* 1982;125:359.
60a. Pappas PG, Pottage JC, Powderly WG, et al. Blastomycosis in patients with the acquired immunodeficiency syndrome. *Ann Intern Med* 1992;116:847–853.
60b. Pappas PG, Threlkeld MG, Bedsole GD, et al. Blastomycosis in immunocompromised patients. *Medicine (Baltimore)* 1993;72:311.
61. Colsky J. Treatment of systemic blastomycosis with 2-hydroxy-stilbamidine. *Arch Intern Med* 1954;93:796.
62. Parker JD, Doto IL, Tosh FE. A decade of experience with blastomycosis and its treatment with amphotericin B. *Am Rev Respir Dis* 1969;99:895.
63. National Institute of Allergy and Infectious Diseases Study Group. Treatment of blastomycosis and histoplasmosis with ketoconazole. Results of a prospective randomized trial. *Ann Intern Med* 1985;103:861.
64. Bradsher RW, Rice DC, Abernathy RS. Ketoconazole therapy for endemic blastomycosis. *Ann Intern Med* 1985;103:872.
65. Dismukes WE, Bradsher RW, Cloud GC, et al. Itraconazole therapy for blastomycosis and histoplasmosis. *Am J Med* 1992;93:489.
66. Cherniss EI, Waisbren BA. North American blastomycosis: a clinical study of 40 cases. *Ann Intern Med* 1956;44:105.
67. Abernathy RS. Clinical manifestations of pulmonary blastomycosis. *Ann Intern Med* 1959;51:707.
68. Lockwood WR, Allison F, Batson BE, et al. The treatment of North American blastomycosis: ten years' experience. *Am Rev Respir Dis* 1969;100:314.
69. Duttera MJ, Osterhout S. North American blastomycosis: a survey of 63 cases. *South Med J* 1969;62:295.
70. Kepron MD, Schoemperlen B, Hershfield ES, et al. North American blastomycosis in central Canada. *Can Med Assoc J* 1972;106:243.

Paracoccidioides

71. Lutz A. Una mycose pseudococcidioidica localizada no boca e observada no Brasil. Contribucao ao conhecimento dos hyphoblastomycoses Americanas. *Brasil Med* 1908;22:121.
72. Almeida F. Estudos comparativos do granuloma coccidioidica nos Estados Unidos a no Brasil. Novo genero para parasito brasilero. *An Fac Med Univ Sao Paulo* 1930;5:3.
73. Padiha-Gonzalvez A. Paracoccidioidomycosis. *Cutis* 1987;40:214.
74. Rippon JW, ed. *Medical mycology*, 3rd ed. Philadelphia: WB Saunders, 1988:506–531.
75. San Blas G, San Blas F, Serrano LE. Host-parasite relationship in the yeastlike form of *P. brasiliensis*. *Infect Immun* 1977;15:343.
76. San Blas G, San Blas F. Variability in cell wall composition in *P. brasiliensis*. A study of two strains. *Sabouraudia* 1982;20:31.
77. Restrepo A. The ecology of *Paracoccidioides brasiliensis*: a puzzle still unsolved. *Sabouraudia* 1985;23:323.
78. Greer DL, Restrepo A. The epidemiology of paracoccidioidomycosis. In: Al Doory Y, ed. *The epidemiology of human mycotic diseases*. Springfield, IL: Charles C Thomas, 1975:117–130.
79. Bouzy E, Winston DJ, Rhodes JC, et al. Paracoccidioidomycosis (South American blastomycosis) in the United States. *Chest* 1977;72:100.
80. Borelli D. *Some ecological aspects of paracoccidioidomycosis; proceedings of the Pan American Symposium on Paracoccidioidomycosis*. Washington, DC: Pan American Health Organization, 1972:59–64.
81. Calle D, Rosero DS, Orozco LC, et al. Paracoccidioidomycosis in Colombia: an ecological study. *Epidemiol Infect* 2001;26:309.
82. Restrepo A. Immune response to *Paracoccidioides brasiliensis* in human and animal hosts. *Curr Top Med Mycol* 1988;2:239.
83. Franco M. Host-parasite relationships in paracoccidioidomycosis. *J Med Vet Mycol* 1986;25:5.
84. Franco M, Montenegro MR. Anatomia patologica. In: Del Negro G, Lacaz CS, Fiorillo AM, eds. *Paracoccidioidomycosis (Blastomicose Sul-Americana)*. Sao Paulo, Brazil: Sarvier Editores, 1982:97–117.
85. Brummer E, Restrepo A, Stevens DA, et al. Murine model of paracoccidioidomycosis. production of fatal acute pulmonary or chronic pulmonary and disseminated disease. Immunological and pathological observations. *J Exp Pathol* 1984;1:241.
86. Restrepo A, Salazar ME, Cano LE, et al. Estrogens inhibit mycelial-to-yeast transformation in the fungus *P. brasiliensis*. Implications for resistance of females to paracoccidioidomycosis. *Infect Immun* 1984;46:346.
87. Loose DS, Stover EP, Restrepo A, et al. Estradiol binds to a receptor-like cytosol-binding protein and initiates a biological response in *P. brasiliensis*. *Proc Natl Acad Sci U S A* 1983;80:7659.
88. Restrepo A, Moncada LH. *Serologic procedures in the diagnosis of paracoccidioidomycosis; proceedings of the International Symposium on Mycoses*. Washington, DC: Pan American Health Organization, 1977.
89. Restrepo A, Velez H. Efectos de la fagocitosis *in vitro* sobre *P. brasiliensis*. *Sabouraudia* 1975;13:10.
90. Calich VLG, Kipnis TL, Mariano M, et al. The activation of the complement system by *P. brasiliensis in vitro*: its opsonic effect and possible significance for an in vivo model of infection. *Clin Immunol Immunopathol* 1979;12:20.
91. McEwen JG, Brummer E, Stevens DA, et al. Effect of murine polymorphonuclear leukocytes on the yeast form of *P. brasiliensis*. *Am J Trop Med Hyg* 1987;36:603.
92. McEwen JG, Sugar AM, Brummer E, et al. Toxic effects of products of oxidative metabolism on the yeast phase form of *P. brasiliensis*. *J Med Microbiol* 1984;18:423.
93. Brummer E, Hanson LH, Restrepo A, et al. *In vivo* and *in vitro* activation of pulmonary macrophages by IFN-γ for enhanced killing of *Paracoccidioides brasiliensis* or *Blastomyces dermatitidis*. *J Immunol* 1988;140:2786.
94. Jimenez BE, Murphy JW. *In vitro* effects of natural killer cells against *Paracoccidioides brasiliensis* yeast phase. *Infect Immun* 1984;46:552.
95. Mussatti CC, Rezkallah-Iwasso MT, Mendes E, et al. *In vivo* and *in vitro* evaluation of cell-mediated immunity in patients with paracoccidioidomycosis. *Cell Immunol* 1978;24:365.
96. Costa PC, Pagnano PMG, Bechelli LM, et al. Lymphocyte transformation test in patients with paracoccidioidomycosis. *Mycopathologia* 1983;84:55.
97. Mota NGS, Rezkallah-Iwasso MT, Peracoli MT, et al. Correlation between cell-mediated immunity and clinical forms of paracoccidioidomycosis. *Trans R Soc Trop Med Hyg* 1985;79:765.
98. Arango M, Oropeza F, Anderson O, et al. Circulating immunocomplexes and *in vitro* cell reactivity in paracoccidioidomycosis. *Mycopathologia* 1982;79:153.
99. Karhawi AS, Colombo AL, Salomao R. Production of IFN-γ is impaired in patients with paracoccidioidomycosis during active disease and is restored after clinical remission. *Med Mycol* 2000;38:225.
100. Castaneda E, Brummer E, Pappagianis D, et al. Regulation of immune responses by T suppressor cells and by serum in paracoccidioidomycosis. *Cell Immunol* 1988;117:1.
101. Jimenez-Finkel BE, Murphy JW. Induction of antigen-specific T suppressor cells by soluble *Paracoccidioides brasiliensis* antigen. *Infect Immun* 1988;56:734.
102. Pena CE. Deep mycotic infections in Colombia. A clinicopathological study of 102 cases. *Am J Clin Pathol* 1967;47:505.
103. Restrepo A, Robledo M, Giraldo R, et al. The gamut of paracoccidioidomycosis. *Am J Med* 1976;61:33.
104. Restrepo A, Gomez I, Cano LE, et al. Treatment of paracoccidioidomycosis with ketoconazole: a three year experience. *Am J Med* 1983;74:48.
105. Vargas J, Recacoechea M. Ketoconazole in the treatment of paracoccidioidomycosis (South American blastomycosis). Experience in 30 cases in Bolivia. *Mycoses* 1988;31:187.
106. Del Negro G, Melo EHL, Rodbard P, et al. Limited adrenal reserve in paracoccidioidomycosis. Cortisol and aldosterone response to 1-24 ACTH. *Clin Endocrinol* 1980;13:553.
107. Abad A, Gomez I, Velez P, et al. Adrenal function in paracoccidioidomycosis: a prospective study in patients before and after ketoconazole therapy. *Infection* 1986;14:22.
108. Restrepo A, Moncada LH. Characterization of the precipitin bands detected in the immunodiffusion test for paracoccidioidomycosis. *Appl Microbiol* 1974;28:138.
109. Kauffman L. *Evaluation of serological tests for paracoccidioidomycosis. Preliminary report; proceedings of the Pan American Symposium on Paracoccidioidomycosis*. Washington DC: Pan American Health Organization, 1972:221–224.
110. Puccia R, Schenkman PA, Travassos LR. Exocellular components of *Paracoccidioides brasiliensis*: identification of a specific antigen. *Infect Immun* 1986;53:199.
111. Mendes-Giannini MJS, Bueno JP, Shikanai-Yasuda MA, et al. Detection of the 43,000-molecular-weight glycoprotein in sera of patients with paracoccidioidomycosis. *J Clin Microbiol* 1989;27:2842.
112. Puccia R, Travassos LIZ. The 43 kDa glycoprotein from the human pathogen *Paracoccidioides brasiliensis* and its deglycosylated form: excretion and susceptibility to proteolysis. *Arch Biochem Biophys* 1991;289:298.
113. Puccia R, Travassos LR. 43-Kilodalton glycoprotein from *Paracoccidioides brasiliensis*: immunochemical reactions with sera from patients with paracoccidioidomycosis, histoplasmosis, or Jorge Lobo's disease. *J Clin Microbiol* 1991;29:1610.
114. Salfelder K, Doehnert G. Paracoccidioidomycosis. Anatomic study with complete autopsies. *Virchows Arch* 1969;348:51.
115. Negroni P. *Prolonged therapy for paracoccidioidomycosis: approaches, complications, and risks; proceedings of the Pan American Symposium on Paracoccidioidomycosis*. Washington DC, Pan American Health Organization, 1977:147–155. PAHO Scientific Publication no. 254.
116. Restrepo A, Gomez I, Cano LE, et al. Posttherapy status of paracoccidioidomycosis treated with ketoconazole. *Am J Med* 1983;74:53.
117. Brummer E, Castaneda E, Restrepo A. Paracoccidioidomycosis: an update. *Clin Microbiol Rev* 1993;6:89.
118. Munera MI, Naranjo MS, Gomez I, et al. Seguimiento postterapia de pacientes con paracoccidioidomicosis tratados con itraconazol. *Medicina Univ Pontificia Bolivariana (Medellín)* 1989;8:33.
119. Naranjo MS, Trujillo M, Munera MI, et al. Treatment of paracoccidioidomycosis with itraconazole. *J Med Vet Mycol* 1990;28:67.
120. Mok WY, Fava-Netto C. Paracoccidioidin and histoplasmin sensitivity in Coari (State of Amazonas), Brazil. *Am J Trop Med Hyg* 1978;27:808.
121. Dietze R, Fowler VG Jr, Steiner TS, et al. Failure of amphotericin B colloidal dispersion in the treatment of paracoccidioidomycosis. *Am J Trop Med Hyg* 1999;60:837.

CHAPTER 274
Dematiaceous Fungi

Jill R. Rosenthal

The dematiaceous fungi are pigmented fungi that have brown or black cell walls in their conidia, mycelia, and sclerotic bodies and form brown to black colonies in culture. The pigment appears to be a form of melanin (1). The taxonomy of this group has been controversial, and many of the organisms appear in the literature under multiple names. Identification is based on the morphological features of conidia and conidiophores in culture; many species can form different types of conidia within a single culture, contributing to morphological confusion.

Cutaneous diseases caused by this group of fungi include chromoblastomycosis, phaeohyphomycosis, and mycetoma. These diseases are characterized by their clinical appearance, the tissue form of the infecting organism, and the etiologic agent. The causative fungi are saprophytes and are usually found in soil or in association with decaying vegetable material. Disease is usually the result of traumatic implantation, such as by a wood splinter, and therefore usually involves an extremity. Both normal and immunocompromised hosts can be affected. Although most of the dematiaceous fungi tend to cause one type of disease, there are rare instances of fungi that usually cause chromoblastomycosis, producing clinical presentations more suggestive of phaeohyphomycosis or mycetoma and vice versa (2–5). This has led some authors to propose that the clinical syndrome produced may depend as much on the interaction between the organism and the host as on the identity of the infective agent (4).

CHROMOBLASTOMYCOSIS

Clinical Manifestations

The most common form of dematiaceous fungal infection is chromoblastomycosis (chromomycosis, verrucous dermatitis), a chronic localized infection of the skin that follows traumatic inoculation of a causative organism. The most common infecting organisms are *Fonsecaea pedrosoi, Fonsecaea compacta, Phialophora verrucosa, Cladosporium carrionii,* and *Rhinocladiella aquaspersa; Exophiala jeanselmei* has also been reported as a cause (6). In the United States, *P. verrucosa* is the most commonly isolated agent; worldwide, *F. pedrosoi* is most common (7,8). The disease occurs most commonly in tropical rural areas but has been reported in Central America, South America, North America, Cuba, Jamaica, Martinique, India, South Africa, Madagascar, Australia, northern Europe, and Great Britain (9, pp. 1205–1206). The most commonly isolated fungi from woody materials, soil, and vegetable material are *F. pedrosoi, C. carrionii,* and *P. verrucosa,* with their frequency in nature corresponding to the frequency with which these agents cause disease; woody plant materials are the most common sources of fungal isolates (10).

Because the dematiaceous fungi are saprophytes found in soil, decomposing vegetation, and particularly decaying wood, and because the disease is acquired by traumatic implantation, chromoblastomycosis is most commonly seen in adult male agricultural workers, who often work barefoot and may receive puncture wounds on the feet (7,9). Lesions most commonly occur on exposed sites such as the feet and lower legs but have been reported on other sites, such as the hands, buttocks, face, neck,

ears, or trunk. Infection is usually limited to the skin and subcutaneous tissue in the vicinity of the initial injury, which may be inconsequential and may pass unnoticed by the patient. There have been no cases of human-to-human transmission (7).

Early descriptions of chromoblastomycosis describe five morphological types of infection, including nodular, tumorous, verrucous, plaque, and cicatricial lesions (11). Possibly these represent different stages of disease or vary with the site of involvement. Chromoblastomycosis begins as a small pink papule, usually on the exposed surface of the lower extremity, that gradually enlarges to form a superficial nodule. In time, the lesion forms a scaly and fissured pink, violaceous, or brownish plaque, which eventually becomes verrucous and may ulcerate with trauma (Fig. 274.1; see also Color Fig. 274.1). Small nodular lesions may develop into larger papillomatous or lobulated tumorous lesions with epidermal debris, crusting, and hyperkeratosis. Markedly verrucous lesions may occur on the sides of the feet (Fig. 274.2; see also Color Fig. 274.2). Ultimately, thick, crusted, tumorous hyperkeratotic masses may result, with ulceration due to trauma or secondary bacterial infection a frequent occurrence. Cicatricial lesions may result after peripheral enlargement with central healing, leading to atrophic scarring. Black dots may be visible on the surface of lesions and represent sites where blood and fungal cells (sclerotic bodies, "copper pennies") are expelled from the skin through transepidermal elimination; these may be sampled for skin scrapings or culture (7). Chromoblastomycosis is usually asymptomatic in the absence of secondary infection. Satellite lesions may result from scratching or, more rarely, may occur via the lymphatic system (12). Hematogenous spread is rare but has been reported to cause brain abscess (9,13). After many years, chronic and recurrent secondary infections may lead to elephantiasis due to lymphatic obstruction (7,9).

Differential Diagnosis

The differential diagnosis includes blastomycosis, cutaneous tuberculosis, leprosy, leishmaniasis, tertiary syphilis, yaws, and halogenoderma. Diagnosis is established by identification of pigmented thick-walled cells in clusters on microscopic examination of tissue scrapings in potassium hydroxide, fungal culture, or biopsy. Histopathologic examination reveals pseudoepitheliomatous hyperplasia with foreign body granulomata with focal abscess formation, chronic fibrosis, and the presence of brownish fungal cells within giant cells, as well as in the stratum corneum, within abscesses, and free in tissue (7,9,14). The brown, thick-walled, septate 5- to 12-μm cells are known variously as *copper pennies, Medlar bodies, sclerotic bodies,* and *muriform cells,* among other names, and represent the tissue form of the causative fungi (7). The septa or cross-walls are seen in two planes; these bodies are seen only in chromoblastomycosis and are not seen in other dematiaceous fungal infections such as phaeohyphomycosis or mycetoma (6,7). Culture of crusts, exudate, pus, or biopsy specimens should be performed on plain Sabouraud's glucose agar and Sabouraud's glucose agar containing cycloheximide and chloramphenicol; verrucous lesions are said to have the highest yield for culture and for the visualization of sclerotic bodies (15). Cultures should be kept at 25°C for at least 6 weeks, because the organisms that cause chromoblastomycosis grow slowly (12). Unlike mycetoma, in which the morphological appearance of the granules yields a clue to identity, the causative fungus in chromoblastomycosis cannot be identified by the appearance of the sclerotic bodies (7). Identification of the causative agent is made by culture morphology and the microscopic appearance of the sporulation patterns. Serologic methods for the detection of complement-fixing and precipitating antibodies can also be used

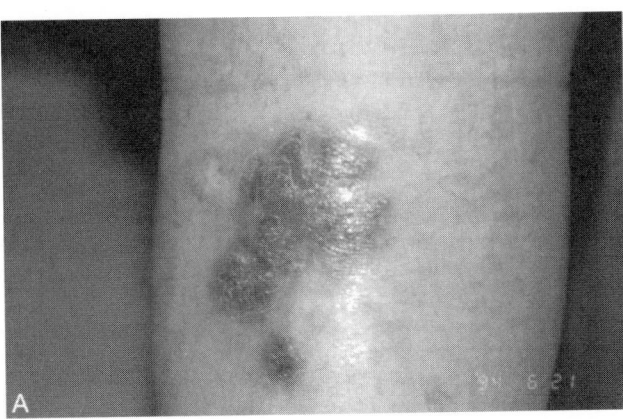 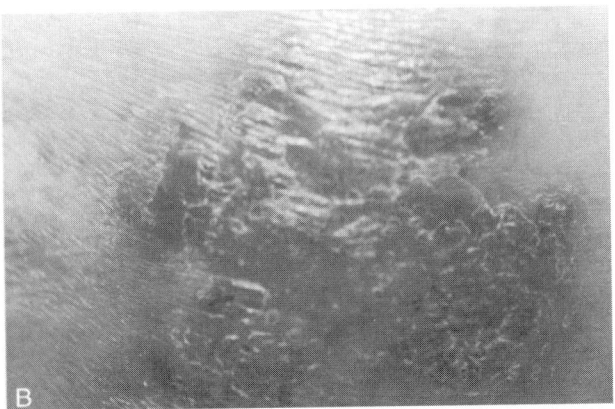

Figure 274.1. (See also Color Fig. 274.1.) Chromoblastomycosis. **A:** Multiple plaques on the lower leg. **B:** Close-up of (A). (Courtesy Nellie Konnikov, M.D., New England Medical Center, Boston, Mass.)

for diagnosis and for assessing response to treatment, although they are not routinely employed in the diagnosis of chromoblastomycosis (7,12,14,16,17).

Treatment

Treatment of chromoblastomycosis is difficult, especially for infections caused by *F. pedrosoi* (18). Therapy for small lesions, if possible, consists of wide and deep excision with skin grafting. With early lesions, excision may be curative. However, most patients present too late in the course to make this practical. Electrosurgical therapy is advocated by some authors and is thought by others to produce a higher risk of recurrence. Cryosurgical destruction or local heat therapy may also be helpful (19–21). Previously reported treatments have included various drugs singly or in combination: intravenous or intralesional amphotericin B, flucytosine, thiabendazole, and ketoconazole (9,18). Development of resistance to flucytosine may be a problem when this

agent is used alone in the treatment of chromoblastomycosis, as it is with other fungal infections. Combination therapy with flucytosine and ketoconazole or amphotericin B appears to be synergistic (7,22,23). Ketoconazole alone is slightly effective in mild disease, but its usefulness is limited by the risk of hepatotoxicity; fluconazole appears not to be useful in the treatment of chromoblastomycosis (23,24). Itraconazole at 200 mg daily for 6 to 24 months is effective in more than 60% of cases, even those due to *F. pedrosoi* infection (18,25,26). Saperconazole, the newest triazole, not yet available in the United States, did well in a small series of patients at doses of 200 mg daily for 6 to 12 months and appears to be promising for the treatment of chromoblastomycosis, with response rates of about 75% (18,27). With additional studies, it may prove more effective than itraconazole, in briefer treatment courses. Rarely, amputation of the affected limb may be required as a last resort.

PHAEOHYPHOMYCOSIS

Phaeohyphomycosis refers to localized subcutaneous or deeper abscesses caused by *E. jeanselmei*, *Wangiella (Exophiala) dermatitidis*, and occasionally other agents. Infecting species include those from the genera *Exophiala*, *Exserohilum*, *Cladosporium*, *Bipolaris*, *Alternaria*, *Curvularia*, and *Wangiella* (28). There are several different clinical syndromes ranging in severity. Infections may occur in both immunocompetent and immunocompromised patients and in animals and humans. On histologic examination, pigmented yeastlike cells, hyphae, and pseudohyphae may be seen in infected tissue; sclerotic bodies, as seen in chromoblastomycosis, and grains, as seen in mycetoma, are absent. Both *E. jeanselmei* and *W. dermatitidis* have been recovered from soil, wood, and other plant materials (14). The agents of phaeohyphomycosis have also been isolated from sewage, shower curtains, toilet bowls, bats, frogs, and wasp nests (29).

Superficial, Cutaneous, and Subcutaneous Phaeohyphomycosis

Superficial phaeohyphomycosis includes tinea nigra and black piedra superficial infections of the stratum corneum of the skin and of the hair, respectively (see Chapter 136). Examples of cutaneous phaeohyphomycosis include dermatomycoses produced by the nondermatophyte molds *Scytalidium* and *Hendersonula*, which produce chronic diseases of the skin and nails clinically

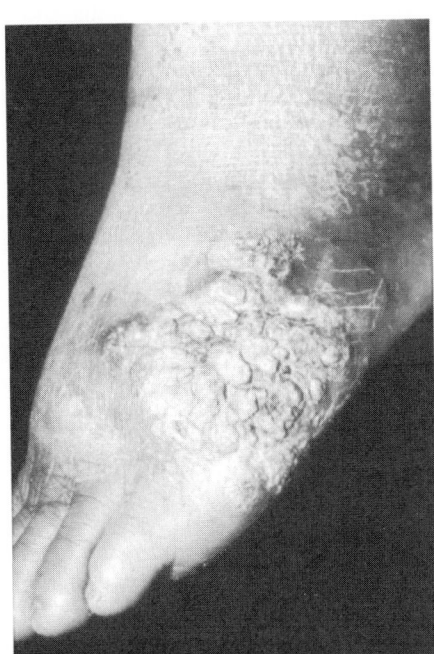

Figure 274.2. (See also Color Fig. 274.2.) Chromoblastomycosis. Verrucous plaques on the lateral aspect of the foot.

similar to the dermatophytoses (6) (see Chapter 136). Colonization of fissured areas on the soles, skin ulcers, or dermatitic skin may also occur with dematiaceous fungi such as *Alternaria, Curvularia, Cladosporium,* and *Aureobasidium* (29). Such colonization is not always pathogenic. These species may rarely cause skin or more invasive infection.

Like other dematiaceous fungal infections, subcutaneous phaeohyphomycosis begins after an abrasion or penetrating injury. Some patients are diabetic, but infections commonly occur in normal hosts as well (29). Lesions of subcutaneous phaeohyphomycosis (phaeohyphomycotic cyst) begin with a firm nodule that may be tender and that may then develop into a large cyst or abscess up to several centimeters in diameter (9). A history of trauma may be obtained, and a wooden splinter is sometimes found in the tissue in association with the cyst (30). Surgical excision is usually the treatment of choice. The most common cause of phaeohyphomycotic cyst is *E. jeanselmei,* although *W. dermatitidis* is more common in Japan (29). Phaeohyphomycotic cysts have been mistaken for ganglion cysts, epidermal cysts, foreign body granulomata, and Baker's cysts (14). Lesions due to *W. dermatitidis* may exhibit more epidermal change, with a scaly or verrucous surface or pustules (14). Diagnosis is established with potassium hydroxide preparation and culture of purulent aspirates, homogenized tissue from excision or biopsy specimens, or skin scrapings (14). As for chromoblastomycosis, cultures should be inoculated onto Sabouraud's glucose agar both with and without cycloheximide and chloramphenicol.

Unusual examples of traumatic inoculations causing phaeohyphomycosis include a mixed phaeohyphomycotic infection caused by *Exserohilum rostratum* and *Curvularia* in a cocaine user and phaeohyphomycosis due to *Curvularia lunata* after an explosion (31,32). *Curvularia geniculata* and *C. lunata* have also been reported to result from football injuries, eventuating in disseminated disease, and to cause fungal keratitis, mycetoma, and prosthetic valve endocarditis (29). Systemic symptoms such as chills, dizziness, and nausea may accompany cutaneous disease (33). If lesions of different morphological appearance are observed, multiple biopsies and cultures are indicated, as illustrated by the report of a patient receiving glucocorticosteroids for sarcoidosis who developed distinct but concurrent lesions of phaeohyphomycosis due to *P. verrucosa* and cutaneous abscess due to *Mycobacterium fortuitum* (34). Cutaneous alternariosis appears to occur primarily in immunocompromised patients receiving systemic corticosteroids (35).

Cutaneous phaeohyphomycosis due to *Hormonema dematioides* has also been reported in an immunocompetent man who developed anular, fungating, ulcerated lesions on the hands after he was cut with barbed wire (36). He was successfully cured with ketoconazole. Other reported agents include *Tetraploa aristata, Phialophora richardsiae, Pleurophoma* species, *Bipolaris spicifera, Phialophora repens, E. rostratum,* and many others (33,37–41). *Exophiala spinifera* has been reported as a cause of phaeohyphomycosis in both humans and cats (42,43). *P. verrucosa,* a common cause of chromoblastomycosis, is a rare cause of subcutaneous phaeohyphomycosis (3). *W. dermatitidis* has also been reported as a cause of onychomycosis of the toenails (44). Phaeohyphomycosis presenting as a leg ulcer caused by *Curvularia pallescens* was reported in a patient receiving low-dose prednisone and methotrexate (45).

Fungal keratitis results from traumatic inoculation of dematiaceous fungi such as *W. dermatitidis,* which also causes cutaneous phaeohyphomycosis and can occur after penetrating injury or ophthalmic surgery (46). Other agents reported to cause fungal keratitis include *E. jeanselmei, Bipolaris hawaiiensis, Exserohilum longirostratum, E. rostratum, Fusarium, Curvularia,* and nondematiaceous agents such as *Aspergillus* and *Candida* (47–51).

Systemic Phaeohyphomycosis

Systemic phaeohyphomycosis is usually an opportunistic infection (29). However, agents causing cutaneous phaeohyphomycosis have also been described as causing aggressive sinus infections in immunocompetent hosts (52–54). Dematiaceous fungi, including *Bipolaris, Exserohilum, Curvularia,* and *Alternaria* species, also appear to be more common causes than *Aspergillus* of allergic fungal sinusitis, an immunoglobulin E–mediated hypersensitivity condition, as opposed to a true invasive infection (55–58). Disseminated *Fusarium* infections can occur in immunosuppressed patients and should be considered in patients with fever and neutropenia who present with myalgias and violaceous necrotic papules, vesicles, pustules, and nodules (59,60). Cerebral phaeohyphomycosis, which occurs in both immunocompetent hosts and immunosuppressed patients, is usually caused by a neurotropic dematiaceous fungus, *Xylohypha bantiana* (previously known as *Cladosporium bantianum* or *Cladosporium trichoides*) (61–64). Fatal cerebral phaeohyphomycosis has also been reported with *Chaetomium globosum* in a renal transplant recipient and with *Ochroconis gallopavum* in a patient with large-cell lymphoma (65,66). Cerebral phaeohyphomycosis has also been caused by *F. pedrosoi,* which usually causes chromoblastomycosis, and by *W. dermatitidis,* which usually causes subcutaneous phaeohyphomycosis and has neurotropic tendencies with systemic infections (67,68). Cerebral phaeohyphomycosis due to *X. bantiana* usually presents only with cerebral lesions, without a known primary extra–central nervous system source, but cutaneous lesions may be seen in patients with disease due to *F. pedrosoi* or other agents that usually involve the skin (63,64,69). The sinuses may be portals of entry for cerebral infection (54). Inhalation of spores followed by hematogenous spread to the brain is another possibility (63). Cerebral phaeohyphomycosis most commonly manifests as brain abscess, resulting in focal symptoms such as hemiparesis, but other symptoms such as headache, visual impairment, ataxia, incoordination, and seizures may be seen as well, and meningeal irritation or frank meningitis may be present (69). The prognosis in cerebral phaeohyphomycosis is poor. Other systemic phaeohyphomycotic infections include pneumonia, tenosynovitis, septic arthritis, esophagitis, endophthalmitis, endocarditis, peritonitis, and osteomyelitis (32,54,70).

Therapy for phaeohyphomycosis involves surgical débridement or excision and systemic antifungal therapy (33,70). Small cutaneous and subcutaneous lesions can be treated with surgery alone. Small cutaneous lesions have occasionally responded to topical imidazoles under occlusion, and localized heat application may also be considered (39). Agents used include ketoconazole, itraconazole, flucytosine, fluconazole, and amphotericin B (33,68,71,72). In general, results are poor, except for small, localized lesions, but itraconazole may be helpful for some patients (28). Keratitis is treated with systemic and topical antifungal agents. There appears to be no effective therapy yet for cerebral phaeohyphomycosis, and the prognosis for this disease is poor (69).

MYCETOMA

Mycetoma (Madura's foot, maduromycosis), a localized chronic infection involving the skin, subcutaneous tissue, and sometimes bone, is characterized by swelling (tumefaction) and discharge of infected grains from draining sinuses (Fig. 274.3). The name *mycetoma* literally means fungal tumor. The process may be due to fungal infection (eumycotic mycetoma, or eumycetoma) or aerobic actinomycetes (actinomycotic mycetoma, or

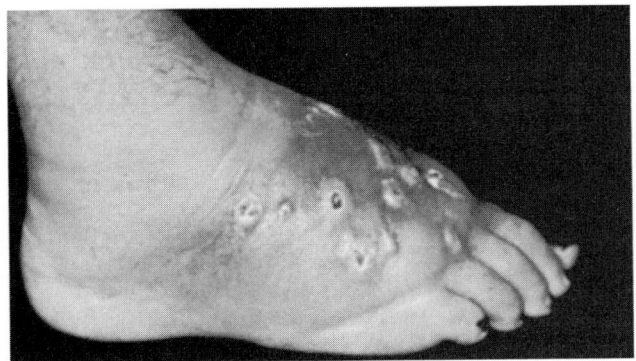

Figure 274.3. Mycetoma of the foot. (Courtesy Victor Newcomer, M.D., Santa Monica, Calif.)

TABLE 274.1.   Appearance of Grains in Mycetoma

Causative organism	Grain appearance
Actinomycetoma	
Nocardia asteroides	White, yellow to orange
Nocardia brasiliensis	Yellow-white
Actinomadura madurae	White to yellow or pink
Actinomadura pelletieri	Red
Streptomyces somaliensis	Yellow-white
Actinomyces israelii	White
Nocardia madurae	White; rarely pink
Mycotic mycetoma	
Pseudallescheria boydii	White to yellow
Madurella grisea	Black
Madurella mycetomatis	Black
Exophiala jeanselmei	Black

actinomycetoma). The various agents causing mycetoma are saprophytes found in soil and decaying vegetation. Infection occurs after traumatic inoculation, such as a puncture by a wooden splinter or a thorn. The condition is most common in tropical and subtropical regions, where people walk barefoot, and is most common in male agricultural workers between the ages of 20 and 50 years. Pathogenicity may be determined by many factors, including the thermal tolerance of the organisms. For example, most strains of *E. jeanselmei* isolated from soil are unable to grow at temperatures warmer than 30°C, in contrast to most specimens isolated from human infections, which grow readily at warmer temperatures (73). The prevalence of the causative agents of eumycetoma and actinomycetoma varies by geographic location and soil type (73). Mycetoma due to *Madurella grisea* has been reported in California. *Pseudallescheria boydii* has been isolated in sewage and has been reported as a cause of mycetoma in sewer workers in the United States (73). The onset of disease may be many years, even several decades, after the initial injury (9).

Worldwide, actinomycotic mycetoma and eumycotic mycetoma occur with about equal frequency (73). This may vary widely by area, however; for example, actinomycotic mycetoma accounts for 98% of cases in Mexico (74). The agents most commonly responsible for causing actinomycotic mycetoma are *Nocardia brasiliensis, Actinomadura (Streptomyces) pelletieri, Streptomyces somaliensis,* and *Actinomadura madurae; Madurella mycetomatis* is the most common cause of eumycetoma (9). In the United States, however, *P. boydii* is the most common cause of eumycotic mycetoma (8). *P. verrucosa,* which commonly causes chromoblastomycosis and rarely phaeohyphomycosis, has been reported as a cause of mycetoma (3). *E. jeanselmei,* which usually causes phaeohyphomycosis, occasionally causes mycetoma. *Aspergillus, Fusarium,* and other agents have also rarely caused mycetoma (73).

Mycetoma begins clinically with the development of firm, painless nodules that enlarge to produce a lumpy swelling. The lesions break down and discharge pus or a serous or serosanguineous drainage containing grains (tiny fungal or bacterial colonies that may have a crystalline matrix), the color and appearance of which may give a clue to the infecting organism (Table 274.1). Multiple sinus tracts may be present, and some may close and reopen or be replaced by new sinuses as the old ones heal with fibrosis. Raised borders or nodules around sinus tracts may be seen with *N. brasiliensis, A. madurae,* or *A. pelletieri,* giving a bumpy appearance; bone involvement is common with these organisms as well (73). *S. somaliensis* tends to produce less bone involvement and is not characterized by raised sinus tract openings (73). With time, infection may spread to deeper tissues,

causing periostitis, osteomyelitis, and infectious arthritis (9). Although progression is slow, marked swelling and deformity may eventually result. Actinomycetoma tends to develop more rapidly than eumycetoma. Systemic spread is extremely unusual, although it may occur in actinomycetoma; spread on the skin may occur rapidly in actinomycetoma, especially when it is caused by *N. brasiliensis* (73). Lesions are most commonly seen on the lower extremities, which are unprotected from trauma. It is thought that repeated punctures or lacerations result in inoculation of the causative organisms, perhaps accounting for the presence of multiple lesions. The back is a common site of infection in Mexico, where people may carry contaminated branches and other materials on their backs without protective clothing (74). In Mexico and in Central and South America, *N. brasiliensis,* which causes the most aggressive form of actinomycetoma, accounts for almost 90% of cases of mycetoma (74).

The differential diagnosis of mycetoma includes chronic osteomyelitis due to bacteria or mycobacteria; other deep fungal infections, such as blastomycosis, coccidioidomycosis, or sporotrichosis; botryomycosis; leishmaniasis; yaws; syphilis; and chromoblastomycosis. Botryomycosis is a bacterial infection in which abscesses also drain granules consisting of clusters of bacteria. It is usually caused by *Staphylococcus aureus* and occasionally by gram-negative bacteria such as *Pseudomonas aeruginosa, Escherichia coli,* or *Proteus* species; Gram stain, biopsy, and culture will distinguish it from actinomycotic mycetoma.

Diagnosis is made by microscopic examination with potassium hydroxide preparation, Gram stain, and acid-fast stains of smears of pus and granules and by culture of the grains. If possible, drug sensitivity testing should be performed. In some instances, serologic evaluation may be helpful. Early lesions may need incision and drainage for appropriate material to be obtained for diagnosis. If no sinuses are present, biopsy may be necessary for diagnosis. Histologic examination reveals granulation tissue with abscess formation and grains. The shape and color of the grains, along with their appearance in tissue on skin biopsy, may be helpful in identifying the causative agent (74). Radiographs of bone should be performed to determine the presence and extent of bone involvement. Actinomycetoma is more likely to invade bone or other structures than is eumycetoma (73).

Treatment of mycetoma is difficult, in part because the condition is usually far advanced by the time the diagnosis is made. Choice of therapy and response are determined by the causative organism, the site of involvement, and the degree of invasion. Specific identification of the etiologic agent is essential to guide therapy; the agents used for actinomycetoma and eumycetoma are different. Actinomycetoma should be treated with antibiotics such as trimethoprim-sulfamethoxazole plus streptomycin, dapsone plus streptomycin, penicillin, tetracycline, and rifampin, and surgical débridement (9). Trimethoprim-sulfamethoxazole with dapsone, sulfadoxine-pyrimethamine with either streptomycin or rifampin, sulfadiazine with tetracycline, and minocycline are regimens found useful by some authors (73,74). Prolonged treatment courses are necessary.

Wide excision may be curative of early, localized lesions of eumycetoma before bone involvement occurs, but relapse rates are high, and surgical therapy must be accompanied by appropriate antibiotic therapy guided by culture and *in vitro* susceptibility testing (74). Eumycotic mycetoma is extremely resistant to medical therapy, in part because the organism is somewhat protected by its grain form in tissue in both eumycetoma and actinomycetoma (75). Ketoconazole in high doses for prolonged courses appears effective in about 60% to 70% of patients with mycetoma caused by *M. mycetomatis* (9,76). However, eumycetoma due to *P. boydii* or acremonium is refractory to therapy, although intravenous miconazole has been helpful in some patients with *P. boydii* (18,73,77). Itraconazole appears less effective than ketoconazole in this condition but may be useful in mycetoma due to *Fusarium* (18,78,79). Amphotericin appears not to be useful, except in occasional infections with *M. grisea* or *M. mycetomatis* (73).

REFERENCES

1. Dixon DM, Polak-Wyss A. The medically important dematiaceous fungi and their identification. *Mycoses* 1991;34:1.
2. Sughayer M, DeGirolami PC, Khettry U, et al. Human infection caused by *Exophiala pisciphila*: case report and review. *Rev Infect Dis* 1991;13:379.
3. Turiansky GW, Benson PM, Sperling LC, et al. *Phialophora verrucosa*: A new cause of mycetoma. *J Am Acad Dermatol* 1995;32:311.
4. Barba-Gómez JF, Mayorga J, McGinnis MR, et al. Chromoblastomycosis caused by *Exophiala spinifera*. *J Am Acad Dermatol* 1992;26:367.
5. Zaharopoulos P, Schnadig VJ, Davie KD, et al. Multiseptate bodies in systemic phaeohyphomycosis diagnosed by fine needle aspiration cytology. *Acta Cytol* 1988;32:885.
6. McGinnis MR, Hilger AE. Infections caused by black fungi. *Arch Dermatol* 1987;123:1300.
7. Milam CP, Fenske NA. Chromoblastomycosis. *Dermatol Clin* 1989;7:219.
8. Morris MI, Gurevitch A, Edwards JE Jr. Dematiaceae and agents of superficial mycoses. In: Gorbach S, Bartlett JG, Blacklow NR, eds. *Infectious diseases*. Philadelphia: WB Saunders, 1992:1937–1941.
9. Hay RJ, Roberts SOB, MacKenzie DWR. Mycology. In: Champion RH, Burton JL, Ebling FJG, eds. *Rook/Wilkinson/Ebling textbook of dermatology*, 5th ed. Boston: Blackwell Scientific Publications, 1992:1127–1216.
10. Okeke CN, Gugnani HC. Studies on pathogenic dematiaceous fungi. 1. Isolation from natural sources. *Mycopathologia* 1986;94:19.
11. Carrion AL. Chromoblastomycosis. *Ann N Y Acad Sci* 1950;50:1255.
12. Rippon JW: Chromoblastomycosis. In: Rippon JW, ed. *Medical mycology: the pathogenic fungi and the pathogenic actinomycetes*, 3rd ed. Philadelphia: WB Saunders, 1988:276–296.
13. Azulay RD, Serruya J. Hematogenous dissemination in chromomycosis. *Arch Dermatol* 1967;95:57.
14. McGinnis MR. Chromoblastomycosis and phaeohyphomycosis: new concepts, diagnosis, and mycology. *J Am Acad Dermatol* 1983;8:1.
15. Zaias N, Rebell G. A simple and accurate diagnostic method in chromoblastomycosis. *Arch Dermatol* 1973;108:545.
16. Vollum DI. Chromomycosis: a review. *Br J Dermatol* 1977;96:454.
17. Espinel-Ingroff A, Shadomy S, Dixon D, et al. Exoantigen test for *Cladosporium bantianum*, *Fonsecaea pedrosoi*, and *Phialophora verrucosa*. *J Clin Microbiol* 1986;23:305.
18. Restrepo A. Treatment of tropical mycoses. *J Am Acad Dermatol* 1994;31:591.
19. Kinbara T, Fukushiro R, Eryu Y. Chromomycosis: report of two cases successfully treated with local heat therapy. *Mykosen* 1982;25:689.
20. Tagami H, Ginaza M, Imaizumi S, et al. Successful treatment of chromoblastomycosis with topical heat therapy. *J Am Acad Dermatol* 1984;10:615.
21. Lubritz RR, Spence JE. Chromoblastomycosis: cure by cryosurgery. *Int J Dermatol* 1978;17:830.
22. Silber JG, Gombert ME, Green KM, et al. Treatment of chromomycosis with ketoconazole and 5-fluorocytosine. *J Am Acad Dermatol* 1983;8:236.
23. Arenas R. Chromoblastomycosis. In: Jacobs PH, Nall L, eds. *Antifungal drug therapy: a complete guide for the practitioner*. New York: Marcel Dekker, 1990:43–51.
24. Diaz M, Negroni R, Montero-Gei F, et al. A Pan American 5-year study of fluconazole therapy for deep mycoses in the immunocompetent host. *Clin Infect Dis* 1992;14[Suppl 1]:568.
25. Tufanelli L, Milburn PB. Treatment of chromoblastomycosis. *J Am Acad Dermatol* 1990;23:728.
26. Restrepo A, Gonzalez A, Gomez I, et al. Treatment of chromoblastomycosis with itraconazole. *Ann N Y Acad Sci* 1988;544:504.
27. Franco L, Gomez I, Restrepo A. Saperconazole in the treatment of systemic and subcutaneous mycoses. *Int J Dermatol* 1992;31:725.
28. Sharkey PK, Graybill JR, Rinaldi MG, et al. Itraconazole treatment of phaeohyphomycosis. *J Am Acad Dermatol* 1990;23:577.
29. Rippon JW. Phaeohyphomycosis. In: Rippon JW. *Medical mycology: the pathogenic fungi and the pathogenic actinomycetes*, 3rd ed. Philadelphia: WB Saunders, 1988:297–324.
30. Kawachi Y, Tateishi T, Shojima K, et al. Subcutaneous phaeomycotic cyst of the finger caused by *Exophiala jeanselmei*: Association with a wooden splinter. *Cutis* 1995;56:41.
31. Lavoie SR, Espinel-Ingroff A, Kerkering T. Mixed cutaneous phaeohyphomycosis in a cocaine user. *Clin Infect Dis* 1993;17:114.
32. Grieshop TJ, Yarbrough D 3rd, Farrar WE. Case report: phaeohyphomycosis due to *Curvularia lunata* involving the skin and subcutaneous tissue after an explosion at a chemical plant. *Am J Med Sci* 1993;305:387.
33. Burges GE, Walls CT, Maize JC. Subcutaneous phaeohyphomycosis caused by *Exserohilum rostratum* in an immunocompetent host. *Arch Dermatol* 1987;123:1346.
34. Faulk CT, Lesher JL. Phaeohyphomycosis and *Mycobacterium fortuitum* abscesses in a patient receiving corticosteroids for sarcoidosis. *J Am Acad Dermatol* 1995;33:309.
35. Chaidemenos GC, Mourellou O, Karakatsanis G, et al. Cutaneous alternariosis in an immunocompromised patient. *Cutis* 1995;56:145.
36. Coldiron BM, Wiley EL, Rinaldi MG. Cutaneous phaeohyphomycosis caused by a rare fungal pathogen, *Hormonema dematioides*: successful treatment with ketoconazole. *J Am Acad Dermatol* 1990;23:363.
37. Markham WD, Key RD, Padhye AA, et al. Phaeohyphomycotic cyst caused by *Tetraploa aristata*. *J Med Vet Mycol* 1990;28:147.
38. Tam M, Freeman S. Phaeohyphomycosis due to *Phialophora richardsiae*. *Australas J Dermatol* 1989;30:37.
39. Dooley DP, Beckius ML, Jeffery BS, et al. Phaeohyphomycotic cutaneous disease caused by *Pleurophoma* in a cardiac transplant patient. *J Infect Dis* 1989;159:503.
40. Straka BF, Cooper PH, Body BA. Cutaneous *Bipolaris spicifera* infection. *Arch Dermatol* 1989;125:1383.
41. Hironaga M, Nakano K, Yokoyama I, et al. *Phialophora repens*, an emerging agent of subcutaneous phaeohyphomycosis in humans. *J Clin Microbiol* 1989;27:394.
42. Kotylo PK, Israel KS, Cohen JS, et al. Subcutaneous phaeohyphomycosis of the finger caused by *Exophiala spinifera*. *Am J Clin Pathol* 1989;91:624.
43. Kettlewell P, McGinnis MR, Wilkinson GT. Phaeohyphomycosis caused by *Exophiala spinifera* in two cats. *J Med Vet Mycol* 1989;27:257.
44. Matsumoto T, Matsuda T, Padhye AA, et al. Fungal melanonychia: ungual phaeohyphomycosis caused by *Wangiella dermatitidis*. *Clin Exp Dermatol* 1992;17:83.
45. Berg D, Garcia JA, Schell WA, et al. Cutaneous infection caused by *Curvularia pallescens*: a case report and review of the spectrum of disease. *J Am Acad Dermatol* 1995;32:375.
46. Levenson JE, Duffin RM, Gardner SK, et al. Dematiaceous fungal keratitis following penetrating keratoplasty. *Ophthal Surg* 1984;15:578.
47. Anandi V, Suryawanshi NB, Koshi G, et al. Corneal ulcer caused by *Bipolaris hawaiiensis*. *J Med Vet Mycol* 1988;26:301.
48. Thomas PA. Mycotic keratitis—an underestimated mycosis. *J Med Vet Mycol* 1994;32:235.
49. Bouchon CL, Greer DL, Genre CF. Corneal ulcer due to *Exserohilum longirostratum*. *Am J Clin Pathol* 1994;101:452.
50. al-Hedaithy SS, al-Kaff AS. *Exophiala jeanselmei* keratitis. *Mycoses* 1993;39:97.
51. Anandi V, George JA, Thomas R, et al. Phaeohyphomycosis of the eye caused by *Exserohilum rostratum* in India. *Mycoses* 1991;34:489.
52. Aviv JE, Lawson W Bottone EJ, et al. Multiple intracranial mucoceles associated with phaeohyphomycosis of the paranasal sinuses. *Arch Otolaryngol Head Neck Surg* 1990;116:1210.
53. Rao A, Forgan-Smith R, Miller S, et al. Phaeohyphomycosis of the nasal sinuses caused by *Bipolaris* species. *Pathology* 1989;21:280.
54. Lawson W, Blitzer A. Fungal infections of the nose and paranasal sinuses. Part II. *Otolaryngol Clin North Am* 1993;26:1037.
55. Cody DT 2nd, Neel HB 3rd, Ferreiro JA, et al. Allergic fungal sinusitis: the Mayo Clinic experience. *Laryngoscope* 1994;104:1074.
56. Manning SC, Schaefer SD, Close LG, et al. Culture-positive allergic fungal sinusitis. *Arch Otolaryngol Head Neck Surg* 1991;117:174.
57. Manning SC, Mabry RL, Schaefer SD, et al. Evidence of IgE-mediated hypersensitivity in allergic fungal sinusitis. *Laryngoscope* 1993;103:717.
58. Friedman GC, Hartwick RWJ, Ro JY, et al. Allergic fungal sinusitis: report of three cases associated with dematiaceous fungi. *Am J Clin Pathol* 1991;96:368.

59. Alvarez-Franco M, Reyes-Mugica M, Paller AS. Cutaneous *Fusarium* infection in an adolescent with acute leukemia. *Pediatr Dermatol* 1992;9:62.
60. Bushelman SJ, Callen JP, Roth DN, et al. Disseminated *Fusarium solani* infection. *J Am Acad Dermatol* 1995;32:346.
61. Sekhon AS, Galbraith J, Mielke BW, et al. Cerebral phaeohyphomycosis caused by *Xylohypha bantiana*, with a review of the literature. *Eur J Epidemiol* 1992;8:387.
62. Borges MC Jr, Warren S, White W et al. Pulmonary phaeohyphomycosis due to *Xylohypha bantiana*. *Arch Pathol Lab Med* 1991;115:627.
63. Aldape KD, Fox HS, Roberts JP, et al. *Cladosporium trichoides* cerebral phaeohyphomycosis in a liver transplant recipient. Report of a case. *Am J Clin Pathol* 1991;95:499.
64. Palaoglu S, Sav A, Basak T, et al. Cerebral phaeohyphomycosis. *Neurosurgery* 1993;33:894.
65. Anandi V, John TJ, Walter A, et al. Cerebral phaeohyphomycosis caused by *Chaetomium globosum* in a renal transplant patient. *J Clin Microbiol* 1989;27:2226.
66. Sides EH 3rd, Benson JD, Padhye AA. Phaeohyphomycotic brain abscess due to *Ochroconis gallopavum* in a patient with malignant lymphoma of a large cell type. *J Med Vet Mycol* 1991;29:317.
67. al-Hedaithy SS, Jamjoom ZA, Saeed ES. Cerebral phaeohyphomycosis caused by *Fonsecaea pedrosoi* in Saudi Arabia. *APMIS* 1988;3[Suppl]:94.
68. Kenney RT, Kwon-Chung KJ, Waytes AT, et al. Successful treatment of systemic *Exophiala dermatitidis* infection in a patient with chronic granulomatous disease. *Clin Infect Dis* 1992;14:235.
69. Salaki JS, Louria DB, Chmel H. Fungal and yeast infections of the central nervous system. A clinical review. *Medicine (Baltimore)* 1984;63:108.
70. Gold WL, Vellend H, Salit IE, et al. Successful treatment of systemic and local infections due to *Exophiala* species. *Clin Infect Dis* 1994;19:339.
71. Vukmir RB, Kusne S, Linden P, et al. Successful therapy for cerebral phaeohyphomycosis due to *Dactylaria gallopava* in a liver transplant recipient. *Clin Infect Dis* 1994;19:714.
72. Noel SB, Greer DL, Abadie SM, et al. Primary cutaneous phaeohyphomycosis. Report of three cases. *J Am Acad Dermatol* 1988;18:1023.
73. Rippon JW. Mycetoma. In: Rippon JW, ed. *Medical mycology: the pathogenic fungi and the pathogenic actinomycetes*, 3rd ed. Philadelphia: WB Saunders, 1988:80–118.
74. Magaña M, Magaña-García M. Mycetoma. *Dermatol Clin* 1989;7:203.
75. Roberts SOB, MacKenzie DWR. Mycology. In: Rook A, Ebling FJG, Wilkinson DS, et al, eds. *Textbook of dermatology*, 4th ed. Boston: Blackwell Scientific Publications, 1986:980–982.
76. Mahgoub ES, Gumaa SA. Ketoconazole in the treatment of eumycetoma due to *Madurella mycetomii*. *Trans R Soc Trop Med Hyg* 1984;78:376.
77. Hay RJ, MacKenzie DWR. Mycetoma (Madura foot) in the United Kingdom: a survey of 44 cases. *Clin Exp Dermatol* 1983;8:553.
78. Mahgoub ES. Mycetoma. In: *Tropical mycoses*. Beerse, Belgium: Janssen Research Council, 1990:50–72.
79. Resnik BI, Burdick AE. Improvement of eumycetoma with itraconazole. *J Am Acad Dermatol* 1995;33:917.

CHAPTER 275
Phycomycetes

Burt R. Meyers, Fernando Borrego, and Alejandra C. Gurtman

The class Zygomycetes consists of two orders containing species pathogenic for humans: Mucorales and Entomophthorales. The order Mucorales is further divided into six genera, of which three, *Mucor, Rhizopus*, and *Absidia*, are the most important; infections with species of *Cunninghamella* and *Mortierella* have been described (1–3), and less commonly, infections with *Saksenaea, Syncephalastrum, Apophysomyces*, and *Thamnidium* (4–8) (Table 275.1). The order Mucorales is associated with mucormycosis and does not include infection with *Entomophthora* organisms. The two main pathogenic genera of Entomophthorales are *Conidiobolus* and *Basidiobolus*. Tropical subcutaneous phycomycosis and rhinoentomophthoromycosis are rather indolent infections associated with nodules and granuloma formation (1,9–11). Mucorales infections usually are rapidly progressive, invading blood vessels, leading to infarction of tissue involving vital organs such as the brain and lung (12–17), and often associated with a fatal outcome.

MICROBIOLOGY AND MORPHOLOGY OF THE MUCORALES

Growth of these fungi on either food or agar is characterized by a white or gray woolly appearance (Fig. 275.1). This growth represents mycelia with multiple nuclei that are nonseptate. All the genera give rise to specialized mycelia known as *conidiophores*, which are sacs filled with asexual spores called *sporangia*. A rhizoid filament-like mycelium that extends into the air is also seen. The genera can be further classified by differences in the origin of the rhizoids and sporangiophores for the genera *Rhizopus* and *Absidia* (Fig. 275.2); the genus *Mucor*, on the other hand, does not produce rhizoids and therefore appears less abundant in culture. The columella, the tip of sporangiophore appearing within the sporangium, differentiates *Cunninghamella* from the other genera, which do not possess this structure.

Colonies of Entomophthorales differ from those of Mucorales, being flat and covered with white fuzz. This order also produces septate hyphae, which differentiate it from the Mucorales, which are nonseptate. The genera can be further differentiated by the presence or absence of zygospores and other changes in conidiophores.

EPIDEMIOLOGY

Mucorales are ubiquitous saprophytes found throughout the world that usually thrive in any organic material. They can affect fruits (including strawberries) and sweet potatoes and account for the mold that grows on moist bread. *Aspergillus* species are often found in hospital environments, whereas Mucorales organisms are not. Mucormycosis involving the skin and subcutaneous tissue was reported in hospitals when contaminated elastic dressings were used (18).

CUNNINGHAMELLA

In 1988, 10 cases of infection secondary to *Cunninghamella* species were reported (19). The fungus is a soil saprophyte that can cause disseminated disease; the only clinical presentation may be fever associated with thrombocytopenia (20). There is only one report of disease without hematogenous spread, which presented as a chronic infection in the skin resembling an entomophthoromycosis infection. Sensitivity to amphotericin B varies (21,22).

Entomophthorales

Entomophthorales organisms are usually found in tropical climates and typically infect immunocompetent hosts. Infections with these organisms have not been described in the Western Hemisphere. Because the fungus grows poorly at 15°C, it has been suggested that in temperate climates it is disseminated only during warm months from its reservoir in reptiles that feed on insects. *Basidiobolus haptosporus* infection probably follows insect bites or minor trauma in children in this environment. Infection with *Conidiobolus coronatus* usually follows inhalation of spores and is observed in adult agricultural workers exposed to tropical rain forest vegetation (23).

Although the organisms infect the nasal mucosa, they usually do not cause tissue infarction, because blood vessels are not invaded. The affinity of these spores for the nasal mucosa has not been adequately described. Invasive disease caused by *Conidiobolus incongruus* has been reported in a granulocytopenic host (24).

TABLE 275.1. Classification of Pathogenic Zygomycetes

Pathogen	Comments
Order 1: Mucorales	
Family 1: Mucoraceae	Rhinocerebral, rhinoorbital/paranasal, cardiac involvement;
Genera: *Absidia, Apophysomyces, Mucor, Rhizomucor, Rhizopus*	pulmonary, gastrointestinal, skin and soft tissue
Pathogenic species: *Absidia corymbifera, Apophysomyces elegans,*	involvement; disseminated disease; osteomyelitis;
Mucor circinelloides, Mucor hiemalis, Mucor racemosus, Mucor	cerebral involvement; occurs in patients with chronic
ramosissimus, Rhizomucor miehei, Rhizomucor pusillus, Rhizopus	renal failure or hemodialysis taking deferoxamine
arrhizus, Rhizopus microsporus, Rhizopus microsporus	
rhizopodiformis	
Family 2: Mortierellaceae	Bovine abortion
Genus: *Mortierella*	
Pathogenic species: *Mortierella wolfii*	
Family 3: Cunninghamellaceae	Disseminated disease, thrombocytopenia
Genus: *Cunninghamella*	
Pathogenic species: *Cunninghamella bertholletiae*	
Family 4: Sakenaeaceae	Subcutaneous infection, disseminated disease, osteomyelitis
Genus: *Saksenaea*	
Pathogenic species: *Saksenaea vasiformis*	
Family 5: Syncephalastraceae	
Genus: *Syncephalastrum*	
Pathogenic species: Not identified to species level	
Family 6: Thamnidiaceae	Chronic cystitis
Genus: *Cokeromyces*	
Pathogenic species: *Cokeromyces recurvatus*	
Order 2: Entomophthorales	
Family 1: Entomophthoraceae	Subcutaneous granuloma; rhinopharyngeal, sinus, and
Genus: *Conidiobolus*	pulmonary involvement
Pathogenic species: *Conidiobolus coronatus, Conidiobolus*	
incongruus	
Family 2: Basidiobiolaceae	Subcutaneous granuloma, adenopathy
Genus: *Basidiobolus*	
Pathogenic species: *Basidiobolus ranarum*	

Source: Adapted from Rinaldi MC. Zygomycosis. *Infect Dis Clin North Am* 1989;3:19–41, with permission.

Mucormycosis has worldwide distribution and usually occurs in association with underlying conditions, including diabetes mellitus with or without ketoacidosis, lymphoid malignancy, burns, severe trauma, prolonged postoperative courses, multiple myeloma, hepatitis, cirrhosis, renal failure (25), steroid therapy, and immunodeficiency states (induced or acquired) (26), as well as use of contaminated Elastoplast bandages (18). Uncontrolled diabetes with hyperglycemia and acidosis is often the setting for the development of serious infection with the Zygomycetes. High levels of glucose impair phagocytosis. De-layed or diminished neutrophil chemotaxis has been described in diabetic patients with ketoacidosis. Other studies *in vitro* have shown that *Rhizopus* favors an acid environment, a temperature of 39°C, and glucose-rich media (27). A normal leukocyte complement is important in preventing mucormycosis, as demonstrated in animal infection (28), because neutropenia reduces resistance to mucormycosis. Bronchoalveolar macrophages prevent spore germination and tissue invasion. In experimentally induced diabetic animal models or those treated with cortisone, phagocytosis is reduced and the macrophages allow spore

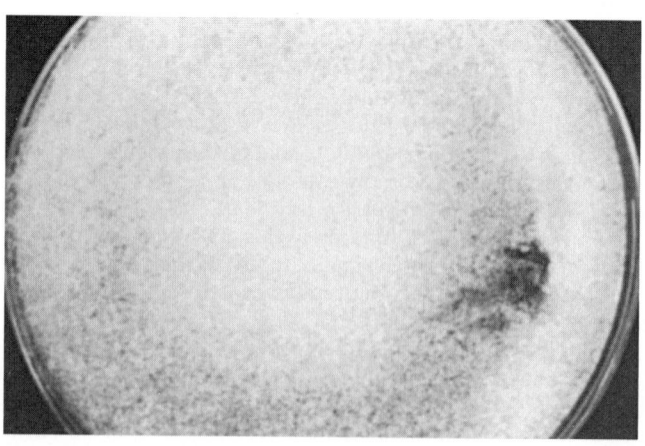

Figure 275.1. Mold-like growth of *Rhizopus* species covering the entire surface of a plate with Sabouraud agar after 48 hours of incubation at 37°C.

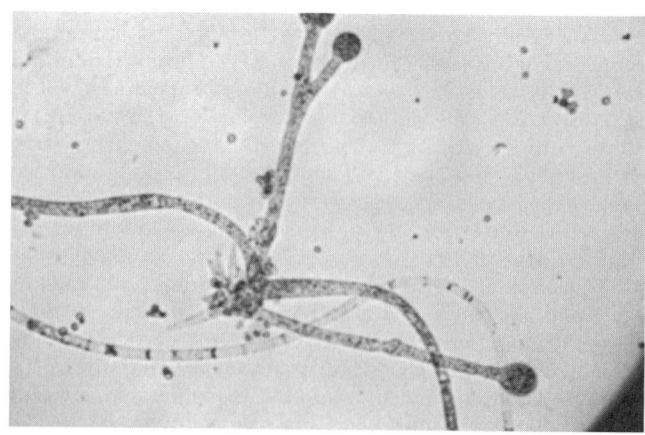

Figure 275.2. Sporangiophores of *Rhizopus* species arising directly from finger-like rhizoids with sporangium-containing spores.

germination and infection (29). Other serum factors (i.e., antibodies) are probably necessary to inhibit spore germination (30).

Infection is probably initiated by the inhalation of asexual sporangiospore spores through the nose and into the sinuses, from where the organism may extend into the cerebrum and retroorbital tissues; spores may enter the lower airways and settle in the alveoli or enter through denuded skin. When they cause infection, these fungi have a predilection for invading blood vessels, leading to venous and arterial thrombosis with subsequent ischemia and gangrene. Spores of Mucorales may also invade bronchi, stomach, and intestines of neutropenic patients.

The clinical states associated with mucormycosis include rhinocerebral-rhinoorbital-paranasal syndrome; pulmonary, gastrointestinal (GI) tract, cardiac, skin, and soft tissue involvement; a disseminated form; osteomyelitis; cerebritis; and chronic renal failure (in patients undergoing hemodialysis receiving deferoxamine).

With Entomophthorales infection, three clinical syndromes have been described: basidiobolomycosis, subcutaneous granuloma infiltrating muscle with lymph gland hyperplasia; rhinoentomophthoromycosis, granulomata of the inferior turbinate with superficial spread without ulceration to the nasopharynx or paranasal sinuses; and pulmonary infection by *C. incongruus*. In none of these cases does tissue destruction occur.

A common antigen is shared by *Absidia, Rhizopus,* and *Mucor* organisms. Although some specific antigens for each genus have been found by immunodiffusion, their role in the diagnosis of acute disease has not been elucidated. Fewer data are available for the Entomophthorales.

CLINICAL SYNDROMES

In patients who have a predisposing factor such as leukemia, malignancy, immunosuppression, including human immunodeficiency virus (HIV) infection or diabetes mellitus, infection may occur in the nasal turbinates, the paranasal sinuses, the palate, and the skin eye or retroorbital area with invasion into brain and cavernous sinus (Fig. 275.3), as well as the GI tract. However, rarely, rhinocerebral infection may occur in a healthy patient (31). Symptoms depend on the areas involved. With the rhinocerebral form, fever, facial and orbital pain, headache, diplopia, loss of vision, and facial or orbital cellulitis may be

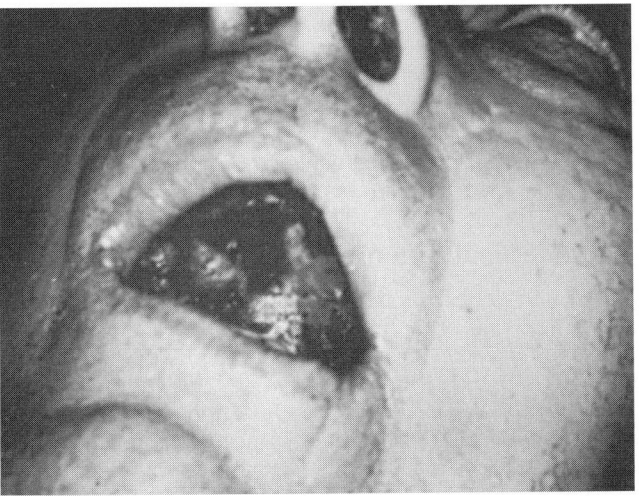

Figure 275.3. Necrosis of the hard palate secondary to invasion by *Rhizopus* species in a renal transplant recipient taking corticosteroids.

noted. Facial anesthesia may be an early clinical sign. Cranial nerve involvement is not uncommon. Black nasal discharge in this setting is often mistaken for dried blood rather than evidence of tissue infarction. Abdominal pain, malabsorption, and GI tract perforation may occur. Black appearing ulceration of the skin at an intravenous site has been noted (32). Careful physical examination of the pharynx, nasal turbinate, and palate for necrotic ulcerations is necessary. Physical signs may include proptosis, chemosis, and retinal infarction; thrombosis of the cavernous sinus or internal carotid artery may occur. Patients may develop seizures and epistaxis. Radiographic examination usually reveals evidence of destruction of the paranasal sinuses or of inflammation; computed tomography (CT) or magnetic resonance imaging (MRI) best reveals involvement of the sinuses and orbital and retroorbital areas.

DIAGNOSTIC PROCEDURES

The diagnosis is best established by direct examination and culture of infected tissue obtained by biopsy, because superficial culture of necrotic material may reveal only colonizing microorganisms; areas from which to obtain biopsy material include the buccal, nasal, and palatal mucosa or paranasal sinuses. Examination of a smear of tissue with direct light without staining may establish the diagnosis within minutes after the biopsy procedure. Morphologically, broad, nonseptate, nonpigmented hyphae 15 to 20 μm in diameter, up to 20 μm long, often with right-angled branching are noted. The hyphae of *Aspergillus* species are smaller and septate and branch at acute angles. Blood culture should be attempted, although the organism is rarely isolated. Spinal tap may reveal pleocytosis, usually with an elevated protein value; the glucose level may be normal. Culture of cerebrospinal fluid is necessary, but the organism has not been isolated from the central nervous system (CNS). In transplant recipients with abdominal pain, gastroscopy is required to rule out GI tract mucor infection.

The differential diagnosis of this acute syndrome in patients who are at risk includes acute sinusitis secondary to *Aspergillus* or *Pseudomonas aeruginosa* infection, because both organisms can invade blood vessels, proceeding to vascular thrombosis and infarction. Malignant tumors, midline lethal granulomata, Burkitt's lymphoma, and noma must be considered. For more indolent disease, the differential diagnosis includes granulomatous infections, including other fungi (i.e., blastomycosis), tuberculosis, syphilis, and leprosy, each of which can produce ulceration and invasion of the nasal turbinate.

THERAPY AND OUTCOME

A lipid formulation of amphotericin B is the drug of choice; the total dose necessary for eradication and cure has not been determined. The liposomes disseminate in organs that are rich in reticuloendothelial cells (33). The empirical dose is 1 to 2 g; in some cases 4 g or more has been necessary to effect a cure. The efficacy of the azole compounds in the treatment of Zygomycetes infections is limited to one experimental model in guinea pigs and few human cases (31,33a). If a patient has evidence of acidosis and hyperglycemia, the clinical condition should be reversed immediately; other supportive therapy may be necessary—intravenous fluids and blood pressure and ventilatory support. Synergy of flucytosine with rifampin and tetracycline has been reported. In some cases, local irrigation of infected sinuses with amphotericin B has been employed. The use of hyperbaric oxygen is suggested, although clinical trials have not determined its efficacy (34,35).

In neutropenic patients, granulocyte colony-stimulating factor (G-CSF) coupled with amphotericin B lipid complex was successful in therapy (36). The azole compounds have limited or poor activity with itraconazole, the most active against basidial strains. Posaconazole, an experimental agent, is active against most strains both *in vitro* (37,38) and in an immunosuppressed mouse model (39). The echinocandins are not active against Zygomycetes.

The activity *in vitro* is related to the incubation time, whereas minimum inhibitory concentration (MIC) determinations, both visual and spectrophotometric, were in good agreement (38). In general *in vitro* tests reveal that Zygomycetes are a heterogenous group regarding antifungal testing (38).

In one study in which all patients had premortem diagnoses, patients with diabetes mellitus tended to survive, whereas those with acute leukemia and transplant recipients did not (12) In another study, Parfrey (14) noted that survival before 1970 was 6% compared with 73% thereafter. Another study reviewing survival in patients with paranasal sinus mucormycosis revealed that survival had increased to 70% from 1970 to 1979, compared with early estimates with lower survival data. It appears that the chance of survival is better for patients who have no underlying disease (75%) or diabetes (60%) than for those who have renal disease (25%); the overall survival rate, including cases before 1960, was 50% in the 179 cases surveyed. The authors noted that surgical débridement or radical resection and amphotericin B therapy significantly increased the chances of survival; 79% of diabetics who received the drug survived, versus 37% of those who did not receive the drug. With amphotericin B and surgery, 81% survived (and 89% of those who also had diabetes). Prognosis was poorer for patients with hemiplegia, facial necrosis, and nasal deformity. Survival was not related to age or sex, laterality of involvement, or x-ray findings (13).

A review of 33 patients with mucormycosis revealed that patients with only rhinoorbital or paranasal involvement had a better prognosis than those with either cerebral or disseminated disease (14). Invasive fungal sinusitis must be differentiated from chronic noninvasive disease, which has also been associated with fungal colonization. In the latter case, cure is usually associated with surgical removal of hyphal masses and draining of sinuses (40). Itraconazole is generally not active against Zygomycetes but has some activity against some *Rhizopus* strains (41,42).

SPECIFIC INFECTIONS

Pulmonary Mucormycosis

Pulmonary mucormycosis is characterized by invasion of the pulmonary vessels, with lung infarction and pneumonia (43,44). Patients with underlying disease (diabetes, leukemia, lymphoma) and allograft recipients are at risk of infection. Spores of Mucorales enter through the nares into the nasal sinus and subsequently to bronchi and lungs. The organism then invades blood vessels, causing pulmonary hemorrhage, infarction, and gangrene. Lymphatics may also be involved; the disease may run an indolent course and produce a solitary nodule on chest radiographs. On histologic section and examination, nonseptate hyphae surrounded by neutrophilic leukocytes are noted.

Clinically there is evidence of pulmonary infarction, pneumonia, lung abscess, or any combination of these. The presentation may be acute and fulminant or subacute. Patients with underlying disease who experience a new episode of chills, fever, and pulmonary infiltrates, especially if they are receiving antibiotics, should be suspected of having fungal infection. Sudden onset of pleuritic chest pain, bloody sputum, and pleural friction rub in this setting is highly suggestive; the x-ray appearance of an infarction with cavitation suggests either *Mucor* or *Aspergillus* species. Usually, the patchy heterogeneous infiltrate progresses, despite antibiotic therapy, into consolidation and cavity formation, often associated with a hemorrhagic pleural effusion. The condition may be complicated by massive hemoptysis and death, the pulmonary vessels being eroded by the fungus; endogenous spread to all organs has been described (45). Severe bacterial superinfection by *Pseudomonas* or *Staphylococcus* has been reported (16). The disease may be less fulminant in diabetic patients, producing a subacute pneumonitis, with or without cavitation (46).

DIAGNOSIS

Pulmonary mucormycosis should be considered when immunocompromised patients have evidence of pulmonary infarction or acute pneumonitis that does not respond to antimicrobial agents. Because Mucorales organisms are rarely seen on Gram stain or isolated from sputum culture, further diagnostic studies may be necessary: bronchoalveolar lavage and bronchoscopy with transbronchial biopsy of lung parenchyma for smear, culture, and histologic examination. Patients who are profoundly thrombocytopenic may require platelet transfusions before undergoing this procedure. On examination of the tissue, large, broad nonseptate hyphae with wide-angled branching suggest Mucorales. Isolates should be sent to the laboratory for plating on blood or Sabouraud agar at 37°C and kept for 10 to 14 days; growth usually occurs within 1 or 2 days. Direct plating of biopsy material on agar increases the yield.

The differential diagnosis includes other infectious agents (fungi, parasites) that produce pulmonary disease in immunocompromised hosts. *Nocardia asteroides* produces acute necrotizing pneumonia, often with cerebral involvement. Examination of sputum and tissue may reveal threadlike, beaded, branching, gram-positive filamentous rods that are also partially acid fast. *Aspergillus* species can invade blood vessels and produce an identical clinical picture. Differentiation can be made only with tissue specimens or culture. Other organisms that cause pneumonia in immunocompromised hosts include *Pneumocystis carinii* and cytomegalovirus. In patients with these infections, pneumonia is diffuse, often associated with dyspnea and hypoxia; cavitation and hemoptysis do not usually occur. *Legionella* species may also produce pulmonary cavitation but this is uncommon.

When *Mucor* infection is suspected, therapy should be instituted promptly with an intravenous liposomal amphotericin B product. In most cases, treatment is empirical; patients receive between 1 and 2 g, and the total dose necessary for cure is not known. The role of neutrophil transfusions has not been studied. In some cases, surgical resection is necessary for cure, especially in nonimmunosuppressed patients (47). Patients have survived even without the administration of amphotericin B (48).

Gastrointestinal Zygomycosis

Patients with underlying conditions such as solid organ transplantation, kwashiorkor, malnutrition, pellagra, amebic colitis, uremia, and typhoid fever are more susceptible to GI tract zygomycosis (49); the incidence is increased in South Africa compared with the rest of the world. Infection may occur in the neonatal period (50). The route of infection is believed to be secondary to ingestion of fungi, which then may colonize or infect the GI tract, especially in patients who have gastric ulcers; one third of patients are children. The stomach and large bowel are the organs most commonly involved; invasion of blood vessels causes ischemia and necrosis, and infarction and perforation may occur (51,52). Symptoms include abdominal pain, diarrhea, hematemesis, and bloody stools. Erosive necrotic ulcers and gangrene, hemorrhages, peritonitis, and bowel infarction are associated. Diagnosis is made by biopsy and cultures; stool and gastric cultures should be obtained, although results are rarely positive. The cause of death is shock secondary to hemorrhagic infarction; most cases have been recognized at autopsy, although more recently a renal transplant recipient was successfully treated.

Cutaneous Zygomycosis

Cutaneous zygomycosis can be primary or secondary and has occurred in patients with burns (53), diabetes mellitus (53), postsurgical wound infections (54), elastic (Elastoplast) bandages (18), or as part of nodular lesions, secondary to hematogenous seeding. Primary cutaneous mucormycosis may follow trauma, especially at an intravenous site in an immunosuppressed patient (32,55). Outcome will depend on the extension and location of the injury (56,57). Diagnosis is based on the demonstration of the fungus in culture or biopsy specimens. Parenteral amphotericin B or a liposomal product or a solution containing 5 mg/mL applied with gauze or by atomization may be required (58). When this therapy is not successful, patients may need aggressive surgical débridement, amputation, or both.

Disseminated Zygomycosis (Rare)

After primary infection in the lungs, the fungi can spread to the CNS, GI tract, spleen, kidneys, and heart. The disseminated form of zygomycosis is more commonly seen in patients with lymphoid malignancies and solid-organ transplant recipients. It is usually fatal, and the diagnosis is often made only at necropsy.

Cardiac Mucormycosis

Endocarditis has been reported without prior cardiac involvement (59), as well as in association with cardiac surgery and infection of prosthetic valves (60); large vegetations with symptoms secondary to subsequent emboli may occur. Diffuse cardiac involvement may occur in patients with underlying diseases. Diagnosis is suggested by echocardiography, because blood cultures rarely propagate the pathogen. Surgical extirpation may be curative.

Septic Arthritis and Osteomyelitis

Osteomyelitis of the femur has been observed secondary to hematogenous spread (61); cranial bone involvement in the absence of rhinocerebral involvement has been described. Recently after trauma, a patient with AIDS developed a cutaneoarticular form of *Cunninghamella* infection (62); bone infection of the ankle secondary to a primary cutaneous infection has also been reported (63).

Brain Abscess

After inadvertent direct intravenous injection of the fungus, the most common presentation is brain abscess (64); 22 cases have been reported in the literature, half of them in intravenous drug users (65). The basal ganglia are most often affected; deep abscesses were noted (66). The clinical presentation includes fever, headaches, and lethargy; hemiparesis and speech disturbances

may be the initial presentation. Most patients died despite attempts at surgery and amphotericin B therapy.

Mucormycosis in Hemodialysis Patients

Mucormycosis has been seen with increased frequency in patients undergoing hemodialysis (67), who received deferoxamine therapy for iron and aluminum overload (19,68). Iron is a growth factor for some bacteria and fungi. Patients who received iron have a greater incidence of infections such as tuberculosis, malaria, brucellosis, and amebiasis (69). Deferoxamine might increase the availability of iron to the fungi, acting as a growth promoter. It is postulated that the microorganism may be unable to synthesize siderophores but has receptors for them; the organism might use deferoxamine as a siderophore as a source of iron. This may be the same mechanism that promotes *Yersinia* infection in these patients (70).

CONCLUSION

Even though the diagnosis, treatment and prognosis of mucormycosis has improved, infection with these organisms still is associated with a high mortality rate. If prognosis and survival are to improve, early diagnosis must be achieved, as well as control of the underlying disorder, aggressive surgery when indicated, and systemic antifungal therapy.

REFERENCES

1. Rinaldi MG. Zygomycosis. *Infect Dis Clin North Am* 1989;3:19.
2. Rippon JW. *Medical mycology: the pathogenic fungi and the pathogenic actinomycetes,* 2nd ed. Philadelphia: WB Saunders, 1988:615–640.
3. Bottone EJ, Weitzman I, Hanna BA. *Rhizopus rhizopodiformis:* emerging etiological agent of mucormycosis. *J Clin Microbiol* 1978;9:530.
4. Pierce PF, Wood MB, Roberts GD, et al. *Saksenaea vasiformis* osteomyelitis. *J Clin Microbiol* 1987;25:933.
5. Axelrod P, Kwon-Chung KJ, Frawley P, et al. Chronic cystitis due to *Cokeromyces recurvatus:* a case report. *J Infect Dis* 1987;155:1062.
6. Padhye AA, Koshi G, Anandi V, et al. First case of subcutaneous zygomycosis caused by *Saksenaea vasiformis* in India. *Diagn Microbiol Infect Dis* 1988;9:69.
7. Meis JPGM, Kullberg B-J, Pruszczynski M, et al. Severe osteomyelitis due to the zygomycete *Apophysomyces elegans. J Clin Microbiol* 1994;32:3078.
8. Huffnagle KE, Southern PM Jr, Byrd LT, et al. *Apophysomyces elegans* as an agent of zygomycosis in a patient following trauma. *J Med Vet Mycol* 1992;30:83.
9. Braude AI. The Zygomycetes. In: Braude AI, Davis CE, Fierer J, eds. *Infectious diseases and medical microbiology,* 2nd ed. Philadelphia: WB Saunders, 1986:597–601.
10. Martinson FD. Phycomycosis (zygomycosis). In: Braude AI, Davis CE, Fierer J, eds. *Infectious diseases and medical microbiology,* 2nd ed. Philadelphia: WB Saunders, 1986:743–748.
11. Burkitt DP, Wilson A, Jelliffe D. Subcutaneous phycomycosis: a review of 31 cases seen in Uganda. *Br Med J* 1964;1:1669.
12. Meyers BR, Wormser G, Hirschman SZ, et al. Rhinocerebral mucormycosis. Diagnosis premortem and therapy. *Arch Intern Med* 1979;139:557.
13. Blitzer A, Lawson W, Meyers BR, et al. Patient survival factors in paranasal sinus mucormycosis. *Laryngoscope* 1980;90:635.
14. Parfrey NA. Improved diagnosis and prognosis of mucormycosis. *Medicine (Baltimore)* 1986;65:113.
15. Lehrer R. Mucormycosis. *Ann Intern Med* 1980;93:108.
16. Meyer RD, Rosen P, Armstrong D. Phycomycosis complicating leukemia and lymphoma. *Ann Intern Med* 1972;77:871.
17. Marchevsky AM, Bottone EJ, Geller SA, et al. The changing spectrum of disease etiology and diagnosis of mucormycosis. *Hum Pathol* 1980;11:457.
18. Gartenberg G, Bottone E, Keusch G, et al. Hospital-acquired mucormycosis (*Rhizopus rhizopodiformis*) of skin and subcutaneous tissue: epidemiology, mycology and treatment. *N Engl J Med* 1978;299:1115.
19. Rex JM, Ginsberg AM, Fries LF, et al. *Cunninghamella bertholletiae* infection associated with deferoxamine therapy. *Rev Infect Dis* 1988;10:1187.
20. McGinnis MR, Walker DM, Dominy IE, et al. Zygomycosis caused by *Cunninghamella bertholletiae. Arch Pathol Lab Med* 1982;106:282.
21. Kolbeck PC, Makhoul RG, Randal Bollinger R, et al. Widely disseminated *Cunninghamella* mucormycosis in an adult renal transplant patient: case report and review of the literature. *Am J Clin Pathol* 1984;83:747.

22. McGinnis MR, Walker DH, Dominy IE, et al. Zygomycosis caused by *Cunninghamella bertholletiae*. *Arch Pathol Lab Med* 1982;106:287.

23. Ng KH, Chin CS, Jalleh RD, et al. Nasofacial zygomycosis. *Oral Surg Oral Med Oral Pathol* 1991;72:685.

24. Walsh TJ, Renshaw G, Andrews J, et al. Invasive zygomycosis due to *Conidiobolus incongruus*. *Clin Infect Dis* 1994;19:423.

25. Hammer GS, Bottone EJ, Hirschman SZ. Mucormycosis in a transplant recipient. *Am J Clin Pathol* 1975;64:389.

26. Cuadrado LM, Guerrero A, Lopez Garcia Asenjo GA, et al. Cerebral mucormycosis in two cases of acquired immunodeficiency syndrome. *Arch Neurol* 1988;1:109.

27. Reinhardt FJ, Kaplan W, Ajello L. Experimental cerebral zygomycosis in alloxan-diabetic rabbits. I. Relationship of temperature tolerance of selected Zygomycetes to pathogenicity. *Infect Immun* 1970;2:404.

28. Artis WM, Fountain JA, Delcher HK, et al. A mechanism of susceptibility to mucormycosis in diabetic ketoacidosis: transferrin and iron availability. *Diabetes* 1982;31:1109.

29. Waldorf AR, Levitz SM, Diamond RD. In vivo bronchoalveolar macrophage defense against *Rhizopus oryzae* and *Aspergillus fumigatus*. *J Infect Dis* 1984;150:752.

30. Waldorf AR, Halde C, Vedros NA. Murine model of pulmonary mucormycosis in cortisone-treated mice. *Sabouraudia* 1982;20:217.

31. Radner AB, Witt MD, Edwards JE Jr. Acute invasive rhinocerebral zygomycosis in an otherwise healthy patient: case report and review. *Clin Infect Dis* 1995;20:163.

32. Meyers B, Papanicolaou G, Bottone EJ, et al. Nosocomial cutaneous phycomycoses in immunocompromised patients—a cluster of patients. Paper presented at the 37th International Conference on Antimicrobial Agents and Chemotherapy; Toronto, Canada; September 1987.

33. Lopez-Berestein G, Fainstein V, Hopfer R, et al. Liposomal amphotericin B for the treatment of systemic fungal infection in patients with cancer: a preliminary study. *J Infect Dis* 1985;151:704.

33a. Van Cutsem J, Van Gerven F, Fransen J, et al. Treatment of experimental zygomycosis in guinea pigs: azoles and amphotericin B. *Chemotherapy* 1989;35:267.

34. Ferguson BJ, Mitchell TG, Moon R, et al. Adjunctive hyperbaric oxygen for treatment of rhinocerebral mucormycosis. *Rev Infect Dis* 1988;10:551.

35. Couch L, Theilen F, Mader JT. Rhinocerebral mucormycosis with cerebral extension successfully treated with adjunctive hyperbaric oxygen therapy. *Arch Otolaryngol Head Neck Surg* 1988;114:791.

36. Walsh TJ, Groll AH. Emerging fungal pathogens: evolving challenges to immunocompromised patients for the twenty first century. *Transplant Infect Dis* 1999;1:247–261.

37. Uchida K, Yokota N, Yamahuchi H. In vitro antifungal activity of posaconazole against various pathogenic fungi. *Int J Antimicrob Agents* 2001;18:167–172.

38. Dannalui E, Meletiadis J, Mouton J, et al. In vitro susceptibilities of Zygomycetes to conventional and new antifungals. *J Antimicrob Chemother* 2003;51:45–52.

39. Sun Q, Najvar LK, Bocangera R, et al. In vivo activity of posaconazole against *Mucor* spp in an immunosuppressed mouse model. *Antimicrob Agents Chemother* 2002;46:2310–2312.

40. Washburn RG, Kennedy DW, Begley MG, et al. Chronic fungal sinusitis in apparently normal hosts. *Medicine (Baltimore)* 1988;67:231.

41. Dannaoui E, Mouton W, Meis JFGM, et al. Efficacy of antifungal therapy in a nonneutropenic murine model. *Antimicrob Agents Chemother* 2002;44:1953–1959.

42. Grant SM, Clissold SP. Itraconazole—a review of its pharmacodynamic and pharmacokinetic properties, and therapeutic use in superficial and systemic mycoses. *Drugs* 1989;37:310.

43. Meyers BR. Pulmonary mucormycosis. In: Braude AI, Davis CE, Fierer J, eds. *Infectious diseases and medical microbiology*, 2nd ed. Philadelphia: WB Saunders, 1986:875–877.

44. Baker RD. Pulmonary mucormycosis. *Am J Pathol* 1956;32:287.

45. Meyer R, Kaplan M, Ong M. Cutaneous lesions in disseminated mucormycosis. *JAMA* 1973;225:737.

46. Murray HW. Pulmonary mucormycosis with massive fatal hemoptysis. *Chest* 1975;68:65.

47. Temeck BK, Benzon DJ, Moskaluk CA, et al. Thoracotomy for pulmonary mycoses in non-HIV immunosuppressed patients. *Ann Thorac Surg* 1994;58:333.

48. Gribetz AR, Chuang MT, Burrows L, et al. *Rhizopus* lung abscess in renal transplant patient successfully treated by lobectomy. *Chest* 1980;77:102.

49. Calle S, Klatsky S. Interstitial phycomycosis (mucormycosis). *Am J Clin Pathol* 1966;45:264.

50. Reimund E, Ramos A. Disseminated neonatal gastrointestinal mucormycosis: a case report and review of the literature. *Pediatr Pathol* 1944;14:385.

51. Knoop C, Antoine M, Vachiery JL, et al. Gastric perforation due to mucormycosis after heart-lung and heart transplantation. *Transplant* 1996;10:170.

52. De Oliveira P, Milech A. A fatal case of gastric mucormycosis and diabetic ketoacidosis. *Endocr Pract* 2002;8:44–46.

53. Bruk HM, Nash G, Foley FD, et al. Opportunistic fungal infection of the burn wound with *Phycomycetes* and *Aspergillus*. *Arch Surg* 1971;102:476.

54. Paparello SF, Parry RL, MacGillivray DC, et al. Hospital-acquired wound mucormycosis. *Clin Infect Dis* 1992;14:350.

55. Adam RD, Hunter G, DiTomasso J, et al. Mucormycosis: emerging prominence of cutaneous infections. *Clin Infect Dis* 1994;19:67–76.

56. Johnson PC, Satter White RK, Monheit JE, et al. Primary cutaneous mucormycosis in trauma patients. *J Trauma* 1987;27:437.

57. Vainrub B, Macarsno A, Mander S, et al. Wound zygomycosis (mucormycosis) in otherwise healthy adults. *Am J Med* 1988;84:546.

58. Green JF, Dhaliwal AS. Cutaneous mucormycosis. *Infect Med* 1987;4:423.

59. Virmani R, Connor DH, McAllister HA. Cardiac mucormycosis. *Am J Clin Pathol* 1982;78:42.

60. Chaudhry R, Venugopal P, Chopra P. Prosthetic mitral valve mucormycosis caused by *Mucor* species. *Int J Cardiol* 1987;17:333.

61. Echols RM, Selinger DS, Hallowell C, et al. *Rhizopus* osteomyelitis: a case report and review. *Am J Med* 1979;66:141.

62. Mostaza JM, Barbado FJ, Fernandez-Martrin J, et al. Cutaneoarticular mucormycosis due to *Cunninghamella bertholletiae* in a patient with AIDS. *Rev Infect Dis* 1989;77:316.

63. Maliwan N, Reyes CV, Rippon JW. Osteomyelitis secondary to cutaneous mucormycosis. Report of a case and a review of the literature. *Am J Dermatol Pathol* 1984;6:479.

64. Pierce PF, Solomon SL, Kaufman L, et al. Zygomycetes brain abscesses in narcotic addicts with serological diagnosis. *JAMA* 1982;248:2881.

65. Freeman Woods K, Hanna BJ. Brain stem mucormycosis in a narcotic addict with eventual recovery. *Am J Med* 1986;80:126.

66. Stave GM, Heimberger T, Kerkering TM. Zygomycosis of the basal ganglia in intravenous drug users. *Am J Med* 1989;86:115.

67. Boelaret JR, Fenves AZ, Coburn JW. Mucormycosis among patients on dialysis. *N Engl J Med* 1989;321:190.

68. Boelaert JR, van Roost GF, Vergauwe PL, et al. The role of desferrioxamine in dialysis-associated mucormycosis: report of three cases and review of the literature. *Clin Nephrol* 1988;29:261.

69. Murray MJ, Murray AB. Adverse effect of iron repletion on infection. *Am J Clin Nutr* 1978;31:700 (abstr).

70. Robins-Browne RM, Prpic JK. Effects of iron and desferrioxamine on infections with *Yersinia enterocolitica*. *Infect Immun* 1985;47:774.

CHAPTER 276
Miscellaneous Fungi

Alan M. Sugar

As experience with immunocompromised and seriously ill hospitalized patients has grown, so has appreciation of the importance of "unusual" fungi in the cause of human disease. Although many "saprophytic" fungi are not described in medical textbooks or journals, the recovery of such microorganisms from clinical specimens must be considered important in the appropriate clinical situation. The patients at greatest risk of developing such infections are those with the most seriously impaired immune systems. The importance of the neutrophil in protection against invasion from these organisms with low virulence is clear, and the role of high doses of corticosteroids in predisposing toward the development of these infections is appreciated. The introduction of monoclonal antibodies such as infliximab has been associated with the development of progressive infections, and as the use of such cytokine inhibition increases, the number and nature of invasive fungal in these patients will no doubt increase as well. Only some of medically important fungi are reviewed here. An encyclopedic reference source is available for the interested reader and for the clinician confronted with a patient infected with one of the rarely recovered fungi (1). Consultation with physicians expert in the diagnosis and management of fungal diseases is encouraged when the less common fungi are found to be involved in the clinical setting.

FUSARIUM SPECIES

These molds are well-known plant pathogens, living in soil worldwide. Although now being encountered more often as agents of invasive infections, *Fusarium* species have been appreciated as rather common etiologic agents recovered from patients with fungal keratitis, mycetoma, and onychomycosis. The following species have been recovered from invasive infection:

Fusarium moniliforme
Fusarium proliferatum
Fusarium oxysporum
Fusarium solani
Fusarium napiforme

Given their widespread distribution in the environment, it is not surprising that the organism can be acquired through direct inoculation. This is the usual mode of transmission of infection in cases of corneal infection, endophthalmitis, continuous ambulatory peritoneal dialysis-associated peritonitis, localized skin disease, and nail infections (2,3). In the immunocompetent host, there is little risk of dissemination of the infection from the initial focus. However, in patients with neutropenia and rarely in those receiving large doses of corticosteroids, disseminated disease has been increasingly recognized (4–9).

Fusarium species grow in the environment and in tissue as molds. The characteristic microscopic appearance is that of narrow septate hyphae, with acute angle branching. By histopathologic criteria, they are indistinguishable from several other fungi, especially *Aspergillus* species. The hyphae are most easily visualized in tissue after staining with periodic acid–Schiff or Gomori methenamine silver.

In the laboratory, *Fusarium* grows rapidly on agar, but cycloheximide inhibits its growth. Mature colonies can produce various pigments depending on the species. The genus derives from the characteristic morphology of the fusiform conidia.

Invasive fusariosis is primarily a disease of neutropenic patients. Thus, patients with leukemia and those undergoing bone marrow transplantation are at greatest risk of developing this mycosis during the neutropenic phase of their therapy. Most often beginning as fever during the neutropenic episode, clinically evident fusariosis is most commonly seen as a pulmonary illness, often with cutaneous manifestations. Blood culture results are often positive in patients with fusariosis, in contrast to the negative blood culture results in patients with aspergillosis. The chest film may demonstrate infiltrates or nodules, but the lesions are best seen by computed tomography of the lungs and are often evident as multiple nodular lesions. Because the organism is acquired through the respiratory tract, it is not surprising to see patients with sinusitis caused by *Fusarium*. Recent evidence implicates the presence of *Fusarium* in water systems as an important predicate of infection in the hospitalized immunocompromised patient (10). Anaissie et al. (10) have demonstrated that various *Fusarium* species can be recovered from hospital water systems and that the fungi can be isolated from shower heads. In addition, the fungi could be aerosolized during use of the shower head. Completing the story is the matching of molecular biotypes of *Fusarium* from patients with those found in the water supply system (10).

Many of the clinical and histopathologic manifestations of fusariosis overlap those of aspergillosis. Given the different antifungal susceptibility patterns of *Aspergillus* and *Fusarium* species, this distinction may be of great clinical utility. However, some features tend to favor one organism over the other. For example, positive blood culture results are distinctly uncommon in patients with aspergillosis but are common in patients with fusariosis (approximately 40%) (6). Skin lesions are also more commonly found in patients with fusarial infection, with up to 79% of such patients developing cutaneous manifestations of the infection (8).

Mortality of patients with invasive fusariosis is high, the causes likely being profound and continuing neutropenia combined with the relative lack of efficacy of amphotericin B (11). However, clinical experience with other antifungal drugs is limited, and some authors still recommend amphotericin B as the drug of first choice in treating disseminated fusariosis (8). Much of the mortality may be explained by the extremely immunocompromised nature of the patients with these infections and the lack of return of normal neutrophil counts. In such a setting, recovery would be exceptional and no antifungal drug can be expected to be efficacious. Liposomal amphotericin B has been reported to be active, perhaps because more amphotericin B can be administered to the patient (12–14). Until more evidence is available, initial therapy should be with amphotericin B. Given the poor results with conventional amphotericin B and that much higher doses of amphotericin B can be delivered with lipid formulations, high-dose amphotericin B therapy administered as either Abelcet (10 to 15 mg/kg per day) or AmBisome (15 to 20 mg/kg per day) could be tried. In addition, the use of other concomitant antifungals, especially an echinocandin such as caspofungin, should be considered. Use of newer azoles (voriconazole, posaconazole, ravuconazole) in combination with amphotericin B should not be routinely used because there is no information about whether this combination will be antagonistic as with the case of amphotericin B and itraconazole (15). The use of granulocyte-macrophage colony-stimulating factor (GM-CSF) or granulocyte colony-stimulating factor (G-CSF) may have some beneficial effects on outcome of treatment, but definitive recommendations can not yet be made. Single-agent therapy with the newer azoles might also be effective, but experience is quite limited.

PSEUDALLESCHERIA/SCEDOSPORIUM

Most recently known by the name *Pseudallescheria boydii*, this fungus is unique in medicine in that it is the sexual (perfect) stage that is most often recovered from human infections. The asexual (imperfect) stage is known as *Scedosporium apiospermum*. Other mycoses are typically caused by the asexual stages of the different fungi. To complicate matters further, the sexual stage of the fungus has been known by the now obsolete names of *Allescheria boydii* and *Petriellidium boydii* and the asexual stage was once called *Monosporium apiospermum*. An additional unique feature of these fungi is the innate resistance to amphotericin B and the need to treat disease with an azole derivative. Reports of various types of infection caused by *Pseudallescheria* and *Scedosporium* are found in the literature, often with no cross-reference to each other in the title of the paper 16-18 (Table 276.1). *Scedosporium prolificans (inflatum)* is the species of *Scedosporium* most commonly recovered from patients infected with this pathogenic fungus.

The disease in immunocompetent patients is largely confined to localized infection, usually initiated as a result of penetrating

---

TABLE 276.1. Pathogenic Species of Pseudallescheria/Scedosporium[a]

Pseudallescheria boydii (Allescheria boydii, Petriellidium boydii)
Scedosporium inflatum (Scedosporium prolificans)
Scedosporium apiospermum (Monosporium apiospermum)

[a]Names in parentheses are obsolete.

trauma. Involvement of the eyes, bones, joints, brain, and subcutaneous tissue has been reported (20–25). Several cases of endocarditis have been reported (26,27). Meningitis has also been reported (20,28,29). Sinusitis and pneumonitis, both as invasive processes and as ones characterized by the formation of fungus balls, resembling in many ways aspergillosis, both occur (30–32). Pulmonary infection typically occurs in patients with chronic obstructive pulmonary disease or other anatomic abnormalities of the lungs and their airways. The infection is marked by an extensive inflammatory response and tissue necrosis.

In immunocompromised patients, such as those with neutropenia and those who have been treated with high-dose corticosteroids, disseminated disease is the rule. The disease usually presents in these situations as fever, accompanied by pulmonary infiltrates, followed by extrapulmonary dissemination, usually to the brain or eye (33,34). As with *Aspergillus* species, vascular invasion occurs.

Infection caused by *Aspergillus* species or *Fusarium* species closely mimics the clinical presentations of infections caused by *Pseudallescheria*. Culture results of lesions are usually positive, but blood culture results are most often negative. The organism appears in tissue as septate hyphae, characterized by acute angle branching, much like *Aspergillus*. Growth in the laboratory occurs in several days, and colonies may progress from a whitish coloration to light or brownish gray. As for all molds, correct speciation is dependent on conidiation and evaluation of the morphology of those conidia and their associated structures.

Therapy for both forms of disease requires adequate surgical débridement whenever possible and the use of an antifungal drug. Because the experience with amphotericin B has been so poor, the azole derivatives have been used, including miconazole (22,35,36), ketoconazole (37,38), fluconazole (19), and itraconazole (39–41). Given the positive anecdotal experience in treating these infections with itraconazole, many experts favor this drug over the more difficult to administer miconazole and the more toxic ketoconazole. The role of the newer azoles, voriconazole, posaconazole, and ravuconazole, in the treatment of invasive infections caused by *Pseudallescheria* is not known, but the agents may be effective based on early work with these drugs. The drug of choice, however, is not known. Various combinations of amphotericin B, azoles, and cytokines have been used in scattered case reports, with no clear evidence for the best management strategy. Consultation with a medical mycologist is desirable to construct an initial treatment regimen and especially for patients not responding to therapy.

TRICHOSPORON

A member of the Cryptococcaceae family, *Trichosporon* species, is being increasingly recognized as a cause of invasive infection in immunocompromised patients, especially those with chemotherapy-induced neutropenia (42–45). Cases of endocarditis in immunocompetent patients (46,47) and of invasive disease in patients with organ transplants, trauma, or acquired immunodeficiency syndrome (AIDS) have also been reported (48–51). However, more commonly in the past, *Trichosporon* species have been recovered from superficial infections of the hair, known as *white piedra*. The principal species of *Trichosporon* recovered from patients with invasive disease is *Trichosporon asahii* formerly called *Trichosporon beigelii* or *Trichosporon cutaneum*. *Trichosporon mucoides* is less commonly recovered from patients with invasive trichosporonosis. Other members of the *Trichosporon* genus include *Trichosporon ovoides*, *Trichosporon inkin*, and *Trichosporon asteroides*. For the most part, these other *Trichosporon* species are recovered from superficial infections of the skin and hair.

Invasive trichosporonosis is characterized by onset during periods of severe neutropenia (absolute neutrophil count less than $100/mm^3$) or other significant immunosuppression. Skin lesions are relatively common, as are positive blood culture results. An interesting and usually helpful finding is the cross-reactivity of the latex agglutination test for cryptococcal antigen (52,53). A positive latex agglutination test result for cryptococcal antigen in a neutropenic patient almost always reflects infection with *Trichosporon* species and not with *Cryptococcus neoformans*.

Blastoschizomyces capitatus was once known as *Trichosporon capitatum* or *Geotrichum capitatum*. It can cause invasive disease in the immunocompromised patient, as well (54). Pulmonary infiltrates are more commonly seen with this organism than with the other two closely related organisms. Patients are usually severely immunosuppressed and therefore have a high mortality rate. Therapy with amphotericin B may be successful if the underlying predispositions can be reversed.

Successful treatment of disseminated trichosporonosis depends in large part on the recovery of an adequate neutrophil count, if neutropenia was an important predisposing condition for the development of this infection. Reports on the utility of amphotericin B in treating invasive trichosporonosis have not been encouraging, and some evidence suggests that azoles, such as fluconazole, might be more effective (55,56). Selection of the most appropriate antifungal drug depends on the clinical situation and should be made, if possible, in consultation with a physician who has experience in treating these types of infections. Based on limited experience in animal models, high-dose amphotericin B (as a lipid formulation) with or without fluconazole may sustain patients until neutrophils reconstitution can be occur (57,58).

MALASSEZIA

Malassezia furfur, also known as *Pityrosporum ovale*, is a lipophilic fungus, growing as a yeast. It is a normal inhabitant on human skin and is the etiologic agent of tinea versicolor. Folliculitis in patients with cancer (59) and seborrheic dermatitis in patients with AIDS are more invasive manifestations of cutaneous disease (60,61). Invasive disease is most commonly manifested as intravenous catheter–associated sepsis, and most cases are in children, especially neonates (62–65), but adults are not immune (63,66). Virtually all of the patients with this invasive form of infection are receiving parenteral lipids. *Malassezia pachydermatis* has also been associated with invasive infection (67).

Because *M. furfur* requires lipids for its growth, special media containing fatty acids must be used in the laboratory for the fungus to be recovered from clinical specimens. The polymerase chain reaction technique has been reported to be useful in documenting spread of the organism within an intensive care unit (68).

Treatment most often requires removal of the infected catheter and discontinuation of the lipid hyperalimentation. Antifungal drugs have not been demonstrated to be absolutely required in every case and an attempt to eliminate the predisposing factors for the infection should be considered the most important therapeutic step. However, in the extremely ill patient with manifestations of sepsis, treatment with amphotericin B would be prudent.

PENICILLIUM MARNEFFEI

This fungus is widely distributed in Southeast Asia, including Vietnam, Thailand, and southern China (69–72). It is most prominently recognized as an important agent of invasive mycosis in human immunodeficiency virus (HIV)–infected patients who have lived or traveled in that endemic area (73–79). As the epidemic of AIDS progresses unabated, the importance of penicilliosis as a cause of significant morbidity and mortality should not be underestimated. In addition to AIDS and other forms of immunocompromise, such as that induced by corticosteroid therapy, lymphoma predisposes to this infection.

The fungus is dimorphic, growing in the environment as a mold and in tissue as a yeastlike organism. In addition to humans, the bamboo rat and its surrounding underground living places have been found to harbor the fungus (70,80). In the yeast-like form, the fungus divides by fission, with the production of characteristic cross-walls, yielding a profile different from that of other more commonly seen fungi. In the laboratory, the fungus can be recognized by the production of a red pigment that surrounds the mold as it grows on agar (82).

The presentation of penicilliosis is that of a chronic infection with the development of fever and weight loss. Skin lesions, cough, and generalized malaise are also often present. On physical examination, the patient is often found to have involvement of multiple organ systems, including lungs (pneumonia), bones (osteolytic lesions), hepatosplenomegaly, diffuse lymphadenopathy, skin (papular or ulcerated lesions), and subcutaneous abscesses. Laboratory evaluation may reveal evidence of anemia or thrombocytopenia. Thus, nothing is pathognomonic of the disease, and appropriate diagnostic tests must be guided by the clinical presentation and the presence of a travel history to the endemic regions.

Diagnosis is made by positive culture of material taken from appropriate lesions, histopathologic examination, and serology (81–83). Preliminary criteria for interpretation of an indirect immunofluorescent antibody test have been proposed (82).

The disease usually responds to therapy. Amphotericin B and itraconazole seem to be the most active agents (84,85). As with other infections in HIV-infected persons, long-term suppressive therapy is thought to be necessary in patients who have had an initial response to antifungal therapy (85,86).

DEMATIACEOUS FUNGI

The fungi placed within this group contain melanin-like pigment in the cell walls of their hyphae, spores, or both. Classification of the organisms and the diseases they cause has generated considerable confusion, as is evident from the profusion of names by which clinical syndromes and the fungi are called. Ajello et al. (87) have proposed the term *phaeohyphomycosis* to cover all infections caused by hyphomycetes that grow in tissue as dark-walled hyphae. However, the definition has been extended over the years to include fungi in other classes. In addition, phaeohyphomycosis is a histopathologic designation and not one that is amenable to easy clinical description of a given disease. The suggestion made by Kwon-Chung and Bennett (88) (that the clinical syndrome followed by the causative organism is a better way to communicate information about these diseases) seems to be one that should be adapted. Many dematiaceous fungi have been recovered from human disease and the list continues to grow (Table 276.2).

The dematiaceous molds typically give rise to infections of the skin and subcutaneous tissues, paranasal sinuses, and central nervous system. Manifestations of the former syndrome are of a single abscess, which can grow quite large. This usually appears at a site of trauma. Sinus involvement presents with a chronic course of nasal congestion and symptoms that may be confused

TABLE 276.2. Some Dematiaceous Fungal Species Associated with Human Disease

Alternaria	*Exophiala*
Aureobasidium	*Exserohilum*
Cladosporium	*Fonsecaea*
Curvularia	*Phialophora*
Dactylaria	*Sarcinomyces*

with allergic sinusitis. The ethmoid sinus is most commonly involved. Facial pain develops, and examination of the sinuses is consistent with a mass filling the cavity. Systemic symptoms are absent. Evaluation with computed tomography or magnetic resonance imaging is useful in demonstrating the extent of the pathologic changes. Central nervous system involvement is usually manifested by the development of a brain abscess. Typical symptoms and signs reflect the anatomic location of the lesions.

For all types of phaeohyphomycosis, diagnosis depends on the visualization of the dark-walled hyphae in tissue and growth of the fungus from culture. The primary treatment has been surgical excision, but the supplemental use of itraconazole may be helpful (89). The most appropriate drug, dose, and duration of medical therapy are unknown.

RHINOSPORIDIUM

Rhinosporidium seeberi causes a localized infection of the mucous membranes (90). The infection is chronic, enlarging for months to years, forming a friable pedunculated polypoid lesion usually in the nose or conjunctiva. In tissue, the organism appears as a thick-walled cyst, from 10 to 200 μm in diameter. In the past, the organism had not been cultured, and confirmation of reports of successful *in vitro* propagation of the organism have not been forthcoming (91,92). However, in tissue culture, the life cycle of the organism can be maintained. The precise classification of this microorganism is in doubt, but it is thought to be a fungus, given the morphology observed in infected tissue. Although the disease is cosmopolitan, most patients have been from India and Sri Lanka. Therapy consists of surgical extirpation of the lesion.

PROTOTHECA

The true classification of this organism is not clear, but it is thought to be an achloric alga. However, most discussions of this organism and protothecosis, the resulting disease, are generally in the context of mycoses. *Prototheca wickerhamii* and *Prototheca zopfii* are the two species that have been recovered from humans with protothecosis. The organism lives in water and soil and causes a rare noncontagious disease, primarily affecting adults. Involvement of skin and soft tissue has been reported (93–96), as has olecranon bursitis (97). The disease has been noted to occur in HIV-infected patients (98,99). The typical skin lesions are papules or plaques, and ulcerations occur, but no systemic symptoms or signs of infection are noted. Diagnosis depends on visualizing the organism in tissue or isolating it in the microbiology laboratory. *Prototheca* species grow within 48 hours on Sabouraud's agar and other agars not containing cycloheximide. Treatment is accomplished by surgical excision of the lesion, if possible. Amphotericin B and tetracycline, alone or in combination, have also been used successfully in some of the reported cases.

REFERENCES

1. Kwon-Chung KJ, Bennett JE. *Medical mycology*. Philadelphia: Lea & Febiger, 1992.
2. Nelson PE, Dignani MC, Anaissie EJ. Taxonomy, biology, and clinical aspects of *Fusarium* species. *Clin Microbiol Rev* 1994;7:479–504.
3. Louie T, el Baba F, Shulman M, et al. Endogenous endophthalmitis due to *Fusarium*: case report and review. *Clin Infect Dis* 1994;18:585–588.
4. Anaissie E, Kantarjian H, Ro J, et al. The emerging role of *Fusarium* infections in patients with cancer. *Medicine (Baltimore)* 1988;67:77–83.
5. Robertson MJ, Socinski MA, Soiffer RJ, et al. Successful treatment of disseminated *Fusarium* infection after autologous bone marrow transplantation for acute myeloid leukemia. *Bone Marrow Transplant* 1991;8:143–145.
6. Rabodonirina M, Piens MA, Monier MF, et al. *Fusarium* infections in immuno-compromised patients: case reports and literature review. *Eur J Clin Microbiol Infect Dis* 1994;13:152–161.
7. Gais AS, Gudnason T, Giebink GS, et al. Disseminated infection with *Fusarium* in recipients of bone marrow transplants. *Rev Infect Dis* 1991;13:1077–1088.
8. Martino P, Gastaldi R, Raccah R, et al. Clinical patterns of *Fusarium* infections in immunocompromised patients. *J Infect* 1994;28[Suppl 1]:7–15.
9. Guarro J, Gen J. Opportunistic fusarial infections in humans. *Eur J Clin Microbiol Infect Dis* 1995;14:741–754.
10. Anaissie EJ, Kuchar RT, Rex JH, et al. Fusariosis associated with pathogenic *Fusarium* species colonization of a hospital water system: a new paradigm for the epidemiology of opportunistic mold infections. *Clin Infect Dis* 2001;33:11871–1878.
11. Anaissie EJ, Hachem R, Legrand C, et al. Lack of activity of amphotericin B in systemic murine fusarial infection. *J Infect Dis* 1992;165:1155–1157.
12. Viviani MA, Cofrancesco E, Boschetti C, et al. Eradication of *Fusarium* infection in a leukopenic patient treated with liposomal amphotericin B. *Mycoses* 1991;34:255–256.
13. Wolff MA, Ramphal R. Use of amphotericin B lipid complex for treatment of disseminated cutaneous *Fusarium* infection in a neutropenic patient. *Clin Infect Dis* 1995;20:1568–1569.
14. Ellis ME, Clink H, Younge D, et al. Successful combined surgical and medical treatment of *Fusarium* infection after bone marrow transplantation. *Scand J Infect Dis* 1994;26:225–258.
15. Sugar AM, Liu X-P. Interactions of itraconazole with amphotericin B in the treatment of murine invasive candidiasis. *J Infect Dis* 1998;177:1660–1663.
16. Hofman P, Saintpaul MC, Garitoussaint M, et al. Disseminated infection due to *Scedosporium apiospermum* in liver transplantations—a differential diagnosis with invasive aspergillosis. *Ann Pathol* 1993;13:332–335.
17. Hopwood V, Evans EGV, Matthews J, et al. *Scedosporium prolificans*, a multi-resistant fungus, from a UK AIDS patient. *J Infect* 1995;30:153–155.
18. Rabodonirina M, Paulus S, Thevenet F, et al. Disseminated *Scedosporium pro-lificans* (*S. inflatum*) infection after single-lung transplantation. *Clin Infect Dis* 1994;19:138–142.
19. Tapia M, Richard C, Baro J, et al. *Scedosporium inflatum* infection in immuno-compromised haematological patients. *Br J Haematol* 1994;87:212–214.
20. Garcia JA, Ingram CW, Granger D. Persistent neutrophilic meningitis due to *Pseudallescheria boydii*. *Rev Infect Dis* 1990;12:959–960.
21. Dellestable F, Kures L, Mainard D, et al. Fungal arthritis due to *Pseudallescheria boydii* (*Scedosporium apiospermum*). *J Rheumatol* 1994;21:766–768.
22. Dworzack DL, Clark RB, Borkowski WJ Jr, et al. *Pseudallescheria boydii* brain abscess: association with near-drowning and efficacy of high-dose, prolonged miconazole therapy in patients with multiple abscesses. *Medicine (Baltimore)* 1989;68:218–224.
23. Hung LH, Norwood LA. Osteomyelitis due to *Pseudallescheria boydii*. *South Med J* 86:231–234, 1993.
24. Bloom PA, Laidlaw DA, Easty DL, et al. Treatment failure in a case of fun-gal keratitis caused by *Pseudallescheria boydii*. *Br J Ophthalmol* 1992;76:367–368.
25. Salitan ML, Lawson W, Som PM, et al. *Pseudallescheria* sinusitis with intracra-nial extension in a nonimmunocompromised host. *Otolaryngol Head Neck Surg* 1990;102:745–750.
26. Welty FK, McLeod GX, Ezratty C, et al. *Pseudallescheria boydii* endocarditis of the pulmonic valve in a liver transplant recipient. *Clin Infect Dis* 1992;1.5:858–860.
27. Raffanti SP, Fyfe B, Carreiro S, et al. Native valve endocarditis due to *Pseu-dallescheria boydii* in a patient with AIDS: case report and review. *Rev Infect Dis* 1990;12:993–996.
28. Peacock JE Jr. Persistent neutrophilic meningitis. *Infect Dis Clin North Am* 1990;4:747–767.
29. Huang HJ, Zhu JY, Zhang YH. The first case of *Pseudallescheria boydii* meningitis in China—electron microscopic study and antigenicity analysis of the agent. *J Tongji Medical Univ* 1990;10:218–221.
30. Watters GW, Milford CA. Isolated sphenoid sinusitis due to *Pseudallescheria boydii*. *J Laryngol Otol* 1993;107:344–346.
31. Hung CC, Chang SC, Yang PC, et al. Invasive pulmonary pseudallescheriasis with direct invasion of the thoracic spine in an immunocompetent patient. *Eur J Clin Microbiol Infect Dis* 1994;13:749–751.
32. Severo LC, Kaemmerer A, Camargo JJ, et al. Actinomycotic intracavitary lung colonization. *Mycopathologia* 1989;108:1–4.
33. Berenguer J, Diaz-Mediavilla J, Urra D, et al. Central nervous system infec-tion caused by *Pseudallescheria boydii*: case report and review. *Rev Infect Dis* 1989;11:890–896.
34. Caya JG, Farmer SG, Williams GA, et al. Bilateral *Pseudallescheria boydii* endoph-thalmitis in an immunocompromised patient. *Wis Med J* 1988;87:11–14.
35. Collignon PJ, Macleod C, Packham DR. Miconazole therapy in *Pseudallescheria boydii* infection. *Australas J Dermatol* 1985;26:129–132.
36. Grigg AP, Phillips P, Durham S, et al. Recurrent *Pseudallescheria boydii* sinusitis in acute leukemia. *Scand J Infect Dis* 1993;25:263–267.
37. Pluss JL, Opal SM. An additional case of pulmonary *Pseudallescheria boydii* improved with ketoconazole therapy. *Chest* 1985;87:843.
38. Galgiani JN, Stevens DA, Graybill JR, et al. *Pseudallescheria boydii* infections treated with ketoconazole. Clinical evaluations of seven patients and *in vitro* susceptibility results. *Chest* 1984;86:219–224.
39. Goldberg SL, Geha DJ, Marshall WF, et al. Successful treatment of simultane-ous pulmonary *Pseudallescheria boydii* and *Aspergillus terreus* infection with oral itraconazole. *Clin Infect Dis* 1993;16:803–805.
40. Walsh M, White L, Atkinson K, et al. Fungal *Pseudallescheria boydii* lung infil-trates unresponsive to amphotericin B in leukaemic patients. *Aust N Z J Med* 1992;22:265–268.
41. Nomdedeu J, Brunet S, Martino R, et al. Successful treatment of pneumonia due to *Scedosporium apiospermum* with itraconazole: case report. *Clin Infect Dis* 1993;16:731–733.
42. Gueho E, Improvisi L, de Hoog GS, et al. *Trichosporon* on humans: a practical account. *Mycoses* 1994;37:3–10.
43. Naum S, Petursson SR, Weinbaum D, et al. Long-term survival after allogenic bone marrow transplantation complicated by trichosporonosis. *South Med J* 1994;87:286–287.
44. Grauer ME, Bokemeyer C, Bautsch W, et al. Successful treatment of a *Tri-chosporon beigelii* septicemia in a granulocytopenic patient with amphotericin B and granulocyte colony-stimulating factor. *Infection* 1994;22:283–286.
45. Pierard GE, Read D, Pierard-Franchimont C, et al. Cutaneous manifestations in systemic trichosporonosis. *Clin Exp Dermatol* 1992;17:79–82.
46. Sidarous MG, O'Reilly MV, Cherubin CE. A case of *Trichosporon beigelii* en-docarditis 8 years after aortic valve replacement. *Clin Cardiol* 1994;17:215–219.
47. Miralles A, Quiroga J, Farinola T, et al. Recurrent *Trichosporon beigelii* endocardi-tis after aortic valve replacement. *Cardiovasc Surg* 1994;2:119–223.
48. Mirza SH. Disseminated *Trichosporon beigelii* infection causing skin lesions in a renal transplant patient. *J Infect* 1993;27:67–70.
49. Ness MJ, Markin RS, Wood RP, et al. Disseminated *Trichosporon beigelii* infection after orthotopic liver transplantation. *Am J Clin Pathol* 1989;92:119–123.
50. Miro O, Sacanella E, Nadal P, et al. *Trichosporon beigelii* fungemia and metastatic pneumonia in a trauma patient. *Eur J Microbiol Infect Dis* 1994;13:604–606.
51. Nahass GT, Rosenberg SP, Leonardi CL, et al. Disseminated infection with *Trichosporon beigelii*. Report of a case and review of the cutaneous and histologic manifestations. *Arch Dermatol* 1993;129:1020–1023.
52. McManus EJ, Jones JM. Detection of a *Trichosporon beigelii* antigen cross-reactive with *Cryptococcus neoformans* capsular polysaccharide in serum from a pa-tient with disseminated *Trichosporon* infection. *J Clin Microbiol* 1985;21:681–685.
53. Melcher GP, Reed KD, Rinaldi MG, et al. Demonstration of a cell wall antigen cross-reacting with cryptococcal polysaccharide in experimental disseminated trichosporonosis. *J Clin Microbiol* 1991;29:192–196.
54. Martino P, Venditti M, Micozzi A, et al. *Blastoschizomyces capitatus*: an emerging cause of invasive fungal disease in leukemia patients. *Rev Infect Dis* 1990;12:570–582.
55. Walsh TJ, Melcher GP, Rinaldi MG, et al. *Trichosporon beigelii*, an emerging pathogen resistant to amphotericin B. *J Clin Microbiol* 1990;28:1616–1622.
56. Anaissie E, Goaslan A, Hachem R, et al. Azole therapy for trichosporonosis: clinical evaluation of eight patients, experimental therapy for murine infection, and review. *Clin Infect Dis* 1992;45:781–787.
57. Anaissie EJ, Hachem R, Karyotakis NC, et al. Comparative efficacies of ampho-tericin B, triazole, and combination of both as experimental therapy for murine trichosporonosis. *Antimicrob Agents Chemother* 1994;38:2541–2544.
58. Kamberi P, Atsuro H, Taskayoshi T, et al. Efficacy of amphotericin B and azoles alone and in combination against disseminated trichosporonosis in neutropenic mice. *Chemotherapy* 1998;44:55–62.
59. Sandin RL, Fang TT, Hiemenz JW, et al. *Malassezia furfur* folliculitis in cancer patients. The need for interaction of microbiologist, surgical pathologist, and clinician in facilitating diagnosis by the clinical microbiology laboratory. *Ann Clin Lab Sci* 1993;23:377–384.
60. Groisser D, Bottone EJ, Lebwohl M. Association of *Pityrosporum orbiculare* (*Malassezia furfur*) with seborrheic dermatitis in patients with acquired immun-odeficiency syndrome (AIDS). *J Am Acad Dermatol* 1989;20:770–773.
61. Ross S, Richardson MD, Graybill JR. Association between *Malassezia furfur* col-onization and seborrheic dermatitis in AIDS patients. *Mycoses* 1994;37:367–370.
62. Sizun J, Karangwa A, Giroux JD, et al. *Malassezia furfur*–related colonization and infection of central venous catheters. A prospective study in a pediatric intensive care unit. *Intensive Care Med* 1994;20:496–499.
63. Barber GR, Brown AE, Kiehn TE, et al. Catheter-related *Malassezia furfur* fungemia in immunocompromised patients. *Am J Med* 1993;95:365–370.
64. Marcon MJ, Powell DA. Human infections due to *Malassezia* spp. *Clin Microbiol Rev* 1992;5:101–191.

65. Weiss SJ, Schoch PE, Cunha BA. *Malassezia furfur* fungemia associated with central venous catheter lipid emulsion infusion. *Heart Lung* 1991;20:87–90.

66. Athar MA, Stafford L. *Malassezia furfur* fungemia: a case report. *Can J Infect Control* 1993;8:63–64.

67. Welbel SF, McNeil MM, Pramanik A, et al. Nosocomial *Malassezia pachydermatis* bloodstream infections in a neonatal intensive care unit. *Pediatr Infect Dis J* 1994;13:104–108.

68. van Belkum A, Boekhout T, Bosboom R. Monitoring spread of *Malassezia* infections in a neonatal intensive care unit by PCR-mediated genetic typing. *J Clin Microbiol* 1994;32:2528–2532.

69. Deng Z, Ribas JL, Gibson DW, et al. Infections caused by *Penicillium marneffei* in China and Southeast Asia: review of eighteen published cases and report of four more Chinese cases. *Rev Infect Dis* 1988;10:640–652.

70. Deng ZL, Yun M, Ajello L. Human penicilliosis marneffei and its relation to the bamboo rat (*Rhizomys pruinosus*). *J Med Vet Mycol* 1986;24:383–389.

71. Jayanetra P, Nitiyanant P, Ajello L, et al. Penicilliosis marneffei in Thailand: report of five human cases. *Am J Trop Med Hyg* 1984;33:637–644.

72. Imwidthaya P. Update of penicilliosis marneffei in Thailand. Review article. *Mycopathologia* 1994;127:135–137.

73. Piehl MR, Kaplan RL, Haber MH. Disseminated penicilliosis in a patient with acquired immunodeficiency syndrome. *Arch Pathol Lab Med* 1988;112:1262–1264.

74. Rokiah I, Ng KP, Soo-Hoo TS. *Penicillium marneffei* infection in an AIDS patient—a first case report from Malaysia. *Med J Malaysia* 1995;50:101–104.

75. Wong KH, Lee SS, Lo YC, et al. Profile of opportunistic infections among HIV-1 infected people in Hong Kong. *Chung Hua I Hsueh Tsa Chih* 1995;55:127–136.

76. Borradori L, Schmit JC, Stetzkowski M, et al. Penicilliosis marneffei infection in AIDS. *J Am Acad Dermatol* 1994;31:843–836.

77. Sirisanthana V, Sirisanthana T. *Penicillium marneffei* infection in children infected with human immunodeficiency virus. *Pediatr Infect Dis* 1993;12:1021–1025.

78. Hilmarsdottir I, Meynard JL, Rogeaux O, et al. Disseminated *Penicillium marneffei* infection associated with human immunodeficiency virus: a report of two cases and a review of 35 published cases. *J Acquir Immune Defic Syndr* 1993;6:466–471.

79. Chiewchanvit S, Mahanupab P, Hirunsri P, et al. Cutaneous manifestations of disseminated *Penicillium marneffei* mycosis in five HIV-infected patients. *Mycoses* 1991;34:245–249.

80. Li JC, Pan LQ, Wu SX. Mycologic investigation on *Rhizomys pruinous senex* in Guangxi as natural carrier with *Penicillium marneffei*. *Chin Med J* 1989;102:477–485.

81. Deng ZL, Connor DH. Progressive disseminated penicilliosis caused by *Penicillium marneffei*. Report of eight cases and differentiation of the causative organism from *Histoplasma capsulatum*. *Am J Clin Pathol* 1985;84:323–327.

82. Yuen KY, Wong SS, Tsang DN, et al. Serodiagnosis of *Penicillium marneffei* infection. *Lancet* 1994;344:444–445.

83. Supparatpinyo K, Sirisanthana T. Disseminated *Penicillium marneffei* infection diagnosed on examination of a peripheral blood smear of a patient with human immunodeficiency virus infection. *Clin Infect Dis* 1994;18:246–247.

84. Supparatpinyo K, Khamwan C, Baosoung V, et al. Disseminated *Penicillium marneffei* infection in southeast Asia. *Lancet* 1994;344:110–113.

85. Supparatpinyo K, Chiewchanvit S, Hirunsri P, et al. An efficacy study of itraconazole in the treatment of *Penicillium marneffei* infection. *J Med Assoc Thail* 1992;75:688–691.

86. Supparatpinyo K, Nelson KE, Merz WG, et al. Response to antifungal therapy by human immunodeficiency virus–infected patients with disseminated *Penicillium marneffei* infections and *in vitro* susceptibilities of isolates from clinical specimens. *Antimicrob Agents Chemother* 1993;37:2407–2411.

87. Ajello L, Georg LK, Steigbigel RT, et al. A case of phaeohyphomycosis caused by a new species of *Phialophora*. *Mycologia* 1974;66:490–498.

88. Kwon-Chung KJ, Bennett JE. *Medical mycology*. Philadelphia: Lea & Febiger, 1992:620–677.

89. Sharkey PK, Graybill JR, Rinaldi MG, et al. Itraconazole treatment of phaeohyphomycosis. *J Am Acad Dermatol* 1990;23:577–586.

90. Thianprasit M, Thagerngpol K. Rhinosporidiosis. *Curr Top Med Mycol* 1989;3:64–85.

91. Levy MG, Meuten DJ, Breitschwerdt EB. Cultivation of *Rhinosporidium seeberi* in vitro: interaction with epithelial cells. *Science* 1986;234:474–476.

92. Krishnamoorthy S, Sreedharan VP, Koshy P, et al. Culture of *Rhinosporidium seeberi*: preliminary report. *J Laryngol Otol* 1989;103:178–180.

93. McAnally T, Parry EL. Cutaneous protothecosis presenting as recurrent chromomycosis. *Arch Dermatol* 1985;121:1066–1069.

94. Goldstein GD, Bhatia P, Kalivas J. Herpetiform protothecosis. *Int J Dermatol* 1986;25:54–55.

95. Nelson AM, Neafie RC, Connor DH. Cutaneous protothecosis and chlorellosis, extraordinary "aquatic-borne" algal infections. *Clin Dermatol* 1987;5:76–87.

96. Modly CE, Burnett JW. Cutaneous algal infections: Protothecosis and chlorellosis. *Cutis* 1989;44:23–24.

97. Demontclos M, Chatte G, Perrinfayolle M, et al. Olecranon bursitis due to *Prototheca wickerhamii*, an algal opportunistic pathogen. *Eur J Clin Microbiol Infect Dis* 1995;14:561–562.

98. Laeng RH, Egger C, Schaffner T, et al. Protothecosis in an HIV-positive patient. *Am J Surg Pathol* 1994;18:1261–1264.

99. Woolrich A, Koestenblatt E, Don P, et al. Cutaneous protothecosis and AIDS. *J Am Acad Dermatol* 1994;31:920–924.

XI

Parasites

Protozoa

CHAPTER 277

Entamoeba histolytica *and Other Intestinal Amebae*

Sharon L. Reed

HISTORY

Dysentery was first well described by Hippocrates, but it was not until 1875 that Losch carefully noted motile trophozoites in the stool of a Russian farmer. He fulfilled Koch's postulates by reproducing dysentery in a dog fed the infected stool and detecting similar parasites in submucosal ulcers at autopsy of the dog and the patient (1). Koch first reported amebic liver abscesses in 1833. The name *Entamoeba histolytica* was coined by Dobell in his 1919 monograph entitled, *The Amoebae Living in Man.* Infection with *Entamoeba* continues to be a public health problem in both developed and developing countries.

CHARACTERISTICS OF THE PATHOGEN

Infection is acquired by the ingestion of environmentally resistant cysts, most often from infected food or water. Cysts of *E. histolytica* range in size from 10 to 20 μm and are characterized by four nuclei with a distinct, central nucleolus. The chitinous cell wall of cysts contributes to their ability to remain viable for up to 1 month in moist conditions (2). Motile trophozoites, which are released from the cysts after exposure to stomach acid, colonize the large intestine. In most patients, infection is asymptomatic, and the trophozoites remain in the bowel and later encyst and complete the life cycle. In few infected patients, trophozoites either invade the bowel locally causing amebic dysentery or enter the bloodstream to cause distant abscesses, particularly of the liver.

EPIDEMIOLOGY

Up to 10% of the world's population is infected with *Entamoeba*, resulting in a morbidity second only to malaria and schistosomiasis (3). Infection is usually spread by fecal-oral transmission of infectious cysts. Although other primates can harbor *E. histolytica*, humans are the primary reservoir of infection, and asymptomatic carriers can excrete up to 15 million cysts per day (2). Recent immigrants, institutionalized patients, and homosexuals are all at higher risk for amebiasis. Clinicians in developed countries should be aware of atypical mechanisms of transmission, including colonic irrigation (4) and imported water (5).

E. histolytica infection can cause either asymptomatic infection or a wide spectrum of clinical disease. Recent studies support the separation of *Entamoeba* into two distinct species: *E. histolytica*, which is capable of invasion, and *Entamoeba dispar*, which is not (6). The cysts of *E. histolytica* and *E. dispar* are identical, making interpretation of early epidemiological studies difficult. Although some surveys reported up to 30% of stool specimens in homosexuals were positive for *E. histolytica* (7), subsequent studies that differentiated *Entamoeba* by isoenzyme analysis found that all harbored *E. dispar* and remained free of invasive amebiasis (8). If untreated, these patients spontaneously cleared the parasite (8,9). These data suggested that *E. dispar* does not cause morbidity, even in patients with acquired immunodeficiency syndrome (AIDS). Thus, *Entamoeba* cysts detected in the stool of a symptomatic patient with AIDS cannot be assumed to be the cause of diarrhea. In longitudinal studies of asymptomatic carriers of *E. histolytica*, only 10% developed invasive amebiasis within 1 year (10). More accurate determinations of the true prevalence of *E. histolytica* and *E. dispar* infection will now be possible with better serologic testing and specific stool antigen-detection tests, which can differentiate *E. histolytica* from *E. dispar* (11).

PATHOGENESIS

Successful invasion by *E. histolytica* trophozoites requires multiple steps, including attachment, degradation of the extracellular matrix to allow bowel invasion, killing of host cells, and evasion of local and systemic immunity. To initiate symptomatic infection, trophozoites within the bowel lumen must penetrate the mucous layer and adhere to the intestinal epithelium. A galactosamine (GalNac) adherence lectin is critical for attachment to colonic mucins, bacteria, and host epithelial cells (12,13), and immunization with the purified lectin has protected gerbils from the development of liver abscesses (14).

The earliest pathologic changes of invasive amebiasis have been best characterized in rodent models where epithelial cells undergo marked microvilli shortening and apical separation before direct contact with trophozoites (15,16). Dissolution of the extracellular matrix is most likely mediated by extracellular cysteine proteinases, enzymes that degrade collagen, laminin, and extracellular matrix macromolecules (17). Clinical isolates from patients with invasive amebiasis release significantly more cysteine proteinase activity, and patients with clinical amebiasis develop an antibody response to the amebic cysteine proteinase, demonstrating that it is released during the course of human infection (18). Cysteine proteinases are encoded by at least seven genes, several of which are present only in *E. histolytica* (19,20). Inhibition of cysteine proteinases in *E. histolytica* trophozoites with inhibitors or antisense prevented or significantly inhibited invasion in human intestinal xenografts (21) or amebic liver abscess formation in mice with severe combined immunodeficiency (22).

After apical separation of epithelial cells, trophozoites can penetrate the interglandular epithelium, erode through the lamina propria, and extend laterally under epithelium that appears normal to produce the classic flask-shaped ulcer (23). Trophozoites are usually detected by standard hematoxylin-eosin (H&E) staining of tissues at the periphery of necrotic tissue. The bright pink staining with periodic acid–Schiff (PAS) stain helps to differentiate trophozoites from phagocytic cells (23) (Fig. 277.1). In amebic liver abscesses, the liver parenchyma is replaced by necrotic debris with few inflammatory cells. Trophozoites are usually detectable only near the capsule.

Although well-established intestinal lesions and amebic liver abscesses are notable for the paucity of acute inflammatory cells, results of experimental animal infection suggest that an early neutrophil infiltrate occurs in both the intestine and the liver (15,24,25). The initial signal to inflammatory cells may be derived from both a direct effect of *E. histolytica* products on leukocyte migration (26) and the local release of chemokines. Coculture of trophozoites with human epithelial and stromal cell lines stimulates an array of potent chemoattractant and proinflammatory chemokines, including interleukin-8 (IL-8), GROα,

granulocyte-macrophage colony-stimulating factor, interleukin-1α (IL-1α), and interleukin-6 (IL-6) (27). When interleukin-1β (IL-1β) and IL-8 gene expression was blocked in intestinal cells by inhibition of the transcription factor, nuclear factor-κB, the local inflammatory response to *E. histolytica* invasion, was significantly decreased in human xenografts (28). Neutrophils may play a role in the first line of defense against acute *E. histolytica* infection. Nonactivated neutrophils are lysed by virulent *E. histolytica* trophozoites *in vitro* (29), but cytokine-activated neutrophils killed amebae (30).

To kill epithelial cells, *E. histolytica* trophozoites must adhere to target cells by the GalNac adherence lectin (31). Cell death can occur within seconds and is associated with increased intracellular calcium (32). Cytotoxicity may be mediated by pore-forming peptides (33), phospholipases (34), or hemolysins (35). *E. histolytica* may also kill cells by inducing apoptosis (36,37).

Once amebae penetrate the mucosa of the bowel, they encounter components of the complement system. To cause a liver abscess, trophozoites must survive invasion through the bloodstream. Indeed, studies of recent clinical isolates from patients with invasive disease revealed that they were resistant to complement-mediated lysis (38). Resistance is mediated in part by the GalNac lectin, which interferes with formation of the membrane attack complex (39). In contrast, *E. dispar* trophozoites are rapidly lysed by fluid-phase–activated components, limiting them to the bowel lumen (38).

The role of cell-mediated immunity in amebiasis is unclear. Activated macrophages kill trophozoites (40), and incubation of immune T cells with amebic antigen stimulates a cytotoxic T-cell response (29) *in vitro*. However, the T-cell–mediated response appears to be suppressed in patients with acute disease (41). Patients with AIDS do not have an increased incidence of severe amebiasis, which suggests that cell-mediated immunity is not critical in controlling initial invasion (42).

Serum antibodies do not appear to be protective, as recurrent invasive amebiasis is rare but does occur. More than 95% of patients with acute amebiasis develop antibodies with titers that correlate best with the length of illness (43). A recent prospective study of the mucosal immune response in amebiasis has revealed that the development of a stool immunoglobulin A (IgA) lectin-specific response protected against colonization with *E. histolytica* (44). Although specific stool IgA antibodies block attachment of trophozoites to epithelial cell monolayers (45), purified extracellular cysteine proteinases and whole parasites cleave secretory IgA (46) and immunoglobulin (IgG) (47) *in vitro*, potentially circumventing the host immune response.

CLINICAL MANIFESTATIONS

Intestinal Amebiasis

ASYMPTOMATIC CYST PASSERS

The most common patient with intestinal amebic infection is an asymptomatic cyst passer. Asymptomatic patients with no biopsy evidence of invasive disease spontaneously stop shedding within 5 months (48). In developed countries, homosexual patients are the highest risk group, although the incidence has dropped from a high of 30% to less than 8%, possibly reflecting safer sexual practices (49). Studies of 100 homosexual patients from London revealed that all patients were carriers of *E. dispar*, had negative amebic serologic test results, and had no histologic evidence of disease (8,50). It is important to identify the rare asymptomatic patient who is harboring *E. histolytica* however. When a group of these patients were followed for 1 year in Durban, South Africa, 10% developed amebic colitis

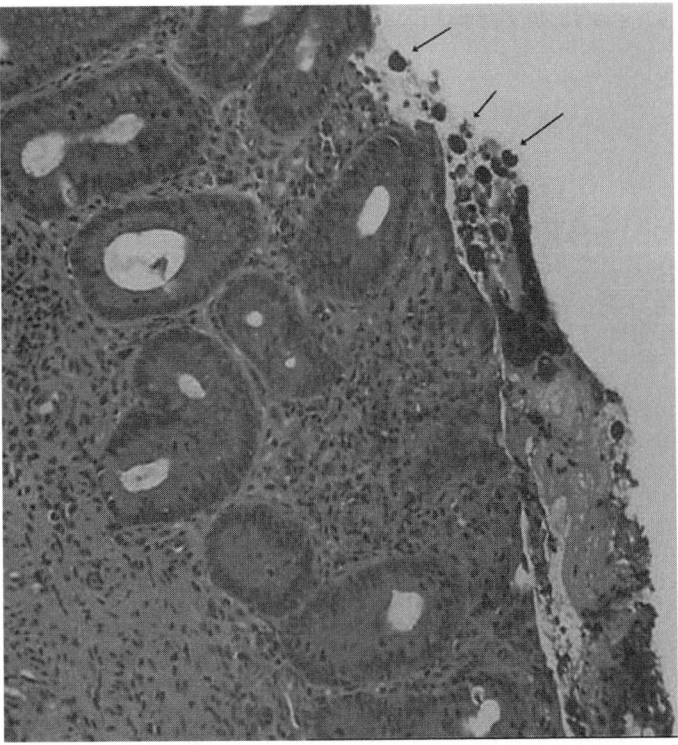

Figure 277.1. Pathology of amebic colitis. The section shows a necrotic ulcer in the large intestine with trophozoites (*arrows*) in the overlying mucus (periodic acid–Schiff stain, ×40).

(10). These patients represent a public health risk but can be identified by positive amebic serology (10) or stool antigen test results (11).

AMEBIC COLITIS

Patients with amebic colitis typically present with a gradual onset of abdominal pain and frequent, watery stools containing blood and mucus. Symptoms of diarrhea, tenesmus, and back pain may be present for 1 to 2 weeks before patients seek medical attention. In contrast to bacterial dysentery, fever is uncommon. More than 80% of patients complain of localized abdominal tenderness (51). Fulminant progression of amebic colitis, an unusual disease that occurs most often in children, is characterized by severe, bloody diarrhea and fever with rapid progression to acute abdominal tenderness (52). More than 60% may have colonic and transmural necrosis on pathologic specimens (53). Ameboma occurs in less than 1% of patients with invasive amebic intestinal disease (51). Although the clinical presentation of a patient with an abdominal mass and radiographic studies with "apple-core" lesions may mimic carcinoma (54), the diagnosis of ameboma can be made by serology and biopsy.

COMPLICATIONS

The most common complication from intestinal amebiasis is peritonitis, which may develop gradually (51). Hemorrhage and strictures of the anus or colon are less common (51). Direct spread of infection can cause perianal cutaneous amebiasis with painful ulcers mimicking squamous cell carcinoma (55).

DIFFERENTIAL DIAGNOSIS

Bacterial etiologies including *Shigella, Campylobacter, Salmonella, Vibrio,* and enteroinvasive *Entamoeba coli* must be ruled out in any patient presenting with dysentery. Lack of fever and paucity of fecal leukocytes are clues to amebiasis. Because amebic colitis may also mimic inflammatory bowel disease, it is particularly important to establish the correct diagnosis by serology or detection of antigen or trophozoites in stools as presumptive therapy with steroids may cause toxic megacolon (56).

Extraintestinal Amebiasis

AMEBIC LIVER ABSCESS

The most common complication of invasive amebiasis is amebic liver abscess (57,58). This condition can be challenging to diagnose because the symptoms may be nonspecific and develop months after leaving an endemic area. Most patients present with less than 10 days of fever and right upper quadrant pain, often radiating to the shoulder (43,59). A tender, enlarged liver is detected in 80% (59). Approximately 10% of patients have no abdominal findings and may present as fever of unknown origin (59). All patients with extraintestinal amebiasis have preceding intestinal infection, but fewer than 30% have active diarrhea at the time of presentation (59). The actual prevalence of asymptomatic colonization may be as high as 72% in these patients, however, when they are evaluated with amebic cultures (60). A smaller subset of patients have a subacute course, presenting with hepatomegaly, weight loss, and anemia of more than 2 weeks' duration.

PLEUROPULMONARY AMEBIASIS

The most common complication of amebic liver abscess is pleuropulmonary involvement, which occurs in 10% to 20% of patients (61). Half may have a small serous pleural effusion. Localized contiguous spread of an abscess into the pleural cavity usually responds to medical therapy alone. Hepatopleural fistula is a rare but dramatic event sometimes accompanied by cough productive of large amounts of necrotic material, which may contain trophozoites. Unless aspiration occurs, medical therapy alone usually elicits a good response. The sudden development of pain and respiratory distress may herald the formation of an empyema, which requires aggressive drainage.

PERITONEAL AMEBIASIS

The second most common complication of amebic liver abscess is rupture into the peritoneum, which occurs in 2% to 5% of patients (59). Because the contents of liver abscesses are sterile, the prognosis is much better than rupture of amebic colitis and the condition usually can be treated with percutaneous catheter drainage (62).

PERICARDIAL AMEBIASIS

The most serious complication of amebic liver abscess is rupture into the pericardium, with a mortality approaching 70% (63). More than two thirds of these patients have abscesses of the left lobe of the liver. Patients usually have a preceding serous effusion but may rapidly deteriorate from cardiac tamponade, even on medical therapy (59). Open drainage may be required because of the development of loculations.

CEREBRAL AMEBIASIS

Cerebral amebiasis is usually diagnosed at autopsy in 1% to 2% of patients in large series (59). Symptoms depend on the size and location of the lesion, but patients can die within 24 hours of cerebellar involvement. Because metronidazole penetrates well into the brain, the incidence of this complication is low.

GENITOURINARY AMEBIASIS

Renal amebiasis can result from rupture of a hepatic abscess, hematogenous spread from lesions in the liver, or extension through the lymphatics. Patients usually respond well to aspiration and medical therapy.

DIAGNOSIS

Microscopic Diagnosis

The identification of motile hematophagous trophozoites of *E. histolytica*, ideally in a wet mount of fresh stool sample or scrapings from the edge of a bowel ulcer, is key to the early diagnosis of amebic colitis. Trophozoites are rapidly killed by drying, water, urine, barium, and several antibiotics. The diagnosis of amebic colitis cannot be made by the presence of quadrinucleate cysts alone because cysts of *E. histolytica* and *E. dispar* are identical and must be reported as "*E. histolytica/dispar*." Additional testing by antigen detection or serology must be performed to identify patients infected with *E. histolytica*.

Stool Antigen Detection

The development of an *E. histolytica*–specific stool antigen test has been a major diagnostic advance. The assay is based on monoclonal antibodies, which recognize epitope differences in the GalNac lectin of *E. histolytica* and *E. dispar* (11). A number of clinical trials in Bangladesh have demonstrated more than 90% correlation with the sensitive but technically difficult tests of polymerase chain reaction (PCR) and culture with isoenzyme determination (64).

Serologic Tests

Amebic serology is very useful in the diagnosis of invasive amebiasis. The most commonly used tests, enzyme-linked immunosorbent assay (ELISA), indirect hemagglutination (IHA), and agar gel diffusion (AGD), are positive in more than 90% of patients with invasive amebiasis, including asymptomatic carriers of E. histolytica (10,65). Because the titer correlates with the duration of disease, up to 10% of patients presenting acutely with amebic liver abscess may have a negative serology, but follow-up studies should turn positive within 2 weeks (43). The diagnosis of acute amebiasis by IHA is problematic because titers can remain positive for years after successful treatment (65). In contrast, ELISA and AGD usually revert to negative within months, so a positive test result is almost always indicative of acute disease.

Radiographic Studies

Noninvasive radiographic studies are critical to the early diagnosis of amebic liver abscess. Ultrasounds typically show a round or oval hypoechoic area contiguous to the liver capsule with significant wall echoes (66). Computed tomography scans (Fig. 277.2) and magnetic resonance imaging scans are also very sensitive procedures for detection of amebic liver abscesses. More than 80% of patients with symptoms for more than 10 days have a single abscess of the right lobe. In contrast, up to half of patients who present acutely have multiple lesions that may require diagnostic aspiration to rule out a bacterial etiology. Imaging studies are useful to identify abscesses of the left lobe of the liver, which increase the risk of rupture into the pericardium. Frequent radiographic studies may be confusing in patients responding well to medical management, because abscesses may actually increase in size during the first 2 weeks (66). More than two thirds of patients will have a normal ultrasound within 6 months, but abnormalities may persist longer than 1 year in 10% (66). Barium studies are relatively contraindicated in the

diagnosis of acute amebic colitis because of the possibility of colonic perforation.

Laboratory Tests

Routine laboratory tests are rarely helpful in the diagnosis of acute amebiasis. More than three fourths of patients with amebic liver abscesses have white blood cell counts greater than 10,000 cells/mm³ (43). Eosinophilia is not associated with amebiasis. The level of alkaline phosphatase is elevated in more than 75% of patients with amebic liver abscess. Transaminases are elevated in less than 50% of patients with amebic liver abscesses, especially in those with acute disease or complications.

TREATMENT

The introduction of imidazoles has dramatically improved the therapy of invasive amebic disease. Metronidazole is well absorbed orally and can be given intravenously. Standard therapy for amebic colitis or liver abscess is 750 mg (10 mg/kg) three times a day for 5 to 10 days, although single-dose therapy of liver abscesses with 2 g of metronidazole, tinidazole, or ornidazole is effective in more than 80% of patients (Table 277.1). The main side effects of metronidazole are nausea, vomiting, and a disulfiram-like effect with alcohol. There is little role for older treatment modalities. Emetine and dehydroemetine have potential cardiovascular and gastrointestinal side effects, and higher relapse rates are associated with chloroquine. With early diagnosis and effective treatment, mortality from uncomplicated amebic liver abscesses has decreased to less than 1%.

Follow-up therapy with a luminal agent is important in all patients with invasive amebiasis because metronidazole is not effective against cysts. Only one luminal agent is available in the United States, paromomycin, although diloxanide furoate and iodoquinol are also quite effective (Table 277.1). Paromomycin is a nonabsorbable aminoglycoside that is active against both cysts and trophozoites (67). Iodoquinol is a halogenated hydroxyquinoline that must be given for a 20-day course. Diloxanide furoate, a substituted acetanilide, has been extensively used outside the United States. All have efficacy rates of 85% to 95% for the eradication of cyst passage. Although all 50 patients with liver abscesses in a South African study rapidly responded to metronidazole, 55% still had cysts in their stool, and 15% developed recurrent invasive disease (60).

Most patients respond dramatically to therapy with metronidazole, with resolution of their fever and abdominal pain within 72 hours (68). Percutaneous drainage should be considered in patients who remain symptomatic. Aspiration should also be performed to rule out a pyogenic abscess, particularly if multiple abscesses are present, for imminent rupture with lesions larger than 12 cm, and to decrease the risk of rupture of an abscess of the left lobe of the liver into the pericardium (69). Percutaneous drainage has proven so successful that open surgery is reserved for bowel perforation.

The two biggest dilemmas in the treatment of amebic infection involve the therapy of asymptomatic cyst passers (particularly in patients with AIDS) and pregnant women. If a patient is asymptomatic, has a negative serology, and the infecting strain can be identified as E. dispar, no treatment is necessary (8). The treatment of pregnant women is problematic because there is anecdotal evidence that invasive amebic disease is more severe, and the drug of choice, metronidazole, has potential teratogenic effects. One approach is careful follow-up of asymptomatic pregnant women

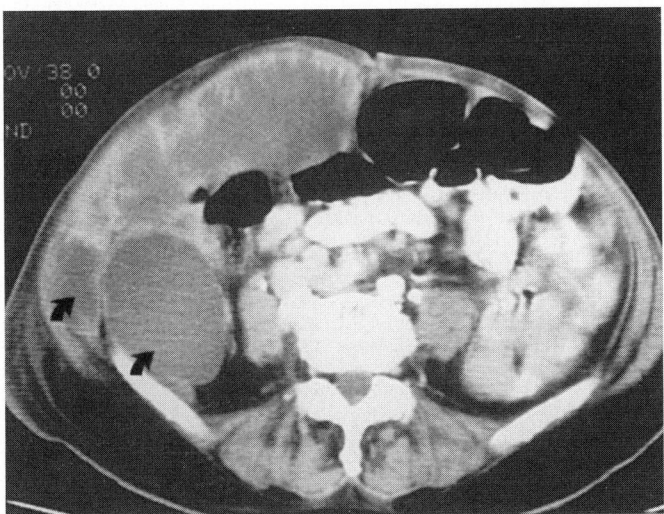

Figure 277.2. Computed tomographic scan of a patient with localized rupture of an amebic liver abscess (arrows). (Courtesy Department of Radiology, UCSD Medical Center.)

TABLE 277.1.   Treatment of Amebiasis

Syndrome	Adult dosage	Pediatric dosage
Asymptomatic cyst passer, luminal agent		
Paromomycin (250-mg tablets)	500 mg t.i.d. × 7 d	30 mg/kg/d in 3 doses × 7 d
Iodoquinol[a] (650-mg tablets)	650 mg t.i.d. × 20 d	20–40 mg/kg/d in 3 doses × 20 d
Diloxanide furoate[a] (500-mg tablets)	500 mg t.i.d. × 10 d	20 mg/kg/d in 3 doses × 10 d
Acute colitis		
Metronidazole (250- or 500-mg tablets)	750 mg t.i.d. × 5–10 d	30–50 mg/kg/d in 3 doses × 5–10 d
plus		
Luminal agent (above)		
Amebic liver abscess		
Metronidazole	750 mg t.i.d. i.v. or p.o. × 5–10 d	30–50 mg/kg/d in 3 doses × 5–10 d
Tinidazole[a]	2 g p.o.	
Ornidazole[a]	2 g p.o.	
plus		
Luminal agent (above)		

[a] Not available in the United States.
i.v., intravenously; p.o., per os; t.i.d., three times a day.

with negative serologies or proven *E. dispar* infections without therapy and reserve treatment with metronidazole for those with invasive disease. Others would treat all pregnant women with "mild to moderate" intestinal disease with paromomycin (70).

PREVENTION OF AMEBIASIS

Transmission of amebiasis could be completely prevented with adequate sanitation, which requires both adequate disposal of human feces and sterilization of water. Cysts are resistant to levels of chlorination used in standard water purification, but filtration and precipitation are effective. Because infected food handlers are a major source of transmission, health education and early treatment of cyst passers and patients with invasive disease is critical. There is no effective chemoprophylaxis for the individual traveler. Risk of infection can be minimized by avoiding unpeeled fruits and vegetables and by using bottled water. Cysts are killed by boiling and by iodination (71).

OTHER INTESTINAL AMEBAE

E. histolytica is the only intestinal ameba that causes human disease. The cysts must be differentiated from *Entamoeba coli*, which are larger (30 to 40 μm) and have up to eight nuclei with eccentric karyosomes. *Entamoeba hartmanni* is smaller (10 to 20 μm) and has a single nucleus. *Endolimax nana* contains a characteristic glycogen-containing vacuole. Infection by intestinal amebae other than *E. histolytica* does not warrant treatment.

REFERENCES

1. Kean BH. A history of amebiasis. In: Ravdin JI, ed. *Amebiasis: human infection by Entamoeba histolytica.* New York: John Wiley & Sons, 1988:1–10.
2. Walsh JA. Prevalence of *Entamoeba histolytica* infection. In: Ravdin JI, ed. *Amebiasis: human infection by Entamoeba histolytica.* New York: John Wiley & Sons, 1988:93–105.
3. Walsh JA. Problems in recognition and diagnosis of amebiasis: estimation of the global magnitude of morbidity and mortality. *Rev Infect Dis* 1986;8(2):228–238.
4. Amebiasis associated with colonic irrigation. *MMWR Morb Mortal Wkly Rep* 1981;30:101–102.
5. Reed SL, Davis CE, Jinich H. Amebiasis from the "miraculous water of Tlacote." *N Engl J Med* 1995;332:687–688.
6. WHO/Pan America Health Organization Expert Consultation on Amoebiasis: Amoebiasis. *WHO Wkly Epidemiol Rep* 1997;72:97–100.
7. William DC, Shookhoff HB, Felman YM, et al. High rates of enteric protozoal infections in selected homosexual men attending a venereal disease clinic. *Sex Transm Dis* 1978;5:155–157
8. Allason-Jones E, Mindel A, Sargeaunt PG, et al. Outcome of untreated infection with *Entamoeba histolytica* in homosexual men with and without HIV antibody. *Br Med J* 1988;297:654–657.
9. Reed SL, Wessel DW, Davis CE. *Entamoeba histolytica* infection and AIDS. *Am J Med* 1991;90:269–270.
10. Gathiram V, Jackson TFHG. A longitudinal study of asymptomatic carriers of pathogenic zymodemes of *Entamoeba histolytica. South Afr Med J* 1987;72:669–672.
11. Haque R, Neville L, Hahn P, et al. Rapid diagnosis of *Entamoeba* infection by using *Entamoeba* and *Entamoeba histolytica* stool antigen detection kits. *J Clin Microbiol* 1995;33:2558–2561.
12. Petri WA, Smith RD, Schlesinger PH, et al. Isolation of the galactose-binding lectin that mediates the in vitro adherence of *Entamoeba histolytica. J Clin Invest* 1987;80:1238–1244.
13. Chadee K, Petri WA, Innes DJ, et al. Rat and human colonic mucins bind to and inhibit adherence lectin of *Entamoeba histolytica. J Clin Invest* 1987;80:1245–1254.
14. Petri WA, Ravdin JI. Protection of gerbils from amebic liver abscess by immunization with the galactose-specific adherence lectin of *Entamoeba histolytica. Infect Immun* 1991;59:97–101.
15. Chadee K, Meerovitch E. The pathology of experimentally induced cecal amebiasis in gerbils (*Meriones unguiculatus*). *Am J Pathol* 1985;119(3):485–494.
16. Takeuchi A, Phillips BP. Electron microscope studies of experimental *Entamoeba histolytica* infections in the guinea pig. I. Penetration of the intestinal epithelium by trophozoites. *Am J Trop Med Hyg* 1975;24:34–48.
17. Keene WE, Pettit MG, Allen S, et al. The major neutral proteinase of *Entamoeba histolytica. J Exp Med* 1986;163:536–549.
18. Reed SL, Keene WE, McKerrow JH. Thiol proteinase expression correlates with pathogenicity of *Entamoeba histolytica. J Clin Microbiol* 1989;27:2772–2777.
19. Reed SL, Bouvier J, Pollack AS, et al. Cloning of a virulence factor of *Entamoeba histolytica*: pathogenic strains possess a unique cysteine proteinase gene. *J Clin Invest* 1993;91:1532–1540.
20. Bruchhaus I, Jacobs T, Leippe M, et al. *Entamoeba histolytica* and *Entamoeba dispar*: differences in numbers and expression of cysteine proteinase genes. *Mol Microbiol* 1996;22:255–263.
21. Zhang Z, Yan L, Wang L, et al. *Entamoeba histolytica* cysteine proteinases with interleukin-1 beta converting enzyme (ICE) activity cause intestinal inflammation and tissue damage in amoebiasis. *Mol Microbiol* 2000;37:5442–5548.
22. Stanley SL, Zhang T, Rubin D, et al. Role of the *Entamoeba histolytica* cysteine proteinase in amebic liver abscess formation in severe combined immunodeficient mice. *Infect Immun* 1995;63:1587–1589.
23. Joyce MP, Ravdin JI. Pathology of human amebiasis; In: Ravdin JI, ed. *Amebiasis: human infection by Entamoeba histolytica.* New York: John Wiley & Sons, 1988:129–146.

24. Brandt H, Perez-Tamayo R. Pathology of human amebiasis. *Hum Pathol* 1970;1:351–384.
25. Chadee K, Meerovitch E. The pathogenesis of experimentally induced amebic liver abscess in the gerbil (*Meriones unguiculatus*). *Am J Pathol* 1984;117:71–80.
26. Chadee K, Moreau F, Meerovitch E. *Entamoeba histolytica*: chemoattractant activity for gerbil neutrophils *in vivo* and *in vitro*. *Exp Parasitol* 1987;64:12–23.
27. Eckmann L, Reed SL, Smith JR, et al. *Entamoeba histolytica* trophozoites induce an inflammatory cytokine response by cultured human cells through the paracrine action of cytolytically released interleukin-1α. *J Clin Invest* 1995;95:55–65.
28. Seydel KB, Li E, Zhang Z, et al. Epithelial cell-initiated inflammation plays a crucial role in early tissue damage in amebic infection of human intestine. *Gastroenterology* 1998;115:1446–1453.
29. Salata RA, Martinez-Palomo A, Murphy CF, et al. Patients treated for amebic liver abscesses develop a cell-mediated immune response effective in vitro against *Entamoeba histolytica*. *J Immunol* 1986;136:2633–2639.
30. Denis M, Chadee K. Human neutrophils activated by Interferon-gamma and tumor necrosis factor-α kill *Entamoeba histolytica* trophozoites *in vitro*. *J Leukoc Biol* 1989;46:270–274.
31. McCoy JJ, Mann BJ, Petri WA. Adherence and cytotoxicity of *Entamoeba histolytica* or how lectins let parasites stick around. *Infect Immun* 1994;62:3045–3050.
32. Ravdin JI, Moreau F, Sullivan JA, et al. Relationship of free intracellular calcium to the cytolytic activity of *Entamoeba histolytica*. *Infect Immun* 1988;56:1505–1512.
33. Leippe M, Sebastian E, Schoenberger OL, et al. Pore-forming peptide of pathogenic *Entamoeba histolytica*. *Proc Natl Acad Science U S A* 1991;88:7659–7663.
34. Long-Krug SA, Fischer KJ, Hysmith RM, et al. Phospholipase A enzymes of *Entamoeba histolytica*: description and subcellular localization. *J Infect Dis* 1985;152:536–541.
35. Jansson A, Gillin F, Kagardt U, et al. Coding of hemolysins within the ribosomal RNA repeat on a plasmid in *Entamoeba histolytica*. *Science* 1994;263:1440–1443.
36. Ragland BD, Ashley LS, Vaux DL, et al. *Entamoeba histolytica*: target cells killed by trophozoites undergo apoptosis which is not blocked by bcl-2. *Exp Parasitol* 1994;79:460–467.
37. Seydel KB, Stanley SL. *Entamoeba histolytica* induces host cell death in amebic liver abscess by a non–Fas-dependent, non–tumor necrosis factor alpha–dependent pathway of apoptosis. *Infect Immun* 1998;66:2980–2983.
38. Reed SL, Gigli I. Lysis of complement-sensitive *Entamoeba histolytica* by activated terminal complement components. Initiation of complement activation by an extracellular neutral cysteine proteinase. *J Clin Invest* 1990;86:1815–1822.
39. Braga L, Ninomiya H, McCoy JJ, et al. Inhibition of the complement membrane attack complex by the galactose-specific adhesin of *Entamoeba histolytica*. *J Clin Invest* 1992;90:1131–1137.
40. Lin Y, Seguin R, Keller K, et al. Tumor necrosis factor alpha augments nitric oxide–dependent macrophage cytotoxicity against *Entamoeba histolytica* by enhanced expression of the nitric oxide synthase gene. *Infect Immun* 1994;62:1534–1541.
41. Salata RA, Martinez-Palomo A, Canales L, et al. Suppression of T-lymphocyte responses to *Entamoeba histolytica* antigen by immune sera. *Infect Immun* 1990;58:2941–3946.
42. Jessurun J, Barron-Rodriguez LP, Fernandez-Tinoco G, et al. The prevalence of invasive amebiasis is not increased in patients with AIDS. *AIDS* 1992;6:307–309.
43. Katzenstein D, Rickerson V, Braude AI. New concepts of amebic liver abscess derived from hepatic imaging, serodiagnosis, and hepatic enzymes in 67 consecutive cases in San Diego. *Medicine* 1982;61:237–246.
44. Haque R, Ali IM, Sack B, et al. Amebiasis and mucosal IgA antibody against the *Entamoeba histolytica* adherence lectin in Bangladeshi children. *J Infect Dis* 2001;183:1787–1793.
45. Carrero JC, Diaz MY, Viveros M, et al. Human secretory immunoglobulin A anti-*Entamoeba histolytica* antibodies inhibit adherence of amebae to MDCK cells. *Infect Immun* 1994;62:764–767.
46. Kelsall BL, Ravdin JI. Degradation of human immunoglobulin A by *Entamoeba histolytica*. *J Infect Dis* 1993;168:1319–1322.
47. Tran VQ, Herdman DS, Torian BE, et al. The neutral cysteine proteinase of *Entamoeba histolytica* degrades IgG and prevents its binding. *J Infect Dis* 1998;177:508–511.
48. Nanda R, Baveja U, Anand BS. *Entamoeba histolytica* cyst passers: clinical features and outcome in untreated subjects. *Lancet* 1984;2:301–303.
49. Sorvillo FJ, Lieb L, Mascola L, et al. Declining rates of amebiasis in Los Angeles County: a sentinel for decreasing acquired immunodeficiency syndrome (AIDS) incidence? *Am J Public Health* 1989;79:1563–1564.
50. Allason-Jones E, Mindel A, Sargeaunt PG, et al. *Entamoeba histolytica* as a commensal intestinal parasite in homosexual men. *N Engl J Med* 1986;315:353–356.
51. Adams EB, MacLeod IN. Invasive amebiasis. I. Amebic dysentery and its complications. *Medicine* 1977;56:315–323.
52. Fuchs G, Ruiz-Palacios G, Pickering LK. Amebiasis in the pediatric population. In: Ravdin JI, ed. *Amebiasis: human infection by Entamoeba histolytica*. New York: John Wiley & Sons, 1988:594–613.
53. Aristizabal H, Acevedo J, Botero M. Fulminant amebic colitis. *World J Surg* 1991;15:216–221.
54. Radke RA. Ameboma of the intestine: an analysis of the disease as presented in 78 collected and 41 previously unreported cases. *Ann Intern Med* 1955;43:1048–1066.
55. Mhlanga BR, Lanoie LO, Norris HJ, et al. Amebiasis complicating carcinomas: a diagnostic dilemma. *Am J Trop Med Hyg* 1992;759:764.
56. Patel AS, DeRidder PH. Amebic colitis masquerading as acute inflammatory bowel disease: the role of serology in its diagnosis. *J Clin Gastroenterol* 1989;11:407–410.
57. Reed SL. Amebiasis: an update. *Clin Infect Dis* 1992;14:385–393.
58. Petri WA, Singh U. Diagnosis and management of amebiasis. *Clin Infect Dis* 1999;29:1119–1125.
59. Adams EB, MacLeod IN. Invasive amebiasis. II. Amebic liver abscess and its complications. *Medicine* 1977;56:325–334.
60. Irusen EM, Jackson TFHG, Simjee AE. Asymptomatic intestinal colonization by pathogenic *Entamoeba histolytica* in amebic liver abscess: prevalence, response to therapy, and pathogenic potential. *Clin Infect Dis* 1992;14:889–893.
61. Ibarra-Perez C. Thoracic complications of amebic abscess of the liver. Report of 501 cases. *Chest* 1981;79:672–677.
62. Ken JG, vanSonnenberg E, Casola G, et al. Perforated amebic liver abscesses: successful percutaneous treatment. *Radiology* 1989;170:195–197.
63. Ibarra-Perez C, Green L, Calvillo-Juarez M, et al. Diagnosis and treatment of rupture of amebic abscess of the liver into the pericardium. *J Thorac Cardiovasc Surg* 1972;64:11–17.
64. Haque R, Ali IKM, Akther S, et al. Comparison of PCR, isoenzyme analysis, and antigen detection for diagnosis of *Entamoeba histolytica* infection. *J Clin Microbiol* 1998;36:449–452.
65. Healy GR. Immunologic tools in the diagnosis of amebiasis: epidemiology in the United States. *Rev Infect Dis* 1986;8:239–245.
66. Ralls PW, Quinn MF, Boswell WD, et al. Patterns of resolution in successfully treated hepatic amebic abscess: sonographic evaluation. *Radiology* 1983;149:541–543.
67. Sullam PM, Slutkin G, Gottlieb AB, et al. Paromomycin therapy of endemic amebiasis in homosexual men. *Sex Transm Dis* 1986;13:151–155.
68. Thompson JE, Forlenza S, Verma R. Amebic liver abscess: a therapeutic approach. *Rev Infect Dis* 1985;7:171–179.
69. vanSonnenberg E, Mueller PR, Schiffman HR, et al. Intrahepatic amebic abscesses: indications for and results of percutaneous catheter drainage. *Radiology* 1985;156:631–635.
70. McAuley JB, Juranek DD. Luminal agents in the treatment of amebiasis. *Clin Infect Dis* 1992;14:1161–1162.
71. Backer H. Field water disinfection. In: Auerbach PS, Geehr EC, eds. *Management of wilderness and environmental emergencies*. St. Louis: C.V. Mosby, 1989:805–829.

CHAPTER 278
Giardia intestinalis

Michael J. G. Farthing

Giardiasis, the most common protozoal infection of the human intestinal tract, is found worldwide. *Giardia intestinalis* is a well established small intestinal pathogen that may cause acute and/or chronic diarrhea and intestinal malabsorption, particularly in young persons. In the developing world however, the parasite is commonly isolated in stool from healthy asymptomatic individuals, which initially created a vigorous debate over whether *Giardia* was a true enteropathogen. *Giardia* cysts, the infective form of the parasite, are widely disseminated in the environment, mainly in surface water and mammalian reservoirs. Although there is evidence to suggest that protective immunity eventually develops, this may not occur until several years after primary exposure, suggesting that in highly endemic environments, multiple exposures are necessary to produce protective immunity. Developing new ways of controlling infection thus constitutes a major challenge for epidemiologists, clinicians, and scientists.

HISTORY

Giardia was probably first seen through a hand lens made by Anton van Leeuwenhoek in the late seventeenth century. At the time, the Dutch microscopist was suffering from chronic diarrhea and saw the organism in his own feces (1). He named it *pissabed*, which in old Dutch approximates "wood louse." Vilem Lambl formally rediscovered the parasite in 1859 and called it *Cercomonas intestinalis*. Some 20 years later, Kunstler identified a similar parasite in amphibians, which he called *Giardia agilis*, after his teacher and mentor, Alfred Giard. The binomial *Giardia lamblia* was introduced by Stiles in 1915, although the most widely accepted names are *G. intestinalis* (humans and some other mammals), *Giardia muris* (rodents), and *G. agilis* (amphibians). The first clear description of the pathogenicity of *Giardia* resulted when Fantham and Porter (2) experimentally infected young animals with cysts from humans and produced diarrhea, and in some instances weight loss. Knowledge of the parasite remained rudimentary until Meyer (3) successfully cultured the parasite axenically in 1976.

CHARACTERISTICS OF THE PATHOGEN

Giardia is a flagellate protozoan (phylum Sarcomastigophora; class Zoomastigophorea; order Diplomonadida). The organism exists in two forms: the motile trophozoite, which cannot survive outside its host, and the cyst, which is the infective form of the parasite that can survive in the environment, particularly in moist, cool conditions (4). The trophozoite has two nuclei and four pairs of flagella. The dorsal surface of the parasite is convex, whereas the ventral surface is concave and occupied predominantly by the ventral disk. This organelle is unique to *Giardia* and is a rigid structure consisting of microtubules, cross-bridges attached to microtubules, and microribbons, which run perpendicularly to both the microtubules and the cross-bridges. The disk contains a variety of cytoskeletal proteins, including the family of giardins, actin, α-actinin, myosin, and tropomyosin. α_1-Giardin has recently been identified structurally and functionally to be an annexin with a typical calcium-binding domain (5).These proteins give the disk flexibility and allow it to change shape, a process that is thought to be important for attachment. The flagella have the usual eukaryotic structure consisting of nine pairs of microtubules with two central single microtubules (6–9). Another distinctive structure in the parasite is the median body. Morphologically, this differs among the three major types of *Giardia*: hammer-claw shaped in *G. intestinalis*, a pair of round bodies in *G. muris*, and teardrop shaped in *G. agilis* (Fig. 278.1). The function of the median body is not known. Studies suggest that two other morphological variants exist: *Giardia psittaci*, which lacks the ventrolateral flange that in other types encircles the ventral disk (10), and *Giardia ardeae*, an isolate from the great blue heron, which has a median body similar to those of *G. muris* and *G. intestinalis*, but a ventral disk and single caudal flagellum more similar to *G. muris*.

The parasite surface membrane has not been well characterized, although there is antigenic diversity between isolates (11,12) and N-acetyl-D-glucosamine is the major glycosyl residue (13). Within the cytoplasm are rough endoplasmic reticulum, glycogen particles, and free ribosomes but no mitochondria or Golgi's bodies. *Giardia* is an aerotolerant anaerobe that uses an iron-sulfur protein and flavin electron transport system for respiration (14). Glycolysis is the major pathway of carbohydrate metabolism, the necessary enzymes being located within the cytosol (15,16). The parasite is unable to synthesize phospholipids and sterols (15), which it acquires by uptake from the intestinal lumen; bile must be a major source (17). *Giardia* is unable

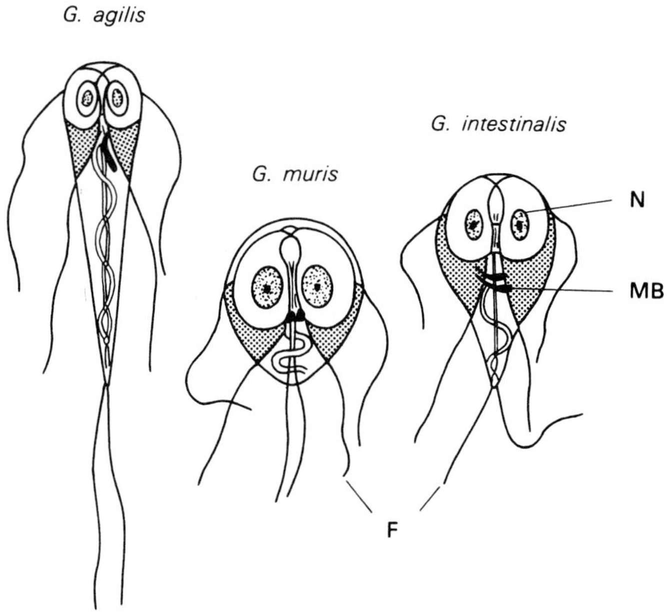

Figure 278.1. Morphological types of *Giardia*. Diagrammatic representation of light microscopic appearances of *Giardia agilis*, *Giardia muris*, and *Giardia intestinalis*. N, nucleus; MB, median body; F, flagellum.

to synthesize purines and pyrimidines but does have respective salvage pathways (18,19).

Although *Giardia* can be grown in culture *in vitro*, its growth requirements have not been clearly defined. The parasite is dependent on nutrients from the intestinal lumen, some of which, including bile salts and biliary lipids, have been shown to stimulate growth (17,20,21). The final stage of the life cycle, encystation, can also be completed *in vitro* after exposure of trophozoites to high concentrations of conjugated bile salts and myristic acid at a neutral pH level. Thus, bile and bile salts may have a dual role in the parasite life cycle, on one hand promoting growth and multiplication while ensuring that the parasite completes its life cycle by encystation. An encystation-specific promoter for glucosamine-6-phosphate isomerase, the first enzyme required for N-acetylgalactosamine synthesis, has recently been identified (22,23).

Although five morphologically distinct forms of the parasite have been identified, it is now well established that diversity exists among different isolates of *G. intestinalis*. Phenotypic variation has been shown by analysis of surface antigens (11,12), isoenzyme analysis (24,25), and metabolic radiolabeling with ^{35}S-methionine (26). In addition, genotypic variation has been shown by restriction fragment length polymorphism, chromosome analysis (27,28), and deoxyribonucleic acid (DNA) fingerprinting (29,30). The relationship between these phenotypic and genotypic variations and the parasite's virulence and their effects on the host immune response have not been determined.

The chemotaxonomy of *Giardia* has been explored using various techniques, including antigen, isoenzyme, and DNA analysis. These approaches have confirmed that *Giardia* isolates differ from one to another, although the sensitivity of the techniques varies. Molecular genetic approaches have shown that human *Giardia* isolates may be subdivided into two major genotypes (31). Some animal isolates have been identified to possess the same genotype providing evidence that giardiasis is likely to be a zoonosis.

EPIDEMIOLOGY

G. intestinalis is found throughout the world, but prevalence is greatest in developing countries where peak rates in childhood can be 25% to 30% (33,34). In the industrialized world, prevalence rarely exceeds 7% (35), although higher rates are reported from some areas of North America and Eastern Europe. Age-specific prevalence rates reported from Africa (36) and the Indian subcontinent (33) rise throughout childhood and begin to fall only during adolescence. Giardiasis is transmitted by water or contaminated food and by direct person-to-person contact. The importance of waterborne spread of giardiasis became apparent in North America (37) during the mid-1960s, when a large number of skiers in Colorado became infected. Since then, numerous waterborne outbreaks have occurred in North America, eastern Europe, and the United Kingdom (38). Interruption of the ancillary water purification procedures can lead to contamination of municipal water supplies and has been shown to account for many of the reported epidemics of waterborne giardiasis. A recent survey in the United States suggests that there may be as many as 2.5 million cases of giardiasis each year (39). Infection is also transmitted in swimming pools, usually after contamination by an infected infant or child.

Person-to-person spread is particularly important in schools, day care centers, and other residential institutions. Infection may be spread during sexual activity, particularly intimate oral-anal contact (40). The ease with which *Giardia* is transmitted from person to person almost certainly relates to the observation that an inoculum of only 10 to 100 cysts is required to initiate infection.

There is increasing evidence to suggest that giardiasis is a zoonosis (41–43). Many wild and domestic animals carry the parasite, which is indistinguishable from the human form, *G. intestinalis*. Molecular genetic analyses have shown extremely close similarity between human and animal isolates. Studies have also shown that the prevalence of *G. intestinalis* is unexpectedly high in domestic cats and dogs (44–46), so these animals may act as a reservoir of infection in both developed and developing communities. Further confirmatory evidence that giardiasis is a zoonosis has been provided by an author-volunteer who successfully infected himself with an isolate obtained from a Gambian giant pouched rat (47).

PATHOGENESIS

Colonization

Colonization may be considered a three-stage process: excystation, adherence, and multiplication. Excystation occurs predominantly in the proximal small intestine; experimental evidence *in vitro* indicates that it is triggered by exposure to gastric acid and pancreatic enzymes (48,49). Intracellular vacuoles have been observed to discharge their contents during excystation, suggesting that hydrolases are required to complete the process (50). Adherence to the epithelium plays a major part in ensuring that the parasite remains within the gut. The ventral disk is traditionally considered the organelle of attachment using a combination of hydrodynamic and mechanical forces (6,7). The disk contains contractile proteins that enable it to alter its shape (Figs. 278.2 and 278.3). Attachment to glass or plastic surfaces can be inhibited by agents that interfere with contractile protein function (51).

A mannose-binding lectin has been identified in the surface membrane of *Giardia*, which like bacterial adhesins, may also mediate attachment to the intestinal epithelium (53,54) (Fig. 278.4).

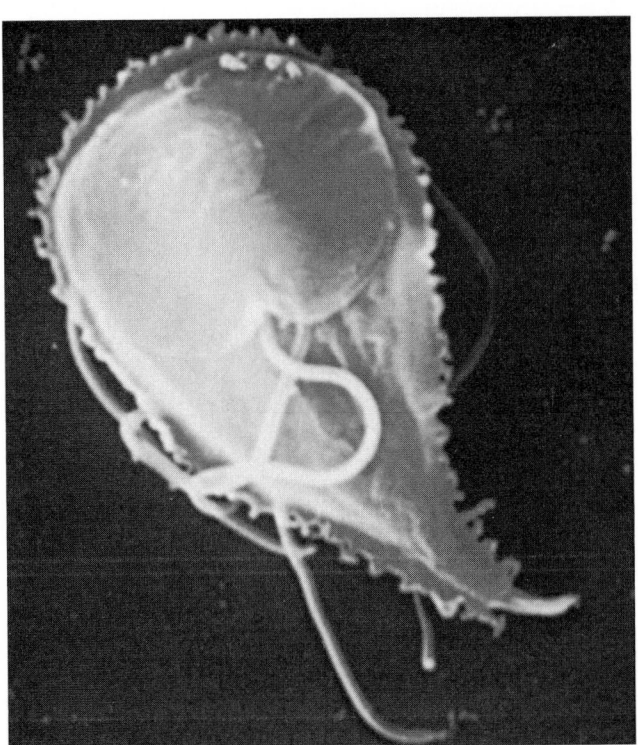

Figure 278.2. Scanning electron micrograph of *Giardia intestinalis* trophozoite showing ventral surface with ventral disk.

This lectin appears to be involved in attachment to isolated enterocytes *in vitro* and is trypsin sensitive (55). However, treatment of disrupted trophozoites with trypsin increases lectin activity, suggesting that the intracellular form of the molecule is a prolectin (53). The lectin appears to be present over the entire parasite surface, having no predilection for the ventral disk. Lectin-mediated attachment may be the primary attachment mechanism before ventral disk-mediated mechanisms can operate.

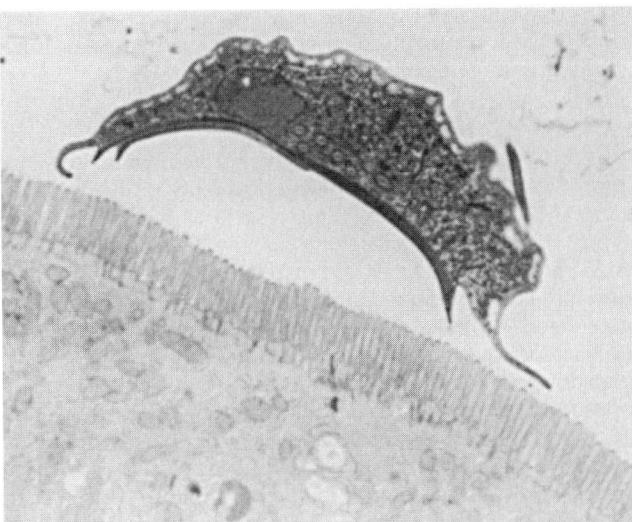

Figure 278.3. Transmission electron micrograph of *Giardia intestinalis* trophozoite in transverse section situated above the human jejunal microvillus membrane.

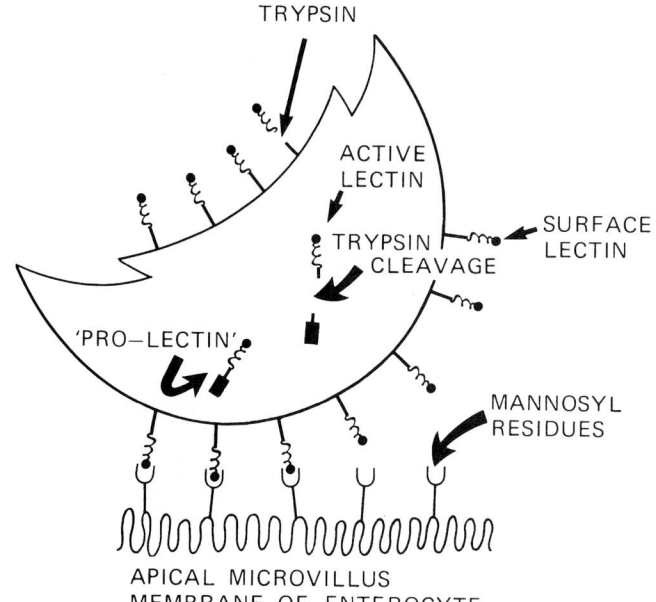

TRYPSIN

ACTIVE
LECTIN

TRYPSIN
CLEAVAGE

SURFACE
LECTIN

'PRO—LECTIN'

MANNOSYL
RESIDUES

APICAL MICROVILLUS
MEMBRANE OF ENTEROCYTE

Figure 278.4. Some characteristics of the mannose-binding lectin of *Giardia intestinalis.*

The parasite multiplies by binary fission, which *in vitro* occurs every 6 to 10 hours. Bile stimulates parasite growth, principally because it contains phospholipid, uptake of which is facilitated by bile salts (17,20). Bile salts are also taken up actively by the parasite by what appears to be an active carrier-mediated transport process (56,57). There is no evidence that the parasite metabolizes bile salts, and why it should take up substantial amounts of these substances remains unknown (58). Interestingly, conjugated bile salts appear to be at least one of the promoting factors for encystation (59).

Mechanisms of Diarrhea, Malabsorption, and Intestinal Damage

A unifying hypothesis that explains the diarrhea and malabsorption of giardiasis is not yet available. Various mechanisms have been proposed, some of which operate in the intestinal lumen and others in the intestinal mucosa (60–63).

LUMINAL FACTORS
The early belief that *Giardia* could prevent absorption by acting as a physical barrier to nutrients seems highly unlikely, largely because of the enormous functional reserve of the small intestine and the relatively small size of the parasite. There is no evidence that *Giardia* produces an enterotoxin by which it might induce water and electrolyte secretion, and there is no evidence that it causes direct epithelial damage by producing cytotoxin; however, bacterial overgrowth has been described in patients from India with giardiasis and in overland travelers (64,65). It has been proposed that these bacteria deconjugate bile salts, leading to impaired lipid solubilization and fat malabsorption. Deconjugated bile salts were found in the luminal fluid of Indian patients with giardiasis (64), although not in patients from the United Kingdom (49). *Giardia* organisms do not themselves deconjugate bile salts, but they may reduce effective intraluminal concentrations by taking them up by active transport (56). It is conceivable that during chronic infection, this process might deplete the bile salt pool, particularly in infants and young children.

Duodenal concentrations of trypsin, chymotrypsin, and lipase have been shown to be reduced in symptomatic patients with giardiasis. This is not due to primary pancreatic insufficiency but to a direct effect of trophozoites on hydrolytic enzyme activity. The mechanism has not been established but may relate to an effect of one of the *Giardia* proteinases (66,67).

MUCOSAL INJURY
Some patients with giardiasis have morphological abnormalities of the intestinal mucosa, namely reduction in villus height and increased numbers of lamina propria and intraepithelial lymphocytes (68–70). Rarely, this can result in subtotal villus atrophy (71). In others, there may be no obvious light microscopic abnormalities, although ultrastructural studies indicate that there can be damage to microvilli. There is a close relationship between the extent of the mucosal damage and the degree of impaired absorption of dietary substrates. The mechanism by which *Giardia* damages the intestinal mucosa has not been determined. There is no evidence that it is a direct effect of the parasite, and invasion of the mucosa is seen only rarely.

Evidence is increasing that immune responses in the intestinal mucosa may be responsible for the abnormalities of villus architecture (72,73). There is evidence from both animal and human studies that the increase in intraepithelial and lamina propria lymphocytes antedates the morphological abnormalities in the villi. There is also a functional counterpart to this observation, because the intensity of the mucosal inflammatory response is related to the impairment of absorptive function. Furthermore, although T-cell–deficient, athymic *(nu/nu)* mice fail to clear the parasite, they sustain substantially less morphological damage than immunocompetent animals (74). Finally, there is now clear evidence that T-cell activation in human fetal small intestine *in vitro* results in villus atrophy (75). The possibility remains, therefore, that sensitization and subsequent activation of mucosal T cells by *Giardia* antigen(s) could account for the mucosal abnormalities, perhaps in the same way that intolerance to gluten and cow's milk protein produces similar effects in susceptible persons. Whether *Giardia* lectin can act as a mitogen and directly activate mucosal T cells remains to be established (52,54).

Immune Responses

Immune responses are important in eradicating the parasite from the intestine during acute infection and in the development of protective immunity (76). Infection is more common in immunodeficiency states, particularly those associated with malnutrition, hypogammaglobulinemia, and human immunodeficiency virus infection.

ANTIBODY
Acute giardiasis is associated with serum immunoglobulin M (IgM), immunoglobulin A (IgA), and immunoglobulin G (IgG) responses. The specific anti-*Giardia* IgM response occurs early in infection and generally declines within 2 to 3 weeks (77,78). Current evidence suggests that an IgM response is present in the vast majority of patients with acute giardiasis, if not in all. Approximately 30% of patients also mount a serum IgA response, which like IgM is present in relatively low titer and is probably short lived (79). As with other acute infections, the IgG response occurs later and may persist for months or even years, particularly in highly endemic areas, where continued exposure to the parasite boosts the specific serum IgG response (33,77). Elevated IgG titers can be found in both infected and noninfected persons in endemic areas, whereas specific anti-*Giardia* IgM is generally found only during current infection, indicating that this antibody response may be helpful in diagnosis.

Occasionally, increased concentrations of total serum IgE have been reported in giardiasis, which in one case was not due to specific anti-*Giardia* IgE, but possibly to food antigens after increased intestinal permeability as a result of the infection (80). Secretory IgA probably has a major role in parasite clearance and in the development of protective immunity. Specific anti-*Giardia* surface IgA has been demonstrated in human jejunal fluid, human milk, and in experimental animals (81,82). During experimental infection, clearance of the parasite relates closely to rising concentrations of surface IgA and IgG in intestinal secretions (83–85), and suckling mice can be protected from experimental *G. muris* infection by immune animals' milk (86).

CELLULAR IMMUNE RESPONSE

The importance of cell-mediated immunity in clearing *Giardia* organisms has been clearly demonstrated in congenitally hypothymic T-cell–deficient mice, which experience prolonged infections with *G. muris* (87). In immunocompetent mice, lymphocyte numbers increase in the small intestinal epithelium, being maximal 2 weeks after the initiation of experimental infection, at which time there is a decrease in the number of trophozoites in the intestine (88). Peyer's patch lymphocytes also proliferate, but their numbers decline after the parasite is eradicated. Results of preliminary studies indicate that both intraepithelial and lamina propria lymphocytes from infected animals are sensitized to *Giardia* antigens (88). Corticosteroids, cyclosporine, and malnutrition increase susceptibility to infection and in some instances prolong the infective period (76).

A similar increase in lymphocyte numbers, including intraepithelial lymphocytes (70,89), has been reported in human jejunal mucosa of patients with giardiasis. Increased numbers of lymphocytes have also been demonstrated in the intestinal lumen in murine giardiasis, where T lymphocytes have been observed in direct contact with trophozoites (90). These lymphocytes may be directly cytotoxic and contribute to parasite eradication. There is also evidence that antibody-dependent, cell-mediated cytotoxicity exists against *Giardia*, involving both T lymphocytes and peripheral blood granulocytes (91).

Giardia Antigens. Various surface antigens have been studied, including an 82- to 88-kd protein that is an immunodominant antigen in human infections (92–94). A 56-kd antigen may also be important, as are other high-molecular-mass *Giardia* polypeptides and proteins of the cytoskeleton, such as the ventral disk protein giardin, which has a molecular mass of 31 kd (95–97). Some *Giardia* surface antigens are excreted or secreted during growth *in vitro*, which may assist immune evasion. In some instances, cyst antigens may be different from the major trophozoite antigens, although a 65-kd antigen has been identified that is common to both cyst and trophozoite (98,99). A *Giardia* heat-shock antigen has also been shown to be important in human giardiasis (100), and failure to produce an antibody response to this antigen may be an important factor leading to persistent infection. Expression of this antigen is now known to occur not only following a temperature shift but also on exposure to the physical and chemical environment found in duodenal fluid (100). This antigen has been recently identified to be homologous with heat-shock protein-70, a highly conserved family of heat shock proteins found throughout the animal kingdom and shown to be important determinants of the host immune response in other bacterial and parasitic infections.

Giardia is able to vary expression of certain of its surface antigens during both experimental and human infection, and this may be a way in which the parasite evades immune clearance. These variant-specific surface proteins (VSPs) constitute a family of related proteins, the expression of which is regulated by the organism (100). Expression of individual VSPs appears to be related to the stage of differentiation and genotype (101). Further evidence is required before it can be established whether this mechanism is relevant in humans *in vivo*. A 170-kd surface antigen may be one such protein (102,103). It has a high cysteine content, and part of the gene encoding this antigen has been cloned and used as a probe to investigate the mechanism of antigenic variation in *Giardia* (104). Current evidence suggests that there are frequent rearrangements at the gene locus of this 170-kd antigen.

A 57-kd antigen has been identified by mouse monoclonal antibody and shown to be immunogenic during human infection (105). This antigen in predominantly cytoplasmic but also expressed at the surface membrane. In children with *acute* giardiasis, IgG and IgA antibodies to this antigen were detected in serum, but in Gambian children with *chronic* giardiasis the IgA response was absent, suggestive that this antigen may be a determinant of immune clearance (106,107).

CLINICAL MANIFESTATIONS

Most persons infected with *Giardia* have no symptoms, and there is little evidence that the parasite does them any harm. This situation is most common in highly endemic areas of the tropics and subtropics. It is probably this observation that led to the commonly held belief during the first half of this century that *Giardia* was a harmless commensal organism. There is no doubt, however, that *Giardia* is an important cause of acute diarrhea, particularly in travelers to endemic areas, in children, and in those involved in waterborne epidemics resulting from contaminated water. The symptom pattern has been well documented in travelers (108,109) (Table 278.1). Symptoms begin 1 to 3 weeks after cysts are ingested. Diarrhea may be watery initially, but it can resolve rapidly. Associated symptoms include nausea, anorexia, and abdominal bloating. Occasionally, allergic manifestations are reported, including arthralgia, myalgia, urticaria, and eosinophilia (80). If their disease is not treated, 30% to 50% of these patients develop persistent diarrhea; half have biochemical evidence of malabsorption with steatorrhea and weight loss (110–113). These symptoms may persist for many weeks, and in children, chronic giardiasis may be confused with celiac disease (114), cow's milk protein enteropathy, and other noninfective causes of intestinal malabsorption.

TABLE 278.1. Symptoms of Acute Giardiasis in Travelers

Clinical features	Aspen, Colorado (*n* = 324) (%)	Former Soviet Union (*n* = 56) (%)
Diarrhea	96	93
Weakness	72	80
Weight loss	62	73
Abdominal pain	61	77
Nausea	60	59
Steatorrhea	57	55
Flatulence	35	—
Vomiting	29	—
Fever	17	—

Source: Data from Moore GT, Cross WM, McGuire D, et al. Epidemic giardiasis at a ski resort. *N Engl J Med* 1969;281:402–407; and Brodsky RE, Spencer HC Jr, Schultz MG. Giardiasis in American travelers to the Soviet Union. *J Infect Dis* 1974;130:319–323, with permission.

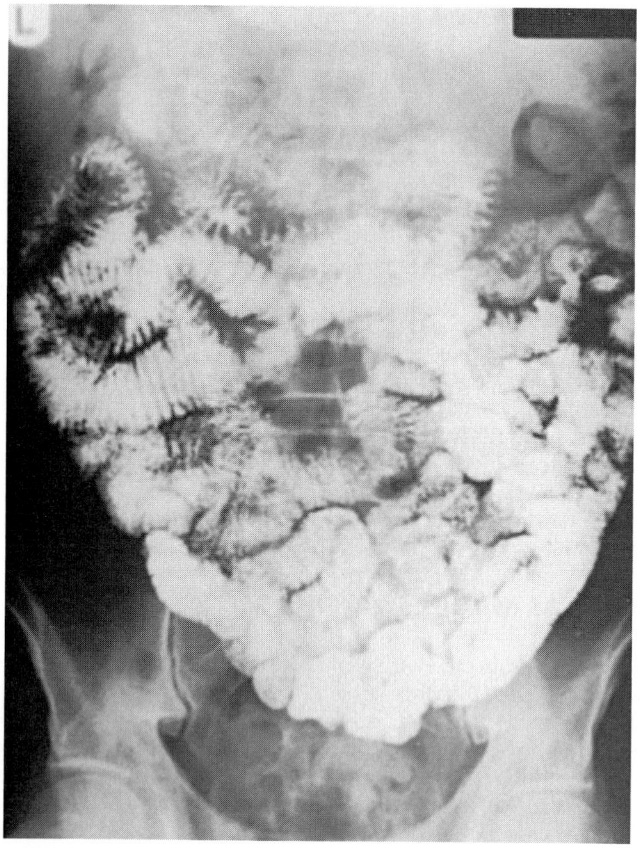

Figure 278.5. Barium follow-through examination in a man with chronic giardiasis and hypogammaglobulinemia, showing diffuse lymphoid nodular hyperplasia throughout the small intestine.

Since the 1920s, it has been alleged that *Giardia* infection can impair growth and development of children (115). This has been confirmed by several hospital-based studies in which retarded growth and weight gain were demonstrated, predominately in preschool children (115,116). Results of community-based studies in the Gambia and Guatemala (34) also suggest that this parasite does have an independent inhibitory effect on growth, although the analyses required to show such an association were complex because all children had other intestinal, respiratory, and systemic infections at the same time.

Immunodeficiency states, particularly hypogammaglobulinemia and malnutrition, are apparently associated with increased susceptibility to giardiasis (117). Although its prevalence is greater in homosexual men and individuals with human immunodeficiency virus infection, unlike cryptosporidiosis, it does not appear to be a major clinical problem for them. However, in hypogammaglobulinemic patients, it may be extremely difficult, if not impossible, to eradicate the infection, despite multiple courses of appropriate antimicrobials, either single agents or combinations. Lymphoid nodular hyperplasia is a common finding in patients with giardiasis and hypogammaglobulinemia (Fig. 278.5).

DIAGNOSIS

Clinical history may now be the most common approach to making a diagnosis of giardiasis, particularly in travelers who have moved from an area of low endemicity to one of high endemicity. Such persons often receive anti-*Giardia* chemotherapy before

---

TABLE 278.2.   Diagnosis of Giardiasis

Clinical history (empirical treatment)
Microscopy: feces, duodenal juice, jejunal biopsy or smear
Immunodiagnosis[a]: serology (IgM, IgA), fecal antigen
DNA probes[a]: fecal *Giardia* DNA

[a]Research techniques.
DNA, deoxyribonucleic acid; IgA, immunoglobulin A; IgM, immunoglobulin M.

a precise microbiologic diagnosis is made and a good clinical response to therapy is often taken as confirmation. The "gold standard" for diagnosis is still the microscopic demonstration of the parasite (cysts, trophozoites, or both) in feces, duodenal fluid, or a jejunal mucosal biopsy specimen. Various immunodiagnostic approaches have also been used, and DNA-based tests are currently under development (Table 278.2).

Microscopy

Although detection of *Giardia* forms in feces is enhanced by cyst concentration techniques, most studies indicate that even after examination of three consecutive specimens on different days, only about 80% of infections are detected (118–120). This probably relates to the highly variable pattern of cyst excretion and the fact that the ability to detect cysts in feces is observer dependent. Although examination of duodenal fluid obtained either by aspiration or by the string test is often put forward as producing a higher diagnostic yield (121), studies suggest that this may not be the case (122). If repeated fecal specimens do not demonstrate the pathogen and the clinical presentation strongly suggests giardiasis, this approach certainly complements fecal microscopy. Trophozoites can also be detected in jejunal mucosal biopsy specimens and impression smears taken from these specimens.

Immunodiagnosis

Serologic responses in giardiasis and the use of immunologic techniques to detect *Giardia* antigen in feces are potentially useful approaches for improving the speed and accuracy of diagnosis in giardiasis (76), although these techniques are still largely restricted to research laboratories. Most patients with giardiasis have an increased specific anti-*Giardia* IgG antibody titer, but this comes relatively late in infection and can persist for many months, possibly years (33,77). The IgG response in giardiasis is, therefore, not helpful in distinguishing past from present infection, and it accounts for the high prevalence of anti-*Giardia* IgG in noninfected persons in endemic areas. The anti-*Giardia* IgM response occurs relatively early in infection and is short-lived, probably lasting only a few weeks (77,78). The anti-*Giardia* IgM response does appear to distinguish current infections from past ones. Specific serum anti-*Giardia* IgA titers, like IgM titers, are lower than those of IgG and can be detected in only about 30% of patients (79). Like the IgM response, however, it is relatively short-lived and so may be useful in identifying patients with current infection.

Several approaches have been used to detect specific *Giardia* antigens in feces by counterimmunoelectrophoresis or enzyme-linked immunosorbent assay (ELISA) (123–125). Several groups have produced encouraging results with sensitivity better than 90%, and a simple commercially available test is now available. A 65-kd *Giardia* antigen has been identified in feces, and its detection has formed the basis of a diagnostic test based on counterimmunoelectrophoresis (99). Whether this approach will survive in a routine diagnostic laboratory remains to be established. Sensitive and specific commercially available ELISAs for *Giardia* antigens have been recently evaluated when sensitivity and specificity are reported to be 87% to 100% (126,127).

Specific DNA probes for *Giardia* are available, although preliminary studies suggest that there may be difficulties in liberating DNA from *Giardia* cysts (128,129). A polymerase chain reaction (PCR)–based assay that amplifies the intergenic spacer region of multicopy ribosomal ribonucleic acid (rRNA) gene followed by nested PCR appears to be a rapid and reliable technique for detecting *Giardia* in stool (130).

TREATMENT

The most widely used drugs to treat giardiasis are the nitroimidazole derivatives (metronidazole, tinidazole), the acridine dyes (mepacrine), and the nitrofurans (furazolidone). The regimens for adults and children are shown in Table 278.3. Unfortunately, none of these drugs is ideal, because they have a variety of unwanted adverse effects, and none is regarded as being safe in pregnancy. The drugs of choice are the nitroimidazole derivatives, because the high-dose, short-treatment regimen is usually acceptable to patients and generally ensures good compliance; however, in some countries, they are not licensed for treatment of giardiasis.

Various other chemotherapeutic agents have been assessed *in vitro*, and some have been used in the clinical setting. The benzimidazole drugs have antigiardial activity that almost certainly relates to their ability to inhibit cytoskeletal function. Albendazole has been shown to have antigiardial activity *in vitro* and recent clinical trial data would support its value in human infection (131). Other drugs such as sodium fusidate (132), D- and D,L-propranolol (133), tricyclic compounds (134), mebendazole (135), mefloquine, doxycycline, and rifampicin have all been shown to have antigiardial activity (136), although the majority have not been subjected to rigorous evaluation in clinical practice. Perhaps the most encouraging new development in antigiardial therapy is the introduction of the broad-spectrum antiparasitic agent, nitazoxanide. Recent clinical studies have confirmed its efficacy and safety and have suggested that its efficacy is similar to that of metronidazole (137,138).

Treatment failures with nitroimidazole derivatives are common in giardiasis, and it is often necessary to give a second course of the drug. Failing this, a second-line drug such as mepacrine can be given alone or in combination with the nitroimidazole derivative. The reason for treatment failures has not been clearly established, although there is increasing evidence that *Giardia* may become relatively resistant to some anti-*Giardia* drugs (139). The development of sensitivity assays *in vitro* should help plan further treatment when infection is difficult to eradicate (140,141). It has been shown that the phenotype and genotype of *Giardia* isolates can change during the course of chronic infection, possibly because of selection of relatively resistant strains after treatment with a nitroimidazole derivative (27).

PREVENTION

Giardia organisms are widely distributed throughout the environment, in water and in human and animal reservoirs. It is unlikely that any single environmental intervention will eradicate the disease. Transmission, however, may be interrupted by ensuring high standards of water purification, it being particularly important not to rely on chlorination alone, because the effect on cyst viability is variable. Travelers to endemic areas should avoid consuming tap water and locally produced soft drinks and ice. Boiling water for 10 minutes destroys cysts, but the opportunity to do so is often not available to travelers.

Person-to-person spread can be controlled by ensuring high standards of personal hygiene and adequate supervision in nurseries and residential institutions. Avoidance of intimate oral-anal contact reduces the risk of transmission during sexual activity. Treating carriers in areas of low endemicity should help to control human reservoirs, although it is doubtful whether this would have any impact whatsoever in highly endemic areas.

There is compelling evidence that breast-feeding protects against giardiasis; this can be partly attributed to passive immunization. Whether active immunization in the form of a vaccine is feasible, or even appropriate, continues to be evaluated. Parenteral immunization with adjuvants can protect experimental animals from challenge with *G. intestinalis*, and the epidemiological evidence in humans that protective immunity does eventually develop, probably over a number of years, suggests that immunologic approaches to prevention are feasible. However,

---

TABLE 278.3. Drug Treatment of Giardiasis

Drug	Dosage	Side effects
Metronidazole	Adults: 1.2-g dose/d × 3 d, or 250 mg t.i.d. × 7 d	Metallic taste, peripheral neuropathy
	Children: 15 mg/kg/d (maximum, 750 mg) × 10 d	Disulfiram-like reaction with alcohol
Tinidazole	2-g single dose 50–75 mg/kg single dose	As for metronidazole
Albendazole	400 mg daily for 5 d	GI disturbance, alopecia, blood disorders
Quinacrine	Adults: 100 mg t.i.d. daily × 7 d	Bitter taste, yellow discoloration of the skin and sclerae
	Children: 2 mg/kg t.i.d. × 7 d	Nausea, vomiting, toxic psychosis, exfoliative dermatitis, exacerbation of psoriasis
Furazolidone	Adults: 100 mg q.i.d. daily for 7–10 d	Nausea, vomiting, hemolysis in patients with glucose-6-phosphate dehydrogenase deficiency
	Children: 2 mg/kg t.i.d. × 10 d	

GI, gastrointestinal; t.i.d., three times daily; q.i.d., four times daily.

why the development of protective immunity following natural infection appears to require repeated exposure to the organism is unclear. It is possible that this is related, at least in part, to the variable antigenic profiles of different *Giardia* isolates. In addition, it is known that the expression of certain *Giardia* antigens can vary during both experimental and human infection, thus providing a way in which the organism may evade the host immune response. Failure to mount an antibody response to *Giardia* heat-shock antigen in children with chronic diarrhea in the Gambia suggests that impaired response may also be a factor. Clearly all of these issues need to be taken into account in planning a vaccine development strategy. Preliminary studies in animal models of giardiasis suggest that a trophozoite-derived vaccine can provide some measure of protection in dogs and cats (143,144).

ACKNOWLEDGMENTS

I am grateful for the financial support of the Wellcome Trust and the Digestive Diseases Foundation.

REFERENCES

1. Dobell CA. The discovery of intestinal protozoa in man. *Proc R Soc Med* 1920;13:1.
2. Fantham HB, Porter A. The pathogenicity of *Giardia lamblia intestinalis* from man to experimental animals. *Br Med J* 1916;2:139.
3. Meyer EA. *Giardia lamblia*: Isolation and axenic cultivation. *Exp Parasitol* 1976;39:101.
4. Feely DE, Erlandsen SL, Chase DG. Structure of the trophozoite and cyst. In: Erlandsen SL, Meyer EA, eds. *Giardia and giardiasis*. New York: Plenum Publishing, 1984:3–31.
5. Bauer B, Engelbrecht S, Bakker-Grunwald T, et al. Functional identification of alpha 1-giardin as an annexin of *Giardia lamblia*. *FEMS Microbiol Lett* 1999;173:147–53.
6. Holberton DV. Attachment of *Giardia*—a hydrodynamic model based on flagellar activity. *J Exp Biol* 1974;60:207.
7. Holberton DV. Fine structure of the ventral disc apparatus and the mechanism of attachment in the flagellate *Giardia muris*. *J Cell Sci* 1973;13:11.
8. Feely DE, Schollmeyer JV, Erlandsen SL. *Giardia*: distribution of contractile proteins in the attachment organelle. *Exp Parasitol* 1982;53:145.
9. Crossley R, Holberton DV. Characterization of proteins from the cytoskeleton of *Giardia lamblia*. *J Cell Sci* 1983;59:81.
10. Erlandsen SL, Bemrick WJ. SEM evidence for a new species, *Giardia psittaci*. *J Parasitol* 1987;73:623.
11. Smith PD, Gillin FD, Kaushal NA, et al. Antigenic analysis of *Giardia lamblia* from Afghanistan, Puerto Rico, Ecuador and Oregon. *Infect Immun* 1982;36:714.
12. Nash TE, Keister DB. Differences in excretory-secretory products and surface antigens among 19 isolates of *Giardia*. *J Infect Dis* 1985;152:1166.
13. Ward HD, Alroy J, Lev BI, et al. Biology of *Giardia lamblia*. Detection of N-acetyl-D-glucosamine as the only surface saccharide moiety and identification of two distinct subsets of trophozoites by lectin binding. *J Exp Med* 1988;167:73.
14. Weinbach EC, Claggett CE, Keister DB, et al. Respiratory metabolism of *Giardia lamblia*. *J Parasitol* 1980;66:347.
15. Jarroll EL, Muller PJ, Meyer EA, et al. Lipid and carbohydrate metabolism of *Giardia lamblia*. *Mol Biochem Parasitol* 1981;2:187.
16. Lindmark DG. Energy metabolism of the anaerobic protozoan *Giardia lamblia*. *Mol Biochem Parasitol* 1980;1:1.
17. Farthing MJG, Keusch GT, Carey MC. Effect of bile and bile salts on growth and membrane lipid uptake by *Giardia lamblia*: possible implications for pathogenesis of intestinal disease. *J Clin Invest* 1985;76:1727.
18. Lindmark DG, Jarroll EL. Pyrimidine metabolism in *Giardia lamblia* trophozoites. *Mol Biochem Parasitol* 1982;5:291.
19. Wang CC, Aldritt S. Purine salvage networks in *Giardia lamblia*. *J Exp Med* 1983;158:1703.
20. Farthing MJG, Varon SR, Keusch GT. Mammalian bile promotes growth of *Giardia lamblia* in axenic culture. *Trans R Soc Trop Med Hyg* 1983;77:467.
21. Keister DB. Axenic culture of *Giardia lamblia* in TYI-S-33 medium supplemented with bile. *Trans R Soc Trop Med Hyg* 1983;77:487.
22. Bertram MA, Meyer EA, Lile JD, et al. A comparison of isoenzymes of five axenic *Giardia* isolates. *J Parasitol* 1983;69:793.
23. Van Keulen H, Steimle PA, Bulik DA, et al. Cloning of two putative *Giardia lamblia* glucosamine 6-phosphate isomerase genes only one of which is transcriptionally activated during encystment. *J Eukaryotic Microbiol* 1998;45:637–642.
24. Jarroll EL, Macechko PT, Steimle PA et al. Regulation of carbohydrate metabolism during *Giardia* encystment. *J Eukaryot Microbiol* 2001;48:22–26.
25. Meloni BP, Lymbery AJ, Thompson RCA. Isoenzyme electrophoresis of 30 isolates of *Giardia* from humans and felines. *Am J Trop Med Hyg* 1988;38:65.
26. Cevallos AM, Morrison AM, Archibald SC, et al. [35S]-methionine biosynthetic radiolabelling of *Giardia lamblia*: basis for a typing system? *Gut* 1989;5:A748.
27. Nash TE, McCutchan T, Keister D, et al. Restriction-endonuclease analysis of DNA from 15 *Giardia* isolates from humans and animals. *J Infect Dis* 1985;152:64.
28. Butcher PB, Clark C, Farthing MJG. *Giardia lamblia* cloned genomic DNA probes: uses in faecal diagnosis and genetic analysis of clinical isolates. *Gut* 1988;29:A722.
29. Butcher PD, Cevallos AM, Carnaby S, et al. Phenotypic and genotypic variation in *Giardia lamblia* isolates during chronic infection. *Gut* 1993;35:51.
30. Carnaby S, Butcher PD, Summerbell CD, et al. Minisatellites corresponding to the human polycore probes 33.6 and 33.15 in the genome of the most "primitive" known eukaryote *Giardia lamblia*. *Gene* 1995;166:167.
31. Thompson RC, Hopkins RM, Homan WL. Nomenclature and genetic groupings of *Giardia* infecting mammals. *Parasitol Today* 2000;16:210–213.
32. O'Handley RM, Olson ME, Fraser D, et al. Prevalence and genotypic characterization of *Giardia* in dairy calves from Western Australia and Western Canada. *Vet Parasitol* 2000;90:193–200.
33. Gilman RH, Brown KH, Visvesvara GS, et al. Epidemiology and serology of *Giardia lamblia* in a developing country: Bangladesh. *Trans R Soc Trop Med Hyg* 1985;79:469.
34. Farthing MJG, Mata L, Urrutia JJ, et al. Natural history of *Giardia* infection of infants and children in rural Guatemala and its impact on physical growth. *Am J Clin Nutr* 1986;43:393.
35. Petersen H. Giardiasis (lambliasis). *Scand J Gastroenterol* 1972;7:44.
36. Oyerinde JPO, Ogunbi O, Alonge AA. Age and sex distribution of infections with *Entamoeba histolytica* and *Giardia intestinalis* in the Lagos population. *Int J Epidemiol* 1977;6:231.
37. Craun GF. Waterborne outbreaks of giardiasis. Current status. In: Erlandsen SL, Meyer EA, eds. *Giardia and giardiasis*. New York: Plenum Publishing, 1984:243–261.
38. Jephcott AE, Begg NT, Baker IA. Outbreak of giardiasis associated with mains water in the United Kingdom. *Lancet* 1986;1:730.
39. Furness BW, Beach MJ, Roberts JM. Giardiasis surveillance—United States, 1992–1997. *MMWR Morb Mortal Wkly Rep* 2000;49:1–13.
40. Owen RL. Direct fecal-oral transmission of giardiasis. In: Erlandsen SL, Meyer EA, eds. *Giardia and giardiasis*. New York: Plenum Publishing, 1984:329–339.
41. Woo PK. Evidence for animal reservoirs and transmission of *Giardia* infection between animal species. In: Erlandsen SL, Meyer EA, eds. *Giardia and giardiasis*. New York: Plenum Publishing, 1984:341–364.
42. Thompson RCA, Meloni BP, Lymbery AJ. Humans and cats have genetically identical forms of *Giardia*: evidence of a zoonotic relationship [Letter]. *Med J Aust* 1988;148:207.
43. Bemrick WJ, Erlandsen SL. Giardiasis—is it really a zoonosis? *Parasitol Today* 1988;4:69.
44. Sykes TJ, Fox MT. Patterns of infection with *Giardia* in dogs in London. *Trans R Soc Trop Med Hyg* 1989;83:239.
45. Winsland JKD, Nimmo S, Butcher PS, et al. Prevalence of *Giardia* in dogs and cats in the United Kingdom: survey of an Essex veterinary clinic. *Trans R Soc Trop Med Hyg* 1989;83:791.
46. Hill SL, Cheney JM, Taton-Allen GF, et al. Prevalence of enteric zoonotic organisms in cats. *J Am Vet Assoc* 2000;216:687–692.
47. Majewska AC. Successful experimental infections of a human volunteer and Mongolian gerbils with *Giardia* of animal origin. *Trans R Soc Trop Med Hyg* 1994;88:360.
48. Bingham AK, Meyer EA. *Giardia* excystation can be induced *in vitro* in acidic solutions. *Nature* 1979;277:301.
49. Rice EW, Schaefer FW. Improved *in vitro* excystation procedure for *Giardia lamblia* cysts. *J Clin Microbiol* 1981;14:709.
50. Hetsko ML, McCaffery JM, Svard SG, et al. Cellular and transcriptional changes during excystation of *Giardia lamblia in vitro*. *Exp Parasitol* 1998;88:172–183.
51. Feely DE, Erlandsen SL. Effect of cytochalasin-B, low Ca++ concentration, iodoacetic acid and quinacrine-HCl on the attachment of *Giardia* trophozoites *in vitro*. *J Parasitol* 1982;68:869.
52. Farthing MJG, Perreira MEA, Keusch GT. Description and characterization of a surface lectin from *Giardia lamblia*. *Infect Immun* 1986;51:661.
53. Lev B, Ward H, Keusch GT, et al. Lectin activation in *Giardia lamblia* by host protease: a novel host-parasite interaction. *Science* 1986;232:71.
54. Ward HD, Lev BI, Kane AV, et al. Identification and characterization of Taglin, a mannose-6-phosphate binding, trypsin-activated lectin from *Giardia lamblia*. *Biochemistry* 1987;26:8669.
55. Inge PMG, Edson CM, Farthing MJG. Attachment of *Giardia lamblia* to mammalian intestinal cells. *Gut* 1988;29:795.
56. Halliday CEW, Inge PM, Farthing MJ. Characterization of bile salt uptake by *Giardia lamblia*. *Int J Parasitol* 1995;25:1089.

57. Das S, Schteingart CD, Hofmann AF, et al. *Giardia lamblia:* evidence for carrier-mediated uptake and release of conjugated bile acids. *Exp Parasitol* 1997;87:133–141.

58. Halliday CEW, Inge PMG, Farthing MJG. *Giardia*-bile salt interactions. *Trans R Soc Trop Med Hyg* 1988;82:428.

59. Gillin FD, Reiner DS, Boucher SE. Small intestinal factors promote encystation of *Giardia lamblia in vitro. Infect Immun* 1988;56:705.

60. Katelaris PH, Farthing MJG. Diarrhoea and malabsorption in giardiasis: a multifactorial process. *Gut* 1992;33:295.

61. Farthing MJG. Pathogenesis of giardiasis. *Trans R Soc Trop Med Hyg* 1993;87 [Suppl 3]:17.

62. Farthing MJG. Molecular pathogenesis of giardiasis. *J Pediatr Gastroenterol Nutr* 1997;24:79–88.

63. Adam RD. Biology of *Giardia lamblia. Clin Microbiol Rev* 2001;14:447–475.

64. Tandon BN, Tandon RK, Satpathy BK, et al. Mechanism of malabsorption in giardiasis: a study of bacterial flora and bile salt deconjugation in upper jejunum. *Gut* 1977;18:176.

65. Tomkins AM, Drasar BS, Bradley AK, et al. Bacterial colonization of jejunal mucosa in giardiasis. *Trans R Soc Trop Med Hyg* 1978;72:33.

66. Katelaris PH, Seow F, Ngu MC. The effect of *Giardia lamblia* trophozoites on lipolysis *in vivo. Parasitology* 1991;103:35.

67. Seow F, Katelaris PH, Ngu MC. The effect of *Giardia lamblia* trophozoites on trypsin, chymotrypsin and amylase *in vitro. Parasitology* 1993;106:233.

68. Yardley JH, Takano J, Hendrix TR. Epithelial and other mucosal lesions of the jejunum in giardiasis. Jejunal biopsy studies. *Bull Johns Hopkins Hosp* 1964;115:389.

69. Hartong WA, Gourley WK, Arvanitakis C. Giardiasis: clinical spectrum and functional-structural abnormalities of the small intestinal mucosa. *Gastroenterology* 1979;77:61.

70. Wright SG, Tomkins AM. Quantification of the lymphocytic infiltrate in jejunal epithelium in giardiasis. *Clin Exp Immunol* 1977;29:408.

71. Levinson JD, Nastro LJ. Giardiasis with total villous atrophy. *Gastroenterology* 1978;74:271.

72. Farthing MJG. Host-parasite interactions in human giardiasis. *Q J Med* 1989;70:191.

73. Scott KG, Logan MR, Klammer GM, et al. Jejunal brush border microvillous alterations in *Giardia muris*–infected mice: role of T lymphocytes and interleukin-6. *Infect Immun* 2000;68:3412–3418.

74. Roberts-Thomson IC, Mitchell GF. Giardiasis in mice. I. Prolonged infections in certain mouse strains and hypothymic (nude) mice. *Gastroenterology* 1978;75:42.

75. MacDonald TT, Spencer J. Evidence that activated mucosal T cells play a role in the pathogenesis of enteropathy in human small intestine. *J Exp Med* 1988;167:1341.

76. Farthing MJG, Goka AKJ. Immunology of giardiasis. *Ballieres Clin Gastroenterol* 1987;1:589.

77. Goka AKJ, Rolston DDK, Mathan VI, et al. Diagnosis of giardiasis by specific IgM antibody enzyme-linked immunosorbent assay. *Lancet* 1986;2:184.

78. Nash TE, Herrington DA, Losonsky GA, et al. Experimental human infections with *Giardia lamblia. J Infect Dis* 1987;156:974.

79. Goka AKJ, Rolston DDK, Mathan VI, et al. Serum IgA response in human *Giardia lamblia* infection. *Serodiagn Immunother* 1989;3:273.

80. Farthing MJG, Chong S, Walker-Smith JA. Acute allergic phenomena in giardiasis. *Lancet* 1984;2:1428.

81. Briaud M, Morichau-Beauchant M, Matuchansky C, et al. Intestinal immune response in giardiasis. *Lancet* 1981;2:358.

82. Miotti PG, Gilman RH, Pickering LK, et al. Prevalence of serum and milk antibodies to *Giardia lamblia* in different populations of lactating women. *J Infect Dis* 1985;152:1025.

83. Snider DP, Gordon J, McDermott MR, et al. Chronic *Giardia muris* infection of anti-IgM–treated mice. I. Analysis of immunoglobulin- and parasite-specific antibody in normal and immunoglobulin-deficient animals. *J Immunol* 1985;135:4153.

84. Snider DP, Underdown BJ. Quantitative and temporal analyses of murine antibody response in serum and gut secretions to infection with *Giardia muris. Infect Immun* 1986;52:271.

85. Heyworth MF. Antibody response to *Giardia muris* trophozoites in mouse intestine. *Infect Immun* 1986;52:568.

86. Andrews JS, Hewlett EL. Protection against infection with *Giardia muris* by milk containing antibody to *Giardia. J Infect Dis* 1981;143:242.

87. Stevens DP, Frank DM Mahmoud AAF. Thymus dependency of host resistance to *Giardia muris* infection: studies in nude mice. *J Immunol* 1978;120:680.

88. Kanwar SS, Ganguly NK, Walia BNS, et al. Enumeration of small intestinal lymphocyte population in *Giardia lamblia* infected mice. *J Diarrhoeal Dis Res* 1984;2:243.

89. Ferguson A, McClure JP, Townley RRW. Intraepithelial lymphocyte counts in small intestinal biopsies from children with diarrhoea. *Acta Paediatr Scand* 1976;65:541.

90. Heyworth MF, Owen RL, Seaman WE, et al. Harvesting of leukocytes from intestinal lumen in murine giardiasis and preliminary characterization of these cells. *Dig Dis Sci* 1985;30:149.

91. Smith PD, Keister DB, Elson CO. Human host response to *Giardia lamblia.* II. Antibody-dependent killing *in vitro. Cell Immunol* 1983;82:308.

92. Edson CM, Farthing MJG, Thorley-Lawson DA, et al. An 88,000 M, *Giardia lamblia* surface protein which is immunogenic in humans. *Infect Immun* 1986;54:621.

93. Einfeld DA, Stibbs HH. Identification and characterization of a major antigen of *Giardia lamblia. Infect Immun* 1984;46:377.

94. Kumkum, Khanna R, Khuller M, et al. Plasma membrane associated antigens of trophozoites of axenic *Giardia lamblia. Trans R Soc Trop Med Hyg* 1988;82:439.

95. Torian BE, Barnes RC, Stephens RS, et al. Tubulin and high-molecular weight polypeptides as *Giardia lamblia* antigens. *Infect Immun* 1984;46:152.

96. Clark JT, Holberton DV. Plasma membrane isolated from *Giardia lamblia:* Identification of membrane proteins. *Eur J Cell Biol* 1986;42:200.

97. Taylor GD, Wenman WM. Human immune response to *Giardia lamblia* infection. *J Infect Dis* 1987;155:137.

98. Gillin FD, Reiner DS, Gault MJ, et al. Encystation and expression of cyst antigens by *Giardia lamblia in vitro. Science* 1987;235:1040.

99. Rosoff JD, Stibbs HH. Isolation and identification of a *Giardia lamblia*–specific stool antigen (GSA 65) useful in coprodiagnosis of giardiasis. *J Clin Microbiol* 1986;23:905.

100. Char S, Cevallos AM, Yamson P, et al. Impaired IgA response to *Giardia* heat shock antigen in children with persistent diarrhoea and giardiasis. *Gut* 1992;34:38–40.

101. Nash TE, Luján HT, Mowatt MR, et al. Variant-specific surface protein switching in *Giardia lamblia. Infect Immun* 2001;69:1922–1923.

102. Aggarwal A, Nash TE. Antigenic variation of *Giardia lamblia in vivo. Infect Immun* 1988;56:1420.

103. Adam RD, Aggarwal A, Lal AA, et al. Antigenic variation of a cysteine-rich protein in *Giardia lamblia. J Exp Med* 1988;167:109.

104. Upcroft JA, Capon AG, Dharmkrong-At A, et al. *Giardia intestinalis* antigens expressed in *Escherichia coli. Mol Exp Parasitol* 1987;26:267.

105. Char S, Shetty N, Elliott EJ, et al. Serum IgA response in children with *Giardia lamblia* infection and identification of an immunodominant 57-kDa antigen. *Parasite Immunol* 1991;13:329.

106. Char S, Cevallos AM, Farthing MJG. An immunodominant antigen of *Giardia lamblia* is a heat shock protein. *Biotechnol Ther* 1992;3:151.

107. Char S, Cevallos AM, Yamson P, et al. Impaired IgA response to *Giardia* heat shock antigen in children with persistent diarrhoea and giardiasis. *Gut* 1992;34:38.

108. Moore GT, Cross WM, McGuire D, et al. Epidemic giardiasis at a ski resort. *N Engl J Med* 1969;281:402.

109. Brodsky RE, Spencer HC, Schultz HG. Giardiasis in American travelers to the Soviet Union. *J Infect Dis* 1974;130:319.

110. Cantor D, Biempica L, Toccalino H, et al. Small intestine studies in giardiasis. *Am J Gastroenterol* 1967;47:134.

111. Tewari SG, Tandon BN. Functional and histological changes of small bowel in patients with *Giardia lamblia* infestation. *Indian J Med Res* 1974;62:689.

112. Rabassa EB Arbelo TF, Guillot CC, et al. Malabsorption por *Giardia lamblia. Rev Cubana Pediatr* 1975;47:247.

113. Wright SG, Tomkins AM, Ridley DS. Giardiasis: clinical and therapeutic aspects. *Gut* 1977;18:343.

114. Cortner JA. Giardiasis: a cause of celiac syndrome. *Am J Dis Child* 1959;98:311.

115. Farthing MJG. Giardiasis: pathogenesis of chronic diarrhea and impact on child growth and development. In: Lebenthal E, ed. *Chronic diarrhea in children.* New York: Raven Press, 1984:253–267.

116. Kay R, Barnes GL, Townley RRW. *Giardia lamblia* infestation in 154 children. *Aust Paediatr* 1977;13:98.

117. Webster ADB. Giardiasis and immunodeficiency diseases. *Trans R Soc Trop Med Hyg* 1980;74:440.

118. Kamath KR, Murugasu R. A comparative study of four methods for detecting *Giardia lamblia* in children with diarrheal illness and malabsorption. *Gastroenterology* 1974;66:16.

119. Madanagopalan N, Prabhakar Rao U, Somasundaram A, et al. A correlative study of duodenal aspirate and feces examination in giardiasis before and after treatment with metronidazole. *Curr Med Res Opin* 1975;3:99.

120. Thornton SA West AH, Du Pont HL, et al. Comparison of methods for identification of *Giardia Lamblia. Am J Clin Pathol* 1983;80:858.

121. Rosenthal P, Liebman WM. Comparative study of stool examinations: duodenal aspiration and pediatric Entero-Test for giardiasis in children. *J Pediatr* 1980;96:278.

122. Goka AKJ, Rolston DDK, Mathan VI, et al. The relative merits of faecal and duodenal juice microscopy in the diagnosis of giardiasis. *Trans R Soc Trop Med Hyg* 1990;84:66.

123. Craft JC, Nelson JD. Diagnosis of giardiasis by counterimmunoelectrophoresis of feces. *J Infect Dis* 1982;145:499.

124. Ungar BLP, Yolken PH, Nash TE, et al. Enzyme-linked immunosorbent assay for detection of *Giardia lamblia* in fecal specimens. *J Infect Dis* 1984;149:90.

125. Green EL, Miles MA, Warhurst DC. Immunodiagnostic detection of *Giardia* antigen in faeces by a rapid visual enzyme-linked immunosorbent assay. *Lancet* 1985;2:691.

126. Aldeen WE, Carroll K, Robison A, et al. Comparison of nine commercially available enzyme-linked immunosorbent assays for detection of *Giardia lamblia* in fecal specimens. *J Clin Microbiol* 1998;36:1338–1340.

127. Fedorko DP, Williams EC, Nelson NA, et al. Performance of three enzyme immunoassays and two direct fluorescence assays for detection of *Giardia*

lamblia in stool specimens preserved in ECOFIZ. *J Clin Microbiol* 2000;38:2781–2783.

128. Butcher PD, Farthing MJG. DNA probes for the faecal diagnosis of *Giardia lamblia* infections in man. *Biochem Soc Trans* 1988;17:363.

129. Butcher PB, Clark C, Farthing MJG. *Giardia lamblia* cloned genomic DNA probes: uses in faecal diagnosis and genetic analysis of clinical isolates. *Gut* 1988;29:A722.

130. Ghosh S, Debnath A, Sil A, et al. PCR detection of *Giardia lamblia* in stool: targeting intergenic spacer region of multicopy rRNA gene. *Mol Cell Probes* 2000;14:181–189.

131. Reynoldson JA, Behnke JM, Gracey M, et al. Efficacy of albendazole against *Giardia* and hookworm in a remote Aboriginal community in the north of Western Australia. *Acta Trop* 1998;71:27–44.

132. Farthing MJG, Inge PMG. Antigiardial activity of the bile salt-like antibiotic sodium fusidate. *J Antimicrob Chemother* 1986;17:165.

133. Farthing MJG, Inge PMG, Pearson RM. Effect of D-propranolol on growth and motility of flagellate protozoa. *J Antimicrob Chemother* 1987;20:519.

134. Hewlett EL, Pearson RD. Antiprotozoal activity of tricyclic compounds. *Science* 1985;230:1063.

135. Al-Waili NS, Al-Waili BH, Saloom KY. Therapeutic use of mebendazole in giardial infections. *Trans R Soc Trop Med Hyg* 1988;82:438.

136. Crouch AA, Seow WK, Whitman LM, et al. Sensitivity *in vitro* of *Giardia intestinalis* to dyadic combinations of azithromycin, deoxycyline, mefloquine, tinidazole and furazolidone. *Trans R Soc Trop Med Hyg* 1990;84:246–248.

137. Rossignol JF, Ayoub A, Ayers MS. Treatment of diarrhea caused by *Giardia intestinalis* and *Entamoeba histolytica* or *E. dispar*: a randomized, double-blind, placebo-controlled study of nitazoxanide. *J Infect Dis* 2001;184:381–384.

138. Ortiz JJ, Ayoub A, Gargala G, et al. Randomized clinical study of nitazoxanide compared to metronidazole in the treatment of symptomatic giardiasis in children from Northern Peru. *Aliment Pharmacol Ther* 2001;15:1409–1415.

139. Boreham PFL, Phillips RE, Shepherd RW. Heterogeneity in the responses of clones of *Giardia intestinalis* to antigiardial drugs. *Trans R Soc Trop Med Hyg* 1987;81:406.

140. Jokipii L, Jokipii AMM. *In vitro* susceptibility of *Giardia lamblia* trophozoites to metronidazole and tinidazole. *J Infect Dis* 1980;141:317.

141. Boreham PF, Phillips RE, Shepherd RW. The sensitivity of *Giardia intestinalis* to drugs *in vitro*. *J Antimicrob Chemother* 1984;14:449.

142. Inge PMG, Farthing MJG. A radiometric assay for antigiardial drugs. *Trans R Soc Trop Med Hyg* 1987;81:345.

143. Olson ME, Morck DW, Ceri H. Preliminary data on the efficacy of a *Giardia* vaccine in puppies. *Can Vet J* 1997;38:777–779.

144. Olson ME, Ceri H, Morck DW. *Giardia* vaccination. *Parasitol Today* 2000;16:213–217.

CHAPTER 279
Malaria and Babesiosis

Kathryn N. Suh and Jay S. Keystone

MALARIA

Historical Perspectives

Malaria has been a scourge of humans for centuries and continues to be a significant social and economic burden in endemic countries. From its speculated origins in Africa, malaria spread through the Mediterranean, Asia, and even to North America, where it was endemic in the United States and Canada during the eighteenth, nineteenth, and early twentieth centuries. Periodic fevers, possibly references to malaria, were described as early as the seventeenth century BC in Chinese, Egyptian, and Hindu writings. In the fifth century BC, Hippocrates described seasonal and geographic features of the illness in his patients in Greece, as well as clinical manifestations of the disease. The association between febrile illness and stagnant marsh water finally gave rise to the term malaria in eighteenth century Italy, in reference to the presumed miasmatic origin of the disease (*malo*, bad; *aria*, air).

Scientific knowledge of malaria was rapidly incremental in the late nineteenth and early twentieth centuries, with recorded observations of the parasite in human blood, and descriptions of its life cycle and mode of transmission. The first half of the twentieth century also heralded new developments in vector control (larvicides, insecticides) and antimalarial chemotherapy and led to optimism that malaria could be successfully eradicated. In 1957 the World Health Organization (WHO) launched its program for global malaria eradication, which was met with varying degrees of success around the world. The revised WHO strategy of 1969 emphasized greater involvement of general health services, in addition to improved malaria surveillance, development of new drugs and insecticides, and novel approaches to vector control. Since then, emphasis has shifted toward malaria prevention and reduction of attributable morbidity and mortality. Roll Back Malaria, a joint program of the WHO, UNICEF, the World Bank, and the United Nations Development Programme, was instituted in 1998 with the goal of reducing the global malaria burden by 50% by the year 2010 (1). The four main components of this program are (a) prompt institution of effective treatment for infected individuals, (b) reduction of mosquito-human contact, (c) prevention of malaria during pregnancy, and (d) timely detection and response to malaria epidemics. The persistence of malaria despite almost 50 years of organized effort to eliminate it is due to many factors, including inadequate provision of health care and public health programs in endemic areas, increasing human migration—both volitional (travel) and forced displacement resulting from wars or other civil unrest—and the increasing prevalence of plasmodial resistance to antimalarial agents and anopheline resistance to insecticides.

The Parasite and Its Life Cycle

Of more than 100 species of plasmodia, only 4 are significant causes of human infection. By far the most important is *Plasmodium falciparum;* not only does this species cause most cases globally, but it is also responsible for almost all malaria deaths. Infection by the other three species—*Plasmodium vivax, Plasmodium ovale,* and *Plasmodium malariae*—are milder and generally not fatal. Although the four species are similar in many respects, there are some important differences in their life cycles and morphological and clinical characteristics (Table 279.1). The life cycle of plasmodia is illustrated in Fig. 279.1.

THE HUMAN PHASE

Human infection has two components: the exoerythrocytic and erythrocytic phases (Fig. 279.1). The exoerythrocytic phase of infection begins with the release of infective sporozoites from the salivary glands of the feeding female mosquito. After entering the circulation, sporozoites rapidly and specifically invade hepatocytes, mediated by the binding of plasmodial circumsporozoite protein (CSP) to highly sulfated regions of hepatic heparan sulfate proteoglycans (2,3). After 1 to 2 weeks of development (depending on the species) as hepatic schizonts, merozoites are released and enter the bloodstream. Hepatic schizonts rupture simultaneously in infections due to *P. falciparum* and *P. malariae,* but in *P. vivax* and *P. ovale* infections, some may remain dormant (hypnozoites) for variable intervals—weeks to years—before releasing merozoites and causing clinical relapse(s) of malaria. The merozoites invade erythrocytes (the erythrocytic phase); *P. falciparum* invades erythrocytes of all ages, whereas *P. vivax* and *P. ovale* preferentially infect young red cells, and *P. malariae* older ones. Red blood cell (RBC) invasion depends on the interaction between merozoite surface proteins and erythrocyte receptors. The erythrocyte-binding antigen EBA 175 of *P. falciparum* binds to glycophorin A on the RBC surface (4) and shares some homology with the Duffy binding protein of *P. vivax,* which is required

TABLE 279.1.   Distinguishing Morphological and Clinical Characteristics of Human Malaria Infection

	Plasmodium falciparum	*Plasmodium vivax*	*Plasmodium ovale*	*Plasmodium malariae*
Morphology				
Trophozoites	Multiple ring forms per PRBC Multiple chromatin dots common	Small, ameboid Double chromatin dot occasionally	Small Single chromatin dot	Small Pigment bands visible
Schizonts	Rarely seen due to sequestering 6–24 merozoites	Visible 12–24 merozoites	Visible 4–12 merozoites	Visible 6–12 merozoites
Gametocytes	Banana shaped; pathognomonic	Round	Round	Round
PRBCs	Infects RBCs of all ages PRBCs are normal size Knobs on EM Maurer's dots Suspect if >2% of RBCs are infected	Infects young RBCs PRBCs are enlarged, irregularly shaped Schüffner's dots	Infects young RBCs PRBCs slightly enlarged with fimbriated edges Schüffner's dots	Infects older RBCs PRBCs small to normal size
Clinical features				
Incubation period	10–14 d	12–18 d	12–18 d	Usually 18–40 d; can be much longer
Duration from infection to onset of symptoms	98% symptomatic by 2 mo, but may be delayed in semiimmune individuals	50% by 2 mo 80% by 1 yr	Up to 3 yr	May be significantly delayed (many years)
Paroxysms (if present)	48 hr	48 hr	48 hr	72 hr
Relapses	No	Common within first 6 mo if hypnozoites untreated	Common within first 6 mo if hypnozoites untreated	No
Other features	Most severe form of malaria, potentially fatal	Most commonly identified species in North America		Most common species in transfusion-related malaria

EM, electron microscopy; PRBCs, parasitized red blood cells; RBCs, red blood cells.

for this species to bind to erythrocytes bearing Duffy blood group determinants (5).

Within the erythrocyte, merozoites begin the process of asexual reproduction. Ring forms, the earliest trophozoites, are visible microscopically (Fig. 279.2A and B); nuclei appear as blue chromatin dots with Giemsa's stain. Characteristics of trophozoites are useful in speciating plasmodia (Table 279.1). As trophozoites develop, they become more irregular in shape, and hemoglobin-degradation products may be visible as pigmented granules within the cytoplasm. The first division of the trophozoite nucleus produces an erythrocytic schizont (Fig. 279.2C). In *P. falciparum* infections, unlike those due to other species, schizonts are rarely seen on peripheral blood films because they are sequestered within the microvasculature. Repeated nuclear division culminates in the release of 6 to 24 merozoites from each schizont. This process of erythrocytic schizogony may be periodic, giving rise to the cyclic fevers classically associated with malaria infection; the periodicity varies depending on the infecting species (Table 279.1). Some merozoites will invade uninfected erythrocytes to begin another cycle of erythrocytic schizogony, whereas others will develop into sexual forms or gametocytes (Fig. 279.2D), which may be visible in peripheral blood 3 to 15 days after the onset of illness.

THE VECTOR (MOSQUITO) PHASE

Anophelines feeding on infected humans ingest male and female gametocytes, which reproduce sexually. Within the mosquito midgut, the male gametocyte gives rise to four to eight microgametes, which fertilize the female and produce an ookinete that is attached to the lining. The ookinete matures into an oocyst; repeated nuclear division produces thousands of sporozoites from each oocyst. Sporozoites are released into the body cavity of the

mosquito and migrate to the salivary glands, where they are infective for humans and initiate another life cycle.

Epidemiology

Malaria is one of the most prevalent human infections in the world. The exact incidence and prevalence are unknown, because of underreporting, inconsistent and erratic methods of diagnosis and reporting, and variable surveillance. An estimated 41% of the world's population (2.3 billion people) lived in malarious regions in 1994; 300 to 500 million cases (34.8 million of which were reported to the WHO) and 1.5 to 2.7 million deaths occur annually (6). More than 90% of deaths occur in sub-Saharan Africa, half in children younger than 5 years. In addition to young children, other populations at high risk of severe morbidity and death include pregnant women—particularly primigravidas—and nonimmune individuals such as travelers and foreign laborers. In epidemics, which often occur in association with civil strife and mass movement of large populations (e.g., refugees), all age-groups may be at risk of severe disease. Malaria is among the most common causes of death reported among refugees (7). Epidemics have also been attributed to changes in climate, agriculture, and industry, however. Overall, an estimated $12 billion in economic revenue is lost each year in Africa because of malaria.

Malaria is transmitted by the night-biting female *Anopheles* mosquito (only females consume blood meals). Relatively few of the many *Anopheles* species are effective vectors for transmission of disease; the predominant species varies depending on locale. Interestingly, anopheline species capable of transmitting malaria are widely distributed in the United States; the two most important are *Anopheles quadrimaculatus* and *Anopheles freeborni*

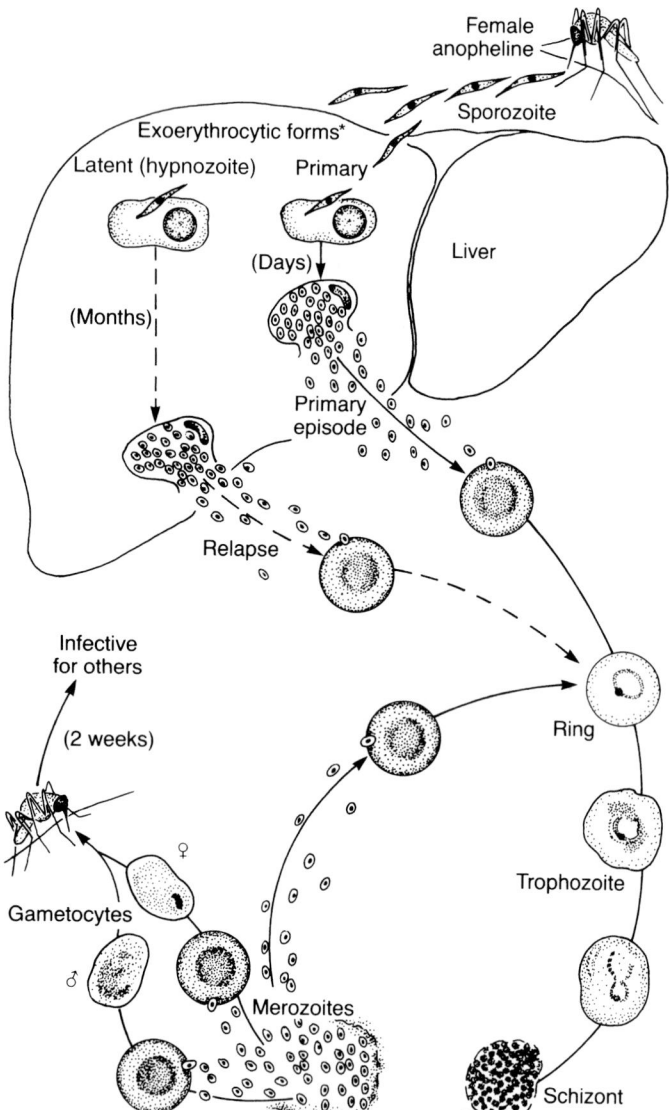

Figure 279.1. The life cycle of plasmodia in humans. *Exoerythrocytic forms are also called tissue *schizonts*.

(8). Malaria transmission from mosquito to human is optimal in warm climates (20°C to 30°C) with relatively high humidity (more than 60%). High humidity not only leads to rain, thereby increasing the number of breeding areas for mosquitoes, but also increases anopheline survival and therefore the likelihood of a mosquito becoming infective for humans. Altitude is also a factor due to temperature change; malaria is rarely acquired at altitudes above 2,000 m.

Geographically, malaria risk is present in 105 countries (Fig. 279.3), albeit to varying degrees; in 13, only *P. vivax* has been reported (Table 279.2). More than 90% of all malaria cases occur in Africa, where *P. falciparum* is the predominant species; *P. falciparum* also predominates in Haiti and the Dominican Republic. Infection by *P. malariae* occurs in these same regions but is relatively uncommon. *P. vivax* infection is rare in Africa; black Africans are relatively resistant to *P. vivax* infection because they lack the Duffy blood group, which is required for erythrocytic invasion by this parasite (9). Both *P. vivax* and *P. falciparum* cause infections in Mexico, Central and South America, the Mediterranean, Southeast Asia, India, and Oceania. Infection by *P. ovale*, which is found mainly in Africa, is relatively

rare. Malaria transmission has been successfully interrupted in Canada, the United States, the Caribbean, most of Europe (except for Armenia, Turkey, and areas of the former Soviet Union), and parts of South America and Asia (Fig. 279.3).

Imported malaria currently accounts for most cases of malaria reported in industrialized nations. In 1997, 1,036 cases were reported in Canada (10), and 1,227 in the United States in 1998 (11). Of the U.S. cases, 60% were acquired in Africa, 20% in Asia (mainly India), and 19% in the Americas. *P. vivax* caused more than one third of all cases and most of those from Asia and the Americas (68% to 78%), whereas *P. falciparum* accounted for most cases from Africa. "Runway" and "airport" malaria have been described (12,13), and outbreaks of autochthonous malaria within the United States are increasingly reported (8). Transfusion-transmitted infection can also occur (14,15); though rare, this has obvious public health implications and in Canada has led to rejection of blood donations from individuals with a history of malaria (14). Plasmodial resistance to antimalarial agents and anopheline resistance to insecticides is discussed in greater detail in the relevant sections of this chapter.

Pathogenesis of Infection

Falciparum malaria differs distinctly from infection by *P. vivax*, *P. ovale*, and *P. malariae*, with respect to both clinical illness and the pathogenesis of infection. Pathogenesis of malaria is best understood for *P. falciparum*, although there continues to be debate regarding the exact mechanisms of disease and much is still unknown. A more thorough understanding of pathogenetic mechanisms may identify targets for the development of new antimalarial therapies.

PATHOGENESIS OF *P. FALCIPARUM* MALARIA

The severe clinical manifestations of *P. falciparum* malaria are attributable to two major factors: (a) cytoadherence, leading to microvascular occlusive phenomena, and (b) release of parasite toxins and stimulation of the inflammatory cytokine cascade. The relative contribution of each mechanism remains unclear, but ample evidence exists in support of both in the pathogenesis of falciparum malaria. In addition, parasitization of RBCs also leads to direct hematologic and metabolic derangements independent of the first two mechanisms.

Cytoadherence. *Cytoadherence* refers to the sequestration of infected erythrocytes in the microvascular circulation, with resultant vasoocclusive phenomena. Parasitized RBCs (PRBCs) may bind to other infected cells (autoagglutination), to uninfected RBCs (rosetting), or to vascular endothelium (16), the latter usually in postcapillary venules of deeper tissues. The most severe clinical consequence of cytoadherence is cerebral malaria, due to adherence of PRBCs to cerebrovascular endothelium (17), although other organs can also be involved. The severity of disease appears to correlate directly with the degree of cytoadherence, particularly rosetting (18). However, severe disease in mice can also result from infection with nonsequestering plasmodial species, suggesting that other virulence mechanisms may be equally important.

Erythrocytes infected with mature parasites lose their normal biconcave shape and become distended, rigid spheres with multiple protrusions or knobs on the cell surface, a result of deposition of parasitic proteins within the RBC. The importance of knobs in causing disease has been demonstrated by the mild clinical illness in monkeys infected with knobless PRBCs (19). An antigenically variable, high-molecular-weight protein encoded by the parasitic *var* gene, known as *P. falciparum* erythrocyte membrane protein 1 (PfEMP1), is one of several polypeptides

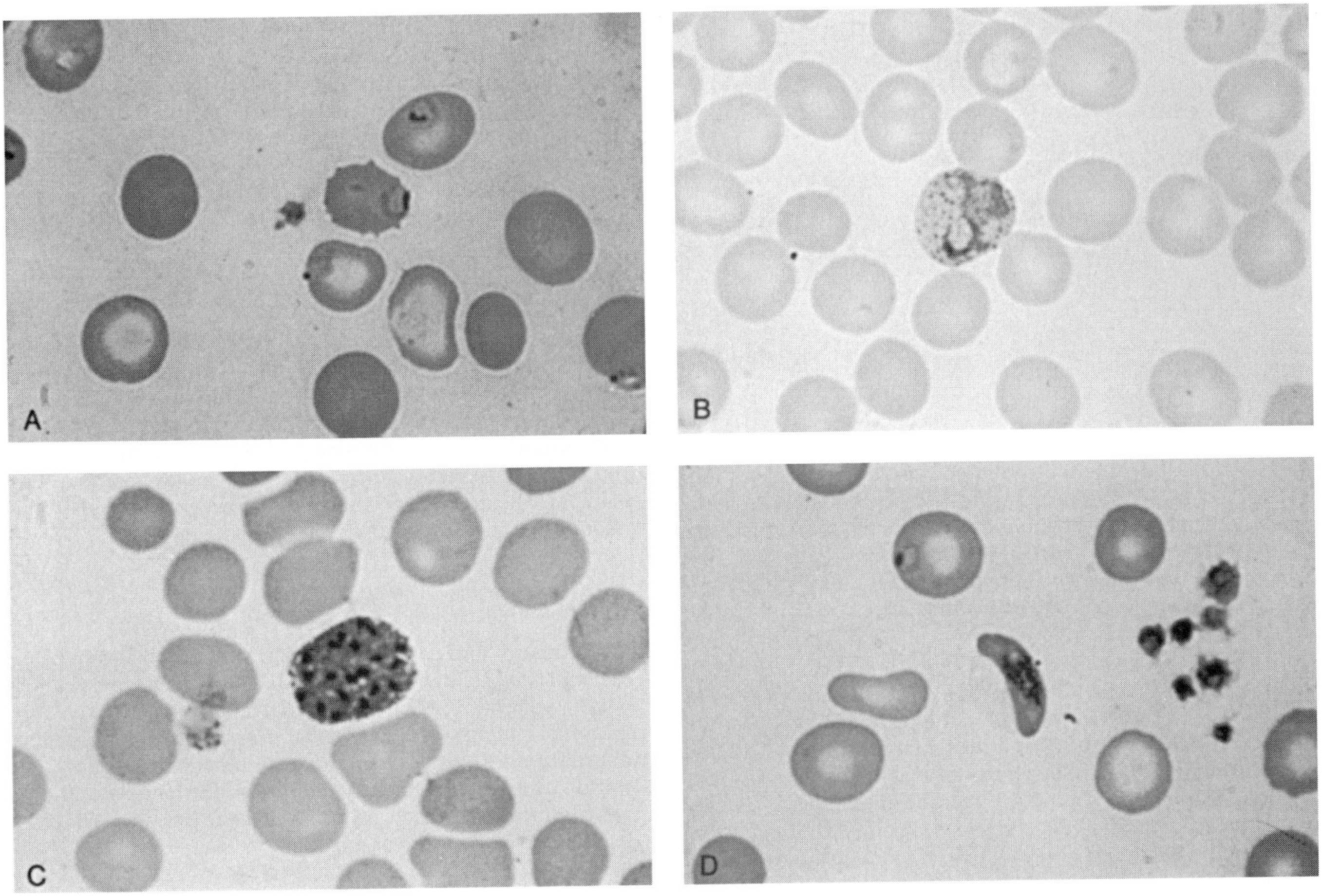

Figure 279.2. Stages in the life cycle of plasmodia that infect humans. **A:** Ring stage of *Plasmodium falciparum.* **B:** Trophozoite of *Plasmodium vivax,* showing Schüffner's dots. Note that the infected erythrocyte is slightly enlarged. **C:** Schizont of *P. vivax,* containing merozoites. **D:** Pathognomonic banana-shaped gametocyte of *P. falciparum.*

expressed on the surface of the RBC knobs and is felt to be the major parasitic adherence ligand (20–22). Other possible adhesins (rifins, rosettins) have also been identified (16,23). PfEMP1 interacts with receptors on a variety of host cells. Several receptors have been identified: chondroitin sulfate and intercellular ad-

hesion molecule-1 (ICAM-1) on endothelium; heparan sulfate, A and B blood group antigens, and complement receptor 1 on RBCs; and the platelet receptors CD36 and platelet-endothelial cell adhesion molecule-1 (also known as CD31) (16,23). Recently, hyaluronic acid has been identified as a major placental receptor

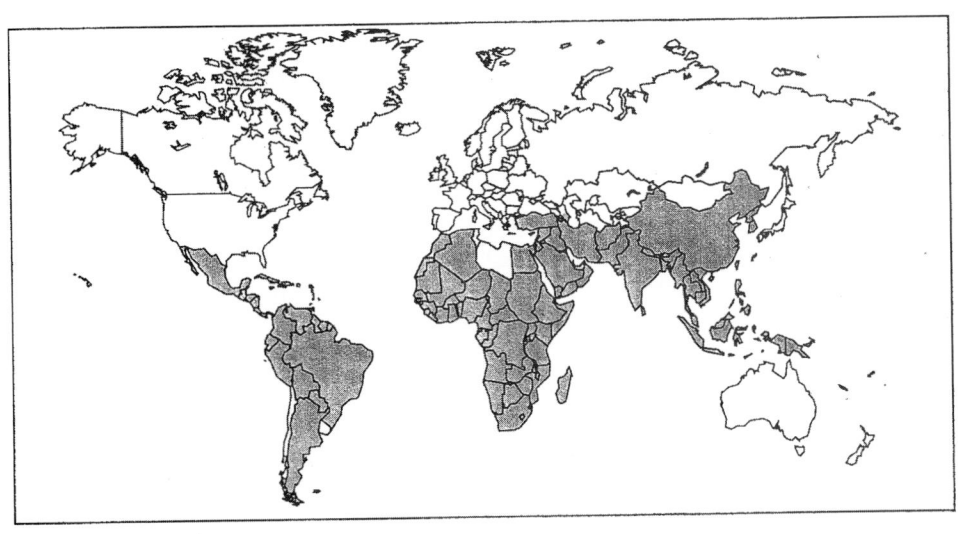

Figure 279.3. Areas of malaria risk. Map is intended as a visual aid only. (From the Centers for Disease Control and Prevention, 2000.)

▨ Countries with Malaria Risk   ☐ Countries with No Malaria Risk

TABLE 279.2.	Countries with *Plasmodium vivax* Infections Only
Continent/world region	**Country**
South America	Argentina
Africa	Algeria, Mauritius
Asia	North Korea, South Korea
Middle East	Iraq, Morocco, Syria
Europe	Armenia, Azerbaijan, Georgia, Turkmenistan, Turkey

Source: Adapted from World Health Organization. World malaria situation in 1994. Parts I–III. *Wkly Epid Rec* 1997;72:269–274, 277–283, 285–290.

(24). Several other putative receptors are under investigation. Unanswered questions include which receptors are most important, the relative contributions of each in the cytoadherence process, and the possibility of synergy between two or more receptors. Research in this area of malaria pathogenesis is clearly evolving, and much more remains to be learned.

Malaria Toxins and Cytokines. Malaria "toxins" and cytokines have also been implicated in the pathogenesis of severe disease. Cytokines are released with schizont rupture. Proteins released from *P. falciparum* trophozoites and schizonts act as toxins, stimulating the inflammatory cascade and leading to overproduction of cytokines (25); glycosylphosphatidylinositol of *P. falciparum* is one such parasite toxin (26). In addition, hemozoin pigment has been shown to induce interleukin-1 (IL-1) and tumor necrosis factor-α (TNF-α) production (27).

High levels of TNF-α, IL-1, and interferon-α (IFN-α) have been found in the circulation of patients with severe malaria (28), and extensive local deposition of cytokines has been demonstrated in fatal cases of cerebral malaria (29). Proposed effects of cytokines, in addition to causing fever, include up-regulation of endothelial receptors and nitric oxide production, and suppression of erythropoiesis (23). Nitric oxide was long ago suggested as one mediator responsible for the manifestations of cerebral malaria (30). Polymorphisms in the TNF promoter region (31) and the nitric oxide synthase promoter (32,33) have been associated with altered susceptibility to severe malaria. However, a randomized trial of anti–TNF-α monoclonal antibodies in severe cerebral malaria has not demonstrated any therapeutic benefit apart from fever reduction (34).

Parasitized Erythrocytes. The rupture of PRBCs causes intravascular hemolytic anemia, which can be severe (blackwater fever) and may lead to hemoglobinuria with secondary acute renal failure. In addition, parasites can consume large amounts of glucose; in conjunction with depleted hepatic glycogen stores and impaired gluconeogenesis, this may lead to significant pretreatment hypoglycemia, which may then be compounded by the effects of quinine therapy.

Host (Genetic) Factors. Genetic factors can affect an individual's susceptibility to infection, illness, and severe disease. In addition to the natural resistance to *P. vivax* infection conferred by a single mutation in the Duffy antigen gene (35), other genetic variations within the human host have been associated with either reduced or enhanced susceptibility to malaria.

Protection conferred against falciparum malaria by heterozygosity for sickle cell disease in Africa has ensured the persistence of this potentially fatal gene (36,37); similarly, glucose-6-phosphate dehydrogenase (G6PD) deficiency and ovalocytosis are also protective against severe malaria (38,39), and α-thalassemia is thought to be, although this has not been proven (40,41). Polymorphisms in the human leukocyte antigen (HLA) B gene (37) and ICAM-1 (42) have also been associated with altered susceptibility to malaria in Africa. Again, much research remains to be done in this area.

PATHOGENESIS OF MALARIA CAUSED BY OTHER PLASMODIA

Cytoadherence does not occur in *P. vivax*, *P. ovale*, and *P. malariae* infections, and microvascular complications do not occur. Symptoms are therefore related only to parasitemia, and illness is generally milder and nonfatal compared with falciparum malaria. Furthermore, because of the propensity of these three species to infect only selected erythrocytes (young or old), massive hemolysis generally does not occur. However, several deaths have been associated with *P. vivax* infection (43).

Immunology

Both humoral and cell-mediated immune responses have been demonstrated following natural infection and administration of malaria vaccines. Although both mechanisms seem to be important in modulating the severity of disease, complete protective immunity does not develop, because repeated infections occur in individuals living in endemic areas. Furthermore, the relative importance of each immune mechanism appears to vary depending on the stage of infection.

PREERYTHROCYTIC IMMUNITY

Murine immunity to malaria has been conferred by induction of antisporozoite antibodies and by cell-mediated immune responses (44). In humans, nonprotective levels of antibody to plasmodial CSP are produced following natural infection (45). However, the main immune effector mechanisms against the preerythrocytic (sporozoite and hepatic) stages of malaria are thought to be mediated by CD8$^+$ T lymphocytes, which produce protective IFN-γ in mice (46). Deoxyribonucleic acid (DNA)–based vaccines using CSP have been shown to induce a CD8$^+$ cell response in humans, without production of detectable levels of CSP antibody (47). Parasites can evade this cell-mediated immune response, however, by interfering with T-cell priming and rendering CD8$^+$ cells unable to produce IFN-γ (48). IFN-γ is also produced by CD4$^+$, natural killer, and $\gamma\delta$ T cells (49–51). Protective, IFN-γ producing CD4$^+$ cells can also be induced by recombinant CSP vaccine (52). Cytokines, particularly IFN-γ, protect against reinfection at the hepatic stage but probably also during the erythrocytic stage (53).

ERYTHROCYTIC IMMUNITY

Protection against the blood stage of malaria infection is mediated by both humoral and cell-mediated responses (44). In natural infection, protection is primarily mediated by antibodies against parasite proteins that are expressed on merozoites and PRBCs (46); such antibodies can inhibit parasite maturation by preventing RBC invasion, mediating PRBC lysis and enhancing phagocytosis (54). Antirosette antibody titers have been found to be lower in children with severe malaria compared with those with uncomplicated disease (18,55). Antibodies do not prevent infection but appear to modulate the course of illness and protect against severe malaria. Cytokines probably also play a protective role at this stage (56) but have the potential to be pathogenic.

IMPLICATIONS FOR VACCINE DEVELOPMENT

Human immune responses in malaria are clearly varied and complex and provide many possible targets for malaria vaccines. The multitude of P. falciparum antigens described to date, their genetic variability, the lack of cross-reactivity among these antigens, and the parasite's proven ability to evade immune defenses have created significant challenges in vaccine development. All of these issues must be considered during the development of an effective vaccine.

Malaria vaccines can aim to either prevent disease altogether, by preventing hepatic invasion by sporozoites or merozoite invasion of RBCs (preerythrocytic vaccines), or prevent severe disease and death (blood stage vaccines); the former might be more suitable for use in nonimmune populations, the latter in individuals living in endemic areas (56). Vaccines against preerythrocytic parasites must ensure compete protection against tissue invasion—one sporozoite can give rise to 30,000 merozoites and cause severe disease—and blood stage immunization, if used in those at greatest risk of severe disease in endemic areas (i.e., children), may prevent them from acquiring natural immunity and only expose them to potentially fatal infection at a later age. Although research is progressing in this field, there are still many obstacles to overcome.

Clinical Manifestations of Malaria

Symptoms of malaria rarely develop before departure from an endemic area; 85% to 90% of infected travelers will become symptomatic only after their return (11,57,58). Most of those with P. falciparum infections present within 4 to 6 weeks of their return (11,58,59). In contrast, P. vivax infections may not become apparent for weeks to several months after return (11,58). Most infections become symptomatic within the first year after return, regardless of the infecting species. The shortest incubation for malaria is approximately 10 days, with the longest up to 40 years (for P. malariae). Symptoms may be mild in semiimmune individuals (immigrants or visitors from highly endemic areas, primarily Africa) and in travelers taking antimalarial chemoprophylaxis (60).

Fever, the hallmark of malaria, occurs in almost all patients and usually in conjunction with other nonspecific symptoms, most commonly chills, headache, and malaise (58,59,61–64). Myalgias and sore throat can be present and may lead to the diagnosis of a viral illness. Nausea and vomiting are the most common gastrointestinal (GI) symptoms, but diarrhea and abdominal pain may also occur. Pulmonary symptoms are uncommon; fewer than 20% of patients complain of cough, and dyspnea and chest pain occur in fewer than 5%.

Classic paroxysms of fever occur only in synchronous infections, in which all intraerythrocytic parasites mature simultaneously. The classic tertian fever, occurring every 48 hours in P. falciparum, P. vivax, and P. ovale infections, and the quartan fever (every 72 hours) associated with P. malariae infection are rare (59). More commonly, fever is hectic, with no discernible pattern; this is the rule in P. falciparum infection. Therefore, fever pattern cannot be relied on to exclude the diagnosis of malaria. The protean symptoms of malaria in addition to the omission (or disregard) of a travel history often lead to an incorrect or delayed diagnosis, sometimes with grave consequences. Semiimmune patients, particularly those from sub-Saharan Africa, are often asymptomatically infected with P. falciparum, and the presence of fever and parasitemia in this group should always raise the suspicion of another diagnosis (65).

The most common physical finding apart from fever (usually higher than 38°C) is splenomegaly, present in one fourth to one

third of patients (58,59,61,64). Other less common findings may include hepatomegaly, jaundice, and abdominal tenderness; rash (urticarial) and pulmonary findings are rare. Lymphadenopathy is not usually a feature of malaria and its presence should suggest another (or additional) diagnosis.

Clinical findings suggestive of severe malaria include a decreased level of consciousness with or without focal neurologic findings, prostration, respiratory distress, and/or pulmonary edema, hypotension, abnormal bleeding, and/or jaundice (66) (Table 279.3). Complications of falciparum malaria usually begin when parasitemia reaches 5% or greater. Severe malaria is a medical emergency; even with timely institution of appropriate antimalarial therapy and advanced medical care, more than 20% of patients die of complications (67). Respiratory and renal failure, hypoglycemia, metabolic acidosis, severe anemia, coma, and secondary bacterial infection may all contribute to death. It is not uncommon for respiratory failure to develop during the recovery phase of a severe infection.

Laboratory and Radiologic Findings

Laboratory findings in malaria are similarly nonspecific and can be summarized based on several case series (58,59,61,67). Hematologic abnormalities include thrombocytopenia (platelet count $<150,000/mm^3$) in 50% to 70% of infected individuals, and anemia (hemoglobin $<12 g/dL$) in one fourth to one third; anemia may worsen as the disease progresses. The total leukocyte count is usually normal or low; leukocytosis is not usually a feature of malaria and is seen in about 5% of cases. Hypoglycemia, especially in the nondiabetic patient, should raise suspicion of malaria, although it is rare on presentation. Electrolyte abnormalities, particularly hyponatremia, can be present, and a metabolic acidosis may be seen in severe malaria but is reversible with treatment. Serum creatinine is elevated (more than 1.2 mg/dL) in fewer than 15% of patients on presentation. Liver function test results are often elevated: lactose dehydrogenase level in approximately 80%, aspartate aminotransferase (AST) in 25% or more, alkaline phosphatase in 20%, and bilirubin in 30% to 40%.

Radiologic investigations are usually noncontributory in uncomplicated malaria, although nonspecific pulmonary infiltrates, increased vascular markings, and pleural effusions have

---

TABLE 279.3. Criteria for Severe Malaria

A history of possible malaria exposure, and no other cause for clinical illness; or, laboratory diagnosis of *Plasmodium falciparum* malaria
And
One or more of the following:
1. Prostration, impaired consciousness, or coma
2. Renal failure
3. Respiratory distress
4. Circulatory collapse or shock
5. Spontaneous bleeding or disseminated intravascular coagulation
6. Repeated generalized seizures
7. Radiographic evidence of pulmonary edema
8. Jaundice
9. Severe anemia
10. Hypoglycemia
11. Metabolic acidosis
12. Hemoglobinuria
13. Parasitemia of >5% in a nonimmune individual

Source: Adapted from World Health Organization. Severe falciparum malaria. *Trans R Soc Trop Med Hyg* 2000;94[suppl 1]:1–90.

been described (68,69). In severe infections with more than 5% parasitemia, findings consistent with noncardiogenic pulmonary edema are common. Computed tomography or magnetic resonance imaging scans may reveal mild brain swelling in cases of cerebral malaria, but focal lesions are unusual (66).

Pathology

Death is almost always caused by infection with *P. falciparum*. Gross autopsy findings include diffuse distribution of malaria pigment (hemozoin), which imparts a gray or brown coloration to affected tissues. Cerebral congestion and edema render the brain pink; intracerebral hemorrhage may be noted, in addition to evidence of PRBC sequestration within the cerebral microvasculature. Pigmentation, congestion, and enlargement of other organs including the spleen, liver, kidneys, and lungs are common. Histologic sections reveal parasitized or ruptured erythrocytes, macrophages, and malarial pigment; glomerulonephritis or immune complex deposition may be evident in the kidney. Placental pathology reveals similar changes, but the placental size may be reduced and parasites are usually concentrated only on the maternal aspect of the placenta.

Diagnosis of Malaria

Rapid accurate diagnosis of malaria is essential to institute appropriate antimalarial therapy. Examination of peripheral blood films is currently the gold standard for diagnosis but requires adequate laboratory facilities and sufficient expertise in reading films. Unfortunately, accurate interpretation of malaria smears remains problematic, particularly in laboratories located outside major referral centers (57,70). Newer diagnostic tests designed to overcome these problems and improve sensitivity include fluorescent microscopy, rapid diagnostic tests (RDTs) for detection of parasite antigens, and molecular methods such as polymerase chain reaction (PCR); each of these tests has its own limitations, however. The sensitivities, specificities, relative merits, and shortcomings of each are shown in Table 279.4.

MALARIA SMEARS

Blood for malaria smears should be obtained using fresh blood from the febrile patient, preferably before therapy is initiated. Both thick and thin smears should be requested. Giemsa's stain is preferred but Wright-Giemsa or Field's stains can also be used. Thick smears are more difficult to read, but are 10 times more

TABLE 279.4.   Summary of Diagnostic Tests for Malaria

Method of detection	Available tests	Sensitivity[a]	Specificity[a]	Advantages	Disadvantages
Blood films					
Direct examination for parasites	Thick and thin smears	80%–90%	>90%	Inexpensive Permits speciation	Time consuming Experience required
Fluorescence microscopy					
Acridine orange staining of parasitic nucleic acids					Sensitivity ↓ with low-level parasitemia Does not permit speciation Special equipment needed for acridine orange methods
	Acridine orange QBC	83%–98% >90%	≥86% ≥90%	Rapid, inexpensive Rapid	Experience required Expensive Cannot archive for future reference Technical problems can occur
Antigen detection					
Detection of histidine-rich protein-2 of *Plasmodium falciparum*				Both are rapid and easy to perform, and interpret	Cannot quantify parasitemia Sensitivity ↓ with low-level parasitemia Does not detect other plasmodial species Prolonged antigenemia after infection
	*Para*Sight-F	84%–95%	>90%	False negative if only mature gametocytes present	High false-positive rate due to rheumatoid factor in earlier versions
	ICT Malaria Pf	90%–100%	>95%		Some reagents require refrigeration
Detection of parasite lactate dehydrogenase	OptiMAL	93%–95%	99%–100%	Detects only viable parasites	Cannot quantify parasitemia Sensitivity ↓ with low-level parasitemia Cannot detect *Plasmodium ovale* or *Plasmodium malariae*
Polymerase chain reaction					
Nucleic acid amplification and detection		90%–100%	About 100%	High sensitivity and specificity	Labor intensive Potential for dead parasites to cause false-positive reactions

[a]Sensitivity and specificity: for blood films, relative to polymerase chain reaction (PCR); for fluorescence microscopy and antigen detection, relative to PCR and/or blood smear; for PCR, relative to blood films.

sensitive than thin smears and are therefore preferred for screening; the smear is considered negative if no parasites are seen after 10 minutes of examination (71). Thin smears allow identification of the infecting species and will at least exclude life-threatening high-level parasitemia. Parasite density (quantification) is reported as the percentage of RBCs infected on a thin smear examined under oil immersion. Smears should be repeated at least twice within 48 hours before malaria is excluded and can be useful for following response to therapy.

Malaria smears are inexpensive and allow rapid, precise identification of the infecting plasmodial species. Disadvantages in addition to those listed include the time (60 minutes) and labor required for preparation and interpretation; in addition, there is often a significant delay in communicating results.

FLUORESCENT MICROSCOPY

Several different fluorescent microscopy techniques are available for the diagnosis of malaria. Acridine orange (AO) methods, including the quantitative buffy coat test in which blood is centrifuged and lysed before staining (commercially available as the QBC, Becton Dickinson, Cockeysville, Maryland), preferentially stain parasitic nucleic acids. Reported sensitivities of AO methods are highly variable, ranging from 41% to 97% depending on parasite density and species (72–75); sensitivity decreases markedly with low-level parasitemia (76,77). A benzothiocarboxypurine procedure, based on the same principle as AO methods, has more than 90% sensitivity and specificity (78). Though rapid, disadvantages include the need for specialized equipment and the inability to speciate plasmodia.

RAPID DETECTION TESTS

Rapid antigen-detection tests are based on the detection of parasite proteins in fingerprick blood samples. Histidine-rich protein 2 (HRP-2), produced only by *P. falciparum,* is the basis of both the *Para* Sight-F (Becton Dickinson) and the ICT Malaria Pf (AMRAD-ICT, Brookvale, Australia) tests. The OptiMAL dipstick (Flow Inc., Portland, Oregon) detects parasite lactate dehydrogenase (pLDH) produced by all four human plasmodia, although to date only *P. falciparum* and *P. vivax* infections can be diagnosed using this method.

The HRP-2–based tests have comparable sensitivities of 84% to 100% and specificities of 81% to 100% (77,79–83). HRP-2 antigenemia can persist for several weeks after infection (27% at 28 days) (79), which can lead to false-positive test results if repeated and therefore limit its use as a "test of cure." Major shortcomings include the inability to diagnose infections caused by non-falciparum species and a marked reduction in sensitivity with low levels of parasitemia (79,81). A newer combined test for both *P. falciparum* and *P. vivax,* the ICT Malaria Pf/Pv (AMRAD-ICT, Sydney, Australia), is also available (84). Test characteristics of the pLDH-based OptiMAL assay are somewhat better (sensitivity 93% to 95%, specificity 99% to 100%) (83,85), although sensitivity is again dependent on parasite density (86). In contrast to the HRP-2–based tests, the pLDH test detects only viable parasites and can be used to assess response to therapy. Some reagents require refrigeration, however, potentially limiting its use in field settings. Regardless, the diagnostic accuracy and simplicity of these tests make them attractive for use both in endemic areas where laboratory facilities and expertise may be lacking and in medical centers in which malaria is infrequently encountered.

MOLECULAR DIAGNOSIS

PCR using various parasite gene targets is more than 90% sensitive compared with standard microscopy (87–89) and can confirm the diagnosis when smears for malaria are negative (90).

Other advantages of PCR include its ability to detect low-level parasitemia that might be missed using other methods (89) and its utility in diagnosing mixed infections. The specialized equipment and the time and labor required make routine use of PCR unfeasible, however.

OTHER DIAGNOSTIC METHODS

Other diagnostic methods studied for malaria diagnosis include automated detection of malaria pigment (91,92) and flow cytometry (93), although neither method has been widely used. Malaria serology is available, although a positive result reflects only previous exposure and is not generally useful in the diagnosis of acute disease.

Treatment

Malaria in the nonimmune individual should be considered a medical emergency, and prompt therapy is essential to maximize survival. Admission to hospital is recommended for all patients with falciparum malaria, and those with severe illness or in whom speciation cannot be determined. Severely ill patients should be admitted to an intensive care unit. If the species cannot be identified, the patient should be assumed to have *P. falciparum* malaria until proven otherwise. Treatment for malaria may be warranted in absence of a laboratory-confirmed diagnosis, given an appropriate exposure history and compatible clinical picture. Supportive care including judicious fluid replacement, antipyretics, and prevention and therapy of complications should be routine.

The antimalarial agents of choice and route of administration depend on the infecting species and the likelihood of drug resistance (Table 279.5 and Figs. 279.4 and 279.5), as well as host factors (e.g., age, pregnancy, and severity of illness). Chloroquine resistance in *P. falciparum,* first detected in the late 1950s, is now widespread (Table 279.5). Chloroquine-resistant *P. vivax* was first reported in Papua, New Guinea, in 1991 (94) and in South America in 1996 (95). Mefloquine resistance first appeared along the Thai-Burmese border in the early 1990s (96) and remains limited to this area (Fig. 279.5). More recently, evidence of primaquine resistance in *P. vivax* has emerged (97). [Readers are referred elsewhere for reviews of chloroquine and primaquine resistance in plasmodia (98,99).]

Treatment guidelines are outlined in Tables 279.6 and 279.7. Currently available antimalarial drugs, their mechanisms of action, and toxicities have been described elsewhere in this text and thus are not discussed in detail here.

TABLE 279.5. Geographic Distribution of Drug-Resistant Malaria

Plasmodium falciparum	
Chloroquine resistant	All areas where *P. falciparum* infection occurs except: Mexico, Dominican Republic, Haiti, Central America west/north of the Panama Canal, Argentina, North Africa, and parts of the Middle East and China
Mefloquine resistant	Thailand, along the Cambodian and Myanmar borders
Pyrimethamine-sulfadoxine (Fansidar) resistant	Amazon Basin, Southeast Asia, Africa
Plasmodium vivax	
Chloroquine resistant	Oceania, Myanmar, Guyana, Colombia, Brazil
Primaquine resistant	Oceania, Southeast Asia, Somalia

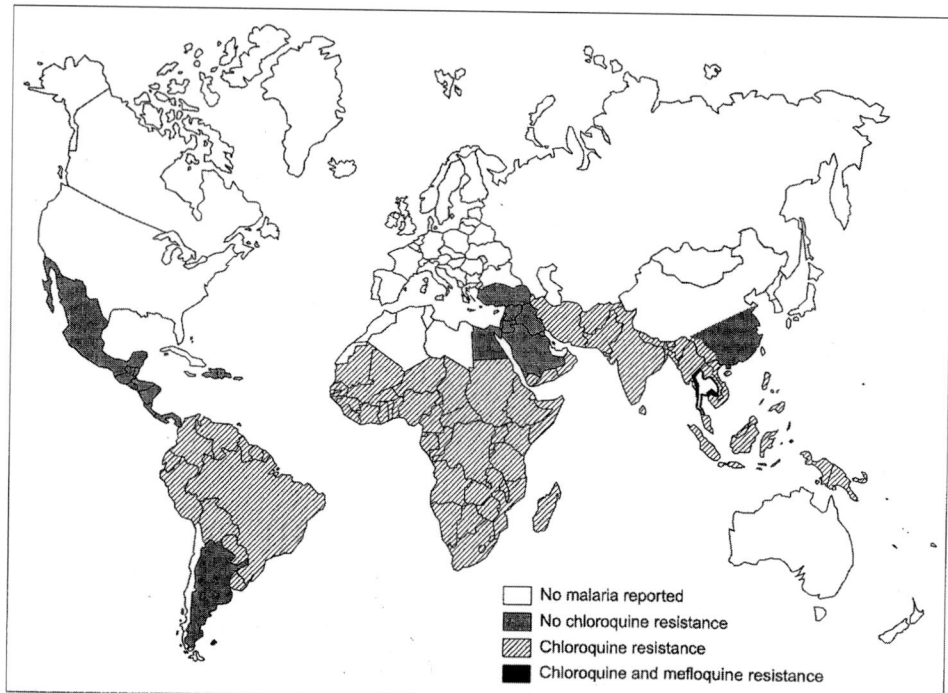

Figure 279.4. Geographic distribution of drug-resistant malaria. Map is intended as a visual aid only. [From Committee to Advise on Tropical Medicine and Travel (CATMAT). Canadian recommendations for the prevention and treatment of malaria among international travelers 2000. *Can Comm Dis Rep* 2000;26(S2):1–42, with permission.]

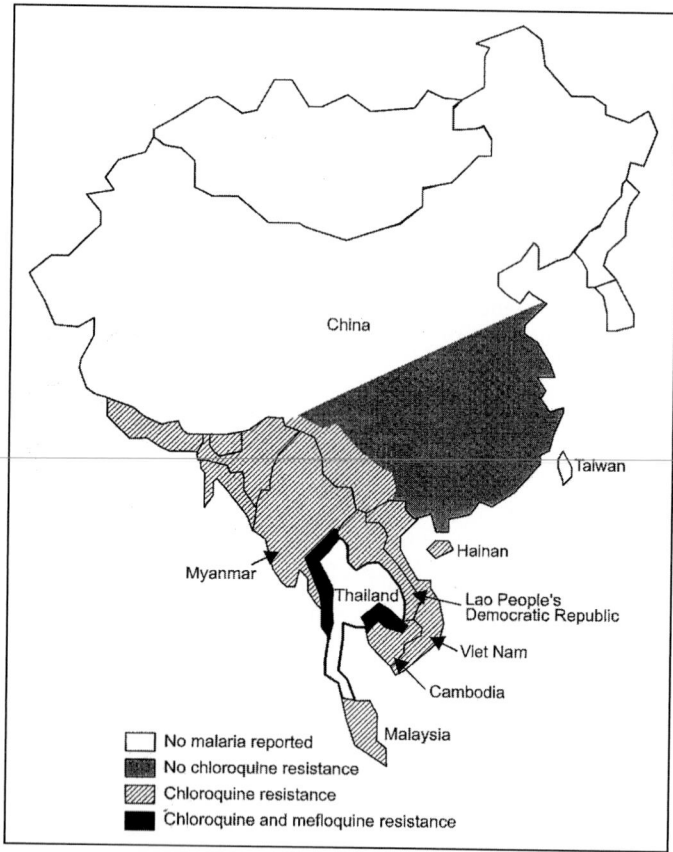

Figure 279.5. Enlarged map of Southeast Asia, showing distribution of malaria resistance. Map is intended as a visual aid only. [From Committee to Advise on Tropical Medicine and Travel (CATMAT). Canadian recommendations for the prevention and treatment of malaria among international travelers 2000. *Can Comm Dis Rep* 2000;26(S2):1–42, with permission.]

TREATMENT OF UNCOMPLICATED FALCIPARUM MALARIA

Chloroquine is the treatment of choice for uncomplicated malaria due to chloroquine-sensitive strains of *P. falciparum*; various equally effective dosing regimens have been used (Table 279.6). Chloroquine is generally well tolerated and safe to use in children and pregnant women.

The combination of atovaquone with proguanil (available as a combination tablet, Malarone, containing 250 mg of atovaquone and 100 mg of proguanil) has been shown to be highly effective for treatment of chloroquine- and mefloquine-resistant *P. falciparum* infections and should be considered the preferred therapy in this setting. Cure rates were equivalent or superior to those obtained with chloroquine alone, pyrimethamine-sulfadoxine (Fansidar) alone, or a combination of both in trials in Peru and the Philippines (100,101) and Africa (102); halofantrine (103,104); mefloquine in Thailand (105); and amodiaquine in Gabon (106). The short (3-day) single daily dose regimen is well tolerated, with few significant adverse effects; the most frequently reported side effect includes GI symptoms, anorexia, and headache. GI side effects may be reduced by taking the drug with food and by dividing the dose. Atovaquone-proguanil is safe for use in children, but there are no data regarding its safety during pregnancy.

Alternative therapy for chloroquine- and mefloquine-resistant falciparum malaria includes quinine in combination with a second agent, the latter to prevent delayed recrudescence of infection. The preferred second agent is either doxycycline (or tetracycline) or pyrimethamine-sulfadoxine (Fansidar, available as a fixed-dose combination tablet containing 25 mg of pyrimethamine and 500 mg of sulfadoxine); for those who cannot tolerate tetracyclines or pyrimethamine-sulfadoxine or in whom these agents are contraindicated, clindamycin may be used. Mefloquine, 1,250 mg once or as two divided doses, is also effective for the treatment of chloroquine-resistant *P. falciparum* infections, but serious neuropsychiatric side effects (seizures and psychosis) can occur in 1:200 to 1:1,700 treatments (107,108), and cardiotoxicity (QT-interval prolongation) is possible. It is not recommended for treatment during pregnancy because of

TABLE 279.6. Oral Treatment of Uncomplicated Malaria

Species	Drug	Adult dose	Pediatric dose
Plasmodium falciparum Chloroquine sensitive	Chloroquine (base)	600 mg, followed by 600 mg 24 hr and 300 mg 48 hr later; Or 600 mg, followed by 300 mg at 6–12, 24, and 36–48 hr	10 mg/kg, followed by 10 mg/kg 24 hr and 5 mg/kg 48 hr later; Or 10 mg/kg, followed by 5 mg/kg at 6–12, 24, and 36–48 hr Note: total dose 25 mg/kg to maximum 1.5 g over 3 d
Chloroquine or mefloquine resistant	Atovaquone-proguanil[a]	4 tablets once daily for 3 d	20 mg/kg atovaquone plus 8 mg/kg proguanil once daily for 3d: 11–20 kg: 1 tablet daily 21–30 kg: 2 tablets daily 31–40 kg: 3 tablets daily >40 kg: 4 tablets daily
	Or Quinine sulphate (base) Plus one of the following[b] Doxycycline	500 mg q8h × 7 d 100 mg b.i.d. × 7 d	7.5 mg/kg (max 500 mg) q8h × 7 d 8 years or older only: 1.5–2.0 mg/kg (max 100 mg) b.i.d × 7 d
	or Pyrimethamine-sulfadoxine[c]	3 tablets once	2–3 mo: ¼ tablet once 4–11 mo: ½ tablet once 12–24 mo: ¾ tablet once 3–4 yr: 1 tablet once 5–9 yr: 1 ½ tablets once 10–11 yr: 2 tablets once 12–13 yr: 2 ½ tablets once 14 yr or older: 3 tablets once
	or Clindamycin	300 mg q6h × 7 d	5 mg/kg (max 300 mg) q8h × 7d
	Or Mefloquine (base)[d]	1,250 mg once; or 750 mg, followed by 500 mg 6–8 hr later	Not recommended
P. vivax Chloroquine and primaquine sensitive	Chloroquine (base) Plus	As above	As above
	Primaquine (base)	15 mg daily × 14 d	0.3 mg/kg (max 15 mg) × 14 d
Chloroquine resistant	Mefloquine (base) Or	As above	Not indicated
	Atovaquone-proguanil; Plus	As above	As above
	Primaquine (base)	As above	As above
Primaquine resistant	Chloroquine (base) Plus	As above	As above
	Primaquine (base)	30 mg daily × 14 d	0.5 mg/kg (max 30 mg) × 14 d
P. ovale	Chloroquine (base) Plus	As above	As above
	Primaquine (base)	15 mg daily × 14 d	0.3 mg/kg (max 15 mg) × 14 d
P. malariae	Chloroquine (base)	As above	As above

Note: See text for contraindications.
[a]One tablet of atovaquone-proguanil (Malarone) contains atovaquone 250 mg and proguanil 100 mg.
[b]The second agent (doxycycline, pyrimethamine-sulfadoxine, or clindamycin) should be given concurrently with or immediately after quinine.
[c]One tablet of pyrimethamine-sulfadoxine (Fansidar) contains pyrimethamine 25 mg and sulfadoxine 500 mg.
[d]Mefloquine should not be used for treatment of mefloquine-resistant *P. falciparum*.

an increased risk of stillbirth (109) or in children weighing less than 5 kg. Halofantrine, though also effective (110), is not available in North America because of its high risk of cardiotoxicity (QT-interval prolongation).

Side effects of treatment with any antimalarial drug include GI upset. Quinine may cause cinchonism (tinnitus, hearing loss, headache, nausea, and vomiting), which is usually reversible, and hypoglycemia because of stimulation of pancreatic insulin secretion. Doxycycline has been associated with esophageal ero-

sions, which can be prevented by drinking adequate fluids with, and avoiding recumbency immediately following, each dose; it is contraindicated in children younger than 8 years and during pregnancy and breast-feeding. Pyrimethamine-sulfadoxine, like other sulfonamide drugs, may lead to hypersensitivity reactions including the potentially fatal Stevens-Johnson syndrome, although these are more likely to occur when used for prophylaxis. The theoretical risk of kernicterus with sulfonamide use during pregnancy has never been proven (111).

TABLE 279.7.   Treatment of Severe Falciparum Malaria

Chloroquine sensitive	Chloroquine base 10 mg/kg i.v. given over 8 hr, followed by 15 mg/kg i.v. over 24 hr
Chloroquine resistant	Quinine dihydrochloride (salt) 20 mg/kg i.v. infused over 4 hr, followed by 10 mg/kg i.v. infused over 4 hr and repeated q8h for up to 72 hr[a]
	Or
	Quinidine gluconate (salt) 24 mg/kg i.v. infused over 4 hr followed by 12 mg/kg i.v. infused over 4 hr and repeated q8h for up to 72 hr; or 10 mg/kg i.v. infused over 1 hr, followed by 0.02 mg/kg/min i.v. as continuous infusion for up to 72 hr[a]
	Plus one of the following[b]
	Doxycycline (i.v. or orally; doses as per Table 279.6)
	Or
	Pyrimethamine-sulfadoxine (doses as per Table 279.6)
	Or
	Clindamycin 10 mg/kg i.v. once, followed by 5 mg/kg i.v. q8h (oral doses as per Table 279.6)

[a]Loading dose of quinine should not be given if the patient has received quinine, quinidine, or mefloquine in the preceding 24 hours. The dose of quinine or quinidine should be reduced by one third to one half on the third day of therapy if there is no improvement or if acute renal failure develops. Regardless of the initial therapy, switch to oral quinine as soon as possible to complete a 7-day course of therapy.
[b]The second agent (doxycycline, pyrimethamine-sulfadoxine, or clindamycin) should be given concurrently with or immediately after quinine-quinidine. A 7-day course of doxycycline or clindamycin, or one dose of pyrimethamine-sulfadoxine, should be given.

TREATMENT OF SEVERE FALCIPARUM MALARIA

Individuals with severe falciparum malaria and those who are unable to take oral medications require parenteral therapy (Table 279.7). Infections by chloroquine-sensitive strains can be treated with intravenous chloroquine, but intravenous quinine (or quinidine) is generally used because of its greater availability. Quinine is preferred over quinidine but is not available in the United States.

Intravenous quinine (or quinidine) should be administered as a loading dose, followed by maintenance therapy. The loading dose of quinine should be omitted in those who have received quinine, quinidine, or mefloquine in the preceding 24 hours. Cardiac monitoring is recommended when quinidine is used, because it can cause prolongation of the QT interval. Regardless of the intravenous therapy used, a 7-day course of therapy should be completed with oral quinine. A second agent (a tetracycline, pyrimethamine-sulfadoxine, or clindamycin) should also be added.

Artemisinin, from the Chinese qinghaosu plant (*Artemisia annua*), and its derivatives artemether and artesunate are not available in North America but are commonly used in Asia and Africa for the treatment of severe malaria in children and adults. The high intraerythrocytic concentration and rapid clearance of parasitemia seen with artemether make it attractive for use, especially as resistance to other antimalarial agents continues to rise. Several randomized clinical trials (112–114) and two recent meta-analyses including these and other studies (115,116) have shown artemesinin derivatives to be as effective as quinine in severe malaria. However, some studies were quite small and caution must be exercised in interpreting the findings of systematic reviews. Artemether can cause hypoglycemia and prolong the QT interval but is generally well tolerated.

Exchange transfusion in severe malaria has conferred a survival benefit in small retrospective studies (117,118); erythrocytapheresis has also been used (119). The rationale for exchange transfusion includes the rapid removal of PRBCs and reduction of parasite burden, removal of circulating toxins and cytokines, and replacement of normal RBCs (66). Indications include parasitemia of more than 30%, or more than 10% in the presence of complications, poor prognosis, or poor response to chemother-

apy (66). There is no role for corticosteroids, anticoagulation, or aggressive diuresis in cerebral malaria (66).

TREATMENT OF *P. VIVAX, P. OVALE,* AND *P. MALARIAE* INFECTIONS

Infections caused by susceptible strains of *P. vivax* and those caused by *P. ovale* and *P. malariae* should be treated with chloroquine (Table 279.6); atovaquone-proguanil is also effective (120–122). Chloroquine and atovaquone-proguanil are effective only against erythrocytic forms of *P. vivax* and *P. ovale*, not their hypnozoites; a 14-day course of primaquine is required to treat these dormant forms. Primaquine should be given only after G6PD deficiency is excluded, to avoid intravascular hemolysis, and should not be used in pregnancy.

Treatment options for resistant *P. vivax* infections include mefloquine or atovaquone-proguanil for chloroquine-resistant strains (followed by primaquine) (121), and high-dose primaquine for treatment of hypnozoites in primaquine-resistant infections (Table 279.6).

Prevention and Control of Malaria

Most cases of imported malaria are preventable. The risk of acquiring malaria is determined by several factors: the region(s) visited; exact destination(s) (urban vs. rural; elevation); the nature of the visit and (business vs. recreation), which in turn determine accommodations (e.g., hotel vs. camping); duration of travel; and time of year (i.e., risk of transmission). Compliance with both personal protective measures and chemoprophylaxis can significantly reduce the risk of acquiring malaria. However, no regimen is 100% effective, and travelers must be aware that they should seek medical attention immediately if fever develops during or after travel. Information regarding malaria risks and prophylaxis are readily available from several reliable sources on the Internet (Table 279.8).

PERSONAL PROTECTION MEASURES

Avoidance or reduction of evening and nocturnal outdoor activity can reduce exposure to night-biting *Anopheles* mosquitoes.

TABLE 279.8. Internet Sources for Information on Malaria Prevention

Organization	Web site/alternate contact
Centers for Disease Control and Prevention, Atlanta, Georgia	*www.cdc.gov/travel* 24-hour malaria information by phone 888-232-3228 or by fax 888-232-3299
Health Canada Travel Medicine Program, Ottawa, Canada	*www.travelhealth.gc.ca* 24-hour malaria information by fax 613-941-3900
Malaria Foundation International	*www.malaria.org*
Shoreland's Travel Health ONLINE	*www.tripprep.com/travinfo frame.asp*
World Health Organization, Geneva, Switzerland	*www.who.int/ith*

If this is impractical, long-sleeved clothing and trousers should be worn, preferably impregnated with permethrin (or deltamethrin). If a secure sleeping environment—ideally an enclosed area with screened windows—is not available, a permethrin-impregnated bed net is recommended (123). Permethrin is safe for use in young children and during pregnancy.

Insect repellants should be used on exposed skin, especially during evening and nighttime hours. N,N-diethyl-3-methylbenzamide (DEET)–containing insect repellants are the most effective. Higher concentrations of DEET increase only the duration of action and do not increase its effectiveness. In general, concentrations higher than 50% offer little advantage to the traveler and can increase the risk of side effects; systemic absorption does occur, and serious adverse effects have been reported rarely, particularly in children (124). DEET is nonteratogenic in animals, but safety data in pregnant women are inconclusive (125). Because of the limited number of chemoprophylactic agents that can be used during pregnancy and in infants, attention to personal protection measures is especially important in these groups if travel cannot be avoided.

CHEMOPROPHYLAXIS

Chemoprophylaxis should be considered for any traveler venturing to a malarious area; selection of an agent depends on the individual risk assessment, resistance patterns, and the presence of any underlying medical conditions that might preclude use of certain agents. Expatriates of malaria-endemic areas should also receive chemoprophylaxis but may consider themselves immune to malaria and are less likely to seek pretravel advice (126–128). Currently recommended prophylactic agents and their doses are listed in Tables 279.9 and 279.10.

For travel to regions with chloroquine-sensitive strains, chloroquine is the agent of choice; it is well tolerated and may be used in children and during pregnancy. At prophylactic doses, retinal toxicity is unlikely to occur.

Mefloquine, doxycycline, and atovaquone-proguanil are the agents of choice for travel to areas with chloroquine-resistant strains. Adverse effects with mefloquine prophylaxis include GI upset and neuropsychologic phenomena (mood change, dizziness, insomnia, headache); they are common (25% to 50%) but often transient. Mefloquine should not be used in travelers with cardiac conduction delays or neuropsychiatric disorders, although the risk of serious neuropsychiatric adverse events (roughly 1: 10,000) is lower than when used for treatment (129). At prophylactic doses, mefloquine is safe for use in the second half of pregnancy (130) and is nonteratogenic. There is little convincing evidence to support an increased risk of spontaneous abortion when used during early pregnancy (111,131), but its use in this setting (and in children less than 5 kg) is not usually recommended; a decision supporting its use will depend on the results of a risk/benefit assessment, always keeping in mind that the risk of falciparum malaria to a nonimmune mother and fetus is considerable. The combination of chloroquine and proguanil is well tolerated and safe in pregnancy (and infants and young children), but much less effective than mefloquine and cannot be recommended. Doxycycline, in addition to the caveats noted earlier, can cause vaginal candidiasis in women, as well as UVA-induced phototoxicity, and is considered effective for prevention of mefloquine-resistant falciparum malaria. Agents considered unsuitable for prophylaxis include pyrimethamine-sulfadoxine, because of the unacceptably high incidence of severe cutaneous reactions at prophylactic doses (132), and azithromycin, which does have

TABLE 279.9. Recommended Agents for Chemoprophylaxis and Standby Therapy

Zone of travel	Chemoprophylaxis		Standby therapy[a]
	Preferred	**Alternatives**	
Chloroquine sensitive	Chloroquine	Mefloquine, doxycycline, or atovaquone-proguanil	Chloroquine if not taking prophylaxis, otherwise atovaquone-proguanil
Chloroquine resistant	Mefloquine, atovaquone-proguanil, or doxycycline	Primaquine, or chloroquine, plus proguanil[b]	Atovaquone-proguanil, or quinine plus doxycycline, or quinine plus pyrimethamine-sulfadoxine
Chloroquine and mefloquine resistant	Doxycycline	None; atovaquone-proguanil may be effective	Atovaquone-proguanil, or quinine plus doxycycline

Note: Atovaquone-proguanil is available as Malarone, and pyrimethamine-sulfadoxine as Fansidar.
[a]Doses of drugs for standby therapy are the same as those listed for treatment in Table 279.6.
[b]Chloroquine plus proguanil is no longer recommended by the Centers for Disease Control and Prevention.

TABLE 279.10.   Recommended Doses of Antimalarial Drugs for Chemoprophylaxis

Agent(s)	Adult dose	Pediatric dose	Duration
Chloroquine (base)	300 mg p.o. every wk	5 mg/kg (max 300 mg) p.o. every wk	Starting 1 wk before entering malaria-endemic region weekly during exposure, and for 4 wk after leaving
Mefloquine (base)	250 mg p.o. every wk	<5 kg: no data, not recommended 5–9 kg: ⅛ tablet p.o. every wk 10–19 kg: ¼ tablet every wk 20–29 kg: ½ tablet every wk 30–45 kg: ¾ tablet every wk >45 kg: 1 tablet every wk	Starting 1 wk before entering malaria-endemic region, weekly during exposure, and for 4 wk after leaving
Doxycycline	100 mg p.o. daily	<8 yr: not recommended ≥8 yr: 1.5 mg/kg (max 100 mg) p.o. daily	Starting 1 d before entering malaria-endemic region, daily during exposure, and for 4 wk after leaving
Atovaquone-proguanil[a]	1 tablet daily	11–20 kg: ¼ tablet p.o. daily 21–30 kg: ½ tablet p.o. daily 31–40 kg: ¾ tablet p.o. daily >40 kg: 1 tablet p.o. daily	Starting 1 d before entering malaria-endemic region, daily during exposure, and for 1 wk after leaving
Primaquine (base)	30 mg p.o. daily	0.5 mg/kg (max 30 mg) p.o. daily	Starting 1 d before entering malaria-endemic region, daily during exposure, and for 1 wk after leaving
Chloroquine (base)	300 mg p.o. every wk	Chloroquine as above;	Chloroquine as above; plus proguanil starting 1 wk before entering malaria-endemic region, daily during exposure, and for 4 wk after leaving
plus proguanil[b]	200 mg p.o. daily	<8 mo: 25 mg p.o. daily 8–36 mo: 50 mg p.o. daily 4–7 yr: 75 mg p.o. daily 8–10 yr: 100 mg p.o. daily 11–13 yr: 150 mg p.o. daily ≥14 yr: 200 mg p.o. daily	

Note: See text for contraindications.
[a] One tablet of atovaquone-proguanil (Malarone) contains atovaquone 250 mg and proguanil 100 mg.
[b] Chloroquine plus proguanil is no longer recommended by the Centers for Disease Control and Prevention.

antimalarial activity but does not provide adequate protection against *P. falciparum.*

In several recent studies, atovaquone-proguanil (Malarone) has been found to be a safe and highly effective prophylactic agent against chloroquine-resistant *P. falciparum* in children and nonpregnant adults living in endemic areas), with overall efficacy rates of 98% (133–135). In nonimmune travelers, the drug combination was shown to have significantly greater tolerability compared with chloroquine plus proguanil or mefloquine (136–138); headache and GI upset were the most common side effects. It may also be effective for prophylaxis against mefloquine-resistant strains but has not yet been approved for this. Studies in endemic regions have also found primaquine to be highly effective against both *P. falciparum* and *P. vivax* infections compared with placebo (139,140), doxycycline (141), and mefloquine (141,142), again with an excellent safety profile. Because both primaquine and atovaquone-proguanil provide causal prophylaxis (i.e., they are active against the liver stages of infection), they may both be discontinued 7 days after the last exposure and compliance with therapy may therefore be improved. Tafenoquine, a new 8-aminoquinoline agent, appears promising (143,144), although further studies are required.

Standby therapy (SBT, self-treatment) has been recommended for those who may be unable to obtain medical care quickly (Table 279.9). SBT is not intended to be curative (although it may be) or to replace the need for medical attention but is a temporizing measure that can be potentially life saving until additional care can be sought. Studies of SBT use among travelers

have shown poor adherence to guidelines for usage and follow-up, however (145).

MALARIA VACCINES

No effective malaria vaccines are available. Human immune responses in vaccine studies to date have been variable and short-lived; new methods of vaccine delivery are being explored. Irradiated sporozoite vaccines confer complete protection against malaria but are not strain specific and are highly impractical (146). Recombinant CSP fused to hepatitis B surface antigen elicited a sufficient antibody response to confer immunity against experimental infection in some but not all subjects (52). However, the vaccine showed poor efficacy in a recent clinical trial (147). Other approaches include immunization against the merozoite surface protein and combination sporozoite and blood stage vaccines (148). Current opinion is that a prime and boost strategy would be more immunogenic than previous approaches (56).

VECTOR CONTROL

Vector (mosquito) control is only one aspect of malaria control. Although still successfully used in some regions of the world, insecticides have for several reasons been inadequate for the global control of malaria. Insecticide resistance is increasingly present in malaria-endemic areas (149), further limiting their use. Although the use of DDT was central to earlier schemes for global eradication of malaria, current malaria control strategies have shifted away from insecticide use, as evidenced by their exclusion from the Roll Back Malaria program.

BABESIOSIS

Babesiosis is a zoonotic, malaria-like illness caused by protozoa of the order Piroplasmidora. The pathogenic role of *Babesia* in domestic animals has long been known; biblical references are suggestive of hemoglobinuria and babesiosis in cattle. The Hungarian pathologist Babes first noted the parasite in the blood of febrile cattle in 1888, but it was not until almost 70 years later (1957) that the first human case was described in an asplenic farmer in Europe (150). In 1969, the first case of babesiosis in an immunocompetent patient was reported in the United States (151). Initially considered to be relatively rare, it is clear that the incidence and distribution of babesiosis are increasing in the United States, as is awareness of this disease.

The Parasite and Its Life Cycle

Of more than 100 species of *Babesia*, most human infections have been attributed to *Babesia divergens* (Europe) and *Babesia microti* (northeastern United States), with their normal hosts being cattle and rodents, respectively.

The life cycle of *B. microti* is depicted in Fig. 279.6. *Babesia* are transmitted by ixodid ticks, mainly *Ixodes dammini* in the United States and *Ixodes ricinus* in Europe. The human phase of infection with *B. microti* begins with the release of sporozoites from infected nymphs or less often adult ticks. The likelihood of transmission is directly proportional to the duration of feeding; tick attachment for more than 24 hours is required. In contrast to malaria, there is no preerythrocytic stage, and sporozoites invade erythrocytes directly. The mechanism of invasion of human RBCs remains unclear, but a erythrocyte C3b receptor appears to be required in rats infected with *Babesia rodhaini* (152). Asexual reproduction by budding produces two to four merozoites, which are sometimes visible on blood films in pairs, or as the characteristic tetrad or "maltese cross" (Fig. 279.7). Rupture of PRBCs releases merozoites, which then infect additional erythrocytes. The resulting hemolysis is not usually massive because this process is asynchronous.

Parasitized erythrocytes are ingested by the tick as it feeds on an infected host. Within the gut, some intraerythrocytic forms

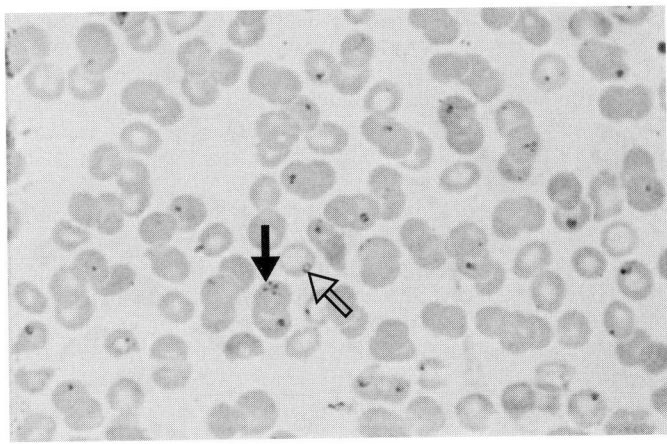

Figure 279.7. *Babesia microti*–infected erythrocytes, from a case of transfusion-transmitted babesiosis. Note the ring form (*open arrow*), and the characteristic tetrad or "Maltese cross" (*closed arrow*).

develop into gametocytes; gametes then fuse to form a zygote. The zygote becomes mobile, leaves the gut, and travels to the salivary glands. Sporogony takes place, producing thousands of infectious sporozoites ready for inoculation into another host.

Epidemiology

Cases of babesiosis have been reported mainly from temperate climates in the United States and Europe. Recently, infections caused by species closely related to *B. microti* have been described in humans: WA-1 in Washington and California (153,154), MO-1 in Missouri (155), and TW-1 in Taiwan (156). In addition, human babesiosis has been reported in Japan (157), Egypt (158), and South Africa (159). In Europe, babesiosis is still rare (approximately 30 cases reported, most in France and the British Isles) and have for the most part involved asplenic individuals infected with *Babesia divergens* (160).

In the United States, both the white-footed deer mouse (*Peromyscus leucopus*) and *I. dammini* are necessary for the persistence

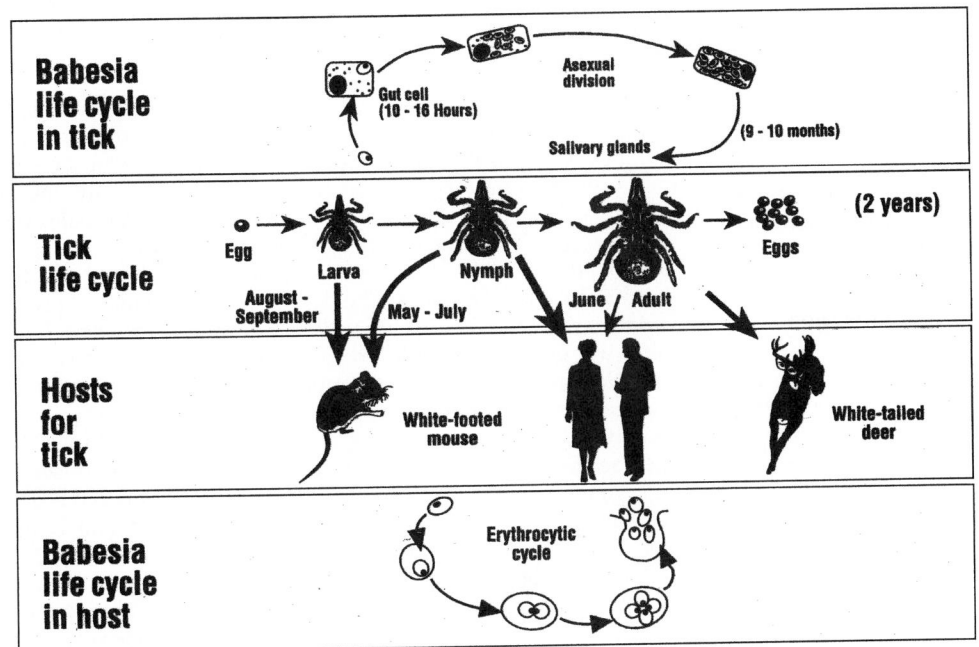

Figure 279.6. The life cycle of *Babesia microti*. (From Boustani MR, Gelfand JA. Babesiosis. *Clin Infect Dis* 1996;22:611–615, with permission.)

of *B. microti*. The estimated prevalence of *B. microti* in engorged (i.e., feeding) *I. dammini* nymphs in nature is 5% (161). Most cases of *B. microti* infection occur during the summer months, coincident with the nymph stage of the *Ixodes* life cycle, and most have been concentrated in the northeastern United States—mainly in New York (Long Island) and Massachusetts (Nantucket Island, hence "Nantucket fever"), but cases have also been described in Connecticut and Rhode Island (162,163), New Jersey (164), and as far west as Wisconsin (165). Seroepidemiological surveys in endemic areas reveal prevalences between 1% and 9% (166–169). Two serosurveys in California revealed prevalence rates of 16% to 20% for WA-1 (154,170), although the specificity of the test used was known to be low. Serologic evidence of co-infection with *Borrelia burgdorferi* (Lyme disease) in individuals diagnosed with either disease is not uncommon, occurring in 4% in residents of Wisconsin and Minnesota (171), 8% on Nantucket Island (172), and 16% in Rhode Island (168).

Transfusion-transmitted *B. microti* infection is well documented, with more than 20 cases reported in the United States (173). Cases are usually related to an asymptomatic donor, and multiple recipients may be infected (174). The risk of transfusion-transmitted disease in endemic areas has not been studied extensively; in Connecticut, the risk has been estimated at 0.17% per unit of packed RBCs (175).

Pathogenesis and Immunology

Little is understood regarding the pathogenesis of babesiosis. In *B. microti* infection, RBC deformability is reduced and the PRBC membrane can become extensively damaged (176); hemolytic anemia may occur as a result of PRBC destruction.

Unlike malaria, naturally acquired babesiosis generates both humoral and cell-mediated immune responses and leads to protective immunity. During the sporozoite stage, IgG antibodies can prevent erythrocyte invasion (177), but immunity in rodents appears to persist even in the absence of antibody production, suggesting that humoral immunity plays a limited role. Serum complement levels are often reduced, presumably because of the formation of circulating immune complexes (178). Cell-mediated immunity conferred by CD4$^+$ helper T cells appears to provide the most resistance to infection (179); in murine models, CD4$^+$-depleted mice are more susceptible to babesiosis (180), and adoptive transfer of immune T cells and to a lesser extent macrophages can render protection to naive mice (181). Soluble mediators such as IFN-γ produced by CD4$^+$ cells and natural killer cells, as well as macrophage-produced TNF-α and nitric oxide, appear to inhibit parasitemia and play a protective role in mice (182,183); however, cytokines may also contribute to the pathogenesis of severe disease.

The importance of an intact spleen in protection against *Babesia* is evident from the increased frequency of severe and fatal disease in asplenic individuals (160,184).

Clinical Manifestations and Laboratory Findings

B. MICROTI INFECTIONS

Asymptomatic or subclinical infection with *B. microti* appears to be common, based on seroprevalence studies. Clinical features of symptomatic disease caused by *B. microti* infection can be summarized from the findings of several case series (185–190). Men appear to be infected more often than women, and the risk of infection is higher with age older than 50 years (188). Patients with previous splenectomies accounted for 12% to 32% of cases in three studies (187,189,190). Symptoms develop after an incubation period of 7 to 28 days following a known tick bite (186),

although a history of the same is present in fewer than 40% of patients. The duration from onset of symptoms to diagnosis is variable, ranging from 1 to 72 days, but most infections are diagnosed within 6 weeks of onset. Therefore, despite the fact that most infections occur between June and August, patients may not present until colder months, when the suspicion of babesiosis is low.

Fatigue and malaise are prominent symptoms, usually in conjunction with fever, shaking chills, or sweats. Myalgias, arthralgias, nausea, anorexia, and headache are other common symptoms. Cough and dyspnea occur in fewer than 20% of patients. Relative bradycardia has been described as a feature of babesiosis (191). Physical findings are usually nonspecific; fever, hepatosplenomegaly, and a cardiac murmur are common. Septic shock is a rare but severe presentation in immunocompetent hosts (192).

Most patients recover uneventfully with or without therapy. Symptoms and parasitemia may be prolonged (weeks to months), especially without treatment, and relapses of disease can occur (163). Complications including congestive heart failure, acute respiratory distress syndrome, disseminated intravascular coagulation, and renal failure can occur in up to 40% of patients (189). Severe disease has been associated with prior splenectomy, advanced age (185), human immunodeficiency virus infection (190,193), underlying malignancy (190), and the presence of anemia (190).

Anemia, leukopenia, and thrombocytopenia are common hematologic abnormalities. Nonspecific elevations of liver function test results are also common. Renal failure is uncommon on presentation.

B. DIVERGENS INFECTIONS

Infection with *B. divergens* tends to be acute and clinically apparent. Based on a review of 29 cases in Europe, acute illness occurs 1 to 3 weeks after a tick bite and is characterized by severe intravascular hemolysis, hemoglobinuria, and jaundice, in addition to other features of babesiosis as described (160). The clinical course and outcomes are more severe than in *B. microti* infection, in part because of the increased incidence of splenectomy in this group. Rapid progression to renal failure and pulmonary edema are common, and mortality is high (38% overall) (160).

Diagnosis

Babesiosis should be suspected in the presence of compatible symptoms and an appropriate exposure history. Examination of Wright's or Giemsa's stained thin blood smears is the most commonly used laboratory method for diagnosis. Organisms may appear as ring forms, or merozoites may be seen as pairs or tetrads (Fig. 279.7). The absence of hemozoin pigment and mature malarial forms (schizonts and gametocytes) should distinguish *Babesia* from malaria. The degree of parasitemia is highly variable, with less than 1% up to 85% parasitemia reported. Parasites are generally visible on thin smears for 3 to 12 weeks (185,190), but parasitemia of 7 months' duration was reported in one splenectomized patient (194).

Immunofluorescent antibody tests are sensitive (88% to 96%) and specific (90% to 100%) (195) and are recommended for serologic diagnosis of babesiosis. Most infected patients have detectable antibody at the time of presentation. A titer of more than 1:64 is considered positive, and a titer of more than 1:256 is diagnostic of acute infection. Titers may decline very slowly (months), however, making the main limitation of this test its inability to distinguish acute infection from prior exposure.

PCR may be particularly useful in cases with mild illness and low-level parasitemia. Detection of parasite DNA using PCR reflects acute or ongoing infection. PCR has been used to demonstrate the prolonged duration of parasitemia in infected individuals (163). Highly sensitive and specific assays have been developed for both *B. microti* and *B. divergens*. However, PCR is not widely available and is not currently a primary method of laboratory diagnosis. Intraperitoneal inoculation of human blood into hamsters is a reliable diagnostic test but is too impractical for routine use.

Treatment

Since first used to successfully treat a case of transfusion-transmitted infection, a 7- to 10-day course of quinine (500 mg base orally every 8 hours) and clindamycin (600 mg orally every 8 hours) has been the treatment of choice for babesiosis (196). Pediatric doses are as shown for malaria (Table 279.6). Severely ill individuals should be treated with intravenous therapy. Treatment can reduce the duration of parasitemia and clinical illness (163) and should be offered to symptomatic individuals and those at high risk of complications.

Treatment failure with quinine and clindamycin can occur. A combination of quinine and azithromycin (500 mg orally twice daily) for 10 days has been successfully used to treat babesiosis in this setting (197). Atovaquone has also been used in conjunction with azithromycin and exchange transfusion to treat one patient in whom quinine and clindamycin failed (198). A combination of atovaquone (750 mg orally every 12 hours) and azithromycin (500 mg on day 1 followed by 250 mg daily) for 7 days was recently shown to be as effective as quinine and clindamycin in a small randomized clinical trial (199). In severe cases, whole-blood exchange transfusion or apheresis may be life saving (198,200,201).

Prevention

The most effective prevention against babesiosis is avoidance of endemic areas during summer months, which should be considered in immunocompromised or asplenic individuals. Personal protection measures, such as use of tick repellents (e.g., DEET) on exposed skin and insecticides (e.g., permethrin) on clothing, and wearing long-sleeved shirts and long pants with legs tucked into socks, can reduce the risk of tick bites. Light-colored clothing may improve detection of ticks. Because ixodid ticks require more than 24 hours of attachment to transmit babesiosis (and Lyme disease), a thorough examination of head and body, and of pets, should be carried out at least once daily; attached ticks should be carefully removed with forceps. No human vaccine exists, and its development is not a priority at this time.

Although the risk of transfusion-transmitted babesiosis is low, this complication has certainly been realized. Currently no policies are in place to reject donors who have a history of babesiosis. Screening donors is fraught with potential problems and is unlikely to be instituted given the rarity of the problem. However, appreciation of babesiosis as one cause of a febrile transfusion reaction in endemic areas may lead to a more rapid diagnosis and reduced morbidity in infected recipients.

REFERENCES

1. The World Bank. *Malaria-at-a-glance*. Washington, DC: The World Bank, 2001.
2. Frevert U, Sinnis P, Cerami C, et al. Malaria circumsporozoite protein binds to heparan sulfate proteoglycans associated with the surface membrane of hepatocytes. *J Exp Med* 1993;117:1287–1298.
3. Pinzon-Ortiz C, Friedman J, Esko J, et al. The binding of the circumsporozoite protein to cell surface heparan sulfate proteoglycans is required for plasmodium sporozoite attachment to target cells. *J Biol Chem* 2001;276:26784–26791.
4. Sim BKL, Chinis CE, Wasniowska K, et al. Receptor and ligand domains for invasion of erythrocytes by *Plasmodium falciparum*. *Science* 1994;264:1941–1944.
5. Adams JH, Sim BKL, Dolan SA, et al. A family of erythrocyte binding proteins of malaria parasites. *Proc Natl Acad Sci U S A* 1992;89:7085–7089.
6. World Health Organization. World malaria situation in 1994. Parts I–III. *Wkly Epid Rec* 1997;72:269–274, 277–283, 285–290.
7. Centers for Disease Control and Prevention. Famine affected, refugee and displaced populations: recommendations for public health issues. *MMWR Morb Mort Wkly Rep* 1992;41(RR13):1–76.
8. Zucker JR. Changing patterns of autochthonous malaria transmission in the United States: a review of recent outbreaks. *Emerg Infect Dis* 1996;2:37–43.
9. Miller LH, Mason SJ, Clyde DF, et al. The resistance factor to *Plasmodium vivax* in blacks: the Duffy blood-group genotype, Fy Fy. *N Engl J Med* 1976;295:302–304.
10. Committee to Advise on Tropical Medicine and Travel (CATMAT). Canadian recommendations for the prevention and treatment of malaria among international travelers 2000. *Can Comm Dis Rep* 2000;26(S2):1–42.
11. Centers for Disease Control and Prevention. Malaria surveillance—United States, 1998. *MMWR Morb Mort Wkly Rep* 2001;50(SS-1):25–43.
12. Conlon CP, Berendt AR, Dawson K, et al. Runway malaria. *Lancet* 1990;335:472–473.
13. Curtis CF, White GB. *Plasmodium falciparum* transmission in England: entomological and epidemiologic data relative to cases in 1983. *J Trop Med Hyg* 1984;87:101–114.
14. Slinger R, Giulivi A, Bodie-Collins M, et al. Transfusion-transmitted malaria in Canada. *CMAJ* 2001;164:377–379.
15. Mungai MW, Kachur SP, Tegtmeier GE, et al. Transfusion-transmitted malaria in the United States, 1963–1998. *Transfusion* 1998;38[Suppl 10]:104S (abstr).
16. Cooke BM, Wahlgren M, Coppel RL. Falciparum malaria: sticking up, standing out and out-standing. *Parasitol Today* 2000;16:416–420.
17. MacPherson GG, Warrell MJ, White NJ, et al. Human cerebral malaria. A quantitative ultrastructural analysis of parasitized erythrocyte sequestration. *Am J Pathol* 1985;119:385–401.
18. Carlson J, Helmby H, Hill AVS, et al. Human cerebral malaria: association with erythrocyte resetting and lack of anti-rosetting antibodies. *Lancet* 1990;336:1457–1460.
19. Langreth SG, Peterson E. Pathogenicity, stability, and immunogenicity of a knobless clone of *Plasmodium falciparum* in Colombian owl monkeys. *Infect Immun* 1985;47:760–766.
20. Su XZ, Heatwole VM, Wertheimer SP, et al. The large diverse gene family *var* encodes proteins involved in cytoadherence and antigenic variation of *Plasmodium falciparum*–infected erythrocytes. *Cell* 1995;82:89–100.
21. Baruch DI, Pasloske BL, Singh HB, et al. Cloning the *P. falciparum* gene encoding PfEMP1, a malarial variant antigen and adherence receptor on the surface of parasitized human erythrocytes. *Cell* 1995;82:77–87.
22. Smith JD, Chitnis CE, Craig AG, et al. Switches in expression of *Plasmodium falciparum var* genes correlate with changes in antigenic and cytoadherent phenotypes of infected erythrocytes. *Cell* 1995;82:101–110.
23. Chen Q, Schlichtherle M, Wahlgren M. Molecular aspects of severe malaria. *Clin Microbiol Rev* 2000;13:439–350.
24. Beeson JG, Rogerson SJ, Cooke BM, et al. Adhesion of *Plasmodium falciparum*–infected erythrocytes to hyaluronic acid in placental malaria. *Nat Med* 2000;6:86–90.
25. Jakobsen PH, Bate CAW, Taverne J, et al. Malaria: toxins, cytokines and disease. *Parasite Immunol* 1995;17:223–231.
26. Schofield L, Hackett R. Signal transduction in host cells by a glycosylphosphatidylinositol toxin of malaria parasites. *J Exp Med* 1993;177:145–153.
27. Pichyangkul S, Saengkrai P, Webster HK. *Plasmodium falciparum* pigment induces monocytes to release high levels of tumor necrosis factor-α and interleukin-1. *Am J Trop Med Hyg* 1994;51:430–435.
28. Kwiatkowski D, Hill AV, Sambou I, et al. TNF concentration in fatal cerebral, non-fatal cerebral, and uncomplicated *Plasmodium falciparum* malaria. *Lancet* 1990;336:1201–1204.
29. Udomsangpetch R, Chivapat S, Viriyavejakul P, et al. Involvement of cytokines in the histopathology of cerebral malaria. *Am J Trop Med Hyg* 1997;57:501–506.
30. Clark IA, Rockett KA, Cowden WB. Proposed link between cytokines, nitric oxide, and cerebral malaria. *Parasitol Today* 1991;7:205–207.
31. McGuire W, Knight JC, Hill AVS, et al. Severe malarial anemia and cerebral malaria are associated with different tumor necrosis factor promoter alleles. *J Infect Dis* 1999;179:287–290.
32. Kun JFJ, Mordmuller B, Lell B, et al. Polymorphism in promoter region of inducible nitric oxide synthase gene and protection against malaria. *Lancet* 1998;351:265–266.
33. Burgner D, Xu W, Rockett K, et al. Inducible nitric oxide synthase polymorphism and fatal cerebral malaria. *Lancet* 1998;352:1193–1194.
34. Kwiatkowski D, Molyneux ME, Stephens S, et al. Anti-TNF therapy inhibits fever in cerebral malaria. *Q J Med* 1993;86:91–98.
35. Tournamille C, Colin Y, Cartron JP, et al. Disruption of a GATA motif in the *Duffy* gene promoter abolishes erythroid gene expression in Duffy-negative individuals. *Nat Genet* 1995;10:224–228.
36. Allison AC. Protection afforded by sickle cell trait against subtertian malarial infection. *BMJ* 1954;1:290–294.

37. Hill AV, Allsopp CE, Kwiatkowski D, et al. Common West African HLA antigens are associated with protection from severe malaria. *Nature* 1991;352:595–600.

38. Ruwende C, Khoo SC, Snow RW, et al. Natural selection of hemi- and heterozygotes for G6PD deficiency in Africa by resistance to severe malaria. *Nature* 1995;376:246–249.

39. Genton B, al-Yaman F, Mgone CS, et al. Ovalocytosis and cerebral malaria [Letter]. *Nature* 1995;378:564–565.

40. Flint J, Hill AV, Bowden DK, et al. High frequencies of α-thalassemia are the result of natural selection by malaria. *Nature* 1986:744–750.

41. Williams TN, Maitland K, Bennett S, et al. High incidence of malaria in α-thalassemic children. *Nature* 1996;383:522–525.

42. Fernandez-Reyes D, Craig AG, Kyes SA, et al. A high frequency African coding polymorphism in the N-terminal domain of ICAM-1 predisposing to cerebral malaria in Kenya. *Hum Mol Genet* 1997;6:1357–1360.

43. Mendis K, Sina BJ, Marchesini P, et al. The neglected burden of *Plasmodium vivax* malaria. *Am J Trop Med Hyg* 2001;64[1-2 Suppl]:97–106.

44. Miller LH, Good MF, Kaslow DC. Vaccines against the blood stages of falciparum malaria. *Adv Exp Med Biol* 1998;452:193–205.

45. Hoffman SL, Oster CN, Plowe CV, et al. Naturally acquired antibodies to sporozoites do not prevent malaria: vaccine development implications. *Science* 1987;237:639–642.

46. Good MF, Doolan DL. Immune effector mechanisms in malaria. *Curr Opin Immunol* 1999;11:412–419.

47. Wang R, Doolan DL, Le TP, et al. Induction of antigen-specific cytotoxic T lymphocytes in humans by a malaria DNA vaccine. *Science* 1998;282:476–480.

48. Plebanski M, Lee EA, Hannan CM, et al. Altered peptide ligands narrow the repertoire of cellular immune responses by interfering with T-cell priming. *Nat Med* 1999;5:565–571.

49. Weiss WR, Sedegah M, Berzofsky JA, et al. The role of CD4+ T cells in immunity to malaria sporozoites. *J Immunol* 1993;151:2690–2698.

50. Doolan DL, Hoffman SL. IL-12 and NK cells are required for antigen-specific adaptive immunity against malaria initiated by CD8+ T cells in the *Plasmodium yoelii* model. *J Immunol* 1999;163:884–892.

51. Rzepczyk CM, Anderson K, Stamatiou S, et al. Gamma delta T cells: their immunobiology and role in malaria infections. *Int J Parasitol* 1997;27:191–200.

52. Stoute JA, Slaoui M, Heppner DG, et al. A preliminary evaluation of a recombinant circumsporozoite protein vaccine against *Plasmodium falciparum* malaria. *N Engl J Med* 1997;336:86–91.

53. Luty AJF, Lell B, Schmidt-Ott R, et al. Interferon-gamma responses are associated with resistance to reinfection with *Plasmodium falciparum* in young African children. *J Infect Dis* 1999;179:980–988.

54. Plebanski M, Hill AVS. The immunology of malaria infection. *Curr Opin Immunol* 2000;12:437–441.

55. Barragan A, Kremsner PG, Weiss W, et al. Age-related buildup of humoral immunity against epitopes for rosette formation and agglutination in African areas of malaria endemicity. *Infect Immun* 1998;66:4783–4787.

56. Doolan DL, Hoffman SL. DNA-based vaccines against malaria: status and promise of the multi-stage malaria DNA vaccine operation. *Int J Parasitol* 2001;31:753–762.

57. Kain KC, Harrington MA, Tennyson S, et al. Imported malaria: prospective analysis of problems in diagnosis and management. *Clin Infect Dis* 1998;27:142–149.

58. Svenson JE, MacLean JD, Gyorkos TW, et al. Imported malaria. Clinical presentation and examination of symptomatic travelers. *Arch Intern Med* 1995;155:861–868.

59. Winters RA, Murray HW. Malaria—the mime revisited: fifteen more years of experience at a New York City teaching hospital. *Am J Med* 1992;93:243–246.

60. Lewis SJ, Davidson RN, Ross EJ, et al. Severity of imported falciparum malaria: effect of taking antimalarial prophylaxis. *BMJ* 1992;305:741–743.

61. Kean BH, Reilly PC. Malaria—the mime. Recent lessons from a group of civilian travellers. *Am J Med* 1976;61:159–164.

62. Gordon S, Brennessel DJ, Goldstein JA, et al. Malaria: a city hospital experience. *Arch Intern Med* 1988;148:1569–1571.

63. Newton JA, Schnepf GA, Wallace MR, et al. Malaria in US Marines returning from Somalia. *JAMA* 1994;272:397–399.

64. Svenson JE, Gyorkos TW, MacLean JD. Diagnosis of malaria in the febrile traveler. *Am J Trop Med Hyg* 1995;53:518–521.

65. Gopinath R, Keystone JS, Kain KC. Concurrent falciparum malaria and *Salmonella* bacteremia in travelers: report of two cases. *Clin Infect Dis* 1995;20:706–708.

66. World Health Organization. Severe falciparum malaria. *Trans R Soc Trop Med Hyg* 2000;94[Suppl 1]:1–90.

67. Murphy GS, Oldfield EC III. Falciparum malaria. *Infect Dis Clin North Am* 1996;10:747–775.

68. Cayea PD, Rubin E, Teixidor HS. Atypical pulmonary malaria. *Am J Roentgenol* 1981;137:51–55.

69. Gozal D. The incidence of pulmonary manifestations during *Plasmodium falciparum* malaria in non immune subjects. *Trop Med Parasitol* 1992;43:6–8.

70. Milne LM, Kyi MS, Chiodini PL, et al. Accuracy of routine laboratory diagnosis of malaria in the United Kingdom. *J Clin Pathol* 1994;47:740–742.

71. Warhurst DC, Williams JE. Laboratory diagnosis of malaria. *J Clin Pathol* 1996;49:533–538.

72. Wongsrichanalai C, Namsiripongpun V, Pronsliapatip J, et al. Sensitivity of QBC malaria test. *Lancet* 1992;340:702–703.

73. Delacollette D, van der Stuyft P. Direct acridine orange staining is not a "miracle" solution to the problems of malaria diagnosis in the field. *Trans R Soc Trop Med Hyg* 1994;88:187–188.

74. Bawden M, Malone J, Slaten D. QBC malaria diagnosis: easily learned and effectively applied in a temporary military field laboratory. *Trans R Soc Trop Med Hyg* 1994;88:302.

75. Lowe BS, Jeffa NF, New L, et al. Acridine orange fluorescence techniques as alternatives to traditional Giemsa staining for the diagnosis of malaria in developing countries. *Trans R Soc Trop Med Hyg* 1996;90:34–36.

76. Gay F, Traore B, Zanoni J, et al. Direct acridine orange fluorescence examination of blood slides compared to current techniques for malaria diagnosis. *Trans R Soc Trop Med Hyg* 1996;90:516–518.

77. Craig MH, Sharp BL. Comparative evaluation of four techniques for the diagnosis of *Plasmodium falciparum* infections. *Trans R Soc Trop Med Hyg* 1997;91:279–282.

78. Cooke AH, Morris-Jones S, Horton J, et al. Evaluation of benzothiocarboxypurine for malaria diagnosis in an endemic area. *Trans R Soc Trop Med Hyg* 1993;87:549.

79. Humar A, Ohrt C, Harrington MA, et al. *Para* Sight-F test compared with the polymerase chain reaction and microscopy for the diagnosis of *Plasmodium falciparum* malaria in travelers. *Am J Trop Med Hyg* 1997;56:44–48.

80. Kilian AHD, Mughusu EB, Kabagambe G, et al. Comparison of two rapid HRP-2 based diagnostic tests for *Plasmodium falciparum*. *Trans R Soc Trop Med Hyg* 1997;91:666–667.

81. Pieroni P, Mills CD, Ohrt C, et al. Comparison of the *Para* Sight-F test and the ICT Malaria PF test with the polymerase-chain reaction for the diagnosis of *Plasmodium falciparum* malaria in travelers. *Trans R Soc Trop Med Hyg* 1998;92:166–169.

82. Tham JM, Lee SH, Tan TMC, et al. Detection and species determination of malaria parasites by PCR: comparison with microscopy and with ParaSight-F and ICT Malaria Pf tests in a clinical environment. *J Clin Microbiol* 1999;37:1269–1273.

83. Jelinek T, Grobusch MP, Schwenke S, et al. Sensitivity and specificity of dipstick tests for rapid diagnosis of malaria in nonimmune travelers. *J Clin Microbiol* 1999;37:721–723.

84. Tijtra E, Suprianto S, Dyer M, et al. Field evaluation of the ICT Malaria P.f/P.v immunochromatographic test for detection of *Plasmodium falciparum* and *Plasmodium vivax* in patients with a presumptive clinical diagnosis of malaria in Eastern Indonesia. *J Clin Microbiol* 1999;37:2412–2417.

85. Palmer CJ, Lindo JF, Klaskala WI, et al. Evaluation of the OptiMAL test for rapid diagnosis of *Plasmodium vivax* and *Plasmodium falciparum* malaria. *J Clin Microbiol* 1998;36:203–206.

86. Iqbal J, Sher A, Hira PR, et al. Comparison of the OptiMAL test with PCR for diagnosis of malaria in immigrants. *J Clin Microbiol* 1999;37:3644–3646.

87. Kain KC, Brown A, Mirabelli L, et al. Detection of *Plasmodium vivax* by polymerase-chain reaction in a field study. *J Infect Dis* 1993;168:1323–1326.

88. Oliveira DA, Shi YP, Oloo AJ, et al. Field evaluation of a polymerase-chain reaction based nonisotopic liquid hybridization assay for malaria diagnosis. *J Infect Dis* 1996;173:1284–1287.

89. Seesod N, Nopparat P, Hedrum A, et al. An integrated system using immunomagnetic separation, polymerase-chain reaction and colorimetric detection for diagnosis of *Plasmodium falciparum*. *Am J Trop Med Hyg* 1997;56:322–328.

90. Rubio JM, Buhigas I, Subirats M, et al. Limited level of accuracy provided by available rapid tests for malaria enhances the need for PCR-based reference laboratories. *J Clin Microbiol* 2001;39:2736–2737.

91. Mendelow BV, Lyons C, Nhlangothi P, et al. Automated malaria detection by depolarization of laser light. *Br J Haematol* 1999;104:499–503.

92. Hanscheid T, Melo-Cristino J, Pinto BG. Automated detection of malaria pigment in white blood cells for the diagnosis of malaria in Portugal. *Am J Trop Med Hyg* 2001;64:290–292.

93. van Vianen PH, van Engen A, Thiathong S, et al. Flow cytometric screening of blood samples for malaria parasites. *Cytometry* 1993;14:276–280.

94. Rieckmann KH, Davis DR, Hutton DC. *Plasmodium vivax* resistance to chloroquine? *Lancet* 1989;2:1183–1184.

95. Phillips EJ, Keystone JS, Kain KC. Failure of combined chloroquine and high-dose primaquine therapy for *Plasmodium vivax* malaria acquired in Guyana, South America. *Clin Infect Dis* 1996;23:1171–1173.

96. Nosten F, ter Kuile F, Chongsuphajaisiddhi T, et al. Mefloquine-resistant falciparum malaria on the Thai-Burmese border. *Lancet* 1991;337:1140–1143.

97. Luzzi GA, Warrell DA, Barnes AJ, et al. Treatment of primaquine-resistant *Plasmodium vivax* malaria. *Lancet* 1992;340:310.

98. Wellems TE, Plowe CV. Chloroquine-resistant malaria. *J Infect Dis* 2001;184:770–776.

99. Collins WE, Jeffery GM. Primaquine resistance in *Plasmodium vivax*. *Am J Trop Med Hyg* 1996;55:243–249.

100. Llanos-Cuentas A, Campos P, Clendenes M, et al. Atovaquone and proguanil hydrochloride compared with chloroquine or pyrimethamine/sulfadoxine for treatment of acute *Plasmodium falciparum* malaria. *Braz J Infect Dis* 2001;5:67–72.

101. Bustos DG, Canfield CJ, Canete-Miguel E, et al. Atovaquone-proguanil compared with chloroquine and chloroquine-sulfadoxine-pyrimethamine for treatment of acute *Plasmodium falciparum* malaria in the Philippines. *J Infect Dis* 1999;179:1587–1590.

102. Mulenga M, Sukwa TY, Canfield CJ, et al. Atovaquone and proguanil versus pyrimethamine/sulfadoxine for the treatment of acute falciparum malaria in Zambia. *Clin Ther* 1999;21:841–852.

103. Bouchaud O, Monlun E, Muanza K, et al. Atovaquone plus proguanil versus halofantrine for the treatment of imported acute uncomplicated *Plasmodium falciparum* malaria in non-immune adults: a randomized comparative trial. *Am J Trop Med Hyg* 2000;63:274–279.

104. Anabwani G, Canfield CJ, Hutchison DB. Combination atovaquone and proguanil hydrochloride vs. halofantrine for treatment of acute *Plasmodium falciparum* malaria in children. *Pediatr Infect Dis J* 1999;18:456–461.

105. Looareesuwan S, Wilairatana P, Chalermarut K, et al. Efficacy and safety of atovaquone/proguanil compared with mefloquine for treatment of acute *Plasmodium falciparum* malaria in Thailand. *Am J Trop Med Hyg* 1999;60:526–532.

106. Radloff PD, Philipps J, Nkeyi M, et al. Atovaquone and proguanil for *Plasmodium falciparum* malaria. *Lancet* 1996;347:1511–1514.

107. Luxemburger C, Nosten F, ter Kuile F, et al. Mefloquine for multidrug-resistant malaria. *Lancet* 1991;338:1268.

108. Weinke T, Trautmann M, Held T, et al. Neuropsychiatric side effects after the use of mefloquine. *Am J Trop Med Hyg* 1991;45:86–91.

109. Nosten F, Vincenti M, Simpson J, et al. The effects of mefloquine treatment in pregnancy. *Clin Infect Dis* 1999;28:808–815.

110. Doorduijn JK, Wismans PJ, Stuiver PC. Halofantrine treatment of *Plasmodium falciparum* malaria. *Ann Intern Med* 1994;120:167.

111. Phillips-Howard PA, Wood D. The safety of antimalarial drugs in pregnancy. *Drug Saf* 1996;14:131–145.

112. Tran TH, Day NPJ, Nguyen HP, et al. A controlled trial of artemether or quinine in Vietnamese adults with severe falciparum malaria. *N Engl J Med* 1996;335:76–83.

113. van Hensbroek MB, Onyiorah E, Jaffar S, et al. A trial of artemether or quinine in children with cerebral malaria. *N Engl J Med* 1996;335;69–75.

114. Danis M, Chandenier J, Doumbo O, et al. Results obtained with i.m. artemether versus i.v. quinine in the treatment of severe malaria in a multicentre study in Africa. *Jpn J Trop Med Hyg* 1996;24[Suppl 1]:93–96.

115. Courval JM, van Hensbroek MB, Murphy S, et al. Meta-analysis of open, randomized trials comparing artemether versus quinine for cerebral malaria in African children. *Jpn J Trop Med Hyg* 1996;24[Suppl]:97–100.

116. Pittler MH, Ernst E. Artemether for severe malaria: a meta-analysis of randomized clinical trials. *Clin Infect Dis* 1999;28:597–601.

117. Alfandari S, Dixmier G, Guery B, et al. Exchange transfusion for severe malaria. *Infection* 2001;29:96–97.

118. Hoontrakoon S, Suputtamongkol Y. Exchange transfusion as an adjunct to the treatment of severe falciparum malaria. *Trop Med Int Health* 1998;3:156–161.

119. Macallan DC, Pocock M, Robinson GT, et al. Red cell exchange, erythrocytapheresis, in the treatment of malaria with high parasitemia in returning travellers. *Trans R Soc Trop Med Hyg* 2000;94:353–356.

120. Looareesuwan S, Viravan C, Webster HK, et al. Clinical studies of atovaquone, alone or in combination with other antimalarial drugs, for treatment of acute uncomplicated malaria in Thailand. *Am J Trop Med Hyg* 1996;54:62–66.

121. Looareesuwan S, Wilairatana P, Glanarongan R, et al. Atovaquone and proguanil hydrochloride followed by primaquine for treatment of *Plasmodium vivax* malaria in Thailand. *Trans R Soc Trop Med Hyg* 1999;93:637–640.

122. Radloff PD, Philipps J, Hutchinson D, et al. Atovaquone plus proguanil is an effective treatment for *Plasmodium ovale* and *Plasmodium malariae* malaria. *Trans R Soc Trop Med Hyg* 1996;90:682.

123. Choi HW, Breman JG, Teutsch SM, et al. The effectiveness of insecticide-impregnated bednets in reducing cases of malaria infection: meta-analysis of published results. *Am J Trop Med Hyg* 1985;52:377–382.

124. Fradin MS. Mosquitoes and mosquito repellents: a clinician's guide. *Ann Intern Med* 1998;128:931–940.

125. McGready R, Hamilton KA, Simpson JA, et al. Safety of the insect repellent N,N-diethyl-M-toluamide (DEET) in pregnancy. *Am J Trop Med Hyg* 2001;65:285–289.

126. dos Santos CC, Anvar A, Keystone JS, et al. Survey of use of malaria prevention measures by Canadians visiting India. *CMAJ* 1999;160:195–200.

127. Castelli F, Matteelli A, Caligaris S, et al. Malaria in migrants. *Parasitologia* 1999;41:261–265.

128. Froude JRL, Weiss LM, Tanowitz HB, et al. Imported malaria in the Bronx: review of 51 cases recorded from 1986 to 1991. *Clin Infect Dis* 1992;15:774–780.

129. Lobel HO, Miani M, Eng T, et al. Long term malaria prophylaxis with weekly mefloquine. *Lancet* 1993;341:848–851.

130. Nosten F, ter Kuile F, Maelankiri L, et al. Mefloquine prophylaxis prevents malaria during pregnancy: a double-blind, placebo-controlled study. *J Infect Dis* 1994;169:595–603.

131. Smoak BL, Writer JC, Keep LW, et al. The effects of inadvertent exposure of mefloquine chemoprophylaxis on pregnancy outcomes and infants of US Army servicewomen. *J Infect Dis* 1997;176:831–833.

132. Miller KD, Lobel HO, Satriale RF, et al. Severe cutaneous reactions among American travelers using pyrimethamine-sulfadoxine (Fansidar) for malaria prophylaxis. *Am J Trop Med Hyg* 1986;35:451–458.

133. Lell B, Luckner D, Ndjave M, et al. Randomised placebo-controlled study of atovaquone plus proguanil for malaria prophylaxis in children. *Lancet* 1998;351:709–713.

134. Shanks GD, Gordon DM, Klotz FW, et al. Efficacy and safety of atovaquone/proguanil as suppressive prophylaxis for *Plasmodium falciparum* malaria. *Clin Infect Dis* 1998;27:494–499.

135. Sukwa TY, Mulenga M, Chisdaka N, et al. A randomized, double-blind, placebo-controlled field trial to determine the efficacy and safety of Malarone (atovaquone/proguanil) for the prophylaxis of malaria in Zambia. *Am J Trop Med Hyg* 1999;60:521–525.

136. van der Berg JD, Duvenage CS, Roskell NS, et al. Safety and efficacy of atovaquone and proguanil hydrochloride for the prophylaxis of *Plasmodium falciparum* malaria in South Africa. *Clin Ther* 1999;21:741–749.

137. Hogh B, Clarke PD, Camus D, et al. Atovaquone-proguanil versus chloroquine-proguanil for malaria prophylaxis in non-immune travellers: a randomized, double-blind study. *Lancet* 2000;356:1888–1894.

138. Overbosch D, Schilthuis H, Bienzle U, et al. Atovaquone-proguanil versus mefloquine for malaria prophylaxis in nonimmune travelers: results from a randomized, double-blind study. *Clin Infect Dis* 2001;33:1015–1021.

139. Fryauff DJ, Baird JK, Basri H, et al. Randomised placebo-controlled trial of primaquine for prophylaxis of falciparum and vivax malaria. *Lancet* 1995;346:1190–1193.

140. Baird JK, Lacy MD, Basri H, et al. Randomized, parallel placebo-controlled trial of primaquine for malaria prophylaxis in Papua, Indonesia. *Clin Infect Dis* 2001;33:1990–1997.

141. Weiss WR, Oloo AJ, Johnson A, et al. Daily primaquine is effective for prophylaxis against falciparum malaria in Kenya: comparison with mefloquine, doxycycline, and chloroquine plus proguanil. *J Infect Dis* 1995;171:1569–1575.

142. Schwartz E, Regev-Yochay G. Primaquine as prophylaxis for malaria in non-immune travelers: a comparison with mefloquine and doxycycline. *Clin Infect Dis* 1999;29:1502–1506.

143. Lell B, Faucher JF, Missinou MA, et al. Malaria chemoprophylaxis with tafenoquine: a randomized study. *Lancet* 2000;355:2041–2045.

144. Shanks GD, Oloo AJ, Aleman GM, et al. A new primaquine analogue, tafenoquine (WR 238605), for prophylaxis against *Plasmodium falciparum* malaria. *Clin Infect Dis* 2001;33:1968–1974.

145. Schlagenhauf P. Standby emergency treatment by travelers. In: Schagenhauf P, ed. *Travelers' malaria.* Hamilton, ON: BC Decker, 2001:446–462.

146. Egan JE, Hoffman SL, Haynes JD, et al. Humoral immune responses in volunteers immunized with irradiated *Plasmodium falciparum* sporozoites. *Am J Trop Med Hyg* 1993;49:166–173.

147. Bojang KA, Milligan PJ, Pinder M, et al. Efficacy of RTS,S/AS02 malaria vaccine against *Plasmodium falciparum* infection in semi-immune adult men in the Gambia: a randomized trial. *Lancet* 2001;358:1927–1934.

148. Sturchler D, Berger R, Rudin C, et al. Safety, immunogenicity, and pilot efficacy of *Plasmodium falciparum* sporozoite and asexual blood-stage combination vaccine in Swiss adults. *Am J Trop Med Hyg* 1995;53:423–431.

149. Roberts DR, Andre RG. Insecticide resistance issues in vector-borne disease control. *Am J Trop Med Hyg* 1994;50[6 Suppl]:21–34.

150. Skrabalo Z, Deanovic Z. Piroplasmosis in man: report of a case. *Doc Med Geogr Trop* 1957;9:11–16.

151. Western KA, Benson GD, Gleason NN, et al. Babesiosis in a Massachusetts resident. *N Engl J Med* 1970;283:854–856.

152. Jack RM, Ward PA. *Babesia rodhaini* interactions with complement: relationship to parasitic entry into red cells. *J Immunol* 1980;124:1566–1573.

153. Quick RE, Herwaldt BL, Thomford JW, et al. Babesiosis in Washington state: a new species of *Babesia? Ann Intern Med* 1993;119:284–290.

154. Persing DH, Herwaldt BL, Glaser C, et al. Infection with a *Babesia*-like organism in northern California. *N Engl J Med* 1995;332:298–303.

155. Herwaldt BL, Persing DH, Precigout EA, et al. A fatal case of babesiosis in Missouri: identification of another piroplasm that infects humans. *Ann Intern Med* 1996;124:643–650.

156. Shih C-M, Liu L-P, Chung W-C, et al. Human babesiosis in Taiwan: asymptomatic infection with a *Babesia microti*–like organism in a Taiwanese woman. *J Clin Microbiol* 1997;35:450–454.

157. Wei Q, Tsuji M, Zamoto A, et al. Human babesiosis in Japan: isolation of *Babesia microti*–like parasites from an asymptomatic transfusion donor and from a rodent from an area where babesiosis is endemic. *J Clin Microbiol* 2001;39:2178–2183.

158. Michael SA, Morsy TA, Montasser MF. A case of human babesiosis (preliminary case report in Egypt). *J Egypt Soc Parasitol* 1987;17:409–410.

159. Bush JB, Isaacson BM, Mohamed AS, et al. Human babesiosis—a preliminary report of 2 suspected cases in South Africa. *S Afr Med J* 1990;78:699.

160. Gorenflot A, Moubri K, Precigout E, et al. Human babesiosis. *Ann Trop Med Parasitol* 1998;92:489–501.

161. Piesman J, Spielman A. Human babesiosis on Nantucket Island: prevalence of *Babesia microti* in ticks. *Am J Trop Med Hyg* 1980;29:742–746.

162. Alward W, Javaid M, Garner J. Babesiosis in a Connecticut resident. *Conn Med* 1990;54:425–427.

163. Krause PJ, Spielman A, Telford SR III, et al. Persistent parasitemia after acute babesiosis. *N Engl J Med* 1998;339:160–165.

164. Eskow ES, Krause PJ, Spielman A, et al. Southern extension of the range of human babesiosis in the eastern United States. *J Clin Microbiol* 1999;37:2051–2052.

165. Steketee RW, Eckman MR, Burgess EC, et al. Babesiosis in Wisconsin. A new focus of disease transmission. *JAMA* 1985;253:2675–2678.

166. Filstein MR, Benach JL, White DJ, et al. Serosurvey for human babesiosis in New York. *J Infect Dis* 1980;141:518–521.

167. Popovsky MA, Lindberg LE, Syrek AL, et al. Prevalence of *Babesia* antibody in a selected blood donor population. *Transfusion* 1988;28:59–61.

168. Krause PJ, Telford SR III, Pollack RJ, et al. Babesiosis: an underdiagnosed disease of children. *Pediatrics* 1992;89:1045–1048.

169. Hilton E, DeVoti J, Benach JL, et al. Seroprevalence and seroconversion for tick-borne disease in a high-risk population in the northeast United States. *Am J Med* 1999;106:404–409.

170. Fritz CL, Kjemtrump AM, Conrad PA, et al. Seroepidemiology of emerging tickborne infectious diseases in a northern California community. *J Infect Dis* 1997;175:1432–1439.

171. Mitchell PD, Reed KD, Hofkes JM. Immunoserologic evidence of coinfection with *Borrelia burgdorferi*, *Babesia microti*, and human granulocytic *Ehrlichia* species in residents of Wisconsin and Minnesota. *J Clin Microbiol* 1996;34:724–727.

172. Wang TJ, Liang MH, Sangha O, et al. Coexposure to *Borrelia burgdorferi* and *Babesia microti* does not worsen the long-term outcome of Lyme disease. *Clin Infect Dis* 2000;31:1149–1154.

173. McQuiston JH, Childs JE, Chamberland ME, et al. Transmission of tick-borne agents of disease by blood transfusion: a review of known and potential risks in the United States [published erratum in *Transfusion* 2000;40:274–284]. *Transfusion* 2000;40:891.

174. Dobroszycki J, Herwaldt BL, Boctor F, et al. A cluster of transfusion-associated babesiosis cases traced to a single asymptomatic donor. *JAMA* 1999;281:927–930.

175. Gerber MA, Shapiro ED, Krause PJ, et al. The risk of acquiring Lyme disease or babesiosis from a blood transfusion. *J Infect Dis* 1994;170:231–234.

176. Boustani MR, Gelfand JA. Babesiosis. *Clin Infect Dis* 1996;22:611–615.

177. Homer MJ, Aguilar-Delfin I, Telford SR III, et al. Babesiosis. *Clin Microbiol Rev* 2000;13:451–469.

178. Benach JL, Habicht GS, Hamburger MI. Immunoresponsiveness in acute babesiosis in humans. *J Infect Dis* 1982;146:369–380.

179. Ruebush MJ, Hanson WL. Thymus dependence of resistance to infection with *Babesia microti* of human origin in mice. *Am J Trop Med Hyg* 1980;29:507–515.

180. Shimada T, Shikano S, Hashiguchi R, et al. Effects of depletion of T cell subpopulation on the course of infection and anti-parasite delayed type hypersensitivity response in mice infected with *Babesia microti* and *Babesia rodhaini*. *J Vet Med Sci* 1996;58:343–347.

181. Meeusen E, Lloyd S, Soulsby EJ. *Babesia microti* in mice: adoptive transfer of immunity with serum and cells. *Aust J Exp Biol Med Sci* 1984;62:551–566.

182. Igarashi I, Waki S, Ito M, et al. Role of CD4$^+$ cells in the control of primary infection with *Babesia microti* in mice. *J Protozool Res* 1994;4:164–171.

183. Rosenblatt-Bin H, Klein A, Srdeni B. Antibabesial effect of the immunomodulator AS101 in mice: role of increased production of nitric oxide. *Parasitol Immunol* 1996;18:297–306.

184. Rosner F, Zarrabi MH, Benach JL, et al. Babesiosis in splenectomized adults: review of 22 reported cases. *Am J Med* 1984;76:696–701.

185. Ruebush TK II, Cassaday PB, Marsh HJ, et al. Human babesiosis on Nantucket Island. *Ann Intern Med* 1977;86:6–9.

186. Ruebush TK II, Juranek DD, Spielman A, et al. Epidemiology of human babesiosis on Nantucket Island. *Am J Trop Med Hyg* 1981;30:937–941.

187. Gombert ME, Goldstein EJC, Benach JL, et al. Human babesiosis. Clinical and therapeutic considerations. *JAMA* 1982;248:3005–3007.

188. Meldrum SC, Birkhead GS, White DJ, et al. Human babesiosis in New York state: an epidemiological description of 136 cases. *Clin Infect Dis* 1992;15:1019–1023.

189. White DJ, Talarico J, Chang H-G, et al. Human babesiosis in New York state. Review of 139 hospitalized cases and analysis of prognostic factors. *Arch Intern Med* 1998;158:2149–2154.

190. Hatcher JC, Greenberg PD, Antique J, et al. Severe babesiosis in Long Island: review of 34 cases and their complications. *Clin Infect Dis* 2001;32:1117–1125.

191. Kim N, Rosenbaum GS, Cunha BA. Relative bradycardia and lymphopenia in patients with babesiosis. *Clin Infect Dis* 1998;26:1218–1219.

192. Dacey MJ, Martinez H, Raimondo T, et al. Septic shock due to babesiosis. *Clin Infect Dis* 2001;33:e37–e38.

193. Benezra D, Brown AE, Polsky B, et al. Babesiosis and infection with human immunodeficiency virus (HIV). *Ann Intern Med* 1987;107:944.

194. Sun T, Tenenbaum MJ, Greenspan J, et al. Morphologic and clinical observations in human infection with *Babesia microti*. *J Infect Dis* 1984;148:239–248.

195. Krause PJ, Telford SR III, Ryan R, et al. Diagnosis of babesiosis: evaluation of a serologic test for the detection of *Babesia microti* antibody. *J Infect Dis* 1994;169:923–926.

196. Wittner M, Rowin KS, Tanowitz HB, et al. Successful chemotherapy of transfusion babesiosis. *Ann Intern Med* 1982;96:601–604.

197. Shih C-M, Wang C-C. Ability of azithromycin in combination with quinine for the elimination of babesial infections in humans. *Am J Trop Med Hyg* 1998;59:509–512.

198. Bonoan JT, Johnson DH, Cunha BA. Life-threatening babesiosis in an asplenic patient treated with exchange transfusion, azithromycin, and atovaquone. *Heart Lung* 1998;27:424–428.

199. Krause PJ, Leport T, Sikand VK, et al. Atovaquone and azithromycin for the treatment of babesiosis. *N Engl J Med* 2000;343:1454–1458.

200. Dorman SE, Cannon ME, Telford SR III, et al. Fulminant babesiosis treated with clindamycin, quinine, and whole-blood exchange transfusion. *Transfusion* 2000;40:375–380.

201. Evenson DA, Perry E, Kloster B, et al. Therapeutic apheresis for babesiosis. *J Clin Apheresis* 1998;13:32–36.

CHAPTER 280
Leishmania

John L. Ho and Warren D. Johnson, Jr.

Few infectious diseases are as complex as leishmaniasis (1–3). An endemic disease of the tropics and subtropics, human leishmaniasis assumes a bewildering variety of forms in the skin. Visceral leishmaniasis (kala-azar, VL) has a more typical presentation. Leishmaniasis threatens 350 million women, men, and children around the world (4,5). The prevalence of leishmaniasis is estimated to be 12 million persons, making this one of the top infectious diseases impacting global health. Leishmaniasis was named after William Boog Leishman who found the amastigotes in the liver of a British soldier who returned from India. Later studies conducted by Charles Nicolle, a 1928 Nobel laureate, at the Institut Pasteur of Tunis characterized human Mediterranean visceral leishmaniasis and cultivated the etiologic agent, *Leishmania infantum*. The amastigotes, or *Leishmania donovani* bodies, are the smallest major parasites of humans, measuring 2 μm and characterized by a nucleus and a rod-shaped kinetoplast (Fig. 280.1A). *Trypanosoma cruzi* amastigotes are indistinguishable, but the type of cells the parasites invade (muscle cells for *T. cruzi*) provides the distinction. *Leishmania* amastigotes are found only in skin Langerhans cells, and tissue macrophages including those in the bone marrow, spleen and Kupffer cells of the liver. The amastigote form is found in mammals and the ingestion of this form by the sandfly vector results in the development of a flagellated promastigote form (Fig. 280.1B), which causes transmission when the female fly feeds again.

GEOGRAPHIC DISTRIBUTION

The family Trypanosomatidae, defined by Doflein in 1901, has two genera, *Trypanosoma* and *Leishmania*, that cause disease in humans. Trypanosomal diseases are restricted in their geographic distribution by the glossinae (tsetse flies) to Africa, and the triatomine bugs to the New World. The sandflies involved in the transmission of leishmaniasis has no such limitations. Although sandflies do not survive in cold climates, rapid air travel and the slow genesis of *Leishmania* infections mean that cases now can be seen anywhere in the world. Leishmaniasis has been reported in at least 88 countries, including Africa, parts of central and south America, Asia, southern Europe; 66 are in the Old World, and 22 are in the New World (4,5) (Fig. 280.2). More than 90% of all cases of visceral leishmaniasis occur in Bangladesh, India, Sudan, Brazil, and Nepal. More than 90% of all cases of cutaneous leishmaniasis occur in Afghanistan, Brazil, Iran, Peru, Saudi Arabia and the Syria. *L. mexicana* is enzootic in Texas and Arizona and human cases of cutaneous leishmaniasis have been documented in Texas as well as an epidemic of leishmaniasis in U.S. hunting hounds (6). More than 90% of mucosal leishmaniasis cases occur in Bolivia and Brazil, but exist throughout Central and South America (4,5).

The clinical aspects of *Leishmania* infections differ depending on where the infections are contracted and the species causing the infection (Table 280.1). Visceral leishmaniasis affects mainly adults in India but in the Mediterranean and Brazil it is a disease of childhood. This may be due in part to the species of *Leishmania* causing infection (see Table 280.1). No animal reservoir has been documented in India, while dogs have epidemiologic importance in the Mediterranean, Brazil, and China. Patients'

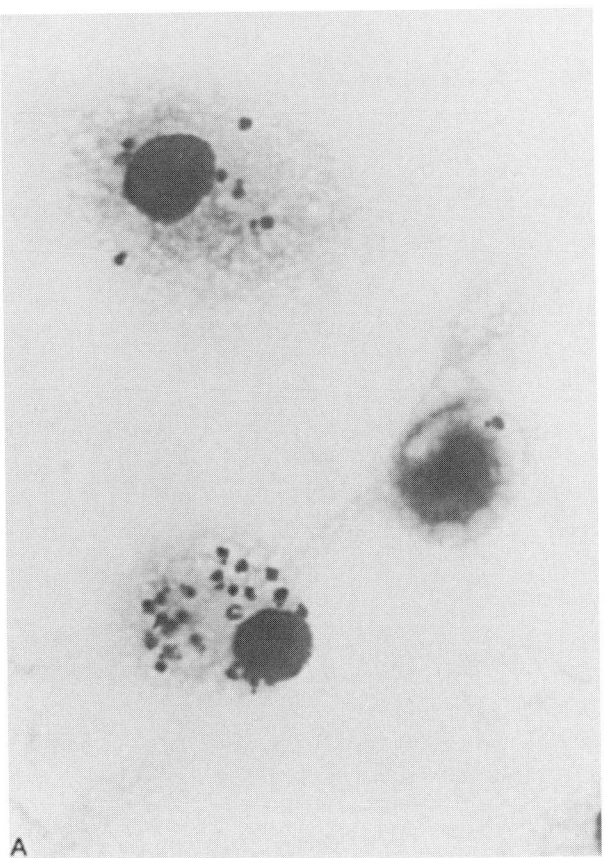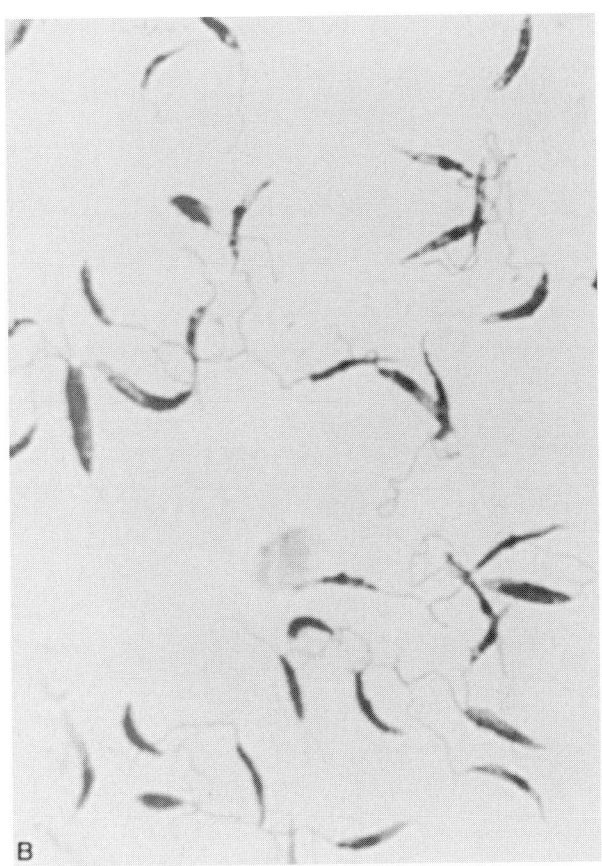

Figure 280.1. **A:** *Leishmania* amastigotes within host macrophages. **B:** Flagellated promastigote leishmanial forms found in the sandfly vector. Promastigote forms also grow when infected tissues are cultivated in blood agar Nicolle-Novy-MacNeal (10% defibrinated rabbit blood in agar) medium at a temperature of 24°C to 26°C. Fresh tissue can be sent to the Centers for Disease Control and Prevention (CDC), Atlanta, GA for culture and speciation with special arrangement.

responses to treatment differ in these locations; Indian leishmaniasis is more difficult to treat and more likely to be resistant to antimony. Cutaneous leishmaniasis also has multiple geographic variants (see Table 280.1) (1–3,7). The classic oriental sore of the Middle East is often a closed, nodular, chronic skin granuloma, although it ulcerates with time. The lesions of Ethiopian cutaneous leishmaniasis may remain closed but gradually increase in diameter. The most common form of cutaneous leishmaniasis in South America is a rapidly ulcerating lesion. A curious and rare form of "anergic" cutaneous disease, called diffuse leishmaniasis consisting of papular lesions throughout the body is being seen especially in Brazil and Ethiopia.

TAXONOMY

Parasites are now grouped into species and subspecies according to a variety of biologic, biochemical (i.e., isoenzymes and antigenic analysis using monoclonal antibodies) and various deoxyribonucleic acid (DNA) typing criteria. Despite these new techniques, the classification of *Leishmania* remains in flux (2,3,8). Furthermore, the taxonomy of *Leishmania* organisms is rarely available at the time of consultation, because it takes weeks to isolate and characterize the organisms. It is important for clinicians who see patients with leishmaniasis to know what species of *Leishmania* are present at a specific area in the world and within a country. For example, in northeastern Brazil the great majority of patients have *L. Viannia braziliensis* infection, which is impor-

tant because it is more resistant to treatment and is the species most commonly associated with mucosal disease. *L. donovani*, the agent of visceral leishmaniasis, a relatively uniform organism is subdivided into several species and discussed as a single entity with important regional differences indicated (see Table 280.1). Cutaneous leishmaniasis is divided into Old World and New World disease and is caused by an array of species giving rise to a spectrum of disease manifestations (see Table 280.1). Mucosal leishmaniasis is caused predominantly by *L. V. braziliensis* and will be discussed separately even though *Leishmania* species causing mucosal disease also cause cutaneous disease (see Table 280.1).

LIFE CYCLE OF *LEISHMANIA* IN SANDFLIES AND IMMUNOLOGIC BASIS OF LEISHMANIASIS

The syndrome of leishmaniasis is caused by the bite of an infected female sandfly. At least 30 species of the genus, *Lutzomyia* in the Americas, and *Phlebotomus* elsewhere in the world, have been identified (Fig 280.3). Sandflies are infected by the taking of a blood meal from an infected mammal. The blood meal is required for egg production, and the fertilized eggs are oviposited in moist soil. The amastigote upon liberation from macrophages transforms into a promastigote and survives within a peritrophic matrix formed around the blood meal in the gut of the sandfly (9). Later, the promastigote escapes the peritrophic matrix to attach to specific ligand(s) on the gut epithelial by lipophosphoglycan

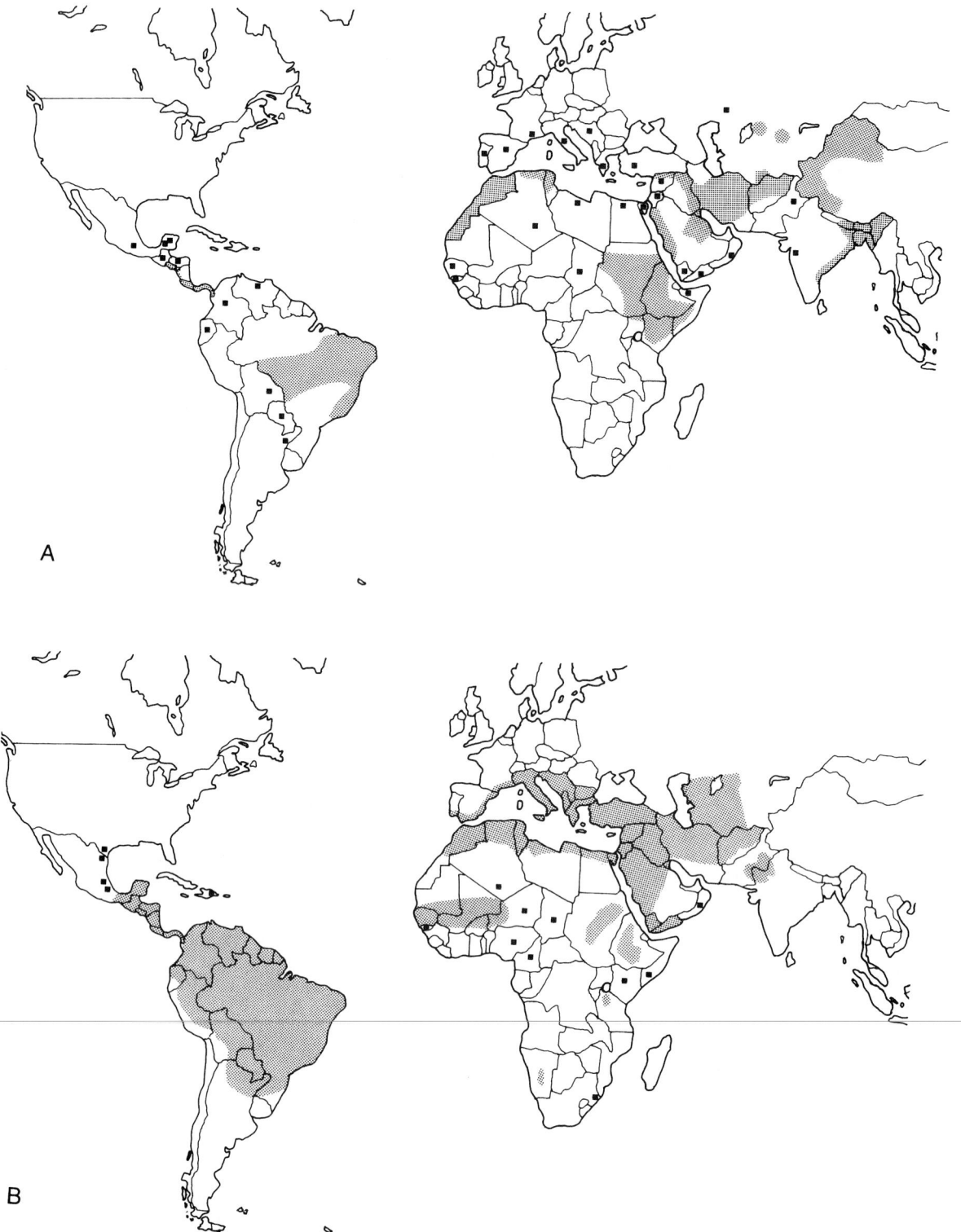

Figure 280.2. A: Visceral leishmaniasis. Cases of visceral leishmaniasis have been reported from the following countries: Afghanistan, Algeria, Argentina, Bangladesh, Bolivia, Brazil, Chad, China, Colombia, Costa Rica, Democratic Yemen, Ecuador, Egypt, El Salvador, Ethiopia, France, Gambia, Greece, Guatemala, Honduras, India, Iran, Iraq, Israel, Italy, Jordan, Kenya, Kuwait, Lebanon, Libyan Arab Jamahiriya, Malta, Mexico, Morocco, Nepal, Nicaragua, Oman, Pakistan, Paraguay, Portugal, Saudi Arabia, Senegal, Spain, Sudan, Syria, Tunisia, Turkey Uganda, former USSR, Venezuela, Yemen, and Yugoslavia. **B:** Cutaneous leishmaniasis. Cases of cutaneous leishmaniasis have been reported from the following countries: Afghanistan, Algeria, Argentina, Belize, Bolivia, Brazil, Burkina Faso, Cameroon, Chad, Colombia, Costa Rica, Democratic Yemen, Dominican Republic, Ecuador, Egypt, Ethiopia, French Guiana, Gambia, Greece, Guatemala, Guyana, Honduras, India, Iran, Iraq, Israel, Jordan, Kenya, Kuwait, Lebanon, Libyan Arab Jamahiriya, Mali, Mauritania, Mexico, Morocco, Nicaragua, Niger, Nigeria, Oman, Pakistan, Panama, Paraguay, Peru, Saudi Arabia, Senegal, Sudan, Suriname, Syria, Tunisia, Turkey, United States, Venezuela, USA, former USSR republics, and Yemen. (**A** and **B** data from Guidelines for Leishmaniasis Control at Regional and Subregional Levels. Geneva, World Health Organization, 1988. (No new map update available 2002.)

TABLE 280.1. Causative Organisms of Leishmaniasis

Cutaneous Leishmaniasis[a]

Old World	New World
Leishmania Leishmaia	*Leishmania L. mexicana*
(*L.*) *tropica*	*Leishmania L. amazonensis*
Leishmania L. major	*Leishmania L. venezuelensis*
Leishmania L. aethiopica	*Leishmania L. garnhami*
Leishmania L tropica	*Leishmania L. pifanoi*
	Leishmania Viannia (V.) braziliensis
	Leishmania V. panamensis
	Leishmania V. guyanensis
	Leishmania V. peruviana

Visceral Leishmaniasis

Old World	New World
L. L. donovani	*L. L. chagasi*
L. L. infantum	*L. L. amazonensis*
L. L. tropica	

Mucosal Leishmaniasis[a]

Old World	New World
L. L. donovani	*Leishmania V. braziliensis*
	Leishmania V. guyanensis
	Leishmania V. panamensis
	Leishmania V. peruviana
	Leishmania L. amazonensis

[a]Rarely, *L. donovani* has been known to cause purely cutaneous disease.

(LPG), the major glycolipid surrounding the entire exterior of the promastigote. The addition of specific sugar side chain to LPG during promastigote development releases the infectious metacyclic promastigote allowing migration to the anterior gut, where they await, poised and ready to infect a mammalian host (10,11).

Studies using in-bred mice infected with *L. major* have led to the identification of morphologically similar but functionally distinct CD4$^+$ T subsets of helper (Th) cell populations as defined by their cytokine production profiles (12–16). Th-1 subset cells produce interleukin-2 (IL-2), interferon-γ (IFN-γ), IL-3, granulocyte-macrophage–colony-stimulating factor (GM-CSF), and IL-12; while Th-2 subset cells produce IL-4, IL-5, IL-7, IL-9, IL-10, and IL-13 (12–14,17). Overproduction of IL-4 and IL-10 inhibits expansion of Th-1 cells and macrophage activation by IFN-γ (14,18,19). In susceptible mice strains, *L. major* infection produces cutaneous disease with a predominance of Th2 cells (12,14), and likely both IL-4 and IL-10 play role in immune suppression and disease outcome (12,13,19–23). In contrast, resis-

tant mice strains that show self-healing lesions when infected with *L. major* demonstrate a Th1 predominant response (14,24). IFN-γ, a Th1 cytokine, is critical for triggering macrophage activation and killing of the parasites (25,26). IL-12 produced by NK cells, dendritic cells, macrophages, and Th1 cells also plays an important role by directing the expansion of Th1 cells and thus, influences the control of *Leishmania* infection (20,24,27,28). In contrast to murine cutaneous leishmaniasis, the immune response of visceral leishmaniasis caused by *L. chagasi* is associated with active suppression of Th1 response rather than an expansion of Th2 cells. The suppression is mediated in part by transforming growth factor-β (TGF-β) and IL-10 (29,30). These murine models showed that *Leishmania* species cause disease with distinct immunologic patterns, and suggest both parasite gene products (*L. major* versus *L. chagasi*) and mouse genetic background (i.e., susceptible or resistant strains) are likely involved in the modulation of the disease immune response. The evolution of Th cell subsets is also influenced by parasite factors and by priming of the innate immunity (12,15,31–34).

CLINICAL MANIFESTATIONS OF LEISHMANIASIS

The complexity of the clinical manifestations and differences in epidemiologic distribution, *Leishmania* species, transmission patterns, immunopathologic mechanisms, and diagnostic conditions necessitate separate sections for visceral, cutaneous, and mucosal (mucocutaneous) leishmaniasis.

Visceral Leishmaniasis or Kala-Azar

Kala-azar is a Hindi term meaning black fever or fatal fever. Visceral leishmaniasis is fatal unless treated and is due to the systemic parasitism of the reticuloendothelial system by *L. donovani*, *L. infantum*, *L. chagasi*, and recently *L. tropica* (see Table 280.1). Worldwide, there appear to be increasing numbers of cases (5). Transmission of the disease appears to be peridomestic in parts of the world, and is reflected by the early age of onset of visceral leishmaniasis, typically less than 5 years in Brazil and ~2 years in Tunisia (35–38). Prospective studies conducted in Brazil found that infection is far greater than disease, at a ratio of 10:1 (37–39). The spectra of outcome following infection consist of symptom-free individual, and a subclinical state in which some children will control the infection while other will evolve into full-blown visceral disease over several months (37,38). Thus, although most disease occurs within 6 months after infection, it may be as long as 9 years. Those infected in the first decade of life are the most vulnerable and malnutrition further increases the risk for disease (37,40). Although visceral leishmaniasis afflicts disproportionately those residing in rural area where agriculture is the main activity, transmission is encroaching urban areas, notably in Brazil and Venezuela (37,41,42).

PATHOGENESIS

During active leishmaniasis, *Leishmania* parasites circulate in patients' blood steam associated with leukocytes. The risk for visceral disease is presumably increased by the immaturity of the immune system at young age and increased by malnutrition (38,40). *Leishmania* antigen-specific B cells provide no protection against disease. Anti-*Leishmania* antibodies are readily detected and antibodies to *Leishmania* K39 antigen is an excellent marker for acute visceral leishmaniasis (43–46). In contrast, there is a T cell immune "defect," manifested by a absent delayed hypersensitivity skin test responses to leishmanial crude

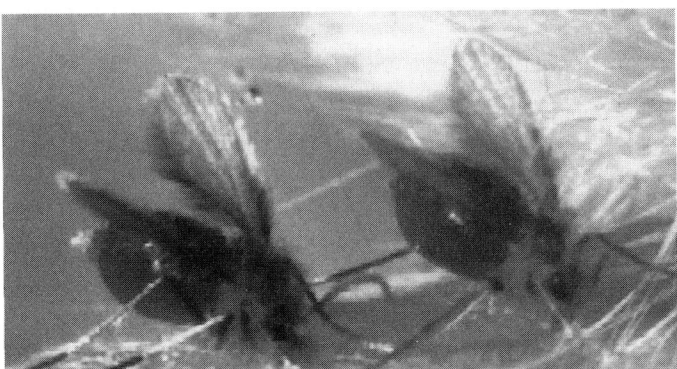

Figure 280.3. Sandfly taking a blood meal. The abdomen is engorged with blood. Courtesy of Dr. Edgar Rowton, Walter Reed Army Institute of Research, Washington, DC 20307.

antigens (47,48). Moreover, peripheral blood mononuclear cells from patients with acute visceral leishmaniasis do not proliferate or produce interferon-γ (IFN-γ) or IL-2 when cultured *in vitro* with leishmanial antigen (47,49–51). In contrast, when challenged with mitogens or unrelated antigens patients' mononuclear cells produce normal amounts of IL-2 and IFN-γ (47,52). Circulating T cells from patients with acute visceral leishmaniasis produce soluble factors that are capable of suppressing antigen-driven lymphocyte proliferation (47). One of the soluble factor is IL-10. *In vitro*, monoclonal antibodies against IL-10 partially reverse the antigen-specific proliferation defect and restore IFN-γ production (49,50). Data suggest IL-10 and IL-12 are the main regulators of the immune dysfunction (49,50,53,54). Upon recovery from the illness, the Th1 cytokines (IFN-γ, IL-2) are elaborated in response to *Leishmania* antigens while Th2 cytokines (IL-5, IL-10) are reduced or absent (49,53). TGF-β may also be involved in the immune suppression because high serum levels are detected in patients during acute visceral disease, and neutralization of IL-10 and TGF-β in mononuclear cell cultures restores IFN-γ production (Nascimento ET, Wilson M, Jeronimo S, Federal University of Rio do Norte, Brazil, and University of Iowa, USA, personal communication). Despite these findings, there is considerable lack of knowledge regarding how the immune dysfunction is triggered and assessing the parasite and host determinants for human disease.

CLINICAL MANIFESTATION

The hallmark of visceral leishmaniasis is fever, hepatosplenomegaly, leukopenia, and thrombocytopenia in an acutely ill immunocompetent patient who is a resident of, or recently arrived from an endemic region. In an immunosuppressed patient, past travel to or emigration from an endemic country may be elicited. The onset of visceral leishmaniasis is insidious with recurrent fever, weakness, weight loss, and in some, small volume episodic diarrhea (55,56), probably caused by infiltration of intestinal macrophages by *Leishmania* amastigotes. On examination, the patient is thin, emphasizing the markedly enlarged liver and spleen. Both organs are firm and non-tender on palpation, although the patient may complain of discomfort resulting from the splenic enlargement. Anemia, thrombocytopenia, and leukopenia are common. Bleeding phenomena, particularly epistaxis, resulting from thrombocytopenia and poor synthesis of coagulation factors from hepatic infiltration by *Leishmania* is present in a fair number of the patients. Hemophagocytosis when present can be confused with hematologic malignancies because a majority of these patients have negative smears in their bone marrow (57). Intercurrent respiratory or intestinal infection or bleeding are the associated events causing death in visceral leishmaniasis. Even with treatment, fatality may be as high as 10% (58). Minor accessory signs of visceral leishmaniasis are increased pigmentation on the face and trunk leading to the term Kala-azar "black fever" frequently seen in India. Lymphadenopathy may be present, especially in the East African and Mediterranean cases. Histologic examination of the liver shows normal hepatocytes but masses of parasites within the Kupffer cells. Slight increases in transpeptidases (transaminases) and alkaline phosphatase levels are common but jaundice is rare. The spleen shows massive parasite involvement making the splenic aspirate a sensitive diagnostic test. Rare complications of established kala-azar are intralobular cirrhosis (Rogers cirrhosis), glomerulonephritis caused by immunoglobulin deposition in the basement membrane, and amyloidosis. The differential diagnosis of visceral leishmaniasis must include the two other major tropical infections that cause hepatosplenomegaly: malaria and schistosomiasis. Hyperimmune malarial splenomegaly is characterized by high immunoglobulin M levels and hepatic

sinusoidal lymphocytosis. Hepatosplenic schistosomiasis associated with *Salmonella* septicemia may closely resemble visceral leishmaniasis, but *Schistosoma mansoni* eggs are present in the stool. The hepatosplenomegaly of visceral leishmaniasis is often so marked that conditions with an equivalent degree of enlargement of these organs, namely leukemias, lymphomas, myelosclerosis, chronic brucellosis, and deposition disorders (Gaucher disease), are part of the differential diagnosis. In early visceral leishmaniasis with modest splenomegaly, typhoid fever and acute malaria must be excluded, as well as a host of fungal, bacterial, rickettsial, and viral infections. Laboratory investigation confirms the presence of a normocytic, normochromic anemia that is often severe. Pancytopenia is usual, with a low white cell count caused by a marked reduction in granulocytes, especially neutrophils. In occasional patients, one or all of these three elements are relatively normal. The serum globulin level is often markedly elevated (4 to 8 g/dL), and electrophoresis shows a polyclonal increase of the immunoglobulin classes.

DIAGNOSIS

With these findings, the clinician must then seek the organism. The safest procedure is bone marrow aspiration. Giemsa-stained smears are prepared from the aspirate and scrutinized for the characteristic amastigotes within macrophages. A definitive diagnosis is established with this procedure in 90% of cases. If the clinical suspicion is strong but bone marrow findings are negative, splenic aspiration is indicated. A fine intramuscular needle attached to a syringe is inserted into the non-mobile spleen and negative pressure is applied. The needle is withdrawn immediately and the aspirated splenic pulp is used to prepare Giemsa-stained slides and to seed cultures. This procedure should not be performed if the platelet count is 80,000/mm³ or less, the prothrombin activity is 60% or more than the control value (59), the spleen is palpable less than 4 cm below the costal margin, or the physician is inexperienced with the technique. The potential risk is that of tearing the splenic capsule, but the value of the procedure, particularly in the evaluation of treatment, is undisputed (60). A liver biopsy examination, a less sensitive procedure may also reveal amastigotes. Fresh specimens of the bone marrow, spleen aspirate or liver biopsy should also be sent to CDC for culture and *Leishmania* speciation. Alternative methods for diagnosis of visceral leishmaniasis not currently commercially available include: examination of Giemsa stained smear of the buffy coat from spun peripheral blood, gene amplification by PCR of tissue sample or of leukocytes from spun peripheral blood (Walter Reed Armed Forces Institute, or the National Institutes of Health), and serologic assays (K39 assay for visceral leishmaniasis, Corixa Corp., Seatlle, WA, USA; indirect fluorescent antibody assay that can distinguish the major *Leishmania* species, CDC, ATL, GA).

Anti-*Leishmania* drugs are often first evaluated in visceral leishmaniasis patients because of the multiplicity of signs, which disappear with successful treatment. Thus, the fever remits; anemia, leukopenia, and thrombocytopenia improve; and the liver and spleen diminish in size. The serum gamma-globulin value takes longer to normalize. Results of the *Leishmania* delayed hypersensitivity skin test become positive. In therapeutic studies, the absence of amastigotes in splenic aspirates is the best guide to treatment success, but it is likely that amastigotes persist silently and indefinitely, as in *Mycobacterium tuberculosis* infection even after successful treatment. In support of this concept is the finding of parasites in the healed cutaneous scars, in the chronic skin rash of leishmania recidivans, and in the skin nodules of patients with post-kala-azar dermal leishmaniasis (61–64).

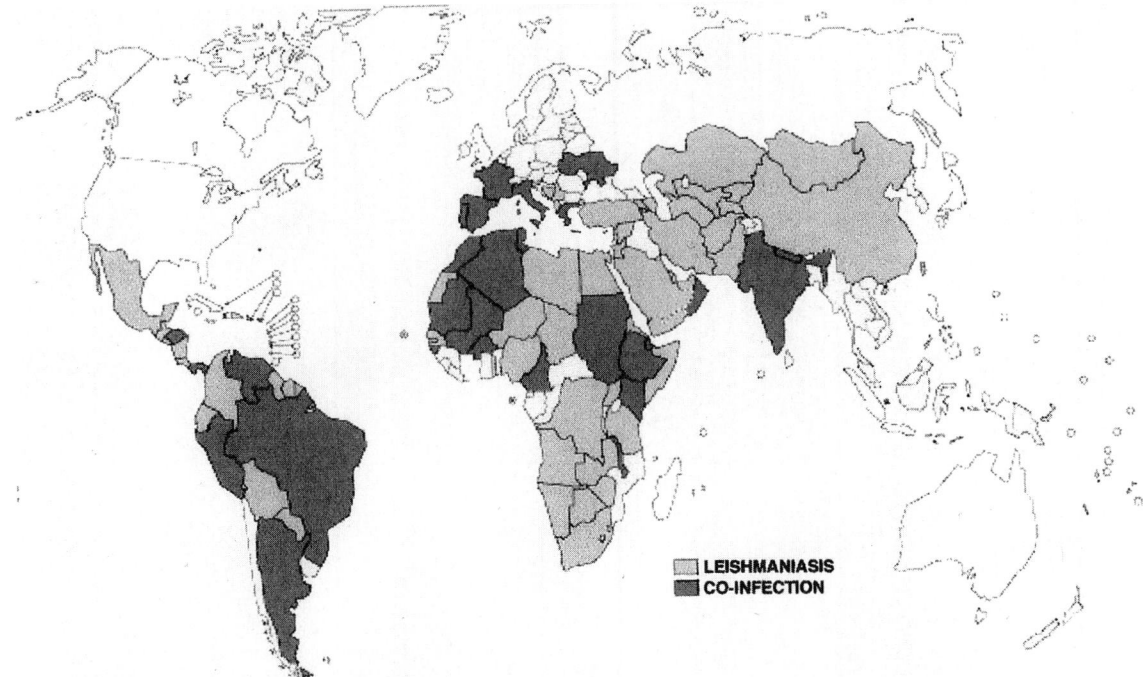

Figure 280.4. Global distribution of *Leishmania* and HIV-1 co-infection. Leishmania endemic countries are in *light shading*, and HIV-1 co-infected are in *dark shading*. (Courtesy of WHO 2000.)

Leishmaniasis in Human Immunodeficiency Virus-1/Acquired Immunodeficiency Disease and the Immunosuppressed Patient

The countries reporting *Leishmania*/human immunodeficiency virus-1 (HIV-1) co-infection to the World Health Organization (WHO) are illustrated in Fig. 280.4 (65). Although cases of *Leishmania*/HIV-1 co-infection have been reported in at least 33 countries worldwide, currently most of the reported cases have originated from France, Italy, Portugal, and Spain. Visceral leishmaniasis is the clinical form most frequently associated with HIV-1/AIDS (~85%) (65,66). Atypical forms of visceral disease including intestinal manifestations should be suspected in a patient with fever, hepatosplenomegaly, adenopathy, or anemia. Other manifestations of leishmaniasis in HIV-1 co-infected patients include simple cutaneous, and mucocutaneous disease while more unusual cutaneous forms or atypical locations have also been observed. Atypical location presentation was more likely in a patient with severe CD4 depletion less than 50/μL. More than 90% of the 682 patients with *Leishmania*/HIV-1 co-infection in a WHO series had CD4 T cell counts less than 200/μL, and only 1% have CD4 T cell counts over 500/μL (65). Clinical manifestation of leishmaniasis in patients immunocompromised by cancer or immunosuppressive agents mimics that of *Leishmania*/HIV co-infection (67–69).

Cutaneous Leishmaniasis

The causative *Leishmania* organisms of New World cutaneous leishmaniasis are divided into the *L. Viannia (V)* subgenera and the *L. Leishmania (L.) mexicana* that include *L. L. amazonensis* and *L. L. mexicana* (see Table 280.1). Old World leishmaniasis is caused predominantly by *L. L. major*, *L. L. tropica*, or *L. L. aethiopica* but on occasion *L. L. donovani* and *L. L. infantum* also can produce cutaneous leishmaniasis (70,71). The most common form of cutaneous leishmaniasis is classic (or simple) cutaneous leishmaniasis, and is the major focus of this section. It consists usually one to three lesions distributed in one bodily region (but may extend to up to three contiguous bodily regions with always less than ten lesions). Other cutaneous manifestation forms are discussed at the end of this section. Two transmission cycle forms of cutaneous leishmaniasis exist: zoonotic and anthroponotic (5). For the zoonotic form of cutaneous leishmaniasis, animals are the reservoir that maintain and disseminate *Leishmania*. This transmission form in the New World is predominately in Latin America but extends from south Texas, United States to northern Argentina, and in the Old World is in southwestern and central Asia, Middle East, and Africa (see Fig 280.2B). Zoonotic cutaneous leishmaniasis in the New World transmitted by diverse *Lutzomyia* species is caused by *L. Viannia* species (especially *L. V. braziliensis*), *L. L. mexicana*, and *L. L. amazonensis* and the reservoirs include small rodents or big animals inhabiting primary forests or secondary forests and is emerging in peridomestic areas. In the Old World, zoonotic cutaneous leishmaniasis is due to *L. L. major*; transmission is mainly by *Phlebotomus papatasi* and its major reservoir is rodents (gerbils). In the anthroponotic form caused by *L. L. tropica*, man is the sole source of infection of the *Phlebotomus sergenti* vector, and is restricted solely to the Old World (see Fig 280.2B).

PATHOGENESIS

Following inoculation of *Leishmania* during the sandfly's blood meal, the promastigotes enter skin Langerhans cells. It is common to find regional adenopathy in early cutaneous leishmaniasis due to *L. V. braziliensis* and *L. L. amazonesis*. Human responses to cutaneous leishmaniasis and mucosal disease caused by *L. V. braziliensis* appear to be much more complex than in-bred murine models. Classic cutaneous disease and mucosal leishmaniasis are associated with high production of IFN-γ and TNF-α (72–74). High levels of TNF-α are detected in serum of patients with cutaneous, diffuse cutaneous and mucosal leishmaniasis (73). How a down-regulated Th1 type response in early cutaneous lesions (less than 60 days of lesion) transits to the immune state seen in late-established ulcer is a mystery (75). These

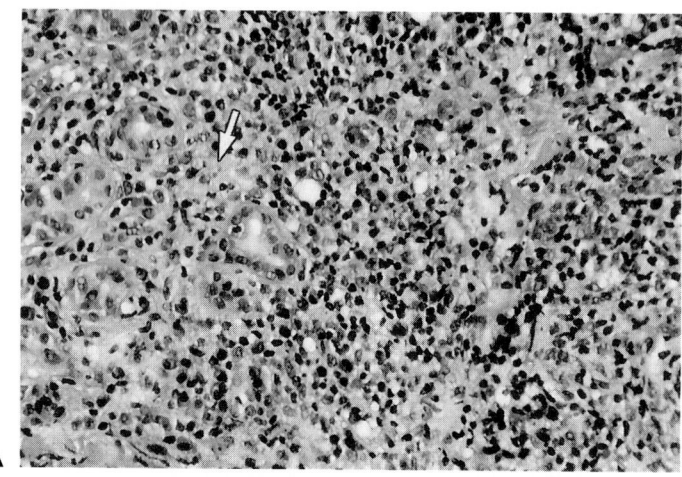

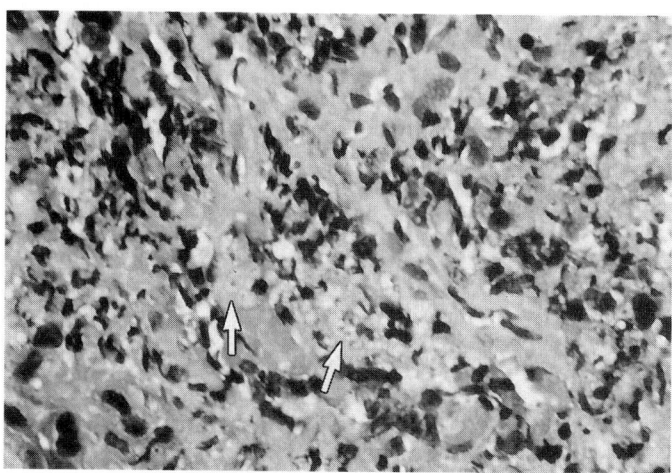

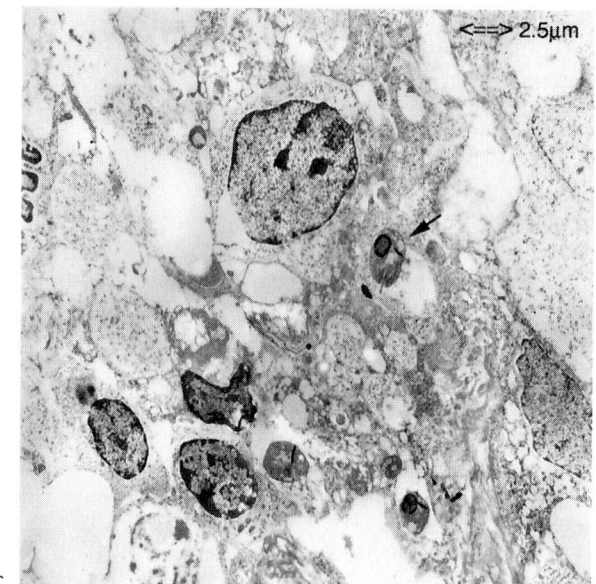

<==> 2.5μm

Figure 280.5. Histology of classic cutaneous leishmaniasis caused by *L. L. braziliensis*. A middle-age university lecturer and cinematographer from New York City traveled in 1999 for 1 week to Costa Rica, stayed overnight in a jungle area and recalled sustaining multiple insect bites. Approximately 1 week after departure she noted irritated skin under the right eye and a second irritation under the chin. At 5 weeks after symptom onset, the lesions evolved to a 5 × 3 cm infraorbital raised hypertrophic lesion covered by a crust, and to a 2 cm² crusted and raised chin lesion. A biopsy specimen of the infraorbital lesion was examined histologically and by culture. *L. L. braziliensis* was identified by culture (CDC, Atlanta, GA). **A:** The skin showed pseudoepitheliomatous hyperplasia with partial epidermal necrosis, and a diffuse, dense dermal mononuclear infiltrate containing foamy histiocytes (hematoxylin and eosin stain, 400x). **B:** Foamy histiocytes contain small round to oval bodies suggestive of amastigotes (1000x). **C:** Electron micrograph showed "*Leishmania*" amastigotes within tissue histiocyte. The amastigote has an eccentrically placed nucleus, glycogen vacuole(s), a kinetoplast DNA seen as the chromatin bar and the remnant of flagellum (courtesy of Mr. Jason Reidy; initial review of the biopsy by Dr. Sameera Husain, Pathology Department, Beth Israel Hospital, New York). The chin lesion healed while the infraorbital lesion diminished (75%) in size during treatment and by 1 week after a course of Pentostam treatment (Sb^V 20 mg/kg), the eschar fell off leaving healed epithelialized skin (diagnosis and treatment, Dr. John L. Ho).

findings are distinctly in contrast to murine models, where a Th1 response is associated with self-healing after *L. major* infection, while the Th2 type response predominance is associated with progressive disease. The in situ immune response of classic cutaneous ulcer is seen as an inflammatory reaction with infiltrates of lymphocytes, plasma cells, and macrophages in a granulomatous reaction (Fig 280.5 and Fig 280.6). Foamy macrophages may be seen, and under high power (and especially stained with Giemsa) these foamy cells are seen as macrophages laden with intracellular Leishmania amastigotes. Biopsy and histologic sections of the very early papular lesion (less than 3 weeks' duration) demonstrate vasculitis with large numbers of lymphocytes invading vascular wall, suggesting an important role of local inflammatory mechanisms in the development of the subsequent ulcer (76). In the *L. L. braziliensis* classic cutaneous ulcer, there is a predominance of helper phenotype cells, higher numbers of memory T cells, and increased tissue cellular expression of IL-1β, TNF-α, IFN-γ, and IL-10 and TGF-β, and messenger ribonucleic acid of IL-12 (77–80). The immune response of human cutaneous leishmaniasis due to *L. major* possesses similarly an adequate Th1 response and IL-10 appears to mediate suppression of the Th1 cellular immunity (81). The in situ findings further support the peripheral blood immune response suggesting that a hyper-Th1 response contributes to the development of the ulcer. This suspicion is further supported by the lack of clinical re-

sponse to anti-leishmania treatment in about half of the patients even when therapy was initiated less than 3 weeks after onset of cutaneous lesions (76).

CLINICAL MANIFESTATIONS

Increases in population migration and tourism have resulted in more cases of cutaneous leishmaniasis appearing outside of endemic regions (Fig 280.7;see Fig 280.2B). Data from the Centers for Disease Control (CDC) on U.S. travelers with cutaneous leishmaniasis suggest the majority (~75%) had traveled to the New World (Barbara Herwaldt, CDC, personal communication). The origin of the disease acquisition in U.S. travelers was from 14 countries, of which 56% of the travelers had traveled to Mexico or Central America, the two most visited areas (82). The bodily distribution of ulcers in these travelers is similar to that of residents in endemic regions: over 30% of the lesions presented in the lower extremities, another 30% in the upper extremities. Delay in diagnosis and treatment is typical for these returned travelers and is in keeping with the authors' experience. Therefore, more medical awareness is needed.

NEW WORLD CUTANEOUS LEISHMANIASIS: *LEISHMANIA VIANNIA* GROUP

The *L. braziliensis* subgenus was renamed *Viannia* to honor the physician who introduced antimonials for the treatment of

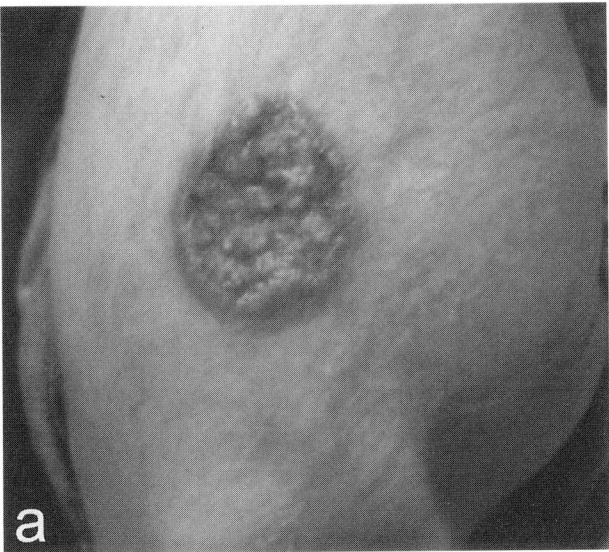
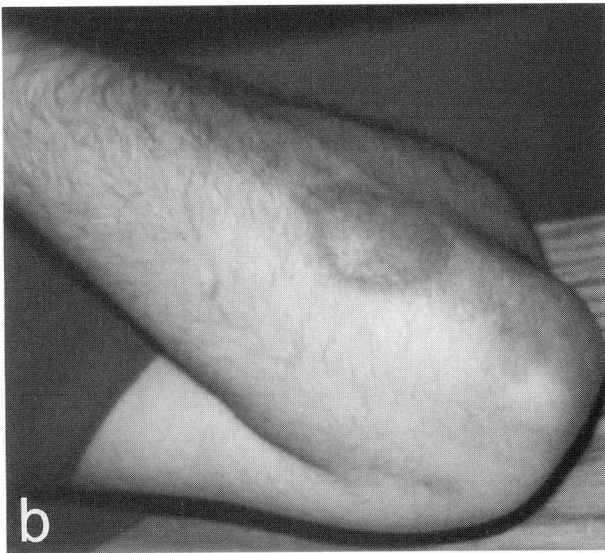

Figure 280.6. Cutaneous leishmaniasis before and after treatment. New York City teacher traveled to Bolivia in 1997 for 2 months and was in the Amazon jungle for 6 weeks working as a tour guide. Cervical adenopathy developed at the end of his stay approximately at the time of noting three papular lesions: ear, back, and forearm. These papules evolved over 6 weeks to appear as verrucous-like lesions with raised edges. **A:** Lesion on the forearm with raised edges and a central granulation tissue with a cauliflower appearance. Biopsy specimen by 8 weeks showed on histologic section a dense superficial and deep dermal perivascular and periadnexal infiltrate of lymphocytes, histiocytes, and some neutrophils and plasma cells. The infiltrate obscured the dermal-epidermal junction. The dermis contained necrotic keratinocytes and parakeratotic scale. On 1000x magnification, numerous small round organisms having eccentrically placed nuclei were seen within histiocytes. Biopsy specimen sent to the CDC for culture was negative; serology by IFA was positive 1:32 titer for *L. braziliensis* and negative for *L donovani*. **B:** Lesion after two courses of Pentostam (Sb^V 20 mg/kg for 20 days, 80 days of observation, followed by a second course of 28 days). The patient had three lesions: 2.5 cm on pinna of the ear, 1 cm on the upper back, and 6 cm on the extensor surface of the forearm. After one course of Pentostam, the ear and back lesions epithelialized (healed). The forearm lesion reduced in size by 50% at 80 of observation after the first course of Pentostam, and a second course was initiated. Photograph was taken before treatment and about 2 weeks after completion of second course of treatment (courtesy of Dr. John L. Ho).

leishmaniasis. The individual parasites merit brief separate consideration. *L. V. braziliensis* is the most destructive in terms of the rapidity of skin ulceration and evidence of metastatic lesions. The skin ulcers tend to be large, deep, and slow to heal. Sometimes active skin and mucosal lesions are seen together. Although lesions are slow to resolve, however spontaneous healing without therapy does occasionally occur. The geographic distribution of *L. V. braziliensis* in Latin America is extensive. It also occurs in countries east of the Andes and has been documented as far north as Belize. Isolation of *L. V. braziliensis* is difficult in the longer duration lesion because it contains scant number of parasites. *L. V. panamensis* causes smaller skin ulcers than those caused by *L. V. braziliensis*, and appears to be less destructive in the skin. However, *L. V. panamensis* can also cause mucosal metastasis. *L. V. guyanensis* initially identified in French Guyana extends to north of the Amazon River. It causes small skin ulcers that are frequently multiple and ascend the lymphatics. These lesions must be differentiated from sporotrichosis. This parasite has been reported in mucosal disease patients. *L. V. peruviana* typically causes a single ulcer that usually self-heal without metastasis and is reported only from the western slopes of the Andes and the Argentine highlands.

L. L. MEXICANA GROUP

Initial work in Mexico defined a self-limited type of cutaneous leishmaniasis that was particularly prevalent in the Yucatan peninsula and that closely resembled dry oriental sore (*L. L. mexicana*), although the ear pinna was involved more frequently and infections at this site tended to last a long time. Later work

in Belém, Brazil, defined a closely related *L. mexicana* subspecies, *L. L. amazonensis*. One very important clinical aspect of *L. L. amazonensis* is that it can cause all of the clinical spectra of leishmaniasis from visceral to classic, disseminated leishmaniasis, and diffuse anergic cutaneous leishmaniasis in the New World. In most patients, *L. L. amazonensis* produce relatively small classic lesions resembling Old World leishmaniasis, which may or may not ulcerate. However, the lesions of diffuse and disseminated cutaneous diseases rarely if ever self-healing are detailed later.

OLD WORLD CUTANEOUS LEISHMANIASIS

L. L. major, *L. L. tropica*, or *L. L. aethiopica* are the major species causing Old World cutaneous leishmaniasis but on occasions *L. L. donovani* and *L. L. infantum* may be the cause. The urban (dry) type of oriental sore caused by *L. L. tropica* presents as a firm, erythematous papule that is usually no larger than 2 to 4 cm and occurs on an exposed part of the body where the female sandfly. As the lesion enlarges, a serous crust forms and the reddish, inflamed border is elevated above the level of the surrounding skin (the so-called volcano sign). Clinical variants include a psoriasiform type with marked scaling and warty hyperkeratosis. The lesion remains static for 4 to 6 months, but fibrosis gradually effects healing, leaving a well defined and characteristic scar. Immunity is usually lifelong. This type of leishmaniasis is frequently contracted in cities of the Middle East leading to a number of epithets for the oriental sore (Aleppo or Bagdad boil, Biskra button). The so-called wet type of Old World leishmaniasis is prone to earlier ulceration, is found principally in rural areas of the

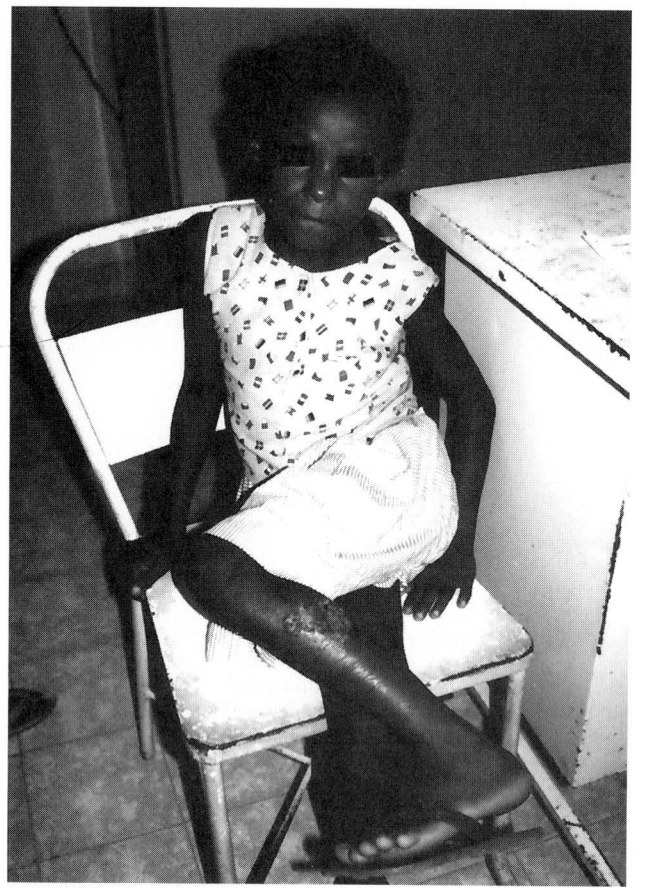

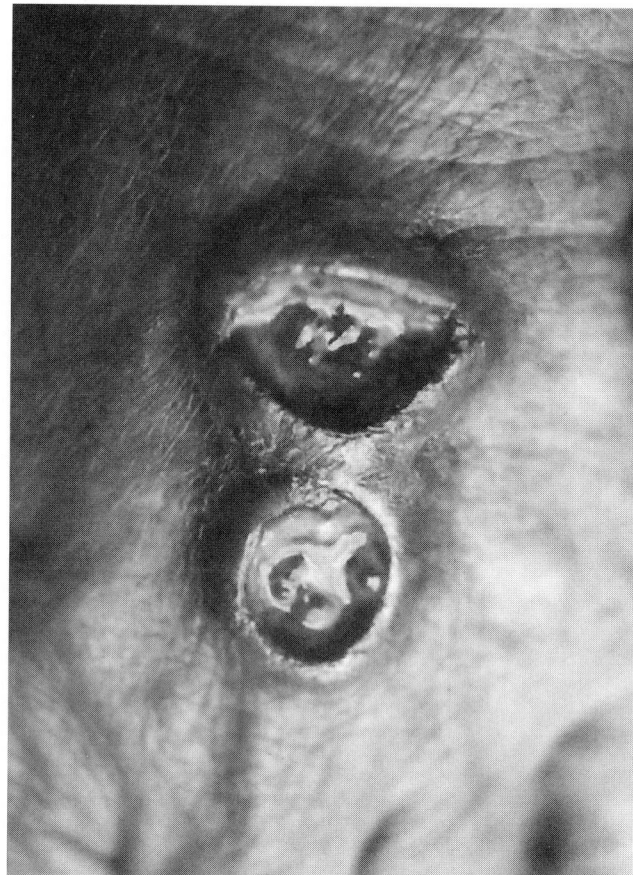

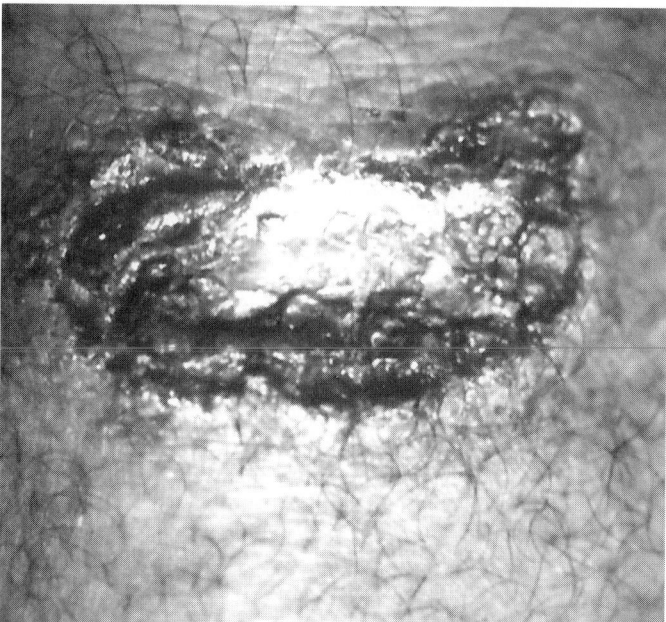

Figure 280.7. Clinical manifestations of classic cutaneous leishmaniasis. **A:** Chronic ulcer on a lower extremity. **B:** Wet ulcer with raised edges and a central clean ulcer with moderate granulation tissue. **C:** A dry ulcer with slightly raised edges and central eschar. Courtesy of Dr. Edgar Carvalho and Investigative Team, Federal University of Bahia, Brazil.

endemic zone, and is caused by *L. L. major*. It must be stressed that these are general distinctions, and rapidly ulcerating lesions can be found that are due to *L. tropica* and vice versa. The ulcer of the wet type is a larger lesion with a granulomatous base and an active, firm, erythematous border. It is slow to heal, but most lesions close within the year. Ethiopian cutaneous leishmaniasis, caused by *L. L. aethiopica*, also presents as a chronic skin granuloma, which may not ulcerate but may persist for many years and gradually extend.

DIAGNOSIS

Skin malignancies may present as ulcers similar to those of leishmaniasis. Biopsy for cutaneous leishmaniasis should always involve the active edge of the lesion to avoid histologic changes produced by necrosis or secondary infection. The histologic findings suggest an inflammatory reaction with mononuclear infiltrate as presented for two cases presented in Figs. 280.5 and 280.6. The granulomatous reaction if present is not diagnostic. The definitive diagnosis requires demonstration of the parasite.

Parasites may be seen in hematoxylin-eosin-stained sections of the biopsy specimen (Fig. 280.7B). Giemsa-stained smears of aspiration or glass slide-imprint of the dermis at the active border of the lesion usually demonstrates parasites or after culture (CDC, Atlanta, GA). Electron microscopy can provide definitive visualization of amastigotes of *Leishmania* (Fig 280.5C). In general, the older the lesion, the more difficult it is to find parasites. Detection of circulating antibodies against *L.V. braziliensis* or other species by indirect fluorescent antibody assay (CDC, Atlanta GA) or gene amplification with speciation may aid in diagnosis.

OTHER CUTANEOUS FORMS OF LEISHMANIASIS

Two forms of relapsing cutaneous lesions following acute disease are PKDL and leishmaniasis recidivans. PKDL, the relapse of leishmaniasis in the skin is frequently documented in India but seen elsewhere (58,83–86). Both *L. L. donovani* and *L. L. infantum* have been isolated from lesions of patients with PKDL (87,88). It is reported to occur in up to 10% or more of Indian visceral leishmaniasis patients after antimonial treatment; although it is much less frequent in East Africa and Brazil (58,83–86). PKDL is described as polymorphic in appearance and may present as hypopigmented or erythematous macules or as nodules resembling leprosy. On biopsy the nodules are especially rich in parasites (87,88). Some 5% to 10% of Old World cutaneous lesions, caused respectively by *L. L. tropica* and *L. L. major*, follow an atypical course, with persistence of an active foci in the form of nodules or as papules in the edge of the healed ulcer. Both types of lesions, called leishmaniasis recidivans, may follow soon or many years after the initial ulcer (61,62,89–92). The longest presentation of leishmaniasis recidivans was 43 years; the recrudescence of a papular lesion may be initiated by trauma or skin irritation

(62,91). Leishmaniasis recidivans though most frequently associated with *L. L. tropica* can be also caused by *L. V. braziliensis* (90). Biopsy of the lesion easily demonstrates amastigotes. The established cases of lupoid leishmaniasis, with well-defined tubercle formation with giant cells, may have scarce parasites on biopsy. The nodular lesions of leishmaniasis recidivans are similar in appearance to lupus vulgaris giving rise to the term lupoid leishmaniasis (92).

Two other forms of acute cutaneous leishmaniasis have been described: diffuse cutaneous leishmaniasis and disseminated leishmaniasis. Diffuse cutaneous leishmaniasis is caused by *L. L. amazonensis* in the New World and *L. L. aethiopica* in the Old World in Ethiopia (93–95). The New World disease is predominately in South American, especially in Brazil, but has also been reported in West Indies, and Mexico (96,97). *L. L. panamensis* from Columbia have been infrequently reported to cause diffuse cutaneous leishmaniasis (98). Diffuse cutaneous leishmaniasis is very rare, and only a few cases are seen yearly in Brazil. Clinically patients with diffuse cutaneous leishmaniasis have multiple non-ulcerative nodules or plaques widespread throughout their body (93,94,99,100). The nodules of diffuse cutaneous leishmaniasis resemble those of lepromatous leprosy and are rich in amastigotes. A new and emerging form of leishmaniasis observed in the northeastern Brazil is disseminated leishmaniasis (101–103). Cases of disseminated leishmaniasis are defined as patients with ten or more mixed type lesions in the same patient located in two or more body regions. These lesions appear as either acneiform, papular, nodular, or ulcerated (Fig 280.8). The prevalence of disseminated leishmaniasis in one surveyed area was estimated to be approximately 2% of all cases of cutaneous leishmaniasis, a number that is at least 20-fold greater than diffuse cutaneous leishmaniasis (101).

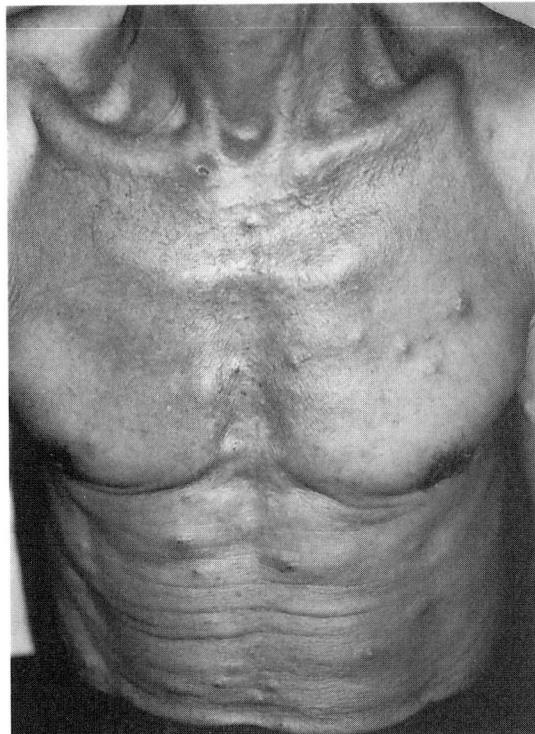 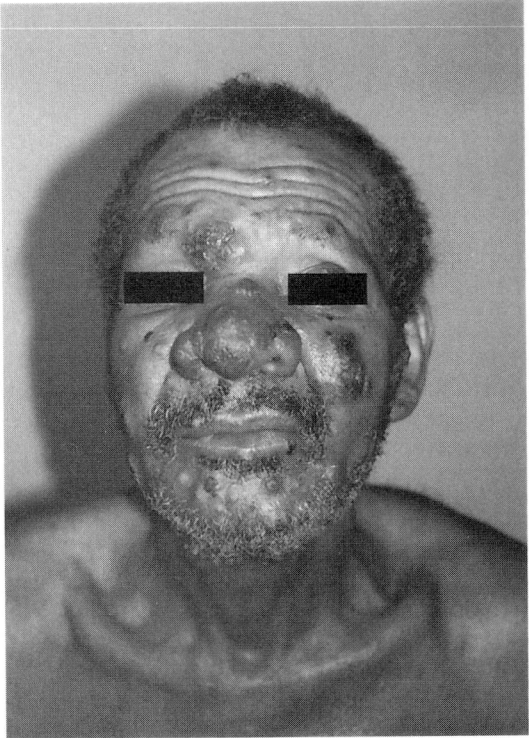

Figure 280.8. Disseminated cutaneous leishmaniasis. Typically patients present with ten or more mixed type lesions in the same patient located in two or more bodily regions. The lesions may appear as either acneiform, papular, nodular and/or ulcerated and are illustrate in this photograph of a patient with disseminated cutaneous leishmaniasis caused by *L. L. braziliensis*. Courtesy of Dr. Edgar Carvalho and Investigative Team, Federal University of Bahia, Brazil.

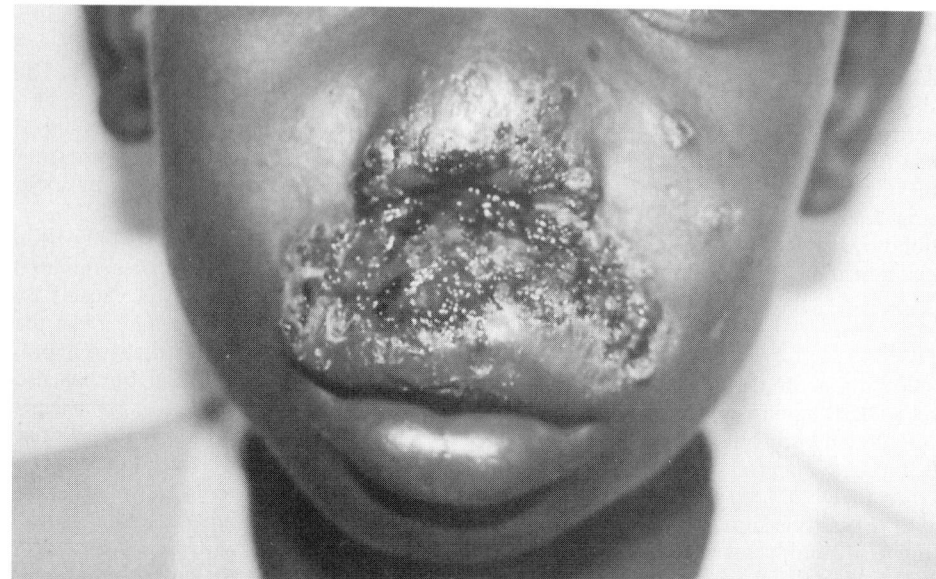

A

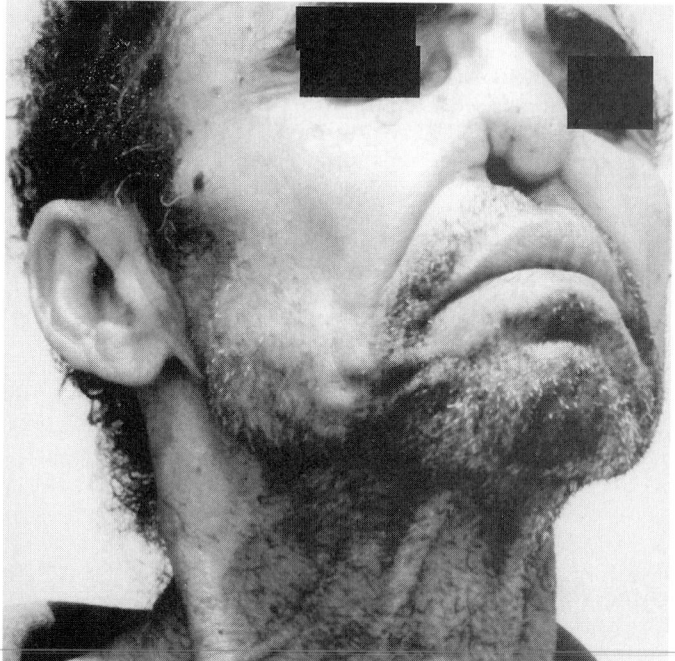

B

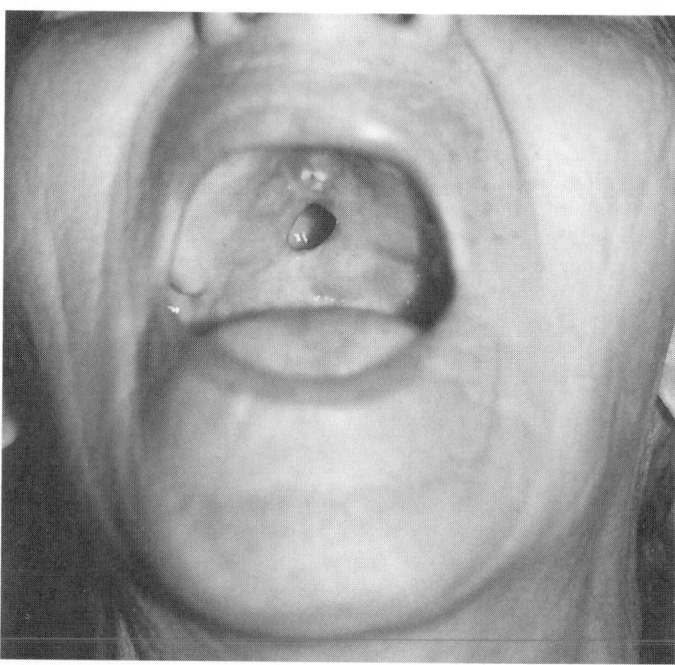

C

Figure 280.9. Mucosal leishmaniasis. **A:** Mucocutaneous lesion involving the lip, nasal mucosa with destruction of the anterior nasal septum. **B:** Severe chronic lesion with destruction of the nasal septum, involvement of the floor of the nose and extension into the sinuses. **C:** Extension of mucosal disease from the posterior nasal passage to the hard palate with perforation of the palate. Courtesy of Dr. Edgar Carvalho and Investigative Team, Federal University of Bahia, Brazil.

Although both *L. L. amazonensis* and *L. L. braziliensis* have been isolated from lesions of patients with disseminated cutaneous leishmaniasis, a recent study identified only *L. L. braziliensis* (101–103).

Mucosal Leishmaniasis

Mucosal leishmaniasis virtually restricted to South America is because of the distribution of the *Leishmania Viannia* group or *L. L. amazonensis* (see Table 280.1) (104–106). Mucosal leishmaniasis is especially common in central Brazil, where *L. V. braziliensis* is the dominant species. It has been estimated that less than 5% of patients in whom a *L. V. braziliensis* primary skin lesion develops will experience mucosal disease (107,108). Onset of disease is typically 5 or more years after the initial lesion but a minority of the cases present with mucosal disease concurrent with

the primary ulcer. The initial symptoms are nasal discharge and obstruction, epistaxis, and in an advanced case tissue coming from the nose. The lesion begins as an erythematous or hyperemic area on the nasal mucosal, usually of the septum. In time, tissue granulomas ensue, followed by ulceration. As the lesion advances, perforation of the nasal septum may occur (109). In more advanced cases, the process can extend from the floor of the nose to the hard and soft palate (Fig 280.9B and C). The pharynx and larynx may be involved, and a hoarse voice is a valuable sign. Tissue destruction can result in loss of the cartilaginous nose or lips (Fig 280.9A). Aspiration pneumonia and laryngeal closure may result in a fatal outcome. Recently, mucosal leishmaniasis has been reported in Sudan caused by *L. L. donovani* (110). Sudanese mucosal leishmaniasis is a chronic infection of the upper respiratory tract or oral mucosa. Although the condition may develop during or after acute visceral leishmaniasis, the Sudanese variant is not preceded or accompanied by a cutaneous lesion. Studies of the immunopathology of mucosal disease compared to classic cutaneous leishmaniasis suggest that mucosal patients significantly over-produce Th1 cytokines (IFNγ and TNFα), have diminished IL-10 levels, and fail to respond to exogenous IL-10 and TGFβ (74). Similarly, *ex vivo* study of PBMC found only one in three mucosal disease patients expressed IL-10 (111).

DIAGNOSIS

At the initial consultation, a careful history must be obtained. A *Leishmania* scar can be located (usually on the limbs) if the patient had American cutaneous leishmaniasis. The risk for developing mucosal diseases increases by having multiple skin lesions, inadequate therapy or no therapy. The diagnosis of mucosal leishmaniasis in endemic regions is made by 1) having a characteristic mucosal lesion, 2) a positive intradermal leishmanin skin test result (100%), and 3) a history of cutaneous leishmaniasis. These criteria have a high predictive value in endemic areas (104). The indirect fluorescent antibody (IFA) assay for *L. L. braziliensis* may be an aid for the diagnosis of mucosal leishmaniasis because it is invariably positive. Histologic examination for the *Leishmania* amastigotes may be positive in only 30% of the patients (109). Culture of tissue biopsy or aspirate specimens using special techniques may be positive in only 50% of attempts (112). In a patient presenting to a physician outside of an endemic area with an exposure history and a skin scar, a presumptive diagnosis of mucosal leishmaniasis can be made based on the following: 1) a positive immunofluorescence antibody result for *L. L. braziliensis*, 2) a compatible histology (even without the finding of amastigotes in tissue, culturable *Leishmania* or *Leishmania* DNA by polymerase chain reaction gene amplification), and 3) exclusion of etiologies that form the differential diagnosis for mucosal leishmaniasis. Histologically, the lesion is infiltrated by inflammatory mononuclear cells (100%); granulomas with epithelioid cells are seen (55%), and seen less often is acanthosis (45%), and pseudo-epitheliomatous hyperplasia (27%) (110). Systemic mycoses are in the differential diagnosis of mucosal leishmaniasis, including lobomycosis and particularly paracoccidioidal-mycosis, which can affect the nasal mucosa in a similar manner but is usually associated with pulmonary lesions. The differential diagnosis also includes cancer, leprosy, tertiary treponematoses, rhinoscleroma, and lethal midline granuloma.

TREATMENT OF LEISHMANIASIS

The treatment of all forms of leishmaniasis remains less than satisfactory but is evolving as new therapies are introduced. Two key questions need to be answered once the diagnosis of leishmaniasis has been made: Does the patient need to be treated? If yes, with what anti-leishmanial agent? All patients with visceral and mucosal leishmaniasis require treatment. The former is invariably fatal if untreated, and the latter is destructive, disfiguring and can progress to airway obstruction or aspiration. New World cutaneous disease due to *L. V. braziliensis* or other *Vianna* species can cause mucosal disease. Therefore, in addition to curing of the primary lesion, a secondary goal is to prevent the future occurrence of mucosal leishmaniasis. Studies found that cutaneous ulcers cause by *L. V. braziliensis* infrequently resolve and self-healing was seen in less than 20% of patients at 5 months after ulcer onset (107,113–116). Old World cutaneous leishmaniasis due to *L. L. major* tends to self-heal, and may not require treatment if it involves a cosmetically unimportant area (discussed later). The choice of drug depends on the disease, the

region or country in which the patient acquired the disease, and the suspected or identified *Leishmania* species. The latter two factors relate to intrinsic differences in the sensitivity of *Leishmania* species to several of the drugs, and to acquired-resistance associated with clinical failure (i.e., antimony resistance in Bihar, India will be discussed later) (117,118). Table 280.2 serves as a guide for the selection for an anti-leishmanial agent. The bases for the recommendations stated in Table 280.2 are derived from published recommendations (55,112,119) and from studies detailed later for each condition and are consistent with our collective experience in the United States and in Brazil. For each patient, additional factors (such as, disease severity/symptoms, immune status, and pregnancy) need to be considered in the selection of the agent, dose, and duration of treatment.

Visceral Leishmaniasis

The first-line therapies for visceral leishmaniasis are pentavalent antimonials or amphotericin. Pentavalent antimonials (Sb^V), which were introduced more than 80 years ago, remain one of the first line drugs for treatment of all forms of leishmaniasis in much of the world because of the accumulated data on its use, its lower cost compared to the newer agents and relative effectiveness (121–123). Pentostam (sodium stibogluconate, 100 mg Sb^V per mL, 10%) is marketed by Wellcome; Specia (Rhodia) makes Glucantime (meglumine antimonate, 85 mg Sb^V per mL, 8.5%). Pentostam is available in the USA from the Drug Service of the CDC (404-639-3679). Glucantime is used in Francophone and Latin American countries. The pentavalent antimony dose and duration currently used owe much to the work of Thakur et al. (60). The current evidence suggest that Sb^V at a dose of 20 mg/kg per day for 28 days should result in clinical cure in most cases of visceral leishmaniasis (119,120,124). The cure rate at the end of treatment in field situations is over 95% in immune competent patients with the exception of Indian cases (118,125). The clinical cure rate may be less in pediatric patients; but all were cured with another first line drug, amphotericin B (126). As a general principle, the evaluation of treatment response is based on clinical criteria, such as absence of fever, regression of hepatosplenomegaly, normalization of hematopoietic parameters, a decrease in serum globulin, and an increase of albumin levels. A test for patient's antibody levels to rK39 before and after therapy may assist in the clinical management of patients, although rK39 assay is at present a research tool (Steven Reed, PhD, Corixa, Seattle, WA) (43–46). After therapy, a repeated bone marrow examination or splenic aspiration to search for *Leishmania* organisms in smears and a culture may be indicated if the clinical response is incomplete. Clinical follow-up for a 2-year period is desirable because approximately 1% or more of initially cured patients may experience relapse (118,125). In general, patients who have a clinical response but have residual parasites at the end of treatment can be re-treated with a second course of Sb^V. Those who relapse after parasitologic "cure" (if not from India), can be retreated with Sb^V or another first-line agent. Clinical resistance to Sb^V in India (particularly from the State of Bihar) may be as high as 60% (118). Pentavalent antimonials should be administered in a single slow intravenous (30 minute) infusion or as an intramuscular injection. The adverse reactions associated with the current pentavalent antimonials are much less serious. They are dose related and include arthralgias, pancreatitis, abnormal liver function test results (aminopeptidases (transaminases), alkaline phosphatase), and prolongation of the ST interval or inversion of the T wave. Clinically silent amylase elevation to several times above normal is not uncommon, and typically return to

TABLE 280.2. Treatment Regimens for Leishmaniasis

Drug	Syndrome	Dosage regimen	Comments
Parenteral			
Pentavalent antimony (intravenous or intramuscular)[a]	VL	20 mg Sb^v kg daily for 28 d	Longer courses of therapy may increase toxic effects.
	CL	20 mg Sb^v kg daily for 20 d	Shorter courses may have merit in some situations.
	ML	20 mg Sb^v kg daily for 28 d	Longer courses do not necessarily improve effectiveness.
Amphotericin B deoxycholate (intravenous)	VL	0.5–1.0 mg/kg on alternate d or daily (total about 15–20 mg/kg)	Range, total dose about 7–20 mg/kg (varies by region and host status).
	CL, ML	Alternative to failed antimony therapy, see comments in text; (total approx. 20–40 mg/kg)	Limited data for CL or ML; efficacy based on VL; consider the toxic.
Lipid formulations of Amphotericin B (intravenous)	VL	2–5 mg/kg daily (total approx. 15–21 mg/kg)	Range, total dose approx. 5–40 mg/kg (varies with host status, failure rates higher for <15 mg)
(intravenous)	CL, ML	See comments in text	Limited data for CL or ML; efficacy based on VL.
Pentamidine isethionate (intravenous or intramuscular)	VL	4 mg/kg on alternate days or three times per week for approx. 15–30 doses	Considered second-line therapy because of toxicity or suboptimal effectiveness
	CL	3 mg/kg on alternate days × 4 doses or 2 mg/kg on alternate days × 7 doses	Based on studies in Columbia (most cases probably caused by *Viannia* subgenus, particularly *L. (V.) panamensis*).
	ML	2–4 mg/kg on alternate days or three times per week for 15 or more doses	Considered second-line therapy.
Paromomycin sulphate[b] (intravenous or intramuscular)	VL	15–20 mg/kg daily for approx. 21 days	Has been used as monotherapy in India and as adjunct to antimony compounds.
	CL	Not currently recommended	
Recombinant interferon gamma (subcutaneous or intramuscular)		100 µg/m² daily or on alternate days (adult dose)	Ineffective against *L. (V.) panamensis* (Colombia) and *L. (V.) braziliensis* (Belize). Sometimes useful as adjunct for difficult cases of VL and other syndromes.
Oral			
Ketoconazole	CL	600 mg daily for 28 d (adult dose)	Consider for *L. mexicana* and *L. (V.) panamensis* and possibly for *L. major*.
Itraconazole	CL	200 mg twice daily for 28 d (adult dose)	Failure rate of at least 75% in Colombia (most cases probably caused by *Viannia* subgenus, particularly *L. (V.) panamensis*).
Dapsone	CL	100 mg twice daily for 6 wk (adult dose)	Promising results obtained in India but not in Colombia (against mostly *L. (V.) panamensis*).
Miltefosine	CL	See comments in text	Efficacy equal to amphotericin B for Indian VL; open trial for New World CL.
Local/topical			
Paromomycin sulphate ointment[c]	CL	Apply twice daily for 10–20 d	Consider especially for *L. major* and *L. mexicana*.
Intralesional Sb^v	CL	Weekly or alternate-day injections×multiple doses	Infiltrate four opposing sides of lesion until base completely blanched.[d]

VL, Visceral leishmaniasis; CL, cutaneous leishmaniasis; ML, mucosal leishmaniasis; Sb^v = pentavalent antimony.

[a]Sodium stibogluconate = 100 mg Sb^v/ml and meglumine antimonate = 85 mg Sb^v/mL; locally made antimony preparations may have different antimony concentrations. Intravenous administration preferable for large volumes. Children, particularly those weighing <20 kg, may benefit from dosing according to body surface area and treating with proportionately >20 mg Sb^v/kg daily.

[b]500 mg paromomycin sulphate corresponds to 350 mg base.

[c]An ointment containing 15% paromomycin and 12% methylbenzethonium chloride in soft white paraffin is modestly effective. Much of the experience has been with *L. major* infection. Methylbenzethonium chloride can cause local inflammation (e.g., burning sensation, pruritus, vesicles). A product containing 10% urea instead is cheaper and better tolerated but less effective.

[d]Depending on number and characteristics of lesions, intralesional therapy may not be practical. Much of the experience with intralesional therapy has been for Old-World disease. Published regimens vary widely in total number of and interval between injections.

Updated and modified with permission from Herwaldt BL. *Lancet* 1999;354:1191–1199. Data from which these recommendations have been derived are discussed in the text reference cited.

normal despite continuation of the antimonials. The development of electrocardiographic abnormalities, particularly conduction defects or arrhythmias, is an indication for stopping treatment (127).

Amphotericin B, a polyene antibiotic first developed as an antifungal agent has selective activity against not only fungi, but also *Leishmania* due to its higher affinity for microbial ergosterol, than for human cell membrane cholesterol (128). The recommended dose and duration of amphotericin B treatment of immune competent patients, either as the deoxycholate or lipid formulation, should achieve near 100% success rate for first treatment (see Table 280.2) (55,128–132). The success is defined by clinical resolution of illness, and absence of parasite on direct examination of Giemsa stained splenic or bone marrow aspirates). Accounting for relapses after initial success, an overall success rate of greater than 98% at 6-months' follow-up is anticipated (128,131,132). Patients who relapse can be retreated with the same amphotericin regimen (118,133,134). Doses of amphotericin B less than 15 mg/kg and given less frequently are associated with failures (118,135,136). The major complication of any amphotericin B preparation is renal dysfunction, which in most patients normalizes after cessation of therapy. Infusion reactions and phlebitis are more associated with deoxycholate amphotericin B. The upper limit of total dose has not been established but a patient with AIDS has received 14 g of amphotericin B (133). Pentamidine is a second-line treatment. In a randomized trial with antimony-resistant Indian visceral leishmaniasis, pentamidine at dose of 4 mg/kg on alternate days three times weekly produced a 98% clinical cure (137). Under therapeutic doses, side effects are estimated to be in the range of 30% to 50% of patients that included skin rashes, hypoglycemia, hypotension, electrocardiography changes, nephrotoxicity and sudden death have been reported (138). The high rates of these toxicities and the stated "suboptimal effectiveness in India" (119) have relegated pentamidine to second-line drug status for the treatment of visceral leishmaniasis. Paromomycin (aminosidine) is an aminoglycoside analog with anti-leishmanial activity (139). The first efficacy trial was conducted against Indian visceral leishmaniasis in which daily intramuscular dose of 16 mg/kg or 20 mg/kg for 21 days resulted in a cure rate of 93% and 97%, respectively (138). Unfortunately, the previous manufacturer has ceased production.

Miltefosin, an alkyl phospholipid also known as hexadecylphosphocholine, is the first effective oral anti-leishmanial agent (119,132,140). A regimen of 100 mg of miltefosine per day (approximately 2.5 mg/kg of body weight) for 4 weeks resulted in a cure rate of 97% (132). Gastrointestinal side effects occurred in 62% of persons under treatment, but none discontinued treatment. The findings are very encouraging. A second orally administered drug, sitamaquine (WR6026) is under clinical trials (141). Recombinant cytokines have been shown to control *Leishmania* in *in vitro* human macrophage assays, and in murine models of leishmaniasis (48). In patients with either refractory or relapsed visceral leishmaniasis, the combination of interferon-gamma (IFN-γ and pentavalent antimony is effective in a majority of patients (125). Human GM-CSF has also been used in conjunction with antimony (142,143).

Treatment of AIDS and visceral leishmaniasis or disseminated forms of leishmaniasis in HIV-1 patients represents a real challenge. It is not uncommon for the patient to respond clinically, but to relapse soon after treatment (133). The relapse is not due to drug resistance but likely due to the inherent immunodeficiency of AIDS (134,144). Therefore, suppression of HIV replication during anti-leishmania treatment with combined highly active anti-retroviral therapy (HAART) should be another aim to control leishmaniasis. The initial response rate of HIV-infected patients to either antimonials or amphotericin appears comparable to that of immune competent patients (134,145). For chronic suppression in those AIDS patients with CD4 T cells less than 200/μL, once-weekly infusion of either antimony, amphotericin B, or oral miltefosine (once available) may be used. However, there are little data as to the upper limit for total dose that can be safely administered (133). Oral agents, such as ketoconazole, itraconazole, dapsone, and allopurinol have limited data for treatment of visceral disease. The treatment of a patient immunosuppressed by agents other than HIV-1 is equally challenging (146).

Cutaneous Leishmaniasis

The decision to treat cutaneous leishmaniasis is based on the *Leishmania* species causing the disease, and the type of cutaneous syndrome. Speciation is critical because *Leishmania* species differ in their potential for mucosal disease. The natural history of the ulcer healing differs between species and there are differences in the intrinsic susceptibility to anti-leishmanial agents. In two studies of *Leishmania* ulcers, 22% or less of the ulcers caused by *L. V. braziliensis* healed by 13 weeks of follow-up; in contrast, 50% to 88% of ulcers caused by *L. L. mexicana* healed by 13 weeks of follow-up (124,147). In the Old World oriental sores due *to L. L. major* that typically self-heal, 34% of the patients had healed by 3 months (148).

Antimony is the first choice for treatment of cutaneous leishmaniasis (55,119,120,149). In Brazil, Sb^v at 20 mg/kg per day for 20 days is the regimen of choice for primary infections mainly due to *L. V. braziliensis*. This regimen and dose is probably adequate for the great majority of *L. V. guyanensis, L. V. panamensis,* and *L. V. peruviana* primary infections. Cure rates after one course of this regimen for cutaneous leishmaniasis due to these species vary from 50% to 97% (147,150–152). A case of American cutaneous leishmaniasis treated with Pentostam is presented in Fig. 280.6 to illustrate the therapeutic response of the lesion. Lower dose regimen of antimony (Sb^v at 5 mg/kg for 20 days) has been reported with cure rates of 47% to 80% (153,154). However, such a lower dose must be chosen with discretion and knowledge of the regional parasitologic response to such regimens (154). In Mexican cutaneous leishmaniasis due to *L. L. mexicana*, daily ampule of antimony ($\sim$7 mg/kg, based on Sb^v 425 mg each vial and assuming 60 kg average weight) was successful at a mean of 25 days (155). For Old World oriental sore due to *L. tropica*, a single 20-day course of Sb^v, at 10 mg/kg per day achieved high rates of cure (120).

After a course of the standard antimony regimen, the patient should be observed for 90 days because many lesions will continue to heal. If the ulcer has not fully healed at this time, and is 50% or more improved, a second course of treatment can be initiated (as in the patient illustrated in Fig. 280.6). If there is still no improvement an alternative agent, such as amphotericin B, should be administered. Factors associated with delayed healing or requirement for more than one course of treatment include multiple lesions, very large lesions (greater than 3 cm), lesions on the leg or trunk (153,154), in children (156), lesions caused by *L. V. braziliensis* and variant cutaneous lesions (discussed later). The addition of intralesional injected granulocyte-macrophage colony stimulating factor (GM-CSF) may hasten wound healing (151). Also, IFN-γ (every other day injection) has been used in conjunction with short courses of antimony (Sb^v for 10 days) (157). Alternative parenteral therapies for treatment of cutaneous leishmaniasis are amphotericin B and pentamidine. They should be used in cases where antimony has failed or is problematic because of significant underlying cardiac arrhythmia or conduction defects because there are limited data on the use of these agents, and comparison studies have not been reported. Amphotericin B, both the deoxycholate and lipid formulation, used in several reports as an alternative to failed antimony therapy have reported mixed results (55,119,158–165). A total of 1.5 to 2 g of either deoxycholate amphotericin B (every other day course of 1 mg/kg) or lipid-formulated amphotericin B (3 mg/kg) should be adequate for cure. Pentamidine tested in open-labeled trials conducted in Columbia reported a 96% cure rate (115,166). The good response against predominant *Vianna* subgroup of *Leishmania* isolates is encouraging but needs confirmation. Data have not been reported on the effectiveness of parenteral paromomycin although it has been used as a topical agent.

The use of oral agents for cutaneous leishmaniasis is attractive, but should be cautioned for use against *L. V. braziliensis* or other species of the *Vianna* group because the data that they can prevent subsequent development of mucosal disease is inadequate. Oral agents including ketoconazole, fluconazole, itraconazole, and dapsone have been used (147,148,167). Oral fluconazole

(200 mg daily for 6 weeks) compared to placebo showed a cure rate 79% versus a self-cure rate of 34%. Oral miltefosine (133 to 150 mg/day for 3 to 4 weeks) in an open label dose comparison trial of Columbian cutaneous leishmaniasis caused by *L. L. mexicana* and *L. V. panamensis* reported an encouraging cure rate of 94% comparable to the 93% cure rate of a historic control using antimony) (168). If comparison trials confirm the preliminary results and tested in New World cutaneous leishmaniasis cause by *L. L. braziliensis* and other *Vianna* species, oral fluconazole and miltefosine will greatly advance the treatment of American cutaneous leishmaniasis. Topical and local therapies have been tested in cutaneous leishmaniasis with mixed results. These include topical paromomycin (15% paromomycin and 12% methylbenzethonium in soft white paraffin) (169,170), local heat (171), and intralesional injection of antimony. Excisional surgery has also been used but it has no role in cutaneous leishmaniasis because satellite lesions can develop after the procedure, and it does not prevent mucosal leishmaniasis.

Variant cutaneous leishmaniasis syndromes include, diffuse "anergic" cutaneous, disseminated cutaneous, lupoid leishmaniasis, leishmaniasis recidivans, and PKDL. Treatment of the complicated variant syndromes of cutaneous leishmaniasis is difficult and failures for almost all of the regimens have been observed (172). Antimony and amphotericin B remain the agents with the most information on their effectiveness and should be used first, though more prolonged courses and higher total doses will be required. Diffuse cutaneous leishmaniasis in both the Old World and the New World, is notoriously difficult to treat (172). IFN-γ plus antimony has been used successfully in Brazil for diffuse cutaneous leishmaniasis (173). Patients with disseminated cutaneous leishmaniasis respond better to antimony than patients with diffuse cutaneous disease but may still require more than one course of treatment. Chronic infections such as lupoid leishmaniasis or leishmaniasis recidivans require Sb^v, at 20 mg/kg per day, for longer periods, and multiple courses. *L. aethiopica* skin infections are relatively resistant to treatment, so the higher dose would have to be used. Alternative treatment with amphotericin B had met with some success in these variant syndromes (163–165).

Mucosal (Mucocutaneous) Leishmaniasis

The current recommendation for treatment of mucosal leishmaniasis is Sb^v, at 20 mg/kg per day for 28 days (55,149,174–176). The activity of the lesion should be assessed clinically during and upon completion of treatment. Signs of persistent activity or non-epithelialization are an indication to continue treatment after an observational interval of 30 to 90 days. In our Brazilian experience, two to three repeated courses of antimony may be required (177). Alternative treatment, such as, amphotericin B may be initiated (149,174–184). Deoxycholate amphotericin B (1 mg/kg per day) or lipid formulated amphotericin B (3 mg/kg per day) to a total of 30 mg/kg or a maximal total dose of 2.5 g should achieve cure of the lesion. However, total doses have ranged from 2 to 5 g in immunocompetent patients; and to over 12 g in HIV-1–infected patients (133,181–184). Pentamidine is a second-line drug and its use is based on clinical data obtained for visceral and cutaneous leishmaniasis, and limited trials (185,186). Pentamidine isethionate is given intramuscularly at 2 to 4 mg/kg per day for up to 15 doses. Itraconazole is a potential drug because of it is given orally, and in an open trial had a reported cure rate of 60% at 3 months after treatment (187). Although still experimental, IFN-γ has been use in conjunction with antimony in a few cases of mucosal leishmaniasis that had failed antimony therapy (188). The pathophysiology of mucosal

leishmaniasis suggests that over-production of host TNF-α may contribute to mucosal destruction. Pentoxifyline, a TNF-α antagonist, has been used in an open-label trial of patients who failed prior course(s) of antimony therapy (189). Pentoxifyline (400 mg three times a day for 30 days) plus antimony (20 mg/kg for 30 days) cured all ten patients studied with mucosal disease (189). The encouraging result from this open-labeled trial is currently being tested in treatment naïve patients with mucosal leishmaniasis (Machado P. and Carvalho E.M., personal communications).

PREVENTION AND THE FUTURE

Additional drug targets and effective oral drug treatment remain a priority in leishmaniasis research. Research is currently directed at select leishmanial targets theoretically unlikely to affect the host (e.g., microtubules and their biosynthesis, folate metabolism, cysteine proteases, and trypanthione reductase) (190). The current encouraging data regarding miltefosine, if confirmed, will greatly advance the treatment of visceral and cutaneous leishmaniasis. Combination anti-*Leishmania* drug regimens should be tested. Lastly, biologic agents, not limited to IFN-γ, GM-CSF, or immune modifiers, such as pentoxifyline should be further evaluated as adjuvants to standard anti-*Leishmania* drug to improve efficacy and/or shorten the duration of treatment, and thereby compliance.

Prevention from transmission of *Leishmania* includes personal and environmental preventive measures, and prophylactic vaccines. Personal prophylaxis in endemic areas should include restricting activity in crepuscular hours when phlebotomines are active. Impregnating clothing and bed nets with repellents, such as pyrethroids, can further reduce transmission (191,192). The use of permethrin-impregnated clothing was shown in a double-blinded, randomized study to reduce the acquisition of leishmaniasis and malaria among Colombian army personnel conducting jungle maneuvers (191). The analysis of vectorborne prevention in the British Army suggest that practical insect avoidance measures, combined with pyrethroid-treated nets and clothing, and DEET-based topical repellents, can achieve near 100% protection against biting arthropods (192). For peridomestic transmission, spraying in and around the home with insecticides may also reduce transmission. However, on a cautionary note, repellents and insecticides are not a panacea. Permethrin and over-the-counter formulations for human lice have already encountered resistance and clinical failures (193,194). Reservoir control measures depend on what is known of the transmission cycle (195). The former Soviet Union has had success in controlling *L. major* transmission by attacking the giant gerbil (*Rhombomys opimus*, the main animal reservoir) and the vector *Phlebotomus papatasi*. Control of infected dogs and the use of pyrethrin-impregnated collars have been advocated. Sole reliance on such measure will not guarantee complete removal of the reservoir(s) because the elimination of infected dogs has been noted with mixed results (196,197).

The current advances in immunologic understanding of leishmaniasis, genetic studies of the parasite, and genome sequencing of *Leishmania* will identify targets for prophylactic vaccines. Attenuated live vaccines have been reported with limited success (198). However, the persistence of the attenuated vaccine parasites at the inoculation site, the slow to healing in some patients, and development of secondary infection have resulted in the abandonment of this approach. A recent large randomized trial of school children with killed whole *L. major* mixed with *M. bovis*-Bacillus-Calmette-Guerin (BCG) vaccine has an overall 2-year protective efficacy of 55% (199). In addition to this approach, genetically modified less virulent *Leishmania* have been engineered to study pathogenesis and maybe vaccine candidates (11, 200). Recombinant subunit protein vaccines and DNA multigenic vaccine are being evaluated in the laboratory (201–205). One caveat is that *Leishmania* is a successful obligate intramacrophage parasite that utilizes an array of strategies for survival. Therefore, effective immune control after the parasite's invasion must target factors involving parasite cell entry and intracellular survival, and contain immunodominant *Leishmania* antigens to elicit cytolytic T cell destruction. Vaccine formulation and delivery may greatly affect immunogenicity and Th profile (202,203,205). Another potentially effective approach is to use sandfly salivary proteins as vaccines (16,206,207). Eliciting an immune response to these proteins may allow an accelerated immune response at the site of *Leishmania* invasion and innate immune elimination and reduce infection. In summary, a preventive vaccine should aim to provide specific anti-*Leishmania* immunity (203) and bystander protection provided by sandfly salivary proteins.

ACKNOWLEDGMENTS

We wish to acknowledge support from the National Institutes of Health for our research, AI22624 (WDJ), AI 16282 (WDJ), AI39606 (JLH) and HL61960 (JLH). This chapter is dedicated to the memory of Philip D. Marsden.

REFERENCES

1. Chang K-P, Bray RS. *Leishmaniasis*. Amsterdam: Elsevier, 1985.
2. Peters W, Killick-Kendrick R, eds. *The Leishmaniases in Biology and Medicine*. London: Academic Press, 1987.
3. Grimaldi G Jr, McMahon-Pratt D. Leishmaniasis and its etiologic agents in the New World: An overview. *Prog Clin Parasitol* 1991;2:73.
4. Desjeux P. Leishmaniasis: public health aspects and control. *Clin Dermatol* 1996;14:417–423.
5. Desjeux P. The increase in risk factors for leishmaniasis worldwide. *Trans Roy Soc Trop Med Hyg* 2001;95:239–243.
6. McHugh CP, Melby PC, LaFon SG. Leishmaniasis in Texas: epidemiology and clinical aspects of human cases. *Am J Trop Med Hyg* 1996;55:547–555.
7. Schnur LF. On the clinical manifestations and parasites of Old World leishmaniasis and *Leishmania tropica* causing visceral leishmaniasis. In: Hart DT, ed. *Leishmaniasis, NATO Advanced Scientific Institute Series*. New York: Plenum Press, 1986:939–943.
8. Desjeux P. Information on the epidemiology and control of leishmaniasis by country and territory. 1991. Geneva: WHO, WHO/Leish/91.30.
9. Pimenta PF, Modi GB, Pereira ST, Shahabuddin M, Sacks DL. A novel role for the peritrophic matrix in protecting *Leishmania* from the hydrolytic activities of the sand fly midgut. *Parasitology* 1997;115:359–369.
10. Pimenta PF, Turco SJ. *Leishmania chagasi*: lipophosphoglycan characterization and binding to the midgut of the sand fly vector *Lutzomyia longipalpis*. *Mol Biochem Parasitol* 2002;121(2):213–224.
11. Turco SJ, Spath GF, Beverley SM. Is lipophosphoglycan a virulence factor? A surprising diversity between *Leishmania* species. *Trends Parasitol* 2001;17:223–226.
12. Hondowicz B, Scott P. Influence of host and parasite factors on the innate immune response and Th2 stability following infection with *Leishmania major*. *Microbes Infect* 1999;1(1):65–71.
13. Launois P, Himmelrich H, Tacchini-Cottier F, Milon G, Louis JA. New insight into the mechanisms underlying Th2 cell development and susceptibility to *Leishmania major* in BALB/c mice. *Microbes Infect* 1999;1(1):59–64.
14. Locksley RM, Pingel S, Lacy D, Wakil AE, Bix M, Fowell DJ. Susceptibility to infectious diseases: Leishmania as a paradigm. *J Infect Dis* 1999;179[Suppl 2]:S305–S308.
15. Menon JN, Bretscher PA. Parasite dose determines the Th1/Th2 nature of the response to Leishmania major independently of infection route and strain of host or parasite. *Eur J Immunol* 1998;28(12):4020–4028.
16. Rogers KA, DeKrey GK, Mbow ML, Gillespie RD, Brodskyn CI, Titus RG. Type 1 and type 2 responses to *Leishmania major*. *FEMS Microbiol Lett* 2002; 209(1):1–7.
17. Matthews DJ, Emson CL, McKenzie GJ, Jolin HE, Blackwell JM, McKenzie AN. IL-13 is a susceptibility factor for Leishmania major infection. *J Immunol* 2000;164(3):1458–1462.
18. Uzonna JE, Bretscher PA. Anti-IL-4 antibody therapy causes regression of chronic lesions caused by medium-dose *Leishmania major* infection in BALB/c mice. *Eur J Immunol* 2001;31(11):3175–3184.
19. Belkaid Y, Hoffmann KF, Mendez S, Kamhawi S, Udey MC, Wynn TA, Sacks DL. The role of interleukin (IL)-10 in the persistence of *Leishmania major* in the skin after healing and the therapeutic potential of anti-IL-10 receptor antibody for sterile cure. *J Exp Med* 2001;194(10):1497–1506.
20. Mattner F, Alber G, Magram J, Kopf M. The role of IL-12 and IL-4 in *Leishmania major* infection. *Chem Immunol* 1997;68:86–109.
21. Himmelrich H, Launois P, Maillard I, Biedermann T, Tacchini-Cottier F, Locksley RM, Rocken M, Louis JA. In BALB/c mice, IL-4 production during the initial phase of infection with *Leishmania major* is necessary and sufficient to instruct Th2 cell development resulting in progressive disease. *J Immunol* 2000;164(9):4819–4825.
22. Chatelain R, Mauze S, Coffman RL. Experimental *Leishmania major* infection in mice: role of IL-10. *Parasite Immunol* 1999;21(4):211–218.
23. Kane MM, Mosser DM. The role of IL-10 in promoting disease progression in leishmaniasis. *J Immunol* 2001;166(2):1141–1147.
24. Park AY, Hondowicz BD, Scott P. IL-12 is required to maintain a Th1 response during *Leishmania major* infection. *J Immunol* 2000;165(2):896–902.
25. Murray HW, Delph-Etienne S. Roles of endogenous gamma interferon and macrophage microbicidal mechanisms in host response to chemotherapy in experimental visceral leishmaniasis. *Infect Immun* 2000;68(1):288–293.
26. Murray HW, Nathan CF. Macrophage microbicidal mechanisms in vivo: reactive nitrogen versus oxygen intermediates in the killing of intracellular visceral *Leishmania donovani*. *J Exp Med* 1999;189(4):741–746.
27. Satoskar AR, Rodig S, Telford SR 3rd, Satoskar AA, Ghosh SK, von Lichtenberg F, David JR. IL-12 gene-deficient C57BL/6 mice are susceptible to *Leishmania donovani* but have diminished hepatic immunopathology. *Eur J Immunol* 2000;30(3):834–839.
28. Stobie L, Gurunathan S, Prussin C, Sacks DL, Glaichenhaus N, Wu CY, Seder RA. The role of antigen and IL-12 in sustaining Th1 memory cells in vivo: IL-12 is required to maintain memory/effector Th1 cells sufficient to mediate protection to an infectious parasite challenge. *Proc Natl Acad Sci USA* 2000;97(15):8427–8432.
29. Wilson ME, Young BM, Davidson BL, Mente KA, McGowan S. The importance TGF-b in murine visceral leishmaniasis. *J Immunol* 1998;161:6148–6155.
30. Murphy ML, Wille U, Villegas EN, Hunter CA, Farrell JP. IL-10 mediates susceptibility to *Leishmania donovani* infection. *Eur J Immunol* 2001;31(10):2848–2856.
31. Lira R, Doherty M, Modi G, Sacks D. Evolution of lesion formation, parasitic load, immune response, and reservoir potential in C57BL/6 mice following high- and low-dose challenge with *Leishmania major*. *Infect Immun* 2000;68(9):5176–5182.
32. Gomes NA, Barreto-de-Souza V, DosReis GA. Early *in vitro* priming of distinct T(h) cell subsets determines polarized growth of visceralizing *Leishmania* in macrophages. *Int Immunol* 2000;12(9):1227–1233.
33. Kebaier C, Louzir H, Chenik M, Ben Salah A, Dellagi K. Heterogeneity of wild *Leishmania major* isolates in experimental murine pathogenicity and specific immune response. *Infect Immun* 2001;69(8):4906–4915.
34. Colmenares M, Kar S, Goldsmith-Pestana K, McMahon-Pratt D. Mechanisms of pathogenesis: differences amongst Leishmania species. *Trans R Soc Trop Med Hyg* 2002;96[Suppl 1]:S3–S7.
35. Ben Salah AB, Ben Ismail R, Amri F, et al. Investigation of the spread of human visceral leishmaniasis in central Tunisia. *Trans R Soc Trop Med Hyg* 2000;94(4):382–386.
36. Jeronimo SM, Teixeira MJ, Sousa A, Thielking P, Pearson RD, Evans TG. Natural history of *Leishmania (Leishmania) chagasi* infection in Northeastern Brazil: long-term follow-up. *Clin Infect Dis* 2000;30(3):608–609.
37. Badaro R, Jones TC, Carvalho EM, et al. New perspectives on a subclinical form of visceral leishmaniasis. *J Infect Dis* 1986b;154(6):1003–1011.
38. Badaro R, Jones TC, Lorenco R, Cerf BJ, et al. A prospective study of visceral leishmaniasis in an endemic area of Brazil. *J Infect Dis* 1986a;154(4):639–649.
39. Pearson RD, Sousa AQ. Clinical spectrum of Leishmaniasis. *Clin Infect Dis* 1996;22(1):1–13.
40. Cerf BJ, Jones TC, Badaro R, et al. Malnutrition as a risk factor for severe visceral leishmaniasis. *J Infect Dis* 1987;156:1030.
41. Cunha S, Freire M, Eulalio C, et al. Visceral leishmaniasis in a new ecological niche near a major metropolitan area of Brazil. *Trans R Soc Trop Med Hyg* 1995;89(2):155–158.
42. Aguilar CM, Fernandez E, Cannova DC, Ferrer E, Cabrera Z, Souza WJ, Coutinho SG. Urban visceral leishmaniasis in Venezuela. *Mem Inst Oswaldo Cruz* 1998;93:15–16.
43. Singh S, Kumari V, Singh N. Predicting kala-azar disease manifestations in asymptomatic patients with latent *Leishmania donovani* infection by detection of antibody against recombinant Kk39 antigen. *Clin Diagn Lab Immunol* 2002;9(3):568–572.
44. Zijlstra EE, Nur Y, Desjeux P, Khalil EA, El-Hassan AM, Groen J. Diagnosing

visceral leishmaniasis with the recombinant K39 strip test: experience from the Sudan. *Trop Med Int Health* 2001;6(2):108–113.

45. Badaro R, Benson D, Eulalio MC, et al. rK39: a cloned antigen of *Leishmania chagasi* that predicts active visceral leishmaniasis. *J Infect Dis* 1996;173(3):758–761.

46. Qu JQ, Zhong L, Masoom-Yasinzai M, et al. Serodiagnosis of Asian leishmaniasis with a recombinant antigen from the repetitive domain of a Leishmania kinesin. *Trans R Soc Trop Med Hyg* 1994;88(5):543–545.

47. Carvalho EM, Bacellar O, Barral A, et al. Antigen-specific immunosuppression in visceral leishmaniasis is cell mediated. *J Clin Invest* 1989;83:860–865.

48. Ho JL, Badaro R, Hatzigeogiou D, Reed SG, Johnson Jr WD. Cytokines in the treatment of leishmaniasis: from studies of immunopathology to patient therapy. *Biotherapy* 1994;7:223–235.

49. Carvalho EM, Bacellar O, Brownell C, Regis T, Coffman RL, Reed SG. Restoration of IFN-gamma production and lymphocyte proliferation in visceral leishmaniasis. *J Immunol* 1994;152(12):5949–5956.

50. Holaday BJ, Pompeu MML, Jeronimo SMB, et al. Potential role of IL-10 in the immunosuppression associated with Kala-azar. *J Clin Invest* 1993;92:2626–2632.

51. Pirmez C, Yamamura M, Uyemura K, Paes-Oliveira M, Conceicao-Silva F, Modlin RL. Cytokine patterns in the pathogenesis of human leishmaniasis. *J Clin Invest* 1993;91:1390–1395.

52. Carvalho EM, Barral A, Pedral-Sampaio, et al. Immunologic markers of clinical evolution in children recently infected with *Leishmania donovani chagasi*. *J Infect Dis* 1992;165:535–540.

53. Bacellar O, D'oliveira A Jr, Jeronimo S, Carvalho EM. IL-10 and IL-12 are the main regulatory cytokines in visceral leishmaniasis. *Cytokine* 2000;12(8):1228–1231.

54. Kharazmi A, Kemp K, Ismail A, et al. T-cell response in human leishmaniasis. *Immunol Lett* 1999;65(1-2):105–108.

55. Berman JD. Human leishmaniasis: clinical, diagnostic, and chemotherapeutic developments in the last 10 years. *Clin Infect Dis* 1997;24(4):684–703.

56. Magill AJ, Grogl M, Gasser RA Jr, Sun W, Oster CN. Visceral infection caused by *Leishmania tropica* in veterans of operation desert storm. *N Engl J Med* 1993;328(19):1383–1387.

57. Gagnaire MH, Galambrun, Stephan JL. Hematophagocytic syndrome: a misleading complication of visceral leishmaniasis in children- a series of 12 cases. *Pediatrics* 2000;106:1–6.

58. Bora D. Epidemiology of visceral leishmaniasis in India. *Natl Med J India* 1999;12(2):62–68.

59. Bryceson A. Splenic aspiration procedure. In: Peters W, Killick-Kendrick R, eds. *The leishmaniases in biology and medicine,* vol. 2. London: Academic Press, 1987:728–729.

60. Thakur CP, Kumar M, Kumar P, et al. Rationalisation of regimens of treatment of kala-azar with sodium stibogluconate in India: a randomised study. *BMJ* 1988;296:1557.

61. Montelius S, Maasho K, Pratlong F, Lebbad M, Gregory L, Akuffo H. Skin rash for 15 years. *Lancet* 1998;352(9138):1438.

62. Marovich MA, Lira R, Shepard M, et al. Leishmaniasis recidivans recurrence after 43 years: a clinical and immunologic report after successful treatment. *Clin Infect Dis* 2001;33(7):1076–1079.

63. Schubach A, Haddad F, Oliveira-Neto MP, Degrave W, Pirmez C, Grimaldi G Jr, Fernandes O. Detection of Leishmania DNA by polymerase chain reaction in scars of treated human patients. *J Infect Dis* 1998;178(3):911–914.

64. Schubach A, Marzochi MC, Cuzzi-Maya T, et al. Cutaneous scars in American tegumentary leishmaniasis patients: a site of *Leishmania (Viannia) braziliensis* persistence and viability eleven years after antimonial therapy and clinical cure. *Am J Trop Med Hyg* 1998;58(6):824–827.

65. Leishmania/HIV coinfection in South-Western Europe 1990-1998: retrospective analysis of 965 cases. WHO 2000. Available at: *www.who.int/emc/leish/2000.42.*

66. Rosenthal E, Marty P, del Giudice P, et al. HIV and *Leishmania* coinfection: a review of 91 cases with focus on atypical locations of *Leishmania*. *Clin Infect Dis* 2000;31:1093–1095.

67. Hernandez-Perez J, Yebra-Bango M, Jimenez-Martinez E, et al. Visceral leishmaniasis (Kala-azar) in solid organ transplantation: report of five cases and review. *Clin Infect Dis* 1999;29:918–921.

68. Alrajhi AA, Saleem M, Ibrahim EA, Gramiccia M. Leishmaniasis of the tongue in a renal transplant recipient. *Clin Infect Dis* 1998;27(5):1332–1333.

69. Iborra C, Caumes E, Carriere J, Cavelier-Balloy B, Danis M, Bricaire F. Mucosal leishmaniasis in a heart transplant recipient. *Br J Dermatol* 1998;138(1):190–192.

70. Ashford RW, Bettini S. Ecology and epidemiology: Old World. In: Peters W, Killick-Kendrick R, eds. *The leishmaniases in biology and medicine,* vol. 1. London: Academic Press, 1987:365–424.

71. Gramiccia M, Ben-Ismail R, Gradoni L, et al. A *Leishmania infantum* enzymatic variant, causative agent of cutaneous leishmaniasis in north Tunisia. *Trans R Soc Trop Med Hyg* 1991;85:370–371.

72. Castes M, Trujillo D, Rojas ME, et al. Serum levels of tumor necrosis factor in patients with American cutaneous leishmaniasis. *Biol Res* 1993;26(1-2):233–238.

73. Bottrel RL, Dutra WO, Martins FA, et al. Flow cytometric determina-

tion of cellular sources and frequencies of key cytokine-producing lymphocytes directed against recombinant LACK and soluble Leishmania antigen in human cutaneous leishmaniasis. *Infect Immun* 2001;69(5):3232–3239.

74. Bacellar O, Lessa H, Schriefer A, et al. Up-regulation of Th1 type response in mucosal leishmaniasis patients. *Infect Immun* 2002;70:6734–6740.

75. Rocha PN, Almeida RP, Bacellar O, et al. Dow-regulation of Th1 type of response in early human American cutaneous leishmaniasis. *J Infect Dis* 1999;180:1731–1734.

76. Machado P, Araujo C, Da Silva AT, et al. Failure of early treatment of cutaneous leishmaniasis in preventing the development of an ulcer. *Clin Infect Dis* 2002;34(12):E69–E73.

77. Barral A, Jesus AR, Almeida RP, et al. Evaluation of T-cell subsets in the lesion infiltrates of human cutaneous and mucocutaneous leishmaniasis. *Parasite Immunol* 1987;9(4):487–497.

78. Pirmez C, Cooper C, Paes-Oliveira M, Schubach A, Torigian VK, Modlin RL. Immunologic responsiveness in American cutaneous leishmaniasis lesions. *J Immunol* 1990;145(9):3100–3104.

79. Melby PC, Andrade-Narvaez FJ, Darnell BJ, Valencia-Pacheco G, Tryon VV, Palomo-Cetina A. Increased expression of proinflammatory cytokines in chronic lesions of human cutaneous leishmaniasis. *Infect Immun* 1994;62(3):837–842.

80. Melby PC, Andrade-Narvaez F, Darnell BJ, Valencia-Pacheco G. In situ expression of interleukin-10 and interleukin-12 in active human cutaneous leishmaniasis. *FEMS Immunol Med Microbiol* 1996;15(2-3):101–107.

81. Louzir H, Melby PC, Ben Salah A, et al. Immunologic determinants of disease evolution in localized cutaneous leishmaniasis due to *Leishmania major*. *J Infect Dis* 1998;177(6):1687–1695.

82. Herwaldt BL, Sokes SL, Juranek DD. American cutaneous leishmaniasis in U.S. travelers. *Ann Intern Med* 1993;118:779–784.

83. Ramesh V, Mukherjee A. Post-kala-azar dermal leishmaniasis. *Int J Dermatol* 1993;32:272–275.

84. Moral L. Post-kala-azar dermal Leishmaniasis and *Leishmania infantum*. *Br J Dermatol* 1999;140(4):760.

85. el Hassan AM, Ghalib HW, Zijlstra EE, et al. Post kala-azar dermal leishmaniasis in the Sudan: clinical features, pathology and treatment. *Trans R Soc Trop Med Hyg* 1992;86(3):245–248.

86. Zijlstra EE, el-Hassan AM. Leishmaniasis in Sudan. Post kala-azar dermal leishmaniasis. *Trans R Soc Trop Med Hyg* 2001;95[Suppl 1]:S59–S76.

87. Sharma MC, Gupta AK, Verma N, Das VN, Saran R, Kar SK. Demonstration of Leishmania parasites in skin lesions of Indian post kala-azar dermal leishmaniasis (PKDL) cases. *J Commun Dis* 2000;32(1):67–68.

88. El Hassan AM, Khalil EA. Post-kala-azar dermal leishmaniasis: does it play a role in the transmission of *Leishmania donovani* in the Sudan? *Trop Med Int Health* 2001;6(9):743–744.

89. Gunduz K, Afsar S, Ayhan S, et al. Recidivans cutaneous leishmaniasis unresponsive to liposomal amphotericin B (AmBisome). *J Eur Acad Dermatol Venereol* 2000;14(1):11–13.

90. Oliveira-Neto MP, Mattos M, Souza CS, Fernandes O, Pirmez C. Leishmaniasis recidiva cutis in New World cutaneous leishmaniasis. *Int J Dermatol* 1998;37(11):846–849.

91. Wortmann GW, Aronson NE, Miller RE, et al. Cutaneous leishmaniasis following local trauma: a clinical pearl. *Clin Infect Dis* 2000;31:199–200.

92. Landau M, Srebrnik A, Brenner S. Leishmaniasis recidivans mimicking lupus vulgaris. *Int J Dermatol* 1996;35(8):572–573.

93. Teklemariam S, Hiwot AG, Frommel D, Miko TL, Ganlov G, Bryceson A. Aminosidine and its combination with sodium stibogluconate in the treatment of diffuse cutaneous leishmaniasis caused by *Leishmania aethiopica*. *Trans R Soc Trop Med Hyg* 1994;88(3):334–339.

94. Badaro R, Johnson WD Jr. The role of interferon-gamma in the treatment of visceral and diffuse cutaneous leishmaniasis. *J Infect Dis* 1993;167[Suppl 1]:S13–S17.

95. Akuffo H, Maasho K, Blostedt M, Hojeberg B, Britton S, Bakhiet M. *Leishmania aethiopica* derived from diffuse leishmaniasis patients preferentially induce mRNA for interleukin-10 while those from localized leishmaniasis patients induce interferon-gamma. *J Infect Dis* 1997;175(3):737–741.

96. Cnudde F, Raccurt C, Boulard F, Terron-Aboud B, Nicolas M, Juminer B. Diffuse cutaneous leishmaniasis with visceral dissemination in an AIDS patient in Guadeloupe, West Indies. *AIDS* 1994;8(4):559–560.

97. Monroy-Ostria A, Fuentes-Fraga I, Garcia-Flores C, Favila-Castillo L. Infection of BALB/c, C57B1/6 mice and F1 hybrid CB6F1 mice with strains of *Leishmania mexicana* isolated from Mexican patients with localized or diffuse cutaneous leishmaniasis. *Arch Med Res* 1994;25(4):401–406.

98. Velez I, Agudelo S, Robledo S, et al. Diffuse cutaneous leishmaniasis with mucosal involvement in Columbia, caused by an enzymatic variant of Leishmania panamensis. *Trans R Soc Trop Med Hyg* 1994;88:199.

99. Costa JML, Saldanha ACR, Melo e Silva AC, et al. Estudo atual da leishmaniose cutanea difusa no Estado do Maranhao. II. Aspectos epidemiologicos, clinico-evolutivos. *Rev Soc Brazil Med Trop* 1992;25:115–123.

100. Barral A, Costa JM, Bittencourt AL, Barral-Netto M, Carvalho EM. Polar and subpolar diffuse cutaneous leishmaniasis in Brazil: clinical and immunopathologic aspects. *Int J Dermatol* 1995;34(7):474–479.

101. Turetz ML, Machado PR, Ko AI, et al. Disseminated leishmaniasis: a new and emerging form of leishmaniasis observed in the northeastern of Brazil. *Clin Infect Dis* 2002 *(in press)*.

102. Carvalho EM, Barral A, Costa JML, Bittencourt A, Marsden P. Clinical and immunopathological aspects of disseminated cutaneous leishmaniasis. *Acta Trop* 1994;56:315–325.

103. Costa JML, Marsden PD, Llanos-Cuentas EA, et al. Disseminated cutaneous leishmaniasis in a field clinic in Bahia, Brazil: a report of eight cases. *J Trop Med Hyg* 1986;89:319–323.

104. Marsden PD. Mucosal leishmaniasis. ("Espundia" or "escomel"). *Trans R Soc Trop Med Hyg* 1986;80:859–867.

105. Almeida RP, Barral-Netto M, De Jesus AM, De Freitas LA, Carvalho EM, Barral A. Biological behavior of *Leishmania amazonensis* isolated from humans with cutaneous, mucosal, or visceral leishmaniasis in BALB/C mice. *Am J Trop Med Hyg* 1996;54(2):178–184.

106. Barral A, Pedral-Sampaio D, Grimaldi Junior G, et al. Leishmaniasis in Bahia, Brazil: evidence that *Leishmania amazonensis* produces a wide spectrum of clinical disease. *Am J Trop Med Hyg* 1991;44(5):536–546.

107. Jones TC, Johnson WD Jr, Barretto AC, et al. Epidemiology of American cutaneous leishmaniasis due to *Leishmania braziliensis*. *J Infect Dis* 1987;156(1):73–83.

108. Netto EM, Marsden PD, Llanos-Cuentas EA, et al. Long-term follow-up of patients with *Leishmania (Viannia) braziliensis* infection and treated with glucantime. *Trans R Soc Trop Med Hyg* 1990;84(3):367–370.

109. Guerreiro JB, Lessa HA, Cruz AA, Rocha H, Barral A, Carvalho EM. Mucosal leishmaniasis: quantitative nasal cytology as a marker of disease activity and indicator of healing. *Ann Otol Rhinol Laryngol* 2000;109:89–94.

110. el-Hassan AM, Zijlstra EE. Leishmaniasis in Sudan. Mucosal leishmaniasis. *Trans R Soc Trop Med Hyg* 2001;95[Suppl 1]:S19–S26.

111. Skeiky YA, Benson DR, Guderian JA, Whittle JA, Bacelar O, Carvalho EM, Reed SG. Immune responses of leishmaniasis patients to heat shock proteins of Leishmania species and humans. *Infect Immun* 1995;63(10):4105–4114.

112. Zajtchuk JT, Casler JD, Netto EM, et al. Mucosal leishmaniasis in Brazil. *Laryngoscope* 1989;99(9):925–939.

113. Velez I, Agudelo S, Hendrickx E, et al. Inefficacy of allopurinol for Colombian cutaneous leishmaniasis: a randomized, controlled trial. *Ann Intern Med* 1997;126:2326.

114. Herwaldt BL, Arana BA, Navin TR. The natural history of cutaneous leishmaniasis in Guatemala. *J Infect Dis* 1992;165:51827.

115. Soto-Mancipe J, Grogl M, Berman JD. Evaluation of pentamidine for the treatment of cutaneous leishmaniasis in Colombia. *Clin Infect Dis* 1993;16(3):417–425.

116. Guderian RH, Chico ME, Rogers MD, Pattishall KM, Grogl M, Berman JD. Placebo controlled treatment of Ecuadorian cutaneous leishmaniasis. *Am J Trop Med Hyg* 1991;45(1):92–97.

117. Croft SL. Monitoring drug resistance in leishmaniasis. *Trop Med Int Health* 2001;6(11):899–905.

118. Sundar S. Drug resistance in Indian visceral leishmaniasis. *Trop Med Int Health* 2001;6(11):849–854.

119. Herwaldt BL. Leishmaniasis. *Lancet* 1999;354(9185):1191–1199.

120. Drugs for parasitic infection. *Med Lett* 2002;April:1–12.

121. Marsden PD. Pentavalent antimonials: old drugs for new diseases. *Rev Soc Bras Med Trop* 1985;18:187.

122. Bryceson A. Therapy in man. In: Peters W, Killick-Kendrick R. eds. *The leishmaniases in biology and medicine*, vol 2. London: Academic Press, 1987:847–907.

123. Berman JD. Chemotherapy for leishmaniasis: biochemical mechanisms, clinical efficacy, and future strategies. *Rev Infect Dis* 1988;10(3):560–586.

124. Herwaldt BL, Berman JD. Recommendations for treating leishmaniasis with sodium stibogluconate (Pentostam) and review of pertinent clinical studies. *Am J Trop Med Hyg* 1992;46(3):296–306.

125. Badaro R, Falcoff E, Badaro FS, et al. Treatment of visceral leishmaniasis with pentavalent antimony and interferon-γ. *N Engl J Med* 1990;322:16.

126. Minodier P, Piarroux R, Garnier JM, Unal D, Perrimond H, Dumon H. Pediatric visceral leishmaniasis in southern France. *Pediatr Infect Dis J* 1998;17(8):701–704.

127. Chulay JD, Spencer HC, Mugambi M. Electrocardiographic changes during treatment of leishmaniasis with pentavalent antimony (sodium stibogluconate). *Am J Trop Med Hyg* 1985;34:702.

128. Coukell AJ, Brogden RN. Liposomal amphotericin B. Therapeutic use in the management of fungal infections and visceral leishmaniasis. *Drugs* 1998;55(4):585–612.

129. Berman JD, Badero R, Thakur CP, et al. Efficacy and safety of lipisomal amphotericin B (AmBisome) for visceral leishmaniasis in endemic developing countries. *Bull WHO* 1998;76:25–32.

130. Berman JD. U.S Food and Drug Administration approval of AmBisome (liposomal amphotericin B) for treatment of visceral leishmaniasis. *Clin Infect Dis* 1999;28(1):49–51.

131. di Martino L, Davidson RN, Giacchino R, et al. Treatment of visceral leishmaniasis in children with liposomal amphotericin B. *J Pediatr* 1997;131(2):271–277.

132. Sundar S, Jha TK, Thakur CP, et al. Phase III trial of oral miltefosine for Indian visceral leishmaniasis. *N Engl J Med* 2002;22:1739–1746.

133. Durand R, Paul M, Pratlong F, et al. *Leishmania infantum*: lack of parasite resistance to amphotericin B in a clinically resistant visceral leishmaniasis. *Antimicrob Agents Chemother* 1998;42(8):2141–2143.

134. Laguna F, Lopez-Velez R, Pulido F, et al. Treatment of visceral leishmaniasis in HIV-infected patients: a randomized trial comparing meglumine antimonate with amphotericin B. Spanish HIV-Leishmania Study Group. *AIDS* 1999;13(9):1063–1069.

135. Sundar S, Agrawal G, Rai M, Makharia MK, Murray HW. Treatment of Indian visceral leishmaniasis with single or daily infusions of low dose liposomal amphotericin B: randomised trial. *BMJ* 2001;323(7310):419–422.

136. Sundar S, Jha TK, Thakur CP, Mishra M, Singh VR, Buffels R. Low-dose liposomal amphotericin B in refractory Indian visceral leishmaniasis: a multicenter study. *Am J Trop Med Hyg* 2002;66(2):143–146.

137. Thakur CP, Kumar M, Pandey AK. Comparison of regimes of treatment of antimony-resistant kala-azar patients: a randomized study. *Am J Trop Med Hyg* 1991;45:435–441.

138. Voringer HF, Arasteh K. Pharmacokinetic optimization in the treatment of *Peumocytis carinii* pneumonia. *Clin Pharmacokinet* 1993;24:388–412.

139. Jha TK, Olliaro P, Thakur CP, et al. Randomised controlled trial of aminosidine (paromomycin) v sodium stibogluconate for treating visceral leishmaniasis in North Bihar, India. *BMJ* 1998;316(7139):1200–1205.

140. Jha TK, Sundar S, Thakur CP, et al. Miltefosine, an oral agent, for the treatment of Indian visceral leishmaniasis. *N Engl J Med* 1999;341(24):1795–1800.

141. Sherwood JA, Gachihi GS, Mugai RK, et al. Phase 2 efficacy trial of an oral 8-aminoquinoline (WR6026) for treatment of visceral leishmaniasis. *Clin Infect Dis* 1994;19:1034–1039.

142. Badaro R, Nascimento C, Carvalho JS, et al. Recombinant human granulocyte-macrophage colony-stimulating factor reverses neutropenia and reduces secondary infections in visceral leishmaniasis. *J Infect Dis* 1994;170(2):413–418.

143. Badaro R, Nascimento C, Carvalho JS, et al. Granulocyte-macrophage colony-stimulating factor in combination with pentavalent antimony for the treatment of visceral leishmaniasis. *Eur J Clin Microbiol Infect Dis* 1994;13[Suppl 2]:S23–S28.

144. Alvar J, Canavate C, Gutierrez-Solar B, et al. Leishmaniasis and human immunodeficiency syndrome. *Clin Microbiol Rev* 1997;10:289–319.

145. Morales MA, Cruz I, Rubio JM, et al. Relapse versus reinfection in patients coinfected with *Leishmania infantum* and human immunodeficiency virus type 1. *J Infect Dis* 2002;185:1533–1537.

146. Choi CM, Lerner EA. Leishmaniasis: recognition and management with a focus on the immunocompromised patient. *Am J Clin Dermatol* 2002;3(2):91–105.

147. Navin TR, Arana BA, Arana FE, Berman JD, Chajon JF. Placebo-controlled clinical trial of sodium stibogluconate (Pentostam) versus ketoconazole for treating cutaneous leishmaniasis in Guatemala. *J Infect Dis* 1992;165(3):528–534.

148. Alrajhi AA, Ibrahim EA, De Vol EB, Khairat M, Faris RM, Maguire JH. Fluconazole for the treatment of cutaneous leishmaniasis caused by *Leishmania major*. *N Engl J Med* 2002;346:891–895.

149. Berman JD. Treatment of New World cutaneous and mucosal leishmaniases. *Clin Dermatol* 1996;14(5):519–522.

150. Romero GA, Guerra MV, Paes MG, Macedo VO. Comparison of cutaneous leishmaniasis due to *Leishmania (Viannia) braziliensis* and *L.(V.) guyanensis* in Brazil: therapeutic response to meglumine antimonate. *Am J Trop Med Hyg* 2001;65(5):456–465.

151. Almeida R, D'Oliveira A, Machado P, et al. Randomized, double-blind study of stibogluconate plus human granulocyte macrophage colony-stimulating factor versus stibogluconate alone in the treatment of cutaneous leishmaniasis. *J Infect Dis* 1999;180:1735–1737.

152. Soto J, Fuya P, Herrera R, Berman J. Topical paromomycin/methylbenzethonium chloride plus parenteral meglumine antimonate as treatment for American cutaneous leishmaniasis: controlled study. *Clin Infect Dis* 1998;26(1):56–58.

153. Oliveira-Neto MP, Schubach A, Mattos M, Goncalves-Costa SC, Pirmez C. Treatment of American cutaneous leishmaniasis: a comparison between low dosage (5 mg/kg/day) and high dosage (20 mg/kg/day) antimony regimens. *Pathol Biol (Paris)* 1997;45(6):496–499.

154. Oliveira-Neto MP, Schubach A, Mattos M, Goncalves-Costa SC, Pirmez C. A low-dose antimony treatment in 159 patients with American cutaneous leishmaniasis: extensive follow-up studies (up to 10 years). *Am J Trop Med Hyg* 1997;57(6):651–655.

155. Vargas-Gonzalez A, Canto-Lara SB, Damian-Centeno AG, Andrade-Narvaez FJ. Response of cutaneous leishmaniasis (chiclero's ulcer) to treatment with meglumine antimonate in Southeast Mexico. *Am J Trop Med Hyg* 1999;61(6):960–963.

156. Palacios R, Osorio LE, Grajalew LF, Ochoa MT. Treatment failure in children in a randomized clinical trial with 10 and 20 days of meglumine antimonate for cutaneous leishmaniasis due to *Leishmania viannia* species. *Am J Trop Med Hyg* 2001;64(3-4):187–193.

157. Arana BA, Navin TR, Arana FE, Berman JD, Rosenkaimer F. Efficacy of a short course (10 days) of high-dose meglumine antimonate with or without interferon-gamma in treating cutaneous leishmaniasis in Guatemala. *Clin Infect Dis* 1994;18(3):381–384.

158. Vardy D, Barenholz Y, Naftoliev N, Klaus S, Gilead L, Frankenburg S. Efficacious topical treatment for human cutaneous leishmaniasis with ethanolic lipid amphotericin B. *Trans R Soc Trop Med Hyg* 2001;95(2):184–186.

159. Torre-Cisneros J, Prada JL, Villanueva JL, Valverde F, Sanchez-Guijo P. Successful treatment of antimony-resistant cutaneous leishmaniasis with liposomal amphotericin B. *Clin Infect Dis* 1994;18(6):1024–1025.

160. Wortmann GW, Fraser SL, Aronson NE, Davis C, Miller RS, Jackson JD, Oster CN. Failure of amphotericin B lipid complex in the treatment of cutaneous leishmaniasis. *Clin Infect Dis* 1998;26(4):1006–1007.

161. Thakur CP, Narain S, Kumar N, Hassan SM, Jha DK, Kumar A. Amphotericin B is superior to sodium antimony gluconate in the treatment of Indian post-kala-azar dermal leishmaniasis. *Ann Trop Med Parasitol* 1997;91(6):611–616.

162. Amato VS, Nicodemo AC, Amato JG, Boulos M, Neto VA. Mucocutaneous leishmaniasis associated with HIV infection treated successfully with liposomal amphotericin B (AmBisome). *J Antimicrob Chemother* 2000;46(2):341–342.

163. Gunduz K, Afsar S, Ayhan S, Kandiloglu AR, Turel A, Filiz EE, Ok UZ. Recidivans cutaneous leishmaniasis unresponsive to liposomal amphotericin B (AmBisome). *J Eur Acad Dermatol Venereol* 2000;14(1):11–13.

164. Roustan G, Jimenez JA, Gutierrez-Solar B, Gallego JL, Alvar J, Patron M. Post-kala-azar dermal leishmaniasis with mucosal involvement in a kidney transplant recipient: treatment with liposomal amphotericin B. *Br J Dermatol* 1998;138(3):526–528.

165. Hashim FA, Khalil EA, Ismail A, el Hassan AM. Apparently successful treatment of two cases of post kala-azar dermal leishmaniasis with liposomal amphotericin B. *Trans R Soc Trop Med Hyg* 1995;89(4):440.

166. Soto J, Buffet P, Grogl M, Berman J. Successful treatment of Colombian cutaneous leishmaniasis with four injections of pentamidine. *Am J Trop Med Hyg* 1994;50(1):107–111.

167. Weinrauch L, Livshin R, El-On J. Ketoconazole in cutaneous leishmaniasis. *Br J Dermatol* 1987;117:666–668.

168. Soto J, Toledo J, Gutierrez P, et al. Treatment of American cutaneous leishmaniasis with miltefosine, an oral agent. *Clin Infect Dis* 2001;33(7):E57–E61.

169. Neva FA, Ponce C, Ponce E, Kreutzer R, Modabber F, Olliaro P. Non-ulcerative cutaneous leishmaniasis in Honduras fails to respond to topical paromomycin. *Trans R Soc Trop Med Hyg* 1997;91(4):473–475.

170. Soto J, Fuya P, Herrera R, Berman J. Topical paromomycin/methylbenzethonium chloride plus parenteral meglumine antimonate as treatment for American cutaneous leishmaniasis: controlled study. *Clin Infect Dis* 1998;26(1):56–58.

171. Navin TR, Arana BA, Arana FE, de Merida AM, Castillo AL, Pozuelos JL. Placebo-controlled clinical trial of meglumine antimonate (glucantime) vs. localized controlled heat in the treatment of cutaneous leishmaniasis in Guatemala. *Am J Trop Med Hyg* 1990;42(1):43–50.

172. Bryceson ADM. Diffuse cutaneous leishmaniasis in Ethiopia. II. Treatment. *Trans R Soc Trop Med Hyg* 1997;64:369–393.

173. Badaro R, Johnson WD Jr. The role of interferon-gamma in the treatment of visceral and diffuse cutaneous leishmaniasis. *J Infect Dis* 1993;167[Suppl 1]:S13–S17.

174. Rocha RAA, Sampaio RN, Guerra M, et al. Apparent glucantime failure in five patients with mucocutaneous leishmaniasis. *Am J Trop Med Hyg* 1980;83:131–139.

175. Franke ED, Wignall S, Cruz ME, et al. Efficacy and toxicity of sodium stibogluconate for mucosal leishmaniasis. *Ann Intern Med* 1990;113:934–940.

176. Franke ED, Llanos-Cuentas A, Echevarria J, et al. Efficacy of 28-day and 40-day regimens of sodium stibogluconate (Pentostam) in the treatment of mucosal leishmaniasis. *Am J Trop Med Hyg* 1994;51(1):77–82.

177. Marsden PD, Sampaio RNR, Carvalho EM, et al: High continuous antimony therapy in two patients with unresponsive mucosal leishmaniasis. *Am J Trop Med Hyg* 1985;4:710.

178. Futado TA, Clinical results in the treatment of American leishmaniasis with oral and intravenous amphotericin. In: Welch H, Marti-Ibanez E, eds. *Antibiotics annual 1959–1960.* New York: Antibiotica, 1960:631–637.

179. Sampaio SAP, Godoy JT, Paiva L, et al. The treatment of American (mucocutaneous) leishmaniasis with amphotericin B. *Arch Dermatol.* 1960;82:627–635.

180. Croft MAJ. Use of amphotericin B in mucocutaneous leishmaniasis. *J Trop Med Hyg* 1976;79:111–113.

181. Marsden PD, Netto EM, Badaro R, Cuba CA, Costa JL, Barreto AC. Apparent cure of a difficult treatment problem in a patient with mucosal leishmaniasis. *Am J Trop Med Hyg* 1986;35(2):449.

182. Rodriguez LV, Dedet JP, Paredes V, Mendoza C, Cardenas F. A randomized trial of amphotericin B alone or in combination with itraconazole in the treatment of mucocutaneous leishmaniasis. *Mem Inst Oswaldo Cruz* 1995;90(4):525–528.

183. Amato VS, Nicodemo AC, Amato JG, Boulos M, Neto VA. Mucocutaneous leishmaniasis associated with HIV infection treated successfully with liposomal amphotericin B (AmBisome). *J Antimicrob Chemother* 2000;46(2):341–342.

184. Nonata R, Sampaio R, Marsden PD. Mucosal leishmaniasis unresponsive to glucantime therapy successfully treated with AmBisome. *Trans R Soc Trop Med Hyg* 1997;91(1):77.

185. Amato V, Amato J, Nicodemo A, Uip D, Amato-Neto V, Duarte M. Treatment of mucocutaneous leishmaniasis with pentamidine isothionate. *Ann Dermatol Venereol* 1998;125(8):492–495.

186. Lopes CF, de Almeida MA. Treatment of mucocutaneous American leishmaniasis with a pentamidine. *Hosp (Rio J)* 1968;73(1):223–231.

187. Amato VS, Padilha AR, Nicodemo AC, et al. Use of itraconazole in the treatment of mucocutaneous leishmaniasis: a pilot study. *Int J Infect Dis* 2000;4(3):153–157.

188. Boattasso O, Cabrine J, Falcoff R. Successful treatment of antimony-resistant American mucocutaneous leishmaniasis. *Arch Dermatol* 1992;128:996–997.

189. Lessa HA, Machado P, Lima F, Cruz AA, Bacellar O, Guerreiro J, Carvalho EM. Successful treatment of refractory mucosal leishmaniasis with pentoxifylline plus antimony. *Am J Trop Med Hyg* 2001;65(2):87–89.

190. Croft SL, Yardley V. Chemotherapy of leishmaniasis. *Curr Pharmaceut Design* 2002;8:319–342.

191. Soto J, Medina F, Dember N, Berman J. Efficacy of permethrin-impregnated uniforms in the prevention of malaria and leishmaniasis in Colombian soldiers. *Clin Infect Dis* 1995;21(3):599–602.

192. Croft AM, Baker D, von Bertele MJ. An evidence-based vector control strategy for military deployments: the British Army experience. *Med Trop (Mars)* 2001;61(1):91–98.

193. Downs AM, Stafford KA, Hunt LP, Ravenscroft JC, Coles GC. Widespread insecticide resistance in head lice to the over-the-counter pediculocides in England, and the emergence of carbaryl resistance. *Br J Dermatol* 2002;146(1):88–93.

194. Speare R, Koehler JM. A case of pubic lice resistant to pyrethrins. *Aust Fam Physician* 2001;30(6):572–574.

195. Marsden PD. Selective primary health care: strategies for control of disease in the developing world. XIV. Leishmaniasis. *Rev Infect Dis* 1984;6:736.

196. Palatnik-de-Sousa CB, dos Santos WR, Franca-Silva JC, et al. Impact of canine control on the epidemiology of canine and human visceral leishmaniasis in Brazil. *Am J Trop Med Hyg* 2001;65(5):510–517.

197. Reithinger R, Davies CR. Is the domestic dog (*Canis familiaris*) a reservoir host of American cutaneous leishmaniasis? A critical review of the current evidence. *Am J Trop Med Hyg* 1999;61(4):530–541.

198. Greenblatt CL. The present and future of vaccination for cutaneous leishmaniasis. In: Misrahi A, Hertman I, Klingberg et al, eds. *Progress in clinical and biological research,* vol 47. *New developments with human and veterinary vaccines.* New York: Alan R. Liss, 1980:259–285.

199. Sharifi I, FeKri AR, Aflatonian MR, et al. Randomised vaccine trial of single dose of killed Leishmania major plus BCG against anthroponotic cutaneous leishmaniasis in Bam, Iran. *Lancet* 1998;351(9115):1540–1543.

200. Papadopoulou B, Roy G, Breton M, et al. Reduced infectivity of a Leishmania donovani biopterin transporter genetic mutant and its use as an attenuated strain for vaccination. *Infect Immun* 2002;70(1):62–68.

201. Jaffe CL. Recent trends in vaccine development and immunization. *Clin Dermatol* 1999;17(3):339–344.

202. Handman E. Leishmaniasis: current status of vaccine development. *Clin Microbiol Rev* 2001;14(2):229–243.

203. Reed SG. Leishmaniasis vaccination: targeting the source of infection. *J Exp Med* 2001;194(3):F7–F9.

204. Gradoni L. An update on antileishmanial vaccine candidates and prospects for a canine leishmania vaccine. *Vet Parasitol* 2001;100(1-2):87–103.

205. Mendez S, Gurunathan S, Kamhawi S, et al. The potency and durability of DNA- and protein-based vaccines against *Leishmania major* evaluated using low-dose, intradermal challenge. *J Immunol* 2001;166(8):5122–5128.

206. Morris RV, Shoemaker CB, David JR, Lanzaro GC, Titus RG. Sandfly maxadilan exacerbates infection with *Leishmania major* and vaccinating against it protects against *L. major* infection. *J Immunol* 2001;167(9):5226–5230.

207. Sacks D, Kamhawi S. Molecular aspects of parasite-vector and vector-host interactions in leishmaniasis. *Annu Rev Microbiol* 2001;55:453–483.

CHAPTER 281
Trypanosoma

James H. Maguire

Four flagellated protozoans of the genus *Trypanosoma* infect human beings. In Africa, *Trypanosoma brucei rhodesiense* and *Trypanosoma brucei gambiense* produce sleeping sickness. *Trypanosoma cruzi*, the agent of Chagas disease, and the nonpathogenic *Trypanosoma rangeli* are endemic to the Americas. Trypanosomes pass through morphologically and physiologically distinct developmental stages in their insect vectors and mammalian hosts. Each stage contains a kinetoplast, a dark-staining structure that consists of tight coils of deoxyribonucleic acid (DNA) lying within the terminal portion of the organism's single mitochondrion (Fig. 281.1).

AFRICAN TRYPANOSOMES

Characteristics of the Pathogen

The two morphologically identical subspecies of *T. brucei*, *T. b. gambiense* in West and Central Africa and *T. b. rhodesiense* in East Africa, cause epidemiologically and clinically distinct patterns of human African trypanosomiasis (1). Within the human or other mammalian host, African trypanosomes assume the fusiform trypomastigote stage, which measures 15 to 40 μm long and is propelled by a single anterior flagellum that extends from a lateral undulating membrane (see Fig. 281.1). Trypomastigotes circulate extracellularly in the blood, lymph, and interstitial fluids and replicate by longitudinal binary fission. Early generations of parasites are long and slender, whereas later generations that are infectious to the tsetse fly vector are short and stumpy. Trypomastigotes are covered by a thick glycoprotein surface coat that undergoes antigenic variation during infection, a process that allows the organism to evade lysis by specific antibodies (2,3).

The blood-sucking tsetse fly vector (genus *Glossina*) ingests trypomastigotes upon taking a blood meal from an infected person or animal. The trypomastigotes transform into procyclic forms that multiply and migrate from the insect's gut to the salivary glands, where they transform into epimastigotes, which also replicate. After about 3 weeks, infective metacyclic trypanosomes develop from the epimastigotes. While feeding, tsetse flies inoculate saliva containing metacyclic forms, which upon entering the mammalian host, transform into blood stream trypomastigotes, replicate locally, and then spread to the bloodstream, lymphatics, and interstitial spaces.

Epidemiology

Transmission of African trypanosomiasis is limited to focal areas of sub-Saharan Africa roughly between latitudes 15 degrees north and 15 degrees south (1,4). An estimated 60 million persons in 36 countries live at risk of being infected. Although about 45,000 cases per year are reported, the actual number of persons affected may be as high as 300 to 500 million (5). Because of successful control programs, the disease had practically disappeared in the early 1960s, but economic constraints and political instability led to relaxing of control efforts and a tremendous increase in the incidence of disease in recent years, especially in parts of Angola, Democratic Republic of Congo, and Sudan,

where the disease is epidemic and the prevalence in some villages exceeds 20% (5).

In West and Central Africa, the tsetse vectors of West African trypanosomiasis include *Glossina palpalis*, *Glossina tachinoides*, and *Glossina fuscipes*, which inhabit forested riverbanks and similar humid areas (1). Human beings in nearby settlements are the major reservoir of infection, although pigs and other domestic animals may harbor the parasite.

T. b. rhodesiense is transmitted by *Glossina morsitans* and related species that live in the sparsely inhabited savannas of East Africa. Wild animals, such as the bushbuck and hartebeest, are important reservoirs, and except under epidemic conditions, human beings become infected when they enter areas of natural transmission to hunt, fish, collect honey, or visit wild game parks. Infection of livestock with *T. b. rhodesiense* and other trypanosomes seriously limits cattle production in Africa.

Reported cases of African trypanosomiasis caused by congenital infection, blood transfusion, and laboratory accident are rare. In the United States from 1967 to 2001, there were 30 cases of East African trypanosomiasis, mostly acquired by travelers to game parks, and eight cases of West African disease, most among African nationals living in the United States (7,8). In 2001, a marked increase in cases of East African trypanosomiasis was noted among travelers to Tanzania; six cases were reported from the United States and a number of others from Canada and Europe (7).

Pathogenesis

An inflamed nodule or trypanosomal chancre forms at the site of the bite, where inoculated parasites multiply extracellularly in the subcutaneous tissue. The organisms spread gradually to the lymphatics, blood stream, and interstitial spaces and continue to replicate. Parasitemia increases until specific host antibodies cause a sharp decline of parasite numbers (2,3). Parasites that have different surface antigen variants escape destruction and give rise to a new wave of parasitemia. Because each organism contains the genetic code for numerous variants, the waves of parasitemia continue to recur for months. Months to years later, the organisms penetrate the central nervous system (CNS).

The mechanisms by which African trypanosomes produce disease are not well understood (9,10). Parasite antigens activate lymphocytes and macrophages, resulting in enlargement of lymph nodes and the spleen and massive production of nonspecific and nonprotective immunoglobulin M (IgM). Circulating immune complexes, lymphokines and kinins, and toxins produced by the parasite may all play a role in the pathogenesis of the illness. Later, lymphocytes and plasma cells form cuffs around blood vessels, especially in the heart and CNS, where parasites are located (Fig. 281.2). Perivascular demyelinization, proliferation of astrocytes, and focal hemorrhages are seen in the brain. Generalized immunosuppression and associated secondary infections are common as the disease progresses. Pancarditis frequently occurs in East African disease.

Clinical Manifestations

The clinical features of African trypanosomiasis vary according to the stage of infection and the subspecies of parasite (7,8,11–13). Without treatment, both infections are invariably fatal. The course of East African disease is more rapid and severe than that of West African disease.

First symptoms appear several days to 2 weeks after the tsetse bite. A tender, red nodule, the trypanosomal chancre, may develop at the site of inoculation in persons infected with *T. b.*

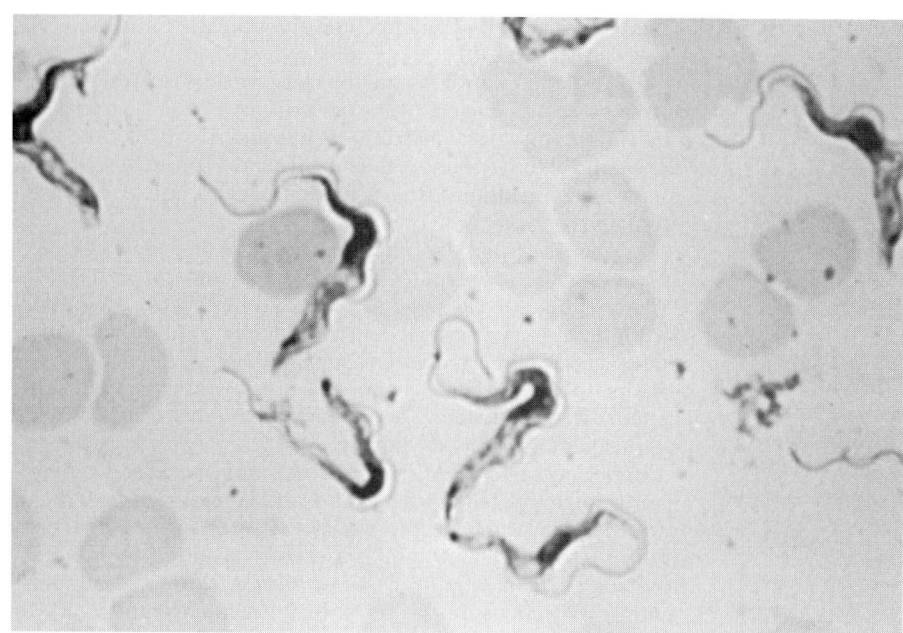

Figure 281.1. Bloodstream trypomastigotes (slender forms) in the peripheral blood of a patient with Gambian sleeping sickness. Note the free flagellum extending from the anterior end and the dotlike, posteriorly situated kinetoplast (approximately 1,200X). (From the teaching collection of the Department of Tropical Public Health, Harvard School of Public Health, Boston, MA, with permission.)

rhodesiense. With systemic dissemination of parasites, patients experience headache, myalgia, malaise, and episodes of fever that recur with each wave of parasitemia. Lymphadenopathy, most notably of posterior cervical nodes (Winterbottom sign), is a more prominent feature of West African trypanosomiasis. Splenomegaly and transient edema of the face and extremities are common, and a diffuse, macular rash or a circinate erythematous rash may be observed in whites.

Anemia, monocytosis, and markedly elevated levels of IgM in the serum are characteristic of both forms of the disease. In East African infections, the signs and symptoms of systemic disease appear within a week or two of inoculation, and the course is often complicated by congestive heart failure or arrhythmias related to myocarditis, by secondary infection, or less commonly, disseminated intravascular coagulation (13). Death caused by *T. b. rhodesiense* occurs within weeks to months, frequently before the CNS is invaded. In contrast, the symptoms of the dis-

seminated phase of Gambian trypanosomiasis are often mild or absent, and the infection may not be recognized for several years until CNS invasion occurs.

The CNS becomes involved within a few months of inoculation in East African disease and after months to several years in West African disease. CNS disease usually progresses gradually over several weeks to months, although occasionally coma and death can occur within a few days. Characteristic symptoms and signs include a persistent headache; inability to concentrate; personality changes; seizures; motor disturbances including tremors, choreoathetosis, and ataxia; and finally coma. Daytime somnolence (sleeping sickness) is due to disruption of normal circadian alternation of sleeping and waking rather than to hypersomnia (14). The cerebrospinal fluid (CSF) is under increased pressure and has elevated protein and IgM concentrations and a predominantly lymphocytic pleocytosis and an occasional morula cell of Mott (plasma cell that contains

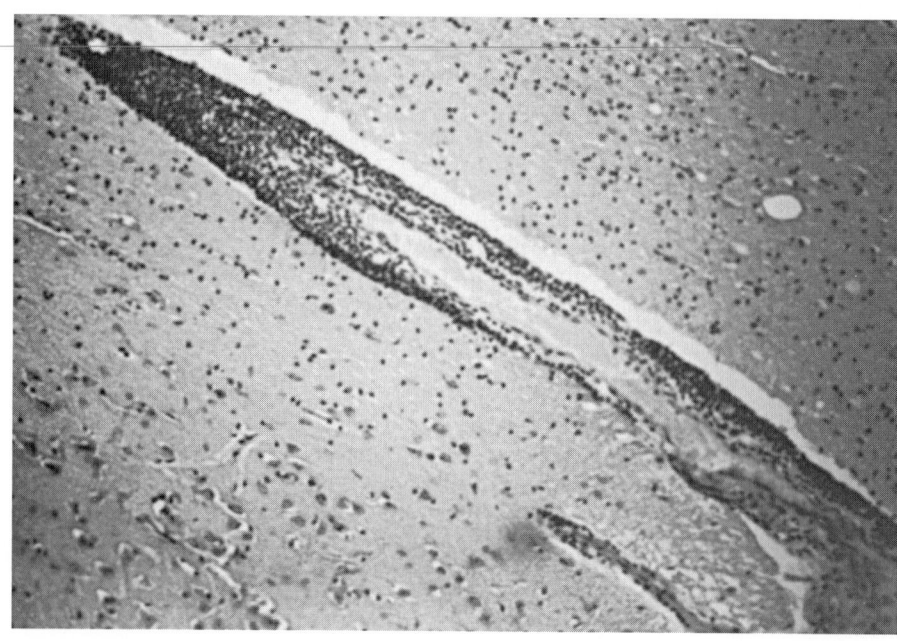

Figure 281.2. Section of human brain from a fatal case of Gambian sleeping sickness. An infiltrate of lymphocytes and plasma cells forms a cuff around the blood vessel. Parasites are rarely seen in tissue sections (approximately 200X). (From the teaching collection of the Department of Tropical Public Health, Harvard School of Public Health; and courtesy of Dr. S. C. Pan, Harvard School of Public Health, Boston, MA, with permission.)

aggregates of immunoglobulin). In time, patients lapse into coma and die with malnutrition and secondary infection or in status epilepticus.

Human immunodeficiency virus (HIV) infection, which is highly prevalent in many parts of sub-Saharan Africa, does not appear to have a major impact on the incidence or severity of African trypanosomiasis (16). HIV-infected persons infected with *T. b. gambiense*, however, may be at higher risk of relapse after treatment with eflornithine, and those infected with *T. b. rhodesiense* may have an unfavorable outcome while receiving melarsoprol (16,17).

Diagnosis

The diagnosis of African trypanosomiasis cannot be made solely on clinical grounds. Early disease may be confused with malaria, Epstein-Barr virus or cytomegalovirus infection, tuberculosis, or lymphoma; late-stage disease mimics psychiatric illness or meningoencephalitis of another infectious cause.

Definitive diagnosis of African trypanosomiasis requires microscopic identification of trypanosomes in the blood, CSF, or fluid aspirated from a chancre or a lymph node (17). Motile trypanosomes can be seen in fresh preparations, and the morphologic characteristics can be further studied in Giemsa- or Wright-stained smears. In the early stage of disease, *T. b. gambiense* is more readily detected in lymph node aspirates and *T. b. rhodesiense* in blood. The sensitivity of parasitologic diagnosis is increased by examining thick blood films, buffy coat preparations from centrifuged microhematocrit tubes, or eluates of blood fractionated on diethylaminoethyl cellulose anion-exchange columns. With all of these techniques, repeated examinations may be necessary because of fluctuating levels of parasitemia. Parasites can be isolated by inoculation of body fluids or tissue into culture media or, in the case of Rhodesian but not Gambian trypanosomiasis, laboratory rodents.

Serologic tests to detect specific antibodies to *T. b. gambiense* have been developed but require parasitologic tests to confirm the diagnosis (17). A card agglutination test for West African trypanosomiasis is widely used for screening rural populations because it is easily performed under field conditions (18). Antigen detection tests and polymerase chain reaction-based assays are under evaluation (19).

In all cases of African trypanosomiasis, the CSF should be examined for evidence of CNS involvement, even if neurologic examination findings are normal. Identification of parasites, increased numbers of mononuclear cells, or an increased protein level indicates CNS invasion.

Treatment

Specific treatment of African trypanosomiasis is most effective in reducing mortality and preventing permanent neurologic damage if administered early in the course of infection, before involvement of the CNS (1,7,11,20). The choice of antitrypanosomal drugs depends on the stage and the geographic origin of infection. Because the drugs are toxic and several different treatment regimens have been proposed, expert advice should be sought before therapy is administered. In the United States, such assistance, as well as several of the antitrypanosomal drugs listed in Table 281.1, can be obtained from the Parasitic Disease Drug Service, Centers for Disease Control and Prevention in Atlanta.

Pentamidine is generally used to treat early stage *T. b. gambiense* infection. Pentamidine causes sterile abscesses when injected intramuscularly, but it can be given safely by slow intravenous infusion over 2 hours. Persons who receive pentamidine

TABLE 281.1. Therapeutic Dosages for Treatment of African and American Trypanosomiasis

Disease and drug	Dose
African trypanosomiasis	
Pentamidine isethionate	Base: 4 mg/kg/d IM or IV × 10 doses
Suramin[a]	0.1 mg(test dose) IV on day 1; followed by 1 gm (or 20 mg/kg/d for children) on days 1, 3, 7, 14, 21
Melarsoprol[a]	3.6 mg/kg IV on days 1, 2, 3, 10, 11, 12, 20, 21, 22
Eflornithine	Adults: 100 mg/kg IV q 6 h × 2 wk
	Children: 150 mg/kg IV q 6 h × 2 wk
American trypanosomiasis	
Nifurtimox[a]	Adults: 8–10 mg/kg/d in four doses PO × 90 d
	Youths 11–16 y: 12.5–15 mg/kg/d in four doses PO × 90 d
	Children <11 y: 15–20 mg/kg/d in four doses PO × 90 d
Benznidazole	5 mg/kg/d PO × 60 d

[a]Available in the United States from the Parasitic Disease Drug Service, Centers for Disease Control and Prevention, Atlanta, Georgia.
IM, Intramuscularly; IV, intravenously; PO, orally.

should be monitored closely for hypotension, hypoglycemia, bone marrow toxicity, and hepatotoxicity. Suramin (Bayer 205) is the drug of choice for early-stage *T. b. rhodesiense* infection. Therapy with suramin should begin with a small test dose to check for idiopathic hypersensitivity reactions to the drug or anaphylactoid reactions related to the action of the drug on *Onchocerca volvulus*, a filarial parasite endemic to parts of Africa. Renal insufficiency, fever, arthralgia, rash, and neuropathy may complicate suramin therapy.

Because neither pentamidine nor suramin crosses the blood-brain barrier, the trivalent arsenical derivative melarsoprol (mel B) is used for late-stage infection due to both species. Before beginning melarsoprol treatment, two doses of pentamidine or a test dose and one full dose of suramin are administered first to clear the bloodstream of trypanosomes. Melarsoprol may cause exfoliative dermatitis, diarrhea, or peripheral neuropathy. Its most serious adverse effect, however, is an encephalopathy in 2% to 10% of persons with a mortality of 10% to 70% (12,20,21). The mechanism of this reactive arsenical encephalopathy is unknown. In West African disease, administration of corticosteroids reduces the incidence by a factor of three, but its effectiveness in preventing encephalopathy in persons with East African disease is not known (7,12,20). In preliminary studies of persons with late-stage *T. b. gambiense* disease, a simplified regimen of melarsoprol (2.2 mg/kg/d for 10 days) based on pharmacokinetic data was as efficacious as the traditional complicated regimen (see Table 281.1); it is not recommended for *T. b. rhodesiense* infections (22).

Rates of failure with melarsoprol have become alarmingly common in several areas where *T. b. gambiense* is endemic (7,22). Eflornithine (difluoromethylornithine), which has excellent CNS penetration and low toxicity, is the treatment of choice for patients with late-stage West African trypanosomiasis who relapse after melarsoprol (21). Side effects include mild and reversible bone marrow depression, diarrhea, and seizures. The high cost of eflornithine and its requirement for multiple intravenous, and issues of availability have restricted its use to infections that are refractory to melarsoprol. Nifurtimox, an oral drug used for treating Chagas disease, when given alone or in combination with other drugs, may prove beneficial in the treatment of relapsed West African trypanosomiasis (7,22). The only effective treatment for late-stage *T. b. rhodesiense* disease is repeat administration of melarsoprol.

All persons treated for African trypanosomiasis should be followed up for a minimum of 2 years for evidence of relapse. The CSF should be examined at the end of treatment and 3, 6, 12, 18, and 24 months later for signs of CNS involvement.

Prevention

The only sure means of preventing infection is by avoiding areas infested by tsetse flies. Tsetse flies are attracted to bright and contrasting colors and can bite through light clothing. Use of repellents, although only partially protective, and wearing heavy, light-colored trousers and long-sleeved shirts reduce the risk of tsetse bites. Pentamidine is no longer recommended as a prophylactic drug because the dose used is not curative, may mask infection until CNS invasion occurs, and promotes the emergence of drug-resistant strains of the parasite.

Strategies for controlling sleeping sickness in West and Central Africa involve systematic surveillance of populations at risk and early detection and treatment of infected persons to reduce the human reservoir of disease (2,5,23). In these regions and in East Africa, vector control efforts are directed at reducing contact between humans and flies by using simple, inexpensive, and nonpolluting technologies such as tsetse traps and screens.

TRYPANOSOMA CRUZI

Trypanosoma cruzi, the protozoan that causes American trypanosomiasis or Chagas disease, is found only in the Americas, where it is transmitted by triatomine bugs to more than 100 different species of wild and domestic animals as well as to human beings (24–26). In contrast to the African trypanosomes, the infective metacyclic trypomastigote stage of *T. cruzi* is discharged in the feces of the infected insect vector during or shortly after it takes a blood meal. Metacyclic trypomastigotes enter through the bite wound or mucous membranes and invade host cells. Within the cell, the parasite loses its flagellum and transforms into a round amastigote 3 to 4 μm in diameter (Fig. 281.3), which replicates by binary fission. After amastigotes have about filled the host cell, they transform into flagellated, motile trypomastig-

otes, which are released into the interstitial spaces and the blood stream on host cell lysis. Trypomastigotes invade other host cells and continue the intracellular multiplication cycle. Trypomastigotes of *T. cruzi* are distinguished from those of African trypanosomiasis by their inability to multiply, their larger kinetoplast (see Figs 281.1 and 281.3), and their C- or S-shaped appearance in blood smears.

Triatomine bugs acquire infection by ingesting blood taken from an infected mammalian host. In the bug's midgut, trypomastigotes transform into epimastigotes, which replicate by binary fission and assume the infective metacyclic stage in the hindgut approximately 2 weeks later.

Infection with *T. cruzi* persists for the life of the host. Escape from phagocytic vacuoles within the host cell, avoidance of antibody-mediated lysis by extracellular trypomastigotes, and other, not completely understood mechanisms allow the parasite to evade the host's immune defenses (3,27). There is no evidence that *T. cruzi* organisms have the kind of surface antigenic variation that occurs in African trypanosomiasis.

Epidemiology

Triatomine bugs, also called reduviid, kissing, or assassin bugs, and sylvatic mammals infected with *T. cruzi* are found throughout warmer regions of the Americas, including southern portions of the United States (24–26). Within this area, an estimated 16 to 18 million persons are infected, and an additional 100 million are at risk of infection. The geographic distribution of human infection and disease is focal: the greatest numbers of infected persons live in Brazil, Bolivia, Argentina, Chile, and Venezuela. Chagas disease is enzootic in the Caribbean. Trinidad and Tobago has reported a small number of human cases. Vector control programs have markedly reduced the incidence of new cases in several countries in South America (3).

The distribution of human infection is affected by the range and habits of the insect vector and by the degree of contact between humans and the vector. Rates of infection are highest in tropical areas where highly domesticated vectors such as *Triatoma infestans*, *Rhodnius prolixus*, and *Panstrongylus megistus* are found. The bugs hide in cracks in the walls and in the thatch of roofs during the day and emerge at night to take their blood meal from sleeping residents. Insect-mediated transmission occurs principally in the impoverished mud-stick houses of rural

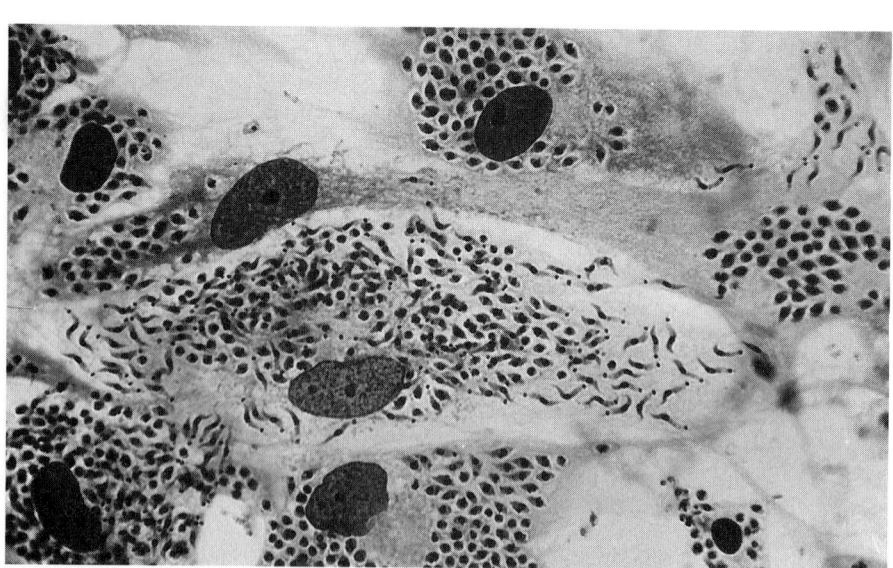

Figure 281.3. Infection of fibroblasts in tissue culture with *Trypanosoma cruzi*. The fibroblast in the center contains elongated trypomastigotes with a prominent posterior kinetoplast. The other fibroblasts contain predominantly round or oval-shaped amastigotes that are in the process of transforming into trypomastigotes (approximately 1,000X).

areas or the slums surrounding large cities to which rural families have migrated. In the United States, only a few autochthonous cases of human infection have been reported (28). The potential for transmission is low in the United States because the vector bugs prefer sylvatic habitats and do not infest houses. It is estimated, however, as many as 100,000 chronically infected immigrants from Latin America are living in the United States (29).

Transmission of *T. cruzi* via blood products from chronically infected donors may lead to infection in as many as 10% to 20% of recipients of a single unit of blood. Serologic screening of donors has dramatically reduced the incidence of transfusion-induced infection in many large Latin American cities with large numbers of immigrants from rural areas (30,31). However, in some endemic areas, reliable serologic screening of blood is not uniformly available, and transfusion-associated Chagas disease is a frequent and serious problem. Transmission of infection from a chronically infected donor of a solid organ or bone marrow transplant has been well documented in Latin America. In the United States, there have been only a few cases of documented transfusion- and transplantation-induced Chagas disease, but the actual number of episodes may be considerably higher because of the large numbers of immigrants from endemic areas of Latin America (32–34). Uniform screening of donors for *T. cruzi* infection is currently under consideration in the United States.

T. cruzi can also be transmitted across the placenta, a phenomenon that occurs in approximately 2% to 5% of pregnancies of chronically infected women (35). Other, less frequent, routes of transmission include ingestion of food contaminated with *T. cruzi* and accidents among laboratory personnel who work with live parasites (26,36).

Pathogenesis

Infection with *T. cruzi* has an initial acute stage that lasts for several weeks and a chronic phase that persists for the life of the host (26). After replicating at the site of entry, large numbers of parasites disseminate via the circulation and infect all types of nucleated cells but preferentially muscle cells, macrophages, and neurons and supporting cells of the central and peripheral nervous systems. Rupture of parasitized cells provokes an intense mononuclear cell inflammatory response and in severe cases causes acute myocarditis, destruction of autonomic ganglia in the heart and gastrointestinal tract, and meningoencephalitis. With development of humoral and cell-mediated immunity, the parasitemia falls to a subpatent level, and the number of parasites in the tissues declines dramatically, which signals an end to the acute phase (37).

Despite the appearance of the immune response, persons remain infected for life with both circulating and intracellular parasites. The majority of chronically infected individuals remain asymptomatic, and tissue damage is limited to small foci of inflammation and scars in various tissues and some loss of autonomic ganglia (37,38). Approximately 10% to 30% of chronically infected persons sustain progressive damage to the heart or gastrointestinal tract that is sufficient to produce clinical disease. Why chronic disease develops in some but not other infected persons is not understood.

In chronic Chagas heart disease, there is a slowly progressive myocarditis that leads to flaccid dilatation of all four chambers and, in some cases, an apical aneurysm. On histologic examination, the heart has widespread destruction of myocardial cells, diffuse fibrosis, edema, and mononuclear cell infiltration of the myocardium, and scarring of the conduction system with fibrous and adipose tissues (37): the pathogenesis of chronic Chagas' disease is largely believed to be due to the persistence of parasites in tissues as demonstrated by in-situ hybridization and other techniques and the resultant inflammatory reaction (26). A less-widely held hypothesis is that the etiology of chronic lesions is an autoimmune process (39). Abnormalities in the coronary microvasculature and focal hypoperfusion may contribute to the myocardial damage (40).

Chronic Chagas gastrointestinal disease is caused by destruction of autonomic ganglia (38). Impaired motility and emptying of the esophagus and the colon lead to hypertrophy and dilatation of these organs, the so-called megasyndromes.

Clinical Manifestations

The acute stage of *T. cruzi* infection is usually asymptomatic or may present as an influenza-like illness (26). Symptoms appear 1 to 2 weeks after exposure to infected triatomine bugs or as long as several months after transfusion of infected blood. There may be a characteristic unilateral edema of the eyelids (Romaña sign) or an indurated erythematous lesion of the skin (chagoma) at the site of inoculation. Acute infection may be accompanied by fever, malaise, generalized lymphadenopathy, and hepatosplenomegaly that last 4 to 8 weeks. The peripheral blood shows increased numbers of lymphocytes, atypical lymphocytes, and trypomastigotes, and parasites can be isolated from the CSF with ease (41). Severe acute myocarditis or meningoencephalitis that is occasionally fatal develops in up to 10% of patients with acute Chagas disease, most commonly young children. Acute transfusion- or transplantation-induced infection may be fulminant and produce life-threatening involvement of the heart and CNS, especially in immunocompromised patients (29–34).

Survivors of the acute stage of infection, whether apparent or inapparent, enter an asymptomatic chronic "indeterminate" stage. The indeterminate stage may last for life, but about 10% to 30% of patients develop chronic myocarditis or gastrointestinal tract disease after several years or decades. An early sign of chronic Chagas myocarditis is an abnormal electrocardiogram with right bundle branch block, which may be present years before symptoms appear (42,43). Symptoms of heart disease appear most frequently in early adulthood or middle age. The most common presentation is biventricular congestive heart failure that is often complicated by systemic and pulmonary thromboembolism (Fig. 281.4). Some patients complain of anginal or atypical chest pain even though coronary angiography shows no lesions (44). Complete atrioventricular block or ventricular arrhythmias may cause syncopal episodes or sudden cardiac death, even in persons with no previous cardiac symptoms. Less than one third of patients with symptomatic chronic Chagas heart disease survive longer than 2 years.

Denervation of the esophagus in Chagas disease leads to a clinical syndrome resembling idiopathic achalasia of the esophagus (Fig. 281.5A) (45). Failure of the lower esophageal sphincter to relax and disordered peristalsis cause dysphagia, regurgitation, recurrent episodes of aspiration pneumonia, and eventually permanent dilatation of the esophagus (megaesophagus). Chagas megacolon resembles Hirschsprung disease of the colon and is characterized by prolonged periods of obstipation and occasionally intestinal obstruction or volvulus. Barium contrast radiographs readily demonstrate megaesophagus, megacolon, and the associated motor disorders (Fig. 281.5B).

Chagas gastrointestinal disease is common south of the Amazon basin but seldom occurs in northern South America or Central America, perhaps because of infection with different strains of *T. cruzi* (46).

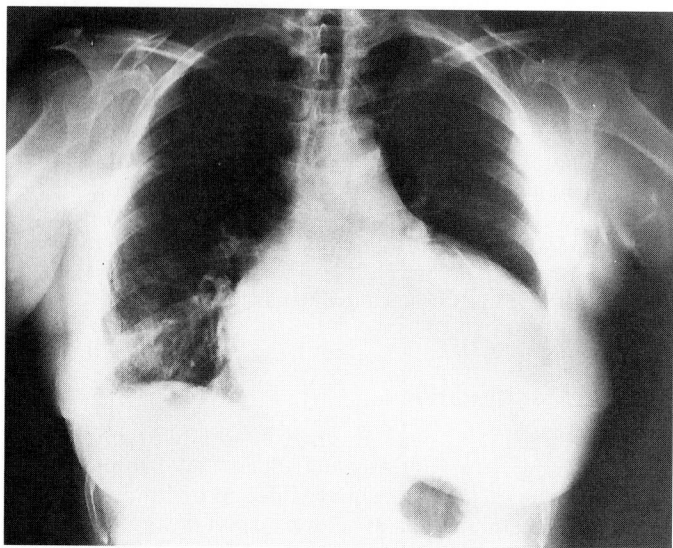

Figure 281.4. Chest radiograph from a 46-year-old woman with chronic Chagas cardiomyopathy. Global enlargement of the heart and clear lung fields are seen.

Persons with acquired immunodeficiency syndrome or persons receiving immunosuppressive therapy may experience an exacerbation of chronic infection (32,34,47). Fever, myocarditis, and skin lesions are common among recipients of cardiac allografts, whereas patients with acquired immunodeficiency syn-

drome frequently have lesions of the CNS that resemble the lesions of cerebral toxoplasmosis or lymphoma by computed tomography or magnetic resonance imaging. Parasites are occasionally seen in blood smears and are readily detected in biopsy specimens of heart, skin, or brain.

Congenital infection with *T. cruzi* leads to abortion or stillbirth, asymptomatic infection, or an acute disease that is apparent at birth or develops within weeks after delivery (35,48). Symptomatic congenital Chagas disease of the newborn is characterized by fever, jaundice, anemia, thrombocytopenia, hepatosplenomegaly, and skin lesions that contain parasites. Death may result from encephalitis, myocarditis, or pneumonitis. Severe disease has been reported in children infected with both *T. cruzi* and human immunodeficiency syndrome at birth (49).

Diagnosis

The diagnosis of acute Chagas disease and congenital Chagas disease is established by detection of trypomastigotes in the peripheral blood (26,50). Wet mounts of whole blood, buffy coat, cord blood or centrifuged serum should be examined microscopically for motile parasites, and smears should be stained with Giemsa or Wright stain. When parasites are not identified by direct observation during the acute stage, they can be isolated by cultivation of blood on Novy-MacNeal-Nicolle, LIT, or another special medium, by animal inoculation, or by xenodiagnosis (allowing laboratory-reared, uninfected triatomine bugs to feed on the patient or the patient's blood and examining them for the presence of trypanosomes 3 to 4 weeks later).

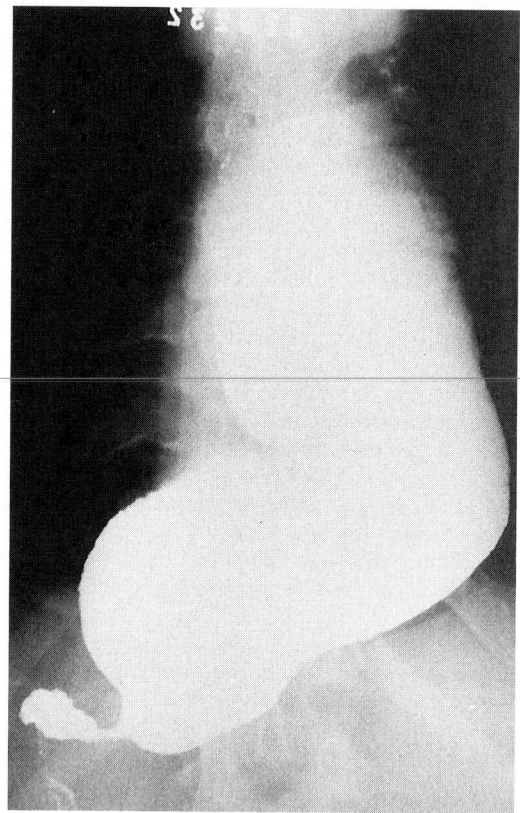

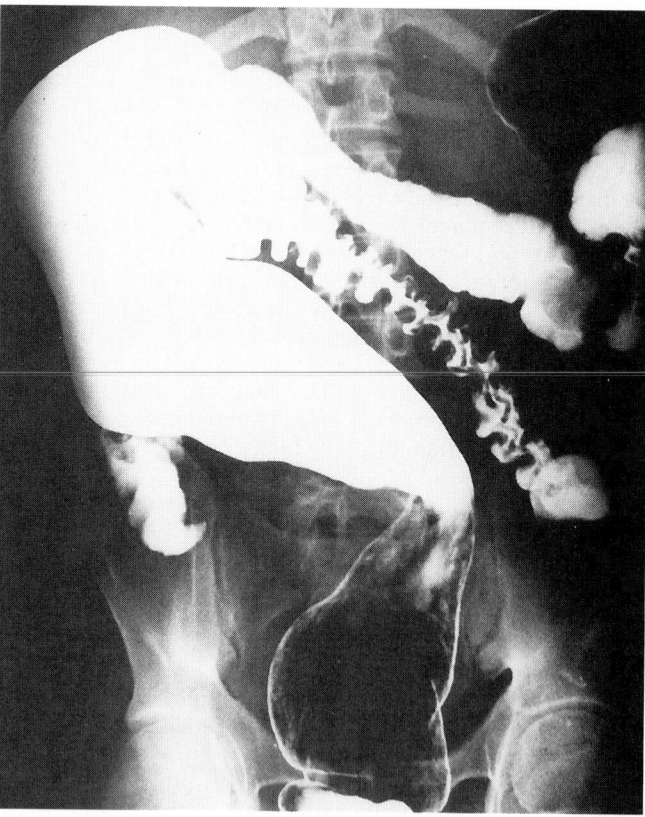

Figure 281.5. A: Radiograph from a patient with Chagas megaesophagus (with barium contrast). Marked dilatation and folding of the esophagus and retention of barium are seen. **B:** Radiograph from a patient with Chagas megacolon (with barium contrast). Marked dilatation of the descending colon and part of the transverse colon and retention of feces are present despite attempts to clear the bowel before the procedure.

Detection of parasites by culture, animal inoculation, or xenodiagnosis does not distinguish acute from chronic infection. In cases with negative smears, recently acquired infection can be demonstrated by the presence of specific IgM antibodies by the enzyme-linked immunosorbent assay or indirect fluorescent antibody test or by observing a fourfold rise of specific immunoglobulin G titers.

Because the parasitemia is subpatent during the chronic stage, the diagnosis usually relies on serologic tests for immunoglobulin G antibody to *T. cruzi*. Indirect fluorescent antibody, enzyme-linked immunosorbent assay, and indirect hemagglutination antibody tests using intact parasites or crude lysates of *T. cruzi* as antigens may attain sensitivities in excess of 98% but are less specific because of cross reactions that occur in persons with mucocutaneous or visceral leishmaniasis or infection with the nonpathogenic *T. rangeli*. Testing with two different assays is recommended for making the diagnosis of chronic Chagas disease (26). Use of purified glycoprotein antigens or recombinant antigens avoids false-positive reactions (51). It is seldom necessary, for clinical purposes, to confirm a serologic diagnosis of chronic *T. cruzi* infection by culture or xenodiagnosis. Assays based on the polymerase chain reaction are more sensitive for detecting parasitemia in the chronic stage of infection than is xenodiagnosis or culture (52).

Treatment

Antitrypanosomal therapy traditionally was indicated only for acute and congenital Chagas disease and for infections in immunocompromised persons (53). The Pan American Health Organization, however, now recommends treatment for all chronically infected persons (26). Because the data on which this recommendation are based on studies of school children, some authorities suggest that treatment be given routinely to chronically infected children under the age of 12 years, but the decision to treat older persons be left to the discretion of the patient and the physician (53,54). Both nifurtimox (Lampit) and benznidazole (Rochagan, see Table 281.1) clear the parasitemia, reduce the severity and duration of the acute illness, and may eradicate the infection in the majority of cases. In several studies, treatment resulted in cure in up to 60% of chronically infected children younger than 12 years of age as documented by conversion of culture, xenodiagnosis and serological tests to negative. Cure of infection should be regarded as certain only when serologic tests, xenodiagnosis, culture, and polymerase chain reaction-based assays fail to demonstrate parasites for several years. There is some evidence that treatment may prevent the complications of chronic Chagas disease (54,55).

The long course of treatment with either nifurtimox or benznidazole (see Table 281.1) requires meticulous monitoring because of the high incidence of adverse effects. Nifurtimox causes severe anorexia and weight loss, and both drugs may cause neuropathy, psychotic reactions, rashes, and gastrointestinal upset.

Treatment of patients with chronic asymptomatic infection entails close clinical observation for complications. Persons in whom symptomatic heart disease develops may require treatment with diuretics, vasodilators, antiarrhythmic agents, pacemakers, or, in selected cases, cardiac transplantation. Both megaesophagus and megacolon can be effectively treated by surgery.

Prevention

No vaccine or chemoprophylactic agent prevents *T. cruzi* infection. Travelers should avoid sleeping in houses or outdoor areas that may be infested with triatomine bugs. Transfusion-induced Chagas disease can be prevented by careful serologic screening of blood donors or by treating donor blood with gentian violet for at least 24 hours before transfusion. Efforts to prevent transmission of *T. cruzi* by triatomine vectors in endemic areas focus on application of insecticides in houses by sprays, fumigant canisters, and impregnated paints; and improvement of housing to discourage colonization by triatomine bugs; and by education and community-based surveillance for reinfestation of houses (26,56). Vector control and screening of blood donors have reduced the incidence of new cases to nearly zero in Chile and Uruguay and much of Argentina, Brazil, and Venezuela. The "Southern Cone" initiative is nearing its goal of eradicating the vector *T. infestans* from an area that accounts for more than two thirds of persons infected with *T. cruzi*, and programs in the Andean and Central American countries are showing great progress (56).

REFERENCES

1. World Health Organization. Control and surveillance of African trypanosomiasis. Report of a WHO Expert Committee. *WHO Tech Rep Ser* 1998;881:1.
2. Vickerman K. Antigenic variation in trypanosomes. *Nature* 1978;273:613.
3. Zambrano-Villa S, Rosales-Borjas D, Carrero JC, Ortiz-Ortiz L. How protozoan parasites evade the immune response. *Trends Parasitol* 2002;18:272.
4. Pepin J, Meda HA. The epidemiology and control of human African trypanosomiasis. *Adv Parasitol* 2001;49:71.
5. African trypanosomiasis or sleeping sickness. Fact sheet no. 259. Geneva: World Health Organization, 2002. Available at *http://www.who.int/inf-fs/en/fact 259.html*. Accessed April 30, 2002.
6. Receveur MC, Le Bras M, Vincendeau P. Laboratory-acquired Gambian trypanosomiasis. *N Engl J Med* 1993;329:209.
7. Moore AC, Ryan ET, Waldron MA. Case records of the Massachusetts General Hospital. Weekly clinicopathological exercises. Case 20-2002. A 37-year-old man with fever, hepatosplenomegaly, and a cutaneous foot lesion after a trip to Africa. *N Engl J Med* 2002;346:2069.
8. Sinha A, Grace C, Alston WK, Westenfeld F, Maguire JH. African trypanosomiasis in two U.S. travelers. *Clin Infect Dis* 1999;29:840.
9. Greenwood BM, Whittle HC. The pathogenesis of sleeping sickness. *Trans R Soc Trop Med Hyg* 1980;74:716.
10. Pentreath VW. Royal Society of Tropical Medicine and Hygiene Meeting at Manson House, London, 19 May 1994. Trypanosomiasis and the nervous system. Pathology and immunology. *Trans R Soc Trop Med Hyg* 1995;89:9.
11. Stitch A, Abel PM, Sanjeev K. Clinical review. Human African trypanosomiasis. *BMJ* 2002;325:201.
12. Haller L, Adams H, Merouze F, et al. Clinical and pathological aspects of human African trypanosomiasis (*T. b. gambiense*) with particular reference to reactive arsenical encephalopathy. *Am J Trop Med Hyg* 1986;35:94.
13. Gear JHS, Miller GB. The clinical manifestations of Rhodesian trypanosomiasis: an account of cases contracted in the Okavango swamps of Botswana. *Am J Trop Med Hyg* 1986;35:1146.
14. Buguet A, Bert J, Tapie P, et al. Sleep-wake cycle in human African trypanosomiasis. *J Clin Neurophysiol* 1993;10:190.
15. Pepin J, Ethier L, Kazadi C, et al. The impact of human immunodeficiency virus infection on the epidemiology and treatment of *Trypanosoma brucei gambiense* sleeping sickness in Nioki, Zaire. *Am J Trop Med Hyg* 1992;47:133.
16. Blum J, Nkunku S, Burri C. Clinical description of encephalopathic syndromes and risk factors for their occurrence and outcome during melarsoprol treatment of human African trypanosomiasis. *Trop Med Int Health* 2001;6:390.
17. Van Meirvenne N. Diagnosis of human African trypanosomiasis. *Ann Soc Belg Med Trop* 1992;72[Suppl 1]:53.
18. Noireau F, Lemesre JL, Nzoukoudi MY, et al. Serodiagnosis of sleeping sickness in the Republic of Congo: comparison of indirect immunofluorescent antibody test and card agglutination test. *Trans R Soc Trop Med Hyg* 1988;82:237.
19. Nantulya VM, Doua F, Molisho S. Diagnosis of human trypanosomiasis, due to *Trypanosoma brucei gambiense* in Central Africa, by the polymerase chain reaction.sleeping sickness using an antigen detection enzyme-linked immunosorbent assay. *Trans R Soc Trop Med Hyg* 2000;94:392.
20. Pepin J, Milord F. The treatment of human African trypanosomiasis. *Adv Parasitol* 1994;33:1.
21. Milord F, Pepin J, Loko L, et al. Efficacy and toxicity of eflornithine for treatment of *Trypanosoma brucei gambiense* sleeping sickness. *Lancet* 1992;340:652.
22. Legros D, Ollivier G, Gastellu-Etchegorry M, et al. Treatment of human African trypanosomiasis—present situation and needs for research and development. *Lancet Infect Dis* 2002;2:437.

23. Rogers DJ, Hendricks G, Slingenbergh JH. Tsetse flies and their control. *Rev Sci Tech* 1994;13:1075.
24. Brener Z, Andrade Z, Barral-Neto M, eds. *Trypanosoma cruzi e Doença de Chagas*, 2nd ed. Rio de Janeiro: Guanabara Koogan, 2000.
25. Marsden PD. The transmission of *Trypanosoma cruzi* to man and its control. In: Croll NA, Cross JH, eds. *Human ecology and infectious disease.* New York: Academic Press, 1983:253–289.
26. World Health Organization. Control of Chagas disease. Second Report of the WHO Expert Committee. *WHO Tech Rep Ser* 2002;905:1.
27. Reed SG. Immunology of *Trypanosoma cruzi* infections. *Chem Immunol* 1998; 70:124.
28. Herwaldt B, Grijalva MJ, Newsome AL, et al. Use of the polymerase chain reaction to diagnose the fifth reported US case of autochthonous transmission of *Trypanosoma cruzi*, in Tennessee, 1998. *J Infect Dis* 2000;181:395.
29. Leiby DA, Herron RM Jr, Read EJ, Lenes BA. *Trypanosoma cruzi* in Los Angeles and Miami blood donors: impact of evolving donor demographics on seroprevalence and implications for transfusion transmission. *Transfusion* 2002;42:549.
30. Schmuniz GA, Zicker F, Cruz JR, Cuchi P. Safety of blood supply for infectious diseases in Latin American countries, 1994–1997. *Am J Trop Med Hyg* 2001;65:924.
31. Schmunis GA. *Trypanosoma cruzi*, the etiologic agent of Chagas' disease: status in the blood supply in endemic and nonendemic countries. *Transfusion* 1991;31:547.
32. Bocchi EA, Bellotti G, Uip D et al. Long-term follow-up after heart transplantation in Chagas' disease. *Transplant Proc* 1993;25:1329.
33. Cimo PL, Luper WE, Scouros MA. Transfusion-associated Chagas' disease in Texas: report of a case. *Tex Med* 1993;89:48.
34. CDC. Chagas disease after organ transplantation—United States, 2001. *MMWR* 2002;51:210.
35. Bittencourt AL. Congenital Chagas' disease, a review. *Am J Dis Child* 1976;130:99.
36. Herwaldt BL. Laboratory-acquired parasitic infections from accidental exposures. *Clin Microbiol Rev* 2001;14:659, 2001.
37. Andrade ZA: Mechanisms of myocardial damage in *Trypanosoma cruzi* infection. *Ciba Found Symp* 1983;99:214.
38. Koberle F. Chagas' disease and Chagas' syndromes: the pathology of American trypanosomiasis. *Adv Parasitol* 1968;6:63.
39. Engman DM, Leon JS. Pathogenesis of Chagas heart disease: role of autoimmunity. *Acta Trop* 2002;81:123.
40. Torres FW, Acquatella H, Condado JA, et al. Coronary vascular reactivity is abnormal in patients with Chagas' heart disease. *Am Heart J* 1995;129:995.
41. Hoff R, Teixeira RS, Carvalho JS, et al. *Trypanosoma cruzi* in the cerebrospinal fluid during the acute stage of Chagas' disease. *N Engl J Med* 1978;298:604.
42. Laranja FS, Dias E, Nobrega G, et al. Chagas' disease: clinical, epidemiologic, and pathologic study. *Circulation* 1956;14:1035.
43. Maguire JH, Hoff R, Sherlock 1, et al. Cardiac morbidity and mortality due to Chagas' disease: prospective electrocardiographic study of a Brazilian community. *Circulation* 1987;75:1140.
44. Hagar JM, Rahimtoola SH. Chagas' heart disease in the United States. *N Engl J Med* 1991;325:763.
45. Tanowitz HB, Simon D, Gumprecht JP, et al. Gastrointestinal manifestations of Chagas' disease. In: Rustgi VK, ed. *Gastrointestinal infections in the tropics.* Basel: S Karger, 1990:56–75.
46. Miles MA, Povoa MM, Prata A, et al. Do radically dissimilar *Trypanosoma cruzi* strains (zymodemes) cause Venezuelan and Brazilian forms of Chagas' disease? *Lancet* 1981;1:1338.
47. Rocha A, de Meneses AC, da Silva AM, et al. Pathology of patients with Chagas' disease and acquired immunodeficiency syndrome. *Am J Trop Med Hyg* 1994;50:261.
48. Freilij H, Altcheh J. Congenital Chagas' disease: diagnostic and clinical aspects. *Clin Infect Dis* 1995;21:551.
49. Freilij H, Altcheh J, Muchinik G. Perinatal human immunodeficiency virus infection and congenital Chagas' disease. *Pediatr Infect Dis J* 1995;14:161.
50. Frasch ACC, Reyes MB, Sánchez DO. Diagnosis of Chagas' disease: present and future. In: *Chagas' disease and the nervous system.* Washington, DC: Pan American Health Organization, 1994:47–53.
51. da Silveira JF, Umezawa ES, Luquetti AO. Chagas disease: recombinant *Trypanosoma cruzi* antigens for serological diagnosis. *Trends Parasitol* 2001;17:286.
52. Britto C, Cardoso MA, Vanni CM, et al. Polymerase chain reaction detection of *Trypanosoma cruzi* in human blood samples as a tool for diagnosis and treatment evaluation. *Parasitology* 1995;110:241.
53. de Castro SL. The challenge of Chagas' disease chemotherapy: an update of drugs assayed against *Trypanosoma cruzi*. *Acta Trop* 1993;53:83.
54. de Andrade AL, Zicker F, de Oliveira RM, et al. Randomized trial of benznidazole in treatment of early *Trypanosoma cruzi* infection. *Lancet* 1996;348:1407.
55. Viotti RC, Vigliano C, Armenti H, Segura E. Treatment of chronic Chagas' disease with benznidazole: clinical and serologic evolution of patients with long-term follow-up. *Am Heart J* 1994;127:151.
56. Schofield CJ, Dias JCP. The southern cone initiative against Chagas disease. *Adv Parasitol* 1999;42:1.

CHAPTER 282
Toxoplasma gondii

Craig Roberts and Rima McLeod

TAXONOMY

Toxoplasma gondii is in the phylum Apicomplexa and the class Sporozoea. Isolates of *T. gondii* have been called strains (e.g., the RH strain or the ME49 strain). There are three main patterns of virulence of *T. gondii* tachyzoites for mice, measured as differences in survival. Restriction fragment length polymorphism patterns and isoenzyme zymodemes are characteristic for each of these three phenotypes of virulence (I, similar to the RH strain of *T. gondii*; II, similar to the ME49 strain of *T. gondii*; and III, similar to the C56 strain of *T. gondii*). Virulence varies (i.e., differences in lethality and for cyst numbers produced in mice); isolates proliferate at different rates in tissue culture and produce different neurologic manifestations (i.e., variable destruction and inflammatory responses) (1,2). The RH strain, the most commonly used laboratory strain, does not undergo gametogenesis in cat intestine and proliferates rapidly.

LIFE CYCLE

T. gondii is an obligate intracellular protozoan parasite that can infect a wide variety of birds and mammals (see Chapter 173). It can enter all host cells. There appears to be a special propensity for cyst formation and recrudescence with tissue destruction in the central nervous system.

In the acute infection, the tachyzoite (formerly called trophozoite and sometimes endozoite) proliferates within cells in many tissues. In persons who have a competent immune system, cyst formation begins about 8 days after infection, and cysts persist for the remainder of the host"s life. The cysts form in many tissues but especially in muscle and brain. The wall of these cysts is derived partly from the host cell. The cysts contain hundreds of the slowly replicating form of the parasite, bradyzoites, which are more resistant than tachyzoites to acid and pepsin. If tissues that contain cysts are ingested by a carnivore, bradyzoites are released from the cyst in the intestine and again disseminate from the intestine to cause acute, and then chronic, infection. Cats, which develop acute infection with tachyzoites and then form cysts as described before for all other hosts, are also the definitive host for the sexual phase of the life cycle (3). After a cat ingests cysts, bradyzoites invade their intestinal cells. After several stages of schizogony, they yield male and female gametes, which fuse and form a zygote. The zygote synthesizes a protective wall and is excreted by the cat as a single-celled, unsporulated oocyst. At 37°C, the excreted oocyst sporulates, dividing three times, which yields eight infectious sporozoites that are still contained within the oocyst wall. The oocyst can remain viable for more than a year in warm, moist soil. When oocysts are ingested by a mammal or bird, sporozoites are released and again infect intestinal epithelial cells, becoming tachyzoites and finally, again, encysted bradyzoites.

STAGE CONVERSION

T. gondii exists as two actively dividing stages, the tachyzoite and the bradyzoite, in intermediate hosts, including humans

Tachyzoite

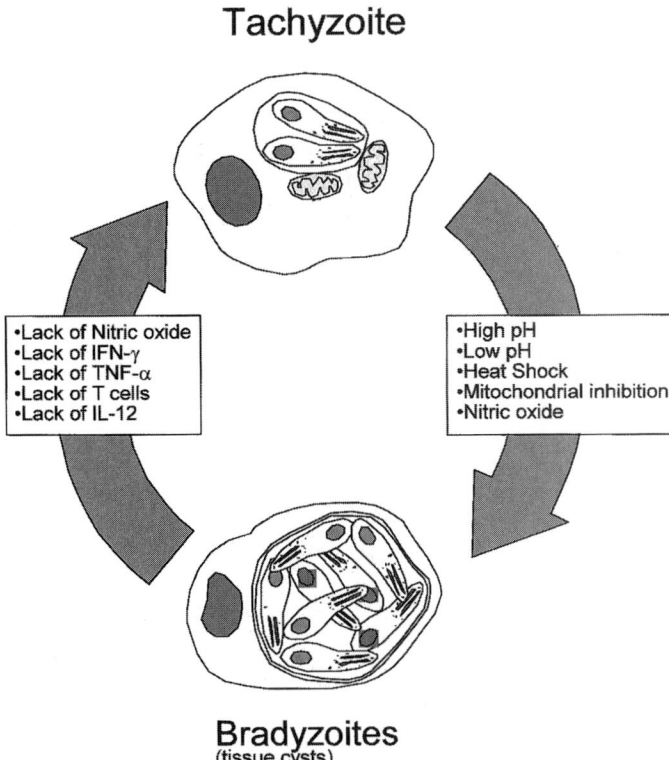

Figure 282.1. Stage conversion between *T. gondii* tachyzoites and brady-zoites. The tachyzoite is the fast dividing form of the parasite that invades host cells and multiplies rapidly within a parasitophorous vacuole surrounded by host cell mitochondria. Tachyzoites can be induced to transform into slowly dividing bradyzoites in vitro by a variety of stresses including altered pH, heat shock, mitochondrial inhibition or exposure to nitric oxide. Bradyzoites can transform into tachyzoites in vivo in the absence of immune factors such as nitric oxide, IFN-γ, TNF-α, IL-12 or T cells. The stimuli that induce the sexual cycle in the intestine of cats remain to be determined.

(see Fig. 282.1). While the process of tachyzoite to bradyzoite conversion facilitates the establishment of a chronic infection, the reverse process is responsible for disease reactivation. *In vitro* studies have demonstrated that tachyzoite conversion to bradyzoite is induced by stress: pH or heat shock, nitric oxide, sodium arsenite, which induces oxidative stress, antimycin A, oligomycin and other inhibitors of mitochondrial function induce bradyzoite formation. It has been hypothesized that elevation of cyclic adenosine monophosphate (cAMP) may be a common factor induced by stress as addition of cAMP or cyclic guanosine monophosphate (cGMP) to tachyzoites can result in stage switch. Relevant stresses that may induce stage switch in *in vivo* include nitric oxide (an inhibitor of mitochondrial function), fever (causing heat shock), and phagosome acidification causing a lowering of pH (4–14).

Impairment of immune function (15–29) allows bradyzoite to tachyzoite conversion *in vitro*, and results in uncontrollable tachyzoite multiplication *in vivo*. For example, in murine models, tumor necrosis factor-α (TNF-α) and interferon-γ (IFN-γ) and T cells are required to prevent disease reactivation. Impaired immune function during acquired immunodeficiency syndrome is responsible for disease reactivation in humans. The cause of persistent reactivation of disease in congenitally infected individuals has not been established definitely.

MORPHOLOGY AND COMPOSITION

Tachyzoites (see Chapter 173, Fig. 173.1A to C) and bradyzoites (see Fig. 173.1D to F) are crescentic and measure approximately 6 × 2 m. Tachyzoites have a nucleus, mitochondria, Golgi apparatus, and endoplasmic reticulum (Fig. 282. 2; see also Fig. 173.1A to C). They have three unit membranes that compose their pellicle (see Fig. 173.1A). Their outer membrane is continuous; their two inner membranes are discontinuous, are closely apposed, and end at internal structures (located at either end of the tachyzoite) called polar rings. These inner membranes have holes called micropores. Under the pellicle, extending from the anterior polar ring almost the length of the tachyzoite, are 22 microtubules (the cytoskeleton). A hollow, truncated cone of fibers, probably microtubules, wound in a spiral (the conoid) is present at the anterior end of the parasite and protrudes as tachyzoites enter host cells. Rhoptries (club-shaped, dense, osmophilic structures with narrow ends that terminate in the conoid), micronemes (osmophilic vesicles between the few rhoptries) (30–33), and a plastid (a multilamellar structure that contains unique extranuclear deoxyribonucleic acid (DNA), related to chloroplasts) (34–40) are characteristic of *Apicomplexa*, and the first two organelles may be important during entry into host cells (19). Electron-dense granules contain proteins that are secreted (41–52). SAG1 is a unique tachyzoite antigen, part of a family of surface antigens (53,54). Temperature-sensitive and drug-resistant mutant tachyzoites have been produced.

Bradyzoites (see Fig. 173.1D to F) are resistant to pepsin, become an oocyst in the week after they are ingested by cats, have unique antigens not present in tachyzoites, have electron-dense rhoptries, and have unique cytoplasmic granules (perhaps stored carbohydrates). Cysts contain bradyzoites (a few to 10,000). The cyst wall is argyrophilic and stains weakly with periodic acid-Schiff stain. Bradyzoites stain well with the periodic acid-Schiff stain. High or low pH, nitric oxide, and other "stresses" lead to tachyzoite to bradyzoite interconversion. A 5-hydroxynaphthoquinone–resistant mutant organism expresses bradyzoite antigens.

Oocysts (see Fig. 173.1H) form after five stages of schizogony (detectable by light microscopy). By the third stage, gametes are either male (microgamete with increased DNA content, a flagellum, and cytoplasm with a nucleus and a mitochondrion) or more abundant female (macrogamete, large, spherical cell with two types of peripheral cytoplasmic granules). These granules contribute to the outer and inner layers of the rigid, impervious oocyst wall. Sporulation, which requires aeration for 1 to 3 days at room temperature, produces eight sporozoites (in two sporocysts) in an oocyst wall. Sporozoites and the inside of the oocyst wall have stage-specific antigens. Drug-resistant mutants incapable of forming oocysts have been identified.

Deoxyribonucleic Acid

The sporozoite contains approximately 0.1 pg of DNA and approximately 8×10^7 base pairs per cell (haploid DNA content) (34). Mitochondrial DNA is approximately 3% of the total DNA. The plastid also contains DNA (36,39). Nucleotide sequences encoding many proteins are known, and complementary DNA and genomic libraries have been produced (9,10,25,30,31,37,38,42–45,48,55–68). Some of the *T. gondii* genes identified have introns. Information about translation as well as transcription has been reviewed (49). An EST project examining complementary DNAs from tachyzoite and bradyzoite complementary DNA libraries

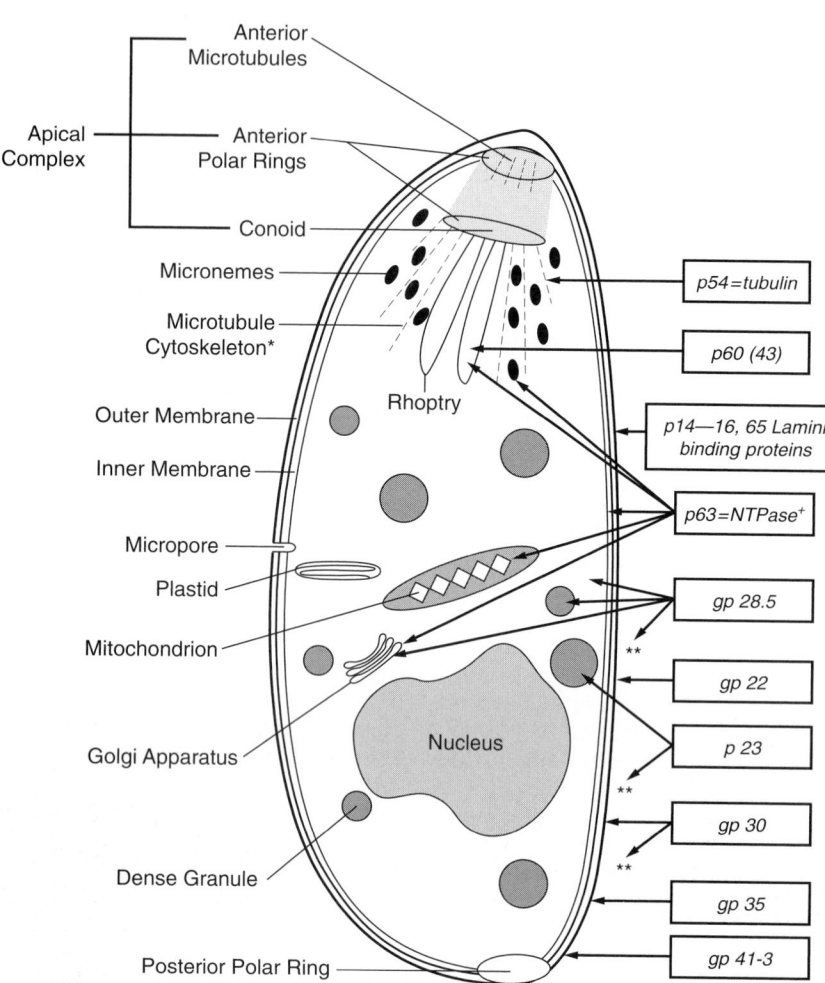

Figure 282.2. Diagrammatic representation of *Toxoplasma gondii* tachyzoite. Representative proteins and glycoproteins are indicated by a square outline that encloses them. Their locations are indicated by arrowheads. NTPase, Nucleoside triphosphate hydrolases. *The cytoskeleton of *T. gondii* is composed of 22 microtubules; these actually extend posteriorly but are indicated schematically in this figure only at the anterior end. **Parasitophorous vacuole. †Locations of adenosine triphosphatase activity, not necessarily the cloned 63-kDa protein. (Redrawn from McLeod R, Mack D, Brown C: *Toxoplasma gondii:* new advances in cellular and molecular biology. *Exp Parasitol* 1991;72:109–121, with permission.)

greatly facilitate understanding of the biology of this parasite. It is estimated that by the end of 2002 the full *T. gondii* DNA sequence will be known.

Ribonucleic Acid

T. gondii ribosomal ribonucleic acid (RNA) has a typical large and small molecule. Its messenger RNA has a 3'-polyadenylated tail. This has been translated in heterologous systems producing *T. gondii* proteins. *T. gondii* has an RNase P that cleaves transfer RNA.

Antigens

The tachyzoite contains many proteins. Many of the antigens and proteins of *T. gondii* have now been named. They are designated with three letters and a number, according to the life cycle stage from which they were isolated, their location within the organism, or their function. The surface antigens of tachyzoites are designated SAG; proteins found within the micronemes, MIC; those in the rhoptries, ROP; and those in the dense granules, GRA. Antigens found in the bradyzoite stage, but not in the tachyzoite stage, are designated BAG (11,51); those secreted by bradyzoites to form the cyst matrix are called MAG. Some of these, their localization, and characteristics of the genes that encode them are shown in Figure 282.2.

SURFACE AND CYST ANTIGENS

A number of antigens have been identified on the surface of tachyzoites and bradyzoites. Two major families have been identified either related to the SAG1 or SAG2 proteins originally identified on the tachyzoite form (54,65). SAG1 and SAG3 have been shown to be important during the invasion process. Thus antibodies to SAG1 reduce but do not completely prevent invasion and parasites lacking this molecule are able to invade host cells. It is likely that the other members of the SAG1 family including SAG3, BSR4 the SRS1-4 proteins, SAG5, SAG5.1 and SAG5.2 also play a role during invasion. SAG3 is common to tachyzoites and bradyzoites while SAG1 and SRS1-3 are present only on tachyzoites and BSR4 is present only on bradyzoites. Four members of the SAG2 family of proteins designated SAG2A and SAG2B-D. SAG2A and B are expressed in tachyzoites, whereas SAG2C and SAG2D are expressed in bradyzoites. SAG4 and SAG4.2 are expressed by bradyzoites and not tachyzoites.

A glycoprotein, CST1 and a cyst matrix molecule designated MAG1 have been identified on the cyst wall which is formed around the bradyzoites.

APICAL ORGANELLE ANTIGENS

A number of proteins have been identified and localized to the micronemes, rhoptries, or dense granules of *T. gondii*. Many of the MIC proteins described have been found to have adhesive properties. For example, MIC2 is secreted early in the invasion process, becomes associated with the apical end of the parasite and binds host cell heparin sulfate proteoglycans. As ROP proteins are released early in invasion they have been implicated in the process of invasion and forming the structure of the parasitophorous vacuole. ROP1 has been noted to enhance parasite invasion and has been called 'penetration enhancing factor.' ROP2 becomes inserted into the parasitophorous vacuole where its cytoplasmic exposed portion appears to hold host cell mitochondria in close proximity. Dense granules release their contents from 10 minutes following invasion. GRA1-8 are specifically targeted to either or both the parsitophorous vacuole or the parasitophorous vacuole network (25,45–47). The functions of these proteins have not been determined, but an additional two dense granule proteins, NTPase I and NTPase II, are secreted into the parasitophorous vacuole where they are involved in purine salvage (41–44).

HEAT SHOCK PROTEINS

T. gondii is known to possess three heat shock proteins HSP70, HSP60, and HSP30 (BAG1) (11,51). HSP30 is expressed by bradyzoites and not tachyzoites, has homology with the small heat shock proteins of plants, and is induced when tachyzoites are stressed *in vitro* to become bradyzoites. HSP60 has two differentially spliced forms which and have been localized to different locations within tachyzoites and bradyzoites. HSP70 normally is expressed by both tachyzoites and bradyzoites but is expressed at high levels during stage conversion in either direction.

INVASION OF HOST CELLS BY TACHYZOITES AND REPLICATION

Attachment of the parasite to the host cell and orientation so that the conoid, positioned at the anterior of the parasite, is in contact with the host cell is prerequisite to invasion. A number of parasite surface molecules including those of the SAG1 family and SAG3 are involved in these processes. When the tachyzoite first makes contact with the host cell, the micronemes release their contents including a number of proteins involved in attachment. The conoid of the parasite protrudes and forms an indentation in the host cell, coinciding with the release of the rhoptries that contain a number of proteins and lipids. A tight junction is formed between the host cell and parasite that moves posteriorly as the parasite enters the cell. The parasitophorous vacuole that contains the parasite is composed of host cell membrane minus a number of proteins that are actively excluded during the process of invasion and rhoptry-derived material (69). The process of invasion is dependent on the parasite cytoskeleton and requires the interaction of actin and myosin (60). Following invasion, the dense granules release their contents which modify the parasitophorous vacuole to support the intracellular survival of the parasite. Host cell mitochondria become closely associated with the cytoplasmic face of the parasitophorous vacuole. The parasitophorous vacuole is resistant to acidification and lysosome fusion (69).

T. gondii organisms then multiply by a type of binary fission called endodyogeny within the parasitophorous vacuole. During division, the nuclear membrane of *T. gondii* remains intact and chromosomes do not condense at metaphase (in contrast to mitosis in higher eukaryotes). Without appreciably disrupting the host cell's function, the tachyzoite divides until the vacuolar membrane and host cell lyse, releasing many tachyzoites. Mutant parasites, mutant host cells, and inhibitors of cellular processes have been used to study biochemical interactions between *T. gondii* and host cells. *T. gondii* needs host cell purines to replicate. The hypoxanthine-guanine phosphoribosyltransferase of *T. gondii* can provide sufficient purine salvage. None of the following host cell processes is needed for replication: synthesis of nucleic acids, proteins, oxidative phosphorylation, and adenosine triphosphate synthesis by mitochondria. The biologic role of host cell lipid synthesis is not known.

METABOLISM

T. gondii tachyzoites have functional mitochondria and an aerobic metabolism, although it has been suggested that bradyzoites may rely more heavily on anaerobic metabolism as they have higher levels of lactate dehydrogenase (LDH) (9,10) and pyruvate kinase activity than tachyzoites. Recent work has demonstrated that *T. gondii* has tachyzoite and bradyzoite specific isoforms of many enzymes including many of those involved in glycolysis (LDH [9,10], enolase [6], and glucose 6 phosphate isomerase). These observations, combined with the presence of amylopectin granules in bradyzoite but not tachyzoite stages, point towards differences in carbohydrate metabolism between life cycle stages. *T. gondii* can not use preformed folates, and thus its dihydrofolate reductase (DHFR) has been targeted by pyrimethamine as an antimicrobial agent (63,70). *T. gondii* has recently been shown to have a shikimate pathway which is sensitive to glyphosate (37). Additional plant-like biochemical pathways have been described which may yield new antimicrobial agents (35–38,40). These include a type-II fatty acid biosynthesis pathway (35,36,38) and isoprenoid biosynthesis (40).

PROPAGATION AND ISOLATION

Isolation of the organism is discussed in Chapter 173. Tachyzoites and bradyzoites can be isolated by use of animal inoculation or tissue culture. Tachyzoites can be maintained in culture, and addition of interferon-γ to the media or change in pH or nitric oxide concentration leads to cyst formation *in vitro*. Velocity and equilibrium sucrose gradient centrifugation is used to purify unsporulated oocysts. The oocyst stage has not been propagated *in vitro*.

IMMUNE RESPONSES TO *TOXOPLASMA GONDII*

Murine models have been instrumental in our understanding of the immune response to *T. gondii* (15–17, 21–27). Severe combined immune deficient (SCID) mice that lack T and B lymphocytes have demonstrated the crucial role for cells of the innate immune system in providing protection in the early stages of infection. Current evidence suggests that IL-12, a product of dendritic cells, neutrophils and macrophages in combination with IL-1, TNF-α, IL-15 and IL-18, stimulate natural killer (NK) cell production of IFN-γ. Following exposure to *T. gondii* lysate, the ability of both murine and human NK cells to kill tumor cells is augmented. NK cell produced IFN-γ is responsible for activation of macrophages which kills intracellular parasites. In murine systems the predominant killing mechanism is through the toxic effects of reactive nitrogen intermediates (RNI). In contrast, this mechanism, although still operative in certain human macrophage populations is likely to be less important where induction of tryptophan degrading enzymes play an important role.

The innate immune response is not only important in early protection against this parasite, but also has an instrumental role in directing the developing adaptive immune response. Thus IL-12 and IL-18 preferentially expand T-helper 1 (Th1) cells rather that T-helper 2 (Th2) cells. Th1 cells further contribute to the ongoing immune response by production of IFN-γ. Th1 cells also provide IL-2 and IL-12, which facilitate the development and expansion of cytotoxic T cells which are capable of lysing *T. gondii*–infected cells. While the major population of cytotoxic T cells in mice is CD8+, both CD4+ and CD8+ cytotoxic T cells have been identified in infected humans. In keeping with these observations, susceptibility to toxoplasmic encephalitis in mice has been precisely mapped and shown to be dependent on MHC class I genes (the products of which interact with CD8+ T cells). MHC Class II genes also play a role in pathogenesis and protection against *T. gondii* in mice. Susceptibility to human disease has been shown to be influenced by MHC class II genes (the products of which interact with CD4+ T cells).

Th2 cell products, such as IL-4 and IL-10, have generally been associated with disease progression due to their ability to counteract the effects of IFN-γ and TNF-α on macrophages. However, recent murine studies have demonstrated that under certain circumstances, these cytokines play an important role in preventing excessive inflammation.

Antibodies have been shown to interfere with the ability of *T. gondii* to invade host cells, and opsonized parasites are killed following complement activation or uptake by macrophages and phagosome acidification. Secretory IgA specific for *T. gondii* is secreted in the intestine and milk of infected mothers. The largely intracellular location of *T. gondii* makes the role for antibodies in protection less important than cell-mediated immunity.

RELATED ORGANISMS

An encysted organism (*Neospora caninum*) that appears similar to *T. gondii* in preparations examined with light microscopy (with electron-dense rhoptries) has been described in tissues from a number of animals, such as dogs and cats, but not in humans. Serologic evidence for infection has been obtained although clinical significance is not known. This organism is serologically distinct from *T. gondii*, however, and no association with disease in humans has been recognized. Other related apicomplexan infections such as malaria, babesiosis, and cryptosporidiosis are discussed in Chapters 279 and 284.

ANTIMICROBIAL SUSCEPTIBILITY TESTING

Studies *in vitro* and *in vivo* (in mice) have demonstrated inhibition of replication of *T. gondii* tachyzoites by pyrimethamine, sulfadiazine (70) (and sulfamerazine and sulfamethazine), and spiramycin. Pyrimethamine and these sulfonamides act synergistically (37,70). Studies *in vitro* (with longer incubation times) and *in vivo* have demonstrated efficacy for clindamycin. The relevance of these data to antimicrobial levels needed for treatment of toxoplasmosis in humans remains to be determined.

SURFACE DECONTAMINATION

Tachyzoites are easily destroyed by desiccation, heat, and pepsin. Cysts are destroyed by cooling below $-20°C$ and heating above $60°C$. Bradyzoites are resistant to pepsin. The oocyst wall is not disrupted by 0.5% ammonium sulfate, sodium hydroxide, or sodium hypochlorite. Disinfection of a cat litter box can be accomplished by burning feces or flushing them in the toilet and then soaking the tray in boiling water for 5 minutes or strong (7%) ammonia for 3 hours. Disposal by drying, surface burial, freezing, chlorine bleach, dilute ammonia, quaternary ammonium compounds, or any general disinfectant cannot be relied on to destroy oocysts.

REFERENCES

1. Grigg ME, Bonnefoy S, Hehl AB, Suzuki Y, Boothroyd JC. Success and virulence in *Toxoplasma* as the result of sexual re-combination between two distinct ancestries. *Science* 2001;294:161.
2. Darde ML, Bouteille B, Pestre-Alexandre M. Isoenzymic characterization of seven strains of *Toxoplasma gondii* by isoelectrofocusing in polyacrylamide gels. *Am J Trop Med Hyg* 1988;39:551.
3. Dubey JP, Swan GV, Frenkel JK. A simplified method for isolation of *Toxoplasma gondii* from the feces of cats. *J Parasitol* 1972;58:1005.
4. Bohne W, Heesemann J, Gross U. Reduced replication of *Toxoplasma gondii* is necessary for induction of bradyzoite-specific antigens—A possible role for nitric oxide in triggering stage conversion. *Infect Immun* 1994;62:1761.
5. Bohne W, Gross U, Ferguson DJ, Heesemann J. Cloning and characterization of a bradyzoite-specifically expressed gene (hsp30/bag1) of *Toxoplasma gondii*, related to genes encoding small heatshock proteins of plants. *Mol Microbiol* 1995;16:1221.
6. Dzierszinski F, et al. Differential expression of two plant-like enolases with distinct enzymatic and antigenic properties during stage conversion of the protozoan parasite *Toxoplasma gondii*. *J Mol Biol* 2001;309:1017.
7. Dzierszinski F, et al. The protozoan parasite *Toxoplasma gondii* expresses two functional plant-like glycolytic enzymes. Implications for evolutionary origin of apicomplexans. *J Biol Chem* 1999;274:24888.
8. Knoll LJ, Boothroyd JC. Isolation of developmentally regulated genes from *Toxoplasma gondii* by a gene trap with the positive and negative selectable marker hypoxanthine-xanthine-guanine phosphoribosyltransferase. *Mol Cell Biol* 1998;18:807–814.
9. Parmley S, Weiss LM, Yang S. Cloning of a bradyzoite-specific gene of *Toxoplasma gondii* encoding a cytoplasmic antigen. *Mol Biochem Parasitol* 1995;73:253.
10. Parmley S, Yang S, Harth G, et al. Molecular characterization of a 65-kilodalton *Toxoplasma gondii* antigen expressed abundantly in the matrix of tissue cysts. *Mol Biochem Parasitol* 1994;66:283.
11. Weiss L, LaPlace D. Development of bradyzoites of *Toxoplasma gondii* in vitro. *J Eukaryot Microbiol* 1994;41:185.
12. Weiss LM, et al. Bradyzoite development in *Toxoplasma gondii* and the hsp70 stress response. *Infect Immun* 1998;66:3295–3302.
13. Yang S, Parmley SF. A bradyzoite stage-specifically expressed gene of *Toxoplasma gondii* encodes a polypeptide homologous to lactate dehydrogenase. *Mol Biochem Parasitol* 1995;73:291.
14. Yang S, Parmley SF. *Toxoplasma gondii* expresses two distinct lactate dehydrogenase homologous genes during its life cycle in intermediate hosts. *Gene* 1997;184:1–12.
15. Brown CR, McLeod R. Class I MHC genes and CD8+ T cells determine cyst number in *Toxoplasma gondii* infection. *J Immunol* 1990;145:3438.
16. Denkers EY, Gazzinelli RT. Regulation and function of T-cell mediated immunity during *Toxoplasma gondii* infection. *Clin Microbiol Rev* 1998;11:569.
17. Gazzinelli RT, Wysocka M, Hayashi S, et al. Parasite-induced IL-12 stimulates early INF-gamma synthesis and resistance during acute infection with *Toxoplasma gondii*. *J Immunol* 1994;153:2533.
18. Herion P, Hernandez-Pando R, Dubremez J-F, Saavedra R. Subcellular localization of the 54-kDa antigen of *Toxoplasma gondii*. *J Parasitol* 1993;79:216.
19. Joiner KA, Dubremez JF. *Toxoplasma gondii*: a protozoan for the nineties. *Infect Immun* 1993;61:1169.
20. Kasper LH, Crabb JH, Pfefferkorn ER. Isolation and characterization of a monoclonal antibody-resistant antigenic mutant of *Toxoplasma gondii*. *J Immunol* 1982;129:1694.
21. Liesenfield O, Kosek J, Remington JS, Suzuki Y. Association of CD4+ T cell–dependent interferon mediated necrosis of the small intestine with genetic susceptibility of mice to peroral infection with *Toxoplasma gondii*. *J Exp Med* 1996;184:597.
22. Luder CG, Gross U, Lopes MF. Intracellular protozoan parasites and apoptosis: diverse strategies to modulate parasite–host interactions. *Trends Parasitol* 2001;17:480.

23. Mack D, Johnson JJ, Roberts C, et al. HLA – Class II genes modify outcome of *Toxoplasma gondii* infection. *Int Parasitol* 1999;29:1351.
24. Mennechet FJD, Kasper LH, Rachiner N, Li W, Vandewalle A, Buzoni-Gatel D. Lamina propria CD4+T lymphocytes synergize with marine intestinal epithelial cells to enhance pro-inflammatory response against an intracellular pathogen. *J Immunol* 2002;168:2988.
25. Mevelec M-N, Chardes T, Mercereau-Puljalon O, et al. Molecular cloning of GRA4, a *Toxoplasma gondii* dense granule protein, recognized by mucosal IgA antibodies. *Mol Biochem Parasitol* 1992;56:227.
26. Mordue PG, Monroy F, La Regina M, Dinarello CA, Sibley LD. Acute toxoplasmosis leads to lethal overproduction of Th 1 cytokines. *J Immunol* 2001; 167:4574.
27. Sharma SD. Immunology of *Toxoplasma gondii* infection. In: Wyler D, ed. *Modern parasite biology: cellular, immunological, and molecular aspects.* New York: WH Freeman, 1990:184–199.
28. Sharma SD, Araujo FG, Remington JS. *Toxoplasma* antigen isolated by affinity chromatography with monoclonal antibody protects mice against lethal infection with *Toxoplasma gondii. J Immunol* 1984;133:2818.
29. Sibley LD, Adams LD, Fukutomi Y, Krahenbuhl JL. Tumor necrosis factor triggers antitoxoplasmal activity of IFN-γ primed macrophages. *J Immunol* 1991;147:2340.
30. Beckers CJM, Dubremetz J-F, Mercereau-Puijalon O, Joiner KA. The *Toxoplasma gondi* rhoptry protein ROP2 is inserted into the parasitophorous vacuole membrane, surrounding the intracellular parasite, and is exposed to the host cell cytoplasm. *J Cell Biol* 1994;127:947.
31. Ajioka J, Fitzpatrick JM, Reitter CP. *Toxoplasma gondii* genomics: shedding light on pathogenesis and chemotherapy. *Exp Rev Mol Med* 2001;1.
32. Ossorio PN, Schwartzman JD, Boothroyd JC. A *Toxoplasma gondii* rhoptry protein associated with host cell penetration has unusual charge asymmetry. *Mol Biochem Parasitol* 1992;50:1.
33. Pfefferkorn ER. Cellular biology of *Toxoplasma gondii*. In: Wyler D, ed. *Modern parasite biology: cellular, immunological, and molecular aspects.* New York: WH Freeman, 1990:26–50.
34. Wilson RJ, et al. Complete gene map of the plastid–like DNA of the malaria parasite *P. falciparum. J Mol Biol* 1996;261:155.
35. Zuther E, Johnson JJ, Haselhorn R, McLeod R, Gornicki P. Growth of *Toxoplasma gondii* is inhibited by aryloryphenoxy propronate herbicides targeting acetyl-CoA carboxylase. *PNAS* 1999;96:13387.
36. Waller RF, et al. Nuclear-encoded proteins target to the plastid in *T. gondii* and *P. falciparum. PNAS* 1998;95:12352.
37. Roberts F, Roberts C, Johnson JJ, et al. Evidence for the shikimate pathway in apicomplexan parasites. *Nature* 1998;393:801.
38. McLeod, R, Muench S, Rafferty J, et al. Triclosan inhibits the growth of *Plasmodium falciparum* and *Toxoplasma gondii* by inhibition of apicomplexa Fab I. *Int J Parasitol* 2001;31:109.
39. Kohler S, et al. A plastid of probable green algal origin in apicomplexa parasites. *Science* 1997;275:1485.
40. Jomaa H, Wiesner J, Sanderbrand S, Altincicek B, et al. Inhibitors of the non-mevalonate pathway of is aprenoid biosynthesis as antimalarial drugs. *Science* 1999;285:5433.
41. Johnson AM, Illana S, McDonald PJ, Asai T. Cloning, expression and nucleotide sequence of the gene fragment encoding an antigenic portion of the nucleoside triphosphate hydrolase of *Toxoplasma gondii. Gene* 1989;85:215.
42. Asai T, Miura S, Sibley D, et al. Biochemical and molecular characterization of nucleoside triphosphate hydrolase isozymes from the parasitic protozoan *Toxoplasma gondii. J Biol Chem* 1995;270:11391.
43. Bermudes D Dubremetz J-F, Achbarou A, Joiner KA. Cloning of a cDNA encoding the dense granule protein GRA3 from *Toxoplasma gondii. Mol Biochem Parasitol* 1994a;68:247.
44. Bermudes D, Peck KR, Afifi MA, et al. Tandemly repeated genes encode nucleoside triphosphate hydrolase isoforms secreted into the parasitophorous vacuole of *Toxoplasma gondii. J Biol Chem* 1994b;269:29252.
45. Cesbron-Delauw MF, Guy B, Torpier G, et al. Molecular characterization of a 23-kilodalton major antigen secreted by *Toxoplasma gondii. Proc Natl Acad Sci USA* 1989;86:7537.
46. Lecordier L, Mercier C, Torpier G, et al. Molecular structure of a *Toxoplasma gondii* dense granule antigen (GRA-5) associated with the parasitophorous vacuole membrane. *Mol Biochem Parasitol* 1993;59:143.
47. Lecordier L, Moleon-Borodowski I, Dubremetz J-F, et al. Characterization of a dense granule antigen of *Toxoplasma gondii* (GRA6) associated to the network of the parasitophorous vacuole. *Mol Biochem Parasitol* 1995;70:85.
48. Mercier C, Lecordier L, Darcy F, et al. Molecular characterization of a dense granule antigen (Gra2) associated with the network of the parasitophorous vacuole in *Toxoplasma gondii. Mol Biochem Parasitol* 1993;58:71.
49. McLeod R, Mack D, Brown C: *Toxoplasma gondii*—New advances in cellular and molecular biology. *Exp Parasitol* 1991;72:109.
50. Miller SA, et al. A conserved subtilisin-like protein TgSUB1 in microneme organelles of *Toxoplasma gondii. J Biol Chem* 2001;276:1.
51. Prince JB, Araujo F, Remington J, et al. Cloning of cDNAs encoding a 28 kilodalton antigen of *Toxoplasma gondii. Mol Biochem Parasitol* 1989;34:3.
52. Sibley LD, Sharma SD: Ultrastructural localization of an intracellular *Toxoplasma* protein that induces protection in mice. *Infect Immun* 1987;55:2137.
53. Burg JL, Perelman D, Kasper L, et al. Molecular analysis of the gene encoding the major surface antigen of *Toxoplasma gondii. J Immunol* 1988;141:3584.
54. Cesbron-Delauw M-F, Tomavo S, Beauchamp P, et al. Similarities between the primary structures of two distinct major surface proteins of *Toxoplasma gondii. J Biol Chem* 1994;269:16217.
55. Boothroyd JC, Burg JL, Nagel SD, et al. Antigen and tubulin genes of *Toxoplasma gondii*. In: Agabian N, Goodman H, Nogueira N, eds. *Molecular strategies of parasitic invasion.* New York: Alan R Liss, 1987:237–250.
56. Donald RGK, Roos DS. Stable molecular transformation of *Toxoplasma gondii*: a selectable dihydrofolate reductase-thymidylate synthase marker based on drug-resistance mutations in malaria. *Proc Natl Acad Sci USA* 1993;90:11703.
57. Fox BA, Bzik DJ. De novo pyrimidine biosynthesis is required for virulence of *Toxoplasma gondii. Nature* 2002;415:926.
58. Grover CM, Thulliez P, Remington JS, Boothroyd JC. Rapid prenatal diagnosis of congenital *Toxoplasma* infection by using polymerase chain reaction and amniotic fluid. *J Clin Microbiol* 1990;28:2297.
59. Kim K, Soldati D, Boothroyd JC. Gene replacement in *Toxoplasma gondii* with chloramphenicol acetyltransferase as selectable marker. *Science* 1993;262:911.
60. Schwartzman JD, Pfefferkorn ER. Immunofluorescent localization of myosin at the anterior pole of the coccidian *Toxoplasma gondii. J Protozool* 1983;30:657.
61. Vasanthakumar G, van Ginkel S, Parish G. Isolation and sequencing of a cDNA encoding the hypoxanthine-guanine phosphoribosyltransferase from *Toxoplasma gondii. Gene* 1994;147:153.
62. Ng HC, Singh M, Jeyaseelan K. Identification of two protein serine/threonine kinase genes and molecular cloning of a *SNF1* type protein kinase gene from *Toxoplasma gondii. Biochem Mol Biol Int* 1995;35:155.
63. Roos D. Primary structure of the dihydrofolate reductase-thymidylate synthase gene from *Toxoplasma gondii. J Biol Chem* 1993;268:6269.
64. Nagel SD, Boothroyd JC. The alpha- and beta-tubulins of *Toxoplasma gondii* are encoded by single copy genes containing multiple introns. *Mol Biochem Parasitol* 1988;29:261.
65. Manger ID, Hehl AB, Boothroyd JC. The surface of *Toxoplasma* tachyzoites is dominated by a family of glycosylphosphatidylinositol–anchored antigens related to SAG1. *Infect Immun* 1998;66:2237.
66. Burg JL, Grover M, Pouletty P, Boothroyd JC. Direct and sensitive detection of a pathogenic protozoan, *Toxoplasma gondii*, by polymerase chain reaction. *J Clin Microbiol* 1989;27:1787.
67. Deroin F, Thulliez P, Candolfi M, et al. Early prenatal diagnosis of congenital toxoplasmosis using amniotic fluid samples and tissue culture. *Eur J Clin Microbiol* 1988;7:423.
68. Sibley LD, Pfefferkorn ER, Boothroyd JC. Development of genetic systems for *Toxoplasma gondii. Parasitol Today* 1993;9:392.
69. Sibley LD, Weidner E, Krahenbuhl JL. Phagosome acidification blocked by intracellular *Toxoplasma gondii. Nature* 1985;315:416.
70. Mack D, McLeod R. A new micromethod to study effects of antimicrobial agents on *Toxoplasma gondii*: Comparison of sulfadoxine and sulfadiazine and study of clindamycin, metronidazole, and cyclosporine A. *Antimicrob Agents Chemother* 1984;26:26.

CHAPTER 283
Pneumocystis carinii*

Walter T. Hughes

Pneumocystis carinii is a unique microbe that is found almost exclusively in the lungs of immunocompromised mammalian hosts. It has not been found outside the animal reservoir, and the only known mode of transmission is from animal to animal by the respiratory route. Most humans are believed to have contracted asymptomatic infection with *P. carinii* in infancy and childhood and to maintain a latent, undetectable infection throughout life. If the host's immunity is compromised, life-threatening *P. carinii* pneumonitis may develop due to re-activation of latent organisms, acquisition of new organisms, or both.

MORPHOLOGY

Three structural forms of *P. carinii* are the cyst, sporozoite, and trophozoite. The cyst, the largest of the three forms, often

*Pneumocystis carinii has been reclassified as a fungus but is included in the section on parasites because the need for reassignment was appreciated too late in the book's production phase.

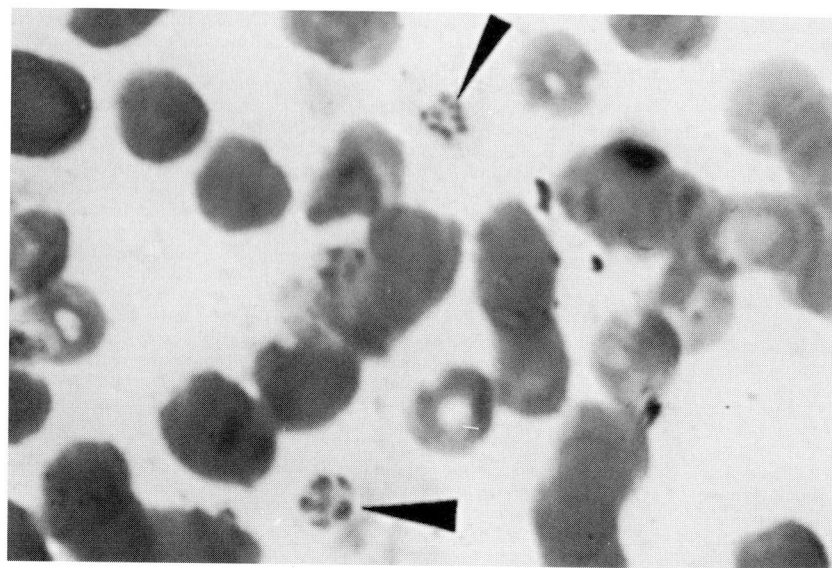

Figure 283.1. Imprint of lung biopsy specimen stained with Giemsa method. Clusters of *Pneumocystis carinii* sporozoites (*arrowheads*) are located within the cyst. The cyst wall does not stain, but an area of rarefaction is usually discernible.

measures 5 to 6 μm in diameter. The fully developed cyst has a thick cell wall, providing a sturdy round, oval, or cup-shaped structure while it is intact. The cyst wall is generally about 0.1 to 0.3 μm thick in most areas, but some sites may be twice that. The sporozoite is an intracystic cell about 1 to 2 μm in diameter. As many as eight sporozoites may be found in the intact cyst. These cells appear fragile and pleomorphic with punctate, eccentric nuclei. The trophozoite (2 to 5 or 6 μm in diameter) is believed to be the excysted sporozoite. The cell wall is thinner than that of the cyst.

The method used for staining preparations of *P. carinii* determines the visibility of the three forms. Polychrome stains such as Giemsa or Wright stain the trophozoites and sporozoites but not the cyst (Fig. 283.1). The Gomori-Grocott methenamine-silver nitrate and toluidine blue O stains color the cysts but do not permit visualization of the sporozoites and trophozoites (Fig. 283.2).

CLASSIFICATION

Early investigators such as Chagas, Carini, and the Delanoes considered the organism a protozoan without question. More recently, Yoneda and coworkers (1) supported the protozoan classification by demonstrating evidence of membrane fusion. Vossen and colleagues (2) also argued that the organism was a protozoan because of the presence of a microtubular system similar to that of the Sporozoa. Jackson and coworkers (3) were unable to detect characteristic fungal protein elongation factor-3 in *P. carinii*. *P. carinii* is susceptible to the antiprotozoan drugs pentamidine (*Trypanosoma, Leishmania* species), trimethoprim-sulfamethoxazole (*Isospora*), pyrimethamine-sulfonamide, atovaquone (Toxoplasma, *Plasmodium* species), and dapsone (*Plasmodium* species). Antifungal drugs in clinical use tested to date (amphotericin B, ketoconazole, fluconazole, itraconazole, gentian violet, nystatin) are ineffective.

Edman and colleagues found the ribosomal ribonucleic acid (RNA) sequences (4), thymidylate synthase (5), and dihydrofolate reductase (6) of *P. carinii* to be more similar to those of the ascomycetes than to those of protozoa. Liu and coworkers (7) compared 26S ribosomal RNA genes in *P. carinii, Saccharomyces cerevisiae*, and *Trypanosoma pyriformis* and found greater resemblance to the yeast than to the protozoan. Analysis of amino acid sequences of β-tubulin showed close matches with certain fungi (8). The cyst form of *P. carinii* has chitin in the cell wall, in common with the fungi (9). Pixley and coworkers (10) concluded that the mitochondrial DNA of *P. carinii* is more like that of fungi than of protozoa. Eriksson (11) reviewed available taxonomic features of *P. carinii* and proposed placement in a new family, Pneumocystidaceae, and a new order, Pneumocystidales (Ascomycota). A major problem in taxonomy is the lack of specific and detailed definitions for protozoa and fungi, in order to properly place *P. carinii*.

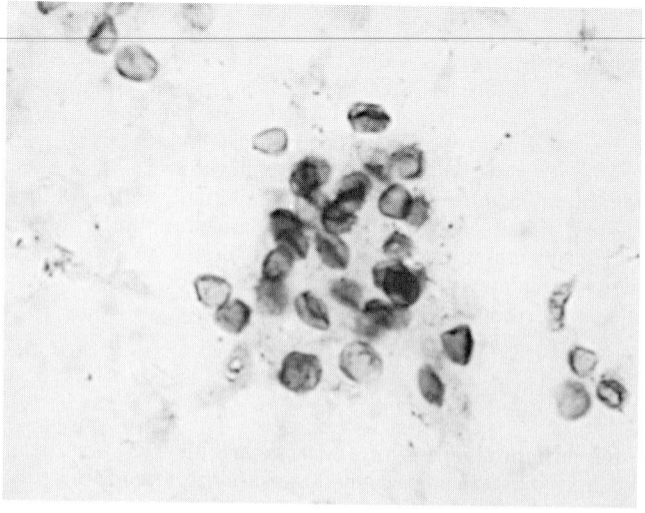

Figure 283.2. Cyst forms of *P. carinii* stained with the Gomori methenamine-silver nitrate method. The dark-staining cysts are 5 to 6 μm in diameter and are usually round- or cup-shaped. The intracystic sporozoites are not seen with this stain.

LIFE CYCLE

The complete life cycle of *P. carinii* has not been firmly established; however, microscopic observations from infections in vivo and propagation of *P. carinii in vitro* provide information on the replicative cycle. The most mature form is the thick-walled cyst containing up to eight sporozoites. Through breaks in the cyst wall, the small sporozoites excyst, after which they are referred to as trophozoites. The mechanism by which the trophozoite proceeds through a replicative system is not known.

GENETIC AND ANTIGENIC STRUCTURE

Several genes and gene fragments have been identified for *P. carinii*, including mitochondrial large subunit ribosomal RNA gene and internal transcribed spacers of the nuclear ribosomal RNA array (12). Genetic heterogeneity has been observed from different host species, suggesting *P. carinii* is host-species specific (13). Some understanding of the antigenic features of *P. carinii* has come from studies using monoclonal antibodies that recognize specific epitopes on *P. carinii* from various animal species, including rats, rabbits, ferrets, and humans (14,15). Evidence shows that organisms derived from humans are different from those of lower animals. Major surface glycoproteins with molecular weights from 95 to 140 kDa are the main protein components of both trophozoites and cysts. These glycoproteins are important factors in host-parasite interactions (16).

REFERENCES

1. Yoneda K, Walzer PD. Attachment of *Pneumocystis carinii* to type 1 alveolar cells studied by freeze-fracture electron microscopy. *Infect Immun* 1983;40:812–815.
2. Vossen MEMH, Beckers PJA, Meuwissen JHETh, Stadhowders AM. Microtubules in *Pneumocystis carinii*. *Z Parasitenkd* 1976;49:291–292.
3. Jackson HC, Colthurst D, Hancock V, et al. No detection of characteristic fungal protein elongation factor EF-3 in *Pneumocystis carinii*. *J Infect Dis* 1991;163:675–677.
4. Edman JC, Kovacs JA, Masur H, et al. Ribosomal RNA sequence shows *Pneumocystis carinii* to be a member of the fungi. *Nature* 1988;334:519–522.
5. Edman U, Edman JC, Lundgren B, Santi DV. Isolation and expression of the *Pneumocystis carinii* thymidylate synthase gene. *Proc Natl Acad Sci USA* 1989;86:6503–6507.
6. Edman JC, Kovacs JA, Masur H, et al. Molecular biology: future effects on taxonomy, diagnosis, and therapy. In: Masur H, moderator. Pneumocystic pneumonia: from bench to clinic. *Ann Intern Med* 1989;111:813–826.
7. Liu Y, Rocourt M, Pan S, et al. Sequence and variability of the 5.8S and 26S rRNA genes of *Pneumocystis carinii*. *Nucl Acids Res* 1992;20:3763–3772.
8. Edlind TD, Bartlett MS, Weinberg GA, et al. The beta-tubulin gene from rat and human isolates of *Pneumocystis carinii*. *Mol Microbiol* 1992;6:3365–3372.
9. Walker AN, Garner RD, Horst MN. Immunocytochemical detection of chitin in *Pneumocystis carinii*. *Infect Immun* 1990;58:412–415.
10. Pixley FJ, Wakefield AE, Banergfi S, Hopkin JM. Mitochondrial gene sequences show fungal homology for *Pneumocystis carinii*. *Mol Microbiol* 1991;5:1347–1351.
11. Eriksson OE. *Pneumocystis carinii*, a parasite in lungs of mammals, referred to a new family and order (Pneumocystidaceae, Pneumocystidales, Ascomycota). *Syst Ascomycetym* 1994;13:165–172.
12. Beard CB, Carter JL, Keely SP, et al. Genetic variations in *Pneumocystis carinii* isolates from different geographic regions: implications for transmission. *Emerg Infect Dis* 2000;6:265–272.
13. Wakefield AE. Genetic heterogeneity in *Pneumocystis carinii*: an introduction. *FEMS Immunol Med Microbiol* 1998;22:5–13.
14. Gigliotti F, Stokes DC, Cheatham AB, et al. Development of monoclonal antibodies to *Pneumocystis carinii*. *J Infect Dis* 1986;154:315–322.
15. Kovacs JA, Helpern JL, Lundgren B, et al. Monoclonal antibodies to *Pneumocystis carinii*: identification of specific antigens and characterization of antigenic difference between rat and human isolates. *J Infect Dis* 1989;159:60–70.
16. Wada, Nakamura Y. Type II major surface glycoprotein family of *Pneumocystis carinii* under the control of novel expression elements. *DNA Res* 1999;6:211–217.

CHAPTER 284

Cryptosporidium, Isospora, Cyclospora, Microsporidia, *and* Dientamoeba

Ynes R. Ortega and Charles R. Sterling

CRYPTOSPORIDIUM

Cryptosporidium is a coccidian parasite that infects humans. First recognized by Tyzzer (1) in 1907 in the gastric glands of asymptomatic laboratory mice, this protozoan was considered a benign commensal organism for nearly 50 years. In 1955, *Cryptosporidium* was first implicated as the cause of disease in animals when it was found in young turkeys with fatal enteritis. Since the 1970s, *Cryptosporidium* has been identified in the gastrointestinal or respiratory tract of most species of animals, including mammals, reptiles, birds, and fish. The parasite is also responsible for major agricultural losses each year (2,3).

Although human cryptosporidiosis was first reported in 1976 (4), appreciation of its pathogenic potential for humans came in the early 1980s, when *Cryptosporidium* was detected in acquired immunodeficiency syndrome (AIDS) patients with severe enteritis (5,6). Subsequent reports of cryptosporidial disease outbreaks in animal handlers and travelers (7,8). demonstrated that it could parasitize the immunocompetent population as well (5,7,9). As familiarity with diagnostic techniques improved, the number of reported cases has continued to increase, and *Cryptosporidium* has become recognized as a common cause of enteritis for both immunocompetent and immunocompromised hosts worldwide (10–14).

Characteristics of the Pathogen

Cryptosporidium (Greek for hidden spore) oocysts have four motile sporozoites with apical complexes; thus, the parasite is assigned to the phylum Apicomplexa, class Sporozoa, subclass Coccidiasina. Although taxonomically related to the other true coccidia, including *Toxoplasma gondii*, *Isospora*, and *Eimeria* species, *Cryptosporidium* has a number of unique features. The *Cryptosporidium* oocyst contains naked sporozoites. The parasite develops just under the host epithelial cell membrane in an intracellular but extracytoplasmic position. Finally, *Cryptosporidium* oocysts are fully sporulated when formed and a distinct population of thin-walled oocysts, comprising about 20% of oocysts formed, has the ability to reinfect the same host (10–14).

Since 1907, approximately 19 species of *Cryptosporidium* have been named for the host in which they were found; however, cross-transmission studies reveal that there is little or no host specificity, and some investigators regard *Cryptosporidium* as a single-species genus. (15) To date, eight Cryptosporidium species have been regarded valid based on their host specificity, pathogenesis and oocyst morphology. *C. parvum* in mammals, *C. muris* in rodents and ruminants, *C. felis* in domestic cats, *C. wrairi* in guinea pigs, *C. baileyi* and *C. melagridis* in birds, *C. serpentis* in reptiles, and *C. nasorum* in fish. *Cryptosporidium parvum* was classified in two basic genotypes. Type I, which to date, infects humans exclusively, and type II that can infect humans and animals. Cryptosporidium species responsible for causing diarrhea in immunocompromised adults and children also include

C. meleagridis, C. muris and *C. felis* (16). Additional genotypes have been described based on the homology of deoxyribonucleic acid (DNA) sequences of various proteins and single-strand ribosomal ribonucleic acid (SS-rRNA). Classification and naming of the subgroups or genotypes associated to human infections are still being worked on.

The *Cryptosporidium* life cycle, like that of other coccidia, can be divided into five stages: excystation (release of infective sporozoites from the oocyst), merogony (asexual replication), gametogony (formation of microgametes and macrogametes), fertilization, and oocyst formation. Infection is initiated by ingestion, or perhaps inhalation, of oocysts. (17) The acid-fast oocyst is 4 to 6 μm in diameter and, when mature (sporulated), contains four thin, motile sporozoites (Fig. 284.1). When ingested, a suture on the oocyst wall dissolves in the small intestine releasing sporozoites that move freely by gliding. They make contact with host enterocytes and enter into a compartment beneath the limiting host cell membrane where they subsequently develop into trophozoites. Asexual multiplication (merogony) results in the formation of type 1 and type 2 meronts (schizonts) that contain eight and four merozoites, respectively. The merozoites closely resemble sporozoites and may reinvade the host cells and reinitiate merogony, or they may differentiate into sexual stages, microgametocytes (male) or macrogametocytes (female), which further differentiate into gametes to initiate fertilization. Fertilized macrogametes develop into oocysts that can either reinfect the host (thin-walled oocysts) or exit the body to infect a new host (thick-walled oocysts) (18).

Epidemiology

The major modes of *Cryptosporidium* transmission appear to be human to human or through contaminated water (10–13,19,20). Transmission by the animal-to-human, human-to-animal, and foodborne routes also occurs (5,14). A small oral inoculum of oocysts is sufficient to cause human illness (21).

Waterborne outbreaks account for the greatest number of cryptosporidiosis cases identified to date in the United States. Contaminated municipal drinking water was responsible for a diarrhea outbreak involving approximately 400,000 cases in Milwaukee, Wisconsin, in 1993 and has been implicated in five other major outbreaks in the United States (20,22,23). Filtration of municipal water can reduce oocyst contamination, but protection is not absolute. The municipal water systems that were implicated in outbreaks included filtration treatment, and small numbers of oocysts have been detected in filtered municipal water in 27% to 54% of municipalities tested (20,24,25). Endemic transmission of *Cryptosporidium* through drinking water has not been demonstrated but is under investigation. Swimming in fresh surface water (i.e., lakes or rivers) or in swimming pools has also been associated with the acquisition of cryptosporidial infection (26–28.) *Cryptosporidium* oocysts have been demonstrated in 65% to 97% of surface water bodies tested (25–27,29,30).

A 1993 diarrhea outbreak in Maine traced to consumption of contaminated apple cider was the first documentation of foodborne *Cryptosporidium* transmission (31). Other foodborne outbreaks associated with consumption of contaminated fresh vegetables (32) and prepared foods (33) were also reported. Human-to-human spread has been responsible for infection in daycare center attendees, household contacts of index cases, hospitalized patients, and health care workers (34–36). Transmission related to animal contact has been well documented in handlers of calves (37,38) and other mammals, particularly neonates (20). Travelers are at increased risk for cryptosporidiosis, probably because of ingestion of contaminated water or possibly food (7). Spread of the parasite by aerosolization and fomites has been suggested but not confirmed.

Cryptosporidiosis has been described in more than 50 countries worldwide (10–13,19). Its true prevalence is currently not known. Surveys of selected populations have revealed rates of infection from 0.6% to 20% in developed countries and 4% to 32% in underdeveloped countries. Higher infection rates appear to be associated with younger age and a warm, humid climate (10–13,19,39). Both sexes are affected equally. Breast-feeding may confer protection, although this remains controversial (19,40). Various serologic surveys have revealed greater than expected rates of seropositivity, suggesting that active or recent infection is common in the general population (41,42).

As of 1986, the Centers for Disease Control and Prevention estimated that 3% to 4% of all AIDS patients had cryptosporidiosis as their AIDS-defining opportunistic infection (43). In later

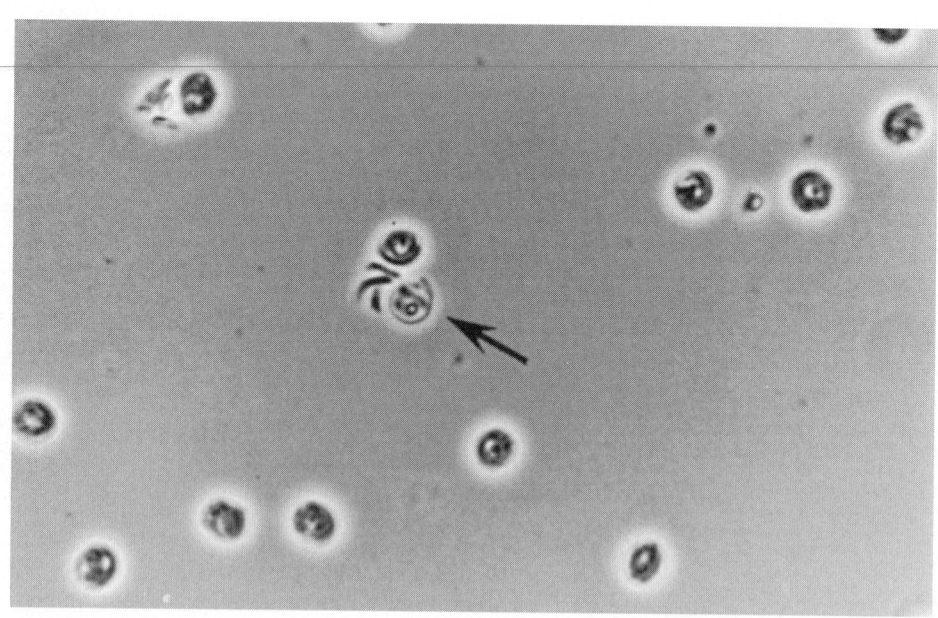

Figure 284.1. Human stool-derived *Cryptosporidium* oocysts. Excysting oocyst (*arrow*) is releasing three of its four sporozoites. (Phase-contrast microscopy 630X.)

studies, the parasite was identified in 15% of patients with AIDS and diarrhea at the National Institutes of Health (44) and in 16% of those at the Johns Hopkins Hospital (45). In Haiti and Africa, up to 50% of AIDS patients are infected (46).

Although an asymptomatic carrier state has been described for *Cryptosporidium*, its frequency is not known (47). Twenty-four percent to 30% of children with cryptosporidiosis who were younger than 3 years of age did not have diarrhea in a Peruvian study (48). Whether cryptosporidiosis in an immunocompromised host represents reactivation of previous infection or infection de novo also remains to be determined (49).

Pathology and Pathogenesis

Evaluation of tissue biopsy specimens obtained primarily from immunocompromised patients provides the basis for most of our understanding of the histopathologic process of cryptosporidiosis (6,50,51). Cryptosporidia are most often seen along the apical surfaces of epithelial cells of the small intestine (Fig. 284.2); however, the parasite has also been detected throughout the alimentary tract, including the esophagus, stomach, small and large intestine (6,50,51); gallbladder and bile and pancreatic ducts; within colonic submucosal vessels (52); and in the respiratory tract (53,54). Histologic changes are nonspecific and mild despite the presence of numerous organisms. They include blunting or complete loss of villi, elongation of crypts, and infiltration of the lamina propria with polymorphonuclear leukocytes, lymphocytes, and plasma cells (55). Histologic changes do not correlate with the degree of clinical symptoms. Ultrastructural studies of infected intestine reveal the parasite ensconced between microvilli and enclosed within a parasitophorous vacuole just under the host cell membrane yet outside the host cytoplasm, a unique "intracellular yet extracytoplasmic" position (10,50,51).

The pathogenic mechanisms in intestinal cryptosporidiosis remain to be fully elucidated. Diminished small intestinal glucose, electrolyte, and water absorption has been demonstrated in conjunction with characteristic histopathologic features of cryptosporidiosis in an animal model (56). Enterotoxic or humoral factors may play a role (57); *in vitro* findings suggest that in-

creased local prostanoid production contributes to impaired enterocyte sodium-coupled glucose transport (58).

Cryptosporidial cholecystitis or cholangitis is a fairly frequent finding in immunocompromised patients with cryptosporidial enteritis. Such patients have marked histopathologic changes in the biliary tract and gallbladder, ranging from acute inflammation to gangrenous necrosis. Cryptosporidia are found adherent to the biliary epithelium and in the bile (50,59). A number of patients with cryptosporidial cholecystitis were also found to have concurrent cytomegalovirus infection of the biliary tract. Pancreatitis has been reported in association with cryptosporidiosis in both immunocompetent and immunocompromised patients (60,61).

Although cryptosporidia have been isolated from sputum, tracheal aspirates, bronchoalveolar lavage fluid, and lung tissue, whether they are pathogens, colonizers, or contaminants from the gastrointestinal tract has not been determined (53,54,62). Cryptosporidial involvement of the biliary and pulmonary tracts has not been described for immunocompetent patients with cryptosporidial infection.

Clinical Manifestations

The hallmark of human cryptosporidiosis in both immunocompetent and immunocompromised hosts is voluminous watery diarrhea (6,63). It is usually accompanied by crampy abdominal pain (often after eating), weight loss, flatulence, and malaise. Nausea, vomiting, myalgias, and fever are less common. Fecal examination reveals *Cryptosporidium* oocysts and mucus but rarely blood or leukocytes. Peripheral blood leukocytosis and eosinophilia are also uncommon. Fat, carbohydrate, and vitamin B_{12} malabsorption is well documented and contributes significantly to the wasting syndrome that is seen in patients with AIDS. Radiographic findings are nonspecific and include mucosal thickening and disordered small bowel motility.

The incubation period for cryptosporidiosis is typically 2 to 14 days. The severity and duration of the illness are determined by the immune status of the host (6,9). In the immunocompetent host, symptoms may have an explosive onset and last 10 to 14 days (9). Clearance of the oocysts (and the potential for

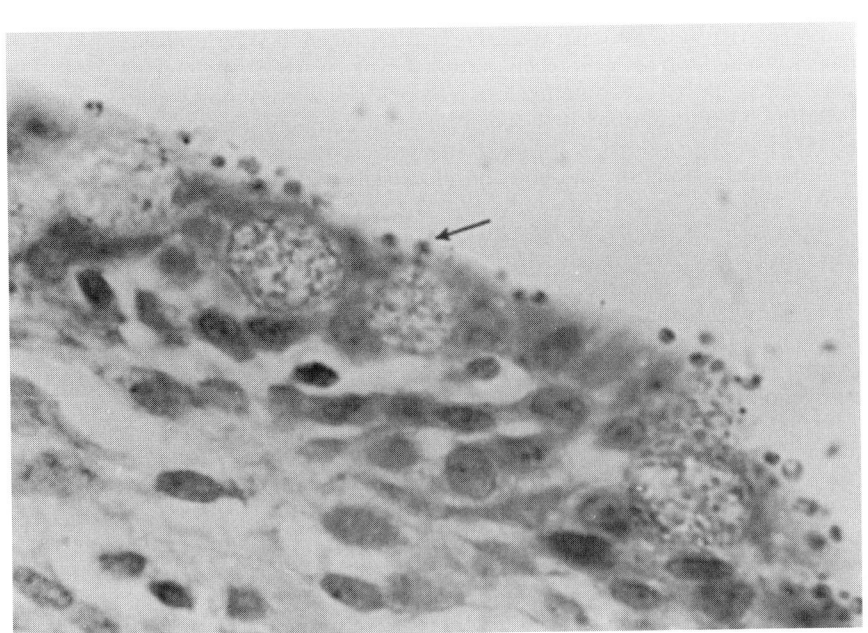

Figure 284.2. Cryptosporidia (*arrow*) studding the small bowel epithelial surface of a patient with AIDS. (Giemsa stain, 450X.)

contagion) may lag behind clinical improvement by 1 to 2 weeks (64).

In immunocompromised persons, including those with AIDS, the disease often develops insidiously; however, as immune competence wanes, clinical symptoms frequently worsen. Patients may experience voluminous (1 to 25 L daily) watery diarrhea, profound weight loss, electrolyte imbalance, and severe dehydration, requiring hospitalization for months, often until they die (6,63,65).

Patients with biliary cryptosporidiosis often have classic signs of cholangitis: right upper quadrant pain, nausea, vomiting, and enteritis (59,66). The serum alkaline phosphatase and γ-glutamyl transpeptidase levels are usually elevated, whereas bilirubin and transaminase values remain normal. On radiographic examination, the gallbladder may be dilated, with thickened walls and luminal irregularities suggestive of sclerosing cholangitis. Patients who underwent cholecystectomy or endoscopic retrograde cholangiopancreatography have been found to have cryptosporidia studding the gallbladder epithelial surface and in the bile. The patients' symptoms improved transiently after either cholecystectomy or endoscopic papillotomy. Pancreatitis complicating cryptosporidial infection has also been described (60,61).

Diagnosis

The diagnosis of cryptosporidial enteritis is made by detection of oocysts in fecal or intestinal biopsy specimens. Since 1981, many staining techniques for detecting the parasite in stool specimens have been popularized (67,68). Most widely accepted have been modified acid-fast stains, which readily distinguish the acid-fast *Cryptosporidium* oocysts from yeasts, which although similar in shape and size are not acid-fast. Data, however, indicate that acid-fast staining lacks sensitivity, especially when stools are formed. Concentration by centrifugation may improve sensitivity.

A direct immunofluorescent antibody stain using monoclonal murine immunoglobulin G to the oocyst wall (Meridian) and enzyme-linked immunosorbent assays for detection of cryptosporidial antigen in stool specimens are now commercially available and in use in some clinical laboratories. Additional diagnostic testing for *Cryptosporidium* spp. involving immunoassays (fluorescent antibody [FA] or enzyme immunoassay [EIA]) is also available (69). Immunofluorescence assays and enzyme-linked immunosorbent assay (ELISA) (70) are available commercially and can be used to identify the organisms. Merifluor® DFA and IFA (Meridian Diagnostics, Cincinnati, OH) (71) were reported to have a 100% specificity and sensitivity. Other kits have been developed for clinical samples such as such as Crypto-Cel IF-DFA (Cellabs, Brookvale, Australia) and ProSpect®-EIA (Alexon, Inc., Ramsey, MN). Water and environmental sample kits are also available including Cryp-a-Glo™ Kits and reagents (Waterborne, New Orleans, LA), Dynabeads® anti-Cryptosporidium (Dynal Biotech, Lake Success, NY), and Hydrofluor™– Combo (Meridian Diagnostics, Cincinnati, OH). PCR has been described, but its possible role and use in a clinical laboratory have not yet been established.

Immunofluorescence and enzyme-linked immunosorbent assays have been developed to detect anticryptosporidial immunoglobulins in serum and various secretions (41,72,73). Both immunocompetent and immunocompromised patients generate immunoglobulin G in response to infection with *Cryptosporidium*. Whereas patients with AIDS seldom generate anticryptosporidial immunoglobulin M, immunocompetent patients usually exhibit an increase in immunoglobulin M antibody early in the course of cryptosporidial infection. Current work at the Centers for Disease Control and Prevention is aimed at identifying *Cryptosporidium* epitopes responsible for the early antibody response that might be useful diagnostically (74).

Treatment

No consistently effective therapy for human cryptosporidiosis is currently known. *In vitro* cultivation of *Cryptosporidium* in tissue culture systems (HCT-8, Caco-2, L292) is being used for screening potential drugs (75–78). Symptomatic small-animal models are being developed but have not been widely accepted. A wide variety of antimicrobial and immunomodulating agents as well as special diets have been tested in an unprecedented fashion on a compassionate basis for AIDS patients with cryptosporidiosis; although most have been unsuccessful, a few have shown limited promise (10,63,79).

Interest in macrolide antibiotics for cryptosporidiosis began with anecdotal reports of responses to spiramycin in the mid-1980s (80). In the first placebo-controlled trial for AIDS-related cryptosporidiosis, oral spiramycin was found to be no more efficacious than placebo, probably owing to poor absorption in the target population (81). Results of a single-blind placebo-controlled trial of intravenous spiramycin suggest that despite modest anticryptosporidial activity, use of this form of the agent is limited by toxic effects. Controlled trials of oral spiramycin in immunocompetent children have provided both positive (82) and negative (83) results, possibly related to inadequate dosing.

The newer macrolide azithromycin may be more promising. Preliminary results of a randomized, double-blind, placebo-controlled crossover trial in AIDS patients suggest that a lactose-free form of oral azithromycin, 900 mg once daily, conferred modest, statistically significant, clinical and parasitologic improvement (84). Preliminary regression analysis of the data suggests a statistically significant decrease in stool oocyst counts in patients who achieved higher serum azithromycin levels (84). Anecdotal reports of improved liver function after treatment with intravenous azithromycin have prompted further study of this route. Pilot clinical trials of the macrolides roxithromycin and clarithromycin for AIDS-related cryptosporidiosis are in progress. Diclazuril and letrazuril benzeneacetonitrile derivatives active against coccidian infection in poultry, were not effective in placebo-controlled trials in AIDS patients (85).

Paromomycin is a nonabsorbable aminoglycoside that concentrates in the colon. Data are conflicting on the efficacy of paromomycin for AIDS-related cryptosporidiosis. In one double-blind, placebo-controlled trial, 1.5 to 2 g/day for 14 days was associated with partial symptomatic and parasitologic responses, consistent with other anecdotal observations (86). However, in an AIDS Clinical Trials Group-sponsored multicenter, double-blind, placebo-controlled trial, paromomycin at 2 g/day for 21 days was associated with no significant benefit relative to placebo (87). Clinical use of paromomycin has been disappointing because clinical response may not correlate with reduction in parasite shedding and response may be transient.

Nitazoxanide (NTZ) is a nitrothiazole benzamide compound with a broad spectrum of antimicrobial activity. In an open-label trial of NTZ at 0.5 to 2 g/day orally for 4 weeks, 43% of patients with AIDS-related cryptosporidiosis had a 50% or greater reduction in diarrheal frequency and/or a significant reduction in oocyst shedding in stool; some patients experienced additional benefit with extended therapy (88).

Given the limitations of antimicrobial chemotherapy for cryptosporidiosis, strategies for immunotherapy are of great interest. Novel therapies, including hyperimmune bovine colostrum, bovine colostral immunoglobulins, and cow's milk globulin, have resulted in both success and failure in humans and animals when they were administered orally (63,89–91). The use of bovine transfer factor also appeared promising, but more investigation is required, including identification of the active component (92). Clinical investigation of various novel immunomodulatory agents including a hyperimmune egg yolk preparation containing high titers of anticryptosporidial antibody have also been evaluated.

Anecdotal reports of AIDS patients experiencing improvement in cryptosporidial enteritis while receiving zidovudine therapy (63,93,94) may be explained by improved immune function rather than specific anticryptosporidial activity.

Cryptosporidiosis in immunocompetent hosts is self-limited, although the enteritis can be severe. In the absence of defined specific therapy, management is generally limited to supportive measures. Cryptosporidiosis in patients with weakened immunity due to exogenous factors such as chemotherapy may resolve if immunoreductive therapy is lessened or interrupted. Cryptosporidiosis in AIDS is commonly chronic and unremitting; supportive measures are often vital, and an attempt at specific anticryptosporidial therapy is usually justified.

Fluid and electrolyte management, with oral or intravenous repletion as needed, is crucial for supportive therapy. AIDS patients with chronic cryptosporidiosis may benefit from parenteral nutrition. Nonspecific antidiarrheal agents such as kaolin plus pectin (Kaopectate), loperamide (Imodium), diphenoxylate (Lomotil), bismuth subsalicylate (Pepto-Bismol), or opiates may provide symptomatic relief, but safety has not been investigated in cryptosporidiosis. The long-acting parenteral somatostatin analog octreotide has provided symptomatic relief in some patients with AIDS and cryptosporidiosis (95), although no consistent benefit was observed in a prospective, multicenter clinical trial (96).

Prevention

The *Cryptosporidium* oocyst is hardy and resistant to many disinfectants used in hospitals and laboratories including 3% hypochlorite solution, iodophor, cresylic acid, benzalkonium chloride, and 5% formaldehyde (10,19). Oocyst infectivity appears to be eliminated by exposure to temperatures above 73°C for 1 minute (97) and reduced by prolonged exposure to undiluted bleach or 5% ammonia. Whether freezing reduces or eliminates infectivity is under study.

Persons who are immunocompromised should be advised that certain activities are risks for cryptosporidiosis and should be avoided. These include unprotected physical contact with infected persons or animals, swimming in pools, and consumption of or swimming in freshwater. Data on the risk associated with the consumption of municipal water are insufficient to recommend preventive measures, but immunocompromised individuals who wish to do so can eliminate the risk for transmission from tap water by boiling it for at least 1 minute, by drinking bottled water from safe sources (such as steam-distilled water), or by the correct use of certain types of water filtration units (20,25).

ISOSPORA BELLI

Human infection with *I. belli* was first described in 1915 (98). Although it has been recognized as a pathogen for many years, much remains to be learned about infection with this parasite.

Characteristics of the Pathogen

I. belli, like *Cryptosporidium* and *Cyclospora*, is a true coccidian. Its oocysts are elliptical and substantially larger (22 to 33 μm by 10 to 15 μm), and each contains two sporocysts. Inside each sporocyst are four sporozoites. Clinical disease is acquired through ingestion of the mature (sporulated) oocyst. The parasite invades host intestinal epithelium and, once in the enterocyte cytoplasm, passes through the asexual (merogony) and sexual (gametogony) phases of its life cycle. Unsporulated oocysts are shed in the feces and must mature outside the host to become infective.

Epidemiology

The prevalence of *I. belli* in humans is not known. It is distributed throughout the world but is more common in tropical and subtropical climates. Endemic areas include Latin America, the Caribbean, Africa, Australia, and Southeast Asia (99–102). In the United States, *I. belli* has been implicated in several institutional outbreaks of diarrhea, as the cause of enteritis in World War II veterans returning from the Pacific, and as a cause of traveler's diarrhea (99–101,103). Isosporiasis has been documented in 0.2% to 1.0% of all AIDS patients in the United States and in 5% to 19% of AIDS patients in Haiti and Africa (101,104,105). The relative infrequency of clinical *I. belli* infection among AIDS patients in the United States may be due to the use of trimethoprim-sulfamethoxazole (TMP-SMX) for *Pneumocystis carinii* prophylaxis. The mode of transmission is not well worked out; acquisition from infected humans, and through contaminated water, is suspected but not confirmed.

Pathology and Pathogenesis

Histopathologic evaluation of small bowel biopsy specimens from infected patients reveals atrophic mucosa, shortened villi, hypertrophic crypts, and infiltration of the lamina propria with inflammatory cells, particularly eosinophils (99,106). Electron microscopic examination has demonstrated parasites within cytoplasmic vacuoles of enterocytes. Extraintestinal isosporiasis is well documented in cats (107) but rarely described in humans. *I. belli* has been identified in the lymph nodes of one patient with AIDS and in the gallbladder lumen of an AIDS patient with acalculous cholecystitis (108,109).

Clinical Manifestations

Signs and symptoms of isosporiasis include watery diarrhea without blood or inflammatory cells, cramping, abdominal pain, anorexia, and weight loss. Low-grade fever may be present. Fat malabsorption is common; peripheral eosinophilia has been documented in some cases. Immunocompetent adults usually have a self-limited diarrheal illness, but there have been case reports of prolonged illness (103). AIDS patients and immunocompetent infants and children often have a chronic or relapsing form of the disease (100,104,110–112).

Diagnosis

Diagnosis is established by finding *Isospora* oocysts in fecal specimens (Fig. 284.3). Like *Cryptosporidium* and *Cyclospora*, they are acid-fast but are easily distinguished by their larger size and ellipsoid shape (Fig. 284.4). *Isospora* organisms may also be identified with a fluorescent auramine stain. Other methods of identifying *Cryptosporidium*, including serologic tests, have not been

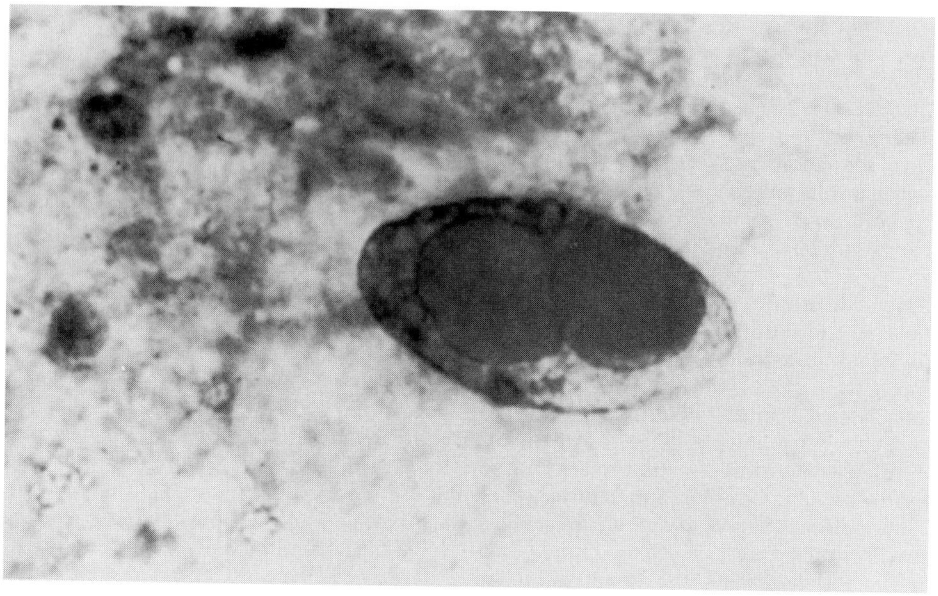

Figure 284.3. Acid-fast *Isospora belli* oocyst in the stained smear of a fecal specimen from a patient with AIDS and diarrhea. (450X.) (Courtesy of Madeleine Boncy, Haitian Study Group on Kaposi's Sarcoma and Opportunistic Infection [GHESKIO], Port-au-Prince, Haiti.)

extended to *Isospora*. *Isospora* oocysts may be shed only intermittently, suggesting that specimen concentration or obtaining multiple specimens may be useful in diagnosis (103).

Treatment

Unlike cryptosporidiosis, isosporiasis promptly responds to therapy. One week of oral double-strength TMP-SMX, 160 mg of TMP and 800 mg of SMX four times a day, usually effects a clinical and parasitologic cure, with response evident, on average, within 3 days (111,113). AIDS patients have a high rate of relapse but respond well to retreatment with TMP-SMX. To prevent relapse, AIDS patients can be maintained with long-term suppressive therapy; double-strength TMP-SMX three times weekly or pyrimethamine, 25 mg, plus sulfadiazine, 500 mg (Fansidar), once weekly appears effective (113). There have been scattered anecdotal reports of response to pyrimethamine alone (114) and to the experimental agents roxithromycin (115) and Diclazuril (116). Results of treatment with metronidazole, quinacrine, and nitrofurantoin have been mixed (99,106,113,117). Controlled studies are needed to establish the precise dose and duration of induction and maintenance therapy. Better alternative therapy is needed.

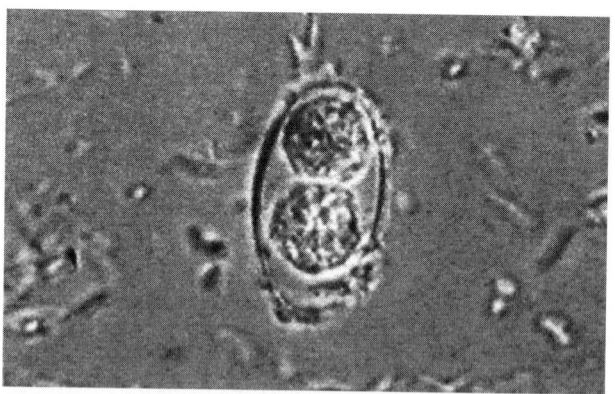

Figure 284.4. *Isospora belli* sporulated oocyst. (Nomarski microscopy 400X.)

CYCLOSPORA

Cyclospora is the newest coccidian to be discovered in humans. Since 1986, and possibly as early as 1979, a unique acid-fast organism resembling a "large *Cryptosporidium*" has been characterized in humans with diarrheal illness (118,119). Although variously termed a coccidian-like body, and a cyanobacterium-like body, similarities between these reports suggested that the same parasite was being described (120–126). Sporulation, excystation, and ultrastructural analyses support the classification of this pathogen as *Cyclospora* (122,124).

Characteristics of the Pathogen

Cyclospora is an intracellular enteric parasite. The genus is in the phylum Apicomplexa, class Sporozoa, subclass Coccidiasina, suborder Eimeriina. The species name *Cyclospora cayetanensis* has been proposed for the human pathogen (124), although the degree of relatedness between *Cyclospora* identified in diverse human cohorts remains under study. *Cyclospora* species reported in several animal hosts appear to be distinct from *Cyclospora* species in humans (122,125). Three other species of *Cyclospora* have been described in non-human primates. Morphologically they are similar to *C. cayetanensis* but different by phylogenetic analysis (127).

The round *Cyclospora* oocysts contain two sporocysts, each containing two sporozoites. *Cyclospora* oocysts identified in human fecal specimens are typically 8 to 10 μm in diameter, distinct from oocysts of *Cryptosporidium* (4 to 6 μm) and *Isospora* (28 × 13 μm). Intracellular stages of *Cyclospora* have been identified in biopsy specimens of infected patients. Asexual stages (meronts type I and II) and sexual stages were observed in parasitic vacuoles in the cytoplasm of epithelial cells of the duodenum and jejunum (128). No animal model is yet available for *Cyclospora*. This would greatly facilitate the understanding of this parasite (120,121,129).

Epidemiology

Human *Cyclospora* appears to be globally distributed, with reports matching its description in residents and travelers from North America, Central America, South America, the

Caribbean islands, Eastern Europe, India, Nepal, Bangladesh, and Southeast Asia (126,130,131). Incidence is seasonal, with most cases reported from Nepal and Peru occurring during the warm, rainy months, and from the United States between May and July (120–122,125). Symptomatic infection occurs in all ages and in immunocompetent and immunocompromised hosts alike. Persons native to endemic areas appear less susceptible to clinical infection, suggesting that previous infection may confer some degree of immunity (121). Prevalence data are limited. In endemic areas, investigators identified *Cyclospora* in 6% to 18% of children aged 1 to 24 months in Lima, Peru, shantytowns, and in 12% of Nepalese children with diarrhea aged 18 to 60 months, but in no Nepalese or Haitian children with diarrhea younger than 18 months (122,132,133). Among Haitian adults with chronic diarrhea, *Cyclospora* was detected in 11% of human immunodeficiency virus (HIV)-seropositive, but none of the HIV-seronegative, patients tested (132). In the United States and England, which have not been considered endemic areas, *Cyclospora* was identified in 0.1% to 0.5% of stool specimens received in three clinical laboratories (125,126,133,134).

There was a surge in non-travel-related cases in the New York City and Palm Beach, Florida, metropolitan areas in May to June 1995, and nearly 1,450 sporadic and cluster-related cases were reported in 20 states, Washington, DC, and two Canadian provinces in May to June 1996 (125,126,135,136). The risk factors involved have not been identified in all cases, although epidemiologic investigation has suggested an association with eating fresh fruits (particularly raspberries) (137), basil (138), and lettuce (139), particularly in association with case clustering.

Although the range of exposure risks for *Cyclospora* infection remains to be defined, humans appear to have contracted *Cyclospora* from contaminated water in outbreaks in Nepal and Chicago (120,140). One case of infection after ingestion of lettuce contaminated with cyanobacterium-like bodies has also been reported (121). Direct transmission from animals or from person to person has not been documented.

Pathology and Pathogenesis

Diarrhea associated with *Cyclospora* infection is typically watery and negative for occult blood or leukocytes, consistent with a noninvasive process (121). Small bowel injury is prominent. Endoscopy reveals duodenal erythema in some patients; histologic features on duodenal (141) and jejunal (142) biopsy include villous atrophy, crypt hyperplasia, and epithelial disarray, with acute and chronic inflammation (128).

Electron microscopic analysis of jejunal biopsy specimens has demonstrated intracytoplasmic parasites within enterocytes, contained within vacuoles toward the luminal poles (128,142). The specific mechanism of intestinal injury remains to be elucidated. Extraintestinal infection (cholangitis) has been suggested in two patients with AIDS (143).

Clinical Manifestations

Symptoms of *Cyclospora* infection commonly include nonbloody diarrhea, cramping, abdominal pain, nausea, anorexia, and weight loss (143–147). In contrast to cryptosporidiosis, fatigue is often a principal complaint, and fever and influenza-like symptoms such as myalgias are common, especially during the first few days. Diarrhea may not be consistently watery but is often described as urgent or explosive. Gastrointestinal symptoms are often intermittent and may not be the first or most prominent symptoms of illness. Malabsorption has been demonstrated in a small series of patients (141). In immunocompetent hosts, illness

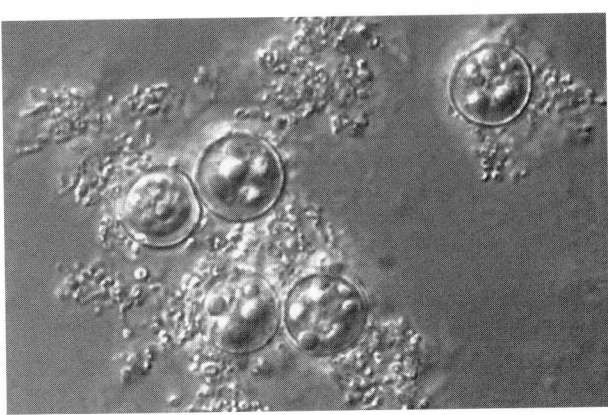

Figure 284.5. *Cyclospora cayetanensis* unsporulated oocysts. (Nomarski microscopy 400X).

is self-limited but may be prolonged, with symptoms typically lasting 2 to 6 weeks if untreated. In AIDS patients, however, untreated *Cyclospora* infection and its symptoms are often chronic or relapsing (132,148).

Diagnosis

Diagnosis of *Cyclospora* infection is established by identifying the oocysts in stool samples. *Cyclospora* oocysts are round and 8 to 10 μm in diameter (Fig. 284.5); on unstained wet preparations, they are nonrefractile and contain globular inclusions (122). Although morphologically quite similar, *Cryptosporidium* oocysts are smaller (4 to 6 μm); and careful measurement permits differentiation. Modified acid-fast staining greatly facilitates detection of *Cyclospora* and should be requested; although the intensity of oocysts staining within a smear is often highly variable, in contrast to *Cryptosporidium*, which stains more homogeneously. A Safranin-based stain with microwave heating stains the oocysts more homogeneously (149). In addition, *Cyclospora* oocysts characteristically autofluoresce blue-green under ultraviolet epifluorescence microscopy, depending on which dichroic filter is used. Direct immunofluorescent stains specific for *Cryptosporidium* do not cross react with *Cyclospora* (122).

Cyclospora oocysts have also been identified in duodenal aspirates and in small bowel biopsy specimens examined by electron microscopy (142).

Treatment

The illness associated with human *Cyclospora* infection responds promptly to oral TMP-SMX, much like isosporiasis, but in contrast to cryptosporidiosis. For adults, TMP at 160 mg and SMX at 800 mg twice daily for 7 days in immunocompetent patients (144,146), and four times daily for 10 days in patients with AIDS (132), has been associated with resolution of symptoms and eradication of *Cyclospora* from stool. Relapse subsequent to therapy is common in AIDS patients but responds to retreatment; long-term suppressive therapy with TMP at 160 mg and SMX at 800 mg three times a week appears to greatly reduce recurrence (132). Ciprofloxacin at 500 mg twice daily for 7 days can also be used to treat cyclosporiasis (150). Further study is needed to define (a) appropriate children's dosages, (b) additional alternative therapy for TMP-SMX–intolerant patients, and (c) whether a smaller TMP-SMX dose than that suggested for adults with AIDS would be as effective in children.

MICROSPORIDIA

Microsporidial organisms are obligate intracellular spore-forming protozoan parasites long recognized as pathogens in mammals, fish, crustaceans, and insects (151). Until the AIDS epidemic, association of human disease with microsporidial infection was rare; first reported in 1959 (152), only eight cases were known until 1985. Subsequently, however, human microsporidial infection associated with varied clinical syndromes, predominantly among HIV-infected persons, has been described with increasing frequency (153–155).

Characteristics of the Pathogen

Microsporidia is the term used to refer to members of the phylum Microspora, order Microsporida. The phylum contains more than 1,000 species within approximately 100 genera. Six genera have been described in human infection (Table 284.1): *Encephalitozoon* include *Encephalitozoon intestinalis*, formerly *Septata intestinalis* (156), *Enterocytozoon, Pleistophora, Nosema,* and the more recently designated *Vittaforma* (one species, *Vittaforma corneae,* formerly *Nosema* corneum [157]) and *Trachipleistophora* (158). *Microsporidia* that have been not been characterized well enough to assign to a genus have been named *Microsporidium* sp.

The Microsporidia are primitive eukaryotes lacking mitochondria and Golgi. Spores contain a coiled polar filament, and sporoplasm, which consists of cytoplasm and one or two nuclei. In the appropriate environment, spores extrude their filament which penetrates a host cell and provides a conduit for the transfer of the sporoplasm into the host cytoplasm. Merogony and sporogony follow. The resultant new spores are released when the host cell ruptures, remaining within the host or passing into the environment (155,159).

Spores are typically ovoid or piriform. Dimensions vary by species and range from 1 to 20 μm in diameter. Microsporidial spores found in humans are relatively small at 1 to 2 μm. Shape, position of nuclei, and number of nuclei and coils of the polar filament also vary. The classification of microsporidian species into various genera is determined by morphologic features and the mode of replication within the host cell (159).

Epidemiology

The majority of microsporidiosis cases have been reported in AIDS patients, including nearly all cases of *Enterocytozoon bieneusi* and all cases of *Encephalitozoon hellem* and *E. intestinalis* (160). Only ten non-HIV-related cases of microsporidiosis have been documented; four of these were in immunocompromised individuals (153–155) (see Table 284.1).

Human microsporidiosis has a worldwide distribution, with cases in HIV-infected patients reported from North and South America, Europe, Africa, Asia, and Australia (153,160). The actual prevalence of microsporidial infection in humans is unknown, because diagnostic techniques are limited, and studies have been few. Microsporidia have been identified in 7.5% to 50% of AIDS patients with previously unexplained diarrhea (161–165). Most (166) but not all (167) studies reveal a strong correlation between intestinal microsporidiosis and clinical enteritis, suggesting that microsporidia, particularly *E. bieneusi,* are an important cause of AIDS-related diarrhea. However, asymptomatic enteric carriage may be common in HIV infection (167).

The modes by which humans become infected with microsporidia are unknown. Spores may be shed in feces, urine, or respiratory secretions of infected humans (152,160). Fecal-oral and sexual modes of transmission from human to human have been proposed (153), but not documented. Microsporidial spores have been identified in surface water (168), but only of species not known to infect humans (169,170). Microsporidia species are found in numerous animal hosts representing most

TABLE 284.1.   Clinical Manifestations of Microsporidia Infection, by Species and Host

Species	Host	
	HIV infected	Non-HIV infected
Encephalitozoon cuniculi	Disseminated infection	Seizures[a]
Encephalitozoon hellem	Keratoconjunctivitis, disseminated infection	—
Encephalitozoon intestinalis[b]	Enteritis, disseminated infection	—
Enterocytozoon bieneusi	Enteritis, cholangitis, respiratory infection	Enteritis[c]
Pleistophora species	Myositis	Myositis[d]
Trachipleistophora hominis	Myositis	—
Nosema connori	—	Disseminated infection[e]
Nosema ocularum		Keratitis[f]
Vittaforma cornea[g]	—	Keratitis[h]
Microsporidium africanum	—	Corneal ulcer[i]
Microsporidium ceylonensis	—	Corneal ulcer[j]

[a]Two cases, one with decreased CD4/CD8 (172,220).
[b]Formerly *Septata intestinalis.*
[c]Two cases, one an organ recipient receiving immunosuppressive therapy (155,221).
[d]One case, cellular immunity impaired (222).
[e]One case, thymic aphasia (223).
[f]One case, immunocompetent (185,224).
[g]Formerly *Nosema corneum.*
[h]One case, immunocompetent (157).
[i]One case, immunocompetent (224).
[j]One case, immunocompetent (225).

phyla and including fish and crustacean species consumed by humans. However, other than several mammalian hosts in which *Encephalitozoon cuniculi* has been identified, the animal reservoirs of microsporidia species pathogenic to humans remain unknown, and zoonotic transmission to humans has yet to be demonstrated.

Pathology and Pathogenesis

Tissue distribution, histopathologic features, and propensity to disseminate vary widely among species of microsporidia recognized in human disease (153,155). Pathophysiologic mechanisms and the full range of organ involvement remain to be elucidated for these organisms. Impaired cellular immunity is a factor in host susceptibility; nearly all cases of human microsporidiosis have been in HIV-infected individuals (155,171).

Human infection with *E. bieneusi* is virtually always limited to intestinal and biliary tissue (172,173). Organisms have been observed from duodenum to colon, in biliary and gallbladder epithelia, and in the pancreatic duct (174). Whereas the greatest density is typically in the duodenum or proximal jejunum (173), predominantly biliary infestation has been reported (164,175,176). Infection is nearly always limited to the epithelial cell layer, with organisms evident within apical cytoplasm. Histopathologic features range from minimal injury to marked epithelial cell dystrophy, vesiculation, and sloughing (176). Intraepithelial and lamina propria mononuclear cell infiltrates are variable. Damage to small intestinal villous architecture may be minimal or extreme with atrophy and crypt elongation and often correlates with the degree of infestation (177). Infection of biliary epithelia has been linked to sclerosing cholangitis, acalculous cholecystitis, and papillary stenosis (176,178), although histopathologic changes are often minimal (155). There have been rare reports of *E. bieneusi* in nasal and tracheobronchial tissue (179).

Human infection with *Encephalitozoon* species is frequently disseminated. *E. intestinalis* is, like *E. bieneusi*, associated with gastroenteritis (180). Small bowel villous atrophy, enterocyte sloughing, and acute inflammatory infiltrates are variably present (180,181). However, in contrast to *E. bieneusi, E. intestinalis* organisms are commonly demonstrable in both the apical and basal enterocyte cytoplasm as well as within macrophages from the lamina propria to the submucosa (180,181). In addition, disseminated *E. intestinalis* infection, with hepatobiliary, bronchial, and renal involvement, has been reported (182,183). *E. intestinalis* has been identified in the urine or respiratory secretions of several patients with enteritis (184), suggesting that disseminated infection is underrecognized.

E. hellem has been identified in superficial corneal and conjunctival epithelia (185–187). Inflammatory changes are variable. Subclinical, systemic infection may accompany ocular disease, with spores demonstrable in respiratory secretions and urine (190). Superficial respiratory epithelial cell infection has been demonstrated in symptomatic tracheitis, bronchiolitis, and sinusitis (187–189). *E. hellem* was demonstrated in the bronchi, kidneys, ureters, bladder, and corneas of a patient with advanced AIDS who died of renal and respiratory failure (190).

E. cuniculi has been identified in hepatocytes and in omental tissue of two AIDS patients with granulomatous hepatitis (191) and peritonitis (192), respectively.

Myositis has been reported associated with *Pleistophora* infection (one AIDS patient [193] and one HIV-seronegative individual with impaired cellular immunity) and with *Trachipleistophora* infection (one AIDS patient [157]). Organisms were demonstrated among atrophic muscle fibers (157,193).

Clinical Manifestations

Clinical features of microsporidiosis include chronic diarrhea, keratoconjunctivitis, myositis, nephritis, hepatitis, sinusitis, and pneumonia (154,155).

Enteritis due to *E. bieneusi* or *E. intestinalis* is the most common clinical manifestation of microsporidiosis in patients with AIDS (161,163). Diarrhea is typically chronic and intermittent, loose to watery, and nonbloody (154,155,161,163). Fecal leukocytes are usually absent. Anorexia, weight loss, and dehydration are common, and findings on D-xylose testing are often abnormal, consistent with malabsorption (163,174). Abdominal cramping, nausea, and vomiting may occur. The density of *E. bieneusi* infestation and associated histopathologic appearance may not correlate with severity of enteritis, and chronic asymptomatic carriage has been documented (167). Concomitant infection with other opportunistic gastrointestinal pathogens, such as *Cryptosporidium* or cytomegalovirus, is often present (165,194).

E. bieneusi and *E. intestinalis* have been implicated in biliary disease, including cholangitis and acalculous cholecystitis (176,182). Patients may present with right upper quadrant pain or intractable nausea. The alkaline phosphatase level is often elevated, whereas bilirubin and transaminase levels are typically normal. Radiologic imaging may reveal dilatation or luminal irregularities of biliary ducts and gallbladder distention or thickening (176).

Although *E. intestinalis* infection has been recognized chiefly in association with intestinal and biliary disease (161), dissemination is underrecognized and extragastrointestinal manifestations remain poorly characterized.

Infection with *E. hellem* in patients with AIDS is most commonly associated with keratoconjunctivitis (186,187). Ocular pain or pruritus, foreign body sensation, lacrimosis, and blurred vision may be present. Infection may be bilateral, and bacterial superinfection has been reported. Isolated cases of bronchitis, nephritis, and cystourethritis associated with *E. hellem* infection have been reported (187). However, asymptomatic or cryptic disseminated infection may be underrecognized.

E. cuniculi has been identified in single cases of hepatitis (191), peritonitis (192), and generalized infection (155), all from HIV-infected patients. *E. cuniculi* has also been reported in two children with seizure disorders (195), one of whom had a decreased CD4/CD8 ratio.

Pleistophora species have been identified in skeletal muscle biopsy specimens in two patients presenting with generalized muscle weakness: a patient with AIDS (193) and an HIV-negative individual with decreased cell-mediated immunity. Creatine kinase and aldolase values were elevated in the former but not the latter case, and electromyography was consistent with inflammatory myopathy in both.

Vittaforma corneae, Nosema ocularum, and *Microsporidium* species not belonging to recognized genera have been identified in rare cases of keratitis with or without iritis in immunocompetent hosts (157) (see Table 284.1).

Diagnosis

Diagnosis of microsporidiosis requires demonstration of organisms in tissue, stool, or body fluids. Electron microscopic examination of tissue specimens remains the "gold standard" for species identification, but improvements in the sensitivity of various staining techniques that employ light microscopy have made testing for microsporidia easier and more accessible (155,176). With use of chromotrope-based stains (trichrome blue stain, Weber chromotrope stain) (196,197), spores appear pink and refractile, and some have a darker staining band along the shorter axis, making them distinct from other stained elements. With chemofluorescence (Uvitex 2B, calcofluor white 2MR), spore walls can be identified with fluorescence microscopy (198). Because nonmicrosporidial elements may be stained and the morphologic appearance is not distinctive, the specificity of chemofluorescence is suboptimal. Giemsa stains (160) are more useful for body fluid specimens than for stool. Immunofluorescent stains for *Encephalitozoon* species are under development (199,200). The relative sensitivity, specificity, and predictive value of the different diagnostic methods have not yet been determined, and the number of negative specimens needed to confirm a true negative result is unknown. Concentration of body fluid specimens may improve yield but has not been consistently helpful for stool specimens (166,197).

Studies suggest that stool examination is as sensitive as endoscopic biopsy for detection of microsporidia (155,165). Still, when microsporidiosis is suspected, despite negative findings on stool examination, small bowel biopsy is advisable. Although microsporidial infestation is frequently densest in the jejunum (165,174), biopsy of the duodenum often provides the diagnosis (163). Colonic biopsy is insensitive for microsporidiosis, although infection may be detected in the terminal ileum (201).

Light microscopic examination of histologic specimens for microsporidia is complicated by the small size of these organisms and the sometimes near-normal appearance of infected tissue (161,163). Hematoxylin-eosin and Giemsa stains are commonly used (160), although tissue Gram stains (e.g., Brown-Brenn) (166) or chromotrope stains (202) may provide increased contrast of microsporidia spores against surrounding tissue. Microsporidia have also been visualized on touch preparations of small intestinal biopsy specimens stained with Giemsa (203).

Encephalitozoon keratoconjunctival infection may be diagnosed with chromotrope or Giemsa staining of scrapings or smears from swabs of cornea or conjunctiva (200,204,205). Examination of urine or sputum for microsporidia may assist in diagnosis, even in the absence of urinary or respiratory symptoms.

Speciation of human microsporidia is useful clinically, because disease manifestations and responsiveness to therapy vary from species to species. However, speciation by light microscopy is difficult owing to the small size and similar shapes of these organisms. Whereas *Encephalitozoon* and *Nosema* species have been successfully cultured (188,205–207), the process is not useful for routine diagnosis. Serologic assays (195,208) and polymerase chain reaction method (207) have been developed.

Treatment

Therapeutic options for human microsporidiosis are few, and their effectiveness appears to vary among species. Controlled studies are lacking, and most of the available information is based on anecdotal data. To date, albendazole (at doses of 400 mg orally twice daily for a minimum of 4 weeks) has been the most successful agent used in the treatment of AIDS-related microsporidiosis; *E. intestinalis* and *E. cuniculi* are susceptible, *E. bieneusi* seems much less responsive (152,207,209). Even in responders, microsporidia may not be eradicated, and chronic maintenance therapy may be required (209). A placebo-controlled, multicenter trial of albendazole for intestinal microsporidiosis is under way. Metronidazole was associated with clinical improvement of *E. bieneusi* enteritis in one study, but parasite infestation was not affected, and subsequent investigations found no benefit (161,209). Atovaquone in patients with *E. bieneusi* infection was associated with improvement in diar-

rhea but limited reduction in parasite burden in one small series (210). Supportive measures to address chronic diarrhea, fluid and electrolyte loss, and malabsorption remain the principal component of management in most cases of intestinal microsporidiosis.

Improvement in *E. hellem* keratoconjunctivitis has been reported with topical fumagillin (211) and oral itraconazole (212) therapy, but controlled trials have not been performed.

DIENTAMOEBA FRAGILIS

D. fragilis was described by Weynon in 1915 and reported as a new species by Jepps and Dobell in 1918 (213). Although it is ubiquitous, *D. fragilis* is often overlooked by standard parasitologic techniques, and it remains poorly understood.

Characteristics of the Pathogen

D. fragilis appears to exist only in the trophozoite form. The lack of a cyst stage may account for the difficulty in identifying it on standard ova and parasite examinations. Although initially assigned to the phylum Sarcodina, it is now considered to be more closely related to the flagellate genera *Histomonas* and *Trichomonas* (214,215). The organism has an ameboid shape and measures 5 to 12 μm in diameter. It is binucleate, with central nuclear granules and cytoplasmic vacuoles.

Epidemiology

D. fragilis has a worldwide distribution, but its true prevalence is not known (215). It has been variously reported to be common and rare. Its frequency appears to be higher in studies that employ preserved stool specimens, permanently stained fecal smears, and multiple stool examinations. In various surveys in the United States, the prevalence of the parasite has ranged from 1.4% to 18.6% (214).

The mode of transmission of *D. fragilis* is not known. Dientamoebiasis rarely occurs in conjunction with the other parasitic enteritides that are typically transmitted by fecally contaminated food and water. Some researchers have suggested that *D. fragilis* may be transmitted by the ova of the human pinworm *Enterobius vermicularis* (215).

Pathology and Pathogenesis

D. fragilis may colonize the cecum and proximal large intestine but does not cause invasive disease. Local irritation has been suggested as the mechanism whereby it produces gastrointestinal symptoms (215).

Clinical Manifestations

Clinical disease occurs in 50% of infected adults and almost all infected children (215). Dientamoebiasis is not known to be more severe or more common in immunocompromised hosts. Symptoms are nonspecific and typically include intermittent diarrhea, cramping, and bloating. Biliary involvement may occur. Peripheral eosinophilia has been documented principally in children (216).

Diagnosis

Diagnosis requires demonstration of the *D. fragilis* trophozoite in stool; it is not detectable by biopsy. Specimens are optimal if they are submitted fresh for immediate processing or preserved in polyvinyl alcohol, sodium acetate-acetic acid-formalin, or Schaudinn fixative; other preservatives, such as formalin alone, may substantially lower the yield (213). Hematoxylin-Kinyoun or trichrome staining of stool smears facilitates detection (217). Multiple specimens obtained on different days may enhance the chances of finding this organism.

Treatment

As yet, no therapy for dientamoebiasis has been approved by the U.S. Food and Drug Administration; however, some benefit has been obtained from treatment with iodoquinol, 650 mg three times daily for 20 days (218); tetracycline, 500 mg four times daily for 10 days (214); or paromomycin, 25 to 30 mg/kg per day in three doses for 7 days (219).

ACKNOWLEDGMENT

This chapter contains information presented in Chapter 292 by Lawrence Davis and Rosemary Soave in the Second Edition of this book.

REFERENCES

1. Abdel-Maksoud NM, Dyab AK, Shatat MA. Immunological and parasitological studies of Cryptosporidium muris, Tyzzer (1907). *J Egypt Soc Parasitol* 1999;29:551–560.
2. Sischo WM, Atwill ER, Lanyon LE, George J. Cryptosporidia on dairy farms and the role these farms may have in contaminating surface water supplies in the northeastern United States. *Prev Vet Med* 2000;43:253–267.
3. Tzipori S, Larsen J, Smith M, Luefl RU. Diarrhoea in goat kids attributed to cryptosporidium infection. *Vet Rec* 1982;111:35–36.
4. Nime FA, Burek JD, Page DL, et al. Acute enterocolitis in a human being infected with the protozoan Cryptosporidium. *Gastroenterology* 1976;70:592–598.
5. Current WL, Reese NC, Ernst JV, et al. Human cryptosporidiosis in immunocompetent and immunodeficient persons. Studies of an outbreak and experimental transmission. *N Engl J Med* 1983;308:1252–1257.
6. Soave R, Danner RL, Honig CL, et al. Cryptosporidiosis in homosexual men. *Ann Intern Med* 1984;100:504–511.
7. Jokipii L, Pohjola S, Jokipii AM. Cryptosporidiosis associated with traveling and giardiasis. *Gastroenterology* 1985;89:838–842.
8. Flanigan TP, Soave R. Cryptosporidiosis. *Prog Clin Parasitol* 1993;3:1–20.
9. Wolfson JS, Richter JM, Waldron MA, et al. Cryptosporidiosis in immunocompetent patients. *N Engl J Med* 1985;312:1278–1282.
10. Fayer R, Ungar BL. Cryptosporidium spp. and cryptosporidiosis. *Microbiol Rev* 1986;50:458–483.
11. Janoff EN, Reller LB. Cryptosporidium species, a protean protozoan. *J Clin Microbiol* 1987;25:967–975.
12. Tzipori S. Cryptosporidiosis in perspective. *Adv Parasitol* 1988;27:63–129.
13. Crawford FG, Vermund SH. Human cryptosporidiosis. *Crit Rev Microbiol* 1988;16:113–159.
14. Soave R, Armstrong D. Cryptosporidium and cryptosporidiosis. *Rev Infect Dis* 1986;8:1012–1023.
15. Tzipori S, Angus KW, Campbell I, et al. Cryptosporidium: evidence for a single-species genus. *Infect Immun* 1980;30:884–886.
16. Xiao L, Bern C, Limor J, et al. Identification of 5 types of Cryptosporidium parasites in children in Lima, Peru. *J Infect Dis* 2001;183:492–497.
17. Hojlyng N, Holten-Andersen W, Jepsen S. Cryptosporidiosis: a case of airborne transmission. *Lancet* 1987;2:271–272.
18. Tzipori S, Griffiths JK. Natural history and biology of Cryptosporidium parvum. *Adv Parasitol* 1998;40:5–36.
19. Navin TR. Cryptosporidiosis in humans: review of recent epidemiologic studies. *Eur J Epidemiol* 1985;1:77–83.
20. Juranek DD. Cryptosporidiosis: sources of infection and guidelines for prevention. *Clin Infect Dis* 1995;21[Suppl 1]:S57–S61.
21. DuPont HL, Chappell CL, Sterling CR, et al. The infectivity of Cryptosporidium parvum in healthy volunteers. *N Engl J Med* 1995;332:855–859.
22. D'Antonio RG, Winn RE, Taylor JP, et al. A waterborne outbreak of cryptosporidiosis in normal hosts. *Ann Intern Med* 1985;103:886–888.
23. MacKenzie WR, Schell WL, Blair KA, et al. Massive outbreak of waterborne cryptosporidium infection in Milwaukee, Wisconsin: recurrence of illness and risk of secondary transmission. *Clin Infect Dis* 1995;21:57–62.
24. Wright MS, Collins PA. Waterborne transmission of cryptosporidium, cyclospora and giardia. *Clin Lab Sci* 1997;10:287–290.
25. Barwick RS, Levy DA, Craun GF, et al. Surveillance for waterborne-disease outbreaks—United States, 1997–1998. *MMWR* 2000;49:1–21.
26. Gallaher MM, Herndon JL, Nims LJ. Cryptosporidiosis and surface water. *Am J Public Health* 1989;79:39–42.
27. Joce RE, Bruce J, Kiely D, Noah ND, et al. An outbreak of cryptosporidiosis associated with a swimming pool. *Epidemiol Infect* 1991;107:497–508.
28. Cryptosporidium infections associated with swimming pools—Dane County, Wisconsin, 1993. *MMWR* 1994;43:561–563.
29. From the Centers for Disease Control and Prevention. Cryptosporidium infections associated with swimming pools-Dane County, Wisconsin, 1993. *JAMA* 1994;272:914–915.
30. Madore MS, Rose JB, Gerba CP, et al. Occurrence of cryptosporidium oocysts in sewage effluents and selected surface waters. *J Parasitol* 1987;73:702–705.
31. Millard PS, Gensheimer KF, Addiss DG, et al. An outbreak of cryptosporidiosis from fresh-pressed apple cider. *JAMA* 1994;272:1592–1596.
32. Foodborne outbreak of cryptosporidiosis—Spokane, Washington, 1997. *MMWR* 1998;47:565–567.
33. From the Centers for Disease Control and Prevention. Foodborne outbreak of diarrheal illness associated with *Cryptosporidium parvum*—Minnesota, 1995. *JAMA* 1996;276:1214.
34. Heijbel H, Slaine K, Seigel B, et al. Outbreak of diarrhea in a day care center with spread to household members: the role of cryptosporidium. *Pediatr Infect Dis J* 1987;6:532–535.
35. Dryjanski J, Gold JW, Ritchie MT, et al. Cryptosporidiosis. Case report in a health team worker. *Am J Med* 1986;80:751–752.
36. Cordell RL, Addiss DG. Cryptosporidiosis in child care settings: a review of the literature and recommendations for prevention and control. *Pediatr Infect Dis J* 1994;13:310–317.
37. Lengerich EJ, Addiss DG, Marx JJ, et al. Increased exposure to cryptosporidia among dairy farmers in Wisconsin. *J Infect Dis* 1993;167:1252–1255.
38. Miron D, Kenes J, Dagan R. Calves as a source of an outbreak of cryptosporidiosis among young children in an agricultural closed community. *Pediatr Infect Dis J* 1991;10:438–441.
39. Caprioli A, Gentile G, Baldassarri L, et al. Cryptosporidium as a common cause of childhood diarrhoea in Italy. *Epidemiol Infect* 1989;102:537–540.
40. Mata L, Bolanos H, Pizarro D, Vives M. Cryptosporidiosis in children from some highland Costa Rican rural and urban areas. *Am J Trop Med Hyg* 1984;33:24–29.
41. Ungar BL, Soave R, Fayer R, Nash TE. Enzyme immunoassay detection of immunoglobulin M and G antibodies to cryptosporidium in immunocompetent and immunocompromised persons. *J Infect Dis* 1986;153:570–578.
42. Ungar BL, Mulligan M, Nutman TB. Serologic evidence of cryptosporidium infection in US volunteers before and during Peace Corps service in Africa. *Arch Intern Med* 1989;149:894–897.
43. Navin TR, Juranek DD. Cryptosporidiosis: clinical, epidemiologic, and parasitologic review. *Rev Infect Dis* 1984;6:313–327.
44. Smith PD, Lane HC, Gill VJ, et al. Intestinal infections in patients with the acquired immunodeficiency syndrome (AIDS). Etiology and response to therapy. *Ann Intern Med* 1988;108:328–333.
45. Laughon BE, Druckman DA, Vernon A, et al. Prevalence of enteric pathogens in homosexual men with and without acquired immunodeficiency syndrome. *Gastroenterology* 1988;94:984–993.
46. Quinn TC, Mann JM, Curran JW, Piot P. AIDS in Africa: an epidemiologic paradigm. *Science* 1986;234:955–963.
47. Roberts WG, Green PH, Ma J, et al. Prevalence of cryptosporidiosis in patients undergoing endoscopy: evidence for an asymptomatic carrier state. *Am J Med* 1989;87:537–539.
48. Ortega YR, Sterling CR, Gilman RH, et al. Cyclospora species—a new protozoan pathogen of humans. *N Engl J Med* 1993;328:1308–1312.
49. Holley HP Jr, Dover C. Cryptosporidium: a common cause of parasitic diarrhea in otherwise healthy individuals. *J Infect Dis* 1986;153:365–368.
50. Guarda LA, Stein SA, Cleary KA, Ordonez NG. Human cryptosporidiosis in the acquired immune deficiency syndrome. *Arch Pathol Lab Med* 1983;107:562–566.
51. Lefkowitch JH, Krumholz S, Feng-Chen KC, et al. Cryptosporidiosis of the human small intestine: a light and electron microscopic study. *Hum Pathol* 1984;15:746–752.
52. Gentile G, Baldassarri L, Caprioli A, et al. Colonic vascular invasion as a possible route of extraintestinal cryptosporidiosis. *Am J Med* 1987;82:574–575.
53. Kocoshis SA, Cibull ML, Davis TE, et al. Intestinal and pulmonary cryptosporidiosis in an infant with severe combined immune deficiency. *J Pediatr Gastroenterol Nutr* 1984;3:149–157.
54. Miller RA, Wasserheit JN, Kirihara J, Coyle MB. Detection of cryptosporidium oocysts in sputum during screening for mycobacteria. *J Clin Microbiol* 1984;20:1192–1193.
55. Current WL, Garcia LS. Cryptosporidiosis. *Clin Lab Med* 1991;11:873–897.
56. Argenzio RA, Liacos JA, Levy ML, et al. Villous atrophy, crypt hyperplasia, cellular infiltration, and impaired glucose-Na absorption in enteric cryptosporidiosis of pigs. *Gastroenterology* 1990;98:1129–1140.

57. Guarino A, Canani RB, Pozio E, et al. Enterotoxic effect of stool supernatant of cryptosporidium-infected calves on human jejunum. *Gastroenterology* 1994;106:28–34.

58. Argenzio RA, Lecce J, Powell DW. Prostanoids inhibit intestinal NaCl absorption in experimental porcine cryptosporidiosis. *Gastroenterology* 1993;104:440–447.

59. Schneiderman DJ, Cello JP, Laing FC. Papillary stenosis and sclerosing cholangitis in the acquired immunodeficiency syndrome. *Ann Intern Med* 1987;106:546–549.

60. Gross TL, Wheat J, Bartlett M, O'Connor KW. AIDS and multiple system involvement with cryptosporidium. *Am J Gastroenterol* 1986;81:456–458.

61. Hawkins SP, Thomas RP, Teasdale C. Acute pancreatitis: a new finding in cryptosporidium enteritis. *BMJ* 1987;294:483–484.

62. Forgacs P, Tarshis A, Ma P, Federman M, et al. Intestinal and bronchial cryptosporidiosis in an immunodeficient homosexual man. *Ann Intern Med* 1983;99:793–794.

63. Mannheimer SB, Soave R. Protozoal infections in patients with AIDS. Cryptosporidiosis, isosporiasis, cyclosporiasis, and microsporidiosis. *Infect Dis Clin North Am* 1994;8:483–498.

64. Jokipii L, Jokipii AM. Timing of symptoms and oocyst excretion in human cryptosporidiosis. *N Engl J Med* 1986;315:1643–1647.

65. Soave R. Cryptosporidiosis and isosporiasis in patients with AIDS. *Infect Dis Clin North Am* 1988;2:485–493.

66. Margulis SJ, Honig CL, Soave R, et al. Biliary tract obstruction in the acquired immunodeficiency syndrome. *Ann Intern Med* 1986;105:207–210.

67. Garcia LS, Bruckner DA, Brewer TC, et al. Techniques for the recovery and identification of cryptosporidium oocysts from stool specimens. *J Clin Microbiol* 1983;18:185–190.

68. Ma P, Soave R. Three-step stool examination for cryptosporidiosis in 10 homosexual men with protracted watery diarrhea. *J Infect Dis* 1983;147:824–828.

69. MacPherson DW, McQueen R. Cryptosporidiosis: multiattribute evaluation of six diagnostic methods. *J Clin Microbiol* 1993;31:198–202.

70. Weitz JC. [Detection of fecal *Cryptosporidium parvum* antigens using an ELISA technique]. *Rev Med Child* 1995;123:330–333.

71. Garcia LS, Shum AC, Bruckner DA. Evaluation of a new monoclonal antibody combination reagent for direct fluorescence detection of giardia cysts and cryptosporidium oocysts in human fecal specimens. *J Clin Microbiol* 1992;30:3255–3257.

72. Campbell PN, Current WL. Demonstration of serum antibodies to cryptosporidium sp. in normal and immunodeficient humans with confirmed infections. *J Clin Microbiol* 1983;18:165–169.

73. Tzipori S, Campbell I. Prevalence of cryptosporidium antibodies in 10 animal species. *J Clin Microbiol* 1981;14:455–456.

74. Moss DM, Bennett SN, Arrowood MJ, et al. Kinetic and isotypic analysis of specific immunoglobulins from crew members with cryptosporidiosis on a U.S. Coast Guard cutter. *J Eukaryot Microbiol* 1994;41:52S–55S.

75. Gargala G, Delaunay A, Li X, et al. Efficacy of nitazoxanide, tizoxanide and tizoxanide glucuronide against cryptosporidium parvum development in sporozoite-infected HCT-8 enterocytic cells. *J Antimicrob Chemother* 2000;46:57–60.

76. Woods KM, Upton SJ. Efficacy of select antivirals against *Cryptosporidium parvum* in vitro. *FEMS Microbiol Lett* 1998;168:59–63.

77. McDonald V, Stables R, Warhurst DC, et al. In vitro cultivation of Cryptosporidium parvum and screening for anticryptosporidial drugs. *Antimicrob Agents Chemother* 1990;34:1498–1500.

78. Arrowood MJ, Mead JR, Xie L, You X. In vitro anticryptosporidial activity of dinitroaniline herbicides. *FEMS Microbiol Lett* 1996;136:245–249.

79. Ritchie DJ, Becker ES. Update on the management of intestinal cryptosporidiosis in AIDS. *Ann Pharmacother* 1994;28:767–778.

80. Moskovitz BL, Stanton TL, Kusmierek JJ. Spiramycin therapy for cryptosporidial diarrhoea in immunocompromised patients. *J Antimicrob Chemother* 1988;22[Suppl B]:189–191.

81. Sterling CR. Cryptosporidiosis: the treatment dilemma. *J Med Microbiol* 2000;49:207–208.

82. Saez-Llorens X, Odio CM, Umana MA, Morales MV. Spiramycin vs. placebo for treatment of acute diarrhea caused by cryptosporidium. *Pediatr Infect Dis J* 1989;8:136–140.

83. Wittenberg DF, Miller NM, van den EJ. Spiramycin is not effective in treating cryptosporidium diarrhea in infants: results of a double-blind randomized trial. *J Infect Dis* 1989;159:131–132.

84. Soave R, Havlir D, Lancaster D, et al. Azithromycin (AZ) therapy of AIDS-related cryptosporidial diarrhea (CD): a multicenter, placebo-controlled, double blind study (Abstr 405). New Orleans: Programs and Abstracts of the 33rd Interscience Conference on Antimicrobial Agents and Chemotherapy, 1993.

85. Soave R, Dieterich DT, Kotler D, et al. Oral diclazuril for cryptosporidiosis (Abstr 520). San Francisco: Programs of the Sixth International Conference on AIDS, 1990.

86. Scaglia M, Atzori C, Marchetti G, et al. Effectiveness of aminosidine (paromomycin) sulfate in chronic Cryptosporidium diarrhea in AIDS patients: an open, uncontrolled, prospective clinical trial. *J Infect Dis* 1994;170:1349–1350.

87. Hewitt RG, Yiannoutsos CT, Higgs ES, et al. Paromomycin: no more effective than placebo for treatment of cryptosporidiosis in patients with advanced human immunodeficiency virus infection. AIDS Clinical Trial Group. *Clin Infect Dis* 2000;31:1084–1092.

88. Davis AJ, Soave R, Dudley RE, et al. Nitazoxanide for AIDS-related cryptosporidial diarrhea: an open-label safety, efficacy and pharmacokinetic study (Abstr LM50). New Orleans: Interscience Conference on Antimicrobial Agents and Chemotherapy, 1996.

89. Saxon A, Weinstein W. Oral administration of bovine colostrum anti-cryptosporidia antibody fails to alter the course of human cryptosporidiosis. *J Parasitol* 1987;73:413–415.

90. Tzipori S, Roberton D, Cooper DA, White L. Chronic cryptosporidial diarrhoea and hyperimmune cow colostrums. *Lancet* 1987;2:344–345.

91. Ungar BL, Ward DJ, Fayer R, Quinn CA. Cessation of cryptosporidium-associated diarrhea in an acquired immunodeficiency syndrome patient after treatment with hyperimmune bovine colostrum. *Gastroenterology* 1990;98:486–489.

92. McMeeking A, Borkowsky W, Klesius et al. A controlled trial of bovine dialyzable leukocyte extract for cryptosporidiosis in patients with AIDS. *J Infect Dis* 1990;161:108–112.

93. Flanigan T, Whalen C, Turner J, et al. Cryptosporidium infection and CD4 counts. *Ann Intern Med* 1992;116:840–842.

94. Greenberg RE, Mir R, Bank S, Siegal FP. Resolution of intestinal cryptosporidiosis after treatment of AIDS with AZT. *Gastroenterology* 1989;97:1327–1330.

95. Cook DJ, Kelton JG, Stanisz AM, Collins SM. Somatostatin treatment for cryptosporidial diarrhea in a patient with the acquired immunodeficiency syndrome (AIDS). *Ann Intern Med* 1988;108:708–709.

96. Romeu J, Miro JM, Sirera G, et al. Efficacy of octreotide in the management of chronic diarrhoea in AIDS. *AIDS* 1991;5:1495–1499.

97. Fayer R. Effect of high temperature on infectivity of *Cryptosporidium parvum* oocysts in water. *Appl Environ Microbiol* 1994;60:2732–2735.

98. Soave R. Cryptosporidiosis and isosporiasis in patients with AIDS. *Infect Dis Clin North Am* 1988;2:485–493.

99. Brandborg LL, Goldberg SB, Breidenbach WC. Human coccidiosis—a possible cause of malabsorption. *N Engl J Med* 1970;283:1306–1313.

100. Lindsay DS, Dubey JP, Blagburn BL. Biology of *Isospora* spp. from humans, nonhuman primates, and domestic animals. *Clin Microbiol Rev* 1997;10:19–34.

101. Sorvillo FJ, Lieb LE, Seidel J, et al. Epidemiology of isosporiasis among persons with acquired immunodeficiency syndrome in Los Angeles County. *Am J Trop Med Hyg* 1995;53:656–659.

102. Prociv P, Luke R, Quayle P. Isosporiasis in the aboriginal population of Queensland. *Med J Aust* 1992;156:115–117.

103. Shaffer N, Moore L. Chronic travelers' diarrhea in a normal host due to *Isospora belli* [letter]. *J Infect Dis* 1989;159:596–597.

104. DeHovitz JA, Pape JW, Boncy M, et al. Clinical manifestations and therapy of *Isospora belli* infection in patients with the acquired immunodeficiency syndrome. *N Engl J Med* 1986;315:87–90.

105. Tarimo DS, Killewo JZ, Minjas JN, et al. Prevalence of intestinal parasites in adult patients with enteropathic AIDS in north-eastern Tanzania. *East Afr Med J* 1996;73:397–399.

106. Trier JS, Moxey PC, Schimmel EM, Robles E. Chronic intestinal coccidiosis in man: intestinal morphology and response to treatment. *Gastroenterology* 1974;66:923–935.

107. Dubey JP, Frenkel JK. Extra-intestinal stages of Isospora felis and I. rivolta (protozoa: eimeriidae) in cats. *J Protozool* 1972;19:89–92.

108. Restrepo C, Macher AM, Radany EH. Disseminated extraintestinal isosporiasis in a patient with acquired immune deficiency syndrome. *Am J Clin Pathol* 1987;87:536–542.

109. Benator DA, French AL, Beaudet LM, et al. *Isospora belli* infection associated with acalculous cholecystitis in a patient with AIDS. *Ann Intern Med* 1994;121:663–664.

110. Forthal DN, Guest SS. *Isospora belli* enteritis in three homosexual men. *Am J Trop Med Hyg* 1984;33:1060–1064.

111. Pape JW, Johnson WD Jr. *Isospora belli* infections. *Prog Clin Parasitol* 1991;2:119–127.

112. Liebman WM, Thaler MM, DeLorimier A, et al. Intractable diarrhea of infancy due to intestinal coccidiosis. *Gastroenterology* 1980;78:579–584.

113. Pape JW, Verdier RI, Johnson WD Jr. Treatment and prophylaxis of *Isospora belli* infection in patients with the acquired immunodeficiency syndrome. *N Engl J Med* 1989;320:1044–1047.

114. Weiss LM, Perlman DC, Sherman J, Tanowitz H, Wittner M. *Isospora belli* infection: treatment with pyrimethamine. *Ann Intern Med* 1988;109:474–475.

115. Musey KL, Chidiac C, Beaucaire G, et al. Effectiveness of roxithromycin for treating *Isospora belli* infection. *J Infect Dis* 1988;158:646.

116. Kayembe K, Desmet P, Henry MC, et al. Diclazuril for *Isospora belli* infection in AIDS. *Lancet* 1989;1:1397–1398.

117. Ma P, Kaufman D, Montana J. *Isospora belli* diarrheal infection in homosexual men. *AIDS Res* 1983;1:327–338.

118. Soave R, Dubey JP, Ramos LJ, Tummings M. A new intestinal pathogen? *Clin Res* 1986;34:533A.

119. Ashford RW. Occurrence of an undescribed coccidian in man in Papua New Guinea. *Ann Trop Med Parasitol* 1979;73:497–500.

120. Outbreaks of diarrheal illness associated with cyanobacteria (blue-green-algae)-like bodies—Chicago and Nepal, 1989 and 1990. *MMWR* 1991;40:325–327.

121. Hoge CW, Shlim DR, Rajah R, et al. Epidemiology of diarrhoeal illness associated with coccidian-like organisms among travellers and foreign residents in Nepal. *Lancet* 1993;341:1175–1179.
122. Ortega YR, Sterling CR, Gilman RH, et al. Cyclospora species—a new protozoan pathogen of humans. *N Engl J Med* 1993;328:1308–1312.
123. Shlim DR, Cohen MT, Eaton M, et al. An alga-like organism associated with an outbreak of prolonged diarrhea among foreigners in Nepal. *Am J Trop Med Hyg* 1991;45:383–389.
124. Ortega YR, Gilman RH, Sterling CR. A new coccidian parasite (Apicomplexa: Eimeriidae) from humans. *J Parasitol* 1994;80:625–629.
125. Soave R. Cyclospora: an overview. *Clin Infect Dis* 1996;23:429–435.
126. Taylor AP, Davis LJ, Soave R. Cyclospora. *Curr Clin Top Infect Dis* 1997;17:256–268.
127. Eberhard ML, da Silva AJ, Lilley BG, et al. Morphologic and molecular characterization of new cyclospora species from Ethiopian monkeys: *C. cercopitheci* sp.n., *C. colobi* sp.n., and *C. papionis* sp.n. *Emerg Infect Dis* 1999;5:651–658.
128. Ortega YR, Nagle R, Gilman RH, et al. Pathologic and clinical findings in patients with cyclosporiasis and a description of intracellular parasite life-cycle stages. *J Infect Dis* 1997;176:1584–1589.
129. Eberhard ML, Ortega YR, Hanes DE, et al. Attempts to establish experimental *Cyclospora cayetanensis* infection in laboratory animals. *J Parasitol* 2000;86:577–582.
130. Long EG, White EH, Carmichael WW, et al. Morphologic and staining characteristics of a cyanobacterium-like organism associated with diarrhea. *J Infect Dis* 1991;164:199–202.
131. Albert MJ, Kabir I, Azim T, et al. Diarrhea associated with Cyclospora Sp. in Bangladesh. *Diagn Microbiol Infect Dis* 1994;19:47–49.
132. Pape JW, Verdier RI, Boncy M, et al. Cyclospora infection in adults infected with HIV. Clinical manifestations, treatment, and prophylaxis. *Ann Intern Med* 1994;121:654–657.
133. Ooi WW, Zimmerman SK, Needham CA. Cyclospora species as a gastrointestinal pathogen in immunocompetent hosts. *J Clin Microbiol* 1995;33:1267–1269.
134. Clarke SC, McIntyre M. The incidence of *Cyclospora cayetanensis* in stool samples submitted to a district general hospital. *Epidemiol Infect* 1996;117:189–193.
135. Outbreaks of *Cyclospora cayetanensis* infection—United States, 1996. *MMWR Morb.Mortal.Wkly.Rep.* 1996;45:549-51.
136. Update: outbreaks of Cyclospora cayetanensis infection—United States and Canada, 1996. *MMWR* 1996;45:611–612.
137. Herwaldt BL, Ackers ML. An outbreak in 1996 of cyclosporiasis associated with imported raspberries. The Cyclospora Working Group. *N Engl J Med* 1997;336:1548–1556.
138. Lopez AS, Dodson DR, Arrowood MJ, et al. Outbreak of cyclosporiasis associated with basil in Missouri in 1999. *Clin Infect Dis* 2001;32:1010–1017.
139. Chalmers RM, Nichols G, Rooney R. Foodborne outbreaks of cyclosporiasis have arisen in North America. Is the United Kingdom at risk? *Commun Dis Public Health* 2000;3:50–55.
140. Rabold JG, Hoge CW, Shlim DR, et al. Cyclospora outbreak associated with chlorinated drinking water. *Lancet* 1994;344:1360–1361.
141. Connor BA, Reidy J, Soave R. Cyclosporiasis: clinical and histopathologic correlates. *Clin Infect Dis* 1999;28:1216–1222.
142. Bendall RP, Lucas S, Moody A, et al. Diarrhoea associated with cyanobacterium-like bodies: a new coccidian enteritis of man. *Lancet* 1993;341:590–592.
143. Sifuentes-Osornio J, Porras-Cortes G, Bendall RP, et al. *Cyclospora cayetanensis* infection in patients with and without AIDS: biliary disease as another clinical manifestation. *Clin Infect Dis* 1995;21:1092–1097.
144. Madico G, Gilman RH, Miranda E, et al. Treatment of cyclospora infections with co-trimoxazole. *Lancet* 1993;342:122–123.
145. Berlin OG, Novak SM, Porschen RK, et al. Recovery of cyclospora organisms from patients with prolonged diarrhea. *Clin Infect Dis* 1994;18:606–609.
146. Hoge CW, Shlim DR, Ghimire M, et al. Placebo-controlled trial of co-trimoxazole for Cyclospora infections among travellers and foreign residents in Nepal. *Lancet* 1995;345:691–693.
147. Wurtz R, Kocka F, Peters CS, et al. Clinical characteristics of seven cases of diarrhea associated with a novel acid-fast organism in the stool. *Clin Infect Dis* 1993;16:136–138.
148. Hart AS, Ridinger MT, Soundarajan R, et al. Novel organism associated with chronic diarrhoea in AIDS. *Lancet* 1990;335:169–170.
149. Visvesvara GS, Moura H, Kovacs-Nace E, et al. Uniform staining of cyclospora oocysts in fecal smears by a modified safranin technique with microwave. *J Clin Microbiol* 1997;35:730–733.
150. Verdier RI, Fitzgerald DW, Johnson WD Jr, Pape JW. Trimethoprim-sulfamethoxazole compared with ciprofloxacin for treatment and prophylaxis of *Isospora belli* and *Cyclospora cayetanensis* infection in HIV-infected patients. A randomized, controlled trial. *Ann Intern Med* 2000;132:885–888.
151. Berg J, Diaz LE, Bender BS. Microsporidia in humans. *Ann Intern Med* 1996;125:522–523.
152. Asmuth DM, DeGirolami PC, Federman M, et al. Clinical features of microsporidiosis in patients with AIDS. *Clin Infect Dis* 1994;18:819–825.
153. Bryan RT, Cali A, Owen RL, Spencer HC. Microsporidia: opportunistic pathogens in patients with AIDS. *Prog Clin Parasitol* 1991;2:1–26.
154. Mannheimer SB, Soave R. Protozoal infections in patients with AIDS. Cryptosporidiosis, isosporiasis, cyclosporiasis, and microsporidiosis. *Infect Dis Clin North Am* 1994;8:483–498.
155. Weber R, Bryan RT, Schwartz DA, Owen RL. Human microsporidial infections. *Clin Microbiol Rev* 1994;7:426–461.
156. Hartskeerl RA, van Gool T, Schuitema AR, et al. Genetic and immunological characterization of the microsporidian septata intestinalis cali, kotler and orenstein, 1993: reclassification to encephalitozoon intestinalis. *Parasitology* 1995;110(Pt 3):277–285.
157. Silveira H, Canning EU. Vittaforma corneae n. comb. for the human microsporidium nosema corneum shadduck, meccoli, davis and font, 1990, based on its ultrastructure in the liver of experimentally infected athymic mice. *J Eukaryot Microbiol* 1995;42:158–165.
158. Hollister WS, Canning EU, Weidner E, et al. Development and ultrastructure of trachipleistophora hominis n.g., n.sp. after in vitro isolation from an AIDS patient and inoculation into athymic mice. *Parasitology* 1996;112(Pt 1):143–154.
159. Cali A. General microsporidian features and recent findings on AIDS isolates. *J Protozool* 1991;38:625–630.
160. Bryan RT, Weber R. Microsporidia. Emerging pathogens in immunodeficient persons. *Arch Pathol Lab Med* 1993;117:1243–1245.
161. Eeftinck Schattenkerk JK, van Gool T, van Ketel RJ, et al. Clinical significance of small-intestinal microsporidiosis in HIV-1- infected individuals. *Lancet* 1991;337:895–898.
162. Kotler DP, Francisco A, Clayton F, et al. Small intestinal injury and parasitic diseases in AIDS. *Ann Intern Med* 1990;113:444–449.
163. Molina JM, Sarfati C, Beauvais B, et al. Intestinal microsporidiosis in human immunodeficiency virus-infected patients with chronic unexplained diarrhea: prevalence and clinical and biologic features. *J Infect Dis* 1993;167:217–221.
164. Orenstein JM, Chiang J, Steinberg W, et al. Intestinal microsporidiosis as a cause of diarrhea in human immunodeficiency virus-infected patients: a report of 20 cases. *Hum Pathol* 1990;21:475–481.
165. Kotler DP, Orenstein JM. Prevalence of intestinal microsporidiosis in HIV-infected individuals referred for gastroenterological evaluation. *Am J Gastroenterol* 1994;89:1998–2002.
166. Weber R, Bryan RT, Owen RL, et al. Improved light-microscopical detection of microsporidia spores in stool and duodenal aspirates. The Enteric Opportunistic Infections Working Group. *N Engl J Med* 1992;326:161–166.
167. Rabeneck L, Gyorkey F, Genta RM, et al. The role of microsporidia in the pathogenesis of HIV-related chronic diarrhea. *Ann Intern Med* 1993;119:895–899.
168. Avery SW, Undeen AH. The isolation of microsporidia and other pathogens from concentrated ditch water. *J Am Mosq Control Assoc* 1987;3:54–58.
169. Hunter PR. Waterborne outbreak of microsporidiosis. *J Infect Dis* 2000; 182:380–381.
170. Cotte L, Rabodonirina M, Chapuis F, et al. Waterborne outbreak of intestinal microsporidiosis in persons with and without human immunodeficiency virus infection. *J Infect Dis* 1999;180:2003–2008.
171. Shadduck JA, Greeley E. Microsporidia and human infections. *Clin Microbiol Rev* 1989;2:158–165.
172. Canning EU, Hollister WS. Enterocytozoon bieneusi (microspora): prevalence and pathogenicity in AIDS patients. *Trans R Soc Trop Med Hyg* 1990;84:181–186.
173. Desportes-Livage I, Chilmonczyk S, Hedrick R, et al. Comparative development of two microsporidian species: *Enterocytozoon bieneusi* and *Enterocytozoon salmonis*, reported in AIDS patients and salmonid fish, respectively. *J Eukaryot Microbiol* 1996;43:49–60.
174. Kotler DP, Reka S, Chow K, Orenstein JM. Effects of enteric parasitoses and HIV infection upon small intestinal structure and function in patients with AIDS. *J Clin Gastroenterol* 1993;16:10–15.
175. Orenstein JM, Tenner M, Kotler DP. Localization of infection by the microsporidian *Enterocytozoon bieneusi* in the gastrointestinal tract of AIDS patients with diarrhea. *AIDS* 1992;6:195–197.
176. Pol S, Romana CA, Richard S, et al. Microsporidia infection in patients with the human immunodeficiency virus and unexplained cholangitis. *N Engl J Med* 1993;328:95–99.
177. Orenstein JM. Microsporidiosis in the acquired immunodeficiency syndrome. *J Parasitol* 1991;77:843–864.
178. McWhinney PH, Nathwani D, Green ST, et al. Microsporidiosis detected in association with AIDS-related sclerosing cholangitis. *AIDS* 1991;5:1394–1395.
179. Weber R, Kuster H, Keller R, et al. Pulmonary and intestinal microsporidiosis in a patient with the acquired immunodeficiency syndrome. *Am Rev Respir Dis* 1992;146:1603–1605.
180. Cali A, Kotler DP, Orenstein JM. Septata intestinalis N. G., N. Sp., an intestinal microsporidian associated with chronic diarrhea and dissemination in AIDS patients. *J Eukaryot Microbiol* 1993;40:101–112.
181. Orenstein JM, Tenner M, Cali A, et al. A microsporidian previously undescribed in humans, infecting enterocytes and macrophages, and associated with diarrhea in an acquired immunodeficiency syndrome patient. *Hum Pathol* 1992;23:722–728.
182. Orenstein JM, Dieterich DT, Kotler DP. Systemic dissemination by a newly recognized intestinal microsporidia species in AIDS. *AIDS* 1992;6:1143–1150.

183. Didier ES, Rogers LB, Orenstein JM, et al. Characterization of encephalitozoon (septata) intestinalis isolates cultured from nasal mucosa and bronchoalveolar lavage fluids of two AIDS patients. *J Eukaryot Microbiol* 1996;43:34–43.
184. Field AS, Hing MC, Milliken ST, Marriott DJ. Microsporidia in the small intestine of HIV-infected patients. A new diagnostic technique and a new species. *Med J Aust* 1993;158:390–394.
185. Cali A, Meisler DM, Lowder CY, Lembach R, et al. Corneal microsporidioses: characterization and identification. *J Protozool* 1991;38:215S–217S.
186. Friedberg DN, Stenson SM, Orenstein JM, et al. Microsporidial kerato-conjunctivitis in acquired immunodeficiency syndrome. *Arch Ophthalmol* 1990;108:504–508.
187. Metcalfe TW, Doran RM, Rowlands PL, et al. Microsporidial keratoconjunctivitis in a patient with AIDS. *Br J Ophthalmol* 1992;76:177–178.
188. Didier PJ, Didier ES, Orenstein JM, et al A. Fine structure of a new human microsporidian, *Encephalitozoon hellem*, in culture. *J Protozool* 1991;38:502–507.
189. Hollister WS, Canning EU, Colbourn NI, et al. Characterization of *Encephalitozoon hellem* (Microspora) isolated from the nasal mucosa of a patient with AIDS. *Parasitology* 1993;107(Pt 4):351–358.
190. Schwartz DA, Bryan RT, Hewan-Lowe KO, et al. Disseminated microsporidiosis (*Encephalitozoon hellem*) and acquired immunodeficiency syndrome. Autopsy evidence for respiratory acquisition. *Arch Pathol Lab Med* 1992;116:660–668.
191. Terada S, Reddy KR, Jeffers LJ, et al. Microsporidan hepatitis in the acquired immunodeficiency syndrome. *Ann Intern Med* 1987;107:61–62.
192. Zender HO, Arrigoni E, Eckert J, et al. A case of *Encephalitozoon cuniculi* peritonitis in a patient with AIDS. *Am J Clin Pathol* 1989;92:352–356.
193. Chupp GL, Alroy J, Adelman LS, et al. Myositis due to pleistophora (microsporidia) in a patient with AIDS. *Clin Infect Dis* 1993;16:15–21.
194. Weber R, Sauer B, Luthy R, et al. Intestinal coinfection with *Enterocytozoon bieneusi* and *Cryptosporidium* in a human immunodeficiency virus-infected child with chronic diarrhea. *Clin Infect Dis* 1993;17:480–483.
195. Bergquist NR, Stintzing G, Smedman L, et al. Diagnosis of encephalitozoonosis in man by serological tests. *BMJ* 1984;288:902.
196. Ryan NJ, Sutherland G, Coughlan K, et al. A new trichrome-blue stain for detection of microsporidial species in urine, stool, and nasopharyngeal specimens. *J Clin Microbiol* 1993;31:3264–3269.
197. van Gool T, Canning EU, Dankert J. An improved practical and sensitive technique for the detection of microsporidian spores in stool samples. *Trans R Soc Trop Med Hyg* 1994;88:189–190.
198. van Gool T, Snijders F, Reiss P, et al. Diagnosis of intestinal and disseminated microsporidial infections in patients with HIV by a new rapid fluorescence technique. *J Clin Pathol* 1993;46:694–699.
199. Aldras AM, Orenstein JM, et al. Detection of microsporidia by indirect immunofluorescence antibody test using polyclonal and monoclonal antibodies. *J Clin Microbiol* 1994;32:608–612.
200. Schwartz DA, Visvesvara GS, Diesenhouse MC, et al. Pathologic features and immunofluorescent antibody demonstration of ocular microsporidiosis (*Encephalitozoon hellem*) in seven patients with acquired immunodeficiency syndrome. *Am J Ophthalmol* 1993;115:285–292.
201. Weber R, Muller A, Spycher MA, et al. Intestinal Enterocytozoon bieneusi microsporidiosis in an HIV-infected patient: diagnosis by ileo-colonoscopic biopsies and long-term follow up. *Clin Invest* 1992;70:1019–1023.
202. Moura H, Schwartz DA, Bornay-Llinares F, et al. A new and improved "quick-hot Gram-chromotrope" technique that differentially stains microsporidian spores in clinical samples, including paraffin-embedded tissue sections. *Arch Pathol Lab Med* 1997;121:888–893.
203. Visvesvara GS, Leitch GJ, Moura H, et al. Culture, electron microscopy, and immunoblot studies on a microsporidian parasite isolated from the urine of a patient with AIDS. *J Protozool* 1991;38:105S–111S.
204. Weber R, Kuster H, Visvesvara GS, et al. Disseminated microsporidiosis due to *Encephalitozoon hellem*: pulmonary colonization, microhematuria, and mild conjunctivitis in a patient with AIDS. *Clin Infect Dis* 1993;17:415–419.
205. Schwartz DA, Visvesvara GS, Leitch GJ, et al. Pathology of symptomatic microsporidial (*Encephalitozoon hellem*) bronchiolitis in the acquired immunodeficiency syndrome: a new respiratory pathogen diagnosed from lung biopsy, bronchoalveolar lavage, sputum, and tissue culture. *Hum Pathol* 1993;24:937–943.
206. Shadduck JA, Meccoli RA, Davis R, et al. Isolation of a microsporidian from a human patient. *J Infect Dis* 1990;162:773–776.
207. De Groote MA, Visvesvara G, Wilson ML, et al. Polymerase chain reaction and culture confirmation of disseminated *Encephalitozoon cuniculi* in a patient with AIDS: successful therapy with albendazole. *J Infect Dis* 1995;171:1375–1378.
208. Weiss LM, Cali A, Levee E, et al. Diagnosis of *Encephalitozoon cuniculi* infection by western blot and the use of cross-reactive antigens for the possible detection of microsporidiosis in humans. *Am J Trop Med Hyg* 1992;47:456–462.
209. Blanshard C, Ellis DS, Tovey DG, et al. Treatment of intestinal microsporidiosis with albendazole in patients with AIDS. *AIDS* 1992;6:311–313.
210. Anwar-Bruni DM, Hogan SE, Schwartz DA, et al. Atovaquone is effective treatment for the symptoms of gastrointestinal microsporidiosis in HIV-1-infected patients. *AIDS* 1996;10:619–623.
211. Diesenhouse MC, Wilson LA, Corrent GF, et al. Treatment of microsporidial keratoconjunctivitis with topical fumagillin. *Am J Ophthalmol* 1993;115:293–298.
212. Yee RW, Tio FO, Martinez JA, et al. Resolution of microsporidial epithelial keratopathy in a patient with AIDS. *Ophthalmology* 1991;98:196–201.
213. Shein R, Gelb A. Colitis due to *Dientamoeba fragilis*. *Am J Gastroenterol* 1983;78:634–636.
214. Kean BH, Malloch CL. The neglected ameba: dientamoeba fragilis. A report of 100 "pure" infections. *Am J Dig Dis* 1966;11:735–746.
215. Yang J, Scholten T. *Dientamoeba fragilis*: a review with notes on its epidemiology, pathogenicity, mode of transmission, and diagnosis. *Am J Trop Med Hyg* 1977;26:16–22.
216. Spencer MJ, Garcia LS, Chapin MR. *Dientamoeba fragilis*. An intestinal pathogen in children? *Am J Dis Child* 1979;133:390–393.
217. Grendon JH, DiGiacomo RF, Frost FJ. *Dientamoeba fragilis* detection methods and prevalence: a survey of state public health laboratories. *Public Health Rep* 1991;106:322–325.
218. Millet V, Spencer MJ, Chapin M, et al. *Dientamoeba fragilis*, a protozoan parasite in adult members of a semicommunal group. *Dig Dis Sci* 1983;28:335–339.
219. Simon M, Shookhoff HB, Terner H, et al. Paromomycin in the treatment of intestinal amebiasis; a short course of therapy. *Am J Gastroenterol* 1967;48:504–511.
220. Matsubayashi M, Koike T, Mikata T, et al. A case of encephalitozoon-like body infection in man. *Arch Pathol* 1959;67:181.
221. Sandfort J, Hannemann A, Gelderblom H, et al. *Enterocytozoon bieneusi* infection in an immunocompetent patient who had acute diarrhea and who was not infected with the human immunodeficiency virus. *Clin Infect Dis* 1994;19:514–516.
222. Ledford DK, Overman MD, Gonzalvo A, et al. Microsporidiosis myositis in a patient with the acquired immunodeficiency syndrome. *Ann Intern Med* 1985;102:628–630.
223. Margileth AM, Strano AJ, Chandra R, et al. Disseminated nosematosis in an immunologically compromised infant. *Arch Pathol* 1973;95:145–150.
224. Pinnolis M, Egbert PR, Font RL, Winter FC. Nosematosis of the cornea. Case report, including electron microscopic studies. *Arch Ophthalmol* 1981;99:1044–1047.
225. Ashton N, Wirasinha PA. Encephalitozoonosis (nosematosis) of the cornea. *Br J Ophthalmol* 1973;57:669–674.

Other Parasites

CHAPTER 285
Intestinal Nematodes

Michael V. Callahan and Davidson H. Hamer

The phylum Nematoda includes both free-living and parasitic species, which are widely distributed in nature. The diseases they cause rank among the most prevalent communicable infections, with more than one billion people worldwide infected (1). The geographic distribution of roundworms in many tropical and subtropical regions closely parallels socioeconomic and sanitary conditions. In certain locales, coinfection with *Ascaris lumbricoides*, *Trichuris trichiura*, and hookworms is common. Although many subjects are asymptomatic, those with a high worm burden, especially children, may suffer significant morbidity including anemia, malnutrition, and impaired physical and cognitive development. Constant reinfection is common in most endemic areas; thus, periodic treatment regimens that result in reductions in parasitic burden may be more practical than attempts to completely eliminate infection.

Understanding the life cycles of roundworms responsible for human infection provides a basis for appreciating the epidemiology of infections and the correlation between clinical findings and pathological effects of infection. The roundworms are true geohelminths, which have no intermediate host but have eggs, or in the case of *Strongyloides*, larva and adults which may survive in soil for days to years. Certain species, such as *Enterobius*, lack

TABLE 285.1. Life Cycle Characteristics of the Major Intestinal Nematodes

Organism	Mode of transmission	Infective stage	Host tissue involved	Final habitat	Typical life span
Trichuris trichiura	Oral	Eggs	Intestine	Cecum, ascending colon	1–2 y
Ascaris lumbricoides	Oral	Eggs	Lung, intestine	Jejunum, ileum	1–2 y
Ancylostoma duodenale	Percutaneous, oral	Filariform larvae	Skin, lung, intestine	Jejunum	5 y
Necator americanus	Percutaneous	Filariform larvae	Skin, lung, intestine	Jejunum	4 y
Enterobius vermicularis	Oral	Eggs	Intestine	Colon	37–93 d
Strongyloides stercoralis	Percutaneous, autoinfection	Filariform larvae	Skin, lung, intestine	Duodenum, jejunum	Unknown

a soil phase and can be readily transmitted from person to person, whereas other species must undergo a cycle of maturation outside of the human host before they are capable of infection. The pathologic consequences of infection with individual nematode species result from interactions between certain stages of the organism and the host's immune responses. Relevant aspects of the life cycles of the major intestinal nematodes are outlined in Table 285.1. Nematodes reproduce sexually; species identification is frequently dependent on the adult worm's morphologic features although many species can be identified by microscopic examination of the ova. With the exceptions of *Strongyloides stercoralis* and *Capillaria philippinensis*, intestinal nematodes are not capable of multiplying within their respective host.

TRICHURIASIS (*TRICHURIS TRICHIURA*)

Trichuris trichiura is commonly known as the whipworm because of the characteristic shape of the adult worm. It is responsible for an estimated one billion human infections worldwide (1), with the greatest frequency in regions that have warm, moist environments. In certain parts of Southeast Asia, sub-Saharan Africa, and some Caribbean island communities, the prevalence of trichuriasis approaches 100% (1–3). Polyparasitism with *Ascaris* and hookworms is common. Children tend to have a greater intensity of infection than do adults living in the same environment and are thus more likely to be symptomatic and to suffer ill consequences.

Life Cycle

Humans are the only recognized host of *T. trichuris*, and infection is acquired by direct transmission through the oral route. Although other species of *Trichuris* have been found in a number of mammalian species, they appear to maintain host specificity with the possible exception of *Trichuris vulpis*, a canine species, which has been rarely described as a cause of human infection (4). Adult worms reside in the cecum and transverse and descending colon; involvement of the sigmoid and rectum occurs in heavy infections. The white to gray-colored female worm has an estimated life span of 1 to 2 years, measures between 35 to 50 mm in length, and produces 3,000 to 10,000 eggs per day (2). When viewed in-situ, the thin whip-like anterior region of the worm appears to disrupt the colonic mucosa; however, minimal epithelial disruption and inflammation are visible on histopathologic examination.

After excretion in feces, the eggs require about 21 days to embryonate and form an infectious first-stage larva. After a new host ingests the embryonated egg, it hatches to release a larva in the small intestine, which subsequently undergoes four molts.

The immature adult is passively transported to the large intestine, where the long, narrow, anterior portion of its body embeds in the intestinal mucosa. The complete cycle takes approximately 90 days from the time of egg ingestion to the production of new ova by mature worms.

Epidemiology

Infection with *T. trichiura* is most common in areas of the world that are impoverished and lack adequate sanitary facilities. Soil pollution by infected human feces is integral to the continued spread of this ubiquitous organism. Infection results from ingestion of embryonated eggs after direct contamination of hands, food, or drink with infested soil or indirect transmission by insects, domestic animals, or dust. Given appropriate conditions, *Trichuris* eggs can survive for prolonged periods in moist soil. The intensity of infection in many individuals is light. Young children tend to have heavier worm burdens and, consequently, are more likely to be symptomatic.

The prevalence of trichuriasis ranges from 1% in the United States, Western Europe, and Japan to as high as 80% in certain regions of the developing world. Treatment and control measures initiated earlier in this century resulted in significant reductions in the prevalence of this infection in the United States (5). Nevertheless, moderate rates of infection persist in rural areas of the Southeast, in young Puerto Rican children, and in recent immigrants.

Clinical Manifestations

Most *T. trichiura* infections are asymptomatic, with the parasite discovered only on routine stool examinations. Heavy, chronic infections tend to occur most frequently in young children, primarily in the 4- to 10-year age range (2). A chronic dysentery syndrome may develop, characterized by protracted bloody diarrhea, abdominal pain, nausea, vomiting, iron deficiency anemia, and protracted tenesmus leading to rectal prolapse (6). Prolonged infections may lead to pica, clubbing, severe malnutrition, stunting of growth, and congestive heart failure secondary to severe anemia. Eosinophilia is relatively uncommon. Specific antihelminthic chemotherapy results in the resolution of these long-term complications, although reinfection is common.

The anemia associated with trichuriasis, although generally less intense than hookworm anemia, may still be severe. Hemorrhage appears to result from local mucosal damage at the site of attachment, but the worm is unable to ingest blood directly because of its capillary esophagus. An estimated 0.005 mL of blood is lost daily for each adult worm (7). Although this rate of blood loss may not be sufficient to cause severe anemia, the presence of malnutrition and polyparasitism may predispose children to its development.

TABLE 285.2. Diagnosis and Treatment of Major Intestinal Nematode Infections

Organism	Type of specimen	Specimen preparation	Size of eggs or larvae (μm)	Drug of choice	Alternative therapies
Trichuris trichiura	Stool	Direct smear or concentration	50–54 × 23	Mebendazole, 100 mg orally (PO) twice daily (bid) × 3 d or albendazole[a] 400 mg PO qd × 3 d	Albendazole[a] 400 mg PO once is effective for milder infections
Ascaris lumbricoides	Stool	Direct smear or concentration	45–70 × 35–50	Mebendazole, 100 mg PO bid × 3 d *or* Albendazole,[a] 400 mg PO once *or* Pyrantel pamoate, 11 mg/kg PO once (max 1 g)	Piperazine citrate, 75 mg/kg bid (max 1 g) by nasogastric tube × 2–3 d until resolution of obstruction
Ancylostoma duodenale Necator americanus	Stool	Direct smear or concentration	55–70 × 35–45	Mebendazole, 100 mg PO bid × 3 d *or* Albendazole,[a] 400 mg PO once	Pyrantel pamoate, 11 mg/kg PO × 3 d (max 1 g)
Enterobius vermicularis	Adhesive tape preparation	Direct microscopy	50–60 × 20–30	Mebendazole, 100 mg PO once *or* Pyrantel pamoate, 11 mg/kg PO once Repeat in 2 wk	Albendazole,[a] 400 mg PO once Repeat in 2 wk
Strongyloides stercoralis	Stool, duodenal aspirate	Concentration or Baermann method	400–500 × 15	Ivermectin, 150–200 μg/kg PO × 1–2 d	Thiabendazole, 25 mg/kg PO bid × 2 d (max 3 g/d)

[a]Drug has received approval from the U.S. Food and Drug Administration only for the treatment of neurocysticercosis and echinococcosis in the United States.

Diagnosis

The diagnosis is established by the demonstration of characteristic lemon-shaped ova on fecal examination (Table 285.2). The ova have a characteristic barrel shape with a thick outer shell and two terminal polar plugs (Fig. 285.1). A simple fecal smear is usually adequate for identification because large numbers of eggs are consistently excreted by infected hosts. Although the diagnosis can usually be made with a single specimen, the evaluation of multiple stools is warranted given the high frequency of coinfection with pathogenic protozoa. Heavy infection with

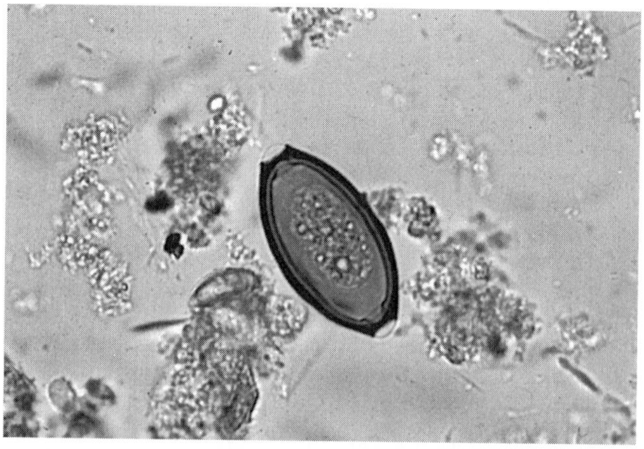

Figure 285.1. *Trichuris trichiura* unembryonated egg. Note the absence of a larva. Embryonization takes place in soil and usually takes 2 to 4 weeks to be completed. (40 × 10 μm.)

T. trichiura can be detected by anoscopic visualization of worms embedded in the rectal mucosa (8).

Treatment

Early chemotherapeutic agents for the treatment of this infection including hexylresorcinol enemas, dithiazanine, and thiabendazole were only partially effective. The benzimidazoles mebendazole and albendazole are currently the treatments of choice for trichuriasis (see Table 285.2). As these drugs are minimally absorbed from the gastrointestinal (GI) tract and therefore well tolerated, they do not require dosage adjustment for weight. Despite a relatively safe therapeutic index, benzimidazoles are not recommended in pregnancy and children younger than 1 year because of possible toxic and teratogenic effects. A 3-day course of mebendazole or albendazole is highly effective, although rare treatment failures may require an additional round of therapy. Single-dose treatment regimens with albendazole are convenient for control programs and may result in significant improvements in physical fitness, appetite, and growth in infected children (9). Although single-dose treatment regimens are useful in milder infections, triple-dose therapy with albendazole is more effective in reducing the prevalence of trichuriasis (10).

Prevention

Sanitary disposal of human feces is vital to the disruption of this parasite's life cycle. Contamination of produce with human excreta used for fertilization also serves to propagate the organism. Although the eggs are relatively resistant to chemical disinfectants, they can be destroyed by exposure to direct sunlight for

12 hours or to temperatures below −80°C and above 40°C for 1 hour.

ASCARIASIS

The roundworm *A. lumbricoides* has a cosmopolitan distribution and is estimated to infect one fourth of the world's population (1). The highest prevalence is in tropical regions, especially in Asia. Although most infections are asymptomatic, *A. lumbricoides* can cause significant morbidity, including pulmonary disease during larval migration, malabsorption, intestinal obstruction, biliary or pancreatic disease, and growth retardation.

The adult worms (Fig. 285.2), which may attain a length of up to 40 cm, reside in the small intestine, mainly in the jejunum and ileum. They maintain their position by continuously moving against peristalsis. The worms secrete an antitrypsin protease, which allows them to utilize proteins ingested by the host.

Life Cycle

Humans are the principal hosts of *A. lumbricoides*, which has no reservoir hosts, although pigs can be infected experimentally. Infection with *Ascaris suum*, the pig ascarid, rarely leads to symptomatic disease (11). Adult worms have an average life span of 1 to 2 years (see Table 285.1). The female worms produce up to 200,000 eggs per day, with the number of eggs produced per worm decreasing as the total intestinal worm load increases (12).

A. lumbricoides larvae, on hatching in the small intestine, penetrate the wall and enter the bloodstream (Fig. 285.3). They must then undergo development in the liver parenchyma, where they feed on "liver pate" before migrating to the lungs. They develop into third-stage larvae, and, after the infected host coughs them up, the larvae return to the small intestine, where they complete their development into mature adult worms. The entire process of worm morphogenesis takes approximately 1 month from the time the egg is ingested until the fertilized mature female adults begin to release eggs. When excreted with feces into warm, well-oxygenated soil, embryonization occurs within 2 to 4 weeks. In cooler climates, embryonization is delayed, allowing the eggs to survive in an unembryonated state for months to years.

Epidemiology

The majority of the estimated billion or more people with ascariasis live in Asia, sub-Saharan Africa, and Latin America. Ascariasis is now rare in the United States although several decades ago, approximately 4 million people were infected, with the greatest prevalence in the rural Southeast (5). Infection with *A. lumbricoides* can occur at any age but, in endemic regions, it is most common in children in the 3- to 14-year age group, who may have prevalence rates of 80% or higher (1). Transmission is by the fecal-oral route, usually via the ingestion of contaminated foods, and is sustained by the high egg output of the female worms and the longevity of eggs in the soil. Changes in the soil environment, such as lower temperature or humidity, may be responsible for seasonal breaks in transmission.

Clinical Manifestations and Pathogenesis

The intensity of the host response to the migrating *A. lumbricoides* larvae relates directly to the level of infection. Asymptomatic worm migration is common in light infections; heavier infestation may result in pulmonary, intestinal, biliary, and pancreatic manifestations. Infection does not result in meaningful protective immunity.

Previously exposed individuals may experience a hypersensitivity reaction during the migration of larvae through lung tissue and tracheobronchial tree. The result is a Löffler-like syndrome characterized by a productive cough, dyspnea, wheezing, and fever, which may be accompanied by angioedema or urticaria (13). Transient pulmonary infiltrates and eosinophilia often occur in association with the respiratory symptoms. In endemic regions such as Saudi Arabia where the transmission of *A. lumbricoides* peaks from March through May, a seasonal pneumonitis has been described (14).

Light infections generally do not elicit any clinical or pathologic reactions in the intestine, although vague, crampy abdominal pain may occur. Large worm burdens can result in intestinal obstruction, which is clinically manifested by diminished bowel sounds, vomiting, abdominal distention, pain, and radiographic evidence of bowel obstruction (15). This complication is most common in young children and is usually localized to the ileum. Additional rare intestinal complications in heavily infected individuals include perforation, volvulus, intussusception, and appendicitis.

Aberrant migration of the worms into the biliary or pancreatic ducts can result in biliary colic, acute cholecystitis, ascending cholangitis, obstructive jaundice, acute pancreatitis, and, rarely, hepatic abscess formation (16,17). Previous cholecystectomy or endoscopic sphincterotomy appear to facilitate invasion of the biliary ducts. Re-invasion of the biliary tree is common upon reinfection of treated subjects, especially in those patients who have undergone endoscopic sphincterotomy.

Intense infections with *A. lumbricoides* in young children may result in malabsorption and malnutrition secondary to anorexia, increased metabolism, and the consumption of essential nutrients by the worms (18). Adverse consequences of these events include stunting of growth, micronutrient deficiencies, steatorrhea, lactose intolerance, and protein-energy malnutrition. Although it is difficult to distinguish the influence of concomitant parasitic, bacterial, and viral infections on the development of these complications in endemic regions, ascariasis clearly plays a role.

Diagnosis

The high egg output (200,000 per day!) by each fertilized female worm makes a direct smear of stools sufficient for diagnosis in the majority of cases (see Table 285.2). Standard stool concentration techniques may be necessary in light infections. The fertilized, unembryonated eggs are oval with a characteristic thick, irregular cortical layer (Fig. 285.4). Egg counts are useful in field studies for estimating worm burden and the response to therapy.

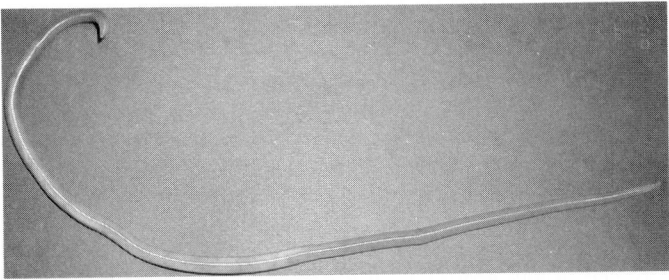

Figure 285.2. Adult female *Ascaris lumbricoides* worm.

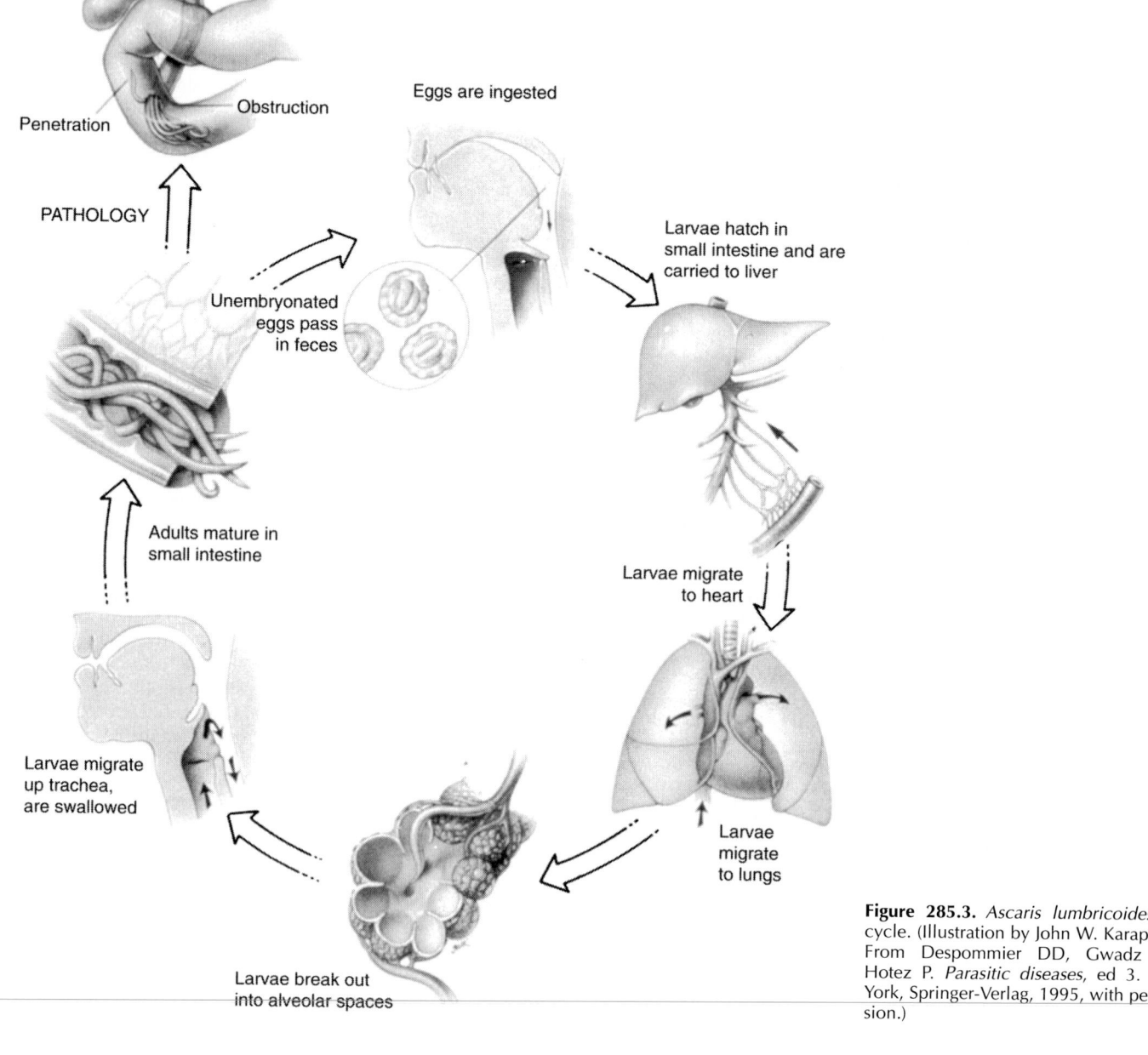

Eggs are ingested

Penetration — Obstruction

PATHOLOGY

Larvae hatch in small intestine and are carried to liver

Unembryonated eggs pass in feces

Larvae migrate to heart

Adults mature in small intestine

Larvae migrate to lungs

Larvae migrate up trachea, are swallowed

Larvae break out into alveolar spaces

Figure 285.3. *Ascaris lumbricoides* life cycle. (Illustration by John W. Karapelou. From Despommier DD, Gwadz RG, Hotez P. *Parasitic diseases,* ed 3. New York, Springer-Verlag, 1995, with permission.)

The diagnosis of biliary or pancreatic ascariasis can be difficult because the worm may exit these tracts after producing symptoms. The adult worm can be extracted by means of endoscopic retrograde cholangiopancreatography (17). Barium studies of the gastrointestinal tract may reveal a luminal filling defect or ingestion of the barium into the adult worm's intestinal tract (19). The combination of shifting infiltrates on serial chest radiographs, peripheral eosinophilia, and presence of ascarid larvae in sputum is diagnostic of pulmonary ascariasis. This syndrome may be confused with strongyloidiasis, hookworm disease, tropical pulmonary eosinophilia, and acute schistosomiasis.

Therapy and Prevention

All cases of intestinal ascariasis should be treated because of the potential for multiple complications. Mebendazole and alben-

dazole are the treatments of choice (see Table 285.2), although single-dose therapy with pyrantel pamoate is also highly effective (20). A 3-day regimen of mebendazole results in nearly a 100% reduction of egg output. No currently available drug affects the larval stages responsible for pulmonary symptoms, although steroids may provide symptomatic relief.

Intestinal obstruction is usually only partial and should be managed supportively with parenteral hydration and nasogastric suction. Piperazine citrate, administered by nasogastric tube, is recommended for the treatment of intestinal obstruction due to *A. lumbricoides.* This agent effectively paralyzes the worms and usually leads to resolution of obstruction in 2 to 3 days. Refractory or complete obstruction may require surgical intervention.

Mass therapy for subjects in endemic regions and treatments targeted at age groups with high prevalences are effective for community control, although complete elimination of ascariasis is difficult because reinfection is common. Periodic deworming

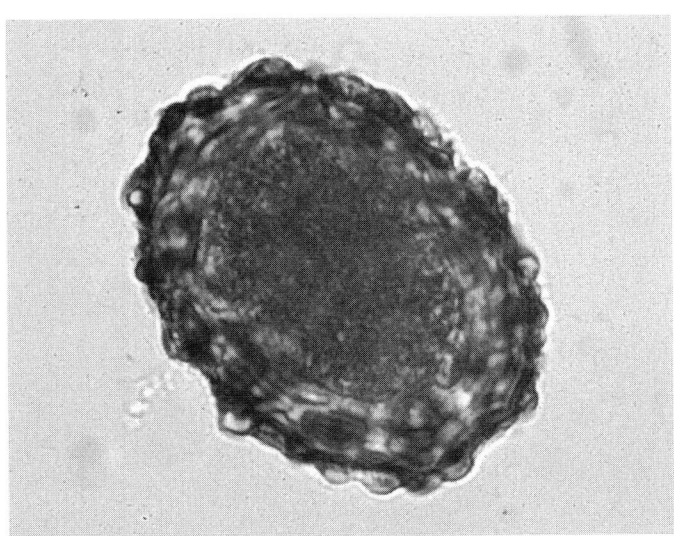

Figure 285.4. *Ascaris lumbricoides* unembryonated egg. Note the absence of a larva. Eggs become embryonated in soil during a 2- to 4-week period, depending on ambient temperatures. (40 × 10 μm.)

in endemic locales leads to significant improvement in growth (18).

Improvements in sanitation, water supplies, and health education are necessary components of a plan to eradicate ascariasis worldwide. The eggs can be destroyed by prolonged exposure to direct sunlight or by temperatures above 40°C but they are relatively resistant to chemical disinfectants and can survive temperatures below 0°C in temperate climates.

HOOKWORMS INFECTION

An estimated 1.3 billion people worldwide are infected with the hookworms *Ancylostoma duodenale* and *Necator americanus* (1). *N. americanus* is more commonly found in the Americas, equatorial Africa, Southeast Asia, Polynesia, and Australia whereas *A. duodenale* is more prevalent in northern Africa and north and southwest Asia (21). Although the distributions of these two species were formerly thought to be discrete, surveys have shown that ranges overlap in parts of Asia, Africa, and South America. *Ancylostoma ceylanicum*, a minor nematode species, which is primarily a pathogen of large felines such as panthers and tigers, uncommonly infects humans in parts of Southeast Asia and Suriname. Although many individuals have light, asymptomatic infections, heavy worm burdens can cause significant gastrointestinal blood loss, iron deficiency anemia, and rarely, death.

Life Cycle

The hookworm life cycle is similar to that of *A. lumbricoides* with the nuance that the penetration of unbroken skin by infective larva initiates the infection (Fig. 285.5). There are no reservoir hosts for either species of hookworm.

The adult worms are small, ranging from 9 to 13 mm in length. Morphologic differences of the mouth parts of adult worms help to differentiate the two species. *N. americanus* adults have two pairs of rounded, chitinized cutting plates, whereas *A. duodenale* adults have two pairs of cutting teeth. The adult worms obtain their nutrients from the consumption of villous tissue and blood sucked directly from their site of attachment to the intestinal mucosa. The *A. duodenale* adult is responsible for the loss of

0.1 to 0.2 mL of blood per day; the adult of *N. americanus* accounts for the loss of 0.01 to 0.02 mL of blood daily through direct ingestion of blood and focal hemorrhages produced at the site of intestinal attachment (22). Proteases and anticoagulants released by the worms play a role in the pathogenesis of the blood loss (23).

Adult females of *A. duodenale* produce up to 30,000 eggs per day, whereas females of *N. americanus* produce 5,000 to 10,000 eggs per day. Eggs passed in the feces contain a segmented ovum that will undergo larval maturation and hatch within 1 to 2 days in soil, if the necessary conditions of temperature and moisture are present (24). The freshly hatched rhabditiform larvae pass through a free-living cycle in the soil during which they molt twice and then become sheathed, filariform larvae that are infectious to humans. If soil conditions are suitable, the larvae can survive for months. Humans are infected by penetration of the skin, most commonly through the feet. Infection with *A. duodenale* may occur by the oral route. The larvae migrate through the venous system to the pulmonary arterial circulation where they cross into the alveoli and then are passively carried up the bronchi to the trachea and larynx. The migrating larvae of *N. americanus* undergo maturation in the lung, whereas those of *A. duodenale* do not. On reaching the pharynx, the larvae are swallowed and reach the small intestine approximately 3 to 5 days from the time of skin penetration. During the next 4 to 6 weeks, the worms become mature. Intestinal survival is an average of 4 years for *N. americanus* and 5 years for *A. duodenale*. In some regions where reinfection is common, the filariform larvae of *A. duodenale* may remain dormant in skeletal muscle and then later complete their development when the external environmental conditions have again become favorable for parasite development in the soil (25).

Epidemiology

The prevalence of hookworm infection varies substantially from region to region, with rates as high as 90% described. The prevalence tends to be higher in rural than in urban areas. The age-specific prevalence in tropical regions peaks in schoolchildren and then levels off in adulthood. Hookworm infections used to be common in the rural southeast of the United States and Puerto Rico, but the frequency has dropped as socioeconomic conditions have improved. Survival of hookworm larvae is optimal in moist, sandy, or loamy soil with ambient temperatures of 24°C to 32°C. The practices of using the same site for defecation and not wearing footwear facilitate infection. Because *A. duodenale* can also be acquired by the oral route, contamination of fresh produce with nightsoil contributes to the transmission of hookworms.

Clinical Manifestations

A dermatitis characterized by intense pruritus, edema, and erythema followed later by a vesiculopapular eruption may occur at the skin entry site of the filariform larvae. This cutaneous manifestation of infection, known as ground itch or coolie's itch, may last as long as 2 weeks and is more common in individuals in endemic areas who are presensitized to hookworms. Although pulmonary symptoms can occur during the larval migration, they tend to be mild in comparison with *A. lumbricoides*, unless the initial infection is heavy, in which case dyspnea and cough may occur (26). During worm maturation in the intestine, there may be abdominal pain, steatorrhea, and an intense peripheral eosinophilia with 1,000 to 4,000 cells per mm³. Lighter worm burdens tend to result in no or only mild symptoms, whereas

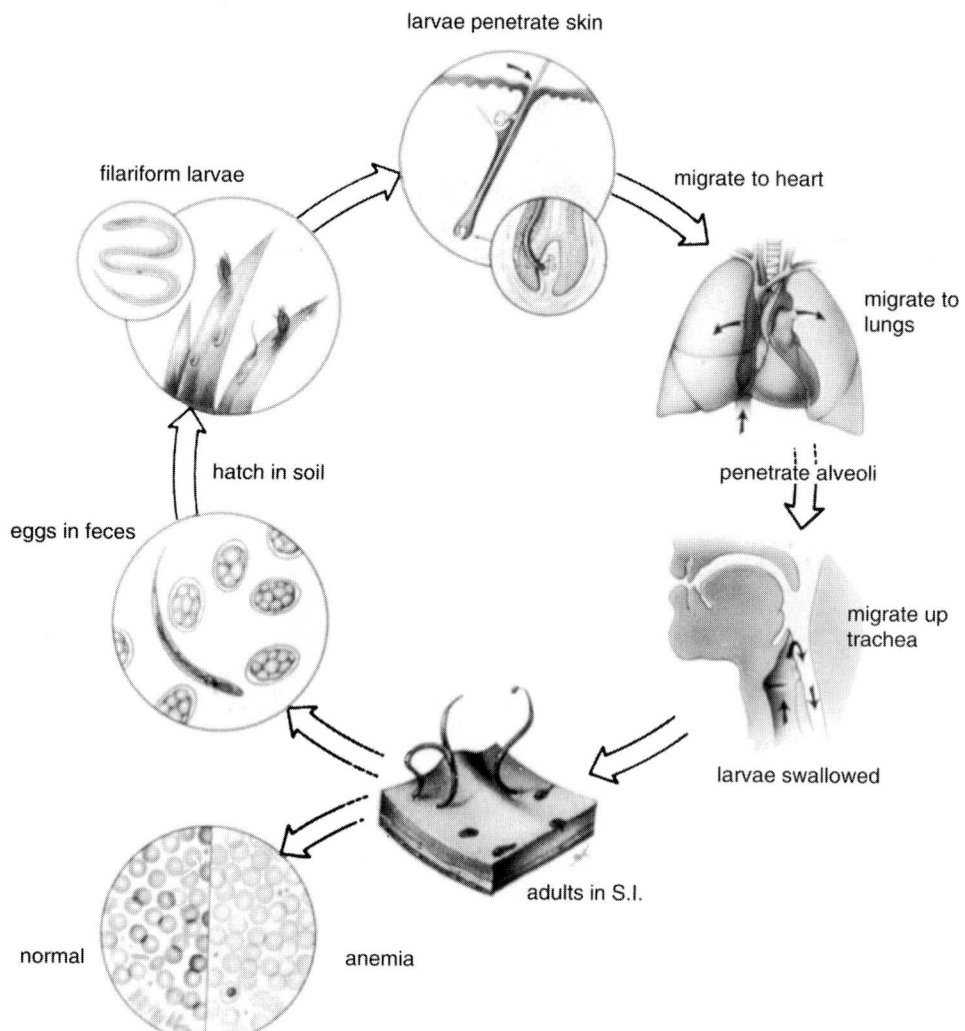

larvae penetrate skin

filariform larvae

migrate to heart

migrate to lungs

penetrate alveoli

migrate up trachea

hatch in soil

eggs in feces

larvae swallowed

adults in S.I.

normal

anemia

PATHOLOGY

Figure 285.5. *Necator americanus* life cycle. (Illustration by John W. Karapelou. From Despommier DD, Gwadz RG, Hotez P. *Parasitic diseases*, ed 3. New York: Springer-Verlag, 1995, with permission.)

heavier infections can be complicated by severe iron deficiency anemia from chronic intestinal blood loss and hypoalbuminemia secondary to a protein-losing enteropathy. These complications are manifested by fatigue, peripheral edema, dyspnea, high-output heart failure, pale skin, and other manifestations of chronic iron deficiency anemia. The hypoproteinemia that results from chronic infection may lead to a kwashiorkor-like state characterized by growth impairment, facial and lower extremity edema, dermatitis, and hair loss. Factors influencing the severity of anemia include the iron content of the individual's diet, the underlying iron stores, and the intensity and duration of infection. Chronic hookworm anemia contributes to physical and intellectual growth retardation.

Diagnosis

The diagnosis is established by the identification of characteristic hookworm eggs in direct stool smears (Fig. 285.6). Concentration techniques may be necessary in light infections (see Table 285.2). Fresh or preserved stool specimens should be examined because the eggs may hatch into rhabditiform larvae, which can be misinterpreted as *Strongyloides* larvae. Such distinctions are critical to the selection of optimal therapeutic agents. Hookworm ova

can be confused with those of *Oesophagostomum* species, which appear identical, or ova of *Trichostrongylus* species, which tend to be much larger. *A. duodenale* and *N. americanus* can be differentiated by the examination of adult worms or third-stage larvae.

Therapy

The main goal of treatment in endemic regions is to reduce the worm burden below the level of clinical significance. Infected people in nonendemic areas should be treated. Mebendazole, albendazole, and pyrantel pamoate are effective treatments for hookworm infections (see Table 285.2). However, the failure of a single-dose regimen of mebendazole suggests that the development of resistance to the benzimidazoles may interfere with the utility of these drugs in the near future (27). The safety of the benzimidazole agents, mebendazole and albendazole, has not been established in infants. Pyrantel pamoate is available as a suspension and is an effective therapy for hookworm infections in infants. Oral iron supplements should be given to rectify the iron deficiency anemia. Chemotherapy of hookworm infections and correction of the associated anemia result in improved physical fitness and catch-up growth in endemic populations (9,28).

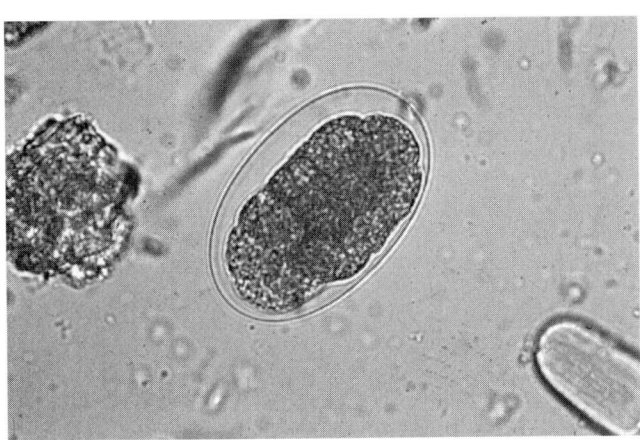

Figure 285.6. Hookworm egg. Sixteen-cell stage of embryonization. (40 × 10 μm.)

Prevention and Control

Three major aspects of prevention include the sanitary disposal of feces, chemotherapy, and public health education (24). Correct use of latrines helps to contain the hookworm larvae. In regions where fresh human fecal matter is used as manure (nightsoil), it should be treated to kill the larvae by composting or through the addition of chemicals such as sodium nitrate, ammonium sulfate, or calcium superphosphate. Protective footwear and education about the mode of transmission may prove helpful in geographic locales where percutaneous rather than oral transmission is more common.

ENTEROBIASIS

Human infection with *Enterobius vermicularis*, the pinworm, dates back many millennia. This organism is found worldwide with a prevalence that is higher in temperate regions than in the tropics. *E. vermicularis* is the most common intestinal nematode in the United States, where an estimated 20 to 42 million people are infected (29). This parasite has managed to persist despite modern advances in hygiene, sanitation, and standards of living. Moderate humidity, dense indoor crowding, and high proportion of school-aged children favor increased prevalence. While infection with pinworms is generally not associated with significant morbidity, it may cause social stigma in certain populations.

Life Cycle

Humans are the only host to *E. vermicularis*; no reservoir host is known. The life cycle is a direct one, beginning with the ingestion of the embryonated eggs. The larvae hatch in the stomach and proximal small intestine, and then migrate to the ileum, cecum, appendix, and colon where they mature to adulthood. Adult females measure 8 to 13 mm in length and survive 37 to 93 days; the males, at 2 to 5 mm in length, are smaller and survive approximately 50 days. After copulation, each female produces approximately 10,000 fertilized, unembryonated ova. Eggs are oviposited at night when gravid females migrate through the rectum to lay their eggs on the perirectal skin. The light eggs are easily dispersed and often settle on nearby surfaces, which serve as fomites to propagate infection. The eggs embryonate rapidly and become infectious within 6 hours of oviposition.

Egg survival is increased under cool and humid conditions. The outer cortex of the eggs contain substances that cause intense itching of the perianal area, leading to scratching and entrapment of eggs under the host's fingernails. The eggs are transmitted directly to the mouth by contaminated hands or food or by exposure to contaminated sites such as soiled bed linen. Once the eggs are swallowed, the life cycle takes 4 to 6 weeks to be completed. Infection may also be maintained non-enterally, whereby larva released from eggs deposited on the perineum migrate in a retrograde fashion back through the rectum to reinitiate the cycle. Freshly hatched larvae may migrate into the vagina, where an aberrant infection may be established.

Epidemiology

Pinworm infection is most common among school-age children in the United States and Europe. Increased rates of infection are associated with high indoor population densities such as in mental health institutions, in families with young children, or among homosexual men. Prevalence rates of 16% to 100% have been described, although some surveys have noted a recent decline in enterobiasis in certain regions (30). Although this infection is generally more common in cooler, temperate climates, it may nevertheless be prevalent in some tropical locales where it may not be restricted to children (31). Persistent infections result from autoinfection or reinfection between family members.

Clinical Manifestations and Pathology

Most infections are asymptomatic. The most common symptom is pruritus ani, which most commonly occurs at night. Infected children may rarely be troubled by insomnia, restlessness, irritability, anorexia, weight loss, and emotional lability (32). Scratching can result in excoriation and secondary infection. Aberrant migration of adult pinworms can lead to vulvovaginitis and an increased frequency of urinary tract infections in prepubertal girls. Ectopic migration followed by the death of the worm and the formation of granulomata has been described in the cervix, uterus, fallopian tubes, ovary, peritoneum, prostate, lung, liver, kidney, and spleen. Although *E. vermicularis* is occasionally found in inflamed appendices, its role in the pathogenesis of appendicitis remains controversial. No significant intestinal disease has been attributed to pinworm infection.

Diagnosis

Identification of adult worms or eggs in specimens taken from the perianal or, less commonly, the vaginal area establishes the diagnosis (Fig. 285.7; see Table 285.2). Following egg-laying, the 5- to 15-mm long adult worms die and may remain temporarily attached to folds of the rectal mucosa. Both adult worms and the distinctive 50-um long ovoid eggs, which have an asymmetrically flattened side, can be identified using a light microscope. In suspected cases, transparent adhesive tape preparations should be taken from the perianal skin shortly after the patient awakens on successive days. If five or more consecutive tape test results are negative, the diagnosis is virtually excluded. Stool specimens provide a diagnosis in only 5% to 15% of infected patients and therefore are not reliable. Eosinophilia is not a feature of enterobiasis.

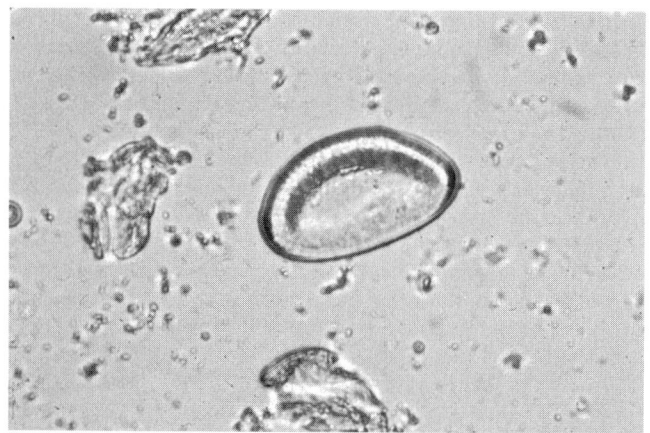

Figure 285.7. *Enterobius vermicularis* embryonated egg. Note larva inside. (40 × 10 μm.)

Treatment

A single dose of mebendazole or pyrantel pamoate is effective (see Table 285.2) and should be repeated in 2 to 3 weeks to eliminate reinfection (20). Albendazole is also effective. All family members or subjects within an institution should be treated simultaneously to eradicate other reservoirs of infection. Parents of infected children should be reassured that this is not a serious infection and should be educated about the importance of careful hygienic measures.

STRONGYLOIDIASIS

Strongyloides stercoralis was first described in the 19th century in French army personnel returning from Indochina. It remains a significant cause of disease in many tropical and subtropical regions and, less commonly, in temperate climates such as North America (33). The unique ability of this nematode to replicate within its host for decades and its potential to cause massive infections with high mortality rates in immunocompromised patients make it a clinically significant pathogen. Although *S. stercoralis* is the usual cause of human strongyloidiasis, *Strongyloides fuelleborni*, an intestinal nematode of old-world primates, may be responsible for occasional human infections in central Africa and New Guinea. The ability of *S. fulleborni* to maintain sustained endogenous infections in humans has not been established.

Life Cycle

S. stercoralis has a complex life cycle with a free-living soil phase and a parasitic phase (Fig. 285.8). The free-living phase is initiated when second-stage, rhabditiform larvae are excreted by an infected host into moist, shaded soil. Under proper conditions, the larvae molt twice to become free-living adult worms. In contrast with the intestinal phase, the free-living cycle is not sustained, and thus is not thought to be a significant factor in the amplification of infection.

The initial infection occurs when humans come in contact with fecally contaminated soil that contains the third stage

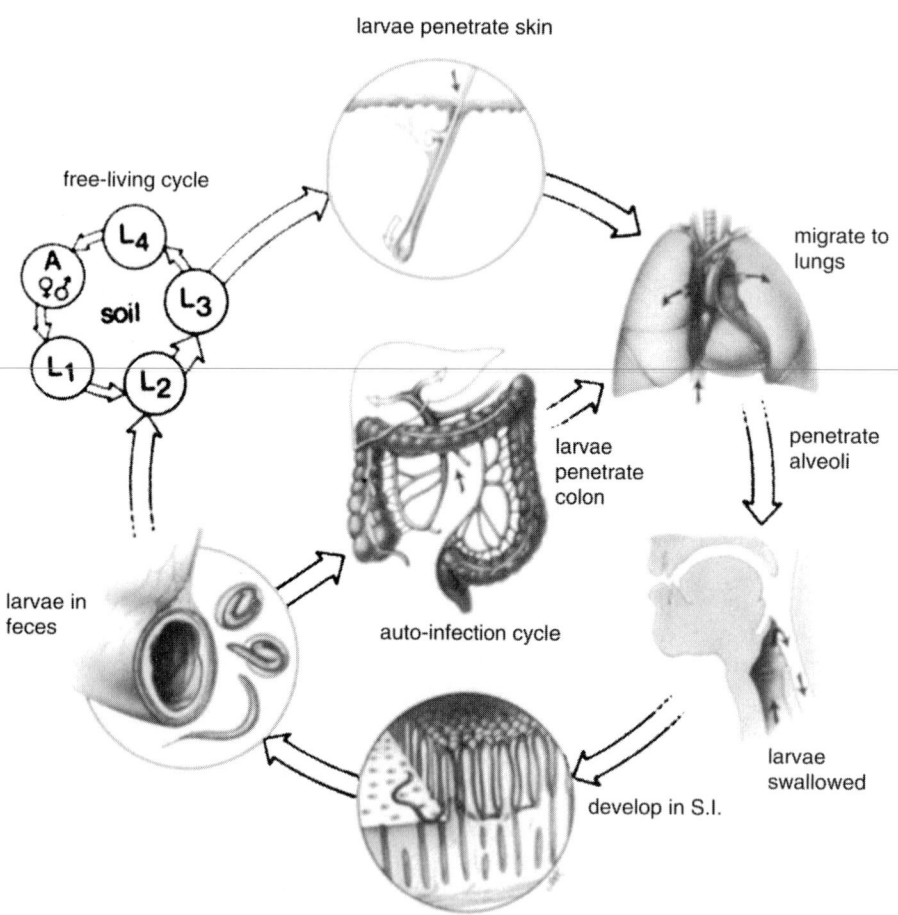

Figure 285.8. *Strongyloides stercoralis* life cycle. (Illustration by John W. Karapelou. From Despommier DD, Gwadz RG, Hotez P. *Parasitic diseases,* ed 3. New York: Springer-Verlag, 1995, with permission.)

filiform larvae. The larvae respond to vibration by penetrating the skin of the host. The larvae are transported through the blood stream to the pulmonary circulation where they penetrate the alveoli, migrate up the tracheobronchial tree to the pharynx, and are then swallowed. The larvae undergo a final molt in the duodenum and upper jejunum to become the 2-mm long gray-white adults. Interestingly, the parasitic host cycle is maintained by adult females, which reproduce by parthenogenesis (i.e., in the absence of male worms). Females release small numbers of eggs into the bowel lumen. The time from initial skin penetration to the excretion of eggs is approximately 25 to 30 days. Eggs quickly hatch within the lumen, releasing first stage larvae; for this reason, ova of *S. stercoralis* are rarely seen in stool samples. The larvae then molt in the colon to become second-stage, rhabditiform larvae, which may be passed in feces to contaminate soil or may undergo an additional molt to form the infectious third-stage, filariform larvae. The filariform larvae are infectious, and can penetrate either the bowel mucosa, resulting in internal autoinfection, or penetrate the perianal skin resulting in external autoinfection. External autoinfection is increased when fecal-contaminated clothes remain in close contact with perianal skin. This process of autoinfection allows *S. stercoralis* to persist in its host for decades. Immunocompromised hosts may harbor many infective larvae in their intestines, which can lead to a hyperinfection syndrome, a difficult to treat and frequently fatal complication of chronic strongyloidiasis.

Epidemiology

S. stercoralis is estimated to infect as many as 100 to 200 million people worldwide. Infection is endemic in many less developed, tropical areas of the world where warmth, moisture, and poor sanitation allow the soil stages to flourish. There is some evidence to suggest that dogs, cats, or monkeys may also serve as nonhuman reservoirs of infection. In the United States, strongyloidiasis can occasionally be found in recent immigrants from Southeast Asia, in rural areas of the Southeast, and in institutionalized settings where personal hygiene and sanitation are inadequate. Accurate estimates of the prevalence of strongyloidiasis are hindered by difficulties identifying the low numbers of larva and near absent ova in routine stool samples. The importance of autoinfection has been emphasized by the detection of symptomatic disease three to four decades after exposure in ex-prisoners of war who had worked on the railroad between Myanmar (formerly Burma) and Thailand during World War II (34).

Clinical Manifestations

The clinical manifestations of strongyloidiasis can be related to stages of the parasite's life cycle, that is, the location and type of symptoms depend on whether the larvae are invading the skin, migrating through the lung, or penetrating the intestinal mucosa. Many infections with *S. stercoralis* are light and often asymptomatic. Gastrointestinal symptoms range from watery diarrhea to constipation, pseudo-obstruction, epigastric pain, and nausea. Children with heavy infections occasionally develop chronic diarrhea, anorexia, malabsorption, abdominal distention, and growth impairment. Infants in Papua New Guinea infected with *S. fuelleborni* may be afflicted by a swollen belly syndrome characterized by persistent diarrhea, ascites, and edema secondary to a protein-losing enteropathy.

Patients with chronic strongyloidiasis may have intermittent urticarial eruptions lasting 1 to 2 days that commonly occur on the buttocks, upper thighs, or lower back. A less common but pathognomonic manifestation, larva currens, is characterized by a fast-moving serpiginous, pruritic rash that migrates at a rate of several centimeters per hour. During the pulmonary phase of larval migration, patients may experience a Löffler-like syndrome with bronchospasm and cough associated with peripheral eosinophilia. Pulmonary strongyloidiasis may be manifested by interstitial infiltrates, lobar pneumonia, and adult respiratory distress syndrome in massive infections (35). Gastrointestinal symptoms of chronic infection can include indigestion, abdominal cramping, intermittent or chronic diarrhea, anal pruritus, and weight loss.

Hyperinfection or disseminated disease may occur in patients who become immunocompromised as a result of hematologic malignancies, chemotherapy, glucocorticoid use, H$_2$-receptor antagonist therapy, and infection with human T-lymphocyte virus-1 (HTLV-1) or human immunodeficiency virus (HIV) (36). Individuals with the hyperinfection syndrome have heavy worm burdens that can lead to intestinal obstruction, respiratory failure, and gram-negative bacteremia or meningitis. These latter complications are believed to result from the carriage of enteric bacteria across the intestines by migrating *S. stercoralis* filariform larvae. Bacteremias due to unusual enteric microorganisms occurring in patients with remote or recent travel histories should raise the question of strongyloidiasis. Hyperinfection is usually fatal if it is not promptly diagnosed and treated.

Diagnosis

The diagnosis is established by demonstrating characteristic, motile rhabditiform larvae in stool or duodenal fluid specimens (see Table 285.2). Concentration techniques such as the Baermann funnel method, fecal culture, and serial sampling are often necessary because larval output is often sporadic and low. The use of duodenal aspirates, mucosal biopsies, or the string test (Enterotest™) can increase the likelihood of diagnosing strongyloidiasis. In contrast to normal hosts, patients with the hyperinfection syndrome may have large numbers of larvae present in sputum, bronchial washings, cerebrospinal fluid, urine, and ascitic fluid.

Patients with acute or chronic infections may have a moderate eosinophilia (10% to 25%), but this is usually absent in cases of hyperinfection. Most infected subjects will have *S. stercoralis*–specific immunoglobulin G detectable by enzyme-linked immunosorbent assays (37). These assays are both sensitive and specific, and are now available in reference laboratories.

Treatment

In recent years, ivermectin has replaced thiabendazole as the drug of choice for treating strongyloidiasis. Ivermectin has proven to be both more effective, to require fewer doses, and to have fewer side effects then thiabendazole (38). Thiabendazole remains a useful alternative choice for treatment; however, its efficacy is variable and its use may be complicated by multiple side effects including nausea, vomiting, dizziness, rash, and hallucinations. Albendazole, which has excellent activity against hookworm, the larvae of which are occasionally confused with *S. stercoralis* larvae, has only modest efficacy in the treatment of strongyloidiasis (39). Patients with the hyperinfection syndrome tend to be refractory to treatment, which may need to be both prolonged and repeated. Intensive supportive therapy, antimicrobial coverage for secondary bacterial infections, and nutritional supplementation are necessary adjuncts to antiparasitic drugs in patients with overwhelming *S. stercoralis* infection.

ZOONOTIC INTESTINAL NEMATODE INFECTIONS

Humans are accidental hosts to the intermediate larval stage of several species of zoonotic intestinal nematodes that may cause symptomatic gastrointestinal disease. Several of these infections are becoming more common in western countries due to an increase in adventure travel and increased popularity of uncooked foods.

Anisakiasis

Anisakiasis is an infection of the stomach or intestine by the larval form of a number of species of marine nematodes that normally infect sea mammals (40). The intermediate larval stage of four genera (*Anisakis, Pseudoterranova, Contracaecum,* and *Thynnascaris*) of the family Anisakidae has been found to cause disease in humans (41). The adult worm of these marine parasites is found in the stomachs or intestines of whales, dolphins, sea lions, and seals. Eggs released by these final hosts hatch in seawater to form free-living larval stages that infect intermediate hosts, usually crustaceans. These are subsequently ingested by fish such as salmon, herring, cod, haddock, and mackerel, or by squid, which serve as transport hosts. Ingestion of the uncooked flesh of the infected fish or squid by the marine mammalian final hosts or humans, who are accidental hosts, leads to infection.

After ingestion of raw or undercooked saltwater fish by humans, the larva embeds itself in the gastric or intestinal mucosa and then dies. The burrowing or dead larva precipitates an intense hypersensitivity reaction characterized by a granulomatous, eosinophilic tissue infiltrate (Fig. 285.9), which is often accompanied by systemic manifestations of an acute al-lergic reaction including urticaria, eosinophilia, elevated serum anti-*Anisakis* IgE, and even anaphylaxis (42). Most symptomatic infections are caused by third-stage larvae of *Anisakis simplex*. Gastric infections are more common than intestinal infections; the esophagus is rarely involved (43). Infection with *Pseudoterranova* species usually involves only the stomach and tends to be milder than disease due to *Anisakis* species, which may cause symptomatic gastric or intestinal infections. Asymptomatic infections with *Pseudoterranova* species may first come to medical attention when the patient coughs up a live or dead worm. This usually occurs within 48 hours of the ingestion of infected fish and may be preceded by a sensation of feeling a worm crawling in the upper esophagus or pharynx.

Gastric anisakiasis is heralded by the abrupt (generally 1 to 12 hours after ingestion of raw fish) onset of severe epigastric pain, nausea, vomiting, and low-grade fever. There is frequently an accompanying leukocytosis with an intense eosinophilia. Endoscopy with removal of the larva provides a means of both diagnosis and treatment.

Intestinal anisakiasis is characterized by intermittent or constant abdominal pain, which may be severe enough to result in peritoneal signs or evidence of a partial bowel obstruction. In contrast to gastric anisakiasis, the symptoms may not appear until 1 to 3 weeks after ingestion of the anisakid larvae. Leukocytosis without eosinophilia may be present. Diagnosis is made when laparotomy is performed for suspected appendicitis or bowel perforation. Intraperitoneal anisakiasis is a rare complication (40).

The annual occurrence of this seafood-associated parasitic infection is greatest in Japan, where the consumption of raw fish is common. Numerous cases were previously described in

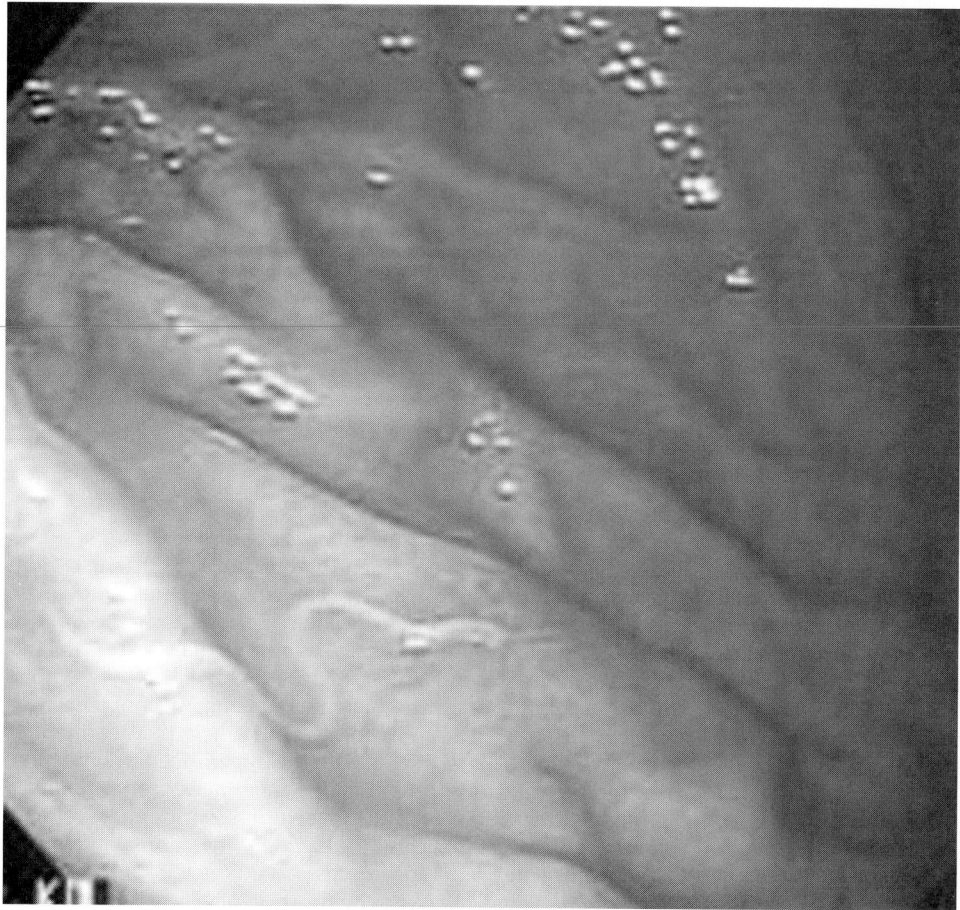

Figure 285.9. Third-stage larva of *Anisakis simplex* burrowing into the gastric mucosa. Surrounding erythema and edema of the mucosa are evident. (Endoscopic view courtesy of Drs. Tomohiro Kato and Itaru O-I, Department of Medicine, Daini Hospital, Tokyo Women's Medical University.)

northern Europe, especially Holland, which were attributed to the ingestion of raw herring. Compulsory treatment of herring has largely eliminated anisakiasis in Holland. However, in Spain an increasing number of cases have been recognized as a result of the consumption of raw anchovies and undercooked fish (42). Although only about 50 cases have been reported from North America, the frequency may be higher as a result of underreporting or milder forms of disease that go unrecognized. Anisakiasis can be prevented by thorough cooking of fish or freezing at −20°C for more than 24 hours. Eviscerating fish as soon as possible after catch may decrease the number of larvae in the fish flesh by not allowing them the opportunity to migrate from the intestinal tract into the edible musculature.

Capillariasis

CAPILLARIA PHILIPPINENSIS
Intestinal disease caused by *C. philippinensis* has been mainly described in coastal regions of the Philippines and Thailand, although scattered cases have been reported from other countries in Southeast Asia and the Middle East (44). Human infection with this zoonotic nematode can result in severe diarrhea with malabsorption, which may be fatal if untreated.

Eggs, passed in the feces of infected patients or by migratory fish-eating birds, embryonate in fresh or brackish water during a 5- to 10-day period. After ingestion of the embryonated eggs by the intermediate fish host, the eggs hatch and release larvae, which mature in the fish intestine in 3 weeks. After consumption of the parasitized fish by the natural definitive host, fish-eating birds, the larva develops into an adult male or female, which copulate and fertilize. Humans are accidental hosts who acquire infection by eating inadequately cooked or raw freshwater fish. The larvae of *C. philippinensis* develop into the 3- to 4-mm thin adult worms in the small intestine 1 to 2 months after ingestion. Adult females appear capable of producing infective larvae in humans, which can lead to an autoinfectious cycle similar to that of *S. stercoralis*. Local outbreaks may occur when feces from humans contaminate local fishing sites or aquaculture establishments. Clinical disease is manifested by borborygmi, abdominal pain, and intermittent diarrhea, which, if left untreated, may progress to voluminous watery diarrhea. Dehydration, weight loss, steatorrhea, and a protein-losing enteropathy may ensue with the eventual development of muscle wasting, anasarca, and electrolyte disturbances. Death may occur in 4 to 6 months in the absence of treatment.

The diagnosis should be suspected in patients in endemic regions with the aforementioned symptoms. Direct microscopic examination of stool or duodenal aspirate may reveal the adult worms, larvae, or eggs. *C. philippinensis* is related to *T. trichiura* and the eggs appear roughly similar, leading to occasional confusion by inexperienced technicians. Mebendazole at a dose of 200 mg twice daily administered for 20 days is the current treatment of choice. Preliminary findings with albendazole are promising.

CAPILLARIA HEPATICA
Hepatic capillariasis is a rare zoonotic infection of humans caused by *Capillaria hepatica*, a parasite of rodents (45). Ingestion of soil or food contaminated with the embryonated eggs of this nematode is followed by hatching of the larvae, which traverse the intestinal wall and migrate to the liver by the portal vein. The larvae mature to adult worms in the liver, which deposit thousands of eggs. An intense granulomatous response may ensue, which leads to prolonged fever, hepatomegaly, leukocytosis with a relative eosinophilia, and progressive hepatic failure. The diagnosis is confirmed by the detection of worms or ova in a liver biopsy specimen. Thiabendazole and albendazole have resulted in clinical improvement or resolution of signs of infection but there is limited experience with these antiparasitic drugs in the treatment of hepatic capillariasis (46).

Trichostrongyliasis

The genus *Trichostrongylus* is distributed worldwide and includes many species that parasitize the intestinal tracts of herbivorous mammals. Human infection has been described in many less developed countries and has been attributed to at least seven different species of *Trichostrongylus* (47). People who care for animals such as sheep and goats are more likely to acquire this rare infection.

Ingestion of infectious larvae on fecally contaminated vegetables or hands is the probable mode of transmission. The filariform larvae penetrate the oral mucosa, pass through the lung, and then fully mature in the small intestine. The intensity of infection in humans is usually low, although high worm burdens have been described (48). Most infections are asymptomatic, although heavy infections may rarely lead to anemia, eosinophilia, and emaciation. Diagnosis is established by the detection of eggs in stool specimens; concentration techniques are needed for lighter infections. The eggs can be confused with those of hookworms, although hookworm eggs tend to be smaller and have more rounded ends. Treatment may be unnecessary in milder infections. Therapy with thiabendazole has been successful in some cases, but resistance has been described. Single-dose therapy with pyrantel pamoate has been effective in cases treated in Japan and Korea, whereas less favorable results have been reported from Iran.

Oesophagostomiasis

Oesophagostomum species, although common parasites of mammals, have rarely been described in humans. Studies in northern Togo and Ghana have found that as many as 30% of the human populations in some villages are infected with *Oesophagostomum bifurcum*, a nematode of monkeys (49). Transmission is presumed to be oral. The larvae and adult worms of this parasite have been found in nodular lesions of the intestinal wall, which can be visualized with ultrasound (50). The eggs of *O. bifurcum* are nearly identical to hookworm eggs, and therefore coproculture with identification of the larvae is needed to establish this diagnosis. Polymerase chain reaction assays have also been developed, which can be used to estimate the prevalence of *O. bifurcum* and *N. americanus* (51). The two anthelmintic drugs, pyrantel pamoate and albendazole, appear to be capable of eliminating adult worms from infected individuals.

REFERENCES

1. Crompton DWT. How much human helminthiasis is there in the world? *J Parasitol* 1999;85:397–403.
2. Bundy DAP, Cooper ES. Trichuris and trichuriasis in humans. *Adv Parasitol* 1989;28:107–173.
3. Stephenson LS, Holland CV, Cooper ES. The public health significance of *Trichuris trichiura*. *Parasitology* 2000;121:S73–S95.
4. Mirdha BR, Singh YG, Samantray JC, Mishra B. *Trichuris vulpis* infection in slum children. *Ind J Gastroenterol* 1988;17:154.
5. Warren KS. Helminthic diseases endemic in the United States. *Am J Trop Med Hyg* 1974;23:723.
6. Gilman RH, Chong YH, Davis C, et al. The adverse consequences of heavy *Trichuris* infection. *Trans R Soc Trop Med Hyg* 1983;77:432–438.
7. Layrisse M, Aparcedo L, Martinez-Torres C, et al. Blood loss due to infection with *Trichuris trichiura*. *Am J Trop Med Hyg* 1967;16:613–619.

8. Kamath KR. Severe infection with *Trichuris trichiura* in Malaysian children. A clinical study of 30 cases treated with stilbazium iodide. *Am J Trop Med Hyg* 1973;22:600–605.

9. Stephenson LS, Latham MC, Adams EJ, et al. Physical fitness, growth and appetite of Kenyan school boys with hookworm, *Trichuris trichiura* and *Ascaris lumbricoides* infections are improved four months after a single dose of albendazole. *J Nutr* 1993;123:1036–1046.

10. Taylor M, Jinabhai CC, Couper I, Kleinschmidt I, Jogessar VB. The effect of different antihelminthic treatment regimens combined with iron supplementation on the nutritional status of school children in KwaZulu-Natal, South Africa: a randomized controlled trial. *Trans R Soc Trop Med Hyg* 2001;95:211–216.

11. Davies NJ, Goldsmid JM. Intestinal obstruction due to *Ascaris suum* infection. *Trans R Soc Trop Med Hyg* 1978;72:107.

12. Sinniah B. Daily egg production of *Ascaris lumbricoides*: the distribution of eggs in the faeces and the variability of egg counts. *Parasitology* 1982;84:167–175.

13. Spillman RK. Pulmonary ascariasis in tropical communities. *Am J Trop Med Hyg* 1975;24:791–800.

14. Gelpi AP, Mustafa A. *Ascaris* pneumonia. *Am J Med* 1968;44:377–389.

15. Blumenthal DS, Schultz MG. Incidence of intestinal obstruction in children infected with *Ascaris lumbricoides*. *Am J Trop Med Hyg* 1975;24:801–805.

16. Khuroo MS, Zargar SA, Mahajan R. Hepatobiliary and pancreatic ascariasis in India. *Lancet* 1990;335:1503–1506.

17. Sandouk F, Haffar S, Zada MM, et al. Pancreatic-biliary ascariasis: experience of 300 cases. *Am J Gastroenterol* 1997;92:2264–2267.

18. Stephenson LS. The contribution of *Ascaris lumbricoides* to malnutrition in children. *Parasitology* 1980;81:221–233.

19. Reeder MM. The radiological and ultrasound evaluation of ascariasis of the gastrointestinal, biliary, and respiratory tracts. *Semin Roentgenol* 1998;33:57–78.

20. Drugs for parasitic infections. Medical Letter March 2000. Available at: *www.medletter.com/freedocs/parasitic.pdf.*

21. Miller TA. Hookworm infection in man. *Adv Parasitol* 1979;17:315–384.

22. Roche M, Layrisse M. The nature and causes of "hookworm anemia." *Am J Trop Med Hyg* 1966;15:1031–1100.

23. Hotez PJ. Hookworm disease in children. *Pediatr Infect Dis J* 1989;8:516–520.

24. Gilles HM. Selective primary health care: strategies for control of disease in the developing world. XVII. Hookworm infection and anemia. *Rev Infect Dis* 1985;7:111–118.

25. Schad GA, Chowdhury AB, Dean CG, et al. Arrested development in human hookworm infections: a adaptation to a seasonally unfavorable external environment. *Science* 1973;180:500–501.

26. Koshy A, Raina V, Sharma MP, et al. An unusual outbreak of hookworm disease in north India. *Am J Trop Med Hyg* 1978;27:42–45.

27. De Clercq D, Sacko, Behnke J, et al. Failure of mebendazole in treatment of human hookworm infections in the southern regions of Mali. *Am J Trop Med Hyg* 1997;57:25–30.

28. Stoltzfus RJ, Albonico M, Tielsch JM, et al. School-based deworming program yields small improvement in growth of Zanzibari school children after one year. *J Nutr* 1997;127:2187–2193.

29. Russell LJ. The pinworm, *Enterobius vermicularis*. *Primary Care* 1991;18:13–27.

30. Vermund SH, MacLeod S. Is pinworm a vanishing infection? Laboratory surveillance in a New York City medical center from 1971 to 1986. *Am J Dis Child* 1988;142:566–568.

31. Haswell-Elkins MR, Elkins DB, Manjula K, et al. The distribution and abundance of *Enterobius vermicularis* in a south Indian fishing community. *Parasitology* 1987;95:339–354.

32. Cook GC. *Enterobius vermicularis* infection. *Gut* 1994;35:1159–1162.

33. Grove DI. Strongyloidiasis: a conundrum for gastroenterologists. *Gut* 1994;35:437–440.

34. Pelletier LL. Chronic strongyloidiasis in World War II far east ex-prisoners of war. *Am J Trop Med Hyg* 1984;33:55–61.

35. Woodring JH. Pulmonary strongyloidiasis: clinical and imaging features. *AJR* 1994;162:537–542.

36. Celedon JC. Systemic strongyloidiasis in patients infected with the human immunodeficiency virus. A report of 3 cases and review of the literature. *Medicine (Baltimore)* 1994;73:256–263.

37. Lindo JF. Prospective evaluation of enzyme-linked immunosorbent assay and immunoblot methods for the diagnosis of endemic *Strongyloides stercoralis* infection. *Am J Trop Med Hyg* 1994;51:175–179.

38. Gann PH, Neva FA, Gam AA. A randomized trial of single- and two-dose ivermectin versus thiabendazole for treatment of strongyloidiasis. *J Infect Dis* 1994;169:1076–1079.

39. Marti H, Haji HJ, Savioli L, et al. A comparative trial of a single-dose of ivermectin versus three days of albendazole for the treatment of *Strongyloides stercoralis* and other soil-transmitted helminth infections in children. *Am J Trop Med Hyg* 1996;55:477–481.

40. Ishikura H, Kikuchi K, Nagasawa K, et al. Anisakidae and anisakidosis. *Prog Clin Parasitol* 1993;3:43–102.

41. World Health Organization. Parasitic zoonoses. Report of a WHO expert committee with the participation of FAO. *WHO Tech Rep Ser* 1979;637:1.

42. López-Serrano MC, Gomez AA, Daschner A, et al. Gastroallergic anisakiasis: findings in 22 patients. *J Gastroenterol Hepatol* 2000;15:503–506.

43. Muguruma N, Okamura S, Okahisa T, et al: *Anisakis* larva involving the esophageal mucosa. *Gastrointest Endosc* 1999;49:653–654.

44. Cross JH, Basaca-Sevilla V. Intestinal capillariasis. *Prog Clin Parasitol* 1989;1:105–119.

45. Choe G, Lee HS, Seo JK, et al. Hepatic capillariasis: first case report in the republic of Korea. *Am J Trop Med Hyg* 1993;48:610–625.

46. Sawamura R, Fernandes MIM Peres CL, et al. Hepatic capillariasis in children: report of 3 cases in Brazil. *Am J Trop Med Hyg* 1999;61:642–647.

47. Wolfe MS. Oxyuris, trichostrongylus, and trichuris. *Clin Gastroenterol* 1978;7:201–217.

48. Ghadirian E, Arfaa F. Present status of trichostrongyliasis in Iran. *Am J Trop Med Hyg* 1975;24:935–941.

49. Pit DSS, Rijcken EM, Raspoort EC, Baeta SM, Polderman AM. Geographic distribution and epidemiology of *Oesophagostomum bifurcum* and hookworm infections in humans in Togo. *Am J Trop Med Hyg* 1999;61:951–955.

50. Storey PA, Spannbrucker N, Yelifari L, et al. Ultrasonographic detection and assessment of preclinical *Oesophagostomum bifurcum*–induced colonic pathology. *Clin Infect Dis* 2001;33:166–170.

51. Verweij JJ, Pit DSS, van Lieshout L, et al. Determining the prevalence of *Oesophagostomum bifurcum* and *Necator americanus* infections using specific PCR amplification of DNA from faecal samples. *Trop Med Int Health* 2001;6:726–731.

CHAPTER 286
Tissue Nematodes

Davidson H. Hamer and David O. Freedman

FILARIASIS

Filarial parasites infect approximately 200 million humans worldwide although mansonellosis is thought to cause insignificant clinical disease. Chronic filariasis, although not responsible for significant mortality, is associated with tremendous suffering and long-term debility in diverse populations, with a resultant adverse socioeconomic impact on afflicted individuals and their communities.

All human infections are caused by filariae of the family Onchocercidae (Table 286.1). The long, thin adult worms reside in the subcutaneous tissues, lymphatics, or peritoneum. Female adults are usually much larger than males because of the large number of larvae contained in the uteri. Sexual reproduction yields microfilariae, the usual diagnostic stage, which migrate in the blood or skin. These microfilariae are ingested by an obligate, bloodsucking arthropod that serves as an intermediate host within which the microfilariae develop into third-stage larvae. These infective larvae escape from the insect at the time of feeding and then migrate within the human host to the tissues or lymphatics, where they develop into adult worms. Generally, repeated and prolonged exposure to infective larvae is required for establishment of human infection. Incubation periods range from 3 to 12 months so a history of remote exposure must be elicited in travelers. Adult worms live for 5 to 15 years but because an individual adult worm cannot multiply within the same host, an increased parasite burden requires ongoing re-infection.

Clinical disease varies between species and results from the host's immune response to either the migrating microfilariae or dying adult parasites. In advanced lymphatic filariasis, bacterial superinfection of compromised vessels plays an important role.

Diethethylcarbamazine (DEC) and ivermectin have been the mainstays of therapy. DEC has a substantial but inconsistent effect against adults of *Loa loa* and the lymphatic filariases so that for these species curative efforts with repeated courses are important to pursue in nonendemic individuals who will not be re-exposed. DEC kills microfilariae of all species except *Mansonella ozzardi* and *Mansonella perstans*. Ivermectin never kills adult filarial parasites but is microfilaricidal to all species except *M. perstans*. Suppression of microfilaria production with either drug

TABLE 286.1. Characteristics of Human Filarial Infections

Organism	Geographic distribution	Habitat of adult worms	Vector	Location of microfilariae	Periodicity of microfilariae
Wuchereria bancrofti	Worldwide, tropics and subtropics	Lymphatic system	Mosquitoes: *Culex, Anopheles, Aedes* sp.	Blood	Nocturnal; South Pacific form is subperiodic
Brugia malayi	Southeast Asia, India, western Pacific	Lymphatic system	Mosquitoes: *Anopheles, Mansonia* sp.	Blood	Nocturnal
Brugia timori	Islands of Timor and Flores	Lymphatic system	Mosquitoes: *Anopheles* sp.	Blood	Nocturnal
Onchocerca volvulus	Africa, Latin America	Subcutaneous tissues	*Simulium* sp. (black flies)	Skin	None
Loa loa	West and Central Africa	Subcutaneous tissues	*Chrysops* sp. (deer flies)	Blood	Diurnal
Mansonella perstans	Africa, Central and South America	Body cavities, mesenteric and retroperitoneal tissues	*Culicoides* sp. (biting midges)	Blood	None
Mansonella streptocerca	West and Central Africa	Subcutaneous tissues	*Culicoides* sp.	Skin	None
Mansonella ozzardi	Caribbean, Central and South America	Subcutaneous tissues	*Culicoides* and *simulium* sp.	Blood	None

may last from weeks to months. Albendazole has significant antifilarial activity but there is not enough data to recommend it as first-line therapy of individual patients although it may be useful in refractory cases.

LYMPHATIC FILARIASIS

Wuchereria bancrofti and *Brugia malayi* are the main causes of lymphatic filariasis in humans, although other minor members of the genus *Brugia*, such as *Brugia timori*, can cause human disease (1). These threadlike nematodes infect approximately 120 million people worldwide (2) and are responsible for a spectrum of disease ranging from asymptomatic infections with microfilaremia to disfiguring lymphatic obstructive disease including elephantiasis.

Life Cycle

The adult worms live in the lumen of lymphatic vessels. The females measure 4 to 10 cm in length; the *W. bancrofti* females are longer than those of *B. malayi*, whereas the males are about 4 and 1.5 cm long, respectively. The adult parasites are thin; the females measure approximately 250 and 150 μm in diameter, respectively. The adult worms reproduce sexually to yield large numbers of microfilariae or first-stage larvae, which migrate into the bloodstream. The microfilariae measure approximately 270 × 9 μm and are ensheathed (Figs. 286.1, 286.2). When mosquitoes take a blood meal from infected humans, they ingest the microfilariae, which then undergo two molts to become infective third-stage larvae during a 10- to 20-day period. The infective larvae are deposited onto the skin during the mosquito's next blood meal. The larvae crawl into the open wound, migrate through the subcutaneous tissues, and finally reach the peripheral lymphatics where they mature into adult worms. Microfilariae are released into the blood stream approximately 6 to 12 months after the infecting bite.

Epidemiology

An estimated 120 million people are infected with *W. bancrofti* (90%) and *B. malayi* (10%). *W. bancrofti*, which has no animal reservoir, is endemic in 76 countries in Africa, South America, the Caribbean, the Indian subcontinent, Southeast Asia, and the western Pacific (see Table 286.1). *B. malayi* is endemic in India, Southeast Asia, and the western Pacific; *B. timori* is localized to the islands of Timor and Flores in the Indonesian archipelago. Newer, more sensitive diagnostic techniques suggest that the number of people with lymphatic filariasis is considerably underestimated. Filarial infections are usually first detected in asymptomatic 5- to 10-year-old children in endemic regions.

W. bancrofti usually shows nocturnal periodicity; microfilariae appear in the peripheral circulation late at night. *Culex* and *Anopheles* mosquitoes transmit this form of *W. bancrofti*, which is mainly present in Africa, India, Southeast Asia, and Latin America. A diurnal form of infection caused by *W. bancrofti* exists in the South Pacific; this is transmitted by day-biting *Aedes* mosquitoes. *B. malayi* infections with nocturnal periodicity, transmitted by *Anopheles* and *Mansonia* mosquito species, are found in areas of India, Sulawesi, Vietnam, and China. A less common subperiodic form characterized by less exaggerated fluctuations in microfilarial blood density is found in areas of Southeast Asia where it

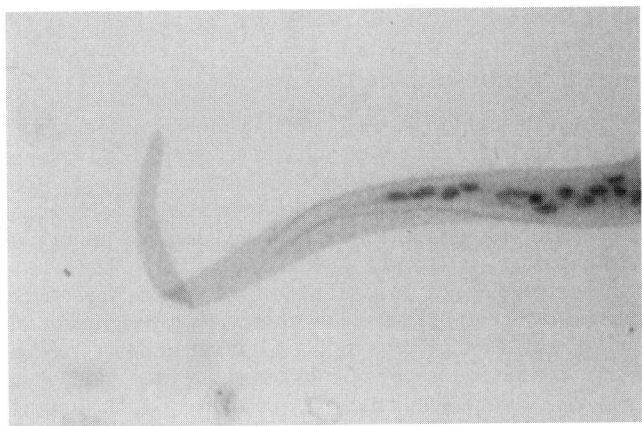

Figure 286.1. *Wuchereria bancrofti* microfilaria. Note that the nuclei are evenly spaced and do not extend to the tip of the tail; the second stage larva is ensheathed in the first-stage cuticle. (Giemsa stain, 100 × 10.)

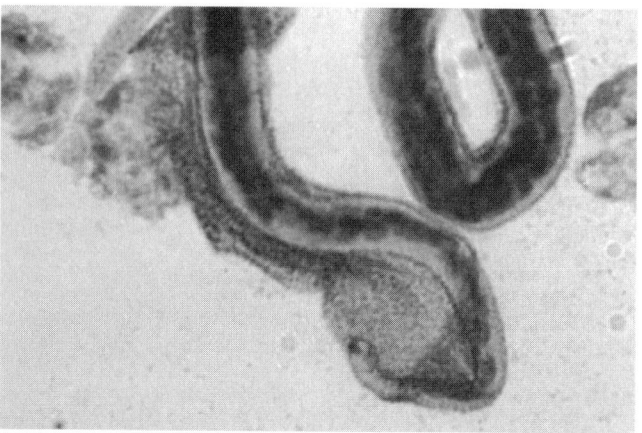

Figure 286.2. *Brugia malayi* microfilaria. Note that the nuclei are unevenly spaced, extending to the tip of the tail and the second-stage larva is ensheathed in the first-stage cuticle. (Giemsa stain, 100 × 10.)

is associated with numerous animal reservoirs. *B. timori* demonstrates nocturnal periodicity and is transmitted by anopheline mosquitoes.

Pathogenesis

Microfilariae in blood do not cause any pathology. The adult worm does not seem to cause blockage of the vessel. The adult lymphatic parasite causes a parasite-specific local inflammatory reaction with both cell-mediated and humoral components, which lead to hypertrophy of the vessel walls (3). This results in vessel dilatation and intraluminal polyposis, which diminish normal lymphatic function. The resulting lymphedema is reversible in its early stages. Following worm death there is necrosis and granulomatous reaction with infiltration of plasma cells, eosinophils, and giant cells. With progression, fibrosis and obstruction of lymph flow within the vessel leads to irreversible elephantiasis of the affected part. At an uncertain point during the clinical evolution of the lymphatic insufficiency, repeated limb bacterial infections in previously damaged vessels may in some individuals become superimposed on other processes. The relative contribution to disease evolution of each of the components and the degree of interindividual variability are incompletely defined at present. Recently, *Wolbachia*, which are symbiotic bacteria coexisting inside filarial worms, have been implicated as factors in filarial inflammation in animal models but relevance in human disease is not yet established (4).

Clinical Manifestations

Most infected individuals remain clinically asymptomatic microfilaria carriers even though sub-clinical lymphatic damage is often present. Those with clinical manifestations present a spectrum of disease including filarial fevers, acute adenolymphangitis, chronic lymphatic obstruction, and tropical pulmonary eosinophilia.

In the early stages of disease a syndrome of filarial fevers characterized by general malaise, low-grade fevers, headaches, and pain associated with lymphangitis or lymphadenitis can occur. Affected lymph nodes may be enlarged and tender, and the skin overlying infected lymphatics may be thickened, firm, tender, and edematous.

Acute episodes of filarial inflammation due to *W. bancrofti* frequently affect the male genitalia and can lead to complications including funiculitis, epididymitis, orchitis, hydrocele, and

elephantiasis of the scrotum. In many areas the most common chronic manifestation of disease is hydrocele with no history of acute inflammatory episodes. A genital examination is mandatory in all males in endemic areas. Chyluria may develop if the obstructed, swollen lymphatic channels rupture into the urinary tract. The legs are more commonly involved than the upper extremities in bancroftian filariasis. In contrast to the common involvement of male genitalia in bancroftian filariasis, brugian filariasis is more likely to present clinically as lymphadenitis and lymphangitis as a result of a predilection of *Brugia* species to involve the superficial inguinal lymphatics. Elephantiasis of the lower extremities involves the entire leg in bancroftian filariasis (Fig. 286.3), whereas the leg above the knee maintains a relatively normal contour in brugian filariasis. Involvement of the upper extremities, breasts, and other areas of the body is relatively infrequent in both forms of lymphatic filariasis. Patients with chronic disease may be microfilaremic but most often are not, having previously cleared their acute infection. Acute attacks of adenolymphangitis may continue even with far advanced lymphedema and may be accompanied by a cellulitis that is bacterial in origin.

Tropical pulmonary eosinophilia is a hypersensitivity syndrome found mainly in southern India, where it is most common in young adult men (5,6). Symptoms include low-grade fever, nocturnal asthma, cough, fatigue, and weight loss.

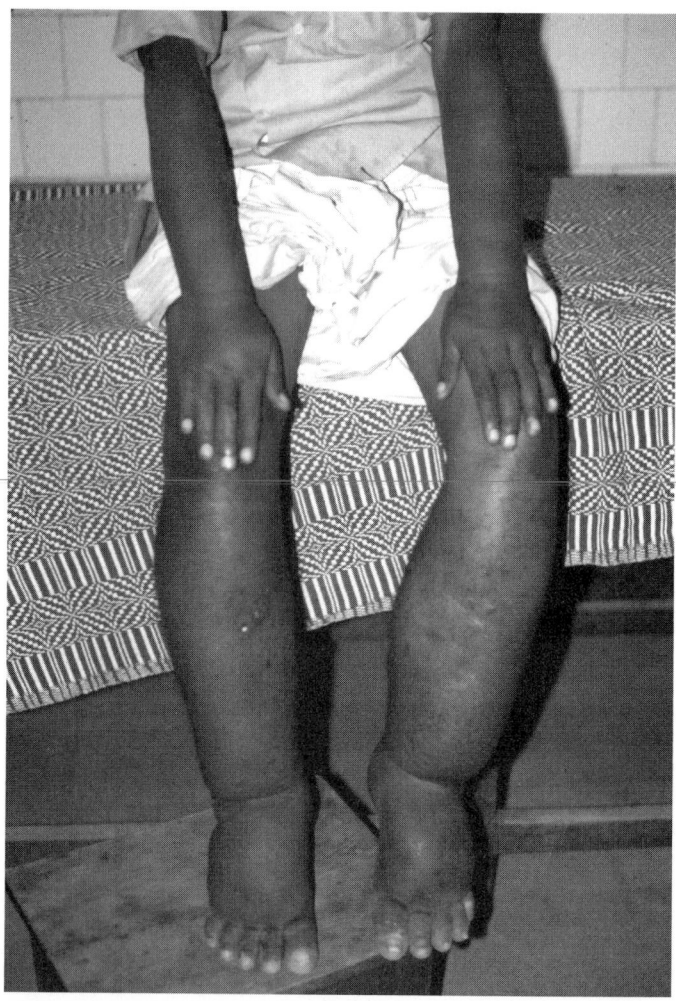

Figure 286.3. Bilateral elephantiasis of the lower extremities, which is prominent from the knees down.

Associated findings include interstitial infiltrates on chest radiographs, marked eosinophilia, and high levels of serum immunoglobulin E. Subjects with this syndrome mount an intense immune response in vitro to the parasite and usually have no circulating microfilariae. If left untreated, tropical pulmonary eosinophilia can result in chronic restrictive lung disease.

Diagnosis

The definitive parasitologic diagnosis is based on the demonstration of microfilariae in blood samples (7). In patients with lymphatic filariasis from regions where nocturnal periodicity is common, blood specimens should be obtained between 10 PM and 2 AM. Microfilariae in blood can be detected by Giemsa-stained thick smears, although this method is generally less sensitive than concentration techniques that use centrifugation (Knotts test) or filtration through a 5 μm polycarbonate membrane filter. Species identification is based on size, staining characteristics of the sheath, and arrangement of nuclei in the tail (see Figs. 286.1 and 286.2). The presence of eosinophilia and elevated titers of specific antifilarial antibodies in serum help support the diagnosis but are only variably present. Antifilarial antibody tests do not distinguish between the eight human filarial species and often cross-react with *Strongyloides* species and other helminths. Antibodies may be present in those with exposure and in those with past but not current infection. Adult worms may be found incidentally in asymptomatic persons in diverse body tissues but lymph node biopsy is not indicated in suspected filariasis unless malignancy is also a concern. An enzyme-linked immunosorbent assay and rapid card test for the detection of circulating antigens of *W. bancrofti* are commercially available but are not approved by the U.S. Food and Drug Administration (FDA) (8,9). Circulating antigen tests are the most sensitive diagnostic modality available for *W. bancrofti* and can be done on serum drawn at any time of day or night (10). Ultrasound techniques have been used to visualize rapidly moving ("dancing") adult worms in the dilated scrotal lymphatics of infected men (11). Such findings are pathognomonic of filarial parasites, but the technique is less sensitive than other modalities. Abnormalities detected by lymphoscintigraphy are not specific for filarial disease (12).

Treatment

Both symptomatic and asymptomatic patients with lymphatic filariasis should be treated with diethylcarbamazine (DEC) (6 mg/kg/day in three divided doses for 2 to 3 weeks). DEC is FDA-approved but at the present time is only available through the Centers for Disease Control (CDC) Drug Service (Telephone 404-639-3670). DEC is non-toxic but dying parasites can cause adverse reactions including fever, chills, headache, dizziness, nausea, vomiting, and arthralgias, which usually occur in the first 24 to 36 hours. The magnitude of the reaction is directly proportional to the number of circulating microfilariae. In those with high levels of microfilaremia, treatment can be initiated with single doses of 50 to 100 mg of DEC on the first 2 days or patients can be pre-medicated with steroids. Adenolymphangitis due to dying adult worms may occur. In individuals who will not be returning to areas of transmission, attempted adulticidal therapy, which requires repeated or prolonged courses of DEC, is recommended. However, less than 25% of patients treated aggressively in this way clear all adult worms (13). If the patient remains microfilaremic, at least two repeat courses at 1-month intervals should be considered. Patients with lymphedema or elephantiasis should receive low-dose DEC daily for at least a year in an attempt to determine whether any reversible component of the chronic disease is present. In trials to date, single dose albendazole has been demonstrated to have adulticidal and microfilaricidal activity in lymphatic filariasis, but appropriate dosing regimens for attempts at prolonged curative treatment of individual patients with albendazole alone or an albendazole plus DEC combination have yet to be determined (14).

Treatment of complications due to chronic lymphatic obstruction is difficult. Limb elevation, massage, use of elastic stockings, and careful skin care with early antimicrobial therapy can help minimize bacterial superinfections of affected limbs (15).

Prevention and Control

Although it may be difficult for residents of endemic areas to avoid mosquito bites, temporary visitors should use repellants and mosquito nets. DEC has some value as a prophylactic agent in a dose of 10 mg/kg on 2 consecutive days each month. Attempts to control the mosquito vectors have failed owing to the development of resistance to insecticides. Yearly mass treatment with single dose albendazole plus DEC or albendazole plus ivermectin is being utilized by the global lymphatic filariasis elimination program to reduce the load of microfilariae in treated individuals and thereby to decrease transmission (16).

ONCHOCERCIASIS

Chronic infection with the parasite *Onchocerca volvulus* is commonly manifested by dermatologic or ocular disease that may progress to disabling dermatitis and blindness. The long-term disability that results from this filarial infection is responsible for a significant negative social and economic impact in endemic areas of equatorial Africa, Latin America, and the Arabian peninsula.

Epidemiology

An estimated 17.7 million people worldwide are infected with *O. volvulus*, most of whom live in equatorial Africa in a broad belt stretching from the Atlantic Coast on the west to the Indian Ocean and Red Sea on the east (see Table 286.1) (17). The greatest number of infected persons is found in Cameroon, Nigeria, the Congo, Uganda, and Ethiopia. Approximately 100,000 individuals suffer from onchocerciasis in Latin America where scattered foci exist in Guatemala, Mexico, Venezuela, Brazil, Colombia, and Ecuador. Onchocerciasis is also endemic in Yemen and southwestern Saudi Arabia.

Humans are the definitive host of this parasite, although similar species are found in other mammals. *O. volvulus* larvae are transmitted to humans by black flies of the genus *Simulium*. The insect vector breeds along free-flowing waterways that have sufficient forest canopy to protect the black flies from excessively intense sun and heat. The black flies deposit their eggs on rocks, sticks, and vegetation along the rapidly flowing bodies of water from which the developing larvae and pupae derive their nutrients. Consequently, onchocerciasis, or river blindness, is clustered around rivers and streams. The disease has a higher prevalence in men than in women in many communities because of greater exposure during daily activities such as fishing, farming, washing, and water collection.

Approximately 1% to 4% of all infected individuals will become blind; however, as many as half of adults in hyperendemic areas may develop this complication. A much higher prevalence of skin disease and other forms of ocular involvement is found in endemic regions than of blindness. The prevalence of infection rises with age such that almost all members of a village may be infected by early adulthood (18). The debilitating effects of chronic dermatitis and severe ocular disease tend to affect adults in their third to fifth decades of life at a time when they are the heads of households. The impact of this disease on some rural communities can be devastating in terms of the severe, personal discomfort and negative economic effects stemming from reduced productivity and time away from work.

Life Cycle

Microfilariae in the skin are ingested by female black flies while they are taking a blood meal from an infected individual. Once ingested, the immature worms penetrate the fly's intestinal wall and migrate to the thoracic flight muscles where they molt twice. The infective third-stage larvae migrate into the proboscis after 6 to 12 days of development and are then deposited on human skin when the fly bites. The larvae enter the bite wound and migrate into the subcutaneous tissues, where they molt twice over several months to become mature male and female worms. The adults become encapsulated in fibrous nodules in the subcutaneous tissue and deeper fascial planes during their growth and maturation. The female adult measures 23 to 50 cm in length and about 250 to 450 μm in diameter; the males are 2 to 5 cm long and 125 to 210 μm wide. After a prepatent period of 9 to 20 months, fertilized female worms release millions of microfilariae during their estimated life span of 8 to 10 years. The microfilariae are motile, are unsheathed, and measure 220 to 360 μm long. The host's immune response to dead and dying microfilaria is responsible for the clinical manifestations of this disease.

Pathophysiology

The skin, lymph nodes, and ocular tissues are the principal sites of infection. More frequent, intensive exposures lead to greater levels of infection. Histopathologic examination of the skin reveals a low-grade, chronic inflammatory process that may progress to dermal atrophy, loss of elastic fibers, and fibrosis (19). Live microfilariae do not appear to induce any host response, whereas the dead worms cause inflammation that increases with severity the longer the infection persists. The nodules containing adult worms, known as onchocercomata, have an outer fibrous capsule, a thin layer of chronic inflammation, and an inner inflammatory cell infiltrate around the adult worm.

A punctate keratitis develops around dead microfilaria in the outer eye, which with long-term, heavy infection progresses to sclerosing keratitis and iridocyclitis, finally culminating in blindness. A chronic, nongranulomatous inflammatory process in other parts of the eye can result in anterior uveitis, chorioretinitis, and optic atrophy (17).

The host reaction to the microfilariae, resulting from cell-mediated immunity to parasite antigens, appears to be the driving force behind the skin and ocular damage. Individuals who manifest the most vigorous immune responses appear more likely to experience severe disease (19). A multiplicity of factors including host inflammatory mediators, especially eosinophils, and parasite antigens contribute to the complex immunopathogenesis of onchocerciasis.

Clinical Manifestations

Intense pruritus and intermittent urticarial or papular eruptions localized to one region of the body and conjunctivitis are early manifestations of disease (20,21) (Fig. 286.4). These may be the only signs and symptoms in nonresidents of endemic areas who

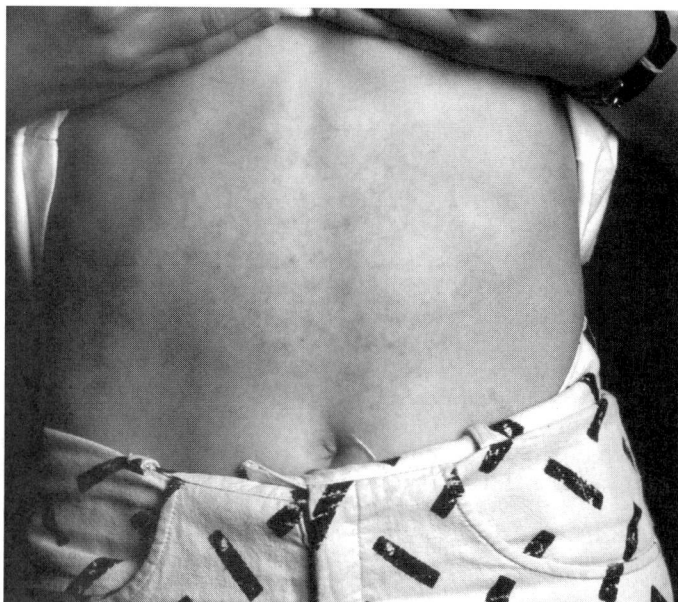

Figure 286.4. White Peace Corps worker with a maculopapular, erythematous rash, which is typically seen in expatriates with onchocercal dermatitis.

usually have lighter infections. Chronic inflammation of the skin can result in hyperpigmentation and, later, a loss of elasticity, a widespread maculopapular rash, hypopigmentation, scaling, and edema. Depigmentation ("leopard skin"), thickening ("elephant skin"), and eventually a shiny, atrophic epidermis ("lizard skin") may develop in long-standing infections. The increased fragility of the skin can lead to areas of breakdown, which places the patient at risk for bacterial super-infection. A classification and grading system of the cutaneous changes of onchocerciasis has been developed in an attempt to standardize interpretation of skin involvement (22). Dermal manifestations of the disease in Africa more commonly involve the lower trunk, buttocks, and lower extremities, whereas they are more prominent around the head and neck in Central America. Lymph node involvement parallels the sites of skin involvement in these two geographic regions. It is usually manifested as non-tender lymphadenopathy although secondary obstructive changes in the groin region can lead to a hanging groin. A hypergic form of onchocerciasis known as *sowda* (meaning "dark" or "black" in Arabic) characterized by hyperpigmentation, papular eruptions, swelling, and regional lymphadenopathy, usually limited to one extremity, is common in Yemen and Sudan, but has also been observed elsewhere in Africa and Latin America. In contrast to *sowda*, in which skin snips reveal few microfilariae, the more common, nonreactive form of onchocerciasis tends to be symmetric with many microfilariae present in skin snips.

Onchocercomata are firm, nontender, and freely mobile subcutaneous or dermal nodules that usually measure 1 to 2 cm. If they are attached to periosteum, the nodules may be immobile. The nodules often occur in clusters in areas where lymphatics converge, including the skull, scapula, intercostal areas, iliac crests, and sacrum (Fig. 286.5). The nodules tend to predominate in the lower part of the body in infected Africans, whereas they are more common in the upper regions of the body in Central Americans.

Early ocular involvement is usually manifested by punctate keratitis and conjunctivitis associated with local irritation and increased tearing. Any part of the eye can be involved from the cornea to the posterior segment, including the retina and optic

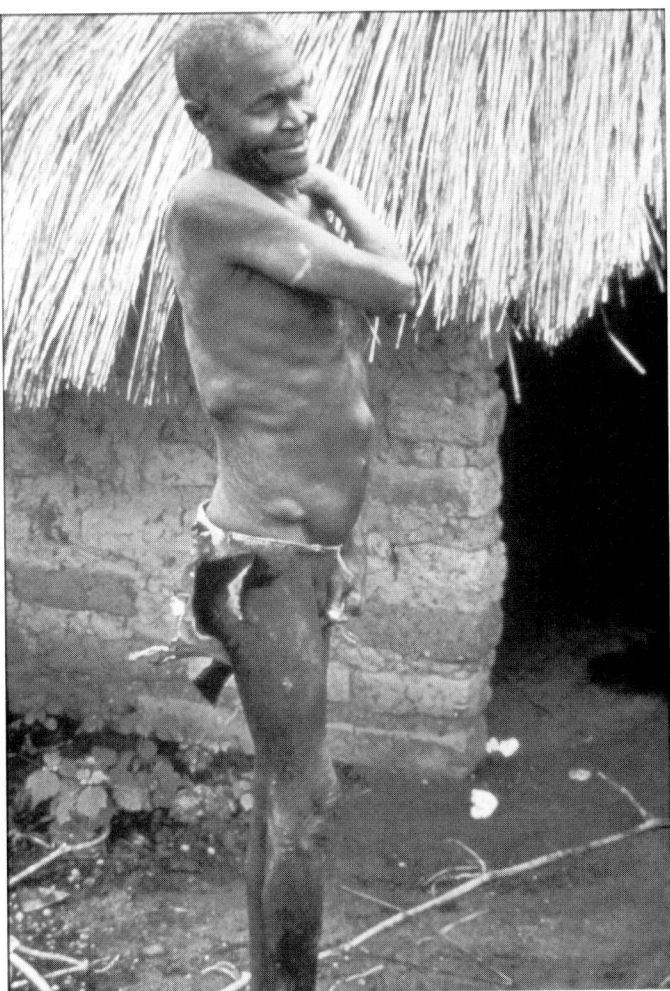

Figure 286.5. A blind man with two large onchocercal nodules on the iliac crest and ribs. (Photograph provided by Dr. D. H. Connor of the Armed Forces Institute of Pathology.)

nerve. Slit-lamp examination may reveal living and dead microfilariae in the cornea, limbus, anterior chamber, retrolental space, vitreous humor, and retina. Additional ophthalmologic manifestations of onchocerciasis include sclerosing keratitis, iridocyclitis, chorioretinitis (which may cause progressive narrowing of visual fields), and optic neuritis and atrophy. Persistent anterior uveitis can lead to meiosis, pupillary distortion, and glaucoma. Sclerosing keratitis, the primary cause of blindness in onchocerciasis, typically develops after decades of infection.

Diagnosis

A clinical diagnosis of onchocerciasis can be made in infected subjects in endemic regions who have typical skin changes, subcutaneous nodules, or ocular lesions. The diagnosis is confirmed by demonstrating *O. volvulus* microfilariae in skin specimens. Samples of skin are usually taken with a corneoscleral biopsy instrument or razor blade from commonly infected sites, such as the upper portion of the body in Central Americans and the lower part in Africans. The skin is weighed and then placed in saline or tissue culture media. Microfilariae that emerge from the skin specimen are counted after incubation at room temperature for 30 minutes to 3 hours. They must be distinguished microscopically from the smaller microfilariae of *M. perstans*. The skin

snips provide a measure of the intensity of infection; less than 10 microfilariae per milligram of skin are present in light infections, whereas more than 100 are found in heavy infections. Skin snips should be taken from several standard sites including the iliac crest, buttocks, calf, and scapula to ensure reliable sampling.

Because the diagnosis of onchocerciasis based on skin snips is highly specific but relatively insensitive, better serologic and molecular diagnostic tests have been sought. Serologic tests, which use a combination of recombinant *O. volvulus* antigens, appear to be useful for determining the seroprevalence of infections (18). In addition, a rapid-format card test for the detection of IgG4 antibodies to antigen Ov16 has been shown to be sensitive and specific for the diagnosis of onchocerciasis in patients in Africa and Latin America (23). Polymerase chain reaction-based tests of skin snips is another highly sensitive approach to diagnosis (24).

Treatment

Although DEC was the standard therapy for nearly half a century, it has largely been supplanted by ivermectin. Ivermectin has been consistently demonstrated to be well tolerated, acceptable to endemic communities, and highly effective in eliminating microfilariae (25,26). Ivermectin is administered as a single oral dose of 150 to 200 μg/kg on an empty stomach at least 2 hours before the next meal. Although many treated subjects have little or no reaction to treatment, some may have increased pruritus, fever, headache, edema, and conjunctivitis or blurring of vision. Adverse reactions usually occur in the first 24 to 48 hours of therapy and last for 5 to 10 days. A minority will develop a maculopapular rash characteristic of the Mazzotti reaction after treatment with ivermectin; more serious reactions such as hypotension or worsening ocular disease are rare. The frequency and severity of adverse reactions to treatment are directly proportional to the intensity of infection. Skin snips should be taken every 6 to 12 months to monitor the response to treatment and to select patients who will need retreatment.

Repeated courses of ivermectin at 6-month intervals lead to a progressive reduction of skin microfilariae counts as well as a decrease in the prevalence of punctate corneal opacities and microfilariae in the anterior chamber of the eye (26,27). The intensity and frequency of adverse reactions diminish with later treatments. Although ivermectin is not macrofilaricidal, three monthly courses of the drug appear to be effective in reducing the numbers of male *O. volvulus* worms, preventing embryogenesis to the microfilarial stage in females, and progressively reducing the numbers of viable female worms (28). Even annual treatment with ivermectin results in an irreversible decline in microfilariae production of about 30% per treatment (29).

Contraindications to ivermectin therapy include pregnancy, breast-feeding during the first 3 months postpartum, age younger than 5 years, central nervous system disorders such as meningitis that may increase the permeability of the blood-brain barrier, and a history of allergy to the drug. If a serious Mazzotti-like reaction occurs during treatment, symptomatic therapy with fluids, antipyretics, antihistamines, and corticosteroids should be used.

Studies in an animal model of onchocerciasis have recently demonstrated that tetracycline has macrofilaricidal activity by virtue of its effect on the parasite's endosymbiont, *Wolbachia* (30). Worm sterilization occurs as a result of the depletion of *Wolbachia* from the worm's tissues. A recent evaluation of doxycycline in combination with ivermectin in humans found that the period of sterility after doxycycline lasted for at least 18 months. In contrast, treatment with ivermectin alone was characterized by recurrence of microfilaremia 12 months after initial treatment (31). Anti-*Wolbachia* plus ivermectin treatment thus holds great promise for the reduction of transmission and potentially the elimination of onchocerciasis in endemic regions.

Suramin has both macrofilaricidal and microfilaricidal activities against *O. volvulus* but it is rarely used because it can cause serious toxic effects. DEC is well tolerated in uninfected persons, whereas severe side effects and complications occur in infected persons as a result of the massive killing of microfilariae during the first few days of treatment. The Mazzotti reaction, an exacerbation of pruritus or rash after a test dose of DEC, is common in heavily infected individuals. Complications of treatment with DEC include fever, intense pruritus, prostration, lymph node swelling and pain, hypotension, and arthralgias (25). Ocular complications include conjunctivitis, keratitis, chorioretinal damage, and optic neuritis. Reactions in the posterior segment of the eye can lead to permanent damage and blindness. Patients treated with DEC should receive escalating doses, and corticosteroids should be considered to help minimize the aforementioned complications. However, as a result of numerous studies in the last two decades demonstrating the efficacy of and improved tolerance to ivermectin therapy for onchocerciasis, DEC should be reserved for patients who cannot take ivermectin.

Surgical removal of nodules containing adult worms should be strongly considered if the nodules are in the head region because of an increased risk for ocular involvement. Nodulectomy has been widely practiced in Latin America but not in Africa, where many nodules are deeper in the subcutaneous tissues or are situated adjacent to bones or joints.

Prevention and Control

No effective prophylactic drugs or vaccines exist. Personal protection measures such as protective clothing and insect repellents and the avoidance of breeding sites of *Simulium* vectors are recommended for visitors to endemic areas. Attempts to eliminate the insect vector with larvicide have been successful in some parts of Africa but have been hampered by the development of larvicidal resistance. Mass treatment with ivermectin has become the principal method for the control of onchocerciasis.

LOIASIS

L. loa is a filarial parasite endemic to the rain forests of equatorial West and Central Africa where an estimated 20 million people are infected (see Table 286.1). Risk is highest in southeastern Nigeria, Cameroon, Gabon, Central African Republic, Equatorial Guinea and the Democratic Republic of Congo (32). Loiasis is transmitted to humans by tabanid flies of the genus *Chrysops*. Adult worms migrate and reside in subcutaneous tissues where they cause transient swellings. They occasionally migrate across the eye, hence the name eyeworm. The adult females measure about 6 cm in length and 0.5 mm in width; the males are 3.2 cm by 0.4 mm. Sheathed microfilariae deposited by the adult females migrate from the subcutaneous tissues to the blood stream (Fig. 286.6). Peak levels of microfilaremia occur at midday. After ingestion in a blood meal by the vector deerfly, the microfilariae develop into infective third-stage larvae, which are released into the bite wound when the fly feeds. The larvae mature to adults in the subcutaneous tissue and reproduce sexually to reinitiate the cycle.

Infected people are frequently asymptomatic despite having heavy microfilaremia and an intense blood eosinophilia.

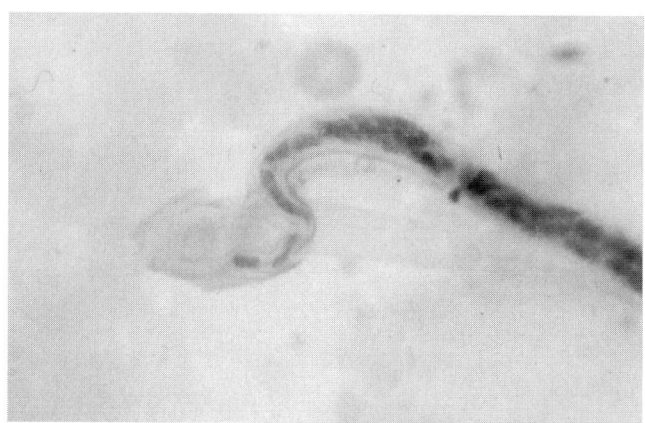

Figure 286.6. *Loa loa* microfilaria. Nuclei are evenly spaced and extend to the tip of the tail; the second-stage larva is ensheathed in the cuticle of the first stage. (Giemsa stain, 100 × 10.)

Migration of the adult worms through subcutaneous tissue results in painful, angioedematous eruptions known as Calabar swellings. The forearms, wrists, and periorbital tissues are most commonly affected. These transient skin swellings last 1 to 2 days; are frequently preceded by localized pain and pruritus; and may be associated with fever, arthralgias, and urticaria. Migration of the adult worm across the conjunctiva and sclera can precipitate an intense conjunctivitis. Visitors to endemic regions who develop loiasis often have exaggerated allergic reactions to the migratory worms characterized by more frequent Calabar swellings and cutaneous symptoms as well as higher levels of eosinophilia, parasite-specific immunoglobulin E, and lymphocyte blastogenic responses to parasite antigen (33,34). However, these individuals are amicrofilaremic 90% of the time. Rare, potentially life-threatening complications include cardiomyopathy, encephalitis, nephropathy, and pulmonary disease. The microfilariae of *L. loa* have been encountered in a variety of aberrant locations including ascites and pleural and joint effusions.

Identification of characteristic microfilariae in thick or thin smears of blood taken during the day and stained with Wright or Giemsa stain establishes the diagnosis of loiasis (see Fig. 286.6). Concentration techniques, as for lymphatic filariasis, may be necessary in patients with low levels of microfilaremia. Short-term visitors are often amicrofilaremic so the diagnosis may need to depend on the characteristic exposure history, clinical presentation, blood eosinophilia, and elevated antifilarial antibody titers. *O. volvulus*, *M. perstans*, *M. ozzardi*, and *M. streptocerca* all cause overlapping syndromes and must, if epidemiologically possible, be ruled out by a complete search for microfilariae in blood and skin. An adult *L. loa* excised while crawling across the conjunctiva or under the skin provides a definitive diagnosis.

DEC (6 to 10 mg/kg/day for 21 days) effectively eliminates microfilariae and is reliably adulticidal in most individuals with repeated courses. One course will cure about half of treated individuals (33). Decisions about retreatment should be based on resolution of symptoms, antifilarial titers and eosinophilia. The latter parameters should slowly decrease with successful therapy but may not return to normal for a year or more. Subjects with high levels of microfilaremia may develop intense allergic reactions to the dying parasites characterized by fever, nausea, urticaria, and rarely encephalitis. In any patient with microfilaremia, a test dose of 25 mg of DEC should be given on day 1 followed by 50 mg the following day and then 400 mg/day for 7 to 21 days. Corticosteroids may be given as an adjunct to decrease the initial inflammatory reaction. With microfilaremia greater than a few hundred microfilariae per milliliter of blood DEC-induced inflammatory reactions to dying microfilariae may progress to encephalopathy and death. If available, apheresis to remove circulating microfilariae can be performed before initiating DEC therapy in these individuals. If this latter option is not available for highly microfilaremic individuals, limited data support the use of albendazole (200 mg twice a day for 21 days) as it appears to be moderately adulticidal but without any effect on the microfilariae (35). Ivermectin is microfilaricidal but has no adulticidal effect and may also cause toxic encephalopathy in highly microfilaremic individuals (36,37). If epidemiologically appropriate, onchocerciasis must be carefully ruled out before the initiation of DEC therapy for loiasis in order to prevent toxicity due to dying *O. volvulus* microfilariae. A 21-day course of albendazole is indicated for those failing multiple courses of DEC (38). DEC has also been used successfully as a prophylactic agent in long-term visitors to endemic regions (39). Migrating adult worms should be surgically removed, especially if they are found in the conjunctiva.

MANSONELLA PERSTANS

M. perstans is found commonly in rain forests in tropical Africa, and less so in Central and South America, and the Caribbean (see Table 286.1). This parasite is transmitted by midges of the *Culicoides* genus with host reservoirs including humans and chimpanzees. The adult worms normally live in the peritoneal cavity of their host but have also been found in pleural and pericardial spaces (40). Unsheathed microfilariae are released into the blood without periodicity. Infected residents of endemic regions are often asymptomatic, although they may have vague joint or cutaneous complaints and eosinophilia. Visitors to endemic areas may develop angioedema, serositis, arthralgia, fever and neurologic manifestations. Demonstration of characteristic microfilariae in blood smears confirms the diagnosis; eosinophilia and positive antifilarial titers are often present. No reliable therapy exists. DEC and ivermectin seem ineffective. Albendazole (400 mg twice a day for 10 days) has given the best results (41). Microfilaremia does not decrease until 30 days or more after treatment.

MANSONELLA STREPTOCERCA

Streptocerciasis is a common filarial infection in parts of Central and West Africa and has recently been found in Uganda as well (see Table 286.1). *M. streptocerca* is transmitted by midges of the genus *Culicoides*. The adult females, which measure approximately 3 cm in length, live in the subcutaneous tissue. The unsheathed microfilariae are about 200 μm long, have a distinctive "shepherd's crook" appearance, and can be found in the skin. Clinical manifestations of infection include pruritus, axillary or inguinal adenopathy, and a chronic dermatitis with hypopigmented macules or papules that resemble those of leprosy but are not anesthetic (42). Skin snips incubated in saline usually reveal the presence of the microfilariae. Caution must be used to avoid confusion with the larger microfilariae of *O. volvulus*. Treatment with DEC (6 mg/kg/day for 2 weeks) is effectively microfilaricidal and adulticidal but may exacerbate the pruritus. Single dose ivermectin (150 μg/kg) is microfilaricidal and concomitantly kills *O. volvulus* microfilariae-these two infections are co-endemic in many areas (43).

MANSONELLA OZZARDI

Mansonelliasis, the filarial infection caused by *M. ozzardi*, is found only in parts of Central and South America and in certain Caribbean islands (see Table 286.1). Midges of the genus *Culicoides* or black flies of the *Simulium* group serve as vectors. The location of adult worms is unclear. The microfilariae in the blood have a characteristic sharp tail and are nonperiodic. Clinical manifestations of this usually asymptomatic infection are ill-defined but may include chronic arthritis and pruritus. Therapy with DEC is generally ineffective (44). Single-dose therapy with ivermectin may be effective, but experience with this agent is limited (45).

DIROFILARIA AND OTHER ZOONOTIC FILARIIDS

Filarial nematodes of the genus *Dirofilaria* are responsible for two syndromes in humans. Transmission of *Dirofilaria immitis* (dog heartworm) larvae from dogs to humans by mosquitoes can lead to the development of a granulomatous pulmonary nodule (46). Subcutaneous dirofilariasis results from the accidental infection of humans by *Dirofilaria repens*, whose natural hosts are dogs and cats, or by *Dirofilaria tenuis*, a parasite of the subcutaneous tissue of raccoons (47).

The larvae of *D. immitis* are commonly found in mosquitoes in urban areas of the United States, especially in the Southeast. Accidental infection of humans has been described in the United States, Japan, Australia, and Western Europe. The adult worms of this parasite are unable to develop fully in humans. Infected individuals are usually asymptomatic, although there may be cough, chest pain, hemoptysis, and fever in up to 44% (46). Chest radiographs commonly reveal a solitary, peripheral pulmonary nodule, most often in the lower lobes, which, when it is excised, will reveal a granulomatous reaction surrounding an intact dead worm or worm fragments within an arteriole. Surgical excision of the nodule, often performed to rule out malignant neoplasm, fulfills the dual purposes of diagnosis and treatment of pulmonary dirofilariasis. Antifilarial serology is unreliable and unproven and peripheral eosinophilia is present in less than 10%. No additional therapy is necessary because this infection is self-limited.

Subcutaneous dirofilariasis is a rare, cosmopolitan infection that is probably acquired by humans from the usual animal host by a mosquito vector. Because humans represent a dead-end host, the larvae are unable to mature to adults, and therefore microfilariae are never observed. Granulomatous, subcutaneous nodules may be found in the conjunctiva, chest wall, and extremities. The lesion develops slowly during many weeks into a nodule that may be painful and erythematous. Diagnosis is made by identification of the worm in biopsy specimens, a procedure that also serves as treatment.

More than 100 filarial species of animals are described. When these parasites accidentally enter humans the larvae quickly die in tissues and on occasion cause an inflammatory response, which comes to clinical attention. Non-human *Brugia*, *Dirofilaria*, *Mansonella* species are most commonly implicated (48). Pathologic identification requires expert consultation.

OTHER TISSUE NEMATODE INFECTIONS

Dracunculiasis

Dracunculiasis, also known as guinea worm disease or dracontiasis, develops after the ingestion of water contaminated with copepods infected with *Dracunculus medinensis*. A chronic skin ulcer from which the adult worm protrudes is the main manifestation of disease. Dracunculiasis is responsible for significant morbidity and decreased agricultural productivity in endemic populations.

EPIDEMIOLOGY

Dracunculiasis remains endemic in rural populations in several countries in sub-Saharan Africa. A worldwide eradication campaign has successfully reduced the incidence of disease from more than 3 million cases in 1986 to less than 100,000 cases in 1999 (49). The prevalence of dracunculiasis exhibits seasonal variation. The frequency of infection increases with age until the second or third decade of life (50). Greater exposure to infected water through agricultural activities or the collection of water for domestic use places certain groups at higher risk for infection. Sources of drinking water such as step wells or ponds that require people to walk down into the water are necessary for continued transmission of this parasite.

LIFE CYCLE

Human infection is acquired after drinking water containing copepods (*Cyclops*) harboring the third-stage larvae of the parasite. The larvae penetrate the intestinal mucosa to reach the retroperitoneum, where they mature into adult worms during a 12-month period. The adult female migrates to the skin surface to form a blister from which a portion of the worm protrudes. Water exposure leads to the release of many first-stage larvae from the wound, which are in turn ingested by copepods. After a period of about 10 days, the larvae mature to a new infective stage. The adult females of *D. medinensis* range from 70 to 120 cm in length; the males, uncommonly observed in infected humans, measure only 3 to 5 cm.

CLINICAL FEATURES

Prodromal symptoms of urticaria, fever, nausea, vomiting, diarrhea, and dysphoria may precede the formation of a skin blister (51). The lesion is initially pruritic and erythematous and then progresses to form a vesicle that may measure several centimeters in diameter. After the blister ruptures, the adult female protrudes to a distance of several centimeters. The ulcers are painful and occur most commonly in the lower extremities (Fig. 286.7), although many other locations are possible. Multiple ulcers may be present, with greater numbers directly correlating with the degree of disability suffered. The adult worm intermittently discharges a milky white fluid containing larvae and is gradually resorbed or completely extruded. The healing process may take many weeks or even months, during which the affected person is incapacitated. Secondary bacterial infections with abscess formation are common complications whereas tetanus is rare. If the ulcer formation occurs during a critical agricultural period or the school year for children, the resulting disability can have significant negative social and economic impact (51,52). The proximity of an ulcer to a joint may lead to arthritis and long-term disability due to joint contractures.

DIAGNOSIS

The clinical picture is diagnostic. Larvae can be seen on microscopic examination of fluid discharged from the ulcer. Attempts to develop serologic tests for the diagnosis of the infection during the prepatent period have been unsuccessful.

TREATMENT

Treatment consists of manually extracting the worm by winding it around a stick with gentle traction. Accidental rupture of the worm will precipitate severe systemic reactions manifested by fever, anaphylaxis, and urticaria with late complications including abscess formation and chronic ulceration. Surgical extraction of the unerupted worm under local anesthesia effectively shortens the removal time and associated period of disability (53). Topical or systemic antimicrobial agents help to relieve ulcer-associated pain, improve healing, and facilitate more rapid removal of worms, although no agent has been found to have curative activity against *D. medinensis* (54). Local care of the wound is necessary to prevent bacterial superinfection. Tetanus immunization is recommended.

PREVENTION

Dracunculiasis can be prevented by teaching people to filter their drinking water through a fine-mesh cloth or nylon filter; to boil their drinking water; to avoid entering drinking water sources when the adult worm is emerging; by providing improved sources of drinking water; and by treating contaminated water supplies with the chemical Temefos monthly during the season of transmission.

Gnathostomiasis

Human gnathostomiasis is a sporadic infection principally caused by *Gnathostoma spinigerum*, although at least four other species of *Gnathostoma* have been found in human infections (55). The disease is endemic in Asia, especially in Japan and Thailand. Humans are accidental hosts who acquire infection by the consumption of the raw or undercooked flesh of freshwater fish or other intermediate hosts that contain the encysted, infective larvae. The consumption of raw, marinated fish in the form of ceviche has resulted in the increased recognition of gnathostomiasis in Mexico, Ecuador, and Peru. The definitive hosts of *G. spinigerum* include dogs, cats, and wild mammals. The adult worms reside in the gastric wall and release eggs, which, after passage into the environment, hatch to release first-stage larvae. These larvae are ingested by an intermediate host of the *Cyclops* genus in which they mature to second- or third-stage larvae that may be ingested by a second intermediate host, usually fish or amphibians. The larvae migrate to the musculature, complete development, and encyst. The life cycle is completed when a definitive host ingests the flesh of the infected second intermediate host.

Initial clinical manifestations, which occur within 24 to 48 hours after ingestion of the parasite, include malaise, fever,

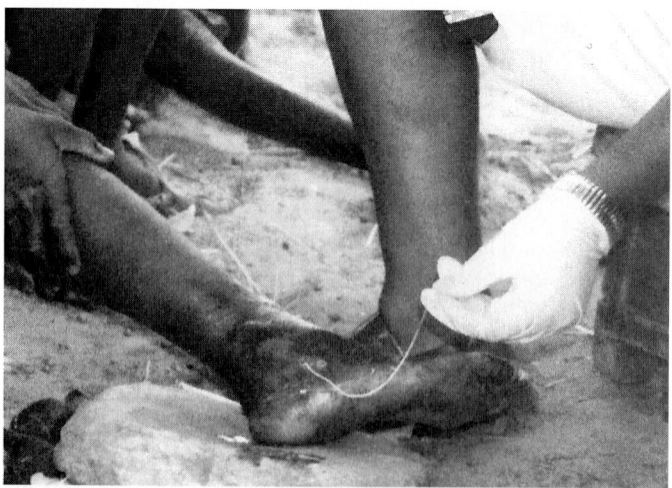

Figure 286.7. A female *Dracunculus* worm emerging from an ulcer on the ankle. (Courtesy of the Carter Center.)

urticaria, nausea, vomiting, diarrhea, and abdominal pain (56). An intense eosinophilia develops in association with the penetration of the gastric or intestinal wall by the larvae. Cutaneous gnathostomiasis, the most common manifestation of infection, may take 3 to 4 weeks to develop. Cutaneous disease is characterized by intermittent episodes of migratory swelling with associated edema, pain, pruritus, and eosinophilia (55). Migrating, immature adult worms are responsible for the subcutaneous eruptions. The episodes last 1 to 2 weeks and may recur at variable intervals. Ocular complications, including anterior uveitis, iritis, intraocular hemorrhage, and even blindness, may occur. Less common sites of visceral involvement include the lung, intestine, bladder, and regions of the ear, nose, and throat.

Infection of the central nervous system (CNS) with *G. spinigerum*, a potentially fatal complication, is manifested by an eosinophilic myeloencephalitis characterized by severe nerve root pain, paralysis, and urinary retention with an associated eosinophilic pleocytosis of the cerebrospinal fluid. Blindness, impairment of visual acuity, paraplegia, and death are potential serious complications of CNS involvement.

Gnathostomiasis should be suspected in patients from an endemic area who have a positive dietary history, migratory skin lesions, and peripheral eosinophilia. Gnathostomal creeping eruptions are frequently confused with those caused by canine or feline hookworms. Most other diseases characterized by subcutaneous swellings can be differentiated on epidemiologic and clinical grounds. Central nervous system gnathostomiasis can be clinically distinguished from eosinophilic meningitis caused by *Angiostrongylus cantonensis*, which tends to be less severe in terms of nerve root and cranial nerve involvement. The definitive diagnosis of gnathostomiasis is dependent on identification of the worms in surgical specimens or body fluids.

Surgical removal of the worm is the most effective treatment for this infection. Supportive therapy should include antiinflammatory agents and analgesics. A number of anthelmintic drugs have been tried but have not proved effective, although albendazole holds some promise (57). Adequate cooking of potentially infected intermediate or transport hosts is needed to prevent infection.

Angiostrongylus cantonensis

Human eosinophilic meningitis is most commonly caused by *A. cantonensis*, a parasite of rats (58,59). The adult worms live in the rat's pulmonary artery and right ventricle. Female adult worms release eggs, which embryonate in pulmonary capillaries. The first-stage larvae penetrate into the alveoli, migrate up the tracheobronchial tree, are swallowed, and are eventually eliminated in the feces. A number of different molluscan species including snails and slugs serve as intermediate hosts. After ingestion by a suitable mollusk, the larvae mature to third-stage larvae, which are ingested by rats. The larvae penetrate the intestinal wall and migrate through the venous system to the pulmonary circulation, from which they migrate to the brain and other organs. The larvae undergo additional maturation in the brain before returning to the lungs to complete the cycle. Humans are accidental hosts who acquire infection by ingesting inadequately cooked or raw snails, freshwater shrimp, or terrestrial crabs. Vegetables or other foods contaminated by the mucus of slugs or planaria may also serve as a source of infection.

Human infection with *A. cantonensis* has been principally found in Southeast Asia and some Pacific islands including Guam, American Samoa, and Hawaii. Sporadic cases have been reported from the Ivory Coast, Cuba, Réunion, and Louisiana (60). Infected patients tend to be young people with a history of exposure to snails, raw fish, or prawns.

Invasion of the brain parenchyma and spinal cord by larval stages of the parasite is responsible for clinical symptoms. After an incubation period of about 1 week, infected patients commonly develop the acute onset of severe headache, nausea, vomiting, lethargy, paresthesias, meningismus, and low-grade fever (61,62). Physical examination may reveal signs of meningeal irritation, cranial nerve palsies, altered mental status, and a temperature less than 38°C. Characteristic cerebrospinal fluid findings include elevated opening pressure, turbid fluid, eosinophilic pleocytosis (often greater than 20% eosinophils), elevated protein concentration, and normal glucose level. Adult worms are recovered from the cerebrospinal fluid in less than 10% of cases. The parasite is occasionally observed in and may be removed from the eye. The diagnosis can be substantiated by demonstrating elevated titers of antibodies to *A. cantonensis* antigens by enzyme-linked immunosorbent assay. In addition, circulating antigens of the parasite can be detected in serum and CSF (63).

No antihelmintic therapy has been proved beneficial in treating neuro-angiostrongyliasis. Supportive treatment with fluids and analgesics is indicated. A course of corticosteroids may be justifiable in severe, life-threatening infections of the central nervous system. However, most persons recover after a period of a few weeks and rarely suffer from chronic neurologic sequelae.

Angiostrongylus costaricensis

Abdominal angiostrongyliasis has mainly been described in children in Central and South America although adults may rarely be infected as well (64,65). The life cycle of *A. costaricensis* is similar to that of *A. cantonensis*. Natural hosts include the cotton rat (*Sigmodon hispidus*) and other rodents. Human infection is probably acquired by the ingestion of infective larvae contained in tissues of the intermediate host, commonly a slug, or by consumption of vegetables contaminated with extruded slug mucus. Consumption of raw mint and ceviche containing mint was associated with an increased risk of abdominal angiostrongyliasis in the only reported outbreak of this infection (65). Ingested larvae develop into adult worms, which reside in mesenteric arterioles, especially in the ileocolic area. Eggs released by the female adult result in eosinophilic granulomata, thrombosis, and arteritis of the intestinal wall. The eggs have not been found in the stool of infected humans.

Infection is clinically manifested by acute right lower quadrant abdominal pain, a tumor-like mass, and peritoneal signs are common signs of infection, which clinically resembles acute appendicitis. Complications include intestinal perforation, obstruction, and gastrointestinal hemorrhage. A visceral larva migrans-like syndrome is a rare complication of the ectopic localization of adult worms in the liver. Marked eosinophilia frequently accompanies the infection. The diagnosis is usually established by histopathologic examination of surgical specimens. Treatment with thiabendazole may be helpful but has not been conclusively demonstrated to be effective. Surgical resection of infected regions of the ileum, appendix, cecum, and ascending colon is often necessary.

REFERENCES

1. Lymphatic filariasis: the disease and its control. Fifth report of the WHO Expert Committee on Filariasis. *WHO Tech Rep Ser* 1992;821:871.
2. Michael E, Bundy DAP, Grenfell BT. Re-assessing the global prevalence and distribution of lymphatic filariasis. *Parasitology* 1996;112:409–428.
3. Freedman DO. Immune dynamics in the pathogenesis of human lymphatic filariasis. *Parasitol Today* 1998;14:229–233.

4. Taylor MJ, Hoerauf A. *Wolbachia* bacteria of filarial nematodes. *Parasitol Today* 1999;15:437–442.

5. Ong RK, Doyle RL. Tropical pulmonary eosinophilia [Review]. *Chest* 1998;113:1673–1679.

6. Teo SK. Tropical pulmonary eosinophilia. *Singapore Med J* 1991;32:118–119.

7. Eberhard ML, Lammie PJ. Laboratory diagnosis of filariasis. *Clin Lab Med* 1991;11:977–1010.

8. More SJ, Copeman DB. A highly specific and sensitive monoclonal antibody-based ELISA for the detection of circulating antigen in bancroftian filariasis. *Trop Med Parasitol* 1990;41:403–406.

9. Weil GJ, Lammie PJ, Weiss N. The ICT filariasis test: a rapid-format antigen test for diagnosis of bancroftian filariasis. *Parasitol Today* 1997;13:401–404.

10. Freedman DO, de Almeida A, Miranda J, et al. Field trial of a rapid card test for *Wuchereria bancrofti* [letter]. *Lancet* 1997;350:1681.

11. Faris R, Hussain O, El Setouhy M, et al. Bancroftian filariasis in Egypt: visualization of adult worms and subclinical lymphatic pathology by scrotal ultrasound. *Am J Trop Med Hyg* 1998;59:864–867.

12. Freedman DO, de Almeida Filho PJ, Besh S, et al. Lymphoscintigraphic analysis of lymphatic abnormalities in symptomatic and asymptomatic human filariasis. *J Infect Dis* 1994;170:927–933.

13. Freedman DO, Plier DA, De Almeida AB, et al. Effect of aggressive prolonged diethylcarbamazine therapy on circulating antigen levels in bancroftian filariasis. *Trop Med Int Health* 2001;6:37–41.

14. Ismail MM, Jayakody RL, Weil GJ, et al. Efficacy of single dose combinations of albendazole, ivermectin and diethylcarbamazine for the treatment of bancroftian filariasis. *Trans R Soc Trop Med Hyg* 1998;92:94–97.

15. Shenoy RK, Kumaraswami V, Suma TK, et al. A double-blind, placebo-controlled study of the efficacy of oral penicillin, diethylcarbamazine or local treatment of the affected limb in preventing acute adenolymphangitis in lymphoedema caused by brugian filariasis. *Ann Trop Med Parasitol* 1999;93:367–377.

16. Ottesen EA. The global programme to eliminate lymphatic filariasis. *Trop Med Int Health* 2000;5:591–594.

17. Burnham G. Onchocerciasis. *Lancet* 1998;351:1341–1346.

18. Bradley JE, Atogho BM, Elson L, Stewart GR, Boussinesq M. A cocktail of recombinant *Onchocerca volvulus* antigens for serologic diagnosis with the potential to predict the endemicity of onchocerciasis infection. *Am J Trop Med Hyg* 1998;59:877–882.

19. Ottesen EA. Immune responsiveness and the pathogenesis of human onchocerciasis. *J Infect Dis* 1995;171:659–671.

20. Gibson DW, Duke BOL, Connor DH. Onchocerciasis: a review of clinical, pathologic and chemotherapeutic aspects, and vector control programs. *Prog Clin Parasitol* 1989;1:57–103.

21. Makunde WH, Salum FM, Massaga JJ, Alilio MS. Clinical and parasitological aspects of itching caused by onchocerciasis in Morogoro, Tanzania. *Ann Trop Med Parasitol* 2000;94:793–799.

22. Murdoch ME, Hay RJ, MacKenzie CD, et al. A clinical classification and grading system of cutaneous changes in onchocerciasis. *Br J Dermatol* 1993;129:260–269.

23. Weil GJ, Steel C, Liftis F, et al. A rapid-format antibody card test for diagnosis of onchocerciasis. *J Infect Dis* 2000;182:1796–1799.

24. Vincent JA, Lustigman S, Zhang S, Weil GJ. A comparison of newer tests for the diagnosis of onchocerciasis. *Ann Trop Med Parasitol* 2000;94:253–258.

25. Greene BM, Taylor HR, Cupp EW, et al. Comparison of ivermectin and diethylcarbamazine in the treatment of onchocerciasis. *N Engl J Med* 1985;313:133–138.

26. Paque M, Munoz B, Greene BM, et al. Community-based treatment of onchocerciasis with ivermectin: safety, efficacy, and acceptability of yearly treatment. *J Infect Dis* 1991;163:381–385.

27. Greene BM, Dukuly ZD, Munoz B, et al. A comparison of 6-, 12-, and 24-monthly dosing with ivermectin for treatment of onchocerciasis. *J Infect Dis* 1991;163:376–380.

28. Duke BOL, Zea-Flores G, Castro J, et al. Effects of three-month doses of ivermectin on adult *Onchocerca volvulus*. *Am J Trop Med Hyg* 1992;46:189–194.

29. Plaisier AP, Soumbey Alley E, Boatin BA, et al. Irreversible effects of ivermectin on adult parasites in onchocerciasis patients in the Onchocerciasis Control Programme in West Africa. *J Infect Dis* 1995;172:204–210.

30. Langworthy NG, Renz A, Mackenstedt U, et al. Macrofilaricidal activity of tetracycline against the filarial nematode *Onchocerca ochenji*: elimination of *Wolbachia* precedes worm death and suggests a dependent relationship. *Proc R Soc Lond B* 2000;267:1063–1069.

31. Hoerauf A, Mand S, Adjei O, Fleischer B, Büttner DW. Depletion of wolbachia endobacteria in *Onchocerca volvulus* by doxycycline and microfilaridermia after ivermectin treatment. *Lancet* 2001;357:1415–1416.

32. Boussinesq M, Gardon J. Prevalences of *Loa loa* microfilaraemia throughout the area endemic for the infection. *Ann Trop Med Parasitol* 1997;91:573–589.

33. Klion AD, Massougbodji A, Sadeler BC, et al. Loiasis in endemic and nonendemic populations: immunologically mediated differences in clinical presentation. *J Infect Dis* 1991;163:1318–1325.

34. Churchill DR, Morris C, Fakoya A, et al. Clinical and laboratory features of patients with loiasis (*Loa loa* filariasis) in the UK. *J Infect* 1996;33:103–109.

35. Klion AD, Massougbodji A, Horton J, et al. Albendazole in human loiasis: results of a double-blind, placebo-controlled trial. *J Infect Dis* 1993;168:202–206.

36. Gardon J, Gardon-Wendel N, Demanga N, et al. Serious reactions after mass treatment of onchocerciasis with ivermectin in an area endemic for *Loa loa* infection. *Lancet* 1997;350:18–22.

37. Gardon J, Kamgno J, Folefack G, et al. Marked decrease in *Loa loa* microfilaraemia six and twelve months after a single dose of ivermectin. *Trans R Soc Trop Med Hyg* 1997;91:593–594.

38. Klion AD, Horton J, Nutman TB. Albendazole therapy for loiasis refractory to diethylcarbamazine treatment. *Clin Infect Dis* 1999;29:680–682.

39. Nutman TB, Miller KD, Mulligan M, et al. Diethylcarbamazine prophylaxis for human loiasis. Results of a double-blind study. *N Engl J Med* 1988;319:752–756.

40. Baird JK, Neafie RC, Lanoie L, et al. Adult *Mansonella perstans* in the abdominal cavity in nine Africans. *Am J Trop Med Hyg* 1987;37:578–584.

41. Duong TH, Kombila M, Ferrer A, et al. Decrease in *Mansonella perstans* microfilaraemia after albendazole treatment. *Trans R Soc Trop Med Hyg* 1998;92:459.

42. Fischer P, Bamuhiiga J, Buttner DW. Occurrence and diagnosis of *Mansonella streptocerca* in Uganda. *Acta Tropica* 1997;63:43–55.

43. Fischer P, Tukesiga E, Buttner DW. Long-term suppression of *Mansonella streptocerca* microfilariae after treatment with ivermectin. *J Infect Dis* 1999;180:1403–1405.

44. Chadee DD, Tilluckdharry CC, Rawlins SC, et al. Mass chemotherapy with diethylcarbamazine for the control of bancroftian filariasis: a twelve-year follow-up in northern Trinidad, including observations on *Mansonella ozzardi*. *Am J Trop Med Hyg* 1995;52:174–176.

45. Nutman TB, Nash TE, Ottesen EA. Ivermectin in the successful treatment of a patient with *Mansonella ozzardi* infection. *J Infect Dis* 1987;156:662–665.

46. Flieder DB, Moran CA. Pulmonary dirofilariasis: a clinicopathologic study of 41 lesions in 39 patients. *Hum Pathol* 1999;30:251–256.

47. Orihel TC, Helentjaris D, Alger J. Subcutaneous dirofilariasis: single inoculum, multiple worms. *Am J Trop Med Hyg* 1997;56:452–455.

48. Orihel TC, Eberhard ML. Zoonotic filariasis. *Clin Microbiol Rev* 1998;11:366–381.

49. Centers for Disease Control and Prevention. Progress toward global dracunculiasis eradication. *MMWR* 2000;49:7315.

50. Abdel-Hameed AA, Ahmed AGM, Elturabi MK, et al. An outbreak of dracunculiasis in central Sudan. *Ann Trop Med Parasitol* 1993;87:5717.

51. Ilegbodu VA, Kale OO, Wise RA, et al. Impact of Guinea worm disease on children in Nigeria. *Am J Trop Med Hyg* 1986;35:962–964.

52. Ilegbodu VA, Ilegbodu AE, Wise RA, et al. Clinical manifestations, disability and use of folk medicine in *Dracunculus* infection in Nigeria. *J Trop Med Hyg* 1991;94:35–41.

53. Rohde JE, Sharma BL, Patton H, et al. Surgical extraction of Guinea worm: disability reduction and contribution to disease control. *Am J Trop Med Hyg* 1993;48:71–76.

54. Magnussen P, Yakubu A, Bloch P. The effect of antibiotic- and hydrocortisone-containing ointments in preventing secondary infections in Guinea worm disease. *Am J Trop Med Hyg* 1994;51:797–799.

55. Diaz Camacho SP, Ramos MZ, Torrecillas EP, et al. Clinical manifestations and immunodiagnosis of gnathostomiasis in Culiacan, Mexico. *Am J Trop Med Hyg* 1998;59:908–15.

56. Rusnak JM, Lucey DR. Clinical gnathostomiasis: case report and review of the English-language literature. *Clin Infect Dis* 1993;16:33–50.

57. Suntharasamai P, Riganti M, Chittamas S, Desakorn V. Albendazole stimulates outward migration of *Gnathostoma spingerum* to the dermis in man. *Southeast Asian J Trop Med Public Health* 1992;23:716–722.

58. Prociv P, Spratt DM, Carlisle MS. Neuro-angiostrongyliasis: unresolved issues. *Int J Parasitol* 2000;30:1295–1303.

59. Koo J, Pien F, Kliks MM. *Angiostrongylus* (*Parastrongylus*) eosinophilic meningitis. *Rev Infect Dis* 1988;10:1155–1162.

60. New D, Little MD, Cross J. *Angiostrongylus cantonensis* infection from eating raw snails. *N Engl J Med* 1995;332:1105–1106.

61. Punyagupta S, Juttijudata P, Bunnag T. Eosinophilic meningitis in Thailand. Clinical studies of 484 typical cases probably caused by *Angiostrongylus cantonensis*. *Am J Trop Med Hyg* 1975;24:921–931.

62. Yii CY. Clinical observations on eosinophilic meningitis and meningoencephalitis caused by *Angiostrongylus cantonensis* on Taiwan. *Am J Trop Med Hyg* 1976;25:233–249.

63. Chye S-M, Yen C-M, Chen E-R. Detection of circulating antigen by monoclonal antibodies for immunodiagnosis of angiostrongyliasis. *Am J Trop Med Hyg* 1997;56:408–412.

64. Loria-Cortes R, Lobo-Sanahuja JF. Clinical abdominal angiostrongylosis. A study of 116 children with intestinal eosinophilic granuloma caused by *Angiostrongylus costaricensis*. *Am J Trop Med Hyg* 1980;29:538–544.

65. Kramer MH, Greer GJ, Quiñonez JF, et al. First reported outbreak of abdominal angiostrongyliasis. *Clin Infect Dis* 1998;26:365–372.

CHAPTER 287
Schistosoma *and Other* Trematodes

Charles H. King and Adel A. F. Mahmoud

Several groups of flukes (flatworms) infect humans and are responsible for significant morbidity. Flukes can be classified clinically by the primary site of involvement in humans (blood, intestines, liver, lungs, brain). Like most other parasitic worms, flukes are characterized by their inability to multiply within the mammalian host. Also, there is a characteristic association between the tissue migratory phase of worm infections and significant peripheral as well as tissue eosinophilia (1).

BLOOD FLUKES: SCHISTOSOMIASIS

History

Human infection with species of the blood flukes (schistosomes) was reported in mummies from ancient Egypt approximately 3,000 to 5,000 years ago, and calcified *Schistosoma haematobium* eggs have been found in tissues dating back to 1250 BC. In modern history, the worms were first identified and described by Theodor Bilharz, who found them while performing autopsies in Cairo, Egypt, in 1852. Five species of *Schistosoma* are currently known to infect humans (Table 287.1): *S. haematobium*, *S. mansoni*, and *S. japonicum* and the less common *S. mekongi* and *S. intercalatum* (2). Infection is endemic in many parts of Africa, the Middle East, Southeast Asia, South America, and the Caribbean. The total number of infected persons is estimated at 200 to 300 million, and those at risk for acquiring infection range from 600 million to 1 billion (3).

Characteristics of the Pathogen

The schistosomes are flatworms (platyhelminths) but differ from other flukes that infect humans in that they have separate sexes. Adult worms inhabit the venous system draining the urinary bladder or intestines. Adult male worms measure approximately 1 to 1.5 cm in length; the flattened sides of the body curve anteriorly to form the gynecophoric canal, in which adult females usually live. Adult females are rounded and longer than males (1.5 to 2.0 cm) and produce several hundred eggs daily. Epidemiologic evidence indicates that the mean life span of adult schistosomes is 5 to 10 years, although case reports document that viable eggs may be detected in excreta of infected persons as long as 40 years after they depart endemic areas. The life cycle of the schistosome is shown in Fig. 287.1.

Epidemiology

Schistosomiasis is a waterborne infection. The infective larvae, called cercariae, are found in freshwater bodies in endemic areas. Cercariae infect humans by penetrating intact skin within a few minutes of contact. On maturation in humans, adult worms begin oviposition. A proportion of the ova pass to the environment through human excreta; if they reach freshwater, eggs hatch, releasing free-swimming miracidia that seek the specific snail intermediate host. After a series of multiplications in the snail, cercariae emerge and must find and penetrate the skin of the

human definitive host within several hours to complete the life cycle of the parasite.

The geographic distribution of schistosomiasis parallels that of the specific snail intermediate host and is dependent on availability of infected humans who, because of their cultural habits or socioeconomic factors, pass their excreta in or close to freshwater bodies. *S. haematobium* infection is endemic in many parts of Africa and the Middle East; *S. mansoni* in Africa, the Middle East, South America, and some Caribbean islands; *S. japonicum* in the Far East; *S. mekongi* in isolated foci in Southeast Asia; and *S. intercalatum* in Central and West Africa (4).

The epidemiology of schistosomiasis in human populations has several characteristic features (5). Infection is gradually acquired as children begin to experience contact with cercariae-contaminated freshwater bodies. Prevalence gradually increases with age until it reaches a peak at approximately 10 to 20 years. The extent of prevalence varies from one endemic community to another and may reach 100% in high-transmission areas. A slight but insignificant decrease in prevalence is usual among persons 30 years and older. Intensity of infection (estimated by egg count in excreta) increases with age, again reaching a maximum at age 15 to 20 years. Thereafter, intensity decreases significantly, so that it is rare to find heavy infection in persons older than 30 years. From this marked reduction of intensity in older persons living in endemic areas, acquisition of protective immunity has been inferred.

Pathogenesis

Disease manifestations due to schistosome infection are a result of the stage of parasite active in the host and its interaction with specific and nonspecific inflammatory and immune responses (6). Multiple studies have demonstrated that only a proportion of infected persons exhibit disease. Most of them are heavily infected, but the relationship of disease to intensity of infection is not exact. There is evidence that other factors, such as host genetics (7), nutrition, and intercurrent infection, participate to varying degrees in determining the susceptibility to and the pathologic outcome of schistosomiasis.

Skin penetration by cercariae and the death of some of these organisms in the subcutaneous tissues result in an eruption called swimmers' itch, which is associated with humoral, cellular, and local infiltrative responses. A serum sickness-like syndrome (acute schistosomiasis or Katayama fever) occurs in some infected individuals at 6 to 8 weeks, particularly those with heavy infection. This syndrome is thought to be due to the formation of antigen-antibody complexes.

The most significant disease manifestations of schistosomiasis follow egg deposition. As mentioned earlier, a proportion of ova escape in excreta; those retained in host tissues elicit a series of immunopathologic reactions. The basic host response to parasite eggs is a delayed-type hypersensitivity granulomatous reaction that far exceeds the size of retained ova. These large granulomata account for some of the early obstructive lesions seen in the lower end of ureters in *S. haematobium*–infected persons and also in the hepatomegaly and interference with portal blood flow seen in *S. mansoni*, *S. japonicum*, and *S. mekongi* infections. Despite multiple immunologic factors that regulate granuloma formation (resulting in smaller granulomatous response in chronically infected persons) (6), another set of more permanent fibrotic responses leads to obstructive and hemodynamic changes that herald significant morbidity (8).

The multicellular, multistage schistosome infection presents the mammalian host with a variety of antigenic stimuli. The host responds at both systemic and local levels. Serum antibodies and

TABLE 287.1.   Clinically Significant Trematode Parasites of Humans

Species	Geographic distribution	Infective stage	Diagnosis	Potential complications
Blood flukes				
Schistosoma haematobium	Africa, Mideast	Cercaria	Urine examination	Hydronephrosis, pyelonephritis, carcinoma
Schistosoma mansoni	Africa, South America, Middle East	Cercaria	Stool examination, biopsy	Portal hypertension, polyposis, splenomegaly
Schistosoma japonicum	Asia, Philippines	Cercaria	Stool examination, biopsy	Seizures, hepatic dysfunction, splenomegaly
Schistosoma mekongi	Southeast Asia	Cercaria	Stool examination, biopsy	As for *S. japonicum*
Schistosoma intercalatum	Africa	Cercaria	Stool and urine examination	Colonic and urinary tract inflammation, prostatitis
Liver flukes				
Clonorchis sinensis	Asia	Metacercaria	Stool examination	Cholangitis, cirrhosis, cholangiocarcinoma
Opisthorchis felineus	Asia, Eastern Europe	Metacercaria	Stool examination	Cholangitis, cirrhosis, cholangiocarcinoma
Opisthorchis viverrini	Asia	Metacercaria	Stool examination	Cholangitis, cirrhosis, cholangiocarcinoma
Fasciola hepatica	Worldwide	Metacercaria	Stool examination	Fever, hepatomegaly, biliary and pharyngeal obstruction
Fasciola gigantica	Africa, Asia	Metacercaria	Stool examination	Fever, hepatomegaly, biliary obstruction
Tissue flukes				
Paragonimus westermani	Asia, Africa, Americas	Metacercaria	Sputum and stool examination	Lung abscess, seizures, gastrointestinal ulceration
Other *Paragonimus* spp.	South and Central America	Metacercaria	Sputum and stool examination, biopsy	Lung and cerebral lesions, tissue abscess
Intestinal flukes				
Fasciolopsis buski	India, Asia	Metacercaria	Stool examination	Intestinal ulceration, diarrhea, ascites
Echinostoma ilocanum	Asia, India, Philippines	Metacercaria	Stool examination	Abdominal pain, diarrhea
Heterophyes heterophyes	Egypt, Asia, India, Philippines	Metacercaria	Stool examination	Diarrhea, central nervous system and cardiac lesions
Metagonimus yokogawai	Asia, Eastern Europe, Spain	Metacercaria	Stool examination	Intestinal ulceration
Nanophyetus salmincola	North America, Siberia	Metacercaria	Stool examination	Nausea, diarrhea, fatigue

sensitized lymphocytes that react with the different stages of schistosomes are detected after infection. It is remarkable that as long as adult worms live in the venous system, no recognition by the host immune or inflammatory responses can be detected in situ. On the other hand, once ova are deposited, the host recognizes their existence, and the sensitized lymphocytes along with other inflammatory cells and antibodies contribute to granuloma formation. Schistosome egg granulomata are dynamic lesions that are tightly controlled, representing the balance between initiating and down-regulating immune mechanisms. Granuloma formation is further complicated by the subsequent development of fibrosis, which is responsible for the more permanent fibroobstructive and hemodynamic changes seen in schistosomiasis.

Like other worm infections that involve migration through host tissues, schistosome infections are characteristically associated with peripheral as well as tissue eosinophilia. This observation has been related to the role of eosinophils as effector cells in mediating host defense to multicellular organisms (9). Both oxidative and nonoxidative mechanisms have been linked with eosinophil-induced destruction of schistosome invading stages (schistosomula) and parasite eggs.

Clinical Manifestations

Specific disease manifestations due to schistosomiasis appear in only a proportion of infected individuals (6). Skin penetration by human schistosomes results in the itchy papular eruption known as swimmers' itch. Acute schistosomiasis manifests

as a febrile illness with lymphadenopathy, hepatosplenomegaly, and eosinophilia. The more characteristic clinical manifestations occur after oviposition. In *S. haematobium* infection, the main features are hematuria, dysuria, and frequency as well as laboratory evidence of proteinuria and hematuria. Thickening and irregularity of urinary bladder wall and obstructive uropathy with hydroureter and hydronephrosis is observed in a significant proportion of infected persons (Fig. 287.2). In *S. mansoni*, *S. japonicum*, and *S. mekongi* infections, the intestinal phase may be associated with abdominal pain and blood in stools. As egg deposition in the liver increases, hepatomegaly, portal hypertension, splenomegaly, and evidence of portosystemic anastomosis may be seen. These individuals remain asymptomatic for a considerable time, retain good liver function, may bleed several times without progressing to hepatic encephalopathy, but finally succumb to the effects of repeated bleeding or liver failure.

Schistosome eggs can be found in virtually any tissue in the human host. The more common sites are the abdominal organs, the lungs, and more rarely, the spinal cord. Transverse myelitis has been reported with chronic *S. haematobium* or *S. mansoni* infection, and jacksonian epilepsy has been reported with *S. japonicum* infection.

Diagnosis

Parasitologic examination of human excreta or tissue remains the standard procedure for diagnosis of schistosomiasis (10). Eggs

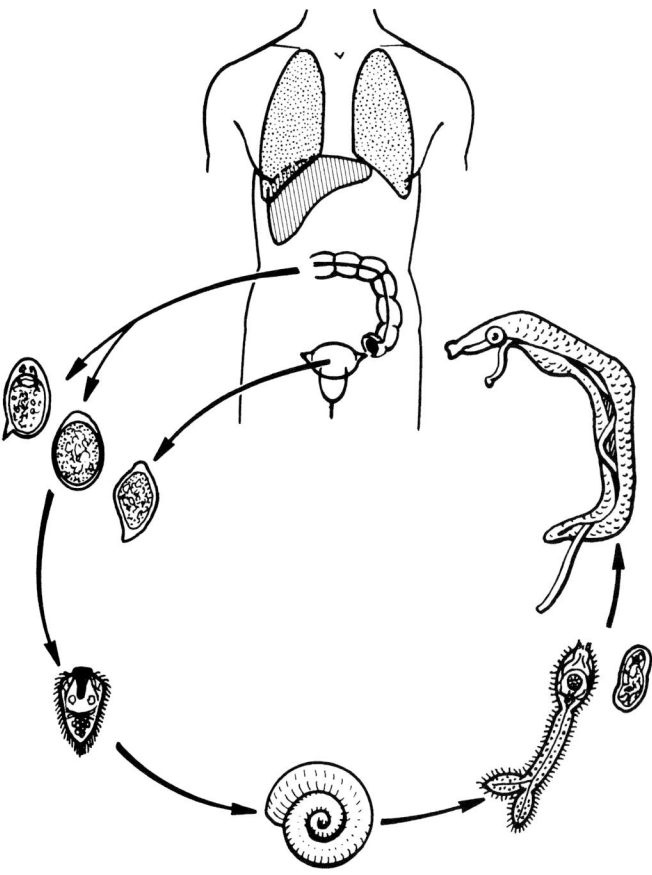

Figure 287.1. The life cycle of schistosomes (counterclockwise): parasite eggs passed into freshwater in human excreta hatch into miracidia that infect the intermediate host, an aquatic snail. Several weeks later, the snail releases free-swimming cercarial forms that seek and penetrate human skin, transforming into immature male or female larvae. Six to 8 weeks later, mature worms complete the cycle by mating in portal or urinary tract veins and releasing eggs into nearby viscera.

can be detected in urine or stools of infected persons by direct examination—or with greater sensitivity by use of concentration and quantitative methods (Fig. 287.3). The recommended procedures are Nuclepore filtration for urine and the Kato thick smear for fecal examination. Serologic testing is a useful adjunct to diagnosis particularly in individuals with early or light infection.

The differential diagnosis of the major clinical features of schistosomiasis is complex because of its protean manifestations. Even the more specific features, such as hematuria, obstructive uropathy, hematemesis, or hepatosplenomegaly, are common manifestations of many diseases. The most helpful aspect for establishing the correct diagnosis is a thorough geographic history. This provides accurate assessment of the possibility of the infection's having been acquired and suggests the likely species of infecting parasite.

Treatment

The drug of choice for treating all species of schistosomes that infect humans is currently praziquantel (11). It is administered orally and is extremely effective in either eliminating adult worms or markedly reducing their numbers. The dose and schedule of praziquantel depend on the *Schistosoma* species. For *S. japonicum* and *S. mekongi*, the recommended dosage is 60 mg/kg of body weight orally in two or three divided doses in 1 day. The recommended dose for *S. haematobium, S. mansoni,* and *S. intercalatum* is 40 mg/kg as a single oral dose. Follow-up stool or urine examinations for viable eggs should be performed several weeks after therapy to ensure successful treatment. Praziquantel treatment may also reverse the pathologic process if it is instituted early in the course of infection. However, the drug has no detectable effect on reversing the established fibro-obstructive lesions seen in chronic schistosomiasis. The side effects and toxicity of praziquantel are remarkably low.

Prevention

The only reliable method of prevention is to avoid any contact with freshwater bodies in areas known to be endemic for schistosomes. This can easily be achieved for visitors to such areas; the local inhabitants, however, are attracted to these water bodies for many purposes, and in many instances they have

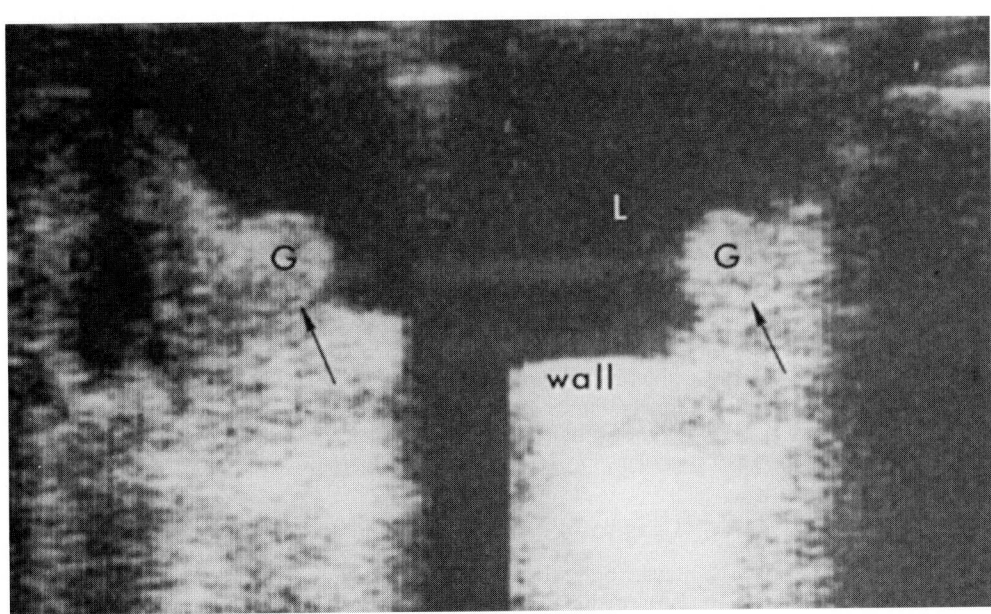

Figure 287.2. Longitudinal and transverse ultrasonographic images of the urinary bladder of a child infected with *Schistosoma haematobium. Arrows* indicate a large granuloma *(G)* protruding from the wall of the bladder into the lumen *(L).*

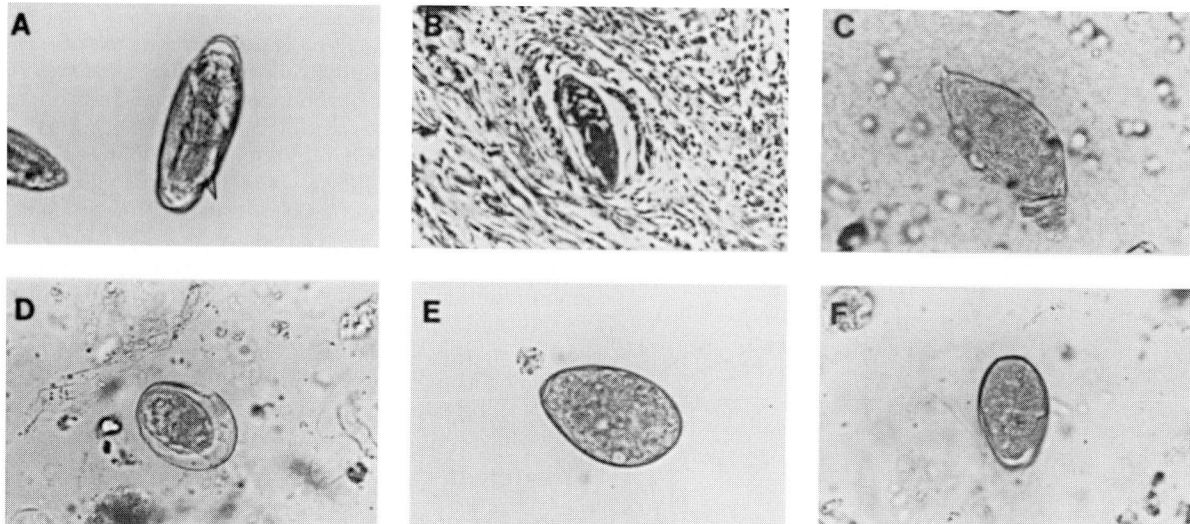

Figure 287.3. Diagnosis of trematode infection. **A** and **B:** Eggs of *Schistosoma mansoni* under high power in stool and tissue specimens. **C** to **F:** Eggs of *Schistosoma haematobium, Schistosoma japonicum, Fasciola hepatica,* and *Paragonimus westermani* in urine *(S.h.)* and stool samples.

no alternative. Another strategy is to stop environmental contamination by excreta of infected persons and so prevent snail infection. In endemic areas, this can be achieved only if cultural and socioeconomic changes are implemented to allow alternative sewage disposal. Several other approaches have been tried, such as the use of widespread chemotherapy and Molluscicides. The availability of praziquantel and other safe, effective, and orally administered antischistosomal agents has encouraged the use of chemotherapy as a strategy for parasite control, and such programs have been reasonably successful. Molluscicides, on the other hand, have proved ineffective except under special circumstances.

The hope for the future prevention and control of schistosomiasis is in vaccine production (12). This is an ambitious goal, but evidence suggests that several characterized, defined parasite antigens are partially protective in experimental animals. Several candidate vaccines are in phase I clinical trials in humans.

OTHER TREMATODES

The other human trematode parasites can be grouped according to site of infection (liver, lung, intestine; see Table 287.1).

Characteristics of the Pathogen

Like schistosomes, the liver, lung, and intestinal flukes of humans have complex life cycles that involve one or more intermediate hosts. Infection is established by ingestion of a larval or metacercarial stage found in freshwater plants, insects, fish, or crustaceans. Humans acquire infection through consumption of raw, pickled, smoked, or undercooked foods containing these larval stages. After ingestion, the larvae hatch in the intestine and migrate to their preferred niche in the host's body.

Epidemiology

The epidemiology of tissue and intestinal fluke infections is determined by the distribution of the aquatic intermediate hosts. Transmission occurs in either tropical or temperate regions, but the distribution of individual fluke species is usually limited in range. For the individual patient, a travel history is important for determining exposure risk. The second important feature that determines the prevalence and intensity of infection is the dietary preference of the definitive human host (i.e., could the patient have consumed uncooked or undercooked food known to harbor infective larvae?).

Pathogenesis

Clinical symptoms of tissue fluke infections are the result of inflammatory response to the parasite or its secretions and, less commonly, to eggs (13). For intestinal flukes, mechanical irritation may also play a role in causing gastrointestinal symptoms such as cramping, diarrhea, and gastrointestinal tract bleeding. In tissue fluke infection, significant symptoms are often noted early, as developing parasites migrate from the intestinal tract into host tissues. Adult flukes range in size from 2 mm (*Heterophyes heterophyes*) to 7.5 cm (*Fasciola*). Experimental animals have been shown to develop strong humoral and cell-mediated immune responses to parasite antigens, and there is some evidence that these responses can alter the course of a challenge tissue fluke infection. The local inflammatory response to tissue flukes often wanes as parasites encyst in host tissues and become surrounded by fibrosis. In the case of the lung fluke *Paragonimus*, the tissue cyst containing the parasite must rupture into airway spaces so that parasite eggs can be expectorated and reach the environment (13). In abortive *Paragonimus* infections, tissue fluke encystment may occur in almost any part of the body, including peritoneum, mesenteric lymph nodes, diaphragm, pleura, heart, reproductive organs, and central nervous system. Secondary effects of parasite migration may include effusions, abscess formation, local granuloma formation, fibrosis, calcification, and phlebitis. Biliary tract infection with liver flukes may result in local stenosis and intrahepatic obstruction. Chronic inflammation of biliary structures appears to predispose to formation of cholangiocarcinoma in older patients.

Diagnosis

Infection with any of these trematodes is diagnosed by detection of parasite eggs in stool or sputum. Eggs are characteristically ovoid, spineless, and operculate (lidded). Tissue flukes and their eggs may also be identified in biopsy material. Serologic tests to assist diagnosis are available for some fluke species; however, the specificity of these tests may be limited. In the setting of acute illness, significant travel history, eosinophilia, and characteristic radiographic or sonographic findings strongly suggest active fluke infection.

Therapy

The drug of choice for liver, lung, and tissue fluke infection is praziquantel, 25 mg/kg of body weight three times a day for 1 or 2 days (14). Efficacy of praziquantel therapy for *Fasciola hepatica* may be limited, and alternative triclabendazole therapy is recommended (15).

Prophylaxis

Prevention of tissue and liver fluke infection depends on avoidance of raw or undercooked foods in endemic areas. Advances in food preparation, freezing, and sewage treatment will help break the cycle of transmission of these parasites. Although developed countries such as Japan, Korea, Thailand, and China have made strides in reducing fluke transmission, technologic progress has been slow in many developing countries, and traditional methods of cultivation and aquaculture continue to foster parasite transmission.

LIVER FLUKES

The Chinese liver fluke *Clonorchis sinensis* and the various *Opisthorchis* species (found in Southeast Asia and Eastern Europe) produce clinically significant infections. (13) Human infection with *F. hepatica* is less common, having been reported in livestock-raising areas of the Americas, Europe, North Africa, and Asia.

Clonorchiasis

Human infection with *C. sinensis* is endemic in China, Taiwan, Hong Kong, Korea, and the countries of Southeast Asia. The adult worm is approximately 15 × 3 mm and inhabits the distal branches of the biliary tree or pancreatic duct. Eggs measure 30 × 14 μm and are passed with the bile into feces. After reaching freshwater, the eggs hatch to infect snails. The miracidium then multiplies by asexual division within this intermediate host. After several weeks, cercariae emerge and encyst to form infectious metacercariae under the scales of freshwater fish. Human consumption of raw, pickled, smoked, or incompletely cooked fish allows living metacercariae to reach the intestine, where they hatch and pass through the ampulla of Vater to mature in the biliary tree.

Disease due to clonorchiasis is often minimal, and many infected persons have no symptoms. Acute symptoms include anorexia, epigastric pain, and diarrhea. With chronic infections, cholangitis, cholelithiasis, pancreatitis, and biliary stricture have been reported. Cholangiocarcinoma, often multicentric, may arise as a late sequel to chronic infection, in some cases long after the infection has cleared. Oral treatment with praziquantel, 25 mg/kg three times a day for 1 or 2 days, is highly effective in eliminating infection (87% to 100% cure) but may not prevent or eliminate the late obstructive complications of infection.

Opisthorchiasis

Opisthorchiasis is due to human infection with the cat and dog liver flukes *Opisthorchis felineus* and *Opisthorchis viverrini*. *O. felineus* is endemic in Southeast Asia, the Siberian lowlands, and Eastern Europe; *O. viverrini* is endemic in Thailand, western Malaysia, and Laos. The life cycle and clinical features of *Opisthorchis* species are similar to those of *Clonorchis* (16) The eggs are distinguished from *Clonorchis* eggs by being somewhat narrower (11 × 30 μm). Praziquantel has been found to be effective in treating established infection.

Fascioliasis

Livestock infection with the liver fluke *F. hepatica* is found worldwide, with humans serving only occasionally as accidental hosts. Infections have been reported in all major sheep- and cattle-raising areas of the world. The metacercariae for this parasite encyst on freshwater plants, and human consumption of aquatic plants (such as wild watercress) harvested from contaminated areas leads to infection. After hatching, developing larvae penetrate the gut wall and enter the peritoneal cavity. The young flukes enter the liver by direct penetration of the capsule to the biliary radicles, where they mature and begin to pass eggs. The prolonged tissue migration of the parasite through host tissues is an important aspect of the pathologic process in the host. During this period, the patient may have prolonged febrile episodes, right upper quadrant pain, hepatomegaly, urticaria, and marked eosinophilia. These symptoms abate once the flukes enter the bile ducts, but low-grade biliary symptoms may persist, and local fibrosis may develop around the mature worm. Maturing worms may occasionally fail to reach the liver and may continue to migrate through the peritoneal tissues and retroperitoneum. Rarely, invasion of the subdural space may lead to eosinophilic meningitis and central nervous system tissue inflammation or destruction.

Currently recommended therapy for fascioliasis is triclabendazole. (15) Therapy may need to be repeated if eggs return in the stool after the first course of treatment.

Lung Fluke and Other *Paragonimus* Infections

Infection with *Paragonimus* species results in fluke encystment in various organs, the most common being the lung fluke infection caused by *Paragonimus westermani* (13). Different strains of *Paragonimus* are common in different areas of the world; infection with *P. westermani* is common in Asia (China, Japan, Korea, Laos, the Philippines, Taiwan, Thailand) but can also be found in West Africa and in South and Central America, including Mexico, Colombia, Costa Rica, and Peru. Humans are infected by consuming raw or undercooked crustaceans, including freshwater crabs and crayfish. Metacercariae hatch in the intestine, penetrate the gut into the peritoneal cavity, and migrate through the diaphragm and pleural space to invade the lung parenchyma. Acute clinical symptoms of infection include abdominal pain, diarrhea, fever, malaise, and urticaria followed by chest pain or pressure, malaise, dyspnea, and night sweats. Chronic symptoms include hemoptysis and abscess formation due to pulmonary hemorrhage and necrosis in the inflammation surrounding the parasite and pulmonary fibrosis and bronchiolar damage as a consequence of chronic inflammation. Secondary inflammatory response may lead to bronchopneumonia, bronchitis, bronchiectasis, atelectasis, and vasculitis of the lung. Imaging studies may demonstrate the migratory pathway in the lungs. Ectopic worm cysts may also be found in the intestines, peritoneal cavity, lymph nodes, pleura, diaphragm, heart, subcutaneous tissues, and central nervous system (17). Diagnosis can be made by examination of expectorated sputum for the characteristic 60×80 to 120 μm ova. If the patient swallows sputum, eggs may also be noted in the stool. Recommended treatment for paragonimiasis is praziquantel, 25 mg/kg three times daily for 2 or 3 days (reported success rate, 89% to 100%) (18). Resolution of lung fluke infection should be monitored for several months by sputum examination and chest radiographs.

Other *Paragonimus* species may favor encystment in different tissues. For example, a syndrome of cerebral hemorrhagic infestation has been described for *Paragonimus mexicanus* in Costa Rica. This syndrome appears to be rare with *P. westermani*. Other significant central nervous system syndromes may include meningitis (acute or chronic); mass lesions; infarction; hemorrhage; and visual disturbances associated with papilledema, nystagmus, or optic atrophy (17). The most frequent presenting symptoms are seizures, headache, and visual disturbances. Diagnosis of central nervous system involvement may be difficult because of the isolated location of these organisms, far from the gastrointestinal tract and bronchial tree. Travel history, serologic tests, and laboratory evidence of active infection provide only presumptive evidence of central nervous system involvement. Definitive diagnosis depends on tissue biopsy to identify the parasite or its eggs in the affected tissues. Optimal therapy of central nervous system fluke involvement is not established. Surgical removal of the parasite in combination with praziquantel therapy has been recommended. Symptoms of central nervous system infection may also require long-term therapy with anticonvulsants, corticosteroids, or ventricular shunting.

INTESTINAL FLUKES

The metacercariae of intestinal flukes infest various freshwater plants (*Fasciolopsis buski*), fish (*H. heterophyes, Metagonimus yokogawai, Nanophyetus salmincola*), and shellfish (*Echinostoma ilocanum*). These parasites are primarily endemic to Southeast Asia, although *Heterophyes* is also found in the Nile delta of Egypt. To date, transmission to humans of the intestinal fluke *N. salmincola* has been limited to the northwestern United States (19). Symptoms of light infection with intestinal flukes are generally mild and limited to the intestine; heavy infection may be associated with severe abdominal pain, diarrhea, intestinal ulceration, and even ascites. Diagnosis of individual intestinal flukes is made by identification of parasite eggs on stool examination. Recommended therapy is praziquantel, as listed before for liver flukes.

REFERENCES

1. King CH, Mahmoud AAF. Schistosomiasis. In: Guerrant RL, Walker DH, Weller PF, eds. *Tropical infectious diseases: principles, pathogens and practice*. Philadelphia: Churchill Livingstone, 1999:1031–1038.
2. Sturrock RF. The schistosomes and their intermediate hosts. In: Mahmoud AAF, ed. *Schistosomiasis*. London: Imperial College Press, 2001:7–83.
3. van der Werf MJ, De Vlas SJ. *Morbidity and infection with schistosomes or soil-transmitted helminths*. Rotterdam: Erasmus University, 2001:1–103.
4. World Health Organization. Schistosomiasis: epidemiological data/geographical distribution. WHO Health Topics, 2002. Available at: *www.who.int/ctd/schisto/epidemio.htm*.
5. Anderson RM. Determinants of infection in human schistosomiasis. In: Mahmoud AAF, ed. *Bailliere's clinical tropical medicine and communicable diseases*. Philadelphia: Baillière Tindall, 1987:279–300.
6. King CL. Initiation and regulation of disease in schistosomiasis. In: Mahmoud AAF, ed. *Schistosomiasis*. London: Imperial College Press, 2001:213–264.
7. Abel L, Demenais F, Prata A, et al. Evidence for the segregation of a major gene in human susceptibility/resistance to infection by *Schistosoma mansoni*. *Am J Hum Genet* 1991;48:959–970.
8. Chen MG, Mott KE. Progress in assessment of morbidity due to *Schistosoma haematobium* infection. *Trop Dis Bull* 1989;86:R1–R36.
9. Mahmoud AAF. Eosonophilia. In: Warren KS, Mahmoud AAF, eds. *Tropical and geographical medicine*, 2nd ed. New York: McGraw-Hill, 1990:65–70.
10. Peters PAS, Kazura JW. Update on diagnostic methods for schistosomiasis. In: Mahmoud AAF, ed. *Balliere's clinical tropical medicine and communicable diseases, schistosomiasis*. London: Bailliere Tindall, 1987:419–433.
11. King CH, Mahmoud AA. Drugs five years later: praziquantel. *Ann Intern Med* 1989;110:290–296.
12. James SL, Colley DG. Progress in vaccine development. In: Mahmoud AAF, ed. *Schistosomiasis*. London: Imperial College Press, 2001:469–495.
13. MacLean JD, Cross J, Mahanty S. Liver, lung and intestinal fluke infections. In: Guerrant RL, Walker DH, Weller PF, eds. *Tropical infectious diseases: principles, pathogens and practice*. Philadelphia: Churchill Livingstone, 1999:1039–1057.
14. Drugs for parasitic infections. *Med Lett Drugs Ther* 2002:1–12. Available at: *www.medletter.com/html/prm.htm#Parasitic*.
15. Richter J, Knipper M, Gobels K, et al. Fascioliasis. *Curr Treat Options Infect Dis* 2002;4:313–317.
16. Upatham ES, Viyanant V, Kurathong S, et al. Morbidity in relation to intensity of infection in *Opisthorchiasis viverrini*: study of a community in Khon Kaen, Thailand. *Am J Trop Med Hyg* 1982;31:1156–1163.
17. Kusner DJ, King CH. Paragonimiasis of the central nervous system. *Semin Neurol* 1993;13:201–208.
18. Mahanty S. Treatment of paragonimiasis. *Curr Treat Opt Infect Dis* 2001;3:351–356.
19. Eastburn RL, Fritsche TR, Terhune CA Jr. Human intestinal infection with *Nanophyetus salmincola* from salmonid fishes. *Am J Trop Med Hyg* 1987;36:586–591.

CHAPTER 288
Cestodes (Tapeworms)

Kaethe Willms

The true tapeworms, class Cestoda, belong to the phylum Platyhelminthes, the most highly specialized of the metazoan parasites (Table 288.1). All adult members of this class are endoparasites of the alimentary tract or associated ducts of vertebrates. Their life cycle includes at least one intermediary host, in which the tapeworm undergoes one phase of development (1,2). In this chapter, only tapeworms that cause significant human disease are discussed: *Taenia solium, Taenia saginata*, Asian *Taenia, Echinococcus granulosus* (hydatid cyst), *Hymenolepis nana*, and *Diphyllobothrium latum*.

Within the Cestoda is the order of the Cyclophyllidea, composed of two families that are of medical importance: the Taeniidae and the Hymenolepididae. Within the Taeniidae are three zoonotic tapeworms for which humans are the only natural definitive host, *T. solium, T. saginata*, and Asian *Taenia*. Their life cycles require at least one intermediary host, in which the tapeworm undergoes one phase of development, the larval stage or metacestode (also called cysticercus, which has no taxonomic value). A fourth zoonosis caused by the taeniid *E. granulosus* has a similar life cycle; domestic dogs and other carnivores are definitive hosts, and a large number of intermediate hosts (including humans) become infected by the larval stage and develop hydatid disease. All four taeniids still cause widespread disease in developing countries and are zoonoses generally associated with ignorance and poverty. Eggs produced in the *T. solium* tapeworm contain the infective embryos that cause human and porcine cysticercosis in many countries of Latin America, South Africa, and Asia (3). *T. saginata* tapeworms are the source of bovine cysticercosis and still represent a major public health risk in developing countries and in developed countries, where raw or undercooked beef is consumed and where localized feedlot epidemics

TABLE 288.1. Classification of Medically Important Cestodes

Phylum					Platyhelminthes	
Class					Cestoda	
Order			Cyclophyllidea			Pseudophyllidea
Family		Taeniidae			Hymenolepididae	Diphyllobothriidae
Genus	*Taenia*		*Echinococcus granulosus*		*Hymenolepis nana*	*Diphyllobothrium latum*
Species	*solium*					
	saginata					

Data from Cheng T. Cestoda. The true tapeworms. In: Cheng TC, ed. *General parasitology*. New York: Academic Press, 1973:474–541; and Schmidt GD. *Handbook of tapeworm identification. Key to the genera taeniidae*. Boca Raton, FL: CRC Press, 1986:221–227.

have been reported (4). The adult and larval stages of all cestodes are endoparasites, which lack a digestive system and are therefore able to live only in the intestine.

TAENIA TAPEWORMS

Tapeworms of the genus *Taenia* are flat and exceptionally long parasites measuring 1.5 to 12 m, depending on the species. All species share several morphologic features: a scolex (head with four suckers) and a rostellum, which may be armed with hooks (*T. solium*) or unarmed (*T. saginata* and Asian *Taenia*) (Fig. 288.1). The scolex is attached to the mucosa in the small intestine of the host. Morphologic evidence obtained from adult cestodes has shown that the worm attaches to intestinal epithelium by the scolex suckers, which engulf the host tissue, lysing and destroying the epithelium and submucosal layer. Inspection of the mucosal wall suggests that the worm survives by alternately attaching suckers and obtaining nutrients from the lysis of epithelial cells (Fig. 288.2). From the scolex emerges the neck, from which strobilization (growth of proglottids) occurs. Each proglottid can be considered an independent reproductive unit because it contains both male and female reproductive organs (Fig. 288.3). The distal proglottids become fertile (gravid proglottids) and contain several thousand eggs, which are at different stages of maturation. Gravid proglottids become detached from the worm and leave the host in feces or by spontaneous migration. When mature eggs are ingested by the intermediate host in contaminated water, food, or fodder, the outer shell of the egg is disrupted by exposure to gastric and intestinal juices and the embryo, called the oncosphere, is released (Fig. 288.4). The oncosphere can traverse the intestinal wall and be transported through the circulation to any organ, where it lodges in the host tissues and develops into a larva or metacestode, a 1- to 2-cm cyst, with an inverted scolex. The larval stage in the intermediate host (cattle or swine) becomes infective for humans in about 8 to 10 weeks. Viable cysticerci ingested by humans from undercooked beef or pork undergo an evagination process in the human intestine, by which the scolex becomes attached to the intestinal wall and matures into a gravid (egg-producing) tapeworm 2 to 6 months after infection. The life cycles of these parasites are entirely dependent on the link between the intermediary host and the definitive host, and any break in this link can end the cycle.

TAENIA SAGINATA (TAENIARHYNCHUS SAGINATUS) (BEEF TAPEWORM)

Life Cycle

The adult tapeworm lives only in the jejunum of humans and so far has never been found naturally in any other host (Fig. 288.5). The worm can measure 4 to 12 m and has been reported to survive up to 30 years in a host. Humans are usually infected with a single *T. saginata* tapeworm. Multiple infections are found only in highly endemic areas (5). In contrast to *T. solium*, the gravid proglottids of *T. saginata* migrate actively in groups of six to eight segments through the anus, and patients report an unpleasant creeping sensation. Segments (proglottids) can be found in underclothing, in bedding, or on the ground. It has been estimated that approximately 50% of the eggs contained in the gravid proglottids are mature and therefore infective. When they are ingested by cattle, digestive enzymes release the oncospheres (embryos), which then traverse the intestinal wall and enter the blood stream or lymphatics, whence they are carried to various tissues and develop into larvae. The larvae are infective for humans if they are ingested in raw or undercooked beef. In cattle, the cysticerci are most commonly found in the heart and masseters, but they can be found dispersed throughout the musculature and in any organ (6).

Epidemiology

As Pawlowski and coworkers pointed out a number of years ago, few studies on the epidemiology of *T. saginata* have been carried out (7). A survey of the literature shows that the situation has not improved significantly. I suggest that this is due to three factors: the difficulties in diagnosing tapeworms in developing countries, the absence of symptoms associated with these intestinal parasites, and the difficulties of carrying out adequate inspection of beef carcasses.

Transmission patterns from humans to the bovine intermediate host have been studied in various locations. The studies of Pawlowski and coworkers in Poland showed clearly that the infective eggs can be disseminated over long distances and can remain infective for many months or even years, particularly under conditions of favorable humidity and low temperatures (4°C to 6°C) (7). The common practice in developing countries of using raw sewage for fertilization of horticultural or agricultural fields is an effective means of dispersing eggs over large geographic areas. *T. saginata* eggs also survive most sewage treatment systems (8). Harrison and coworkers described the appearance of cases of bovine cysticercosis in Scotland in a group of farms in which sewage sludge had been applied to farm pastures (9).

It has been estimated that a tapeworm carrier releases between six and nine proglottids daily, each containing about 100,000 eggs, about half of which are probably mature and therefore infective. One infected person may therefore contaminate the environment with more than a half-million eggs per day. The studies of Silverman have shown that under certain climatic conditions, taeniid eggs can survive for many months (10). The transmission of *T. saginata* from animals to humans depends on the habit of eating raw or undercooked beef. It has been

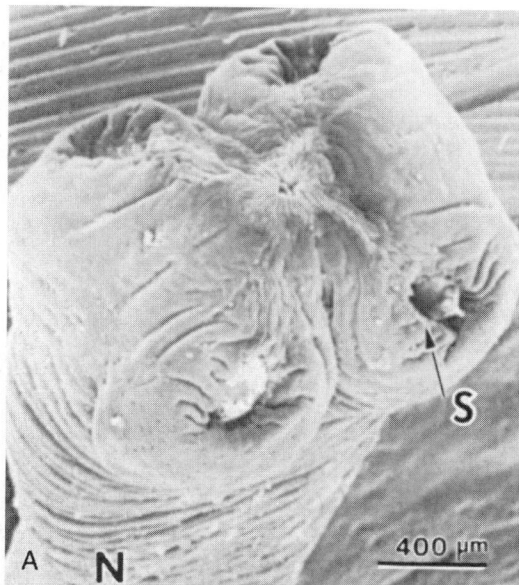

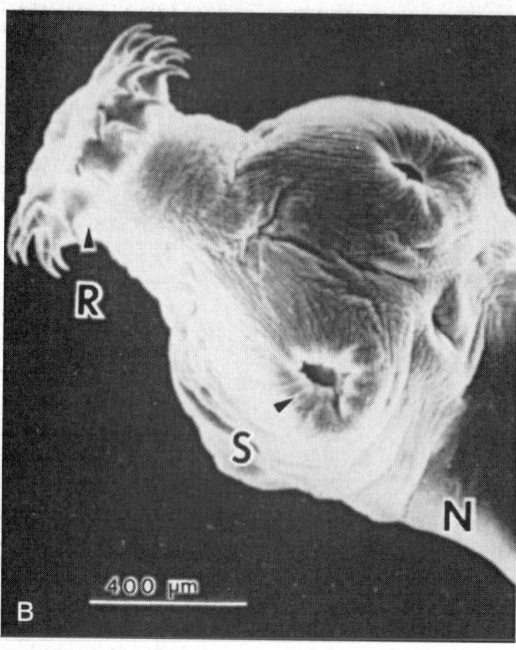

Figure 288.1. Scanning electron micrographs of *Taenia* scolices. **A:** *T. saginata*. *S*, Sucker; *N*, neck. **B:** *T. solium*. *R*, Rostellum with double row of hooks; *S*, sucker; *N*, neck. (**A**, Courtesy of Dr. Juan Pedro Laclette, Instituto de Investigaciones Biomédicas, UNAM, Mexico. **B**, By permission of Fondo de Cultura Economica, Mexico.)

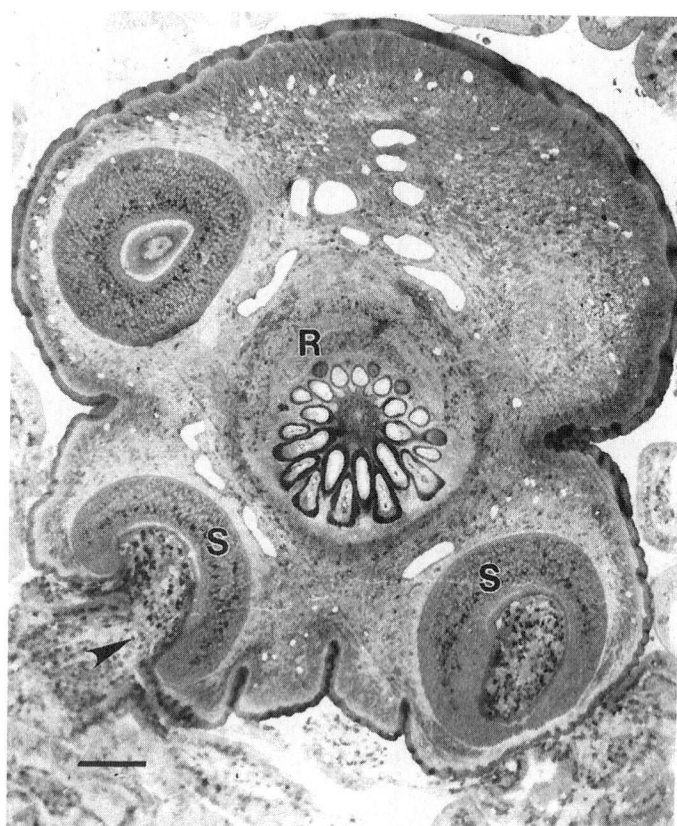

Figure 288.2. Section of mucosal wall of an experimentally infected golden hamster showing 5-day-old *Taenia solium* in situ. Rostellum (*R*) and the suckers (*S*) grasping the epithelium at the base of the villi (*arrowhead*). Space bar = 100 μm. (Courtesy of Kaethe Willms.)

disposed of on open ground, used to fertilize, or even used for medicinal purposes (12), both *T. saginata* and *T. solium* continue to flourish.

Clinical Manifestations

One of the many paradoxes of taeniasis is the relative absence of symptoms in the definitive host. The symptoms that are usually recorded are vague and include abdominal pain, nausea, weakness, weight loss, increased appetite, headache, constipation, dizziness, pruritus ani, and excitation. The presence of the tapeworm can often be detected by the carrier, who observes proglottids in the stool or senses their active migration through the anus. Many infections may go unnoticed, however (5). Lenoble and Dumontier described the unusual case of the perforation of the small intestine due to a *T. saginata* infection, the first case reported in the literature in 20 years (13).

Diagnosis

T. saginata can be suspected by clinical history in a patient who ingests raw beef and who describes elimination of tapeworm segments in stool or active migration of segments through the anus. The diagnosis can be further confirmed by the finding in feces of *Taenia* species eggs or proglottids with more than 12 uterine branches. When the whole worm is retrieved after treatment and an unarmed scolex can be identified, a definite

confirmed that the infection rate in humans is closely related to the frequency of ingesting raw beef (11).

Geographic Distribution

T. saginata worms can be found worldwide in countries where cattle are raised for human consumption. The frequency of beef tapeworm has decreased in developed countries owing to stricter meat inspection practices, better hygiene, and significantly better sanitary facilities. In developing countries, particularly in pastoral societies and rural areas, where sanitary installations are not an element of the culture and where human excrement is

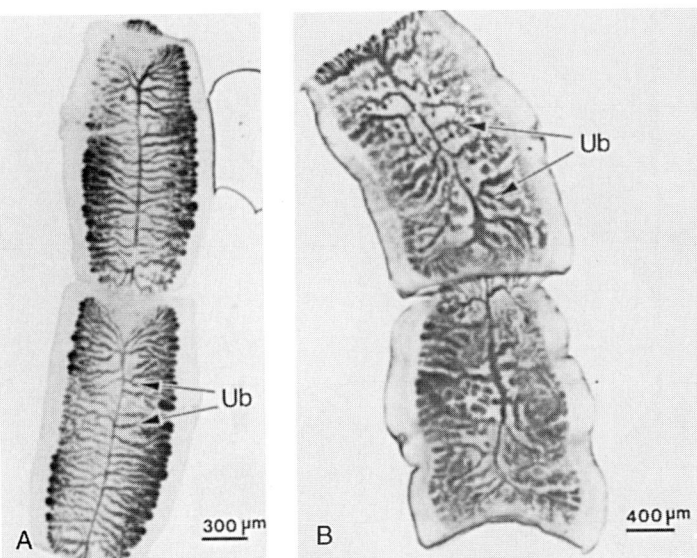

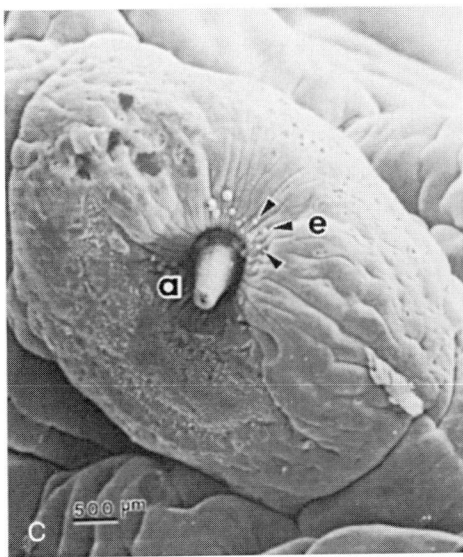

Figure 288.3. Gravid proglottid segments from *T. saginata* (**A**) and *T. solium* (**B**). Cleared in glycerol and mounted on a slide. *Ub*, Uterine branches. (**A** and **B** courtesy of Sylvia Paz Diaz Camacho.) **C:** Scanning electron micrograph of *T. solium* proglottid, showing genital atrium *(a)* and eggs *(e)* on surface *(arrows)*. (Courtesy of Dr. Juan Pedro Laclette, Instituto de Investigaciones Biomédicas, UNAM, Mexico.)

diagnosis can be established. The most effective method reported for diagnosis of *Taenia* species eggs is the perianal swab (14), or the adhesive tape method, which detects 85% to 95% of eggs from *T. saginata* infections (15). Other methods reveal between 20% and 80%, depending on the experience of the laboratory. Most parasitologists recommend carrying out three serial stool examinations to increase the probability of detecting taeniid eggs.

The other methods, some of which have been in use for many years (16–19) are not as reliable as the Graham method for *T. saginata*. However, this method is not dependable for detection of *T. solium* eggs, probably because the proglottids of this tapeworm do not migrate spontaneously. This fact should be kept in mind for patients who live in areas where both pork and beef are consumed and when the specific diagnosis is of consequence, because of the potential risk posed by infections with the *T. solium* tapeworm, the only agent of cysticercosis in humans.

Treatment

See the later section on treatment of *Taenia* tapeworms.

Prevention and Control of *Taenia saginata* Taeniasis

Prevention and control of taeniasis are based on health education, diagnosis, and treatment. Health education should be directed to alerting the population to the risk associated with eating raw or undercooked beef, particularly in countries where meat inspection is haphazard or nonexistent. One of the most frequent vectors of beef tapeworm in developed countries has been infected laborers, who introduce epizootic feedlot cysticercosis (4,20). Immigration and movement of people from infected to uninfected areas have increased much during the past years, increasing the risk for these zoonoses to become established in countries where they had been rare.

ASIAN *TAENIA*

Studies on the epidemiologic patterns of taeniasis in Asia indicate the existence of a distinct species of *Taenia* infecting humans. This cestode is closely related to *T. saginata*, having an unarmed scolex, a large number of uterine branches, and a posterior protuberance (21). Genetic characterization of this cestode

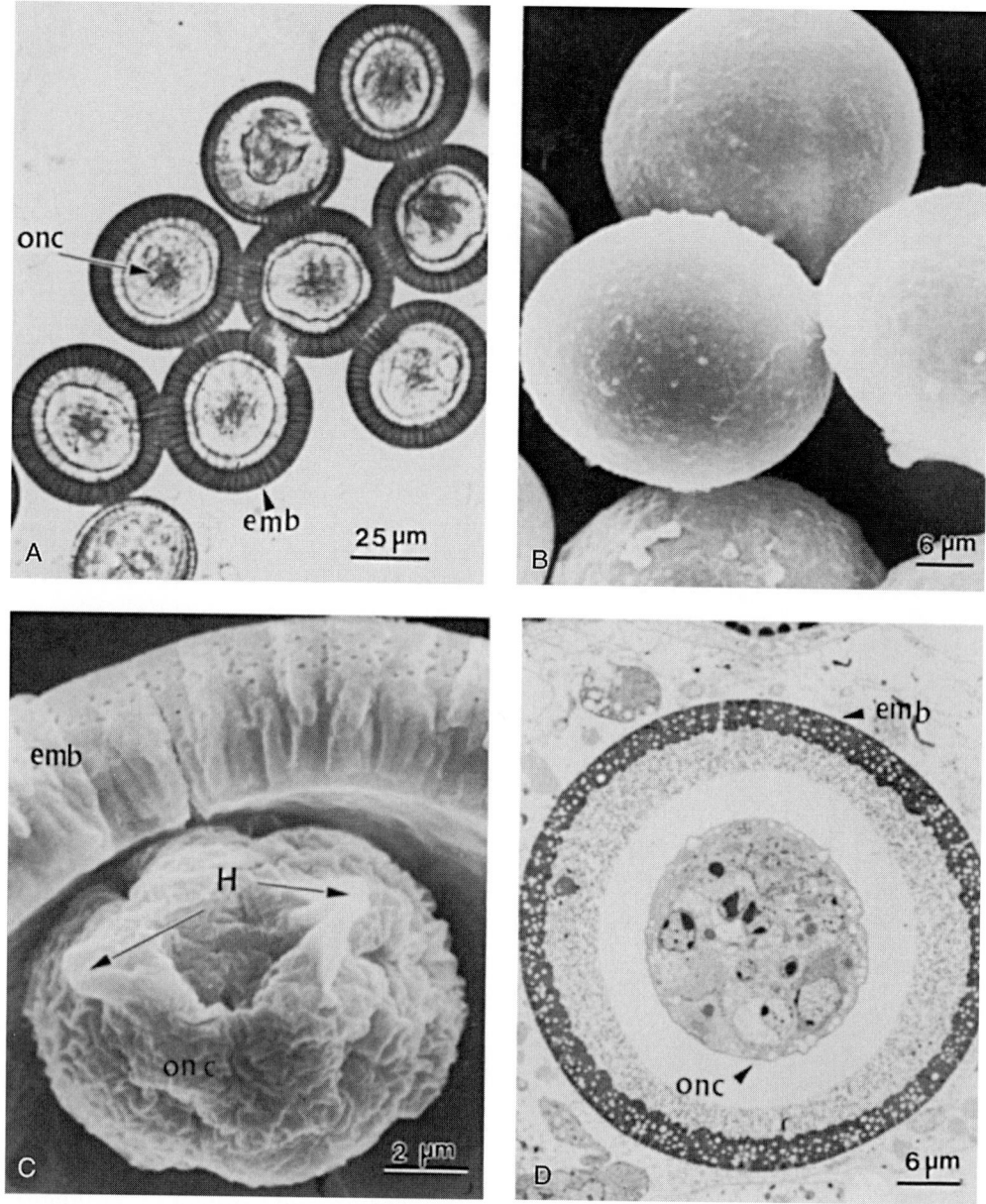

Figure 288.4. *Taenia* spp. eggs. **A:** Light microscopic appearance of eggs obtained from concentration-flotation method (*onc*, oncosphere or hexacanth embryo; *emb*, embryophore shell). **B:** Scanning electron micrograph of *T. solium* eggs. (**B** from Flisser A, Willms K, Laclette JP, et al, eds. *Cysticercosis.* New York: Academic Press, 1982.) **C:** Scanning electron micrograph of an open *T. solium* egg, showing outer embryophore shell *(emb)* and oncosphere *(onc)* covered by membrane. *H*, Oncospheral hooks. (**C** courtesy of Dr. Juan Pedro Laclette, Instituto de Investigaciones Biomédicas, UNAM, Mexico.) **D:** Transmission electron micrograph of *T. solium* egg. Section stained with lead citrate and uranyl acetate (*emb*, embryophore shell; *onc*, oncosphere tissue). (**D** courtesy of Dr. Juan Pedro Laclette, Instituto de Investigaciones Biomédicas, UNAM, Mexico.)

supports its close relation to *T. saginata* (22). This cestode, originally described in Taiwanese aborigines (23), has also been recorded in Korea, Indonesia, the Philippines, and Thailand and is now referred to as Asian *Taenia*. It is viscerotropic and infects mainly the liver of pigs and cattle. Humans become infected by the ingestion of raw meat and viscera. The most frequent clinical signs are passing proglottids in feces, pruritus ani, nausea, abdominal pain, dizziness, increased appetite, and headache. The reported frequencies of this taeniasis in Asia and the South Pacific basin are high and have important public health implications. However, the close relationship of Asian *Taenia* to

T. saginata makes it unlikely to be an important cause of human cysticercosis.

TAENIA SOLIUM (PORK TAPEWORM)

Life Cycle

Under natural conditions, the *T. solium* tapeworm is found only in the small intestine of humans. It can be 1.5 to 8 m long and has been reported to survive for up to 25 years. As shown in

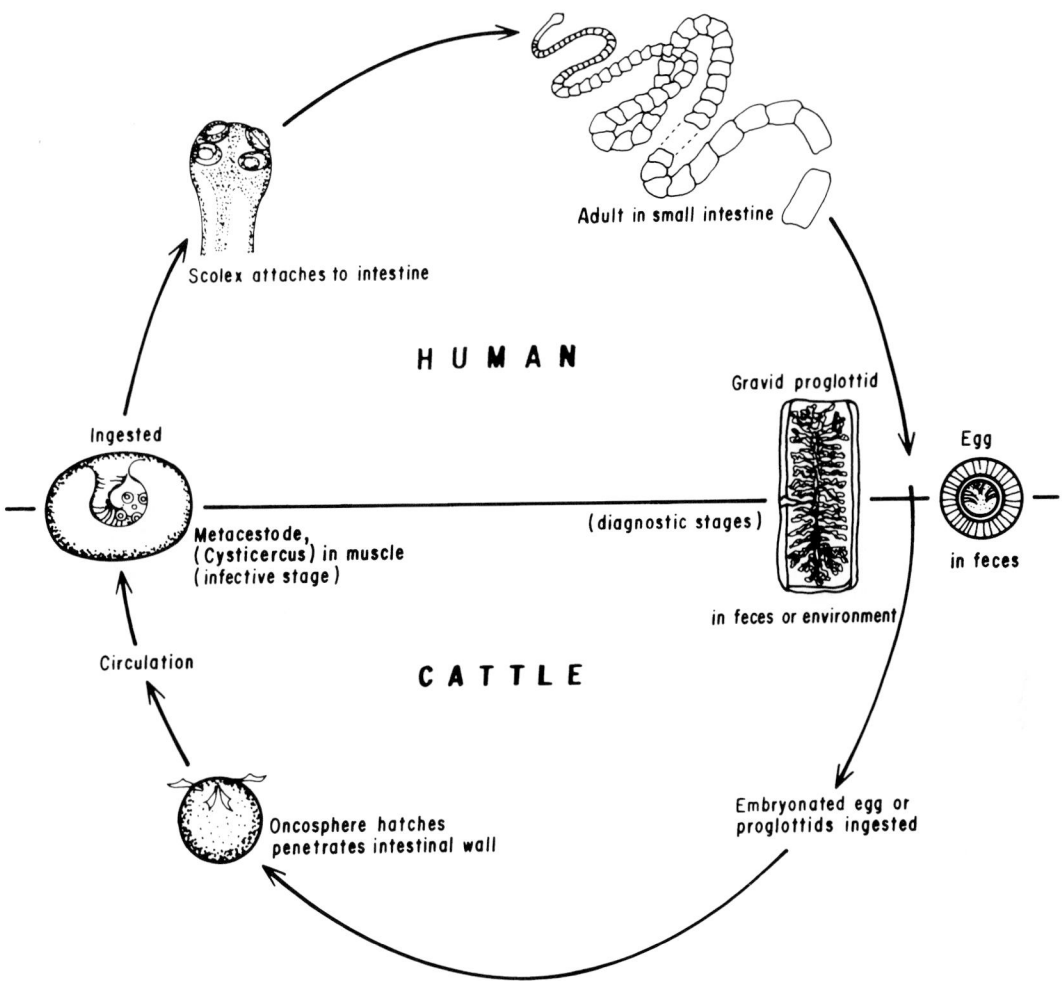

Figure 288.5. Life cycle of *Taenia saginata*.

Fig. 288.1, it has an armed scolex (head), that is, a rostellum bearing two rows of hooks that vary between 22 and 32. The scolex attaches to the intestinal mucosa, from which it derives its nutrients. Growth of the worm (strobilization) proceeds from the distal end of the scolex neck, producing an ever-increasing number of proglottids. As the distal proglottids mature, they become filled with eggs, oncospheres (embryos) surrounded by a keratin-like shell (see Fig. 288.4). The eggs contained in the gravid proglottids have reached different degrees of maturation when the segments are detached from the worm and passively voided in the feces.

Each gravid proglottid contains approximately 50,000 eggs, and because it is estimated that each worm releases four to five proglottids per day, a person with *T. solium* tapeworm is depositing 250,000 eggs a day into the environment. Although not all of the eggs may be infective on release from the host, they may, like other taeniid eggs, mature and survive in humid pastures or sewage for many months. *T. solium* eggs are morphologically indistinguishable from eggs of other *Taenia* species.

When *T. solium* eggs are ingested by their natural intermediate host, the pig, the egg shell or embryophore, made of keratin blocks, becomes progressively disaggregated due to the effects of pepsin and pancreatin (24), and the oncosphere is released. The activated oncosphere penetrates the intestinal wall and is then transported through the blood or lymphatics to the tissues.

In the interstitial tissues, the oncosphere develops into a larva (metacestode), a process that takes approximately 8 weeks. The larva is an oval vesicle filled with fluid and measuring 0.2 to 2 cm in diameter, with an invaginated scolex, which in the adult tapeworm has four suckers and an armed rostellum. The outer tissue of this bladder, the tegument, which is in direct contact with the host tissue, is a syncytium made up of microtrichia covered by a glycocalyx.

In the porcine host, most of the larvae are found in striated muscle masses; in heavily infected animals, they are also in the central nervous system (CNS) (25). The life cycle of the parasite (Fig. 288.6) is completed when a human ingests viable cysticerci in raw or undercooked pork. The cyst undergoes an evagination process in the intestinal lumen, by which the scolex, rostellum, and suckers are actively extruded from several membranes and are then capable of attaching to the intestinal wall of the definitive host (26).

Morphology and Biochemistry

Since the earliest studies of the ultrastructure of larval and adult tapeworms of many species, the tegumental (protoplasmic) nature of the body covering has been established (27). Because tapeworms lack an alimentary tract, this tegumentary surface is the principal tissue through which the parasite interacts with the

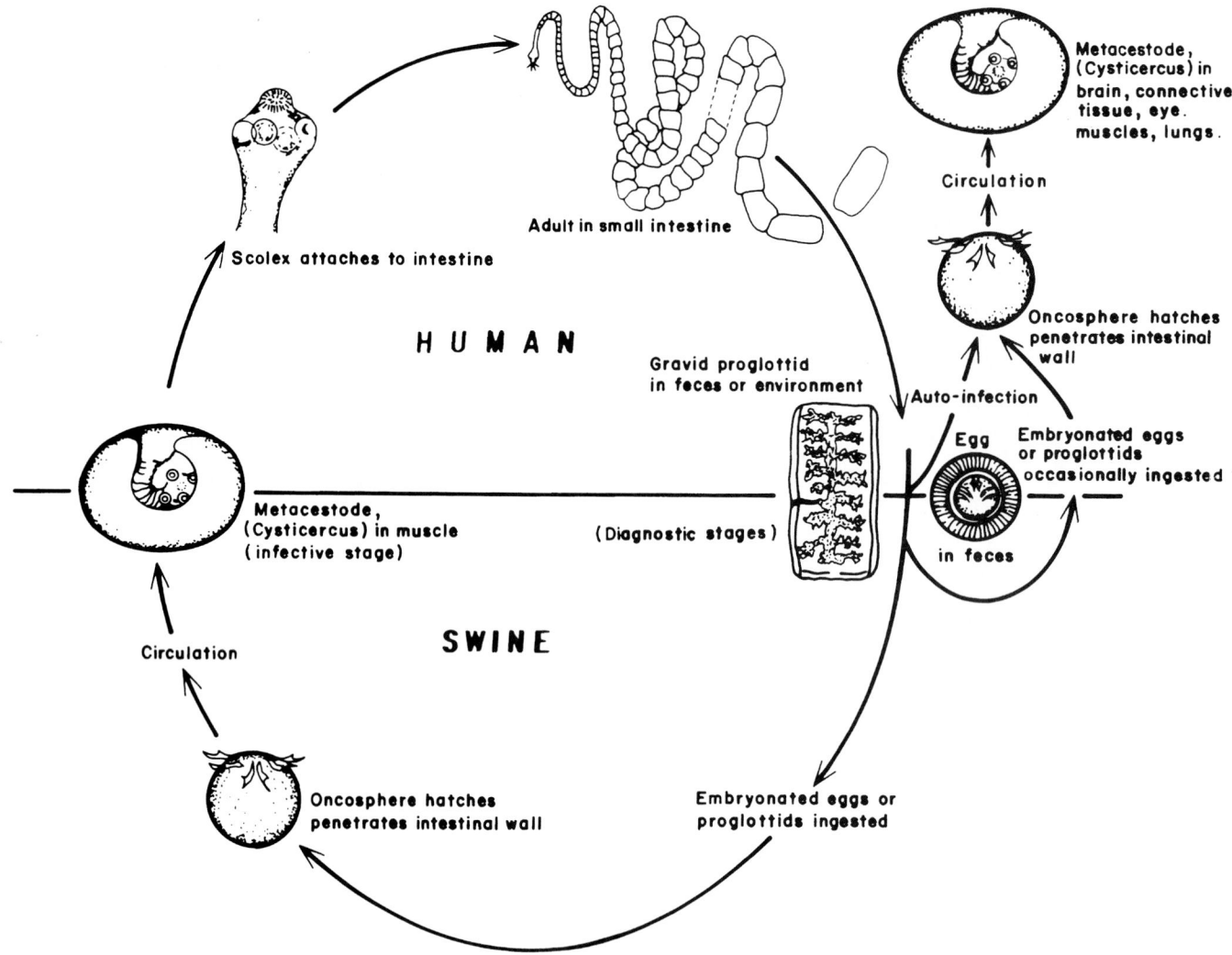

Figure 288.6. Life cycle of *Taenia solium.*

host. Although the number of known tapeworm species is impressive (close to 4,000), the basic morphologic character of their tegumentary surfaces has been shown to be similar: a continuous protoplasmic band, joined to cell bodies (tegumentary cytons) by cytoplasmic processes and separated from the rest of the parasite wall by a basement membrane. All cestode tegumentary surfaces have a brush border covered by microvilli or microtrichia, structures that are in contact with the host tissue and, in the case of the metacestode (larva), make up the host-parasite interface.

Differential Diagnosis of *Taenia solium* and *Taenia saginata* Infestations

There seems to be general agreement that *T. solium* goes undiagnosed for various reasons: the infected person is not aware of harboring a tapeworm; the infection causes few symptoms and in more primitive or less educated communities is not considered a disease worth treating; few developing countries have the facilities and trained personnel to establish an accurate diagnosis at the primary health care level; the methods presently available for diagnosis of taeniid eggs in stool specimens are not optimal (14–19). In addition, *T. solium* eggs are identical to *T. saginata* eggs, so that treatment, when given, is seldom followed up by specific identification of the voided tapeworm.

Nevertheless, taeniasis can be diagnosed on the basis of the following findings:

1. A careful clinical history and questioning of patients about ingestion of raw beef or pork (particularly sausages).
2. Discharging of proglottids or worm segments in the stool (loose gravid proglottids in underclothing or bedclothes are indicative of *T. saginata*).
3. Coprologic analysis: three serial stool examinations on three consecutive days by use of perianal swabs (14) or the method of Graham (15) if *T. saginata* is suspected or the method of Faust (16), Ritchie (17), or Kato (18) if *T. solium* is suspected. If proglottids become available, an effort should be made to fix them and count the uterine branches under the microscope. If the number of branches is 12 or fewer, it can be assumed that the patient has *T. solium*. The patient should be advised that he or she is a potential risk to other humans, instructed on hygiene measures, and treated as soon as possible. The patient should also be asked to recover the tapeworm (taking all safety precautions and using gloves and a disposable or autoclavable container) and bring it into the laboratory for definitive diagnosis.

From the medical point of view, the specific diagnosis and treatment of *Taenia* species infestations are important, because the eggs of *T. solium* and *T. saginata* are indistinguishable, the former being the cause of human cysticercosis (see Fig. 288.6). Although the identification of the scolex and some morphologic features of the proglottids allows precise diagnosis of the tapeworm species, this is frequently not possible. Well-preserved proglottids and trained personnel, which many countries do not have, are required. In addition, when the proglottids are macerated, it is virtually impossible to establish a definitive diagnosis. Two promising new techniques for the detection of taeniid antigens in stool specimens have been worked out by several groups: (a) antigen capture and detection by enzyme-linked immunosorbent assay (ELISA) (28–30), and (b) the preparation of specific deoxyribonucleic acid (DNA) probes for the detection of *Taenia* eggs in stool, which promise rapid, highly sensitive and specific assays that could eventually be used for epidemiologic surveys (31).

Treatment of *Taenia* Tapeworms

Praziquantel is a broad-spectrum and efficient anthelmintic drug. It has been shown to have a high cure rate (32) in the elimination of intestinal cestodes and in the past 10 years has been used successfully in the treatment of human neurocysticercosis (NCC). It should be used only under medical supervision in patients suspected of having NCC. Its use is also contraindicated for pregnant women, children younger than 2 years, and cirrhosis patients. The recommended dose for treatment of tapeworm in adults is between 2.5 and 10 mg/kg given in a single dose (33).

Albendazole is a potent anthelmintic drug with unique broad-spectrum activity indicated in multiple parasitosis. It should not be used in patients with hypersensitivity to the drug, children younger than 2 years or during pregnancy owing to the embryotoxic and teratogenic effects, which have been observed in experimental animals. The recommended dose for treatment of tapeworms is 6.6 mg/kg (two doses of 200 mg each per day on 3 consecutive days) (34).

Niclosamide is effective in 85% to 95% of cases (14). It is contraindicated during the first trimester of pregnancy. The dose per adult is 2 g (four tablets) in a single dose, chewed and swallowed with water, preferably after fasting or some hours after a light meal. For children weighing between 11 and 34 kg, the recommended dose is 1 g. Children younger than 2 years of age are given 0.5 g in one dose, the tablets ground to powder and mixed with water. Niclosamide is tolerated well, and less than 10% of patients report nausea, vomiting, abdominal pain, or exanthema, which are transitory. If the species of *Taenia* has not been determined, it is recommended that the drug be followed by a laxative 1 hour later to ensure expulsion of the worm.

HUMAN CYSTICERCOSIS

Human cysticercosis is caused by the development of *T. solium* oncospheres to the larval stage, or cysticercus, in the interstitial tissues of humans. Because the oncospheres are transported passively from the intestinal wall through the circulation, they can lodge in almost any tissue, but cysticerci are most frequently found in brain, skeletal muscle, and subcutaneous tissues. By far the most important clinicopathologic picture is the one these parasites produce in the CNS. Cysticercosis is the most common parasitosis affecting the CNS and a major cause of neurological disease (35). It is considered an emerging public health problem and been reported to be increasing in countries that receive immigrants from countries where the tapeworm is endemic (36).

Immune Response

There is no doubt that human cysticercosis is accompanied by a humoral immune response, which can be measured in serum and, in the case of NCC, often in cerebrospinal fluid (CSF). Various studies have shown that most seropositive patients have antibodies to several parasite components (37), and the results of Grogl and colleagues (38) indicated that some patients' sera recognize up to 31 antigenic polypeptides in an immunoblot assay. Although the sensitivity of several immunoenzyme tests has been considerably improved in the past few years, there is a recurring problem of patients with a certified diagnosis of NCC who do not have demonstrable serum antibody titers. The reasons for this are not yet clear, but they are more probably due to the severity of the disease and the immune status of the patient than to differences in method.

As Schantz analyzed in a review, negative serum reactions are often found in patients with calcified cysts, others in cases with one or a few viable cysts in early infections (39). On the other hand, patients with severe cases of NCC—with associated inflammatory processes, involvement of meninges, vasculitis, and increased intracranial pressure, among others—almost always have detectable levels of serum and CSF antibodies (40,41).

Pathology

The pathologic process of NCC is determined by the localization of the parasite in the CNS and by the inflammatory reaction it induces in brain tissue. Macroscopic analysis of brain sections from patients with parenchymatous NCC detects a large variety of localizations (Fig. 288.7) and various degrees of inflammatory infiltrate, which can range from negligible to severe exudative or granulomatous lesions. In early inflammatory lesions, the infiltrates are composed of multifocal groups of lymphocytes, plasma cells, and eosinophils located in a fibrous connective tissue capsule surrounding the parasite. The severity of the reaction appears to be associated with the degree of damage or deterioration of the parasite tissue. As hyalinization and calcification of the parasite progress, the inflammatory infiltrate is found inside the parasite, and mononuclear cells, eosinophils, and polymorphonuclear neutrophils can be observed. The final stages of this process are characterized by the appearance of epithelioid and multinucleated giant cells, which persist until the complete calcification of the parasite.

The composition of the inflammatory exudate clearly suggests the elicitation of a local immune response to this parasite. Recent studies in NCC patients have shown that brain granulomas are clearly associated with Th1 and Th2 profiles (42). Other pathologic lesions secondary to the inflammatory response are vasculitis, fibrinoid necrosis, and ischemic necrosis of the neighboring vessels, which may be due to the deposition of immune complexes.

Clinical Manifestations

The clinical manifestations of NCC are secondary to location, number of cysts, and inflammatory response of the host. The clinical signs and symptoms are generally the result of the inflammatory host response to the cysticerci in the brain tissue. The neurologic picture it produces is complex and pleomorphic; often, it can be asymptomatic (43).

Several studies have pointed out that most viable cysts are accompanied by little or no inflammatory infiltrate and that symptoms appear only after a latent period of several years. The classic description of Dixon and Lipscomb (44), who studied 450 British soldiers returning from India, found that the average time

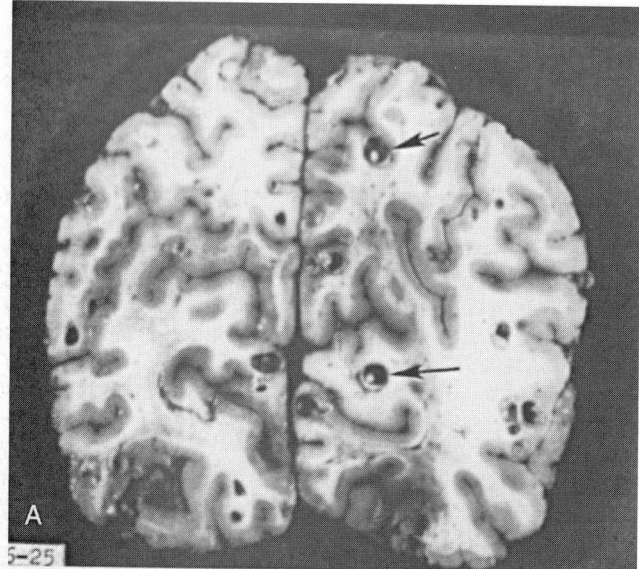

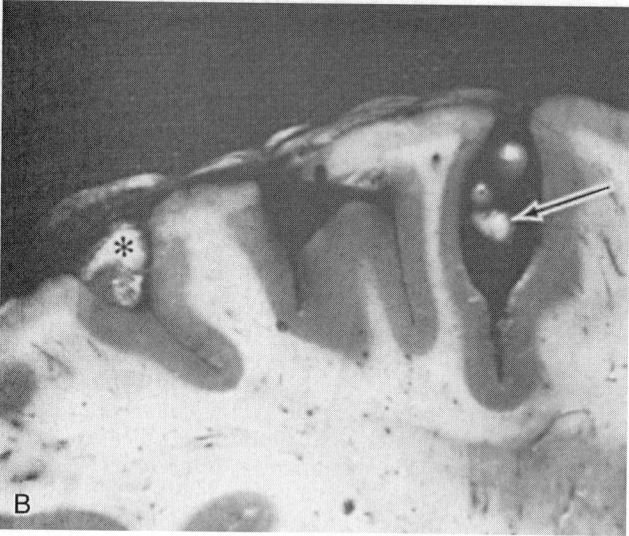

Figure 288.7. A: Coronal section of human brain showing multiple parenchymatous cysticerci (*arrows*). **B:** Cortical cysticerci: calcified cyst (*asterisk*); viable cyst (*arrow*). (**A** and **B** courtesy of Dr. Alfonso Escobar Izquierdo, Instituto de Investigaciones Biomédicas, UNAM, Mexico.)

granulomata or calcified cysts that are fortuitously detected on radiographs. In other cases, viable, translucent larvae have been seen with computed tomography (CT) in persons without symptoms.

The symptoms of patients with parenchymal cysts are varied, but most induce epilepsy that includes focal or generalized seizures (30% to 92%) and headache. Cysticercosis has been recognized as a major cause of late-onset epilepsy in several endemic countries (45–47).

When parasites lodge in the ventricular cavities, they may become trapped in lateral ventricles, the fourth ventricle (by far the most frequent ventricular location), or the aqueduct. If the cyst is free, it may cause little inflammatory reaction. The clinical manifestations are the result of obstruction of CSF circulation, which can give rise to hydrocephalus (see Fig. 288.8). Acute hydrocephalus is a syndrome characterized by increased intracranial pressure, headache, vomiting, impaired vision, dizziness, and ataxia. Papilledema and mental disturbances are also common in patients with hydrocephalus. The syndrome progresses if the hydraulic problem is not resolved with a ventricular shunt, causing progressive loss of consciousness, decerebration, and death. Cysticerci that lodge in the fourth ventricle exhibit a syndrome of progressive hydrocephalus, with headache, nausea, vomiting, and papilledema associated with disturbances in the cerebellar functions (dizziness, vertigo, and loss of equilibrium and motor coordination). In other cases, the cyst adheres to the base of the fourth ventricle, inducing an inflammatory response with ependymitis characterized by signs of brain dysfunction.

Cysticerci found in the basal cisternae are frequently in clumps or of the racemose type. The racemose cysticercus is a large membranous cyst measuring up to 5 cm in diameter. It often does not have a visible scolex, but it is certainly derived from a taeniid because it has the ultrastructural morphologic feature of taeniid tegumentary bladder walls. The work of Rabiela and coworkers (48) has shown by serial sections that these racemose forms do contain vestiges, or sometime whole scolices, unequivocally belonging to the species *T. solium*. For reasons that are at present not understood, the parasite located in the ventricles frequently becomes of the racemose type.

In cases in which the inflammatory process advances or increases, it can induce vasculitis or neuritis with local or distant ischemic phenomena, all of which are responsible for further brain damage and functional deterioration.

Cysticerci located in the subarachnoid space are in close contact with the CSF, and it is assumed that the parasites reach the meninges from the ventricles. This form of NCC is almost always associated with severe inflammatory infiltrates, which eventually give a clinical picture of chronic basal meningitis. This complication gives rise to one of the most frequent signs of NCC: increased intracranial pressure, without focal deficits, which can progress rapidly and cause death if it is not treated. On CT examination, they can be confused with parenchymal cysts.

Diagnosis

NCC should be suspected when the patient is known to live or to have lived in an endemic zone or country or has a clinical history of taeniasis or a family member who does; when there is chronic, persistent, atypical headache that is resistant to ordinary treatment, or seizures in young adults; when there are neurologic symptoms associated with increased intracranial pressure (papilledema); or when a nonsenile person exhibits mental deterioration. CT is the most useful study and in most cases is virtually

between their return from the endemic area and the appearance of symptoms was 4.8 years. Various authors have reported the existence of asymptomatic NCC; however, to date, no data have been published on the frequency or distribution of such cases. Escobedo has estimated from his experience in Mexico that approximately one third of NCC patients are asymptomatic (43).

The principal sites and approximate frequency of brain cysticerci are as follows (43): parenchyma, approximately 60%; subarachnoid space, meningobasal and cortical, approximately 40%; ventricular system, approximately 10%; mixed areas, more than 50%; spine, approximately 1%. Parenchymal cysts can be single or multiple. The majority of these larvae, when viable, are 1 or 2 cm in diameter, are filled with fluid, and have an invaginated scolex (Fig. 288.8). They are observed in children and young adults and frequently cause no symptoms. It is surmised that a proportion of these infections are resolved spontaneously by the patients' immune response, leaving small

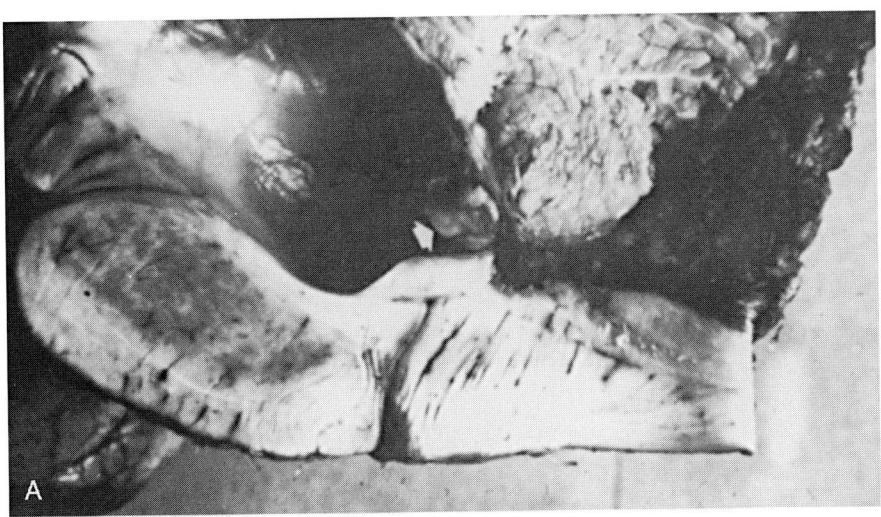

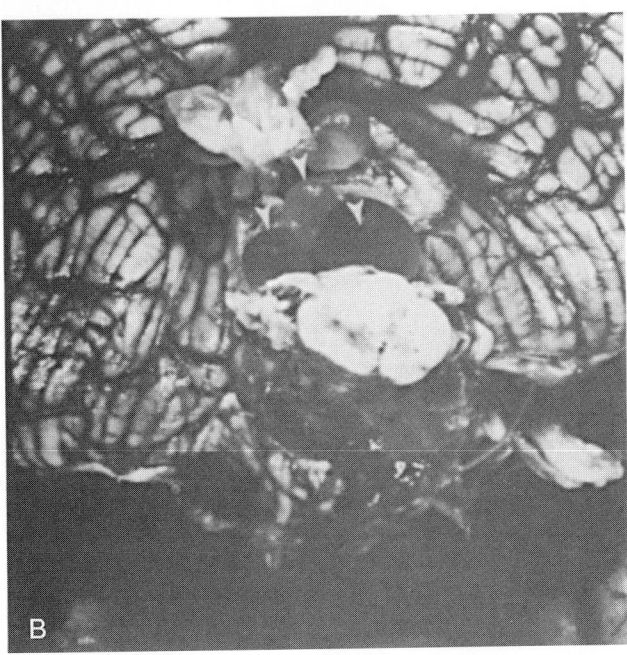

Figure 288.8. A: Cysticercus lodged in aqueduct of fourth ventricle (*arrow*). **B:** Cysticercus racemosus in posterior fossa. *Arrows* point to various lobules of this cyst. (**A** and **B** courtesy of Dr. Alfonso Escobar Izquierdo, Instituto de Investigaciones Bìomédìcas, UNAM, Mexico.)

diagnostic (49) (Fig. 288.9). In some cases, contrast enhancement is necessary.

Subarachnoid or intraventricular cysts are difficult to detect by CT, and other imaging studies must be carried out. Magnetic resonance imaging has turned out to be another powerful technique with a high resolution; parenchymal cysts are clearly outlined in the brain section. The equipment and its cost still limit the study to developed countries; and to a few centers in developing countries where the organism is endemic.

CSF analysis is useful and shows lymphocytic pleocytosis and elevated protein content in most cases, eosinophilia in about 50% of cases, and decreased glucose level in about 25% of cases (50).

Immunodiagnostic Procedures

Great progress has been made in the development of immunoenzymatic methods for the diagnosis of human cysticercosis. Several ELISAs have been developed. Reproducibility and sensitivity are greatest when larval bladder fluid is used as antigen.

The test detects 80% to 90% of seropositive cases in endemic areas and as many as 95% of seropositive cases in nonendemic areas (51,52). Indirect hemagglutination is also a sensitive serologic test when bladder fluid is used as antigen and a useful test in countries where enzyme products for the ELISA are more difficult to obtain (51).

By using a combination of ELISA and immunoblotting (enzyme-linked immunoelectrotransfer blot assay), Gottstein and colleagues have been able to identify specific antibodies against *T. solium* in 92% of serum samples and 100% of CSF samples from patients with cysticercosis (53). An additional enzyme-linked immunoelectrotransfer blot assay based on affinity of purified glycoprotein antigens and lentil lectin has reported a 98% sensitivity and 100% specificity in detecting antibodies in serum and CSF from patients with confirmed cysticercosis. It is also capable of discriminating cysticercosis from other infections and from no infection (54). Enzyme-linked immunoelectrotransfer blot assay has been used successfully in numerous field trials (55,56). Serodiagnosis with these methods has been extremely useful in epidemiologic studies, and they do aid in the diagnosis of individual cases of suspected NCC. However, definitive

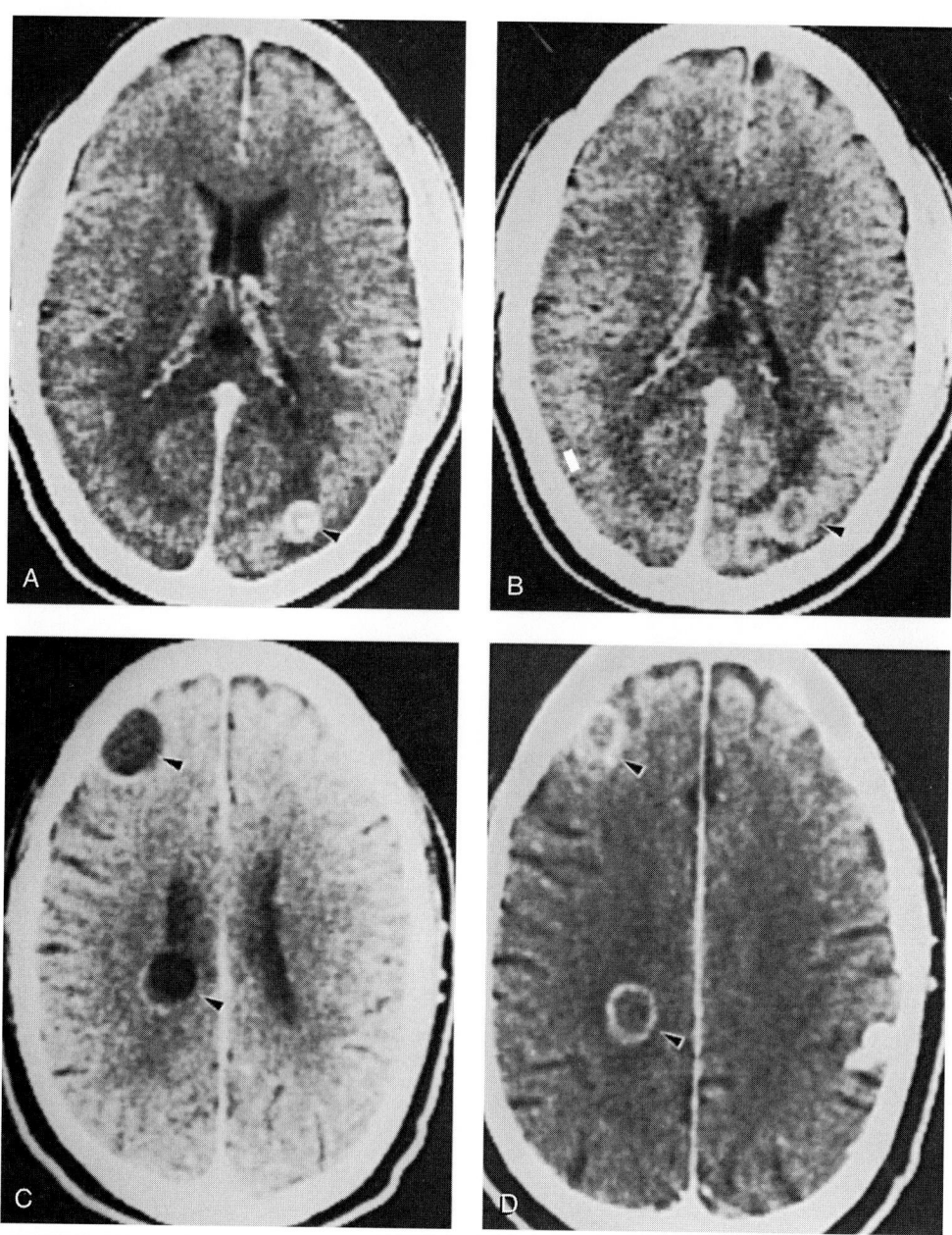

Figure 288.9. CT scan images. **A:** A patient with an occipital cyst (*arrow*). **B:** Same patient as in **A,** 8 months later, without treatment, showing inflammatory reaction but no reduction in size of lesion. **C:** Patient with two parenchymatous cysts showing as hypodense round areas (*arrows*). **D:** Same patient 4 months after treatment with praziquantel; both lesions are surrounded by an inflammatory infiltrate and are reduced in size. (**A** to **D** courtesy of Dr. Jesus Rodriguez, Instituto Nacional de Neurologia y Neurocirugia, "Manuel Velasco Suarez," Mexico City.)

diagnosis can be carried out only by CT or magnetic resonance imaging techniques.

Treatment

Praziquantel has been shown by various workers in different countries to be an effective drug against parenchymal NCC (33,57,58). Clinical and radiographic improvements have been shown in 70% to 90% of patients with parenchymal cysts (33). The drug is less effective for patients with chronic arachnoiditis, for whom only 47% remission is reported. The patients are treated with 50 mg/kg daily for 15 days. About 2 or 3 days after the treatment is started, a strong inflammatory reaction occurs, with increased protein levels and cells in CSF, headaches, exacerbation of neurologic symptoms, and edema around cystic lesions, which can be detected by CT. These reactions can be suppressed with steroids and usually last 2 or 3 days. Clinical evidence of improvement is observed about 3 months after treatment.

Albendazole, an imidazole, has been used in several trials and is as effective as praziquantel for parenchymal lesions (59). It has the additional advantage of being considerably less expensive than praziquantel and should be particularly useful in endemic countries where economy is an important factor in health care. The effective dosage tested by Sotelo and coworkers was 15 mg/kg per day for 1 week (59). A review of clinical trials indicates that both praziquantel and albendazole are effective drugs in the treatment of parenchymal NCC; albendazole is also effective in the treatment of large subarachnoid cysts (60).

A "single-day" treatment schedule with praziquantel has been shown to be effective and with similar results to those obtained with 1- and 2-week schedules: a total dose of 75 mg/kg of praziquantel divided into three administrations of 25 mg/kg each given at 2-hour intervals, followed 5 hours later by 20 mg of dexamethasone intramuscularly, with the same dose repeated the next 2 days. A high plasma concentration of praziquantel is obtained, exposing the parasites for longer periods to the cysticidal drug. Dexamethasone is administered 5 hours later, at a time when most of the praziquantel has been cleared from the blood. The advantage for the patient is a shorter treatment period, lower cost and the drugs are given sequentially reducing pharmacologic interference (61).

Extraparenchymal lesions affecting basal or lateral cisternae, lesions caused by Cysticercus racemosus, and calcified cysts do not improve with praziquantel or albendazole. These types of NCC require surgery for extirpation of the parasite or insertion of valves to drain CSF and relieve increased intracranial pressure due to hydrocephalus. The specialized surgical techniques are beyond the scope of this chapter (43).

Several studies have reported good responses to symptomatic therapy alone, the long-term results being similar to those obtained after anthelmintic drugs. No long-term control studies have been carried out to ascertain the benefits of one schedule over the other (35; Cochrane review, cited in AC White).

Epidemiology of Taeniasis/Cysticercosis

The epidemiology of this zoonosis is intimately dependent on the life cycle of the parasite: the adult tapeworm stage, found only in humans; the metacestode or larval stage in the intermediate host, which causes human and porcine cysticercosis; and the egg stage, which is infective and found in the tapeworm proglottids in the intestine of humans or dispersed in the environment, in sewage, or in pastures or other locations, depending on the defecation habits of the local population.

A large number of publications in the past 10 years from a number of endemic countries indicate that human NCC is a significant public health problem in Latin America, Asia, and Africa (5,62–69). There is ever-increasing evidence that this disease is now emerging in nonendemic countries, particularly in the United States, because of increased immigration of persons from endemic countries. T. solium carriers have been identified among domestic employees from Latin America, and a large number of cases of NCC have been found among immigrants, mostly acquired in their native countries (70–74).

Clinical data indicate that as many as 10% of CT studies carried out at the National Institute for Neurology and Neurosurgery in Mexico between 1976 and 1981 were diagnosed as cases of intracranial cysticercosis, or NCC (75). These results are in stark contrast to the prevalence of NCC reported in 1970, when it constituted only 0.08% of all cases seen in a neurologic department in a 12-year period (76).

Autopsy reports published in the past 20 years indicate that NCC has not diminished in most countries where the tapeworm is endemic (5). A review of 20,206 autopsies carried out at the General Hospital in Mexico City between 1953 and 1984 revealed 481 cases of NCC (2.38%), of which only 189 (32.29%) were from persons who actually died of NCC, emphasizing again the large number of asymptomatic or relatively benign cases of this disease (77).

Transmission Patterns

As Mackiewicz (78) pointed out, the low probability of an egg's developing into an adult has been resolved in the cestodes by three basic strategies: (a) evolution of life cycles interpolated into host biology, (b) presentation of infective stages that increase probability of contact between host and parasite, and (c) increase in reproductive potential. Successful direct cycles are rare and confirm that a key element of cestode survival is the two (or three) host life cycles. Another central element of cestode transmission is the passive incorporation of cestodes into intermediate hosts or through the food chain. In the context of these basic strategies, the life cycles of T. solium and T. saginata are easily understood, particularly with regard to the transmission of the infection from the adult infective tapeworm eggs to the natural intermediate host.

In the case of T. solium, there is no doubt that pigs become infected by ingesting infected human feces. In pastoral or rural communities where sanitary installations do not exist, defecation on open ground is an accepted practice. In small villages or hamlets where pigs are kept as domestic animals, they are usually left to wander and feed freely on garbage and excrement. Aluja has described a widespread practice that consists of having the latrine drain into the pigpen, serving a twofold purpose of feeding the pigs and eliminating the fecal material without a drainage system (79). Although the development of high-technology farming practices has significantly decreased the number of cysticercotic pigs in large urban slaughterhouses, the life cycle continues to be supported in small rural villages and hamlets, where modern health education is often pitted against century-old cultural patterns (49). Studies show that porcine cysticercosis can be found in as many as 48% of pigs in villages where no meat inspection is carried out (80).

Transmission from Human to Human

There are two processes by which infective eggs from a tapeworm carrier can be transmitted to a human intermediary host: ingestion of contaminated food and water and ingestion of eggs from hands contaminated by fecal material. Other mechanisms, such as inhalation of airborne eggs, ingestion of infected insects, and autoinfection by reverse peristalsis, have been suggested but not proved (5). Little is known about the dynamics of transmission from human to human.

Common features in three epidemiologic studies were poverty, poor personal hygiene and sanitary facilities, the common practice of defecation on open ground, the rearing of domestic pigs that are left free to roam and scavenge through the town and adjacent fields, and the absence of meat inspection at local slaughtering facilities. An important observation derived from these epidemiologic studies carried out in rural villages was a clustered distribution of tapeworm carriers in one house or in neighboring houses. These clusters were associated with significantly higher seropositivity rates to tapeworm antigens in individuals living with a tapeworm carrier. Several studies confirm that seropositive persons are significantly clustered within households in which a member had a history of passing proglottids. The data suggest that transmission from human to human in rural settings is mainly intradomiciliary (64–66,80,82).

Persons who live in daily close contact with a T. solium tapeworm carrier, under poor to fair hygiene conditions, may be exposed to frequent minimal doses of tapeworm egg antigens and eventually develop immune resistance to oncosphere infection. This possibility is a reasonable assumption, based on the results of experimental work carried out in other taeniids (83–85). Animals reared from birth in close association with the infected definitive host demonstrate the lightest infection patterns in the intermediate host population (5).

Molinari and associates have shown that immunization of hogs with cysticercal antigens induces an immune response leading to degeneration and destruction of cysticerci in heavily infected animals (86). Very recent experimental evidence from the Mexican group of Sciutto and coworkers has shown that epitopes shared between the murine T. crassiceps and T. solium confer protection in mice through a prominent Th1 response (87).

Such results are encouraging, particularly in relation to the possibility of developing vaccines, which could be used to protect swine in high-risk areas.

Prevention

T. solium has been successfully eradicated in many European and North American countries by strict meat inspection practices, health education, hygiene, and widespread sanitary installations. In some central European countries, taeniasis was eradicated by massive treatment of the population with anthelmintic drugs, a measure that diminished the egg reservoir in the environments Unfortunately, not all of these measures are immediately applicable in many developing countries. Health education through schools, television, and other programs involving the local population are among the measures suggested by an ad hoc World Health Organization committee. The development of local task forces for the detection, treatment, and proper elimination of tapeworms in small rural communities is a feasible goal and should certainly be considered in areas where porcine cysticercosis is known to exist or where seropositivity of the population to *T. solium* antigens is high (more than 3% or 4%) (66). In addition, Pawlowski (34) and Warren and colleagues (88) have recommended large-scale anthelmintic treatment of the population in endemic areas. Intervention trials carried out in several countries by administration of praziquantel to the population have significantly decreased the prevalence of *T. solium* tapeworms in communities (66,89). In spite of the success of these trials, treatment should not be undertaken without strict medical supervision owing to the risk of nonsymptomatic persons with

NCC responding to anthelmintic drugs (90). Reports describing resistance to anthelmintic drugs in livestock and human schistosomiasis (91,92) should also be given serious consideration, and the detection and treatment of individual cases should be encouraged instead.

ECHINOCOCCUS GRANULOSUS

E. granulosus belongs to the family Taeniidae (see Table 288.1) and is the cause of zoonotic infections by the adult tapeworm found in canids (dogs and other carnivores) and by the larval stage, which produces cystic hydatid disease, found in humans but also in a wide range of mammalian species (93).

Life Cycle

The adult worm is small, measuring between 2 and 7 mm (Figs. 288.10, 288.11). The scolex bears four suckers and a rostellum with two rows of hooks, one small and one large. The scolex attaches to the mucosa of the small intestine (Fig. 288.12) by burrowing into submucosal cryptae. Each worm has between two and seven proglottids, the average number being three. The genital pore in all *Echinococcus* species opens laterally. The penultimate segment is mature, containing the eggs, which are

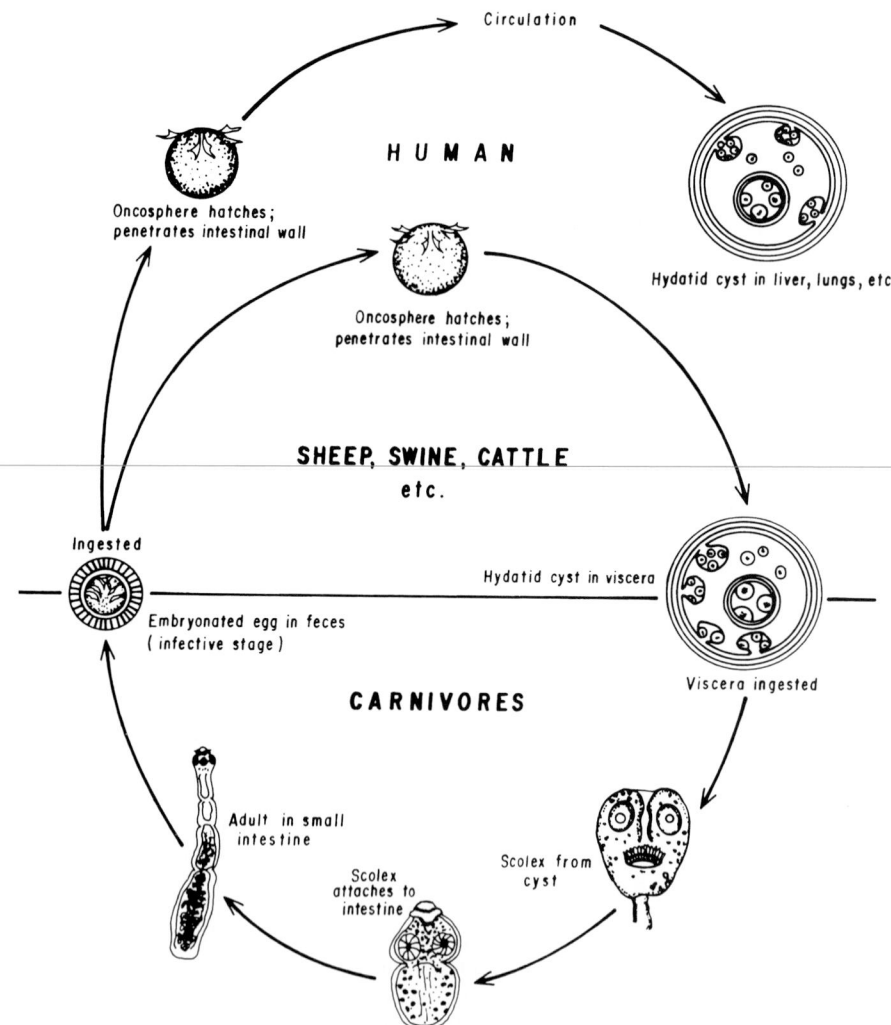

Figure 288.10. Life cycle of *Echinococcus granulosus.*

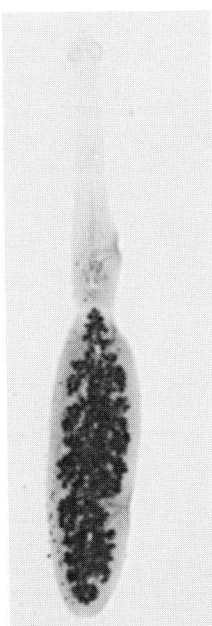

Figure 288.11. Whole adult worm (strobila) of *E. granulosus* (origin: Argentina), stained with carmine. (Courtesy of Dr. Peter M. Schantz, Centers for Disease Control and Prevention, Atlanta.)

ovoid and measure about 30 to 40 μm in diameter. The egg contains the hexacanth embryo (oncosphere) surrounded by the embryophore, a keratin shell, similar to the one found in *T. solium* and *T. saginata*, which also gives it a characteristic dark, striated appearance.

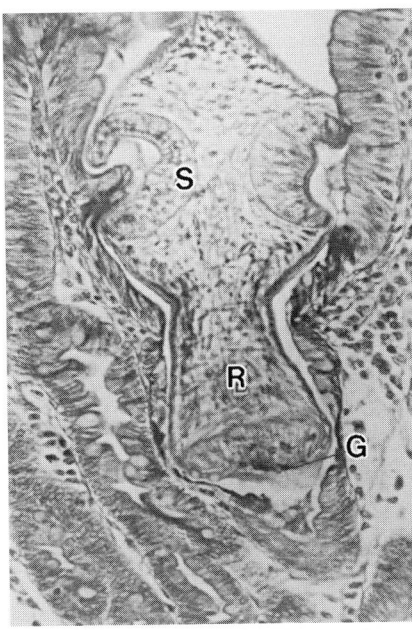

Figure 288.12. Section of mucosal wall of an experimentally infected dingo (*Canis familiaris dingo*) showing 35-day-old *Echinococcus granulosus* in situ. Rostellum (*R*) extended into crypt of Lieberkühn and the suckers (*S*) grasping the epithelium at the base of the villi. *G*, Rostellar gland. (Magnification, 40X.) (From Thompson RCA. Biology and systematics of *Echinococcus*. In: Thompson RCA, Lymbery AJ, eds. *Echinococcus and hydatid disease*. Oxford: CAB International, 1995:1–50.)

The adult worm parasitizes a wide range of *Canidae* (carnivores): domestic dogs, wolves, coyotes, jackals, and foxes. When proglottids from infected animals are released into the environment, the infective eggs can survive for long periods under suitable conditions of temperature and humidity (94,95).

The intermediate host acquires the infection by ingestion of infective eggs. Under the action of gastric and intestinal enzymes, the oncosphere is released and penetrates the intestinal wall and is transported to the liver or other organs. When the oncosphere reaches its final location, it develops into the larval stage or metacestode, commonly known as the hydatid cyst. The growth time of this cyst is variable but may take several months. Some cysts produce protoscolices and are known as fertile cysts; others do not and are classified as sterile cysts. The life cycle (see Fig. 288.10) is completed when a suitable definitive host ingests raw meat with cysts containing viable protoscolices. These evaginate in the upper duodenum, attach to the intestinal mucosa, and develop into sexually mature tapeworms approximately 6 to 8 weeks after infection.

The list of intermediate hosts for *E. granulosus* is long. Suffice it to say that it is maintained primarily in a domestic cycle with the domestic dog as definitive host and sheep the most important intermediate host. Other domestic ungulates, such as cattle, pigs, goats, horses, and camels, are susceptible hosts and may become infected in diverse geographic areas. There exists also a sylvatic cycle involving wolves and moose in North America (96,97), foxes and horses in Argentina (98), and jackals and wild ruminants in Kenya (99). Among the taeniids that parasitize humans, *E. granulosus* probably has the lowest host specificity of all, both the adult tapeworm and the hydatid cyst (93).

Epidemiology and Control

The spread and maintenance of this zoonosis in rural areas are facilitated by the widespread practice of feeding dogs the viscera of home-slaughtered sheep. Humans acquire hydatid cyst by coming in close contact with infected dogs passing infective eggs in feces. Infective eggs can also be ingested through contaminated water or food. As has been discussed in previous sections, taeniid eggs are resistant to environmental factors and survive particularly well in humid, temperate climates. Desiccation and high temperatures appear to be among the few factors that affect their viability.

The geographic distribution of the disease is cosmopolitan in countries of temperate climates: southern South America, the Mediterranean coast, southern and central Russia, central Asia, Australia, and parts of Africa (100). In Turkana, Kenya, the highest incidence of clinically recognized hydatid disease has been reported by Nelson (101), with 198 surgical cases per 100,000 people in 1986. Combining serodiagnosis and mobile ultrasonography, they were able to establish a prevalence of 5% to 10% of persons infected with hydatid cyst. In the United States, autochthonous transmission occurs in Alaska, California, Utah, Arizona, and New Mexico (100).

HUMAN HYDATID DISEASE

Pathology

After penetration of the oncosphere through the intestinal mucosa, the embryo reaches the tissues and develops into a cyst. Most human infections are acquired from the pastoral strain (domestic strain) and produce a single cyst. The most common site is the liver (65%), followed by the lungs (25%), but cysts can also

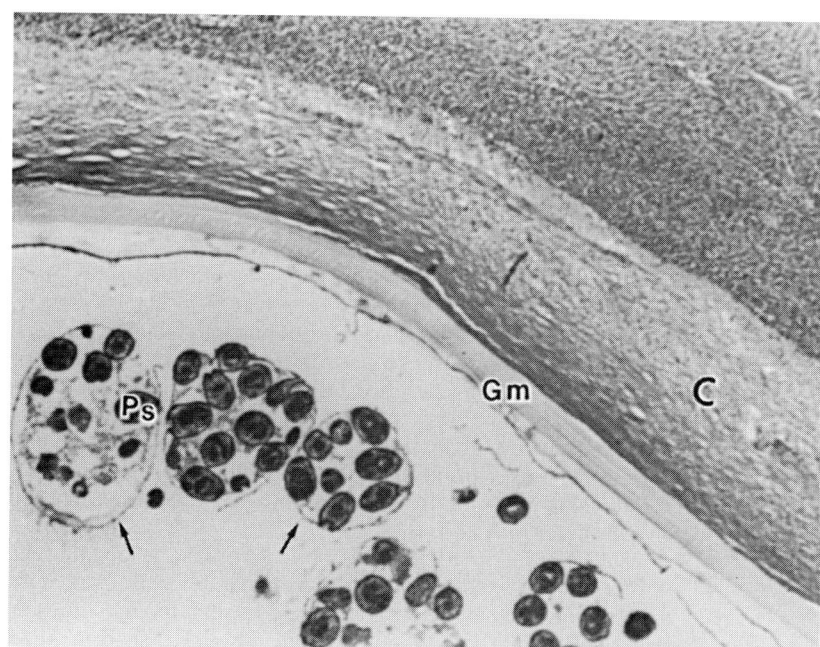

Figure 288.13. Histologic section of *E. granulosus* hydatid cyst from sheep liver showing protoscolices (*Ps*) in brood capsules (*arrows*), germinative membrane (*Gm*), and host capsule (*C*). (Courtesy of Dr. Peter M. Schantz, Centers for Disease Control and Prevention, Atlanta.)

be found in the spleen, bone, kidneys, heart, and CNS. Cysts from the sylvatic strain of this cestode tend to localize in the lungs and cause a less severe disease than the domestic strain (100). The growth rate of cysts is variable and can range from 1 to 5 cm a year. Transverse sections of the cyst reveal a nonnucleated laminated white membrane about 1 mm thick and an internal germinal membrane 10 to 15 μm thick with nucleated cells (see Fig. 288.12). Progressive growth of the cyst is accompanied by the formation of a host connective tissue capsule. Secondary cysts can be generated from the germinal wall of fertile cysts, which contain several hundred to thousands of invaginated, infective protoscolices (Fig. 288.13). The slowly growing cyst can be tolerated well until its size causes malfunction. Hydatid cysts containing up to 15 L of fluid have been reported and may contain up to 2 million protoscolices, each one of which can develop into a sexually mature worm if it is ingested by an appropriate definitive host. The major risk for patients with hydatid cysts is accidental rupture of the cyst wall. The sudden, massive release of cyst fluid can precipitate allergic reactions that can range from mild to fatal anaphylaxis. Dissemination of protoscolices may generate multiple secondary hydatid cysts.

Immune Response to Hydatid Cyst

In 1967 Capron and coworkers described a major precipitin band by immunoelectrophoresis found in serum of animals infected with *E. granulosus* (102). This precipitation band was termed arc 5 and has since been demonstrated to be the immunodominant and most specific antigen of this larval cestode. Its presence in a patient's serum is virtually diagnostic of *Echinococcus* species (103). Schantz and coworkers later demonstrated that arc 5 could also be found in some patients with NCC; however, this poses differential diagnostic problems only in countries where both infections coexist (104). Several studies have demonstrated that the more recently developed enzyme-linked immunoelectrotransfer blot tests are capable of discriminating between serologic reactions to hydatidosis and human cysticercosis (105).

ELISAs developed by Coltorti for the detection of arc 5 have shown a high efficiency (106). One of the major drawbacks of

serologic tests for detection of hydatid cyst is that about a third of the patients with proven disease are seronegative. Studies carried out by Craig and colleagues in Turkana, Kenya, have shown that clinically normal persons living in a highly endemic area had a significantly higher titer of antibodies (by ELISA) to oncospheral antigens than did clinically normal persons living in a nonendemic area (107). The authors speculated that these differences could be due to the presence, in the endemic areas, of a large number of infected persons who do not develop cystic disease and may, in fact, be exhibiting some degree of protective immunity. Such observations may be important for the eventual development and application of a preventive vaccine in high-risk endemic areas.

Clinical Manifestations

The clinical manifestations depend on the site and size of the hydatid cyst. They can be variable. The interval between infection and the appearance of symptoms can range from months to years, depending on the growth rate and situation of the cyst. Hepatic cysts may manifest as liver enlargement, with or without a palpable mass, right-sided epigastric pain, nausea, and vomiting. Rupture or leakage may cause allergic reactions and, if massive, may lead to anaphylactic shock.

Unilocular liver cysts can survive for many years in the patient and may be accidentally discovered on radiographs, particularly when the cyst wall is calcified. It is assumed that most infections are acquired during childhood and are not detected until adult life (108).

Diagnosis

A history of exposure to sheepdogs in endemic areas and the presence of a cystlike mass in the liver or lung supports the diagnosis of hydatid disease. CT and ultrasonography are the methods of choice for detailed characterization of the cyst. Closed aspiration of cysts should never be attempted because accidental spillage or rupture may cause anaphylaxis or secondary cysts. In lung infections, protoscolices may sometimes be demonstrated in bronchial lavage fluid or sputum. Eosinophilia is present in less than 25% of cases.

Serologic tests are useful and are diagnostic when results are positive, although a significant percentage of patients do not have circulating antibodies. Whenever possible, such sera should be tested for circulating antigen or circulating immune complexes, as described in the previous section.

Therapy

Surgical removal of the hydatid cyst still remains the most effective treatment (100). In cases of inoperable hydatid cysts, or when the general condition of the patient precludes surgery, albendazole, 10 to 15 mg/kg per day for 1 month, or mebendazole, 50 to 150 mg/kg per day for 3 months, may be administered, although the results are unpredictable. Okelo in Turkana, Kenya, has reported encouraging results with albendazole in series of patients with large inoperable cysts and extensive secondary involvement (109). The treatment schedule was 10 mg/kg per day in two divided doses for 8 weeks. Albendazole is also recommended for the prevention of recurrent secondary disease.

Prevention and Control

At present, preventive measures depend mainly on diminishing the infection rate in domestic dogs by avoiding the practice of feeding them sheep offal (viscera) and by periodic mass treatment of dogs with praziquantel (5 mg/kg) in endemic areas. For the prevention of human hydatid disease, measures such as careful personal hygiene and avoidance of infected dogs are essential. Health education and the strict enforcement of meat inspection and proper disposal of infected livestock should be carried out.

In some endemic countries, official control programs against *E. granulosus* are being carried out and maintained as recommended by the World Health Organization. A control program that has been in operation for more than 30 years has almost extinguished this parasite from New Zealand. The main features of the program were education and systematic deparasitization (dosing) of dogs (110). However, the disease still persists in many parts of the world, with alarming increases in the number of human cases reported in Bulgaria, Kazakhstan, and China (111).

A control program being carried out in Turkana, Kenya, includes case detection of human disease by ultrasonography and serologic tests; treatment of humans with surgery and albendazole; elimination of stray dogs; and registration of remaining dogs for treatment with praziquantel (112).

HYMENOLEPIS NANA

H. nana belongs to the family Hymenolepididae. It was originally described in rats and mice but was later found in humans.

Life Cycle

Among the Cyclophyllidea, it is the only tapeworm that is capable of completing the whole life cycle in one host, but it also sometimes uses the two-host life cycle. The length of the adult worm is inversely proportional to the number of individual worms present in the intestine. Its average length is between 2 and 3 cm. The scolex has four suckers and an armed rostellum with a single row of eight to 30 hooks. The scolices are attached to the small intestine, and gravid proglottids rupture in the lumen, releasing the embryonated eggs, which have a diameter of 40 to 50 μm. The eggs can hatch in the intestine and lodge between the mucosal microvilli until they develop into cysticercoids. These continue to develop into adult worms, a process that takes 15 to 20 days, when again they begin to release infective eggs.

Epidemiology

Hymenolepiasis is a parasitic disease of populations living under conditions of poor hygiene and is particularly prevalent in children from developing countries with tropical and subtropical climates. The disease is acquired by ingestion of infected mice feces, which contaminate water and food in such areas. Infected children may also contaminate others with infective eggs passed on dirty hands.

H. nana is found mainly in children younger than 8 years. Its prevalence is particularly high in rural communities, where hygiene and sanitation facilities are poor (113). Experimental work carried out in different laboratories indicates that *H. nana* infections induce humoral immunity (114) and probably have an important cellular immune component (115), responses that could account for the decreased prevalence of this parasitosis in adults living in endemic areas. Experimental evidence indicates that immunoglobulin E and mast cells participate in the expulsion of *H. nana* adults from the intestine of mice (116).

Clinical Manifestations

Symptoms are mild (vague abdominal distress) in light infections. Children with multiple infections, however, can have severe disease with abdominal pain, nausea, vomiting, weight loss, diarrhea, and irritability. Erosion of the intestinal mucosa can occur in massive infections.

Diagnosis

The diagnosis can be made on coprologic analysis of serial stool samples by identification of the eggs (which differ from the taeniid egg in that they lack a striated outer embryophore). Adult worms, which can also be found in multiple infections, can be identified by their size and armed scolex.

Treatment

The treatment of choice is niclosamide, 2 g daily for 5 days consecutively. Praziquantel has also been used with good effect, in a single dose of 20 mg/kg (117).

Prevention

Health education and careful personal hygiene, particularly for children, should diminish the frequency of this parasitosis.

DIPHYLLOBOTHRIUM LATUM (BROAD FISH TAPEWORM) LIFE CYCLE

D. latum belongs to the order of the Pseudophyllidea (see Fig. 288.13 and Table 288.1). In contrast to the taeniid tapeworms, Diphyllobothriidae organisms require two intermediate hosts to complete their life cycle and in addition have a free-swimming life stage that takes place in freshwater.

The scolex of *D. latum* is variable in shape, with distinct bothria, narrow, deep and not connected by an apical groove (2). Adult worms have been reported as long as 6 to 9 m with 3,000 to 4,000 proglottids that are wider than long. A single worm can produce about 1 million eggs per day. Von Bonsdorff and Bylund have reported the release of 20 to 40 million eggs per day per worm carrier (118). Expelled eggs are not completely mature and lie dormant in water after passing from the host. They become fully mature within 8 to 12 days. The egg hatches in water and releases the embryo, known as the coracidium, which is a free-swimming form. The coracidium must then be ingested within 4 or 5 days by its first intermediate host a copepod (nonspecific microcrustacean). In this host it becomes an oncosphere and bores through the intestinal wall of the copepod to reach the coelomic cavity, where it metamorphoses into a procercoid larva, measuring about 500 to 600 μm. When the infected microcrustacean is ingested by a fish, the procercoid dislodges and penetrates the intestinal wall of the fish and eventually situates itself in the muscle or one of various viscera. There it develops into a plerocercoid, which may remain viable for the lifetime of the fish. Plerocercoids are visible to the naked eye and measure about 1 to 5 cm. Many freshwater fish species are affected: pike, perch, turbot, ruff, and rainbow trout in Chile, whitefish and salmon in the United States. The life cycle (see Fig. 288.13) is completed when a human or other definitive host ingests raw or undercooked fish. The most suitable definitive host is humans, and the parasite seems to establish itself only in areas where its life cycle includes humans. Other final hosts are dogs, cats, pigs, wolves, foxes, and bears, among others. Worms develop in the small intestine and begin laying eggs about 1 month after infection. They may live for a number of years.

Epidemiology

D. latum is found in various terrestrial and marine fish-eating carnivores. The adult tapeworm also parasitizes humans, and infections have been reported in the subarctic and temperate regions of the Eurasian continent, in the area from the Siberian rivers Yenisei and Ob to the Baltic Sea. There is a high prevalence in the northern European areas of Russia, Volga basin, and Finland. It is also found in the lake districts of northern Italy and western Switzerland and around the Danube River. Immigration has transported the disease to freshwater lakes in North and South America.

Clinical Manifestations

Symptoms include abdominal pain, weight loss, and a unique form of pernicious anemia, which, although not common, is caused by the special capacity of *D. latum* for taking up vitamin B_{12} in the proximal small intestine.

Diagnosis

Diagnosis can be made in persons who report eating raw or undercooked fish by serial stool examinations for proglottids and eggs, which are oval and have a characteristic operculum on one pole.

Treatment

Treatment is a single dose of niclosamide, 2 g, or praziquantel, 5 to 10 mg/kg.

Prevention

Prevention can be achieved by avoiding the ingestion of raw or undercooked fish in endemic areas. The direct drainage of sewage into freshwater lakes or rivers should also be prevented.

ACKNOWLEDGMENT

The author is indebted to Dr. Julio Sotelo for his revision and constructive criticism of the section on human cysticercosis and treatment; to Dr. Jaime Martuscelli for his generous help in revising the manuscript; and to Drs. Jesus Rodriguez Carbajal, Alfonso Escobar Izquierdo, Juan Pedro Laclette, and Peter Schantz for many of the figures included in this chapter. To my long-time collaborator, Marie Therese Merchant, acknowledgment is given for her fine work in the preparation of the photographic material.

REFERENCES

1. Cheng TC. Cestoda. The true tapeworms. In Cheng TC, ed. *General parasitology.* New York: Academic Press, 1973:474–541.
2. Schmidt GD. *Handbook of tapeworm identification. Key to the genera Taeniidae.* Boca Raton, FL: CRC Press, 1986:221–227.
3. Mahajan RC. Geographic distribution of human cysticercosis. In: Flisser A, Willms K, Laclette JP, et al, eds. *Cysticercosis: present state of knowledge and perspectives.* New York: Academic Press, 1982:39–46.
4. Schultz MG, Halterman LG, Rich AB, et al. An epizootic of bovine cysticercosis. *J Am Vet Med Assoc* 1969;155:1708.
5. Gemmel MM, Matyas Z, Pawlowski Z, et al, eds. *Guidelines for the surveillance, prevention, and control of taeniasis/cysticercosis.* Geneva: World Health Organization, 1983.
6. Slais J. *The morphology and pathogenicity of the bladder worms: Cysticercus cellulosae and Cysticercus bovis.* Prague: Academia, 1970.
7. Pawlowski ZS. Epidemiology of *Taenia saginata* infection. In: Hisser A, Willms K, Laclette JP, et al, eds. *Cysticercosis: present state of knowledge and perspectives.* New York: Academic Press, 1982:69–85.
8. Burger HJ, Wilkens S. Infections of cattle with *Cysticercus bovis* and sarcocystic spp. on pastures irrigated with sewage plant effluent. *Mol Biochem Parasitol Suppl* 1982;274.
9. Harrison LJ, Holt K, Sewell MM. Serum antibody levels to *Taenia saginata* in cattle grazed on Scottish pastures. *Res Vet Sci* 1986;40:344.
10. Silverman PH. The longevity of eggs of *Taenia pisiformis* and *Taenia saginata* under various conditions. *Trans R Soc Trop Med Hyg* 1956;50:8.
11. Lisowska M. Epidemiological analysis of *Taenia saginata* taeniasis in Poznan [in Polish]. Poznan, Poland: Academy of Medicine, 1979. Thesis.
12. Heinz HJ, Klintworth GK. Cysticercosis in the aetiology of epilepsy. *S Afr J Med Sci* 1965;30:32.
13. Lenoble E, Dumontier C. Perforations du grele et parasitoses intestinales. A propos d'un cas de péritonite par perforation du grêle associéeàun *Taenia saginata. J Chir (Paris)* 1988;125:350.
14. Pawlowski ZS, Schultz MG. Taeniasis and cysticercosis (*Taenia saginata*). *Adv Parasitol* 1972;10:269.
15. Graham CF. A device for the diagnosis of *Enterobius* infection. *Am J Trop Med Hyg* 1941;21:159.
16. Faust EC, D'Antoni JS, Odom V, et al. A critical study of clinical laboratory techniques for the diagnosis of protozoan, cyst and helminth eggs in faeces. *Am J Trop Med Hyg* 1938;18:169.
17. Ritchie LS. An ether sedimentation technique for routine stool examinations. *Bull US Army Dept* 1948;8:326.
18. Martin LK, Beaner P. Evaluation of Kato thick-smear technique for quantitative diagnosis of helminth infections. *Am J Trop Med Hyg* 1968;17:382.
19. David ED, Lindquist WD. Determination of the specific gravity of certain helminth eggs using sucrose density gradient centrifugation. *J Parasitol* 1982;68:916.
20. McAninch NH. Case report. An outbreak of cysticercosis in feedlot cattle. *Can Vet J* 1974;15:120.
21. Eom KS, Rim HJ. Morphologic descriptions of *Taenia asiatica* sp. *Korean J Parasitol* 1993;31:1.
22. Bowles J, McManus DP. Genetic characterization of the Asian *Taenia*, a newly described taeniid cestode of humans. *Am J Trop Med Hyg* 1994;50:33.
23. Fan PC, Chung WC, Lin CY, Chan CH. Clinical manifestations of taeniasis in Taiwan aborigenes. *J Helminthol* 1992;66:118.
24. Webbe G. The hatching and activation of taeniid ova in relation to the development of cysticercosis in man. *Z Trop Parasitol* 1967;18:354.

25. Hernandez-Jauregui PA, Marquez-Monter H, Sastré-Ortiz S. Cysticercosis of the central nervous system in hogs. *Am J Vet Res* 1973;34:451.

26. Merchant MT, Aguilar L, Avila G, Robert L, Flisser A, Willms K. *Taenia solium*: description of the intestinal transplantation sites in experimental hamster infections. *J Parasitol* 1998;84:681–685.

27. Lumsden R, Voge M, Sogandares-Bernal F. The metacestode tegument: Fine structure, development, topochemistry and interactions with the host. In: Hisser A, Willms K, Laclette JP, et al, eds. *Cysticercosis: present state of knowledge and perspectives.* New York: Academic Press, 1982:307–361.

28. Allan JC, Craig PS, Garcia Noval J, et al. Coproantigen detection for immunodiagnosis of echinococcosis and taeniasis in dogs and humans. *Parasitology* 1992;104:347.

29. Maass M, Delgado E, Knobloch J. Isolation of an immunodiagnostic *Taenia solium* coproantigen. *Trop Med Parasitol* 1992;43:201.

30. Allan JC, Mencos F, Garcia Noval J, et al. Dipstick dot ELISA for the detection of *Taenia* coproantigens in humans. *Parasitology* 1993;107:79.

31. Chapman A, Vallejo V, Mossie KG, et al. Isolation and characterization of species-specific DNA probes from *Taenia solium* and *Taenia saginata* and their use in an egg detection assay. *Clin Microbiol* 1995;33:1283.

32. Groll E. Praziquantel for cestode infections in man. *Acta Trop* 1980;37: 293.

33. Pawlowski ZS. Efficiency of low doses of praziquantel in taeniasis. *Acta Trop* 1989;48:83.

34. Horton J. Albendazole: a review of anthelmintic activity and safety in humans. *Parasitology* 2000;121:113–132.

35. White AC. Neurocysticercosis: updates on epidemiology, patogénesis, diagnosis and management. *Annu Rev Med* 2000;51:187–206.

36. Schantz PM, Wilkins PP, Tsang VCW. Immigrants, imaging, and immunoblots: the emergence of neurocysticercosis as a major public health problem. In: Scheld WM, Craig WA, Hughes JM, eds. *Emerging infections*, 2nd ed. Washington DC: American Society of Microbiology, 1998:213–242.

37. Grogl M, Estrada JJ, MacDonald G, et al. Antigen-antibody analysis in neurocysticercosis. *J Parasitol* 1985;71:433.

38. Schantz PM. Improvements in the serodiagnosis of helminthic diseases. *Vet Parasitol* 1987;25:95.

39. Corona T, Pascoe D, Gonzalez-Barranco D, et al. Anticysticercosis antibodies in serum and cerebrospinal fluid in patients with cerebral cysticercosis. *J Neurol Neurosurg Psychiatry* 1986;49:1044.

40. McCormick GF, Zee CS, Heiden J. Cysticercosis cerebri: review of 127 cases. *Arch Neurol* 1982;39:534.

41. Escobar A, Nieto D. Parasitic diseases. In: Minckler J, ed. *Pathology of the nervous system*, vol 3. New York: McGraw-Hill, 1972:2503–2521.

42. Restrepo BI, Alaverz JI, Castano JA, et al. Brain granulomas in neurocysticercosis patients are associated with a Th1 and Th2 profile. *Infect Immun* 2001;69:4554–4560.

43. Escobedo F. Neurosurgical aspects of neurocysticercosis. In: Schmidek HH, Sweet WH, eds. *Operative neurosurgical techniques. Indications, methods and results.* Orlando, FL: Grune & Stratton, 1988:93–102.

44. Dixon H, Lipscomb F. Cysticercosis: an analysis and follow-up of 450 cases. Medical Resource Council Special Report 299. London: Her Majesty's Stationery Office, 1961.

45. White AC. Neurocysticercosis: a major cause of neurological disease worldwide. *Clin Infect Dis* 1997;24:101.

46. Garcia HH, Gilman R, Martinez M, et al. Cysticercosis as a major cause of epilepsy in Peru. The Cysticercosis Working Group in Peru. *Lancet* 1993;342:197.

47. Carpio A, Escobar, A, Hauser WA. Cysticercosis and epilepsy: a critical review. *Epilepsia* 1998;39:1025–1040.

48. Rabiela MT, Rivas-Hernández A, Castillo-Medina S et al. Pruebas morfológicas de que *Cysticercus cellulosae* y *Cysticercus racemosus* son larvas de *Taenia solium*. *Arch Inest Med (Mex)* 1985;16:83.

49. Rodriguez-Carbajal J, Boleaga-Duran B, Dorfsman J. Cerebral cysticercosis. The role of computed tomography (CT) in the diagnosis of neurocysticercosis. *Childs Nerv Syst* 1987;3:199.

50. Del Brutto OH, Sotelo J. Neurocysticercosis: an update. *Rev Infect Dis* 1988;10:1075.

51. Larralde C, Laclette JP, Owen CS, et al. Reliable serology of *Taenia solium* cysticercosis with antigens from cyst vesicular fluid: ELISA and hemagglutination tests. *Am J Trop Med Hyg* 1986;35:965.

52. Baily GG, Mason PR, Trijssener FE. Serological diagnosis of neurocysticercosis: evaluation of ELISA tests using cyst fluid and other components of *Taenia solium* cysticerci as antigens. *Trans R Soc Trop Med Hyg* 1988;82:295.

53. Gottstein B Zini D, Schantz PM. Species-specific immunodiagnosis of *Taenia solium* cysticercosis by ELISA and immunoblotting. *Trop Med Parasitol* 1987;38:299.

54. Tsang VC, Brand JA, Boyer AE. An enzyme-linked immunoelectrotransfer blot assay and glycoprotein antigens for diagnosing human cysticercosis (*Taenia solium*). *J Infect Dis* 1989;159:50.

55. Montenegro T, Gilman RH, Castillo R, et al. The diagnostic importance of species specific and cross-reactive components of *Taenia solium, Echinococcus granulosus* and *Hymenolepis nana*. *Rev Inst Med Trop Sao Paulo* 1994;36: 327.

56. Schantz PM, Sarti E, Plancarte A, et al. Community-based epidemiological investigations of cysticercosis due to *Taenia solium*: comparison of serological screening tests and clinical findings in two populations in Mexico. *Clin Infect Dis* 1994;18:879.

57. Botero D, Castaño S. Treatment of cysticercosis with praziquantel in Colombia. *Am J Trop Med Hyg* 1982;31:810.

58. Vasconcelos D, Cruz-Segura H, Mateos-Gomez H, et al. Selective indications for the use of praziquantel in the treatment of brain cysticercosis. *J Neurol Neurosurg Psychiatry* 1987;50:383.

59. Cruz I, Cruz ME, Carrasco F, Horton J. Neurocysticercosis: optimal dose treatment with albendazole. *J Neurol Sci* 1995;133:152–154.

60. Sotelo J, Jung H. Pharmakocinetic optimization of the treatment of neurocysticercosis. *Clin Pharmacokinet* 1998;34:503–515.

61. Jung H, Medina R, Castro N, et al. Pharmacocinetic study of praziquantel administered alone and in combination with cimetidine in a single.day therapeutic regimen. *Antimicrob Agents Chemother* 1997;41:1256–1259.

62. Fan PC, Chung WC, Chan CH, et al. Studies on taeniasis in Taiwan. V Field trial on evaluation of therapeutic efficacy of mebendazole and praziquantel against taeniasis. *Southeast Asian J Trop Med Public Health* 1986;17:82.

63. Sarti-Gutierrez EJ, Schantz PM, Lara-Aguilera R, et al. *Taenia solium* taeniasis and cysticercosis in a Mexican village. *Trop Med Parasitol* 1988;29:194.

64. Keilbach N, Aluja AS, Sarti E. A programme to control taeniasis/cysticercosis (*T. solium*). Experiences in a Mexican village. *Acta Leidensia* 1989;57:181.

65. Diaz Camacho S, Candil Ruiz A, Beltran Uribe M, et al. Serology as an indicator of *Taenia solium* tapeworm infections in a rural community of Mexico. *Trans R Soc Trop Med Hyg* 1990;84:563.

66. Diaz Camacho S, Candil Ruiz A, Suate Peraza V, et al. Epidemiological study and control of *Taenia solium* infections with praziquantel in a rural village of Mexico. *Am J Trop Med Hyg* 1991;45:522.

67. Kong Y, Ch SY, Cho MS, et al. Seroepidemiological observations of *Taenia solium* cysticercosis in epileptic patients in Korea. *J Korean Med Sci* 1993;8: 145.

68. Thomson AJ. Neurocysticercosis-Experience at the teaching hospital of the University of Cape Town. *S Afr Med J* 1993;83:332.

69. Spina Franca A, Livramento JA, Machado LR. Cysticercosis of the central nervous system and cerebrospinal fluid. Immunodiagnosis of 1573 patients in 63 years (1929–1992). *Arq Neuropsiquiatr* 1993;51:16.

70. Schantz PM, Moore AC, Munoz JL, et al. Neurocysticercosis in an Orthodox Jewish community in New York City. *N Engl J Med* 1992;327:692.

71. Locally acquired neurocysticercosis-North Carolina, Massachusetts, and South Carolina, 1989-1991. *MMWR* 1992;41:1.

72. Ehnert KL, Roberto RR, Barrett L, et al. Cysticercosis: first 12 months of reporting in California. *Bull Pan Am Health Organ* 1992;26:165.

73. Sorvillo FJ, Waterman SH, Richards FO, Schantz PM. Cysticercosis surveillance: Locally acquired and travel related infections and detection of intestinal tapeworm carriers in Los Angeles County. *Am J Trop Med Hyg* 1992;47: 365.

74. Dietrichs E, Tyssvang T, Aanonsen NO, Bakke SJ. Cerebral cysticercosis in Norway. *Acta Neurol Scand* 1993;88:296.

75. Rodriguez Carbajal J. La cisticercosis humana en Mexico. Diagnóstico radiológico. *Gac Med Mex* 1988;124:198.

76. Macias Sanchez R, Rodriguez Trujillo F, Ordoñez Martinez S. Cisticercosis cerebral: Anatomia patológica y correlación anatomoclinica. *Neurol Neurochir Psychiatry* 1970;11:271.

77. Villagran Uribe J, Olvera Rabiela JE. Cisticercosis humana: Estudio clinico y patologico de 481 casos de autopsia. *Patologia (Mex)* 1988;26:149.

78. Mackiewicz JS. Cestode transmission patterns. *J Parasitol* 1988;74:60.

79. Aluja AS. Frequency of porcine cysticercosis in Mexico. In: Flisser A, Willms K, Laclette JP, et al, eds. *Cysticercosis: present state of knowledge and perspectives.* New York: Academic Press, 1982:53–62.

80. The marketing of cysticercotic pigs in the Sierra of Peru. The Cysticercosis Working Group in Peru. *Bull WHO* 1993;71:223.

81. Sarti E, Schantz PM Plancarte A, et al. Epidemiological investigation of *Taenia solium* taeniasis and cysticercosis in a rural village of Michoacan State, Mexico. *Trans R Soc Trop Med Hyg* 1994;88:49.

82. Sarti E, Schantz PM, Plancarte A, et al. Prevalence and risk factors for *Taenia solium* taeniasis and cysticercosis in humans and pigs in a village in Morelos, Mexico. *Am J Trop Med Hyg* 1992;46:677.

83. Musoke AJ, Williams JF. Immunological response of the rat to infection with *Taenia taeniaeformis*: protective antibody response to implanted parasites. *Int J Parasitol* 1976;6:265.

84. Sewell MMH, Gallie GJ. Immunological studies on experimental infections with the larval stage of *Taenia saginata*. In: Soulsby EJL, ed. *Parasitic zoonoses. Clinical and experimental studies.* New York: Academic Press, 1974:187–193.

85. Rickard MD. Immunization against infection with larval taeniid cestodes using oncospheral antigens. In: Flisser A, Willms K, Laclette JP, et al, eds. *Cysticercosis: present state of knowledge and perspectives.* New York: Academic Press, 1982:633–646.

86. Molinari JL, Meza R, Tato P. *Taenia solium*: cell reactions to the larva (*Cysticercus cellulosae*) in naturally parasitized, immunized hogs. *Exp Parasitol* 1983;56:327.

87. Toledo A, Fragoso G, Rosas G et al. Two epitopes shared by *Taenia crassiceps* and *Taenia solium* confer protection against murine *T. crassiceps* cysticercosis along with a prominent Th1 response. *Infect Immun* 2001;69:1766–1773.

88. Warren KS, Bundy DAP, Anderson RM, et al. *Helminth infections, Health Sector Priorities Review.* Washington, DC: The World Bank, 1989.

89. Sarti E, Schantz PM, Avila G, Ambrosio J, Medina-Santillán R, Flisser A. Mass treatment against human taeniasis for the control of cysticercosis: a

population-based intervention study. *Trans R Soc Trop Med Hyg* 2000;94:85–89.

90. Flisser A, Madrazo I, Plancarte A, et al. Neurological symptoms in occult neurocysticercosis after single taeniacidal dose of praziquantel. *Lancet* 1993;342:748.

91. Jackson F. Anthelmintic resistance—the state of play. *Br Vet J* 1993;149:123.

92. Brindley PJ. Drug resistance to schistosomiasis and other anthelmintics of medical significance. *Acta Trop* 1994;56:213.

93. Eckert J, Gemmel MA, Soulsby EJL, eds. *Guidelines for surveillance, prevention and control of echinococcosis/hydatidosis.* Geneva: World Health Organization, 1981.

94. Sweatman GK, Williams RJ. Survival of *Echinococcus granulosus* and *Taenia hydatigena* eggs in two extreme climatic regions of New Zealand. *Res Vet Sci* 1963;4:199.

95. Laws GF. Physical factors influencing survival of taeniid eggs. *Exp Parasitol* 1968;22:227.

96. Rausch RL, Nelson GS. A review of the genus *Echinococcus rudolphi,* 1801. *Ann Trop Med Parasitol* 1963;57:127.

97. Rausch RL. Life cycle patterns and geographic distribution of *Echinococcus* species. In: Thompson RCA, Lymbery AJ, eds. *Echinococcus and hydatid disease.* Oxford: CAB International, 1995:89–134.

98. Schantz PM, Lord RD, de Zavaleta O. *Echinococcus* in the South American red fox (*Dusicyon culpaeus*) and the European hare (*Lepus europaeus*) in the province of Neuquen, Argentina. *Ann Trop Med Parasitol* 1972;66:479.

99. Eugster RO. *Contribution to the epidemiology of echinococcosis/hydatidosis in Kenya (East Africa) with special reference to the Kajiado District* (PhD thesis). Zurich: University of Zurich, 1978.

100. Schantz PM. Larval cestodiasis. In: Hoeprich PD, Jordan MC, eds. *Infectious diseases. A modern treatise of infectious processes,* 4th ed. Philadelphia: JB Lippincott, 1989:829–841.

101. Nelson GS. Hydatid disease: research and control in Turkana, Kenya. 1. Epidemiological observations. *Trans R Soc Trop Med Hyg* 1986;80:177.

102. Capron A, Vernes A, Biguet J. Le diagnostic immunoelectrophoretique de l'hydatidose. In: Conder J, ed. *Le kyste hydatique du foie.* Lyon, France: SIMEP, 1967:27–40.

103. Schantz PM. Improvements in the serodiagnosis of helminthic zoonoses. *Vet Parasitol* 1987;25:95.

104. Schantz PM, Shanks D, Wilson M. Serologic cross-reactions with sera from patients with echinococcosis and cysticercosis. *Am J Trop Med Hyg* 1980;21:609.

105. Moro PL, Guevara A, Verstegui MM, et al. Distribution of hydatosis and cysticercosis in different Peruvian populations as demonstrated by an enzyme-linked immunoelectrotransfer blot (EITB) assay. *Am J Trop Med Hyg* 1994;51:851.

106. Coltorti EA. Standardization and evaluation of an enzyme immunoassay as a screening test for the seroepidemiology of human hydatidosis. *Am J Trop Med Hyg* 1986;35:1000.

107. Craig PS, Zeyle E, Romig T. Hydatid disease: research and control in Turkana. II. The role of immunological techniques for the diagnosis of hydatid disease. *Trans R Soc Trop Med Hyg* 1986;80:183.

108. Amman R, Eckert J. Clinical diagnosis and treatment of echinococcosis in humans. In: Thompson RCA, Lymbery AJ, eds. *Echinococcus and hydatid disease.* Oxford: CAB International, 1995:411–463.

109. Okelo GBA. Hydatid disease: research and control in Turkana, III. Albendazole in the treatment of inoperable hydatid disease in Kenya—a report on 12 cases. *Trans R Soc Trop Med Hyg* 1986;80:193.

110. Lawson JR, Roberts MG, Gemmel MA, et al. Population dynamics in echinococcosis and cysticercosis: economic assessment of control strategies for *Echinococcus granulosus, Taenia ovis* and *Taenia hydatigena. Parasitology* 1988;97:177.

111. Eckert J, Conraths FJ, Tackmann K. Echinococcosis: an emerging or reemerging zoonosis? *Int J Parasitol* 2000;30:1283–1294.

112. Macpherson CNL, Wachira TM, Zeyle E, et al. Hydatid disease: research and control in Turkana, IV. The pilot control programme. *Trans R Soc Trop Med Hyg* 1986;80:196.

113. Mason PR, Patterson BA. Epidemiology of *Hymenolepis nana* infections in primary school children in urban and rural communities in Zimbabwe. *J Parasitol* 1994;80:245.

114. Ito A, Honey RD, Scanlon T, et al. Analysis of antibody responses to *Hymenolepis nana* infection in mice by the enzyme-linked immunosorbent assay and immunoprecipitation. *Parasite Immunol* 1988;10:265.

115. Palmas C, Bortolette G, Conchedda M. Immunological memory and lymphoblast migration in mice infected with *Hymenolepis nana. Z Parasitenkd* 1986;72:397.

116. Watanabe N, Nawa Y, Okamoto K, Kobayashi A. Expulsion of *Hymenolepis nana* from mice with congenital deficiencies of IgE production or of mast cell development. *Parasite Immunol* 1994;16:137.

117. Bouree P. Intérêt du praziquantel, un cure unique, comme traitement de *Taenia saginata* et de *Hymenolepis nana. Pathol Biol (Paris)* 1988;36:759.

118. von Bonsdorff B, Bylund G. The ecology of *Diphyllobothrium latum. Ecol Dis* 1982;1:21.

CHAPTER 289
Arthropods

Andrew Spielman, Mitchell Wachtel,
and Richard J. Pollack

Although many diverse hematophagous arthropods transmit a great variety of pathogenic microorganisms, these jointed-legged creatures themselves directly compromise human health. Entomologic discussions in public health, however, generally focus on vectorborne infections while only peripherally treating arthropods themselves as agents of disease. Such treatments only infrequently include comprehensive analyses of the direct entomologic causes of human disease. Accordingly, we describe the arthropods that persistently infest people with a focus on the mites, lice, fleas, and myiasis-producing flies and the conditions that they cause. We also describe features of the stings caused by certain Hymenoptera and of the bites of spiders (1). When considering complaints by patients of purported chronic infestations, the clinician should make every reasonable attempt to sample and have identified the etiologic agent. When neither the agent is discovered nor relief is offered by presumptive treatment, delusional parasitosis or other psychoses should be considered (2,3). Our objective is to present a body of information that is useful in the practice of medicine and particularly adapted for temperate parts of the world.

SCABIES

The ovoid mite that causes scabies, due to *Sarcoptes scabiei,* is colorless and less than 1 mm long (4). Human scabies infestations perpetuate solely in human skin, forming characteristic sinuous burrows in the stratum corneum. Adult females periodically emerge from these burrows and crawl on their eight legs over the surface of the skin.

Epidemiology

Although no population-based estimates of the prevalence of scabies in temperate parts of the world have yet become available, risk may be appreciable. Some 2% to 5% of patients treated by dermatologists suffer from this infestation. In 1983, for example, scabies was the second most common diagnosis in a San Francisco hospital (5, p36). The condition is far more frequent, however, in the tropics. Immigrant children from lesser developed nations should therefore be examined routinely for this condition (6). As many as 300 million cases of scabies are said to occur annually throughout the world (7).

Because scabies mites die within 2 days when they are isolated from a human host, transmission depends mainly on direct contact between hosts rather than on fomite transfer through contaminated clothing or bedding. Crowding promotes outbreaks. A secondary attack rate of 38% prevails among household contacts, providing a rationale for presumptive community treatment. Scabies affects people of any age but decreases in people older than 40 years. Although scabies infestations frequently burden African villagers, black people appear less susceptible to infection than are others (8).

Nosocomial infections commonly occur in nursing homes and mental hospitals, where health care providers suffer certain occupational risk. Norwegian scabies, discussed later, may pose a particular threat in such settings because of the absence of the characteristic pruritus and the highly infectious nature of the infestation.

Zoonotic scabies frequently afflicts people who experience intimate contact with dogs and where sanitation is poor. Although human disease most commonly results from such canine infection, cats, horses, pigs, and pigeons have also been implicated as sources of infestation (9,10). The incubation period of zoonotic scabies is shorter than that of the anthroponosis and is self-limited owing to the failure of these mites to propagate in human skin. Repeated infestations are common, however.

Pathogenesis and Histopathology

The inflammatory skin lesions of scabies derive from cell-mediated and humoral immune hypersensitivity responses to the mite's saliva and feces. The immunoglobulin E level tends to be elevated. Although infection is generally silent for some 4 to 6 weeks in people infected for the first time, symptoms may appear almost immediately after subsequent reinfestation (11, p53) (12). The papular pruritic eruption of scabies derives from immune sensitivity and often bears no relation to the location of the mites. Pruritic nodules may be present for several months after the infestation is eliminated.

For the most part, the burrows of these mites are mainly confined to the stratum corneum of the skin. The blind ends of burrows that contain adult females, however, generally extend into the stratum malpighii. Spongiosis, developing near the mite, may result in vesicle formation. A variable eosinophilic infiltrate characterizes the lesion. Even if no mite is discovered, the mere presence of eggs in the horny layer is pathognomonic for scabies. Papules are characterized by a nonspecific inflammatory reaction that includes no eosinophils and is free of mites.

Chronic nodules, which similarly contain no mites, are characterized by a dense mononuclear infiltrate that may or may not include eosinophils. The walls of adjacent blood vessels may be thickened.

Norwegian or crusted scabies may develop in immuno-compromised or mentally-impaired patients. Administration of steroids may induce crusted scabies (13), and this has been treated with ivermectin (14). Residents of the tropics, however, seem to suffer this syndrome spontaneously. Numerous mites lying in multiple subcorneal burrows characterize biopsy specimens of the crusts of Norwegian scabies. Such lesions are generally characterized by hyperkeratosis, acanthosis, and a marked dermal cellular infiltrate.

Disease Relationships

Scabies is characterized by intense pruritus, often worse at night or after a hot shower. (15) In the usual form of the disease, the symmetric, papulovesicular lesions, 2 to 3 mm in diameter, may be accompanied by macules, pustules, and scaly plaques. Burrows measure 3 to 15 mm and appear as irregular, fine black threads that are often difficult to find (Fig. 289.1).

Scabies lesions are confined to the flexor surfaces of the interdigital spaces in two thirds of patients; nearly nine tenths suffer at least one lesion in these sites. Other affected sites include the breasts, periumbilicus, belt line, buttocks, thighs, penis, scrotum, elbows, feet, ankles, and anterior axillary folds. In children and infants, lesions may appear on any skin surface. In addition, the disease may be present in children as a bullous lesion. Scabies may also appear as a blistering eruption (16,17).

Norwegian scabies is characterized by widespread erythema, hyperkeratosis, and crusting but little or no itching (18–20).

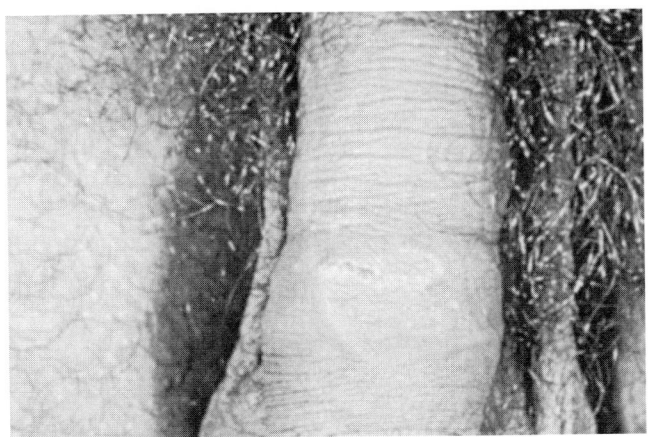

Figure 289.1. Sinuous burrow of scabies mite in a characteristic site.

No discrete burrows are evident. Nail involvement is common. Alopecia, generalized hyperpigmentation, pyoderma, and eosinophilia may also occur.

Other atypical forms of the disease may occur (11, p53). Patients with a high level of hygiene may develop "scabies of the cultivated." Although burrows are evident in only 7% of such patients and findings may be scant, the patient continues to be infectious. Corticosteroids may suppress symptoms, thereby resulting in a misdiagnosis of fungal infection or impetigo. In nodular scabies, indurated nodules that may be pigmented develop on the groin or axilla but generally contain mites after the first month. Even when treated, infestations may continue for more than a year despite therapy.

Patients infected by human immunodeficiency virus tend to develop papulosquamous lesions in skin cleavage lines, similar to those seen in pityriasis rosea. Other findings tend not to be seen, but Norwegian scabies has been reported (21,22).

Zoonotic scabies produces papulovesicular erythematous, pruritic lesions, usually around the waist or on the arms (11, p53). No burrows are present. Excoriation from the intense pruritus may produce secondary bacterial infection that confuses the clinical picture. The bleeding that derives from the excoriation constitutes a useful clinical clue to the presence of scabies. Epidemics of poststreptococcal glomerulonephritis have been associated with scabies and secondary bacterial infection (7).

Diagnosis

Scabies is a highly polymorphic disease, well deserving its reputation as a great imitator, a descriptor once reserved for syphilis (12). An index of suspicion must be maintained with any patient presenting with pruritus, particularly if more than one household contact suffers from the condition. Primary care physicians more frequently overdiagnose than underdiagnose scabies (23).

Definitive diagnosis requires discovery of the mites, scybala, or eggs (5, p4). Burrows are present in virtually all North American patients and should be sought in the web spaces between the fingers; on the wrists and elbows; and on the sides of the hands, feet, and ankles. Topical application of liquid tetracycline, followed after several minutes by alcohol, causes the burrows to fluoresce yellow-gray with a Wood lamp. Other methods of detecting the burrows include the use of mineral oil to alter the refractive index of the stratum corneum, the ink test, in which ink wiped over an affected area is permitted to penetrate the burrows and the excess wiped away, epiluminiscence microscopy and high magnification videodermatoscopy (24–26).

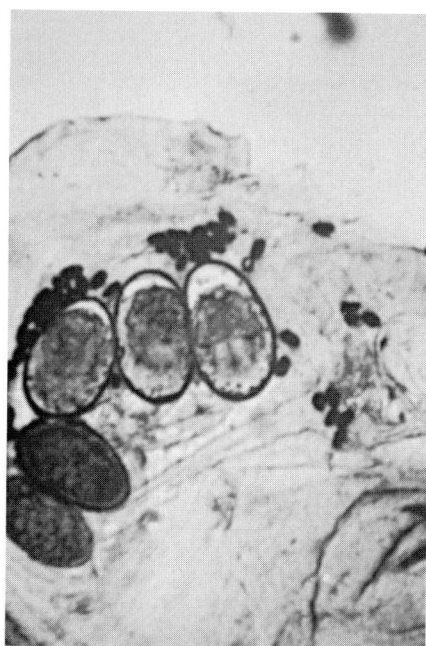

Figure 289.2. Eggs and feces of a scabies mite in a skin scraping.

The mites, their scybala, or their eggs can be demonstrated by any of various methods. An epidermal shave biopsy or superficial scraping involves placing a drop of sterile mineral oil at the anterior end of a suspected burrow, scraping the epidermal surface with a No. 15 blade, and examining the scrapings microscopically (Fig. 289.2). A magnifying glass may be used to detect the mite within its burrow. It appears as an oval, white object that is darkly pigmented caudally. The mite can be extracted with a needle point and examined under a microscope. An incident light microscope can be used to identify the mites *in vivo* (26). In the absence of burrows, a scraping or a shave biopsy of the papulovesicular lesions may yield definitive diagnostic material.

For patients with Norwegian scabies, examination of the crust is diagnostic (11, p53). In zoonotic scabies, scrapings of the vesicles into mineral oil often provides diagnostic material. Mites or their products will not always be found, unfortunately, and diagnosis must then rest on clinical features of the lesion.

On the other hand, a diagnosis of scabies does not exclude other conditions. Other pruritic and nonpruritic dermatologic and venereal diseases may be present as well.

Treatment

Although lindane has been the most frequently used scabicide in the United States (27), permethrin formulations have largely displaced lindane because of toxicity concerns (28). Permethrin is highly effective and relatively nontoxic (29,30). In a double-blind prospective study, for example, 91% of patients treated with 95% permethrin remained free of lesions 1 month after therapy began. The comparable figure for 1% lindane was only 45%, apparently because these mites have developed physiologic resistance against this long-used insecticide.

A single application of permethrin generally eliminates living scabies mites. The presence of persisting antigens, however, may continue to provoke allergic reactions even months after the mites have been destroyed. Of course, treatment cannot preclude reinfestation, particularly among the homeless, whose close

contacts often cannot be identified and treated in a timely fashion (5 pp44,53). Treatment with calamine lotion or antihistamines generally reduces the urticaria, but a brief course of steroid therapy may occasionally be required. Patients infected by human immunodeficiency virus may require repeated treatment. Secondary bacterial infections should be treated with topical antibiotics or, when lesions are extensive or adenitis is present, with systemic therapy.

Orally administered ivermectin appears to be effective as a scabicide. At 1 month after administration of a single dose of ivermectin, 70% of 23 originally scabies-infected subjects remained scabies free (31). Benzyl benzoate, on the other hand, eliminated these mites in only 48% of 21 randomized subjects. Ivermectin appears to be effective in treating Norwegian scabies (32). This drug has the advantage of simplicity of application and apparent absence of irritation.

Alternative scabicides, including benzyl benzoate, crotamiton cream (Eurax), or sulfur ointment, may be preferred for infants, pregnant women, or nonsupervised mass treatments. For infants, monosulfiram is applied at diagnosis and after a day and a week. Sulfur dermatitis may result. If sulfur ointments are used, alcohol must be avoided because of the possibility of a disulfiram-type reaction. For Norwegian scabies or for nail involvement, a keratolytic agent, such as salicylic acid, may be required before the scabicide is applied. Repeated treatment may be required. For patients with human immunodeficiency virus (HIV) and crusted scabies, a combination of topical benzoyl benzoate and oral ivermectin has been found effective in one clinical trial (33). The treatment of crusted scabies may require a combination of oral ivermectin, 5% permethrin cream, and a keratolytic agent (34).

DUST MITES

House dust mites are minute sarcoptiform organisms that feed mainly on exfoliated human danders (35). Of the various dust mites, *Dermatophagoides pteronyssinus* and *Dermatophagoides farinae* most commonly cause human disease. All life history stages are similar. The mites are too small to be seen in situ.

Epidemiology

The abundance of dust mites correlates with the quantity of accumulated human dander; their antigens, carried in house dust, directly induce bronchoconstriction in affected asthmatic patients (36,37). Dust mites dehydrate when the ambient relative humidity falls below 60% (38,39). *D. pteronyssinus* requires exceptionally humid conditions, whereas *D. farinae* is somewhat more tolerant to drying. For this reason, dust mites rarely become abundant at high altitudes or during the winter months. Mite antigens, however, persist in the absence of living mites. Certain housing features permit dust mites to become abundant, particularly inadequate moisture seals in older homes, excessively tight sealing in newer homes, and the presence of fitted carpets (40). Mites and their secretory products tend to accumulate in carpeting, bedding, mattresses, and upholstered furniture.

Disease Relationships

Three major kinds of antigens derive from dust mites. Those designated Der p I, Der p II, and Der p III are associated with *D. pteronyssinus*; Der f I is associated with *D. farinae*. Der I and II are the best characterized (41–43), and Der p III has been cloned and sequenced (44). Der I antigens are associated with mite feces, whereas the Der II moieties are associated with the bodies of these mites; both become airborne in house dust (45). In sensitized people, these proteins induce an allergic immunoglobulin E–mediated response. In addition, vascular permeability is increased by exposure to the serine proteases that are contained in mite feces (46,47). Such exposure, at least in rats, provokes non-immunoglobulin E-mediated mast cell degranulation (46). Intradermal injection of mite antigen induces expression of the endothelial leukocyte adhesion molecule-1 in susceptible patients, leading to the development of inflammatory cell infiltrates (48). Ratios of helper to suppressor T cells are altered, and the expression of CD23 on B cells and the serum levels of interleukin-2 are increased in asthmatic children subjected to bronchial allergen provocation (49).

Exposure to dust mite allergens is associated with asthma (50), atopic dermatitis (51), or perennial rhinitis and conjunctivitis (52–55). Such a dust mite etiology is particularly well supported in the case of asthma (56). Although asthma was initially associated with childhood disease, adults appear to suffer a similar spectrum of disease (57). Early childhood exposure seems crucial in the development of these conditions (58).

Patients with atopic dermatitis experience elevated serum immunoglobulin E levels (59). Immunoglobulin E receptors in epidermal Langerhans cells (60) present mite antigen to helper T lymphocytes (61). The risk for atopic dermatitis is greatest in patients who have previously experienced chronically itchy skin and at least three other important signs, including involvement of skin creases or cheeks (in children younger than 10 years), history of asthma or hay fever (or atopy in children younger than 4 years), history of general dry skin in the previous year, visible flexural eczema (or eczema of the cheeks or forehead and outer limbs in children younger than 4 years), and onset in children younger than 2 years unless the child is younger than 4 years (62,63). Laboratory tests are available but not required for presumptive diagnosis.

Mite-associated rhinitis and conjunctivitis can be separated from the more common pollen-related allergies by their non-seasonal nature and by the presence of a reactive skin test result or antibody against mite antigen (52,53). The characteristic symptoms are useful in diagnosis, particularly when they are aggravated by the patient's house-cleaning activities. Perennial rhinitis is not associated with nasal polyps. Nasal provocation tests can be used to support the diagnosis (38). Dust mite-specific immunoglobulin G levels are elevated, for example, in patients suffering from chronic rhinosinusitis (64).

Treatment

Although specific therapy for atopic disease lies beyond the scope of this discussion, certain general comments are appropriate. Immunotherapy for asthma appears to be a safe and effective treatment of dust mite allergy when it is provided under optimal conditions in certain patients (65). Exposure to antigen should be minimized by enclosing pillows and mattresses in plastic covers, washing bedding at least once a week, removing carpeting from the bedroom, and reducing upholstered furniture to a minimum. Humidity should be reduced by use of air conditioners and dehumidifiers; outdoor ventilation should be maximized whenever the weather permits (66). The mites can be destroyed by directly applying chemical acaricides, such as a pyrethroid or tannic acid. Airborne dust can be reduced by the use of portable air filters or, when the patient is absent from the room, by the use of vacuum cleaners. These measures, properly used, generally reduce the symptoms of house dust allergy.

TICKS

Except in the case of certain residents of Africa who sleep on the ground, people encounter hard (ixodid) ticks far more often than soft (argasid) ticks. Indeed, the few soft ticks that are present in temperate parts of the world are generally closely restricted to the nests of rodents. Hard ticks attach firmly to their hosts and feed continuously for 3 to 10 days; soft ticks attach lightly, mainly on sleeping hosts, and detach within 20 minutes or so. A wide array of viral, rickettsial, bacterial, and protozoal infectious agents are tickborne, and certain of these are discussed elsewhere in this volume.

Tick saliva contains a complex of chemicals. A thrombin inhibitor, ixin, and an antithromboplastin, ixodin, are present in the salivary glands of *Ixodes ricinus* (67). An apyrase component of the saliva of a soft tick, *Ornithodoros moubata*, that inhibits platelet aggregation (68) has been dubbed moubatin (69). An anticoagulant peptide, which affects factor Xa, is also present (70). This pharmacologically active secretion includes a diverse array of other components that alter humoral and cell-mediated immunity and cytokine function and that suppress various immunoregulatory and immune effector pathways of the host (71,72). Antitick salivary components are antigenic in human hosts (73).

Deer Ticks

The emergence of Lyme disease, human babesiosis, human granulocytic ehrlichiosis (HGE) and tickborne encephalitis (TBE) in parts of North America and Eurasia (74) has stimulated an intense interest in ticks and an investment in medical attention directed at these hematophagous organisms. The diagnosis and therapy of these infections is discussed elsewhere in this volume. Only certain members of the genus *Ixodes* appear to serve as vectors of these zoonotic infections (75). The deer tick *Ixodes dammini* in the eastern United States (which differs from southern *Ixodes scapularis*) and similar *Ixodes pacificus* ticks in the West affect human health in North America. Related ticks (*I. ricinus* and *Ixodes persulcatus*) do so in the Old World. The term *Ixodes scapularis*, however, frequently is used to designate members of vector as well as non-vector populations. Deer serve as the definitive hosts for these ticks; their larval and nymphal stages feed mainly on mice (Fig. 289.3), which serve as the main reservoirs of the pathogens. *Ixodes* ticks attach firmly, feeding for several days

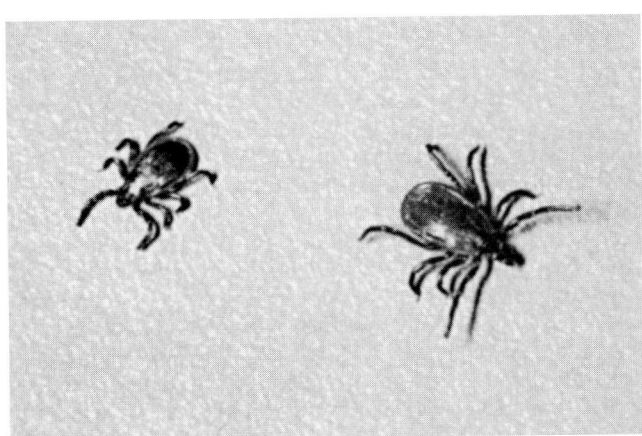

Figure 289.3. Adult female (*right*) and male (*left*) deer ticks. Note the long mouthparts of the female and her light coloring posteriorly. Males rarely attach to human hosts, and then only lightly.

or more and engorging most markedly toward the end of the period of attachment. Adult *I. dammini* ticks quest for hosts from October through April, larvae from August through September, and nymphs mainly from May into July. All developmental stages of these ticks attack people.

These *Ixodes* ticks thrive solely where deer are numerous, particularly at the brushy margins of forested sites. In the eastern United States, people are most frequently attacked by the nymphal stage of the deer tick. Although the physical presence of a tick on a person's body is generally distressing, immediate attention is required because of the possibility of consequent microbial infection.

To prevent transmission of the agents of Lyme disease or babesiosis, ticks should be removed from the skin promptly and at least during the first 2 days of attachment, before their rapid phase of engorgement commences. They should be detached by firm traction, with care taken to remove as much of the tick as possible by use of a forceps applied close to the point of attachment to the skin. Although some rotational movement may help dislodge the mouthparts intact, retention of a fragment of the feeding apparatus is inconsequential. The use of heat, burning, or chemical treatment merely delays removal of an attached tick and does not facilitate the process. Dead ticks pose little danger.

The agents of Lyme disease and human babesiosis enter the saliva of the vector tick only after approximately 2 days of attachment, and saliva is the vehicle of transmission. Spirochetes are delivered to the skin of the host, rather than directly to the blood vasculature, where they remain for 2 days or more (76). The site of attachment of a tick should therefore be disinfected, as with an antiseptic such as tincture of iodine (76).

Where the risk of Lyme disease, human babesiosis or HGE is great, any poppy seed-sized tick (about 2 mm in diameter) that becomes distended with blood should be considered a potential source of infection (77). A person bitten by such a tick during May through July should be alert to the possibility of infection if the tick had been feeding for at least 2 days. Presumptive treatment of Lyme disease remains an attractive option. Ticks found attached to a person between October and April would generally be adult deer ticks, and spirochetes generally infect approximately two thirds of such ticks (78). Because nymphal deer ticks may be relatively scarce (79), because they are generally not infected by spirochetes, and because they are not apt to be noticed before becoming infectious, presumptive treatment of tick bite may be futile (81). Doxycycline administration soon after discovery of an attached tick, however, appears to prevent Lyme disease (81a).

Dog and Wood Ticks

Of the various kinds of ticks that attack residents of the North American continent, dog and wood ticks (of the genus *Dermacentor*) are the most ubiquitous. Wood ticks (*Dermacentor andersoni*) are indigenous to mountainous regions of the West, and dog ticks (*Dermacentor variabilis*) infest more coastal sites. Interestingly, the range of the mountain species seems to be diminishing, whereas that of the lowland species is increasing. Where they are abundant, both of these ticks transmit rickettsial infection (Rocky Mountain spotted fever), and either may cause tick paralysis.

The adult stage of the dog tick (Fig. 289.4) feeds mainly on dogs and that of the wood tick on wood-chuck or marmots. Larvae and nymphs feed on voles and sometimes mice. All trophic stages feed early in the summer, but only the adult stage attacks people.

Dog ticks infest grassy sites where dogs are numerous. Adults quest most frequently near sources of carbon dioxide, as where

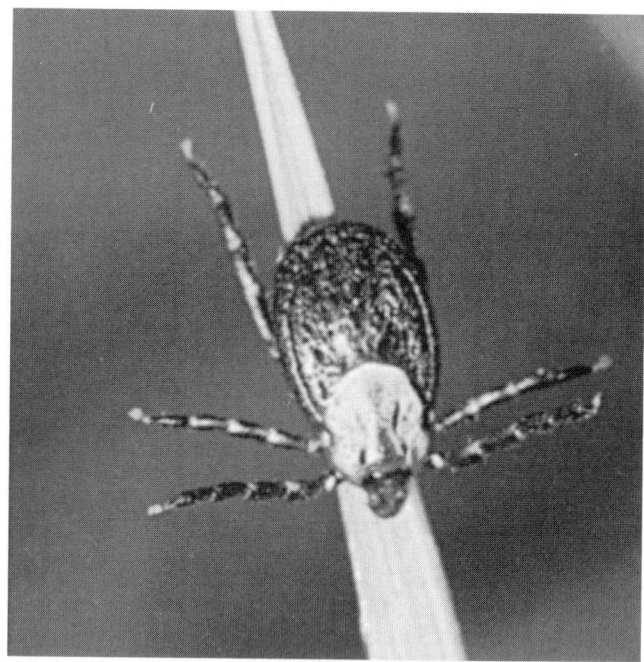

Figure 289.4. Adult female dog tick. Note the short mouthparts and white sculpturing on the dorsal plate. This plate covers the entire body of a male.

automobiles pause on a hill or park on a sandy site; such gaseous emanations suggest the presence of large hosts.

As in the case of deer ticks, attached dog or wood ticks should be promptly removed by gentle traction. In contrast to deer ticks, however, these ticks come away readily and always remain intact. To avoid contamination by the agent of spotted fever, such ticks should be handled by means of forceps or while wearing rubber gloves. The site of attachment should be disinfected, as with such a substance as tincture of iodine.

Except in southeastern sections of the United States, ticks that are 6 mm or longer and that feed during the summer months should be considered to be dog or wood ticks. Because spotted fever is infrequent, presumptive antibiotic treatment after removal of such a tick seems inadvisable.

Lone Star Ticks

Lone star ticks (*Amblyomma americanum*) may be abundant locally in forested portions of the southeastern United States and in isolated foci as far north as southern Rhode Island. Although these ticks are incompetent as vectors for the agent of Lyme disease, they may transmit a distantly related and mildly pathogenic *Borrelia* (82). Deer serve as the main host population throughout the entire life cycle of these ticks, and any stage may attack human hosts. They become abundant solely where deer are abundant. These ticks may be associated with a transient condition that resembles Lyme disease.

As in the case of *Ixodes* deer ticks, lone star ticks attach so firmly to their hosts that their mouthparts frequently remain in place after the body of the tick is removed. This condition, however, appears to be innocuous. Massive infestations by larval lone star ticks occur when people walk near the site where an egg mass has been deposited and recently has hatched. Infestations by these "seed ticks" can cause considerable discomfort and may be confused with that of the deer ticks that transmit Lyme disease.

LICE

The human pediculiases include infestations by head lice (*Pediculus humanus capitis*), body lice (*Pediculus humanus humanus*), and pubic lice (*Pthirus pubis*) (11 p53). These insects are dorsoventrally flattened and lack wings. The three body regions of the head and body lice are clearly demarcated. The central thorax bears the three pairs of clawed legs. The seven abdominal segments have lateral lobes. All stages of development appear similar morphologically. Unlike many other arthropods, lice are host-specific. Thus, human lice solely infest people. People may transiently be affected by lice of other animals, and this generally occurs when in direct contact with such infested animals and dens.

The mouth of a louse is a toothed tubular structure, the haustellum, which remains invaginated within the head until feeding begins and contains the feeding apparatus. Blood is the sole food and is aspirated through a pair of stylets. A third such stylet directs the highly antigenic and antihemostatic saliva into the skin of the host. Copious quantities of feces are discharged onto the skin of the host during feeding, thereby providing the vehicle of transmission for louse-borne typhus and relapsing fever.

Pubic lice are crablike and about as broad as they are long. They are shorter than the other anthroponotic lice, and their body appears more fused. Their appendages are unique in that the claws of the forelegs are more slender than the others, enabling this louse to grasp pubic and facial hairs.

Epidemiology

Head lice most commonly infest the head hair of children. Some 0.3% of North American black children, as opposed to 10% of whites, appear to be infested (83). Direct contact seems to be the most important means of transmission. Although fomites such as shared headgear and grooming implements have long been considered to be the primary means of facilitating louse transfer, the significance of such inanimate objects is now in question. Because head lice feed several times each day, their survival off a host is limited to about a day or less.

In contrast to head lice, body lice mainly infest indigent people who remain clothed for extended periods. These insects tend to remain sequestered in the seams and between layers of clothing except when feeding (Fig. 289.5) (5 p45). Body lice are trans-

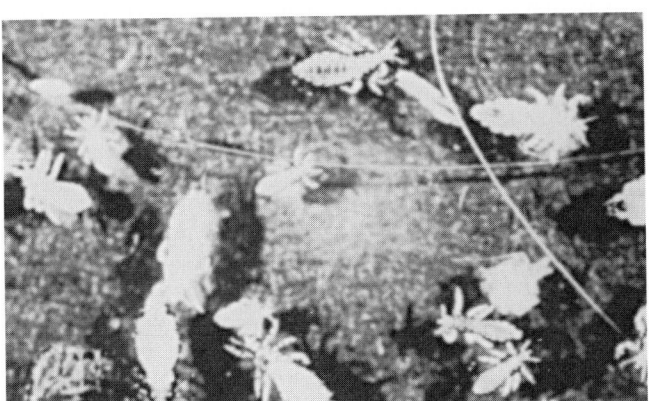

Figure 289.5. Body lice and nits concentrated in the seams of clothing. (From Parish LC, Schwartzman RM, Nutting WB, eds. *Cutaneous infestations of man and animals.* New York: Praeger Publishers, 1983, with permission.)

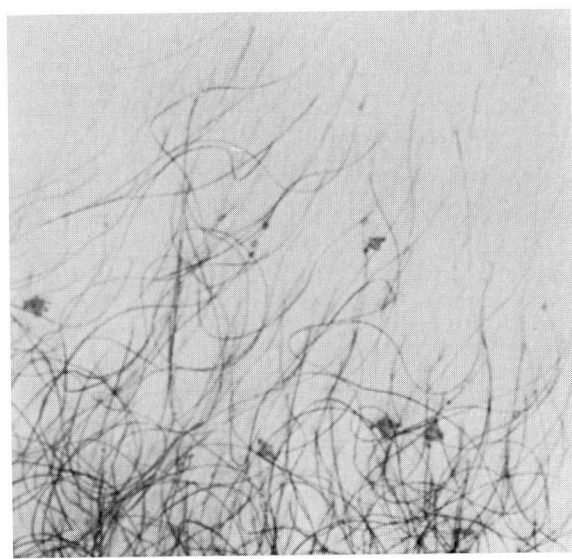

Figure 289.6. Pubic lice and nits infesting pubic hairs. (From Domonkos AN, Arnold HL Jr. *Diseases of the skin,* 7th ed. Philadelphia: WB Saunders, 1982:556, with permission.)

mitted mainly by direct contact between people and by exchange of contaminated clothing and bedding.

Pubic lice mainly infest the hair of the pubis of sexually active people (Fig. 289.6) but also the eyelashes, facial hair, and axillae and less often the scalp hair in the case of children. Venereal contact provides the main, but not the only, means of transmission.

Histopathology

Early histologic changes after the bites of lice include dermal edema and a mild perivascular lymphocytic, eosinophilic, and neutrophilic infiltrate (11 p53). The edema is less prominent than that after other insect bites. Late changes include a lymphocytic histiocytic infiltrate with minimal edema.

Disease Relationships

The saliva of body lice and to a lesser extent head lice produces an intensely pruritic, 2- to 3-mm, erythematous, maculopapular eruption (Fig. 289.7) forming hours to days after feeding. Hives may appear immediately, with flare and wheal formation. Excoriation may produce secondary changes and infection, including crust formation and regional adenopathy. The bites may be inapparent to the patient. A hemorrhagic component is occasionally present, presumably promoted by the salivary product.

An erythematous, maculopapular rash on the scalp, the nape of the neck, and the shoulders may occasionally result from the bites of head lice, but most infestations seem asymptomatic. Secondary changes due to excoriation may include crusting, matting of hair, oozing, and bacterial infection. Although the lice may seldom be seen during a cursory examination, nits are more readily apparent. Hair casts, seborrheic material, and other debris are frequently misidentified as head louse eggs (84,85).

Chronic infestation by body lice may result in generalized hyperpigmentation and a characteristic lichenification known as vagabond's disease.

The particularly intense pruritus due to the bites of pubic lice mainly affects pubic, perineal, inguinal, and lower abdominal sites as well as the axillae and eyelids. The rash may present

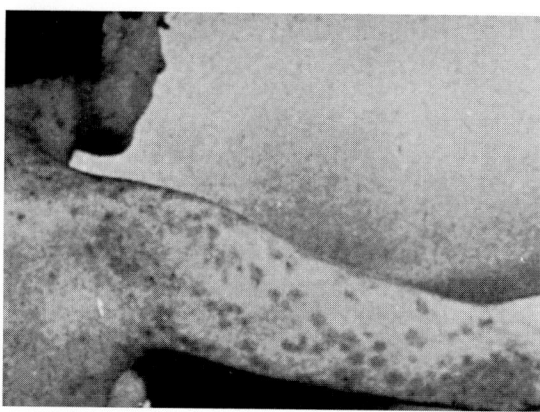

Figure 289.7. Macules due to chronic exposure to the bites of body lice. (From Domonkos AN, Arnold HL Jr. *Diseases of the skin*, 7th ed. Philadelphia: WB Saunders, 1982:557, with permission.)

as blue-gray macules, a syndrome known as maculae ceruleae (85). Excoriation may produce secondary changes, but secondary infection is less likely than with body or head lice. Nits would virtually always be present, and the lice would be visible with the aid of a magnifying lens. Infestations of the eyelids may present with a blepharoconjunctivitis and occasionally with a serosanguineous discharge at the conjunctival margins. Adult lice may be evident at the eyelash roots.

Other sexually transmitted diseases should be considered whenever pubic lice are discovered. Whereas an infestation in a juvenile may suggest abuse (86), more innocent means of transfer are possible. A child with pubic lice should be evaluated for other signs of abuse, and referred to a child protection agency if warranted.

Treatment

Treatment for head lice should be considered solely when live lice are discovered. Discriminating live nits from those that have died or hatched requires specialized training, and should not be attempted by the clinician. The presence of dead and hatched nits frequently misleads patients into repeated applications of the lousicide in the mistaken belief that the prior treatment has failed.

Head lice may be eliminated by mechanical removal of lice and their eggs with special fine-toothed combs or other implements, or by topical applications of insecticide. Non-prescription pediculicidal formulations based on synthetic pyrethroids and natural pyrethrins are relatively safe and can often be effective if applied twice, with an interval of 10 days between treatments. Resistance to pyrethroids has been documented (87). If live lice persist following application of pyrethroids, then prescription pediculicidal formulations of malathion or lindane should be considered. Infested children, as well as those who are incorrectly labeled as infested, are frequently sent home from school under a policy known as "No Nits." The resulting school absenteeism seems far more disruptive than is the medical burden, and these policies are unsupported by scientific scrutiny (84,88).

Infestations of body lice are eliminated mainly by more frequent laundering or changing of clothing and linens, supplemented by topical application of pediculicide when needed. Disinsection of all clothing and bedding is crucial; clothing should be placed loosely in a clothes dryer for 30 minutes or more at a temperature of at least 65°C. If lice or louse eggs are found clinging to body hair, individual patients may then be

treated from head to foot with pyrethroid-based or lindane-based pediculicides. Mass treatment of affected populations in disaster situations has required application of dust formulations of any of a variety of insecticides.

Infestations of pubic lice may be eliminated by applications of pyrethroid-containing shampoo, by mechanical removal of lice and their eggs, and also by shaving the affected region. For eyelid infestations, 1% yellow mercuric acid ointment, four times daily for two weeks, has been found effective (89).

FLEAS

Fleas are wingless, laterally compressed insects, 1 to 4 mm long, that are equipped with powerful jumping legs. In developed regions of the world, the human flea *Pulex irritans* and the cat flea *Ctenocephalides felis* most commonly attack people. The chigoe flea *Tunga penetrans* may do so where conditions are more primitive. The minute, caterpillar-like larvae develop where the host sleeps and feed mainly on the dried pellets of nondigested blood that the adults defecate while feeding. The spatial and seasonal distribution of fleas is limited by the tendency of their larvae to desiccate. Where houses are centrally heated, fleas cannot survive the winter except when the host sleeps on a moist surface, such as a concrete floor. Fleas may live for 1 to 4 months when they are isolated from hosts and for a year or more when suitable hosts are present. Fleas transmit the agents of plague, *Yersinia pestis*, and of murine typhus, *Rickettsia typhi*, as well as the rat tapeworm *Hymenolepis diminuta* and the dwarf tapeworm *Hymenolepis nana*.

Disease Relationships

The bites of fleas induce a pruritic papular urticaria composed of wheals or firm papules with occasional bullae distributed on characteristic parts of the body (20). The eruption occurs mainly on the lower legs when the feet and ankles are exposed. In children having intimate contact with domestic animals, lesions may occur over the whole body. A generalized allergic response may occur. Extreme pruritus results in secondary changes that may include bacterial infection. Other insects, including bedbugs and mosquitoes, may produce a similar dermatitis. Basophils have been implicated in the production of such lesions (90). Histologic changes include intercellular and intracellular edema of the stratum malpighii with occasional vesicle formation, a chronic perivascular dermal infiltrate, usually of the superficial and midcorium. Eosinophils are generally prominent. The microscopic appearance of the lesion may mimic prurigo simplex, except that the presence of eosinophils suggests a papular urticaria. Without sensitization, or with hyposensitization, the clinical and histologic appearances become less pronounced, and the lesion is then mildly edematous with a mild mononuclear perivascular infiltrate (91).

The chigoe or jigger flea *T. penetrans* may infest travelers who walk barefoot or in sandals in rural sites in the Americas, Africa, and India. The fertilized female penetrates the stratum corneum of the skin, generally in crevices, such as beneath the margins of toenails. The lesion initially appears as a dark furuncular pinpoint that enlarges within 2 weeks as the flea swells to the size of a pea. The lesion is painful but self-limiting. If the flea is permitted to remain in situ, a 0.5-cm section of skin will eventually slough. Developing chigoe fleas should be removed as soon as possible by means of a sterile needle.

Flea infestations may be detected most readily in the host's bedding. Both adults and larvae may be evident (92). Most often, cat fleas are responsible for infestations that affect residents of North America.

Treatment

Treatment of bites consists of antipruritics and antihistamines. Secondary bacterial infections may be treated with local antibiotics or, if extensive, by systemic therapy.

Flea infestations should be treated mainly by cleaning the nesting site of the host and by ensuring that all bedding is clean and dry. Diverse new insecticide formulations are labeled for use on animal bedding and also directly on pets, but because the toxicity profiles of some of these products differ markedly between cats and dogs, the labels should be scrutinized. Recurrence of the flea infestation may result from a new infestation, ineffective treatment, or resistance against the insecticide that was used. Insect growth regulators, such as methoprene, prevent maturation of fleas and other arthropods.

MYIASIS-PRODUCING FLIES

The term myiasis designates a group of infections produced by the maggots of certain flies. The myiases include those that produce traumatic, furuncular, intestinal, creeping, and ocular disease (20,93).

The traumatic myiases that affect non-necrotic tissue are produced by "primary screw-worm" flies, *Cochliomyia hominivorax* in the New World and *Chrysomyia bezziana* in the Old World. Lesions that are generally confined to necrotic tissue are due to the secondary screw-worm flies. The green bottle fly *Lucilia sericata* is the most common cause of such secondary screw-worm fly infection. These conditions are produced by the larvae of brightly metallic flies that do not feed or feed solely on vegetable products in their adult stage and whose larvae develop solely in animal products or in the feces of carnivores. The dull, grayish flies that are anthropophilic as adults are associated with vegetable products as larvae and do not cause traumatic myiasis. The striped, redmarked flesh flies, such as *Wohlfahrtia vigil*, may occasionally produce an adventitious lesion involving nonnecrotic tissue.

Traumatic myiasis occurs after the skin has been breached, as by a wound or secondary to a condition such as cancer. An infestation by a primary screw-worm fly would endanger deep tissues and produce a large and suppurating lesion. Although primary screw-worm flies occur mainly in tropical regions, flesh flies are common in North America and Europe. Infections by secondary screw-worm flies may even benefit the host by débriding necrotic tissue and by a bacteriostatic effect, and larvae of such flies have intentionally been used for this purpose (94). Some systemic illness may result from a screw-worm infection. Prevention involves adequate wound débridement and protection of incompetent or unconscious people. Applying an occlusive covering, by restricting access to air, induces larvae to exit the wound (95,96).

The secondary screw-worm flies may produce a range of complications in unconscious patients, ranging from a trivial colonization of a tracheotomy tube to a variety of serious complications including oronasal destruction. With restriction by bone or cartilage, pain, edema, and purulent discharge may be seen. Aural myiasis may be complicated by deafness, tinnitus, infection, and perforation of the eardrum, and nasal myiasis by penetration of the cribriform plate or bloody exudates (97). Maggot removal may require endoscopy. Genitourinary or anorectal destruction may occur. Entry into the urinary tract occurs when larvae hatched at the urethral meatus migrate into the bladder;

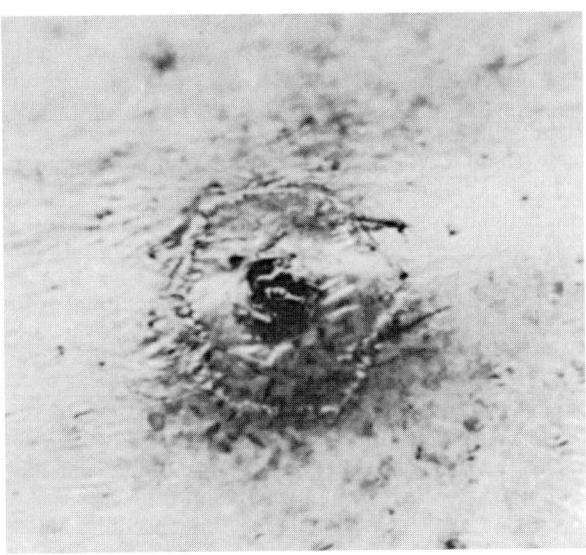

Figure 289.8. Furuncular myiasis due to the human botfly. The posterior end of the warble *Dermatobia hominis* can be seen, with the shiny black spiracles in the center of the dermal lesion. (Courtesy of the Armed Forces Institute of Pathology. Photograph no. N-49503.)

the larvae are then passed in the urine. Clinical manifestations range from urinary distress to bladder and urethral pain, dysuria, and priapism. A diagnosis of urinary myiasis requires certainty that the specimen container had previously been free of flies or their larvae.

In Central and South America, furuncular myiasis is caused by *Dermatobia hominis* (the human botfly) (98,99). The larvae of these flies penetrate unbroken skin and produce a boil-like lesion on which breathing holes may be evident (Fig. 289.8). Botfly infections occur after the female fly attaches her eggs to the underside of some other insect that she captures while following a large mammal. After a period of embryonization, these eggs hatch in response to the moist heat of the skin of another host. The larva then penetrates the skin to form a flask-shaped boil. Larvae mature in about a month to emerge and pupate in the soil. Extraction of younger maggots may require surgical excision, but pressure generally suffices after the larva begins to mature. Injection of lidocaine into the lesion may facilitate removal (100). In the case of concomitant cellulitis, where surgical excision may be hazardous, a venom extractor is one alternative (101).

Another form of furuncular myiasis may afflict people traveling in Africa. Adult female tumbu flies, *Cordylobia anthropophaga*, deposit as many as 100 eggs on urine- or sweat-contaminated clothing. The problem most frequently derives from underclothing that has been laundered traditionally by washing in a stream and drying in the open air. The eggs become embryonated within 2 days and remain viable for approximately 2 weeks. Contact with warm, moist skin causes the larvae to emerge and penetrate the victim's skin. Numerous boils may result, from which larvae emerge within 9 days. Tourists should require that their clothes be ironed if they have been traditionally laundered in endemic regions.

Creeping myiasis is due mainly to horse botflies, *Gasterophilus intestinalis* (20), which deposit their eggs on the flanks of horses and hatch in response to contact with the animal's tongue. The "Lady Godiva" syndrome results when larvae hatch against the bare legs of a rider. The larvae then migrate through the skin, producing pruritic tunnels that are narrow and raised. Differential diagnosis includes subdermal migrating eruptions caused by helminths. Biopsies are most diagnostic if samples are taken from skin just beyond the burrow. The burrows appear to be intraepidermal or subepidermal and may contain debris and desquamated cells in addition to larvae. Although surrounding tissues may appear unaffected, polymorphonuclear leukocytes and eosinophils may be present.

Acute ocular conjunctivitis may result from infestation by the sheep botfly *Oestrus ovis* (93). Ovipositing adult flies "strike" their eggs into the eyes of sheep and, on occasion, people. Motile maggots may be evident in the inflamed area and may invade both the anterior and the posterior chambers. They may be extracted most readily from the anterior chamber. In the posterior chamber, maggots may cause retinal detachment or invade the optic nerve. Acute vitrectomy and photocoagulation have successfully been applied (102,103).

Diagnoses of intestinal myiasis tend to be highly controversial (93). Such a complaint is generally stimulated when maggots are noted in an asymptomatic patient's stool, but this is often due to the rapidly developing maggots of flesh flies that were larviposited on the stool a few hours earlier. Genuine intestinal myiasis is infrequent and generally due to the rattail maggots of a drone fly, *Eristalis tenax*. The pathognomonic appearance of the maggot is suggested by its common name. Whereas acute enteritis is the most common complaint, obstruction occasionally results. Before a diagnosis of intestinal myiasis is rendered, however, a fresh stool specimen should be carefully collected in fly-free conditions.

The fly responsible for each myiasis infestation should be identified. Maggots may be placed in 70% ethanol and delivered to a reference laboratory. To facilitate identification, living maggots may be sent to a specialist to be reared to maturity. Except as indicated before, treatment involves removal of maggots from the host.

SPIDERS

Of the numerous kinds of spiders that have been recognized, including 100 or so that tend to attack people, human disease in general is generated solely by the bites of those in the genera *Latrodectus*, *Loxosceles*, and *Chiracanthium* (104). Because as many as 80% of attributed spider bites actually appear to have resulted from other causes (105), diagnosis of spider bite is best limited to episodes in which the offending organism can be examined. Identification may be possible even when the spider has been damaged.

Spiders have two body compartments and eight legs. With few exceptions, they are insectivorous. Venom is delivered through the fangs and is generated by specialized poison glands. Spiders spin webs by means of spinnerets located posteriorly on their ventral surfaces.

Widow Spiders

In the United States, black widow spiders range throughout the East Coast (*Latrodectus mactans*), through the midwestern and southwestern states (*Latrodectus hesperus*), and from east Texas to the East Coast (*Latrodectus variolus*); the red (*Latrodectus bishopi*) and brown (*Latrodectus geometricus*) widow spiders are found in Florida. (104,106–108). Females (males do not bite people) are black and ornamented ventrally by a red hourglass or circular markings (Fig. 289.9). Males and immature spiders are the more colorful. Adult females can attain more than 1 cm in length, males about 0.5 cm. Widow spiders have eight eyes, with the lateral pairs widely separated. Their webs vary in size and are spun close to the ground.

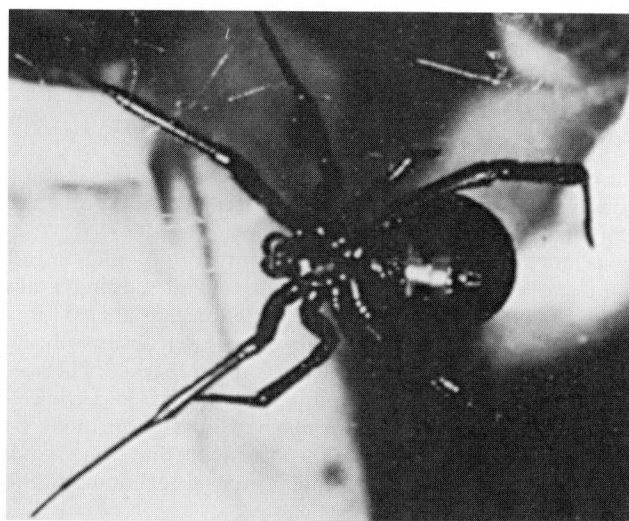

Figure 289.9. Black widow spider. Note the ventral hourglass marking. (From Wong RC, Hughes SE, Voorhees JJ. Spider bites. *Arch Dermatol* 1987;123:98–104, with permission. Copyright 1987, American Medical Association, with permission.)

EPIDEMIOLOGY

Widow spiders live in a variety of sites: behind stones, logs, shutters, windows, and doors and in such littered sites as dumps, barns, and sheds. In the past, widow spiders commonly bit men on the penis while they were seated in an outdoor privy. The vibrations caused by the urine stream striking its web stimulated the spider as would its insect prey. Today, however, bites most commonly occur when a hand or foot disturbs the web, when a child plays with the spider, or when the spider is trapped against a part of the body.

PATHOPHYSIOLOGY

The venom of widow spiders is an oily yellow fluid containing a mixture of components. Six active components have molecular masses varying from 5 to 130 kDa. Experimental envenomation has resulted in necrosis of a wide variety of organs, but the main effects in vivo relate to the neurotoxic aspects of the venom. The toxin causes acetylcholine, epinephrine, and central nervous system transmitters in presynaptic terminals to release to exhaustion. Antivenin readily blocks the action of the venom.

SYMPTOMS

Local symptoms are minimal; bite pain ranges from a sharp pinprick to none. A pair of small red marks demarcate the fang entrance sites. Slight erythema and edema may also be present.

Nonetheless, within an hour, a dull, cramping, often severe pain and numbness begin to spread from the bite to the entire torso. Generalized muscle cramping and pain result. The abdominal pain is often most prominent; it may be so severe as to be confused with a surgical abdomen, but the history, generalized muscle spasm, and absence of tenderness and distention should point the clinician toward the correct diagnosis. The pain begins to recede after 3 hours but may continue for 2 days. Other symptoms include tachycardia, headache, diaphoresis, salivation, weakness, fever, vomiting, backache, respiratory distress, priapism, impotence, urinary retention, anxiety, increased deep tendon reflexes, proteinuria, paresthesia, hypertension, fetal positioning, and burning (especially of the plantar surfaces). These symptoms generally resolve spontaneously after a few days but may last 1 week to several months. The course may be complicated by renal, cardiac, or respiratory failure; shock; convulsions; and cerebral hemorrhage. Patients who are younger than 16 years or older than 60 years and those with chronic diseases are at greatest risk.

DIAGNOSIS

The most secure diagnosis rests on the identification of the spider. If this is not possible, the patient may be able to select the spider from illustrations. In many cases, however, the history, the physical signs, and the course of the disease form the basis of the diagnosis.

TREATMENT

Tetanus prophylaxis should be administered. The wound should be cleansed. Placing an ice cube on the wound, except when antivenin is administered, will reduce pain at the site.

Hospitalization and antivenin administration are recommended for patients younger than 16 years or older than 60 years, pregnant women, patients suffering from chronic disease, and those with particularly severe symptoms. Vital signs should be closely monitored for the first 12 hours. Hypertension may be severe, but it is usually asymptomatic (109). Methocarbamol, diazepam, calcium gluconate, or magnesium sulfate may be useful. Pain control may require morphine sulfate but is usually accomplished with acetaminophen for hospitalized patients. Vigorous exercise has also been said to be of some help. Antivenin can significantly shorten the duration of pain (110).

Although various insecticides destroy spiders, reinfestation frequently occurs. Gloves and long sleeves should be worn in cleaning infested sites.

Necrotic Arachnidism

Severely necrotic spider bite most frequently results from the bites of recluse spiders of the genus *Loxosceles* (104,111,112). For the various New World species, human disease is most often associated with *Loxosceles reclusa* in the United States and *Loxosceles laeta* in South and Central America. *L. laeta* spiders have established potentially dangerous infestations in the United States (113). The brownish recluse spiders are distinguished by a fiddle-shaped mark on their dorsal surface and three pairs of eyes arrayed in a curved row (Fig. 289.10). Their legs may span 5 cm,

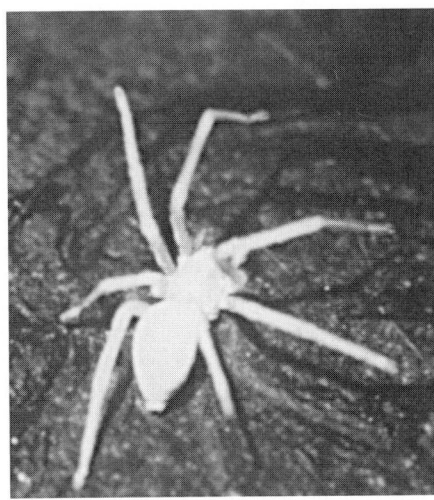

Figure 289.11. The *Chiracanthium* garden spider. (From Wong RC, Hughes SE, Voorhees JJ. Spider bites. *Arch Dermatol* 1987;123:98–104. Copyright 1987, American Medical Association, with permission.)

and their bodies more than 1 cm. Females are slightly larger than males, but both bite if disturbed. They spin a funnel-shaped web in dark, secluded locations.

Other necrotic lesions result from the bite of a garden spider, *Chiracanthium mildii* (Fig. 289.11), that was introduced into the United States from Europe during the 1940s. This greenish gray hunting spider has become the most common domestic spider in much of North America. It tends to invade homes in the fall. Garden spiders' tubelike webs may be seen in crevices near windows and porches.

EPIDEMIOLOGY

In out-of-door locations, recluse spiders seek prey beneath rocks and boards and in caves (104,111). Indoors, these spiders prefer dark and dry locales, such as closets, garages, storage spaces, areas under furniture, and piled rubbish. Garden spiders seek their prey in more exposed locations. These spiders bite mainly when trapped against a person's body, and bites are generally inflicted when a person is dressing. Necrotic arachnidism, therefore, most commonly affects the face, neck, and hands.

PATHOPHYSIOLOGY

The venom of recluse spiders is a clear, viscous fluid containing hyaluronidase, phospholipase D (sphingomyelinase D), an esterase, alkaline phosphatase, and a protease (104). The component responsible for dermatonecrosis is unknown but may be sphingomyelinase D, which would interact with erythrocyte and endothelial cell membranes and cause secondary prostaglandin activation.

Various host factors may contribute to the development of the lesion. Age and size of the patient affect severity. Sites having little subcutaneous tissue are most vulnerable.

Microscopic examination reveals a progression to necrosis with subsequent scarring. Neutrophils promote the lesion. Dermatonecrosis may result from platelet aggregation and vascular thrombosis. In severe bites, early changes include dermal edema; arteriolar thrombosis; a polymorphonuclear and eosinophilic infiltrate with possible leukocytoclasis; erythrocyte extravasation; and separation of the dermis and epidermis. Marked necrosis with ulceration follows. A mononuclear infiltrate is seen after several weeks. Granulation tissue underlies the necrotic area. Ultimately, scar formation results.

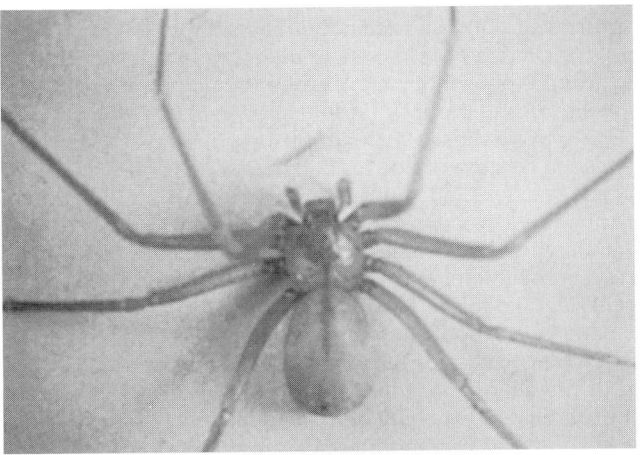

Figure 289.10. Brown recluse spider. Note the fiddle-shaped dorsal marking. (From Wong, Hughes SE, Voorhees JJ. Spider bites. *Arch Dermatol* 1987;123:98–104, with permission. Copyright 1987, American Medical Association, with permission.)

DISEASE RELATIONSHIPS

Clinical manifestations of necrotic arachnidism are highly variable, ranging from mild pain and erythema to local skin necrosis and systemic viscerocutaneous disease. The bite is frequently painless and the resulting lesion consequently not associated with the spider.

In mild cases, the bite site becomes indurated and erythematous and is mildly painful and pruritic. An ischemic zone of pallor may surround the lesion. These changes occur within hours of envenomation and resolve in several days. Many investigators believe that the mild lesions are the predominant manifestation of recluse spider bites. In general, if necrosis has not developed within 3 days, no scar formation will occur.

More severely affected patients characteristically experience only pain and pruritus for the first 8 to 24 hours. A blue-gray macular halo subsequently develops. A pustule or bulla may also be present at the inoculation site. The generally irregular lesion is often surrounded by erythematous, edematous, and purpuric skin. Progression to necrosis, eschar formation, and ulceration often follows. These changes may be accompanied by edema of the affected limb or portion of the torso. The first changes of severe lesions generally occur within the first day and almost always within the first 3 days (114). Healing and scar formation may take 6 months. Dermonecrotic lesions are often accompanied by a diffuse eruption of variable appearances. Local complications may include chronic pain, secondary infection, repeated failure of skin grafts, a pyoderma granulosa-like reaction, and upper extremity functional impairment (115,116).

The severity and frequency of systemic manifestations are proportional to the size of the lesion. Systemic signs usually appear within 3 days. Mild systemic reactions include leukocytosis, malaise, headache, arthralgia, myalgia, proteinuria, hematuria, vomiting, diarrhea, and generalized urticaria. Severe complications include anuria, delirium, shock, hemolysis, disseminated intravascular coagulation, and coma. All persons with necrosis larger than 1 cm should be screened for hemolysis, renal failure, and disseminated intravascular coagulation. The presence of systemic complications is an indication for hospitalization.

DIAGNOSIS

When the offending spider has not been captured, diagnosis must be presumptive. An increasingly painful plaque with central pallor and surrounding erythema may be suggestive, but the initial signs are sufficiently nonspecific to preclude anything but retrospective diagnosis.

Differential diagnosis involves exclusion of the bites of other arthropods, infections, vasculitides, embolic phenomena, burns, and trauma. Examination of the history and careful exclusion of other diagnostic possibilities may be helpful.

A passive hemagglutination inhibition test detects venom in fluid expressed from the bite as long as 1 day after the bite (117). A thymidine uptake in vitro test is also available, but it requires acute- and convalescent-phase serum and may take as long as a month to complete. (118)

TREATMENT

Mildly necrotic lesions and those with necrotic areas less than 2 cm across may require only pain medications, antihistamines, sterile dressings, tetanus prophylaxis, ice, and elevation of the affected limb (119). Although a variety of steroid preparations and protocols have been suggested for more serious lesions, clear-cut evidence of their benefit is lacking. Because it is an inhibitor of neutrophils, dapsone has been suggested (120,121). A prospective study demonstrated more rapid healing after administration of dapsone and excision of the necrotic lesion after 6 weeks in place of immediate excision (122). Administration of antivenin

may be helpful. Systemic symptoms warrant hospitalization and treatment of complications. Surgical excision of skin lesions is best reserved for stabilized, non-enlarging lesions. Steroids are indicated in severe skin lesions, loxoscelism, and small children. Dapsone may be used in adults who have been screened for glucose-6-phosphate dehydrogenase deficiency. Topical nitroglycerin can decrease the enlargement of ulcers (123). The specific treatment of these complications is beyond the scope of this chapter.

BEES AND WASPS

The stinging insects belong to the order Hymenoptera, a diverse taxon that includes the ants, bees, wasps and numerous entomophagous parasitoids. People are stung mainly by members of two superfamilies, Apoidea and Vespoidea (124). The Apoidea includes the honeybees and bumblebees, familiar insects that frequently lose their venom apparatus in the course of stinging. Although they generally attack people only when disturbed, the Africanized bees that have invaded North America are readily provoked. The Vespoidea includes a myriad of yellow jackets, whose abdomens are marked with alternating black and yellow bands; the hornets, whose bodies are black but with a white-marked face; and the paper wasps, brownish insects with long legs. Yellow jackets place their roughly spherical paper-covered nests in trees, under the eaves or within the walls of buildings and within burrows in the ground, and other paper wasps suspend their flat uncovered nests from the eaves of buildings and within hollow walls. Adult Vespoidea generally feed on nectar, and their larvae are fed insects. They are attracted to sugary substances and to meat, leading to their unwelcome appearance at picnics and garbage dumps. Vespoidea retain their stings and can sting repeatedly. Approximately 40 United States residents die each year of anaphylaxis induced by the stings of these insects (2); between 0.5% and 3.3% of the population is allergic (125–127). The majority of stings attributed to bees, however, are more likely caused by yellow jacket wasps.

Pathophysiology

Stinging insects rapidly and efficiently deliver venom into the skin. Honeybees, for example, expel 90% of their venom sac within 20 seconds (128). Venoms of different insects are biochemically and immunologically distinct (129,130), necessitating use of an array of skin tests and individualized venom immunotherapies for allergic people. Venom allergens have been classified into group I (phospholipases), group II (hyaluronidases), group I1 (melittin), and group V (vespid antigen 5) (131–136).

The phospholipase A, toxin of these insects is particularly interesting because it induces both hemolysis and edema (137). Allergic reactions, of course, are mediated by immunoglobulin E antibodies to venom constituents. The pathogenesis of insect sting anaphylaxis is complex, involving plasminogen, the contact system, complement activation, mast cell activation, and basophil degranulation (138–141). Despite its many components, the pathogenesis of insect sting anaphylaxis seems fundamentally similar to that of other forms of anaphylaxis. The intensity of the allergic reaction to the sting of an insect increases with subsequent exposure only in about 10% of patients, limiting the utility of venom immunotherapy in those whose initial reaction is mild (142). In other respects, age, the nature of the patient's anaphylactic symptoms, and duration of the interval between stings all contribute to the natural history of the disease (143).

Disease Relationships and Treatment

Diagnosis of an insect sting is rarely ambiguous. The patient presents with a painful, erythematous, and edematous lesion and relates a history of contact with the offending insect. The condition generally resolves spontaneously within a few hours. Cold compresses and analgesics offer some relief. More extensive local reactions occur, developing in 2 days and lasting as long as a week. Aspirin, antihistamines, and cold compresses may be of use; prednisone may be used if the reaction is particularly disabling.

Anaphylaxis due to insect stings can strike at any age and result from a sting delivered anywhere on the body. The clinical symptoms are variable. Cutaneous signs include generalized urticaria, flushing, and angioedema. Upper airway edema or bronchospasm can result in respiratory failure and shock. Primary vascular collapse occurs in a fourth of all cases of fatal anaphylaxis and may be accompanied by cardiac symptoms (144). Diarrhea, nausea, vomiting, abdominal pain, tenesmus, and uterine contractions are uncommon. Symptoms usually appear within 20 minutes of a sting but may be delayed for as long as 3 days (145). Although diagnosis is generally unambiguous, the differential diagnosis may require the exclusion of pulmonary embolism, acute myocardial infarction, cardiac arrhythmia, foreign body aspiration, acute asthma, hereditary angioedema, seizure disorder, and vasovagal reactions. The treatment of this disorder is identical to that for anaphylaxis due to other causes. Epinephrine hydrochloride is immediately administered subcutaneously; intravenous injections, if needed, are diluted tenfold. Antihistamines may also be administered. Other therapeutic modalities that may be of use include vasopressors, oxygen, and aerosol bronchodilators. Fluid resuscitation may also be required. Airway maintenance is vital and may require intubation.

Skin tests for detecting allergy to hymenopterous antigen can be used to guide specific immunotherapy for patients who have reacted systemically. Although the current criteria for assessing risk generally fail to predict how a patient will react to an insect sting (146), supplementary laboratory studies improve predictability (147). Immunotherapy appears to be safe and effective (143,148,149).

A few commonsense preventive measures are in order. People who have experienced an anaphylactic response should carry and learn to use epinephrine kits when exposure seems likely. Neutral-colored clothing should be worn. Patients should not walk barefoot and should wear long pants and gloves when gardening. Cosmetics, perfumes, and hair sprays, which attract wasps, should be avoided. Such a patient, of course, should avoid the site where a previous sting was experienced unless the nest has been identified and destroyed.

FIRE ANTS

The fire ants illustrate the direct effects of these ubiquitous insects on human health. The fire ants *Solenopsis richteri* and *Solenopsis invicta* that were introduced into Alabama in 1918 have become abundant in at least 13 southern states in the United States, the Virgin Islands, and Puerto Rico (150). Although sensitivity to cold has limited their range (151), cold-resistant forms have been identified, and this may permit invasion of more northerly sites (152). Their expansion has displaced other relatively more docile ants. Thirty percent to 60% of urban residents who live within the range of these ants report being stung each year (153,154). In the southwestern United States, fire ants are the most important cause of insect hypersensitivity (155). Although their effects on

human health are important, these insects burden agriculture by stinging animals, eating seeds, and creating mounds that interfere with the operation of farm machinery (156).

These red-brown, 2- to 5-mm-long ants construct their nests in mounds that may be 50 cm across (157). Such a colony can include 200,000 members, communicating with the outside world through a system of tunnels extending some 25 m from the center of the mound. Fire ant colonies are constructed in such open sites as fields, yards, or pastures (158). Stings generally result from direct human contact with their mounds; as many as 10,000 stings have been received in a single such encounter (157).

Disease Relationships and Treatment

Before stinging, fire ants fasten themselves to their victim by their prominent mandibles. Their bodies then pivot around their heads, successively delivering numerous stings by means of a caudally placed stinging apparatus. This tubular, modified ovipositor serves as an extension of the duct of their venom glands (159,160). The wheal and flare reaction that develops 30 minutes to an hour thereafter resolves within another 30 minutes. A sterile pustule generally forms about a day later (159,161). Pustule formation is induced by the piperidine component of fire ant venom (162–164). Two, 6-di-substituted piperidines compose 99% of the alkaloid fraction of this secretion, which in turn composes 95% of the insect's venom. Piperidines possess hemolytic, bactericidal, and cytotoxic properties and have been implicated in the alternative complement pathway. No available treatment for pustules appears to be effective (161).

Systemic reactions occur in 16% of people who have been stung by fire ants, and anaphylaxis in approximately 2% (165). Symptoms and signs of a systemic reaction occur within 30 to 45 minutes after the sting and include urticaria, chest tightness, pruritus, dysphagia, abdominal cramping, nausea, vomiting, diarrhea, and wheezing (161,166). Symptoms and signs of anaphylaxis differ little from those described elsewhere. Neurologic reactions, including syncope, convulsions, confusion, mononeuropathy, and seizures, have infrequently been reported (167). Treatment for these complications is specific to the syndrome.

As with other insects, protein makes up less than 5% of fire ant venom and is responsible for both the systemic and the anaphylactic responses. *S. richteri* has at least three allergen components (168), and *S. invicta* has at least four (169).

Although an ideal immunotherapy would be based on the venom itself as antigen, such secretions are difficult to harvest because their volume is so small. Instead, whole-body extracts are used to treat sensitivity to ants. In one such experiment, 65 subjects who received immunotherapy were compared with 11 nontreated subjects (170). Anaphylaxis followed ant stings in a tenth of these subjects, regardless of treatment. Despite these inconclusive results, expert opinion tends to support immunotherapy (170,171). Definitive studies in the form of double-blinded placebo trials have yet to be produced, however. A new therapy, rush immunotherapy combined with conventional whole body extract immunotherapy has shown great promise (172).

CONCLUSION

The human environment is dynamic, and novel pathogens continue to emerge (173). The resulting list of "new diseases" includes numerous vector-borne infections of major public health importance. The arthropods that directly affect human health are subject to similar change. Fire ants, Africanized bees, a European wasp, the several newly introduced mosquitoes, and the garden spider, for example, have invaded North America during the past century. The future will surely bring other pathogenic arthropods into contact with these and other residents of the temperate zone. New strategies for ameliorating the effects of such contact will be required.

REFERENCES

1. Natural history of insect sting allergy. *Allergy Proc* 1989;10:97.
2. Koo J, Gambla C. Delusions of parasitosis and other forms of monosymptomatic hypochondriacal psychosis. General discussion and case illustrations. *Dermatol Clin* 1996;14:429–438.
3. Trabert W. 100 years of delusional parasitosis. Meta-analysis of 1,223 case reports. *Psychopathology* 1995;28(5):238–246.
4. Mellenby K. *Scabies.* Hampton, England: EW Classey, 1972.
5. Green RW. Infestations: Scabies and lice. In: Brickner P, ed. *Health care of homeless people.* New York: Springer-Verlag, 1985:33–55.
6. Jenista JA, Chapman D. Medical problems of foreign-born adopted children. *Am J Dis Child* 1987;141:298.
7. Reid AF, Poonking T. Epidemic scabies and associated acute glomerulonephritis in Trinidad. *Bull Pan Am Health Organ* 1988;22:103.
8. Alexander AM. Role of race in scabies infestation. *Arch Dermatol* 1987;114:627.
9. Chakrabari A. Human notoedric scabies from contact with cats infested with *Notoedres cati. Int J Dermatol* 1978;25:646.
10. Regan AM, Metersky ML, Craven DE. Nosocomial dermatitis and pruritus caused by pigeon mite infestation. *Arch Intern Med* 1987;147:2185.
11. Parish LC, Nutting WB, Schwartzman RM. *Cutaneous infestations of man and animals.* New York: Praeger Publishers, 1983.
12. Arlian LG. Biology, host relations and epidemiology of *Sarcoptes scabiei. Annu Rev Entomol* 1989;34:139.
13. Marleire V, Roul S, Labreze C, et al. Crusted (Norwegian) scabies induced by use of topical corticosteroids and treated successfully with ivermectin. *J Pediatr* 1999;135:122–124.
14. Jaramillo-Ayerbe F, Berrio-Munoz J. Ivermectin for crusted Norwegian scabies induced by use of topical steroids. *Arch Dermatol* 1998;134:143–145.
15. Orkin M, Maibach HI. This scabies pandemic. *N Engl J Med* 1978;298:496.
16. Pereiro M, Roson E, Sanchez Aguilar D, et al. Scabies presenting as a blistering eruption. *Cutis* 2001;68:279–281.
17. Said S, Jay S, Kang J, et al. Localized bullous scabies. Uncommon presentation of scabies. *Am J Dermatopathol* 1993;15:590–593.
18. Dick GF, Burgdorf WHC, Gentry WC Jr. Norwegian scabies in Blooms syndrome. *Arch Dermatol* 1979;115:212.
19. Wolf R, Krakowski A. Atypical crusted scabies. *J Am Acad Dermatol* 1987;17:434.
20. Binford CH, Connor DH, eds. *Pathology of tropical and extraordinary diseases,* vol II. Washington DC: Armed Forces Institute of Pathology, 1976:626–630.
21. Glover A, Young L, Goltz AW. Norwegian scabies in acquired immunodeficiency syndrome: Report of a case resulting in death from associated sepsis. *J Am Acad Dermatol* 1987;16:396.
22. Sadick N, Kaplan MH, Pahwa SG, et al. Unusual features of scabies complicating human T-lymphotropic virus type III infection. *J Am Acad Dermatol* 1986;15:486.
23. Pariser RJ, Pariser DM. Primary care physicians' errors in handling cutaneous disorders: a prospective survey. *J Am Acad Dermatol* 1987;17:239.
24. Chouela E, Abeldano A, Pellerano G, et al. Diagnosis and treatment of scabies: a practical guide. *Am J Clin Dermatol* 2002;3:9–18.
25. Lacarrubba F, Musumeci ML, Caltabiano R, et al. High-magnification videodermatoscopy: a new noninvasive diagnostic tool for scabies in children. *Pediatr Dermatol* 2001;18:439–441.
26. Haas N. A simple vital microscopy aid for the detection of scabies mites. *Z Hautkr* 1987;62:1395.
27. Mussen JE. Lindane: a prudent approach. *Arch Dermatol* 1987;123:1008.
28. Solomon LM, Fahrner L, West DP. Gamma benzene hexachloride toxicity: a review. *Arch Dermatol* 1977;113:353.
29. Taplin D, Rivera A, Walker JG, et al. A comparative trial of three treatment schedules for the eradication of scabies. *J Am Acad Dermatol* 1983;9:550.
30. Taplin D, Meinking TL, Porcelain SL, et al. Permethrin 5% dermal cream: a new treatment for scabies. *J Am Acad Dermatol* 1983;9:550.
31. Glaziou P, Cartel JL, Alzieu P, et al. Comparison of ivermectin and benzyl benzoate for treatment of scabies. *Trop Med Parasitol* 1993;44:331.
32. Aubin F, Humber P. Ivermectin for crusted (Norwegian) scabies. *N Engl J Med* 1995;332:612.
33. Alberici F, Pagani L, Ratti G, et al. Ivermectin alone or in combination with benzyl benzoate in the treatment of human immunodeficiency virus-associated scabies. *Br J Dermatol* 2000;142:969–972.
34. Taplin D, Meinking TL. Treatment of HIV-related scabies with emphasis on the efficacy of ivermectin. *Semin Cutan Med Surg* 1997;16:123.
35. Wharton GW. House dust mites. *J Med Entomol* 1976;12:577.
36. Kifuji K, McCullough J, Ownby DR. Relationship between dust mite allergen and human IgA in house dust samples. *Ann Allergy* 1993;70:219.
37. M'Raihi L, Charpin D, Thibaudon M, Vervloet D. Bronchial challenge to house dust can induce immediate bronchoconstriction in allergic asthmatic patients. *Ann Allergy* 1990;65:485.
38. Platts-Mills TA, Chapman MD. Dust mites: immunology, allergic disease, and environmental control. *J Allergy Clin Immunol* 1987;80:755.
39. Pollart S, Chapman MD, Platts-Mills TA, et al. House dust mite and dust control. *Clin Rev Allergy* 1988;6:23.
40. Hyndman SJ, Brown DI, Ewan PW, et al. Humidity regulation in the management of asthma patients sensitized to house dust mites. *Q J Med* 1994;87:367.
41. Lind P. Purification and partial characterization of two major allergens from the house dust mite *Dermatophagoides pteronyssinus. J Allergy Clin Immunol* 1985;76:753.
42. Yasueda H, Mita H, Yiu Y, et al. Isolation and characterization of two allergens for *Dermatophagoides farinae. Int Arch Allergy Appl Immunol* 1986;81:214.
43. Heymann PW, Chapman MD, Aalberse RC, et al. Antigenic and structural analysis of group II allergens (Der f II and Der p II) from house dust mites (*Dermatophagoides* spp). *J Allergy Clin Immunol* 1989;83:1055.
44. Smith WA, Chua KY, Kuo MC, et al. Cloning and sequencing of the *Dermatophagoides pteronyssinus* group III allergen, Der p III. *Clin Allergy* 1994;24:220.
45. de Blay F, Heymann PW, Chapman MD, et al. Airborne dust mite allergens: comparison of group II allergens with group I mite allergen and cat allergen Fel d I. *J Allergy Clin Immunol* 1991;88:919.
46. Stewart GA, Boyd SM, Bird CH, et al. Immunobiology of the serine protease allergens from house dust mites. *Am J Ind Med* 1994;25:105.
47. Maruo K, Akaike T, Matsumarua Y, et al. Triggering of the vascular permeability reaction by activation of the Hageman factor-prekallikrein system by house dust mite proteinase. *Biochim Biophys Acta* 1991;1074:62.
48. Leung DY, Pober JS, Cotran RS. Expression of endothelial-leukocyte adhesion molecule-1 in elicited late phase allergic reactions. *J Clin Invest* 1991;87:1805.
49. Schmitt M, Niggemann B, Kleinau I, et al. Lymphocyte subsets, sIL2-r and sICAM-1 in blood during allergen challenge tests in asthmatic children. *Pediatr Allergy Immunol* 1993;4:208.
50. Duff AL, Platts-Mills TA. Allergens and asthma. *Pediatr Clin North Am* 1992;39:1277.
51. Casimeir GJ, Duchatheau J, Gossart B, et al. Atopic dermatitis: role of food and house dust mite allergens. *Pediatrics* 1993;92:252.
52. Dart JK, Buckley RJ, Monnickendan M, Prasad J. Perennial allergic conjunctivitis: definition, clinical characteristics and prevalence. *Trans Ophthalmol Soc UK* 1986;105:513.
53. Warner JO. Low-dose sublingual therapy in patients with allergic rhinitis due to house dust mite (Editorial). *Clin Allergy* 1986;16:387.
54. Scadding GK, Brostoff J. Low-dose sublingual therapy in patients with allergic rhinitis due to house dust mite. *Clin Allergy* 1986;16:483.
55. Liu CM, Shun CT, Song HC, et al. Investigation into allergic response patients with chronic sinusitis. *J Formos Med Assoc* 1992;91:252.
56. Platts-Mills TA. How environment affects patients with allergic disease: indoor allergens and asthma. *Ann Allergy* 1994;72:381.
57. Gelber LE, Seltzer LH, Bousoukis JK, et al. Sensitization and exposure to indoor allergens as risk factors for asthma among patients presenting to hospital. *Am Rev Respir Dis* 1993;147:572.
58. Sporik R, Holgate St, Platts-Mills TA, et al. Exposure to housedust mite allergen (Der p 1) and the development of asthma in childhood: a prospective study. *N Engl J Med* 1990;323:502.
59. Leung DYM. Role of IgE in atopic dermatitis. *Curr Opin Immunol* 1993;5:956.
60. Wang B, Rieger A, Kilgus O, et al. Epidermal Langerhans cells from normal human skin bind monomeric IgE via FceRL. *J Exp Med* 1992;175:1353.
61. Muddle G, van Reijsen FC, Bolan GF, et al. Allergen presentation by epidermal Langerhans' cells from patients with atopic dermatitis is mediated by IgE. *Immunology* 1990;69:335.
62. Collof MJ. Exposure to house dust mites in homes of people with atopic dermatitis. *Br J Dermatol* 1992;127:322.
63. Hunter JAA, Herd RM. Recent advances in atopic dermatitis. *Q J Med* 1994;87:323.
64. Armenaka MC, Grizzanti JN, Oriel B, Rosentreich DL. Increased immune reactivity to house dust mites in adults with chronic rhinosinusitis. *Clin Exp Allergy* 1993;23:669.
65. Bousquet J. Specific immunotherapy in asthma: is it effective? *J Allergy Clin Immunol* 1994;94:1.
66. Corey JP. Environmental control of allergens. *Otolaryngol Head Neck Surg* 1994;111:340.
67. Hoffman A, Walmann P, Tiesener G, et al. Isolation and characterization of a thrombin inhibitor from the tick *Ixodes ricinus. Pharmazie* 1991;46:209.
68. Ribeiro JM, Endris TM, Endris R. Saliva of the soft tick, *Ornithodoros moubata,* contains anti-platelet and apyrase activities. *Comp Biochem Physiol A Comp Physiol* 1991;100:109.
69. Waxman L, Connolly TM. Isolation of an inhibitor selective for collagen-stimulated platelet aggregation from the soft tick *Ornithodoros moubata. J Biol Chem* 1993;268:5445.

70. Vlasuk GP. Structural and functional characterization of tick anticoagulant peptide (TAP): a potent and selective inhibitor of blood coagulation factor Xa. *Thromb Haemost* 1993;70:212.

71. Wikel SK, Ramachandra RN, Bergman DK. Tick-induced modulation of the host immune response. *Int J Parasitol* 1994;24:59.

72. Kubes M, Fuchsberger N, Labuda M, et al. Salivary gland extracts of partially fed *Dermacentor reticulatus* ticks decrease natural killer cell activity in vitro. *Immunology* 1994;82:113.

73. Schwartz BS, Nadelman RB, Fish D, et al. Entomologic and demographic correlates of anti-tick saliva antibody in a prospective study of tick bite subjects in Westchester County, New York. *Am J Trop Med Hyg* 1993;48:50.

74. Spielman A. The emergence of Lyme disease and human babesiosis in a changing environment. *Ann NY Acad Sci* 1994;740:146.

75. Spielman A. Lyme disease and human babesiosis: evidence incriminating vector and reservoir hosts. In: Englund P, Scher A, eds. *The biology of parasitism.* New York: Alan R Liss, 1988:147–165.

76. Shih C-M, Pollack RJ, Telford SR III, Spielman A. Delayed dissemination of Lyme disease spirochetes from the site of deposition in the skin of mice. *J Infect Dis* 1992;166:827.

77. Matushchka F-R, Spielman A. The vector of the Lyme disease spirochete. *N Engl J Med* 1992;327:54.

78. Treatment of Lyme disease. *Med Lett* 1989;31:57.

79. Smith RP, Lacombe EH, Rand PW, et al. Diversity of tick species biting humans in an emerging area for Lyme disease. *Am J Public Health* 1992;82:66.

80. Spielman A, Wilson ML, Levine JF, et al. Ecology of *Ixodes dammini*-borne human babesiosis and Lyme disease. *Annu Rev Entomol* 1988;30:439.

81. Steere AC, Taylor E, McHugh G, Logigian EL. The overdiagnosis of Lyme disease. *JAMA* 1993;269:1812.

81a. Nadelman RB, Nowakowski J, Fish D, et al. Prophylaxis with single-dose doxycycline for the prevention of Lyme disease after an *Ixodes scapularis* tick bite. *N Engl J Med* 2001;345:79–84.

82. Rich SM, Armstrong PM, Smith RD, et al. Lone star tick-infecting borreliae are most closely related to the agent of bovine borreliosis. *J Clin Microbiol* 2001;39:494–497.

83. Lane AT. Scabies and head lice. *Pediatr Ann* 1987;16:51.

84. Pollack RJ, Kiszewski AE, Spielman A. Overdiagnosis and consequent mismanagement of head louse infestations in North America. *Pediatr Infect Dis J* 2000;19:689–693.

85. Baker RS, Feingold M. Phthirus pubis (pubic louse) blepharitis. *Am J Dis Child* 1985;138:1079.

86. Akinner CJ, Viswalingam ND, Goh BT. Phthirus pubis infestation of the eyelids: a marker for sexually transmitted diseases. *Int J STD AIDS* 1995;6:451–452.

87. Pollack RJ, Kiszewski A, Armstrong P, et al. Differential permethrin susceptibility of head lice sampled in the United States and Borneo. *Arch Pediatr Adolesc Med* 1999;153:969–973.

88. Williams LK, Reacher A, MacKenzie WR, et al. Lice, nits, and school policy. *Pediatrics* 2001;107:1011–1015.

89. Ashkenazi I, Desatnik HR, Abraham FA. Yellow mercuric oxide: a treatment of choice for phthiriasis palpebrarum. *Br J Ophthalmol* 1991;75:356–358.

90. Halliwell REW, Schemmer KR. The role of basophils in the immunopathogenesis of hypersensitivity to fleas (*Ctenocephalides felis*) in dogs. *Vet Immunol Immunopathol* 1987;15:203.

91. Lever WF, Schaumberg-Lever G. *Histopathology of the skin.* Philadelphia: JB Lippincott, 1983:209.

92. Burns DA. The investigation and management of arthropod bite reactions acquired in the home. *Clin Exp Dermatol* 1987;12:114.

93. James MT. *The flies that cause myiasis in man.* Washington DC: US Department of Agriculture, 1947.

94. Sherman RS, Pechter EA. Maggot therapy: a review of the therapeutic applications of fly larvae in human medicine, especially for treating osteomyelitis. *Med Vet Entomol* 1988;2:225–230.

95. Brewere TF, Wilson ME, Gonzalez E, et al. Bacon therapy and furuncular myiasis. *JAMA* 1993;270:2087–2088.

96. Schulte C, Schunk M, Krebs B. One catches not only mice with bacon. An atraumatic treatment for cutaneous myiasis. *Dtsch Med Wochenschr* 2002;127:266–268.

97. Finlay GA, Brown JS, Marcus LC, et al. Nasal myiasis—a "noso"comial infection. *Infect Dis Clin Prac* 1999;8:218–220.

98. Farrell LD, Wong RK, Manders EK, et al. Cutaneous myiasis. *Am Fam Physician* 1987;35:127.

99. Kleeman FJ. *Dermatobia hominis* comes to Boston. *N Engl J Med* 1983;308:847.

100. Nunzi E, Rongioletti F, Rebora A. Removal of *Dermatobia hominis* larvae. *Arch Dermatol* 1986;122:140.

101. Boggild AK, Keystone JS, Kain KC. Furuncular myiasis: a simple and rapid method for extraction of intact dermatobia hominis larvae. *Clin Infect Dis* 2002;35:336–338.

102. Gjotterberg M, Ingemansson SO. Intraocular infestation by reindeer warble fly larva: an unusual indication for acute vitrectomy. *Br J Ophthalmol* 1988;106:880.

103. Laborde RP, Kaufman HE, Beyey WB. Intracorneal ophthalmomyiasis. Case report. *Arch Ophthalmol* 1988;72:420.

104. Wong RC, Hughes SE, Voorhees JJ. Spider bites. *Arch Dermatol* 1987;123:98.

105. Parrish HM. Analysis of 460 fatalities from venomous animals in the United States. *Am J Med Sci* 1964;254:129.

106. Moss HS, Binder LS. A retrospective review of the black widow spider envenomation. *Ann Emerg Med* 1987;16:188.

107. Kobernick M. Black widow spider bite. *Am Fam Physician* 1984;29:241.

108. Timms PK, Gibbons RB. Latrodectism—effects of the black widow spider bite. *West J Med* 1986;144:315.

109. Woestman R, Perkin R, Van Stralen D. The black widow: is she deadly to children? *Pediatr Emerg Care* 1996;12:360.

110. Clark RF, Wethern-Kestner S, Vance MV, Gerkin R. Clinical presentation and treatment of black widow spider envenomation: a review of 163 cases. *Ann Emerg Med* 1992;21:782–787.

111. Young VI, Pin P. The brown recluse spider bite. *Ann Plast Surg* 1988;20:447.

112. Bernstein B, Ehrlich F. Brown recluse spider bites. *J Emerg Med* 1986;4:457.

113. Levi HE, Spielman A. The biology and control of the South American brown spider, *Loxosceles laeta* (Nicolet), in a North American focus. *Am J Trop Med Hyg* 1964;13:132.

114. King LE, Rees RS. Treatment of brown recluse spider bites. *J Am Acad Dermatol* 1986;14:691.

115. Delozier JB, Reaves L, King LE, Rees RS. Brown recluse spider bites of the upper extremity. *South Med J* 1988;81:181.

116. Pennell TC, Babu SS, Meredith JW. The management of snake and spider bites in the southeastern United States. *Am Surg* 1986;53:198.

117. Finke JH, Campbell J, Barrett JT. Serodiagnostic test for *Loxosceles reclusa* bites. *Clin Toxicol* 1974;7:375.

118. Berger RS, Millikan LE, Conway F. An in vitro test for *Loxosceles reclusa* spider bites. *Toxicon* 1973;11:465.

119. Rees R, Campbell D, Rieger E, et al. The diagnosis and treatment of brown recluse spider bites. *Ann Emerg Med* 1987;16:654.

120. Pennell TC, Babu SS, Meredith JW. The management of snake and spider bites in the southeastern United States. *Am Surg* 1987;51:198.

121. King LE, Rees RS. Dapsone treatment of a brown recluse bite. *JAMA* 1983;250:648.

122. Rees RS, Altenbern P, Lynch JB, et al. Brown recluse spider bites: a comparison of early surgical excision vs dapsone and delayed surgical excision. *Ann Surg* 1985;202:659.

123. Forks TP. Brown recluse spider bites. *J Am Board Fam Pract* 2000;13:415–423.

124. Barnard JH. Studies of 400 Hymenoptera sting deaths in the United States. *J Allergy Clin Immunol* 1973;52:259.

125. Chaffee FH. The prevalence of bee sting allergy in allergic population. *Acta Allergol* 1970;25:292.

126. Golden DBK. Epidemiology of allergy to insect venoms and stings. *Allergy Proc* 1989;16:103.

127. Charpin D, Birnbaum J, Vervloet D. Prevalence of allergy to *Hymenoptera* stings in different samples of the general population. *J Allergy Clin Immunol* 1992;90:331.

128. Schumacher MJ, Tveten MS, Egen NB. Rate and quantity of delivery of venom from honeybee stings. *J Allergy Clin Immunol* 1994;93:831.

129. Mueller U, Elliot W, Reisman RE, et al. Comparison of biochemical and immunologic properties of venoms from the four hornet species. *J Allergy Clin Immunol* 1981;67:290.

130. Juarez C, Blanca M, Miranda A, et al. Specific IgE antibodies to vespids in the course of immunotherapy with *Vespula germanica* administered to patients sensitized to *Polistes dominulus*. *Allergy* 1992;47:299.

131. Levine MI, Lockey RF, eds. *Monograph on insect allergy,* 2nd ed. American Academy of Allergy and Immunology, Committee on Insects. Pittsburgh: Dave Lambert Associates, 1986.

132. Hoffman DR. Allergens in *Hymenoptera* venom XV: the immunologic basis of vespid venom cross-reactivity. *J Allergy Clin Immunol* 1985;75:611.

133. Hoffman DR. Allergens in *Hymenoptera* venom XIII: isolation and purification of protein components from three species of vespid venoms. *J Allergy Clin Immunol* 1985;75:599.

134. King TP. Antigenic cross reactivity of venom proteins from hornets, wasps, and yellow jackets. *J Allergy Clin Immunol* 1985;75:621.

135. Hoffman DR. Allergens in *Hymenoptera* venom XVI: studies of the structures and cross-reactivities of vespid venom phospholipases. *J Allergy Clin Immunol* 1986;78:337.

136. Hoffman DR, Dove DE, Moffit JE, et al. Allergens in *Hymenoptera* venom XXI: cross-reactivity and multiple reactivity between fire ant venom and bee and wasp venoms. *J Allergy Clin Immunol* 1988;82:828.

137. Ho CL, Hwang LL, Chen CT. Edema-inducing activity of a lethal protein with phospholipase A1 activity isolated from the black-bellied hornet (*Vespa basalis*) venom. *Toxicon* 1993;31:605.

138. van der Linden PW, Hack CE, Struyvenberg A, et al. Controlled insect-sting challenge in 55 patients: correlation between activation of plasminogen and the development of anaphylactic shock. *Blood* 1993;82:1740.

139. van der Linden PW, Hack CE, Eerenberg AJ, et al. Activation of the contact system in insect-sting anaphylaxis: association with the development of angioedema and shock. *Blood* 1993;82:1732.

140. van der Linden PW, Hack CE, Poortman J, et al. Insect-sting challenge in 138 patients: relation between clinical severity of anaphylaxis and mast cell activation. *J Allergy Clin Immunol* 1992;90:110.

141. van der Linden PW, Hack CE, Kerckhaert JA, et al. Preliminary report: complement activation in wasp-sting anaphylaxis. *Lancet* 1990;336:904.

142. Reisman RE. Natural history of insect sting allergy: relationship of severity of symptoms of initial sting anaphylaxis to re-sting reactions. *J Allergy Clin Immunol* 1992;90:335.

143. Reisman RE. Stinging insect allergy. *Med Clin North Am* 1992;76:883.

144. Delage C, Irey NS. Anaphylactic deaths: a clinicopathologic study of 43 cases. *J Forensic Sci* 1972;17:525.

145. Lockey RF, Turkeltaub PC, Baird-Warren A, et al. The *Hymenoptera* study I, 1979-1982: Demographics and history - Sting data. *J Allergy Clin Immunol* 1988;82:370.

146. van der Linden PG, Hack CE, Struyvenberg A, et al. Insect challenge in 324 subjects with a previous anaphylactic reaction: current criteria for insect-venom hypersensitivity do not predict the occurrence and the severity of anaphylaxis. *J Allergy Clin Immunol* 1994;94:151.

147. Li JTC, Yunginger JW. Management of insect sting hypersensitivity. *Mayo Clin Proc* 1992;67:1988.

148. Day JH, Buckeridge DL, Welsh AC. Risk assessment in determining systemic reactivity to honeybee stings in sting-threatened individuals. *J Allergy Clin Immunol* 1994;93:691.

149. Muller U, Helbling A, Berchold E. Immunotherapy with honeybee venom and yellow jacket venom is different regarding efficacy and safety. *J Allergy Clin Immunol* 1992;89:529.

150. Lofgren CS. History of imported fire ants in the United States. In: Lofgren CS, Vandermeer RD, eds. *Fire ants and leaf-cutting ants: biology and management.* Boulder, CO: Westview Press, 1986:36–37.

151. Stafford CT, Hoffman DR, Rhoades RB. Allergy to imported fire ants. *South Med J* 1989;82:1520.

152. Vandermeer RK, Lofgren CS, Alvarez FM. Biochemical evidence for hybridization in fire ants. *Fla Entomol* 1985;68:501.

153. de Shazo RD, Griffing C, Kwan TH, et al. Dermal hypersensitivity reactions to imported fire ants. *J Allergy Clin Immunol* 1984;74:841.

154. Clemnes DI, Sterling RE. The imported fire ant: dimensions of the urban problem. *South Med J* 1975;68:113.

155. Stablein JJ, Lockey RF. Adverse reactions to ant stings. *Clin Rev Allergy* 1987;5:161.

156. Revkin AC. March of the fire ants. *Discover* 1989;10:70.

157. Diaz JD, Lockey RF, Stablein JJ, Mines HK. Multiple stings by imported fire ants (*Solenopsis invicta*) without systemic effects. *South Med J* 1989;82:775.

158. Hibel JA, Clore ER. Prevention and primary care treatment of stings from imported fire ants. *Nurse Pract* 1992;17:65.

159. Rhoades RB, Schafer WL, Schmid WH, et al. Hypersensitivity to the imported fire ant. A report of 49 cases. *J Allergy Clin Immunol* 1975;56:84.

160. Rhoades RB, Schafer WL, Newman M, et al. Hypersensitivity to the imported fire ant in Florida. Report of 104 cases. *J Fla Med Assoc* 1977;64:247.

161. de Shazo RD, Butcher BT, Banks WA. Reactions to the sting of the imported fire ant. *N Engl J Med* 1990;323:462.

162. Blum MS, Walker JR, Callahan PS, Novak AF. Chemical insecticidal and antibiotic properties of fire ant venom. *Science* 1958;128:306.

163. Bufkin DC, Russell FE. A study of the venom of the imported fire ant: physiopharmacology, chemistry and therapeutics. *Proc West Pharmacol Soc* 1974;17:223.

164. Rhoades AB. *Medical aspects of the imported fire ant.* Gainesville, FL: University Presses of Florida, 1977.

165. Stafford CT, Hutto LS, Rhoades RB, et al. Imported fire ants as a health hazard. *South Med J* 1989;82:1515.

166. Adamski DB. Assessment and treatment of allergic response to stinging insects. *J Emerg Nurs* 1990;16:77.

167. Candiotti KA, Lamas AM. Adverse neurological reactions to the sting of the imported fire ant. *Int Arch Allergy Immunol* 1993;102:417.

168. Jacobsen RS, Hoffman DR. Structural studies of imported fire ant venom allergens. *J Allergy Clin Immunol* 1989;83:232.

169. Hoffman DR, Dalton DE, Jacobson RS. Allergies in *Hymenoptera* venom: isolation of four allergens from imported fire ants (*Solenopsis invicta*) venom. *J Allergy Clin Immunol* 1988;82:818.

170. Freeman TM, Hylander R, Ortiz A, Martin ME. Imported fire ant immunotherapy: Effectiveness of whole body extracts. *J Allergy Clin Immunol* 1992;90:210.

171. Triplet RF. Sensitivity to imported fire ants: successful treatment with immunotherapy. *South Med J* 1973;66:477.

172. Tankersley MS, Walker RL, Butler WK, Hagan LL, Napoli DC, Freeman TM. Safety and efficacy of an imported fire ant rush immunotherapy protocol with and without prophylactic treatment. *J Allergy Clin Immunol* 2002;109:556–562.

173. Spielman A. A commentary on research needs for monitoring and containing emergent vector-borne infections. *Ann NY Acad Sci* 1994;740:457.

Index

Note: Page numbers followed by *f* indicate figures; page numbers followed by *t* indicate tables.

Urinalysis
  and appendicitis, 745
Urinary antigen assay
  for detection of *Legionella*, 475
Urinary antigen test
  for *Legionella pneumophila*, 1739
Urinary carrier state, 627
Urinary catheters
  and infection prevention, 1146
  management of, 381
Urinary infections
  Salmonella, 627
  and trimethoprim-sulfamethoxazole
    (TMP-SMX), 249
Urinary leukocytes
  detection of, 866
Urinary myiasis, 2407
Urinary tract infection (UTI), 133, 396, 861
  and adolescence, 862
  bacterial virulence factors, 863
  and cancer patients with cellular immunity
    defeciencies, 1109
  and *Candida*, 2201
  catheter-associated, 869
    treatment for, 870
  causative pathogens of, 861
  cause of, 1611
  and children, 864
  clinical manifestations of, 864
  community-acquired, 863
  complicated, 865
    clinical manifestations of, 865
  diagnosis of, 865
  and elderly, 864
  epidemiology of, 862
  from *Escherichia coli*, 861
  and hospitals, 1711
  host defense mechanisms in, 864
  laboratory tests for
    selection of, 866
  pathogenesis of, 863
  polymyxin B for, 282
  prevalence of, 862
  prevention of, 870
  and *Pseudomonas*, 1711
  rapid tests for, 866
  recurrent, 863
  risk factors, 863
  risk of acquisition of, 381
  segmented cultures of, 874f
  from *Staphylococcus aureus*, 862
  from *Staphylococcus saprophyticus*, 861
  statistics for, 382
  treatment of, 257, 866
  urine culture for, 865
  associated with vesicoureteral reflux, 862
  white blood cell count for, 819f
Urine
  and coccidioidomycosis, 2235
  collection, 133
  culture of, 865
    methods, 866
  storage of, 133
Urine tests
  for HIV, 1025
Urokinase
  for empyema, 550
Urologic procedures
  antimicrobial prophylaxis for, 393
Uropathogenic *Escherichia coli*, 863
US. *See* Ultrasound (US)
Uterine cervical infections, 948
Uterine gas gangrene, 832
  symptoms of, 832
Uterine infections
  as cause of premature labor and delivery, 952

Uterus
  infection of, 955
  operative removal of, 956
  soft tissue damage, 952
UTI. *See* Urinary tract infection (UTI)
Uveitis, 340
  with *Campylobacter*, 1689
  etiologic agent of, 1720

V

Vaccination
  poliomyelitis, 2041
Vaccine(s)
  to activate T lymphocytes, 42
  for adenovirus, 501
  administration of, 371
  and adult respiratory distress syndrome,
    1901
  adverse reactions, 372
  for anthrax, 1462
  against Argentine hemorrhagic fever,
    2138
  bacterial, for special populations, 379
  for cholera
    killed oral, 665
    live attenuated, 665
  constituents of, 371
  for herpes simplex virus, quest for, 911
  and Group B *Streptococcus* immunization,
    1620
  for HIV, 1040
    development of, 2092
  for human papillomavirus, 926
  for influenza, 469
    development of, 501
  for influenza A, 447
  integrating multiple
    for travelers, 408
  for long-term travelers, 408
  for measles, 1183
  pneumococcal, 446, 1608
  for poliovirus infection, 2045
  for Q fever, 1888
  and refugees, 374
  simultaneous administration of, 373
  for specific populations or special
    indications, 377
  for travelers, 406, 406t
  viral, 447
  for yellow fever, 2112
  and zoonotic infections, 1427
Vaccine-associated paralytic polio (VAPP),
  1352, 2043
Vaccine-derived poliovirus (VDPV), 1352,
  2045
Vaccine information
  sources of, 371
  web sites, 371
Vaccine products
  available in United States, 372t
Vaccine schedules, 371
Vaccine versus immune globulin
  and travel, 407
Vaccinia, 1983. *See also* Smallpox, vaccine
  diagnosis of, 1013
  and eyelid infection, 1242
Vaccinia immunoglobulin (VIG), 1984
  and smallpox, 1210
Vacuolar myelopathy, 1357
  clinical features of, 1357
  diagnosis of, 1357
  pathology of, 1357
  treatment for, 1357
Vacuum sealing technique
  and foot ulcer management, 1161

Vagina
  examination of, 929
  flora, 1769
    and *Bacteroides*, 1787
  normal state of, 944
Vaginal candidiasis
  and pregnancy, 946t
  recurrent, 945
    and HIV-infected women, 1092
  treatment for, 945, 1093
Vaginal colpotomy, 939
Vaginal discharge
  examination of, 944
Vaginal hysterectomy
  antibiotic recommendations for, 393
Vaginal microbicides
  and HIV prevention, 1051
Vaginal pH
  test for, 929
Vaginal secretions, 929
  gram stain examination of, 930
Vaginitis, 944
  allergic, 930
  diagnosis of, 137, 945f
  diagnostic tests for, 930
  pathogens of, 883t
  therapy for, 944
Vaginosis, bacterial. *See* Bacterial vaginosis
  (BV)
Valacyclovir
  absorption of, 300
  adverse effects of, 302
  antiviral activity of, 300
  chemistry of, 300
  clinical indications of, 300
  for cytomegalovirus, 1548
  distribution of, 300
  elimination of, 300
  for genital herpes, 909, 909t
  for herpes gladiatorum, 1911
  for herpes labialis, 301, 1911
  for herpes simplex virus (HSV), 300, 301,
    1913
  for herpes simplex virus (HSV) with HIV,
    1010
  for herpesvirus infection, 300
  for herpes zoster, 302, 1202
  mechanism of action, 300
  for pregnancy and genital herpes, 910
  for recurrent genital herpes, 910
  risk of transmission of genital herpes
    simplex virus (HSV) infection, 911
  for varicella-zoster virus, 1202
  for varicella-zoster with HIV, 1010
Valganciclovir
  absorption, distribution, and elimination
    of, 304
  adverse effects of, 305
  for AIDS patients with cytomegalovirus
    retinitis, 305
  chemistry, mechanism of action, and
    antiviral activity of, 304
  clinical indications of, 305
  for cytomegalovirus, 501, 1116
  and liver transplant patients, 1137
  for pneumonitis with HIV, 992
  resistance to, 305
  for viral pneumonia, 501
Valley fever, 2227
Valve replacement surgery, 1563
Vancomycin, 233
  absorption of, 235
  administration and dosing of, 235
  adverse effects of, 236
  allergic reactions to, 236
  alternative for, 249